Table of Logarithms

Natural Numbers	0	1	2	3	4	5	6	7	8	9
10	0000	0043	0086	0128	0170	0212	0253	0294	0334	0374
11	0414	0453	0492	0531	0569	0607	0645	0682	0719	0755
12	0792	0828	0864	0899	0934	0969	1004	1038	1072	1106
13	1139	1173	1206	1239	1271	1303	1335	1367	1399	1430
14	1461	1492	1523	1553	1584	1614	1644	1673	1703	1732
15	1761	1790	1818	1847	1875	1903	1931	1959	1987	2014
16	2041	2068	2095	2122	2148	2175	2201	2227	2253	2279
17	2304	2330	2355	2380	2405	2430	2455	2480	2504	2529
18	2553	2577	2601	2625	2648	2672	2695	2718	2742	2765
19	2788	2810	2833	2856	2878	2900	2923	2945	2967	2989
20	3010	3032	3054	3075	3096	3118	3139	3160	3181	3201
21	3222	3243	3263	3284	3304	3324	3345	3365	3385	3404
22	3424	3444	3464	3483	3502	3522	3541	3560	3579	3598
23	3617	3636	3655	3674	3692	3711	3729	3747	3766	3784
24	3802	3820	3838	3856	3874	3892	3909	3927	3945	3962
25	3979	3997	4014	4031	4048	4065	4082	4099	4116	4133
26	4150	4166	4183	4200	4216	4232	4249	4265	4281	4298
27	4314	4330	4346	4362	4378	4393	4409	4425	4440	4456
28	4472	4487	4502	4518	4533	4548	4564	4579	4594	4609
29	4624	4639	4654	4669	4683	4698	4713	4728	4742	4757
30	4771	4786	4800	4814	4829	4843	4857	4871	4886	4900
31	4914	4928	4942	4955	4969	4983	4997	5011	5024	5038
32	5051	5065	5079	5092	5105	5119	5132	5145	5159	5172
33	5185	5198	5211	5224	5237	5250	5263	5276	5289	5302
34	5315	5328	5340	5353	5366	5378	5391	5403	5416	5428
35	5441	5453	5465	5478	5490	5502	5514	5527	5539	5551
36	5563	5575	5587	5599	5611	5623	5635	5647	5658	5670
37	5682	5694	5705	5717	5729	5740	5752	5763	5775	5786
38	5798	5809	5821	5832	5843	5855	5866	5877	5888	5899
39	5911	5922	5933	5944	5955	5966	5977	5988	5999	6010
40	6021	6031	6042	6053	6064	6075	6085	6096	6107	6117
41	6128	6138	6149	6160	6170	6180	6191	6201	6212	6222
42	6232	6243	6253	6263	6274	6284	6294	6304	6314	6325
43	6335	6345	6355	6365	6375	6385	6395	6405	6415	6425
44	6435	6444	6454	6464	6474	6484	6493	6503	6513	6522
45	6532	6542	6551	6561	6571	6580	6590	6599	6609	6618
46	6628	6637	6646	6656	6665	6675	6684	6693	6702	6712
47	6721	6730	6739	6749	6758	6767	6776	6785	6794	6803
48	6812	6821	6830	6839	6848	6857	6866	6875	6884	6893
49	6902	6911	6920	6928	6937	6946	6955	6964	6972	6981
50	6990	6998	7007	7016	7024	7033	7042	7050	7059	7067
51	7076	7084	7093	7101	7110	7118	7126	7135	7143	7152
52	7160	7168	7177	7185	7193	7202	7210	7218	7226	7235
53	7243	7251	7259	7267	7275	7284	7292	7300	7308	7316
54	7324	7332	7340	7348	7356	7364	7372	7380	7388	7396

Natural Numbers	0	1	2	3	4	5	6	7	8	9
55	7404	7412	7419	7427	7435	7443	7451	7459	7466	7474
56	7482	7490	7497	7505	7513	7520	7528	7536	7543	7551
57	7559	7566	7574	7582	7589	7597	7604	7612	7619	7627
58	7634	7642	7649	7657	7664	7672	7679	7686	7694	7701
59	7709	7716	7723	7731	7738	7745	7752	7760	7767	7774
60	7782	7789	7796	7803	7810	7818	7825	7832	7839	7846
61	7853	7860	7868	7875	7882	7889	7896	7903	7910	7917
62	7924	7931	7938	7945	7952	7959	7966	7973	7980	7987
63	7993	8000	8007	8014	8021	8028	8035	8041	8048	8055
64	8062	8069	8075	8082	8089	8096	8102	8109	8116	8122
65	8129	8136	8142	8149	8156	8162	8169	8176	8182	8189
66	8195	8202	8209	8215	8222	8228	8235	8241	8248	8254
67	8261	8267	8274	8280	8287	8293	8299	8306	8312	8319
68	8325	8331	8338	8344	8351	8357	8363	8370	8376	8382
69	8388	8395	8401	8407	8414	8420	8426	8432	8439	8445
70	8451	8457	8463	8470	8476	8482	8488	8494	8500	8506
71	8513	8519	8525	8531	8537	8543	8549	8555	8561	8567
72	8573	8579	8585	8591	8597	8603	8609	8615	8621	8627
73	8633	8639	8645	8651	8657	8663	8669	8675	8681	8686
74	8692	8698	8704	8710	8716	8722	8727	8733	8739	8745
75	8751	8756	8762	8768	8774	8779	8785	8791	8797	8802
76	8808	8814	8820	8825	8831	8837	8842	8848	8854	8859
77	8865	8871	8876	8882	8887	8893	8899	8904	8910	8915
78	8921	8927	8932	8938	8943	8949	8954	8960	8965	8971
79	8976	8982	8987	8993	8998	9004	9009	9015	9020	9026
80	9031	9036	9042	9047	9053	9058	9063	9069	9074	9079
81	9085	9090	9096	9101	9106	9112	9117	9122	9128	9133
82	9138	9143	9149	9154	9159	9165	9170	9175	9180	9186
83	9191	9196	9201	9206	9212	9217	9222	9227	9232	9238
84	9243	9248	9253	9258	9263	9269	9274	9279	9284	9289
85	9294	9299	9304	9309	9315	9320	9325	9330	9335	9340
86	9345	9350	9355	9360	9365	9370	9375	9380	9385	9390
87	9395	9400	9405	9410	9415	9420	9425	9430	9435	9440
88	9445	9450	9455	9460	9465	9469	9474	9479	9484	9489
89	9494	9499	9504	9509	9513	9518	9523	9528	9533	9538
90	9542	9547	9552	9557	9562	9566	9571	9576	9581	9586
91	9590	9595	9600	9605	9609	9614	9619	9624	9628	9633
92	9638	9643	9647	9652	9657	9661	9666	9671	9675	9680
93	9685	9689	9694	9699	9703	9708	9713	9717	9722	9727
94	9731	9736	9741	9745	9750	9754	9759	9763	9768	9773
95	9777	9782	9786	9791	9795	9800	9805	9809	9814	9818
96	9823	9827	9832	9836	9841	9845	9850	9854	9859	9863
97	9868	9872	9877	9881	9886	9890	9894	9899	9903	9908
98	9912	9917	9921	9926	9930	9934	9939	9943	9948	9952
99	9956	9961	9965	9969	9974	9978	9983	9987	9991	9996

PROPORTIONAL PARTS (columns 1–9 accompany each section of the table)

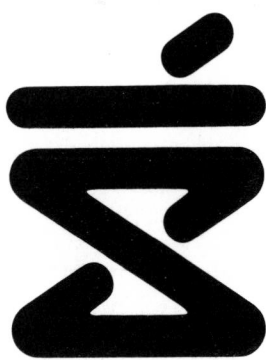

PRESENTED TO

Bruce Fetcher
U of A   ID. # 162793

by the

SHOPPERS DRUG MART.

ASSOCIATE/OWNERS

Ph. # 922-3433

Each Shoppers Drug Mart is owned and operated by a Pharmacist known as an Associate, and we are located in every province throughout Canada.

We, the Associates of Shoppers Drug Mart, take this opportunity to wish you the best of luck and success in your new career as a Pharmacist.

Remington's Pharmaceutical Sciences

17

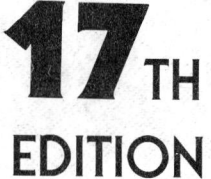

17TH
EDITION

Remington's

ALFONSO R GENNARO
*Editor, and Chairman
of the Editorial Board*

Pharmaceutical Sciences

1985

MACK PUBLISHING COPMANY

Easton, Pennsylvania 18042

Remington's Pharmaceutical Sciences . . . *a treatise on the theory and practice of the pharmaceutical sciences, with essential information about pharmaceutical and medicinal agents; also a guide to the professional responsibilities of the pharmacist as the drug-information specialist of the health team . . . A textbook and reference work for pharmacists, physicians, and other practitioners of the pharmaceutical and medical sciences.*

EDITORS

Alfonso R Gennaro, *Chairman*

Grafton D Chase

Melvin R Gibson

C Boyd Granberg

Stewart C Harvey

Robert E King

Alfred N Martin

Thomas Medwick

Ewart A Swinyard

Gilbert L Zink

AUTHORS

The 109 chapters of this edition of *Remington's Pharmaceutical Sciences* were written by the editors, by members of the Editorial Board, and by other authors listed on pages ix to xi.

Production Manager

Christine L Bailey

Directors

William A Thawley, 1980–1983

Allen Misher 1984–1985

Seventeenth Edition—1985

Published in the 165th year of the
PHILADELPHIA COLLEGE OF PHARMACY AND SCIENCE

Remington Historical / Biographical Data

The following is a record of the editors and the dates of publication of successive editions of this book, prior to the 13th Edition known as *Remington's Practice of Pharmacy* and subsequently as *Remington's Pharmaceutical Sciences*.

First Edition, 1886 Joseph P Remington
Second Edition, 1889
Third Edition, 1897
Fourth Edition, 1905

Fifth Edition, 1907 Joseph P Remington
Sixth Edition, 1917 *Assisted by*
    E Fullerton Cook

Seventh Edition, 1926

Editors
  E Fullerton Cook
  Charles H LaWall

Eighth Edition, 1936

Editors *Associate Editors*
  E Fullerton Cook   Ivor Griffith
  Charles H LaWall   Adley B Nichols
    Arthur Osol

Ninth Edition, 1948 *Editors*
  E Fullerton Cook
  Eric W Martin

Tenth Edition, 1951 *Editors*
  E Fullerton Cook
  Eric W Martin

Eleventh Edition, 1956

Editors *Associate Editors*
  Eric W Martin   E Emerson Leuallen
  E Fullerton Cook   Arthur Osol
    Linwood F Tice
    Clarence T Van Meter

Twelfth Edition, 1961

Editors *Assistant to the Editors*
  Eric W Martin   John E Hoover
  E Fullerton Cook
  E Emerson Leuallen
  Arthur Osol
  Linwood F Tice
  Clarence T Van Meter

Thirteenth Edition, 1965

Editor-in-Chief
  Eric W Martin
Editors
  Grafton D Chase   Robert E King
  Herald R Cox   E Emerson Leuallen
  Richard A Deno   Arthur Osol
  Alfonso R Gennaro   Ewart A Swinyard
  Stewart C Harvey   Clarence T Van Meter
    Managing Editor
    John E Hoover

Fourteenth Edition, 1970

Chairman, Editorial Board
  Arthur Osol
Editors
  Grafton D Chase   Robert E King
  Richard A Deno   Alfred N Martin
  Alfonso R Gennaro   Ewart A Swinyard
  Melvin R Gibson   Clarence T Van Meter
  Stewart C Harvey   Bernard Witlin
    Managing Editor
    John E Hoover

Fifteenth Edition, 1975

Chairman, Editorial Board
  Arthur Osol
Editors
  John T Anderson   C Boyd Granberg
  Cecil L Bendush   Stewart C Harvey
  Grafton D Chase   Robert E King
  Alfonso R Gennaro   Alfred N Martin
  Melvin R Gibson   Ewart A Swinyard
    Managing Editor
    John E Hoover

Sixteenth Edition, 1980

Chairman, Editorial Board
  Arthur Osol
Editors
  Grafton D Chase   Robert E King
  Alfonso R Gennaro   Alfred N Martin
  Melvin R Gibson   Ewart A Swinyard
  C Boyd Granberg   Gilbert L Zink
  Stewart C Harvey

Editorial Board Members and Editors

Alfonso R Gennaro, PhD / *Philadelphia College of Pharmacy and Science*—Director of Graduate Studies and Professor of Chemistry. Chairman of the Editorial Board and Editor, *Remington's Pharmaceutical Sciences*.

Grafton D Chase, PhD / *Philadelphia College of Pharmacy and Science*—Professor of Chemistry; Chairman, Department of Chemistry, Editor, Part 4, *Radioisotopes in Pharmacy and Medicine*. Author, Chapters 28, 29.

Melvin R Gibson, PhD / *Washington State University College of Pharmacy*—Professor of Pharmacognosy. Editorial Board member. Editor, Part 9, *Pharmaceutical Practice*. Author, Chapters 1, 4.

C Boyd Granberg, PhD / *Drake University College of Pharmacy*—Dean and Professor of Pharmacy. Editor, Part 1, *Orientation*. Author, Chapter 7.

Stewart C Harvey, PhD / *University of Utah School of Medicine*—Professor of Pharmacology. Editorial Board member. Editor, Part 6, *Pharmaceutical and Medicinal Agents*. Author, Chapters 37, 40, 42, 45 to 49, 51, 63, 64; Coauthor, Chapters 38, 43, 52.

Robert E King, PhD / *Philadelphia College of Pharmacy and Science*—Professor of Industrial Pharmacy. Editorial Board member. Editor, Part 8, *Pharmaceutical Preparations and Their Manufacture*. Coauthor, Chapter 86.

Alfred N Martin, PhD / *University of Texas at Austin College of Pharmacy*—Sublett Professor of Pharmaceutics, Drug Dynamics Institute. Editorial Board member. Editor, Part 2, *Pharmaceutics*. Coauthor, Chapter 21.

Thomas Medwick, PhD / *Rutgers University*—Professor and Chairman, Department of Pharmaceutical Chemistry. Editorial Board member. Editor, Part 3, *Pharmaceutical Chemistry*, and Part 5, *Testing and Analysis*. Coauthor, Chapter 30.

Ewart A Swinyard, PhD / *University of Utah*—Professor Emeritus of Pharmacology, College of Pharmacy and School of Medicine. Editorial Board member. Editor, Part 6, *Pharmaceutical and Medicinal Agents*. Author, Chapters 41, 44, 50, 55 to 62, 65, 67, 72; Coauthor, Chapter 68.

Gilbert L Zink, PhD / *Philadelphia College of Pharmacy and Science*—Associate Professor of Biology, Editor, Part 7, *Biological Products*. Author, Chapter 73.

Authors

The following contributors to the Seventeenth Edition of *Remington's Pharmaceutical Sciences* served as authors or coauthors, along with the editors and members of the Editorial Board, of the 109 chapters of this book.

Hamed P Abdou, PhD / Director of Product Quality Control, E R Squibb & Sons; Author of Chapter 34, *Instrumental Methods of Analysis* and Chapter 35, *Dissolution*.

John Adams, PhD / Vice President, Scientific & Professional Relations, Pharmaceutical Manufacturers Association; Author of Chapter 8, *Research*.

Mary Celeste Alessandri, BA / Free Lance Writer; Coauthor of Chapter 26, *Drug Nomenclature and United States Adopted Names*.

Joan Anderson, MSc / Clinical Assistant Professor of Pharmacy, Philadelphia College of Pharmacy & Science; Coauthor of Chapter 99, *Patient Communication*.

Howard C Ansel, PhD / Professor of Pharmacy & Dean, School of Pharmacy, University of Georgia; Author of Chapter 101, *The Prescription*.

Kenneth E Avis, DSc / Goodman Professor and Chairman, Department of Pharmaceutics, College of Pharmacy, University of Tennessee; Author of Chapter 85, *Parenteral Preparations*.

Leonard Bailey, PhD / Associate Professor of Pharmaceutical Chemistry, Rutgers University College of Pharmacy; Author of Chapter 33, *Chromatography*.

Thomas Blake, RPh / Director, Regulatory Drug Affairs, Pharmaceutical Division, Ciba-Geigy Corp; Author of Chapter 5, *Pharmacists in Industry*.

Lawrence H Block, PhD / Professor of Pharmaceutics, Duquesne University College of Pharmacy; Author of Chapter 88, *Medicated Applications*.

Joseph B Bogardus, PhD / Associate Director, Pharmaceutical Research & Development, Bristol Myers Co; Coauthor of Chapter 18, *Reaction Kinetics*.

John A Bosso, PharmD / Associate Professor of Clinical Pharmacy, College of Pharmacy, University of Utah; Coauthor of Chapter 36, *Diseases: Manifestations and Pathophysiology*.

Arthur A Cammarata, PhD / Professor of Physical Medicinal Chemistry, School of Pharmacy, Temple University; Author of Chapter 15, *Thermodynamics*.

Alan Cheung, PharmD / Deputy Director, Pharmacy Service, Veterans' Association, Washington DC; Coauthor of Chapter 96, *Long-Term Care Facilities*.

Joseph L Ciminera, DSc / Director, Biometrics Long Term Planning, Merck Sharp & Dohme Research Laboratories; Author of Chapter 10, *Statistics*.

Anthony J Cutie, PhD / Director of Pharmaceutics & Industrial Pharmacy, Professor of Pharmaceutics, Anna and Marie Schwartz College of Pharmacy; Coauthor of Chapter 93, *Aerosols*.

Ara Der Marderosian, PhD / Professor of Pharmacognosy, Philadelphia College of Pharmacy & Science; Author of Chapter 66, *Pesticides*.

Anthony R DiSanto, PhD / Director, Clinical Biopharmaceutics/New Formulation Development, The Upjohn Co; Author of Chapter 77, *Bioavailability and Bioequivalency Testing*.

Clarence A Discher, PhD / Professor Emeritus, Rutgers University; Author of Chapter 23, *Inorganic Pharmaceutical Chemistry*.

Barry N Eigen, MBA / President, Sickroom Service, Milwaukee WI; Author of Chapter 104, *Health Accessories*.

Clyde R Erskine, BSc / Director, Corporate Quality Assurance, SmithKline Beckman Corporation; Author of Chapter 83, *Quality Assurance and Control*.

Lorraine Evans, BS, H(ASCP) / Clinical Pathology, Bristol-Myers Co; Coauthor of Chapter 32, *Clinical Analysis*.

Joseph L Fink III, BS(Pharm), JD / Assistant Dean & Professor, College of Pharmacy, University of Kentucky; Coauthor of Chapter 107, *Laws Governing Pharmacy*.

Michael R Franklin, PhD / Professor of Pharmacology, College of Pharmacy & School of Medicine, University of Utah, Author of Chapter 54, *Enzymes*.

Donald G Fraser, PharmD / Director of Medical & Clinical Affairs, Reid-Provident Laboratories; Author of Chapter of 103, *Utilization and Evaluation of Clinical Drug Literature*.

James W Freston, MD, PhD / Professor & Chairman, Department of Medicine, University of Connecticut; Coauthor of Chapter 36, *Diseases: Manifestations and Pathophysiology*.

Philip P Gerbino, PharmD / Professor of Clinical Pharmacy, Philadelphia College of Pharmacy & Science; Coauthor of Chapter 99, *Patient Communication*.

Thomas J Gildea, BSc / Manager, Data Quality Assurance & Scientific Computing, G D Searle & Company; Coauthor of Chapter 11, *Computer Science*.

Robert L Giles, BA / Vice President & General Manager, Glenn Beall Engineering Co, Gurnee IL; Coauthor of Chapter 81, *Plastic Packaging Material*.

Harold N Godwin, MS / Professor & Director of Pharmacy, University of Kansas; Author of Chapter 95, *Institutional Patient Care*.

Frederick J Goldstein, PhD / Professor of Pharmacology, Philadelphia College of Pharmacy & Science; Coauthor of Chapter 71, *Pharmacological Aspects of Drug Abuse*.

Larry D Grieshaber, PhD / Veterans Administration Medical Center, St Louis MO; Coauthor of Chapter 3, *Ethics*.

Frank E Halleck, PhD / Corporate Director for Scientific Affairs, American Sterilizer Corporation; Coauthor of Chapter 79, *Sterilization*.

William I Higuchi, PhD / Distinguished Professor & Chairman, Department of Pharmaceutics, College of Pharmacy, University of Utah; Coauthor of Chapter 21, *Particle Phenomena and Coarse Dispersions*.

Norman F H Ho, PhD / Professor of Pharmaceutics, College of Pharmacy, University of Michigan; Coauthor of Chapter 21, *Particle Phenomena and Coarse Dispersions*.

Daniel A Hussar, PhD / Remington Professor of Pharmacy, Philadelphia College of Pharmacy & Science; Author of Chapter 100, *Patient Compliance* and Chapter 102, *Drug Interactions*.

Joseph B Jerome, PhD / Secretary Emeritus, United Adopted Names Council; Coauthor of Chapter 26, *Drug Nomenclature—United States Adopted Names*.

*Lloyd Kennon, PhD / Associate Professor Industrial Pharmacy Program Director, Arnold & Marie Schwartz College of Pharmacy & Health Sciences; Coauthor of Chapter 13, *Molecular Structure, Properties, and States of Matter*.

Adelbert M Knevel, PhD / Professor of Medicinal Chemistry & Associate Dean, School of Pharmacy & Pharmacal Sciences, Purdue University; Author of Chapter 78, *Separation*.

Harry B Kostenbauder, PhD / Associate Dean for Research, College of Pharmacy, University of Kentucky; Author of Chapter 18, *Reaction Kinetics*.

Richard Kronenthal, PhD / Director of Research, Ethicon Inc; Author of Chapter 105, *Surgical Supplies*.

Austin H Kutscher, DDS / Professor of Dentistry (in Psychiatry) and Director, New York State Psychiatric Institute Dental Service, School of Dental & Oral Surgery, Columbia University; Author of Chapter 109, *Dental Services*.

Eric J Lien, PhD / Professor of Pharmacy & Pharmaceutics, School of Pharmacy, University of Southern California; Coauthor of Chapter 13, *Molecular Structure, Properties, and States of Matter*.

Joseph A Linkewich, PharmD / Director, Pharmacy Service, Jeanes Hospital, Philadelphia 19111, PA; Author of Chapter 69, *Adverse Effects of Drugs*.

* Deceased

Carl J Lintner, PhD / Lintner Associates, Kalamazoo MI; Author of Chapter 82, *Stability of Pharmaceutical Products.*

Mark A Longer, BSc / Research Assistant, School of Pharmacy, University of Wisconsin; Coauthor of Chapter 92, *Sustained Release Drug Delivery Systems.*

Werner Lowenthal, PhD / Professor of Pharmacy & Pharmaceutics, School of Pharmacy, Commonwealth University of Virginia; Author of Chapter 9, *Metrology and Calculation* and Coauthor of Chapter 68, *Pharmaceutical Necessities.*

John D Mullins, PhD / Director, Pharmaceutical Services, Alcon Laboratories, Fort Worth TX; Author of Chapter 87, *Ophthalmic Preparations.*

Marvin C Myer, PhD / Professor of Pharmaceutics and Associate Dean for Graduate & Research Programs, College of Pharmacy, University of Tennessee; Author for Chapter 14, *Complexation.*

Maven J Myers, JD, PhD / Dean of Health Sciences & Professor of Pharmacy Administration, Philadelphia College of Pharmacy & Science; Coauthor of Chapter 3, *Ethics.*

J G Nairn, PhD / Professor of Pharmacy, Faculty of Pharmacy, University of Toronto; Author of Chapter 84, *Solutions, Emulsions, Suspensions, and Extractives.*

Paul J Niebergall, PhD / Professor of Pharmaceutics & Director for Pharmaceutical Development, Medical University of South Carolina; Author of Chapter 17, *Ionic Solutions and Electrolytic Equilibria.*

Steven J Padula, MD / Instructor, Department of Medicine, University of Connecticut Health Center; Coauthor of Chapter 36, *Diseases: Manifestations and Pathophysiology.*

Richard W Pecina, PhD / President, Richard W Pecina & Associates, Waukegan IL; Coauthor of Chapter 81, *Plastic Packaging Materials.*

G Briggs Phillips, PhD / Senior Vice President for Scientific Affairs, Health Industries Manufacturers Association; Coauthor of Chapter 79, *Sterilization.*

Nicholas G Popovich, PhD / Associate Professor of Pharmacy Practice, School of Pharmacy & Pharmacal Sciences, Purdue University; Author of Chapter 94, *Ambulatory Patient Care.*

Stuart C Porter, PhD / COLORCON Inc, Author of Chapter 91, *Coating of Pharmaceutical Dosage Forms.*

James W Ravin, MBA / Professor of Pharmacy Administration, College of Pharmacy, University of Michigan; Author of Chapter 108, *Pharmaceutical Economics and Management.*

Edward W Rippie, PhD / Professor of Pharmaceutics, College of Pharmacy, University of Minnesota; Author of Chapter 12, *Calculus* and of Chapter 89, *Powders.*

Joseph R Robinson, PhD / Professor of Pharmacy, School of Pharmacy, University of Wisconsin; Coauthor of Chapter 92, *Sustained Drug Delivery Systems.*

Frank Roia, PhD / Dean of Students and Professor of Biology, Philadelphia College of Pharmacy & Science; Author of Chapter 74, *Immunizing Agents and Diagnostic Skin Antigens.*

Douglas E Rollins, MD, PhD / Associate Professor of Medicine, School of Medicine & College of Pharmacy, University of Utah; Author of Chapter 39, *Clinical Pharmacokinetics.*

G Victor Rossi, PhD / Vice President for Academic Affairs and Professor of Pharmacology, Philadelphia College of Pharmacy & Science; Author of Chapter 31, *Biological Testing* and Coauthor of Chapter 71, *Pharmacological Aspects of Drug Abuse.*

Paul G Sanders, MS / Consulting Biostatistician, G D Searle & Co; Coauthor of Chapter 11, *Computer Science.*

Hans Schott, PhD / Professor of Pharmaceutics, School of Pharmacy, Temple University; Author of Chapter 20, *Colloidal Dispersions* and of Chapter 22, *Rheology.*

Joseph B Schwartz, PhD / Professor of Pharmaceutics, Philadelphia College of Pharmacy & Science; Coauthor of Chapter 90, *Oral Solid Dosage Forms.*

John J Sciarra, PhD / Executive Dean & Professor of Industrial Pharmacy, Arnold & Marie Schwartz College of Pharmacy & Health Sciences; Coauthor of Chapter 93, *Aerosols.*

John H Shinkai, PhD / Associate Professor of Pharmaceutical Chemistry, Rutgers University; Coauthor of Chapter 24, *Organic Pharmaceutical Chemistry.*

Richard H Shough, PhD / Associate Dean and Professor, College of Pharmacy, University of Oklahoma; Author of Chapter 75, *Allergenic Extracts.*

Frederick P Siegel, PhD / Professor of Pharmacy, College of Pharmacy, University of Illinois; Author of Chapter 80, *Tonicity, Osmoticity, Osmolality, and Osmolarity.*

Anthony P Simonelli, PhD / Professor of Pharmaceutics, School of Pharmacy and Institute of Material Science, University of Connecticut; Coauthor of Chapter 21, *Particle Phenomena and Coarse Dispersions.*

Larry M Simonsmeier, BS, PharmD / Dean & Associate Professor, College of Pharmacy, Washington State University; Coauthor of Chapter 107, *Laws Governing Pharmacy.*

Milton W Skolaut, BSc / Director, Department of Pharmacy, Duke University Hospital; Author of Chapter 6, *Pharmacists in Government.*

Robert D Smyth, PhD / Vice President, Research Support, Bristol-Myers Co; Coauthor of Chapter 32, *Clinical Analysis.*

Theodore D Sokoloski, PhD / Professor of Pharmacy, College of Pharmacy, Ohio State University; Author of Chapter 16, *Solutions and Phase Equilibria.*

Glenn Sonnedecker, PhD / Professor, History of Pharmacy, School of Pharmacy, University of Wisconsin; Author of Chapter 2, *Evolution of Pharmacy.*

Frederick J Spencer, MB, BS, MPH / Professor & Chairman, Department of Preventative Medicine, School of Medicine, Medical College of Virginia; Author of Chapter 97, *The Pharmacist and Public Health.*

James Swarbrick, DSc, PhD / Professor & Chairman, Division of Pharmaceutics, School of Pharmacy, University of North Carolina; Coauthor of Chapter 21, *Particle Phenomena and Coarse Dispersions.*

Anthony R Temple, MD / Medical Director, McNeil Consumer Products; Author of Chapter 106, *Poison Control.*

John P Tischio, PhD / Director, Clinical Drug Testing, Pragma Bio-Tech Inc; Author of Chapter 70, *Pharmacogenetics.*

Salvatore J Turco, PharmD / Professor of Pharmacy, Temple University; Coauthor of Chapter 86, *Intravenous Mixtures.*

John W Turczan, BS / NMR Spectroscopist, Food & Drug Administration, Brooklyn NY; Coauthor of Chapter 30, *Analysis of Medicinals.*

Vincent S Venturella, PhD / Senior Technical Fellow, Roche Research Center, Hoffman-LaRoche Inc; Author of Chapter 25, *Natural Products.*

Peter H Vlasses, PharmD / Associate Director, Clinical Pharmacology & Associate Professor of Medicine, Thomas Jefferson University College of Medicine; Coauthor of Chapter 96, *Long-Term Care Facilities.*

Albert J Wertheimer, PhD / Professor & Director, Department of Graduate Studies in Social & Administrative Pharmacy, College of Pharmacy, University of Minnesota; Author of Chapter 98, *The Patient: Behavioral Determinants.*

Dean D Withrow, PhD / Associate Professor of Pharmacology, School of Medicine, University of Utah; Coauthor of Chapter 39, *Basic Pharmacokinetics;* Chapter 43, *Cardiovascular Drugs;* and Chapter 52, *Hormones.*

Murray Zanger, PhD / Professor of Chemistry, Philadelphia College of Pharmacy & Science; Author of Chapter 27, *Structure-Activity Relationship and Drug Design.*

George Zografi, PhD / Professor, School of Pharmacy, University of Wisconsin; Author of Chapter 19, *Interfacial Phenomena.*

Preface to the First Edition

The rapid and substantial progress made in Pharmacy within the last decade has created a necessity for a work treating of the improved apparatus, the revised processes, and the recently introduced preparations of the age.

The vast advances made in theoretical and applied chemistry and physics have much to do with the development of pharmaceutical science, and these have been reflected in all the revised editions of the Pharmacopoeias which have been recently published. When the author was elected in 1874 to the chair of Theory and Practice of Pharmacy in the Philadelphia College of Pharmacy, the outlines of study which had been so carefully prepared for the classes by his eminent predecessors, Professor William Procter, Jr, and Professor Edward Parrish, were found to be not strictly in accord, either in their arrangement of the subjects or in their method of treatment. Desiring to preserve the distinctive characteristics of each, an effort was at once made to frame a system which should embody their valuable features, embrace new subjects, and still retain that harmony of plan and proper sequence which are absolutely essential to the success of any system.

The strictly alphabetical classification of subjects which is now universally adopted by pharmacopoeias and dispensatories, although admirable in works of reference, presents an effectual stumbling block to the acquisition of pharmaceutical knowledge through systematic study; the vast accumulation of facts collected under each head being arranged lexically, they necessarily have no connection with one another, and thus the saving of labor effected by considering similar groups together, and the value of the association of kindred subjects, are lost to the student. In the method of grouping the subjects which is herein adopted, the constant aim has been to arrange the latter in such a manner that the reader shall be gradually led from the consideration of elementary subjects to those which involve more advanced knowledge, whilst the groups themselves are so placed as to follow one another in a natural sequence.

The work is divided into six parts. Part I is devoted to detailed descriptions of apparatus and definitions and comments on general pharmaceutical processes.

The Official Preparations alone are considered in Part II. Due weight and prominence are thus given to the Pharmacopoeia, the National authority, which is now so thoroughly recognized.

In order to suit the convenience of pharmacists who prefer to *weigh solids* and *measure liquids*, the official formulas are expressed, in addition to parts by weight, in *avoirdupois weight* and *apothecaries' measure*. These equivalents are printed in *bold type* near the margin, and arranged so as to fit them for quick and accurate reference.

Part III treats of Inorganic Chemical Substances. Precedence is of course given to official preparation in these. The descriptions, solubilities, and tests for identity and impurities of each substance are systematically tabulated under its proper title. It is confidently believed that by this method of arrangement the valuable descriptive features of the Pharmacopoeia will be more prominently developed, ready reference facilitated, and close study of the details rendered easy. Each chemical operation is accompanied by equations, whilst the reaction is, in addition, explained in words.

The Carbon Compounds, or Organic Chemical Substances, are considered in Part IV. These are naturally grouped according to the physical and medical properties of their principal constituents, beginning with simple bodies like cellulin, gum, etc, and progressing to the most highly organized alkaloids, etc.

Part V is devoted to Extemporaneous Pharmacy. Care has been taken to treat of the practice which would be best adapted for the needs of the many pharmacists who conduct operations upon a moderate scale, rather than for those of the few who manage very large establishments. In this, as well as in other parts of the work, operations are illustrated which are conducted by manufacturing pharmacists.

Part VI contains a formulary of Pharmaceutical Preparations which have not been recognized by the Pharmacopoeia. The recipes selected are chiefly those which have been heretofore rather difficult of access to most pharmacists, yet such as are likely to be in request. Many private formulas are embraced in the collection; and such of the preparations of the old Pharmacopoeias as have not been included in the new edition, but are still in use, have been inserted.

In conclusion, the author ventures to express the hope that the work will prove an efficient help to the pharmaceutical student as well as to the pharmacist and the physician. Although the labor has been mainly performed amidst the harassing cares of active professional duties, and perfection is known to be unattainable, no pains have been spared to discover and correct errors and omissions in the text. The author's warmest acknowledgments, are tendered to Mr A B Taylor, Mr Joseph McCreery, and Mr George M Smith for their valuable assistance in revising the proof sheets, and to the latter especially for his work on the index. The outline illustrations, by Mr John Collins, were drawn either from the actual objects or from photographs taken by the author.

Philadelphia, October, 1885   JPR.

Preface to the Seventeenth Edition

A number of trite phrases may be penned to recognize the 100th anniversary of Remington's Pharmaceutical Sciences (nee Practice of Pharmacy); "The Second Hundred Years," "One Century Down and Still Counting," etc. It is remarkable, due to the "faddish" philosophy of the American public, *not* excluding the scientific community, that a building, a park, a national treasure, or a book manages to survive for even one lifetime. Why is "Remington" alive and well going into its second century? It is for the reader to provide an answer.

In the year 1885, Joseph Price Remington, then Dean of the Philadelphia College of Pharmacy, published the first edition, as the sole author. He edited and authored five additional revisions in 1889, 1894, 1905, 1907, and 1917 until his death in 1918. The Seventh edition was produced by two of Remington's colleagues, who in their own right were men of stature in the reaches of pharmacy, and was published in 1926.

The two aforementioned authors, E Fullerton Cook and Charles H LaWall, also were coeditors of the 8th edition published in 1936. Over 30 contributors assisted with this latter edition, the editors recognizing that due to the burgeoning growth of pharmacy, one or two authors could no longer cope with the extensive coverage necessary to compile such a comprehensive text.

When his coauthor, Dean LaWall, died in 1937 Professor Cook began efforts to convince the heirs to the Remington copyright that perpetuation of the book would best be accomplished by assigning the copyright to PCP&S. This was finalized in 1940 with the stipulation that a Remington Chair of Pharmacy be established at the College and funded through the income from the sale of the book. Due to the intervention of World War II the 9th edition was not published until 1948 with Dr Eric Martin and Professor Cook as coeditors. With the death of Dr Cook in 1961, Dr Martin assumed the burden of sole editorship. Having been associated with Remington since the 9th edition, Dr Martin was up to the task.

With the 13th edition Dr Martin recognized the need to alter again the composition of the editorial staff and a separate editor was appointed for each of the 9 Parts and a separate author(s) for each of the 100 chapters. The wisdom of this organization has been proved by its successful implementation for the 13th through 17th editions.

It is noteworthy to reproduce one sentence from the Preface of the 13th edition, but to add an additional phrase (in italics) to contemporize the statement.

"This textbook has gradually evolved from a practical manual for the retail pharmacist into a comprehensive, treatise covering the scientific foundations of pharmaceutical research, development, control, manufacture, *and clinical and community practice.*"

The 14th, 15th, and 16th editions of Remington were prepared under the able guidance of Dr Arthur Osol, one who had been associated with his predecessors since the time of LaWall. Under his direction the philosophy of the book was transformed from an essentially scientific/industrial/academic view of pharmacy to one which also incorporated the more contemporary role of the Clinical and Community Practitioner.

Generally, the seventeenth edition is organized as its immediate predecessors adhering to the concept of division into 9 Parts, each subdivided into several chapters. Every chapter in the book has been revised, rewritten, and updated where necessary.

Only one completely new chapter appears, *Dissolution* (Chapter 35) authored by Dr Hamed Abdou. The editors deemed the existing Section and Chapter headings were adequate to incorporate the essential new material covering the science and practice of pharmacy as required by the philosophy of this text.

When a great number of authors contribute individual chapters to compile this rather large tome, it is inevitable that duplication of concepts will be found. Not that duplication is without merit, but excessive repetition serves no pedagogical purpose and should be avoided when possible. During revision, the several chapters which constitute the first five parts were thoroughly reviewed to eliminate unessential duplication of material and thus recover space sorely needed for new material. Perhaps the reader may still uncover a few pockets of duplication, but the editors have determined it is essential to remain.

A number of halftone photographs have been deleted entirely, or replaced by schematic drawings or "blow-apart" drawings which better explain the construction or operation of a piece of equipment or apparatus.

Practically all the structural formulas depicted in the drug monographs have been replaced with standard USAN structures, when available, for uniformity and clarity. At the discretion of the editors many systematic chemical names, which appeared directly beneath the structural formulas in the monographs, have been deleted if the names were merely the inverted form of the previously listed name; a space-saving concept without loss of information.

All CAS Registry numbers and molecular formulas were checked and molecular weights recalculated by computer to insure accuracy to the number of significant figures indicated.

This edition will contain about 100 pages of additional material besides that gained through streamlining the several chapters. It is estimated that almost 200 pages of new material has been incorporated in the book with an actual physical increase of fewer than 100 pages.

The number of authors has increased by 7 from the previous edition to a total of 97 for the 109 chapters. A new member of the Editorial Board, Dr Thomas Medwick of Rutgers University, is to be welcomed. Dr Medwick supplements the expertise of the other members of the Board with his extensive experience in the area of Pharmaceutical Chemistry.

In Part 2, Pharmaceutics, the chapters on *Drug Information* (Chapter 7), *Statistics* (Chapter 10), *Computer Science* (Chapter 11), *Structure, Properties, and States of Matter* (Chapter 13), *Complexation* (Chapter 14), and *Reaction Kinetics* (Chapter 18) have been revised extensively. For Part 3, Pharmaceutical Chemistry, all of the chapters essentially have been rewritten, many by new authors with interesting and pertinent concepts, such as the prediction of pK from the structural formula for a molecule, in Chapter 24, *Organic Pharmaceutical Chemistry*. Chapters 30 and 32 to 34 are completely redone by new authors and Chapter 35 is the new addition, *Dissolution*, in Part 5.

A portion of the information presented in Part 6 has been rearranged for a neater pharmacological grouping of some of the drugs presented, to reflect current thinking and uses. Every monograph in this section has been thoroughly dissected and updated to confirm uses, dosages, and dosage forms. The section of each chapter which deals with general information of the specific drug classes has been amplified to provide the pharmacist with additional, useful, fundamental information.

In Part 8 a number of new authors bring fresh, contemporary concepts to the section on *Pharmaceutical Preparations and their Manufacture.* Two chapters in this section bear new names to better describe the entire gamut of drug dosage forms included. These are Chapter 90, *Oral Solid Dosage Forms*, to replace the title, *Tablets, Capsules, and Pills* of RPS16 and *Sustained Release Drug Delivery Systems* (Chapter 92) in place of *Prolonged Action Pharmaceuticals* of the previous edition.

The wisdom of creating an editorial board to share the burden of producing a voluminous text has been demonstrated admirably during the preparation of the 17th Edition. Each of the section editors worked diligently to maintain a smooth flow of manuscripts, proofs, etc and to prod the very few recalcitrants so that deadlines could be met. Every editor also doubled as an author of one or more chapters. Although these individuals are mentioned elsewhere, it certainly would be remiss not to do so again: Dr C Boyd Granberg of Drake University for Part 1; Dr Alfred Martin of the University of Texas at Austin for Part 2; Dr Thomas Medwick of Rutgers University for Parts 3 and 5; Dr Grafton D Chase of the Philadelphia College of Pharmacy & Science, Part 4; Drs Stewart C Harvey and Ewart A Swinyard of the University of Utah for Part 6; Dr Gilbert L Zink, Part 7 and Dr Robert E King, Part 8, both of the Philadelphia College of Pharmacy & Science; and finally Dr Melvin R Gibson of the Washington State University for Part 9. Special note must be given to the stalwarts, Drs Harvey and Swinyard, for their meticulous, comprehensive, and faithful attention to the section comprising almost a third of the book. A job very well done.

For the preparation of the index and many interesting discussions related to the philosophy of indexing, a grateful acknowledgement to Mr John E Hoover, a name not entirely unfamiliar to the masthead of previous editions of this book.

The Mack Publishing Company, through Messers James and Paul Mack have been exceptionally supportive for many years and have continued with that support during the tenure of this editor. Their staff is competent, cooperative, and tolerant of the many requests made of them.

A R GENNARO
Chairman of The Editorial Board

Table of Contents

Index

C Boyd Granberg, PhD

Dean and Professor of Pharmacy
College of Pharmacy
Drake University
Des Moines, IA 50311

CHAPTER 1

Scope

Melvin R Gibson, PhD
Professor of Pharmacognosy, College of Pharmacy
Washington State University
Pullman, WA 99164

Pharmacy has been defined[1] as that profession which is concerned with the art and science of preparing from natural and synthetic sources suitable and convenient materials for distribution and use in the treatment and prevention of disease. It embraces a knowledge of the identification, selection, pharmacologic action, preservation, combination, analysis, and standardization of drugs and medicines. It also includes their proper and safe distribution and use, whether dispensed on the prescription of a licensed physician, dentist, or veterinarian, or, in those instances where it may legally be done, dispensed or sold directly to the consumer.

The word pharmacy is derived from the Greek word *pharmakon*, meaning medicine or drug. A pharmacist, then, is the person of drugs, or, the expert on drugs. He is the *only* expert on drugs, for expertise regarding drugs requires knowledge in depth in all the facets of pharmacy as outlined in the definition of the term pharmacy above.

The physician, dentist, and veterinarian may prescribe drugs and be primarily interested in the effect of those drugs on the patient, their therapeutic value, and toxicology. The nurse may administer the drug and be concerned with dosage forms, routes of administration, and toxic manifestations. But the pharmacist *is the only expert on drugs*. It is his legally granted responsibility to handle drugs. It is his professional responsibility to know *all about* those drugs. No educational program other than that in pharmacy provides the background to understand completely all there is to understand about drugs. The pharmacist, and the pharmacist alone, is in that unique position of embracing complete drug expertise.

Pharmacy Careers

Most persons when thinking of pharmacy tend to think first of the community pharmacist. And this generalization is numerically justified. It is estimated there are 156,958 licensed pharmacists now in practice. About 74% are community pharmacists, 19% are hospital pharmacists, and the rest are in other areas of the profession.[2]

The *community pharmacist* in the US is a unique hybrid of businessman and professional. Born out of the necessity for back-up income, the business aspects of some pharmacies now all but inundate and obscure the primary unit of the pharmacy—the prescription laboratory. The supermarket and cut-rate pharmacies may be important factors in forcing a future dichotomy of pharmacy practice into stores selling merchandise and professionally oriented pharmacies of the Pharmaceutical Center type. An extensive coverage of the current practice of pharmacy and its future may be found in Chapter 4.

Hospital pharmacy, the practice of pharmacy in private and government-owned hospitals, is emerging as one of the most important areas of pharmacy practice. The number of pharmacists in the hospitals of the future will increase for three principal reasons:

1. There will be an increase in population.
2. There will be a greater utilization of hospitals by those who need hospitalization and, hence, will receive better medical care. Hospitalization insurance, both private- and government-sponsored, will foster this trend. There is little question that more adequate care of the sick by government-sponsored programs will increase greatly in the years ahead requiring more of all medical facilities.
3. The pharmacist in the hospital will be given a greater role in all aspects of the use and monitoring of the use of drugs; this is related to the health manpower shortage brought about by the two conditions mentioned above. Current trends of progressive hospitals make the need for pharmacists per hospital much greater than ever before, because of their involvement in assuring better and safer[3] use of drugs.

A very active American Society of Hospital Pharmacists with special studies, imagination, and zeal vigorously promotes this vital aspect of American pharmacy. A comprehensive study of hospital pharmacy may be found in Chapter 95.

Wholesale pharmacy offers opportunities for a limited number of pharmacists. Like most wholesalers, the pharmacy wholesaler serves as the middleman between manufacturer and community pharmacist. Because of the special nature of the products handled and their legal restrictions, all wholesale drug firms employ registered pharmacists in supervisory capacities. These wholesale firms may specialize in a broad range of products sold in a pharmacy, both prescription and nonprescription drugs as well as merchandise items, or sometimes they deal in a limited line of quick-moving items.

Whatever their scope, the wholesale drug firms play a vital role in assuring the community pharmacist of a quick and convenient source of supplies from a multiplicity of manufacturers. This makes possible better service by the pharmacist to his patients of those drugs which may be vital to the patient's welfare. It also lessens the community pharmacist's financial burden of carrying large volumes of stock and the necessity of negotiations with hundreds of manufacturers. Recently, the larger wholesalers have assumed advisory roles to pharmacists in providing them with information and consultants on store redecorating and remodeling. The Pharmaceutical Center concept described in Chapter 4 is a project of one wholesaler, McKesson Drug Company.

Industrial pharmacy offers opportunities to pharmacists of all educational levels. The greatest number of pharmacists are involved in marketing and administration. The medical service representative, or pharmaceutical sales representative who is in contact with physicians and pharmacists regarding his company's products may or may not be a pharmacist. But the most effective use is made of a pharmaceutically trained pharmaceutical sales representative because he is the only person educated as an expert on drugs. Some manufacturers employ pharmacists almost exclusively in this capacity; others do not.[4] The shortage of pharmacists is usually given as the reason why companies do not employ more pharmacists as pharmaceutical sales representatives. This can be a rewarding career for persons with the right personality and inclinations.[5] It also is sometimes a stepping-stone to supervisory positions in sales and to integration into the administrative and sales structure of a pharmaceutical firm.

Pharmacists with master's degrees in business or additional bachelor's degrees in law find opportunities in the pharmaceutical industry in the marketing, sales, and legal departments. Production and quality control supervisory positions in the industrial plant are often held by pharmacists with bachelor's degrees. Research and development personnel often have advanced degrees, but not necessarily so. A more complete discussion of pharmacists in industry may be found in Chapter 5.

Government service offers opportunities to pharmacists in various capacities. They may serve as noncommissioned officers and commissioned officers in the Army, Navy, and Air Force. Also, they may serve as commissioned officers in the United States Public Health Service, which furnishes pharmacists for the Coast Guard and Bureau of Prisons. Civil Service appointments are available for pharmacists in various capacities: in the Drug Enforcement Administration of the Department of Justice, National Institutes of Health, Social Security Administration, Food and Drug Administration, Department of Labor, Department of Agriculture, and various other areas. See Chapter 6.

Pharmaceutical education offers an opportunity for pharmacists with advanced degrees in any of the professional specialties. Expanding enrollments in colleges to meet the manpower needs of the future offer opportunities for careers in college teaching. Higher salaries, more freedom for research and writing, independence of action, and cultural surroundings in pharmaceutical education make teaching attractive. Persons interested in a future in pharmaceutical education should read the issues of the *American Journal of Pharmaceutical Education*.[6]

For a limited number of pharmacists with writing and editing talent, *pharmaceutical journalism* offers rewarding experiences. National, regional, state, and industrial publications require a pharmaceutical background for their effective publishing, editing, and writing.

Organizational management also offers an opportunity for those pharmaceutically educated persons who wish to be officers of national and state associations and boards of pharmacy. With the increase in number of pharmacists, the responsibilities of associations and boards will increase and be complicated by the greater involvement of state and federal governments in health care. The demand for such personnel will be limited, but persons with organizational interests and talents will be in great demand and will play important roles in the *future of pharmacy* in this country.

Pharmaceutical Education

The first school in the US to include pharmacy in the title of one of its professors was the Medical School of the College of Philadelphia in 1789. Pharmacy at this institution was taught by physicians for physicians. Prior to the founding of the Philadelphia College of Pharmacy in 1821, only a few attempts to provide instruction in pharmacy for pharmacists had been made.[7]

The education in medicine and law as in pharmacy evolved from entirely apprenticeship training to the current extensive collegiate education. At the beginning of the century, minimal standards for colleges of pharmacy which were members of the AACP (known as the American Conference of Pharmaceutical Faculties prior to 1925) were unspecified until 1904 when grade school plus a 40-week course was the requirement. This was increased to grade school plus 50 weeks to be done in two years in 1907. In 1908 the one year of high school plus a two-year course was the requirement which was changed to two years of high school prerequisite in 1918. The entrance

to pharmacy curricula prerequisite was raised to high school graduation in 1923. In 1925 the pharmacy curriculum was increased to three years and the PhG degree given, four years in 1932 with the BS (or BS in Pharmacy) degree, and five years in 1960 giving the BS in Pharmacy (or BPharm) degree. This is the minimal degree required for licensure and for entry into the profession.

Most colleges of pharmacy today offer the five-year program which is often so formulated that either the first year or the first two years may be taken at junior colleges or liberal arts colleges. Three years is the usual requirement for registration in a college of pharmacy. The state of California requires four years of registration in a college of pharmacy for those applying for registration in that state. If all five years are not to be taken at an institution where pharmacy is taught, students are strongly advised to communicate with the college of pharmacy they are to enter to insure that their prepharmacy curriculum meets the prerequisite requirements for entrance into the formal pharmacy instruction years.

In addition to the minimal degrees (BPharm or BS) for licensure and entry into the profession, some schools offer the PharmD degree either as the minimal degree for that institution, as a second choice for their students, as an add-on degree for the baccalaureate degree, or a combination of the last two options. The July 1, 1983, American Council on Pharmaceutical Education report of accredited degree programs lists 43 schools and colleges of pharmacy offering only the baccalaureate degree, six offering only the PharmD degree, and 23 offering both degrees.[8] This report also lists seven schools and colleges which now offer only the baccalaureate degree but have PharmD programs proposed for accreditation by the Council.

Pharmaceutical educators and pharmacy practitioners are divided on the issue as to whether there should be two entry degree programs. They are aso divided as to which degree it should be. The PharmD taken as a single unit usually requires six years. If the PharmD degree is pursued as an additional degree to the baccalaureate, the time required is usually more than one year and has been as long as three additional years. More commonly the program is now approximately two additional years. Requirements for PharmD degrees vary considerably from school to school and it is only recently that accreditation standards have been considerably clarified.

In general, PharmD degrees require different lower level courses as prerequisite to the greater amount of clinical exposure of the student and the ancillary courses which support the clinical experience. It is assumed that a good PharmD program better prepares students for hospital practice. Whether it offers advantages in other pharmacy practice settings is debatable.

The undergraduate curriculum in pharmacy is intended to prepare men and women for the profession of pharmacy. *The Pharmaceutical Curriculum*[9] defines this:

Undergraduate education in pharmacy is intended to prepare men and women for the profession of pharmacy. Stated in another way, it trains students to think and act like pharmacists. These general objectives need to be comprehended in light of the activities which are required (1) to recognize, identify, select, procure, create, process, standardize, stabilize, fabricate, test, evaluate, and preserve all substances of whatever kind and combinations used in preventive, palliative, and curative medicine, and (2) to distribute them to other members of the health professions and to the public. No single individual today engages in all of these activities, but every pharmacist has to do with one or more of them. Out of these specific activities arise a number of others, such as (1) acting as the informed and readily accessible adviser to health-service personnel and the health-seeking public; (2) contributing to the continuing improvement in professional service and sharing his contributions freely with other professionals; (3) assisting in training the manpower for the profession of pharmacy; and (4) evaluating the numerous proposals for social and political improvement and actively supporting those which his informed judgment can approve.

The curriculum is divided into a number of areas to provide the future pharmacist with the background to achieve the goals quoted above.

General Education—One of the principal objectives of the extension of the curriculum to five years in 1960 was to provide the pharmacy student with more general education so that he could, as a practicing pharmacist, more easily take his place in society as a more well-rounded individual whose formal education was not so completely monolithic. As the pressures for more pharmacists in the future become more apparent, there well may be arguments presented to reverse the upward historical trend in the length of time required to educate a pharmacist. History has shown that more educational requirements have consistently attracted more students, not less. There are no ways to test the increased caliber of the students attracted by a longer, more well-rounded education, but those who have seen the progress of pharmaceutical education over the years have expressed subjective judgment that the general caliber of pharmacy students has increased along with increased educational requirements.

The pharmacist of the future will need in his ever-increasing responsibilities to evince ever-increasing intellectual powers to meet the demand of moral, political, and social problems. Only a broad general education can provide the background for that responsibility.

Prerequisite Courses—Any professional curriculum must be based upon a firm foundation of basic courses. To provide the background for the professional pharmacy courses, the basic courses can be classified into the physical sciences and mathematics, and the biological sciences. It is generally agreed that to be able to present many of the professional courses in pharmacy on a professional plane it is necessary to build upon a firm foundation of the principles of mathematics, chemistry, and physics. The applications of these principles find their way into many of the professional pharmacy courses.

As the future pharmacist becomes less product-oriented and more patient-oriented his education will shift necessarily to a greater biological orientation. The basic biological courses dealing with the fundamental phenomena of biological systems will play an ever-increasing role in his background for professional education.

Students of pharmacy often fail to recognize the importance of prerequisite courses in the physical sciences, mathematics, and biological sciences in their search for "instant relevance." These courses are rightly taught most commonly by non-pharmacists. "Rightly" because the complexity of the pure sciences today can be taught best by specialists in those pure sciences. Once the fundamentals of these sciences are entrenched in the mind of the pharmacy student, he often fails to recognize from whence they came in his application of them in his professional courses.

Professional Courses—These vary in scope and content in the different schools and colleges of pharmacy. In recent years many institutions have made and are now making serious attempts to gear their curricula more closely to the demands of the future pharmacist.

Basic to all pharmacy professional curricula are offerings in *pharmacognosy*, the study of the biology, biochemistry, and commerce of natural drugs; *pharmacology*, the study of the action and use of drugs; *pharmaceutical chemistry*, the application of basic organic and inorganic chemistry to pharmaceuticals and the relation of these principles to drug use; *pharmacy* (*pharmaceutics*), the broad term which includes offerings in introductory pharmacy, calculations, preparations, techniques, dispensing pharmacy, physical pharmacy, and biopharmaceutics (defined as the study of the influence of formulation on the therapeutic activity of a drug product[10]); *clinical pharmacy*, which has been defined by Tyler[11] as "... that division of pharmacy which deals with patient care with particular emphasis on drug therapy. In practice it is patient oriented and includes not only the dispensing of required medication but also advising the patient on the proper use of all medications, both prescribed and patient selected. It also utilizes the pharmacist as an information source for members of the medical and other health professions on all matters pertaining to drugs and their dosage forms"; and *pharmacy administration* which deals with the principles and practices of business and law as they apply to pharmacy practice. Not yet generally accepted among the basic professional areas of pharmacy is the area of behavioral sciences of pharmacy. Undoubtedly, the socioeconomic problems of pharmacy are part of its heritage and future. Just what part this area will play in pharmaceutical education is yet to be determined.

Opportunities for undergraduate students to specialize in certain professional areas beyond the core of courses are becoming increasingly prevalent in pharmaceutical education. Most prominent among the areas of specialization will be hospital pharmacy and research. Pharmacy faculties who have determined what core material is necessary for *all* pharmacists have supported various programs aimed at better preparing the student for specific special functions among the variety of career opportunities available to the pharmaceutically educated individual. A greater trend for this type of education specialization is foreseen in the future.

The American Foundation for Pharmaceutical Education—No discussion of pharmaceutical education, no matter how brief, would be complete without appropriate credit to the American Foundation for Pharmaceutical Education (AFPE). The AFPE was incorporated in 1942. Its objectives are set forth as follows:[12]

The principal objectives of the American Foundation for Pharmaceutical Education, in brief, are: (1) To encourage and assist in providing improved educational standards and facilities for the adequate training of competent personnel in the practice of pharmacy and all related fields; (2) to supply the pharmaceutical and allied manufacturing industries, hospitals, government agencies, college faculties and other professional fields with technically and scientifically trained personnel; (3) to help colleges develop strong undergraduate programs; (4) to support graduate work in properly qualified colleges; and (5) to encourage scientific research as a necessary component of graduate work and as special projects.

The AFPE derives its income from individuals, former Fellows, and the voluntary contributions of the drug trade and allied manufacturing industries.

The accomplishments of the AFPE in the interest of pharmaceutical education are impressive and are summarized for the 1943–1982 period in Table I.

Table I—Summary Report of AFPE Grants in Support of Education—1943–1982[12]

Graduate Fellowships (1946–82)	$5,068,000
Undergraduate Scholarships (1943–78)	1,048,000
Student Recruitment Programs (1944–47; 1955–79)	645,000
World War II Aid to Colleges (1944–46)	97,000
American Journal of Pharmaceutical Education (1945–82)	423,000
Pharmacy Teachers' Seminar (1949–78)	283,500
American Council on Pharmaceutical Education (1945–82)	1,201,000
The Pharmaceutical Survey (1946–50)	178,000
Visiting Lecturers Program (1966–73)	72,000
Education Survey (AACP) (1967–69)	62,000
Interinstitutional Pharmacology Program (1968–72)	52,000
Commission on Pharmacy (1972–73)	30,000
Council of Sections Special Projects Program (AACP) (1979–82)	30,000
Pharmacy Education Profile System (1980–82)	20,000
Feasibility Study—AACP Coordinated Multicentered Research Project (1981–82)	11,600
Grand Total	$9,221,100

The support of pharmaceutical education by the AFPE has become a vital necessity for progress of pharmaceutical education and, hence, of the profession itself.

Licensure Requirements

The practice of pharmacy within each state is regulated by the laws of that state. This includes the regulation of licensure for pharmacy practice. To practice pharmacy in any state, a pharmacist must be a registered pharmacist (RPh) in that state. A "registered pharmacist" is also known as a "licensed pharmacist." Administration of pharmacy laws and the granting of registration to practice pharmacy are authorities vested in each state board of pharmacy. A graduate of any accredited college of pharmacy is eligible to take the examination for registration in any of the 50 states in the US providing he fulfills the requirements of the state. (See special California educational requirement below.) In recent years, these examinations have been oriented more toward the application of theoretical material to actual practice than to an examination of fact and theory alone.

A pharmacist registered in one of the 47 reciprocating states (California, Florida, and Hawaii are nonreciprocating states) may gain registration in most of the other reciprocating states by fulfilling the reciprocity requirements of the other states. Information about the reciprocity requirements of individual states may be obtained from the National Association of Boards of Pharmacy, One East Wacker Drive, Suite 2210, Chicago, IL 60601.

Licensing in the nonreciprocating states is governed by each state's regulations which usually involve, in addition to fulfilling residence and internship requirements, the taking of each state's complete licensure examination. Reciprocating states sometimes waive all but that part of the licensing examination which deals with state law. California also requires a minimum of *four years* registration *in an accredited college of pharmacy*, whereas the requirement for all other states is a degree in pharmacy from an accredited college of pharmacy. Colleges of pharmacy vary in their recommended programs allowing one or two years to be taken in junior or liberal arts colleges for the student to make normal progress toward graduation.

Additional information regarding pharmacy regulations may be found in Chapter 107.

Accredited Colleges of Pharmacy

The following colleges hold membership in the American Association of Colleges of Pharmacy and were accredited by the American Council on Pharmaceutical Education as of July 1, 1983:

Alabama	Auburn University, School of Pharmacy, Auburn
	Samford University, School of Pharmacy, Birmingham
Arizona	University of Arizona, College of Pharmacy, Tucson
Arkansas	University of Arkansas for Medical Sciences, College of Pharmacy, Little Rock
California	University of California, San Francisco, School of Pharmacy, San Francisco
	University of the Pacific, School of Pharmacy, Stockton
	University of Southern California, School of Pharmacy, Los Angeles
Colorado	University of Colorado, School of Pharmacy, Boulder
Connecticut	University of Connecticut, School of Pharmacy, Storrs
District of Columbia	Howard University, College of Pharmacy and Pharmacal Sciences, Washington
Florida	Florida Agricultural and Mechanical University, College of Pharmacy and Pharmaceutical Sciences, Tallahassee
	University of Florida, College of Pharmacy, J. Hillis Miller Health Center, Gainesville

Georgia	Mercer University, Southern School of Pharmacy, Atlanta
	University of Georgia, College of Pharmacy, Athens
Idaho	Idaho State University, College of Pharmacy, Pocatello
Illinois	University of Illinois at Chicago, College of Pharmacy, Chicago
Indiana	Butler University, College of Pharmacy, Indianapolis
	Purdue University, School of Pharmacy and Pharmacal Sciences, West Lafayette
Iowa	Drake University, College of Pharmacy, Des Moines
	The University of Iowa, College of Pharmacy, Iowa City
Kansas	University of Kansas, School of Pharmacy, Lawrence
Kentucky	University of Kentucky, College of Pharmacy, Lexington
Louisiana	Northeast Louisiana University, School of Pharmacy, Monroe
	Xavier University of Louisiana, College of Pharmacy, New Orleans
Maryland	University of Maryland, School of Pharmacy, Baltimore
Massachusetts	Massachusetts College of Pharmacy and Allied Health Sciences, Boston Campus, Boston
	Northeastern University, College of Pharmacy and Allied Health Professions, Boston
Michigan	Ferris State College, School of Pharmacy, Big Rapids
	University of Michigan, College of Pharmacy, Ann Arbor
	Wayne State University, College of Pharmacy and Allied Health Professions, Detroit
Minnesota	University of Minnesota, College of Pharmacy, Minneapolis
Mississippi	University of Mississippi, School of Pharmacy, University
Missouri	St. Louis College of Pharmacy, St. Louis
	University of Missouri—Kansas City, School of Pharmacy, Kansas City
Montana	University of Montana, School of Pharmacy and Allied Health Sciences, Missoula
Nebraska	Creighton University, School of Pharmacy and Allied Health Professions, Omaha
	University of Nebraska, College of Pharmacy, Omaha
New Jersey	Rutgers, The State University of New Jersey, College of Pharmacy, Piscataway
New Mexico	University of New Mexico, College of Pharmacy, Albuquerque
New York	Long Island University, Arnold and Marie Schwartz College of Pharmacy and Health Sciences, Brooklyn
	St. John's University, College of Pharmacy and Allied Health Professions, Jamaica
	State University of New York at Buffalo, School of Pharmacy, Buffalo
	Union University, Albany College of Pharmacy, Albany
North Carolina	University of North Carolina at Chapel Hill, School of Pharmacy, Chapel Hill
North Dakota	North Dakota State University, College of Pharmacy, Fargo
Ohio	Ohio Northern University, College of Pharmacy and Allied Health Sciences, Ada
	The Ohio State University, College of Pharmacy, Columbus
	University of Cincinnati, College of Pharmacy, Cincinnati
	University of Toledo, College of Pharmacy, Toledo
Oklahoma	Southwestern Oklahoma State University, School of Pharmacy, Weatherford
	University of Oklahoma, College of Pharmacy, Oklahoma City
Oregon	Oregon State University, School of Pharmacy, Corvallis
Pennsylvania	Duquesne University, School of Pharmacy, Pittsburgh
	Philadelphia College of Pharmacy and Science, Philadelphia
	Temple University, School of Pharmacy, Philadelphia
	University of Pittsburgh, School of Pharmacy, Pittsburgh
Puerto Rico	University of Puerto Rico, College of Pharmacy, Medical Science Campus, San Juan
Rhode Island	University of Rhode Island, College of Pharmacy, Kingston

South Carolina	Medical University of South Carolina, College of Pharmacy, Charleston
	University of South Carolina, College of Pharmacy, Columbia
South Dakota	South Dakota State University, College of Pharmacy, Brookings
Tennessee	University of Tennessee Center for Health Sciences, College of Pharmacy, Memphis
Texas	Texas Southern University, School of Pharmacy, Houston
	University of Houston, College of Pharmacy, Houston
	The University of Texas at Austin, College of Pharmacy, Austin
Utah	University of Utah, College of Pharmacy, Salt Lake City
Virginia	Virginia Commonwealth University, School of Pharmacy, Medical College of Virginia, Richmond
Washington	University of Washington, School of Pharmacy, Seattle
	Washington State University, College of Pharmacy, Pullman
West Virginia	West Virginia University, School of Pharmacy, Medical Center, Morgantown
Wisconsin	University of Wisconsin—Madison, School of Pharmacy, Madison
Wyoming	University of Wyoming, School of Pharmacy, Laramie

References

1. Deno RA, *et al: The Profession of Pharmacy*, 2nd ed, Lippincott, Philadelphia, 1, 1966.
2. *1981 Census of Pharmacists*, NABP, Chicago 1981.
3. Lader L: *Look:* 76, Nov. 26, 1968.
4. Gibson MR: *Am J Pharm Educ 23:* 461, 1959.
5. Smith MC: *Principles of Pharmaceutical Marketing*, 3rd ed, Lea & Febiger, Philadelphia, 400, 1983.
6. Lyman RA, *et al* (eds): *Am J Pharm Educ*, 1937–present.
7. Sonnedecker G: *Kremers and Urdang's History of Pharmacy*, 4th ed, Lippincott, Philadelphia, 227, 1976.
8. Colleges and Schools of Pharmacy Accredited Degree Programs, July 1, 1983, American Council on Pharmaceutical Education, Chicago.
9. Blauch LE, Webster GL: *The Pharmaceutical Curriculum*, Am Council Educ, Washington, DC, 47, 1952.
10. Wagner JG: *Drug Intel 2:* 31, 1968.
11. Tyler VE: *Am J Pharm Educ 22:* 764, 1968.
12. *40 Years of Service to Pharmacy, 1982 Progress Report*, American Foundation for Pharmaceutical Education, Fair Lawn, NJ, 3, 1982.
13. *Ibid*, p 7.

CHAPTER 2

Evolution of Pharmacy

Glenn Sonnedecker, PhD

Professor, History of Pharmacy
School of Pharmacy, University of Wisconsin
Madison, WI 53706

Pharmacy in some guise has been inseparable from mankind's history since it fulfils one of our most basic needs. As man made his way through remote times or places, he shielded himself against disease as best he could, reaching out, often blindly, toward the resources of nature but in the process gradually elaborating pharmaceutical theories, techniques, and implements. The person supplying this essential service may not be recognizable always as a pharmacist in our sense of the term; conversely, the pharmacist as such has been designated in a variety of ways throughout the ages. However designated, it is above all the community practitioner of pharmacy who comes within the focus of this short socio-historical essay.

Primitive Probings—How people fend off disease depends largely on how they define its cause. In the world still are millions who see the patient as a victim of evil forces or of a god's anger, who see disease as punishment for sin. So we can imagine, in the absence of much surviving evidence, how terrifying and supernatural seemed the afflictions of primitive people in the dawn of history. Afflictions that came in such mysterious ways and with such uncanny effects certainly called for supernatural as well as natural countermeasures.

Thus the healing practitioner, whether shaman or priest, had best know how to command the resources of the spirit world and know what substances from the natural world convey or reinforce the countervailing powers. From such blind empirical groping, extending over many millennia, it came to be appreciated that some herbs were more powerful than others, whether with or without incantations. Yet, up to the present moment, there have been people who sought healing not from medication but from religion; indeed, most patients rely partly—and wholly when medical science fails—on their faith. Nevertheless, the changing relationship between empiricism (later, science) and religion is one significant strand in the history of therapeutics through antiquity and into the Middle Ages.

Antiquity

By the second millennium BC the civilizations of Babylonia and Egypt had produced the small clay tablets and the long scrolls (see Fig 2-1) that survive as the oldest pharmaceutical records known. They show that these river-valley peoples knew, however crudely, many of the basic forms of drug administration employed today (eg, gargles, suppositories, inhalations, poultices, ointments) and knew hundreds of different substances used as drugs (eg, asafoetida, dates, garlic, castor beans, hellebore). In application, the theurgical and magical potentiation of the medications may never have been thrust aside entirely by practitioners in the ancient Near East, although the emphasis varied with the ebb and flow of civilization.

When no pressing need for specialization was felt, pharmacy and medicine have tended to coalesce, and a steadily progressive development of two cleanly separated fields scarcely can be traced before the late Middle Ages. However, from fragmentary pharmacomedical records so far deciphered, it appears that at one time, at least, a Babylonian class of preparers of remedies and cosmetics was quartered in a special street, and westward in Egypt the collectors, preparers, and conservators of drug resources became more specialized and separated than had been supposed before recent studies.

Within another millennium the Greeks living around the Aegean Sea and on its islands, nourished by the intellectual produce of the fertile basins of the Nile and the Tigris and Euphrates, burst the old mold and created a distinctive intellectual life that today still commands admiration. Greek medicine was no exception.

Looking nature full in the face, without being blinded either by the divine or by the customary, Greek intellectuals sought rational explanations of everything. In the medical field perhaps this was exemplified best by the followers of Hippocrates (born ca 460 BC on Cos). Their best writings and practices showed the fundamentals of scientific method—observation and classification, rejection of unsupported theory and superstition, and a cautious generalization and induction that remained open to critical discussion and revision.

This produced less rather than more reliance on drug therapy among many practitioners, and in neither the drug armamentarium nor the cadre of pharmacomedical workers were advances as startling as might be expected.

Hippocratic insistence on rational treatment of the indi-

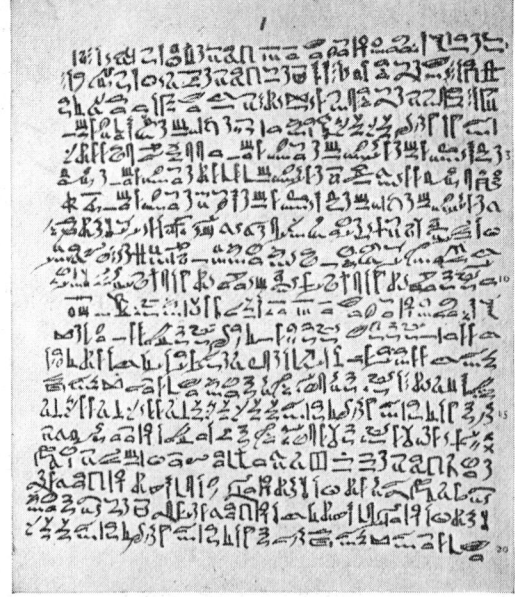

Fig 2-1. Since the dawn of recorded history, the pharmaceutical efforts of mankind against disease are attested on scroll, stone, parchment, and paper. Illustrated is an excerpt from one of the most important pharmaceutical records of the ancient Near East, a papyrus more than 21 yards long, largely filled with information on drugs of the Egyptians. (Ebers Papyrus, about 1500 BC)

Middle Ages

With the advent of Christianity the healing temples of Asklepios eventually fell into disuse. During the medieval millennium, however, religious medicine within Christian concepts gave the healing power of faith and divine intervention new scope. Moreover, the practice of pharmacy and medicine in the Western world largely passed from the hands of lay practitioners to clerics, under the impact of cultural barbarization and political fragmentation.

Monasteries became the centers of intellectual life, including pharmacomedical study as well as practice. Greco-Roman treatises were preserved, and fragments and epitomes, handwritten in Latin, were passed about as a basis for health services. Two widely used treatises on simple drugs were a condensate from Galen's medical writings, perhaps compiled by Gariopontus in the 11th century, and the herbal of a so-called Pseudo-Apuleius (an anonymous work from the 6th century or earlier, influenced by Dioscorides). The monks often cultivated medicinal plants outside the monastery, as well as collecting them from the countryside. Inside was an "armarium pigmentarium," a room where the drugs were kept, to which a laboratory sometimes was added. Some monastic laboratories were renowned for expert distillation of aromatic and cordial waters.

As a guide to preparing compound drugs, two traditional types of Latin compilations, which evolved into modern counterparts, were the "Antidotaria" (similar to dispensatories) and the "Receptaria" (more modest formularies). It was a practical literature for both medicine and pharmacy, copied by scribes who added, omitted, and revised to suit local needs.

During the second half of the European Middle Ages, pharmacy gradually moved outside the monasteries, became better separated from medicine, and began to evolve independent standards and responsibilities in the more urbanized centers. This trend becomes noticeable early in Italy, Spain, and France, which provided transit points for drugs and for pharmacomedical knowledge flowing along Mediterranean trade routes from the more advanced Islamic civilization.

Scholars working in Islamic lands after the 8th century assimilated old Greco-Roman wisdom more thoroughly than could be done in Europe; the best of them produced a pharmacomedical amalgam of their own which became influential and authoritative in Europe after their treatises were translated into Latin (11th and 12th centuries).

For pharmacy, the Arabic influence was important also because we can discern the rise of the qualified pharmacist (al-Saidalani) as a separate functionary, beginning around Baghdad not later than the first half of the 9th century. The richer Arabic materia medica and more refined and elegant polypharmacal modes of administering drugs (as compared with antiquity) intensified the need for a specialist in pharmaceutical work. Thus, pharmacy reflected a general elaborative tendency of Arabic intellectualism.

Therapeutic effectiveness advanced only modestly, however, and the rationale of drug therapy, which was chiefly botanic, remained congealed in the Galenic mold of humoural pathology.

By the 12th century public pharmacies probably had begun to appear in the south of Italy and France and perhaps elsewhere. Some pharmacies apparently remained under church control since information about them appears in old monastic documents. Hospitals, however, were being secularized under municipal authority by the 13th century. While it is debated to what extent modern pharmacy—as part of a governmentally supervised system of health care—grew directly from monastic medicine, it is clear that the influence was pervasive.

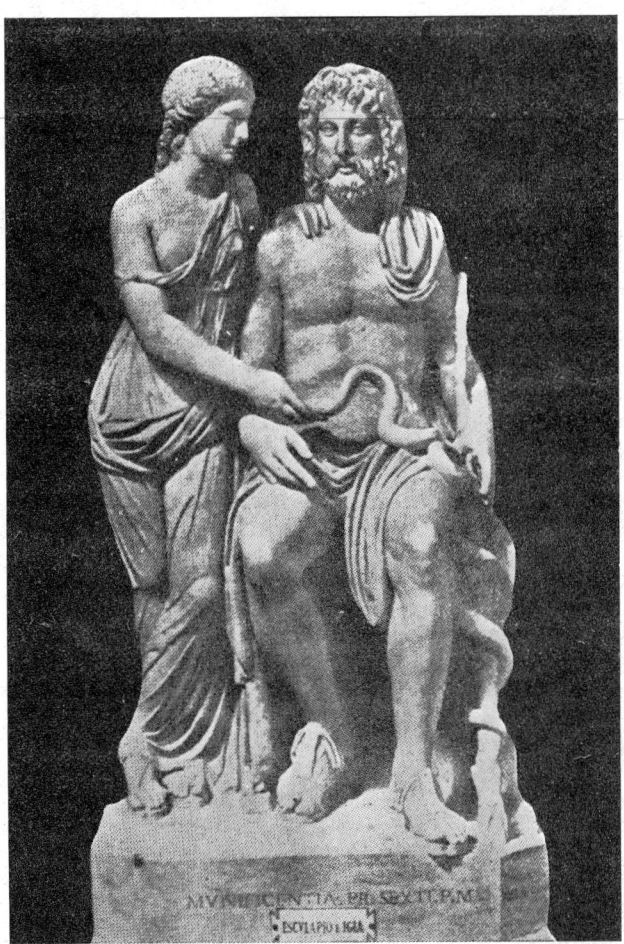

Fig 2-2. The god Asklepios and his daughter Hygeia with a sacred serpent, are shown in this classical statue. Together they healed the afflicted of ancient Greece who sought their supernatural aid, and from them arose the international symbols of pharmacy and medicine still used today. (From Osler W: *Evolution of Modern Medicine*, Yale Univ. Press, New Haven, 1922.)

vidual did not require rejection of religion but it did place the supernatural in a separate category of the patient's resources, and the practitioner himself typically relied on his natural resources whether for explanation, diagnosis, or treatment. This so limited the scope of claimed effectiveness that we are not surprised to find that ancient Greeks, rich and poor alike, streamed into the temples for aid when lay medicine failed, as it often did.

Beginning in the 7th century before Christ, the wise and kind Asklepios gradually superseded Apollo as the greatest of the healing gods. At the touch of his hand or staff or of the tongue of his sacred serpent, miraculous things happened to the afflicted. Medical practitioners were tolerant; indeed, in Asklepios they saw symbolic embodiment of an ideal perfection of their calling which reality could never be. The staff of Asklepios, entwined by a sacred serpent, gradually emerged as the official symbol of medicine around the world. On the right hand of Asklepios, helping to minister to the afflicted, stood Hygeia, one of his daughters, her arm entwined by a serpent and holding a bowl, now thought to have contained a healing potion. In modern times her bowl entwined by the serpent gradually emerged as the official symbol of pharmacy throughout most of the Western world and by the mid-20th century had come into prominence in the United States. How the virgin goddess and her divine, powerful father were envisioned may be seen in the classical statue depicted as Fig 2-2.

The Pharmacists' Code of Genoa, As Revised 1407

from *Historiae Patriae Monumenta* . . . (Vol 18, col 674*ff*); adapted from a translation.   See Reynolds RL *Am J Pharm Educ 5:* 330, 1941.

We fix and ordain that no outsider may take over, conduct or hold a pharmacy (or house or warehouse for a drug business) unless he has been licensed by the Master Pharmacists ["Speciarii"].

Nor shall any pharmacist break the rules of the profession under penalty.

No one save a licensed pharmacist may sell at retail syrups, elixirs, pills or other pharmacist's preparations.   Except that merchants from overseas may sell small consignments of pharmaceutical materials.

Pharmacists are expected to keep their shops open during business hours.   However, shops must be closed Sundays, Feasts of the Apostles and San Lorenzo's day.   Save, however, that on such holy days they shall keep a [dispensing] window open at one table of only two palms size.

No quantity of arsenic or poisons may be sold, given away, allowed to be used or transferred except by a Master Pharmacist or his licensed employee who may be in charge.   A pharmacist's son of over twenty years of age, trained in the profession, may suffice in such a case.

Since in the pharmacist's profession no personal advantages or prerogatives may be permitted, but only that whoever is best and produces the best products should be esteemed, and so that each may have incentive to improve and grow steadily from good to better: We fix and ordain that no pharmacist shall dare or presume to place or stamp, or cause to be placed or stamped, the label of another pharmacist on any bottle or pill-box.   Rather, every pharmacist having or wishing to have a trade-mark which he might make, affix or stamp—or have made, affixed or impressed—on bottles and pill-boxes of preparations and other goods, may have such a trade-mark made or placed or impressed, but it must be different from every other pharmacist's mark.

No pharmacist may fill the bottle or pill-box bearing the label of any other pharmacist.   If a purchaser comes with a bottle or box bearing another pharmacist's label, such label must be taken off or scratched over and the second pharmacist must affix his own label or trademark.

All materials from which remedies are compounded must be kept in the windows of the shop, in view of the public, continuously for eight days after the compound has been mixed.

No Turk or Tartar slave may be taught how to be a pharmacist. Other slaves may be taught the profession, but they may not be left in charge of shops even if they have been liberated, nor may they hold guild offices.

We fix and ordain—to prevent any pharmacist from having temptation or reason for sinning, and to keep them from raising prices higher than is becoming—that no pharmacist may keep shop in partnership or agreement with any physician.   All pharmacists must swear an oath before the Masters of the Craft, each year, to observe completely and precisely the letter and spirit of this prohibition.

No one may peddle drugs, pills, or elixirs through the streets or from door to door, unless specially licensed.   Sailors, mariners, and merchants coming from overseas may, however, seek purchasers for small consignments of pharmacist's wares.

No pharmacist or agent may receive, purchase, take, or accept as gift any merchandise from a city inspector or agent of such inspector or city warehouse supervisor.

By the 13th century the lay practice of pharmacy had developed sufficiently in the Kingdom of the Two Sicilies to justify legislation.   These edicts became so influential elsewhere that they have been called the "magna charta" of pharmacy.   This was part of serial health legislation (completed by 1240) that provided for the separation of pharmacy from medicine, for official supervision, and for obligating the pharmacist by oath to prepare drugs reliably, according to skilled art, in a uniform, suitable quality.   Two further provisions placed a legal limitation on the number of pharmacies and on the prices of drugs.

Some of the responsibilities and some of the problems of a late-medieval pharmacist in Genoa are suggested by the code reproduced in the box on this page.   A further glimpse of an acceptable pharmacist in 15th-century Italy can be seen in

requirements stated by a contemporary physician, Saladin di Asculo.   In his . . . *Compendium for Pharmacists* he said that a pharmacist must know Latin to understand the pharmaceutical literature and the physicians' prescriptions.   His main task is to prepare drugs (by such processes as rubbing, levigating, infusing, decocting, and distilling) and to compound and preserve them well.   A pharmacist should be mature and modest, a pious and honest man, with compassion toward the poor.   He must not be avaricious, and ask only reasonable fees.   He must not be unskilled; he neither keeps deteriorated drugs in his shop nor substitutes one drug for another against the patient's interest or the physician's expressed wish.   If a young and inexperienced physician chooses unsuitable drugs on occasion, the pharmacist should "advise the physician to prescribe more placable and better ones. . . ." A pharmacist needs at hand at least six books, to practice his art properly, for which Saladin particularly recommended treatises on simple drugs by Avicenna and Serapion, on synonyms by Simon Januensis, and on compound drugs by Pseudo-Mesuë and Nicolaus.

The late Middle Ages strengthened pharmacy functionally, legally, and as an independent calling.   Often it was organized and disciplined within early guilds.   This development was uneven, regionally, and was periodically marred by friction (usually jurisdictional disputes) with medicine on one side or with spicers, grocers, or the like, on the other.*

Modern Europe

During the Renaissance, medicine moved more boldly outside the rather rigid framework of clerical and Arabic scholasticism.   A year after Columbus reached America there was born in a Swiss village a boy who would become a medical iconoclast of far-reaching influence on the practice of pharmacy.   Paracelsus, as he was later called, introduced the idea of the body as a chemical laboratory and railed against outmoded authorities.   Through the Paracelsians, his followers, alchemical processes became more widely applied in pharmacy, chemicals were used more boldly for internal therapy, and extraction of medicinally active "quintessences" from nature's resources became a goal.   Thus eventually the chemical role of the pharmacist overshadowed his more traditional art rooted in botanic science.

Through mastery of practical chemistry the best European pharmacists of the early modern period made discoveries important not only to drug therapy but also to the youthful science of chemistry (Fig 2-3).   The specialized development of sciences basic to pharmacy of the later 18th and 19th centuries would be needed, however, to generate the therapeutic revolution that meanwhile has replaced most of the centuries-old accretion of materia medica.

The scope and importance of guilds for pharmacy had varied markedly with the social circumstance of various cultural areas, but even in Italy and France they were being superseded by the 18th century.   In their place rose modern professional societies, which also offered varying degrees of self-government.   Frequently, they either opened schools of pharmacy or encouraged established institutions of higher learning to do so.   The traditional entrance to pharmacy through prolonged apprenticeship (often four to eight years as apprentice and clerk) gradually was modified by academic study.   For example, pharmacy gained a better-defined place among scientific professions in Prussia when in 1725 obligatory examinations based on academic standards were instituted.   During the later 18th century, private institutes for formal education in pharmacy arose on German territory,

---

* Apparently some interchange of titles and of personnel among these groups occurred (at least in certain regions) until a clearer structuring of pharmacy and related occupations took place after the Middle Ages.

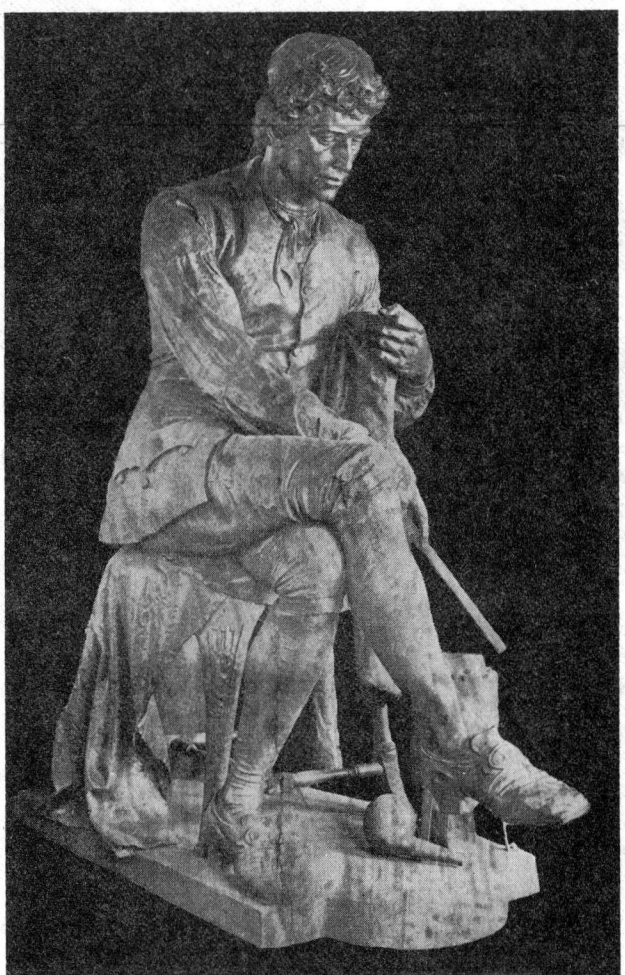

Fig 2-3. This monument in Stockholm memorializes Carl Wilhelm Scheele, one of the most distinguished of the 18th-century pharmacist-chemists who made important contributions to science. Scheele discovered oxygen (a year before Priestley) and chlorine; he paved the way to the isolation of tungsten, manganese, and molybdenum; and through his method of isolating organic acids, he opened a new era of organic chemistry. These and many other discoveries were made in the pharmacies where he worked.

leading to establishment of required pharmacy curricula in the regular universities, first in Bavaria (1808), then in other German states. In Italy by the early 19th century academic study and examination were required for pharmacy throughout the peninsula. About the same time, French legislation provided six higher schools of pharmacy for the country (1803), although there had been local and uneven development of academic courses there since the 16th century.

The maturing of West European pharmacy during the 17th century had given its best qualified practitioners a part in the early organized activities of science and its periodical literature. The pattern was set and ambitions nurtured for purely pharmaceutical organizations, and then specialized pharmaceutical periodicals, such as a German annual (f 1780) and Trommsdorff's *Journal der Pharmacie* (f 1793), and the French *Journal de la société des pharmaciens de Paris* (f 1797).

Pharmaceutical manuals and reference works that began to come from the pens of pharmacists themselves by the 16th century also signalized a profession ascendant. The proliferation of formulas and the risk of varying composition in compound drugs of the same name stimulated a trend toward drug standardization. This was expressed in the adoption of the *Dispensatorium* of Valerius Cordus (1546) as official for the imperial city of Nuremberg, followed by other local pharmacopeias still in the 16th century. Still earlier (1499), the *Nuovo receptario* was published as a standard for the city-state of Florence, but its "officiality" rested on guild rather than on government authority—a reminder that the question of defining the term "pharmacopeia" affects pharmacopeial history.

Descendants of this literature would be used eclectically by American practitioners, especially the British pharmacopeias. The *Pharmacopoeia Londinensis* (1st ed, 1618), intended for the whole realm of England, was the first for so large a political unit. (Earlier pharmacopeias had been for Continental city-states or principalities.) Several British dispensatories, based on this and other pharmacopeias, made the dispensatory seem almost a British specialty. Duncan's *Edinburgh New Dispensatory* provided the basis for the first dispensatory published on American soil, the *American Dispensatory* (1806), compiled by John Redman Coxe, a Philadelphia physician.

Symptomatic of the *laissez-faire* development in Britain, which hindered orderly professional structuring, was the fact that the original apothecaries evolved into legally recognized medical practitioners (confirmed, 1703, by the Rose case). Although these general practitioners only slowly gave up drug dispensing (mostly in the present century), during the 19th century a modern profession of pharmacy was fashioned anew out of the "chymists" and "druggists." Education as well as organization was created through the present Pharmaceutical Society of Great Britain (founded 1841, after the old Society of Apothecaries of London, f 1617, had become preoccupied with the medical ambitions of its members). The now-traditional designation of the British practitioner as a "chemist-and-druggist" (rather than apothecary or pharmacist) finds explanation in his unusual antecedents.

A dominant pharmaceutical influence from England, until long after the Revolution, helped shape the particular character of American pharmacy, fed by the availability of literature in the mother tongue, the immigration of ideas as well as men, and the heavy import of British drugs.

American Pharmacy*

In New England the settler often had to serve as their own physician and pharmacist. As the frontier moved amoeba-like west and south, a primitive battle against disheartening health conditions repeated itself again and again. In an emergency someone with a greater medical experience was sought, perhaps the clergyman or the teacher. But the settler could meet many contingencies with some medical lore picked up from the Indians, a few store-bought remedies that were either imports or imitations of those popular in England, and a household herbal or medical book. Some brought over the volumes called *Countrey Contentments*, or *The English Huswife* and *The English Husbandman*, written by that prolific literary figure Gervase Markham. Others had *The English Physician* from the pen of that raucous medical figure, Nicolas Culpeper. English herbals, such as those by John Parkinson and by John Gerarde, often guided the colonial cultivation and use of medicinal plants.

In larger settlements individuals appeared who called themselves physician or apothecary—a title self-bestowed, often signifying little more than a bold medical pretension and courage. There were also a few persons, especially after the Revolution in the few maturing cities, who had qualified in

* The discussion of American pharmacy is adapted in part from an address at an Evening Meeting of the Pharmaceutical Society of Great Britain by Sonnedecker G *Pharm J 176:* 171, 1956, which is utilized here with permission of the publisher.

Europe by professional experience and training. Both the qualified and the unqualified practitioners ordinarily practiced pharmacy as well as medicine. Their public pharmaceutical shops served as a base for medical practice, like the shops of the so-called apothecaries in 18th-century England. It was a pattern only slowly outgrown in New England as in the Olde.

The physician–pharmacist, whatever his knowledge or lack of it, multiplied his kind through a system of indentured apprenticeship imported from the mother country. The word "system" may be too strong, for a system already decadent in Europe had to be transplanted without the organized controls and standards that gave it measurable meaning within the old guilds.

By the early 19th century pharmacy began to show some independence from medicine. Here and there medical practice was disappearing from public drug shops into private offices. More pharmacists from abroad were venturing to America. Some Americans who had trained under a physician–pharmacist came to specialize increasingly in pharmaceutical service. A few of the drug merchants, importers, or operators of general stores grew more knowledgeable and ambitious as opportunity for pharmaceutical service grew. The need for higher competence and standards was felt particularly among the so-called "druggists," men who imported drugs, developed small-scale manufacturing, operated a dispensing shop, and distributed drugs wholesale to physicians and to the general stores at country crossroads. These men began the long process of professionalization by helping to found the first associations and schools.

At first the independence of pharmacy and a feeling of interdependence among its practitioners were nurtured entirely through local associations. These "colleges," as they were called, sprang up in a few highly developed urban centers during the second quarter of the 19th century, setting a pattern for others later on. In the local associations, formerly isolated dispensers found mutual encouragement for improving their knowledge, technique, and ethical standards.

Pharmaceutical Organizations

As iron rails fanned out across the states and better communications tied towns more closely together, larger pharmaceutical organizations flourished and the pioneering local associations declined in importance. In 1852 the local associations were instrumental in founding the American Pharmaceutical Association (APhA). It in turn fostered pharmaceutical associations in the individual states. Most of the state associations in the present United States were born during the last 30 years of the 19th century. Today, their combined membership far exceeds that of any single national organization. The activities of state associations embrace all aspects of dispensing pharmacy, although as a generality the main orientation has tended to be commercial.

The professional interests of pharmacists have always centered in the American Pharmaceutical Association. Its membership lies open to any pharmacy graduate who wishes to foster its aims. Kremers and Urdang succinctly characterized the role of the APhA in saying:

It represented, defended and promoted, during the decades in which the calling gained its distinctive shape, all fields of pharmaceutical enterprise and interest, the scientific and educational as well as the commercial, the ethical, and the legal. It always has been the guardian, although not always the initiator, of all progressive movements concerning American pharmacy.

The initiative was increasingly divided after the end of the 19th century, as organized pharmacy splintered and developed more specialized organizations. Some of these offshoots remained affiliated or closely oriented to the mother society; others went separate, sometimes divergent ways. For ex-

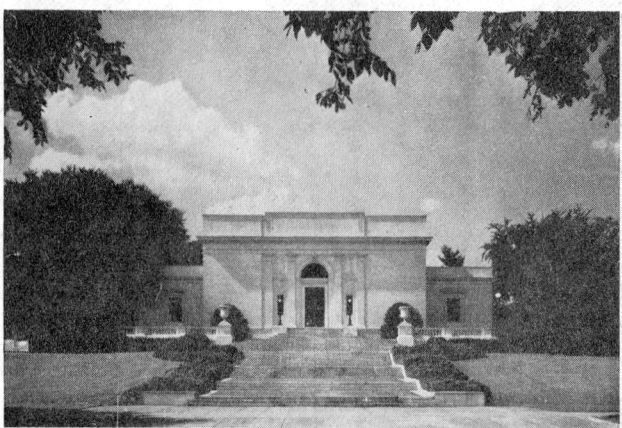

Fig 2-4. The headquarters building of the American Pharmaceutical Association in Washington, DC (dedicated in 1934) symbolizes the professional development and aspirations of American pharmacy. The Association (founded in 1852) was the first national organization of pharmacy in the US.

ample, the American Pharmaceutical Association could not focus sufficiently on economic interests to satisfy pharmacy owners, for whom a free economic system offered perplexing problems in the late 19th century. Therefore, such problems have been dealt with since 1898 through the National Association of Retail Druggists (NARD), which limits its active membership to pharmacy owners. The NARD has demonstrated the compelling need for organized cooperation on questions of business and finance, just as the APhA has done in the professional and scientific sphere (see Fig 2-4).

The fact that these two major national organizations have never contained more than a minority of the pharmacists in community practice illustrates a chronic organizational problem persisting since the 19th century. For the group-conscious segment of practicing pharmacists, this problem has been painfully intensified by periodic disharmony between the NARD and the APhA, ranging from erratic coordination of effort to open clashes, especially after the 1940s. The roots of this organizational dilemma have never been carefully evaluated, but the record implies an inadequate definition of the respective commercial and professional spheres of action and influence, ineffective diplomacy, and fundamental differences as to the goals of American pharmacy.

Less dissension, although only a tenuous coordination, has characterized the relations of 20-odd national societies, councils, and conferences that have come to serve the branches of dispensing pharmacy, manufacture, wholesale distribution, education, and legal control. With such a compartmented subdivision of power and functions, organized effort remained "uncoordinated, oft-times in conflict," concluded The Pharmaceutical Survey of 1946–1949. Two avenues for the exchange and harmonizing of varied views are the House of Delegates of the APhA and the National Drug Trade Conference.

Education

The associations of pharmacists have been instrumental in erecting an educational system, which must nourish every viable profession. Local pharmaceutical associations that sponsored the early pioneering instruction during the second quarter of the 19th century drew a certain stimulus from the burgeoning public interest in education generally, from the lead taken by medicine, and from a popular fascination with science at the time. The Philadelphia College of Pharmacy launched instruction in 1821, the same year it was founded as the first local association. It was 20 years before a similar beginning in England, because in the mother country the cord of professional continuity had been broken, and pharmacy still steered an unsteady course in the crosscurrents of her particular historical circumstance.

In America by the end of the Civil War, five of the seven local associations were offering some academic instruction to those apprentices who had the desire, time, and money for formal schooling. Classes usually were held at night in rented rooms. There were no laboratories. Finances were uncertain. The pharmacists who controlled the new schools saw their purpose largely as a "rounding-off" and systematizing of the traditional apprenticeship. Students heard series of lectures in chemistry and in materia medica—and later on in pharmacy, as the inadequacies of the apprenticeship were more frankly faced. The evolution of the instructional pattern closely paralleled that in England. Moreover, the most popular textbooks were of British origin. The lack of an American literature was a gap not quickly closed; and competent British texts not only were at hand in the mother tongue but probably were preferred also because French and German works tended to be more theoretical.

The early association schools in urban centers made their fundamental contribution by establishing an educational system, by raising the sights of pharmacy, and by sending into the more sparsely settled areas some graduates who might serve as foci around which professional endeavors could crystallize. However, perhaps not more than 1 in 20 of those entering pharmacy before the 1860s were able or willing to obtain a diploma.

After the war between the states came an upsurge in the founding of schools. At least 83 schools of various types opened their doors to pharmacy students during the 1800s, and about 60 of them survived the century. A student could choose among a wide array of standards, degrees, and curricula. Within this wild, mixed growth emerged an entirely new outlook for American pharmaceutical education, when it began to make connection with vigorous general institutions of higher learning.

The first significant break from the old pattern had come in 1868 when the state University of Michigan established a pharmacy course. It was infused with laboratory work. It demanded practically the full time of the student. It ignored the traditional apprenticeship requirement. The consequences were revolutionary as one state university after the other put pharmacy into its constellation of curricula.

This developing structure represented a promise rather than its fulfilment. For nowhere in the USA at the end of the 19th century, among all the states and schools, was any *formal* professional education actually required for licensure. The first half of the present century brought sweeping changes. There was a consolidation and reintegration of pharmaceutical education, on the plane largely set by the schools of pharmacy in state universities. Cooperation and reasonable uniformity among the schools replaced the rugged individualism and wide disparity. The United States was growing up culturally, and nationally. The era of westward expansion had come to an end, and the more uniform social conditions emerging among the states, across this 3000-mile expanse, made it easier to cooperate in setting and in maintaining standards.

When a new student walked through the door of a pharmacy school in 1900 he was expected to have at least an elementary school preparation—although standards of the different schools varied widely. In little more than two decades, recognized pharmacy schools would erase a severe handicap to adequate instruction by agreeing upon high-school graduation as an entrance prerequisite. In 1900 the pharmacy student commonly took a two-year course of study, but he could find schools where he would graduate after studying only 40 weeks or so. The University of Wisconsin was already pioneering the four-year course, as an optional curriculum to the two-year

course. After another three decades, all recognized schools agreed to make the four-year course a minimum standard (1932).

A five-year course was adopted as the minimum, after sharp controversy, for all students entering accredited schools after the spring of 1960. Thereafter, some schools experimented with longer or different programs that led to a Doctor of Pharmacy degree (first initiated in 1950 at the University of Southern California), encouraged by findings of The Pharmaceutical Survey of 1946–49. These extended programs tended to place more emphasis upon biological sciences to foster the kind of professional practice that came to be called "clinical pharmacy."

Pharmaceutical education at large also was responding to changes that had occurred in the pharmaceutical field and in the needs of medical care. The curricular trend increasingly emphasized studies and clinical experience that would permit the pharmacist an authoritative role aimed at maximizing the safe and effective utilization of both prescription and nonprescription products. Studies gradually deemphasized were those designed for the traditional, central function of drug making, which after mid-century had become outmoded in community practice.

If American pharmacy had begun to move in a new direction, questions remained about the education course to be followed: the length of the curriculum, the extent of specialization, the degrees to be awarded. One response was to appoint a Study Commission on Pharmacy, under the aegis of the American Association of Colleges of Pharmacy. Its report in 1975 helped to focus the debate and efforts toward clarifying pharmacy's goals, although it by no means resolved the issues.

As professional education lengthened beyond the standard baccalaureate degree, apprehensions arose that it might undermine research education in pharmacy, which offered career opportunities beginning in 1902 when the first Doctor of Philosophy degree associated with a school of pharmacy (University of Wisconsin) was awarded.

A hesitant growth of graduate departments gained more momentum after the early 1930s. During the subsequent three decades, the number of postgraduate students undertaking pharmaceutical research specialties multiplied about 15-fold, by 1963–1964 numbering 1339 in 54 schools and by 1982 increasing to 2927.

Since 1932 an accrediting agency, the American Council on Pharmaceutical Education, has been active in maintaining standards of pharmaceutical education and fostering improvements. Because of modern demands on schools of pharmacy, both at the undergraduate and at the graduate levels, the tendency since the early part of this century has been toward strengthening the educational system rather than expanding it and toward consolidation of independent schools with general institutions of higher learning.

Legal Controls

While the development of pharmaceutical education represented one of the efforts to help everyone more effectively take advantage of the liberty and opportunity of young America, legal controls then seemed to smack of oppressive restriction, if not even of class distinction. But the British *laissez-faire* spirit, so congenial to American conditions, was gradually attenuated during the 19th century without being lost.

In most states the original laws that effectively defined American pharmacy for the first time and delimited its practice were adopted in the period between 1870 and 1900. Earlier attempts to regulate pharmacy by local and state laws typically were not enforced sufficiently to support the development of professional standards.

After the Civil War the APhA promulgated a model state pharmacy act and fostered the founding of state pharmaceutical associations, which frequently played a key role in securing passage of a pharmacy law in the individual states. These laws were sufficiently disparate to make reciprocity of licenses difficult, if not impossible. The need to develop and coordinate a system expediting the transfer of pharmacists from one state to another therefore was one of the principal functions that gave life to the National Association of Boards of Pharmacy (f 1904).

In modern form the state pharmacy acts mainly establish standards for pharmacists and pharmacies (and for other conditions of drug dispensing), typically leaving to additional legislation the setting of standards for drug products as such (including particularly the ramifications of adulteration and misbranding).

Early state regulation in this latter field proved to be gravely inadequate, thus increasing social pressures after the turn of the century for federal legislation. The movement led by the physician–chemist Harvey W. Wiley, which culminated in the Federal Food and Drug Act of 1906, was strengthened by exposés of bad conditions in the food industry and, later, of uncontrolled quackery that infested much of the patent-medicine industry. The federal law repeatedly has had strengthening revision and amendment (notably 1938, 1952, and 1962), supplemented by a separate statute governing biological products (since 1902; modified 1944 and 1972).

Because of the abuse of narcotics, and the enigma and thraldom of addiction, the Federal (Harrison) Narcotic Act was passed in 1914, placing the United States in the vanguard of nations pledged to build an effective control mechanism, based on international agreement and cooperation. The problem flared anew during the 1960s with an increase in the number and types of drug dependencies. This culminated in the Drug Abuse Act of 1970, which both consolidated and revised the federal legal controls against nonmedicinal use of drugs that had evolved since the 1914 enactment. State laws analogous both to the national narcotic law and to the food and drug law were adopted in most states, protecting against intrastate violators who are constitutionally beyond the reach of federal agents.

This complex of laws, evolving into their modern form during the past century, has relied on pharmacists to fulfil important responsibilities and, in so doing, has helped to create a professionalized role for pharmacists in society. These legal controls are supplemented by the self-control represented by professional ethics.

The Ethics of Pharmacy

Characteristic of professions is a common concern with collective self-discipline of the group. As part of the *quid pro quo* for certain legal prerogatives granted to the profession by society, the practitioner has accepted responsibilities for an ethical standard of conduct going beyond conformity with law or technical skill. This has seemed particularly needful in health professions, such as pharmacy, where the services meet one of mankind's basic needs and where the patient often has no reliable means of judging the standard of service for himself.

In a profession this ethical obligation cannot be superseded by passage of laws; no matter how wide the net may be woven for controlling a profession through force (law), an area of activities always remains for control through voluntary self-discipline (ethics). For the pharmacist that means essentially a willingness to help assure that a patient, at whatever time or place, may assume that a qualified practitioner invariably will use his professional knowledge in the best interests of the patient and of society—within a framework of interlaced technical, legal, and ethical standards of practice.

The American Pharmacist's Professional Oath*

At this time, I vow to devote my professional life to the service of mankind through the profession of pharmacy.

I will consider the welfare of humanity and relief of human suffering my primary concerns.

I will use my knowledge and skills to the best of my ability in serving the public and other health professionals.

I will do my best to keep abreast of developments and maintain professional competency in my profession of pharmacy.

I will obey the laws governing the practice of pharmacy and will support enforcement of such laws.

I will maintain the highest standards of moral and ethical conduct.

I take these vows voluntarily with the full realization of the trust and responsibility with which I am empowered by the public.

In pharmacy, as in other health professions, the ethical standards have been expressed through a professional oath and a professional code (historically, these two forms sometimes hybridize). The oath ordinarily is brief and general, intended to obligate and inspire the pharmacist to abide by applicable laws, codified ethics, and the dictates of conscience and religious principles.

The ancient Hippocratic Oath is a classical example in the health field. A modern version is still administered, internationally, to neophytes of the medical profession, and a pharmaceutical version has had some usage in the pharmaceutical profession. The oath gradually gaining wider use in American pharmacy has been developed by the American Association of Colleges of Pharmacy. It is administered in various states either upon graduation from a school of pharmacy or upon conferral of the state license to practice.

The codes of ethics, compared with an oath, have been much more detailed and explicit. In well-elaborated form, a code provides an operational blueprint of the norms of professional conduct, a concrete recital of desirable and undesirable actions having recognized impact on the profession's character and functional reliability. If a codified ethos becomes too abstract or idealized—for the sake of brevity or of avoiding public acknowledgment of problem areas—the document becomes correspondingly handicapped as a practical instrument of self-government. An alternative (as employed by American medicine, for example) supplements a relatively concise and generalized code with a manual of currently valid interpretations and case histories concerning individual clauses or principles contained in the basic public-oriented document.

In American pharmacy professional ethics were first codified (1848) by the first association, the Philadelphia College of Pharmacy. Four years later the American Pharmaceutical Association, still in the year of founding, promulgated the document antecedent to the present Code of Ethics. At first too far ahead of its time for general application, the Code was given renewed life through major revisions in 1922, 1952, and 1969.

The APhA's Code has been considered the basic guide and document for American pharmacists, although pharmaceutical manufacturers, wholesalers, and other specialized groups have sufficiently specialized problems to make separate codes seem necessary. Even among practicing pharmacists themselves, there are sufficiently divergent interests and ideas so that some organizations have adopted their own version of the

---

* As revised 1983, developed and approved, 1963, by the American Association of Colleges of Pharmacy. For suggestions on use of the oath, see Bowers RA *Am J Pharm Educ 28:* 269, 1964. A noteworthy change in the current version of the oath is omission of explicit reference to the Code of Ethics of the American Pharmaceutical Association.

code of ethics—although ordinarily based on or harmonized with the principles codified by the APhA.

American pharmacy had not developed an effective program for encouraging compliance and adjudicating violations as a corollary of its well-developed sense of professional ethics. Symptomatic of a new level of maturity in 1968, the APhA inaugurated a Judicial Board to take responsibility in this field. Moreover, several state pharmaceutical associations since mid-century developed a mechanism for doing so (eg, New York and Wisconsin), while other states experimented with using the regulatory power of state boards to enforce ethical standards (eg, Louisiana and Connecticut). Despite machinery for self-disciplinary proceedings, the rarity of its use seems to imply a trend among pharmacists—probably shared by other professions—toward depending on government to set and enforce standards of professional conduct.

Pharmacists differ on what these standards should be and how to achieve uniform compliance, yet they have been united in recognizing, through centuries, that scientific competence becomes meaningful only when the practitioner's services are mediated by a sense of social responsibilities.

Mixed Trends

The legal and ethical controls, a more uniform education and competence among practitioners, organizational structuring, the solidification of group-consciousness concerned with norms of responsibility and performance—all these suggest a professional maturing of American pharmacy during the past century. Countervailing influences have been an almost complete loss of the practitioner's central function of preparing medications from their individual constituents, and a commercializing development.

Although the large-scale industrialization of producing drugs had occurred already in the 19th century, the disappearance of prescription compounding, tailored to the individual patient, occurred mainly between the 1920s and the 1960s. Thus, while drugs became dramatically more effective during the present century, the practicing pharmacist lost much of his creative identification with the prescriptions he dispensed. At the same time, the multiplicity and complexness of the new materia medica gave the practitioner more potential as an expert advisor on pharmaceutical products to other health practitioners and, in a different sense, to lay patrons. Although by mid-century this role had become well defined as an objective, the transition into practice developed only slowly as a national trend (within a broad concept of "clinical pharmacy").

A corollary of this advisory function was the emergence of another goal: making the American pharmacy a center of health-education literature for the laity. Begun in an organized way through a collaborative project (1940) with the American Social Hygiene Association, such service has been fostered, meanwhile, by the APhA, as sporadic funds permit. The scope and effectiveness of "the community pharmacy as a community health education center" was given its most definitive test by the Association through a grant from the US Public Health Service (1963).

Two other trends that helped to blunt the impact of the withdrawal of the preparation of drugs from pharmacies, into remote manufacturing laboratories, were the rising number of prescriptions dispensed and some retrenching in the number of pharmacies. For example, prescriptions that nationally numbered close to 165,000,000 in 1931, had risen to at least 741,400,000 in 1963, and to more than 1.46 billion in 1982. Reflected in these estimates are such changes as less physician dispensing, greater economic prosperity, and more prescribing of drugs individually (ie, fewer medications compounded with multiple active ingredients). While the estimated number of prescriptions nationally was increasing

about $4\frac{1}{2}$ times, the number of retail pharmacies was steadily decreasing in relation to the population—from about 1 to 3360 persons (1960) to about 1 to 4500 persons (1976). Even so, the average patronage potential is not large compared with other highly developed Western countries. It was an unused capacity in the average American prescription department that permitted pharmacy to fulfil the increased demand for pharmaceutical service without comparable increases in facilities.

The trend toward larger establishments since World War II reflected more directly the influence of the concept of a supermarket or variety store, which could have a pharmacy as one of its units. A drift toward this type of "drugstore" design has not been resisted as strongly in America as it has among pharmacists in other highly developed countries, partly because of a tradition here associating drug dispensing with a general store, a concept with roots in early America, and associating the practitioner with extensive nonpharmaceutical work as an accepted norm.

An equally noteworthy countertrend (countertrends have not been uncommon in American pharmacy) runs in the direction of devoting a higher proportion of the pharmacy to health-related services. For example, in 1930 fewer than 1% of all pharmacies were estimated to be receiving half or more of their dollar volume from the prescription department. During the period up to the 1960s, this percentage probably rose to somewhere between 12 and 25% of all pharmacies (although there is a lack of agreement or verification of the exact figure). By the mid-1970s, prescription practice constituted at least 50% of total dollar volume as an average among independent community pharmacies. But when chain-stores are included, the average overall is considerably lower (eg, 32.1% of dollar volume in 1976).

These developments as a whole remind us that the community practice of pharmacy in America has retained its variegated nature even though evolving to a new level and character.

The concise compass of an introductory essay limits discussion largely to an overview of this segment of the pharmacist's history. Even within this scope, the individual pharmacists who most decisively shaped or altered the course of pharmacy's history have had to remain in the background. The lives of some of them have been briefly reported in biographical sketches in the 13th edition of this book (p. 20).

For accounts of the rise of smaller specialties within the profession, of the contributions from pharmacists to science and society, and of the development of the drug trade and industry, the reader may consult more specialized or more comprehensive historical writings. The section *Bibliographic Notes* below provides one key to finding many of these publications in libraries.

The American pharmacist, like his counterpart in other countries, has earned increasing responsibilities within the legal structure regulating society. The extent to which pharmaceutical accomplishments have been given a place by historians in the record of man's endeavor permits practitioners and laity alike to appreciate the persisting and essential contribution of pharmacy.

Bibliographic Notes

History

Besides giving recognition to sources on which the above historical essay is based, these references suggest further readings and reference materials. English-language publications are cited unless there is no approximate counterpart of a foreign-language publication. For those with deeper historical interests, bibliographies in some of the publications mentioned will lead to more specialized and often more meaningful literature.

A few general guides to the historical literature are: Glenn Sonnedecker, JH Hoch, and Wolfgang Schneider, *Some Pharmaco-Historical Guidelines to the Literature*, American Institute of the History of Pharmacy, Madison, WI, 1959 (also in *Am J Pharm Educ*, **23**, 143 (1959)); *Index-Catalogue of the Library of the Surgeon-General's Office*, US Army, Washington, DC, 4 series, 1880–1936; E-H Guitard, *Manuel d'Histoire de la Littérature pharmaceutique*, Paris, 1942; *Bibliography of the History of Medicine*, National Library of Medicine, USPHS, Bethesda, MD, No. 1 (1965), *et seq.* (annual; includes pharmacy); *Current Work in the History of Medicine*, quarterly from The Wellcome Historical Medical Library, London, since 1954 (includes pharmacy internationally); "Bibliography of the History of Medicine of the United States and Canada," annually 1939–1966 in *Bulletin of the History of Medicine* (includes pharmacy section); E-H Guitard, *Index des Travaux d'Histoire de la Pharmacie de 1913 à 1963*, Société d'Histoire de la Pharmacie, Paris, [1968]; "Pharmaziegeschichtliche Rundschau" (GE Dann, ed), Vol I, 1954–1957, *et seq* (historical abstracts) as periodic supplement to the *Pharmazeutische Zeitung*. Glenn Sonnedecker and Alex Berman, *Some Bibliographic Aids for Historical Writers in Pharmacy*, American Institute of the History of Pharmacy, Madison, WI, 1958; and David L Cowen, *America's Pre-Pharmacopeial Literature*, American Institute of the History of Pharmacy, Madison, WI, 1961. *ISIS Cumulative Bibliography*, Mansell, London, 1971 (and continuations; includes pharmacy).

The book of most comprehensive scope in English is *Kremers and Urdang's History of Pharmacy*, revised by Glenn Sonnedecker, Lippincott, Philadelphia, 1976 (see "Glossary" and "Appendix 6" as well as "Notes and References" for bibliographic material). Hermann Schelenz, *Geschichte der Pharmazie*, Berlin, 1904, republished by Oscar Rothacker, Berlin, 1961, a monumental reference work, is now outdated in many details but richly documented to the earlier literature. Erwin H Ackerknecht, *Therapeutics from the Primitives to the 20th Century*, Hafner, New York, ca 1973 (from German edition, 1970) is the only general overview of its scope. For illustrations, see particularly W-H Hein and DA Wittop Koning, *Bildkatalog zur Geschichte der Pharmazie*, ns Bd 33, *Veröffentlichungen der Internationalen Gesellschaft für Geschichte der Pharmazie*, Stuttgart, 1969.

On antiquity: The most definitive paper of general scope on Egypt is by Frans Jonckheere, "Le 'Préparateur de Remèdes' dans l'Organisation de la Pharmacie égyptienne," Deutsche Akademie der Wissenschaften zu Berlin, Institut für Orientforschung, Veröffentlichung Nr 29, Berlin, 1955 (Sonderdruck aus "Aegyptologische Studien . . ."). CD Leake, *The Old Egyptian Medical Papyri*, Lawrence, KS, 1952, gives an overview of the documents; and for a first-hand impression of the papyrus most important pharmaceutically, see B Ebbell, *The Papyrus Ebers*, Copenhagen, 1937. Henry Sigerist, *A History of Medicine, Vol 1: Primitive and Archaic Medicine*, New York, 1955, is the best general survey. On Mesopotamia, an excellent book of breadth, relevant to pharmacy, is by Martin Levey, *Chemistry and Chemical Technology in Ancient Mesopotamia*, Amsterdam (Van Nostrand, distributor, Princeton), 1959; on Assyria, see monographs by Reginald C Thompson. The best sociohistorical view of its scope in English is Henry E Sigerist, *A History of Medicine, Vol II: Early Greek, Hindu and Persian Medicine*, Oxford University Press, New York, 1961; more specifically on pharmacy are J Berendes, *Die Pharmacie bei den alten Culturvölkern*, 2 vols, Halle aS, 1891 and Alfred Schmidt, *Drogen und Drogenhandel im Altertum*, Leipzig, 1924. The Hippocratic treatises have been translated into English by WHS Jones and ET Withington, *Hippocrates*, 4 vols, London, 1923–1931, while a compilation on Hippocratic drugs was published by Johann H Dierbach, *Die Arzneimittel des Hippokrates . . .*, Heidelberg, 1824. For modern scholarship, from a different viewpoint, see Jerry Stannard, "Hippocratic Pharmacology," *Bull Hist Med*, **35**, 497 (1961); see also his "Materia Medica and Philosophical Theory in Aretaeus," *Sudhoffs Arch Gesch Med Naturw*, **48,** 27 (1964). For a first-hand impression of the classical materia medica, see, eg, the three translations: Robert T Gunther, ed., *The Greek Herbal of Dioscorides*, Oxford, 1934, republished Hafner Publ Co, New York, 1959; Francis Adams, trans, *The Seven Books of Paulus Aegineta . . .*, 3 vols, Sydenham Society, London, 1844–1847; and WG Spencer, trans, *Celsus, De Medicina*, 3 vols, Loeb Classical Library, London and Cambridge, MA, 1935–1938. On Greek temple medicine, see Ch Kerenyi, *Le Medecin divin*, Basle, 1948, and EJ Edelstein and L Edelstein, *Asclepius, A Collection and Interpretation of the Testimonies*, 2 vols, Baltimore, 1945.

On the Middle Ages: For a general survey of *medieval Islam* and its influence, see Lucien Leclerc, *Histoire de la Médecine Arabe*, 2 vols, Paris, 1876; also Donald Campbell, *Arabian Medicine and Its Influence on the Middle Ages*, 2 vols, London, 1926, and Cyril Elgood, *A Medical History of Persia and the Eastern Caliphate*, Cambridge, England, 1951. Much has been translated or written about Arabic materia medica and drug therapy, to which the principal key is a bibliographic volume by Sami K Hamarneh, published in 1964 by the Internationale Gesellschaft für Geschichte der Pharmazie, Stuttgart, 1964. Of Hamarneh's other publications, see especially *Origins of Pharmacy and Therapy in the Near East* (1973); also of much general interest is "The Rise of Professional Pharmacy in Islam," *Medical History*, **6,** 59 (1962); and for a detailed view into 10th-century Spain (with a useful bibliography), see SK Hamarneh and G Sonnedecker, *A Pharmaceutical View of Abulcasis al-Zahrawi in Moorish Spain*, EJ Brill, Leiden, 1963. Important works by Max Meyerhof include several on materia medica, such as his monographs on al-

Ghâfiqî, Publication No 4, The Egyptian University Faculty of Medicine, Cairo, 1932, on al-Beruni in *Studien zur Geschichte des Naturwissenschaften und der Medizin*, Vol 3, Berlin, 1943, pp 159–208, and his four articles in *Ciba Symposia*, 6, Nos 5 and 6 (1944). See likewise the writings of Martin Levey, such as *The Medical Formulary or Agrabadhin of al-Kindi*, University of Wisconsin Press, Madison, [ca 1965]. For *medieval Europe*, a volume still not superseded (although outdated in details) is George F Fort, *Medical Economy During the Middle Ages . . .*, New York, 1883; see also, David Riesman, *The Story of Medicine in the Middle Ages*, New York, 1935. A valuable guide and commentary is by Henry E Sigerist, "The Latin Medical Literature of the Early Middle Ages," *J Hist Med*, **13**, 127 (1958). Of more specifically pharmaceutical interest: The definitive work on the renowned pharmacomedical edicts in the Kingdom of the Two Sicilies is by Wolfgang-Hagen Hein and Kurt Sappert, *Die Medizinalordnung Friedrichs II. Eine pharmaziehistorische Studie*, Internationale Gesellschaft für Geschichte der Pharmazie, Eutin, 1957. In the periodical literature, note particularly the writings of Alfons Lutz (eg, "Der verschollene frühsalernitanische Antidotarius magnus . . . ," *Veröffentlichungen der Internationalen Gesellschaft für Geschichte der Pharmazie*, ns V 16, Stuttgart, 1960, pp 97–133, with a rich bibliography), and of Rudolf Schmitz (eg, ". . . Apothekerstandes im Hoch- und Spät-Mittelalter," *ibid*, Vol 13, 1958, pp 157–165) and "Ueber deutsche mittelalterliche Quellen zur Geschichte von Pharmazie und Medizin," *Deut Apotheker-Ztg*, **100,** 980 (1960). Writings of unusual value and clarity in English-language literature are by GE Trease, such as "The Spicers and Apothecaries of the Royal Household in the Reigns of Henry III, Edward I and Edward II," in *Nottingham Mediaeval Studies*, **3,** 19 (1959) and abridged in *Pharm J*, 4 April 1949, pp 246–248. Sister Mary Francis Xavier [Welhoefer], *Statutes of the Guild of Physicians, Apothecaries and Merchants in Florence (1313–1316); a Brief Commentary, with an Introduction and Translation*, unpublished PhD dissertation, University of Wisconsin, 1935, is uniquely useful, even though dated as to many details. On medieval European materia medica, see Henry E Sigerist, "Materia Medica in the Middle Ages," *Bull Hist Med*, **7,** 417 (1939) and his "Studien und Texte zur frühmittelalterlichen Rezeptliteratur," *Studien zur Geschichte der Medizin*, V 13, Leipzig, 1923, pp 187 *ff*; probably the earliest pharmacist's textbook and manual has been translated into German by Leo Zimmermann, *Saladini de Asculo . . . Compendium aromatariorum*, Leipzig, 1919 (for Hebrew, see Suessmann Muntner, ed, Tel-Aviv, 1953).

On modern Europe: For a reliable and concise medical overview, see Erwin Ackerknecht, *A Short History of Medicine*, Ronald Press Co, New York, 1955; supplemented for detailed reference by Fielding H Garrison, *An Introduction to the History of Medicine*, 4th ed, Philadelphia, 1929; republished 1960 (note the bibliographic essays of Appendix III). Some international survey volumes on pharmacy, with particular reference to the modern period, are listed by Sonnedecker and Berman, *Some Bibliographic Aids . . .* (cited above). A gap has been closed, meanwhile, by Leslie G Matthews, *History of Pharmacy in Britain*, E & S Livingstone Ltd., Edinburgh and London, 1962, and Cecil Wall, HC Cameron, and EA Underwood, *A History of the Worshipful Society of Apothecaries of London, Vol I: 1617–1815*, Oxford University Press, London, 1963. There is not yet a history both up-to-date and dealing comprehensively with European pharmacy; general bibliographic guides, such as those cited at the beginning of this essay, will yield books and monographs from particular topical and national viewpoints. Especially rich in European history are the publications of the International Society for the History of Pharmacy, 1927 to date, to which a partial key has been published by Herbert Hügel, *Die Veröffentlichungen der Internationalen Gesellschaft für Geschichte der Pharmazie 1953–1965; Eine Bibliographie*, ns Bd. 29 of the Veröffentlichungen, Stuttgart, 1967.

On the United States: The standard volume in English, *Kremers and Urdang's History of Pharmacy*, revised by Glenn Sonnedecker, Lippincott, Philadelphia, 1976, devotes approximately two-thirds of the main text to the United States; and its bibliographies open up a wide range of other American literature. Noteworthy are the anniversary issues of *Druggists Circular*, **51** (Jan 1907), and *Pharmaceutical Era*, **16,** No 27 [Dec 31] (1896). An article drawn upon in the preceding chapter is my address, "Structure and Stress of American Pharmacy," *Pharm J*, 14 April 1956, pp 3–8. A useful bibliography still in print is by George Griffenhagen, *Bibliography of Papers Published by the American Pharmaceutical Association that were presented before the Association's Section on Historical Pharmacy, 1904–1967*, American Institute of the History of Pharmacy, Madison, WI, nd (includes subject and author indexes; emphasizes American history, but by no means restricted thereto). The "Pharmacy" section of the annual bibliography in the *Bulletin of the History of Medicine*, previously offered an important key to the literature, which was cumulated in *Bibliography of the History of Medicine of the United States and Canada*, Genevieve Miller, ed, Johns Hopkins, Baltimore, 1964; see also other "General Guides" listed (supra). Also noteworthy is the "Bookshelf" section of *Pharmacy in History* (a quarterly of the American Institute of the History of Pharmacy) and the sections on "History and Ethics," Sociology and Economics," and "Literature," in *International Pharmaceutical Abstracts*.

On ethics: For cross-sections from the history of the American expression of pharmaceutical ethics, see Charles La Wall, "Pharmaceutical Ethics," *J APhA*, **10,** 895 and 961 (1921); George F Archambault, "Ethical

Standards . . . ," *Bull Am Soc Hosp Pharm*, **13**, 446 (1956); for a Catholic viewpoint, William L Wolkovich, *Norms of Conduct for Pharmacists* (17 Loring Street), Hudson, MA, 1962; from a sociologist, Isador Thorner, "Pharmacy: The Functional Significance of an Institutional Pattern," *Am J Pharm Ed*, **6**, 305 (1942), or *Social Forces*, **20**, 321 (1942), and Urdang's commentary, *Am J Pharm Ed*, **6**, 319 and 617 (1942); Karl L Kaufman, "Ethics for the Pharmacy Student," *Am J Pharm Educ*, **17**, 225 (1953); Theodore Greiner, "The Ethics of Drug Research on Human Subjects," *J New Drugs*, **2**, 7 (1962); Allen I White, "The Development of Professional Morality in Pharmacy Students," *Am J Pharm Ed*, **17**, 222 (1953); Frank Arnal, "International Code of Ethics for Pharmacists," in *Commission de l'Exercice de la Pharmacie d'Officine: Rapports, Federation Internationale Pharmaceutique*, Brussels, 1958, pp 157–168.

A Chronology for Pharmacists

The dating of events often involves uncertainties, approximations, and questions of meaning that are not apparent in a concise table such as that below. Particularly, dates before the 18th century often are unverifiable or estimated.

BC
2000? **Earliest formulary** known in history (Sumerian).
1500 **Ebers Papyrus,** Egyptian manuscript pertaining to pharmacy and therapy.
460 **Hippocrates,** famous Greek physician, born.
350 **Diocles** wrote an important treatise on materia medica.
372 **Theophrastus** (372–285), the "father of botany," born.
AD
50 **Dioscorides** wrote an important book on materia medica.
130 **Galen** born, Roman physician who experimented with compounded drugs.
350 **Cosmas** and **Damian,** who became patron saints of pharmacy and medicine, martyred.
857 **Johann Mesue Senior,** Arabian physician (777–857) dies.
925 **Rhazes,** Persian physician (865–925) dies.
1035 **Avicenna** (980–1035), physician and philosopher dies.
1178 **Mention of pharmacists in French records.**
1180 **Guild of Pepperers** already active in London.
1225 **Apothecary shop** established at Cologne.
1297 **Guild of Pharmacists** organized in Bruges.
1345 **Apothecary shops** have been established in London.
1348 **The Black Death**—Great Plague struck Europe.
1480 **Poison law** enacted by James I of Scotland.
1499 **Guild pharmacopoeia** published in Florence, Italy.
1529 **Paracelsus** (1493–1541) published his first treatise.
1546 **Nuremburg Pharmacopoeia** (Dispensatory of Valerius Cordus), perhaps the first to be "official."
1589 **Galileo** demonstrated the **law of falling bodies.**
1604 **Louis Hébert,** first pharmacist to settle in North America.
1617 **Society of Apothecaries** in London organized.
1618 **First London pharmacopoeia** published.
1620 **Pilgrims** settled at Plymouth, MA.
1628 **Harvey** published his book on the **circulation of the blood.**
1646 **William Davis** operating apothecary shop, probably one of the first in America (Boston).
1665 **Sir Isaac Newton** discovered the **law of gravitation.**
1680 **Leeuwenhoeck** discovered **yeast** plants.
1703 English **apothecaries authorized to prescribe** as well as dispense.
1715 **Bartram's Botanical Gardens** established at Philadelphia. First tabulation of relationship between chemical substances issued by French pharmacist E Fr Geoffroy.
1736 **First law related to pharmacy** in America enacted in Virginia.
1752 **First hospital pharmacy** in America established at Pennsylvania Hospital in Philadelphia.
1762 **Antoine Baumé** publishes his *Élémens de Pharmacie* in France.
1765 **John Morgan** becomes influential advocate of **prescription writing** in United States.
1773 **Scheele** isolates **oxygen** about 1773, **Priestley** by 1774.
1774 **Scheele** discovers **chlorine.**
1776 **Declaration of Independence;** position of Apothecary-General created in army of the patriots.
1776 **Christopher Marshall,** famous American pharmacist, makes medicines for wounded soldiers.
1777 **Collège de Pharmacie** established in Paris.
1783 **Pilâtre de Rozier,** a pharmacist, makes **first human flight** in a balloon.
1785 **Withering** publishes his treatise on **digitalis; Fowler** introduces **Fowler's Solution.**
1787 **Ergot** introduced in obstetrics by **Paullitzsky.**
1790 **First United States patent law** passed. Elisha Perkins took out first medical patent in 1796.
1793 **Plague** strikes Philadelphia.
1793 **Trommsdorff's** *Journal der Pharmacie* founded; first professional-scientific journal devoted to **pharmacy.**
1798 **Jenner** publishes his work on **vaccination.**
1805 German pharmacist **Sertürner** reports isolation of **morphine.**

1809 *Journal de Pharmacie et de Chimie* founded; first published as *Bulletin de Pharmacie.*
1811 **Iodine** discovered by **Courtois,** a French pharmacist.
1818 French pharmacist-chemists **Caventou** and **Pelletier** isolated **strychnine.**
1820 **Quinine** isolated by **Pelletier** and **Caventou.**
1820 **First edition of United States Pharmacopoeia** published.
1821 **Philadelphia College of Pharmacy** founded as first local association and school of pharmacy, USA.
1823 **Massachusetts College of Pharmacy** founded.
1825 **First American professional journal of pharmacy** published, *American Journal of Pharmacy.*
1826 **Bromine** discovered by French pharmacist **Balard. Ethyl alcohol** synthesized by **Hennel.**
1828 **Wöhler synthesizes urea,** thus bridging gulf between organic and inorganic chemistry.
1829 **New York College of Pharmacy** founded.
1831 **Chloroform** prepared independently by **Liebig** and by **Soubeiran.**
1832 **Codeine** isolated by French pharmacist **Pierre Robiquet.**
1834 **Carbolic acid** and **aniline** prepared by German pharmacist **F F Runge.**
1842 **Crawford Long** performed **first operation under anesthesia** using ether.
1843 **Oliver Wendell Holmes** points out that puerperal fever is contagious.
1848 First **American code of pharmaceutical ethics** prepared by Philadelphia College of Pharmacy.
1848 **First drug import law** enacted by Congress to curb adulterations.
1852 **American Pharmaceutical Association** founded as first national organization.
1852 **Darwin** publishes his *Origin of Species.*
1865 First **International Pharmaceutical Conference** in Brunswick, Germany.
1868 **University of Michigan** opens pharmacy course that will have far-reaching influence in modernizing American pharmaceutical education.
1883 First **National Retail Druggists Association** founded.
1888 First **National Formulary** issued by American Pharmaceutical Association.
1890 **Serum therapy** introduced by **von Behring** and **Kitasato.**
1893 **Aspirin** discovered by **A Eichengrün** and **Felix Hoffman.**
1895 **Roentgen** discovered **X rays.**
1898 **Radium** discovered by the **Curies.**
1898 **National Association of Retail Druggists** founded in USA.
1899 **Walter Reed** proved mosquitoes carry **yellow fever.**
1900 **American Association of Colleges of Pharmacy** founded.
1902 **First International Pharmacopoeial Conference** held at Brussels; **first American PhD** supervised in pharmacy granted at University of Wisconsin.
1906 **Federal Food and Drug Act** passed, USA.
1910 **Paul Ehrlich** and **S Hata** introduce **arsphenamine** ("606") in widespread clinical trial.
1912 First Assembly of **International Pharmaceutical Federation** (The Hague).
1922 **Banting** and **Best** isolate **insulin.**
1928 **Sir Alexander Fleming** discovers **penicillin,** the first antibiotic.
1935 **Prontosil,** the first "sulfa" drug, introduced by **G Domagk.**
1937 **American Journal of Pharmaceutical Education** founded; first periodical devoted to pharmaceutical education.
1938 **League of Nations Commission on International Pharmacopoeial Standards** held conferences. Important revision of Federal Food and Drug Act (USA).
1940 First clinical **trials of penicillin** by Florey and Chain.
1942 **American Society of Hospital Pharmacists** founded.
1944 Antibiotic activity of **streptomycin** announced.
1945 **Atomic energy** released for use in warfare and medicine.
1947 **Medical Service Corps** created in US Army, with pharmacy represented by special group of commissioned officers.
1948 **First Pan American Congress of Pharmacy and Biochemistry.**

1949   **Cortisone and ACTH** introduced for rheumatic arthritis.   Influence for change initiated by analysis and suggested reforms from Pharmaceutical Survey (USA).

1951   **First International Pharmacopoeia,** World Health Organization.

1952   **Chlorpromazine** introduced into psychiatry, thus opening the field of psychopharmacology.

1955   **Salk poliomyelitis vaccine** released for general use.

1959   **Synthetic modifications of natural penicillin** introduced; **American Society of Pharmacognosy** founded.

1962   Important amendments of the Federal Food, Drug and Cosmetic Act.

1973   US Supreme Court decision (No 72-1176) holds that states may require that licensed pharmacists have **ownership-control of pharmacies.**

1975   Official **drug standardization program unified** by US Pharmacopeia absorbing National Formulary.   Report by Study Commission on Pharmacy (AACP) gives impetus to trend toward drug information and **counseling role** of pharmacists.

1977   Clinical trials of adenine arabinoside against herpes raise prospect of **controlling viral diseases.**

1982   **Specialty certification** begins in American pharmacy with the board certification of sixty-three pharmacists in the field of nuclear pharmacy.

CHAPTER 3

Ethics

Maven J Myers, JD, PhD
Dean of Health Sciences and Professor of Pharmacy Administration
Philadelphia College of Pharmacy and Science
Philadelphia PA 19104

Larry D Grieshaber, PhD
Veterans Administration Medical Center
St Louis MO 63125

The quest to systematically construct an ethical framework for Western civilization was begun over 2000 years ago by Socrates. Socrates approached ethics as a science; i.e., as being ". . .governed by principles of universal validity, so that what was good for one was good for all, and what was my neighbor's duty was my duty also." [1] Acceptance of this Socratic approach has proven burdensome. After two thousand years of effort mankind universally adheres to not even one ethical principal.

Even relatively narrow and homogeneous segments of society such as religious groups have difficulty formulating and enforcing rules for ethical behavior. For professional groups the task is especially difficult. One of the problems faced by professional groups is that they cannot begin their quest for ethical principles from a common theological base. Even the predominantly Judeo-Christian background of American pharmacists does not provide a strong starting point because of the number of sects within that background. One striking example of interdenominational difference that has raised ethical issues in our health care system arises from the belief of Jehovah's Witness. Official doctrine of Jehovah's Witness does not permit the transfusions of blood on the basis of a biblical interpretation. The life-saving nature of transfusion, their widespread use, and placing a high value on life-saving medical techniques by society have caused the courts to become involved in several cases where the religious belief of a Jehovah's Witness is in conflict with the prevailing ethics of American society. Without the underpinning of a uniform theological belief, it is difficult to find ethical principles that are acceptable to an entire group.

No set of ethical principles no matter how carefully thought out or how well constructed can provide the individual professional with guidance each time he is faced with a decision about his client(s), or peers, or society. Life events are not precisely repetitive in every detail. There are people who believe that because each situation is different, each decision requires separate analysis of relevant factors, possible outcomes of available actions, and weighing of right and wrong. This philosophical position is appropriately called situational ethics.

Given these seemingly insurmountable obstacles, is it possible to develop a viable set of ethical principles of a profession? Indeed, is it even desirable to develop such a set of principles?

The Case for Professional Ethics

In this discussion, *professional ethics* is used only to denote ". . . . the set of ethical principles perceived only by the professionals themselves to be appropriate for their professional behavior." [2] In other contexts the term might be used to denote those ethical principles to which society believes any individual claiming professional status should subscribe. So inseparable are professional ethics and the social context in which they are spawned and applied, that any discussion such as this one taken out of the social context is incomplete. A Utopian approach to formulating professional codes of ethics would integrate professional and societal goals. "Provisions of an ideal code would mesh with the rules of the ideal social system, which would maximize and fairly distribute the benefits of social labor under contemporary conditions." [3] What is to be gained by a unilateral development of a set of ethical principles (or code of ethics) by a profession to which it expects its members to abide?

First, a code of ethics makes the decision-making process more efficient. In opposition to situation ethicists, Veach claims,

". . . Yet if those who must resolve the ever-increasing ethical dilemmas in medicine—including patients, family members, physicians, nurses, hospital administrators, and public policy-makers—treat every case as something entirely fresh, entirely novel, they will have lost perhaps the best way of reaching solutions: to understand the general principles of ethics and face each new situation from a systematic ethical stance." [4]

Clinical practice predisposes pharmacists to a situationalist approach to ethics through its emphasis on individual differences in response to therapeutic regimens. However, some guidelines exist for adjusting drug therapy in patients with compromised renal or hepatic function, electrolyte or hormonal imbalance, and other pathophysiological abnormalities. Therapeutic guidelines give us a place to begin solving a clinical problem. Rules of morality serve the same purpose.

"They may at least act as rules-of-thumb for handling easy cases. They may at least summarize ethical reasoning that has gone before by others who have found themselves in somewhat similar situations. They may at least serve as guidelines for formulating thinking about the problem at hand." [5]

Second, individual professionals may occasionally need guidelines for directing their professional behavior. Each decision made by a professional requires that he call upon both his store of technological information as well as upon his own sense of right and wrong. Confrontation with situations about which an individual professional has not considered in great detail will almost assuredly arise. Where he can find no apparent theological or personal ethical principles to apply, he might turn to professional ethics for guidance.

Finally, professional ethics establish a pattern of behavior which clients come to expect for members of the profession. Assuming that the role of a professional code of ethics is to establish a pattern of behavior among the members of the profession, the consistency of the behavior should become evident to the clients of a profession. Once a consistent pattern of behavior is discerned by clients, they expect that behavior to remain constant. Their expectations become part

Code of Ethics

American Pharmaceutical Association[25]

Preamble

These principles of professional conduct for pharmacists are established to guide the pharmacist in his relationship with patients, fellow practitioners, other health professionals, and the public.

Section 1

A pharmacist should hold the health and safety of patients to be of first consideration; he should render to each patient the full measure of his ability as an essential health practitioner.

Section 2

A pharmacist should never condone the dispensing, promoting or distributing of drugs or medical devices, or assist therein, which are not of good quality, which do not meet standards required by law or which lack therapeutic value for the patient.

Section 3

A pharmacist should always strive to perfect and enlarge his professional knowledge. He should utilize and make available this knowledge as may be required in accordance with his best professional judgment.

Section 4

A pharmacist has the duty to observe the law, to uphold the dignity and honor of the profession, and to accept its ethical principles. He should not engage in any activity that will bring discredit to the profession and should expose, without fear or favor, illegal or unethical conduct in the profession.

Section 5

A pharmacist should seek at all times only fair and reasonable remuneration for his services. He should never agree to or participate in transactions with practitioners of other health professions or any other person under which fees are divided or which may cause financial or other exploitation in connection with the rendering of his professional services.

Section 6

A pharmacist should respect the confidential and personal nature of his professional records; except where the best interest of the patient requires or the law demands, he should not disclose such information to anyone without proper patient authorization.

Section 7

A pharmacist should not agree to practice under terms or conditions which tend to interfere with or impair the proper exercise of his professional judgment and skill, which tend to cause a deterioration of the quality of his service or which require him to consent to unethical conduct.

Section 8

A pharmacist should strive to provide information to patients regarding professional services truthfully, accurately, and fully, and should avoid misleading patients regarding the nature, cost, or value of the pharmacist's professional services.

Section 9

A pharmacist should associate with organizations having for their objective the betterment of the profession of pharmacy; he should contribute of his time and funds to carry on the work of these organizations.

---

of the relationship they establish with the profession. For example, a patient who has had several interactions with pharmacists may observe the confidentiality with which his records are treated. He comes to expect this behavior of his pharmacist and upon observing directly (or vicariously through his social contacts) the same behavior on the part of other pharmacists, he comes to identify maintenance of confidentiality as a behavior characteristic of pharmacists. Once a behavior becomes part of the concept of the public concerning that profession it becomes part of the basis for the interaction between professions and society and between professional and clients.

To better understand the role of and necessity for ethics in professions, one must first look at the characteristics of professions.

Professional Characteristics

Specialized Knowledge and Social Utility—The first group of professional characteristics is the existence of a specialized body of knowledge, possession and utilization of which enable the practitioner to perform a highly useful social function. It will be observed that all occupations, except criminals, provide some positive benefit to society and are based on specialized knowledge. Thus, the functions performed by a garbage collector are important to the health of society and, through experience, garbage collectors likely have gained some knowledge which permits them to perform their functions more efficiently than the inexperienced layman.

Generally, the professions are more socially useful than other occupations; however, social utility alone does not make an occupation a profession. The social utility of an occupation must be based on the possession and utilization of a specialized body of knowledge.

An applied body of knowledge may be composed of knowledge of a manual skill or intellectual knowledge. It is the latter which is of primary significance as a criterion for professions. Thus, the pharmacist is not considered a professional because he can rapidly type a prescription label. Rather, the relevant professional function involved in this operation is the pharmacist's knowledge about drugs and patients which permits him (among other things) to advise patients and prescribers concerning drug therapy, detect drug interactions, select appropriate product sources, and exercise professional judgment. These are functions based on intellectual knowledge rather than knowledge of a manual skill.

The exercise of proper judgment is a key element in this first group of professional characteristics. Traditionally, professional services are rendered to an individual rather than to a group. Using the specialized body of knowledge of the profession and the intellectual abilities of the professional practitioner, the practitioner makes a judgment as to the best course of treatment for the particular individual.

The first group of professional characteristics is related to ethics in that a major function of the ethics of a profession is to increase the social value of the profession by encouraging the development, acquisition, and proper utilization of the specialized knowledge of the profession.

Attitudes and Professional Behavior—The second group of characteristics of a profession is the possession by its practitioners of a set of attitudes which influences their professional behavior. The basic component of this set of attitudes is altruism, an unselfish concern for the welfare of others. Marshall summarized this thought in the following words:

> The professional man, it has been said, does not work in order to be paid: he is paid in order that he may work. Every decision he takes in the course of his career is based on his sense of what is right, not on his estimate of what is profitable.[6]

In the development of professions, one finds a strong historical base for altruism. In Greece and Rome the functions of the lawyer were not performed by specially trained advocates but by (presumably unpaid) friends of the litigants. The physician in the Roman Empire was not a free-lance practitioner but a slave attached to a rich man's household. When training for the professions became formalized in the universities of the Middle Ages, not only were the universities controlled by the church but professional men were required to take religious orders. Thus, one would expect to find that the early professionals did not practice for personal financial gain.

The contemporary bases for altruism as a characteristic of professions already have been alluded to. The professions are concerned with matters that are vital to the health or well-being of their patients. In practicing a profession the practitioner employs highly specialized technical knowledge—knowledge which the patient or client does not possess. Because of the patient's lack of knowledge, opportunity exists for exploitation of the patient by the professional. Because of the vital nature of professional services, the consequences to the patient of such exploitation are severe. Thus, the smooth functioning of the professions requires that the practitioner consider the needs of the patient as paramount, relegating the material needs of the practitioner to an inferior position.

Social Sanction—What might be thought of as a third group of professional characteristics, although they are actually the resultant effect of the two groups previously discussed, is social sanction. Ultimately, whether or not an occupation is a profession depends, to a large degree, on whether society views it as a profession. One measure of social sanction is the granting of exclusive rights of practice through the licensing power of the state. While such licensing attempts to protect the public from incompetent practitioners, frequently it also creates a relationship of trust between society and the professionals.

The extent of this trust also is a measure of the degree of social sanction; however, it is measured by a lack of the exercise of sovereign power. Given the legal monopoly inherent in professional licensing, the failure of society to impose further controls on the profession by implication sanctions the performance and self-regulation of the profession.

Another measure of social sanction is the status, income, and power with which society rewards the professional. Thus, given either the altruistic goal of service to mankind or the egoistic goals of status, income, or power, a means of goal achievement is professionalization of the occupation. This professionalization is accomplished through adherence on the part of practitioners to ethical precepts which encourage

qualitative increases in, for example, pharmacists' occupational role performance.

Desire To Be A Professional—Many occupations seek to be classified as professional. The designation implies that the practitioners of the occupation are performing an essential function in society. As Parsons has noted, "many of the most important features of our society are to a considerable extent dependent on the smooth functioning of the professions".[7]

Other reasons, derived from the first, and perhaps more significant in contemporary society, also provide motivation to an occupational group seeking classification as a profession. Smith observed:

> We trust our health to the physician, our fortune and sometimes our life and reputation to the lawyer and attorney. Such confidence could not safely be reposed in people of a very mean or low condition.[8]

Because of the importance of the professional functions and the inability of the receiver of these functions to assess the quality of service, a relationship of trust must exist between the professional and the patient.

Smith recognized, and society in general appears to have agreed, that if the professional is to place the interest of the patient above the immediate pecuniary gain of the professional, the professional must enjoy an income sufficiently high so that the gain from exploiting an individual patient becomes an insignificant part of the total income of the professional. Thus, the average income of the professional usually is higher than that of the nonprofessional.

It has been pointed out that in the evolution of professions those most likely to engage in the professions were aristocrats or men of leisure. Professions thus evolved as occupations connected with high status. The functional relationship of professions to society reinforces the status position of the professions, while the status itself acts as a motivating factor in the drive of an occupation to gain recognition as a profession.

A third relevant motivating factor is man's desire for power. Within the sphere of his professional activities, the professional exercises an authoritative power over his patient. As explained by Greenwood:

> (T)he professional dictates what is good or evil for the client, who has no choice but to accede to professional judgement. Here the premise is that, because he lacks the requisite theoretical background, the client cannot diagnose his own needs or discriminate among the range of possibilities for meeting them.[9]

Thus, the functional relationship of the professions to social progress places them in an important position in the social framework. The desire to serve a highly useful function in society is one of the main stimuli to professional behavior. Flowing from the important positions the professions occupy in society are the income, status, and power possessed by professional practitioners. The extent to which these goals are achieved is intimately related to the degree to which an occupation can validate its claim to being a profession.

Is Pharmacy a Profession?—Several studies have been done in an attempt to ascertain whether various occupations are professions. The most prominent study was done by Carr-Saunders and Wilson and the results were reported in their book, *The Professions.*[10]

After a careful examination of pharmacy practice (1933), no definitive conclusion as to the professional status of pharmacy was reached, primarily because of the commercial elements of pharmacy. More recent studies have produced similar results. In studies by Montague[11], Smith[12], Smith and Knapp[13], and Denzin and Mettlin[14], pharmacy was consistently found to fall short of full professional status. However, all professions can be found to fall short of being a complete profession in at least a few respects. Pharmacy has a legitimate claim to a theoretical body of knowledge, to a growing degree of socially sanctioned decision-making authority, and to a commitment of service functions as articulated by a code of ethics and an oath sworn to by many persons entering the profession. Therefore, pharmacists can and do demand professional standing.

Pharmacy Oath and Ethical Code—An oath of allegiance and a code of ethics constitute the formal declarations of ethics of most professions. Swearing an oath is symbolically a formal step in the professional socialization process. While pharmacists are not legally required to pledge themselves to such an oath, the oath is commonly administered at commencement exercises or licensure ceremonies. The current pharmacy oath (approved by the Board of Directors of the American Association of Colleges of Pharmacy and shown on page 22) is quite different from its historic ancestor, the Hippocratic Oath. Whereas the Hippocratic Oath emphasizes collegial allegiance to the profession, the pharmacy oath emphasizes the societal duty of the pharmacist. The pharmacist pledges to make the "welfare of humanity" and "relief of human suffering" his primary concerns. This implies an individual commitment to the patient and a collective commitment to society. While the pharmacist pledges to behave in a moral and ethical manner, the oath does not define that behavior.

The foundation of all ethical behavior is the basic precept "Do good and avoid evil." The ethics of pharmacy attempt to relate this basic precept to the practice of pharmacy. An initial problem, as pointed out by Barber, is "to specify how such rules are to be applied in the everyday, real-life, concrete situations that present us with ethical dilemmas.[16]

A first step in this specification is the codification of more particularized principles relating the basic ethic to pharmaceutical practice. Such a code "makes explicit what man already knows implicitly. It puts at his fingertips a concrete expression of principles already familiar to him . . ."[17] The ostensible purpose then of a professional code of ethics is a clear statement of ethical principles which should serve as guidelines for daily professional behavior. It should be noted, however, that the development of professional codes of conduct has been interpreted as a self-serving device that serves more to contribute to the high social standing of professions than to provide practitioners with solid guidelines for decision-making.[18]

Larson sees the concepts of ethicality and community as being "indissolubly related. In fact, profession is more often defined as *an occupation which tends to be colleague-oriented*, rather than client-oriented."[19] In this light, the development of a code of ethics might be seen as an attempt to ensure the marketability of the product of a profession by maintaining its quality and to minimize public intervention in the profession by establishing internal standards of conduct to be affirmed and enforced only by members of the profession.

The skepticism about professional codes of ethics is grounded in the speculation about professional motives. The critics question the good faith efforts of professionals to self-regulate. No one can divine unstated motives; one can, however, discern significant concern for public welfare in the codes developed by many professions.

The first code of ethics for pharmacists in the US was adopted in 1848 by the Philadelphia College of Pharmacy. Having believed that they had "erected a standard of scientific attainments, which there is a growing disposition on the part of candidates for the profession to reach," the code was adopted because of a desire "that in relation to professional conduct and probity, there should be a corresponding disposition to advance . . . ."[20]

When the American Pharmaceutical Association (APhA) was founded in 1852 it adopted a code of ethics modeled after that of the Philadelphia College of Pharmacy. The code of

---

> # Oath of a Pharmacist
>
> ## *American Association of Colleges of Pharmacy* [15]
>
> At this time, I vow to devote my professional life to the service of mankind through the profession of pharmacy. I will consider the welfare of humanity and relief of human suffering my primary concerns. I will use my knowledge and skills to the best of my ability in serving the public and other health professionals.
>
> I will do my best to keep abreast of developments and maintain professional competency in my profession of pharmacy. I will obey laws governing the practice of pharmacy and will support enforcement of such laws. I will maintain the highest standards of moral and ethical conduct. I take these vows voluntarily with the full realization of the trust and responsibility with which I am empowered by the public.

the APhA, the national professional society of pharmacists, is generally recognized as establishing the guidelines of conduct for American pharmacists.

Initially, members of the Association were required to subscribe to the code, but in 1855 "the obligation to subscribe to the APhA code as a prerequisite of membership was dropped and the code itself disappeared from the literature for over half a century."[21] Relating the 1852 code to 20th-century pharmacy, Sletten observed:

> The old code obviously referred to a by-gone day. The colleges had taken over many of the educational functions of the apothecary and planned to take over most of the remainder. Uniformity of performance among pharmacists was to be engendered by a uniform educational program among the schools, examinations, and a common ethical code. The USP and NF had now become official standards. In addition, the growth of pharmaceutical manufacturers had greatly advanced product uniformity. No doubt the emphasis on fraud and quackery were thought to be inappropriate for the current situation. In addition, the old code had long been dormant in its written form. Rather than merely to give it renewed publicity, a new code reflecting more closely the current ideals of the APhA could be drawn up.[22]

The revised code adopted by the Association in 1922 with modifications in 1952 was divided into three parts: the pharmacist in his relations to (1) the public, (2) other health practitioners, and (3) other pharmacists and the profession. Although the code was quite detailed, there was a need for an authoritative interpretation of its broad provisions as well as a mechanism to secure adherence to its principles. Thus, in 1966 there was established within the framework of APhA:

> A judicial board with full powers to discipline members and render advisory opinions and interpretative statements, reprimanding, suspending or expelling a member in any category for violation of the obligations of the constitution or bylaws, or for unprofessional conduct.[23]

In 1967 the APhA convened a Conference on Ethics. The sentiments expressed by the conferees likely reflect the thinking of the leadership of American pharmacy concerning the form and role of professional ethics in pharmacy's future.

> It was generally agreed that the Association and the profession require a code of ethics stated in broad principles with the APhA Judicial Board applying the principles to specific situations. Further, it was proposed that the new code of ethics encourage and guide the pharmacist in the performance of his professional duty rather than present him with nothing more than a compilation of "thou shalt nots."
> The most important aim of the new code of ethics was considered to be the protection of the public—not the profession . . . .
> (T)he new code should be general rather than specific, positive rather than negative and should stress the integrity and professional judgment of the individual pharmacist.[24]

In response to the sentiments expressed at the 1967 Conference on Ethics, the Judicial Board began to rewrite the profession's code of ethics. The code of ethics adopted by the Association in 1969, amended in 1975, is shown on page 20.

Following the adoption of the new code in 1969, the Judicial Board has issued advisory opinions and has taken formal action against pharmacists alleged to have violated the code. However, in 1979, bylaw changes were approved by which the Judicial Board was deleted as an elected unit of APhA. Under the revised bylaws, a judicial board may be appointed to render a specific opinion.[26]

Functional Performance

A principal factor contributing to the importance of professions is the functions they perform based on the possession and utilization of a specialized body of knowledge. On the one hand, the patients of the professional do not possess this body of knowledge; therefore, they must trust that the professional does. On the other hand, the ability of the professional to serve his patients as well as the income, status, and power of the professional are dependent on the ability to perform his professional functions.

Thus, a profession serves itself and society by giving high-quality performance in its professional role. A principal feature of ethics is to encourage a high level of role performance. Professional ethics are concerned not merely with the moral conduct of the practitioner in his professional relations but also with the function the profession performs and the quality of this performance.

Pharmacy has been only partially successful in fulfilling its potential function. As noted in the Millis Commission Report:

> (P)harmacy must be described as being both effective and efficient in developing, manufacturing, and distributing drug products . . . . However, the system of pharmacy cannot be described as either effective or efficient in developing, organizing and distributing knowledge and information about drugs.[27]

The precept that "A pharmacist should always strive to perfect and enlarge his professional knowledge" has, with minor changes, been part of pharmacy's code of ethics since its 1922 revision. The increased institutionalization of training for professions through colleges, formalized internship programs, and state licensing examinations does not decrease the significance of this ethic.

However, the main tool of the professions (knowledge) is being constantly expanded and changed and, in some cases, the function of the profession itself is being modified. In recent years the institutionalized training structure of pharmacy has become more aware of the gap which may exist between initial competence and continuing competence and through voluntary or compulsory continuing education is making a strong effort to reduce this gap.

The position of pharmacy (and thus of individual pharmacists) in our society depends on the service the profession renders to the members of society. However, the mere possession of the requisite technical knowledge makes no contribution to the well-being of society unless this knowledge is used for the benefit of the pharmacist's patients. Thus, the pharmacist is directed to "utilize and make available this knowledge as may be required in accordance with his best professional judgment."

While proper functioning of the professional in his role is important, of equal importance are the functions of the pharmacist as "an essential health practitioner." Thus, even though a practitioner performs his function with great technical competence, his role and the role of his occupation in society depend on the contribution of his function to the achievement of society's objectives. Pharmacy's function has, over the period of its existence, undergone changes, and the

stated ethics of the profession have been modified to reflect these changes.

Thus, in 1852, when a main function of the pharmacist was compounding medicinal agents into dosage forms, the pharmacist was told that his first duty "after duly preparing himself for his profession" was "to procure good drugs and preparations . . . ." In 1922, when the community pharmacist received many of his drugs already manufactured into dosage forms, the primary object of pharmacy was expanded and redefined as "the service it can render to the public in safeguarding the handling, sale, compounding, and dispensing of medicinal substances." The 1952 revision of the code expanded this to include the storage of drugs.

The current code still proscribes "the dispensing . . . of drugs . . . which are not of good quality" and offering for sale any drugs or medical devices that "lack therapeutic value"; however, the functional role of the pharmacist is now introduced with the broad statement that: "A pharmacist should hold the health and safety of patients to be of first consideration; he should render to each patient the full measure of his ability as an essential health practitioner."

While the proper performance of the physical act of dispensing drugs requires a high degree of skill and is an important function in society, the broad function expressed in the first section of the code indicates a belief that pharmacy's contribution to society can be more than that which is embodied in the physical act of dispensing drugs.

Thus, the professional ethics of pharmacy seek not only to encourage the adequate performance of the existing accepted role of the pharmacist but also to facilitate the expansion of this role to increase the functional contribution of pharmacy to society.

Relationship of Trust

In writing about the relation between professionalism and social structure, Marshall explained the necessity of the existence of a relationship of trust between the professional and the patient:

> Ethical codes are based on the belief that between professional and client there is a relationship of trust, and between buyer and seller there is not . . . .
> There are two reasons for this. One is that professional service is not standardized. It is unique and personal . . . . It is hardly possible to be satisfied with a doctor or a lawyer unless one likes and respects him as a man . . . . These essential qualities cannot be specified in a contract, they cannot be bought. They can only be given . . . .
> The second reason for the relationship of trust . . . is the ignorance of the client. He often hardly knows what to ask for, let alone how it can be provided. He must surrender all initiative and put himself in his lawyer's hands or under his doctor's orders.[6]

These reasons justify the extension of the scope of professional ethics, beyond the technical performance of an occupational role, to the personal characteristics of the practitioner. Thus, we find that: "A pharmacist has the duty to observe the law . . . . He should not engage in any activity that will bring discredit to the profession . . . ."

Offenses directly related to the professional role, such as the illegal sale of narcotics by a pharmacist or falsification of claims for prepaid prescription insurance, clearly violate the ethic. The ethic, however, is not limited to such offenses but, presumably, includes all conduct which reflects adversely on the trustworthiness of a practitioner.

Ideal of Service—The necessity of a relationship of trust to the smooth functioning of the professions also imposes other restrictions on the professional practitioner. As the first section of the code dictates, "A pharmacist should hold the health and safety of patients to be of first consideration." Thus, the ideal of service embodied in the professional ethic places the financial gain of the professional in a position secondary to the service he renders. As Kohn expressed it:

(T)he professions in the finest sense do actually get their inspiration from a motive other than the money-getting motive .... The earning of a livelihood is naturally the result of competent practice of a profession. But that is not its prime purpose in the best sense. The prime purpose is the perfection of a service ....[28]

This altruistic subordination of the personal gain of the practitioner to the best interest of the patient is a dominant factor in distinguishing professions from other occupations. This subordination of the private interest of the practitioner does not mean that the professional must be oblivious to materialistic goals. A distinction should be made between the total professional income and his income from a given patient transaction. With respect to the latter, the professional ethic requires that the needs and welfare of the patient are superior to the immediate financial interest of the practitioner. Such an ethic is, however, difficult to adhere to unless the total professional income is at a satisfactory level.

Indirect Remuneration—One of the main ethics derived from the required altruistic attitude is a prohibition on indirect remuneration of the practitioner. According to Carr-Saunders and Wilson:

The fiduciary relationship between professional and client involves certain restrictions on the professional man's methods of charging. It requires that the practitioner shall be financially disinterested in the advice he gives, or, at least, that the possibility of conflict between duty and self-interest shall be reduced to a minimum.[29]

The 1848 code of the Philadelphia College of Pharmacy declared it unjust to medicine and injurious to the public for an apothecary to allow "any physician a percentage or commission on his prescriptions." Through various mutations, this prohibition has continued through the present code.

The obvious dangers of a prescriber standing to profit (whether through a direct commission, percentage rental in a prescriber-owned building, or other mechanisms) from having the prescriptions he writes dispensed in a given pharmacy include the possible denying to the patient of freedom of choice of pharmacist and the ordering of unnecessary medication by the prescriber.

The bases of the prohibition against fee-splitting can also be interpreted as discouraging certain widely used practices, such as gifts to prescribers at Christmas or other occasions and even the granting of a professional discount to prescribers on their purchases in a pharmacy. There is a thin line which separates these practices from ethical gestures of friendship or professional respect and the unethical practice of attempting to influence the prescriber to steer his patients to a particular pharmacy.

Although the code specifically prohibits "arrangements with practitioners of other health professions" involving fee-splitting or other methods of patient exploitation, the indirect remuneration ethic is not limited to arrangements with other health professionals. The code also prohibits splitting of fees for professional services with persons in addition to health professionals, such as granting rebates to operators of nursing homes or extended-care facilities.

Conflict of Interest—By the very nature of the professional relationship and the trust that is required, conflict of interest situations which could lead to patient exploitation are inevitable. A distinction should be made between those conflicts which are inherent in the professional relationship and those which are voluntarily created by the practitioner. The former require restraint by the professional to insure that there is no patient exploitation. The latter, since they are an unnecessary part of the professional relationship, should be avoided.

For example, if a pharmacist receives a prescription written generically for reserpine, he must exercise his professional judgment to determine which of the available reserpine products he will dispense. Depending on his method of charging for his professional services, the pharmacist might make more profit from dispensing one brand of reserpine than from another. Although this conflict could be avoided by the use of the professional fee, the choice among available reserpine products is a part of the professional service of the pharmacist and requires that he restrain his profit motive to dispense the product which best satisfies the patient's needs rather than the product which is most profitable.

An unnecessary part of the community pharmacist's professional relationship would be an ownership interest in a drug repackaging firm which distributes reserpine or other products which he could use to dispense generic prescriptions. The conflict of interest in this latter case differs from that in the former in that the ownership interest is a voluntarily acquired conflict which is not necessary to the proper performance of the professional.

To avoid these potential conflicts of interest, a pharmacist likely should not have an influential ownership interest in a company which distributes products that he would use to dispense prescriptions written generically.

The mere existence of unnecessary action which could result in patient exploitation can do much to destroy the public's trust in pharmacists, regardless of whether or not exploitation occurs. To avoid these problems, the pharmacist should refuse to participate in any unnecessary scheme whereby his professional judgment may become clouded by considerations of personal financial gain.

Commercial Practices—The relationship of trust that must exist between professional and patient also imposes restrictions on the methods used by the professional to attract patients. According to Carr-Saunders and Wilson:

When the position of trust is regarded as extending to a profession as a whole, it is seen that certain common commercial practices are incompatible with the rendering of professional services; and from these practices the professional man is required to abstain. In particular professional men may only compete with one another in reputation for ability, which implies that advertisement, price-cutting, and other methods familiar to the business world are ruled out.[30]

If the patient is to have the required degree of trust in the professional whose services he utilizes, the primary motivating factor in determining patronage must be the quality of service, and not its price. In the commercial world, advertising has two basic purposes: to inform a consumer who has already decided to purchase of the availability of a product or service and to stimulate demand for the product or service. In the professional environment the use of advertising for the former purpose usually is allowed within reasonable limits while for the latter purpose advertising is generally discouraged.

The Federal Trade Commission, however, has strongly suggested that efforts to deter price advertising of prescriptions may be unlawful practices under the FTC Act.[31] In 1972 the APhA recognized that "Patients have a right to know upon request the cost of pharmaceutical service ... prior to the providing of such service ...."[32] This resulted in the elimination in 1975 of the prohibition in the Code of Ethics against the solicitation of professional practice by means of advertising and its replacement with the new Section 8 prohibiting misleading patients about cost or value.

In 1976 the US Supreme Court declared unconstitutional a Virginia statute which made it unlawful to advertise prescription prices.[33] The Court held that such prohibitions violate the right to freedom of speech.

Emerging Conflicts

The conflict between the personal interests of the professional and his duty to subordinate this interest to the best interest of his patient presents one of the major unresolved problems of the professions. In addition, changing patterns in pharmacy and health-care delivery present additional ethical conflicts.

The traditional unit of professional service has been the individual. Thus, professional services have not been mass produced, but each rendering of a service is specifically tailored to the individual needs of a specific patient. In general, the ethics of professions have evolved on the basis of primacy of the individual with the general welfare of society relegated to a secondary position. Marshall has summarized the situation as follows:

The professional man cannot spread his services . . . . He is unable to go in for mass production and is forbidden to offer cheap lines for slender purses. Since he works for a limited market it is not surprising that he should choose one which is solvent and concentrate on the wealthy individual client. In other words he must find an employer, and the general public was not organized for his employment . . . . (T)his state of affairs led to a maldistribution of professional services in terms of social need, a maldistribution due to economic motives among professional men but not necessarily implying any disloyalty to the principle that service must not be sacrificed to profit . . . . Big-scale social activities only became possible when the initiative was taken by the state and the local authorities, by public corporations and rich charities. And by that time the professions had built up their tradition of individualism, which meant not so much the pursuit of individual self-interest as the service of individual clients in a relationship of individual trust. They were therefore disinclined to press for the establishment of corporate agencies for the distribution of professional services and reluctant to work for them when they appeared.[6]

The correction of this maldistribution likely can be effected only with structural changes in the health-care system and a resulting alteration of the professional–patient relationship. A system appears to be emerging in which frequently someone other than the recipient of the service provides the payment to the professional. The resulting third-party-payment programs likely will produce a system in which the third party exercises some control over the professional practice.

For example, traditionally the pharmacist has considered as confidential information about a patient which is contained in his prescription files and patient record cards. However, if a third party is to pay the prescription charges for a patient, the third party usually will require access to the information contained in these records.

The increasing incidence of pharmacists not practicing in the community pharmacy environment gives some indication of the nature of the problem. Thus, the problems relating to professional ethics which are encountered by the institutional pharmacist, the industrial pharmacist, or the pharmacist functioning in an administrative capacity frequently are quite different from those encountered by the pharmacist in community practice.

Emerging systems of health care as well as other factors indicate the likelihood that an increased percentage of health practitioners will have an employee rather than an independent status. As with third-party payment, this can present situations in which the professional's duty to his patient is in conflict with his duty to his employer. Although this is not a new situation for pharmacy, the changing nature of the employer may present additional conflicts. Traditionally, the employed pharmacist has been an employee of another pharmacist in a community pharmacy. However, with increasing frequency the employer is a nonpharmacist—a corporate chain of pharmacies, an industrial corporation, a hospital, or a government agency. Thus, the pharmacist–pharmacist employment relationship, with the attendant obligation of both employer and employee to adhere to pharmacy's ethics, is being replaced in many instances with a pharmacist–nonpharmacist employment relationship, in which only the pharmacist is obligated to adhere to the profession's ethical precepts.

Encouraging Adherence

One characteristic of ethics is that they are a mechanism of self-regulation for a profession. As Sonnedecker expressed:

However far governmental regulation of pharmacy may reach, room remains for a set of moral expectations and injunctions in some form—for an institutionalized action pattern that makes it normal for the pharmacist to accept social responsibilities going beyond legal compulsion.[34]

Thus, in the primary sense ethics are not enforced by law, but they are adhered to because of an "institutionalized action pattern that makes it normal for the pharmacist to accept social responsibilities . . . ." The strengthening of this institutionalized action pattern leads to the advancement of the profession through its own self-regulation. A failure of this system necessitates government intervention in order to maintain pharmacy standards at a level required for the protection of the public health.

Reasons for Ethical Failures—As developed in previous sections, adherence to the ethics of pharmacy by a practitioner frequently is an example of enlightened self-interest. Thus, by all practitioners maintaining high professional standards, the profession as a whole advances and each practitioner benefits. There appear to be two reasons why this enlightened self-interest does not always occur.

The first is lack of knowledge: ignorance on the part of practitioners of the existence or meaning of pharmacy's ethical precepts.

The second reason relates to a concentration on short-run goals. Thus, a pharmacist might prostitute the heritage of the profession which has accumulated over the centuries by, for example, advertising low prescription prices to attract patronage. In doing so, the pharmacist takes a calculated risk that he will be able to continue profitably prostituting the profession and that the overall effects of his actions will not be felt until succeeding generations take over the profession.

This type of ethical failure is much more difficult to correct and, likely, the optimum approach would be to prevent its occurrence rather than attempting to deal with it after it has occurred. To a considerable extent, this is a purpose of pharmacy education. As Bullough observed:

It seems obvious that professional status for the individual is achieved only after long training . . . . One of the chief purposes of such training is to initiate the candidate into a set of professional attitudes and controls, to give him a professional conscience.[35]

The reference groups with which an individual identifies can have a profound effect on his actions. If the group as a whole accepts the ethical standards, an individual who desires further association with the group (or fears disassociation from the group) will be likely to conform to the group standard. The effect of increasing the reference groups which accept the ethical standards of the profession likely is cumulative, since as more ethical groups emerge there is a smaller probability that a pharmacist will select a nonethical group as his reference group.

Sanctions—In spite of these actions, there still will remain a small proportion of pharmacists who do not adhere to the ethical precepts. Sanctions against members of this group by the professional association can range from censure to revocation of membership. The imposition of such sanctions must, of course, be in accordance with the member's right to due process.

Potentially, the result of disciplinary action may be to increase, rather than decrease, the nonconformity of the offender. As Toby has noted:

The status degradation inherent in punishment makes it more difficult to induce the offender to play a legitimate role instead of a nonconforming one. Whatever the offender's original motivations for nonconformity, punishment adds to them by neutralizing his fear of losing the respect of the community—he has already lost it.[36]

An additional limitation on sanctions by professional associations is the general limitation of their effect to members of the association. Thus, an association obviously cannot revoke the membership of a nonmember. In many cases, those most likely to commit offenses against the ethical code are not likely to have acquired membership in the professional association. A further deficiency is the failure of many members of the profession to expose unethical practice. In a study of discipline in the American Medical Association it was observed that:

First and foremost, the Committee found apathy, substantial ignorance, and a lack of a sense of individual responsibility by physicians as a whole. The latter is demonstrated by the "hear no evil, see no evil" attitude of many doctors and through the complaints which are received concerning physicians when the complaining physician later refuses to testify or give a deposition.[37]

In spite of the deficiencies of self-regulation, there remains much that can be done within pharmacy to increase the service contribution of pharmacists through ethics. The situation was summarized by the late Dean LaWall when he described pharmacy as:

(A) highly specialized calling, which may rise to the dignity of a true profession or sink to the level of the lowest commercialism, according to the ideals, the ability, and the training of the one who practices it.[38]

References

1. Tomlin EWF: *The Western Philosophers: An Introduction*, Harper and Row, New York, 1963.
2. Veach RM: *A Theory of Medical Ethics*, Basic Books, New York, 6, 1981.
3. Kultgen J: *Bus and Prof Ethics J 1:* 65, 1982
4. Veach RM: *Case Studies in Medical Ethics*, Harvard University Press, Cambridge, 1, 1977.
5. Veach RM: *A Theory of Medical Ethics*, 310.
6. Marshall TH: *Can J Econ Political Sci 5:* 325, 1939.
7. Parsons T: *Social Forces 17:* 457, 1939.
8. Smith A: *An Inquiry into the Nature and Causes of the Wealth of Nations*, Collier, New York, 107, 1937.
9. Greenwood E, in Noscow S, Form WH, eds: *Man, Work and Society*, Basic Books, New York, 210, 1962.
10. Carr-Saunders AM, Wilson PA: *The Professions*, Oxford University Press, Oxford, 141–144, 1933.
11. Montague JB: *J APHA NS8:* 228–230, 1968.
12. Smith MC: *Am J Pharm Educ 34:* 16–32, 1970.
13. Smith MC, Knapp DA: *Pharmacy, Drugs and Medical Care*, Williams and Wilkins, Baltimore, 1972.
14. Denzin NR, Mettlin CJ: *Soc Forces 46:* 357–382, 1968.
15. *Apharmacy Weekly 22*, April 1, 1983.
16. Barber B: *J APhA NS8:* 137, 1968.
17. Guilano C: *J APhA NS3:* 73, 1963.
18. Kultgen, *op cit*
19. Larson MS: *The Rise of Professionalism*, University of California Press, Berkley, 226, 1977.
20. *Am J Pharm 20:* 148, 1848.
21. *J APhA NS3:* 65, 1963.
22. Sletten CA: *The Social Structure and Ideology of Organized Pharmacy*, unpublished PhD dissertation, Harvard Univ., 329–330, 1959.
23. *J APhA NS6:* 293, 1966.
24. *J APhA NS8:* 142, 1968.
25. *Apharmacy Weekly 40*, Oct. 2, 1976.
26. *Am Pharmacy NS19:* 200, 1979.
27. *Pharmacists for the Future: The Report of the Study Commission on Pharmacy*, Health Administration Press, Ann Arbor, MI, 58, 1975.
28. Kohn RD: *Ann Am Acad Political Sci 101 (May):* 1, 1922.
29. Carr-Saunders AM, Wilson PA: *op cit* 426.
30. *Ibid*, 432.
31. *J APhA NS15:* 668, 1975.
32. *Ibid.*, 677.
33. Virginia State Board of Pharmacy *et al.*, v Virginia Citizens Consumer Council, Inc., *et al.*, 425 US 748 (1976).
34. Sonnedecker G: *Am J Pharm 133:* 243, 1961.
35. Bullough VL: *The Development of Medicine as a Profession*, Hafner, New York, 2, 1966.
36. Toby J: *J Criminal Law Criminol Police Sci 55:* 332, 1964.
37. *Report of the Medical Disciplinary Committee to the Board of Trustees*, AMA, Chicago, 52, 1961.
38. LaWall CH: *Four Thousand Years of Pharmacy*, Lippincott, Philadelphia, 1920.

CHAPTER 4

Pharmacists in Practice

Melvin R Gibson, PhD

Professor of Pharmacognosy
College of Pharmacy, Washington State University
Pullman, WA 99164

The Pharmacist and the Pharmacy

The pharmacist and his function in the last quarter century have undergone dramatic changes in both personal orientation and professional activity. He is no longer a handmaiden of medicine filling secret prescriptions containing medication of often questionable value requiring manipulative arts and techniques. Today, he is a professional in his own right—a partner in the health team who handles drugs of great potency and value manufactured by a highly sophisticated industry. He handles these drugs in open consultation with physicians and patients with the confidence his advanced knowledge as an expert on drugs demands that he should.

In this last quarter century, also, there has been a marked increase in the type and quantity of convenience goods distributed by pharmacies, some of which have no relation to health. It is this commercialization of pharmacy which has created many of the problems now faced by the profession. Not the least part of this problem is the public image of pharmacy practice. The late distinguished pharmaceutical educator, Dr Rufus A Lyman (himself a physician and staunch Presbyterian) said, "There is commercialism in medicine and in the Presbyterian Church, as well as in pharmacy. The only difference is that commercialism in pharmacy is on display on every main street in the country."

Displayed as it is and exploited as it is, commercialization of pharmacy has created problems at all levels of pharmaceutical engagement. The glimmer of a reverse trend to strictly professional practice will be discussed later in this chapter.

The commercialization of retail pharmacy, whether motivated by a desire to be of greater service or by profits, has yet failed to completely besmirch the image of the pharmacist as a dedicated professional who holds the respect of the community at large and of the business and professional persons of our towns and cities. The pharmacist is still the professional on main street most accessible to the public whose image remains as that of a reliable person with whom the public can talk in confidence on a variety of subjects and who does not send a bill for this counsel. He is the person who is active in community affairs and often a community leader in worthwhile projects as well as giving generously of his time and efforts for the community good.

The separation of professional and business functions is today clouded in the public's mind. They are also clouded in the minds of many pharmacists. It is often easier to slip into commercialism than to develop the professional aspects of pharmaceutical practice. White[1] put it this way:

Observations made throughout my thirty years in the profession suggest that motivation rather than education is the quality most lacking when pharmacists fail to achieve important new goals. The demands made day after day in a routine job allow the years to slip by without time taken for a self-analysis or a periodic evaluation of one's business. Soon both pharmacist and pharmacy have slipped into a decadence from which there is no easy escape.

Pharmacy is at a critical era in its history. At the center of interest is the pharmacist himself. He is fairly well paid. In a survey of 904 pharmacies[2] in 1982, the average salary of the proprietor or manager was $30,381 with the average net profit before taxes of $15,265. For self-employed proprietors the total income before taxes would be $45,646. He is in a big profession with drug store sales, chains and independents combined, reaching a level of more than $21 billion in 1981.[3] He is well educated. A five-year curriculum is a minimum, and some curricula require six years (see Chapter 1). The rest of this chapter will deal with the pharmacist, his practice, his problems, and his challenges; in short, where he is, what he is doing, and what he can do to affect his future in this critical period of the profession.

The Pharmacist and His Principal Roles

The Pharmacist, the Prescription, and the OTC Drugs—Hager[4] has said, "Adequate communication of information about drugs to persons who need such information by persons who are in a position and are qualified to supply that information is today a most important factor in the improvement of the health, strength, and vigor of the people of this country."

The people who know most about drugs are pharmacists. That is their province; that is their responsibility. Primary in this responsibility are prescription drugs. The physician must diagnose; he must prescribe. But the pharmacist handles that all-important commodity—the drug that alleviates or cures. His approach to the handling of this important commodity must not be taken lightly. In some instances he may be a consultant to the physician on drugs. But before he can really function as a partner with the physician in therapy, both his training and experience must be so directed. *Now his most important service* can be rendered to the person who wants and needs it most—the patient. Every new prescription should be discussed privately with the patient. Every prescription renewal which the pharmacist believes needs discussing with the patient should be discussed in private.[5]

The pharmacist is not in a position to discuss diagnoses and the ramifications of diseases. However, he is capable of discussing the drug as a drug with the patient. He does know how the drug is taken. He does know the side reactions of it which may be of concern to the patient. He does know its stability under various conditions. He does know its toxicity and dosage. He does understand its route of administration. He is an expert on drugs. The physician is not. The information which the pharmacist is able to supply can be of great assurance, interest, and need to the patient.

The second most important responsibility the pharmacist has to the patient is in the area of over-the-counter (OTC) drugs. The pharmacist's responsibility in this regard is well summarized by Penna[6] in his address to the Conference of Teachers of Pharmacy of the American Association of Colleges of Pharmacy:

The necessity that practicing pharmacists take on a more professional attitude toward non-prescription medication is practically axiomatic. Likewise, the need which exists on behalf of the public for such professional pharmaceutical activity is self-evident. We see in the area of non-prescription medication, a new field of professional involvement, a new endeavor where the pharmacist can perform professional functions without first receiving instructions from a physician.

In handling a case dealing with self-diagnosis and a non-prescription drug, the pharmacist has the total responsibility for all the professional decisions. He decides which products he carries in his pharmacy. He decides whether or not a patient has accurately self-diagnosed his condition. The pharmacist decides whether or not to recommend that the patient consult a physician or recommend a product, and finally, the pharmacist makes the decision as to which product to recommend in a given case.

These decisions—all professional acts—are the reasons why pharmacists must take a more active and professional interest in non-prescription medication. These decisions are also the reasons why pharmacists in increasing numbers are becoming more involved in this specialty—they recognize the potential for professional service, the need and the professional satisfaction which are inherent in the specialty of non-prescription medication.

Certainly non-prescription medication will play an ever-increasing role in the medical treatment of the future. Self-diagnosis and self-medication will continue to increase as the public becomes more knowledgeable about diseases and drugs. While this is intrinsically good and will have an immediate effect on reducing the physician work load, self-diagnosis and medication must be subject to professional guidance. The pharmacist who is available, accessible, knowledgeable and concerned is the logical choice for the individual on whom this responsibility should fall.

With greater pharmacist–patient orientation and patient drug-record-keeping the pharmacist becomes the only person who has *all* the information regarding the patient's drug consumption, prescription and nonprescription. He must use that information about drug consumption, coupled with his own singular drug expertise, to advise the patient and, if necessary, the patient's physician so that the patient benefits most and does not suffer from the multiple-drug therapy from prescription and nonprescription drugs.

The Pharmaceutical Center—Probably no event in the recent history of pharmacy has caught more dramatically the imagination of the professionally minded student than the Pharmaceutical Center concept. It was originally the 1960 realization of the dream of one man, Eugene V. White of Berryville, VA. Through the promotion of the American Pharmaceutical Association and McKesson Drug Company, the Pharmaceutical Center has become a thriving concept of the epitome of professional pharmacy practice. Its most eloquent evangelist is Mr. White himself.[7]

The professional store devoted almost exclusively to handling prescriptions is not new. It has its counterpart all over Europe. But the need for multipurpose retail establishments of all kinds in a rapidly developing and often sparsely settled US made the multipurpose pharmacy (business and professional) the common trend in this country. The trend of overcommercialization often outweighed the professional development until the pharmacist found himself the educational product of professionalism and the in-practice victim of overcommercialization. This dichotomy between education and practice led to the disillusion of many young pharmacists.

The disillusionment of Mr. White brought forth the Pharmaceutical Center. Figs 4–1 & 4–2 illustrate interior and exterior views of such centers.

A departure from the usual strictly prescription store, the Pharmaceutical Center is an innovation not only in pharmacy interiors but also in the pharmacist–patient relationship. Placed in a relaxed and professional setting, and devoid of merchandise on display, the pharmacist has as his primary interest the patient and what he, the pharmacist, can do to serve the patient's best health interests. As Mr. White has emphasized in his many talks on the subject, a Pharmaceutical Center cannot be successful without the genuine interest of the pharmacist in the health needs of the patient. This pharmacist–patient relationship must be genuine, personal,

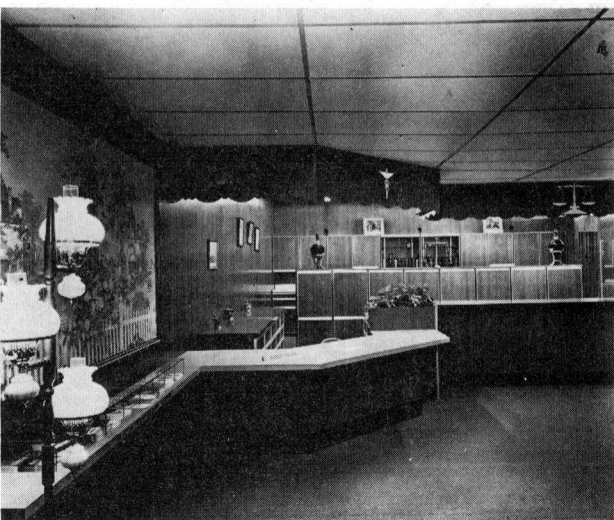

Fig 4–1. Pharmaceutical Center, John J. Eshleman, owner, San Jose.

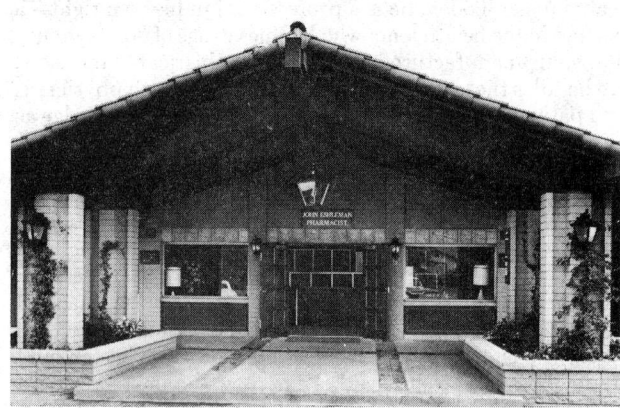

Fig 4–2. Pharmaceutical Center (courtesy, McKesson Drug Company).

and performed in the interest of the patient's welfare. There is no place for commercialism in such an establishment. The author of this chapter has even suggested[5] that all Pharmaceutical Centers have a consultation room so that each new prescription, and refills where indicated, should be discussed with the patient by the pharmacist.

The Pharmaceutical Center is the setting for the practice of pharmacy in its most professional context. Without the merchandise as a prop for financial security, it should not be entered into without thorough evaluation of prescription volume. But more important an evaluation is that of the sincerity of the pharmacist in his motives. The success of the Pharmaceutical Center is most determined by the dedication of the pharmacist to the best interests of the patients requiring his services.

What might be considered the creed of the Pharmaceutical Center has been expressed by an owner of such a center, Mr Ralph S Kuhn of Dolyestown, PA[7]:

Society creates a profession because of the need of the services rendered by said profession. Such a profession will only live so long as it renders the services required by the society that created it. Therefore, a profession is a trust and a privilege given by society to render a specialized service for members of society. If the profession refuses to recognize its responsibility or exploits its trust, then society will find other means for acquiring the necessary services. Pharmacists must be made to realize that they have not been fulfilling the very purpose for which they exist. They have been very cleverly diverted from doing the will of pharmacy to doing the will of the self-schooled, diabolical and articulate huckster and merchandiser. If pharmacy were fulfilling its obligation to society, we would not have to fight for ourselves because they would do it for us and do it better.

In small communities there will always be the need for a multipurpose pharmacy to serve the needs of the people and supply the pharmacist with diversified sources of income. These can be attractive, profitable establishments meeting the needs of these communities (Fig 4-3).

In metropolitan areas the large diverse-product pharmacies will continue to be part of the pharmacy picture (Fig 4-4). There is something undeniably attractive about wide selections of many lines of merchandise open for public view and selection. The supermarket pharmacy will find its place in shopping centers and metropolitan centers. However, as the Pharmaceutical Center concept gains public acceptance and appreciation, it is predicted that the dichotomy between merchandising and strictly professional practice will become more evident. This is seen in the rapidly growing areas of the West Coast. The US eventually may see the pattern which exists in Europe—one class of pharmacy devoted to merchandise, another devoted strictly to professional practice.

Patient Orientation—The breakaway of the professional practice of pharmacy from the business image will neither be quick nor easy. However, it is believed by many that such a separation is critical for the survival of pharmacy as a professional entity. It is believed that the deciding factor in the emergence of a new professional image will depend upon the ability of the pharmacist to alter his image from that of simply a purveyor of drugs and merchandise to one of being a purveyor of advice and counsel both to the patient and to the public at large. The pharmacist's role as a consultant on drugs to the physician is often not well developed. The pharmacist has often viewed himself as subservient to the physician and his almighty prescription. In the future health-care picture the pharmacist will need to become a full-time partner to the physician, for he is the only expert on drugs today. This is expertise which is not being effectively utilized in the average pharmacy.

Where there is the greatest need for counsel and advice on drugs is to the patient. To emerge as a full-fledged professional, the pharmacist must divest himself of the image and practice of product-orientation and become patient-oriented. A more detailed presentation of this subject may be found in Chapters 94, and 97–100.

The pharmacist is in a unique position in the community. He is usually the best-educated and -informed person on main street. He is the most "available" professional. No appointments are necessary to talk with him. He doesn't charge for his advice. This unique availability is appreciated and deserved by the public, but it is not always utilized to its fullest by the pharmacist as a means of service to the public.

The orientation of the pharmacist to the patient is often impersonal and businesslike. The patient is quick to sense this and to form his impression of the pharmacist as a result. The "business" impression tags the pharmacist as a business man rather than as a professional. One needs only to observe the functioning of a successful physician or attorney to know why they enjoy the prestige and confidence of people in general. In their functioning they have an intense *interest* in *you* and *your* problems—or they seem to. The *professional* pharmacist must also exhibit this interest and concern.

The physician sees his patient as a body of order and disorder. The attorney sees his client as an accumulation of personal and business assets and liabilities. The pharmacist should see his patient as a consumer of a multiplicity of drugs, the subject of numerous physician proddings and administrations. In this regard the pharmacist, like the physician and the attorney, is unique. He sees one specialized aspect of a person's functioning. However, unlike the physician and the attorney, he often does not put this information to use for the good of the patient or client.

The pharmacist *alone* knows what drugs a patient is taking—nonprescriptions, old prescriptions, new prescriptions,

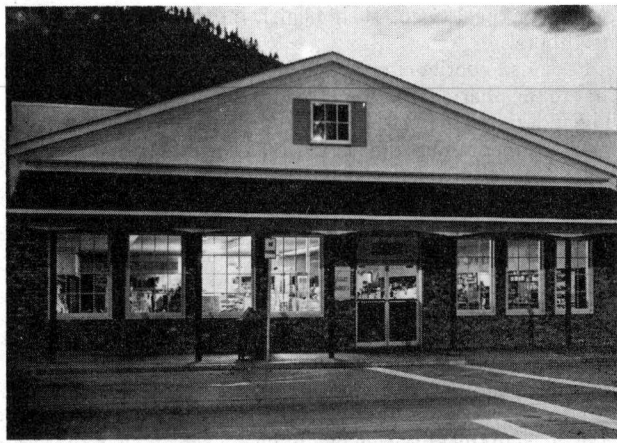

Fig 4-3.   Valley Pharmacy, Ron and Wayne Doane, owners, Cashmere, WA (population: 1,950).

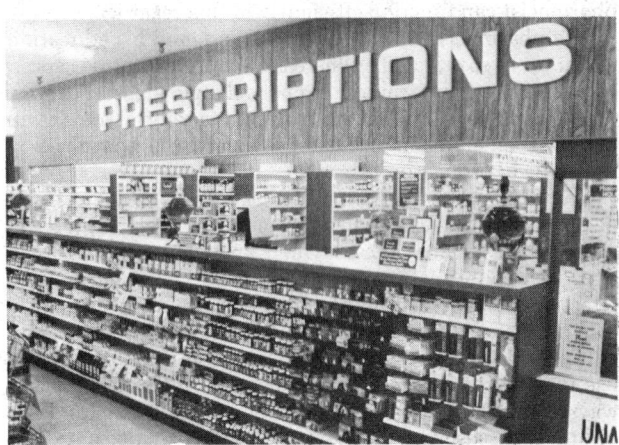

Fig 4-4.   Walgreens Drugs, Chicago, IL.

or multiple prescriptions from different physicians. In this age of specialization a patient may be seeing several physicians at one time. Physicians' ethics, the reason for which seems somewhat obscure, seem to militate against mutual consultation on what each is doing for an individual patient. This often complicates the medication picture and may lead to serious drug interactions and untoward side effects. The *pharmacist knows this*. He must take steps in the patient's interest to use his drug knowledge to aid the physicians in their drug regimen for individual patients.

Another peculiarity of medical practice seems to be the lack of follow-up of patients. Unless a physician knows a patient very well he will usually make no effort to recontact a patient. The patient must always take the initiative to contact the physician. Often, a patient may have a prescription refilled for years without the knowledge of the physician. The *pharmacist knows this*. Both the physician and the patient should be informed of dangers which may result from such a practice. The pharmacist is in a unique position to recommend a revisit to a physician. Often that is all that is needed. There is a natural reluctance in all of us to go to a physician.

Not only can the pharmacist be of great value to the patient in suggesting revisits to a physician for medication purposes but he also can be of great assistance to a person who needs a physician's care. Americans are an independent lot. They like "to do things themselves," whether this be car repair, home repairs, building, or picture framing. The "do it yourself" industry is tremendous. The same applies to medication. A survey a few years ago indicated that about $\frac{1}{3}$ of the people in the US got their health information from their neighbors!

Persons experiencing some physical problem often come first to the pharmacist. He is readily available and accessible. The individual may be only in need of advice or he may be in need of either minor or major medical attention. In any event, the pharmacist can be of considerable value to the individual, and also of assistance to the physician. Minor complaints often can be helped with nonprescription items, thus saving the physician's time from unnecessary patient visitations.

Advice on *when* a patient should see a physician can be most valuable. Many patients wait too long, until their condition becomes so complex as to be dangerous to the patient and to require considerable time of the physician. In a conference at the University of Michigan in 1967[8] it was recognized by physicians that the pharmacist can be of considerable assistance to the physician by intelligent screening of physical complaints of persons seeking the advice of the pharmacist. Often in the past the pharmacist has been reluctant to assume this responsibility. With his education properly oriented, the pharmacist can function efficiently in this regard.

The pharmacist is not a diagnostician, and his education will never be so oriented. Whereas he cannot diagnose cancer, he can certainly inform others of the danger signs of cancer. The pharmacist's optimal functioning as a referral source will become even more important as his expertise is recognized by the medical profession.

The pharmacist can serve also as an important referral person to health facilities in a community as well as a referral agent to physicians. Few laymen know about and how to approach county, state, and federal health agencies. The effective utilization of these facilities can be enhanced greatly by a pharmacist who has the information regarding these facilities and recognizes in his patients the desirability of their use for persons in need of such agencies. There are many ways[9] a pharmacist can help the lay person understand the nature of disease and understand what he can do to protect his own health through an intelligent understanding of health and disease and what factors are brought into play in both instances.

The *Survey of Sickness*[10] found that three out of four people who felt ill did not go to their physician. They made a self-diagnosis of their condition. There is evidence that such self-diagnosis can be disastrously wrong. Teeling-Smith pointed out that the pharmacist can be a most effective source of "health publicity." The APhA in an extensive survey[11] proved that pharmacists could be an effective source of information and literature regarding health.

As early as 1928 Surgeon General Cumming[12] recognized the important role pharmacists can play in educating the public in community health.

The usually strategic position and the familiar association of the drug store with medical matters in the popular mind place pharmacists in a position to render a material service to the community in connection with public health activities. It is the privilege, as well as the duty, of pharmacists to cooperate with public health agencies in the dissemination of reliable information concerning the public health and to assist the public health authorities especially as relates to communicable diseases and the protection of biological products.

It should be recognized that in any attempt at pharmacist–patient professional orientation there must be a genuine and personal interest by the pharmacist in the patient. Without such interest the association will be unsuccessful. In the words of the former Food and Drug Administration Commissioner Goddard,[13] the pharmacist must cooperate to see that the public is "well cared for—and *cared about*."

Nursing Homes and Long-Term Health Care Facilities

The US Public Health Service[14] defines a nursing home as "a facility or unit which is equipped for the accommodation of individuals not requiring hospital care but needing nursing care and related medical services."

The long-term health care facilities are varied and essential as custodial institutions for those unable to care for themselves. They bridge the gap between nursing homes and self-care facilities.

The aged population in this country is about 22 million and increasing at the rate of about 1000 a day. Medicare and various forms of insurance provide hospitalization for large numbers of the aged population. This strain on hospital facilities finds partial respite with the growing nursing home and long-term health care facilities. The future strain on hospital facilities will demand a tremendous increase in the number of hospitals and also a concomitant increase in nursing home and long-term health care facilities.

Hospital pharmacy and the role of the pharmacist in long-term health care facilities are outlined in Chapters 95 and 96.

Problems in Pharmacy Practice

Pharmacy, like any profession, has its problems. Those mentioned here are limited to those not mentioned elsewhere in this chapter but still having a direct bearing on the practice of pharmacy itself.

Continuing Education—Pharmacy has begun to face up to the problem of continuing education. The rapid advances in medicine and in drug therapy dictate that the pharmacist keep abreast of developments in his science after his formal education is completed. To do otherwise is to deny his patients full benefits of modern science. As Bowers has said,[15] "Nothing less than the welfare of the profession and the health of the public is involved."

In recent years there has been considerable interest by practitioners and educators, both in medicine and in pharmacy, in the desirability, if not the necessity, of continuing education. As a result, there have been developed numerous conferences, seminars, lectures, special television and telephone programs, and correspondence courses aimed at keeping the practicing pharmacist abreast of the changing scene in the practice of pharmacy. In 1973 the American Association of Colleges of Pharmacy and the American Pharmaceutical Association formed a Joint Task Force on Continuing Competence in Pharmacy. The following quotation is from the introductory statement of the final report from the Task Force.[16]

For many years reliance has been placed on the processes of registration and licensure as means of assuring competence of health professionals to serve the public. In the process of using these screening mechanisms, it has been assumed with rare exceptions that an individual initially registered or licensed would continue to possess competence to practice. This assumption is now being questioned not only by many members of the professions but also by the general public.

The issue of continuing competence of professionals to practice is influenced by various factors, such as the rapid and numerous scientific and technological developments during the past several decades, the increasing numbers of persons seeking health care, the changing patterns in the management and delivery of health care, and the growing recognition of the need to protect the public from unqualified personnel, a recognition that is shared by an expanding proportion of the health professionals themselves, including members of the profession of pharmacy.

The Task Force concluded:[17]

1. In the interests of the public welfare, pharmacists should be subject to evaluation and relicensure at periodic intervals.
2. Although participation in continuing education does not itself automatically assure that the practitioner is thereby maintaining his competence, at this stage in the development of means to assure continuing competence it is the most effective method available by which the practitioner may update and enrich his qualifications.
3. When adequate standards for continuing competence have been developed, and when appropriate and valid techniques for measurement and evaluation of professional competence have been devised, demonstrated proof of continuing competence should be a requirement for relicensure.

The Task Force recommended:[18]

> For the present and until additional methods of assuring continuing competence of pharmacists are developed, reliance should be placed on continuing education. In view of the need for this reliance for the indefinite future, imaginative and innovative programs of continuing education should be developed; and an effective organization for and adequate financing of continuing education should be accorded a high priority.

At the college level great strides have been made in the area of continuing education not only in developing the various types of programs but in assigning faculty personnel to the program, sometimes on a full-time basis. However, one of the major problems in developing continuing education at the college level has often been the lack of financial resources to mount or to maintain the programs. In some instances the state pharmaceutical associations have assumed some of the responsibilities for program development. The National Association of Boards of Pharmacy has been involved in attempting to coordinate efforts within the states because some states now require continuing education credits as a prerequisite for relicensure.

There are two very real problems facing pharmacy in regard to continuing education. The first is the matter of how such programs are to be adequately financed and the second is the quality of such programs. Both problems will not be easy to solve. At present, the programs are usually financed by the colleges alone or in cooperation with the state associations, by the pharmacists involved in the programs, by pharmaceutical manufacturers, or by a combination of these. Proper financial backing has not been achieved. The quality of the programs reflects this lack of adequate support. The second problem is a reflection, in part, of the first. Too often continuing education programs are uncoordinated, one-shot programs aimed at plugging the gap in what is considered to be an area which requires updating. Too often the audience to which the program is directed is such a diversified group, both in educational background and in professional interest, to make participation by the practitioner an exercise in futility. There needs to be a serious study made of the needs of pharmacists at all levels and a coordinated program to see that these needs are met. Such a program would require a long-range and expensive study before the implementation of the program could occur. Whereas the goals of continuing education are admirable and desirable, at present programs are falling far short of accomplishing the need which the pharmacist has to keep current in his field. It is the opinion of the author that the profession would be hard pressed to prove that participation in the current programs gives the pharmacist the right to practice and the lack of participation in the programs should deny him that right. The American Council on Pharmaceutical Education, on request of the profession, began in 1977 to certify providers of continuing pharmaceutical education in the US in an effort to assure quality programs.

The profession of medicine is met with the same problems. In 1967 President Johnson's National Advisory Commission on Health Manpower recommended that relicensure in medicine be based on continuing education. In 1974 Senator Edward Kennedy, health committee subcommittee chairman, tried unsuccessfully to institute federal licensure of physicians based on periodic examination. He still favors the concept and will push hard for it in any national health insurance plan, a spokesman says. There is also the possibility of enforcing continuing medical education by federal regulation, according to an officer of the Federation of State Medical Boards who states there are rumors that the federal health bureaucracy wants to set minimum competency standards that physicians would be required to meet in order to treat Medicare and Medicaid patients.[19]

Pharmacy may well see the handwriting on the wall for itself as it becomes more involved in government payment for the pharmacist's services.

The preparation for a lifetime of continuing education must begin while the student is in college. He must be given the responsibility while a student to learn the tools and techniques of self-education. Cartter[20] has underlined this need in his statement, "The standard commencement ceremony, with its invitation to lifelong self-education, has too often been an initiation ceremony for which the initiates have no real preparation."

The Professional Fee and Third-Party Payment—In the rapidly developing US there developed in its early history a type of pharmacy practice which was unique—and necessary. Sparse population made prescription pharmacies economically unfeasible. Merchandise became the economic backstop for the pharmacist. The relationship of this merchandise to health and drugs was sometimes real, sometimes not. Often the needs of the community determined the inventory. After all, the commercial outlets in frontier America were few. The American pharmacist has been loathe to give up the economic backstop of "up-front" merchandise. Just as he has too often spent an inordinate amount of his time with up-front things, so his orientation toward prescription drugs has been commodity-oriented. Prescriptions have been priced on the cost of the commodity. It is now recognized that he, unlike any other professional, has been selling "things" and giving away his most valuable property—his professional expertise on drugs. This expertise is in no way related to the price of the drug.

As the necessity in more populated areas for the merchandise-prescription dual-purpose store diminishes, this country has witnessed the advent of the supermarket drugstore, the cut-rate drugstore, and other mass merchandisers. The community pharmacist has lost ground in his attempts to compete successfully with these operations. He will probably continue to do so. His recourse is to a greater involvement in prescription practice and the professional promotion of expertise on drugs and de-emphasis of his product orientation. By emphasizing his professional function to the public and other members of the health team, he is on firm ground to charge a professional fee for prescriptions. This should be a common fee for all prescriptions regardless of cost to him. The products would be dispensed at cost plus a set professional fee determined on the basis of the cost of the operation of his pharmacy, including professional services rendered. The rationale of this practice is presented in an excellent article by Myers,[21] and in other articles by Myers.[22-25]

This country has seen only the beginning of health insurance plans which include prescriptions and the involvement of the state and federal government in this "third-party" payment trend for prescriptions and other health services. Whether private or public, these plans will continue to insist on getting prescriptions priced at the lowest possible denomination. The pharmacist in the future more than ever will need to justify his profits on prescriptions. His most legitimate recourse is his professional fee for professional services he renders. He will be forced to become service-oriented rather than product-oriented. This well may be the most effective catalyst to his functioning more effectively in the area for which he is best trained—professional service.

Pharmacy Technicians—It is possible that health manpower will be a critically short commodity in the future. Whether pharmacists will be in that category is yet to be proved. Yet, there is a segment of the profession which believes we must have technicians trained to help the pharmacist. Just what they will do is as yet not determined to the satisfaction of many people. However, everyone seems disturbed that his functions will neither be adequately defined nor contained. Some educators believe that colleges of pharmacy should train these technicians before community colleges preempt the privilege and pharmaceutical education has no control. Others believe that pharmaceutical education should have no part of the training. Some legalists and state boards of pharmacy believe that any technician produced should be licensed; others believe that to license would only give a foothold to prerogatives which would go beyond training.

This author can only advise that the community pharmacist's greatest need is to concentrate more on his professional functions and less on merchandising. In so doing he could make better use of his time and education. If he needs a technician he might consider training him to sell those items out front which don't need his expertise. He also might spend some time recruiting students for pharmaceutical education. The colleges are far from full of top-notch students!

The pharmaceutical profession might be advised to gain a lesson from nursing. It has three categories of registered nurses (associate, diploma, and baccalaureate)—all are RNs, and their problems have multiplied rather than diminished as a result of recognizing various levels of education. It will take generations to bring up the educational standards in nursing to where they should be.

Pharmaceutical education and pharmaceutical practice have been on the upward path for many years. The profession should be wary of vested interests who may wish to see pharmacy's future prostituted for selfish gain.

Women in Pharmacy—Forty years ago women in pharmacy were almost a curiosity. In 1959 10% of the students enrolled in first-degree programs in colleges of pharmacy were women. Ten years ago the percentage was 24%.[26] In 1982 the number was 47% of the total enrollment,[27] an unexpected increase in the number of women entering pharmacy. Dickson and Rodowskas did not predict such a percentage of enrollees (47.39%) until the year 2000.[28] A number of studies have been made regarding the role of women in pharmacy and the overall impact which this increase in numbers may have on the profession.[29–34]

Several factors need to be taken into consideration regarding the effect a greater percentage of women practitioners will have on the practice of pharmacy. Studies of the career patterns for professional women indicate they are frequently less productive than professional men in terms of full-time equivalent years of professional practice.[35] This is primarily because of their shorter professional career life due to their movement in and out of the active labor force according to the dictates of their family home life and home responsibilities.

Some have questioned whether women will choose to become owners and managers of retail stores. Will they choose to take active leadership roles in professional associations? Will they choose to remain part-time employees putting their family responsibilities foremost? Another question also arises as to whether women will be willing to work for less wages if they want only limited professional careers. Will this negatively affect the salary structure of all pharmacists? On the negative side of some of these questions one need only look at the low salaries of nurses and secretaries. On the positive side, women in hospital pharmacy have shown considerable leadership and professional activity with little variance in salary compared to men.

Future studies of the role of women in pharmacy may reveal answers to these unknown factors. But it is very clear that women will play an increasingly important role in pharmacy practice as their number increases. The Department of Health and Human Services reports that by the year 2000 there will be more than twice the number of women in actual pharmacy practice than there are today.[36]

The Future of Pharmacy and Professional Trends

I think a keynote for the function of pharmacy might be best expressed in the words of Surgeon General W. H. Stewart.[37] "We have more to offer than we are delivering. We have more people to serve than we are serving."

Bernzweig of the USPHS has placed the responsibility for the future of pharmacy in more direct terms.[38]

Apparently, the major affliction facing pharmacists . . . is a disease of near epidemic proportions, which might be labeled *professional inertia*. Its chief symptom is a general attitude of indifference to what is going on . . . unfortunately, too many community pharmacists today . . . just don't seem to care. This laissez-faire attitude poses a real danger, for unless these individuals begin to enlarge their horizons and strive for greater professional identity not only their *skills* but their *services* will soon become obsolete!

The increase in this country's population is a certainty. The shortage of personnel in many health professions is also a certainty. This shortage will be particularly critical in the medical profession. The health professions will need to find answers to the problem of treating those who are ill and advising those who are well. To do this, the health professionals will need to start talking to each other more often and more productively. There will need to be a realignment of responsibilities and a coordination of those responsibilities. The maximum use will need to be made of the education and experience of all in the health professions. Pharmacists should not let this challenge go unheeded.

It has been mentioned before in this chapter that the pharmacist will need to change his orientation from product to patient. The physician sees a patient as an organism of functioning and malfunctioning parts. The pharmacist should see the patient as a consumer of a multiplicity of drugs and respondent to those drugs. The pharmacist of the future must emerge as a consultant on drugs to the public. He must maintain current records of his patients which indicate the total regimen of drug consumption by the patient, both prescribed and nonprescribed drugs. The records must further indicate any untoward reactions of these patients to drugs and/or physical conditions which preclude the use of certain drugs. Such "patient profiles" are now required by some states.

The pharmacist of the future will need to take a more active role in health education of the public. He is the most accessible of all health professionals and is in the position of knowing most about the patient's general health problems, and even his economic status, which may have a direct bearing on his total health. His pharmacy can effectively serve as a distribution center for the free literature made available by a multiplicity of health agencies. The pharmacist can serve as an effective referral agent for patients in need of the services of county, state, and federal health units.

In case of disaster the pharmacist should be prepared in supplies and technical orientation to be an effective source of assistance in emergencies and recognize his responsibilities to organized disaster programs.

The pharmacist of the future should take a more active role in poison control programs. He should be the most readily accessible source of emergency information and be able to use organized poison control centers for the most efficient benefit of those in need of such services.

The pharmacist should take full advantage of his potential to be of assistance to nursing homes and other long-term care facilities so that they have the appropriate pharmaceutical services. His role in these facilities is discussed in Chapter 96.

These are some of the opportunities which await the community pharmacist in the immediate future. The opportunities for greater service open to hospital pharmacists are discussed in Chapter 95.

The Pharmacy and its Products

Personnel and Drug Statistics

The National Association of Boards of Pharmacy[39] estimates that there are 156,958 licensed pharmacy practitioners in the US. Of these, approximately 74% are in community practice, 19% in hospital pharmacy practice, and the rest in education, manufacturing, or other pursuits.

In this chapter primary concern has been with the community pharmacist. Community pharmacy viewed on a nationwide scale is big business. In 1982 pharmacists in US pharmacies dispensed 1.5 billion prescriptions.[40] The average retail price of a prescription rose 11.3% in 1982 over the 1981 figures ($10.34 in 1981 compared with $11.51 in 1982).[41] This amounted to total prescriptions sales of $9.9 billion.[42] The total sales of all merchandise and prescriptions in 1982 was $42.7 billion.[43]

Evolution and Trends

The American pharmacy has been a unique entity that developed out of a necessity for multipurpose community needs in a rapidly growing frontier country. Sparse population dictated low prescription volume necessitating income from merchandise which may or may not have been related to the expertise of the pharmacist. This "up-front" merchandise remains a necessary source of income for pharmacies with a prescription volume insufficient to support the pharmacy. In earlier days when shopping hours for all but "necessary" stores were limited both on a daily basis and on Sundays, pharmacies were the only merchandise stores open evenings and Sundays. This brought pressure on pharmacists to carry an extensive number of items which the public wished to have available at odd hours when other stores were closed. Pharmacists responded by expanding their lines of merchandise as a convenience for their customers, not without considerable profit to themselves.

If some modern pharmacists complain about the diverse products found in some pharmacies today and bemoan the exploitation of merchandising by many chain pharmacies, they have only to look to their predecessors in the profession for the mold out of which these commercial establishments have developed.

Of the total $42.7 billion in drugstore sales in 1982, the chains (four stores or more) account for 56%. The stores in the one-to-three store category account for 44% based on estimates of the National Association of Chain Drug Stores.[32] In 1982 chain stores had an average sales increase compared to 1981 of 10%. Other retail pharmacies had only a 3% increase in 1982.[44] Chains represent about 30% of the community pharmacies in the US, but as indicated above, they account for 56% of the volume of drugstore sales.[45]

In 1961 there were approximately 5,052 pharmacies belonging to chains and 49,000 classified as independents. Two decades later the chain units almost tripled to 14,000 while the independents dropped to 36,900.[46] Obviously, the trend is toward more chain stores which capture more of the retail market. This presents a challenge to pharmacists in independent pharmacies to provide services and counseling to their patients which they do not find in chain stores. Such accommodations as delivery at all hours and charge accounts are usually taken for granted. However, the greatest assets which the pharmacist should have are his acquaintance and caring for the patients whose prescriptions he dispenses and whose confidence he maintains on a personal basis as their authority on drugs. They should look upon him as their counselor of first resort on all health matters. It has been shown by a poll conducted by Louis Harris and Associates, Inc. that people are willing to pay for such counseling by the pharmacist.[47] They also pay by their continued patronage of a pharmacist who takes a personal and genuine interest in their well being. This appreciation for care and concern is seen most prominently in the elderly. The great increase in the number of elderly in future decades is well documented. The pharmacist in an independent setting not only has the greater opportunity to be of service to his patients, but he also will find it more personally rewarding as a career as shown by a survey of chain and independent pharmacists.[48]

Wherever the place of practice, the future of pharmacy practice portends to be a healthy and robust profession with a bright future for all who are part of it.

References

1. White AI. *Washington-Alaska Pharmacist 9:* 8, 1967.
2. *The Lilly Digest*, Lilly, Indianapolis, 1983.
3. Waldo DR, Gibson RM. National Health Expenditures 1981, *Health Care Financing Review 4:* 19, US Health Care Financing Administration, Washington, DC, 1982.
4. Hager GP. *J APhA NS5:* 72, 1965.
5. Gibson MR. *J APhA NS6:* 632, 1966.
6. *APhA Newsletter 7(12):* 1, 1968.
7. White EV. *J APhA NS5:* 532, 1965.
8. Deno RA., ed: *Proc Pharmacy-Medicine-Nursing Conf Health Educ*, U. of Michigan, 1967.
9. Gibson MR. *Am J Pharm Educ 36:* 189, 1972.
10. Teeling-Smith G. *J APhA NS6:* 22, 1966.
11. Griffenhagen GB. *The Pharmacy as a Health Center*, APhA, Washington, DC, 1964.
12. Cumming HS. *J APhA 17:* 325, 1928.
13. Goddard, JL. *J APhA NS6:* 358, 1966.
14. *Nursing Home Standards Guide*, USDHEW, Washington, DC, 1, 1961.
15. Bowers RA. *Am J Pharm Educ 23:* 4, 1959.
16. *Final Report*, AACP/APhA Task Force on Continuing Competence in Pharmacy, AACP/APhA, Washington, DC, 1, 1974.
17. *Ibid:* 13.
18. *Ibid:* 14.
19. Frederick L. *Med World News 18:* 51, 1977.
20. Cartter AM, in Lee CBT (ed): *Improving College Teaching*, Am. Council Educ., Washington, DC, 113, 1967.
21. Myers MJ. *Am J Pharm 140:* 101, 1968.
22. Myers MJ. *J APhA NS8:* 628, 1968.
23. *Ibid:* 632.
24. *Ibid:* 636.
25. *Ibid:* 639.
26. Orr JE. *Am J Phar Ed. 37:* 138, 1973.
27. Chasin SH. *ibid. 47:* 168, 1983.
28. Dickson WM, Rodowskas CA. *JAPhA 13:* 631, 1973.
29. Schwirian PM. *ibid.* 618, 1973.
30. Ginzberg E. *Am Phar NS21:* 22, 1981.
31. Pachin L, Dickson M. *Contemp Phar Pract 5:* 183, 1982.
32. Kirk KW, Shepherd MD. *Am Phar NS23:* 19, 1983.
33. Chi J. *Drug Topics 127:* 32, 1983.
34. Tash, RH, Dickson WM, Rodowskas CA. *JAPhA NS13:* 622, 1973.
35. *Ibid.*
36. Chi J. *loc cit.*
37. Stewart WH. *JAPhA NS7:* 366, 1967.
38. Bernzweig EP. *Bull Ontario Coll Pharm 17:* 61, 1968.
39. *1981 Census of Pharmacists*, NABP, Chicago, 1981.
40. Glaser M: *Drug Topics* (April 18): 34, 1983.
41. *Ibid.*
42. *Ibid.*
43. Glaser M, Chi J: *ibid.* (July 4): 2, 1983.
44. Cardinale V. *ibid.* (June 6): 42, 1983.
45. *Ibid.*
46. Mrtek RJ. *ibid.* (April 19): 124, 1982.
47. Smith DL. *Am Pharm 23:* 58, 1983.
48. Glaser M, Chi J. *loc. cit.*

CHAPTER 5

Pharmacists in Industry

Thomas Blake, RPh
Director, Regulatory Drug Affairs
Pharmaceutical Division, Ciba-Geigy Corporation
Summit, NJ 07901

The pharmacist's multidisciplinary scientific background, business training, and sense of accuracy and control make him uniquely qualified to serve in the pharmaceutical industry. No matter where he may be located in the corporate structure, the pharmacist often calls on his training in the health sciences in order to render judgments that will ensure the safety and well-being of the people for whom his company's products are intended. By virtue of his training in many scientific disciplines, he can work very effectively within an organization encompassing a broad range of specialties. In short, the pharmaceutical scientist is inherently capable of understanding the facets of a complex health-related industry and of filling the many roles that exist therein . . . roles that are far more numerous and of greater importance than generally realized.

Profile of the Industry

A prescription pharmaceutical company, as well as its close relatives, proprietary drugs and toiletries companies, is a complex operation. Under its roof come together for common purpose a team of scientists and technicians representing virtually all of the sciences. Further contributions to the corporate effort are made by management executives, lawyers, accountants, engineers, systems analysts, writers, salesmen, and many others whose skills and talents maintain the viability of this unique business enterprise.

Why is the pharmaceutical industry different or unique? Many reasons, but five in particular.

Product Categories—The products of the pharmaceutical industry, more than those of any other major industry, can intimately affect the lives, health, welfare, and happiness of humans. The extent to which this is so is reflected in the *Physicians' Desk Reference*. The Product Classification Index of this volume contains 151 different therapeutic categories ranging from Allergens and Antibiotics to Vitamins and X-Ray Contrast Media. Under the Generic and Chemical Name Index are listed more than 1200 separate and different drugs.

Scientific Disciplines—The pharmaceutical industry depends for its existence on scientists, including pharmacists, who encompass a tremendous breadth of science and technology. Some of the various scientific disciplines and functions required include: chemistry, for quality control and the synthesis and processing of essential ingredients; pharmacology and toxicology, for drug screening and safety testing; biochemistry, for tracing drug metabolism and absorption; physical pharmacy, for pharmaceutical research and process development; information science, for technical documentation and support; medicine, for clinical testing; and biostatistics, for accurate scientific evaluation.

Among the scientists involved in these various activities the pharmacist is unusual; his training touches on many of these sciences and functions, and this extensive background, with and without additional training in pharmacy or other specialties, gives him broad career opportunities in the industry. Two specific examples are Science Information/Regulatory Affairs and Pharmaceutical Research and Development, areas wherein the pharmacist's broad academic training often is extremely valuable because it spans across the safety and efficacy of drugs, and their synthesis, formulation, manufacture, analysis, and testing.

Quality Regulation—The operations of the pharmaceutical industry are under the constant scrutiny of various federal and state agencies, each of which has its own set of regulations to be adhered to. These regulations, coupled with the industry's own sense of responsibility, result in manufacturing operations conducted at the highest level of quality. This, in turn, leads to career opportunities for those scientists charged with maintaining this level of quality.

At each step from their inception to their clinical disposition, prescription and other drugs are covered by government rules, regulations, and guidelines. There are regulations governing the way animal studies are performed and recorded (Good Laboratory Practices) and regulations that set standards for clinical testing (Good Clinical Practices). Government approval to market new drugs requires manufacturers to submit Investigational New Drug Applications and New Drug Applications. The manner in which drugs are processed is likewise controlled (Current Good Manufacturing Practices), with guidelines specified for such things as isolation of production equipment, sampling and quality assurance, sterility validation, permissible tolerances, standards of purity, inventory control, and packaging and labeling. Special methods of record keeping as well as production quotas are applied to those drugs, "Controlled Substances," capable of being abused.

The manufacturers of proprietary drugs and toiletries (often called over-the-counter or OTC products) also develop products to high standards and comply with regulations covering their making and marketing. True, proprietary manufacturers do not often synthesize brand-new drug substances and they, therefore, usually do not engage in the chemical research or biological screening associated with new drug entities. Nevertheless, the proprietary side of the industry does carry on extensive and important research in such areas as pharmacokinetics, drug delivery systems, pharmacology, and toxicology, some of which leads to innovations requiring New Drug Applications.

Proprietary manufacturers also do in-depth studies on the actions of dermatologicals and toiletries. These programs are designed to develop new products, to evaluate their effectiveness, to establish their safety, and to provide scientific support for their label claims.

Obviously, then, the fact that a drug or toiletry preparation is available without a prescription in no way exempts it from rigorous testing before it is released to the consumer. Detailed monographs covering the safety, efficacy, and testing of all proprietary medicines in this country are, or soon will be, available as a result of a comprehensive program of evaluation carried out by industry and the Food and Drug Administration.

Clearly, in the regulatory milieu surrounding the pharmaceutical industry, company decisions affecting both prescription and proprietary preparations are thoroughly checked and checked again. And just as clearly, the scientific efforts required to comply with the various sets of regulations are crucial elements of drug company operations carried out by pharmaceutically trained scientists and other personnel.

Research and Development—Research and Development contribute to the uniqueness of the pharmaceutical industry. R&D takes place, of course, in other industries; but in the prescription drug industry and, to a large extent, in the proprietary and toiletry industries, R&D is the birthplace of virtually all new products and a goodly number of innovations.

The course a potential prescription or proprietary product must take from inception to consumer is arduous and, from an investment viewpoint, often risky. For each newly discovered compound a very reliable method of synthesis and extraction must be worked out, standards of purity defined, and techniques devised to determine the short- and long-term fate of the substance and its metabolites in biological systems. Extensive animal testing profiles the toxicity of the drug and reveals through sophisticated screening techniques its gross pharmacological effects. Pharmaceutical development scientists must design dosage forms that are compatible with both the chemistry of the compound and the biological target site(s) and that also deliver, usually within a specific time, the proper dose of the drug. Stability testing establishes the shelf life of the product and detects changes in formulation during storage. Reliable and efficient methods of manufacturing the drug are developed. Rigorous control measures, themselves the result of specialized investigations, are applied to the process and to the product, ensuring that specifications for the finished drug lie within well-defined limits.

The crucial determinant of a drug's safety and effectiveness is its performance in carefully conducted clinical studies, which proceed after the compound's animal toxicity has been established and suitable protocols for tests in humans have been developed. Clinical studies can cover one or more phases, depending upon how much data already exist as to the drug's safety and efficacy in humans.

R&D expenditures further contribute to the uniqueness of the pharmaceutical industry. Because of the very nature of the product, the R&D effort in pharmaceuticals generally accounts for a much larger share of the corporate dollar than does R&D in other businesses. Of the 1976 dollar spent on ethical pharmaceutical R&D by the (then) 127 member firms of the Pharmaceutical Manufacturers Association (PMA), 68 cents went to basic and applied research for the advancement of scientific knowledge and the development of new products and related services, 17 cents was spent on modifying and improving existing products, and 15 cents was used for international R&D.

These firms made a significant R&D investment—nearly 44% of their US pharmaceutical R&D money—on such important functions as process development; dosage formulation and stability testing; animal toxicology; and bioavailability studies. The remainder of their R&D money spent in this country went to clinical evaluation (20%), biological screening and testing (19%), and synthesis and extraction (17%).

The commitment by the pharmaceutical industry to the search for new and better prescription and proprietary medicines and toiletries thus is significant by whatever measure applied, especially considering that less than 1% of money spent for the endeavor is government provided; nearly all funding for the industry's research activities is from the profits generated by sales of existing products.

Statistical Data—Size and diversity are other interesting characteristics of the industry. There are literally thousands of pharmaceutical establishments, all registered with the FDA. However, the *Physicians' Desk Reference* lists 242 firms and the *Over-the-Counter Review List* consists of 62. Thus, there are about 300 major pharmaceutical companies. Some develop and manufacture a diversity of products covering many treatment areas; others specialize in limited therapeutic areas, such as dermatological or ophthalmic preparations.

In terms of the number of employees, the pharmaceutical industry, while not a giant, certainly is of a respectable size. Total domestic employment by the industry—ethical and proprietary—is more than 200,000. A significant percentage are R&D scientists and engineers with at least a four-year college education in their respective fields. Recent data from PMA member firms show that of all their R&D personnel, 20% hold doctoral degrees, 10% have masters and 21% have bachelors. The remainder are technicians and assistants with specialized training.

There are more than 4400 licensed pharmacists employed in the industry. With respect to total time devoted to careers, their principal activities are, in declining order: detailing, managerial functions, research, and development, and processing functions.

The final lines in this Profile of the Industry are perhaps best drawn in a textbook edited by C M Lindsay:

We have not been poorly served by the pharmaceutical industry during the century of its existence—even during the lengthy period when little regulation or supervision by government was practiced. The industry has provided us with a host of drugs which have revolutionized the practice of medicine, and it has provided them at prices that have steadily declined relative to the consumer price index. Although profits have been substantial, for the most part they have been reinvested in research and development making possible a future even freer of disease then the present. Legislation and regulation in this area must proceed with an eye ever-fixed on the potential impact of new policy on that future as well.

Education of Industrial Pharmacists

As of 1978, most (about 80%) of the pharmacists in industry held the four-year baccalaureate degree, the reason being that these individuals matriculated and entered industry prior to the establishment of five- and six-year degrees in pharmacy. More than 1 of every 6 (16.1%) *registered* pharmacists, and, most likely, at least 1 of every 3 of the total number of pharmacists employed in industry, is the possessor of a pharmacy

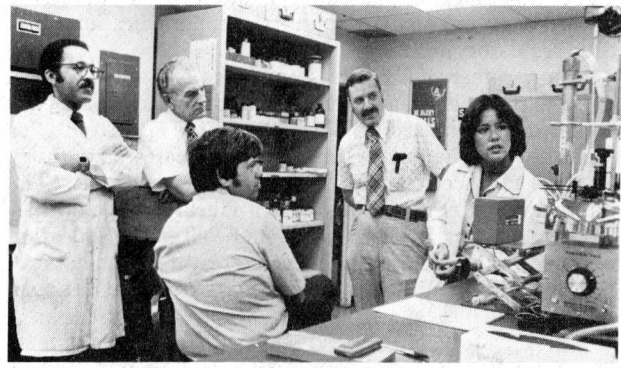

Fig 5-1. The broad-based scientific training of the pharmacist qualifies him to choose a career from among many areas in the pharmaceutical industry. Here, pharmacists from Quality Assurance, Product Development, and Physical Testing discuss a complex stability problem (courtesy, Vick Divisions Research and Development).

degree above the baccalaureate level. Most of the graduate pharmacy degrees are in pharmaceutics, pharmaceutical (medicinal) chemistry, pharmacology, and pharmacy administration. A significant number hold advanced degrees in other areas, such as the MBA.

The student interested in a career in the pharmaceutical industry is fortunate in that many schools of pharmacy in this country offer courses at the undergraduate and graduate levels in the principles of industrial pharmacy.

Undergraduate academic instruction in industrial pharmacy can include such topics as application of pharmaceutics, pharmacokinetics, and bioavailability; preformulation testing; formulation of solid, liquid, semisolid and other dosage forms, and stability testing; principles of processing, such as tableting, encapsulating, filling, molding, and sterile technique; principles of quality control; and key regulatory aspects of the industry, including New Drug Regulations and Current Good Manufacturing Practices. In some schools, students can acquire hands-on experience in manufacturing facilities operated by the school itself, during which time they actually develop and manufacture a range of preparations, including some sterile products, for patients in state and other institutions.

Those students contemplating industrial careers more oriented to the business side of the operation will benefit from such undergraduate courses as drug information, economics, commercial law, business administration, advertising and marketing, and accounting. Some pharmacy schools offer undergraduate programs leading to combined degrees in pharmacy and business and many business-oriented pharmacy graduates obtain MBA training.

Many pharmacy students are offered the benefits of industrial on-site training programs prior to graduation. An example of one such program is the Pharmaceutical Industry Summer Internship Program sponsored by the Student American Pharmaceutical Association and the National Pharmaceutical Council. It permits selected fourth-year pharmacy students to spend that summer employed as interns (actually externs) by participating pharmaceutical companies. The student rotates through several divisions of a company. Though specific assignments vary among companies, most expose the student to applied research, formulation, quality control, manufacturing, marketing, and regulatory affairs.

Postgraduate study for those interested in industry encompasses the more specialized activities of pharmaceutical and related industries. Opportunities for such graduate study are numerous. Courses available center on the various areas of basic pharmaceutics; medicinal chemistry; biological courses such as biochemistry, pharmacology, and drug metabolism and detoxification; pharmaceutical manufacturing and engineering; pharmaceutical marketing (including drug advertising); research and industrial communications; and drug regulatory affairs.

In any career, but more especially in one founded on a multidisciplined science such as pharmacy, advanced education and specialized training enhance the opportunity for success. The pharmacist contemplating a career in industry can take advanced courses on a full- or part-time basis. The pharmacist in industry obtains such education from on-the-job training, and from extension and continuing education courses given by many academic and private organizations. He can also take advanced university courses on a part-time or sabbatical basis.

Opportunities for Pharmacists in Industry

Research and Development

The quest by industry for new and better medicines is a team effort wherein Research and Development brings together a diversity of scientific talents directed toward the

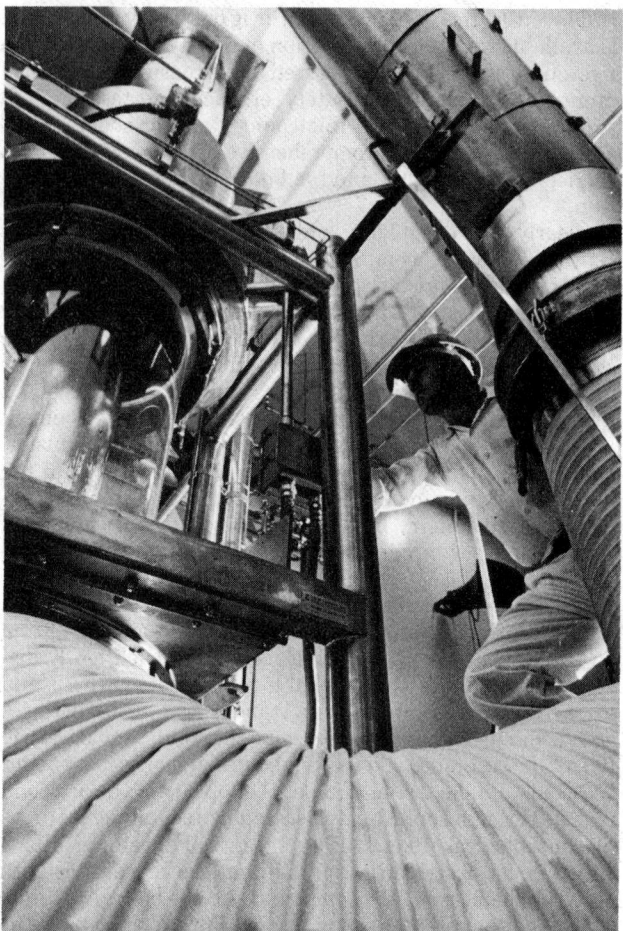

Fig 5-2. Pharmacists in Process Improvement work closely with Production and Product Development to streamline methods used to manufacture pharmaceuticals, as is the case here with column film-coating of tablets (courtesy, Merck Sharp & Dohme).

achievement of therapeutic goals. (Some companies have one staff for Research, another for Development; others have a single staff to handle both functions.)

At the research level, investigations are undertaken that may result in the discovery and understanding of new active ingredients, the development of a drug delivery mechanism, or a basic innovation in an OTC drug or toiletry system.

Development, in turn, has as its purpose the creation, from Research's discoveries as well as Development's own innovations, of dosage forms and other drug and toiletry formulations that are bioavailable, stable, and esthetic and that can be manufactured reproducibly on a large scale to high standards. Those in Development also utilize new technology to improve existing preparations.

Further, the overall data generated in R&D, along with data from the biological and clinical testing areas, provide the extensive documentation that supports the safety, effectiveness, and reliability of pharmaceutical preparations.

In all these areas of R&D can be found scientists who originated their undergraduate academic training in pharmaceutical sciences, with many going on to further specialize in pharmacy and other disciplines. Their pharmaceutical training allowed them to gain a broad and substantial background at the undergraduate level and this, in turn, permitted them a choice of many interesting specialties at the graduate level.

In research, for instance, those who were attracted to medicinal chemistry can be found synthesizing new drug entities, then perfecting the means for purifying the compounds.

Similarly, pharmacy students with an interest in biochemistry are among the biological scientists working at the interface between chemistry and biology to discover valuable naturally occurring agents and to elucidate their roles in biological processes—prostaglandins in inflammation, for example.

The pharmaceutical curriculum has spawned other specialists in industry: microbiologists and immunologists involved in vaccine research; pharmacologists and toxicologists conducting initial drug screening and safety testing in animals; analytical chemists devising the means for characterizing new substances; pharmacokineticists tracing the route of the drug and its metabolites through biological systems; and pharmaceutical scientists investigating drug delivery systems.

R&D scientists with pharmaceutical training also play important roles in designing, developing, and evaluating over-the-counter products by delving into systems affecting absorption, biotransformation, and target-site activity of drug and cosmetic ingredients.

In the development area, the pharmaceutical scientist is called on to develop esthetic and stable formulations, with associated manufacturing procedures, that will effectively deliver drug and toiletry ingredients. In so doing he must often solve problems of stability, taste, odor and appearance, preservation, bioavailability, and manufacturability. Such formulations include regular tablets, capsules, and syrups and suspensions for oral use; sustained release and other special drug delivery systems and devices; ampuls, multidose vials, and intravenous solutions for parenteral administration; suppositories, creams, and douches for rectal and vaginal treatment; dermatological creams, ointments, gels, lotions and aerosols; ophthalmic, otic, and nasal preparations; and variants of many of these.

Pharmacists at all degree levels, along with nonpharmacists, participate in Development and they find that development of a formulation and manufacturing procedure requires the application of broad, multidisciplinary knowledge and experience. Information is used from almost all the undergraduate and graduate courses in the pharmacy curriculum to meet the challenges of product development. As examples, inorganic and organic chemistry techniques are used to remove bitter impurities, to optimize absorptivity, and to improve the stability of drugs; other techniques from physical pharmacy are used to develop improved dispersion, compression, and in-process control procedures in manufacturing.

Throughout the development stage emphasis is on discovering and correcting problems in all the areas mentioned above before the dosage form is exposed to wide use. The development process is applied to new pharmaceuticals and also to provide improvements in existing products and manufacturing methods. Development further is an important function in cosmetics and proprietary medicines since the design of the formulation can have a vital effect on the absorption and activity of both drug and cosmetic, and on their acceptance by consumers.

Expressed broadly, responsibilities of pharmaceutical scientists and others in Development include:

1. Establishment of those physiochemical properties of drug substances and dosage forms that will influence potency, uniformity, stability, and bioavailability.
2. Preparation of Clinical Materials for the study of safety and effectiveness (see separate section following).
3. Development of the final formulations and full-scale manufacturing processes and controls for all products, regardless of the route of administration.
4. Improvement of existing preparations and processes from the standpoint of absorption, activity, and safety; cost or product elegance; and quality.
5. Scientific investigation of product stability, including the making of recommendations for storage conditions and setting of expiration dates for old and new products.
6. Evaluation of new raw materials and their specifications—colors, flavors, excipients, solvents, preservatives, etc—with respect to potential value in pharmaceutical and toiletry formulations.

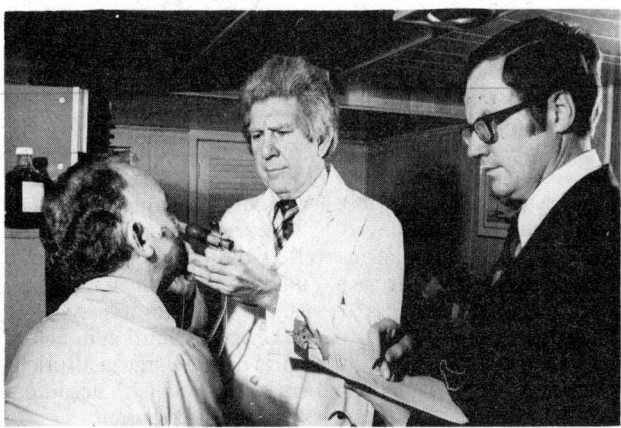

Fig 5-3. Industry pharmacists who are Clinical Research Associates monitor studies in progress. Here, a pharmacist monitors the protocol of a clinical investigation designed to measure nasal airway resistance before and after the administration of a proprietary colds preparation by a clinical investigator (courtesy, Vick Divisions Research and Development).

7. Scientific evaluation of new equipment and new or improved processes, and the determination of their effect on product quality prior to routine use in pharmaceutical production.
8. Investigation into the suitability and possible improvement of proposed packaging materials and containers.
9. Development of information from the foregoing for submission to the FDA and other regulatory agencies.

Some further examples of the projects developmental pharmacists might be called on to undertake are: to develop an oral-route drug release system that corrects variations in blood drug levels due to erratic gastric absorption; to overcome bitterness or burning sensations produced by some drugs; to eliminate leaching of a potentially harmful packaging resin into the product; to protect a hydrolytically sensitive drug from degradation; to insure the sterility of a parenteral solution too sensitive to be heated; to establish the uniform flow and dosage of powdered ingredients with high static charge into encapsulating machinery; to adapt improved production equipment to existing formulas, or vice-versa; and a great deal more.

Without the proper degree of pharmaceutical development, important prescription and proprietary drugs of today— antimetabolites, hormones, analgesics, anti-inflammatories, antibiotics, dermatologicals, and many others—would have encountered significant problems and delays in becoming as reliably available and acceptable as they now are to the millions who need them.

The *Clinical Materials Section*, usually a part of the Pharmaceutical Development Group, provides the formulations for clinical trials and often for animal studies as well. In some companies the Clinical Materials Section is responsible for the manufacture of products to undergo clinical testing; in others, this is done by the Pharmaceutical Development Group. Almost all companies, however, assign to the Clinical Materials Section these responsibilities: confirming from the quality control data that the batch meets called-for specifications; inventorying and controlling the distribution of test material; shipping the material to the clinical investigators; and receiving and inspecting any test material returned from the site of the trial.

Within the Clinical Materials Section the clinical materials pharmacist plays a key role. It is a role that fits closely with pharmacy's tradition as the dispenser of medication. The clinical materials pharmacist must properly understand the projected use of the test drug, control its dispensing (distribution to clinical testing sites), keep orderly records, and closely control its inventory and storage. If, in addition, the clinical materials pharmacist is responsible for the preparation of clinical supplies, then he must make use of his training in compounding, formulation, manufacturing techniques, proper packaging, and related scientific principles.

The clinical materials pharmacist does not, as a rule, need a graduate degree. He must be a good coordinator because he is often the link between Product Development and Clinical Testing. Thus, he does need a solid grasp of the methods and techniques employed in the preparation and quality control of the materials as well as those used in the actual clinical testing of drugs. Finally, the clinical materials pharmacist will find his job easier to perform if he has had some experience with systems of drug distribution in health care facilities; clinical testing often is done in large institutions and can involve sizable numbers of subjects with accompanying problems in the logistics of drug distribution.

Analytical Research and Quality Control and Assurance

Historically, Analytical Research and Quality Control and Assurance evolved out of the necessity to monitor and control the various phases involved in the production of quality pharmaceuticals. These controls included: tests for the identity and purity of the active and inactive agents; in-process analyses to ensure proper production procedures; analysis of the final product to guarantee that it met all specifications; and inspection of the container labeling and other packaging material for accuracy and adherence to specifications.

The Analytical Research Department has classically developed the techniques needed to assay the ingredients and the finished product, and to determine its stability. Quality Control and Assurance samples in-process materials, packaging materials, and the final product, and then analyzes the final product and all its associated components. In the late 60s and early 70s Analytical Research and Quality Control and Assurance began to take on added responsibilities. With increasing frequency, methods for measuring drugs and metabolites in biological fluids are being developed by Analytical Research. Quality Control and Assurance has added the goal of assuring that the operational procedures in the manufacture of pharmaceuticals, as well as the components of a product, meet good manufacturing specifications and that they also provide built-in deterrents to manufacturing quality problems such as contamination, mix-up, and excessive variation.

The Analytical Research Group is generally responsible for these important functions:

1. Developing methods for the analysis of raw materials, chemical intermediates, and active and other ingredients of the product. Often this must be accomplished in the presence of other interfering ingredients, necessitating the design of special techniques to remove or avoid them. Today's analytical researcher must devise techniques that will specifically measure complex and potent active molecules, sometimes at the microgram (10^{-6} g) level in a finished formulation, or in the case of impurities, down to the nanogram (10^{-9} g) and picogram (10^{-12} g) levels.

2. Development of analytical methods to determine stability, including finding out how the active components degrade, identifying and measuring degradation products, and selectively analyzing for the amount of intact, active species remaining over time after storage at ambient and accelerated conditions.

3. Development of methods to identify and quantify the presence and the metabolism of drugs in biological systems. Projects in this area have grown with the increasing interest in pharmacokinetics and the growing emphasis on bioavailability. The analyst is confronted with the challenge of detecting often minute amounts of drug and its metabolites among the many interfering agents and confounding variables that can exist in biological fluids.

To aid in doing these important and difficult projects, the analytical researcher must receive training in, and utilize, sensitive analytical techniques such as mass spectroscopy, X-ray crystallography, high-pressure and other advances in plate, gas, and liquid chromatography, and electron microscopy.

In this new era of intensified emphasis on *Quality Control and Assurance*, those involved in this area are attempting to approach the state of "zero" defects in all key aspects of pharmaceutical operations. To do this they concentrate on identifying potential production problems before they occur; they seek to assure high quality operations on an ongoing basis; and they work to improve the techniques designed to reveal whether the finished product conforms to all specifications and to FDA and Industry Good Manufacturing Practices.

In some companies the two functions, Control and Assurance, are separate. But whether separate or combined, the major responsibilities include:

1. Inspection, analysis, and approval of raw materials and processing intermediates, and of all final products manufactured for biological and clinical testing and for commercial sale. Quality control chemists utilize methods often developed by the Analytical Research Group and, where needed, these chemists adapt the methods for higher speed repetitive use.

2. Checking for freedom from microbiological contamination in nonsterile products, and testing for sterility in all sterile products.

3. Examining and approving packages, including monitoring of the product run to prevent mix-ups in labels, lot numbers, and products.

4. Developing procedures and checks to assure adherence to Good Manufacturing Practices (and now Good Laboratory Practices) in all key areas of plant operations, such as proper storage of raw materials, synthesis of drugs, preparation of biological and clinical test supplies, maintenance of laboratory animals and proper research records in all laboratories, manufacture of final products, maintaining careful inventory control, and much more.

The recent expansions in the functions and importance of Analytical Research and Quality Control and Assurance have greatly increased the responsibilities of those working in this area and also have meant many more career opportunities in the industry.

Pharmaceutical Production

Pharmacists make excellent candidates for positions of responsibility in Pharmaceutical Production because their technical training in the preparation of drugs is highly relevant to the production process, as is their penchant for accuracy and their strong sense of responsibility concerning the handling of drugs. The pharmaceutical scientist in production may have responsibilities in planning, equipment evaluation, processing operations, packaging, and inventory control.

The production process begins with the Production Planning Group, whose members often include pharmacists. This group determines if the plant has the necessary staff and equipment to manufacture the quantity of product requested by Marketing. If so, the group then arranges to establish production schedules and coordinate the production run with other departments involved, such as Synthesis, Pharmaceutical Research and Development, Sales, Purchasing, Quality Control, Shipping and Receiving, and Engineering. Only then can the actual processing of the product begin.

Most pharmaceutical production facilities are divided into functional areas corresponding to the various dosage forms. Since each dosage form requires specialized production equipment and techniques, there may be separate areas of production for tablets, capsules, liquids, ointments, parenterals, etc.

In each of these areas drugs are manufactured in stages wherein specific operations are performed—weighing, mixing, granulating, tableting, sterilization, homogenization, and packaging. Certain operations, in turn, are specialized in themselves, requiring their own physical operations, equipment, support personnel, and level of expertise.

Essentially, the basic steps in the manufacture of most dosage forms consist of assuring the availability of proper compounding and packaging equipment, gathering and carefully weighing or metering raw materials, processing them by various means, forming these into a finished preparation, and packaging and labeling the product and getting it into cartons.

As an example of specialized dosage form procedures, consider tablets.

- Ingredients that have been cleared by Quality Control are stored and subsequently weighed in a location segregated for that purpose to eliminate the possibility of contamination.
- From there, components are blended. The type of blender used is determined by such factors as batch size and whether the contents are wet or dry, uniform or heterogeneous. The mixture may then be granulated to the desired particle size by the accepted wet or dry methods. In some instances newer techniques permit direct compression without granulating.
- After another inspection and release by Quality Control, the material is fed into tablet presses which are capable of speeds up to 1000s of tablets per minute. They can turn out homogeneous tablets, two- or three-layer tablets, and compression-coated tablets, as well as tablets in special shapes and sizes from the delicate ones to the large bolus sizes for livestock.
- Tablets must be checked frequently for potency and controlled for such factors as hardness, thickness, and weight; also, the machines must be kept adjusted to narrow tolerances. Other important in-process test parameters might include friability, rate of dissolution, and moisture content. Coating of tablets primarily is by fluid-bed or pan coating.
- On the packaging line, tablets cleared by Quality Control are counted mechanically or electronically as they go into waiting containers, and labels verified. Far from being a purely routine function, the packaging operation requires total accountability of all components used in the process. A shortage or overage of tablets or labels or containers can signal a potential problem in Good Manufacturing Practices. A final quality control evaluation is made before the product is released for storage and shipment.

Many in-process controls exist in pharmaceutical production to assure the integrity and uniformity of the final product. Examples include inspection of tablets and capsules for integrity and proper size; checks for freedom from particulate matter—essential for parenterals; and control of particle size and rheology of emulsions and dispersions. Other controls are applied across most levels of production, regardless of dosage form. At the end of the run all production materials must be properly accounted for before a product lot can be released.

The manufacture of "Controlled Substances" requires its own particular controls—special records, restricted access to production areas, and, in some instances, adherence to production quotas established by the government.

In addition, quality assurance personnel independently monitor production and see to it that quality control procedures are carried out properly. These quality assurance people also examine the interface of production with other functions to avert quality control problems. Their many responsibilities include determining whether shipping and storage are carried out with the required level of attention to such factors as temperature and humidity; monitoring plant environment (dust, solvents, hazardous wastes); and checking that sampling procedures are reliable and used appropriately. The numerous quality assurance procedures in pharmaceutical production—from creation of the drug to its final disposition—thus are subject to constant checking so that any discrepancies will be discovered in time to permit corrective action.

A Process Development Group, allied closely with Product Development, is responsible for improving the mechanics of the production line so as to reduce costs, or improve product quality, or, hopefully, both. By adjusting formulas, revising methods, and adapting equipment, workers in process development improve the operation and solve production problems.

Scientific Information and Regulatory Affairs

Some pharmacists in industry, especially, perhaps, those with a literary and regulatory bent, find satisfying careers in Scientific Information and Regulatory Affairs. *Scientific Information Specialists* are individuals skilled in literature search and information organization. They work to supply the various scientific disciplines in the company with scientific information of both general and specific interest. In some companies these specialists also evaluate the relevance of the information before sending it on; they also may be the central source for all information a company develops about the chemistry, safety, efficacy, and other properties of its products. Such information ultimately finds its way into package inserts, promotional material, FDA submissions, and elsewhere.

The specialists in *Regulatory Affairs* monitor new regulations and regulatory information for the company and obtain and write up the scientific information that must be submitted to various regulatory bodies such as the Food and Drug Administration, Environmental Protection Agency, and The Consumer Product Safety Commission. They also may serve as liaison between the company and these agencies. Obviously, these individuals must work closely with all the scientific disciplines represented in the company, as well as with the Legal Department.

In some companies Scientific Information and Regulatory Affairs are combined into one department; in others, they are separate. But either way, some pharmacists find these functions particularly attractive because both the information and regulatory areas require people who have broad scientific training and who can integrate and apply their knowledge to pharmaceutical and related problems. Thus, here is another place in industry where the pharmacist can capitalize on his training as a scientific generalist. Almost the entire spectrum of pharmaceutical education is utilized since the modern scientific literature and regulatory aspects in industry span many scientific areas.

Other Opportunities

Clinical/Medical Testing—Once a drug has passed appropriate tests in animals it moves on to Clinical Testing, the extent of which is determined by the amount of data already at hand as to the drug's safety and efficacy in humans. The various types of Clinical Testing are:

1. *Clinical Pharmacology*—evaluates the pharmacological actions of the compound in humans, preferred route of administration, and safe dosage range.
2. *Exaggerated Use*—therapeutic and side effects at high dose levels or dose frequencies.
3. *Broad Clinical Trials*—safety and effectiveness in managing the target disease or conditions.
4. *Postmarketing*—for some potent or complex new drugs there are postmarketing trials which accumulate experience from the clinical use of the drug in broad populations.

Physicians, dentists, and other personnel in the Medical Department oversee Clinical Testing. They design appropriate experimental protocols; select qualified clinical investigators; monitor studies in progress; coordinate activities with institutional review committees; collect and interpret test data; and, along with representatives from other areas in R&D and Management, decide on sending a drug to market. They also provide considerable input to drug labeling: package inserts in the case of prescription items and label claims and cautions for proprietary medicines. Postmarketing drug surveillance and investigations of reports of adverse drug reactions likewise fall within the purview of the Medical Department.

While the physicians and dentists in the Medical Department are directly responsible for the design, execution, and evaluation of clinical studies, they are aided in this endeavor by clinical research associates. The clinical research associate, who is a scientist but not a physician, has a proficiency in human pharmacology and toxicology, along with a thorough knowledge of relevant FDA regulations, a good grounding in statistics, and skill in clinical study design. The clinical re-

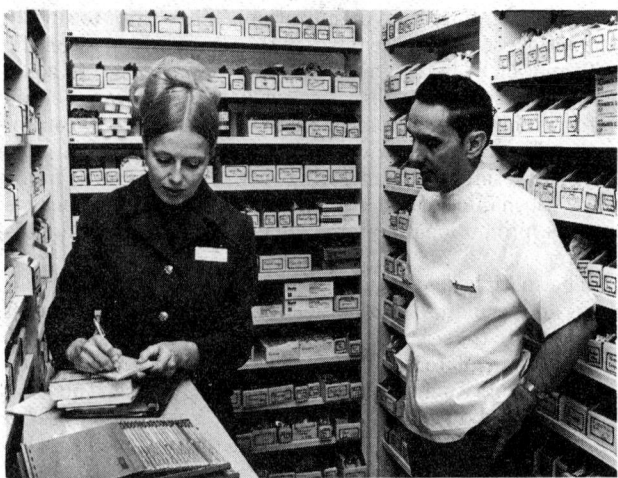

Fig 5-4.   Pharmacists who serve as professional sales representatives communicate accurate and comprehensive product information to health-care professionals.   Such "detailing" insures that products are used with full understanding by those who prescribe and dispense them (courtesy, Merck Sharp & Dohme).

search associate helps the staff physician in charge of the project to develop a clinical protocol that contains the fine details of how the evaluation of the drug in humans shall proceed.   These details include the nature of the drugs and the dosages to be studied; the type of subjects who are or are not suitable for the trials; clinical, chemical, and other tests to be run; records to be kept; duration of the study; etc.   The clinical associate will then often visit the test site with the physician to thoroughly review details of the protocol with the clinical investigator and his staff.   The clinical associate returns to the clinical site during the course of the study to monitor the progress of the trials and assure that procedures and records are in proper order.

The position carries many responsibilities and those clinical associates with pharmaceutical training find, with added training and experience in the area, that their pharmaceutical background has given them a broad and thorough appreciation of pharmacology, toxicology, and drug biotransformation, interaction, and administration—all important in clinical trials of new drugs.   For those who have had clinical pharmacy training, their knowledge of clinical testing, clinical chemistry, clinical study design, patient handling, and institutional routine is especially useful.

Other Medical Areas—Pharmacists with additional medical training and experience also hold important positions within *Medical Promotion*, *Medical Services*, and *Medical Information Departments*.   These departments usually are involved in communicating the results of clinical testing to individual physicians, to various clinics and institutions, and to medical seminars, journals, etc.   Personnel in these departments also aid such groups in utilizing drugs to their best advantage.   Pharmaceutical and clinical pharmacy training provide good backgrounds for all these positions.

Aside from the physician, the pharmacist has possibly the broadest perspective about the mode of action and interaction of drugs, the target diseases, the patients, and the details of biological and clinical testing.   The need for scientists such as pharmacists to fulfill these important staff responsibilities in clinical areas has been growing, both in industry and in government.

Biostatistics—Biostatistics, a specialty that attracts some pharmacists, is an integral part of both research and clinical testing.   The biostatistician is especially valuable in the pharmaceutical industry because in the scientific studies of today's prescription and proprietary drugs the findings must not only be medically and biologically sound, they must be reproducible and mathematically reliable; in short, any differences claimed in drug activities must stand the test of statistical validity.

In research studies as well as in clinical testing the biostatistician applies his expertise whenever data are generated, in order to determine whether the results are meaningful.   This specialist also helps design the research study or clinical trial so that it can have an optimum chance of achieving its objectives.

The pharmacist who wishes to enter the field of biostatistics has a head start by virtue of his broad scientific training.   However, he will need for career satisfaction in this specialty training in those areas of particular applicability to biostatistics.   They include: design of experimentation; multivariate analysis of variance; categorical data analysis; theory of probability; statistical methods of bioassay; sampling techniques; nonparametric statistics; life tables; and computer programming.

Sales and Marketing—Most pharmaceutical companies employ professional representatives who represent the company and its products to physicians, dentists, pharmacists, and other health care personnel.   The pharmaceutical *sales representative* must be able to sell a product professionally; that is, by presenting the product's good features and its adverse effects in fair balance so that the physician or dentist knows when to use it and when not to; how to administer it for maximal benefit; what clinical signs to look for to confirm benefits or to detect adverse effects; and how to handle the adverse effects if they occur.   The many pharmaceutical sales personnel who perform in this manner find that physicians and dentists welcome their visits and consider the information thereby received to be a useful resource in the operation of their practices.   Pharmaceutical sales personnel also present product information and conduct seminars before groups in hospitals, at professional meetings, and elsewhere.

The product lines of many companies span across a wide range of drugs; broad scientific knowledge thus is required if the professional representative is to understand such a wide range of information and effectively communicate it to health care professionals.   The pharmacist's training accordingly serves as an excellent foundation for this important position within the industry.

In a pharmaceutical company *marketing* encompasses advertising and promotion, marketing research, professional services, product distribution, and marketing itself.   Those who specialize in pharmaceutical marketing must understand not only the technical aspects of the product and how it should be sold to the health profession, they also must know how to operate a business so that it is profitable, maintains growth, and builds a positive, long-lasting reputation for quality, performance, and dependability.   Pharmacists who pursue careers in marketing often have prior experience in pharmaceutical sales; many hold advanced degrees in business.   Pharmaceutical marketing is truly an interesting area for the individual who is business oriented and who likes to deal with both scientific and commercial problems.

Summary

The pharmaceutical industry which, by broad definition, includes the makers of prescription, veterinary, and proprietary drugs, and cosmetics and toiletries, offers many career opportunities in various scientific disciplines.   Individuals trained as undergraduates in pharmacy find that their broad-based background in the sciences, sometimes with advanced training in pharmacy or in other areas, permits them to move in numerous career directions.   Pharmaceutically trained scientists can be found serving in various industry capacities: Research and Development, Pharmaceutical Production, Analytical Research and Quality Control and

Assurance, Scientific Information and Regulatory Affairs, Clinical Testing, Professional Relations, Sales and Marketing, Management, and more.

To put it succinctly: Few other professions offer to the individual with basic training in the pharmaceutical sciences such a variety of potential careers in so many different areas. In some of these areas the pharmaceutical scientist needs little or no additional training; in others his broad-based pharmacy training provides an excellent foundation to integrate and effectively use added education and training in other specialties.

For the pharmacist in industry the opportunities are many; the responsibilities are important; and the careers are rewarding.

Bibliography

Prices and Profits in the Pharmaceutical Industry, PMA, Washington, DC, 1976.

US Industrial Outlook 1978, US Department of Commerce, USGPO, 1978.

Annual Survey Report, Research and Development Activities: Ethical Pharmaceutical Industry, 1976, PMA, Washington, DC, 1977.

Survey of Corporate Research: What 600 Companies Spend for Research, Business Week, June 27, 1977.

Research and Development in Industry, 1975, NSF 77-324, USGPO, 1977.

New Products Parade, 1977–1978, Paul De Haen, Inc, New York, 1978.

Burns JJ: The biological knowledge gap. From *Advances in Chemistry*, Series 108, Am Chem Soc, 1971.

Numbers of Establishments, FDA Office of Planning and Evaluation, USDHEW, Washington, DC, 1977.

Lindsay CM: *The Pharmaceutical Industry: Economics, Performance, and Government Regulation*, Wiley, New York, 1978.

Survey, 1976: American Council on Pharmaceutical Education.

Lachman L, *et al: Theory and Practice of Industrial Pharmacy*, 2nd ed, Lea & Febiger, Philadelphia, 1977.

Weaver LC, *et al:* Members Report for the AACP-Academy of Pharmaceutical Sciences Joint Committee on Pharmacy Graduate Education, *Am J Pharm Ed 39:* 152, May 1975.

Kelly ET, Herman CM: An evaluation of the PMA-coordinated industry program for pharmacy administration faculty. Presented at the AACP Annual Meeting, August 1977.

Rodowskas CA, Dickson WM: The pharmacy manpower information project: a profile of the profession. Presented at the Annual Meeting of the APhA, San Francisco, 1975.

Survey of Pharmacists in Industry, PMA, Washington, DC, 1978.

Questions and Answers About the US Drug Industry, PMA, Washington, DC, 1977.

CHAPTER 6

Pharmacists in Government

Milton W Skolaut, BSc

Director, Department of Pharmacy
Duke Hospital
Duke University Medical Center
Durham, NC 27710

The emphasis on health services for the population of the US has increased the importance of pharmacist participation in health programs. Many new doors have been opened for careers in the clinical practice of pharmacy in federal hospitals, outpatient clinics, extended-care facilities, administrative, or health-related programs.

Pharmacists have a unique and broad-based education which will allow them to function effectively in a new and broader scope than ever before. Certain pharmacists, oriented to patients by their education rather than to products, can fulfill a rewarding career in a federal hospital or related health program. All pharmacists have a wide range of opportunities for rewarding careers in health programs requiring the pharmacist's basic knowledge.

Career Opportunities

Career opportunities in the federal services are unlimited for the pharmacist with an excellent educational background and armed with a desire to serve. A continual supply of new commissioned officers are required by the Army, Navy, Air Force, and Public Health Service.

Pharmacists' opportunities for civil service employment are available in the Veterans Administration; Department of Health and Human Services; Department of Commerce; Department of Labor; and Department of Justice. The Department of Health and Human Services offers civil service positions in the Food and Drug Administration, National Institutes of Health, Social Security Administration, and Office of Equal Opportunity. The Department of Justice utilizes pharmacists in the Drug Enforcement Administration.

While it is not compulsory to have pharmacists in some of these positions, the fact that their talents are made available has contributed measurably to the efficiency and quality of the service rendered in a number of important governmental activities.

More and more it becomes evident to those who study the structure and function of government that there are certain positions of responsibility and trust where pharmaceutical training is of special usefulness.

Often pharmacists who come into the military or civilian service as pharmacists find that the logical line of advancement takes them out of actual dispensing or compounding of drugs and medicines and leads them into administrative positions. This is, of course, comparable to what takes place in private practice and in the drug industry. The heads of large government agencies have found pharmacists invaluable in administrative positions because of their broad knowledge and experience in the professional and scientific phases of pharmaceutical practice. These individuals also recognize that the pharmacist has a unique training and knowledge to prepare him for an ever-increasing clinical role in a partnership with practicing physicians. In government service, as well as in private industry, it is the ability of the individual to adapt himself to expanding services and new applications of his professional training and techniques which marks him for promotion and assignment to tasks of continually wider importance.

Recruitment—Broadly speaking, the positions in government service which require pharmaceutical training can be classified into *military* and *civilian* pursuits. In the military, the services of pharmacists are provided either by enlistment or commissioning of qualified persons and also, to a more limited extent, through civil service employment.

In the nonmilitary phases of government service pharmacists are recruited through the Civil Service Commission. The Public Health Service largely depends on its commissioned corps for the professional services of pharmacists, although it also calls on civil service for recruitment when necessary.

Armed Forces Requirements—While the Armed Forces are in a position to set up their medical services without reference to civilian pharmacy requirements, the modern tendency is to follow the standards of civilian pharmacy to the greatest extent possible, adapting them to the exigencies of military situations as indicated. Service community hospitals and medical centers maintained by the Army, Navy, and Air Force make use of the same type of facilities and services found in civilian hospitals.

The pharmaceutical service in mobile units, such as those of the Navy and Air Force, and such as is required when armies are on the move, like every other phase of medical care, is adapted to the requirements of the armed forces which are being served.

Although the Medical Service Corps of the Army, Navy, and Air Force stem from the Medical Service Corps Act of 1947, each service is governed to a considerable extent by the provisions of the Officer Personnel Act of 1947. It is this latter Act which establishes rank structure and promotion procedure which are designed to place all officers on common ground within their services, but not necessarily on common ground with their contemporaries of sister services.

Qualifications of Applicants—Anyone aspiring to make a professional career of service in the Armed Forces must bear in mind that professional knowledge by itself will not characterize him as a good officer. He must have other qualifications to fit him as a commissioned officer. These include ability to exhibit cooperation, judgment, leadership, promotion potential, and management effectiveness. The extent to which he possesses these is determined by selection boards within the respective services.

Applicants for a direct reserve commission as a pharmacist must be citizens of the US, of good moral character, physically and professionally qualified, and at least 21 years of age. Individuals must possess a baccalaureate degree in pharmacy from an institution accredited by the American Council on Pharmaceutical Education and be licensed to practice pharmacy in one of the states or territories of the US or the District of Columbia.

Army

Revolutionary War—As far back as 1775 the Continental Congress established a hospital for the Army with an apothecary as one of the officers. In 1776 the Congress created the office of "druggist." He was to "receive and deliver all medicines, instruments, and shop furniture of the United States," and in 1777, when the Continental Congress reorganized the medical department, it divided the country into four districts and stated that there should be "one apothecary general for each district whose duty it shall be, to receive, prepare, and deliver medicines, and other articles of his department to the hospitals and Army, as shall be ordered by the director general."

During the Revolutionary War, a central laboratory was established to manufacture the pharmaceutical products needed in the Army which were prepared and compounded mostly in the shop of the apothecary general at Carlisle, PA. The first apothecary general of the Army was Andrew Craigie. This led to the publication of the first pharmacopeia in America, the *Lititz Pharmacopoeia*, which was prepared for use in the military hospitals.

Civil War—During the Civil War, the purchase and distribution of medicines was in the hands of medical officers. Pharmacists were employed in the volunteer regiments; however, their rank and pay were unsatisfactory. In peacetimes, no progress was made in providing for pharmaceutical service in the Army which came anywhere near the equivalent of such service in civilian life.

The American Pharmaceutical Association took cognizance of this situation in 1894 by appointing a "Committee on The Status of Pharmacists in the Service of the United States." The title of this committee was later changed to the "Committee on Status of Pharmacists in Government Service."

Spanish–American War—The Committee on Status of Pharmacists in Government Service was active during the Spanish–American War in endeavoring to secure commissions for pharmacists in the National Guard of the various states. In 1900 it succeeded in having the State of New York pass an act which assigned a pharmacist to each regiment in the National Guard with the rank of lieutenant, but this law was repealed in 1901.

World War I—It is quite understandable that in the absence of emergencies the interest of civilian pharmacists in serving in a military capacity has never been very great. Accordingly, there was very little activity on the part of the Committee on Status of Pharmacists in Government Service until the advent of World War I. It had become a matter of routine for the Army to train personnel to dispense drugs and to provide for noncommissioned grades for such personnel. All of the pharmaceutical service in the Army was given under the direction of medical officers.

World War I was probably the first occasion for the drafting of pharmacists in sufficiently large numbers to cause concerted action to improve their rank and assignment in the Armed Forces. Not only did this stimulate the APhA Committee on Status of Pharmacists in Government Service to become more active, but it also caused the formation of a separate organization known as the National Pharmaceutical Service Association, which urged the organization of a *Pharmacy Corps* in the Medical Department of the Army, and led Congressman Edmonds of Pennsylvania, in 1917, to introduce a bill in the House of Representatives to accomplish this.

The public hearing on this measure assembled one of the largest groups of pharmacists and pharmaceutical educators ever brought together to sponsor such legislation. The hearing focused attention on the fact that the basic education of pharmacists would have to be brought to a 4-year college level in order for the profession to receive consideration in the matter of commissioning its members directly from civilian

life. The bill did not reach the stage of action by the House of Representatives. However, a number of pharmacists were commissioned in the *Sanitary Corps* of the Medical Department of the Army during World War I, and they were assigned to supervise pharmaceutical and medical supply procurement. An effort was also made to place pharmacists, who were obtained by the Army through the draft, in positions where their pharmaceutical background could be utilized.

In 1920 the Army organized a *Medical Administrative Corps* in which it commissioned men with various backgrounds in the ancillary medical professions and with experience in medical supply and administration who could relieve medical officers of many nonmedical duties, thus freeing them for more strictly medical services.

World War II—When the United States became involved in the second world war, and the Selective Service draft again brought into the service a very large number of pharmacists, the pressure on the part of the profession for providing a separate *Pharmacy Corps* became more and more pronounced, and in 1942 Congressman Carl Durham of North Carolina, who had introduced a bill to establish a Pharmacy Corps in the Army, succeeded in having it passed. This bill provided specific assignments for a limited number of commissioned pharmacists and for the transfer of all officers in the Medical Administrative Corps to the Pharmacy Corps. The Bill became a law on July 12, 1943, but the Corps was never properly organized or implemented during the war years because of strong opposition to it on the part of the Medical Department of the Army supported by the War Department.

Army Medical Service Corps

The unsatisfactory situation, with respect to organization and proper utilization of the Pharmacy Corps, which existed at the end of World War II was finally resolved by the passage of new legislation in 1947. This legislation provided for a *Medical Service Corps* in both Army and Navy and the consolidation within this Corps of the Pharmacy Corps, the Medical Administration Corps, and the Sanitary Corps. The Act creating the Corps is known as Public Law 337 of the 80th Congress and became a law on August 4, 1947. The Air Force activated a Medical Service Corps on July 1, 1949.

Organization of the Medical Service Corps—The Corps is divided into four major Sections: *Pharmacy, Supply, and Administration; Sanitary Engineering; Optometry;* and *Medical Allied Sciences.* The Corps consists of officers trained in 24 career fields, with many related occupational specialties. In addition to pharmacy these disciplines include hospital administration, biochemistry, optometry, nutrition, psychology, bacteriology, engineering, management, etc., all vitally necessary to the proper function of the Army medical service.

Pharmacy Officers—Pharmacists by their background, diversified professional training in the sciences and management, together with their close working relationships with the medical profession, make an ideal source of officer material for the army medical team headed by the physician whose mission is the preservation of the health of the Army.

Pharmacy officers have complete charge of supervision, training, and administration of enlisted and civilian personnel and, in general, concern themselves with the orderly management of pharmacies in Army treatment facilities. Pharmacy officers may expect to have a challenging and rewarding professional career in the US Army. The practice of pharmacy in the Army community hospitals and Medical Centers is at a high professional level. In addition to outpatient dispensing activities, the majority of these facilities feature intravenous admixture services and unit dose programs. Clinical involvement, particularly in the area of nuclear and hematology-oncology pharmacy, is rapidly expanding. The opportunity also exists for the pharmacy officer to broaden his career utilization into the area of materiel management, supply functions, and administration.

Graduate level education is available to selected career pharmacy officers leading to Master of Science and Doctor of Philosophy degrees.

Table I indicates salary schedules in effect in 1982.

Navy

The US Navy organization for medical care is considerably different from that of the Army because of the nature of the basic service rendered by this branch of the Armed Forces. It does have some training stations and medical centers in various parts of the United States and its possessions, and here the general pattern of excellent pharmaceutical service in hospitals is followed.

However, medical service on ships takes on a different form, and only the larger units of the aircraft carrier class carry major equipment and personnel for complete medical service. The smaller units rely on emergency facilities, and the Navy, since its formal beginning in 1775, has relied on a *Hospital Corps* which is trained specifically to care for the sick and injured.

In the early days of the Navy it was the practice to buy stocks of drugs from pharmacies and to have such prescriptions as were compounded made up by the surgeon's assistants, who were in many cases trained pharmacists.

In 1894 the APhA Committee on Status of Pharmacists in Government Service reported that graduates of schools of pharmacy were assigned to the position of apothecary in the Navy following examination by a board of medical officers. In 1898 an Act of Congress was passed providing for the establishment of a Hospital Corps in the Navy consisting of pharmacists, hospital stewards, and hospital apprentices in the US Navy, and it authorized the Secretary of the Navy to appoint 25 pharmacists with the rank, pay, and privileges of warrant officers. This Act was approved on June 17, 1898.

It was not until 1916 that any worthwhile progress was made in improving the status of pharmacists in the Navy. In that year the Naval Appropriation Act provided that pharmacists could, after 6 years of service as warrant officers, be commissioned as chief pharmacists "after passing satisfactorily such examinations as the Secretary of the Navy may prescribe."

During World War II, pharmacists enlisting in the Navy were assigned to the Hospital Corps and were advanced in both noncommissioned and commissioned grades for duties involving first aid, minor surgery, general hospital work, prescription compounding, chemical analysis, and bacteriological work.

Navy Medical Service Corps

When the Medical Service Corps Act was passed in 1947, the Surgeon General of the Navy provided for a Pharmacy Section in the Medical Service Corps and a number of pharmacists have been commissioned for service in this Section. The US Navy Medical Service Corps is organized in six sections: *Supply and Administration; Medical and Allied Sciences; Pharmacy; Optometry; Podiatry;* and *Medical Specialist.*

Commissioned pharmacists have been used in the Navy as instructors for hospital corpsmen and as chiefs of pharmacy service in naval hospitals. Pharmacists who have entered upon graduate study and have special qualifications have also been commissioned in the Allied Sciences Section of the Medical Service Corps of the Navy.

Table I indicates salary schedules in effect in 1982.

Table I—Approximate Monthly Basic Salaries of Commissioned Officers [a]

Pay grade	Entrance pay	Over 2 yrs	Over 4 yrs	Over 10 yrs	Over 20 yrs
01-2nd Lt	1098	1143	1382	1382	1382
02-1st Lt	1265	1382	1716	1752	1752
03-Captain	1451	1623	1919	2196	2361
04-Major	—	1902	2029	2305	2731
05-Lt Colonel	—	—	2326	2397	3155
06-Colonel	—	—	—	2712	3488

[a] Approximate salaries in effect October 1, 1982. In addition, nontaxable allowances as follows: Subsistence $98.17/month and monthly rental allowances with dependents: 01-$290.70; 02-$361.80; 03-$406.50; 04-$452.10; 05-$506.70; 06-$556.80. Salaries listed above are for comparison only—actual salaries are adjusted annually.

Air Force

The United States Air Force Medical Service was activated on July 1, 1949. Although young in comparison with other federal medical services, the Air Force Medical Service has developed and matured rapidly. Pharmacists actively participated in the development of an excellent Air Force Medical Service.

In March 1965 the Medical Service Corps was reorganized into a Medical Service Corps and a Biomedical Sciences Corps. The pharmacist commissioned officers assigned to pharmacy duties were transferred to the Biomedical Sciences Corps. Pharmacy officers assigned to medical administration and medical supply duties remain in the Medical Service Corps.

The Biomedical Sciences Corps (BSC) consists of allied health specialists serving in 15 areas of responsibility. Pharmacists assigned to nonpharmacy functions in the Medical Service Corps were offered the opportunity to enter the pharmacy component of the professionally oriented Biomedical Sciences Corps. Many graduate pharmacists are utilized by the Air Force as Civil Service employees, but the majority of pharmacists in the Air Force are serving as commissioned officers in the Biomedical Sciences Corps.

Air Force Biomedical Sciences Corps

The objectives of the BSC program are to provide a management structure for more efficient career planning and development and to formulate long-range programs for the most effective utilization of allied health professionals within the Air Force Medical Service.

The 15 authorized specialties that now comprise the Corps are pharmacy, optometry, biomedical laboratory sciences, bioenvironmental engineering, medical entomology, clinical psychology, social work, health physics, dietetics/nutrition, occupational therapy, physical therapy, speech therapy, podiatry, audiology, and aerospace physiology.

The chief of the BSC is assigned to the USAF Surgeon General's Office and monitors the activities of the various specialties. The specialty groups in turn are directed by their respective associate chiefs.

The pharmacy component of the BSC is responsible for promoting and instituting professionally oriented pharmacy services in Air Force medical facilities. Through proper utilization and supervision of highly trained Air Force pharmacy technicians serving in the dispensing function, pharmacists are made available to implement unit-dose drug distribution and centralized pharmacy-supervised intravenous additive services in Air Force hospitals. Air Force pharmacists devote an extensive amount of effort to promoting rational drug therapy through participation in the policy formulating activities of pharmacy and therapeutics committees. The clinical orientation of Air Force pharmacists reflects the progressive leadership and direction of the BSC. Assignments for Air Force pharmacists are authorized at numerous medical facilities located both overseas and in the continental United States. In addition, the Air Force allows selected BSC officers to further their education in some of the finest civilian and military schools in the nation.

The United States Air Force offers unlimited opportunities to its pharmacy officers. The satisfying fulfillment of personal objectives and professional goals coupled with the chance to serve one's country honorably and distinctively represent a much sought after but seldom realized blend of human endeavor.

Table I indicates salary schedules in effect in 1982.

Department of Health and Human Services

The United States Public Health Service of the Department of Health and Human Services is an outgrowth of the *Marine Hospital Service* which was established in 1798 to provide hospital service and medical treatment for American merchant seamen. Pharmacists were employed in the Marine hospitals from the beginning under various titles including apothecaries, hospital stewards, pharmacists, and chemists. Those employed in the early days of the Marine Hospital Service under the title of apothecaries were engaged fully in pharmaceutical work except for such administrative duties as were part of the operation of the pharmacy.

In 1870 the Marine Hospital Service was reorganized as a national hospital system with centralized administration under a medical officer, the supervising surgeon, who was later given the title of Surgeon General. The first career service for civilian employees in the federal government was created by regulations put into effect in 1873. This paved the way for the statutory establishment of the Commissioned Corps of the Public Health Service in 1889. The reorganization of the 1870s marked the beginning of preventive medicine in the Service. Congress provided for a Reserve Corps in 1918.

Until the turn of the present century, physicians and pharmacists were the only professionally trained persons employed in the Service hospitals and health activities. Pharmacists have been employed in the Service since its very beginning, under a variety of designations, ie, apothecary, hospital-steward, pharmacist and chemist, pharmacist, and medical purveyor, each designation comprising one or more grades. Graduation in pharmacy before appointment was first required in 1897.

A betterment of special import to pharmacy resulted from the approval on April 9, 1930, of the "Parker Act" which provided for the coordination of public health activities of the government. This law included provision for the appointment of pharmacists in the commissioned corps with promotion up to and including the grade corresponding to Army Captain. A further and substantial improvement in the status and opportunity for pharmacists in the Service occurred upon the approval of the Public Health Service Act of 1944 (Public Law 410—78th Congress). Under this Act the promotion limitation was lifted and pharmacists may now be promoted to the Director Grade corresponding to that of Army Colonel.

The *Public Health Service* (PHS) is the principal health agency of the federal government. Stated in the broadest possible terms, the mission of the Public Health Service is to protect and advance the health of the American people. The Assistant Secretary for Health—with overall responsibility for the direction of PHS—serves as the Department of Health and Human Services Secretary's principal advisor on health and provides leadership and guidance on all health and health-related activities, including research and development; education and training; and the organization, financing, and delivery of health care services.

The Public Health Service is comprised of civil servants and officers of the Commissioned Corps. The latter is composed of physicians, dentists, nurses, pharmacists, and other health professionals with graduate level training who volunteer for service in PHS.

With regard to the basic organization of the Service, the major components are the five line agencies: the Alcohol, Drug Abuse, and Mental Health Administration; the Center for Disease Control; the Food and Drug Administration; the Health Resources and Services Administration; and the National Institutes of Health.

The *Alcohol, Drug Abuse, and Mental Health Administration* (ADAMHA) develops policies and programs for the treatment and prevention of alcohol, drug abuse, and mental health problems. It conducts clinical and biochemical research in its own laboratories and provides assistance in establishing and operating alcohol, drug abuse, and mental health programs. ADAMHA's responsibilities are shared by its three component Institutes: the National Institute on Alcohol Abuse and Alcoholism, the National Institute on Drug Abuse, and the National Institute of Mental Health.

The *Center for Disease Control* (CDC) assists state and local health authorities and other health-related organizations in preventing and controlling diseases, improving the performance of clinical and Public Health laboratories, and improving occupational safety and health. It maintains surveillance of diseases and undertakes to prevent the importation of diseases. CDC provides assistance in the control and prevention of diseases and surveys the immunization status of the population. It develops new methods for testing and preventing communicable and vector-borne diseases and conducts a program for improving the performance of clinical laboratories.

The *Food and Drug Administration* protects the public health of the Nation as it may be impaired by foods, drugs, biological products, cosmetics, medical devices, radiation-emitting products, poisons, pesticides, and food additives. It insures that foods are safe and wholesome; that drugs, medical devices, and biological products are safe and effective; and that cosmetics are harmless.

The *Health Resources and Services Administration* (HRSA) provides leadership with respect to the identification and deployment of personnel and to educational, physical, financial, and organizational resources in the achievement of optimal health services for the people of the United States.

In addition, the agency serves as a national focus for programs and health services, with emphasis on achieving the integration of service delivery and public and private financing systems to assure their responsiveness to the needs of all Americans. HRSA administers health service delivery programs supported by project grants or contracts and provides or arranges for personal health services, including both hospital and outpatient care, to designated beneficiaries.

The *National Institutes of Health* (NIH) provides leadership and direction to programs designed to improve the health of the people of the United States. It conducts and supports research in the causes, diagnosis, prevention, and cure of diseases in man, in the processes of human growth and development, in the biological effects of environmental contaminants, and in related sciences. It supports the training of research personnel, the construction of research facilities, and the development of other research resources.

Activities of Pharmacists—There are 450 commissioned pharmacy officers and about 100 Civil Service pharmacists in the US Public Health Service assigned to clinical, administrative, and research positions in the various agencies. A brief summary of the programs with pharmacists follows.

The *Indian Health Service* operates 86 large health centers and more than 300 field clinics to provide comprehensive health care to 500,000 American Indians and Alaskan Natives.

The objective of the pharmacy services program is to utilize fully pharmacists' knowledge and skills in providing preventive health care and curative health services to the Indians and to assure that quality drugs are properly used in each health facility and in each Indian home.

The records indicate that the first practicing hospital pharmacist was employed in the Indian Hospital at Mt. Edgecumbe, AK, in October 1950. Today, pharmacists are assigned to a majority of the facilities with full- or part-time physicians.

Indian Health pharmacy services utilize the total knowledge and skills of pharmacists in ambulatory primary care, clinical pharmacy services for hospitalized patients, and the distribution of drug products within the hospital. Pharmacists have primary responsibility in diagnosing and treating the outpatient for certain acute diseases, in managing the condition of the outpatient with certain diagnosed chronic diseases, and in exercising independent judgment as to the care of such patients. In carrying out his primary care responsibilities the pharmacist obtains a history and vital signs, requests laboratory tests, performs certain physical diagnostic techniques, evaluates the data, and determines the treatment plan.

Pharmacists provided primary care for more than 10% of all ambulatory patients.

Inpatient pharmacy services include obtaining a medication and related history upon admission, attending physician working rounds, making daily pharmacy rounds to monitor the drug therapy and to prevent adverse drug effects, offering patient education, attending nursing reports at change of nursing shifts, and counseling on discharge.

National Institutes of Health Clinical Center—The Clinical Center is a 14-story, 516-bed research hospital located in Bethesda, MD. The Center is designed to bring scientists working in 1100 laboratories into close proximity with clinicians caring for patients so bench investigators and physicians may collaborate on problem diseases.

The primary mission of the Clinical Center is to provide the specialized forms of hospital care necessary for Institute studies. The illnesses under study are the ones common in people throughout the nation. Ranging from the common cold to cancer, the widespread maladies being investigated reflect a public health mission—to accomplish the most for the greatest number.

The pharmacy department of the Clinical Center consists of three separate subunits designed organizationally as Services, each under the immediate supervision of a Service Chief. Pharmacists assigned to the Pharmacy Service fill outpatient prescriptions, dispense drugs for inpatients, bulk compound pharmaceuticals, prepare sterile ophthalmic solutions, fill orders for intravenous solutions containing additives, and furnish specific drug information as requested by physicians. In addition to routine hospital pharmacy services, this Service conducts a clinical pharmacy program on the patient unit, along with a drug information service and a patient-oriented drug distribution system.

Pharmacists assigned to the Pharmaceutical Development Service are engaged in activities to assist the clinical investigator in the development and stability of suitable dosage forms of clinical drugs for investigational use. Such dosage forms are not usually commercially available and, if they are, they may be altered for a specific clinical investigational study.

Practice at the Clinical Center Pharmacy Department provides an opportunity to practice hospital pharmacy in an environment wherein productive medical research can be expected to flourish.

The *Food and Drug Administration*, a regulatory agency of the federal government, protects the public health of the nation as it may be impaired by foods, drugs, cosmetics, therapeutic devices, hazardous household substances, poisons, pesticides, food additives, flammable fabrics, and various other types of consumer products.

Pharmacists working in the Bureau of Biologics Standards play a vital role in the federal control of biologic products through activities such as: (1) reviewing manufacturers' methods of preparing and testing biologicals; (2) performing a variety of control tests on biologicals produced by the manufacturers; (3) reviewing labeling for biologicals; and (4) performing inspections of manufacturers' facilities.

Pharmacists assigned to the Bureau of Drugs are working in such areas as the review of data relating to the pharmacological aspects of drugs, laboratory analysis, and the collection of samples for enforcement purposes and the inspection of manufacturers' facilities.

The *Division of Hazardous Substances and Poison Control* furnishes information on formulation, estimated toxicity, symptomatology and suggested treatment of household products and medicines to 500 Poison Control Centers for use by the physician in an emergency. This information is derived from industry, literature, federal agencies, and case reports.

Pharmacy officers are assigned the responsibilities of reviewing and evaluating the formulations, symptomatology, and treatment recommended by the manufacturer.

The *Bureau of Radiological Health* has primary responsibility for protecting the public against radiation hazards. The several pharmacy officers assigned to the Bureau have graduate degrees in radiological health and work in such areas as enforcement of radiation equipment standards, control and improvements of radiopharmaceuticals, calculation of radiation exposure to the population, and program administration.

The Public Health Service has a number of one-year hospital pharmacy residency positions at the Clinical Center (National Institutes of Health) and the Indian Health Service Hospitals, all of which are accredited by the American Society of Hospital Pharmacists.

The Service has a Commissioned Officer Student Training and Extern Program (COSTEP) in which students are brought on active duty between school years or at another free period of time. The assignment is generally for about three months.

The following is a partial listing of other programs that utilize Public Health Service pharmacists: US Coast Guard, Bureau of Prisons, Community Health Service, National Health Service Corps, Health Maintenance Organization Service, Bureau of Quality Assurance, and the National Institute of Occupational Safety and Health.

Table I indicates salary schedules in effect in 1982.

Veterans Administration

Rapid expansion of the Veterans Administration began immediately following World War II, with the tremendous increase in the veteran population. Today the Veterans Administration operates 166 hospitals and 200 outpatient clinics with more than 700 pharmacists providing professional pharmacy service to these facilities.

VA Department of Medicine and Surgery

With the reorganization of the Veterans Administration and the passage of Public Law 293 in 1946, provisions were made for a chief pharmacist in the Department of Medicine and Surgery, and basic educational requirements were established for pharmacists.

The director of the Pharmacy Service, along with a staff in the Washington office, is responsible for developing overall professional procedures and policies for pharmacy operations. He evaluates the effectiveness and operating efficiency of the pharmacies as a part of the medical care program, ensuring operation in keeping with the principles and practices of the profession of pharmacy.

Training—In-service training is planned and conducted to keep all pharmacists abreast of trends in the field of pharmacy and related technical sciences. Under the present program pharmacists are sent to institutes on hospital pharmacy sponsored by the American Society of Hospital Pharmacists; intra-VA pharmacy conferences are scheduled and held in various localities throughout the United States; chief pharmacists from smaller hospitals and clinics are sent for training periods to larger teaching hospitals to benefit from modern trends and developments in professional practices; staff personnel are detailed to other hospitals or clinics for indoctrination periods in administrative and professional procedures and given opportunities to assume sole responsibility for their application. In-service training programs are subject to continuing review and are changed or adapted to suit special needs or advances in pharmacy and medicine.

Recognizing the need for highly trained specialists in the field of hospital pharmacy, the Veterans Administration conducts a program of hospital pharmacy residency training. The residency is a 2-year combined course established at a hospital in cooperation with the graduate school of a university. It consists of clinical experience in hospital and outpatient pharmacy with assigned duties of the highest professional level including pharmaceutical research. The resident also is given general orientation in hospital administration and pharmacy's relationship to other professional and administrative services. Approximately half of the resident's time is devoted to hospital and clinic training and the remainder in attending college classes at the graduate level to satisfy the requirements for the degree of Master of Science or Doctor of Pharmacy (PharmD).

Opportunity is also offered to pharmacy college graduates to train as pharmacy interns in some VA hospitals. During the 1-year program, training and clinical experience under supervision of registered pharmacists is provided. The training program meets the standards for hospital pharmacy internships adopted by the American Society of Hospital Pharmacists. Although given primarily for specialized training in hospital pharmacy, a VA hospital pharmacy internship will meet the practical experience requirements of most state boards of pharmacy for registration.

Applications for residencies and internships are made directly to the hospital offering this program. Information on the current programs available may be obtained from the Director, Pharmacy Service, VA Central Office, Washington, DC 20420.

Duties and Responsibilities—Pharmacists perform a full range of professional pharmacy duties and are an integral part of the medical team. Organizationally, the pharmacy service is at the same level as other professional specialties.

In hospitals and clinics, pharmacists are expected to give indoctrination and refresher training courses. They also prepare lectures and demonstrations for the nursing staff covering topics such as storage of drugs, drug usage, methods of administration, pharmaceutical arithmetic and conversions, percentage solutions, and calculating doses. Topics such as prescription writing, drug usage, posology, and incompati- ... may be assigned for presentation at training sessions ... ical staff. At hospitals with medical residency and ... pharmacists may be called on to prepare ... and interns as part of the formal training ... ists work with the medical staff in ... pharmacy contribution to the

... to hospital and clinic ... mmittees, usually ... as chairman

and other designated medical consultants, formulate drug policy, recommend drugs for standard pharmacy stock, and determine which drugs will be added to the formulary and the scope of information to be included.

Pharmacists are responsible for maintaining a working library of standard pharmaceutical references and a current file of pertinent data from professional journals and drug manufacturers' literature.

Guided by general policies established in Central Office, chief pharmacists establish procedures, methods, and working schedules for pharmacy operations. The pharmacy functions vary in each institution, but many include the unit-dose concept of drug dispensing, intravenous drug additives, and clinical pharmacy services. The chief pharmacist coordinates pharmacy activities with other medical services or clinics. With the cooperation of the personnel office, he selects suitable professional and nonprofessional personnel, initiates promotions, and prepares performance ratings.

Qualifications—To be eligible for appointment, all applicants must have completed at least a 4-year course in pharmacy and have a bachelor's, master's, or doctor's degree from an approved school. The applicant must also be currently registered as a pharmacist in one of the states or territories of the United States or in the District of Columbia. Appointments are made from Civil Service registers established by competitive examinations. The examination consists of rating the applicant on the basis of his education and experience as a registered pharmacist, including the breadth, variety, difficulty, and complexity of his work, and on his demonstrated ability to supervise.

Appointments—Appointments of registered pharmacists are generally made at the staff pharmacist level, and higher grade vacancies are usually filled by promotion of qualified on-duty VA pharmacists. This provides a maximum of opportunity for career development.

Staff pharmacist positions are generally classified at Grades GS-9 and GS-11, GS-9 being a staff pharmacist with limited responsibilities; it is essentially a training position preparing the employee for the next higher grade level. The GS-11 position applies to a staff pharmacist performing a full range of pharmacy duties as a specialist or generalist.

Chief pharmacist positions are usually classified in Grades GS-11 to GS-14, depending on the extent of the activity and the responsibilities of the position. There are a limited number of administrative positions in Grades GS-14 and GS-15, which are usually filled by promotion of pharmacists within the Veterans Administration.

Benefits—Pharmacists in the Veterans Administration receive numerous benefits afforded by federal employment, including paid vacations, sick leave pay, low-cost group life insurance, health insurance, and an excellent retirement plan. Salary is based on the standard federal work week of 40 hours.

Other Federal Agencies

The Drug Enforcement Administration employs registered pharmacists in its inspection service since this work requires much of the knowledge received in pharmaceutical education and subsequent training. Many of these positions are available in the field rather than in the main office in Washington, DC. They involve the inspection of all types of records, including prescriptions, and the detection of the illicit distribution of narcotic and controlled drugs.

State, County, and Municipal Government Agencies

In addition to employment in federal government agencies dealing with regulation of the distribution of drugs, there are numerous opportunities for similar service with state departments of health, state boards of pharmacy, state bureaus of controlled drugs, state and county welfare administration departments, and similar agencies where activities such as those described above are carried on at the state and county levels. This applies also to the larger municipalities.

The coordination of municipal, state, and federal enforcement procedures with regard to drugs, especially as this pertains to regulation of controlled drugs and dangerous drugs and poisons, opens a great opportunity for the employment of pharmacists who may be especially interested in regulatory activities. Very often pharmacists who start in federal positions and acquire considerable experience at that level have opportunity to take over administrative functions of a similar nature in state and municipal agencies where coordination is greatly enhanced by the past experience at the federal level.

The administrative functions of state, county, and local organizations having to do with the enforcement of health and welfare regulations frequently include specific duties that require a background of pharmaceutical training.

Many of these agencies deal with such matters as disease prevention and medical care. A recently increasing function of state governments is the administration of welfare medical care programs. In carrying out this function state and local appropriations are augmented or matched by federal appropriations to an ever-increasing extent. In such instances pharmacists are frequently employed to supervise the administration of pharmaceutical services in welfare medical care programs, especially those which involve what has become known as "vendor payments" for prescription drugs and pharmaceutical services.

These agencies usually appoint advisory committees consisting of representatives of the various health professions, including pharmacy, to aid in developing and enforcing their programs.

Some pharmacists, as well as other health personnel, are employed by these agencies on a full-time basis and are usually designated as pharmacy advisors or consultants. State welfare agencies which are called on to pay for millions of prescriptions supplied annually to indigent or medically indigent and aging patients at government expense will employ such consultants on a full- or part-time basis or will create positions under civil service for pharmacists in order to provide for an expert review of the pricing of prescriptions so as to keep them within the range of payment prescribed by the agency.

These pharmacists are expected to give advice on the best methods of reducing drug costs to the welfare agency. They are also expected to work with medical consultants and members of the medical profession in devising such limitations and extension of medical care services as may be indicated.

Government service, while usually not as remunerative as employment in industry, has certain compensations in the form of retirement benefits, medical services, annual and sick leave, and other benefits which constitute attractions. In recent years there has also been a tendency on the part of government agencies to provide time for formal education in various specialties, thus enabling the incumbents of these positions to improve their status.

The Department of Labor as well as the US Civil Service Commission are usually good sources of information for openings in government positions.

CHAPTER 7

Drug Information

C Boyd Granberg, PhD
Dean and Professor of Pharmacy
College of Pharmacy, Drake University
Des Moines, IA 50311

The pharmacist is in constant need of information concerning drugs, pharmaceutical products, and disease states. The rate at which professional and scientific information is accumulating threatens to make even the recent pharmacy graduate obsolescent within a few years unless he is familiar with the literature of the field and uses it regularly. In seeking desired information, the pharmacist makes use of the knowledge of others. That knowledge is either written in books or journals or transmitted by oral communication or by electronic device. The pharmacist shares, through the scientific literature, knowledge of the physical, chemical, biological, and health care sciences.

Pharmacy also has its own extensive and expanding body of knowledge which rightfully can be referred to as the *literature of pharmacy*.

Not only the pharmacist engaged in the delivery of pharmaceutical services but the undergraduate and graduate student, as well as the pharmacist in industry, research, and other vocational areas, depends on the literature to know what has already been achieved. The forms of the literature which each of these groups uses often overlap, but each also has its own specialties, categories, and peculiarities.

The techniques and the technologies of information retrieval are changing constantly; thus, not only is the pharmaceutical literature a vast field, but the pharmacist interested in keeping up-to-date or in searching information must be aware of these new methodologies and retrieval devices and know how to use them.

Prior to the mid-17th century, written communication among scientists was accomplished by books, diaries, and correspondence. The books dealing with drugs and medicines were formularies, dispensatories, and a variety of treatises which became the sources of the material which was compiled into the first books of recognized official standards for drugs and medicines, the pharmacopeias.

The 17th century has been termed the period of scientific revolution. Not only was there the birth of experimental science, but scientists organized themselves into the first scientific societies in the modern tradition, established the first scientific periodicals, and began to write scientific papers instead of the books which hitherto had been their only outlets. Thus, the 17th century also is recognized as the era in which *scientific literature* was established.

In the US the historical development of pharmaceutical literature paralleled the universal development of scientific literature. Pharmaceutical periodicals were slow to evolve in this country. The first such journal was established in 1825 by the Philadelphia College of Pharmacy.

Sonnedecker[1] and Cowen[2] have provided a chronology of the evolution of the American pharmaceutical literature.

The Literature Search

The method used to conduct either a limited search or a general survey of the pharmaceutical literature depends both on the information being sought and on whether the searcher is a pharmacy practitioner, an undergraduate or a graduate student, or a researcher.

Grogan[3] has grouped various kinds of consultations of the literature into a series of approaches and divides literature into *primary* and *secondary* sources.

Primary sources are those which record the original reports of scientific, technological, or professional investigations. The material presented is new knowledge and constitutes the most recent and up-to-date information. Forms in which such reports are published include periodicals, research reports, conference proceedings, reports of scientific expeditions, official publications, patents, standards, trade literature, and theses and dissertations. Because primary sources are widely scattered and the information they contain is often difficult to locate, it becomes necessary and desirable to gather much of the information from the primary sources into more organized and convenient forms.

Secondary sources contain second-hand information, but they are more widely and easily available to searchers. They include periodicals, indexing and abstracting services, citation indexes, computerized search services, reviews of progress, reference books (encyclopedias, dictionaries, handbooks, tables, formularies), treatises, monographs, compendia, and textbooks.

Organizing the Search—To use the literature efficiently and effectively, the searcher must know the library and how to use it. Libraries differ in their physical arrangements, the extent of their holdings, and the services they offer to users. The *card catalog* is the key to the resources available in any library, and librarians are anxious to assist library patrons in understanding and using it, as well as all other resources of the library.

The individual beginning a search of the literature should have an organized system of search and record keeping. A haphazard, unplanned, and careless search technique will lead to unnecessary mechanical labor.

The investigator must be sure he knows what he is looking for. Basic assumptions about the topic should be guaranteed correct. Definitions should be precise, and formulas, equations, or other data pertinent to the search should be checked for accuracy. Knowing what use is to be made of information helps determine the references which are needed and ensures effective use of the library. If a problem can be phrased as a series of questions, they may offer clues to the solution of the problem.

- Is the information sought a definition of some word or idea not found in an ordinary dictionary or encyclopedia?
- Is it a numerical or statistical fact or a particular procedure?
- Are you looking for evidence to support an argument?
- Do you seek trends?
- Are you interested in finding all there is to know about a disease or a new drug?
- Are you looking for a chemical, biological, or other procedure you want to try to duplicate?

The information necessary to answer these and other questions requires a different approach to the literature search, and the questions can serve as a working outline for the library project.

The searcher should compile a list of keywords, phrases, or topical headings to assist in the search of the card catalog, the indexes, the bibliographies, etc. It may be necessary to revise the list once the search has begun, but a final list should be adhered to strictly to avoid overlooking and missing a pertinent reference. If the search requires a check of several volumes of a series of abstract or index services, a record should be kept of volumes checked to avoid duplication or missing one or more volumes.

Prior to the actual search, the librarian should be asked if there are *guides to the literature* appropriate to the search. These aids include not only lists of references about a topic or discipline but also, in some instances, discussion of the functions and the uses of various types of literature. They offer a starting point for the search and will help to decide on the kinds of materials needed from the library. A representative list of such guides useful for searching the literature follows:

Andrews T, Oslet J: *Am J Hosp Pharm 32:* 85, 1975.
Bottle RT: *The Use of Biological Literature*, 2nd ed, Butterworth, 1972.
Bottle RT, ed: *The Use of Chemical Literature*, 3rd ed, Butterworth, 1979.
Gates JK: *Guide to the Use of Books and Libraries*, 4th ed, McGraw, 1979.
Pritchard A: *A Guide to Computer Literature: An Introductory Survey of the Sources of Information*, 2nd ed, Linnet, 1972.
Sewell W: *Guide to Drug Information*, Drug Intl Pubns, 1976.
Sheehy EP: *Guide to Reference Books*, 9th ed, Am Lib Assoc, 1976.
The Standard Periodical Directory, 8th ed, Oxbridge, 1982.
Ulrich's International Periodicals Directory, 21st ed, Bowker, 1982.

Before proceeding to search for references, a recording form should be devised. The use of a uniform system will force the searcher to note all available data at the time the reference is first encountered and will eliminate time-consuming second visits to a particular source. Fig. 7-1 shows a sample form. The space headed "File" in the upper right-hand corner indicates the desirability of keeping references filed as they are accumulated. Filing all references in one alphabetical list by authors or some other means will not allow the searcher to keep a proper perspective of the study as a whole. Rather, files should be developed and references classified into as many categories as necessary. By filing the references as they are gathered, one is able to spot subproblems or subtopics as the study advances and is able to identify and to discard duplications and to note shortages of references in particular areas.

Two maxims to be observed in conducting a library search are (1) begin with the most recent sources first and (2) begin with the most general, obvious, and available sources and work to the particular, differential, and specific. It will serve no good purpose to seek information on a new drug in the 1950 literature if the drug was not introduced until 1980. The more recent bibliographies are likely to cite earlier ones and to repeat many of the earlier references. Likewise, it will be a serious waste of time and effort to read all issues of a medical journal to find out about a particular disease if all knowledge about the disease has been published in a recent book.

Time can be saved by minimizing movement from place to place as much as possible. All work at the card catalog or with the index/abstract services should be completed before going into the stacks to look up specific references. If you are not permitted in the stacks, avoid wasting time at the loan desk waiting for books by having enough work to keep busy.

On occasion, a reference which seems to be of benefit proves to be of no value on more complete reading and examination; note of this should be made to avoid alluding to the reference again. On other occasions, a reference proves to be of such value that a personal copy of the article is desired. If reprints are available one may be ordered from the author; if not

File_____

Book Title_____
_____

Author(s)/Editor(s)_____
_____

Publisher_____City____Year____

Article Title_____
_____

Author(s)/Editor(s)_____
_____

Periodical Title_____
_____

Volume____Number____Page(s)____Date____

Abstract:

Fig. 7-1. A sample reference recording form.

available, permission should be obtained from the periodical or from the author to photocopy the article.

At other times, books or periodicals needed for reports or research may not be available locally but may be borrowed from other libraries. An extensive system of interlibrary loans has been developed among libraries in the US, and most libraries can arrange either for a loan or a photocopy of the desired reference. Public Law 94-553, a general revision of the copyright statute, became effective on January 1, 1978, and places certain restrictions on the reproduction of copyrighted works. The law is complex, and users should consult with the librarian to know what is authorized and what is proscribed.

Primary Sources

As important as books are to the researcher they are not the most popular reference sources. That distinction is held by *periodicals*, also referred to as *journals*, *serials*, *magazines*, *bulletins*, etc. They are published as issues (eg, weekly, monthly, or quarterly) and as volumes (eg, annually).

The advantage of periodicals over books is the reduction in the time lag between a discovery or an idea and its publication.

Periodicals also contain information of a more personal and contemporary nature than could or should be expected in reference books of any kind. For example, editorials and other commentaries, books reviews, announcements and current news items, and even advertisements are logical and important components of many pharmaceutical periodicals.

The popularity of the scientific periodical is reflected in the number of such journals which have made their appearance in the last 150 years. It was stated earlier that the scientific journal did not appear as part of the scientific literature until the mid-17th century and that the periodical did not become a part of the American pharmaceutical literature until 1825 when the Philadelphia College of Pharmacy instituted the *Journal of the Philadelphia College of Pharmacy*, the earliest publication of its kind which is still in existence. Gross estimates place the number of scientific, technical, and professional periodicals between 30,000 and 100,000 titles. There may be as many as 1000 journals which qualify as a part of the pharmaceutical literature. If one assumes the printing of an average of 50 articles per journal per year, there are 50,000 articles being published annually in the pharmaceutical journals. Theoretically, because many of these manuscripts have been accepted for publication through a referee system, these 50,000 articles have an important contribution to make to the profession.

Interestingly, the result of this abundance is that as the number of periodicals increases—ostensibly better to inform the scientific or professional community—the actual use of the periodicals decreases; people just do not have time to read all of the magazines which are available.

Classification

Just as the scientific literature can be classified into primary and secondary sources, so too can the periodicals. *Primary* periodicals print only reports of original research. *Secondary* journals cull from the primary sources that portion of the original research which fits their needs and then condense, interpret, and print that which serves their purposes.

Periodicals can be classified on the basis of the publisher: journals are published by academic, scientific, or professional associations, governmental bodies, research institutes, commercial firms, and individuals. Another classification is geographic, based on whether the publication is local, state, regional, or national in distribution. In fact, several American publications go beyond national boundaries and are distributed internationally; examples are the *American Journal of Hospital Pharmacy*, the *Journal of Pharmaceutical Sciences*, and the *American Journal of Pharmaceutical Education*.

A useful classification of periodicals is an arbitrary one based on scope; ie, scientific, professional, or commercial.

Scientific periodicals are those scholarly publications which report original research; they are sometimes referred to as research journals. The standards for articles are very high, and manuscripts are accepted for publication after being reviewed by experts in the field, through the referee system. Such journals commonly have an editorial board of eminent scientists who determine editorial policy. Scientific periodicals important to the field of pharmacy include:

Journal of Natural Products, formerly *Lloydia*, The Lloyd Library and Museum and Am Soc Pharmacog, bimonthly.
Journal of Pharmaceutical Sciences, APhA, monthly.
Science, AAAS, weekly.

Professional periodicals may also publish the results of original research. The research, however, is less technically and scientifically oriented than that reported in the scientific journals and has a more practical bias, with the results of the research more devoted to the practice aspects of the profession than to the scientific. Frequently, periodicals in this category are published by professional associations and are the official voice of the society. Some of the prestigious professional periodicals in pharmacy are:

American Journal of Hospital Pharmacy, ASHP, monthly.
American Journal of Pharmaceutical Education, AACP, 4 times a year.
American Journal of Pharmacy, Phila. Coll. Pharm. Sci., quarterly.
American Pharmacy, formerly *Journal of the American Pharmaceutical Association*, APhA, monthly.
Canadian Pharmaceutical Journal, Can. PhA, monthly.
Pharmacy in History, Am. Inst. Hist. Pharm., quarterly.
Pharmacy Times, Pharmacy Times, Inc., monthly.
Scientific American, Scientific American, Inc., monthly.

Commercial periodicals form the basis of the trade literature and are produced by the industry or by publishing houses. These periodicals vary considerably in form and include such publications as magazines designed for circulation to the practitioner, house organs, price and product catalogs, promotional literature, and customers' handbooks. A few of the many available in pharmacy are:

American Druggist, The Hearst Corp., monthly.
Chain Drug Review, Racher Press Inc., monthly.
Drug and Cosmetic Industry, Harcourt Brace Jovanovich, monthly.
Drug Topics, Medical Economics Co., semimonthly.
Medical Marketing and Media, C P S Communications, monthly.
NARD Journal, NARD, monthly.
The Gold Sheet (Quality Control Reports), F-D-C Reports, Inc., monthly.
The Green Sheet (Weekly Pharmacy Reports), F-D-C Reports, Inc., weekly.
The Pink Sheet (F-D-C Reports), F-D-C Reports, Inc., weekly.

Those publications listed in the various categories above are intended to be only a representative sampling of those available and not a comprehensive catalog. Conspicuous by their absence from the lists are the publications in the various disciplines in pharmacy and the journals which are especially important to the clinical practice of pharmacy. The former are too numerous to list, and a rather complete list of the latter will be found in Appendix A, Chapter 103

Secondary Sources

Bibliographies—A library search should begin with the most general available resources—i.e., books. In many areas of science and technology the lists of available books are referred to as *bibliographies*. In pure terms a bibliography is a list of books only; in practice, however, some so-called bibliographies include pamphlets, articles from periodicals, audiovisual records, and other printed material as well as books. Librarians often use the term "generic books" which means any record in permanent or near-permanent form. The card catalog of a library is, in essence, a bibliography.

Bibliographies also vary in form and in the depth of their coverage. Some are selective, annotated (i.e., accompanied by explanatory comment), and evaluative lists, while others are comprehensive, broad-based, and retrospective. The librarian will often need to be consulted to determine which bibliographies are available and are the most suitable in a particular circumstance.

The list below is a sampling of bibliographies of the pharmaceutical and associated literature.

Andrews T: *Bibliography of Drug Abuse, Including Alcohol and Tobacco*, Libraries Unlimited, 1977; suppl., 1977–1980, 1981.
Cohon MS, Rice BS, and Noble V: *Concepts in Clinical Pharmacology: Information Sources in Pharmacy and Pharmacology*, Scope (The Upjohn Co.), 1979.
Hall VB, Schwerzel SW: *Index to Sources of Data and Statistics in Pharmacy and the Health Field*, APhA, 1981.
Jackson EC: Books for pharmacy college libraries. *Am J Pharm Educ*, Part I, *33:* 246, 1969; Part II, *33:* 441, 1969.
Piermatti P, Hill BM, and Snow B: *A Basic Booklist for Pharmaceutical Education*, Am Assoc Coll Phcy, 1983.
Zachert MJK, Thomasson CL: Bibliography of books and reference works relating to the professional courses in the pharmaceutical curriculum. *Am J Pharm Educ 27:* 266, 1963; *27:* 361, 1963.

Several additional bibliographies of use to the pharmacy student or to the practitioner have been listed by Hellums.[4]

Encyclopedias—Although there are no encyclopedias available for the specialty of pharmacy, the multivolume encyclopedias written for the layman frequently contain articles about the general aspects of the profession. Because of the time lag in getting such works into print, the information found in these encyclopedias is usually out-of-date. Supplements to and revisions of encyclopedias appear with varying frequency in an attempt by editors and publishers to keep the information in them as current as possible.

Special-subject encyclopedias are available in most of the basic and applied sciences. In addition to the information each contains, encyclopedias may also have bibliographic references. The encyclopedias most useful are:

Considine DM, ed: *Van Nostrand's Scientific Encyclopedia*, 5th ed, Van Nostrand Reinhold, 1976.

Gray P: *Encyclopedia of Biological Sciences*, 2nd ed, Van Nostrand Reinhold, 1970.
Considine DM: *The Encyclopedia of Chemistry*, 4th ed, Van Nostrand Reinhold.
Kirk RE, Othmer DF: *Encyclopedia of Chemical Technology*, vols 1–12, 3rd ed, Wiley, 1978–1980.
McGraw-Hill Encyclopedia of Science and Technology, 15 vols, 5th ed, McGraw, 1982.

Dictionaries—No reference work is better known and more familiar in form to the student than the dictionary. Pharmacy students should have in their personal library, in addition to a current abridged dictionary such as *Webster's New Collegiate Dictionary* (rev ed, Merriam-Webster, 1977), a medical dictionary, preferably illustrated. Selection may be made from

Blakiston's Gould Medical Dictionary, 4th ed, McGraw-Hill, 1979.
Critchley M, ed: *Butterworths Medical Dictionary*, 2nd unabr ed, Butterworth, 1980.
Dorland's Illustrated Medical Dictionary, 26th ed, Saunders.
Dox I, Melloni BJ, and Eisner, GM: *Mellon's Illustrated Medical Dictionary*, Williams & Wilkins, 1979.
Stedman's Medical Dictionary, 24th ed, Williams & Wilkins, 1981.

Of special interest to graduate students preparing to pass a foreign language examination are the translating dictionaries such as the DeVries' works *German-English Science Dictionary* and *French-English Science Dictionary*. An example of a more ambitious translating dictionary is *Steinbichler's Lexikon für die Apothekenpraxis in sieben Sprachen* (*Steinbichler's Seven Language Dictionary for the Pharmaceutical Practice*, Govi-Verlag GmBH, 1967) with equivalent pharmaceutical terms in German, English, French, Spanish, Italian, Greek, and Russian.

Other dictionaries which should be familiar to pharmacists are:

Buckingham J et al., eds: *Dictionary of Organic Compounds*, 7 vols, 5th ed, Methuen Inc., 1982.
Haensch G, Haberkamp De Anton G: *Dictionary of Biology*, 2nd ed, Elsevier, 1981.
Hawley GG: *The Condensed Chemical Dictionary*, 10th ed, Van Nostrand Reinhold, 1981.
Steen EB: *Abbreviations in Medicine*, 4th ed, Saunders, 1978.
Steen EB: *Dictionary of Biology*, Barnes & Noble, 1975.
USAN and the USP Dictionary of Drug Names, 21st ed US Pharmacopeial Conv Inc, 1984. See also Chapter 26.

Handbooks—A handbook is a compilation of facts and figures in a form which can be consulted with ease, usually a one-volume work. Frequently, the information and scientific data which they contain are in tabular form for easy reference. Other titles applied to works of this kind are *manual, data book, reference book, companion, benchbook, sourcebook, tables*, or *vade mecum*.

Handbooks are a convenient and practical source of quantitative, quick-reference, reliable information. They are revised and updated often to insure that the data are authoritative and current.

Examples of handbooks are:

Bailey AE, et al., eds: *Tables of Physical and Chemical Constants*, 14th ed, Longman, 1973.
Berkow R, ed: *Merck Manual of Diagnosis and Therapy*, 14th ed, Merck, 1982.
Buchanan RE, Gibbons NE: *Bergey's Manual of Determinative Bacteriology*, 8th ed, Williams & Wilkins, 1974.
Condon EW, Odishaw H, eds: *Handbook of Physics*, 2nd ed, McGraw-Hill, 1967.
Knoben JE, et al., eds: *Handbook of Clinical Drug Data*, 4th ed, Drug Intl Pubns, 1979.
Ritschel WA: *Handbook of Basic Pharmacokinetics*, 2nd ed, Drug Intl Pubns, 1980.
Weast RC: *Handbook of Chemistry and Physics*, 63rd ed, Chemical Rubber Co., 1982.

Directories and Yearbooks—Directories are lists of names and addresses which serve to supply information about persons, organizations, or places. These lists are updated with

regularity and, if revised annually, the title frequently uses the term *yearbook*.

There are trade and industrial directories, directories of individuals such as scientists and technologists, and directories of scientific, technological, and professional associations.

Hayes EN: *Hayes' Druggist Directory*, 1983 ed, Hayes, 1983.

The yearbooks included in the list below are annual surveys of events related to the pharmaceutical or allied sciences. These basically are review publications which provide a retrospective look at advances or accomplishments of the previous year in a particular field or on a specific subject. They usually have such titles as "Advances of . . . ," "Progress in . . . ," "Annual Review of . . . ," etc. Some are published at time intervals other than annually.

Bean HS, et al., eds: *Advances in Pharmaceutical Sciences*, vol 5, Academic, 1982.
Creger WP, et al., eds: *Annual Review of Medicine*, Annual Reviews, annual.
Elliott HW, et al., eds: *Annual Review of Pharmacology*, Annual Reviews, annual.
Ellis GP, West GB: *Progress in Medicinal Chemistry*, vol 18, Elsevier, 1981.
Garattini S, et al.: *Advances in Pharmacology and Chemotherapy*, vol 19, Academic, 1982.
Harper NJ, Simmons AB, eds: *Advances in Drug Research*, vol 12, Academic, 1978.
Hess HJ, ed: *Annual Reports in Medicinal Chemistry*, vol 17, Academic, 1983.
Hollister LE, Shand DG, eds: *Year Book of Drug Therapy*, Year Bk Med, annual.
Jucker E: *Progress in Drug Research*, vol 26, Brikhauser, 1982.
Snell EE, et al., eds: *Annual Review of Biochemistry*, vol 52, Annual Reviews, 1983.

Pharmacopeias and Formularies

Books of standards for drugs and devices, known as pharmacopeias and formularies, are collectively referred to as the *drug compendia*.

A *pharmacopeia* or a *formulary* is a book containing a list of medicinal substances (drugs) and/or articles (devices) with descriptions, tests, and formulas for preparing the same, selected by some *recognized authority*. The recognized authority which issues the books of standards in most countries is governmental, but in the US both the national pharmacopeia and the national formulary have been published by private organizations.

Official Compendia—The drug compendia are subclassified as *official* or *nonofficial*. The former are those compilations of drugs and devices which have been recognized as legal standards of purity, quality, and strength by a governmental agency of the country of origin. In the US legal recognition of drug standards did not occur until 1906 when the congress enacted the first Food and Drug Act. With the passage of this law, both *The United States Pharmacopeia*, published originally in 1820 under the authority of the United States Pharmacopeial Convention (an independent, nonprofit organization incorporated in 1900) and *The National Formulary*, established in 1888 under the auspices of the American Pharmaceutical Association, received full legal recognition by the US government. The fact that both the USP and the NF have been published by private initiative but have had the impact of law made these books unique.

In July 1974 the American Pharmaceutical Association and the United States Pharmacopeial Convention announced that the latter group had purchased *The National Formulary* from the APhA. The APhA carried through with publication of the 1975 edition of the formulary but the USP Convention assumed responsibility for supplements to the 1975 issue and for other services such as the NF Reference Standard Program and associated laboratory services.

Sonnedecker[5] has provided a complete account of the origin and development of each book. Through 1975, the history of the USP has been printed in abstract in each revision and the history of the NF has been published in more detail in each edition. Briefly, whereas the USP was originally published and revised by physicians, with pharmacists gaining a stronghold only with the 1883 (6th) revision, the NF was always a project of pharmacy. The periodic revision of each compendium has been possible only with the cooperation, support, and assistance of the pharmaceutical, the medical, and the other health professions.

Revisions of both compendia occurred at 10-year intervals through 1940, when both sponsoring authorities invoked a plan of continuous revision wherein a new book was published every five years. The USP is published as revisions; thus, the 20th revision, official in 1980, was the 21st pharmacopeia. The NF was published as editions; thus, the 15th and last edition of the NF (official in 1980) was the 15th formulary.

The USP and the NF, during their concurrent years of publication, cooperated to fulfill their mutual objective: the provision of standards which serve as the basic measures of strength, quality, purity, packaging, and labeling of drugs to ensure that the American public receives pharmaceutical products of uniform and consistent quality and strength. Committees on scope and admission, composed both of pharmacists and of physicians, selected the drugs and articles to be included in each book, guided by principles guaranteeing the therapeutic value of the selected medicinal agents and devices. For details concerning the revision process and other information relative to the structure, the format, and the general principles which guide the revision process, the reader is referred to the most recent copy of each book.

Foreign Pharmacopeias and Formularies—Pharmacopeias and formularies are generally national in origin and scope. Among the foreign English-language compendia with which the American student or practitioner of pharmacy should be familiar are:

British Pharmacopoeia 2 vols, 2nd ed, Pharm Soc Great Britain, 1980; addendum, 1983.
British National Formulary, Pharm Soc Great Britain, 1983.
The Pharmaceutical Codex (incorporating the British Pharmaceutical Codex), 11th ed, Pharm Press, 1979.

There have been hopes that a supranational pharmacopeia could be authorized and published which would serve to consolidate drug standards. In 1951 the World Health Organization (WHO) published the *Pharmacopoeia Internationalis* (PhI), a compilation in two volumes (vol 2, 1955; suppl, 1959) designed as a collection of standards which could serve as references for the establishment of international standards. A second edition of this work, *Specifications for the Quality Control of Pharmaceutical Preparations*, was published in 1967. The third edition will appear in five volumes; vol 1 was published in 1979 and vol 2 in 1981. Because the initiating authority (WHO) does not have official jurisdiction in any country, these standards do not have legal status in any country and there remains a need for a compendium which is a legal and binding authority.

To meet this need, a Council of Europe was established in 1964 and included seven countries whose Council of Ministries adopted a resolution to establish a European pharmacopeia. The seven countries which signed the document and thereby made the proposed pharmacopeia legal and binding for all were Belgium, France, the Federal Republic of Germany, Italy, Luxembourg, The Netherlands, and the United Kingdom. Later, Switzerland was accepted as the eighth member

of the European Pharmacopoeial Commission which began in 1964 to prepare a European pharmacopoeia. The initial work, *European Pharmacopoeia*, vol 1, was published in 1969. Volume 2 appeared in 1971, a supplement was offered in 1973, and vol 3 was published in 1975 (Pharm. Press, London). *European Pharmacopoeia, Nineteen Eighty to Eighty-two, Part 1*, 2nd ed, was published by Maisonneuve France in 1980.

Nonofficial Drug Compendia—Secondary reference sources not subject to categorization in the preceding sections are textbooks, treatises, and monographs, which are often referred to as books in the field (or discipline). There are subtle but recognizable differences among these three forms.

The *treatise* is a comprehensive, exhaustive, systematic, sometimes critical approach to a broad topic or to a whole field of knowledge. A treatise is extensively documented and generally is written for the specialist.

The *monograph*, by contrast, is a written account of a single topic. The monograph usually includes recent information, and there is an attempt to be systematically comprehensive without including background and historical data such as would be found in a treatise. The monograph, too, may be documented.

The *textbook* serves the prime function of presenting the principles of a topic or discipline in such a way that the information is used as the basis for instruction in the subject. Because authors of textbooks have the privilege of selecting those principles which they wish to include in the book, textbooks are written at different levels of sophistication and comprehension. Also, because textbooks concentrate on principles rather than on the details of last-minute developments in a field, they may be useful over a long period of time and require only infrequent revision. Documentation is generally an important part of the textbook.

A variation on the basic textbook is the programmed or self-instructional text. Although relatively rare as yet in pharmacy, there are such texts available in the areas of pharmaceutical calculations and medical terminology.

The textbooks a pharmacy student acquires during the collegiate program should serve as the basis of a collection for a personal drug information library. If the student adds to this primary collection by careful selection of new books as they come to the market and if the student replaces older editions of textbooks at regular intervals, he can build a personal library which is useful to him in his role as drug information specialist. The following list can serve as a guide in developing a reference collection of drug information sources:

Accepted Dental Therapeutics (Am Dent Assoc), a compilation of the Council on Dental Therapeutics of the American Dental Association, is intended as a handbook on dental therapeutics. The editions include information on drugs of recognized value in dentistry, drugs of recent origin whose value in dentistry has not been established, and older drugs which may still be in use but whose value is considered questionable. There are sections on the general principles of medication, on therapeutic aids, and on therapeutic guides. The book is indexed.

AMA Drug Evaluations (5th ed, Publ Sci Group, Inc, 1983) is a comprehensive listing by therapeutic classifications of both old and new single-entity drugs and combinations. The original evaluations were prepared by the medical profession and ". . . may be favorable, unfavorable, or both, depending on the merits of the preparation." Each therapeutic classification is introduced by a general statement, and the information given for each drug listed includes an appraisal, actions and uses, adverse reactions, contraindications, dosage, routes of administration, and the available preparations, with their sizes, strengths, known sources of supply, and trade or brand names. This publication indexes by trade name as well as by generic name and includes structural formulas for some single-entity drugs.

American Drug Index (Lippincott), published annually, is prepared as an alphabetical listing of single-entity and combination drugs cross-referenced by generic, brand, and chemical names. The cross-referencing feature allows one to find combinations of drugs if only one ingredient is known. The monographs list the name of the product, the manufacturer,

---

* The preferred spelling in the US now eliminates the diphthong oe and uses the simplified spelling. In other countries, however, the diphthong is still used.

the use and the dosage, the dosage forms available, and their size and strength.

American Druggist Blue Book (Hearst Corp), an annual price list of drug products and devices, giving for each item its manufacturer, its National Drug Code (if any), the available sizes, and the wholesale and retail prices. The listing is alphabetical by trade and generic name. Additional information in the book includes: a product identification guide in color; a controlled substances manual; professional product information; a manufacturers' index; and tables of various information. A supplement limited mainly to prescription and health-related products is issued in October. Computerized product and price information is available.

American Hospital Formulary Service (ASHP) is a single bound volume of both old and new single-entity and combination drugs with three bound supplements per year; the listing is by pharmacologic action and therapeutic indications; the information includes nonproprietary and/or trade names; the structural formula and the systematic chemical name; chemical and physical properties of the product; the mode of action, when known; therapeutic indications, side effects, cautions, and contraindications; dosage and use; and dosage forms available.

Clin-Alert (Sci Eds, Inc) is a unique abstract service which provides current information on drug reactions, drug interactions, and related therapeutic hazards. Published semimonthly, the information is collected from leading medical journals. Quarterly cumulative indexes and a special binder are provided to subscribers. Back issues from 1962 are available singly or as hardbound volumes, and there is a five-year cumulative index (1977–1981).

Drug Topics Red Book (Medical Economics), promoted as the pharmacist's guide to products and prices, is an annual price list of drug products, giving their manufacturer, available sizes and strengths, and wholesale and retail prices. The listing is alphabetized by trade and by generic name, plus a list of products by manufacturer. Additional information in the book includes: emergency procedures; a pharmacists' reference section; drug interactions; product identification (full-color and size reproductions of selected dosage forms); manufacturers' catalogs; and a list of manufacturers. Supplements are provided.

Drug Interactions (4th ed, Hansten PD, Lea & Febiger, 1979) is a guide to drug-drug interactions and to the effects of drugs on clinical laboratory results, presented in a form which makes the data easily accessible and convenient to use. The entries are extensively supplied with citations from the primary literature. The two divisions of the book are a section dealing with drug-drug interactions covering 10 specific pharmacologic groups of drugs and a miscellaneous section; part two deals with the effects of drugs on laboratory tests and describes effects of drugs on 15 types of blood, serum, or plasma tests, 12 types of urine tests, and a miscellaneous group of tests. In the index the interactions are categorized as being of major, moderate, or minor clinical significance.

Drugs in Current Use and New Drugs (Modell W, Springer Publ Co) is an annual alphabetical listing by generic name of drugs commonly used or referred to in the literature with cross-references to trade and chemical names. The monographs indicate actions and uses, warnings, administration, preparations available, and antidotes against poisoning when these are available.

Facts and Comparisons (Boyd JR, Kastrup EK, Facts & Comparisons, Inc.), a useful, looseleaf publication, is a constantly updated service wherein the products are grouped according to use rather than being listed alphabetically or by manufacturer. This arrangement permits easy comparison of related products. Much of the information is presented in a tabular format which also facilitates comparison of products. Pertinent data are presented on actions, indications, warnings, interactions, contraindications, precautions, adverse reactions, prescribing, and dosage. A unique feature is a cost index, a wholesale cost ratio between two or more comparable products. An alphabetical index is included. Monthly revision pages are available. In 1977 the drug information in *Facts and Comparisons* was made available also in microfiche format, and in 1978 a bound, hard-cover book was published.

Handbook of Non-Prescription Drugs (7th ed, APhA, 1982) is a handbook which contains 32 chapters dealing with specific classes of home remedies. There are charts and tables which give the formulas for over 1500 different over-the-counter products. There are a product index and a cross-referenced index of manufacturers.

Merck Index (10th ed, Merck & Co, Inc, 1983) is an encyclopedia which lists approximately 10,000 single-entity chemicals; approximately 8000 structural or line formulas are given. The alphabetical listing includes the chemical name, other names, chemical formula, chemical activity, medical and other uses, literature references, dosage, and veterinary use, if any. A cross-referenced index contains more than 60,000 listings, including brand names.

Merck Manual of Diagnosis and Therapy (2 vols, 14th ed, Berkow, R, ed, Merck, 1982) is a handbook used often as a textbook and designed primarily to assist medical practitioners. The format is an alphabetical arrangement of general disease categories in sections with chapters related to specific conditions within the general category. Volume 1 covers general medicine, and volume 2 is devoted to obstetrics, gynecology, pediatrics, and genetics. There is a section on prescriptions with a representative selection of drugs. The prescriptions are classified therapeutically according to the system devised by the American Society of Hospital Pharmacists. A comprehensive index is provided.

Modern Drug Encyclopedia and Therapeutic Index (16th ed, Yorke, 1981) is a compendium of pharmaceutical data arranged in an alphabetical listing by generic drug name or by the primary ingredient of combination products; multiple combination products are listed under their trade names. The monographs stress nomenclature, descriptions, indications, contraindications, dosage and administration, trade names, dosage forms available, and manufacturers. There are three indexes: therapeutic, manufacturers', and general. Supplements to each edition are issued regularly.

National Drug Code Directory, 1982 (USGPO, 1983). Divided into two volumes and four sections, this directory contains the only complete list of drug products marketed in the US.

Pediatric Dosage Handbook (1980 ed, Shirkey HC, APhA), a manual for physicians, dentists, and pharmacists, is intended as a guide to the determination of average or generally recognized doses for children and infants. A general discussion of concepts of pediatric dosage is followed by a table of drugs used in pediatric practice with information on their doses, cautions, contraindications, and available dosage forms.

PharmIndex (Skyline Publ.) is a monthly reference to pharmaceutical products, both old and new, with complete data including costs and prices. There is a four-way cross-indexing of products by trade name, manufacturer, generic composition, and therapeutic use. Investigational drugs not yet on the market are indexed, and articles which review the pharmacology and chemistry of classes of drugs are printed regularly.

Physicians' Desk Reference (Medical Economics) is an annual publication, intended primarily for physicians, providing essential prescription information on major pharmaceutical products as prepared by the manufacturers in consultation with a medical consultant. The color-coded sections of the book are: a manufacturers' index (white); a product name index (pink); a product category index (blue); a generic and chemical name index (yellow); a product identification section (actual size, full-color reproductions of selected dosage forms and products) (gray); a product information section (white); and diagnostic product information (green). New or revised information is published periodically in supplements.

Remington's Pharmaceutical Sciences (17th ed., Mack Publ. Co., 1985), the most comprehensive work in the area of the pharmaceutical sciences, is a textbook revised every 5 years. First published in 1886, the volumes are encyclopedic in their coverage of the pharmaceutical sciences and are well illustrated. The book is indexed adequately.

United States Pharmacopeia Dispensing Information, 1983, 2 vols (US Pharmacopeial Conv, 1982). Volume I contains drug information for the health care provider; volume II contains advice for the patient. Monographs for drugs are listed alphabetically by established name or by family group. Monographs directed to patient information correspond directly to those in the health provider section. An annual publication updated bimonthly through *USP DI Update.*

Other books which should be considered in building a reference library include:

Arena JM: *Poisoning: Toxicology-Symptoms-Treatment*, 4th ed, Thomas, 1979.

Brobeck JR, ed: *Best & Taylor's Physiological Basis of Medical Practice*, 10th ed, Williams & Wilkins, 1979.

Goodman LS, Gilman A: *The Pharmacological Basis of Therapeutics*, 6th ed, Macmillan, 1980.

Gosselin R, *et al: Clinical Toxicology of Commercial Products*, 4th ed, Williams & Wilkins, 1976.

Hartshorn EA, ed: *Drug Interactions Update 1982*, ASHP, 1983.

Hassan WE, Jr.: *Hospital Pharmacy*, 4th ed, Lea & Febiger, 1981.

Hoover JE, ed: *Dispensing of Medication*, 8th ed, Mack Publ. Co., 1976.

Kaluzny EL: *Pharmacy Law Digest: 1980–1981*, Douglas-McKay, 1980.

Martin AN *et al*, eds: *Physical Pharmacy:* Physical Chemical Principles in the Pharmaceutical Sciences, 3rd ed, Lea & Febiger, 1983.

Modell W: *Drugs of Choice, 1982–1983*, Mosby, 1982.

Notari RE: *Biopharmaceutics and Clinical Pharmacokinetics: An Introduction*, 3rd ed, Dekker, 1980.

Rowland M, Tozer TN: *Clinical Pharmacokinetics: Concepts and Applications*, Lea & Febiger, 1980.

Shirkey HC: *Pediatric Drug Handbook*, Saunders, 1977.

Smith MC, Knapp DA: *Pharmacy, Drugs and Medical Care*, 3rd ed, Williams & Wilkins, 1981.

Sonnedecker G: *Kremers and Urdang's History of Pharmacy*, 4th ed, Lippincott, 1976.

It is no longer uncommon for the pharmacist even in the most interior areas of the US to receive prescriptions written in a foreign country. The mobility with which American citizens move about the world and the constantly increasing travel of people of all nationalities make all pharmacists potential recipients of prescriptions for drugs not common in this country. The following reference sources are of help in identifying foreign drug products. (See also Chapter 103).

Compendium of Pharmaceuticals and Specialties, 17th ed, Can PhA, 1982.

Index Nominum 1982, 11th ed, Swiss Pharm Soc, 1983.

Negwer M: *Organic-Chemical Drugs and Their Synonyms*, Drug Intl Pubns, 1984.

Reynolds JEF, ed: *Martindale: The Extra Pharmacopoeia*, 28th ed, Pharm. Press, 1982.

Index and Abstract Services

Index Services—When one considers the vast collection of books and periodicals identified or implied in the foregoing discussions and when one considers the steady increase in the annual volume of the scientific literature, the thought of embarking on a literature search is intimidating. Fortunately, tools have been devised to facilitate information retrieval.

Responsible periodicals, as books, are indexed, usually on a volume-year basis. They may include a separate author index and an index of titles of articles or of subjects and titles. The periodical indexes often are cumulated to cover a period of years, frequently a 10-year span (decennial index).

There are, however, journals which do not provide an index. For these periodicals, and for those which do index, there are *index services* available which provide annual and/or cumulated indexes for a group of periodicals, sometimes running into the thousands of titles, usually related to a particular field or discipline.

Index services are used to locate a given article, the writings of a particular author, or material on a given topic. Therefore, to be adequate, an index service must be accurate, must index topics according to subject headings which are in current usage, and must be devised to reduce to a minimum the time lag between the publication of an article and the appearance of the reference in an index. Lastly, the index service must be comprehensive. One of the dangers of index services is that material may not get into the index, thus denying certain information to those who seek it.

The information available from an index is limited to bibliographic references: the title of the article and the author(s), the title of the periodical in which the article is printed with the volume, the page(s), and the date of publication.

There is no index service available which is exclusively for the pharmaceutical sciences. A service which is of use to pharmacy is *Index Medicus*, the only national index service covering the life sciences. The current index is a continuation of one which began in 1879; since 1960 it has been published by the National Library of Medicine. Published monthly, the index is arranged alphabetically by authors and by subject headings. The monthly issue contains references to more than 20,000 journal articles cited under one or more of 7500 index terms as well as the names of the authors. More than 2700 selected biomedical journals are the source of the cited articles. The monthly issues are cumulated annually in *Cumulated Index Medicus*.

Index Medicus publishes annually under the title "Medical Subject Headings" (MeSH) a controlled list of those subject headings used to reference the articles it indexes. Researchers should construct their own list of search keywords, phrases, or topical headings in accord with the MeSH thesaurus in order to be efficient and accurate in their search.

The *Bibliography of Medical Reviews* is included in *Index Medicus*. It contains many review articles selected from periodicals regularly indexed in *Index Medicus*. Annual and multiyear cumulations are published separately.

Abridged Index Medicus is a bibliographical service available also from the National Library of Medicine's computerized store of data. It cites articles from more than 100 key English-language journals in clinical medicine. An annual cumulation is available.

Beginning in 1958, the Institute for Scientific Information located in Philadelphia began publication of a weekly magazine known as *Current Contents*. Today, the publication is issued in six editions covering agriculture, biology, and the environmental sciences; the behavioral and social sciences; engineering, technology, and applied sciences; the physical, chemical, and earth sciences; the life sciences; and clinical practice. The last two sections are of special interest in the pharmaceutical sciences.

Current Contents/Life Sciences reproduces the tables of contents from more than 1100 journals concerned with medicine, physiology, pharmacology, biochemistry, microbiology, and therapeutics. Each weekly issue contains a subject index and an author index with an address directory to facilitate the ordering of reprints. Also available is a service (OATS—*Original Article Text Service*) which allows the Institute to supply on request from a patron either a photocopy of or the actual article cut from the original journal.

Current Contents/Clinical Practice reproduces the tables of contents from more than 790 journals covering the practice of medicine and the allied health sciences, some of which are also included in *Current Contents/Life Sciences*.

Other services available from the Institute for Scientific Information which are of assistance to pharmaceutical researchers are:

Science Citation Index is a multidisciplinary index covering more than 3000 journals of the scientific literature. It is published six times a year and is cumulated annually and at 5-year intervals. The four indexes included are: (1) the author index, also called the *Source Index*; (2) the *Citation Index*, an alphabetical list of authors whose works were cited in the source items; (3) the *Permuterm Subject Index* which gives access to each source item by pairing the significant words from the item's title; and (4) the *Corporate Index*, a collection of current authors under the name of their organizations. An *Abridged Edition* which indexes more than 500 journals is also available.

Pharmaceutical News Index is a monthly, looseleaf citation providing access to information from pharmaceutical, cosmetics, and medical devices newsletters and special publications. It is the exclusive index for five FDC publications. The index is available from the Database Company of Louisville, KY.

ADIS Publications. Inpharma, *Reactions*, and *Drugs* are authoritative and comprehensive sources reporting on: the current international drug literature; on adverse drug reactions, interactions, drug overdose, and abuse and dependency; and on new and major drug evaluations, respectively. *Inpharma* is published weekly with monthly, semiannual, and annual indexes. *Reactions* is published twice a month and supplies quarterly and annual cumulated indexes. *Drugs* comes out monthly and reports from a database of more than 1500 journals.

Although not an index service in the usual meaning of the term, a useful service to assist pharmacy students and practitioners in the search for new drug information is *Unlisted Drugs*. This monthly listing of new drugs which are not yet in the standard reference sources is published by the Pharmaceutical Section of the Special Libraries Association and is classified as an index because of the literature references which are an integral part of each entry. The lists are arranged systematically by experimental or code numbers and/or by the name of the drug. The information recorded is limited to the composition, action, and dosage of the drug; the manufacturer; and literature references. The monthly issues are indexed semiannually, with the latter index being cumulated.

Abstract Services—The index services have the limitation of supplying only bibliographic information in their citations. Of added value are those citations which in addition to the bibliographic data supply summaries of the articles cited. These publications are known as *abstract services*.

The abstract services must have the qualifications for excellence as mentioned under index services. In addition, the summaries which are published must be accurate and in sufficient detail so that those reading them will know whether it will be worth their time to consult the original article. Also, the abstracts themselves must be indexed properly to provide quick and easy information retrieval. The most familiar form is a journal devoted to abstracts. These serial publications may be produced at any time interval—weekly, biweekly, and monthly being common. The indexes of abstract services are cumulated at varying intervals, eg, semiannually, annually, quinquennially, or decennially.

The abstract services most useful in retrieving information in the pharmaceutical and related sciences are *Biological Abstracts*, *Chemical Abstracts*, *Excerpta Medica*, *International Pharmaceutical Abstracts*, and *Dissertation Abstracts*.

Published since 1926, currently by BioSciences Information Service (BIOSIS), *Biological Abstracts* is a comprehensive abstracting and indexing journal reporting on the world's literature in theoretical and applied biology, *exclusive of clinical medicine*. Five indexes are published in each issue, and these are cumulated semiannually. The five are: (1) author index (personal or corporate names); (2) subject index (specific words); (3) concept index (broad subject concepts); (4) biosystematic index (taxonomic categories); and (5) generic index (genus-species names). In 1978, *Serial Sources for the BIOSIS Data Base* replaced the *BIOSIS List of Serials* as the source of those serials which contribute to the database of all BIOSIS services.

The most comprehensive of all indexing and abstracting services, *Chemical Abstracts*, has been published since 1907 by the American Chemical Society. Issued weekly and including abstracts from more than 11,000 periodicals, this truly is the key to the world's chemical literature. In addition to periodicals, *Chemical Abstracts* covers symposia, dissertations, technical reports, books, pamphlets, and patents. Abstracts are classified according to 80 chemical subject groups. Decennial indexes were prepared during the years 1907–1956; since then, cumulative indexes have been issued quinquennially. An *Index Guide* has been published at approximately 18-month intervals since 1982.

Although published in Amsterdam, *Excerpta Medica*, a comprehensive abstracting service for medicine and the allied health sciences, is printed in English. The service has been available since 1947. The abstracts are issued monthly in sections; the number of sections has increased regularly over the years as the life sciences have expanded; currently (1983) there are 43 sections. Many libraries will subscribe only to those sections which are useful to students, teachers, or researchers in a particular specialty, eg, endocrinology, pediatrics, ophthalmology, hematology, etc. There are author and subject indexes in each issue, and these are cumulated on an annual basis.

Excerpta Medica also publishes *Adverse Reactions Titles* and the *Drug Literature Index*. The former is a monthly indexed bibliography of the biomedical literature reporting adverse reactions or similar side effects caused by drugs or other biologically active compounds. The latter is issued twice a month and is a bibliography of all articles reviewed by Excerpta Medica and which contain a significant mention of drugs and other biologically active substances.

The most recent of the abstracting/indexing services and the one directed specifically to the pharmaceutical sciences is *International Pharmaceutical Abstracts*. The publication was started in 1964 and is sponsored by the American Society of Hospital Pharmacists. Described as the key to the world's literature of pharmacy, the journal is published twice a month. A subject index is included in each abstract issue. Cumulative subject and author indexes are published twice annually. A three-year (1978–1980) cumulative subject and author index is available. A second three-year index was planned for 1983.

Arranged under 25 controlled subject headings, nearly 6000 abstracts are printed annually from a list of more than 470 pharmaceutical, medical, and related journals published around the world. In 1970 the publication went to a computerized abstracting and indexing system, and in 1973 the IPA Information System was introduced, making available a variety of printed, microform, and computerized services to patrons from the automated data bank of *International Pharmaceutical Abstracts*. The IPA database is available online through Lockheed's DIALOG, the National Library of Medicine's TOXLINE, and the Bibliographic Retrieval Services (see next section).

An often overlooked source of information from the primary literature are the dissertations and theses required by most universities of candidates for graduate degrees. While it is true that much of value from these sources is often published later in the established research journals and thus appears in the popular abstract/index services, many dissertations are not published.

In an effort to bring these sources to the attention of potential users and to make them more accessible, University Microfilms of Ann Arbor, MI, publishes *Dissertation Abstracts*. This is a monthly compilation of abstracts of doctoral dissertations from more than 160 cooperating universities and colleges in the US and Canada. The abstracts, prepared by the authors, are available either on microfilm or as photocopies and are published in two sections; section B is devoted to the sciences and engineering.

The titles are arranged under broad subject headings, and there are annual author and subject indexes.

The theses have been placed in a computer file, and searches of the more than 130,000 theses dating back to 1938 may be requested. The automated system is called DATRIX (Direct Access to Reference Information).

Computerized Retrieval Services

Computerized Retrieval Services—The enormous task of indexing and abstracting the world's scientific literature would have become physically impossible had it not been for the development of the computer. The mechanization of the extracting, classifying, and storing of the literature has made possible the fast and accurate retrieval of information.

The first computerized national bibliographic service was initiated in 1964 by the National Library of Medicine. The system, MEDLARS (*Med*ical *L*iterature *A*nalysis and *R*etrieval *S*ystem), was developed to achieve rapid bibliographic access to the library's collection of biomedical information. Persons studying or working in the health sciences now have online access, using computer terminals, to the literature by means of this computerized system. Based on a computer at the National Library of Medicine in Bethesda, MD, MEDLARS is available through a nationwide telephone-based communications network to users in more than 1900 universities, medical schools, hospitals, government agencies, and commercial organizations. It is also available in a number of foreign countries.

MEDLARS contains some 6,000,000 references to journal articles and books in the health sciences published after 1965. Most of these references have been published via MEDLARS in *Index Medicus* or in other printed NLM indexes and bibliographies. This same computer system also makes it possible for an individual user to search the store of references and to produce a list of them pertinent to a specific question.

References may be retrieved by searching on one or a combination of the 14,000 designated Medical Subject Headings (MeSH) used by NLM in indexing and cataloging materials. It is also possible to search for references by using words appearing in titles and abstracts. The ability of the computer to search rapidly through a large number of references to determine which meet the specified criteria results in an individualized bibliography that would not be possible except by the most laborious and time-consuming manual search.

The requestor may ask that the complete record be printed out for each reference retrieved—including the subject headings and abstract—or that a less detailed format include only the elements necessary to locate the item: author, title, and publication source.

There are some 20 online databases available through MEDLARS; among these are:

MEDLINE, which contains approximately 800,000 references to biomedical journal articles published in the current and three preceding years. An English abstract, if published with the article, is frequently included. The articles are obtained from 3000 journals published in the US and foreign countries. Coverage of previous periods (back to 1966) is provided by backfiles searchable online that total some 3,500,000 references. MEDLINE can also be used to update a search periodically. The search formulation is stored in the computer and each month, when new references are added to the database, the search is processed automatically and the results mailed from NLM.

TOXLINE (TOXicology Information OnLINE) is a bibliographic database covering the pharmacological, biochemical, physiological, environmental, and toxicological effects of drugs and other chemicals. Almost all references in TOXLINE have abstracts and/or indexing terms and Chemical Abstracts Service (CAS) Registry Numbers. The TOXLINE database contains more than 1.4 million references. TOXLINE contains recent references, while older information is available in the backfiles.

CHEMLINE is an online chemical dictionary with more than 500,000 records. It contains chemical names, synonyms, CAS Registry Numbers, molecular formulas, NLM file locators, and limited ring structure information. CHEMLINE assists the user in searching the other MEDLARS databases by providing synonyms and CAS Registry Numbers, the use of which can significantly increase retrieval in those databases. CHEMLINE can also be searched to locate classes of chemical substances.

RTECS is an online, interactive version of the National Institute of Occupational Safety and Health (NIOSH) publication, *Registry of Toxic Effects of Chemical Substances*. It contains basic acute and chronic toxicity data for more than 60,000 potentially toxic chemicals. Records include toxicity data, chemical identifiers, exposure standards, and status under various federal regulations and programs. The file can be searched by chemical identifiers, type of effect, or other criteria.

TDB (Toxicology Data Bank) is composed of approximately 4000 comprehensive, peer-reviewed records describing chemical substances. It contains toxicological, pharmacological, environmental, occupational, manufacturing, and use information, as well as chemical and physical properties. Compounds selected for description in TDB include regulated chemicals, high volume production/exposure chemicals, chemicals found in waste sites, and drugs and pesticides exhibiting high toxicity potential.

AVLINE (AudioVisuals OnLINE) contains citations to more than 11,000 audiovisual teaching packages covering a wide range of subject areas in the health sciences. In some cases, review data such as rating, audience levels, instructional design, specialties, and abstracts are included. Procurement information on titles is provided.

Private, commercial computerized retrieval systems have been developed and marketed by:

MICROMEDEX, Inc, Englewood, CO. The *Drugdex* system is a computer-generated microfiche information system which makes available consultations regarding drug therapy to subscribers to the system. The database, which consists of drug evaluations and drug consults, is accessed by generic products, brand/trade name products, disease state, pharmacologic class, and organ system. In answer to specific drug and disease state inquiries, the system provides consultation reports (drug consults) suitable for inclusion in a patient's chart. Drug evaluations contain information on dosage, pharmacokinetics, contraindications, precautions, adverse reactions, drug interactions, IV incompatibilities, clinical applications, therapeutic indications, comparative efficacy, and patient instructions. The data are referenced to the primary sources of information.

MICROMEDEX also publishes *Emergindex*, a system designed to provide users with group professional opinions on current topics in acute care medicine, including arrhythmia managements, clinical reviews, differential reviews, emergency techniques, clinical abstracts, and prehospital care.

Poisindex is an emergency information system also offered by MICROMEDEX, Inc. The system provides ingredient information on more than 300,000 commercial, pharmaceutical, industrial, and botanical items. Information on management of a poison includes symptoms, pharmacology, toxicology, and treatment procedures.

deHaen Systems. A specialized, computerized retrieval service of interest to individuals or organizations involved in pharmacy education, drug information centers, and pharmaceutical research and marketing is the deHaen line of drug information systems and publications. Produced and marketed by Paul deHaen International, Inc. of Englewood, CO, the deHaen systems provide a comprehensive indexing and abstracting of the world's drug-related literature. Instead of the commonly used format of an author's and/or narrative abstract, the deHaen systems provide standardized, structured excerpts from the literature. Important and relevant predetermined data elements are extracted from the literature reviewed. The deHaen systems include reports from more than 1000 national and international journals.

The four major deHaen drug information systems are currently available on computer generated microfiche and, in addition, will soon be available in online computer format. A brief description of each of the four systems follows:

Drugs in Prospect. This system provides reports of newly synthesized compounds exhibiting some type of pharmacological activity. The system is published bimonthly on computer-generated microfiche and monthly as a paper publication called *Early Awareness.* On an annual basis, between 1500 and 2000 reports are published. The system includes a comprehensive, cumulative index.

Drugs in Research. This system provides reports of investigational drugs involved both in preclinical and clinical studies. The group of drugs involved in clinical studies is limited to those drugs which have not received marketing approval in the US from the FDA. The system is published bimonthly on computer-generated microfiche. Between 8000 and 10,000 reports are published annually. The system includes a comprehensive, cumulative index.

Drugs in Use. This system provides reports of drugs involved in clinical studies, regardless of the world marketing status of the drugs. The system is published quarterly on computer generated microfiche. Between 6000 and 8000 reports are published annually, and the system has a comprehensive, cumulative index.

ADRIS provides reports of adverse drug reactions and drug interactions as excerpted from clinical studies of investigational and approved drugs. The system is published quarterly on computer generated microfiche. ADRIS is provided as a cumulative (since 1980) database and thus contains more then 10,000 reports. Approximately 3000 new reports are added each year and added to the cumulative index.

deHaen also markets print publications as follows:

Nonproprietary Name Index, a comprehensive and cumulative index of drugs introduced in the US since 1941 and in major foreign countries since 1969. The information is cross-indexed for rapid access and extensive referencing.

New Product Survey is divided into two components. The annual component provides a five-year summary of newly marketed drugs worldwide, and the monthly component provides information on newly marketed drugs on a more current basis.

New Drug Analysis-USA. This annual publication provides a five-year analysis of new drugs introduced in the US, including information on marketing statistics, trends, and other projections.

New Drug Analysis-Europe and Japan, an annual publication, provides a five-year analysis of new drugs introduced in major European countries and Japan.

Bibliographic Retrieval Services. This online search service has more than 50 database files available to users. The science/medicine files include MEDLINE, International Pharmaceutical Abstracts, and those of BioSciences Information Service, Chemical Abstracts, and the National Technical Information Service. In addition to the online search capability, the system offers private database services; automatic, monthly update information; and a service which provides online access to the *Abridged Index Medicus.*

Dialog Information Services, Inc. This subsidiary of the Lockheed Corporation provides access to more than 170 databases. Among the databases useful to pharmacy are those from BioSciences Information Service, National Technical Information Service, Chemical Abstracts, Institute for Scientific Information, University Microfilms, Pharmaceutical News Index, Excerpta Medica, International Pharmaceutical Abstracts, and the National Library of Medicine. Special services for customers include the opportunity for an automatic search each time a selected file is updated, the opportunity to receive full text of selected documents on line, and the opportunity to use some of the databases in the classroom at special reduced rates.

SDC Search Service. Through the ORBIT Information Retrieval System, access to bibliographic and full-text records are available to users from more than 80 databases. These include those available from Chemical Abstracts, BioSciences Information Service, the US Government Printing Office, and the National Technical Information Service. Full abstracts or summaries of original documents can be received. Automatic updates are also available.

AMA/NET (a part of the GTE Telenet Medical Information Network). This system, a cooperative venture between the American Medical Association and the GTE Corporation, originally featured four databases: Drug Information, Disease Information, Socioeconomic Bibliographic Information, and Medical Procedure Coding and Nomenclature. MED/MAL is an additional feature which permits instant transmission of written messages between subscribers. The drug information base,

online program is a part of a more extensive computerized medical information system titled GTE Telenet Medical Information Network (MINET). The data included in the DIB were extracted solely from *AMA Drug Evaluations.*

The Iowa Drug Information Service is a specialized and unique drug information retrieval program organized in 1965 by the University of Iowa College of Pharmacy. The service is described as "A central repository for an organized body of specialized information relating to drugs and drug therapy . . . and is the input-duplication center and coordinating unit for a network of subscribing institutions."

The subscriber receives on a monthly basis microfilmed articles on microfiche and a set of microfiche indexes pertaining to the drugs and to the disease conditions reported in the articles. All English-language articles concerning drugs and drug therapy published in more than 156 American and foreign pharmaceutical and medical journals are covered by the service.

In addition to the drug or disease condition, the index record lists the title of the article, the authors, the source, the microfilm number of the total article, and *descriptors.* The last are identified as ". . . a term used to describe or define the contents, structure, and results reported in an article. There are 93 descriptor definitions . . . . A maximum of 33 descriptors are assigned to any one article." Computer searches of the data base are available to subscribers on request.

PHARMASCOPE is a monthly digest of pharmaceutical information published by Transpharma, Inc., Huntington Station, NY. Each issue contains one section devoted to scientific data on recently synthesized or discovered drugs. The abstracts also include information on drugs undergoing pharmacologic and/or clinical testing and have citations to the primary sources. A selected list of recent US patents is printed. A second section in each issue has the trade name, composition, indications, administration, and manufacturer's name of each new pharmaceutical product as it is marketed in the US and a listing of recent new drug applications approved by the FDA. A semiannual index is provided.

Computerized retrieval services are expensive to implement and to maintain. While some are supported wholly or are subsidized in part by governmental agencies, users of the systems must pay for the costs of use either on a fee-for-service charge, a computer time charge, a subscription, or a combination of these methods.

In addition to the expense involved in automated retrieval systems, a general limitation is that the search terms used are specific and restricted; hence, certain searches cannot be made and some pertinent references may not be retrieved.

Other Sources

Although the periodical is the main primary source of scientific, technical, and professional information and the book is the principal secondary source, there are other forms of information which provide the latest discoveries, theories, and thoughts of the world's scientists. These include government documents, research reports, and papers presented at conferences and meetings.

As communication media, these items have the advantage of making the contents of the papers and reports immediately available to those who are in attendance at the meeting or who otherwise receive copies of the reports. The disadvantages of such communicative devices are their limited distribution and the difficulty of getting the information into the established indexing/abstracting services.

Government Publications—The US government is probably the world's chief producer of research reports and the world's foremost printer and distributor of technical and scientific information. These activities are carried out through the US Government Printing Office (USGPO) and its Division of Public Documents and through the National Technical Information Service of the Department of Commerce.

Since 1895 the US has made available information on the publications of the various branches, departments, agencies, and bureaus of the federal government.

The *Monthly Catalog of United States Government Publications* contains the titles of publications and instructions for ordering them. Titles included are arranged alphabetically by publishing office. The entries are indexed both monthly and semiannually, and the index includes subject entries, some title entries, the name of the agency issuing the document (if the agency name is used in the title), and the series title, if any. Quinquennial cumulative indexes are also available.

A less comprehensive listing is the *Selected List of United States Government Publications*. Available free from the Superintendent of Documents of the USGPO's Documents Division, the brochure, issued biweekly, gives titles and prices of the more important government publications which are on sale. The entries are annotated to show the scope of each publication.

Those government publications which are distributed at no cost to the public generally are available from the issuing agency. Individuals or corporate bodies may purchase other publications directly from the Superintendent of Documents, from the National Technical Information Service (which is located in Springfield, VA), or from the several retail bookstores operated around the country by the Division of Public Documents. Additionally, more than 1350 US libraries have been designated official depositories for government documents, and these libraries are eligible to receive selected categories of documents on a regular basis.

The National Technical Information Service is ". . . the central source for the public sale of Government-sponsored research and development reports, and other Government analyses prepared by Federal agencies, their contractors or grantees." The agency publishes semimonthly *Government Reports Announcements*, a catalog of reports, analyses, and translations arranged in 22 subject fields. Field 6, Biological and Medical Sciences, includes the subgroups of biochemistry, biology, clinical medicine, microbiology, pharmacology, and toxicology. Field 7 is chemistry. In addition to its print services, NTIS offers a broad selection of computerized and machine-readable services.

Government Reports Index is published concurrently with *Government Reports Announcements* and indexes each issue of the latter by corporate author, subject, personal author, contract number, and accession/report number.

The Library of Congress compiles numerous valuable bibliographies and issues a number of periodical publications of a bibliographical nature, such as *Guide to the World's Abstracting & Indexing Services in Science & Technology*, *Union List of Serials in Libraries of the United States and Canada*, *New Serial Titles* (supplements *Union List of Serials*), and *Directory of Information Resources in the United States*.

A wide variety of other government-generated catalogs, reports, abstracts, and indexes, too numerous to mention here, are also available. Many of these are listed in the *Monthly Catalog*.

Patents—Patents are a source of up-to-date technological and scientific information. Although difficult to use at times because of their length, their complexity, and the peculiarities of the legal terminology in which they are written, these documents often provide the very latest chemical or technical information, data which are not available from any other source.

In the US, as in many other countries, the proper government agency (US Patent Office) issues weekly a list of newly granted patents, in numerical order, with name and subject indexes. The *Official Gazette of the US Patent Office* has been issued continuously since 1872.

As mentioned previously, *Chemical Abstracts* has a patent index and reports new chemical information from the patent literature. Information on how to obtain copies of patents from the US Patent Office is also printed in the first January issue of *Chemical Abstracts*.

Audiovisual Materials—The audiovisual materials available to the health professions in the form of tape and disc recordings, films, filmstrips, film loops, TV tapes, cassettes, etc., are mainly for teaching purposes. These nonprint materials are available from a variety of educational and commercial sources. Frequently not subject to critical review prior to distribution, the quality of these materials has varied greatly.

In an effort to improve the quality and use of these materials, the National Library of Medicine has established in Atlanta, GA, the National Medical Audiovisual Center. The Center acquires and distributes audiovisual materials; consults and assists in the development of audiovisual materials and systems; conducts research, training, and experiments in the production of audiovisual materials; provides reference services in audiovisual technology and information; and in other ways strives to improve the quality and use of learning materials in the health field.

Another problem with audiovisual materials is that the bibliographical aids to such materials are limited. Film distribution companies, industrial and manufacturing companies, and some libraries maintain catalogs of films and other audiovisual materials which they distribute, but these are widely scattered and difficult to correlate.

The Library of Congress issues quarterly as a special part of the comprehensive *Library of Congress Catalogs* the catalog titled *Motion Pictures and Filmstrips* which is arranged alphabetically by title with a subject index. See also the reference to AVLINE under *Computerized Retrieval Systems*.

References

1. Sonnedecker G. *Kremers and Urdang's History of Pharmacy*, 4th ed, Lippincott, Philadelphia, 287, 1976.
2. Cowen DL. *America's Pre-pharmacopeial Literature*, Am. Inst. Hist. Pharm., Madison, WI, 1961.
3. Grogan D. *Science and Technology, An Introduction to the Literature*, Bingley, London, 14–18, 1970.
4. Hellums BA. *A Manual to the Literature of Pharmacy*, Univ. Miss., University, MS, 35–42, 1968.
5. Sonnedecker G. *Kremers and Urdang's History of Pharmacy*, 4th ed, Lippincott, Philadelphia, Chap. 15, 1976.

CHAPTER 8

Research

William W Bromer PhD

Introduction

Science and technology, at one time accepted as the solution to all of mankind's problems, are being questioned by many groups. In fact, some groups believe that science in the developed countries has progressed too far and too fast, resulting in a decrease rather than an increase in the quality of life. Many governments perceive the necessity for prohibiting and controlling certain types of scientific research. But whatever one's view of science is, one fact is apparent: Society must rely in part on continued scientific research to help alleviate the problems of society and improve the quality of life. Nowhere is this more apparent than in the medical sciences.

One of the main functions of the pharmaceutical industry is to create products. Products are defined as drugs, devices, or services that have a perceived impact on health care systems. This chapter illustrates how biology, the science of life and life processes, can be utilized to develop new products that will fulfill the needs of mankind.

In most instances, products result from a stepwise or evolutionary process based on incremental additions to knowledge or technology or on increased definition of a need. Products of this type can be foreseen to some extent and are amenable to planned research and development. For example, if the cause of a disease has been identified as an infection by a microorganism, a search can be undertaken for an agent that will prevent or cure the infection.

However, in some instances, the etiology of a disease is unknown in spite of intensive investigation. In the latter situation, the pathway to a satisfactory cure or method of prevention cannot be foreseen or forecast. Products in such cases may be developed from careful investigations, from a "revolutionary" new approach, or from a serendipitous finding.

No matter how a pharmaceutical product arises, its development is generally dependent on the vast and growing background of scientific knowledge generated by a diversity of research organizations; universities, private institutes, governmental laboratories, and industrial research all play a highly significant role in developing new knowledge which provides the basis for a new product. This new knowledge may involve improved scientific methodology and instrumentation, increased understanding of a disease state, or significant advances in basic science. In some instances a new potential product may emerge directly from research organizations other than the industrial laboratories.

The Role of Research in Pharmacy and Medicine

A century ago, pioneer women gathered and dried herbs for "doctoring"; a housewife zealously guarded her bag of herbs when her family moved west. Boneset tea reduced fevers, peppermint relieved an aching tooth or a colicky baby, and foxglove was used to revive a failing heart. Even 50 years ago, drug materials were derived only from natural products such as menthol, from peppermint, used for treatment of coughs

and colds. More recently, chemical research on the isolation, identification, and synthesis of drugs has yielded many important drug substances which are both effective and specific.

Until World War I, most synthetic drugs and chemicals used in the US were discovered and produced in Europe. When supplies were curtailed by the war, the impetus was provided for the establishment of an independent chemical and pharmaceutical industry in the US. Accordingly, production of chemicals and drugs was undertaken and was the stimulus for the development of industrial research. In the following years, the US pharmaceutical industry made major contributions through discovery and development of new drugs and assumed a place of leadership in the world.

Discovery and development of the sulfonamides, antibiotics, and other anti-infective agents dramatically reduced the death rates from a number of infectious diseases. A large proportion of the deaths from these diseases occur prior to adulthood; consequently, these lives are lost before the individuals mature and take their places in productive activities. Principally because of the use of drugs, the tuberculosis death rate between 1945 and 1978 has declined from 39 per 100,000 people to 1 per 100,000 people. More recently, acute leukemia, a disease almost always fatal, has achieved a five-year, 50% survival rate by the use of a combination of anticancer drugs.

A number of classes of drugs have marked effects on the quality of life without significantly affecting longevity. Compounds that control pain are illustrative. The development of reliable oral contraceptive therapy has made intelligent family planning possible. Tranquilizers and other central nervous system drugs have made an important contribution to the control of mental diseases and the restoration of mental patients to normal activities. Diuretics and drugs which alleviate arthritis also have improved the quality of life.

Many important examples of the impact of drugs on health and longevity may be cited. Much of the credit can go to research, along with the development, production, and distribution facilities of the pharmaceutical industry. Important contributions, particularly in basic research, also originate in academic and government laboratories. Among the major drugs discovered and/or developed in the US are insulin, sulfa drugs, penicillins and broad-spectrum antibiotics, cortisone and other steroid compounds, isoniazid for the treatment of tuberculosis, diuretics, and the tranquilizers.

Of the 1071 new single-chemical entities introduced as drugs in the US in the period 1940–1981, the US pharmaceutical industry was the country of origin for 681 (64%). Out of approximately 40 therapeutic drug classes, anti-infective (191), cardiovascular (85), hormone (88), and gastrointestinal (68) drugs accounted for more than 40% of the single-chemical entities.

These significant contributions to the national health and welfare have been achieved through effective collaboration of researchers in the biological and physical sciences. The pharmaceutical industry is an outstanding example of successful collaboration between scientists of these disciplines.

* This chapter was revised and updated by Dr John G Adams, VP of The Pharmaceutical Manufactures's Association, retired. His contribution is gratefully acknowledged.

Chemists and other physical scientists have been predominantly responsible for synthesis, isolation, and characterization of medicinal agents. However, the biological scientists have played an equally essential role in originating meaningful screening and testing models and in the overall evaluation of new agents.

Qualified specialists in many fields—pharmacy, physics, statistics, chemistry, biology, engineering, pharmacology, physiology, medicine, and many others—take part in the tremendous research effort in pharmaceuticals. Cooperation is a major feature of today's scientific investigations. Multidisciplinary "teams" are essential in industrial research requiring collaboration and effective communication. Sometimes a hundred or more scientists are involved in developing a compound into a useful drug. The major objective of research in the pharmaceutical industry is to produce safe drugs which prevent, cure, or ameliorate disease. Other important research goals leading to this major objective include:

To understand the molecular bases of biological mechanisms in health and disease.
To develop new biological testing procedures relevant to human medicine.
To develop a quantitative understanding of physical or electronic interactions of drugs with key biological systems, leading to the rational design of drugs.
To understand the absorption, transport, and mode of action of drugs.
To develop drugs of low toxicity, reproducible delivery, and high specificity for a given pathological state.

Research Organizations

The pharmaceutical industry is a leader among all US industries in the support of research and development. A significant portion of every sales dollar is devoted to drug research activities. For instance, US pharmaceutical companies over the years 1967 to 1980 devoted to research and development each year an average of more than 11% of their total US domestic sales revenues.

The industry finances almost all (99%) of its research and development with its own funds; no other industry spends as high a percentage of R&D funds for basic and applied research.

Research expenses in the pharmaceutical industry have grown from $50 million in 1950 to about $1.9 billion in 1980. Planned expenditures for 1982 were well over $2 billion. Scientists and supporting personnel in industrial R & D activities totaled about 2000 in 1940 as compared with more than 25,000 in 1982.

The academic community continues to play a vital role in the development of new drugs. Its role has been in the initial clinical evaluation of new drugs, development of biochemical or physiological rationale for new drug design, basic understanding of disease states, and the training of scientists.

Observations of clinicians often lead to the discovery of new uses for drugs. Chlorpromazine, originally synthesized as an antihistamine, was found to be useful as a tranquilizer. The clinical use of this compound, and of other CNS drugs, has resulted in a marked reduction in the number of the mentally ill needing hospitalization.

Research in the academic community has been supported to a major extent by agencies of the US government, such as the US Public Health Service, the National Institutes of Health, and the National Science Foundation. The pharmaceutical industry also contributes financial support to academic laboratories where research of general or specific interest to the industry is conducted.

Institutes established by government funds or private endowment—such as the Sloan–Kettering Institute, Shrine Children's Hospitals, the National Institutes of Health, and the Centers for Disease Control—pursue basic and applied research in many fields related to the public health. Many hospitals also maintain research clinics and/or privately or publicly endowed foundations to pursue causes and treatment of specific diseases, a related group of diseases, diseases endemic to a certain geographic area, or the group of diseases affecting a certain organ of the body. Since research does not depend on the vending of items or services, it is not immediately self-supportive and must necessarily be supported by public as well as private funds.

The Search for New Drugs

From about the 3rd century BC to the early 20th century most useful drugs—morphine, quinine, digitalis, ergot, atropine, to name a few—were derived from plant sources, and their therapeutic uses were based on ancient serendipitous discoveries. As the abilities of chemists to synthesize, isolate, and characterize new compounds grew and as biologists learned more about the action of drugs and about biological mechanisms in health and disease, the search for new drugs gradually took on a more rational basis. Today, useful drugs arise from natural products, from chemical synthesis, or from combinations of both sources by means of approaches that vary in a complete spectrum between serendipitous discovery and rational synthesis.

Natural Products—Organic chemists and biochemists derive natural products from plant and animal sources; in the latter category microbial and marine organisms are often considered separately from ordinary domestic animals. In addition to the plant alkaloids mentioned earlier, some of the important natural products include antibiotics, steroid and peptide hormones, vitamins, enzymes, prostaglandins, and pheromones. In the search for most natural products serendipity plays a relatively large role, although rational biological inputs based on deficiency syndromes, replacement therapy, or known biological effects clearly influence the development of these drugs. Nutritionists, endocrinologists, pharmacologists, microbiologists, biochemists, physiologists—all play a vital role in understanding the underlying biological mechanisms. Antibiotics, steroids, and prostaglandins provided fertile new fields for chemical modification, leading in all three cases to drugs more useful than the parent compounds.

Synthetic Drugs—Organic chemists in the pharmaceutical industry synthesize hundreds of new compounds every week. In most cases, the chemist has specific reasons for synthesizing a particular compound, usually based on theoretical considerations, medicinal chemistry, biological mechanisms, or a combination of all three.

One of the major factors leading to a more rational approach to new drugs has been improved knowledge of biochemical mechanisms. In the past three decades the biological sciences have undergone a major redirection toward molecular understanding of biological systems. In other words, biology is much more chemically oriented and is slowly becoming more physically oriented. For example, molecular biology, biochemical pharmacology, and molecular pathology are fields of research which were not established a few decades ago. It is important to understand the broad implications of this trend for research in the modern pharmaceutical industry.

As knowledge evolves of the molecular bases for normal and pathological functions, more specific hypotheses also evolve regarding which molecular mechanism may be beneficially controlled by drugs. The search for new drugs still involves a generous measure of serendipity, but a more rational approach has gradually developed. For example, a discovery in basic biological research may lead to a hypothesis that a certain chemical mediator, a particular enzyme, or perhaps a specific receptor plays a key role in a pathological condition.

Candidate drugs are designed and synthesized partly on the basis of known mediators, hormones, metabolites, or substrates. Initial screening of hundreds or perhaps thousands of compounds may be rapidly accomplished by use of *in vitro* enzymatic or receptor test systems. Typically, several unique active lead compounds emerge, which are studied in a variety of biologic systems, either confirming or refuting the original hypothesis. Whether or not a promising new drug is born, the extensive biological characterization often reveals an unexpected action for one or more of the compounds. This unusual finding frequently leads to a new biological concept, a new series of compounds, and another promising new drug.

Because of the awesome complexity of biological macromolecules, progress in quantitative understanding of physical or electronic interactions of drugs with key biological systems has been slow and tortuous. Nonetheless, steady progress is being made in quantum chemical and molecular orbital calculations, in computer science, and in free energy models which should lead eventually to accurate predictions of the optimum chemical structure for a new drug.

Partly spurred by FDA requirements, pharmaceutical research has become increasingly interested in what happens to drugs after their administration. In some cases the metabolic products of the drug formed *in vivo* are biologically active, giving new clues to the chemist for further structural modifications. Some research efforts are underway to design *prodrugs*, which do not become therapeutically active until modified by a known metabolic system of the recipient. Possible advantages of this approach include reduction of general cytotoxicity, better internal control of active drug, or longer duration of action.

Although progress has been made, the relative lack of detailed chemical and physical understanding of complex biological systems in healthy and diseased states will continue to be the chief limitation to the rational design of new drug entities.

Functions of Research Scientists

Some industrial research laboratories are organized according to the disciplines of the scientists, e.g., departments of organic chemistry or pharmacology; other companies may use a project-team style wherein chemists, biologists, and pharmacologists are organized into an administrative unit for the purpose of discovering drugs useful for a particular disease state. Irrespective of the organizational style, problems in drug discovery and development have become so complex that a multidisciplinary approach to research is nearly always used. For the sake of simplicity, this section will outline the functions of scientists with particular backgrounds who play leading roles in pharmaceutical research; however, the reader should understand that drug development is a cooperative venture among all scientists.

Organic Chemistry—As noted previously, organic chemists synthesize new drug candidates as well as isolate and characterize natural products, such as alkaloids. In each case there is interest in the complex relationships between chemical structure and pharmacologic action.

The search for chemical structures which exhibit physiologic activity is a difficult goal of organic chemical research. Compounds are submitted to screening for numerous types of biologic and pharmacologic action. Observation of interesting and repeatable biological activity opens pathways for additional chemical research effort in the expansion of the series and often leads to significant new medicinal products.

The pharmacologic activity of a compound is an involved function of the structure, and very small changes may profoundly modify the pharmacologic effect. These structural modifications may involve replacing one group with another at a specific point in the molecule, shifting the same group from place to place in the parent molecule, saturating valence bonds, or modifying the acidity or basicity.

Slight changes sometimes completely reverse the action of the compound, as is the case when the terminal methyl group of 1-methylamyl-ethyl-barbituric acid is moved one carbon atom nearer the nucleus to form 1,3-dimethylbutyl-ethyl-barbituric acid. The latter compound produces convulsions and is fatal in small doses. These convulsions can be neutralized and the animal's life saved by a dose of the sedative isomer.

Many of the currently used antispasmodics, anticonvulsants, local anesthetics, nonnarcotic analgesics, ataractics, chemotherapeutic agents, and hypnotics have been products of this approach.

Another research style is to identify, isolate, and purify compounds from biologically active mixtures. The determination of the structure of a biologically active molecule provides a two-fold benefit to pharmacy and medicine. It makes possible research leading to synthesis and modification of the structure. Changes in structure are usually accompanied with changes in biologic activity, and occasionally vast improvement is accomplished.

Our present knowledge of adrenal corticosteroids began with the study of the various components in an extract of the adrenal cortex. These were characterized as to structure and studied clinically. Eventually, cortisone was synthesized from bile acids. Today, some synthetic analogues of cortisone are available which are superior therapeutically to the naturally occurring steroids.

The tetracyclines are a clinically important group of antibiotics. The first of these, 7-chlorotetracycline, was isolated in 1948 from *Streptomyces aureofaciens*. Shortly thereafter, a group of scientists isolated 5-hydroxytetracycline from *Streptomyces rimosus*, and in 1953 its structure was established. Once the chemical structure of this antibiotic was known, the way was opened for systematic variation of the basic nucleus in order to obtain new drugs with improved properties.

The catalytic removal of chlorine from 7-chlorotetracycline gave tetracycline itself, which proved to be superior to either of the above-mentioned antibiotics, and has displaced them to a considerable extent. Although tetracycline has subsequently been isolated from a *Streptomyces* species, this useful antibiotic is more readily prepared by the semisynthetic method.

Studies on the structure and synthesis of penicillins led to the development of the semisynthetic penicillins and later to cephalosporins. Some of the new compounds have made possible major improvements in antibiotic therapy.

Total synthesis is made possible by knowledge of chemical structures and, in some instances, is important economically in reducing the cost of the drug. Chloramphenicol, which can be obtained from cultures of *Streptomyces Venezuelae*, combats bacteria-produced typhoid dysentery and Rocky Mountain spotted fever. A commercially feasible chemical synthesis has replaced the fermentation process for production of the antibiotic.

Many of the water-soluble vitamins are produced commercially in large amounts by chemical synthesis. In addition, the total synthesis of compounds such as penicillin, tetracycline, insulin, and lysergic acid, although not economical, nevertheless represents outstanding contributions to the science of organic chemistry.

Microbiology—Since the discovery and development of penicillin during World War II, the search for new antibiotics among the metabolic products of microorganisms has constituted a major research effort in the pharmaceutical industry. The proven clinical usefulness of antibiotics in treating many bacterial infections has fully justified this effort.

Microbiologists have searched among a wide variety of fungi and bacteria looking for antibiotic substances. In this search, microorganisms from plant tissues, animal sources, the sea, many types of soil, and from many other ecologic niches have been examined. More than 1000 antibiotic substances have been detected and at least partially characterized. A combination of microbiological and chemical methods is required to distinguish the new antibiotics from the host of older ones which have already been discovered.

After a culture has been found to produce a new antibiotic, microbiologists then turn their attention to the biosynthesis of the compound, seeking to improve yields in order to produce quantities of the compound for testing and evaluation. An effort is also made to understand biosynthetic pathways, to further improve yields, and to facilitate the biosynthetic production of the isotope-labeled antibiotic for pharmacologic and toxicologic evaluation.

New antibiotics are being evaluated for application in an increasing number of disease conditions. Tests are conducted to determine activity of new antibiotics against a variety of yeasts, molds, and protozoa, as well as against normal and antibiotic-resistant bacterial pathogens. The antibacterial drugs have contributed to major advances in the control of bacterial and other microbial diseases. However, impetus for continued research is provided by problems of drug resistance, patient sensitivity, and the inability to control certain infections.

Microbiologists are concerned not only with the microorganisms which produce antibiotics, but also with the microbial pathogens which the antibiotics are expected to control. The mode of transmission of disease and the pathogenicity, virulence, and invasiveness of the infectious microorganisms are under investigation.

A newly recognized problem in drug resistance involves the transfer of drug resistance among gram-negative bacteria by means of an episome bearing one or more antibiotic resistance factors. Agents that prevent the emergence of the resistance factor, or that prevent its transfer, may be sought, or future research may be directed toward agents that enhance host resistance.

An integration of microbiologic research and organic chemical research resulted in the production of a series of semisynthetic penicillins and cephalosporins. These antibiotics are chemically modified derivatives of biosynthetically produced antibiotics, which possess improved spectra of action or other advantageous chemical and biological properties.

Biochemistry and Physiology—Research in biochemistry includes investigations on the specific physiologic action of substances affecting the life processes; i.e., the mode of action of biologically active compounds. Biochemists are involved in the isolation, purification, and characterization of small and large biologically active molecules.

Biochemistry is concerned also with the underlying biochemical processes which are involved in the wonderfully complex metabolism of living things: the energy-yielding systems, the systems for the synthesis of small molecules, and the processes for the synthesis of proteins, nucleic acids, and other macromolecules. Normal metabolic patterns are determined, and efforts are made to define the abnormal conditions that occur in various disease states.

Biochemists are becoming more concerned with the search for biomedical rationale to guide medicinal chemists in the design of drugs more selective for specific aspects of disease. Knowledge of the structure and biochemical function of coenzymes has stimulated the chemist to synthesize a large number of analogues of coenzymes, some of which have proved to be useful compounds in the chemotherapy of cancer.

Increasing emphasis is being placed on studies of enzymatic processes such as those related to the biosynthesis of cholesterol, fatty acids, and triglycerides; regulation and control of protein and nucleic acid synthesis; absorption processes; and biochemical mechanisms in central nervous processes.

The increasing sophistication of research demands that an understanding of the molecular bases of diseases emerge as a primary goal. This knowledge will strongly influence both the methodology of testing new drugs and the choice or design of compounds to be tested.

Targets, or receptor locations where drugs act, are recognized and, in some instances, may be isolated and characterized. Some of the receptor systems under investigation include those for catecholamines, opiates, and steroid and peptide hormones. Recent discovery of the *enkephalins*, natural brain polypeptides which bind the opiate receptor, has opened new horizons in CNS pharmacology. This information will be useful in acquiring new knowledge of the interaction between drugs and their receptor sites and in understanding the requirements for specific spatial orientation of essential structural features of drugs. Drug design will also make provision for those characteristics which will assure absorption, transport to the receptor site, and elimination of the therapeutic agent.

During recent years, the importance of high blood levels of cholesterol and certain other lipids in experimental and clinical atherosclerosis has focused attention on drugs that may influence the metabolic synthesis and disposition of these substances. A few of these drugs are beginning to be available, and more may be expected. Many years of careful study may be required before it is possible to demonstrate that such drugs prevent or ameliorate the problems of hardening of the arteries; however, there is some hope that such degeneration may respond to treatment with new drugs.

The acute problems that are associated with atherosclerosis are caused by a formation of thrombi. Various approaches are being applied to this problem; eg, platelet agglutination, the first step in the formation of a clot, is being studied. Some factors that stimulate agglutination are recognized, and compounds may be found to counteract this influence. Enzymes which are capable of dissolving a recently formed blood clot, such as streptokinase and urokinase, have been approved for marketing. The known anticoagulant properties of aspirin are under intensive study as a means to prevent recurrence of coronary thrombi.

Biochemical investigations on the structure and function of deoxyribonucleic acid (DNA), the genetic code, and the synthesis of nucleic acids and proteins have given us knowledge which has illuminated the paths of scientists interested in virology, immunology, genetics, cancer research, and indeed, all scientists interested in fundamental biological processes. Recombinant DNA research holds significant promise as a source of scarce or valuable human proteins such as growth hormone, antibodies, interferon, and insulin.

Physiology, especially reproductive physiology, is of interest to the industry because of the demand for drugs to regulate fertility and the concern about the effects of drugs on the fetus. Many species of laboratory animals, including subhuman primates, are being used for physiological studies. Reproductive physiologists are urging the use of primates for studies, drawing upon the likelihood of greater similarity in primates and man than, for example, in rodents and man.

Major advances have been made in the field of gastrointestinal physiology; many new GI polypeptide hormones have been isolated and characterized and their primary functions have been determined. Evidence for many years pointed to the existence of gastric (H2) receptors for histamine in addition to the vascular receptors. Recently, new drugs have been designed to block specifically the H2 receptor and have been marketed for use in the treatment of peptic ulcer.

A major objective of biologic research is the design of satisfactory model disease systems in animals that will give reliable predictions of the safety and efficacy of new drugs in humans. Tests for antibiotic activity against bacteria and fungi are done first *in vitro*, after which animal tests using standardized, controlled experimental infections are conducted. The establishment of reliable experimental bacterial infections has facilitated the development of new antibacterial agents. More recently, new methods of establishing experimental fungal infections have led to the discovery of new antifungal compounds.

Virology—The search for antiviral agents has depended on the development of both *in vitro* and *in vivo* testing procedures. Development of methodology for propagation and assaying of viruses in tissue culture has led to more precise procedures of testing compounds for antiviral activity. Recent research findings, in which some biochemical events involved in viral multiplication have been determined, provide insight into several possibilities for drug interference. These include:

1. Interference with viral attachment or penetration of the cell.
2. Interference with viral-induced enzymes responsible for replication of viral nucleic acid.
3. Interference with assembly of viral components.
4. Induction of faulty coding with production of nonfunctional components.

An increasing number of antiviral compounds are being discovered. For example, 5-iodo-2′-deoxyuridine, vidarabine, and trifluridine are effective in treating herpes infections of the eye, and amantadine has been found useful in influenza A virus infections. Chemotherapeutic prevention or treatment of more viral diseases may be expected as new antiviral substances are developed.

Tissue culture techniques have made possible the production of large quantities of viruses for vaccine manufacture. This method of culture, which was utilized for a variety of virus vaccines, is now being focused on the study of other viral problems.

New and improved vaccines represent a major objective of biologic research. New separation methods developed in biochemistry and physical chemistry have been applied to the isolation and purification of viruses, and have led to preparation of highly purified and concentrated vaccines. Such vaccines are more effective and produce markedly less side reactions.

Immunology—Recent research has focused attention on various aspects of immunity other than those concerned with the use of prophylactic vaccines. A number of important diseases such as arthritis and multiple sclerosis appear to be manifestations of autoimmune phenomena. Antibodies appear to be formed against body constituents; these antibodies then combine with the tissue containing the antigen and cause degeneration. For these diseases, suppression of immune phenomena or induction of immune tolerance may be of great importance. More detailed knowledge of the immune system has permitted a search for drugs which either enhance or inhibit the immune response. A much clearer picture of the molecular basis of allergy heightens the probability that additional helpful drugs will be found to alleviate allergic reactions.

Biologic and immunologic research has also been directed to the problem of cancer. The existence of tumor-specific antigens in both virus- and chemically induced tumors, as well as new evidence for host reactions to the tumor, increase the possibility of useful immunologic approaches to cancer.

One of the most important developments in the past decade has been the isolation and production of monoclonal antibodies. These agents can be used to identify tumor-specific antigens and thus serve as powerful *in vitro* diagnostic tools.

The technique can be applied to other antigens as well. It is also possible that these substances can be developed as carrier systems for drugs by virtue of their ability to deliver the antibody-drug complex directly to the antigen-producing cell or tissue.

Pharmacology—Pharmacologic research plays two important roles in its contribution to pharmacy and medicine. The pharmacologist designs and operates model systems for detecting and evaluating the activity of compounds for control of diseases such as those of the central nervous system, the gastrointestinal tract, the cardiovascular bed, and the endocrine organs. Following the discovery of a new drug, the dosage, toxicity, mode of action, metabolism, and fate of that drug in the body must be determined.

Intact animals, whole organs, isolated tissue, or purified enzyme and receptor systems may be used in modern pharmacology. The classic pharmacologic methods are undergoing rapid changes to more automated and more biochemically oriented methods. The elevation or depression of such important metabolic substances as acetylcholine, histamine, and catecholamines is used as a guide for drug studies. Such biochemical measurements and highly automated methods of recording behavioral responses are employed jointly in the study of CNS drugs.

It is rare to find a potent new drug which does not have side effects in some individuals. The pharmacologist, on the basis of experimental work on a variety of species of laboratory animals, must predict an effective human dose which hopefully will produce a minimum of side effects. He must also be able to tell the physician or the clinical pharmacologist who first administers the drug to humans what form of toxicity might appear, what abnormal conditions in the patient would contraindicate use of the drug, and how other drugs administered simultaneously might affect the recommended dosage schedule.

An important part of pharmacology is the study of drug absorption, distribution, metabolism, and excretion. Rational drug therapy requires a thorough knowledge of the kinetics of these processes after intravenous and/or oral administration of the drug. Initial studies in animals are often performed with radioactive forms of the drug to determine the amounts of drug and its metabolites which appear in blood, urine, and tissues. Animal models can be used to determine the manner in which a living organism assimilates a drug; however, human pharmacokinetic studies are essential to determine the fate of the compound in man; ie, is it accumulated in specific organs, is it excreted into bile or urine, and is it metabolized? To determine the concentration of drugs in biological fluids or tissues requires special separation techniques as well as sensitive, accurate, and precise instrumental measurements. Accurate quantitation and identification of the drug and its metabolites often require the use of modern chromatographic techniques coupled with the mass spectrograph.

Toxicology—In order to be certain that a new drug is safe, detailed studies are made of the effects of varying doses and of prolonged administration of that drug. The pharmacologist provides acute toxicity data. The toxicologist must then refine the acute toxicity measurement in laboratory animals and begin chronic studies. The latter are conducted in a variety of species, at several dosage levels of the drug, and over periods of time ranging up to two years.

During the test period, animals are observed carefully for all adverse symptoms. At the end of this period, and occasionally during its progress, animals are sacrificed, and their vital tissues, such as liver, heart, kidney, intestine, brain, etc., are removed and studied grossly and microscopically by a competent pathologist.

In addition to gross and microscopic pathology, biochemical and physiologic responses are measured as an indication of liver function, kidney function, endocrine function, etc.

During recent years, metabolic investigations have become more sophisticated and have been brought to bear on the comparative effects of drugs on various animals and man. In some instances, the metabolism of drugs or the therapeutic effects of drugs vary from species to species. Such variability can be the basis for differences in toxicity as well as differences in efficacy. For these reasons, increasing emphasis is being given to studies of comparative metabolism in man and animals to determine which laboratory animal handles the drug in a manner similar to man. Selection of that species for extensive toxicity testing should increase confidence that the toxic reactions which may occur in man will have been predicted by the animal tests.

Reproductive studies to determine the potential effects of the new drug on the reproductive processes and on subsequent generations are performed. Teratological studies are done to determine whether or not the new drug affects the fetus. Special toxicity tests have been designed to detect specific toxic reactions, such as nerve damage resulting in hearing loss.

Toxicologic studies are assuming increasing importance in the world of pharmacy and medicine. As knowledge and skills increase, and ability to measure toxic reactions improves, we will be able to assure greater safety and efficacy of new drugs.

Physical Chemistry—Modern research in pharmacy and medicine is supported and expedited by instrumentation. Modern instruments make possible the rapid and accurate measurement of physical and chemical properties of molecules. Separation and characterization of molecules sometimes are possible today in a matter of hours or days, whereas only a decade or two ago such work often required days, weeks, or even months.

Examples of the specialized physicochemical methods that are applicable to the research directed at the isolation, characterization, and chemical study of large molecules are the use of the ultracentrifuge and buoyant density techniques, which have been extremely useful in the study of DNA and RNA structure and function. The electron microscope is a valuable instrument for the study of large nucleic acid or protein molecules, viruses, and organized structures of microorganisms and tissues.

Structure studies in organic chemistry, electrometric titration, polarography, and spectrophotometry in the ultraviolet, visible, or infrared make possible the identification of chemical groups within the molecule.

Nuclear magnetic resonance spectra identify chemical groups and indicate the nature of neighboring chemical groups in the molecule. Mass spectroscopy permits determination of the molecular weight and empiric formula of an organic molecule, and of the major fragments of the molecule. With this information it is often possible to deduce the entire structure of a molecule rapidly and precisely.

X-ray crystallographic analysis enables the physical chemist to determine the precise position of each atom of a molecule as it exists in the crystalline form. Optical rotatory dispersion and circular dichroism techniques are becoming useful in determining the conformation of molecules in solutions.

Physicochemical studies are directed not only at the chemical groups and stereochemical configuration of biologically active molecules, but on a more sophisticated level, calculations are being undertaken which describe molecules in terms of energy and electron distributions, and which approximate the influence of the chemical environment on these distributions.

The spatial and electronic conformation of drugs, and the changes in conformation which occur in various environments, govern the absorption, transport, distribution, and reaction with the receptor site. If description of molecules in these functional terms is achieved, correlation of electronic structure

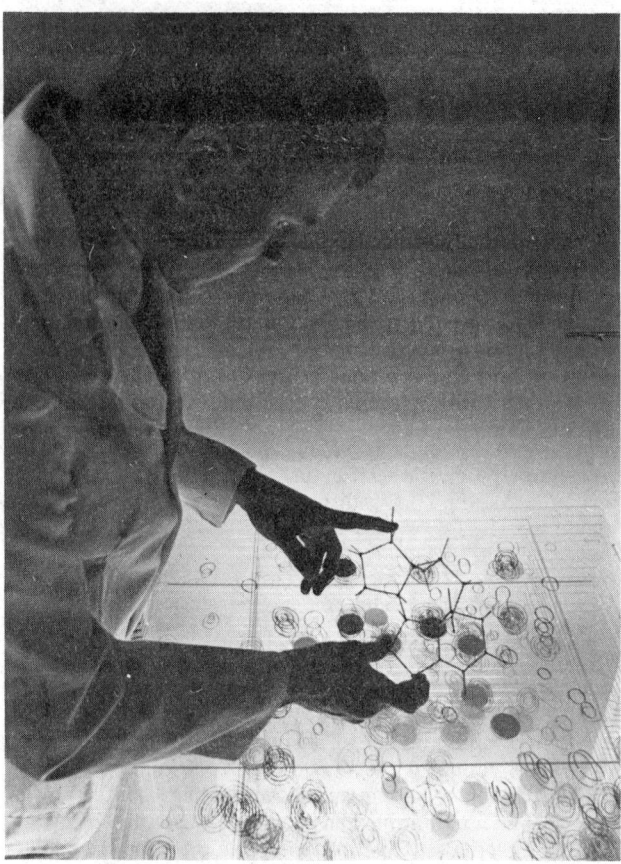

Fig 8-1.   The three-dimensional structures of drug molecules. The X-ray crystallographer solves the molecular structure of a compound through the use of automated data collection systems and computerized treatment of diffraction data. Information on preferred conformations as well as absolute configuration is readily obtained (courtesy, Lilly).

with function may be possible, and the design of safer, specific, and more effective drugs on a rational basis may occur.

Information Science—Throughout the preceding sections, the interdependence between chemical and biological information has been stressed. In many projects, so many data are needed that their generation and analysis become a limiting factor. The laboratory computer has become an invaluable tool to solve these problems. All the major analytical instrumentation can be or has been computerized to integrate areas, calculate, and print out readable reports. Computer-assisted chemistry and computer graphics have also added a new dimension in structure and activity relationships. The computer has also permitted constant monitoring and analysis of many animal studies. On-line signal processing allows the investigator to interact more fully with his experiments. Automation often permits collection of many more data points with a resulting increase in accuracy. The computer has replaced the calculator for statistical analysis and evaluation of laboratory and clinical data. Time-sharing computer terminals are required by many scientists to do their jobs effectively. Sophisticated software packages are available commercially or may be developed in house.

Attention should also be directed to another development that is continuing and is affecting the researcher. Formerly, the individual scientist subscribed personally to a few journals and depended on a scientific library for coverage of additional new scientific findings. With the tremendous growth of the scientific and patent literature and the emergence of interdisciplinary investigations, the individual must depend on new ways to stay abreast of the literature. Personal perusal of literature is still important; however, increasing use is being made of various kinds of alerting services and facilities, many of them computer-based, for retrieval or retrospective search of pertinent information.

Drug Development

Before a new drug candidate can proceed to toxicologic or clinical evaluation, considerable analytical chemical development is required to lay the ground work for subsequent quality control and stability studies. Drug standards are established and analytical methods for the bulk drug and for the proposed final product are devised. Tentative chemical, physical, and biological specifications of the candidate drug are established.

Simultaneously with analytical development, pharmacists and pharmaceutical chemists begin formulation studies toward the goal of a stable, highly acceptable product which delivers the correct amount of drug in a reproducible, effective manner. Sometimes a new drug must be chemically modified (eg, esterified) to provide a form that is pharmaceutically acceptable and effective. Considerable judgment and forethought are involved in choosing necessary excipients. Accelerated and long-term stability studies are started to estimate the conditions in which the product will be stable.

Clinical Research

If a compound has desirable activity in an experimental testing system, and appears to be safe upon toxicologic examination, it becomes a candidate for clinical trial.

Two more tasks must be accomplished before clinical trial. First, the pharmaceutical chemist must put the compound in a suitable stable dosage form. The stabilization of a product must preclude physical or chemical change (discoloration, precipitation, or decomposition). The active compound must be available for absorption and transport to the site of action. The components of the pharmaceutical form must be compatible and must provide an elegant product to the physician or the patient.

Because of the many physical forms in which pharmaceuticals are presented, the research necessary is broad in scope, and involves not only the principles of physical pharmacy but requires the application of principles from the allied fields of chemistry and biology.

The second task at this stage is to file an Investigational New Drug Application (IND) with the Food and Drug Administration (FDA). The IND is, in fact, a document which gives a full description of the new drug, where and how it is manufactured, all quality control information and standards, stability, analytical methods, pharmacology, toxicology, documentation of efficacy in animals, the physicians (and their qualifications) who will be doing the clinical studies, and complete protocols of the proposed clinical studies.

A new drug is administered to man for the first time by a physician. This investigator is often a professor at a leading medical school and a recognized authority in some special medical area.

The first trial of a drug in man is done with great caution

and on a very limited basis. This study, called Phase I, is devoted primarily to ascertaining the safety in the human. When these limits have been established and are found acceptable, the drug is made available to a larger number of practicing specialists for the Phase II study, which is principally concerned with the determination of efficacy in patients.

If, after Phase II, the drug still looks promising, it is distributed more widely to selected practicing physicians in the Phase III study. The purpose at this stage is to secure data from a larger number of patients on efficacy and incidence of side effects.

Finally, before the new drug can be marketed, a New Drug Application (NDA) must be filed with the FDA and approval obtained. The NDA contains most of the information included in the IND, which has been revised and updated, as well as all the results of the clinical studies proving safety and efficacy. Most all clinical, laboratory, and patient history data are processed on computers. These medical data are updated in computerized retrieval systems and are designed to provide timely information during the FDA review. These systems also provide an additional information resource for pre- and postmarketing queries. Only after FDA approval of the NDA can distribution and marketing of the new drug begin.

Depending on the nature of the disease, some drugs require such a massive and expensive clinical trial that a drug company could not afford to undertake it. One such study is funded by the Heart, Lung and Blood Institute and is called the Lipid Research Clinics Program. The trial is designed to determine whether lowering plasma cholesterol in asymptomatic but hypercholesterolemic subjects will indeed decrease the incidence of coronary heart disease. This $80 million study, over a seven-year period, required careful screening of more than one-half million persons to select 3800 for the trial.

The clinical research effort on a new drug represents the culmination of many years of effort by large numbers of scientists of many disciplines and skills. It is the proving ground on which the intelligence, creativity, and perseverance of laboratory researchers comes to fruition. Of the candidate drugs that come to clinical research, only a few survive as safe and effective items to be added to the clinical armamentarium. When this successful conclusion is achieved, the real beneficiary is the recipient of the new drug who may be able to live a longer and more healthful life.

Bibliography

Annual Survey Report Ethical Pharmaceutical Industry Operations, PMA, Washington, DC, 1981–1982, Unpublished.

Fed Proc 28(1): 160–215, 1969.

Chemistry, A New Look, WA Benjamin, Inc, New York, 1966.

Baldry PE: *The Battle Against Bacteria*, Cambridge, London, 1965.

Stewart GT: *The Penicillin Group of Drugs*, Elsevier, New York, 1965.

Davis BD, *et al.: Microbiology*, Hoeber, New York, 1967.

Drug Discovery, Advances in Chemistry Series 108: Am Chem Soc, Washington, DC, 1971.

Clarke FH, ed: *How Modern Medicines Are Developed*, Futura Publ. Co Inc, Mount Kisco, New York, 1977.

PART 2

Pharmaceutics

Alfred N Martin, PhD

Coulter R Sublett Professor
Drug Dynamics Institute
College of Pharmacy
University of Texas
Austin, TX 78712

CHAPTER 9

Metrology and Calculation

Werner Lowenthal, PhD

Professor of Pharmacy and Pharmaceutics and Professor of Educational Development and Planning
School of Pharmacy, Medical College of Virginia, Virginia Commonwealth University
Richmond, VA 23298

The first technical operation which the student of pharmacy must learn is the manipulation of balances and weights. This entails a study of the various systems of weights and measures, their relationships, and a mastery of the mathematics involved. This chapter considers the fundamental principles of metrology underlying the testing, manufacturing, and compounding of pharmaceutical preparations, under three headings, as follow:

Weights and Measures—an accumulation of facts concerning the various systems, with tables of conversion factors and practical equivalents. The relationships among the various systems of weights and measures are clarified.

Weighing and Measuring—a discussion of the various types of balances, particularly prescription balances, and methods of using, testing, and protecting them; also of various devices and methods of their use for measuring large or small volumes of fluids.

Density and Specific Gravity—a consideration of the mass/volume ratio of a substance (density), and the ratio of the weight (mass) of one substance to the weight (mass) of another substance taken as the standard (specific gravity).

Weights and Measures

Weight is a measure of the gravitational force acting on a body and is directly proportional to its mass. The latter, being a constant based on inertia, never varies, whereas weight varies slightly with latitude, altitude, temperature, and pressure. The effect of these factors is not usually considered unless very precise weighings and large quantities are involved.

Measure is the determination of the volume or extent of a body. Temperature and pressure have a pronounced effect, especially on gases and liquids. These factors are, therefore, considered when making precision measurements.

All standard weights and measures in this country are derived from or based on the United States National Prototype Standards of the Meter and the Kilogram, made of platinum–iridium, in the custody of the National Bureau of Standards at Washington, DC.

History of Weights and Measures

A brief outline of the origin of the many systems of weights and measures may help in remembering essential distinctions between them. The sense of the weight of a body cannot be conveyed intelligibly to the mind unless a means of comparison is chosen. As weight is the measure of the gravitational force of a body, so this force is expressed in terms of standards of resistance, which exactly balance the body and keep it in equilibrium when used with a mechanical device constructed for this specific purpose. Such standards are termed *weights* and the mechanical devices are called *balances* or *scales*.

The standards which have been chosen by various nations are arbitrary, and instances are common where different standards are in use at the same time in the same country. Many of the ancient standards are clearly referable to variable parts of the human body, as nail, foot, span, pace, cubit (length of the forearm), and fathom or faethm (stretch of the arms). In the history of metrology three periods may be traced:

1. The *Ancient* period, during which the old classical standards originated, terminated with the decline of the Roman Empire. It is interesting to note that the unit of distance used at the present day by all nations in maritime measurements is the *nautical* or *meridian* mile or $\frac{1}{60}$ of a degree of the earth's equatorial circumference, and that this is exactly equal to 1000 Egyptian fathoms or 4000 Egyptian cubits. These Egyptian measurements, which have persisted for more than 4000 years, were based on astronomical or meridian measurements which were imperishably recorded in the great Pyramid of Ghizeh, whose perimeter is exactly 500 fathoms, or $\frac{1}{2}$ nautical mile.

2. The *Medieval* period extended to the 16th century. During this period the old standards were lost, but their names were preserved, and European nations adopted various independent standards.

3. The *Modern* period extends from the 16th century to the present. Since the 17th century the efforts of most enlightened nations have been directed toward scientific accuracy and simplicity, and during the present century toward international uniformity.

Historical metrology is also referred to as *Documentary Metrology*, which is concerned with the study of monuments and records of ancient periods, and *Inductive Metrology*, which is concerned with the accumulation of data concerning the measurement of large numbers of objects which have been referred to as standards but which have no exact measure except by statutory regulation.

The English Systems—In Great Britain, in 1266, the 51st Act of the reign of Henry III declared "that by the consent of the whole realm of England the measure of the King was made—that is to say, that an English silver penny called the sterling, round and without clipping, shall weigh *thirty-two grains of wheat*, well dried and gathered out of the middle of the ear; and twenty pence (pennyweights) do make an ounce and twelve ounces a pound, and eight pounds do make a gallon of wine, and eight wine gallons do make a bushel, which is the eighth of a quarter."

The 16-oz lb (*avoirdupois pound*), undoubtedly of Roman origin, was introduced at the time of the first civilization of the British island. The word "haberdepois," according to Gray, was, however, first used in English laws in 1303. A statute of Edward I (AD 1304) states "that every *pound* of money or of *medicines* is of *twenty shillings weight*, but the pound of all other things is *twenty-five shillings weight*. The *ounce of medicines* consists of *twenty pence*, and the *pound* contains *twelve* ounces (the Troy Pound), but in other things the pound contains *fifteen* ounces, in both cases the ounce weighing twenty pence."

These laws unfold the theory of the ancient weights and measures of Great Britain, and reveal the standards, i.e., a natural object, grains of wheat; a difference existed then between the Troy and the avoirdupois pound, but the weights now in use are $\frac{1}{16}$ heavier than those of Edward I, owing to the change subsequently made in the value of the coin by the sovereign; in addition to this, the true pennyweight standard was lost, and in the next revision of the weights and measures the present troy and avoirdupois standards were adopted.

The *troy weight* is of still earlier origin. The great fairs of the 8th and 9th centuries were held at several French cities, including Troyes, the gathering place of traders from all countries. Coins were frequently so mutilated that they were sold by weight, and the standard weight of Troyes for selling coin was adopted for precious metals and medicines in all parts of Europe. The troy ounce and the avoirdupois ounce were originally intended to have the same weight, but after the revision it was found that the avoirdupois ounce was lighter by $42\frac{1}{2}$ gr than the troy ounce. The subsequent adoption of troy weight by the London College of Physicians in 1618, on the recommendation of Sir Theodore Turquet de la Mayerne, who compiled their first Pharmacopoeia, has entailed upon all apothecaries who are governed by British customs, to this day, the very great inconvenience of buying and selling medicines by one system of weights (the *avoirdupois*) and compounding them by another (the *apothecary* or *troy*).

In the next century efforts were made toward reforming the standards, and the Royal Society, in 1736, began the work, which ended in the preparation, under the direction of the House of Commons, by Mr Bird, of the standard "yard" and standard "pound" troy in 1760. Copies of these were prepared and no intentional deviation has been made since. In 1816, on account of the growing popularity of the French Metric System, and in view of the desirability of securing a standard which could easily be recovered in case of loss or destruction and which should be commensurable with a simple unit, steps were taken in England to secure these advantages. The labors of English scientists led to the adoption of the *Imperial* measures and standards, which were legalized January 1, 1826, and are now in use in Great Britain, thus introducing another element of confusion into an already complicated subject.

In this system the *yard* is equivalent to 36 in., and its length was determined by comparison with a pendulum beating seconds of mean time, in a vacuum, at the temperature of 62°F at the level of the sea in the latitude of London, which length was found to be 39.1393 in. The *pound troy* (containing 5760 gr) was determined by comparison with a given measure of distilled water under specified conditions. Thus, a cubic inch of distilled water was weighed with brass weights in air at 62°F, the barometer at 30 in., and it weighed 252.458 gr. The standard for measures of capacity in Great Britain (either dry or liquid) is the *Imperial gallon*, which contains 10 lb avoir (each 7000 gr) of distilled water weighed in air at 62°F, the barometer standing at 30 in. The *bushel* contains 8 such gal.

Washington, in his first annual message to Congress, January, 1790, recommended the establishment of uniformity in currency, weights, and measures. Action was taken with reference to the currency, and recommendations were made by Jefferson, then Secretary of State, for the adoption of either of the currently used English systems or a decimal system. However, nothing was accomplished until in 1819–1820 when efforts were again made in the United States to secure uniformity in the standards which were in use by the several states. Finally, after a lengthy investigation, the Secretary of the Treasury, on June 14, 1836, was directed by Congress to furnish each state in the Union with a complete set of the revised standards, and thus we have the *troy pound* (5760 gr), the *avoirdupois pound* (7000 gr), and the *yard* (36 in.) all identical with the British standards; but the US *gallon* is quite different, the old wine gallon of 231 cu in., containing 58,372.2

gr of distilled water at its maximum density, weighed in air at 62°F, the barometer standing at 30 in., being retained, while the bushel contained 77.274 lb of water under the same conditions, thus making the dry quart about 16% greater in volume than the liquid quart.

In 1864 the use of the metric measures was legalized in Great Britain, but not made compulsory, and in 1866 the United States followed the same course. By *the United States law of July 28, 1866, all lengths, areas, and cubic measures are derived from the international meter equivalent to 39.37 in.* Since 1893 the United States Office of Standard Weights and Measures has been authorized to derive the yard from the meter, 1 yd equals $^{3600}/_{3937}$ m, *and the customary weights are referred to the kilogram* by Executive order approved April 5, 1893. Capacities were to be based on the equivalent, 1 cu dm equals 1 L, the decimeter being equal to 3.937 in. The gallon still remains at 231 cu in. and the bushel contains 2150.42 cu in. This makes the liquid quart equal to 0.946 L and the dry quart 1.1013 L, while the Imperial quart is 1.1359 L. The customary weights are derived from the international kilogram, based on the value that 1 avoir lb = 453.5924277 g and that $^{5760}/_{7000}$ avoir lb equals 1 troy lb.

Avoirdupois weight is in general use in the United States for commercial purposes, including the buying and selling of drugs on the large scale and occasionally on prescription orders.

The Metric System—The idea of adopting a scientific standard for the basis of metrology, which could be accurately reverified, was suggested by a number of individuals after the Renaissance. Jean Picard, the French astronomer, in the 17th century proposed to take as a unit the length of a pendulum beating 1 sec of time at sea level, at a latitude of 45°.

James Watt, the English inventor, in 1783 first suggested the application of decimal notation, and the commensurability of weight, length, and volume. The French National Assembly in 1790 appointed a committee to decide the preferability of the pendulum standard or a terrestrial measure of some kind as a basis for the new system. The committee reported in 1791 in favor of the latter, and commissions were appointed to measure an arc of meridian and to perfect the details of the commensurability of the units and of nomenclature. However, certain inaccuracies were inherent in the early standards and they do not bear to each other the intended exact relationships. The present accepted standards are defined in publications of the National Bureau of Standards.

In its original conception the meter was the fundamental unit of the metric system, and all units of length and capacity were to be derived directly from the meter which was intended to be equal to one ten-millionth of the earth's quadrant. Furthermore, it was originally planned that the unit of mass, the kilogram, should be identical with the mass of a cubic decimeter of water at its maximum density. At present, however, the units of length and mass are defined independently of these conceptions.

For all practical purposes calibration of length standards in industry and scientific laboratories is accomplished by comparison with the material standard of length: the distance between two engraved lines on a platinum–iridium bar, the international prototype meter, which is kept at the International Bureau of Weights and Measures.

The kilogram is independently defined as the mass of a definite platinum–iridium standard, the *International Prototype Kilogram*, which is also kept at the International Bureau of Weights and Measures. The *Liter* is defined as the volume of a kilogram of water, at standard atmospheric pressure, and at the temperature of its maximum density, approximately 4°C. The meter is thus the fundamental unit on which are based all metric standards and measurements of length and area, and of volumes derived from linear measurements.

Of basic scientific interest is the fact that on October 14, 1960, the 11th General Conference on Weights and Measures, meeting in Paris, adopted a new international definition for the standard of length: the meter is now defined as the length equal to 1,650,763.73 wavelengths of the orange–red light of the krypton-86 isotope. This standard will be used in actual measurements only when extreme accuracy is needed.

The kilogram is the fundamental unit on which are based all metric standards of mass. The L is a secondary or derived unit of capacity or volume. The L is larger by about 27 ppm than the cube of the tenth of the meter, ie, the cu dm—that is 1 L = 1.000027 cu dm.

The conversion tables in this publication which involve the relative length of the yard and meter are based upon the relation: 1 m = 39.37 in., contained in the act of Congress of 1866. From this relation it follows that 1 in. = 25.40005 mm (nearly).

In recent years engineering and industrial interests the world over have urged the adoption of the simpler relation, 1 in. = 25.4 mm exactly, which differs from the preceding value by only 2 ppm. This simpler relation has not as yet been officially adopted by either Great Britain or the United States, but is in wide industrial use.

In the United States, the abbreviation *cc* still persists in general use and is taken as synonymous for the more correct term *mL*. USP IX and NF IV adopted the term *milliliter* with its abbreviated form *mil*, but it proved so unpopular in practice that the following Pharmacopeial Convention directed the return to the older term cubic centimeter (cc). In 1955 USP XV and NF X, however, once again adopted the term milliliter with the abbreviation *ml*.

National jealousies and the natural antipathy to changing established customs interfered greatly with the adoption of the metric system during the early part of the 19th century. At present the metric system is in use in every great country of the world. In the US and and Great Britain it is legalized for reference to and definition of other standards, is in exclusive use by nearly all scientists, and by increasing segments of industry and the public. In the US the metric system was legalized in 1866, but not made compulsory, and in the same year the international prototype meter and kilogram were adopted as fundamental standards.

The US silver coinage was based upon the metric system, the half dollar being exactly $12\frac{1}{2}$ g and the quarter and the dime being of the proportionate weights.

Since 1875 there has been established and maintained an International Bureau of Weights and Measures, with headquarters at Paris. This Bureau is managed by an International Committee on which all civilized countries are represented. One object of the committee is to make and provide prototypes of the meter and kilogram for the subscribing nations; approximately 40 such copies have been prepared.

The US prototype standards of both the meter and the kilogram mass, constructed of a platinum–iridium alloy, were brought from Paris in 1890 and are now in the custody of the Bureau of Standards at Washington, DC. They have been reproduced and distributed by our own government to the various states having bureaus needing such replicas. The original US prototype meter was taken back to Paris in 1957 for reverification and was found to have altered only 3 parts in 100,000,000 after 67 years of use. Thus, there was no demonstrable change within the limits of experimental error.

Adoption of the krypton-86 wavelength of light definition for the meter gives the different countries the means to check their prototype meter bars without returning them to Paris at periodic intervals for comparison with the international meter bar.

Orthography and Reading

Orthography—There are two methods of orthography of the metric units in use. In one of these, the original French, the units are spelled me*tre*, li*tre*, gram*me;* in the other, proposed by the American Metric Bureau, the units are spelled met*er*, lit*er*, and gram. In the USP and the NF for three decades after the original adoption of the metric system, met*er* and lit*er* were adopted but the French gram*me* was used. Now these official compendia use the spelling gram.

Reading—Some difficulty is usually experienced by those unfamiliar with the metric system in reading the quantities. In the linear measures in pharmacy centimeters and millimeters are almost exclusively used; thus, 0.05 m would not be read five hundredths of a meter, but 5 centimeters (5 cm); if

the millimeter column contains a unit, as in 0.055 m it is read fifty–five millimeters (55 mm), in preference to fifty-five thousandths of a meter.

Fractions of a millimeter must be read decimally, as, 0.0555 m, fifty-five and five-tenths millimeter (55.5 mm). In measures of capacity, cubic centimeters (cc) or milliliters (mL), are used exclusively for quantities of less than a liter, the terms half liter, quarter liter, 100 milliliters, and one milliliter are denoted by 500 mL, 250 mL, 100 mL, and 1 mL; with water the milliliter is considered equivalent to a gram. In weight, when the quantity is relatively large, and in commercial transactions, the *kilogram* is abbreviated to *kilo*, when less than a *kilogram* and not less than a *gram*, the quantity is read with the gram for the unit; 2000 g would be read either as two thousand grams or as two kilos, and 543 g would be read five hundred and forty-three grams, while 2543 g is sometimes read two kilos and five hundred and forty-three grams, although twenty-five hundred and forty-three grams is usually preferred. For quantities below the gram, decigram and centigram are not usually used, but milligram has been regarded as the most convenient unit. With the increase in the use of extremely small doses of very potent drugs and the wide application of more delicate analytical procedures, the term microgram (mcg, μg, or γ), for thousandths of a milligram, is frequently used to designate quantities up to 999 μg (less than 1.000 mg).

Both the metric and English systems of weights and measures are in use in the United States, even though the metric system has now all but replaced the English system; the pharmacist must have a practical knowledge of both.

Weights

The Metric System of Weight

The USP of 1890 adopted the metric system of Weights and Measures to the exclusion of all others except for equivalent dosage statements, and the British Pharmacopoeia of 1914 did likewise. In 1944 the Council on Pharmacy and Chemistry of the American Medical Association adopted the metric system exclusively. The advantages of the metric or decimal system, and its simplicity, brevity, and adaptability to everyday needs are now universally conceded.

Fractional and Multiple Prefixes—In many experimental procedures, including some in the pharmaceutical sciences, very small (and occasionally very large) quantities of weight, length, volume, time, radioactivity, etc are measured. To avoid use of numbers with many zeros in such cases, the National Bureau of Standards recognizes prefixes to be used to express fractions or multiples of the International System of Units (SI) established in 1960 by the General Conference on Weights and Measures (see foregoing discussion). The recognized prefixes, which in use are adjoined to an appropriate unit (as, for example, in such quantities as nanogram, picomole, microcurie, microsecond, megavolt) are defined in Table I.

Table II lists some metric weights. The prefixes, which indicate multiples, are of Greek derivation—deka, 10; hecto,

Table I—Prefixes for Fractions and Multiples of SI Units

Fraction	Prefix	Symbol	Multiple	Prefix	Symbol
10^{-1}	deci	d	10	deka	da
10^{-2}	centi	c	10^2	hecto	h
10^{-3}	milli	m	10^3	kilo	k
10^{-6}	micro	μ	10^6	mega	M
10^{-9}	nano	n	10^9	giga	G
10^{-12}	pico	p	10^{12}	tera	T
10^{-15}	femto	f	10^{15}	peta	P
10^{-18}	atto	a	10^{18}	exa	E

Table II—Metric Weight

1 microgram	μg	=	0.000,001	g
1 milligram	mg	=	0.001	g
1 centigram	cg	=	0.01	g
1 decigram	dg	=	0.1	g
1 gram	g	=	1.0	g
1 dekagram	dag	=	10.0	g
1 hectogram	hg	=	100.0	g
1 kilogram	kg	=	1000.0	g

Note—The abbreviation μg or mcg is used for microgram in pharmacy rather than gamma (γ) as in biology.

100; kilo, 1000. Fractions of the units are expressed by Latin prefixes—deci, $\frac{1}{10}$; centi, $\frac{1}{100}$; milli, $\frac{1}{1000}$.

Only a few of the most convenient denominations are employed in practical work. Whole numbers from 1 to 1000 are usually expressed in terms of grams while the kilogram is used as the unit for larger quantities. Quantities between 1 milligram and 1 gram are usually referred to in terms of milligrams; microgram (μg or mcg) is used in quantitative analysis, biological studies, and for minute dosage statements.

The English Systems of Weight

In the United States both the avoirdupois and apothecaries systems of weight measurement are still sometimes used in the handling of medicines.

It must be emphasized that *the pharmacist may buy his drugs by avoirdupois and dispense by apothecary weight.* These two systems differ thus:

1 **pound** avoirdupois = **7000 gr** and is abbreviated **lb.**
1 **pound** apothecary = **5760 gr** and is abbreviated **lb apoth.**
1 **ounce** avoirdupois = **437.5 gr** and is abbreviated **oz.**
1 **ounce** apothecary = **480 gr** and is abbreviated ℥.

The *grain* avoirdupois is exactly the same as the *grain* apothecary. The apothecary pound is therefore 1240 gr *lighter* than the avoirdupois pound, and the apothecary ounce is therefore 42.5 gr *heavier* than the avoirdupois ounce.

The abbreviations of the denominations of apothecary weight are represented by the signs ℥, ounce; ʒ, dram; ℈, scruple; and gr, grain; these have long been in use but may possibly be mistaken for one another in rapid or careless writing. The abbreviations or signs of avoirdupois weight differ from those of apothecary weight, and care should be used not to confound them; they are lb (sometimes written #), pound; oz, ounce; gr, grain. Tables III, IV, and V show three English systems of weight.

Jewelers evaluate precious stones with troy weight, which is very similar to apothecary weight. The apothecary and troy grain, ounce, and pound are identical, but the ounces are subdivided differently. The *carat*, used by jewelers, is equal to 3.168 troy grains or 4 carat grains. When used to express

Table III—Avoirdupois Weight

Pound		Ounces		Grains
lb 1	=	16	=	7000
		oz 1	=	**gr** 437.5

Note—2000 lb = 1 ton and 2240 lb = 1 long ton.

Table IV—Apothecary Weight

Pound		Ounces		Drams		Scruples		Grains
lb 1	=	12	=	96	=	288	=	5760
		℥ 1	=	8	=	24	=	480
				ʒ 1	=	3	=	60
						℈ 1	=	**gr** 20

Table V—Troy Weight

Pound		Ounces		Pennyweights (Pwt)		Grains
lb 1	=	12	=	240	=	5760
		℥ 1	=	20	=	480
				Pwt 1	=	**gr** 24

Note—The abbreviation lb refers to the avoirdupois pound of 7000 gr unless further qualified, as in the headings of Tables IV and V. The apothecary pound is sometimes abbreviated ℔.

Table VI—Metric Linear Measure

1 millimicron (or nanometer)	(mμ) (nm)	=	0.000,000,001 m (0.001 μ; 10^{-9} m; 10 Å)
1 micron (or micrometer)	(μ) (μm)	=	0.000,001 m (0.001 mm; 10^{-6} m; 10,000 Å)
1 millimeter	(mm)	=	0.001 m
1 centimeter	(cm)	=	0.01 m
1 decimeter	(dm)	=	0.1 m
1 meter	(m)	=	1.0 m
1 dekameter	(dam)	=	10.0 m
1 hectometer	(hm)	=	100.0 m
1 kilometer	(km)	=	1000.0 m

Note—While the meter (m) is observed to be the initial unit, it is seldom necessary to use it in pharmaceutical practice, and the same holds true for a number of the above measures. The micrometer (μm), millimeter (mm), and the centimeter (cm) are employed in the description of many official drugs. Measurements pertaining to spectrometric and colorimetric tests and assays of many official drugs are recorded in micrometers (μm) or the equivalent microns (μ) for infrared and in nanometers (nm) or the equivalent millimicrons (mμ) for ultraviolet and visible wavelengths of light, respectively.

the fineness of gold 1 carat signifies $\frac{1}{24}$ part. A 14-carat ring is $\frac{14}{24}$ pure gold.

As indicated in the footnote to Table VI, a number of special metric system units are used in various pharmacopeial and nonofficial descriptions, tests, and assays of drugs and other substances to express linear measurements of very small dimension. These units and their symbols or abbreviations are listed in Table X, together with their equivalents in terms of the other metric units and the inch.

Measures

Systems of Measure

Two systems of linear measure are used in the United States—English and metric—and two systems of liquid measure—apothecary (also called the wine measure and US liquid measure) and metric. The units of the English system of linear measure (inch, foot, yard, mile) are too well known to be described here. The units of the metric systems of linear and liquid measure, and of the apothecary (wine, US liquid) system of liquid measure, with their respective equivalents, are given in Tables VI, VII, and VIII.

Table VII—Metric Liquid Measure

1 microliter	(μL)	=	0.000001	l
1 milliliter	(mL)	=	0.001	l
1 centiliter	(cL)	=	0.01	l
1 deciliter	(dL)	=	0.1	l
1 liter	(L)	=	1.0	l
1 dekaliter	(daL)	=	10.0	l
1 hectoliter	(hL)	=	100.0	l
1 kiloliter	(kL)	=	1000.0	l

Note—The Standard of Capacity is the *liter*, which is the volume of 1 kg of distilled water at its maximum density (approx. 4°C). Microliters (μL) are used to measure volumes of solutions used in chromatographic procedures for the separation and quantitative determination of some official drugs.

Table VIII—Apothecary or Wine Measure (US)

Gallon	Pints	Fluidounces	Fluidrams	Minims
Cong 1 =	8 =	128 =	1024 =	61,440
	O. 1 =	16 =	128 =	7,680
		f℥ 1 =	ℨ 8 =	480
			f℥ 1 =	ℳ 60

Table IX—Imperial Measure (British)

Gallon	Pints	Fluidounces	Fluidrams	Minims
Cong 1 =	8 =	160 =	1280	76,800
	O. 1 =	20 =	160	9,600
		fl℥ 1 =	8 =	480
			fl℥ 1 =	ℳ 60

Note—O. is the abbreviation for the Latin word *Octarius;* Cong, for the Latin word *Congius.* The gill, which is ¼ pint, is obsolete but is occasionally found in old family recipes. 31 US gallons equal 1 barrel.

Pharmacists who fill Canadian or British prescriptions should also be familiar with the substantially different British imperial liquid measure system, the units of which, and their equivalents, are given in Table IX.

The following facts concerning the US system of liquid measure, Table VIII, should be noted:

1. The apothecary fluidounce of distilled water weighs 454.6 gr at 25°C (77°F).
2. The apothecary pint contains 16 fl℥.
3. The US gallon contains 128 fl℥ or 231 cu in. One gallon of distilled water weighs 8.337 avoir lb at 62°F. The US pint therefore weighs 1.04 avoir lb and the pound of distilled water measures only 0.96 pt. *One pound does not measure 1 pt.*

The following facts concerning the imperial system, Table IX, should be noted:

1. The imperial fluidounce of distilled water weighs 437.5 gr at 15.6°C (60°F). It therefore weighs 1 avoir oz.
2. The imperial pint contains 20 fl℥.
3. The imperial gallon contains 160 fl℥. One gallon of distilled water weighs 10 avoir lb. 16 fl℥ in this system therefore weigh 1 avoir lb.

From the above statements we deduce the following

1. The US fluidounce and minim are larger than the imperial fluidounce and minim. One US minim or fluidounce equals 1.04 imperial minims or fluidounces.
2. The imperial pint and gallon are much larger than the US pint and gallon.

It is, therefore, inaccurate to use measuring devices calibrated in the US system in measuring quantities directed in English prescriptions when the imperial measure is intended, and, conversely, devices calibrated in the imperial system should not be used to measure quantities directed in US prescriptions when the US measure is intended. For example, Canadian pharmacists using American graduates should calculate percentage solutions on the basis of 454.6 gr of distilled water to the fluidounce. This is one more argument in favor of adoption internationally by all pharmacists of the metric system of weights and measures.

The Relationships of Weights and of Measures

When the systems of weights and measures in use in this country are studied, the lack of close relation between the different units is at once appreciated. Nevertheless, if the following statements are carefully memorized, many pharmaceutical problems will be greatly simplified.

1. The pharmacist may buy merchandise, sell over the counter, weigh himself, calculate postage, etc, by avoirdupois weight which contains *437.5 gr in 1 oz.*
2. He may dispense prescriptions and compound formulas by apothecary weight which contains *480 gr in 1 oz.*
3. One apothecary fluidounce of water weighs *455 gr* at 25°C. Since 480 ℳ weigh 455 gr, then 1 ℳ weighs 455/480 = 0.95 gr.

> 1 ℳ does *not* weigh 1 gr
> 1 fl℥ does *not* weigh 1 oz avoir.

Practical Equivalents

Tables of weights and measures and a table of practical equivalents should be kept in a conspicuous and convenient place in the prescription department, and the following equivalents, which are given with practical accuracy, should be committed to memory. Other equivalents may be calculated from these.

Linear Measure

1 meter	= **39.4 in.** (39.37 in.)	
1 inch	= 2.54 cm = **25 mm** (25.4 mm)	
1 micron	= **1/1000 mm** = 10^{-6} m = 1/25,000 in.	

Liquid Measure

1 milliliter	= **16.2 ℳ** (16.23 ℳ)
1 fluidounce	= **30 mL** (29.57 mL)
1 pint	= **473 mL**
1 gallon	= **3785 mL**

Weight

1 kilogram	= **2.2 lb**
1 pound avoir	= **454 g** (453.59 g)
1 ounce avoir	= **28.4 g** (28.35 g)
1 ounce apoth	= **31.1 g**
1 gram	= **15.4 gr** (15.432 gr)
1 grain	= **65 mg**

The USP *Table of Metric Doses with Approximate Apothecary Equivalents* is reproduced on the front inside cover of this book, along with information concerning its permissible uses.

Table XIV gives the *exact* equivalents of metric, avoirdupois, and apothecary weights and measures.

Approximate Measures

In apportioning doses for a patient the practitioner is usually compelled to order the liquid medicine to be administered in certain quantities that have been established by custom, and estimated as follows:

1 tumblerful	f℥ viii	240 mL
1 teacupful	f℥ iv	120 mL
1 wineglassful	f℥ ii	60 mL
2 tablespoonfuls	f℥ i	30 mL

Table X—Equivalent Linear Measurements

Unit	in.	mm	μm	nm	Å
1 in. (inch)	1	25.4	25,400	2.54×10^7	2.54×10^8
1 mm (millimeter)	0.0394	1	1000	10^6	10^7
1 μm (micrometer) or μ (micron)	3.94×10^{-5}	10^{-3}	1	1000	10,000
1 nm (nanometer or millimicron)	3.94×10^{-8}	10^{-6}	10^{-3}	1	10
1 Å (angstrom unit)	3.94×10^{-9}	10^{-7}	10^{-4}	0.1	1

Table XI—Converting Metric Quantities to Quantities in Avoirdupois Weight at 25°C

Grams to Grains, etc. (Product Measured)

g/l	gr/fl℥ oz av	gr/fl℥ gr	gr, etc./pt oz av	gr, etc./pt gr	gr, etc./gal lb av	gr, etc./gal oz av	gr, etc./gal gr
1	..	0.45	..	7.3	..	..	58.2
2	..	0.91	..	14.5	..	..	116.4
3	..	1.36	..	21.8	..	..	174.6
4	..	1.82	..	29.1	..	..	232.7
5	..	2.27	..	36.4	..	..	290.9
6	..	2.73	..	43.6	..	..	349.1
7	..	3.18	..	50.9	..	..	407.3
8	..	3.64	..	58.2	..	1	28.0
9	..	4.09	..	65.5	..	1	86.2
10	..	4.55	..	72.7	..	1	144.3
20	..	9.09	..	145.5	..	2	288.7
30	..	13.64	..	218.2	..	3	433.0
40	..	18.18	..	290.9	..	5	139.9
50	..	22.73	..	363.7	..	6	284.2
60	..	27.27	..	436.4	..	7	428.6
70	..	31.82	1	71.6	..	9	135.4
80	..	36.37	1	144.3	..	10	279.8
90	..	40.91	1	217.1	..	11	424.1
100	..	45.46	1	289.8	..	13	131.0
200	..	90.91	3	142.1	1	10	262.0
300	..	136.37	4	431.9	2	7	393.0
400	..	181.83	6	284.2	3	5	86.5
500	..	227.29	8	136.6	4	2	217.5
600	..	272.74	9	426.4	4	15	348.5
700	..	318.20	11	278.7	5	13	42.0
800	..	363.66	13	131.0	6	10	173.0
900	..	409.11	14	420.9	7	7	304.0
1000	1	17.07	16	273.1	8	4	435.0

Note—It should be particularly noted that the table given above gives conversion figures for use at 25°C, the average temperature of the dispensary. One fluidounce of water weighs 454.6 gr at 25°C. A similar table was printed in the appendix of the USP XIV, but it gave conversion figures for use at 4°C at which temperature 1 fl℥ of water weighs 456.4 gr. For practical purposes the difference between the two tables is negligible.

1 tablespoonful	f℥ iv	15 mL
1 dessertspoonful	f℥ ii	8 mL
1 teaspoonful	f℥ i	5 mL
½ teaspoonful	f℥ ss	2 mL

Note—1 drop, through a popular error, is considered to be 1 minim. This is incorrect as "drops" are variable. See also page 82.

In almost all cases the modern teacups, tablespoons, dessertspoons, and teaspoons, after careful tests, are found to average 25% greater capacity than the theoretical quantities just given. The physician and the pharmacist should therefore recommend the use of accurately graduated medicine droppers, teaspoons, glasses, and other devices, which may be procured at a small cost (Fig 9-1).

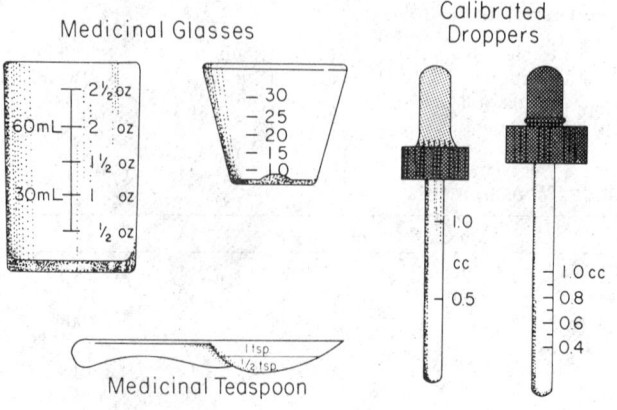

Fig 9-1.

Table XII—Converting Metric Quantities to Quantities in Apothecary Measures

mL to ♏, etc. (Product Measured)

mL/L	♏/fl℥	♏, etc./pt fl℥	♏, etc./pt ♏	♏, etc./gal pt	♏, etc./gal fl℥	♏, etc./gal ♏
1	0.48	..	7.68	..	..	61
2	0.96	..	15.36	..	..	123
3	1.44	..	23.04	..	..	184
4	1.92	..	30.72	..	..	246
5	2.40	..	38.40	..	..	307
6	2.88	..	46.09	..	..	369
7	3.36	..	53.76	..	..	430
8	3.84	..	61.44	..	1	12
9	4.32	..	69.12	..	1	73
10	4.80	..	76.80	..	1	134
20	9.60	..	153.60	..	2	269
30	14.40	..	230.40	..	3	403
40	19.20	..	307.20	..	5	58
50	24.00	..	384.00	..	6	192
60	28.80	..	460.80	..	7	326
70	33.60	1	57.60	..	8	461
80	38.40	1	134.40	..	10	115
90	43.20	1	211.20	..	11	250
100	48.00	1	288.00	..	12	384
200	96.00	3	96.00	1	9	288
300	144.00	4	384.00	2	6	192
400	192.00	6	192.00	3	3	96
500	240.00	8	....	4	..	....
600	288.00	9	288.00	4	12	384
700	336.00	11	96.00	5	9	288
800	384.00	12	384.00	6	6	192
900	432.00	14	192.00	7	3	96
1000	480.00	16	....	8	..	...

Table XIII—Converting Metric Quantities to Quantities in Apothecary Weights

Parts per 1000 to grains, etc, per pound avoirdupois

Grams per Kilogram	Grains and Apothecaries Ounces per Pound Avoirdupois oz	Grains and Apothecaries Ounces per Pound Avoirdupois gr	Grains and Ounces Avoirdupois per Pound Avoirdupois oz	Grains and Ounces Avoirdupois per Pound Avoirdupois gr
1	..	7	..	7.0
2	..	14	..	14.0
3	..	21	..	21.0
4	..	28	..	28.0
5	..	35	..	35.0
6	..	42	..	42.0
7	..	49	..	49.0
8	..	56	..	56.0
9	..	63	..	63.0
10	..	70	..	70.0
20	..	140	..	140.0
30	..	210	..	210.0
40	..	280	..	280.0
50	..	350	..	350.0
60	..	420	..	420.0
70	1	10	1	52.5
80	1	80	1	122.5
90	1	150	1	192.5
100	1	220	1	262.5
200	2	440	3	87.5
300	4	180	4	350.0
400	5	400	6	175.0
500	7	140	8	...
600	8	360	9	262.5
700	10	100	11	87.5
800	11	320	12	350.0
900	13	60	14	175.0
1000	14	280	16	...

Approximate Dose Equivalents

For many years the apothecaries' system of weights and measures was widely used by physicians and pharmacists when considering the doses of medicinal substances, and it was customary to translate these apothecaries' doses into relatively exact amounts when the metric equivalents were mentioned. Today, however, a united effort is being made to establish doses primarily in the metric system and to select for these doses the metric quantities which produce the desired therapeutic effect, without considering the relation of these metric figures to the corresponding quantities in any other system of weights and measures.

Table XIV—Exact Equivalents of Weights and Measures

Metric, Avoirdupois, and Apothecary

Weights: grains	Weights: Apothecary oz	Weights: Apothecary gr	Weights: Avoirdupois lb	Weights: Avoirdupois oz	Weights: Avoirdupois gr	Metric Weight and Measure, g or mL[a]	Measures: Fluid oz	Measures: Fluid min	Measures: fl oz and Fract
15432.4	32	72.4	2	3	119.9	**1000**	33	391.1	33.815
15360.0	**32**	...	2	3	47.5	995.311	33	314.9	33.656
15060.5	31	180.5	2	2	185.5	975.906	**33**	...	**33**
15046.5	31	166.5	2	2	171.5	**975**	32	465.3	32.969
14880.0	**31**	...	2	2	5.0	964.208	32	290.1	32.604
14660.7	30	260.7	2	1	223.2	**950**	32	59.5	32.124
14604.1	30	204.1	2	1	166.6	946.333	**32**	...	**32**
14400.0	**30**	...	2	..	400.0	933.104	31	265.2	31.553
14274.9	29	354.9	2	..	274.9	**925**	31	133.7	31.279
14147.8	29	227.8	2	..	147.8	916.700	**31**	...	**31**
14000.0	29	80.0	**2**	..	...	907.185	30	324.6	30.676
13920.0	**29**	...	1	15	357.5	902.001	30	240.4	30.501
13889.1	28	449.1	1	15	326.6	**900**	30	207.9	30.433
13691.4	28	251.4	1	15	128.9	887.187	**30**	...	**30**
13562.5	28	122.5	**1**	**15**	...	878.835	29	344.4	29.718
13503.3	28	63.3	1	14	378.3	**875**	29	282.2	29.588
13440.0	**28**	...	1	14	315.0	870.897	29	215.6	29.449
13235.0	27	275.0	1	14	110.0	857.614	**29**	...	**29**
13125.0	27	165.0	**1**	**14**	...	850.486	28	364.3	28.759
13117.5	27	157.5	1	13	430.0	**850**	28	356.4	28.742
12960.0	**27**	...	1	13	272.5	839.794	28	190.8	28.397
12778.6	26	298.6	1	13	91.1	828.041	**28**	...	**28**
12731.7	26	251.7	1	13	44.2	**825**	27	430.6	27.897
12687.5	26	207.5	**1**	**13**	...	822.136	27	384.1	27.800
12480.0	**26**	...	1	12	230.0	808.690	27	165.9	27.346
12345.9	25	345.9	1	12	95.9	**800**	27	24.9	27.052
12322.3	25	322.3	1	12	72.3	798.469	**27**	...	**27**
12250.0	25	250.0	**1**	**12**	...	793.787	26	504.0	26.842
12000.0	**25**	...	1	11	187.5	777.587	26	141.1	26.294
11960.1	24	440.1	1	11	147.6	**775**	26	99.1	26.206
11865.9	24	345.9	1	11	53.4	768.896	**26**	...	**26**
11812.5	24	292.5	**1**	**11**	...	765.437	25	423.8	25.883
11574.3	24	54.3	1	10	199.3	**750**	25	173.3	25.361
11520.0	**24**	...	1	10	145.0	746.484	25	116.2	25.242
11409.5	23	369.5	1	10	34.5	739.323	**25**	...	**25**
11375.0	23	335.0	**1**	**10**	...	737.088	24	443.7	24.924
11188.5	23	148.5	1	9	251.0	**725**	24	247.5	24.516
11040.0	**23**	...	1	9	102.5	715.380	24	91.4	24.190
10953.1	22	393.1	1	9	15.6	709.750	**24**	...	**24**
10937.5	22	377.5	**1**	**9**	...	708.738	23	463.6	23.966
10802.6	22	242.6	1	8	302.6	**700**	23	321.7	23.670
10560.0	**22**	...	1	8	60.0	684.277	23	66.5	23.139
10500.0	21	420.0	**1**	**8**	...	680.389	23	3.4	23.007
10496.7	21	416.7	1	7	434.2	680.177	**23**	...	**23**
10416.8	21	336.8	1	7	354.3	**675**	22	396.0	22.825
10080.0	**21**	...	1	7	17.5	653.173	22	41.7	22.087
10062.5	20	462.5	**1**	**7**	...	652.039	22	23.3	22.049
10040.4	20	440.4	1	6	415.4	650.604	**22**	...	**22**
10031.0	20	431.0	1	6	406.0	**650**	21	470.2	21.980
9645.2	20	45.2	1	6	20.2	**625**	21	64.4	21.134
9625.0	20	25.0	**1**	**6**	...	623.690	21	43.2	21.090
9600.0	**20**	...	1	5	412.5	622.070	21	16.8	21.035
9584.0	19	464.0	1	5	396.5	621.031	**21**	...	**21**
9259.4	19	139.4	1	5	71.9	**600**	20	138.6	20.289
9187.5	19	67.5	**1**	**5**	...	595.340	20	63.0	20.131
9127.6	19	7.6	1	4	377.6	591.458	**20**	...	**20**
9120.0	**19**	...	1	4	370.0	590.966	19	472.0	19.983
8873.6	18	233.6	1	4	123.6	**575**	19	212.9	19.444
8750.0	18	110.0	**1**	**4**	...	566.991	19	82.8	19.173
8671.2	18	31.2	1	3	358.7	561.885	**19**	...	**19**
8460.0	**18**	...	1	3	327.5	559.863	18	447.2	18.932
8487.8	17	327.8	1	3	175.3	**550**	18	287.1	18.598
8312.5	17	152.5	**1**	**3**	...	538.641	18	102.7	18.214
8214.8	17	54.8	1	2	339.8	532.312	**18**	...	**18**
8160.0	**17**	...	1	2	285.0	528.759	17	422.3	17.880
8102.0	16	422.0	1	2	227.0	**525**	17	361.3	17.753
7875.0	16	195.0	**1**	**2**	...	510.291	17	122.5	17.255
7758.5	16	78.5	1	1	321.0	502.739	**17**	...	**17**
7716.2	16	36.2	1	1	278.7	**500**	16	435.6	16.907
7680.0	**16**	...	1	1	242.5	497.656	16	397.5	16.828
7437.5	15	237.5	**1**	**1**	...	481.942	16	142.4	16.297
7330.4	15	130.4	1	..	330.4	**475**	16	29.8	16.062
7302.1	15	102.1	**1**	..	302.1	473.167	**16**	...	**16**
7200.0	**15**	...	1	..	200.0	466.552	15	372.6	15.776

Weights: grains	Weights: Apothecary oz	Weights: Apothecary gr	Weights: Avoirdupois lb	Weights: Avoirdupois oz	Weights: Avoirdupois gr	Metric Weight and Measure, g or mL[a]	Measures: Fluid oz	Measures: Fluid min	Measures: fl oz and Fract
7000.0	14	280.0	**1**	..	...	453.592	15	162.3	15.338
6944.6	14	224.6	..	15	382.1	**450**	15	104.0	15.217
6845.7	14	125.7	..	15	283.2	443.594	**15**	...	**15**
6720.0	**14**	...	..	15	157.5	435.449	14	347.8	14.725
6562.5	13	322.5	..	**15**	...	425.243	14	182.2	14.379
6558.8	13	318.8	..	14	433.8	**425**	14	178.2	14.371
6389.3	13	149.3	..	14	264.3	414.021	**14**	...	**14**
6240.0	**13**	...	..	14	115.0	404.345	13	322.9	13.673
6172.9	12	412.9	..	14	47.9	**400**	13	252.4	13.526
6125.0	12	365.0	..	**14**	...	396.893	13	202.0	13.421
5932.9	12	172.9	..	13	245.4	384.448	**13**	...	**13**
5787.1	12	27.1	..	13	99.6	**375**	12	326.6	12.681
5760.0	**12**	...	..	13	72.5	373.242	12	298.1	12.621
5687.5	11	407.5	..	**13**	...	368.544	12	221.9	12.462
5476.6	11	196.6	..	12	226.6	354.875	**12**	...	**12**
5401.3	11	121.3	..	12	151.3	**350**	11	400.8	11.835
5280.0	**11**	...	..	12	30.0	342.138	11	273.3	11.569
5250.0	10	450.0	..	**12**	...	340.194	11	241.7	11.504
5020.2	10	220.2	..	11	207.7	325.302	**11**	...	**11**
5015.5	10	215.5	..	11	203.0	**325**	10	475.1	10.990
4812.5	10	12.5	..	**11**	...	311.845	10	261.6	10.545
4800.0	**10**	...	..	10	425.0	311.035	10	248.4	10.518
4629.7	9	309.7	..	10	254.7	**300**	10	69.3	10.144
4563.8	9	243.8	..	10	188.8	295.729	**10**	...	**10**
4375.0	9	55.0	..	**10**	...	283.495	9	281.4	9.586
4320.0	**9**	...	..	9	382.5	279.931	9	223.6	9.466
4244.0	8	403.9	..	9	306.4	**275**	9	143.5	9.299
4107.4	8	267.4	..	9	169.9	266.156	**9**	...	**9**
3937.5	8	97.5	..	**9**	...	255.146	8	301.3	8.628
3858.1	8	18.1	..	8	358.1	**250**	8	217.8	8.454
3840.0	**8**	...	..	8	340.0	248.828	8	198.7	8.414
3651.0	7	291.0	..	8	151.0	236.583	**8**	...	**8**
3500.0	7	140.0	..	**8**	...	226.796	7	321.1	7.669
3472.3	7	112.3	..	7	409.8	**225**	7	292.0	7.608
3360.0	**7**	...	..	7	297.5	217.724	7	173.9	7.362
3194.7	6	314.7	..	7	132.2	207.010	**7**	...	**7**
3086.5	6	206.5	..	7	24.0	**200**	6	366.2	6.763
3062.5	6	182.5	..	**7**	...	198.557	6	341.0	6.710
2880.0	**6**	...	..	6	255.0	186.621	6	149.0	6.311
2738.3	5	338.3	..	6	113.3	177.437	**6**	...	**6**
2700.7	5	300.7	..	6	75.7	**175**	5	440.4	5.918
2625.0	5	225.0	..	**6**	...	170.097	5	360.9	5.752
2400.0	**5**	...	..	5	212.5	155.517	5	124.1	5.259
2314.9	4	394.9	..	5	127.4	**150**	5	34.7	5.072
2281.9	4	361.9	..	5	94.4	147.865	**5**	...	**5**
2187.5	4	267.5	..	**5**	...	141.748	4	380.7	4.793
1929.0	4	9.0	..	4	179.0	**125**	4	108.9	4.227
1920.0	**4**	...	..	4	170.0	124.414	4	99.4	4.207
1825.5	3	385.5	..	4	75.5	118.292	**4**	...	**4**
1750.0	3	310.0	..	**4**	...	113.398	3	400.6	3.835
1543.2	3	103.2	..	3	230.7	**100**	3	183.1	3.381
1440.0	**3**	...	..	3	127.5	93.310	3	74.5	3.155
1388.9	2	428.9	..	3	76.4	**90**	3	20.8	3.043
1369.1	2	409.1	..	3	56.6	88.719	**3**	...	**3**
1312.5	2	352.5	..	**3**	...	85.049	2	420.4	2.876
1234.6	2	274.6	..	2	359.6	**80**	2	338.5	2.705
1157.4	2	197.5	..	2	282.4	**75**	2	257.3	2.536
1080.3	2	120.3	..	2	205.3	**70**	2	176.2	2.367
960.0	**2**	...	..	2	85.0	62.207	2	49.7	2.104
925.9	1	445.9	..	2	50.9	**60**	2	13.9	2.029
912.8	1	432.8	..	2	37.8	59.146	**2**	...	**2**
875.0	1	395.0	..	**2**	...	56.699	1	440.3	1.917
771.6	1	291.6	..	1	334.1	**50**	1	331.5	1.691
617.3	1	137.3	..	1	179.8	**40**	1	169.2	1.353
480.0	**1**	...	..	1	42.5	31.1035	1	24.9	1.052
463.0	..	...	..	1	25.5	**30**	1	6.9	1.014
456.380	..	...	..	1	18.88	29.5729	**1**	...	**1**
437.5	..	...	..	**1**	...	28.350	..	460.15	0.959
385.8	..	...	..	..	...	**25**	..	405.78	0.845
308.6	..	...	..	..	...	**20**	..	324.62	0.676
154.3	..	...	..	..	...	**10**	..	162.31	0.338
15.4324	..	...	..	..	...	**1**	..	16.23	0.0338
1	..	...	..	..	...	0.06480	..	1.0517	0.0022
0.9508	..	...	..	..	...	0.06161	..	**1**	0.0021

[a] *Note*—The abbreviation "mL" for milliliter may be used interchangeably with "cc" for cubic centimeter since they are practically identical.
The values given for the relation of weight to measure and *vice versa*, are for water at the temperature of 4°C (39.2°F) *in vacuo*. See page 71.

Table XIV—Continued

From 480 grains down

Grains	Metric Weight and Measure, g or mL [a]	Minims (of Water at 4°C)
480 (1 ℥)	31.103	504.8
478.4	31	503.2
475.4	30.805	500
463.0	30	486.9
456.4	29.573	480 (1 f℥)
450	29.160	473.3
447.5	29	470.7
437.5 (1 oz av)	28.350	460.2
432.1	28	454.5
427.9	27.725	450
420 (7 ʒ)	27.216	441.7
416.7	27	438.2
401.2	26	422.0
399.3	25.876	420
390	25.272	410.2
385.8	25	405.8
380.3	24.644	400
370.8	24.028	390
370.4	24	389.5
360 (6 ʒ)	23.328	378.6
354.9	23	373.3
342.3	22.180	360
339.5	22	357.1
330	21.384	347.1
324.1	21	340.9
313.8	20.331	330
308.6	20	324.6
300 (5 ʒ)	19.440	315.5
293.2	19	308.4
285.2	18.483	300
277.8	18	292.2
270	17.496	284.0
262.4	17	275.9
256.7	16.635	270
246.9	16	259.7
240 (4 ʒ)	15.552	252.4
231.5	15	243.5
228.2	14.786	240.0
218.75 (½ oz av)	14.175	230.1
216.1	14	227.2
210	13.608	220.9
200.6	13	211.0
199.7	12.938	210.0
185.2	12	194.8
180 (3 ʒ)	11.664	189.3
171.1	11.090	180.0
169.8	11	178.5
154.3	10	162.3
150	9.720	157.8
142.6	9.242	150.0
138.9	9	146.1
123.5	8	129.8
120 (2 ʒ)	7.776	126.2
114.1	7.393	120.0
109.375 (¼ oz av)	7.087	115.0
108.0	7	113.6
100	6.480	105.2
95.1	6.161	100.0
92.6	6	97.4
80	5.184	84.1
77.2	5	81.2
76.1	4.929	80.0
61.7	4	64.9
60 (1 ʒ)	3.888	63.1
57.0	3.697	60.0
54.6875 (⅛ oz av)	3.544	57.5
50	3.240	52.6
47.5	3.081	50.0
46.3	3	48.7
42.8	2.772	45.0
40	2.592	42.1
38.0	2.464	40.0
33.3	2.156	35.0
30.9	2	32.5

From 30 grains down

Grains	Metric Weight and Measure, g of mL [a]	Minims (of Water at 4°C)
30 (½ ʒ)	1.944	31.55
28.52	1.848	30
23.77	1.540	25
20	1.296	21.04
19.02	1.232	20
15.4324	1	16.23
15	0.972	15.78
14.26	0.924	15
14	0.907	14.72
13.31	0.863	14
13	0.842	13.67
12.36	0.801	13
12	0.778	12.63
11.41	0.739	12
11	0.713	11.57
10.46	0.678	11
10	0.648	10.52
9.51	0.616	10
9	0.583	9.46
8.56	0.554	9
8	0.518	8.41
7.72	0.5	8.12
7.61	0.493	8
7	0.454	7.37
6.66	0.431	7
6	0.389	6.31
5.70	0.370	6
5	0.324	5.26
4.75	0.308	5
4	0.259	4.20
3.80	0.246	4
3	0.194	3.15
2.85	0.185	3
2	0.130	2.11
1.90	0.123	2
1	0.06480	1.0518
0.9508	0.06161	1

From 5 grains down

Milligrams (mg)	Grains
324	5
292	4½
259	4
227	3½
194	3
162	2½
130	2
97	1½
65	1
60.7	15/16
58.3	9/10
56.7	7/8
52.6	13/16
51.8	4/5
48.6	3/4
44.5	11/16
40.5	5/8
36.4	9/16
32.4	½
28.3	7/16
25.9	2/5
24.3	3/8
20.2	5/16
16.2	¼
12.1	3/16
8.1	⅛
4.0	1/16
3.2	1/20
2.6	1/25
2.2	1/30
1.8	1/36
1.6	1/40
1.3	1/50
1.1	1/60
1.0	1/64
0.6	1/100
0.5	1/128
0.4	1/160
0.3	1/210
0.2	1/320
0.1	1/640

[a] *Note*—The abbreviation "mL" for milliliter may be used interchangeably with "cc" for cubic centimeter since they are practically identical.

It should be emphasized that exact alternative formulas in the avoirdupois system of weights and measures are *not* obtained by using approximate equivalents but for the purpose of compounding should be calculated with the use of the conversion tables printed as Tables XI–XIV. These give the exact proportionate amounts required to produce an identical formula in the English system. For example, the quantities used to make a formula for 1000 mL are frequently converted into quantities required to make 2 pt. Two pints do not equal 1000 mL and therefore all ingredients must be calculated in the same ratio as 2 pt to 1000 mL.

Weighing and Measuring

Having studied the several systems of weights and measures, one may now learn to apply his knowledge to the *weighing* and *measuring* of pharmaceuticals. The former process requires the use of the *balance*, or, for manufacturing purposes, *scales*, and the latter process requires the use of the *measure*, the *graduate*, and the *pipet*. Since the successful performance of many of the operations in pharmacy depends on a thorough knowledge of the principles of the balance and a correct understanding of its care and use, and since weighing is nearly always the preliminary step in any compounding, it will be discussed first.

There is a relativity of accuracy in weighing (or measuring) which must not be overlooked and which may be illustrated by giving consideration to the following graded list: coal, salt, sugar, epsom salt, penicillin G, morphine, digoxin, vitamin B_{12}, and radium. One of the most important things for the pharmacist to learn is the degree of tolerance or error permissible in weighing or measuring any particular ingredient.

The empiric weighing and measuring methods of the kitchen, embodied in such concepts as a handful, a pinch, or "sweeten to suit your taste," have no place in pharmacy. Accurate work can be accomplished only by means of suitable apparatus.

Weighing

In pharmacy, weighing usually refers to the ascertaining of a definite weight of material to be used in compounding a prescription or manufacturing a dosage form.

The *balance* may be defined as an instrument for determining the relative weights of substances, and should be *correctly selected* for the specific task at hand, *skillfully used*, *carefully protected from injury*, and *periodically checked*, if accurate results are to be obtained. Of even greater importance is its *construction*. Standards for balances are given by the National Bureau of Standards.[1]

Construction of the Balance

For systematic consideration pharmaceutical balances may be classified as follows: (1) single-beam, equal-arm, (2) unequal arm, (3) compound lever, and (4) torsion.

Single-Beam Equal-Arm Balances—The principle on which these balances (or scales) operate is clearly evident in the construction of the classical two-pan analytical balance. This type of balance has a metallic lever or beam, divided into two equal arms at the center by a knife edge, on which it is supported. At exactly equal distances from this point of support, and situated in the same plane, are placed the end knife edges; these suspend the pans which carry the substances to be weighed. A properly constructed balance of this type should meet the following requirements:

1. When the beam is in a horizontal position, the center of gravity should be slightly below the point of support, or central knife edge, and perpendicular to it.

The relative sensitiveness of the balance depends on the fulfilment of this principle, which may be roughly illustrated by forcing a pin through the center of a circular piece of pasteboard; if the edge of the pasteboard is touched slightly, it does not oscillate at all, but revolves around the center to a degree corresponding to the impulse given it. In this position it illustrates neutral equilibrium. If the pin is removed and inserted at a very short distance above the center, and the edge of the pasteboard touched as before, it will oscillate slowly, corresponding to a very sensitive beam, the point of support being *slightly* above the center of gravity as in the balance; if the pin is again removed and inserted far above the center, and the same impulse imparted to the edge, it will oscillate quickly, illustrating stable equilibrium characteristic of a beam which comes to rest quickly and is not particularly sensitive. Unstable equilibrium may be illustrated by balancing the disk so that the point of support is below the center. The slightest touch then causes it to reverse its position completely and finally come to rest with the center of gravity below the point of support.

2. The end knife edges must be exactly equal distances from the central knife edge; they all must be in the same plane, and the edges absolutely parallel to each other.

It is very apparent that the conditions of a good prescription balance cannot be satisfied if there is inequality in the length of the arms of the beam. The distance from the central knife edge to the one on the left must be exactly the same as the distance from the central knife edge to the one on the right, otherwise unequal weights would be required to establish equilibrium. If the central knife edge is placed either above or below a line drawn so that it connects the end knife edges, the loading of the pans will either cause the beam to cease oscillating, or will diminish the sensitiveness in proportion to the load. If the knife edges are not parallel, the weight of a body will not be constant upon every part of the pan, but will be greater if placed near the edge on one side, and correspondingly less at a point directly opposite.

3. The beam should be inflexible, but as light in weight as possible, and the knife edges in fine balances should bear upon agate planes.

Rigidity of the beam is necessary because any serious deflection caused by a loading of the pans would lower the end knife edges and thus accuracy in weighing would be impossible. The beam should not be heavier than necessary because the sensitiveness of the balance would be thereby lessened, and to diminish friction which constantly increases with the age and use of a balance, the bearings of the knife edges should

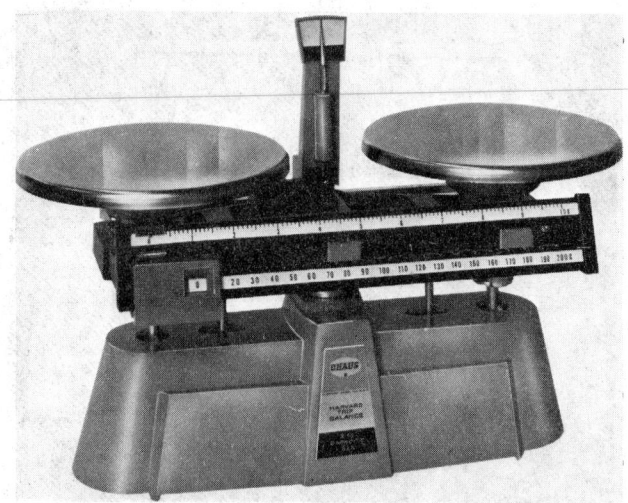

Fig 9-2. Single-beam equal-arm balance (courtesy, Ohaus).

be agate planes, which are polished flat pieces of the very hard mineral called agate.

A single-beam equal-arm balance with two rider beams, one graduated to 10 g in increments of 0.1 g, and the other to 200 g in increments of 10 g, is shown in Fig 9-2.

Unequal-Arm Balances—This type of balance is preferred for laboratory work when large amounts are to be weighed. The lever principle upon which these scales are constructed is based on the law of physics that at equilibrium the force applied at one end of the lever multiplied by the length of the arm (distance from the fulcrum to the point where the force is applied) must be equal to the product of the force acting at the opposite end of the lever and the length of the other arm. The inequality in the length of the arms of this beam permits the convenient use of movable weights upon the graduated longer arm of the beam, thus dispensing with the use of small weights, which are liable to be lost. This scale (Fig 9-3) is of great advantage in laboratory or manufacturing work because it is particularly adapted for weighing liquids, a sliding tare being set on one beam for the weight of the container, while other sliding weights can be adjusted to the weight of liquid desired. These are available with the beams graduated either in the avoirdupois or metric system.

Compound-Lever Balances—The principle of the compound lever was first applied in the construction of balances by Robervahl, of Paris, about AD 1660. It was skillfully adopted for both prescription balances and the general counter and platform scales. The principal objection to this type of balance, when compared with single-beam balances, consists in the multiplicity of points of contact and suspension, thus necessarily increasing friction and the liability to disarrangement; however, their general convenience has made them

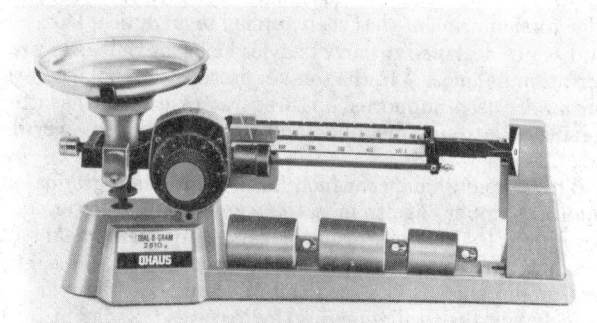

Fig 9-3. Manufacturing laboratory scale and weights (courtesy, Ohaus).

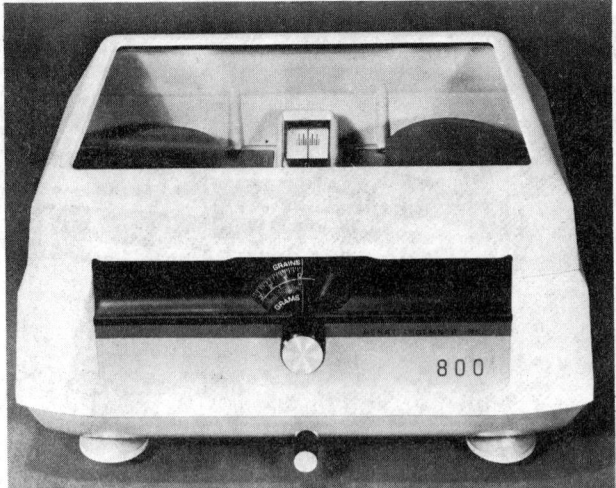

Fig 9-4. Troemner/800 prescription balance (courtesy, Troemner).

popular. The principle of the compound lever balance, with the arrangement of the levers as formerly utilized in a prescription balance, is shown in RPS-14, Fig. 29, page 88.

Torsion Balances—A simple illustration of the principle of torsion is afforded by tying a stout piece of cord to a firm support and inserting a lead pencil in the middle of the cord between the strands, at right angles to it. If the free end of the cord is tightly stretched, and the effort is made to turn the lead pencil over, it will at once be noticed that resistance is offered, and if the pencil is released, it at once flies back to its original position.

Torsion is the term applied to this method of twisting. The principle of supporting the beam of a balance on a tightly stretched wire, with the view of doing away with knife edges and diminishing friction, occupied the attention of inventors for years. In 1882 Prof Roeder and Dr Springer contrived an ingenious torsion balance which gave promise of valuable results. Two illustrations of this original balance were shown on page 54 of the first edition of *Remington's Practice of Pharmacy* in 1885. Improvements have greatly increased its efficiency; the most important difficulty in applying the principle—that of torsional resistance—was overcome by the device of placing a weight just above the center of gravity, torsional resistance having the tendency to keep the beam in a horizontal position, while the elevation of a weight above the center of gravity, by its tendency to produce unstable equilibrium, exercises an opposite effect—that of inclining the beam to be top-heavy, and therefore to tip on either side. If now the weight is made adjustable, by mounting it upon a perpendicular screw, so that it can be raised or lowered, it is possible to arrange these opposite forces so that one exactly neutralizes the other. In this manner sensitivity is obtained. The torsion principle has been applied to analytical balances and scales designed to carry heavier loads, as well as to prescription balances. In the torsion prescription balance two beams are used, supported on three frames, each of the latter having a flattened metallic band stretched tightly over its edge.

The Torsion balance, which has a rider beam graduated upon the upper edge from $\frac{1}{8}$ to 15 gr and on its lower edge from 0.01 to 1.0 g, furnishes a very convenient means of weighing small quantities without having to use small weights. One model, the DRX-2 (see Fig 9-5), includes a "damper" to quickly halt the oscillations and a direct-reading dial instead of a rider beam. A recent model of the Troemner balance (Fig 9-4) has the metric scale on the upper edge of the rider beam and the apothecary scale on the lower edge.

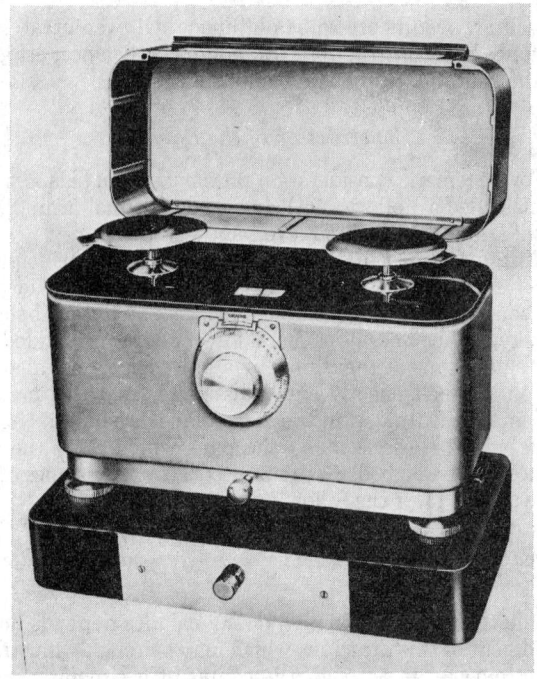

Fig 9-5. Torsion DRX2 prescription balance on balance stand (courtesy, Torsion).

The prescription balances may be placed upon a base containing a drawer which can be used for holding weights, powder papers, etc.

Prescription Balances

There were two common types of prescription balances. One type, no longer available, used the compound lever principle with steel on agate bearings. The type now used utilizes the taut wire frame or torsion principle (Figs 9-4 and 9-5). Such balances are manufactured to meet the requirements of the National Bureau of Standards Class A prescription balances. A Class A prescription balance has a maximum maintenance sensitivity of about 6 mg with no load and with a load of 10 g on each pan, ie, addition of the 6-mg weight to one pan causes the indicator or the rest point to be shifted not less than one division on the index plate. The class A balance is used to weigh quantities up to 120 g depending on the stated capacity, and subject to the physical limit of the amount of the material that can be placed on the pan. All prescription departments must have a Class A balance.

Requirements of Prescription Balances—A prescription balance should meet the following general requirements:

1. It should be constructed so as to support its full capacity without developing undue stresses, and should not be thrown out of adjustment by repeated weighings of the capacity load. (The capacity of the balance will be seen on the metal plate attached to the balance.) If the capacity of the balance is not stated, it is assumed to be at least 15 g ($\frac{1}{2}$ oz). The new Class A balances usually have a capacity of 120 g (4 oz).

2. The removable pans of a prescription balance should be of equal weight. If the pans show any difference in weight, they should be adjusted. Pans with any appreciable corrosion or wear should be refinished or replaced.

3. A prescription balance should have a leveling device, usually leveling feet or screws, so that the balance can be adjusted to a level position. A balance that does not have these is not entitled to be designated as a prescription balance.

4. The balance that has a rider or poise should have, at the end of the scale, a stop which halts the rider at the "zero" reading. The reading edge of the rider should be parallel to the graduations on the beam.

5. The indicator points, when there are two on the balance, should be sharp, and their ends should not be separated by more than 1 mm (0.04 in.) when the scale is in balance. The distance from the face of the index plate to the indicator pointer or pointers should be small (1 mm or less) to protect the operator against making errors resulting from parallax since

it is unlikely that the eye of the operator will be exactly in line with the indicator and the division on the index plate. The indicating elements as well as the lever system of the balance should be protected against drafts. The balance should have a lid which allows a weighing to be made when the lid is closed.

6. A prescription balance must have a mechanical means for arresting the oscillation of the mechanism.

Testing Balances—Having stated the essential points in the construction of the balance, some of the tests which are always applied by manufacturers before approving a balance will now be described. These tests may be applied by any intelligent and careful person to satisfy himself with regard to the construction and character of a balance, the origin, history, or condition of which is in doubt. The prescription balance, being one of the most delicate and important of the instruments in use by the pharmacist, is selected for illustration.

The following is a simplified statement of the most important tests. Additional tests are carried out by the National Bureau of Standards, by manufacturers, and by local and state testing agencies.

A Class A prescription balance meets the following four basic tests. Use a set of *test weights* and keep the rider on the weighbeam at zero unless directed to change its position.

1. *Sensitivity Requirement*—Level the balance, determine the rest point, place a 6-mg weight on one of the empty pans and again determine the rest point. Repeat the operation with a 10-g weight in the center of each pan. The rest point is shifted not less than one division of the index plate each time the 6-mg weight is added.

2. *Arm Ratio Test*—This test is designed to check the equality of length of both arms of the balance. Determine the rest point of the balance with no weight on the pans. Place in the center of each pan 30 g of test weights and determine the rest point. If the second rest point is not the same as the first, place a 20-mg weight on the lighter side; the rest point should move back to the original place on the index plate scale or farther.

3. *Shift Tests*—These tests are designed to check the arm and lever components of the balance.

a. Determine the rest point of the indicator without any weights on the pans.

b. Place one of the 10-g weights in the center of the left pan, and place the other 10-g weight successively toward the right, left, front, and back side of the right pan, noting the rest point in each case. If in any case the rest point differs from the rest point determined in (a), add the 10-mg weight to the lighter side; this should cause the rest point to shift back to the rest point determined in (a) or farther.

c. Place a 10-g weight in the center of the right pan, and place a 10-g weight successively toward the right, left, front, and back side of the left pan, noting the rest point in each case. If in any case the rest point is different from that obtained with no weights on the pans, this difference should be overcome by addition of the 10-mg weight to the lighter side.

d. Make a series of observations in which both weights are simultaneously shifted to off-center positions on their pans, both toward the outside, both toward the inside, one toward the outside and the other toward the inside, both toward the back, and so on until all combinations have been checked. If in any case the rest point differs from that obtained with no weights on the pan the addition of the 10-mg weight to the lighter side should overcome this difference.

A balance which does not measure up to these tests *must* be corrected.

4. *Rider and Graduated Beam Tests*—Determine the rest point for the balance with no weight on the pans. Now place on the left pan the 500-mg test weight and move the rider to the 500-mg point on the beam. Now determine the rest point. If it is different from the zero rest point, add a 6-mg weight to the lighter side. This should bring the rest point back to its original position or farther. Repeat this test, using the 1-g test weight and moving the rider to the 1-g division on the beam. If the rest point is different it should be brought back at least to the zero rest point position by addition of 6 mg to the lighter pan. If the balance does not meet this test, the weighbeam graduations or the rider *must* be corrected.

Protecting Balances—The necessity for protecting the delicate mechanism of a balance is frequently overlooked, notwithstanding the possibility of having a precision apparatus irretrievably ruined by lack of care in using or cleaning it or in protecting it while at rest. The position chosen for the balance or scales should be on a level and firm counter, desk, or table, where it will be subjected to little risk of injury from dampness, dust, or corrosive vapors, and where the knife edges will not be liable to become dulled by jarring or other vibrations.

In the analytical class of balances, protection is afforded by enclosing them in glass cases having sash doors in the front, sides, or in the back. They are protected against injury from vibration by a lever for elevating or locking the beam, so that the knife edges are not in contact with any surface whatever. To prevent injury from jarring while the balance is in use, by a weight falling on the pan, or other accident, the finest balances are provided with pan supports, which break the fall and serve the additional purpose of quickly arresting the beam, thus saving time while weighing.

In using a prescription balance neither the weights nor the substance that is to be weighed should be placed on the scale pans while the beam is free to oscillate. The desired weight should be placed upon one scale pan (usually the one on the right-hand side) and an amount of the substance to be weighed, approximately the desired weight, placed upon the opposite pan. The beam should be released by means of the lever and if the substance is in excess, the beam should be locked and a small portion removed and the beam again released and the oscillations observed. This procedure should be repeated until the correct amount is obtained. In case of a deficiency of the substance to be weighed the reverse procedure is followed until the correct amount is obtained. With practice this can be done very deftly and very quickly and the sensitiveness of the balance retained for years.

Substances which act on metals, such as iodine, and those which are adhesive, such as the extracts, should not be weighed directly upon the scale pans, but upon counterpoised watch crystals, or, if these are not at hand, upon glazed paper, care being taken to balance the papers before weighing the substance. In cleaning the scales great care should be exercised; polishing powders should be used sparingly; a portion is very apt to find its way into crevices and elude detection until an attempt is made to adjust the scales, when the increased weight of one of the sides of the beam leads to its discovery. Frequent cleaning with soft leather is generally sufficient to keep a balance in good order; but if through neglect it becomes necessary to use more active measures, some simple polishing powder for the metal work, with soapsuds for nickel plate, and simple brushing for the lacquered brass, is all that is necessary.

As the pans are subjected to more wear and tear than any other part of the balance, it is economical to use *solid* rather than *plated* pans because constant friction wears off the plating and the additional cost for replating soon absorbs the difference in price. Equipped in this way, and with agate bearings, a prescription balance is durable and really cheap because it will remain for a long time fully equal to the most exacting demands.

Weights Used in Pharmacy

The weights used by the pharmacist are a very important part of his equipment, and care in their selection and examination is necessary. False economy is particularly to be avoided, as the use of cheap, inaccurate weights must lead ultimately to serious consequences. Prescription weights, so worn that the characters on their faces had disappeared, have been found in use in pharmacies by official inspectors, and, on the contrary, weights have been found with bits of hardened extract and dirt almost entirely obscuring their characters. An unused set of standard weights should be kept on hand, so that at least once a year the weights in daily use can be tested and adjusted or rejected if necessary. The standard weights should be used also when the balance is tested. The set should contain the following weights in a well-fitted box with forceps: two 20-g or two 30-g, two 10-g, one 1-g, one

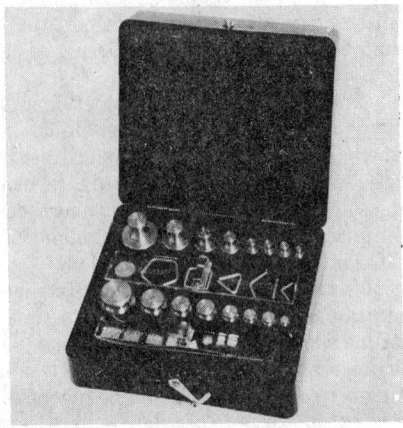

Fig 9-6.   Metric and apothecary weight set (courtesy, Troemner).

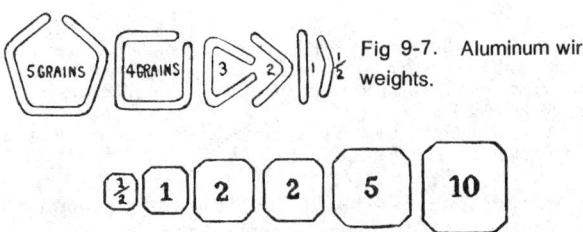

Fig 9-7.   Aluminum wire weights.

Fig 9-8.   Aluminum grain weights.

500-mg, one 20-mg, one 10-mg, and one 6-mg weights; all adjusted to NBS tolerances for analytical or Class P weights.

Metric Weights—For weighing larger quantities, japanned iron weights are available. They are preferably hexagonal in shape, to distinguish them from the round avoirdupois weights. Sets of brass weights, usually in the range of 10–1000 g, fitted into holes of appropriate size in a block of plastic ("block weights"), are especially convenient for many weighing operations. For prescription compounding accurate sets of weights ranging from 10 mg to 50 g are available. A set containing both metric and apothecary weights is shown in Fig. 9-6.

For analytical purposes, metric weights are used exclusively; usually the highest weight is 100 g, the lowest 1 mg. The weights, from 1 g upward, are of brass, finely lacquered, or of nonmagnetic stainless steel or rhodium-plated bronze. The smaller weights are made of squares of platinum foil or aluminum foil with one edge turned up, to permit them to be easily handled with the forceps. Fractions of a milligram are weighed by means of the rider on the graduated beam of the balance.

In analytical work and in using the Class A balance in prescription work, the weights should never be handled with the fingers but always with the forceps which accompany an accurate set of weights. In the more expensive sets of weights the forceps are tipped with bone or ivory to prevent the wearing away of the weights during handling. With proper care the accuracy of a fine set of weights may be maintained for years.

Common Avoirdupois Weights—These are usually made of iron, and are flat and circular, japanned to prevent rusting; these form a pyramidal pile, and range from ½ oz to 4 lb; they may be adjusted if found to be incorrect by adding to or diminishing the amount of lead which is hammered into a depression in the base of each. These weights are sometimes made of brass in this form, and sometimes of zinc; the latter, however, are brittle and unserviceable. For general use in the pharmacy, the cylindrical weights, known technically as "block weights," are preferable. The advantages of block weights are that the gaps left by missing weights are readily noticed and that the greater part of the surface of the weight is protected from the action of corrosive vapors when not in use.

Apothecary Weights—These may be had either as "block weights" or the less desirable flat forms. The round, flat, brass "dram" weights, which have the denomination stamped distinctly on their faces in raised characters, are still used but should be replaced. Undoubtedly the best grain weights are the aluminum wire weights. These are more easily and quickly distinguished from one another than any other form, and there is less likelihood of dangerous mistakes than from the flat weights, where the denomination is stamped on the face, often faintly, and is liable to be obliterated by constant use or by corrosive contact. The number of sides in the wire weights at once gives the denomination (Fig 9-7). The aluminum grain weights, cut out of aluminum plates, are preferred to the flat, brass grain weights because they are less liable to corrosive action. They are usually more accurately adjusted; the corners of the weights are clipped, and each weight is usually pressed into a curved form so that it may be picked up easily (Fig 9-8).

Measuring

In pharmacy, measuring usually refers to the exact determination of a definite volume of liquid. Many types of apparatus are used in this operation, depending on the kind and quantity of liquid to be measured and the degree of accuracy required. For NBS requirements for graduates see ref. 2.

Measuring Large Quantities

Glass measures are preferred for measuring liquids, for, although subject to breakage, they can more accurately indicate volume because of the transparency of glass.

The Meniscus—When an aqueous or alcoholic liquid is poured into a graduate, surface forces cause its surface to become concave, ie, that portion in contact with the vessel is drawn upward. This phenomenon is known as the formation of a *meniscus* (Fig 9-9), and in determining the volume of a liquid *the reading must be made at the bottom of this meniscus*. This regulation has been established by the NBS and all glass measuring vessels are graduated on this basis. Liquids with large contact angles, eg, mercury, form an inverted meniscus, and the reading is then made at the top of the curved surface (see Fig 9-9).

Procedure—Pharmaceutical manufacturers package their liquid preparations in glass or plastic containers equipped with a plastic screw cap. These containers serve as a stock bottle from which liquids may be poured directly into a graduate.

The procedure for pouring liquid from screw-capped containers is that the cap is removed and placed on the counter while the transfer of liquid is made. While holding the

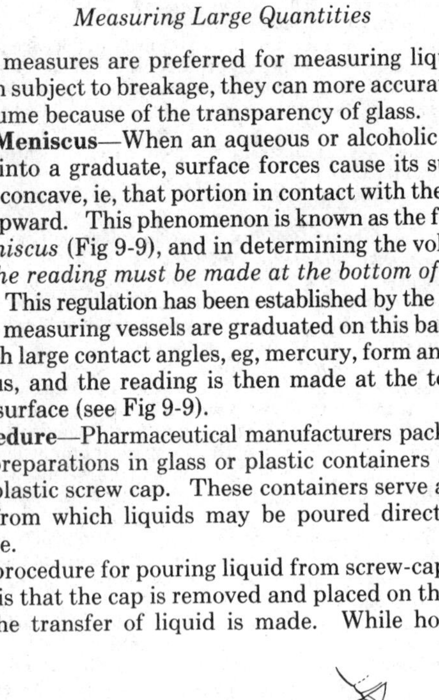

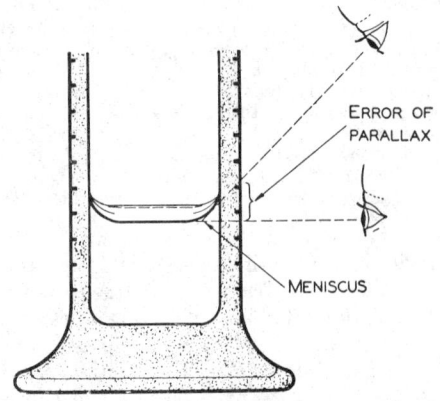

Fig 9-9.   Error of measurement due to parallax.

graduate in the left hand, the original container is grasped with the label in such a position that, after pouring, any excess of liquid will not soil the label if it should run down the side of the bottle. The graduate is raised and held so that the graduation point to be read is on a level with the eye, and the liquid is measured. The extension of the graduating mark into a circle which passes entirely around the graduate is an improvement which obviates the necessity of placing the graduate upon a level place, as the corresponding mark upon the opposite side may be seen through the glass and the graduate easily leveled even when held in the hand.

The cap is replaced and the bottle may be returned to the counter or shelf. Finally the liquid is poured into the bottle or mortar, for dispensing or compounding.

Metallic measures nearly cylindrical in shape, but slightly wider at the bottom, are generally used for measuring liquids when the quantity is over a pint. A set usually consists of five (gallon, half-gallon, quart, pint, and half-pint) of these measures. Those made of tinned iron, or of the enameled sheet iron called agate ware, are greatly inferior to those made of *tinned copper* or *stainless steel*. Tinned iron measures soon become rusty and, although a protection is afforded if enameled, particles of the enamel chip off and the exposed iron soon contaminates the liquids measured in them. The first cost of copper or stainless steel measures is greater than tinned iron, but they are far more durable. Care must be taken to protect them from blows which will cause dents as these may be serious enough to detract from the accuracy of the measures. Cylindrical metric measures, usually made of monel metal or stainless steel, having a diameter just half their height are available in various sizes. Such containers are relatively expensive but their resistance to corrosion and wear is a tremendous advantage. Copper, of course, should not be used where it is likely to catalyze oxidation.

Graduated Glass Measures—These are nearly always used for quantities of 500 mL or 1 pt or less, and are of two forms—*conical* and *cylindrical* (Figs 9-10 and 9-11). The conical graduate is suitable for some measurements because of the greater ease with which it can be handled, but cylindrical measures are more accurate because of their uniform and smaller average diameter. Thus, while the error in volume caused by a deviation of ±1 mm in reading the meniscus in a graduated cylinder remains constant along the height of the uniform column, the same deviation causes a progressively larger error in a conical graduate because the diameter and, therefore, the volume of the 1-mm column increases along its vertical axis. It is safe to assume that practically all good-grade modern graduates comply with the NBS requirements for internal diameters at stated volumes.

A study[3] indicated that, to improve accuracy, the lower portions of graduates should not be used and, therefore, should not be marked. A composite tabulation (Table XV) shows the calculated and the assigned blank portions of graduates. Elimination of the lower markings on graduates

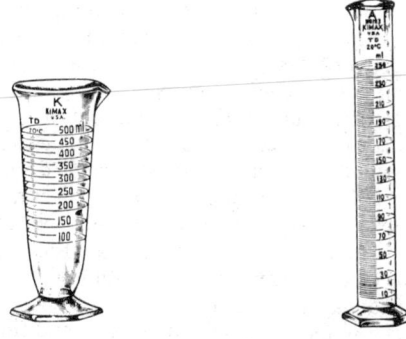

Fig 9-10. Glass conical graduate (courtesy, Owens-Illinois).

Fig 9-11. Glass cylindrical graduate (courtesy, Owens-Illinois).

was suggested, and in 1955 the NBS specifications for graduates utilized this principle.[2] The NBS Handbook states:

A graduate shall have an initial interval that is not subdivided, equal to not less than one-fifth and not more than one-fourth of the capacity of the graduate.

For accurate measurement of volumes less than 1.5 mL a graduated pipet or a graduated dropper could be used.

Effect of Liquid and Container—It is difficult to measure accurately when pouring from a completely filled bottle because of the uneven flow of the liquid. After the first portion of the liquid is removed the shape of the bottle does not influence the ease of pouring to any appreciable extent unless the neck is extremely narrow.

Viscous liquids pour slowly but their accurate measurement is not difficult. Experiments showed that when glycerin is poured into a graduate without letting the liquid run down the inside surface, the precision of measurement can be very high. Naturally, the chance of hitting the inner surface is greater with smaller than with larger graduates. The increase in possible deviation is then caused by the slow movement of the viscous liquid to the desired mark.

Viscous liquids introduce another factor: drainage time. Graduates are calibrated to contain or deliver indicated volumes within specified limits. Aqueous, alcoholic, and hydroalcoholic liquids can be drained from a graduate in ½ min so completely that the delivered and contained volumes are fairly close. When 25 mL of glycerin was measured in the same cleaned and dried cylinders, the received volume measured 23.7 mL after the same time period.

The viscosity factor might be altered when another liquid is to be mixed with the glycerin by measuring and mixing both liquids in a suitable graduate.

Silicone-treated glassware, which is now frequently used, drains completely in a few seconds.

Measuring Small Quantities

For measuring smaller quantities of liquids, graduated glass tubes of small diameter should be used. The narrower bore permits greater distances between the graduations on the apparatus, and therefore greater accuracy in making the reading is achieved. For example, with a buret the pharmaceutical chemist can estimate volumes to the nearest $1/100$ mL.

Pipets and similar apparatus are more accurate and convenient than very small graduates. The graduations on very small graduates are necessarily in the very small lowest portion of a comparatively tall measure. Now, if it is desired to measure 1 mL or 10 ♏ of a volatile oil in a graduate the surface which the oil must traverse when this measure is inverted is so great that probably 20% of the oil will be left adhering to the measure. In those instances of liquid preparations where

Table XV—Unmarked (Unreliable) Portions of Graduates

| Capacity of graduate, mL | Calculated blanks (1951) | | NBS blanks (1965), mL |
	2.5%[a] allowed, mL	5%[a] allowed, mL	
5	3.0	1.5	1
10	4.4	2.2	2
25	11.8	5.9	5
50	15.8	7.9	10
100	20.9	10.5	20
250	36.3	18.2	50
500	66.5	33.2	100
1000	....	....	200

[a] Calculations by Goldstein and Mattocks[3] based on deviation of ±1 mm from graduation mark and allowable errors of 2.5 and 5%.

the smaller liquid is miscible with the larger quantity of diluting liquid, the graduate may be rinsed and this loss recovered, but inconveniences are largely overcome and greater accuracy secured by the use of a pipet.

In administering small quantities of liquids, the very convenient *drop* is almost always used. It should be emphasized that *1 drop is not equivalent to 1 ♏* and that *60 drops are not equivalent to 1 fl dr.* This impression doubtless arose from the fact that 60 ordinary drops of *water* are about equal to 1 fl dr, but the volume of a drop of fluid depends on many factors, including density, temperature, viscosity, surface tension, and the size and nature of the orifice from which it is dropped. Thick viscous liquids, such as the mucilages and the syrups, necessarily produce large drops because the drop adheres to the surface of the glass as long as its weight does not overcome its power of adhesion, while chloroform, a mobile liquid, having very little adhesion to the dropping surface—produces very small drops. The greater the surface tension, the larger will be the drop, and the greater the extent of surface to which the drop adheres, the larger, proportionally, will be the drop.

A "normal" or "standard" drop measure was recommended by the Brussels Conference of 1902 for international adoption. This dropper is recognized in the USP.

Medicine Dropper

The pharmacopeial medicine dropper is 3 mm in external diameter at its delivery end, and when held vertically delivers 20 drops of water, the total weight of which is between 0.9 g and 1.1 g (at 25°). In using a medicine dropper, one should keep in mind that few medicinal liquids have the same surface and flow characteristics as water, and therefore the size of drops varies materially from one preparation to another.

When drops are specified on a prescription, the usual custom has been to employ an "eye dropper," but the standard dropper should now be supplied. It is particularly important to use the standard or a specially calibrated dropper for administering potent medicines when accuracy is required.

A standard teaspoon has not yet received acceptance.

Teaspoon

Agreement has not been reached on a standard official teaspoon, in spite of the need for such a standard measure in connection with compounding and labeling liquid medicines. For household purposes, an American Standard Teaspoon has been established by the American National Standards Institute* as containing 4.93 ± 0.24 mL. In view of the almost universal practice of employing teaspoons ordinarily available in the household for the administration of medicine, the teaspoon may be regarded as representing 5 mL.

It must be kept in mind that the actual volume delivered by a teaspoon of any given liquid is related to the latter's viscosity and surface tension, among other influencing factors.

The Human Factor—The human factor of carefulness is of paramount importance in every pharmaceutical operation in which accuracy is essential. The basic necessities for accurate measurement of liquids require (1) accurate technical equipment, (2) careful manipulation, (3) good vision, and (4) a steady hand.

---

* American National Standards Institute, 1430 Broadway, New York, NY 10018.

Density and Specific Gravity

Several terms are used to express the mass (weight) of equal volumes of different substances.

Absolute density is the ratio of the mass of an object, determined in or referred to a vacuum, at a specified temperature, to the volume of the object at the same temperature. This relationship is expressed mathematically as:

$$\frac{\text{mass in grams (in a vacuum)}}{\text{volume in milliliters}} = \text{absolute density}$$

Apparent density differs from absolute density only in that the mass of the object is determined in air, which mass is influenced by the difference in the buoyant effect of air on the object being weighed and on the standard masses (weights) used for comparison (if the object and masses are made of the same material, or have the same density, there will be no difference in the buoyant effect, and the apparent density will be identical with the absolute density).

Relative density is an expression sometimes employed to indicate the mass of 1 mL (not cc, which is very slightly different) of a standard substance, such as water, at a specified temperature, relative to water at 4°C taken as unity. Thus, at 4°C the relative density of water is 1.0000, while its absolute density at the same temperature is 0.999973.* To convert a relative density of water to absolute density, the former should be multiplied by 0.999973.

Specific gravity may be defined as the ratio of the mass of a substance to the mass of an equal volume of another substance taken as the standard. For gases, the standard may be hydrogen or air; for liquids and solids, it is water. From what has been stated, it is obvious that in a determination of specific gravity there will be, in general, a difference in the result if the masses (weights) are determined in air or in vacuum; if determined in, or referred to, a vacuum, the result is a *true specific gravity* (sometimes called *absolute specific gravity*), while if the masses are determined in air, the calculated result is an *apparent specific gravity*. The difference between these specific gravities is, as a rule, very small. A very important variable in specific gravity determinations is temperature, and this is doubly important because both the temperature of the substance under examination and the temperature of the standard may be different. The common practice with regard to the determination of specific gravity is that defined by the USP as follows:

Unless otherwise stated, the specific gravity basis is 25°/25°, i.e., the ratio of the weight of a substance in air at 25° to that of an equal volume of water at the same temperature.

But it is not always convenient, or desirable, to determine the weight of both the substance and the water at 25°, or even to determine the weight of the substance at the same temperature as that at which the water is weighed. Thus, the substance may be weighed at 25°, and compared with the weight of an equal volume of water at 4°, in which case the specific gravity is reported as being on a 25°/4° basis; in the case of theobroma oil, which is solid at 25°, the specific gravity is determined on a 100°/25° basis, and for alcohol it is determined on a 15.56°/15.56° basis because many years ago the US Government adopted 60°F (15.56°C) as the temperature at which alcoholometric measurements are to be made in connection with the Government's control of alcoholic liquids.

It is apparent that a completely informative statement of specific gravity must indicate the temperature of the substance under examination, as well as that of the equal volume of water (the temperatures are commonly shown as a ratio, with the temperature of the water always being indicated in the denominator). Furthermore, it should be stated whether

---

* Water attains its maximum absolute density of 0.999973 at 3.98°C.

the determinations of mass (weight) were made on an "in vacuum" or "in air" basis, in which latter case the material of construction of the weights should also be indicated (since the buoyant effect of air on weights depends on their volume).

Calculations

The principle underlying the determination of the specific gravity of either a liquid or a solid is the same; it is to find the ratio of the mass (weight) of the substance to that of an equal volume of water.

This may be expressed by a simple relationship:

$$\text{Specific gravity} = \frac{W_s}{W_w}$$

where W_s = weight of substance and W_w = weight of equal volume of water.

The following relationships and examples illustrate important applications of specific gravity data.

Reducing Metric Fluid Measure to Weight

1 mL of liquid with a sp gr of 1 weighs 1 g
1 mL of liquid with a sp gr of x weighs x g
Vol. in mL $\times$ sp gr = weight in g

Example: What is the weight in g of 1 L of chloroform having a sp gr of 1.48?

No. of mL $\times$ sp gr = weight in g
$1000 \times 1.48 = 1480$ g

Density

Density is defined as the mass of a substance per unit volume. It has the units of mass over volume.

Specific gravity is the ratio of the weight of a substance in air to that of an equal volume of water. It does not have any units.

In the metric system both density and specific gravity may be numerically equal, although the density figure has units. In the English system, density and specific gravity are not numerically equal; eg, the density of water is 62.4 lb/ft^3 and the specific gravity is 1. This shows the convenience of the metric system. The equations for calculating density, weight, and volume are as follows:

$$\text{Density} = \frac{\text{weight}}{\text{volume}}$$

$$\text{Weight} = \text{density} \times \text{volume}$$

$$\text{Volume} = \frac{\text{weight}}{\text{density}}$$

Given any two variables, the third one can be calculated.

Examples

1.   A pharmacist weighs out 2 kg of glycerin (density, 1.25 g/mL). What is the volume of the glycerin? Remember to convert to like units; eg, kg to g.

$$\text{Volume} = \frac{2000 \text{ g}}{1.25 \text{ g/mL}} = 1600 \text{ mL}$$

2.   What is the weight of 60 mL of oil whose density is 0.9624 g/mL?

$$\text{Weight} = 60 \text{ mL} \times 0.9624 \text{ g/mL}$$

$$= 57.7 \text{ g}$$

3.   Calculate the weight of 30 mL of sulfuric acid whose density is 1.8 g/mL.

$$\text{Weight} = 1.8 \text{ g/mL} \times 30 \text{ mL} = 54 \text{ g}$$

4.   If a prescription order requires 25 g of concentrated hydrochloric acid (density, 1.18 g/mL), what volume should the pharmacist measure?

$$\text{Volume} = \frac{25 \text{ g}}{1.18 \text{ g/mL}} = 21.2 \text{ mL}$$

Problems

(answers on page 102)

1.   What is the weight in grams of 1 L of alcohol (density, 0.816 g/mL)?
2.   What is the volume (mL) of 1 lb of glycerin whose density is 1.25 g/mL?
3.   What volume does 65 g of an acid whose density is 1.2 g/mL occupy?

Calculation

Pharmaceutical dispensing and compounding calculations utilize simple arithmetic. The errors that may arise are often due to carelessness, as in improper placing of decimal points, or incorrect conversion from one system of measurement to another, or to uncertainty concerning the system of measurement to be used. Before proceeding with any calculation it is imperative that the problem presented (in a prescription, chart order, formula, etc) be read carefully, the information given and that required be identified, and the procedure to be used in the calculation selected.

Often several steps are necessary to solve problems. Shortcuts should not be taken unless one is certain they are proper. Many problems can be solved by the method of "ratio and proportion," but if the student understands the problem, he may use any method that will give him the correct answer. Many problems can be solved by more than one procedure, and if the student finds a procedure that is more logical to him and gives the correct answer, he should use it. The solutions to sample problems used here should, therefore, generally be considered suggestive rather than the only way to solve a given type of problem.

Before the student reads this part of the chapter and attempts to solve the problems, he should be thoroughly familiar with, and understand, the information in the preceding part of this chapter.

Mathematical Principles

A few mathematical principles (eg, common decimal fractions, exponents, powers, and roots, significant figures, and logarithms) will be reviewed; these are areas where students often become careless or have forgotten skills. Following this, various types of practical pharmaceutical problems that the

pharmacist may be required to solve are discussed and solutions are given. Where practical, rules for solving these problems are given. No attempt is made to elaborate on any mathematical theory.

The problems generally consist in determining the quantity

or quantities of material(s) required to compound prescriptions properly and make products used to aid the compounding of prescriptions. The materials used to compound prescription orders may be pure or mixtures of substances in varying strengths. The strengths of mixtures may be denoted in different ways. Conversions may be necessary between systems of varying strengths or between different measuring systems. At the end of each section, sample problems are given for the student to solve, the answers to which appear on page 102.

Because of the decreasing importance of the apothecary system, the metric system will be emphasized. Chemicals and preparations most likely will be bought in the avoirdupois or metric systems. Prescription orders are filled in the system indicated on the order, usually the apothecary or metric systems.

The student should become familiar with the terminology used in writing prescription orders such as Latin words and abbreviations used in giving directions to the pharmacist and patient. The prescriber may occasionally use Roman numerals instead of Arabic numerals. Students, therefore, must be familiar with these even if the practice is declining.

Significant Figures

Weighings and measurements can be carried out with only a certain maximum degree of accuracy; the result is always approximate due to the many sources of error such as temperature, limitations of the instruments employed, personal factors, etc. The pharmacist must achieve the greatest accuracy possible with his equipment, but it would be erroneous to claim that he has weighed 1 mg of a solid on a Class A prescription balance, which has a sensibility reciprocal of 6 mg, or that he has measured 76.32 mL of a liquid in a 100-mL graduate, which can be read only to 1 mL. When quantities are written, the numbers should contain only those digits which are "significant" within the precision of the instrument.

Significant figures are digits which have practical meaning. In some instances zeros are significant; in other instances they merely indicate the order of magnitude of the other digits by locating the decimal point. For example, in the measurement 473 mL all the digits are significant, but in the measurement 4730 mL the zero may or may not be significant. In the weight 0.0316 g the zeros are not significant but only locate the decimal point. In any result the last significant figure is only approximate, but all preceding figures are accurate. When 473 mL is recorded, it is understood that the measurement had been made within ±0.5 mL or somewhere between 472.5 and 473.5 mL. The student should stop to consider the full implications of this, specifically that the measurement is subject to a maximum error of

$$\frac{0.5}{473} \times 100 = \text{(approx) } 0.1\% \text{ or 1 part in 1000}$$

A zero in a quantity such as 473.0 mL is a significant figure and implies that the measurement has been made within the limits 472.95 mL and 473.05 mL or with a possible error of

$$\frac{0.05}{473} \times 100 = \text{(approx) } 0.01\% \text{ or 1 part in 10,000}$$

Thus, 473 is correct to the nearest mL, 473.0 is correct to the nearest 0.1 mL.

Rules

1. *When adding or subtracting, retain in the sum or remainder no more decimal places than the least number entering into the calculations.* For example:

11.5 g	11.50 g
2.65 g	2.65 g
3.49 g	3.49 g
17.64 g	17.64 g
Answer: 17.6 g	*Answer:* 17.64 g

In the first column 11.5 g was weighed to 0.1 g or with an accuracy of ±0.05 g. Although the other two weighings were made with an accuracy of ±0.005 g, the sum can be expressed properly only to one decimal place.

In the second column 11.50 g was weighed to the nearest 0.01 g or with an accuracy of ±0.005 g. Since all weighings were made with this degree of accuracy, the sum may be stated as in the example, 17.64 g.

Retain all figures possible until all the calculations are completed and then retain only the significant figures for the answer. Additions or subtractions involving both large and small quantities, each expressed with maximum significance, are often useless. For example, if one were to add 1.2 and 0.041 g, the physical sum would be 1.2 g, regardless of the fact that the two numbers add numerically to 1.241. To express the physical sum as 1.241 g would convey an erroneous degree of accuracy with which the quantity was known.

2. *When multiplying or dividing, retain in the answer no more significant figures than the least number entering into the calculation.*

Table XVI

Weight, g		Equivalent used, gr/g		Equivalent weight, gr	Significant figures
4.522	×	15.432	=	69.78	4
4.522	×	15.43	=	69.77	4
4.522	×	15.4	=	69.6	3
4.522	×	15	=	69	2

The meaning of this rule may be illustrated by the use of equivalents during conversions from one measuring system to another. Table XVI gives different equivalent values and the number of significant figures to which the answer is correct. Always use an equivalent which will give the desired degree of accuracy. Repeated multiplication of an approximation increases the error progressively; therefore, retain all figures during calculations and drop insignificant figures as the final step.

Fractions

Common Fractions

An example of a common fraction is ⅜. It is read as "three-eighths" and indicates three parts divided by eight parts of the same thing. The units with both numbers must be the same. If a pharmacist measures ⅜ of a fluidounce into a graduate, he measures 3 drams, out of 8 drams (a fluidounce contains 8 drams).

The following principles should be applied when using common fractions:

1. The value of a fraction is not altered by multiplying or dividing both numerator and denominator by the same number.
2. Multiplying the numerator or dividing the denominator by a number, multiplies the fraction by that number.
3. Dividing the numerator or multiplying the denominator by a number, divides the fraction by that number.
4. To add or subtract fractions, form fractions with the *lowest common denominator*, perform the arithmetical operation, and reduce to the lowest common denominator.
5. To multiply fractions, multiply all numbers above the line to form the new numerator and multiply all numbers below the line to form the new denominator. Cancel if possible to simplify and reduce to the lowest common denominator.
6. To divide by a fraction, multiply by the reciprocal of the fraction.

Decimal Fractions

Fractions with the power of 10 as denominator are known as *decimal fractions* and are written by omitting the denominator and inserting a decimal point in the numerator as many places from the last number on the right as there are ciphers of 10 in the denominator.

The following principles should be applied when using decimal fractions:

1. When adding or subtracting decimals, keep the decimal points under each other.
2. When multiplying decimals, proceed as with whole numbers, then place the decimal point in the product as many places from the 1st number on the right as the sum of the decimal places in the multiplier and the multiplicand.
3. When dividing by a decimal fraction, move the decimal point to the right, in both divisor and dividend, as many places as it is to the left in the divisor to form a whole number in the divisor; proceed as with whole numbers. The decimal point in the quotient should be placed immediately above the decimal point in the dividend.
4. When converting a common fraction into a decimal fraction, divide the numerator by the denominator and place the decimal point in the correct place.
5. When converting a decimal fraction into a common fraction, place the entire number, as numerator, over the power of 10 containing the same number of ciphers of 10 as there are decimal places. Cancel if possible, to simplify.

Exponents, Powers, and Roots

In the expression $2^4 = 16$, the following names are given to the terms: 16 is called the *power* of the *base* 2, and 4 is the *exponent* of the power. If the exponent is 1, it is usually omitted. The following laws should be recalled:

1. The product of two or more powers of the same base is equal to that base with an exponent equal to the sum of the exponents of the powers; eg, $2^5 \times 2^3 = 2^8$.
2. The quotient of two powers of the same base is equal to that base with an exponent equal to the exponent of the dividend minus the exponent of the divisor; eg, $2^8 \div 2^3 = 2^5$.
3. The power of a power is found by multiplying the exponents; eg, $(2^8)^3 = 2^{24}$.
4. The power of a product equals the product of the powers of the factors; eg, $(2 \times 3 \times 4)^2 = 2^2 \times 3^2 \times 4^2$.
5. The power of a fraction equals the power of the numerator divided by the power of the denominator; eg,

$$\left(\frac{2}{3}\right)^2 = \frac{2^2}{3^2}$$

6. The root of a power is found by dividing the exponent of the power by the index of the root; eg,

$$\sqrt[3]{3^6} = 3^{6/3} = 3^2$$

7. Any number other than 0 with exponent 0 equals 1; eg, $2^0 = 1$.
8. A number with a negative exponent equals 1 divided by the number with a positive exponent equal in numerical value to the negative exponent; eg,

$$2^{-4} = \frac{1}{2^4}$$

Logarithms

To facilitate the solution of involved and lengthy problems, *logarithms* (*logs*) were invented. Many calculations, which are difficult by ordinary arithmetical processes, are rapidly and easily performed with the aid of logs.

The log of a number is the exponent of the power to which a given base must be raised in order to equal that number. John Napier, of Scotland, who discovered logs over three centuries ago, used the Natural Log Number, 2.71828+, as the base. Henry Briggs, using Napier's discovery a few years later, introduced 10 as the base, which is the most convenient for practical purposes. Napier's system is called natural logs and Brigg's system is called common logs. In this latter system the natural numbers are regarded as powers of the base 10 and the corresponding exponents are the logs. For example,

$$Y = a^x, \text{ taking logs}$$

$$\log_a Y = x$$

$$8 = 2^3$$

$$\log_2 8 = 3$$

$$100 = 10^2$$

$$\log_{10} 100 = 2$$

$$25 = 10^{1.3979} \text{ or } \log_{10} 25 = 1.3979$$

This reads log to the base 10 of 25 equals 1.3979.

$$2 = 10^{0.3010} \text{ or } \log_{10} 2 = 0.3010$$

Laws and Rules

The following laws, governing the use of logs, are based on the laws of exponents, and hence hold for any log system.

1. The log of a product equals the *sum* of the log of the component numbers; eg, for 25×2

$$\log (25 \times 2) = \log 25 + \log 2$$

$$= \log 10^{1.3979} + \log 10^{0.3010}$$

$$= 1.3979 + 0.3010 = 1.6989$$

2. The log of a quotient equals the log of the numerator minus the log of the denominator; eg, for $25 \div 2$,

$$\log (25 \div 2) = \log 25 - \log 2 = \log 10^{1.3979} - \log 10^{0.3010}$$

$$= 1.3979 - 0.3010 = 1.0969$$

3. The log of a power of a number equals the log of the number multiplied by the exponent of the power; eg, for $(25)^{12}$,

$$\log (25)^{12} = 12 \log 25 = 12 \times 1.3979 = 16.7748$$

4. The log of a root of a number equals the log of the number divided by the index of the root; eg, for $\sqrt{25}$,

$$\log \sqrt{25} = \frac{\log 25}{2} = \frac{1.3979}{2} = 0.6990$$

5. The log of a negative power of a number equals the reciprocal of the number multiplied by the exponent of the power; eg $(5)^{-2}$,

$$\log (5)^{-2} = 2 \log \frac{1}{5} = 2 \times \bar{1}.301 = \bar{2}.602$$

The logs of 1, 10, 0.01, etc are integers, but for numbers between these the logs will consist of two parts: an integral part called the characteristic and a fractional part called the mantissa. Thus,

10^2	$= 100$		$\log 100$	$= 2$
10^1	$= 10$		$\log 10$	$= 1$
10^0	$= 1$		$\log 1$	$= 0$
10^{-1}	$= 0.1$		$\log 0.1$	$= -1$
10^{-2}	$= 0.01$		$\log 0.01$	$= -2$

The log of a number between 100 and 1000 has 2 for a characteristic plus a fraction, the log of a number between 0.1 and 0.01 has -2 for a characteristic plus a fraction, and so on. The mantissa of a log must always be positive, whereas the characteristic may be either positive or negative.

Every number may be regarded as the product of two numbers, one being 10 with a positive or negative exponent and the other being some number between 1 and 10. For example,

$$760 = 10^2 \times 7.6 = 10^2 \times 10^{0.8808}$$

$$\therefore \log 760 = \log 10^2 + \log 7.6 = 2.8808$$

$$0.076 = 10^{-2} \times 7.6 = 10^{-2} \times 10^{0.8808}$$

$$\therefore \log 0.076 = \log 10^{-2} + \log 7.6 = -2 + 0.8808$$

This is written $\overline{2}.8808$ (or $8.8808 - 10$).

The characteristic is made a positive number by subtracting the -2 from 10 to give a characteristic of $8 \ldots -10$. The -10 is put after the mantissa. From the above explanation the following rules are derived:

1. The characteristic of a number greater than 1 is one unit less than the number of figures to the left of the decimal point; e.g., for 1000 the characteristic is 3.
2. The characteristic of a number less than 1 is one unit more than the number of ciphers between the decimal point and the first significant figure; eg, for 0.001 the characteristic is -3.
3. If the characteristic of a log is positive, the integral part of the corresponding number contains one more figure than the number of units in the characteristic; eg, if the characteristic equals 2, the corresponding number lies between 100 and 1000.
4. If the characteristic of a log is negative, the number of zeros between the decimal point and the first significant figure is one less than the number of units in the characteristic; eg, if the characteristic is -2, the corresponding number lies between 0.01 and 0.001.
5. Numbers which are related to each other by some power of 10 possess logs with the same mantissa; eg, $\log 760 = 2.8808$ and $\log 76 = 1.8808$.

Obtaining the Log of a Number

The characteristic of a log is determined readily by inspection of the natural number, but to obtain the mantissa a table of logs must be used. These tables vary in accuracy according to the number of decimal places to which the mantissa is expanded. For most calculations four places are satisfactory.

Under the heading *Natural Numbers* (referred to as N) on the inside front cover, the first two figures of the number are given down the column on the left, while the third figure (from 0 to 9) is given across the top. The mantissa for large numbers or numbers falling between three-place ones may be found by the process of interpolation. For example,

1. Find the log of 273.

Under N find 27 and along the top line find the third number, 3. Across from 27 and under 3 the mantissa for 273 (4362) is found. No interpolation is necessary. By inspection (see Rule 1) the characteristic is 2. Then log $273 = 2 + .4362 = 2.4362$.

2. Find the log of 0.08206.

Under N find 82 and along the top find the next number, 0. Now 8206 falls between 820 and 821 ($^6/_{10}$ of the difference). The mantissa for 820 is 9138 and the mantissa for 821 is 9143. The difference between these two mantissas is 5, and $^6/_{10}$ of 5 is 3. The mantissa for 8206 is therefore 9138 $+ 3 = 9141$. By inspection (see Rule 2) the characteristic is -2. Then log $0.08206 = -2 + 0.9141 = 8.9141 - 10$ or $\overline{2}.9141$.

The process of finding a number between two other numbers is known as interpolation. It is based on the assumption that the mantissa varies directly with the number. This is not quite true. Many log tables supply the proportionate parts to facilitate interpolation (see the chart on the right of the log table inside the front cover).

Obtaining the Antilog of a Number

To find the number corresponding to a given log, the reverse procedure of that discussed above is employed. The first step is to find figures corresponding to the mantissa (interpolation may be necessary). The last step is to place the decimal point

in the correct position, following Rules 3 and 4. The following examples demonstrate the method:

1. Find the number corresponding to the log 3.8357.

In the log table, 8357 is found across from 68 and under 5. The figures required are therefore 685. Since the characteristic is 3 (Rule 3), the log 3.8357 is the number 6850.

2. Find the number corresponding to the log 0.4351.

In the log table, 4351 is found to fall between 4346 and 4362, the difference being 16. 4351 is 5 units more than 4346 or $^5/_{16}$ of the difference between the two mantissas. The log table gives 272 as the antilog of 4346, to which $^5/_{16}$ or 0.31 must be added. Adding on the 0.3 to the fourth place, the required figures are 2723. Since the characteristic is zero, the required number is 2.723.

Antilogarithm of a Negative Number

Finding the antilog of a negative number is easy when you remember that the mantissa is always *positive*. Thus, the first step is to convert the negative mantissa to a positive one. For example: $\log X = -3.523$

1. Add -1 to the characteristic, so that it becomes -4.
2. Add $+1$ to the mantissa, so that it becomes 0.477 ($+1.0000 - 0.523 = +0.477$)
3. The result is:

$$\log X = \overline{4}.477$$

From the log table the antilog of 0.477 is 3.0, so that the antilog of $\overline{4}.477$ is 3.0×10^{-4}. Hence, if $\log X = -3.523$, then $X = 3.0 \times 10^{-4}$.

Example:

1. Using the Henderson-Hasselbalch equation, find the ratio of ionized to unionized drug at a pH of 3.0. The pK_a of the drug is 7.4.

$$pH = pK_a + \log \frac{[\text{Salt}]}{[\text{Acid}]}$$

$$pH - pK_a = \log \frac{[\text{Salt}]}{[\text{Acid}]}$$

$$3.0 - 7.4 = -4.4 = \overline{5}.6 = \log \frac{[\text{Salt}]}{[\text{Acid}]}$$

$$3.98 \times 10^{-5} = \frac{[\text{Salt}]}{[\text{Acid}]}$$

Logarithmic Calculations

Representative problems illustrated below show the rapidity and simplicity of calculations with logs.

1. Find the value of $8.52 \times 36.4 \times 0.0056$.

To multiply, add logs of the numbers.

$$\log 8.52 \quad = 0.9304$$

$$\log 36.4 \quad = 1.5611$$

$$\underline{\log 0.0056 \quad = \overline{3}.7482}$$

$$\log \text{number} = 0.2397$$

To find the natural number corresponding to log number 0.2397, take the antilog.
Answer: antilog $0.2397 = 1.737$.

2. Find the fifth root of 0.00475.

To find the nth root of a number, divide the log of the number by the index of the root.

$$\log \sqrt[5]{0.00475} = \tfrac{1}{5} \log 0.00475 = \tfrac{1}{5} (\overline{3}.6767) =$$

$$\tfrac{1}{5} (7.6767 - 10) = 1.5353 - 2 \text{ or } \overline{1}.5353$$

To find the natural number corresponding to the log number $\overline{1}.5353$, take the antilog.
Answer: antilog $\overline{1}.5353 = 0.343$.

3.   Find the value of,

$$\frac{6.062 \times 10^{23}}{0.08206 \times 293.1 \times 760,000}$$

Remember: to multiply, add the logs of the numbers; to divide, subtract the logs of the numbers:

log 6.062	= 0.7826		log 0.08206	= $\bar{2}$.9141
log 10^{23}	= 23.		log 293.1	= 2.4670
			log 760,000	= 5.8808
log numerator = 23.7826				
			log denominator	= 7.2619

Log value: 23.7826 − 7.2619 = 16.5207.
Answer: antilog 16.5207 = 3.32×10^{16}.

4.   The pH of a solution is the log of the reciprocal of the hydrogen-ion concentration. If the concentration of H$^+$ ions in a solution is 2.57×10^{-4} g-ion/L, what is the pH?

$$pH = \log\frac{1}{[H^+]} = \log\frac{1}{2.57 \times 10^{-4}} = \log\frac{10^4}{2.57}$$

Taking logs,

$$pH = \log 10^4 - \log 2.57 = 4 - 0.4099 = 3.59$$

Problems

1.   The rate of creaming of an emulsion may be calculated by Stokes' law:

$$-V = \frac{2gr^2(d_2 - d_1)}{9\eta}$$

If d_1 = 0.88 g/mL, d_2 = 1.32 g/mL, g = 980.6 cm/sec^2, r = 10^{-3} cm, and η = 1.14 poise, find the rate, V.

2.   The surface tension (S) of a liquid may be found by the Capillary Rise Method using the formula

$$S = \frac{1}{2}hdgr$$

where h is the height of the liquid in the capillary, d is the density of the liquid, g is the acceleration of gravity, and r is the radius of the capillary. Find S when h = 2.62 cm, d = 2.43 g/mL, g = 980.6 cm/sec^2, and r = 0.021 cm.

3.   Using the Henderson-Hasselbalch equation, find the ratio of ionized to unionized drug at a pH of 1.5. The pK$_a$ of the basic drug is 9.6.

Pharmaceutical Problems

The student who has knowledge of algebra and has studied the previous sections of this chapter and Roman numerals and Latin abbreviations used on prescription orders for directions to the pharmacist and patient by the prescriber should have sufficient knowledge to solve the routine problems he may encounter in a pharmacy. The various symbols and abbreviations and their meanings should be well understood. Explanation of practical problems, representative of those one faces in practice, are presented below. Practice problems follow each section and the answers to these problems are found at the end of this chapter (page 102).

To solve each problem properly, the following procedure is suggested:

1.   Analyze the problem carefully so that all data are clearly fixed in the mind; determine what is given and what is called for.
2.   Select the most direct method of solving the problem. Not all problems can be solved properly in one step. Look up doses, equivalents, and abbreviations when you are not sure.
3.   Prove or check the result.

Addition

Review weighing and measuring systems discussed earlier in this chapter.

The expression "weighable or measurable quantities" means pounds, ounces, drams, quarts, pints, fluidounces, etc. For example, it is not practical to weigh 300 gr or measure 50 fl oz, since neither a 300-gr weight nor a 50-fl oz graduate is commonly available. These are converted to 5 drams, and 1 qt, 1 pt, 2 fl oz, respectively, which are weighable and measurable quantities.

Rules

1.   Add like quantities. If, in the metric system, the quantities are not alike, change to a common unit. For the apothecary or avoirdupois systems, place in columns of like quantities arranged in descending order of magnitude toward the right.
2.   In the apothecary or avoirdupois systems, add together the smaller quantities first, then advance to the next higher units in these systems.
3.   Always extract the next higher unit, wherever possible,

to simplify the answer, which should be stated in weighable or measurable quantities.
4.   When adding decimals, keep the decimal points directly under each other.
5.   When adding fractions, reduce to the lowest common denominator, add the resulting numerators, and reduce the fraction, if possible, by canceling.

Examples

1.   Add 3 kg, 33 g, 433 mg.

Convert to a common unit. The gram is convenient because it is the unit of weight.

3 kg	=	3 × 1000 g	= 3000	g
33 g	=		33	g
433 mg	=	433 mg ÷ 1000	= 0.433	g
			3033.433	g

2.   Add 4 pounds, 3 ounces, 1 dram, 59 grains and 5 pounds, 10 ounces, 7 drams, 2 grains (apoth).

℔	℥	ʒ	gr
4	3	1	59
5	10	7	2
9	13	8	61

Explanation:

61 grains = 1 dram + 1 grain (60 gr = 1 ʒ)

Add 1 dram to the next column:

8 + 1 = 9 drams = 1 ounce + 1 dram (8 ʒ = 1 ℥)

Add 1 ounce to the next column:

13 + 1 = 14 ounces = 1 pound + 2 ounces (12 ℥ = 1 ℔)

Add 1 pound to the next column:

9 + 1 = 10 pounds.

Answer: 10 ℔, 2 ℥, 1 ʒ, 1 gr.

3.   Add the following volumes: 5 gal, 3 pt, 2 fl oz and 2 pt, 3 fl oz, 4 fl dr.

Write out in proper sequence of the units in the measuring system and arrange the numbers given in the problem under each other.

Thus,

gal	pt	fl oz	fl dr
5	3	2	
	2	3	4
5	5	5	4

Note: 5 pt = 2 qt + 1 pt (2 pt = 1 qt).
Answer: 5 gal, 2 qt, 1 pt, 5 fl oz, 4 fl dr.

Problems

1. Add 25 mg, 25 g, 210 mg, 2 kg, 1.75 g, 215 mg, 454 g, and 30 mg.
2. The following quantities of a drug were removed from a container: 31 g, 225 g, 855.6 g, and 45.4 g. What is the total weight removed from the container?
3. What is the weight of powder formed by mixing together 1ʒ, 175 gr of Drug A, 87.5 gr of Drug B, and 6ʒ, 55 gr of Drug C? Give the answer in weighable quantities.
4. Add ʒxi, ʒvi, Ɵii, gr xiv and ʒvii, ʒv, Ɵii, gr x. Give the answer in weighable quantities.
5. Each unit of a mixture contains the following drugs: ⅕ gr of Drug M, ¹/₉₀ gr of Drug N, ⅙ gr of Drug P, and 2½ gr of Drug Q. What is the total weight of each unit?
6. The inventory card shows the following amounts of a syrup: 3 gal, 2½ qt, 6 pt, 8 fl oz, 19 fl oz. What is the total volume in stock (in measurable quantities)?

Subtraction

Rules

1. Subtract only like quantities. If the quantities are not alike, change to a common unit (metric system) or place in columns of like quantities or units arranged in descending order of magnitude toward the right (avoirdupois and apothecary systems).
2. In the apothecary and avoirdupois systems, begin with the smallest quantities and advance to the largest.
3. When necessary, reduce larger quantities to smaller ones and place in the proper column.
4. Treat common and decimal fractions as indicated under *Addition.*

Examples

1. Subtract 1 pt, 4 fl oz, 6 fl dr from 2 gal.

The problem may be solved as follows: divide 1 gal into 4 qt, leaving 1 gal in its column; divide 1 of the 4 qt into 2 pt, leaving 3 qt; divide 1 pt into 16 fl oz, leaving 1 pt; divide 1 fl oz into 8 fl dr, leaving 15 fl oz.

gal	qt	pt	fl oz	fl dr
1	3	1	15	8
		1	4	6
1	3	0	11	2

Answer: 1 gal, 3 qt, 0 pt, 11 fl oz, 2 fl dr.

2. Subtract 285 mL from 1 L. Convert to a common unit.

$$1 \text{ L} = 1000 \text{ mL} \qquad \begin{array}{r} 1000 \text{ mL} \\ -\ 285 \text{ mL} \\ \hline 715 \text{ mL} \end{array}$$

Answer: 715 mL.

Problems

1. How much is left in a 5 L container after the removal of 895 mL?
2. A pharmacist buys 1 oz of Drug C. At intervals he uses the following quantities to compound prescription orders: ʒii, ʒss, Ɵii, 56 gr, and 48 gr. How much of Drug C remains?

3. A bottle contains 1 pt of a liquid; 8 fl oz and 6 fl dr were removed. How much of the liquid remains?
4. A pharmacist buys 5 g of a potent drug and at different times dispenses 0.2 g, 0.85 g, 90 mg, and 150 mg on prescription orders. How much of the drug remains?

Multiplication

Rules

1. The product has the same denomination as the multiplicand.
2. If the multiplicand is composed of different denominations in the metric system, form a common unit before multiplying and reduce the product to measurable units. In the apothecary or avoirdupois systems, arrange the quantities in descending order of magnitude toward the right, and multiply. Extract the next higher units, beginning with the smallest unit, and place in the proper columns, proceeding to the left.
3. Multiply fractions and decimals as in any arithmetic problem, and reduce fractional quantities to measurable or weighable units.

Examples

1. Multiply 4 pt, 7 fl oz, and 3 fl dr by 4.

Begin with the smallest unit, working from right to left. When it becomes necessary, change the product to the next higher unit, writing only the remainder, if there is any, under the unit multiplied as follows:

pt	fl oz	fl dr
4	7	3
		× 4
16	28	12

12 fl dr = 1 fl oz + 4 fl dr remainder

28 fl oz + 1 fl oz = 29 fl oz = 1 pt + 13 fl oz remainder

16 pt + 1 pt = 17 pt = 2 gal + 1 pt remainder

Answer: 2 gal, 1 pt, 12 fl oz, 4 fl dr.

2. What will be the *total weight* of the ingredients in a prescription order for 25 units, each unit containing 0.4 g of Solid F, 0.01 g of Solid G, and 5 mg of Solid H? First, convert to a common unit; eg, grams.

0.4 g + 0.01 g + 0.005 g = 0.415 g total weight of 1 unit

0.415 g/unit × 25 units = 10.375 g total weight of all units

3. Multiply 22.4 mL by 2.65.

$$\begin{array}{r} 22.4 \text{ mL} \\ \times\ 2.65 \\ \hline 59.36 \text{ mL} \end{array}$$

Problems

1. Multiply 48.5 mL by 3.24.
2. A certain preparation is to contain 0.0325 g of a chemical in each mL of solution. How much must be weighed out to make 5 L of the solution?
3. How much cod liver oil is necessary to make 2500 capsules, each containing 0.33 mL?
4. A formula calls for 1 pt, 3 fl oz, 4 fl dr of an oil. How much is required to make 15 times the formula quantity? Give amounts in measurable quantities.
5. How many mg are used to make 1500 units, each of which contains 250 μg of a drug?

Division

Rules

1. The quotient always has the same denomination as the dividend.
2. If the dividend is composed of different denominations, form a common unit in the metric system before dividing and reduce the quotient to weighable or measurable quantities. In the apothecary or avoirdupois systems arrange as under *Multiplication* and, begin division with the largest quantity at the left, convert the remainder, if any, into the next lower units and add to the next column before proceeding with the division.
3. Treat fractions, and decimals as under *Multiplication*.

Examples

1. Divide 3 L by 25.

$$3 \text{ L} = 3000 \text{ mL}$$

$$\frac{3000 \text{ mL}}{25} = 120 \text{ mL}$$

2. Divide 10 gal, 3 pt, 8 fl oz by 8.

$$\begin{array}{c|ccc} & \text{gal} & \text{pt} & \text{fl oz} \\ \hline 8 & 10 & 3 & 8 \end{array}$$

$$\frac{10 \text{ gal}}{8} = 1 \text{ gal} + 2 \text{ gal remainder}$$

$$2 \text{ gal} = 16 \text{ pt}$$

Place 16 pt in the next column.

$$16 \text{ pt} + 3 \text{ pt} = 19 \text{ pt}$$

$$\frac{19 \text{ pt}}{8} = 2 \text{ pt} + 3 \text{ pt remainder}$$

$$3 \text{ pt} = 48 \text{ fl oz}$$

Place 48 fl oz in the next column.

$$48 \text{ fl oz} + 8 \text{ fl oz} = 56 \text{ fl oz}$$

$$\frac{56 \text{ fl oz}}{8} = 7 \text{ fl oz}$$

Answer: 1 gal, 2 pt, 7 fl oz or 1 gal, 1 qt, 7 fl oz.

The alternative method is to reduce all quantities to a small unit such as fl oz, divide, and convert to measurable quantities.

$$(10 \text{ gal} \times 128 \text{ fl oz/gal}) + (3 \text{ pt} \times 16 \text{ fl oz/pt}) + 8 \text{ fl oz} = 1336 \text{ fl oz}$$

$$\frac{1334 \text{ fl oz}}{8} = 167 \text{ fl oz}$$

Extract the largest units possible (convert to measurable quantities).

167 fl oz	39 fl oz
− 128 fl oz = 1 gal	− 32 fl oz = 2 pt = 1 qt
39 fl oz remainder	7 fl oz remainder

Answer: 1 gal, 1 qt, 7 fl oz.

3. A pharmacist buys an 8-ounce container of a drug. How many 5-gr capsules can be made from the contents?

a. The pharmacist usually purchases by the avoirdupois system. The first step is to convert ounces to grains.

$$437.5 \text{ gr/oz} \times 8 \text{ oz} = 3500 \text{ gr}$$

b. Since 3500 gr are available and each capsule contains 5 gr, divide the total amount by 5 gr.

$$\frac{3500 \text{ gr}}{5 \text{ gr}} = 700$$

Therefore, 700 5-gr capsules can be made.

Problems

1. How many 65-mg capsules can be made from 50 g of a drug?
2. How many 15-minim capsules can be filled from 5 fl oz of an oil?
3. The dose of a drug is 0.1 mg. How many doses are contained in 15 mg of the drug?
4. The dose of a drug is $\frac{1}{150}$ gr. How many doses are obtainable from 1 gr of the drug?
5. How many 325-mg capsules of a drug can be filled from a 454-g amount?

Conversion

As long as the student knows the interrelationships of the various units within the different weighing and measuring systems (eg, 20 gr = 1Ә, 3Ә = 1Ʒ, etc; 1000 mg = 1 g, etc), there are only three conversions necessary for him to memorize in order to convert between the apoth, avoir, and metric systems. These are:

$$1 \text{ gr (avoir)} = 1 \text{ gr (apoth)}$$

$$15.43 \text{ gr} = 1 \text{ g}$$

$$16.23 \text{ m} = 1 \text{ mL}$$

Learn them!

With these three conversions the student is able to derive all other necessary conversions.

Review conversions within the apothecary system.

Various equalities within the apothecary system may be calculated. The number of grains in a dram, grains in a pound, etc may be calculated as follows:

1.

$$20 \text{ gr/Ә} \times 3 \text{Ә/Ʒ} = 60 \text{ gr/Ʒ}$$

$$60 \text{ gr/Ʒ} \times 8 \text{ Ʒ/Ʒ} \times 12 \text{ Ʒ/lb} = 5760 \text{ gr/lb}$$

Cancel the units. If they do not cancel properly, something has been left out.

2.

$$1 \text{ gr (apoth)} = 1 \text{ gr (avoir)}$$

Since 1 gr (apoth) = 1 gr (avoir), the number of grains in one system equals the number of grains in the other system; eg, 480 gr (apoth) = 480 gr (avoir).

Convert 1 Ʒ (apoth) to weighable quantities in the avoir system

$$20 \text{ gr/Ә} \times 3 \text{ Ә/Ʒ} \times 8 \text{ Ʒ/Ʒ} = 480 \text{ gr/Ʒ (apoth)}$$

$$480 \text{ gr (apoth)} = 480 \text{ gr (avoir)}$$

$$437.5 \text{ gr} = 1 \text{ oz avoir}$$

$$\begin{array}{r} 480.0 \text{ gr} \\ - 437.5 \text{ gr} \\ \hline 42.5 \text{ gr} \end{array}$$

Answer: 1 Ʒ (apoth) = 1 oz, 42.5 gr (avoir).

3. Conversions in the metric system are made by moving the decimal point. Moving the decimal point to the right gives a larger number and a smaller unit notation; eg,

$$1.000 \text{ g} = 1.000. \text{ mg}$$

Moving the decimal point to the left gives a smaller number and a large unit notation; eg,

$$1 \text{ g} = 0.001. \text{ kg,}$$

$$1000 \text{ g} = 1.000. \text{ kg}$$

The same procedure is valid for volume measurements in the metric system.

4. Conversions between the apothecary and metric weight systems are based on the fact that 15.43 gr = 1 g, which may be restated as 15.43 gr/g or 1 g/15.43 gr.

a. How many mg equal 1 gr?

$$\frac{1.000\ g}{15.43\ gr} = 0.0648\ g/gr = 64.8\ mg/gr\ or\ 64.8\ mg = 1\ gr$$

Cancel units.

b. How many grams are in 1 ℥?

$$\frac{1.000\ g}{15.43\ gr} \times 480\ gr/℥ = 31.11\ g/℥$$

c. How many grams are in 1 oz (avoir)? *Remember:* 1 gr (apoth) = 1 gr (avoir).

$$\frac{1.000\ g}{15.43\ gr} \times 437.5\ gr/oz = 28.35\ g/oz$$

d. Other weight conversions are then found in a similar manner.

5. Conversions between the apothecary and metric measuring systems are based on the fact that 16.23 ♏ = 1 mL, which may be restated as 16.23 ♏/mL or 1 mL/16.23 ♏.

a. How many mL are in 1 fl oz?

$$60\ ♏/fl\ dr \times 8\ fl\ dr/fl\ oz = 480\ ♏/fl\ oz$$

$$480\ ♏/fl\ oz \times \frac{1\ mL}{16.23\ ♏} = 29.57\ mL/fl\ oz$$

$$or\ 29.57\ mL = 1\ fl\ oz$$

6. *Remember:* 1 g = 1 mL = 1 cc for practical purposes, but 1 gr does *not* equal 1 ♏. This means that the student can convert easily between solids and liquids in the metric system but *not* in the apothecary system.

Rules

1. The USP states that for prescription compounding one uses exact equivalents rounded to three (3) significant figures.

2. To calculate quantities required in pharmaceutical formulas, the USP directs use of exact equivalents.

3. In converting doses the USP uses approximate equivalents. Use USP tables wherever possible.

Examples

1. Convert 1 pt, 4 fl oz into mL.

First, convert into fl oz.

$$16\ fl\ oz/pt + 4\ fl\ oz = 20\ fl\ oz$$

Second, convert fl oz to mL.

$$1\ fl\ oz = 29.6\ mL\ (as\ calculated\ above)$$

$$20\ fl\ oz \times 29.6\ mL/fl\ oz = 592\ mL$$

Answer: 1 pt, 4 fl oz = 592 mL.

2. What is the weight of 1200 g in the apothecary system?

$$1\ g = 15.43\ gr$$

$$1200\ g \times 15.43\ gr/g = 18,516\ gr$$

Convert to weighable quantities.

$$480\ gr = 1\ ℥$$

$$480\ gr/℥ \times 38\ ℥ = 18,240\ gr$$

$$\begin{array}{r} 18,516\ gr \\ -\ 18,240\ gr \\ \hline 276\ gr \end{array} \quad (38\ ℥),\ 38\ ℥ = 3\ ℔,\ 2\ ℥\ (12\ ℥ = 1\ ℔)$$

$$\begin{array}{r} -\ 240\ gr \\ \hline 36\ gr \end{array} \quad (60\ gr = 1\ ʒ),\ (4\ ʒ)$$

Answer: 3 ℔, 2 ℥, 4 ʒ, 36 gr (apoth).

3. Convert 1 pound (apoth) into grams.

$$\frac{1\ g}{15.43\ gr} \times 480\ gr/℥ = 31.11\ g/℥$$

$$1\ ℔ = 12\ ℥$$

$$12\ ℥ \times 31.11\ g/℥ = 373.3\ g/℔$$

4. Convert 25 gr to grams.

$$25\ gr \times \frac{1\ g}{15.43\ gr} = 1.62\ g$$

5. Convert 50 grams to grains.

$$50\ g \times 15.43\ gr/g = 771\ gr$$

Problems

1. Convert:
    a. 6.50 grains into milligrams.
    b. $^{3}/_{10}$ grain into milligrams.
    c. 3½ apoth ounces into grams.
    d. 2 ℥ into mg.
    e. 3½ avoir ounces into grams.
    f. 1 lb into grams.

2. Convert:
    a. 550 g into weighable quantities in the avoir system.
    b. 450 mg into grains.
    c. 550 g into weighable quantities in the apoth system.
    d. 100 μmg into grains.
    e. 1 kg into lb (avoir).

3. Convert the following doses into metric weights:
    a. $^{1}/_{100}$ gr.
    b. $^{1}/_{320}$ gr.
    c. $^{1}/_{6}$ gr.
    d. 5 gr.
    e. 20 gr.

4. Convert:
    a. 200 ♏ into mL.
    b. 3 fl dr into mL.
    c. 8 fl oz into mL.
    d. 1 pt into mL.
    e. 5 ♏ into mL.
    f. 0.1 mg into gr.
    g. 5 mg into gr.

5.
    a. How many gr are in 1 ℥?
    b. How many drams are in 1 ℥?
    c. How many grains are in 1 oz (avoir)?
    d. How many gr are in ½ ℔ (apoth)?
    e. Convert 250 gr to weighable quantities in the apothecary system.

Household Equivalents

Common household equivalents are found on page 73. These are used to interpret the prescriber's instructions to the patient. The teaspoonful is usually indicated by the symbol ℥ or 5 mL, although 1 ℥ does not equal 5 mL. The problem of "the teaspoonful" has been discussed by Morrell and Ordway.[4] For practical purposes, a teaspoonful is equal to 5 mL and 1 ℥ in the directions to the patient on the prescription means 1 teaspoonful; therefore there are 6 teaspoonful quantities in 1 fluidounce (5 mL × 6 = 30 mL).

For purposes of solving most compounding and dispensing problems, the exact equivalents found on pages 75 and 76 rounded to three significant places should be used.

Dosage Calculations

Over the past years various rules for calculating infants' and children's dosages have been devised. All these rules give only approximate dosages because they erroneously assume that the child is a small adult. Some of these rules are still used because as yet no absolute method of calculating an infant's or child's dose has been found. Children are sometimes more susceptible than adults to certain drugs. Doses for infants and children, where they are known, may be found in the USP, the APhA booklet entitled *Pediatric Dosage Handbook*, edited by HS Shirkey and textbooks on pediatrics.[5–7] Doses should not be calculated when it is possible to obtain the actual infant's or child's dose.

Rules for Infants' and Children's Doses

1. *Young's Rule* (for children 2 years and older).

$$\frac{Age\ (yr)}{Age\ (yr) + 12} \times adult\ dose = child's\ dose\ (approx)$$

2. *Clark's Rule.*

$$\frac{Weight\ (lb)}{150} \times adult\ dose = child's\ dose\ (approx)$$

3. *Fried's Rule* (for infants up to 2 years old).

$$\frac{Age\ (months)}{150} \times adult\ dose = infant's\ dose\ (approx)$$

Additional discussions on formulas used in calculating infant and children's dosages can be found in a handbook by Ritschel.[8]

Rules for Calculating Dosage on Prescriptions

1. To find the amount of an ingredient/dose in a compound prescription order, divide the total amount of ingredient prescribed by the number of doses.

2. To find the total amount of an ingredient used to compound a prescription, multiply the amount/dose prescribed by the total number of doses. On a prescription, when the instructions to the pharmacist includes the expression, D.T.D. No. ... (ie, send ... such doses), it instructs the pharmacist to multiply the dose (amount of drug) stated in the order by the number indicated in the expression, D.T.D. No. ....

3. The *Square Meter Surface Area Method* relates the surface area of individuals to dose. It is thought that this may be a more realistic way of relating dosages (see Crawford, *et al*,[9] Talbot, *et al*,[10] and Butler and Richie[11]).

$$\frac{Body\ surface\ area\ of\ child}{Body\ surface\ area\ of\ adult} \times adult\ dose = child's\ dose\ (approx)$$

The average body surface area for an adult has been given as 1.73 square meters (m²); hence,

$$\frac{Body\ surface\ area\ of\ child\ (m^2)}{1.73\ m^2} \times adult\ dose =$$

$$child's\ dose\ (approx)$$

The body surface area for individuals may be found in various reference sources such as the previously mentioned APhA booklet, and in drug dosage data by Shirkey.[12] Talbot, *et al*,[10] includes a chart which relates weight to body surface area. Wagner[13] presents a discussion on dosage of drugs.

Many drugs have doses stated as *so much drug/m² body surface area* and may be calculated as follows:

Amount of drug/m² × body surface area (m²) = individual's dose

Many physiological functions are proportional to body surface area, such as metabolic rate and kidney function.

4. Drug doses are often stated in *mg/kg body weight* and may be calculated as follows:

$$mg/kg \times body\ weight\ (kg) = individual's\ dose$$

This is the most common way of determining children's doses.

5. Drug doses also may be stated in *units;* e.g., vitamins A and D, penicillin, and hormones. This means that a certain quantity of biologic activity of that drug is called 1 unit. When the term unit is used in connection with a drug, the calculations involved are the same as those for more familiar weight or volume notations. The USP often standardizes the unit for such drugs so that the expression "USP Units" is used. This means the units are calculated, based on a USP assay procedure and reference standard.

Examples

1. The adult dose of a drug is 5 gr. What is the dose for a 3-year-old child?

Use Young's Rule:

$$Child's\ dose\ (approx) = \frac{3}{3 + 12} \times 5\ gr = 1\ gr$$

2. Determine the dose for each ingredient contained in 1 dose of the following prescription.

℞

Solid A	300 mg
Solid B	150 mg
Solid C	200 mg

D.T.D. No 12 M ft capsules.

The directions to the pharmacist request him to make and send 12 capsules containing the three solids in the amounts indicated. Thus, the dose of each ingredient is as stated in the prescription.

3. How much of each ingredient is used in compounding the following prescription?

℞

Drug E	7.2 g
Drug F	0.24 g
Drug G	1.2 g

M ft capsules no 24.

In this prescription the prescriber requests that 24 capsules be made from the three ingredients. The amounts of the ingredients requested are considerable and drugs usually do not have doses of 7.2 g or 1.2 g, so that division of the amounts by the number of doses (24) is required. The pharmacist should check a textbook or compendium to confirm the average adult dose.

Drug E:	7.2 g ÷ 24	= 0.300 g
Drug F:	0.24 g ÷ 24	= 0.010 g
Drug G:	1.2 g ÷ 24	= 0.050 g

4. What is the dose for a 40-lb child if the average adult dose of the medicament is 10 mg?

Use Clark's Rule:

$$Child's\ dose\ (approx) = \frac{40}{150} \times 10\ mg = 2.67\ mg$$

5. What is the dose for an 8-month-old infant if the average adult dose of a drug is 250 mg?

Use Fried's Rule:

$$Infant's\ dose\ (approx) = \frac{8}{150} \times 250\ mg = 13.3\ mg$$

6. If the average adult dose of a drug is 50 mg, what is the dose for a child that has a body surface area equal to 0.57 m²?

Child's dose (approx) $= \dfrac{0.57}{1.73} \times 50 \text{ mg} = 16.5 \text{ mg}$

7. A prescription calls for 10 units of a drug to be taken 3 times a day. How much will the patient have taken after 7 days?

10 units/dose × 3 doses/day × 7 days = 210 units

8. If 250 units of an antibiotic weighs 1 mg, how many units are in 15 mg?

250 units/mg × 15 mg = 3750 units

9. If the dose of a drug is 0.5 mg/kg of body weight/24 hr, how many g will a 33-lb infant receive per 24 hr and per week?

33 lb = 15 kg

0.5 mg/kg/24 hr × 15 kg = 7.5 mg/24 hr = 0.0075 g/24 hr

0.0075 g/24 hr × 7 days = 0.0525 g/wk

10. A patient is to receive 260 μg of a drug four times a day for 14 days. How many $\frac{1}{250}$-gr tablets must be dispensed?

$\frac{1}{250}$ gr × 64.8 mg = 260 μg

$\frac{1}{250}$-gr tablet × 4/day × 14 days = 56 tablets

11. An antibiotic is available as an injection containing 10 mg antibiotic/mL. How many mL are needed for an infant weighing 8 kg, the dose being 1.4 mg/kg of body weight?

1.4 mg/kg × 8 kg = 11.2 mg needed

10 mg:1 mL::11.2 mg:Y mL

Y = 1.12 mL needed for the infant

12. A preparation for coughs contains 1.5 g of an expectorant per 100 mL. How many gr of the expectorant are there in a teaspoonful?

1 teaspoonful = 5 mL

1.5 g:100 mL::D g:5 mL

D = 0.075 g/5 mL

0.075 g × 15.4 gr/g = 1.12 gr/5 mL

Problems

1. Calculate the dose for each ingredient in the following prescription.

℞
Chemical J .... 10 mg
Chemical K .... 50 mg
Chemical L .... 300 mg
M ft capsules   D.T.D. No 14.

2. Calculate the dose of each ingredient in the following prescription.

℞
Drug Q .... 10.5 g
Drug R .... 6.3 g
Make 21 doses.

3. An 8-fl oz prescription contains 6 fl dr of a tincture. If 1 teaspoonful 4 times a day is prescribed, how much tincture does the patient take/dose and how much does he take daily?

4. How many 0.3-mL doses are contained in 15 mL of a solution?

5. If 1 mg of a hormone equals 22.5 units, how many mg are required to obtain 1 unit?

6. What is the dose of a drug for a 9-month-old infant if the average adult dose is 25 mg?

7. What is the dose of a drug for a 6-year-old child if the average adult dose is 1½ gr?

8. What is the dose of a drug for a child that weighs 28 lb if the average adult dose is 100 mg?

9. What is the dose of a drug for an individual that has a 1.21 m² body surface area? The average adult dose is 400,000 units.

10. What is the dose of a medicament for a child that weighs 66 lb if the dose is stated as 2.5 mg/kg body weight?

11. What is the dose of a drug for an average adult patient if the dose of the drug is 45 mg/m²?

12. If a bottle contains 80 units of a drug/mL, how many mL must the patient take to get a 60-unit dose? If the bottle contains 10 mL total volume of the drug solution, how many days' supply will the patient have if he uses 60 units daily?

13. A 10-mL ampul contains a 2.5% solution of a drug. How many mL are needed to give a dose of 150 mg?

14. The dose of an antibiotic is 75 mg for a child. How much of a flavored suspension containing 125 mg antibiotic/5 mL must be given to the child per dose?

15. How many gr of a drug are there in each teaspoonful of a syrup that contains 0.5% of the drug?

Remember: It is always better to look up the dose of drugs in textbooks or compendia than to rely on memory or equations.

Reducing and Enlarging Formulas

Rules

1. Determine the total weight or volume of ingredients and convert, if necessary, to the system of the quantities desired. The quantities in the original and new formulas will have the same ratio.

2. To reduce formulas in the metric system, divide by a power of 10 by moving the decimal place to the left the required number of places for each ingredient; to enlarge formulas, multiply by a power of 10 by moving the decimal place to the right the required number of places.

Examples

1. The formula for a syrup is

Drug M .... 140 g
Sucrose .... 450 g
Purified Water, q.s., to make .... 1000 mL

a. To find the quantities required for 100 mL, move the decimal place to the left since only $\frac{1}{10}$ of the original formula quantity is needed.

14.0. .... 14 g

45.0. .... 45 g

100.0. .... 100 mL

b. What quantities are required to compound 60 mL of the syrup?

The new formula required $^{60}/_{1000}$ or 0.06 parts of the quantities in the original formula (1000 mL). Multiply the original quantities by 0.06 to get the new quantities.

Drug M .... 0.06 × 140 g = 8.4 g
Sucrose .... 0.06 × 450 g = 27.0 g
Purified Water, to ...... 0.06 × 1000 mL = 60.0 mL

2. Calculate the amounts needed for 100 g of antiseptic powder as follows:

Solid A	2 g
Solid B	1 g
Solid C	7 g
Solid D	25 g
Solid E	115 g
	150 g

The original formula calls for a total of 150 g and the new one for 100 g. Form the following ratio to determine the quantities for the new formula:

$$\frac{100 \text{ g}}{150 \text{ g}} = 0.667$$

Each ingredient must be multiplied by 0.667 to reduce the original formula of 150 g to 100 g of finished product.

Solid A	2 g × 0.667 = 1.33 g
Solid B	1 g × 0.667 = 0.667 g
Solid C	7 g × 0.667 = 4.67 g
Solid D	25 g × 0.667 = 16.7 g
Solid E	115 g × 0.667 = 76.7 g
	100.067 g

3. Prescriptions, where the instruction to the pharmacist calls for making a certain number of doses of an ingredient or mixture of several ingredients, are a type of formula enlargement. The expression usually used is D.T.D., which means send such doses (see Table I, Chapter 101). Occasionally the prescriber will not use this expression, but inspection of amounts of the ingredients indicates that this is what is desired. For example,

R

Solid H	50	mg
Solid K	150	mg
Liquid N	0.2 mL	

M ft capsules, D.T.D. no 24.

The pharmacist checked the individual doses of the ingredients and found them to be slightly below the average adult dose, confirming that the prescriber wanted the quantities listed to be multiplied by 24.

Ingredients	Amounts	Multiplier	New amounts
Solid H	50 mg	× 24	1200 mg or 1.2 g
Solid K	150 mg	× 24	3600 mg or 3.6 g
Liquid N	0.2 mL	× 24	4.8 mL

Problems

1. The formula for a liquid preparation is

Liquid C	35	mL
Solid B	9	g
Liquid R	2.5	mL
Liquid P	20	mL
Purified water, sufficient to make	100	mL

Calculate the quantities of the ingredients to make 2.5 L.

2. The formula for an ointment is

Solid G	1 ℥
Liquid D	30 ℳ
Solid M	3 ℨ
Ointment base, sufficient to make	1 ℔

Calculate quantities of the ingredients for 2 lb.

3. How much of each of the three solids and how much purified water are needed to properly compound the following prescription order?

R

Solid N	0.1 mg
Solid Q	2.5 mg
Solid R	150.0 mg
Purified water, qs, to	5 mL

M ft solution, D.T.D. no 48.

4. How much of each ingredient is required to compound 90 mL of the following product?

Solid S	7.5 g	
Solid T	25	g
Oil C	350	mL
Alcohol	250	mL
Purified water, q.s., to	1000	mL

Ratio and Proportion

This arithmetical procedure often can be used to solve various pharmaceutical compounding and dispensing problems.

A ratio states the relation of one quantity to another and may be written as a common fraction (implying division) or with a colon between the two numbers. For example, three parts compared with four parts is written $\frac{3}{4}$ or $3:4$ and is stated, "three is to four." The ratio is $\frac{3}{4}$, $3:4$, or three is to four. Any units may be substituted for "parts" but the value of the ratio does not change. The units must be the same.

Two equal ratios that are set equal to each other result in an equation which is called a proportion. For example, $\frac{3}{4} = \frac{15}{20}$, $3:4::15:20$, or "three is to four as fifteen is to twenty" are ways of writing and stating that 3 and 4 form the same ratio or fraction as 15 and 20.

The first and last terms of a proportion are called the extremes, and the second and third terms are called the means.

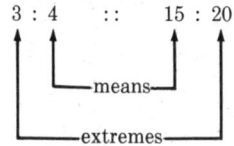

Rules

The following statements are true for any proportion.

1. The product of the means equals the product of the extremes.

2. The product of the means divided by one extreme gives the other extreme.

3. The product of the extremes divided by one mean gives the other mean. Therefore, if any three terms of a proportion are known, the fourth may be found by simple calculation.

In solving problems involving proportions the following procedure may be used.

First—Let the unknown quantity be represented by X and let it be the fourth term.

Second—Let the third term be that number in the question which expresses the same kind of value (unit) as is expected in the answer.

Third—Arrange the remaining two quantities in the same ratio as the third term and X. Thus the first and second terms will express the same kind of values (units) and the third and fourth terms will express the same kind of values. If the answer sought (X) is to be greater than the third term, the second term will be larger than the first, and vice versa.

Fourth—To solve for X, divide the product of the means by the known extreme. Cancel to simplify. Since the first and second terms form a ratio, common factors may be removed without altering the ratio; and since the first and third terms are actually numerators of equal fractions, they can be divided by the same number without changing the proportion.

Example

100 g of a drug cost $1.80. How much will 25 g cost?

If the three quantities in the problem, namely 100 g, $1.80, and 25 g are considered, it will be seen readily that 100 g bears the same relation to 25 g as $1.80 does to the unknown quantity to be calculated. In other words, the quantities and prices form equal ratios. The following proportion can be made:

$$100 \text{ g} : 25 \text{ g} :: \$1.80 : \$X$$

There are three known terms in the statement and X, the unknown term. Arithmetically the product of the means must equal the product of the extremes. Therefore, if one of the extremes is unknown, it may be calculated by dividing the product of the means by the known extreme.

$$X = \frac{25 \text{ g} \times \$1.80}{100 \text{ g}} = \$0.45$$

While the proportion is preferably set down as given above, it may be stated in several other ways. These are given below merely to show their relationship to the original form. It may be stated as two equal ratios in equation form:

$$\frac{100 \text{ g}}{25 \text{ g}} = \frac{\$1.80}{X}$$

Keeping in mind the basic three rules, it is also possible to place the unknown quantity, X, in either the first, second, or third position as long as the relationship of the three known terms is not altered. Thus, the problem may be written as,

$$25 \text{ g} : 100 \text{ g} :: X : \$1.80 \text{ (Rule 3)}$$
$$\frac{25 \text{ g} \times \$1.80}{100 \text{ g}} = \$0.45$$

or

$$\$1.80 : X :: 100 \text{ g} : 25 \text{ g} \text{ (Rule 3)}$$
$$\frac{\$1.80 \times 25 \text{ g}}{100 \text{ g}} = \$0.45$$

or

$$X : \$1.80 :: 25 \text{ g} : 100 \text{ g} \text{ (Rule 2)}$$
$$\frac{\$1.80 \times 25 \text{ g}}{100 \text{ g}} = \$0.45$$

Obviously, the method of ratio and proportion can be used to solve more involved problems.

Problems

1. If a drug costs \$3.00/g, how much would 65 mg cost? How much would 5 gr cost?
2. One pound of a chemical cost \$7.65. What is the cost of sufficient chemical needed to make 10,000 capsules containing 0.2 g of the chemical?

See also the preparation of isotonic solutions by proportion, Chapter 79.

Percentage

Percent, written as %, means per hundred. Fifteen percent is written 15% and means $^{15}/_{100}$, 0.15, or 15 parts in a total of 100 parts. Percent is a type of ratio and has no units. Thus 10% of 1500 tablets is $^{10}/_{100} \times 1500$ tablets = 150 tablets.

To change percent to a fraction the percent number becomes the numerator and 100 is the denominator. To change a fraction to percent, put the fraction in a form having 100 as its denominator; multiply by 100 so that the numerator becomes the percent.

$$^1/_2 = \frac{50}{100}; \quad \frac{50}{100} \times 100 = 50\%$$

$$^1/_8 = \frac{12.5}{100}; \quad \frac{12.5}{100} \times 100 = 12.5\%$$

Calculations involving percentages are continually encountered by pharmacists. He must be familiar, not only with the arithmetic principles, but also with certain compendial interpretations of the different type percentages involving solutions and mixtures.

The USP states:

Percentage concentrations of solutions are expressed as follows:
Percent weight in weight—(w/w) expresses the number of g of a constituent in 100 g of solution.
Percent weight in volume—(w/v) expresses the number of g of a constituent in 100 mL of solution, and is used regardless of whether water or another liquid is the solvent.
Percent volume in volume—(v/v) expresses the number of mL of a constituent in 100 mL of solution.
The term *percent* used without qualification means, for mixtures of solids, percent weight in weight; for solutions or suspensions of solids in liquids, percent weight in volume; for solutions of liquids in liquids, percent volume in volume; and for solutions of gases in liquids, percent weight in

volume. For example, a 1 percent solution is prepared by dissolving 1 g of a solid or 1 mL of a liquid in sufficient of the solvent to make 100 mL of the solution.

In the dispensing of prescription medications, slight changes in volume owing to variations in room temperature may be disregarded.

Ratio Strength

This is another manner of expressing strength. Such phrases as "1 in 10" are understood to mean that 1 part by volume of a liquid is to be diluted with, or 1 part by weight of a solid dissolved in, sufficient of the solution to make the finished solution 10 parts by volume. For example, a 1:10 solution means 1 mL of a liquid or 1 g of a solid dissolved in sufficient solvent to make 10 mL of solution. It can be converted to percent by:

$$1 \text{ g} : 10 \text{ mL} :: X \text{ g} : 100 \text{ mL}$$

$X = 10$ g in 100 mL of solution which is 10%

The expression "parts per thousand" (e.g., 1–5000) always means parts weight in volume when dealing with solutions of solids in liquids and is similar to the above expression. A 1–5000 solution means 1 g of solute in sufficient solvent to make 5000 mL of solution. This can be converted to percent by:

$$1 \text{ g} : 5000 \text{ mL} :: X \text{ g} : 100 \text{ mL}$$

$X = 0.02$ g in 100 mL solution which is 0.02%

The expression "trituration" has two different meanings in pharmacy. One refers to the process of particle-size reduction, commonly by grinding or rubbing in a mortar with the aid of a pestle. The other meaning refers to a dilution of a potent powdered drug with a suitable powdered diluent in a definite proportion by weight. It is the second meaning that is used in this chapter. When a pharmacist refers to a "1 in 10 trituration" he means a mixture of solids composed of 1 g of drug plus sufficient diluent (another solid) to make 10 g of mixture of *dilution*. In this case the "1 in 10 trituration" is actually a solid dilution of a drug with an inert solid. The strength of a trituration may also be stated as percent *w/w*.

Thus, the term trituration has come to mean a solid dilution of a potent drug with a chemically and physiologically inert solid.

The meanings implied by the USP statements under *Percentage* are illustrated below with a few examples of the three types of percentages.

Weight-in-Volume Percentages

This is the type of percent problem encountered on prescriptions. The preparation of these solutions is very simple if the student will keep in mind that for practical purposes the calculation is made on the basis that 1 ʒ (apoth) of solvent weighs 455 gr, or 1 mL of solvent weighs 1 g. The density of the solvent or solution is *not* required in these calculations, and is assumed to be one. The volume occupied by the solute is not considered in *w/v* problems. The volume of the solvent is *not* known because sufficient solvent is added to make a given or known final volume.

Examples

1. Prepare 1 fl oz of a 10% solution.

Since this is a solution of a solid in a liquid, this is a *w/v* solution. Therefore, 455 gr/fʒ is taken as the base.

$$455 \text{ gr/fʒ} \times \% \text{ (decimal)} \times \text{no. of fʒ} = \text{gr solute}$$

$$455 \text{ gr/fʒ} \times 0.10 \times 1 \text{ fʒ} = 45.5 \text{ gr solute}$$

45.5 gr is dissolved in sufficient purified water to make 1 fʒ of solution.

2.   How much of a drug is required to compound 4 fl oz of a 3% solution in alcohol?

$$455 \text{ gr/f}ʒ \times \% \text{ (decimal)} \times \text{no. of f}ʒ = \text{gr solute}$$

$$455 \text{ gr/f}ʒ \times 0.03 \times 4 \text{ f}ʒ = 54.6 \text{ gr drug}$$

It should be emphasized that the percentage of solute is calculated from 455 gr/fʒ of water because this is the only way in which solutions of identical percentage strength can be prepared in both the metric and apothecary systems.

3.   How much 0.9% solution of sodium chloride can be made from ½ ʒ of NaCl?

$$480 \text{ gr/}ʒ \div 2 = 240 \text{ gr in } \tfrac{1}{2} ʒ$$

$$455 \text{ gr/f}ʒ \times \% \text{ (decimal)} \times \text{no. of f}ʒ = \text{gr solute}$$

$$455 \text{ gr/f}ʒ \times 0.009 \times Y \text{ f}ʒ = 240 \text{ gr}$$

$$Y = \frac{240 \text{ gr}}{455 \text{ gr/f}ʒ \times 0.009} = 58.6 \text{ f}ʒ = 1 \text{ qt, 1 pt, 10.6 f}ʒ$$

In the metric system the following equation can be used to calculate the quantity of solute necessary to prepare a given percent w/v solution.

$$\text{mL of solution} \times \% \text{ (decimal)} = \text{g solute required}$$

4.   How many grams of a drug are required to make 120 mL of a 25% solution?

Remember: percent w/v is indicated.

$$\text{mL of solution} \times \% \text{ (decimal)} = \text{g solute required}$$

$$120 \text{ mL} \times 0.25 = 30 \text{ g of drug}$$

5.   How would you prepare 480 mL of a 1 in 750 solution of an antiseptic?

Remember: percent w/v is indicated.
1 in 750 means 1 g of the antiseptic dissolved in sufficient solvent to make 750 mL solution.
By ratio and proportion,

$$1 \text{ g} : 750 \text{ mL} : : U \text{ g} : 480 \text{ mL}$$

$$U = 1 \text{ g} \times 480 \text{ mL}/750 \text{ mL} = 0.64 \text{ g antiseptic needed}$$

Dissolve 0.64 g of antiseptic in sufficient solvent to make 480 mL solution.

6.   How much of a substance is needed to prepare 1 L of a 1:10,000 solution?

$$1 : 10,000 \text{ means 1 g of a substance in 10,000 mL of solution}$$

$$1 \text{ L} = 1000 \text{ mL}$$

By ratio and proportion,

$$1 \text{ g} : 10,000 \text{ mL} : : V \text{ g} : 1000 \text{ mL}$$

$$V = 1 \text{ g} \times 1000 \text{ mL}/10,000 \text{ mL} = 0.1 \text{ g substance needed}$$

7.   How would you prepare 120 mL of 0.25% solution of neomycin sulfate? The source of neomycin sulfate is a solution which contains 1 g neomycin sulfate/10 mL.

a. $0.25 \text{ g} : 100 \text{ mL} : : Y \text{ g} : 120 \text{ mL}$
     $Y = 0.3 \text{ g drug needed}$
b. $1 \text{ g} : 10 \text{ mL} : : 0.3 \text{ g} : V \text{ mL}$
     $V = 3 \text{ mL}$ of the stock solution needed. Add sufficient purified water to make 120 mL.

Problems

1.   How would you make 3 fl oz of a 12.5% solution?
2.   How many liters of a 4% solution can be made from 4 oz of a solid?
3.   How many liters of an 8% solution can be made from 500 g of a solid?
4.   How many grams of a drug are needed to make 4 L of a 1 in 500 solution?

Weight-in-Weight Percentages

For this type of problem, remember that there are 480 gr in an apothecary ounce (480 gr/ʒ). Density must be considered in some of these problems. If a weight-in-weight solution is requested on a prescription both the solute and solvent must be weighed, or the solute and the solvent may be measured if their densities are taken into consideration in determining the volumes. Since the solutions are made to a given weight, a given volume is not always obtainable; e.g., 4 ʒ does *not* equal 4 f ʒ and 100 g of solution does *not* equal 100 mL. For the apothecary system, the following equation may be used to calculate the grains of solute required.

$$480 \text{ gr/}ʒ \times \% \text{ (decimal)} \times \text{no. of } ʒ = \text{gr solute required}$$

Examples

1.   What weights of solute and solvent are required to make 2 ʒ of a 3% w/w solution of a drug in 90% alcohol?

$$480 \text{ gr/}ʒ \times \% \text{ (decimal)} \times \text{number of } ʒ$$
$$= \text{gr solute required}$$

$$480 \text{ gr/}ʒ \times 0.03 \times 2 ʒ = 28.8 \text{ gr of drug required}$$

$$480 \text{ gr/}ʒ \times 2 ʒ = 960 \text{ gr}$$

$$\begin{array}{r} 960.0 \text{ gr} \\ -\underline{\ 28.8 \text{ gr}} \\ 931.2 \text{ gr solvent} \end{array}$$

2.   The solubility of boric acid is 1 g in 18 mL of water at 25°C. What is the percentage strength, w/w, of a saturated solution?

1 g of boric acid + 18 mL of water make a saturated solution, 18 mL of water weighs 18 g; hence, the weight of solution is 19 g. The amount of boric acid present is 1 g in 19 g solution; therefore, the following proportion can be set up:

$$1 \text{ g} : 19 \text{ g} : : X \text{ g} : 100 \text{ g}$$

$$X = 1 \text{ g} \times 100 \text{ g}/19 \text{ g} = 5.26 \text{ g}/100 \text{ g or } 5.26\%$$

3.   How many grams of a chemical are needed to prepare 200 g of a 10% w/w solution?

10% w/w means 10 g solute in 100 g total solution. If 100 g solution contains 10 g of solute, there are 90 g of solvent (100 g solution − 10 g solute = 90 g solvent). The following proportion may be set up

$$10 \text{ g} : 100 \text{ g} : : M \text{ g} : 200 \text{ g}$$

$$M = 10 \text{ g} \times 200 \text{ g}/100 \text{ g} = 20 \text{ g solute needed}$$

4.   How would you make 240 mL of a 2% w/w solution of a drug in alcohol. The density of alcohol is 0.816 g/mL.

a.   First, convert 240 mL to weight. *Remember:* alcohol is the solvent and it has a density different from that of water.

$$\text{Density} = \text{weight/volume}$$

$$\text{Weight} = \text{density} \times \text{volume}$$

$$\text{Weight} = 0.816 \text{ g/mL} \times 240 \text{ mL} = 195.8 \text{ g (196 g)}$$

b.   2% w/w means 2 g solute in 100 g solution. In this problem the final weight of solution is not known; 240 mL (196 g) of alcohol represents the solvent only. The solvent is 98% w/w of the total solution, so that the following proportion may be set up:

$$2 \text{ g} : 98 \text{ g} : : N \text{ g} : 196 \text{ g}$$

$$N = 2 \text{ g} \times 196 \text{ g}/98 \text{ g} = 4.00 \text{ g}$$

c.   Dissolve 4.00 g of the drug in 240 mL alcohol. The resulting solution will be 2% w/w and have a volume slightly larger than 240 mL because of the volume displacement of the drug.

5.   How much of a 5% w/w solution can be made from 1 oz avoir of a chemical?

480 gr/ʒ × % (decimal) × no. of ʒ = gr of solute

$$1 \text{ oz av} = 437.5 \text{ gr}$$

$$\text{no. of } ʒ = \frac{\text{gr of solute}}{(480 \text{ gr/ʒ} \times \% \text{ as a decimal fraction})}$$

$$= \frac{437.5 \text{ gr}}{480 \text{ gr/ʒ} \times 0.05} = 18.2 \text{ ʒ} = 1 \text{ ℔}, 6.2 \text{ ʒ}$$

6. How many mL of a 70% *w/w* solution having a density of 1.2 g/mL will be needed to prepare 600 mL of a 10% *w/v* solution?

a. 10 g:100 mL::Z g:600 mL
    Z = 60 g of drug needed
b. 70 g:100 g::60 g:T g.
    T = 85.7 g of 70% *w/w* solution needed.
c. Volume = Weight/Density = 85.7 g/1.2 g/mL = 71.4 mL of the 70% *w/w* solution needed.

Compounding problems involving solid preparations (such as mixtures of powder) and semisolid preparations (such as ointments, creams, and suppositories) are also percent *w/w*. For example:

1. How much drug is required to make 2 ʒ of a 10% ointment?

Since this preparation is an ointment, percent *w/w* is indicated.

480 gr/ʒ × % (decimal) × no. of ʒ = gr drug

480 gr/ʒ × 0.10 × 2 ʒ = 96 gr = 1 ʒ, 1 ϴ, 16 gr drug

The same procedure could be used for mixtures of powders, suppository masses, etc. Instead of using units in the various measuring systems, quantities can be indicated "by parts" similar to percent *w/v* solutions. The term "parts" can then mean any unit in any measuring system, as long as the units are kept constant. For example:

2.

℞
Solid A	0.5 part
Powder B	3.0 parts
Powder C, qs, to	30 parts

How many g of each of the three ingredients are required to make 30 g of the product?

Since the product is a mixture of powders, percent *w/w* is indicated. In the above prescription order the total product is 30 parts because Powder C is used to "qs to" or "make up to" 30 parts. Therefore, 0.5 g of Powder A and 3.0 g of Powder B are needed

Powder A	0.5 g	
Powder B	+ 3.0 g	
	3.5 g	

Total product	30.0 g	
	− 3.5 g	
	26.5 g	Powder C needed

3.

℞
Solid D	3.0 parts
Solid E	6.0 parts
Ointment Base Q	30.0 parts

How much of each ingredient is needed to make 60 g of the ointment?

Solid D	3.0 parts
Solid E	6.0 parts
Base Q	30.0 parts
	39.0 parts total

Since a total of 60 g is needed, the following proportions can be made:

39 Parts total in ℞:60 g total needed::3.0 parts Solid D:X g

X = 60 g × 3.0 parts/39 parts = 4.62 g Solid D needed

39 Parts:60 g::6.0 parts:Y g

Y = 60 g × 6.0 parts/39 parts = 9.23 g Solid E needed

4.62 g Solid D	60.00 g Total
+ 9.23 g Solid E	− 13.85 g
13.85 g	46.15 g Base Q needed

The amount of ointment base needed can also be calculated by the above ratio and proportion method.

4. What is the percent strength of a salt solution obtained by diluting 100 g of a 5% solution to 200 g?

a. Since the solutions are expressed by weight, percent *w/w* is indicated. 5% *w/w* means 5 g active ingredient plus 95 g solvent to make 100 g solution.
b. 100 g solution is diluted to 200 g by the addition of water. The solvent was not stated, so it is assumed to be purified water, and 100 mL of water = 100 g.
c. The original 5 g active ingredient is now in 200 g solution; thus, the following proportion can be set up:

5 g:200 g::X g:100 g

X = 5 g × 100 g/200 g = 2.5 g/100 g = 2.5%

When liquids are incorporated into ointments they should be weighed to give a % *w/w* formulation, but often they are measured, with lesser accuracy, on a % volume per weight basis.

Problems

1. How much of the drug and solvent are needed to compound the following prescription?

℞
Compound A	6% *w/w*
Solvent, qs, to make	4 ʒ

2. How many grams of solute are needed to prepare 240 g of a 12% *w/w* solution?
3. How many kg of a 20% *w/w* solution can be made from 1 kg of the solute?
4. How would you prepare, using 120 mL of glycerin (density, 1.25 g/mL), a solution that is 3% *w/w* with respect to a drug?
5. How much of each substance is needed to prepare a total of 24 g of the following suppository mass?

Compound K	0.3 g
Solid H	0.15 g
Suppository base, qs, to	2.0 g

6. How would you prepare 500 mL of a 15% *w/w* aqueous solution?
7. How much of each of the ingredients is required to make 1 kg of the following mixture?

Powder P	1 part
Powder Q	8 parts
Powder R	12 parts
Powder S	15 parts
	36 parts

8. How much of each ingredient is required to prepare the following ointment?

℞
Coal Tar Solution	10%
Hydrophilic Ointment, qs, to	30 g

Volume-in-Volume Percentages

A direct calculation of percentage from the total volume is made, neglecting slight shrinkages which may occur and making up to the desired volume with the diluent. The following equation is based on the fact that 480 minims = 1 fl oz may be used.

480 ♏/fl oz × % (decimal) × number of fl oz

$$= \text{minims of drug}$$

Examples

1.   How much of a liquid is needed to make 6 fl oz of a hand lotion containing 0.5% *v/v* of the liquid?

480 ♏/fl oz × % (decimal) × no. of fl oz = ♏ of drug

480 ♏/fl oz × 0.005 × 6 fl oz = 14.4 ♏ of liquid needed

Add sufficient lotion to 14.4 ♏ of the liquid to make 6 f♌ of the product.

2.   How much 90% alcohol is required to compound 500 mL of a 10% alcohol mixture? In *v/v* mixtures, percentage is directly proportional to volume.

a.   Since alcohol, a liquid, is mixed with water, percent *v/v* is indicated. Assume no shrinkage.
b.   500 mL of the 10% solution contains the following amount of alcohol:

10 mL:100 mL::X mL:500 mL

$$X = 10 \text{ mL} \times 500 \text{ mL}/100 \text{ mL} = 50 \text{ mL alcohol}$$

c.   90% alcohol contains 90 mL alcohol in 100 mL solution. 50 mL of pure alcohol is needed; therefore, the following proportion may be set up:

90 mL:100 mL::50 mL:Y mL

$$Y = 100 \text{ mL} \times 50 \text{ mL}/90 \text{ mL} = 55.5 \text{ mL of 90\% alcohol needed}$$

Problems

1.   How many minims of a liquid are needed to make 4 f♌ of a 12.5% *v/v* solution?
2.   How much purified water should be added to 1 L of alcohol (95% *v/v*) to make 50% *v/v* alcohol?
3.   What is the percentage strength, weight in weight, of a liquid made by dissolving 16 g of a salt in 30 mL of water?
4.   How much drug will be required to prepare 1 fl oz of a 2.5% solution?
5.   What is the percentage, weight in weight, of sugar in a syrup made by dissolving 5 kg of sugar in 8 kg of water?
6.   How many g of a drug are required to prepare 120 mL of a 12.5% aqueous solution?
7.   How much drug is needed to compound a liter of a 1–2500 aqueous solution?
8.   A solution contains 37% of active ingredient. How much of this solution is needed to prepare 480 mL of an aqueous solution containing 2.5% of the active ingredient?
9.   How much of a drug is required to make 2 qt of a 1–1200 solution?

Stock Solutions

In order to facilitate the dispensing of certain soluble substances, the pharmacist frequently prepares or purchases solutions of high concentration. Portions of these concentrated solutions are diluted to give required solutions of lesser strength. These concentrated solutions are known as stock solutions. This procedure is satisfactory if the substances are stable in solution or if the solutions are to be used before they decompose.

In the case of potent substances, a properly prepared stock solution permits the pharmacist to obtain accurately a quantity of solid which might otherwise be difficult to weigh. In the case of frequently prescribed salt solutions, a stock solution readily provides the required amount of salt without the necessity of weighing and dissolving it every time.

Stock solutions may be of various concentrations depending on the requirements for use. The stock solutions should be properly labeled and fractional parts needed to make various strengths also may be listed as a further convenience. Typical concentrations might be:

♏ mL = 1 mL;   %;   by parts;   ratio strength;   100 mL = 1 g

There is a type of compounding and dispensing problem that involves the concept of stock solutions. This problem involves the patient diluting a dose from the prescription order to a given volume to obtain a solution of desired concentration.

For example, how many grams of a salt are required to make 90 mL of a stock solution, 5 mL of which makes a 1–3000 solution when diluted to 500 mL?

a.   Determine how many g are in 500 mL of a 1–3000 solution.

1 g:3000 mL::X g:500 mL

$$X = 1 \text{ g} \times 500 \text{ mL}/3000 \text{ mL} =$$
$$0.167 \text{ g salt in 500 mL of 1–3000 solution}$$

b.   The 0.167 g in the dilute solution came from the 5 mL of the original stock solution (prescription order). The following proportion can be used:

0.167 g:5 mL::Y g:90 mL

$$Y = 0.167 \text{ g} \times 90 \text{ mL}/5 \text{ mL} = 3.01 \text{ g salt}$$
$$\text{needed to make the original 90 mL of stock solution}$$

Problems

1.   How much of a drug is needed to compound 120 mL of a prescription order such that when 1 teaspoonful of the solution is diluted to 1 qt, a 1–750 solution results?
2.   How many grams of a drug are needed to make 240 mL of a solution of such strength that when 5 mL is diluted to 2 qt, a 1–2500 solution results?
3.   An ampul of solution of an anti-inflammatory drug contains 4 mg of drug/mL. What volume of the solution is needed to prepare a liter of solution that contains 2 μg of the drug/mL?

Parts Per Million

An expression that is occasionally used in the compounding prescriptions is *parts per million* (ppm). This is another way of expressing concentration, particularly concentrations of very dilute preparations. A 1% solution may be expressed as 1 part/100, a 0.1% solution is 0.1 part/100 or 1 part/1000. A 1 ppm solution contains 1 part of solute/1 million parts of solution; 5 ppm is 5 parts solute/1 million parts solution, and so on. Remember that the two parts must have the same units, except in the metric system where 1 g = 1 mL of water.

Sodium fluoride is a drug that may be prescribed by a dentist as a preventative for tooth decay in children. It is used only in very dilute solutions due to the drug's toxicity and because only minute quantities are needed.

℞
   Sod Fluoride, qs
   Purified water, qs 60 mL
Make soln such that when 1 ♌ is diluted to 1 glassful of water a 2 ppm soln results.
Sig: 1 ♌ in a glassful of water daily.

The mathematics to solve this compounding problem is easy once the steps for calculating the answer are outlined. This problem should be worked "backwards."

a.   The amount of NaF needed is not known.
b.   One glassful of water has a volume of 240 mL. The concentration of NaF in 240 mL is 2 ppm.
c.   The NaF solution poured into the glass came from a teaspoonful dose (1 ♌), which is equal to 5 mL.
d.   The 5-mL dose came from the prescription order bottle containing a NaF solution.

Now let us put it in numbers:

a. 240 mL contains 2 ppm NaF.

$$2\ g : 1{,}000{,}000\ mL : : X\ g : 240\ mL$$

$$X = 2\ g \times 240\ mL/1{,}000{,}000\ mL = 0.00048\ g$$

b. The 0.00048 g NaF in the glass came from the teaspoonful dose; therefore, the teaspoonful (5 mL) contained 0.00048 g NaF.
c. The 5 mL came out of the original prescription order bottle (60 mL).

$$5\ mL : 0.00048\ g : : 60\ mL : Y\ g$$

$$Y = 0.00048\ g \times 60\ mL/5\ mL = 0.00576\ g$$

The pharmacist would weigh out 5.76 mg (actually, he would weigh out a larger quantity and take an aliquot part) and qs to 60 mL.

Another variation of this problem is where the prescriber requests the concentration in terms of fluoride ion (F^-). In this case the atomic weight of F^- and molecular weight of NaF are used in the calculation. If the request called for 2 ppm fluoride, the initial calculations would be the same as above and an additional step would be added at the end. The 5.76 mg would now represent the weight of fluoride ion needed. This must be converted to weight of NaF. The molecular weight of NaF is 42 and the atomic weight of fluorine is 19. The following proportion can be set up:

$$5.76\ mg : 19 : : Z\ mg : 42$$

$$Z = 5.76\ mg \times 42/19 = 12.7\ mg$$

Problems

1. How many mg of NaF are needed in the following prescription?

R̸
  Sodium Fluoride
  Purified water, qs to 90 mL
  M ft solution such that when 1 ℥ is dild to 1 glassful of water a 3 ppm NaF soln results.

Dilution and Concentration

Stock solutions can be diluted to make a product that has a lower concentration; also, mixtures of powders or semisolids (eg, ointments) can be diluted to give a product of lower concentration of the drug(s). The diluent is an inert solid or semisolid or base which does not contain any active ingredients. For example, how much of a diluent must be added to 50 g of a 10% ointment to make it a 5% ointment?
1. How many g of active ingredient is in 50 g of 10% ointment?

$$10\ g : 100\ g : : V\ g : 50\ g$$

$$V = 10\ g \times 50\ g/100\ g = 5\ g$$

2. How many g of a 5% ointment can be made from 5 g of active ingredient?

$$5\ g : 100\ g : : 5\ g : W\ g$$

$$W = 100\ g \times 5\ g/5\ g = 100\ g$$

3. How many g of base must be added to the 50 g of the original 10% ointment?

$$\begin{array}{ll} 100\ g & 5\%\ ointment \\ -\ \underline{50\ g} & 10\%\ ointment \\ 50\ g & base \end{array}$$

The term trituration was used previously to mean a dilute powder mixture of a drug. It is often necessary to further dilute this mixture in order to obtain the required amount of drug. For example, how much of a 1 in 10 trituration of a potent drug contains 200 mg of the drug?
1. A 1 in 10 trituration means 1 g of drug in 10 g of mixture or 1 g of drug plus 9 g diluent. *Remember:* mixtures of solids are percent *w/w*. The following proportion can be made:

$$1\ g : 10\ g : : 0.2\ g : T\ g$$

$$T = 10\ g \times 0.2\ g/1\ g = 2\ g$$

2. How much diluent must be added to 10 g of a 1:100 trituration to make a mixture that contains 1 mg of drug in each 10 g of the final mixture?

a. Determine the amount of drug in 10 g of trituration.

$$1\ g : 100\ g : : M\ g : 10\ g$$

$$M = 1\ g \times 10\ g/100\ g = 0.1\ g$$

b. Determine the amount of mixture that can be made from 0.1 g (100 mg) of drug.

$$1\ mg : 10\ g : : 100\ mg : N\ g$$

$$N = 10\ g \times 100\ mg/1\ mg = 1000\ g$$

c. Determine the amount of diluent needed.

$$\begin{array}{l} 1000\ g\ total\ mixture \\ -\ \underline{\ \ 10\ g\ trituration} \\ 990\ g\ diluent \end{array}$$

Occasionally it is necessary for a pharmacist to increase the strength of a product. For example, a prescription calls for 50 g of a 10% ointment. The pharmacist only has a 5% ointment and the pure ingredient available. How much of the 5% ointment and the pure ingredient are needed to compound the prescription?
1. Determine the amount of ingredient needed to compound the prescription by setting up the following proportion:

$$10\ g : 100\ g : : Q\ g : 50\ g$$

$$Q = 10\ g \times 50\ g/100\ g = 5\ g$$

This means that there are 45 g (50 g − 5 g = 45 g) of the base (90% of the total).

2. Determine the amount of ingredient in 50 g of a 5% ointment by forming the following proportion:

$$5\ g : 100\ g : : R\ g : 50\ g$$

$$R = 5\ g \times 50\ g/100\ g = 2.5\ g$$

This means that there are 47.5 g of the base.

3. Determine the amount of 5% ointment needed.

47.5 g base : 50 g total 5% ointment : :
  45 g base needed : S g of 5% ointment

$$S = 50\ g \times 45\ g/47.5\ g = 47.4\ g$$

4. Determine the amount of active ingredient.

$$\begin{array}{l} 50.0\ g\ total\ ointment\ required \\ -\ \underline{47.4\ g\ 5\%\ ointment\ required} \\ 2.6\ g\ active\ ingredient\ required \end{array}$$

Mix 2.6 g active ingredient with 47.4 g of 5% ointment to give 50 g of 10% ointment.

Normality

Occasionally solutions of a required normality are requested by prescribers. The pharmacist then must apply his knowledge gained in quantitative chemistry.

1. How much sodium bicarbonate powder is needed to prepare 60 mL of a 0.07 N solution of $NaHCO_3$?

   a. A 1N solution of $NaHCO_3$ contains 84 g/L
   $$84 \text{ g.}:1N::Wg:0.07N$$
   $$W = 5.88 \text{ g/L}$$

   b. $5.88 \text{ g} \times \dfrac{60 \text{ mL}}{1000 \text{ mL}} = 0.353 \text{ g } NaHCO_3 \text{ needed.}$

Problems

1. The following prescription order was received in a pharmacy. If the only R cream available is a 10% concentration, how much of the 10% cream and how much diluent are required to compound the prescription?

   R

   R Cream 3% .... 30 g

2. How many grams of a 1:100 trituration contains 100 μg of the active ingredient?
3. How many grams of a 1:1000 dilution can be made from 1 g of a 1:25 trituration?
4. How many grams of a 5% sulfur ointment and pure sulfur are needed to prepare 60 g of a 7.5% sulfur ointment?
5. A prescription calls for 240 mL of a 0.1N HCl solution. How many mL of concentrated HCl are needed to make this solution?
Note: Concentrated HCl is 37%, has a density of 1.2 g/mL and a mole wt of 36.5.

Mixing Different Strengths

Rules

1. The sum of the products obtained by multiplying a series of quantities by their respective concentrations equals the product obtained by multiplying a concentration by the sum of the quantities. For example, the sum of the products, obtained by multiplying the individual weights or volumes of a series of preparations by the concentration of a given ingredient contained in each preparation, is equal to the product obtained by multiplying the total weight of the series of preparations by the percentage of the given ingredient resulting from a homogeneous mixture of the same series of preparations.
2. When mixing products of varying strengths, the units and type of percent (w/w, w/v, v/v) must be kept constant.

Examples

1. What is the percent of alcohol in a mixture made by mixing 5 L of 25%, 1 L of 50%, and 1 L of 95% alcohol?

   a. Determine the total amount of alcohol in the 3 solutions and the total amount of solution (1 L = 1000 mL). Assume additivity of volumes on mixing.

$$
\begin{aligned}
25\% \times 5000 \text{ mL} &= 1250 \text{ mL}\\
50\% \times 1000 \text{ mL} &= \ \ 500 \text{ mL}\\
95\% \times \underline{1000 \text{ mL}} &= \underline{\ \ 950 \text{ mL}}\\
7000 \text{ mL} \quad & \ \ 2700 \text{ mL}
\end{aligned}
$$

   b. Determine the percent of alcohol in the mixture. There is a total of 2700 mL of alcohol in 7000 mL of total solution.

$$2700 \text{ mL}:7000 \text{ mL}::X \text{ mL}:100 \text{ mL}$$

$$X = 2700 \text{ mL} \times 100 \text{ mL}/7000 \text{ mL} = 38.6 \text{ mL}$$

Because 38.6 mL of alcohol are in 100 mL, a 38.6% solution is formed

2. What is the strength of a mixture obtained by mixing 50 g of a 5%, 100 g of a 7.5%, and 40 g of a 10% ointment?

   a.

$$
\begin{aligned}
5\ \ \% \times \ \ 50 \text{ g} &= \ \ 2.5 \text{ g}\\
7.5\% \times 100 \text{ g} &= \ \ 7.5 \text{ g}\\
10\ \ \% \times \underline{\ \ 40 \text{ g}} &= \underline{\ \ 4.0 \text{ g}}\\
190 \text{ g} \quad & \ \ 14.0 \text{ g}
\end{aligned}
$$

   b. There is a total of 14.0 g of active ingredient in 190 g of total mixture.

$$14 \text{ g}:190 \text{ g}::W \text{ g}:100 \text{ g}$$

$$W = 14 \text{ g} \times 100 \text{ g}/190 \text{ g} = 7.37 \text{ g}$$

Since there are 7.37 g of active ingredient in 100 g of the mixture, a 7.37% preparation results.

Problems

1. What percent of a drug is contained in a mixture of powder consisting of 0.5 kg, containing 0.038% of a drug, and 10 kg, containing 0.043% of a drug?
2. What is the strength of a mixture produced by combining the following lots of alcohol: 2 L of 95%, 2 L of 50%, and 7 L of 60% alcohol?
3. What is the percent of drug content in the following mixture: 2 kg of 3%, 300 g of 2.5%, and 500 g of 4.2% resin?

Alligation Alternate

Alligation is a rapid method of calculation which is useful to the pharmacist. The name is derived from the Latin *alligatio*, meaning the act of attaching and hence refers to lines drawn during calculation to bind quantities together. This method is used to find the proportions in which substances of different strengths or concentrations must be mixed in order to yield a mixture of desired strength or concentration. When the proportion is found, a calculation may be performed to find the exact amounts of the substances required.

Rules

1. The substance with a higher value than that required is the one with the lower amount.
2. The gain in value or amount of one substance balances the loss in value or amount of another substance.

Examples

1. In what proportion must a preparation containing 10% of drug be mixed with one containing 15% of drug, to produce a mixture of 12% drug strength?

The 10% drug is 2% too weak and the 15% drug is 3% too strong. Therefore, the excess in strength of 3 parts of the stronger can be calculated to just balance the deficiency of 2 parts of the weaker drug. Set up the problem in this manner:

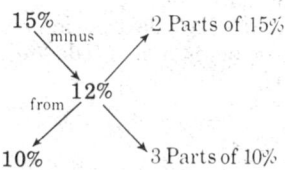

The desired percent or concentration is placed in the center, the lower percentage is placed on the left side below the center, and the higher percentage is placed on the left side above the center. The figure obtained by subtracting 10% from 12% is placed opposite the 15% on the right side and that obtained by subtracting the 12% from 15% is placed opposite the 10% figure on the right side.

Then, mixing 2 parts of 15% drug preparation with 3 parts of 10% drug preparation will produce a drug mixture of the desired 12% strength.

2. In what proportion must 30% alcohol and 95% alcohol be mixed to make 500 mL of 50% alcohol. Set up the problem in the following manner:

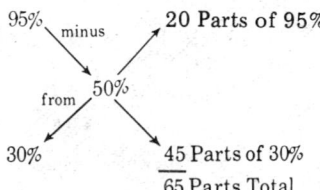

In a total of 65 parts, 20 parts of 95% alcohol + 45 parts of 30% alcohol are needed. Since the total parts is proportional to 500 mL, the following proportion can be made:

$$65 \text{ parts} : 500 \text{ mL} :: 20 \text{ parts} : V \text{ mL}$$

$$V = 500 \text{ mL} \times 20 \text{ parts}/65 \text{ parts} = 154 \text{ mL}$$

The amount of 30% alcohol can be found by a similar proportion, or by subtracting 154 mL from 500 mL:

```
  500 mL    total
- 154 mL    95% alcohol
  346 mL    30% alcohol
```

Thus, when 154 mL of 95% alcohol and 346 mL of 30% alcohol are mixed, 500 mL of 50% alcohol results (assuming there is no contraction in volume on mixing).

3.   How many grams of an ointment containing 0.18% of active ingredient must be mixed with 50 grams of an ointment containing 0.14% of active ingredient to make a product containing 0.15% of active ingredient?

a.

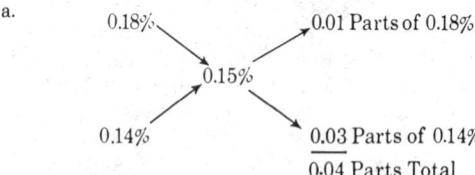

b.   0.03 parts is proportional to 50 g.

$$0.03 \text{ parts} : 50 \text{ g} :: 0.01 \text{ parts} : U \text{ g}$$

$$U = 50 \text{ g} \times 0.01 \text{ part}/0.03 \text{ part} = 16.7 \text{ g}$$

Problems

1.   How much of an ointment containing 12% drug, and how much ointment containing 16% drug must be used to make 1 kg of a product containing 12.5% drug?

2.   In what proportion should 50% alcohol and purified water be mixed to make a 35% alcohol solution? (The purified water is 0% alcohol.)

Note: This problem may be solved by a method other than alligation as was shown above.

3.   How many grams of 28% *w/w* ammonia water should be added to 500 g of 5% *w/w* ammonia water to produce a 10% *w/w* ammonia concentration?

4.   How many mL of 20% dextrose in water and how many mL of 50% dextrose in water are needed to make 1 L of 35% dextrose in water?

Proof Spirit

For tax purposes, the US government calculates the strength of pure or absolute alcohol (herein referred to as C_2H_5OH) by means of *proof degrees*. 100 proof spirit contains 50% (by volume) or 42.49% (by weight) of C_2H_5OH, and its specific gravity is 0.93426 at 60°F/60°F. Thus, 2 proof degrees equals 1% (by volume) of C_2H_5OH. One proof gallon is 1 gal of 50% (by volume) of C_2H_5OH at 15.56°C (60°F). In other words, a proof gallon is a gallon that contains ½ gal of C_2H_5OH. A proof gallon is 100 proof.

The term *10 degrees under proof* (10° up) signifies that 100 volumes of the spirit contains 90 volumes of proof spirit plus 10 volumes of water, and *30 degrees over proof* (30° op) in-

dicates that 100 volumes diluted with water yields 130 volumes of proof spirit. To prepare proof spirit, 50 volumes of C_2H_5OH are mixed with 53.71 volumes of water to allow for the contraction which occurs to yield 100 volumes of product.

The terms *proof strength*, *proof gallon*, *proof spirit*, etc. are used so that the tax is levied only on the actual quantity of C_2H_5OH contained in any mixture. It is therefore sometimes necessary for the pharmacist to convert alcohol purchased to proof strength to compute tax refunds or convert proof strengths to percent for compounding purposes.

A quantity of solution that contains ½ gal of C_2H_5OH is said to contain 1 proof gal. Proof gallons may be calculated by the following two equations:

$$\text{Proof gal} = \frac{\text{gal} \times \% \ v/v \text{ strength}}{50\% \ v/v}$$

$$\text{Proof gal} = \frac{\text{gal} \times \text{proof strength}}{100 \text{ proof}}$$

The second equation is the same as the first because proof strength is always twice the % *v/v* strength.

With these equations, given any two variables the third can be calculated.

Examples

1.   What is the taxable alcohol in 1 pt of Alcohol USP?

$$1 \text{ pt} = \tfrac{1}{8} \text{ gal (8 pt = 1 gal)}$$

Alcohol USP is 95% *v/v*; therefore,

$$\text{Proof gal} = \frac{\text{gal} \times \% \text{ strength}}{50\%} = \frac{\tfrac{1}{8} \text{ gal} \times 95\%}{50\%} = 0.2375 \text{ proof gal}$$

2.   How much Diluted Alcohol USP can be made from 1 qt of alcohol labeled ½ proof gallon?

Diluted Alcohol USP is 49% *v/v*; therefore,

$$\text{Proof gal} = \frac{\text{gal} \times \% \text{ strength}}{50\%}$$

$$\text{gal} = \frac{0.5 \text{ proof gal} \times 50\%}{49\%} = 0.510 \text{ gal}$$

Problems

1.   How many proof gallons are there in 1 qt of a preparation that is labeled 75% *v/v* alcohol?

2.   How many proof gallons are there in a pint of an elixir that contains 14% alcohol?

3.   How much Diluted Alcohol USP can be made from 1 gal of 190 proof alcohol?

Saturated Solutions

Occasionally it is necessary for a pharmacist to make saturated solutions. Solubility in the USP and NF is expressed as the number of milliliters of a solvent that will dissolve 1 g of a solid; eg, 1 g dissolves in 0.5 mL of water. In other words, if 1 g of a solid is dissolved in 0.5 mL of water, a saturated solution results. An example will illustrate this.

How much of a drug is needed to make 120 mL of a saturated solution if 1 g of the drug dissolves in 7.5 mL?

The following proportion may be made:

$$1 \text{ g} : 7.5 \text{ mL} :: X \text{ g} : 120 \text{ mL}$$

$$X = 1 \text{ g} \times 120 \text{ mL}/7.5 \text{ mL} = 16 \text{ g}$$

When 16 g of the drug are dissolved in 120 mL of water, a saturated solution results which has a volume greater than 120 mL because the solid will take up a certain volume. Only 120 mL would be dispensed.

What is the % w/w of the above solution?

$$120 \text{ g (mL) solvent} + 16 \text{ g solute} = 136 \text{ g}$$

of total solution weight. There is 16 g of solute in 136 g of solution; therefore,

$$16 \text{ g}:136 \text{ g}::P \text{ g}:100 \text{ g}$$

$$P = 16 \text{ g} \times 100 \text{ g}/136 \text{ g} = 11.8 \text{ g}$$

in 100 g of solution; therefore, this is a 11.8% w/w solution.

Problems

1. What is the solubility of a chemical if a saturated solution is 0.5% w/w?
2. How many grams are needed to make 500 mL of a saturated solution if 1 g of the solute is soluble in 14 mL of solvent?

Milliequivalents

See Chapter 17 for additional discussion on electrolytic equilibria.

The quantities of electrolytes administered to patients are usually expressed by the term *milliequivalents* (mEq). The reason that weight units (mg, g) are not used is that the electrical activity of the ions, which in this instance is important, may be best expressed as mEq.

A mEq is $\frac{1}{1000}$ of an *equivalent* (Eq). An Eq is the weight of a substance which combines with or replaces one gram-atomic weight (g-at wt) of hydrogen. In pharmacy the terms equivalent and equivalent weight (Eq wt) have been used interchangeably. For practical purposes an Eq wt is the weight in grams of an atom or radical divided by the valence of the atom or radical. For example, the g at wt of potassium (K) is 39.102 (approx. 39). The Eq wt is calculated by dividing 39 g by the valence of K (which is 1), giving 39 g/1 = 39 g-Eq wt. The mEq of K is the Eq wt divided by 1000. Thus, 39 g/1000 = 0.039 g = 39 mg. One mEq of K^+ (ion) combines with 1 mEq of Cl^- to give 1 mEq of KCl. The mEq of KCl is 74.5 mg (1 mEq K^+ is 39 mg + mEq Cl^- is 35.5 mg).

Water of hydration contributes to the molecular weight (mol wt) of a compound but *not* to the valence, and the total mol wt is used to calculate mEq.

Examples

1. Calcium (Ca^{2+}) has a gram-atomic wt of 40.08. What is the mEq wt?

Determine the Eq wt:

$$\text{gram-atomic wt/valence} = \text{Eq wt}$$

$$40.08 \text{ g}/2 = 20.04 \text{ g}$$

Determine the mEq wt:

$$\text{Eq wt}/1000 = \text{mEq wt}$$

$$20.04 \text{ g}/1000 = 0.02004 \text{ g} = 20.04 \text{ mg}$$

2. A solution that contains 409.5 mg of NaCl/100 mL has how many mEq of Na^+ and Cl^-?

$$\text{mEq wt of NaCl} = 58.5 \text{ mg}$$

$$\text{mEq} = \frac{409.5 \text{ mg}}{58.5 \text{ mg/mEq}} = 7 \text{ mEq}$$

of NaCl which dissociates to 7 mEq of Na^+ and 7 mEq of Cl^-.

3. A prescription order calls for a 500 mL solution of potassium chloride to be made so that it will contain 400 mEq of K^+. How many grams of KCl (mol wt: 74.5) are needed?

$$\text{Eq wt} = \text{g mol wt/valence}$$

$$\text{Eq wt} = 74.5 \text{ g/L} = 74.5 \text{ g}$$

$$\text{mEq of KCl} = \text{Eq wt}/1000$$

$$\text{mEq of KCl} = 74.5 \text{ g}/1000 = 0.0745 \text{ g} = 74.5 \text{ mg}$$

1 mEq of KCl yields 1 mEq of K^+; 400 mEq of KCl yields 400 mEq of K^+:

$$\begin{array}{r} 74.5 \text{ mg KCl/mEq} \\ \times\, 400 \text{ mEq} \\ \hline 29800 \text{ mg KCl} \end{array}$$

Dissolve 29.8 g of KCl in sufficient purified water to make 500 mL. This solution will yield 400 mEq of K^+.

4. How many mEq of K^+ are in a 250-mg tablet of potassium phenoxymethyl penicillin (mol wt: 388.5; valence: 1)?

$$\text{Eq wt} = \text{g-mol wt/valence}$$

$$\text{Eq wt} = 388.5 \text{ g/L} = 388.5 \text{ g}$$

$$\text{mEq wt} = \text{Eq wt}/1000$$

$$\text{mEq wt} = 388.5 \text{ g}/1000 = 0.3885 \text{ g} = 388.5 \text{ mg}$$

$$\frac{250 \text{ mg/tablet}}{388.5 \text{ mg/mEq}} = 0.644 \text{ mEq } K^+/\text{tablet}$$

5. How many mEq of Mg are there in 10 mL of a 50% Magnesium Sulfate Injection? The mol wt of $MgSO_4 \cdot 7H_2O$ is 246.

a. 50% solution means 5 g $MgSO_4 \cdot 7H_2O$ in 10 mL.

b. $\text{Eq wt} = \dfrac{\text{g-mol wt}}{\text{Valence}} = \dfrac{246 \text{ g}}{2} = 123 \text{ g}$

$$\text{mEq wt} = \frac{\text{Eq wt}}{1000} = 0.123$$

c. $\text{Total mEq} = \dfrac{5 \text{ g}}{0.123 \text{ g/mEq}} = 40.7 \text{ mEq in the 10 mL.}$

6. A vial of Sodium Chloride Injection contains 3 mEq/mL. What is the percentage strength of this solution? Mol wt of NaCl is 58.5.

a. 3 mEq/mL = 300 mEq/100 mL
b. mEq wt of NaCl is 58.5 mg
    58.5 mg/mEq × 300 mEq/100 mL = 17550 mg/100 mL or 17.6% solution.

Problems

1. What is the mEq wt of ferrous ion (Fe^{2+}) which has a g atomic wt of 55.85 g?
2. What is the mEq wt of sodium phosphate ($Na_2HPO_4 \cdot 7H_2O$)?
3. How many mEq of Na are in 60 mL of an 5% solution of sodium saccharin (g mol wt: 241 g; valence: 1)?
4. How many mEq of Ca^{2+} are there in a 600-mg calcium lactate pentahydrate (g mol wt: 308.30 g) tablet?
5. How many mEq of sodium are there in a 5 gr sodium bicarbonate tablet? Mol wt of $NaHCO_3$ is 84 and the valence is 1.
6. How many mEq of Na are there in 500 mL of $\frac{1}{3}$ normal saline solution? Normal saline solution contains 9 g NaCl/l; mol wt NaCl is 58.5.
7. How much KCl is needed to make a pt of syrup that contains 10 mEq of K^+ in each tablespoonful? Mol wt of KCl is 74.5.

Temperature

Rules

The relationship of Centigrade (C) and Fahrenheit (F) degrees is

$$9(°C) = 5(°F) - 160$$

where °C is the number of degrees Centigrade and °F is the number of degrees Fahrenheit.

Examples

1. Convert 77°F into °C.

$$9(°C) = 5(°F) - 160$$

$$9(°C) = 5(77) - 160$$

$$°C = \frac{385 - 160}{9} = 25°C$$

2. Convert 10°C into °F.

$$9(°C) = 5(°F) - 160$$

$$9(10) = 5(°F) - 160$$

$$\frac{90 + 160}{5} = °F = 50°F$$

Problems

1. Convert
   a. 30°C into °F
   b. 100°C into °F
   c. 37°C into °F
   d. 120°F into °C

References

1. *NBS Handbook 44*, 1980, *Specifications, Tolerances, and Other Technical Requirements for Weighing and Measuring Devices;* US Dept. of Commerce, Natl. Bur. Standards, Government Printing Office, Washington, DC.
2. *Ibid:* 4-270.
3. Goldstein SW, Mattocks AM: *Professional Equilibrium and Compounding Accuracy (pamphlet)*, APhA, Washington, DC, 1967.
4. Morrell CA, Ordway EM: *Drug Std 22:* 216, 1954.
5. Shirkey HC, Dosage (posology) in Shirkey HC, ed: *Pediatric Therapy*, 5th ed, Mosby, St. Louis, 19–33, 1975.
6. Benitz WE and Tatro DS: *The Pediatric Drug Handbook*, Yearbook Medical Publishers, 1981.
7. Nelson JD: *Pocketbook of Pediatric Antimicrobial Therapy*, 4th ed, Jodane Publishing Co., Dallas, 1981.
8. Ritschel WA: *Handbook of Basic Pharmacokinetics*, 2nd ed, Drug Intelligence Publications, Hamilton, Chap 23 Dosage in Children, pp 296–310, 1980.
9. Crawford JD, *et al: Pediatrics 5:* 783, 1950.
10. Talbot NB, *et al:* Metabolic Homeostasis. A Syllabus for Those Concerned with the Care of Patients, Harvard Univ Press, Cambridge 1959.
11. Butler AM, Richie RH: *New Engl J Med 262:* 903, 1960.
12. Shirkey HC, in Nelson WE, ed: *Textbook of Pediatrics*, 10th ed, Saunders, Philadelphia, 287, 1713, 1975.
13. Wagner J: *Drug Intel 2:* 144, 1968.

Answers To Problems

Density

1. 816 g
2. 363 mL
3. 54.2 mL

Logarithms

1. $V = -0.000084$ cm/sec or -8.4×10^{-5} cm/sec
2. $S = 65.5$ dynes/cm
3. $\dfrac{[\text{Unionized}]}{[\text{Ionized}]} =$

7.94×10^{-7}

Addition

1. 2481.23 g or 2.48123 kg
2. 1157 g or 1.157 kg
3. 2 ʒ, 3 ʒ, 17½ gr
4. 1 ℔, 7 ʒ, 4 ʒ, 2 Ə, 4 gr
5. 27⁹/₉₀ gr
6. 4 gal, 2 qt, 11 fl oz

Subtraction

1. 4105 mL or 4.105 L
2. 143½ gr
3. 7 fl oz, 2 fl dr
4. 3.71 g

Multiplication

1. 157.14 mL
2. 162.5 g
3. 825 mL
4. 2 gal, 1 qt, 4 fl oz, 4 fl dr
5. 375,000 µg or 375 mg

Division

1. 769 capsules + 15 mg remainder
2. 160 capsules
3. 150 doses
4. 150 doses
5. 1396 capsules + 300 mg remainder

Conversions

1. a. 421 mg
   b. 19.4 mg
   c. 109 g
   d. 7776 mg
   e. 99.2 g
   f. 454 g
2. a. 1 lb, 3 oz, 173 gr

   b. 6.94 gr
   c. 1 ℔, 5 ʒ, 5 ʒ, 26 gr
   d. 0.00154 gr
   e. 2.2 lb
3. a. 0.648 mg
   b. 0.203 mg
   c. 10.8 mg
   d. 0.325 or 0.324 g
   e. 1.299 or 1.296 g
4. a. 12.3 mL
   b. 11.1 mL
   c. 237 mL
   d. 473 mL
   e. 0.309 mL
   f. 0.00154 gr
   g. 0.0772 gr
5. a. 480 gr
   b. 8 ʒ
   c. 437½ gr
   d. 2880 gr
   e. 4 ʒ, 10 gr

Dosage Calculation

1. D.T.D. No. 14 means, send 14 such doses. Assuming the doses have been checked, they are for chemicals, J, K, and L (10 mg, 50 mg, and 300 mg, respectively).
2. Drug Q: 0.5 g
   Drug R: 0.3 g
3. 7.5 ♏/dose; 30 ♏/day
4. 50 doses
5. 0.0444 mg
6. 1.5 mg
7. ½ gr
8. 18.7 mg
9. 280,000 units
10. 75 mg
11. 77.9 mg
12. 0.75 mL contains 60 units;
13. 13⅓-day supply.
13. 6 mL
14. 3 mL
15. 0.386 gr

Reducing and Enlarging

1. Liquid C   875   mL
   Solid B   225   g
   Liquid R   62.5 mL
   Liquid P   500   mL
2. Solid G   24 ʒ or 3 ʒ
   Liquid D   720 ♏ or 1 fʒ, 4 fʒ
   Solid M   72 ʒ or 9 ʒ
3. Solid N   4.8 mg
   Solid Q   120   mg
   Solid R   7.2 g
   Add sufficient purified water to make 240 mL solution
4. Solid S   0.675 g
   Solid T   2.25   g
   Oil C   31.5   mL
   Alcohol   22.5   mL

Ratio and Proportion

1. 65 mg costs 19½¢ ($0.20);
5 gr costs 97.4¢ ($0.97)
2. $33.70

Percentage

w/v Solutions

1. Dissolve 171 gr (2 ʒ, 2 ᴲ, 11 gr) in sufficient solvent to make
    3 f ʒ
2. 2.84 L
3. 6.25 L
4. 8 g

w/w Products

1. Compound A   115 gr or 1 ʒ, 2 ᴲ, 15 gr
    Solvent   3 ʒ, 365 gr
2. 28.8 g
3. 5 kg
4. Dissolve 4.64 g of drug in 120 mL (150 g) of glycerin
5. Compound K   3.6 g
    Solid H   1.8 g
    Base   18.6 g
6. Dissolve 88.2 g of the solute in 500 mL of purified water
    Dispense 500 mL
7. Powder P   27.8 g
    Powder Q   222.2 g
    Powder R   333.3 g
    Powder S   416.7 g
8. 3 g or mL of coal tar solution; 27 g of hydrophilic ointment

Percent (*v/v*, *w/v*, and *w/w*)

1. 240 ᵐ
2. 900 mL
3. 34.8% *w/w*
4. 11.4 gr
5. 38.5% *w/w*
6. 15 g
7. 0.4 g
8. 32.4 mL of a 37% solution
9. 1.57 g

Stock Solutions

1. 30.2 g
2. 36.3 g
3. 0.5 mL

Parts per Million

1. 13 mg

Dilution and Concentration

1. 9 g of 10% cream and 21 g of diluent (base)
2. 0.01 g
3. 40 g
4. 58.42 g of 5% ointment + 1.58 g of sulfur
5. 1.98 mL

Mixing Products of Different Strengths

1. 0.0428%
2. 64.6%
3. 3.16%

Alligation Alternate

1. 875 g of 12% ointment and 125 g of 16% ointment
2. 35 parts of 50% alcohol and 15 parts of purified water
3. 139 g of 28% ammonia water
4. 500 mL each of the 20% and 50% solutions are needed

Proof Spirit

1. 0.375 proof gal
2. 0.035 proof gal
3. 1.94 gal

Saturated Solutions

1. 1 g in 199 mL
2. 35.7 g of solute

Milliequivalents

1. 27.925 mg/mEq
2. 89.3 mg/mEq
3. 12.5 mEq
4. 3.9 mEq
5. 3.86 mEq Na
6. 25.6 mEq Na
7. 23.8 g

Temperature

1. a. 86°F
    b. 212°F
    c. 98.6°F
    d. 48.9°C

CHAPTER 10

Statistics

Lila Knudsen Randolph, * BS

Mathematical Statistician
Office of the Assistant Commissioner for Planning
US Food and Drug Administration

Joseph L Ciminera, ScD

Director, Biometrics, Long Range Planning
Merck Sharp & Dohme Research Laboratories
West Point, PA 19486

In this chapter an attempt will be made to acquaint the student with the nature of the statistical approach as it applies to pharmacy and pharmacological problems, especially biological assay. However, within this division of statistics there are large gaps as yet unexplored and all that is attempted here is an aerial photograph with telescopic views of a few of the most important landmarks. A list of books and articles is given at the end of the chapter as recommended reading for the student who wishes to learn more about this field of statistics.

There are two parts to the definition of the word statistics.

1. Statistics are a collection of data or numbers, such as the number of cases of diabetes per state per year, or the number of capsules in a bottle.
2. Statistics is logic which makes use of mathematics in the science of collecting, analyzing and interpreting data for the purpose of making decisions.

In this chapter we shall deal with the second part of this definition.

Statistics is fundamentally logic and common sense. It is neither a collection of formulas that can be applied to patch up deficiencies in experiments nor a panacea for all the weaknesses of the data. The data cannot be improved simply by applying statistical analysis to them; the resulting analysis is no better than the data themselves. Definite, sweeping conclusions cannot be drawn from a small amount of poor data just because several weeks were spent in making an involved statistical analysis of them.

It is true that there are a great many mathematical formulas in statistics, but logic and reasoning are the true core of this subject. The underlying fundamental ideas in an experiment must be thoroughly investigated. There are different statistical formulas to be used depending on the assumptions made. Each situation must be approached individually, the assumptions set forth, the possible causes of variation enumerated and the problem at hand stated as clearly as possible. Dr RA Fisher, who was one of the most prominent statisticians in England, has said that a question clearly stated is a problem half solved.

It must be clearly realized at the outset that all nature is inherently variable. One often hears the comparison "as alike as two peas." Actually even peas vary and no two would be *exactly* alike in size, shape, color, maturity, blemishes, etc. If an experimenter makes several independent measurements on the length of a table, no matter how accurately the measurements are made, he will find that they are not all alike.

Statistics recognizes this variability in nature and takes it into account in planning how the data should be gathered. In the analysis of the data gathered, it utilizes this inherent

variation by making allowances for it in the interpretation of the results.

The practice of the statistical method may be divided into four parts: (1) design of the experiment, (2) collection of data, (3) analysis of data collected, and (4) interpretation of the analysis. The four parts are inextricably woven together. The plan or design used and the subsequent methods of gathering data under this design to answer the question posed should be considered carefully so as to avoid biases (unintentional or otherwise) that would erroneously influence results; the data then should be analyzed by the proper methods; and an interpretation of the analysis should be made to furnish a sound answer to the question stated. This is the ideal approach. Often, however, the materials already have been gathered before the problem is stated. Even in such cases the interpretation and analysis always should be made with full consideration of any biases that may have entered because of the manner of obtaining the data. In no instance should an interpretation be made without considering the manner of collection.

Design of the Experiment and Collection of Data

Collection of data always involves either the planning or *design of an experiment*, sampling, or complete census. In the collection of data a sample is generally taken except, of course, in such instances as a complete census of the population of the United States. Sometimes a sample is inadvertently taken when it is not the intention to take a sample, as when a questionnaire is sent out to every pharmacist in the state. There will always be some people who do not respond to a questionnaire and anything less than 100% response will constitute a sample.

In the following breakdown according to the type of data sampled, the sampling method is not limited to the field in which the illustration is given. An attempt has been made to give only the broadest type of illustrations in the brief chapter allotted to statistics and yet cover as many types of data as possible.

Questionnaire Type of Response—Suppose questionnaires on the sales of some drugs were sent to all the pharmacists in a state and only 50% of the questionnaires were returned; thus only a sample of the pharmacists would be taken, and any results tabulated from such a sample would be biased in that those who did not return the questionnaire would not be represented. It has been definitely shown that persons who respond to questionnaires have different characteristics, and possibly different environments, from those who do not respond. In the hypothetical case just mentioned, perhaps sales of the drug were so large that reporting an accurate figure was just too much work, so the questionnaire was left unanswered. Possibly in another community there were

---

* Deceased.

no sales of the drug, so the pharmacist did not bother to return the questionnaire. The statistician does not know which is the case. A bias thus enters into the results and the direction and amount of the bias are unknown.

However, there are questionnaire techniques worked out by mathematical statisticians that could have been employed to reduce and sometimes eliminate the bias in the sample of the pharmacists' responses. These same mathematical statisticians have also worked out methods of obtaining not only the average response to the question asked, but also the limits within which the average response might have occurred due to sampling of pharmacists. If only a certain amount of money is available for the survey or questioning there are techniques for obtaining the best design for the limited sampling program with a minimum of error. If, on the other hand, results within certain limits of error are desired regardless of cost, a sampling design can be used which will meet these specifications.

The public opinion polls use certain statistical sampling techniques continuously. These workers have obtained from the Census Bureau and other sources the percentages of men, women, and children in the United States, in various income groups, in certain nationality groups, and in many other types of population groups. Their samples are designed to contain the same proportions in these various groups as are in the population. However, instead of sending questionnaires by mail, interviewers are assigned certain quotas of definite types of people to interview and the interviewers fill out the questionnaire for each person while asking the questions.

It is impossible to elaborate fully here on the various methods of sampling such as area sampling, sampling with probability proportionate to size, etc. The purpose is rather to create an awareness to the problems of sampling, and, more important, to show that a design can be used that will give the limits of error of the result for any given expenditure of funds. A few references will be given at the end of this chapter for those interested in this type of sampling. There are other errors in the questionnaire type of response that may introduce bias, such as the way in which the question is stated, the order of the questions, and the actions of the interviewer.

Sampling in the Chemical Laboratory—Gathering data is accomplished in another manner in the laboratory even though it is still sampling. Sampling of the material to be chemically analyzed, sampling of reagents (if any) used, sampling of laboratory personnel used, sampling of conditions in general (such as, possibly, room temperature, room humidity, equipment, etc). Various such factors may contribute some variation to the final results, depending on which factors are important in the method of analysis involved. It has been shown that results differ even from laboratory to laboratory, though sometimes to a very minute extent. However, sampling of the material usually contributes the most variation and this factor usually can be controlled easily.

By way of illustration, several samples may be taken of a large lot of digitalis leaves for the chemical determination of acid-insoluble ash in the lot. In order to represent the lot truly, the samples must be taken from different parts of the lot to insure that every part of the lot is represented in some sample. Naturally, ash determinations from five samples taken from the same part of a lot will probably check each other more closely than if the five samples are taken from entirely different parts of the lot, but the former five samples will not give the best average ash value for the lot. The more heterogeneous the lot, the more effort should be expended in being sure that every part of the lot is represented by a sample. It might be that the leaves having the most ash are in the bottom of the lot; samples all taken from the top then would give too low an estimate of average ash content of the lot.

Another aspect of sampling in a chemical determination is the sampling of the chemist or chemists who perform the chemical analysis. If a single chemist makes several check determinations on portions taken from the same sample of thoroughly mixed substance, one expects the results to check more closely than if several chemists had made these check determinations. However, the true reproducibility of a method can be indicated only in terms of how closely an analyst at one laboratory can check an analyst at another laboratory on exactly the same material. Thus, due to slight differences in technique, one chemist might always obtain higher results than another chemist. The sampling of chemists might thus have some effect on the results and the method reproducibility.

Sampling in the Biological Laboratory—It should be realized that a biological experiment on, for example, the temperature response of rabbits to pyrogens constitutes a sample of the infinitely possible number of combinations of results that could be obtained from all possible rabbits, laboratories, and technicians. Different breeds of rabbits may give different results. Differences between results from two or more laboratories are usually greater than differences between results obtained by two or more technicians at the same laboratory. Season of the year, temperature, and humidity sometimes cause differences as well as other factors—possibly lack of clarity in the write-up of the method. In biological experimentation the differences between individual animals are likely to be large so that the results of an experiment repeated at the same laboratory may give results different from those obtained the first time. The use of statistical procedures will give an estimate of the amount of variation to be expected under identical conditions. As in the questionnaire problem already mentioned, it is important to know not only the average but also the standard error of that average. Then one can estimate how close is the agreement obtained between results of repetitions of the experiment and just how far off the results might be because of some inherent factor causing variation in the assay.

Frequently, methods are tested for their accuracy and precision by conducting collaborative studies of these methods in several laboratories. Collaborative studies are also made to evaluate a lot of a drug to be used as a reference standard, eg, USP Insulin Reference Standard, etc. From such a collaborative study it is necessary to determine what differences can be expected between laboratories. Fig 10-1 shows the results of a collaborative assay on a working standard of calcium penicillin[1] plotted according to the potencies obtained from several assays at different laboratories. The laboratories are lettered A through R. The average for all the laboratories combined is indicated by the long horizontal line in the center

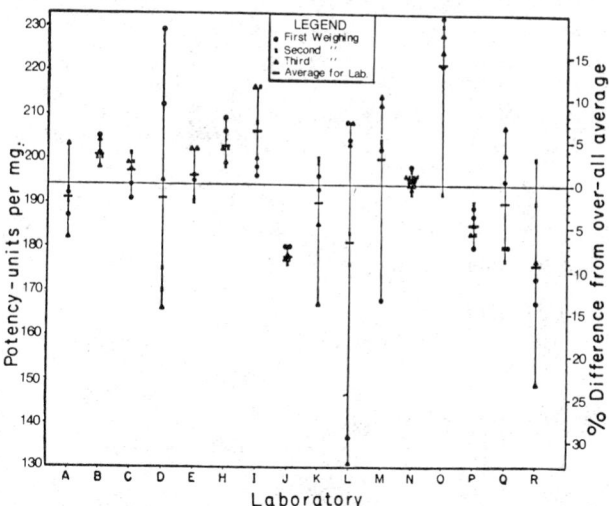

Fig 10-1. A chart illustrating the variation between laboratories of collaborative assays on working standard calcium penicillin.

of the chart. Short horizontal lines indicate the averages for each laboratory. Note that some laboratories show very little variation of their individual assay results about the average for that laboratory, eg, laboratory J has an overall variation of only about 2% as measured on the right-hand scale. However, the average result of that laboratory is almost 10% below the overall average of all the laboratories. Note also the results from laboratories B, H, I, and P. Compare the variation of the results from laboratory N with that of the results from laboratory L.

Statistics should be used in setting up the design for a single experiment so that biases will not influence the results. This point may be illustrated by an extreme example—something that no experimenter would do. A technician wishes to compare two drugs as to their effects on the growth of rats. He uses 30 rats from a single cage and puts the first 15 rats caught on drug No 1 and the last 15 caught on drug No 2. Naturally, the first 15 rats caught are less lively than the last 15 and because they are less lively they very likely differ in size and nervous temperament from the last 15 rats. Thus the results are biased from the very beginning and one drug is "favored" merely by the method of choosing the animals to be used on each drug. Obviously, some method entirely free from subjective influences (unconscious or conscious) should be used. A table of random numbers[2-4] could be used or a series of numbered metal-edged disks could be shaken and picked out of a hat in some objective manner.

Suppose, for example, one wishes to choose 16 rats, numbered in the order they are taken from the cage, from 1 to 16. Four doses are to be administered. Four consecutively numbered disks are shaken in a container and one selected without looking; then the disks are shaken again and another selected, etc. In this way the order of the doses is randomized. These are labeled a, b, c, and d. Then 16 disks numbered from 1 to 16 are shaken and disks are selected without looking and without replacement. Suppose the first four numbers selected are 12, 2, 15, and 10. Dose a will be given to the twelfth animal chosen from the cage, dose b to the second, dose c to the fifteenth, etc., until all 16 animals have been assigned doses.

Another aspect of sampling in a biological laboratory involves the choice of doses of a drug to be used in an experiment to determine the relationship between dose and response. In administering a single dosage of a drug to a group of animals an average response is noted (the type of response depends on the drug administered). However, there is variation between individual animals. If 10 or 12 different doses are administered to suitably chosen animals, one might obtain a relationship between dosage and response of individual ani-

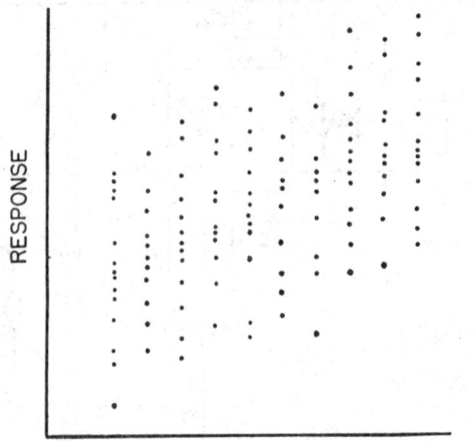

Fig 10-2. Typical relationship between dosage and response of individual animals.

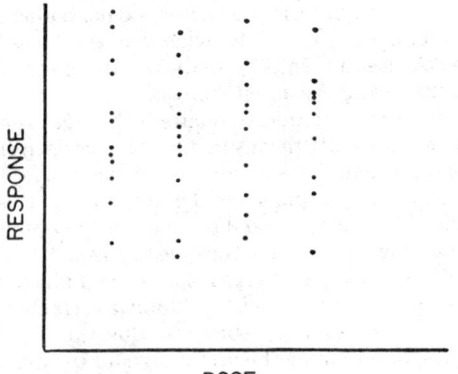

Fig 10-3. Partial relationship between dosage and response—a section of Fig 10-2 with the dosage scale enlarged.

mals as shown in Fig 10-2. The larger the dose, the higher the average response elicited. However, if the choosing (sampling) of doses had been such that only the four doses in the central portion of Fig 10-2 had been administered, the dosage response relationship would look entirely different as shown in Fig 10-3.

In Fig 10-2 a very definite relationship between dosage and response is shown, while in Fig 10-3, which is part of the same data, there appears to be no relationship merely because the dosages chosen were not far enough apart and did not cover the proper range in order to represent the true picture adequately.

In biological assay it is often advantageous to design the dosage schedule to take advantage of the fact that there is less variation within a litter than between litters, or that there is a trend in the response of a single animal to several consecutive doses of a drug. This can be illustrated by an epinephrine assay (see RPS-14, 1970, p 633) wherein a single dog is given 16 consecutive doses, the order of which is determined by a Latin square design, illustrated by the following pattern:

$$
\begin{array}{cccc}
A & D & B & C \\
D & C & A & B \\
B & A & C & D \\
C & B & D & A
\end{array}
$$

Note that each letter occurs only once in each row and each column of the square. A Latin square design was applied to an assay involving two levels of doses of the standard (high and low doses s_H and s_L, respectively), and two levels of doses of the unknown (u_H and u_L). The dosage schedule is given in Table I. In this type of design each dose occurs once in each order of administration (eg, u_H is given first of four doses but once, s_H is given first but once, etc). In such an assay equal doses of epinephrine given a dog elicit a smaller and smaller rise in blood pressure with each succeeding dose.

In all biological experimentation the design should be planned so that differences in treatment do not coincide with differences in weight, sex, litters, dates of administration, etc. Animals should be assigned to doses at random, and the availability of certain designs should be realized. Fisher[5] has written an excellent book on planning or designing of exper-

Table I—Typical Dosage Schedule for Epinephrine Assay
Using a Latin Square Design

	First dose	Second dose	Third dose	Fourth dose
First group	u_L	s_H	u_H	s_L
Second group	s_H	s_L	u_L	u_H
Third group	u_H	u_L	s_L	s_H
Fourth group	s_L	u_H	s_H	u_L

iments. He explains fully the various types of designs mentioned here. Another book on design of experiments is by Cochran and Cox.[6] It goes into great detail and gives at least 150 of the most useful experimental designs with complete directions for the analysis of data obtained using any of the designs described therein.

Clinical Type of Data—Certain designs are available for the planning of an experiment or, rather, the purposive sampling involved in setting up an experiment. In the early days of penicillin a clinical experiment on 300 patients was conducted to determine why injections of some penicillins caused pain while others of the same penicillin did not. Data had been gathered hit or miss as penicillin was administered in the hospital. Potency, site of injection, and amount of pain produced were recorded. However, no conclusions could be drawn from the data because the subjective responses of the patients were confounded with the site of injection and the potency. There was no pattern for comparison of responses of the same individual to the different penicillins. A design was set out using a "balanced incomplete block" type of experimental design involving 30 patients with 3 sites of injection for each patient, and the grouping of the commercial penicillin into 6 different concentration levels. The design of the experiment was taken from Table XVII, design No 1, in the tables by Fisher and Yates,[3] which is given there as:

abc	aef	bef
abd	bcf	cde
ace	bde	cdf
adf		

Since there are only ten groups of letters, this design could be used for ten patients only. However, to increase the precision of the results and also to investigate whether the order of injection affected the pain response, two more groups of ten patients were added making 30 patients in all with three repetitions of the design as given above. The first group of patients received the injection in one order of site of injection (B, T, D), the second group received them in another order (T, D, B), and the third group still another order (D, B, T). Patients were randomized in assigning the set of doses and locations of administration to be used. The manner in which the design was utilized in this experiment is given in Table II, together with the results from each injection on each patient.[7]

The results can be plotted as shown in Fig 10-4 and because of the efficient design little formal statistical analysis is necessary for the demonstration of the evident trend. A calculation of averages, as shown by the horizontal lines plotted on the chart, shows that as potency of the penicillin increased the pain produced decreased.

Design and Conduct of Clinical Trials—Proof of efficacy and safety of new drugs or treatments requires testing in human subjects. This is best achieved by carrying out controlled clinical trials. A clinical trial is said to be controlled when it is designed and carried out in such a manner that the results reflect the true action of the treatments.

The usual procedure is to compare the effects of the treatment with those of a concurrently tested control or placebo. When this is not feasible, drug efficacy may be assessed by testing graded doses of drug and establishing a dosage–response relation. Implicit also is the assurance that the trial includes sufficient and adequate sampling to allow projection of the trial's results to other future patients. The results cannot be projected beyond the types of severity of disease, and the ages and sex of the patients included in the trial.

The distribution among treatments of variables such as age, sex, differences in diagnosis, and initial severity of disease may be controlled by stratification. Where this is not feasible, patients should be assigned to treatments at random, and allowances made for the effects of the variables using suitable

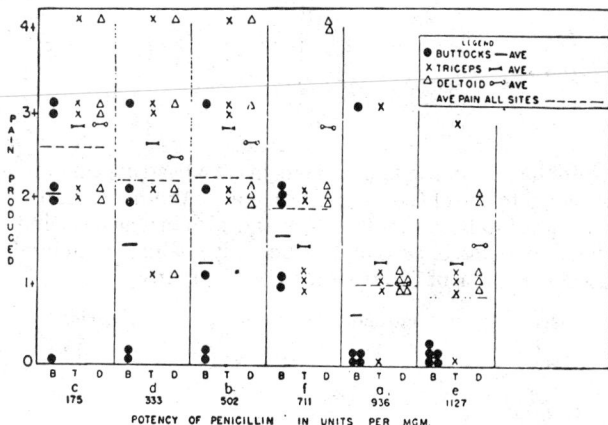

Fig 10-4. Clinical study of relationship of pain produced at site of injection and potency of penicillin sodium.

Table II—Balanced Incomplete Block Type of Experimental Design

Showing Site of Injection[a] and Degree of Pain[b]

Patient	Sample and potency					
	a 936 units per mg	b 502 units per mg	c 175 units per mg	d 333 units per mg	e 1127 units per mg	f 711 units per mg
Order No. 1						
1	B-0	T-3+	D-2+	...	...	...
2	B-3+	T-4+	...	D-3+	...	...
3	B-0	...	T-4+	...	D-2+	...
4	B-0	...	...	T-1+	...	D-2+
5	B-0	...	...	...	T-3+	D-4+
6	...	B-1+	T-2+	...	...	D-2+
7	...	B-0	...	T-2+	D-1+	...
8	...	B-3+	...	...	T-1+	D-2+
9	...	...	B-3+	T-3+	D-2+	...
10	...	...	B-3+	T-4+	...	D-4+
Order No. 2						
11	T-0	D-2+	B-0	...	...	...
12	T-1+	D-4+	...	B-0	...	...
13	T-1+	...	D-3+	...	B-0	...
14	T-3+	...	...	D-4+	...	B-2+
15	T-1+	...	...	...	D-1+	B-2+
16	...	T-3+	D-3+	...	...	B-2+
17	...	T-2+	...	D-3+	B-0	...
18	...	T-2+	...	...	D-1+	B-1+
19	...	...	T-3+	D-1+	B-0	...
20	...	...	T-3+	D-2+	...	B-1+
Order No. 3						
21	D-1+	B-0	T-2+	...	...	...
22	D-1+	B-2+	...	T-3+	...	...
23	D-1+	...	B-2+	...	T-1+	...
24	D-1+	...	...	B-3+	...	T-2+
25	D-1+	...	...	...	B-0	T-1+
26	...	D-2+	B-2+	...	...	T-1+
27	...	D-3+	...	B-2+	T-1+	...
28	...	D-2+	...	...	B-0	T-1+
29	...	...	D-2+	B-0	T-0	...
30	...	...	D-4+	B-2+	...	T-2+

[a] B: buttocks; T: triceps; D: deltoid.
[b] 0: no pain; 1+: very slight pain; 2+: slight pain; 3+: moderate pain; 4+: severe pain.

statistical methods. A restricted randomization procedure is useful if it is desired to assure about an equal number of patients on all treatment groups as patients enter the trial. This is illustrated below for a completely randomized design in which 15 patients are allocated at random, 5 to each of 3 treatments:

A	B	C
3	1	2
6	5	4
8	9	7
12	10	11
14	13	15

Note that the individual patients in each triad are randomly assigned to one of the three treatments. Another example is shown below for a simple crossover design in which the individual patients in each of five successive pairs are randomly assigned to one of two treatment order groups:

Group	Patient	Period 1	Period 2
	1		
	4		
I	5	A	B
	7		
	10		
	2		
	3		
II	6	B	A
	8		
	9		

The latter design may be more efficient than a completely randomized design since each patient acts as his own control, thus eliminating patient-to-patient variability. However, this advantage may be offset if drug carry-over effects are present, or if the severity of the disease wanes in the second period to the point where treatment differences no longer can be demonstrated.

In order to be certain that the random allocation is strictly followed, and to remove subjective bias on the part of both the patient and the clinical investigator in assessing the effects of the treatments, the clinical trial should be carried out blind. A double-blind trial is one in which neither the patient nor the physician is made aware of the nature of treatment administered.

In order to keep the study blind, all treatments must be put up in identical-appearing dosage forms. This may require a great deal of ingenuity on the part of the pharmacist called upon to prepare such dosage forms, especially with respect to the taste of liquid preparations to be administered orally. In some instances characteristic side effects of the drugs make it impossible to keep a study blind. In these situations we must rely more heavily on objective measures of response, and less on subjective measures.

Federal regulations require that drugs shipped to clinical investigators must be properly labeled with the name of the drug. In order to keep the study blind, a suggested procedure is to use a two-part tear-off label.

One part is glued to the container and reveals only the patient's study number, the period number, and directions for taking the drug; the tear-off part shows the identity of the drug. The name of the drug is overlaid with a water-washable or erasable ink so as not to reveal the identity of the drug to the physician. This portion of the label is torn off and stapled to the back of the clinical form. The physician is instructed to break the code for an individual patient, if necessary, by washing off or erasing the overlaid ink. However, when this is done, the patient must be considered as a treatment failure.

A less satisfactory procedure, which however does not require an ink overlay, is to have a disinterested individual tear off the identifying portion of the labels before the clinical material is turned over to the clinical investigator. The identifying labels are placed in individual opaque sealed envelopes that are identified only with the patient's study number and the period number.

These then would be handled in the same fashion as the labels with the ink overlay. The unopened envelopes serve as evidence that the study was carried out blind. The phy-sician is instructed to number the patients serially as they enter the trial, and assign them to treatment with the container having the same number, starting with the container for period 1. The drug allocation code is not revealed to the clinician until the study is completed.

To facilitate computerization and statistical evaluation, the results of clinical trials should be recorded on precoded clinical forms. Data pertinent to clinical trials include subjective and objective measures of the course of the disease, laboratory determinations, and adverse reactions.

Subjective measures are exemplified by such determinations as severity of pain, degree of hyperemia, and the patient's or the physician's overall assessment of the effectiveness of treatment. Body weight and body temperature are examples of objective measures.

Laboratory determinations usually include such measures as complete blood count, liver function tests, and analyses on urine and stool specimens. The occurrence of adverse effects may be recorded as ascertained by inquiry or as volunteered by the patient. It is informative also to determine the severity as well as the frequency of occurrence of adverse effects, and whether or not the physician feels they were drug related.

Generally, it is more difficult to evaluate clinical data than laboratory animal data. Some of the contributing factors are (1) failure of patients to take the medication as directed, and to report for examination at stated intervals; (2) the use of ancillary or concomitant medications by the patients; and (3) incomplete data caused by patients dropping out of the study for various reasons. These factors are more prevalent among outpatients than among hospitalized patients. A trial secretary can be of great help in assuring the completeness and accuracy of clinical forms.

Analysis of Data Collected

Analysis usually consists of graphing the data, applying some statistical formula or formulas to the data, and drawing inferences from the results. Terminology plays a very important part in the statistical method, but unfortunately there is a lack of standardization among various statistical texts. In this text the terminology used will be similar to that given by Youden.[8]

Graphs—There are various types of graphs including:

1. The bar graph or histogram, such as Fig 10-8.
2. The "pie chart" in which various sized pieces of pie represent percentages to be compared as part of a whole, sometimes called polar coordinates.
3. A graph in which one variable Y is plotted against another variable X, sometimes called rectangular coordinates. Since graphing and graphs are well known, the subject need not be elaborated on here. Suffice it to say that it is usually necessary to plot the data, sometimes in several ways before beginning the statistical analysis. The graphic plot can sometimes show the types of analysis to be applied and relationships between various parts of the data.

The Average or Mean—Suppose from a population or universe a sample of n observations is taken as usual in order to determine some of the characteristics of the population. A chemist, for example, may make n determinations on a lot of digitalis leaves in order to be able to estimate the ash content of that lot. The sample of n determinations can be designated by:

$$x_1, x_2, x_3, \ldots, x_n$$

The sample mean, $\bar{x}$, can be calculated by:

$$\bar{x} = \frac{x_1 + x_2 + x_3 + \ldots + x_n}{n} = \frac{\Sigma x_i}{n}$$

where i goes from 1 to n.

This sample mean is an estimate of μ, the actual mean of the population or, in this case, the lot of digitalis leaves.

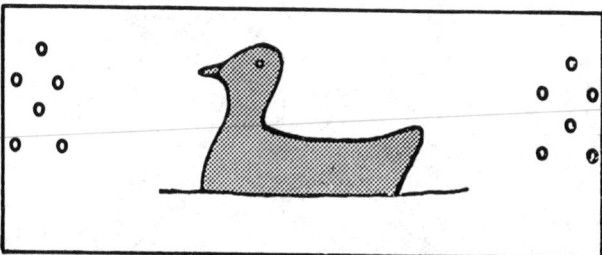

Fig 10-5. *On an average the duck was dead.* A hunter fired both barrels of a shotgun at a duck. The first hit 2 ft in front, the second hit 2 ft behind. On an average the duck was dead. What the hunter really wanted was meat on the table. In duck hunting one wants to keep trying until a single shot hits the mark. But in estimating purity by a chemical test the best estimate is usually the average.

Example I—A series of data on the acid-insoluble ash content of digitalis leaves is given as follows:

4.1	4.4	4.0
4.3	4.2	4.7
4.9	4.6	4.4

$n = 9$. The sum of these 9 values is 39.6.

$$\text{The average} = \bar{x} = \frac{\Sigma x_i}{n} = \frac{39.6}{9} = 4.4$$

This example is given mainly to illustrate the symbols employed.

Fig 10-5 is taken from an article by Stearns[9] and illustrates one instance where an average has no meaning.

Frequency Distributions—There are many types of variation patterns in nature. These patterns are called frequency distributions of data. The most common of these is the normal (or bell-shaped) curve in which most of the observations fall near the average and the greater the distance from the average in either direction the fewer the observations. This is illustrated by the frequency curve shown in Fig 10-6. This type of curve is sometimes called the normal curve of error, or *normal probability curve*. Many statistical formulas and interpretations are based on the assumption of a normal frequency curve distribution of data.

Although the normal distribution is the most common, there are many other types of frequency curves such as the *U-shaped curve* for which there is a classic illustration. In getting a distribution of the amount of sunlight for each day over a period of time it was found that many days were entirely sunny and many days were entirely cloudy but that fewer days fell in between these two extremes so that the distribution of amount of sunlight was shaped like a U as shown in Fig 10-7. There are also other types of distribution curves such as the *Poisson, binomial, t, chi-square* distribution, etc.

It is possible to ascertain the distribution of data from a given experiment. It can be approximated roughly by means of a bar chart as shown in the following problem:

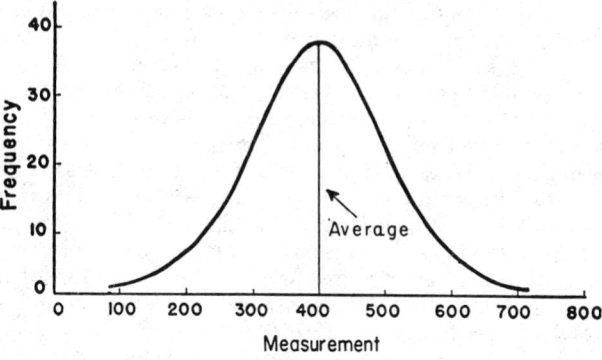

Fig 10-6.   The normal probability curve.

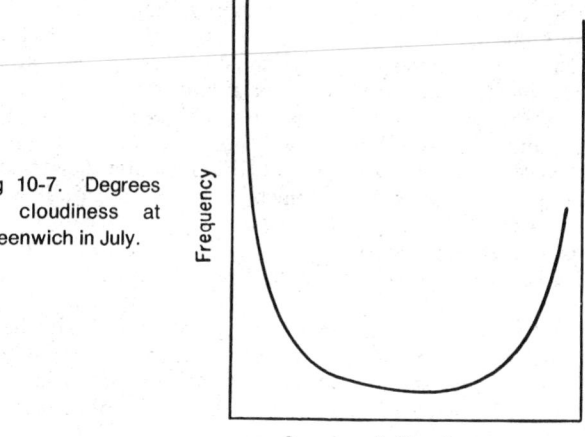

Fig 10-7. Degrees of cloudiness at Greenwich in July.

Example II—The weights of 50 rats at weaning were as follows:

30 g	47 g	37 g	29 g	38 g
32	42	32	30	34
34	32	33	37	36
39	33	45	40	35
43	41	35	32	41
36	27	28	35	30
38	28	41	37	34
41	36	32	30	37
31	31	35	28	25
26	49	34	34	33

These weights can be assembled in the following groups with the frequency of occurrence in each group tabulated.

Weight group	Frequency
24–25 g	1
26–27	2
28–29	4
30–31	6
32–33	8
34–35	9
36–37	7
38–39	3
40–41	5
42–43	2
44–45	1
46–47	1
48–49	1

This can be plotted in the form of a bar chart as shown in Fig. 10-8.

Measures of Variation—There are statistical formulas for measuring the variation that exists in nature as well as the man-made variation. The simplest measure of variation is the *range*. It is the difference between the highest value and

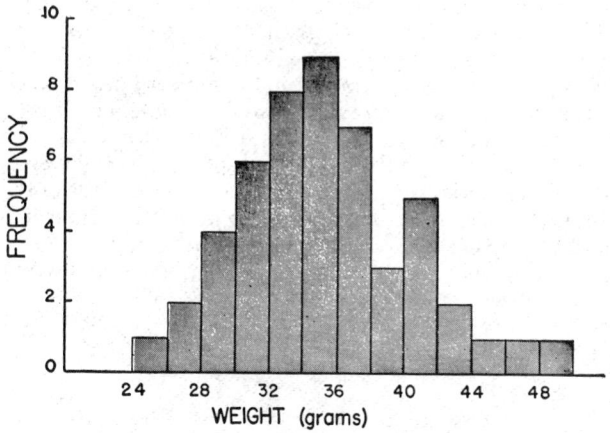

Fig 10-8.   Bar chart showing frequency distribution of weights of 50 rats at weaning (data in *Example II*).

the lowest value in a series of observations. For Example I the range would be $4.9 - 4.0 = 0.9$; for Example II, $49 - 25 = 24$. The range is most valuable in small series of observations, usually for n less than 10. Dixon and Massey[4] have an excellent dissertation on the use of the range.

The *standard deviation* is the measure of variation most commonly used. When $n = 2$, the range and the standard deviation are equally as efficient. For n greater than ten, the standard deviation gives a much better estimate of the variation than the range. The two are quite closely related, especially for sample sizes less than ten. See Table XIII for the average number of standard deviations in the average range.

The standard deviation of the population is usually designated by σ, and the standard deviation of the sample by s, where s is an estimate of σ. The standard deviation of a sample is calculated by getting the differences of each observation from the mean and putting them in the following formula:

$$s = \sqrt{\frac{(x_1 - \bar{x})^2 + (x_2 - \bar{x})^2 + (x_3 - \bar{x})^2 + \ldots + (x_n - \bar{x})^2}{n - 1}}$$

The formula can be given in several forms, some of which are easier to calculate:

$$s = \sqrt{\frac{\Sigma(x_i - \bar{x})^2}{n - 1}} = \sqrt{\frac{\Sigma x_i^2 - (\Sigma x_i)^2/n}{n - 1}}$$

Using the data in Example I, $n = 9$, the sum of the nine observations (Σx_i) is 39.6. The sum of the squares of the observations is:

$$\Sigma x_i^2 = (4.1)^2 + (4.3)^2 + \ldots + (4.4)^2 = 174.92$$

Putting these values in the formula:

$$s = \sqrt{\frac{\Sigma x_i^2 - (\Sigma x_i)^2/n}{n - 1}}$$

$$s = \sqrt{\frac{174.92 - (39.6)^2/9}{9 - 1}} = \sqrt{\frac{174.92 - 174.24}{8}} = 0.29$$

The $n - 1$ in the denominator of the formula for the standard deviation is called the degrees of freedom, sometimes abbreviated DF, and for the standard deviation is one less than the number of observations.

The standard deviation also can be estimated by using the range as will be shown later. There are tables showing the number of standard deviations contained in the range depending on n, the sample size.

In a normal distribution one standard deviation measured both above and below the population average includes about $2/3$ of the number of observations in the whole distribution; two standard deviations measured off on each side of the average includes about 95% of the observations. In fact, tables of the normal probability curve* have been calculated to show the multiple (sometimes fractional) of the standard deviation on either side of the average which would include any desired proportion of the observations (see Fig 10-9 and also the bottom line of Table III). It is from such tables and graphs that probabilities can be derived. Note that the title of Fig 10-9 is "normal probability curve," and that the center line at the hump of the curve is the population average, μ. More accurately, this represents the frequency of distribution of standardized values expressed as

---

* One of the most complete tables of this kind can be found in Pearson.[10] Other tables can be found in almost any statistical text such as Snedecor and Cochran, Rider, Fisher, etc. (see *Bibliography*), or in Fisher and Yates.[3]

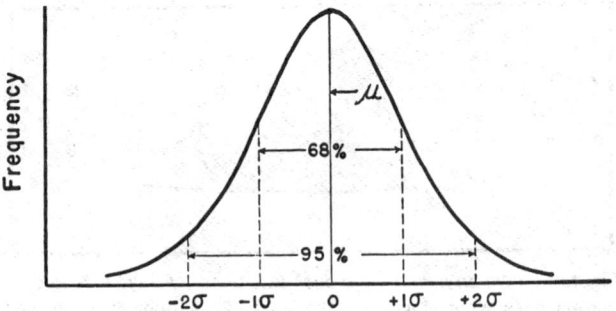

Fig 10-9. The normal probability curve showing standard deviation units around the average.

$$\frac{\mu_i - \mu}{\sigma}$$

Then the area under the normal probability curve will be 1, and the mean and standard deviation will be 0 and 1, respectively. The vertical dotted lines divide the distribution into standard deviation units or sigma (σ) units. (The standard deviation of the infinite parent population is usually denoted by sigma (σ) while the standard deviation of the sample of n observations is denoted by s.) Thus, if 95% of the observations in this distribution are between 2σ above the average and 2σ below the average, only 5% of the observations will be beyond these limits (which are called the 95% confidence limits) and an observation would have a 5% probability of occurrence beyond these limits.

Also, in the bottom line of Table III which applies to an infinitely large sample, the limits indicated by the population average $\pm 2.326\sigma$ (i.e., two tails) include all but 2% ($P = 0.02$) of the observations. Only 1% ($P = 0.01$) is *above* $\mu + 2.326\sigma$, using one tail of the distribution. Likewise, 1% ($P = 0.01$) is below the lower limit, $\mu - 2.326\sigma$. Both Fig. 10-9 and Table III are theoretical distributions. More complete tables of the normal probability distribution are available in statistical texts and books of tables previously referred to.

The standard deviation gives a measure of the variation of *individual observations* around the average. A comparable measure of variation of *averages* of samples about their average is called the *standard error of an average*. It can be calculated from the standard deviation, s, and the number of observations, n.

$$\text{Standard error of the average} = s_{\bar{x}} = \frac{s}{\sqrt{n}}$$

A shortcut (and only approximate) method of estimating the standard error of the average is to divide the range by the number of observations.

$$s_{\bar{x}} = \frac{\text{range}}{n}$$

This method can be used only if n is less than ten.

The square of the standard deviation is called the *variance*. The square of the standard error of the average is called the *variance of the average*. By means of mathematical statistics, it is possible to derive the variance for almost any statistic which can be expressed by a formula. There is not only the variance of an average but also the variance of a weighted average, regression coefficient, etc. Each statistic also has its own distribution about its true value; tables of the normal curve sometimes can be applied to a particular statistic.

Suppose an infinitely large box contains marbles of differing weights with an average weight of 50 g and the individual weights of the marbles have a normal distribution and a standard deviation of 9 g. If 1000 samples of 4 marbles each are taken from the box, the average for each of the 1000 samples recorded, and the standard deviation of these averages

Table III—The _t_ Table

Distribution of t Giving Both the Two-Sided or Two-Tailed Probability and the One-Sided or One-Tailed Probability According to Degrees of Freedom

	One Tail							
	P 0.4	P 0.3	P 0.2	P 0.1	P 0.05	P 0.025	P 0.01	P 0.005
				Two Tails				
DF	P 0.8	P 0.6	P 0.4	P 0.2	P 0.1	P 0.05	P 0.02	P 0.01
1	0.325	0.727	1.376	3.078	6.314	12.706	31.821	63.657
2	0.289	0.617	1.061	1.886	2.920	4.303	6.965	9.925
3	0.277	0.584	0.978	1.638	2.353	3.182	4.541	5.841
4	0.271	0.569	0.941	1.533	2.132	2.776	3.747	4.604
5	0.267	0.559	0.920	1.476	2.015	2.571	3.365	4.032
6	0.265	0.553	0.906	1.440	1.943	2.447	3.143	3.707
7	0.263	0.549	0.896	1.415	1.895	2.365	2.998	3.499
8	0.262	0.546	0.889	1.397	1.860	2.306	2.896	3.355
9	0.261	0.543	0.883	1.383	1.833	2.262	2.821	3.250
10	0.260	0.542	0.879	1.372	1.812	2.228	2.764	3.169
11	0.260	0.540	0.876	1.363	1.796	2.201	2.718	3.106
12	0.259	0.539	0.873	1.356	1.782	2.179	2.681	3.055
13	0.259	0.538	0.870	1.350	1.771	2.160	2.650	3.012
14	0.258	0.537	0.868	1.345	1.761	2.145	2.624	2.977
15	0.258	0.536	0.866	1.341	1.753	2.131	2.602	2.947
16	0.258	0.535	0.865	1.337	1.746	2.120	2.583	2.921
17	0.257	0.534	0.863	1.333	1.740	2.110	2.567	2.898
18	0.257	0.534	0.862	1.330	1.734	2.101	2.552	2.878
19	0.257	0.533	0.861	1.328	1.729	2.093	2.539	2.861
20	0.257	0.533	0.860	1.325	1.725	2.086	2.528	2.845
21	0.257	0.532	0.859	1.323	1.721	2.080	2.518	2.831
22	0.256	0.532	0.858	1.321	1.717	2.074	2.508	2.819
23	0.256	0.532	0.858	1.319	1.714	2.069	2.500	2.807
24	0.256	0.531	0.857	1.318	1.711	2.064	2.492	2.797
25	0.256	0.531	0.856	1.316	1.708	2.060	2.485	2.787
26	0.256	0.531	0.856	1.315	1.706	2.056	2.479	2.779
27	0.256	0.531	0.855	1.314	1.703	2.052	2.473	2.771
28	0.256	0.530	0.855	1.313	1.701	2.048	2.467	2.763
29	0.256	0.530	0.854	1.311	1.699	2.045	2.462	2.756
30	0.256	0.530	0.854	1.310	1.697	2.042	2.457	2.750
40	0.255	0.529	0.851	1.303	1.684	2.021	2.423	2.704
60	0.254	0.527	0.848	1.296	1.671	2.000	2.390	2.660
120	0.254	0.526	0.845	1.289	1.658	1.980	2.358	2.617
∞	0.253	0.524	0.842	1.282	1.645	1.960	2.326	2.576

calculated, this figure would agree very well with the population standard error of the average as calculated from

$$\sigma_{\bar{x}} = \frac{\sigma}{\sqrt{n}} = \frac{9}{\sqrt{4}} = 4.5 \text{ g}$$

Also the averages of the 1000 samples of 4 marbles each would be distributed normally about the true average (50 g) and have a standard error of the average equal to 4.5 g. This means that the averages of about ⅔ of the 1000 samples (about 670) would occur between 50 + 4.5 g and 50 − 4.5 g (or between 54.5 and 45.5 g).

The normal probability tables would apply to the distribution of these averages. About 95% of the averages would occur between the average plus or minus two standard errors of the average. Therefore, beyond these "two sigma" limits on either side of the grand average only about 5% (ie, 100% minus 95%) of the averages will occur. If, sometime in the future, a sample of 4 marbles is drawn from the box the chances are about 5 in 100 or 1 in 20 that the average for this sample will be below 41 g or above 59 g, ie,

$$50 - 2(4.5) = 41$$
$$50 + 2(4.5) = 59$$

and 1 chance in 100 that the average for this sample will be below 38.4 g or above 61.6 g, ie,

$$50 - 2.57(4.5) = 38.4$$
$$50 + 2.57(4.5) = 61.6$$

The factors to be used in multiplying the standard error of the average and the probability attached to each factor (eg, 95 or 99%) can be found in any table of the normal probability distribution or normal curve of error as it is sometimes called. This table is usually included in any statistical text or book of statistical tables.[3] The factors are given here in the bottom line of Table III.

Probability—Usually the capital letter _P_ (for probability) is used in statistics to indicate the chances a given result would occur by random sampling from a specific population. If it is found rarely enough (usually $P = 0.05$, 5% of the time, or 1 time in 20), it is considered unlikely that the sample was taken from that population and it is said to be significantly different.

Confidence Limits—This terminology is used to denote limits around a sample average, $\bar{x}$, that would encompass the true average of the population, μ, a given percentage of the time. These confidence limits are obtained using the standard error of the sample average, $s_{\bar{x}}$, and a _t_ value (see Table III) corresponding to the degrees of freedom, $n - 1$, and the probability one wishes to associate with the confidence limits.

Upper confidence limit $= \bar{x} + ts_{\bar{x}}$

Lower confidence limit $= \bar{x} - ts_{\bar{x}}$

where $s_{\bar{x}} = s/\sqrt{n}$.

The confidence statement could be written:

$$\bar{x} - ts_{\bar{x}} < \mu < \bar{x} + ts_{\bar{x}}$$

If t corresponds to $P = 0.05$, the population average, μ, lies between these confidence limits 95% of the time, ie, if such intervals are computed in repeated samples of n observations, 95% of such intervals would include μ.

The t distribution is proper when the sample standard deviation is used; then the normal curve of error does not apply. It can be seen, however, that as n increases, the t value approaches the value obtained using the normal distribution.

Suppose, however, that in the example above, the population average, μ, and population standard deviation, σ, were unknown and that instead of 1000 samples of 4, there was only 1 sample of 4;

$$n = 4$$
$$\bar{x} = 50$$
$$s_{\bar{x}} = 4.5$$

and we wish to know the limits within which the true average (μ) of the population would occur 95% of the time. The t table is entered on the row corresponding to the degrees of freedom ($n - 1$ or 3 in this case), and $P = 0.05$ for two tails to obtain $t = 3.182$. Using the equations given for upper and lower confidence limits, we obtain

$$\bar{x} + ts_{\bar{x}} = 50 + 3.182(4.5) = 64.3$$

$$\bar{x} - ts_{\bar{x}} = 50 - 3.182(4.5) = 35.7$$

Thus 95% of the time the confidence limits of 35.7 to 64.3 would include the true average of the box. These limits would be called the confidence limits for $P = 0.95$. Note that these are much larger limits than if knowledge of the standard deviation were based on 1000 samples of 4.

It can also be stated that $2\frac{1}{2}\%$ of the time the true average will be below the confidence interval, and $2\frac{1}{2}\%$ of the time above. These are generally referred to as "the tails," and t tables are given for one tail as well as for two tails. Table III is for both two tails and one tail. Note that the probabilities for one tail are just half of those for two tails. Confidence limits can be made smaller by taking a larger sample and thus reducing the size of the standard error of the mean. This is an illustration of how chance operates in sampling procedures because of the inherent variability of nature. A similar use of sigma limits is applied to biological assays in stating confidence limits for the potency of a drug. In general the probability accompanying the confidence limits indicates the probability that the true figure will be within these limits.

Standard deviations and confidence limits can also be obtained for a percentage. For instance, if questionnaires were sent out to 100 pharmacists asking if they handled a certain new drug, and if 20% of them replied they did and 80% replied they did not, it is possible to calculate or find the confidence limits of that percentage or the limits which would include the true percentage of all pharmacists carrying that drug. The standard deviation could be calculated:

$$s = \sqrt{\frac{pq}{n}} = \sqrt{\frac{0.20(0.80)}{100}} = 0.04$$

where p is the percentage as a decimal fraction equal to $= 0.20$, $q = 1 - p = 0.80$, and $n =$ size of sample $= 100$.

Thus the 2-sigma limits ($P = 0.95$) would be 12% and 28%. This, however, is an approximation. More accurate confidence limits for percentages have been tabled by Clopper and Pearson, Snedecor and Cochran, Geigy, and others. A condensed form is given in Table IV where it can be seen that the confidence limits for the example are actually 13 and 29%.

Weighted Average—There are instances where a *grand average* of several averages is desired, such as in collaborative work on a method. The formula given above for the calculation of the average assumes equal weights for all observations. This formula could be used for determining a grand average of several averages if all are determined with the same precision. The precision of an average is dependent on the amount of variation as well as the number of observations and is given by the formula for the *variance of an average*, which is

$$s_{\bar{x}}^2 = s^2/n$$

(*Note*—Variance is the square of the standard deviation and the variance of an average is the square of the standard error of the average.) The more precise an average, the smaller its standard error. Therefore, the *weight* attached to any one average is the reciprocal of the variance of that average.

$$W = \frac{1}{s_{\bar{x}}^2} = \frac{n}{s^2}$$

The formula for the grand average of two averages then becomes:

$$\bar{x} = \frac{W_1\bar{x}_1 + W_2\bar{x}_2}{W_1 + W_2}$$

where:

$\bar{x} =$ grand average
$\bar{x}_1$ and $\bar{x}_2$ are two individual averages
W_1 and W_2 are weights for $\bar{x}_1$ and $\bar{x}_2$, respectively

This formula can be extended in the same manner for more than two averages:

$$\bar{x} = \frac{\Sigma W_i \bar{x}_i}{\Sigma W_i}$$

where, as before, Σ indicates a summation.

Table IV—Confidence Limits for Binomial Distribution[a]

$P = 0.95$ for two limits (both upper and lower)

$P = 0.975$ for only one limit (either upper or lower)

% Failures in sample	Size of sample						
	10	20	30	50	100	250	1000
0	0 31	0 17	0 12	0 7	0 4	0 1	0 0
10	0 45	1 32	2 27	3 22	5 18	7 14	8 12
20	3 56	6 44	8 39	10 34	13 29	15 26	18 23
30	7 65	12 54	15 49	18 45	21 40	24 36	27 33
40	12 74	19 64	23 59	26 55	30 50	34 46	37 43
50	19 81	27 73	31 69	36 64	40 60	44 56	47 53

[a] Adapted from Mainland[14]

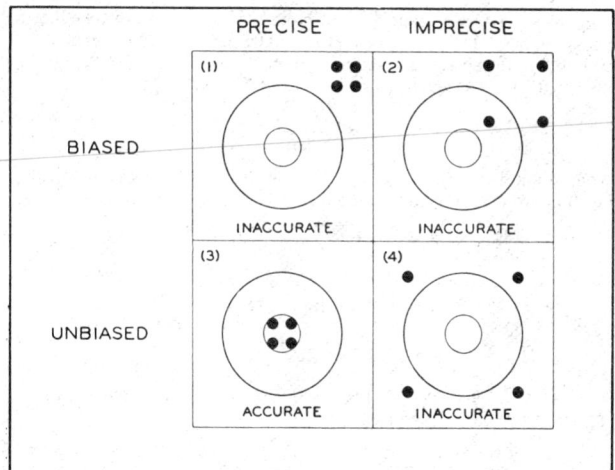

	PRECISE	IMPRECISE
BIASED	(1) INACCURATE	(2) INACCURATE
UNBIASED	(3) ACCURATE	(4) INACCURATE

Fig 10-10. Diagram illustrating bias, precision, and accuracy. The shots on targets (1) and (2) are biased; in both cases the shots cluster away from the bull's eye. The clusters on targets (3) and (4) are both unbiased; the center of each cluster is on the bull's eye. The shots on targets (1) and (3) are precise; both sets are bunched together. The shots on targets (2) and (4) are widely scattered, hence imprecise. Only the shots on target (3) are accurate, ie, precise and unbiased (courtesy, Lilly).

Example III—A few students each made several determinations of the total alkaloids in a single lot of belladonna leaves; however, a different number of determinations was made by each student. The standard deviation was determined for each student's determinations.

Student	n	Average	Std dev
1	10	0.40	0.05
2	5	0.31	0.07
3	4	0.53	0.05
4	7	0.36	0.02

The best estimate of the average total alkaloid content of this lot of belladonna leaves will be given by the weighted average.

Student	n	Average $\bar{x}$	Weight W	Product $W\bar{x}$	Product $n\bar{x}$
1	10	0.40	4,000	1600	4.00
2	5	0.31	1,020	316	1.55
3	4	0.53	1,000	848	2.12
4	7	0.36	17,500	6300	2.52
Sum	26		24,120	9064	10.19

$$\bar{x} = \frac{\Sigma W_i \bar{x}_i}{\Sigma W_i} = \frac{9064}{24,120} = 0.376$$

If only $\bar{x}$ and n had been given for each student and the variances (also the standard deviations) were assumed to be equal, the weights would be the number of observations and

$$\bar{x} = \frac{\Sigma n_i \bar{x}_i}{\Sigma n_i} = \frac{10.19}{26} = 0.392$$

There are instances where a weighted average is the best to use, and other instances where the actual weights that should be assigned are unknown even though both the number of observations, n, in each group and the standard deviation, s, of these observations are given. The weight in itself should be a measure of the *accuracy*, not the *precision*, of an average. Sometimes it may be that the number of determinations is large because for some reason the analyst suspected that his first results were incorrect and therefore he repeated the determinations. The standard error, although calculated from both n and s does not necessarily give a measure of the *accuracy* of an average; it may give only the *precision*.

Bias, Precision, and Accuracy—The *bias* (or *systematic error*) of a method is indicative of its tendency to measure something other than what was intended, while its *precision* (or *reproducibility*) refers to the agreement among repeated measurements. The comprehensive term, *accuracy*, refers to the closeness of such measurements to the "true" magni-

tude concerned. In other words, accuracy shows how closely a method measures what it is supposed to measure, while precision shows only how closely many measurements agree. An accurate method of measurement is both precise and unbiased. Given a sample which is known to contain 100 mg of iodine, five determinations by an accurate method might range from 99.5 to 100.5 mg of iodine, while five by an unbiased but imprecise method might range from 95.0 to 105.0 mg. (However, because averages are more precise than individual measurements the average of a large number (eg, 100) of determinations by the second method would be just as accurate as the average of a few (eg, 5) by the first method.) Five measurements made by a biased but precise method might possibly range from 85 to 86 mg of iodine, while five made by a method which is both biased and imprecise might range from 80 to 90 mg. The bias of approximately 15 mg in these last two methods cannot be "averaged out" merely by making additional determinations.

The interrelations of bias, precision, and accuracy are clearly illustrated in Fig 10-10 (taken from illustrations by Eisenhart[12] and Stearns[9]). A detailed discussion of these topics is presented by Eisenhart.[12]

Interpretation of the Analysis

There are three types of significance tests that are quite generally used: the t test, χ^2 test, and the F test, or analysis of variance.

The t Test of Significance—If two samples are to be compared to see if they are drawn from the same population, i.e., whether they are samples of the same thing or whether they are "significantly" different, the t test can be used as a means of comparison. (This is the same t we used in calculating confidence limits.) A significant difference means that a real difference *may* exist. It does not *prove* that it exists, but is an indication that the difference may be real and that the two samples may be drawn from entirely different populations. (The t test also can be used to compare a sample and a population.) The formula is:

$$t = \frac{\text{difference}}{\text{standard error of difference}}$$

For calculation purposes we can use

$$t = \frac{\bar{x}_1 - \bar{x}_2}{s} \sqrt{\frac{n_1 n_2}{n_1 + n_2}}$$

where:

$\bar{x}_1$ = mean of first sample of n_1 observations
$\bar{x}_2$ = mean of second sample of n_2 observations

and:

$$s^2 = \frac{\Sigma x_{1i}^2 - (\Sigma x_{1i})^2/n_1 + \Sigma x_{2i}^2 - (\Sigma x_{2i})^2/n_2}{n_1 + n_2 - 2}$$

where:

Σx_{1i}^2 is sum of squares of observations in first sample
Σx_{1i} is sum of observations in first sample
Σx_{2i}^2 is sum of squares of observations in second sample
Σx_{2i} is sum of observations in second sample
s^2 is the pooled variance of the two samples

Example IV—Suppose one sample of four and one sample of five are taken, respectively, from each of two lots of amobarbital capsules and the milligrams of amobarbital are determined in each capsule and it is desired to determine whether or not there is a significant difference between the two samples. Do they come from different lots or populations? It is assumed that there is no difference between them (the null hypothesis), and the probability that they could have been drawn from the same population is found. If this probability is small enough, there is said to be a statistically "significant" difference.

Sample 1	Sample 2
	9.8
10.1	9.6
13.6	10.1
12.5	11.4
11.4	9.1
$\Sigma x_{1i} = 47.6$	$\Sigma x_{2i} = 50.0$
$\Sigma x_{1i}^2 = 573.18$	$\Sigma x_{2i}^2 = 502.98$
$\bar{x}_1 = 11.90$	$\bar{x}_2 = 10.00$
$n_1 = 4$	$n_2 = 5$

$$s^2 = \frac{573.18 - (47.6)^2/4 + 502.98 - (50.0)^2/5}{4 + 5 - 2}$$

$$= \frac{573.18 - 566.44 + 502.98 - 500.00}{7} = \frac{9.72}{7} = 1.3886$$

$$s = 1.18$$

$$t = \frac{\bar{x}_1 - \bar{x}_2}{s}\sqrt{\frac{n_1 n_2}{n_1 + n_2}}$$

$$= \frac{11.90 - 10.00}{1.18}\sqrt{\frac{4(5)}{4 + 5}}$$

$$= 1.61(1.49) = 2.40$$

The degrees of freedom involved in the pooled standard deviation are seven, $DF = (n_1 - 1) + (n_2 - 1)$. In the t table (see Table III), for $P = 0.05$ and $DF = 7$ (two tails) the value of t given is 2.365. The value of t calculated is greater than this. Therefore, since the probability of these two samples being drawn from the same population is less than 0.05, we conclude that they were drawn from different populations. (This conclusion may be wrong 5 times in 100). It can be stated that there is a statistically significant difference between the two samples. To determine whether the average of sample 1 was *greater* than the average of sample 2, the "one tail" portion of the t table is used. Of course, one must decide before making the test whether one tail or two tails should be used, depending on the question to be answered.

For $DF = 7$ and $P = 0.05$ (one tail) Table III shows $t = 1.895$. Our calculated value of $t = 2.40$ is greater than the tabled value, and we conclude that the average of Sample 1 (11.90) is statistically significantly greater than the average of Sample 2 (10.00).

The standard error of the difference could be estimated crudely using the range:

standard error of difference

$$= \sqrt{\left(\frac{\text{Range}_1}{n_1}\right)^2 + \left(\frac{\text{Range}_2}{n_2}\right)^2}$$

$$= \sqrt{\left(\frac{13.6 - 10.1}{4}\right)^2 + \left(\frac{11.4 - 9.1}{5}\right)^2}$$

$$= \sqrt{(0.875)^2 + (0.460)^2} = 0.986$$

thus, t:
$$= \frac{\bar{x}_1 - \bar{x}_2}{\text{standard error of difference}}$$

$$= \frac{11.90 - 10.00}{0.986} = 1.93$$

However, now the value of t is smaller than the value from the table, which was 2.365, and we conclude that we have no proof that they were drawn from different populations.

This was an example of a borderline significance test, and the crude estimate of the standard error of the difference may be the cause of the difference between the two tests. When the significance test is not borderline, the results using the range give a good approximation to those using the standard deviation, provided n_1 and n_2 are less than 15.

One of the assumptions made in carrying out the t test is that the variances for the two samples being compared are homogeneous. If this assumption is violated, we carry out a weighted t test.

Suppose one sample of six and one sample of seven gave the following results:

Sample 1	Sample 2
	15
6	10
7	5
3	20
6	4
4	11
4	9
$\Sigma x_{1i} = 30$	$\Sigma x_{2i} = 74$
$\Sigma x_{1i}^2 = 162$	$\Sigma x_{2i}^2 = 968$
$n_1 = 6$	$n_2 = 7$
$\bar{x}_1 = 5.0$	$\bar{x}_2 = 10.6$
$s_1^2 = 2.40$	$s_2^2 = 30.95$

Using the procedure described in Example XIII, page 118, it can be shown that $s_1^2 \neq s_2^2$. The values of t at $P = 0.05$ for five and six degrees of freedom for s_1^2 and s_2^2, respectively, are 2.571 and 2.447 (see Table III). The weights for each sample are calculated from:

$$W_i = \frac{s_i^2}{n_i}$$

so that W_1 and W_2 equal $2.40/6 = 0.40$ and $30.95/7 = 4.42$, respectively. The standard error of the difference between sample means is given by:

$$\text{S.E.}_{\bar{x}_1 - \bar{x}_2} = \sqrt{W_1 + W_2} = \sqrt{0.40 + 4.42} = 2.2$$

and the weighted t is:

$$t_W = \frac{|\bar{x}_1 - \bar{x}_2|}{\text{S.E.}_{x_1 - x_2}} = \frac{|5.0 - 10.6|}{2.2} = 2.55$$

where $|\bar{x}_1 - \bar{x}_2|$ = absolute (positive) difference. The critical value of t_W at $P = 0.05$ is given by:

$$t^*_W = \frac{W_1 t_1 + W_2 t_2}{W_1 + W_2}$$

$$= \frac{(0.40)(2.571) + (4.42)(2.447)}{0.40 + 4.42} = 2.46$$

Since the calculated value of t_W (2.55) is greater than the critical value of t^*_W (2.46), we conclude that the two samples are drawn from different populations (ie, are statistically significantly different at $P \leq 0.05$).

The t test also may be applied to paired (sometimes referred to as correlated) data. Such data occur when pairs of subjects or test units matched on the basis of certain characteristics (eg, age, sex, etc) are assigned at random, one to each treatment or condition to be tested, or when the same subject or test unit is assigned to each treatment given in random order. The objective is to remove the inherent variability from test unit to test unit, and thus obtain a more sensitive comparison. The formula for computational purposes is:

$$t = \frac{\bar{d}}{s}\sqrt{n}$$

where:

$\bar{d}$ = mean of the differences, $x_1 - x_2$, of the n pairs of observations

$$s^2 = \frac{\Sigma d_i^2 - (\Sigma d_i)^2/n}{n - 1}$$

where:

Σd_i^2 = the sum of squares of the n differences
Σd_i = sum of the n differences
n = number of differences or pairs of observations

Example V—Duration of loss of righting reflex (min) was measured in 16 mice following treatment with a barbiturate administered in the morning and the afternoon on two different occasions, the order of giving the morning or the afternoon dose being randomized in each mouse. It was desired to test the null hypothesis that the duration of loss of righting reflex is the same in the morning and the afternoon.

Mouse no	am x_1	pm x_2	Difference $d = x_1 - x_2$
1	75	73	2
2	86	89	-3
3	93	89	4
4	87	79	8
5	91	95	-4
6	87	81	6
7	76	77	-1
8	83	89	-6
9	87	82	5
10	95	91	4
11	91	87	4
12	86	86	0
13	83	78	5
14	76	69	7
15	82	78	4
16	93	88	5

$$\Sigma d_i = 40$$
$$\Sigma d_i^2 = 354$$
$$\bar{d} = 2.5$$
$$n = 16$$

$$s^2 = \frac{354 - (40)^2/16}{16 - 1} = \frac{354 - 100}{15} = 16.9333$$

$$s = 4.11$$

$$t = \frac{\overline{d}}{s}\sqrt{n} = \frac{2.5}{4.11}\sqrt{16} = \frac{2.5(4)}{4.11} = 2.43$$

$$DF = n - 1 = 16 - 1 = 15$$

In the t table (see Table III), for $P = 0.05$ and $DF = 15$ (two tails) the value of t given is 2.131. The value of t calculated is greater than this. Therefore, since the probability of the morning and afternoon values being the same is less than 0.05, we conclude that they are different. Apparently, the duration of loss of righting reflex in mice tested on the barbiturate in the morning was longer than when tested in the afternoon.

The Chi-Square Tests of Significance—The chi-square test can assume many different forms. In one form it tests agreement between expected frequencies and frequencies observed. Of course, there are many ways of stating what you expect.

$$\chi^2 = \sum \frac{(\text{observed frequency} - \text{expected frequency})^2}{\text{expected frequency}}$$

Example VI—In tossing a coin, 50% tails and 50% heads are expected. Suppose a coin is tossed 40 times and 25 heads and 15 tails are obtained, whereas 20 heads and 20 tails are expected. Is the coin biased or weighted in some way?

$$\chi^2 = \frac{(25 - 20)^2}{20} + \frac{(15 - 20)^2}{20} = 2.5$$

Again the degrees of freedom associated with χ^2 are one less than the number of categories. Here $\chi^2 = 2.5$ with one degree of freedom. The greater the disagreement between expected and observed, the larger the χ^2. See Table V for probabilities of getting this value or larger. For one degree of freedom the probability of getting a value larger than 2.5 is somewhere between $P = 0.20$ and $P = 0.10$. In order to say that we had a statistically significant departure from the expected values, χ^2 would have to be larger than 3.84 which is the value for $P = 0.05$ at one degree of freedom. A value of χ^2 larger than 6.64 for one degree of freedom would indicate a statistically highly significant ($P < 0.01$) departure from the expected.

The chi-square test may be used for comparing two percentages in a 2×2 or fourfold contingency table:

Example VII—Following are the survival rates for drug-treated and control pigs with swine dysentery:

Treatment	Survived	Died	Total
Drug	$a = 25$	$b = 14$	$a + b = 39$
Controls	$c = 21$	$d = 22$	$c + d = 43$
Totals	$a + c = 46$	$b + d = 36$	$N = 82$

The survival rates for the drug-treated and control pigs are $p_D = 25/39 = 64\%$ and $p_C = 21/43 = 49\%$, respectively. To test the null hypothesis that there is no difference in the survival rates of drug-treated and control pigs, we calculate

$$\chi^2 = \frac{(|ad - bc| - N/2)^2 N}{(a + b)(c + d)(a + c)(b + d)} =$$

$$\frac{(|25 \cdot 22 - 14 \cdot 21| - 82/2)^2 82}{(39)(43)(46)(36)} = 1.36$$

Table V—The Chi-Square Table[a]

Probability

DF	P = 0.20	P = 0.10	P = 0.05	P = 0.01
1	1.64	2.71	3.84	6.64
2	3.22	4.61	5.99	9.21
3	4.64	6.25	7.82	11.34
4	5.99	7.78	9.49	13.28
5	7.29	9.24	11.07	15.09
6	8.56	10.64	12.59	16.81
7	9.80	12.02	14.07	18.48
8	11.03	13.36	15.51	20.09
9	12.24	14.68	16.92	21.67
10	13.44	15.99	18.31	23.21
20	25.04	28.41	31.41	37.57
30	36.25	40.26	43.77	50.89

[a] Adapted from Fisher and Yates.[3]

where $|ad - bc|$ is the absolute (i.e., positive) difference of $ad - bc$.

The degrees of freedom associated with an $R \times C$ contingency table = $(R - 1)(C - 1)$, so that for a 2×2 contingency table we have one degree of freedom. Table V shows that for one degree of freedom the probability of getting a value of χ^2 larger than the calculated value 1.36 is greater than $P = 0.20$. Since P is not equal to or less than 0.05, we conclude that there is insufficient evidence to indicate that the survival rates for the drug-treated and control pigs are different.

The chi-square test for comparing two correlated percentages for paired data takes a somewhat different form:

Example VIII—Two different types of penicillin were given to each of 22 patients in random order on successive occasions, and the presence or absence of a detectable blood level was determined:

		Type II +	−	Totals
Type I	+	$a = 6$	$b = 10$	16
	−	$c = 2$	$d = 4$	6
Totals		8	14	22

The percentage of patients with detectable blood levels for the two forms of penicillin are $p_I = 16/22 = 73\%$ and $p_{II} = 8/22 = 36\%$. To test the null hypothesis that there is no difference in the percentage of patients with detectable blood levels for the two forms of penicillin, we calculate

$$\chi^2 = \frac{(|b - c| - 1)^2}{b + c} = \frac{(|10 - 2| - 1)^2}{10 + 2} = \frac{49}{12} = 4.08$$

In Table V, for $P = 0.05$ and $DF = 1$, the value of χ^2 given is 3.84. The value of χ^2 calculated is greater than this. Therefore, since the probability of the percentages for type I and type II penicillin being the same is less than 0.05, we conclude that they are different.

Reference is made to sets of tables for determining significance of χ^2 for a fourfold table without any calculations. These tables are self explanatory and were published by Mainland.[13,14] An excellent discussion of χ^2 is given by Dixon and Massey,[15] and a series of articles on χ^2 are given in *Biometrics* (Dec., 1954).

Nonparametric Tests of Significance—The validity of the t test for comparing two means depends to some extent (especially for small samples) on the assumptions that the two populations sampled are approximately normally distributed and have essentially equal variances. The procedure for unequal variances has been discussed previously (page 114). Statistical procedures that do not depend on the assumption of normality are called nonparametric tests. Three commonly used procedures are the Rank Sum test for unpaired data, and the Signed-Rank Sum and Statistical Sign tests for paired data.

Rank Sum Test of Significance—After the n_1 and n_2 observations are arranged in order of size, the combined values are ranked from 1, for the lowest, to $(n_1 + n_2)$ for the highest, and the sum of the ranks T of the n_1 observations in the smaller sample is computed. Values which are tied are given average ranks. We also calculate $T' = n_1(n_1 + n_2 + 1) - T$, and enter Table VI with n_1, n_2, and T or T', whichever is smaller. If the calculated T (or T') is equal to or less than the tabled value, we reject the null hypothesis at the significance level P.

Example IX—Data were available on the duration of loss of righting reflex (min) for 10 mice given a standard barbiturate and for 11 mice given a test barbiturate:

Standard drug	Rank	Test drug	Rank
96	4.5	0	1
109	8	91	2
126	13	92	3
130	15	96	4.5
130	15	99	6
148	17	103	7
153	18	117	9
158	19	118	10
169	20	119	11
Died	21	120	12
		130	15
$T = \overline{150.5}$			$n_2 = \overline{11}$
$n_1 = $ 10			

$$T' = n_1(n_1 + n_2 + 1) - T = 10(10 + 11 + 1) - 150.5 = 69.5$$

Table VI—The Rank Sum Table[a]

Values of T or T', Whichever is Smaller, Significant at the 10%, 5%, and 1% Levels

n_2	P	4	5	6	7	8	9	10	11	12	13	14	15	16	17	18	19	20
8	0.10	15	23	31	41	51												
	0.05	14	21	29	38	49												
	0.01	11	17	25	34	43												
9	0.10	16	24	33	43	54	66											
	0.05	14	22	31	40	51	62											
	0.01	11	18	26	35	45	56											
10	0.10	17	26	35	45	56	69	82										
	0.05	15	23	32	42	53	65	78										
	0.01	12	19	27	37	47	58	71										
11	0.10	18	27	37	47	59	72	86	100									
	0.05	16	24	34	44	55	68	81	96									
	0.01	12	20	28	38	49	61	73	87									
12	0.10	19	28	38	49	62	75	89	104	120								
	0.05	17	26	35	46	58	71	84	99	115								
	0.01	13	21	30	40	51	63	76	90	105								
13	0.10	20	30	40	52	64	78	92	108	125	142							
	0.05	18	27	37	48	60	73	88	103	119	136							
	0.01	14	22	31	41	53	65	79	93	109	125							
14	0.10	21	31	42	54	67	81	96	112	129	147	166						
	0.05	19	28	38	50	62	76	91	106	123	141	160						
	0.01	14	22	32	43	54	67	81	96	112	129	147						
15	0.10	22	33	44	56	69	84	99	116	133	152	171	192					
	0.05	20	29	40	52	65	79	94	110	127	145	164	184					
	0.01	15	23	33	44	56	69	84	99	115	133	151	171					
16	0.10	24	34	46	58	72	87	103	120	138	156	176	197	219				
	0.05	21	30	42	54	67	82	97	113	131	150	169	190	211				
	0.01	15	24	34	46	58	72	86	102	119	136	155	175	196				
17	0.10	25	35	47	61	75	90	106	123	142	161	182	203	225	249			
	0.05	21	32	43	56	70	84	100	117	135	154	174	195	217	240			
	0.01	16	25	36	47	60	74	89	105	122	140	159	180	201	223			
18	0.10	26	37	49	63	77	93	110	127	146	166	187	208	231	255	280		
	0.05	22	33	45	58	72	87	103	121	139	158	179	200	222	246	270		
	0.01	16	26	37	49	62	76	92	108	125	144	163	184	206	228	252		
19	0.10	27	38	51	65	80	96	113	131	150	171	192	214	237	262	287	313	
	0.05	23	34	46	60	74	90	107	124	143	163	182	205	228	252	277	303	
	0.01	17	27	38	50	64	78	94	111	129	147	168	189	210	234	258	283	
20	0.10	28	40	53	67	83	99	117	135	155	175	197	220	243	268	294	320	348
	0.05	24	35	48	62	77	93	110	128	147	167	188	210	234	258	283	309	337
	0.01	18	28	39	52	66	81	97	114	132	151	172	193	215	239	263	289	315

when $n_1 > 20$ and $n_2 > 20$, significance values are given to a good approximation by

$$n_1(n_1 + n_2 + 1)/2 - z \sqrt{n_1 n_2 (n_1 + n_2 + 1)/12}$$

where z is 1.64 for the 10% level, 1.96 for the 5%, and 2.58 for the 1%. The probability figures given are for a two-tailed test. For a one-tailed test, P is halved.

[a] Adapted from Tate and Clelland.[16]

Entering Table VI with $n_1 = 10$, $n_2 = 11$, and $T' = 69.5$, we find that the calculated T' value 69.5 is less than the tabulated value 73 for $P = 0.01$. Therefore, since the probability of the standard drug and test drug values being the same is less than 0.05 (actually, it is less than 0.01), we conclude that they are different. This test compares the medians of the two populations sampled. The median of an ordered set of observations is defined as the middlemost value for an odd number of observations, and as the average of the two middlemost values for an even number of observations. Thus, the median for the standard drug is $(130 + 148)/2 = 139$ and the median for the test drug is 103.

Signed-Rank Sum Test of Significance—The differences between the n paired values are ranked in order of absolute size from 1, for the lowest, to n, for the highest, ignoring zero differences. Tied values are assigned an average rank. After the differences are ranked, the signs of the differences are attached to the ranks, and the sum of the positive ranks and of the negative ranks are obtained. We enter Table VII with $n =$ the number of non-zero differences and the sum T of positive or negative ranks, whichever is smaller. When the calculated T is equal to or less than the tabled T, the null hypothesis is rejected at the significance level P.

Example X—The procedure is illustrated for data given in Example V:

Differences	Signed-Ranks
2	2
−3	−3
4	6
8	15
−4	−6

Differences	Signed-Ranks
6	12.5
−1	−1
−6	−12.5
5	10
4	6
4	6
0	ignore
5	10
7	14
4	6
5	10

Sum of positive ranks = 97.5
Sum of negative ranks = 22.5 = T
$n = 15$

Entering Table VII with $n = 15$ and $T = 22.5$, we find that the calculated T value 22.5 is less than the tabulated value 25 for $P = 0.05$. Therefore, since the probability of the morning and afternoon values being the same is less than 0.05, we conclude that they are different.

Statistical Sign Test of Significance—Count the number of positive differences (b) and the number of negative differences (c), ignoring zero differences, and calculate;

$$\chi^2 = \frac{(|b - c| - 1)^2}{b + c}$$

where $|b - c|$ is the absolute (ie, positive) difference $b - c$. This is referred to the chi-square table (see Table V) with

Table VII—The Signed-Rank Sum Table [a]

Values of T for Signed-Rank Test, Significant at the 10%, 5%, and 1% Levels

	P		
n	0.10	0.05	0.01
5	0		
6	2	0	
7	3	2	
8	5	3	0
9	8	5	1
10	10	8	3
11	14	10	5
12	17	13	7
13	21	17	9
14	25	21	12
15	30	25	16
16	35	29	19
17	41	34	23
18	47	40	27
19	53	46	32
20	60	52	37
21	67	58	43
22	75	65	49
23	83	73	55
24	91	81	61
25	100	89	68
26	110	97	75
27	120	106	83
28	130	116	91
29	141	126	100
30	152	136	109

when $n > 30$, use

$$T = n(n + 1)/4 - 1 - Z\sqrt{n(n + 1)(2n + 1)/24}$$

where Z is 1.64 for the 10% level, 1.96 for the 5%, and 2.58 for the 1%. The probability figures given are for a two-tailed test. For a one-tailed test, P is halved.

[a] Adapted from Tate and Clelland.[16]

$DF = 1$, the test being essentially the same as the chi-square test for correlated percentages illustrated in Example VIII.

Example XI—The procedure is illustrated for the data given in Examples V and X:

$$b = \text{number of positive differences} = 11$$

$$c = \text{number of negative differences} = 4$$

$$\chi^2 = \frac{(|b - c| - 1)^2}{b + c} = \frac{(|11 - 4| - 1)^2}{11 + 4} = \frac{36}{15} = 2.40$$

Table V shows that for one degree of freedom the probability of getting a value of χ^2 larger than the calculated value 2.40 is between $P = 0.10$ and $P = 0.20$. Since P is not equal to or less than 0.05, we conclude that there is insufficient evidence to indicate that the morning and afternoon values are different. This conclusion is not in agreement with that of the t test and the Signed-Rank test. The reason for this is that the Statistical Sign test considers only the sign of the difference and not the magnitude, and thus is a less sensitive test in borderline situations such as this one.

Hotelling's T^2 Test of Significance—This is a multivariate generalization of the t test. For example, if we measure standing and supine, systolic and diastolic blood pressure in two treated groups, we may want a single test of the null hypothesis that the two groups have the same average blood pressures with respect to all four measurements. The procedure is too complex to illustrate and discuss here for other than two variables, and the reader is referred to Hicks[17] for a more detailed discussion of the problem.

Example XII—Sitting systolic and diastolic blood pressure (mm Hg) was measured in 14 patients; in 7 patients after treatment with placebo, and in 7 patients after treatment with an antihypertensive drug. The blood pressure is recorded as systolic/diastolic and is symbolized as S/D.

$n_1 = 7$ Placebo	$n_2 = 7$ Drug
150/100	130/90
180/120	140/100
140/100	150/100
180/110	150/110
180/90	140/90
190/110	130/90
170/120	130/90

Variable		
S	$\Sigma S_1 = 1,190$	$\Sigma S_2 = 970$
	$\Sigma S_1^2 = 204,300$	$\Sigma S_2^2 = 134,900$
D	$\Sigma D_1 = 750$	$\Sigma D_2 = 670$
	$\Sigma D_1^2 = 81,100$	$\Sigma D_2^2 = 64,500$
S,D	$\Sigma S_1 D_1 = 127,900$	$\Sigma S_2 D_2 = 93,200$
S	$\overline{S}_1 = 1,190/7$	$\overline{S}_2 = 970/7$
	$= 170.0$	$= 138.6$
	$[S_1^2] = 204,300 -$	$[S_2^2] = 134,900 -$
	$(1,190)^2/7$	$(970)^2/7$
	$= 2000.00$	$= 485.71$
D	$\overline{D}_1 = 750/7$	$\overline{D}_2 = 670/7$
	$= 107.1$	$= 95.7$
	$[D_1^2] = 81,100 -$	$[D_2^2] = 64,500 -$
	$(750)^2/7$	$(670)^2/7$
	$= 742.86$	$= 371.43$
S,D	$[S_1 D_1] = 127,900 -$	$[S_2 D_2] = 93,200 -$
	$(1,190)(750)/7$	$(970)(670)/7$
	$= 400.00$	$= 357.14$

t test for systolic blood pressure alone:

$$t = \frac{\overline{S}_1 - \overline{S}_2}{\sqrt{\left(\frac{[S_1^2] + [S_2^2]}{n_1 + n_2 - 2}\right)\left(\frac{1}{n_1} + \frac{1}{n_2}\right)}} =$$

$$\frac{170.0 - 138.6}{\sqrt{\left(\frac{2000.00 + 485.71}{7 + 7 - 2}\right)\left(\frac{1}{7} + \frac{1}{7}\right)}} = 4.08$$

$$DF = n = n_1 + n_2 - 2 = 7 + 7 - 2 = 12$$

$$P < 0.01$$

t test for diastolic blood pressure alone:

$$t = \frac{\overline{D}_1 - \overline{D}_2}{\sqrt{\left(\frac{[D_1^2] + [D_2^2]}{n_1 + n_2 - 2}\right)\left(\frac{1}{n_1} + \frac{1}{n_2}\right)}} =$$

$$\frac{107.1 - 95.7}{\sqrt{\left(\frac{742.86 + 371.43}{7 + 7 - 2}\right)\left(\frac{1}{7} + \frac{1}{7}\right)}} = 2.19$$

$$DF = n = n_1 + n_2 - 2 = 7 + 7 - 2 = 12$$

$$0.02 < P < 0.05$$

T^2 test for both systolic and diastolic blood pressure:

$$d_1 = \frac{\overline{S}_1 - \overline{S}_2}{\sqrt{\frac{1}{n_1} + \frac{1}{n_2}}} = \frac{170.0 - 138.6}{\sqrt{\frac{1}{7} + \frac{1}{7}}} = 58.80$$

$$d_2 = \frac{\overline{D}_1 - \overline{D}_2}{\sqrt{\frac{1}{n_1} + \frac{1}{n_2}}} = \frac{107.1 - 95.7}{\sqrt{\frac{1}{7} + \frac{1}{7}}} = 21.35$$

$$a_{11} = \frac{1}{n}([S_1^2] + [S_2^2]) = \frac{1}{12}(2000.00 + 485.71) = 207.14$$

$$a_{12} = \frac{1}{n}([S_1 D_1] + [S_2 D_2]) = \frac{1}{12}(400.00 + 357.14) = 63.10$$

$$a_{22} = \frac{1}{n}([D_1^2] + [D_2^2]) = \frac{1}{12}(742.86 + 371.43) = 92.86$$

$$T^2 = \frac{d_1^2 a_{22} - 2 d_1 d_2 a_{12} + d_2^2 a_{11}}{a_{11} a_{22} - a_{12}^2}$$

$$= \frac{(58.80)^2(92.86) - 2(58.80)(21.35)(63.10) + (21.35)^2(207.14)}{(207.14)(92.86) - 3,981.61} = 16.85$$

In order to test the significance of this result, we make use of the fact that:

$$F = \left(\frac{n - p + 1}{np}\right) T^2 = \left[\frac{12 - 2 + 1}{(12)(2)}\right] (16.85) = 7.72$$

where p = number of variables = 2.

This follows the F distribution with degrees of freedom $f_1 = p = 2$, and $f_2 = n - p + 1 = 11$. We enter the F table (see Table VIII) with $f_1 = 2$, $f_2 = 11$, and $F = 7.72$, and find that the calculated F value 7.72 is larger than the interpolated F value 7.30 for $P = 0.01$. Therefore, since the probability of the average systolic and diastolic blood pressures of the placebo and drug-treated patients being the same is less than 0.05 (actually, it is less than 0.01), we conclude that they are different.

The F Test of Significance—To compare the variances of samples from two populations, the calculation is made:

$$F = s_1^2/s_2^2 \text{ with } s_1^2 > s_2^2$$

where:

$$s_1^2 = \frac{\Sigma x_{1i}^2 - (\Sigma x_{1i})^2/n_1}{n_1 - 1} = \text{larger variance}$$

$$s_2^2 = \frac{\Sigma x_{2i}^2 - (\Sigma x_{2i})^2/n_2}{n_2 - 1} = \text{smaller variance}$$

To test for significance, the F ratio is referred to the F table (see Table VIII) with $f_1 = n_1 - 1$ and $f_2 = n_2 - 1$ degrees of freedom. The null hypothesis that the two variances are the same is rejected at the $2P$ level of significance.

Example XIII—Two treatments showed the following results:

	A	B
	6	15
	4	4
	3	10
	7	10
	6	5
	4	11
		9
Σx_i	30	64
Σx_i^2	162	668
n_i	6	7
s_i^2	2.40	13.81
f_i	5	6

$$F = s_1^2/s_2^2 = 13.81/2.40 = 5.75$$

$$f_1 = n_1 - 1 = 7 - 1 = 6$$

$$f_2 = n_2 - 1 = 6 - 1 = 5$$

Entering Table VIII with $f_1 = 6$ and $f_2 = 5$ degrees of freedom, we find that the tabulated values of F are 4.95 and 6.98 for $P = 2 (0.05) = 0.10$ and $P = 2 (0.025) = 0.05$, respectively. Thus, the probability of getting a value of F larger than the calculated value 5.75 is between $P = 0.05$ and $P = 0.10$. Since P is not equal to or less than 0.05, we conclude that there is insufficient evidence to indicate that the two variances are different.

In the test described and exemplified above, both variances were identified as random sampling errors. In some situations (eg, analysis of variance described in Example XV), only one variance can be so identified. The F test then is made by always placing the random sampling error in the denominator, regardless of the size of the other variance. We then use the probability values directly from the F table and do not multiply them by 2.

If we desire to compare the variances from paired data, the F test described above would be inappropriate. Instead, we proceed as exemplified below.

Example XIV—A characteristic was measured before and after aging for each of ten items. Is the variability changed with aging?

Item no.	Before aging	After aging
1	8.3	9.3
2	8.4	10.9
3	14.9	13.2
4	14.2	12.8
5	12.5	16.0
6	15.0	15.2
7	17.1	16.8
8	19.2	16.2
9	22.0	17.9
10	18.9	18.9
	$\Sigma x_B = 148.5$	$\Sigma x_A = 147.2$

$$\Sigma x_B^2 = 2{,}393.81 \qquad \Sigma x_A^2 = 2{,}252.72$$

$$\Sigma x_B x_A = 2{,}298.92$$

$$[x_B^2] = 2{,}393.81 - (148.5)^2/10$$
$$= 188.59$$

$$[x_A^2] = 2{,}252.72 - (147.2)^2/10$$
$$= 85.94$$

$$[x_B x_A] = 2{,}298.92 - (148.5)(147.2)/10$$
$$= 113.00$$

$$t = \frac{([x_B^2] - [x_A^2])\sqrt{n - 2}}{2\sqrt{[x_B^2][x_A^2] - [x_B x_A]^2}} =$$

$$\frac{(188.59 - 85.94)\sqrt{8}}{2\sqrt{(188.59)(85.94) - (113.00)^2}} = 2.476$$

$$DF = n - 2 = 10 - 2 = 8$$

In the t table (see Table III), for $P = 0.05$ and $DF = 8$ (two tails), the value of t given is 2.306. The value of t calculated is greater than this. Therefore, since the probability of the variance before and after aging being the same is less than 0.05, we conclude that they are different. Apparently, the variability decreased after aging.

Multiple Comparison Procedures—If three or more samples are to be compared to see if they are all drawn from the same population, the analysis of variance (a sort of multiple t test) can be used as a means of comparison.

Example XV—Groups of three subjects each were given one of ten food regimens and showed the following weight gains (lb):

	A	B	C	D	E	F	G	H	I	J	(t = 10 regimens)
	2	1	2	4	9	3	6	7	4	4	
	3	2	4	8	8	8	5	6	4	6	
	2	0	1	7	11	6	6	6	7	6	
											Sums
Σx_i	7	3	7	19	28	17	17	19	15	16	$\Sigma x = 148$
Σx_i^2	17	5	21	129	266	109	97	121	81	88	$\Sigma x^2 = 934$
n_i	3	3	3	3	3	3	3	3	3	3	$N = 30$
$n_i - 1$	2	2	2	2	2	2	2	2	2	2	$\Sigma(n_i - 1) = 20$
$\bar{x}_i$	2.3	1.0	2.3	6.3	9.3	5.7	5.7	6.3	5.0	5.3	

Analysis of Variance

Source of variation	Degrees of freedom	Sums of squares	Mean squares	F ratio
Among regimens	$t - 1 = 9$	160.54	17.81	8.22
Within regimens	$\Sigma(n_i - 1) = 20$	43.33	$s^2 = 2.17$	
Total	$N - 1 = 29$	203.87		

These are unpaired data, and this type study is referred to as a completely randomized experiment. There are only two sources of variation; the variation among regimens and the variation within regimens, as indicated in the analysis of variance table. The breakdown of the degrees of freedom is self-explanatory. The sums of squares are obtained as follows:

$$\text{Total S.S.} = \Sigma x^2 - (\Sigma x)^2/N = 934 - (148)^2/30 = 203.87$$

Table VIII—The F Table [a]

10%, 5%, 2.5%, and 1% Points for the Distribution of F

		f_1 Degrees of freedom (for greater mean square)														
f_2	P	1	2	3	4	5	6	7	8	9	10	20	30	40	60	120	∞
5	0.10	4.06	3.78	3.62	3.52	3.45	3.40	3.37	3.34	3.32	3.30	3.21	3.17	3.16	3.14	3.12	3.10
	0.05	6.61	5.79	5.41	5.19	5.05	4.95	4.88	4.82	4.77	4.74	4.56	4.50	4.46	4.43	4.40	4.36
	0.025	10.01	8.43	7.76	7.39	7.15	6.98	6.85	6.76	6.68	6.62	6.33	6.23	6.18	6.12	6.07	6.02
	0.01	16.26	13.27	12.06	11.39	10.97	10.67	10.45	10.27	10.15	10.05	9.55	9.38	9.29	9.20	9.11	9.02
10	0.10	3.28	2.92	2.73	2.61	2.52	2.46	2.41	2.38	2.35	2.32	2.20	2.16	2.13	2.11	2.08	2.06
	0.05	4.96	4.10	3.71	3.48	3.33	3.22	3.14	3.07	3.02	2.98	2.77	2.70	2.66	2.62	2.58	2.54
	0.025	6.94	5.46	4.83	4.47	4.24	4.07	3.95	3.85	3.78	3.72	3.42	3.31	3.26	3.20	3.14	3.08
	0.01	10.04	7.56	6.55	5.99	5.64	5.39	5.21	5.06	4.95	4.85	4.41	4.25	4.17	4.08	4.00	3.91
15	0.10	3.07	2.70	2.49	2.36	2.27	2.21	2.16	2.12	2.09	2.06	1.92	1.87	1.85	1.82	1.79	1.76
	0.05	4.54	3.68	3.29	3.06	2.90	2.79	2.71	2.64	2.59	2.54	2.33	2.25	2.20	2.16	2.11	2.07
	0.025	6.20	4.76	4.15	3.80	3.58	3.41	3.29	3.20	3.12	3.06	2.76	2.64	2.58	2.52	2.46	2.40
	0.01	8.68	6.36	5.42	4.89	4.56	4.32	4.14	4.00	3.89	3.80	3.36	3.20	3.12	3.05	2.96	2.87
20	0.10	2.97	2.59	2.38	2.25	2.16	2.09	2.04	2.00	1.96	1.94	1.79	1.74	1.71	1.68	1.64	1.61
	0.05	4.35	3.49	3.10	2.87	2.71	2.60	2.51	2.45	2.39	2.35	2.12	2.04	1.99	1.95	1.90	1.84
	0.025	5.87	4.46	3.86	3.51	3.29	3.13	3.01	2.91	2.84	2.77	2.46	2.35	2.29	2.22	2.16	2.09
	0.01	8.10	5.85	4.94	4.43	4.10	3.87	3.71	3.56	3.45	3.37	2.94	2.77	2.69	2.61	2.52	2.42
25	0.10	2.92	2.53	2.32	2.18	2.09	2.02	1.97	1.93	1.89	1.87	1.72	1.66	1.63	1.59	1.56	1.52
	0.05	4.24	3.39	2.99	2.76	2.60	2.49	2.40	2.34	2.28	2.24	2.01	1.92	1.87	1.82	1.77	1.71
	0.025	5.69	4.29	3.69	3.35	3.13	2.97	2.85	2.75	2.68	2.61	2.30	2.18	2.12	2.05	1.98	1.91
	0.01	7.77	5.57	4.68	4.18	3.86	3.63	3.46	3.32	3.21	3.13	2.70	2.54	2.45	2.36	2.27	2.17
30	0.10	2.88	2.49	2.28	2.14	2.05	1.98	1.93	1.88	1.85	1.82	1.67	1.61	1.57	1.54	1.50	1.46
	0.05	4.17	3.32	2.92	2.69	2.53	2.42	2.33	2.27	2.21	2.16	1.93	1.84	1.79	1.74	1.68	1.62
	0.025	5.57	4.18	3.59	3.25	3.03	2.87	2.75	2.65	2.57	2.51	2.20	2.07	2.01	1.94	1.87	1.79
	0.01	7.56	5.39	4.51	4.02	3.70	3.47	3.30	3.17	3.06	2.98	2.55	2.38	2.29	2.21	2.11	2.01
40	0.10	2.84	2.44	2.23	2.09	2.00	1.93	1.87	1.83	1.79	1.76	1.61	1.54	1.51	1.47	1.42	1.38
	0.05	4.08	3.23	2.84	2.61	2.45	2.34	2.25	2.18	2.12	2.08	1.84	1.74	1.69	1.64	1.58	1.51
	0.025	5.42	4.05	3.46	3.13	2.90	2.74	2.62	2.53	2.45	2.39	2.07	1.94	1.88	1.80	1.72	1.64
	0.01	7.31	5.18	4.31	3.83	3.51	3.29	3.12	2.99	2.88	2.80	2.37	2.20	2.11	2.02	1.92	1.81
60	0.10	2.79	2.39	2.18	2.04	1.95	1.87	1.82	1.77	1.74	1.71	1.54	1.48	1.44	1.40	1.35	1.29
	0.05	4.00	3.15	2.76	2.53	2.37	2.25	2.17	2.10	2.04	1.99	1.75	1.65	1.59	1.53	1.47	1.39
	0.025	5.29	3.93	3.34	3.01	2.79	2.63	2.51	2.41	2.33	2.27	1.94	1.82	1.74	1.67	1.58	1.48
	0.01	7.08	4.98	4.13	3.65	3.34	3.12	2.95	2.82	2.72	2.63	2.20	2.03	1.93	1.84	1.73	1.60
120	0.10	2.75	2.35	2.13	1.99	1.90	1.82	1.77	1.72	1.68	1.65	1.48	1.41	1.37	1.32	1.26	1.19
	0.05	3.92	3.07	2.68	2.45	2.29	2.18	2.09	2.02	1.96	1.91	1.66	1.55	1.50	1.43	1.35	1.25
	0.025	5.15	3.80	3.23	2.89	2.67	2.52	2.39	2.30	2.22	2.16	1.82	1.69	1.61	1.53	1.43	1.31
	0.01	6.85	4.79	3.95	3.48	3.17	2.96	2.79	2.66	2.56	2.47	2.03	1.86	1.76	1.66	1.53	1.38
∞	0.10	2.71	2.30	2.08	1.94	1.85	1.77	1.72	1.67	1.63	1.60	1.42	1.34	1.30	1.24	1.17	1.00
	0.05	3.84	3.00	2.60	2.37	2.21	2.10	2.01	1.94	1.88	1.83	1.57	1.46	1.39	1.32	1.22	1.00
	0.025	5.02	3.69	3.12	2.79	2.57	2.41	2.29	2.19	2.11	2.05	1.71	1.57	1.48	1.39	1.27	1.00
	0.01	6.64	4.60	3.78	3.32	3.02	2.80	2.64	2.51	2.41	2.32	1.87	1.69	1.59	1.47	1.32	1.00

[a] Adapted from Snedecor and Cochran[18] and from Bliss and Calhoun.[19]

Among regimens S.S. $= \dfrac{(\Sigma x_1)^2}{n_1} + \dfrac{(\Sigma x_2)^2}{n_2} + \ldots + \dfrac{(\Sigma x_{10})^2}{n_{10}} - \dfrac{(\Sigma x)^2}{N}$

$= \dfrac{(7)^2}{3} + \dfrac{(3)^2}{3} + \ldots + \dfrac{(16)^2}{3} - \dfrac{(148)^2}{30}$

$= 160.54$

Within regimens S.S. $= 203.87 - 160.54 = 43.33$

The mean squares are obtained by dividing the sums of squares by their corresponding degrees of freedom. The mean square within regimens, s^2, is the pooled variance for the ten samples. Since this is the only variance that can be identified as random sampling error (the mean square among regimens has in addition a component due to the variability among regimens), it becomes the denominator in the F ratio, so that:

$$F = \frac{\text{mean square among regimens}}{\text{mean square within regimens}} = \frac{17.81}{2.17} = 8.22$$

To test for significance, the F ratio is referred to the F table (see Table VIII) with $f_1 = t - 1 = 9$ and $f_2 = \Sigma(n_i - 1) = 20$ degrees of freedom. We find that the calculated value 8.22 is larger than the tabulated value 3.45 for $P = 0.01$. Therefore, since the probability of these ten samples being drawn from the same population is less than 0.05 (actually, it is less than 0.01), we conclude that they are not all the same (i.e., not all the means are equal).

However, this conclusion in itself is not very helpful. One is generally interested in making multiple comparisons, to determine which means are different from each other and which are not. The general procedure is to list the ranked means from lowest to highest and underline the means which are not statistically significantly different from each other. Sometimes brackets or parentheses are used instead of an underline. The procedure is carried out by calculating a 5% allowance, which is defined as the critical difference between means which allows one to reject the null hypothesis ($\mu_i = \mu_j$) and accept the alternative hypothesis ($\mu_i \neq \mu_j$) for any two sample means $\bar{x}_i$ and $\bar{x}_j$ at $P = 0.05$. To calculate the 5% allowance we need the following:

s^2 = pooled variance from the analysis of variance.

DF = degrees of freedom for the pooled variance from the analysis of variance.

n_i, n_j = the number of observations from which the means $\bar{x}_i$ and $\bar{x}_j$ were determined, respectively.

t = a critical value at $P = 0.05$ which depends upon the DF and the degree of conservatism desired as exemplified by the multiple comparison procedures described below:

Least Significant Difference Procedure—For this procedure:

$$\text{5\% allowance} = t \sqrt{s^2(1/n_i + 1/n_j)}$$

where t is the value of t from Table III (two tails). This is the least conservative procedure, and assures that the probability that any one comparison is judged to be significant by chance alone is 5%. However, the probability of one or more comparisons being judged significant would be greater than 5%. Applied to the results of Example XV, we have:

$$s^2 = 2.17$$

$$n_i, n_j = 3,3$$

$$DF = 20$$

Table IX—The Q Table[a]

Upper 5% Points, Q, in the Studentized Range

DF	2	3	4	5	6	7	8	9	10	11	12	13	14	15	16	17	18	19	20
												k (Number of treatments)							
10	3.15	3.88	4.33	4.66	4.91	5.12	5.30	5.46	5.60	5.72	5.83	5.93	6.03	6.12	6.20	6.27	6.34	6.41	6.47
11	3.11	3.82	4.26	4.58	4.82	5.03	5.20	5.35	5.49	5.61	5.71	5.81	5.90	5.98	6.06	6.14	6.20	6.27	6.33
12	3.08	3.77	4.20	4.51	4.75	4.95	5.12	5.27	5.40	5.51	5.61	5.71	5.80	5.88	5.95	6.02	6.09	6.15	6.21
13	3.06	3.73	4.15	4.46	4.69	4.88	5.05	5.19	5.32	5.43	5.53	5.63	5.71	5.79	5.86	5.93	6.00	6.06	6.11
14	3.03	3.70	4.11	4.41	4.64	4.83	4.99	5.13	5.25	5.36	5.46	5.56	5.64	5.72	5.79	5.86	5.92	5.98	6.03
15	3.01	3.67	4.08	4.37	4.59	4.78	4.94	5.08	5.20	5.31	5.40	5.49	5.57	5.65	5.72	5.79	5.85	5.91	5.96
16	3.00	3.65	4.05	4.34	4.56	4.74	4.90	5.03	5.15	5.26	5.35	5.44	5.52	5.59	5.66	5.73	5.79	5.84	5.90
17	2.98	3.62	4.02	4.31	4.52	4.70	4.86	4.99	5.11	5.21	5.31	5.39	5.47	5.55	5.61	5.68	5.74	5.79	5.84
18	2.97	3.61	4.00	4.28	4.49	4.67	4.83	4.96	5.07	5.17	5.27	5.35	5.43	5.50	5.57	5.63	5.69	5.74	5.79
19	2.96	3.59	3.98	4.26	4.47	4.64	4.79	4.92	5.04	5.14	5.23	5.32	5.39	5.46	5.53	5.59	5.65	5.70	5.75
20	2.95	3.58	3.96	4.24	4.45	4.62	4.77	4.90	5.01	5.11	5.20	5.28	5.36	5.43	5.50	5.56	5.61	5.66	5.71
24	2.92	3.53	3.90	4.17	4.37	4.54	4.68	4.81	4.92	5.01	5.10	5.18	5.25	5.32	5.38	5.44	5.50	5.55	5.59
30	2.89	3.48	3.84	4.11	4.30	4.46	4.60	4.72	4.83	4.92	5.00	5.08	5.15	5.21	5.27	5.33	5.38	5.43	5.48
40	2.86	3.44	3.79	4.04	4.23	4.39	4.52	4.63	4.74	4.82	4.90	4.98	5.05	5.11	5.17	5.22	5.27	5.32	5.36
60	2.83	3.40	3.74	3.98	4.16	4.31	4.44	4.55	4.65	4.73	4.81	4.88	4.94	5.00	5.06	5.11	5.15	5.20	5.24
120	2.80	3.36	3.69	3.92	4.10	4.24	4.36	4.47	4.56	4.64	4.71	4.78	4.84	4.90	4.95	5.00	5.04	5.09	5.13
∞	2.77	3.32	3.63	3.86	4.03	4.17	4.29	4.39	4.47	4.55	4.62	4.68	4.74	4.80	4.84	4.89	4.93	4.97	5.01

[a] Adapted from Snedecor and Cochran.[18]

$t = 2.086$ from Table III for 20 DF and $P = 0.05$ (two tails)

5% allowance $= t \sqrt{s^2(1/n_i + 1/n_j)} =$

$$2.086 \sqrt{2.17(1/3 + 1/3)} = 2.51$$

Thus, any two means differing by 2.51 or more are judged to be different.

Ranked Means

B	A,C		I	J	F,G	D,H		E
1.0	2.3		5.0	5.3	5.7	6.3		9.3

or, $(BAC) \ (IJFGDH) \ (E)$.

Any two means underscored by the same line (or included in the same parentheses) do not differ statistically at $P = 0.05$.

Any two means *not* underscored by the same line (or *not* included in the same parentheses) are statistically significantly different at $P \leq 0.05$.

Studentized Range Procedure—For this method

$$5\% \text{ allowance} = \frac{Q}{\sqrt{2}} \sqrt{s^2(1/n_i + 1/n_j)}$$

where Q is the Studentized Range value for k treatments from Table IX. This is one of the most conservative procedures, and assures that the probability of one or more comparisons being judged significant by chance alone is 5%. Applied to the results of Example XV, we have:

$Q = 5.01$ from Table IX for $k = 10$ treatments, 20 DF, and $P = 0.05$.

5% allowance $= \dfrac{Q}{\sqrt{2}} \sqrt{s^2(1/n_i + 1/n_j)} =$

$$\frac{5.01}{\sqrt{2}} \sqrt{2.17(1/3 + 1/3)} = 4.26$$

Thus, any two means differing by 4.26 or more are judged to be different.

Ranked Means

B	A,C		I	J	F,G	D,H		E
1.0	2.3		5.0	5.3	5.7	6.3		9.3

or, $(BACI) \ (ACIJFGDH) \ (JFGDHE)$.

Duncan's New Multiple Range Procedure—For this method:

$$5\% \text{ allowance} = \frac{t_k}{\sqrt{2}} \sqrt{s^2(1/n_i + 1/n_j)}$$

where t_k are values for 2,3, - - - - , k treatments obtained from Table X. The critical values will be $A_2, A_3, \text{- - - -}, A_k$, depending upon how many means are included in the range of ranked means being compared. This is next to the least conservative procedure. Applied to the results of Example XV, we have:

5% allowance $= \dfrac{t_k}{\sqrt{2}} \sqrt{s^2(1/n_i + 1/n_j)} =$

$$\frac{t_k}{\sqrt{2}} \sqrt{2.17(1/3 + 1/3)}$$

Table X—The Multiple Range Table[a]

Values of t_k for Duncan's New Multiple Range Test at the 5% Level of Significance

DF	2	3	4	5	6	8	10	14	20
				k (Number of treatments)					
10	3.15	3.30	3.37	3.43	3.46	3.47	3.47	3.47	3.48
12	3.08	3.23	3.33	3.36	3.40	3.44	3.46	3.46	3.48
14	3.03	3.18	3.27	3.33	3.37	3.41	3.44	3.46	3.47
16	3.00	3.15	3.23	3.30	3.34	3.39	3.43	3.45	3.47
18	2.97	3.12	3.21	3.27	3.32	3.37	3.41	3.45	3.47
20	2.95	3.10	3.18	3.25	3.30	3.36	3.40	3.44	3.47
24	2.92	3.07	3.15	3.22	3.28	3.34	3.38	3.44	3.47
30	2.89	3.04	3.12	3.20	3.25	3.32	3.37	3.43	3.47
60	2.83	2.98	3.08	3.14	3.20	3.28	3.33	3.40	3.47
100	2.80	2.95	3.05	3.12	3.18	3.26	3.32	3.40	3.47
∞	2.77	2.92	3.02	3.09	3.15	3.23	3.29	3.38	3.47

[a] Adapted from Duncan.[20]

Table XI—The t_D Table [a]

Values of t_D for Dunnett's Procedure for Comparing Several Treatments with a Control at the 5% Level of Significance
(Use $P = 0.10$ values for a one-tailed test and $P = 0.05$ values for a two-tailed test)

DF	P	\multicolumn{8}{c}{k (Number of treatments, excluding the control)}							
		2	3	4	5	6	7	8	9
10	0.10	2.15	2.34	2.47	2.56	2.64	2.70	2.76	2.81
	0.05	2.57	2.76	2.89	2.99	3.07	3.14	3.19	3.24
11	0.10	2.13	2.31	2.44	2.53	2.60	2.67	2.72	2.77
	0.05	2.53	2.72	2.84	2.94	3.02	3.08	3.14	3.19
12	0.10	2.11	2.29	2.41	2.50	2.58	2.64	2.69	2.74
	0.05	2.50	2.68	2.81	2.90	2.98	3.04	3.09	3.14
13	0.10	2.09	2.27	2.39	2.48	2.55	2.61	2.66	2.71
	0.05	2.48	2.65	2.78	2.87	2.94	3.00	3.06	3.10
14	0.10	2.08	2.25	2.37	2.46	2.53	2.59	2.64	2.69
	0.05	2.46	2.63	2.75	2.84	2.91	2.97	3.02	3.07
15	0.10	2.07	2.24	2.36	2.44	2.51	2.57	2.62	2.67
	0.05	2.44	2.61	2.73	2.82	2.89	2.95	3.00	3.04
16	0.10	2.06	2.23	2.34	2.43	2.50	2.56	2.61	2.65
	0.05	2.42	2.59	2.71	2.80	2.87	2.92	2.97	3.02
17	0.10	2.05	2.22	2.33	2.42	2.49	2.54	2.59	2.64
	0.05	2.41	2.58	2.69	2.78	2.85	2.90	2.95	3.00
18	0.10	2.04	2.21	2.32	2.41	2.48	2.53	2.58	2.62
	0.05	2.40	2.56	2.68	2.76	2.83	2.89	2.94	2.98
19	0.10	2.03	2.20	2.31	2.40	2.47	2.52	2.57	2.61
	0.05	2.39	2.55	2.66	2.75	2.81	2.87	2.92	2.96
20	0.10	2.03	2.19	2.30	2.39	2.46	2.51	2.56	2.60
	0.05	2.38	2.54	2.65	2.73	2.80	2.86	2.90	2.95
24	0.10	2.01	2.17	2.28	2.36	2.43	2.48	2.53	2.57
	0.05	2.35	2.51	2.61	2.70	2.76	2.81	2.86	2.90
30	0.10	1.99	2.15	2.25	2.33	2.40	2.45	2.50	2.54
	0.05	2.32	2.47	2.58	2.66	2.72	2.77	2.82	2.86
40	0.10	1.97	2.13	2.23	2.31	2.37	2.42	2.47	2.51
	0.05	2.29	2.44	2.54	2.62	2.68	2.73	2.77	2.81
60	0.10	1.95	2.10	2.21	2.28	2.35	2.39	2.44	2.48
	0.05	2.27	2.41	2.51	2.58	2.64	2.69	2.73	2.77
120	0.10	1.93	2.08	2.18	2.26	2.32	2.37	2.41	2.45
	0.05	2.24	2.38	2.47	2.55	2.60	2.65	2.69	2.73
∞	0.10	1.92	2.06	2.16	2.23	2.29	2.34	2.38	2.42
	0.05	2.21	2.35	2.44	2.51	2.57	2.61	2.65	2.69

[a] Adapted from Dunnett.[21,44]

Values of t_k from Table X for $k = 2$ to 10 treatments, 20 *DF*, and $P = 0.05$ give the following allowances:

k	t_k	A_k
2	2.95	2.51
3	3.10	2.64
4	3.18	2.70
5	3.25	2.76
6	3.30	2.81
7	3.34	2.84
8	3.36	2.86
9	3.38	2.87
10	3.40	2.89

Thus, the critical difference between E and B is 2.89 because the range includes ten means; the critical difference between E and H is 2.64 because the range includes three means; etc.

Ranked Means

B	A,C		I	J	F,G	D,H		E
1.0	2.3		5.0	5.3	5.7	6.3		9.3

or, (BAC) $(IJFGDH)$ (E).

Dunnett's Procedure—The three procedures previously described are appropriate when it is desired to compare all possible pairs of means. Dunnett considered the problem when the objective of the study is to compare several treatments with a standard or control. In his method

$$5\% \text{ allowance} = t_D \sqrt{s^2(1/n_i + 1/n_j)}$$

where t_D is Dunnett's t_D value for k treatments (excluding the standard or control) obtained from Table XI. Like the Stu-

dentized Range procedure, this is one of the most conservative procedures, and assures that the probability of one or more comparisons between treatments and a standard or control being judged significant by chance alone is 5%. The one-tail values (listed in tables for $P = 0.10$) are used when the objective of the study is to select only those treatments that have higher (or lower) means than the standard or control; the two-tail values (listed in the table for $P = 0.05$) are used when the objective of the study is to select those treatments that are different from the standard or control. Of course, the decision to carry out a one-tailed or a two-tailed test must be made before the study begins.

In Example XV, suppose J is a standard regimen, and it is desired to determine which regimens show different weight gains from J. We would proceed as follows:

$t_D = 3.07$ from Table XI for $k = 9$ treatments, 20 *DF*, and $P = 0.05$ (two-tails)

$$5\% \text{ allowance} = t_D \sqrt{s^2(1/n_i + 1/n_j)} =$$
$$3.07 \sqrt{2.17(1/3 + 1/3)} = 3.68$$

Thus, any regimen mean that differs from the mean for regimen J by 3.68 or more is judged to be different from J.

Ranked Means

B	A,C	I	J	F,G	D,H	E
1.0	2.3	5.0	5.3	5.7	6.3	9.3

We would conclude that B showed a statistically significant smaller weight gain than J, that E showed a statistically significantly larger weight gain than J, and that there was insufficient evidence to indicate that the other regimens were different from J.

In the same example, if regimen A is a control group and we knew beforehand that all of the other regimens had to be at least as good as the control or better, it may be desired to select those regimens that are statistically significantly better. We would proceed as follows:

$t_D = 2.60$ from Table XI for $k = 9$ treatments, 20 DF, and $P = 0.10$ (this corresponds to a one-tail $P = 0.05$)

5% allowance $= t_D \sqrt{s^2(1/n_i + 1/n_j)} =$
$$2.60 \sqrt{2.17(1/3 + 1/3)} = 3.12$$

Thus, any regimen mean that is larger than the mean for regimen A by 3.12 or more is judged to be better than A.

Ranked Means

B	A,C	I	J	F,G	D,H	E
1.0	2.3	5.0	5.3	5.7	6.3	9.3

It can be concluded that $F, G, D, H,$ and E showed a statistically significantly better weight gain than A, and that there is insufficient evidence to indicate that $B, C, I,$ and J were any better than A.

Comparison of Several Variances—The multiple comparison procedures discussed previously can be used also to compare three or more variances. The procedure is illustrated below for data given by Finney,[22] and applying Duncan's New Multiple Range test to an analysis of variance procedure suggested by Levene.[23]

To test for significance, the F ratio is referred to the F table (see Table VIII) with $f_1 = t - 1 = 3$ and $f_2 = \Sigma(n_i - 1) = 34$ degrees of freedom. We see that the calculated value 8.12 is larger than the tabulated value 4.4 (interpolated from the values 4.51 and 4.31 for $f_1, f_2 = 3,30$ and 3,40, respectively) for $P = 0.01$.

Therefore, since the probability of these four results being drawn from the same population is less than 0.05 (actually, it is less than 0.01), we conclude that they are not all the same. To apply Duncan's New Multiple Range test, we need:

$s \quad = \sqrt{1.6129} = 1.270$
$k \quad = $ number of variances $= 4$
$DF = 34$
$t_k \quad = $ values interpolated from Table X for $k = 2$ to 4 variances, 34 DF, and $P = 0.05$
$R_k \quad = t_k s = $ critical values for ranges of 2 to 4 ranked means.

Then, these give the critical values R_k:

k	(2)	(3)	(4)
t_k	2.88	3.03	3.11
R_k	3.658	3.848	3.950

The ranked $\overline{Z}_i$ and replication numbers are:

A	D	B	C
1.604	1.924	3.305	4.244
(11)	(9)	(11)	(7)

We next calculate:
$$(\overline{Z}_i - \overline{Z}_j)' = (\overline{Z}_i - \overline{Z}_j) \sqrt{2(n_i n_j)/(n_i + n_j)}$$

Thus, for $C - A$, it follows that:

Dose
(International Units of vitamin D)

	A (0.64)		B (1.28)		C (2.15)		D (4.30)		(t = 4 doses)
x	Z	x	Z	x	Z	x	Z	
2	0.64	4	3.36	8	4.29	14	2.56	
0	2.64	9	1.64	17	4.71	14	2.56	
2	0.64	4	3.36	6	6.29	13	3.56	
4	1.36	13	5.64	14	1.71	19	2.44	
0	2.64	3	4.36	17	4.71	17	0.44	
5	2.36	7	0.36	16	3.71	17	0.44	
3	0.36	4	3.36	8	4.29	20	3.44	
4	1.36	4	3.36			18	1.44	
2	0.64	10	2.64			17	0.44	
6	3.36	12	4.64					
1	1.64	11	3.64					Sums
Σx_i	29		81	86		149			
n_i	11		11	7		9		$N = 38$
$\overline{x}_i$	2.64		7.36	12.29		16.56		
ΣZ_i	17.64		36.36		29.71		17.32	$\Sigma Z = 101.03$
ΣZ_i^2	38.5456		140.5456		137.4287		46.2224	$\Sigma Z^2 = 362.7423$
$\overline{Z}_i$	1.604		3.305		4.244		1.924	
$n_i - 1$	10		10		6		8	$\Sigma(n_i - 1) = 34$

The procedure also illustrates the modifications required for Duncan's New Multiple Range test when $n_i \neq n_j$ (ie, unequal number of observations in each sample).

Example XVI—Line test scores (bounded so that they could only vary from 0 to 24) were obtained in groups of rachitic rats given four graded doses of Vitamin D. There was some indication that rats on the lowest and on the highest dose varied less than rats on the two middle doses. Are these differences statistically significant? where:

$x_i = $ the individual line test scores

$Z_i = |x_i - \overline{x}_i| = $ the individual absolute (ie, positive) differences between the line test scores in a dose group, and the average line test score for that group.

An analysis of variance is carried out using the Z's in exactly the same manner as was described in Example XV.

Analysis of variance (Z's)

Source of variation	DF	S.S.	M.S.	F
Among doses	$t - 1 = $ 3	39.2967	13.0989	8.12
Within doses	$\Sigma(n_i - 1) = 34$	54.8387	$s^2 = $ 1.6129	
Total	$N - 1 = 37$	94.1354		

$(C - A)' = (C - A) \sqrt{2(n_i n_j)/(n_i + n_j)} =$
$$(4.244 - 1.604) \sqrt{2(7)(11)/18} = 7.719$$

Similarly, for the other differences we obtain:

$$(C - D)' = 6.510$$
$$(C - B)' = 2.746$$
$$(B - A)' = 5.642$$
$$(B - D)' = 4.345$$
$$(D - A)' = 1.007$$

To test for significance, we compare these to the critical values R_k:

Test sequences	Result
1. $(C - A)' > R_4, (C - D)' > R_3, (C - B)' \ne R_2$	(BC)
2. $(B - A)' > R_3, (B - D)' > R_2$	
3. $(D - A)' \ne R_2$	(AD)

The final result is: $(AD)(BC)$

The interpretation is that doses A and D have the same variances, doses B and C have the same variances, and doses A and D have smaller variances than doses B and C.

Linear Correlation and Linear Regression—Thus far problems involving only a single measurement or variable per test unit have been considered. There are many problems involving the relation between two or more variables measured in the same unit. For simplicity, only linear relations between two variables will be discussed. The procedures are usually referred to as linear correlation (or simply, correlation) and linear regression (or simple regression). Discussions involving several variables and non-linear relations may be found in Snedecor and Cochran[18].

There are two distinct types of problems or relations. In one type, exemplified by the stature of fathers and sons, there is no mathematical relation between the two variables. In this type problem one is interested usually in determining the direction and degree or strength of the relationship between the two variables and in estimating a value of either in terms of the other. Although a strong association may be observed, this does not necessarily imply that a cause and effect relation exists. In the second type, there is a mathematical relationship between the two variables, one of which is designated the independent variable (usually considered to be measured without error) and the other the dependent variable. An example of the latter would be the response observed (dependent variable) for graded doses (independent variable) of a drug.

Example XVII—To illustrate a problem of the first type, consider the data given in example XIV on page 118. In that problem measures made in ten items before aging (x_B) and after aging (x_A) are given:

Item no.	x_B	x_A
1	8.3	9.3
2	8.4	10.9
3	14.9	13.2
4	14.2	12.8
5	12.5	16.0
6	15.0	15.2
7	17.1	16.8
8	19.2	16.2
9	22.0	17.9
10	18.9	18.9
	$\Sigma x_B = 148.5$	$\Sigma x_A = 147.2$

$$\Sigma x_B{}^2 = 2{,}393.81 \quad \Sigma x_A{}^2 = 2{,}252.72$$

$$\Sigma x_B x_A = 2{,}298.92$$

Then

$$[x_B{}^2] = \Sigma x_B{}^2 - (\Sigma x_B)^2/n$$

$$= 2{,}393.81 - (148.5)^2/10$$

$$= 188.59$$

$$[x_A{}^2] = \Sigma x_A{}^2 - (\Sigma x_A)^2/n$$

$$= 2{,}252.72 - (147.2)^2/10$$

$$= 85.94$$

$$[x_B x_A] = \Sigma x_B x_A - (\Sigma x_B)(\Sigma x_A)/n$$

$$= 2{,}298.92 - (148.5)(147.2)/10$$

$$= 113.00$$

The sign of $[x_B x_A]$ determines the direction of the relationship between x_B and x_A. In this example, the sign is positive, indicating a positive relation between x_B and x_A.

The association or correlation between x_B and x_A is measured by the correlation coefficient:

$$r = [x_B x_A]/\sqrt{[x_B{}^2][x_A{}^2]}$$

$$= +113.00/\sqrt{(188.59)(85.94)}$$

$$= +0.89$$

The value of r can vary from -1 (indicating perfect negative correlation), through 0 (indicating no correlation), to $+1$ (indicating perfect positive correlation). The value of the correlation coefficient has no physical dimension.

A more quantitative measure of association is the slope or regression coefficient, which measures the change in value of one variable per unit change of the other variable. There are two regression coefficients, $b_{x_B \cdot x_A}$ and $b_{x_A \cdot x_B}$. The two slopes are not the same, except when $r = \pm1$. They are estimated from:

$$b_{x_A \cdot x_B} = [x_B x_A]/[x_A{}^2]$$

$$= 113.0/85.94 = 1.3149$$

$$= \text{change in } x_B \text{ per unit change in } x_A$$

$$b_{x_A \cdot x_B} = [x_B x_A]/[x_B{}^2]$$

$$= 113.0/188.59 = 0.5992$$

$$= \text{change in } x_A \text{ per unit change in } x_B$$

To test whether the correlation coefficient (or equivalently, either slope) is statistically significantly different from zero, the following procedure is employed:

$$s^2{}_{x_A \cdot x_B} = \frac{[x_B{}^2] - [x_B x_A]^2/[x_A{}^2]}{n - 2}$$

$$= \frac{188.59 - (113.0)^2/85.94}{8} = 5.0012$$

$$s^2{}_{x_A \cdot x_B} = \frac{[x_A{}^2] - [x_B x_A]^2/[x_B{}^2]}{n - 2}$$

$$= \frac{85.94 - (113.0)^2/188.59}{8} = 2.2790$$

$$s^2{}_{b_{x_B \cdot x_A}} = s^2{}_{x_B \cdot x_A}/[x_A{}^2]$$

$$= 5.0012/85.94 = 0.0582$$

$$s^2{}_{b_{x_A \cdot x_B}} = s^2{}_{x_A \cdot x_B}/[x_B{}^2]$$

$$= 2.2790/188.59 = 0.0121$$

The t-tests are carried out as follows

$$t = b_{x_B \cdot x_A}/\sqrt{s^2{}_{b_{x_B \cdot x_A}}}$$

$$= 1.3149/\sqrt{0.0582} = 5.45$$

$$t = b_{x_A \cdot x_B}/\sqrt{s^2{}_{b_{x_A \cdot x_B}}}$$

$$= 0.5992/\sqrt{0.0121} = 5.45$$

$$DF = n - 2 = 10 - 2 = 8$$

In the t table (see Table III), for $P = 0.05$ (two tails) and $DF = 8$, the value of t given is 2.306. The value of t calculated is greater than this. Therefore, since the probability of the correlation coefficient (or either slope) being equal to zero is less than 0.05 (actually, it is less than 0.01), it can be concluded that it is (and the slopes are) different from zero. Values of x_B are positively correlated with values of x_A (and vice versa).

To determine the proportion of the variance of x_B that can be attributed to the linear regression on x_A, the calculation is:

$$r^2 = (0.89)^2 = 0.79 \text{ or } 79\%$$

The same would be true for x_A.

It may be desired to plot the values of x_A vs x_B as in Fig. 10-11. Note that separate regression lines are plotted; one for estimating values after storage (A) from those before storage, the other for estimating values before storage (B) from those after storage. The least squares regression lines are given by:

$$\hat{x}_A = \bar{x}_A + b_{x_A \cdot x_B}(x_B - \bar{x}_B)$$

$$= 147.2/10 + 0.5992(x_B - 148.5/10)$$

$$= 5.82 + 0.5992\, x_B$$

$$\hat{x}_B = \bar{x}_B + b_{x_B \cdot x_A}(x_A - \bar{x}_A)$$

$$= 148.5/10 + 1.3149\,(x_A - 147.2/10)$$

$$= -4.51 + 1.3149\, x_A$$

These are called least squares regression lines because they are derived mathematically in such a manner that the sums of squares of the differences between observed and estimated values will be at a minimum.

For clarity, and to conserve space, 95% confidence limits will be estimated and illustrated for x_A only. The variance for an *average* estimated value of x_A for a given value of x_B is given by:

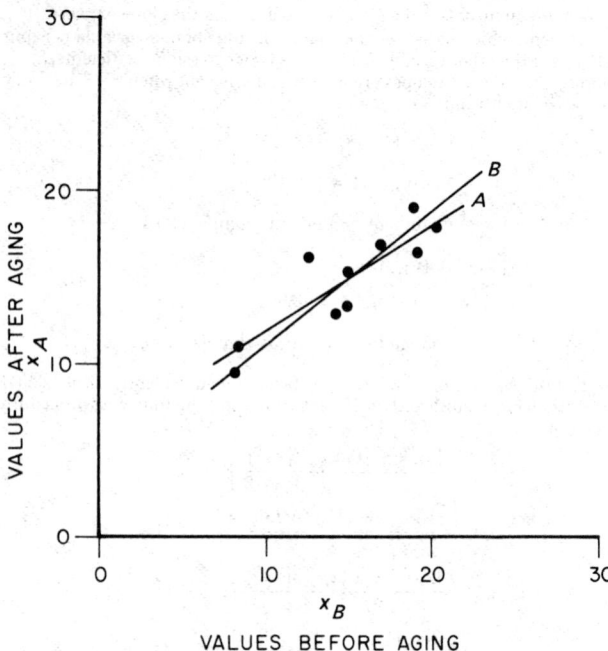

Fig 10-11.   Regression lines for measure in ten items before and after aging.

$$s^2_{\hat{x}_A} = s^2_{x_A \cdot x_B}\{1/n + (x_B - \bar{x}_B)^2/[x_B{}^2]\}$$

Thus, for $x_B = 10$, $\hat{x}_A = 5.82 + 0.5992(10) = 11.8$

$$s^2_{\hat{x}_A} = 2.2790\,[1/10 + (10 - 14.85)^2/188.59] = 0.5122$$

The 95% confidence limits are given by:

$$\hat{x}_L, \hat{x}_U = \hat{x}_A \pm 0.05t_8\sqrt{s^2_{\hat{x}_A}}$$

$$= 11.8 \pm 2.306\,\sqrt{0.5122} = 11.8 \pm 1.7 = 10.1, 13.5$$

Similar calculations for other values of x_B will give the inner parabolic confidence lines shown in Fig 10-12.

The variance of a *single* new estimate of x_A for a given value of x_B is given by:

$$s^2_{\hat{x}_A} = s^2_{x_A \cdot x_B}\{1 + 1/n + (x_B - \bar{x}_B)^2/[x_B{}^2]\}$$

$$= 2.2790\,[1 + 1/10 + (10 - 14.85)^2/188.59] = 2.7912$$

The 95% confidence limits are given by

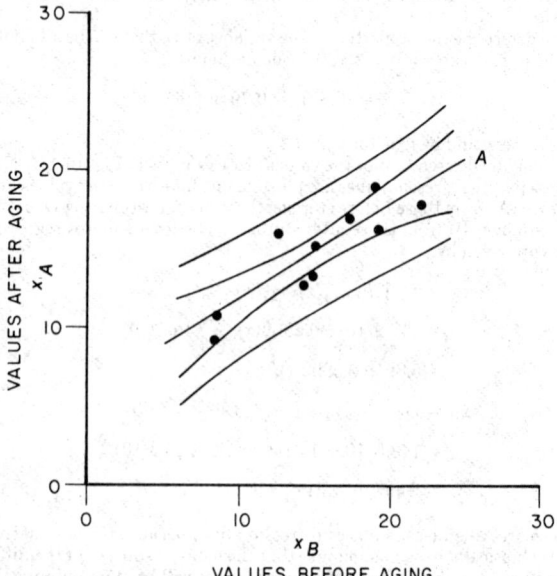

Fig 10-12.   Regression line and 95% confidence limits for determining values after storage from those before storage.

$$\hat{x}_L, \hat{x}_U = 11.8 \pm 2.306\sqrt{2.7912} = 11.8 \pm 3.9 = 7.9, 15.7$$

Similar calculations for other values of x_B will give the outer parabolic confidence lines shown in Fig 10-12. These limits should include 95% of all observed individual values.

Example XVIII—To illustrate a problem of the second type, consider the following measures of the reciprocal log virus titer (y) for purified polio virus Type I at various hours (x) of inactivation.

Reciprocal log Virus Titer	Time in Hours
y	x
8.1	0
5.9	17
5.7	24
4.7	30
3.6	41.25
2.8	47.5
$\Sigma y = 30.8$	$\Sigma x = 159.75$

$$n = 6$$

$$\bar{y} = 5.1333 \quad \bar{x} = 26.625$$

$$\Sigma y^2 = 175.80 \quad \Sigma x^2 = 5722.8125$$

$$\Sigma xy = 659.6$$

$$[y^2] = \Sigma y^2 - (\Sigma y)^2/n = 175.80 - (30.8)^2/6 = 17.6933$$

$$[x^2] = \Sigma x^2 - (\Sigma x)^2/n = 5722.8125 - (159.75)^2/6 = 1469.4688$$

$$[xy] = \Sigma xy - (\Sigma x)(\Sigma y)/n = 659.6 - (159.75)(30.8)/6$$

$$= -160.45$$

In this illustration, x is assumed to be measured without error, and is referred to as the independent variable, while y is subject to statistical variation, and is referred to as the dependent variable.

The sign of $[xy]$ is negative, indicating a negative relation between y and x; the y values decrease with increasing values of x.

The slope of the least squares regression line is estimated from:

$$b = b_{y \cdot x} = \text{slope} = [xy]/[x^2]$$

$$= -160.45/1469.4688 = -0.1092$$

Thus, the reciprocal log virus titer is estimated to decrease by 0.1092 units per hour of inactivation.

The y intercept (ie, the value of y at $x = 0$) is estimated from:

$$a = \bar{y} - b\bar{x} = 5.1333 - (-0.1092)(26.625)$$

$$= 8.0408$$

The regression line is given by:

$$\hat{y} = \bar{y} + b(x - \bar{x}) = \bar{y} - b\bar{x} + bx = a + bx$$

$$= 8.0408 - 0.1092x$$

and is shown plotted in Fig. 10-13.

The results may be summarized in a regression analysis table:

Sources of variation	Regression analysis			
	DF	S.S.	M.S	F
Linear Regression	1	17.5194	17.5194	403
Residual Error	4	0.1739	$0.0435 = s^2_{y \cdot x}$	
Total	5	17.6933		

The degrees of freedom for total, linear regression and residual error are $n - 1$, 1, and $n - 2$, respectively. The sums of squares for total, linear regression and residual error are given by $[y^2]$, $[xy]^2/[x^2]$, and $[y^2] - [xy]^2/[x^2]$, respectively.

Entering Table VIII with $f_1 = 1$ and $f_2 = 4$ degrees of freedom, we find that tabulated values of F are not shown for f_2 less than 5. However, when $f_1 = 1$, we can make use of the relation that $t = \sqrt{F} = \sqrt{403} = 20.075$. In the t table (see Table III), for $P = 0.05$ (two tails) and $DF = 4$, the value of t given is 2.776. The value of t calculated is greater than this. Therefore, since the probability of the slope being equal to zero is less than 0.05 (actually, it is less than 0.01), it is concluded to be different from zero.

In problems of this type, the investigator usually is interested in estimating the value of x for a given value of y. Unlike problems of the first type, it is not necessary to determine x from a separate slope of the relation of x upon y. Instead, estimation is made by inverse interpolation from:

$$\hat{x} = \bar{x} + \frac{x - \bar{y}}{b}$$

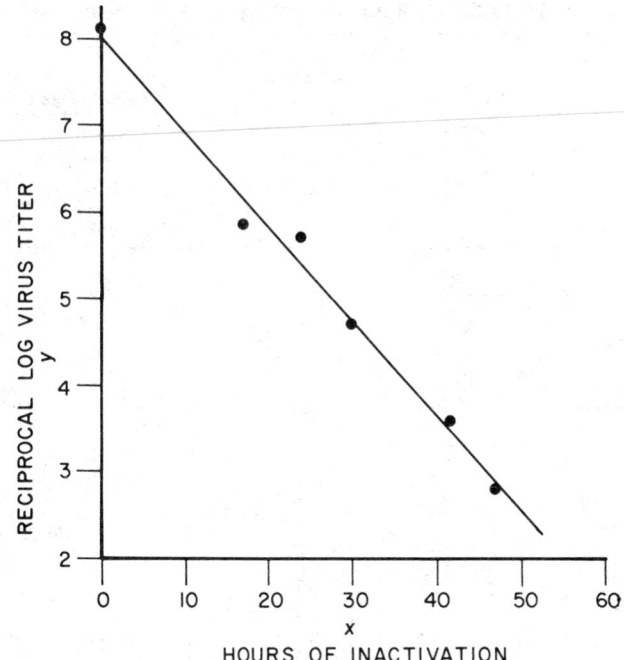

Fig 10-13.   Regression line for reciprocal log virus titer vs hours of inactivation for pure polio virus Type I.

For example, to estimate the number of hours of inactivation required to obtain a reciprocal log virus titer of 4.0, one uses:

$$\hat{x} = 26.625 + \frac{4.0 - 5.1333}{-0.1092} = 37.0 \text{ hours}$$

To estimate 95% confidence limits, first a quantity:

$$g = \frac{t^2 s^2_{y \cdot x}}{b^2 [x^2]} = \frac{(2.776)^2 (0.0435)}{(-0.1092)^2 (1469.4688)} = 0.0191$$

is calculated and then Fieller's Theorem is applied to obtain:

$$\hat{x}_L, \hat{x}_U = \hat{x} + \frac{g}{1-g}(\hat{x} - \overline{x})$$

$$\pm \frac{t}{b(1-g)} \sqrt{s^2_{y \cdot x} \left[\frac{1-g}{n} + \frac{(\hat{x} - \overline{x})^2}{[x^2]} \right]}$$

$$= 37.0 + \frac{0.0191}{0.9809}(37.0 - 26.625)$$

$$\pm \frac{2.776}{(-0.1092)(0.9809)}$$

$$\times \sqrt{0.0435 \left[\frac{0.9809}{6} + \frac{(37.0 - 26.625)^2}{1469.4688} \right]}$$

$$= 37.0 + 0.20 \pm 2.63 = 34.6, 39.8$$

Thus, it can be stated with 95% confidence that it will require 34.6 to 39.8 hours of inactivation to achieve a reciprocal log virus titer of 4.0.

Example XIX—The problem of how to proceed when replicate values of y are available at each value of x, is ilustrated for the data given in the thyroid assay in Table XX on page 134. To determine the regression line for the standard thyroid preparation alone, the variables are:

$$N_s = 55$$
$$\Sigma y_s = 664.5 \qquad\qquad \overline{x}_s = -0.167$$
$$\Sigma x_s = -9.17 \qquad\qquad [x^2]_s = 3.5724$$
$$\overline{y}_s = 12.08 \qquad\qquad [xy]_s = 11.9893$$

Then, the calculation is made:

$$b_s = 11.9893/3.5724 = 3.3561$$

$$[y^2] = (10.0)^2 + - - - + (12.2)^2 - (664.5)^2/55 = 265.7818$$

$$D^2 = \frac{(197.2)^2}{18} + \frac{(232.3)^2}{19} + \frac{(235.3)^2}{18} - \frac{(664.5)^2}{55} = 48.1345$$

$$s^2_{y \cdot x} = \frac{[y^2] - D^2}{\Sigma(n_i - 1)} = \frac{265.7818 - 48.1345}{52} = 4.1855$$

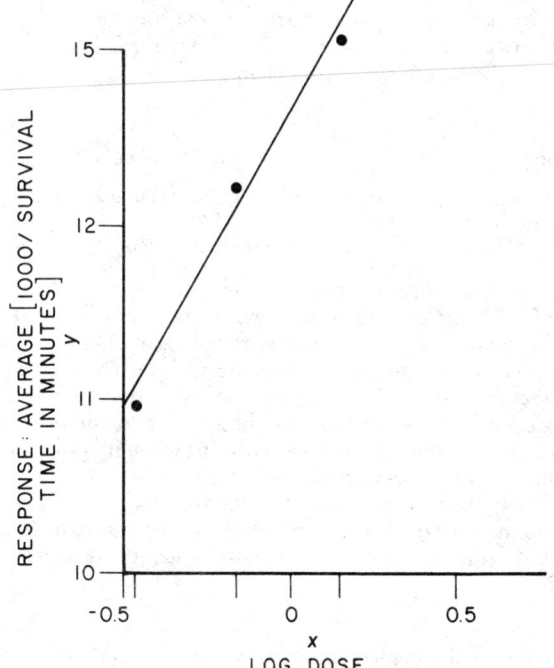

Fig 10-14.   Regression line for response vs log dose for standard thyroid preparation.

The regression line is given by:

$$\hat{y} = 12.08 + 3.3561 [x_s - (-0.167)]$$

$$= 12.64 + 3.3561 x_s$$

and is plotted in Fig 10-14.

$$t = b/\sqrt{s^2_{y \cdot x}/[x^2]}$$

$$= 3.3561/\sqrt{4.1855/3.5724} = 3.10$$

$$DF = \Sigma(n_i - 1) = 52$$

In the t table (see Table III), for $P = 0.05$ (two tails) and $DF = 52$, the value of t is about 2.01. The value of t calculated is greater than this. Therefore, since the probability of the slope being equal to zero is less than 0.05 (actually it is less than 0.01), one must conclude that it is different from zero.

Rejection of Aberrant Observations—It is common practice among chemists and others working in the physical sciences to make observations in duplicate or triplicate. This is usually for the purpose both of obtaining a more accurate result and also detecting mistakes in dilution, weighing, etc. It is quite a common practice to reject the most extreme of the three results if it appears to disagree with the others.

Youden[24,25] of the National Bureau of Standards, a chemist as well as a statistician, made a study of this problem of rejection of observations in an attempt to answer two questions:

1. If the extreme observation of triplicates is always rejected when only normal variation is present, how accurate is the result? Is the average of the two closest observations as good an estimate as the average of all three?

2. By how much should the outlying observation of triplicates differ from the other two in order to be reasonably assured that this difference is due to a blunder rather than normal variation?

He found that by rejection of the outlying observation not only was the variation greatly underestimated but the mean was biased. If a group of 20 samples of three observations each was considered and in each sample the extreme observation was rejected, this operation increased the variation among the averages of the 20 samples.

If one wished to follow a simple rule of rejection[24,25] of observations in samples of three so as to reject not more than 5% of the extreme observations arising from normal variation, a rejection ratio of D/d greater than 20 would be required.

$$D/d = 20$$

where

D = difference between the most extreme observation and its closest neighbor

d = difference between two closest observations

In the USP there is an excellent chapter on the *Design and Analysis of Biological Assays* in which are included some tests for rejection of such observations as may be out of line. Some of the same tests and some others are also given by Dixon and Massey.[26] Two definite criteria are given, one for rejecting single suspect observations in one group and the other for rejecting a whole group of observations when it is suspect as compared with three or more other groups.

To use the first criterion, arrange the observations in the group in order of their magnitude and number them from 1 to n beginning with the supposedly erratic observation, thus

$$y_1, y_2, y_3 \ldots y_n$$

where y_1 is the suspect observation. If there are 3–7 observations in the group, calculate

$$G_1 = \frac{y_2 - y_1}{y_n - y_1}$$

If there are 8–13 observations in the group, and the smallest value seems suspect, again arrange them in order from lowest to highest and calculate

$$G_2 = \frac{y_3 - y_1}{y_{n-1} - y_1}$$

If the largest value is open to suspicion as possibly being aberrant, arrange the observations in order from highest to lowest and number them, always labeling the suspect observation y_1.

If there are 14–24 observations, follow the same procedure, but use the statistic

$$G_3 = \frac{y_3 - y_1}{y_{n-2} - y_1}$$

If the calculated value of G_1, G_2, or G_3 is larger than the tabled value for the desired probability of occurring by chance, it can be assumed that the observation does not truly belong to the group and the observation is rejected. The values of G_1, G_2, and G_3 for a probability $P = 0.01$ that an outlier could occur at either end or $P = 0.02$ that it would occur only at one end is given in the right-hand column of Table XII. This same criterion could be used for testing whether the largest or smallest average in a group of averages differs significantly from the remainder of the averages.

Example XX—Suppose among the gains in weight of six rats after a feeding experiment one weight was found to be much less than the other five. Can that observation be discarded? The six gains in weight are: 36, 40, 38, 42, 20, and 39.

Rearrange these in order from smallest to largest and label $y_1 \ldots y_6$, where $n = 6$.

y_1	20
y_2	36
y_3	38
y_4	39
y_5	40
y_6	42

$$G_1 = \frac{y_2 - y_1}{y_6 - y_1} = \frac{36 - 20}{42 - 20} = \frac{16}{22} = 0.727$$

Referring to the value of G_1 for $n = 6$ in the table, $G_1 = 0.644$ for $P = 0.01$.

Table XII—Criteria for Testing Extreme Value

Statistic	n, Number of observations	Critical values
$G_1 = \dfrac{y_2 - y_1}{y_n - y_1}$	3	.976
	4	.846
	5	.729
	6	.644
	7	.586
$G_2 = \dfrac{y_s - y_1}{y_{n-1} - y_1}$	8	.780
	9	.725
	10	.678
	11	.638
	12	.605
	13	.578
$G_3 = \dfrac{y_3 - y_1}{y_{n-2} - y_1}$	14	.602
	15	.579
	16	.559
	17	.542
	18	.527
	19	.514
	20	.502
	21	.491
	22	.481
	23	.472
	24	.464

Since the calculated value of G_1 is larger than this value, reject the value of 20 and work with the remaining five values.

The second criterion for an aberrant observation as given in the USP compares the variation or range between various groups. It is a test for the homogeneity of the ranges (the range is again the highest value in a group minus the lowest value) and is for the purpose of locating outliers within one group of values. This method and its accompanying table are presented in considerable detail in the USP.

Caution to Be Observed in Interpretation of Results—Again it must be repeated that the purposes and assumptions made in designing the experiment or assay must be kept in mind while interpreting the results. One must not be overwhelmed by the calculations into believing that the use of statistics covers all the weak points in the experiment. As Francis Galton said:

"It is always well to retain a clear geometric view of the facts when we are dealing with statistical problems, which abound with dangerous pitfalls, easily overlooked by the unwary, while they are cantering gaily along upon their arithmetic."

It is unwise to draw sweeping conclusions from one experiment.

Quality-Control Methods—A very short explanation is given here regarding the quality-control methods that were developed primarily by Dr Walter Shewhart of the Bell Telephone Laboratories. A more complete explanation can be found in two short publications of the American Standards Association[27,28] and many texts, including Dixon and Massey.[29]

The quality-control method for variables involves plotting the data as dots on a graph with the variable measured on the vertical axis and time (hours, days, etc) on the horizontal axis. The "control" is maintained by inserting on the chart the grand average and control limits which have been calculated from accumulated experience and drawn on the chart as parallel horizontal lines as shown in Fig 10-15. When all the dots fall within the limits, the results are said to be in a state of "statistical control." When a dot falls outside the limits, trouble is indicated.

In a control chart usually each dot is an average for a sample consisting of, eg, four observations. The standard error of the average is then calculated for each group of four obser-

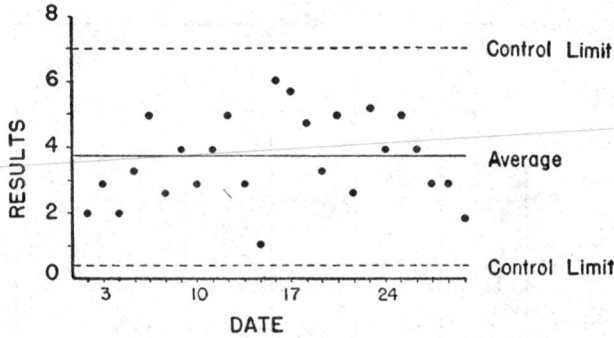

Fig 10-15.   A typical quality control chart.

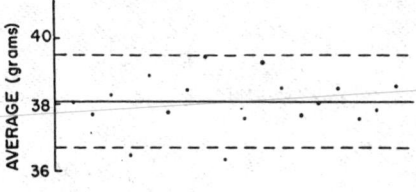

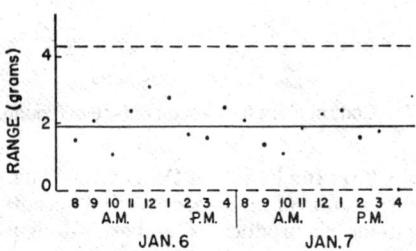

Fig 10-16.   Quality control charts for data from Table XV.

vations, and an average value for the standard error of the average is obtained. Let us designate this by $s_{\bar{x}}$. The grand average of all the averages plotted is also calculated and is labeled $\bar{\bar{x}}$. The "3-sigma" control limits used on the control chart can be obtained from:

$$\text{Upper limit} = \bar{\bar{x}} + 3s_{\bar{x}}$$
$$\text{Lower limit} = \bar{\bar{x}} - 3s_{\bar{x}}$$

Thus it can be seen that the control chart technique is a graphic means of investigating whether or not the variation exhibited over a very short period of time is the same as the variation that occurs over a long period of time. If the two variations are identical and all of the plotted dots fall within the control limits, the experiments or processes that produced the data are said to be in a state of "statistical control."

It is possible to calculate the control limits by using the range in each group of four, eg, instead of calculating the standard deviation. This is because, on the average, for samples of less than ten, the range and the standard deviation are very closely related. Given the number of observations in the sample the standard deviation can be calculated by dividing the range by the appropriate figure given in Table XIII for the size of sample, n. The factors for calculating 3-sigma limits from the range are given as Column A_2 in Table XIV.

Control charts using 3-sigma limits can be obtained by the use of figures given in Table XIV. The formulas are as follows:

Upper limit for averages = $\bar{\bar{x}} + A_2\bar{R}$
Lower limit for averages = $\bar{\bar{x}} - A_2\bar{R}$
Upper limit for ranges = $D_4\bar{R}$
Lower limit for ranges = $D_3\bar{R}$
Where $\bar{R}$ = average range

These calculated limits are drawn on the charts as described above.

Example XXI—A drug manufacturing concern keeps a record of the uniformity of the machine that is filling a given weight of a drug into ampuls. Samples of the finished product are taken at definite time intervals.

Table XIII—Calculation of Standard Deviation from Range

Size of sample (n)	Average number of standard deviations in the average range (d)
2	1.128
3	1.693
4	2.059
5	2.326
6	2.534
7	2.704
8	2.847
9	2.970
10	3.078

Table XIV—Factors for 3-Sigma Limits [a]

Size of sample (n)	Factors for $\bar{R}$ chart		Factor for $\bar{X}$ chart
	D_3	D_4	A_2
2	0	3.27	1.880
3	0	2.57	1.023
4	0	2.28	0.729
5	0	2.11	0.577
6	0	2.00	0.483
7	0.08	1.92	0.419
8	0.14	1.86	0.373
9	0.18	1.82	0.337
10	0.22	1.78	0.308

[a] This table contains parts of the tables in Appendix 1 of Z1.3—1958.[2]

The data are accumulated and arranged into groups of 4 ampuls according to the order in which they were taken from a filling machine. The average and the range are computed for each group of 4 as given in Table XV according to the time the samples are taken. The resulting quality-control charts are given in Fig 10-16.

Table XV—Calculations for a Quality Control Chart
On Averages and Ranges for Samples of 4 from a Filling Machine

Time	Average (g)	Range (g)	Time	Average (g)	Range (g)
Jan. 6			Jan. 7		
8 am	38.1	1.5	8 am	37.6	2.1
9 am	37.6	2.1	9 am	39.1	1.4
10 am	38.3	1.1	10 am	38.5	1.1
11 am	36.5	2.4	11 am	37.7	1.9
12 M	38.9	3.1	12 M	38.1	2.3
1 pm	37.8	2.8	1 pm	38.5	2.4
2 pm	38.5	1.7	2 pm	37.6	1.6
3 pm	39.4	1.6	3 pm	37.9	1.8
4 pm	36.4	2.5	4 pm	38.6	1.0

Grand average = $\bar{\bar{x}}$ = 38.1
Average range = $\bar{R}$ = 1.9
Control limits[a] for average = $\bar{\bar{x}} \pm A_2\bar{R}$ = 38.1 ± 0.729(1.9)
Upper limit = 39.49
Lower limit = 36.71
Control limits[b] for range, are $D_3\bar{R}$ and $D_4\bar{R}$ or 0(1.9) and 2.28(1.9) which equal 0 and 4.33, respectively.

[a] A_2 is the factor for using the range to calculate 3-sigma limits for the average (ie, 3 times the standard error of the average). See Table XIV for N = 4.
[b] D_2 and D_4 are the factors for using the range to calculate 3-sigma limits for the range (ie, 3 times the standard error of the range). These values are taken from Table XIV. In two instances the point plottings fell below the lower control limit, indicating a lower average fill than one might expect, ie, there is a lack of statistical control.

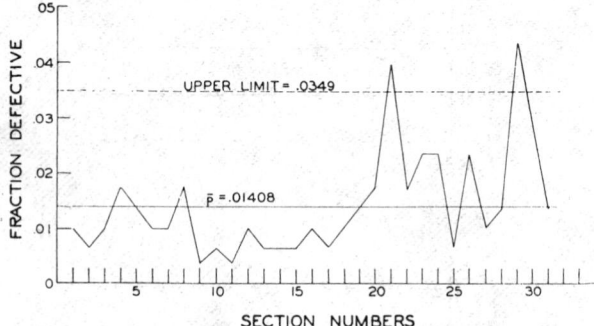

Fig 10-17.   Control chart for fraction defective (courtesy, Lilly).

Control Chart for Fraction Defective—This chart may be applied to results of an inspection that accepts or rejects individual items of a product.   The chart is designed with the same objectives in mind as the $\bar{x}$ and $\bar{R}$ charts.   Its most effective use is in the improvement of quality, although it also discloses the presence of assignable causes of variation.   It provides management with an effective quality history. Fraction defective, p, may be defined as the ratio of the number of defective articles found in any inspection or series of inspections to the total number of articles actually inspected.   This is expressed nearly always as a decimal fraction (see Fig 10-17).   The formula for the control limits on a fraction defective chart is

$$\bar{p} \pm 3\sqrt{\frac{\bar{p}(1-\bar{p})}{n}}$$

In the minds of pharmaceutical personnel, defective pieces are usually in the nature of minor blemishes such as scratches on tablets or air bubbles in gelatin capsules.   These do not affect the therapeutic quality of the product.

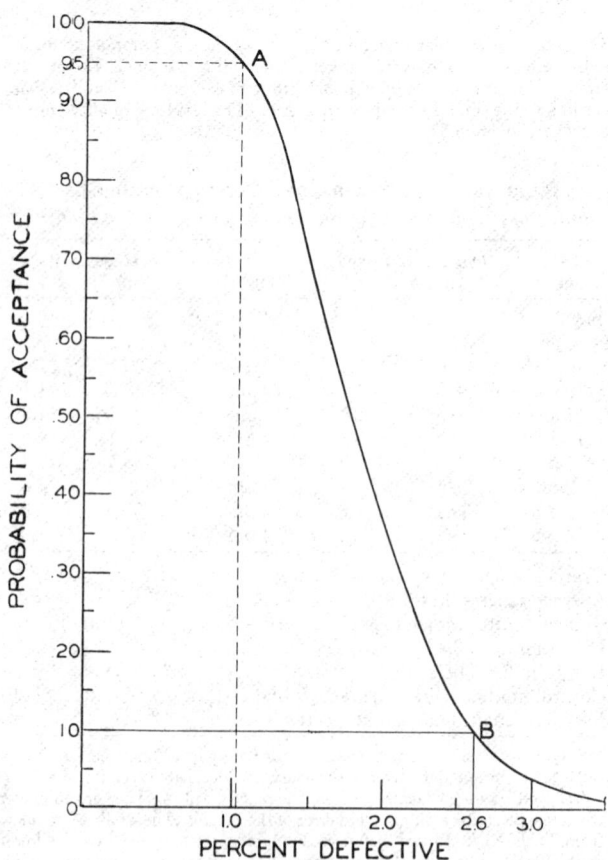

Fig 10-18.   Operating characteristic curve.

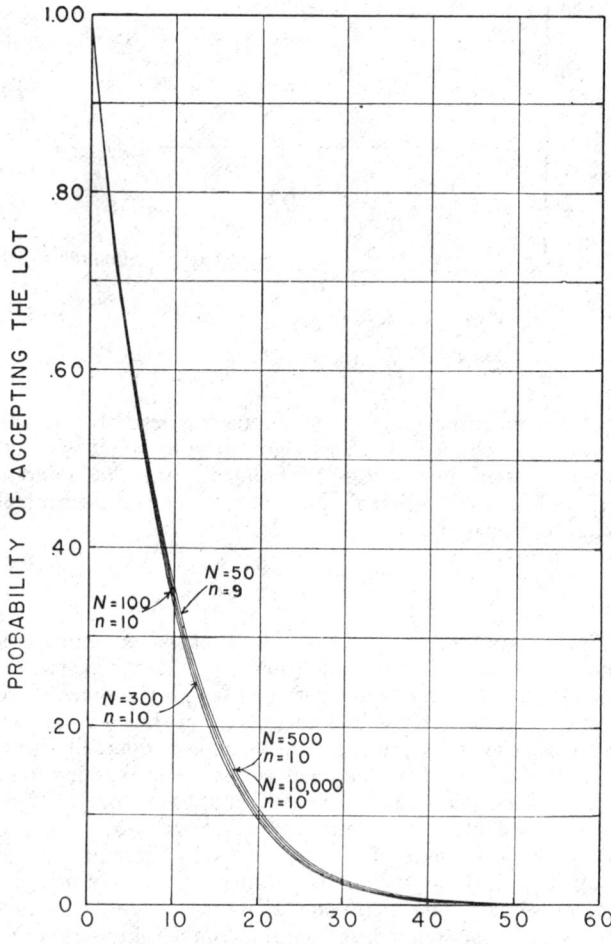

PERCENT OF CONTAMINATED UNITS IN THE LOT

Fig 10-19.   Operating characteristic curves for several lot sizes (N) and sample size (n) of about 10 units.   The lot is passed if there are no contaminated units in the sample tested.[29]

Example XXII—A department head in a capsule department of a large pharmaceutical house keeps a control on the number of defective capsules found in sections (approximately 19,000 capsules are in each section) of large lots of capsules (see Table XVI).   In instances where the point plottings fall above the upper control limit this indicates that a greater number of defects are present than one might expect, ie, there is lack of statistical control.   These sections of production are given special sortings and action is taken at the machine to correct causes of bad quality.

The sample size, n, is 300 capsules from each section and typical data are given in Table XVI, and plotted in Fig 10-17.

It should be noted that Sections 21 and 29 appear to be out of control. These sections were given 100% sortings.   Approximately 4.5% defective capsules were removed from each section.

Another type of chart for attributes can be used that often has advantages over the $\bar{p}$ chart.   If sample sizes are constant, it is convenient to use a control chart for number of defectives or a chart for $n\bar{p}$.   Control limits for this chart are

Control limits for $n\bar{p} = n\bar{p} \pm 3\sqrt{n\bar{p}(1-\bar{p})}$

Acceptance Sampling—Acceptance sampling has become one of the major fields of statistical quality control.   It is used in many phases of manufacturing such as inspection of incoming materials, process inspection at various points in the manufacturing operations, and final inspection of the finished product.   Sampling inspection usually is used in lieu of 100% inspection for several reasons: (1) the cost of 100% inspection is prohibitive; (2) 100% inspection is fatiguing and may result in the inspectors making errors; (3) the inspection operation may involve destructive testing; and (4) a statistical sampling plan well applied may give better quality assurance than 100% inspection.   In sampling one must consider the laws of probability.   There are certain risks involved, namely, the risk of rejecting good quality material and the risk of accepting bad

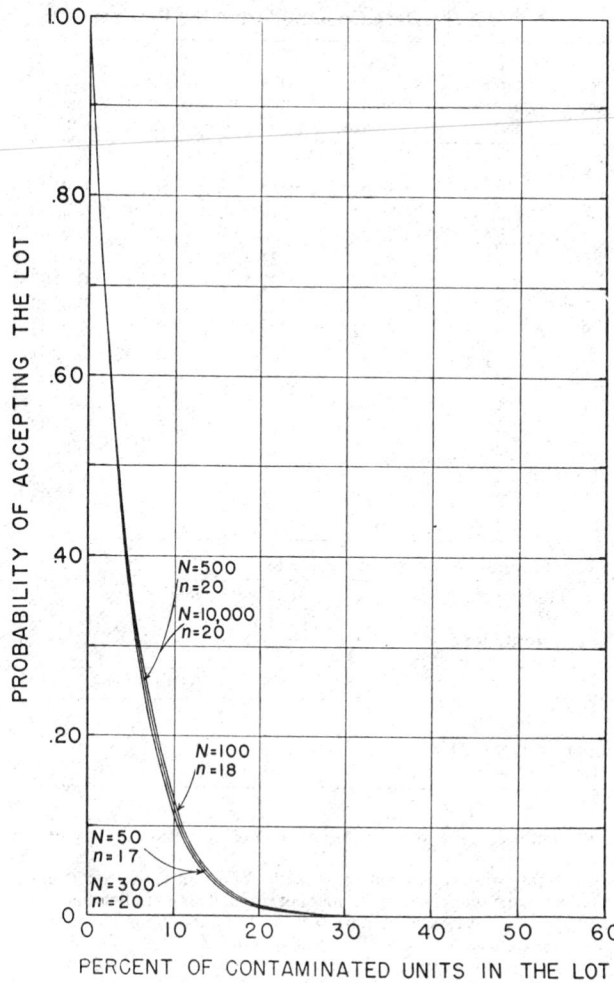

Fig 10-20. Operating characteristic curves for several lot sizes (*N*) and sample size (*n*) of about 20 units. The lot is passed if there are no contaminated units in the sample tested.[30]

merchandise. Sampling plans can be designed and applied in such a manner as to reduce these risks to a minimum and, over a period of time, give assurance of quality products.

The graph illustrating the performance of a sampling plan (ie, ability to discriminate between acceptable and unacceptable lots) is called an *operating characteristic curve*. For any given quality of submitted material it is possible to determine the probability of acceptance.

Example XXIII—The following is an example of a *Statistical Sampling Plan*. A pharmaceutical manufacturing company receives empty bottles of a particular size from a supplier in lots of 20,000 bottles each. The drug firm would like the producer to submit material that is 1.0% defective or less most of the time, or specifically 95% of the time. See point *A*, Fig 10-18. However, the pharmaceutical firm has agreed to take one chance in ten of accepting a lot that is 2.6% defective. See point *B*, Fig 10-18.

The acceptance sampling plan that complies with these specifications is as follows. Take a random sample of 540 bottles. Inspect the bottles for defectives. If zero to nine bottles are found defective, accept the lot; if ten or more defectives are found, reject the lot. The operating characteristic curve for this plan is illustrated in Fig 10-18.

One can also see that using this sampling plan, submitted lots having 0.5% defective will be accepted about 99 times in 100 (probability of acceptance = 0.99) and thus rejected about one time in 100. Submitted lots having 1.75% defective will be accepted 50 times in 100 (probability of acceptance = 0.50) and rejected half the time.

For every sampling plan there is an operating characteristic (OC) curve. In fact there is an OC curve for every standard governing acceptance or rejection of drugs, foods, or materials of any kind. There are OC curves for the manufacturing process and for the inspectional process of every drug in the USP.

In sampling varying sized lots of material having from 50 to 10,000 units in a lot, the size of the sample taken should not be proportional to the size of the lot, or even proportional to the square root of the size of the lot. Fig 10-19[34] shows the closely agreeing operating characteristic curves for lot sizes $N = 50$ to $N = 10,000$ and the respective sample sizes $n = 9$, $n = 10$ that should be taken from these lots. If the sample size is to be increased to around 20, Fig 10-20[34] shows the lot sizes $N = 50$ to $N = 10,000$ and their respective sample sizes $n = 17$ to $n = 20$ that should be used in order to have the operating characteristic curves relatively constant.

Statistics in Biological Testing

The statistical study of biological investigations or *biometrics* is a well-established tool. A few examples of its application to biological assaying will be presented.

Calculation of a Dose Response Curve

It is a well-known fact that the physiological response to a drug varies with the size of the dose given. Many investigators have found that this relationship is usually typified by an S-shaped dose response curve, as illustrated in Fig 10-21. At a low dosage there is no effect, but as the dosage increases the effect becomes more pronounced until beyond a certain dosage there is no further increase in the effect.

The dose response curve is the foundation of much biological experimentation, however there are many different ways of making use of it. Although the dose response curve is sigmoid or S-shaped, over a certain range in the center the dose response curve sometimes approximates a straight line. The use of some function such as logarithm or square root of the variable instead of the variable itself is called a transformation. There are transformations (changes in scale) that have been used to linearize even greater portions of the dose response curve. In these instances when it can be expressed as

a straight line, the equation of that line can be calculated easily. The steepness of this line is called the slope and is usually designated by *b*. The intercept of this line on the vertical axis (*y* axis) is designated by *a*. The equation of such a line is then

$$y = a + bx$$

where

$$b = \frac{\Sigma xy - \bar{x}\Sigma y}{\Sigma x^2 - \bar{x}\Sigma x}$$

$$a = \bar{y} - b\bar{x}$$

The term Σxy indicates the sum of the products of *x* and *y*. (*Note*—this is entirely different from the product of the sums which would be indicated by $\Sigma x \Sigma y$). In a vitamin A assay, for instance, the response here is the gain in weight of the rat over a designated period of time after a definitely stated depletion period. For this assay the gain in weight is plotted against the logarithm of the dose to obtain a linear dose response curve. In most biological assays the logarithm of the dose is used instead of the dose. Also, the statistical calculations are facilitated if the doses are chosen so that the intervals between the logarithms of the doses are equal.

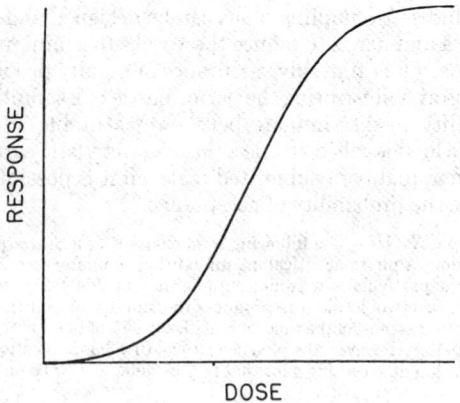

Fig 10-21. A typical dose response curve.

Example XXIV—For determining a log dose response curve on NF Reference Cod Liver Oil Standard, four dosage levels of this standard are given, one dosage level to each of four groups of rats. There are 12 male rats in each group, representing four male rats from each of 12 litters. The rats conformed to the specifications given in the USP XIV assay for vitamin A. The resulting gains in weight in grams are tabulated as responses* in Table XVII. The four doses used were 0.794, 1.26, 2.00, and 3.17 units daily and their logarithms are 9.9–10, 0.1, 0.3, and 0.5, respectively. (For our purposes we will use 9.9–10 as −0.1.) For each rat the log dose and response are given. There are four rats from each litter. The results are plotted in Fig 10-22.

Evaluation of Biological Assays

A biological assay is a means of estimating the strength of a drug (generally by comparison to a standard of the same drug) by using some living organism. There are several types of biological assay, from a statistical viewpoint:

1. Assays which use the direct determination of threshold or lethal dose (eg, USP XVIII Digitalis Pigeon Assay).
2. Assays which give a measurable response (eg, gain in weight of rats

---

* For more explicit details see the section on Vitamin A in the chapter on *Biological Testing* in RPS-13, page 1600.

Table XVI—Data Collected from the Process

Section number	Number defectives	Fraction defective	Section number	Number defectives	Fraction defective
1	3	0.01	17	2	0.0067
2	2	0.0067	18	3	0.01
3	3	0.01	19	4	0.0133
4	5	0.0167	20	5	0.0167
5	4	0.0133	21	12	0.04
6	3	0.01	22	5	0.0167
7	3	0.01	23	7	0.0233
8	5	0.0167	24	7	0.0233
9	1	0.0033	25	2	0.0067
10	2	0.0067	26	7	0.0233
11	1	0.0033	27	3	0.01
12	3	0.01	28	4	0.0133
13	2	0.0067	29	13	0.0433
14	2	0.0067	30	9	0.03
15	2	0.0067	31	4	0.0133
16	3	0.01			

$$\bar{p} = \frac{\text{Total number of defectives}}{\text{Total number inspected}} = \frac{131}{31 \times 300} = \frac{131}{9300} = 0.01408$$

Control limits for $\bar{p} = \bar{p} \pm 3 \sqrt{\dfrac{\bar{p}(1 - \bar{p})}{n}}$

$$= 0.01408 \pm 3 \sqrt{\frac{0.01408(1 - 0.01408)}{300}}$$

Upper limit = 0.0349
Lower limit = 0

in a vitamin A assay, or diameter of zone of inhibition in a penicillin assay).
3. Assays which give an all or none type of response wherein an individual animal either responds or does not respond, or an individual object passes or does not pass a set mark (eg, the number of animals that show a decrease in blood pressure of at least 10 mm Hg).
4. Assays which utilize a time factor (eg, the duration of cure of polyneuritis in rats on a vitamin B₁ assay).

In a biological assay the potency of the drug may be measured as a percentage of the standard, or in terms of some es-

Table XVII—Log dose Response Curve for Vitamin A Assay

Litter no.	Log dose x	Response y	Log dose x	Response y	Log dose x	Response y	Log dose x	Response y
1	−0.1	4	0.1	24	0.3	35	0.5	43
2	−0.1	24	0.1	55	0.3	46	0.5	60
3	−0.1	18	0.1	45	0.3	50	0.5	58
4	−0.1	8	0.1	30	0.3	38	0.5	54
5	−0.1	15	0.1	28	0.3	48	0.5	47
6	−0.1	28	0.1	40	0.3	57	0.5	62
7	−0.1	36	0.1	49	0.3	49	0.5	57
8	−0.1	38	0.1	53	0.3	67	0.5	85
9	−0.1	30	0.1	57	0.3	59	0.5	71
10	−0.1	20	0.1	47	0.3	60	0.5	59
11	−0.1	25	0.1	38	0.3	53	0.5	62
12	−0.1	10	0.1	31	0.3	40	0.5	48

$n = 48$
$\Sigma x = 9.6$
$\Sigma x^2 = 4.32$

$\Sigma y = 2061$

$\Sigma xy = 557.7$

$\bar{x} = 0.2000$

$\bar{y} = 42.9375$

$$\text{Slope} = b = \frac{\Sigma xy - \bar{x}\Sigma y}{\Sigma x^2 - \bar{x}\Sigma x} = \frac{557.7 - 0.2000(2061)}{4.32 - 0.2000(9.6)} = 60.625$$

$$\text{Intercept} = a = \bar{y} - b\bar{x} = 42.9375 - 60.625(0.2000) = 30.8125$$

Equation of log dose response curve:

$$\text{Response} = 30.8125 + 60.625 \text{ times log dose}$$

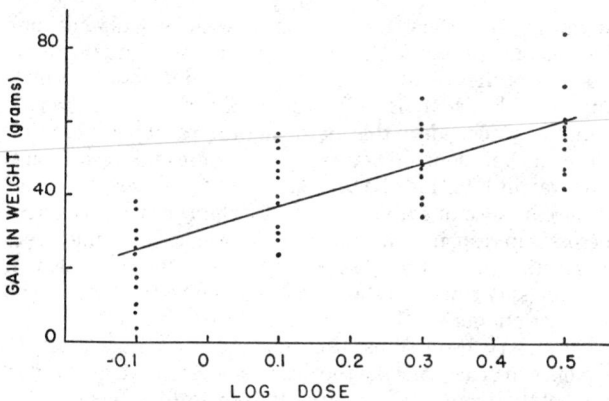

Fig 10-22. Log dose response curve for vitamin A assay (data given in Table XVII).

tablished unitage. In recent years it has been increasingly evident that not only should the potency be obtained but also some measure of the reproducibility of the assay such as the standard error of the assay or the confidence limits for the potency. This can be accomplished if the design of the assay is such that it takes into account all the causes of variation within one laboratory.

The calculated error of an assay and the confidence limits for a potency can estimate errors that can be shown to cause variations *within* the assay. Ordinarily, it can neither take into account the errors of weighing and measuring of the material (which are sizable in some assays, notably penicillin), nor can it take into account the differences between materials used in each laboratory, between samples of the lot to be assayed or, most important, between assayists. The assayist *cannot* state, on the basis of the calculated error of the assay, that the lot assayed was, say, 650 ± 20 units per mg. He *can* say that, if he repeated the assay many times under the same conditions using the same "made-up" solutions, this calculated error could be used to estimate the unavoidable variation in his own series of results.

The statistical evaluation of the biological assays of USP XVII, also their procedures and calculations, as well as the basis of the official chapter on *Design and Analysis of Biological Assays* (retained in USP as a general chapter) have been described in publications by Bliss.[31,32]

Direct Determinations of the Threshold Dose

Digitalis Assay—As given in USP XVIII potency is determined by injecting suitably diluted tincture into randomly selected, anesthetized pigeons at 5-min intervals until the pigeons die of cardiac arrest. The dilution of the Standard Preparation of Digitalis and the preparation to be assayed shall be such that the estimated fatal dose of each preparation per kg of pigeon shall be contained in 15 mL. In the data in Table XVIII the estimated fatal dose of the standard is 0.975 ml. Six pigeons are assigned at random to the standard and six to the unknown. The number of doses (1 mL of the diluted material for each kg of pigeon at 5-min intervals) necessary to produce death in each pigeon is also given. As stated in the USP XVIII, the average number of doses for each material must be not less than 13 or greater than 19 to have a valid assay.

To calculate the potency of the preparation assayed in USP Digitalis Units per mL find the average number of doses of the test and standard solutions which were injected and designate these $\bar{v}_u$ and $\bar{v}_s$, respectively.

The potency of the unknown is given by the formula

$$\text{Potency} = P_* = \bar{v}_s R / \bar{v}_u$$

Table XVIII—Digitalis Pigeon Assay

	No of doses		Dilutions
	Std.	Unknown	
	14	16	6½ mL of std preparation
	13	17	per 100 mL of test
	16	15	dilution (0.975 mL/15 mL)
	15	17	7 mL of preparation to be
	15	18	assayed per 100 mL of test
	12	15	dilution for unknown (1.05
Sum	85	98	mL/15 mL)
Average	14.2	16.3	

$$f_u = f_s = 6$$
$$\Sigma v_s = T_s = 85 \qquad\qquad \bar{v}_s = 14.2$$
$$\Sigma v_u = T_u = 98 \qquad\qquad \bar{v}_u = 16.3$$
$$\Sigma v^2 = 14^2 + 13^2 + \ldots + 15^2 = 2823$$

$R = 6\frac{1}{2}/7 = 0.928$

Potency $= P_* = \bar{v}_s R / \bar{v}_u = 14.2(0.928)/16.3 = 0.808$

$s^2 = \{\Sigma v^2 - T_s^2/f_s - T_u^2/f_u\}/(f_s + f_u - 2)$
$\quad = \{2823 - (85)^2/6 - (98)^2/6\}/(6 + 6 - 2)$
$\quad = \{2823 - 1204.17 - 1600.67\}/10 = 1.816$

$C = \bar{v}_u^2/(\bar{v}_u^2 - s^2 t^2/f_u)$

From the t table for 10 degrees of freedom and $P = 0.05$ for two tails, $t = 2.228$. Inserting the proper values in the formula for C:

$C = (16.3)^2/\{(16.3)^2 - 1.816(2.228)^2/6\}$
$\quad = 265.69/\{265.69 - 1.5024\} = 1.0057$

$L = 2\sqrt{(C-1)(CP_*^2 + R^2 f_u/f_s)}$
$\quad = 2\sqrt{(1.0057 - 1)\{1.0057(0.808)^2 + (0.928)^2(6/6)\}}$
$\quad = 2\sqrt{0.0057\{0.6566 + 0.8612\}} = 2\sqrt{0.008651}$
$\quad = 2(0.0930) = 0.1860$

Confidence limits ($P = 0.05$) for the potency in USP units

$X_{P*} = CP_* \pm \frac{1}{2}L = 1.0057(0.808) \pm \frac{1}{2}(0.1860)$
$\quad = 0.81206 \pm 0.0930$
$\quad = 0.9056 \text{ and } 0.7196$

A more acceptable general procedure utilizes log-tolerances, as follows:

	Log of no. of doses	
	Std.	Unknown
	1.15	1.20
	1.11	1.23
	1.20	1.18
	1.18	1.23
	1.18	1.26
	1.08	1.18
Σx	6.90	7.28
Σx^2	7.9458	8.8382
n	6	6
$\bar{x}$	1.150	1.213

$M = \bar{x}_S - \bar{x}_T = 1.150 - 1.213 = -0.063$

Potency $= P_* = R$ antilog $M = 0.928(0.865) = 0.803$

Pooled $s^2 = \dfrac{7.9458 - (6.90)^2/6 + 8.8382 - (7.28)^2/6}{6 + 6 - 2} = 0.001593$

S.E.$(M) = \sqrt{s^2(1/n_S + 1/n_T)} = \sqrt{0.001593(1/6 + 1/6)} = 0.0230$

Confidence limits ($P = 0.05$) for the potency

$X_{P*} = R$ antilog $[M \pm t \cdot \text{S.E.}(M)]$
$\quad = 0.928$ antilog $[-0.063 \pm 2.228(0.0230)]$
$\quad = 0.928$ antilog $(-0.012, -0.114)$
$\quad = 0.928(0.973, 0.769)$
$\quad = 0.903 \text{ and } 0.714$

where R is the ratio of the number of mL of standard preparation to the number of mL of assay preparation in 100 mL of their respective test dilutions.

Calculate the square of the standard error of the threshold dose. This is referred to as the error variance since variance is merely the square of the standard deviation.

$$s^2 = \{\Sigma v^2 - T_s^2/f_s - T_u^2/f_u\}/(f_s + f_u - 2)$$

where $T_s = \Sigma v_s$ and $T_u = \Sigma v_u$ and v designates each individual threshold dose.

f_s = number of animals on the standard
f_u = number of animals on the unknown

Notice that the formula for s^2 is merely the pooled variances for the responses to the standard and unknown since the variance for the standard would be

$$s^2 = \frac{\Sigma v_s{}^2 - (\Sigma v_s)^2/n_s}{n_s - 1}$$

if v_s is used instead of x as on page 110.

The confidence interval is denoted by L in USP XVIII and the value of t used is that corresponding to a probability of $P = 0.05$. The value: potency $+ \frac{1}{2}L$ is the upper confidence limit and the value: potency $- \frac{1}{2}L$ is the lower confidence limit. The formula given for L in USP XVIII for the digitalis assay is

$$L = 2 \sqrt{(C - 1)(CP_*{}^2 + R^2 f_u/f_s)}$$

where

$$C = \bar{v}_u{}^2/(\bar{v}_u{}^2 - s^2 t^2/f_u)$$

and P_* is the assayed potency in USP units.

If L exceeds 0.30 USP Digitalis Unit, repeat the assay or inject more pigeons with one or both preparations until the confidence interval is 0.30 or less. The confidence limits ($P = 0.05$) for the potency in USP units are:

$$X_{P*} = CP_* \pm \frac{1}{2}L$$

Example XXV—The calculation of the potency and the confidence limits of the assay within one laboratory is given in Table XVIII. An alternate and more acceptable general procedure utilizing log tolerances is also described.

Assays Based on a Log Dose Response Curve

Statistics can best be applied to those assays in which two or more doses of the standard are run simultaneously with two or more doses of the unknown and the log dose response curve is calculated from both standard and unknown.

Potency of an unknown is usually calculated as a certain percent of the standard. It thus can be obtained by getting the antilog of the difference between the logarithms of the doses of the unknown and of a standard having the same response (since a quotient is a difference in terms of logarithms). It has been found that when the logarithm of the dose is plotted against some function of the response the result is a straight line. Much has been written on this subject by various writers. Among the first were Gaddum,[33] Trevan,[34] and Bliss.[35]

It will suffice to say that when the logarithm of the dose is plotted against some function of the response, two parallel straight lines are obtained (as shown in Fig 10-23), one for the standard material and one for the assay material (for which a dosage based on an assumed potency was used). Then, since the potency of the unknown is the antilog of the difference between the logarithms of the doses for standard and for unknown, the potency can be calculated from the horizontal distance between the lines. The parallel lines are usually fitted to the observations by least squares (so called because it mathematically minimizes the sum of the squares of the

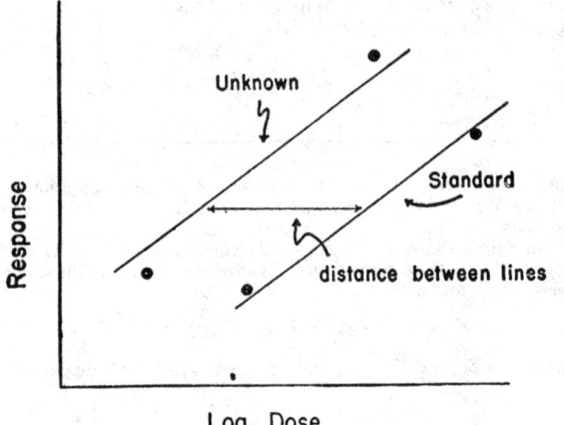

Fig 10-23.   A graph of the data from a typical assay.

distances from the observed points to the calculated line). The calculated error of an assay is, then, some quantitative measure of the scatter of the observed points about the lines but depends also on the slope of the lines. At least two assumptions are made in this mathematical reasoning. The first is that the relationship between the log dose and the response is a straight line, and the second is that equal percentage increases in dose of standard and of unknown will give equal increases in response (ie, that the unknown has the same effect as the standard). Both these assumptions should be tested, and no assay run until they are known to be true within the range recommended for the assay.

Various types of transformations have been used for the response in order to make the dose response curve linear over most of its range. Dose is usually transformed by using log dose; although in some assays, eg, most microbiological assays, no transformations are necessary. Some authors recommend using a logarithmic transformation for the response in a vitamin D assay and others do not. All of the assays having an "all or none" type of response require some transformation for the response. For this purpose the probit, the logit, and the angular transformations are recommended by various authors. The *probit transformation* is the most common. *Probit* is an abbreviation for "probability unit." Probits are derived from the standard deviation units in a table of the normal probability curve. A 50% response is equivalent to the left-hand half of the area under the normal curve in Fig 10-9 and to a standard deviation unit of zero. Since probits are obtained by adding 5 to the standard deviation units, a 50% response corresponds to a probit of 5. As can also be seen from Fig 10-9, a 16% ($\frac{1}{2}$ of the difference between 100% and 68%) response corresponds to a standard deviation unit of about -1 and a probit of approximately 4. A 2.5% response corresponds approximately to a standard deviation unit of -2 and a probit of 3. A 97.5% response corresponds to a standard deviation unit of $+2$ and a probit of 7 (see Table XIX).

The probit method is essentially a modification of the methods used by Gaddum[33] and Trevan.[34] The logarithm of the dose is used and the response is transformed to probits. There are many refinements that have been made for a very accurate determination of potency and standard error of the assay in using the probit method by Bliss[35] and further outlined by Miller, *et al*,[36] and by Finney.[37] They advocate plotting the empirical probits vs log dose and fitting two parallel straight lines (one for standard and one for unknown) to the points by means of a straightedge. The expected probit for each dose is read from the graph. The corrected probit and the weights to be attached to each observation are read from a series of tables. However, a short-cut procedure will be given here using only the empirical probits and their weights in the calculations. The procedure they give from that point on is essentially the same as is given in Example XXVI.

Thyroid Assay—This assay, although not official, serves to illustrate the generalized "least-squares" procedure for estimating the potency and 95% confidence limit for a quantitative graded-response assay.

In this assay three graded doses of a standard thyroid preparation and four graded doses of a solubilized test thyroid preparation were given to mice, and the survival time was measured after the mice were placed in airtight containers. For statistical reasons the response was measured as

$$y = \frac{1000}{\text{survival time in minutes}}$$

Actually, six equally spaced log doses of each preparation were tested on an equal number of mice. Data from the original assay were omitted to illustrate the generalized procedure to be used for unbalanced assays.

Table XIX—Empirical Probits

For Use with Percentage Responses in "All or None" Assays[a]

%	0	1	2	3	4	5	6	7	8	9
0	...	2.674	2.946	3.119	3.249	3.355	3.445	3.524	3.595	3.659
10	3.718	3.773	3.825	3.874	3.920	3.964	4.006	4.046	4.085	4.122
20	4.158	4.194	4.228	4.261	4.294	4.326	4.357	4.387	4.417	4.447
30	4.476	4.504	4.532	4.560	4.587	4.615	4.642	4.668	4.695	4.721
40	4.747	4.773	4.798	4.824	4.849	4.874	4.900	4.925	4.950	4.975
50	5.000	5.025	5.050	5.075	5.100	5.126	5.151	5.176	5.202	5.227
60	5.253	5.279	5.305	5.332	5.358	5.385	5.413	5.440	5.468	5.496
70	5.524	5.553	5.583	5.613	5.643	5.674	5.706	5.739	5.772	5.806
80	5.842	5.878	5.915	5.954	5.994	6.036	6.080	6.126	6.175	6.227
90	6.282	6.341	6.405	6.476	6.555	6.645	6.751	6.881	7.054	7.326

[a] From Bliss.[38]

It can be shown that for the doses selected, the log dose response lines for the standard and test preparations are linear and parallel within the limits of experimental error of the assay. Accordingly parallel log dose response lines can be fitted to the data from the equations

$$y_S = \bar{y}_S + b_c(x - \bar{x}_S)$$

$$y_T = \bar{y}_T + b_c(x - \bar{x}_T)$$

where y is response, x is log dose, and b_c is the common slope. The potency of the test preparation relative to the standard is then calculated from

$$R = \text{antilog } M = \text{antilog } \left(\bar{x}_S - \bar{x}_T \frac{\bar{y}_S - \bar{y}_T}{b_c} \right)$$

The variance, s^2, is generally estimated from the variability "within doses" and the 95% confidence limits are calculated from

$$R_L, R_U = \text{antilog } (M_L, M_U)$$

where

$$M_L, M_U = \bar{x}_S - \bar{x}_T + \left(M - \bar{x}_S + \bar{x}_T \pm \right.$$

$$\left. \frac{t}{b_c}\sqrt{s^2[(1-g)(1/n_S + 1/n_T) + (M - \bar{x}_S + \bar{x}_T)^2/[x^2]]} \right) \Big/ (1-g)$$

The value of t is obtained from a t table for degrees of freedom $= \Sigma(n_i - 1)$, and g is calculated from

$$g = \frac{t^2 s^2}{b_c^2 [x^2]}$$

A value of $g < 0.05$ may be ignored. As g approaches unity, the assay becomes less valid. A value of $g > 1$ indicates a completely invalid assay due to either too flat a slope, b_c, or to unusually high variability within doses, s^2.

The example given in Table XX shows the calculations of the thyroid assay.

Estrogen Assay—The estrogen assay is described in the chapter on *Biological Testing* in RPS-14, page 639. It is one of the "all or none" type of assays.

Example XXVI—An example of a 3-level assay is given below demonstrating the application of, first, the probit method to this type of assay, then the angular transformation method. The assay is designed so that the intervals between the log doses are equal on both standard and unknown although the method of calculation given here can be used even if they are not equal.

The data obtained from the assay and the dosages given each group of 16 animals are included with the calculations for the probit method given in Table XXII. Probits and their weights are given in Tables XIX and XXI.

Table XXII gives the generalized form for calculations that can be used even if the number of animals is not equal on all the doses and the differences between consecutive log doses are not equal for standard and unknown. It can also be used on any number of doses although only three doses are used in the example.

Various short-cut procedures have been used to shorten the arithmetical calculations for the probit method but these will not be enumerated here. There is another method that has been suggested; namely, the use of the angular transformation instead of the probit transformation.

The *angular transformation* is stated by the formula:

$$p = \sin^2\theta$$

where p is the percentage response and θ is the transformed value in degrees. See Table XXIII.

The same estrogenic assay can be evaluated by the angular transformation method. A partial table of the angular transformation of proportions to angles is given in Table XXIII. The method of calculation and formulas for a 3-dose assay using this procedure are given in Table XXIV. Note that, in order to use the formulas given in this table, the three-dose assay must be designed so that the number of animals, n, on each dose is the same and the differences between consecutive log doses are equal. In this example, $n = 16$ and the difference between log doses = 0.15.

Here it is assumed that R, the ratio of corresponding doses of standard and unknown, is unity. When this is not the case, the potency must be multiplied by R.

Four-point Symmetric Assay—The following formulas apply to a percentage response assay using the angular transformation in which only two doses are used on each of the standard and the unknown.

$$V = U_H + U_L - S_H - S_L$$

$$W = U_H - U_L + S_H - S_L$$

$$M = \frac{iV}{W}$$

$$\text{Potency} = \text{antilog } \left(2 + \frac{iV}{W} \right)$$

$$\text{Standard error of the assay} = 131.9 \frac{i(\text{potency})}{W^2\sqrt{n}}\sqrt{W^2 + V^2}$$

Eight-point Symmetric Assay—The following formulas apply to a percentage response assay using the angular transformation in which four doses are used on each of the standard and the unknown:

$$V = U_L + U_M + U_G + U_H - (S_L + S_M + S_G + S_H)$$

$$W = 3(S_H - S_L + U_H - U_L) + (S_G - S_M + U_G - U_M)$$

$$M = \frac{5iV}{W}$$

$$\text{Potency} = \text{antilog } \left(2 + \frac{5iV}{W} \right)$$

$$\text{Standard error of the assay} = 933 \frac{i(\text{potency})}{W^2\sqrt{n}}\sqrt{W^2 + 5V^2}$$

Insulin Injection Assay—In the USP the assay of Insulin Injection makes use of the twin crossover rabbit test using four equal groups of six or more rabbits each. Two dilutions are made of each of the standard and the unknown. Standard dilution 1 contains 1.0 USP Insulin unit in each mL and Standard dilution 2 contains 2.0 USP Insulin units in each mL. The two assay dilutions contain similar amounts on the

Table XX—Thyroid Assay

	Standard thyroid			Test thyroid			
Dose (mg/mouse)	0.333	0.683	1.400	1.000	2.050	4.200	8.620
log dose, x	−0.48	−0.17	0.15	0.00	0.31	0.62	0.94
Response, y	10.0	10.6	13.7	10.9	12.3	9.3	11.2
	9.4	9.9	14.7	9.9	10.6	13.2	14.1
	14.9	12.7	16.4	14.3	10.5	12.7	10.6
	9.1	12.3	11.8	10.8	11.9	12.5	14.5
	11.6	15.2	10.2	9.3	11.8	12.3	15.4
	10.2	16.1	13.7	8.8	8.6	14.3	11.9
	11.9	10.8	14.9	9.6	9.9	10.5	12.7
	12.0	12.3	12.8	9.0	15.6	8.3	12.8
	13.2	12.3	16.7	9.2	14.5	10.3	11.4
	11.9	13.3	15.2	7.6	11.6	10.5	12.5
	10.5	11.6	9.7	10.2	15.4	11.1	14.1
	11.9	9.7	12.8	10.6	10.5	11.2	13.5
	16.4	15.6	12.7	9.0	11.9	11.0	10.8
	6.5	12.2	12.0	8.7	12.2	13.3	11.4
	10.2	10.0	14.3	7.6	10.1	11.0	11.8
	9.2	11.6	11.6	7.5	8.1	18.5	13.5
	9.3	11.2	9.9	7.8	10.9	14.1	13.3
	9.0	12.7	12.2	10.2	7.1	11.0	11.8
		11.9		11.8	12.2	10.5	14.9
				9.4	9.4	10.0	10.8
				7.8	9.0	11.0	14.9
				8.8	9.5	12.3	14.9
				10.3	9.4	12.0	9.3
				7.9	10.6		
Σy_i	197.2	232.0	235.3	227.0	263.6	270.9	292.1
n_i	18	19	18	24	24	23	23
$\bar{y}_i$	10.96	12.21	13.07	9.46	10.98	11.78	12.70

$n_S = 55$	$n_T = 94$
$\Sigma y_S = 664.5$	$\Sigma y_T = 1053.6$
$\Sigma x_S = -9.17$	$\Sigma x_T = 43.32$
$\bar{y}_S = 12.08$	$\bar{y}_T = 11.21$
$\bar{x}_S = -0.167$	$\bar{x}_T = 0.461$
$N = 149$	$\Sigma y = 1718.1$

$$[x^2]_S = 18(-0.48)^2 + 19(-0.17)^2 + 18(0.15)^2 - (-9.17)^2/55 = 3.5724$$
$$[x^2]_T = 24(0.00)^2 + 24.(0.31)^2 + 23(0.62)^2 + 23(0.94)^2 - (43.32)^2/94 = 11.5063$$
$$[xy]_S = (-0.48)(197.2) + (-0.17)(232.0) + (0.15)(235.3) - (-9.17)(664.5)/55 = 11.9893$$
$$[xy]_T = (0.00)(227.0) + (0.31)(263.6) + (0.62)(270.9) + (0.94)(292.1) - (43.32)(1053.6)/94 = 38.6953$$
$$[xy] = [xy]_S + [xy]_T = 11.9893 + 38.6953 = 50.6846$$
$$[x^2] = [x^2]_S + [x^2]_T = 3.5724 + 11.5063 = 15.0787$$
$$b_c = [xy]/[x^2] = 50.6846/15.0787 = 3.3613$$

$$M = \bar{x}_S - \bar{x}_T - \frac{\bar{y}_S - \bar{y}_T}{b_c} = -0.167 - 0.461 - \frac{12.08 - 11.21}{3.3613} = -0.887$$

Relative potency = R = antilog M = antilog (-0.887) = antilog $(9.113 - 10)$ = 0.13 or 13% of standard

$$[y^2] = (10.0)^2 + (9.4)^2 + \cdots + (9.3)^2 - (1718.1)^2/149 = 742.5980$$

$$D^2 = \frac{(197.2)^2}{18} + \cdots + \frac{(292.1)^2}{23} - \frac{(1718.1)^2}{149} = 200.6287$$

$$s^2 = \frac{[y^2] - D^2}{\Sigma(n_i - 1)} = \frac{742.5980 - 200.6287}{142} = 3.8167$$

$$g = \frac{t^2 s^2}{b_c^2 [x^2]} = \frac{(1.98)^2(3.8167)}{(3.3613)^2(15.0787)} = 0.0878$$

$$M_L, M_U = \bar{x}_S - \bar{x}_T + \left(M - \bar{x}_S + \bar{x}_T \pm \frac{t}{b_c} \sqrt{s^2\{(1-g)(1/n_S + 1/n_T) + (M - \bar{x}_S + \bar{x}_T)^2/[x^2]\}} \right) \Big/ (1-g)$$

$$= -0.628 + \left(0.259 \pm \frac{1.98}{3.3613} \sqrt{3.8167\,[0.9122(1/55 + 1/94) + (-0.259)^2/15.0787]} \right) \Big/ 0.9122$$

$$= -0.628 + \frac{(-0.259 \pm 0.202)}{0.9122}$$

$$= -0.628 - 0.505, \; -0.628 - 0.062$$

$$= -1.133, \; -0.690$$

R_L, R_U = lower and upper 95% confidence limits
   = antilog (M_L, M_U) = antilog $(-1.133, -0.690)$
   = antilog $(8.867 - 10, 9.310 - 10)$
   = 0.074, 0.20 or 7.4% and 20% of standard

Thus, the solubilized thyroid test preparation is estimated to be 13% as potent as the standard thyroid preparation, with 95% confidence limits of 7.4% and 20%.

Table XXI—Weighting Coefficients for Use with Probits[a]

Probit	Weighting coefficient	Probit
5.0	0.6366	5.0
5.1	0.6343	4.9
5.2	0.6274	4.8
5.3	0.6161	4.7
5.4	0.6005	4.6
5.5	0.5810	4.5
5.6	0.5579	4.4
5.7	0.5316	4.3
5.8	0.5026	4.2
5.9	0.4714	4.1
6.0	0.4386	4.0
6.1	0.4047	3.9
6.2	0.3703	3.8
6.3	0.3359	3.7
6.4	0.3020	3.6
6.5	0.2691	3.5
6.6	0.2375	3.4
6.7	0.2077	3.3
6.8	0.1799	3.2
6.9	0.1544	3.1
7.0	0.1311	3.0
7.1	0.1103	2.9
7.2	0.0918	2.8
7.3	0.0756	2.7
7.4	0.0617	2.6
7.5	0.0498	2.5
7.6	0.0398	2.4
7.7	0.0314	2.3
7.8	0.0246	2.2
7.9	0.0190	2.1

[a] From Bliss.[38]

basis of the assumed potency. Specific instructions as to choice of animals, feeding schedules, and other details are given. Two injections are given each group of rabbits, the "Second injection being made on the day after the First injection or not more than one week later," according to the following schedule:

Group	First injection	Second injection
1	Standard dilution 2	Assay dilution 1
2	Standard dilution 1	Assay dilution 2
3	Assay dilution 2	Standard dilution 1
4	Assay dilution 1	Standard dilution 2

At 1 hr and $2\frac{1}{2}$ hr from the time of injection, blood samples are obtained from the marginal ear vein. The response in this assay is the sum of the blood sugar concentration at 1 hr and $2\frac{1}{2}$ hr. The "y" values used to calculate the assay results are the individual differences.

Group	Differences	Individual response y	Total response T
1	Standard 2 − Assay 1	y_1	T_1
2	Assay 2 − Standard 1	y_2	T_2
3	Assay 2 − Standard 1	y_3	T_3
4	Standard 2 − Assay 1	y_4	T_4

The number of rabbits in each group is f and

$$T_a = -T_1 + T_2 + T_3 - T_4$$
$$T_b = T_1 + T_2 + T_3 + T_4$$

The logarithm of the relative potency is

$$M' = ci\, T_a/T_b = 0.301\, T_a/T_b$$

The potency in USP units = antilog (M' + log of the assumed potency) where i = the interval in logarithms between successive log doses = log $2 = 0.301$ and $c = c' = 1$.

The confidence interval of the log potency M' is determined as given in the USP

$$L = 2\sqrt{(C-1)(CM'^2 + c'i^2)}$$

where $c'i^2$ is equal to 0.09062 since $c' = 1$ and $i = 0.301$ and

$$C = T_b{}^2/(T_b{}^2 - s^2 t^2 N)$$

where t^2 is the square of the value from the t table for $n = 4(f-1)$ degrees of freedom.

$$s^2 = \{\Sigma y^2 - \Sigma T_i{}^2/f\}/n$$

C is often little greater than unity. The more precise the assay the more nearly C approaches 1.

The upper and lower confidence limits in logarithms at a single laboratory are, respectively:

$$X_M = \log R + CM' + \tfrac{1}{2}L \text{ and } \log R + CM' - \tfrac{1}{2}L$$

where R is assumed potency.

For an insulin assay, if the confidence interval in logarithms is more than 0.082 (which corresponds to 95% confidence limits of about ±10% of the computed potency), the assay should be repeated until the combined data of two or more assays meet this acceptable limit.

Example XXVII—A typical USP Insulin Assay* follows:

S_1 = 1 USP unit per mL
S_2 = 2 USP units per mL
U_1 = 4 mg per 100 mL   (assumed potency equals 25 units per mg)
U_2 = 8 mg per 100 mL   (assumed potency equals 25 units per mg)

Dose per rabbit = 0.40 mL in all cases.
Response is sum of blood sugar at 1 hr and $2\frac{1}{2}$ hr
y = response to high dose minus response to low dose

$T_a = -T_1 + T_2 + T_3 - T_4 = +239 - 113 - 170 + 210 = 166$
$T_b = T_1 + T_2 + T_3 + T_4 = -239 - 113 - 170 - 210 = -732$
$M' = 0.301\, T_a/T_b = 0.301(166)/-732 = -0.06825$
log of assumed potency = log 25 = 1.3979
potency in USP units = antilog (M' + log of assumed potency)
           = antilog ($-0.06825 + 1.3979$) = 21.4 units per mg

$N = 24$ and $f = 6$ animals in a group
$t = 2.086$ for $n = 4(f-1)$ or 20 degrees of freedom
$t^2 = 4.351$
$t^2 N = 104.424$
$\Sigma y^2 = (25)^2 + (20)^2 + \ldots + (24)^2 = 25468$
$\Sigma T_i{}^2/f = [(239)^2 + (113)^2 + (170)^2 + (210)^2]/6$
       $= 142890/6 = 23815$
$s^2 = \{\Sigma y^2 - \Sigma T_i{}^2/f\}/n$
    $= \{25468 - 23815\}/20 = 82.65$
$s^2 t^2 N = 82.65\ (104.424) = 8630.64$
$C = T_b{}^2/(T_b{}^2 - s^2 t^2 N) = (-732)^2/\{(-732)^2 - 8630.64\}$
    $= 1.01637$
$CM'^2 = 1.01637\ (-0.06825)^2 = 0.00473$
$CM'^2 + c'i^2 = 0.00473 + 0.09062 = 0.09535$
$L^2/4 = (C-1)(CM'^2 + c'i^2) = 0.01637\ (0.09535)$
    $= 0.0015609$
$L/2 = \sqrt{0.0015609} = 0.03951$
$X_M = \log R + CM' \pm \tfrac{1}{2}L$
Upper limit $X_M = 1.3979 - 0.06937 + 0.03951 = 1.3680$
Lower limit $X_M = 1.3979 - 0.06937 - 0.03951 = 1.2890$
Then obtaining the antilogarithms of the X_M:
          Upper limit = 23.3
          Lower limit = 19.4

Thus, the calculated potency is 21.4 units per mg and the upper and lower 95% confidence limits are respectively 23.3 and 19.4 units per mg.

Vitamin D Biological Assay—The official Vitamin D assay is used as an illustration of the calculations involved in a 3-point (2 doses of standard and 1 dose of unknown) littermate bioassay. The following example uses data from a vitamin D assay* in which three animals from each of eight litters of rats had been placed at random on the proper diets

---

* The data in the Insulin Injection Assay example given were kindly furnished by Dr RL Grant, US Food and Drug Administration. (See Table XXV.)
* The data for the Vitamin D Assay were kindly furnished by Dr Leo Friedman, US Food and Drug Administration.

Table XXII—Probit Method of Calculation

A Three-Dose Assay Having an All or None Type of Response

Dose	Log dose x	Re-sponse	%	Probit y	Weight[a] w	wx	wy
			Standard				
8.9	0.95	5/16	31.2	4.51	9.328	8.8616	42.0693
12.6	1.10	8/16	50.0	5.00	10.186	11.2046	50.9300
17.8	1.25	12/16	75.0	5.67	8.632	10.7900	48.9434
			Unknown				
8.9	0.95	2/16	12.5	3.85	6.200	5.8900	23.8700
12.6	1.10	6/16	37.6	4.68	9.808	10.7888	45.9014
17.8	1.25	11/16	68.8	5.49	9.328	11.6600	51.2107

	Standard	Unknown
Σw	28.146	25.336
Σwx	30.8562	28.3388
$\bar{x} = \Sigma wx/\Sigma w$	1.09629	1.11852
Σwy	141.9427	120.9821
$\bar{y} = \Sigma wy/\Sigma w$	5.04309	4.77511
Σwx^2	34.2311	32.0382
Σwxy	157.1681	137.1815
$[wx^2] = \Sigma wx^2 - \bar{x}\Sigma wx$	0.4038	0.3407
$[wxy] = \Sigma wxy - \bar{y}\Sigma wx$	1.5575	1.8606

Combining Standard and Unknown

$$\Sigma[wx^2] = [wx^2]_S + [wx^2]_U = 0.7445$$
$$\Sigma[wxy] = [wxy]_S + [wxy]_U = 3.4181$$

$$b_c = \frac{\Sigma[wxy]}{\Sigma[wx^2]} = 4.5911$$

$$M = \bar{x}_S - \bar{x}_U - \frac{1}{b_c}(\bar{y}_S - \bar{y}_U) = -0.08060$$

$$s_M = \frac{1}{b_c}\sqrt{\frac{1}{\Sigma w_S} + \frac{1}{\Sigma w_U} + \frac{(\bar{y}_S - \bar{y}_U)^2}{b_c\Sigma[wxy]}} = 0.0614$$

Potency = antilog $(2 + M) = 83.1$

Approximate 95% confidence limits for $DF = 4$

$$L_{95} = \text{antilog}\{M \pm ts_M\}$$
$$= \text{antilog}\{-0.0806 \pm 2.78(0.0614)\}$$

Lower limit = antilog $(2 - 0.2513) = 56.1$

Upper limit = antilog $(2 + 0.0901) = 123.0$

[a] Weights are from Table XXI times number of animals tested.

after the specified depletion procedure. The graded degrees of healing (y = individual response) as found are shown in Table XXVI. Two doses of the standard were used (the highest dose twice the lowest dose) and one dose of the unknown.

This is the Design 2,1 (2 doses of the standard and 1 of the unknown) as shown in the USP in the section on *Design and Analysis of Biological Assays*, from which it is seen (with slightly different notation):

Design	Row	Factorial coefficients			e_i	T_i
		s_1	s_2	u_1		
2,1	a	−1	−1	2	6	T_a
	b	−1	1	0	2	T_b

For computing	Equation no.	Constant	Value in design		
			2,1	3,2	4,3
M'	8,10	c	1/2	5/6	7/6
L	25,28	c'	3/4	25/12	49/12

Table XXIII—Angular Transformation

Transformation of Percentages to Angle Theta[a]

%	0	1	2	3	$P = \sin^2\theta$ 4	5	6	7	8	9
0	0	5.7	8.1	10.0	11.5	12.9	14.2	15.3	16.4	17.5
10	18.4	19.4	20.3	21.1	22.0	22.8	23.6	24.4	25.1	25.8
20	26.6	27.3	28.0	28.7	29.3	30.0	30.7	31.3	31.9	32.6
30	33.2	33.8	34.4	35.1	35.7	36.3	36.9	37.5	38.1	38.6
40	39.2	39.8	40.4	41.0	41.6	42.1	42.7	43.3	43.9	44.4
50	45.0	45.6	46.1	46.7	47.3	47.9	48.4	49.0	49.6	50.2
60	50.8	51.4	51.9	52.5	53.1	53.7	54.3	54.9	55.6	56.2
70	56.8	57.4	58.1	59.3	60.0	60.7	61.3	62.0	62.7	
80	63.4	64.2	64.9	65.6	66.4	67.2	68.0	68.9	69.7	70.6
90	71.6	72.5	73.6	74.7	75.8	77.1	78.5	80.0	81.9	84.3

[a] From Fisher and Yates.[39]

Note—For 100% response, angle theta is 90.

Table XXIV—Angle Theta Method of Calculation

Three-Dose Assay Having All or None Type of Response

Log dose	Response	θ
	Standard	
0.95	5/16	$S_L = 34.0$
1.10	8/16	$S_M = 45.0$
1.25	12/16	$S_H = 60.0$
	Unknown	
0.95	2/16	$U_L = 20.7$
1.10	6/16	$U_M = 37.8$
1.25	11/16	$U_H = 56.0$

n = number of animals on each dose = 16
i = difference between log doses = 1.25 − 1.10
    = 1.10 − 0.95 = 0.15
$V = U_H + U_m + U_L - S_H - S_M - S_L = -24.5$
$W = U_H + S_H - U_L - S_L = 61.3$

$$M = \frac{4iV}{3W} = \frac{4(0.15)(-24.5)}{3(61.3)} = -0.079934$$

Potency = antilog $(2 + M)$ = antilog (1.920066) = 83.2
$Z = \sqrt{3W^2 + 2V^2} = \sqrt{3(61.3)^2 + 2(24.5)^2} = 111.7$

Standard error of assay = $\dfrac{1224.385\, iZ}{W^2 \sqrt{n}}$ (potency) =

$$\frac{124.385(0.15)111.7}{(61.3)^2\sqrt{16}}(83.2) = 11.5$$

Approximately 95% confidence limits for $DF = 4$
L_{95} = potency ± t (standard error of assay)
    = 83.2 ± 2.78 (1.5)
    Upper limit = 115.2
    Lower limit = 51.2

Note—The above formulas apply only to a three-dose assay.

In this table are shown the coefficients to be used in multiplying the totals for s_1, s_2, and u_1 (or u) in order to get T_a and T_b. Thus,

$$T_a = 2T_u - T_1 - T_2$$
$$T_b = T_2 - T_1$$

The equation for the log-relative potency of the unknown before adjustment for its assumed potency is

$$M' = ci\, T_a/T_b$$

where $c = \frac{1}{2}$ from the above table and i = log (high dose/low dose) = log 2 = 0.30103 for this assay.
The equation for the variance as given in the USP is

$$s^2 = \{\Sigma y^2 - \Sigma T_r^2/k - \Sigma T_t^2/f + T^2/N\}/(k-1)(f-1)$$

where k = number of different doses given = 3
    f = number of rows (litters) = 8
    $N = kf$
    T_t = total for each dose
    T_r = total for each row (litter)

Table XXV—An Insulin Injection Assay

Group	Rabbit	Response Dilution 2	Response Dilution 1	y
1	7	122	147	− 25
(S_2 & U_1)	52	81	101	− 20
	62	105	152	− 47
	73	168	213	− 45
	77	87	131	− 44
	80	57	145	− 58
		(650)	(889)	−239 = T_1
2	29	111	124	− 13
(S_1 & U_2)	45	111	134	− 23
	50	121	137	− 16
	72	171	198	− 27
	75	158	177	− 19
	90	177	192	− 15
		(849)	(962)	−113 = T_2
3	30	90	117	− 27
(U_2 & S_1)	47	169	197	− 28
	54	101	130	− 29
	74	158	184	− 26
	78	201	233	− 32
	84	157	185	− 28
		(876)	(1046)	−170 = T_3
4	36	115	139	− 24
U_1 & S_2	46	104	151	− 47
	63	151	190	− 39
	66	124	158	− 34
	76	166	208	− 42
	87	140	164	− 24
		(800)	(1010)	−210 = T_4
Total				−732

The confidence limits for the log potency are given in the USP as follows:

$$X_M = \log R + CM' \pm \frac{1}{2}L$$

where R is the ratio of corresponding dose of the standard and of the unknown or the assumed potency of the unknown and where

$$L = 2\sqrt{(C-1)(CM'^2 + c'i^2)}$$

and

$$C = T_b^2/(T_b^2 - e_b f s^2 t^2)$$

where e_b and c' are given in the same table with the factorial coefficients.

Table XXVII shows a systemized calculation of this assay.

For the Vitamin D Biological Assay, if C is negative, the assay is invalid. Here, C is positive. Thus the assay yields as the potency of the unknown 109% of the standard with

Table XXVI—Vitamin D Assay

	Response to low dose of standard s_1	Response to high dose of standard s_2	Response to unknown u	Totals T_r
Litter No. 1	1.00	3.75	4.37	9.12
Litter No. 2	2.00	3.37	2.50	7.87
Litter No. 3	2.12	3.75	2.00	7.87
Litter No. 4	3.25	4.50	2.75	10.50
Litter No. 5	2.50	4.50	4.00	11.00
Litter No. 6	1.75	4.00	2.25	8.00
Litter No. 7	2.00	4.50	4.00	10.50
Litter No. 8	1.37	3.37	4.00	8.74
Totals T_t	$T_1 = 15.99$	$T_2 = 31.74$	$T_u = 25.87$	$T = 73.60$

Table XXVII—Vitamin D Assay Calculations

$T_a = 2T_u - T_1 - T_2 = 2(25.87) - 15.99 - 31.74 = 4.01$
$T_b = T_2 - T_1 = 31.74 - 15.99 = 15.75$
$M' = ciT_a/T_b = 0.5(0.30103)(4.01)/15.75 = 0.0383$
$R = 1 \therefore M = M'$
$\Sigma y^2 = \Sigma(y_1^2 + y_2^2 + \ldots + y_N^2) = (1.00^2 + 2.00^2 + \ldots + 4.00^2) =$
  252.8070
$T^2/N = (73.60)^2/24 = 225.7067$
$\Sigma T_t^2/f = \{(15.99)^2 + (31.74)^2 + (25.87)^2\}/8 = 241.5456$
$\Sigma T_r^2/k = \{(9.12)^2 + (7.87)^2 + \ldots + (8.74)^2\}/3 = 229.6453$
$s^2 = (252.8070 - 229.6453 - 241.5456 + 225.7067)/14 = 0.5231$
$t^2 = 4.601$ using tabled t value for $(k-1)(f-1)$ degrees of
  freedom
$e_b f s^2 t^2 = 2(8)(0.5231)(4.601) = 38.5085$
$C = T_b^2/(T_b^2 - e_b f s^2 t^2) = (15.75)^2/\{(15.75)^2 - 38.5085\} = 1.1838$
$\quad L^2/4 = (C-1)(CM'^2 + c'i^2) = 0.1838[1.1838(0.0383)^2 +$
  $\quad\quad 0.75(0.30103)^2]$
  $\quad\quad = 0.1838[0.001736 + 0.067964] = 0.01281$
$\quad L/2 = \sqrt{0.01281} = 0.1132$
$L = 0.2264$
Potency (%) = antilog $(2 + M')$ = antilog $(2 + 0.0383) = 109\%$
$X_M = CM' \pm L/2$
Upper limit $X_M = 1.1838(0.0383) + 0.1132 = 0.1585$
Lower limit $X_M = 1.1838(0.0383) - 0.1132 = 9.9321 - 10$
Obtaining the antilogarithms of the X_M and converting to %
  Upper limit = 144%
  Lower limit = 86%

An alternate and more general procedure is as follows:
Let the doses of standard be 2 and 4 (ie, log-doses x_{S_1} and x_{S_2} equal to 0.30103 and 0.60206, respectively). Let the dose of unknown be the geometric mean of the doses for the standard, 2.8284 [i.e., antilog $(0.30103 + 0.60206)/2$ = antilog 0.45154 = antilog x_T]. Then

$\bar{x}_S$	$= [8(0.30103) + 8(0.60206)]/16 = 7.22472/16 = 0.45154$
$\bar{x}_T$	$= 0.45154$
$\bar{y}_S$	$= (15.99 + 31.74)/16 = 47.73/16 = 2.98312$
$\bar{y}_T$	$= 25.87/8 = 3.23375$
$[x^2]_S$	$= 8(0.30103)^2 + 8(0.60206)^2 - (7.22472)^2/16 = 0.36247$
$[xy]_S$	$= (0.30103)(15.99) + (0.60206)(31.74) -$
	$\quad (7.22472)(47.73)/16$
	$= 2.37061$
b	$= [xy]_S/[x^2]_S = 2.37061/0.36247 = 6.54016$
M	$= \bar{x}_S - \bar{x}_T - (\bar{y}_S - \bar{y}_T)/b$
	$= 0.45154 - 0.45154 - (2.98312 - 3.23375)/6.54016$
	$= 0.03832$
Potency	$=$ antilog M = antilog $0.03832 = 1.09$ or 109%
g	$= \dfrac{t^2 s^2}{b^2[x^2]_S} = \dfrac{(4.601)(0.5231)}{(6.54016)^2(0.36247)} = 0.1552$

Since $\bar{x}_S = \bar{x}_T$, the estimate of M_L, M_U (see Table XX) reduces to

$$M_L, M_U = (M \pm t/b\sqrt{s^2\{(1-g)(1/n_S + 1/n_T) + M^2/[x^2]_S\}})/(1-g)$$

$$= \left(0.03832 \pm \frac{2.145}{6.54016} \right.$$
$$\left. \times \sqrt{.5234\left\{0.8448\left(\frac{1}{16} + \frac{1}{8}\right) + \frac{(0.03832)^2}{0.36247}\right\}} \right) \Big/ 0.8448$$

$$= -0.06781, 0.15853$$

95% confidence limits for the potency = antilog (M_L, M_U)
$\quad\quad\quad$ = antilog $(-0.06781, 0.15853)$
$\quad\quad\quad$ = 0.86 and 1.44, or 86% and
$\quad\quad\quad\quad$ 144%

---

upper and lower 95% confidence limits of 144% and 86%, respectively, of the standard.

Evaluation of a Microbiological Assay—In most microbiological assays it has been found that there is a linear relationship between the *dose* and the response instead of (as in most biological assays) a linear relationship between the *log dose* and the response. Thus instead of fitting two parallel lines to the log dose response data and calculating the potency as the anti logarithm of the horizontal distance between these two lines as in biological assays, in microbiological assays two

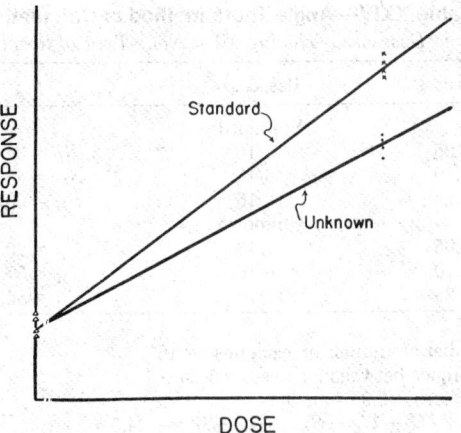

Fig 10-24. A typical microbiological vitamin assay. △ indicates responses to blank; ✕ indicates responses to standard; ● indicates responses to unknown.

straight lines are used which intersect at a "common-zero" point and the potency is calculated as the ratio of the slopes of these two lines. See Fig 10-24 for a graphic illustration of the results of a microbiological assay.

The statistical evaluation of a microbiological assay has been developed by Wood and Finney[40,41] but the calculations are rather complicated as applied to the usual procedure for a microbiological assay and will not be described here. However, one simple type of calculation which they give for a "common-zero 3-dose assay" will be described with a cautioning statement as to its use. When the dose of the standard and the unknown are taken as two arbitrary units of the respective preparations and the same number, n, of tubes (observations) are run on the blank, the standard and the unknown, the formulas for the potency and the standard error of the assay are rather simple. This assay is called a "common-zero 3-dose" assay since the blank is common to both dose response lines, and the blank, standard, and unknown together constitute three doses.

The uninitiated must exercise great caution in using this type of assay since so many factors in the assay itself may affect one point on the curve and not others. From the point of view of the vitamin assayist, it is safer to run several levels of both standard and unknown.

Let $\bar{y}_0$, $\bar{y}_s$, and $\bar{y}_u$ represent the mean responses to the blank, the standard, and the unknown, respectively. Let R represent the average range in response to each dose, as calculated from the data, and D, the average number of standard deviation units in the range. Then the ratio of the potency of the unknown to the potency of the standard is equal to

$$B = \frac{\bar{y}_u - \bar{y}_0}{\bar{y}_s - \bar{y}_0}$$

and the standard error of the assay is given by

$$s_B = \frac{R\sqrt{1 - B + B^2}}{D(\bar{y}_s - \bar{y}_0)\sqrt{2n}}$$

There are other designs for microbiological assays which together with the so-called "common-zero 3-point assay design" are given by Wood and Finney.

The range can be used in estimating the standard error of the assay[42] (and also the confidence limits) for other biological assays by substituting the range divided by the appropriate tabled factor (see Table XIII) for the number of standard deviations in the range, given the number of observations, n.

An article by Knudsen[43] explains calculations of potency, standard error of the assay, control-chart procedures as used in microbiological assay, and the operating characteristic curves for various types of assay procedures where acceptance or rejection of the lot is based on the results of one to three assays.

References

1. Welch H, *et al: J APhA Sci Ed 35:* 102, 1946.
2. Tippett LC: *Random Sampling Numbers* (Tracts for Computers No. 15), Cambridge, London, 1927.
3. Fisher RA, Yates F: *Statistical Tables for Biological, Agricultural, and Medical Research*, Hafner, New York, 134, Table XXXIII, 1963.
4. Dixon WJ, Massey FJ, Jr.: *Introduction to Statistical Analysis*, McGraw-Hill, New York, 366, Table I, 1957.
5. Fisher RA: *The Design of Experiments*, 4th ed, Oliver & Boyd, Edinburgh, 1953.
6. Cochran WG, Cox GM: *Experimental Design*, 2nd ed, Wiley, New York, 1957.
7. Herwick RP, *et al: J Am Med Assoc 127:* 74, 1945.
8. Youden WJ: *Statistical Methods for Chemists*, Wiley, New York, 1951.
9. Stearns EI: *Chem Met Eng 53:* 119, 1946.
10. Pearson L, ed: *Tables for Statisticians and Biometricians*, part I, University College, London, 1930.
11. Mainland D: *Can J Res 26 (E):* 1, 1948.
12. Eisenhart C: *Photogrammetric Eng 18:* 3, 1952.
13. Mainland D: *Science 116:* 592, 1952.
14. Mainland D: *Can J Res 26(E):* 1 1948.
15. Dixon WJ, Massey FJ, Jr.: *Introduction to Statistical Analysis*, McGraw-Hill, New York, 221, 1957.
16. Tate MW, Clelland RC: *Nonparametric and Shortcut Statistics*, Interstate Print. & Publ., Inc., Danville, IL, 137, Table L, 1957.
17. Hicks CR: *Ind Quality Control 11:* 1, 1955.
18. Snedecor GW, Cochran WG: *Statistical Methods*, Iowa State Univ. Press, Ames, IA, 560–567, Table A-14, 1967.
19. Bliss CI, Calhoun DW: *An Outline of Biometry*, Yale Cooperative Corp., New Haven, CT, Table IX, 1954.
20. Duncan DB: *Biometrics 11:* 1, 1955.
21. Dunnett CW: *Am Statist Assoc J 50:* 1096, 1955.
22. Finney DJ: *Statistical Method in Biological Assay*, Hafner, New York, 71, 1964.
23. Levene H: *Contributions to Probability and Statistics*, Stanford Univ. Press, Stanford, CA, 278–292, 1960.
24. Youden WJ: *Sci Monthly 77:* 143, 1953.
25. Youden WJ: *Natl Bur Std (US) Tech News Bull 33 (July):* 1949.
26. Dixon WJ, Massey FJ, Jr.: *Introduction to Statistical Analysis*, McGraw-Hill, New York, 275, 1957.
27. *Control Chart Method of Controlling Quality during Production* (Std. Z1.3), Am. Std. Assoc., New York, 1958.
28. *Guide for Quality Control* (Std. Z1.1), Am. Std. Assoc., New York, 1958.
29. Dixon WJ, Massey FJ, Jr.: *Introduction to Statistical Analysis*, McGraw-Hill, New York, 130, 237, 1957.
30. Knudsen LF (now Randolph LK): *J APhA Sci Ed 38:* 332, 1949.
31. Bliss CI: *Drug Std 24:* 33, 1956.
32. Bliss CI: *Biometrics 12 (June):* 491, 1956.
33. Gaddum JH: *Med Res Council Spec Rept Ser 183:* 1933.
34. Trevan JW: *Proc Roy Soc (London) Ser B 101:* 483, 1927.
35. Bliss CI: *Ann Appl Biol 22:* 134, 307, 1935.
36. Miller LC, *et al: J APhA 28:* 644, 1939.
37. Finney DJ: *Probit Analysis*, 2nd ed, Cambridge, London, 65, 1952.
38. Bliss CI: *Quart J Pharm Pharmacol 11:* 195, 1938.
39. Fisher RA, Yates F: *Statistical Tables for Biological, Agricultural, and Medical Research*, Oliver & Boyd, Edinburgh, 74, 75, Table X, 1963.
40. Wood EC, Finney DJ: *Quart J Pharm Pharmacol 19:* 112, 1946.
41. Finney DJ: *Quart J Pharm Pharmacol 18:* 77, 1945.
42. Randolph LK: *J APhA Sci Ed 41:* 438, 1952.
43. Knudsen LF (now Randolph LK): *Ann NY Acad Sci 52:* 889, 1950.
44. Dunnett CW: *Biometrics 20:* 482, 1964.

Bibliography

Experimental Design

Brownlee KA: *Industrial Experimentation*, Chem. Publ. Co., Inc., Brooklyn, NY, 1947.
Cochran WC, Cox GM: *Experimental Designs*, 2nd ed, Wiley, New York, 1957.
Finney DJ: *Experimental Design and Its Statistical Basis*, Univ. Chicago Press, Chicago, 1955.
Fisher RA: *Statistical Methods for Research Workers*, 12th ed, Oliver & Boyd, Edinburgh, 1958.
Mainland D: *The Treatment of Clinical and Laboratory Data*, Oliver & Boyd, Edinburgh, 1938.
Snedecor GW, Cochran WG: *Statistical Methods*, 6th ed, Iowa State Univ. Press, Ames, IA, 1967.
Steel JM, ed: *Methods in Medical Research*, Yearbook, Chicago, 1954.

Statistical Quality Control

Dodge HF, Romig HF: *Sampling Inspection Tables*, Wiley, New York, 1951.
Duncan AJ: *Quality Control and Industrial Statistics*, Richard D. Irwin, Inc., Homewood, IL, 1953.
Grant EL: *Statistical Quality Control*, 2nd ed, McGraw-Hill, New York, 1952.

Sampling

Cochran WG: *Sampling Techniques*, Wiley, New York, 1963.
Deming WE: *Some Theory of Sampling*, Wiley, New York, 1961.
Hansen MH, Hurwitz WH: *Ann Math Statist 14:* 333, 1943.
Smith JG, Duncan AJ: *Fundamentals of Theory of Statistics*, vol I, McGraw-Hill, New York, Chaps. II, III, 1944.
Yates F: *Sampling Methods for Censuses and Surveys*, Hafner, New York, 1953.

Biological Assay

Berkson J: *J Am Statist Assoc 48:* 565, 1953.
Bliss CI: Cattell M: *Ann Rev Physiol 5:* 479, 1943.
Bliss CI: *The Statistics of Bioassay with Special Reference to the Vitamins*, Academic, New York, 1952.
Bliss CI: *Am Scientist 45:* 449, 1957.
Burn JH: *Biological Standardization*, Oxford Univ. Press, New York, 1950.
Finney DJ: *Statistical Method in Biological Assay*, 2nd ed, Hafner, New York, 1964.
Finney DJ: *Probit Analysis*, 3rd ed, Cambridge, London, 1971.
Mather K: *Statistics in Biology*, 3rd ed, Interscience, New York, 1947.

General

Armitage P: *Sequential Medical Trials*, Blackwell Sci. Publ., Oxford, England, 1959.
Bennett CA, Franklin NL: *Statistical Analysis in Chemistry and the Chemical Industry*, Wiley, New York, 1954.
Brownlee KA: *Statistical Theory and Methods in Science and Engineering*, Wiley, New York, 1960.
Croxton FE, Cowden DJ: *Applied General Statistics*, Prentice-Hall, New York, 1955.
Davies OL: *The Design and Analysis of Industrial Experiments*, Hafner, New York, 1954.
Hoel PC: *An Introduction to Mathematical Statistics*, 2nd ed, Wiley, New York, 1962.
Natrella MG: *Experimental Statistics* (Natl. Bur. Std. Hdbk. 91), USGPO, Washington, DC, 1963.

CHAPTER 11

Computer Science

Thomas J Gildea

Manager
Data Quality Assurance and Scientific Computing

Paul G Sanders

Consulting Biostatistician
G D Searle & Co
Skokie, IL 60077

Computer technology has become a factor in such widely diverse areas as journalism, art, politics, manufacturing production control, and most fields of science. The medical sciences, especially, reflect the impact of this new technology. Its pervasiveness may be illustrated in the applications listed in Table I.

While these glamorous uses often generate headlines, the greatest use for computers in the health sciences is still as a data transformer and retriever in research and as a record keeper in business. Thus, the risk/benefit analysis for a potential new pharmaceutical product is likely to be based on computer-tabulated data; later, the presence of that drug on the pharmacist's shelf when needed will be assured by a computer-directed distribution system.

The rapid growth and pervasiveness of the computer *revolution* tend to mask the basic simplicity of computing and data processing concepts; the heart of the matter is to collect data and data aggregates and perform prespecified operations on these collected *data* to yield *information*. The data may be as simple as entering an account number at a remote teller device or as complex as the coded transmission of planetary photographs from space vehicles. Data size may range from the magnetic sense strip on the back of a credit card to the results of the 1980 US Census. Having been collected, data can then be manipulated by classification, sorting, summarization, calculation, recording, storing or any combination of these. The processing time may range from the instantaneous in the case of industrial process control or life support applications, to hours or days for complex simulations (psychological research and econometric modeling) or census applications. In spite of the wide variations of uses, all computing

and data processing can be analyzed by the simple model

$$INPUT \rightarrow PROCESS \rightarrow OUTPUT$$

abbreviated I–P–O. Data are gathered, processed by prespecified operations and an information product or output is produced.

History of Computing

The concept of machine assistance in the processing of data is certainly not modern; indeed the abacus, a computational tool extensively used in the Orient was developed sometime around 450 BC. Seventeenth and eighteenth century scientists, Leibniz, Pascal, and others designed and, in some cases, built calculating machines to solve specific problems. Most notable of these efforts was the *analytical engine* designed by Charles Babbage in 1833. While falling short of a working model due to engineering limitations, the design laid the groundwork for the development of modern computers. Another advance of note was the development of the electrical tabulating machine by Herman Hollerith in 1888; this machine used electrical rather than mechanical power and introduced punched cards to code and process data. The basic punched card as a coding medium survives to this day and the company Hollerith founded eventually became IBM.

In the early 1940's, Howard Aiken and his associates at Harvard used the basic design strategies of Charles Babbage and successfully built the first digital computer; the Mark I was electromechanical and not very efficient, but it worked. Simultaneously, designers at the Moore School of Engineering at University of Pennsylvania used the work of Atanasoff of Iowa State University to produce the first completely electronic digital computer in 1946. These efforts eventually yielded the Univac I which was used by the Census Bureau in 1951 to process the 1950 Census and by the Columbia Broadcasting System in forecasting the results of the 1952 presidential election and by the first commercial user, General Electric in 1953. IBM introduced its first commercial computer in 1956, quickly establishing a dominance they *still* enjoy. These early models, or *first generation* computers, were characterized by dependence on vacuum tubes as electronic components. The tubes were expensive, unreliable, consumed a great deal of power and generated much heat. The discovery and development of the transistor launched the *second generation* of computers and began the trend of declining size and cost and rapidly increasing performance. The *third generation* continued using semiconductor technology

Table I—Applications of Computer Technology in Various Medical and Biological Science Settings

Setting	Computer application
Intensive Care Unit	Monitor EKG's.
Clinical Laboratory	Return laboratory results on-line together with costs for billing.
Psychological Laboratory	Monitor and control behavioral tests in animals.
Community Pharmacy	Preparation of prescription histories, accounting for patient's tax returns, and checking prescriptions for potentially adverse combinations.
Diagnostic Clinic	Relieve medical personnel of tedious chore of taking patient histories.

and Large Scale Integration (LSI), and some believe that today we are in the *fourth generation* with Very Large Scale Integration (VLSI) characterized by microchips and desk top components. The desk top personal computers belong to this latest generation.

Despite the evolutionary change in components with corresponding dramatic changes in size, price and performance, every computer designed adheres to the basic I–P–O model. Each design phase has addressed the volume and velocity aspects of the data. In this accelerating information age machines are being designed to manipulate more data faster and more accurately, the same design problems the computing pioneers were solving.

Hardware

Computers are generally classified as digital, analog or hybrid depending on the manner in which they treat data. Digital computers operate with discrete coded symbols for words and numbers; analog computers operate on continuously varying quantities, usually voltages. Hybrid computers combine characteristics of both analog and digital to accomplish their processing, however, all three classes are amenable to I–P–O analysis. While the analog computer is of importance in research and process control applications, this discussion will focus on the digital computer which is far more prevalent. Most laboratory systems today have analog to digital converters that transform the continuous voltages of an instrument into digital signals to be operated on by a digital laboratory computer. Therefore the use of analog computers has decreased markedly in recent years.

At the heart of a computer is an assemblage of electronic devices which are either *on* or *off* and representing two digits, 0 and 1. An advantage of this *bi*nary digi*t* (bit) is the fact that its value is independent of size (vacuum tube, transistor or chip) and, in combination with adjacent bits, forms the basis of an elementary coding scheme to represent data. One bit can represent the quantities 0 or 1, two bits the quantities 0, 1, 2, 3 with n bits being able to represent a number up to 2^n-1. The coding scheme used varies between manufacturers and, as a general purpose scheme, must allow for the codification of non-numeric data such as characters of the alphabet or special symbols such as ?, !, @. Binary coding schemes are not new, having been used in telegraphy for many years and they lend themselves well to computer representation of data. An early decision a computer designer must make is the type of coding to be employed, with two codes, ASCII and EBCDIC, predominating. The American Standard Code for Information Interchange (ASCII) is basically a seven bit code. That is, each unique combination of seven consecutive bits corresponds to a specific number, letter or symbol. The Extended Binary Coded Decimal Interchange Code (EBCDIC) is an 8-bit code developed by IBM. Current standards use 8-bit codification schemes and the ASCII code has been mapped into an 8-bit set called ASCII-8; so the basic unit of computation is a set of 8 contiguous bits (sometimes referred to as a byte) coded in ASCII-8 or EBCDIC. Examples of several numbers using these codes are found in Table II.

Having decided on a binary based coding scheme for data, a computer designer must then decide on a computer word length. A computer *word* is the basic unit of operation in a computing system and is composed of a fixed number of contiguous bits. The size of the word determines the number of data types a computer may use, the number of operations a computer can support, and the overall *size of the computer*. Word size is generally used to classify computers. Since the predominant coding schemes for data are 8-bit (ASCII-8 and EBCDIC), the most common word lengths are generally

multiples of 8 bits, 8, 16, 32 and 64 being the most common. Microcomputers use 8 or 16-bit; minicomputers generally 16 or 32-bit while maxicomputers usually have 64-bit words. Early personal computers used an 8-bit word and current introductions are using the 16-bit architecture. Scientific computation requires longer word lengths to support numerical size and precision while commercial systems can generally be well supported by a shorter word length. This basic unit of activity, word length, is generally dictated by the basic design purpose of the computer.

Computing systems, historical and contemporary, can conveniently be analyzed in terms of their physical and non-physical components, hardware and software. *Hardware* refers to all the tubes, relays, transistors, components, circuits and cabinets that comprise a computing system. The term equally applies to all machinery (*peripherals* like printers, cathode ray tubes (CRT's), plotters, etc) associated with or connected to it. *Software* generally refers to *programs* which are executed on the hardware. Programs are sequential, computational steps which are coded for implementation by a computer. A computer by itself is useless without software, needing programs to accomplish general, as well as specialized, tasks. Software is further categorized as being either *systems* software or *applications* software. Systems software is a collection of programs that coordinate the activities of the machinery internally and with the outside world. Application software are programs that are designed to run on a machine to solve particular problems. A program to schedule jobs on a computer belongs to system software while a program to estimate pharmacokinetic parameters exemplifies applications software. In current technology a number of systems software functions is embedded in the hardware of the computer so some of these distinctions are beginning to blur and some authors refer to these hardware/software components as *firmware*.

What is generally referred to and understood as a computer is actually a complicated collection of electrical circuitry and electronic components called a *Central Processing Unit* (CPU) housed in an impressive looking cabinet. The essential work of computation takes place in the CPU and generally there are a number of associated devices used to store or input data into the CPU. The CPU, as the center of intelligence and activity in the computer, is responsible for controlling tasks, manipulating data and coordinating the associated hardware. The CPU is organized to perform these tasks using three basic units: a control unit, an arithmetic-logic unit, and primary storage. The control unit supervises the overall activity of the CPU by fetching, and interpreting program instructions one by one and sending the appropriate control signals to the various units for action or execution. Every computer has a basic set of coded instructions (eg, addition, subtraction, comparison, moving of data) that can be executed by that system. Decodification by the control unit identifies the physical and logical pathways to be taken, as well as the data which must be routed along that pathway. The arithmetic-logic unity (ALU) contains the necessary electronic circuitry to control all logical and arithmetic operations. The basic arithmetic operations are addition, subtraction, multiplication and division, while operations of logic are primarily comparison tasks to test equality, types of inequality or system conditions. Because of the design and circuitry, these operations (each operation is referred to as an execution cycle) are generally accomplished at extremely high rates, in some machines as high as 50,000,000 per second.

The third component of the CPU is main or primary storage and it contains all the coded data *and* instructions necessary to execute a currently running program. Because of its components and electrical circuits, locations in primary storage or memory can be accessed at incredible speeds. Because of its complexity, storage is generally an expensive part of a

Table II—Computer Codes

	ASCII	ASCII - 8	EBCDIC
1	011 0001	0101 0001	1111 0001
2	011 0010	0101 0010	1111 0010
3	011 0011	0101 0011	1111 0011
A	100 0001	1010 0001	1100 0001
B	100 0010	1010 0010	1100 0010
C	100 0011	1010 0011	1100 0011
P	101 0000	1011 0000	1101 0111
Q	101 0001	1011 0001	1101 1000
R	101 0010	1011 0010	1101 1001
?	011 1111	0101 1111	0110 1111
=	011 1101	0101 1101	0111 1110

computer system. Memory is actually the organized structure of the bistable components (bits) discussed earlier and is organized into bytes or words, depending on the system design and architecture. This organization allows each byte or each word to have a specific physical and logical location to be *addressed* by the control unit. Each byte or word is like a bank of mailboxes at the post office—discrete units with unique locations and unique numbers or addresses. Some of these physical locations are reserved for special purposes such as systems software coded into an area of primary storage or memory. These areas, which are specially protected and inaccessible to programmers are called Read Only Memory (ROM). The non-reserved areas of memory are called Random Access Memory (RAM) and may be used by any executing program for reading or writing during execution of that program.

To execute a program, the control unit must load the coded program in specific areas of memory. In addition, the data to be processed are also loaded into specific areas of memory. The control unit then fetches each program instruction, step by step, decodes the instruction, identifies the *addresses* of the data elements needed for the instruction and dispatches the decoded instruction and data addresses to the ALU. The ALU performs the indicated operation (multiplication or exponentiation, for example) on the addressed data elements and stores the result in an address which has also been provided by the control unit. On completion of this task, *control* is returned to the control unit to fetch the next program instruction. The speed and combination of these basic steps enables the computer to perform extraordinary feats of data management, logic and computation.

Input-Output

Much of the previous discussion has focused on the P (processing) of the I–P–O model. While processing is the critical factor, it is meaningless without efficient and effective input (I) resources to make data and programs available to process. A record of the data used and the results of data processed must also be available in the form of output (O) consisting of numbers, words, graphical material or signals. Because of the fact that the CPU is code dependent and that memory stores data and instructions in coded form, it becomes clear that the primary purpose of *Input* and *Output* (I/O) is the codification and decodification of data for transfer to the CPU. I/O devices can generally be classified as *general* or *special* purpose. General purpose devices are not specific to any one application, while special purpose devices are designed and employed to satisfy the needs of a particular application. The ubiquitous *IBM punched card* is a product of a prototypical general purpose device—the keypunch. The *automated teller* used by most savings institutions is an example of such a keypunch, but it finds little utility outside of that industry. The basic purpose of the newer devices remains the same, however, and that is to convert data found in its raw form into a series of ASCII or EBCDIC characters to be processed and reconverted to original or other form for consumption as information.

The earliest general purpose input devices were the teletypewriter and the Hollerith keypunch card, owing both to their coding properties and the prevalence of their usage prior to the introduction of computers. The keypunch machine which codes the Hollerith card and the teletypewriter actually work on the same principle and these principles are in use in computer terminals and personal computers even today. These early devices use a typewriter-like keyboard which essentially had two types of keys, data and function. Depressing a key causes an electrical contact to be made and this contact is then converted to a coded pulse which either punches holes in a card or transmits coded signals over a communications line. Data keys are converted into their corresponding letters, numbers or symbols while function keys perform special operations specific to the data entry operation (eg, advancing a card, testing a communications line, etc.). These early devices and their evolutionary counterparts continue in heavy use today although the use of cards is diminishing rapidly.

Hollerith cards were also heavily used as an early general purpose output device. Recomputed or computer generated data were decoded and punched into cards by a card punching machine. The great advantage here was that the cards produced from one program or from one system could be used as input into another program or system. This concept has been greatly refined and amplified with the introduction of magnetic tapes and disk storage. Another early output device still much used today is the line printer. The document it prints is used as a permanent record and ready reference of calculations or word processing. Computer printouts are low cost and may contain a large amount of data, conveniently formatted for readability and interpretation. However, as the volume and velocity of data handling has increased, large printed reports have fallen into disfavor. Microfilm and graphics have become more popular as efficient techniques for storing, analyzing and interpreting large amounts of data.

Some devices can be used extensively as both input and output devices. Punched cards were used early on, however, they were eclipsed in popularity by magnetic tape and storage devices such as magnetic drums and disks. Magnetic tape was favored because of low cost, the ability to store large amounts of data in a small physical space, and its general reliability. Magnetic drums and disks are more expensive, however, they store vast quantities of data which are more directly accessed by a computer. These multiple purpose devices are often referred to as a secondary storage as they can hold programs and data for use by more than one program for future use. Personal computers rely heavily on a disk technology called *floppy disks* as both a storage device for data and programs and a tool for dissemination of programs and data.

Software

Early computers required that their logic and relay circuits be set manually prior to each computer run. This manual process was time consuming, tedious, subject to extensive scheduling problems and prone to human error. Because of the great expense of purchase and maintenance, it became important to devise methods to increase the efficiency of computer usage. The results of these efforts were the development of *operating systems* and *application programming languages*. Operating systems are generally specific with each computer manufacturer and are designed to optimize the time of processing data through a manufacturer's computer by scheduling tasks, assigning specific input and output devices, and providing utility programs that can be shared by most applications programs. Early operating systems were designed to interact with tasks which were batched together, scheduled and executed when the required resources became available. Today's operating systems provide direct user access to a computer's resources and this *on-line* access has been reflected in new utilities and functions (eg, communications between tasks, text editors, etc.).

Applications programs languages grew out of early attempts to codify the manual setting of switches and relays. Early languages required the direct codification of machine instructions on a step by step basis and required extensive knowledge of the computing machine. Later languages became more oriented toward the problem to be solved, rather than to the machine used to solve the problem; FORTRAN (FORmula TRANslator), COBOL (COmmon Business Oriented Language) and ALGOL (ALGOrithmic Oriented Languages) enabled people who were more familiar with applications problems to design computer based algorithms to solve these application problems without being familiar with the machine configuration. Each of these languages is distinguished by the description of the problem-solving steps in a formal, problem-oriented language which are then codified by an input device, interpreted by a program called a compiler and translated into machine language for execution. These languages gave rise to the applications programming industry and now provide for the development of computer programs that can be shared by many computer users. Of particular interest here is that generic solutions to problems are now being produced and programs common to industries and applications are being developed by third parties and sold to computer users. Collections of computer programs such as the Statistical Analysis System (SAS), Statistical Package for the Social Sciences (SPSS) and the Biomedical Programs (BMDP) have been developed to provide researchers with a readily available library of reliable, standardized, statistical programs for data analysis. Collections of programs for the management of hospitals including the ordering, recording, checking and dispensing of medications have been developed as Hospital Information Systems; accounting programs for the maintenance of inventory of drug wholesalers and retailers is yet another example. It is expected that these third parties will play an increasing role in the development and dissemination of computer applications software in the future, especially prescription record and accounting programs in the community pharmacy.

Networks

As the user base of computers expanded, the necessity to physically accommodate more users and devices became clear. Much effort resulted in computer designs better able to handle the increased number and speed of I/O devices. As applications increased beyond capacity and as prices dropped, multiple systems were employed in companies to help organize activities. As these multiple systems became more geographically dispersed, it became necessary to use segments of the telecommunications industry (eg, local and long distance telephone lines) for communications. The US Defense Department, in 1968, in an effort to link widely scattered researchers and research sites, developed the ARPA net, a specialized telecommunications network specifically designed to enable different computers to communicate with each other. The 1970's and 1980's saw the development of Value Added Networks, which, in addition to communications, also provided a wide variety of computer resources and services to network users. Projections of future usage indicate that computer based networks will grow in importance for resource sharing and become a prime vehicle for information sharing among the scientific community.

A problem with this distributed *computer* revolution and the attendant growth in the number of machines, programs and users, was the integrity of data being used. Companies often found themselves with the embarrassing predicament of having two divisions or departments producing reports with conflicting results. Because of this problem, companies have begun to manage data and information as a corporate asset in much the same fashion as inventory and personnel. Central to this philosophy was a Data Base Management System (DBMS) which is a collection of programs to manage a central repository of data, allowing access by multiple users while maintaining security and providing a common interface to applications programs requiring those data in the DBMS. This common interface concept was further developed by Value Added Networks and other users of telecommunications networks to provide information services for users or subscribers. The National Library of Medicine was an early developer of an on-line, remote data base which could be accessed by a variety of users. Current data bases are maintained for financial and stock information, special interest information, as well as a number of pharmacy related data bases for product information, patient education or drug interaction information.

Personal Computers

The growth and importance of the personal computer revolution was aptly recognized in 1983 as TIME Magazine's Man (Machine) of the year. The seeds of this productivity were sown in the 1960's with the introduction and acceptance of the minicomputer, especially in the laboratory environment where researchers often found themselves configuring various components of a computer system to suit their laboratory needs. In parallel, there was growing acceptance of time sharing services and network usage by "non" data processing people. As the size and price of components dropped, hobby kits were introduced in 1976, and in 1978 Apple Computer and Radio Shack shocked the world by introducing fully packaged *personal computers*. In price and design, personal computers are targeted for the single user with functionality sharply defined by the amount of data and the size of programs to be processed. Although designed for personal use and hailed as a *liberator* of the user from the tyrannies of central data processing and the expenses of time sharing, there is much evidence that the personal computer use and rationale is evolving strongly toward centralized systems to access data bases and to communicate with other users and shared resources. Third party software houses have joined forces with personal computer manufacturers to provide low cost, *turnkey* systems for a variety of applications; many systems have been and are being developed to aid in pharmacy management in the clinical as well as in the retail setting.

A nagging frustration of early personal computer owners was the proprietary nature of most hardware and software. It was difficult, if not impossible to interface system components from different manufacturers and virtually impossible to use systems or applications software with different computer lines. These frustrations have largely been addressed by arriving at prescribed and *de facto* standards. Manufacturers of computers and computer peripherals gradually agreed on communications standards (eg, S-100 bus) to enable the transfer of data from the CPU of one manufacturer to the peripheral device of another, using a common bus or communications architecture. Standards of the Electrical Industry Association (RS-232 protocol) for transfer of data between terminal and communications equipment were adopted to enable communications between personal computers and with mainframe computers over telecommunications lines. In the mid 1970's, Digital Research Associates introduced the CP/M *operating system* which could execute on machines from different manufacturers using similar architecture. An operating system is the basic system software required to execute tasks on a CPU. Having such a standard enabled a tremendous degree of sharing and transportability of systems and applications software among personal computer users.

The introduction of the Apple, and the IBM PC created *de facto* market place standards for both hardware and software. Personal older products were adapted to become compatible with these manufacturers' products primarily because of the overwhelming number of their users. MS/DOS, an operating system developed by MICROSOFT INC, and selected by IBM for its PC, is generally acknowledged to be the industry standard for 16-bit machines. Future software and hardware products will probably be developed in reference to 1) the IBM market, 2) the Apple market or 3) the *all others* market.

Computers & Pharmaceutical Science

Pharmaceutical science has, as has the rest of the world, been dramatically impacted by computer technology and data processing concepts. Originally a curiosity and labor saver, computer based systems are absolute necessities in the development, distribution and dispensing of pharmaceutical products. They provide the controls and documentation necessary in a regulated industry and provide the competitive edge in the market place. We will explore some of the applications of these systems in the practice of pharmaceutical science.

Pharmaceutical Industry

The discovery and development of new chemical entities, drugs, is essentially a market driven process. Public health data on disease states, current medications, prescription profiles, provider information and population demographics are the data that are processed to yield information on desirable new products. This early collection and processing of information is essentially computer based and generally consists of collecting data from diverse sources. Once the target market is selected the search for a safe and effective substance can begin.

This early drug discovery phase is extremely dependent on data processing and computerized systems are essential in this process. Exhaustive searches of the scientific literature must be made on computerized data bases and these searches must be collated with the results from similar searches on patent and test article files. A new discipline, Computer Aided (Assisted) Drug Design, (CADD) is gradually emerging as a key element in the discovery process. This computer based process searches extremely large sets of molecular configurations and allows a chemist to select or design a configuration with specified properties. Heavy use is made in CADD of computer graphics to explore the spatial molecular relations from virtually any viewpoint with respect to precise bond energies and angles, molecular configurations, and interactions of a drug molecule with the active site of an enzyme or the lattice structure of genetic molecules.

Ascertaining the efficacy and safety of test substances has become computer dependent. Screening tests to evaluate effectiveness are essential to identification of *good* drugs, but are also important in the effective utilization of resources by identifying *bad* drugs as early as possible and storing the results of these screens for later referral. Computer based systems for planning, analysis, and the scheduling of resources play a vital role in organizing the testing process. Study protocols on a computer coordinate the acquisition and analysis of data and subject the results to predefined and data dependent analyses. The storage of test results is necessary for regulatory purposes but also input for definition of future research protocols or in structure/activity research.

The toxicology and pathology functions of safety assessment have seen a great degree of computerization and a number of commercially available systems are now offered. These current systems are designed to facilitate the planning and control of animal studies and to collect data specified in study protocols. Researchers generally interact with these systems 'on-line' using a computer terminal. Data are collected by instrumentation and transferred electronically to a host computer—or entered manually by a lab technician. At the conclusion of the study, the computerized data are then available for computer based statistical analysis and report generation.

After a product has been characterized biologically and chemically, it is ready for product formulation and design. These activities are heavily dependent on instrumentation and the use of computers. Many experimental processes and batch applications are machine controlled and they lend themselves well to integration with computer systems in order to control the processes and record the data. Integration of the instrument and computer components can occur at essentially two levels: at the instrument level or at the computer level. Because of current sophistication in design and components, and the decreased size of circuits, many analytical instruments are provided with microprocessors as an integral part of the device. These embedded processors control the process application, adjust or react to experimental conditions or results, and translate and gather data for transfer and analysis. Some of these processors are programmable and allow the researchers a great deal of flexibility while others are confined to predesigned functions.

At the computer level instruments which produce output signals may be connected directly via cable to a separate computer for coordination and control. This approach provides a greater degree of flexibility and independence but at a price. The essential elements of either approach are analog to digital and digital to analog converters, computer controlled clocks, a basic communication link for receiving and transmitting control and data signals, and a storage device to store data and control programs. The integrated components design of machine and computer is neat, generally inexpensive and gives a great degree of independence to the researchers. Most of these systems do need, however, to be linked to other systems to transmit data for storage or analysis. The *connected* design provides greater benefits at the organizational level by being instrument independent, providing a greater amount of program and machine resources and, in general, by the ability of the computer to interface with many machines simultaneously. A third alternative is emerging as personal computers are now being packaged with specific instruments to provide the best of both worlds. This trend will, no doubt, increase in popularity in the future.

In the final phase in the development of a new pharmaceutical product are the clinical trials conducted to prove the safety and efficacy of the product in human populations. Computers are used to randomly assign patients to various treatment groups and to generate the necessary labels and control sheets of the dispensed treatments; case report forms (CRF's) are used to collect demographic, diagnostic and treatment data for each subject and these forms are then codified and entered into a data base for further analysis. During the course of the clinical trial various management reports are generated by the data base system to provide information on the progress of the trial, number of patients enrolled and any non-treatment specific trends. At the end of a trial a number of analyses and reports must be prepared for submission to regulators (FDA) for their review and, hopefully, for the approval of the test drug. Essential to these reports are statistical analyses of the trial results. Because of the data management tasks and the variety and sophistication of the statistical tests that need to be done, this statistical process is almost entirely computer based and the Statistical Analysis System (SAS), a collection of computer

based statistical programs, is the predominant package used in this phase.

Word processing and computer generated graphics are computer based applications that are used heavily in clinical trials, their use is very evident in other areas as well. Word processing is basically a set of programs to allow an operator to create and edit printed documents electronically. The operator generally interacts with the word processing system through a CRT terminal which allows the person to create, preview, and/or edit a document. Documents are stored on a disk device and are transmitted to a letter quality printer to produce a paper (hard) copy. The advantage is obvious—changes can be made in a matter of seconds without having to manually retype an entire document. The system works well with memos, letters or lengthy manuscripts (such as this chapter).

Computer generated graphics are rapidly becoming more affordable and more acceptable as their quality increases. With computer generated graphics the computer is used to compress data into highly stylized graphical elements for display on plotting devices or on special purpose graphics tubes. (Popular examples are the arcade and home video games which execute a program with data supplied by the player's paddle or joystick to create and manipulate images on a TV screen.) These graphs can convey complex ideas and relationships in lieu of reams of printed reports. Line plots of concentration vs time provide neat pharmacokinetic profiles, and comparative line plots can easily illustrate the superior properties of one substance over another. Graphics capabilities are rapidly being developed in micro as well as maxicomputer systems and their use as design, analytical and discussion aids are increasing dramatically.

The marketing and sales efforts of pharmaceutical companies have also become heavily computer dependent. Market identification was alluded to earlier; market development is another task that becomes possible with the aid of a computer. Reams of market and use data can be easily compressed to identify specific geographic or functional areas for attention. The definition and staffing of sales territories are more and more being accomplished with a computer, and the field support of sales staff is yet another application. Inventory and order control is now automated and systems for providing the detail person with sales and marketing strategy or for *in the field* computer aided instruction are in the design stages. A very important role accomplished in these areas is the monitoring of usage patterns and the recording of adverse experience data. Because of the data diversity and the need to react quickly, these systems, too, are computerized.

Computers in the Pharmacy

The practice of pharmacy began to feel the effects of the computer revolution in the early 1970's. Large drug wholesalers and drug chains began to develop inventory and distribution models on computers and some major clinical pharmacies began to experiment with computer based prescription and drug interaction programs. The popularity and sophistication of these programs grew rapidly as many of them enjoyed broad usage via computer time sharing networks and were eventually sold or leased as packaged products.

The introduction of Hospital Information Systems (HIS) in the mid-1970's culminated a trend already begun to formalize and control ordering, dispensing, charging, and inventorying in clinical pharmacies. In the HIS environment a pharmaceutical order or prescription is entered into a computer terminal by a physician. This order is logged for control purposes and is transmitted by the computer to a terminal in the clinical pharmacy. On receipt, the pharmacist

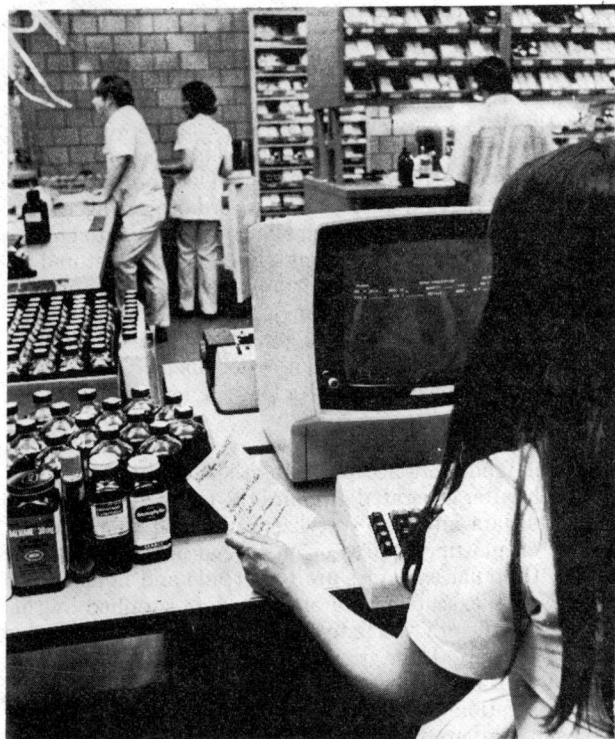

Fig 11-1.   An IBM communications terminal shown in use in a hospital pharmacy where it is a part of a system that provides a safeguard against overdosing, relief from clerical detail for the pharmacist, and data available for research (courtesy, IBM).

need only be concerned with screening and processing the order, as the patient identification has already been validated and the drug has been verified in reference to that clinic's formulary. The pharmacist then uses the computerized data bases available through the HIS to check for potential drug interactions, allergies, appropriateness of dosage and form, and previous therapeutic profile. As the drug is dispensed a label for the medication is printed and the order is confirmed in the system. After the medications are delivered to the appropriate locations, the activity is confirmed by a member of the nursing staff to track compliance and control of the medication process. Concurrent with the dispensing, a charge for the medication, computed from the standard price list, is written to the patient's account at the same time that the drug inventory file reflects the dispensing of that medication. The patient account is presented to the patient on discharge and the status of the inventory file is regularly produced for the pharmacy management to monitor inventory and to place orders at prespecified inventory levels. Fig 11-1 illustrates the use of a computer terminal in the hospital pharmacy.

Community pharmacies now employ mini and microcomputers for the dispensing of drugs, to check for possible drug interactions, and to update family medication records. The small personal computer is also used in the community pharmacy for inventory control and cash flow management. Inventory control systems are crucially important to the community pharmacy to avoid the expenses of overstocking, of stock shortages, and to balance inventory levels to expected usage rates and shelf lives of individual products.

Large chains usually maintain their own proprietary systems. Third party reimbursements are becoming a larger portion of the professional pharmaceutical service and these charges have dramatic effects on cash flow management. Computer systems now exist for the preparation of third party claims. These systems keep track of approved drugs, approved dosages, and charges; all of which may differ from

agency to agency. A patient identifies these insurers and the prescription is then screened to see if it agrees with the guidelines. After dispensing, a computer generated invoice is prepared for reimbursement. The quality control check done by the computer minimizes review time, lessens risk of return and ensures prompt payment from the insurer. A variety of other systems are available to the pharmacists to assist in their practice, including drug information data bases, indexes for pharmacy journals and publications, and computer based information services covering new companies, new products and new markets.

Computers in Pharmacy Education

As in all education areas today, computers continually are playing a greater role. In addition to computer science electives, today's pharmacy student can expect to find computer based courses in every facet of pharmacy education. Considerable progress has been made in computer assisted education in the basic sciences, for example at Ohio State University and the University of Illinois. A wide variety of courses in the basic and clinical sciences are available to enable the student to step through a learning sequence or to interact with a simulation of a physiological or clinical situation. Students in biodynamics and pharmacokinetics learn early the necessity of computer based tools in modeling and curve fitting; NONLIN, a program developed at Upjohn and NLIN developed at the University of Wisconsin have found great popularity in solving these problems. In practice pharmacies (eg, University of Nebraska and University of Texas) undergraduate students are exposed to the use and application of various computer based tools in the clinical and community pharmacy. In the future it is expected that computer based instruction will play an even larger role in education as the trend to continuing professional education and development among health care providers continues to grow.

Epilog

The 1965 edition of Remington's Pharmaceutical Sciences did not contain a single reference to "computers." The coverage in this edition, which only shows the tip of the iceberg, indicates the dynamic growth and impact of computers on the pharmaceutical sciences. This trend is certain to continue. As computer technology is integrated into almost all phases of our society, scenes like that shown in Fig 11-2 will become common.

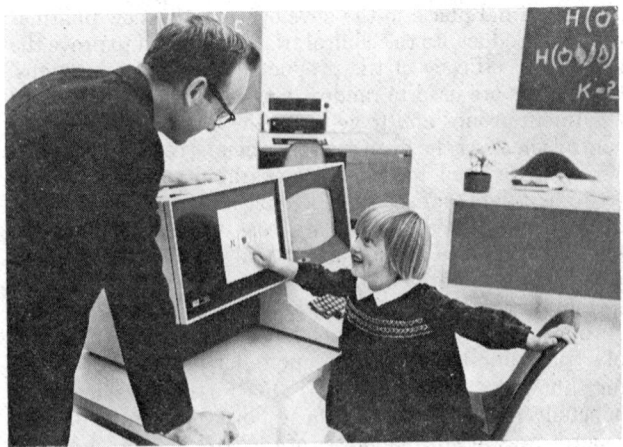

Fig 11-2.   Computer-assisted instruction. The kindergartener is learning the concept of number from a computer-controlled console. This technology, still in a developmental stage, will do much to amplify the abilities of good teachers (courtesy, IBM).

The day of *artificial intelligence* (from robot chess players to automated laboratories) has not arrived. Nevertheless, systems like SYNCHEM are rapidly evolving a new realm of thinking machines. This system has proven to be almost human-like in its successes and failures at finding efficient organic synthesis routes.

The critical element in securing the advantages offered by computers is the availability of people who can define and implement systems. The pure logic of the computer places unusual stress on the need for communication between the user and the implementer of systems. The attitude of the user—scientist or professional—toward the computer is crucial. The pharmacist, as a health care professional and scientist, will be called upon by his clients and associates for information, instruction and advice about computers. This chapter and the associated references should provide the needed introduction to the exciting and rapidly advancing field of computer science.

Bibliography

Gear WC: *Computer Organization and Programming*, McGraw-Hill, New York, 1974.

Hellerman H: *Digital Computer System Principles*, McGraw-Hill, New York, 1967.

Levy HM and Eckhouse, Jr, RH: *Computer Programming and Architecture The VAX-11*, Digital Equipment Corporation, Massachusetts, 1980.

Ralston A, Editor, and Meek, CL, Asst. Editor: *Encyclopedia of Computer Science*, Petrocelli/Charter, New York, 1976.

CHAPTER 12

Calculus

Edward G Rippie, PhD

Professor of Pharmaceutics
College of Pharmacy, University of Minnesota
Minneapolis, MN 55455

Students of pharmacy, in common with students of the natural sciences in general, are frequently concerned with the mathematical analysis of dynamic or kinematic processes for the purpose of understanding the manner in which they function. Observations of such systems often yield data which represent or which must be interpreted in terms of a continuously changing property or component of the system.

This chapter is intended as an introduction to the fundamental concepts and techniques of calculus which are necessary for the adequate mathematical description of systems in such a state of flux. Emphasis will be given to the development of these concepts within a format as uncluttered with formalism and/or complex notation as is possible. For this reason, conditions and limitations required for complete mathematical rigor will be omitted when they do not contribute to a basic understanding of fundamental principles, as they will be applied within the scope of this chapter.

Subjects discussed are limited to those which will be of most use to the undergraduate pharmacy student during his course of study. When greater detail or broader coverage is required, it may be obtained by selective reading from any of the rather large number of excellent calculus texts available.

Functions and Their Limits

The Concept of the Functional Relationship between Variables—Whenever two or more variable quantities are in some way interrelated, such that the value or values any one of them can assume is determined by the values of the others, they are said to be *functions* of each other. Occasionally, the relationships between such real-valued variables can be expressed by a mathematical equation or set of equations. The expressions comprising these equations then define the functional relationships between the variables and are themselves called *functions*. The equation

$$m = x^2 + 2xy + y^2 \qquad (1)$$

explicitly expresses m as a function of x and y. This equation also can be written symbolically as $m = f(x,y)$, where the right-hand term simply signifies that m is a function of x and y without specifying the exact nature of the relationship.

In this case, however, f is defined by Eq 1 to denote a particular algebraic expression. If x and y are allowed to take values a and b, respectively, m assumes the value $f(a,b)$. Different functions of x and y may be designated as $g(x,y)$ or $h(x,y)$ to distinguish them from each other. The letters g and h represent no function in particular unless so defined.

In an equation containing n number of variables, any $n-1$ of them arbitrarily can be assigned numerical values and are called *independent variables*. The value(s) of the remaining variable is thus fixed and it is designated the *dependent variable*.

A function is said to be *single-* or *multiple-valued* depending on the number of values it has for each set of values given the independent variables. Thus, in Eq 1, m is a single-valued function of x and y. If, however, the equation is solved for x, where $x = \pm m^{1/2} - y$, two values of x result from every positive value of m. x is therefore a double-valued function for $m > 0$, but only a single-valued function of y.

Graphing of Functions—In order to better visualize relationships between variables, it is often desirable to represent them pictorially by means of a *graph*. Graphs drawn in two dimensions can show the mutual behavior pattern of any two variables. While graphs also can be constructed so as to give a three-dimensional perspective, they will not be considered here.

The coordinate system used for construction of a graph is selected arbitrarily and is generally chosen so as to simplify the figure. Since the functions encountered in this chapter are relatively simple, rectangular coordinates will be used unless otherwise stated.

A single point on a graph denotes a value for each of the two variables represented on the axes. Thus, if $y = f(x)$, associated pairs (x,y) can be generated corresponding to values of x and y which satisfy the equation. If the values are plotted on a graph, the resulting points, one for each pair (x,y), lie on a curve which depicts the function.

With the careful selection of a few points, the curve can be sketched without need of calculating points at short intervals over the entire curve. Good choices of points include intercepts (where the curve crosses the axes) and points of discontinuity. Special features such as symmetry and asymptotes are also useful guides.

Example 1—Consider the equation $y = 1/x$. It can be seen that the curve has no intercepts but rather approaches the axes asymptotically. Also, the sign of y is always the same as that of x, indicating that the curve lies within the first and third quadrants of the graph. Consequently, because $1/x$ is undefined at $x = 0$, the function must be discontinuous (Fig 12-1).

A table of coordinates, as shown in Fig 12-1, is a useful aid in the plotting of a graph and reduces the possibility of error.

Increments of Variables and Functions—If an independent variable x is changed by an increment Δx, the variable assumes a new value $x + \Delta x$ which may be either greater or less than before, depending on the sign of Δx. If $y = f(x)$,

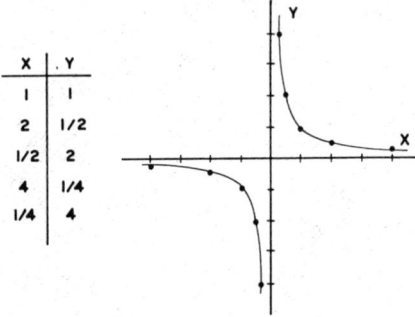

X	Y
1	1
2	1/2
1/2	2
4	1/4
1/4	4

Fig 12-1. A plot of the equation y = 1/x.

the dependent variable y will undergo a corresponding change Δy so that $y + \Delta y = f(x + \Delta x)$. While the incremental change Δy is a direct result of the change in x, its magnitude and sign are determined by the functional relationship between x and y, and on the values of x and Δx. Thus

$$\Delta y = f(x + \Delta x) - f(x) \qquad (2)$$

derives from expression $\Delta y = f(x + \Delta x) - y$.

Example 2—Let $y = x(x - 1) = f(x)$, and calculate the increment Δy when x changes from 1 to 3. In this case, $x = 1$ and $\Delta x = 2$ correspond to the initial value of x and the incremental change in x, respectively. Thus

$$\Delta y = (x + \Delta x)(x + \Delta x - 1) - x(x - 1)$$

$$= \Delta x^2 + 2x\Delta x - \Delta x$$

Substituting for x and Δx, Δy is found to be 6. This may also be seen from Fig 12-2.

The Concept of the Limit of a Function—A necessary concept to the understanding of calculus is that of the *limit* (abbreviated lim) of a function. Allow the independent variable x, of a function $y = f(x)$, to assume a sequence of values successively closer to some number a. The dependent variable will then assume a corresponding set of values. The function $f(x)$ is said to approach a limit b as x approaches a, if the absolute difference between $f(x)$ and b can be made arbitrarily small by choosing x sufficiently close in value to a. This is written symbolically as

$$\lim_{x \to a} f(x) = b$$

Although the formal definition of the limit must be modified in some cases, the numbers a and b can take any set of values from $-\infty$ to ∞.

Example 3—Calculate the limit of the function $y = 1 - x^2$ as $x \to 2$. It is apparent in this case that as x assumes values close to 2, y can be made to approach -3; thus

$$\lim_{x \to 2} (1 - x^2) = -3$$

Example 4—Consider again the function $y = 1/x$, discussed in Example 1, and calculate its limit as $x \to 0$. Here, the choice of positive values of x near zero results in large values of y which increase without bound as $x \to 0$. The limit of $1/x$ as $x \to 0$ is thus infinity (∞). If x is allowed to approach zero from negative values, the limit is found to be negative infinity. These results can be written in the form

$$\lim_{x \to 0} (1/x) = \infty; \ \lim_{-x \to 0} (1/x) = -\infty$$

where $x \to 0$ means that x approaches zero through positive values of x and $-x \to 0$ means that x approaches zero through negative values of x, and can be visualized from Fig 12-1. It is apparent from this discussion that the function $1/x$ is *discontinuous* at the point $x = 0$.

The Properties of Limits—When finding the limits of relatively complex functions, it is frequently useful to break them down into simpler functions whose limits are more easily calculated. The following rules are necessary for such manipulations and also serve to reinforce the basic concept of a limit.

Consider a sequence of functions, $F_1, F_2, F_3, \ldots, F_n$, having a common independent variable x, and which possess limits as x approaches any value in the interval $-\infty \leq x \leq \infty$.

Rule 1

$$\lim (F_1 + F_2 + \ldots + F_n) = \lim F_1 + \lim F_2 + \ldots + \lim F_n$$

Rule 2

$$\lim (F_1.F_2.\ldots.F_n) = \lim F_1.\lim F_2.\ldots.\lim F_n$$

Rule 3

$$\lim (F_1/F_2) = \lim F_1/\lim F_2$$

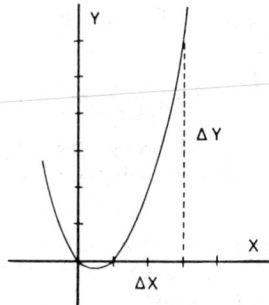

Fig 12-2. A plot of the equation y = x(x − 1) = f(x), including the increment Δy when x changes from 1 to 3.

if $\lim F_2 \neq 0$.

Rule 4

$$\lim (F_1{}^r) = (\lim F_1)^r$$

where r may be a fractional number as well as an integer.

Example 5—Evaluate the limit of the function $(x^2 - x + 6)/(x^3 + 1)$ as $x \to 2$. The problem may be simplified by applying Rules 3 and 1 in succession. Thus

$$\lim_{x \to 2} (x^2 - x + 6)/(x^3 + 1) = \lim_{x \to 2} (x^2 - x + 6) \Big/ \lim_{x \to 2} (x^3 + 1)$$

$$= \left[\lim_{x \to 2} (x^2) - \lim_{x \to 2} (x) + \lim_{x \to 2} (6)\right] \Big/ \left[\lim_{x \to 2} (x^3) + \lim_{x \to 2} (1)\right]$$

$$= (4 - 2 + 6)/(8 + 1) = 8/9$$

When Rule 3 is applied to evaluate the limit of a quotient, it may be found that the quotient of limits has the *indeterminate* form 0/0. This result implies that the function is undefined at the limiting value of the independent variable. In spite of this, however, the function may possess a well-defined limit which can be determined if the proper technique is used.

Example 6—Consider the function $(1 - x)/(1 - x^2) = f(x)$. The limit of $f(x)$ as $x \to 1$ can be seen to be indeterminate if computed in the usual way. However, if the function is placed in the form $1/(1 + x)$, the limit can be seen to equal $1/2$.

The concept of the limit of quotients is fundamental to an understanding of calculus, a subject which results in the frequent encounter with indeterminate forms. As will be seen, the problem of indeterminacy is resolved in these cases by defining the limiting behavior in terms of specific functions.

Exercises

1. Given $f(x) = 1 - 3x^2$, calculate $f(1)$, $f(a)$, and $f(b - 1)$.

2. Given $f(y) = y - 1/y$ and $g(x) = x^2$, express $f[g(x)]$ in terms of x.

3. By graphing, show that the curves in Fig 12-1 are symmetrical about the lines $y = x$, and $y = -x$.

4. Given $y = 6x - x^2$, calculate Δy if $x = 1$ and $\Delta x = 0.1$.

5. Calculate the following limits:

   a. $\lim_{x \to 1} (x^2 - 3x + 2)$

   b. $\lim_{x \to 2} [(x^2 - 1)(1 - 1/x)]$

   c. $\lim_{x \to 0} [(1 - x)/(3x^2 + 2)]^3$

   d. $\lim_{x \to 2} [(3x - 6)/(2 - x)]$

6. Given $y = 1/x$, calculate $\Delta y/\Delta x$ in terms of x and Δx. What is the limit of this expression for $\Delta y/\Delta x$ when $x = 1$, and $\Delta x \to 0$?

7. The binding of drugs by various tissue proteins can frequently be described by "site" models. In the simplest of these, where only one type of binding site exists, the average

number of drug molecules, r, bound per molecule of protein is given by the following equation:

$$r = \frac{nK(D)}{1 + K(D)}$$

where n is the number of binding sites per protein molecule; K is the binding constant; and (D) is the concentration of unbound drug.

   a.   Classify the quantities in this equation as constants, dependent variables, or independent variables.
   b.   Graph r as a function of (D).
   c.   Determine the limit of r as $(D) \rightarrow \infty$.

  8.   The equation in Exercise 7 is not linear but can be rearranged into the following linear forms.

$$1/r = 1/nK(D) + 1/n$$

$$(D)/r = 1/nK + (D)/n$$

$$r/(D) = nK - rK$$

Data for the binding of a drug to serum albumin is given in the table below.

r	(D) moles/L $\times 10^5$	r	(D) moles/L $\times 10^5$
1.0	0.5	2.4	4.0
1.5	1.0	2.7	9.0
2.0	2.0	2.9	29.0

   a.   What are the dependent and independent variables in the three linear equations above?
   b.   In terms of n and K, what are the slopes of these equations?
   c.   In terms of n and K, what are the y intercepts of these equations?
   d.   What is the x intercept of the third equation in the set?
   e.   Plot the data above in terms of each of the equations and determine the numerical values of n and K from the plots.

The Derivative of a Function

The Derivative as a Limit—The *derivative* of a function $y = f(x)$ is defined formally as the limit of $\Delta y/\Delta x$ as $\Delta x \rightarrow 0$, over intervals where $f(x)$ is differentiable. It is apparent that as $\Delta x \rightarrow 0$, Δy also approaches zero and that the expression

$$\lim_{\Delta x \rightarrow 0} (\Delta y/\Delta x)$$

is in an indeterminate form. When the limit exists, it may be taken out of the indeterminate form by substitution of an expression in x and Δx for the quantity Δy.

Inasmuch as the derivative of a function of x is another related function of x, its value will depend on x. This is implicit in the following notation, which will be used in subsequent work. If $y = f(x)$, the derivative of $f(x)$ with respect to x is

$$dy/dx = \lim_{\Delta x \rightarrow 0} (\Delta y/\Delta x) = f'(x) \tag{3}$$

The mechanism for finding the derivative of a function is simple in principle. Starting with the definition (Eq 3) it is necessary first to find Δy, in terms of x and Δx, for the particular function under consideration. This is accomplished by means of Eq 2 so that

$$dy/dx = \lim_{\Delta x \rightarrow 0} \left(\frac{f(x + \Delta x) - f(x)}{\Delta x} \right) \tag{4}$$

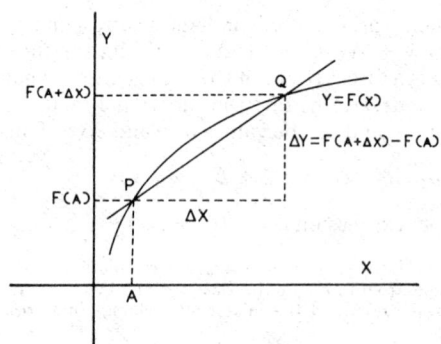

Fig 12-3.   A portion of the graph of the function y = f(x), where f(a) denotes the derivative of f(x) at a point where x = a.

After carrying out the necessary algebra to obtain $[f(x + \Delta x) - f(x)]/\Delta x$ explicitly, it only remains to take the limit as $\Delta x \rightarrow 0$. The value of the resulting derivative can be obtained for any desired value of x by simple substitution.

Example 7—Find the derivative of y with respect to x, (dy/dx), for the function $y = x^2 - 3x$. What is the value of $f'(x)$ when $x = 2$? Calculating Δy from Eq 2,

$$\Delta y = (x + \Delta x)^2 - 3(x + \Delta x) - x^2 + 3x = 2x\,\Delta x - 3\Delta x + \Delta x^2$$

Dividing by Δx,

$$\Delta y/\Delta x = 2x - 3 + \Delta x$$

Taking the limit as $\Delta x \rightarrow 0$,

$$\lim_{\Delta x \rightarrow 0} (\Delta y/\Delta x) = \lim_{\Delta x \rightarrow 0} (2x - 3 + \Delta x) = 2x - 3$$

The derivative, dy/dx, is therefore equal to $2x - 3$ for all values of x. The value of the derivative, $f'(x)$, when $x = 2$ is 1.

Graphical Interpretation of the Derivative—The derivative of a function of a single variable, $y = f(x)$, has been defined analytically, in the previous section, as a new function $dy/dx = f'(x)$. The limiting process leading to the derivative can be visualized easily by the use of a graph. Consider the curve in Fig 12-3 to represent a portion of the graph of the function $y = f(x)$, and let $f'(a)$ denote the derivative of $f(x)$ at the point where $x = a$. Then by definition,

$$f'(a) = \lim_{\Delta x \rightarrow 0} \left(\frac{f(a + \Delta x) - f(a)}{\Delta x} \right)$$

The expression $[f(a + \Delta x) - f(a)]/\Delta x$ represents the slope of a line through the Points P and Q. However, as $\Delta x \rightarrow 0$, the Point Q moves down the curve toward P, and the line drawn through P and Q becomes tangential to the curve at Point P. Thus when the limit of $\Delta y/\Delta x$ as $\Delta x \rightarrow 0$ is computed for $x = a$, it is numerically equal to the slope of a line tangent to the curve at point P. For this reason the derivative is said to be the slope of the curve, and as a function of x it can be computed for all values (subject to certain limitations not discussed here) of x.

The Derivative as a Rate of Change—The derivative also may be interpreted physically as the rate of change of one quantity with respect to another. For example, the quotient $\Delta m/\Delta t$ may denote the change in mass of a growing plant over a time interval Δt and therefore represents the average rate of growth for that period. However, the derivative dm/dt is the rate of change of mass at a point in time and represents the instantaneous rate of growth.

The concept of an instantaneous rate of change can be applied to any two variables, one of which changes as a function of the other. Examples of pairs of such related variables which are frequently encountered are distance–time, drug blood level–time, radiation intensity–distance, chemical change–time, and pH as a function of added acid or base.

Example 8—The probability of disintegration of an unstable nucleus, within a given time interval, is independent of its past history and the chemical state of the atoms. Given a large number, N, of similar unstable nuclei, the rate at which they disintegrate can be approximated in terms of an instantaneous rate, dN/dt. This rate is proportional to the number of intact nuclei at any given instant. Therefore, a differential equation for radiodecay can be written in terms of N, dN/dt, and a proportionality constant, λ, as follows:

$$dN/dt = -\lambda N$$

Exercises

9. Calculate the derivative (dy/dx, ds/dt, dm/dn) of the following functions:

   a. $y = 2x^3 - 5$
   b. $s = t/(1 - t)$
   c. $m = n^5$

10. Compute the value of dy/dx for Exercise 9a, when $x = 0, 1, -3, a$.
11. Show that the rate of change of volume of a cube with respect to the length of an edge is three times the surface area of one of its sides.
12. If the rate of loss of drug by degradation from an elixir with time is equal numerically to $\frac{1}{1000}$ the concentration of the drug at any given time, express the rate of loss as a function of concentration.

The Process of Differentiation

Origin of the Rules for Differentiation—As has been shown, the process of differentiation, wherein the derivative of a function is determined, follows logically from the formal definition of the derivative, Eq 4. The procedure, however, can become involved and time consuming even when applied to relatively simple functions. For this reason general rules for differentiation have been developed which greatly simplify matters. These rules arise directly from the application of the methods of the previous section to generalized functions. Several frequently used rules are given in Table I. While the rules presented are general, the derivations are subject to certain limitations not discussed here.

Table I—Rules for Differentiation[a]

Rule	Function	Derivative
	Primary rules[b]	
1	$y = x^n$	$dy/dx = nx^{n-1}$
2	$y = ku$	$dy/dx = k(du/dx)$
3	$y = u + v$	$dy/dx = du/dx + dv/dx$
4	$y = u \cdot v$	$dy/dx = u(dv/dx) + v(du/dx)$
5	$y = u/v$	$dy/dx = \dfrac{v(du/dx) - u(dv/dx)}{v^2}$
6	$y = f(z)$, $z = g(x)$	$dy/dx = (dy/dz)(dz/dx)$
7	$y = e^u$	$dy/dx = e^u(du/dx)$
8	$y = \ln u$	$dy/dx = (du/dx)/u$
	Secondary rules	
9	$y = k$	$dy/dx = 0$
10	$y = x$	$dy/dx = 1$
11	$y = kx$	$dy/dx = k$
12	$y = u^n$	$dy/dx = nu^{n-1}du/dx$
13	$y = e^x$	$dy/dx = e^x$
14	$y = \ln x$	$dy/dx = 1/x$

[a] Definitions: the variables y, u, and v are functions of x, the independent variable; k and n are constants; e is the base of the natural logarithms, designated by "ln."
[b] Several of these rules are in themselves special cases of more general rules.

Higher-Order Derivatives—It was shown earlier that the derivative of a function of x is itself, in general, also a function of x. If this *first derivative* is differentiated, a *second derivative* is obtained which is also a function of x. Thus when the process of differentiation is repeated again and again, a succession of higher-order derivatives is obtained, the original function alone determining the number of successive derivatives which may be found. These higher-order derivatives are denoted by the following symbols.

1st derivative: $dy/dx = f'(x)$
2nd derivative: $d^2y/dx^2 = f''(x)$
3rd derivative: $d^3y/dx^3 = f'''(x)$
nth derivative: $d^ny/dx^n = f^{(n)}(x)$

Example 9—Find all the derivatives of the function $y = x^3 - x + e^x$.

$$dy/dx = 3x^2 - 1 + e^x$$
$$d^2y/dx^2 = 6x + e^x$$
$$d^3y/dx^3 = 6 + e^x$$
$$d^ny/dx^n = e^x \text{ where } n \geq 4.$$

It is often desirable to find the high and/or low points of a function analytically and to determine their identity as *maxima* or *minima*. If a function has a lesser value immediately to both sides of a point, that point denotes a *relative maximum* value of the function. Similarly, a *relative minimum* exists if the function has a higher value immediately to both sides of a point. Such relative maximum and minimum points do not necessarily represent the greatest or least values taken by the function, and there is no limit to the number of maxima and minima a function can possess.

Both maximum and minimum points are located on the curve where the slope, and hence the first derivative of the function, is equal to zero. This is a necessary but not a sufficient requirement for the existence of maxima or minima points over intervals where the first derivative exists.

The second derivative, which represents the rate of change of slope with distance along the curve, is useful in identifying maxima and minima over intervals where it exists. As a maximum is approached from small values of the independent variable, the slope decreases, becomes zero, and then becomes negative. Therefore, the second derivative would possess a negative value at a maximum point on the curve. By the same reasoning, the second derivative is positive at a minimum point.

Let $y = f(x)$ possess continuous first and second derivatives. Then if

$$(a, f(a)) \text{ is a maximum point; } f'(a) = 0, f''(a) < 0$$
$$(a, f(a)) \text{ is a minimum point; } f'(a) = 0, f''(a) > 0$$

If the second derivative is equal to zero, the point may be neither a maximum nor a minimum but may be a point of inflection at which the line changes its direction of curvature. This will be the case if the third derivative is not zero.

Example 10—A drug, B, forms a 1:3 complex with a macromolecule, A, according to the expression:

$$(AB_3) = K(A)(B)^3$$

Given: $K = 1.6 \times 10^2$ L³/moles³ and (A) held constant at $0.2\,M$, at what rate (moles/mole) is (AB_3) increasing with added drug at a free drug concentration of 0.1 mole/L?

$$d(AB_3)/d(B) = 3K(A)(B)^2 = 0.96$$

At what rate is this rate changing per added mole of drug at this concentration?

$$d^2(AB_3)/d(B)^2 = 6K(A)(B) = 19.2 \text{ L/mole}$$

Example 11—The Van Slyke equation for buffer capacity, β, is a function of hydrogen ion concentration, the dissociation constant, K_a, of the buffer acid, and the buffer concentration, C, as follows:

$$\beta = \frac{2.3C\,K_a[H^+]}{(K_a + [H^+])^2}$$

Determine the pH at which the buffer capacity is a maximum. This would correspond to the hydrogen ion concentration at which $d\beta/d[H^+]$ is zero. This can be found by differentiating β with respect to $[H^+]$. The numerator is found to be:

$$2.3C(K_a + [H^+])^2 K_a - 2K_a[H^+](K_a + [H^+])$$

Since this quantity must also equal zero at the maximum, it can be seen that: $K_a = [H^+]$. Therefore the pH numerically equals pK_a at the point of maximum buffer capacity.

Exercises

13. Derive Rules 1 through 8 for differentiation.

14. Deduce Rules 9 through 14 as special cases of certain of the primary rules listed.

15. Derive a general rule for which Rules 4 and 5 are special cases.

16. Calculate the derivatives of the following functions:

a. $y = x^3 - 3x + 1/x - 6$

b. $y = x^{1/2}/(1 + x^2)$

c. $y = e^{x^2}$

d. $y = \ln(1 + x^2)$

17. If $y = e^z$, $z = 1 - x^2$, calculate dy/dx.

18. Find du/dt if

$$u = (e^{3t} - 3 \ln t)^{5/2}.$$

19. Find all the successive derivatives of the function

$$y = x^5/5 + x^3/3 + x.$$

20. In the titration of a monobasic weak acid, the pH rises as the fraction, F, of acid titrated increases. At what value of F is the rate of change of pH, with respect to F, a minimum?

$$F = K_a/[(H^+) + K_a]$$

21. Compound A is converted to compounds B and C according to the steps:

$$A \xrightarrow{k_1} B \xrightarrow{k_2} C$$

If $dA/dt = -k_1A$ and $dC/dt = k_2B$, calculate the ratio A/B when B is at its maximum concentration.

$$k_1 = 0.25 \text{ sec}^{-1}, \qquad k_2 = 1.75 \text{ sec}^{-1}$$

Partial Differentiation

The Partial Derivative—Differentiation has been defined and discussed thus far only in terms of its application to functions of a single independent variable. The concept of the derivative, however, can be generalized and extended to include functions of several variables.

Whereas a function of a single variable can be visualized as a curve in two-dimensional space, a function of two independent variables can be represented by a surface in three-dimensional space. Similarly, functions of $n - 1$ independent variables can be abstractly conceived as "surfaces" in n-dimensional space. If all but one independent variable is held constant, an n-dimensional surface is reduced to a curve in two dimensions.

The slope of such a curve represents the rate of change of the function with respect to the retained variable, as all the other variables are held at their particular, arbitrarily selected values. This slope may be determined by taking the derivative of the function with respect to the selected variable while holding all the other variables constant.

Such a derivative is termed a *partial derivative* since it represents the rate of change of the function with respect to only a part (one) of the independent variables.

The partial derivative of a function $y = f(x_1, x_2, \ldots, x_k)$, of k independent variables $(x_1, x_2, \ldots, x_k)$, with respect to the variable x_1 is defined as

$$\partial y/\partial x_1$$

$$= \lim_{\Delta x_1 \to 0} \left(\frac{f(x_1 + \Delta x_1, x_2, \ldots, x_k) - f(x_1, x_2, \ldots, x_k)}{\Delta x_1} \right) \quad (5)$$

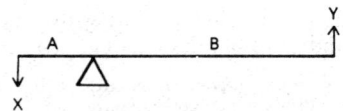

Fig 12-4. A lever—*A* and *B*: arm lengths; *X* and *Y*: distances traveled by the tips of the left and right arms, respectively.

Example 12—Find the partial derivatives of the function $u = x^3 - 2xy + y^2$ with respect to both x and y. That is, find $\partial u/\partial x$ and $\partial u/\partial y$, where all independent variables are considered as constants except the one with respect to which the derivative is taken. Thus,

$$\partial u/\partial x = 3x^2 - 2y; \qquad \partial u/\partial y = -2x + 2y$$

Example 13—The volume of a right circular cylinder is given by the equation $V = \pi r^2 h$, where r is the radius of curvature and h is the height. Find the rate of change of height with respect to radius at constant volume. Expressing the height in terms of r and V,

$$h = \frac{V}{\pi r^2}; \qquad \partial h/\partial r = \frac{-2V}{\pi r^3}$$

Example 14—The pressure-volume product, PV, of an ideal gas is given as a function of the absolute temperature, T, in terms of the gas constant, R, and the number of moles, n. Find $\partial P/\partial T$.

$$PV = nRT$$

Solving for pressure

$$P = nRT/V$$

Thus

$$\partial P/\partial T = nR/V$$

Total Differentials and Total Derivatives—It was shown previously that if $y = f(x)$, the rate of change of y with respect to x is equal to the derivative, $dy/dx = f'(x)$. Upon rearrangement, $dy = f'(x)\,dx$, where dy is defined as the *differential* of y, and dx as the differential of x. The quantities dx and dy may be intuitively thought of as the "potentials" for change of x and y, respectively.

Consider a lever, as shown in Fig 12-4, having arms of length a and b. Let x represent the distance traveled by the tip of the left arm and y that traveled by the right arm. The relationship between x and y is given by the expression $y = bx/a$, and the differential of y is defined by the equation $dy = f'(x)dx = (b/a)dx$. It is clear from Fig 12-4 that the "potential" for a change in y is in direct proportion to that for x, and is in the ratio b/a.

The differential of a function of k independent variables $(x_1, x_2, \ldots, x_k)$ is itself a function of the k dx_i's and is referred to as the *total differential*. If $y = f(x_1, x_2, \ldots, x_k)$, the total differential of y is defined by the expression

$$dy = \frac{\partial y}{\partial x_1}\,dx_1 + \frac{\partial y}{\partial x_2}\,dx_2 + \ldots + \frac{\partial y}{\partial x_k}\,dx_k \quad (6)$$

Each term of the type $(\partial y/\partial x_i)dx_i$ represents the contribution of the ith independent variable to dy, and is sometimes called a *partial differential*.

Example 15—Find the total differential of $u = xyz$. From Eq 6, the total differential is given by

$$du = (\partial u/\partial x)dx + (\partial u/\partial y)dy + (\partial u/\partial z)dz$$

Substituting for $\partial u/\partial x$, $\partial u/\partial y$, $\partial u/\partial z$;

$$du = yzdx + xzdy + xydz$$

Let the k variables, x_i, of Eq 6 not be independent, but rather let them be functions of a single independent variable t. This implies that y is a function of t only and can be expressed in the form $y = g(t)$. While the derivative of y with respect to t then could be computed directly, it is frequently more convenient to calculate dy/dt by a different method.

If Eq 6 is divided through by the differential of t, dy/dt is obtained in the form

$$\frac{dy}{dt} = \frac{\partial y}{\partial x_1} \cdot \frac{dx_1}{dt} + \frac{\partial y}{\partial x_2} \cdot \frac{dx_2}{dt} + \ldots + \frac{\partial y}{\partial x_k} \cdot \frac{dx_k}{dt} \quad (7)$$

and is defined as the *total derivative* of y with respect to t. Eq 7 therefore permits dy/dt to be calculated without the need to express y explicitly in terms of t.

Higher-Order Partial Derivatives—The first partial derivatives of the function $y = f(x_1, x_2, \ldots, x_k)$ are themselves functions of the variables x_i. As such, they can be differentiated further, to yield higher partial derivatives, without regard to the identity of the variable of the first partial differentiation. Thus, the first partial derivatives ($\partial y/\partial x_1$, $\partial y/\partial x_2, \ldots, \partial y/\partial x_k$) yield *second partial derivatives* ($\partial^2 y/\partial x_i \partial x_j$, where i may or may not equal j). Third and higher partial derivatives can be obtained also and are designated by the following notation:

$$\frac{\partial}{\partial x_i}\left(\frac{\partial y}{\partial x_j}\right) = \frac{\partial^2 y}{\partial x_i \partial x_j}$$

$$\frac{\partial}{\partial x_1}\left(\frac{\partial^2 y}{\partial x_i \partial x_j}\right) = \frac{\partial^3 y}{\partial x_1 \partial x_i \partial x_j} \text{ etc.}$$

When the given function y and all the partial derivatives up to and including the nth are continuous, the order of differentiation is immaterial in computing the nth partial derivative.[1] This condition is satisfied in most cases encountered in pharmacy.

Example 16—Given the function $u = xy^3 + x^3y$, calculate $\partial^4 u/\partial x^4$.

$$\partial u/\partial x = y^3 + 3x^2y$$

$$\partial^2 u/\partial x^2 = 6xy$$

$$\partial^3 u/\partial x^3 = 6y$$

$$\partial^4 u/\partial x^4 = 0$$

Example 17—Given the function $u = x^2y^2z^2$, calculate $\partial^3 u/\partial z \partial y \partial x$, and $\partial^3 u/\partial x \partial y \partial z$ and verify their equality.

$$\frac{\partial u}{\partial z} = 2x^2y^2z, \qquad \frac{\partial^2 u}{\partial y \partial z} = 4x^2yz, \qquad \frac{\partial^3 u}{\partial x \partial y \partial z} = 8xyz$$

$$\frac{\partial u}{\partial x} = 2xy^2z^2, \qquad \frac{\partial^2 u}{\partial y \partial x} = 4xyz^2, \qquad \frac{\partial^3 u}{\partial z \partial y \partial x} = 8xyz$$

Example 18—Fick's first law of diffusion in one dimension defines the flux, J, (rate of mass transport per unit area) as a function of the diffusion constant, D, and the concentration gradient, $\partial c/\partial x$.

$$J = -D(\partial c/\partial x)$$

In general, the concentration at any given point along the x axis will be a function of time. This may be deduced from Fick's law since the quantity of material crossing a plane of unit area at point x in time dt is $J dt$. The corresponding quantity crossing a similar plane of point $x + dx$ is:

$$\left[J + \left(\frac{\partial J}{\partial x}\right)dx\right]dt$$

The difference between these quantities represents the rate of change of material with time in the zone of volume dx.

$$dcdx = Jdt - \left[J + \left(\frac{\partial J}{\partial x}\right)dx\right]dt$$

$$dcdx = -\left(\frac{\partial J}{\partial x}\right)dxdt$$

The time dependence of concentration can be seen to be:

$$\frac{\partial c}{\partial t} = -\frac{\partial J}{\partial x}$$

Taking the derivative of Fick's first law with respect to distance yields:

$$\frac{\partial J}{\partial x} = -D\frac{\partial^2 c}{\partial x^2}$$

Substitution of this result into the previous equation yields Fick's second law.

$$\frac{\partial c}{\partial t} = D\frac{\partial^2 c}{\partial x^2}$$

Example 19—Fick's second law of diffusion relates the change of concentration, c, with respect to time to the diffusion coefficient, D, and to the second partial derivative of concentration with respect to distance.

$$\partial c/\partial t = D(\partial^2 c/\partial x^2)$$

Calculate $\partial c/\partial t$ when $x = 2$ cm, $D = 0.15$ cm^2 sec^{-1}, and $c = 3x^3 - f(t)$.

$$\partial c/\partial x = 9x^2; \qquad \partial^2 c/\partial x^2 = 18x$$

Therefore

$$\partial c/\partial t = (0.15)(18)(2) = 5.4 \text{ moles L}^{-1} \text{ sec}^{-1}$$

Exercises

22. Given $u = x^2 + y^2 + z^2$, show that

$$x\frac{\partial u}{\partial x} + y\frac{\partial u}{\partial y} + z\frac{\partial u}{\partial z} = 2u$$

23. Find $\partial u/\partial x$ and $\partial u/\partial y$ if $u = e^{x^2y^2}$.
24. Calculate the value of $\partial A/\partial u$ when $u = 1$ and $v = 2$ for the function $A = (u^2v + v^2u)^2$.
25. Given $M = x^3y^3$, calculate the numerical value of

$$xy\left(x\frac{\partial^3 M}{\partial x^2 \partial y} + y\frac{\partial^3 M}{\partial x \partial y^2}\right)\bigg/9M$$

26. Find the total differential of $u = e^{xyz}$.
27. Derive Eq 7 from the definitions of the derivative and partial derivative, and independent of Eq 6.
28. Find the total derivative of the function $u = \ln(xyz)$ if; $x = t, y = t^2, z = t^3$.
29. Find the total derivative of the function $u = xy^2z^3$ if; $x = 1/t, y = e^t, z = \ln t$.
30. Determine the ratio $(\partial^2 u/\partial x^2)/(\partial^2 u/\partial y^2)$ in terms of x and y if $u = (xyz)^{1/2}$.
31. Find all the second partial derivatives of $u = xe^y$.
32. The heat capacity of a physical system is defined in thermodynamics as the derivative of the heat absorbed with respect to the absolute temperature. The molar heat capacities of an ideal gas at constant pressure, C_p, and constant volume, C_v, are related by the expression:

$$C_p - C_v = P(\partial V/\partial T)$$

Using the ideal gas law, show that

$$C_p - C_v = R.$$

Indefinite Integration

The Indefinite Integral—The observation that the derivative $dy/dx = f'(x)$ of the function $y = f(x)$ can be found through the application of a formal set of procedures suggested that the inverse also may be true. This process, wherein a function is found when only its derivative is known, is called *integration*.

In particular, the function $f(x) + C$ is defined as the *indefinite integral* of $f'(x)$, where C is the *constant of integration* and where $f'(x)$ is the first derivative of $f(x)$. The term indefinite integral arises from the fact that unless certain information in addition to $f'(x)$ is given, the constant of integration may take on any value whatever.

The process of integration is denoted symbolically as follows:

$$y = \int dy = \int f'(x)dx = f(x) + C \qquad (8)$$

The symbol $\int$ is called the integral sign and indicates that the function following it (the integrand) is to be integrated. The differential term to the right of the integrand determines the variable of integration. A useful check on the accuracy of any integral consists of taking the derivative of the integral. The result must equal the integrand.

Basic Rules for Integration—The rules which follow are

the result of the definition of integration applied to the rules of differentiation listed in this chapter.

Rule 1

$$\int du = u + C$$

where u is any function and C is an arbitrary constant.

Rule 2

$$\int u^n du = u^{n+1}/(n+1) + C, \text{ if } n \neq -1$$

Rule 3

$$\int ku\,dx = k\int u\,dx$$

where u is a function of x and k is a constant.

Rule 4

$$\int (u+v)dx = \int u\,dx + \int v\,dx$$

where u and v are functions of x.

Rule 5

$$\int e^u\,du = e^u + C$$

Rule 6

$$\int du/u = \int d\ln u = \ln u + C$$

Methods of Integration—The method of *integration by parts* is derived directly from Rule 4 for the differentiation of the product of functions.

Given the functions $u(x)$ and $v(x)$, the derivative of the product $u \cdot v$ with respect to x is $d(uv)/dx = u(dv/dx) + v(du/dx)$. Multiplying by dx and rearranging,

$$udv = d(uv) - vdu$$

Integrating both sides,

$$\int u\,dv = uv - \int v\,du \qquad (9)$$

Eq 9 defines the procedure used in this method of integration. It is applied when the integral resulting from the exchange of integrand and differential is easier to integrate than the original integral. That is, when $\int v\,du$ is simpler than $\int u\,dv$.

Example 20—Determine $\int xe^x dx$ by the method of parts. Let $x = u$ and $e^x dx = dv$, then it follows that $du = dx$ and $v = e^x$. By substitution into Eq 9,

$$\int xe^x dx = xe^x - \int e^x dx = xe^x - e^x + C$$

Integrals which do not lend themselves to solution by simple rules or the method of parts can be evaluated frequently by a *change of variable* of integration. That is, a complicated integral which is a function of x may be transformed into a simple function of u by the substitution of a suitable function $u(x)$ into the original integral. This method is explained easily by means of an example.

Example 21—Evaluate the integral $\int 2xe^{x^2}dx$. Let $u = x^2$ and substitute into the integral. Since $du = 2xdx$,

$$\int 2xe^{x^2}dx = \int e^u du = e^u + C = e^{x^2} + C$$

Example 22—Evaluate the integral, $\int xdx/(x^2 - 2)$. Let $u = x^2 - 2$, then $du = 2xdx$. Thus,

$$\frac{xdx}{(x^2-2)} = \frac{1}{2}\int du/u = \frac{1}{2}\int d\ln u$$

$$= \frac{1}{2}\ln u + C = \frac{1}{2}\ln(x^2-2) + C$$

An integral having an integrand in the form of a rational fraction, whose denominator can be factored, is often subject to simplification by *partial fractions*. In this method the original integrand is broken into a sum of fractions whose denominators are factors of the original denominator. Consider the following example.

Example 23—Evaluate the integral, $\int (x-2)dx/(x^2 - 2x - 3)$. It is necessary to first write the integrand in the partial fractional form as follows:

$$\frac{x-2}{x^2-2x-3} = \frac{x-2}{(x+1)(x-3)} = \frac{M}{(x+1)} + \frac{N}{(x-3)}$$

M and N are constants having values such that the equality is satisfied. Thus, $M(x-3) + N(x+1) = x-2$, since the numerators resulting from the above equation must be equal. Equating coefficients of like powers of x, it may be seen that:

$$M + N = 1; \qquad -3M + N = -2$$

Solving these equations simultaneously, M and N are found to equal $\frac{3}{4}$ and $\frac{1}{4}$, respectively. Substituting into the original integral,

$$\int \frac{(x-2)dx}{x^2-2x-3} = \int\left[\frac{M}{(x+1)} + \frac{N}{(x-3)}\right]dx$$

$$= \frac{3}{4}\int\frac{dx}{(x+1)} + \frac{1}{4}\int\frac{dx}{(x-3)}$$

$$= \frac{3}{4}\ln|x+1| + \frac{1}{4}\ln|x-3| + C$$

Example 24—Given the general expression for the rate of a third order reaction:

$$\frac{dx}{dt} = k(a-x)(b-x)(c-x)$$

where $k, a, b,$ and c are constants, place the equation in a form where it can be easily integrated. This can be done by defining constants $A, B,$ and C such that:

$$\frac{dx}{(a-x)(b-x)(c-x)} = \frac{Adx}{(a-x)} + \frac{Bdx}{(b-x)} + \frac{Cdx}{(c-x)}$$

By placing the right hand terms over a common denominator and adding:

$$(b-x)(c-x)A + (a-x)(c-x)B + (a-x)(b-x)C = 1$$

Equating the coefficients of powers of x on both sides of this equation, three equations are obtained.

$$A + B + C = 0$$
$$A(b+c) + B(a+c) + C(a+b) = 0$$
$$Abc + Bac + Cab = 1$$

Solving these simultaneously for $A, B,$ and C:

$$A = (a^2 - ab - ac + bc)^{-1}$$
$$B = (b^2 - ab - bc + ac)^{-1}$$
$$C = (c^2 - ac - bc + ab)^{-1}$$

Thus, the first of the three terms in the integral becomes:

$$(a^2 - ab - ac + bc)^{-1}\ln\frac{(a)}{a-x}$$

The remaining two terms have the same form.

The methods of integration presented here represent but a few of those available. They will, however, be adequate for the solution of most of the problems encountered in undergraduate pharmacy.

As mentioned earlier, the constant of integration can be determined if certain information in addition to the integrand is provided. Such information is usually given in the form of *boundary conditions*, which have the effect of fixing the value of C.

Example 25—Determine the integral of $dy/dx = x^2 - x$, if it is known that $y = 0$, if and when $x = 1$. It is first necessary to find the indefinite integral.

$$y = \int(x^2 - x)dx = x^3/3 - x^2/2 + C$$

Applying the boundary conditions to the indefinite integral; when $y = 0$ and $x = 1$,

$$y = 0 = \frac{1}{3} - \frac{1}{2} + C, \qquad \therefore C = \frac{1}{6}$$

The desired integral is thus,

$$y = x^3/3 - x^2/2 + \frac{1}{6}$$

Example 26—Consider the equation for the rate of radioactive decay, as presented in *Example 8*. Given $N_0 = 10\ \mu c$ at time zero, find an equation for N at any time t. Rearranging the equation to separate the variables:

$$\int dN/N = -\lambda \int dt$$

Integrating:

$$\ln N = -\lambda t + C$$

Substituting in the boundary conditions:

$$C = \ln N_0; \qquad \ln N = \ln N_0 - \lambda t$$

Exercises

33. Evaluate the following integrals:

a. $\int d(x - e^x \ln x)$

b. $\int (x^7 - x^{-3})^2 d(x^7 - x^{-3})$

c. $\int 8x^3 dx$

d. $\int (x^3 + 2x^2 - 7) dx$

e. $\int 2e^x dx$

f. $\int dx/(1 + x)$

34. Integrate the following:

a. $dy/dx = (x - 3)(x + 5)$

b. $du/dt = e^t - 1/t$

35. Find the following integrals by the method of parts:

a. $\int x^2 e^x dx$ (*Hint:* apply the method twice in succession)

b. $\int 7xe^{-2x} dx$

c. $\int \ln x \, dx$

36. Evaluate the following integrals by change of variable:

a. $\int x^2(x^3 - 1)^{1/2} dx$

b. $\int (x - 1)(x^2 - 2x)^{-1/2} dx$

37. Evaluate the following integral, $\int x(x^2 - 1)^{-1} dx$, by the method of partial fractions. Check the answer by the method of change of variable.

38. Write and integrate an equation which describes the rate of production of product in the following bimolecular reaction. The starting concentrations of A and B are unequal and that of C is zero.

$$A + B \rightarrow C$$

39. Find y in terms of x for the following.

a. $dy/dx = e^x$ if $y = 0$ when $x = 0$.

b. $dy/dx = x^3 + 5$, if $y = 20$ when $x = 2$.

Definite Integration

The Definite Integral—Integrals obtained by reversing the process of differentiation are indefinite to the extent that the values of the constants of integration are unknown. This indeterminacy can be removed either by the application of boundary conditions, as discussed previously, or by taking the difference between two values of the indefinite integral, thereby eliminating the constant of integration. The latter method gives rise directly to the *definite integral*.

Consider the indefinite integral of the function $f'(x)$.

$$y = \int f'(x) dx = f(x) + C$$

Let x assume values a and b, and denote the corresponding values of y by y_a and y_b. It then follows that the difference, $y_b - y_a$, is given by

$$y_b - y_a = f(b) - f(a) = \frac{\int f'(x) dx - \int f'(x) dx}{(x = b) \qquad (x = a)} \quad (10)$$

The last term in Eq 10 is an integral whose value is completely determined by the function $f(x)$ and by the numbers

a and b. For this reason it is termed the definite integral and is denoted by the equation

$$\int_a^b f'(x) dx = \frac{\int f'(x) dx - \int f'(x) dx}{(x = b) \qquad (x = a)} = f(b) - f(a) \quad (11)$$

This expression provides a link between the concept of the indefinite integral and that of the definite integral. The first term in Eq 11 denotes the integral of the function $f'(x)$ from the *lower limit of integration*, a, to the *upper limit of integration*, b.

The Relationship of Integration to Summation—One of the most important concepts of integral calculus is that of the relationship of the definite integral to a sum. As will be shown later, this concept may be applied in understanding the calculation of the areas under irregular curves. In general terms, it may be used to compute the sum of the product of a function and infinitesimal increments of its independent variable over a given interval.

Let $f'(x)$ be any continuous and single-valued function in the interval from $x = a$ to $x = b$. Divide the interval $a \leqslant x \leqslant b$ into n segments of length Δx_i, and let x_i be the division point between segments i and $i + 1$. Define the limit L as follows:

$$L = \lim_{\substack{n \to \infty \\ \Delta x_i \to 0}} \sum_{i=1}^{n} f'(x_i) \Delta x_i \quad (12)$$

The mean value theorem of derivatives states[2] that

$$f(q) - f(p) = f'(x_j) \cdot (q - p) \quad (13)$$

where $f'(x)$ is the derivative of $f(x)$ and where x_j is a suitably chosen point interior to the interval $p \leqslant x \leqslant q$. It is important to point out that while the location of x_j, such that Eq 13 holds true, will vary depending on $f(x)$ and on the interval $q - p$, x_j will always satisfy the condition $p \leqslant x_j \leqslant q$.

Let p and q represent the initial and final points of the segment Δx_i; that is, let $q - p = \Delta x_i$. Therefore, in the limit as $\Delta x_i \to 0$, $x_j \to x_i$. Eq 13 thus may be combined with Eq 12 in the form

$$L = \lim_{\substack{n \to \infty \\ \Delta x_i \to 0}} \sum_{i=1}^{n} [f(x_i) - f(x_{i-1})]$$

$$= \lim_{\substack{n \to \infty \\ \Delta x_i \to 0}} ([f(x_1) - f(x_0)] + [f(x_2) - f(x_1)] + \ldots$$

$$+ [f(x_n) - f(x_{n-1})])$$

All terms except $f(x_0)$ and $f(x_n)$ cancel in the above sum so that $L = f(x_n) - f(x_0)$. Since $x_0 = a$ and $x_n = b$, this may be written

$$L = f(b) - f(a) \quad (14)$$

Combining Eqs 11, 12, and 14, it may be shown that

$$\int_a^b f'(x) dx = \lim_{\substack{n \to \infty \\ \Delta x_i \to 0}} \sum_{i=1}^{n} f'(x_i) \Delta x_i \quad (15)$$

Eq 15 explicitly defines the relationship between summation and integration. Further, it shows that sums of the kind indicated can be evaluated as definite integrals; this is a distinct advantage in most instances.

Interpretation of the Definite Integral as an Area—It is often necessary to calculate the area of a region bounded by an irregular line. Such a figure is exemplified by the surface of the xy plane bounded by the curve $y = f'(x)$, the x axis, and the lines $x = a$ and $x = b$. This region can be divided into n segments of width Δx_i and area approximated by $f'(x_i) \Delta x_i$, as shown in Fig 12-5. When the areas of the n rectangles are summed, they approximate the area of the figure. In general,

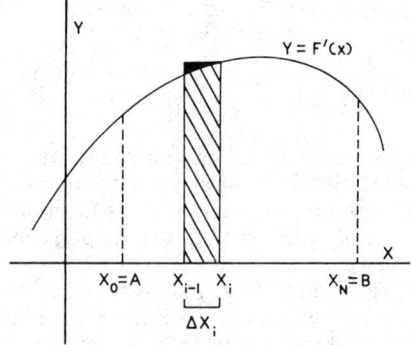

Fig 12-5.   A plot of the calculation of the area of a region bounded by an irregular line.

any portions of $f'(x)$ lying below the x axis generate negative values and must be taken into account in this interpretation. An error arises due to the inclusion and/or exclusion of small regions (shown in Fig 12-5 in solid black) in the sum.   However, in taking the limit of the sum, as the number of rectangles increases without bound and as their width approaches zero, the error vanishes.   The area of the figure is thus,

$$\text{Area} = \lim_{\substack{n \to \infty \\ \Delta x_i \to 0}} \sum_{i=1}^{n} f'(x_i)\Delta x_i = \int_a^b f'(x)dx$$

It can be seen from this expression that the computation of the given area involves only the evaluation of the definite integral of $f'(x)$ between the limits a and b.

Calculation of Definite Integrals—The following rules regarding the algebra of definite integrals may be deduced directly from either Eq 11 or Eq 15 by inspection.

Rule 1

$$\int_a^c g(x)dx = \int_a^b g(x)dx + \int_b^c g(x)dx$$

where a, b, and c are points along the x axis.

Rule 2

$$\int_a^b kg(x)dx = k \int_a^b g(x)dx$$

where k is a constant.

Rule 3

$$\int_a^b (g(x) + h(x))dx = \int_a^b g(x)dx + \int_a^b h(x)dx$$

The general method of evaluation of definite integrals follows from their definition as expressed in Eq 11,

$$\int_a^b f'(x)dx = f(b) - f(a)$$

where $f(x) + C$ is the indefinite integral of $f'(x)$.   The problem may be resolved into two stages: (1) finding the indefinite integral of the given integrand and (2) computing the difference in value of the indefinite integral between its upper and lower limits of integration.

A number of methods for accomplishing Step 1 have been presented and discussed.   Only one of these, the method of change of variable, need be developed further here.   Consider a function $f'(x)$ which is to be integrated following a change in variable such that

$$f'(x) = g'(u)$$

where $u = t(x)$.   It should be noted that, in the expression $\int_a^b f'(x)dx$, a and b refer to values of the independent variable x.   When the variable of integration is changed from x to u, the limits of integration must also be changed corresponding to u, thus

$$\int_a^b f'(x)dx = \int_{t(a)}^{t(b)} g'(u)du$$

The need to change limits can be overcome if, following indefinite integration, the indefinite integral is rewritten in terms of the original independent variable.   This is generally time consuming, however, and is not recommended.

Example 27—Rewrite the integral $y = \int_1^2 x(x^2 + 5)^3dx$ with the change of variable $u = x^2 + 5$.   Since $du = 2xdx$, $u = 6$ when $x = 1$, and $u = 9$ when $x = 2$, the integral may be transformed as follows:

$$y = \frac{1}{2} \int_1^2 (x^2 + 5)^3 2xdx = \frac{1}{2} \int_6^9 u^3du$$

Step 2 in the evaluation of the definite integral consists of determining the difference $f(b) - f(a)$ in Eq 11.   For convenience of notation, $f(b) - f(a)$ is written $f(x)|_a^b$.

Example 28—Complete the evaluation of the integral presented in Example 24.

$$\frac{1}{2} \int_6^9 u^3du = \frac{1}{8} u^4\Big|_6^9 = (9^4 - 6^4)/8 = \frac{5265}{8}$$

Example 29—Evaluate the integral, $\int_1^e \ln x \, dx$, by the method of parts. The definite integral must be found first.   Let $u = \ln x$ and $dv = dx$; then $du = dx/x$ and $v = x$.

$$\int \ln x \, dx = x \ln x - \int dx = x \ln x - x + C$$

$$\int_1^e \ln x \, dx = x \ln x - x \Big|_1^e = (e - e) - (0 - 1) = 1$$

Example 30—The material ejected from an aerosol spray can is cooled by the combined effects of evaporation of propellant and adiabatic expansion of the gas.   Work is done by the expanding gas but little heat, if any, enters the gas due to the short time period for the event.   Such a process, if reversible, is described in thermodynamics by the equation:

$$C_pdT = RTdP/P$$

where C_p, P, R, and T are as defined in Example 14 and Exercise 32. Given that the initial and final pressures and temperatures are P_a, T_a and P_b, T_b, respectively, integrate the equation in terms of these quantities.

Separating variables and indicating the limits of integration we obtain:

$$\int_{T_a}^{T_b} dT/T = R/C_p \int_{P_a}^{P_b} dP/P$$

Changing the variables to logarithmic form:

$$\int_{\ln T_a}^{\ln T_b} d \ln T = R/C_p \int_{\ln P_a}^{\ln P_b} d \ln P$$

The definite integral is thus:

$$\ln (T_b/T_a) = R/C_p \ln (P_b/P_a)$$

Approximate Numerical Integration—While the definite integral can be found for most of the functions encountered in pharmacy, this is not always the case.   The function to be integrated may not be known explicitly but instead may be represented only as a table of data.   It is also possible that the indefinite integral can not be expressed in terms of known functions.   In such cases, calculation of the definite integral by means of Eq 11 is impossible and an alternate method must be used.   The need to find the indefinite integral can be avoided by the use of Eq 15 which equates the definite integral to a sum involving the integrand itself.

As illustrated in Fig 12-5, the integral can be interpreted as an area which can be approximated by adding the areas of rectangles of width Δx_i and height $f'(x_i)$.   If this could be done exactly according to the requirements of Eq 15, where each Δx_i is infinitesimally small, an exact numerical value of the integral would be obtained.   Obviously, such a summation of an infinite number of terms cannot be performed.   Instead, an approximate value may be computed by dividing the interval, $b - a$, into n small equal increments, $(b - a)/n = \Delta x$.   In general, $f'(x)$ will vary in value over each small increment and, therefore, some means must be devised to obtain a representative value.   In Fig 12-5 this was done by selecting the ordinate at the right side of the interval Δx_i.   In this instance the solid black area represents an error in estimating the true incremental area. Such an error usually can be reduced by taking the average of the ordinates at the extremities of the segment as the height of the rectangle.   The resulting incremental area is that of a trapezoid formed by joining the points $(x_{i-1}, f'(x_{i-1}))$ and $(x_i, f'(x_i))$ by a straight line and the method is termed the *trapezoidal rule*.

Applying the trapezoidal rule, the sum in Eq 15 is approximated by the sum:

$\frac{1}{2}[f'(a) + f'(a + \Delta x)]\Delta x + \ldots$

$\qquad + \frac{1}{2}[f'(a + (n-1)\Delta x) + f'(b)]$

$$= \frac{b-a}{2n}[f'(a) + 2f'(a + \Delta x) + \ldots$$

$$\qquad + 2f'(a + (n-1)\Delta x) + f'(b)] \quad (16)$$

This equation may be applied directly to tabular data if the abscissa points are equally spaced. If not, the method may still be used but each trapezoid must be treated separately.

The desired integral may be determined, in most cases, to any degree of accuracy by choosing Δx suitably small. While other methods such as Simpson's rule are available for approximate integration, they essentially consist of alternate methods of assigning values to the height of the incremental rectangles and are not discussed here. In particular cases, one method may give a more accurate estimate than another for the same choice of n.

Example 31—Evaluate $\int_0^1 e^{-x^2} dx$ by the trapezoidal rule setting $n = 10$. The required sum as given by Eq. 16 is:

$[1 + 2(.99) + 2(.96) + 2(.91) + 2(.85) + 2(.78) + 2(.70)$

$\qquad + 2(.61) + 2(.53) + 2(.44) + 0.37]/20 = 0.75$

Multiple Integrals—The counterpart of the process of successive differentiation is the process of repeated or iterated integration. As was shown previously, the definite integral of $f(x)$ over a particular interval of x can be envisaged as an area between the curve and the x axis. Similarly, the double integral $\int\int_R f(x,y) dx dy$, over a particular region, R, in x and y, can be interpreted as a volume between the surface, $f(x,y)$, and the plane of the x and y axes. Physical interpretations are also possible for double integrals. Given suitable boundary conditions, the equation for the acceleration of an object may be integrated to give its velocity and, subsequently, the velocity equation integrated to obtain the distance traveled by the object over a given period of time. While triple and higher integrals may be computed they will not be discussed here. The following examples will further define multiple integrals and illustrate the procedure for their evaluation by iterated integration.

Example 32—Evaluate the double integral, $\int_1^3 \int_0^1 x dx^2$. This may be written as $\int_1^3 [\int_0^1 x dx] dx$.

$$\int_0^1 x dx = x^2/2 \big|_0^1 = \frac{1}{2}; \qquad \frac{1}{2} \int_1^3 dx = x/2 \big|_1^3 = 1$$

Example 33—Evaluate the double integral, $\int_0^2 \int_0^x (x+y) dy dx$. This may be written as $\int_0^2 [\int_0^x (x+y) dy] dx$.

$$\int_0^x (x+y) dy = xy + y^2/2 \big|_0^x = 3x^2/2; \qquad 3/2 \int_0^2 x^2 dx = x^3/2 \big|_0^2 = 4$$

Note that a partial integration, holding x constant, occurs first.

Exercises

40. Calculate the area bounded by the curve $y = x^2$, the y axis, and the line $y = 4$, and which lies in the first quadrant.

41. Calculate the value of the following integrals.

  a. $\displaystyle\int_1^{10} (1 + \ln x) dx$

  b. $\displaystyle\int_1^3 (x^3 - 1) dx$

  c. $\displaystyle\int_0^1 x e^{x^2} dx$

  d. $\displaystyle\int_1^3 (5 - 3y^2) dy$

42. Calculate a numerical value for t given

$$\int_0^t y dy = 4 \int_0^{\ln 3} e^x dx$$

43. Calculate the value of g if

$$2.303 \int_{-\infty}^0 e^z dz = \int_g^5 (6 - x)^{-1} dx$$

44. Show that

$$\int_1^5 d \ln a \neq \int_1^5 da/a$$

45. Evaluate the integral in Exercise 41a, setting $n = 10$, 20.

46. Verify by computation that the double integral $\int_0^x \int_0^2 (x + y) dx dy$ is not equal to the double integral in Example 33 from which it was obtained by reversing the order of integration.

47. In any physical or chemical equilibrium, the equilibrium constants, K_1 and K_2, corresponding to temperatures T_1 and T_2 are related by the following function.

$$d \ln K / dT = \Delta H^\circ / RT^2$$

where ΔH° is the standard enthalpy change and R is the gas constant. Assuming ΔH° to be a constant, integrate this equation to obtain the well known van't Hoff equation:

$$\log\left(\frac{K_2}{K_1}\right) = \frac{\Delta H^\circ}{2.3R}\left(\frac{T_2 - T_1}{T_1 T_2}\right)$$

48. In graphically determining the value of ΔH°, using the van't Hoff equation, it is common to plot $\ln K$ vs $1/T$. Show that the differential form of the equation in Exercise 47 may be written as:

$$\frac{d \ln K}{d(1/T)} = -\frac{\Delta H^\circ}{R}$$

Integrate this equation and verify your answer with Exercise 47.

Laplace Transformation

Differential Equations—Although they have not been referred to as such, we have derived, integrated, and otherwise worked with *differential equations* throughout much of this chapter. They differ from the familiar equations of algebra and trigonometry in that they contain the *differentials* of variables and, frequently, the variables themselves together with various constants. The equation $dN/dt = -\lambda N$, given in Example 8 is a differential equation.

Finding the solutions to algebraic or trigonometric equations can be accomplished by a variety of familiar techniques. Such a solution results in an identity when substituted into the original equation and is said to satisfy the equation.

We have found the solutions to differential equations by integrating them. These solutions do not contain differentials but instead are functions of the variables which were contained in the original differential equation. If such a solution is substituted into the respective differential equation, an identity will result in a manner analogous to the case of algebraic equations. This can be easily verified for some of the examples and exercises worked previously, eg Exercises 34 and 39 and Example 25. The relationship between the solutions of algebraic and differential equations suggests that the solutions to differential equations might be found by the relatively simple methods of algebra if differential equations could be transformed into algebraic equations. A transformation of this type would eliminate the need to integrate in the usual sense. Fortunately, Laplace transformations will frequently do this.

The Laplace Transform—Given a function, $f(t)$, which can be Laplace transformed, then its Laplace transform, $\bar{f}(s)$, is defined as follows.

$$\bar{f}(s) = \int_0^\infty f(t) e^{-st} dt \qquad (17)$$

Since we are transforming a function of t into a function of a new variable s, the process consists essentially of a change of variable. As shown earlier in this chapter, the use of a change of variable to facilitate integration ultimately requires an inverse change of variable to express the final solution in terms of the original variable. Although it is possible to define the inverse Laplace transformation formally and to compute

Table II—Laplace Transforms and Their Inverses

Functions $f(t)$	Laplace Transforms $\bar{f}(s)$
1	$1/s$
A	A/s
t	$1/s^2$
$\dfrac{t^{n-1}}{(n-1)!}$	$\dfrac{1}{s^n}\ (n = 1,2,\ldots)$
t^m	$m!/s^{m+1}$
e^{-at}	$1/(s+a)$
te^{at}	$1/(s+a)^2$
$\dfrac{1}{a}(1 - e^{-at})$	$1/s(s+a)$
$\dfrac{1}{a}e^{-(b/a)t}$	$1/(as+b)$
$\dfrac{(B - Aa)e^{-at} - (B - Ab)e^{-bt}}{b - a}\ (b \neq a)$	$(As + B)/(s + a)(s + b)$
$\dfrac{1}{b-a}(e^{-at} - e^{-bt})$	$1/(s + a)(s + b)$
$e^{-at}[A + (B - Aa)t]$	$(As + B)/(s + a)^2$
$-\dfrac{1}{PQR}[P(Aa^2 - Ba + C)e^{-at}$ $+ Q(Ab^2 - Bb + C)e^{-bt}$ $+ R(Ac^2 - Bc + C)e^{-ct}]$ $(P = b - c, Q = c - a, R = a - b)$	$(As^2 + Bs + C)/$ $(s + a)(s + b)(s + c)$
$\left[\dfrac{1}{ab} + \dfrac{1}{a(a - b)}e^{-at} - \dfrac{1}{b(a - b)}e^{-bt}\right]$	$1/s(s + a)(s + b)$
$\dfrac{1}{a}t - \dfrac{1}{a^2}(1 - e^{-at})$	$1/s^2(s + a)$
$\dfrac{B}{ab} - \dfrac{Aa - B}{a(a - b)}e^{-at} + \dfrac{Ab - B}{b(a - b)}e^{-bt}$	$(As + B)/s(s + a)(s + b)$
$\dfrac{B}{ab} - \dfrac{a^2 - Aa + B}{a(b - a)}e^{-at} + \dfrac{b^2 - Ab + B}{b(b - a)}e^{-bt}$	$(s^2 + As + B)/s(s + a)(s + b)$
$t^r e^{-at}$	$r!/(s + a)^{r+1}$
$e^{-at}\cos bt$	$(s + a)/[(s + a)^2 + b^2]$
$e^{-at}\sin bt$	$b/[(s + a)^2 + b^2]$
$t^r e^{-at}\cos bt$	$(-1)^r d^r/ds^r\{(s + a)/$ $[(s + a)^2 + b^2]\}$
$t^r e^{-at}\sin bt$	$(-1)^r d^r/ds^r\{b/[(s + a)^2 + b^1]\}$
$\dfrac{2}{a\sqrt{\pi}}e^{-a^3 t}\displaystyle\int_0^{a\sqrt{1}} e^{\lambda^3}\,d\lambda$	$\dfrac{1}{\sqrt{s}(s + a^2)}$
$\dfrac{1}{t}(e^{bt} - e^{at})$	$\log \dfrac{s - a}{s - b}$
$\sin bt$	$\dfrac{b}{s^2 + b^2}$
$\cos bt$	$\dfrac{s}{s(s^2 + b^2)}$

it analytically in many cases, this will not be necessary here. Instead, the inverse transformation of $\bar{f}(s)$ simply will be taken as $f(t)$ as implicitly stated in Eq 17.

It should be mentioned that s is a complex variable consisting of real and imaginary parts. This fact may be encountered by the reader in various reference texts used in conjunction with this chapter. However, for our purposes, no use will be made of the complex nature of s and it can be regarded as a real-valued quantity.

The Laplace transform of a function can be determined using Eq 17, provided the function is of a type that is transformable. Two examples will be worked out to provide a basis for understanding the transformation. In general, however, fairly extensive tables of transformations and their inverses are provided in handbooks of chemistry and physics and in other compilations of mathematical tables.

Example 34—Find the Laplace transform of a constant. Let the constant equal k. Thus:

$$\bar{k} = \int_0^\infty ke^{-st}dt = -(k/s)e^{-st}\Big|_0^\infty$$

$\bar{k}$ is therefore equal to k/s.

Example 35—Find the Laplace transform of the variable t. From Eq 17 we obtain:

$$\bar{t} = \int_0^\infty te^{-st}dt$$

Table III—Laplace Transforms of Derivatives

Derivative	Laplace Transform
dy/dt	$s\bar{y} - y_0$
d^2y/dt^2	$s^2\bar{y} - sy_0 - \dot{y}_0$
d^3y/dt^3	$s^3\bar{y} - s^2y_0 - s\dot{y}_0 - \ddot{y}_0$

Integrating by the method of parts we obtain:

$$\int_0^\infty te^{-st}dt = [-(t/s)e^{-st} - (1/s^2)e^{-st}]\Big|_0^\infty = 1/s^2$$

Many differential equations of importance in pharmacy are classified as ordinary, linear differential equations with constant coefficients and are subject to various boundary conditions. This type of differential equation often can be solved easily using Laplace transformations and has the following general form.

$$a_n\frac{d^ny}{dt^n} + \ldots + a_2\frac{d^2y}{dt^2} + a_1\frac{dy}{dt} + a_0y = g(t) \qquad (18)$$

$a_0, a_1, \ldots, a_n$ are constants and $g(t)$ is a function of t. Equations of this type are frequently encountered with the compartmental models used to approximate the pharmacokinetic behavior of drugs in the body.

Solution of Differential Equations Using Laplace Transforms—From a comparison of Eq 18 with Table II, it can be seen in general that a differential equation of that type can be converted into an equation devoid of differentials if the transformations given in Table III are also used. This is actually the first step in finding the solution to the differential equation. Step two consists of solving the resultant equation in s explicitly for $\bar{y}(s)$. Step three, largely a matter of trial and error, is to place the algebraic expression for $\bar{y}(s)$ in a form found in a table of transforms. The function $y(t)$ is then read directly from the table and may be verified by substitution into the original differential equation. In the remainder of this chapter, $y(t)$ and $\bar{y}(s)$ will be abbreviated as y and $\bar{y}$, respectively.

Two simple rules of algebra are sufficient to establish the relationship between a differential equation and its transform. (1) The Laplace transform of a sum of functions is equal to the sum of the Laplace transforms of the functions. Thus: $\overline{x + y + z} = \bar{x} + \bar{y} + \bar{z}$, where x, y, and z are functions of t. (2) The Laplace transform of a constant times a function is equal to the constant times the transform of the function. Thus: $\overline{ky} = k\bar{y}$.

Example 36—Find the solution of the following expression if $y = 4$ when $t = 0$.

$$2dy/dt - 13y = 0$$

Taking the Laplace transforms of all terms we obtain:

$$-2y_0 + 2s\bar{y} - 13\bar{y} = 0$$

Solving for $\bar{y}$ and substituting $y_0 = 4$:

$$\bar{y} = \frac{8}{2s - 13}$$

Referring to Table II, the inverse transformation is found to be:

$$y = 4e^{(13/2)t}$$

Example 37—Simple harmonic motion consists of a linear vibration about a central point such that the acceleration toward the point is proportional to the displacement from the point. It is, therefore, defined by the equation

$$d^2y/dt^2 = -k^2y,$$

where the proportionality constant is taken as k^2 for convenience, as will be seen. Find an expression for the displacement, y, as a function of time given that: at $t = 0$; $y = y_0 = 0$, and $\dot{y} = \dot{y}_0 = \frac{dy}{dt} = 1$.

After Laplace transformation the differential equation has the form:

$$s^2\bar{y} - sy_0 - \dot{y}_0 = -k^2\bar{y}$$

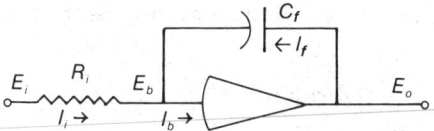

Fig 12-6. Electronic integration.

Solving for $\bar{y}$ and substituting for y_0 and $\dot{y}_0$:

$$\bar{y} = 1/(s^2 + k^2) = 1/(s - k)(s + k)$$

From Table II it can be seen that:

$$y = 1/k \sin(kt)$$

It is apparent from these examples that the use of Laplace transforms reduces the problem of solving differential equations to simple algebra. Secondly, the solutions which result automatically take into account the initial boundary conditions. This is equivalent to finding the definite integral.

Physical Methods of Integration

Integration of certain functions has been previously discussed, wherein an explicit definite or indefinite function is obtained by analytical mathematical methods. However, in some cases in which the integral can be expressed as a voltage which is a function of time, integration can be accomplished physically using an electrical circuit.

Consider the diagram in Fig 12-6. An input voltage, E_i, as a function of time is integrated, producing an output voltage, E_o, also a function of time and which is the integral. A high impedance operational amplifier, symbolized by the cone in the diagram, amplifies the input voltage with a change in sign and feeds it back through a capacitor. As a consequence of this arrangement, the following equations can be written.

$$I_i + I_f = I_b$$

$$I_f = C_f\frac{d(E_o - E_b)}{dt}$$

$$I_i - (E_i - E_b)/R_i$$

$$\therefore \frac{E_i - E_b}{R_i} + C_f\frac{d(E_o - E_b)}{dt} = I_b$$

Since, for reasons of physics, E_o and I_b are negligible:

$$dE_o = \frac{-E_i dt}{R_i C_f}$$

Integrating this expression, it can be seen that:

$$E_o = \frac{-1}{R_i C_f}\int_o^t E_i dt$$

Exercises

49. Calculate the Laplace transforms of dy/dt, d^2y/dt^2, and d^3y/dt^3 using the method of integration by parts.

50. By inductive reasoning, write an expression for d^ny/dt^n using the results obtained from Exercise 49.

51. Solve the equations in Exercise 36 using Laplace transforms. Tables of transforms from other sources may be needed.

52. The plasma concentration, C, of a drug is expected to correspond to the following differential equation

$$dC/dt = bC - ae^{-gt},$$

following intravenous injection of a drug. Find C as a function of time given that a, b, and g are constants and that $C = 0$ at time zero.

Answers to Exercises

1. $-2, 1 - 3a^2, -3b^2 + 6b - 2$
2. $x^2 - 1/x^2$
4. 0.39
5. $0, \frac{3}{2}, \frac{1}{8}, -3$
6. $\Delta y/\Delta x = -1/(x^2 + x\Delta x), -1$
7. a. n and K are constants, r is the dependent variable, and (D) is the independent variable.
    c. n
8. a. $1/r, 1/(D); (D)/r, (D); r/(D), r$
    b. $1/nK, 1/n, -K$
    c. $1/n, 1/nK, nK$
    d. n
    e. $n = 3, K = 10^5$
9. $6x^2, (1 - t)^{-2}, 5n^4$
10. $0, 6, 54, 6a^2$
12. $d(\text{drug})/dt = -(\text{drug})/1000$
16. $3x^2 - 3 - x^{-2}$,
    $$\frac{(1 + x^2)/2x^{1/2} - 2x^{3/2}}{(1 + x^2)^2},$$
    $2xe^{x^2}$,
    $2x/(1 + x^2)$
17. $dy/dx = e^z(-2x) = -2xe^{1-x^2}$
18. $(5/2)(e^{3t} - 3\ln t)^{3/2}(3e^{3t} - 3t^{-1})$
19. $x^4 + x^2 + 1, 4x^3 + 2x, 12x^2 + 2, 24x, 24, 0 \ldots 0$
20. $1/2$
21. 7
23. $2xy^2e^{x^2y^2}, 2x^2ye^{x^2y^2}$
24. 96
25. 4
26. $du = yze^{xyz}dx + xze^{xyz}dy + xye^{xyz}dz$
28. $6/t$
29. $-t^{-2}e^{2t}\ln^3 t + 2t^{-1}e^t\ln^3 t + 3t^{-2}e^{2t}\ln^2 t$
30. y^2/x^2
31. $\partial^2u/\partial x^2 = 0, \partial^2u/\partial y^2 = xe^y, \partial^2u/\partial x\partial y = \partial^2u/\partial y\partial x = e^y$

33. $x - e^x\ln x + C, (x^7 - x^{-3})^3/3 + C, 2x^4 + C,$
    $x^4/4 + 2x^3/3 - 7x + C, 2e^x + C, \ln(1 + x) + C$
34. $y = x^3/3 + x^2 - 15x + C, u = e^t - \ln t + C$
35. $x^2e^x - 2xe^x + 2e^x + C, -xe^{2x}/2 - e^{2x}/4 + C,$
    $x\ln x - x + C$
36. $2(x^3 - 1)^{3/2}/9 + C, (x^2 - 2x)^{1/2}/4 + C$
38. $kt = \dfrac{1}{(a - b)}\ln\dfrac{b(a - x)}{a(b - x)}$
39. $y = e^x - 1, y = x^4/4 + 5x + 6$
40. $16/3$
41. $23.03, 18, (e - 1)/2, -16$
42. ± 4
43. -4
49. See Table III
50. $\overline{d^ny/dt^n} = s^n\overline{y} - s^{n-1}y_0 - s^{n-2}(dy/dt)_0 - \ldots - (d^{n-1}y/dt^{n-1})_0$, where: $(dy/dt)_0 = \dot{y}_0$
52. $C = (a/(b - g))(e^{-gt} - e^{-bt})$

References

1. Sokolnikoff IS. *Advanced Calculus*, McGraw-Hill, New York, 87–89, 1939.
2. Smail LL. *Calculus*, Appleton-Century-Crofts, New York, 98, 1949.

Bibliography

Bres L: *Calculus*, vol 2, Holt, Rinehart and Winston, New York, 1969.

Daniels F: *Mathematical Preparation for Elementary Physical Chemistry*, McGraw-Hill, New York, 1928.

Lang S: *A Complete Course in Calculus*, Addison-Wesley, Reading, 1968.

Salas SL, Hille E: *Calculus: One and Several Variables*, 2nd ed, vol I and II, Wiley, New York, 1974.

Strum RD, Ward JR: *Laplace Transformation Solutions of Differential Equations: A Programmed Text*, Prentice-Hall, New Jersey, 1968.

Taylor AE: *Advanced Calculus*, 3rd ed John Wiley & Sons, Inc. New York, 1983.

Wylie, CR, JR: *Advanced Engineering Mathematics*, 3rd ed. McGraw-Hill, New York, 1966.

CHAPTER 13

Molecular Structure, Properties, and States of Matter

Eric J Lien, PhD

Professor of Pharmacy/Pharmaceutics and Biomedicinal Chemistry
School of Pharmacy, University of Southern California
Los Angeles, CA 90033

Lloyd Kennon, PhD*

Associate Professor and Industrial Pharmacy Program Director
Arnold and Marie Schwartz College of Pharmacy and Health Sciences
Long Island University, Brooklyn, NY 11201

The many significant advances in the pharmaceutical sciences in recent years are in large part attributable to the accelerated development of knowledge of the molecular structure and physicochemical properties of drugs, and to the correlation of this knowledge with that of the nature of biological reactions of drugs. In this chapter are discussed fundamental principles of atomic and molecular structure and of certain physicochemical properties which are basically important in the pharmaceutical sciences.

Atomic Structure

Atoms and Elementary Particles—The word atom is derived from the Greek word *atomos*, indivisible; the atoms were believed to be the minute indivisible particles of which all material things were made. The search for the ultimate particle has been a continuous effort since the time of Democritus. Before the discovery of mesons and hyperons, the structure of matter was believed to be much simpler. The nucleus was thought to consist of protons and neutrons, and to form an atom only electrons needed to be added in external shells. Therefore, protons, neutrons, and electrons were considered as the elementary particles.

During the past three decades nuclear physics has progressively probed atoms from their periphery to their center. The search for ultimate units of nuclear structure by means of experiments consisting in large part of bombarding nuclei with high-energy particles has revealed a spectrum of over 100 species, most of them unstable. Some of these particles are listed in Table I. The proton is no longer considered an ultimate particle, but is believed to be made up of particles called *quarks* (from "three quarks for Muster Mark," in James Joyce's *Finnigans Wake*). One theory of quark structure of protons calls for nine kinds of quarks (along with antiquarks) and eight kinds of *gluons* (analogous to photons) to hold the quarks together. Whether these and other elementary particles are all composed of yet simpler elements remains to be investigated.[1]

L de Broglie in 1924 raised the question that if light waves show corpuscular character, should not particles also show wave character? Now it is generally accepted that in the case of a photon there are two fundamental equations to be obeyed: $E = h\nu$ and $E = mc^2$, where E is the energy, h is Planck's constant, ν is the frequency, and c is the speed of light. Combining both equations we have $h\nu = mc^2$ or $\lambda = c/\nu = h/mc = h/p$, where p is the momentum of the proton.

De Broglie proposed that a similar equation should govern the wavelength of the electron wave. It is interesting to note that X-ray diffraction is a good example of the utilization of the wave property of electromagnetic radiation.

More recently, scattering of slow neutrons has been employed to provide information about the structure and dynamic properties of biological structures, eg, myoglobin and membranes.[2]

Dalton's Atomic Theory—In 1808 Dalton proposed his atomic theory on the basis of three generalizations; namely, the Law of Conservation of Mass, the Law of Definite Proportions, and the Law of Multiple Proportions. The essential parts of the theory can be summarized as follows:

1. All elements are composed of very small, discrete, indivisible particles called atoms.
2. All atoms of any one element are identical. Modern structural theory tells us that electronic differences between the atoms of an element may occur, but these differences arise as a consequence of electronic excitation. The lowest energy state of an atom is more appropriate for purposes of classification.
3. The atoms of no two elements are alike.
4. Atoms undergo no fundamental change in chemical reactions. There are subtle changes in the electronic character of atoms, although this does not change the identity of an atom.
5. Compounds are formed when atoms of two or more different elements combine to form a molecule.
6. In general, atoms combine in simple ratios.

Periodic Table—The periodic classification of the elements is one of the most striking advances in generalizing many isolated facts; moreover, it contributes tremendously to the strength of the atomic theory and extends it to new sets of facts. The periodic table serves as an easily learned summary of almost limitless information about the chemical nature of the elements; it is of prime importance to students of pharmaceutical sciences as well as to students of chemistry.

After the publication of the independent researches of Mendeléev and Meyer in 1869, the *Periodic Law* was well established. The *Periodic Table* is an arrangement of the elements in accordance with the periodic law (see inside back cover). The present arrangement is essentially the same as that of Mendeléev, although there are now minor variations due to the incorporation of new elements and modern data. A few terms should be carried in mind for a thorough understanding of the table.

Atomic number (Z) is the positive charge of the nucleus expressed as multiples of the electronic charge e.

Atomic weight is the average weight expressed in atomic weight units of the natural atoms of an element existing as a mixture of isotopes in the same ratio as found in nature. An atomic weight unit, used in chemistry, is exactly $1/16$ the average mass of the oxygen isotopes taken in the same ratio as

---

* Deceased.

Table I—Subatomic Particles

Group	Particles	Relative mass (electron = 1)	Electric charge	Mean life-time (sec)
Heavy particles	α-Particle (He^{2+}, α)	7348	+2	stable
	Triton (T, ^{3}H)	5451	+1	3.8×10^8
	Deuteron (D, d, ^{2}H)	3674	+1	stable
	Neutron (n)	1837	0	7.2×10^2
	Proton (p, ^{1}H)	1837	+1	stable
Hyperons	Λ° Particle	~2181	0	2.5×10^{-10}
	$\Sigma^\pm$ Particle	~2326	±1	$\Sigma^+\ 0.8 \times 10^{-10}$ $\Sigma^-\ 1.6 \times 10^{-10}$
	$\Xi^\pm$ Particle	~2580	±1	1.3×10^{-10}
Mesons	K meson (K$^\pm$)	966	±1	1.2×10^{-8}
	K meson (K$^\circ$)	974	0	$10^{-9} - 10^{-10}$
	Pi meson ($\pi^\pm$)	273	±	2.6×10^{-8}
	Pi meson (π°)	264	0	1.9×10^{-16}
	Mu meson ($\mu^\pm$)	209 ± 2	±1	2.2×10^{-6}
Leptons	Electrons (e$^-$, β^-)	1	−1	stable
	Positron (e$^+$, β^+)	1	+1	stable
	Neutrino (ν)	0.01	0	stable
	Photons (γ)	0	0	stable

they occur in nature. One atomic weight unit is equivalent to 1.000272 atomic mass unit.

An *isotope* is one of a group of nuclides of the same element (same Z), having the same number of protons in the nucleus but differing in the number of neutrons, resulting in different mass numbers.

A *nuclide* is any one of the more than 1000 species of atoms and is characterized by the number of protons and neutrons in the nucleus.

Bohr's Theory of Atomic Structure—In 1913 Bohr proposed a theory of atomic structure for the problem of atomic spectra. His picture of the atom had the extranuclear electrons revolving around the nucleus in definite orbits. These orbits were assigned principal quantum numbers 1, 2, 3, ... n, counting outward from the nucleus.

When an electron absorbs a definite increment or quantum of energy, it is promoted to an orbit of higher energy (excited state), and when it falls back to the original orbit, it emits radiation energy. The energy of the various levels in the atom can be related to the frequency of radiation which is emitted from or absorbed by the atom. This relationship is expressed by

$$\Delta E = E_2 - E_1 = h\nu \tag{1}$$

where ΔE is the difference of the energy in ergs between two levels, h is Planck's constant (6.624×10^{-27} erg sec), and ν is the frequency. Since the frequency is equivalent to the speed of light c divided by the wavelength, Eq 1 can be written as

$$\Delta E = hc/\lambda \tag{2}$$

When the electrons possess the lowest energy possible, the atom is said to be in its *ground state*.

The energy of an electron in an orbit is given by

$$E = \frac{-2\pi^2 Z^2 m e^4}{n^2 h^2} \tag{3}$$

where Z is the atomic number, m is the mass of the electron (9.1×10^{-28} g), e is the charge of the electron in electrostatic units (4.8×10^{-10} esu), n is the principal quantum number, and h is Planck's constant. One can calculate the radiation energy emitted when an electron falls from n_2 orbit to n_1 orbit by Eq 4

$$E_2 - E_1 = \frac{2\pi^2 Z^2 m e^4}{h^2} \left(\frac{1}{n_1^2} - \frac{1}{n_2^2} \right) \tag{4}$$

When n_2 is ∞, Eq 4 gives the energy required for ionization. For example, the ionization potential of the hydrogen atom can be calculated as

$$E_\infty - E_1 =$$

$$\frac{2 \times (3.14)^2 \times (1)^2 \times 9.1 \times 10^{-28} \times (4.8 \times 10^{-10})^4}{(6.624 \times 10^{-27})^2} \times$$

$$\left(\frac{1}{(1)^2} - \frac{1}{(\infty)^2} \right)$$

$$= 2.18 \times 10^{-11} \text{ erg} =$$

$$\frac{2.18 \times 10^{-11} \text{ erg}}{1.60 \times 10^{-12} \text{ erg/electron volt (ev)}}$$

$$= 13.6 \text{ ev}$$

It is interesting to note that the quantum theory is founded on the principle that the energy of an atom or molecule does not change continuously but only by some definite whole number unit of energy referred to as a quantum.

Modern Model of Atomic Structure—After Bohr published his theory, there was a period of intense activity by theoreticians and experimental physicists. Based on mathematical principles and considerable experimental data, a more definite picture of atomic structure emerged. The modern interpretation of the atom is more elaborate than the

Table II—Electronic Configurations of Some Elements in Their Ground States

Atomic no	Elements	n = 1, K, l = 0, 1s	n = 2, L, l = 0, 2s	n = 2, L, l = 1, 2p	n = 3, M, l = 0, 3s	n = 3, M, l = 1, 3p	n = 3, M, l = 2, 3d	n = 4, N, l = 0, 4s	n = 4, N, l = 1, 4p	n = 4, N, l = 2, 4d	n = 4, N, l = 3, 4f	
1	H	1										
2	He	2										
3	Li	2	1									
4	Be	2	2									
5	B	2	2	1								
6	C	2	2	2								
7	N	2	2	3								
8	O	2	2	4								
9	F	2	2	5								
10	Ne	2	2	6								
11	Na				1							
12	Mg				2							
13	Al				2	1						
14	Si	Neon core			2	2						
15	P				2	3						
16	S				2	4						
17	Cl				2	5						
18	Ar				2	6						
19	K							1				Beginning of 1st long period
20	Ca							2				
21	Sc						1	2				
22	Ti						2	2				
23	V						3	2				
24	Cr						5	1				
25	Mn						5	2				1st transition series
26	Fe	Argon core					6	2				
27	Co						7	2				
28	Ni						8	2				
29	Cu						10	1				
30	Zn						10	2				
31	Ga						10	2	1			
32	Ge						10	2	2			
33	As						10	2	3			
34	Se						10	2	4			
35	Br						10	2	5			
36	Kr						10	2	6			

original idea of Bohr. Four quantum numbers are used to describe the energy levels or orbitals of each electron.

The *principal quantum number n* is an approximate measure of the size of the electron cloud; ie, the order of magnitude of the potential energy. It has the values 1, 2, 3, ... 7, corresponding to the K, L, M, ... Q shells of electrons.

The *azimuthal quantum number l* is related to the shape of the electron cloud, indicating whether it is a spherical, dumbbell-shaped, or of more complex geometry. It may have values of $0, 1, 2, \ldots (n-1)$, corresponding, respectively, to the terms s, p, d, f, used by spectroscopists. For example, a $4d$ electron would have an n number of 4 and an l value of 2.

The *magnetic quantum number* m_l is related to the orientation of the electron cloud in space. It has values of $0, \pm 1, \pm 2, \ldots \pm l$. For a spherical cloud there is only one orientation. However, the dumbbell-shaped orbital, for example, could be oriented in three different directions corresponding to the x, y, and z axes of a set of Cartesian coordinates.

The *spin quantum number s* (or m_s) gives the orientation of the magnetic component of an electron. There are only two discrete ways an electron can interact with an external magnetic field: like a tiny magnet, it can either line up in the direction of the field or it can orient itself in the opposite direction. The electron's magnetic moment was at first pictured as being due to the rotation of the electron on its axis, and for this reason an electron was said to exhibit spin. The two spin quantum numbers $s = +\frac{1}{2}$ and $s = -\frac{1}{2}$ were used to describe the two observable spin states.

Considerable progress has been made in the last few years in the application of quantum mechanical and molecular orbital theories in studying drug-receptor interactions and in correlating chemical structure with pharmacological activities of drugs.

Electronic Configuration of the Elements—Two rules are of extreme importance in explaining the building up of electronic shells of elements (as shown in Fig 13-1 and Table II).

The *Pauli exclusion principle* states that an atom cannot exist in a state where two electrons in the same energy level or orbital have the same set of four quantum numbers. This is analogous to the principle in classical physics that no two bodies can be in the same place at the same time. Thus two electrons in the K shell have the same principal, azimuthal, and magnetic quantum numbers ($n = 1$, $l = 0$, $m_l = 0$), and different spin quantum numbers ($s = +\frac{1}{2}$ and $-\frac{1}{2}$).

Hund's rule of maximum multiplicity states that when orbitals are of the same energy electrons distribute themselves one to each orbital so as to maintain parallel spins. For example, oxygen with an atomic number of 8, possesses 8 electrons. Two electrons are in the K shell ($1s^2$), and 6 are in the L shell. In the L shell 2 electrons fill the $2s$ orbitals ($2s^2$) and the remaining 4 fill the $2p$ orbitals ($2p^4$).

According to Hund's rule, 3 electrons occupy $2p_x$, $2p_y$, and

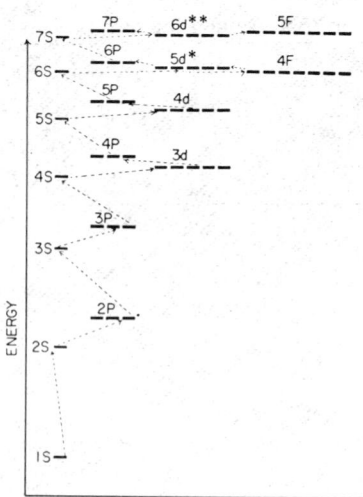

Fig 13-1.   Atomic energy levels and the order of filling of orbitals: (*) a single 5*d* electron is added before the 4*f* orbitals can be filled; (**) one or more 6*d* electrons must be added before the 5*f* orbitals can be filled.

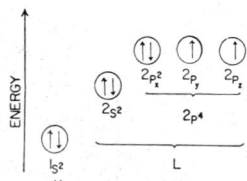

Fig 13-2.   The electronic configuration of an oxygen atom.

$2p_z$ orbitals and spin in the same direction (indicated by the direction of the arrow in Fig 13-2); the fourth electron can pair up with any one of these 3 electrons (say $2p_x$).   The electronic configuration for oxygen atom can be expressed as $1s^2\, 2s^2\, 2p_x{}^2\, 2p_y\, 2p_z$.

The Uniqueness of Carbon

Since organic chemistry is concerned mainly with carbon and its compounds, closer attention is warranted to the kinds of bonds exhibited by the carbon atom.

Carbon (and, to a much lesser extent, boron and beryllium) is in a special class.   Although only the twelfth most abundant element on earth, its compounds far outnumber those of the remainder of the periodic table *combined*.   The exact number of existing carbon compounds is probably unknown and the theoretical number is infinite.   For example, the number of known hydrides of carbon is about 2300, while the next most prolific member (boron) of this period in the periodic table can boast of only seven!   This uniqueness stems from the simple fact that carbon is capable of bonding with itself in many unusual modes.

Carbon Bonds

Ordinarily, carbon is said to exhibit a valence of four.   Thus it can combine with four other monovalent atoms or groups or with four other carbon atoms in a linear or cyclic fashion with or without branching, or any combination thereof:

Also, carbon atoms can unite to each other or to other atoms such as nitrogen, oxygen, or sulfur by means of multiple bonds.

To compound the situation further, the structural diagrams just presented are not flat objects, but are three-dimensional. For example, a six-membered carbon ring may have several configurations, such as:

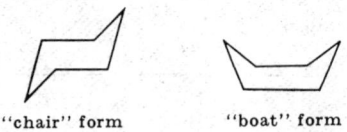

"chair" form   "boat" form

This feature alone could essentially double the number of compounds of this type.

Hybridization—What is so unusual about the constitution of the carbon atom that allows so many diverse compounds? Simply stated, the reason is *hybridization*, and a review of the electronic configuration of the atom is required to explain what hybridization is and how it is attained.   The extranuclear configuration of an isolated carbon atom is $1s^2 2s^2 2p_x{}^1 2p_y{}^1 2p_z{}^0$, which means that there are two electrons in the 1s level, two in the 2s level, and two in the 2p level, but since the two 2p electrons reside in different subshells (p_x and p_y) they are unpaired.   Since only unpaired valence electrons are capable of bonding, it would be expected that carbon should exhibit a valence of two.   However, in every instance (except for possibly carbon monoxide) carbon combines with four univalent atoms or groups.

Bond formation is a stabilizing (exothermic) process and there is a tendency to form as many bonds as possible, even if the resulting molecular orbitals bear little resemblance to the atomic orbitals which exist in the isolated or *ground* state of an atom.   A carbon atom must be elevated or *excited* (energetically) to assume a valence state of four and to do this four unpaired electrons must be created.   This feat can be accomplished by promoting one electron from the 2s level to the vacant $2p_z$ level and thus the resulting extranuclear electronic configuration becomes $1s^2 2s^1 2p_x{}^1 2p_y{}^1 2p_z{}^1$.   More than enough energy is available during the process of bond formation to excite the 2s electron.   Four unpaired electrons are now available for bonding purposes.

It might now be expected that carbon could form two different types of bonds, *viz*, three bonds of a type using p orbitals ($2p_x$, $2p_y$, $2p_z$) and a fourth bond utilizing the 2s orbital. This is contrary to known fact—all four bonds are equivalent so far as bond energy and bond length are concerned.

The simplest two-dimensional picture of such a carbon atom, as noted in the diagram of the molecule dichloromethane, CH_2Cl_2, would be as in *A*:

```
        Cl                        Cl
        |                         |
   H──C─Cl                  H──C──H
        |                         |
        H                         Cl
        A                         B
```

However, it can readily be observed that if the molecule was flat, it should exist in the two isomeric forms, *A* and *B*.   Since only one dichloromethane is known (and for other, more convincing, reasons) the structure as depicted is spatially incorrect.   In 1874 LeBel and van't Hoff demonstrated, using the concept of stereoisomerism, that a carbon atom assumes a *tetrahedral* configuration.   That is, each covalent bond is directed to a corner of a regular tetrahedron:

109.5°

To more clearly illustrate the three-dimensional aspect of this arrangement, the usual two-dimensional diagram is better shown as follows:

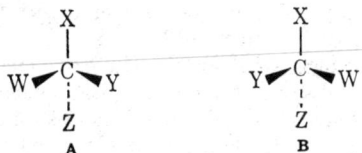

in which a solid line is understood to be in the plane of the paper, a broken line extends behind the plane, and solid arrowheads extend in front of the plane. Study of the many kinds of three-dimensional organic models is very beneficial in the understanding of this concept. A cursory look at such models (or the diagram) indicates that A and B are not identical (not superimposable) but are in reality isomers. This situation is known as *stereoisomerism* and the phenomenon essentially doubles the number of possible compounds of this particular type.

Since the resultant bonds are comprised of one s and three p electrons and are neither of the spherical s or linear p configuration, but some combination thereof, they are said to be *hybridized*. This *tetrahedral* or sp^3 hybridization can be explained by the tendency for unshared electrons to get as far from each other as possible (Pauli *exclusion* principle) and for four bonds the tetrahedral configuration satisfies this requirement. Covalent bonds, beside having characteristic bond length and energy, are also associated with direction in space.

Another peculiarity is associated with carbon-to-carbon bonding. Beside the aforementioned tetrahedral or sp^3 hybridization, two other possibilities are known to occur in the bonding of two carbon atoms; trigonal or sp^2 and linear (digonal) or sp hybridization.

Alkenes are examples of the sp^2 type, the hybrid orbitals being directed toward the corners of an equilateral triangle. This permits the hybrid orbitals to be as far removed from each other as possible. An unhybridized p orbital also exists perpendicular to the plane of the sp^2 orbitals:

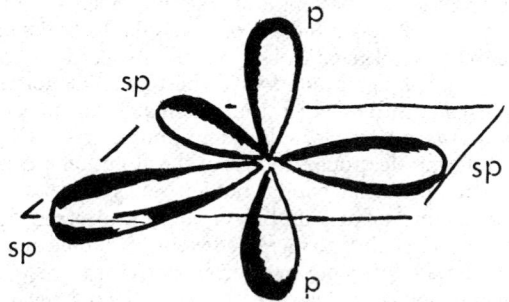

The union of two carbon atoms of this type produces a multiple bond, involving two electron pairs (a *double bond*), shown at the bottom of this page. Overlap of the sp^2 orbitals forms a sigma (σ) bond and the p orbital overlap produces a pi (π) bond. A carbon-carbon double bond is not composed of two similar bonds, as might be interpreted from the usual notation of C=C, which is used. Each bond is a distinct and separate entity and many physical and chemical properties confirm this feature. All of the sigma bonds lie in the same plane, but the pi bonds project above and below the plane as is evident from the previous diagram. As might be expected, because of the added "cementing" properties of the extra electrons, the carbon atoms of a multiple bond are held more closely. Thus the carbon-carbon bond distance for a double bond is 1.34 Å in ethylene compared to 1.54 Å for the single carbon-carbon bond of ethane.

Another interesting situation occurs due to the configuration of the sigma-pi double bond. Reference to the preceding illustration of the completed molecule shows that groups a, b, c, and d are in the same plane and, by reversing the two

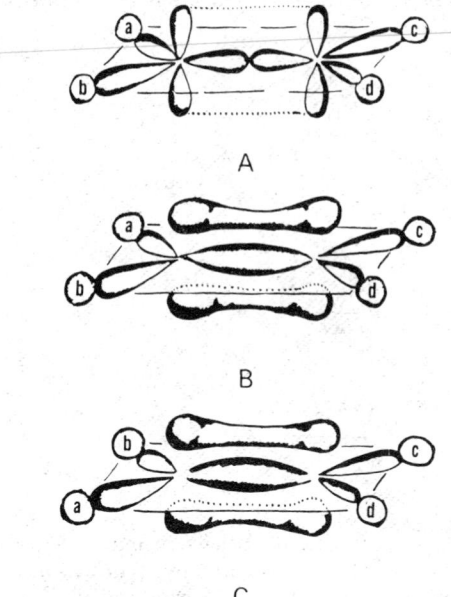

A

B

C

substituent groups at either end of the molecule (as in B and C), we have now generated an isomer—a *geometric* isomer. Again, this phenomenon leads to a doubling of the number of compounds of this particular type.

A third variety of hybridization that exists involves the coalition of one s and one p electron (sp). The resulting two sp orbitals produced are directed axially, 180° apart and 90° removed from the plane of the unhybridized p orbitals:

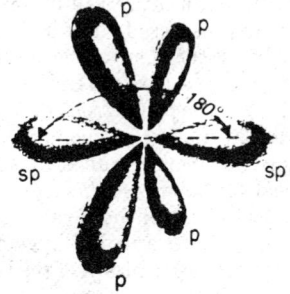

A combination of two carbon atoms exhibiting sp hybridization along the sp axis will yield carbon-carbon triple bonds:

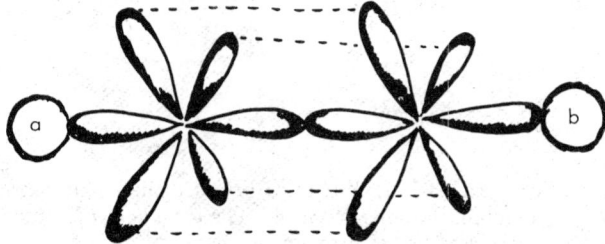

The p orbitals form a cylindrical sheath about the sigma bond. For a carbon-carbon triple bond the interatomic distance is smaller than a single or double bond, being 1.20 Å. Isomerism (geometric or stereoisomerism) is not possible with a triple bond as the substituents, a and b, are located axially.

Delocalization—Benzene represents a large series of compounds exhibiting a kind of bonding which is perhaps as unique and different from the usual carbon-carbon bond types as is carbon from the rest of the periodic table. Although the six annular carbon atoms are bonded to each other via sp^2

orbitals (as with ethylene), the resultant molecule does not behave as an unsaturated compound. Although the compound is depicted as having a conjugate system of three double bonds (*B*, *C*, and *D*),

the benzene molecule does not behave chemically like a simple conjugated diene. Reactions normally occur by substitution of a hydrogen atom rather than the expected addition to the double bond. Also two simple disubstitution products would be expected:

However, only one disubstitution product is known. Benzene, therefore, must exhibit an entirely different kind of bonding than those previously discussed. It is believed that the p orbitals, above and below the plane of the benzene ring, overlap in *both* directions and each electron can participate in several bonds. The ability of the pi electrons to be active in joining several atoms results in stronger bonds and a more stable molecule. This phenomenon of *delocalization* of electrons results in a delocalization or *resonance* energy of stability.

Due to the delocalization of the electrons only one type of bond exists and the classic alternate arrangement of single and double bonds between carbon atoms of the benzene molecule is misleading and incorrect. The carbon-carbon bond dis-

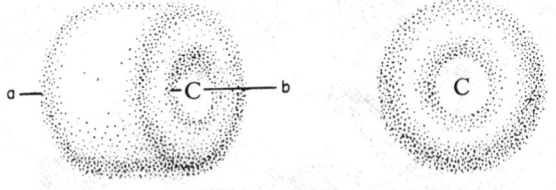

axial view

tance for benzene is 1.39 Å, lying between the single- and double-bond interatomic distance. The term *delocalization* better describes the resultant molecular orbital picture of benzene, rather than the concept of resonance. The term *resonance* may imply a rapid alternation between two or among several structural forms, which is totally incorrect.

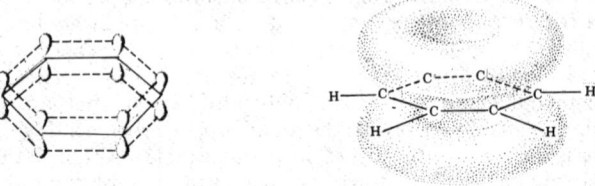

Delocalization (resonance) stabilization is evidenced by many organic compounds which contain multiple bonds. Just as a lowering of energy results from the formation of molecular orbitals whereby electrons are associated with two positive nuclei, a further lowering results if a molecular orbital is formed by utilizing several nuclei. This *extra* energy lowering increases the stability of a compound and the net energy difference derived from summing bond energies and that of the heat of combustion of the molecule is termed resonance or delocalization energy. Several types of organic compounds, other than benzene, exhibit delocalization:

$$\left[R-C \begin{smallmatrix} \nearrow O \\ \searrow O \end{smallmatrix} \right]^{-} \qquad CH_2\text{===}CH\text{ ===}CH\text{ ===}CH_2$$

carboxylate ion   1,3-Butadiene

Delocalization accounts for the stability of *aromatic* compounds such as naphthalene, anthracene, pyridine, pyrimidine, thiophene, furan, etc. *Aromaticity* has become synonymous with the unusual stability and chemical behavior of benzene-like compounds. A quantum mechanical treatment of cyclic, conjugated systems indicates that aromaticity exists in those rings associated with (4n + 2) pi electrons, where n is an integer. Thus rings having 6, 10 or 14π electrons may be aromatic (if they are planar), while those of 4, 8 or 12π electrons cannot. While the supporting mathematical theory is beyond the scope of this chapter, chemical evidence easily suggests that compounds such as pyridine, thiophene, or furan do behave as benzene, while cyclooctatetraene—although a cyclic, conjugate system—behaves merely as a typical conjugated alkene and does not show the exceptional stability of an aromatic compound.

Carbon-Heteroatom Bonds

Practically all of the foregoing material pertains to the structure of a carbon-to-carbon or carbon-to-hydrogen bond. A majority of the compounds normally included in the area of organic chemistry also contain *heteroatoms* (atoms other than carbon and hydrogen) and the mode of bonding between carbon and the heteroatoms is of great importance. A rigorous treatment of this subject is well outside the limits of this chapter but several general observations are in order. Carbon forms a typical sigma bond with the univalent nonmetals (halogens) and with other electronegative polyvalent elements such as oxygen, nitrogen, sulfur, and phosphorus. Because of the differing electronegativities of the atoms on either side of the sigma bond, the bond is not entirely symmetrical and the slightly uneven distribution of bonding electrons causes an asymmetry leading to increased values of dipole moments with increased difference in electronegativities.

Multiple bonds can also exist between the polyvalent elements and carbon. Typical of this group is the carbonyl function (=C=O), an example of sp² hybridization. The carbon atom is joined to two other atoms and the oxygen atom by sigma bonds; the remaining p orbital of the carbon overlaps a p orbital of oxygen to form a typical π bond. Thus carbon and oxygen are joined by a double bond. Each of the three sigma bonds radiating from the carbon atom is at an angle of 120°, and the carbonyl portion and the two atoms to which it is attached lie in the same plane.

The electrons of the carbonyl double bond join two elements of quite different electronegativity and hence are not shared equally, the electron cloud being pulled more strongly toward the electronegative oxygen atom. As the π electrons are of a lower energy than sigma electrons, they are more easily influenced by the electronegative oxygen atom. This effect is much more pronounced with multiple bonds than for a single (sigma) bond and results in the occurrence of a permanent polarity. Therefore, aldehydes and ketones (which contain the carbonyl function) exhibit fairly large dipole moments (2.3–2.75 D) because of the polarity of the carbonyl group as shown below. A lower-case delta (δ) indicates that a *fractional* charge of appropriate sign resides on the designated atoms:

$$\overset{\delta^+}{R}—\overset{\delta^-}{C}=\overset{}{O}$$
$$\underset{R}{|}$$

The structure of the carbonyl group largely determines the physical and chemical properties of aldehydes and ketones. Similar analogies can be drawn for carbon-to-sulfur and carbon-to-nitrogen multiple bonds.

Although carbon usually bonds to other elements by covalent-type linkages, several examples of ionic type bonds are known (carbanion $R_3C:^-$ and carbonium ion R_3C^+), but these are very short-lived and are primarily useful in explaining the *mechanism* of various organic reactions via intermediates of transient existence.

Noncarbon Bonds

The magnitude of the number of organic compounds is not due solely to the intricacies shown in carbon-to-carbon and carbon-to-heteroatom bonds. The electronegative elements, especially nitrogen and oxygen, impart their individualities such that a carbon-to-oxygen or carbon-to-nitrogen bond can participate in new types of bonds not previously discussed. As an example, the *hydrogen bond* or *bridge* can cause intermolecular association which can lead to an apparent increase in molecular weight or is the reason for a drug binding to certain sites of activity. Formation of *chelates, clathrates,* coordination complexes, etc. also extends the number of compounds which would be possible if only classic types of bonding existed between elements. Chapter 14 deals in depth with the concepts mentioned in this paragraph, and the reader is referred there for more information.

Molecular Structure

A molecule is the smallest possible quantity of a substance. It is composed of two or more atoms; eg, N_2, O_2, $CHCl_3$, H_2SO_4. There is a chemical bond between atoms when the forces acting between them are strong enough to give an aggregate with sufficient stability to make it convenient for the chemist to consider the aggregate as an independent molecular species. Different types of chemical bonds will be discussed in the following sections.

Covalent Bonds—When two electrons of two atoms are paired and localized in the space between the two atoms, a covalent bond results. The paired electrons (with opposed spins) will then occupy the new molecular orbital encompassing the two atoms. It should be noted that the electron pair held jointly by two atoms is considered to do double duty by completing a stable electronic configuration for each atom.

For instance, in the case of methane, the carbon atom, with its 2 inner electrons and its outer shell of 8 shared electrons, has assumed the stable 10-electron configuration of neon; and the hydrogen atoms have achieved the configuration of helium. Covalent bonds and ionic bonds are found in both organic and inorganic chemistry.

Hybridization of Atomic Orbitals—The ground state of the carbon atom has the electron distribution $1s^2\,2s^2\,2p^2$. Hence it might be expected to be bivalent. However, in all stable compounds carbon is found to have a valence of 4.

To account for this fact, Pauling proposed that the atomic orbitals about an atom may "mix" to form hybrid orbitals. Thus, if one of the $2s$ electrons of carbon is promoted to a $2p$ orbital, the $2s$ and three $2p$ orbitals may merge to form four

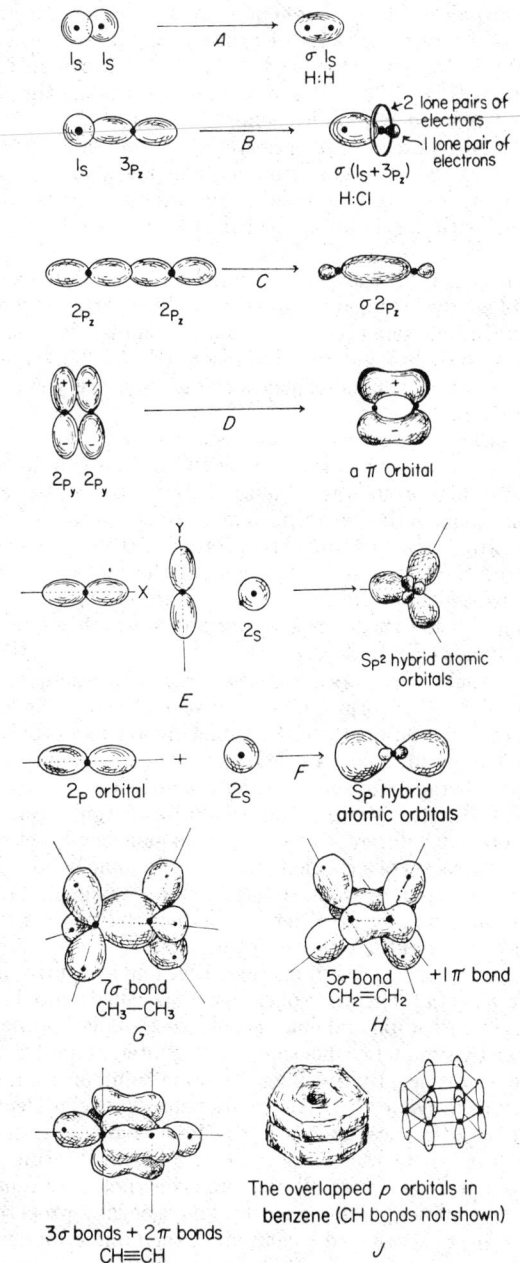

Fig 13-3.   Formation of molecular orbitals from the overlap of atomic orbitals.

sp^3 hybrid orbitals containing 1 electron each. This process enables carbon to form four stable covalent bonds instead of only two. The new set of orbitals are called *hybrid atomic orbitals*. They are designated as sp^3, indicating that they are made by mixing one s and three p orbitals. For instance, in methane (CH_4), the four hydrogen atoms lie at the corners of a regular tetrahedron, and in ethane, (C_2H_6), one CH_3 takes the place of one H in methane (Fig 13-3G).

Two other types of hybridizations are useful in describing unsaturated compounds. Mixing an s orbital with two p orbitals gives three equivalent sp^2 hybrids. These *trigonal* orbitals lie in a plane and are symmetrical about axes separated by 120° (Fig 13-3E). Hybridization of one s and one p orbital gives a pair of *linear*, or sp, orbitals (Fig 13-3F).

Sigma (σ) and Pi (π) Bonds—Covalent bonds may be distinguished by the type of atomic orbitals used in forming the bonds or by the kind of resultant molecular orbitals. The most common covalent bonds are formed from electrons of s

and p atomic orbitals. A σ bond results from the overlap of a pair of s orbitals (Fig 13-3A); the overlap of an s and a p orbital (Fig 13-3B); or the head-on overlap of p orbitals from two atoms (Fig 13-3C). The σ bond thus formed is the classical single bond of organic chemistry (Fig 13-3G).

When singly occupied p lobes overlap side-by-side, a π bond results (Fig 13-3D). This can only take place, however, if a σ bond already exists between the two atoms. A π bond associated with a σ bond is termed a double bond (Fig 13-3H).

Furthermore, if the two σ-bonded atoms each have two pairs of singly occupied p lobes oriented properly, they may overlap in four separate zones. Two π bonds now form in addition to the σ bond already present (Fig 13-3I). This is the classical triple bond of such substances as acetylene and cyanide ion.

In benzene the six carbon atoms are joined together in a hexagonal plane by bonds involving sp^2 orbitals (Fig 13-3E). The molecular orbitals are localized between the nuclei of the carbon atoms in the hexagon. The third sp^2 orbital of each carbon atom overlaps with the s orbitals of the hydrogens to form the C—H bonds in the plane of the molecule. The unhybridized $2p_z$ orbitals of the six carbon atoms extend above and below the plane and overlap to form the nonlocalized π bonds (Fig 13-3J).

Interatomic distances decrease appreciably to achieve the overlap needed to form π bonds between atoms. The *bond distance* is characteristic of the atoms involved and the type of bond between them. Table III gives the bond energy and the bond distance for some covalent bonds.

Polar Bonds: Partial Ionic Bond and Ionic Bond— There are many different types of partial ionic bonds between the two extremes of a covalent bond and an ionic bond. The tendency of a pair of atoms to form an ionic or a partial ionic bond is measured by the difference in their abilities to attract an electron, or in their *electronegativities*.

If a molecule acts as if it has a positive and a negative pole (ie, has a partial separation of charge), it is called a dipole. A molecule with dipolar bonds is said to be polar, while an electrically symmetric molecule is designated nonpolar.

The electronegativity values for some common elements are listed in Table IV. The relationship between electronegativity differences and the partial ionic character is shown in Table V. It is interesting to point out that fluorine, the most electronegative of all elements, has not only unique chemical qualities but also important physiological properties. In very low doses fluorides can reduce the number of dental caries by well over 50%, while in excessive doses mottled enamel may result during the period of tooth formation. Lithium, a metal of very low electronegativity has, on the other hand, been used in the treatment of manic depressive disor-

Table IV—Electronegativity Values for Some Elements[a]

F	4.0	I	2.4	Be	1.5
O	3.5	P	2.1	Mg	1.2
N	3.0	H	2.1	Li	1.0
Cl	3.0	B	2.0	Ca	1.0
Br	2.8	Si	1.8	Na	0.9
S	2.5	Sn	1.7	K	0.8
C	2.5	Al	1.5	Cs	0.7

[a] Adapted from Pauling.[5b]

ders. Both the carbonate and citrate are the salt forms used clinically (see Chapters 23 and 59).

Dipole Moment— The process by which dipoles arise is known as polarization. The total polarization P can be written as

$$P = P_i + P_o + P_a \qquad (5)$$

The induced or electronic polarization P_i represents the shift of the electron cloud due to the influence of an electric field or an electromagnetic wave such as light. The induced molar polarization P_i can be determined from molar refraction measurements using the D-line of a sodium lamp since the permanent dipole cannot follow an electromagnetic wave of such high frequency:

$$P_i = \frac{n_D^2 - 1}{n_D^2 + 2} \cdot \frac{M}{d} = MR \qquad (6)$$

Eq 6 is known as the Lorenz–Lorentz equation, where n_D is the refractive index of the liquid measured with the D-line of a sodium lamp, M is the molecular weight, d is the density, and MR is the molar refraction.

One can also calculate the induced molar polarization from the electron group refractions given by Smyth, or from the Atomic Refractivities compiled by Fajans (see Ref 6 and Table VI). For example, the molar refraction of methyl acetate

$$(CH_3—C—O—CH_3)$$
$$\overset{\|}{O}$$

can be calculated as follows:

	Na-D
$3 \times C = 3 \times 2.42$	$= 7.26$
$6 \times H = 6 \times 1.10$	$= 6.60$
$1 \times {=}O = 1 \times 2.21$	$= 2.21$
$1 \times {—}O{—} = 1 \times 1.64$	$= 1.64$
	Total $= 17.71$

or,

$$MR = \frac{n_D^2 - 1}{n_D^2 + 2} \cdot \frac{M}{d}$$

$$= \left[\frac{(1.3593)^2 - 1}{(1.3593)^2 + 2}\right] \cdot \left[\frac{74.08}{0.928}\right] \text{ (at } 20°)$$

$$= 17.57$$

An apparent correlation between the activity of chloramphenicol analogues, as determined by microbial kinetics, and the group refraction of their aromatic substituents has been reported.

In Eq 5 P_o is the orientation polarization due to the permanent dipole, and P_a is the atomic polarization, which may be neglected for practical purposes since it is only 5–10% of P_i. The orientation polarization P_o arises from the separation of charges due to the difference in electronegativities of the atoms.

Using an electromagnetic wave of much lower frequency

Table III—Covalent Bond Energy

Bond	Bond energy, ΔH kcal/mole	Bond distance Å
H—H	103.2[a]	0.74[c]
H—Cl	102.1[a]	1.27[c]
O—H	109.4[a]	0.96[b]
N—H	92.2[a]	1.01[b]
C—H	98.2[a]	1.09[b]
C—Cl	78[a]	1.77[b]
Cl—Cl	57.8[a]	1.99[c]
C—C	80[a]	1.54[b]
C=C	130[a]	1.33[b]
C≡C	193[a]	1.20[b]
C=O	152[b]	1.21[b]

[a] From Pitzer.[3]
[b] From Fieser and Fieser.[4]
[c] Pauling.[5a]

Table V—The Difference in Electronegativities and Ionic Character of Some Chemical Bonds[a]

Bond	Electronegativity difference, $X_a - Z_b$	Partial ionic character, %
C—H	0.4	4
I—Br	0.4	4
I—Cl	0.6	9
O—H	1.4	30
C—F	1.5	44
Si—F	2.2	70
Be—F	2.5	79
K—F	3.2	92

[a] cf, Pauling.[5c]

Table VI—Atomic and Group Refractions for Sodium-D Light

Element	Na_D cc	Element	Na_D cc
C	2.42	N in	
H	1.10	Aliphatic oximes	3.93
O in OH	1.52	R—CONH$_2$	2.65
O in ester OR	1.64	R—CONHR′	2.27
O=	2.21	R—CONR′R″	2.71
F	1.22	NO$_2$ group in	
Cl	5.96	Alkyl nitrates	7.59
Br	8.86	Alkyl nitrites	7.44
I	13.90	Nitroparaffins	6.72
S in SH	7.69	Aromatic nitro	
S in R S	7.97	compounds	7.30
S in RCNS	7.91	Nitramines	7.51
S in R S	8.11	NO group in	
N in		Nitrites	5.92
Hydroxylamines	2.48	Nitrosamines	5.37
Hydrazines	2.47	Structural units	
RNH$_2$	2.32	Double bond	1.73
RNHR′	2.49	Triple bond	2.40
RNR′R″	2.84	3-membered ring	0.71
ArNH$_2$	3.21	4-membered ring	0.48
ArNHR	3.59	Oxirane	
ArNRR′	4.36	Terminal	2.02
R—C≡N	3.05	Non-terminal	1.85
Ar—C≡N	3.79	Conjugation—(cf, Ref 6)	

than the frequency of light, such as a radio wave, one can measure the total polarization since the permanent dipole as well as the electron cloud can follow the alternation of direction of the radio wave. In other words one can calculate P from dielectric constant and molar volume (M/d) measurements:

$$P = \frac{\epsilon - 1}{\epsilon + 2} \cdot \frac{M}{d} \tag{7}$$

From Eqs 5–7, Debye's equation (Eq 8) for a pure compound, the Clausius-Mossotti equation (Eq 9), and by neglecting P_a, we have

$$P = \frac{4}{3} \pi N_A \left(\alpha + \frac{\mu^2}{3kT} \right) \tag{8}$$

$$P_i = \frac{4}{3} \pi N_A \alpha \tag{9}$$

$$P_o = P - P_i = \frac{4}{3} \pi N_A \frac{\mu^2}{3kT} \tag{10}$$

where N_A is Avogadro's number, α is the induced polarizability (a measure of the ease of polarization by an electric field), μ is the dipole moment (esu-cm), k is the Boltzmann constant, and T is the absolute temperature. It should be noted that molar refraction is a molar property and induced polarizability is a molecular property.

Eq 8 can be written as

$$P = a + b/T \tag{11}$$

where $a = 4\pi N_A \alpha/3 = P_i$, $b = 4\pi N_A \mu^2/9k$. Since Eq 11 is a linear equation, by plotting values of P at several temperatures (calculated from dielectric constant measurements) vs $1/T$, one can compute α and P_i from the intercept and the permanent dipole moment (μ) of the compound from the slope b. This procedure is usually applied to gases.

For a pure liquid one can obtain the total polarization P according to Eq 7 and the induced polarization P_i from refractive index and molar volume measurements at a constant temperature (Eq 6). Regardless of the manner of obtaining P_i, the final equation for the calculation of the dipole moment, usually expressed in Debye units, is the same (Eq 12). One Debye unit (D) is equivalent to 10^{-18} esu-cm.

$$\mu = \sqrt{\frac{9kb}{4\pi N_A}} = 0.0128 \times 10^{-18} \sqrt{b} =$$
$$0.0128 \times 10^{-18} \sqrt{(P - P_i)T} \text{ (esu-cm)} =$$
$$0.0128 \sqrt{(P - P_i)T} \text{ (Debye units)} \tag{12}$$

There are other equations for calculating dipole moments from measured values of the dielectric constant, refractive index, and density of liquids. However, for pure liquids the results are not very satisfactory. The dipole moment of medicinal substances is usually measured in a nonpolar solvent, eg, benzene, cyclohexane, heptane, or in a solvent with some polarity but without resultant moment, eg, dioxane.

It has been suggested that, in order to eliminate the inaccuracies that arise from treating the solvent in a different way than solutions, only the results of measurements on dilute solutions be used.

Correlations of biological activity with dipole moment have been reported for the insecticidal activity of chlorophenothane (DDT) isomers, the cholinesterase inhibitory activity of N-alkylsubstituted amides, and the respiratory stimulation activity of cyclic ureas and cyclic thioureas. Investigations have shown that high dipole moment enhances CNS stimulatory activity or toxicity while low dipole moment favors anticonvulsant or CNS depression activity. The use of dipole moment as a parameter in drug receptor interaction and quantitative structure-activity relationship studies has recently been reviewed by Lien et al.[7]

When the electronegativities of the bonded atoms are quite different, a formal electron pair bond can no longer exist. The bonding electron pair is now associated exclusively with the more electronegative atom and an *anion* is formed. The atom which has lost its electron becomes positively charged and a *cation* is formed.

Coordinate Covalent Bonds—A coordinate covalent bond is formed when only one atom donates both electrons. For example, the unshared electron pair on the nitrogen atom of an amine can serve to form such a bond with a proton or trimethyl boron:

Since the nitrogen suffers a loss of negative charge and the boron atom gains an equivalent negative charge, it is more realistic to depict the complex molecule as

$$R'—\overset{\overset{\displaystyle R''}{|}}{\underset{\underset{\displaystyle R}{|}}{N}}{}^{\delta+}{-}\hspace{-0.5em}-\hspace{-0.5em}-\overset{\overset{\displaystyle CH_3}{|}}{\underset{\underset{\displaystyle CH_2}{|}}{B}}{}^{\delta-}{—}CH_3$$

Amine oxides are other examples of coordinate covalent compounds:

$$R'—\overset{\overset{\displaystyle R''}{|}}{\underset{\underset{\displaystyle R}{|}}{N}}{\rightarrow}O \qquad or \qquad R'—\overset{\overset{\displaystyle R''}{|}}{\underset{\underset{\displaystyle R}{|}}{N}}{}^{\oplus}{—}O^{\ominus}$$

Because oxygen is far more electronegative than boron (see Table IV), the ionic character of the *N*-oxide is more pronounced than that of the N—B bond. This is evidenced by the relatively high melting point, high solubility in water, and low solubility in nonpolar solvents of the amine oxides. One can also infer the polar character by a comparison of dipole moments: 6.2 *D* for KCl (ion pairs), 5.02 *D* for trimethylamine oxide, and 3.92 *D* for the trimethylamine–trimethylboron complex.

Chelates—The term chelate (Greek, *chela*, claw) describes this class of compounds appropriately. Chelates consist of a partial ring of atoms which close up by holding a given atom, usually a metal, in a molecular claw. The compounds capable of forming a ring structure with a metal are designated as *ligands*.

Due to the range of normal bond angles, 5- and 6-member rings are most stable. The 5-membered ring is usually the most stable for a ring of single bonds only, whereas 6-member rings have maximum stability when there are two double bonds in the ring. The copper chelate of salicylaldehyde (I) and the calcium chelate of ethylenediamine-tetraacetic acid (EDTA, II) are some examples:

I

$$Na^{\oplus}\;{}^{\ominus}O—\overset{\overset{\displaystyle O}{\|}}{C}—CH_2—N—CH_2—CH_2—N—CH_2—\overset{\overset{\displaystyle O}{\|}}{C}—O^{\ominus}\;Na^{\oplus}$$

II   M = Metal ion

(III)

Cisplatin (III), a platinum coordination compound with the ammine groups at the *cis*-position, has been used in the treatment of testicular and ovarian tumors in combination with other anticancer drugs (see Chapter 63). Its major side effect is renal toxicity which can be lessened by using diuretics.

Some biologically important compounds (eg, chlorophyll, hemoglobin, peroxidases, cytochromes, oxidases, ascorbic acid oxidase, tyrosinase, polyphenoloxidase, laccase, phosphatase, carboxylases, insulin, and cyanocobalamin) are naturally occurring chelates. Tetracyclines are also capable of forming chelates with metals. Chelating agents may be used for a number of purposes, such as sequestration of metals, stabilization of drug preparations vulnerable to oxidation in the presence of trace of metals, and for the treatment of heavy metal poisoning.

Molecular Bonds—Several classes of compounds contain *intermolecular coordinate covalent bonds*, eg, "sandwich" compounds, charge transfer complexes, and the molecular addition compounds. These types of bonds are referred to as *molecular bonds* for brevity.

Metallocenes—In 1951 Kealy and Pauson accidentally discovered ferrocene by oxidizing cyclopentadienemagnesium bromide with anhydrous ferric chloride in ether solution. Ferrocene has aromatic character and is an unusually stable iron-containing orange product with the formula $C_{10}H_{10}Fe$, that melts at 174° and boils at 249°; it is soluble in common organic solvents but insoluble in water. The generally accepted structure of ferrocene was first proposed by Woodward and his co-workers in 1952. X-ray and electron diffraction studies have shown that the iron is packed between two parallel cyclopentadienyl rings, like a sandwich (IV).

The solubility, volatility, and other properties of metallocenes are due to the covalent character of the molecular bonds. This indicates that each cyclopentadienyl ion donates an electron pair to the metal ion. Ferrocene is diamagnetic, hence the six $3d$ electrons of iron are paired up to make available two open $3d$ orbitals. A large number of metallocenes have been prepared and studied since the discovery of ferrocene.

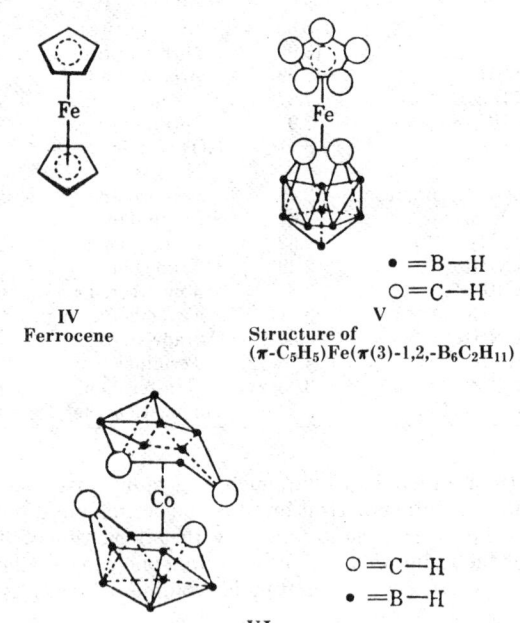

$\bullet = B—H$
$\bigcirc = C—H$

IV
Ferrocene

V
Structure of
$(\pi\text{-}C_5H_5)Fe(\pi(3)\text{-}1,2,\text{-}B_6C_2H_{11})$

$\bigcirc = C—H$
$\bullet = B—H$

VI
Structure of the $(B_7C_2H_2)_2\,Co^-$ ion obtained from $B_7C_2H_{11}{}^{2-}$ and Co^{1+}

Several different aromatic rings (e.g., indene, azulene, benzene, and others) will also form metallocenes. In many metallocenes, CO or NO molecules are found in place of one of the aromatic rings, and the metal may be Cr or Mn, as well as Fe. Metallocenes undergo most of the typical aromatic reactions. It has been shown that daily oral administration of ferrocene produced hemosiderosis with an unusually high, dose-related accumulation of iron in dogs. A decrease in hemoglobin, packed cell volume, and erythrocyte count occurred within 4 weeks in dogs receiving 300 mg/kg of ferrocene. This and higher dosage resulted in cirrhosis, which was considered to be an effect of the hydrocarbon moiety.

Recent work has opened up a new field of research which combines polyhedral carborane and transition metal chemistry. Several families of polyhedral species are now known in which a transition metal resides in the polyhedral surface (V, VI)

Charge-Transfer Complexes—Certain substances combine in a 1:1 molar ratio to form crystalline addition products. The molecular addition compound is held together by weak forces, such as van der Waals (dipole–dipole, dipole–induced dipole, induced dipole–induced dipole), ion–dipole, and even hydrogen bonds. Polynitroaromatic compounds, such as trinitrobenzene and picric acid, are well known for their ability to form charge-transfer complexes (pi complexes) (VII, VIII).

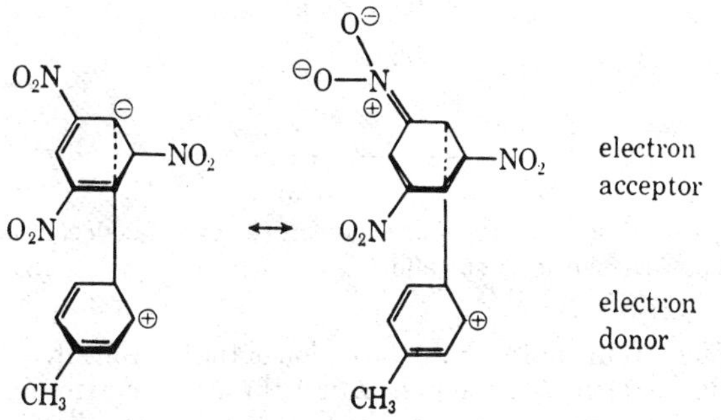

VII
1,3,5-Trinitrobenzene: toluene complex

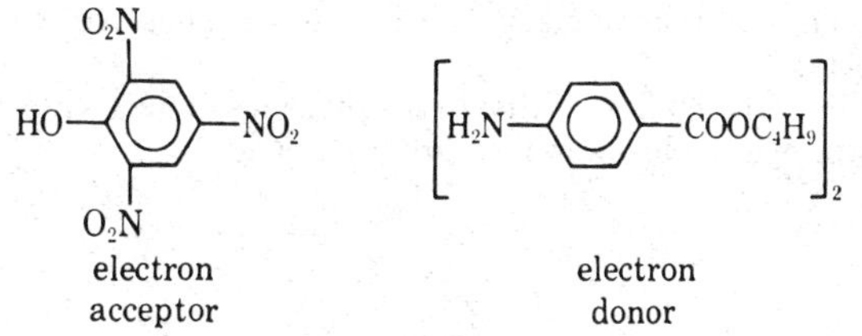

electron
acceptor

electron
donor

VIII
Butesin picrate

Caffeine complexes with various drugs, such as sodium benzoate, sodium salicylate, sulfonamides, barbiturates and 5-chlorosalicylic acid.

Aromatic Sigma (σ) Bond Complexes—Aromatic compounds react with $HCl.AlCl_3$ or $HF.BF_3$ to produce salts that ionize in highly polar nonaqueous solvents, eg, liquid hydrogen fluoride or sulfuric acid:

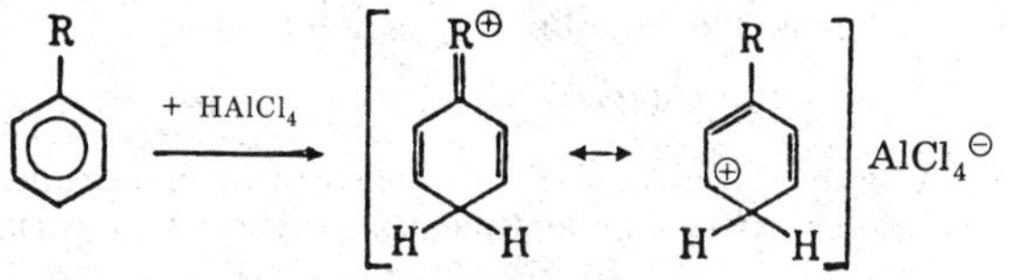

Using NMR spectroscopy Olah, *et al.*[8] detected the *p*-anisonium and the 2,4,6-trimethylphenonium ions produced by ionizing β-*p*-anisyl ethyl chloride and β-mesityl ethyl chloride, respectively, in SbF_5—SO_2 at −70° to −60°C:

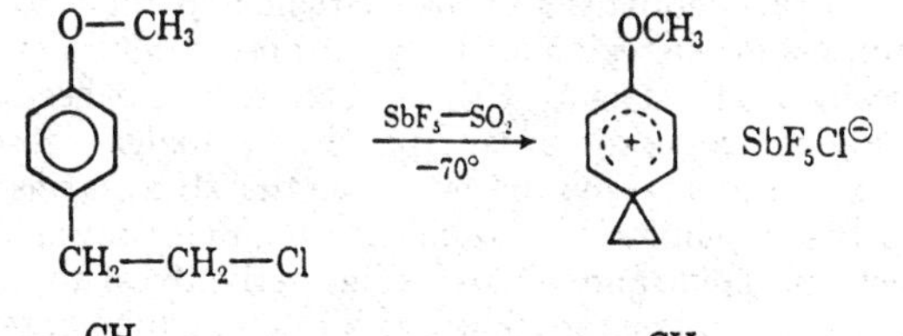

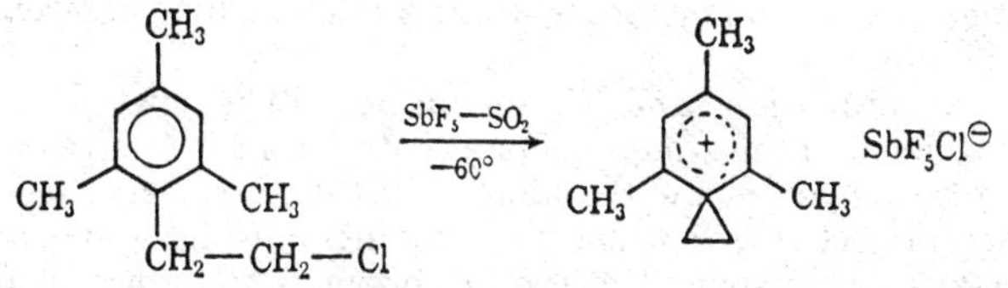

Sigma complexes are molecular complexes resulting from the rupture of a sigma bond (eg, H—$AlCl_4$, $ArCH_2CH_2$—Cl); they also occur in Friedel–Crafts reactions. Since they are reactive toward water, no practical pharmaceutical uses have been made of these complexes. Refer to Chapter 14 for a more extensive treatment of *complexation.*

Stereoisomerism—Early in 1874 van't Hoff envisaged a double bond by joining two tetrahedra at two corners, and correctly predicted that unsymmetrically substituted derivatives of ethylene should exist in two stereochemical forms, or as a pair of *cis* and *trans* isomers. From our previous dis-

cussion of σ and π bonds, we know that in an alkene, rotation about the σ bond is restricted by the overlap of *p* orbitals comprising the π bond.

The stereoisomerism due to the rigid configuration about a double bond or other rigid structure such as a ring is known as *geometric isomerism.* It is interesting to note that in the case of the synthetic estrogens, the *cis*-isomer of diethylstilbestrol is unstable and has less than one-tenth the activity of the *trans*-isomer. One should note the structural similarity between *trans*-diethylstilbestrol and estradiol.

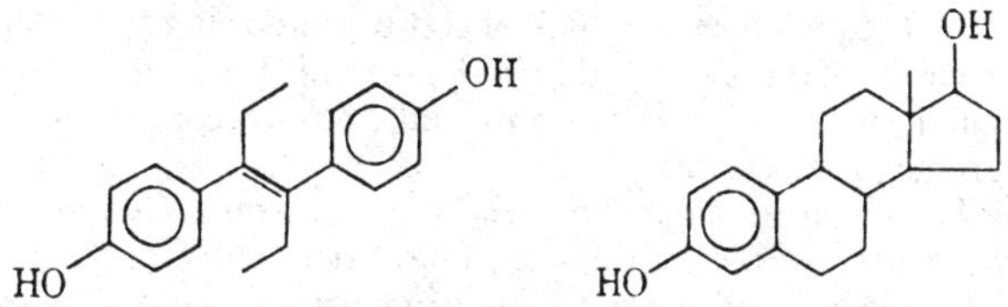

trans-Diethylstilbestrol   **Estradiol**

It has been reported that tamoxifen, a drug that structurally resembles *trans*-diethylstilbestrol, showed arrest or reduction of breast tumor growth rate in 77% of patients given 20 mg of the drug orally twice daily. The compound is believed to block estrogen receptor sites.

Due to the presence of symmetry, the type of geometric isomerism occurring in substituted ethylenes is not usually associated with optical activity; some other site in the molecule ordinarily gives rise to optical isomerism.

Another type of geometric isomerism is found in ring compounds, the ring taking the place of the rigid double bond. For example, *trans*-2-phenylcyclopropylamine is more stable than the *cis*-isomer and is a potent monoamine oxidase inhibitor.

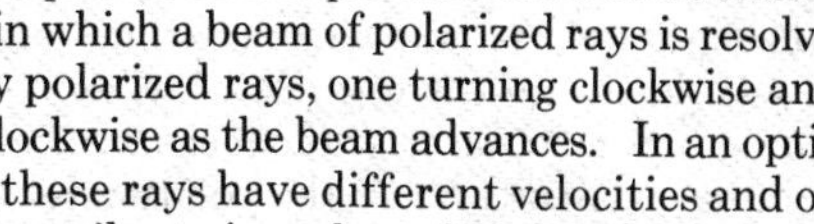

trans-2-Phenylcyclo-
propylamine
(Tranylcypromine)

cis-2-Phenylcyclo-
propylamine

A substance that rotates the plane of polarized light is said to be optically active. *Optical rotation* may be considered as a consequence of the phenomenon of circular double refraction in which a beam of polarized rays is resolved into two circularly polarized rays, one turning clockwise and the other counterclockwise as the beam advances. In an optically active medium these rays have different velocities and on recombination they vibrate in a plane different from that of the incident ray.

The necessary and sufficient condition for a molecule to show optical activity is that the molecule should be dissymmetric (ie, the molecule should not be superimposable with its mirror image); in other words, it should be *chiral.* Although many optically active compounds have asymmetric carbon atoms (carbon atoms bearing four different groups), not all compounds possessing asymmetric carbon atoms are optically active. For example, *meso*-tartaric acid has two asymmetric carbon atoms, but it is optically inactive due to the presence of a plane of symmetry within the molecule.

Optical isomerism due to restricted rotation (eg, as with tetra-*ortho*-substituted biphenyls and dissymmetric polyphenyls) is well documented in Eliel's book *Stereochemistry of Carbon Compounds* (McGraw-Hill). Atoms other than carbon can serve as a center of asymmetry. For instance, optically active *N*-oxides, quaternary ammonium compounds, sulfonium and selenonium salts, sulfoxides, and sulfinic esters have been resolved.

Enantiomorphs—Molecules whose mirror images are nonsuperimposable are called enantiomorphs, enantiomers, or optical antipodes. Enantiomorphs have identical physicochemical properties in an optically inactive environment; they rotate the plane of polarized light to the same degree but in opposite directions.

The measurement of optical rotation is useful for the purpose of identifying and/or assaying an optically active substance. The *specific rotation* is defined as:

$$[\alpha]_D^t = \frac{\alpha}{l(g/v)}$$

where D stands for the D-line of sodium vapor lamp, t is the temperature, α is the rotation in degrees, l is the length of the cell in decimeters (1 dm = 10 cm), and g/v is the concentration in grams per milliliter.

When equal amounts of *dextro*- and *levo*-isomers are mixed a *racemic modification* arises. They are denoted as (d,l) or $(\pm)$. Racemic modifications occur in most organic syntheses; they also may be obtained by racemization of a pure enantiomer. In a racemic modification the substance in bulk is not optically active, even though the individual molecule is optically active. The overall rotation is zero due to the cancellation of rotations with equal magnitude but different signs.

Diastereoisomers—Stereoisomers which are not mirror images of each other are called diastereoisomers. Diastereoisomerism exists when a given structural formula has at least two asymmetric atoms:

CHO CHO CHO CHO

H—C—OH HO—C—H HO—C—H H—C—OH

H—C—OH HO—C—H H—C—OH HO—C—H

CH₂OH CH₂OH CH₂OH CH₂OH

(−) Erythrose (+) Erythrose (−) Threose (+) Threose

Enantiomorphs   Enantiomorphs

Diastereoisomers

Optical Rotatory Dispersion (ORD)—Optical rotatory dispersion involves the measurement of the angle of optical rotation at various wavelengths. Usually greater rotational angles are obtained at shorter wavelengths. The source of light consists of a xenon arc, and a monochromator to isolate the desired wavelength in the ultraviolet region. A photomultiplier and photometer are used to measure the intensity after the light has passed through the polarimeter.

As the wavelength of the polarized light is varied, the absolute value of rotation may increase continuously, so that the plot of $[\alpha]$ vs λ is a plain curve (Line A, Fig 13-4). On the other hand, the rotation may change direction either from left to right or right to left, and show one or more maxima and minima.

The appearance of a maximum and a minimum in a plot of specific rotation vs wavelength is referred to as *single Cotton effect* (Line B, Fig 13-4), while the appearance of several maxima and several minima is referred to as a *multiple Cotton*

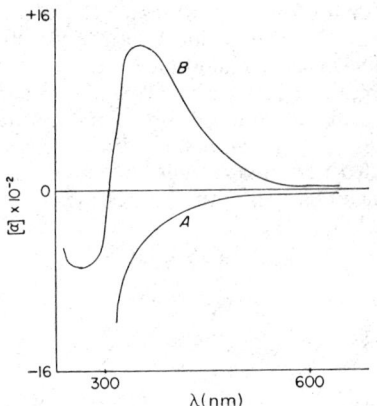

Fig 13-4. Rotatory dispersion curves: (*A*) levorotatory plain curve; (*B*) positive simple Cotton effect.

effect. If in approaching the region of the Cotton effect from long wavelengths, one passes first through a maximum and then through a minimum, the Cotton effect is called "positive," but if the minimum is reached first and then the maximum at shorter wavelength, it is called a "negative" Cotton effect.

The Cotton effect is due to the presence of an asymmetric center near a chromophoric group, such as;

\C=O
/

in the optically active molecule which has unequal absorption of right and left circularly polarized light. ORD is useful for the study of the stereochemistry of natural products, ketosteroids, and for the analysis of randomly coiled and helical configurations of polypeptide chains.

Circular Dichroism (CD)—A CD curve is a plot of the molecular ellipticity $[\theta]$ vs the wavelength λ. The CD effect results from the fact that the right circularly polarized ray is differently *absorbed* from the left circularly polarized beam of light. The molecular ellipticity is defined as

$$[\theta] = 3{,}300 \cdot \Delta\epsilon, \qquad \Delta\epsilon = \epsilon_L - \epsilon_R$$

where $\Delta\epsilon$ is the differential dichroic absorption and ϵ_L and ϵ_R are the molar extinction coefficients for the left and right rays.

If in a dichrograph the oscillating crystal is correctly oriented, the plane-polarized beam of light passed through the instrument can be resolved into right and left components. These are then passed through the optically active medium. When these unequally absorbed circular components are recombined in the region of electronic absorption, they give elliptically polarized light. CD measurements have been used for studying drug–protein binding with 52 analgesics, sedatives, and antidepressive drugs. From this study it was suggested that a plane-ring system with high electron density (eg, benzdiazepine and dibenzazepine derivatives) appeared to be an essential factor for strong binding to human serum albumin.

Configuration and Conformation—The spatial arrangement of the groups about a central atom is referred to as the *configuration* of the atom. Three dimensional models, their projections, or perspective drawings must be used to illustrate the difference between stereoisomers. The particular shape that a molecule assumes by free rotation about single bonds is referred to as its conformation.

It may be thought that an ethane molecule may have an infinite number of conformations because of rotation about the C—C bond; however, only a few conformations are possible which will make the molecular energy a minimum. The conformational preferences of some diastereoisomers have been determined from NMR studies.

For a series of diastereoisomers involving a substituted phenylethyl skeleton, when the alkyl groups attached to each asymmetric center are small (e.g., methyl), both *gauche* and

$$(CH_3 \overset{2}{-}CHOH \overset{3}{-} CH - C_6H_5)$$
$$|$$
$$CH_3$$

(gauche)   (gauche)

trans conformers (rotamers) have substantial populations because of the relatively low rotational barriers. Newman projection formulas are used for the illustrations. In these projection formulas, the molecules are viewed from front to back in the direction of the bond linking the asymmetric carbon atoms. In the following formulas, the center of the circle represents C_2 and the circle represents C_3 of 3-phenyl-2-butanol

(trans or anti)   (trans or anti)
Erythro-3-phenyl-   Threo-3-phenyl-
2-butanol   2-butanol

When the alkyl groups are large (eg, isopropyl), steric interactions cause the bulky groups to prefer a *trans* orientation; the vicinal hydrogens are then *trans* in the *erythro* but *gauche*

(trans or anti)   (gauche)
2,5-Dimethyl-4-phenyl-3-hexanol

in the *threo* isomers. For a more detailed discussion of potential energy barriers in various systems, the student should consult Eliel's book (see above).

The preferred conformation of serotonin has been calculated using molecular orbital theory. Complementary fea-

Calculated preferred conformation of serotonin

tures of the serotonin receptor have been postulated and the relationship of serotonin in its preferred conformation to the serotonin antagonist, LSD, has been presented as an explanation of LSD's antagonism.

Intermolecular Binding Forces

An understanding of intermolecular and intramolecular binding forces is very important in many different aspects of

pharmaceutical sciences, such as in the manufacture of various preparations, in stability studies, and in the design of new drugs. A knowledge of these forces is not only essential for predicting some physicochemical properties of various dosage forms, but also indispensable for the interpretation of drug action at the molecular level and for structure–activity correlations.

Martin's classification[9] for various types of forces will be used in the following discussion.

Repulsive and Attractive Forces—Intermolecular repulsive forces exist when two dipolar molecules are brought close together "head-to-head" or "tail-to-tail," or when any two molecules are brought so close that their nonbonding electronic clouds interpenetrate. Otherwise, two molecules having opposite charges closer together than the like charges will attract each other. When the repulsive and the attractive forces are equal, the potential energy of the two molecules is a minimum and an equilibrium will be established. Similar forces may exist in the same molecule (intramolecular) as well as between different molecules. Only intermolecular forces will be discussed here.

Van der Waals Forces—Due to electrostatic attraction, dipolar molecules tend to align themselves with neighboring molecules so that the negative pole of one molecule points towards the positive pole of the next, eg,

$$\overset{\leftarrow}{O} = C < \dots \overset{\leftarrow}{N}R_3$$

This type of attraction is known as a *dipole–dipole* interaction and has a force of 1–7 kcal/mole. Dipole–dipole forces vary inversely as the 4th power of the distance between molecules, $F \propto (1/d^4)$.

The importance of the permanent dipole attractions in the stabilization of an α-helix has been pointed out. The electric dipoles in an α-helix add to one another along the direction of the axis. Two helices that wind in the same direction will, therefore, repel each other and two that wind in opposite directions will attract each other.

Permanent dipoles can induce a transient electric dipole in nonpolar molecules and produce *dipole–induced dipole* or Debye forces. These interactions involve a force of about 1–3 kcal/mole.

When any two atoms belonging to different molecules are brought sufficiently close together, *induced dipole–induced dipole* or London attractions arise. In this case, the force is about 0.5–1 kcal/mole. These forces originate from molecular internal vibrations. The temporary dipoles which this vibration creates in the constituent atoms induce dipoles in neighboring atoms of other molecules, and this process results in a net attraction.

This type of force is responsible for the liquefaction of nonpolar gases. London forces vary inversely as the 7th power of the distance between molecules, $F \propto (1/d^7)$.

Hydrogen Bonds—When a hydrogen atom holds two other atoms, a hydrogen bond (hydrogen bridge) is formed. The two bonds attached to the same hydrogen cannot both be covalent bonds. The H-bond must be in part ionic. Indeed, the hydrogen bond is usually formed only between electronegative atoms. In addition, the atoms capable of forming H-bonds have at least one unshared electron pair.

Without hydrogen bonds this world would be much different, since water would boil at a temperature far below 0°. The surprisingly high boiling point of H_2O (100°) compared to H_2S (−60.7°) and H_2Se (−41.5°) can be attributed to the higher H-bonding ability of oxygen, which in turn is due to its smaller volume and higher electron density as compared to S and Se.

The most common atoms capable of forming H-bonds are F, O, N, and to a lesser degree Cl and S. There is also some evidence that hydrogen attached to a triply bonded carbon (eg, HCN, HC≡CH, or CHCl$_3$) forms H-bonds. The strength of most H-bonds ranges from 1–7 kcal/mole:

H-bond	Bond strength (kcal/mole)
F—H...F	7
O—H...O	4.5–7.6
O—H...N	4–7
C—H...π electrons	2–4
C—H...O	2–3
N—H...O	2–3
N—H...N	1.3

The strength of the H-bond depends on the solvent as well as the state. For instance, the H-bond strength of O-H ... O for (CH$_3$COOH)$_2$ as a vapor is 7.64 kcal/mole, while that of (CH$_3$COOH)$_2$ in benzene is 4.85 kcal/mole. In water the H-bond has been estimated to have an energy of 4.5 kcal/mole; in ice the bond strength is 6 kcal/mole. Hydrogen bonding is responsible for the higher boiling point of a carboxylic acid compared with that of its ester. This is due to the fact that in the free acid dimerization can occur by H-bonding, while this is impossible for an ester.

Hydrogen bonding is also responsible for the high solubility of polyhydroxy compounds, such as sugars, in water. During the replication of DNA molecules, hydrogen bonds between base pairs are broken and rematched.

Various physical methods may be used to study H-bonding, such as molecular weight determination, and IR and NMR spectroscopy.

Ion-Dipole and Ion-Induced Dipole Forces—Ion pairs in the solid state have bond strengths comparable to or even stronger than covalent bonds (100–200 vs 50–150 kcal/mole). However, in a biological system, due to hydration and the large amount of inorganic salts present for ion-exchange, the bond strength would be substantially weakened to the neighborhood of 5 kcal/mole.

When an ionic bond is reinforced by the simultaneous presence of other forces, such as hydrogen bonding, the bond becomes stronger (10 kcal/mole for

$$\begin{array}{ccc} H & & O \\ | & & \diagdown \\ -N^{\oplus} & \ominus & C- \\ \diagup \diagdown & & \diagup \\ H & H \cdots O & \end{array}).$$

An ion pair can attract a dipole or induce a dipole in a neighboring nonpolar molecule. The strength of an *ion-dipole* bond (eg, R$_4$$\overset{\oplus}{N}$ ..... $\overset{}{N}$R$_3$) is about 1–7 kcal/mole, and that of an *ion-induced* dipole (eg, $\overset{\oplus}{K}$—$\overset{}{I}$ ... I—I) would be somewhat weaker.

Hydrophobic Interactions—The association of nonpolar groups with each other in aqueous solution, arising because of the tendency of water molecules to exclude nonpolar molecules, is known as a hydrophobic interaction, or "hydrophobic bonding." The word hydrophobic is really a misnomer. It implies that the nonpolar molecule dislikes water; in fact, it is water that dislikes the nonpolar molecule.

The formation of hydrophobic bonds is favored because of an entropy effect. Before the formation of a hydrophobic bond, water molecules are arranged in an ordered fashion around exposed nonpolar groups. When hydrophobic interactions occur, the order is disrupted and results in a favorable entropy change. The entropy change is great enough to overcome the enthalpy for the interaction of the nonpolar groups, and hence the free energy is negative and the process is spontaneous. The strength of hydrophobic interactions has been reported to be 0.37 kcal/mole per CH$_2$ group.

A side chain of C$_{14}$ which binds with another nonpolar

counterpart would have a bond strength of 5.2 kcal/mole. This bond, being stronger than an ionic bond or other weak forces in the biological system, may then dominate the mode of binding of a complicated drug molecule. The importance of hydrophobic interactions in stabilizing protein structure, drug–protein binding, transport and storage of drugs, and drug–receptor interaction has been noted in recent years. More practical applications as well as further theoretical study should be expected in the future. Refer to Chapter 14, *Complexation*, for further details.

Additive Physical Properties

The division of physical properties into additive, constitutive, and colligative can be found in many textbooks. Additive physical properties depend on the number and kind of atoms in a molecule. Such additivity enables one to calculate many molecular values from a few fundamental constants. The best example is the calculation of molecular weights from atomic weights. The additive nature of molar refractions has been utilized for the calculation of induced polarization (see *Dipole Moment*).

Molar Volume—The term molar volume is self-explaining. It is defined as the molecular weight divided by the density of a liquid (molar volume = MW/d). Using statistical analysis, it has been shown that the additivity of molar volume is better fulfilled at ordinary temperatures (20°) rather than at the boiling point of each individual substance. This is an interesting result, since from the *Principle of Corresponding States* it might be expected that additivity would hold better at the boiling point.

In the homologous series of nonbranched primary derivatives the accuracy of a calculation of molar volume is relatively good. The deviations increase gradually with polysubstituted derivatives, 1,1-bis derivatives, *ortho* derivatives, and branched isomers; nevertheless, the additive scheme can serve as a first approximation.

Partition Coefficients and the π Constant—In the early theory of narcosis, lipid solubility was regarded as the most important factor for the inhibition of cell activity. At the beginning of this century Meyer and Overton proposed that narcotic efficiency parallels the coefficient for the partition of a drug between oil and water. Although this theory cannot explain the mechanism of narcotic action, it does explain at least the mode of transport to nerve tissues.

It is more logical to use partition coefficients rather than solubility in a single solvent for structure–activity correlations since in a biological system one is dealing with a heterogeneous system rather than a simple solution. Partition coefficients have been used in the study of drug absorption, distribution, metabolism, toxicity, and structure–activity correlation.

It has been shown that the partition coefficients for a given compound in two different solvent systems (eg, ether/water, octanol/water) are related as follows: $\log P_1 = a \log P_2 + b$, where a and b are constants. This suggests that one can use the results from one set of solvents to predict results in a second set.

Hansch's group[12–16] has systematically extended use of partition coefficients, measured from octanol/water, to serve as a measure of the ease of random walk of organic molecules through various lipoprotein barriers and/or as a measure of the hydrophobic binding with protein such as bovine serum albumin. From the partition coefficients of a variety of derivatives of the type X—C$_6$H$_4$OCH$_2$COOH, X—C$_6$H$_5$, and C$_6$H$_5$(CH$_2$)$_n$—X, the substituent constants (π) for the aromatic and the aliphatic function (X) have been determined.

The π constant is defined as $\pi = \log P_X - \log P_H$, where P_X is the partition coefficient of a derivative and P_H is that of the

Table VII—π Constants for Some Functional Groups[a]

Function X	Aromatic system[b]	Aliphatic system
H—	0	0
F—	0.13	−0.17
Cl—	0.76	0.39
Br—	0.94	0.60
I—	1.15	1.00
CH_3—	0.50	0.50
$CH{\equiv}C$—		0.48
$CH_2{=}CH$—		0.70
C_2H_5—	1.00	1.00
$CH_2{=}CCH_3$		1.00
$CH_2{=}CHCH_2$—		1.20
$n\text{-}C_3H_7$—	1.50	1.50
$i\text{-}C_3H_7$—	1.30	1.30
$n\text{-}C_4H_9$—	2.00	2.00
$sec\text{-}C_4H_9$—	1.80	1.80
$t\text{-}C_4H_9$—	1.68	1.68
$cyclo\text{-}C_3H_5$—		1.21
$cyclo\text{-}C_5H_9$—	2.14	2.14
$cyclo\text{-}C_6H_{11}$—	2.51	2.51
adamantyl	3.30	
C_6H_5—	2.13	2.13
—$(CH_2)_3$—	1.04	
—$(CH_2)_4$—	1.39	
—$(CH)_4$—	1.24	
—CF_3	1.07	
—CH_2OH	−1.03	−0.66
—CH_2COOH	−0.72	−0.76
—COOH	−0.28	−1.26
—$CONH_2$	−1.49	−1.71
—$COOCH_3$	−0.01	−0.27
—$COCH_3$	−0.55	−0.71
—CN	−0.57	−0.84
—OH	−0.67	−1.16
—OCH_3	−0.02	−0.47
—OCH_2COOH	−0.86	
—$OCOCH_3$	−0.64	−0.91
$CH{=}NNHCONH_2$	−0.85	
$CH{=}NNHCSNH_2$	−0.27	
$O\text{-}\beta\text{-glucose}$	−2.84	
—NH_2	−1.23	−1.19
—$N(CH_3)_2$	−0.18	−0.32
—NO	−0.12	
—NO_2	−0.28	−0.82
—$NHCOCH_3$	−0.97	
—$NHCOC_6H_5$	0.72	
—$N{=}NC_6H_5$	1.69	
—$NHCONH_2$	−1.01	
—$N(CH_3)_3^{+}$	−5.96	
—SCH_3	0.62	
—SCF_3	1.58	
—SO_2CH_3	−1.26	
—SO_2CF_3	0.93	
—SF_5	1.50	
—SO_2NH_2	−1.82	

[a] Adapted from Refs 10–14.
[b] From $X\text{—}C_6H_5$ or $X\text{—}C_6H_4OCH_2COOH$ system, for different positions in the latter system slightly different values were reported in the original paper (Ref 10). In cases where strong interaction between two functioins can occur (eg, in phenol or aniline series), different π values should be used.

parent compound. It is found that, although π varies continuously for a given function depending on its electronic environment, the variation is generally small; it is therefore called additive–constitutive.

The application of log P and the additive–constitutive nature of π constants for the correlation of biological activity with chemical structure has been illustrated in many cases. Table VII lists the constants for some important functional groups. One can calculate many log P values from a few constants. The method of calculation can be illustrated with the drug diphenhydramine:

$$\Sigma\pi = +4.26 \quad +0.30 \quad -0.98 \quad +0.50 \quad -0.32$$

$$3.76 = \text{calc log } P$$
$$3.40 = \text{obs log } P$$

Good correlation has been reported for the hypnotic action of barbiturates in mice and their log P values:

$$\text{Activity} = \log 1/C = -0.438\,(\log P)^2 + 1.579 \log P + 1.926 \tag{13}$$

n	r	s	$\log P_0$
13	0.969	0.098	1.80

In Eq 13, C represents the moles of drug per kilogram of test animal producing hypnosis in 50% of the animals, n is the number of drugs tested, r is the correlation coefficient, and s is the standard deviation. It is interesting to note that the dependence of activity on log P is parabolic, and the optimum lipohydrophilic character (log P_0) is not much different from those of alcohols or carbamates (all around 2.0).

A linear relationship between the binding of penicillin derivatives by human serum and the π constant has been reported:

$$\log (B/F) = 0.488\Sigma\pi - 0.627 \quad \begin{array}{ccc} n & r & s \\ 79 & 0.924 & 0.134 \end{array} \tag{14}$$

In Eq 14, B/F is the ratio of bound penicillin/free penicillin and $\Sigma\pi$ represents the sum of π values for the attached substituents on the side-chain R–:

Table VIII shows the common intermolecular forces by which

Table VIII—The Common Functional Groups Present in Different Neurotransmitters

Neurotransmitter	Dipole and/or H-bonding	van der Waals and/or hydrophobic	Ionic
Acetylcholine (Ach)			
Epinephrine			
Dopamine			
Serotonin			
Histamine			
γ-Aminobutyric Acid (GABA)			

various neurotransmitters may bind to their receptors. They all have positively charged nitrogen atoms (under physiological conditions) separated from a dipolar function by two carbon atoms.

X-ray Analyses

In recent years the number of compounds of medicinal value that have been isolated from plant and animal sources and by purely synthetic means has increased astronomically. In addition to the many compounds isolated, the more sophisticated isolation techniques now available to the chemist have extended his capabilities of exploring biological molecules heretofore thought too complex to understand or investigate. The pharmaceutical chemist is thus faced with the task of identifying the chemical structure of a large number of complex materials in order to understand their biological functions.

For many of the compounds the chemist may rely on standard spectroscopic methods, ie, IR, UV, NMR, and ORD, together with other chemical measurements to elucidate molecular structure. Newer methods, especially mass spectroscopy, are emerging as useful means of elucidating the structures of complex organic materials. In many instances these approaches have shortcomings, as they provide only fragmentary evidence about various portions of the molecule, which must be pieced together to get the picture of the whole compound. See also Chapter 34.

One of the most powerful of all techniques, when it can be used, is that of X-ray crystallographic analysis. Using this method, the three-dimensional structure of a molecule can be determined without relying on any chemical information.

The maximum resolution that can be obtained through an ordinary light microscope under the most favorable conditions is about 2000 Å. This limitation is primarily imposed by the wavelength of the illumination. However, other forms of radiation capable of giving atomic resolution (1 Å or less) exist; *viz*, electron beams, neutrons, and X-rays. Lenses have been constructed only for the first of these radiations, and at best they have a resolving power of about 6 Å. This resolution is insufficient to measure the distances between atoms. It is possible, however, to study the details of molecules without lenses, by means of diffraction experiments. Of the three radiations, X-rays have proved to be the most useful and fruitful for studying molecular structure.

Crystalline State

Atoms and molecules tend to organize themselves into their most favorable thermodynamic state, which under certain conditions results in their appearance as crystals. This form is characterized by a highly ordered arrangement of the molecules, associated with which is a three-dimensional periodicity. The repeating three-dimensional patterns, ideally depicted as lattices, are essential for X-ray structural analysis. For a brief discussion of the crystalline state and various crystal systems see RPS-15, pages 184–185.

X-Ray Diffraction

In 1912 von Laue and two of his students, Friedrich and Knipping, carried out an experiment with X-rays that opened the door to crystallographic structural analysis. They allowed a beam of nonhomogeneous X-rays to pass through a crystal of copper sulfate pentahydrate, and recorded by means of photographic plates the diffracted X-ray beam. A diagram of the experimental setup is shown in Fig 13-5.

The results showed that X-rays which had been discovered by Roentgen less than two decades earlier had wave characteristics (wavelength: approximately 1 Å). Since a crystal

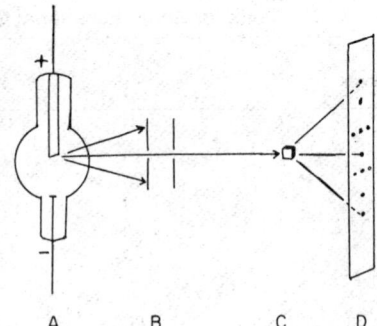

Fig 13-5.   Diagram of Laue experiment: (*A*) X-ray tube; (*B*) lead slits; (*C*) crystal; (*D*) photographic plate.

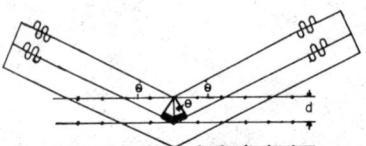

Fig 13-6.   Bragg condition for reflection.

is composed of a regular array of atoms with interatomic separations of the Angstrom (Å) range, they were able to show that the diffraction pattern obtained on the plates was due to the crystal acting as a three-dimensional diffraction grating towards the X-rays.

This discovery led Bragg to make use of X-rays for the study of the internal structures of crystals. He considered that X-rays are reflected from planes of atoms within the crystal lattice. The reflections from a particular family of planes will only occur at a particular angle of incidence and reflection. The essential condition for reflection is diagramed in Fig 13-6. In this figure the "crests" of the two incident waves will stay in phase if the thickened portion of the path (as shown in the diagram) of one wave is an integral multiple (*n*) of the wavelength (λ). The condition for reflection is given by the well-known Bragg equation:

$$\frac{\lambda}{2} = d_{nh,nk,nl} \sin \theta$$

The equation is satisfied only when $n = 1, 2, 3, \ldots$. If n is not a whole number, there will be destructive interference between the diffracted waves.

In any crystal there are an infinite number of families of planes that can be constructed. These planes are usually denoted by their Miller indices (hkl), *cf* Fig 13-7. These indices dictate the spacing between the planes (d_{hkl}) for a particular crystal. Since the highest value of θ that is theoretically possible to measure is 90° (reflected beam comes back along the incident beam's path), the number of planes (highest order) that one is capable of orienting in a diffracting position is limited by the wavelength of the radiation.

The planes that are accessible for a particular wavelength (X-ray) can be brought into a diffracting position by the proper orientation of the crystal relative to the collimated beam. In turn, many sets of planes can be recorded on a photographic plate by the movement of the crystal, such that each of the

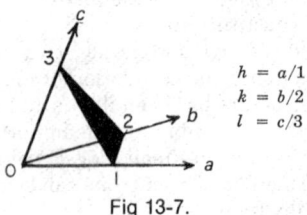

$h = a/1$
$k = b/2$
$l = c/3$

Fig 13-7.

planes will come into its diffracting position. In diffraction photographs, in which the crystal has been oscillated about an axis relative to the incident radiation, the various spots on the film arise from reflections from different planes, and each spot can be indexed, according to the Miller indices of the respective plane, by its location on the film. The spacing between the various spots enables one to derive the distances and angles between the primitive translations, ie, the unit-cell dimensions.

In most cases little information can be gleaned from a knowledge of the unit-cell dimensions alone. In order to learn about the crystal and molecular structure it is necessary to consider the intensities of the Bragg reflections. For a discussion of factors influencing these intensities and methods of measuring the latter see RPS-15, pages 186–189. Refer to Chapter 34, also.

Application of X-Ray Diffraction

Molecular Weight—The measurement of the unit-cell parameters provides a means of accurately determining molecular weights of compounds. The density of a crystal can be obtained by means of flotation in mixtures of suitable liquids, the density of which is altered by dilution until it matches that of the crystal.

The density (g/cm^3) is proportional to the molecular weight of the material in the unit cell. The relationship is

$$\text{Mol Wt} = \frac{\text{Density} \times V_{\text{cell}} \times N_a}{Z}$$

where N_a is Avogadro's number (6.023×10^{23}) and Z is the number of molecules in the unit cell. The unit-cell volume (V_{cell}) can be measured to a very high degree of accuracy. The number of molecules in the unit cell (Z) must be a whole number, with values of 1, 2, 4, and 8 being the most common among organic materials. When there is a high degree of solvation, it is necessary to approximate the amount of liquid bound by another means.

Identification of Materials—Every compound that is crystalline will give a characteristic X-ray diffraction pattern. These patterns can be very useful for identification purposes, and also for quantitative analysis of solid mixtures (see Chapter 34). They also have been utilized to a great extent by the pharmaceutical industry for the identification and classification of polymorphic and solvated forms of drugs. The powder method, in which the specimen is ground to a fine powder which contains minute crystals oriented in every possible direction and a large number have their Bragg planes in correct orientation for reflection, is a valuable technique when quick comparisons of different forms are to be made and also when quantitative work is done. An example of such a comparison between the hydrated and anhydrous form of theophylline is shown in Fig 13-8.

Extraction of quantitative information from diffraction patterns permits measurements of the physical and chemical stability of solid dosage forms. The kinetics of phase transformations are easily obtained by following the disappearance and/or appearance of various diffraction maxima corresponding to certain solid states as a function of time. One can easily visualize how this can be accomplished for theophylline hydrate by looking at the patterns in Fig 13-8.

Structure Determination—The body of substances of medicinal value whose structures were primarily elucidated by X-ray diffraction techniques is quite large. They range in molecular size from penicillin, to vitamin B$_{12}$, on up to the globular proteins. The structural determinations, in most instances, have played a major role in uncovering the secrets associated with the biological functions of the various molecules. A photograph of the ribonuclease molecule as deter-

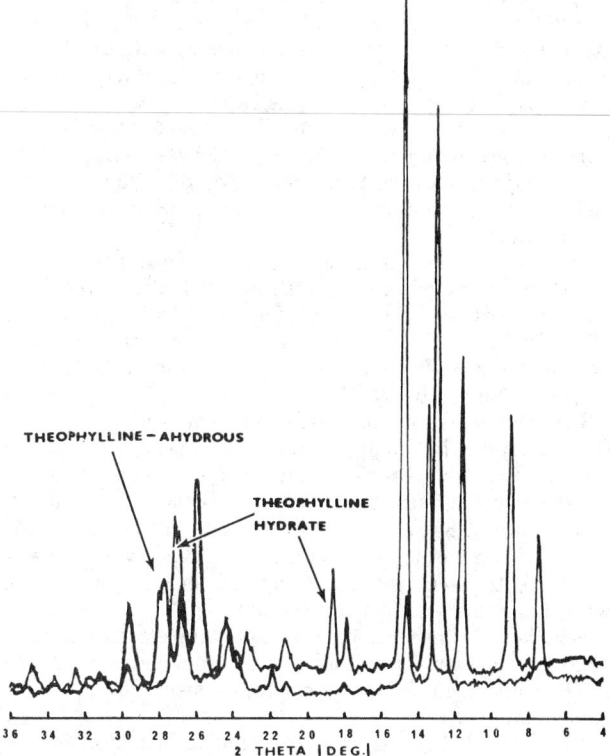

THEOPHYLLINE – AHYDROUS

THEOPHYLLINE HYDRATE

2 THETA (DEG.)

Fig 13-8. A tracing of the powder diffraction patterns of theophylline monohydrate and an anhydrous form.

mined by the X-ray studies of Kartha, Bello, and Harker is shown in Fig 13-9.

There are also large numbers of macromolecules of biological importance which do not form three-dimensional crystals in the usual sense, but will form fibers. The bundles of molecules in the fiber are aligned with respect to one another in a somewhat crystalline manner. These materials give X-ray diffraction patterns that have proved very useful in deriving molecular information. By fitting models to the X-ray pattern, many valuable biological polymers have had their secrets exposed. The two best examples are the α-helices of keratin and the double helix of deoxyribonucleic acid.

Intramolecular Bonding and Configurations—The precise determination of a crystal structure enables the bond lengths and angles between the various atoms to be deter-

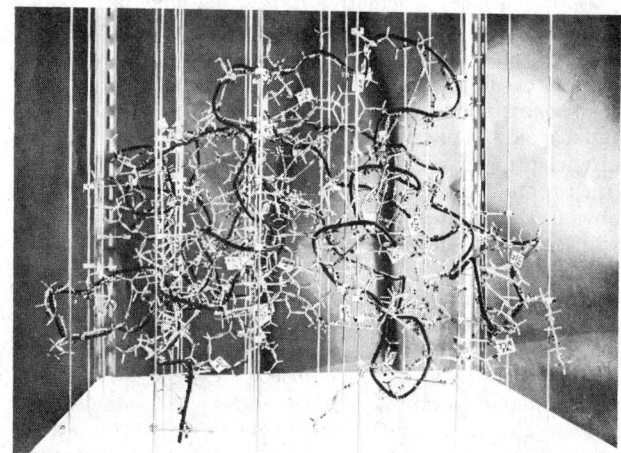

Fig 13-9. Model of bovine ribonuclease derived from x-ray data. Snakelike tube marks the backbone of the protein (courtesy, Dr G Kartha).

mined accurately. This information is extremely valuable in the further understanding of how various chemical substituents influence the valence states and configurations of a molecule. With such knowledge, structure–activity relationships that are of fundamental interest to the medicinal chemist have much more depth. The observed bond orders also serve as experimental criteria by which theoretical models can be judged. It is also possible to compare quantum mechanical calculations relating drug interaction with actual observation.

Intramolecular steric effects that tend to distort molecules are easily unraveled by the scrutiny of their structures. It is possible to distinguish between repulsive and attractive effects of substituents. The torsional angles about various bonds can be calculated from the atomic positions and are extremely helpful in correlating NMR data to structure.

In recent years the combination of X-ray and neutron diffraction studies has enabled information on the bonding and nonbonding electrons within a molecule to be clearly delineated. Neutron diffraction experiments enable atomic nuclei in a crystal to be accurately positioned; on the other hand X-rays locate the electron clouds. Both types of data can be combined to calculate 3-dimensional electron density maps with the inner core electrons around each atom subtracted; this makes the unshared pairs and bonding electrons clearly visible. The atomic positions derived from neutron data are used for phases in calculating electron-density maps with the X-ray data.

Refer to Chapter 34 for additional information on the physical methods discussed in this chapter.

States of Matter

The aim of this section is to discuss both generalities and specifics, most of which are not explicitly related to dosage forms because the latter will be discussed in other chapters. Some of the principles should be useful to have in mind when dosage forms and their manufacture and processing are studied by the product development pharmacist. It should be noted that due to the range of subjects covered by the section title it was necessary to take an eclectic approach in developing mostly qualitative discussions. The goal has been not to produce a difficult in-depth section but rather one which presents an overview of the significant states—mostly macroscopic—of matter.

Normally, matter exists in one of three states: solid, liquid, or gas. Although it is not pharmaceutically important, two other states of matter exist: one is the plasma state in which matter exists as a hot gaseous cloud of atoms and electrons; the other, a more speculative state which may have only a momentary existence, is one having characteristics of a superdense supermetal. This transient state is produced when material is subjected to very high pressures such as those used to make diamonds by compressing graphite.

To avoid the pitfalls of semantics, there is no need to call attention to other systems of classification because for all practical purposes it is convenient to think only of the most obvious three states. These states are actually a continuum with two common factors determining the position on the "scale of states."

The first factor is the intensity of intermolecular forces of all kinds: solids have the strongest forces; gases, the weakest. The other common factor is temperature. Obviously, as the temperature of substances is raised, they tend to pass from solid to liquid to gas. When the phrase "as temperature is increased" is used it should be remembered that this is a relative phrase. Even at what is called room temperature, some of the effects of a temperature increase are present because room temperature is far above absolute zero.

As a point of historical interest, note that Lavoisier, the late

great "father of modern chemistry," thought of heat as a type of matter and held the view even in the 18th century that the three states of aggregation differ only with respect to how much heat they "contain." Although not all are satisfied with this phraseology, the term *enthalpy* (or *heat content*) is still used in thermodynamics.

Thinking further back to the ancient Greek philosophers and their original four elements (earth, air, fire, and water) note again the great significance attached to heat. Although their concepts of the nature of matter were not exactly right, they recognized heat as an integral part of the scheme of things; nothing could be truer. Heat, a vital form of energy, the mirror of molecular motion, is *the* form of energy of greatest importance to mankind.

As alluded to above, there is no clear line of demarcation between the states of matter, but the following arbitrary division may make the approach this section takes more coherent.

Changes of State

As a solid becomes a liquid and then a gas, heat is absorbed and the enthalpy or heat content increases as the material passes through these phase changes. Thus, the enthalpy of a liquid is greater than that of its solid, and the enthalpy of a gas is greater than that of its liquid, because heat is absorbed when melting and vaporization occur. The *entropy* (a measure of the degree of total molecular randomness) also increases as materials go from solid to liquid to gas.

It is the balance of enthalpy, entropy, and temperature which determines if changes proceed spontaneously or not. Obviously, if systems tend to settle to states of lowest energy, it means that enthalpy and entropy considerations may counteract each other. Much of thermodynamics is concerned with explaining and quantitating the changes which systems undergo.

Latent heat is heat absorbed when a change of state takes place without a temperature change, as when ice turns to water at 0°. This example is one in which the heat required to produce the change of state is designated the *heat of fusion*. The counterpart, the *heat of vaporization*, is used when a change of state from liquid to gas is involved.

As molecules of a liquid in a closed evacuated container continually leave the surface and go into the free space above it, some molecules return to the surface, depending on their concentration in the vapor. Ultimately, a condition of equilibrium is established, and the rate of escape equals the rate of return. The vapor is then saturated and the pressure is known as the vapor pressure.

Vapor pressure depends on the temperature, but not on the amounts of liquid and vapor as long as equilibrium is established and both liquid and vapor are present. Heat is absorbed in the vaporization process and, therefore, the vapor pressure increases with temperature. As the temperature is raised further, the density of the vapor increases, and that of the liquid decreases. Ultimately, the densities equal each other and liquid and vapor cannot be distinguished. The temperature at which this happens is called the critical temperature, and above it there can be no liquid phase.

A very important process that involves a change of state—from liquid to vapor and back to liquid—is that of *distillation*, the theory and methods of which are discussed in RPS-14, pages 184–188.

Solids also have vapor pressures which depend on temperature. When a solid is converted directly into gas, it is said to sublime. Sublimation pressures of solids are much lower than those of liquids at any given temperature. When a solid is transformed directly into a liquid, two types of melting may be distinguished. The first is the crystalline type in which a rigid solid becomes a liquid during which procedure two

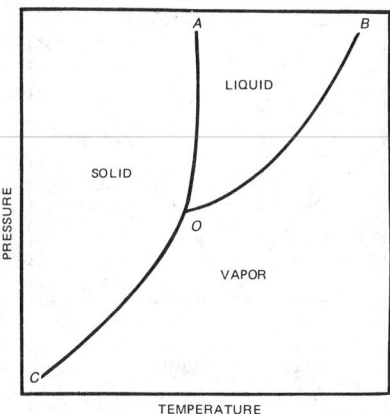

Fig 13-10.   Phase diagram to illustrate the principle of sublimation.

phases are present; the bulk of the solid or its inner parts are not really changing.   The second type is amorphous melting. This involves an intermediate plastic-like condition which envelops the whole mass; the viscosity decreases and a state of liquidity follows.   Crystalline melting involves more definite melting points and latent heats than does amorphous melting.

Sublimation

All solids have some tendency to pass directly into the vapor state.   At a given temperature each solid has a definite, though generally small, vapor pressure; the latter increases with rise in temperature.   *Sublimation* is the term applied to the process of transforming a solid to vapor without intermediate passage through the liquid state; in pharmaceutical manufacturing the process commonly includes also the condensation of the vapor back to the solid state.

A solid sublimes only when the pressure of its vapor is below that of the *triple point* for that substance.   The triple point here referred to is the point, having a definite pressure and temperature, at which the solid, liquid, and vapor phases of a chemical entity are able to coexist indefinitely.   If the pressure of vapor over the solid is above that of the triple point, the liquid phase will be produced before transformation to vapor can proceed.   Fig 13-10 depicts a phase diagram illustrating the principle involved.   The line *OA* indicates the melting point of the solid form of a substance at various pressures; only along this line can both solid and liquid forms exist together in equilibrium.   To the left only the solid form is stable and to the right only the liquid form remains permanently.   The line *OB* shows the vapor pressure of the liquid form of the substance at various temperatures; it is called the vapor-pressure curve of the liquid and represents the conditions of temperature and vapor pressure for coexistence of liquid and vapor phases.   Above this line only the liquid phase exists permanently; below it only vapor occurs.   The line *OC* represents the vapor pressure of the solid at various temperatures; it is designated as the sublimation curve of the solid and represents the conditions of temperature and vapor pressure for the coexistence of solid and vapor phases.   To the left of this line only solid can exist, to the right only the vapor form is stable.   The intersection of the three lines, point *O*, is the triple point.   It is apparent from the diagram that at pressures of vapor below that of the triple point it is possible to pass directly from the vapor to the solid state, and *vice versa*, simply by changing the temperature.   At pressures above the triple point the liquid phase must intervene in transformations between solid and vapor phases, in a closed system.   Since the melting point of a solid is commonly taken at 1 atmos of pressure, it is evident that if the triple point

pressure is less than 1 atmos, fusion of the solid form will occur on heating in a closed vessel; if, on the other hand, the triple point pressure is greater than 1 atmos, the solid form cannot be melted by heating at atmospheric pressure.

In a current of air, however, the conditions are somewhat different; some solids that melt when heated in a closed system now sublime appreciably even at ordinary temperatures because the vapor pressure of the solid does not attain the triple-point pressure.   Thus, camphor, naphthalene, *p*-dichlorobenzene, and iodine, all of which have a triple-point pressure below 1 atmos, will vaporize in a current of air but melt when heated in a closed system.

Critical Point

The critical point, by way of a general definition, is expressed as a certain value of temperature or pressure (or molar volume) above which or below which certain physical changes will not take place or certain states of being will not exist.   At these points, some properties are constant and are referred to as the critical temperature, pressure, or volume.   At the usual critical point, the properties of liquid and gas are identical and the phase diagram curve of *P* vs *T* ends.   (Phase diagrams will be discussed later.)   When a liquid changes to a vapor, increased disorder or randomness and, therefore, increased entropy results.   At the critical temperature, the entropy of vaporization is zero as is the enthalpy of vaporization since the gas and liquid are indistinguishable.

Although the gas–liquid critical point is the one most discussed, there are others.   Each critical point marks the disappearance of a state.   Note that most liquids behave similarly not only at their critical temperatures but also at equal fractions of their critical temperatures.   For example, the normal boiling points of many liquids are approximately equal fractions (about 60%) of their critical temperatures (in absolute temperature degrees).

Visualization of Changes of State

This section is to serve as an introduction to the following one entitled *Eutectics*.

When a pure substance cools and is transformed from a liquid to a solid, a graph (Fig 13-11) of its (decreasing) temperature vs time is continuous.   At the temperature at which solid crystallizes out (that is, the melting point) the cooling curve becomes horizontal.   The same is true at the boiling point, the temperature of a liquid at which the continuing application of heat no longer raises the temperature, but rather converts the liquid into vapor; it is the point where the

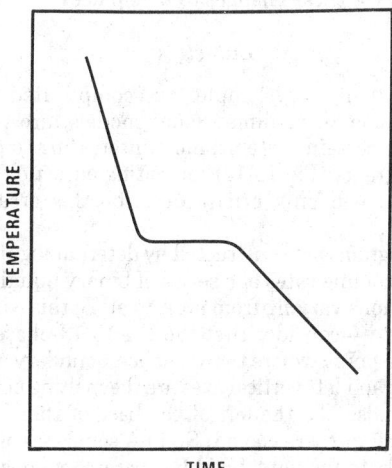

Fig 13-11.   A single change of state as shown by a slowing of the cooling rate.

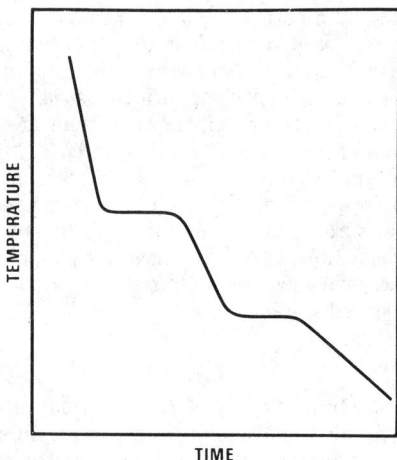

Fig 13-12.   Two changes of state with resulting temporary decreases in cooling rate.

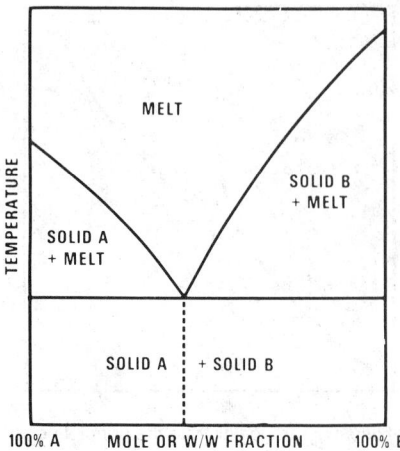

Fig 13-13.   Simple phase diagram of system showing eutectic point; see text for details.

vapor pressure of the liquid (or the sum of its components) equals that of the atmosphere above the liquid.

Increasing the pressure above the liquid or adding solutes, raises the boiling point and *vice versa*. These plateaus observed at certain specific temperatures are due to the release of the heats of fusion or vaporization. Similarly when solutions are cooled, the slope of the cooling curve (Fig 13-12) changes when one of the components starts to crystallize out. Although a very horizontal plateau may not be formed as in the case of pure materials, the change in slope indicates precipitation of one of the components. If the same plateaus are formed when binary solutions of varied composition are cooled, it indicates that both components of the binary solution are coming out together. The temperature at which this occurs is the *eutectic temperature*, and the composition is generally called a *eutectic*.

Normally, cooling curves *per se* are converted to phase diagrams to facilitate visualization of the interrelationships as phase changes take place. If instead of a minimum point or eutectic, a maximum point is observed, it may indicate that the components are reacting to form a solid compound which can exist in equilibrium with the melt over a range of compositions.

It is undoubtedly true that many unknown phase equilibria exist. Thus when conditions are changed, as for example when a process is scaled up in a manufacturing process, different phase changes may take place and produce different final products. The pharmaceutical use of heterogeneous materials such as waxes and fats certainly provides ample opportunity for these changes to take place.

Eutectics

Although many very complex and complicated diagrams, including some three-dimensional models, are needed to characterize certain systems, most interesting to pharmacy are the diagrams (Fig 13-13) indicating eutectic formation. This section will only briefly describe this area of technology.

Phase diagrams are constructed by determining the melting points and cooling rates of a series of binary liquid solutions of compositions varying from all A to all B; this will be illustrated shortly—consider first the Fig 13-13 phase diagram *per se*. The points where the V-shaped boundary of the melt hit the right and left vertical axes are the melting points of the pure materials. To the left of the base of the V (ie, when solutions rich in A are cooled) Solid A separates as the temperature falls; to the right, Solid B separates as shown. Thus, the left arm of the V is the curve which represents the temperature conditions under which various liquid mixtures are

in equilibrium with Solid A, and the right arm of the V is that curve which shows which mixtures are in equilibrium with Solid B.

At the point of the V both Solid A and Solid B are in equilibrium with the liquid; this point, the lowest temperature at which any of the infinite possible combinations of liquid solutions of A and B will freeze (or the lowest melting point of any possible mixture of Solids A and B) is called the eutectic point. Only at this point is the composition of the solid the same as that of the solution from which it is separating; this does *not* necessarily mean that the composition of the eutectic is a chemical compound of A and B. Thus, at the eutectic point, both A and B come out together in a constant proportion.

The eutectic composition is, however, a simple two-phase mixture, but when made *in situ* it has a very fine-grained structure which could impart to it different properties (eg, solubility or gastrointestinal absorption rate) as compared to a gross mixture of the same composition. The structure is very-fine-grained because the crystallization was very intimate since crystals of both phases were formed simultaneously. This is quite a different situation than one in which only one component is separating. It is important to remember that one can be only at one place on a phase diagram at any one time; ie, the diagram describes what a *particular* system is like at a certain temperature, which components are in the liquid and/or solid state, and the proportions of each.

As mentioned above, the diagrams are constructed from information obtained on the cooling rates of binary solutions. Consider again a cooling curve analysis in which temperature vs time are plotted. The curves change slope to form plateaus when any solid phase separates out; the plateaus tend to become more horizontal as absolute temperatures are lower because the intensity of radiation and conduction are lessened. A final plateau results, of course, when the whole liquid mass (or the last of it) solidifies. Thus, if a molten liquid having a composition lying *between*, eg, pure A and the eutectic were cooled, the following would be observed in a plot of temperature vs time (Fig 13-12): first T drops with time; then Solid A will come out of solution, release its heat of fusion, and thus slow the cooling rate to produce the first (upper) plateau; the temperature then starts to drop more sharply again as enough A comes out of solution, and the system changes composition until it contains only the eutectic composition; when the eutectic composition is reached, the second solid (B) also coprecipitates, and the temperature remains constant (lower plateau) until all of the A and B have solidified after which, of course, the temperature will be able to drop further. If the system being cooled started as the eutectic composition, only

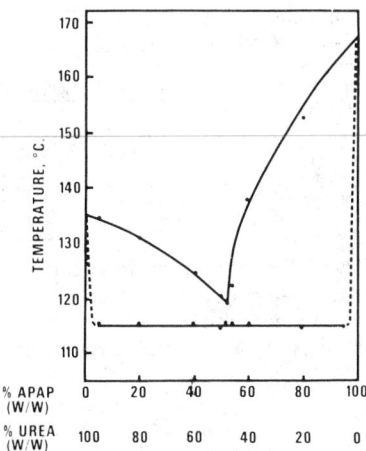

Fig 13-14. Phase diagram of the urea:acetaminophen (APAP) (46%:54%) eutectic melting in the 110°–115° range (courtesy, Goldberg, *et al*[17]).

the lower break and plateau would be observed; ie, a pure material and a eutectic would have similarly shaped cooling diagrams. This should be clear from the discussion. Note then that a phase diagram can be constructed by studying a number of cooling curves made on a series of mixtures of known composition. To do this, the temperatures at which cooling rate changes are noted are plotted against each particular composition studied. Note that Fig 13-13 is idealized in that no solid–solid solution of A and B is formed. If the two components are somewhat soluble in each other, the diagram would differ by having two thin solution areas along the left and right axes; such are partly in evidence in Fig 13-14.

Two pharmaceutical examples of eutectic formation are these. The first concerns a mixture of two common antipyretic–analgesic compounds: aspirin and acetaminophen. There has always been some "magic" associated with eutectic formation and, indeed, since such a binary composition does melt at a lower temperature than other combinations, the eutectic probably does have weaker bonding forces if any, and, being very fine grained also, it is more rapidly soluble. It is known that many drug compounds form eutectics and the aspirin–acetaminophen (APAP) eutectic (37% APAP by weight) does dissolve more quickly than a simple mixture of the two of the same composition. Since a formed eutectic is created under equilibrium conditions of intimate mixing as noted, the contact of the two compounds is much closer than that achievable by simply mixing the dry powders. The increase in dissolution rate obtained by using the eutectic may result in a greater speed of physiological absorption.

The second example is illustrated in Fig 13-14. It was found that urea and acetaminophen formed a eutectic containing approximately 46% urea and 54% acetaminophen (by weight) which melted in the 110°–115° range.

Gases

Aerosols—Gases *per se* are used directly in dosage forms in the field of aerosols. Although this subject, including the use of the so-called liquefied propellants, is covered elsewhere, note that pressure packs often use nitrogen, nitrous oxide, and carbon dioxide to expel the contents from their containers. The latter two gases are much more soluble in water so that some aeration (which may be desired) of the material discharged will take place.

In water, carbon dioxide is about six times as soluble as nitrogen, and nitrous oxide is about four times as soluble as nitrogen. Thus, if it is desired to have some of the gas dissolve in the product, either nitrous oxide or carbon dioxide can be used. In organic solvents and in fatty materials such as found in emulsions, nitrous oxide is somewhat more soluble than carbon dioxide. There is not a great deal of difference in solubility properties, however, but the possibility exists that the pH lowering effect of carbon dioxide as it forms carbonic acid may be as undesirable as a carbonate precipitation in an alkaline product.

Inhalers—Inhalers are classified as being one of two types. The first may be called a *surface* type; ie, the volatile material *per se* resides on the surface of the pledget. This represents a conventional adsorption situation; it is easy to appreciate the fact that the more surface area the pledget has the greater the surface area of the material exposed to the airflow and the greater the opportunity for volatilization. Hence, a larger or more loosely packed pledget will cause a larger dose to emanate from an inhaler than a smaller or tightly packed pledget.

It is convenient to make this type of inhaler if the volatile material itself is a liquid. The doses produced stay relatively high because the pledget charge is being depleted according to a zero-order scheme. This is reasonable because the volatile material has formed a multimolecular (as distinguished from a monomolecular) layer on the pledget surfaces; thus, even though molecules are stripped off, the surface area and hence the dose remain essentially unchanged. However, as some areas of the pledget are denuded, the total exposed surface area of the volatile material decreases, and so does the dose.

The second inhaler type may be termed a *solution* type: ie, the volatile material is dissolved in a suitable nonvolatile solvent, and this solution is placed on the pledget. The situation may be taken as an example of the operation of Raoult's and Henry's laws, ie, the vapor pressure of the components is proportional in some way to their concentrations. To keep the vapor pressure contribution of the solvent low in order to enhance the vapor pressure of the solute, a solvent of very low vapor pressure is used as the vehicle.

In this inhaler type the exposed surface area of the material does not change as the inhaler is used; what does change is the concentration of the volatile material in the solvent. Thus the dose gradually decreases according to a first-order scheme as the drug concentration decreases. Of course, the nature of the pledget and the inhaler body exert some effect here also, because if the airflow through the inhaler and the pledget does not permit volatilization of the material, insignificant, low doses will result.

If the drug is a volatile solid, the solution-type inhaler should be made because solids do not lend themselves to easy pledget-charging procedures even if a volatile solvent such as ether is used to deliver the material to the pledget during manufacturing.

Further amplification and clarification of the surface- and solution-type classification of inhalers might be achieved by considering the existing analogy to chromatographic systems. The surface-type inhaler corresponds to adsorption chromatography with the material being initially adsorbed on a carrier and then desorbed by a passing stream of liquid or gas. The solution-type inhaler corresponds to partition chromatography in which material in a solvent is supported by some medium, partitioned between its original solvent and a passing stream of gas or liquid, and thus removed.

Another point of significance concerns the relationship of the volatile active ingredient to the solvent. An increase in dose should result when the active ingredient is dissolved in solvents which cause it to deviate more positively from Raoult's law. Thus, the less the solute–solvent interaction and the greater the solute–solute interaction, the more pronounced will be the tendency toward volatilization of the solute. Using relative solubility as a gauge of such interaction, one would expect greater doses of a volatile solid from, eg, dibutyl phthalate (if it were less soluble in it) than from benzyl salicylate (if it were more soluble in it) at the same concentrations.

Although it might seem that the vapor pressure of the drug and additives would assume a position of primary importance, this does not appear to be the case. Vapor pressure values represent an equilibrium situation, whereas what is involved in the inhaler cases is a process controlled by factors affecting rates of volatilization.

Although it is true that volatile materials usually have appreciable vapor pressures, it is not generally true that a compound with a vapor pressure value of, eg, twice that of another compound will volatilize twice as fast. Besides this fact, inhaler recovery times may be essentially zero and no equilibration time may be needed. Also, no dosage drops would be noted with the surface-type inhaler and no regular (ie, linear with concentration) dosage drops would be noted with the solution-type inhaler if the vapor pressure were the controlling factor.

Unfortunately (from the standpoint of not having a more straightforward system to analyze), equilibrium and rate concepts are inextricably mixed in the present situation. This easily can lead to the basically incorrect tendency to try to predict kinetic data from thermodynamic values. However, because vaporization is relatively unencumbered with entropy and orientation factors, rates of volatilization are often qualitatively proportional to the equilibrium properties of the materials involved.

Equimolar quantities of the following compounds, allowed to evaporate at room temperature under the same conditions, will complete the evaporation process in this order: ether, acetone, chloroform, carbon tetrachloride, ethyl acetate, water. This order corresponds both to the materials' vapor pressures and boiling points.

To further becloud the cause-and-effect relationship, the very magnitude of the numbers (the concentrations in mole fractions) is such that the partial vapor pressure of a volatile solid may increase proportionately with the mole fraction. Hence, although vapor pressure concepts should not be neglected in inhaler development, it is the rates of volatilization which must be controlled or modified. For more information and experimental data on inhalers see Kennon and Gulesich.[18]

Relative Humidity—In the production of effervescent products, one of the most vital factors to be considered is the use of controlled humidity conditions. It is well known that the effective control of humidity is closely related to the success or failure of attempts to produce effervescent products.

It is useful to bring to light some of the facets of this area of technology. Two factors predominate when one views the situation: the effective concentration of water in the air and temperature. In chemical reactions, particularly the kind involved here, the effect of temperature on an equilibrium condition is not very significant when compared to the influence manifested by concentration. Certainly, water of hydration, crystallization, or simple adsorption (which is tenacious at room temperature) does not disappear at temperatures under 100°F. What *is* effective and influential, however, in keeping and increasing such additional moisture on solids is the *concentration* of water in the air.

The concept proposed here is that considerations based purely on relative humidity will probably be unfruitful. For purposes of illustration, note Table IX; it shows the amounts of water which are found under conditions encountered during the development of effervescent products.

The following points may be drawn from this information. A 10% relative humidity (RH) at 36°C is equivalent to 25% RH at room temperature. Either of these conditions represents a fairly dry day, but certainly not a very dry day. Therefore, although heating air surely lowers its RH, it probably does not

Table IX—Moisture Content (g/m^3) Existing at the Conditions Noted

Temperature	Relative humidity (%)			
	10	15	25	40
RT (22°C or 72°F)	1.9	2.9	4.8	7.7
Hot (36°C or 97°F)	4.1	6.2	10.3	16.5

lower the ability of the water in the air to cause trouble. Regardless of the temperature of processing rooms, experience has shown that water concentrations represented by the 72°F, 10–15% RH should not be exceeded if minimum difficulties are desired.

Liquids

The liquid state may be considered an intermediate one entered into as matter goes from solid to gas. Liquids have neither the strong cohesive forces of solids nor the weak ones of gases; hence, they are also intermediate in that they have neither the orderliness of a crystal nor the randomness of a gas. One might then consider a liquid a highly compressed gas or slightly released solid.

Due to the concept of molecular motion, there must be some free space in liquids. Also, if the motion is completely random, some spaces may be larger than others at a particular point in time. Thus, liquids may have holes, and this concept has explained phenomena such as the expansion of volume that materials undergo upon fusion (holes are created), diffusion in liquids, viscosity (movement of holes in the opposite direction of the viscous flow), and density decreases as temperature rises (the solubility of holes increases). It might be said that liquids are solutions of holes in material, whereas gases are solutions of matter in free space.

With respect to fluid mechanics, a fluid can be considered a material which cannot sustain shear forces when in static equilibrium; this is the distinguishing factor separating solids and fluids, the latter of which may be gases or liquids. This movement under the slightest stress is sometimes called "no sideways friction." It can be seen in operation in the case where a sailor standing watch near the gangplank of a docked ship can step on a mooring rope and cause the ship to move toward the dock.

Liquids, just as gases, take the shape of their container, but only the lower part of it as the liquid occupies a definite volume; gases expand to fill their entire container. Intermolecular spaces are greater in a gas than in a liquid so that they can be compressed. Relative to gases, both liquids and solids are quite incompressible. They can be considered already compressed due to the stronger intermolecular forces.

After a fluid is set in motion, it comes to rest because of the internal friction caused by the molecules sliding over each other; this resistance to flow is called viscosity and, as is well known, can be quantified. To effect good quantification with viscometers, normal, smooth (laminar or layer) flow is needed. With excessive stirring, at a so-called critical velocity, the fluid becomes turbulent, and instrumental measurements are difficult to effect. As the temperature of fluids increases, viscosity decreases. In general, also, as pressure increases, viscosity increases.

Because fluids have some structure, they may change upon standing so that when one is considering viscous behavior, the recent past history of the sample may have great effects. Thixotropy is the term used for liquids which flow freely if recently stirred, but gel on standing. Solids also flow but more slowly even under minor stresses, including those produced by their own weight. The wavy, bumpy surface of tarred roads, particularly seen on hills, is a result of a flow phenomenon.

Of interest also is the cluster theory of liquids, the main concept being that localized order exists but does not extend to a great distance. One property explained by this visualization is that as the temperature rises, the clusters disintegrate and viscosity decreases; another is that transmitting momentum through a liquid is not due only to molecular movements, but due to the transmissions of elastic waves through the groups of semistationary clusters. It is possible that the cluster theory affords another way of looking at pharmaceutical complexes in solution.

Complexes

As mentioned above, in addition to structure in solvents it is also possible for solutes to create a structure of a sort within the solvent. Thus, it has been shown that benzocaine in water solution with caffeine exhibits a much reduced rate of hydrolysis. In a somewhat similar vein it also has been noted that different salts of the same compound (eg, hydrochloride vs nitrate) may exhibit different stability characteristics. Similarly, it has been shown that saccharin in certain chlorpromazine hydrochloride solutions enhances the light-stability of the drug. It appears that such changes are due to the fact that the ionic environment may form a protective molecular "overcoat" or loose ionic atmosphere complex around the drug.

Liquid Crystals

Lipids, when heated, usually do not pass directly from a crystalline to an isotropic structure, but rather they assume intermediate liquid crystal phases. Most interesting pharmaceutically and physiologically is that these structures are, undoubtedly, intimately involved in the structure and, hence, the function of membranes and cells.

All biological systems are basically aqueous, and it is particularly in such systems that lyotropic mesomorphism (the formation of liquid crystal phases in the presence of water) takes place. In other words, the lipid phases undergo transformations involving crystal, liquid crystal, and liquid forms, and it is these changes which are mediators of the various physiological absorption, transport, storage, and excretory functions of cells. Many *in vitro* studies of biologically significant lipids have been carried out in attempts to elucidate the mechanisms of their interaction and behavioral properties in aqueous systems.

Liquid crystals differ from solids and gases in that they have some freedom to move and to take on many different shapes while yet maintaining a high degree of order through quite long distances, relatively speaking. In the laboratory, liquid crystals can be prepared from one component by heat treatments (thermotropic systems) or from one or more components by adding controlled amounts of water or other polar solvents (lyotropic mesomorphism). Note that the only molecules of significance here are asymmetric and have a definite long direction so that their orientation "3-D wise" is essential. This should be remembered throughout the discussion.

For present purposes three types of liquid crystal phases will be described briefly so that at least some appreciation for this particular state of matter may be gained. The phases are generally characterized as being nematic, smectic, or cholesteric.

Nematic molecules (Fig 13-15) are set in parallel arrangements and have restricted rotation about at least one axis. The molecules are parallel or nearly so. One might picture this as a long box filled with pencils with the latter being able to roll. Overall, the system might be considered to be thread- or cable-like. Another picture would be that of a group of logs going through a pipe. There is overlap of the pencils or logs somewhat as the cars in an auto race.

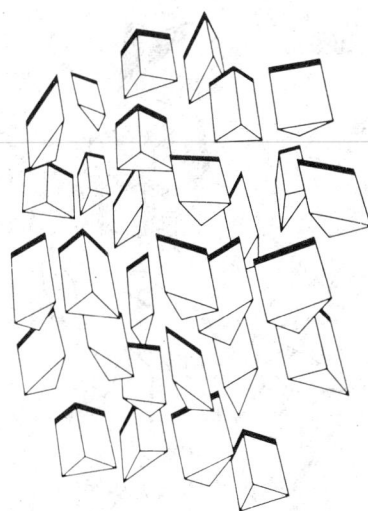

Fig 13-15. The nematic phase of a liquid crystal; see text for details (based on Fergason and Brown[19]).

The smectic or "two-dimensional" crystal (Fig 13-16) has its molecules arranged in layers with their long axes essentially normal (ie, at right angles) to the plane of the layers. Their centers of gravity are then mobile in two directions in their plane, and the molecules can rotate about one axis. Overall, one could consider the arrangement layerlike with the degree of order just described in each layer.

The smectic arrangement is similar to the nematic in that there is still essentially only one axis of rotation, except in this case there is no overlap. The logs go through the pipe as a member of a group; that is, it would be like a series of drag races in which no one wins and all are tied. Each successive group, however, does not follow the same paths as the others; that is, within any one group there may be equal spacings sideways between the long axes or there may not be. Note also that the thickness of the layers is about the same as the length of the molecules.

The cholesteric arrangement (Fig 13-17) is to some extent a combination of the nematic and smectic wherein the layers are nematic but, in addition, certain layering formations which resemble the smectic phase are incorporated. In essence, the result is a helical, twisting repetition of the nematic phase which, corkscrewlike, slowly changes head direction (for example, the lead end of the pencil) as one proceeds to examine

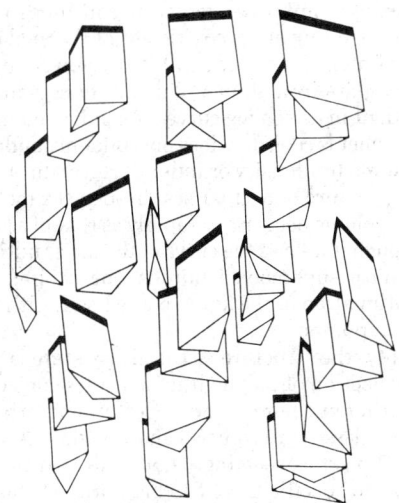

Fig 13-16. The smectic liquid crystal phase (based on Fergason and Brown[19]).

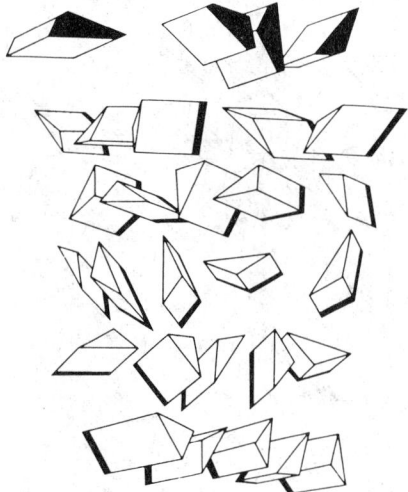

Fig 13-17.   A 180° turn of the molecules in the cholesteric liquid crystal phase (based on Fergason and Brown[19]).

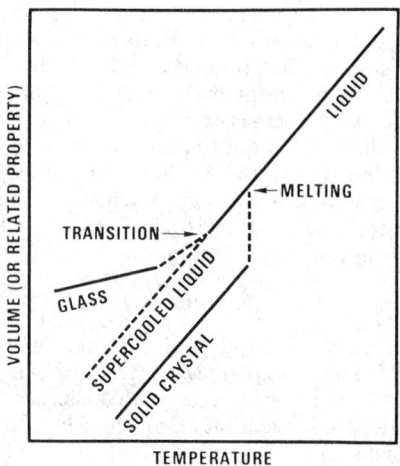

Fig 13-18.   Composite cooling curve of liquids forming glass, super-cooled liquid, and solid crystal states; see text for explanation.   For a more detailed discussion, see Dietz.[20]

underlying layers of molecules.   The cholesteric arrangement is, *in toto*, much thicker than a smectic layer.

All three structures, as alluded to, are involved in building cells, and each type can (when viewed totally) form curved surfaces, membranes, or any other required micelle-like shapes.   Some workers constructed cell models utilizing these structures and showed how the mechanics of many cellular functions can be visualized using the known properties of liquid crystals.

The Glassy State

Although glass is usually thought of as a specific, nonconducting, transparent solid, it actually is a *type* of solid matter. It can be considered neither a typical solid nor liquid.   The atoms of most solid states are generally structurally strictly ordered, whereas glassy materials are highly disordered. Glasses may, however, have some short-range order just as polymers do.   Another characteristic of glasses is that they do not have specific melting points but slowly and gradually become liquids when they are heated.   Sometimes glasses are considered supercooled liquids, but this is not strictly accurate.

A graph of volume vs temperature for most substances shows that the volume of a liquid decreases as the crystallization temperature is approached.   If solidification is accomplished by crystallization, the volume decreases sharply at the freezing point, after which it continues to decrease gradually depending on its coefficient of thermal expansion. This type of behavior is not exhibited when solidification is followed by glass formation.   The uniqueness of the glassy state is evident in its cooling curve.   As indicated in Fig 13-18, as a glass-former is cooled, it does not suddenly undergo a large drop in volume (or density or index of refraction) at any particular temperature or as it passes through the melting point, nor does its volume decrease as rapidly as that of a supercooled liquid although it follows the curve of the latter initially during cooling.   With supercooled liquids, the cooling curve is a simple continuation of the liquid curve itself, with no melting or transition points.

Atomically, the structure of the glassy state is marked by a random selection of polyhedral molecules considered to be linked together at their corners.   Certain materials are easy to cast into a glassy state, others can be made glassy with great difficulty, and some, seemingly not at all.   At present there seems to be no specific theory to help predict this behavior. Materials which do form glasses seem, however, to have a very high viscosity at their melting point; this inhibits the forma-

tion of an ordered structure.   In addition, non-glass-formers tend to have large energy differences between the ordered form of the solid and the disordered liquid.   Thus, the low-energy, ordered form of the solid tends to be developed. Obviously, the energetic tendencies here are balanced by entropy factors which tend to favor states of minimum order.

Although the most well-known glass-formers are the metal oxides, many other materials can exist in the glassy state; even steel can be so cast if it is very, very quickly cooled.   This technique produces glasses as the materials become solid before they have a chance to develop a crystalline structure. With regard to crystal formation, note that in a crystallization process, when concentrated solutions of the material to be crystallized are cooled slowly, larger and more perfect crystals form.

Incomplete or imperfect crystallization, whether due to technique or to the nature of the material itself (for example, natural and synthetic high polymers), often causes the formation of crystallites, glasses, or liquid crystals.   Crystallites have no recognizable regular crystal pattern but yet are, in a sense, incipient crystals.   Many shapes and arrangements are possible such as globular, rows or clouds of globules, threads, cylinders, or rods.

Solids

The most significant physical property of the solid state is the high degree of order in which substances such as metals and minerals exist.   The structure may be crystalline and lattice-like or noncrystalline, such as in plastic, glass, or gels which are not lattice-like or only partly so.   These latter materials do have, however, much more order than liquids and gases.   These materials also have, in varying degree, some plastic and elastic properties wherein some resistance to applied stresses exists, but when the stress reaches a certain intensity, either flow or fracture ensues.

Although different classifications exist, four major different types of bonds hold solids together; the strong bonds impart higher melting points to substances.   In order of decreasing strength, the bond types are metallic, ionic (salts), valence (diamond), and molecular (many organic compounds).   Thus, in some solids, the atoms or molecules or ions may be arranged in a regularly repeating pattern (crystalline state), whereas other solids are considered noncrystalline or amorphous if they do not have this characteristic of regularity.   Although there is some blurring of the division, in general, metals, minerals, rocks, and alloys are examples of the former class and glass, wood, ceramics, and plastics are examples of the latter.

Alloys are an example of a mixed solid having characteristics of regularity but being intermediate between strictly crystalline and amorphous. They are metal substances consisting of two or more elements not counting the trace amounts of materials which make any element less than 100% pure. Alloys are solid solutions of one of two types. In the interstitial type, the smaller solute atoms occupy the interstices between the solvent atoms; the overall structure is quite like the parent or solvent metal. The other type is the substitutional one and all atoms occupy (ie, contribute to building) a common lattice.

In general, alloys are stronger and harder than purer metals. This is probably due to the fact that both dislocations and the perfectly regular crystal structure of pure metals permit the planes of the crystals to slip over each other. These processes are inhibited in alloys because the resident or solute atoms interact with the dislocations and with the regular sections so that any lattice distortions produced make slipping more difficult.

A process that also depends on the internal structure and possibilities for partial shifting of it is annealing. It is based on the concept that a ductile metal becomes harder and less workable as cold work is done on it. Finally, a point is reached where cracking is imminent. To restore the original ductility, the metal is heated and slowly cooled. The temperatures used just permit the relaxation of the overstrained areas. A visualization might consider this a type of partial recrystallization or atomic rearrangement.

Polymorphism

Polymorphism, the existence of one or more crystalline and/or amorphous forms, is a characteristic of most solid substances. As applied to crystals it refers to the different crystal structures the same chemical compound may have. The various forms also usually have different X-ray diffraction patterns, melting points, and most important pharmaceutically, different solubilities.

Particularly in many cases in which dissolution in the gastrointestinal tract is the rate-limiting factor in absorption, differing solubilities may have a great effect, either good or bad. Different polymorphic forms are produced, depending on such factors as storage temperature, recrystallization solvent *per se*, and the rate of cooling (and hence the rate of crystallization) of the solvent. It appears that all organic materials exist in several polymorphic forms with the number of forms found depending on the effort spent searching! In the field of drugs, polymorphs of such diverse molecules as cortisone and prednisolone to aspirin have been found. As an example of the latter case, two different aspirin polymorphs form depending on whether the material is crystallized from 95% alcohol or *n*-hexane. The two forms have different melting points but most important, the form produced from the hexane dissolves in water much more quickly.

References

1. Feynman RP: *Science 183:* 601, 1974.
2. Schoenborn BP: *Chem Eng News*, Jan 24, 1977, p 31.
3. Pitzer KS: *J Am Chem Soc 70:* 2140, 1948.
4. Fieser LF, Fieser M: *Introduction to Organic Chemistry*, Heath, Boston, inside back cover, 1957.
5. Pauling LC: *The Nature of the Chemical Bond*, 3rd ed, Cornell Univ Press, Ithaca, NY, 1960—(*a*) 225–6; (*b*) 93; (*c*) Chap 3.
6. Fajans K: *Physical Methods of Organic Chemistry*, vol 1, part II, 2nd ed, Interscience, NY, 1162, 1949.
7. Lien EJ, *et al:* *J Pharm Sci 71:* 641, 1982.
8. Olah GA, *et al:* *J Am Chem Soc 89:* 711, 1967.
9. Martin AN, *et al:* *Physical Pharmacy*, 3rd ed, Lea & Febiger, Philadelphia, 58–61, 1983.
10. Fujita T, *et al:* *J Am Chem Soc 86:* 5175, 1964.
11. Iwasa J, *et al:* *J Med Chem 8:* 150, 1965.
12. Hansch C, Anderson SM: *J Org Chem 32:* 2583, 1967.
13. Hansch C, Anderson SM: *J Med Chem 10:* 745, 1967.
14. Hansch C, *et al:* *J Med Chem 16:* 1207, 1973.
15. Hansch C, *et al:* *J Med Chem 20:* 304, 1977.
16. Hansch C: *Farmaco 23:* 293, 1968.
17. Goldberg AH, *et al:* *J Pharm Sci 55:* 482, 1966.
18. Kennon L, Gulesich JJ: *J Pharm Sci 51:* 278, 1962.
19. Fergason JL, Brown GH: *J Am Oil Chemists' Soc 45:* 120, 1968.
20. Dietz ED: *Sci Technol* 10 (*Nov*): 1968.

CHAPTER 14

Complexation

Marvin C Meyer, PhD

Professor of Pharmaceutics and Associate Dean for Graduate and Research Programs
College of Pharmacy, University of Tennessee Center for the Health Sciences
Memphis, TN 38163

The most general definition of *complex formation* considers a *complex* to represent the association of two or more species, each capable of independent existence. Further, a *complex* is said to be present when the association of these species is such that they are in closer proximity than would be expected on the basis of a random distribution. Complexation is a broad topic which includes a consideration of bonding forces and physicochemical properties. The formation of a *complex* can alter the solubility, partitioning characteristics, or stability of a drug. Certain *complexes* are useful in drug product formulation, while others can affect the bioavailability of a drug, as well as change the pharmacokinetic and pharmacodynamic properties of drugs. In addition, certain therapeutic agents are useful because they are either in the form of a *complex*, or result in the formation of a *complex* following administration. The objective of this chapter is to provide a survey of the phenomena of complexation, with an emphasis on *complexes* of importance in pharmacy and medicine.

The complex formed by the association of two molecules of an organic acid in solution consists of atoms held together by normal covalent bonds, shown by a dash between the various elements. However, two molecules of the acid are joined by *hydrogen bonds*, illustrated as dotted lines, which are neither covalent, coordinate, nor ionic, but are the result of a *dipole–dipole* attraction between negative oxygen and positive hydrogen.

$$CH_3-C\overset{\displaystyle O\cdots H-O}{\underset{\displaystyle O-H\cdots O}{}}C-CH_3$$

Such bonds may be of the *ion–dipole, dipole–dipole, dipole–induced dipole*, or even of the *covalent* or *coordinate* type. The term complex is now usually extended to cover a multitude of compounds in which the bonding is simple, intricate, or a combination thereof.

Classification—Classification of complex compounds according to a rigid set of conventions is a difficult, if not impossible, task. For example, a type of complex compound (*Inclusion Compounds*) has been investigated that is considered a *no-bond* complex. For such complexes there is no evidence for the existence of bonding forces responsible for joining two or more molecules to form a somewhat stoichiometric combination.

In order to facilitate discussion of complexation, some form of classification is useful. One approach is to characterize complexes on the basis of bonding forces. Three subdivisions can be included: *true-bond* types, in which the union between the components can be explained in the classical manner; *weak-bond* types, or those exhibiting attraction due to van der Waals' forces, hydrogen bonding, etc; and *no-bond* types, which include the *inclusion compounds*. A second approach is to group complexes according to the type of complex which is formed.

The following classification of complex compounds, representing a hybrid arrangement of types of bonds and compounds, will be used in this chapter.

Metal Complexes
  Inorganic Complexes
  Chelates
  Olefin Complexes
Molecular Complexes
  Aromatic Complexes (Charge-Transfer)
  Hydrogen-Bonded Complexes
No-Bond (Inclusion) Complexes
  Clathrates
  Channel-Lattice Types
  Intercalation "Compounds"
Ion-Exchange Compounds

Ion-exchange materials are also included, although in many instances they may not be regarded as complexes. In addition, the latter portion of the chapter will emphasize the interactions between drugs and proteins. This special type of complex can have a variety of significant effects on the pharmacodynamics and pharmacokinetics of a drug. Several other types of interactions, such as adsorption of drugs to solid surfaces, and interactions between drugs and surface-active agents will be covered in other chapters.

Metal Complexes

This category can be subdivided into the inorganic and aromatic types.

Inorganic Complexes—Stable "molecular compounds" can be formed by the union of two simple molecules in which the atoms already seem to be exerting their maximum possible valencies. The custom was to indicate the formula for the "molecular compound" by writing the components side by side, eg, $2KI.HgI_2$ or $2KCl.MgCl_2$. However, upon examination of solutions of these "double salts," the former salt was found to yield only three ions, and the latter a total of seven. The formulation of the mercuri compound was then changed to $K_2[HgI_4]$ and the HgI_4^{2-} ion, resulting from the reaction

$$HgI_2 + 2I^- = HgI_4^{2-}$$

was termed a *complex* ion, and the salts *complex* salts. However, analogous ions such as SO_4^{2-} or CrO_4^{2-} are not regarded as complex, again pointing to the somewhat loose definition attributed to this term.

Werner, in 1891, postulated his famous coordination theory, which helped to explain some of the deviations from the classic valency theories for compounds of the above-mentioned type. According to Werner:

1. There are two types of valences: (*a*) primary (ionic) and (*b*) secondary (coordinate).
2. The same type of anion, radical, or molecule may be held by either or both types of valence.
3. For each *central atom* or ion there is a fixed number (*coordination number*) of nonionic valences. The coordinated atoms or groups occupy the *first sphere* or *coordination sphere*. Other atoms are said to be in the *second* or *ionization sphere*.
4. Neutral molecules, as well as ions, may satisfy the nonionic valences.
5. The nonionic valences are directed toward definite positions in space (this explains the existence of stereoisomers of many coordinate complexes). These postulates can be illustrated by the following compound.

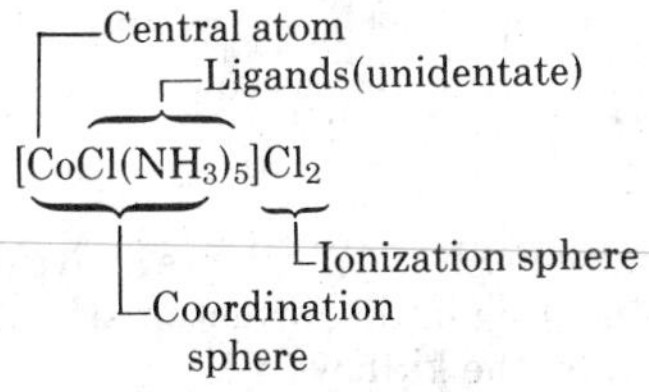

Central atom
Ligands(unidentate)

$[CoCl(NH_3)_5]Cl_2$

Ionization sphere
Coordination
sphere

In solution this compound will ionize to form $[CoCl(NH_3)_5]^{2+}$ and $2Cl^-$ ions. The chloride ion in the coordination sphere is not precipitated by silver nitrate. The groups that combine with the central atom, by any type of bonding, are known as *ligands*. The type of bonding between the metal and ligand may be electrostatic or covalent. However, whether the bonding is ionic, covalent, or intermediate, the function of the ligand is always that of donating electrons to the central atom. The *coordination number* is the maximum number of atoms or groups that can combine, in the coordination sphere, with the central atom (usually an even number). Ligands that have more than one electron pair available for coordination with the central ion are said to be bi-, tri-, or poly-*dentate*. In Fig 14-1a the central atom, M, has a coordination number of 4 and the ligands A, A′, A″, A‴ are *unidentate*, while in Fig 14-1b ligands A-A′ and A″-A‴ are *bidentate*.

Compound (a) would be referred to as a metal complex and (b) as a *chelate*. Groups which occupy more than one coordination position in a complex and form a ring with the central ion and are termed *chelates* (Greek, *claw*).

Many groups have the ability to coordinate with the central atom, and the following illustrates the order of decreasing affinity of coordinating groups:

$—O^-$(enolate ion); $—NH_2$(amine); $—N{=}N—$(azo);

$\rangle N$(ring nitrogen); $—COO^-$(carboxylate ion);

$—O—$(ether); and $—CO—$(carbonyl)

More recently, the *crystal field theory*, originally applied to crystals, has been employed to elucidate the structure of coordination compounds. A complete discussion is beyond the scope of this chapter, but the essence of the theory is that the five *d* orbitals of the central atom, which are of equal energy in the gaseous metal atom, are split by the presence of the electrostatic field due to the ligands, and acquire different energies. Quantitative energy calculations can be made in many cases, and a number of physical and chemical properties can be correlated, such as stability of the complex, magnetic properties, rates and mechanism of reaction, etc.

Perhaps the most familiar members of the nonchelate type of metal complexes (*unidentate ligands*) are: $[Ag(CN)_2]^-$ and $[Cu(CN)_3]^{2-}$ in electrodeposition of silver and copper from aqueous solution; $[Ag(NH_3)_2]^+$ formed in the solution of insoluble silver halides in ammonia; $[Fe(CNS)]^{2+}$ occurring at the end point of the titration with NH_4CNS using ferric alum indicator; use of fluoride or phosphate to form a soluble complex with iron; polyphosphates in water-softening to complex calcium and magnesium and the gravimetric determination of potassium as the chloroplatinate or cobaltinitrite.

In addition, platinum complexes have recently become important as a new class of antineoplastic agents. The most widely employed complex of this type is *cisplatin*. The drug

is believed to enter the cell intact, with subsequent removal of the chloride ions by hydrolysis, resulting in the formation of two active ligand sites.

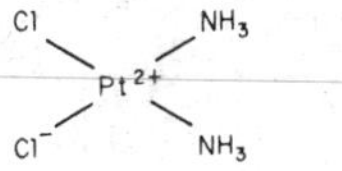

$Cl_2H_6N_2Pt$
cis-dichlorodiamine-
platinum

Chelates—The *chelate* type of metal complex is of great importance, especially in the pharmaceutical field. Chelation refers to the coordination of a metal with a polydentate ligand (Fig 14-1b). The complex so formed may result in precipitation of the metal or the formation of a stable, soluble compound. If the ligand forms a stable, water-soluble metal chelate, it is said to be a *sequestering* agent. *Sequestration* (Latin, *sequestrare*, to remove) is the suppression of a property or reaction of a metal without removal of that metal from the system or phase by any process of precipitation or extraction and is usually accomplished by chelation.

Materials such as citric acid have been long and extensively used for the purpose of sequestering metals in living systems, foods, beverages, and cosmetics. Metallic complexes of bivalent cation. with tartrates and citrates exist in a 1:1 molar ratio of tartrate or citrate to the metal. Salts of citric acid are required to form complexes of the bivalent metals; free citric or tartaric acid will, however, complex trivalent iron, but the ratio of metal to citrate or tartrate is dependent on the acid concentration. The structures of such complexes have been the subject of much study and are still not completely resolved.

The interaction between tetracycline and various cations such as calcium, iron, zinc, magnesium, and aluminum is another well known example of complexation. The result is a decreased absorption of the drug due to the formation of a poorly water-soluble species.

Sequestration has two important pharmaceutical uses: in analysis and in removal or deactivation of unwanted ions in solution. Mention has been made of the use of unidentate ligands (fluoride and cyanide ions, etc) as complexing agents, but polydentate agents are much more important for sequestering purposes. One compound, ethylenediaminetetraacetic acid (EDTA, (ethylenedinitrilo)tetraacetic acid,

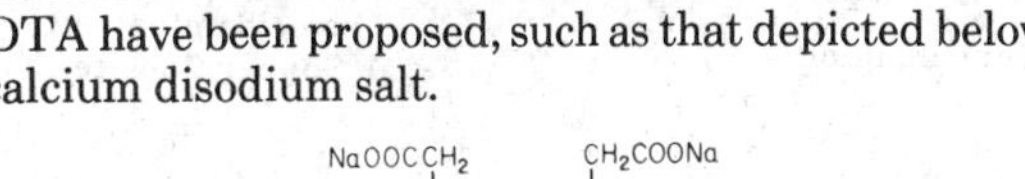

$HOOC—CH_2$ $CH_2—COOH$
$N—CH_2—CH_2—N$
$HOOC—CH_2$ **EDTA** $CH_2—COOH$

edetic acid) has been studied and employed extensively in the pharmaceutical field. EDTA has two nitrogen and four oxygen donor groups, and thus is termed hexadentate. Most of the official drugs containing calcium and the zinc content of zinc stearate are analyzed by titration with a standard EDTA solution. Several structures for the calcium complex of EDTA have been proposed, such as that depicted below for the calcium disodium salt.

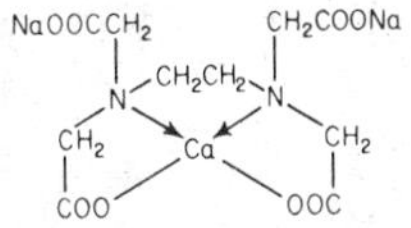

A general term given to the aminopolycarboxylic acids, such as EDTA, is *Complexons*. The following formulas illustrate two such compounds.

Complexon II is EDTA and Complexon III or B is the sodium salt of EDTA.

There are many pharmaceutical applications of EDTA (and other sequestering agents); for example, in antibiotic, anti-

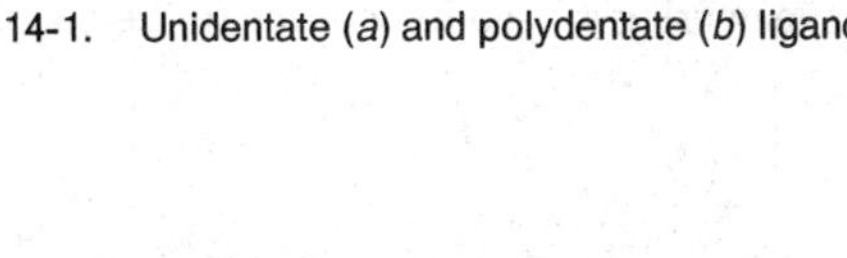

Fig 14-1.   Unidentate (*a*) and polydentate (*b*) ligands.

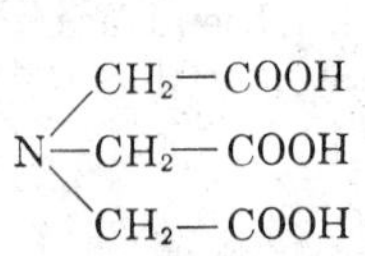

Complexon I
(nitrilotriacetic acid)

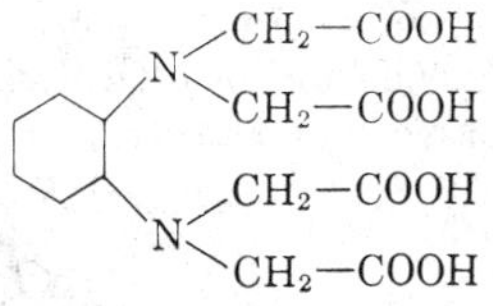

Complexon IV
(1,2-cyclohexylenedinitrilo)-
tetraacetic acid

histamine, sulfonamide, epinephrine, anesthetic, and barbiturate preparations to prevent discoloration due to traces of metals; in cosmetic creams or lotions containing unsaturated fatty acids and alcohols to prevent oxidation catalyzed by trace metals; in alkaline bottle-washing compositions to avoid precipitation of metal hydroxides; in the stabilization of ascorbic acid, hydrogen peroxide, gum and resin preparations, formaldehyde, essential oils, folic acid, and hyaluronidase; and as a cleaning agent to retain the efficiency of filters in processes where the filter cloth becomes blocked by precipitation and occlusion of polyvalent metallic salts.

Among the best known therapeutic uses for chelating agents is the treatment of intoxication from heavy metals (eg, lead, mercury, iron, copper, zinc, and arsenic). The treatment of lead poisoning involves the use of CaNa$_2$EDTA. The calcium is displaced by lead in the intoxicated patient. In contrast, Na$_2$EDTA administration may result in depletion of body calcium stores, and this form of EDTA can be used in the treatment of hypercalcemia. The observation that a particular agent can complex or chelate another species *in vitro* does not necessarily indicate its efficacy *in vivo*. For example, mercury can displace calcium, and can be chelated by CaNa$_2$EDTA, but this agent is not effective as an antidote for mercury poisoning. This may be due to mercury being highly bound to reactive sites in the body, or the failure of the ionic EDTA to penetrate to the sites of the body where the mercury is localized.

Dimercaprol (BAL) is an effective chelator for mercury, as well as arsenic. Since the 1:1 complex of dimercaprol:mercury is insoluble in water, dosages of dimercaprol are designed to achieve a plasma concentration such that the formation of the water-soluble and readily excreted 2:1 complex occurs.

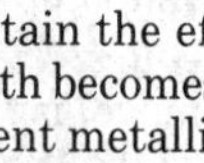

$$CH_2CHCH_2OH$$
$$\underset{SH}{|}\quad\underset{SH}{|}$$

This drug may also be employed in conjunction with EDTA in the treatment of lead poisoning.

Penicillamine chelates copper, mercury, zinc, and lead and has an advantage that it is effective when administered orally. The drug has been employed in the treatment of hepatolenticular degeneration (Wilson's disease), and acts by promoting the excretion of copper in patients with a deficiency of ceruloplasmin, a plasma protein which normally binds copper.

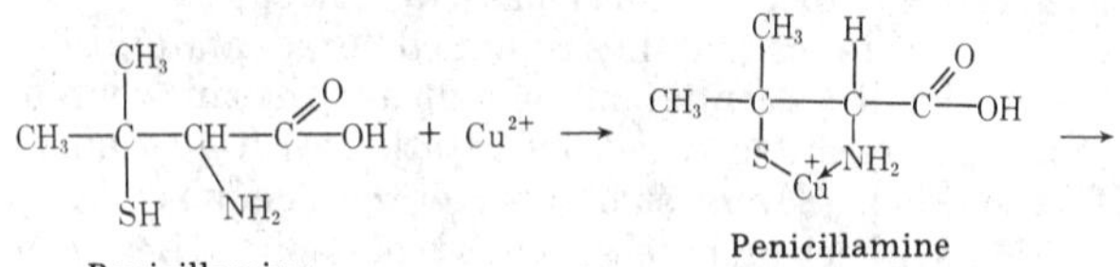

Penicillamine

Penicillamine
1:1 Copper Chelate

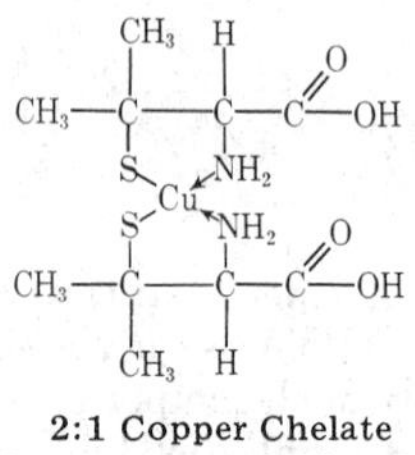

2:1 Copper Chelate
Forms water-soluble salts

Deferoxamine, available as the mesylate salt, is an effective agent in the treatment of iron intoxication. The three seg-

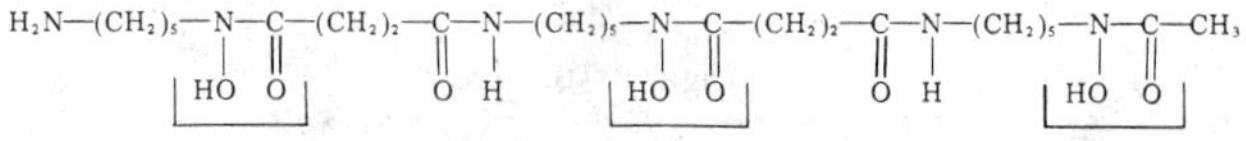

Deferoxamine

ments of the molecule shown above are active in the chelation of ferric ions, resulting in the formation of a chelate which is readily excreted by the kidneys.

Metal chelates are also important in analytical pharmacy, as already indicated for EDTA. Dithizone (diphenylthio-

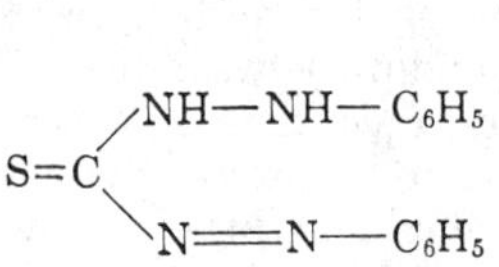

dithizone

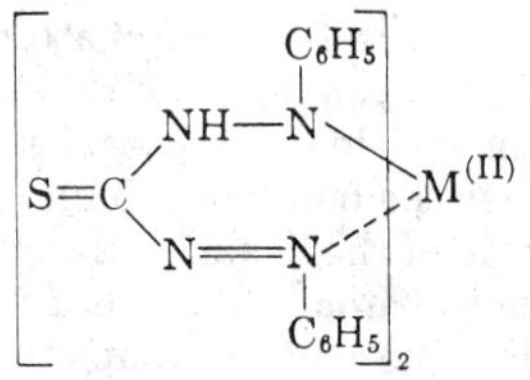

dithizone—divalent
metal complex

carbazone) forms colored complexes with many metals and is useful in the estimation of trace quantities of lead and zinc (see Chapter 30). These two complexes are soluble in carbon tetrachloride or chloroform and can be extracted from aqueous solution, and determined colorimetrically, whereas the metal ions alone would not be extractable.

The complex of ferrous iron with *o*-phenanthroline or barium diphenylamine sulfonate is used as an indicator in titrations utilizing ceric sulfate. Nickel forms the well-known red complex with dimethylglyoxime. Aluminum and magnesium salts are often precipitated as their 8-hydroxyquinoline complexes.

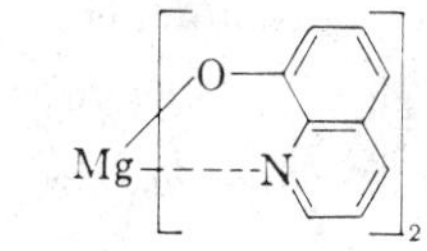

magnesium 8-hydroxyquinoline complex

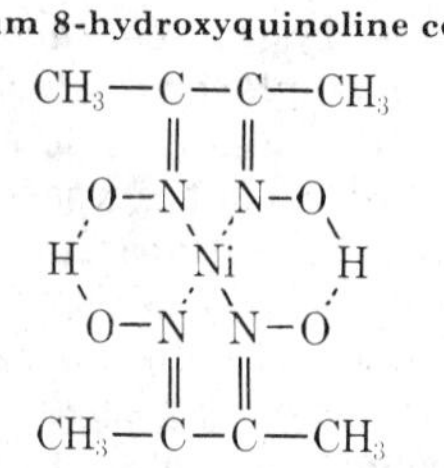

nickel dimethylglyoxime complex

Biological materials are often dependent on formation of metal chelates. The stabilization of insulin with zinc; the iron in heme, magnesium in chlorophyll, and cobalt in vitamin B$_{12}$ are examples of systems in which metal chelate complexes are essential for biologic activity. Many enzymes contain metals which are essential for the activity of the enzyme system. Removal of the metal, or lack of the metal, can inactivate the enzyme and therefore trace amounts of copper, cobalt, zinc, manganese, and molybdenum are required in human nutrition.

Olefin Complexes—A third kind of metal complex is known as the olefin type. One of the best known is *ferrocene* or dicyclopentadienyl iron. A single covalent bond appears to link the metal to the plane of each ring. The modern theories of bonding (atomic orbital and molecular orbital) acknowledge the existence of spatially directed valences when two atoms are brought together, this arising because of the engagement of electronic orbits originally separate in each atom. (Refer to Chapters 13 and 24 for an extensive discussion of bonding.)

In ferrocene, and other complexes of this nature, one π electron of each ring is used in bonding to the metal atom and

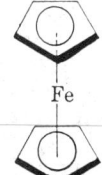

Butesin Picrate

the resultant rings now have the 4n + 2 pi electron configuration (n = 1) and exhibit aromatic character, as evidenced by lack of reaction with maleic anhydride and of certain spectral characteristics. An ionic-type bond is not indicated for ferrocene-like substances as they are nonelectrolytes. Due to the layer structure of the ring–metal complexes they are often referred to as "sandwich" compounds. Many metals also form complexes with straight-chain unsaturation. A complex of platinum with ethylene or styrene is known, and iron, palladium, mercury, silver, iridium complexes are quite stable.

Little direct application of the metal–olefin complexes to the pharmaceutical field is in evidence at the present time. These complexes, however, are thought to enter into the polymerization of ethylene and propylene to form the well-known polyethylene and polypropylene.

Molecular Complexes (Addition Compounds)

Complexes formed by the union of two organic molecules by other than covalent bonds generally utilize hydrogen bonds or other electrostatic forces in their formation. For the purpose of this presentation it is expedient to consider such molecular complexes in either of two categories: (1) charge-transfer complexes; (2) hydrogen-bonded complexes.

Charge-Transfer Complexes—This type of complex functions by sharing of π electrons. The complexing agent, usually a polynitro aromatic hydrocarbon, must by nature be an electron acceptor and, to some degree, be capable of accepting a negative charge from the nucleus of the agent being complexed. Other theories involve the presence of a dipole-induced dipole, dipole–dipole, or ionic complex (a donor molecule shares an electron pair with the acceptor by a process similar to a Lewis acid–base interaction). It is evident that the bonding structures in these complexes are not yet clearly defined.

In some cases proof of the existence of such complexes is quite simple to demonstrate. If picric acid is distributed between a chloroform–water mixture and increasing concentrations of an aromatic compound, soluble only in chloroform (such as naphthalene), is added, the concentration of picric acid in the chloroform layer increases and that in the aqueous layer decreases. The picric acid–naphthalene complex that is formed causes an increase in picric acid concentration in the organic phase.

Various physical studies such as solubility measurements, distribution studies, vapor pressure measurements, melting point–composition relationships, spectral characteristics, dipole moment measurements, and viscosity isotherms have been helpful in elucidating the nature of aromatic complexes.

The most common type of aromatic complex exists between the aromatic hydrocarbons and polynitro compounds, usually formed in a 1:1 ratio. Picric acid, styphnic acid, and *sym*-trinitrobenzene form complexes with many polynuclear, aromatic hydrocarbons. The stability of the complex appears to be governed by two factors: the number of electron-attracting groups on the nitro compound and by the ring complexity and presence of electron-releasing groups on the second component.

A well-known example of such a complex in use in pharmacy today is butesin picrate, a local anesthetic, consisting of a complex of two molecules of butyl *p*-aminobenzoate with one molecule of picric acid.

Hydrogen-Bonded Complexes—A large number of compounds containing the —O—H or —N—H linkage exhibit hydrogen bonding (for a discussion of the hydrogen bond, see page 217). Abnormalities of physical constants such as boiling point of alcohols, carboxylic acids, and amines provides evidence for such bonding. Dimethyl ether and ethanol both have the same molecular formula, C_2H_6O, and hence the same molecular weight, but ethanol boils at a temperature over 100° higher than that of ether. This phenomenon is easily explained by the presence of hydrogen bonding with ethanol, which increases its *apparent* molecular weight. The hydrogen bond is considered an example of dipole–dipole interaction in which the "positive" hydrogen atoms of one molecule are electrostatically attracted to the "negative" oxygen atoms of a second molecule, thus:

Hydrogen bonds are relatively weak bonds, having about 10% of the strength of an ordinary covalent bond. The solubility of water-soluble organic compounds is achieved by solvation involving hydrogen bond formation.

Complexation will occur only if intermolecular hydrogen bonds are formed. It is equally possible, with compounds such as salicylic acid, for several intramolecular species to exist.

The pharmaceutical literature dealing with hydrogen bonding is extensive, and even a cursory treatment is beyond the range of this chapter. A brief discussion of a few examples of this kind of bonding must suffice.

Saccharin forms water-soluble complexes with theophylline, caffeine, and various amides and phenols. The stability and appearance of pharmaceutical preparations such as aqueous solutions of benzocaine, tetracaine, or procaine are enhanced by the formation of complexes with caffeine. Caffeine is also known to complex, eg, with sulfonamides, *p*-aminobenzoic acid, and phenobarbital. The complexes aminophylline (theophylline ethylenediamine), theophylline sodium acetate, theobromine sodium salicylate, citrated caffeine, and caffeine sodium benzoate are well-known medicinal agents. Fig 14-2 illustrates the delayed absorption of theophylline in a subject who received the drug as a 2:1 complex with phenobarbital, compared to theophylline given as a simple physical mixture with phenobarbital and to theophylline given alone.

Polymeric materials such as polyethylene glycols, polyvinylpyrrolidone, and sodium carboxymethylcellulose, which may be present in suspensions, ointments, emulsions, suppositories, and some solid dosage forms, have also been shown

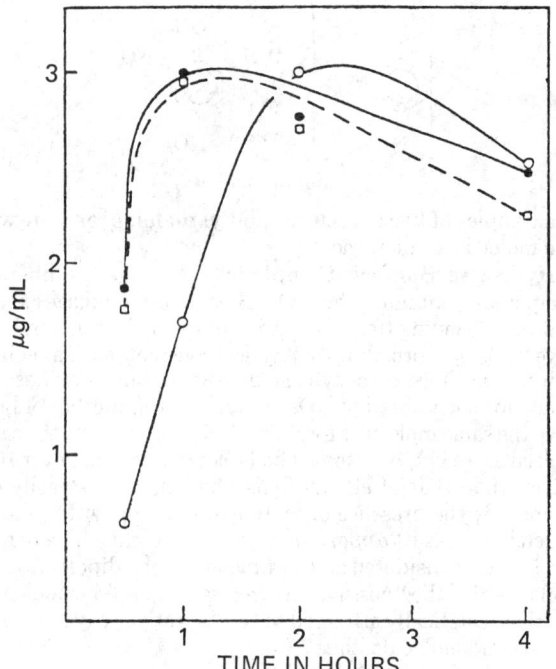

Fig 14-2.   Theophylline serum levels in a subject following a 100 mg oral dose of theophylline.   Key: ● alone; ☐ mixed with phenobarbital; ○ complexed with phenobarbital.   (From Bettis, *et al*[1]).

to complex with a wide variety of drugs. Such interactions may result in solubilization, precipitation, a change in the "effective" concentration, or an alteration in bioavailability.

Changes in the physicochemical properties of drugs due to complexation can also affect the release of the drug from topically applied dosage forms. For example, the inclusion of 10% w/w salicylic acid in various ointment bases containing benzocaine has been shown to increase, decrease, or not affect the diffusion of the benzocaine from the ointment, depending on the nature of the ointment base. The observed effects were attributed to the formation of a benzocaine–salicylic acid complex, with properties different from those of the parent compound.

No-Bond (Inclusion) Complexes

As previously stated, the inclusion compounds or complexes are characterized by the lack of adhesive forces between the components of the complex. They arise from the ability of one compound spatially to enclose another. It is not possible, in most cases, to predict the formation of an inclusion compound between two selected components.

Clathrates—Inclusion compounds, which are formed by the envelopment of a molecule of a "guest" compound in the cage-like hollow space formed by combination of several molecules of the "host" compound, are known as *clathrates* (Latin, *clathri*, lattice). This type of compound is frequently nonstoichiometric. Clathrates can be depicted by ⒸM), in which the molecular component M is trapped during the formation of cage C from molecules or other complexes which exist in the same solution with it. One component may be a solid, liquid, or gas retained within the cages of the host; it may be released by dissolving, heating, or grinding the clathrate. Such complexes are usually prepared by crystallization of the host substance from a solution containing the guest component.

In the formation of such a compound four factors are involved: (1) there is no apparent means of linking C and M;

(2) component C must be capable of cage formation; (3) M must be replaceable by other molecules that fit into the cages (but not by chemically analogous compounds if their molecules are of unsuited size); (4) the ratio of the cage-forming component C to the number of cavities available to contain M limits the composition, but the composition may vary since not all cavities may be occupied.

Many applications for this novel type of complex have already been demonstrated. Because of the ability of hydroquinone to clathrate inert gases, krypton-85 (radioactive, a β-emitter) can be successfully trapped to provide a solid, easily handled source of the gas. Thiophene can be removed from benzene using Werner complexes as the clathrate host. Synthetic metal-alumino silicates, advertised as "molecular sieves," are available; these materials can be used to store gaseous, volatile, and toxic materials, to dry gases, and to separate gaseous mixtures. It is also possible to "load" the host material of the sieve with substances such as volatile oils, germicidal agents, detergents, and pesticides and provide a convenient, dry material for ease of formulation. The clathrated guest can later be removed by some simple, physical process.

Channel-Lattice Complexes—This type of inclusion complex occurs primarily when the host component crystallizes in such a way as to form channel-like spaces in the crystal lattice. The guest molecule then must be of a shape which will fit into the voids or channels in the lattice. Urea, amylose, the zeolites, and other compounds will complex other materials in this fashion. Since the channels are formed by crystallization of the host, in spring-like spirals, the nature of the guest component is usually limited to long, unbranched, straight-chain compounds. Urea will complex *n*-octane, but not *iso*-octane. Choleic acids also function as host components in which the guest components are held in canals situated lengthwise to the crystals. Digitonin–cholesterol complexes are examples of the choleic acid type of complex.

The potential and present applications of the channel-lattice complexes are many. Separation of petroleum products, prevention of oxidation (vitamin A palmitate is successfully complexed with urea and thereby protected), separation of optical isomers (several host compounds have steric features that allow complexation of only one enantiomorph of a racemic mixture), and many analytical uses are illustrative of such applications. The well-known starch–iodine color has been shown to involve formation of an inclusion compound of iodine in the central channel of the screw-like starch molecule. Other compounds such as the flavones, coumarin, benzophenone, benzamide, and barbituric acid are also capable of giving the blue iodine-addition compound.

Intercalation Compounds—Although termed "compounds" in the scientific literature, this type of material closely resembles charge-transfer complexes. For a typical complex, the *intercalant*, or guest material, is diffused between layers of carbon atoms, hexagonally oriented, as in graphite, to form alternate monoatomic or monomolecular layers of guest and host. The resulting complex of charged sheets, caused by the transfer of electrons between host and guest, is metallic in nature and exhibits properties markedly different from either constituent.

A wide range of chemical species can be intercalated into graphite depending on the direction of electron transfer. Alkali metals and earths donate electrons, whereas halogen acids or other electrophiles remove electrons from the carbon host.

Uses for this type of complex are currently quite limited, but since the potential exists to form "compounds" with extremely large surface-to-volume ratios, a promising future in catalysis or other phenomena requiring exposure of tremendous surface area is evident.

Ion-Exchange Compounds

As mentioned previously, ion-exchange phenomena may not strictly belong in a chapter on complexation. However, since ion exchange is regarded as both an absorption and adsorption process, there is some rationale for its inclusion.

Three theories, all of which may be simultaneously applicable, are proposed to explain ion-exchange processes.

1. **Crystal-Lattice Theory**—If an ionic solid is considered to be completely dissociated, the surface ions are bound to the lattice with a lower binding energy than are internal ions of the same species since the surface ions are not completely surrounded by ions of the opposite charge. When the solid is placed in a polar solvent, extensive solvation of the surface ions further reduces their binding energy with the result that marked dissociation from the lattice occurs. Addition of a foreign electrolyte may then cause an exchange process between the surface ions and those of the same charge of the foreign electrolyte. The ease of replacement at a fixed number of exchange sites is proportional to a number of factors, including the nature of the forces binding the surface ion to the lattice, the charge of the exchange ion, the concentration of exchange ions, the accessibility of lattice ions, the sizes of the two ions, and the solubility effects.

2. **Double-Layer Theory**—The presence of two rigid charged layers at the surface of the exchanging material is assumed in this theory; the inner layer is fixed, the outer diffuse, with no sharp boundary. The concentration of ions at the diffuse layer is in equilibrium with those in solution. Addition of a foreign ion to the solution upsets the equilibrium and some of the new ions will enter the outer, diffuse layer, by exchange. In the double-layer exchange mechanism the number of exchange sites is not fixed, being dependent both on the concentration of the foreign ion being exchanged and on the pH of the solution.

3. **Donnan Membrane Theory**—In this theory the interface between the solid, exchange material and liquid is considered a membrane exhibiting an unequal distribution of charges on either side; diffusion through the membrane establishes equilibrium. Disruption of the equilibrium by addition of a foreign electrolyte necessitates a rebalancing, with subsequent exchange of ions through the membrane.

All of the theories are similar, as they require that the exchange must observe the laws of electrical neutrality; they differ in the postulated position and origin of the exchange site. This exchange site is a fixed, nondiffusible, ionic grouping capable of forming an ionic bond with small, diffusible ions of opposite charge.

Modern ion-exchange materials are usually synthetic, being formed from an inert, insoluble polymer of high molecular weight containing suitable ionic groupings as integral parts of the polymer structure. However, such natural materials as clays, zeolites, and ultramarines are still used to advantage. The resins are of the cation-exchange type (formed with acidic groups as part of the polymer) or anionic type (with basic exchange groups). The exchange groups may be of varying degrees of basicity or acidity, selected to suit the intended application. Amino groups are usually the reactive sites of the anion type of exchange resins, while sulfonic acid, carboxylic acid, or phenolic groups are reactive sites in cation exchange resins.

All exchange materials have a finite capacity for exchange limited by the number of exchange sites available. After a period of use the exchange process ceases because of the loss of exchange sites; the material then must be regenerated by a reversal of the exchange technique. For example, if a resin is used to soften water through replacement of sodium ions on the resin with calcium or magnesium ions from the water, the process will eventually stop when sodium ions are no longer available. If the resin is now treated with a concen-

trated solution of sodium ions, reversal of the process occurs, resulting in replacement of calcium by sodium and regeneration of the ion-exchange material.

It is imperative that the pharmacist caution patients on low-salt or salt-free diets to avoid use of water treated by home water softeners, since the sodium content may approach 60 mg per 8-oz glass of water, for an initial hardness of 30 grains per gallon (an average value).

There are many pharmaceutical and medical uses for ion-exchange materials, besides that of their important use in water conditioning. For example, they are employed in the purification of alkaloids, vitamins, hormones, serological solutions, and viruses. Potassium penicillin may be converted to the sodium salt and streptomycin sulfate to the chloride by processes of ion exchange.

Ion-exchange principles have also been used in the development of controlled-release dosage forms (see Chapter 92). For example, in one product, a cationic drug (eg, dextromethorphan) is bound to a nonabsorbable ion-exchange polymer, which is subsequently coated by a semipermeable coating. The gradual release of the drug occurs when ions such as potassium and sodium present in the gastrointestinal tract diffuse through the coating and displace the bound drug.

Some therapeutic applications of ion-exchange compounds include: use of kaolin, a natural ion-exchange material, in diarrhea; removal of body potassium in hyperkalemia, with cation exchangers such as sodium polystyrene sulfonate; bulk laxative action of resins that swell in the gastrointestinal tract; removal of waste materials in impaired kidney function; anion-exchange resins which remove bile acids from the intestinal tract to prevent irritation of the bowel.

This latter application may also result in a decreased absorption of certain acidic drugs (eg phenylbutazone, warfarin, phenobarbital) and thus it is recommended that such drugs should be administered 1 hr before or 4–6 hr after the ion-exchange resin to reduce any effect on the bioavailability of these drugs.

Complex Equilibria

The formation of a complex may significantly affect the physicochemical properties of the drug and/or complexing agent. When the complex results from the interaction of a drug and protein, such as albumin or globulin, the pharmacodynamics and pharmacokinetics of the drug may also change, as will be discussed in a later section.

Typically, complexation is described as an equilibrium reaction between drug (D) and complexing agent (C),

$$m(D) + n(C) \underset{\rightleftharpoons}{\overset{K_s}{}} (D)^m (C)^n$$

where m and n refer to the stoichiometry of the complex. Further, an equilibrium, association, or stability constant (K_s) is used to characterize the strength of the complex, eg, for an $m:n$ complex,

$$K_s = \frac{(D_m C_n)}{(D)^m (C)^n}$$

The quantitation of complex formation involves the determination of the values of m, n and K_s. Several of the commonly employed experimental techniques to study complex formation also serve to illustrate the effects of complexation. Changes in the solubility of a drug, or changes in the distribution of a drug between two immiscible phases, can occur when a drug is complexed. For example, Fig 14-3 illustrates a system which initially contains a suspension of p-hydroxybenzoic acid. When no ethyltheophylline is present, the concentration of acid is equal to the intrinsic solubility of the acid in water. As the ethyltheophylline concentration is in-

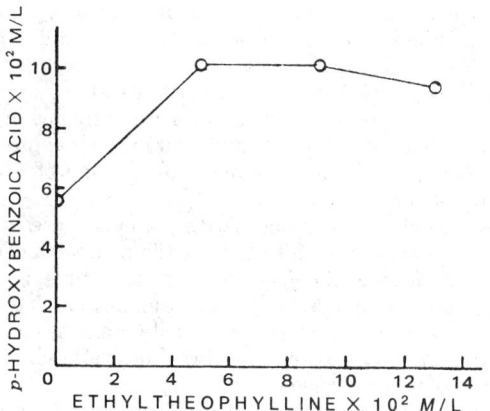

Fig 14-3. The apparent solubility of *p*-hydroxybenzoic acid in water at 30° as a function of complex formation with ethyltheophylline[2].

creased, the amount of total acid (free and complexed) increases until the solution is saturated with respect to both free acid and complex. As additional ethyltheophylline is added, there is no change in the total dissolved acid concentration, since newly formed complex precipitates. Finally, the total concentration of acid decreases with the addition of more ethyltheophylline, at a point where there is no longer any undissolved acid, as the acid in solution is complexed and precipitated. Of course, if the complex itself is totally insoluble, the amount of acid present in solution would remain unchanged with the addition of complexing agent, since the complex would precipitate as it was formed, up to the point where all excess acid was in solution. Thereafter, the acid concentration would begin to decrease as additional complexation occurred. Similarly, one can determine the distribution of a drug and drug-complex between two immiscible phases, as a function of the extent of complexation, and the solubility of the complexing agent and drug-complex in each of the phases.

As stated earlier, the formation of a complex may increase, decrease or have no effect on the stability of a given drug. Thus, the rate of drug degradation has also been employed to evaluate the extent to which the drug is complexed by a second agent. For example, Fig 14-4 illustrates an increase in the degradation rate of dicloxacillin as a result of the formation of a 1:1 complex between the drug and sucrose.

Other studies have demonstrated enhanced stability of certain drugs, such as local anesthetic esters in the presence of caffeine, and greater stability of epinephrine in the presence of boric acid, which acts by chelating metal ions which can catalyze oxidation.

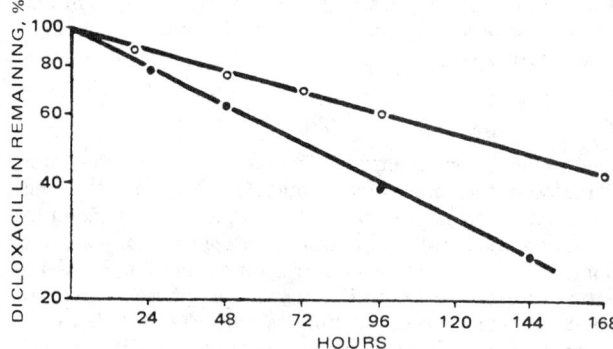

Fig 14-4. Change in potency of sodium dicloxacillin monohydrate, during aging in a 0.01 *M* solution at pH 7, 45°. Key: O, in absence of sucrose; and ●, in presence of 0.0175 *M* sucrose.[4]

Protein Binding

Many types of biochemical and pharmacologic processes involve interactions between specialized functional proteins and lower molecular weight compounds such as drugs. Examples include enzyme–substrate complexes and drug–receptor complexes, in which there is considerable structural specificity. Also of importance are interactions between small molecules and protein constituents of blood. This latter type of interaction has been the subject of extensive research. Most drugs are bound to some extent by plasma proteins such as albumin, globulin, α_1-acid glycoprotein or lipoproteins. It is generally known that such binding can influence the disposition of a drug in the body in terms of distribution and elimination, as well as affect the pharmacodynamic properties of a drug. Other related interactions between a drug and erythrocytes, blood vessels, or tissue binding sites may also be of great importance, but have not been studied as extensively. Binding studies involving plasma proteins have progressed more rapidly because of the availability of purified proteins. In contrast, studies of the binding of drugs to tissues is much more difficult since attempts to isolate the binding species result in a destruction of their integrity.

A large number of publications describing protein binding studies are found in the literature. The studies resulted, either directly or indirectly, from the desire to answer one or more fundamental questions relating to protein binding: "How many? How tightly? Where? Why? What of it?" Thus, many of the reported studies were physical–chemical in nature and were oriented to determining:

1. The maximum number of small molecules which could be bound by a protein molecule.
2. The magnitude of the association constant or constants which characterized the association.
3. The chemical and conformational nature of the binding sites on the protein.
4. The nature of the intermolecular forces which were responsible for interaction.

Other studies attempted to assess the importance of protein binding as it relates to the action and fate of specific drugs in the body.

Mass Law Expressions—Protein binding, like other types of complexation, results from reversible associations and can be described by conventional mass law expressions. It should be recognized, however, that a protein is a macromolecule composed of many hundreds of amino acids linked together to form the primary protein structure.

It is the side-chains of the composite amino acids that possess the functional groups which are responsible for attracting and binding small molecules. For example, epsilon amino groups of certain of the many lysine residues and phenolic hydroxyl groups of some tyrosine residues have been implicated in the binding of a number of drugs by albumin.

It is apparent that many and varied sites, capable of binding, can exist on the same macromolecule. Mass law expressions used to treat and interpret data are, therefore, somewhat more complicated than those encountered in more familiar situations such as the ionization of weak electrolytes. Many studies have demonstrated that the sites can be divided into classes with different binding abilities but that, usually, sites within a class possess the same intrinsic affinity for a small molecule. Fundamental studies are designed to gain some idea about the classes of sites involved, the number of sites in a particular class, and the strength of binding to a site.

The simplest case involves a reversible interaction to form a 1:1 protein–small molecule complex; ie,

$$\text{Protein} + \text{Drug} \underset{\rightleftarrows}{\overset{K}{}} \text{Protein:Drug}$$

The mass law expression, defining this behavior, is

$$K = \frac{(PD)}{(P)(D)} \qquad (1)$$

where K = association constant, (PD) = concentration of the 1:1 complex, (P) = concentration of unbound protein, and (D) = concentration of unbound small molecule.

Experimental methods used to study binding behavior usually permit determination of the concentrations of bound and unbound small molecule. The total concentration of protein is usually known or can be determined readily. It is convenient, for the purpose of data treatment, to define an experimentally determinable quantity, r, as the average number of small molecules bound per mole of protein; ie, for a 1:1 complex,

$$r = \frac{(PD)}{(P)_t} \qquad (2)$$

where $(P)_t$ = total concentration of protein in the binding system. The quantity r can be defined in terms of K and (D) by the following expression:

$$r = \frac{K(D)}{1 + K(D)} \qquad (3)$$

A more complex case is the interaction of a small molecule species with two sites on the protein. The simplest situation here is that involving two sites that belong to the same class and behave independently; ie, both sites possess the same intrinsic affinity for the small molecule and the binding of a small molecule to one site does not influence the binding behavior of the remaining site. It should be recognized that three identifiable complexes can result from this situation. For convenience, these can be symbolized by $-PD$, $DP-$, and DPD. Unbound protein is symbolized by $-P-$ to indicate that two sites can participate. The appropriate relationship becomes:

$$r = \frac{2K(D)}{1 + K(D)} \qquad (4)$$

In the general case of n equivalent and independent sites,

$$r = \frac{nK(D)}{1 + K(D)} \qquad (5)$$

The terms n and K are known as *binding parameters* with n being the number of sites in a class and K being the intrinsic association constant that characterizes the strength of the binding between the small molecule and a site in the class under consideration.

Suppose, as a further extension, that two entirely different classes of sites exist on the protein molecule and that, as before, all sites are independent and sites within a class are equivalent.

An expression for r for this case can be derived,

$$r = \frac{n_a K_a(D)}{1 + K_a(D)} + \frac{n_b K_b(D)}{1 + K_b(D)} \qquad (6)$$

which describes binding to n_a sites in the "a" class, characterized by an intrinsic association constant K_a for that class of sites. Similarly, the "b" class of sites is also described by a set of binding parameters, n_b and K_b.

A general expression which describes binding to "i" different classes of sites is

$$r = \sum_{i=1}^{i} \frac{n_i K_i(D)}{1 + K_i(D)} \qquad (7)$$

Experimental Methods—A variety of approaches have been employed to study protein binding. Some of these are based on changes in the physicochemical properties of the small molecule and/or the protein when binding occurs.

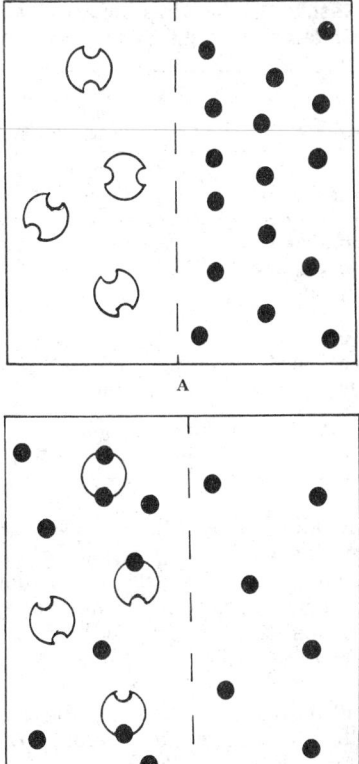

Fig 14-5. An equilibrium dialysis experiment. The large open symbols represent protein molecules. The small enclosed circles represent molecules of a low molecular weight compound capable of being protein-bound. A: Before equilibration; B: after equilibration.

Examples include changes in the solubility, partitioning, or spectral properties of the interactants. More typically, binding studies involve the use of some type of barrier membrane which retains protein and permits free passage of the unbound small molecule. The two most common techniques are equilibrium dialysis and ultrafiltration. The dialysis method is illustrated in Fig 14-5. The two sides of the dialysis cell are separated by a semipermeable membrane, such as cellophane. A protein solution is placed on one side and a solution of drug, usually in a physiological buffer, is placed on the other side. The membrane is impermeable to the protein and drug bound to the protein, while unbound drug freely diffuses across the membrane. Following an equilibration period, samples are withdrawn from both sides of the cell and assayed for drug content. If binding has occurred, the total drug concentration (free and bound) will be greater on the protein side than on the side without protein (free only). At equilibrium the concentration of free drug will be the same on both sides of the membrane, as shown in Fig 14-5. Table I illustrates typical data which could be obtained during a study of the binding of a small molecule, caffeine, to a purified plasma protein (albumin) obtained from an animal source.

Another widely used technique is ultrafiltration. Here, a solution containing protein and small molecule is filtered through a membrane that is impermeable to the protein and protein-bound complexes, using centrifugation, pressure or vacuum. A small volume of filtrate is collected and assayed to yield the concentration of unbound small molecule, and the unfiltered portion is assayed to obtain the total concentration of unbound and bound species. A number of devices based on this principle are now commercially available to facilitate the determination of free drug concentration in blood samples

Table I—Results Obtained in a Study of the Binding of Caffeine by Bovine Serum Albumin

	Solution within membrane	Solution outside membrane
Volume	10 mL	10 mL
Concentration of albumin	$2.8 \times 10^{-4}\,M$	0
Concentration of caffeine before equilibration	0	$1 \times 10^{-4}\,M$
Concentration of caffeine after equilibration	0.7×10^{-4}	0.3×10^{-4}
Concentration of unbound caffeine is, therefore	0.3×10^{-4}	0.3×10^{-4}
Concentration of bound caffeine is, therefore	0.4×10^{-4}	0

$$r = \frac{0.4 \times 10^{-4}}{2.8 \times 10^{-4}} = 0.143$$

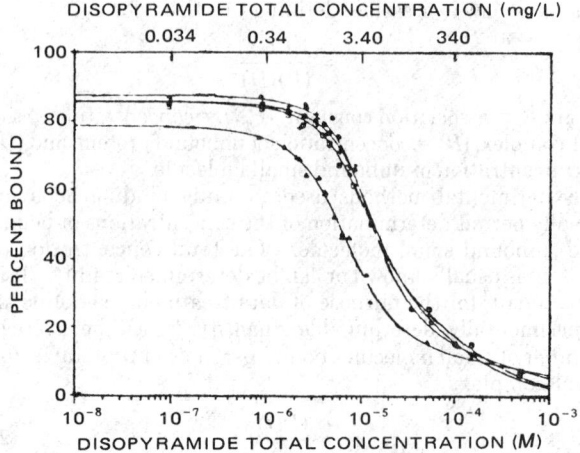

Fig 14-6. Percentage of disopyramide bound to protein in serum from four normal volunteers, using equilibrium dialysis. (After Lima, *et al*[4]).

obtained from individuals who have received treatment with specific drugs. It should be emphasized that while the principles involved in the use of dialysis and filtration techniques are relatively simple, careful attention must be paid to possible errors, such as binding of the drug to the membrane, which can result in erroneous calculations of the binding parameters.

Experimental Results—Many investigators report the results of protein binding studies in terms of the fraction of total small molecule present in bound form. This fraction is usually symbolized by β; ie,

$$\beta = \frac{(D)_b}{(D)_t}$$

where $(D)_b$ is the concentration of bound small molecule and $(D)_t$ is the total concentration of small molecule in the protein–small molecule system. For example, for the data of Table I:

$$\beta_{\text{caffeine}} = \frac{0.4 \times 10^{-4}}{0.7 \times 10^{-4}} = 0.571$$

which means, of course, that 57.1% of the caffeine in the protein compartment is present in the form of a protein complex. It should be emphasized, however, that β is not a constant but changes depending on both the concentration of protein and small molecule in the system under study and that a β value does not provide a reflection of the intrinsic affinity of a small molecule for a protein. This can be appreciated readily by considering a binding system in which only one class of sites on the protein participates in the binding. The binding behavior for such a case is described by Eq 5, which in a slightly different form is

$$\frac{(D)_b}{(P)_t} = \frac{nK(D)}{1 + K(D)} \tag{8}$$

It is instructive to define β in terms of n and K,

$$\beta = \frac{1}{1 + \dfrac{(D)}{n(P)_t} + \dfrac{1}{nK(P)_t}} \tag{9}$$

It is apparent from Eq 9 that β exhibits a dependency on both the protein and small molecule concentrations and can, for the same binding system, vary depending on the design of the experiment. If, for example, a system is studied that contains a relatively low protein concentration and a relatively high small molecule concentration, then a low β value will result. Conversely a high β value would be generated if the protein concentration is large compared to the small molecule concentration.

Thus *in vitro* binding studies, which use protein or drug

concentrations that are either lower or higher than the concentrations normally present *in vivo*, may result in calculated values for β that are of limited value in gaining insight into the effect of protein binding *in vivo*. Similarly, binding studies conducted *in vitro*, with a physiologically realistic protein concentration, may not be applicable to the prediction of binding *in vivo* for patients with hypoproteinemia. Further, it should be recognized that *in vitro* binding studies involving a purified protein may exhibit a binding profile that is different from that present *in vivo*, when the drug must compete with metabolites or endogenous materials for the available binding sites.

A good example of the magnitude of changes in β with drug concentration is shown in Fig 14-6 for disopyramide. Recent studies have demonstrated significant intersubject differences in the binding of this drug, which is primarily bound to plasma α_1-acid glycoproteins. Further, the value of β ranges from approximately 90% at relatively low plasma drug concentrations, to about 20% at elevated drug concentrations. It should be obvious that a single value for β cannot be employed to characterize the protein binding of disopyramide.

In addition to intersubject differences in binding, certain disease states have been shown to affect the protein binding of a variety of drugs. For example, phenytoin binding has been shown to be lower in uremic patients, and in general, drug binding declines in such patients. Patients with liver dysfunction may also exhibit altered protein binding, although specific effects are less well defined compared to renal disease. Obviously, conditions resulting in hypoalbumenia will also decrease the binding of drugs which interact with albumin.

A more meaningful way to characterize binding behavior is by the binding parameters, n and K. A knowledge of these values permits the calculation of β at any protein–small molecule combination. An approach to determining n and K values might be intuitively anticipated by examining Eq 5, for as (D) becomes very large, r approaches n; ie, the protein becomes saturated with small molecule. Determination of r at very high concentrations of small molecule relative to that of the protein would be expected to yield an estimate of n. With a knowledge of n, K could be determined from studies conducted under concentration conditions well below those resulting in saturation. Unfortunately, this approach is not usually practical or possible because solubility limitations frequently preclude attainment of very high concentrations of many low-molecular-weight compounds. It is, therefore, necessary to use indirect graphical methods to obtain estimations of n and K. Eq 5, for example, can be rearranged to the form

$$1/r = 1/nK(D) + 1/n \qquad (10)$$

This form of the binding equation was first proposed by Klotz who suggested that a plot of $1/r$ vs $1/(D)$ should yield, in the case of binding by one class of sites on a protein, a straight line with the ordinate intercept being $1/n$ and the slope, $1/nK$. One disadvantage of the "Klotz plot" is that experimental points obtained at low (D) values are excessively weighted and the plot can mask behaviors that might occur at high values of (D). For example, participation of a second class of sites with a lower K might not be apparent if the data are treated by a Klotz plot. Scatchard, therefore, recommended a different plot based on a different rearrangement of Eq 5:

$$r/(D) = nK - Kr \qquad (11)$$

A "Scatchard plot" results when $r/(D)$ is plotted as a function of r. In the case of one class of binding sites such a plot should be linear with a slope of $-K$ and extrapolation to the abscissa yields an intercept with the value of n (when $r/(D) = 0, r = n$). Furthermore, extrapolation to the ordinate yields an intercept with the value of nK (when $r = 0, r/(D) = nK$). Participation of secondary classes of sites is quite apparent when data are presented as a Scatchard plot. Such an occurrence is manifested by marked upward curvature of the plot. It can be shown from Eq 7 that when more than one class of sites are responsible for binding, curvature should result and that the ordinate and abscissa intercepts are $\Sigma\, nK$ and $\Sigma\, n$.

Unfortunately, many drugs appear to be bound to more than one class of binding sites, and the Scatchard and Klotz plots may be inaccurate for the estimation of the binding parameters because of the difficulty inherent in characterizing a nonlinear relationship. Recent reviews of protein binding should be consulted for a discussion of alternate methods employed for more accurate data treatment.

Extent of Occurrence—Two protein binding review articles, published during the period of 1968–1976, cited in excess of 850 references. Most drugs that have been studied have exhibited at least some affinity for plasma proteins. A brief summary of a few of the major drugs which have been evaluated are given in Table II. This summary demonstrates the wide range of binding which can occur. Of course, the caution expressed in the previous section regarding the use of single values for percent binding should be kept in mind when considering these data.

Significance—It has long been suggested that it is the free, unbound drug concentration which is responsible for the pharmacologic action of a drug. This can be appreciated by considering the lack of permeability of bound drug across a biologic membrane to a site of action, or the binding of a drug resulting in a hindrance of the interaction between the drug and a receptor site or enzyme. This concept can explain for some drugs why there may appear to be a lack of relationship between total plasma drug concentration and pharmacologic response. Of course, if the percent of drug bound remains relatively constant over the range of drug concentrations normally present in the body, free and total drug concentrations may both parallel drug action. It should be noted that most analytical procedures employed to determine drug concentrations in blood or plasma actually measure total (bound and free) drug concentration, unless some type of dialysis or filtration procedure is used to separate the free drug.

The distribution of a drug within the body will also be affected by binding. If a drug is confined primarily to the vascular space, it is said to have a relatively low volume of distribution. Such a drug may be very polar, and thus, have difficulty diffusing across biologic membranes. Or, the drug may be highly bound to plasma proteins, with the resulting formation of a drug–protein complex that cannot diffuse across such membranes. In the case of a drug which is highly

Table II—Percent Binding of Drugs to Plasma Proteins

% Bound	Drug
99	Warfarin
95	Furosemide
	Amitryptyline
	Chlorpromazine
	Dicloxacillin
93	Propranolol
	Tolbutamide
	Valproic Acid
90	Digitoxin
	Indomethacin
	Phenytoin
	Sulfisoxazole
70	Quinidine
	Erythromycin
65	Tetracycline
	Hydrochlorothiazide
60	Meperidine
50	Lidocaine
	Phenobarbital
45	Methotrexate
25	Digoxin
20	Cimetidine
	Ampicillin
15	Procainamide
0	Isoniazid

bound to the plasma proteins, and negligibly bound to sites in the extravascular space, the apparent volume of distribution may approach a lower limit of approximately 3 L, which is the plasma volume for an average man. In contrast, if a drug is less completely bound to plasma proteins, and/or is significantly bound to tissue proteins, the drug will exhibit a large apparent volume of distribution. The net result is that for equivalent doses, a drug with a low apparent volume of distribution will exhibit higher plasma drug concentrations than a drug with a higher apparent volume of distribution, assuming all other pharmacokinetic factors are equivalent. The binding and distribution characteristics of a drug are of importance because the site of drug action is usually not within the systemic circulation. For example, the use of chemotherapy in the treatment of tumors may depend on the diffusion of the drug into the tumor cells. Further, the degree of binding will influence the distribution of a drug into the lymph and the cerebral spinal fluid.

Martin[5] has provided, by means of a simple model, an excellent quantitative visualization of the potential effects of binding in plasma on drug distribution in the body. His model was essentially that of a large dialysis system at equilibrium; i.e., he assumed that drug in the body was distributed into two compartments: plasma with a volume of 3 L and a second compartment composed of the remaining body water with a volume of 39 L.

Martin further assumed that binding occurred only in the plasma compartment and resulted from the interaction between albumin, present at a concentration of $5 \times 10^{-4}\, M$, with drug to form nondiffusible 1:1 complexes. As in a dialysis system, unbound drug was considered to be in equilibrium between the two compartments. He then performed calculations related to the binding of four hypothetical drugs whose interactions with albumin could be characterized by associ-

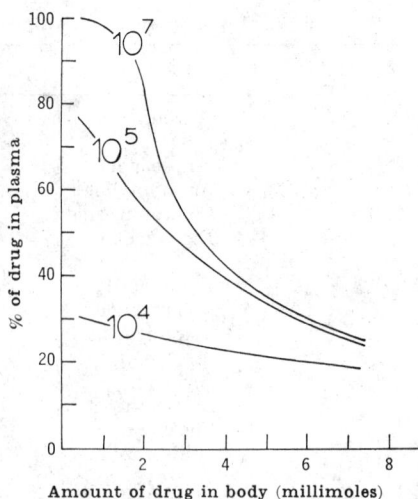

Fig 14-7. A plot, based on theoretical considerations, which illustrates the potential influence of plasma-binding on the distribution of drug between plasma and other aqueous compartments in the body. Each curve represents a different value of K (after Martin[5]).

ation constants (K) of 10^4, 10^5, 10^6, and 10^7 L mole^{-1}, respectively. For each drug he assumed a concentration of unbound drug (D) and calculated, first, the total concentration of drug in plasma (D)$_t$ by an equation directly derivable from Eq 9:

$$(D)_t = (D) \left\{ 1 + \frac{(P)_t}{1/K + (D)} \right\} \qquad (12)$$

He then calculated for each value of (D): (a) the amount of drug in the body = 39 (D) + 3 (D)$_t$; (b) percent of drug free in the body = 42 (D) × 100/(39(D) + 3(D)$_t$); and (c) percent of drug in plasma = 3(D)$_t$ × 100/(39(D) + 3(D)$_t$). The results of such calculations were presented in graphical form such as those illustrated by Figs 14-7 and 14-8.

It is apparent from these representative theoretical curves that binding can influence drug distribution in the body and that the magnitude of the effect will depend on both the strength of association and the dosage of drug. For example,

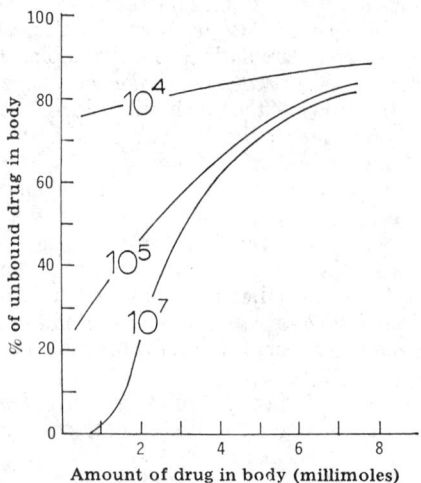

Fig 14-8. A plot based on theoretical considerations, which illustrates the potential influence of plasma-binding on the distribution of drug between bound and unbound forms in the body. Each curve represents a different value of K (after Martin[5]).

a strongly bound drug such as that with a K of 10^7 will, at low dosage levels, be concentrated primarily in the plasma compartment. However, at higher dosage levels, the fraction of drug in the plasma will be markedly reduced.

Martin also emphasized another characteristic attributable to the plasma binding of drugs with a high affinity for proteins; that there is a dosage range within which small increases in dose result in relatively large increases in the amount of drug in the body that is not bound. He noted that this behavior can have interesting manifestations on dose–response characteristics and pharmacokinetic properties of such drugs. His treatment additionally emphasizes that binding to plasma proteins will have an appreciable effect on drug distribution only if the strength of binding is quite high. For example, with a drug having a K of 10^4, the "fraction bound" in plasma can be 83.4% but, nevertheless, 73% of the total dose is present in the body in the unbound form.

It must be emphasized, however, that this model ignores any effect of binding in the nonvascular space. Thus, while it is useful to illustrate changes in drug disposition which may occur as a result of protein binding in the vascular space, it cannot be employed quantitatively to predict drug disposition *in vivo*. For example, Martin's treatment indicates an increase in the apparent volume of distribution as the fraction of drug bound to the plasma proteins decreases with increasing amount of drug in the body. However, if the binding is very similar in both the vascular and nonvascular space, changes in binding will have no effect on the apparent volume of distribution. Similarly, if the extent of binding in the nonvascular space is the predominant consideration, a decrease in this binding can result in a decrease in the apparent volume of distribution.

Protein binding may also have an effect on the elimination of a drug from the body. Hepatic elimination and renal elimination, including both glomerular filtration and active secretion, depend on free, unbound drug concentration in the plasma. The magnitude of the effect of binding will be determined by how efficiently the eliminating organ acts on the drug. For example, if nearly all of the drug is removed from the blood as it circulates through the kidney or liver, the drug is said to be highly extracted, and the elimination process may actually be governed by the rate at which the drug is presented to the organ, ie, rate of blood flow. For such drugs which are efficiently eliminated (eg, propranolol), a decrease in the extent of protein binding will have little effect on the clearance of the drug from the blood. However, if the drug is poorly extracted by the eliminating organ, an increase in the fraction of drug in the unbound form can increase the clearance of the drug (eg, warfarin, phenytoin). A good example of the effect of binding on elimination kinetics has recently been reported for disopyramide. As was shown in Fig 14-6, the fraction of drug bound ranges from approximately 20–90% for plasma concentrations which may be present in patients receiving this drug. Because more drug is unbound at higher plasma concentrations, it has been shown that the apparent volume of distribution and clearance of total drug increase significantly at higher drug concentrations. One of the results of this finding is that disopyramide plasma concentrations show less than proportional increases with increasing dose of drug.

Competitive Binding—Many studies have demonstrated that two different compounds can compete for the same protein binding sites. Thus, the fraction of a drug which is bound at a given concentration may decrease when a second compound or competitor is introduced into the system. A simple equation can be developed to illustrate this situation. Assume a single binding site which can interact with a drug (D) and a competitor (C), with the binding of each being characterized by association constants K_D and K_C, respectively:

$$(D) + (P) \underset{\rightleftarrows}{\overset{K_D}{}} (PD)$$

$$(C) + (P) \underset{\rightleftarrows}{\overset{K_C}{}} (PC)$$

then,

$$r_D = \frac{(D)_b}{(P)_t} = \frac{(PD)}{(P) + (PD) + (PC)}$$

$$= \frac{K_D(D)}{1 + K_D(D) + K_C(C)} \qquad (13)$$

This equation is identical to Eq 5, except for the $K_C(C)$ term. The relationship predicts that the moles of drug bound per mole of protein (r_D) will decrease as the $K_C(C)$ term increases. Thus the extent of displacement will depend on both the competitor concentration and the affinity of the competitor for the binding site(s).

While it is often easy to demonstrate competitive binding *in vitro*, the displacement of bound drug by a competitor species *in vivo* is a more complicated situation. For example, the displacement may occur in the plasma, the tissues or both. When bound drug is displaced the increase in the unbound fraction will result in changes in the distribution of the drug within the body, and may also influence the elimination of the drug, as discussed earlier. Further, the fraction of drug and competitor bound may change significantly, but to different degrees, as a function of their concentration. Finally the rates of elimination of the drug and the competitor will effect their relative concentrations, and there can be large intersubject variability in the extent to which a given compound is protein bound.

The following are examples of a few drug–drug interactions which have been reported to represent displacement of bound drug by a second therapeutic agent: elevation of serum digoxin concentrations, due at least in part to displacement of tissue-bound drug by quinidine; displacement of phenytoin by acidic drugs such as salicylates, valproic acid, sulfonylureas, and phenylbutazone; and the displacement of protein-bound warfarin by phenylbutazone, resulting in an increased anticoagulant effect. Circulating endogenous compounds, eg, bilirubin, which are bound to protein can also be displaced by drugs. Thus salicylates, sulfonamides, and phenylbutazone can increase unbound bilirubin plasma concentrations and result in increased diffusion of bilirubin into the CNS (kernicterus). This situation is of particular importance for indi-

viduals, such as neonates, with limited or impaired bilirubin conjugating processes. Two other types of competitive binding have also been noted, which can lead to artifacts in the interpretation of binding data. Heparin is frequently employed in the collection of blood samples. Heparin can contribute to an apparent increase in plasma free fatty acid concentrations, and the latter compounds can displace protein-bound drug. Similarly, certain blood collection devices made of rubber or plastic may contain additives such as plasticizers which are released when in contact with the blood. These compounds can compete with certain drugs, particularly basic drugs like quinidine, lidocaine, and propranolol, for protein binding sites. The result may be artificially elevated free drug concentrations, or increased uptake of the drug into the erythrocyte, resulting in measured plasma drug concentrations that are erroneously low.

In summary, the characterization of interactions between drugs and protein binding sites continues to be an area of active research. The determination of the strength and extent of the interaction is now routinely determined as part of the pharmacologic investigations of the properties of new therapeutic agents. The degree to which such interactions contribute to the pharmacokinetic and pharmacodynamic properties of a drug, and the potential for displacement of protein-bound drug by other compounds, is most significant for those drugs which are highly bound to plasma and/or tissue binding sites.

References

1. Bettis JW, *et al: Am J Hosp Pharm 30:* 240, 1973.
2. Higuchi T, *et al:* in Reilley CN, ed: *Advances in Analytical Chemistry and Instrumentation*, Wiley-Interscience, New York, 133–140, 1975.
3. Hem SL, *et al: J Pharm Sci 62:* 267, 1973.
4. Lima JJ, *et al: J Pharmacol Exp Ther 219:* 741, 1981.
5. Martin BK: *Nature 207:* 274, 1965.

Bibliography

Connors KA, *et al: J Pharm Sci 55:* 772, 1965.
Gibaldi M, *et al: Pharmacokinetics.* 2nd ed Marcel Dekker, Inc, New York, 1982.
Martin AN, *et al: Physical Pharmacy.* 3rd ed Lea & Febiger, Philadelphia, 1983.
Meyer MC, *et al: J Pharm Sci 57:* 895, 1968.
Rowland M, *et al: Clinical Pharmacokinetics*, Lea & Febiger, Philadelphia, 1980.
Vallner JJ: *J Pharm Sci 66:* 447, 1977.

CHAPTER 15

Thermodynamics

Arthur Cammarata, PhD

Professor of Physical Medicinal Chemistry
School of Pharmacy, Temple University
Philadelphia, PA 19140

The term *thermodynamics* implies literally an area of science concerned with mechanical action produced by heat. Historically, the subject of thermodynamics developed as a consequence of efforts to produce an efficient heat engine, but early in the development it became evident that the concepts of thermodynamics were of much greater generality. It is now recognized, notably through the efforts of Gibbs,[1] that chemical and physical changes can be interpreted in terms of the energy requirements for these processes and that the energy changes accompanying such transformations are predictable through the use of thermodynamic principles. Since pharmaceutical scientists are primarily interested in the energy changes accompanying a chemical or physical conversion, *energetics* is a more descriptive word for the content of this chapter. Further discussion than is possible here can be found in texts.[2,3]

Heat—A person can sense whether an object is hot or cold either visually or by contact with the object. A bar of metal removed from a furnace may glow red, and as it cools the color dulls progressively until there is no visual evidence that the bar is still hot. If the bar is touched, however, the resulting sensation indicates immediately whether the bar is hot or cool. If the hot bar of metal is placed in contact with a cooler one, after a short period of time both bars will be found to be equally warm. Heat has been lost from the hot bar and gained by the cold bar, and this transfer of heat stops when the bars are of equivalent warmth; ie, when *thermal equilibrium* is established.

The transfer of heat from one object to another is analogous to a system in which two compartments separated by a porous membrane contain differing levels of water. The compartment having the higher water level loses water to the second compartment until the water level on both sides of the membrane is the same; ie, in this case, until hydrostatic equilibrium is established. Using this analogy, it could be said that a hot substance contains an amount of heat Q_H which is greater than the amount of heat Q_C contained by a cold substance,

$$Q_H > Q_C \tag{1}$$

For every small increment of heat lost from the hot substance, $-dQ_H$, a corresponding amount of heat must be gained by the cold substance, $+dQ_C$,

$$-dQ_H = +dQ_C \tag{2}$$

When heat is no longer transferred, the two substances are in thermal equilibrium, so that

$$Q_H - \Delta Q_H = Q_C + \Delta Q_C \tag{3}$$

where ΔQ is the total amount of heat that has been transferred. A representation of the conditions suggested by Eqs 1 to 3 is shown in Fig 15-1.

Temperature—While varying amounts of heat may be experienced through the senses, a more accurate measure is needed if quantitative relationships between heat and other forms of energy are to be developed. A measure of heat is called *temperature* and the instrument used in the measurement of temperature is a *thermometer*. To arrive at a graduated indication of the heat of a substance, known as a *temperature scale*, a property of a substance that varies as the substance is heated or cooled may be used. The thermal expansion or contraction of gases and liquids is useful in this regard. The temperature scale used in thermodynamics is derived using a gas thermometer, while liquid thermometers are used in most practical situations. It is seldom realized, however, that the graduations found on a liquid thermometer are based on temperatures determined with a gas thermometer; i.e., liquid thermometers are calibrated against a gas thermometer.

Consider the problem of measuring the temperature of a liquid with a thermometer. According to Eq 3, the heat of the liquid and the heat of the thermometer are the same only after thermal equilibrium has been established. But, in order for thermal equilibrium to be attained, the liquid will have gained or lost an amount of heat ΔQ. This would seem to indicate that the temperature measured by the thermometer is not the true temperature of the liquid. However, if the heat contained by the liquid, Q_L, is very much greater than the amount of heat that has to be exchanged with the thermometer, ΔQ_T, to attain thermal equilibrium

$$Q_L \gg \Delta Q_T \tag{4}$$

the measured temperature may be considered the true temperature of the liquid.

Thus, introducing Eq 4 into Eq 3, when the liquid is initially cooler than the thermometer

$$Q_L = Q_T - \Delta Q_T \tag{5}$$

and, when, the liquid is initially hotter than the thermometer,

$$Q_L = Q_T + \Delta Q_T \tag{6}$$

The liquid functions as a *heat reservoir* in much the same way as the Atlantic Ocean is a heat reservoir when an ice cube is dropped into it. The ice cube melts, but the ocean is still as warm as it was initially.

For example, a gas thermometer may be used to measure the heat of the liquid. This thermometer may be a cylinder containing a gas, and the pressure of the gas provides an in-

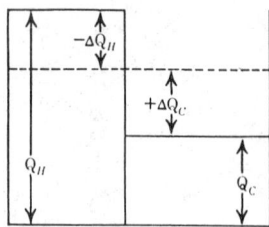

Fig 15-1. The conditions preceding (—) and following (- - -) the transfer of heat.

dication of the heat of the liquid. If the liquid is hot, the pressure of the gas is high; if the liquid is cold, the pressure of the gas is low. Because the gas pressure is directly related to the heat of the liquid, one may say that there is a linear relation between the pressure P and the heat of the liquid Q_L,

$$P = aQ_L + b \tag{7}$$

Since the heat of a substance is said to be given by its temperature, t, it may also be stated that there is a linear relationship between heat and temperature, so that

$$Q_L = ct + d \tag{8}$$

The substitution of Eq 8 into Eq 7 gives the relationship between pressure and temperature:

$$P = kt + I \tag{9}$$

Hence, as Fig 15-2 shows, a plot of P against t is a straight line of slope k having an intercept on the P-axis given by I.

Pressure is measured in units of atmospheres, but to this point no indication has been provided of the units for temperature. Temperature units may be defined by measuring the pressure of the gas when the gas thermometer is immersed in a mixture of ice and water and, subsequently, in boiling water (at sea level). For each pressure reading there is a corresponding temperature, according to Eq 9, so that at the *boiling point*

$$P_b = kt_b + I \tag{10}$$

while at the *ice point*

$$P_i = kt_i + I \tag{11}$$

By taking the difference between Eqs 10 and 11, a relation is obtained which gives the number of pressure units corresponding to a set number of temperature units between the boiling and ice points of water

$$P_b - P_i = k(t_b - t_i) \tag{12}$$

Thus, by defining $t_i = 0$ and $t_b = 100$, pressure is related to a temperature scale of 100 units. This is the centigrade or Celsius scale, and temperatures measured in these units are given the symbol °C. Alternatively, the definition $t_i = 32$ and $t_b = 212$ could be made, in which pressure is related to a temperature scale of 180 units. This is known as the Fahrenheit scale and these units are given the symbol °F.

The Celsius and Fahrenheit temperature scales are related by the equation

$$\frac{°C - 0}{°F - 32} = \frac{100}{180} \tag{13}$$

so that temperature measured in °F can be converted to °C using Eq 13 written in the form

$$°C = \frac{5}{9}(°F - 32) \tag{14}$$

Alternatively, temperature measured in °C can be converted to °F using the equation

$$°F = \frac{9}{5}°C + 32 \tag{15}$$

A more meaningful temperature scale, from a physical standpoint, is one which would avoid assigning negative heats to substances that are much colder than the ice point of water. Eq 9 can be used as a basis for constructing a temperature scale fulfilling this requirement by setting the condition that when the pressure is zero the temperature is also zero. This new scale, called the *absolute* temperature scale, is thus based on the relation (Boyle's law)

$$P = kT \tag{16}$$

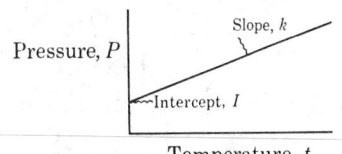

Fig 15-2. The linear relationship between temperature and pressure.

in which T is the temperature according to this scale. The absolute temperature scale is also known as the Kelvin scale, and the units are given the symbol °K. Each unit of the Kelvin scale is taken to be equal in magnitude to a Celsius unit, so that interconversions between the two scales are readily accomplished using

$$T(°K) = t(°C) + 273.16 \tag{17}$$

By international agreement, the terminal constant in Eq 17 is the number of Celsius units between absolute zero ($T = 0$ °K) and the *triple point* of water, ie, the temperature where water in all its forms (solid, liquid, and gas) at a pressure of 1 atm is in a state of equilibrium.

Heat Capacity—It is known from Eq 3 that in order for two substances, A and B, to come to thermal equilibrium a total amount of heat ΔQ must be transferred between them; ie,

$$-\Delta Q_A = +\Delta Q_B \tag{18}$$

The heat that is transferred is the difference of the heat content at a stage preceding the heat transfer Q_I and the heat content after thermal equilibrium has been established Q_F. This difference can be determined by a measurement of temperature alone since, by the use of Eq 8,

$$Q_F - Q_I = C_v(T_F - T_I) \tag{19}$$

or

$$\Delta Q = C_v \Delta T \tag{20}$$

The absolute temperature scale is used for reasons already discussed. The constant C_v in Eqs 19 and 20 is characteristic of a substance and is termed its *heat capacity*. Since the magnitude of this constant is proportional to the quantity of material present, it is convenient to define a heat capacity/unit mass of substance. The unit of mass may be 1 g or 1 mole of material. In the former case *specific heat* has been defined; in the latter case *molal heat capacity* has been defined.

The subscript v attached to the constant in Eqs 19 and 20 designates that the temperature change of a substance is measured under conditions such that the substance underwent no change in volume. A gas contained in a closed cylinder, for example, maintains a constant volume as its temperature is varied, since the walls of the cylinder limit the expansion of the gas. In many instances, however, a change in temperature causes a change in the volume of a material. For example, a glass of water at 70°C (158°F) contains a greater volume of water than when it is at 10°C (50°F). As, under ordinary circumstances, this expansion takes place against the constant pressure of the atmosphere, it is appropriate to ask whether there is a difference between heat capacities determined under conditions of constant volume (C_v) and heat capacities determined under conditions of constant pressure (C_p).

For convenience, consider a closed cubic container containing a gas to have one of its faces in contact with a face of a second cubic vessel containing an equivalent amount of the same gas (Fig 15-3). Assume that one of the containers is at a higher temperature than the other, and let the lower temperature container have a movable piston for one of its faces.

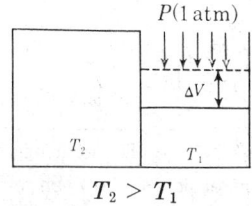

$$P(1 \text{ atm})$$

$$T_2 > T_1$$

Fig 15-3. A constant-volume container in contact with a constant-pressure container. The dotted line indicates the position of the movable piston after thermal equilibrium is established between the containers.

As heat is transferred to the container of lower temperature, the piston is forced to rise against the constant pressure of the atmosphere due to the thermal expansion of the gas within this container. Hence, when thermal equilibrium is established between the vessels, the container with the movable piston will have the gas confined in a larger volume than it had initially.

Making use of Eq 18, it may be said that to attain equilibrium an amount of heat given by Eq 21 has been transferred between the containers.

$$-\Delta Q_v = +\Delta Q_P \tag{21}$$

However, for the constant-pressure container, a portion of the total heat absorbed was absorbed by the gas and another portion was used in moving the piston against the atmosphere. This may be represented by

$$\Delta Q_P = \Delta Q_p + \Delta Q_w \tag{22}$$

where ΔQ_p is the heat absorbed by the gas and ΔQ_w is the heat used in moving the piston. Substitution of Eq 22 into Eq 21 yields

$$-\Delta Q_v = \Delta Q_p + \Delta Q_w \tag{23}$$

Since heat capacities refer only to the heat absorbed by a substance, Eq 20 may be substituted into Eq 23 to obtain

$$C_v \Delta T = C_p \Delta T + \Delta Q_w \tag{24}$$

or

$$C_v = C_p + \frac{\Delta Q_w}{\Delta T} \tag{25}$$

Thus, heat capacities determined at constant volume differ from heat capacities determined at constant pressure by an amount corresponding to the heat absorbed to move against the atmosphere/degree temperature change.

Work—By definition, work W is the force F needed to move an object a given distance, Δs, and the equation relating work to force and distance is

$$W = F \Delta s \tag{26}$$

The container discussed in the previous section whose piston moved against a constant pressure was doing work, since the pressure P exerted on the face of the piston has units of force/unit area. Thus, if A is the area of the piston, the work done by the piston is

$$W = PA \Delta s \tag{27}$$

or, recognizing that the change in volume ΔV is given by $A \Delta s$:

$$W = P \Delta V \tag{28}$$

Since heat is required to perform this work, it can be said that

$$W = \Delta Q_w \tag{29}$$

and, therefore,

$$\Delta Q_w = P \Delta V \tag{30}$$

It should be noted that Eq 29 is the mathematical form of Joule's statement that heat and *mechanical work* are interconvertible. Mechanical work is the work done on or by a system.

For an ideal gas where

$$PV = nRT \tag{31}$$

a change in the volume of the gas when the pressure is maintained constant necessarily implies a change in temperature. That is, when there is a volume change of an ideal gas, Eq 31 can be written

$$P \Delta V = nR \Delta T \tag{32}$$

when the pressure P and the number of moles of gas n are maintained constant. The quantity R is the gas constant (0.0821 L-atm/°K-mole, 1.99 cal/°K-mole). Thus, substituting Eq 32 into Eq 30, it is found that Eq 25 may be given by

$$C_v = C_p + nR \tag{33}$$

For the more general case where the state of a substance (solid, liquid, or gas) does not have to be specified, Eq 30 can be substituted into Eq 23 to obtain

$$-\Delta Q_v = \Delta Q_p + P \Delta V \tag{34}$$

or, from Eq 28,

$$-\Delta Q_v = \Delta Q_p + W \tag{35}$$

First Law of Thermodynamics—From the concepts of heat, temperature, and work which have been developed, and which are summarized by Eqs 34 and 35, the first basic law of thermodynamics can be obtained. In its simplest form, the *first law of thermodynamics* states that *energy may be converted from one form to another, but it cannot be created or destroyed.* Another way of saying this is to state that the first law recognizes the *Law of Conservation of Energy* and deals with all forms of energy as they appear either as heat or work.

Before presenting the mathematical form of the first law, it is suitable at this point to redefine certain of the terms appearing in Eq 34. For the heat absorbed at constant volume ΔQ_v, a new quantity ΔE, called the *internal energy*, will be defined such that

$$\Delta E = E_F - E_I = \Delta Q_v \tag{36}$$

In Eq 36, E_I is the internal energy of a substance at an initial temperature T_I and E_F is the internal energy of the same substance at a second final temperature (where equilibrium may be established) T_F. This new quantity can be determined by a knowledge of heat capacities since the substitution of Eq 20 into Eq 36 provides the relation

$$\Delta E = C_v \Delta T \tag{37}$$

Substituting Eq 36 into Eq 34, there is obtained

$$-\Delta E = \Delta Q_p + P \Delta V \tag{38}$$

which is given equivalently by

$$(E_F - E_I) + P(V_F - V_I) = -\Delta Q_p \tag{39}$$

Grouping the terms of Eq 39 yields

$$(E_F + PV_F) - (E_I + PV_I) = -\Delta Q_p \tag{40}$$

and if another quantity H, called *enthalpy*, is defined by

$$H = E + PV \tag{41}$$

Eq 40 can be written

$$\Delta H = H_F - H_I = -\Delta Q_p \qquad (42)$$

Since the negative sign in Eq 42 signifies a heat loss, a change in sign would designate that heat is being absorbed. Thus, it could be said that enthalpy, defined by

$$\Delta H = H_F - H_I = \Delta Q_p \qquad (43)$$

(note the change in sign), represents heat *absorbed* at constant pressure, and this heat can be obtained from a knowledge of heat capacities using the relation

$$\Delta H = C_p \Delta T \qquad (44)$$

Eqs 36 and 43 are presented to emphasize that in thermodynamics internal energy and enthalpy are terms used in place of the word heat since these terms specify, by definition, the conditions under which heat is measured.

For the condition where heat is absorbed at constant pressure, Eq 40 can be written

$$(E_F + PV_F) - (E_I + PV_I) = \Delta H \qquad (45)$$

or, in a form equivalent to Eq 38,

$$\Delta E = \Delta H - P\Delta V \qquad (46)$$

The *First Law of Thermodynamics* may be obtained by removing the restriction of constant pressure from the right side of Eq 46,

$$\Delta E = DQ - DW \qquad (47)$$

In Eq 47, DQ and DW still represent heat and work, respectively, but they are written in this manner to designate that the conditions for their measurement are to be specified before the equation is used. In essence, the reason DQ and DW can remain unspecified is that for any set of conditions one wishes to impose on a given system, the system can always be compared to a second system maintained at a constant volume. One such comparison is made in Fig 15-3 for the imposed condition of constant pressure.

In applying the First Law to a given experimental situation, it is necessary to note initially whether the experimental system exchanges heat with or can do work on its surroundings. A material in a perfectly insulated thermos bottle, for example, cannot exchange heat with its surroundings and under these *adiabatic* conditions $DQ = 0$. When heat can be exchanged with the surroundings,

$$DQ = C\Delta T \qquad (48)$$

and a subscript p or v is applied to the molar heat capacity depending on whether the exchange occurs at constant pressure or constant volume.

Work can be done under conditions of constant pressure or constant volume, so that to take into account these two possibilities

$$DW = P\Delta V + V\Delta P \qquad (49)$$

When the pressure is constant $\Delta P = 0$ and

$$DW = P\Delta V \qquad (50)$$

whereas, when the volume is constant $\Delta V = 0$ and

$$DW = V\Delta P \qquad (51)$$

A collapsed metal container caused to return to its original shape by increasing the pressure within it does not have its internal volume changed but yet it does work against the surroundings.

An alternative form for Eq 49 can be given by assuming that the work is done on or by an ideal gas. By use of the ideal gas law,

Table I—Some Relations Obtained Using the First Law
$$\Delta E = DQ - DW$$

Conditions	Relation
Constant pressure ($\Delta P = 0$)	$\Delta H = C_p \Delta T$
Constant volume ($\Delta V = 0$)	$\Delta E = C_v \Delta T - V\Delta P$
Constant volume; no work ($DW = 0$)	$\Delta E = C_v \Delta T$
Adiabatic ($DQ = 0$)	$\Delta E = -DW$
Constant temperature ($\Delta T = 0$); ideal gas	$\Delta E = 0; DQ = DW$
Adiabatic; constant pressure	$\Delta E = -P\Delta V$

$$DW = (nR\Delta T)_p + (nR\Delta T)_v \qquad (52)$$

so that at constant pressure or constant volume

$$DW = nR\Delta T \qquad (53)$$

With Eqs 48, 49, and, for an ideal gas, 53, the appropriate form of the First Law can be deduced for a variety of experimental conditions. However, in applying these relations care must be taken in recognizing whether the First Law is to refer to a substance or to a process involving the substance. For example, at constant temperature (ie, $\Delta T = 0$) the internal energy of an ideal gas is given by

$$\Delta E = C\Delta T - nR\Delta T \qquad (54)$$

or

$$\Delta E = 0 \qquad (55)$$

If the ideal gas is allowed to expand against a constant pressure while at a constant temperature, then

$$\Delta E = 0 = DQ - DW \qquad (56)$$

or

$$DQ = P\Delta V \qquad (57)$$

In Table I some expressions obtained by the use of the First Law are shown.

Thermochemistry—The study of the heat effects accompanying chemical reactions and certain physical processes such as solution or change of state is called thermochemistry. Thermochemical data are usually obtained by carrying out reactions in calorimeters and measuring the heat absorbed or evolved according to the temperature change of a surrounding weighed amount of water. Heat changes measured in closed calorimeters, where the volume remains constant, correspond to ΔE, while heat changes measured in open calorimeters, where the pressure remains constant, correspond to ΔH. When, during the course of a reaction, there is no change in volume, or only a very small change, $\Delta E = \Delta H$. Thus, it is possible to express thermochemical data in terms of ΔE or ΔH for any specific reaction or process. If the process is *exothermic* (ie, is accompanied by the evolution of heat) ΔE or ΔH has a negative value; conversely, if the process is *endothermic* (ie, is accompanied by the absorption of heat) ΔE or ΔH has a positive value.

Heat of Combustion—The heat evolved when 1 gram-formula weight of a substance undergoes combustion with oxygen to form water and carbon dioxide is called the *heat of combustion*. The reactants and products of the combustion are considered to be in the form that they would ordinarily be at 25°C and 1 atmos pressure. These conditions constitute the *standard state* of the substances involved in the reaction. Thus, the combustion of ethanol in an atmosphere of oxygen to form water and carbon dioxide in an open calorimeter corresponds to the equation

$$C_2H_5OH\ (l) + 3O_2\ (g) = 2CO_2\ (g) + 3H_2O\ (l);$$
$$\Delta H°_{298} = -326{,}700\ cal$$

where the state of the substances, gaseous g or liquid l, is indicated in parenthesis. Since the substances are in their standard states, the heat measured for the process ΔH has affixed to it a superscript degree sign and a subscript designating the temperature in °K chosen as standard.

Hess's Law of Heat Summation—In 1840 Hess pointed out that the heat absorbed (or evolved) in a given chemical reaction is the same whether it takes place in one step or in several steps. This principle has wide utility, since it provides a means of calculating heat quantities that cannot be determined directly by experiment.

A good illustration of the use of Hess's Law is provided by the calculation of the heat of reaction of carbon (as graphite) when it undergoes combustion to carbon monoxide. This heat of combustion is difficult to measure experimentally because of the complication of the simultaneous formation of carbon dioxide and the incomplete reaction of carbon. It is relatively much easier to measure the heat of combustion of carbon

$$C(graphite) + O_2\ (g) = CO_2\ (g);\ \Delta H°_{298} = -94,052\ cal$$

and of carbon monoxide

$$CO\ (g) + \frac{1}{2}O_2\ (g) = CO_2\ (g);\ \Delta H°_{298} = -67,636\ cal$$

and to obtain the desired quantity by subtracting the second equation from the first

$$C(graphite) + \frac{1}{2}O_2\ (g) = CO\ (g);\ \Delta H°_{298} = -26,416\ cal$$

Heat of Formation —The *heat of formation*, symbolized $\Delta H°_f$, of a substance is the heat evolved when 1 gram-formula weight of the substance is produced from its constituent elements, the reactants and product being taken as in their standard states. The heat of reaction of carbon and oxygen in forming carbon dioxide is properly a heat of combustion as well as a heat of formation. In calculating heats of reaction by Hess's Law, one usually obtains the heats of formation of the respective products and reactants from tables (*cf*, Table II) and arrives at the heat of reaction using the relation

$$\Delta H° = \Sigma\Delta H°_{f,products} - \Sigma\Delta H°_{f,reactants} \qquad (58)$$

where Σ designates that the sum of $\Delta H°_f$ for each of the products or the reactants is taken. As an example, consider the calculation of the heat of reaction for the production of acetic acid from methane and carbon dioxide

$$CH_4\ (g) + CO_2\ (g) = CH_3CO_2H\ (l)$$

$$\begin{array}{ccc} \Delta H°_f = & \Delta H°_f = & \Delta H°_f = \\ -17,889 & -94,052 & -116,400 \\ cal & cal & cal \end{array}$$

The heat of reaction is found to be

$$\Delta H° = (-116,400\ cal) - [(-17,889\ cal) + (-94,052\ cal)]$$

or

$$\Delta H° = -4,459\ cal$$

Thus, if the reaction was to occur as written there would be an evolution of 4,459 cal of heat.

Table II—Heats of Formation for Some Compounds at 25°C

Compound	$\Delta H°_f$, kcal/mole
$H_2O\ (l)$	-68.317
$H_2O\ (g)$	-57.798
$NO\ (g)$	21.600
$CO\ (g)$	-26.415
$CO_2\ (g)$	-94.052
$CH_4\ (g)$	-17.889
$C_2H_5OH\ (l)$	-66.356
$CH_3CO_2H\ (l)$	-116.4

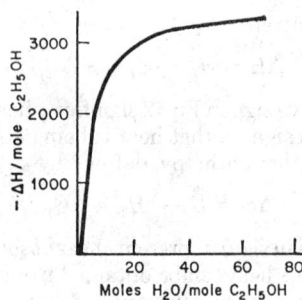

Fig 15-4.   Integral heat of solution of ethyl alcohol in water (0°C).

Heat of Solution—When a specified amount, conventionally 1 gram-formula weight, of a solute is dissolved in a solvent, a quantity of heat called the *heat of solution* is evolved or absorbed. The heat of solution of a given solute–solvent system is generally not constant but varies with the volume of the solvent to which a specified amount of solute is added. Fig 15-4 illustrates the variation in the amount of heat evolved when 1 gram-formula weight of ethanol is added to differing amounts of water.

There are three ways of expressing heats of solution, and each of these may be determined from plots such as is shown in Fig 15-4. The *integral heat of solution* is the heat absorbed when 1 gram-formula weight of solute is dissolved in enough water to form a solution of specified concentration. In Fig 15-4, this is the value of ΔH for any given dilution of the alcohol solution. The *differential heat of solution* is the heat absorbed when a quantity of solute so small as to cause no significant change in concentration is added to a solution of a specified concentration. This quantity is obtained from the slope of the curve in Fig 15-4 at any specified dilution of the alcohol solution. The *heat of solution at infinite dilution* is the maximum value the heat of solution approaches as the volume of solvent is increased. The practically constant value approached in Fig 15-4 gives this quantity for an alcohol solution.

Heats of dilution are obtained from integral heats of solution by taking the difference between the integral heats of solution of two specified concentrations of a solute–solvent system. Compounds that form a hydrate with water have their *heat of hydration* given by the difference between the integral heats of solution of the solvated and nonsolvated solute.

Second Law of Thermodynamics—While all forms of energy can be converted completely into heat, only a fraction of heat energy can be converted into work. The efficiency of this latter conversion is the concern of the Second Law of Thermodynamics. From a theoretical consideration of a reversible cycle of operations performed on a machine whereby heat is converted into work, Carnot (1824) showed that the maximum proportion of work that can be obtained from heat is governed by the following equation, which constitutes a mathematical expression of the Second Law of Thermodynamics.

$$w_{max} = q_2\frac{(T_2 - T_1)}{T_2} \qquad (59)$$

In this equation w_{max} is the maximum work that can be obtained from q_2 units of heat supplied at absolute temperature T_2 to the "boiler" of a hypothetical engine of perfect mechanical efficiency with a "condenser" maintained at absolute temperature T_1. The fraction of heat converted into work—the so-called maximum theoretical efficiency of the process—is expressed by the ratio

$$\frac{w_{max}}{q_2} = efficiency \qquad (60)$$

The dependence of this efficiency on the temperature difference $T_2 - T_1$, as well as on the boiler temperature T_2, is illustrated by the following calculations of the maximum work obtainable from 1000 cal of heat supplied to a steam engine operating at (a) a boiler temperature of 100° and a condenser temperature of 25° and at (b) a boiler temperature of 150° (superheated steam) and a condenser temperature of 25°.

Substituting in Eq 59:

(a) $\quad w_{\max} = 1000 \dfrac{(373.1 - 298.1)}{373.1} = 201 \text{ cal}$

(b) $\quad w_{\max} = 1000 \dfrac{(423.1 - 298.1)}{423.1} = 295 \text{ cal}$

The greater efficiency of conversion of heat into work when the boiler temperature is high explains why superheated steam (steam under pressure) yields more work than the same amount of heat supplied as steam at a temperature of 100°. In either case the heat that is not converted to work is retained in the condenser system; none of it is destroyed. If the condenser temperature is reduced, more heat will be converted to work. Thus, if the temperature *could* be maintained continuously at absolute zero—which is, of course, a practical impossibility—all of a given quantity of heat supplied to the boiler could be converted to work.

Entropy—While the total amount of energy (and mass) in the universe is believed to be constant, none of it being created or destroyed, all the chemical and physical processes that occur spontaneously result in a decrease in the proportion of energy that is available for doing work or, conversely, an increase in the proportion of energy that is unavailable for doing work. (The reason why spontaneous processes occur is that the energy of the reacting system is at a higher level than it is when the process is completed.) The possibility is suggested that at some distant time in the future the energy of the universe will be unavailable for doing work because all of it has been degraded to a common level of intensity.

An important thermodynamic quantity that measures the increase in unavailable energy accompanying spontaneous reactions is *entropy*. For a reversible process in which heat DQ_{rev} at absolute temperature T is absorbed by a system (as when a substance changes from one physical state to another), the change in entropy, ΔS, is defined by the relationship

$$\Delta S = \frac{DQ_{\text{rev}}}{T} \qquad (61)$$

This equation may be used to calculate the increase in entropy when a definite amount of water, eg, 1 mole, at a temperature of 100°, is converted to steam at the same temperature. In this case DQ_{rev} is the amount of heat required to vaporize 18.02 g (1 mole) of water, which is 18.02 times 539.7 cal, the latter quantity being the number of calories required to vaporize 1 g of water at its normal boiling point. Substituting in Eq 61:

$$\Delta S = \frac{18.02 \times 539.7}{373.1} = 26.1 \text{ cal/°K}$$

The increase in entropy accompanying the melting of ice at 0° may be calculated similarly

$$\Delta S = \frac{18.02 \times 79.7}{273.1} = 5.26 \text{ cal/°K}$$

Entropy may be defined as the capacity factor of isothermally unavailable energy; when multiplied by the reference temperature, the product measures the amount of energy unavailable for doing work at the specified temperature. Entropy is sometimes described as being a measure of the randomness, disorder, or "mixed-upness" of a system. In every spontaneous process there is an increase in entropy and hence of the randomness or disorder of the system. To illustrate this aspect of entropy, consider the three states of matter—solid, liquid, and gas. The solid state of any substance represents the highest degree of orderliness of the molecules (or atoms or ions) composing the substance; when it is converted to a liquid by heating, the orderliness of arrangement of the molecules (or atoms or ions) is destroyed and their distribution becomes more random; when the liquid is converted to a gas, there results still greater disorder or mixed-upness of the molecules. The increase in randomness is expressed quantitatively in the examples above for calculating increase in entropy accompanying change of state.

When the temperature of a substance is raised by heating, without changing the state of the substance, the motion of the molecules (or atoms or ions) becomes more disordered, that is, the entropy is increased. To calculate the entropy change, the process may be considered as a series of steps in which an infinitesimal change of temperature, dT, increases entropy by an infinitesimal amount dS, according to the equation

$$dS = \frac{CdT}{T} \qquad (62)$$

where C is the molar heat capacity (essentially the heat absorbed in raising the temperature of 1 mole of the substance through 1°). The similarity of this equation to Eq 61 is obvious. In order to apply this equation to a finite process it must be used in its integral form

$$\Delta S = S_2 - S_1 = 2.303 \, C \log \frac{T_2}{T_1} \qquad (63)$$

As an example of the application of this equation, the increase in entropy of 1 mole (18.02 g) of water when it is heated from 10 to 20° may be calculated. As the specific heat of water is approximately 1 cal/g, it may be assumed that the molar heat capacity of water is 18.02 times the specific heat. The complete calculation is

$$\Delta S = 18.02 \times 2.303 \log \frac{293}{283}$$

$$= 0.62 \text{ cal/°K/mole}$$

Reversible Processes—The concept of a *reversible process*, used in a thermodynamic sense, is quite different from that of a *reversible reaction*, applied to chemical reactions. A reversible process, whether physical or chemical in nature, is one in which a system that has been displaced from equilibrium only minutely by an infinitesimal force may be restored to equilibrium by applying an infinitesimal force in the opposite direction. Any other manner of conducting the process results in more or less irreversibility of the process.

The work obtained by the isothermal expansion of an ideal gas under different conditions of irreversibility may be compared with the work obtained on reversible expansion to illustrate both the distinction between an irreversible and a reversible process and the difference in their respective quantitative effects. Consider 1 liter (L) of an ideal gas, maintained at a constant temperature of 0°C (273.1°K) and at an initial pressure of 10 atm, enclosed in a cylinder with a weightless, frictionless piston (capable of being locked in position) on which various weights may be placed, the atmosphere above the piston evacuated, and the piston released to permit expansion of the gas. On expansion the gas performs work equivalent to $P\Delta V$, where P is the *resisting* pressure (produced by the weights on the piston), and ΔV is the increase in volume on expansion. Five different ways of expanding the gas from its initial volume of 1 L to a final volume of 10 L will be considered, and the work obtained in each case calculated.

1. The gas is permitted to expand from 1 L to 10 L without any weights being placed on the piston.

$$w = P\Delta V = 0 \times (10 - 1) = 0 \text{ L-atm}$$

2. Weights equivalent to 1 atm pressure are placed on the piston, which is released, so that the gas expands to 10 L.

$$w = 1 \times (10 - 1) = 9 \text{ L-atm}$$

3. Weights equivalent to 2 atm pressure are placed on the piston, the gas expanding to 5 L (Boyle's law). The weights are then reduced to 1 atm, so that the gas expands to the final volume of 10 L.

$$w = \Sigma P \Delta V = 2 \times (5 - 1) + 1 \times (10 - 5)$$
$$= 13 \text{ L-atm}$$

4. Weights equivalent to 5 atm are placed on the piston, the gas expanding to 2 L; the weights are reduced to 2 atm, with an expansion of gas to 5 L; finally, the weights are reduced to 1 atm, with expansion to 10 L.

$$w = \Sigma P \Delta V = 5 \times (2 - 1) + 2 \times (5 - 2) + 1 \times (10 - 5)$$
$$= 16 \text{ L-atm}$$

5. On the basis of the foregoing evidence that the amount of work obtained increases with the load on the piston, it may be deduced that the maximum work will be obtained when the piston load is successively reduced so that it is always infinitesimally less than the pressure of the gas in the cylinder. The process is continued until the infinitesimal increases in volume bring the final volume of gas to 10 L. Such a process is reversible. The total work obtained in the process can be calculated exactly by the expression

$$w_{\max} = nRT \int_{V_i}^{V_f} dV/V = 2.303 \, nRT \log \frac{V_f}{V_i}$$

where V_f is the final volume, V_i is the initial volume, and n is the number of moles of gas enclosed in the cylinder (1/2.241). Substituting numerical values

$$w_{\max} = \frac{1}{2.241} \times 2.303 \times 0.08205 \times 273.1 \times \log \frac{10}{1}$$
$$= 23.02 \text{ L-atm}$$

Free-Energy and Work Functions—What force causes a physical or chemical change to occur spontaneously? Nearly a century ago it was believed that chemical change occurred in the direction of evolution of heat. While this is often true, it is not always the case, for some spontaneous reactions take place with absorption of heat. For systems of constant internal energy (E) and volume, change will occur in the direction in which entropy is increased. But what thermodynamic criteria determine the course of a reaction when temperature and pressure are constant, as is the case with most chemical reactions, or when temperature and volume are constant?

These criteria may be established by introducing two additional thermodynamic quantities: the *Helmholtz free energy* or *work function*, symbolized A (German, *arbeit*, work), and the *Gibbs free energy*, now designated G but formerly (and sometimes still) symbolized by F. Consider the internal energy, E, of a system to consist of a part, A, available for doing work, and the remainder unavailable for performing work, at temperature T. The latter quantity is represented by the product TS (see *Entropy*, page 203). Symbolically,

$$E = A + TS \tag{64}$$

and

$$A = E - TS \tag{65}$$

For systems at constant volume and temperature the driving force of any physical or chemical change resides in the component of the internal energy available for doing work, namely A. The validity of this statement may be developed mathematically as follows. When a system undergoes change, Eq 65 may be written

$$\Delta A = \Delta E - \Delta (TS) \tag{66}$$

at constant temperature this becomes

$$\Delta A = \Delta E - T \Delta S \tag{67}$$

If for ΔE is substituted its equivalent, $DQ - DW$, from the

First Law of Thermodynamics (Eq 47), we obtain

$$\Delta A = DQ - DW - T \Delta S \tag{68}$$

Since, in a reversible process, where maximum work is obtained, $DQ = T\Delta S$ (Eq. 61), the preceding equation may be simplified to

$$\Delta A = -w_{\text{rev}} \tag{69}$$

or

$$-\Delta A = w_{\text{rev}} \tag{70}$$

This equation indicates that useful work may be obtained when a system undergoes any change in which A at the beginning of the change is greater than A when the change is completed. This decrease of A, as expressed by either Eq 69 or 70, is a measure both of the capacity of a system to do work and of the driving force impelling the system to undergo spontaneous change in the direction of diminishing its *work capacity* or *function*. For systems at constant temperature and constant volume, a reaction will occur spontaneously only if ΔA has a negative value (or $-\Delta A$ has a positive value), signifying a loss in the capacity of the system to do work.

If a system at constant temperature increases in volume while under constant atmospheric pressure, the capacity of the system for doing work is reduced by an amount equivalent to the work of expansion against the atmosphere. The *net* work that can be obtained is given by

$$w_{\text{net}} = w_{\text{rev}} - P\Delta V \tag{71}$$

Of course, if the volume of the system decreases while it is undergoing a reaction at constant temperature and pressure, the ΔV term is negative, indicating that work equivalent to $P\Delta V$ is done *on* the system, thereby increasing the capacity of the system for doing work, that is, making w_{net} larger than w_{rev}.

The quantity w_{net} may now be correlated with a thermodynamic function known as *Gibbs free energy*, designated G (or F). This function is formally defined as

$$G = H - TS \tag{72}$$

Since

$$H = E + PV \tag{73}$$
$$G = E + PV - TS \tag{74}$$

When a system undergoes a change at constant pressure and temperature, the change of free energy, designated ΔG, is

$$\Delta G = \Delta E + P\Delta V - T\Delta S \tag{75}$$

Replacing ΔE by $DQ - DW$, and equating $T\Delta S$ with DQ, we obtain

$$\Delta G = -w_{\text{rev}} + P\Delta V \tag{76}$$

With signs reversed this becomes

$$-\Delta G = w_{\text{rev}} - P\Delta V \tag{77}$$

Comparing this with Eq 71, it is apparent that

$$-\Delta G = w_{\text{net}} \tag{78}$$

For systems at constant pressure and temperature, it is the quantity $-\Delta G$, commonly called the *decrease in free energy* of a process, that measures both the net capacity of a system for doing work and the driving force impelling the system to undergo spontaneous change in the direction of diminishing free energy. If the system undergoes no change in volume, it is obvious that w_{net} equals w_{rev}, and that ΔG and ΔA must be equal.

Some Free-Energy Relationships—Lack of knowledge of absolute values of Gibbs free energy makes it necessary to refer differences in G to some standard state. In dealing with chemical reactions it is convenient to use for reference the *standard free-energy change*, symbolized ΔG°, for a hypothetical reaction in which reactants in their standard states are converted to products in their standard states; the standard state is, commonly, one gram-mole of substance at 1 atm pressure at 25°.

A very useful equation for calculating the standard free-energy change when the equilibrium constant for a reaction is known is the following:

$$\Delta G^\circ = -2.303 RT \log K \tag{79}$$

Conversely, K may be calculated for any reaction for which ΔG° is known.

When the standard electromotive force of an electrochemical cell operating reversibly is known, the standard free energy of the chemical reaction occurring in the cell may be calculated by the relationship

$$\Delta G^\circ = -nFE^\circ \tag{80}$$

where n is the number of electrons transferred in the reaction, F is the faraday (96,500 coulombs), and E° is the standard electromotive force of the cell.

Chemical Potential—In the foregoing discussion of thermodynamic quantities no consideration was given to changes in the number of moles of chemical reactants and products, or exchanges of matter with surroundings; the systems were considered *closed*. In *open systems*, however, cognizance must be taken of changes in free energy (or internal energy) resulting from variations of the number of moles and exchanges of matter with surroundings. This may be done by using a quantity μ, introduced by Gibbs and called by him the chemical potential, which is defined as

$$\mu_1 = \left(\frac{\partial G}{\partial n_1}\right)_{T,P,n_2,n_3,\ldots} \tag{81}$$

This partial differential expression states that the chemical potential of Substance 1 in a mixture of Substances $1, 2, 3, \ldots$ is equal to the rate of change in Gibbs free energy of the system with the number of moles n_1 of Substance 1 when temperature, pressure, and the number of moles of all other substances in the system are held constant. The product $\mu_1 \cdot dn_1$ then represents the change of free energy produced by dn_1 moles of Substance 1. The summation of such changes for all the different substances in the system, represented as $\Sigma \mu dn$, provides for open systems the necessary correction for changes in free energy resulting from changes in the number of moles of components in the system.

Some Thermodynamic Calculations—The following problems, and their solutions, illustrate the application of the thermodynamic principles discussed in preceding sections.

Problem 1—One mole of liquid water is vaporized reversibly at 100° and 1 atm pressure. The heat of vaporization under these conditions is 539.7 cal/g. Calculate DQ, DW, ΔH, ΔE, ΔA, ΔG, and ΔS.

The heat of vaporization per gram multiplied by the molecular weight represents the heat absorbed in the process; since the process occurs at constant pressure the heat absorbed is ΔQ_p which, according to Eq 43, is equal to ΔH. Thus

$$\Delta Q_p = \Delta H = 539.7 \times 18.02 = 9725 \text{ cal/mole}$$

The work performed is the increase in volume of the system resulting from vaporization of the water, against a constant pressure of 1 atm. Then

$$w = P\Delta V = P(V_{\text{vap}} - V_{\text{liq}}) \cong PV_{\text{vap}}$$

While the work performed may be calculated using this equation, it is more readily calculated, when the result is to be expressed in calories, as follows:

$$w \cong PV_{\text{vap}} \cong RT = 1.987 \times 373.1 = 741 \text{ cal/mole}$$

$$\Delta E = DQ - DW = \Delta H - P\Delta V = 9725 - 741 = 8984 \text{ cal/mole}$$

$$\Delta S = \frac{DQ}{T} = \frac{\Delta H}{T} = \frac{9725}{373.1} = 26.0 \text{ cal/°/mole}$$

$$\Delta A = \Delta E - T\Delta S = 8984 - (373.1 \times 26.0) = -741 \text{ cal/mole}$$

The quantity ΔA may be calculated also from the relationship

$$\Delta A = -w_{\text{rev}} = -(741) = -741 \text{ cal/mole}$$

Finally

$$\Delta G = \Delta E + P\Delta V - T\Delta S$$
$$= 8984 + 741 - (373.1 \times 26.0) = 0 \text{ cal/mole}$$

Problem 2—The equilibrium constant, K_p, for the reaction $2H_2(g) + O_2(g) \rightarrow 2H_2O(g)$ at 2000° K is 1.55×10^7, the partial pressures being expressed in atmospheres. Calculate the standard free-energy change for the reaction, assuming ideal behavior of all the gases.

$$\Delta G^\circ = -RT \ln K_p$$
$$= -2.303 \times 1.987 \times 2000 \log 1.55 \times 10^7$$
$$= -65,800 \text{ cal}$$

Problem 3—The electromotive force of a galvanic cell consisting of a zinc electrode immersed in zinc sulfate solution of unit activity and a copper electrode immersed in cupric sulfate solution of unit activity is 1.100 v, at 25°. Calculate ΔG° for the cell reaction

$$Zn + Cu^{2+} \rightarrow Zn^{2+} + Cu$$

In this reaction two electrons are transferred, hence $n = 2$, and

$$\Delta G^\circ = -2 \times 96,500 \times 1.100 = -212,300 \text{ joules}$$

The calorie equivalent may be calculated from the relationship

$$1 \text{ cal} = 4.184 \text{ joules}$$

or

$$\Delta G^\circ = -\frac{212,300}{4.184} = -50,741 \text{ cal}$$

Miscellaneous Thermodynamic Relationships—The following differential forms of certain equations introduced earlier in this chapter are useful in the study of reversible processes in which the only work done is pressure–volume work.

$$dE = DQ - DW = TdS - PdV \tag{82}$$

$$dH = dE + d(PV) = dE + PdV + VdP \tag{83}$$

$$dG = dH - d(TS) = dH - TdS - SdT \tag{84}$$

From these equations may be obtained, by appropriate substitutions in the equations, the following:

$$dH = VdP + TdS \tag{85}$$

$$dG = VdP - SdT \tag{86}$$

At constant pressure these become

$$\left(\frac{\partial H}{\partial S}\right)_P = T \tag{87}$$

$$\left(\frac{\partial G}{\partial T}\right)_P = -S \tag{88}$$

At constant temperature Eq. 86 yields

$$\left(\frac{\partial G}{\partial P}\right)_T = V \tag{89}$$

and for an ideal gas

$$\left(\frac{\partial G}{\partial P}\right)_T = \frac{nRT}{P} \tag{90}$$

rearranging prior to integrating between G_2 and P_2 and G_1 at P_1

$$dG = nRT \frac{dP}{P} \tag{91}$$

then integrating

$$G_2 - G_1 = \Delta G = 2.303 \, nRT \log \frac{P_2}{P_1} \qquad (92)$$

Third Law of Thermodynamics—In discussing entropy as a measure of the disorder or randomness of a system it was pointed out that entropy increased (1) with change of state from solid to liquid to gas and (2) with increase of temperature in any given state. The most orderly arrangement of any substance would be expected to be that of a perfect crystal when its temperature is absolute zero; under these conditions the entropy is, according to the Third Law of Thermodynamics, zero. Since it is impossible to reach absolute zero, a better statement of the Law is that the entropy of a perfect crystal approaches zero as the temperature approaches absolute. The importance of this law lies in the fact that it provides the basis for calculating absolute values of entropy of pure substances from measurements of their heat capacity; if the absolute entropies and heats of formation of substances are known it is possible to calculate their Gibbs free-energy values and from these to calculate the equilibrium constants for various physical and chemical reactions.

The Clapeyron Equation—An important thermodynamic relationship between the variables of vapor pressure and temperature in any equilibrium between two phases of a substance was developed by Clapeyron in 1834. To derive this equation it is convenient to consider a liquid in equilibrium with its vapor at temperature T and pressure P equal to the vapor pressure of the liquid at the specified temperature. At constant temperature and pressure the Gibbs free energy of the liquid, G_1, must be equal to that of the vapor, G_v:

$$G_1 = G_v \qquad (93)$$

If the temperature is raised to $T + dT$, the pressure must be increased to $P + dP$ to correspond to the vapor pressure at the higher temperature, to maintain the two phases in equilibrium. The free energy of both liquid and vapor is increased, but since the two phases are in equilibrium, the increase must be the same for both, so that

$$dG_1 = dG_v \qquad (94)$$

The change of free energy of a pure substance with pressure and temperature being defined by

$$dG = VdP - SdT \qquad (95)$$

Eq 94 may be written

$$V_1 dP - S_1 dT = V_v dP - S_v dT \qquad (96)$$

rearranging

$$\frac{dP}{dT} = \frac{S_v - S_1}{V_v - V_1} \qquad (97)$$

Since Eq 61 applies,

$$S_v - S_1 = \Delta S = \frac{\Delta H_{vap}}{T} \qquad (98)$$

where ΔH_{vap} is the molar heat of vaporization (the heat absorbed by 1 mole of liquid during vaporization), substitution into Eq 97 yields

$$\frac{dP}{dT} = \frac{\Delta H_{vap}}{T(V_v - V_1)} \qquad (99)$$

This is the Clapeyron equation, which relates dP/dT, the rate of change of vapor pressure with temperature, to the heat of vaporization of a liquid and to the molar volume of the liquid (V_1) and of the vapor (V_v) at temperature T and pressure equal to the vapor pressure.

The Clapeyron equation is not limited, however, to the equilibrium between a liquid and its vapor in the process of

vaporization; it applies, with suitable modifications, to the equilibrium between a solid and a gas phase (as in sublimation), a solid and a liquid phase (as in melting or fusion), and between two crystalline forms, distinguished as 1 and 2, of a solid (as in the transition of one form to the other). The applicable equations are

Sublimation $$\frac{dP}{dT} = \frac{\Delta H_{sub}}{T(V_v - V_s)} \qquad (100)$$

Fusion $$\frac{dP}{dT} = \frac{\Delta H_{fus}}{T(V_1 - V_s)} \qquad (101)$$

Transition $$\frac{dP}{dT} = \frac{\Delta H_{trans}}{T(V_2 - V_1)} \qquad (102)$$

The Clausius–Clapeyron Equation—Clausius placed the Clapeyron equation on a sound thermodynamic basis—dependent on the Second Law of Thermodynamics—and also introduced certain simplifications applicable to the vaporization and sublimation forms of Clapeyron's equation. Clausius assumed that the vapor obeys Boyle's ideal gas law and that the molar volume of the liquid, V_1, or of the solid, V_s, in the sublimation equation, may be neglected in comparison with the volume of a mole of vapor, V_v. Eq 99 then may be written

$$\frac{dP}{dT} = \frac{P\Delta H_{vap}}{RT^2} \qquad (103)$$

which is commonly called the Clausius–Clapeyron equation.

This equation is equivalent to

$$\frac{d \ln P}{dT} = \frac{\Delta H_{vap}}{RT^2} \qquad (104)$$

the integral of which is, in Naperian logarithm form

$$\log P = \frac{-\Delta H_{vap}}{2.303 \, RT} + \text{constant} \qquad (105)$$

This integral form of the Clausius–Clapeyron equation indicates that a plot of $\log P$ against $1/T$ yields a straight line, a fact observed some time before the Clausius–Clapeyron equation was known. The slope of the line, $-\Delta H_{vap}/2.303 \, R$, provides a graphical method for calculating ΔH_{vap}. When the equation is integrated between the limits P_2 at T_2 and P_1 at T_1, it becomes

$$\log \frac{P_2}{P_1} = \frac{\Delta H_{vap}(T_2 - T_1)}{2.303 \, RT_2 T_1} \qquad (106)$$

This equation may be used either to calculate the heat of vaporization when the vapor pressure is known at two temperatures (assuming that the heat of vaporization remains constant over the temperature interval), or the vapor pressure at a specified temperature if it is known at another temperature and the heat of vaporization is known and remains constant.

The Clapeyron and the Clausius–Clapeyron equations, in various forms, may be used to calculate a variety of pressure–temperature data, some of which have already been mentioned. The equations are used also to calculate the theoretical value of the molal boiling-point elevation constant and the molal freezing-point depression constant for dilute solutions (see Chapter 16, pages 223–224).

References

1. *The Collected Works of J Willard Gibbs*, Yale Univ Press, New Haven, CT, 1928; reprinted 1948.
2. Klotz IM: *Chemical Thermodynamics*, Benjamin, New York, 1964.
3. Lewis GN, Randall M: *Thermodynamics*, 2nd ed (revised by Pitzer KS, Brewer L), McGraw-Hill, New York, 1961.

CHAPTER 16

Solutions and Phase Equilibria

Theodore D Sokoloski, PhD

Professor of Pharmacy, College of Pharmacy
Ohio State University
Columbus, OH 43210

Solutions and Solubility

A solution is a chemically and physically homogeneous mixture of two or more substances. The term solution generally denotes a homogeneous mixture that is liquid even though it is possible to have homogeneous mixtures which are solid or gaseous. Thus it is possible to have solutions of solids in liquids, liquids in liquids, gases in liquids, gases in gases, and solids in solids. The first three of these kinds of solutions are most important in pharmacy and ensuing discussions will be concerned primarily with them.

In discussing solutions it is customary to consider them as members of a particular class of dispersions of one substance in another substance. Depending on the size of the dispersed particle they are classified as *true solutions*, *colloidal solutions*, or *suspensions*. If sugar is dissolved in water, it is supposed that the ultimate sugar particle is of molecular dimensions and that a *true solution* is formed. On the other hand if very fine sand is mixed with water, a *suspension* of comparatively large particles, each consisting of many molecules, is obtained. Between these two extremes lie *colloidal solutions*, the dispersed particles of which are larger than those of true solutions but smaller than the particles present in suspensions. In this chapter only true solutions will be discussed.

It is possible to classify broadly all solutions as one of two types. In the first type, although there may be a lesser or greater interaction between the dispersed substance (the solute) and the dispersing medium (the solvent), the solution phase contains the same chemical entity as found in the solid phase and thus, upon removal of the solvent, the solute is recovered unchanged. One example of this type of solution would be sugar dissolved in water where, in the presence of sugar in excess of its solubility, there is an equilibrium between sugar molecules in the solid phase with sugar molecules in the solution phase. A second example of this kind of a solution would be the dissolving of silver chloride in water. Admittedly, the solubility of this salt in water is small, but it is finite. In this case the solvent contains silver and chloride ions and the solid phase contains the same material. Removal of solvent yields initial solute.

In the second type of solution the solvent contains a compound which is different from that in the solid phase. The difference between the compound in the solid phase and solution is due generally to some chemical reaction that has occurred in the solvent. An example of this type of solution would be dissolving aspirin in an aqueous solvent containing some basic material capable of reacting with the acid aspirin. Now the species in solution would not only be undissociated aspirin, but aspirin also as its anion, whereas the species in the solid phase is aspirin in only its undissociated acid form. In this situation, if the solvent were removed part of the sub-stance obtained (the salt of aspirin) would be different from what was initially present in the solid.

Solutions of Solids in Liquids

Reversible Solubility without Chemical Reaction—From the pharmaceutical standpoint solutions of solids in liquids, with or without accompanying chemical reaction in the solvent, are of the greatest importance, and many quantitative data on the behavior and properties of such solutions are available. This discussion will be concerned with definitions of solubility, the rate at which substances go into solution, and with temperature and other factors which control solubility.

Solubility—When an excess of a solid is brought into contact with a liquid, molecules of the former are removed from its surface until equilibrium is established between the molecules leaving the solid and those returning to it. The resulting solution is said to be saturated at the temperature of the experiment, and the extent to which the solute dissolves is referred to as its *solubility*. The extent of solubility of different substances varies from almost imperceptible amounts to relatively large quantities, but for any given solute the solubility has a constant value at constant temperature.

Under certain conditions it is possible to prepare a solution containing a larger amount of solute than is necessary to form a saturated solution. This may occur when a solution is saturated at one temperature, the excess of solid solute removed, and the solution cooled. The solute present in solution, even though it may be less soluble at the lower temperature, does not always separate from the solution and there is produced a *supersaturated solution*. Such solutions, formed by sodium thiosulfate and potassium acetate, for example, may be made to deposit their excess of solute in one of the following ways: (1) by vigorous shaking, (2) by scratching the side of the vessel in contact with the solution, or (3) by introducing into the solution a small crystal of the solute.

Methods of Expressing Solubility—When quantitative data are available, solubilities may be expressed in many ways. For example, the solubility of sodium chloride in water at 25°C may be stated in the following ways:

1. 1 g of sodium chloride dissolves in 2.786 mL of water. (An approximation of this method is used by the USP.)

2. 35.89 g of sodium chloride dissolves in 100 mL of water.

3. 100 mL of a saturated solution of sodium chloride in water contains 31.71 g of solute.

4. 100 g of a saturated solution of sodium chloride in water contains 26.47 g of solute.

5. 1 liter of a saturated solution of sodium chloride in water contains 5.425 moles of solute. This also may be stated: a saturated solution of sodium chloride in water is 5.425 molar with respect to the solute.

The author acknowledges the kind assistance of Dr Gordon L Flynn, University of Michigan, in the revision of parts of this chapter.

In order to calculate *3* from *1* or *2* it is necessary to know the density of the solution, in this case 1.198 g/mL. To calculate *5*, the number of grams of solute in 1000 mL of solution (obtained by multiplying the data in (*3*) by ten) is divided by the molecular weight of sodium chloride, namely, 58.45.

Several other concentration expressions are used. Molality is the number of moles of solute in 1000 g of solvent and could be calculated from the data in *4* by subtracting grams of solute from grams of solution to obtain grams of solvent, relating this to 1000 g of solvent, and dividing by molecular weight to obtain moles. Mole fraction is the fraction of the total number of moles present which are moles of one component. Mole % may be obtained by multiplying mole fraction by 100. Normality refers to the number of g-Eq of solute dissolved in 1000 mL of solution.

In pharmacy, use also is made of three other concentration expressions. Percent by weight (% w/w) is the number of grams of solute per 100 g of solution and is exemplified by *4* above. Percent weight in volume (% w/v) is the number of grams of solute per 100 mL of solution and is exemplified by *3* above. Percent by volume (% v/v) is the number of milliliters of solute in 100 mL of solution, referring to solutions of liquids in liquids. The USP indicates that the term "percent," when unqualified, means percent weight in volume for solutions of solids in liquids and percent by volume for solutions of liquids in liquids.

When in pharmacopeial texts it has not been possible, or in some instances not desirable, to indicate exact solubility, a descriptive term has been used. The following table indicates the meaning of such terms:

Descriptive terms	Parts of solvent for 1 part of solute
Very soluble	Less than 1
Freely soluble	From 1 to 10
Soluble	From 10 to 30
Sparingly soluble	From 30 to 100
Slightly soluble	From 100 to 1000
Very slightly soluble	From 1000 to 10,000
Practically insoluble, or insoluble	More than 10,000

Rate of Solution—It is possible to define quantitatively the rate at which a solute goes into solution. The simplest treatment is based on a model depicted in Fig 16-1. A solid particle dispersed in a solvent is surrounded by a thin layer of solvent having a finite thickness, *l* in cm. The layer is an integral part of the solid and is thus characteristically referred to as the "stagnant layer." This means that regardless of how fast the bulk solution may be stirred the stagnant layer remains a part of the surface of the solid, moving wherever the particle moves. The thickness of this layer may get smaller as stirring of the bulk solution increases, but it is important to recognize that this layer will always have a finite thickness however small it may get.

Using Fick's First Law of Diffusion the rate of solution of the solid can be explained, in the simplest case, as the rate at which a dissolved solute particle diffuses through the stagnant layer to the bulk solution. The driving force behind the movement of the solute molecule through the stagnant layer is the difference in concentration that exists between the concentration of the solute, C_1, in the stagnant layer at the surface of the solid and its concentration, C_2, on the farthest side of the stagnant layer (see *Diffusion in Liquids*, page 221). The greater this difference in concentration ($C_1 - C_2$), the faster the rate of solution.

According to Fick's Law, the rate of solution is also directly proportional to the area of the solid, *A* in cm², exposed to solvent and inversely proportional to the length of the path through which the dissolved solute molecule must diffuse.

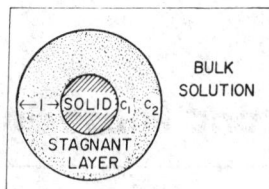

Fig 16-1.   Physical model representing the dissolution process.

Mathematically, then, the rate of solution of the solid is given by

$$\text{Rate of solution} = \frac{DA}{l}(C_1 - C_2) \qquad (1)$$

where *D* is a proportionality constant called the diffusion coefficient in cm²/sec. In measuring the rate of solution experimentally, the concentration C_2 is held small compared to C_1 and hence considered to have a negligible effect on the rate. Furthermore, C_1 is most often the saturation solubility of the solute. Hence Eq 1 is simplified to

$$\text{Rate of solution} = \frac{DA}{l}(\text{saturation solubility}) \qquad (2)$$

Eq 2 quantitatively explains many of the phenomena commonly observed that affect the rate at which materials dissolve.

1.   Small particles go into solution faster than large particles. For a given mass of solute, as we make the particle size smaller, the surface area per unit mass of solid increases and Eq 2 shows that as area increases, the rate must proportionally increase. Hence, if a pharmacist wishes to increase the rate of solution of a drug, he should decrease its particle size.

2.   Stirring a solution increases the rate at which a solid dissolves. This is because the thickness of the stagnant layer depends on how fast the bulk solution is stirred; as stirring rate increases, the length of the diffusional path decreases. Since the rate of solution is inversely proportional to the length of the diffusional path, the faster the solution is stirred, the faster the solute will go into solution.

3.   The more soluble the solute, the faster is its rate of solution. Again, Eq 2 predicts that the larger the saturation solubility, the faster the rate.

4.   With a viscous liquid, the rate of solution is slowed. This is because the diffusion coefficient is inversely proportional to the viscosity of the medium; the more viscous the solvent, the slower the rate of solution.

Heat of Solution and Temperature Dependency of the Solubility Process—Turning from the kinetic aspects of dissolution, this discussion will be concerned with the situation where there is thermodynamic equilibrium between solute in its solid phase* and the solute in solution. As defined earlier, the concentration of solute in solution at equilibrium is the saturation solubility of the substance.

When a solid (*A*) dissolves in some solvent two steps may be considered as occurring: the solid absorbs energy to become a liquid and then the liquid dissolves.

$$A_{(\text{solid})} \rightleftarrows A_{(\text{liquid})} \rightleftarrows A_{(\text{solution})}$$

For the overall dissolution the equilibrium existing between solute molecules in the solid and solute molecules in solution may be treated as any equilibrium. Thus, for a solute *A* in equilibrium with its solution we can write,

$$A_{(\text{solid})} \rightleftarrows A_{(\text{solution})}$$

Using the Law of Mass Action we can define an equilibrium constant for this system just as any equilibrium constant may be written. Thus,

$$K_{\text{eq}} = \frac{a_{(\text{solution})}}{a_{(\text{solid})}}$$

---

* It is assumed that there is an amount of solid material in excess of the amount that can go into solution; hence a solid phase is always present.

where a denotes activity of the solute in each phase. Since the activity of a solid is defined as unity,

$$K_{eq} = a_{(solution)}$$

Because the activity of a compound in dilute solution is approximated by its concentration and because this concentration is the saturation solubility, K_S, we can use the van't Hoff Equation* which defines the relationship between an equilibrium constant (here, solubility) and absolute temperature. This relation is

$$\frac{d \log K_S}{dT} = \frac{\Delta H}{2.3RT^2} \qquad (3)$$

where $d \log K_S/dT$ is the change of $\log K_S$ with a unit change of absolute temperature, T; ΔH is a constant which in this situation is the heat of solution for the overall process (solid $\rightleftarrows$ liquid $\rightleftarrows$ solution); and R is the gas constant, 1.99 cal/mole/deg. Eq 3, a differential equation, may be solved to give

$$\log K_S = -\frac{\Delta H}{2.3RT} + J \qquad (4)$$

where J is a constant. A more useful form of this equation is

$$\log \frac{K_{S,T_2}}{K_{S,T_1}} = \frac{\Delta H(T_2 - T_1)}{2.3RT_1T_2} \qquad (5)$$

where K_{S,T_1} is the saturation solubility at absolute temperature T_1 and K_{S,T_2} is the solubility at temperature T_2. Through the use of Eq 5, if ΔH and the solubility at one temperature are known, the solubility at any other temperature may be calculated.

Effect of Temperature—As is evident from Eq 4, the solubility of a solid in a liquid is dependent on the temperature. If in the process of solution heat is absorbed (as evidenced by a reduction in temperature), ΔH is by convention positive and the solubility of the solute will increase with increasing temperature. Such is the case for most salts, as is shown in Fig 16-2. In this figure the solubility of the solute is plotted as ordinate and the temperature as abscissa, and the line joining the experimental points represents the solubility curve for that solute.

If a solute gives off heat during the process of solution (as evidenced by an increase in temperature), ΔH is by convention negative and solubility decreases with increase in temperature. This is the case with calcium hydroxide and, at higher temperatures, with calcium sulfate.† When heat is neither absorbed nor given off, the solubility is not affected by variation of temperature as is nearly the case with sodium chloride.

Solubility curves are usually continuous as long as the chemical composition of the solid phase in contact with the solution remains unchanged, but if there is a transition of the solid phase from one form to another, a break will be found in the curve. Such is the case with $Na_2SO_4 \cdot 10H_2O$ which dissolves with absorption of heat up to a temperature of 32.4° at which point there is a transition of the solid phase to anhydrous sodium sulfate, Na_2SO_4, which dissolves with evolution of heat. This change is evidenced by increased solubility of the hydrated salt up to 32.4°, but above this temperature the solubility decreases.

These temperature effects are what would be predicted from Eq 4. When the heat of solution is negative, signifying that energy is released during dissolution, the relation between

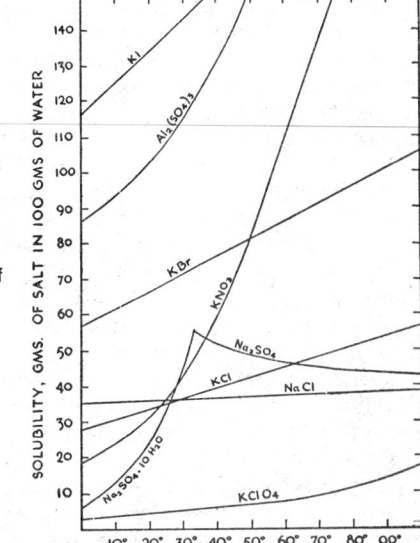

Fig 16-2.   Effect of heat on solubility.

$\log K_S$ and $1/T$ is typified in Fig 16-3A, where as $1/T$ increases, $\log K_S$ increases. We see that with increasing temperature (T itself actually increases as you go to the left in Fig 16-3A) there is a decrease in solubility. On the other hand, when the heat of solution is positive—that is, when heat is absorbed in the solution process—the relation between $\log K_S$ and $1/T$ is typified in Fig 16-3B. Here, as temperature increases ($1/T$ decreases), the solubility increases.

Effect of Salts on the Solubility of Nonelectrolytes—The solubility of a nonelectrolyte, in water, is generally either decreased or increased by the addition of an electrolyte; it is only rarely that the solubility is not altered. When the solubility of the nonelectrolyte is decreased, the effect is referred to as "salting out"; if it is increased, it is described as "salting in." Inorganic electrolytes commonly decrease solubility, though there are some exceptions to the generalization.

Salting out occurs because the ions of the added electrolyte interact with water molecules and thus in a sense reduce the amount of water available for solution of the nonelectrolyte. (Refer to the section on *Thermodynamics of the Solution Process*, p 215, for another view). The greater the degree of hydration of the ions the more the solubility of the nonelectrolyte is decreased. If, for example, one compares the effect of equivalent amounts of lithium chloride, sodium chloride, potassium chloride, rubidium chloride, and cesium chloride (all of which belong to the family of alkali metals and are of the same valence type), it is observed that lithium chloride

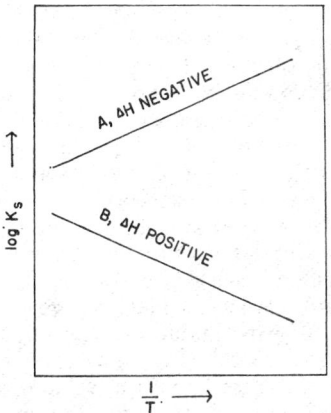

Fig 16-3.   Typified relationship between the logarithm of the saturation solubility and the reciprocal of the absolute temperature.

---

*For a more complete treatment of the van't Hoff Equation, see Ref 1, p 113.
†Because of the slight solubility of these substances their solubility curves are not included.

decreases the solubility of a nonelectrolyte to the greatest extent and that the salting out effect decreases in the order given. This is also the order of the degree of hydration of the cations; lithium ion, being the smallest ion and therefore having the greatest density of positive charge per unit of surface area (see also Chapter 13, *Electronegativity Values*), is the most extensively hydrated of the cations while cesium ion is hydrated the least. Salting out is encountered frequently in pharmaceutical operations.

Salting in commonly occurs when either the salts of various organic acids or organic-substituted ammonium salts are added to aqueous solutions of nonelectrolytes. In the first case the solubilizing effect is associated with the anion and in the second with the cation. In both cases the solubility increases as the concentration of added salt is increased. The solubility increase may be relatively great, sometimes amounting to several times the solubility of the nonelectrolyte in water.

Solubility of Solutes Containing Two or More Species—In cases where the solute phase consists of two or more species (as in an inorganic salt), when the solute goes into solution, the solution phase often contains each of these species as discrete entities. For some such substance, *AB*, we can then write the following for the solution process:

$$AB_{(solid)} \rightleftharpoons A_{(solution)} + B_{(solution)}$$

Since there is an equilibrium between the solute and saturated solution phases, the Law of Mass Action defines an equilibrium constant, K_{eq}:

$$K_{eq} = \frac{a_{A(solution)} \cdot a_{B(solution)}}{a_{AB(solid)}} \quad (6)$$

where $a_{A(solution)}$, $a_{B(solution)}$ and $a_{AB(solid)}$ are the activities of *A* and *B* in solution and of *AB* in the solid phase. Recall from our earlier discussion that the activity of a solid is defined as unity, and that in a very dilute solution (eg, where we have a slightly soluble salt), concentrations may be substituted for activities; Eq 6 then becomes

$$K_{eq} = C_A C_B$$

where C_A and C_B are the concentrations of *A* and *B* in solution. K_{eq} in this situation has a special name, the *solubility product*, K_{SP}. Thus,

$$K_{SP} = C_A C_B \quad (7)$$

This equation will hold true theoretically only for slightly soluble salts.

As an example of this type of solution, consider the solubility of silver chloride. We can write for silver chloride

$$K_{SP} = [Ag^+][Cl^-]$$

where the brackets [ ] designate concentrations.

This constant, K_{SP}, is known as the solubility product; at 25° it has a value of 1.56×10^{-10}, the concentration of silver and chloride ions being expressed in moles/liter. The same numerical value applies also to solutions of silver chloride containing an excess of either silver or chloride ions. If the silver-ion concentration is increased by the addition of a soluble silver salt, the chloride-ion concentration must decrease until the product of the two concentrations is again numerically equal to the solubility product. In order to effect the decrease in chloride-ion concentration, silver chloride is precipitated and hence its solubility is decreased. In a similar manner an increase in chloride-ion concentration by the addition of a soluble chloride effects a decrease in the silver-ion concentration until the numerical value of the solubility product is attained. Again this decrease in silver ion concentration is brought about by the precipitation of silver chloride.

The solubility of silver chloride in a saturated aqueous solution of the salt may be calculated by assuming that the concentration of silver ion is the same as the concentration of chloride ion, both expressed in moles/liter, and that the concentration of dissolved silver chloride is numerically the same since each silver chloride molecule gives rise to one silver ion and one chloride ion. Since

$$[dissolved\ AgCl] = [Ag^+] = [Cl^-]$$

the solubility of AgCl is equal to $\sqrt{1.56 \times 10^{-10}}$, which is 1.25×10^{-5} mole per liter. Multiplying this by the molecular weight of silver chloride (143) we obtain a solubility of approximately 1.8 mg/liter.

For a salt of the type $PbCl_2$ the solubility product expression takes the form

$$[Pb^{2+}][Cl^-]^2 = K_{SP}$$

while for As_2S_3 it would be

$$[As^{3+}]^2[S^{2-}]^3 = K_{SP}$$

because from the Law of Mass Action we have

$$PbCl_{2(solid)} \rightleftharpoons Pb^{2+}_{(solution)} + 2Cl^-_{(solution)}$$

and

$$As_2S_{3(solid)} \rightleftharpoons 2As^{3+}_{(solution)} + 3S^{2-}_{(solution)}$$

For further details of methods of using solubility product calculations, the reader is referred to books on qualitative or quantitative analysis, or on physical chemistry.

Recall that the solubility product principle is valid for aqueous solutions of slightly soluble salts, provided the concentration of added salt is not too great. Where the concentrations are high, deviations from the theory occur and these have been explained by assuming that in such solutions the nature of the solvent has been changed. Frequently deviations may also occur as the result of the formation of complexes between the two salts. An example of increased solubility by virtue of complex-ion formation is seen in the effect of solutions of soluble iodides on mercuric iodide. According to the solubility product principle it might be expected that soluble iodides would decrease the solubility of mercuric iodide, but because of the formation of the more soluble complex salt K_2HgI_4 which dissociates as follows:

$$K_2HgI_4 \rightleftharpoons 2K^+ + (HgI_4)^{2-}$$

the iodide ion no longer functions as a common ion.

Practical applications of the solubility product principle are found in qualitative and quantitative analysis whenever an excess of a precipitant is added in order to diminish, by common ion effect, the solubility of the precipitate.

It is possible to formulate some general rules regarding the effect of the addition of soluble salts to slightly soluble salts where the added salt does not have an ion common to the slightly soluble salt. If the ions of the added soluble salt are not highly hydrated (see *Effect of Salts on the Solubility of Nonelectrolytes*), the solubility product of the slightly soluble salt will increase because the ions of the added salt tend to decrease the interionic attraction between the ions of the slightly soluble salt. On the other hand, if the ions of the added soluble salt are hydrated, water molecules become less available and the interionic attraction between the ions of the slightly soluble salt increases with a resultant decrease in solubility product. Another way of considering this effect is discussed later (*Thermodynamics of the Solution Process*).

The effect of temperature is in general what we would expect; increasing the temperature of the solution results in an increase of the solubility product.

Solubility Following a Chemical Reaction—Thus far in this chapter discussion has been concerned with solubility that comes about because of interplay of entirely physical forces. The dissolution of some substance resulted from overcoming the physical interactions between solute molecules and solvent molecules by the energy produced when a solute molecule interacted physically with a solvent molecule. The solution process can, however, also be facilitated by a chemical reaction. Almost always the chemical enhancement of solubility in aqueous systems is due to the formation of a salt following an acid–base reaction.

An alkaloidal base, or any other nitrogenous base of relatively high molecular weight, is generally slightly soluble in water, but if the pH of the medium is reduced by addition of acid, the solubility of the base is increased, considerably so as the pH continues to be reduced. The reason for this increase in solubility is that the base is converted to a salt, which is relatively soluble in water. Conversely, the solubility of a salt of an alkaloid or other nitrogenous base is reduced as pH is increased by addition of alkali.

The solubility of slightly soluble acid substances is, on the other hand, increased as the pH is increased by addition of alkali, the reason again being that a salt, relatively soluble in water, is formed. Examples of acid substances whose solubility is thus increased are acetylsalicylic acid, theophylline, theobromine, the sulfonamides, and the barbiturates. Conversely, the solubility of salts of the same substances is decreased as the pH decreases.

Among some inorganic compounds a somewhat similar behavior is observed. Tribasic calcium phosphate, $Ca_3(PO_4)_2$, for example, is almost insoluble in water, but if an acid is added its solubility increases rapidly with decrease in pH. This is because hydrogen ions have such a strong affinity for phosphate ions, to form nonionized phosphoric acid, that the calcium phosphate is dissolved in order to release phosphate ions. Or, stated in another way, the solubilization is an example of a reaction in which a strong acid (which is the source of the hydrogen ions) displaces a weak acid.

In all the examples cited above solubilization occurs as the result of an interaction of the solute with an acid or a base. Compounds which do not react with either acids or bases are, on the other hand, but slightly if at all influenced in their aqueous solubility by variations of pH. Such effects as may be observed are generally due to ionic "salt effects."

It is possible to quantitatively analyze solubility following an acid–base reaction by considering solubility as a two-step process. We will first use as an example an organic acid, designated as HA, that is relatively insoluble in water. Its two-step dissolution can be represented as

$$HA_{(solid)} \rightleftharpoons HA_{(solution)}$$

followed by

$$HA_{(solution)} \rightleftharpoons H^+_{(solution)} + A^-_{(solution)}$$

The equilibrium constant for the first step is the solubility of HA ($K_S = [HA]_{solution}$), just as we developed earlier when no chemical reaction took place, and the equilibrium constant for the second step is the dissociation constant of the acid:

$$K_a = \frac{[H^+][A^-]}{[HA]}$$

Since the total amount of compound *in solution* is the sum of nonionized and ionized forms of the acid, we can designate the total solubility $S_{t(HA)}$ as

$$S_{t(HA)} = [HA] + [A^-] = [HA] + K_a\frac{[HA]}{[H^+]} \quad (8)$$

Since $K_S = [HA]$, Eq 8 becomes

$$S_{t(HA)} = K_S\left(1 + \frac{K_a}{[H^+]}\right) \quad (9)$$

Eq 9 is very useful since it equates the total solubility of an acid drug with the hydrogen-ion concentration of the solvent. If the water solubility K_S and the dissociation constant K_a are known, the total solubility of the acid may be calculated at various hydrogen-ion concentrations. Eq 9 quantitatively shows us how the total solubility of the acid increases as the hydrogen-ion concentration decreases (that is, as the pH increases).

It is possible to develop an equation similar to Eq 9 for the solubility of a basic drug, B, such as a relatively insoluble nitrogenous base (an alkaloid, for example) at various hydrogen-ion concentrations. The solubility of the base in water may be represented in two steps, as

$$B_{(solid)} \rightleftharpoons B_{(solution)}$$

$$B_{(solution)} \rightleftharpoons BH^+_{(solution)} + OH^-_{(solution)}$$

Again, if K_S is the solubility of the free base in water and K_b is its dissociation constant,

$$K_b = \frac{[BH^+][OH^-]}{[B]}$$

the total solubility of the base in water $S_{t(B)}$ is given by

$$S_{t(B)} = [B] + [BH^+] = [B] + \frac{K_b[B]}{[OH^-]} =$$

$$K_S\left(1 + \frac{K_b}{[OH^-]}\right) \quad (10)$$

It is convenient to rewrite Eq 10 in terms of hydrogen-ion concentration by making use of the dissociation constant for water,

$$K_W = [H^+][OH^-] = 1 \times 10^{-14}$$

Eq 10 then becomes

$$S_{t(B)} = K_S\left(1 + \frac{K_b}{K_W/[H^+]}\right) = K_S\left(1 + \frac{K_b[H^+]}{K_W}\right) \quad (11)$$

Eq 11 quantitatively shows how the total solubility of the base increases as the hydrogen-ion concentration of the solvent increases. If K_S and K_b are known, it is possible to calculate the total solubility of a basic drug at various hydrogen-ion concentrations using this equation.

Eqs 9 and 11 have assumed that the salt formed following a chemical reaction is infinitely soluble. This is, of course, not an acceptable assumption as suggested and demonstrated by Kramer and Flynn.[3] Rather, for an acidic or basic drug there should be a pH at which *maximum solubility* occurs where this solubility is, of course, still a sum of the solution concentrations of the free and salt forms of the drug at that pH. Using a basic drug, B, as the example, this would mean that a solution of B, at pH values greater than the pH of maximum solubility, would be saturated with free base form but not with the salt form and the use of Eq 11 would be valid for the prediction of solubility. On the other hand, at pH values less than the pH of maximum solubility, the solution would be saturated with salt form and Eq 11 is no longer really valid. Since in this situation the total solubility of the base, $S_{t(B)}$ is

$$S_{t(B)} = [B] + [BH^+]_s$$

where the subscript s designates a solution saturated with salt, the correct equation to use at pH values less than the pH maximum would be

$$S_{t(B)} = [BH^+]_s\left(1 + \frac{[OH^-]}{K_b}\right) = [BH^+]_s\left(1 + \frac{K_W}{K_b[H^+]}\right) \quad (12)$$

An equation similar to Eq 12 can likewise be developed for an acidic drug at pHs greater than its pH of maximum solubility.

Modes of Effecting Solution of Solids at the Prescription Counter—The method usually employed by the pharmacist when soluble compounds are to be dissolved in water in compounding a prescription is one which requires the use of the mortar and pestle. The ordinary practice is to crush the substance into fragments in the mortar with the pestle and pour the solvent on it, meanwhile stirring with the pestle until solution is effected. If definite quantities are used, and the whole of the solvent is required to dissolve the given weight of the salt, a portion only of the solvent should be added at first, and when this is saturated the solution is poured off and a fresh portion of solvent added. This operation is repeated until the solid is entirely dissolved; the solutions are then mixed. Other methods of effecting solution are to shake the solid with the liquid in a bottle or flask, or to apply heat to the substances in a suitable vessel. Substances vary greatly in the rate at which they dissolve; some are capable of producing a saturated solution quickly, others require several hours for attainment of saturation. All too often in their haste to prepare a saturated solution pharmacists fail to obtain the required degree of solution of solute.

With hygroscopic substances like pepsin, silver protein compounds, and some others, the best method of effecting solution in water is to place the substance directly upon the surface of the water and then stir vigorously with a glass rod. If the ordinary procedure, such as using a mortar and pestle, is employed with these substances, gummy lumps are formed which are exceedingly difficult to dissolve.

The *solubility* of chemicals and the *miscibility* of liquids are important physical factors for the pharmacist to know, as they often have a bearing on the intelligent and proper filling of prescriptions. Mainly for the information of the pharmacist, the USP provides tabular data indicating the degree of solubility or miscibility of many official substances.

Determination of Solubility—For the pharmacist and pharmaceutical chemist the question of solubility is of paramount importance. Not only is it necessary to know solubilities in connection with the preparation and dispensing of medicines, but such information is necessary to effect separation of substances in qualitative and quantitative analysis. Furthermore, the accurate determination of the solubility of a substance is one of the best methods for determining its purity.

The details of the determination of the solubility are markedly affected by the physical and chemical characteristics of the solute and solvent and also by the temperature at which the solubility is to be determined. Accordingly it is not possible to describe a universally applicable method but, in general, the following must be observed in solubility determinations.

1. Purity of both the dissolved substance and the solvent is essential, since impurities in either affect the solubility to a greater or lesser extent.
2. Constancy of temperature must be accurately maintained during the course of the determination.
3. Complete saturation must be attained.
4. Accurate analysis of the saturated solution and correct expression of the results are imperative.

Consideration should be given also to the varying rates of solution of different compounds, and to the marked effect of the degree of fineness of the particles on the time required for the saturation of the solution.

Many of the solubility data of USP have been determined with regard to the exacting requirements mentioned above.

Phase Solubility Analysis—The procedure of *Phase Solubility Analysis* is one of the most useful and accurate methods for the determination of the purity of a substance.

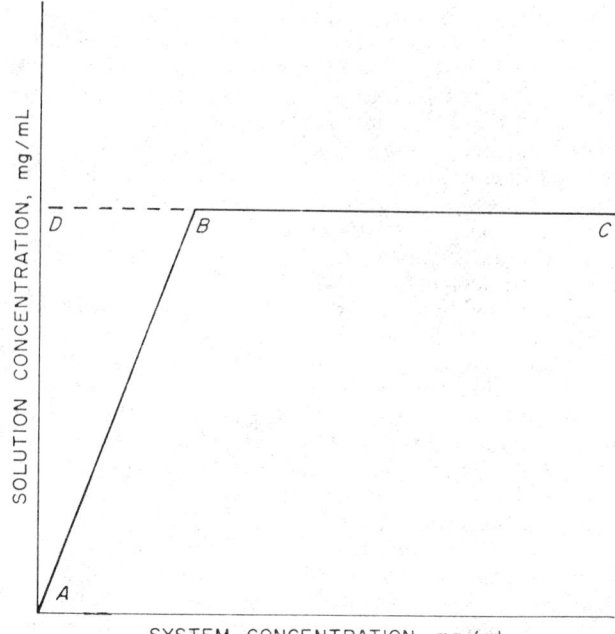

Fig 16-4.   Phase solubility diagram for a pure substance.

It involves the application of precise solubility methods to the principle that constancy of solubility, in the same manner as constancy of melting point, indicates that a material is pure or free from foreign admixture. It is important to recognize that the technique can be used to obtain the exact solubility of the pure substance without the necessity for the experimental material itself to be pure.

The method is based on the thermodynamic principles of heterogeneous equilibria which are among the soundest of theoretical concepts of chemistry. Thus it is not dependent on any assumptions regarding kinetics or structure of matter, but applicable to all species of molecules, and is sufficiently sensitive to distinguish between optical isomers unless they be present in the ratio of 1:1. The requirements for an analysis are simple since the equipment needed is basic to most laboratories and the quantities of substances required are small.

The standard solubility method consists of five steps:

1. Mixing, in separate systems, increasing amounts of a substance with measured amounts of a solvent.
2. Establishment of equilibrium for each system at identical constant temperature and pressure.
3. Separation of the solid phase from the solutions.
4. Determination of the concentration of the material dissolved in the various solutions.
5. Plotting the concentration of the dissolved material per unit of solvent (y-axis, or solution concentration) against the mass of material per unit of solvent (x-axis or system concentration).

The solubility method has been established on the sound theoretical principles of the Gibbs phase rule: $F = C - P + 2$, which relates C, the number of components, F, the degrees of freedom (pressure, temperature, and concentration), and P, the number of phases for a heterogeneous equilibrium. Since solubility analyses are carried out at constant temperature and pressure, a pure solid in solution would show only one degree of freedom, because only one phase is present at concentrations below saturation. This is represented by section Ab in Fig 16-4. For a pure solid in a saturated solution at equilibrium (Fig 16-4, BC), two phases are present, solid and solution; there is no variation in concentration and thus, at constant temperature and pressure, no degrees of freedom.

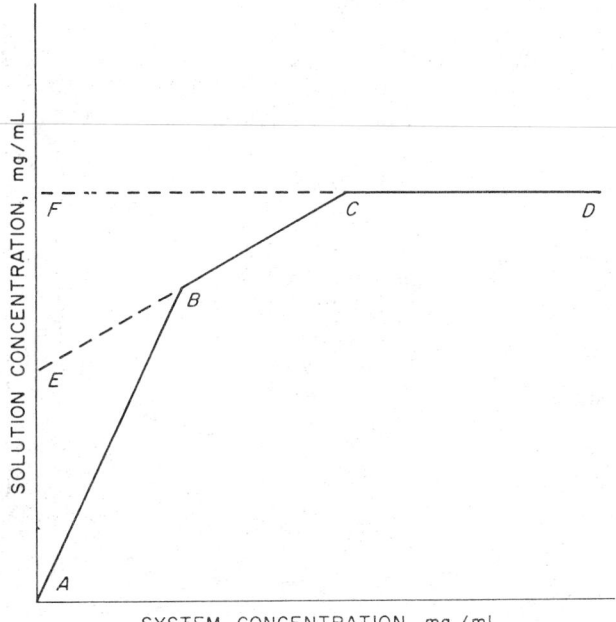

Fig 16-5.   Type of solubility curve obtained when a substance contains one impurity.

Solutions of Liquids in Liquids

Binary Systems—Under this title the following types of liquid-pairs may be recognized.

1. Those which are completely soluble in each other in all proportions. Examples: alcohol and water; glycerin and water; alcohol and glycerin.
2. Those which are soluble in each other in definite proportions. Examples: phenol and water; ether and water; nicotine and water.
3. Those which are imperceptibly soluble in each other in any proportion. Examples: castor oil and water; liquid petrolatum and water.

The mutual solubility of liquid pairs of type 2 has been extensively studied and found to show interesting regularities. If a series of tubes containing varying but known percentages of phenol and water are heated (or cooled if necessary) just to the point of formation of a homogeneous solution, and the temperatures at such points noted, there will be obtained, upon plotting the results, a curve similar to that in Fig 16-6.[4] On this graph the area inside the curve represents the region where mixtures of phenol and water will separate into two layers, while in the region outside of the curve homogeneous solutions will be obtained. The maximum temperature on this curve is called the *critical solution temperature*, that is, the temperature above which a homogeneous solution occurs regardless of the composition of the mixture. For phenol and water the critical solution temperature occurs at a composition of 34.5% phenol in water.

Temperature vs composition curves as depicted in Fig 16-6 provide much useful information in the preparation of homogeneous mixtures of substances showing mutual solubility behavior. At room temperature (here assumed to be 25°), by drawing a line parallel to the abscissa at 25°, we find that we can actually prepare two sets of homogeneous solutions, one containing from 0 to about 7.5% phenol and the other containing phenol from 72 to about 95% (the limit of solubility of phenol). At compositions between 7.5 and 72% phenol at 25° two liquid layers or phases will separate. In sample tubes containing a concentration of phenol in this two-layer region at 25° the lower layer will always be phenol-rich and always contain 72% phenol while the upper layer will be water-rich and always contain 7.5% phenol. These values are obtained by interpolation of the two points of intersection of the line drawn at 25° with the experimental curve. As it may be deduced, at other temperatures, the composition of the two layers in the two-layer region is determined by the points of intersection of the curve with a line (called the "tie line") drawn parallel to the abscissa at that temperature. The relative amounts of the two layers or phases, phenol-rich and

The curve *ABC* of Fig 16-4 represents the type of solubility diagram obtained for: (1) a pure material, (2) equal amounts of two or more materials having identical solubilities, or (3) a mixture of two or more materials present in the unique ratio of their solubilities. These latter two cases are rare and often may be detected by a change in solvent system.

Section *BC* of Fig 16-4 since it has no slope, usually indicates purity. If, however, this section *does* exhibit a slope, its numerical value indicates the fraction of impurity present. Point *D* is the actual solubility of the pure substance.

A representative type of solubility curve which is obtained when a substance contains one impurity is illustrated in Fig 16-5. Here, at *B*, the solution becomes saturated with one component. From *B* to *C* there are two phases present: a solution saturated with Component I (usually the major component) containing also some Component II (usually the minor component), and a solid phase of Component I. The one degree of freedom revealed by the slope of the line *BC* is the concentration of Component II, which is the impurity (usually the minor component). A mixture of *d* and *l* isomers in any ratio other than 1:1 would have such a curve, as would any simple mixtures in which the solubilities are independent of each other.

The section *CD* indicates that the solvent is saturated with both components of the two-component mixture. Here, three phases are present; a solution saturated with both components and the two solid phases. No variation of concentration is possible, hence no degree of freedom is possible (indicated by the lack of slope of section *CD*). The distance *AE* on the ordinate represents the solubility of the major component, and the distance *EF* the solubility of the minor component.

The fact that the equilibration process is time-consuming, requiring as long as three weeks in certain cases, is offset by the fact that all of the sample can be recovered after a determination. This adds to the general usefulness of the method, particularly in cases where the substance is expensive or difficult to obtain. A use for the method other than the determination of purity or of solubility is to obtain especially pure samples by recovering the solid residues at system concentration corresponding to points on section *BC* in Fig 16-5. Thus, the method is useful not only as a quantitative analytical tool, but also as a procedure for purification.

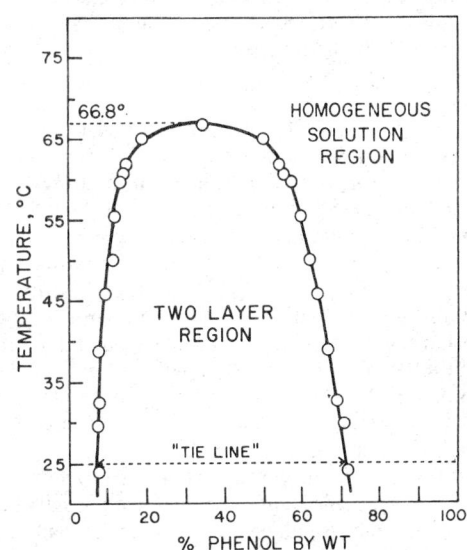

Fig 16-6.   Phenol-water solubility.[4]

water-rich in this example, will depend on the concentration of phenol added. As expected, the proportion of phenol-rich layer relative to the water-rich layer increases as the concentration of phenol added increases. For example, at 20% phenol in water at 25° there would be more of the water-rich layer than of phenol-rich layer while at 50% phenol in water there would be more of the phenol-rich layer. The relative proportion of each layer may be calculated from such tie lines at any temperature and composition as well as the amount of phenol present in each of the two phases. To determine how these calculations are made and for further discussion of this topic the student should consult Ref 1, page 79.

A simple and practical advantage in the use of phase diagrams is pointed out by Martin, Swarbrick, and Cammarata.[1] Based on diagrams such as Fig 16-6, they point out that the most concentrated stock solution of phenol that perhaps should be used by pharmacists is one containing 76% *w/w* phenol in water (equivalent to 80% *w/v*). At room temperature this mixture is a homogeneous solution and will remain homogeneous to around 3.5°, at which temperature freezing occurs. It should be noted that Liquefied Phenol USP contains 90% *w/w* phenol and freezes at 17°. This means that if the storage area in the pharmacy falls to about 63°F, the preparation will freeze resulting in a stock solution no longer convenient to use.

In the case of phenol and water the mutual solubility increases with increase in temperature and the critical solution temperature occurs at a relatively high point. In a certain number of cases, however, the mutual solubility increases with decrease in temperature and the critical solution temperature occurs at a relatively low value. Most of the substances which show lower critical solution temperatures are amines, as, for example, triethylamine with water.

In addition to pairs of liquids which show *either* upper or lower critical solution temperatures, there are other pairs which show *both* upper and lower critical solution temperatures and the mutual solubility curve is of the closed type. An example of this type of liquid pair is found in the case of nicotine and water, the curve for which is shown in Fig 16-7. Mixtures of nicotine and water represented by points within the curve will separate into two layers, but mixtures represented by points outside of the curve are perfectly miscible with each other.

In a discussion of solutions of liquids in liquids it is evident that the distinction between the terms solute and solvent loses its significance. For example, in a solution of water and glycerin, which shall be considered to be the solute and which the solvent? Again in cases where two liquids are only partially soluble in each other the distinction between solute and solvent might easily be reversed. In such cases the term solvent is usually given to the constituent present in larger quantity.

Ternary Systems—The addition of a third liquid to a binary liquid system to produce a ternary or three-component system can result in several possible combinations.

If the third liquid is soluble in only one of the two original liquids or if its solubility in the two original liquids is markedly different, the mutual solubility of the original pair will be decreased. An upper critical solution temperature will be elevated and a lower critical solution temperature lowered. On the other hand, the addition of a liquid having roughly the same solubility in both components of the original pair will result in an increase in their mutual solubility. An upper critical solution temperature then will be lowered and a lower critical solution temperature elevated.

An equilateral triangle graph may be used to represent the situation in which a third liquid is added to a partially miscible liquid pair, the third liquid being miscible with each member of the original pair. In this type of graph, each side of the triangle represents 0% of one of the components and the apex

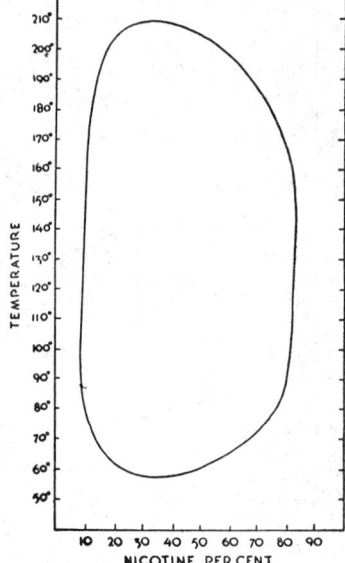

Fig 16-7. Nicotine-water solubility.

opposite that side represents 100% of that component. The reader is referred to texts on experimental physical chemistry for details of the construction and use of graphs of this type.

Two other possibilities exist in ternary liquid systems: that in which two components are completely miscible and the third is partially miscible with each, and that in which all combinations of two of the three components are only partially miscible.

Solutions of Gases in Liquids

Nearly all gases are more or less soluble in liquids. One has but to recall the solubility of carbon dioxide, of hydrogen sulfide, and of air in water as common examples of this type of solution.

The amount of gas dissolved in a liquid in general follows **Henry's law,** which states that *the weight of gas dissolved by a given amount of a liquid at a given temperature is proportional to its pressure.* Thus, if the pressure is doubled, twice as much gas will dissolve as at the initial pressure. The extent to which a gas is dissolved in a liquid, at a given temperature, may be expressed in terms of the *solubility coefficient*, which is the volume of gas measured under the conditions of the experiment, that is absorbed by one volume of the liquid. The degree of solubility is also sometimes expressed in terms of the *absorption coefficient*, which is the volume of gas, reduced to standard conditions, dissolved by one volume of liquid under a pressure of one atmosphere.

Although Henry's law expresses fairly accurately the solubility of slightly soluble gases, it deviates considerably in the case of very soluble gases such as hydrogen chloride and ammonia. Such deviations are most frequently due to chemical interaction of solute and solvent.

The solubility of gases in liquids *decreases* with *rise of temperature* and in general also when salts are added to the solvent, the latter effect being referred to as the "salting out" of the gas.

Solutions of gases are potentially dangerous when exposed to warm temperatures because of the liberation and expansion of the dissolved gas which may cause the container to burst. Bottles containing such solutions (eg, strong ammonia solution) should be cooled before opening if practical, and the stopper should be covered with a cloth before attempting its removal.

Thermodynamics of the Solution Process

In the discussions under this heading solute will be assumed to be in the liquid state, hence the heat of solution ($\Delta H'$) is a term different from that in Eq 3 (ΔH). The heat of solution for a solid solute going into solution as defined in Eq 3 is the net heat effect for the overall dissolution

$$A_{(solid)} \rightleftarrows A_{(liquid)} \rightleftarrows A_{(solution)}$$

We will consider only the process

$$A_{(liquid)} \rightleftarrows A_{(solution)}$$

and assume that the solute is a liquid (or a supercooled liquid in the case of a solid) at temperatures close to room temperature where the energy needed for melting (heat of fusion) is not being considered.

For a physical or chemical reaction to occur spontaneously at a constant temperature and pressure, the net free energy change, ΔG, for the reaction should be negative (see Chapter 15). Furthermore, we know that the free energy change is dependent on heat-related enthalpy ($\Delta H'$) and order-related entropy (ΔS) factors as seen in the equation

$$\Delta G = \Delta H' - T\Delta S \qquad (13)$$

where T is the temperature. Recall also that the relation between free energy, and the equilibrium constant, K, for a reaction is given by

$$\Delta G = -RT \ln K \qquad (14)$$

Eqs 13 and 14 certainly apply to the solution of a drug. Since we have seen that solubility is in reality an equilibrium constant, Eq 14 indicates that the greater the negative value of ΔG, the greater will be the solubility.

The interplay of these two factors, $\Delta H'$ and ΔS in Eq 13, determines the free energy change and hence whether or not dissolution of a drug will occur spontaneously. Thus, if in the solution process $\Delta H'$ is negative and ΔS positive, dissolution is favored since ΔG will be negative.

Since the heat of solution is quite significant in the dissolution process one must look at its origin.* The mechanism of solubility involves severing of the bonds that hold the ions or molecules of a solute together, the separation of molecules of solvent to create a space in the solvent into which the solute can be fitted, and the ultimate response of solute and solvent to whatever forces of interaction may exist between them. In order to sever the bonds between molecules or ions of solute in the liquid state energy must be supplied, as is the case also when molecules of solvent are to be separated. If heat is the source of energy it is apparent that both processes require absorption of heat. Solute–solvent interaction, on the other hand, is generally accompanied by evolution of heat since the process occurs spontaneously. In effecting solution there is, accordingly, a heat-absorbing effect and a heat-releasing effect to be considered beyond those required to melt a solid. If there is no, or very little, interaction between solute and solvent, the only effect will be that of absorption of heat to produce the necessary separations of solute and of solvent molecules or ions. If there is a significant interaction between solute and solvent, the amount of heat in excess of that required to overcome the solute–solute and the solvent–solvent forces is liberated. If the opposing heat effects are equal, there will be no change of temperature. When $\Delta H'$ is zero, and there is no volume change, an *ideal solution* is said to exist since the solute–solute, solvent–solvent, and solute–solvent interactions are the same. For such an ideal solution, the

solubility of a solid can be predicted from its heat of fusion (the energy needed to melt the solid) at temperatures below its melting point. The student is referred to Ref 1, page 281 to see how this calculation is made.

When the heat of solution has a positive (energy absorbed) or negative (energy liberated) value, the solution is said to be a *nonideal solution*. A negative heat of solution favors solubility while a positive heat works against dissolution.

The magnitude of the various attractive forces involved between solute, solvent, and solute-solvent molecules may vary greatly and thus could lead to varying degrees of positive or negative enthalpy changes in the solution process. The reason for this is that the molecular structure of the various solutes and solvents determining the interactions can themselves vary greatly.[†]

The solute–solute interaction that must be overcome can vary from the strong ion–ion interaction (as in a salt) to the weaker dipole–dipole interaction (as in nearly all organic medicinals that are not salts) to the weakest induced dipole-induced dipole interaction (as with naphthalene).

The attractive forces in the solvent that must be overcome are, most frequently, the dipole–dipole interaction (as found in water or in acetone) and the induced dipole–induced dipole interaction (as in liquid petrolatum).

The energy-releasing solute–solvent interactions that must be taken into account may be one of four types. In decreasing energy of interaction these are ion–dipole interactions (eg, a sodium ion interacting with water), dipole–dipole interactions (eg, an organic acid dissolved in water), dipole–induced dipole interaction[‡] (eg, an organic acid dissolved in carbon tetrachloride), and induced dipole–induced dipole interactions (eg, naphthalene dissolved in benzene).

Since the energy-releasing solute–solvent interaction should approximate the energy needed to overcome the solute-solute and solvent–solvent interactions, it is apparent why it is not possible to dissolve a salt like sodium chloride in benzene. The interaction between the ions and benzene does not supply enough energy to overcome the interaction between the ions in the solute and therefore gives rise to a positive heat of solution. On the other hand, the interaction of sodium and chloride ions with water molecules does provide an amount of energy approximating the energy needed to separate the ions in the solute and the molecules in the solvent.

Consideration must next be given to entropy effects in dissolution processes. Entropy is an indicator of the disorder or randomness of a system. The more positive the entropy change (ΔS), the greater is the increase in the randomness or disorder of the reaction system and the more favorably disposed is the reaction. Unlike $\Delta H'$, the entropy change (an entropy of mixing) in an ideal solution is not zero but has some positive value since there is an increase in the disorderliness or entropy of the system upon dissolution. Thus, in an ideal solution with $\Delta H'$ zero and ΔS positive, ΔG would have a negative value and the process therefore would be spontaneous.

In a nonideal solution, on the other hand, where $\Delta H'$ is not zero, ΔS can be equal to, greater than, or less than the entropy of mixing found for the ideal solution. In a nonideal solution with an entropy of mixing equal to that of the ideal solution, we have what is called a "regular solution." Regular solutions usually occur with nonpolar or weakly polar solutes and solvents. Such solutions are accompanied by a positive enthalpy change implying the solute–solvent molecular interaction is less than the solute–solute and solvent–solvent molecular interactions. Regular solutions are amenable to rigorous physical chemical analysis which will not be covered in this

---

* For an excellent and more complete discussion of the interactions and driving forces underlying the dissolution process, see Higuchi.[2]

[†] For a discussion of these effects, see Ref 1, p 41.
[‡] This subject will be discussed later.

chapter but which can be found in outline form in Ref 1, page 282.

The possibility exists in a nonideal solution that the entropy change is greater than that for an ideal solution. Such a solution occurs when there is an association among solute, or solvent, molecules. In essence then the dissolution process occurs when one begins at a relatively ordered (low entropy) state and progress to a disorderly (high entropy) state. The overall entropy change is positive, greater than that of the ideal case, and favorable to dissolution. As may be expected, the enthalpy change in such a solution is positive since association in a solute or solvent must be overcome. The facilitated solubility of citric acid (an unsymmetrical molecule) as compared to inositol (a symmetrical molecule), may be explained on the basis of such a favorable entropy change.[2]

The solubility of citric acid is greater than of inositol. Yet, on the basis of their heats of solution, inositol should be more soluble. One may regard this phenomenon in another way. The reason for the higher solubility of citric acid is that although there is no hindrance in the transfer of a citric acid molecule as it goes from the solute phase to the solution phase, when the structurally unsymmetrical citric acid attempts to return to the solute phase from solution, it must assume an orientation that will allow ready interaction with polar groups already oriented. If it does not have the required orientation it will not readily return to the solute but it will remain in solution, thus bringing about a solubility larger than expected on the basis of heat of solution.

On the other hand, the structurally symmetrical inositol, as it leaves the solution phase, can interact with the solute phase without requiring a definite orientation; all orientations are equivalent. Hence, inositol can enter the solute phase without hindrance and we therefore see no facilitation of its solubility.

In general, unsymmetrical molecules tend to be more soluble than symmetrical molecules.

The third type of nonideal solution occurs where there is an entropy change less than that expected of an ideal solution. Such nonideal behavior can occur with polar solutes and solvents. In a nonideal solution of this type there is significant interaction between solute and solvent. As may be expected, the enthalpy change ($\Delta H'$) in such a solution is negative and favors dissolution, but this effect is tempered by the unfavorable entropy change occurring at the same time. The reason for the lower than ideal entropy change can be visualized where the equilibrium system is more orderly and has a lower entropy than that expected for an ideal solution. The overall entropy change of solution would thus be less and not favorable to dissolution. We might, at least grossly, rationalize the lower-than-expected solubility of lithium fluoride on the basis of this phenomenon. Lithium fluoride, in comparison with other alkali halides has a solubility lower than would be expected based solely on enthalpy changes. Because of the small size of ions in the salt there may be considerable ordering of water molecules in the solution. This effect must of course lead to a lowered entropy and an unfavorable effect on solubility. The effect of soluble salts on the solubility of nonelectrolytes (p 209) or slightly soluble salts (p 210) may be considered a result of an unfavorable entropy effect.

Pharmaceutical Solvents

Our discussion will now focus on solvents available to pharmacists and in particular on the interactions and properties that these solvents have. It is most important that the pharmacist get a real understanding of the possible differences in solubility of a given solute in different solvents since he is most often called on to select a solvent in which the solute is soluble. An understanding of the properties of solvents will allow the intelligent or intuitive selection of suitable solvents.

Molecular Interactions in Solvents

The solvent–solvent interaction is, in pharmaceutical solvents, always made up of a dipole–dipole interaction (Keesom Force) and an induced dipole–induced dipole interaction (London Force). It is important to keep in mind that both forces are always present; the contribution that each of these forces makes toward the overall attractive force depends on the structure of the solvent molecule. Some solvents have interactions which predominantly involve the Keesom Force (water, for example), while others are predominantly composed of the London Force (chloroform, for example); usually, both forces will be found.

Dipole–Dipole Forces—The unequal sharing of the electron pair between two atoms due to a difference in the electronegativity of the atoms brings about a separation of the positive and negative centers of electricity in the molecule, causing it to become polarized, that is to assume a partial ionic character. The molecule is then said to be a *permanent dipole* and the substance is described as being a *polar compound*.

The greater the difference in the electronegativity of the constituent atoms, the greater the inequality of sharing of the electron pair, the greater the distance between the positive and negative centers of electricity in the molecule, and the more polar the resulting molecule. The character of the bonds being intermediate between those existing in nonpolar compounds and those occurring in ionic salts, it is to be expected that the properties of polar compounds should be intermediate between those of the two other classes. Such is, in fact, generally the case.

Coordinate covalent compounds are all very strongly polar because both of the electrons constituting the bonding pair have been contributed by a donor atom, which in effect loses an electron and becomes positively charged, while the acceptor atom may be considered to gain an electron and become negatively charged.

While, in general, the electronegativity of different kinds of atoms is different, and the expectation is, therefore, that all molecules containing two or more different atoms will be polar, many such molecules are actually nonpolar. Thus, while the electronegativity of chlorine is appreciably different from that of carbon, the molecule of carbon tetrachloride, CCl_4, is nonpolar because the symmetrical arrangement of chlorine atoms about the carbon atom is such as to cancel the effects of the difference in the electronegativity of the constituent atoms. The same is true in the case of methane, CH_4, and for hydrocarbons generally. But the molecules CH_3Cl, CH_2Cl_2, and $CHCl_3$ are definitely polar because of the unsymmetrical distribution of the forces within the molecule. A knowledge of the degree of polarity of various molecules is usually available in the measurement of the *dipole moment*, μ, of the molecules. This quantity is defined as the product of one of the charges on the molecule and the distance between the two average centers of positive and negative electricity. Measurements of the dipole moment of a substance are made, when possible, on the vapor of the substance but when this is not possible a dilute solution of the substance in a nonpolar solvent is employed. Table I lists the values of the dipole moment for a number of substances.

As was stated previously, the molecules of nonpolar substances are characterized by weak attractions for one another, while molecules of polar substances exhibit a relatively strong attraction which is all the more powerful the greater the dipole moment. The reason for this is readily apparent; the dipoles tend to align themselves so that the opposite charges of two different molecules are adjacent. They affect each other in

Table I—Dipole Moments

Substance	Electrostatic units ($\mu \times 10^{18}$)
Water	1.85
Acetone	2.8
Methyl alcohol	1.68
Ethyl alcohol	1.70
Phenol	1.70
Ethyl ether	1.14
Aniline	1.51
Nitrobenzene	4.19
o-Dinitrobenzene	6.0
m-Dinitrobenzene	3.8
p-Dinitrobenzene	0.3
Benzene	0
Methane	0
Methyl chloride	1.86
Dichloromethane	1.58
Chloroform	1.05
Carbon tetrachloride	0
Carbon monoxide	0.11
Carbon dioxide	0
Oxygen	0
Hydrogen	0
Hydrogen chloride	1.03
Hydrogen bromide	0.78
Hydrogen iodide	0.38
Hydrogen sulfide	0.95
Hydrogen cyanide	2.93
Ammonia	1.49

somewhat the same manner as do two bar magnets the opposite poles of which are adjacent. While thermal agitation tends to break up the alignment or association of the dipoles, there is, nevertheless, a resultant significant intermolecular force present.

Induced Dipole–Induced Dipole Forces—It is of interest to inquire at this point what force does exist between the molecules of compounds which are nonpolar, eg, those which have zero dipole moment. If some attractive force did not exist, the molecules could not be expected to cling together, as in the solid and liquid states. Though the attraction is relatively slight, there is a force that arises from momentary polarization of the molecules because of electronic oscillations which are continuously taking place within the molecules. The *temporary dipoles* thus produced induce opposite polarizations in adjacent molecules and the net effect is that there is a small but definite attractive force between the molecules to keep them together in the liquid and solid states. This attraction resulting from mutual polarization is commonly referred to as the London Force and as an induced dipole–induced dipole force.

The Hydrogen Bond—The attraction between oppositely charged ends of two dipoles is accentuated when the positive end of one dipole contains a hydrogen atom and the negative end of the other dipole contains an atom of fluorine, oxygen, or nitrogen. In such instances the nucleus of the hydrogen atom—which is a proton—appears to be able to bind together the negative end of the molecule of which it is a part with the negative end of the adjacent molecule. This may be represented as shown in Fig 16-8.

Since the proton is the smallest positively charged atomic particle it can draw together two negatively charged atoms or ions more closely than can any other—and necessarily larger—positively charged particle. Not more than two negative atoms are capable of being attracted at any given instant, as is evident from the Fig 16-8, where a third negative atom is shown to be physically restricted from direct contact with the proton. Water is an excellent example of a substance the molecules of which are associated through the formation of such a bond—called the *hydrogen bond*. An illustration of such bonding in the case of water may be represented as:

$$\underset{\displaystyle |}{H} \quad \underset{\displaystyle |}{H} \quad \underset{\displaystyle |}{H}$$
$$H{-}O{-}{-}{-}H{-}O{-}{-}{-}H{-}O$$

in which each dotted line represents the bond or "bridge" established by the hydrogen of one molecule of water with the oxygen of another molecule of water. It is to be noted that the water molecule is pictured as a bent, rather than as a linear, molecule (H—O—H). This is in accord with the bond angles imposed by the directional character of the bonding orbitals making up the molecule (see Chapter 24). By virtue of its kernel containing six unneutralized protons, not only the valence electrons of the oxygen but also those of the hydrogen atoms are so strongly attracted to the oxygen atom as to make the latter negatively charged, while the rest of the molecule is charged positively.

The hydrogen bond is not a strong bond, but it plays an important role in determining the properties of substances in which it occurs. For example, it is primarily responsible for the unusual properties of water. If the substance H_2O followed the course of the related substances H_2Te, H_2Se, and H_2S, in so far as the physical properties of these latter substances are concerned, the freezing point of water would be about $-100°$ and its boiling point about $-80°$. The unexpectedly high values actually observed are attributed to hydrogen bonding between molecules of water; to break such bonds, as for example in vaporizing water in the form of single H_2O molecules during the process of boiling, more energy is required than would be necessary if the water molecules were not linked by hydrogen bonds.

The molecules of at least the low-molecular-weight alcohols are similarly joined by hydrogen bonds to form a lattice-like structure.

Another example of the manner in which the hydrogen bond functions is seen in the case of carboxylic acids. Such acids usually exist in dimeric form, the two molecules being joined by hydrogen bonding, which may be depicted as

$$
\begin{array}{ccc}
 & OH{-}{-}{-}{-}{-}{-}O & \\
RC & & CR \\
 & O{-}{-}{-}{-}{-}{-}HO &
\end{array}
$$

This tendency is so pronounced in the case of acetic acid that even in the vapor state the substance exists in dimeric aggregation.

Classification of Solvents

On the basis of the forces of interaction occurring in solvents we may broadly classify solvents as one of three types:

1. *Polar solvents*—those made up of strong dipolar molecules having hydrogen bonds (water and hydrogen peroxide).
2. *Semipolar solvents*—those also made up of strong dipolar molecules but which do not form hydrogen bonds (acetone and amyl alcohol).
3. *Nonpolar solvents*—those made up of molecules having a small or no dipolar character (benzene, vegetable oil, and mineral oil).

Naturally there are many solvents that can fit into more than one of these broad classes; for example, chloroform is a weak dipolar compound but is generally considered nonpolar

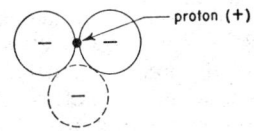

Fig 16-8. Hydrogen bonding.

in character, and glycerin could be considered a polar or semipolar solvent even though it can form hydrogen bonds.

Types

Water—Water is a very unique solvent. Besides being a highly associated liquid, giving rise to its high boiling point, it has another very important property; it has a high dielectric constant. Dielectric constant (ϵ) indicates the effect that a substance has, when it acts as a medium, on the ease with which two oppositely charged ions may be separated. The higher the dielectric constant of a medium, the easier it is to separate two oppositely charged species in that medium. The dielectric constants of a number of liquids are given in Table II. The values listed are relative to a vacuum which by definition has a dielectric constant of unity. According to Coulomb's Law the force of attraction (F) between two oppositely charged ions is

$$F = \frac{Z_1 Z_2}{\epsilon r^2} \qquad (15)$$

where Z_1 and Z_2 are the charges on the ions, r is the distance separating the oppositely charged ions, and ϵ is the dielectric constant of the medium. Eq 15 indicates that the force of interaction between the oppositely charged ions is inversely proportional to the dielectric constant of the medium. Thus, the interaction force between a sodium and chloride ion in water at a distance r would be $\frac{1}{80}$ that of the same ions in a vacuum separated the same distance. Looking at this example in another way, Coulomb's Law suggests that it is much easier to keep sodium and chloride ions apart in water than in a vacuum. Consider another example: the relative ease with which the ions of sodium chloride may be kept apart the same distance in water as compared to olive oil would stand in the ratio of 80/3.1; that is, it is 80/3.1 times easier to keep these ions apart in water than it is in olive oil. The high solubility of salts in solvents like water and glycerin can be explained on the basis of their high dielectric constant. In general also, the more polar the solvent, the greater its dielectric constant.

There is a very close relationship between dielectric constant and the two types of interactions found in all solvents; that is, the dipole–dipole interaction (Keesom) and the induced dipole–induced dipole interaction (London). The dielectric constant is related to these two forces through a quantity called *total molar polarization*, P, which is a measure of the relative ease with which a charge separation may be made within a molecule. The total molar polarization is given by the equation,*

$$P = \frac{\epsilon - 1}{\epsilon + 2} \cdot \frac{M}{D} \qquad (16)$$

where ϵ is the dielectric constant of the substance, M is the molecular weight, and D is the density of the substance. Total molar polarization is in turn composed of two terms:

$$P = P_\alpha + P_\mu = \frac{4}{3} \pi N \alpha + \frac{4}{3} \pi N \left(\frac{\mu^2}{3kT} \right) \qquad (17)$$

where $P_\alpha = 4/3 \, \pi N \alpha$ is the contribution due to induced polarization (the London contribution), and where

$$P_\mu = \frac{4}{3} \pi N \left(\frac{\mu^2}{3kT} \right)$$

is the contribution due to the permanent dipole (the Keesom contribution), N is Avogadro's Number, α is a constant called the polarizability (related to the induced dipole), μ is the dipole moment, k is the Boltzmann constant (1.38×10^{-16} erg/

* For further details, see Ref 1, p 114.

Table II—Dielectric Constants (at 20°)

Hydrogen cyanide	116.
Water	80.
Glycerin	46.
Ethylene glycol	41.
Methyl alcohol	33.
Ethyl alcohol	25.
n-Propyl alcohol	22.
Acetone	21.
Aniline	7.0
Chloroform	5.0
Castor oil	4.6
Ethyl ether	4.3
Octyl alcohol	3.4
Olive oil	3.1
Benzene	2.2
Turpentine oil	2.2
Carbon tetrachloride	2.2
Octane	1.9

mole/deg), and T is the absolute temperature. Grouping all constant terms, it is possible to rewrite Eq 17 as

$$P = A + B/T$$

and substituting Eq 16, we get

$$\frac{\epsilon - 1}{\epsilon + 2} \cdot \frac{M}{D} = A + \frac{B}{T} \qquad (18)$$

The first term on the right-hand side of Eq 18 is the contribution to the dielectric constant of the London dispersions; it is not temperature dependent. The second term on the right-hand side of the equation is the contribution to the dielectric constant of the Keesom dispersions. This latter contribution is temperature dependent because the contribution from the permanent dipole depends on the dipoles aligning themselves, which tendency is opposed by thermal agitation. Thus, it is apparent from Eq 18 (and from common sense) that as temperature increases the dielectric constant of dipolar solvents will tend to decrease.

Eq 18 also indicates that solvents that have large dipole moments tend to have large dielectric constants because of the contribution of the P_μ term. Water, which has a very large dielectric constant, is estimated to have $\frac{2}{3}$ of its molecular interaction due to a dipole–dipole interaction and $\frac{1}{3}$ due to the induced dipole–induced dipole interaction. On the other hand, compounds such as benzene with a dipole moment of zero will have small dielectric constants since the P_μ term will drop out of Eq 18.

Before leaving the topic of water, there is an important concept that should be considered that has been introduced to pharmaceutical systems.[5] It must be recognized that pharmacists are frequently concerned with dissolving relatively nonpolar drugs in aqueous or mixed polar aqueous solvents. To understand what may be happening in such cases, factors concerned with the entropic effects arising from interactions originating with the nonpolar solutes must be considered. Previously we had noted the favorable entropic effect on dissolution that was due to the disruption of associations occurring among solute or solvent molecules. Now we consider the effects on solubility due to solute interactions in the solution phase. Since the solutes under discussion are relatively nonpolar, the interactions are of the London Force type or a *hydrophobic association*. This hydrophobic association in aqueous solutions may cause significant structuring of water with a resultant ordered or low entropy system unfavorable to solution. As we intuitively know, the aqueous solution of an essentially nonpolar molecule is not a favorable process. It should be stressed that this is due to not only an unfavorable enthalpy change but may also be due to an unfavorable entropy change generated by water structuring.

Such an unfavorable entropy change is quite significant in the solution process. As an example of this effect, the aqueous solubility of a series of alkyl p-aminobenzoates shows a ten million-fold decrease in solubility in going from the one carbon analogue to the twelve carbon analogue. These findings clearly demonstrate the considerable effect that hydrophobic associations can have.

Alcohols—Alcohol itself as a solvent is next in importance to water. It has an important advantage over water in the fact that preparations made with it keep almost indefinitely, while many aqueous solutions of organic substances soon hydrolyze and become worthless. A further advantage is that growth of microorganisms does not occur in solutions containing alcohol in not too low a concentration.

Resins, volatile oils, alkaloids, glycosides, etc. are dissolved by alcohol, while many therapeutically inert principles, like gum, albumin, and starch, are insoluble in it, for which reason it is all the more useful as a "selective" solvent. Mixtures of water and alcohol, in proportions varying to suit specific cases, are extensively used. They are often referred to as *hydroalcoholic* solvents.

Glycerin is an excellent solvent, although its range is not as extensive as that of water or alcohol. In higher concentrations it has preservative action. It dissolves the fixed alkalies, a large number of salts, and vegetable acids, pepsin, tannin, some active principles of plants, etc., but it also dissolves gum, soluble carbohydrates, starch, etc., and thus its solutions are generally "loaded" with inert constituents. It is also of special value as a simple solvent as in phenol glycerite, or where the major portion of the glycerin is simply added as a preservative and stabilizer of solutions that have been prepared with other solvents (see *Glycerites*).

Propylene glycol, which has been widely used as a substitute for glycerin, is miscible with water, with acetone, and with chloroform in all proportions. It is soluble in ether and will dissolve many essential oils but is immiscible with fixed oils. It is claimed to be as effective as ethyl alcohol in its power of inhibiting mold growth and fermentation.

Isopropyl alcohol possesses solvent properties similar to those of ethyl alcohol, and is used instead of the latter in a number of pharmaceutical manufacturing operations. It has the advantage over ethyl alcohol in that the commonly available product contains not over 1% of water, while ethyl alcohol contains about 5% water, which is often a disadvantage. Isopropyl alcohol is employed in some liniment and lotion formulations. It cannot be taken internally.

General Properties—Low molecular weight and polyhydroxy alcohols form associated structures through hydrogen bonds just as in the case of water. When the carbon atom content of an alcohol rises above five, generally only monomers are then present in the pure solvent. Although alcohols have high dielectric constants compared to other types of solvents,

they are small compared to water. As we have seen, the solubility of salts in a solvent should be paralleled by its dielectric constant. That is, as the dielectric constant of a series of solvents increases, the probability of dissolving a salt in the solvent increases. This behavior is observed for the alcohols. Table III, taken from Higuchi,[2] shows how the solubility of salts follows alcohol dielectric constant.

As mentioned earlier, absolute alcohol is rarely used pharmaceutically in the pure state. However, hydroalcoholic mixtures such as elixirs and spirits are frequently encountered. A very useful generalization is that the dielectric properties of a mixed solvent such as water and alcohol can be approximated as the weighted average of the properties of the pure components. Thus, a mixture of 60% alcohol (by weight) in water should have a dielectric constant approximated by

$$\epsilon_{(mixture)} = 0.6(\epsilon_{(alcohol)}) + 0.4(\epsilon_{(water)})$$

$$\epsilon_{(mixture)} = 0.6(25) + 0.4(80) = 47$$

The dielectric constant of 60% alcohol in water is experimentally found to be 43, which is in close agreement with that just calculated. The dielectric constant of glycerin is 46, close to the 60% alcohol mixture. We would, therefore, expect a salt like sodium chloride to have about the same solubility in glycerin as in 60% alcohol. The solubility of sodium chloride in glycerin is 8.3 g/100 g solvent and in 60% alcohol about 6.3 g/100 g solvent. This agreement would be even closer if comparisons were made on a volume rather than weight basis. At least qualitatively we can then say that the solubility of a salt in a solvent or a mixed solvent very closely follows the dielectric constant of the medium or, conversely, that the polarity of mixed solvents is paralleled by their dielectric constant based on salt solubility.

Although the dielectric constant is useful in interpreting the effect of mixed solvents on salt solubility, it cannot properly be applied to the effect of mixed solvents on the solubility of nonelectrolytes. We saw earlier that unfavorable entropic effects can occur upon dissolution of relatively nonpolar nonelectrolytes in water. Such an effect due to hydrophobic association considerably affects solubility. Yalkowsky, et al.,[5] have used cosolvent systems to increase the solubility of nonelectrolytes in polar solvents where the cosolvent system essentially brings about a reduction in structuring of solvent. Thus, by increasing, in a positive sense, the entropy of solution by using cosolvents, it was possible to increase the solubility of the nonpolar molecule. Using as an example the solubility of alkyl p-aminobenzoates in propylene glycol-water systems, Yalkowsky and co-workers report that it is possible to increase the solubility of the nonelectrolyte by several orders of magnitude by increasing the fraction of propylene glycol in the aqueous system. It is found that the logarithm of the solubility is linearly related to the fraction of propylene glycol added by the equation

$$\log S_f = \log S_{f=0} + \epsilon f$$

where S_f is the solubility in the mixed aqueous system containing the volume fraction f of nonaqueous cosolvent, $S_{f=0}$ is the solubility in water, and ϵ is a constant (not dielectric constant) characteristic of the system under study. Specifically, when a 50% solution of propylene glycol in water was used, there was a thousand-fold increase in solubility of dodecyl p-aminobenzoate in comparison to pure water.

In a series of studies Martin and coworkers[6] have made attempts to predict solubility in mixed solvent systems through an extension of "regular" solution theory. The equations are logarithmic in nature and can reduce in form to the equations of Yalkowsky and coworkers.[5]

Acetone and Related Semipolar Materials—Even though acetone has a very high dipole moment (2.8×10^{-18}

Table III—Solubilities of Potassium Iodide and Sodium Chloride in Several Alcohols and Acetone [a]

Solvent	g KI/ 100 g solvent	g NaCl/ 100 g solvent
Water	148	35.9
Glycerin	. . .	8.3 (20°)
Glycol	50	7.1 (30°)
Methanol	17	1.4
Acetone	2.9	. . .
Ethanol	1.88	0.065
Propanol	0.44	0.0124
Isopropanol	0.18	0.003
Butanol	0.20	0.005
Pentanol	0.089	0.0018

[a] All measurements at 25° unless otherwise indicated.

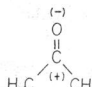

Fig 16-9.   The charge separation in acetone.

esu), as a pure solvent it does not form associated structures. This is evidenced by its low boiling point (57°) in comparison with the boiling point of the lower molecular weight water (100°) and ethanol (79°). The reason why it does not associate is because the positive charge in its dipole does not reside in a hydrogen atom (Fig 16-9), precluding the possibility of its forming a hydrogen bond. However, if some substance which is capable of forming hydrogen bonds, such as water or alcohol, is added to acetone, a very strong interaction through hydrogen bonding will occur (see *Mechanism of Solvent Action* which follows below). Some substances which are semipolar and similar to acetone are aldehydes, low-molecular-weight esters, other ketones, and nitro-containing compounds.

Nonpolar Solvents—In this class of solvents are found fixed oils such as vegetable oil, petroleum benzin, carbon tetrachloride, benzene, and chloroform. On a relative basis there is a wide range of polarity among these solvents; for example, benzene has no dipole moment while that of chloroform is 1.05×10^{-18} esu. But even the polarity of these compounds normally classified as nonpolar is still in line with the dielectric constant of the solvent. The relation between these quantities is best seen through a quantity called *molar refraction*. The molar refraction, R, of a compound is given by

$$R = \frac{n^2 - 1}{n^2 + 2} \cdot \frac{M}{D} \qquad (19)$$

where n is the refractive index of the liquid, M is its molecular weight, and D is its density. The similarity between Eq 19 and Eq 16 is to be noted, and indeed in refractive index measurements using very long wavelengths of light, $n^2 = \epsilon$. Thus, molar refraction under these conditions approximates total molar polarization. Since in the more nonpolar solvents there is generally no dipole moment, μ, total molar polarization reflects polarization due only to the induced dipoles possible. Thus

$$P_\alpha = \frac{n^2 - 1}{n^2 + 2} \cdot \frac{M}{D} = \frac{\epsilon - 1}{\epsilon + 2} \cdot \frac{M}{D} = \frac{4}{3} \pi N \alpha \qquad (20)$$

It is evident from Eq 20 that the refractive index of a nonpolar compound reflects its relative polarity. For example, the more polar benzene ($\epsilon = 2.2$) has a higher refractive index, 1.501, than the less polar hexane ($\epsilon = 1.9$), whose refractive index is 1.375.

It should be emphasized again that when a solvent (such as chloroform) has highly electronegative halogen atoms attached to a carbon atom also containing at least one hydrogen atom, such a solvent will be capable of forming strong hydrogen bonds with solutes which are polar in character. Thus, through the formation of such hydrogen bonds such solvents will dissolve polar solutes. For example, it is possible to dissolve alkaloids in chloroform.

Mechanism of Solvent Action

A solvent may function in one or more of several ways. When an ionic salt is dissolved, as by water for example, the process of solution involves separation of the cations and anions of the salt with attendant orientation of molecules of solvent about the ions. Such orientation of solvent molecules about the ions of the solute—a process called *solvation* (*hydration* if the solvent is water)—is possible only when the solvent is highly polar, whereby the dipoles of the solvent are attracted to and held by the ions of the solute. The solvent

must also possess the ability to keep the solvated, charged ions apart with a minimum requirement of energy. The role of the dielectric constant in keeping this energy to a minimum has been discussed earlier.

A polar liquid such as water may exhibit solvent action also by virtue of its ability to break a covalent bond in the solute and bring about ionization of the latter. For example, hydrogen chloride dissolves in water and functions as an acid as a result of the following reaction:

$$HCl + H_2O \rightarrow H_3O^+ + Cl^-$$

The ions formed by this preliminary reaction of breaking the covalent bond are subsequently maintained in solution by the same mechanism as in the case of ionic salts.

Still another mechanism by which a polar liquid may act as a solvent is that involved when the solvent and solute are capable of being coupled through hydrogen bond formation. The solubility of the low-molecular-weight alcohols in water, for example, is attributed to the ability of the alcohol molecules to become part of a water-alcohol association complex:

$$\begin{array}{ccccccc} & H & & R & & H & & R \\ & | & & | & & | & & | \\ H—&O&------H——&O&------H——&O&------H——&O \end{array}$$

As the molecular weight of the alcohol increases, it becomes progressively less polar, and less able to compete with water molecules for a place in the lattice-like arrangement formed through hydrogen bonding; high-molecular-weight alcohols are, therefore, poorly soluble or insoluble in water. When the number of carbon atoms in a normal alcohol reaches five, solubility in water is materially reduced.

When the number of hydroxyl groups in the alcohol is increased, its solubility in water is generally greatly increased; it is principally, if not entirely, for this reason that such high-molecular-weight compounds as sugars, gums, many glycosides, and such synthetic compounds as the polyethylene glycols are very soluble in water.

The solubility of ethers, aldehydes, ketones, acids, and anhydrides in water—and in other polar solvents—is also largely attributable to the formation of an association complex between solute and solvent by means of the hydrogen bond. While the molecules of ethers, aldehydes and ketones, unlike those of alcohols, are not themselves associated—because of the absence of a hydrogen atom that is capable of forming the characteristic hydrogen bond—the substances are nonetheless more or less polar because of the presence of a strongly electronegative oxygen atom which is capable of association with water through hydrogen bond formation. Acetone, for example, dissolves in water in all likelihood principally because of the following type of reaction:

$$(CH_3)_2CO + H_2O \rightarrow (CH_3)_2CO \cdots H—O \overset{\displaystyle H}{\underset{\displaystyle |}{|}}$$

The maximum number of carbon atoms which may be present per molecule while retaining water solubility is approximately the same as with the alcohols.

Although nitrogen is less electronegative than oxygen and thus tends to form weaker hydrogen bonds, it is observed that amines are more or at least as soluble as alcohols containing an equivalent chain length. The reason for this is that alcohols form two hydrogen bonds with a net interaction of 12 kcal/mole. Primary amines can form three hydrogen bonds; two amine protons are shared with the oxygens of two waters, and the nitrogen accepts one water proton. The net interaction for the primary amine is between 12 and 13 kcal/mole and hence it shows an equal or greater solubility in comparison with corresponding alcohols.

Table IV—Demonstration of Solubility Rules

Chemical compound	Solubility[a]
Aniline, $C_6H_5NH_2$	28.6
Benzene, C_6H_6	1430
Benzoic acid, C_6H_5COOH	275
Benzyl alcohol, $C_6H_5CH_2OH$	25
1-Butanol, C_4H_9OH	12
t-Butyl alcohol, $(CH_3)_3COH$	Miscible
Carbon tetrachloride, CCl_4	2000
Chloroform, $CHCl_3$	200
Fumaric acid, trans-butenedioic acid	150
Hydroquinone, $C_6H_4(OH)_2$	14
Maleic acid, cis-butenedioic acid	5
Phenol, C_6H_5OH	15
Pyrocatechol, $C_6H_4(OH)_2$	2.3
Pyrogallol, $C_6H_3(OH)_3$	1.7
Resorcinol, $C_6H_4(OH)_2$	0.9

[a] *Note*—The above solubility table gives number of milliliters of water required to dissolve 1 g of solute.

The solvent action of nonpolar liquids involves a somewhat different mechanism. Because they are unable to form dipoles with which to overcome the attractions between ions of an ionic salt, or to break a covalent bond to produce an ionic compound, or to form association complexes with a solute, nonpolar liquids are incapable of dissolving polar compounds. They can only dissolve, in general, other nonpolar substances in which the bonds between molecules are weak. The forces involved are usually of the induced dipole–induced dipole type. Such is the case when one hydrocarbon is dissolved in another, or an oil or a fat is dissolved in petroleum ether. Sometimes it is observed that a polar substance such as alcohol will dissolve in a nonpolar liquid such as benzene. This apparent exception to the preceding generalization may be explained by the assumption that the alcohol molecule induces in the benzene molecule a temporary dipole which forms an association complex with the solvent molecules. A binding force of this kind is referred to as a *permanent dipole–induced dipole force.*

Some Useful Generalizations—The preceding discussion indicates that enough is known about the mechanism of solubility to be able to formulate some generalizations concerning this important physical property of substances. Because of the greater importance of organic substances in the field of medicinal chemistry, certain of the more useful generalizations with respect to organic chemicals are presented here in summary form. It should be remembered, however, that the phenomenon of solubility usually involves several variables, and that there may be exceptions to general rules.

One general maxim which holds true in most instances is: *the greater the structural similarity between solute and solvent, the greater the solubility.* Thus phenol is almost insoluble in petroleum benzin but is very soluble in glycerin.

Organic compounds containing polar groups capable of forming hydrogen bonds with water are soluble in water, providing that the molecular weight of the compound is not too great. It is easily demonstrated that the polar groups OH, CHO, COH, CHOH, CH_2OH, COOH, NO_2, CO, NH_2, and SO_3H tend to increase the solubility of an organic compound in water. On the other hand, nonpolar or very weak polar groups, such as the various hydrocarbon radicals, reduce solubility; the greater the number of carbon atoms in the radical, the greater the decrease in solubility. Introduction of halogen atoms into a molecule in general tends to decrease solubility because of increased molecular weight without a proportionate increase in polarity.

The greater the number of polar groups, the greater is the solubility of a compound, provided that the size of the rest of the molecule is not altered; thus pyrogallol is much more soluble in water than is phenol. The *relative positions* of the groups in the molecule also influence solubility; thus, in water, resorcinol (*m*-dihydroxybenzene) is more soluble than pyrocatechol (*o*-dihydroxybenzene), and the latter is more soluble than hydroquinone (*p*-dihydroxybenzene).

Polymers and compounds of high molecular weight are generally insoluble or only very slightly soluble.

High melting points are frequently indicative of low solubility for organic compounds. One reason for high melting points is *association* of molecules; this cohesive force tends to prevent dispersion of the solute in the solvent.

The *cis* form of an isomer is more soluble than the *trans* form. See Table IV.

Solvation, which is evidence of the existence of a strong attractive force between solute and solvent, enhances the solubility of the solute, provided there is not a marked ordering of the solvent molecules in the solution phase.

Acids, especially strong acids, usually produce water-soluble salts when reacted with nitrogen-containing organic bases.

Colligative Properties of Solutions

Up to this point we have been concerned with dissolving a solute in a solvent. Having brought about the dissolution, the solution, quite naturally, has a number of properties that are different from that of the pure solvent. Of very great importance are the *colligative properties* that a solution possesses.

The colligative properties of a solution are those that depend on the *number* of solute particles in solution, irrespective of whether these are molecules or ions, or large or small. Ideally, the effect of a solute particle of one species is considered to be the same as that of an entirely different kind of particle, at least in dilute solution. Practically, there may be differences which may become substantial as the concentration of the solution is increased.

The colligative properties which will be considered in this chapter are:

1. Osmotic pressure.
2. Vapor-pressure lowering.
3. Boiling-point elevation.
4. Freezing-point depression.

Of the four colligative properties, all of which are related, osmotic pressure has the greatest direct importance in the pharmaceutical sciences. It is the property that largely determines the physiologic acceptability of a variety of solutions used for therapeutic purposes. As the property of prime importance, it will be considered first. Afterward the other colligative properties, one of which is much used in pharmacy because it provides an estimate of osmotic pressure, will be studied.

Osmotic-Pressure Elevation

Diffusion in Liquids—Although the property of diffusion is most marked in gaseous systems, it is not limited to such systems. That molecules or ions in liquid systems possess this same freedom of movement may be demonstrated by carefully placing a layer of water on a concentrated aqueous solution of any salt. In time it will be observed that the boundary between solvent and solution gradually widens since salt moves into the water layer and water migrates from its layer into the salt solution below. Eventually the composition of the new solution will become uniform throughout. This experiment indicates that *substances tend to move or diffuse from regions of higher concentration to regions of lower concentrations* so that differences in concentration eventually disappear.

Osmosis—In carrying out the experiment just described, it is impossible to distinguish between the diffusion of the solute and that of the solvent. However, by separating the solution and the solvent by means of a membrane that is permeable to the solvent, but not to the solute (such a membrane is referred to as a *semipermeable membrane*), it is possible to demonstrate visibly the diffusion of solvent into the concentrated solution since volume changes will occur. In a similar manner, if two solutions of different concentration are separated by a membrane, the solvent will move from the solution of lower solute concentration to the solution of higher solute concentration. This diffusion of solvent through a membrane is called *osmosis*.

There is a difference between the activity or escaping tendency of the water molecules found in the solvent and salt solution separated by the semipermeable membrane. Since *activity*, which is related to water concentration, is higher on the pure solvent side, water moves from solvent to solution in order to equalize escaping tendency differences. The difference in *escaping tendency* gives rise to what is referred to as the *osmotic pressure* of the solution which might be visualized as follows. A semipermeable membrane is placed over the end of a tube and a small amount of salt solution is placed over the membrane in the tube. The tube is then immersed in a trough of pure water so that the upper level of the salt solution is initially at the same level as the water in the trough. With time solvent molecules will move from solvent into the tube. The height of the solution will rise until the *hydrostatic pressure* exerted by the column of solution is equal to the *osmotic pressure*.

Osmotic Pressure of Nonelectrolytes—From quantitative studies with solutions of varying concentration of a solute that does not ionize, it has been demonstrated that *osmotic pressure is proportional to the concentration of the solute*, ie, twice the concentration of a given nonelectrolyte will produce twice the osmotic pressure in a given solvent.*

Furthermore, the osmotic pressures of solutions of different nonelectrolytes are proportional to the number of molecules in each solution. Stated in another manner, the osmotic pressures of two nonelectrolyte solutions of the same molal† concentration are identical. Thus a solution containing 34.2 g of sucrose (mol wt 342) in 1000 g of water has the same osmotic pressure as a solution containing 18.0 g of anhydrous dextrose (mol wt 180) in 1000 g of water. These solutions are said to be *iso-osmotic* with each other because they have identical osmotic pressures.

A study of the results of osmotic-pressure measurements on different substances led the Dutch chemist Jacobus Henricus van't Hoff, in 1885, to suggest that the solute in a solution may be considered as being analogous to the molecules of a gas and the osmotic pressure as being produced by the bombardment of the semipermeable membrane by the molecules of solute. According to van't Hoff's theory the osmotic pressure of a solution is equal to the pressure which the dissolved substance would exert in the gaseous state if it occupied a volume equal to the volume of the solution. From this it follows that just as in the case of a gas there is a proportionality between pressure and concentration of dissolved substance. This proportionality is well illustrated by the values of the osmotic pressure of solutions of sucrose at 0° as determined by the Earl of Berkeley and E G J Hartley and shown in Table V.

In column PV of the foregoing table a quantitative confirmation, at least for fairly dilute solutions, of van't Hoff's oversimplified though useful generalization is shown by the constancy of the values of the product PV. The student will recall that the product of the pressure and the volume of a gas, at constant temperature, is likewise constant (Boyle's law).

Van't Hoff also deduced that the osmotic pressure must be proportional to the absolute temperature, just as in Charles'

---

* This is not strictly true in solutions of fairly high solute concentration, but does hold quite well for dilute solutions.
† A molal solution is one that contains the mol wt in grams of a given solute in 1000 g of solvent. A 2-molal solution contains twice the gram-molecular weight; a 0.1 molal, 1/10 the gram-molecular weight in 1000 g of solvent.

Table V—Osmotic Pressure of Sucrose Solutions

Conc. (g/L), C	Vol. in L in which 1 g mole is dissolved, V^a	Pressure in atmos P	P/C	PV
10.00	34.2	0.65	0.065	22.2
20.00	17.1	1.27	0.064	21.7
45.00	7.60	2.91	0.065	22.1
93.75	3.65	6.23	0.067	22.7

^{a} The figures in this column were obtained by calculating the volume of solution in which 342 (mol wt) g of sucrose would be dissolved.

law for gases, which deduction was confirmed by the experiments of several workers. From this it follows that the equation $PV = nRT$ is valid for dilute solutions of nonelectrolytes just as a similar equation is valid for gases. However, even as Boyle's law does not apply to gases under high pressures and at low temperatures, so van't Hoff's equation for osmotic pressure does not apply in concentrated solutions. For a more thorough discussion of osmotic pressure the student is referred to books on physical chemistry.

Osmotic Pressure of Electrolytes—In discussing the generalizations concerning the osmotic pressure of solutions of nonelectrolytes it was stated that the osmotic pressures of two solutions of the same molal concentration are identical. This generalization, however, cannot be made for solutions of electrolytes, ie, acids, alkalies, and salts.

Van't Hoff pointed out that the osmotic pressures of solutions of electrolytes, particularly of the extensively ionized group, are considerably greater than the osmotic pressures of solutions of nonelectrolytes of the same molal concentration. This anomaly remained unexplained until 1887 when Svante August Arrhenius proposed a hypothesis to account for the abnormal osmotic pressures of solutions of electrolytes. Arrhenius advanced the theory that in aqueous solution, acids, bases, and salts may be considered to be dissociated or ionized into positively and negatively charged particles or ions and that the increased osmotic pressure of such solutions is due to increased number of particles formed in the process of ionization. For example, sodium chloride is assumed to be ionized as follows:

$$NaCl \rightarrow Na^+ + Cl^-$$

It is evident that each molecule of sodium chloride that is ionized produces two ions and, if sodium chloride is completely ionized, there will be twice as many particles as would be the case if it were not ionized at all. Furthermore, if each ion has the same effect on osmotic pressure as a molecule, it might be expected that the osmotic pressure of the solution would be twice that of a solution containing the same molal concentration of nonionizing substance. Study of osmotic pressure data indicates that in very dilute solutions of salts which yield two ions the pressure is very nearly twice that of solutions of equivalent concentrations of solutes that do not ionize.

For solutions which yield more than two ions as, for example, the following:

$$K_2SO_4 \rightarrow 2K^+ + SO_4^{2-}$$

$$FeCl_3 \rightarrow Fe^{3+} + 3Cl^-$$

it is to be expected that the complete dissociation of the molecules would give rise to osmotic pressures that are three and four times, respectively, the pressure of solutions containing an equivalent quantity of a nonionized solute. Accordingly, the equation $PV = nRT$, which may be employed to calculate the osmotic pressure of a dilute solution of a nonelectrolyte, may also be applied to dilute solutions of electrolytes if it is changed to $PV = inRT$, where the value of i approaches the number of ions produced by the ionization of the strong electrolytes cited in the preceding examples. For weak electrolytes i represents the total number of particles, ions and molecules together, in the solution, divided by the number of molecules that would be present if the solute did not ionize. The experimental evidence indicates that in dilute solutions at least, the osmotic pressures approach the predicted values. It should be emphasized, however, that in more concentrated solutions of electrolytes the deviations from this simple theory are considerable, due to interionic attraction, solvation, and other factors that need not be discussed here. For further information the reader is referred to standard texts on physical chemistry.[7,8]

Biological Aspects of Osmotic Pressure—Osmotic pressure experiments were made as early as 1884 by the Dutch botanist Hugo de Vries in his study of plasmolysis. This term is applied to the contraction of the contents of plant cells placed in solutions of comparatively high osmotic pressure. The phenomenon is caused by the osmosis of water out of the cell through the practically semipermeable membrane surrounding the protoplasm. If suitable cells, for example, the epidermal cells of the leaf of *Tradescanta discolor*, are placed in a solution of higher osmotic pressure than that of the cell contents, water flows out of the cell, causing the contents to draw away from the cell wall. On the other hand, if the cells are placed in solutions of lower osmotic pressure, water enters the cell, producing an expansion which, however, is limited by the rigid cell wall. By immersing cells in a series of solutions of varying solute concentration, a solution may be found in which plasmolysis is barely detectable or is absent. The osmotic pressure of such a solution is then the same, or very nearly the same, as that of the cell contents and it is then said that the solution is *isotonic* or, more exactly, *isoosmotic* with the cell contents. Solutions of greater concentration than this are said to be *hypertonic* and solutions of lower concentration are said to be *hypotonic*.

Red blood cells or erythrocytes have been similarly studied by immersion into solutions of varying concentration of different solutes. When introduced into water or into sodium chloride solutions containing less than 0.90 g of solute per 100 mL, human erythrocytes swell, and often burst, because of the diffusion of water into the cell and the fact that the cell wall is not sufficiently strong to resist the pressure. This phenomenon is referred to as *hemolysis*. If the cells are placed in solutions containing more than 0.90 g of sodium chloride per 100 mL, they lose water and shrink. By immersing the cells in a solution containing exactly 0.90 g of sodium chloride in 100 mL, no change in the size of the cells is observed; since in this solution the cells maintain their "tone," the solution is said to be *isotonic* with human erythrocytes. For the reasons indicated it is desirable that solutions to be injected into the blood should be made isotonic with erythrocytes. The manner in which this may be done is described in Chapter 80.

Distinction Between Isoosmotic and Isotonic—The terms isoosmotic and isotonic are not to be considered as being equivalent, although often a solution may be described as being both isoosmotic and isotonic. If a plant or animal cell is in contact with a solution that has the same osmotic pressure as the cell contents, there will be no net gain or loss of water by either solution *provided* the cell membrane is impermeable to all solutes that are present. Since the volume of the cell contents remains unchanged, the "tone" or normal state of the cell is maintained, and the solution in contact with the cell may be described not only as being isoosmotic with the solution in the cell but also as being isotonic with it. If, however, one or more of the solutes in contact with the membrane can pass through the latter, it is evident that the volume of the cell contents will change, thus altering the "tone" of the cell; in this case the two solutions may be isoosmotic, yet not be isotonic.

It is possible that some substances used in an injection dosage form can cause hemolysis of red blood cells, even when their concentrations are such as to produce solutions theoretically isoosmotic with the cells, because the solutes diffuse through the membrane of the cells. For example, a 1.8% solution of urea has the same osmotic pressure as a 0.9% solution of sodium chloride, but the former solution produces hemolysis of red blood cells; obviously the urea solution is not isotonic with the cells. To determine whether or not a solution is isotonic with erythrocytes, it is necessary to determine the concentration of solute at which the cells retain their normal size and shape. A simple method for doing this was devised by Setnikar and Temelcou,[9] who determined the concentration of a solution at which red blood cells maintained a volume equal to that occupied in an isotonic solution of sodium chloride; the red cell volumes were determined by centrifuging suspensions of them in different solutions, using a hematocrit tube.

Vapor-Pressure Lowering

When a nonvolatile solute is dissolved in a liquid solvent the vapor pressure of the solvent is lowered. This easily can be qualitatively described by visualizing solvent molecules on the surface of the solvent which normally could escape into the vapor being replaced by solute molecules which have little if any vapor pressure of their own. For ideal solutions of nonelectrolytes the vapor pressure of the solution follows Raoult's law,

$$P_A = X_A P_A^\circ \qquad (21)$$

where P_A is the vapor pressure of the solution, P_A° is the vapor pressure of the pure solvent, and X_A is the mole fraction of solvent. This relationship states that the vapor pressure of the solution is proportional to the number of molecules of solvent in the solution. Rearranging Eq 21 gives

$$\frac{P_A^\circ - P_A}{P_A^\circ} = (1 - X_A) = X_B \qquad (22)$$

where X_B is the mole fraction of the solute. This equation states that the lowering of vapor pressure in the solution relative to the vapor pressure of the pure solvent—what is called simply the *relative vapor-pressure lowering*—is equal to the mole fraction of the solute. The *absolute* lowering of vapor pressure of the solution is defined by

$$P_A^\circ - P_A = X_B P_A^\circ \qquad (23)$$

Example—Calculate the lowering of vapor pressure and the vapor pressure, at 20°, of a solution containing 50 g of anhydrous dextrose (mol wt 180.16) in 1000 g of water (mol wt 18.02). The vapor pressure of water at 20°, in absence of air, is 17.535 mm.

First, the lowering of vapor pressure is to be calculated, using Eq 23, in which X_B is the mole fraction of dextrose, defined by

$$X_B = \frac{n_B}{n_A + n_B}$$

where n_A is the number of moles of solvent and n_B is the number of moles of solute. Substituting numerical values

$$n_B = \frac{50}{180.2} = 0.278$$

$$n_B = \frac{1000}{18.02} = 55.5$$

$$X_B = \frac{0.278}{55.5 + 0.278} = 0.00498$$

the lowering of vapor pressure is

$$P_A^\circ - P_A = 0.00498 \times 17.535$$

$$= 0.0873 \text{ mm}$$

the vapor pressure of the solution is

$$P_A = 17.535 - 0.0873$$

$$= 17.448 \text{ mm}$$

Measurement of Vapor Pressure—The preceding example emphasizes the need for an accurate method of measuring vapor pressure, and especially of small differences of pressure between a solvent and its solutions. Vapor pressure may be determined directly with a suitable manometer or, under certain conditions, by observing the direct depression of the level of mercury in a tube long enough to have an evacuated space above the mercury. A differential manometer, one arm of which is connected to the solution and the other to the solvent, improves the accuracy of measurement. The *isopiestic method*, which is capable of very good precision and accuracy, is based on the principle that if two solutions containing the same solvent are placed side by side in a closed space (preferably evacuated to hasten equilibration) solvent will distil from the solution of higher vapor pressure into the one of lower pressure until both solutions have the same pressure, when they are said to be *isopiestic* (Gr, equal pressure). If the equilibrated solutions are analyzed, and one contains a reference solute of known effect on the vapor pressure of the solvent, it is possible to calculate the vapor pressure of the "unknown" solution.

Boiling-Point Elevation

In consequence of the fact that the vapor pressure of any solution of a nonvolatile solute is less than that of the solvent, the boiling point of the solution—which is the temperature at which the vapor pressure is equal to the applied pressure (commonly 760 mm)—must be higher than that of the solvent. This is clearly evident in Fig 16-10.

The relationship between the elevation of boiling point and the concentration of nonvolatile, nonelectrolyte solute may be derived from the Clausius–Clapeyron equation (Eq 106 in Chapter 15), which is

$$\frac{dP}{dT} = \frac{P \cdot \Delta H_{vap}}{RT^2} \tag{24}$$

Replacing the differential expression dP/dT by $\Delta P / \Delta T_b$, where ΔP is the lowering of vapor pressure and ΔT_b is the elevation of boiling point, and introducing $P_A°$, the vapor pressure of the solvent at its boiling point T_0, results in

$$\frac{\Delta P}{\Delta T_b} = \frac{P_A° \cdot \Delta H_{vap}}{RT_0^2} \tag{25}$$

Since the lowering of vapor pressure in an ideal solution is

$$\Delta P = X_B P_A° \tag{26}$$

substitution of this equation into Eq 25 with rearrangement to provide a solution for ΔT_b gives

$$\Delta T_b = \frac{RT_0^2}{\Delta H_{vap}} X_B \tag{27}$$

This equation may be used to calculate the elevation of boiling point if the concentration of solute is expressed as the mole fraction. A more common expression, however, is in terms of the molality m (the number of gram-moles of solute per 1000 g of solvent), which relationship is derived as follows:

$$X_B = \frac{n_B}{n_A + n_B} = \frac{m}{1000/M_A + m} \cong \frac{m}{1000/M_A} \tag{28}$$

In these equations M_A is the molecular weight of the solvent. When the solutions are dilute, so that m is small, it may be neglected in the denominator (but not in the numerator!) to give the approximate equivalent in Eq 28. Substituting this equivalent into Eq 27 gives

$$\Delta T_b = \frac{RT_0^2 M_A m}{1000 \Delta H_{vap}} \tag{29}$$

Grouping the constants into a single term results in

$$\Delta T_b = K_b m \tag{30}$$

where

$$K_b = \frac{RT_0^2 M_A}{1000 \Delta H_{vap}} \tag{31}$$

and is called the molal boiling-point elevation constant.

The value of this constant for water, which boils at 373.1° K, has a heat of vaporization of 539.7 cal/g and a molecular weight of 18.02, is

$$K_b = \frac{1.987 \times 373.1^2 \times 18.02}{1000 \times 18.02 \times 539.7} = 0.513° \tag{32}$$

Notwithstanding that K_b is called a molal boiling-point elevation constant, it should not be interpreted as the actual rise of boiling point for a 1-molal solution. Such solutions are generally too concentrated to exhibit the ideal behavior assumed in deriving the equation for calculating the theoretical value of the constant. In dilute solutions, however, the actual boiling-point elevation, *calculated to a 1-molal basis*, approaches the theoretical value, the closer the more dilute the solution.

The elevation of boiling point of a dilute solution of a nonelectrolyte solute may be used to calculate the mol wt of the latter. In a solution containing w_B g of solute of M_B in w_A g of solvent the molality m is

$$m = \frac{1000 \, w_B}{w_A M_B} \tag{33}$$

substituting this into Eq 30 and rearranging gives

$$M_B = \frac{K_b 1000 \, w_B}{w_A \Delta T_b} \tag{34}$$

The accurate determination of boiling point requires that cognizance be taken of the following potential sources of error: (1) superheating of the liquid; (2) change of concentration of solution as solvent passes into vapor phase; (3) change of boiling point with variation of atmospheric pressure; (4) variation of temperature with position of thermometer or other temperature-measuring device (if placed in vapor above a solution the thermometer measures the boiling point of condensing solvent and not of solution); (5) inaccuracy resulting from use of uncalibrated or improperly calibrated thermometer.

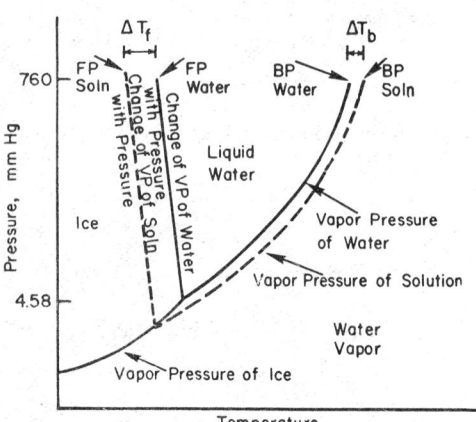

Fig 16-10. Vapor-pressure-temperature diagram for water and an aqueous solution, illustrating elevation of boiling point and lowering of freezing point of the latter.

Freezing-Point Depression

The freezing point of a solvent is defined as the temperature at which the solid and liquid forms of the solvent coexist in equilibrium at a fixed external pressure, commonly 1 atm (760 mm of mercury). At this temperature the solid and liquid forms of the solvent must have the same vapor pressure, for if this were not so the form having the higher vapor pressure would change into that having the lower vapor pressure.

The freezing point of a solution is the temperature at which the solid form of the pure solvent coexists in equilibrium with the solution at a fixed external pressure, again commonly 1 atm. Since the vapor pressure of a solution is lower than that of its solvent, it is obvious that solid solvent and solution cannot coexist at the same temperature as solid solvent and liquid solvent; only at some lower temperature, where solid solvent and solution do have the same vapor pressure, is equilibrium established. A schematic pressure–temperature diagram for water and an aqueous solution, not drawn to scale and exaggerated for the purpose of more effective illustration, shows the equilibrium conditions involved in both freezing-point depression and boiling-point elevation (Fig 16-10).

The freezing-point lowering of a solution may be quantitatively predicted for ideal solutions, or dilute solutions which obey Raoult's law, by mathematical operations similar to (though somewhat more complex than) those used in deriving the boiling-point elevation constant. The equation for the freezing point lowering, ΔT_f, is

$$\Delta T_f = \frac{RT_0^2 M_A m}{1000 \Delta H_{fus}} = K_f m \tag{35}$$

where

$$K_f = \frac{RT_0^2 M_A}{1000 \Delta H_{fus}} \tag{36}$$

The value of K_f for water, which freezes at 273.1°K and has a heat of fusion of 79.7 cal/g, is

$$K_f = \frac{1.987 \times 273.1^2 \times 18.02}{1000 \times 18.02 \times 79.7} = 1.86° \tag{37}$$

The molal freezing-point depression constant is not intended to represent the freezing-point depression for a 1-molal solution, which is too concentrated for the premise of ideal behavior to be applicable. In dilute solutions the freezing-point depression, calculated to a 1-molal basis, approaches the theoretical value, the agreement between experiment and theory being the better the more dilute the solution.

The freezing point of a dilute solution of a nonelectrolyte solute may be used, as with the boiling point, to calculate the molecular weight of the solute. The applicable equation is

$$M_B = \frac{K_f 1000 \, w_B}{w_A \Delta T_f} \tag{38}$$

The molecular weight of organic substances soluble in molten camphor may be determined by observing the freezing point of a mixture of the substance with camphor. This procedure, called the *Rast method*, utilizes camphor because it has a very large molal freezing-point depression constant, about 40°; since the constant may vary with different lots of camphor and with variations of technique, the method should be standardized using a solute of known molecular weight.

Freezing-point determinations have the advantage over boiling-point determinations of greater accuracy and precision by virtue of the larger magnitude of the former; thus, in the case of water the molal freezing-point depression is approximately 3.5 times greater than the molal boiling-point elevation. Potential sources of error in the determination of freezing point include: (1) supercooling of the liquid; (2) in-crease of concentration of solution if solvent crystallizes out of it; (3) loss of heat by transfer to surrounding freezing bath; (4) liberation of latent heat on crystallization of solid solvent; (5) inaccuracy resulting from use of uncalibrated or improperly calibrated thermometer or other temperature-measuring device.

Reasonably accurate determinations of freezing points may be made by the Beckmann method, which utilizes the Beckmann differential thermometer, which permits temperature readings to ±0.001°. The most accurate measurements are obtained by a method in which the difference in temperature between two systems, one of liquid solvent in equilibrium with solid solvent and the other of solution in equilibrium with solid solvent, is determined with a multiple-junction thermocouple and potentiometer.

Relationship between Osmotic Pressure and Vapor-Pressure Depression

The lowering of vapor pressure and the development of osmotic pressure in a solution are both manifestations of the basic condition that the free energy of solvent molecules in the pure solvent is greater than the free energy of solvent molecules in the solution. Consequently, solvent molecules will spontaneously transfer, if given an opportunity, from solvent to solution until equilibrium conditions are established. The transfer can take place either through a membrane permeable only to solvent molecules or, if such contact between solvent and solution is not available, by distillation of solvent from pure solvent to solution if access through a vapor phase is provided.

If an experiment is performed with two sets of vessels containing solution and solvent, as illustrated in Fig 16-11, differing only in that the long tube of one set has a semipermeable membrane attached to its lower end while in the other a hypothetical membrane separates the vapor phases; in time the same hydrostatic pressure should develop in both cases. For a definite volume, eg, a mole, of solvent transferred to the solution by distillation the change of free energy, ΔG, in the process is

$$\Delta G = RT \ln \frac{P_A}{P_A°} \tag{39}$$

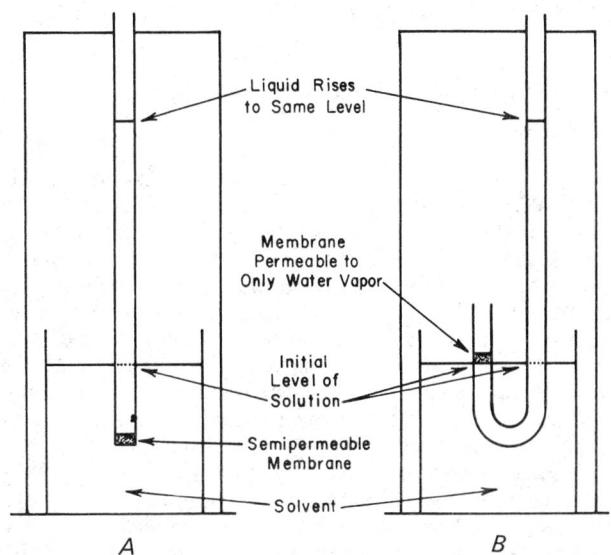

Fig 16-11. Transfer of solvent to equal volumes of solution. *A*: Osmotically through a semipermeable membrane separating solution and solvent. *B*: By distillation of solvent through a membrane separating solution and solvent vapor.

where P_A is the vapor pressure of the solution and $P_A°$ is the vapor pressure of the solvent.

For the transfer of the same volume of solvent by osmosis the free energy change is

$$\Delta G = -\overline{V}_A \pi \qquad (40)$$

where $\overline{V}_A$ is the partial molal volume of solvent (the volume of 1 mole of solvent in the solution) and π is the osmotic pressure of the solution. Since the free energy change is the same in both processes

$$-\overline{V}_A \pi = RT \ln \frac{P_A}{P_A°} \qquad (41)$$

rearranging the equation yields

$$\pi = \frac{RT}{\overline{V}_A} \ln \frac{P_A°}{P_A} \qquad (42)$$

With this equation the osmotic pressure of a solution may be calculated if its vapor pressure and the partial molal volume of the solvent are known, not only when the solution is sufficiently dilute that Raoult's law is obeyed but also when the concentration is so high as to introduce substantial deviation from the law.

From Eq 42, which has some resemblance to van't Hoff's empirical equation $\pi V = nRT$ for dilute solutions, the latter equation may be derived as follows. If a solution is sufficiently dilute to correspond to Raoult's law, we know

$$P_A = X_A P_A° = (1 - X_B)P_A° \qquad (43)$$

and then Eq 42 may be written

$$\pi = -\frac{RT}{\overline{V}_A} \ln (1 - X_B) \qquad (44)$$

When X_B is small (as in a dilute solution), the term $-\ln (1 - X_B)$ can be shown to be approximately equal to X_B, so that

$$\pi = \frac{RT}{\overline{V}_A} X_B \qquad (45)$$

In dilute solutions the approximations $X_B = n_B/n_A$ (where n_B and n_A are the moles of solute and solvent, respectively) and $\overline{V}_A = V/n_A$ (where V is the volume of solution) may be introduced, yielding

$$\pi V = n_B RT \qquad (46)$$

which is van't Hoff's equation.

Ideal Behavior and Deviations from Ideal Behavior

In setting out to derive mathematical expressions for colligative properties such phrases as "for ideal solutions" or "for dilute solutions" were used to indicate the limitations of the expressions. Samuel Glasstone defines an ideal solution as "one which obeys Raoult's law over the whole range of concentration and at all temperatures" and gives as specific characteristics of such solutions their formation only from constituents which mix in the liquid state without heat change and without volume change. These characteristics reflect the fact that addition of solute to a solvent produces no change in the forces between molecules of the solvent. Thus the molecules have the same *escaping tendency* in the solution as in the pure solvent and the vapor pressure above the solution is proportional to the ratio of the number of solvent molecules in the surface of the solution to the number of the molecules in the surface of the solvent—which is the basis for Raoult's law.

Any change in intermolecular forces produced by mixing the components of a solution may result in deviation from ideality; such a deviation may be expected particularly in solutions containing both a polar and a nonpolar substance. Solutions of electrolytes, except at high dilution, are especially prone to depart from ideal behavior, even though allowance is made for the additional particles that result from ionization. When solute and solvent combine to form solvates, the escaping tendency of the solvent may be reduced in consequence of the reduction in the number of free molecules of solvent; thus, a negative deviation from Raoult's law is introduced. On the other hand, the escaping tendency of the solvent in a solution of nonvolatile solute may be increased because the cohesive forces between molecules of solvent are reduced by the solute; this results in a positive deviation from Raoult's law.

While few solutions exhibit ideal behavior over a wide range of concentration, most solutions behave ideally at least in high dilution, where deviations from Raoult's law are negligible.

Comparison of Colligative Properties—In view of the established interrelationships of the colligative properties of ideal solutions or very dilute real solutions, it is possible to predict by calculation the magnitude of all these properties of such solutions if the concentration of the nonelectrolyte solute is given; also, if the magnitude of one of the properties, say the freezing point, is known for a solution of unspecified concentration, it is possible to calculate the vapor pressure, boiling point and osmotic pressure, provided the solution is ideal or sufficiently dilute to show negligible deviation from ideality. To what upper limit of concentration a nonideal solution remains "sufficiently dilute" to show ideal behavior is difficult to specify; the answer depends at least in part on the degree of agreement expected between experimental and theoretical values. Certainly a 1-molal concentration is much too concentrated for a nonideal solution to show conformance with ideal behavior; even in 0.1-molal concentration deviations are significant and for some purposes may be excessive.

In dealing with colligative properties of solutions that do not behave ideally, caution should be exercised in attempting to predict the magnitude of other colligative properties from one that has been determined experimentally. Earlier an equation was derived for calculating the vapor pressure of a solution from its osmotic pressure, or *vice versa*, this equation being valid even with solutions showing substantial departures from ideal behavior; the equation is limited, however, to comparison of these colligative properties at the same temperature. The degree of deviation from ideal behavior for one colligative property will be exactly the same for another only when the temperature is the same for both. It does not follow that the degree of deviation of the colligative properties of a given nonideal solution will be the same for all the properties since at least two of these (freezing point and boiling point) must be determined at quite different temperatures. While in dilute solutions the intermolecular (and/or interionic) forces and interactions *may* change little over the temperature interval between freezing and boiling, in concentrated solutions the change *may* be marked. In the absence of adequate knowledge about the forces and interactions involved, only by experiment can one establish the magnitude of the colligative properties of other than very dilute nonideal solutions. It is important to keep this in mind in estimating the osmotic pressure of a nonideal solution at body temperature from a freezing point determined some 37° lower. While in many cases—possibly the majority of them—such an estimate is warranted by virtue of essential constancy of the various forces and interactions over a wide range of temperature, this is not always the case and the estimate may be significantly inaccurate.

Colligative Properties of Electrolyte Solutions—Earlier in this chapter attention was directed to the increased osmotic pressure observed in solutions of electrolytes, the enhanced effect being attributed to the presence of ions, each of which acts, in general, in the same way as a molecule in developing osmotic pressure. Similar magnification of vapor-pressure lowering, boiling-point elevation, and freezing-point depression occurs in solutions of electrolytes. Thus, at a given constant temperature the abnormal effect of an electrolyte on osmotic pressure is paralleled by abnormal lowering of vapor pressure; the other colligative properties are, subject to variation of effect with temperature, comparably intensified. In general the magnitude of each colligative property is proportional to the total number of particles (molecules and/or ions) in solution.

With strong electrolytes, most of which are commonly assumed to be 100% ionized, the magnitude of effect is determined primarily by the concentration of ions, which concentration may readily be calculated as the product of the molal concentration and the number of ions produced by ionization of each "molecule" (2 ions from such substances as $NaCl$ and $MgSO_4$; 3 from $CaCl_2$ and Na_2SO_4; 4 from $FeCl_3$ and Na_3PO_4; etc.). While in *very* dilute solutions the osmotic pressure, vapor-pressure lowering, boiling-point increase, and freezing-point depression of solutions of electrolytes approach values 2, 3, 4, etc. times greater (depending on the type of strong electrolyte) than in solutions of the same molality of nonelectrolyte, thus confirming the hypothesis than an ion has the same primary effect as a molecule on colligative properties, two other effects are observed as the concentration of electrolyte is increased. The first effect results in *less* than 2-, 3-, or 4-fold intensification of a colligative property; this reduction is ascribed to interionic attraction between the positively and negatively charged ions, in consequence of which the ions are not completely dissociated from each other and do not exert their full effect in lowering vapor pressure, etc. This deviation generally increases with increasing concentration of electrolyte. The second effect intensifies the colligative properties and is attributed to the attraction of ions for solvent molecules (called solvation or, if water is the solvent, hydration), which holds the solvent in solution and reduces its escaping tendency, with consequent enhancement of the vapor-pressure lowering; solvation may also reduce interionic attraction and thereby further lower the vapor pressure. These factors (and possibly others) combine to effect a progressive reduction in the molal values of colligative properties as the concentration of electrolyte is increased to 0.5 to 1 molal, beyond which the molal quantities either increase, sometimes quite abruptly, or remain almost constant.

Activity and Activity Coefficient

Various mathematical expressions are employed to relate properties of chemical systems (equilibrium constants, colligative properties, pH, etc) to the stoichiometric concentration of one or more molecular, atomic, or ionic species. In deriving such expressions it is either stated or implied that they are valid only as long as intermolecular, interatomic, and/or interionic forces may be ignored or remain constant, under which restriction the system may be expected to behave ideally. But intermolecular, interatomic, and/or interionic forces do exist, and not only do they change as a result of chemical reaction but also they change with variation in the concentration or pressure of the molecules, atoms, or ions under observation. In consequence, mathematical expressions involving stoichiometric concentrations or pressures generally have limited applicability. The conventional concentration terms, while providing a count of molecules, atoms, or ions per unit volume, afford no indication of the physical or chemical activity of the species measured, and it is this activity that determines the physical and chemical properties of the system.

In recognition of this, Gilbert N Lewis introduced both the quantitative concept and methods for evaluation of activity as a true measure of the physical or chemical activity of molecular, atomic, or ionic species, whether in the state of gas, liquid, or solid, or whether present as a single species or in a mixture. Activity may be considered loosely as a corrected concentration or pressure which takes into account not only the stoichiometric concentration or pressure but also any intermolecular attractions or repulsions, interactions between solute and solvent in solution, association, and ionization; thus, activity measures the net effectiveness of a chemical species. Because only relative values of activity may be determined, a *standard state* must be chosen for quantitative comparisons to be made; indeed, because activity measurements are needed for many different types of systems several standard states must be selected. The specifications for all these standard states are beyond the scope of this book; they are given in Lewis and Randall.[10] It will suffice to mention, since we are concerned mainly with solutions, that the standard state for the solvent is pure solvent, while for the solute it is a hypothetical solution with free energy corresponding to unit molality under conditions of ideal behavior of the solution.

Definitions—The relationship of activity to concentration is measured in terms of the activity coefficient, expressed as

$$m\gamma = a \qquad (47)$$

where m is the molal concentration, γ is the activity coefficient, and a is the activity. The activity coefficient may be variously determined, as by measurement of colligative properties, electromotive force, solubility, distribution coefficients, etc; procedural details are given in Lewis and Randall's work. For a strong electrolyte the *mean ionic activity coefficient*, designated $\gamma_{\pm}$, provides a measure of the deviation of the electrolyte from ideal behavior. The mean ionic activity coefficients of several strong electrolytes at various concentrations, but at constant temperature (25°), are given in Table VI. It is characteristic of the electrolytes that the coefficients at first decrease with increasing concentration, pass through a minimum, and finally increase with increasing concentration of electrolyte. A partial interpretation of this complex behavior is given in the preceding section. The variation of activity coefficients with temperature, for several concentrations of solutions of sodium chloride, is given in Table VII.

Debye-Hückel Theory—In 1923 Debye and Hückel presented a theory for evaluating the activity coefficient of an ion in solution, expressed mathematically by the equation

$$-\ln \gamma_i = \frac{e^3 z_i^2}{(\epsilon k T)^{3/2}} \sqrt{\frac{2\pi N\mu}{1000}} \qquad (48)$$

where

γ_i = activity coefficient of ion species i
e = charge on an electron
z_i = valence of ion i
ϵ = dielectric constant of the medium
k = Boltzmann constant
T = absolute temperature
N = Avogadro number
μ = ionic strength = $\frac{1}{2}\Sigma m_i z_i^2$ (μ is not to be confused with dipole moment used earlier)

Transferring to 10-base logarithms, and substituting the numerical values for the constants, this equation becomes, for water at 25°,

$$\log \gamma_i = -0.509 \, z_i^2 \sqrt{\mu} \qquad (49)$$

Table VI—Mean Ionic Activity Coefficients of Electrolytes at 25°

Molality	NaCl	KCl	KBr	KI	NaOH	HCl	H_2SO_4	$CaCl_2$
0.001	0.966	0.965	0.965	0.965	. . .	0.966	0.830	0.89
0.002	0.953	0.952	0.952	0.951	. . .	0.952	0.757	0.85
0.005	0.929	0.927	0.927	0.927	. . .	0.928	0.639	0.79
0.01	0.904	0.901	0.903	0.905	. . .	0.904	0.544	0.72
0.02	0.875	. . .	0.872	0.88	. . .	0.875	0.453	0.66
0.05	0.823	0.815	0.822	0.84	0.818	0.830	0.340	0.57
0.1	0.780	0.769	0.777	0.80	0.766	0.796	0.265	0.52
0.2	0.730	0.719	0.728	0.76	0.727	0.767	0.209	0.47
0.5	0.68	0.651	0.665	0.71	0.693	0.758	0.154	0.52
1.0	0.66	0.606	0.625	0.68	0.679	0.809	0.132	0.71
2.0	0.67	0.576	0.602	0.69	0.698	1.01	0.128	0.79
4.0	0.78	0.579	0.622	0.75	0.888	1.76	0.170	2.93
6.0	0.99	. . .	. . .	. . .	1.28	. . .	0.257	11.1

Table VII—Temperature Variation of Mean Ionic Activity Coefficients of Sodium Chloride

Molality	0°	10°	25°	40°	60°	80°	100°
0.1	0.781	0.781	0.778	0.774	0.766	0.757	0.746
0.2	0.731	0.734	0.732	0.728	0.721	0.711	0.698
0.5	0.671	0.677	0.679	0.678	0.671	0.660	0.644
1.0	0.637	0.649	0.656	0.657	0.654	0.641	0.622
2.0	0.630	0.652	0.670	0.678	0.676	0.663	0.641
3.0	0.660	0.691	0.719	0.728	0.726	0.712	0.687
4.0	0.717	0.757	0.791	0.802	1.799	0.777	0.746

and for the mean ionic activity coefficient

$$\log \gamma_\pm = -0.509 \, z_+ z_- \sqrt{\mu} \tag{50}$$

where z_+ is the valence of the cation and z_- is the valence of the anion. The significance of the ionic strength, μ, will be discussed in the next section.

The Debye-Hückel theory is a limiting law applicable to very dilute solutions of electrolytes; large deviations are encountered as the ionic strength of the solution increases. Even in dilute solutions deviations occur with electrolytes containing higher valence ions.

Ionic Strength—The usual expressions of concentration—molarity, molality, mole fraction, etc—take no cognizance of the intensity of the electrical field in a solution of a strong electrolyte, which is an important variable in evaluating interionic forces. To take this into account, Lewis and Randall in 1921 proposed its evaluation in terms of ionic strength, μ, defined mathematically as

$$\mu = \tfrac{1}{2} \Sigma m_i z_i^2 \tag{51}$$

where m_i is the molality of ion i, z_i is its valence, and Σ is the summation of the product of molality and the square of the valence of each ion in the solution. Ionic strength, being a measure of the intensity of the electrical field in a solution, provides a basis for evaluating electrostatic interaction between ions. It already has been shown that the mean ionic activity coefficient is a function of ionic strength; so also are such diverse phenomena as solubilities of sparingly soluble salts (including proteins), rates of ionic reactions, effects of salts on pH of buffers, electrophoresis of proteins, etc.

The greater effectiveness of ions of higher charge type on a specific property, compared with the effectiveness of the same number of singly charged ions, generally coincides with the ionic strength calculated by Eq 51. The variation of ionic strength with the valence (charge) of the ions comprising a strong electrolyte should be noted. For electrolytes composed of univalent cations and univalent anions, called uniunivalent or 1–1 electrolytes, the ionic strength is identical with molality. For bivalent cation and univalent anion (biunivalent or 2-1) electrolytes, or univalent cation and bivalent anion (unibi-

valent or 1-2) electrolytes, the ionic strength is in all cases three times the molality. For bivalent cation and bivalent anion (bibivalent or 2-2) electrolytes, the ionic strength is four times the molality. These relationships are evident from the following numerical illustration.

Example—Calculate the ionic strength of 0.1-molal solutions of NaCl, Na_2SO_4, $CaCl_2$, and $MgSO_4$, respectively. For

$$NaCl \quad \mu = \tfrac{1}{2}(0.1 \times 1^2 + 0.1 \times 1^2) = 0.1$$
$$Na_2SO_4 \quad \mu = \tfrac{1}{2}(0.2 \times 1^2 + 0.1 \times 2^2) = 0.3$$
$$CaCl_2 \quad \mu = \tfrac{1}{2}(0.1 \times 2^2 + 0.2 \times 1^2) = 0.3$$
$$MgSO_4 \quad \mu = \tfrac{1}{2}(0.1 \times 2^2 + 0.1 \times 2^2) = 0.4$$

Practical Applications of Colligative Properties

One of the most important pharmaceutical applications of colligative properties is in the preparation of isotonic intravenous and isotonic lacrimal solutions, the details of which are discussed in Chapter 80.

Other applications of the colligative properties are found in experimental physiology. One such application is in the immersion of tissues in salt solutions, which are isotonic with the fluids of the tissue, in order to prevent changes or injuries that may arise from osmosis.

The colligative properties of solutions also may be used in determining the molecular weight of solutes or, in the case of electrolytes, the extent of ionization. The method of determining molecular weight depends on the fact that each of the colligative properties is altered by a constant value when a definite number of molecules of solute is added to a solvent. For example, in dilute solutions the freezing point of water is lowered at the rate of 1.855° for each gram molecular weight of a nonelectrolyte dissolved in 1000 g of water.* The constant 1.855° is commonly called the *molal freezing-point depression* of water. To find the molecular weight of a nonelectrolyte, therefore, all that is necessary is to determine the

---

* These constants apply only to solutions that are considerably more dilute than 1 molal; a substantial deviation would be observed if a 1-molal solution were to be used.

freezing point of a dilute aqueous solution of known concentration of the nonelectrolyte, and, by proportion, to calculate the quantity that would produce, theoretically, a depression of 1.855° when 1000 g of water is used as solvent. If the substance is insoluble in water, it may be dissolved in another solvent, in which case, however, the freezing-point depression of a solution corresponding to a gram molecular weight of the solute in 1000 g of solvent will be some value other than 1.855°. In the case of benzene, for example, this value is 5.12°; for carbon tetrachloride, it is 2.98°; for phenol, 7.27°; and for camphor, about 40° (see *Freezing-Point Depression*, in this chapter).

The boiling-point elevation may be used similarly for determining molecular weights. The boiling point of water is raised at the rate of 0.52° for each gram molecular weight of solute dissolved in 1000 g of water,* the corresponding values for benzene, carbon tetrachloride, and phenol being 2.57°, 4.88°, and 3.60°, respectively. The observation of vapor-pressure lowering and osmotic pressure likewise may be used to calculate molecular weights.

To determine the extent to which an electrolyte is ionized it is necessary to know its molecular weight, as determined by some other method, and then to measure one of the four colligative properties. The deviation of the results from similar values for nonelectrolytes is then used in calculating the extent of ionization.

References

1. Martin AN, *et al: Physical Pharmacy*, Lea & Febiger, Philadelphia, 1983.
2. Higuchi T, in Lyman R: *Pharmaceutical Compounding and Dispensing*, Lippincott, Philadelphia, 159, 1949.
3. Kramer SF, Flynn GL: *J Pharm Sci 61:* 1896, 1972.
4. Campbell AN, Campbell AJR: *J Am Chem Soc 59:* 2481, 1937.
5. Yalkowsky, SH: *Techniques of Solubilization of Drugs*, Marcel Dekker, New York, 91, 1981.
6. Martin, A, *et al: J. Pharm. Sci*, 71: 849, 1982.
7. Daniels F, Alberty RA: *Physical Chemistry*, 4th ed, Wiley, New York, 1975.
8. Glasstone S: *Textbook of Physical Chemistry*, Van Nostrand, New York, 1946.
9. Setnikar I, Temelcou O: *JAPhA Sci Ed 48:* 628, 1959.
10. Lewis GN, Randall M (Pitzer KS, Brewer L, eds): *Thermodynamics*, 2nd ed, McGraw-Hill, New York, 1961.

CHAPTER 17

Ionic Solutions and Electrolytic Equilibria

Paul J Niebergall, PhD

Professor of Pharmaceutics & Director
Pharmaceutical Development Center
Medical University of South Carolina
Charleston, SC 29425

Electrolytes

In the preceding chapter, attention was directed to the colligative properties of nonelectrolytes, or substances whose aqueous solutions do not conduct electricity. Substances whose aqueous solutions conduct electricity are known as electrolytes, and are typified by inorganic acids, bases, and salts. In addition to the property of electrical conductivity, solutions of electrolytes exhibit anomalous colligative properties.

Colligative Properties

In general, for nonelectrolytes, a given colligative property of two equimolal solutions will be identical. This generalization, however, cannot be made for solutions of electrolytes.

Van't Hoff pointed out that the osmotic pressure of a solution of an electrolyte is considerably greater than the osmotic pressure of a solution of a nonelectrolyte of the same molal concentration. This anomaly remained unexplained until 1887 when Arrhenius proposed a hypothesis which forms the basis for our modern theories of electrolyte solutions.

This theory postulated that when electrolytes are dissolved in water they split up into charged particles known as ions. Each of these ions carries one or more electrical charges, with the total charge on the positive ions (cations) being equal to the total charge on the negative ions (anions). Thus, although a solution may contain charged particles, it remains neutral. The increased osmotic pressure of such solutions is due to the increased number of particles formed in the process of ionization. For example, sodium chloride is assumed to dissociate as follows:

$$Na^+Cl^- \xrightarrow{H_2O} Na^+ + Cl^-$$

It is evident that each molecule of sodium chloride that is dissociated produces two ions and, if dissociation is complete, there will be twice as many particles as would be the case if it were not dissociated at all. Furthermore, if each ion has the same effect on osmotic pressure as a molecule, it might be expected that the osmotic pressure of the solution would be twice that of a solution containing the same molal concentration of a nonionizing solute.

Osmotic pressure data indicate that, in very dilute solutions of salts which yield two ions, the pressure is very nearly double that of solutions of equimolal concentrations of nonelectrolytes. Similar magnification of vapor-pressure lowering, boiling-point elevation and freezing-point depression occurs in dilute solutions of electrolytes.

Van't Hoff defined a factor i as the ratio of the colligative effect produced by a concentration m of electrolyte, divided by the effect observed for the same concentration of nonelectrolyte, or

$$i = \frac{\pi}{(\pi)_0} = \frac{\Delta P}{(\Delta P)_0} = \frac{\Delta T_b}{(\Delta T_b)_0} = \frac{\Delta T_f}{(\Delta T_f)_0} \qquad (1)$$

in which π, ΔP, ΔT_b, and ΔT_f refer to the osmotic pressure, vapor-pressure lowering, boiling-point elevation, and freezing-point depression, respectively, of the electrolyte. The terms $(\pi)_0$, etc. refer to the nonelectrolyte of the same concentration. In general, with strong electrolytes (those assumed to be 100% ionized), the van't Hoff factor is equal to the number of ions produced when the electrolyte goes into solution (2 for NaCl and $MgSO_4$, 3 for $CaCl_2$ and Na_2SO_4, 4 for $FeCl_3$ and Na_3PO_4, etc).

In *very* dilute solutions the osmotic pressure, vapor-pressure lowering, boiling-point elevation, and freezing-point depression of solutions of electrolytes approach values 2, 3, 4, or more times greater (depending on the type of strong electrolyte) than in solutions of the same molality of nonelectrolyte, thus confirming the hypothesis that an ion has the same primary effect as a molecule on colligative properties. It bears repeating, however, that two other effects are observed as the concentration of electrolyte is increased.

The first effect results in less than 2-, 3-, or 4-fold intensification of a colligative property; this reduction is ascribed to interionic attraction between the positively and negatively charged ions, in consequence of which the ions are not completely dissociated from each other and do not exert their full effect on vapor pressure and other colligative properties. This deviation generally increases with increasing concentration of electrolyte.

The second effect intensifies the colligative properties and is attributed to the attraction of ions for solvent molecules (called solvation, or, if water is the solvent, hydration), which holds the solvent in solution and reduces its escaping tendency, with consequent enhancement of the vapor-pressure lowering; solvation also reduces interionic attraction and thereby further lowers the vapor pressure.

Conductivity

The ability of metals to conduct an electric current results from mobility of electrons in the metals. This type of conductivity is called *metallic* conductance. On the other hand, various chemical compounds—notably acids, bases, and salts—conduct electricity by virtue of ions present or formed, rather than by electrons. This is called *electrolytic* conductance, and the conducting compounds are electrolytes. While the fact that certain electrolytes conduct electricity in the molten state is important, their behavior when dissolved in a solvent, particularly in water, is of greater concern in pharmaceutical science.

The electrical conductivity (or conductance) of a solution of an electrolyte is merely the reciprocal of the resistance of

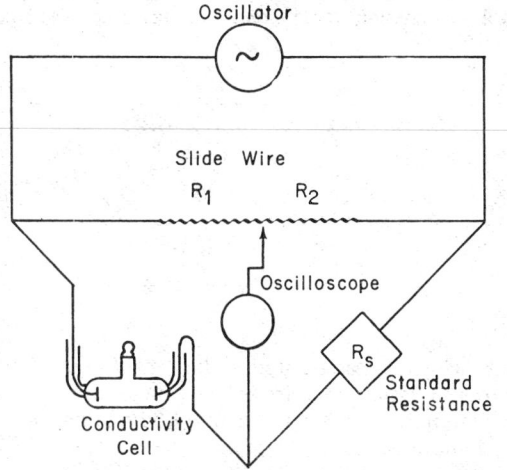

Fig 17-1. Alternating current Wheatstone bridge for measuring conductivity.

the solution. Hence, to measure conductivity is actually to measure electrical resistance, commonly with a Wheatstone bridge apparatus, and then to *calculate* the conductivity. Fig 17-1 is a representation of the component parts of the apparatus. The solution to be measured is placed in a glass or quartz cell having two inert electrodes, commonly made of platinum or gold and coated with spongy platinum to absorb gases, across which passes an alternating current generated by an oscillator at a frequency of about 1000 Hz. The reason for using alternating current is to reverse the electrolysis that occurs during flow of current and which would cause polarization of the electrodes and lead to abnormal results. The size of the electrodes and their distance apart may be varied to reduce very high resistance and increase very low resistance in order to increase the accuracy and precision of measurement; thus, solutions of high conductance (low resistance) are measured in cells having small electrodes relatively far apart while solutions of low conductance (high resistance) are measured in cells with large electrodes placed close to each other (electrolytic resistance, like metallic resistance, varies directly with the length of the conducting medium and inversely with its cross-sectional area). The known resistance required for the circuit is provided by a resistance box containing calibrated coils; the balancing of the bridge may be achieved by sliding a contact over a wire of uniform resistance until no (or minimum) current flows through the circuit, as detected either visually with a cathode-ray oscilloscope or audibly with earphones. The resistance, in ohms, is calculated by the simple procedure used in the Wheatstone bridge method; the reciprocal of this is the conductivity, the units of which are *reciprocal ohms* (also called *mhos*). As the numerical value of the conductivity will vary with the dimensions of the conductance cell, the value must be calculated in terms of *specific conductance*, L, which is the conductance in a cell having electrodes of 1 sq cm cross-sectional area and 1 cm

apart. If the dimensions of the cell used in the experiment were known, it would be possible to calculate the specific conductance. But this information is actually not required, because it is possible—and much more convenient—to calibrate a cell by measuring in it the conductivity of a standard solution of known specific conductance and then calculating a "cell constant" which, since it is a function only of the dimensions of the cell, can be used to convert all measurements in that cell to specific conductivity. Solutions of known concentration of pure potassium chloride are used as standard solutions for this purpose.

Equivalent Conductance—In studying the variation of conductance of electrolytes with dilution it is essential to make allowance for the degree of dilution in order that the comparison of conductances may be made for identical amounts of solute. This may be achieved by expressing conductance measurements in terms of *equivalent conductance*, Λ, which is obtained by multiplying the specific conductance, L, by the volume in milliliters, V_e, of solution containing 1 g-eq of solute. Thus,

$$\Lambda = LV_e = \frac{1000L}{C} \qquad (2)$$

where C is the concentration of electrolyte in the solution in g-Eq/L, ie, the normality of the solution. For example, the equivalent conductance of 0.01 N potassium chloride solution, which has a specific conductance of 0.001413 mho/cm may be calculated in either of the following ways:

$$\Lambda = 0.001413 \times 100,000 = 141.3 \text{ mho cm}^2/\text{eq}$$

or,

$$\Lambda = \frac{1000 \times 0.001413}{0.01} = 141.3$$

Strong and Weak Electrolytes—It is customary to classify electrolytes broadly as *strong electrolytes* and *weak electrolytes*. The former category includes solutions of strong acids, strong bases, and most salts; the latter includes weak acids and bases, primarily organic acids and amines, and a few salts. The usual criterion for distinguishing between strong and weak electrolytes is the extent of ionization; thus, an electrolyte existing entirely or very largely as ions is considered a strong electrolyte, while one that is a mixture of a substantial proportion of molecular species along with ions derived therefrom is a weak electrolyte. For the purposes of this discussion, classification of electrolytes as strong or weak will be on the basis of certain conductance characteristics exhibited in aqueous solution.

The equivalent conductances of a number of electrolytes, at different concentrations, are given in Table I and for certain of these electrolytes again in Fig 17-2, where the equivalent conductance is plotted against the square root of concentration. By plotting the data in this manner a linear relationship is observed for strong electrolytes, while a steeply rising curve is noted for weak electrolytes; this difference is a characteristic

Table I—Equivalent Conductances at 25°

g-Eq/L	HCl	HAc	NaCl	KCl	NaI	KI	NaAc
Inf. dil.	426.1	390.6[a]	126.5	149.9	126.9	150.3	91.0
0.0005	422.7	67.7	124.5	147.8	125.4	...	89.2
0.001	421.4	49.2	123.7	146.9	124.3	...	88.5
0.005	415.8	22.9	120.6	143.5	121.3	144.4	85.7
0.01	412.0	16.3	118.5	141.3	119.2	142.2	83.8
0.02	407.2	11.6	115.8	138.3	116.7	139.5	81.2
0.05	399.1	7.4	111.1	133.4	112.8	135.0	76.9
0.1	391.3	5.2	106.7	129.0	108.8	131.1	72.8

[a] The equivalent conductance at infinite dilution for acetic acid, a weak electrolyte, was obtained by adding the equivalent conductances of hydrochloric acid and sodium acetate and subtracting that of sodium chloride (see text for explanation).

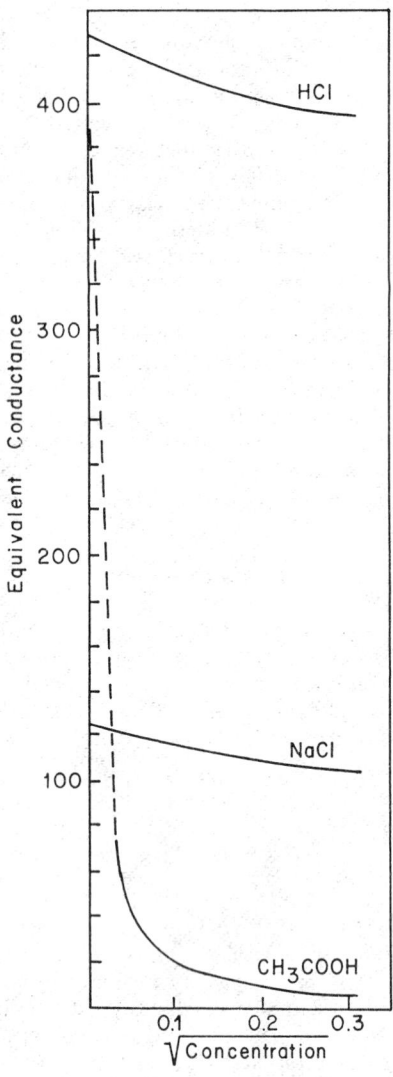

Fig 17-2.   Variation of equivalent conductance with square root of concentration.

Table II—Equivalent Ionic Conductivities at Infinite Dilution, at 25°

Cations	l_0	Anions	l_0
H^+	349.8	OH^-	198.0
Li^+	38.7	Cl^-	76.3
Na^+	50.1	Br^-	78.4
K^+	73.5	I^-	76.8
NH_4^+	61.9	Ac^-	40.9
$\frac{1}{2}Ca^{2+}$	59.5	$\frac{1}{2}SO_4^{2-}$	79.8
$\frac{1}{2}Mg^{2+}$	53.0		

ion with which it is associated. Thus, if the equivalent conductances of various ions are known, the conductance of any electrolyte may be calculated simply by adding the appropriate ionic conductances. Since the fraction of current carried by cations (*transference number* of the cations) and by anions (transference number of anions) in an electrolyte may be determined readily by experiment, ionic conductances are known. Table II gives the equivalent ionic conductances at infinite dilution of some cations and anions. But it is not necessary to have this information in order to calculate the equivalent conductance of an electrolyte, for Kohlrausch's law permits the latter to be calculated by adding and subtracting values of Λ_0 for appropriate electrolytes. For example, the Λ_0 for acetic acid may be calculated as follows:

$$\Lambda_0(CH_3COOH) = \Lambda_0(HCl) + \Lambda_0(CH_3COONa) - \Lambda_0(NaCl)$$

which is equivalent to,

$$l_0(H^+) + l_0(CH_3COO^-) = l_0(H^+) + l_0(Cl^-) + l_0(Na^+) + \\ l_0(CH_3COO^-) - l_0(Na^+) - l_0(Cl^-)$$

This method is especially useful for calculating Λ_0 for weak electrolytes such as acetic acid. As is evident from Fig. 17-2, the Λ_0 value for acetic acid cannot be determined accurately by extrapolation because of the steep rise of conductance in dilute solutions. For strong electrolytes, on the other hand, the extrapolation can be made very accurately. Thus, in the example above, the Λ_0 values for HCl, CH_3COONa and NaCl are all easily determined by extrapolation since the substances are strong electrolytes. Substitution of these extrapolated values, as given in Table II, yields a value of 390.6 for the Λ_0 of CH_3COOH.

Ionization of Weak Electrolytes—When Arrhenius introduced his theory of ionization he proposed that the degree of ionization, α, of an electrolyte is measured by the ratio,

$$\alpha = \Lambda/\Lambda_0 \qquad (4)$$

where Λ is the equivalent conductance of the electrolyte at any specified concentration of solution and Λ_0 is the equivalent conductance at infinite dilution. As strong electrolytes were not then recognized as being 100% ionized, and interionic interference effects had not been evaluated, he believed the equation to be applicable to both strong and weak electrolytes. Since we now know that apparent variation of ionization of strong electrolyte arises from change of mobility of ions at different concentrations rather than from varying ionization, the equation is not applicable to strong electrolytes; it does provide, however, a generally acceptable approximation of the degree of ionization of weak electrolytes, for which deviations resulting from neglect of activity coefficients and of some change of ionic mobilities with concentration are for most purposes negligible. The following example illustrates the use of the equation to calculate the degree of ionization of a typical weak electrolyte.

Example—Calculate the degree of ionization of $1 \times 10^{-3} N$ acetic acid, the equivalent conductance of which is 48.15 mho cm²/Eq. The equivalent conductance at infinite dilution is 390.6 mho cm²/Eq.

which distinguishes strong and weak electrolytes. The interpretation of the steep rise in the equivalent conductance of weak electrolytes is that the degree of ionization increases with dilution, becoming complete at infinite dilution; interionic interference effects generally have a minor role in the conductivity of weak electrolytes. With strong electrolytes, which usually are completely ionized, the increase in equivalent conductance results not from increased ionization but rather from diminished ionic interference as the solution is diluted, in consequence of which ions have greater freedom of mobility, ie, increased conductance.

The value of the equivalent conductance extrapolated to infinite dilution (zero concentration), designated by the symbol Λ_0, has special significance. It represents the equivalent conductance of the completely ionized electrolyte when the ions are so far apart that there is no interference with their migration due to interionic interactions. It has been shown, by Kohlrausch, that the equivalent conductance of an electrolyte at infinite dilution is the sum of the equivalent conductances of its component ions at infinite dilution, expressed symbolically as,

$$\Lambda_0 = l_0(cation) + l_0(anion) \qquad (3)$$

The significance of Kohlrausch's law is that each ion, at infinite dilution, has a characteristic value of conductance that is independent of the conductance of the oppositely charged

$$\alpha = \frac{48.15}{390.6} = 0.12$$

$$\% \text{ ionization} = 100\alpha = 12\%$$

The degree of dissociation can also be calculated using the van't Hoff factor, i, and the following equation:

$$\alpha = \frac{i-1}{v-1} \tag{5}$$

where v is the number of ions into which the electrolyte dissociates.

Example—A $1.0 \times 10^{-3}\ N$ solution of acetic acid has a van't Hoff factor equal to 1.12. Calculate the degree of dissociation of the acid at this concentration.

$$\alpha = \frac{i-1}{v-1} = \frac{1.12-1}{2-1} = 0.12$$

This result agrees with that obtained using equivalent conductance and Eq 4.

Modern Theories

The Arrhenius theory explains why solutions of electrolytes conduct electricity, why they exhibit enhanced colligative properties, and is essentially satisfactory for solutions of weak electrolytes. Several deficiencies, however, do exist when it is applied to solutions of strong electrolytes: it does not explain the failure of strong electrolytes to follow the law of mass action as applied to ionization; discrepancies exist between the degree of ionization calculated from the van't Hoff factor and the conductivity ratio for strong electrolyte solutions having concentrations greater than about 0.5 M.

These deficiencies can be explained by the following observations:

1. When molten, strong electrolytes are excellent conductors of electricity. This suggests that these materials are already ionized in the crystalline state. Further support for this is given by X-ray studies of crystals, which indicate that the units comprising the basic lattice structure of strong electrolytes are ions.
2. Arrhenius neglected the fact that ions in solution, being oppositely charged, tend to associate through electrostatic attraction. In solutions of weak electrolytes, the number of ions is not large and it is not surprising that electrostatic attractions do not cause appreciable deviations from theory. In dilute solutions, in which strong electrolytes are assumed to be 100% ionized, the number of ions is large, and interionic attractions become major factors in determining the chemical properties of these solutions. These effects should, and do, become more pronounced as the concentration of electrolyte or the valence of the ions is increased.

It is not surprising, therefore, that the Arrhenius theory of partial ionization involving the law of mass action and neglecting ionic charge does not hold for solutions of strong electrolytes. Neutral molecules of strong electrolytes, if they do exist in solution, must arise from interionic attraction rather than from incomplete ionization.

Activity and Activity Coefficients—Due to increased electrostatic attractions as a solution becomes more concentrated, the concentration of an ion becomes less efficient as a measure of its net effectiveness. A more efficient measure of the physical or chemical effectiveness of an ion is known as its *activity*, which is a measure of an ion's concentration related to its concentration at a universally adopted reference standard state. The relationship between the activity and the concentration of an ion can be expressed as,

$$a = m\gamma \tag{6}$$

where m is the molal concentration, γ is the activity coefficient, and a is the activity. The activity also can be expressed in terms of molar concentration, c, as,

$$a = fc \tag{7}$$

where f is the activity coefficient on a molar scale. In dilute solutions (below 0.01 M) the two activity coefficients are identical for all practical purposes.

The activity coefficient may be determined in various ways, such as measurement of colligative properties, electromotive force, solubility, distribution coefficients, etc. For a strong electrolyte, the mean ionic activity coefficient, $\gamma_\pm$, or $f_\pm$, provides a measure of the deviation of the electrolyte from ideal behavior. The mean ionic activity coefficients on a molal basis for several strong electrolytes are given in Table VII. It is characteristic of the electrolytes that the coefficients at first decrease with increasing concentration, pass through a minimum, and finally increase with increasing concentration of electrolyte. A partial explanation of this complex behavior, which still is incompletely understood, is given in the preceding chapter.

Ionic Strength—As noted in the preceding chapter, the concept of ionic strength μ, which is a measure of the intensity of the electrical field in a solution, provides a basis for evaluating electrostatic interactions between ions. Ionic strength may be expressed as,

$$\mu = \frac{1}{2}\Sigma c_i z_i^2 \tag{8}$$

where z_i is the valence of ion i. The mean ionic activity coefficient is a function of ionic strength; so also are such diverse phenomena as solubilities of sparingly soluble substances, rates of ionic reactions, effects of salts on pH of buffers, electrophoresis of proteins, etc.

The greater effectiveness of ions of higher charge type on a specific property, compared with the effectiveness of the same number of singly charged ions, generally coincides with the ionic strength calculated by Eq 8. The variation of ionic strength with the valence (charge) of the ions comprising a strong electrolyte should be noted.

For electrolytes composed of univalent cations and univalent anions (called uniunivalent or 1-1 electrolytes), the ionic strength is identical with molarity. For bivalent cation and univalent anion (biunivalent or 2-1) electrolytes, or univalent cation and bivalent anion (unibivalent or 1-2) electrolytes, the ionic strength is three times the molarity. For bivalent cation and bivalent anion (bibivalent or 2-2) electrolytes, the ionic strength is four times the molarity. These relationships are evident from the following example.

Example—Calculate the ionic strength of 0.1 M solutions of NaCl, Na_2SO_4, $MgCl_2$, and $MgSO_4$, respectively. For,

$$NaCl \quad \mu = \frac{1}{2}(0.1 \times 1^2 + 0.1 \times 1^2) = 0.1$$

$$Na_2SO_4 \quad \mu = \frac{1}{2}(0.2 \times 1^2 + 0.1 \times 2^2) = 0.3$$

$$MgCl_2 \quad \mu = \frac{1}{2}(0.1 \times 2^2 + 0.2 \times 1^2) = 0.3$$

$$MgSO_4 \quad \mu = \frac{1}{2}(0.1 \times 2^2 + 0.1 \times 2^2) = 0.4$$

The ionic strength of a solution containing more than one electrolyte is the sum of the ionic strengths of the individual salts comprising the solution. For example, the ionic strength of a solution containing NaCl, Na_2SO_4, $MgCl_2$ and $MgSO_4$, each at a concentration of 0.1 M, is 1.1.

Debye–Hückel Theory—The Debye–Hückel equations on page 227, applicable only to very dilute solutions (about 0.02 μ), may be extended to somewhat more concentrated solutions (about 0.1 μ) in the simplified form:

$$\log f_i = \frac{-0.51\, z_1^2 \sqrt{\mu}}{1 + \sqrt{\mu}} \tag{9}$$

The mean ionic activity coefficient for aqueous solutions of electrolytes at 25° can be expressed as,

$$\log f_\pm = \frac{-0.51\, z_+ z_- \sqrt{\mu}}{1 + \sqrt{\mu}} \tag{10}$$

in which z_+ is the valence of the cation and z_- is the valence of the anion. When the ionic strength of the solution becomes

**Table III—Values of Some Salting-Out Constants for
Various Barbiturates at 25°**

Barbiturate	KCl	KBr	NaCl	NaBr
Amobarbital	0.168	0.095	0.212	0.143
Aprobarbital	0.136	0.062	0.184	0.120
Barbital	0.092	0.042	0.136	0.088
Phenobarbital	0.092	0.034	0.132	0.078
Vinbarbital	0.125	0.036	0.143	0.096

high (approximately 0.3 to 0.5), these equations become inadequate and a linear term in μ is added. This is illustrated for the mean ionic activity coefficient:

$$\log f_\pm = \frac{-0.51\, z_+ z_- \sqrt{\mu}}{1 + \sqrt{\mu}} + K_s \mu \qquad (11)$$

in which K_s is a "salting-out" constant empirically chosen for each salt. This equation is valid for solutions with ionic strength up to approximately 1.

Salting-Out Effect—The aqueous solubility of a slightly soluble organic substance generally is affected markedly by the addition of an electrolyte. This effect is particularly noticeable when the electrolyte concentration reaches 0.5 M or higher. If the aqueous solution of the organic substance has a dielectric constant lower than that of pure water, its solubility is decreased and the substance is "salted out." The use of high concentrations of electrolytes such as ammonium sulfate or sodium sulfate for the separation of proteins by differential precipitation is perhaps the most striking example of this effect. The aqueous solutions of a few substances such as hydrocyanic acid, glycine, and cystine have a higher dielectric constant than that of pure water, and these substances are "salted in." These phenomena can be expressed empirically as,

$$\log S = \log S_0 \pm K_s m \qquad (12)$$

in which S_0 represents the solubility of the organic substance in pure water and S is the solubility in the electrolyte solution. The slope of the straight line obtained by plotting $\log S$ vs m is positive for "salting in" and negative for "salting out." In terms of ionic strength this equation becomes,

$$\log S = \log S_0 \pm K_s' \mu \qquad (13)$$

where $K_s' = K_s$ for univalent salts; $K_s' = K_s/3$ for unibivalent salts; and $K_s' = K_s/4$ for bivalent salts. The "salting-out" constant depends on temperature as well as the nature of both the organic substance and the electrolyte. The effect of electrolyte and of the organic substance can be seen in Table III. In all instances, if the anion is constant, the sodium cation has a greater "salting-out" effect than the potassium cation, probably due to the higher charge density of the former. Although the reasoning is less clear, it appears that for a constant cation, chloride anion has a greater effect than bromide anion upon the "salting-out" phenomenon.

Acids and Bases

Arrhenius defined an acid as a substance that yields hydrogen ions in aqueous solution and a base as a substance that yields hydroxyl ions in aqueous solution. Except for the fact that hydrogen ions neutralize hydroxyl ions to form water, no complementary relationship between acids and bases (such as that between oxidants and reductants, for example) is evident in Arrhenius' definitions for these substances; rather, their oppositeness of character is emphasized. Moreover, no account is taken of the behavior of acids and bases in nonaqueous solvents. Also, while acidity is associated with so elementary a particle as the proton (hydrogen ion), basicity is attributed to so relatively complex an association of atoms

as the hydroxyl ion. It would seem that a simpler concept of a base could be devised.

Proton Concept of Acids and Bases—In pondering the objections to Arrhenius' definitions, Brønsted and Bjerrum in Denmark and Lowry in England developed and in 1923 announced a more satisfactory, and more general, theory of acids and bases. According to this theory an acid is a substance capable of yielding a proton (hydrogen ion), while a base is a substance capable of accepting a proton. This complementary relationship may be expressed by the general equation;

$$\underset{\text{acid}}{A} \rightleftharpoons H^+ + \underset{\text{base}}{B}$$

The pair of substances thus related through mutual ability to gain or lose a proton is called a *conjugate acid–base pair.* Specific examples of such pairs are;

Acid	Base
$HCl \rightleftharpoons H^+ + Cl^-$	
$CH_3COOH \rightleftharpoons H^+ + CH_3COO^-$	
$NH_4^+ \rightleftharpoons H^+ + NH_3$	
$HCO_3^- \rightleftharpoons H^+ + CO_3^{2-}$	
$H_2PO_4^- \rightleftharpoons H^+ + HPO_4^{2-}$	
$H_2O \rightleftharpoons H^+ + OH^-$	
$H_3O^+ \rightleftharpoons H^+ + H_2O$	
$Al(H_2O)_6^{3+} \rightleftharpoons H^+ + Al(H_2O)_5OH^{2+}$	

It is apparent that not only molecules but also cations and anions may function as acids or bases.

The complementary nature of the acid–base pairs listed is reminiscent of the complementary relationship of pairs of oxidants and reductants where, however, the ability to gain or lose one or more electrons—rather than protons—is the distinguishing characteristic.

Oxidant	Reductant
$Fe^{3+} + e^- \rightleftharpoons Fe^{2+}$	
$Na^+ + e^- \rightleftharpoons Na$	
$\frac{1}{2}I_2 + e^- \rightleftharpoons I^-$	

These examples of acid–base pairs and oxidant–reductant pairs represent, however, reactions that are possible in principle only. Ordinarily acids will not release free protons any more than reductants will release free electrons; both protons and electrons, respectively, can only be *transferred* from one substance (an ion, atom, or molecule) to another. Thus, it is a fundamental fact of chemistry that oxidation of one substance will occur only if reduction of another substance occurs simultaneously. Stated in another way, electrons will be released from the reductant (oxidation) only if an oxidant capable of accepting electrons (reduction) is present. For this reason oxidation–reduction reactions must involve two conjugate oxidant–reductant pairs of substances:

$$\text{oxidant}_1 + \text{reductant}_2 \rightleftharpoons \text{reductant}_1 + \text{oxidant}_2$$

where subscript 1 represents one conjugate oxidant–reductant pair and subscript 2 represents the other.

Similarly, an acid will not release a proton unless a base capable of accepting it is simultaneously present; this means that any actual manifestation of acid–base behavior must involve interaction between two sets of conjugate acid–base pairs, represented as:

$$\underset{\text{acid}_1}{A_1} + \underset{\text{base}_2}{B_2} \rightleftharpoons \underset{\text{base}_1}{B_1} + \underset{\text{acid}_2}{A_2}$$

In such a reaction, which is called *protolysis* or a *protolytic reaction*, A_1 and B_1 constitute one conjugate acid–base pair and A_2 and B_2 the other; the proton given up by A_1 (which thereby becomes B_1) is transferred to B_2 (which becomes A_2).

When an acid, such as hydrochloric, is dissolved in water, a protolytic reaction occurs.

$$HCl + H_2O \rightleftharpoons Cl^- + H_3O^+$$
$$\text{acid}_1 \quad \text{base}_2 \quad \text{base}_1 \quad \text{acid}_2$$

The ionic species H_3O^+, called *hydronium* or *oxonium* ion, is always formed when an acid is dissolved in water; very often, for purposes of convenience, this is written simply as H^+ and is called hydrogen ion, although the "bare" ion is practically nonexistent in solution.

When a base, eg, ammonia, is dissolved in water the reaction of protolysis is as follows:

$$NH_3 + H_2O \rightleftharpoons NH_4^+ + OH^-$$
$$\text{base}_1 \quad \text{acid}_2 \quad \text{acid}_1 \quad \text{base}_2$$

The proton theory of acid–base function makes the concept of hydrolysis superfluous. When, for example, sodium acetate is dissolved in water, this acid–base interaction occurs.

$$CH_3COO^- + H_2O \rightleftharpoons CH_3COOH + OH^-$$
$$\text{base}_1 \quad \text{acid}_2 \quad \text{acid}_1 \quad \text{base}_2$$

In an aqueous solution of ammonium chloride the reaction is,

$$NH_4^+ + H_2O \rightleftharpoons NH_3 + H_3O^+$$
$$\text{acid}_1 \quad \text{base}_2 \quad \text{base}_1 \quad \text{acid}_2$$

Transfer of protons (protolysis) is not limited to dissimilar conjugate acid–base pairs. In the preceding examples H_2O sometimes behaves as an acid and at other times as a base; such an amphoteric substance is called, in Brønsted's terminology, an *amphiprotic substance*.

Electron-Pair Concept of Acids and Bases—While the proton concept of acids and bases provides a more general definition for these substances, it does not indicate what the basic reason is for proton transfer, nor does it explain how such substances as sulfur trioxide, boron trichloride, stannic chloride, and carbon dioxide—none of which is capable of donating a proton—can behave as acids. Both deficiencies of the proton theory are avoided in the more inclusive definition of acids and bases proposed by Lewis in 1923. According to Lewis, who in 1916 proposed that sharing of a pair of electrons by two atoms established a bond (covalent) between the atoms, an acid is a substance capable of sharing a pair of electrons made available by another substance called a base, thereby forming a coordinate covalent bond. The base is the substance that donates a share in its electron pair to the acid. The following equation illustrates how Lewis' definitions explain the transfer of a proton (hydrogen ion) to ammonia to form ammonium ion.

$$H^+ + \ :\!\overset{\displaystyle H}{\underset{\displaystyle H}{\ddot{N}}}\!:\!H \ \rightarrow \ \left[\overset{\displaystyle H}{\underset{\displaystyle H}{H\!:\!\ddot{N}\!:\!H}} \right]^+$$

The reaction of boron trichloride, which according to the Lewis theory is an acid, with ammonia is similar, for the boron lacks an electron pair if it is to attain a stable octet configuration, while ammonia has a pair of electrons which may be shared, thus,

$$\overset{\displaystyle Cl}{\underset{\displaystyle Cl}{Cl\!:\!\ddot{B}}} + \ :\!\overset{\displaystyle H}{\underset{\displaystyle H}{\ddot{N}}}\!:\!H \ \rightarrow \ \overset{\displaystyle Cl \ H}{\underset{\displaystyle Cl \ H}{Cl\!:\!\ddot{B}\!:\!\ddot{N}\!:\!H}}$$

Leveling Effect of a Solvent—When the strong acids $HClO_4$, H_2SO_4, HCl, and HNO_3 are dissolved in water the solutions—if they are of identical normality and are not too concentrated—all have about the same hydrogen ion concentration, indicating the acids to be of about the same strength. The reason for this is that each one of the acids undergoes practically complete protolysis in water.

$$HCl + H_2O \rightarrow Cl^- + H_3O^+$$
$$\text{acid}_1 \quad \text{base}_2 \quad \text{base}_1 \quad \text{acid}_2$$

This phenomenon, called the leveling effect of water, occurs whenever the added acid is stronger than hydronium ion; such a reaction manifests the tendency of proton transfer reactions to proceed spontaneously in the direction of forming weaker acid and weaker base.

Since the strongest acid that can exist in an amphiprotic solvent is the conjugate acid form of the solvent, any stronger acid will undergo protolysis to the weaker solvent acid. Since $HClO_4$, H_2SO_4, HCl, and HNO_3 are all stronger acids than hydronium ion, they are converted in water to hydronium ion.

When the strong bases sodium hydride, sodium amide, and sodium ethoxide are dissolved in water, each reacts with water to form sodium hydroxide; these reactions illustrate the leveling effect of water on bases. Since hydroxide ion is the strongest base that can exist in water, any base stronger than hydroxide undergoes protolysis to hydroxide.

Intrinsic differences in the acidity of acids become evident if they are dissolved in a relatively poor proton acceptor such as anhydrous acetic acid. Perchloric acid ($HClO_4$), a strong acid, undergoes practically complete reaction with acetic acid,

$$HClO_4 + CH_3COOH \rightarrow ClO_4^- + CH_3COOH_2^+$$
$$\text{acid}_1 \quad \text{base}_2 \quad \text{base}_1 \quad \text{acid}_2$$
$$\text{(strong)} \quad \text{(strong)} \quad \text{(weak)} \quad \text{(weak)}$$

but sulfuric acid and hydrochloric acid behave as weak acids. It is because perchloric acid is a very strong acid when dissolved in glacial acetic acid that it has found many important applications in analytical chemistry as a titrant for a variety of substances which behave as bases in acetic acid (see *Titrimetric Assays Utilizing Nonaqueous Solvents* in Chapter 30). Because of its ability to differentiate acidity of different acids, it is called a *differentiating solvent for acids*, this property resulting from its relatively weak proton-acceptor tendency. A solvent that differentiates basicity of different bases must have weak proton-donor tendency; it is called a *differentiating solvent for bases*. Typical of solvents in this category is liquid ammonia. Solvents that have both weak proton-donor and proton-acceptor tendencies are called *aprotic solvents* and may serve as differentiating solvents for both acids and bases; they have little if any action on solutes and serve mainly as inert dispersion media for the solutes. Useful aprotic solvents are benzene, toluene, and hexane.

Ionization of Acids and Bases—Acids and bases are commonly classified as strong or weak acids and strong or weak bases according as they are extensively or slightly ionized in aqueous solutions. If, for example, 1 N aqueous solutions of hydrochloric acid and acetic acid are compared, it is found that the former is a better conductor of electricity, reacts much more readily with metals, catalyzes certain reactions more efficiently, and possesses a more acid taste than the latter. Both solutions, however, will neutralize identical amounts of alkali. A similar comparison of 1 N solutions of sodium hydroxide and ammonia reveals the former to be more "active" than the latter, although both solutions will neutralize identical quantities of acid.

The differences in the properties of the two acids is attributed to differences in the concentration of hydrogen (more accurately hydronium) ion, the hydrochloric acid being ionized to a greater extent and therefore containing a higher concentration of hydrogen ion than acetic acid. Similarly, most of the differences between the sodium hydroxide and ammonia solutions are attributed to the higher hydroxyl-ion concentration in the former.

The ionization of incompletely ionized acids may be considered a reversible reaction of the type,

$$HA \rightleftharpoons H^+ + A^-$$

where HA is the molecular acid and A^- is its anion. An equilibrium expression based on the law of mass action may be applied to the reaction, thus;

$$K_a = \frac{[H^+][A^-]}{[HA]} \tag{14}$$

where K_a is the ionization or dissociation constant, and the brackets signify concentration. For any given acid in any specified solvent and at any constant temperature, K_a remains relatively constant as the concentration of acid is varied, provided the acid is weakly ionized; with increasingly stronger acids, however, progressively larger deviations occur.

Although the strength of an acid is commonly measured in terms of the ionization or dissociation constant defined in Eq 14, the process of ionization is probably never as simple as shown above. A proton simply will not detach itself from one molecule unless it is simultaneously accepted by another molecule. When an acid is dissolved in water, the latter acts as a base, accepting a proton (Brønsted's definition of a base) by donating a share in a pair of electrons (Lewis' definition of a base). This reaction may be written,

$$\underset{\text{acid}_1}{HA} + \underset{\text{base}_2}{H_2O} \rightleftharpoons \underset{\text{base}_1}{A^-} + \underset{\text{acid}_2}{H_3O^+}$$

Application of the law of mass action to this reaction gives,

$$K = \frac{[H_3O^+][A^-]}{[HA][H_2O]} \tag{15}$$

since $[H_2O]$ is a constant this equation may be written,

$$K_a = \frac{[H_3O^+][A^-]}{[HA]} \tag{16}$$

This equation is identical with Eq 14 because $[H_3O^+]$ is numerically equal to $[H^+]$.

Acids which are capable of donating more than one proton are termed polyprotic. The ionization of a polyprotic acid occurs in stages and can be illustrated by considering the equilibria involved in the ionization of phosphoric acid:

$$H_3PO_4 + H_2O \rightleftharpoons H_2PO_4^- + H_3O^+$$

$$H_2PO_4^- + H_2O \rightleftharpoons HPO_4^{2-} + H_3O^+$$

$$HPO_4^{2-} + H_2O \rightleftharpoons PO_4^{3-} + H_3O^+$$

Application of the law of mass action to this series of reactions gives,

$$K_1 = \frac{[H_2PO_4^-][H_3O^+]}{[H_3PO_4]} \tag{17}$$

$$K_2 = \frac{[HPO_4^{2-}][H_3O^+]}{[H_2PO_4^{-1}]} \tag{18}$$

$$K_3 = \frac{[PO_4^{3-}][H_3O^+]}{[HPO_4^{2-}]} \tag{19}$$

If the three expressions for the ionization constants are multiplied together, an overall ionization, K, can be obtained:

$$K = K_1K_2K_3 = \frac{[PO_4^{3-}][H_3O^+]^3}{[H_3PO_4]} \tag{20}$$

Each of the successive ionizations is suppressed by the hydronium ion formed from preceding stages according to Le Chatelier's principle. The successive dissociation constants always decrease in value, since successive protons must be removed from species that are always more negatively charged. This can be seen from the data in Table IV, in which K_1 for phosphoric acid is approximately 100,000 times greater than K_2, which is in turn approximately 100,000 times greater than K_3. Although successive dissociation constants are always smaller, the difference is not always as great as it is for phosphoric acid. Tartaric acid, for example, has $K_1 = 9.12 \times 10^{-4}$ and $K_2 = 4.27 \times 10^{-5}$.

Ionization of a base can be illustrated by using the specific substance NH_3 for an example. According to Brønsted and Lewis, when the base NH_3 is dissolved in water, the latter acts as an acid, donating a proton to NH_3, which accepts it by offering a share in a pair of electrons on the nitrogen atom. This reaction is written,

$$\underset{\text{base}}{NH_3} + \underset{\text{acid}}{H_2O} \rightleftharpoons NH_4^+ + OH^-$$

The equilibrium expression for this reaction is;

$$K = \frac{[NH_4^+][OH^-]}{[NH_3][H_2O]} \tag{21}$$

with $[H_2O]$ constant this expression may be written,

$$K_b = \frac{[NH_4^+][OH^-]}{[NH_3]} \tag{22}$$

Ionization of Water—Although it is a poor conductor of electricity, pure water does ionize through a process known as *autoprotolysis*, in the following manner:

$$2H_2O \rightleftharpoons H_3O^+ + OH^-$$

Application of the law of mass action to this reaction gives the following:

$$K = \frac{[H_3O^+][OH^-]}{[H_2O]^2} \tag{23}$$

where K is the equilibrium constant for the reaction. Since the concentration of H_2O (molecular water) is very much greater than either the hydronium ion or hydroxyl ion concentrations, it can be considered to be constant and can be combined with K to give a new constant, K_w, known as the *ion product* of water, and Eq 23 becomes;

$$K_w = [H_3O^+][OH^-] \tag{24}$$

The numerical value of K_w varies with temperature; at 25° it is approximately equal to 1×10^{-14}.

Since the autoprotolysis of pure water yields one hydronium ion for each hydroxyl ion produced, $[H_3O^+]$ must be equal to $[OH^-]$. At 25° each has a value of 1×10^{-7} moles/liter ($1 \times 10^{-7} \times 1 \times 10^{-7} = K_w = 1 \times 10^{-14}$). A solution in which $[H_3O^+]$ is equal to $[OH^-]$ is termed a *neutral* solution.

If an acid is added to water, the hydronium ion concentration will be increased and the equilibrium between hydronium and hydroxyl ions will be *momentarily* disturbed. To restore equilibrium, some of the hydroxyl ions, originally present in the water, will combine with a *part* of the added hydronium ions to form nonionized water molecules until the product of the concentrations of the two ions has been reduced to 10^{-14}. When equilibrium is again restored, the concentrations of the two ions will no longer be equal. If, for example, the hydronium ion concentration is 1×10^{-3} N when equilibrium is established, the concentration of hydroxyl ion will be 1×10^{-11} (the product of the two concentrations being equal to 10^{-14}). Since $[H_3O^+]$ is much greater than $[OH^-]$, the solution is said to be *acid* or *acidic*.

In a similar manner, the addition of an alkali to pure water

Table IV—Dissociation Constants in Water at 25°

Substance		K
Weak Acids		
Acetic		1.75×10^{-5}
Acetylsalicylic		3.27×10^{-4}
Barbital		1.23×10^{-8}
Barbituric		1.05×10^{-4}
Benzoic		6.30×10^{-5}
Benzyl penicillin		1.74×10^{-3}
Boric	K_1	5.8×10^{-10}
Caffeine		1×10^{-14}
Carbonic	K_1	4.31×10^{-7}
	K_2	4.7×10^{-11}
Citric (1H$_2$O)	K_1	7.0×10^{-4}
	K_2	1.8×10^{-5}
	K_3	4.0×10^{-7}
Dichloroacetic		5×10^{-2}
Ethylenediaminetetra-acetic acid (EDTA)	K_1	1×10^{-2}
	K_2	2.14×10^{-3}
	K_3	6.92×10^{-7}
	K_4	5.5×10^{-11}
Formic		1.77×10^{-4}
Glycerophosphoric	K_1	3.4×10^{-2}
	K_2	6.4×10^{-7}
Glycine	K_1	4.5×10^{-3}
	K_2	1.7×10^{-10}
Lactic		1.39×10^{-4}
Mandelic		4.29×10^{-4}
Monochloroacetic		1.4×10^{-3}
Oxalic (2H$_2$O)	K_1	5.5×10^{-2}
	K_2	5.3×10^{-5}
Phenobarbital		3.9×10^{-8}
Phenol		1×10^{-10}
Phosphoric	K_1	7.5×10^{-3}
	K_2	6.2×10^{-8}
	K_3	2.1×10^{-13}
Picric		4.2×10^{-1}
Propionic		1.34×10^{-5}
Saccharin		2.5×10^{-2}
Salicylic		1.06×10^{-3}
Succinic	K_1	6.4×10^{-5}
	K_2	2.3×10^{-6}
Sulfadiazine		3.3×10^{-7}
Sulfamerazine		8.7×10^{-8}
Sulfapyridine		3.6×10^{-9}
Sulfathiazole		7.6×10^{-8}
Tartaric	K_1	9.6×10^{-4}
	K_2	4.4×10^{-5}
Trichloroacetic		1.3×10^{-1}
Weak Bases		
Acetanilide		4.1×10^{-14} (40°)
Ammonia		1.74×10^{-5}
Apomorphine		1.0×10^{-7}
Atropine		4.5×10^{-5}
Benzocaine		6.0×10^{-12}
Caffeine		4.1×10^{-14} (40°)
Cocaine		2.6×10^{-6}
Codeine		9×10^{-7}
Ephedrine		2.3×10^{-5}
Morphine		7.4×10^{-7}
Papaverine		8×10^{-9}
Physostigmine	K_1	7.6×10^{-7}
	K_2	5.7×10^{-13}
Pilocarpine	K_1	7×10^{-8}
	K_2	2×10^{-13}
Procaine		7×10^{-6}
Pyridine		1.4×10^{-9}
Quinine	K_1	1.0×10^{-6}
	K_2	1.3×10^{-10}
Reserpine		4×10^{-8}
Strychnine	K_1	1×10^{-6}
	K_2	2×10^{-12}
Theobromine		4.8×10^{-14} (40°)
Thiourea		1.1×10^{-15}
Urea		1.5×10^{-14}

momentarily disturbs the equilibrium between hydronium and hydroxyl ions; to restore equilibrium, some of the hydronium ions originally present in the water will combine with part of the added hydroxyl ions to form nonionized water molecules. The process continues until the product of the hydronium and hydroxyl ion concentrations is again equal to 10^{-14}. Assuming that the final hydroxyl ion concentration is $1 \times 10^{-4}\,N$, the concentration of hydronium ion in the solution will be 1×10^{-10}. Since [OH$^-$] is much greater than [H$_3$O$^+$], the solution is said to be *basic* or *alkaline*.

Relationship of K_a and K_b—A particularly interesting and useful relationship between the strength of an acid and its conjugate base, or a base and its conjugate acid, exists. For illustration, consider the strength of the base NH$_3$ and its conjugate acid NH$_4^+$, in water. The behavior of NH$_3$ as a base is expressed by,

$$NH_3 + H_2O \rightleftharpoons NH_4^+ + OH^-$$

for which the equilibrium, as formulated earlier is;

$$K_b = \frac{[NH_4^+][OH^-]}{[NH_3]} \qquad (25)$$

The behavior of NH$_4^+$ as an acid is represented by,

$$NH_4^+ + H_2O \rightleftharpoons NH_3 + H_3O^+$$

the equilibrium constant for which is,

$$K_a = \frac{[NH_3][H_3O^+]}{[NH_4^+]} \qquad (26)$$

Multiplying Eqs 25 and 26:

$$K_aK_b = \frac{[NH_3][H_3O^+][NH_4^+][OH^-]}{[NH_4^+][NH_3]} \qquad (27)$$

It is obvious that the product,

$$K_w = K_a . K_b \qquad (28)$$

where K_w is the ion product of water as defined in Eq 24.

The utility of this relationship, which is a general one for any conjugate acid–base pair, is evident from the following deductions: (1) the strength of an acid may be expressed in terms either of K_a or of K_b of its conjugate base, and *vice versa;* (2) the K_a of an acid may be calculated if the K_b of its conjugate base is known, and *vice versa;* (3) the stronger an acid is, the weaker its conjugate base, and *vice versa.*

Bases which are capable of interacting with more than one proton are termed polyacidic, and can be illustrated by the following:

$$PO_4^{3-} + H_2O \rightleftharpoons HPO_4^{2-} + OH^-$$

$$HPO_4^{2-} + H_2O \rightleftharpoons H_2PO_4^- + OH^-$$

$$H_2PO_4^- + H_2O \rightleftharpoons H_3PO_4 + OH^-$$

Applying the law of mass action to this series of reactions, and utilizing the concepts outlined in Eqs 25–28, it becomes obvious that the relationship between the various K_a and K_b values for phosphoric acid are,

$$K_w = K_{a1} \times K_{b3} = K_{a2} \times K_{b2} = K_{a3} \times K_{b1} \qquad (29)$$

where K_{a1}, K_{a2}, and K_{a3} refer to the equilibria given by Eqs 17, 18, and 19, respectively; K_{b1}, K_{b2}, and K_{b3} refer to the reaction of PO$_4^{3-}$, HPO$_4^{2-}$, and H$_2$PO$_4^-$, respectively, with water.

Electronegativity and Dissociation Constants—Table IV gives the dissociation constants of several weak acids and weak bases, in water, at 25°. As pointed out previously, strong acids and strong bases do not obey the law of mass action, so that dissociation constants cannot be formulated for these strong electrolytes.

From an inspection of this table it is evident that great variations occur in the strength of weak acids and weak bases. The effect of various substituents on the strength of acids and bases depends on the electronegativity of the substituent atom or radical. For example, the substitution of one chlorine atom into the molecule of acetic acid increases the degree of ionization of the acid; substitution of two chlorine atoms further increases the degree of ionization, and introduction of three chlorine atoms produces a still stronger acid. The explanation of this effect of chlorine is as follows: Acetic acid ionizes primarily because the oxygen atom adjacent to the hydrogen atom of the carboxyl group has a stronger affinity for electrons than has the hydrogen atom; the result is that when acetic acid is dissolved in water the polar molecules of the latter have a stronger affinity for the hydrogen of acetic acid than has the latter. The acetic acid ionizes as a consequence of this difference in affinities. When an atom of chlorine is introduced into the acetic acid molecule, forming $ClCH_2COOH$, the electrons in the molecule are very strongly attracted to the chlorine because of its relatively high electronegativity; the bond between the hydrogen and the oxygen in the carboxyl group is thereby weakened and the degree of ionization increased. Introduction of two, or of three, chlorine atoms further weakens the bond and increases the strength of the acid. On the other hand, substitution of chlorine into the molecule of ammonia reduces the strength of the base because of its decreased affinity for hydrogen ion.

Ionic Strength and Dissociation Constants—Most solutions of pharmaceutical interest are in a concentration range such that the ionic strength of the solution may have a marked effect on ionic equilibria and observed dissociation constants. One method of correcting dissociation constants for solutions with an ionic strength up to about 0.3 is to calculate an apparent dissociation constant, pK_a' as follows:

$$pK_a' = pK_a + \frac{0.51\,(2Z-1)\,\sqrt{\mu}}{1+\sqrt{\mu}} \qquad (30)$$

in which pK_a is the tabulated thermodynamic dissociation constant, Z is the charge on the acid and μ is the ionic strength.

Example—Calculate pK_2' for succinic acid at an ionic strength of 0.1. Assume that pK_2 is 5.63. The charge on the acid species is −1.

$$pK_2' = 5.63 + \frac{0.51\,(-2-1)\,\sqrt{0.1}}{1+\sqrt{0.1}}$$

$$= 5.63 - 0.37 = 5.26$$

Determination of Dissociation Constants—Although the dissociation constant of a weak acid or base can be obtained in a wide variety of ways including conductivity measurements, and ultraviolet or visible absorption spectroscopy, the most widely used method is potentiometric pH measurement (see discussion under *Potentiometry*, page 245). The simplest method involving potentiometric pH measurement is based on the measurement of the hydronium ion concentration of a solution containing equimolar concentrations of the acid and a strong-base salt of the acid. The principle of this method is evident from inspection of Eq 16; when equimolar concentrations of HA (the acid) and A^- (the salt) are present, the dissociation constant, K_a, is numerically equal to the hydronium ion concentration (also, the pK_a of the acid is equal to the pH of the solution). Although this method is simple and rapid, the dissociation constant obtained is not sufficiently accurate for many purposes.

In order to obtain the dissociation constant of a weak acid with a high degree of accuracy and precision, a dilute solution of the acid (about 10^{-3} to 10^{-4} M) is titrated with a strong base, and the pH of the solution taken after each addition of base. The resulting data can be handled in a wide variety of ways, perhaps the best of which is the method proposed by Benet and Goyan.[2] The proton balance equation (see discussion on page 240) for a weak acid, HA, being titrated with a strong base such as KOH, would be:

$$[K^+] + [H_3O^+] = [OH^-] + [A^-] \qquad (31)$$

in which $[K^+]$ is the concentration of the base added. Eq 31 can be rearranged to give,

$$Z = [A^-] = [K^+] + [H_3O^+] - [OH^-] \qquad (32)$$

When a weak monoprotic acid is added to water, it can exist in the unionized form, HA, and in the ionized form, A^-. After equilibrium is established, the sum of the concentrations of both species must be equal to C_a, the stoichiometric (added) concentration of acid or,

$$C_a = [HA] + [A^-] = [HA] + Z \qquad (33)$$

The term, [HA], can be replaced using Eq 16 to give

$$C_a = \frac{[H_3O^+]Z}{K_a} + Z \qquad (34)$$

which can be rearranged to,

$$Z = C_a - \frac{Z[H_3O^+]}{K_a} \qquad (35)$$

According to Eq 35, if Z, which is obtained from the experimental data using Eq 32 is plotted vs the terms $Z[H_3O^+]$, a straight line results with a slope equal to $1/K_a$, and an intercept equal to C_a. In addition to obtaining an accurate estimate for the dissociation constant, the stoichiometric concentration of the substance being titrated is also obtained. This is of importance when the substance being titrated cannot be purified, or has an unknown degree of solvation. Similar equations can be developed for obtaining the dissociation constant for a weak base.[2]

The dissociation constants for diprotic acids can be obtained by defining P as the average number of protons dissociated per mole of acid or,

$$P = Z/C_a \qquad (36)$$

and,

$$\frac{[H_3O^+]^2P}{(2-P)} = K_1K_2 + \frac{K_1\,[H_3O^+]\,(1-P)}{(2-P)} \qquad (37)$$

A plot of Eq 37 should yield a straight line with a slope equal to K_1 and an intercept of K_2; dividing the intercept by the slope yields K_2.

Micro Dissociation Constants—The dissociation constants for polyprotic acids, as determined by potentiometric titration, are generally known as macro or titration constants. Since we know that carboxyl groups are stronger acids than protonated amino groups there is no difficulty in assigning K_1 and K_2 as determined by Eq 37 to the carboxyl and amino groups respectively of a substance such as glycine hydrochloride. In other chemicals or drugs such as phenylpropanolamine, in which the two acidic groups are the phenolic and the protonated amino group, the assignment of dissociation constants is more difficult. This is due to the fact that, in general, both groups have dissociation constants of equal magnitude. Thus there will be two ways of losing the first proton and two ways of losing the second, resulting in four possible species in solution. This can be illustrated using the convention of assigning a + to a positively charged group, a 0 to an uncharged group, and a − to a negatively charged group. Thus +0 would represent the fully protonated phenylpropanolamine, +− the dipolar ion, 00 the uncharged molecule, and 0− the phenolate anion. The total ionization scheme can therefore be written,

The micro constants are related to the macro constants as follows,

$$K_1 = k_1 + k_2 \qquad (38)$$

$$K_1 K_2 = k_1 k_3 = k_2 k_4 \qquad (39)$$

It can be seen from Eq 38 that unless k_1 or k_2 is very much smaller than the other, the observed macro constant is a composite of the two and cannot be assigned to one or the other acidic group in a nonambiguous way.

Methods for determining k_1 are given by Riegelman[3] and Niebergall, et al.[4] Once k_1, K_1 and K_2 have been determined, all of the other micro constants can be obtained from Eqs 38 and 39.

pH

The numerical values of hydronium-ion concentration may vary enormously; for a normal solution of a strong acid the value is nearly 1, while for a normal solution of a strong base it is approximately 1×10^{-14}; ie, a variation of 100,000,000,000,000 between these two limits. Because of the inconvenience of dealing with numbers that vary so greatly, Sørenson, in 1909, proposed that hydronium ion concentration be expressed in terms of the logarithm (log) of its reciprocal. To this value he assigned the symbol pH. Mathematically it is written,

$$pH = \log \frac{1}{[H_3O^+]} \qquad (40)$$

and since the logarithm of 1 is zero, the equation may also be written,

$$pH = -\log[H_3O^+] \qquad (41)$$

from which it is evident that pH may also be defined as the negative logarithm of the hydronium ion concentration. In general, this type of notation is used to indicate the negative logarithm of the term that is preceded by the "p," which gives rise to the following:

$$pOH = -\log[OH^-] \qquad (42)$$

$$pK = -\log K \qquad (43)$$

Thus, taking logarithms of Eqs 26 and 28 gives,

$$pK_a + pK_b = pK_w \qquad (44)$$

$$pH + pOH = pK_w \qquad (45)$$

The relationship of pH to hydronium-ion and hydroxyl-ion concentrations may be seen in Table V.

Table V—Hydronium Ion and Hydroxyl Ion Concentrations

	pH	Normality in terms of hydronium ion	Normality in terms of hydroxyl ion
	0	1	10^{-14}
	1	10^{-1}	10^{-13}
Increasing acidity	2	10^{-2}	10^{-12}
	3	10^{-3}	10^{-11}
	4	10^{-4}	10^{-10}
	5	10^{-5}	10^{-9}
	6	10^{-6}	10^{-8}
Neutral point	7	10^{-7}	10^{-7}
	8	10^{-8}	10^{-6}
	9	10^{-9}	10^{-5}
Increasing alkalinity	10	10^{-10}	10^{-4}
	11	10^{-11}	10^{-3}
	12	10^{-12}	10^{-2}
	13	10^{-13}	10^{-1}
	14	10^{-14}	1

The following examples illustrate the conversion from exponential to "p" notation:

1. Calculate the pH corresponding to a hydronium ion concentration of 1×10^{-4} g-ion/L.

Solution:

$$pH = \log \frac{1}{1 \times 10^{-4}}$$

$$= \log 10,000 \text{ or } \log (1 \times 10^{+4})$$

$$\log (1 \times 10^{+4}) = +4$$

$$pH = 4$$

2. Calculate the pH corresponding to a hydronium ion concentration of 0.000036 N (or g-ion/L) (Note—This is more frequently written as a number multiplied by a power of 10, thus, 3.6×10^{-5} for 0.000036.)

Solution:

$$pH = \log \frac{1}{3.6 \times 10^{-5}}$$

$$= \log 28,000 \text{ or } \log (2.8 \times 10^{+4})$$

$$\log (2.8 \times 10^{+4}) = \log 2.8 + \log 10^{+4}$$

$$\log 2.8 = +0.44$$

$$\log 10^{+4} = +4.00$$

$$pH = 4.44$$

This problem may also be solved as follows:

$$pH = -\log (3.6 \times 10^{-5})$$

$$\log 3.6 = +0.56$$

$$\log 10^{-5} = -5.00$$

$$= -4.44 = \log (3.6 \times 10^{-5})$$

$$pH = -(-4.44) = +4.44 = 4.44$$

The following examples illustrate the conversion of "p" notation to exponential notation:

1. Calculate the hydronium ion concentration corresponding to a pH of 4.44.

Solution:

$$pH = \log \frac{1}{[H_3O^+]}$$

$$4.44 = \log \frac{1}{[H_3O^+]}$$

$$\frac{1}{[H_3O^+]} = \text{antilog of } 4.44 = 28,000 \text{ (rounded off)}$$

$$[H_3O^+] = \frac{1}{28,000} = 0.000036 \text{ or } 3.6 \times 10^{-5}$$

This calculation may also be made as follows:

$$+4.44 = -\log [H_3O^+]$$

$$\text{or } -4.44 = +\log [H_3O^+]$$

In finding the antilog of -4.44 it should be kept in mind that the mantissa (the number to the right of the decimal point) of a log to the base 10 (the common or Briggsian logarithm base) is *always positive* but that the characteristic (the number to the left of the decimal point) may be *positive* or *negative*. As the entire log -4.44 is negative, it is obvious that we cannot look up the antilog of -0.44. However, the number -4.44 may also be written $(-5.00 + 0.56)$ or, as more often written, $\bar{5}.56$, where the bar across the characteristic indicates that it alone is negative, while the rest of the number is positive. Looking up the antilog of 0.56 we find it to be 3.6 and as the antilog of -5.00 is 10^{-5}, it follows that the hydronium-ion concentration must be 3.6×10^{-5}.

2. Calculate the hydronium-ion concentration corresponding to a pH of 10.17.

Solution:

$$10.17 = -\log [H_3O^+]$$

$$-10.17 = \log [H_3O^+]$$

$$-10.17 = (-11.00 + 0.83) = \overline{11}.83$$

The antilog of $0.83 = 6.8$
The antilog of $-11.00 = 10^{-11}$
The hydronium-ion concentration is therefore $6.8 \times 10^{-11} N$.

In the section on acid–base equilibria it was shown that the hydronium-ion concentration of pure water, at 25°, is 1×10^{-7} N, corresponding to a pH of 7.* This figure is, therefore, designated as the neutral point and all values below a pH of 7 represent acidities, the smaller the number, the greater the acidity. Values above 7 represent alkalinities, the larger the number the greater the alkalinity. The pH scale usually runs from 0 to 14, but mathematically there is no reason why negative numbers or numbers above 14 should not be used. In practice, however, such values are never encountered because solutions which might be expected to have such values are too concentrated to be extensively ionized or the interionic attraction is so great as to materially reduce ionic activity.

It should be strongly emphasized that the generalizations stated concerning neutrality, acidity, and alkalinity hold exactly only when: (1) the solvent is water; (2) the temperature is 25°; and (3) there are no other factors to cause deviation from the simply formulated equilibria underlying the definition of pH given in the preceding discussion.

Species Concentration

When a weak acid, H_nA, is added to water, $n + 1$ species including the un-ionized acid can exist. After equilibrium is established, the sum of the concentrations of all species must be equal to C_a, the stoichiometric (added) concentration of acid. Thus, for a triprotic acid H_3A:

$$C_a = [H_3A] + [H_2A^-] + [HA^{2-}] + [A^{3-}] \quad (46)$$

In addition, the concentrations of all acidic and basic species in solution vary with pH, and can be represented solely in terms of equilibrium constants and the hydronium-ion concentration. These relationships may be expressed as in Eqs 47 and 48:

---

* The pH of the purest water obtainable, so-called "superconductivity" water, is 7.0 when the measurement is carefully made under conditions to exclude carbon dioxide and prevent errors inherent in the measuring technique (such as acidity or alkalinity of the indicator). Upon agitating this water in the presence of carbon dioxide in the atmosphere the value drops rapidly to 5.7, which is the pH of nearly all distilled waters that have been exposed to the atmosphere for even a short time.

$$[H_nA] = [H_3O^+]^n C_a/D \quad (47)$$

$$[H_{n-j}A^{-j}] = [H_3O^+]^{n-j} K_1 \ldots K_j C_a/D \quad (48)$$

in which n represents the total number of dissociable hydrogens in the parent acid, j is the number of protons dissociated, C_a is the stoichiometric concentration of acid, and K represents the acid dissociation constants. The term D is a power series in $[H_3O^+]$ and K, starting with $[H_3O^+]$ raised to the nth power. The last term is the product of all the dissociation constants. The intermediate terms can be generated from the last term by substituting $[H_3O^+]$ for K_n to obtain the next to last term, then substituting $[H_3O^+]$ for K_{n-1} to obtain the next term, etc, until the first term is reached. The following examples show the denominator, D, to be used for various types of acids:

$$H_3A: \quad D = [H_3O^+]^3 + K_1[H_3O^+]^2 + K_1K_2[H_3O^+] + K_1K_2K_3 \quad (49)$$

$$H_2A^-: \quad D = [H_3O^+]^2 + K_1[H_3O^+] + K_1K_2 \quad (50)$$

$$HA^{2-}: \quad D = [H_3O^+] + K_a \quad (51)$$

The numerator, in all instances, is C_a multiplied by the term from the denominator that has $[H_3O^+]$ raised to the $n - j$ power. Thus, for diprotic acids such as carbonic, succinic, tartaric, etc,

$$[H_2A] = \frac{[H_3O^+]^2 C_a}{[H_3O^+]^2 + K_1[H_3O^+] + K_1K_2} \quad (52)$$

$$[HA^-] = \frac{K_1[H_3O^+] C_a}{[H_3O^+]^2 + K_1[H_3O^+] + K_1K_2} \quad (53)$$

$$[A^{2-}] = \frac{K_1K_2 C_a}{[H_3O^+]^2 + K_1[H_3O^+] + K_1K_2} \quad (54)$$

Example—Calculate the concentrations of all succinic acid species in a $1.0 \times 10^{-3} M$ solution of succinic acid at pH 6.0. Assume that $K_1 = 6.4 \times 10^{-5}$ and $K_2 = 2.3 \times 10^{-6}$.

Eqs 52–54 have the same denominator, D, which can be calculated as follows:

$$D = [H_3O^+]^2 + K_1[H_3O^+] + K_1K_2$$

$$= 1.0 \times 10^{-12} + 6.4 \times 10^{-5} \times 1.0 \times 10^{-6} + 6.4 \times 10^{-5} \times 2.3 \times 10^{-6}$$

$$= 1.0 \times 10^{-12} + 6.4 \times 10^{-11} + 14.7 \times 10^{-11}$$

$$= 21.2 \times 10^{-11}$$

Therefore,

$$[H_2A] = \frac{[H_3O^+]^2 C_a}{D} =$$

$$\frac{1.0 \times 10^{-12} \times 1.0 \times 10^{-3}}{21.2 \times 10^{-11}} = 4.7 \times 10^{-6} M$$

$$[HA^-] = \frac{K_1[H_3O^+] C_a}{D} =$$

$$\frac{6.4 \times 10^{-11} \times 1.0 \times 10^{-3}}{21.2 \times 10^{-11}} = 3.0 \times 10^{-4} M$$

$$[A^{2-}] = \frac{K_1K_2 C_a}{D} =$$

$$\frac{14.7 \times 10^{-11} \times 1.0 \times 10^{-3}}{21.2 \times 10^{-11}} = 6.9 \times 10^{-4} M$$

Proton Balance Equation

In the Brønsted–Lowry system the total number of protons released by acidic species must equal the total number of protons consumed by basic species. This results in a very useful relationship known as the proton balance equation (PBE), in which the sum of the concentration terms for species that form by proton consumption is equated to the sum of the concentration terms for species that are formed by the release of protons. The PBE forms the basis of a unified approach to pH calculations, since it is an exact accounting of all proton transfers occurring in solution.

When HCl is added to water, for example, it dissociates yielding one Cl^- for each proton released. Thus, Cl^- is a species formed by the release of a proton. In the same solution, and actually in all aqueous solutions,

$$2H_2O \rightleftharpoons H_3O^+ + OH^-$$

where H_3O^+ is formed by proton consumption and OH^- is formed by proton release. Thus, the PBE is,

$$[H_3O^+] = [OH^-] + [Cl^-] \tag{55}$$

In general, the PBE can be formed in the following manner:

1. Start with the species added to water.
2. Place all species that can form when protons are released on the right side of the equation.
3. Place all species that can form when protons are consumed on the left side of the equation.
4. Add $[H_3O^+]$ to the left side of the equation and $[OH^-]$ to the right side of the equation. These result from the interaction of two molecules of water as shown above.

Example—When H_3PO_4 is added to water, the species $H_2PO_4^-$ forms with the release of one proton, HPO_4^{2-} forms with the release of 2 protons, and PO_4^{3-} forms with the release of 3 protons to give the following PBE:

$$[H_3O^+] = [OH^-] + [H_2PO_4^-] + 2[HPO_4^{2-}] + 3[PO_4^{3-}] \tag{56}$$

Example—When Na_2HPO_4 is added to water, it dissociates into 2 Na^+ and 1 HPO_4^{2-}. The sodium ion is neglected in the PBE since it is not formed from the release or consumption of protons. The species HPO_4^{2-}, however, may react with water to give $H_2PO_4^-$ with the consumption of 1 proton, H_3PO_4 with the consumption of 2 protons, and PO_4^{3-} with the release of 1 proton to give the following PBE:

$$[H_3O^+] + [H_2PO_4^-] + 2[H_3PO_4] = [OH^-] + [PO_4^{3-}] \tag{57}$$

Calculations

The pH of solutions of acids, bases, and salts may be calculated using the concepts presented in the preceding sections.

Strong Acids or Bases

When a strong acid such as HCl is added to water, the following reactions occur:

$$HCl + H_2O \rightarrow H_3O^+ + Cl^-$$

$$2H_2O \rightleftharpoons H_3O^+ + OH^-$$

The proton balance equation for this system would be,

$$[H_3O^+] = [OH^-] + [Cl^-] \tag{58}$$

In most instances ($C_a > 4.5 \times 10^{-7}\,M$) the $[OH^-]$ would be negligible compared to the $[Cl^-]$ and the equation simplifies to,

$$[H_3O^+] = [Cl^-] = C_a \tag{59}$$

Thus, the hydronium-ion concentration of a solution of a strong acid would be equal to the stoichiometric concentration of the acid. This would be anticipated, since strong acids are generally assumed to be 100% ionized.

The pH of a 0.005 M solution of HCl is therefore calculated as follows:

$$pH = -\log 0.005 = 2.30$$

In a similar manner the hydroxyl ion concentration for a solution of a strong base such as NaOH would be,

$$[OH^-] = [Na^+] = C_b \tag{60}$$

and the pH of a 0.005 M solution of NaOH would be,

$$pOH = -\log 0.005 = 2.30$$

$$pH = pK_w - pOH = 14.00 - 2.30 = 11.70$$

Weak Acids or Bases

If a weak acid, HA, is added to water, it will equilibrate with its conjugate base, A^-, as follows:

$$HA + H_2O \rightleftharpoons H_3O^+ + A^-$$

Accounting for the ionization of water gives the following proton balance equation for this system:

$$[H_3O^+] = [OH^-] + [A^-] \tag{61}$$

The concentration of A^- as a function of hydronium-ion concentration can be obtained as shown previously to give,

$$[H_3O^+] = [OH^-] + \frac{K_a C_a}{[H_3O^+] + K_a} \tag{62}$$

Algebraic simplification yields,

$$[H_3O^+] = K_a \frac{(C_a - [H_3O^+] + [OH^-])}{([H_3O^+] - [OH^-])} \tag{63}$$

In most instances for solutions of weak acids, $[H_3O^+] \gg [OH^-]$ and the equation simplifies to give,

$$[H_3O^+]^2 + K_a[H_3O^+] - K_a C_a = 0 \tag{64}$$

This is a quadratic equation* which yields

$$[H_3O^+] = \frac{-K_a + \sqrt{K_a^2 + 4K_a C_a}}{2} \tag{65}$$

since $[H_3O^+]$ can never be negative. Furthermore, if $[H_3O^+]$ is less than 5% of C_a, Eq 64 is simplified further to give,

$$[H_3O^+] = \sqrt{K_a C_a} \tag{66}$$

It is generally preferable to use the simplest equation to calculate $[H_3O^+]$. However, when $[H_3O^+]$ is calculated, it must be compared to C_a in order to determine whether the assumption $C_a \gg [H_3O^+]$ is valid. If the assumption is not valid, the quadratic equation should be used.

Example—Calculate the pH of a $5.00 \times 10^{-5}\,M$ solution of a weak acid having a $K_a = 1.90 \times 10^{-5}$.

$$[H_3O^+] = \sqrt{K_a C_a}$$

$$= 1.90 \times 10^{-5} \times 5.00 \times 10^{-5}$$

$$= 3.08 \times 10^{-5}\,M$$

Since C_a [(5.00 × 10⁻⁵ M)] is not much greater than $[H_3O^+]$, the quadratic

---

* The general solution to a quadratic equation of the form,

$$aX^2 + bX + c = 0$$

is,

$$X = \frac{-b \pm \sqrt{b^2 - 4ac}}{2a}$$

equation (Eq 65) should be used:

$$[H_3O^+] = \frac{-1.90 \times 10^{-5} + \sqrt{(1.90 \times 10^{-5})^2 + 4(1.90 \times 10^{-5} \times 5.00 \times 10^{-5})}}{2}$$

$$= 2.26 \times 10^{-5} \ M$$

$$pH = -\log(2.26 \times 10^{-5}) = 4.65$$

Note that the assumption $[H_3O^+] \gg [OH^-]$ is valid. The hydronium ion concentration calculated from Eq 66 has a relative error of 36% when compared to the correct value obtained from Eq 65.

When a salt obtained from a strong acid and a weak base—eg, ammonium chloride, morphine sulfate, pilocarpine HCl, etc—is dissolved in water, it dissociates as follows:

$$BH^+X^- \xrightarrow{H_2O} BH^+ + X^-$$

in which BH^+ is the protonated form of the base B, and X^- is the anion of a strong acid. Since X^- is the anion of a strong acid, it is too weak a base to undergo any further reaction with water. The protonated base, however, can act as a weak acid to give,

$$BH^+ + H_2O \rightleftharpoons B + H_3O^+$$

Thus Eqs 65 and 66 are valid with C_a being equal to the concentration of the salt in solution. If K_a for the protonated base is not available, it can be obtained by dividing K_b for the base B, into K_w.

Example—Calculate the pH of a 0.026 M solution of ammonium chloride. Assume that K_b for ammonia is 1.74×10^{-5} and K_w is 1.00×10^{-14}.

$$K_a = \frac{K_w}{K_b} = \frac{1.00 \times 10^{-14}}{1.74 \times 10^{-5}} = 5.75 \times 10^{-10}$$

$$[H_3O^+] = \sqrt{K_a C_a}$$

$$= \sqrt{5.75 \times 10^{-10} \times 2.6 \times 10^{-2}}$$

$$= 3.87 \times 10^{-6} \ M$$

$$pH = -\log(3.87 \times 10^{-6}) = 5.41$$

Since C_a is much greater than $[H_3O^+]$ and $[H_3O^+]$ is much greater than $[OH^-]$, the assumptions are valid and the value calculated for pH is sufficiently accurate.

Weak Bases

When a weak base, B, is dissolved in water it ionizes to give the conjugate acid as follows:

$$B + H_2O \rightleftharpoons BH^+ + OH^-$$

The proton balance equation for this system is,

$$[BH^+] + [H_3O^+] = [OH^-] \qquad (67)$$

Substituting $[BH^+]$ as a function of hydronium concentration and simplifying, in the same manner as shown for a weak acid, gives,

$$[OH^-] = K_b \frac{(C_b - [OH^-] + [H_3O^+])}{([OH^-] - [H_3O^+])} \qquad (68)$$

If $[OH^-] \gg [H_3O^+]$, as is generally true,

$$[OH^-]^2 + K_b[OH^-] - K_b C_b = 0 \qquad (69)$$

which is a quadratic with the following solution,

$$[OH^-] = \frac{-K_b + \sqrt{K_b^2 + 4K_b C_b}}{2} \qquad (70)$$

If $C_b \gg [OH^-]$, the quadratic equation simplifies to,

$$[OH^-] = \sqrt{K_b C_b} \qquad (71)$$

Once $[OH^-]$ is calculated, it can be converted to pOH, which can be subtracted from pK_w to give pH.

Example—Calculate the pH of a $4.50 \times 10^{-2} \ M$ solution of a weak base having $K_b = 2.00 \times 10^{-4}$. Assume that $K_w = 1.00 \times 10^{-14}$.

$$[OH^-] = \sqrt{K_b C_b}$$

$$= \sqrt{2.00 \times 10^{-4} \times 4.50 \times 10^{-2}}$$

$$= \sqrt{9.00 \times 10^{-6}} = 3.00 \times 10^{-3} \ M$$

Both assumptions are valid:

$$pOH = -\log 3.00 \times 10^{-3} = 2.52$$

$$pH = 14.00 - 2.52 = 11.48$$

When salts obtained from strong bases and weak acids—eg, sodium acetate, sodium sulfathiazole, sodium benzoate, etc—are dissolved in water, they dissociate as follows:

$$Na^+A^- \xrightarrow{H_2O} Na^+ + A^-$$

in which A^- is the conjugate base of the weak acid, HA. The Na^+ undergoes no further reaction with water. The A^-, however, acts as a weak base to give,

$$A^- + H_2O \rightleftharpoons HA + OH^-$$

Thus, Eqs 70 and 71 are valid with C_b being equal to the concentration of the salt in solution. The value for K_b can be obtained by dividing K_a for the conjugate acid, HA, into K_w.

Example—Calculate the pH of a 0.05 M solution of sodium acetate. Assume K_a for acetic acid is equal to 1.75×10^{-5} and $K_w = 1.00 \times 10^{-14}$.

$$K_b = \frac{K_w}{K_a} = \frac{1.00 \times 10^{-14}}{1.75 \times 10^{-5}}$$

$$= 5.71 \times 10^{-10}$$

$$OH^- = \sqrt{K_b C_b} = \sqrt{5.71 \times 10^{-10} \times 5.0 \times 10^{-2}}$$

$$= 5.34 \times 10^{-6} \ M$$

Both assumptions are valid.

$$pOH = -\log(5.34 \times 10^{-6}) = 5.27$$

$$pH = 14.00 - 5.27 = 8.73$$

Ampholytes

Substances such as $NaHCO_3$ and NaH_2PO_4 are termed *ampholytes*, and are capable of functioning both as acids and bases. When an ampholyte of the type NaHA is dissolved in water, the following series of reactions can occur:

$$Na^+HA^- \xrightarrow{H_2O} Na^+ + HA^-$$

$$HA^- + H_2O \rightleftharpoons A^{2-} + H_3O^+$$

$$HA^- + H_2O \rightleftharpoons H_2A + OH^-$$

$$2H_2O \rightleftharpoons H_3O^+ + OH^-$$

The total proton balance equation for the system is,

$$[H_3O^+] + [H_2A] = [OH^-] + [A^{2-}] \qquad (72)$$

Substituting both $[H_2A]$ and $[A^{2-}]$ as a function of $[H_3O^+]$ (see Eqs 52 and 54), yields

$$[H_3O^+] + \frac{[H_3O^+]^2 C_s}{[H_3O^+]^2 + K_1[H_3O^+] + K_1K_2} =$$
$$\frac{K_w}{[H_3O^+]} + \frac{K_1K_2C_s}{[H_3O^+]^2 + K_1[H_3O^+] + K_1K_2}$$

This gives a fourth-order equation in $[H_3O^+]$, which can be simplified using certain judicious assumptions to,

$$[H_3O^+] = \sqrt{\frac{K_1K_2C_s}{K_1 + C_s}} \qquad (73)$$

In most instances, $C_s \gg K_1$ and the equation further simplifies to,

$$[H_3O^+] = \sqrt{K_1K_2} \qquad (74)$$

and $[H_3O^+]$ becomes independent of the concentration of the salt. A special property of ampholytes is that the concentration of the species HA^- is at a maximum at the pH corresponding to Eq 74.

When the simplest amino acid, glycine hydrochloride, is dissolved in water, it acts as a diprotic acid and ionizes as follows:

$$^+NH_3CH_2COOH + H_2O \rightleftharpoons {}^+NH_3CH_2COO^- + H_3O^+$$

$$^+NH_3CH_2COO^- + H_2O \rightleftharpoons NH_2CH_2COO^- + H_3O^+$$

The form, $^+NH_3CH_2COO^-$, is an ampholyte since it can also act as a weak base as follows:

$$^+NH_3CH_2COO^- + H_2O \rightleftharpoons {}^+NH_3CH_2COOH + OH^-$$

This type of substance, which carries both a charged acidic and a charged basic moiety on the same molecule is termed a *zwitter ion*, and since the two charges balance each other, the molecule acts essentially as a neutral molecule. The pH at which the *zwitter-ion* concentration is at a maximum is known as the isoelectric point, which can be calculated from Eq 74.

On the acid side of the isoelectric point, amino acids and proteins are cationic and incompatible with anionic materials such as the naturally occurring gums used as suspending and/or emulsifying agents. On the alkaline side of the isoelectric point, amino acids and proteins are anionic and incompatible with cationic materials such as benzalkonium chloride.

Salts of Weak Acids and Weak Bases

When a salt such as ammonium acetate (which is derived from a weak acid and a weak base) is dissolved in water, it undergoes the following reactions:

$$BH^+A^- \xrightarrow{H_2O} BH^+ + A^-$$

$$BH^+ + H_2O \rightleftharpoons B + H_3O^+$$

$$A^- + H_2O \rightleftharpoons HA + OH^-$$

The total PBE for this system is,

$$[H_3O^+] + [HA] = [OH^-] + [B] \qquad (75)$$

Replacing $[HA]$ and $[B]$ as a function of $[H_3O^+]$, gives,

$$[H_3O^+] + \frac{[H_3O^+]C_s}{[H_3O^+] + K_a} = [OH^-] + \frac{K_a'C_s}{[H_3O^+] + K_a'} \qquad (76)$$

in which C_s is the concentration of salt; K_a is the ionization constant of the conjugate acid formed from the reaction between A^- and water; and K_a' is the ionization constant for the protonated base, BH^+. In general, $[H_3O^+]$, $[OH^-]$, K_a, and K_a' are usually smaller than C_s and the equation simplifies to

$$[H_3O^+] = \sqrt{K_aK_a'} \qquad (77)$$

Example—Calculate the pH of a 0.01 M solution of ammonium acetate. The ammonium ion has a K_a equal to 5.75×10^{-10}, which represents K_a' in Eq 77. Acetic acid has a K_a of 1.75×10^{-5}, which represents K_a in Eq 77:

$$[H_3O^+] = \sqrt{1.75 \times 10^{-5} \times 5.75 \times 10^{-10}}$$
$$= 1.05 \times 10^{-7}$$
$$pH = -\log(1.05 \times 10^{-7}) = 6.98$$

Note that all of the assumptions are valid.

Buffers

The terms *buffer*, *buffer solution*, and *buffered solution*, when used with reference to hydrogen ion concentration or pH, refer to the ability of a system, particularly an aqueous solution, to resist change of pH on adding acid or alkali, or on diluting it with solvent.

If acid or base is added to water, the pH of the latter is changed markedly, for water has no ability to resist change of pH; it is completely devoid of buffer action. Even a very weak acid such as carbon dioxide changes the pH of water, decreasing it from 7 to 5.7 when the small concentration of carbon dioxide present in air is equilibrated with pure water. This extreme susceptibility of distilled water to change of pH on adding very small amounts of acid or base is often of great concern in pharmaceutical operations. Solutions of neutral salts such as sodium chloride similarly lack ability to resist change of pH on adding acid or base; such solutions are called unbuffered.

Characteristic of buffered solutions, which undergo small changes of pH on addition of acid or base, is the presence either of a weak acid and a salt of the weak acid, or a weak base and a salt of the weak base. An example of the former system is acetic acid and sodium acetate; of the latter, ammonium hydroxide and ammonium chloride. From the proton concept of acids and bases discussed earlier it is apparent that such buffer action involves a conjugate acid–base pair in the solution; it will be recalled that acetate ion is the conjugate base of acetic acid, and that ammonium ion is the conjugate acid of ammonia (the principal constituent of what is commonly called ammonium hydroxide).

The mechanism of action of the acetic acid–sodium acetate buffer pair is that the acid, which exists largely in molecular (nonionized) form, combines with hydroxyl ion that may be added to form acetate ion and water, thus,

$$CH_3COOH + OH^- \rightarrow CH_3COO^- + H_2O$$

while the acetate ion, which is a base, combines with hydrogen (more exactly hydronium) ion that may be added to form essentially nonionized acetic acid and water, represented as,

$$CH_3COO^- + H_3O^+ \rightarrow CH_3COOH + H_2O$$

As will be illustrated later by an example, the change of pH is slight as long as the amount of hydronium or hydroxyl ion added does not exceed the capacity of the buffer system to neutralize it.

The ammonia–ammonium chloride pair functions as a buffer because the ammonia combines with hydronium ion that may be added to form ammonium ion and water, thus,

$$NH_3 + H_3O^+ \rightarrow NH_4^+ + H_2O$$

and ammonium ion, which is an acid, combines with added hydroxyl ion to form ammonia and water, as,

$$NH_4^+ + OH^- \rightarrow NH_3 + H_2O$$

Again, the change of pH is slight if the amount of added hydronium or hydroxyl ion is not in excess of the capacity of the system to neutralize it.

Besides these two general types of buffers, a third appears to exist. This is the buffer system composed of two salts, as monobasic potassium phosphate, KH_2PO_4, and dibasic potassium phosphate, K_2HPO_4. This is not, however, a new type of buffer; it is actually a weak-acid–conjugate-base buffer in which an ion, $H_2PO_4^-$, serves as the weak acid, and HPO_4^{2-} is its conjugate base. When hydroxyl ion is added to this buffer the following reaction takes place:

$$H_2PO_4^- + OH^- \rightarrow HPO_4^{2-} + H_2O$$

and when hydronium ion is added the following occurs:

$$HPO_4^{2-} + H_3O^+ \rightarrow H_2PO_4^- + H_2O$$

It is apparent that the mechanism of action of this type of buffer is essentially the same as that of the weak-acid–conjugate-base buffer composed of acetic acid and sodium acetate.

Calculations—A buffer system composed of a conjugate acid–base pair, NaA − HA (such as sodium acetate and acetic acid) would have a PBE of,

$$[H_3O^+] + [HA] = [OH^-] + [A^-] \quad (78)$$

Replacing [HA] and [A⁻] as a function of hydronium ion concentration, gives,

$$[H_3O^+] + \frac{[H_3O^+]C_b}{[H_3O^+] + K_a} = [OH^-] + \frac{K_aC_a}{[H_3O^+] + K_a} \quad (79)$$

where C_b is the concentration of the salt, NaA, and C_a is the concentration of the weak acid, HA. This equation can be rearranged to give,

$$[H_3O^+] = K_a \frac{(C_a - [H_3O^+] + [OH^-])}{(C_b + [H_3O^+] - [OH^-])} \quad (80)$$

In general, both C_a and C_b are much greater than $[H_3O^+]$, which is in turn much greater than $[OH^-]$, and the equation simplifies to,

$$[H_3O^+] = \frac{K_aC_a}{C_b} \quad (81)$$

or, expressed in terms of pH, as,

$$pH = pK_a + \log \frac{C_b}{C_a} \quad (82)$$

This equation is generally called the Henderson–Hasselbalch equation.

This equation applies to all buffer systems formed from a single conjugate acid–base pair, regardless of the nature of the salts. For example, it applies equally well to the following buffer systems: ammonia–ammonium chloride; monosodium phosphate–disodium phosphate; phenobarbital–sodium phenobarbital; etc. In the ammonia–ammonium chloride system, ammonia is obviously the base and the ammonium ion is the acid (C_a equal to the concentration of the salt); in the phosphate system, monosodium phosphate is the acid and disodium phosphate is the base; in the phenobarbital buffer system, phenobarbital is the acid and the phenobarbital anion is the base (C_b equal to the concentration of sodium phenobarbital).

As an example of the application of this equation, the pH of a buffer solution containing acetic acid and sodium acetate, each in 0.1 M concentration, may be calculated. The K_a of acetic acid, as defined above, is 1.8×10^{-5}, at 25°.

Solution:

First, the pK_a of acetic acid is calculated:

$$pK_a = -\log K_a = -\log 1.8 \times 10^{-5}$$
$$= -\log 1.8 - \log 10^{-5}$$
$$= -0.26 - (-5) = +4.74$$

Substituting this value into Eq 82,

$$pH = \log \frac{0.1}{0.1} + 4.74 = +4.74$$

The Henderson–Hasselbalch equation predicts that any solutions containing the same molar concentration of acetic acid as of sodium acetate will have the same pH. Thus, a solution of 0.01 M concentration of each will have the same pH, 4.74, as one of 0.1 M concentration of each component. Actually, there will be some difference in the pH of the solutions, for the *activity coefficient* of the components varies with concentration; for most practical purposes, however, the approximate values of pH calculated by the Henderson–Hasselbalch equation are satisfactory. It should be pointed out, however, that the buffer of higher concentration of each component will have a much greater capacity for neutralizing added acid or base; this point will be discussed further under *Buffer Capacity.*

The Henderson–Hasselbalch equation is useful also for calculating the ratio of molar concentrations of a buffer system required to produce a solution of specific pH. As an example, suppose that an acetic acid–sodium acetate buffer of pH 4.5 is to be prepared. What ratio of the buffer components should be used?

Solution:

Rearranging Eq 82, which is used to calculate the pH of weak acid-salt type buffers, we obtain

$$\log \frac{[\text{base}]}{[\text{acid}]} = pH - pK_a$$
$$= 4.5 - 4.76 = -0.24 = (9.76 - 10)$$
$$\frac{[\text{base}]}{[\text{acid}]} = \text{antilog of } (9.76 - 10) = 0.575$$

The interpretation of this result is that the *proportion* of sodium acetate to acetic acid should be 0.575 mole of the former to 1 mole of the latter to produce a pH of 4.5. A solution containing 0.0575 mole of sodium acetate and 0.1 mole of acetic acid per liter would meet this requirement, as would also one containing 0.00575 mole of sodium acetate and 0.01 mole of acetic acid per liter. The actual concentration selected would depend chiefly on the desired buffer capacity.

Buffer Capacity—The ability of a buffer solution to resist changes in pH upon addition of acid or alkali may be measured in terms of *buffer capacity.* In the preceding discussion of buffers, we have seen that, in a general way, the concentration of acid in a weak-acid–conjugate-base buffer determines the capacity to "neutralize" added base, while the concentration of salt of the weak acid determines the capacity to neutralize added acid. Similarly, in a weak-base–conjugate-acid buffer the concentration of the weak base establishes the buffer capacity toward added acid, while the concentration of the conjugate acid of the weak base determines the capacity toward added base. When the buffer is equimolar in the concentrations of weak acid and conjugate base, or of weak base and conjugate acid, it has equal buffer capacity toward added strong acid or strong base.

Van Slyke, the biochemist, introduced a quantitative expression for evaluating buffer capacity. This may be defined as the amount, in gram-equivalents (g-Eq) per liter, of strong acid or strong base, required to be added to a solution to change its pH by 1 unit; a solution has a buffer capacity of 1 when 1 l requires 1 g-Eq of strong base or acid to change the pH 1 unit (in practice, considerably smaller increments are measured, expressed as the ratio of acid or base added to the change of pH produced). From this definition it is apparent that the smaller the pH change in a solution caused by the addition of a specified quantity of acid or alkali, the greater is the buffer capacity of the solution.

The following numerical examples illustrate certain basic principles and calculations concerning buffer action and buffer capacity.

Example 1—What is the change of pH on adding 0.01 mole of NaOH to 1 l of 0.10 M acetic acid?

(a)   Calculate the pH of a 0.10 molar solution of acetic acid:

$$[H_3O^+] = \sqrt{K_a C_a} = 1.75 \times 10^{-4} \times 1.0 \times 10^{-1} = 1.33 \times 10^{-3}$$

$$pH = -\log 1.33 \times 10^{-3} = 2.88$$

(b)   On adding 0.01 mole of NaOH to a liter of this solution, 0.01 mole of acetic acid is converted to 0.01 mole of sodium acetate, thereby decreasing C_a to 0.09 M, and $C_b = 1.0 \times 10^{-2}\ M$. Use of the Henderson–Hasselbalch equation gives

$$pH = 4.76 + \log \frac{0.01}{0.09} = 4.76 - 0.95 = 3.81$$

The pH change is, therefore, 0.93 unit. The buffer capacity as defined above is calculated to be

$$\frac{\text{moles of NaOH added}}{\text{change in pH}} = 0.011$$

Example 2—What is the change of pH on adding 0.1 mole of NaOH to 1 l of buffer solution 0.1 M in acetic acid and 0.1 M in sodium acetate?

(a)   The pH of the buffer solution before adding NaOH is

$$pH = \log \frac{[\text{base}]}{[\text{acid}]} + pK_a$$

$$= \log \frac{0.1}{0.1} + 4.76 = 4.76$$

(b)   On adding 0.01 mole of NaOH per liter to this buffer solution, 0.01 mole of acetic acid is converted to 0.01 mole of sodium acetate, thereby decreasing the concentration of acid to 0.09 M and increasing the concentration of base to 0.11 M. The pH is calculated as follows:

$$pH = \log \frac{0.11}{0.09} + 4.76$$

$$= 0.086 + 4.76 = 4.85$$

The change of pH in this case is only 0.09 unit, about $^1/_{10}$ the change in the preceding example. The buffer capacity is calculated as

$$\frac{\text{moles of NaOH added}}{\text{change of pH}} = \frac{0.01}{0.09} = 0.11$$

Thus the buffer capacity of the acetic acid–sodium acetate buffer solution is approximately 10 times that of the acetic acid solution.

As is in part evident from the preceding examples, and may be further evidenced by calculations of pH changes in other systems, the degree of buffer action, and therefore the buffer capacity, are dependent on the kind and concentration of the buffer components, the pH region involved, and the kind of acid or alkali added.

Strong Acids and Bases as "Buffers"—In the foregoing discussion, buffer action was attributed to systems of (1) weak acids and their conjugate bases, (2) weak bases and their conjugate acids, and (3) certain acid-base pairs which can function in the manner either of (1) or (2).

The ability to resist change in pH on adding acid or alkali is possessed also by relatively concentrated solutions of strong acids and strong bases. If to 1 L of pure water having a pH of 7.0 is added 1 mL of 0.01 M hydrochloric acid, the pH is reduced to about 5.0. If the same volume of the acid is added to 1 L of 0.001 M hydrochloric acid, which has a pH of about 3, the hydronium ion concentration is increased only about 1% and the pH is reduced hardly at all. The nature of this buffer action is quite different from that of the true buffer solutions. The very simple explanation is that when 1 mL of 0.01 M HCl, which represents 0.00001 g-Eq of hydronium ions, is added to the 0.0000001 g-Eq of hydronium ions in 1 L of pure water, the hydronium-ion concentration is increased 100-fold (equivalent to 2 pH units), but when the same amount is added to the 0.001 g-Eq of hydronium ions in 1 L

of 0.001 M HCl, the increase is only 1/100 the concentration already present. Similarly, if 1 mL of 0.01 M NaOH is added to 1 L of pure water, the pH is increased to 9, while if the same volume is added to 1 L of 0.001 molar NaOH, the pH is increased almost immeasurably.

In general, solutions of strong acids of pH 3 or less, and solutions of strong bases of pH 11 or more, exhibit this kind of buffer action by virtue of the relatively high concentration of hydronium or hydroxyl ions present. The USP includes among its *Standard Buffer Solutions* a series of hydrochloric acid buffers, covering the pH range 1.2 to 2.2, which also contain potassium chloride; the salt does not participate in the buffering mechanism, as is the case with salts of weak acids, instead it serves as a nonreactive constituent required to maintain the proper electrolyte environment of the solutions.

Determination of pH

Colorimetry

A relatively simple and inexpensive method for determining the approximate pH of a solution depends on the fact that some conjugate acid base pairs (indicators) possess one color in the acid form and another color in the base form. Assume that the acid form of a particular indicator is red, while the base form is yellow. The color of a solution of this indicator will range from red when it is sufficiently acid to yellow when it is sufficiently alkaline. In the intermediate pH range (the transition interval) the color will be a blend of red and yellow depending upon the ratio of the base to the acid form. In general, although there are slight differences between indicators, color changes apparent to the eye cannot be discerned when the ratio of base to acid form, or acid to base form exceeds 10:1. The use of Eq 82 indicates that the transition range of most indicators is equal to the pK_a of the indicator ±1 pH unit, or a useful range of approximately 2 pH units. Standard indicator solutions can be made at known pH values within the transition range of the indicator, and the pH of an unknown solution determined by adding the indicator to it and comparing the resulting color with the standard solutions. Details of this procedure can be found in RPS-14. Another method for using these indicators is to apply them to thin strips of filter paper. A drop of the unknown solution is placed on a piece of the indicator paper and the resulting color is compared to a color chart supplied with the indicator paper. These indicator papers are available in a wide variety of pH ranges.

Potentiometry

Electrometric methods for the determination of pH are based on the fact that the difference of electrical potential between two suitable electrodes dipping into a solution containing hydronium ions depends on the concentration (or activity) of the latter. Development of a potential difference is not a specific property of hydronium ions; a solution of any ion will develop a potential proportional to the concentration of that ion if a suitable pair of electrodes is placed in the solution.

The relationship between the potential difference and concentration of an ion in equilibrium with the electrodes may be derived as follows. When a metal is immersed into a solution of one of its salts, there is a tendency for the metal to go into solution in the form of ions. This tendency is spoken of as the *solution pressure* of the metal and is comparable to the tendency of sugar molecules, for example, to dissolve in water. The metallic ions in solution tend, on the other hand, to become discharged by forming atoms, this effect being proportional to the *osmotic pressure* of the ions. In order for an atom of a metal to go into solution as a positive ion, electrons, equal in number to the charge on the ion, must be left behind on the metal electrode with the result that the latter becomes negatively charged. The positively charged ions in solution, however, may become discharged as atoms by taking up electrons from the metal electrode. Depending on which effect predominates, the electrical charge on the electrode will be either positive or negative and may be quantitatively expressed by the following equation proposed by Nernst in 1889:

$$E = \frac{RT}{nF} \ln \frac{p}{P} \tag{83}$$

where,

E = potential difference or electromotive force
R = the gas constant = 8.316 joules
T = absolute temperature
n = valence of the ion
F = the Faraday of electricity = 96,500 coulombs
p = osmotic pressure of the ions
P = solution pressure of the metal

Inasmuch as it is impossible to measure the potential difference between one electrode and a solution with any degree of certainty, it is customary to use two electrodes and to measure the potential difference between them. If two electrodes both of the same metal are separately immersed in solutions containing ions of that metal, at osmotic pressure p_1 and p_2, respectively, and connected by means of a tube containing a nonreacting salt solution (a so-called "salt-bridge"), the potential developed across the two electrodes will be equal to the difference between the potential differences of the individual electrodes, thus,

$$E = E_1 - E_2 = \frac{RT}{nF} \ln \frac{p_1}{P_1} - \frac{RT}{nF} \ln \frac{p_2}{P_2} \tag{84}$$

Since both electrodes are of the same metal $P_1 = P_2$ and the equation may be simplified to,

$$E = \frac{RT}{nF} \ln p_1 - \frac{RT}{nF} \ln p_2 = \frac{RT}{nF} \ln \frac{p_1}{p_2} \tag{85}$$

In place of osmotic pressures it is permissible, for dilute solutions, to substitute the concentrations c_1 and c_2 which were found (see Chapter 16, page 222) to be proportional to p_1 and p_2. The equation then becomes,

$$E = \frac{RT}{nF} \ln \frac{c_1}{c_2} \tag{86}$$

If either c_1 or c_2 is known, it is obvious that the value of the other may be found if the potential difference, E, of this cell can be measured.

For the determination of hydronium-ion concentration or pH an electrode at which an equilibrium between hydrogen gas and hydronium ion can be established must be used in place of metallic electrodes. Such an electrode may be made by electrolytically coating a strip of platinum, or other noble metal, with platinum black and saturating the latter with pure hydrogen gas. This device then functions as a *hydrogen electrode*. Two such electrodes may then be set up as shown in Fig 17-3.

In this diagram one electrode dips into solution A which is of known hydronium-ion concentration and the other electrode dips into solution B containing an unknown concentration of hydronium ion. The two electrodes and solutions, sometimes called half-cells, are then connected by a bridge of neutral salt solution which has no significant effect on the solutions which it connects. The potential difference across the two electrodes is measured by means of a potentiometer P. If the concentration, c_1, of hydronium ion in solution A is one normal, Eq 86 simplifies to

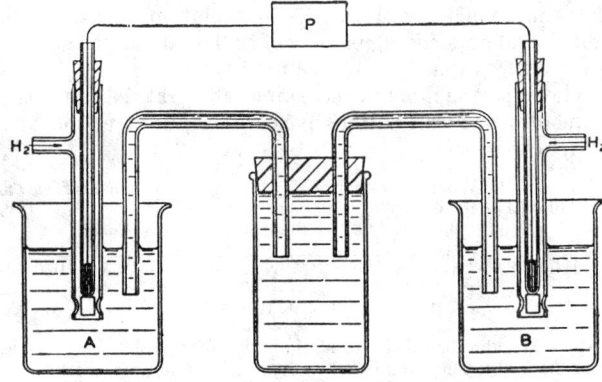

Fig 17-3.   Hydrogen-ion concentration chain.

$$E = \frac{RT}{nF} \ln \frac{1}{c_2} \tag{87}$$

or in terms of Briggsian logarithms,

$$E = 2.303 \frac{RT}{nF} \log_{10} \frac{1}{c_2} \tag{88}$$

If for $\log_{10} 1/c_2$ there is substituted its equivalent pH, the equation becomes,

$$E = 2.303 \frac{RT}{nF} \text{pH} \tag{89}$$

and finally by substituting numerical values for R, n, and F, and assuming the temperature to be 20°, the following simple relationship is derived:

$$E = 0.0581 \text{ pH or pH} = \frac{E}{0.0581} \tag{90}$$

The hydrogen electrode dipping into a solution of known hydronium-ion concentration, called the *reference electrode*, may be replaced by a calomel electrode, one type of which is shown in Fig 17-4. The elements of a calomel electrode are mercury and calomel in an aqueous solution of potassium chloride; the potential of this electrode is constant, regardless of the hydronium-ion concentration of the solution into which

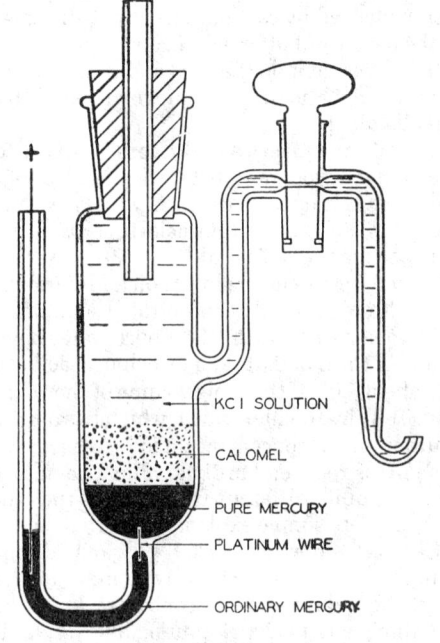

Fig 17-4.   Calomel electrode.

it dips. The potential depends on the equilibrium which is set up between mercury and mercurous ions from the calomel, but the concentration of the latter is governed, according to the solubility product principle, by the concentration of chloride ions which are mainly derived from the potassium chloride in the solution. Therefore the potential of this electrode varies with the concentration of potassium chloride in the electrolyte.

Because the calomel electrode always indicates voltages which are higher, by a constant value, than those obtained when the normal hydrogen electrode chain shown in Fig 17-3 is used, it is necessary to subtract, from the observed voltage, the voltage due to the calomel electrode itself. As the magnitude of this voltage depends on the concentration of potassium chloride in the calomel electrode electrolyte, it is necessary to know the concentration of the former. For most purposes a saturated potassium chloride solution is used which has a potential difference of 0.2488 v. Accordingly, before using Eq 85 for the calculation of pH from the voltage of a cell made up of a calomel and a hydrogen electrode dipping into the solution to be tested, 0.2488 v must be subtracted from the observed potential difference. Expressed mathematically, Eq 91 is used for calculating pH from the potential difference of such a cell.

$$\text{pH} = \frac{E - 0.2488}{0.0581} \tag{91}$$

In measuring the potential difference between the electrodes, it is imperative that very little current be drawn from the cell, for with current flowing the voltage changes, owing to polarization effects at the electrode. Because of this it is not possible to make accurate measurements with a voltmeter which requires appreciable current to operate it. In its place is used a potentiometer which does not draw a current from the cell being measured or, as in most potentiometers in use today, electronic amplification of the voltage developed at the electrodes is effected.

There are many limitations to the use of the hydrogen electrode. For example, it cannot be used in solutions containing strong oxidants such as ferric iron, dichromates, nitric acid, peroxide, and chlorine or reductants such as sulfurous acid and hydrogen sulfide. It is also affected by the presence of organic compounds which are fairly easily reduced. Furthermore, the hydrogen electrode cannot be successfully used in solutions containing cations that fall below hydrogen in the electrochemical series. Erratic results are also obtained in the measurement of unbuffered solutions unless special precautions are taken. Moreover, hydrogen electrodes are troublesome to prepare and maintain. Since other electrodes, more convenient to use, are now available, the hydrogen electrode is today rarely used. Nevertheless, the hydrogen electrode is the ultimate standard for pH measurements.

To avoid some of the difficulties with the hydrogen electrode, the *quinhydrone* electrode was introduced and was popular for a long time, particularly for measurements of acid solutions. The unusual feature of this electrode is that it consists of a piece of gold or platinum wire or foil dipping into the solution to be tested, in which has been dissolved a small quantity of quinhydrone. A calomel electrode may be used for reference, just as in determinations with the hydrogen electrode.

Quinhydrone consists of an equimolecular mixture of quinone and hydroquinone; the relationship between these substances and hydrogen-ion concentration is as follows:

Quinone + 2 hydrogen ions + 2 electrons ⇌ hydroquinone

In a solution containing hydrogen ions the potential of the quinhydrone electrode is logarithmically related to hydronium-ion concentration if the ratio of the hydroquinone concentration to that of quinone is constant and practically equal to one. This ratio is maintained in an acid solution containing an excess of quinhydrone and measurements may be made quickly and accurately however, quinhydrone cannot be used in solutions more alkaline than pH 8.

An electrode which, because of its simplicity of operation and freedom from contamination or change of the solution being tested, has replaced both the hydrogen and quinhydrone electrodes is the glass electrode. It functions by virtue of the fact that when a thin membrane of a special composition of glass separates two solutions of different pH there is developed across the membrane a potential difference which depends on the pH of both solutions. If the pH of one of the solutions is known, the other may be calculated from the voltage measurement. In practice the glass electrode usually consists of a bulb of the special glass fused to the end of a tube of ordinary glass. Inside the bulb is placed a solution of known pH, in contact with an internal silver–silver chloride or other electrode; this glass electrode and another reference electrode are immersed in the solution to be tested and the potential difference is measured. A potentiometer providing electronic amplification of the small current produced is employed; the modern instruments available permit reading the pH directly and provide also for compensation of variations due to temperature in the range of 0–50° and to the small but variable asymmetry potential inherent in the glass electrode.

Pharmaceutical Significance

In the broad realm of knowledge concerning the preparation and action of drugs few, if any, variables are so important as pH. For the purpose of this presentation, four principal types of pH-dependence of drug systems will be discussed: (1) solubility, (2) stability, (3) activity, and (4) absorption.

Drug Solubility

If a salt, NaA, is added to water to give a concentration C_s, the following reactions occur:

$$\text{Na}^+\text{A}^- \xrightarrow{\text{H}_2\text{O}} \text{Na}^+ + \text{A}^-$$

$$\text{A}^- + \text{H}_2\text{O} \rightleftharpoons \text{HA} + \text{OH}^-$$

If the pH of the solution is lowered, more of the A^- would be converted to the un-ionized acid, HA, in accordance with Le Chatelier's principle. Eventually a pH will be obtained, below which the amount of HA formed exceeds its aqueous solubility, S_0, and the acid will precipitate from solution. This pH, below which precipitation occurs, can be designated as pH_p. At this point, at which the amount of HA formed just equals S_0, a mass balance on the total amount of drug in solution yields,

$$C_s = [\text{HA}] + [\text{A}^-] = S_0 + [\text{A}^-] \tag{92}$$

Replacing $[A^-]$ as a function of hydronium ion concentration gives,

$$C_s = S_0 + \frac{K_a C_s}{[\text{H}_3\text{O}^+]_p + K_a} \tag{93}$$

where K_a is the ionization constant for the conjugate acid, HA, and $[\text{H}_3\text{O}^+]_p$ refers to the hydronium ion concentration above which precipitation will occur. This equation can be rearranged to give,

$$[\text{H}_3\text{O}^+]_p = K_a \frac{S_0}{C_s - S_0} \tag{94}$$

Taking logarithms gives,

$$\text{pH}_p = pK_a + \log \frac{C_s - S_0}{S_0} \tag{95}$$

Thus, the pH below which precipitation occurs can be seen to be a function of the amount of salt added initially, the pK_a and the solubility of the free acid formed from the salt.

The analogous equation for salts of weak bases and strong acids (such as pilocarpine hydrochloride, cocaine hydrochloride, codeine phosphate, etc) would be,

$$pH_p = pK_a + \log \frac{S_0}{C_s - S_0} \tag{96}$$

in which pK_a refers to the protonated form of the weak base.

Example—Below what pH will free phenobarbital begin to precipitate from a solution initially containing 1.3 g of sodium phenobarbital/100 mL at 25°? The molar solubility of phenobarbital is 0.0050 and its pK_a is 7.41. The molecular weight of sodium phenobarbital is 254.

The molar concentration of salt initially added is,

$$C_s = \frac{g/L}{\text{mol wt}} = \frac{13}{254} = 0.051\ M$$

$$pH_p = 7.41 + \log \frac{0.051 - 0.005}{0.005}$$

$$= 7.41 + 0.96 = 8.37$$

Example—Above what pH will free cocaine begin to precipitate from a solution initially containing 0.0294 mole/liter? The pK_b of cocaine is 5.59, and its molar solubility is 5.60×10^{-3}.

$$pK_a = pK_w - pK_b = 14.00 - 5.59 = 8.41$$

$$pH_p = 8.41 + \log \frac{0.0056}{0.0294 - 0.0056}$$

$$= 8.41 + (-0.63) = 7.78$$

Drug Stability

One of the most diversified and fruitful areas of study is the investigation of the effect of hydrogen-ion concentration on the stability, or in more general terms the reactivity, of pharmaceutical systems. The evidence for enhanced stability of systems when these are maintained within a narrow range of pH, as well as of progressively decreasing stability as the pH departs from the optimum range, is abundant. Stability (or instability) of a system may result from gain or loss of a proton (hydrogen ion) by a substrate molecule—often accompanied by an electronic rearrangement—which reduces (or increases) the reactivity of the molecule. Instability results when the substance desired to remain unchanged is converted to one or more other, unwanted, substances. In aqueous solution, instability may arise through the catalytic effect of acids or bases, the former by transferring a proton to the substrate molecule, the latter by accepting a proton.

Specific illustrations of the effect of hydrogen-ion concentration on the stability of medicinals are myriad; only a few will be given here, these being chosen to show the importance of pH adjustment of solutions that require sterilization. Morphine solutions are not decomposed during 60-min exposure at a temperature of 100° if the pH is less than 5.5; neutral and alkaline solutions, however, are highly unstable. Minimum hydrolytic decomposition of solutions of cocaine occurs in the range of pH of 2 to 5; in one study a solution of cocaine hydrochloride initially at a pH of 5.7 remained stable during 2 months (although the pH dropped to 4.2 in this time), while another solution buffered to about pH 6 underwent approximately 30% hydrolysis in the same time. Similarly, solutions of procaine hydrochloride containing some hydrochloric acid showed no appreciable decomposition; when dissolved in water alone, 5% of the procaine hydrochloride hydrolyzed, while when buffered to pH 6.5 from 19 to 35% underwent decomposition by hydrolysis. Solutions of thiamine hydrochloride may be sterilized by autoclaving without appreciable decomposition if the pH is below 5; above this, thiamine hydrochloride is unstable.

The stability of many disperse systems, and especially of certain emulsions, is often pH-dependent. Information concerning specific emulsion systems, and the effect of pH upon them, may be found in Chapter 21.

Drug Activity

Drugs that are weak acids or weak bases, and hence may exist in ionized or nonionized form (or a mixture of both), may be active in one form but not in the other; often such drugs have an optimum pH range for maximum activity. Thus, mandelic acid, benzoic acid, and salicylic acid have pronounced antibacterial activity in nonionized form but have practically no such activity in ionized form; accordingly, these substances require an acid environment to function effectively as antibacterial agents. For example, sodium benzoate is effective as a preservative in 4% concentration at pH 7.0, in 0.06 to 0.1% concentration at pH 3.5 to 4.0, and in 0.02 to 0.03% concentration at pH 2.3 to 2.4. Other antibacterial agents, on the other hand, are active principally if not entirely in cationic form; included in this category are the acridines and quaternary ammonium compounds.

Drug Absorption

The degree of ionization and lipoid solubility of a drug are two important factors that determine rate of absorption of drugs from the gastrointestinal tract and, indeed, their passage through cellular membranes generally. Drugs that are weak organic acids or bases, and which in nonionized form are soluble in lipids, are absorbed through cellular membranes by virtue, apparently, of the lipoidal nature of the membranes. Completely ionized drugs, on the other hand, are absorbed poorly, if at all. Rates of absorption of a variety of drugs are related to their ionization constants and in many cases may be quantitatively predicted on the basis of this relationship. Thus, not only the degree of the acidic or basic character of a drug but consequently also the pH of the physiological medium (gastric or intestinal fluid, plasma, cerebrospinal fluid, etc) in which a drug is dissolved or dispersed—since this pH determines the extent to which the drug will be converted to ionic or nonionic form—become important parameters of drug absorption. Further information concerning factors influencing drug absorption is given in Chapter 37.

References

1. Sedam RL, *et al*: *J Pharm Sci 54*: 215 (1965).
2. Benet LZ, Goyan JE: *J Pharm Sci 54*: 1179 (1965).
3. Riegelman S, *et al*: *J Pharm Sci 51*: 129 (1962).
4. Niebergall PJ, *et al*: *J Pharm Sci 61*: 232 (1972).

Bibliography

Freiser H, Fernando Q: *Ionic Equilibria in Analytical Chemistry*, Wiley, New York, 1966.

CHAPTER 18

Reaction Kinetics

Harry B Kostenbauder, PhD
Associate Dean for Research, College of Pharmacy
University of Kentucky
Lexington, KY 40506

Joseph B Bogardus, PhD
Assistant Professor, College of Pharmacy
University of Kentucky
Lexington, KY 40500

Reaction kinetics is the study of rate of chemical change and the way in which this rate is influenced by conditions of concentration of reactants, products, and other chemical species which may be present, and by factors such as solvent, pressure, and temperature. Reaction kinetics permits formulation of models for the intermediate steps through which reactants are converted to other chemical compounds, and is a powerful tool in elucidation of mechanisms by which chemical reactions proceed. In application to pharmaceutics, such information permits a rational approach to stabilization of drug products and prediction of shelf-life and optimum storage conditions.

The treatment presented in this chapter is intended as a general introduction to the subject of reaction kinetics. A comprehensive review of experimental approaches and interpretation of data, and a compilation of information relative to studies on pharmaceuticals, has been published by Garrett.[1]

Reaction Rate and Reaction Order

The rate of a reaction is the velocity with which a reactant or reactants undergo chemical change. The first quantitative study of a rate of reaction was performed in 1850 by Wilhelmy, who observed the velocity of hydrolysis (inversion) of sucrose to glucose and fructose in aqueous solution, under the catalytic influence of acid. The equation for the overall reaction is:

$$C_{12}H_{22}O_{11} + H_2O \rightarrow C_6H_{12}O_6 + C_6H_{12}O_6$$

Sucrose   **Glucose**   **Fructose**

The rate at which the concentration of sucrose, designated c, decreases with time, t, was found to be proportional to the concentration of unhydrolyzed sucrose. The change may be expressed in the notation of calculus by the differential equation

$$-dc/dt = kc \tag{1}$$

where $-dc/dt$ is the velocity (rate) with which the concentration of sucrose *decreases* (the minus sign indicates a decrease) as it undergoes hydrolysis, and k is a constant called the *velocity constant* or *rate constant*.

The term *reaction order* refers to the way in which concentration of a reactant, or reactants, influences the rate of a chemical reaction.

First-Order Reactions—When the rate of a reaction is proportional to the first power of the concentration of a reactant and may be expressed mathematically in the form of Eq 1, the reaction is said to be first-order with respect to the reactant.

The hydrolysis of sucrose is not strictly first-order since the rate varies also with the concentration of water. The amount of water required for hydrolysis of sucrose is so small, however, relative to the large quantity present, that there is no significant change in the concentration of water; for practical purposes, therefore, the concentration of water is constant.

It may be noted here that the rate constant k for the hydrolysis of sucrose increases with the hydrogen-ion concentration of the medium because of the catalytic effect of hydrogen ion on the reaction.

Eq 1 may be written

$$\frac{dc}{c} = -kdt \tag{2}$$

which, on integration, yields in natural logarithm form

$$\ln c = -kt + \text{constant} \tag{3}$$

or in common logarithm form

$$\log c = -\frac{kt}{2.303} + \text{constant} \tag{4}$$

Both Eqs 3 and 4 will be recognized as producing straight lines if $\ln c$ or $\log c$ is plotted against t; this is an identifying characteristic of reactions in which the rate of reaction is proportional to the concentration of a single reactant, that is, of a *first-order reaction* (see Fig 18-1). The rate constant k

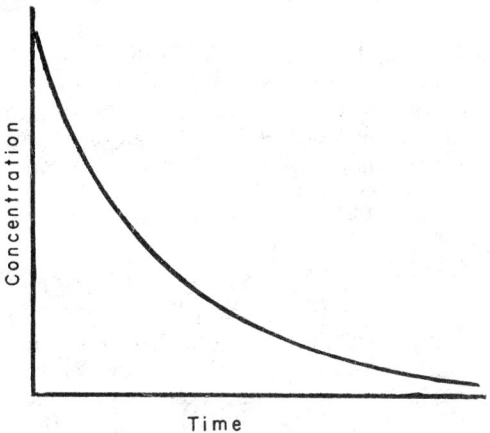

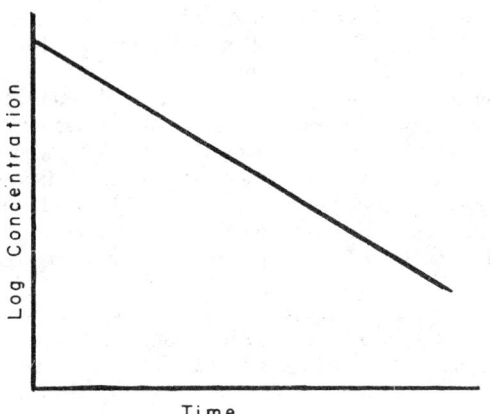

Fig 18-1. A first-order reaction. *Top:* concentration vs time plot; *bottom:* log concentration vs time plot.

may be readily calculated from the slope of the line, which is $-k/2.303$.

Concentration is usually expressed in moles/liter and time in seconds, although other convenient units may be employed. The rate constant, k, for a first-order reaction has units of reciprocal time (time^{-1}).

If Eq 4 is integrated between the limits of concentration c_0 at the beginning of the reaction when time is zero and when the concentration is c at a later time t, Eq 5 is obtained

$$\log \frac{c_0}{c} = \frac{k}{2.303} t \tag{5}$$

which on rearrangement becomes

$$k = \frac{2.303}{t} \log \frac{c_0}{c} \tag{6}$$

A modification of this equation, in which a is the initial amount of reactant and x is the amount that has reacted in time t, is

$$k = \frac{2.303}{t} \log \frac{a}{a-x} \tag{7}$$

Eq 6 may be used to calculate k for first-order reactions when both the concentration at the beginning of the reaction (c_0) and at elapsed time t are known. Sometimes c_0 is either not known or is not a suitable reference concentration, in which cases the concentrations c_1 at time t_1 and c_2 at a later time t_2 are used to calculate k by the following modification of the preceding equation

$$k = \frac{2.303}{t_2 - t_1} \log \frac{c_1}{c_2} \tag{8}$$

A useful exponential form of Eq 6, when the latter is written in natural logarithm notation, is

$$c = c_0 e^{-kt} \tag{9}$$

Although reaction rates may be quantitatively expressed in terms of numerical values of k, for many purposes a more useful expression is in terms of the *half-life* of a reaction, which is the time, $t_{1/2}$, required for half of the substance (reactant) to undergo reaction. Writing Eq 6 in the form

$$k = \frac{2.303}{t_{1/2}} \log \frac{c_0}{c_0/2} = \frac{0.693}{t_{1/2}} \tag{10}$$

it is apparent that

$$t_{1/2} = \frac{0.693}{k} \tag{11}$$

From Eq 11 it is obvious that, for first-order reactions, a constant time interval is required for disappearance of one-half of the substance present at the beginning of the interval, irrespective of the concentration of the substance. Thus, in a first-order reaction, 50% of an initial amount of reactant remains after the first half-life period, 25% after the second, 12.5% after the third, and so on.

It can also be shown by an expression similar to Eq 10 that the time interval required for loss of *any* specified fraction of the reactant will be constant irrespective of the concentration of reactant. Thus, a term sometimes used in studies of drug stability is the time required for loss of 10% of the original concentration, or time required for concentration to decrease to 90% of the original concentration. This interval is referred to as $t_{0.90}$.

It is apparent also that an infinite period of time would be required for all of the substance to undergo reaction. It is thus impossible to measure first-order reaction rates to completion of the reaction, and plots such as those of Fig 18-1 can not be extrapolated to zero concentration. It might be noted, however, that if a first-order reaction is followed through 10 half-lives, less than 0.1% of the original concentration of

reactant remains. In practical studies of rate of reaction it is common to study the change of concentration with time through two or three half-life periods.

First-order rate processes are not restricted to chemical reactions. The passive diffusion of drugs across biological membranes, and processes of drug absorption, distribution, metabolism, and excretion can often be shown to occur at rates proportional to the concentration of drug and thus be described as first-order rate processes. Rate of growth of microorganisms and rate of killing or inactivation of microorganisms by heat or chemical agents are usually first-order processes.

Second-Order Reactions—A second-order reaction is one in which the experimentally determined rate of reaction is found to be proportional to the concentration of each of two reactants or to the second power of the concentration of one reactant. If substances A and B undergo reaction at a rate proportional to the concentration of each (c_A and c_B, respectively) we may write

$$-\frac{dc_A}{dt} = -\frac{dc_B}{dt} = k \cdot c_A c_B \tag{12}$$

If a and b represent the molar concentrations of A and B at the start of the reaction, and x is the number of moles of each which has reacted at time t the reaction rate, dx/dt, may be expressed as

$$\frac{dx}{dt} = k(a-x)(b-x) \tag{13}$$

If the initial concentrations of A and B are equal, Eq 13 simplifies to

$$\frac{dx}{dt} = k(a-x)^2 \tag{14}$$

On integration

$$\frac{1}{(a-x)} = k \cdot t + \text{constant} \tag{15}$$

The constant may be evaluated by substituting 0 for x when $t = 0$, so that

$$k = \frac{1}{t} \cdot \frac{x}{a(a-x)} \tag{16}$$

If the initial concentrations of A and B are not equal, integration of Eq 13, by partial fractions, and evaluation of the integration constant, gives

$$k = \frac{2.303}{t(a-b)} \log \frac{b(a-x)}{a(b-x)} \tag{17}$$

A reaction is second-order if on substitution of the required analytical data into Eq 16 or 17 (whichever applies) constant values of k at different times of reaction are obtained. Alternatively, a plot of $x/a(a-x)$ vs t (see Eq 16) will result in a straight line when a equals b in a second-order reaction; when a is not equal to b a plot of $\log b(a-x)/a(b-x)$ vs t (see Eq 17) will give the straight line, if the reaction is second-order.

An example of a second-order reaction in which two reactants are involved is the saponification of an ester, such as ethyl acetate, in alkaline solution.

$$CH_3COOC_2H_5 + OH^- \rightarrow CH_3COO^- + C_2H_5OH$$

The course of this reaction may be followed by determining by titration, at specified times, the decrease in concentration of hydroxide ions as these are consumed in the reaction.

When only one reactant is involved in a second-order reaction, Eqs 14, 15 and 16 apply. A reaction of this type is the decomposition of hydrogen iodide, which in the gaseous state undergoes the reaction

$$2HI \rightarrow H_2 + I_2$$

The reaction rate in this case is expressed by

$$-\frac{dc_{HI}}{dt} = k \cdot c_{HI}^2 \qquad (18)$$

The half-life of a second-order reaction has significance only when a single reactant or when two reactants, each at the same initial concentration, are involved. In both these cases the time, $t_{1/2}$, required for half of the reactant or reactants (at equal concentration) to undergo reaction may be calculated from Eq 15 to be

$$t_{1/2} = \frac{1}{ka} \qquad (19)$$

It is obvious that while the half-life for a first-order reaction (see Eq 11) is independent of the concentration of the reactant, it varies inversely as the initial concentration of reactant in a second-order reaction.

First- and second-order reactions are by far the most common types of rate processes encountered in consideration of drug stability. If a reaction is of higher order than first-order, it is often convenient to adjust experimental conditions so that the concentrations of all but one of the reactants remain constant throughout the experiment. If, for example, the concentration of hydroxide ion in the saponification of an ester is in great excess of the concentration of ester, or if a buffer system is employed to control hydroxide-ion concentration, then the concentration of hydroxide ion is essentially invariant throughout the course of the experiment.

The observed rate of the reaction therefore depends only on the changing concentration of the ester, and the reaction is said to be *apparent first-order* or *pseudo first-order*. The apparent first-order rate constant thus obtained is $k(OH^-)$ and, of course, is different for each hydroxide-ion concentration. The actual rate constant, k, can be obtained easily by dividing the experimentally determined apparent first-order rate constant, $k(OH^-)$, by the concentration of hydroxide ion maintained throughout the study.

In the study of complex reactions, it is often desirable to use this approach of maintaining the concentration of all but one of the reactants constant to facilitate determination of the dependency of reaction rate on each of the reactants in turn.

Third-Order Reactions—A third-order reaction is one in which the experimentally determined rate of reaction is found to be proportional to the concentration of each of three reactants, or proportional to the concentration of one of two reactants and to the second power of the concentration of the other, or proportional to the third power of the concentration of a single reactant. Third-order reactions are very rare.

For the case of a reaction between one molecule each of A, B, and C, at molar concentrations a, b, and c, respectively, the rate equation is

$$-\frac{dc_A}{dt} = -\frac{dc_B}{dt} = -\frac{dc_C}{dt} = k \cdot c_A c_B c_C \qquad (20)$$

Using the notation of Eq 13, this becomes

$$\frac{dx}{dt} = k(a-x)(b-x)(c-x) \qquad (21)$$

When $a = b = c$

$$\frac{dx}{dt} = k(a-x)^3 \qquad (22)$$

On integration

$$\frac{1}{2(a-x)^2} = k \cdot t + \text{constant} \qquad (23)$$

Evaluating the constant by substituting 0 for x when $t = 0$, we obtain

$$k = \frac{1}{2t}\left[\frac{1}{(a-x)^2} - \frac{1}{a^2}\right] \qquad (24)$$

Zero-Order Reactions—In some reactions the rate is independent of the concentration of reactant or reactants, and such reactions are termed *zero-order* reactions. Photochemical reactions—in which the rate-determining factor is the light intensity, rather than the concentration of reactant—are examples of reactions which may be found to be zero-order. In such cases the rate is expressed as

$$-dc/dt = k \qquad (25)$$

If a compound for which decomposition in solution is first-order is present in excess of its maximum solubility (a suspension), the concentration of reactant in solution will be invariant so long as there is excess solid reactant present, and the observed reaction rate will be of the form of Eq 26,

$$-dc/dt = k \cdot c_s \qquad (26)$$

where c_s is a constant. Such reactions are *apparent zero-order* reactions.

Complex Reactions—Many chemical reactions are not simple reactions of zero-, first-, second-, or third-order. Often they consist of a combination of two or more reactions; sometimes the overall reaction can be characterized as one of these orders, but the rate equation may be a complicated function involving first-, second-, or third-order intermediate steps. Experiment may indicate a reaction order which is nonintegral, or fractional, when reactions are complex. Nevertheless, concentrations of the various reactants usually can be controlled to permit determination of the order of a reaction with respect to each reactant, and by this means integral reaction order with respect to each component can be established.

Among complicating factors that may be involved in the kinetic study of a complex reaction are *simultaneous reactions*, *consecutive reactions*, and *opposing reactions*.

Simultaneous Reactions—Consider a substance, A, that is simultaneously converted into B and C, each at characteristic rates:

$$A \xrightarrow{k_1} B$$

$$A \xrightarrow{k_2} C$$

The equation for rate of disappearance of A is the first-order equation

$$-\frac{dc_A}{dt} = k_1 c_A + k_2 c_A = (k_1 + k_2)c_A \qquad (27)$$

On integration and arrangement in exponential form we obtain

$$c_A = c_{A_0} e^{-(k_1 + k_2)t} \qquad (28)$$

where c_{A_0} is the initial concentration of A at $t = 0$ and c_A is the concentration at time t.

The equation for rate of formation of B is given by

$$\frac{dc_B}{dt} = k_1 c_A = k_1 c_{A_0} e^{-(k_1 + k_2)t} \qquad (29)$$

Integrating and arranging in exponential form

$$c_B = -\frac{k_1 c_{A_0}}{(k_1 + k_2)} e^{-(k_1 + k_2)t} + \text{constant} \qquad (30)$$

setting $c_B = 0$ when $t = 0$

$$\text{constant} = \frac{k_1 c_{A_0}}{(k_1 + k_2)} \qquad (31)$$

then

$$c_B = \frac{k_1 c_{A_0}}{(k_1 + k_2)}[1 - e^{-(k_1+k_2)t}] \qquad (32)$$

since $c_A + c_B + c_C = c_{A_0}$ (initial concentration of A) it follows that

$$c_C = \frac{k_2 c_{A_0}}{(k_1 + k_2)}[1 - e^{-(k_1+k_2)t}] \qquad (33)$$

Inspection of Eqs. 32 and 33 shows that the fraction of A ultimately converted to B (at infinite time) is $k_1/(k_1 + k_2)$; the fraction converted to C is $k_2/(k_1 + k_2)$.

Consecutive Reactions—If two first-order reactions occur consecutively, thus

$$A \xrightarrow{k_1} B \xrightarrow{k_2} C$$

the rate equations for each substance are

$$-\frac{dc_A}{dt} = k_1 c_A \qquad (34)$$

$$-\frac{dc_B}{dt} = -k_1 c_A + k_2 c_B \qquad (35)$$

$$\frac{dc_C}{dt} = k_2 c_B \qquad (36)$$

If at $t = 0$ we set $c_A = c_{A_0}$, $c_B = 0$, and $c_C = 0$, Eq. 33 on integration and arrangement in exponential form becomes

$$c_A = c_{A_0} e^{-k_1 t} \qquad (37)$$

substituting for c_A in Eq 35 and integrating

$$c_B = \frac{k_1 c_{A_0}}{(k_2 - k_1)}[e^{-k_1 t} - e^{-k_2 t}] \qquad (38)$$

since $c_A + c_B + c_C = c_{A_0}$ (initial concentration of A)

$$c_C = c_{A_0}\left[1 + \frac{1}{(k_1 - k_2)}(k_2 e^{-k_1 t} - k_1 e^{-k_2 t})\right] \qquad (39)$$

Opposing Reactions—The rate equation for an opposing (reversible) first-order reaction, represented by

$$A \underset{k_2}{\overset{k_1}{\rightleftharpoons}} B$$

may be expressed thus

$$\frac{dc_A}{dt} = -k_1 c_A + k_2 c_B \qquad (40)$$

At equilibrium the velocity of the forward reaction, $k_1 c_A$, is equal to the velocity of the reverse reaction, $k_2 c_B$, and $dc_A/dt = 0$. If the initial concentration of A is designated c_{A_0}, and the concentrations of A and B at equilibrium are c_{A_e} and c_{B_e}, respectively, then

$$\frac{c_{B_e}}{c_{A_e}} = \frac{c_{A_0} - c_{A_e}}{c_{A_e}} = \frac{k_1}{k_2} = K \qquad (41)$$

where K is the equilibrium constant of the reaction.

Effects on Reaction Rate

Temperature

The application of heat to increase the rate of a chemical reaction is a common laboratory procedure. The rate of most solvolytic reactions of pharmaceuticals is increased roughly 2- to 3-fold by a 10°C increase in temperature in the vicinity of room temperature.

Arrhenius noted, in 1889, that the variation with temperature of the rate constant of chemical reactions could be expressed by the equation

$$k = s e^{-E_a/RT} \qquad (42)$$

where E_a is the Arrhenius *activation energy* (the difference

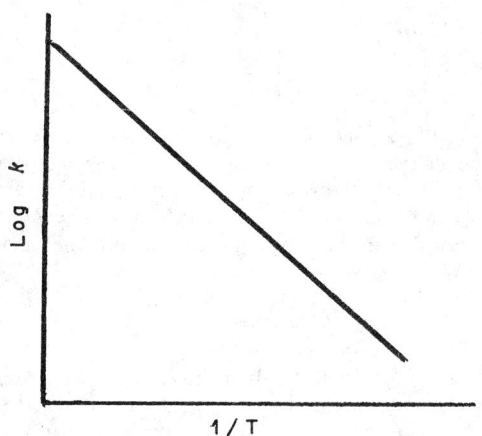

Fig 18-2. Variation of rate constant with temperature, illustrating the applicability of Arrhenius equation.

between the average energy of reactive molecules and the average energy of all molecules), $e^{-E_a/RT}$ is the Boltzmann factor which represents the fraction of molecules having the energy E_a, s is a constant called the frequency factor, R is the gas constant (1.987 cal/°K.-mole), and T is the absolute temperature.

In logarithmic form the Arrhenius equation becomes

$$\log k = \log s - \frac{E_a}{2.303\, RT} \qquad (43)$$

If this equation is valid—and it is for a large number of reactions—a straight line is obtained on plotting $\log k$ against the reciprocal of the absolute temperature. E_a may be calculated from the slope of the line, which is $-E_a/2.303\, R$; the intercept on the $\log k$ axis is $\log s$ (see Fig 18-2).

On differentiating the natural logarithm form of Eq 43 with respect to temperature

$$\frac{d \ln k}{dT} = \frac{E_a}{RT^2} \qquad (44)$$

and on integration between the limits k_2 and k_1 at temperatures T_2 and T_1

$$\log \frac{k_2}{k_1} = \frac{E_a}{2.303R}\left(\frac{T_2 - T_1}{T_1 T_2}\right) \qquad (45)$$

which equation makes it possible to calculate E_a for a reaction when the rate constants are known at two temperatures or to calculate the rate constant at one temperature if E_a and the rate constant at another temperature are known.

Most solvolytic reactions of pharmaceuticals exhibit activation energies in the range of 8 to 20 kcal/mole. Using Eq 45 and the appropriate activation energy one can readily calculate that a reaction having an activation energy of 8 kcal/mole would show an increase of approximately 1.5-fold in k for a temperature increase from 25° to 35°; a reaction having an activation energy of 20 kcal/mole would show an increase of 3.0-fold in k for a similar temperature increase.

When two molecules undergo chemical interaction, it is reasonable to suppose that they must first come close enough to each other to effect a "collision" and then, if conditions are right, undergo a rearrangement of certain electrons to form the bonds characteristic of new molecules. This means that while "collision" is a prerequisite for interaction, not all collisions lead to chemical change. If all collisions did lead to reaction, all chemical reactions would occur with great rapidity since collision frequencies are very high. The explanation is that the colliding molecules must possess at least the amount of energy E_a before reaction can occur. This energy, called the activation energy, must be sufficient to overcome the mutual repulsion of the interacting molecules and enable them

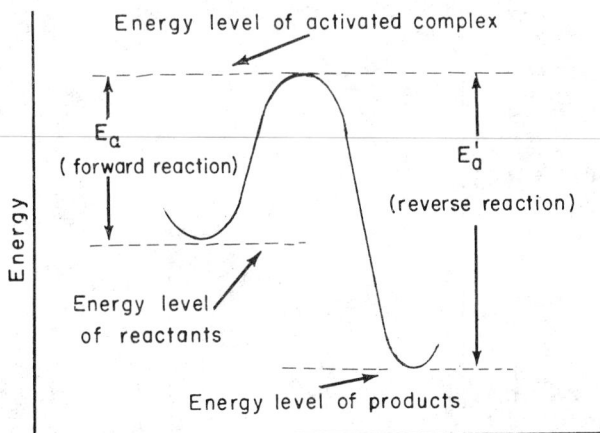

Fig 18-3.   Relation between activation energy and energy levels of reactants, products, and activated complex.

to approach each other close enough to effect certain bond ruptures and simultaneously establish new bonds characteristic of the products. The greater this energy requirement is, the smaller the proportion of colliding molecules that will have the necessary energy, and the slower will be the reaction.

In the Arrhenius equation, s is a factor related to frequency of collisions, and $e^{-E_a/RT}$ is the probability that at temperature T a collision will occur with sufficient energy to provide a "successful" collision.

It would appear that in the reaction

$$A + B \rightleftharpoons [AB]^* \rightarrow products$$

there is an activated complex or transition state, represented by $[AB]^*$, which is not a complex in the usual sense but involves a critical intermediate geometric configuration in which the bonds of the reactants are weakened and the bonds of the products begin to form; if the complex has sufficient energy to effect the changes, the reaction proceeds; if it has not, it reverts to the state of the separate reactants.

The question arises as to the significance of energy of activation in first-order reactions, where only one kind of molecule undergoes chemical change and collision with, or close proximity to, a molecule of different species is not involved. Here again only those molecules that possess energy equal to the activation energy can react. Molecules can acquire the added energy by collisions of the proper kind; hence collisions do play an important role also in reactions involving a single molecular species.

The concept of energy of activation, in relationship to the energy of the reactants and of the products, is illustrated in Fig 18-3.

Other Effects

Specific Acid and Specific Base Catalysis—The term *specific acid catalysis* refers to catalysis by the hydrated proton or hydrogen ion, and *specific base catalysis* refers to catalysis by the hydroxide ion.

If the rate of hydrolysis of an ester such as ethyl acetate is studied at constant pH in a strongly buffered solution, the rate of disappearance of intact ester will be an apparent first-order reaction. If the reaction is studied in solutions buffered at several different pH values in a sufficiently acid pH region, a different apparent first-order rate constant will be observed for each pH value.

The observed rate depends on the concentration of both the ester and hydrogen ion and is actually a second-order reaction, although at a constant hydrogen-ion concentration it is an apparent first-order reaction.

$$k_{observed} = k_1(H^+) \tag{46}$$

The observed apparent first-order rate constant determined in buffered solution is therefore proportional to hydrogen-ion concentration. The variation in observed rate constant with pH can be illustrated by taking logarithms of Eq 46.

$$\log k_{observed} = \log k_1 + \log (H^+) \tag{47}$$

$$\log k_{observed} = \log k_1 - pH \tag{48}$$

Thus a plot of logarithm $k_{observed}$ vs pH should be linear with a slope of -1.

Similarly, if the same hydrolysis reaction is studied in buffered solution at several pH values in a sufficiently alkaline region of the pH scale, the observed apparent first-order rate constants will be found to vary with hydroxide-ion concentration.

$$k_{observed} = k_2(OH^-) \tag{49}$$

$$\log k_{observed} = \log k_2 + \log (OH^-) = \log k_2 + \log \frac{K_w}{(H^+)} \tag{50}$$

$$\log k_{observed} = \log k_2 + \log K_w + pH \tag{51}$$

A plot of logarithm $k_{observed}$ vs pH would be a straight line with a slope of $+1$.

The complete rate expression for hydrolysis of the compound described above at all pH values would therefore be

$$-dc/dt = [k_1(H^+) + k_2(OH^-)]c \tag{52}$$

At any specified pH value

$$k_{observed} = k_1(H^+) + k_2(OH^-) \tag{53}$$

The complete logarithm $k_{observed}$ vs pH profile would be similar to that illustrated in Fig. 18-4 for the hydrogen-ion- and hydroxide-ion- (specific acid and specific base) catalyzed hydrolysis of the ester atropine. The pH at which the minimum rate of hydrolysis is observed is a function of the relative magnitude of the specific rate constants k_1 and k_2.

In the atropine example the minimum rate of hydrolysis is at pH 3.7. If for a specific chemical species $k_1 = k_2$, the expected minimum rate of reaction for that species would be expected to occur at pH 7 (for a temperature of 25°, at which $pK_w = 14$, and $(H^+) = (OH^-)$ at pH 7.0).

At pH values below the minimum in the plot of logarithm

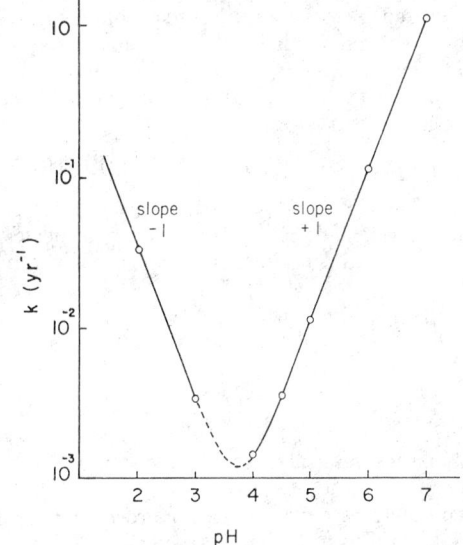

Fig 18-4.   Apparent first-order rate of hydrolysis of atropine as a function of pH at 30°. The reaction is an illustration of specific hydrogen- and hydroxide-ion catalysis (courtesy, data, Kondritzer and Zvirblis[2]).

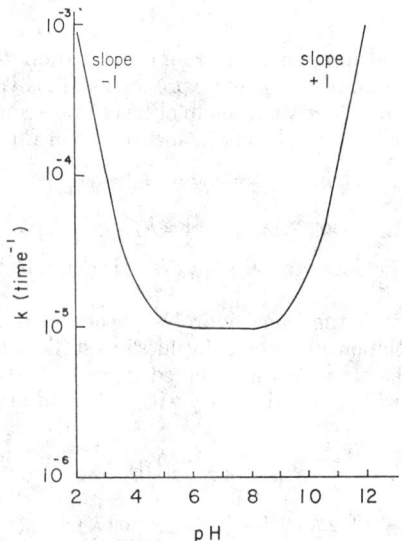

Fig 18-5.   Apparent first-order rate of decomposition as a function of pH for a hypothetical case where $k_{H^+} = k_{OH^-} = 1 \times 10^{-1}$, $k_0 = 1 \times 10^{-5}$. The uncatalyzed reaction predominates in the pH region 5–9.

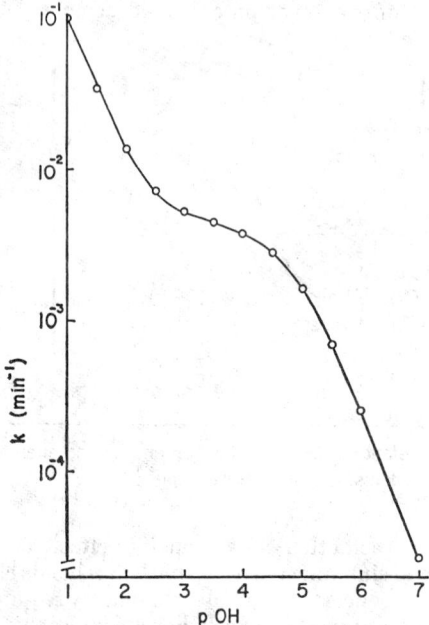

Fig 18-6.   Apparent first-order rate of hydrolysis of procaine as a function of hydroxide-ion concentration at 40° (courtesy, Higuchi, *et al*[3]).

$k_{observed}$ vs pH, the hydrogen-ion-catalyzed reaction is much more significant than the hydroxide-ion-catalyzed reaction, and the plot has a slope of −1. At pH values above the minimum in the plot, the hydroxide-ion-catalyzed reaction is the much more important reaction and the plot has a slope of +1.

If a reaction is catalyzed not only by hydrogen ion and hydroxide ion, but also by the solvent (also called the uncatalyzed reaction), the logarithm $k_{observed}$ vs pH plot might appear as in Fig 18-5, indicating a flat region where the rate of reaction is apparently not pH-dependent. In this region the solvent reaction is much more important than that of either the hydrogen ion or hydroxide ion. The apparent first-order rate constant for such a reaction is

$$k_{observed} = k_0 + k_1(H^+) + k_2(OH^-) \qquad (54)$$

For compounds which are weak acids or weak bases, and can therefore exist in both ionized and nonionized species, the pH rate profiles become more complex. Often both the ionized and nonionized species are subject to decomposition and catalysis by hydrogen and hydroxide ion, but each of the drug species may react at a different rate. For example, hydrolysis of the weakly basic drug procaine can be represented by the following reactions:[2]

$$-dc/dt = k_1(OH^-)(Pr) + k_2(OH^-)(PrH^+) \qquad (55)$$

where Pr is the nonionized procaine molecule and PrH$^+$ is the protonated form. The concentration of each species can be related to the total procaine concentration by the relationships:

$$(Pr) = \frac{(OH^-)}{K_b + (OH^-)} \cdot (\text{Total Procaine});$$

$$(PrH^+) = \frac{K_b}{K_b + (OH^-)} \cdot (\text{Total Procaine}) \qquad (56)$$

where K_b is the classical dissociation constant for the weak base procaine.

The complete rate expression for procaine hydrolysis is therefore, from Eqs 55 and 56,

$$-dc/dt = \left[\frac{k_1(OH^-)^2}{K_b + (OH^-)} + \frac{k_2(OH^-)K_b}{K_b + (OH^-)} \right] c \qquad (57)$$

The pH dependency of procaine hydrolysis is illustrated graphically in Fig 18-6 by a plot of logarithm $k_{observed}$ vs pOH for the pH region 7–13.

General Acid and General Base Catalysis—Acid and base catalysis is not restricted to hydrogen ion and hydroxide ion. Undissociated acids and bases can often be demonstrated to produce a catalytic effect, and in some instances metal ions and various anions can serve as catalysts.

Mutarotation of glucose in acetate buffer is catalyzed by hydrogen ion, hydroxide ion, acetate ion, and undissociated acetic acid. Also, the rate of barbiturate hydrolysis in ammonia buffers is increased by increasing buffer concentration at constant pH as a result of catalysis by NH$_3$. Hydrolysis of the amide function of chloramphenicol exhibits, in addition to solvent and specific acid–base catalysis, general acid–base catalysis in phosphate and citrate buffers. General acid–base catalysis is to be anticipated if there is evidence of a significant solvent catalysis as illustrated in the pH-rate profile of Fig 18-5.

Ionic Strength—In general the effects of increasing concentrations of electrolytes on reaction rate can be predicted by consideration of the influence of ionic strength on interionic attraction. The Debye–Hückel equation may be used to demonstrate that increased ionic strength would be expected to decrease rate of reaction involving interaction between oppositely charged ions, and increase rate of reaction between similarly charged ions. Thus, the hydrogen-ion-catalyzed hydrolysis of sulfate esters is inhibited by increasing electrolyte concentration.

$$ROSO_3^- + H_2O \xrightarrow{H+} ROH + HSO_4^-$$

Reactions between ions and dipolar molecules, and reactions between neutral molecules, are generally less sensitive to ionic strength effects than are reactions between ionic compounds. However, reactions which result in formation of oppositely charged ions as products may exhibit considerable increase in rate with increasing ionic strength.

Dielectric Constant of Solvent—Reactions involving ions of opposite charge are accelerated by solvents of low dielectric constant. The rate of hydrogen-ion-catalyzed hydrolysis of sulfate esters, for example, is much greater in low-dielectric-constant solvents such as methylene chloride than in water.

Reactions between similarly charged species are favored by high-dielectric-constant solvents. Reactions between neutral molecules which produce a highly polar transition state, such as reaction of triethylamine with ethyl iodide to produce a quaternary ammonium salt, will also be enhanced by high-dielectric-constant solvents.

Hydrolysis (Solvolysis)—Hydrolysis of esters such as procaine, aspirin, and atropine represents one of the more common types of drug instability. Ester hydrolysis is both hydrogen- and hydroxide-ion catalyzed, although the catalysis which is important from the viewpoint of drug product stability depends upon the specific compound and the pH of the solution. Amides are generally more stable than esters but are subject to catalysis by hydrogen and hydroxide ions, and often by general acids and bases. Some examples of the kinds of functional groups subject to hydrolytic cleavage and species shown to be catalysts for the reactions are presented below.

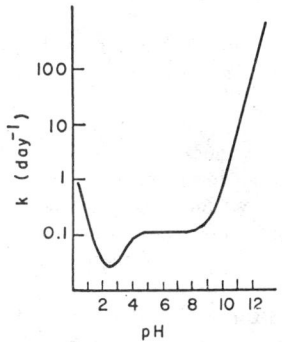

Atropine

Hydrolysis of the ester function of atropine is typical of ester hydrolysis in that the only important reactions are catalysis by hydrogen ion and hydroxide ion. Fig 18-4 illustrates a pH-rate profile which might be considered typical for such a reaction. Below pH 3 the principal reaction is hydrogen-ion-catalyzed hydrolysis of the protonated form of atropine. Above pH 5 the principal reaction is hydroxide-ion-catalyzed hydrolysis of the same species. Maximum stability at 30° is at pH 3.7.

Aspirin

Hydrolytic cleavage of aspirin to salicylic acid and acetic acid was studied by Edwards, who obtained the interesting pH-rate profile reproduced in Fig 18-7. The unusual pH-rate profile obtained for aspirin was attributed to a reaction of the form

$$-dc/dt = k_1(H^+)(HA) + k_2(H^+)(A^-) +$$
$$k_3(OH^-)(A^-) + k_0(A^-) \quad (58)$$

where HA represents undissociated aspirin and A^- represents aspirin anion. The pH-independent anion hydrolysis indi-

Fig 18-7. Apparent first-order rate of hydrolysis of aspirin as a function of pH at 17° (courtesy, Edwards[4]).

cated for the pH region 5–9 has been attributed to intramolecular catalysis by orthocarboxylate anion, rather than to general acid–base catalysis by water. It is principally this intramolecular catalysis which is responsible for the high instability of aqueous solutions of aspirin in the pharmaceutically useful pH range. Fersht and Kirby[5] represented the intramolecular carboxylate ion reaction as a general base catalysis of attack by a water molecule. Other nucleophiles such as ethanol, the terminal hydroxyl of polyethylene glycol, and the lysine ε-amino function in serum albumin can participate in this reaction in the same manner as water. Thus from as-

pirin in ethanol solution ethyl acetate appears as a product, in polyethylene glycol a polyethylene glycol acetate is formed, and in a solution containing serum albumin (both *in vitro* and *in vivo*) aspirin produces an acetylated serum albumin. Whitworth, *et al*[6] reasoned that an aspirin solution prepared in a polyethylene glycol solvent containing no free hydroxyl groups would provide an aspirin solution of improved stability. They used acetylated PEG 400 as a solvent for aspirin and demonstrated that in such a solvent less than 1% aspirin loss occurred after 30 days at 45°.

Chloramphenicol

Chloramphenicol decomposition below pH 7 proceeds primarily through hydrolytic cleavage of the amide function. The reaction may be represented as

$$-dc/dt = [k_0 + k_1(H^+) + k_2(OH^-) +$$
$$k_{HB}(HB) + k_B(B)]c \quad (59)$$

In addition to hydrogen- and hydroxide-ion catalysis there is an uncatalyzed (or water) reaction, and there may be general acid–base catalysis, represented above by the buffer species HB and B. In general, rate of hydroxide-ion-catalyzed hydrolysis of amides is greater than rate of hydronium-ion-catalyzed hydrolysis. Amides are generally much more stable than esters.

Penicillins and cephalosporins are important exceptions to this rule because the amide bond is part of a strained four-membered ring (beta-lactam). The decomposition of these compounds in aqueous solution is catalyzed by hydrogen ion, solvent, hydroxide ion, sugars, and many buffer species. Maximum stability occurs at about pH 7, but beta-lactam antibiotics are too unstable to be formulated as solutions. For example, a buffered aqueous solution of penicillin G under refrigeration has a useful life of only about one week. Formation of the penicillenic acid by water-catalyzed rearrangement in acidic and neutral solutions is thought to be the first step in the degradation process.[7]

Barbiturate hydrolysis involves hydroxide-ion attack on both the undissociated acid and the ionized species. Hy-

Unionized Barbiturate

Ionized Barbiturate

Additional Products

drogen-ion-catalyzed hydrolysis is not observed in the pH range of interest in pharmaceutical products.

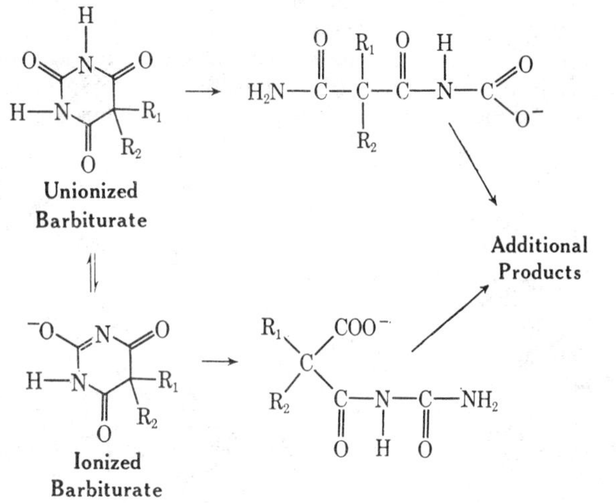

$$-dc/dt = k_1(OH^-)(HP) + k_2(OH^-)(P^-) \qquad (60)$$

Modest buffer catalysis has been observed in ammonia buffers. Cleavage of the ring system leads to loss of pharmacologic activity, with further decomposition of the initial acyclic products.

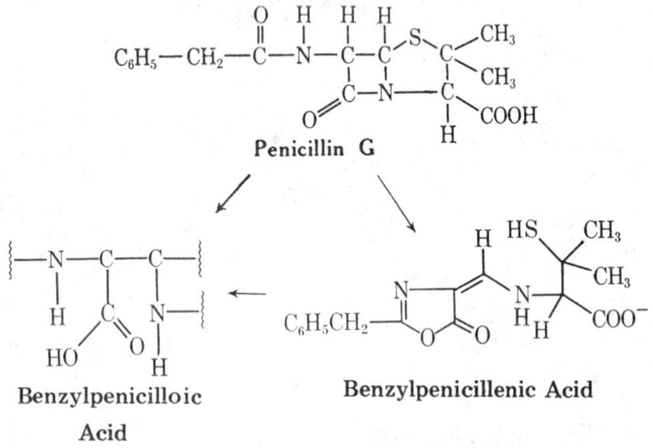

Penicillin G

Benzylpenicilloic Acid

Benzylpenicillenic Acid

Racemization—The acid-catalyzed racemization of epinephrine, with loss of characteristic pharmacologic activity of epinephrine, is illustrative of an additional type of drug decomposition which may be encountered.

Oxidation—Compounds such as phenols, aromatic amines, aldehydes, ethers, and unsaturated aliphatic compounds are subject to oxidation upon exposure to air or oxidizing chemicals. Epinephrine, ascorbic acid, phenothiazines, and vitamin A are examples of important pharmaceutical products which are readily oxidized.

Of particular concern are oxidations which occur when solutions are exposed to atmospheric oxygen. Such reactions are termed autoxidation (or self-oxidation) and are complex reactions which proceed via what is termed a free-radical mechanism. A free radical is a highly unstable (highly reactive) species containing an unpaired electron. Autoxidation reactions are autocatalytic in that free-radical reactions generate additional free radicals, causing a chain reaction. A technique utilized to protect pharmaceuticals susceptible to autoxidation is to include in the formulation agents which will

react readily with free radicals, but which will terminate the chain-propagation either by forming relatively stable radicals (resonance stabilized) or by forming products which do not include additional free radicals.

Photochemical Decomposition—Numerous dyes and drugs are subject to photochemical decomposition. Light-catalyzed oxidations and reductions of photoexcited species are common, and are often mechanistically complex reactions involving free-radical intermediates. Pharmaceuticals such as riboflavin and phenothiazines are examples of common drugs which are extremely light sensitive.

Interaction between Components—Because drugs are often combined in solution with buffers, antioxidants, flavoring agents, antimicrobial preservatives, and other drugs, potential interaction between components of a formulation must be considered in pharmaceutical formulation development. Some obvious interactions, such as possibility of reaction of a drug having a primary amino function with an aldehyde such as vanillin to produce a Schiff base can be predicted, but a number of interesting, less-well-recognized, reactions have been encountered.

In addition to buffer species acting as general acid–base catalysts, as previously indicated, some buffer species undergo specific interactions with drug molecules to form new chemical compounds. The formation of amides, in aqueous solution, between amines such as benzocaine and buffers such as citric acid has been observed.

The aromatic function of procaine reacts with glucose to form procaine N-glycoside; also, phenylethylamine reacts with dehydroacetic acid to form a Schiff base-type compound. Catechols have been shown to catalyze penicillin hydrolysis.

It has been demonstrated that bisulfite, an agent commonly employed to protect epinephrine against oxidative decomposition, is capable of inducing epinephrine degradation through attack on the optically active side chain.

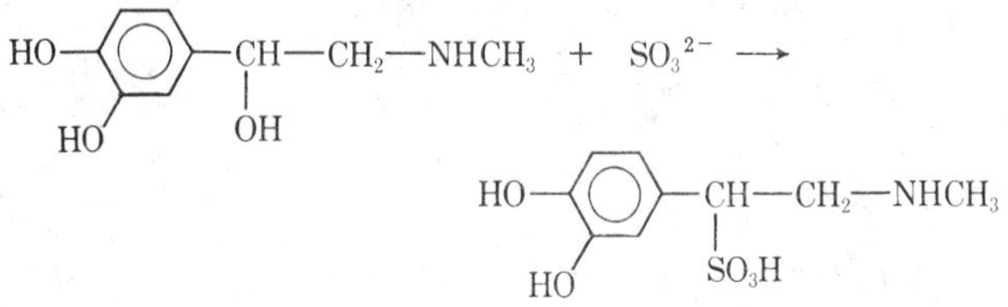

Although a solution of folic acid alone is stable to light, a combination of riboflavin and folic acid showed rapid loss of folic acid through formation of a coupled oxidation–reduction system in which riboflavin was photoreduced with folic acid being utilized as reducing substrate and being itself irreversibly oxidized. In the dark and in the presence of oxygen, the riboflavin was regenerated, and when the solution was again irradiated the cycle was repeated with further destruction of folic acid. The riboflavin is termed a *photosensitizer* in this reaction and would cause the decomposition not only of folic acid but also of ascorbic acid or any other easily oxidized substrate.

The presence of micellar surfactants and certain high-molecular-weight polymers commonly employed in pharmaceuticals also has been shown to lead to decreased drug stability in some cases. Both nonionic and anionic surfactants, as well as polymers such as polyvinylpyrrolidone, accelerate the photodecomposition of riboflavin in aqueous solution. Nonionic surfactants are capable also of increasing the rate of hydrolysis of sulfate esters which may be incorporated in or on the micellar surface.

Drug Stabilization

Some drug decomposition reactions, such as photolytic and oxidative reactions, are relatively easy to avoid by protection of components from light to protect against photodecomposition or exclusion of oxygen and use of chain-terminating reagents or free-radical scavengers to terminate free-radical-mediated reactions. Solvolysis reactions, however, can not be stopped by such procedures, but several techniques may be employed to retard reactions sufficiently to permit formulation of a suitable drug product. The following approaches may be useful in attempts to retard solvolytic reactions.

Selection of Optimum pH, Buffer, and Solvent—Consideration of the mechanism of the reaction and the way in which the reaction rate is influenced by pH, buffer species, and solvent permits selection of the optimum conditions for drug stability. Often, however, ideal conditions for maximum stability may be unacceptable from the viewpoint of pharmaceutically acceptable formulation or therapeutic efficacy, and it may be necessary to prepare a formulation with conditions less than optimum for stability of the drug. If a suitable compromise between conditions for maximum stability and conditions for a pharmaceutically acceptable formulation can not be achieved, techniques such as those described below may be useful in retarding solvolysis reactions.

Specific Complexing Agents—The technique of stabilization by formation of complexes in solution was introduced by Higuchi and Lachman, who demonstrated that the rate of hydrolysis of the ester function of benzocaine was significantly retarded in the presence of caffeine, a reagent with which the benzocaine formed a soluble complex. It was further demonstrated that in these systems the complexed drug did not hydrolyze at all, and that the observed rate of hydrolysis could be ascribed to the concentration of the free or uncomplexed drug which was in equilibrium with the drug complex.

Boric acid chelation of the catechol function of epinephrine stabilizes epinephrine against attack by bisulfite and sulfite.

Surfactants—It has been demonstrated that the incorporation of benzocaine into surfactant micelles could significantly retard the rate of ester hydrolysis. Nonionic and anionic surfactants retarded the hydroxide-ion-catalyzed hydrolysis, but cationic surfactants somewhat increased the rate of hydroxide-ion-catalyzed hydrolysis. Similar observations have been reported for a number of drugs which are sufficiently lipophilic to be solubilized by surfactant micelles.

Suspensions—If the solubility of a labile drug is reduced, and the drug prepared in a suspension form, the rate at which the drug degrades will be related only to the concentration of drug in solution, rather than to the total concentration of drug in the product. Thus it has been demonstrated that penicillin G procaine suspensions degraded at a rate proportional to the low concentration of penicillin in solution. Since the penicillin in solution was in equilibrium with excess solid penicillin G procaine, the penicillin concentration in solution was constant and the observed order of reaction was apparent zero-order.

Refrigeration—Storage at temperatures below room temperature will usually retard solvolytic reactions. Storage in the frozen state is generally an effective means of retarding degradative reactions, though there are notable exceptions. Sodium ampicillin dissolved in 5% dextrose solution, for example, showed approximately 10% decomposition after 4 hours storage at 5° and more than 13% loss after storage for the same period in the frozen state at −20°.

Stability Testing of Pharmaceutical Products

If a product is sufficiently stable to be marketed, it would require relatively long storage at room temperature, or actual temperature at which it will be stored prior to ultimate use, to permit observation of the rate at which the product degrades under normal storage conditions.

To avoid this undesirable delay in evaluating potential formulations, the manufacturer attempts to predict stability under conditions of room temperature, or actual storage conditions, through use of data for rate of decomposition obtained at several elevated temperatures. This prediction is accomplished through use of an Arrhenius plot to predict from high-temperature data the rate of product breakdown to be expected at actual storage conditions. The methods and facilities for accomplishing these predictions have been reviewed and will not be discussed here.

Prediction based on data obtained at elevated temperature is generally satisfactory for solution dosage forms. Success is more uncertain when nonhomogeneous products are involved. Suspensions of drugs may not provide linear Arrhenius plots because there is often the possibility that the solid phase which exists at elevated temperature may not be the same solid phase which exists at room temperature, and differences in solubility of the several solid phases which may exist can invalidate the usual Arrhenius plots.

Such difficulties should be anticipated when polymorphic crystal forms or several different solvates are known to exist. Also, when solid dosage forms such as tablets are subjected to high temperatures, changes in the quantity of moisture in the product may greatly influence the stability of the product.

Arrhenius plots also suffer limitations in application to reactions which have relatively low activation energies, and therefore are not greatly accelerated by increase in temperature. While it is usually desirable to determine drug stability by analyzing samples for the amount of intact drug remaining—in instances where there is very little drug decomposition, and particularly when it is not convenient to accelerate the reaction by increasing temperature—it is sometimes advantageous to determine initial reaction rates from determination of amount of reaction product formed.

Since manufacturers are most interested in the time required to produce just a few percent breakdown in their product, it is not uncommon for them to employ terminology such as $t_{.90}$ or $t_{.95}$, which is the time required for the drug to decompose to 90% or 95%, respectively, of original potency. This terminology is completely analogous to the terminology $t_{1/2}$, or $t_{.50}$, used to represent the half-life period.

An Arrhenius-type plot, analogous to that illustrated in Fig 18-2, can be obtained by plotting logarithm of time required for the specified fractional decomposition vs reciprocal of absolute temperature. The time required for the product to decrease in potency to 90% of original potency at room temperature then can be obtained directly from the plot.

References

1. Garrett ER, in Bean HS, et al: *Advances in Pharmaceutical Sciences*, vol 2, Academic, New York, 2–94, 1967.
2. Kondritzer AA, Zvirblis P: *J APhA Sci Ed 46:* 531, 1957.
3. Higuchi T, et al: *J APhA Sci Ed 39:* 405, 1950.
4. Edwards LJ: *Trans Faraday Soc 46:* 723, 1950.
5. Fersht AR, Kirby AJ: *J Am Chem Soc 89:* 4857, 1967.
6. Whitworth CA, et al: *J Pharm Sci 62:* 1184, 1973.
7. Yamana, T, et al: *J Pharm Sci 66:* 861, 1977.

Bibliography

Connors KA: *Reaction Mechanisms in Organic Analytical Chemistry* Wiley, New York, 1973.
Martin AN, et al: *Physical Pharmacy*, 3rd ed, Lea & Febiger, Philadelphia, 1983, Chap 14.
Lachman L, DeLuca P, in Lachman L, et al: *The Theory and Practice of Industrial Pharmacy*, 2nd ed, Lea & Febiger, Philadelphia, 32–77, 1976.

CHAPTER 19

Interfacial Phenomena

George Zografi, PhD

Professor, School of Pharmacy
University of Wisconsin
Madison, WI 53706

The study of interfacial phenomena is concerned with the properties of molecules situated at or very near the boundary between immiscible phases, generally called the interface or the interfacial region. In systems of pharmaceutical and medicinal interest the number of situations where multiphase systems, and thus interfaces, occur is quite great.

Consider, as examples, the variety of heterogeneous dosage forms such as suspensions (solid dispersed in liquid), emulsions (liquid in liquid), foams (vapor in liquid or solid), and powders (solid in vapor), as well as the contact of drug molecules with various interfaces during transport from the dosage form, passage through biologic membranes, and accumulation at the cellular site of activity.

Interfacial Forces and Energetics

In the bulk portion of each phase, molecules are attracted to one another equally in all directions, such that no resultant forces are acting on any one molecule. The strength of these forces determines whether a substance exists as a vapor, liquid, or solid at a particular temperature and pressure.

At the boundary between phases, however, molecules are acted upon unequally since they are in contact with other molecules exhibiting different forces of attraction. For example, the primary intermolecular forces in water are due to hydrogen bonds, whereas those responsible for intermolecular bonding in hydrocarbon liquids, such as mineral oil, are due primarily to the London dispersion forces.

Because of this, molecules situated at the interface contain potential forces of interaction which are not satisfied relative to the situation in each bulk phase. In liquid systems such unbalanced forces can be satisfied by spontaneous movement of molecules from the interface into the bulk phase. This leaves fewer molecules per unit area at the interface (greater intermolecular distance) and reduces the actual contact area between dissimilar molecules.

Any attempt to reverse this process by increasing the area of contact between phases, ie, bringing more molecules into the interface, causes the interface to resist expansion and to behave as though it is under a tension everywhere in a tangential direction. The force of this tension per unit length of interface generally is called the interfacial tension, except when dealing with the air–liquid interface, where the terms surface and surface tension are used.

To illustrate the presence of a tension in the interface, consider an experiment where a circular metal frame, with a looped piece of thread loosely tied to it, is dipped into a liquid. When removed and exposed to the air, a film of liquid will be stretched entirely across the circular frame, as when one uses such a frame to blow soap bubbles. Under these conditions (Fig 19-1A), the thread will remain collapsed. If now a heated needle is used to puncture and remove the liquid film from within the loop (Fig 19-1B), the loop will spontaneously stretch into a circular shape.

The result of this experiment demonstrates the spontaneous reduction of interfacial contact between air and the liquid

remaining and, indeed, that a tension causing the loop to remain extended exists parallel to the interface. The circular shape of the loop indicates that the tension in the plane of the interface exists at right angles or normal to every part of the looped thread. The total force on the entire loop divided by the circumference of the circle, therefore, represents the tension per unit distance of surface, or the surface tension.

Just as work is required to extend a spring under tension, work should be required to reverse the process seen in Figs 19-1A and B, thus bringing more molecules to the interface. This may be seen quantitatively by considering an experiment where tension and work may be measured directly. Assume that we have a rectangular wire with one movable side (Fig 19-2). Assume further that by dipping this wire into a liquid, a film of liquid will form within the frame when it is removed and exposed to the air. As seen earlier in Fig 19-1, since it comes in contact with air, the liquid surface will tend to contract with a force, F, as molecules leave the surface for the bulk. To keep the movable side in equilibrium, an equal force must be applied to oppose this tension in the surface. We then may define the surface tension, γ, of the liquid as $F/2l$, where $2l$ is the distance of surface over which F is operating ($2l$ since there are two surfaces, top and bottom). If the surface is expanded by a very small distance, Δx, one can then estimate that the work done is:

$$W = F\Delta x \quad (1)$$

and, therefore,

$$W = \gamma 2l\Delta x \quad (2)$$

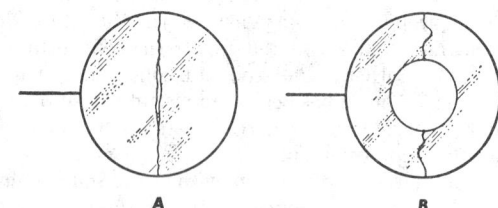

Fig 19-1.   A circular wire frame with a loop of thread loosely tied to it: (A) a liquid film on the wire frame with a loop in it; (B) the film inside the loop is broken.[1]

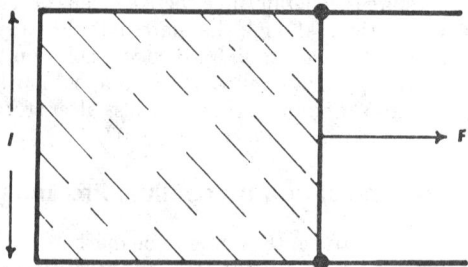

Fig 19-2.   A movable wire frame containing a film of liquid being expanded with a force, F.

Since

$$\Delta A = 2l\Delta x \qquad (3)$$

where ΔA is the change in area due to the expansion of the surface, we may conclude that

$$W = \gamma \Delta A \qquad (4)$$

Thus, the work required to create a unit area of surface, known as the surface free energy/unit area, is equivalent to the surface tension of a liquid system, and the greater the area of interfacial contact between phases, the greater the free-energy increase for the total system. Since a prime requisite for equilibrium is that the free energy of a system be at a minimum, it is not surprising to observe that phases in contact tend to reduce area of contact spontaneously.

Liquids, being mobile, may assume spherical shapes (smallest interfacial area for a given volume), as when ejected from an orifice into air or when dispersed into another immiscible liquid. If a large number of drops are formed, further reduction in area can occur by having the drops coalesce, as when a foam collapses or when the liquid phases making up an emulsion separate.

Surface tension is expressed in units of dynes/cm, while surface free energy is expressed in ergs/cm^2. Since an erg is a dyne-cm, both sets of units are equivalent.

Values for the surface tension of a variety of liquids are given in Table I, while interfacial tension values for various liquids against water are given in Table II. Other combinations of immiscible phases could be given but most heterogeneous systems encountered in pharmacy usually contain water. Values for these tensions are expressed for a particular temperature. Since an increased temperature increases the thermal energy of molecules, the work required to bring molecules to the interface should be less, and thus the surface and interfacial tension will be reduced. For example, the

Table I—Surface Tension of Various Liquids at 20°

Substance	Surface tension, dynes/cm
Mercury	476
Water	72.8
Glycerin	63.4
Oleic acid	32.5
Benzene	28.9
Chloroform	27.1
Carbon tetrachloride	26.8
1-Octanol	26.5
Hexadecane	27.4
Dodecane	25.4
Decane	23.9
Octane	21.8
Heptane	19.7
Hexane	18.0
Perfluoroheptane	11.0
Nitrogen (at 75°K)	9.4

Table II—Interfacial Tension of Various Liquids against Water at 20°

Substance	Interfacial tension, dynes/cm
Decane	52.3
Octane	51.7
Hexane	50.8
Carbon tetrachloride	45.0
Chloroform	32.8
Benzene	35.0
Mercury	428
Oleic acid	15.6
1-Octanol	8.51

surface tension of water at 0°C is 76.5 dynes/cm and 63.5 dynes/cm at 75°C.

As would be expected from the discussion so far, the relative values for surface tension should reflect the nature of intermolecular forces present; hence, the relatively large values for mercury (metallic bonds) and water (hydrogen bonds), and the lower values for benzene, chloroform, carbon tetrachloride, and the n-alkanes. Benzene with π electrons exhibits a higher surface tension than the alkanes of comparable molecular weight, but increasing the molecular weight of the alkanes (and hence intermolecular attraction) increases their surface tension closer to that of benzene. The lower values for the more nonpolar substances, perfluoroheptane and liquid nitrogen, demonstrate this point even more strongly.

Values of interfacial tension should reflect the differences in chemical structure of the two phases involved; the greater the tendency to interact, the less the interfacial tension. The 20-dynes/cm difference between air–water tension and that at the octane–water interface reflects the small but significant interaction between octane molecules and water molecules at the interface. This is seen also in Table II, by comparing values for octane and octanol, oleic acid and the alkanes, or chloroform and carbon tetrachloride.

In each case the presence of chemical groups capable of hydrogen bonding with water markedly reduces the interfacial tension, presumably by satisfying the unbalanced forces at the interface. These observations strongly suggest that molecules at an interface arrange themselves or orient so as to minimize differences between bulk phases.

That this occurs even at the air–liquid interface is seen when one notes the relatively low surface-tension values of very different chemical structures such as the n-alkanes, octanol, oleic acid, benzene, and chloroform. Presumably, in each case, the similar nonpolar groups are oriented toward the air with any polar groups oriented away toward the bulk phase. This tendency for molecules to orient at an interface is a basic factor in interfacial phenomena and will be discussed more fully in succeeding sections.

Solid substances such as metals, metal oxides, silicates, and salts, all containing polar groups exposed at their surface, may be classified as high-energy solids, whereas nonpolar solids such as carbon, sulfur, glyceryl tristearate, polyethylene, and polytetrafluoroethylene (Teflon) may be classified as low-energy solids. It is of interest to measure the surface free energy of solids; however, the lack of mobility of molecules at the surface of solids prevents the observation and direct measurement of a surface tension. It is possible to measure the work required to create new solid surface by cleaving a crystal and measuring the work involved. However, this work not only represents free energy due to exposed groups but also takes into account the mechanical energy associated with the crystal (ie, plastic and elastic deformation and strain energies due to crystal structure and imperfections in that structure).

Also contributing to the complexity of a solid surface is the heterogeneous behavior due to the exposure of different crystal faces, each having a different surface free energy/unit area. For example, adipic acid, $HOOC(CH_2)_4COOH$, crystallizes from water as thin hexagonal plates with three different faces, as shown in Fig 19-3. Each unit cell of such a crystal contains adipic acid molecules oriented such that the hexagonal planes (faces) contain exposed carboxyl groups, while the sides and edges (A and B faces) represent the side view of the carboxyl and alkyl groups, and thus are quite nonpolar. Indeed, interactions involving these different faces reflect the differing surface free energies.[2]

Other complexities associated with solid surfaces include surface roughness, porosity, and contamination produced during recrystallization of the solid. In view of all these complications, surface free energy values for solids, when re-

Table III—Values of γ_{sv} for Solids of Varying Polarity

Solid	γ_{sv} (dynes/cm)
Teflon	19.0
Paraffin	25.5
Polyethylene	37.6
Polymethyl methacrylate	45.4
Nylon	50.8
Indomethacin	61.8
Griseofulvin	62.2
Hydrocortisone	68.7
Sodium Chloride	155
Copper	1300

ported, should be regarded as average values, often dependent on the method used and not necessarily the same for other samples of the same substance.

In Table III are listed some approximate average values of γ_{sv} for a variety of solids, ranging in polarity from Teflon to copper, obtained by various indirect techniques.

Adhesional and Cohesional Forces

Of prime importance to those dealing with heterogeneous systems is the question of how two phases will behave when brought in contact with each other. It is well known, for instance, that some liquids, when placed in contact with other liquid or solid surfaces, will remain retracted in the form of a drop (known as a lens), while other liquids may exhibit a tendency to spread and cover the surface of this liquid or solid.

Based upon concepts developed to this point, it is apparent that the individual phases will exhibit a tendency to minimize the area of contact with other phases, thus leading to phase separation. On the other hand, the tendency for interaction between molecules at the new interface will offset this to some extent and give rise to the spontaneous spreading of one substance over the other.

In essence, therefore, phase affinity is increased as the forces of attraction between different phases (adhesional forces) become greater than the forces of attraction between molecules of the same phase (cohesional forces). If these adhesional forces become great enough, miscibility will occur and the interface will disappear. The present discussion is concerned only with systems of limited phase affinity, where an interface still exists.

A convenient approach used to express these forces quantitatively involves the use of the terms work of adhesion and work of cohesion.

The work of adhesion, W_a, is defined as the energy per cm^2 required to separate two phases at their boundary and is equal but opposite in sign to the free energy/cm^2 released when the interface is formed. In an analogous manner the work of cohesion for a pure substance, W_c, is the work/cm^2 required to produce two new surfaces, as when separating different phases, but now both surfaces contain the same molecules. This is equal and opposite in sign to the free energy/cm^2 released when the same two pure liquid surfaces are brought together and eliminated.

By convention, when the work of adhesion between two substances, A and B, exceeds the work of cohesion for one substance, eg, B, spontaneous spreading of B over the surface of A should occur with a net loss of free energy equal to the difference between W_a and W_c. If W_c exceeds W_a, no spontaneous spreading of B over A can occur. The difference between W_a and W_c is known as the spreading coefficient, S; only when S is positive will spreading occur.

The values for W_a and W_c (and hence S) may be expressed in terms of surface and interfacial tensions, when one considers that upon separation of two phases, A and B, γ_{AB} ergs

of interfacial free energy/cm^2 (interfacial tension) are lost, but that γ_A and γ_B ergs/cm^2 of energy (surface tensions of A and B) are gained; upon separation of bulk phase molecules in an analogous manner, $2\gamma_A$ or $2\gamma_B$ ergs/cm^2 will be gained. Thus,

$$W_a = \gamma_A + \gamma_B - \gamma_{AB} \qquad (5)$$

and

$$W_c = 2\gamma_A \text{ or } 2\gamma_B \qquad (6)$$

For B spreading on the surface of A, therefore,

$$S_B = \gamma_A + \gamma_B - \gamma_{AB} - 2\gamma_B \qquad (7)$$

or

$$S_B = \gamma_A - (\gamma_B + \gamma_{AB}) \qquad (8)$$

Utilizing Eq 8 and values of surface and interfacial tension given in Tables I and II, S can be calculated for three representative substances—decane, benzene, and oleic acid—on water at 20°.

Decane: $S = 72.8 - (23.9 + 52.3) = -3.4$

Benzene: $S = 72.8 - (28.9 + 35.0) = 8.9$

Oleic Acid: $S = 72.8 - (32.5 + 15.6) = 24.7$

As expected, relatively nonpolar substances such as decane exhibit negative values of S, whereas the more polar materials yield positive values; the greater the polarity of the molecule, the more positive the value of S. The importance of the cohesive energy of the spreading liquid may be noted also by comparing the spreading coefficients for hexane on water and water on hexane:

$$S_{H/W} = 72.8 - (18.0 + 50.8) = 4.0$$

$$S_{W/H} = 18.0 - (72.8 + 50.8) = -105.6$$

Here, despite the fact that both liquids are the same, the high cohesion and air–liquid tension of water prevents spreading on the low-energy hexane surface, while the very low value for hexane allows spreading on the water surface. This also is seen when comparing the positive spreading coefficient of hexane to the negative value for decane on water.

To see whether spreading does or does not occur, a powder such as talc or charcoal can be sprinkled over the surface of water such that it floats; then, a drop of each liquid is placed on this surface. As predicted, decane will remain as an intact drop, while hexane, benzene, and oleic acid will spread out, as shown by the rapid movement of solid particles away from the point where the liquid drop was placed originally.

An apparent contradiction to these observations may be noted for hexane, benzene, and oleic acid when more of each substance is added, in that lenses now appear to form even though initial spreading occurred. Thus, in effect a substance does not appear to spread over itself.

It is now established that the spreading substance forms a monomolecular film which creates a new surface having a lower surface free energy than pure water. This arises because of the apparent orientation of the molecules in such a film so that their most hydrophobic portion is oriented towards the spreading phase. It is the lack of affinity between this exposed portion of the spread molecules and the polar portion of the remaining molecules which prevents further spreading.

This may be seen by calculating a final spreading coefficient where the new surface tension of water plus monomolecular film is used. For example, the presence of benzene reduces the surface tension of water to 62.2 dynes/cm so that the final spreading coefficient, S_F, is

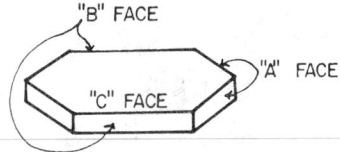

Fig 19-3.   Adipic acid crystal showing various faces.[2]

$$S_F = 62.2 - (28.9 + 35.0) = -1.7$$

The lack of spreading exhibited by oleic acid should be reflected in an even more negative final spreading coefficient, since the very polar carboxyl groups should have very little affinity for the exposed alkyl chain of the oleic acid film. Spreading so as to form a second layer with polar groups exposed to the air would also seem very unlikely, thus leading to the formation of a lens.

Wetting Phenomena

In the experiment described above it was shown that talc or charcoal sprinkled onto the surface of water float despite the fact that their densities are much greater than that of water. In order for immersion of the solid to occur, the liquid must displace air and spread over the surface of the solid; when liquids cannot spread over a solid surface spontaneously, we say that the solid is not wetted.

An important parameter which reflects the degree of wetting is the angle which the liquid makes with the solid surface at the point of contact (Fig 19-4). By convention, when wetting is complete, the contact angle is zero; in nonwetting situations it theoretically can increase to a value of 180°, where a spherical droplet makes contact with solid at only one point.

In order to express contact angle in terms of solid–liquid–air equilibria, one can balance forces parallel to the solid surface at the point of contact between all three phases (Fig 19-4), as expressed in the following equation,

$$\gamma_{SV} = \gamma_{SL} + \gamma_{LV} \cos \theta \qquad (9)$$

where γ_{SV}, γ_{SL}, and γ_{LV} represent the surface free energy/unit area of the solid–air, solid–liquid, and liquid–air interfaces, respectively. Although difficult to use quantitatively because of uncertainties with γ_{SV} and γ_{SL} measurements, conceptually the equation, known as the Young equation, is useful because it shows that the loss of free energy due to elimination of the air–solid interface by wetting is offset by the increased solid–liquid and liquid–air area of contact as the drop spreads out.

The $\gamma_{LV} \cos \theta$ term arises as the horizontal vectorial component of the force acting along the surface of the drop, as represented by γ_{LV}. Factors tending to reduce γ_{LV} and γ_{SL}, therefore, will favor wetting, while the greater the value of γ_{SV} the greater the chance for wetting to occur. This is seen in

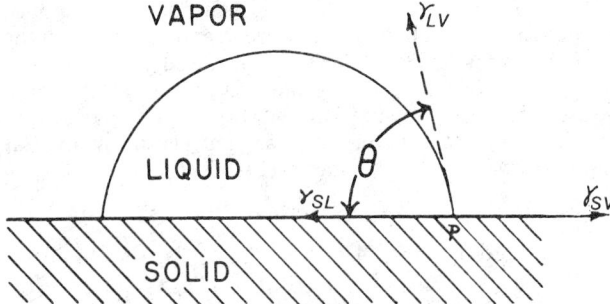

Fig 19-4.   Forces acting on a nonwetting liquid drop exhibiting a contact angle of θ.[3]

Table IV—Contact Angle on Paraffin and Nylon for Various Liquids of Differing Surface Tension

Substance	Surface tension, dynes/cm	Contact angle Paraffin	Nylon
Water	72.8	105°	70°
Glycerin	63.4	96°	60°
Formamide	58.2	91°	50°
Methylene iodide	50.8	66°	41°
α-Bromonaphthalene	44.6	47°	16°
tert-Butylnaphthalene	33.7	38°	spreads
Benzene	28.9	24°	"
Dodecane	25.4	17°	"
Decane	23.9	7°	"
Nonane	22.9	spreads	"

Table V—Critical Surface Tensions of Various Polymeric Solids

Polymeric Solid	γ_c, Dynes/cm at 20°
Polymethacrylic ester of ϕ'-octanol	10.6
Polyhexafluoropropylene	16.2
Polytetrafluoroethylene	18.5
Polytrifluoroethylene	22
Poly(vinylidene fluoride)	25
Poly(vinyl fluoride)	28
Polyethylene	31
Polytrifluorochloroethylene	31
Polystyrene	33
Poly(vinyl alcohol)	37
Poly(methyl methacrylate)	39
Poly(vinyl chloride)	39
Poly(vinylidene chloride)	40
Poly(ethylene terephthalate)	43
Poly(hexamethylene adipamide)	46

Table IV for the wetting of a low-energy surface, paraffin (hydrocarbon), and a higher energy surface, nylon, (polyhexamethylene adipamide). Here, the lower the surface tension of a liquid, the smaller the contact angle on a given solid, and the more polar the solid, the smaller the contact angle with the same liquid.

With Eq 9 in mind and looking at Fig 19-5, it is now possible to understand how the forces acting at the solid-liquid-air interface can cause a dense nonwetted solid to float if γ_{SL} and γ_{LV} are large enough relative to γ_{SV}.

The significance of reducing γ_{LV} was first developed empirically by Zisman when he plotted $\cos \theta$ vs the surface tension of a series of liquids and found that a linear relationship, dependent on the solid, was obtained. When such plots are extrapolated to $\cos \theta$ equal to one or a zero contact angle, a value of surface tension required to just cause complete wetting is obtained. Doing this for a number of solids, it was shown that this surface tension (known as the critical surface tension, γ_c) parallels expected solid surface energy γ_{SV}; the lower γ_c, the more nonpolar the surface.

Table V indicates some of these γ_c values for different surface groups, indicating such a trend. Thus, water with a

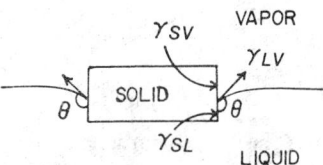

Fig 19-5.   Forces acting on a nonwettable solid at the air+liquid+solid interface: contact angle θ greater than 90°.

surface tension of about 72 dynes/cm will not wet polyethylene (γ_c = 31 dynes/cm), but heptane with a surface tension of about 20 dynes/cm will. Likewise, Teflon (polytetrafluoroethylene) (γ_c = 19) is not wetted by heptane but is wetted by perfluoroheptane with a surface tension of 11 dynes/cm.

One complication associated with the wetting of high-energy surfaces is the lack of wetting after the initial formation of a monomolecular film by the spreading substance. As in the case of oleic acid spreading on the surface of water, the remaining liquid retracts because of the low-energy surface produced by the oriented film. This phenomenon, often called autophobic behavior, is an important factor in many systems of pharmaceutical interest since many solids, expected to be wetted easily by water, may be rendered hydrophobic if other molecules dissolved in the water can form these monomolecular films at the solid surface. Wetting phenomena in the presence of dissolved molecules will be discussed more fully in a later section.

Capillarity

Because water shows a strong tendency to spread out over a polar surface such as clean glass (contact angle 0°), one would expect to observe the meniscus which forms when water is contained in a glass vessel such as a pipet or buret. This behavior is accentuated dramatically if a fine-bore capillary tube is placed into the liquid (Fig 19-6); not only will the wetting of the glass produce a more highly curved meniscus, but the level of the liquid in the tube will be appreciably higher than the level of the water in the beaker.

The spontaneous movement of a liquid into a capillary or narrow tube due to surface forces is defined as capillarity and is responsible for a number of important processes involving the penetration of liquids into porous solids. In contrast to water in contact with glass, if the same capillary is placed into mercury (contact angle on glass: 130°), not only will the meniscus be inverted (see Fig 19-7), but the level of the mercury in the capillary will be lower than in the beaker. In this case one does not expect mercury or other *nonwetting* liquids to easily penetrate pores unless external forces are applied.

To quantitate the factors giving rise to the phenomenon of capillarity, let us consider the case of a liquid which rises to a height, h, above the bulk liquid in a capillary having a radius, r. If (as shown in Fig 19-6) the contact angle of water on glass is zero, a force, F, will act upward and vertically along the circle of liquid–glass contact. Based upon the definition of surface tension this force will be equal to the surface tension, γ, multiplied by the circumference of the circle, $2\pi r$. Thus,

$$F = \gamma 2\pi r \tag{10}$$

This force upward must support the column of water, and since the mass, m, of the column is equal to the density, d, multiplied by the volume of the column, $\pi r^2 h$, the force W opposing the movement upward will be

$$W = mg = \pi r^2 dgh \tag{11}$$

where g is the gravity constant.

Equating the two forces at equilibrium gives

$$\pi r^2 dgh = \gamma 2\pi r \tag{12}$$

so that

$$h = \frac{2\gamma}{rdg} \tag{13}$$

Thus, the greater the surface tension and the finer the capillary radius, the greater the rise of liquid in the capillary.

If the contact angle of liquid is not zero (as shown in Fig 19-8), the same relationship may be developed, except the

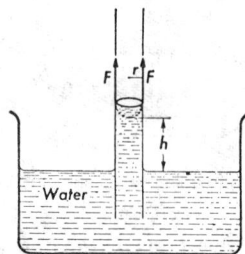

Fig 19-6. Capillary rise for a liquid exhibiting zero contact angle.[1]

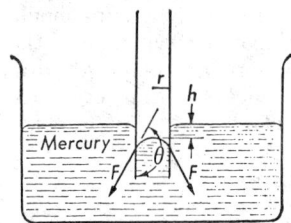

Fig 19-7. Capillary fall for a liquid exhibiting a contact angle, θ, which is greater than 90°.[1]

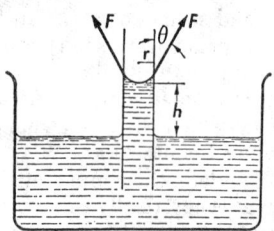

Fig 19-8. Capillary rise for a liquid exhibiting a contact angle, θ, which is greater than zero but less than 90°.[1]

vertical component of F which opposes the weight of the column is $F \cos \theta$ and, therefore,

$$h = \frac{2\gamma \cos \theta}{rdg} \tag{14}$$

This indicates the very important fact that if θ is less than 90°, but greater than 0°, the value of h will decrease with increasing contact angle until at 90° ($\cos \theta = 0$), $h = 0$. Above 90°, values of h will be negative, as indicated in Fig 19-7 for mercury. Thus, based on these equations we may conclude that capillarity will occur spontaneously in a cylindrical pore even if the contact angle is greater than zero, but it will not occur at all if the contact angle becomes 90° or more.

Pressure Differences across Curved Surfaces

From the preceding discussion of capillarity another important concept follows. In order for the liquid in a capillary to rise it must develop a higher pressure than the lower level of the liquid in the beaker. However, since the system is open to the atmosphere, both surfaces are in equilibrium with the atmospheric pressure. In order to be raised above the level of liquid in the beaker and produce a hydrostatic pressure equal to hgd, the pressure just below the liquid meniscus, in the capillary, P_1, must be less than that just below the flat liquid surface, P_0, by hgd, and therefore,

$$P_0 - P_1 = hgd \tag{15}$$

Since, according to Eq 14,

$$h = \frac{2\gamma \cos \theta}{rgd}$$

then

Table VI—Ratio of Observed Vapor Pressure to Expected Vapor Pressure of Water at 25° with Varying Droplet Size

P/P'	Droplet size, μm
1.001	1
1.01	0.1
1.1	0.01
2.0	0.005
3.0	0.001
4.2	0.00065
5.2	0.00060

[a] P is the observed vapor pressure and P' is the expected value for "bulk" water.

$$P_0 - P_1 = \frac{2\gamma \cos \theta}{r} \qquad (16)$$

For a contact angle of zero, where the radius of the capillary is the radius of the hemisphere making up the meniscus,

$$P_0 - P_1 = \frac{2\gamma}{r} \qquad (17)$$

The consequences of this relationship (known as the Laplace equation) are important for any curved surface when r becomes very small and γ is relatively significant. For example, a spherical droplet of air formed in a bulk liquid and having a radius, r, will have a greater pressure on the inner concave surface than on the convex side, as expressed in Eq 17.

Another direct consequence of what Eq 18 expresses is the fact that very small droplets of liquid, having highly curved surfaces, will exhibit a higher vapor pressure, P, than that observed over a flat surface of the same liquid at P'. The equation expressing the ratio of P/P' to droplet radius, r, and surface tension, γ, is called the Kelvin equation where:

$$\log P/P' = \frac{2\gamma M}{2.303RT\rho r} \qquad (18)$$

and M is the molecular weight, R the gas constant in ergs per mole per degree, T is temperature and ρ is the density in g/cm^3. Values for the ratio of vapor pressures are given in Table VI for water droplets of varying size. Such ratios indicate why it is possible for very fine water droplets in clouds to remain uncondensed despite their close proximity to one another.

This same behavior may be seen when measuring the solubility of very fine solid particles since both vapor pressure and solubility are measures of the escaping tendency of molecules from a surface. Indeed, the equilibrium solubility of extremely small particles has been shown to be greater than the usual value noted for coarser particles; the greater the surface energy and smaller the particles, the greater this effect.

Adsorption

Vapor Adsorption on Solid Surfaces

It was suggested earlier that a high surface or interfacial free energy may exist at a solid surface if the unbalanced forces at the surface and the area of exposed groups are quite great.

Substances such as metals, metal oxides, silicates, and salts—all containing exposed polar groups—may be classified as high-energy or hydrophilic solids; nonpolar solids such as carbon, sulfur, polyethylene, or Teflon (polytetrafluoroethylene) may be classified as low-energy or hydrophobic solids (Table III). Whereas liquids satisfy their unbalanced surface forces by changes in shape, pure solids (which exhibit no surface mobility) must rely on reaction with molecules either in the vapor state or in a solution which comes in contact with the solid surface to accomplish this.

Vapor adsorption is the simplest model demonstrating how solids reduce their surface free energy in this manner.

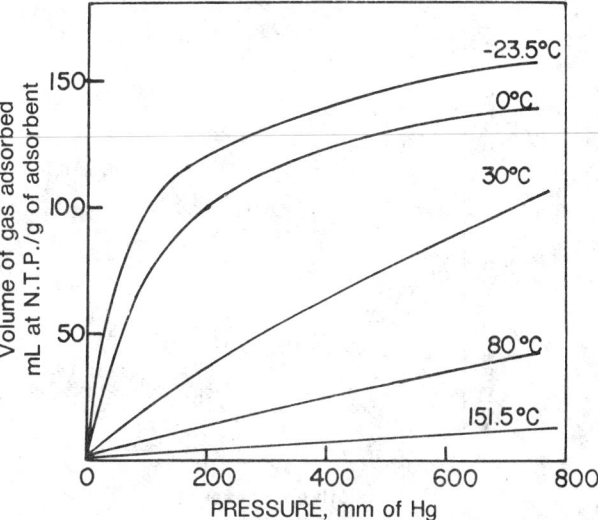

Fig 19-9.   Adsorption isotherms for ammonia on charcoal.[4]

Depending on the chemical nature of the adsorbent (solid) and the adsorbate (vapor), the strength of interaction between the two species may vary from strong specific chemical bonding to interactions produced by the weaker more nonspecific London dispersion forces. Ordinarily, these latter forces are those responsible for the condensation of relatively nonpolar substances such as N_2, O_2, CO_2, or hydrocarbons.

When chemical reaction occurs, the process is called chemisorption; when dispersion forces predominate, the term physical adsorption is used. Physical adsorption occurs at temperatures approaching the liquefaction temperature of the vapor, whereas, for chemisorption, temperatures depend on the particular reaction involved.

In order to study the adsorption of vapors onto solid surfaces one must measure the amount of gas adsorbed/unit area or unit mass of solid, at different pressures of gas. Since such studies usually are conducted at constant temperature, plots of volume adsorbed vs pressure are referred to as adsorption isotherms. If the physical or chemical adsorption process is monomolecular, the adsorption isotherm should look like those shown in Fig 19-9. Note the significant increase in adsorption with increasing pressure, followed by a leveling off. This leveling off is due either to a saturation of available specific chemical groups, as in chemisorption, or to the entire available surface being covered by physically adsorbed molecules. Note also the reduction in adsorption with increasing temperature which occurs because the adsorption process is exothermic. Often in the case of physical adsorption at low temperatures, after adsorption levels off, a marked increase in adsorption occurs, presumably due to multilayered adsorption. In this case vapor molecules essentially condense upon themselves as the liquefaction pressure of the vapor is approached. Fig 19-10 illustrates the type of isotherm one generally sees with multilayered physical adsorption.

In order to have some quantitative understanding of the adsorption process and to be able to compare different systems, two factors must be evaluated; it is important to know (1) what the capacity of the solid is or what the maximum amount of adsorption is under a given set of conditions and (2) what the affinity of a given substance is for the solid surface or how readily does it adsorb for a given amount of pressure? In effect, this second term is the equilibrium constant for the process.

A significant development along these lines was introduced by Langmuir when he proposed his theory of monomolecular adsorption. He postulated that for adsorption to occur a solid must contain uniform adsorption sites, each capable of holding

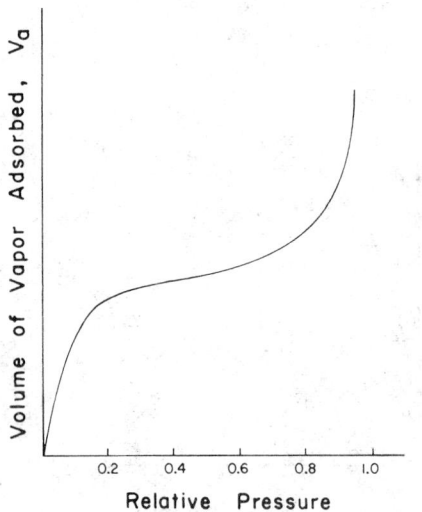

Fig 19-10. Typical plot for multilayer physical adsorption of a vapor on a solid surface.

a gas molecule. Molecules colliding with the surface may bounce off elastically or they may remain in contact for a period of time. It is this contact over a period of time that Langmuir termed adsorption.

Two major assumptions were made in deriving the equation: (1) only those molecules striking an empty site can be adsorbed, hence, only monomolecular adsorption occurs, and (2) the forces of interaction between adsorbed molecules are negligible and, therefore, the probability of a molecule adsorbing onto or desorbing from any site is independent of the surrounding sites.

The derivation of the equation is based upon the relationship between the rate of adsorption and desorption, since at equilibrium the two rates must be equal. Let μ equal the number of molecules striking each sq cm of surface/sec. From the kinetic theory of gases

$$\mu = \frac{p}{(2\pi mkT)^{1/2}} \qquad (22)$$

where p is the gas pressure, m is the mass of the molecule, k is the Boltzmann gas constant, and T is the absolute temperature. Thus, the greater p, the greater the number of collisions. Let α equal the fraction of molecules which will be held by the surface; then $\alpha\mu$ is equal to the rate of adsorption on the bare surface. However, if θ is the fraction of the surface already covered, the rate of adsorption actually will be

$$R_a = \alpha\mu(1 - \theta) \qquad (23)$$

In a similar manner the rate of molecules leaving the surface can be expressed as

$$R_d = \gamma\theta \qquad (24)$$

where γ is the rate at which molecules can leave the surface and θ represents the number of molecules available to desorb. The value of γ strongly depends on the energy associated with adsorption; the greater the binding energy, the lower the value of γ. At equilibrium, $R_a = R_d$ and

$$\gamma\theta = \alpha\mu(1 - \theta) \qquad (25)$$

Isolating the variable term, p, and combining all constants into k, the equation can be written as

$$\theta = \frac{kp}{1 + kp} \qquad (26)$$

and, since θ may be expressed as

$$\theta = \frac{V_a}{V_m} \qquad (27)$$

where V_a is the volume of gas adsorbed and V_m is the volume of gas covering all of the sites, Eq. 26 may be written as

$$V_a = \frac{V_mkp}{1 + kp} \qquad (28)$$

A test of fit to this equation can be made by expressing it in linear form:

$$\frac{p}{V_a} = \frac{1}{V_mk} + \frac{p}{V_m} \qquad (29)$$

The value of k is, in effect, the equilibrium constant and may be used to compare affinities of different substances for the solid surface. The value of V_m is valuable since it indicates the maximum number of sites available for adsorption. In the case of physical adsorption the maximum number of sites is actually the total surface area of the solid and, therefore, the value of V_m can be used to estimate surface area if the volume and area/molecule of vapor are known.

Since physical adsorption most often involves some multilayered adsorption, an equation, based on the Langmuir equation, the B.E.T. equation, is normally used to determine V_m and solid surface areas. Eq 30 is the B.E.T equation:

$$V_a = \frac{V_mcp}{(p_0 - p)[1 + (C - 1)(p/p_0)]} \qquad (30)$$

where c is a constant and p_0 is the vapor pressure of the adsorbing substance.[5] The most widely used vapor for this purpose is nitrogen, which adsorbs nonspecifically on most solids near its boiling point at $-195°$ and appears to occupy about 16 Å^2/molecule on a solid surface.

Adsorption from Solution

By far one of the most important aspects of interfacial phenomena encountered in pharmaceutical systems is the tendency for substances dissolved in a liquid to adsorb to various interfaces. Adsorption from solution is generally more complex than that from the vapor state because of the influence of the solvent and any other solutes dissolved in the solvent. Although such adsorption is generally limited to one molecular layer, the presence of other molecules often makes the interpretation of adsorption mechanisms much more difficult than for chemisorption or physical adsorption of a vapor. Since monomolecular adsorption is so widespread at all interfaces, we will first discuss the nature of monomolecular films and then return to a discussion of adsorption from solution.

Insoluble Monomolecular Films

It was suggested above that molecules exhibiting a tendency to spread out at an interface might be expected to orient so as to reduce the interfacial free energy produced by the presence of the interface. Direct evidence for molecular orientation has been obtained from studies dealing with the spreading on water of insoluble polar substances containing long hydrocarbon chains, eg, fatty acids.

In the late 19th century Pockels and Rayleigh showed that a very small amount of olive or castor oil—when placed on the surface of water—spreads out, as discussed above. If the amount of material was less than could physically cover the entire surface only a slight reduction in the surface tension of water was noted. However, if the surface was compressed between barriers, as shown in Fig 19-11, the surface tension was reduced considerably.

Devaux extended the use of this technique by dissolving

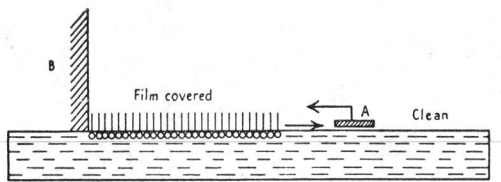

Fig 19-11.   Insoluble monomolecular film compressed between a fixed barrier, *B*, and a movable barrier, *A* (courtesy, Osipow[6]).

small amounts of solid in volatile solvents and dropping the solution onto a water surface.   After assisting the water-insoluble molecules to spread, the solvent evaporated, leaving a surface film containing a known amount of solute.

Compression and measurement of surface tension indicated that a maximum reduction of surface was reached when the number of molecules/unit area was reduced to a value corresponding to complete coverage of the surface.   This suggested that a monomolecular film forms and that surface tension is reduced upon compression because contact between air and water is reduced by the presence of the film molecules.   Beyond the point of closest packing the film apparently collapses very much as a layer of corks floating on water would be disrupted when laterally compressed beyond the point of initial physical contact.

Using a refined quantitative technique based on these studies, Langmuir[7] spread films of pure fatty acids, alcohols, and esters on the surface of water.   Comparing a series of saturated fatty acids, differing only in chain length, he found that the area/molecule at collapse was independent of chain length, corresponding to the cross-sectional area of a molecule oriented in a vertical position.   He further concluded that this molecular orientation involved association of the polar carboxyl group with the water phase and the nonpolar acyl chain out towards the vapor phase.

In addition to the evidence for molecular orientation, Langmuir's work with surface films revealed that each substance exhibits film properties which reflect the interactions between molecules in the surface film.   This is best seen by plotting the difference in surface tension of the clean surface, γ_0, and that of the surface covered with the film, γ, vs the area/molecule, A, produced by film compression (total area ÷ the number of molecules).   The difference in surface tension is called the surface pressure, π, and thus,

$$\pi = \gamma_0 - \gamma. \tag{31}$$

Fig 19-12 depicts such a plot for a typical fatty acid monomolecular film.   At areas greater than 50 Å^2/molecule the molecules are far apart and do not cover enough surface to reduce the surface tension of the clean surface to any extent

and thus the lack of appreciable surface pressure.   Since the molecules in the film are quite free to move laterally in the surface, they are said to be in a two-dimensional "gaseous" or "vapor" state.

As the intermolecular distance is reduced upon compression, the surface pressure rises because the air–water surface is being covered to a greater extent.   The rate of change in π with A, however, will depend on the extent of interaction between film molecules; the greater the rate of change, the more "condensed" the state of the film.

In Fig 19-12, from 50 Å^2 to 30 Å^2/molecule, the curve shows a steady increase in π, representative of a two-dimensional "liquid" film, where the molecules become more restricted in their freedom of movement because of interactions.   Below 30 Å^2/molecule the increase in π occurs over a narrow range of A, characteristic of closest packing and a two-dimensional "solid" film.

The extent of molecular interaction in the film also can be ascertained by measuring the surface viscosity, just as one might measure the viscosity or consistency of a three-dimensional gas, liquid, or solid.   Surface viscosity represents the resistance to movement exhibited by surface-film molecules under the influence of a force tangential to the interface. In effect, one measures the flow of one oriented molecule past another and, therefore, the resistance produced by interaction between film molecules.

Any factor tending to increase polarity or bulkiness of the molecule—such as increased charge, number of polar groups, reduction in chain length, or the introduction of aromatic rings, side chains, and double bonds—should reduce molecular interactions, while the longer the alkyl chain and the less bulky the polar group, the closer the molecules can approach and the stronger the extent of interaction in the film.   Both the change in π with A and surface viscosity values at any area/molecule reflect these expected effects.

Soluble Films and Adsorption from Solution

If a fatty acid exhibits highly "gaseous" film behavior on an aqueous surface, we should expect a relatively small change in π with A over a considerable range of compression.   Indeed, for short-chain compounds—eg, lauric acid (12 carbons) and decanoic acid—not only is the change in π small with decreasing A but at a point just before the expected closest packing area the surface pressure becomes constant without any collapse.

If lauric acid is converted to the laurate ion, or if a shorter chain acid such as octanoic acid is used, spreading on water and compression of the surface produces no increase in π; the more polar the molecule (hence, the more "gaseous" the film), the higher the area/molecule where a constant surface pressure occurs.

This behavior may be explained by assuming that polar molecules form monomolecular films when spread on water but that, upon compression, they are caused to enter the aqueous bulk solution rather than to remain as an intact insoluble film.   The constant surface pressure with increased compression arises because a constant number of molecules/unit area remain at the surface in equilibrium with dissolved molecules.   The extent of such behavior will be greater for substances exhibiting weaker intermolecular interaction and greater water solubility.

Starting from the other direction, it can be shown that short-chain acids and alcohols (when dissolved in water) reduce the surface tension of water, thus producing a surface pressure, just as with insoluble films (see Eq 31).   That dissolved molecules are accumulating at the interface in the form of a monomolecular film is suggested from the similarity in behavior to systems where slightly soluble molecules are spread on the surface.   For example, compressing the surface

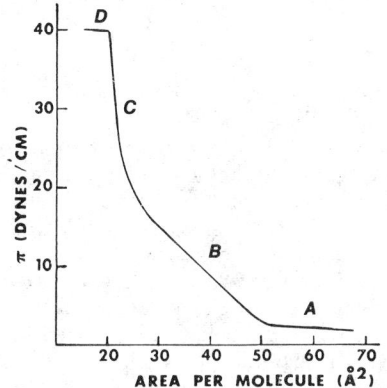

Fig 19-12.   A surface pressure–area curve for an insoluble monomolecular film: Region *A*, "gaseous" film; Region *B*, "liquid" film; Region *C*, "solid" film; Region *D*, film collapse.

of a solution containing "surface-active" molecules has no effect on the initial surface pressure, whereas increasing bulk-solution concentration tends to increase surface pressure, presumably by shifting the equilibrium between surface and bulk molecules.

At this point we may ask, why should water-soluble molecules leave an aqueous phase and accumulate or "adsorb" at an air–solution interface? Since any process will occur spontaneously if it results in a net loss in free energy, such must be the case for the process of adsorption.

A number of factors will produce such a favorable change in free energy. First, the presence of the oriented monomolecular film reduces the surface free energy of the air–water interface. Second, the hydrophobic group on the molecule is in a lower state of energy at the interface, where it no longer is as surrounded by water molecules, than when it is in the bulk-solution phase. Increased interaction between film molecules also will contribute to this process.

A further reduction in free energy occurs upon adsorption because of the gain in entropy associated with a change in water structure. Water molecules, in the presence of dissolved alkyl chains are more highly organized or "ice-like" than they are as a pure bulk phase; hence, the entropy of such structured water is lower than that of bulk water.

The process of adsorption requires that the "ice-like" structure "melt" as the chains go to the interface and, thus, an increase in the entropy of water occurs. The adsorption of molecules dissolved in oil can occur but it is not influenced by water structure changes and, hence, only the first factors mentioned are important here.

It is very rare that significant adsorption can occur at the hydrocarbon–air interface since little loss in free energy can occur by bringing hydrocarbon chains with polar groups attached to this interface; however, at oil–water interfaces the polar portions of the molecule can interact with water at the interface, leading to significant adsorption.

Thus, whereas water-soluble fatty acid salts are adsorbed from water to air–water and oil–water interfaces, their undissociated counterparts, the free fatty acids, which are water insoluble, form insoluble films at the air–water interface, are not adsorbed from oil solution to an oil–air interface, but show significant adsorption at the oil–water interface when dissolved in oil.

From this discussion it is possible also to conclude that adsorption from aqueous solution requires a lower solute concentration to obtain the same level of adsorption if the hydrophobic chain length is increased or if the polar portion of the molecule is less hydrophilic. On the other hand, adsorption from nonpolar solvents is favored when the solute is quite polar.

Since soluble or adsorbed films cannot be compressed, there is no simple direct way to estimate the number of molecules/ unit area coming to the surface under a given set of conditions. For relatively simple systems it is possible to estimate this value by application of the Gibbs equation, which relates surface concentration to the surface-tension change produced at different solute activities. The derivation of this equation is beyond the scope of this discussion, but it arises from a classical thermodynamic treatment of the change in free energy when molecules concentrate at the boundary between two phases. The equation may be expressed as

$$\Gamma = -\frac{a}{RT}\frac{d\gamma}{da} \tag{32}$$

where Γ is the moles of solute adsorbed/unit area; R is the gas constant; T is the absolute temperature; and $d\gamma$ is the change in surface tension with a change in solute activity, da, at activity a. For dilute solutions of nonelectrolytes, or for electrolytes when the Debye–Hückel equation for activity coefficient is applicable, the value of a may be replaced by solute

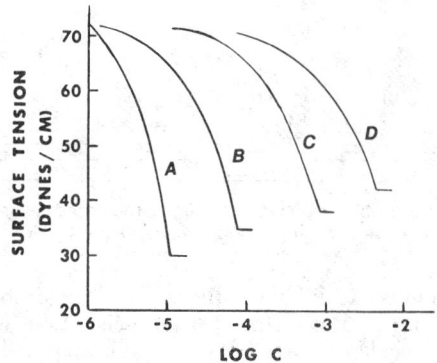

Fig 19-13. The effect of increasing chain length on the surface activity of a surfactant at the air–aqueous solution interface (each figure depicted to differ by two methylene groups with A, the longest chain, and D, the shortest).

concentration, c. Since the term dc/c is equal to $d \ln c$, the Gibbs equation is often written as

$$\Gamma = -\frac{1}{RT}\frac{d\gamma}{d \ln c} \tag{33}$$

In this way the slope of a plot of γ vs $\ln c$ multiplied by $1/RT$ should give Γ at a particular value of c. Fig 19-13 depicts typical plots for a series of water-soluble surface-active agents differing only in the alkyl chain length. Note the greater reduction of surface tension that occurs at lower concentrations for longer chain-length compounds. In addition, note the greater slopes with increasing concentration, indicating more adsorption (Eq 33), and the abrupt leveling of surface tension at higher concentrations. This latter behavior reflects the self-association of surface-active agent to form micelles which exhibit no further tendency to reduce surface tension. The topic of micelles will be discussed in Chapter 20.

If one plots the values of surface concentration, Γ, vs concentration, c, for substances adsorbing to the vapor-liquid and liquid-liquid interface, using data such as those given in Fig 19-13, one generally obtains an adsorption isotherm shaped like those in Fig 19-9 for vapor adsorption. Indeed, it can be shown that the Langmuir equation (Eq 28) can be fitted to such data when written in the form:

$$\Gamma = \frac{\Gamma_{max} k'c}{1 + k'c}$$

where Γ_{max} is the maximum surface concentration attained with increasing concentration and k' is related to k in Eq 28. Combining Eqs 32 and 34 leads to a widely used relationship between surface tension change Π (see Eq 31) and solute concentration, c, known as the Syszkowski equation:

$$\Pi = \Gamma_{max} RT \ln (1 + k'c) \tag{35}$$

Mixed Films

It would seem reasonable to expect that the properties of a surface film could be varied greatly if a mixture of surface-active agents were in the film. As an example, consider that a mixture of short- and long-chain fatty acids would be expected to show a degree of "condensation" varying from the "gaseous" state, when the short-chain substance is used in high amount, to a highly condensed state when the longer chain substance predominates. Thus, each component in such a case would operate independently by bringing a proportional amount of film behavior to the system.

More often, the ingredients of a surface film do not behave independently, but, rather, interact to produce a new surface film. An obvious example would be the combination of organic amines and acids which are oppositely charged and would be expected to interact strongly.

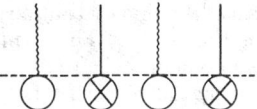

Fig 19-14.   A mixed monomolecular film.   ⊗: a long-chain ion; O: a long-chain nonionic compound.

In addition to such polar-group interactions, chain–chain interaction will strongly favor mixed condensed films. An important example of such a case occurs when a long-chain alcohol is introduced along with an ionized long-chain substance. Together the molecules form a highly condensed film despite the presence of a high number of like charges. Presumably this occurs as seen in Fig 19-14, by arranging the molecules so that ionic groups alternate with alcohol groups; however, if chain–chain interactions are not strong, the ionic species often will be displaced by the more nonpolar un-ionized species and "desorb" into the bulk solution.

On the other hand, sometimes the more soluble surface-active agent produces surface pressures in excess of the collapse pressure of the insoluble film and displaces it from the surface. This is an important concept because it is the underlying principle behind cell lysis by surface-active agents and some drugs, and behind the important process of detergency.

Adsorption on Solid Surfaces From Solution

Adsorption to solid surfaces from solution may occur if the dissolved molecules and the solid surface have chemical groups capable of interacting. Non-specific adsorption also will occur if the solute is surface active and if the surface area of the solid is high. This latter case would be the same as occurs at the vapor-liquid and liquid-liquid interfaces. As with adsorption to liquid interfaces, adsorption to solid surfaces from solution generally leads to a monomolecular layer, often described by the Langmuir equation. However, as Giles[8] has pointed out, the variety of combinations of solutes and solids, and, hence the variety of possible mechanisms of adsorption, can lead to a number of more complex isotherms. In particular, adsorption of surfactants and polymers, of great importance in a number of pharmaceutical systems (see

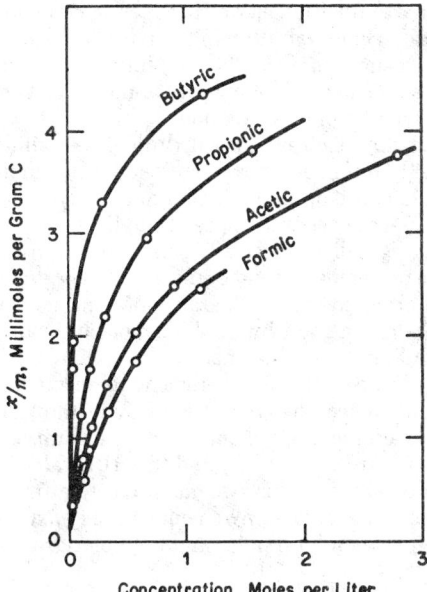

Fig 19-15.   The relation between adsorption and molecular weight of fatty acids (courtesy, Weiser[9]).

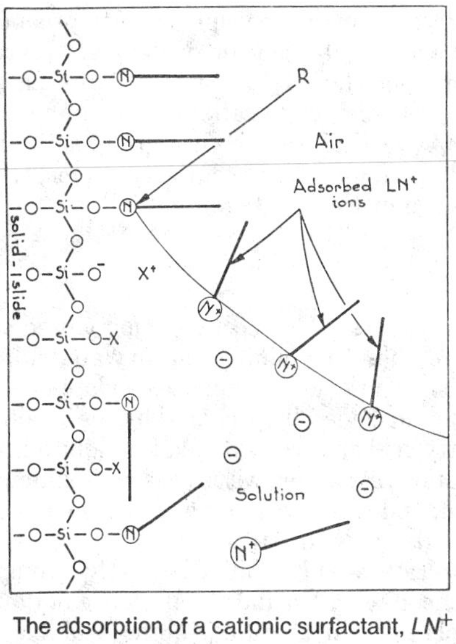

Fig 19-16.   The adsorption of a cationic surfactant, LN^+, onto a negatively charged silica or glass surface, exposing a hydrophobic surface as the solid is exposed to air.[10]

Chapters 20 and 21), is still not well understood on a fundamental level, and may on some occasions even be multilayered.

Adsorption from solution may be measured by separating solid and solution and either estimating the amount of adsorbate adhering to the solid or the loss in concentration of adsorbate from solution.

In view of the possibility of solvent adsorption, the latter approach really only gives an apparent adsorption. For example, if solvent adsorption is great enough, it is possible to end up with an increased concentration of solute after contact with the solid; here, the term negative adsorption is used.

Solvent not only influences adsorption by competing for the surface but, as discussed in connection with adsorption at liquid surfaces, the solvent will determine the escaping tendency of a solute; eg, the more polar the molecule, the less the adsorption that occurs from water. This is seen in Fig 19-16, where adsorption of various fatty acids from water onto charcoal increases with increasing alkyl chain length or nonpolarity. It is difficult to predict these effects but, in general, the more chemically unlike the solute and solvent and the more alike the solid surface groups and solute, the greater the extent of adsorption. Another factor which must be kept in mind is that charged solid surfaces, such as polyelectrolytes, will strongly adsorb oppositely charged solutes. This is similar to the strong specific binding seen in gas chemisorption and it is characterized by significant monolayer adsorption at very low concentrations of solute. See Fig 19-16 for an example of such adsorption.

Surface-Active Agents

Throughout the discussion so far, examples of surface-active agents (surfactants) have been restricted primarily to fatty acids and their salts. It has been shown that both a hydrophobic portion (alkyl chain) and a hydrophilic portion (carboxyl and carboxylate groups) are required for their surface activity, the relative degree of polarity determining the tendency to accumulate at interfaces. It now becomes important to look at some of the specific types of surfactants available and to see what structural features are required for different pharmaceutical applications.

The classification of surfactants is quite arbitrary, but one based on chemical structure appears best as a means of introducing the topic. It is generally convenient to categorize surfactants according to their polar portions since the non-polar portion is usually made up of alkyl or aryl groups. The major polar groups found in most surfactants may be divided as follows: (1) anionic, (2) cationic, (3) amphoteric, and (4) nonionic. As we shall see, the last group is the largest and most widely used for pharmaceutical systems, so that it will be emphasized in the discussion that follows.

Types

Anionic Agents—The most commonly used anionic surfactants are those containing carboxylate, sulfonate, and sulfate ions. Those containing carboxylate ions are known as soaps and are generally prepared by the saponification of natural fatty acid glycerides in alkaline solution. The most common cations associated with soaps are sodium, potassium, ammonium, and triethanolamine, while the chain length of the fatty acids ranges from 12 to 18.

The degree of water solubility is greatly influenced by the length of the alkyl chain and the presence of double bonds. For example, sodium stearate is quite insoluble in water at room temperature, whereas sodium oleate under the same conditions is quite water soluble.

Multivalent ions, such as calcium and magnesium, produce marked water insolubility, even at lower alkyl chain lengths; thus, soaps are not useful in hard water which is high in content of these ions. Soaps, being salts of weak acids, are subject also to hydrolysis and the formation of free acid plus hydroxide ion, particularly when in more concentrated solution.

To offset some of the disadvantages of soaps, a number of long-alkyl-chain sulfonates, as well as alkyl aryl sulfonates such as sodium dodecylbenzene sulfonate, may be used; the sulfonate ion is less subject to hydrolysis and precipitation in the presence of multivalent ions. A popular group of sulfonates, widely used in pharmaceutical systems, are the dialkyl sodium sulfosuccinates, particularly bis-(2-ethylhexyl) sodium sulfosuccinate, best known as Aerosol OT. This compound is unique in that it is both oil and water soluble and hence forms micelles in both phases. It reduces surface and interfacial tension to extremely low values and acts as an excellent wetting agent in many types of solid dosage forms.

A number of alkyl sulfates are available as surfactants, but by far the most popular member of this group is sodium lauryl sulfate, which is widely used as an emulsifier and solubilizer in pharmaceutical systems. Unlike the sulfonates, sulfates are susceptible to hydrolysis which leads to the formation of the long-chain alcohol, so that pH control is most important for sulfate solutions.

Cationic Agents—A number of long-chain cations, such as amine salts and quaternary ammonium salts, are often used as surface-active agents when dissolved in water; however, their use in pharmaceutical preparations is limited to that of antimicrobial preservation rather than as surfactants. This arises because the cations adsorb so readily at cell membrane structures in a nonspecific manner, leading to cell lysis (eg, hemolysis), as do anionics to a lesser extent. It is in this way that they act to destroy bacteria and fungi.

Since anionic and nonionic agents are not as effective as preservatives, one must conclude that the positive charge of these compounds is important; however, the extent of surface activity has been shown to determine the amount of material needed for a given amount of preservation. Quaternary ammonium salts are preferable to free amine salts since they are not subject to effect by pH in any way; however, the presence of organic anions such as dyes and natural polyelectrolytes is an important source of incompatibility and such a combination should be avoided.

Amphoteric Agents—The major group of molecules falling into this category are those containing carboxylate or phosphate groups as the anion and amino or quaternary ammonium groups as the cation. The former group is represented by various polypeptides, proteins, and the alkyl betaines, while the latter group consist of natural phospholipids such as the lecithins and cephalins. In general, long-chain amphoterics which exist in solution in zwitterionic form are more surface-active than ionic surfactants having the same hydrophobic group since in effect the oppositely charged ions are neutralized. However, when compared to nonionics, they appear somewhere between ionic and nonionic.

Nonionic Agents—The major class of compounds used in pharmaceutical systems are the nonionic surfactants since their advantages with respect to compatibility, stability, and potential toxicity are quite significant. It is convenient to divide these compounds into those that are relatively water insoluble and those that are quite water soluble.

The major type of compounds making up this first group are the long-chain fatty acids and their water-insoluble derivatives. These include (1) fatty alcohols such as lauryl, cetyl (16 carbons), and stearyl alcohols; (2) glyceryl esters such as the naturally occurring mono-, di-, and triglycerides; and (3) fatty acid esters of fatty alcohols and other alcohols such as propylene glycol, polyethylene glycol, sorbitan, sucrose, and cholesterol. Included also in this general class of nonionic water-insoluble compounds are the free steroidal alcohols such as cholesterol.

To increase the water solubility of these compounds and to form the second group of nonionic agents, polyoxyethylene groups are added through an ether linkage with one of their alcohol groups. The list of derivatives available is much too long to cover completely, but a few general categories will be given.

The most widely used compounds are the polyoxyethylene sorbitan fatty acid esters which are found in both internal and external pharmaceutical formulations. Closely related compounds include polyoxyethylene glyceryl, and steroidal esters, as well as the comparable polyoxypropylene esters. It is also possible to have a direct ether linkage with the hydrophobic group as with a polyoxyethylene–stearyl ether or a polyoxyethylene–alkyl phenol. These ethers offer advantages since, unlike the esters, they are quite resistant to acidic or alkaline hydrolysis.

Besides the classification of surfactants according to their polar portion, it is useful to have a method that categorizes them in a manner that reflects their interfacial activity and their ability to function as wetting agents, emulsifiers, solubilizers, etc. Since variation in the relative polarity or nonpolarity of a surfactant significantly influences its interfacial behavior, some measure of polarity or nonpolarity should be useful as a means of classification.

One such approach assigns a hydrophile–lipophile balance number (HLB) for each surfactant and, although developed by a commercial supplier of one group of surfactants, the method has received wide-spread application. The HLB value, as originally conceived for nonionic surfactants, is merely the percentage weight of the hydrophilic group divided by five in order to reduce the range of values. On a molar basis, therefore, a 100% hydrophilic molecule (polyethylene glycol) would have a value of 20.

Thus, an increase in polyoxyethylene chain length increases polarity and, hence, the HLB value; at constant polar chain length, an increase in alkyl chain length or number of fatty acid groups decreases polarity and the HLB value. One immediate advantage of this system is that to a first approximation one can compare any chemical type of surfactant to another type when both polar and nonpolar groups are different.

HLB values for nonionics are calculable on the basis of the proportion of polyoxyethylene chain present; however, in order to determine values for other types of surfactants it is necessary to compare physical chemical properties reflecting polarity with those surfactants having known HLB values.

Relationships between HLB and phenomena such as water solubility, interfacial tension, and dielectric constant have been used in this regard. Those surfactants exhibiting values greater than 20 (eg, sodium lauryl sulfate) demonstrate hydrophilic behavior in excess of the polyoxyethylene groups alone. For actual values of HLB see Table XVI in Chapter 21.

Pharmaceutical Applications

The specific use of surface-active agents in pharmaceutical formulations and manufacturing when applicable will be discussed more fully in later chapters dealing with these more applied topics. The three major uses of surfactants are as wetting, solubilizing, and emulsifying agents. Solubilization and emulsification are discussed thoroughly in Chapters 20 and 21, respectively, and therefore will not be presented here. The problems of wetting in pharmaceutical systems are important from a number of points of view and are not presented in any detail elsewhere. Consequently, we shall conclude this chapter with an examination of the wetting of pharmaceutical solids by liquids and how surface-active agents influence such behavior.

Consider a free powder of drug placed into a gelatin capsule. After oral administration, as it comes in contact with the gastric fluid and the gelatin dissolves, the powder must become immersed in the liquid and assume the original particle size distribution. In order for this to occur, liquid must displace air and spread over the surface of the solid. If this wetting does not occur, powder will float as shown in Fig 19-5. It will also tend to agglomerate. That the lack of wetting of solids administered as powders in capsules influences the rate at which drug dissolves in the stomach is well documented. For example, marked increases have been shown in the dissolution rate of phenobarbital when polysorbate 80, in increasing amount, is placed into simulated gastric juice; the rate of dissolution is proportional to the reduction in surface tension of the solution.

A second problem is the inability of powder agglomerates, such as tablets, to break apart when immersed in a liquid. In addition to strong bonding between granules which may prevent disintegration, the presence of air between and in the granules, plus a hydrophobic surface to begin with, often produce a lack of solvent penetration and wetting. For example, the presence of hydrophobic tablet lubricants such as magnesium and aluminum stearate was shown to decrease dissolution rates of salicylic acid from tablets, whereas the addition of sodium lauryl sulfate overcame this difficulty by increasing the wettability of the tablet. It has been demonstrated that removal of air from tablets produced the same effect on wetting as did a surfactant.

Other situations involving wetting behavior of interest to pharmacists include the dispersion of powders to prepare pharmaceutical suspensions and the introduction of polymeric solids into biological systems, eg contact lenses, parts of artificial organs or implants containing drug intended for slow release and long-acting effects.

Wetting Agents—As described in the section dealing with wetting by pure liquids, many solids have critical surface tensions, γ_c, much lower than 72 dynes/cm, the surface tension of water. From the Young equation (Eq 9), we can see that when γ_{LV} and γ_{SL} are reduced, the contact angle is also reduced. Therefore, if water-soluble surfactants are added which adsorb significantly to the vapor-liquid and solid-liquid interface the wetting of such a solid should be facilitated. Table VII indicates the effect of increasing concentration of the surfactant Aerosol OT on surface tension and on the contact angle of water against magnesium stearate, a hydro-

Table VII—Effect of Aerosol OT Concentration on the Surface Tension of Water and the Contact Angle of Water with Magnesium Stearate

Concentration, $m \times 10^6$	γ_{sv}	θ
1.0	60.1	120°
3.0	49.8	113°
5.0	45.1	104°
8.0	40.6	89°
10.0	38.6	80°
12.0	37.9	71°
15.0	35.0	63°
20.0	32.4	54°
25.0	29.5	50°

phobic tablet lubricant. Presumably, Aerosol OT is a good wetting agent because it adsorbs significantly to the vapor-liquid and solid-liquid interfaces before forming micelles. This apparently is due to the irregular molecular shape which makes it difficult to pack into micelles, thus allowing a relatively higher monomer concentration available for adsorption. The manner in which adsorption to the solid–liquid interface occurs, however, is important. If a surfactant adsorbs on the surface of a solid with polar groups oriented towards the aqueous solution, for example, the surface should appear more polar, thus increasing the apparent critical surface tension of a solid and producing wetting.

As a general rule, however, adsorption onto polar solid surfaces often occurs with polar groups attracted to the solid and the hydrocarbon groups oriented towards the aqueous solution. For example, aqueous solutions of long-chain amines, despite their low surface tensions do not wet glass or silica below their critical micelle concentration (cmc), whereas pure water does.

Since glass is negatively charged, the cationic amines should adsorb as shown in Fig 19-16. If, however, the concentration of surfactant is raised near to or above its cmc, a bimolecular layer with polar groups exposed to the aqueous solution occurs and cationic amine solutions wet glass; this provides the polar surface required for aqueous wetting.

Another complication occurs when surfactant adsorbs since this reduces the bulk concentration of the advancing liquid drop, which in turn may raise the air–liquid surface tension to a value above the solid critical surface tension. We may conclude, therefore, that the best wetting agents to use produce low air–liquid surface tension and interfacial tension, and are not readily adsorbed by the solid so as to produce nonwetting behavior.

Pore Penetration—Wetting and surface behavior are particularly important when air in a very fine pore or capillary must be displaced by penetrating solvent, as depicted in Fig 19-17. The rate at which a liquid penetrates a small cylindrical capillary of radius r is, according to Poiseuille's law (see Chapter 22):

$$\frac{dl}{dt} = \frac{Pr^2}{8\eta l} \qquad (36)$$

where l is the distance of penetration, t is the time, η is the viscosity of the liquid, and P is the driving pressure. It has been shown that for fine capillaries the driving pressure is the

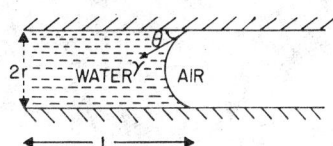

Fig 19-17.   A nonwetting liquid situated in a capillary or pore.[11]

Table VIII—Parameters Characterizing the Salicylic Acid–Polyethylene System as a Function of Polysorbate 80 Concentration

Solvent, 0.1 M K$_2$HPO$_4$ in % polysorbate	$\theta°$	Cos θ	γ_L, dyne/ cm	γ_L Cos θ	$Q/t^{1/2}$ * × 10^6 g/sec$^{1/2}$
0	98	−0.156	59.0	−9.20	1.32
0.001	97	−0.139	42.6	−5.92	1.60
0.005	93	−0.070	44.0	−3.08	1.94
0.01	87	+0.052	38.4	2.00	2.22
0.05	59	+0.515	38.2	19.67	4.26
0.10	46	+0.695	40.0	27.80	5.20

* $Q/t^{1/2}$ is proportional to drug-release rate.

capillary pressure produced by the curved surfaces of the capillary. Thus assuming that there are cylindrical pores in Eq 36 one can substitute for P by using Eq 16 and obtain an expression for the rate of penetration:

$$\frac{dl}{dt} = \frac{\gamma \cos \theta \, r}{4\eta l} \qquad (37)$$

From Eq 37 it is apparent that an increase in r or $\gamma \cos \theta$ will favor greater penetration of pores, while increased viscosity will reduce penetration. Thus in order to bring about penetration one must cause the value of $\gamma \cos \theta$ to be positive ($\theta <$ 90°) and as large as possible, without increasing viscosity. It is apparent, therefore, that a decrease in γ of the penetrating fluid is much less important than is a direct effect on the solid surface so as to reduce the contact angle. The diffusion-controlled release of drugs from polyethylene tablets used for delayed-release purposes was found to be dependent on the penetration of solvent into pores of the tablet. Table VIII shows that the release rate of salicylic acid increases with the addition of surface-active agent. It is interesting that, as suggested above, the increase in penetration rate is not due to changes in surface tension because these values are fairly constant after 0.001% polysorbate 80. Rather, note the significant effect directly on the contact angle with each increase in polysorbate 80 concentration. Presumably the polysorbate 80 is adsorbing on the solid surface and making it more polar and, thus, more wettable by water. Looking at Eq 9, this means that the term $\gamma_{SV} - \gamma_{SL}$ has been reduced.

References

1. Semat H: *Fundamentals of Physics*, 3rd ed, Holt-Rinehart-Winston, New York, 1957.
2. Michaels AS: *J Phys Chem 65:* 1730, 1961.
3. Zisman WA: *Advan Chem Ser 43:* 1, 1964.
4. Titoff Z: *Z Phys Chem 74:* 641, 1910.
5. Lowell S: *Introduction to Power Surface Area*, Wiley-Interscience, New York, 1979.
6. Osipow LI: *Surface Chemistry: Theory and Industrial Applications*, Reinhold, New York, 1962.
7. Langmuir I: *J Am Chem Soc 39:* 1848, 1917.
8. Giles CH: *Anionic Surfactants*, ed EH Lucassen-Reynders Marcel Dekker, New York, 1981, Ch 4.
9. Weiser HB: *A Textbook of Colloid Chemistry*, Elsevier, New York, 1949.
10. Ter Minassian-Saraga L: *Advan Chem Ser 43:* 232, 1964.
11. Washburn EW: *Phys Rev 17:* 273, 374, 1921.

Bibliography

Adamson AW: *Physical Chemistry of Surfaces*, 4th ed, Interscience, New York, 1982.
Davis JT, Rideal EK: *Interfacial Phenomena*, 2nd ed, Academic, New York, 1963.
Hiemenz, PC: *Principles of Colloid and Surface Chemistry*, Marcel Dekker, New York, 1977.
Shaw DJ: *Introduction to Colloid and Surface Chemistry*, Butterworths, London, 1968.

CHAPTER 20

Colloidal Dispersions

Hans Schott, PhD

Professor of Pharmaceutics
School of Pharmacy, Temple University
Philadelphia, PA 19140

Historical Background

The term *colloid*, derived from the Greek word for glue, was applied *ca* 1850 by the British chemist Thomas Graham to polypeptides such as albumin and gelatin, to vegetable gums such as acacia, starch and dextrin, and to inorganic compounds such as gelatinous metal hydroxides and Prussian blue (ferric ferrocyanide). These compounds did not crystallize, and diffused very slowly when dissolved or dispersed in water. They could be separated from ordinary solutes such as salts and sugar, called "crystalloids," as the latter diffused through the fine pores of dialysis membranes made from animal gut which retained the "colloids." "Crystalloids" crystallized readily from solution.[1–3]

Von Weimarn was the first to identify colloidality as a state of subdivision of matter rather than as a category of substances. Many of Graham's "colloids," especially proteins, have been crystallized. Moreover, von Weimarn was able to prepare all "crystalloids" investigated in the colloidal state. Colloidal dispersions by the condensation method resulted from high relative supersaturation, which produced a large number of small nuclei.[1–4] For instance, clear, transparent solidified jellies were prepared by cooling aqueous solutions of $CaCl_2$, $Ba(SCN)_2$, and $Al_2(SO_4)_3$ and aqueous-alcoholic solutions of NaCl, KCl, NH_4Cl, KSCN, NaBr, and NH_4NO_3 which were nearly saturated at room temperature.[4]

Colloid chemistry became a science in its own right around 1906, when Wolfgang Ostwald wrote the booklet "The World of the Neglected Dimensions." In it, he focused on colloidal systems as a state of matter that has disperse phases intermediate in size between small molecules or ions in solution and large, visible particles in suspension. Otwald became the first editor of the journal *Kolloid-Zeitschrift* in 1907. The studies of colloidal systems and surface or interfacial phenomena (Chapter 19) are intimately related. The properties of colloidal dispersions are largely governed by the nature of the surface of their particles. The division of the American Chemical Society specializing in colloidal systems and interfaces is called the "Division of Colloid and Surface Chemistry," while the pertinent session of the Gordon Research Conferences is called "Chemistry at Interfaces."

Colloid and surface chemistry deals with an unusually wide variety of industrial and biological systems. A few examples are catalysts, lubricants, adhesives, latexes for paints, rubbers and plastics, soaps and detergents, clays, packaging films, cigarette smoke, liquid crystals, cell membranes, mucous secretions, and aqueous humors.

Definitions and Classifications

Colloidal Systems and Interfaces

Colloidal dispersions consist of at least two discrete phases, namely, one or more disperse, dispersed or internal phases and a continuous or external phase called the *dispersion medium* or *vehicle*. What distinguishes colloidal dispersions from solutions and coarse dispersions is the particle size of the disperse phase. Systems in the colloidal state contain one or more substances that have at least one dimension in the range of 10 to 100 Å (1 Angstrom unit = 10^{-8} cm = 10^{-10} m) or 1–10 nm (1 nanometer = 10^{-9} m) at the lower end, and a few microns (μ) or micrometers (μm) at the upper end (1 μ or 1 μm = 10^4 Å = 10^{-6} m). Thus blood, cell membranes, the thinner nerve fibers, milk, rubber latex, fog, and beer foam are colloidal systems. Some types of materials, such as many emulsions, and oral suspensions of most organic drugs, are coarser than true colloidal systems but exhibit similar behavior. Even though serum albumin, acacia and povidone form true or molecular solutions in water, the size of the individual solute molecules places such solutions in the colloidal range (particle size > 10 Å).[1,2,3,5–8]

The following features distinguish colloidal dispersions from coarse suspensions. Disperse particles in the colloidal range are usually too fine to be visible in a light microscope, because at least one dimension measures 1 μm or less. They are often visible in the ultramicroscope and always in the electron microscope. Coarse suspended particles are frequently visible to the naked eye and always in the light microscope. Colloidal particles, as opposed to coarse particles, pass through ordinary filter paper but are retained by dialysis or ultrafiltration membranes. Because of their small size, colloidal dispersions undergo little or no sedimentation or creaming: Brownian motion maintains the disperse particles in suspension (see below).

Except for high polymers, most soluble substances can be prepared either as low-molecular-weight solutions, or as colloidal dispersions or coarse suspensions depending on the choice of the dispersion medium and the dispersion technique.[4,7]

Because of the small size of colloidal particles, appreciable fractions of their atoms, ions or molecules are located in the boundary layer between a particle and air (surface) or between a particle and a liquid or solid (interface). The ions in the surface of a sodium chloride crystal and the water molecules in the surface of a rain drop are subjected to unbalanced forces of attraction, whereas the ions or molecules in the interior of the materials are surrounded by similar ions or molecules on all sides, with balanced force fields. Thus a surface free energy component is added to the total free energy of colloidal particles, which becomes relatively more important as the particles become smaller, ie, as greater fractions of their ions, atoms or molecules are located in their surface or interfacial region. Hence the solubility of very fine solid particles and the vapor pressure of very small liquid droplets are larger than the corresponding values of coarse particles and large drops of the same materials, respectively.

Specific Surface Area—Decreasing particle size increases the surface-to-volume ratio, which is expressed as the specific surface area A_{sp}, namely, the area A (cm^2) per unit volume V

Table I—Effect of Comminution on Specific Surface Area of a Volume of $4\pi/3$ cm³, Divided into Uniform Spheres of Radius R

Number of spheres	R	A_{sp} cm²/cm³
1	1 cm	3
10^3	0.1 cm = 1 mm	3×10
10^6	0.1 mm	3×10^2
10^9	0.01 mm = 10 μm	3×10^3
10^{12}	1 μm	3×10^4
10^{15}	0.1 μm	3×10^5
10^{18}	0.01 μm	3×10^6
10^{21}	10 Å = 1 nm	3×10^7
10^{23}	1 Å	3×10^8

Shaded region corresponds to colloidal particle size range.

(1 cm³) or per unit mass M (1 gram). For a sphere, $A = 4\pi r^2$ and $V = 4/3 \pi r^3$. If the density, d, of the material is expressed in g/cm³, the specific surface area is

$$A_{sp} = \frac{A}{V} = \frac{4\pi r^2}{4/3\pi r^3} = \frac{3}{r} \text{ cm}^2/\text{cm}^3 = \frac{3}{r} \text{ cm}^{-1}$$

or

$$A_{sp} = \frac{A}{M} = \frac{A}{Vd} = \frac{4\pi r^2}{4/3\pi r^3 d} = \frac{3}{rd} \text{ cm}^2/\text{g}$$

Table I illustrates the effect of comminution on the specific surface area of $4\pi/3$ cm³ of a material consisting initially of one sphere of 1 cm radius. As the material is broken up into an increasingly larger number of smaller and smaller spheres, its specific surface area increases commensurately.

The solid adsorbents activated charcoal and kaolin have specific surface areas of about 6×10^6 cm²/g and 10^4 cm²/g, respectively. One gram of activated charcoal, because of its extensive porosity and internal voids, has an area equal to ⅙ acre.

In conclusion, colloidal systems by definition are those polyphasic systems where at least one dimension of the disperse phase measures between 10 or 100 Å and a few microns. The term "colloidal" designates a state of matter characterized by submicroscopic dimensions rather than certain substances. Any dispersed substance with the proper dimension or dimensions is in the colloidal state.

Physical States of Disperse and Continuous Phases

A useful classification of colloidal systems (systems in the colloidal particle size range) is based on the state of matter of the disperse phase and the dispersion medium, ie, whether they are solid, liquid or gaseous.[2,3,8] Table II summarizes the various combinations and lists examples. A *sol* is the colloidal dispersion of a solid in a liquid or gaseous medium. Prefixes designate the dispersion medium, such as hydrosol, alcosol, aerosol for water, alcohol and air, respectively. Sols are fluid. If the solid particles form bridged structures possessing some mechanical strength, the system is called a gel (hydrogel, alcogel, aerogel).

Interaction Between Disperse Phase and Dispersion Medium

A second useful classification of colloidal dispersions, originated by Ostwald, is based on the affinity or interaction between the disperse phase and the dispersion medium.[2,3,8] It refers mostly to solid-in-liquid dispersions. According to this classification, colloidal dispersions are divided into the two broad categories of lyophilic and lyophobic. Some soluble, low-molecular-weight substances have molecules with both tendencies, forming a third category called association colloids.

Lyophilic Dispersions—Where there is considerable attraction between the disperse phase and the liquid vehicle, ie, extensive solvation, the system is said to be *lyophilic* (solvent-loving). If the dispersion medium is water, the system is said to be *hydrophilic*. Such solids as bentonite, starch, gelatin, acacia and povidone swell, disperse or dissolve spontaneously in water.

Hydrophilic colloidal dispersions can be further subdivided as follows: (a) True solutions, formed by water-soluble polymers (acacia and povidone). (b) Gelled solutions, gels or jellies if the polymers are present at high concentrations and/or at temperatures where their water solubility is low. Examples of such hydrogels are relatively concentrated solutions of gelatin and starch, which set to gels on cooling, or of methylcellulose, which gel on heating. (c) Particulate dispersions, where the solids do not form molecular solutions but remain as discrete though minute particles. Bentonite and microcrystalline cellulose form such hydrosols.

Lipophilic or oleophilic substances have pronounced affinity for oils. Oils are nonpolar liquids consisting mainly of hydrocarbons, with few polar groups and low dielectric constants. Examples are mineral oil, benzene, carbon tetrachloride, vegetable oils (cottonseed or peanut oil) and essential oils (lemon or peppermint oil). Substances which form *oleophilic* colloidal dispersions include polymers like polystyrene and unvulcanized or gum rubber which dissolve molecularly in benzene, magnesium or aluminum stearate which dissolve or disperse in cottonseed oil, and activated charcoal which forms sols or particulate dispersions in all oils.

Because of the high affinity or attraction between the dispersion medium and the disperse phase, lyophilic dispersions

Table II—Classification of Colloidal Dispersions According to State of Matter

Disperse Phase	Dispersion Medium (Vehicle)		
	Solid	Liquid	Gas
Solid	Zinc oxide paste (zinc oxide + starch in petrolatum). Toothpaste (dicalcium phosphate or calcium carbonate with sodium carboxymethylcellulose binder). Pigmented plastics (titanium dioxide in polyethylene).	Sols: Bentonite Magma NF. Trisulfapyrimidines Oral Suspension USP. Magnesia and Alumina Oral Suspension USP. Tetracycline Oral Suspension USP.	Solid aerosols: Smoke, dust. Epinephrine bitartrate inhalation. Isoproterenol Sulfate Aerosol.
Liquid	Absorption bases (aqueous medium in Hydrophilic Petrolatum USP). Emulsion bases (oil in Hydrophilic Ointment USP). Butter.	Emulsions: Mineral Oil Emulsion. Soybean oil in water emulsion for IV feeding. Milk. Mayonnaise.	Liquid aerosols: Mist, fog. Nasal relief sprays (naphazoline hydrochloride solution). Betamethasone Valerate Aerosol. Povidone-Iodine Aerosol.
Gas	Solid foams (foamed plastics and rubbers). Pumice.	Foams. Carbonated beverages. Effervescent salts in water.	No colloidal dispersions.

form spontaneously when the liquid vehicle is brought into contact with the solid phase. They are thermodynamically stable and reversible, ie, they are easily reconstituted even after the dispersion medium has been removed from the solid phase.[2,3,5,7]

Lyophobic Dispersions—When there is little attraction between the disperse phase and the dispersion medium, the dispersion is said to be *lyophobic* (solvent-hating). *Hydrophobic* dispersions consist of particles that are not hydrated, so that water molecules interact with or attract one another in preference to solvating the particles. They include aqueous dispersions of oleophilic materials such as polystyrene or gum rubber (latex), steroids and other organic lipophilic drugs, paraffin wax, magnesium stearate, and of cottonseed or soybean oil (emulsion). While lipophilic materials are generally hydrophobic, materials like sulfur, silver chloride and gold form hydrophobic dispersions without being lipophilic. Water-in-oil emulsions are lyophobic dispersions in lipophilic vehicles.

Because of the lack of attraction between the disperse and the continuous phase, lyophobic dispersions are intrinsically unstable and irreversible. Their large surface free energy is not lowered by solvation. The dispersion process does not take place spontaneously, and once the dispersion medium has been separated from the disperse phase, the dispersion is not easily reconstituted. The dividing line between hydrophilic and hydrophobic dispersions is not very sharp. For instance, gelatinous hydroxides of polyvalent metals such as $Al(OH)_3$ and $Mg(OH)_2$, and clays such as bentonite and kaolin, possess some characteristics of both.[2,3,5]

Association Colloids—Organic compounds which contain large hydrophobic moieties together with strongly hydrophilic groups in the same molecule are said to be amphiphilic. While the individual molecules are generally too small to bring their solutions into the colloidal size range, they tend to associate in aqueous or oil solutions into aggregates called micelles. Because micelles are large enough to qualify as colloidal particles, such compounds are called association colloids.

Lyophobic Dispersions

Most of the discussion of lyophobic dispersions deals with hydrophobic dispersions or hydrosols (hydrophobic solids or liquids dispersed in aqueous media) because water is the most widely used vehicle. They comprise aqueous dispersions of insoluble organic and inorganic compounds which usually have low degrees of hydration. Organic compounds which are preponderantly hydrocarbon in nature and possess few hydrophilic or polar groups are insoluble in water and hydrophobic.

Hydrophobic dispersions are intrinsically unstable. The most stable state of such systems contains the disperse phase coalesced into large crystals or drops, so that the specific surface area and surface free energy are reduced to a minimum. Therefore, mechanical, chemical or electrical energy must be supplied to the system to break up the disperse phase into small particles, providing for the increase in surface free energy resulting from the parallel increase in specific surface area. Furthermore, special means must be found to stabilize hydrophobic dispersions, preventing the otherwise spontaneous coalescence or coagulation of the disperse phase after it has been finely dispersed.

Preparation and Purification of Lyophobic Dispersions

Colloidal dispersions are intermediate in size between true solutions and coarse suspensions. They can be prepared by aggregation of small molecules or ions until particles of colloidal dimensions result (condensation methods), or by reducing coarse particles to colloidal dimensions through comminution or peptization (dispersion methods).

Dispersion Methods—The first method, *mechanical disintegration* of solids and liquids into small particles and their dispersion in a fluid vehicle, is frequently carried out by input of mechanical energy via shear or attrition. Equipment such as colloid and ball mills, micronizers and, for emulsions, homogenizers is described in Chapters 84 and 89 and in Ref 10. Dry grinding with inert, water-soluble diluting agents also produces colloidal dispersions. Sulfur hydrosols may be prepared by triturating the powder with urea or lactose followed by shaking with water.[9]

Ultrasonic generators provide exceptionally high concentrations of energy. Successful dispersion of solids by means of ultrasonic waves can only be achieved with comparatively soft materials such as many organic compounds, sulfur, talcum, and graphite. Where fine emulsions are mandatory, such as soybean oil-in-water emulsions used for intravenous feeding, emulsification by ultrasound waves is the method of choice.[10] The formation of aerosols is described in Chap 93.

It should be reiterated that hydrosols of hydrophobic substances are intrinsically unstable. While mechanical disintegration may break up the disperse phase into colloidal particles, the resultant dispersions tend towards separation of that phase. Recrystallization, coagulation or coalescence causes the disperse particles to become progressively coarser and fewer, ultimately resulting in the separation of a macroscopic phase. To avoid this, stabilizing agents must be added during or shortly after the dispersion process (see below). For instance, lecithin may be used to stabilize soybean oil emulsions.

Peptization is a second method for preparing colloidal dispersions. The term, coined by Graham, is defined as the breaking up of aggregates or secondary particles into smaller aggregates or into primary particles in the colloidal size range. Particles which are not formed of smaller ones are called "primary." Peptization is synonymous with *deflocculation*. It can be brought about by the removal of flocculating agents, usually electrolytes, or by the addition of deflocculating or peptizing agents, usually surfactants, water-soluble polymers or ions which are adsorbed at the particle surface.[3,5,8,9]

The mechanisms of the following examples are explained in subsequent sections. When powdered activated charcoal is added to water with stirring, the aggregated grains are broken up only incompletely and the resultant suspension is gray and translucent. The addition of 0.1% or less of sodium lauryl sulfate or octoxynol disintegrates the grains into finely dispersed particles forming a deep black and opaque dispersion. Ferric or aluminum hydroxide freshly precipitated with ammonia can be peptized with small amounts of acids which reduce the pH below the isoelectric points of the hydroxides (see below). Even washing the gelatinous precipitate of $Al(OH)_3$ with water tends to peptize it. In quantitative analysis, the precipitate is therefore washed with dilute solutions of ammonium salts that act as flocculating agents, rather than with water.

Condensation Methods—The preparation of sulfur hydrosols is employed to illustrate condensation or aggregation methods. Sulfur is insoluble in water but somewhat soluble in alcohol. When an alcoholic solution of sulfur is mixed with water, a bluish white colloidal dispersion results. In the absence of added stabilizing agents, the particles tend to agglomerate and precipitate on standing. This technique of dissolving the material in a water-miscible solvent such as alcohol or acetone and producing a hydrosol by precipitation with water is applicable to many organic compounds, and has been used to prepare hydrosols of natural resins like mastic and of stearic acid.

For sulfur, another less common physical method is to introduce a current of sulfur vapor into water. Condensation produces colloidal particles. Alternatively, the very fine powder produced by condensing sulfur vapor on cold solid surfaces (sublimed sulfur or flowers of sulfur) can be dispersed in water by addition of a suitable surfactant to produce a hydrosol.

Chemical methods include the reaction between hydrogen sulfide and sulfur dioxide, eg, by bubbling H_2S into an aqueous SO_2 solution:

$$2\ H_2S + SO_2 \rightarrow 3\ S + 2\ H_2O$$

The same reaction occurs when aqueous solutions containing sodium sulfide and sulfite are acidified with an excess of sulfuric or hydrochloric acid. Another reaction is the decomposition of sodium thiosulfate by sulfuric acid, using either very dilute or very concentrated solutions to obtain colloidally dispersed sulfur:

$$H_2SO_4 + 3\ Na_2S_2O_3 \rightarrow 4\ S + 3\ Na_2SO_4 + H_2O$$

Both reactions also produce pentathionic acid, $H_2S_5O_6$, as a by-product. The preferential adsorption of the pentathionate anion at the surface of the sulfur particles confers a negative electric charge on the particles, stabilizing the sol (see below).[3,7-9] When powdered sulfur is boiled with a slurry of lime, it dissolves with the formation of calcium pentasulfide and thiosulfate. Subsequent acidification produces the colloidal "milk of sulfur," which on washing and drying yields Precipitated Sulfur USP (see Chapter 83).

Sols of ferric, aluminum, chromic, stannic and titanium hydroxides or hydrous oxides are produced by hydrolysis of the corresponding chlorides or nitrates:

$$AlCl_3 + 3\ H_2O \rightleftharpoons Al(OH)_3 + 3\ HCl$$

Hydrolysis is promoted by boiling the solution and/or by adding a base to neutralize the acid formed.

Double decompositions producing insoluble salts can lead to colloidal dispersions. Examples are silver chloride and nickel sulfide:

$$NaCl + AgNO_3 \rightarrow AgCl + NaNO_3$$

$$(NH_4)_2S + NiCl_2 \rightarrow NiS + 2\ NH_4Cl$$

Compare also the preparation of White Lotion, which contains precipitated zinc sulfide and sulfur (Chapter 65). Reducing salts of gold, silver, copper, mercury, platinum, rhodium and palladium with formaldehyde, hydrazine, hydroxylamine, hydroquinone or stannous chloride produces hydrosols of the metals. These are strongly colored, eg, red or blue.[1,3,8,9]

Radioactive Colloids—Colloidal dispersions containing radioactive isotopes find increasing diagnostic and therapeutic application in nuclear medicine. Radioactive colloids that accumulate in tumors and/or lesions or emboli, indicating their location and size, may be used as diagnostic aids. Radioactive colloids with a particle size of about 300 Å, injected intravenously, locate mainly in the reticuloendothelial systems of liver, spleen and other organs and are used in scintillation imaging. The radiation emitted by the colloids is made visible by stationary or scanning devices which show the location, size and shape of the organ being investigated, as well as any tumors within. Radiocolloids are useful in anticancer radiation therapy because of their low solubility, radiation characteristics, and their ability to accumulate and remain located in certain target organs or tumors.[11]

Colloidal gold Au 198 is made by reducing a solution of gold ([198]Au) chloride either by treatment with ascorbic acid or by heating with an alkaline glucose solution. Gelatin is added as a protective colloid (see below). The particle size ranges from 50 to 500Å with a mean of 300 Å. The color of the sol is cherry-red in transmitted light. Violet or blue sols have excessively large particle sizes and should be discarded. Col-

loidal gold is used as a diagnostic and therapeutic aid (see Chapter 29). The half-life of [198]Au is 2.7 days.

Technetium 99m sulfur colloid is prepared by reducing sodium pertechnetate ^{99m}Tc with sodium thiosulfate. The product, a mixture of technetium sulfide and sulfur in the colloidal particle size range, is stabilized with gelatin. It is used chiefly in liver, spleen and bone scanning. Its half-life is 6.0 hr.

Microspheres of gelatin or human serum albumin can be prepared in fairly narrow particle-size ranges from 100–200 Å through 45–55 μm. A variety of β- and γ-emitting radionuclides such as ^{131}I, ^{99m}Tc, [113m]In, or ^{51}Cr can be incorporated to label the microspheres. Such products have been used to scan heart, brain, urogenital and gastrointestinal tracts, liver, and in pulmonary perfusion and inhalation studies.[11]

Organic compounds that are weak bases, such as alkaloids, are usually much more soluble at lower pH values where they are ionized than at higher pH values where they exist as the free base. Increasing the pH of their aqueous solutions well above their pKa may cause precipitation of the free base. Organic compounds which are weak acids, such as barbiturates, are usually much more soluble at higher pH values where they are ionized than at lower pH values where they are in the un-ionized acid form. Lowering the pH of their solutions well below their pKa may cause precipitation of the un-ionized acid. Depending on the supersaturation of the un-ionized acids or bases and on the presence of stabilizing agents, the resultant dispersions may be in the colloidal range.

Kinetics of Particle Formation—When the solubility of a compound in water is exceeded, its solution becomes supersaturated and the compound may precipitate or crystallize. The rate of precipitation, the particle size (whether colloidal or coarse), and the particle size uniformity or distribution (whether a narrow distribution and nearly monodisperse or homodisperse particles, or a broad distribution and polydisperse or heterodisperse particles) depend on two successive and largely independent processes, nucleation and growth of nuclei.

When a solution of a salt or of sucrose is supercooled, or when a chemical reaction produces a salt in a concentration exceeding its solubility product, separation of the excess solid from the supersaturated solution is far from instantaneous. Clusters of ions or molecules called nuclei must exceed a critical size before they become stable and capable of growing into colloidal size crystals. These embryonic particles have much more surface for a given weight of material than large and stable crystals, resulting in higher surface free energy and greater solubility.

Whether *nucleation* takes place depends on the *relative supersaturation*. If C is the actual concentration of the solute before crystallization has set in, and C_s is its solubility limit, $C - C_s$ is the supersaturation and $(C - C_s)/C_s$ is the relative supersaturation. Von Weimarn recognized that the rate or velocity of nucleation (number of nuclei formed per liter per second) is proportional to the relative supersaturation. Nucleation seldom occurs at relative supersaturations below 3. The foregoing statement refers to homogeneous nucleation, where the nuclei are clusters of the same chemical composition as the crystallizing phase. If the solution contains solid impurities, such as dust particles in suspension, these may act as nuclei or centers of crystallization (heterogeneous nucleation).[2,4,7-9]

Once nuclei have formed, the second process, *crystallization*, begins. Nuclei grow by accretion of ions or molecules from solution forming colloidal or coarser particles until the supersaturation is relieved, ie, until $C = C_s$. The rate of crystallization or growth of nuclei is proportional to the supersaturation. The appropriate equation,

$$\frac{dm}{dt} = \frac{A_{sp}D}{\delta}(C - C_s)$$

is similar to the Noyes-Whitney equation governing the dissolution of particles (see Chapter 35) except that $C < C_s$ for the latter process, making dm/dt negative. In both equations, m is the mass of material crystallizing out in time t, D is the diffusion coefficient of the molecules or ions of the solute, δ is the length of the diffusion path or the thickness of the liquid layer adhering to the growing particles, and A_{sp} is their specific surface area. The presence of dissolved impurities may affect the rate of crystallization and even change the crystal habit, provided that these impurities are surface-active and become adsorbed on the nuclei or growing crystals.[2,3,4,7-9]

Von Weimarn found that the particle size of the crystals depends strongly on the concentration of the precipitating substance. At a very low concentration and slight relative supersaturation, diffusion is quite slow because the concentration gradient is very small. Sufficient nuclei will usually form to relieve the slight supersaturation locally. Crystal growth is limited by the small amount of excess dissolved material available to each particle. Hence, the particles cannot grow beyond colloidal dimensions. This condition is represented by points A, D, and G of the schematic plot of von Weimarn (Fig 20-1). At intermediate concentrations, the extent of nucleation is somewhat greater but much more material is available for crystal growth. Coarse crystals rather than colloidal particles result (points B, E, or H).

At high concentrations, nuclei appear so quickly and in such large numbers that supersaturation is relieved almost immediately, before appreciable diffusion occurs. The high viscosity of the medium also slows down diffusion of excess dissolved ions or molecules, retarding crystal growth without substantially affecting the rate of nucleation. A large number of very small particles results which, because of their proximity, tend to link, producing a translucent gel (points C and F). On subsequent dilution with water, such gels usually yield colloidal dispersions.

Thus, colloidal systems are usually produced at very low and high concentrations. Intermediate values of supersaturation tend to produce coarse crystals. Low solubility is a necessary condition for producing colloidal dispersions. If the solubility of the precipitate is increased, for instance by heating the dispersion, a new family of curves will result, similar in shape to ABC, DEF, and GHI of Fig 20-1, but displaced upwards (towards larger particle sizes) and to the right (towards higher concentrations).[3,4,6,9]

Condensation methods generally produce polydisperse sols because nucleation continues while established nuclei grow. The particles in the resultant dispersion grew from nuclei formed at different times and had different growth periods. The formation of monodisperse sols requires special techniques.[2,5,6,8]

A feature of Fig 20-1 is that aging increases the particle size. Curves ABC, DEF, and GHI correspond to increasing times after mixing the reagents. Typical ages are 10–30 min, several hours, and weeks or years, respectively. This gradual increase in particle size of crystals in their mother liquor is a recrystallization process called *Ostwald ripening*. Very small particles have a higher solubility than large particles of the same substance owing to their greater specific surface area and higher surface free energy. In a saturated solution containing precipitated particles of the solute in a wide range of particle sizes, the very smallest particles dissolve spontaneously and the material deposits onto the large particles. The growth of the large crystals at the expense of the very small ones occurs because this process lowers the free energy of the dispersion. As mentioned above, the most stable system is the suspension of a few coarse crystals, whereas the colloidal dispersion of a great many fine particles of the same substance is intrinsically less stable.

The spontaneous coarsening of colloidal dispersions on aging is accelerated by a relatively high solubility of the precipitate and can be retarded by lowering the solubility or by adding traces of surface-active compounds which are adsorbed at the particle surface. For instance, barium sulfate precipitated by mixing concentrated solutions of sodium sulfate and barium chloride is largely in the colloidal range and passes through filter paper. The colloidal particles gradually grow in size by Ostwald ripening, forming large crystals which can be removed quantitatively by filtration. Heating the aqueous dispersion speeds up this recrystallization by increasing the solubility of barium sulfate in water. The addition of ethyl alcohol lowers the solubility, retarding Ostwald ripening so that the dispersion remains in the colloidal state for years.

Another process by which particles in colloidal dispersions grow in size is by agglomeration of individual particles into aggregates. This process, called coagulation, is discussed below.

Purification of Hydrosols by Dialysis and Ultrafiltration

Many hydrosols contain low molecular-weight, water-soluble impurities. Inorganic dispersions often contain salts formed by the reaction producing the disperse phase. Salts are especially objectionable in the case of hydrophobic dispersions because they tend to coagulate such dispersions. Protein solutions often contain salts added as part of the separation procedure. The blood of patients with renal insufficiency contains excessive concentrations of urea and other low-molecular-weight metabolites and salts. These dissolved impurities of small molecular size are removed from the colloidal dispersions by means of membranes with pore openings smaller than the colloidal particles.

Membranes—Conventional filter papers are permeable to colloidal particles as well as to small solute molecules. Among the early membranes capable of retaining colloidal particles but permeable to small solute molecules were pig's bladder and parchment. Most membranes in current use consist of cellulose, cellulose nitrate prepared from collodion, cellulose acetate or synthetic polymers, and are available in a variety of shapes, gauges, and pore sizes. *Gel cellophane* is most widely used. It consists of sheets or tubes of cellulose made by extruding cellulose xanthate solutions (viscose) through slit or annular dies into a sodium bisulfate/sulfuric acid bath which decomposes the xanthate, precipitating the regenerated cellulose in a highly swollen or gel state. If the cellulose film were permitted to dry after purification and washing with water, it would crystallize and shrink excessively,

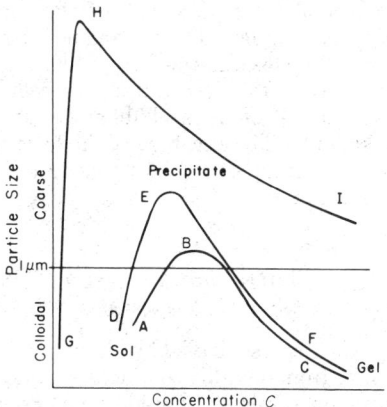

Fig 20-1. Effect of the concentration of the precipitating material and of aging on particle size.[4] Curves ABC, DEF, and GHI correspond to increasing aging. Both axes are on a logarithmic scale.

losing most of its extensive pore structure and turning somewhat brittle. The film is therefore impregnated with glycerin
before drying. Glycerin remains in the film rather than
evaporating like water. It reduces the shrinkage and blocks
crystallization. This action prevents the collapse of the porous gel structure and plasticizes the film, keeping it flexible.
A typical dialysis tube made from sausage casing swells to
about twice its thickness in water and has an average pore
diameter of 34 Å. While the pore structure of cellophane films
used in dialysis and ultrafiltration causes retention of colloidal
particles but permits the passage of small solute molecules,
osmotic membranes are only permeable to water and retain
small solute molecules as well as colloidal particles.

Dialysis—The colloidal dispersion is placed inside a sac
made of sausage casing dipping in water. The small solute
molecules diffuse out into the water while the colloidal material remains trapped inside because of its size. The rate of
dialysis is increased by increasing the area of the membrane,
by stirring, and by maintaining a high concentration gradient
across the membrane. For the latter purpose, the water is
replenished continuously or at least frequently. A membrane
configuration which provides a particularly extensive transfer
area for a given volume of dispersion is the hollow fiber. A
typical fiber measures 175 μm inside diameter and 225 μm
outside diameter. The dispersion to be dialyzed is circulated
inside a bundle of parallel fibers while water is circulated
outside the fibers throughout the bundle. Dialysis of the
diffusing species takes place across the thin fiber wall. Dialysis is used in the laboratory to purify sols and to study
binding of drugs by proteins, as well as in some manufacturing
processes.

Electrodialysis—If the low-molecular-weight impurities
to be removed are electrolytes, the dialysis can be speeded up
by applying an electric potential to the sol which produces
electrolysis. An electrodialyzer (Fig 20-2) is divided into three
compartments by two dialysis membranes supported by
screens. The two outer compartments, in which the two
electrodes are placed, are filled with water while the sol is
placed into the center compartment. Under the influence of
the applied potential, the anions migrate from the sol into the
anode (right) compartment while the cations migrate into the
cathode compartment. Low-molecular-weight nonelectrolyte
solutes diffuse into either compartment.

Colloidal particles are usually charged and therefore tend
to migrate towards the membrane sealing off the compartment
with the electrode of opposite charge. The combination of
electrophoresis (see below) and gravitational sedimentation
produces the accumulation of negatively charged sol particles
shown in Fig 20-2. Hence the supernatant liquid can be
changed by decantation. This process, which may be used
to speed up electrodialysis, is called *electrodecantation*.[1,3,9]

Ultrafiltration—When a sol is placed in a compartment
closed by a dialysis membrane and pressure is applied, the
liquid and the small solute molecules are forced through the
membrane while the colloidal particles are retained. This
process, called ultrafiltration, is based on a sieving mechanism
in which all components smaller than the pore size of the filter

membrane pass through it. The pressure difference required
to push the dispersion medium through the ultrafilter is
provided by gas pressure applied on the sol side or by suction
on the filtrate side. The membrane is usually supported on
a fine wire screen.[3,9]

As ultrafiltrate is being removed, the sol becomes more
concentrated because a constant amount of disperse particles
is confined to a decreasing volume of liquid. Some dissolved
small molecules or ions are left in the sol together with the
residual water. To avoid the increase in concentration of the
colloidal particles and remove the dissolved impurities completely, the ultrafiltrate squeezed from the sol is replenished
continuously or intermittently with an equal volume of water.
During ultrafiltration, solids tend to accumulate on and near
the membrane. To prevent this buildup and maintain uniform composition throughout the sol, it is stirred.

Bundles of hollow fibers are used for ultrafiltration in the
laboratory and on large scale. To withstand higher pressures,
the wall thickness of the fibers used in ultrafiltration is usually
greater than that of fibers used exclusively for dialysis. When
hollow fibers are fouled by excessive accumulation of solids
on the inner wall, they are cleaned by backflushing with water
or ultrafiltrate.

Hemodialysis—The blood of uremic patients is dialyzed
periodically in "artificial kidney" dialyzers to remove urea,
creatinine, uric acid, phosphate and other metabolites, and
excess sodium and potassium chloride. The dialyzing fluid
contains sodium, potassium, calcium, chloride and acetate ions
(the latter are converted in the body to bicarbonate), dextrose
and other constituents in the same concentration as normal
plasma. Since it contains no urea, creatinine, uric acid,
phosphate nor any of the other metabolites normally eliminated by the kidneys, these compounds diffuse from the patient's blood into the dialyzing fluid until their concentration
is the same in blood and fluid. Sodium and potassium chloride diffuse from blood to fluid because of their higher initial
concentration in the blood, and continue to diffuse until the
concentration is equalized. The volume of dialyzing fluid is
much greater than that of blood. The great disparity in volume and the replenishment of dialyzate with fresh fluid ensure
that the metabolites and the excess of electrolytes are removed
almost completely from the blood. Hemodialysis is also
employed in acute poisoning cases.

Plasma proteins and blood cells cannot pass through the
dialysis membrane because of their size. Edema resulting
from water retention can be relieved by ultrafiltration through
the application of a slight pressure on the blood side or a
partial vacuum on the fluid side.

The three geometries used to circulate the blood and the
dialyzing fluid in a countercurrent fashion are a coil of flattened cellulose tubing wound concentrically with a supporting
mesh screen around a core, a stack of flat cellulose sheets
separated by ridged or grooved plates, and hollow fibers. The
regenerated cellulose used in the former two is precipitated
from a cuprammonium solution. The hollow cellulose acetate
fibers have an outside diameter of about 270 μm and a wall
thickness of 30 μm.[12] The advantage of hollow fibers is their
compactness. A bundle of 10,000 fibers 18 cm long has a
surface area of 1.4 m^2.

Particle Shape, Optical, and Transport Properties of Lyophobic Dispersions

Hydrophobic materials handled by pharmacists in aqueous
dispersion range from metallic conductors to inorganic precipitates to organic solids and liquids which are electric in-
sulators. Despite the great diversity of the hydrophobic
disperse phase, their hydrosols have certain common characteristics.

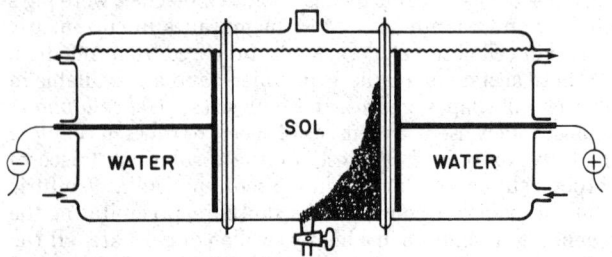

Fig 20-2. Electrodialyzer showing electrodecantation.

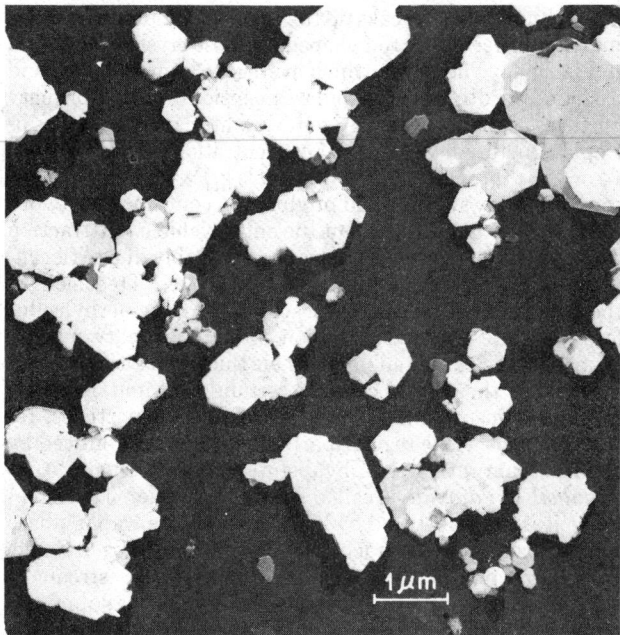

Fig 20-3. Transmission electron micrograph of a well crystallized, fine–particle kaolin. Note hexagonal shape of the clay platelets (courtesy, John L. Brown, Engineering Experiment Station, Georgia Institute of Technology).

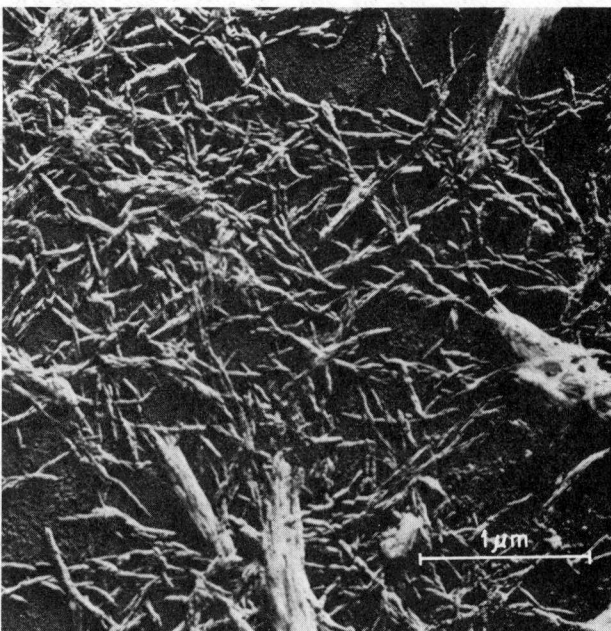

Fig 20-4. Transmission electron micrograph of Avicel RC-591 thickening grade microcrystalline cellulose. The needles are individual cellulose crystallites; some are aggregated into bundles (courtesy, FMC Corporation; Avicel is a registered trademark of FMC Corporation).

Particle Shape and Particle Size Distribution—Both of these properties depend on the chemical and physical nature of the disperse phase and on the method employed to prepare the dispersion. Primary particles exist in a great variety of shapes. Their aggregation produces an even greater variety of shapes and structures. Precipitation and mechanical comminution generally produce randomly shaped particles unless the precipitating solids possess pronounced crystallization habits or the solids being ground possess strongly developed cleavage planes. Precipitated aluminum hydroxide gels and micronized particles of sulfonamides and other organic powders have typical irregular random shapes. An exception is bismuth subnitrate. Even though its particles are precipitated by hydrolyzing bismuth nitrate solutions with sodium carbonate, its particles are lath-shaped. Precipitated silver chloride particles have a cubic habit which is apparent under the electron microscope. Lamellar or plate-like solids in which the molecular cohesion between layers is much weaker than within layers frequently preserve their lamellar shape during mechanical comminution, because milling and micronization break up stacks of thin plates in addition to fragmenting plates in the lateral dimensions. Examples are graphite, mica, and kaolin. Fig 20-5 shows a Georgia crude clay as mined. Processing yields the refined, fine-particle kaolinite of Fig 20-3. Similarly, macroscopic asbestos and cellulose fibers consist of bundles of microscopic and submicroscopic fibrils. Mechanical comminution or beating splits these bundles into the component fibrils of very small diameters as well as cutting them shorter.

Microcrystalline cellulose is a fibrous thickening agent and tablet additive made by selective hydrolysis of cellulose. Native cellulose consists of crystalline regions where the polymer chains are well aligned and in registry, with maximum interchain attraction by secondary valence forces, called crystallites, and of more disordered regions having lower density and reduced interchain attraction and crystallinity, the so-called "amorphous" regions. During treatment with dilute mineral acid, the acid penetrates the amorphous regions relatively fast and hydrolyzes the polymer chains into water-soluble fragments. If the acid is washed out before it

penetrates the crystalline regions appreciably, the crystallites remain intact. Wet milling and spray-drying the aqueous suspension produces spongy and porous aggregates of rod-shaped or fibrillar bundles shown in Fig 20-6. These aggregates, averaging 100 μm in size, were embrittled by the acid treatment and lost the elasticity of the native cellulose. They are well compressible and capable of undergoing plastic deformation, a property important in tableting. Their porosity permits the aggregates to absorb liquid ingredients while still remaining a free-flowing powder, thus preventing these liquids from reducing the flowability of the granulation or direct-

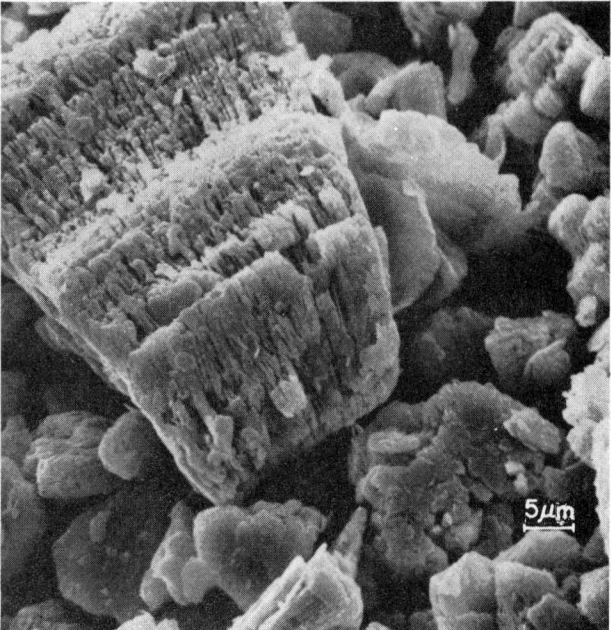

Fig 20-5. Scanning electron micrograph of a crude kaolin clay as mined. Processing yields the fine particle material of Fig 20-3 (courtesy, John L. Brown, Engineering Experiment Station, Georgia Institute of Technology).

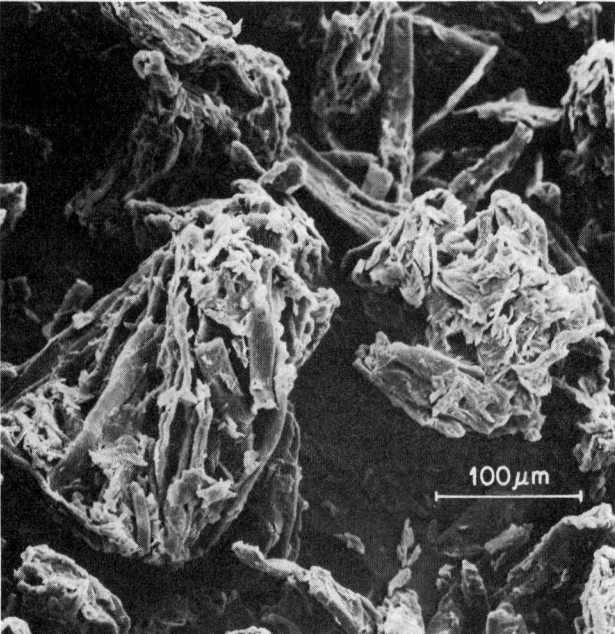

Fig 20-6.   Scanning electron micrograph of Avicel PH-102 tableting grade microcrystalline cellulose. The aggregates of fiber bundles are porous and compressible (courtesy, FMC Corporation; Avicel is a registered trademark of FMC Corporation).

compression mass during tableting. The swelling of the cellulosic particles in water speeds up the disintegration of the ingested tablets.

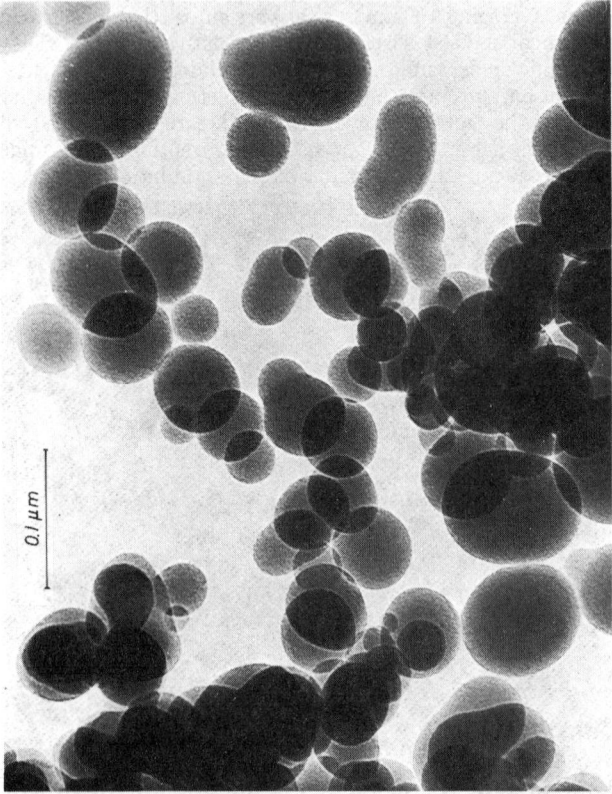

Fig 20-7.   Transmission electron micrograph of Aerosil OX 50, ground and dusted on. The spheres are translucent to the electron beam, causing overlapping portions to be darker owing to increased thickness (courtesy, Degussa AG of Hanau, West Germany; Aerosil is a registered trademark of Degussa). The suffix 50 indicates the specific surface area in m²/g.

Additional shear breaks up the aggregated bundles into the individual, needle- or rod-shaped cellulose crystallites shown in Fig 20-4. The latter, which average 0.3 μm in length and 0.02 μm in width, are of colloidal dimensions. These primary particles act as suspending agents in water, producing thixotropic structured vehicles. At concentrations above 10%, e g 14 or 15%, the cellulose microcrystals gel water to ointment consistency by swelling and producing a continuous network of rods extending throughout the entire vehicle. Attraction between the elongated particles is presumably due to flocculation in the secondary minimum (see below). Treatment of the microcrystalline mass with sodium carboxymethylcellulose facilitates its disintegration into the primary needle-shaped particles and enhances their thickening action.

While in the special cases of certain clays and cellulose, comminution produces lamellar and fibrillar particles, respectively, as a rule regular particle shapes are produced by condensation rather than by disintegration methods. *Colloidal silicon dioxide* is called fumed or pyrogenic silica because it is manufactured by high-temperature, vapor-phase hydrolysis of silicon tetrachloride in an oxy-hydrogen flame, ie, a flame produced by burning hydrogen in a stream of oxygen. The resultant white powder consists of submicroscopic spherical particles of rather uniform size (narrow particle size distribution). Different grades are produced by different reaction conditions. Relatively large, single spherical particles are shown in Fig 20-7. Their average diameter is 50 nm (500 Å), corresponding to the comparatively small specific surface area of 50 m²/g. Smaller spherical particles have correspondingly larger specific surface areas; the grade with the smallest average diameter, 5 nm, has a specific surface area of 380 m²/g. During the manufacturing process, the finer-grade particles tend to sinter or grow together into chain-like aggregates resembling pearl necklaces or streptococci (see Fig 20-8).

Since fumed silica is amorphous, its inhaled dust causes no silicosis. The spheres of colloidal silicon dioxide are nonporous. While the density of the spherical particles is 2.13 g/cm³, the bulk density of their powder is a mere 0.05 g/cm³; the powder is extremely light. This results in two pharmaceutical and cosmetic applications for colloidal silicon dioxide. It is used to increase the fluffiness or bulk volume of powders. Even more than microcrystalline cellulose, its high porosity enables it to absorb a variety of liquids from fluid fragrances to viscous tars, transforming them into free-flowing powders that can be incorporated into tablets or capsules. The porosity in colloidal silicon dioxide is due entirely to the enormous void space between the particles, which themselves are solid.

When these ultrafine particles are incorporated at levels as low as 0.1–0.5% into a powder consisting of coarse particles or granules, they coat the surface of the latter and act as tiny ball bearings and spacers, improving the flowability of the powder and eliminating caking. This action is important in tableting. Moreover, colloidal silicon dioxide improves tablet disintegration.

The surface of the particles contains siloxane (Si—O—Si) and silanol (Si—OH) groups. When colloidal silicon dioxide powder is dispersed in nonpolar liquids, the particles tend to adhere to one another by hydrogen bonds between their surface groups. With finer grades of colloidal silicon dioxide, the spherical particles are linked together into short chain-like aggregates as shown in Fig 20-8, thus agglomerating into loose three-dimensional networks which increase the viscosity of the liquid vehicles very effectively at levels as low as a few percent. These hydrogen-bonded structures are torn apart by stirring but rebuilt while at rest, conferring thixotropy to the thickened liquids.

The grades which consist of relatively large and unattached spherical particles, such as those of Fig 20-7, are less efficient

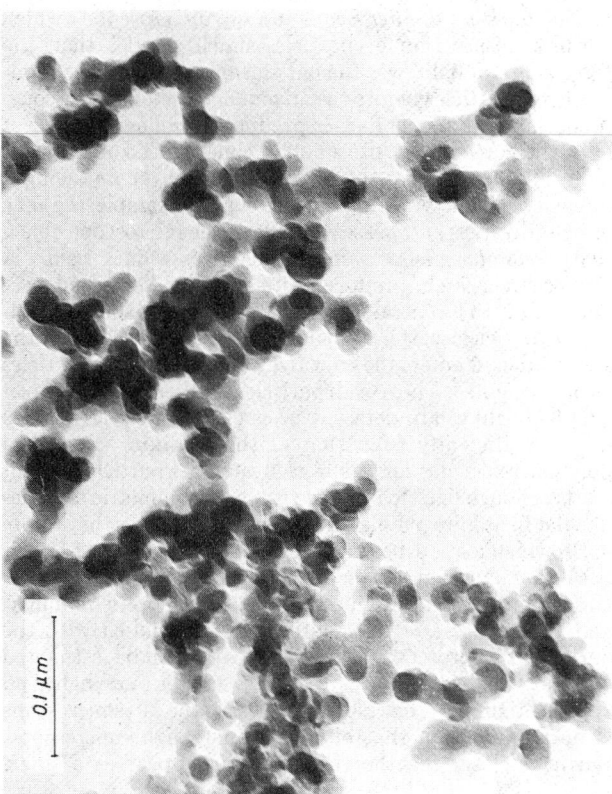

Fig 20-8. Transmission electron micrograph of Aerosil 130, ground and dusted on. The spheres are fused together into chain-like aggregates (courtesy, Degussa AG of Hanau, West Germany; Aerosil is a registered trademark of Degussa). The suffix 130 gives the specific surface area in m²/g.

thickening agents as they lack the high specific surface area and the asymmetry of the finer grades, which consist of short chains of fused spherical particles. In the latter category is Aerosil 200, the grade most widely used as a pharmaceutical adjuvant, whose primary spheres, which are extensively sintered together, have an average diameter of 12 nm. At levels of 8–10%, it thickens liquids of low polarity such as vegetable and mineral oils to the consistency of ointments, imparting considerable yield values to them. The consistency of ointments thickened with colloidal silicon dioxide is not appreciably reduced at higher temperatures. Incorporation of colloidal silicon dioxide into ointments and pastes, such as those of zinc oxide, also reduces the syneresis or *bleeding* of the liquid vehicles.

Hydrogen-bonding liquids like alcohols and water solvate the silica spheres, reducing the hydrogen bonding between particles. These solvents are gelled at silica levels of 12–18% or higher.

Latexes of polymers are aqueous dispersions prepared by emulsion polymerization. Their particles are spherical because polymerization of solubilized liquid monomer takes place inside spherical surfactant micelles which swell because additional monomer keeps diffusing into the micelles. Examples include latex-based paints. Some *clays* grow as plate-like particles possessing straight edges and hexagonal angles, eg bentonite and kaolin (see Fig 20-3). Other clays have lath-shaped (nontronite) or needle-shaped particles (attapulgite).

Emulsification produces spherical droplets to minimize the oil-water interfacial area. Cooling the emulsion below the melting point of the disperse phase freezes it in the spherical shape. For instance, paraffin can be emulsified in 80° water; cooling to room temperature produces a hydrosol with spherical particles.

Sols of viruses and globular proteins, which are hydrophilic, contain compact particles possessing definite geometric shapes. Poliomyelitis virus is spherical, tobacco mosaic virus is rod-shaped, while serum albumin and the serum globulins are prolate ellipsoids of revolution (football-shaped).

Dispersion methods produce sols with wide particle size distributions. Condensation methods *may* produce essentially monodisperse sols provided specialized techniques are employed. Monodisperse polystyrene latexes are available for calibration of electron micrographs (see Fig 20-3). Biologic hydrophilic polymers, such as nucleic acids and proteins, form largely monodisperse particles, as do more highly organized structures such as lipoproteins and viruses.

Electron Microscopy—Because of their size, particles in the middle and lower colloidal size range are too small for direct microscopic observation. The ordinary *light microscope* has a resolving power of about 2000 Å (0.2 µm), ie, it cannot reveal or distinguish structural details or particles which are separated by smaller distances. Two particles which are closer together would appear as one.

The resolving power is directly proportional to the wavelength of the radiation. The *electron microscope*, developed in the late 1930s, employs electrons with a wavelength of about 0.1 Å and has a resolving power of about 5 Å. This value is limited by lens aberrations rather than by the wavelength. The "lenses" used to focus the electron beam are magnetic fields. The electrons transmitted through the object produce an image that is focused and projected with the aid of additional electromagnetic lenses onto a fluorescent screen or photographic plate. Electrons can travel unhindered only in high vacuum. Therefore, only specimens with negligible vapor pressure can be observed. Hydrosols must be thoroughly dried beforehand. If the sample appears flocculated, flocculation may have existed in the original sol or it may have been caused by drying. The electron beam may also alter the sample.

Another shortcoming of the *transmission electron microscope* is that the image is due to differences in transparency to electrons. Transparency depends on the thickness and on the atomic number of the atoms forming the specimen. Organic materials containing only atoms of low atomic numbers, namely, hydrogen, carbon, oxygen and nitrogen, are almost equally and highly transparent. Their pictures show little contrast. Materials containing heavy metal atoms produce better images. Larger objects are cut into very thin slices by means of microtomes for examination with a transmission electron microscope.

The *shadow-casting* technique is used to give a three-dimensional effect to transmission electron micrographs and to improve the contrast. Chromium, gold or other metals are evaporated in vacuum at a small and known angle to the specimen. The shadows cast by salient features of the specimen, ie, the areas behind those features which are not covered by chromium, provide the electron micrograph with relief (see Figs 20-3 and 20-4). From the length of the shadow and from the angle of vaporization, it is possible to calculate the height of the particle. For instance, the sample of Fig 20-3 was shadowed at an 18° angle. Tan 18° = ⅓ is the ratio of particle thickness to length of shadow. The few spherical particles with diameters of 0.25 µm belong to a monodisperse polystyrene latex which was added to the sample to verify magnification and shadow angle.

Replication is a technique for studying the surface structure of a specimen. A thin, uniform carbon film is deposited onto the sample by vacuum evaporation. This replica film is then separated from the sample and examined with the electron microscope.[5,6]

The *scanning electron microscope*, developed during the late 1960s, uses an electron source and electromagnetic lenses to condense and focus the electron beam, just like the transmission electron microscope. A narrow, finely focused, high-energy primary electron beam is made to impinge on the specimen surface. Back-scattered electrons, as well as emitted secondary electrons, photons and X-rays produced by impact ionization, are collected by a scintillation detector which produces an emission current. The current is amplified and regulates the intensity of a spot of light on a cathode-ray tube display. The incident beam is moved across the specimen surface by scanning coils while the display spot moves in synchronism across the display tube in TV fashion. The surface of the specimen is scanned by a raster or series of lines, each of which corresponds to a narrow surface strip. The brightness and contrast of each point observed on the display tube is related to a surface detail of the specimen and depends on the atomic number of the material being scanned, the angle which the surface element makes with respect to the incident beam, and on the shape, thickness and position of the surface element. Protrusions, holes and edges show up more distinctly than flat surfaces. The surface structure displayed on the cathode ray tube is recorded by photographing its screen. The details of surface structure and the unusually great depth of focus of scanning electron micrographs are illustrated by Figs 20-5 and 20-6.

The magnifying power of the scanning electron microscope ranges approximately from 40 to 100,000. The magnification is easily adjusted by changing the length of the scan line on the specimen relative to the length of the display line on the screen, which remains constant. For instance, if the beam scans a 1 mm × 1 mm specimen area and the image is displayed on a 10 cm × 10 cm screen, the magnification is 100. Reducing the area scanned to 0.1 mm × 0.1 mm increases the magnification to 1,000.

Unlike the transmission electron microscope, the scanning electron microscope examines surfaces regardless of the thickness of the specimens. It requires none of the lengthy specimen preparation techniques used with the former.[13]

Light Scattering by Colloidal Particles—The optical properties of a medium are determined by its refractive index. When the refractive index is uniform throughout, light will pass the medium undeflected. Whenever there are discrete variations in the refractive index caused by the presence of particles or by small-scale density fluctuations, part of the light will be scattered in all directions. An optical property characteristic of colloidal systems, called the *Tyndall beam*, is familiar to everyone in the case of aerosols. When a narrow beam of sunlight is admitted through a small hole into a darkened room, the presence of the minute dust particles suspended in air is revealed by bright flashing points.

A beam of light striking a particle polarizes the atoms and molecules of that particle, inducing dipoles which act as secondary sources and reemit weak light of the same wavelength as the incident light. This phenomenon is called *light scattering*. The scattered radiation propagates in all directions away from the particle. In a bright room, the light scattered by the dust particles is too weak to be noticeable.

Colloidal particles suspended in a liquid also scatter light. When an intense, narrowly defined beam of light is passed through a suspension, its path becomes visible because of the scattering of light by the particles in the beam. This Tyndall beam becomes most visible when viewed against a dark background in a direction perpendicular to the incident beam. The magnitude of the turbidity or opalescence depends on the nature, size and concentration of the particles. When clear mineral oil is dispersed in an equal volume of a clear aqueous surfactant solution, the resultant emulsion is milky white and opaque due to light scattering. Microemulsions, where the emulsified droplets are about 400 Å in diameter, ie, much smaller than the wavelength of visible light, are transparent and clear to the naked eye.

The *dark-field microscope* or *ultramicroscope*, which permits observation of particles much smaller than the wavelength of light, was the only means of detecting submicroscopic particles before the advent of electron microscopy. A special cardioid condenser produces a hollow cylinder of light and converges it into a hollow cone focused on the sample. The sample is at the apex of the cone, where the light intensity is high. After passing through the sample, the cone of light diverges and passes outside of the microscope objective. A homogeneous sample thus gives a dark field. A similar effect can be produced with a regular Abbe condenser outfitted with a central stop and a strong light source. Colloidal particles scatter light in all directions. Some of the scattered light enters the objective and shows up the particles as bright spots. Thus, even particles smaller than the wavelength of light can be detected, provided their refractive index differs sufficiently from that of the medium. Dissolved polymer molecules and highly solvated gel particles do not scatter enough light to become visible. Asymmetric particles like flat bentonite platelets give flashing effects as they rotate in Brownian motion, because they scatter more light with their basal plane perpendicular to the light beam than edgewise. Brownian motion, sedimentation, electrophoretic mobility, and the progress of flocculation can be studied with the dark-field microscope. Polydispersity can be estimated qualitatively because larger particles scatter more light and appear brighter. The resolving power of the ultramicroscope is no greater than that of the ordinary light microscope. Particles closer together than 0.2 μm appear as a single blur.

Turbidity may be used to measure the concentration of dispersed particles in two ways. In *turbidimetry*, a spectrophotometer or photoelectric colorimeter is used to measure the intensity of the light transmitted in the incident direction. Turbidity τ is defined by an equation analogous to Beer's law for the absorption of light (see Chapter 34),[5,6,8] namely,

$$\tau = \frac{1}{l} \ln \frac{I_0}{I_t}$$

where I_0 and I_t are the intensities of the incident and transmitted light beams, and l is the length of the dispersion through which the light passes.

If the dispersion is less turbid, the intensity of light scattered at 90° to the incident beam is measured with a *nephelometer*. Both methods require careful standardization with suspensions containing known amounts of particles similar to those to be measured. The concentration of colloidal dispersions of inorganic and organic compounds and of bacterial suspensions can thus be measured by their turbidity.

The turbidity or Tyndall effect of hydrophilic colloidal systems like aqueous solutions of gums, proteins and other polymers is far weaker than that of lyophobic dispersions. These solutions appear clear to the naked eye. Their turbidity can be measured with a photoelectric cell/photomultiplier tube and serves to determine the molecular weight of the solute.

The theory of light scattering was developed in detail by Lord Rayleigh. For white nonabsorbing nonconductors or dielectrics like sulfur and insoluble organic compounds, the equation obtained for spherical particles whose radius is small compared to the wavelength of light λ is[5-8]

$$I_s = I_0 \frac{4\pi^2 n_0^2 (n_1 - n_0)^2}{\lambda^4 d^2 c} (1 + \cos^2 \theta)$$

I_0 is the intensity of the unpolarized incident light; I_s is the intensity of light scattered in a direction making an angle θ

with the incident beam and measured at a distance d. The scattered light is largely polarized. The concentration c is expressed as the number of particles per unit volume. The refractive indices n_1 and n_0 refer to the dispersion and the solvent, respectively.

Since the intensity of scattered light is inversely proportional to the fourth power of the wavelength, blue light ($\lambda \cong$ 4500 Å) is scattered much more strongly than red light ($\lambda \cong$ 6500 Å). With incident white light, colloidal dispersions of colorless particles appear blue when viewed in scattered light, i.e., in lateral directions such as 90° to the incident beam. Loss of the blue rays due to preferential scattering leaves the transmitted light yellow or red. Preferential scattering of blue radiation sideways accounts for the blue color of the sky, sea, cigarette smoke, and diluted milk and for the yellow-red color of the rising and setting sun viewed head-on.

The particles in pharmaceutical suspensions, emulsions and lotions are generally larger than the wavelength of light λ. When the particle size exceeds $\lambda/20$, destructive interference between light scattered by different portions of the same particle lowers the intensity of scattered light and changes its angular dependence. Rayleigh's theory was extended to large and to strongly absorbing and conducting particles by Mie and to nonspherical particles by Gans.[1,3,5-8] By using appropriate precautions in experimental techniques and in interpretation, it is possible to determine an average particle size and even the particle size distribution of colloidal dispersions and coarser suspensions by means of turbidity measurements.[12]

Diffusion and Sedimentation—The molecules of a gas or liquid are engaged in a perpetual, random thermal motion which causes them to collide with one another and with the container wall billions of times per second. Each collision changes the direction and the velocity of the molecules involved. Dissolved molecules and suspended colloidal particles are continuously and randomly buffeted by the molecules of the suspending medium. This random bombardment imparts to solutes and particles an equally unceasing and erratic movement called *Brownian motion*, after the botanist Robert Brown who first observed it under the microscope with an aqueous pollen suspension. The Brownian motion of colloidal particles mirrors on a magnified scale the random movement of the molecules of the liquid or gaseous suspending medium, and represents a three-dimensional random walk.

Solute molecules and suspended colloidal particles undergo rotational and translational Brownian movement. For the latter, Einstein derived the equation

$$\bar{x} = \sqrt{2Dt}$$

where $\bar{x}$ is the mean displacement in the x-direction in time t and D is the *diffusion coefficient*. Einstein also showed that for spherical particles of radius r under conditions specified in Chapter 22 for the validity of Stokes' law and Einstein's law of viscosity,

$$D = \frac{RT}{6\pi\eta rN}$$

where R is the gas constant, T the absolute temperature, N Avogadro's number, and η the viscosity of the suspending medium.

The diffusion coefficient is a measure of the mobility of a dissolved molecule or suspended particle in a liquid medium. Representative values at room temperature, in cm²/sec, are 4.7×10^{-6} for sucrose and 6.1×10^{-7} for serum albumin in water. With a diffusion coefficient of 1×10^{-7} cm²/sec, Brownian motion causes a particle to move by an average distance of 1 cm in one direction in 58 days, by 1 mm in 14 hrs, and by 1 μm in 0.05 sec. Smaller molecules diffuse faster in a given medium. Assuming spherical shape, the radius of a

serum albumin molecule is 35 Å and that of a sucrose molecule 4.4 Å. The ratio of the radii of the two molecules 35/4.4 = 7.9, is nearly identical with the inverse ratio of their diffusion coefficients in water, $4.7 \times 10^{-6}/6.1 \times 10^{-7} = 7.7$, in agreement with the above equation. Diffusion coefficients of steroids and other molecules of similar size dissolved in absorption bases based on petrolatum are generally in the 10^{-10} to 10^{-8} cm²/sec range. Steroids have only slightly higher molecular weights than sucrose. Their much smaller diffusion coefficients are due to the much higher viscosity of the vehicle.

Brownian motion and convection currents maintain dissolved molecules and small colloidal particles in suspension indefinitely. As the particle size and r increase, the Brownian motion decreases; $\bar{x}$ is proportional to $r^{-1/2}$. Provided that the density of the particle d_P and of the liquid vehicle d_L are sufficiently different, larger particles have a greater tendency to settle out when $d_P > d_L$ or to rise to the top of the suspension when $d_P < d_L$ than smaller particles of the same material.

The rate of *sedimentation* is expressed by the Stokes' equation given in Chapter 22, which can be rewritten as

$$h = \frac{2(d_P - d_L)r^2 g t}{9\eta}$$

where h is the height through which a spherical particle settles in time t and g is the acceleration of gravity. The rate of sedimentation is proportional to r^2. Thus, with increasing particle size, the Brownian motion diminishes while the tendency to sediment increases. The two become equal for a critical radius when the distance h through which the particle settles equals the mean displacement $\bar{x}$ due to Brownian motion in the same time interval t.[15] In most pharmaceutical suspensions, sedimentation prevails. Intravenous vegetable oil emulsions do not tend to cream because the mean droplet size, ca 0.5 μm, is smaller than the critical radius.

Passive diffusion caused by a concentration gradient and carried out through Brownian motion is important in the release of drugs from topical preparations (see Chapter 88) and in the gastrointestinal absorption of drugs (see Chapter 37).

Viscosity—Most lyophobic dispersions have viscosities not much greater than that of the liquid vehicle. This holds true even at comparatively high volume fractions of the disperse phase unless the particles form continuous network aggregates throughout the vehicle, in which case yield values are observed. Most O/W and W/O emulsions have specific viscosities not much greater than those predicted by Einstein's modified law of viscosity (see Eq 11 of Chapter 22 and text). For instance, emulsions containing 40% v/v of the internal phase generally have viscosities only three to five times higher than that of the continuous phase. By contrast, the apparent viscosities of lyophilic dispersions, especially of polymer solutions, are several orders of magnitude greater than the viscosity of the solvent or vehicle even at concentrations of only a few percent solids. Lyophilic dispersions are also generally much more pseudoplastic or shear-thinning than lyophobic dispersions (see Chapter 22).

Electric Properties and Stability of Lyophobic Dispersions

Difference between Lyophilic and Lyophobic Dispersions—*Lyophilic* or solvent-loving solids are called hydrophilic if the solvent is water. Owing to the presence of high concentrations of hydrophilic groups, they dissolve or disperse spontaneously in water as far as is possible without breaking covalent bonds. Among hydrophilic groups are ionized ones which dissociate into highly hydrated ions like carboxylate, sulfonate or alkylammonium ions, and organic functional groups like hydroxyl, carbonyl, amino, and imino which bind water through hydrogen bonding.

The free energy of dissolution or dispersion, ΔG_s, of hydrophilic solids includes a large negative (exothermic) heat or enthalpy of solvation, ΔH_s, and a large increase in entropy, ΔS_s. Since $\Delta G_s = \Delta H_s - T\Delta S_s$, ΔG_s has a large negative value: the dissolution of hydrophilic macromolecules and the dispersion of hydrophilic particulate solids in water occur spontaneously (see Chapter 16), overcoming the parallel increases in surface area and surface free energy. Dissolution and dispersion take place so that water can come into contact and interact with the hydrophilic groups of the solids (enthalpy of solvation), and to increase the number of available configurations of the macromolecules and particles (entropy increase).

The van der Waals energies of attraction between dissolved macromolecules or dispersed hydrophilic solid particles are smaller than ΔG_s and are, therefore, insufficient to cause separation of a solid polymer phase or agglomeration through flocculation or coagulation of the dispersed particles. Furthermore, the hydration layer surrounding dissolved macromolecules and dispersed particles forms a barrier preventing their close approach.

Hydrophobic solids and liquids such as organic compounds consisting largely of hydrocarbon portions with few if any hydrophilic functional groups, like cholesterol and other steroids, and some nonionized inorganic substances like sulfur, are hydrated slightly or not at all. Hence they do not disperse or dissolve spontaneously in water: ΔG_s is positive because of a positive (endothermic) ΔH_s term, making the reverse process (agglomeration) the spontaneous one. Aqueous dispersions of such hydrophobic solids or liquids can be prepared by physical means which supply the appropriate energy to the system (see above). They are unstable, however. The van der Waals attractive forces between the particles cause them to aggregate, since the solvation forces which promote dispersal in water are weak. If aqueous dispersions of hydrophobic solids are to resist reaggregation (coagulation and flocculation), they must be stabilized. Stabilizing factors include electric charges at the particle surface (due to dissociation of ionogenic groups of the solid or pertaining to adsorbed ions such as ionic surfactants) and the presence of adsorbed macromolecules or nonionic surfactants. These stabilizing factors do not alter the intrinsic thermodynamic instability of lyophobic dispersions: ΔG_s is still positive so that the reverse process of phase separation or aggregation is energetically favored over dispersal. They establish kinetic barriers which delay the aggregation processes almost indefinitely; the dispersed particles cannot come together close enough for the van der Waals attractive forces to produce coagulation.[5,8] These stabilization mechanisms are discussed below.

The reductions in surface area and surface free energy accompanying flocculation or coagulation are small because irregular solid particles, being rigid, touch only at a few points upon aggregation. The loose initial contacts may grow with time by sintering or recrystallization. Sintering consists of the "fusion" of primary particles into larger primary particles which propagates from initial small areas of contact. This recrystallization process is spontaneous because it decreases the specific surface area of the disperse solid and the surface free energy of the dispersion. Sintering is analogous to Ostwald ripening, the recrystallization process of transferring solid from colloidal to coarse particles discussed above. Low solubility and the presence of adsorbed surface-active substances retard both processes.

Origin of Electric Charges—Particles can acquire charges from several sources. In *proteins*, one end group of the polypeptide chain and aspartic and glutamic acid units contribute carboxylic acid groups, which are ionized into carboxylate ions in neutral to alkaline media. The other chain end group and lysine units contribute amino groups, arginine units contribute guanidine groups, and histidine units contribute imidazole groups. The nitrogen atoms of these groups become protonated in neutral to acid media. For electroneutrality, these cationic groups require anions, such as Cl^- if hydrochloric acid was used to make the medium acid and to supply the protons. The neutralizing ions, called counterions, dissociate from the ionogenic basic functional groups and can be replaced by other ions of like charge: they are not an integral part of the protein particle but are located in its immediate vicinity. The alkylammonium, guanidinium and imidazolium ions, which are attached to the protein molecule by covalent bonds, confer a positive charge to it. In neutral and alkaline media, Na^+, K^+, Ca^{2+}, and Mg^{2+} are among the counterions neutralizing the negative charges of the carboxylate groups. The latter are covalently attached to and constitute an integral part of the protein particle, conferring a negative charge to it.

At an intermediate pH value, which ranges from 4.5 to 7 for the various proteins, the carboxylate anions and the alkylammonium, guanidinium, and imidazolium cations neutralize each other exactly. There is no need for counterions since the ionized functional groups which are an integral part of the protein molecule are in exact balance. At this pH value, called the *isoelectric point*, the protein particle or molecule is neutral: its electric charge is neither negative nor positive but zero.[5]

Many other organic polymers contain ionic groups and are, therefore, called *polyelectrolytes* (polymeric electrolytes or salts). Natural polysaccharides of vegetable origin such as acacia, tragacanth, alginic acid and pectin contain carboxylic acid groups, which are ionized in neutral to alkaline media. Agar and carrageen, as well as the animal polysaccharides heparin and chondroitin sulfate, contain sulfuric acid hemiester groups, which are strongly acidic and ionize even in acid media. Cellulosic polyelectrolytes include *sodium carboxymethylcellulose*, while synthetic carboxylated polymers include *carbomer*, a copolymer of acrylic acid.

Aluminum hydroxide, $Al(OH)_3$, is dissolved by acids and alkalis forming aluminum ions, Al^{3+}, and aluminate ions, $[Al(OH)_4]^-$, respectively. In neutral or weakly acid media, at acid concentrations too low to cause dissolution, an aluminum hydroxide particle has some positive charges attributable to incompletely neutralized positive Al^{3+} valences. The portion of the surface of an aluminum hydroxide particle represented schematically below has one such positive charge neutralized by a Cl^- counterion:

In weakly alkaline media, at base concentrations too low to transform the aluminum hydroxide particles completely into aluminate and dissolve them, they bear some negative charges due to the presence of a few aluminate groups. The portion of the particle surface represented schematically below has one such negative group neutralized by a Na^+ counterion:

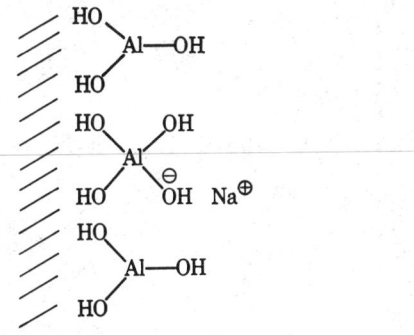

At a pH of 8.5–9.1,[16,17] there are neither $[Al(OH)_2]^+$ nor $[Al(OH)_4]^-$ ions in the particle surface but only neutral $Al(OH)_3$ molecules. The particles have zero charge and therefore need no counterions for charge neutralization. This pH is the isoelectric point. In the case of inorganic particulate compounds such as aluminum hydroxide, it is also called zero point of charge.

Bentonite clay is a lamellar aluminum silicate. Each lattice layer consists of a sheet of hydrated alumina sandwiched between two silica sheets. Isomorphous replacement of Al^{3+} by Mg^{2+} or of Si^{4+} by Al^{3+} confers net negative charges to the thin clay lamellas in the form of cation-exchange sites resembling silicate ions built into the lattice. The counterions producing electroneutrality are usually Na^+ (sodium bentonite) or Ca^{2+} (calcium bentonite). The zero point of charge is probably close to that of quartz, silica gel and other silicates, namely, at a pH of about 1.5–2.

Silver iodide sols can be prepared by the reaction

$$AgNO_3 + NaI \rightarrow AgI(s) + NaNO_3$$

In the bulk of the silver iodide particles, there is a 1:1 stoichiometric ratio of Ag^+ to I^- ions. If the reaction is carried out with an excess silver nitrate, there will be more Ag^+ than I^- ions in the surface of the particles. The particles will thus be positively charged and the counterions surrounding them will be NO_3^-. If the reaction is carried out using an exact stoichiometric 1:1 ratio of silver nitrate to sodium iodide or with an excess sodium iodide, the surface of the particles will contain an excess I^- over Ag^+ ions.[5,6,8] The particles will be negatively charged, and Na^+ will be the counterions surrounding the particles and neutralizing their charges.

An additional mechanism through which particles acquire electric charges is by the adsorption of ions,[6–8] including ionic surfactants.

Electric Double Layers—The surface layer of a silver iodide particle prepared with an excess of sodium iodide contains more I^- than Ag^+ ions, whereas its bulk contains the two ions in exactly equimolar proportion. The aqueous solution in which this particle is suspended contains relatively high concentrations of Na^+ and NO_3^-, a lower concentration of I^-, and traces of H^+, OH^-, and Ag^+.

The negatively charged particle surface attracts positive ions from the solution and repels negative ions: the solution in the vicinity of the surface contains a much higher concentration of Na^+, which are the counterions, and a much lower concentration of NO_3^- ions than the bulk of the solution. A number of Na^+ ions equal to the number of excess I^- ions in the surface (ie, the number of I^- ions in the surface layer minus the number of Ag^+ ions in the surface layer) and equivalent to the net negative surface charge of a particle are pulled towards its surface. These counterions tend to stick to the surface, approaching it as closely as their hydration spheres permit (Helmholtz double layer), but the thermal agitation of the water molecules tends to disperse them throughout the solution. As a result, the layer of counterions surrounding the particle is spread out. The Na^+ concentra-

tion is highest in the immediate vicinity of the negative surface, where they form a compact layer called the Stern layer, and decreases with distance from the surface, throughout a diffuse layer called the Gouy-Chapman layer: the sharply defined negatively charged surface is surrounded by a cloud of Na^+ counterions required for electroneutrality. The combination of the two layers of oppositely charged ions constitutes an electric double layer. It is illustrated in the top part of Fig 20-9. The horizontal axis represents the distance from the particle surface in both the top and bottom parts.

The electric potential of a plane is equal to the work against electrostatic forces required to bring a unit electric charge from infinity (in this case, from the bulk of the solution) to that plane. If the plane is the surface of the particle, the potential is called surface or ψ_0 potential, which measures the total potential of the double layer. This is the thermodynamic potential which operates in galvanic cells. On moving away from the particle surface towards the bulk solution in the direction of the horizontal axis, the potential drops rapidly across the Stern layer because the Na^+ ions in the immediate vicinity of the surface screen Na^+ ions farther removed, in the diffuse part of the double layer, from the effect of the negative surface charge. The decrease in potential across the Gouy-Chapman layer is more gradual. The diffuse double layer gradually comes to an end as the composition approaches that of the bulk liquid where the anion concentration equals the cation concentration, and the potential approaches zero asymptotically. In view of the indefinite end point, the thickness δ of the diffuse double layer is arbitrarily assigned the value of the distance over which the potential at the boundary between the Stern and Gouy-Chapman layers drops to $1/e = 0.37$ of its value.[5–8] The thickness of double layers usually ranges from 10 to 1000 Å. It decreases as the concentration of electrolytes in solution increases, more rapidly for counterions of higher valence. δ is approximately equal to the reciprocal of the Debye-Hückel theory parameter κ discussed in Chapters 17 and 21.

Of practical importance, because it can be measured experimentally, is the electrokinetic or ζ (zeta) potential. In aqueous dispersion, even relatively hydrophobic inorganic particles and organic particles containing polar functional groups are surrounded by a layer of water of hydration attached to them by ion-dipole and dipole-dipole interaction. When a particle moves, this shell of bound water and all ions located inside it move along with the particle. Conversely, if water or a solution flows through a fixed bed of these solid particles, the hydration layer surrounding each particle remains stationary and attached to it. The electric potential at the plane of shear or slip separating the bound water from the free water is the ζ potential. It does not include the Stern layer and only that part of the Gouy-Chapman layer which lies outside the hydration shell. The various potentials are shown on the bottom part of Fig 20-9.

Stabilization by Electrostatic Repulsion—When two uncharged hydrophobic particles are in close proximity, they attract each other by van der Waals secondary valences, mainly by London dispersion forces. For individual atoms and molecules, these forces decrease with the seventh power of the distance between them. In the case of two particles, every atom of one attracts every atom of the other particle. Because the attractive forces are nearly additive, they decay much less rapidly with the interparticle distance as a result of this summation, approximately with the second or third power (see Chapter 21, particularly Eqs 13–16). Since energies of attraction are equal to force x distance, they decrease approximately with the first or second power of the distance. Therefore, whenever two particles approach each other closely, the attractive forces take over and cause them to adhere. Coagulation occurs as the primary particles aggregate into increasingly larger secondary particles or flocs.

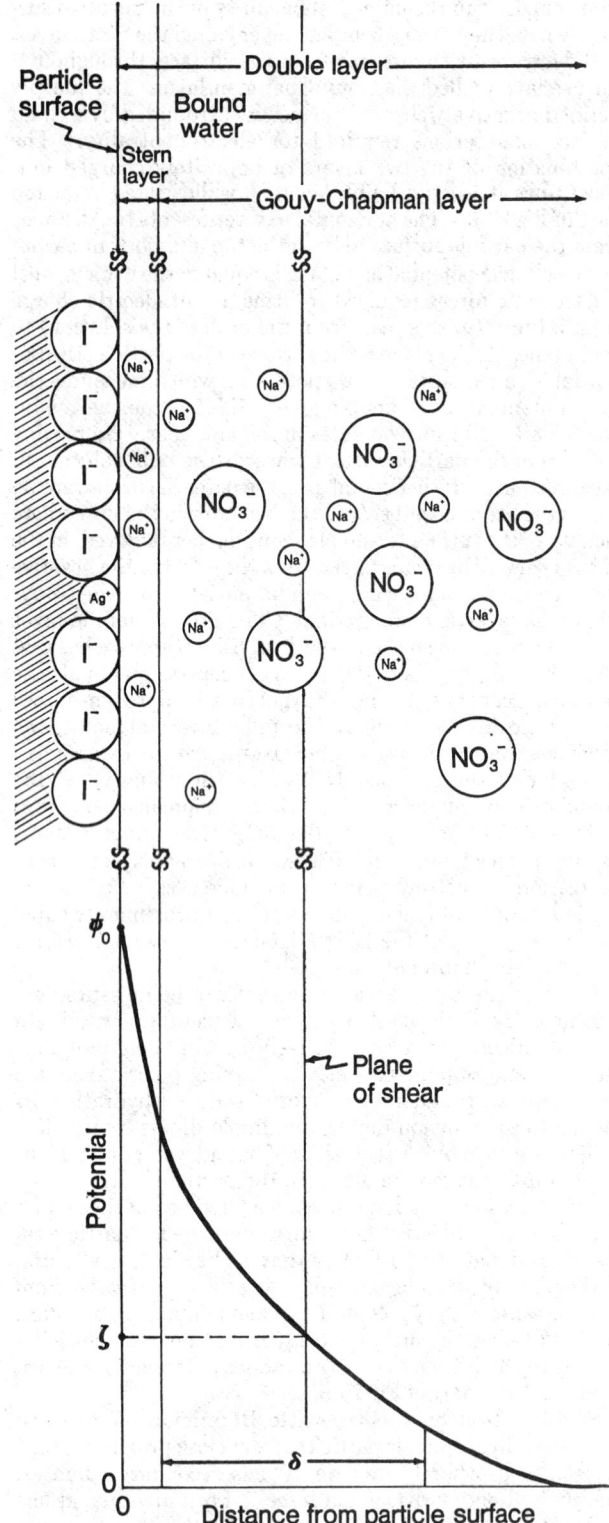

Fig 20-9. Electric double layer at the surface of a silver iodide particle (upper part) and the corresponding potentials (lower part). The distance from the particle surface, plotted on the horizontal axis, refers to both the upper and lower parts.

If the dispersion consists of two kinds of particles with positive and negative charges, respectively, the electrostatic attraction between oppositely charged particles is superimposed on the attraction by van der Waals forces, and coagulation is accelerated. If the dispersion contains only one kind, as is customary, all particles have surface charges of the same sign and density. In that case, electrostatic repulsion tends

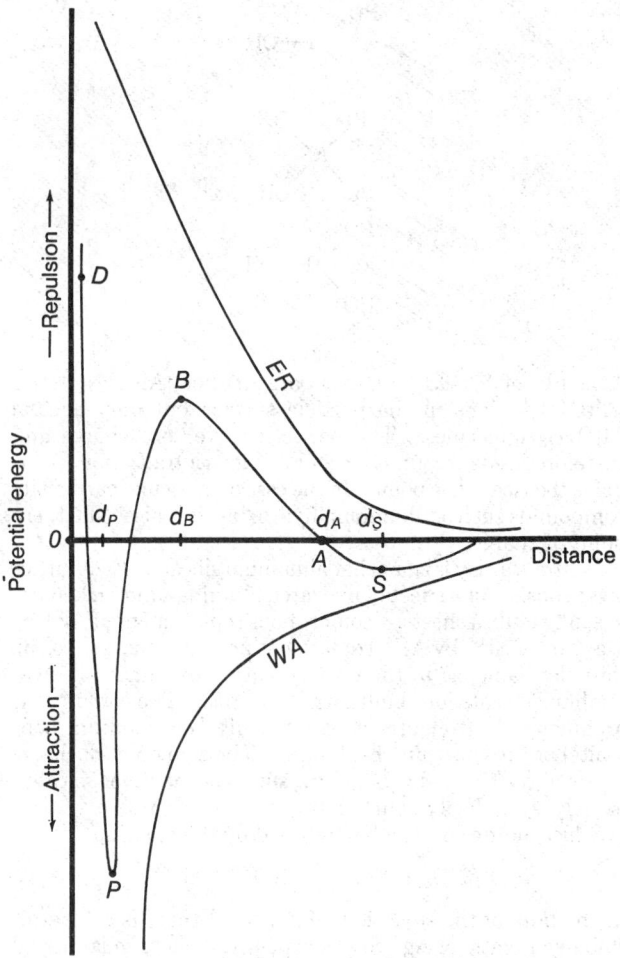

Fig 20-10. Curves representing the van der Waals energy of attraction (*WA*), the energy of electrostatic repulsion (*ER*), and the net energy of interaction (*DPBAS*) between two identical charged particles, as a function of the interparticle distance.

to prevent the particles from approaching closely enough to come within effective range of each other's van der Waals attractive forces, thus stabilizing the dispersion against interparticle attachments or coagulation. The electrostatic repulsive energy has a range of the order of δ.

A quantitative theory of the interaction between lyophobic disperse particles was worked out independently by Derjaguin and Landau in the USSR and by Verwey and Overbeek in the Netherlands in the early 1940s.[1,5–8,18] The so-called DLVO theory predicts and explains many but not all experimental data. Its refinement to account for discrepancies is still continuing.

The DLVO theory is summarized in Fig 20-10, where curve *WA* represents the van der Waals attractive energy which decreases approximately with the second power of the interparticle distance, and curve *ER* represents the electrostatic repulsive energy which decreases exponentially with distance. Because of the combination of these two opposing effects, attraction predominates at small and large distances whereas repulsion may predominate at intermediate distances. Negative energy values indicate attraction, and positive values repulsion. The resultant curve *DPBA*, obtained by algebraic addition of curves *WA* and *ER*, gives the total, net energy of interaction between two particles.

The interparticle attraction depends mainly on the chemical nature and particle size of the material to be dispersed. Once these have been selected, the attractive energy is fixed and cannot readily be altered. The electrostatic repulsion depends on ψ_0 or the density of the surface charge and on the thickness of the double layer, both of which govern the magnitude of the ζ potential. Thus, stability correlates to some extent with this potential.[5] The ζ potential can be adjusted within wide limits by additives, especially ionic surfactants, water-miscible solvents, and electrolytes (see below). If the absolute value of the ζ potential is small, the resultant potential energy is negative and van der Waals attraction predominates over electrostatic repulsion at all distances. Such sols coagulate rapidly.

The two identical particles whose interaction is depicted in Fig 20-10 have a large (positive or negative) ζ potential resulting in an appreciable positive or repulsive potential energy at intermediate distances. They are on a collision course because of Brownian motion, convection currents, sedimentation, or because the dispersion is being stirred.

As the two particles approach each other, the two atmospheres of counterions surrounding them begin to interpenetrate or overlap at point A corresponding to the distance d_A. This produces a net repulsive (positive) energy because of the work involved in distorting the diffuse double layers and in pushing water molecules and counterions aside, which increases if the particles approach further. If the particles continue to approach each other even after most of the intervening solution of the counterions between them has been displaced, the repulsion between their surface charges increases the net potential energy of interaction to its maximum positive value at B. If the height of the potential energy barrier B exceeds the kinetic energy of the approaching particles, they will not come any closer than the distance d_B but move away from each other. A net positive potential energy of about 25 kT units usually suffices to keep them apart, rendering the dispersion permanently stable; k is the Boltzmann constant and T is the absolute temperature. At $T = 298°K$, this corresponds to 1×10^{-12} erg. The kinetic energy of a particle is of the order of kT.

On the other hand, if their kinetic energy exceeds the potential energy barrier B, the particles continue to approach each other past d_B, where the van der Waals attraction becomes increasingly more important compared to the electrostatic repulsion. Therefore, the net potential energy of interaction decreases to zero and then becomes negative, pulling the particles still closer together. When the particles touch, at a distance d_P, the net energy has acquired the large negative value P. This deep minimum in potential energy corresponds to a very stable situation in which the particles adhere. Since it is unlikely that enough kinetic energy can be supplied to the particles or that their ζ potential can be increased sufficiently to cause them to climb out of the potential energy well P, they are attached permanently to each other. When most or all of the primary particles agglomerate into secondary particles by such a process, the sol coagulates.

Any closer approach of two particles than the touching distance d_P is met with a very rapid rise in potential energy along PD because the solid particles would interpenetrate each other, causing atomic orbitals to overlap (Born repulsion).

Coagulation of Hydrophobic Dispersions—The height of the potential energy barrier and the range over which the electrostatic repulsion is effective (or the thickness of the double layer) determine the stability of hydrophobic dispersions. Both factors are reduced by the addition of electrolytes. The transition between a coagulating and a stable sol is gradual and depends on the time of observation. By using standard conditions, however, it is possible to classify a sol as either coagulated or coagulating, or as stable or fully dispersed.

To determine the value of the coagulating concentration of a given electrolyte for a given sol, a series of test tubes is filled with equal portions of the sol. Identical volumes of solutions of the electrolyte, of increasing concentration, are added with vigorous stirring. After some time at rest (eg, 2 hrs), the mixtures are agitated again. After an additional, shorter rest period (eg, $\frac{1}{2}$ hr), they are inspected for signs of coagulation. The tubes can be classified into two groups, one showing no signs of coagulation and the other showing at least some signs, eg, visible flocs. Alternatively, they can be classified into one group showing complete coagulation and the other containing at least some deflocculated colloid left in the supernatant. In either case, the separation between the two classes is quite sharp. The intermediate agitation breaks the weakest interparticle bonds and brings small particles in contact with larger ones, thus increasing the sharpness of separation between coagulation and stability. After repeating the experiment with a narrower range of electrolyte concentrations, the coagulation value c_{CV} of the electrolyte, ie, the lowest concentration at which it coagulates the sol, is established with good reproducibility.[5,6,8]

Typical c_{CV} data for a silver iodide sol prepared with an excess of iodide are listed in Table III. The following conclusions can be drawn from the left half of Table III:

1. The c_{CV} does not depend on the valence of the anion, since nitrate and sulfate of the same metal have nearly identical values.
2. The differences among the c_{CV}'s of cations with the same valence are relatively minor. However, there is a slight but significant trend of decreasing c_{CV} with increasing atomic number in the alkali and in the alkaline earth metal groups. Arranging these cations in the order of decreasing c_{CV} produces the *Hofmeister* or *lyotropic series*. It governs many other colloidal phenomena, including the effect of salts on the temperature of gelation and the swelling of aqueous gels and on the viscosity of hydrosols, the salting out of hydrophilic colloids, the cation exchange on ion-exchange resins, and the permeability of membranes towards salts. The series is also observed in many phenomena involving only small atoms or ions and true solutions, including the ionization potential and electronegativity of metals, the heats of hydration of cations, the size of the hydrated cations, the viscosity, surface tension, and infrared spectra of salt solutions, and the solubility of gases therein. For monovalent cations, the lyotropic series is

$$Li^+ > Na^+ > K^+ > NH_4^+ > Rb^+ > Cs^+$$

A similar lyotropic series exists for anions.[3,5–7]

The lithium ion has a higher c_{CV} than the cesium ion because it is more extensively hydrated, so that Li^+ (aq), including the hydration shell, is larger than Cs^+ (aq). Owing to its smaller size, the hydrated cesium ion can approach the negative particle surface more closely than the hydrated lithium ion. Moreover, because of its greater electron cloud, the Cs^+ ion is more polarizable than the Li^+ ion. Therefore, it is more strongly adsorbed in the Stern layer, which makes it a more effective coagulating agent.

Table III—Coagulation Values for Negative Silver Iodide Sol[a]

Electrolyte	c_{CV}, mM/L	Electrolyte	c_{CV}, mM/L
LiNO$_3$	165	AgNO$_3$	0.01
NaNO$_3$	140	$\frac{1}{2}$ (C$_{12}$H$_{25}$NH$_3$)$_2$SO$_4$	0.7
$\frac{1}{2}$ Na$_2$SO$_4$	141	Strychnine nitrate	1.7
KNO$_3$	136	$\frac{1}{2}$ Morphine sulfate	2.5
$\frac{1}{2}$ K$_2$SO$_4$	138		
RbNO$_3$	126		
Mean	141		
Mg(NO$_3$)$_2$	2.60	Quinine sulfate	0.7
MgSO$_4$	2.57		
Ca(NO$_3$)$_2$	2.40		
Sr(NO$_3$)$_2$	2.38		
Ba(NO$_3$)$_2$	2.26		
Zn(NO$_3$)$_2$	2.50		
Pb(NO$_3$)$_2$	2.43		
Mean	2.45		
Al(NO$_3$)$_3$	0.067		
La(NO$_3$)$_3$	0.069		
Ce(NO$_3$)$_3$	0.069		
Mean	0.068		

[a] From Ref 1 and unpublished data.

3. The coagulation values depend primarily on the valence of the counterions, decreasing by one to two orders of magnitude for each increase of one in their valence (Schulze-Hardy rule). According to the DLVO theory, the coagulation values vary inversely with the sixth power of the valence of the counterions. For mono-, di-, and trivalent counterions, they should be in the ratio

$$\frac{1}{1^6} : \frac{1}{2^6} : \frac{1}{3^6} \quad \text{or} \quad 100 : 1.6 : 0.14$$

The mean c_{CV}'s of Table III are 141 : 2.45 : 0.068, or 100 : 1.7 : 0.05, in satisfactory agreement with the DLVO theory.

The following conclusion can be drawn from the right half of Table III:

4. The cations on the right side of Table III constitute obvious exceptions to the preceding. Ag^+ is the potential-determining counterion. *Potential-determining ions* are those whose concentration determines the surface potential. When silver nitrate is added to the negative silver iodide dispersion, some of its silver ions are incorporated into the negatively charged surface of the particles and lower the magnitude of their charge by reducing the excess of I^- ions in the surface. Thus, silver salts are exceptionally effective coagulating agents because they reduce the magnitude of the ψ_0 as well as of the ζ potential. Indifferent salts, which reduce only the latter, require much higher salt concentrations for comparable reductions in the ζ potential. The other potential-determining ion of silver iodide is I^-. Alkali iodides have higher c_{CV}'s than 141 millimole/liter because they supply iodide ions which enter the surface layer of the silver iodide particles and increase its excess of I^- over Ag^+ ions, thereby making ψ_0 more negative. Bromide and chloride ions act similarly but less effectively.

The principal potential-determining ion for proteins is H^+; those for aluminum hydroxide are OH^- (and hence H^+) and Al^{3+}, but also Fe^{3+} and Cr^{3+} which form mixed hydroxides with Al^{3+}.

5. The cationic surfactant in Table III and the alkaloidal salts, which also behave as such, constitute the second exception to the Schulze-Hardy rule. Surface-active compounds contain hydrophilic and hydrophobic moieties in the same molecule, the latter being hydrocarbon portions which by themselves are water-insoluble. Their dual nature causes these compounds to accumulate in interfaces. Dodecylammonium and alkaloidal cations displace inorganic monovalent cations from the Stern layer of a negatively charged silver iodide particle because they are attracted to it not only by electrostatic forces like sodium ions but also by van der Waals forces between their hydrocarbon moieties (dodecyl chains in the case of the dodecylammonium ions) and the solid. Because they are strongly adsorbed from solution onto the surface and do not tend to dissociate from it, surface-active cations are very effective in reducing the ζ potential of the negative silver iodide particles, ie, they have lower c_{CV} than purely inorganic cations of the same valence.

6. Anionic surfactants like those containing lauryl sulfate ions also have a tendency to be adsorbed at solid-liquid interfaces. However, because of electrostatic repulsion between the negatively charged surface of silver iodide particles whose surface layer contains an excess iodide ions and the surface-active anions, adsorption usually does not occur below the critical micelle concentration (see below). If such adsorption does occur, it increases the density of negative charges in the particle surface, raising the c_{CV} of anionic surfactants above that corresponding to their valence.

Ionic solids with surface layers containing the ionic species in near proper stoichiometric balance, and most water-insoluble organic compounds have relatively low surface charge densities. They adsorb ionic surfactants of like charge from solution even at low concentrations, which increases their surface charge densities and the magnitude of their ζ potentials, stabilizing their aqueous dispersions.

The addition of water-miscible solvents such as alcohol, glycerin, propylene glycol or polyethylene glycols to aqueous dispersions lowers the dielectric constant of the medium. This reduces the thickness of the double layer and, therefore, the range over which electrostatic repulsion is effective, and lowers the size of the potential energy barrier. Addition of solvents to aqueous dispersions tends to coagulate them. At concentrations too low to cause coagulation by themselves, solvents make the dispersions more sensitive to coagulation by added electrolytes, ie, they lower the c_{CV}'s.

Progressive addition of the salt of a counterion of high valence reduces the ζ potential of colloidal particles gradually to zero. Eventually, the sign of the ζ potential may be inverted and its magnitude may increase again, but in the opposite direction. The ψ_0 and ζ potentials of aqueous sul-

famerazine suspensions are negative above their isoelectric points; those of bismuth subnitrate are positive. As discussed in Chapter 21, the addition of Al^{3+} to the former and of PO_4^{3-} to the latter in large enough amounts inverts the sign of their ζ potentials; their ψ_0 potentials remain unchanged. Surface-active ions of opposite charge may also produce such charge inversion.

The superposition of the van der Waals attractive energy with its long-range effectiveness and the electrostatic repulsive energy with its intermediate-range effectiveness frequently produces a shallow minimum (designated S in Fig 20-10) in the resultant energy-distance curve at interparticle distances d_S several times greater than δ. If this minimum in potential energy is small compared to kT, Brownian motion prevents aggregation. For large particles such as those of many pharmaceutical suspensions and for particles which are large in one or two dimensions (rods and plates), the *secondary minimum* may be deep enough to trap them at distances d_S from each other. This requires a depth of several kT units. Such fairly long-range and weak attraction produces loose aggregates or flocs which can be dispersed by agitation or by removal or reduction in the concentration of flocculating electrolytes.[1,6-8,18] This reversible aggregation process involving the secondary minimum is called *flocculation*. By contrast, aggregation in the deep primary minimum P, called *coagulation*, is irreversible.

Stabilization by Adsorbed Surfactants—As discussed in Chapter 19, surfactants tend to accumulate at interfaces because of their amphiphilic nature. This process is an *oriented physical adsorption*. Surfactant molecules arrange themselves at the interface between water and an organic solid or liquid of low polarity in such a way that the hydrocarbon chain is in contact with the surface of the solid particle or sticks inside the oil droplet while the polar headgroup is oriented towards the water phase. This orientation removes the hydrophobic hydrocarbon chain from the bulk of the water, where it is unwelcome because it interferes with the hydrogen bonding among the water molecules, while leaving the polar headgroup in contact with water so that it can be hydrated.

Fig 20-11A shows schematically that at low surfactant concentration and low surface coverage, the hydrocarbon chains of the adsorbed surfactant molecules lie flat against the solid surface. At higher surfactant concentrations, the surfactant molecules are adsorbed in the upright position to permit the adsorption of more surfactant per unit surface area. Fig 20-11B shows a nearly close-packed monolayer of adsorbed surfactant molecules. The terminal methyl groups of their hydrocarbon tails are in contact with the hydrophobic surface and the hydrocarbon tails are in lateral contact with each other. London dispersion forces promote attraction between both types of adjoining groups. The polar headgroups protrude into the water and are hydrated.

The adsorption of ionic surfactants increases the charge density and the ζ potential of the disperse particles. These two parameters are low for organic substances lacking ionic or strongly polar groups. The increase in electrostatic repulsion among the nonpolar organic particles due to adsorption of surface-active ions stabilizes the dispersion against coagulation. This "charge stabilization" is described by the DLVO theory.

Most water-soluble nonionic surfactants are polyoxyethylated (see Chapter 19): Each molecule consists of a hydrophobic hydrocarbon chain combined with a hydrophilic polyethylene glycol chain, eg $CH_3(CH_2)_{15}(OCH_2CH_2)_{10}OH$. Hydration of the 10 ether groups and of the terminal hydroxyl group renders the surfactant molecule water-soluble. It adsorbs at the interface between a hydrophobic solid and water, with the hydrocarbon moiety adhering to the solid surface and the polyethylene glycol moiety protruding into the water, where it is hydrated. The particle surface is thus surrounded

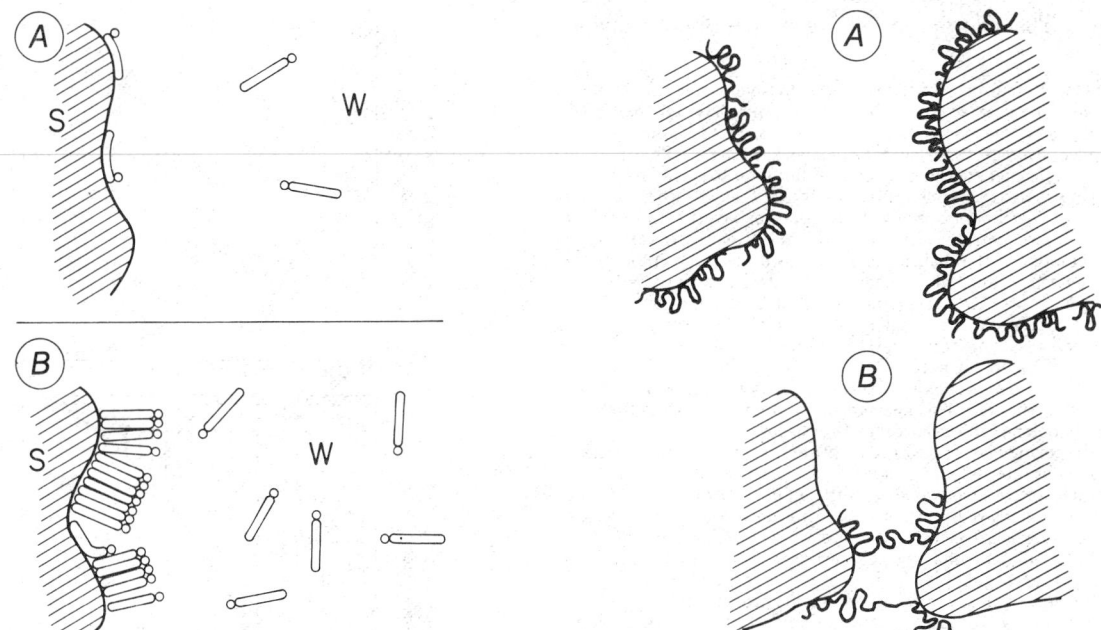

Fig 20-11.   Schematic representation of the physical adsorption of surfactant molecules at a hydrophobic solid (S)/water (W) interface. Cylindrical portions and spheres represent hydrocarbon chains and polar headgroups of the surfactant molecules, respectively.   (A) low surfactant concentration/low surface coverage; (B) near critical micelle concentration/surface coverage near saturation.

Fig 20-12.   Protective action (A) and sensitization (B) of sols of hydrophobic particles by adsorbed polymer chains.

by a thin layer of hydrated polyethylene glycol chains. This hydrophilic shell forms a steric barrier which prevents close contact between particles and, hence, coagulation ("steric stabilization"). Nonionic surfactants also reduce the sensitivity of hydrophobic dispersions towards coagulation by salts, ie, they increase the coagulation values.[19]

In a flocculated dispersion, groups of several particles are agglomerated into flocs. Frequently, the particles of a floc are in physical contact. When a surfactant is added to a flocculated sol, the dissolved surfactant molecules become adsorbed at the surface of the particles. Surfactant molecules tend to pry apart flocs by wedging themselves between the particles at their areas of contact. This action opens up for surfactant adsorption additional surface area that was previously blocked by adhesion of another solid surface. The breaking up of flocs or secondary particles is defined above as deflocculation or peptization.

Ophthalmic suspensions should be deflocculated because the large particle size of flocs causes eye irritation. Parenteral suspensions should be deflocculated to prevent flocs from blocking capillary blood vessels and hypodermic syringes, and to reduce tissue irritation. Deflocculated suspensions tend to cake, however, ie, the sediment formed by gravitational settling is compact and may be hard to disperse by shaking. Caking in oral suspensions is prevented by controlled flocculation as discussed in Chapter 21.

Stabilization by Adsorbed Polymers—Water-soluble polymers are adsorbed at the interface between water and a hydrophobic solid if they have some hydrophobic groups that limit their water solubility and render them amphiphilic and, hence, surface-active. Such polymers also tend to accumulate at the air-water interface and lower the surface tension of the aqueous phase. A high concentration of ionic groups in polyelectrolytes tends to eliminate surface activity and the tendency to adsorb at interfaces, because the polymer is excessively water-soluble. An example is *sodium carboxymethylcellulose*. *Polyvinyl alcohol* is very water-soluble due

to the high concentration of hydroxyl groups and does not adsorb extensively at interfaces. Polyvinyl alcohol is manufactured by the hydrolysis of polyvinyl acetate, which is water-insoluble. Incomplete hydrolysis of, say, only 85% of the acetyl groups produces a copolymer which is water-soluble but surface-active as well. Other surface-active polymers include methylcellulose, hydroxypropyl cellulose, high-molecular-weight polyethylene glycols (polyethylene oxides), and proteins. The surface activity of proteins is due to the presence of hydrophobic groups in the side chains at concentrations too low to cause insolubility in water. Proteins are denatured upon adsorption at air-water and solid-water interfaces.

The long, chain-like polymer molecules are adsorbed from solution onto solid surfaces in the form of loops projecting into the aqueous phase, as shown in Fig 20-12*A*, rather than lying flat against the solid substrate. Only a small portion of the chain segments of an adsorbed macromolecule is actually in contact with and adheres directly to the surface. Because of its great length, however, there are enough of such areas of contact to anchor the adsorbed macromolecule firmly onto the solid. Fig 20-11 is drawn on a much more expanded scale than Fig 20-12.

The sol particles are surrounded by a layer consisting of the adsorbed polymer chains, the water of hydration associated with them, and water trapped mechanically inside the chain loops. This sheath is an integral part of the particle surface. The layers of adsorbed polymer prevent the particles from approaching each other closely enough for the interparticle attraction by London dispersion forces to produce coagulation. These forces are effective only over very small interparticle distances of less than twice the thickness of the adsorbed polymer layer.

The mechanisms of *steric stabilization* by which adsorbed nonionic macromolecules prevent coagulation of hydrophobic sols (*protective action*) are also operative in the stabilization of sols by nonionic surfactants. The difference between adsorbed nonionic surfactants and adsorbed polymers is that the hydrophilic polyethylene glycol moieties of the adsorbed surfactant molecules protruding into water resemble the chain ends of the adsorbed macromolecules rather than their looped segments. The following protective mechanisms are operative:

1. The layer of adsorbed polymer and enmeshed water surrounding the particles forms a *mechanical* or *steric barrier* between them that prevents the close interparticle approach necessary for coagulation. At dense surface coverage, these layers are somewhat elastic. They may be dented by a collision between two particles but tend to spring back.

2. When two particles approach so closely that their adsorbed polymer layers overlap, the chain loops of the two opposing layers compress and mix with or interpenetrate each other. The resulting restriction to the freedom of motion of the chain segments in the overlap region produces a negative entropy change which tends to make the free energy change for the reduction in interparticle distance required for coagulation positive. The reverse process of disentanglement of the two opposing adsorbed polymer layers resulting from separation of the particles occurs because it is energetically more favorable. The particles are thus prevented from coagulation by *entropic repulsion* through the mechanism of *entropic stabilization* of the sol. This mechanism predominates when the concentration of polymer in the adsorbed layer is low.

3. As the polymer layers adsorbed on two approaching particles overlap and compress or interpenetrate each other, more polymer segments become crowded into a given volume of the aqueous region between the particles. The increased polymer concentration in the overlap region causes a local increase in osmotic pressure, which is relieved by an influx of water. This influx to dilute the polymer loops pushes the two particles apart, preventing coagulation.

4. If the adsorbed polymer has some ionic groups, stabilization by electrostatic repulsion or charge stabilization described above is added to the three steric stabilization mechanisms to prevent a close interparticle approach and, hence, coagulation.

5. The adsorption of water-soluble polymers changes the nature of the surface of the hydrophobic particles to hydrophilic, resulting in an increased resistance of the sol to coagulation by salts.[20]

The water-soluble polymers whose adsorption stabilizes hydrophobic sols and protects them against coagulation are called *protective colloids*. *Gelatin* and *serum albumin* are the preferred protective colloids for stabilizing parenteral suspensions because of their biocompatibility. These two polymers, as well as casein (milk protein), dextrin (partially hydrolyzed starch) and vegetable gums like acacia and tragacanth are metabolized in the human body. Cellulose derivatives and most synthetic protective colloids such as *povidone* are not biotransformed. Because of this and because of their large molecular size, polymers pertaining to the last two categories are not absorbed but excreted intact when they are administered in an oral dosage form.

A semiquantitative assessment of the stabilizing efficiency of protective colloids is the *gold number*, developed by Zsigmondy. It is the largest number of milligrams of a protective colloid which, when added to 10 mL of a special standardized gold sol, just fails to prevent the change in color from red to blue on addition of 1 mL of 10% NaCl solution. The gold sol contains 0.0058% gold with a particle size of about 250 Å. Coagulation by sodium chloride causes the color change. Representative gold numbers are 0.005–0.01 for gelatin, 0.01 for casein, 0.02–0.5 for egg albumin, 0.15–0.5 for acacia, and 1–7 for dextrin.[8,9] Gelatin is a more effective protective colloid than acacia and dextrin because the presence of some hydrophobic side groups makes it more surface active and causes more extensive adsorption from solution. Other protective numbers are based on different hydrophobic disperse solids, eg, silver, Prussian blue, sulfur, ferric oxide. The ranking of different protective colloids depends somewhat on the substrate. When formulating a disperse dosage form, one should measure the protective action on the actual solid hydrophobic phase to be dispersed as a sol.

Sensitization is the opposite of protective action, namely, a decrease in the stability of hydrophobic sols. It is brought about by some protective colloids, at concentrations well below those at which they exert a protective action. A protective colloid may, at very low concentrations, flocculate a sol in the absence of added salts and/or lower the coagulation values of the sol.

In the case of nonionic polymers or of polyelectrolytes with charges of the same sign as the sol, flocculation is the result

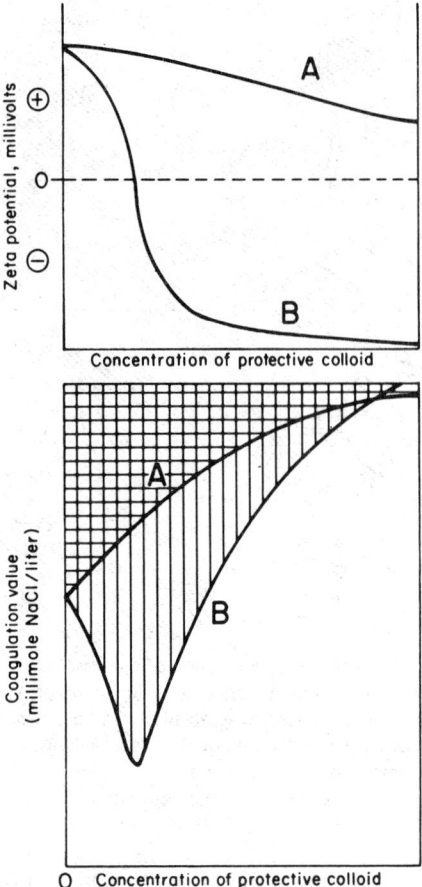

Fig 20-13. Protective action and sensitization: Polymer A exerts protective action at all concentrations while Polymer B sensitizes at low concentrations and stabilizes at high concentrations. Horizontal and vertical hatching indicates region of flocculation for a sol treated with various concentrations of Polymers A and B, respectively. Clear region underneath indicates sol is deflocculated.

of the bridging mechanism illustrated in Fig 20-12B. At very low polymer concentrations, there are not nearly enough polymer molecules present to cover each sol particle completely. Since the particle surfaces are largely bare, a single macromolecule may be adsorbed on two particles, bridging the gap between them and pulling them close together. Flocs of several particles are formed when one particle is bridged or connected to two or more other particles by two or more polymer molecules adsorbed jointly on two or possibly even three particles. Such flocculation usually occurs over a narrow range and at very low values of polymer concentrations. At higher concentrations, when enough polymer is available to cover the surface of all particles completely, bridging is unlikely to occur and the adsorbed polymer stabilizes or peptizes the sol.[20]

The nonionic Polymer A of Fig 20-13 stabilizes the sol at all concentrations. Neither sensitization by bridging nor by charge neutralization is observed. The reason that Polymer A lowers the positive ζ potential of the sol slightly is that increasing amounts of adsorbed polymer chains gradually shift the plane of shear outwards, away from the positively charged surface. If Polymer A were a cationic polyelectrolyte, the ζ potential–protective colloid concentration plot would gradually rise with increasing polymer adsorption rather than drop.

If the polymer has ionic groups of charge opposite to the charge of the sol particles, limited adsorption neutralizes the charge of the particles, reducing their ζ potential to near zero.

With stabilization by electrostatic repulsion thus inoperative, and steric stabilization ineffective because of low surface coverage with adsorbed polymer, the sol either coagulates by itself or is coagulated by very small amounts of sodium chloride. At higher polymer concentrations and more extensive adsorption, charge reversal of the particles to the sign of the charge of the polyelectrolyte reactivates charge stabilization and adds steric stabilization, increasing the coagulation value of the sol well above the initial value before polymer addition.

For example, a partly hydrolyzed polyacrylamide with about 20% of ammonium acrylate repeat units is an anionic polyelectrolyte. At the ppm level, the polymer flocculates aluminum hydroxide sols at a pH of 6–7, where the sols are positively charged and the polyelectrolyte is fully ionized. At a polymer concentration of 1:10,000, the sol becomes negatively charged because extensive polymer adsorption introduces an excess of —COO^- groups over =Al^+ ions into the particle surface. Steric stabilization plus electrostatic repulsion make the sol more stable against flocculation by salts than it was before the polyacrylamide addition.

Polymer B in Fig 20-13 illustrates this example. The curve in the lower plot indicates sensitization, with the coagulation value of sodium chloride lowered by as much as 60%. Zeta potential measurements can distinguish between sensitization by bridging and by charge neutralization. The charge reversal caused by adsorption of Polymer B shown in the upper plot pinpoints charge neutralization as the cause of sensitization. If Polymer B had a ζ potential–polymer concentration plot similar to Polymer A, sensitization would be ascribed to bridging.

Even water-soluble polymers which are too thoroughly hydrophilic to be adsorbed by hydrophobic sol particles can stabilize those sols. Their thickening action slows down Brownian motion and sedimentation, giving the particles less opportunity to come into contact and hence retarding flocculation.

Electrokinetic Phenomena—When a dc electric field is applied to a dispersion, the particles move towards the electrode of charge opposite to that of their surface. The counterions located inside their hydration shell are dragged along while the counterions in the diffuse double layer outside the plane of slip, in the free or mobile solvent, move towards the other electrode. This phenomenon is called *electrophoresis*. If the charged surface is immobile, as is the case with a packed bed of particles or a tube filled with water, application of an electric field causes the counterions in the free water to move towards the opposite electrode, dragging solvent with them. This flow of liquid is called *electroosmosis*, and the pressure produced by it, *electroosmotic pressure*. Conversely, if the liquid is made to flow past charged surfaces by applying hydrostatic pressure, the displacement of the counterions in the free water produces a potential difference between the two ends of the tube or bed called *streaming potential*.

The three phenomena depend on the relative motion of a charged surface and of the diffuse double layer outside the plane of slip surrounding that surface. The major part of the diffuse double layer is within the free solvent and can, therefore, move along the surface.[5-8] All three electrokinetic phenomena measure the identical ζ potential, which is the potential at the plane of slip.

The particles of pharmaceutical suspensions and emulsions are visible in the microscope or ultramicroscope, as are bacteria, erythrocytes and other isolated cells, latex particles, and many contaminant particles in pharmaceutical solutions. Their ζ potential is conveniently measured by *microelectrophoresis*. A potential difference E applied between two electrodes dipping into the dispersion and separated by a distance d produces the potential gradient or field strength E/d, expressed in v/cm. From the average velocity v of the particles, measured with the eyepiece micrometer of a microscope and a stopwatch, the ζ potential is calculated by the Smoluchowski equation

$$\zeta = \left(\frac{4\pi\eta}{D}\right)\left(\frac{v}{E/d}\right) = \left(\frac{4\pi\eta}{D}\right)u$$

The electrophoretic mobility $u = v/(E/d)$ is the velocity in a potential gradient of 1 v/cm. Particle size and shape do not affect the ζ potential according to the above equation. However, if the particle radius is comparable to δ or smaller (in which case the particles cannot be detected in a microscope), the factor 4 is replaced by 6. The viscosity η and the dielectric constant D refer to the aqueous medium in the double layer and cannot be measured directly.[21] Using the values for water at 25°, expressing the velocity in microns/sec and the electrophoretic mobility in (microns/sec)/(volts/cm), and converting into the appropriate units reduces the Smoluchowski equation to $\zeta = 12.9\ u$, with ζ given in millivolts (mV). If the particle surface has appreciable conductance, the ζ potential calculated by this equation may be low.[6,21] Dispersions of hydrophobic particles with ζ potentials below 20–30 mV are frequently unstable and tend to coagulate. On the other hand, values as high as ±180 mV have been reported for the ζ potential.[1,5]

The chief experimental precautions in microelectrophoresis measurements are:

1. Electroosmosis causes liquid to flow along the walls of the cell containing the dispersion. This in turn produces a return flow in the center of the cell. The microscope must be focused on the stationary boundary between the two liquid layers flowing in opposite directions in order to measure the true velocity of the particles.

2. Only in very dilute dispersions is it possible to follow the motion of single particles in the microscope field and to measure their velocity. Since the ζ potential depends largely on the nature, ionic strength, and pH of the suspending medium, dispersions should be diluted not with water but with solutions of composition identical to their continuous phase, eg, with their own serum separated by ultrafiltration or centrifugation. The Zeta-Meter is a commercial microelectrophoresis apparatus of easy, fast and reproducible operation.

When the particles cannot be observed individually with a microscope or ultramicroscope, other electrophoresis methods are employed.[5,8,22,23] In *moving boundary electrophoresis*, the movement of the boundary formed between a sol or solution and the pure dispersion medium in an electric field is studied. If the disperse phase is colorless, the boundary is located by the refractive index gradient (Tiselius apparatus, used frequently with protein solutions). If several species of particles or solutes with different mobilities are present, each will form a boundary moving with a characteristic velocity. Unlike microelectrophoresis, this method permits the identification of different colloidal components in a mixture, the measurement of the electrophoretic mobility of each, and an estimation of the relative amounts present.

Zone electrophoresis theoretically permits the complete separation of all electrophoretically different components, requires much smaller samples than moving boundary electrophoresis, and can be performed in simpler and less expensive equipment. The method avoids convection by supporting the solution in an inert and porous solid like filter paper, cellulose acetate membrane, agar, starch or polyacrylamide gels cut into strips, or disks or columns of polyacrylamide gel.

A strip of filter paper or gel is saturated with a conducting buffer solution and a few microliters of the solution being analyzed is deposited as a spot or narrow band. A potential difference is applied between the ends of the strip which are in contact with the electrode compartments. The spot or band spreads and unfolds as each component migrates towards one or the other electrode at a rate determined primarily by its electrophoretic mobility. Evaporation of water due to the heating effect of the electric current may be minimized by immersing the strip in a cooling liquid or sandwiching it between impervious solid sheets. After a sufficient time has elapsed to afford good separation, the strip is removed and dried. The position of the spots or bands corresponding to the individual components is detected by color reactions or radioactive counting.

Zone electrophoresis is applied mainly in analysis and for small-scale preparative separations. It does not permit mobility measurements. Because several samples can be analyzed simultaneously (in parallel strips or gel columns), because only minute amounts of sample are needed, and because the equipment is simple and easy to operate, zone electrophoresis is widely used to study the proteins in blood serum, erythrocytes, lymph and cerebrospinal fluid, saliva, gastric and pancreatic juices, and bile.

Immunodiffusion combined with electrophoresis is called *immunoelectrophoresis*.[22,24] The proteins in a fluid, including the antigens, are first separated by gel electrophoresis. A longitudinal trench is then cut along one or both sides of the gel strip near the edge in the direction of the electrophoresis axis. The trench is filled with the antibody solution. On standing, antibody and antigen proteins diffuse in all directions, including towards each other. Precipitation occurs along an elliptical arc (precipitin band) wherever an antigen meets its specific antibody. The precipitin bands are either visible directly or may be developed by staining. Since diseases frequently produce abnormal electrophoretic patterns in body fluids, zone electrophoresis and immunoelectrophoresis are convenient and powerful diagnostic techniques.

Isoelectric focusing[23,25] is a novel method using electrophoresis to separate proteins according to their isoelectric points. At pH values equal to their isoelectric points, proteins do not migrate in an electric field because their net charge is zero. In a liquid column on which a pH gradient is imposed, different species arrange themselves so that the protein with the highest isoelectric point will be located nearest to the cathode, which is immersed in the solution of a strong base. The protein with the lowest isoelectric point will be located nearest to the anode, which is immersed in the solution of a strong acid. The other proteins settle into intermediate positions, where the pH values are intermediate and equal to their isoelectric points.

Hydrophilic Dispersions

Most liquid disperse systems of pharmaceutical interest are aqueous. Therefore, most lyophilic colloidal systems discussed below consist of hydrophilic solids dissolved or dispersed in water. Most of the products mentioned below are official in the USP or NF, where more detailed descriptions may be found, also elsewhere in this text.

Hydrophilic colloids can be divided into particulate and soluble materials. The latter are water-soluble linear or branched polymers dissolved molecularly in water. Their aqueous solutions are classified as colloidal dispersions because the individual molecules are in the colloidal particle size range, exceeding 50 or 100 Å. Particulate or corpuscular hydrophilic colloidal dispersions are formed by solids which swell and are peptized in water but whose primary particles do not dissolve or break down into individual molecules or ions. One subdivision of particulate hydrophilic colloids is comprised of dispersions of cross-linked polymers whose linear, uncross-linked analogues are water-soluble.

Particulate Hydrophilic Dispersions

The disperse phase of these sols consists of solids which in water swell and break up spontaneously into particles of colloidal dimensions. The disperse particles have high specific surface areas and are, therefore, extensively hydrated. They

have characteristic shapes. If the attraction between individual particles is strong, the dispersions have yield values at relatively low solids content.

Bentonite is an aluminum silicate crystallizing in a layer structure (see above), with individual lamellas 9.4 Å thick. Their top and bottom surfaces are sheets of oxygen ions from silica plus an occasional sodium ion neutralizing a silicate ion-exchange site. The clay particles consist of stacks of these lamellas. Water penetrates inside the stacks between lamellas to hydrate the oxygen ions, causing extensive swelling. Bentonite particles in bentonite magma consist of single lamellas and packets of a few lamellas with intercalated water. The specific surface area amounts to several hundred square meters per gram. *Kaolin* also has a layer structure, but does not swell in water because water does not intercalate between individual lattice layers. Kaolin plates dispersed in water are, therefore, much thicker than those of bentonite, ca 0.04–0.2 μm. In kaolin, hydrated alumina lattice planes alternate with silica planes. Thus, one of the two external surfaces of a kaolin plate consists of a sheet of oxygen ions from silica, the other is a sheet of hydroxide ions from hydrated alumina. Both surfaces are well hydrated. Magnesium aluminum silicate (*Veegum*) is a clay similar to bentonite but contains magnesium; it is white whereas bentonite is gray.

Additional hydrophilic particles producing colloidal dispersions in water are listed below. *Colloidal silicon dioxide* consists of roughly spherical particles covered with siloxane and silanol groups (pages 278–279). *Titanium dioxide* is a white pigment with excellent covering power due to its high refractive index. *Microcrystalline cellulose* (page 277) is hydrophilic because of the hydroxyl and ether groups in the surface of the cellulose crystals. Gelatinous precipitates of hydrophilic compounds such as *aluminum hydroxide gel*, *aluminum phosphate gel*, and *magnesium hydroxide* consist of coarse flocs produced by agglomeration of the colloidal particles formed in the initial stage of the precipitation. They possess large internal surface areas, which is one of the reasons why the first two are used as substrates for adsorbed vaccines and toxoids.

Cross-linked Polymers—The polymers discussed below are polyelectrolytes, ie, they contain ionic groups and would be soluble in water in the absence of cross-linking. For instance, *sodium polystyrene sulfonate* is a copolymer of about 92% styrene and 8% divinylbenzene, which is sulfonated and neutralized to produce the cation-exchange resin

Chains a–b and c–d are water-soluble linear polymer chains. They are cross-linked or bound together via a phenylene group as shown. There are many such cross-links tieing every chain to two or more other chains, so that every atom in a grain of ion-exchange resin is bound to every other atom by primary, covalent bonds. The grains swell in water until the cross-links are strained but do not dissolve, because this would involve the rupture of primary valence bonds. Swelling renders the ion-exchange sites in the interior of a grain accessible to the gastrointestinal fluids. Partial exchange of Na^+ by K^+ followed by excretion of the used resin in the feces reduces hyperkalemia resulting from acute renal failure. Partial replacement of Na^+ by H^+ could reduce acidosis.

Cholestyramine resin is an anion-exchange resin containing the same backbone of cross-linked polystyrene, but substituted with $—CH_2—N^+(CH_3)_3Cl^-$ instead of sodium sulfonate. Part of the chloride anions is exchanged or replaced by bile salt anions, which are thus eliminated in the feces bound to the resin grains rather than reabsorbed. *Colestipol hydrochloride* is another orally administered anion-exchange resin used to increase the fecal excretion of bile salts. It is an extensively cross-linked, insoluble but permeable copolymer made from diethylenetriamine, tetraethylenepentamine, and epichlorohydrin. Strong cation- and anion-exchange resins are used as sustained-release vehicles for basic and acid drugs, respectively (see Chapter 92).

Polycarbophil is a copolymer of acrylic acid cross-linked with a small amount of divinyl glycol. The weakly acidic carboxyl groups are not ionized in the strongly acid environment of the stomach but only in the more nearly neutral intestines. Therefore, swelling by osmotic influx of water occurs mostly in the intestines, where imbibition of water decreases the fluidity of stools associated with diarrhea. Among natural polymers, tragacanth consists of $1/3$ of a water-soluble fraction, tragacanthin, and $2/3$ of a gel fraction called bassorin which swells in water but does not dissolve. Starch consists of $1/6$ of a fraction, soluble in hot water, called amylose. The remainder, amylopectin, merely absorbs water and swells. It owes its insolubility to extensive branching rather than cross-linking.

Soluble Polymers as Lyophilic Colloids

Most hydrophilic colloidal systems used in dosage forms are molecular solutions of water soluble, high molecular weight polymers. The polymers are either linear or slightly branched but not cross-linked.

Classifications—According to their origin, water-soluble polymers are divided into three classes. *Natural polymers* include polysaccharides (acacia, agar, heparin sodium, pectin, sodium alginate, tragacanth, xanthan gum) and polypeptides (casein, gelatin, protamine sulfate). Of these, agar and gelatin are only soluble in hot water.

Cellulose derivatives are produced by chemical modification of cellulose obtained from wood pulp or cotton to produce soluble polymers. *Cellulose* is an insoluble, linear polymer of glucose repeat units in the ring or pyranose form joined by β-1,4 glucosidic linkages. Each glucose repeat unit (except for the two terminal ones) contains a primary hydroxyl group on the No 6 carbon and two secondary hydroxyls on No 2 and 3 carbons. The primary hydroxyl is more reactive. Chemical modification of cellulose consists in reactions or substitutions of the hydroxyl groups. The extent of such reactions is expressed as *degree of substitution* (DS), namely, the number of substituted hydroxyl groups per glucose residue. The highest value is DS = 3.0. Fractional values are the rule because the DS is averaged over a multitude of glucose residues. A DS value of 0.6 indicates that some glucose repeat units are unsubstituted while others have one or even two substituents.

Soluble cellulose derivatives are listed below. The DS values correspond to the pharmaceutical grades. The groups shown are the replacements for the hydrogen atoms of the cellulosic hydroxyls. Official derivatives are *methylcellulose* (DS = 1.65–1.93), $—O—CH_3$ and *sodium carboxymethyl-*

cellulose (DS = 0.60–1.00), $—O—CH_2—COO^-Na^+$. *Hydroxyethyl cellulose* (DS $\cong$ 1.0), $—O—(CH_2CH_2—O)_nH$ and *hydroxypropyl cellulose* (DS $\cong$ 2.5) are manufactured by the addition of ethylene oxide and propylene oxide, respectively, to alkali-treated cellulose. The value of n is about 2.0 for the former and not much greater than 1.0 for the latter. *Hy-*

$$—O—\left(CH—CH_2—O\right)_n H$$
$$\qquad\quad | $$
$$\qquad\quad CH_3$$

droxypropyl methylcellulose is prepared by reacting alkali-treated cellulose first with methyl chloride to introduce methoxy groups (DS = 1.1–1.8) and then with propylene oxide to introduce propylene glycol ether groups (DS = 0.1–0.3). In general, the introduction of hydroxypropyl groups into cellulose reduces the water solubility somewhat while promoting the solubility in polar organic solvents like short-chain alcohols, glycols and some ethers.

The molecular weight of native cellulose is so high that soluble derivatives of approximately the same degree of polymerization would dissolve too slowly, and their solutions would be excessively viscous even at concentrations of 1% and less. Controlled degradation is used to break the cellulose chains into shorter segments, reducing the viscosity of the solutions of the corresponding soluble derivatives. Commercial grades of a given cellulose derivative such as sodium carboxymethylcellulose come in various molecular weights or viscosity grades as well as with various degrees of substitution, offering the pharmacist a wide selection.

Official cellulose derivatives which are insoluble in water but soluble in some organic solvents include *ethylcellulose* (DS = 2.2–2.7), $—O—C_2H_5$; *cellulose acetate phthalate* (DS = 1.70 for acetyl and 0.77 for phthalyl); and *pyroxylin* or cellulose nitrate (DS $\cong$ 2), $—O—NO_2$. *Collodion*, a 4.0% w/v solution of pyroxylin in a mixture of 75% (v/v) ether and 25% (v/v) ethyl alcohol, constitutes a lyophilic colloidal system.

The third class, water soluble *synthetic polymers*, consists mostly of vinyl derivatives including *polyvinyl alcohol*, *povidone* or polyvinylpyrrolidone, and *carbomer* (*Carbopol*), a copolymer of acrylic acid. High molecular weight polyethylene glycols are also called *polyethylene oxides*.

A second classification of hydrophilic polymers is based on their charge. *Nonionic* or uncharged polymers include methylcellulose, hydroxyethyl and hydroxypropyl cellulose, ethylcellulose, pyroxylin, polyethylene oxide, polyvinyl alcohol and povidone. *Anionic* or negatively charged *polyelectrolytes* include the following carboxylated polymers: acacia, alginic acid, pectin, tragacanth, xanthan gum and carbomer at pH values leading to ionization of the carboxyl groups; sodium alginate and sodium carboxymethylcellulose; also polypeptides at pH values above their isoelectric points, eg, sodium caseinate. A stronger acid group is sulfuric acid, which exists as a monoester in agar and heparin and as a monoamide in heparin. *Cationic* or positively charged *polyelectrolytes* are rare. Examples are polypeptides at pH values below their isoelectric points. Protamines are strongly basic due to a high arginine content, with isoelectric points around pH 12, eg protamine sulfate.

Gel Formation—As described in Chapter 22 and illustrated in Fig 22-7-*A*, the flexible chains of dissolved polymers interpenetrate and are entangled because of the constant Brownian motion of their segments. The chains writhe and forever change their conformations. Each chain is encased in a sheath of solvent molecules that solvate its functional groups. In the case of aqueous solutions, water molecules are hydrogen-bonded to the hydroxyl groups of polyvinyl alcohol, hydroxyl groups and ether links of polysaccharides, ether links of polyethylene oxide or polyethylene glycol, amide groups of polypeptides and povidone, and carboxylate groups of anionic polyelectrolytes. The envelope of water of hydration prevents chains segments in close proximity from touching and attracting one another by interchain hydrogen bonds and van der Waals forces as they do in the solid state. The slippage of solvated chains past one another when the solution flows is lubricated by the free solvent between their solvation sheaths.

Factors that lower the hydration of dissolved macromolecules reduce or thin out the sheath of hydration separating adjacent chains. When the hydration is low, contiguous chains tend to attract one another by secondary valence forces including hydrogen bonds and van der Waals forces. Hydrophobic bonding makes an important contribution to interchain attraction between polypeptide chains even in solution. Van der Waals forces and hydrogen bonds thus establish weak and reversible cross-links between chains at their points of contact or entanglement, bringing about phase separation or precipitation.

Most water-soluble polymers have higher solubilities in hot than in cold water and tend to precipitate on cooling, as the sheaths of hydration surrounding adjacent chains become too sparse to prevent interchain attraction. Dilute solutions separate into a solvent phase practically free of polymer and a viscous liquid phase containing practically all of the polymer but still a large excess of solvent. This process is called *simple coacervation* and the polymer-rich liquid phase a *coacervate*.[26] If the polymer solution is concentrated enough and/or the temperature low enough, cooling causes the formation of a continuous network of precipitating chains attached to one another through weak cross-links consisting of interchain hydrogen bonds and van der Waals forces at the points of mutual contact. Segments of regularly sequenced polymer chains even associate laterally into crystalline bundles or crystallites. Irregular chain structures as found in random copolymers, randomly substituted cellulose ethers and esters, and highly branched polymers like acacia prevent crystallization during precipitation from solution. Chain entanglements provide the sole temporary cross-links in those cases. The network of associated polymer chains immobilizes the solvent and causes the solution to set to a gel. Gelatinous precipitates or highly swollen flocs may separate when cooling more dilute polymer solutions.

Besides the chemical nature of polymer and solvent, the three most important factors causing phase separation, precipitation and gelation of polymer solutions are temperature, concentration and molecular weight. Lower temperatures, higher concentrations and higher molecular weights promote gelation and produce stronger gels.

For a typical *gelatin*, 10% solutions acquire yield values and begin to gel at about 25°, 20% solutions at about 30°, and 30% solutions at about 32°. The *gelation* is reversible: the gels liquefy when heated above these temperatures. Gelation is rarely observed above 34° regardless of concentration, so that gelatin solutions do not gel at 37°. Conversely, gelatin will dissolve readily in water at body temperature. The gelation temperature or gel point of gelatin is highest at the isoelectric point, where the attachment between adjacent chains by coulombic attraction or ionic bonds between carboxylate ions and alkylammonium, guanidinium or imidazolium groups is most extensive. Since the carboxyl groups are not ionized at gastric pH, interchain ionic bonds are practically nonexistent, and interchain attraction is limited to hydrogen bonds and van der Waals forces. The gelation temperature or the melting point of gelatin gels depends more strongly on temperature and concentration than on pH.[27] The combination of an acid pH considerably below the isoelectric point and a temperature of 37° completely prevents the gelation of gelatin solutions. Conversely, these two conditions promote rapid dissolution of gelatin capsules in the stomach. Agar and pectic acid solutions set to gels at only a few percent of solids.

Unlike most water-soluble polymers, methylcellulose, hydroxypropyl cellulose and polyethylene oxide are more soluble in cold than in hot water. Their solutions therefore tend to gel on heating (*thermal gelation*).

When dissolving powdered polymers in water, temporary gel formation often slows the process down considerably. As water diffuses into loose clumps of powder, their exterior frequently turns to a cohesive gel of solvated particles encasing dry powder. Such blobs of gel dissolve very slowly because of their high viscosity and the low diffusion coefficient of the macromolecules. Especially for large-scale dissolution, it is helpful to disperse the polymer powder in water before it can agglomerate into lumps of gel. In order to permit dispersion to precede hydration and to prevent temporary gel formation, the polymer powders are dispersed in water at temperatures where the solubility of the polymer is lowest. Most polymer powders, such as sodium carboxymethylcellulose, are dispersed with high shear in *cold* water before the particles can hydrate and swell to sticky gel grains agglomerating into lumps. Once the powder is well dispersed, the solution is heated with moderate shear to about 60° for fastest dissolution. Because methylcellulose hydrates most slowly in hot water, the powder is dispersed with high shear in ⅕ to ⅓ of the required amount of water heated to 80–90°. Once the powder is finely dispersed, the rest of the water is added cold or even as ice, and moderate stirring causes prompt dissolution. For maximum clarity, fullest hydration and highest viscosity, the solution should be cooled to 0°–10° for about an hour.

The following are two alternative methods for preventing the formation of gelatinous lumps upon addition of water. The powder is prewetted with a water-miscible organic solvent such as ethyl alcohol or propylene glycol that does not swell the polymer, in the proportion of from three to five parts solvent to each part of polymer. If other nonpolymeric powdered adjuvants are to be incorporated into the solution, these are dry-blended with the polymer powder. The latter should comprise ¼ or less of the blend for best results.

A pharmaceutical application of *gelation* in a nonaqueous medium is the manufacture of *Plastibase* or *Jelene*, which consists of 5% of a low-molecular-weight polyethylene and 95% of mineral oil. The polymer is soluble in mineral oil above 90°, which is close to its melting point. When the solution is cooled below 90°, the polymer precipitates and causes gelation. The mineral oil is immobilized in the network of entangled, and adhering, insoluble polyethylene chains which probably even associate into small crystalline regions. Unlike petrolatum, this gel can be heated to about 60° without substantial loss in consistency.

Large increases in the concentration of polymer solutions may lead to precipitation and gelation. One way of effectively increasing the concentration of aqueous polymer solutions is to add inorganic salts. The salts will bind part of the water of the polymer solution in order to become hydrated. Competition for water of hydration dehydrates the polymer molecules and precipitates them, causing gelation. This phenomenon is called *salting out*. Because of its high solubility in water, ammonium sulfate is often used by biochemists to precipitate and separate proteins from dilute solution. To the pharmacist, salting out usually represents an undesirable problem. It is reversible, however, and subsequent addition of water redissolves the precipitated polymers and liquefies their gels. Salting out may cause the polymer to separate as a concentrated and viscous liquid solution or simple coacervate rather than as a solid gel.

The effectiveness of electrolytes to salt out, precipitate or gel hydrophilic colloidal systems depends on how extensively the electrolytes are hydrated. The *Hofmeister* or *lyotropic series* arranges ions in the order of increasing hydration and increasing effectiveness in salting out hydrophilic colloids. The series, for monovalent cations, is

$$Cs^+ < Rb^+ < NH_4^+ < K^+ < Na^+ < Li^+$$

and for divalent cations,

$$Ba^{2+} < Sr^{2+} < Ca^{2+} < Mg^{2+}$$

This series also arranges the cations in the order of decreasing coagulating power or increasing coagulation values for negative hydrophobic sols (see Table III) and of increasing ease of their displacement from cation exchange resins: K^+ displaces Na^+ and Li^+. For anions, the lyotropic series in the order of decreasing coagulating power and decreasing effectiveness in salting out is

$$F^- > citrate^{3-} > HPO_4^{2-} > tartrate^{2-} >$$
$$SO_4^{2-} > acetate^- > Cl^- > NO_3^- > ClO_3^- >$$
$$Br^- > ClO_4^- > I^- > CNS^-$$

Iodides and thiocyanates and to a lesser extent bromides and nitrates actually tend to increase the solubility of polymers in water, salting them in.[1,3,5–7,9] These large polarizable anions destructure water, reducing the extent of hydrogen bonding among water molecules and thereby making more of the hydrogen-bonding capacity of water available to the solute. Most salts except nitrates, bromides, perchlorates, iodides and thiocyanates raise the temperature of precipitation or gelation of most hydrophilic colloidal solutions or their gel melting points. Exceptions among hydrophilic colloids are methylcellulose, hydroxypropyl cellulose and polyethylene oxide whose gelation temperatures or gel points and gel melting points are lowered by salting out.

Hydrophobic aqueous dispersions are coagulated by electrolytes at $0.0001–0.1$ M concentrations (see Table III). Moreover, the coagulation is irreversible, ie, removal of the coagulating salt does not allow the coagulum to be redispersed, because the hydrophobic sols are intrinsically unstable. By contrast, most hydrophilic sols require electrolyte concentrations of 1 M or higher for precipitation. Their precipitation or gelation can be reversed, and the polymer redissolved by removing the salt through dialysis or by adding more water. Hydrophilic colloids disperse or dissolve spontaneously in water, and their sols are intrinsically stable.

Most of the hydrophilic and water-soluble polymers mentioned above are only slightly soluble or insoluble in alcohol. Addition of alcohol to their aqueous solutions may cause precipitation or gelation because (i) alcohol is a nonsolvent or precipitant, lowering the dielectric constant of the medium, and (ii) alcohol tends to dehydrate the hydrophilic solute. Alcohol lowers the concentrations at which electrolytes salt out hydrophilic colloids. Phase separation through the addition of alcohol to an aqueous polymer solution may cause coacervation, ie, the separation of a concentrated viscous liquid phase, rather than precipitation or formation of a gel. Sucrose also competes for water of hydration with hydrophilic colloids, and may cause phase separation. However, most hydrophilic sols tolerate substantially higher concentrations of sucrose than of electrolytes or alcohol. Lower viscosity grades of a given polymer are usually more resistant to electrolytes, alcohol and sucrose than grades of higher viscosity and higher molecular weights.

Whenever hydrophilic colloidal dispersions undergo irreversible precipitation or gelation, chemical reactions are involved. Neither dilution with water nor heating nor attempts to remove the gelling or precipitating agent by washing or dialysis will liquefy those gels or redissolve the gelatinous precipitates formed at lower polymer concentrations. Carboxyl groups are not ionized in strongly acid media. If a polymer owes its solubility to the ionization of these weakly acid groups, reducing the pH of its solution below 3 may lead to precipitation or gelation. This is observed with such carboxylated polymers as many gums, sodium carboxymethyl-cellulose and carbomer. Hydrogen carboxymethylcellulose swells and disperses but does not dissolve in water. Neutralization to higher pH values returns the carboxyl groups to their ionized state and reverses the gelation or precipitation.

Only the sodium, potassium, ammonium and triethanolammonium salts of carboxylated polymers are well soluble in water. In the case of carboxymethylcellulose, salts with heavy metal cations (silver, copper, mercury, lead) and trivalent cations (aluminum, chromic, ferric) are practically insoluble. Salts with divalent cations, especially of the alkaline earth metals, have borderline solubilities. Generally, higher degrees of substitution tend to increase the tolerance of the carboxymethylcellulose to salts.

Precipitation or gelation occur due to metathesis when inorganic salts of heavy or trivalent cations are mixed with alkali metal salts of carboxylated polymers in solution. For instance, if a soluble copper salt is added to a solution of sodium carboxymethylcellulose, the double decomposition can be written schematically as

$$R_1COO^-Na^+ + R_2COO^-Na^+ + CuSO_4 \longrightarrow$$

R_1 and R_2 represent two carboxymethylcellulose chains which are cross-linked by a chelated copper ion. Dissociation of the cupric carboxylate complex is negligible.

Association Colloids

Solution Properties and Micelle Formation of Surfactants

Surface activity characterizes compounds which, while soluble in a given liquid, tend to accumulate in the interfaces between this liquid and air, another immiscible liquid, or a solid. Because of their high concentration in these interfaces, surface-active compounds lower the corresponding interfacial tensions or free energies. This discussion deals mainly with aqueous media, where some soluble high polymers such as methylcellulose and vinyl methyl ether–maleic anhydride copolymer and many small molecules such as soaps and quaternary ammonium salts are surface-active. Because the small molecules in dilute solutions tend to associate into aggregates (micelles) of equivalent diameters in the 30–100 Å range, ie, of colloidal dimensions, they are called *association colloids*. Other names are *surfactants* or *surface-active agents*.[6,28–30]

Surfactants are amphiphiles because they contain a hydrocarbon (hydrophobic and lipophilic) portion and one or more ionic or otherwise strongly hydrophilic groups in the same molecule (see Chapters 19 and 21). This dual nature causes them to be preferentially adsorbed at air-water, oil-water, and solid-water interfaces, forming oriented monolayers in which the hydrophilic groups are in the aqueous phase and the hydrocarbon chains are pointed towards the air, in contact with the solid surface, or immersed in the oil phase.

As increasing amounts of a solid surfactant are dissolved in a beaker full of water and its concentration in solution increases, its monolayers adsorbed at the air-water and glass-water interfaces become more and more crowded until they are so tightly packed that further occupancy requires excessive compression of the surfactant molecules already in the two monolayers (saturation adsorption, see Chapter 19). Further increments in the amount of dissolved surfactant beyond that concentration cause amounts equivalent to the new molecules to aggregate into micelles. This process begins at a characteristic concentration called the *critical micelle concentration*

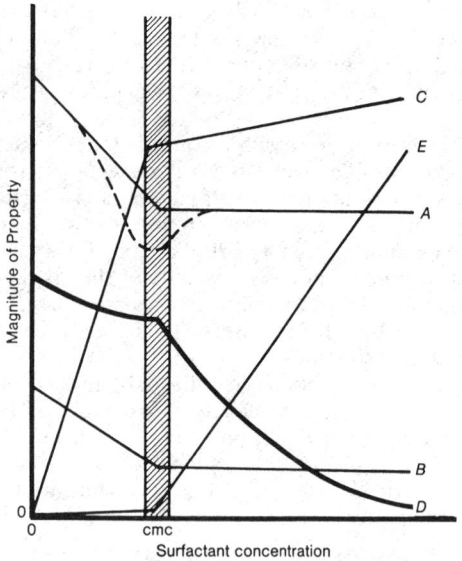

Fig 20-14.   Effect of surfactant concentration and micelle formation on various properties of the aqueous solution of an ionic surfactant. *A:* Surface tension; *B:* interfacial tension; *C:* osmotic pressure; *D:* equivalent conductivity; *E:* solubility of compound with very low solubility in pure water. (Courtesy, Schott H, Martin AN, in Dittert LW, ed: *American Pharmacy*, 7th ed, Lippincott, Philadelphia, Chap 6, 1974).

(cmc). From then on, the concentration of monomeric or nonassociated surfactant molecules hardly increases, rising only slightly above the cmc, but the concentration of micellar or associated molecules increases in direct proportion to the increase in overall surfactant concentration. In dilute solutions, the micelles are approximately of the same size; increments in surfactant concentration merely increase their number.

The magnitudes of several properties of surfactant solutions are plotted against concentration in Fig 20-14. All curves undergo profound changes in slope over a narrow range of concentration which defines the cmc. The reason is that the bulk of the surfactant molecules present at concentrations in excess of the cmc are aggregated into micelles. Since the number of solute particles increases much more slowly with concentration above the cmc than below it, so do the colligative properties like osmotic pressure. The surface and interfacial tensions of surfactant solutions decrease rapidly until the cmc is reached, but remain nearly constant at higher concentrations. Surface-active impurities sometimes produce a minimum in the surface tension–concentration curve in the vicinity of the cmc, shown as a dotted line in curve *A* of Fig 20-14. The equivalent conductivity of ionic surfactant solutions, obtained by dividing the specific electric conductivity by the concentration expressed as equivalents/cm^3, decreases at a faster rate above the cmc than below. This indicates that micelles transport electricity more slowly than nonassociated surfactant ions.[28,30]

The partial molal volume of the surfactant and the relative viscosity and turbidity of its solutions increase faster with increasing concentration above the cmc than below it. Aggregates, because of their larger size, engender more resistance to flow than nonassociated surfactant molecules. The higher turbidity results from the increased amount of light scattered by the comparatively large micelles. However, to the naked eye, solutions above and below the cmc appear equally clear. The rate of increase of the refractive index of surfactant solutions with concentration is higher below than above the cmc.

The shape of micelles formed in dilute surfactant solutions

is approximately spherical (see Fig 20-15*A*). The polar headgroups of the surfactant molecules are arranged in an outer spherical shell whereas their hydrocarbon chains are oriented towards the center, forming a spherical core for the micelle. The hydrocarbon chains are randomly coiled and entangled; the micellar interior has a nonpolar, liquid-like character resembling a liquid normal paraffin such as dodecane. In the micelles of polyoxyethylated nonionic surfactants, the polyoxyethylene moieties are oriented outwards and permeated by water while the hydrocarbon moieties form an "oil droplet" core as in ionic micelles (see Fig 20-15*B*).[28–33]

This arrangement is energetically favorable all around. The hydrophilic headgroups, located externally, are in contact with water and remain extensively hydrated. The hydrocarbon moieties are removed from the aqueous medium and partly shielded from contact with water by the polar headgroups. They no longer interfere with hydrogen bonding among water molecules. This interference is the reason why surfactant molecules are pushed out of aqueous media towards interfaces. The hydrocarbon tails of the surfactant molecules, located in the interior of the micelle, interact with one another by weak London–van der Waals forces (hydrophobic bonding).

Micelles are not static aggregates but dissociate, regroup, and reassociate rapidly. The half-life of micelles of ionic surfactants in the absence of additives is a small fraction of one second. Nonionic micelles dissociate much less rapidly.

Representative values of the critical micelle concentration and of the aggregation number, ie, the number of surfactant molecules/micelle, are listed in Table IV.[28,31–34] Cmc values depend primarily on whether the surfactant is ionic or nonionic. The lateral electrostatic repulsion of the charged headgroups located in the periphery of ionic micelles is an obstacle to micelle formation, deferring it to higher surfactant concentrations. Whether the surfactant is anionic (negatively charged headgroups) or cationic (positively charged headgroups) is of secondary importance in determining the cmc. The addition of simple salts reduces these repulsive forces and, therefore, lowers the cmc of ionic surfactants.

Within a homologous series, the cmc decreases regularly with increasing length of the hydrocarbon chain and, therefore, with increasing surface activity of the surfactant (Traube's rule). As is seen in Table IV, each additional methylene group approximately halves the cmc. For polyoxyethylated nonionic surfactants, the cmc increases with increasing hydrophile-lipophile balance (defined in Chapter 21) and with decreasing temperature.

The size of a micelle or its aggregation number is governed largely by geometric factors. The radius of the hydrocarbon core cannot exceed the length of the extended hydrocarbon chain of the surfactant molecule. Therefore, increasing the chain length or ascending a homologous series increases the aggregation number of spherical micelles. For surfactants whose hydrocarbon portion is a single normal alkyl chain, the maximum aggregation numbers consistent with spherical shape are approximately 27, 39, 54, 72, and 92 for C_8, C_{10}, C_{12}, C_{14}, and C_{16}, respectively. The micelles of sodium lauryl sulfate in the saline solution and of the nonionic surfactants of Table IV are too large to be spherical. The nonionic surfactants form larger micelles at the higher temperature because of lower hydration, ie, the system is moving in the direction of the cloud point. Micellar diameters range from 25 Å for sodium octane sulfonate to 60 Å for the equivalent spherical diameter of the 10 ethylene oxide adduct of dodecanol at 25°. The micelles are thus at the lower end of the particle size range for colloids.

On increasing the surfactant concentration beyond a few percent, on adding electrolytes in the case of ionic surfactants, and on raising the temperature in the case of nonionic sur-

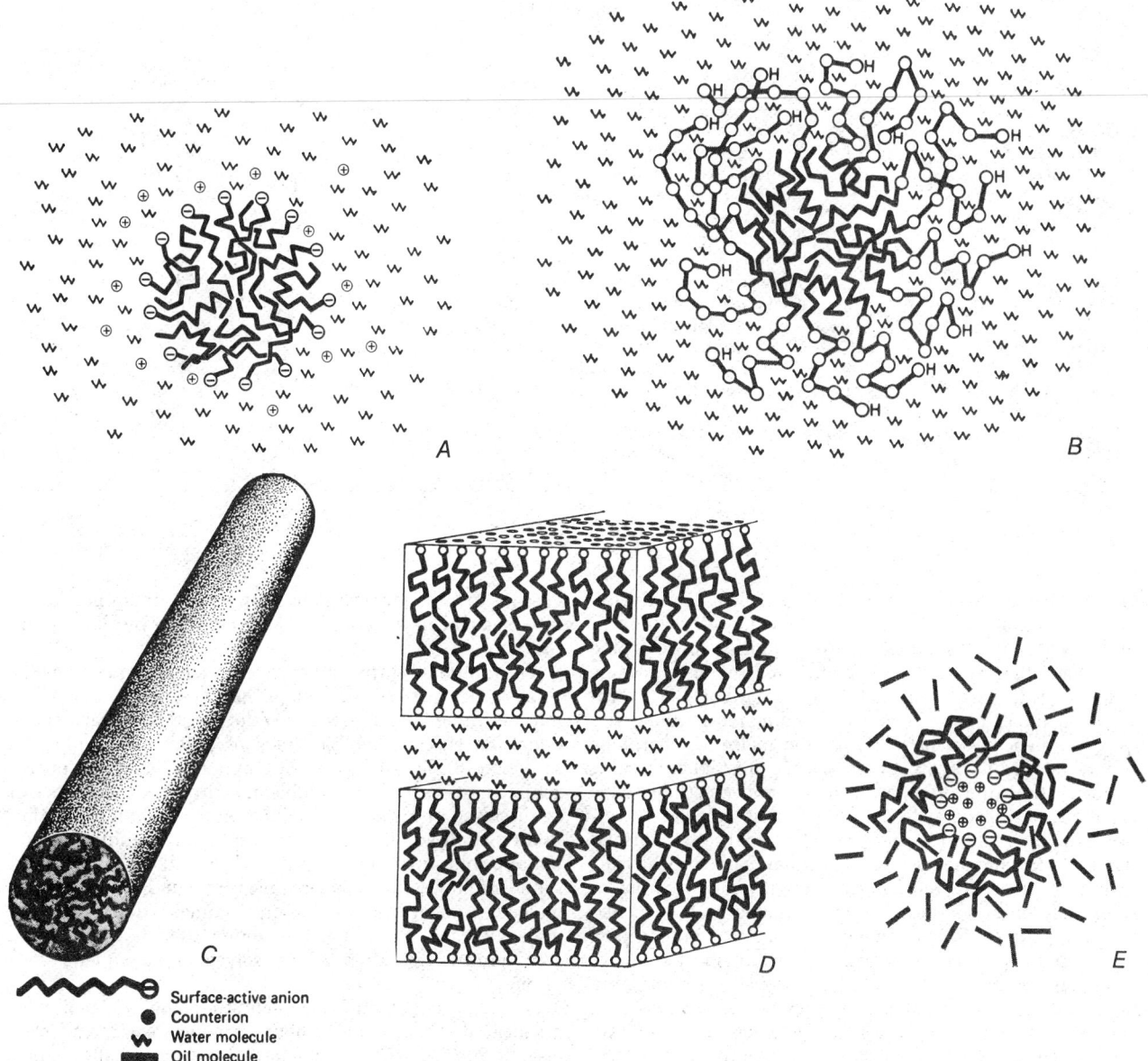

Surface-active anion
● Counterion
ᴡ Water molecule
▬ Oil molecule

Fig 20-15.   Different types of micelles.   *A:* Spherical micelle of an anionic surfactant; *B:* spherical micelle of a nonionic surfactant; *C:* cylindrical micelle of an ionic surfactant; *D:* lamellar micelle of an ionic surfactant; *E:* reverse micelle of an anionic surfactant in oil. (Courtesy: Schott H, Martin AN, in Dittert LW, ed: *American Pharmacy*, 7th ed, Lippincott, Philadelphia, Chap 6, 1974.)

factants, the micelles increase in size. Being too large to remain spherical, they change to ellipsoidal, to cylindrical, and finally to lamellar shapes. In cylindrical micelles, the polar headgroups form the periphery and the hydrocarbon tails fill the interior of cylinders (Fig 20-15C). In lamellar micelles, the surfactant molecules are arranged in parallel bimolecular sheets with a tail-to-tail orientation, ie, the hydrocarbon tails form the inner layer. Water is stratified between sheets, hydrating the external polar headgroups (Fig 20-15D). In both types of micelles, the hydrocarbon tails are randomly coiled and in a liquid-like state.[15,30]

In concentrated aqueous solutions containing 20% or more surfactant, cylindrical micelles often line up parallel and arrange themselves into hexagonal arrays. Likewise, lamellar micelles are often parallel and equidistant from each other, with the intervening water layers of equal thickness. These ordered solutions are birefringent and quite viscous. They are in the liquid crystalline or mesomorphic state, ie, they are liquids which have some of the properties of crystalline solids.

Since the membrane and the protoplasm of cells may be in the liquid crystalline state, such structures are of biological importance.

Oil-soluble surfactants such as heavy-metal soaps, sodium dioctylsulfosuccinate, and sorbitan monoesters form aggregates when dissolved in hydrocarbons, chlorinated hydrocarbons, and other nonaqueous liquids of low polarity. These micelles are inverted or turned inside out (see Fig 20-15E): the hydrocarbon tails are oriented outwards into the oil phase while the polar headgroups are in the center of the micelle, where water can be solubilized. Because the bulky headgroups are in the center, the aggregation numbers of such reverse micelles are small, usually between 3 and 20.[35]

Drugs as Association Colloids

Association into micelles is of importance in the case of surface-active drugs. The following are examples of drugs that behave as cationic or anionic surfactants; they are sur-

Table IV—Critical Micelle Concentrations and Micellar Aggregation Numbers of Various Surfactants in Water at Room Temperature

Structure	Name	CMC, mM/L	Surfactant molecules/ micelle
$n\text{-}C_{11}H_{23}COOK$	Potassium laurate	24	50
$n\text{-}C_8H_{17}SO_3Na$	Sodium octant sulfonate	150	28
$n\text{-}C_{10}H_{21}SO_3Na$	Sodium decane sulfonate	40	40
$n\text{-}C_{12}H_{25}SO_3Na$	Sodium dodecane sulfonate	9	54
$n\text{-}C_{12}H_{25}OSO_3Na$	Sodium lauryl sulfate	8	62
$n\text{-}C_{12}H_{25}OSO_3Na$	Sodium lauryl sulfate[a]	1	96
	Sodium di-2-ethylhexyl sulfosuccinate	5	48
$n\text{-}C_{10}H_{21}N(CH_3)_3Br$	Decyltrimethylammonium bromide	63	36
$n\text{-}C_{12}H_{25}N(CH_3)_3Br$	Dodecyltrimethylammonium bromide	14	50
$n\text{-}C_{14}H_{29}N(CH_3)_3Br$	Tetradecyltrimethylammonium bromide	3	75
$n\text{-}C_{14}H_{29}N(CH_3)_3Cl$	Tetradecyltrimethylammonium chloride	3	64
$n\text{-}C_{12}H_{25}NH_3Cl$	Dodecylammonium chloride	13	55
$n\text{-}C_{12}H_{25}O(CH_2CH_2O)_8H$	Octaoxyethylene glycol monododecyl ether	0.13	132
$n\text{-}C_{12}H_{25}O(CH_2CH_2O)_8H^{b}$		0.10	301
$n\text{-}C_{12}H_{25}(CH_2CH_2O)_{12}H$	Dodecaoxyethylene glycol monododecyl ether	0.14	78
$n\text{-}C_{12}H_{25}O(CH_2CH_2O)_{12}H^{b}$		0.091	116
$t\text{-}C_8H_{17}\text{-}C_6H_4\text{-}O(CH_2CH_2O)_{9.7}H$	Decaoxyethylene glycol mono-p,t-octylphenyl ether (octoxynol 9)	0.27	100

[a] Interpolated for physiologic saline, 0.154 M NaCl.
[b] At 55°C instead of 20°C.

face-active and associate into micelles: Antibacterials (hydrochlorides of acridines, benzalkonium chloride, cetylpyridinium chloride), tranquilizers (hydrochlorides of reserpine and phenothiazine derivatives), local anesthetics (procaine hydrochloride, tetracaine hydrochloride, dibucaine hydrochloride, lidocaine hydrochloride), nonnarcotic analgesics (propoxyphene hydrochloride), narcotic analgesics (morphine sulfate, meperidine hydrochloride), some prostaglandin salts, antimuscarinic drugs (propantheline bromide, methantheline bromide, methixene hydrochloride), cholinergic agents (pilocarpine hydrochloride and other alkaloidal salts), antihistamines (pyrilamine maleate, tripelennamine hydrochloride, chlorcyclizine hydrochloride, diphenhydramine hydrochloride), anthelmintics (lucanthone hydrochloride), and antibiotics (sodium fusidate, some penicillins, and cephalosporins).[36] In the presence of common surfactants, surface-active drugs may form mixed micelles, ie, aggregates containing molecules of both compounds. The properties (composition, cmc, aggregation number) of mixed micelles are frequently a weighted average of the corresponding properties of the individual surfactants.[28,30]

According to the *Ferguson principle*, the toxicity to microorganisms or the therapeutic efficacy of a drug depends on its chemical potential or thermodynamic activity rather than on its concentration. If the external phase to which the drug was administered, eg, blood or gastrointestinal fluid, is in equilibrium with the internal phase where the receptor site is located (eg, tissue or bacteria), the chemical potential of the drug in both phases is the same (see Chapter 15). For drugs capable of associating into micelles, the therapeutically active species are the nonassociated molecules. Micelles are mere reservoirs for monomeric drug molecules into which they dissociate on dilution. Thus, according to the Ferguson principle, no increase in efficacy can be expected by raising the blood level of such drugs or their concentration in the gastrointestinal fluid above their cmc, because the chemical potential of the nonassociated molecules remains nearly constant.

Micellar Solubilization [30,37-47]

The pharmacists Engler and Dieckhoff discovered, in the 19th century, that water-insoluble materials like tars and cresols could be dissolved in concentrated aqueous solutions

of soaps to form clear solutions as opposed to milky emulsions. The mechanism was elucidated 30 years later by Hartley and McBain.[37]

The interior of surfactant micelles formed in aqueous media consists of hydrocarbon tails in liquid-like disorder. The micelles resemble minuscule pools of liquid hydrocarbon like dodecane surrounded by shells of polar headgroups, as sketched in Figs 20-15A–D. Compounds which are poorly soluble in water but well soluble in hydrocarbon solvents can be dissolved inside micelles, ie, they are brought into solution in an overall aqueous medium. In fact, if an aqueous surfactant solution is in contact with a bulk solid or liquid water-insoluble, oil-soluble organic compound, the surfactant molecules penetrate into the organic mass, detach organic molecules and form micelles around them. The organic compound is thus gradually dissolved in the aqueous medium.

Being hydrophobic and oleophilic, the solubilized molecules are located primarily in the hydrocarbon core of the micelles (see Fig 20-16A). Even water-insoluble drugs usually contain polar functional groups such as hydroxyl, carbonyl, ether, amino, amide, and cyano. Upon solubilization, these hydrophilic groups locate on the periphery of the micelle among the polar headgroups of the surfactant in order to become hydrated (see Fig 20-16B). For instance, when cholesterol or dodecanol is solubilized by sodium lauryl sulfate, their hydroxyl groups penetrate between sulfate ions and are even bound to them by hydrogen bonds, while their hydrocarbon portions are immersed among the dodecyl tails of the surfactant which make up the core of the micelle.

Micelles of polyoxyethylated nonionic surfactants consist of an outer shell of hydrated polyethylene glycol moieties and a core of hydrocarbon moieties (see Fig 20-16B). Compounds like phenol, cresol, benzoic acid, salicylic acid, and esters of p-hydroxybenzoic and p-aminobenzoic acids have some solubility in water and in oils but considerable solubility in liquids of intermediate polarity like ethanol, propylene glycol or aqueous solutions of polyethylene glycols. When solubilized by nonionic micelles, they are located in the hydrated outer polyethylene glycol shell as shown in Fig 20-16C. Since these compounds have hydroxyl or amino groups, they frequently form complexes with the ether oxygens of the surfactant by hydrogen bonding.[28,41,42,44,46]

Solubilization is generally nonspecific: any drug which is

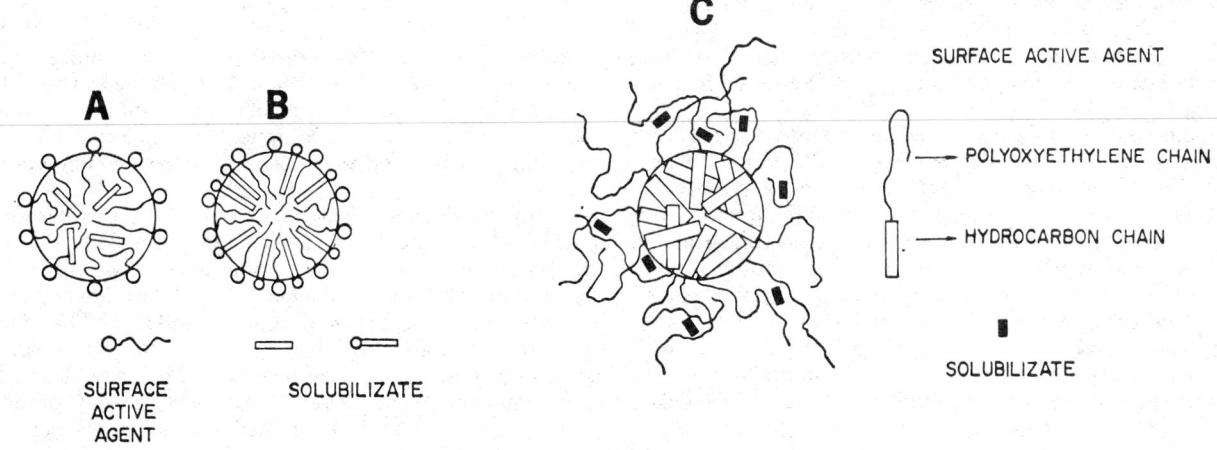

Fig 20-16.   The locations of solubilizates in spherical micelles.   A: Ionic surfactant (solubilized molecule has no hydrophilic groups); B: ionic surfactant (solubilized molecule has a hydrophilic group); C: nonionic surfactant (polar solubilizate). (Courtesy,   Shinoda K, *et al: Colloidal Surfactants*, Academic, New York, Chap 2, 1963.)

appreciably soluble in oils can be solubilized. Each has a solubilization limit, comparable to a limit of solubility, which depends on temperature and on the nature and concentration of the surfactant. Hartley distinguishes two categories of solubilizates. The first consists of comparatively large, asymmetrical and rigid molecules forming crystalline solids, such as steroids and dyes. These do not blend in with the normal paraffin tails which make up the micellar core; because of dissimilarity in structure, they remain distinct as solute molecules. They are sparingly solubilized by surfactant solutions, a few molecules/micelle at saturation (see Table V). The number of carbon atoms in the micellar hydrocarbon core required to solubilize a molecule of steroid or dye at saturation is of the same order of magnitude as the number of carbon atoms of bulk liquid dodecane or hexadecane per molecule of steroid or dye in their saturated solutions in these liquids.

Since solubilization depends on the presence of micelles, it does not take place below the cmc. It can, therefore, be used to determine the cmc, particularly when the solubilizate is a dye or another compound easy to assay. Plotting the maximum amount of a water-insoluble dye solubilized by aqueous surfactant, or the absorbance of its saturated solutions, versus the surfactant concentration produces a straight line which intersects the surfactant concentration axis at the cmc.

Above the cmc, the amount of solubilized dye is directly proportional to the number of micelles and, therefore, proportional to the overall surfactant concentration. Below the cmc, no solubilization takes place. This is represented by Curve E of Fig 20-14.

The second category of compounds to be solubilized are often liquid at room temperature and consist of relatively small, symmetrical, and/or flexible molecules such as many constituents of essential oils. These molecules mix and blend in freely with the hydrocarbon portions of the surfactants in the core of the micelles, so as to become indistinguishable from them. Such compounds are extensively solubilized and in the process usually swell the micelles: they augment the volume of the hydrocarbon core and increase the number of surfactant molecules per micelle. Their solubilization frequently lowers the cmc.

Pharmaceutical Applications of Micellar Solubilization—Saponated cresol solution, which consists of 49% v/v of cresol solubilized in concentrated aqueous sodium or potassium soap solution, is the oldest official preparation making use of solubilization. Hexachlorophene liquid soap contains 0.24% w/w of hexachlorophene solubilized in an 11% solution of a potassium soap. Both are clear liquids. With the advent of nonionic surfactants, it became possible to formulate solubilized preparations for internal use. Polyoxyethylated surfactants with hydrophile-lipophile balance numbers (defined in Chapter 19) between 13 and 18 are the most widely used solubilizing agents. Among them are polysorbate 80, polysorbate 20, and to a lesser extent polyoxyl 40 stearate and octoxynol 9.

Many water-insoluble drugs are formulated as clear, aqueous solutions by processes of micellar solubilization.[41,42,44,46,47] For example, adrenal cortical hormones, including cortisol, prednisolone and their acetates, cortisone acetate, and fluorometholone are solubilized by polysorbate 80 in ophthalmic solutions. The fat-soluble vitamins A alcohol and palmitate, D, E and its acetate, and K are solubilized in aqueous media by polyoxyethylated surfactants. In this state, they are often more stable than when molecularly dissolved in vegetable oils. Antibiotics of low water-solubility like chloramphenicol, tyrothricin, griseofulvin, and amphotericin B are readily solubilized by aqueous solutions of nonionic surfactants, as are sulfonamides of low water-solubility like sulfapyridine, sulfisoxazole, and sulfaethidole. Other poorly soluble drugs which have been solubilized by nonionic surfactants include nonnarcotic analgesics and antipyretics (aspirin, acetanilid, and phenacetin), barbiturates (phenobarbital, secobarbital and others whose soluble sodium salts

Table V—Micellar Solubilization Capacities of Different Surfactants for Estrone [a]

Surfactant	Concentration range, molarity	Temp, °C	Moles surfactant/ mole solubilized estrone
Sodium laurate	0.025–0.023	40	91
Sodium oleate	0.002–0.35	40	53
Sodium lauryl sulfate	0.004–0.15	40	71
Sodium cholate	0.09–0.23	20	238
Sodium deoxycholate	0.007–0.36	20	476
Diamyl sodium sulfosuccinate	0.08–0.4	40	833
Dioctyl sodium sulfosuccinate	0.002–0.05	40	196
Tetradecyltrimethylammonium bromide	0.005–0.08	20	45
Hexadecylpyridinium chloride	0.001–0.1	20	32
Polysorbate 20	0.002–0.15	20	161
Polysorbate 60	0.0008–0.11	20	83

[a] Courtesy, Sjöblom L, in Shinoda K, ed: *Solvent Properties of Surfactant Solutions*, Dekker, New York, Chap 5, 1967.

are unstable and sometimes irritant), anticoagulants (dicumarol, ethyl biscoumacetate), and alkaloidal and glycosidal drugs (cinchona and tropane alkaloids, cardiac glycosides) whose extraction from plant material is facilitated by polysorbates.

Iodine and nitrofurazone are solubilized by octoxynol 9, the former possibly through complexation with the ether oxygens.[41] Polysorbate 80 solubilizes coal tar and Peruvian balsam. Tinctures (eg, benzoin, and lemon) and elixirs (eg, phenobarbital, and terpin hydrate and codeine) can be diluted with water after polysorbate 20 or 80 has been added to solubilize the drugs, resinous components and essential oils which would otherwise come out of solution. Essential oils consist largely of terpenes and their oxygenated derivatives, which fall into Hartley's second category of solubilizates. One gram of micellar polysorbate can solubilize between 0.10 and 0.25 g of essential oil, depending on the nature and content of its polar constituents.[44]

Ichthammol is a dark and very viscous liquid derived from a shale oil, which in turn is produced by destructive distillation of bituminous schists. Sulfonation of the distillate and neutralization with ammonia converts a portion into ammonium alkyl- and arylsulfonates, which are anionic surfactants. When mixed with water, they dissolve, form micelles, and solubilize the water-insoluble portion. Bile salts, the sodium salts of cholic acid and its derivatives, are anionic surfactants. Their solubilization of monoglycerides is an important step in the digestion of triglycerides.

Oil-soluble, water-insoluble drugs are often more stable when solubilized by surfactant micelles in water than when molecularly dissolved in oils. On oral and parenteral administration, they are frequently better absorbed from the aqueous vehicle. The surfactant solutions may be diluted below the cmc by body fluids, causing the solubilized drugs to precipitate. However, the precipitated drugs have very small particle sizes because their dispersions are stabilized by the surfactants. This results in fast and complete absorption. Solubilization of lipophilic drugs by micellar bile salts may play an important role in their intestinal absorption.[48]

Drugs which are sufficiently soluble in water to be effective in the absence of surfactants may have their availability and activity lowered by micellar solubilization. For instance, solubilization of parabens and other preservatives which are somewhat soluble in water reduces their antimicrobial effectiveness: the preservatives are partitioned between the micelles and water. The solubilized fraction is inactive against microorganisms; the fraction molecularly dissolved in water, which is active, has its concentration lowered by solubilization. Such observations have also been made for the antibacterial chloroxylenol in the presence of polyoxyethylated nonionic surfactants. While the total amount dissolving in aqueous solutions was increased manyfold by micellar solubilization, the bactericidal activity of such saturated solutions was no greater than that of a saturated solution of chloroxylenol in pure water. Chloroxylenol solubilized by micelles was inactive.[41,46]

The fact that phenols are complexed by polyoxyethylated surfactants through specific binding via hydrogen bonds may have contributed to their inactivation.[44,46] Such binding is stronger than nonspecific micellar solubilization. On the other hand, antibacterials like thymol, resorcinol, n-hexylresorcinol and trichlorophenol had their solubility in aqueous media as well as their antibacterial activity enhanced by micellar soaps and sodium lauryl sulfate. Anionic surfactants have some antibacterial activity of their own. Overall, several of the studies based on anionic and nonionic surfactants indicated an increase in the activity of a variety of antimicrobial drugs of high and low water solubility, antibiotics, and preservatives at low surfactant concentration and a reduction in activity at high surfactant concentration.[46]

Microemulsions[49,50]

Microemulsions are liquid dispersions of water and oil that are made homogeneous, transparent, and stable by the addition of relatively large amounts of a surfactant and a cosurfactant. *Oil* is defined as a liquid of low polarity and low miscibility with water, eg, toluene, cyclohexane, mineral or vegetable oils.

Microemulsions are intermediate in properties between micelles containing solubilized oils and emulsions. While emulsions are lyophobic and unstable, microemulsions are on the borderline between lyophobic and lyophilic colloids. True microemulsions are thermodynamically stable.[51] Therefore, they are formed spontaneously when oil, water, surfactants, and cosurfactants are mixed together. The unstable emulsions require input of considerable mechanical energy for their preparation, which may be supplied by colloid mills, homogenizers or ultrasonic generators.

Both emulsions and microemulsions may contain high volume fractions of the internal phase. For instance, some O/W systems contain 75% (v/v) of oil dispersed in 25% water, although lower internal phase volume fractions are more common.

At low surfactant concentrations, viz, low multiples of the cmc, micelles are spheres (Figs 20-15 A, B, and E) or ellipsoids. When an oil is solubilized by micelles in water, it blends into the micellar core formed by the hydrocarbon tails of the surfactant molecules (Fig 20-16A) and swells the micelles.

Spherical or ellipsoidal micelles are nearly monodisperse, and their mean diameters are in the range of 25 to 60 Å. Microemulsion droplets also have a narrow droplet size distribution with a mean diameter range of approximately 60 to 1,000 Å. Since the droplet diameters are less than $1/4$ of the wavelength of light (4,200 Å for violet and 6,600 Å for red light), microemulsions scatter little light and are, therefore, transparent or at least translucent.

Emulsions have very broad droplet size distributions. Only the smallest droplets, with diameters of about 1,000 to 2,000 Å, are below the resolving power of the light microscope. The upper size limit is 25 or 50 μm (250,000 or 500,000 Å). Because emulsion droplets are comparable in size, or larger than the wavelength of visible light, they scatter it more or less strongly depending on the difference in refractive index between oil and water. Thus, most emulsions are opaque.

The three disperse systems—micellar solutions, microemulsions, and emulsions—can be of the O/W (oil-in-water) or W/O type. Aqueous micellar surfactant solutions can solubilize oils and lipid-soluble drugs in the core formed by their hydrocarbon chains. Likewise, oil-soluble surfactants like sorbitan monooleate and docusate sodium form "reverse micelles" in oils (Fig 20-15E) capable of solubilizing water in the polar center. The solubilized oil in the former micelles and the solubilized water in the latter may in turn enhance the micellar solubilization of oil-soluble and water-soluble drugs, respectively.

Oil-soluble drugs have been incorporated into O/W emulsions by dissolving them in the oil phase before emulsification (see Chap 21 and Ref 52). By the same token, it may be possible to dissolve oil-soluble drugs in a vegetable oil and make an oral or parenteral O/W microemulsion. The advantage of such microemulsion systems over conventional emulsions is their smaller droplet size and superior shelf stability. Aqueous micellar solutions[53] and O/W microemulsions[54] have both been used as aqueous reaction media for oil-soluble compounds.

Emulsions and micellar solutions of oils solubilized in aqueous surfactant solutions consist of three components, oil, water and surfactant. Microemulsions generally require a 4th component, called *cosurfactant*. Commonly used cosurfactants are linear alcohols of medium chain length, which are

Table VI—Microemulsion Formulations

Compound	Function	Content in microemulsions, % O/W	W/O
Sodium lauryl sulfate	Surfactant	13	10
1-Pentanol	Cosurfactant	8	25
Xylene	Oil	8	50
Water		71	15

sparingly miscible with water. Since the cosurfactants as well as the surfactants are surface-active, they promote the generation of extensive interfaces through the spontaneous dispersion of oil in water, or vice-versa, resulting in the formation of microemulsions. The large interfacial area between oil and water permits the extensive formation of a mixed interfacial film consisting of surfactant and cosurfactant. This film is called the "interphase" because it is thicker than the surfactant monolayers formed at oil-water interfaces in emulsions. The interfacial tension at the oil-water interface in microemulsions approaches zero, which also contributes to their spontaneous formation. According to another viewpoint, microemulsions are regarded as micelles extensively swollen by large amounts of solubilized oil.

Typical formulations for an O/W and a W/O microemulsion are shown in Table VI. The ratio, g surfactant/g solubilized or emulsified oil or water is in the range of 2–20 for micellar solutions and 0.01–0.1 for emulsions. Microemulsions have intermediate values: The ratios for the formulations in Table VI are near unity. In industrial formulations, the ratios are closer to 0.1 to reduce costs. Microemulsions are used in such diverse applications as floor polish and agricultural pesticide formulations and in tertiary petroleum recovery. The use of O/W microemulsions as aqueous vehicles for oil-soluble drugs to be administered by the oral or parenteral route is worth investigating.

Chemical Incompatibilities Involving Hydrophilic Polymers and Surfactants

Ionic surfactants and polyelectrolytes sometimes exhibit chemical incompatibilities in aqueous solution among themselves and with ionizable drugs. Because of the dual hydrophilic and hydrophobic nature of ionic surfactants and because of the large number of ionic groups in a single molecule of a polyelectrolyte, precipitation effects involving these two classes of compounds frequently occur even at low concentrations and are extensive.

Micelles of nonionic surfactants and, to a lesser extent, water-soluble polymers with a multiplicity of hydroxyl or ether groups tend to bind drug molecules which contain phenolic or other hydroxyl groups or un-ionized carboxyl groups and possess some solubility in water. This binding, which occurs mainly through hydrogen bonding, may reduce the effectiveness or bioavailability of such drugs (see above). Otherwise, nonionic surfactants and polymers are generally compatible with most drugs and adjuvants in aqueous solutions.

Basic drugs, cationic surfactants and cationic polyelectrolytes are generally incompatible with anionic surfactants and with acid drugs and anionic polyelectrolytes in their ionized forms. The following equation schematically represents a typical precipitation reaction involving a carboxylate, eg, sodium stearate or glycocholate, sodium salicylate or aminosalicylate, sodium alginate or carboxymethylcellulose. Alkyl sulfates and aryl sulfonates undergo similar reactions, as does tannic acid because of a high concentration of phenolic hydroxyl groups. If R_1 through R_5 are relatively hydrophobic organic moieties (although R_3 and/or R_4 and/or R_5 may be hydrogen atoms), two low-molecular-weight surface-active

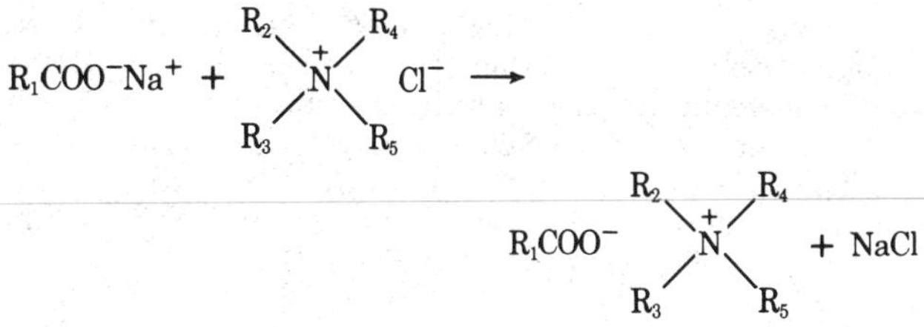

compounds are involved in this precipitation reaction. It should be remembered that most, if not all, basic organic drugs behave as cationic surfactants at pH values low enough to produce substantial ionization. They lower the surface tension of water, aggregate into micelles, have a pronounced tendency to become adsorbed at interfaces of lipophilic organic solids or tissues and water, and precipitate from aqueous solutions in the presence of anionic surface-active compounds. The precipitates consist of carboxylates (or alkyl sulfates or alkylaryl sulfonates) of the mono-, di-, tri-, or tetraalkyl or tetralkylaryl ammonium cations. They form and are held together by the ionic primary valence bond and by hydrophobic bonding between R_1 and R_2 through R_5.

The same type of precipitation reaction takes place if R_1 represents a polymer molecule with many carboxylate (or sulfate) groups and/or if R_2 represents a polymer molecule with many basic nitrogen groups. There are four possibilities: (i) anionic surfactant + cationic surfactant; (ii) anionic polyelectrolyte + cationic surfactant; (iii) anionic surfactant + cationic polyelectrolyte; (iv) anionic polyelectrolyte + cationic polyelectrolyte. Charge neutralization in the first three cases generally produces gelatinous precipitates. In the last instance, where hydrophilic sols or polyelectrolytes of opposite charge are involved, either a gelatinous precipitate or droplets of a viscous liquid phase may separate. The droplets, which tend to coalesce, constitute a *complex coacervate*. Complex coacervates differ from simple coacervates, obtained by the phase separation of a single polymer, in that heating or dilution with water does not reverse the complex coacervation because it involves a chemical reaction.[1] Complex coacervates formed between two oppositely charged hydrophilic sols, such as solutions of gelatin at a pH below its isoelectric point and of acacia, are used in the NCR microencapsulation process described in Chapter 90. A few examples of complex coacervate formation have also been reported for combinations (i) and (ii).

Aqueous dispersions of sodium bentonite are also incompatible with basic drugs or cationic surface-active agents. Chemisorption involving the silicate cation-exchange sites of the clay takes place according to the schematic reaction:

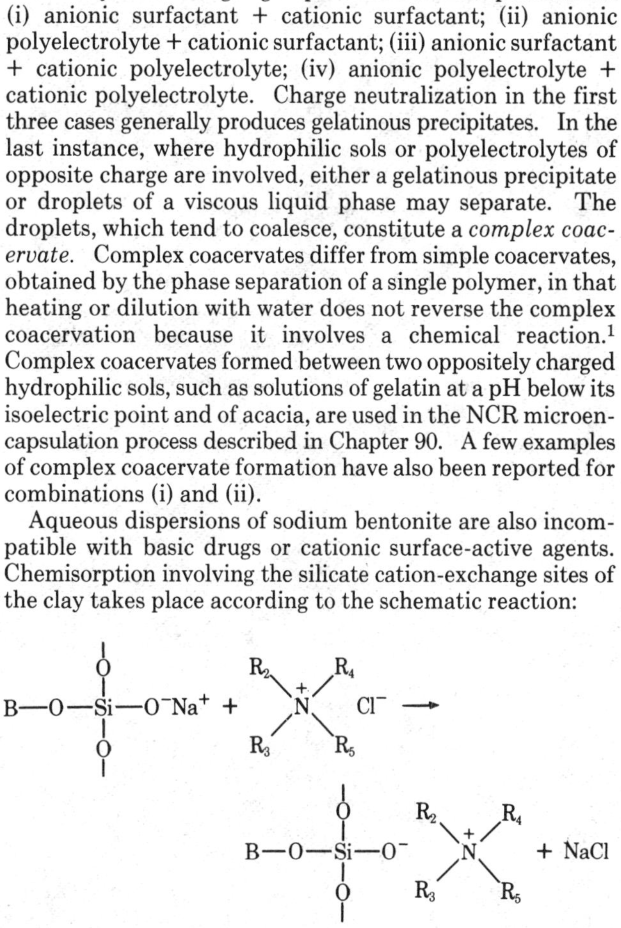

where B represents part of a bentonite lamella. The cationic drug is bound to the surface of the lamella by the ionic bond and by van der Waals forces attracting its hydrophobic organic groups R_2 through R_5 to the clay surface. Cationic drugs chemisorbed on bentonite coagulate the dispersed clay and are excreted in the feces together with the clay rather than being absorbed in the gastrointestinal tract. Bentonite chemisorbs basic drugs extensively because of its high cation-exchange capacity, 0.7–1 milliequivalent/gram. Even kaolin, with the lower cation exchange capacity of 0.01–0.1 milliequivalents/gram, should not be taken simultaneously with a basic drug to avoid chemisorption of the latter.

Chemical incompatibilities involving anionic polyelectrolytes and polyvalent cations are discussed above, in the section on *Hydrophilic Dispersions*, *Gel Formation*.

References

1. Kruyt HR: *Colloid Science*, vols I and II, Elsevier, Houston, 1952 and 1949.
2. Vold MJ, Vold RD: *Colloid Chemistry*, Reinhold, New York, 1964.
3. McBain JW: *Colloid Science*, Heath, Boston, 1950.
4. von Weimarn PP, in Alexander J, ed: *Colloid Chemistry*, vol I, Chemical Catalog Co (Reinhold) New York, 1926. See also *Chem Rev 2:* 217, 1926.
5. Mysels KJ: *Introduction to Colloid Chemistry*, Wiley-Interscience, New York, 1959.
6. Shaw DJ: *Introduction to Colloid and Surface Chemistry*, 2nd ed, Butterworths, London, 1970.
7. Vold RD, Vold MJ: *Colloid and Interface Chemistry*, Addison-Wesley, Reading, MA., 1983.
8. Hiemenz PC: *Principles of Colloid and Surface Chemistry*, Dekker, New York, 1977.
9. Weiser HB: *A Textbook of Colloid Chemistry*, 2nd ed, Wiley, New York, 1949.
10. Lachman L, *et al:* *Theory and Practice of Industrial Pharmacy*, 2nd ed, Lea & Febiger, Philadelphia, 1976.
11. Tubis M, Wolf W, ed: *Radiopharmacy*, Wiley-Interscience, New York, 1976.
12. Gutch CF, Stoner MH: *Review of Hemodialysis*, C. V. Mosby Co, St. Louis, 1975.
13. Reimschuessel AC: *J Chem Ed 49:* A 413 and A 449, 1972.
14. Groves MJ, Freshwater DC: *J Pharm Sci 57:* 1277, 1968.
15. Schott H, Martin AN, in Dittert LW, ed: *American Pharmacy*, 7th ed, Lippincott, Philadelphia, 1974.
16. Parks GA: *Chem Rev 65:* 177, 1965.
17. Schott H: *J Pharm Sci 66:* 1548, 1977.
18. Sonntag H, Strenge K: *Coagulation and Stability of Disperse Systems*, Halstead, New York, 1972.
19. Ottewill RH, in Schick MJ, ed: *Nonionic Surfactants*, Dekker, New York, 1967.
20. Vincent B: *Adv Colloid Interface Sci 4:* 193, 1974.
21. Davies JT, Rideal EK: *Interfacial Phenomena*, 2nd ed, Academic, New York, 1963.
22. Bier M, ed: *Electrophoresis*, vols I and II, Academic, New York, 1959 and 1967.
23. Shaw DJ: *Electrophoresis*, Academic, New York, 1969.
24. Cawley LP: *Electrophoresis and Immunoelectrophoresis*, Little-Brown, Boston, 1969.
25. Catsimpoolas N, ed: *Isoelectric Focusing and Isotachophoresis*, *Ann NY Acad Sci 209:* June 15, 1973.
26. Morawetz H: *Macromolecules in Solution*, 2nd ed, Wiley-Interscience, New York, 1975.
27. Veis A: *The Macromolecular Chemistry of Gelatin*, Academic, New York, 1964.
28. Shinoda K, *et al:* *Colloidal Surfactants*, Academic, New York, 1963.
29. Moilliet JL, *et al:* *Surface Activity*, 2nd ed, Van Nostrand, Princeton, NJ, 1961.
30. Rosen MJ: *Surfactants and Interfacial Phenomena*, Wiley-Interscience, New York, 1978.
31. Schick, MJ, ed: *Nonionic Surfactants*, Dekker, New York, 1967.
32. Jungermann E, ed: *Cationic Surfactants*, Dekker, New York, 1970.
33. Linfield WM, ed: *Anionic Surfactants*, vols I and II, Dekker, New York, 1976.
34. Mukerjee P, Mysels KJ: *Critical Micelle Concentrations of Aqueous Surfactant Systems*, NSRDS-NBS 36, Nat Bur Stand, Washington, 1970.
35. Fowkes FM, in Shinoda K, ed: *Solvent Properties of Surfactant Solutions*, Dekker, New York, 1967.
36. Florence AT: *Adv Colloid Interface Sci 2:* 117, 1968.
37. McBain JW, in Kraemer EO, ed: *Advances in Colloid Science*, vol I, Interscience, New York, 1942.
38. Klevens HB: *Chem Rev 47:* 1, 1950.
39. Winsor PA: *Solvent Properties of Amphiphilic Compounds*, Butterworths, London, 1954.
40. McBain MEL, Hutchinson E: *Solubilization and Related Phenomena*, Academic, New York, 1955.
41. Mulley BA, in Bean HS, *et al:* *Advances in Pharmaceutical Sciences*, vol I, Academic, New York, 1964.
42. Swarbrick JW: *J Pharm Sci 54:* 1229, 1965.
43. Shinoda K, in Shinoda K, ed: *Solvent Properties of Surfactant Solutions*, Dekker, New York, 1967.
44. Sjöblom L, in Shinoda K, ed: *Solvent Properties of Surfactant Solutions*, Dekker, New York, 1967.
45. Nakagawa T, in Schick MJ, ed: *Nonionic Surfactants*, Dekker, New York, 1967.
46. Elworthy PH, *et al:* *Solubilization by Surface-Active Agents*, Chapman & Hall, London, 1968.
47. Florence AT, in Yalkowsky SH, ed: *Techniques of Solubilization of Drugs*, Dekker, New York, 1981.
48. Gibaldi M: *Fed Proc 29:* 1343, 1970.
50. Prince, LM: *Microemulsions—Theory and Practice*, Academic, New York 1977.
50. Shinoda K, Friberg S: *Adv Colloid Interface Sci 4:* 281, 1975.
51. Overbeek JThG: *Disc Faraday Soc 65:* 7, 1978.
52. Davis SS, in Bundgaard H, Hansen AB and Kofod H, ed: *Optimization of Drug Delivery*, Alfred Benzon Symposium 17, Munksgaard, Copenhagen, 1982.
53. Fendler JH, Fendler EJ: *Catalysis in Micellar and Macromolecular Systems*, Academic, New York, 1975.
54. Mackay RA: *Adv Colloid Interface Sci 15*, 131, 1981.

CHAPTER 21

Particle Phenomena and Coarse Dispersions

William I Higuchi, PhD

Distinguished Professor and Chairman
Department of Pharmaceutics
College of Pharmacy
University of Utah, Salt Lake City, UT 84112

James Swarbrick, DSc, PhD

Professor and Chairman
Division of Pharmaceutics
School of Pharmacy, University of North Carolina at Chapel Hill
Chapel Hill, NC 27514

Norman F H Ho, PhD

Professor of Pharmacy, College of Pharmacy
The University of Michigan
Ann Arbor, MI 48104

Anthony P Simonelli, PhD

Professor of Pharmaceutics
School of Pharmacy & Institute of Material Science
University of Connecticut
Storrs, CT 06268

Alfred Martin, PhD

Coulter R Sublett Professor
Drug Dynamics Institute, College of Pharmacy
University of Texas
Austin, TX 78712

Understanding particle phenomena and concepts of dispersion techniques is important in many areas of pharmaceutics and biopharmaceutics. In the formulation and manufacture of dosage forms such as powders, capsules, tablets, suspensions, emulsions, and aerosols, knowledge of particle technology is essential. Also, it is becoming increasingly important to consider such factors as particle size and degree of deaggregation in drug utilization by the patient.

This chapter will discuss the formation of suspensions and emulsions, and the time behavior involving flocculation, coalescence, crystal growth, and caking. The "theory" is intended to give readers qualitative or semiquantitative guidelines, rather than quantitative directions for manufacturing procedures. Many of the equations and concepts presented cannot be used directly for the purpose of formulation; rather they are meant to provide understanding of the interactions involved in the preparation of, for example, an emulsion or a suspension.

For the purposes of the present discussion, a dispersed system will be regarded as a two-phase system in which one phase is distributed as particles or droplets in the second, or continuous, phase. Since each phase can exist in solid, liquid, or gaseous state, there are nine possible combinations. However, since gases are miscible in all proportions, there are in reality only eight combinations. The treatment will be restricted to a discussion of those solid–liquid and liquid–liquid dispersions that are of pharmaceutical significance, namely, suspensions and emulsions. In these systems the dispersed phase is frequently referred to as the discontinuous or internal phase, and the continuous phase is called the external phase or dispersion medium.

All dispersions may be classified into three groups on the basis of the size of the dispersed particles. Chapter 20 deals with one such group—colloidal dispersions—in which the size of the dispersed particles is in the range of approximately 10 Å to 0.5 μm. Molecular dispersions, the second group in this classification, are discussed in Chapters 16 and 17. The third group, consisting of *coarse dispersions* in which the particle size exceeds 0.5 μm, is the subject of this chapter. Knowledge of coarse dispersions is essential for the preparation of both pharmaceutical suspensions (solid–liquid dispersions) and emulsions (liquid–liquid dispersions).

The Dispersion Step

The pharmaceutical formulator is primarily concerned with producing a smooth, uniform, easily flowing (pouring or spreading) suspension or emulsion, one in which dispersion of particles can be effected with minimum expenditure of energy.

In preparing suspensions, particle–particle attractive forces among powder particles present a problem. These forces may be overcome by the high shearing action of such devices as the colloid mill, or by use of surface-active agents. The latter greatly facilitate wetting of lyophobic powders and assist in the removal of surface air that shearing alone may not remove; thus the clumping tendency of the particles is reduced. Moreover, lowering of the surface free energy by the adsorption of these agents directly reduces the thermodynamic driving force opposing dispersion of the particles.

In emulsification a similar situation exists. Frequently high shear rates are necessary for dispersion of the internal phase into fine droplets. The shear forces are opposed by forces operating to resist distortion and subsequent breakup of the droplets. Again surface-active agents help greatly by lowering interfacial tension, which is the primary reversible component resisting droplet distortion. Surface-active agents also may play an important role in determining whether an oil-in-water or a water-in-oil emulsion preferentially survives the shearing action.

For thermodynamic reasons, once the process of dispersion begins there develops simultaneously a tendency for the system to revert to an energetically more stable state, manifested by flocculation, coalescence, sedimentation, crystal growth, and caking phenomena. If these physical changes are not inhibited or controlled, successful dispersions will not be achieved or will be lost during shelf life.

Wetting

Wetting of a solid by a liquid is best illustrated by the behavior of a small droplet of liquid placed on a flat surface of a solid. If the droplet spreads over the solid, the liquid is said to wet the solid completely, and the contact angle, θ, measured through the liquid is zero (see Fig 21-1). The term nonwetting is somewhat arbitrary but may be applied to a liquid when θ

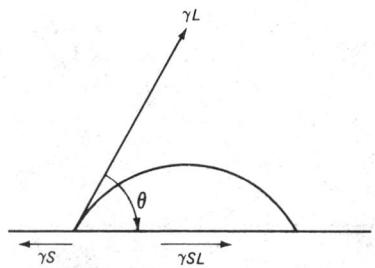

Fig 21-1. A drop of liquid on a flat solid surface. Forces and the contact angle, θ, are shown.

> 90°. For the nonspreading region, $0 < \theta < 90°$, the term partial wetting may be applied.

For a better understanding of the wetting process, the Young equation

$$\gamma_S = \gamma_{SL} + \gamma_L \cos\theta \qquad (1)$$

deduced from analysis of the force vectors (see Fig 21-1) at equilibrium may be instructive. Here γ_S, γ_{SL}, and γ_L are the surface tension of the solid, the interfacial tension of the solid liquid, and the surface tension of the liquid, respectively. Rearranging Eq 1 gives

$$\cos\theta = \frac{\gamma_S - \gamma_{SL}}{\gamma_L} \qquad (2)$$

which states the dependence of θ on γ_S, γ_{SL}, and γ_L. From this equation it is obvious that wetting is favored if γ_S is large, γ_L is small, and γ_{SL} is small. Complete wetting results if the right-hand side of Eq 2 equals one.

The practical significance of wetting may be illustrated by the preparation of methylprednisolone suspensions. Micronized methylprednisolone is not wetted ($\theta > 90°$) by water in the absence of a surfactant, but if a small amount of polysorbate 80 is added the contact angle is reduced to nearly zero and a fine dispersion may be prepared.

Low-Energy Solids—The particle surface of many organic substances is hydrophobic because there are few polar functional groups in the molecules of the substances. For such low-energy solids the surface tension may be relatively small, in the range of 20 to 40 ergs/cm². From Eq 2 it is evident that such surfaces will be poorly wetted by highly polar liquids (of relatively large surface tension) such as water or glycerin. Less polar liquids wet the surfaces more readily. Table I shows that as γ_L decreases, θ decreases in accordance with Eq 2.

Wetting agents are surface-active substances used to reduce contact angle and thus improve wetting. They function by adsorbing at air/liquid and solid/liquid interfaces, reducing both γ_L and γ_{SL}. Eq 2 shows that for wetting of low-energy solids by water, reduction of γ_L is necessary even when γ_{SL} is small.

High-Energy Solids—Metals, silica, clay minerals, and water-insoluble salts are among the substances with γ_S values ranging from several hundred to thousands of ergs/cm².

Table I—Contact Angles of Various Liquids at 20° on Low-Energy Solids

	Paraffin	Polyethylene
Water ($\gamma_L = 73$)	108	94
Glycerol ($\gamma_L = 63$)	96	79
Formamide ($\gamma_L = 58$)	91	77
Bis(2-ethylhexyl) phthalate ($\gamma_L = 31$)	36	5
Benzene ($\gamma_L = 29$)	24	spreads
n-Hexadecane ($\gamma_L = 28$)	28	spreads
Di(n-octyl)ether ($\gamma_L = 28$)	23	spreads
n-Decane ($\gamma_L = 24$)	7	spreads

Hence, clean surfaces of such solids are generally much more wettable by solvents listed in Table I. As Zisman has pointed out, however, there are instances when a relatively low-energy liquid does not spread on a high-energy solid.[1] This behavior occurs when molecules of the liquid or a constituent in it adsorb on the high-energy surface. Sometimes surface contamination of high-energy surfaces by hydrophobic materials significantly lowers γ_S, with the result that wetting does not occur; for example, very low concentrations of cationic surface-active agents render glass nonwetting toward water.

Intermolecular Forces

All interactions involving molecules and ions, and aggregates of molecules and ions include both attractive and repulsive forces. These forces depend on the nature of species, the distance of separation, the orientation of the molecules, and the nature of the medium.

Ion–Ion Electrostatic Interactions—The interionic interaction of two polarizable ions (see Fig 21-2) obeys the following laws:

$$\text{Energy} = E = \frac{q_1 q_2}{\epsilon r} \qquad (3)$$

and

$$\text{Force} = F = -\frac{q_1 q_2}{\epsilon r^2} \qquad (4)$$

where q_1 and q_2 are the charges on ions 1 and 2, respectively, r is the distance of separation of the ions, and ϵ is the dielectric constant of the medium. As can be seen, if q_1 and q_2 are of the same sign, the force, F, is negative and therefore repulsive in nature. On the other hand, if the charges are of opposite sign, the interaction is attractive. It should be noted that the distance dependence for this situation is inversely proportional to the first power in r for E and second power for F. This difference in the distance dependence results from the fact that

$$E = \int_{-\infty}^{r} F dr \qquad (5)$$

which states that the energy is equal to the work, W, of bringing together the two ions from infinity to a distance r from each other.

An example calculation for sodium chloride can be used to illustrate the magnitude of the ion–ion interaction. For the sodium chloride molecule in the vapor state, r is about 2.5×10^{-8} cm, $q_{Na^+} = -q_{Cl^-} = $ electronic charge $= 4.8 \times 10^{-10}$ esu (electrostatic units), and the dielectric constant may be assumed to be unity. Therefore,

$$W = \frac{(4.8 \times 10^{-10})^2}{2.5 \times 10^{-8}} \approx 10^{-11} \text{ erg/ion pair}$$

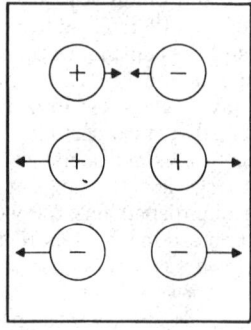

Fig 21-2. Interionic interactions of two polarizable ions. Like charges repel and unlike charges attract.

or

$$W = 120{,}000 \text{ cal/mole}$$

since

$$\text{cal/mole} = \frac{(\text{erg/molecule})N_0}{4.18 \times 10^7 \text{ ergs/cal}}$$

The value for the work, W, represents the amount of work required to separate one mole of sodium chloride molecules in the vapor state into one mole of sodium and one mole of chloride ions.

Other Electrostatic Interactions—In addition to the ion–ion interaction other electrostatic interactions may be possible involving ions, dipoles, and induced dipoles.

A permanent dipole moment exists in a molecule when the "center of gravity" of the negative charges does not coincide with that for the positive charges.

The field of an ion or permanent dipole temporarily may polarize molecules which may not have a permanent dipole. When this occurs, the resulting polarization leads to an induced dipole in the molecule.

Various pair combinations of ions, permanent dipoles, and induced dipoles give rise to higher order electrostatic interactions such as the ion–dipole, the ion–induced dipole, the dipole–dipole, and dipole–induced dipole. These interactions are weaker and generally more short-range than the ion–ion interaction, the distance dependence for the energies ranging from r^{-2} to r^{-6} (see Table II). Furthermore, all of these interactions usually are directionally dependent.

Hydrogen-Bonding—A hydrogen atom attached to an electronegative atom such as oxygen or nitrogen effectively produces a dipole with a highly exposed positive end. As a result, the proton end can participate in unusually strong dipole–dipole interactions with other strongly electronegative centers. Each water molecule has two such hydrogen-bonding protons and therefore water molecules in liquid water and ice are highly associated. The hydrogen-bonding capabilities of water also partially explain its unusually good solvating ability for other polar molecules.

London Dispersion Forces—These attractive forces arise from the fact that at any given instant the electron distribution around an atomic nucleus may not be symmetrical and consequently this leads to the formation of a temporary dipole moment. Such temporary dipoles in neighboring atoms are correlated so as to produce an effective induced dipole–induced dipole interaction.

The characteristics of the dispersion forces are that they are approximately additive, they are not directionally dependent, and they follow the $1/r^6$ dependence in energy. As will be seen later, the London Forces, along with hydrogen-bonding forces, are generally the most important in describing the intermolecular and the interparticulate behavior of nonionic compounds in solutions and dispersions.

Born Repulsive Forces—If molecules or ions are brought very close together, the outer electron clouds of the atoms will begin to overlap. This gives rise to a mutual repulsive force that increases very rapidly ($\sim 1/r^{12}$) as the atoms are brought

closer together such as one might expect when two hard rubber balls touch and are pressed together.

Particle–Particle Interactions

The interaction between particles may be analyzed by the same type of forces responsible for interatomic and intermolecular interactions. Let us consider first the interaction of two arbitrary particles as shown in Fig 21-3.

The kinds of interactions contributing to the particle–particle binding energies are:

1. The various electrostatic contributions (attractive and repulsive).
2. The London dispersion forces between the atoms of one particle with those in the other (attractive).
3. The covalent bonds (attractive).
4. The Born repulsion forces.

The latter two can contribute only when the two particles are touching.

A rigorous quantitative treatment of the above contributions to particle–particle binding is beyond the scope of this text. However, considerable insight into the magnitude, nature, and the applications of these forces can be gained by "order of magnitude" theoretical calculations using approximate theories and simplified models.

Charge–Charge Interactions—Let us examine the possibility of electrostatic interactions between two particles, A and B (see Fig 21-3). While contributions from charge–dipole, charge–induced dipole, and dipole–dipole interactions between an atom, ion, or molecule of one particle and that in the other may occur, generally these are probably of much less importance than the charge–charge interactions. Therefore, as a first approximation let us consider only the charge–charge forces between the two particles.

The energy of coulombic interaction may be written as the summation of Eq 3 (assuming $\epsilon = 1$) over all possible ion–pair combinations between the two particles; ie,

$$E = \sum_{i=1}^{M} \sum_{j=1}^{N} \frac{q_i q_j}{r_{ij}} \tag{6}$$

where q_i is the charge on the ith ion in Particle A which contains M ions, q_j is the charge on the jth ion in Particle B which contains N ions, and r_{ij} is the distance between ions i and j. If it is assumed that the particles are spheres and that charges on each sphere are uniformly distributed, Eq 6 simply reduces

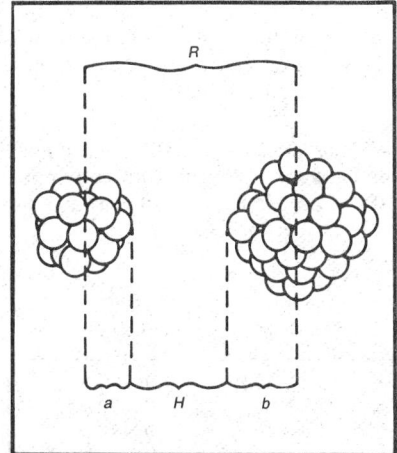

Fig 21-3. Parameters used to describe the interactions between particles where a and b are the particle radii of the particles involved, R is the intercenter distance of separation of the two particles, and H is the distance of separation between the two surfaces of the interacting particles.

Table II—Distance Dependence of Various Electrostatic Interactions

Type interaction	Distance dependence	
	Force	Energy
Ion–ion	$1/r^2$	$1/r$
Ion–dipole	$1/r^3$	$1/r^2$
Dipole–dipole	$1/r^4$	$1/r^3$
Dipole–induced dipole	$1/r^7$	$1/r^6$
London dispersion forces	$1/r^7$	$1/r^6$

to

$$E = \frac{Q_A Q_B}{R} \qquad (7)$$

where Q_A and Q_B are the net charges on Particles A and B and R is the intercenter distance between the two spheres (see Fig 21-4). The corresponding equation for the force is

$$F = \frac{-Q_A Q_B}{R^2} \qquad (8)$$

It is both instructive and useful at this point to examine the magnitude of maximum energies and forces that might arise from purely electrostatic contributions and compare them to the gravitational forces on the particles. The maximum charge on a given particle in air is limited by the electric breakdown field of about 60 esu, which corresponds to a charge of

$$Q = 60a^2 \qquad (9)$$

where a is the radius of the sphere.

Table III tabulates the results of calculations for E and F based on Eqs 7–9 for different-sized particles. It must be kept in mind that these values represent the *maximum* electrostatic interaction limited by surface electrical discharge in air.

It can be noted that for small particles, electrostatic effects may be important. For example, two 1-μm particles with the same maximum charge may repel each other with a force that is 20,000 times greater than the gravitational force, D. These calculations explain why certain dry powders that become charged during trituration in the mortar defy the laws of gravity. Interestingly, as the particle size is reduced, this phenomenon increases in accordance with the predictions of Table III, which shows that the relative importance of the electrostatic force as compared to the gravitational force should increase with decreasing particle size.

London Dispersion Forces—The London dispersion force contribution to the particle–particle interaction may be estimated by summing the attraction over all possible atom pair combinations between the two particles (see Fig 21-5). Thus, we may write

$$E = \sum_{i=1}^{M} \sum_{j=1}^{N} \epsilon_{ij} \qquad (10)$$

or

$$E = \sum_{i=1}^{M} \sum_{j=1}^{N} \frac{k_{ij}}{r_{ij}} \qquad (11)$$

where k_{ij}, the London constant, is characteristic of the atom pair involved and is a function of the polarizabilities and the ionization energies of the atoms.

Table III—*Maximum* Electrostatic Energy and Force of Interaction between Uniformly Charged Spheres Near Contact[a] (R $\simeq$ 2a and Field = 60 esu) as a Function of Particle Size[b]

Radius (cm)	Electrostatic		Gravitational force (dynes)
	Energy (ergs)	Force (dynes)	
10^{-4} (1 μm)	1.8×10^{-9}	9×10^{-6}	4.1×10^{-9}
10^{-3}	1.8×10^{-6}	9×10^{-4}	4.1×10^{-6}
10^{-2}	1.8×10^{-3}	9×10^{-2}	4.1×10^{-3}
10^{-1} (1 mm)	1.8	9	4.1
1	1.8×10^3	9×10^2	4.1×10^3

[a] For these calculations the particles are assumed to be touching. These values approximately apply for particles not touching if distances of separation are not comparable to the particle radius.

[b] Density of 1 is assumed.

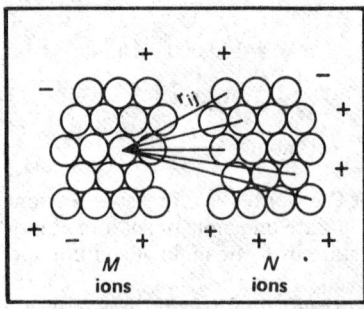

Fig 21-4. Electrostatic interactions between two particles containing M_i and N_j ions, respectively. The distance r_{ij} is the distance between the *i*th ion of one particle and the *j*th ion of the other particle.

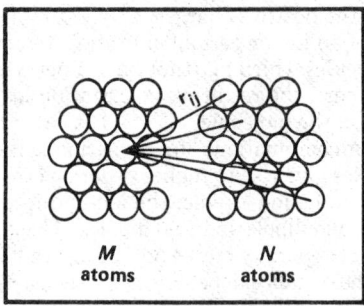

Fig 21-5. The London dispersion force contribution to the particle–particle interaction. This may be estimated by summing the attraction over all possible atom-pair combinations between the two particles, containing M and N atoms, respectively. The above illustrates the interaction of the *i*th atom of one particle with j atoms of the other particles where *i* and *j* are 1, 2, 3, 4, 5, etc.

In the case of two equal-sized spheres of the same substance the summations in Eq 11 may be transformed to double integrals and the following equation is obtained for energy:

$$E = \frac{-A}{6} \left[\frac{2a^2}{R^2 - 4a^2} + \frac{2a^2}{R^2} + \ln \left(\frac{R^2 - 4a^2}{R^2} \right) \right] \qquad (12)$$

where $A = \pi^2 n^2 k$, n is the number of atoms/cm^3, k is the London dispersion force constant, R is the particle–particle intercenter distance, and a is the radius of the sphere. A more rigorous equation may be deduced which takes into account the so-called "retardation effect," but it would not significantly contribute to the present discussion.

It is worthwhile to present the limiting forms of Eq 12. First, when R is much greater than $2a$ (ie, when the intercenter distance is large compared to the sphere diameter), one can show that the energy and force would be inversely proportional to the 6th and 7th power of R, respectively. On the other hand, when the closest distance, H, between the surfaces of the two spheres is much smaller than the sphere radius, one can show that

$$E = \frac{-Aa}{12H} \qquad (13)$$

and

$$F = \frac{Aa}{12H^2} \qquad (14)$$

where $H = R - 2a$ and $H <<< a$ (see Fig 21-3).

In order to gain an appreciation for the magnitude of the London attraction between two particles one can compute the energies and forces using Eqs 13 and 14 employing the appropriate values for A. Table IV gives a list of A values. These may be used in the present calculations. As can be seen from the A values, the London forces do not differ too greatly among materials with widely differing properties. The results

Table IV—Tabulation of A Values

Material	$A \times 10^{12}$ ergs
H_2O	0.31
Paraffin	0.35
Polyethylene	0.50
Polystyrene	0.63
Fe	1.4
Graphite	1.6
Silica	1.8
Rutile	2.1
Mercury	2.9

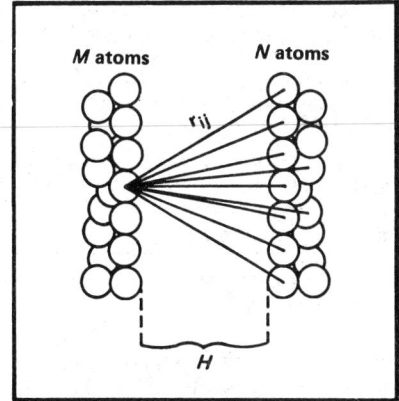

Fig 21-6.   The interaction of two particles based on the flat-plate model. For symbolism, see Figs 3 and 5.

of using Eqs 13 and 14 and an A value of 10^{-12} erg are presented in Table V for two distances of separation, 5×10^{-8} and 5×10^{-7} cm. For other A values the reader may make the appropriate adjustments using Table IV information. The H value of 5×10^{-8} should be a reasonable limiting distance of closest approach (within a factor of two) for two atoms involved in the contact of the two macroscopic spheres.

An examination of the results presented in Tables III and V reveals several important relationships. First, as was the case with electrostatic interactions, London forces decrease much more slowly than the gravitational forces with decreasing particle size. Thus, as can be seen at a distance of separation of 5 Å, 1-μm particles exhibit London attractive forces that are approximately one million times stronger than gravity, but 1-mm particles have approximately the same forces. For this reason fine particles tend to be "stickier" than coarse particles.

Secondly, the London attractive forces decrease more slowly than the electrostatic forces with decreasing particle size. Thus, a 10-fold decrease in particle size corresponds to only a 10-fold decrease in the London forces but to a 100-fold decrease in electrostatic forces. Thus, for 1-μm particles or smaller, it is likely that London forces are always more important than electrostatic forces when the particles are near contact. However, as the distance of separation is increased, the electrostatic forces remain relatively constant while the London forces decrease rapidly. For example, as the distance of separation is changed from 5 to 50 Å, the London forces are decreased by a factor of a hundred while the electrostatic forces for all particles in Table III essentially remain constant. Thus, electrostatics may play an important role in the flow behavior of powders in which the particles are separated sufficiently during handling; eg, during mixing operations. However, once the powder particles are sufficiently packed, London forces should dominate.

It appears that the above relationships have not always been adequately emphasized in the literature. Texts which discuss electrostatic and London forces limit their discussion to molecular interactions in solutions and in solid crystals and do not apply them to solid particulate interactions. This leaves the impression that London forces are only important in the absence of electrostatic forces, which is obviously not true in solid particle–particle interactions.

Nonspherical Particles—The above discussion was restricted to uniform spheres which do not generally represent real powders. Real powder particles are also subject to both plastic and elastic deformation which would provide larger areas of contact between them. The actual situation for powders would be expected to lie somewhere between the interaction between uniform spheres and that for parallel plates and is much more complicated than either of the above cases. Thus, for example, the interaction of two contacting cubes in contrast to that for two spheres, also depends upon their relative orientation (face to face, face to edge, corner to face, edge to edge, etc). In addition to the mutual orientation and shape effects for real powders, one must consider the particle-size distribution and the important factor of whether or not the particle is deformable (plastic and/or elastic) under the prevailing conditions.

It would be beyond the scope of this text to attempt detailed considerations of the above factors. However, in order to gain an appreciation for the magnitudes of the possible London force interactions between real powder particles it is helpful to examine the limiting case of two interacting flat plates (see Fig 21-6).

For two parallel flat surfaces separated by a distance, H, the equations for the London Force interacting energy and force/unit area are

$$E = \frac{-A}{12\pi H^2} \tag{15}$$

and

$$F = \frac{+A}{6\pi H^3} \tag{16}$$

Table VI tabulates the results of calculations for the same two distances of separation used in Table V for comparison purposes.

Tables V and VI show that suitably oriented flat plates or

Table V—London–van der Waals' Energies and Forces for Spheres as a Function of Particle Size (assuming $A = 10^{-12}$)[a]

Radius (cm)	Energy (ergs)		Force (dynes)		
	$H = 5$ Å	$H = 50$ Å	$H = 5$ Å	$H = 50$ Å	Gravity
10^{-5}	1.7×10^{-11}	1.7×10^{-12}	3.3×10^{-4}	3.3×10^{-6}	4.1×10^{-12}
10^{-4}	1.7×10^{-10}	1.7×10^{-11}	3.3×10^{-3}	3.3×10^{-5}	4.1×10^{-9}
10^{-3}	1.7×10^{-9}	1.7×10^{-10}	3.3×10^{-2}	3.3×10^{-4}	4.1×10^{-6}
10^{-2}	1.7×10^{-8}	1.7×10^{-9}	3.3×10^{-1}	3.3×10^{-3}	4.1×10^{-3}
10^{-1}	1.7×10^{-7}	1.7×10^{-8}	3.3	3.3×10^{-2}	4.1

[a] Average thermal energy = $kT = 4 \times 10^{-14}$ erg.

Table VI—London–van der Waals' Energies and Forces for Parallel Plates[a] as a Function of Contact Area (assuming $A = 10^{-12}$)

Area (cm²)	Energy (ergs)		Force (dynes)	
	$H = 5$ Å	$H = 50$ Å	$H = 5$ Å	$H = 50$ Å
10^{-12}	1×10^{-11}	1×10^{-13}	5×10^{-4}	5×10^{-7}
10^{-10}	1×10^{-9}	1×10^{-11}	5×10^{-2}	5×10^{-5}
10^{-8}	1×10^{-7}	1×10^{-9}	5	5×10^{-3}

[a] Forces and energies are applicable to cubes with a linear dimension of the square root of the area listed.

cubical particles may exhibit interactions several orders of magnitude greater than those for rigid spheres of the same size.

Adsorption and Interfacial Energetics

Because there are unsatisfied intermolecular forces at interfaces, adsorption of molecules can occur there; when it does the free energy of the system is lowered. Consider the unfavorable situation of a system involving a paraffin oil/water interface. Paraffin/paraffin interactions and water/water interactions are such that the molecules of the two phases prefer to remain with their own kind (Fig 21-7A). At the interface between the phases there is a shortage of both water molecules and paraffin molecules; however, if surfactant molecules, for example of sodium dodecyl sulfate, are present a more favorable situation develops. Some of the surfactant molecules move to the interface, their polar portions reaching toward and into the water phase and their hydrophobic tails orienting toward the paraffin oil phase (Fig 21-7B). Maximum free-energy lowering, the best compromise for all components of the system, results.

Gibbs Adsorption Equation—The relationship between interfacial tension and adsorption is important and should be examined (see also Chapter 19, page 263).

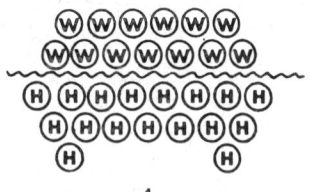

A

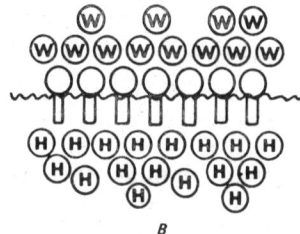

B

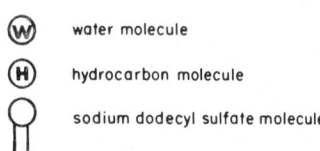

Ⓦ water molecule

Ⓗ hydrocarbon molecule

🪥 sodium dodecyl sulfate molecule

Fig 21-7. Addition of a surface-active agent such as sodium dodecyl sulfate (SDS) lowers the energy of the oil-water interface by adsorption of the SDS molecules as shown. A, Energetically unfavorable without SDS; B, energetically favorable with SDS.

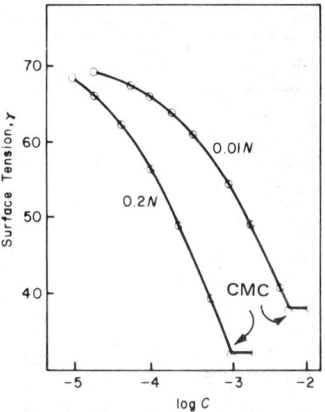

Fig 21-8. Surface tension of sodium lauryl sulfate solutions at 40° in 0.01 and 0.2 N NaCl.

Consider a two-component system containing a solvent and a nonionic solute, with the latter adsorbing at an interface between the solvent phase and another phase. The Gibbs equation for this system may be written

$$\Gamma = -\frac{a}{RT}\left(\frac{d\gamma}{da}\right)_T = -\frac{1}{RT}\left(\frac{d\gamma}{d \ln a}\right)_T \qquad (17)$$

In this equation Γ is the surface excess of solute, in moles/cm², γ is the interfacial tension, a is the activity of the solute in moles/liter, R is the universal gas constant (8.3143×10^7 erg/deg/mole), and T is the absolute temperature. For practical purposes involving surface-active solutes, Γ is essentially equal to moles of solute adsorbed per cm².

Eq 17 shows that the amount of solute adsorbed is simply related to the negative slope of the γ versus $\ln a$ curve. Thus, by measurements of γ, if an air/liquid or liquid/liquid interface is involved, Γ may be determined. This experimental approach is not suitable for a solid/liquid interface. Fig 21-8 depicts plots of γ versus log C for the aqueous sodium lauryl sulfate/air system at 40°. According to Eq 17, as the concentration of surfactant increases, γ decreases. If it may be assumed that the activity coefficient is constant, then $d \ln a = d \ln C = 2.303\ d \log C$. This assumption is probably reasonable, especially in the presence of excess electrolyte, up to the critical micelle concentration (CMC) (see Chapter 20) if pre-micellar association does not occur. Beyond the CMC the curve levels off because with micelle formation the activity, a, of the surfactant changes very little with increasing C.

To calculate Γ, at 40°, (the moles of solute per unit area) near the CMC one may take the limiting slope, $d\gamma/d \log C$ just before the CMC. For the 0.2N sodium chloride solution in Fig 21-8 the slope is approximately -30, and

$$\Gamma = \frac{30}{2.303\ RT} = 5 \times 10^{-10}\ \text{moles/cm}^2$$

and the area per molecule = 30×10^{-16} cm². As this corresponds to a diameter of 6 to 7 Å for the adsorbed molecule, these results show that at the solution/air interface there is probably a relatively compact monolayer of sodium lauryl sulfate molecules near the CMC.

Eq 17 may also be written in an integral form that expresses γ as a function of Γ and a, thus

$$\gamma = \gamma_0 - \int_o^a \frac{RT\Gamma}{a}\ da \qquad (18)$$

where γ_0 is the interfacial tension in the absence of the solute ($a = 0$). This alternative representation of the Gibbs equation states that γ may be obtained by means of Eq 18 through a determination of the area under the curve $RT\Gamma/a$ versus a. A highly active surfactant would begin to adsorb appreciably at a low concentration (activity). Hence $RT\Gamma/a$ would be large even when a is small. Therefore the integral $\int_0^a RT\Gamma\,da/a = \int_0^a RT\Gamma\,d\ln a$ would be appreciable, and a large reduction, $\gamma_0 - \gamma$, would be achieved even at low concentrations of the surfactant. Thus (see Fig 21-8) it can be said that in $0.2N$ sodium chloride, excluding the regions beyond the CMC, sodium lauryl sulfate is about ten times more surface-active than in $0.01N$ sodium chloride, ie, for the $0.2N$ sodium chloride the same $\gamma_a - \gamma$ and the same extent of adsorption (Γ) are observed at one-tenth the concentration of the surfactant.

Adsorption of a Surfactant—Surface-active substances (surfactants) are those that adsorb or tend to concentrate at interfaces. Conventional soaps, detergents (ionic and non-ionic), gums, and finely divided solids belong in this category. These materials adsorb at interfaces, the amount of adsorption generally increasing with increasing solution activity, a.

Fig 21-9 shows an adsorption isotherm that is similar to the one found for adsorption of a surfactant at the air/liquid or solid/liquid interface. Here C (moles/liter), rather than a, has been plotted on the x-axis. The initial slope of the Γ versus C curve is usually a measure of the inherent affinity of single molecules of surfactant for the adsorption site. Therefore, the greater the affinity the sooner (at low C or a) the adsorption begins. Maximum adsorption (plateau in Fig 21-9) usually occurs for one of two reasons: (1) all adsorption sites have become occupied by surfactant molecules, or (2) owing to micelle formation at the critical micelle concentration (CMC) the activity, a, becomes almost constant even while C continues to increase.

Experimental determinations of adsorption isotherms are easily carried out for solid/liquid systems when the solid is sparingly soluble in the solvent. Generally a given weight of adsorbent is equilibrated with a given volume of solution containing the surface-active agent. Analysis of the solution before and after equilibration gives the amount adsorbed. If the surface area of the adsorbent is known from an independent experiment, then Γ and the area per molecule may be calculated. For monolayers of low-molecular-weight (<500) surfactants, the area per molecule at maximum coverage is usually in the range of 20 to 50 Å^2, which is consistent with molecular geometries.

Table VII gives the results of adsorption experiments carried out by Roseman[2] in which 100-mg portions of hydroxyapatite [Ca$_{10}$(PO$_4$)$_6$(OH)$_2$] were equilibrated with 100 mL of dodecylammonium chloride (DAC) solutions of different concentrations. Fig 21-10 is a plot of the data. The plateau portion of this figure indicates that 0.6 millimole of DAC was adsorbed per gram of hydroxyapatite. The surface area of the sample was found to be 60 m^2/g, and it was calculated that each adsorbed DAC molecule occupied 16 Å^2.

As noted previously, the Gibbs equation may be used to

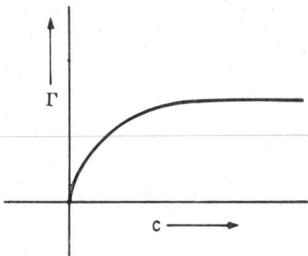

Fig 21-9.   A typical adsorption isotherm. Γ is moles adsorbed/cm^2 and C is moles/liter in the bulk solution.

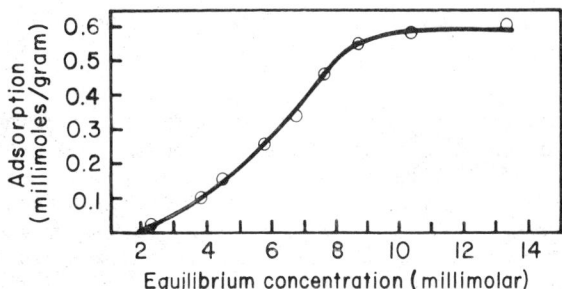

Fig 21-10.   Adsorption of dodecylammonium chloride on hydroxyapatite at 30°.

determine Γ and the area per molecule for the liquid/air interface. This approach may be used also for adsorption at liquid/liquid interfaces, except that interfacial tension, rather than surface tension, must be measured as a function of surfactant concentration.

When the plateau in the adsorption isotherm is the result of saturation of adsorption sites, a relatively compact monolayer of surfactant is formed. In some instances, however, multilayer adsorption occurs. Such adsorption is generally assumed when the area per molecule, calculated from Γ, is appreciably less than 20 Å^2, the lower limit for a single molecular layer. Also, when multilayer adsorption occurs, isotherms are usually more complex than that shown in Fig 21-9. For example, sodium lauryl sulfate and dodecylammonium chloride appear to pack as monolayers on barium sulfate and calcium fluoride surfaces in water. On aluminum oxide and titanium oxide, however, these agents appear to adsorb by a multilayer mechanism at certain pH values. A multilayer mechanism can describe adsorption of cationic agents on glass. At low concentrations these surfactants adsorb with their hydrophobic tails extending into the water phase; a second layer forms at higher concentrations, with the ionic portions in the aqueous phase.

Fig 21-11 shows the adsorption isotherm for dodecylammonium chloride on alumina. The complex curve suggests that at least two layers are formed near the CMC; the first inflection point in the curve probably represents the beginning of the second layer.

The CMC phenomenon is very important because it limits the "ultimate surface activity" of surfactants; the greater the CMC the better the surfactant. The CMC prevents most surfactants from providing zero or negative interfacial tensions (and therefore spontaneous emulsification), as evident in Eq 18. If sufficiently high activity could be attained, γ would become zero or negative. Aerosol OT is a good wetting agent, probably because its irregular shape makes micelle formation difficult. Hence, its CMC in water is relatively high, and low γ_L and γ_{SL} values are obtained with it.

The CMC of many surfactants is lowered by mixed micelle formation with other molecules (Fig 21-12). Long-chain al-

Table VII—Adsorption of Dodecylammonium Chloride on 100 mg of Hydroxyapatite in Water at 30°. Solution volume = 100 mL

Initial Conc. (millimolar)	Equil. Conc. (millimolar)	Millimoles Adsorbed/100 Mg
1.52	1.34	0.0018
3.76	2.77	0.0099
4.98	3.50	0.0148
7.33	4.81	0.0252
9.07	5.68	0.0339
11.3	6.73	0.046
13.3	7.77	0.055
15.2	9.36	0.058
18.3	12.3	0.060

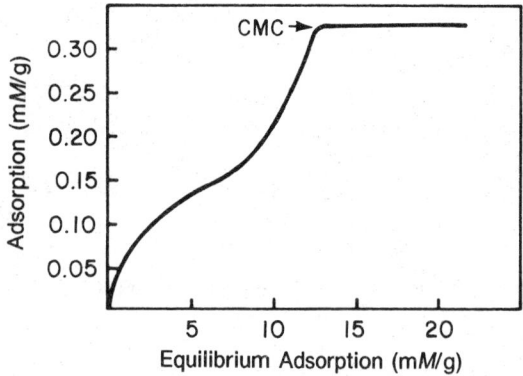

Fig 21-11.   Adsorption isotherm for dodecylammonium chloride on alumina at 20°.

cohols, amines, and esters may participate in mixed micelle formation with ionic and nonionic surfactants. The lowering of the CMC may be considerable. A consequence of this may be reduced surface activity unless these additives are equally proficient in enhancing surface activity by mixed surface-film formation. Thus, in the preparation of emulsions, either impurities in the oil or the oil itself may lower the CMC of the surfactant by incorporation into the micelles, and the surface activity of the agent may then be quite different from what it is in water alone.

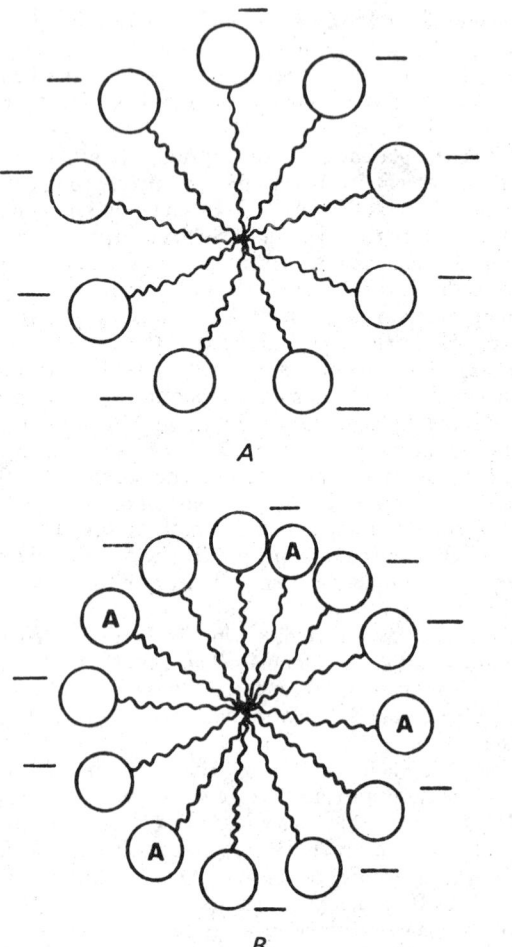

Fig 21-12.   Incorporation of long-chain alcohol molecules can lower the energy of a micelle, thus lowering the critical micelle concentration. A, Micelle of anionic molecules (higher energy); B, mixed micelle: anion + alcohol (A) molecules (lower energy).

Adsorption of surfactants at interfaces may be greatly influenced by the chain length, branching, and nature of the polar head group(s) in the surfactant molecule; the pH; the temperature; added salt in solution; and the nature of the interface-forming phases.

Adsorption of Polymers—Polymeric materials, such as suspending agents, are used in most dispersed pharmaceutical products. Several unique features characterize adsorption of polymers. The polymer consists of a skeleton molecular structure to which is attached, periodically along the skeleton, functional groups of different activity than the rest of the molecule; these groups adsorb at the interface. Neighboring segments may be adsorbed to form a "train" in the interface, or "loops" may form that extend into the solution. The adsorbed anchor groups at the two ends of the loop bind the loop to the interface. The interaction energy between the anchor group and the adsorbent need not be large to produce very extensive adsorption. This is a consequence of the multiple anchor groups. It is not probable that random thermally induced fluctuations would remove all anchor groups simultaneously, even if the individual anchor group interacts with only 4 or $5 kT$ energy. Many anchor groups may be attached to the loop section of the molecule and cannot adsorb at the same interface. However, they have the potential of adsorbing at the interface of a neighboring solid particle.

The nature of the train-loop configuration of adsorbed polymers causes the amount of polymer adsorbed per unit of surface area to increase extremely rapidly with increase in polymer concentration until the surface coverage of the solid is nearly complete. Above this plateau level further adsorption may be negligible. The adsorption often is nearly irreversible, very little being removed by repeated washing.

As polymer adsorbs, the free energy of interaction between neighboring loops becomes strong enough to arrest adsorption. In a good solvent this interaction is stronger than in a poor solvent; therefore, the adsorbed layer will contain more polymer when the adsorption is from a poor solvent. Conversely, in a good solvent long loops tend to cause the polymer to desorb because of the large free energy of interaction of polymer loops in close proximity. Similarly, the configuration of the molecule and the extension of the loops are dependent on solvent quality. Loops in a poor solvent tend to coil and to extend less distance from the interface than those in a good solvent. Again the controlling factor is the magnitude of the interaction of neighboring loops.

Particles in Liquid Systems

The behavior of particles dispersed in a liquid medium is subject to essentially the same forces as those described for powders although the results can be different due to the presence of the liquid. For example, as will be seen, the electrical forces in aqueous media between particles can play a more important role than in powders under certain conditions.

Effect of Charges—A solid particle or a droplet of an immiscible liquid may be electrically charged because an excess of ions of one sign may be present at the interface. The charge-conferring ions may be a constituent of the particle itself, impurity ions from the external-phase liquid, or surfactant ions preferentially adsorbed at the interface.

The particle charge gives rise to a surface potential, ψ_0, at the surface of the particle (see Fig 21-13). The potential will drop to zero at some distance away from the surface depending on the concentration of the counter-ions in the external-phase bulk. The region in which the influence of the surface charge is appreciable is called the electrical double-layer region.

The double layer may be visualized as being made up of two parts. The specific adsorption of counter-ions in the Stern

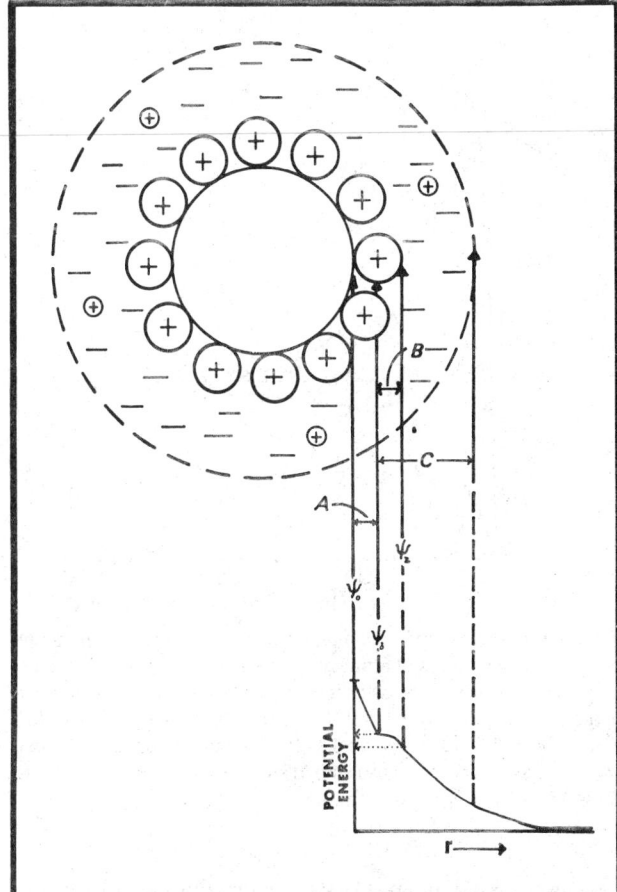

Fig 21-13.   The electrical double layer and the symbols used to describe the potential at various points. A: The Stern layer, B: the plane of shear, and C: the sphere of influence of the diffuse double layer.

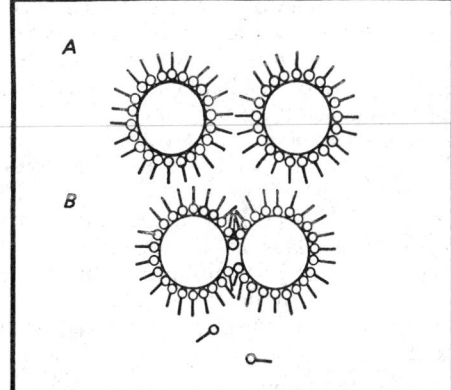

Fig 21-14.   The interaction of two particles coated with surfactant molecules. A: Particles separated by a distance which is large as compared to the size of the adsorbed surfactant molecules; B: particles at a close distance where repulsive forces arise when surfactant molecules are squeezed together and/or desorbed.

Layer comprises the first part, the thickness of which is of the order of ionic dimensions. The potential drop across this region is $\psi_0 - \psi_\delta$. The second part is called the diffuse double layer across which the potential drop is ψ_δ. The thickness of the diffuse double layer is given by the Debye-Hückel quantity $1/\kappa$.

$$1/\kappa = \left(\frac{\epsilon k T}{4\pi e^2 \Sigma n_i z_i^2}\right)^{1/2} \qquad (19)$$

where ϵ is the dielectric constant in the diffuse double-layer region, k is the Boltzmann constant, T is the absolute temperature, e is the electronic charge, n_i is the bulk concentration of ion i, and z_i is its valence.

According to Eq 19 a 1% aqueous sodium chloride solution at room temperature gives $1/\kappa = 8$ Å, a 0.01% solution gives $1/\kappa = 80$ Å, a 1×10^{-4}% solution gives $1/\kappa = 800$ Å, etc. These calculations show that the electrical influence among particles in aqueous media is relatively short-range compared to that involving powder particles which, as predicted by Eqs 3 and 4, extend to distances of the order of particle dimensions.

In nonpolar media n, the bulk ionic concentration, is usually very small. Therefore, $1/\kappa$ values of the order of centimeters are sometimes encountered, and in such cases the distances of electrical influence approach those encountered in powders. This frequently leads to the "electrostatic" problems in such systems. Antistatic agents are helpful in these situations by reducing $1/\kappa$ and by relieving the buildup of charge.

Eq 19 also shows that polyvalent counterions are much more effective than monovalent ions in reducing the double-layer thickness. A 2–2 electrolyte is about four times more effective than a 1–1 electrolyte in reducing the diffuse double-layer thickness.

Zeta Potential—When a charged particle suspended in a liquid is placed in an electrical field, it will migrate towards the electrode with the opposite charge. The ions in the Stern Layer and the bound solvent molecules are also carried along with the particle. Thus, the plane of shear (see Fig 21-13) is very close to the Stern Layer but slightly farther away from the particle surface. While the exact relationship between the zeta potential, ψ_z, and ψ_δ is not clear, it is generally supposed that ψ_δ and ψ_z are of the same order of magnitude, the latter being slightly smaller. If, in addition, ψ_0 is small ($\gtrsim 50$ mV) and there is little special counterion-binding tendency at the interface, the zeta potential will also reflect the ψ_0 value and the changes in it. The surface potential, ψ_o, is related to the surface charge density, the number of charges per unit area, by the Gouy-Chapman diffuse electrical double layer theory.

As will be seen in the next section, when electrical repulsion is present, the flocculation behavior of suspensions and emulsions strongly depends upon the surface charge on the particles which is reflected in the magnitude of ψ_z. Generally when ψ_z is of the order of 25 mV or less, the system becomes kinetically unstable to flocculation and aggregation or coalescence may take place.

Particle Interactions in Liquids—According to the theory of the stability of lyophobic colloids (particles in liquid media) a number of forces are at play in determining the overall interaction among particles. Consideration of these interaction forces is helpful in understanding the dispersion process as well as aggregation and coalescence behavior of dispersed particles. At relatively large distances of separation ($\gtrsim 10$ Å) the primary forces are the London dispersion forces of attraction and the electrical repulsive forces resulting from the interaction of the diffuse double layers of the particles. The electrolyte flocculation behavior of suspensions and emulsions is frequently attributed to the interplay of the electrical and the dispersion forces.

Other forces of repulsion should also be considered, particularly at close distances of approach between the particles. These are the repulsive contributions due to the surfactant molecules themselves, arising from steric hindrance (see Fig 21-14). Particles at very close distances of approach may be kept apart by this mechanism and by the resistance of the adsorbed agents from being displaced (desorbed) from the interface. When surfactant desorption is involved, work must be done against those same forces that are responsible for the interfacial-tension lowering. Barriers to particle–particle aggregation and/or droplet coalescence are also set up by adsorption of polymers and finely divided solids. Lyophilic polymers often provide thick films ($\gtrsim 100$ Å) that effectively prevent close approach of the particles.

London Dispersion Forces of Attraction—As previously stated, the London dispersion forces are generally regarded as short-range and relatively weak. However, considering the large number of molecules in a suspension particle or an emulsion droplet, one finds that the aggregate attraction between two particles may be significant even at surface separation distances (H) of the order of 100 Å.

Eq 20 gives the attraction energy between two spheres according to theory:

$$V_A = -\frac{A'a_1a_2}{6(a_1+a_2)}\left(\frac{\lambda}{\lambda H + 3.54\pi H^2}\right) \quad (20)$$

where a_1 and a_2 are the radii of the spheres, λ is the London wavelength, usually taken as 10^{-5} cm, and A' is the effective Hamaker's constant.

Diffuse Double-Layer Repulsion—When two spherical particles of the same size are close enough so that their electric double layers are appreciably overlapping, a substantial repulsion may arise. Eq 21 may be used to estimate the repulsive potential energy, V_R, as a function of the distance of separation:

$$V_R = \frac{\epsilon a_1 a_2 \psi_0^2}{(a_1+a_2)} \ln\left[1 + \exp(-\kappa H)\right] \quad (21)$$

where ϵ is the dielectric constant of the double-layer region, a_1 and a_2 are the radii of the spheres, ψ_0 is the surface potential, and H is the shortest distance of separation between the surfaces of the spheres. Eq 21 was derived for the case in which the double-layer thickness, $1/\kappa$, is small compared to the radius of the smaller particle. This generally would be a good assumption for most situations in which water is the continuous phase and for particle sizes down to ca 100 Å. The equation is only applicable for small ψ_0 values, viz $\psi_0 \gtrsim 25$ mV. If larger ψ_0 values are involved, it may be more appropriate to substitute ψ_δ for ψ_0 in Eq 21.

Interactions between Adsorbed Layers—As two particles with adsorbed polymer approach each other, the loops of polymer extending from neighboring particles interact. The generic term for stabilization produced by these interactions is "steric stabilization." The interactions are essentially the same as would occur with an increase in concentration of the polymer in solution. The conformations available in one loop will be reduced by the presence of another loop; therefore entropy decreases. A decrease in entropy increases the free energy, so a repulsion develops between the two particles. Since the quality of the solvent affects the excluded volume, it also influences the magnitude of the repulsion at a given distance of separation between the particles. Obviously, two loops cannot interpenetrate without "squeezing out" solvent. Thus, as two particles approach, the loops of adsorbed polymers must replace polymer–solvent interactions with polymer–polymer interactions. Again the quality of the solvent determines the enthalpy changes that occur.

The influence of solvent quality has been studied and verified,[3] but efforts to distinguish experimentally between enthalpic and entropic stabilization have been less successful. Use of model systems to describe particle–particle interactions has improved, but the models are not adequate to explain all observations. One of the simple models for the potential energy of entropic and enthalpic repulsion V_s,[4] which attempts to embody the aforementioned concepts, is expressed by

$$V_S = \frac{4\pi k T \overline{V}_S^2}{3\overline{V}_1}\psi_1\left(1 - \frac{\theta}{T}\right)\left(\delta - \frac{H}{2}\right)^2\left(3r + 2\delta + \frac{H}{2}\right) \quad (22)$$

where k is the Boltzmann constant, T is the absolute tem-

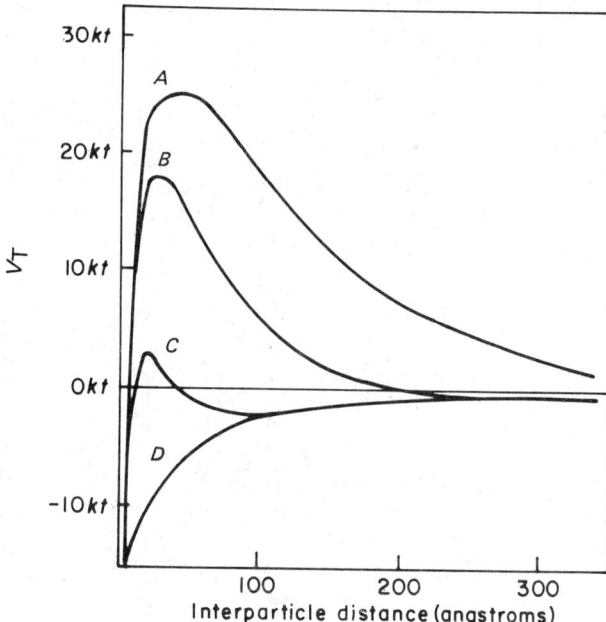

Fig 21-15. The net interaction of two spherical particles considering only the London forces of attraction and electrical repulsion (kt units) as a function of the interparticle distance (Å) for two equally sized particles of 0.1 μm. A: $\kappa = 2 \times 10^6$, B: $\kappa = 4 \times 10^6$, C: $\kappa = 10^7$, and D: $\kappa \geq 2 \times 10^7$. The peaks represent the maximum potential, V_{tmax}. These calculations used the following values: $A = 10^{-13}$ ergs, $\psi_0 = 25$ mV, and $\lambda = 10^{-5}$ cm.

perature, θ is a temperature parameter (Flory temperature), ψ_1 is an entropy term for solvent-polymer interaction, δ is the thickness of the adsorbed polymer layer, r is the radius of the bare particle, $\overline{V}_S$ is the volume fraction of adsorbed polymer in the overlap region, and $\overline{V}_1$ is the molecular volume of the solvent molecules. When the interparticle distance, H, is less than 2δ, V_S is greater than 0; for $H \geq 2\delta$, $V_S = 0$. For additional examples and information see references 5 to 14, at the end of this chapter.

Total Interaction—The net interaction of two spherical particles is given by,

$$V_{total} = V_A + V_R + V_S \quad (23)$$

Considering only the London forces of attraction and the electrical repulsion,* Fig 21-15 shows plots of V_{total} for two particles of equal size ($a_1 = a_2 = 0.1$ μm) at different ionic strengths, in water. At low ionic strengths, where $1/\kappa$ is large (see Eq 19), electrical repulsion dominates at most distances, and V_{total} is positive for all distances beyond the first few angstroms; the maximum potential, V_{max}, is large, ~25 kT. As the salt concentration is increased ($\kappa = 4 \times 10^6$, ca 0.10% NaCl), V_{max} decreases and a minimum develops in the potential energy curve at H $\simeq$ 150 Å. This minimum is called the secondary minimum, V_{min}, which, although small in the present example, could be of substantial depth for larger particles. At high salt concentrations ($\kappa = 10^7$ to 2×10^7, ca 1% NaCl), the repulsion is almost completely eliminated and only attraction persists. The influence of particle size on the total potential energy is shown in Fig 21-16. The energy barrier tends to increase with increasing particle size.

In an aqueous solution at higher concentrations of elec-

*Sample numerical calculations of the potential energy of repulsion, of the potential energy of attraction, and of adsorbed polymer repulsion are given in Appendix B of a communication by Schneider, Stavchansky, and Martin (*Am J Pharm Ed 42:* 280, 1978).

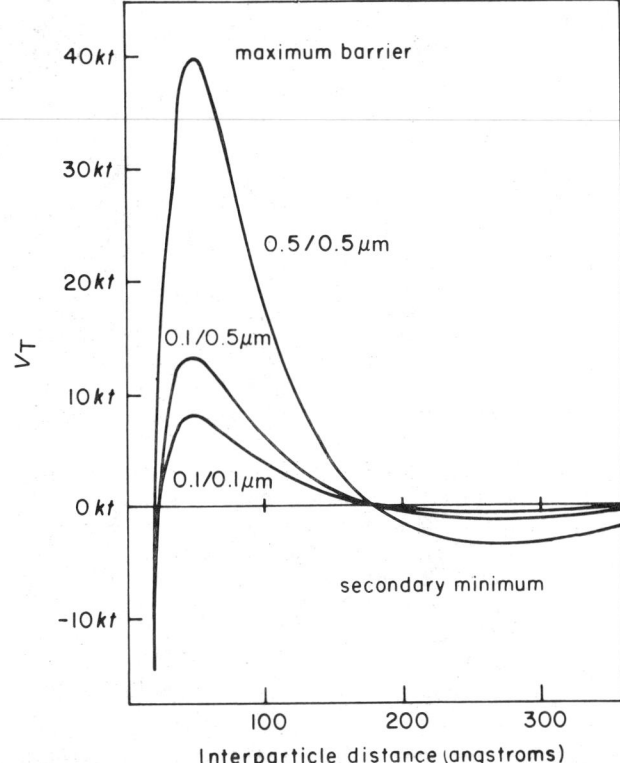

Fig 21-16.   Influence of particle size on total potential energy of interaction. $A = 5 \times 10^{-13}$ erg, $\psi = 25$ mV, and $\kappa = 2 \times 10^6$ cm^{-1}.

trolytes, the double-layer thickness may be so small that it will have no significant effect on the stability of a sterically stabilized system,[5] eg, a double layer of a few angstroms thickness would have little influence when the polymer loops extend into the solution 30 or more angstroms, ie, $1/\kappa < \delta$. As suggested earlier, electrolytes may produce flocculation in the presence of adsorbed polymer, but the flocculation may not be the result of their effect on the double layer. The use of electrophoretic mobility to determine the charge on the particle must be viewed with apprehension when adsorbed polymer is present. The extending loops cause the hydrodynamic shear plane to be moved out from the particle surface; thus, a much lower value of the zeta potential will be observed than would be justified for the charge distribution in the double layer. The presence of other solvents may affect the Stern layer.[6] Also, changes of the dielectric constant of the liquid and of the solvent quality are not independent factors.

An anchor group on the polymer may form a weak bond and be an inefficient anchor.[5] Such a polymer could desorb during interparticle collisions. This is designated "displacement flocculation." The kinetics of this should depend on the size of the adsorption interaction energy. Also, the addition of smaller molecules that could compete for and displace the polymer from the adsorption sites would be a controlling factor for the effectiveness of the polymer. One should be alert to these possibilities.

A possible mechanism of polymer action is that the polymer could prevent the particles from entering into the deep potential energy well illustrated in Fig 21-16, resulting from the combination of the van der Waals attraction and the double-layer repulsions.[7] The relative thickness of the double layer and the adsorbed polymer layer would determine whether steric repulsion prevented entry into the primary minimum. If properly balanced, the net effect of the two terms could be to change the primary minimum to a shallow minimum by preventing closer approach of the particles.

Thereby the adsorbed polymer would lead to a condition in which redispersion would be readily accomplished. Definitive work in this area is lacking, but this possibility should be considered.

Charged particles approaching another charged surface must overcome a potential energy barrier before a successful collision is achieved. This mechanism of particle-particle collision has been used to explain a number of phenomena which include the adhesion of cells, flocculation of charged phospholipid vesicles (or liposomes), and the interaction between particles in blood and surfaces of prosthetic materials. The electrical properties of the interfacial barrier are largely responsible for the slow dissolution rates of cholesterol particles (or cholesterol gallstones) in the presence of negatively charged micelles. The dissolution rates are enhanced manyfold in the presence of high electrolyte concentrations, neutralizing amines and quaternary ammonium compounds. Hence, the dissolution of cholesterol gallstones by perfusion of the gallbladder with sodium cholate micellar solutions is interfacial barrier-controlled in the absence of salt and is aqueous diffusion layer-controlled in sodium chloride solutions.

Flocculation Kinetics

Rapid Flocculation—In the absence of any repulsive barrier ($V_{\text{Total}} = 0$) and when it is controlled only by Brownian motion diffusion, the flocculation rate of a monodispersed suspension is given by the Smoluchowski equation:

$$\frac{dN}{dt} = -4\pi DRN^2 \qquad (24)$$

where dN/dt is the disappearance rate of particles/cc, R is the distance between the centers of the two particles in contact, N is the number of particles per mL, and D is the diffusion coefficient. Eq 24 shows that the flocculation reaction is bimolecular, the rate being proportional to the square of the particle concentration. If D is replaced by the Einstein relation, $D = kT/6\pi\eta a$, and $R = 2a$, the Smoluchowski rate constant for rapid flocculation is predicted by

$$K = 4\pi DR = \frac{4kT}{3\eta} \qquad (25)$$

The time, $t_{1/2}$, required to reduce the total number of particles to one-half the original number is given by

$$t_{1/2} = \frac{3\eta}{4kTN} \qquad (26)$$

Here, η is the viscosity of the liquid medium and N is the initial concentration of particles (number of particles per cc).

It is well known that agitation promotes flocculation but appears to have little influence in the initial stages of the flocculation. In the simplest case (see Fig 21-17) consider the particles in a laminar shear field with a velocity gradient, g, so that other particles are swept into the sphere of action of a central particle. The increase in the flocculation rate is evident when the collisions caused by the movement of the liquid and by Brownian motion are added. By comparing the probability of laminar shear collision, J, with the probability of Brownian collision, I,

$$J/I = \frac{\eta a^3 g}{2kT} \qquad (27)$$

the measure of the relative contributions of these types of motions to flocculation is found. Table VIII shows that for small colloidal particles collisions caused by agitation are few compared to those caused by Brownian motion unless the shear gradient is very high. It also shows the transition between the region of colloidal dispersion, where Brownian

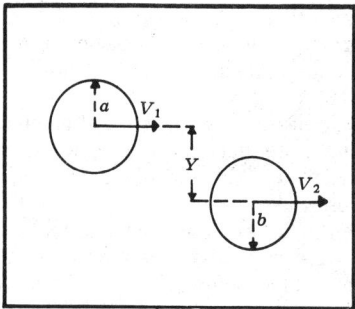

Fig 21-17. The influence of shear upon aggregation rate. If $V_1 > V_2$, collision will occur. Also, any other particle whose center is within the target area $4\pi a^2$ will collide if its velocity is less than Particle 1. The velocity gradient, G, is given by $(V_1 - V_2)/Y$; V_1 is the velocity of Molecule 1 and V_2 is the velocity of Molecule 2.

Table VIII—Relative Contribution of Shear-Induced Flocculation to the Brownian-Motion-Induced Flocculation [a]

Radius (μm)	Brownian motion only [b] ($t_{1/2}$)	Brownian and laminar shear motions	
		g (sec^{-1})	J/I [c]
0.05	0.95 sec	659	1/1000
		6,590	1/10
		65,900	1
0.5	950 sec	659	10/1
5.0	264 hr	659	1000/1

[a] Concentration of particles is 0.1% in water at 25°.
[b] Calculated using Eq 26.
[c] Calculated using Eq 27.

motion is predominant, and the region of suspensions, where agitation may govern flocculation.

Slow Flocculation (Energy Barrier)—When an energy barrier such as the electrical one discussed in the previous section is present, the flocculation rates may be much smaller than those predicted by Eq 24. When shear effects in the medium are negligible, one may write

$$G_{12} = \frac{2kT}{3\eta W_{12}}\left(\frac{1}{a_1} + \frac{1}{a_2}\right)(a_1 + a_2)N_1N_2 \qquad (28)$$

where G_{12} is the sticking rate of two particles of radii a_1 and a_2 with concentrations of N_1 and N_2, respectively. The factor W_{12} accounts for the energy barrier and is given by

$$W_{12} = 2\int_2^\infty \exp(V_{\text{Total}}/kT)\frac{dS}{S^2} \qquad (29)$$

where $S = 2R/(a_1 + a_2)$, R is the intercenter distance between the two particles, and V_{Total} is the potential energy function.

When V_{Total} is primarily the result of the diffuse double-layer repulsion and the London attraction, V_{Total} may be expressed by Eqs 20 and 21 for aqueous media.

The above indicates that the sticking rates of particles can be calculated in the following way: Eqs 20, 21 and 22 are used to calculate V_T at all distances of separation. The values of V_T as a function of S can also be obtained from Fig 21-15. The V_T's obtained by either method are substituted into Eq 29 and numerically integrated between limits to obtain W_{12}. Substituting this value for W_{12} in Eq 28 permits G_{12} to be calculated and G' is obtained from Eq 30.

Fig 21-18 gives the results of calculation with Eqs 20, 21, 22, 28 and 29. The quantity G' is defined by

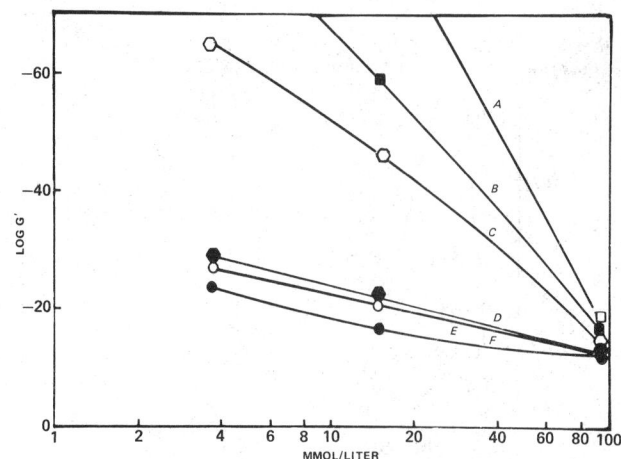

Fig 21-18. The calculated rates of aggregation of 0.1 μm, 0.5 μm, and 1 μm particles with themselves and with larger particles as a function of concentration of a 1–1 electrolyte in solution. ψ_0 is 25 mv and A' is 1×10^{-13} ergs. A: 1.0/1.0 μm; B: 0.5/1.0 μm; C: 0.5/0.5 μm; D: 0.1/1.0 μm; E: 0.1/0.5 μm; F: 0.1/0.1 μm.

$$G' = \frac{G_{12}}{N_1N_2} = \frac{2kT}{3\eta W_{12}}\left(\frac{1}{a_1} + \frac{1}{a_2}\right)(a_1 + a_2) \qquad (30)$$

It can be seen how electrolyte concentration may markedly increase the preference for the aggregation (or coalescence) of small particles with each other or with large particles. Thus, when $\kappa \simeq 2$ to 4×10^6 for $\psi_0 \simeq 25$ mV, it can be seen (Fig 21-18) that the rate of aggregation (or coalescence) of 0.1-μm particles with themselves or larger particles may be 10 to 30 orders of magnitude greater than that for two 0.5-μm particles.

Crystal Growth

Particles in suspensions may undergo dissolution and recrystallization, in part because of the recognized variation of solubility with particle size, expressed mathematically as

$$S = S_\infty \exp\left(\frac{2\gamma M}{r\rho RT}\right) \qquad (31)$$

where S is the solubility of a spherical crystal of radius r, S_∞ is the solubility of an infinitely large crystal ($r = \infty$), M is the molecular weight, ρ is the density, γ is the crystal/solvent interfacial tension, R is the gas constant, and T is the absolute temperature. Only approximations can be obtained with this equation, because the particles are not spheres, and γ values are different for different crystal faces. Table IX shows the magnitude of particle size effects on the solubility for reasonable values of M, γ, and ρ. It is evident that with particles smaller than 1 μm, S values become appreciably greater than that for a coarse crystal, hence the tendency for very fine particles to dissolve and for coarse crystals to grow at the expense of the former. This difference in solubility explains why difficulty is encountered in preparing and stabilizing suspensions of very fine particles of certain substances.

Table IX—Solubility of Small Particles

r (μm)	S
0.01	$7\,S_\infty$
0.10	$1.12\,S_\infty$
1.0	$1.01\,S_\infty$
10	$1.001\,S_\infty$

$M = 500$; $\gamma = 30$ ergs/cm^2; $\rho = 1$

Growth rates of drug crystals may be significantly retarded by use of certain agents that appear to function by adsorption at surface steps and kinks. Tweens and Triton X-100 at very low concentrations (0.005%) significantly retard growth of methylprednisolone crystals in aqueous media. Gelatin and polyvinylpyrrolidone, at concentrations <0.10%, retard crystal growth of sulfathiazole in water.[8]

Other reasons may exist for the dissolution and recrystallization phenomenon. Because of the molecular complexity of many drugs, polymorphic forms other than the thermodynamically stable one may crystallize; these are always more soluble than the stable form. Steroids, sulfonamides, barbiturates, chloramphenicol palmitate, and many other drugs exhibit polymorphism. Solvate formation is another route by which more energetic crystal forms may develop. Also, during milling of a powder a significant amount of amorphous material may be produced, which would be more soluble than the crystalline material. Crystal habit effects are important only if particle sizes are small. Finally, temperature fluctuations in a dispersed system can create a situation whereby the system may be undersaturated for a period of time, then supersaturated for a period, and so on. These changes favor disappearance of small crystals, with concomitant growth of large ones.

Suspensions

A pharmaceutical suspension may be defined as a coarse dispersion containing finely divided insoluble material suspended in a liquid medium. Suspension dosage forms are given by the oral route, injected intramusculary or subcutaneously, applied to the skin in topical preparations, and used ophthalmically in the eye. They are an important class of dosage form. Since some products are occasionally prepared in a dry form, to be placed in suspension at the time of dispensing by the addition of an appropriate vehicle, this definition is extended to include these products.

There are certain criteria that a well-formulated suspension should meet. The dispersed particles should be of such a size that they do not settle rapidly in the container. However, in the event that sedimentation occurs, the sediment must not form a hard cake. Rather, it must be capable of redispersion with a minimum effort on the part of the patient. Additionally, the product should be easy to pour, pleasant to take, and resistant to microbial attack.

The three major problem areas associated with suspensions are (1) adequate dispersion of the particles in the vehicle, (2) settling of the dispersed particles, and (3) caking of these particles in the sediment so as to resist redispersion. Much of the following discussion will deal with the factors that influence these processes and the ways in which they can be minimized.

Interfacial Properties

When considering the interfacial properties of dispersed particles, two factors must be taken into account, regardless of whether the dispersed phase is solid or liquid. The first relates to an increase in the free energy of the surface as the particle size is reduced and the specific surface increased. The second deals with the presence of an electrical charge on the surface of the dispersed particles.

Surface Free Energy—When solid and liquid materials are reduced in size, they tend to agglomerate or stick together. This clumping, which can occur in either air or a liquid medium, is an attempt by the particles to reduce the excess surface free energy of the system. The increase in surface free energy is related to the increase in surface area produced when the particle size is decreased. It may be expressed as follows:

$$\Delta F = \gamma \Delta A \qquad (32)$$

where ΔF is the increase in surface free energy in ergs, ΔA is the increase in surface area in cm^2, and γ is the interfacial tension, in dynes/cm, between the dispersed particle or droplet and the dispersion medium. The smaller ΔF is, the more thermodynamically stable is the suspension of particles. A reduction in ΔF often is effected by the addition of a wetting agent which is adsorbed at the interface between the particle and the vehicle, thereby reducing the interfacial tension.

Unfortunately, while the particles remain dispersed, or deflocculated, and settle relatively slowly, they can form a hard cake at the bottom of the container when they eventually settle. Such a sediment can be extremely difficult to redisperse.

Surface Potential—As discussed earlier in this chapter, both attractive and repulsive forces exist between particles in a liquid medium. The balance achieved between these opposing forces determines whether or not two particles approaching each other actually make contact or are repulsed at a certain distance of separation.

While much of the theoretical work on electrical surface potentials in dispersed systems has been carried out on lyophobic colloids, the theories developed in this area have been applied to suspensions and emulsions.[9]

Flocculation and Deflocculation—Zeta potential ψ_z is a measurable indication of the potential existing at the surface of a particle. When ψ_z is relatively high (25 mV or more), the repulsive forces between two particles exceed the attractive London forces. Accordingly, the particles are dispersed and are said to be *deflocculated*. Even when brought close together by random motion or agitation, deflocculated particles resist collision due to their high surface potential.

The addition of a preferentially adsorbed ion whose charge is opposite in sign to that on the particle leads to a progressive lowering of ψ_z. At some concentration of the added ion the electrical forces of repulsion are lowered sufficiently that the forces of attraction predominate. Under these conditions the particles may approach each other more closely and form loose aggregates, termed flocs. Such a system is said to be *flocculated*.

Some workers restrict the term *flocculation* to the aggregation brought about by chemical bridging; aggregation involving a reduction of repulsive potential at the double layer is referred to as *coagulation*. Other workers regard flocculation as aggregation in the secondary minimum of the potential energy curve of two interacting particles and coagulation as aggregation in the primary minimum. In the present chapter the term *flocculation* is used for all aggregation processes, irrespective of mechanism.

The continued addition of the flocculating agent can reverse the above process, if the zeta potential increases sufficiently in the opposite direction. Thus, the adsorption of anions onto positively charged deflocculated particles in suspension will lead to flocculation. The addition of more anions can eventually generate a net negative charge on the particles. When this has achieved the required magnitude, deflocculation may occur again. The only difference from the starting system is that the net charge on the particles in their deflocculated state is negative rather than positive. Some of the major differences between suspensions of flocculated and deflocculated particles are presented in Table X.

Table X—Relative Properties of Flocculated and Deflocculated Particles in Suspension

Deflocculated	Flocculated
1. Particles exist in suspension as separate entities.	Particles form loose aggregates.
2. Rate of sedimentation is slow, since each particle settles separately and particle size is minimal.	Rate of sedimentation is high, since particles settle as a floc, which is a collection of particles.
3. A sediment is formed slowly.	A sediment is formed rapidly.
4. The sediment eventually becomes very closely packed, due to weight of upper layers of sedimenting material. Repulsive forces between particles are overcome and a hard cake is formed which is difficult, if not impossible, to redisperse.	The sediment is loosely packed and possesses a scaffold-like structure. Particles do not bond tightly to each other and a hard, dense cake does not form. The sediment is easy to redisperse, so as to reform the original suspension.
5. The suspension has a pleasing appearance, since the suspended material remains suspended for a relatively long time. The supernatant also remains cloudy, even when settling is apparent.	The suspension is somewhat unsightly, due to rapid sedimentation and the presence of an obvious, clear supernatant region. This can be minimized if the volume of sediment is made large. Ideally, volume of sediment should encompass the volume of the suspension.

Settling and Its Control

In order to control the settling of dispersed material in suspension, the pharmacist must be aware of those physical factors that will affect the rate of sedimentation of particles under ideal and non-ideal conditions. He must also be aware of the various coefficients used to express the amount of flocculation in the system and the effect flocculation will have on the structure and volume of the sediment.

Sedimentation Rate

The rate at which particles in a suspension sediment is related to their size and density and the viscosity of the suspension medium. Brownian movement may exert a significant effect, as will the absence or presence of flocculation in the system.

Stokes' Law—The velocity of sedimentation of a uniform collection of spherical particles is governed by Stokes' law, expressed as follows:

$$v = \frac{2r^2(\rho_1 - \rho_2)g}{9\eta} \qquad (33)$$

where v is the terminal velocity in cm/sec, r is the radius of the particles in cm, ρ_1 and ρ_2 are the densities (g/cm^3) of the dispersed phase and the dispersion medium, respectively, g is the acceleration due to gravity (980.7 cm/sec^2) and η is the Newtonian viscosity of the dispersion medium in poises (g/cm sec). Stokes' law holds only if the downward motion of the particles is not sufficiently rapid to cause turbulence. Furthermore, an implicit assumption to Stoke's law is that the particle exceeds the critical radius, which is expressed by

$$r_c \geq \left[\frac{40 \, kT}{\pi g(\rho_1 - \rho_2)}\right]^{1/4} \qquad (34)$$

where r_c is the critical radius in cm in which gravity is the dominant force, kT is the thermal energy. For example, the critical radius for latex polymer spheres of $\rho_1 = 1.05$ g/cm^3 is 3.2 μm in water at 25°, while r_c for gold particles of $\rho_1 = 19.3$ is 0.74 μm. Most drugs have densities between 1 and 1.5. On the other hand, latex and gold particles which are smaller than their r_c will settle in a more random fashion due to the increasing influence of thermal forces acting upon the particle to impart Brownian movement. It is estimated that, in the limit, when the particles are less than the critical radius, r_c*, thermal forces will be sufficiently dominant over gravitational forces so that the particles are constantly in Brownian motion. The r_c* is estimated by use of the expression,

$$\frac{2(r_c^*)^2(\rho_1 - \rho_2)}{9\eta} < 1.16 \times 10^{-6} \text{ cm/sec} \qquad (35)$$

Thus, the r_c* values are 0.33 μm for latex particles and 0.017 μm for gold particles. Micelles and small phospholipid vesicles do not settle unless they are subjected to centrifugation.

While conditions in a pharmaceutical suspension are not in strict accord with those laid down for Stokes' law, Eq 33 provides those factors that can be expected to influence the rate of settling. Thus, sedimentation velocity will be reduced by decreasing the particle size, provided the particles are kept in a deflocculated state. The rate of sedimentation will be an inverse function of the viscosity of the dispersion medium. However, too high a viscosity is undesirable, especially if the suspending medium is Newtonian rather than shear-thinning (see Chapter 22), since it then becomes difficult to redisperse material which has settled. It also may be inconvenient to remove a viscous suspension from its container.

According to Stokes' law, the rate of sedimentation will be reduced if the difference in the densities (ρ_1 and ρ_2) of the dispersed particles and the continuous phase can be decreased. This is rarely possible in practice, and will not be discussed further.

Brownian Movement—When the size of particles undergoing sedimentation is reduced to approximately 2 μm, random Brownian movement is observed and the rate of sedimentation departs markedly from the theoretical predictions of Stokes' law. The actual size at which Brownian movement becomes significant depends on the density of the particle as well as the viscosity of the dispersion medium. However, at the lower limit of the coarse-size range, the dispersed particles may remain suspended for a prolonged period of time due to this phenomenon.

Effect of Flocculation—In a deflocculated system containing a distribution of particle sizes, the larger particles naturally settle faster than the smaller particles. The very small particles remain suspended for a considerable length of time, with the result that no distinct boundary is formed between the supernatant and the sediment. Even when a sediment becomes discernible, the supernatant remains cloudy.

When the same system is flocculated (in a manner to be discussed later), two effects are immediately apparent. First, the flocs tend to fall together so that a distinct boundary between the sediment and the supernatant is readily observed; second, the supernatant is clear, showing that the very fine particles have been incorporated into the flocs. The initial rate of settling in flocculated systems is determined by the size of the flocs and the porosity of the aggregated mass. Under these circumstances it is perhaps better to use the term *subsidence*, rather than sedimentation.

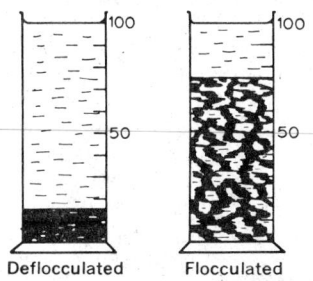

Fig 21-19. Sedimentation parameters of suspensions. Deflocculated suspension: $F_\infty = 0.15$. Flocculated suspension: $F = 0.75$; $\beta = 5.0$.

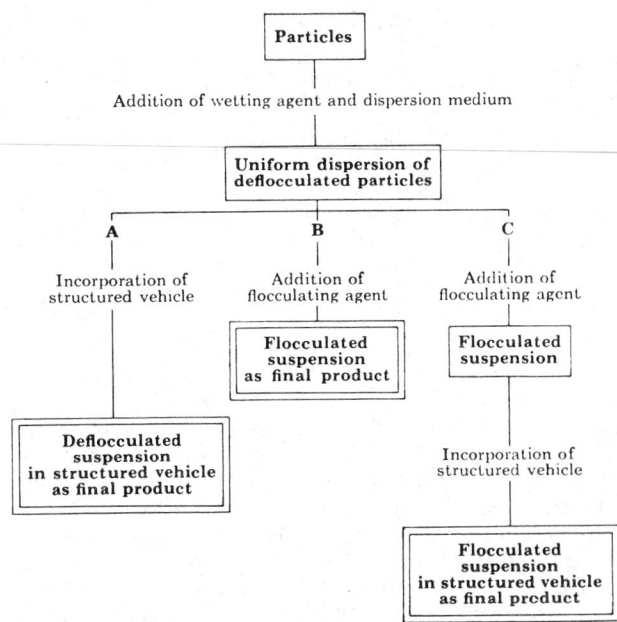

Fig 21-20. Alternative approaches to the formulation of suspensions.

Quantitative Expressions of Sedimentation and Flocculation

Frequently, the pharmacist needs to assess a formulation in terms of the amount of flocculation in the suspension and to compare this with that found in other formulations. The two parameters commonly used for this purpose are outlined below.

Sedimentation Volume—The *sedimentation volume, F,* is the ratio of the equilibrium volume of the sediment, V_u, to the total volume of the suspension, V_0. Thus,

$$F = V_u/V_0 \qquad (36)$$

As the volume of suspension which appears occupied by the sediment increases, the value of F, which normally ranges from nearly 0 to 1, increases. In the system where $F = 0.75$, for example, 75% of the total volume in the container is apparently occupied by the loose, porous flocs forming the sediment. This is illustrated in Fig 21-19. Obviously, in a particular suspension, if F can be made to approach closer to unity, the product becomes more acceptable, since the volume of supernatant (undoubtedly regarded as unsightly) is being progressively reduced. When $F = 1$, no sediment is apparent even though the system is flocculated. This is the ideal suspension for, under these conditions, no sedimentation will occur. Caking also will be absent. Furthermore, the suspension is esthetically pleasing, there being no visible, clear supernatant.

Degree of Flocculation—A better parameter for comparing flocculated systems is the *degree of flocculation, β,* which relates the sedimentation volume of the flocculated suspension, F, to the sedimentation volume of the suspension when deflocculated, F_∞. It is expressed as

$$\beta = F/F_\infty \qquad (37)$$

The degree of flocculation is, therefore, an expression of the increased sediment volume resulting from flocculation. If, for example, β has a value of 5.0 (Fig 21-19), this means that the volume of sediment in the flocculated system is five times that in the deflocculated state. The flocs are quite porous and the desirable scaffold-like structure is present. If a second flocculated formulation results in a value for β of say 6.5, this latter suspension obviously is preferred, if the aim is to produce as flocculated a product as possible. As the degree of flocculation in the system decreases, β approaches unity, the theoretical minimum value.

Formulation of Suspensions

The formulation of a suspension possessing optimal physical stability depends on whether the particles in suspension are to be flocculated or to remain deflocculated. One approach involves use of a structured vehicle to keep deflocculated particles in suspension; a second depends on controlled flocculation as a means of preventing cake formation. A third,

a combination of the two previous methods, results in a product with optimum stability. The various schemes are illustrated in Fig 21-20.

Dispersion of Particles—The dispersion step has been discussed earlier in this chapter. Surface-active agents commonly are used as wetting agents; maximum efficiency is obtained when the HLB value lies within the range of 7–9. A concentrated solution of the wetting agent in the vehicle may be used to prepare a slurry of the powder; this is diluted with the required amount of vehicle. Alcohol and glycerin may be used sometimes in the initial stages to disperse the particles, thereby allowing the vehicle to penetrate the powder mass.

Only the minimum amount of wetting agent should be used, compatible with producing an adequate dispersion of the particles. Excessive amounts may lead to foaming or impart an undesirable taste or odor to the product. Invariably, as a result of wetting, the dispersed particles in the vehicle are deflocculated.

Structured Vehicles—Structured vehicles are generally aqueous solutions of polymeric materials, such as the hydrocolloids, which are usually negatively charged in aqueous solution. Typical examples are methylcellulose, carboxymethylcellulose, acacia, bentonite, and Carbopol. The concentration employed will depend on the consistency desired for the suspension which, in turn, will relate to the size and density of the suspended particles. They function as viscosity-imparting suspending agents and, as such, reduce the rate of sedimentation of dispersed particles, in accordance with Stokes' law. It should be noted, however, that Stokes' law applies strictly only to Newtonian fluids; the majority of suspending agents used in practice are non-Newtonian.

The rheological properties of suspending agents are considered elsewhere (Chapter 22). Ideally, these form pseudoplastic or plastic systems which undergo shear-thinning. Some degree of thixotropy is also desirable. Non-Newtonian materials of this type are preferred over Newtonian systems because, if the particles eventually settle to the bottom of the container, their redispersion is facilitated by the vehicle thinning when shaken. When the shaking is discontinued, the vehicle regains its original consistency and the redispersed particles are held suspended. This process of redispersion, facilitated by a shear-thinning vehicle, presupposes that the deflocculated particles have not yet formed a cake. If sedimentation and packing have proceeded to the point where considerable caking has occurred, redispersion is virtually impossible.

Controlled Flocculation—When using this approach (see Fig 21-20, B and C), the formulator takes the deflocculated, wetted dispersion of particles and attempts to bring about flocculation by the addition of a flocculating agent; most commonly, these are either electrolytes, polymers, or surfactants. The aim is to *control* flocculation by adding that amount of flocculating agent which results in the maximum sedimentation volume.

Electrolytes are probably the most widely used flocculating agents. They act by reducing the electrical forces of repulsion between particles, thereby allowing the particles to form the loose flocs so characteristic of a flocculated suspension. Since the ability of particles to come together and form a floc depends on their surface charge, zeta potential measurements on the suspension as an electrolyte is added provide valuable information as to the extent of flocculation in the system.

This principle is illustrated by reference to the following example, taken from the work of Haines and Martin.[10] Particles of sulfamerazine in water bear a negative charge. The serial addition of a suitable electrolyte, such as aluminum chloride, causes a progressive reduction in the zeta potential of the particles. This is due to the preferential adsorption of the trivalent aluminum cation. Eventually, the zeta potential will reach zero and then become positive as the addition of $AlCl_3$ is continued.

If sedimentation studies are run simultaneously on suspensions containing the same range of $AlCl_3$ concentrations, a relationship is observed (Fig 21-21) between the sedimentation volume, F, the presence or absence of caking, and the zeta potential of the particles. In order to obtain a flocculated, noncaking suspension with the maximum sedimentation volume, the zeta potential must be controlled so as to lie within a certain range (generally less than 25 mV). This is achieved by the judicious use of an electrolyte.

A comparable situation is observed when a negative ion such as PO_4^{3-} is added to a suspension of positively charged particles such as bismuth subnitrate. Ionic and nonionic surfactants and lyophilic polymers also have been used to flocculate particles in suspension. Polymers, which act by forming a "bridge" between particles, may be the most effi-

cient additives for inducing flocculation. Thus, it has been shown that the sedimentation volume is higher in suspensions flocculated with an anionic heteropolysaccharide than when electrolytes were used.

Work by Matthews and Rhodes,[11-13] involving both experimental and theoretical studies, has confirmed the formulation principles proposed by Martin and Haines. The suspensions used by Matthews and Rhodes contained 2.5% w/v of griseofulvin as a fine powder together with the anionic surfactant sodium dioxyethylated dodecyl sulfate (10^{-3} molar) as a wetting agent. Increasing concentrations of aluminum chloride were added and the sedimentation height (equivalent to the sedimentation volume, see page 315) and the zeta potential recorded. Flocculation occurred when a concentration of 10^{-3} molar aluminum chloride was reached. At this point the zeta potential had fallen from −46.4 mV to −17.0 mV. Further reduction of the zeta potential, to −4.5 mV by use of 10^{-2} molar aluminum chloride did not increase sedimentation height, in agreement with the principles shown in Fig 21-21.

Matthews and Rhodes then went on to show, by computer analysis, that the DLVO theory (see page 284) predicted the results obtained, namely, that the griseofulvin suspensions under investigation would remain deflocculated when the concentration of aluminum chloride was 10^{-4} molar or less. Only at concentrations in the range of 10^{-3} to 10^{-2} molar aluminum chloride did the theoretical plots show deep primary minima, indicative of flocculation. These occurred at a distance of separation between particles of approximately 50 Å, and led Matthews and Rhodes to conclude that coagulation had taken place in the primary minimum.

Schneider *et al*[14] have published details of a laboratory investigation (suitable for undergraduates) that combines calculations based on the DLVO theory carried out with an interactive computer program with actual sedimentation experiments performed on simple systems.

Flocculation in Structured Vehicles—The ideal formulation for a suspension would seem to be when flocculated particles are supported in a structured vehicle. The advantages of such a combination, in view of the previous discussion, should be obvious to the reader.

As shown in Fig 21-20 (under C), the process involves dispersion of the particles and their subsequent flocculation. Finally, a lyophilic polymer is added to form the structured vehicle. In developing the formulation, care must be taken to ensure the absence of any incompatibility between the flocculating agent and the polymer used for the structured vehicle. A limitation is introduced here, in that virtually all the structured vehicles in common use are hydrophilic colloids, and these carry a negative charge. This means that an incompatibility arises if the charge on the particles is originally negative. Flocculation in this instance requires the addition of a positively charged flocculating agent or ion; in the presence of such a material, the negatively charged suspending agent may coagulate and lose its suspendibility. This situation does not arise with particles that bear a positive charge, as the negative flocculating agent which the formulator must employ is compatible with the similarly charged suspending agent.

One approach, outlined in Fig 21-22, has universal utility. Here, regardless of the sign of the initial charge on the particle, a positively charged agent is adsorbed onto the particles. Flocculation is then brought about by means of an anionic flocculant which is compatible with the hydrophilic colloid used to keep the flocs in suspension.

Chemical Stability of Suspensions—Particles that are completely insoluble in a liquid vehicle are unlikely to undergo most chemical reactions leading to degradation. However, most drugs in suspension have a finite solubility, even though this may be of the order of fractions of a microgram per mL.

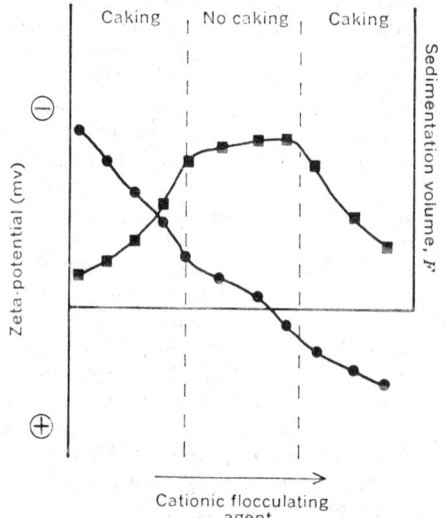

Fig 21-21. Typical relationship between caking, zeta potential, and sedimentation volume, as a positively charged flocculating agent is added to a suspension of negatively charged particles. ●: zeta potential; ■: sedimentation volume.

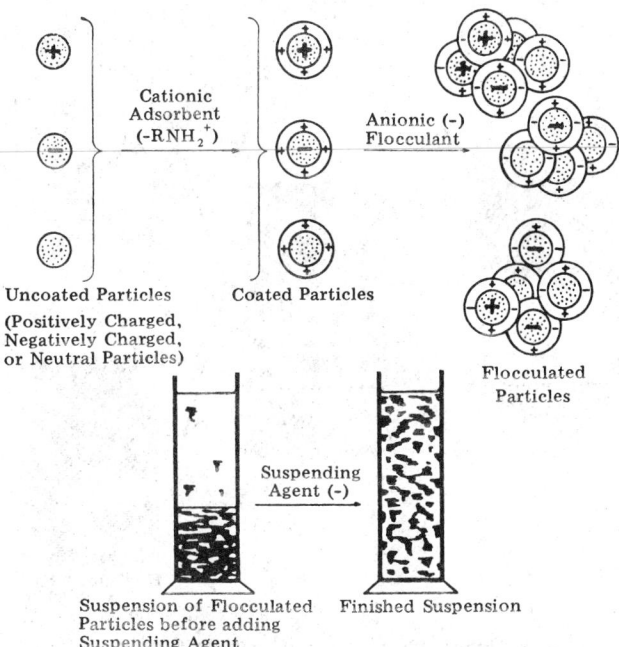

Fig 21-22.   Sequence of steps involved in the preparation of a stable suspension, regardless of the initial charge on the particles.[21]

As a result, the material in solution may be susceptible to degradation. Little work has been performed to quantitate and predict the chemical stability of suspended materials.

However, Tingstad and co-workers[16] developed a simplified method for determining the stability of drugs in suspension. The approach is based on the assumptions that (1) degradation takes place only in the solution and is first order, (2) the effect of temperature on drug solubility and reaction rate conforms with classical theory, and (3) dissolution is not rate-limiting on degradation.

Preparation of Suspensions—The small-scale preparation of suspensions may be readily undertaken by the practicing pharmacist with the minimum of equipment. It is probably true to say that any suspension will only be as good as the initial dispersion of the particles. This preliminary step is best carried out, therefore, by trituration in a mortar, the wetting agent being added in small increments to the powder. Once the particles have been wetted adequately, the slurry may be transferred to the final container. The next step depends on whether the deflocculated particles are to be suspended in a structured vehicle, flocculated, or flocculated and then suspended. Regardless of which of the alternative procedures outlined in Fig 21-20 is employed, the various manipulations can be carried out easily in the bottle, especially if an aqueous solution of the suspending agent has been prepared beforehand.

If the structured vehicle has a high consistency, it may be advisable to leave the slurry in the mortar and add the suspending agent there. Gentle trituration ensures complete dispersion of the powder throughout the vehicle. The final product is then transferred to the container.

For a detailed discussion of the methods used in the large-scale production of suspensions, see the relevant section in Chapter 83.

Emulsions

An emulsion is a dispersed system containing at least two immiscible liquid phases. The majority of conventional emulsions in pharmaceutical use have dispersed particles ranging in diameter from 0.1–100 μm. As with suspensions, emulsions are thermodynamically unstable as a result of the excess free energy associated with the surface of the droplets. The dispersed droplets, therefore, strive to come together and reduce the surface area. In addition to this flocculation effect, also observed with suspensions, the dispersed particles can coalesce, or fuse, and this can result in the eventual destruction of the emulsion. In order to minimize this effect a third component, the *emulsifying agent*, is added to the system to improve its stability. The choice of emulsifying agent is critical to the preparation of an emulsion possessing optimum stability. The efficiency of present-day emulsifiers permits the preparation of emulsions which are stable for many months and even years, even though they are thermodynamically unstable.

Emulsions are widely used in pharmacy and medicine, and emulsified materials can possess advantages not observed when formulated in other dosage forms. Thus, certain medicinal agents having an objectionable taste have been made more palatable for oral administration when formulated in an emulsion. The principles of emulsification have been applied extensively in the formulation of dermatological creams and lotions. Intravenous emulsions of contrast media have been developed to assist the physician in undertaking X-ray examinations of the body organs while exposing the patient to the minimum of radiation. Considerable attention has been directed towards the use of sterile, stable intravenous emulsions containing fat, carbohydrate, and vitamins all in one preparation. Such products are administered to patients unable to assimilate these vital materials by the normal oral route.

Emulsions offer potential in the design of systems capable of giving controlled rates of drug release and of affording protection to drugs susceptible to oxidation or hydrolysis. There is still a need for well-characterized dermatological products with reproducible properties, regardless of whether these products are antibacterial, sustained-release, protective, or emollient lotions, creams, or ointments. The principle of emulsification is involved in an increasing number of aerosol products.

The pharmacist must be familiar with the types of emulsions and the properties and theories underlying their preparation and stability; such is the purpose of the remainder of this chapter. Microemulsions, which can be regarded as isotropic, swollen micellar systems are discussed in Chapter 84.

Emulsion Type and Means of Detection

A stable emulsion must contain at least three components; namely, the dispersed phase, the dispersion medium, and the emulsifying agent. Invariably, one of the two immiscible liquids is aqueous while the second is an oil. Whether the aqueous or the oil phase becomes the dispersed phase depends primarily on the emulsifying agent used and the relative amounts of the two liquid phases. Hence, an emulsion in which the oil is dispersed as droplets throughout the aqueous phase is termed an oil-in-water, O/W, emulsion. When water is the dispersed phase and an oil the dispersion medium, the emulsion is of the water-in-oil, W/O, type. Most pharmaceutical emulsions designed for oral administration are of the O/W type; emulsified lotions and creams are either O/W or

W/O, depending on their use. Butter and salad creams are W/O emulsions.

Recently, so-called *multiple* emulsions have been developed with a view to delaying the release of an active ingredient. In these types of emulsions three phases are present, ie, the emulsion has the form W/O/W or O/W/O. In these "emulsions within emulsions," any drug present in the innermost phase must now cross two phase boundaries to reach the external, continuous, phase.

On theoretical grounds the volume of the dispersed phase can constitute up to approximately 75% of the total volume of the emulsion. However, the assumptions on which this figure is based (namely, that the droplets are rigid spheres of uniform size) are not realized in practice. Accordingly, the volume of the dispersed phase can exceed this value. There comes a point, however, at which the volume of continuous phase is insufficient to contain the dispersed phase. Either the emulsion breaks, or it inverts, whereupon the internal phase now becomes the continuous phase, and *vice versa*. This change in type with increasing phase volume is frequently accompanied by a marked change in viscosity.

It is important for the pharmacist to know the type of emulsion he has prepared or is dealing with, since this can affect its properties and performance. Unfortunately, the several methods available can give incorrect results, and so the type of emulsion determined by one method should always be confirmed by means of a second method.

Dilution Test—This method depends on the fact that an O/W emulsion can be diluted with water and a W/O emulsion with oil. When oil is added to an O/W emulsion or water to a W/O emulsion, the additive is not incorporated into the emulsion and separation is apparent. The test is greatly improved if the addition of the water or oil is observed microscopically.

Conductivity Test—An emulsion in which the continuous phase is aqueous can be expected to possess a much higher conductivity than an emulsion in which the continuous phase is an oil. Accordingly, it frequently happens that when a pair of electrodes, connected to a lamp and an electrical source, are dipped into an O/W emulsion, the lamp lights due to passage of a current between the two electrodes. If the lamp does not light, it is assumed that the system is W/O.

Dye-Solubility Test—The knowledge that a water-soluble dye will dissolve in the aqueous phase of an emulsion while an oil-soluble dye will be taken up by the oil phase provides a third means of determining emulsion type. Thus, if microscopic examination shows that a water-soluble dye has been taken up by the continuous phase, we are dealing with an O/W emulsion. If the dye has not stained the continuous phase, the test is repeated using a small amount of an oil-soluble dye. Coloring of the continuous phase confirms that the emulsion is of the W/O type.

Formation and Breakdown of Dispersed Liquid Droplets

An emulsion exists as the result of two competing processes, namely, the dispersion of one liquid throughout another as droplets, and the combination of these droplets to reform the initial bulk liquids. The first process increases the free energy of the system, while the second works to reduce the free energy. Accordingly, the second process is spontaneous and continues until breakdown is complete; ie, the bulk phases are reformed.

It is of little use to form a well-dispersed emulsion if it quickly breaks down. Similarly, unless adequate attention is given to achieving an optimum dispersion during preparation, the stability of an emulsion system may be compromised from the start. Dispersion is brought about by well-designed

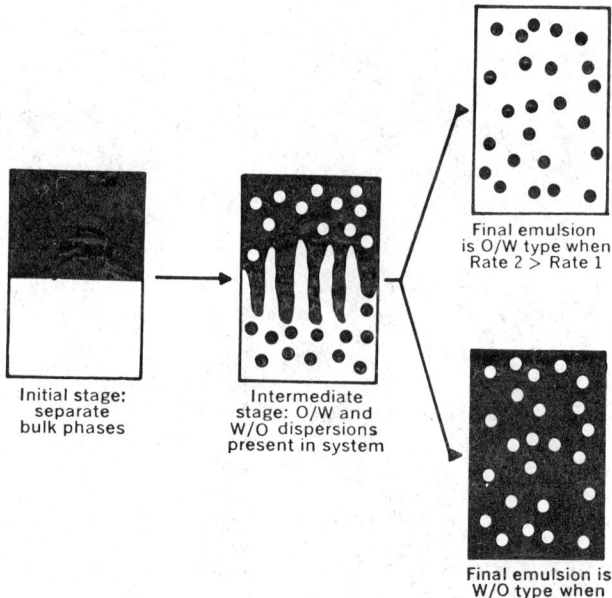

Fig 21-23. Effect of rate of coalescence on emulsion type. Rate 1: O/W coalescence rate; Rate 2: W/O coalescence rate. ●: oil; O: water. For an explanation of Rates 1 and 2, refer to the discussion of Davies on p 323.

and well-operated machinery, capable of producing droplets in a relatively short period of time. Such equipment is discussed in Chapter 84. The reversal back to the bulk phases is minimized by utilizing those parameters which influence the stability of the emulsion once it is formed.

Dispersion Process To Form Droplets—Consider two immiscible liquid phases in a test tube. The heavier phase lies below the second liquid and the system is thermodynamically stable. In order to disperse one liquid as droplets within the other, the interface between the two liquids must be disturbed and expanded to a sufficient degree so that "fingers" or threads of one liquid pass into the second liquid, and *vice versa*. These threads are unstable, and become varicosed or beaded. The beads separate and become spherical, as illustrated in Fig 21-23. Depending on the agitation or the shear rate used, larger droplets are also deformed to give small threads, which in turn produce smaller drops.

The time of agitation is important. Under normal conditions, the mean size of droplets decreases rapidly in the first few seconds of agitation. The limiting size range is generally reached within 1 to 5 min, and results from the number of droplets coalescing being equivalent to the number of new droplets being formed. It is uneconomical to continue agitation any further.

The liquids may be agitated or sheared by several means. Shaking is commonly employed, especially when the components are of low viscosity. Intermittent shaking is frequently more efficient than continual shaking, possibly because the short time interval between shakes allows the thread which is forced across the interface time to break down into drops which are then isolated in the opposite phase. Continuous, rapid agitation tends to hinder this breakdown to form drops. A mortar and pestle is employed frequently in the extemporaneous preparation of emulsions. It is not a very efficient technique and is not used on a large scale. Improved dispersions are achieved by the use of high-speed mixers, blenders, colloid mills and homogenizers. Ultrasonic techniques also have been employed and are described in Chapter 84.

The phenomenon of spontaneous emulsification, as the name implies, occurs without any external agitation. There is, however, an internal agitation arising from certain physicochemical processes that affect the interface between the two bulk liquids. For a description of this process, see Davies and Rideal (*Bibliography*).

Coalescence of Droplets—Coalescence is a process distinct from flocculation (aggregation), which commonly precedes it. While flocculation is the clumping together of particles, coalescence is the fusing of the agglomerates into a larger drop, or drops. Coalescence is usually rapid when two immiscible liquids are shaken together, since there is no large energy barrier to prevent fusion of drops and reformation of the original bulk phases. When an emulsifying agent is added to the system, flocculation still may occur but coalescence is reduced to an extent depending on the efficacy of the emulsifying agent to form a stable, coherent interfacial film. It is therefore possible to prepare emulsions that are flocculated, yet which do not coalesce. In addition to the interfacial film around the droplets acting as a mechanical barrier, the drops also are prevented from coalescing by the presence of a thin layer of continuous phase between particles clumped together.

Davies[17] showed the importance of coalescence rates in determining emulsion type; this work is discussed in more detail on page 323.

Emulsifying Agent

The process of coalescence can be reduced to insignificant levels by the addition of a third component—the emulsifying agent or emulsifier. The choice of emulsifying agent is frequently critical in developing a successful emulsion, and the pharmacist should be aware of (1) the desirable properties of emulsifying agents, (2) how different emulsifiers act to optimize emulsion stability, and (3) how the type and physical properties of the emulsion can be affected by the emulsifying agent.

Desirable Properties

Some of the desirable properties of an emulsifying agent are that it should (1) be surface-active and reduce surface tension to below 10 dynes/cm, (2) be adsorbed quickly around the dispersed drops as a condensed, nonadherent film which will prevent coalescence, (3) impart to the droplets an adequate electrical potential so that mutual repulsion occurs, (4) increase the viscosity of the emulsion, and (5) be effective in a reasonably low concentration. Not all emulsifying agents possess these properties to the same degree; in fact, not every good emulsifier necessarily possesses all these properties. Further, there is no one "ideal" emulsifying agent because the desirable properties of an emulsifier depend, in part, on the properties of the two immiscible phases in the particular system under consideration.

Interfacial Tension—Lowering of interfacial tension is one way in which the increased surface free energy associated with the formation of droplets, and hence surface area, in an emulsion can be reduced (Eq 32). Assuming the droplets to be spherical, it can be shown that

$$\Delta F = \frac{6\gamma V}{d} \tag{38}$$

where V is the volume of dispersed phase in mL and d is the mean diameter of the particles. In order to disperse 100 mL of oil as 1-μm (10^{-4}-cm) droplets in water when $\gamma_{O/W} = 50$ dynes/cm, requires an energy input of

$$\Delta F = \frac{6 \times 50 \times 100}{1 \times 10^{-4}} = 30 \times 10^7 \text{ ergs}$$

$$= 30 \text{ joules or } 30/4.184 = 7.2 \text{ cal}$$

The system attempts to lose this excess surface free energy

to its surroundings by coalescence of the droplets. These grow in size and decrease in number until one large drop (the original bulk phase) is formed. This has minimum surface area in contact with the second phase and the surface free energy is now at a minimum. However, an emulsifying agent which is adsorbed as a monolayer at an interface lowers surface tension in accordance with the Gibbs' equation (Eq 17).

In the above example the addition of an emulsifier that will reduce γ from 50 to 5 dynes/cm will reduce the surface free energy from 7.2 to around 0.7 cal. Likewise, if the interfacial tension is reduced to 0.5 dyne/cm, a common occurrence, the original surface free energy is reduced a hundredfold.

While the above calculations are an oversimplification of the total energies involved in emulsification, they do show that a reduction of interfacial tension by the addition of an emulsifying agent can help to maintain the surface area generated during the dispersion process.

Film Formation—The major requirement of a potential emulsifying agent is that it readily form a film around each droplet of dispersed material. The main purpose of this film—which can be a monolayer, a multilayer, or a collection of small particles adsorbed at the interface—is to form a barrier which prevents the coalescence of droplets that come into contact with one another. For the film to be an efficient barrier, it should possess some degree of surface elasticity and should not thin out and rupture when sandwiched between two droplets. If broken, the film should have the capacity to reform rapidly.

Electrical Potential—The origin of an electrical potential at the surface of a droplet has been discussed earlier in the chapter. Insofar as emulsions are concerned, the presence of a well-developed charge on the droplet surface is significant in promoting stability by causing repulsion between approaching drops. This potential is likely to be greater when an ionized emulsifying agent is employed.

Concentration of Emulsifier—The main objective of an emulsifying agent is to form a condensed film around the droplets of the dispersed phase. An inadequate concentration will do little to prevent coalescence. Increasing the emulsifier concentration above an optimum level achieves little in terms of increased stability. Apart from a possible increase in viscosity, there is little advantage in having a large excess present; indeed, it may produce such undesirable effects as foaming. In practice the aim is to use the minimum amount consistent with producing a satisfactory emulsion.

It frequently helps to have some idea of the amount of emulsifier required to form a condensed film, one molecule thick, around each droplet. Suppose we wish to emulsify 50 g of an oil, density = 1.0, in 50 g of water. The desired particle diameter is 1 μm. Thus,

Particle diameter = 1 μm = 1×10^{-4} cm

Volume of particle = $\frac{\pi d^3}{6}$ = 0.524×10^{-12} cm^3

Total number of particles in 50 g

$$= \frac{50}{0.524 \times 10^{-12}} = 95.5 \times 10^{12}$$

Surface area of each particle = πd^2 = 3.142×10^{-8} cm^2

Total surface area = 3.142×10^{-8}

$$\times 95.5 \times 10^{12} = 300 \times 10^4 \text{ cm}^2$$

If the area each molecule occupies at the oil/water interface is 30 Å^2 (30 $\times 10^{-16}$ cm^2), we require

$$\frac{300 \times 10^4}{30 \times 10^{16}} = 1 \times 10^{21} \text{ molecules}$$

A typical emulsifying agent might have a molecular weight

Table XI—Factors Influencing Emulsion Viscosity[18]

1. Internal phase
   a. Volume concentration (ϕ); hydrodynamic interaction between globules; flocculation, leading to formation of globule aggregates.
   b. Viscosity (η_1); deformation of globules in shear.
   c. Globule size, and size distribution, technique used to prepare emulsion; interfacial tension between the two liquid phases; globule behavior in shear; interaction with continuous phase; globule interaction.
   d. Chemical constitution.
2. Continuous phase
   a. Viscosity (η_0), and other rheological properties.
   b. Chemical constitution, polarity, pH; potential energy of interaction between globules.
   c. Electrolyte concentration if polar medium.
3. Emulsifying agent
   a. Chemical constitution; potential energy of interaction between globules.
   b. Concentration, and solubility in internal and continuous phases; emulsion type; emulsion inversion; solubilization of liquid phases in micelles.
   c. Thickness of film adsorbed around globules, and its rheological properties, deformation of globules in shear; fluid circulation within globules.
   d. Electroviscous effect.
4. Additional stabilizing agents
   Pigments, hydrocolloids, hydrous oxides; effect on rheologic properties of liquid phases, and interfacial boundary region.

of 1000. Thus, the required weight is

$$\frac{1000 \times 10^{21}}{6.023 \times 10^{23}} = 1.66 \text{ g}$$

To emulsify 10 g of oil would require 0.33 g of the emulsifying agent, etc. While the approach is an oversimplification of the problem, it does at least allow the formulator to make a reasonable estimate of the required concentration of emulsifier.

Emulsion Rheology—The emulsifying agent and other components of an emulsion can affect the rheologic behavior of an emulsion in several ways and these are summarized in Table XI. It should be borne in mind that the droplets of the internal phase are deformable under shear and that the adsorbed layer of emulsifier affects the interactions between adjacent droplets and also between a droplet and the continuous phase.

The means by which the rheological behavior of emulsions can be controlled have been discussed by Rogers.[19]

Mechanism of Action

Emulsifying agents may be classified in accordance with the type of film they form at the interface between the two phases. Such a classification is summarized in Table XII.

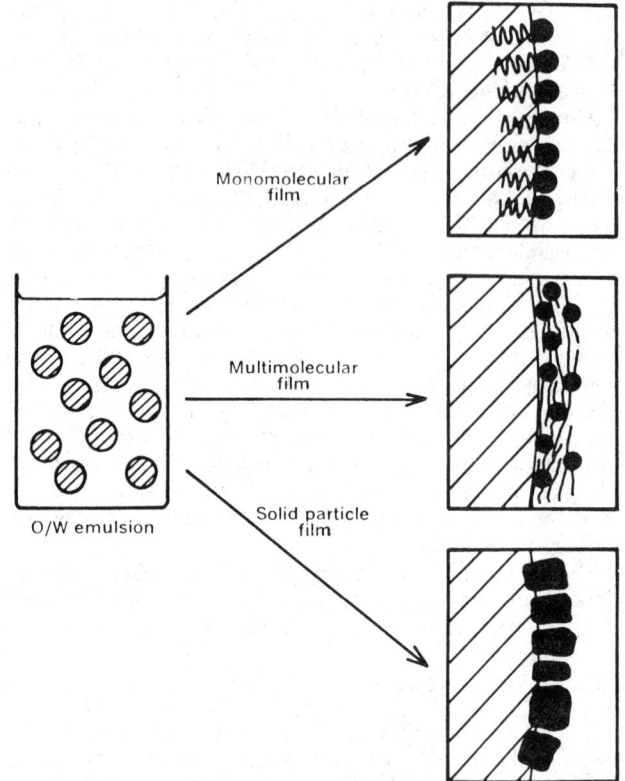

Fig 21-24. Types of films formed by emulsifying agents at the oil/water interface. Orientations are shown for O/W emulsions. ▨: oil; ☐: water.

Monomolecular Films—Those surface-active agents which are capable of stabilizing an emulsion do so by forming a monolayer of adsorbed molecules or ions at the oil/water interface (Fig 21-24). In accordance with Gibbs' law (Eq 17) the presence of an interfacial excess necessitates a reduction in interfacial tension. This results in a more stable emulsion because of a proportional reduction in the surface free energy. Of itself, this reduction is probably not the main factor promoting stability. More significant is the fact that the droplets are surrounded now by a coherent monolayer which prevents coalescence between approaching droplets. If the emulsifier forming the monolayer is ionized, the presence of strongly charged and mutually repelling droplets increases the stability of the system. With un-ionized, nonionic surface-active agents, the particles may still carry a charge; this arises from adsorption of a specific ion or ions from solution.

Multimolecular Films—Hydrated lyophilic colloids form multimolecular films around droplets of dispersed oil (Fig 21-24). The use of these agents has declined in recent years

Table XII—Mechanism of Action of Emulsifying Agents

Type of film	Example	Mechanism
Monomolecular	Potassium laurate Polyoxyethylene sorbitan monooleate	Coherent, flexible film formed by surface-active agents. These agents also lower interfacial tension markedly, and this contributes to stability of emulsion. Are widely used, especially the nonionic type. Depending on the particular agent(s) chosen, can prepare O/W or W/O emulsions.
Multimolecular	Acacia Gelatin	Strong, rigid film formed, mostly by hydrocolloids which produce O/W emulsions. Interfacial tension is not reduced to any degree; stability due mainly to strength of interfacial film.
Solid Particle	Bentonite Graphite Magnesium hydroxide	Film formed by solid particles that are small in size compared to the droplet of dispersed phase. Particles must be wetted by both phases to some extent in order to remain at the interface and form a stable film. From either O/W or W/O emulsions, depending on method of preparation.

Table XIII—Classification of Emulsifying Agents

Type	Type of film	Examples
Synthetic (surface-active agents)	Monomolecular	*Anionic:* Soaps Potassium laurate Triethanolamine stearate Sulfates Sodium lauryl sulfate Alkyl polyoxyethylene sulfates Sulfonates Dioctyl sodium sulfosuccinate *Cationic:* Quaternary ammonium compounds Cetyltrimethylammonium bromide Lauryldimethylbenzylammonium chloride *Nonionic:* Polyoxyethylene fatty alcohol ethers Sorbitan fatty acid esters Polyoxyethylene sorbitan fatty acid esters
Natural	Multimolecular	*Hydrophilic colloids:* Acacia Gelatin
	Monomolecular	Lecithin Cholesterol
Finely divided solids	Solid particle	*Colloidal clays:* Bentonite Veegum *Metallic hydroxides:* Magnesium hydroxide

because of the large number of synthetic surface-active agents available which possess well-marked emulsifying properties. While these hydrophilic colloids are adsorbed at an interface (and can be regarded therefore as "surface-active"), they do not cause an appreciable lowering in surface tension. Rather, their efficiency depends on their ability to form strong, coherent multimolecular films. These act as a coating around the droplets and render them highly resistant to coalescence, even in the absence of a well-developed surface potential. Furthermore, any hydrocolloid not adsorbed at the interface increases the viscosity of the continuous aqueous phase; this enhances emulsion stability.

Solid Particle Films—Small solid particles that are wetted to some degree by both aqueous and nonaqueous liquid phases act as emulsifying agents. If the particles are too hydrophilic, they remain in the aqueous phase; if too hydrophobic, they are dispersed completely in the oil phase. A second requirement is that the particles are small in relation to the droplets of the dispersed phase (Fig 21-24).

Chemical Types

Emulsifying agents may also be classified in terms of their chemical structure; there is some correlation between this classification and that based on the mechanism of action. For example, the majority of emulsifiers forming monomolecular films are synthetic, organic materials. Most of the emulsifiers that form multimolecular films are obtained from natural sources and are organic. A third group is composed of solid particles, invariably inorganic, that form films composed of finely divided solid particles.

Accordingly, the classification adopted divides emulsifying agents into *synthetic, natural,* and *finely dispersed solids* (Table XIII). A fourth group, the *auxiliary materials* (Table XIV), are weak emulsifiers. The agents listed are designed to illustrate the various types available; they are not meant to be exhaustive.

Synthetic Emulsifying Agents—This group of surface-active agents which act as emulsifiers may be subdivided into anionic, cationic, and nonionic, depending on the charge possessed by the surfactant.

Anionics—In this subgroup the surfactant ion bears a negative charge. The potassium, sodium, and ammonium salts of lauric and oleic acid are soluble in water and are good O/W emulsifying agents. They do, however, have a disagreeable taste and are irritating to the gastrointestinal tract; this limits them to emulsions prepared for external use. Potassium laurate, a typical example, has the structure:

$$CH_3(CH_2)_{10}COO^-\quad K^+$$

Solutions of alkali soaps have a high pH; they start to precipitate out of solution below pH 10 because the unionized fatty acid is now formed, and this has a low aqueous solubility. Further, the free fatty acid is ineffective as an emulsifier and so emulsions formed from alkali soaps are not stable at pH values less than about 10.

The calcium, magnesium, and aluminum salts of fatty acids, often termed the metallic soaps, are water insoluble and result in W/O emulsions.

Another class of soaps are salts formed from a fatty acid and an organic amine such as triethanolamine. While these O/W emulsifiers are also limited to external preparations, their alkalinity is considerably less than that of the alkali soaps and they are active as emulsifiers down to around pH 8. These agents are less irritating than the alkali soaps.

Sulfated alcohols are neutralized sulfuric acid esters of such fatty alcohols as lauryl and cetyl alcohol. These compounds are an important group of pharmaceutical surfactants. They are used chiefly as wetting agents, although they do have some value as emulsifiers, particularly, when used in conjunction with an auxiliary agent. Probably the most frequently used compound is sodium lauryl sulfate:

$$CH_3(CH_2)_{10}CH_2OSO_3^-\quad Na^+$$

Table XIV—Auxiliary Emulsifying Agents[15]

Product	Source and composition	Principal use
Bentonite	Colloidal hydrated aluminum silicate	Hydrophilic thickening agent and stabilizer for O/W and W/O lotions and creams
Cetyl alcohol	Chiefly $C_{16}H_{33}OH$	Lipophilic thickening agent and stabilizer for O/W lotions and ointments
Glyceryl monostearate	$C_{17}H_{35}COOCH_2CHOHCH_2OH$	Lipophilic thickening agent and stabilizer for O/W lotions and ointments
Magnesium hydroxide	$Mg(OH)_2$	Hydrophilic stabilizer for O/W emulsions
Methylcellulose	Series of methyl esters of cellulose	Hydrophilic thickening agent and stabilizer for O/W emulsions; weak O/W emulsifier
Silica gel	Hydrous oxide of silica	Hydrophilic stabilizer used in the preparation of ointments
Sodium alginate	The sodium salt of alginic acid, a purified carbohydrate extracted from giant kelp	Hydrophilic thickening agent and stabilizer for O/W emulsions
Sodium carboxymethylcellulose	Sodium salt of the carboxymethyl esters of cellulose	Hydrophilic thickening agent and stabilizer for O/W emulsions
Stearic acid	A mixture of solid acids from fats, chiefly stearic and palmitic	Lipophilic thickening agent and stabilizer for O/W lotions and ointments. Forms a true emulsifier when reacted with an alkali
Stearyl alcohol	Chiefly $C_{18}H_{37}OH$	Lipophilic thickening agent and stabilizer for O/W lotions and ointments
Tragacanth	Dried gummy exudation from species of *Astragalus*, containing a soluble portion and an insoluble portion that swells in water	Hydrophilic thickening agent and stabilizer for O/W emulsions; weak O/W emulsifier
Veegum	Colloidal magnesium aluminum silicate	Hydrophilic thickening agent and stabilizer for O/W lotions and creams

Sulfonates are a class of compounds in which the sulfur atom is connected directly to the carbon atom, giving the general formula

$$CH_3(CH_2)_n CH_2SO_3^- \quad Na^+$$

Sulfonates have a higher tolerance to calcium ions and do not hydrolyze as readily as the sulfates. A widely used surfactant of this type is dioctyl sodium sulfosuccinate.

Cationics—The surface activity in this group resides in the positively charged cation. These compounds have marked bactericidal properties. This makes them desirable in emulsified anti-infective products such as skin lotions and creams. The pH of an emulsion prepared with a cationic emulsifier lies in the pH 4–6 range. Since this includes the normal pH of the skin, cationic emulsifiers are advantageous in this regard also.

Cationic agents are weak emulsifiers and are generally formulated with a stabilizing or auxiliary emulsifying agent such as cetostearyl alcohol. The only group of cationic agents used extensively as emulsifying agents are the quaternary ammonium compounds. An example is cetyltrimethylammonium bromide:

$$CH_3(CH_2)_{14}CH_2N^+(CH_3)_3 \quad Br^-$$

Cationic emulsifiers should not be used in the same formulation with anionic emulsifiers as they will interact. While the incompatibility may not be immediately apparent as a precipitate, virtually all of the desired antibacterial activity will generally have been lost.

Nonionics—These undissociated surfactants find widespread use as emulsifying agents when they possess the proper balance of hydrophilic and lipophilic groups within the molecule. Their popularity is based on the fact that, unlike the anionic and cationic types, nonionic emulsifiers are not susceptible to pH changes and the presence of electrolytes. The number of nonionic agents available is legion; the most frequently used are the glyceryl esters, polyoxyethylene glycol esters and ethers, and the sorbitan fatty acid esters and their polyoxyethylene derivatives.

A glyceryl ester, such as glyceryl monostearate, is too lipophilic to serve as a good emulsifier; it is widely used as an auxiliary agent (Table XIV) and has the structure

$$CH_2OOCC_{17}H_{35}$$
$$|$$
$$CHOH$$
$$|$$
$$CH_2OH$$

Sorbitan fatty acid esters, such as sorbitan monopalmitate (Span 40, Atlas Division of ICI Americas, Inc),

[*R* is $(C_{15}H_{31})COO$]

are nonionic oil-soluble emulsifiers that promote W/O emulsions. The polyoxyethylene sorbitan fatty acid esters, such as polyoxyethylene sorbitan monopalmitate (Tween 40, Atlas Division of ICI (Americas) Inc), are hydrophilic water-soluble derivatives that favor O/W emulsions.

[Sum of w, x, y, and z is 20,
R is $(C_{15}H_{31})COO$]

Polyoxyethylene glycol esters, such as the monostearate,

$$C_{17}H_{35}COO(CH_2OCH_2)_n H$$

are widely used also.

Very frequently, the best results are obtained from blends of nonionic emulsifiers. Thus, an O/W emulsifier such as Tween 40 customarily will be used in an emulsion with a W/O emulsifier such as Span 40. When blended properly, the nonionics produce fine-textured stable emulsions.

Natural Emulsifying Agents—Of the numerous emulsifying agents derived from natural (ie, plant and animal) sources, consideration will be given only to acacia, gelatin, lecithin, and cholesterol. Many other natural materials are only sufficiently active to function as auxiliary emulsifying agents or stabilizers.

Acacia is a carbohydrate gum that is soluble in water and forms O/W emulsions. Emulsions prepared with acacia are stable over a wide pH range. Because it is a carbohydrate it is necessary to preserve acacia emulsions against microbial attack by the use of a suitable preservative. The gum can be precipitated from aqueous solution by the addition of high concentrations of electrolytes or solvents less polar than water, such as alcohol.

Gelatin, a protein, has been used for many years as an emulsifying agent. Gelatin can have two isoelectric points, depending on the method of preparation. So-called Type A gelatin, derived from an acid-treated precursor, has an isoelectric point of between pH 7 and 9. Type B gelatin, obtained from an alkali-treated precursor, has an isoelectric point of approximately pH 5. Type A gelatin acts best as an emulsifier around pH 3, where it is positively charged; on the other hand, Type B gelatin is best used around pH 8, where it is negatively charged. The question as to whether the gelatin is positively or negatively charged is fundamental to the stability of the emulsion when other charged emulsifying agents are present. In order to avoid an incompatibility, all emulsifying agents should carry the same sign. Thus, if gums (such as tragacanth, acacia, and agar) which are negatively charged are to be used with gelatin, Type B material should be used at an alkaline pH. Under these conditions the gelatin is similarly negatively charged.

Lecithin is a phospholipid which, because of its strongly hydrophilic nature, produces O/W emulsions. It is liable to microbial attack and tends to darken on storage.

Cholesterol is a major constituent of wool alcohols, obtained by the saponification and fractionation of wool fat. It is cholesterol that gives wool fat its capacity to absorb water and form a W/O emulsion.

Finely Dispersed Solids—This group of emulsifiers forms particulate films around the dispersed droplets and produces emulsions which, while coarse-grained, have considerable physical stability. It appears possible that any solid can act as an emulsifying agent of this type, provided it is reduced to a sufficiently fine powder. In practice the group of compounds used most frequently are the colloidal clays.

Several colloidal clays find application in pharmaceutical emulsions; the most frequently used are bentonite, a colloidal aluminum silicate, and Veegum (*Vanderbilt*), a colloidal magnesium aluminum silicate.

Bentonite is a white to gray, odorless, and tasteless powder that swells in the presence of water to form a translucent suspension with a pH of about 9. Depending on the sequence of mixing it is possible to prepare both O/W and W/O emulsions. When an O/W emulsion is desired, the bentonite is first dispersed in water and allowed to hydrate so as to form a magma. The oil phase is then added gradually with constant trituration. Since the aqueous phase is always in excess, the O/W emulsion type is favored. To prepare a W/O emulsion, the bentonite is first dispersed in oil; the water is then added gradually.

While Veegum is used as a solid particle emulsifying agent, it is employed most extensively as a stabilizer in cosmetic lotions and creams. Concentrations of less than 1% Veegum will stabilize an emulsion containing anionic or nonionic emulsifying agents.

Auxiliary Emulsifying Agents—Included under this heading are those compounds which are normally incapable themselves of forming stable emulsions. Their main value lies in their ability to function as thickening agents and thereby help stabilize the emulsion. Thus, tragacanth is sometimes combined with acacia to increase the consistency of the aqueous phase of an O/W emulsion. Agents in common use are listed in Table XIV.

Emulsifying Agents and Emulsion Type

For a molecule, ion, colloid, or particle to be active as an emulsifying agent, it must have some affinity for the interface between the dispersed phase and the dispersion medium. With the mono- and multilayer films the emulsifier is in solution and, therefore, must be soluble to some extent in one or both of the phases. At the same time it must not be overly soluble in either phase, otherwise it will remain in the bulk of that phase and not be adsorbed at the interface. This balanced affinity for the two phases also must be evident with finely divided solid particles used as emulsifying agents. If their affinity, as evidenced by the degree to which they are wetted, is either predominantly hydrophilic or hydrophobic, they will not function as effective wetting agents.

The great majority of the work on the relation between emulsifier and emulsion type has been concerned with surface-active agents that form interfacial monolayers. The present discussion, therefore, will concentrate on this class of agents.

Hydrophile–Lipophile Balance—As the emulsifier becomes more hydrophilic, its solubility in water increases and the formation of an O/W emulsion is favored. Conversely, W/O emulsions are favored with the more lipophilic emulsifiers. This led to the concept that the type of emulsion is related to the balance between hydrophilic and lipophilic solution tendencies of the surface-active emulsifying agent.

As described in Chapter 19, surface-active agents are *amphiphiles* in which the molecule or ion contains both hydrophilic and lipophilic portions. Griffin[20] developed a scale based on the balance between these two opposing tendencies. This so-called *HLB scale* is a numerical scale, extending from 1 to approximately 50. The more hydrophilic surfactants have high HLB numbers (in excess of 10), while surfactants with HLB numbers from 1 to 10 are considered to be lipophilic. Surfactants with a proper balance in their hydrophilic and lipophilic affinities are effective emulsifying agents since they concentrate at the oil/water interface. The relationship between HLB values and the application of the surface-active agent is shown in Table XV. Some commonly used emulsifiers and their HLB numbers are listed in Table XVI. The utility of the HLB system in rationalizing the choice of emulsifying agents when formulating an emulsion will be discussed in a later section.

Rate of Coalescence and Emulsion Type—Davies[17] indicated that the type of emulsion produced in systems prepared by shaking is controlled by the relative coalescence rates of oil droplets dispersed in the oil. Thus, when a mixture of oil and water is shaken together with an emulsifying agent, a multiple dispersion is produced initially which contains oil dispersed in water and water dispersed in oil (Fig 21-23). The type of the final emulsion which results depends on whether the water or the oil droplets coalesce more rapidly. If the O/W coalescence rate (Rate 1) is much greater than W/O coalescence rate (Rate 2), a W/O emulsion is formed since the dispersed water droplets are more stable than the dispersed oil droplets. Conversely, if Rate 2 is significantly faster than Rate 1, the final emulsion is an O/W dispersion because the oil droplets are more stable.

According to Davies, the rate at which oil globules coalesce when dispersed in water is given by the expression

Table XV—Relationship between HLB Range and Surfactant Application

HLB range	Use
0–3	Antifoaming agents
4–6	W/O emulsifying agents
7–9	Wetting agents
8–18	O/W emulsifying agents
13–15	Detergents
10–18	Solubilizing agents

Table XVI—Approximate HLB Values for a Number of Surfactants

Generic or chemical name	Trademark	HLB
Sorbitan trioleate	Span 85,[a] Arlacel 85[a]	1.8
Sorbitan tristearate	Span 65[a]	2.1
Propylene glycol monostearate (pure)		3.4
Sorbitan sesquioleate	Arlacel C[a]	3.7
Glycerol monostearate		3.8
Sorbitan monooleate	Span 80[a]	4.3
Propylene glycol monolaurate	Atlas G-917,[a] Atlas G-3851[a]	4.5
Sorbitan monostearate	Arlacel 60[a]	4.7
Glyceryl monostearate (self-emulsifying)	Aldo 28, Tegin[b]	5.5
Sorbitan monopalmitate	Span 40,[a] Arlacel 40[a]	6.7
Sorbitan monolaurate	Span 20,[a] Arlacel 20[a]	8.6
Polyoxyethylene lauryl ether	Brij 30[a]	9.5
Gelatin		9.8
Methocel 15		10.5
Polyoxyethylene monostearate	Myrj 45[a]	11.1
Polyethylene glycol 400 monostearate	S-541l[c]	11.6
Triethanolamine oleate (Trolamine)		12.0
Polyoxyethylene alkyl phenol	Igepal CA-630[d]	12.8
Tragacanth		13.2
Polyoxyethylene sorbitan monolaurate	Tween 21[a]	13.3
Polyoxyethylene castor oil	Atlas G-1794[a]	13.3
Polyoxyethylene sorbitan monooleate	Tween 80[a]	15.0
Polyoxyethylene sorbitan monopalmitate	Tween 40[a]	15.6
Polyoxyethylene sorbitan monolaurate	Tween 20[a]	16.7
Polyoxyethylene lauryl ether	Brij 35[a]	16.9
Polyoxyethylene monostearate	Myrj 52[a]	16.9
Sodium oleate		18.0
Sodium lauryl sulfate		40.0

[a] Atlas, Division of ICI Americas, Inc.
[b] Goldschmidt.
[c] Glycol.
[d] General Aniline.

$$\text{Rate 1} = C_1 e^{-W_1/RT} \quad (39)$$

The term C_1 is a collision factor which is directly proportional to the phase volume of the oil relative to the water, and is an inverse function of the viscosity of the continuous phase (water). W_1 defines an energy barrier made up of several contributing factors that must be overcome before coalescence can take place. First, it depends on the electrical potential of the dispersed oil droplets, since this affects repulsion. Second, with an O/W emulsion, the hydrated layer surrounding the polar portion of emulsifying agent must be broken down before coalescence can occur. This hydrated layer is probably around 10 Å thick with a consistency of butter. Finally, the total energy barrier depends on the fraction of the interface covered by the emulsifying agent.

Eq 40 describes the rate of coalescence of water globules dispersed in oil, namely

$$\text{Rate 2} = C_2 e^{-W_2/RT} \quad (40)$$

Here, the collision factor C_2 is a function of the water/oil phase volume ratio divided by the viscosity of the oil phase. The energy barrier W_2 is, as before, related to the fraction of the interface covered by the surface-active agent. Another contributing factor is the number of —CH$_2$— groups in the emulsifying agent; the longer the alkyl chain of the emulsifier, the greater the gap that has to be bridged if one water droplet is to combine with a second drop.

Davies[17] showed that the HLB concept is related to the distribution characteristics of the emulsifying agent between the two immiscible phases. An emulsifier with an HLB of less than 7 will be preferentially soluble in the oil phase and will favor formation of a W/O emulsion. Surfactants with an HLB value in excess of 7 will be distributed in favor of the aqueous phase and will promote O/W emulsions.

Preparation of Emulsions

Several factors must be taken into account in the successful preparation and formulation of emulsified products. Usually, the type of emulsion (ie, O/W or W/O) is specified; if not, it probably will be implied from the anticipated use of the product. The formulator's attention is focused primarily on the selection of the emulsifying agent, or agents, necessary to achieve a satisfactory product. With experience, he should be able to select an effective emulsifier with the minimum of experimentation. At the same time, he has to take steps to ensure that no incompatibilities occur between the various emulsifiers and the several components commonly present in pharmaceutical emulsions. Finally, the pharmacist must be able to prepare the product in such a way as not to prejudice his formulation. This requires not only a knowledge of the available methods of small-scale preparation, but a possession of the necessary practical skills.

Selection of Emulsifying Agents

The selection of the emulsifying agent, or agents, is of prime importance in the successful formulation of an emulsion. In addition to its emulsifying properties, the pharmacist must ensure that the material chosen is nontoxic and that the taste, odor, and chemical stability are compatible with the product. Thus, an emulsifying agent which is entirely suitable for inclusion in a skin cream may be unacceptable in the formulation of an oral preparation due to its potential toxicity. This consideration is most important when formulating intravenous emulsions.

The HLB System—With the increasing number of available emulsifiers, particularly the nonionics, the selection of emulsifiers for a product was essentially a trial-and-error procedure. Fortunately, the work of Griffin[20,21] provided a

Table XVII—Required HLB Values for Some Common Emulsion Ingredients

Substance	W/O	O/W
Acid, stearic	...	17
Alcohol, cetyl	...	13
Lanolin, anhydrous	8	15
Oil, cottonseed	...	7.5
mineral oil, light	4	10–12
mineral oil, heavy	4	10.5
Wax, beeswax	5	10–16
microcrystalline	...	9.5
paraffin	...	9

Table XVIII—Nonionic Blends having HLB Values of 10.5

Surfactant blend[a]	HLB	Required amounts (%) to give HLB = 10.5
Span 65	2.1	34.4
Tween 60	14.9	65.6
Arlacel 60	4.7	43.2
Tween 60	14.9	56.8
Span 40	6.7	57.3
Tween 40	15.6	42.7
Arlacel C	3.7	48.5
Brij 35	16.9	51.5

[a] Atlas.

logical means of selecting emulsifying agents. Griffin's method, based on the balance between the hydrophilic and lipophilic portions of the emulsifying agent, is now widely used and has come to be known as the *HLB system*. It is used most in the rational selection of combinations of nonionic emulsifiers, and we shall limit our discussion accordingly.

As shown in Table XV, if an O/W emulsion is required, the formulator should use emulsifiers with an HLB in the range of 8–18. Emulsifiers with HLB values in the range of 4–6 are given consideration when a W/O emulsion is desired. Some typical examples are given in Table XVI.

Another factor is the presence or absence of any polarity in the material being emulsified, since this will affect the polarity required in the emulsifier. Again, as a result of extensive experimentation, Griffin evolved a series of "required HLB" values; ie, the HLB value required by a particular material if it is to be emulsified effectively. Some values for oils and related materials are contained in Table XVII. Naturally, the required HLB value differs depending on whether the final emulsion is O/W or W/O.

Fundamental to the utility of the HLB concept is the fact that the HLB values are algebraically additive. Thus, by using a low HLB surfactant with one having a high HLB it is possible to prepare blends having HLB values intermediate between those of the two individual emulsifiers. Naturally, one should not use emulsifiers that are incompatible. The following formula should serve as an example.

O/W Emulsion

Liquid petrolatum (Required HLB 10.5) .... 50 g
Emulsifying agents .... 5 g
    Span 80 (HLB 4.3)
    Tween 80 (HLB 15.0)
Water, qs .... 100 g

By simple algebra it can be shown that 4.5 parts by weight of Span 80 blended with 6.2 parts by weight of Tween 80 will result in a mixed emulsifying agent having the required HLB of 10.5. Since the formula calls for 5 g, the required weights are 2.1 g Span 80 and 2.9 g Tween 80. The oil-soluble Span is dissolved in the oil and heated to 75°; the water-soluble Tween is added to the aqueous phase which is heated to 70°. At this point the oil phase is mixed with the aqueous phase and the whole stirred continuously until cool.

The formulator is not restricted to Span 80 and Tween 80 to produce a blend with an HLB of 10.5. Table XVIII shows the various proportions required, using four other pairs of emulsifying agents, to form a blend of HLB 10.5. When carrying out preliminary investigations with a particular material to be emulsified, it is advisable to try several pairs of emulsifying agents. Based on an evaluation of the emulsions produced, it becomes possible to choose the best combination.

Occasionally, the required HLB of the oil may not be known, in which case it becomes necessary to determine this parameter. Various blends are prepared to give a wide range of HLB mixtures and emulsions are prepared in a standard-ized manner. The HLB of the blend used to emulsify the best product, selected on the basis of physical stability, is taken to be the required HLB of the oil. The experiment should be repeated using another combination of emulsifiers to confirm the value of the required HLB of the oil to within, say, ±1 HLB unit.

There are methods for finding the HLB value of a new surface-active agent. Griffin[21] developed simple equations which can be used to obtain an estimate with certain compounds. It has been shown that the ability of a compound to spread at a surface is related to its HLB. In another approach a linear relation between HLB and the logarithm of the dielectric constant for a number of nonionic surfactants has been observed. An interesting approach has been developed by Davies[17] and is related to his studies on the relative rates of coalescence of O/W and W/O emulsions (page 323). According to Davies, hydrophilic groups on the surfactant molecule make a positive contribution to the HLB number, whereas lipophilic groups exert a negative effect. Davies calculated these contributions and termed them HLB Group Numbers (Table XIX). Provided the molecular structure of the surfactant is known, one simply adds the various group numbers in accordance with the following formula:

$$\text{HLB} = \Sigma(\text{hydrophilic group numbers}) -$$
$$m(\text{group number}/-CH_2-\text{ group}) + 7$$

where m is the number of $-CH_2-$ groups present in the surfactant. Poor agreement is found between the HLB values calculated in this manner and the experimental values obtained by Griffin.

Later, Davies and Rideal[22] attempted to relate HLB to the C_{water}/C_{oil} partition coefficient and found good agreement for a series of sorbitan surfactants. Schott[23] showed, however,

Table XIX—HLB Group Numbers[22]

	Group number
Hydrophilic groups	
$-SO_4^-Na^+$	38.7
$-COO^-K^+$	21.1
$-COO^-Na^+$	19.1
N (tertiary amine)	9.4
Ester (sorbitan ring)	6.8
Ester (free)	2.4
$-COOH$	2.1
Hydroxyl (free)	1.9
$-O-$	1.3
Hydroxyl (sorbitan ring)	0.5
Lipophilic groups	
$-CH-$	
$-CH_2-$	
CH_3-	−0.475
$=CH-$	
Derived groups	
$-(CH_2-CH_2-O)-$	+0.33
$-(CH_2-CH_2-CH_2-O)-$	−0.15

that the method does not apply to polyoxyethylated octyl-phenol surfactants. Schott concluded that "so far, the search for a universal correlation between HLB and another property of the surfactant which could be determined more readily than HLB has not been successful." Lowenthal[24] carried out a statistical multiregression analysis of HLB for a series of polyoxyethylene polyoxypropylene surfactants. He obtained an equation describing the relationship between HLB, percent polyoxyethylene, and the molecular weight of the polyoxy-propylene part of the molecule.

The observant reader will have already realized that the HLB system gives no information as to the *amount* of emul-sifier required. Having once determined the correct blend, the formulator must prepare another series of emulsions, all at the same HLB, but containing increasing concentrations of the emulsifier blend. Usually, the minimum concentration giving the desired degree of physical stability is chosen.

Mixed Emulsifying Agents—Emulsifying agents are frequently used in combination since a better emulsion is usually obtained. This enhancement may be due to several reasons, one or more of which may be operative in any one system. Thus, the use of a blend or mixture of emulsifiers may (1) produce the required hydrophile–lipophile balance in the emulsifier, (2) enhance the stability and cohesiveness of the interfacial film, and (3) affect the consistency and feel of the product.

The first point has been considered in detail in the previous discussion of the HLB system.

With regard to the second point, Schulman and Cockbain in 1940 showed that combinations of certain amphiphiles formed stable films at the air/water interface. It was postu-lated that the complex formed by these two materials (one, oil-soluble; the other, water-soluble) at the air/water interface was also present at the O/W interface. This interfacial complex was held to be responsible for the improved stability. For example, sodium cetyl sulfate, a moderately good O/W emulsifier, and elaidyl alcohol or cholesterol, both stabilizers for W/O emulsions, show evidence of an interaction at the air/water interface. Furthermore, an O/W emulsion prepared with sodium cetyl sulfate and elaidyl alcohol is much more stable than an emulsion prepared with sodium cetyl sulfate alone.

Elaidyl alcohol is the *trans* isomer. When oleyl alcohol, the *cis* isomer, is used with sodium cetyl sulfate, there is no evi-dence of complex formation at the air/water interface. Sig-nificantly, this combination does not produce a stable O/W emulsion either. Such a finding strongly suggests that a high degree of molecular alignment is necessary at the O/W in-terface to form a stable emulsion.

Finally, some materials are added primarily to increase the consistency of the emulsion. This may be done to increase stability or improve emolliency and feel. Tragacanth is fre-quently added to thicken the external phase of emulsions prepared with acacia. Cetyl alcohol, stearic acid, and beeswax are also added to formulations to improve the consistency of the oil phase.

When using combinations of emulsifiers, care must be taken to ensure their compatibility, as charged emulsifying agents of opposite sign are likely to interact and coagulate when mixed.

Small-Scale Preparation

Traditionally, emulsions have been prepared by the phar-macist using a mortar and pestle. Today, this tool is being replaced by the use of electric mixers and hand homogenizers which, rightly so, are recognized now as normal equipment in a contemporary pharmacy.

Mortar and Pestle—This approach is invariably used only for those emulsions that are stabilized by the presence of a multimolecular film (eg, acacia, tragacanth, agar, chondrus) at the interface. There are two basic methods for preparing emulsions with the mortar and pestle. These are the *Wet Gum* (or so-called *English*) *Method* and the *Dry Gum* (or so-called *Continental*) *Method*.

The Wet Gum Method—In this method the emulsifying agent is placed in the mortar and dispersed in water to form a mucilage. The oil is added in small amounts with contin-uous trituration, each portion of the oil being emulsified before adding the next increment. Acacia is the most frequently used emulsifying agent when preparing emulsions with the mortar and pestle. When emulsifying a fixed oil, the optimum ratio of oil:water:acacia to prepare the initial emulsion is 4:2:1. Thus, the preparation of 60 mL of a 40% cod liver oil emulsion requires the following:

Cod liver oil	24 g
Acacia	6 g
Water, qs	60 mL

The acacia mucilage is formed by adding 12 mL of water to the 6 g of acacia in the mortar and triturating. The 24 g of oil is added in increments of 1–2 g and dispersed. The product at this stage is known as the *primary emulsion*, or *nucleus*. The primary emulsion should be triturated for at least 5 min, after which sufficient water is added to produce a final volume of 60 mL.

The Dry Gum Method—In this method, preferred by most pharmacists, the gum is added to the oil, rather than the water as with the wet gum method. Again, the approach is to pre-pare a primary emulsion from which the final product can be obtained by dilution with the continuous phase. If the emulsifier is acacia and a fixed oil is to be emulsified, the ratio of oil:water:gum is again 4:2:1.

Provided dispersion of the acacia in the oil is adequate, the dry gum method can almost be guaranteed to produce an ac-ceptable emulsion. Because there is no incremental addition of one of the components, the preparation of an emulsion by this method is rapid.

With both methods the oil:water:gum ratio may vary, depending on the type of oil to be emulsified and the emulsi-fying agent used. The usual ratios for tragacanth and acacia are shown in Table XX.

The preparation of emulsions by both the wet and dry gum methods can be carried out in a bottle rather than a mortar and pestle.

Other Methods—An increasing number of emulsions are being formulated with synthetic emulsifying agents, especially of the nonionic type. The components in such a formulation are separated into those that are oil-soluble and those that are water-soluble. These are dissolved in their respective solvents by heating to about 70–75°. When solution is complete, the two phases are mixed and the product is stirred until cool. This method, which requires nothing more than two beakers, a thermometer, and a source of heat, is necessarily used in the preparation of emulsions containing waxes and other high-melting-point materials that must be melted before they can

Table XX—Usual Ratios of Oil, Water, and Gum Used to Produce Emulsions

System	Acacia	Tragacanth
Fixed oils (excluding liquid petrolatum and linseed oil)	4	40
Water	2	20
Gum	1	1
Volatile oils, plus liquid petrolatum and linseed oil	2–3	20–30
Water	2	20
Gum	1	1

be dispersed in the emulsion. The relatively simple methodology involved in the use of synthetic surfactant-type emulsifiers is one factor which has led to their widespread use in emulsion preparation. This, in turn, has led to a decline in the use of the natural emulsifying agents.

Hand homogenizers and blenders are being used more widely by practicing pharmacists for preparing emulsions. With hand homogenizers an initial rough emulsion is formed by trituration in a mortar or shaking in a bottle. The rough emulsion is then passed several times through the homogenizer. A reduction in particle size is achieved as the material is forced through a narrow aperture under pressure. A satisfactory product invariably results from the use of a hand homogenizer and overcomes any deficiencies in technique. Should the homogenizer fail to produce an adequate product, the formulation, rather than the technique, should be suspected.

For a discussion of the techniques and equipment used in the large scale manufacture of emulsions, see Chapter 84.

Stability of Emulsions

There are several criteria which must be met in a well-formulated emulsion. Probably the most important and most readily apparent requirement is that the emulsion possess adequate physical stability; without this, any emulsion soon will revert back to two separate bulk phases. In addition, if the emulsified product is to have some antimicrobial activity (eg, a medicated lotion), care must be taken to ensure that the formulation possesses the required degree of activity. Frequently, a compound exhibits a lower antimicrobial activity in an emulsion than, say, in a solution. Generally, this is because of partitioning effects between the oil and water phases, which cause a lowering of the "effective" concentration of the active agent. Partitioning has also to be taken into account when considering preservatives to prevent microbiological spoilage of emulsions. Finally, the chemical stability of the various components of the emulsion should receive some attention, since such materials may be more prone to degradation in the emulsified state than when they exist as a bulk phase.

In the present discussion, detailed consideration will be limited to the question of physical stability. Reviews of this topic have been published by Garrett[25] and Kitchener and Mussellwhite.[26] For information on the effect that emulsification can have on the biologic activity and chemical stability of materials in emulsions, see Wedderburn,[27] Burt,[28] and Swarbrick.[29]

The physical stability of an emulsion depends on many factors, some of which have been discussed. Thus, the various properties of an emulsifying agent (see page 319) are all considered desirable because each makes a contribution to the physical stability of the emulsion.

The three major phenomena associated with physical stability are (1) the upward or downward movement of dispersed droplets relative to the continuous phase, termed *creaming* or *sedimentation*, respectively; (2) the aggregation and possible coalescence of the dispersed droplets to reform the separate, bulk phases; and (3) inversion, in which an O/W emulsion inverts to become a W/O emulsion, and *vice versa*.

Creaming and Sedimentation—Creaming is the upward movement of dispersed droplets relative to the continuous phase, while sedimentation, the reverse process, is the downward movement of particles. In any emulsion one process or the other takes place, depending on the densities of the disperse and continuous phases. This is undesirable in a pharmaceutical product where homogeneity is essential for the administration of the correct and uniform dose. Furthermore, creaming, or sedimentation, brings the particles closer together and may facilitate the more serious problem of coalescence.

The rate at which a spherical droplet or particle sediments in a liquid is governed by Stokes' law (Eq 33). While other equations have been developed for bulk systems, Stokes' equation is still useful since it points out the factors that influence the rate of sedimentation or creaming. These are the diameter of the suspended droplets, the viscosity of the suspending medium, and the difference in densities between the dispersed phase and the dispersion medium.

Usually, only the use of the first two factors is feasible in affecting creaming or sedimentation, although a few successful attempts have been made to equalize the densities of the oil and aqueous phases, to reduce the rate of movement to zero. Reduction of particle size contributes greatly towards overcoming or minimizing creaming, since the rate of movement is a square-root function of the particle diameter. There are, however, technical difficulties in reducing the diameter of droplets to below about 0.1 μm. The most frequently used approach is to raise the viscosity of the continuous phase, although this can be done only to the extent that the emulsion still can be removed readily from its container and spread or administered conveniently.

Aggregation and Coalescence—Even though creaming and sedimentation are undesirable, they do not necessarily result in the breakdown of the emulsion, since the dispersed droplets retain their individuality. Furthermore, the droplets can be redispersed with mild agitation. More serious to the stability of an emulsion are the processes of aggregation and coalescence. In aggregation (flocculation) the dispersed droplets come together but do not fuse. Coalescence, the complete fusion of droplets, leads to a decrease in the number of droplets and the ultimate separation of the two immiscible phases. Aggregation precedes coalescence in emulsions; however, coalescence does not necessarily follow from aggregation. Aggregation is, to some extent, reversible. While not as serious as coalescence, it will accelerate creaming or sedimentation, since the aggregate behaves as a single drop.

While aggregation is related to the electrical potential on the droplets, coalescence depends on the structural properties of the interfacial film. In an emulsion stabilized with surfactant-type emulsifiers forming monomolecular films, coalescence is opposed by the elasticity and cohesiveness of the films sandwiched between the two droplets. In spite of the fact that two droplets may be touching, they will not fuse until the interposed films thin out and eventually rupture. Multilayer and solid-particle films confer on the emulsion a high degree of resistance to coalescence, due to their mechanical strength.

Particle-size analysis can reveal the tendency of an emulsion to aggregate and coalesce long before any visible signs of instability are apparent. The methods available have been reviewed by Groves and Freshwater.[30]

Inversion—An emulsion is said to invert when it changes from an O/W to a W/O emulsion, or *vice versa*. Inversion sometimes can be brought about by the addition of an electrolyte or by changing the phase–volume ratio. For example, an O/W emulsion having sodium stearate as the emulsifier can be inverted by the addition of calcium chloride, because the calcium stearate formed is a lipophilic emulsifier and favors the formation of a W/O product.

Inversion often can be seen when an emulsion, prepared by heating and mixing the two phases, is being cooled. This takes place presumably because of the temperature-dependent changes in the solubilities of the emulsifying agents.

Little quantitative work has been carried out on the process of inversion; nevertheless, it would appear that the effect can be minimized by using the proper emulsifying agent in an adequate concentration. Wherever possible, the volume of the dispersed phase should not exceed 50% of the total volume of the emulsion.

Bioavailability from Coarse Dispersions

In recent years, considerable interest has focused on the ability of a dosage form to release drug following administration to the patient. Both the rate and extent of release are important. Ideally, the extent of release should approach 100%, while the rate of release should reflect the desired properties of the dosage form. For example, with products designed to have a rapid onset of activity, the release of drug should be immediate. With a long-acting product, the release should take place over several hours, or days, depending on the type of product used. The rate and extent of drug release should be reproducible from batch to batch of the product, and should not change during shelf life.

The principles on which biopharmaceutics is based are dealt with in some detail in Chapters 37, 38 and 39. While most published work in this area has been concerned with the bioavailability of solid dosage forms administered by the oral route, the rate and extent of release from both suspensions and emulsions is important and so will be considered in some detail.

Bioavailability from Suspensions—On theoretical grounds, one would expect orally administered dispersion-type dosage forms to be at least as bioavailable as the same drug formulated as a tablet or capsule. Frequently suspensions may be expected to demonstrate improved bioavailability. This is because the suspension already contains discrete drug particles, whereas tablet dosage forms must invariably undergo disintegration in order to maximize the necessary dissolution process. Frequently, antacid suspensions are perceived as being more rapid in action and therefore more effective than an equivalent dose in the form of tablets. Bates *et al.*[31] observed that a suspension of salicylamide was more rapidly bioavailable, at least during the first hour following administration, than two different tablet forms of the drug; these workers were also able to demonstrate a correlation between the initial *in vitro* dissolution rates for the several dosage forms studied and the initial rates of *in vivo* absorption. A similar argument can be developed for hard gelatin capsules, where the shell must rupture or dissolve before drug particles are released and can begin the dissolution process. Such was observed by Antal and co-workers[32] in a study of the bioavailability of several doxycycline products, including a suspension and hard gelatin capsules. Meyer *et al.*[33] studied sulfadiazine bioavailability in 16 male volunteers, using the drug in solution, suspension and two different tablets to determine whether there was any statistical difference in the rate and level of absorption. It was concluded that the suspension showed neither better nor worse bioavailability characteristics, and was equivalent to the solution and tablet dosage forms. Sansom and coworkers[34] found mean plasma phenytoin levels higher after the administration of a suspension than when an equivalent dose was given as either tablets or capsules. It was suggested that this might have been due to the suspension having a smaller particle size.

In common with other products in which the drug is present in the form of solid particles, the rate of dissolution and thus potentially the bioavailability of the drug in a suspension can be affected by such factors as particle size and shape, surface characteristics, and polymorphism. Strum *et al.*[35] conducted a comparative bioavailability study involving two commercial brands of sulfamethiazole suspension (product A and product B). Following administration of the products to 12 normal subjects and taking blood samples at predetermined times over a period of 10 hours, the workers found no statistically significant difference in the extent of drug absorption from the two suspensions. The absorption rate, however, differed, and from *in vitro* studies it was concluded that product A dissolved faster than product B and that the former contained more particles of smaller size than the latter, differences that may be responsible for the more rapid dissolution of particles in product A. Product A also provided higher serum levels in *in vivo* tests half an hour after administration. The results showed that the rate of absorption of sulfamethiazole from a suspension depended on the rate of dissolution of the suspended particles, which in turn was related to particle size. Previous studies[36,37] have shown the need to determine the dissolution rate of suspensions in order to gain information as to the bioavailability of drugs from this type of dosage form.

The viscosity of the vehicle used to suspend the particles has been found to have an effect on the rate of absorption of nitrofurantoin but not the total bioavailability. Thus Soci and Parrott were able to maintain a clinically acceptable urinary nitrofurantoin concentration for an additional two hours by increasing the viscosity of the vehicle[38].

Bioavailability from Emulsions—There are indications that improved bioavailability may result when a poorly absorbed drug is formulated as an orally administered emulsion. However, little study appears to have been made in direct comparison of emulsions and other dosage forms such as suspensions, tablets, and capsules; thus it is not possible to draw unequivocal conclusions as to advantages of emulsions. If a drug with low aqueous solubility can be formulated so as to be in solution in the oil phase of an emulsion, its bioavailability may be enhanced. It must be recognized, however, that the drug in such a system has several barriers to pass before it arrives at the mucosal surface of the gastrointestinal tract. For example, with an oil-in-water emulsion, the drug must diffuse through the oil globule and then pass across the oil/water interface. This may be a difficult process, depending on the characteristics of the interfacial film formed by the emulsifying agent. In spite of this potential drawback, Wagner and co-workers[39] found that indoxole, a nonsteroidal anti-inflammatory agent, was significantly more bioavailable in an oil-in-water emulsion than in either a suspension or a hard gelatin capsule. Bates and Sequeira[40] found significant increases in maximum plasma levels and total bioavailability of micronized griseofulvin when formulated in a corn oil/water emulsion. In this case, however, the enhanced effect was not due to emulsification of the drug in the oil phase *per se* but more probably because of the linoleic and oleic acids present having a specifical effect on gastrointestinal motility.

References

1. Fox HF, Zisman WA, *et al*: *J Phys Chem 59:* 1097, 1955.
2. Roseman TJ: PhD Thesis, University of Michigan, 1967.
3. Napper DH: *Ind Eng Chem PRD 9:* 467, 1970.
4. Ottewill RH, Walker T: *Kolloid Zeit Zeit Polymere 227:* 108, 1968.
5. Napper DH, Netschey A: *J Coll Interface Sci 37:* 528, 1971.
6. Fleer GJ, *et al*: *J Kolloid Zeit Zeit Polymere 250:* 689, 1972.
7. Lyklema J: *Adv Coll Interface Sci 2:* 65, 1968.
8. Mehta SC, *et al*: Unpublished data. Also see *J Pharm Sci 59:* 633, 1970.
9. Hiestand EN: *J Pharm Sci 53:* 1, 1964.
10. Haines BA, Martin A: *J Pharm Sci 50:* 228, 753, 756, 1961.
11. Matthews BA, Rhodes CT: *J Pharm Pharmacol 20* Suppl: 204S, 1968.
12. Matthews BA, Rhodes CT: *J Pharm Sci 57:* 569, 1968.
13. Matthews BA, Rhodes CT: *J Pharm Sci 59:* 521, 1970.
14. Schneider W, *et al*: *Am J Pharm Ed 42:* 280, 1978.
15. Swarbrick J: In *American Pharmacy*, 7th ed, Chap 7, Lippincott, Philadelphia, 1974.
16. Tingstad J, *et al*: *J Pharm Sci 62:* 1361, 1973.
17. Davies JT: *Proc Intern Congr Surface Activity*, 2nd, London, 1957, page 426.

18. Sherman P: In *Emulsion Science*, Chap 4, Academic, New York, 1968.
19. Rogers JA: *Cosmet Toilet 93:* 49, July, 1978.
20. Griffin WC: *J Soc Cos Chem 1:* 311, 1949.
21. Griffin WC: *J Soc Cos Chem 5:* 249, 1954.
22. Davies JT, Rideal EK: *Interfacial Phenomena*, Chap 8, Academic, New York, 1961. Davies JT: *Proc Intern Congr Surface Activity*, 2nd, London, 1957, p 426.
23. Schott J: *J Pharm Sci 60:* 649, 1971.
24. Lowenthal W: *J Pharm Sci 57:* 514, 1968.
25. Garrett ER: *J Pharm Sci 54:* 1557, 1965.
26. Kitchener JA, Mussellwhite PR: In *Emulsion Science*, Chap 2, Academic, New York, 1968.
27. Wedderburn DL: In *Advances in Pharmaceutical Sciences*, vol. 1, 195–268, Academic, London, 1964.
28. Burt BW: *J Soc Cosm Chem 16:* 465, 1965.
29. Swarbrick J: *J Soc Cosm Chem 19:* 187, 1968.
30. Groves MJ, Freshwater DC: *J Pharm Sci 57:* 1273, 1968.
31. Bates TR, *et al: J Pharm Sci 58:* 1468, 1969.
32. Antal EJ, *et al: J Pharm Sci 64:* 2015, 1975.
33. Meyer MC, *et al: J Pharm Sci 67:* 1659, 1978.
34. Sansom LN, *et al: Med J Aust* 1975(2): 593.
35. Strum JD, *et al: J Pharm Sci 67:* 1659, 1978.
36. Bates TR, *et al: J Pharm Sci 62:* 2057, 1973.
37. Howard SA, *et al: J Pharm Sci 66:* 557, 1977.
38. Soci MM, Parrott EL: *J Pharm Sci 69:* 403, 1980.
39. Wagner JG, *et al: Clin Pharmacol Ther 7:* 610, 1966.
40. Bates TR, Sequeira JA: *J Pharm Sci 64:* 793, 1975.

Bibliography

Davies JT, Rideal EK: *Interfacial Phenomena*, Academic, New York, 1963.
Kruyt HR: *Colloid Science*, vols I and II, Elsevier, New York, 1949, 1952.
Osipow LI: *Surface Chemistry*, Reinhold, New York, 1962.
Mysels KJ: *Introduction to Colloid Chemistry*, Interscience, New York, 1959.
Ho NFH: PhD Thesis, University of Michigan, Ann Arbor, 1967.
Hiemenz PC: *Principles of Colloidal and Surface Chemistry*, Marcel Dekker, New York, 1977.
Matijevic E, ed: *Surface and Colloid Science*, vols 1–4, Wiley, New York, 1971.
Cadle RD: *Particle Size*, Reinhold, New York, 1965.
Herdan G: *Small Particle Statistics*, 2nd ed, Academic, New York, 1960.
Parfitt G: *Dispersion of Powders in Liquids*, Applied Science, 1973.
Adamson AW: *Physical Chemistry of Surfaces*, 4th ed, Wiley-Interscience, New York, 1980.
Fowkes FM, ed: *Hydrophobic Surfaces*, Academic, New York, 1969.
Verwey EJW, Overbeek JThG: *Theory of Stability of Lyophilic Colloids*, Elsevier, New York, 1948.
Emulsion Technology, Chemical Publ Co, Brooklyn, 1946.
Sherman P: *Rheology of Emulsions*, Macmillan, New York, 1963.
Becher P: *Emulsions: Theory and Practice*, 2nd ed, Reinhold, New York, 1965.
Vold RD, Vold MJ, *Colloid and Interface Chemistry*, Addison-Wesley, Reading, Mass, 1983.

CHAPTER 22

Rheology

Hans Schott, PhD

Professor of Pharmaceutics, School of Pharmacy
Temple University
Philadelphia, PA 19140

Rheology is the branch of physics which deals with deformation and flow of matter. It is important in many fields. To the physiologist, rheology governs the circulation of blood and lymph through capillaries and large vessels, flow of mucus, bending of bones, stretching of cartilage, contraction of muscles, and spreading of the gluteal region when sitting down. To the physician, the fluidity of solutions to be injected with hypodermic syringes or infused intravenously, flexibility of tubing used in catheters, extensibility of gut, action of fecal softeners, and strength of sutures and ligatures are important rheological properties. To the pharmacist, rheology is important in the flow of emulsions through colloid mills and pumps, working of ointments on slabs or roller mills, trituration of suspensions in mortar and pestle, and mechanical properties of glass or plastic containers and of rubber closures. To the consumer, rheology comes into play when he squeezes toothpaste from a collapsible tube, spreads lotion on his skin or butter on a slice of bread or paint on a surface, writes with a pen, sprays liquids from atomizers or aerosol cans, chews food, hits balls with racket, paddle, bat, or club, jumps on a trampoline or off a diving board, swims, and lies down in bed and compresses the stuffing and metal springs in the mattress.

From the rheological viewpoint, systems are solid if they preserve shape and volume, liquid if they preserve their volume, and gaseous if neither shape nor volume remains constant when forces are applied to them. Of the three systems, the transport properties of gases, described by the kinetic theory of gases, are best understood, but they are of minor importance in pharmacy.

Ideal solids are deformed when stresses are applied to them but regain their original shape completely when the stresses are released. The ability to restore their shape is called elasticity. Similarly, liquids can be compressed to somewhat smaller volumes, but assume their original volumes when the pressure is released. The dividing line between solids and liquids is not clear-cut. As explained below, some systems which behave as elastic solids when subjected to small stresses and/or to moderate stresses of short duration will undergo permanent deformation, resembling very viscous liquids, if the stresses are larger and/or applied for longer periods of time.

Fundamentals

The concepts and quantitative aspects of rheology are described in this section.

Elastic Solids

When a ball (rubber ball, steel ball bearing, or baseball) is dropped on the floor or hit with a bat, it is temporarily flattened. After the impact, the original spherical shape is restored. When we pull on a rubber band, steel spring, or muscle, they stretch or extend. On release, they resume their original length. This behavior, characteristic of solids, is called elasticity.

The force F producing the deformation, or the equal and opposite restoring force in the deformed solid, divided by the area A over which F is applied, is called stress. In the stretching process, A is the cross-sectional area of the filaments, and the deformation is said to be in tension. Other modes of deformation are by bending or flexure, torsion, compression, and shear. The deformation or strain of the stretched filaments, or their elongation, is the difference between their length while under tension, L_s, and their original length, L_o, which is equal to the length after the stress is released, expressed as a fraction of the original length, namely, $(L_s - L_o)/L_o$.

For an ideal elastic solid, the stress is directly proportional to the strain. In tension:

$$\frac{F}{A} = E\left(\frac{L_s - L_o}{L_o}\right) \qquad (1)$$

This relationship, called *Hooke's law*, is obeyed by real solids at moderate stresses and strains sustained for short periods of time. The proportionality constant E, called the *modulus of elasticity* or *Young's modulus*, is a measure of the stiffness, hardness, or resistance to elongation. There is also a modulus of shear or rigidity and a compression or bulk modulus. *Tensile compliance* is the reciprocal of Young's modulus, or the ratio of strain to stress.

In the CGS system, the units of stress are dyne/cm^2 or, since force = mass × acceleration, (g cm/sec^2)/cm^2 = g/cm sec^2. Since strain is dimensionless, Young's modulus has the same dimensions as stress. Modulus values for solids important in appliances, as packaging materials, and in physiology are listed in Table I.

Fig 22-1 shows representative stress-strain curves in tension, also called load-elongation curves. The cross-sectional area of a fiber or cylinder becomes smaller as the solid is

Table I—Values of Modulus of Elasticity of Representative Solids at Room Temperature

Material	Young's modulus, dyne/cm^2
Steel	2.2×10^{12}
Glass	$6 \ \times 10^{11}$
Silk, viscose rayon	1.5×10^{11}
Polystyrene	3.4×10^{10}
Polyethylene (low density)	2.4×10^{9}
Rubber (vulcanized)	$2 \ \times 10^{7}$
Tooth enamel	4.7×10^{11}
Bone	2.2×10^{11}
Tendon	1.3×10^{9}
Muscle	$6 \ \times 10^{6}$
Soft tissue	7.5×10^{4}
Gelatin gels	
10% solids	2.4×10^{5}
20% solids	1.0×10^{6}
30% solids	1.5×10^{6}

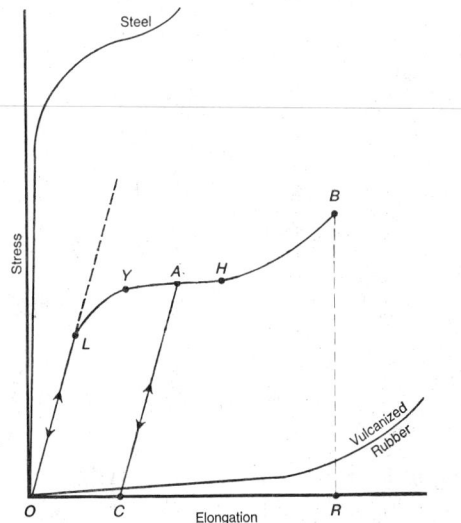

Fig 22-1. Stress-strain curves in tension. Loads or tensile stresses are corrected for actual cross-sectional areas.

stretched. Therefore, to calculate the actual or true tensile stresses, the forces are divided by $A_s = A_o L_o / L_s$; subscripts o designate the original dimensions and s those at each appropriate elongation. Stress-strain curves are often plotted with the strain or extension, the dependent variable, on the abscissa[1-5] while consistency or flow curves (see below) are usually plotted with stress, the independent variable, on the abscissa.[1,2,5-8] The practice followed here is to plot stress on the ordinate for both stress-strain and consistency[5,9] curves, in order to make modulus and viscosity, respectively, the slopes rather than the reciprocal slopes of these curves.

The characteristic portions in the representative stress-strain curve $OLYAHB$ in Fig 22-1 are as follows.[2-4] Hooke's law of proportionality between stress and strain is obeyed throughout the linear portion OL. The elastic modulus of the solid is the slope of OL or the tangent of the angle LOC. The material behaves elastically up to the yield point Y, where the stress is called *yield stress*. When stresses below the yield stress are applied to the sample and then released, it stretches and contracts along the same curve OLY.

Beyond Y, the material behaves as a plastic rather than as an elastic solid. Along the (nearly) horizontal portion YAH, the material is ductile: it flows or creeps under practically constant stress like a viscous liquid. If the stress is released at A, the sample retracts along AC. The nonrecoverable deformation OC is called *permanent set*. Many materials undergoing such "cold flow" are strengthened by some change in structure, causing an upturn HB in the stress-strain curve. This is called work (or strain) hardening. It may result from the elimination of flaws,[1] from a reduction in crystal size as in the case of metals,[2] or from reversible crystallization on stretching as in the case of homopolymer elastomers.[4]

At B, the sample ruptures; R is the elongation at (or: to) break or the ultimate elongation, and the stress corresponding to B is the ultimate strength or tensile strength. These values, as well as the load-elongation curve beyond Y, depend on the rate at which the sample is stretched.

The area $OLYAHBRCO$ under the stress-strain curve is the energy or work required to break or rupture the material. It measures its toughness or brittleness. Glass is hard because of its high elastic modulus. Owing to the absence of a yield point and to a very low elongation to break, it is brittle as opposed to steel, which undergoes work hardening, has a high elongation to break, and is tough. Plastics are medium hard or soft. Those which exhibit comparatively high elongations at break, like polyethylene but unlike polystyrene, are tough.

Vulcanized rubbers are tough even though they are soft (low elastic modulus) because their elongation to break is very high, 600 to 800%.

Liquids

Compressive stresses are the only kind of stresses which liquids can support and from which they recover. All other stresses produce infinite deformation if applied long enough, so that the elastic and shear moduli of liquids are zero.

Cutting a sheet of paper or of metal with scissors or shears, and the deformation before severance, is called *shear*. Pushing a deck of playing cards sideways is also deformation in shear. In Fig 22-2, the upper of the two metal plates held together by a rivet is pulled by a tangential force F while the lower plate is held stationary. *Shear stress* τ is F divided by the cross-sectional area A of the rivet parallel to the force. The *shear strain* or deformation in shear γ is the displacement y divided by the height x of the sheared or deformed portion of the rivet, as shown in Fig 22-2C. It equals the tangent of the displacement angle θ which, at low θ values, is approximately equal to θ expressed in radians.

$$\gamma = \frac{y}{x} = \tan \theta \cong \theta \qquad (2)$$

One can imagine a liquid contained between two very large, parallel plates as being divided into a stack of very thin, parallel layers much like a deck of cards, as shown in Fig 22-3. Shear is applied to the liquid by pulling or pushing the top plate with a constant force F while holding the bottom plate stationary. The velocities of the liquid layers are represented by the arrows in Fig 22-3, whose length measures the magnitude of the velocities and which point in the direction of flow (y-direction). The top liquid layer, in contact with the moving plate, adheres to it and moves with the same velocity as the plate. The second layer, adjacent to the top one, is dragged along by friction, but its velocity is reduced somewhat by the resistance of the layers beneath it. Each layer is pulled forward by the layer moving above it but is held back by the layer underneath it, over which it moves and which it drags along. The farther the liquid layers are from the moving plate, the smaller their velocities. The bottom layer adheres to the stationary plate and has zero velocity. Thus, the velocity of the liquid layers increases in the direction x perpendicular to the direction of flow y.

In due time, all layers except the bottom one undergo infinite deformation. What distinguishes one liquid from an-

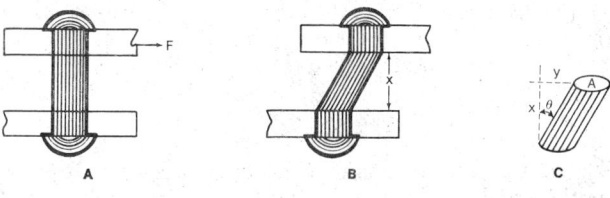

Fig 22-2. Effect of shear on a rivet.

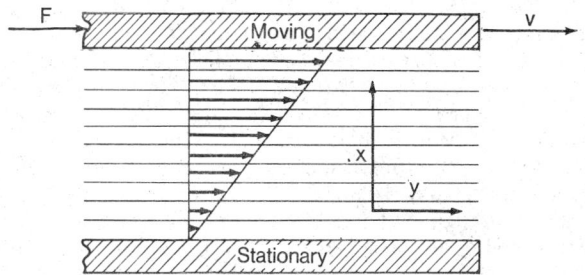

Fig 22-3. Laminar flow of a liquid contained between two parallel plates.

**Table II—Approximate Shear Rate Levels for
Pharmaceutical Operations**

Operation	Rate of shear, sec^{-1}
Pouring from a bottle	50
Spreading lotion on skin, levigating ointment on slab with spatula	400–1000
Injecting through hypodermic syringe	4000
Dispensing nasal spray from plastic squeeze bottle	20,000
Processing in colloid mill	10^5–10^6

other is the rate at which the deformation increases with time. This is called *rate of* (deformation in) *shear*. It is represented by $\dot{\gamma}$, which is the derivative of γ with respect to time t. An equivalent definition for $\dot{\gamma}$ is as the *velocity gradient*, ie, the rate at which the velocity v changes with the distance x perpendicular to the direction of flow.

$$\dot{\gamma} = \frac{d\gamma}{dt} = \frac{dv}{dx} \qquad (3)$$

The rate of shear or velocity gradient $\dot{\gamma}$ indicates how fast the liquid flows when a shear stress is applied to it. Its unit according to both definitions is sec^{-1}, since γ is dimensionless, velocity is expressed in cm/sec, and x in cm.

Eq 3 is illustrated by calculating the rate of shear when lotion is rubbed into the skin. If the hand (moving surface) slides across the skin (stationary surface) with a velocity $v = 45$ cm/sec, and if the thickness of the lotion film is $x = 0.05$ cm, the rate of shear is $\dot{\gamma} = (45 \text{ cm/sec})/0.05 \text{ cm} = 900 \text{ sec}^{-1}$. For a given force and a constant viscosity, the rate of shear is uniform throughout the layer of lotion. Characteristic $\dot{\gamma}$ values for pharmacy-related operations are listed in Table II. Even for a given operation, the shear rate can vary within wide limits, depending on the dimensions of the equipment and the speed at which it is operated.

The flow of liquids by parallel layers moving past each other and dragging adjacent layers along is called *laminar* or *streamline flow*. At higher velocities and/or if the plates have rough surfaces, eddies or swirls develop. This regimen is called *turbulent flow;* it is described quantitatively in chemical engineering texts.

Newtonian Flow—Newton[2] observed that the shear stress τ, or force F divided by the area A of the plate, is directly proportional to the rate of shear or velocity gradient. The proportionality constant is called (coefficient of) *viscosity*, η, while its reciprocal is called *fluidity*.

$$\tau = \frac{F}{A} = \eta\dot{\gamma} \qquad (4)$$

Viscosity or internal friction is the resistance to the relative motion of adjacent layers of liquid. According to Eq. 4, it is calculated as the ratio of shear stress to rate of shear. In the CGS system, viscosity is defined as the tangential force per unit area in dyne/cm^2 required to maintain a difference in velocity of 1 cm/sec between two parallel layers of liquid 1 cm apart. Its unit is therefore dyne/cm^2 sec^{-1} or g/cm sec, which is called a *poise*. Because many common liquids including water have viscosities of the order of $^1/_{100}$ of a poise, their viscosity is often expressed in *centipoises*. Representative values are listed in Table III.

Flow through cylindrical pipes or capillaries is laminar at low velocities and/or for small tube radii and/or viscous liquids. The liquid layers are very thin cylinders concentric with the duct.[2] During flow, they telescope past one another as shown in Fig 22-4A. The arrows in Fig 22-4B represent the

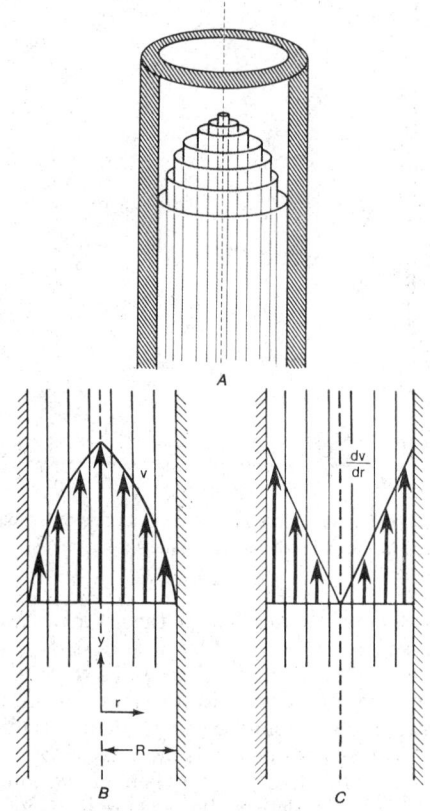

Fig 22-4.   Laminar flow of a liquid through a cylindrical duct. *A:* three-dimensional view of telescoping layers; *B:* cross-section showing radial distribution of velocity; *C:* cross-section showing radial distribution of velocity gradient (Part *A*, courtesy, Schott H, Martin AN. In Dittert L, ed: *American Pharmacy*, 7th ed, Lippincott, Philadelphia, Chap 6, 1974).

velocity v of the individual cylindrical layers of radius r; v is maximum in the center of the tube and decreases in the radial direction, ie, in the direction r (previously x) perpendicular to the direction of flow y. The velocity is zero in the outermost liquid layer adjacent and adhering to the wall, whose radius is equal to the inside radius of the tube R. In the center of the tube, where v is maximum, the velocity gradient dv/dr

**Table III—Newtonian Viscosities and Activation Energies
for Viscous Flow** [a]

Material	Temperature, °C	Viscosity, poise	Activation energy for viscous flow, kcal/mole
Water	20	0.0100	4.2
	50	0.0055	3.4
	99	0.0028	2.8
Ethanol:			
absolute	20	0.0120	3.3
	50	0.0070	3.3
40% *w/w*	20	0.0291	6.8
	50	0.0113	5.3
Benzene	20	0.0065	2.5
	50	0.0044	2.5
Ethyl ether	20	0.0024	1.65
Glycerin:			
anhydrous	20	15.00	12.5
95% *w/w*	20	5.45	10.6
Castor oil	20	10.3	13.2

[a] At 1 atm pressure.

$= \dot{\gamma}$ is zero. This is shown in Fig 22-4C, where the arrows represent $\dot{\gamma}$; it is maximum at the wall.

If V is the volume of liquid flowing through a cylindrical tube of radius R in time t, the volumetric flow rate is V/t, and the shear rate at the wall is

$$\dot{\gamma}_{wall} = \frac{4}{\pi R^3}\left(\frac{V}{t}\right) \qquad (5)$$

The shear stress is zero in the center of the tube and maximum at the wall:

$$\tau_{max.} = \frac{R\Delta P}{2L} \qquad (6)$$

The liquid is made to flow through the tube by pressure, either caused by its own weight (hydrostatic) or produced by a pump. This pressure is used to overcome the viscous friction of the liquid, and is converted into heat. The pressure drop along a length L of tube, ΔP, is the difference in the pressure at the beginning and at the end of that length.

Viscosity is shear stress divided by rate of shear. Since both vary in the x-direction perpendicular to the direction of flow, both must be taken at the same location. Using the values at the wall of a cylindrical tube, dividing Eq 6 by Eq 5 and rearranging gives:

$$\frac{V}{t} = \frac{\pi R^4 \Delta P}{8L\eta} \qquad (7)$$

This is *Poiseuille's law*, found experimentally by this French physician while studying the flow of liquids through capillary tubes representative of blood vessels. The poise is also named in his honor. In the CGS system, pressure is expressed in dyne/cm^2 and V/t in cm^3/sec.

In the human body, the pumping action of the heart supplies the driving pressure for the flow of blood, which is the difference between the arterial and venous pressure.[10] Digitalis increases the force of contraction of the heart muscle and makes the heart a more efficient pump. This increases ΔP and hence the rate of flow of blood V/t. Vasodilator drugs like nitroglycerin or amyl nitrite increase the radius of blood vessels by relaxing the vascular smooth muscles. Since the flow rate varies with the fourth power of the radius of the blood vessel, a mere 5% increase in radius causes a 22% increase in the flow rate at constant blood pressure, because $(1.05)^4 = 1.22$.

The viscosity of simple liquids, ie, pure liquids consisting of small molecules and solutions where solute and solvent are small molecules, depends only on composition, temperature, and pressure. It increases slowly with increasing pressure and fast with decreasing temperature. For solutions of solid solutes, the viscosity usually increases with concentration. Simple liquids follow Newton's law (Eq 4) of direct proportionality between shear stress and rate of shear, so that their viscosity does not depend on either. This is called *Newtonian flow behavior*. The liquids listed in Table III and their viscosities are Newtonian.

The flow curves or consistency curves of Newtonian liquids, like those of Fig 22-5, are straight lines going through the origin. Viscosity is the slope of such a line or the tangent of the angle it makes with the horizontal axis. Of the two liquids shown in Fig 22-5, A has a higher viscosity than B because $\alpha > \beta$, so that $\eta_A = \tan \alpha > \eta_B = \tan \beta$. $\eta_A = \tau_2/\dot{\gamma}_2 = \tau_1/\dot{\gamma}_1$, and $\eta_B = \tau_1/\dot{\gamma}_3 = \tau_3/\dot{\gamma}_2$. A given shear stress τ_1 produces a greater rate of shear $\dot{\gamma}_3$ in the more fluid liquid B than $\dot{\gamma}_1$ in the more viscous liquid A. Alternatively, to produce a given rate of shear $\dot{\gamma}_2$ in the two liquids requires a higher shear stress τ_2 for the more viscous liquid A than τ_3 for the more fluid liquid B. Some texts plot consistency curves with shear stress on the horizontal axis and rate of shear on the vertical axis.[1,2,8] The slope of those plots represents fluidity; viscosity is the reciprocal slope.

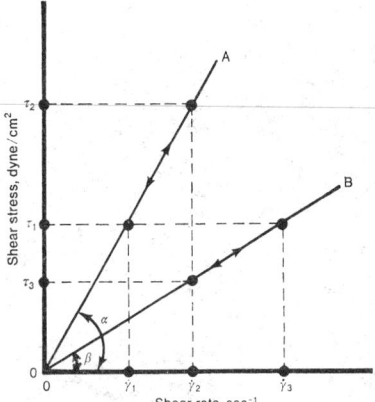

Fig 22-5.   Consistency or flow curves of two Newtonian liquids.

The variation of viscosity with temperature is often described by an *Arrhenius equation*

$$\eta = Ae^{E/RT} \qquad (8)$$

or,

$$2.303 \log \eta = 2.303 \log A + E/RT \qquad (8a)$$

where A and E are constants, T is the absolute temperature, and R is the gas constant. Values of E, the *activation energy* for viscous flow, are listed in Table III. Large values of E indicate that the viscosity decreases fast with rising temperature. According to Eq 8a, plots of $\log \eta$ vs the reciprocal of the absolute temperature should be straight lines with slopes of $E/2.303\,R$. For associated, eg, hydrogen-bonded, liquids such plots are often somewhat curved.

According to the "*hole theory*," liquids contain vacancies or holes which are essential to flow. The activation energy is largely used to form these holes.[11] E is about $\frac{1}{3}$ to $\frac{1}{4}$ of the latent heat of vaporization for nonassociated liquids.

Time-Independent Non-Newtonian Behavior—

Pseudoplasticity—Many colloidal systems, especially polymer solutions and flocculated solid/liquid dispersions, become more fluid the faster they are stirred. This shear-thinning behavior is called *pseudoplasticity*.[6,8,9,12–14] It is an example of non-Newtonian flow behavior because the viscosity is not constant (at constant temperature and composition) as required by Newton's law of viscous flow (Eq 4), but decreases with increasing shear. The shear rate increases faster than the shear stress, making the flow curve of Fig 22-6 concave towards the shear rate axis.

There is an apparent viscosity for each value of shear rate or shear stress, which can be expressed in two different ways. At Point P in Fig 22-6, the apparent viscosity can be taken as

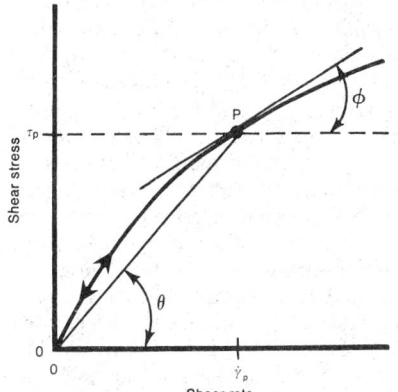

Fig 22-6.   Flow curve of a pseudoplastic liquid.

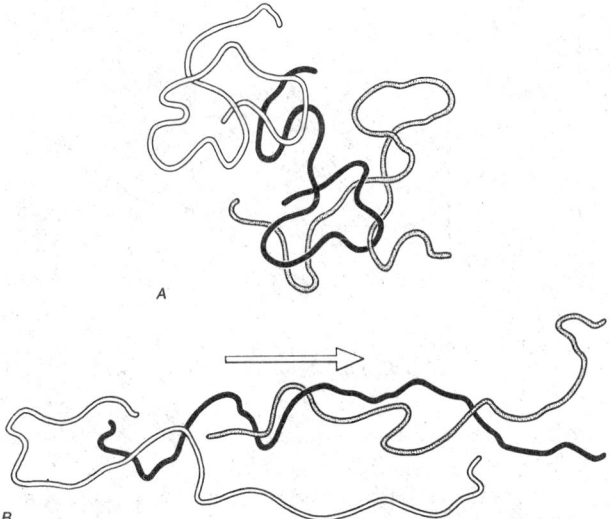

Fig 22-7.   Three randomly coiled polymer chains in solution. *A:* At rest; *B:* in shear field (courtesy, Schott H, Martin AN. In Dittert L, ed: *American Pharmacy*, 7th ed, Lippincott, Philadelphia, Chap 6, 1974).

the slope of the secant to the flow curve at P, or $\tan \theta$, which is the viscosity of a Newtonian liquid whose flow curve passes through P.[6,13] This is equal to the ratio $\tau_P/\dot{\gamma}_P$.[8,9] The second method[14] defines the apparent viscosity as the slope of the tangent to the flow curve at P, ie, $d\tau_P/d\dot{\gamma}_P = \tan \phi$. Since both θ and ϕ decrease with increasing shear stress or shear rate, so does the viscosity.

The causes for pseudoplastic flow are the progressive breakdown of structure in the liquid medium by increasing shear, and the rebuilding of structure by Brownian motion. In the case of polymer solutions, the entanglement of macromolecules and the immobilization of solvent by the entangled macromolecules provide the structure. The flexible, thread-like molecules of, say, methylcellulose or polyvinylpyrrolidone in aqueous solution are constantly buffeted by the surrounding water molecules in thermal agitation. This causes continuous motion of chain segments by translation, and by rotation around bonds between the carbon and oxygen atoms which make up the polymer backbone. These thermal fluctuations are random, so that the polymer chains form loose coils of roughly spherical shapes which are permeated by water. The coiled macromolecules, in constant segmental motion, become entangled (see Fig 22-7A). The polymer chains are encased in sheaths of water of hydration. Additional water is mechanically trapped inside the open coils.

Upon the application of shear, a unidirectional laminar motion is superimposed on the random thermal motion of the water molecules and chain segments. The randomly coiled, entangled polymer chains tend to disentangle themselves and to align themselves in the direction of flow, as shown in Fig 22-7B. The viscosity of the solution—its resistance to flow—depends on the size and shape of the flow units. Shear affects these in three ways: (1) The polymer chains uncoil progressively and become streamlined or elongated, offering less resistance to flow than the original, approximately spherical, shapes; (2) simultaneously, the amount of water trapped inside the coils and dragged along decreases; and (3) the chains become gradually more disentangled. The latter two phenomena reduce the size of the flow unit; all three increase with increasing shear and reduce the viscosity.

At each rate of shear, there is an average equilibrium degree of entanglement and alignment of the macromolecules, resulting from competition between the shear-induced disentanglement and alignment of chains which releases trapped water, and the entanglement and random (i.e., spherical) coiling tendency caused by Brownian motion which entraps water inside the coils. The rate of entanglement and randomization by Brownian motion is constant, while the rate of disentanglement and alignment increases with increasing shear. Therefore, the viscosity diminishes as the shear increases.

Dispersions of flocculated solid particles are pseudoplastic if the particle-particle bonds are too weak to withstand the applied shear stresses. This occurs if particles are flocculated in the secondary minimum (see Chapter 20), or in the case of lamellar clays like sodium bentonite and kaolin. The platelets of these clays have positively charged edges and negatively charged faces. The electrostatic bonds between the edges and faces of different platelets produce a house-of-cards structure in the aqueous suspension which entraps and immobilizes large amounts of water. Aggregates of randomly shaped particles also entrap water in the interparticle voids.

Shear progressively breaks up these aggregates at a rate which increases with increasing shear stress, releasing increasing amounts of trapped water. Brownian motion tends to rebuild the aggregates at a rate which is independent of shear. There is an average equilibrium size for the aggregates at each rate of shear which decreases with increasing shear, resulting in a decrease in the resistance to flow, or viscosity, as the shear increases.

At extremely low shear rates, well below 1 sec^{-1}, the rate of disentanglement and alignment of polymer chains and the rate of breaking up of aggregates of particles under the influence of shear are negligible compared to the rate of entanglement and randomization of polymer chains and to the rate of aggregation of particles produced by Brownian motion, respectively. Hence the flow units are neither noticeably deformed nor reduced in size by shear, and the systems exhibit Newtonian flow, with a constant and high viscosity designated as the *lower Newtonian* or *zero-shear viscosity*, η_0.[2,8]

At very high shear rates, the dissolved polymer chains are wholly disentangled and well aligned in the direction of flow, and the aggregates of particles are broken up as far as possible. There is no residual structure left which can be broken up by further increments in shear rate: The viscosity levels off at a constant value called the *upper Newtonian viscosity*, η_∞. Turbulent flow and shear-induced rupture of polymer chains may set in before the upper Newtonian regime is reached. As can be seen in Fig 22-8, η_∞ is considerably lower than η_0. The value of the non-Newtonian viscosity observed at intermediate shear rates, including those encountered in most practical situations, depends on the amount of residual structure. It is therefore called *structural viscosity*.[1,2,13,14]

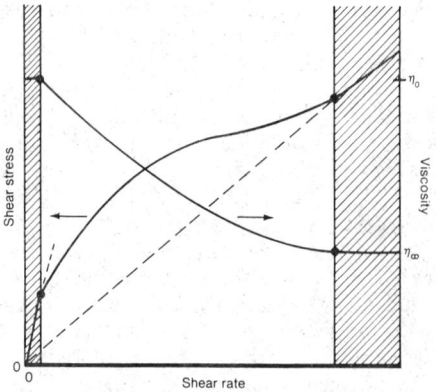

Fig 22-8.   The three flow regions of a pseudoplastic liquid. Shaded areas refer to lower (left) and upper (right) Newtonian regions; center area represents pseudoplastic behavior.

Dilatancy—The opposite behavior, *shear-thickening* or an increase in viscosity with increasing shear, called *dilatancy*,[2,6–9,12–14] is rare. It is shown by concentrated dispersions of particles which do not tend to aggregate or stick together, provided the amount of liquid present is not much larger than that needed to fill the voids between the particles. Sediments of suspensions from which the supernatant liquid has been decanted are sometimes dilatant. When such a concentrated suspension is poured or stirred slowly, there is just enough liquid to lubricate the slipping of particle past particle, and the viscosity is low. When stirred fast, the particles get into each other's way, block each other and bunch up rather than slipping past each other. Large voids form between the unevenly clustered particles, and as the liquid seeps into these, the suspension appears dry—as if the suspended solids had expanded or become dilated (see sketches in Ref 12 and Ref 14). This phenomenon, which results in progressive viscosity increases, becomes more severe with increasing shear. When high shear is followed by low shear or rest, the bunched-up particles separate again, the interparticle void volume decreases, and the viscosity drops as the suspension appears again wet. Wet sand offers small resistance to slow flow or penetration, but stiffens and appears dry when deformed fast.

Among the few systems reported[14] to exhibit dilatant flow are suspensions of starch in water, aqueous glycerin or ethylene glycol containing about 40–50% *v/v* starch, and concentrated suspensions of inorganic pigments in water and in fluid nonpolar liquids with enough surfactant added to deflocculate the disperse phase completely, e.g., red iron oxide (12% *v/v* in water or 18% *v/v* in carbon tetrachloride), zinc oxide (30% *v/v* in water or 33% *v/v* in carbon tetrachloride), barium sulfate (39% *v/v* in water), and titanium dioxide (30–50% *v/v* in water).

Pseudoplastic and dilatant liquids frequently follow the empirical *power law* (*Ostwald-de Waele equation*)[1,2,5,6,8,9] over wide ranges of shear rates:

$$\dot{\gamma} = K\tau^n \tag{9}$$

or

$$\log \dot{\gamma} = \log K + n \log \tau \tag{9a}$$

For power-law liquids, a plot of $\log \dot{\gamma}$ vs. $\log \tau$ is a straight line of slope n. This equation has the advantage of representing the flow behavior in terms of only two constants, K and n. It has the disadvantage of all power laws, namely, the dimensions of K depend on the value of n.[2] Moreover, the power-law curve does not go through the origin, whereas pseudoplastic and dilatant flow curves always do.

The exponent n is an index of the deviation from Newtonian flow behavior. For $n = 1$, $K = 1/\eta$, and Newton's law (Eq 4) results. For pseudoplasticity, $n > 1$ and for dilatancy, $n < 1$. The more n differs from unity, the more non-Newtonian is the flow behavior, ie, the faster will the viscosity decrease or increase with increasing shear.

Yield Value, Elasticity, and Plasticity—Other materials, called semisolids, do not flow at low shear stresses but undergo reversible deformation like elastic solids. When a characteristic shear stress, called the yield value or *yield stress*, is exceeded, they flow like liquids. Yield stresses are usually caused by structural networks extending throughout an entire system. To break such a network requires stresses equal to or exceeding the yield stress. Smaller stresses produce no flow but only elastic deformation. When the yield stress is exceeded, the network is partly ruptured and flow occurs.

There are two classes of semisolid materials with yield stresses, gels and pastes; the distinction between the two is not sharp.

Gels—Gels or jellies are characterized by a comparatively high degree of elasticity. They undergo rather large elastic deformations at shear stresses below the yield value, from which they recover their shape when the stresses are removed.[6,13] Recoverable deformations of 10–30% are not unusual, especially for polymer gels. Clay gels are less elastic and more like pastes.

Two types of gels are of pharmaceutical importance. *Gels of colloidal clays*, especially of sodium bentonite whose plate-like particles have strong edge-to-face attraction, are discussed first. Their elastic deformability is limited. Their elastic modulus or rigidity and their yield value are not particularly sensitive to changes in temperature. However, the presence of flocculating or deflocculating agents affects these parameters markedly. When subjected to shear stresses well above their yield values, these gels break down to smooth and free-flowing sols.

The second type comprises *aqueous gels of organic polymers* such as gelatin, agar, pectin, methylcellulose, and high-molecular-weight polyethylene glycol. Nonaqueous gels such as natural rubber in benzene are of little pharmaceutical importance.

Solutions of gelatin in water and/or glycerin set to gels on cooling and melt on heating. The gelation temperature and the melting point for a given gel are close together; gelation is a reversible process. Gelatin gels are used in pharmacy as *glycerogelatins* and as *suppository bases*. The gelation temperature or melting point of gelatin-water systems is in the range of 20–40°. It increases with increasing gelatin content and with increasing gelatin molecular weight, as does the solution viscosity above the gelation temperature and the gel rigidity below it. While the modulus and the ultimate strength of aqueous gels increase with increasing gelatin content, the elongation at break is not much affected.[5] Gel strength and rigidity are highest at the *isoelectric point*, where cross-linking by salt bridges between amino or guanidino and carboxylate groups is most extensive. While typical aqueous gelatin gels contain 20–45% solids, pectin and agar form strong gels at room temperature which contain only 1–4% solids.

The high viscosity of polymer solutions is largely due to the entanglement of the long, thread-like molecules. The polymer chains are surrounded by a hydration layer, ie, a sheath of water molecules attracted to the polar groups of the macromolecules by secondary valence bonds. Being encased in a solvation sheath largely prevents a polymer chain from forming attachments with neighboring chains at points of entanglement through secondary valence bonds. When the solution is made to flow, the chains slip past one another rather freely and tend to disentangle themselves. If the solvent action decreases, eg, through lowering the temperature or by adding alcohol or another water-miscible nonsolvent to aqueous solutions of gelatin, pectin or agar, the hydration sheath around the dissolved macromolecules becomes thinner. Therefore, some entangled polymer chains come into direct contact with one another at crossover points, where they form attachments by secondary valence bonds. These weak and temporary crosslinks between segments of adjacent polymer chains offer some resistance to the slippage of polymer chains past one another when shear is applied. When enough of these interchain links are formed to establish a three-dimensional network throughout a solution, it sets to a gel. Methylcellulose and high-molecular-weight polyethylene glycol are more soluble in cold than in hot water. They are less extensively hydrated at higher temperatures. Therefore, their solutions gel on heating and melt on cooling.

Polymer gels are strong and elastic. When subjected to shear stresses well in excess of their yield values, they tend to rupture or crumble rather than to flow. Only gels which are weak by virtue of being close to their gelation temperature or of having low solids contents liquefy to sols and flow under the effect of high shear stresses.

The official gels (Aluminum Hydroxide Gel, Aluminum Phosphate Gel) are aqueous suspensions of gelatinous precipitates. They are not gels according to the rheological meaning of the word, but rather are thixotropic liquids.

Plastic Materials—When suspensions of particles which tend to agglomerate or stick together are so concentrated that continuous bridges of particles extend throughout the entire suspension volumes, forming three-dimensional networks, they acquire yield values. Such *pastes* have little elasticity. They cannot recover their shape except from very small deformations. At stresses above their yield values, pastes turn into free-flowing liquids. This type of behavior is called *plasticity;* plastic materials are sometimes called *Bingham bodies* or *semisolids.*[1,2,5-9,12-14]

Brownian motion builds up the networks in gels and pastes and restores them when they have been ruptured by stresses higher than their yield stresses. Thixotropy is often observed. The addition of surfactants or other deflocculating agents to pastes or clay gels often lowers or eliminates the yield value by reducing the attraction among the particles, thereby weakening the three-dimensional structure. Deflocculation also lowers the apparent viscosity of pastes and suspensions.[14]

Examples of plastic materials are ointments and pastes including those of Chapters 40 and 88, creams, salves, cataplasms, cerates, butter and margarine, dough, putties, and modeling clay. The following are advantages of yield values: Ointments, clay slips (potter's clay made into a dough with water), and butter do not drip from fingers, spatulas, and knives but hold their shape until sheared by spreading pressures which exceed their yield values, whereupon they flow and spread. Toothpaste does not sink into the toothbrush under its own weight. Bread dough and potter's clay preserve their shape when put into the baking oven.

Fig 22-9 shows the flow curves for two plastic systems. System *B* has a lower yield value than System *A* and Newtonian behavior at stresses above the yield value; $BC\tau_{yield}$ is a straight line of inclination θ, so that the *plastic viscosity* of *B*, ie, its viscosity above the yield value, is the slope of this line or $\tan \theta$:

$$\eta_{plastic} = \frac{\tau - \tau_{yield}}{\dot{\gamma}} \qquad (10)$$

This is equivalent to moving the origin of the flow curve from zero stress to the yield stress, and treating System *B* as a Newtonian liquid at stresses beyond. Semisolids with high yield values are described as "hard." When their plastic viscosity is high, they are described as "stiff."[15]

Some Bingham bodies have flow curves which deviate from

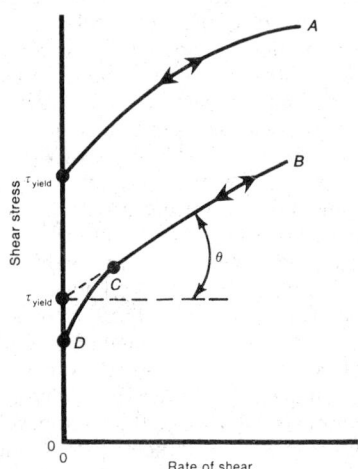

Fig 22-9.   Flow curves of two plastic systems.

straight lines at stresses close to the yield stress, such as the portion *CD* in the flow curve of System *B*, where flow occurs even below the yield stress. This phenomenon is called *plug flow* because the material moves in chunks or as a plug rather than by laminar motion, often through slippage at the wall of the duct. In such cases, the yield value is usually obtained by extrapolating the linear portion *BC* to the stress axis.

System *A* is pseudoplastic above its yield stress. This type of flow behavior is frequently observed with suspensions thickened with dissolved polymers, where the vehicle itself is shear-thinning.

Time-Dependent Non-Newtonian Behavior—In the previous discussion, pseudoplastic and plastic behavior was seen to arise from competition between the detachment of entanglement links among dissolved macromolecules or the rupturing of van der Waals links among dispersed particles by shear, and the reestablishment of such links by Brownian motion. The balance between breakdown and restoration of links shifts more and more towards breakdown as the shear increases. Reduction in interchain or interparticle links results in smaller flow units and lower apparent viscosity. It was tacitly assumed that the system adapts itself to changing shear "instantaneously," ie, so fast that by the time the instrumental conditions had been changed to higher or lower shear and readings are taken, the equilibrium between breakdown and restoration of links at the new shear had already been reached, producing flow units of the new average equilibrium size and the corresponding new apparent viscosity. Points representing pairs of $\dot{\gamma}$, τ values determined at increasing and at decreasing shear rates or shear stresses in Figs 22-5, 6, and 9 fall on the same single curves. It is immaterial whether a given shear rate was reached by increasing or decreasing the speed of the viscometer. This is the meaning of the double arrows on these curves.

If the suspension is viscous and/or the particles are large and heavy, their Brownian motion is too slow to restore broken interparticle links "instantaneously." Likewise, the entanglements of polymer chains are slow to be reestablished by Brownian motion if their solution is viscous. If the rate of link restoration by Brownian motion is lower than the rate of link breakdown by shear, the apparent viscosity decreases even while the system is under constant shear, as the size of the particle aggregates or the extent of macromolecular entanglement is progressively reduced. Furthermore, the apparent viscosity at a given shear rate is lower if the system was recently stirred at high speeds than if that shear rate was approached from low speeds or from rest.

The extreme behavior is an isothermal, reversible sol $\rightleftharpoons$ gel transformation produced by rest and by shear, respectively. For example, an aqueous dispersion of 8% w/w sodium bentonite sets to a gel within an hour or two after preparation when undisturbed, but flows and can be poured within many minutes after it had been stirred above the yield value. After prolonged rest it reverts to a gel as the Brownian motion rebuilds the house-of-cards structure throughout the material.

Such materials, whose consistency depends on the duration of shear as well as on the rate of shear, are said to be thixotropic or to exhibit *thixotropy.*[1,5-9,12-14] Their apparent viscosity depends not only on temperature, composition, and rate of shear or shear stress but on the previous shear history and time under shear.

Thixotropy in a shear-thinning liquid is shown in Fig 22-10. Starting with the system at rest (at the origin *O*) and gradually increasing the speed of the viscometer produces the "up" branch *ODAB* of the flow curve. After the maximum shear rate $\dot{\gamma}_1$ and shear stress τ_3 corresponding to point *B* have been reached, the speed of the instrument is reduced. If there is not enough time for Brownian motion to regenerate completely the structure torn down at the high speed, the liquid

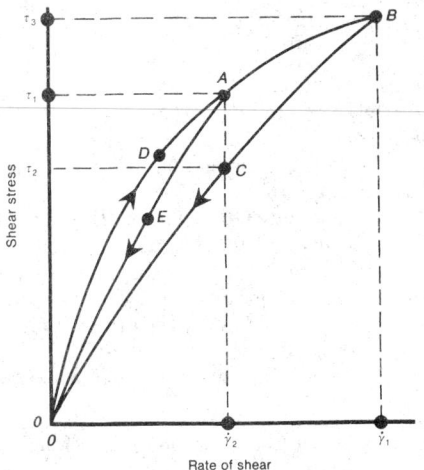

Fig 22-10.   Flow curves of a shear-thinning liquid exhibiting thixotropy.

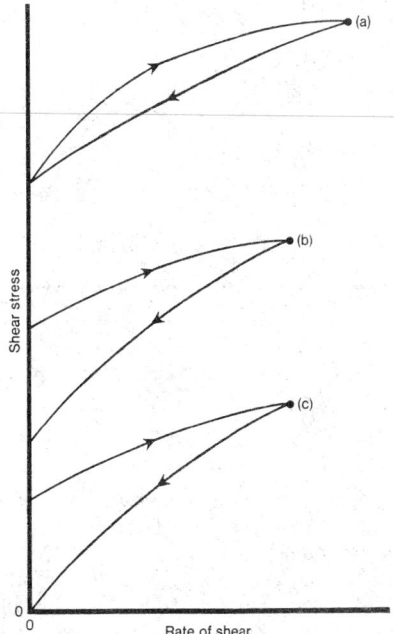

Fig 22-12.   Flow curves of plastic systems exhibiting thixotropy (see text).

will be less viscous and the "down" branch of the flow curve, *BCO*, is lower than the "up" branch. Thus, the shear stress required to maintain the rate of shear $\dot{\gamma}_2$ has been reduced from τ_1 to τ_2, and the apparent viscosity has dropped from $\tau_1/\dot{\gamma}_2$ to $\tau_2/\dot{\gamma}_2$. This contrasts with the flow curve of Fig 22-6, where the "up" and "down" branches coincide.

When starting from rest, if the speed is not increased all the way up to $\dot{\gamma}_1$ but only to $\dot{\gamma}_2$ corresponding to point *A* in Fig 22-10 and then decreased, the "down" branch is *AEO:* Since the maximum speed is lower than previously, less structure is broken down and the apparent viscosity is not reduced by as much.

If the liquid in the instrument is kept at rest for a sufficient time period after it was subjected to the shear cycle *ODABCO*, Brownian motion rebuilds its structure, restoring its original high consistency. Starting from rest, the flow curve is again *ODABCO*. If no rest period is allowed and the shear cycle is repeated as soon as the "down" branch is completed, the next "up" branch is below *ODAB*, say, *OFB* in Fig 22-11. A third shear cycle following immediately after the second may give the "up" branch *OGB*. The "down" branch *BCO* may be curved as in Fig 22-10 or straight as in Fig 22-11. If the build-up of structure is very slow, there may be no structure left after the third shear cycle. In that case, the "up" branch coincides with the straight "down" branch *BCO* and the liquid has become Newtonian. This is only temporary because the

flow curve reverts to *OABCO* of Fig 22-11 after a prolonged rest period.

Thixotropy is frequently superimposed on plastic flow behavior. The yield value may disappear after one or more shear cycles, as in curve *c* of Fig 22-12; it may be reduced as in curve *b* (sometimes called *false body* behavior[7,9]), or it may remain unaltered as in curve *a*.

The difference between the "up" and "down" branches of a flow curve illustrates a common phenomenon called *hysteresis*. The area enclosed by the two branches (eg, areas *ODAEO* and *ODABCO* in Fig 22-10) or by the two branches and the stress axis (as in Fig 22-12 *b* and *c*) is called the *hysteresis loop*.[5,6,8,12,14] Its size is a measure of the extent of thixotropic breakdown in the structure of the system. In Fig 22-11, the areas enclosed by the two branches of the flow curves representing successive shear cycles become progressively smaller: *OABCO* > *OFBCO* > *OGBCO*. This parallels a decrease in the amount of structural breakdown of the system as each cycle leaves intact less residual structure which can be broken down in the next cycle. When no structure remains, the Newtonian flow curve *OCBCO* of Fig 22-11 results. The absence of hysteresis in the flow curves of Figs 22-6 and 9 is due to another cause: The rebuilding of structure by Brownian motion is as fast or faster than the shear-induced structural breakdown or the response time of the viscometer.

Thixotropy can be represented quantitatively by the area of the hysteresis loop,[6,8,12,14] by a coefficient of thixotropic breakdown (Eq 12; also Eq 94 of Ref 6, Eq 25 of Ref 12, or Eq 31 of Ref 14), or by the decay of shear stress or apparent viscosity as a function of time at constant rate of shear.[6,8,9,14] The latter method is illustrated in Fig 22-13. When a system is stirred at a constant shear rate, it eventually reaches constant or equilibrium values for shear stress and apparent viscosity. This is shown by the levelling off of the curve. Equilibration at a given shear rate may take half an hour or longer.

Thixotropy is particularly useful in the formulation of pharmaceutical suspensions and emulsions. These must be poured easily from containers, which implies low viscosity. Low viscosity, however, causes rapid settling of solid particles in suspensions and rapid creaming of emulsions. According to Stokes' equation (see Chapter 21), the rate of sedimentation

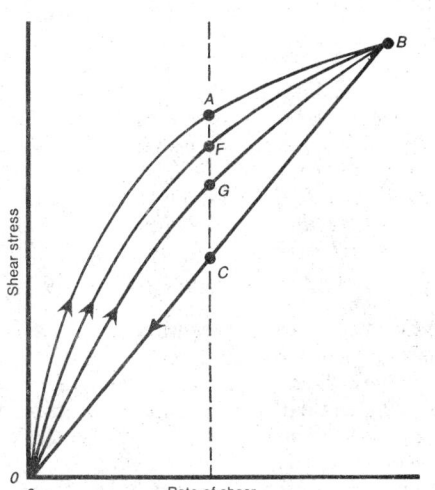

Fig 22-11.   Flow curves representing successive shear cycles for a thixotropic, shear-thinning liquid.

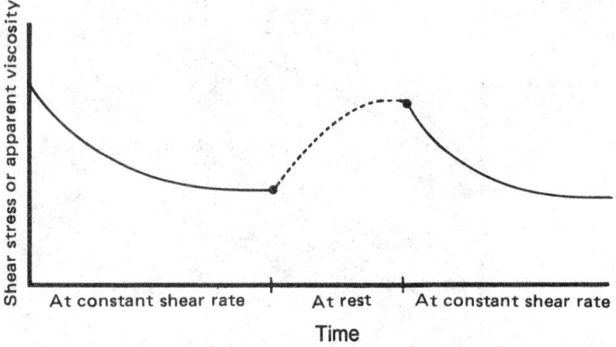

Fig 22-13.   Time dependence of shear stress or of apparent viscosity of a thixotropic system.

is inversely proportional to the viscosity of the medium. Solid particles which have settled out frequently stick together, producing a sediment difficult to redisperse ("caking or claying"). Creaming in emulsions is a first step towards coalescence. Thixotropy can be used to solve this dilemma. A thixotropic agent such as sodium bentonite magma, other colloidal clays (magnesium bentonite, attapulgite), colloidal silicon dioxide, or microcrystalline cellulose is incorporated into the suspensions or emulsions to confer a high apparent viscosity or even a yield value. High viscosities retard sedimentation and creaming while yield values prevent them altogether; since there is no flow below the yield stress, the apparent viscosity at low shear becomes infinite. When it is desired to pour some of the suspension or emulsion from its container, it is shaken well, at shear stresses considerably above the yield value. The agitation breaks down temporarily the thixotropic structure such as the house-of-cards scaffold of bentonite, reducing the yield value to zero and lowering the apparent viscosity. This makes for easy pouring. Back on the shelf, the viscosity slowly increases again and the yield value is restored as Brownian motion rebuilds the house-of-cards structure of bentonite. This prevents sedimentation and claying of the suspended particles and creaming of the emulsion droplets; the disperse particles again become trapped in the plastic matrix. The optimum flow curve for such formulations is that of Fig 22-12c.

Once the links among suspended particles or the entanglements among dissolved polymer chains have been broken by shear, their restoration by Brownian motion is slow if the suspensions or solutions are viscous. In such cases slow flow, gentle agitation or moderate and rhythmic vibration may accelerate the rebuilding of the structure, ie, the restoration of the links between particles or macromolecules by Brownian motion. Low shear rates thus hasten the reappearance of high apparent viscosities or onset of gelation in thixotropic sols. In the case of sheared dispersions of bentonite, gentle vibration or rotation of the beaker speeds up the rebuilding of the house-of-cards structure. Such an increase in apparent viscosity or the advent of a yield value by gentle agitation is called *rheopexy*.[2,7-9,13,14]

Rheology of Dispersions

Many pharmaceutical preparations are dispersions of solids or liquids in liquid or semisolid vehicles, and their usefulness often depends on their flow properties. Few disperse systems are Newtonian. Most exhibit non-Newtonian flow behavior, some of it time-dependent.

Einstein's Law of Viscosity—This is the simplest equation derived to describe the flow behavior of dispersions.[1,2,5-8,12-14] Unfortunately, it applies only to Newtonian and idealized systems.

$$\eta_{\text{spec}} = \frac{\eta_{12}}{\eta_1} - 1 = \frac{\eta_{12} - \eta_1}{\eta_1} = 2.5\,\phi \qquad (11)$$

The Newtonian viscosities η_{12} and η_1 are those of the dispersion and of the liquid vehicle or solvent, respectively; η_{spec} represents the specific viscosity of the dispersion, ie, the increase in viscosity of the dispersion over that of the solvent, expressed as a multiple of the viscosity of the solvent. ϕ is the volume fraction of the disperse phase: Blood contains 45% v/v of red and 1% v/v of white cells; the corresponding ϕ values are 0.45 and 0.01. The viscosity of dispersions obeying Einstein's law depends only on the viscosity of the solvent and on the volume of solvent replaced by the disperse phase, but not on the size of its particles.

The following conditions were imposed in the derivation of Eq 11:

1.   Gravitational and inertial effects are negligible, and turbulence is absent.
2.   The particles are large compared to the solvent molecules, or the discontinuities between the solvent molecules are negligible compared to the size of the dispersed particles: The solvent is a continuous medium. This condition is fulfilled by pharmaceutical dispersions.
3.   The particles are small compared to the dimensions of the viscometer (gap between the coaxial cylinders or diameter of the capillary).
4.   The particles are unsolvated, smooth and rigid spheres. Examples are glass beads, polymer latex particles, and many spores and fungi. Emulsion droplets are deformable and the liquid inside them can circulate. This decreases the distortion of the flow pattern around the droplets and reduces the numerical constant in Eq 11 below 2.5. Rigid anisometric particles offer increased resistance to flow, raising the constant above 2.5. If the solvation layer of solvated spherical particles is included in ϕ, their dispersions may obey Eq 11. Examples are solutions of globular proteins at their isoelectric point, where their net electric charge is zero.
5.   The particles do not interact, ie, neither attract nor repel one another. Most dispersions consist of particles of like charge. The increase in the viscosity of dispersions due to interparticle electrostatic repulsion is called *electroviscous effect*. It can be minimized or swamped by adding salts to aqueous dispersions.
6.   The dispersions are so dilute that the distortion of the laminar streamlines of the solvent at the surface of one particle does not overlap and reinforce the distortions around its neighbors. At higher concentrations, the perturbation of laminar flow produced by one particle reaches into the fields of other particles. This produces additional resistance to flow and increases η_{spec} and η_{12} above the values given by Eq 11. Pharmaceutical dispersions are too concentrated to satisfy this condition.

All deviations from these conditions result in higher dispersion viscosities than those calculated by Einstein's law except that, when the disperse phase is fluid, the calculated viscosity is too high. An example of an extreme positive deviation is found in aqueous sodium bentonite dispersions. Their specific viscosity is about 70 times greater than that calculated from Eq 11. The particles are thin plates, deviating considerably from spherical shape. They are hydrated, and their negatively charged faces attract the positively charged edges but repel the negatively charged faces of other particles. Polymer solutions with their thread-like, highly solvated and entangled macromolecules also deviate considerably from Einstein's law. Several modifications, derived to broaden its stringent conditions, express the specific viscosity as a polynomial in ϕ. In one modification, the term $14.1\,\phi^2$ is added to the right side of Eq 11 to take into account the increased resistance to flow due to overlapping and reinforcing of streamline distortions ruled out by condition 6. This extends the use of the modified Eq 11 to more concentrated dispersions.[2,5-7,12]

Other Equations—Many theories, models, and empirical equations were developed to describe the flow behavior of non-Newtonian systems.[16] Two successful approaches to the flow of pseudoplastic dispersions and polymer solutions are mentioned below. The *impulse theory* of Goodeve and Gillespie is based on Williamson's concept of pseudoplasticity.[5] Some of the shear is used to rupture links between particles (thixotropic effect), while the remainder is used to produce higher shear rates by transfer of momentum from a moving layer to an adjacent layer which moves more slowly (Newtonian effect).[17]   Cross derived his equation by comparing the rates of rupture of interparticle links by shear and by Brownian motion with the rate of formation of links by Brownian motion for a particulate dispersion or polymer solution in steady shear.[5,18]   Both approaches result in equations containing a small number of constants which can be evaluated from experimental data with comparative ease and which have physical significance.   The equations are applicable to a wide variety of pseudoplastic systems and fit the experimental data over a wide range of shear rates.   Sherman discusses the rheology of emulsions in detail.[5,19]

Viscoelasticity

Viscoelastic materials exhibit viscous flow combined with elastic deformation when stressed.   They range from steel springs or rubber bands which are primarily elastic but creep or undergo cold flow under large and prolonged stresses to viscous liquids which recoil at the cessation of high speed stirring or fast extrusion.

When a viscoelastic material is deformed to a given strain, and just enough stress is applied to maintain this strain, the stress decreases gradually as the material flows, creeps or relaxes.   The more extensive this creep, the less pronounced is the return to the original shape when the stress is removed.   The stress decays progressively as the material undergoes relaxation through viscous flow.   The time required for the stress to decay to $1/e = 36.8\%$ of its initial value is a characteristic property of the material called *relaxation time; e* is the basis of natural logarithms.   The relaxation time equals the ratio of viscosity to Young's modulus.[1-9]

Most viscoelastic materials have a range of relaxation times rather than a single value at any one temperature.   If the mean relaxation time of the material is very long compared to the time scale of the measurement, the material behaves as an elastic solid.   If the mean relaxation time is very short compared to the time of observation or measurement, it cannot be observed, and the material behaves as a viscous liquid.   When the mean relaxation time and the time scale of measurement are of comparable orders of magnitude, the material is viscoelastic.   Silicone putty ("Silly Putty") has a comparatively short mean relaxation time at room temperature.   It bounces, behaving like an elastic solid when the time of "measurement" or of application of stress is short, but flows and shows little elasticity when slowly stretched.[13]

Viscoelastic materials frequently contain high concentrations of long-chain molecules, eg, melts and gels and concentrated solutions of polymers.   When subjected to stresses for short times, such assemblies of randomly coiled and entangled macromolecular chains act as elastic networks.   Crosslinks and solid particles ("fillers") and any residual crystalline domains present in such materials enhance the elastic behavior.   Upon release of the stress, the original shapes are restored with little permanent deformation or creep.   Most of the mechanical energy put into the systems is then recovered.

If the polymeric material remains under applied stress for increasingly longer periods of time, the macromolecular chains are progressively uncoiled and disentangled.   Chain segments slip past one another and the system flows.   If fillers are present, chain segments adsorbed on the surface of these solid particles are detached.   Any crystalline regions which had existed in the unstressed material are torn apart.   Thus, while the system is subjected to continuing stress, its deformation or strain becomes increasingly greater and more permanent.   Only a small fraction of the deformation is recovered when the stress is finally released.   Most of the applied mechanical energy is dissipated as heat due to intersegmental friction.

This behavior approaches that of a purely viscous liquid.

Viscoelasticity is widespread even among liquids and plastic materials which seem to lack elasticity or stringiness to the touch, especially if they are tested at small deformations.   Higher deformations or rates of shear approaching use conditions frequently rupture the elastic network in these materials, causing the loss of the elastic components from their rheological properties.   For instance, fluid emulsions are often slightly viscoelastic at very low shear due to flocculation of the disperse droplets and interlinking of the flocs; they flow readily and lose all recovery properties under slightly higher shear.[19]   Davis determined the viscoelastic properties of oleaginous, emulsion, and absorption-type ointment bases by creep measurements.[20]

Biorheology

Two examples of the application of rheology to biological systems are the flow properties of blood and mucus.

Hemorheology—Blood is a very concentrated suspension whose flow properties are important as well as unusual.   The *Fahraeus-Lindqvist effect*[10] consists of a lowering in the apparent viscosity of blood flowing through capillaries compared to the same blood flowing through larger vessels.   Three possible contributory causes are:

1.   The hematocrit value is lower for blood in capillaries.   For instance, blood flowing through a capillary of $50\mu m$ diameter has only 70% of the red blood cells of blood flowing through large vessels.
2.   Red blood cells are biconcave discs with an average diameter, d, of $7.5\,\mu m$.   Their size is by no means negligible compared to the radius R of capillaries.   This leads to a reduction in the apparent viscosity by a factor of $(1 + d/R)^2$ according to the so-called *sigma effect*.[10]
3.   The *tubular pinch effect* consists of an accumulation of red cells in an annular region located at a distance of about 60% of the tube radius from the tube axis during laminar flow of blood through cylindrical capillaries.   Almost colorless plasma flows in the vicinity of the capillary wall.[10]   Blood flowing in the center of the tube is also deficient in red cells.   This phenomenon is commonly observed when suspensions of spherical or asymmetric particles flow through ducts whose diameter is only a low multiple of the particle size.

Rheology of Mucus—Mucus is a viscoelastic, gel-like, stringy slime secreted by cells of the mucous membranes lining the respiratory tract (nose, trachea, bronchi, bronchioles), gastrointestinal tract, and the uterus.   Glycoproteins are the main polymeric constituents of mucus and are chiefly responsible for its consistency.   The glycoprotein molecules are cross-linked by disulfide bridges and further joined by hydrogen bonds, electrostatic bonds, hydrophobic bonds, and chain entanglement.   The elasticity and viscosity of mucus are due to a three-dimensional gel network of these macromolecular chains, which are sometimes associated into fibrils.[21]

Normal functions of mucus depend on its rheological properties.   Pathological conditions are reflected by changes in these properties.   Tracheal or *bronchial mucus* protects the lining of the respiratory tract from foreign particles by trapping and removing them.   Mucus has pronounced pseudoplasticity.[22]   The cilia of the cells lining the mucosal surface beat with a frequency of about 20 vibrations/sec, which corresponds to a shear rate of about $100\ sec^{-1}$.[21,23]   This action maintains the mucus relatively fluid in the immediate vicinity of the mucosal surface and permits it to flow.   Farther removed from the surface and the cilia, the apparent viscosity of the mucus film increases markedly, enabling it to retain contaminating particles.

Bronchitis and bronchial asthma cause an abnormal thickening of the mucus, increasing its viscosity and elasticity.   Among expectorants are *mucolytic agents* (see Chapter 44), which function by liquefying or reducing the viscoelastic consistency of mucus.   Potassium iodide and sodium thiocyanate break the structure of water, thereby reducing hydrophobic bonding between glycoprotein chains. Urea and guanidine hydrochloride disrupt hydrogen bonds between these macromolecules in addition to reducing hydrophobic interactions. N-Acetylcysteine and dithiothreitol break disulfide bridges that cross-link glycoprotein molecules by reducing disulfide to thiol groups. Proteolytic enzymes such as chymotrypsin and trypsin also liquefy mucus.[23–26]

The consistency of *cervical mucus* changes markedly during the menstrual cycle. During the period of ovulation, the mucus is "thin" and easily penetrated by spermatozoa. At other times, the mucus forms a dense, three-dimensional network almost impenetrable to sperm. One of the effects of progestagen contraceptives is to thicken the cervical mucus. In pregnancy, cervical mucus is a highly viscous gel which occludes the cervical canal, thus providing an effective barrier against bacteria.[21,23]

One of the adverse effects of *cystic fibrosis* is the accumulation of thick mucus in lungs, pancreas, and intestine ("mucoviscidosis").

The viscoelastic properties of synovial fluid are largely due to hyaluronic acid.[27] Inflammatory joint diseases reduce the concentration and/or molecular weight of this biopolymer and thereby alter the flow properties of the fluid.[28]

Select Pharmaceutical Systems

Powders and granulated solids are the only type of materials omitted from this chapter whose flow properties are important to dosage forms. Their rheology is discussed in Chapter 21 and by Neumann.[29] Martin *et al.*,[12] and Sherman[5] have reviewed the literature of the rheology of pharmaceutical systems. The three case histories described below illustrate some important and typical problems as well as the complexity of such systems, and show how each ingredient can affect the flow properties of the entire formulation.

Effect of Additives on the Rheology of Ointments

Kostenbauder and Martin[15] determined the effect of various components of ointments on the rheological properties of petrolatum. With the aid of a Stormer viscometer, they measured the up and down curves of petrolatum containing various ingredients for two different maximum shear rates, 125 and 210 sec^{-1}. The down curves were straight lines which were extrapolated to the shear stress axis to obtain yield values. Plastic viscosities were calculated from their slopes by

Eq 10. A *thixotropic index* was defined[6,12,14,15] by,

$$M = (\eta_{\text{plastic, 125 sec}^{-1}} - \eta_{\text{plastic, 210 sec}^{-1}})/\ln(210/125) \quad (12)$$

The higher the value of M, the more extensive the thixotropic breakdown of the ointment structure by shear.

The following conclusions can be drawn from the data of Table IV, which summarizes their results. Incorporation of white wax made petrolatum harder (increased its yield value) and stiffer. The plastic viscosity increased logarithmically with the percentage of white wax. The addition of mineral oil had the opposite effect on petrolatum. When increasing concentrations of the particulate solid zinc oxide were incorporated into a 70:30 mixture of petrolatum and mineral oil, the yield value went through a minimum at 10% zinc oxide while the plastic viscosity and the thixotropic index increased monotonically.

In the three series of tests involving the addition of mineral oil or white wax to petrolatum, or the addition of zinc oxide to a mixture of petrolatum and mineral oil, the yield value was affected more strongly by the change in composition than either the plastic viscosity or the thixotropic index.

Sensory assessment of the spreadability of ointments can be correlated with their rheological properties.[30] In consultation with dermatologists, Kostenbauder and Martin divided ointments into three categories according to their consistency. Class I consists of ophthalmic ointments, which are the softest. Their flow properties should be similar to those of ointments No 5 and 6 of Table IV. Class II includes the common medicated ointments which are soft yet stiff enough to remain in place upon application to the skin. Their flow properties are represented by ointments No 3 and 4 of Table IV. Class III consists of protective ointments, which must be hard and stiff enough to remain in place even when applied to moist, ulcerated areas. Representative flow properties for this class are not listed.[15]

The Role of Thixotropy in Injectable Depot Preparations

An ingenious application of thixotropy is illustrated by the work of Ober *et al*[31] involving depots of procaine penicillin G, a form of penicillin of relatively low water solubility. Its prolonged action on intramuscular injection of concentrated aqueous suspensions is due in part to the low solubility of the compound, and in part to the fact that these suspensions tend to form compact and cohesive deposits which retard dissociation of the complex and release of the penicillin. Comparable amounts of the compound administered by intramus-

Table IV—Rheological Properties of Ointments Based on Petrolatum[15]

	Composition, %			Rheological properties				
No	White petrolatum	Mineral oil	White wax	$\tau_{\text{yield}}{}^a$ dyne / cm^2	$\eta_{\text{plastic}}{}^a$ poise	$\tau_{\text{yield}}{}^b$ dyne / cm^2	$\eta_{\text{plastic}}{}^b$ poise	M^c dyne sec / cm^2
1	80	0	20	27,400	120	33,900	66	100
2	90	0	10	14,200	60	14,900	40	40
3	100	0	0	9,900	38	11,600	26	23
4	90	10	0	4,000	30	5,400	20	21
5	80	20	0	900	31	2,500	18	26
6	70	30	0	800	23	2,000	14	17
			ZnO^d					
7	70	30	0	800	23	2,000	14	17
8	66.5	28.5	5	200	33	1,700	18	29
9	63	27	10	0	36	1,500	21	29
10	59.5	25.5	15	3,700	38	6,600	20	35
11	56	24	20	4,700	43	6,500	24	35

^{a} Maximum shear rate 125 sec^{-1}.
^{b} Maximum shear rate 210 sec^{-1}.
^{c} Thixotropic index, defined by Eq 12.
^{d} Zinc oxide replaces white wax in lines 7–11.

cular injection of dilute aqueous suspensions formed no de-pots, maintaining therapeutically effective blood levels for much shorter periods of time because of fast dispersion and absorption.

Aqueous suspensions containing between 40 and 70% w/v of milled or micronized procaine penicillin G plus small amounts of sodium citrate and polysorbate 80 were thixotropic pastes. Ober and co-workers measured their flow properties with a coaxial-cylinder viscometer capable of producing shear rates up to 2000 sec^{-1}, approaching those produced by injection through hypodermic syringes. The yield values and the areas of the hysteresis loop of the pastes were found to increase with increasing specific surface area and increasing concentration of the powder. Apparent viscosities above the yield value were low. The pastes recovered their original flow properties completely within minutes of being sheared at the highest speed in the viscometer.

As the specific surface area of the powders and the yield values and hysteresis loop areas of their suspensions increased continually, the tendency to plug hypodermic needles went through a minimum. Suspensions of the coarsest and finest powders were troublesome, plugging needles relatively frequently. Suspensions containing powders of intermediate particle size caused little or no plugging. Suspensions of coarser powders probably plugged the needles because aggregates of a few particles were large enough to block the ducts. The finest powders caused plugging by imparting excessively high yield values to the suspensions, so that they could not be extruded at shear stresses corresponding to the maximum pressure applied to the syringes.

Prolonged therapeutic action of the suspensions depended directly on the formation of compact, spherical deposits at the site of the injection. These depots resisted disintegration by the tissue fluids because of their high consistency. By presenting a small surface to these fluids, they retarded the release of the penicillin. The formation of cohesive and spherical depots in turn depended on high yield values and rapid thixotropic recovery of these yield values after the injection of the suspensions into the muscle tissue.

Thus, the prolonged therapeutic action of procaine penicillin G suspensions was determined entirely by their rheological properties. Low yield values and small hysteresis loop areas, produced by low specific surface areas and/or low concentrations of the powders, caused the suspensions to spread and disperse at the site of the injection rather than forming depots. This resulted in rapid release and absorption of the penicillin and short duration of therapeutically effective blood levels. Excessively high yield values and large hysteresis loops, produced by very high specific surface areas and/or high concentrations of the powders, made injection of the suspensions difficult or impossible because of plugging. Yield values which were low enough to permit extrusion of the suspensions through the hypodermic needles yet high enough to produce compact, spherical depots, combined with rapid thixotropic recovery of paste structure and yield values at the site of the injection to strengthen the depots, led to penicillin blood levels which remained above the minimum effective concentration for at least 4 days.

Self-Bodying Action of Mixed Emulsifiers

O/W emulsions of mineral oil, stabilized with surfactants like sodium lauryl sulfate, cetrimide (cetyl or tetradecyl trimethylammonium bromide) or cetomacrogol 1000, a nonionic polyoxyethylated surfactant based on hexadecanol with an average of 20–24 ethylene oxide units, are fluid liquids. Their low viscosity may lead to creaming and coalescence. The British Pharmacopoeia and the British Pharmaceutical Codex list Emulsifying Waxes, which are combinations of any one of these surfactants with cetostearyl alcohol, a mixture of 77%

stearyl alcohol, 21% cetyl alcohol, and lower homologs. The mixed emulsifier system surfactant-fatty alcohol produces a *self-bodying action*. It thickens the emulsions to consistencies ranging from fluid liquids to stiff, viscoelastic semisolids, depending on the total percentage and on the proportion of the mixed emulsifiers. The optimum proportion of fatty alcohol to surfactant for maximum thickening is 9:1. Myristyl and cetyl alcohols are also effective in producing viscous and stable emulsions in combination with any one of the three surfactants. Lauryl alcohol and lower homologs and stearyl alcohol, on the other hand, contribute little or no bodying and stabilizing action.

The mechanism of this self-bodying action was elucidated by Barry et al[32] and by Talman.[33] A representative ointment contains 1 part surfactant, 9 parts cetostearyl alcohol, 30 parts mineral oil, and 60 parts water. The fatty alcohol is melted and dispersed in the mineral oil preheated to 60–70°. This blend is slowly stirred into the aqueous surfactant solution preheated to the same temperature. The mixture is then cooled fast to room temperature while being stirred. This causes it to stiffen to a creamy consistency.

The concentration of cetostearyl alcohol in the mineral oil exceeds its solubility. At the higher temperature, the alcohol distributes itself between the oil phase and the water phase containing surfactant micelles, ie, the excess alcohol migrates from the oil to the water. It interacts with the aqueous surfactant to produce a liquid crystalline phase or *mesophase*, which is probably smectic due to lamellar micelles, and which forms a submicroscopic gel-like network structure throughout the aqueous phase. On cooling, this gel network retains its liquid crystalline character: Cooling is carried out too fast to permit phase equilibration. The network may be reinforced by solidified cetostearyl alcohol. As the gel structure is in the continuous phase, it confers viscoelasticity, a high apparent viscosity, thixotropy, and sometimes a yield value to the emulsion. These rheological properties prevent creaming of the oil droplets which are trapped and more or less immobilized in the mesh of liquid crystals plus precipitated fatty alcohol. Emulsions of mineral oil in water stabilized with the mixed emulsifier system comprising fatty alcohol and surfactant owe their consistency and stability mostly to the liquid crystalline gel network in the aqueous, continuous phase. The fact that the emulsifiers also form condensed mixed films at the O/W interface does not suffice to fully stabilize the emulsions. At low concentrations of fatty alcohol, they were fluid and prone to creaming and breaking.

The droplets of mineral oil in the emulsions produced with the Emulsifying Waxes were small, with mean diameters of about 1 μm. They were agglomerated, more so at higher emulsifier concentrations. Microscopic examination between crossed Nicol prims showed the aggregated droplets to be embedded in and held together by an anisotropic, filamentous matrix. With increasing concentration of the mixed emulsifier system, the emulsions changed from mobile liquids to semisolid creams. Their apparent viscosity increased; their thixotropy, represented by the area of the hysteresis loop, became more extensive, and their compliance was lowered, indicating that they became more viscoelastic.

The ionic surfactants sodium lauryl sulfate and cetrimide had a more effective bodying action when combined with cetostearyl alcohol than did the nonionic polyoxyethylated surfactant. Aqueous solutions of the two ionic surfactants penetrated bulk cetostearyl and cetyl alcohols rapidly above 46–47° to form liquid crystals, whereas cetomacrogol solutions penetrated the fatty alcohols only slowly even at 60–70°. During the emulsification process involving a fatty alcohol and the ionic surfactants, the development of a liquid crystalline phase in the aqueous medium took place mostly at the high temperature employed during mixing, so that the self-bodying action was largely complete soon after the emulsion had been cooled to room temperature. Most of the self-bodying action of emulsions made with cetostearyl alcohol and cetomacrogol, on the other hand, took place very slowly on storage at room temperature. To develop comparable consistency, the mixed emulsifier system comprising the nonionic surfactant had to be employed at higher concentrations than the mixed systems comprising either of the two ionic surfactants.

Techniques for Rheological Measurements

This section outlines the basic aspects of some of the most frequently used instruments. Detailed descriptions are given in specialized texts.[3,5,8,12]

Techniques for Measuring the Mechanical Properties of Solids

Tensile properties such as yield point, ultimate strength, elongation to break, Young's modulus, and energy to break are determined with tensile testers, eg, those manufactured by the Instron Corp., Canton, MA, or Testing Machines Inc., Amityville, NY.

A flat specimen, cut into an appropriate (eg, dumbbell) shape, is attached to two clamps. One clamp is stationary. It is connected to an electro-mechanical transducer which translates the applied force into an electric signal, eg, through a change in the electric resistance of a strain-gage wire. The other clamp is moved at a controlled speed by a motor, thereby stretching the sample. An x-y recorder plots stress versus time or strain, tracing curves such as those in Fig 22-1. The sample can also be subjected to programmed stress cycles, held at constant stress while the strain or creep is being recorded, or held at constant elongation while the stress decay is being measured.

Viscometers for Liquids and Semisolids

A wide variety of viscometers is available commercially. It is necessary to select one suitable for the range of viscosities encountered in a given application. The instrument must provide the required rheological information over the desired range of shear, time under shear, and temperature. This should be combined with ease of operation, good reproducibility, and relatively low cost.

The danger inherent in measuring the apparent viscosity of a material at a single rate of shear instead of covering a wide range[6] is illustrated in Fig 13 of Ref 12. A Newtonian and a pseudoplastic liquid as well as two plastic materials of different yield values and different plastic viscosities all have the same apparent viscosity at 200 sec^{-1} and 4000 dyne/cm^2, which is the point of intersection of their consistency curves. Measuring the apparent viscosity over a range of shear rates but maintaining the material for only short times at each shear rate can also give misleading results by missing thixotropic effects. The latter are usually detected by measuring the consistency first at increasing shear rates and, after reaching the desired maximum value, at decreasing shear rates. This cycle may be repeated until the up and down curves coincide or until they undergo no further changes. Curves like those of Figs 22-5, 6, 9, 11, or 12 may result, establishing the difference between thixotropic and nonthixotropic behavior. An alternate technique is to keep the material at a constant shear rate for a given period of time and to observe the decay, if any, of the shear stress required to maintain this shear rate. This may be interspersed with periods at rest, as shown in Fig 22-13.

One of the two principal methods for measuring viscosity is based on the rate of flow of a liquid through an orifice or a duct of simple geometry. The other method depends on the resistance to rotation of a metallic body in contact with or

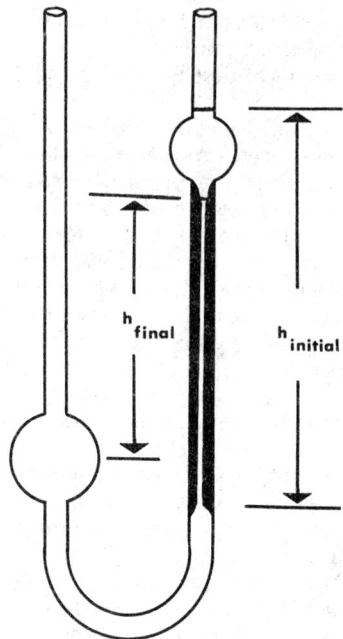

Fig 22-14. Glass capillary viscometer (courtesy, Schott H, Martin AN. In Dittert L, ed: *American Pharmacy*, 7th ed, Lippincott, Philadelphia, Chap 6, 1974).

immersed in the liquid. A third method, based on the velocity of a metal sphere rolling or falling through the liquid under the effect of gravity, or of an air bubble rising through the liquid, is not described here because of its limited use. Its principle is given by Stokes' equation discussed in Chapter 21.

Capillary Viscometer—The glass capillary Cannon-Fenske, Ubbelohde, and Ostwald viscometers are the most popular instruments based on the first method. The duct is a cylindrical capillary, and the driving force causing the liquid to flow through it is its weight. Thus, ΔP in Poiseuille's law (Eq 7) is replaced by the hydrostatic pressure hdG of a liquid column of height h and density d; G is the acceleration of gravity. A standard volume of the liquid is transferred into the viscometer. Liquid is then drawn into the upper reservoir bulb of the instrument by suction (see Fig 22-14). The efflux time t required for the liquid level to fall from the upper to the lower benchmark, emptying the upper reservoir, is measured with a stopwatch. The height h is the difference between the liquid levels in the two arms of the viscometer. It decreases as liquid flows through the capillary, but its time-averaged value is constant for a given viscometer containing a constant volume of liquid.

After replacing ΔP by hdG in Eq 7 and rearranging it, an instrumental constant $K = \pi R^4 hG/8LV$ can be separated, reducing Eq 7 to

$$\eta = Ktd \qquad (13)$$

Calibration of the viscometer consists in determining the constant K with a liquid of known viscosity and density by measuring the efflux time t.

The major portion of the potential energy represented by the hydrostatic pressure head is dissipated in overcoming the viscous resistance against flow in the capillary tube, ie, the friction of layer slipping past concentric layer. This portion is converted into heat. However, a small portion of the potential energy is required to accelerate the liquid as it enters the capillary from the reservoir (*kinetic energy correction*). Another small amount is used up in converging the streamlines from the broad reservoir into the narrow capillary and in spreading the streamlines upon issuing from the capillary (entrance or end effects, also called *Couette correction*).[2,5,6,8,13]

The liquid used to calibrate the viscometer should have approximately the same flow time t as the unknown, in order to minimize these two corrections when using Eq 13. It is not even necessary to evaluate K. It suffices to measure the flow time t_1 for the reference liquid of known viscosity η_1 and density d_1, and to compare it with the flow time t_2 for the liquid of density d_2 whose viscosity η_2 is to be determined. The equation

$$\eta_2 = \left(\frac{t_2 d_2}{t_1 d_1}\right)\eta_1 \qquad (14)$$

gives the unknown viscosity.

A range of glass capillary viscometers of different diameters is available for liquids of different viscosity. The efflux times should exceed 200 sec to minimize the kinetic energy correction and the possible error when starting and stopping the stopwatch. The usual glass capillary viscometers afford viscosity measurements at only one time-averaged value of shear rate. A range of shear rates can be covered when external pressure must be applied to force a viscous liquid through a narrow capillary. A variety of capillary extrusion viscometers operating under pressure are commercially available.[8]

Rotational Viscometers—These instruments depend on the fact that a solid rotating body immersed in a liquid is subjected to a retarding force due to the viscous drag, which is proportional to the viscosity of the liquid. The advantages of rotational viscometers are that the shear rate can be varied over a wide range of values, and that continuous measurements at a given shear rate or shear stress can be made for extended periods of time, affording measurements of the time-dependency as well as of the shear-dependency of the viscosity.

The entire liquid sample is in shear for as long as the rotational viscometer is being operated. Its temperature rises progressively as the energy used to overcome its viscous resistance is transformed into heat. The higher the viscosity, the greater the heat buildup. Since the viscosity of liquids depends strongly on temperature, accurate temperature control is essential. Rotational viscometers have arrangements for circulating water from a constant-temperature bath past the liquid sample, eg, around the cup. In capillary viscometers, only a small portion of the test liquid is sheared at any given moment, and the measurements are intermittent. Despite the minimal heat buildup, glass capillary viscometers are usually operated in constant-temperature baths.

Coaxial-Cylinder Viscometers—In Couette-type or coaxial-cylinder viscometers, the material is contained in the annular gap between an inner cylindrical bob or spindle and an outer, concentric cylindrical cup. In the *Stormer viscometer*, the cup is stationary. The bob or rotor is driven by weights suspended at the end of a pulley to which the shaft of the bob is connected. The shear stress is varied by applying different weights. The weights fall freely. The shear rate is measured as the speed of rotation of the bob: The number of revolutions per minute (rpm) is determined by means of a revolution counter connected to the shaft of the bob, and a stopwatch. The instrument is stopped between readings while the pulley is rewound and the weights are changed. This makes it poorly suited for the study of thixotropic materials of short recovery times.

In the more advanced and versatile *Haake Rotovisco*, the cup is likewise fixed. The bob is rotated at a constant though adjustable speed which can be varied to cover four decades of rpm or shear rates. The torque on the rotating bob required to maintain a constant speed of rotation against the viscous drag of the liquid is measured with a dynamometer consisting

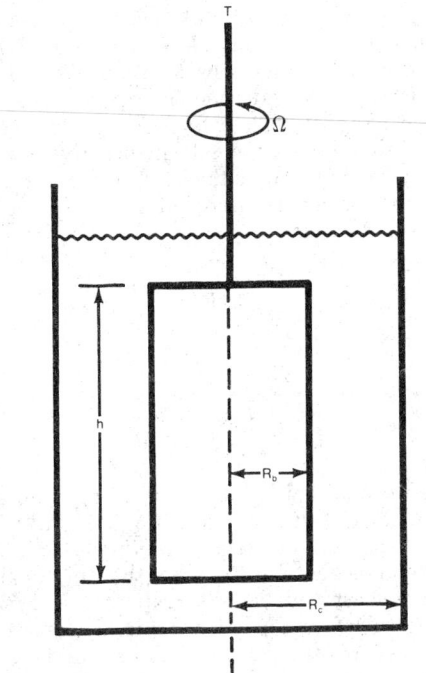

Fig 22-15.   Geometry of a coaxial-cylinder viscometer.

of a torsion spring interposed between the motor and the bob. Torque is the product of the force producing the rotation times the length of the lever or the perpendicular distance between the axis of rotation and the line along which the force acts. The deflection or twist of the spring generates an electric signal by means of a potentiometer. The shear stress is read as the deflection of a needle on the torque scale or plotted on the vertical scale of an *x-y* recorder where the horizontal scale represents the rpm.

In another concentric-cylinder viscometer, the outer cup is rotated at a constant though adjustable speed. The torque on the bob is measured as the deflection or twist of the torsion wire from which the bob is suspended. This is the principle of the *MacMichael viscometer*.

The geometry of a coaxial-cylinder viscometer is shown in Fig 22-15. The viscosity is calculated[2,5,6,8,14] by means of the *Margules equation*,[2,8]

$$\eta = \frac{\left(\dfrac{1}{R_b{}^2} - \dfrac{1}{R_c{}^2}\right)}{4\pi h}\left(\frac{T}{\Omega}\right) = K\left(\frac{S}{\text{rpm}}\right) \qquad (15)$$

where η is the Newtonian viscosity, or the apparent viscosity of a non-Newtonian material, R_b and R_c the radii of bob and cup, respectively; h is the height of the bob immersed in the liquid, T the torque, and Ω the angular velocity in radians/sec; Ω times $60/2\pi$ or 9.55 equals rpm. This conversion factor and the instrumental constants are combined to give the calibration factor K, which can be determined experimentally for each combination of bob and cup by means of a Newtonian calibrating liquid of known viscosity. S is the number of divisions on the torque scale.

Eq 15 was derived for two coaxial cylinders of infinite length. The *end effect* is the traction on both end surfaces of the bob if it is completely immersed in the liquid, or on its bottom surface if it is only partly immersed. It is corrected approximately by using the calibration factor K. The shear rate is lower at the ends of the bob than in the gap between cup and bob. Therefore, pseudoplastic liquids have higher apparent viscosities in the end zones, and this procedure is not accurate for them. Another approximate correction for the end effect consists in adding an increment Δh to the height

h of the bob to arrive at an effective height. For a partly immersed bob with a flat bottom, Δh is frequently of the order of $0.1h$. The added height can be determined experimentally for each material by filling the annular gap to different depths of immersion of the bob. The ratio T/Ω is plotted against the height or depth of immersion h. The negative intercept of this usually straight line with the h axis represents Δh.[5,8]

The shear stress in the material at a given radius R is expressed by the equation

$$\tau = \frac{T}{2\pi R^2 h} \qquad (16)$$

The rate of shear is given by

$$\dot{\gamma} = \frac{2\Omega}{R^2\left(\dfrac{1}{R_b{}^2} - \dfrac{1}{R_c{}^2}\right)} \qquad (17)$$

R varies between R_c and R_b. Since R_b is the smallest value of R, and R^2 is in the denominator in Eqs 16 and 17, shear stress and rate of shear are maximum at the surface of the bob or inner cylinder where $R = R_b$. R_c is the largest value of R and, therefore, shear stress and shear rate have their minimum values at the wall of the cup or outer cylinder, where $R = R_c$. Making these substitutions into Eqs 16 and 17 gives the maximum and minimum values for τ and $\dot{\gamma}$.

A disadvantage of the Couette viscometers is that the shear rate is not uniform at a given rpm but varies across the annular gap. Couette viscometers have several bobs and/or cups. The variation of the shear rate across the gap can be minimized by choosing a combination with a small gap. Two precautions are recommended when studying suspensions. The gap should be 10–100 times wider than the diameter of the largest particles. The cylinder surfaces should be roughened for fine particles and ribbed or knurled for coarse particles to cause some of the particles to be entrapped and carried around with the rotating cylinder. Otherwise, fluid suspending medium separates at the moving surface and its viscosity, rather than the viscosity of the entire suspension, is being measured.[5,8]

Brookfield Synchro-Lectric Viscometer—This instrument measures the viscous traction on a spindle rotating in the liquid, which is contained in a beaker: $1/R_c{}^2$ is essentially zero, and the rate of shear varies widely throughout the sample. There are various models equipped with either four or eight fixed speeds. Each instrument has a set of interchangeable cylindrical spindles or discs of different diameters, to be used for liquids of different viscosities. The spindle is driven by a synchronous motor through a beryllium-copper torsion spring. Different models have springs of different degrees of stiffness and are suitable for different viscosity ranges. The degree to which the spring is wound at a given rpm is indicated by a pointer on a dial calibrated in torque units. Multiplying the dial reading by the constant appropriate for the spindle and for the rpm gives the apparent viscosity of the liquid in centipoises at that rpm. A guard can be mounted around the spindle to prevent it from being deflected laterally and thereby cause misalignment of the shaft. The viscometer spindle can be inserted not only into beakers in the laboratory but also into kettles, reactors and mixing tanks in the plant. Thus, the viscometer can be adapted for continuous in-line viscosity measurements as well as for recording and/or controlling viscosities.

Cone-and-Plate Viscometers—These instruments consist of a rotating cone with a very obtuse angle and a stationary lower flat plate. The plate is raised until the apex of the cone just touches its surface. The liquid fills the narrow triangular gap between cone and plate (see Fig 22-16). Its surface tension prevents it from spreading on the plate. The plate is maintained at a constant temperature by circulating water.

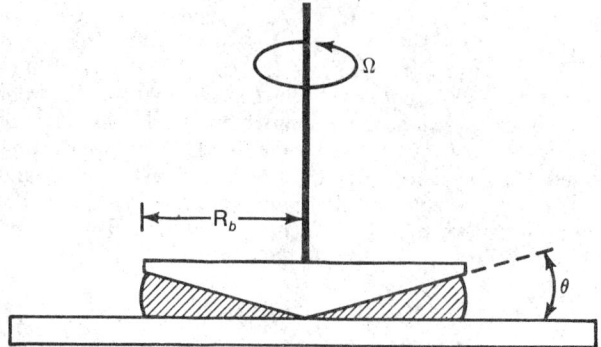

Fig 22-16.   Geometry of a cone-and-plate viscometer.

The cone is driven at controlled speeds which can be varied continuously. The viscous drag on the rotating cone exerts a torque on a dynamometer which is proportional to the shear stress. The angle θ formed by cone and plate is usually less than 3° and the average gap width is less than 2 mm. This results in a uniform rate of shear throughout the sample, given by Ω/θ. An added advantage of the instrument is that sample volumes smaller than 0.5 cm^3 are required. For small values of θ in radians, the Newtonian viscosity, or the apparent viscosity for non-Newtonian materials, is[5,8,9]

$$\eta = \left(\frac{3\theta}{2\pi R_b{}^3}\right)\left(\frac{T}{\Omega}\right) \qquad (18)$$

where T and Ω are as defined for Eq. 15 and R_b is the maximum cone radius. Cone-and-plate viscometers are manufactured by Ferranti Electric Inc (Ferranti-Shirley viscometer) and by Brookfield Engineering Laboratories Inc. The Haake Rotovisco also has a cone-and-plate attachment.

Comparison between Instruments—When a material is to be studied over a wide range of shear rates, more than one viscometer may be used because each individual instrument may have too limited a range. When the flow curves are plotted as maximum shear stress versus maximum rate of shear, instruments of different dimensions and even based on different principles produce a single curve for a given material at a given temperature. Maximum shear stress and maximum rate of shear are measured at the surface of the bob in coaxial-cylinder viscometers (Eqs 16 and 17 with $R = R_b$) and at the wall of the capillary in capillary viscometers (Eqs 6 and 5). When studying a material with two viscometers, it is advisable to use both instruments in the range of overlapping shear rates to ensure that the corresponding flow curves do indeed coincide. When flow curves are plotted as torque units versus rpm, they depend on the geometry of the viscometer.

Other Instruments—

Penetrometers—In the case of semisolids or very viscous liquids, a cone or needle attached to a holding rod is released and plunges vertically into the sample under the influence of its own or added weight. The depth of penetration within a given time interval, eg, 10 sec, is used to rate the consistency of the material.[5,8,12] The results cannot be translated into viscosity and yield values.

Measurement of Viscoelasticity—Measurements of viscosity are best made over a wide range of shear rates including values comparable to use conditions (*cf* Table II). The most valuable information from viscoelastic measurements, on the other hand, is obtained at small strains, where the structure of the material under investigation is preserved. Large strains and high shear rates tend to disrupt elastic network structures.

The parameters for describing and the instrumentation for measuring viscoelasticity are outside the scope of this chapter. Refs 5, 8, 34, and especially 35 should be consulted.

References

1. Houwink R: *Elasticity, Plasticity and Structure of Matter*, 2nd ed, Harren Press, Washington, DC, 1953.
2. Reiner M: *Deformation, Strain and Flow*, 2nd ed, Interscience, New York, 1960.
3. Nielsen LE: *Mechanical Properties of Polymers*, Reinhold, New York, 1962.
4. Billmeyer FW: *Textbook of Polymer Science*, 2nd ed, Wiley-Interscience, New York, 1971.
5. Sherman P: *Industrial Rheology*, Academic, London and New York, 1970.
6. Green H: *Industrial Rheology and Rheological Structures*, Wiley, New York, 1949.
7. Hermans JJ: *Flow Properties of Disperse Systems*, Interscience, New York, 1953.
8. Van Wazer JR, *et al: Viscosity and Flow Measurement*, Interscience, New York, 1963.
9. Wilkinson WL: *Non-Newtonian Fluids*, Pergamon, New York, 1960.
10. Ruch TC, Patton HD: *Physiology and Biophysics*, Saunders, Philadelphia, 1965.
11. Ree T, Eyring H. In Eirich FR, ed: *Rheology*, vol 2, Academic, New York, 1958.
12. Martin AN, *et al.* In Bean HS, *et al*, eds: *Advances in Pharmaceutical Sciences*, vol 1, Academic, London and New York, 1964.
13. Mysels KJ: *Introduction to Colloid Chemistry*, Wiley-Interscience, New York, 1959.
14. Fischer EK: *Colloidal Dispersions*, Wiley, New York, 1950.
15. Kostenbauder HB, Martin AN: *J APhA Sci Ed 43:* 401, 1954.
16. Chaffey, CE: *J Colloid Interface Sci 56:* 495, 1976.
17. Gillespie T: *J Colloid Interface Sci 15:* 219, 1960 and *22:* 554, 1966.
18. Cross MM: *J Colloid Interface Sci 20:* 417, 1965 and *33:* 30, 1970.
19. Sherman P: *Emulsion Science*, Academic, London and New York, 1968.
20. Davis SS: *J Pharm Sci 58:* 412 and 418, 1969.
21. Litt M, *et al: Biorheology 13:* 37, 1976.
22. Gilboa A, Silberberg A: *Biorheology 13:* 59, 1976.
23. Davis SS, *et al: Biorheology 12:* 225, 1975.
24. Khan MA, *et al: Biochim Biophys Acta 444:* 369, 1976.
25. "Workshop on Cough & Expectoration," *Eur J Respir Dis 61*, Supplement 110, 1980: Davis SS, 141; Loefdahl C-G, Odeblad E, 113; Richardson PS, 67.
26. Chantler EN, *et al*, eds: *Mucus in Health & Disease*—II, Plenum, New York, 1982: Silberberg A, Meyer FA, 53; Marriott C, *et al*, 85, 89; Puchelle E, *et al*, 397.
27. Ribitsch V, Schurz J: *Rheol Acta 18:* 139, 1979; *21:* 81, 1982.
28. Altmann S, Zeidler H: *Rheol Acta 16:* 378, 1977; *18:* 151, 1979; *19:* 642, 1980.
29. Neumann BS. In Bean HS, *et al*, eds: *Advances in Pharmaceutical Sciences*, vol 2, Academic, London and New York, 1967.
30. Barry BW, Meyer MC: *J Pharm Sci 62:* 1349, 1973.
31. Ober SS, *et al: J APhA Sci Ed 47:* 667, 1958.
32. Barry BW, *et al: J Pharm Sci 62:* 1954, 1973 and previous publications listed as references.
33. Talman FAJ, Rowan EM: *J Pharm Pharmacol 22:* 338, 1970 and previous publications listed as references.
34. Thurston GB, Martin AN: *J Pharm Sci 67:* 1499, 1978.
35. Ferry JD: *Viscoelastic Properties of Polymers*, 2nd ed, Wiley, New York, 1970.

PART 3

Pharmaceutical Chemistry

Thomas Medwick, PhD

College of Pharmacy
Rutgers—The State University
Busch Campus
New Brunswick, NJ 08903

CHAPTER 23

Inorganic Pharmaceutical Chemistry

Clarence A Discher, PhD

Professor Emeritus
Rutgers University
New Brunswick, NJ

Basis of Chemical Reactions

Although many subatomic particles have been identified during recent decades, only the protons and neutrons of the nucleus of an atom and the extranuclear electrons will be considered here.

Each atom of an element is uniquely described by two pure numbers, its atomic number and its atomic weight. The atomic number gives the number of protons present in the nucleus and therefore its positive charge. Since the ground state atom must be neutral this in turn defines the number of extranuclear electrons. The difference between the atomic number and the atomic weight of a given *isotope* of an element defines the number of neutrons in the nucleus. (Atomic weights in the tables are not whole numbers because they represent the weighted average of the atomic weights of all isotopes present.)

The electrons are arranged in major quantum groups (energy levels, orbitals) occupying the space about the nucleus. Each electron is assigned four quantum numbers: the principle quantum number, n, describes the relative position of an energy level with respect to the other energy levels present; the subquantum number, l, describes the different electron distributions possible for a given value of n; the magnetic quantum number, m_l, is best described as the magnetic contribution to the angular momentum due to the movement of the electrons in space; the magnetic spin quantum number, m_s, is the magnetic component contributed by the spin of the electron. The permitted values for n are $1, 2, 3, \ldots$, for l are $0, 1, 2, \ldots (n-1)$, for m_l are $-l, \ldots 0, \ldots +1$, and for $m_s \pm \frac{1}{2}$. Returning to the subquantum number l; when l is 0 the electrons occupying the suborbital are known as s electrons, when l is 2, p electrons, when 3, d electrons, and when 4, f electrons. Thus if 2 electrons occupy suborbital 0 of major quantum group 3, they are represented as $3s^2$.

In assigning electrons to the atom the Aufbau Principle is used. It is an application of Quantum Theory, Hund's Rules, and the Pauli Exclusion Principle. Simply stated, a given entering electron must occupy the lowest unoccupied energy level of the atom. In other words, each electron must have a unique set of quantum numbers.

As a result of the above process, all atoms except hydrogen and the inert gases, have one or more completely occupied lower major quantum groups and have the suborbitals of their highest major quantum group only partially filled. The electrons of this outer, partially filled, energy level give each element its distinct chemical properties. These are the valence electrons.

Chemical reactions entail the removal of valence electrons, adding electrons to a partly filled valence shell, or sharing a pair of valence electrons between two atoms. Most atoms attempt to achieve a rare gas outer shell, $(ns^2$ or $ns^2np^6)$, by these processes. The energy required for the removal of the electron of least energy is known as the first ionization potential. It is unique for each element. The metals have low ionization potentials and therefore readily form cations. Nonmetals have high ionization potentials.

The attraction of a nucleus for electrons is termed its electronegativity. Metals have low electronegativities (they are electropositive), while nonmetals (especially the halogens) have high electronegativities. This allows the latter to attract additional electrons to form anions.

When atoms with widely differing electronegativities react, eg, sodium, 0.93, and chlorine, 3.98, an electron transfer takes place. The one valence electron of sodium $(3s^1)$ enters the incompletely filled $(3s^23p^5)$ valence shell of the chlorine. Sodium now has an inert gas (Ne) electron structure with a +1 charge. The chlorine achieves the argon structure with a −1 charge. There is no formal electron-pair bond between the two entities. A crystal of sodium chloride consists of equal numbers of sodium and chloride ions held in place by the interaction of the spherically symmetrical positive cation field and the spherically symmetrical negative anion field. These ionic (electrostatic) compounds are characterized by high boiling and melting points and most are water soluble.

If two reacting atoms have similar electronegativities, eg, two hydrogen atoms, a sharing of electrons takes place. One electron is donated to the bond from an incompletely filled suborbital of each atom. A covalent bond is formed by the overlap of the two atomic orbitals involved. With the formation of the bond a molecule results. The bonding electrons are no longer restricted to their atomic orbitals. They are now free to move in a molecular orbital between the two atoms in what is known as a σ molecular orbital.

When the electronegativities of the two atoms involved in the formation of a covalent bond are not identical the atom with the higher electronegativity tends to attract the electrons of the molecule more strongly than its partner. This leads to polarization of the molecule; a dipole results. The extent of polarization is directly proportional to the difference in electronegativities. Such bonds are said to have partial ionic character.

In practice only the most electropositive atoms reacting with the most electronegative atoms result in purely electrostatic compounds, and only atoms with equal electronegativities form purely covalent bonds. Those bonds formed from elements between these extremes have partial covalent or partial electrostatic character.

Atoms with orbitals occupied by an unshared pair of electrons can share this electron pair with an atom lacking two or more electrons in its valence shell. The bond formed is said to be a coordinate covalent bond. Once this bond has been formed it can not be distinguished from an ordinary covalent bond; the difference lies only in the manner of formation. The formation of the ammonium ion from an ammonia molecule, which has an unshared electron pair, and a hydrogen ion, which has an empty s-orbital, illustrates this type of reaction.

Covalent compounds have low melting and boiling points, and are usually insoluble in water. Solubility in water can be induced by introducing an acid or base group into the molecule. Reaction with base or acid will now give a soluble salt.

Other types of bonding exist. Those of interest are weakly bonded; the compounds formed decompose more readily than the electrostatic and covalent types. Hydrogen bonding (bridging) is quite common. Dipole-dipole bonding is also possible; very weak associations result.

Complexes are compounds or ions formed when an atom or cation, *central unit*, acts as a center about which anions or molecules, *ligands*, arrange themselves. The central unit is said to have a *coordination number* equal to the number of complexing ligands. The maximum number of ligands which can arrange themselves about the central unit is known as its *maximum coordination number*; it is a function of the size of the central unit. Usual maximum coordination numbers are 2, 4, 6, or 8. The number of ligands which can coordinate with the central unit is also a function of ligand size. Thus, even though the maximum coordination number of aluminum is six, only four of the relatively large chloride ions can be accommodated as ligands, eg, $[AlF_6]^{3-}$ vs $[AlCl_4]^{1-}$ (See Chapter 14).

The bonding involved in the formation of complexes can be coordinate covalent or electrostatic. Bonds depending on permanent dipoles are also common, eg, hydrates.

Nomenclature

The great advances in chemistry during the past several decades have made necessary constant revision of systems of nomenclature, designed to give precise information with respect to the composition of chemical compounds. Whereas oil of vitriol and lunar caustic at one time were useful names, today they must be looked upon as trivial.

Classical Nomenclature—Prior to elucidation of the structure of coordination complexes, the naming of compounds was handled reasonably well through the utilization of nonnumerical prefixes and suffixes and Latin or Greek numerical prefixes. In general the main function of these prefixes and suffixes was to indicate the oxidation state of elements of variable valence, although some were intended to connote structural characteristics.

Systematic nomenclature must consider two problems; order of citation and stoichiometry. Order of citation is usually well defined; for salts and salt-like compounds the most electropositive element is named first, eg, sodium chloride. For nonmetals the International Union of Pure and Applied Chemistry (IUPAC) recommends the following order of citation:

B, Si, C, Sb, As, P, N, H, Se, S, I, Br, Cl, O, F.

Cations with a single oxidation state are simply named as the element. If a cation has two oxidation states the suffix *-ous* is used to indicate the lower oxidation state, eg, mercur*ous*, and the suffix *-ic* for the higher oxidation state, eg, mercur*ic*. (Obviously this system breaks down when an element exists in more than two oxidation states.) The simple anions are named using the suffix *-ide*. While the newer Stock system of nomenclature uses only the English names of the elements, classical nomenclature uses the stems of the Latin names in identifying the cations of copper, gold, tin, lead, and iron.

For the oxygenated anions a system of prefixes and suffixes was developed to indicate the oxidation state of the central atom. These are illustrated in Table I using the chlorine anions.

Sometimes one or more oxygen atoms of the anion are replaced by another element. The stem of the name of the substituting element is used as a prefix to the name for the fully oxygenated anion, eg, $Na_2S_2O_3$, sodium thiosulfate, Na_3AsS_4, sodium thioarsenate (sodium tetrathioarsenate).

In addition to variable oxidation numbers, oxygenated acids

Table I—Nomenclature for Oxygenated Acids and Salts

Cl Oxid state	Acid formula	Acid name	Anion name
−1	HCl	*Hydro*chloric acid	chlor*ide*
+1	HClO	*Hypo*chlor*ous* acid	*hypo*chlor*ite*
+3	$HClO_2$	Chlor*ous* acid	chlor*ite*
+5	$HClO_3$	Chloric acid	chlor*ate*
+7	$HClO_4$	*Per*chloric acid	*per*chlor*ate*

(and their salts) present two other nomenclature problems: (1) variation in the degree of hydration of the parent acid anhydride, and (2) the naming of the different salts arising from partial neutralization of polyprotic acids. Table II shows the prefixes used for naming the different phosphoric acids (P^{5+}).

For salts of diprotic acids the salt resulting from neutralization of only one proton per acid molecule is named by using the prefix *bi-* or the words hydrogen or acid with the anion, eg, $NaHCO_3$, sodium bicarbonate, acid carbonate, or hydrogen carbonate. The latter is preferred. Several methods have been devised for the triprotic acids. These are shown in Table III. It should be noted that while sodium phosphate is a correct chemical name for Na_3PO_4, the compendia uses this name for monohydrogen phosphate. Due to very strongly basic reaction of the solutions of Na_3PO_4 and other tertiary phosphates, the pharmacist must be especially alert when using containers labelled sodium phosphate.

It is evident from Table III that the numerical Greek prefixes hemi-, mono-, sesqui-, di-, tri-, tetra-, penta-, hexa-, hepta-, octa-, ennea- (nona-), and deca-, are also used in naming compounds. In fact there are compounds, eg, N_2O_4, dinitrogen tetraoxide, which must be named using numerical prefixes since modern systems of nomenclature are unable to precisely identify them.

Stock Nomenclature—Classical nomenclature is satisfactory for simpler compounds involving atoms with one or two oxidation states. It can not indicate proper stoichiometry when atoms having three or more oxidation states are involved. The Stock system of nomenclature attempts to overcome the problem.

In the Stock system simple cations are named as the element followed by its oxidation state, expressed in Roman numerals enclosed in parentheses, eg, Fe^{2+}, iron(II), Fe^{3+}, iron(III), Fe^{6+}, iron(VI). Simple anions use the suffix *-ide* as before. However, complex anions are named using the stem of the name of the central unit and the suffix *-ate* followed by its oxidation state, in Roman numerals, enclosed in parentheses. The ligand(s) involved are cited before the central unit of the complex. If two or more different ligands are present they are cited in alphabetical order, ignoring Greek prefixes. The number of each of the individual ligands involved is indicated by the use of Greek numerical prefixes. These latter rules also govern the citing of ligands associated with complex cations. The preferred nomenclature for common ligands is given in Table IV.

Table II—Nomenclature for the Phosphoric Acids

Water molecules	Resultant acid	Name
$H_2O + \frac{1}{2}P_2O_5$	HPO_3	*Meta*phosphoric acid
$2H_2O + P_2O_5$	$H_4P_2O_7$	*pyro*phosphoric acid *di*phosphoric acid
$3H_2O + P_2O_5$	H_3PO_4	*ortho*phosphoric acid phosphoric acid[a]
$5H_2O + 3P_2O_5$	$H_5P_3O_{10}$	*tri*phosphoric acid

[a] The phosphoric acid of commerce and science is orthophosphoric acid.

Table III—Nomenclature of the Phosphate Salts

Formula	NaH_2PO_4	Na_2HPO_4	Na_3PO_4
Preferred name	sodium dihydrogen phosphate	sodium monohydrogen phosphate	sodium phosphate
Other names	monobasic sodium phosphate	dibasic sodium phosphate	tribasic sodium phosphate
	primary sodium phosphate	secondary sodium phosphate	tertiary sodium phosphate
USP XX	monobasic sodium phosphate	dibasic sodium phosphate	. . .

Table IV—Nomenclature for Common Ligands

Ligand	Preferred prefix	Ligand	Preferred prefix
H_2O	aqua	HS^-	mercapto
NH_3	ammine	S^{2-}	thio (sulfo)[a] (sulfido)
CO	carbonyl	S_2^{2-}	disulfido
F^-	fluoro	SO_3^{2-}	sulfito
Cl^-	chloro	SO_4^{2-}	sulfato
Br^-	bromo	$S_2O_3^{2-}$	thiosulfato
I^-	iodo	NO^-	nitrosyl
O^{2-}	oxo (oxy)	ONO^-	nitrito
O_2^{2-}	peroxo (peroxy)	NO_2^-	nitro
OH^-	hydroxo (hydroxy)	CN^-	cyano
$C_2O_4^{2-}$	oxalato	SCN^-	thiocyanato
$NH_2CH_2CH_2NH_2$	ethylenediamine, or en	NCS^-	isothiocyanato

[a] Forms in parentheses are also used.

Stock names are not used for complex anions with well established classical names. These include sulfate, sulfite, nitrate, nitrite, carbonate, phosphate, thiosulfate, cyanate, and thiocyanate.

Ewens-Bassett—Sometimes it is advantageous to cite the charge on a complex ion rather than the oxidation state of the central unit. The Ewens-Bassett system gives the charge of the complex ion in Arabic numerals enclosed in parentheses, after the name. Other than this, the rules for naming a compound are similar to the Stock system. Thus, the common ferrocyanide ion, $[Fe(CN)_6]^{4-}$, becomes hexacyanoferrate(II) using Stock nomenclature, and hexacyanoferrate(−4) using the Ewens-Bassett system. Table V gives some examples of modern nomenclature.

A more thorough review of inorganic nomenclature may be found in Discher[1] or Huheey.[2] A comprehensive report on the subject will be found in Report of the Commission on Nomenclature of Inorganic Chemistry, issued by IUPAC.[3]

The Periodic Table and Families of Elements

The periodic table constitutes a valuable tool which systematizes the physical and chemical properties of the elements. A table is shown in the back cover of this textbook.

The utility of the periodic table lies in its ability to provide clues to the physical and chemical behavior of the elements and their compounds. Mendeleev could predict the existence of unknown elements of his time, and their behavior, eg, eka-silicon, now known as germanium. A knowledge of periodic relationships enabled atomic scientists to successfully postulate the properties of unknown post-uranic elements so that procedures could be designed for their recovery from atomic reaction products.

Based on periodic law, the periodic table arranges the elements into horizontal rows with the same outermost partly filled major quantum groups and into vertical columns which have elements with the same valence electron structures. As a result, in any given vertical group (family) the members exhibit similar behavior patterns. Differences are a matter of degree, depending upon atomic radius and the type of closed shell underlying the valence electron(s).

The vertical groups of the periodic table are identified by the Roman numerals, I to VIII, except for the inert gases which are assigned as Group 0. Each group divides into two subfamilies, A and B. In this chapter the "typical elements" will be designated the A subgroup, eg, I-A, the alkali metals, and the transition element members of the family will be designated the B subgroup. Group VIII is not divided into A and B subgroups. It consists of three triads of elements. The members of a given triad are remarkably similar in both physical and chemical properties, eg, the first triad, cobalt, nickel, and iron.

Hydrogen $(1s^1)$ and helium $(1s^2)$ constitute the first row of the periodic table. While helium is clearly the first member of Group 0, hydrogen is customarily placed at the head of both Group I-A, the alkalies, and Group VII-A, the halogens. Like

Table V—Examples of Modern Nomenclature

Formula	Classical name	Stock name	Ewens-Bassett[a]
$K_2[HgI_4]$	potassium mercuric iodide	potassium tetraiodomercurate(II)	(−2)
$[Ag(NH_3)_2]^+$	silver ammonia ion	diamminesilver(I) ion	(+1)
$Na_3[Au(S_2O_3)_2]$	sodium gold thiosulfate	sodium dithiosulfatoaurate(I)	(−3)
$[Fe(H_2O)_6]Cl_3$	hydrated ferric chloride	hexaaquairon(III) chloride	(+3)
$BiOCl$	bismuthyl chloride	bismuth(III) chloride oxide	[c]
$[Ni(CO)_4]$	nickel carbonyl	tetracarbonyl nickel(0)	[c]
$[(NH_3)_5CoO_2Co(NH_3)_5]^{4+}$	. . .	decammine-μ-peroxodicobalt(III) ion[b]	(+4)
$Na_2[Fe(CN)_5(NO)].2H_2O$	sodium nitroprusside	sodium pentacyanonitrosylferrate(III) dihydrate	(−2)

[a] This number, as shown, substitutes for the Roman numeral of the Stock name.
[b] This ion illustrates the use of μ to indicate a bridging structure, in this case the peroxo group.
[c] Not applicable.

the alkali metals, it exists as the monovalent cation, H^+, but like the halogens, it can also exist as the monovalent anion, H^-, the hydride ion.

Many of the vertical groups of the periodic table have common names. Group 0, the inert gases, Group I-A, the alkali metals, Group II-A, the alkaline earths, and Group VII-A, the halogens, have already been identified. Additional named groups are Group VI-A, the chalcogens, Group I-B, the coinage elements, and Group II-B, the volatile elements.

Those elements in which a d-orbital is partially filled, starting at Group III-B and ending at Group II-B, are known as transition elements. Horizontal similarities exist to a varying degree in the transition elements, especially in the lower oxidation states. As an example, the element palladium, to the left of silver, forms an insoluble chloride, $PdCl_2$, which is soluble in ammonia.

The lanthanides and actinides (inner transition elements) are fourteen member families in which f orbitals have one to fourteen electrons. Each family has very strong horizontal similarities since the electrons in the partly filled external s, p, and d orbitals are identical for most.

Because the energy levels of the electrons in the d and f orbitals of the transition elements and the inner transition elements, respectively, differ only slightly, these elements give rise to colored compounds. The energy emitted when an excited electron falls to a vacant lower level within the d or f orbitals is that of radiation in the visible range of light.

Starting at the upper right corner of the periodic table, as one proceeds down and to the left, the elements assume increasing metallic character; they become more basic, and less electronegative (more electropositive). The simple anions become less stable; the simple cations more stable. Thus, it may be said the nonmetals occupy the upper right area of the periodic table and the metallic elements are found to the left and toward the bottom. The so-called "heavy metals" are found in the two bottom rows. Metallic elements, for the most part, are protein precipitants, the major exception being the alkali metals. Being protein precipitants, metals, especially heavy metals, are toxic, eg, Ba, Tl, Pb, Hg, are violent poisons.

From the above it is obvious there must be an area in the periodic table where the elements are equally acidic and basic, that is, *amphoteric*. If a line is drawn diagonally through hydrogen and beryllium and through aluminum, germanium, antimony, and polonium, the elements on the line and some adjacent to it, are amphoteric. Thus, as a base aluminum forms compounds such as aluminum chloride, and equally well, as an acid it forms sodium aluminate.

In every "typical" element family the first member of the family can be quite unlike the other members. It more closely resembles the second member of the adjacent group to the right. These diagonally related elements are known as "diagonals" or "bridge" elements. They are:

IA	IIA	IIIA	IVA	VA	VIA	VIIA
Li	Be	B	C	N	O	F
Na	Mg	Al	Si	P	S	Cl

Beryllium and aluminum constitute a bridge pair. Beryllium fluoride is water soluble (but poorly ionized) while the fluorides of magnesium and the other alkaline earths are sparingly soluble. Unlike magnesium and the alkaline earths, beryllium readily acts as the central ion of complexes, both in the solid state and in solution. Like aluminum, beryllium is amphoteric, gives rise to alums, catalyses the Friedel-Craft reaction, etc.

Tables VI to XVII summarize some useful properties and facts concerning the groups of the periodic table. The second and third row "triads" of Group VIII and the lanthanides and actinides are not included in these tables because they present no important applications in pharmacy and medicine.

The orbital electrons are important since they predict the possible oxidation states, the shielding of the nuclear charge, and the polarizability for each element. Those oxidation states which have been identified for each element are also listed.

The atomic radius and the ionic radii give an indication of the relative size of the members of a family. The negative ions of an element are always larger than the neutral atom; the positive ions are always smaller. Because of the increasing effective nuclear charge for a given element, cations of higher charge are always smaller than those with a lower charge. This is important since it gives an indication of the effective coordination number of cations and atoms as central units of complexes.

The ionization potential* is a measure of the energy required to remove an electron by overcoming the attractive force of the nucleus. It is related to atomic size; removal of the first, (I), electron from beryllium and barium requires 9.3 ev and 5.2 ev, respectively. Because the removal of one electron effectively increases the nuclear charge by one unit, the second, (II), ionization potential is about double that of the first, 18.2 ev and 9.95 ev for beryllium and barium, respectively.

Electronegativity, discussed previously, gives an indication of the type of bonding resulting when two atoms react. It gives an indication of the extent of polarization in covalent compounds. It is also used to determine the order of citation in the naming of binary compounds (page 350).

---

* This use of the word potential is improper; ionization potential is a measure of energy.

Elements of Group 0

Because the inert gases were unknown at the time, Mendeleev made no provision for them in his proposed atomic table. With their subsequent discovery Group 0 seemed the most appropriate designation. The group fits very nicely into Mendeleev's arrangement. Its presence explains the extreme transition of properties in going from the very electronegative halogen family to the very electropositive alkali metal family. This shift in properties in going from halogen to inert gas to alkali metal is clearly shown by the change in the valence

electron structures:

$$(n-1)s^2(n-1)p^5$$
$$\rightarrow (n-1)s^2(n-1)p^6 \rightarrow (n-1)s^2(n-1)p^6ns^1.$$

All Group 0 elements except radon occur in the atmosphere. Helium also occurs in commercial quantities in certain natural gases in southwestern United States. Argon, neon, krypton,

Table VI—The Elements of Group O [a]

Element	Helium	Neon	Argon	Krypton	Xenon	Radon
Symbol	He	Ne	Ar	Kr	Xe	Rn
Atomic number	2	10	18	36	54	86
Atomic weight [b]	4.003	20.18	39.95	83.80	131.3	(222) [d]
Orbital electrons	$1s^2$	$[He]2s^22p^6$	$[Ne]3s^23p^6$	$[Ar]3d^{10}4s^24p^6$	$[Kr]4d^{10}5s^25p^6$	$[Xe]4f^{14}5d^{10}6s^26p^6$
Atomic radius (Å)	1.80	1.60	1.92	2.00	2.20	2.29
Ionization potential [c] ev	24.6	21.6	15.8	14.0	12.1	10.7
% by volume in air	5×10^{-4}	15×10^{-4}	0.94	11×10^{-5}	9×10^{-6}	...

[a] Physical data are from *Comprehensive Inorganic Chemistry*, J C Bailar, ed, Pergamon Press, 1973. Atomic and ionic radii from Pauling, *Nature of the Chemical Bond*, 3rd ed, Cornell University Press, 1960 and modified by the work of R D Shannon and C T Prewitt, *Acta Crystallogr* **B25**, 925 (1969). *Handbook of Chemistry and Physics*, Chemical Rubber Publishing Co, 1961.

[b] Given to four significant figures.

[c] First ionization potential unless otherwise noted.

[d] Atomic weights in parenthesis are not exactly known.

The above apply to Tables VI–XVII.

and xenon are produced from liquid air by fractional distillation. Helium is similarly produced from the natural gases named above. Radon is recovered from the natural decay products of radium.

The inert gases are monoatomic and are colorless, odorless gases under ordinary conditions of temperature and pressure. They vary widely in atomic mass and atomic volume. These differences are reflected in the values of their physical constants (Table VI).

Each inert gas, except helium, is characterized by an outermost electron shell of the "inert gas" structure, ns^2np^6 (Table VI). Helium has the $1s^2$ structure; the ns^2 structure is achieved in many stable cations, eg, Pb^{2+}. Since all electrons are paired, the chemical inertness of the group is predictable and is reflected in terms of peak ionization potentials and various other characteristics. However, under unusual reaction conditions, there is evidence of hydrate formation. Some relatively stable fluorides, eg, XeF_2, XeF_4, and XeF_6, a crystalline sodium perxenate, and possibly a perkryptate,

are known. However, in comparison with other elements, those of Group 0 are still logically classed as chemically inert.

Helium, because of its low density and low solubility in blood is used to prepare synthetic airs (page 372).

Argon is relatively plentiful since it is a by-product of the fractionation of liquid air for the production of oxygen and nitrogen. It is used as an inert atmosphere for industrial processes in which nitrogen, the usual inert atmosphere, reacts with the materials present.

Krypton and xenon have been investigated for possible use as anesthetics. However, the sparsity of these elements in nature imposes severe limitations on such use. ^{133}Xe is used for diagnostic studies both by inhalation and intravenous injection.

Radon is used instead of radium in the treatment of certain types of cancer. Sealed tubes containing the gas are embedded in the tissues to be treated. Both radium and radon emit alpha particles in the first stage of their radioactive decay.

Elements of Group I

The elements of this group, (Tables VII and VIII), are characterized by having only one valence electron, ns^1. The subgroups differ in that Group I-A has an underlying, stable, inert gas shell, $(n-1)s^2(n-1)p^6ns^1$, while in Group I-B this has been replaced by a completed d-shell, $(n-1)d^{10}ns^1$.

These elements are strongly metallic, giving rise to cations, M^+. Since electrons can be removed from the underlying d-shell, Group I-B elements can exhibit higher positive oxidation states, M^{2+}, and M^{3+}.

Table VII—Elements of Group I-A

Element	Hydrogen	Lithium	Sodium	Potassium	Rubidium	Cesium	Francium
Symbol	H	Li	Na	K	Rb	Cs	Fr
Atomic number	1	3	11	19	37	55	87
Atomic weight	1.008	6.94_1	22.99	39.10	85.47	132.91	(223)
Orbital electrons	$1s^1$	$[He]2s^1$	$[Ne]3s^1$	$[Ar]4s^1$	$[Kr]5s^1$	$[Xe]6s^1$	$[Rn]7s^1$
Oxidation states	$-1,+1$	+1	+1	+1	+1	+1	+1
Atomic radius (Å)	0.37	1.50	1.86	2.31	2.44	2.62	...
Ionic radius (Å)	$1.36(-1)$ [a]	$0.60(+1)$	$0.95(+1)$	$1.33(+1)$	$1.48(+1)$	$1.69(+1)$	$1.76(+1)$
Ionic (hydrated) radius (Å)	...	3.40	2.76	3.32	2.28	2.28	...
Ionization potential	13.527	5.39	5.14	4.34	4.18	3.89	...
Electronegativity, [b] ev	2.1	0.98	0.93	0.82	0.82	0.79	0.7
% of earth's crust	0.127	6.5×10^{-3}	2.8	2.6	3.1×10^{-2}	7×10^{-4}	...

[a] Hydride ion; figure in parenthesis is oxdation state.

[b] Pauling scale.

Table VIII—The Elements of Groups I-B and II-B

Element	Copper	Silver	Gold	Zinc	Cadmium	Mercury
Symbol	Cu	Ag	Au	Zn	Cd	Hg
Atomic number	29	47	79	30	48	80
Atomic weight	63.54	107.87	196.97	65.38	112.4	200.5_9
Orbital electrons	$[Ar]3d^{10}4s^1$	$[Kr]4d^{10}5s^1$	$[Xe]4f^{14}5d^{10}6s^1$	$[Ar]3d^{10}4s^2$	$[Kr]4d^{10}5s^2$	$[Xe]4f^{14}5d^{10}6s^2$
Oxidation states	+1,+2	+1,+2	+1,(+2),+3	+2	+2	+1,+2
Atomic radius (Å)	1.40	1.70	1.70	1.40	1.60	1.50
Ionic (crystal) radii (Å)	0.96(+1)	1.26(+1)	1.37(+1)	. . .	. . .	1.27(+1)
	0.72(+2)	0.89(+2)	0.99(+3)	0.88(+2)	1.09(+2)	1.16(+2)
Ionization potential, ev	7.724	7.574	9.223	6.92	8.99	10.42
Electronegativity	1.90	1.93	2.54	1.65	1.69	2.00
% of earth's crust	10^{-4}	10^{-8}	10^{-9}	1.3×10^{-2}	1.5×10^{-5}	ca 10^{-6}

Elements of Group I-A

This group comprises the most reactive of all the metallic elements; activity increasing with atomic number. The cations of these elements are chemically stable; the free elements are not found in nature. The single positive charge of the nucleus is effectively screened by the inert gas shell, thus these cations have little or no polarizing effect on anions and molecules and therefore do not form complexes.

The hydroxides give alkaline solutions, alkalinity increasing with atomic number. Alkali metal salts of common inorganic and organic acids are ionic, usually colorless, and with few exceptions, readily soluble in water. Aqueous solutions of the salts are neutral to strongly basic depending on the strength of the anion as a Brønsted base (page 371). Most distinguishing properties of the salts and their solutions are due to the anion present rather than the cation, eg, if colored, the anion is responsible.

The cations hydrate in aqueous media, the degree of solvation decreases with increasing atomic number. In the crystalline state only lithium and sodium regularly form hydrates. Potassium and ammonium salts, (below), are rarely hydrated; if hydrated, the water is usually associated with the anion.

Sodium and Potassium

Except for those properties due to mass and degree of hydration, sodium and potassium compounds are remarkably similar. Sodium salts are more frequently selected for use on a strictly economic basis. In addition, because of the lower atomic weight of sodium, there are usually more reactive units per gram when using sodium salts. (Greater hydration of the sodium versus the potassium salts may partially or entirely erase this latter advantage.) Despite the foregoing factors, subtle differences often favor use of the potassium salt. Generally a given potassium salt is more soluble in nonpolar solvents. Potassium salts are generally less deliquescent (hygroscopic) than the corresponding sodium salt, eg, potassium permanganate is used rather than the deliquescent sodium permanganate. Finally, the living cell differentiates between the two cations; sodium is the cation of the extracellular fluids, while potassium is the cation of the intracellular fluids.

Sodium compounds are widely used in pharmacy and medicine. With a few exceptions, eg, sodium chloride in electrolyte replenishers, the therapeutic activity is referable to the anionic component of the salt. Sodium is commonly the cation of choice to optimize the pharmaceutical utility of organic medicaments, eg, methiodal sodium, phenobarbital sodium, sodium citrate.

Because of the propensity of sodium ion to promote retention of water in the tissues, sodium salts are used with caution in the treatment of cardiac and renal conditions in which edema is a problem. Some drugs, eg, hydrochlorothiazide, promote excretion of potassium ion to an extent requiring auxiliary dietary intake of potassium, usually as the chloride or gluconate. Potassium ion has a diuretic effect.

Rubidium and Cesium

Rubidium and its cation are very similar in behavior to potassium. Neither rubidium nor cesium find application in pharmacy and medicine at this time.

Lithium

Being a bridge element, the behavior of this element and its compounds is often decidedly different from that of the other members of the alkali family. At room temperature the free metal is much less reactive with water; on burning it forms the normal oxide rather than the peroxide. Lithium carbonates and phosphates are only slightly water soluble. Its chloride is soluble in organic solvents. Lithium salts are highly hydrated. In all of these properties lithium resembles magnesium, and to some extent calcium, more closely than sodium.

Lithium has no normal physiological role. In its former therapeutic applications, eg, lithium bromide, the activity was inherent in the anion. However, because of the toxic character of the lithium ion, as revealed by use of lithium chloride in salt substitutes, continued use of these lithium compounds is not justified. Currently Lithium Carbonate, USP XX, has been found valuable in the treatment of hypomanic and manic states. However, these patients must be carefully monitored for blood lithium levels because of the toxicity of the cation.

Ammonia and Ammonium Compounds

Ammonia [NH_3] coordinates readily with a proton to form the ammonium ion [NH_4]$^+$. This ion displays many of the properties of the alkali metal ions. Its salts show striking resemblances to potassium and rubidium salts, with which they are commonly isomorphous. The relationship extends to solubilities as evidenced by the general water-solubility of ammonium salts of inorganic and organic acids, but the low water-solubility of such salts as the bitartrate, chloroplatinate, and perchlorate. However, there are important differences.

"Ammonium hydroxide" (mainly a solution of ammonia molecules in water) is feebly basic. The equilibrium,

$$NH_3 + H_2O \rightleftharpoons NH_4^+ + OH^-$$

lies strongly to the left unless the hydroxyl ion is removed by neutralization. Solutions of ammonium salts are acidic rather than basic.

Ammonium salts commonly used therapeutically include the carbonate (page 372), chloride, and bromide. The bromide is used as a central depressant. Both the chloride and carbonate are common ingredients in expectorant preparations.

In aqueous solution form, ammonia is used in pharmacy as a mild alkalizer. It is often preferred to the alkali bases because of its volatility, any excess being detected by its odor and readily removed by heat. The ammonia in household use contains 10% NH_3 and is known as 16° ammonia (degrees Baumé, a concentration term).

Elements of Group I-B

These elements have been known in antiquity. Because they occur in the free metallic state, are relatively easy to recover from their ores, and are very malleable, they have been used throughout historical times to make decorative vessels and jewelry. They have been employed for centuries as a measure of monetary wealth and for the fabrication of coins, hence the family name, coinage metals.

These elements and their compounds are strikingly different from those of Group I-A. Colored compounds are numerous. The hydroxides and many of the simple salts are insoluble in water. All readily act as the central unit of complexes. The soluble compounds of these elements are toxic. A summary of important characteristics is given in Table VIII.

Copper

Of the monovalent compounds, copper(I) oxide, Cu_2O, and copper(I) chloride, Cu_2Cl_2, are most frequently used. Important copper(II) (cupric) salts are the oxide, CuO, and sulfate, $CuSO_4.5H_2O$. Copper compounds are toxic.

Copper is an essential trace element. Small quantities enhance the physiological utilization of iron. It occurs in the respiratory pigment, hemocyanin, in many enzymes and is widely distributed in foods.

Copper compounds have been used in a variety of medicinal applications. Copper(II) sulfate pentahydrate is the only officially cited copper compound at this time. The radioactive ^{64}Cu isotope has been employed in mineral metabolism studies. Copper(II) sulfate is the basis for Fehling's and Benedict's Solutions, the classical test solutions for reducing sugars. Various copper compounds find commercial application as fungicides, and insecticides and are particularly effective algaecides.

Silver

With the exception of the nitrate and fluoride, the common salts of silver in the +1 oxidation state are insoluble or only slightly soluble in water. Many, including the oxide, react with and dissolve in ammonia water; the iodide and sulfide are important exceptions. Silver also forms a +2 series of salts. Silver has an oligodynamic action. Water distilled in contact with silver metal remains sterile over long periods of time.

Because of the ability of silver ion to precipitate protein and chloride in the affected tissue silver compounds, eg, silver nitrate, are employed to provide local germicidal action.

Silver is slowly released from these *in situ* precipitates to give lasting germicidal action. Cosmetic problems can result because of discoloration due to the photosensitivity of silver ion.

Preparations containing silver or silver compounds in colloidal solution were once widely used as topical antiseptics. A present day survivor is Mild Silver Protein. To reduce brittleness some silver chloride (5%) is formed in silver nitrate by adding hydrochloric acid or potassium chloride. The product, Toughened Silver Nitrate, is cast into sticks and used as a styptic.

The ready reducibility of silver ion to elemental silver gives rise to various instability problems and incompatibilities. Since silver compounds are light sensitive, they must be protected by the use of light-resistant containers. The soluble silver salts are toxic. However, the toxicity is usually limited, owing to local precipitation of adherent layers of silver protein and silver chloride.

Gold

Two series of gold compounds exist, eg, AuCl, gold(I) chloride (aurous chloride), and $AuCl_3$, gold(III) chloride (auric chloride). Gold readily acts as the center for the formation of complexes, eg, $Na_3[Au(S_2O_3)_2]$, sodium dithiosulfatoaurate(I), sodium dithiosulfatoaurate(−3), gold sodium thiosulfate.

Chemically gold salts are characterized by instability to heat, light, and even very mild reducing agents. Simple gold(I) salts can undergo "autoxidation," giving rise to finely divided metal and the corresponding gold(III) compound. The stability of the gold ions is improved by complexation. This is particularly true if a sulfur linkage is available. Because of the ease of reduction gold compounds must be handled with exceptional care and, if possible, dispensed separately.

At the present time, gold compounds are employed in the treatment of lupus erythematosus and rheumatoid arthritis. Aurothioglucose and Gold Sodium Thiomalate are listed in the USP. Since these gold compounds are poorly absorbed orally, parenteral administration is required. Dimercaprol is used as an antidote if the patient shows signs of gold toxicity. Efforts are underway to develop orally effective gold compounds. One such compound, *S*-triethylphosphine gold 2,3,4,6-tetra-*O*-acetyl-1-thio-β-D-glucopyranoside, is undergoing clinical testing at this time.

The radioactive isotope, ^{198}Au, is employed therapeutically in the treatment of certain malignancies (Chapter 29).

Elements of Group II

Each element in this group is characterized by the presence of two s electrons in the outermost orbital. Subgroup II-A elements have a $(n − 1)s^2(n − 1)p^6ns^2$ outer electron structure except for the small beryllium atom whose structure is $1s^22s^2$. Subgroup II-B differs in that its underlying electron structure is the filled *d*-orbital, $(n −1)d^{10}ns^2$.

Elements of Group II-A

While this group is called the alkaline earth group, there is some question whether magnesium, and especially beryllium, should be included under that title.

Except for amphoteric beryllium, these elements are strictly metallic. Like the alkali metals, because of chemical reactivity, they do not occur free in nature. They function uniformly in the +2 oxidation state (Table IX). The similarity existing between calcium, strontium, and barium is especially striking.

Calcium, strontium, and barium react readily with water to form hydroxides with the simultaneous evolution of hydrogen. Magnesium reacts similarly but only at elevated temperatures. The hydroxides of beryllium and magnesium are insoluble in water, that of beryllium is amphoteric. Although less soluble than the alkali hydroxides, the hydroxides of calcium, strontium, and barium give strongly basic solutions. The carbonates, phosphates, sulfates, and fluorides are insoluble; they are important in analytical work.

Except for hydrate formation the three heavier members of the family do not form complex ions. Magnesium forms a few crystalline complexes of the type K_2MgF_4.

Beryllium

Being amphoteric, this element appears both as simple salts and berylates. The cation complexes readily, eg, $[Be(H_2O)_4]^{2+}$, $[Be(NH_3)_4]^{2+}$.

Being a bridge element, beryllium resembles aluminum in its behavior. This similarity is so striking that many early workers considered beryllium a lighter member of the aluminum family before Mendeleev correctly placed it in Group II.

While its ionic diameter is considerably greater than that of beryllium, the higher +3 charge on the aluminum ion results in a polarizing ability similar to that of beryllium. Both elements dissolve in caustic alkalis and both form a protective coating on their surface when placed in nitric acid. The halides of both elements have similar solubilities in organic solvents. Both elements act as Lewis acids and give rise to alums.

Beryllium metal and its compounds are extremely toxic when ingested, inhaled, or absorbed through the skin. None of its compounds are employed as therapeutic agents.

Magnesium

This is a relatively abundant element that is chemically active. The cation, Mg^{2+}, is stable under all conditions ordinarily met in pharmaceutical practice.

Magnesium compounds are employed for a variety of purposes in therapeutics. Many of its insoluble compounds are used as gastric antacids, (page 371). The hydroxide and sulfate are used as cathartics, (page 373), and the sulfate, as an anticonvulsant. A concentrated solution of the sulfate is often applied topically for its anti-inflammatory action. Toxic manifestations following magnesium administration are relatively rare; calcium gluconate given intravenously is an effective antidote. The stearate is employed as a lubricant in the preparation of compressed tablets. The artificial radioactive isotope ^{27}Mg, has been employed in research involving photosynthesis.

Calcium

Calcium is a relatively reactive metal whose cation is stable. However, soluble calcium salts undergo metathesis with soluble borates, carbonates, citrates, oxalates, phosphates, sulfates, and tartrates to yield insoluble calcium compounds. These reactions often lead to pharmaceutical incompatibilities.

Calcium is indispensible to life. Calcium, and to a much lesser degree, magnesium, is the cation of hydroxyapatite, the major constituent (98%) of the bones and teeth. Calcium is essential to many physiological processes. Therapeutic categories represented by official calcium compounds include: antacid (page 371), and calcium replenishers.

Calcium is frequently the cation of choice to carry therapeutically active anions, eg, calcium aminosalicylate, calcium cyclobarbital. In some instances this is referable to better physical characteristics of the calcium compound; in others it is a deliberate attempt to avoid an unnecessary intake of sodium. The artificial radioactive ^{45}Ca isotope has been employed in studies involving mineral metabolism.

Strontium

The behavior of this element is very similar to calcium. Ingested, its distribution is similar to that of calcium. At this time it has no application in pharmacy or medicine. In the

Table IX—The Elements of Group II-A

Element	Beryllium	Magnesium	Calcium	Strontium	Barium	Radium
Symbol	Be	Mg	Ca	Sr	Ba	Ra
Atomic number	4	12	20	38	56	88
Atomic weight	9.012	24.31	40.08	87.62	137.3	226.03
Orbital electrons	$[He]2s^2$	$[Ne]3s^2$	$[Ar]4s^2$	$[Kr]5s^2$	$[Xe]6s^2$	$[Rn]7s^2$
Oxidation states	+2	+2	+2	+2	+2	+2
Atomic radius (Å)	0.90	1.70	1.74	1.92	1.98	. . .
Ionic (crystal) radius (Å) (coordination number 6)	0.31(+2)[a]	0.65(+2)	0.99(+2)	1.13(+2)	1.35(+2)	1.43(+2)
Ionization potential, ev (II)[b]	9.3	7.6	6.1	5.7	5.2	5.252
	18.2	15.0	11.9	11.0	9.95	10.099
Electronegativity	1.57	1.31	1.00	0.95	0.89	0.9
% of earth's crust	6×10^{-4}	2.1	3.6	0.03	0.025	1.3×10^{-10}

[a] Coordination number 4.
[b] Second ionization potential.

past it has been used as the carrier cation for therapeutically active anions, eg, strontium bromide.

Barium

Chemically this element is the most active of Group II-A. Its cation is stable under all ordinary conditions. Barium hydroxide is soluble and is a strong base. Because of this it often finds application in analytical and synthetic operations.

In sharp contrast to the lighter members of Group II-A all barium compounds that are soluble either in water or in dilute acid are poisonous. The most readily available antidote for barium ingestion is magnesium sulfate (Epsom Salt).

With the exception of barium sulfate, which finds use as a radiopaque (page 373), barium compounds are not employed as medicinal agents. Barium hydroxide lime is employed as a carbon dioxide absorber (page 372). Artificial radioactive isotopes of barium have been employed in pharmacokinetic investigations.

Elements of Group II-B

Because zinc, cadmium, and mercury (Table VIII) have comparatively low boiling points, 907°, 768°, 357°, respectively, they are frequently referred to as the volatile metals. The common oxidation state is +2, but mercury also exists in the +1 state. This latter state is achieved by the formation of a covalent, two electron bond between two mercury atoms. Thus the mercury(I) ion (mercurous) is always written Hg_2^{2+}. The filled $(n-1)d^{10}$ orbital is stable in this family. Unlike Group I-B there are no oxidation states involving loss of a d-electron. There is increasing covalent character in the salts of these elements, eg, fused zinc chloride conducts while the mercury chlorides do not.

These elements readily complex with most common ligands and concentrated solutions exhibit autocomplexation. Only zinc is sufficiently amphoteric to form a stable oxygen complex, ZnO_2^{2-}, the zincate ion.

Zinc

All soluble zinc salts show some degree of hydrolysis,

$$Zn^{2+} + 2H_2O \rightleftharpoons [Zn(OH)]^+ + H_3O^+$$

Thus, all zinc salts of weak Brønsted bases show an acid reaction.

Zinc has many therapeutic applications in the treatment of various external surfaces of the body (page 371) and in conditions such as wound healing and taste acuity. Strong zinc sulfate solution is used as an emetic; its emetic action is so rapid that little or no zinc salt is absorbed.

Zinc is present in all living organisms; it is widely distributed in foods. It is an essential trace element and an essential component of carbonic anhydrase and other enzymes.

Zinc compounds soluble in water or in the gastric fluid, eg, ZnO, may be poisonous. There is a relatively wide margin of safety between the required intake and toxic intake. The most readily available antidote is sodium bicarbonate (baking soda).

Artificial radioactive isotopes of zinc have been employed in studies of mineral metabolism.

Cadmium

This element is truly intermediate in properties to zinc and mercury. Soluble cadmium compounds are astringent; $CdSO_4$ has been used both as a topical astringent and for eye infections. Cadmium sulfide has been introduced for the treatment of seborrheic dermatitis (page 371). A disease found in Japan, known as itai-itai, is believed to be caused by drinking water contaminated with cadmium.

Mercury

This member of the family is a true metal. As indicated previously, it alone of the family has two series of salts.

Mercury and its compounds are extremely toxic. Mercury metal, because of its low boiling point, has an appreciable vapor pressure even at room temperatures. If mercury is spilled it should be recovered immediately. Mercury that falls into cracks and other difficult to clean places is best removed by covering with powdered sulfur, allowing several days for conversion to sulfide, and then vacuuming. All common mercury salts are poisonous. The best antidote for mercury poisoning, particularly the bichloride, is Sodium Formaldehyde Sulfoxylate (NF XV), (Chapter 68). Egg albumen may be used in an emergency if the poisoning is discovered shortly after ingestion. The white of one egg should be administered for each 250 mg of mercuric chloride ingested. Emesis should be induced promptly thereafter.

In former years, metallic mercury was important therapeutically as a cathartic and parasiticide, but it has been largely replaced by more efficacious and less toxic medicaments. Surviving mercury compounds are used largely for their germicidal effect, eg, ammoniated mercury and yellow mercuric oxide. Yellow mercuric oxide, with a K_{sp} of 3×10^{-26}, is an extremely insoluble compound. Mercury also survives in some organomercury compounds, eg, meralluride, nitromersol.

The radioactive nuclides ^{197}Hg and ^{203}Hg are used in a diagnostic capacity (Chapter 29).

Elements of Group III

This group of the periodic table includes some thirty-six elements which, on the basis of external electron structure, divide into the usual Group III-A (Table X) with five elements, and Group III-B with thirty-one elements. Subgroup III-B further divides into the usual transition elements (Table XI), the lanthanides (fourteen elements) and actinides (fourteen elements). (See the periodic table on the back cover.) The lanthanide cerium, as cerium(IV), is a widely used analytical reagent. Since the lanthanides and actinides have no applications in pharmacy further discussion is unnecessary.

The members of this family are very reactive and do not appear in nature in the free state. They have no known biological role.

Table X—The Elements of Group III-A

Element	Boron	Aluminum	Gallium	Indium	Thallium
Symbol	B	Al	Ga	In	Tl
Atomic number	5	13	31	49	81
Atomic weight	10.81	26.98	69.72	114.8	204.3_7
Orbital electrons	$[He]2s^22p^1$	$[Ne]3s^23p^1$	$[Ar]3d^{10}4s^24p^1$	$[Kr]4d^{10}5s^25p^1$	$[Xe]4f^{14}5d^{10}6s^26p^1$
Oxidation states	+3	(+1),+3	+1,+2,+3	+1,+3	+1,+3
Atomic radius (Å)	0.82	1.25	1.26	1.44	2.0
Ionic (crystal) radii (Å)	...	...	1.90(+1)	1.90(+1)	1.64(+1)
(coordination number 6)	0.20(+3)[a]	0.675(+3)	0.76(+3)	0.94(+3)	1.03(+3)
Ionization potential, ev	8.30	5.95	6.0	5.8	6.1
(II)[b]	25.15	18.82	20.4	18.8	20.3
(III)[b]	37.92	28.44	30.6	27.9	29.7
Electronegativity	2.04	1.61	1.81	1.78	1.62
% of earth's crust	3×10^{-4}	8.13	1.5×10^{-3}	10^{-5}	ca 10^{-4}

[a] Coordination number 4.
[b] Second & third ionization pot.

Elements of Group III-A

In this family of elements an electron appears in the p orbital of the valence shell for the first time; each element has the structure ns^2np^1. Theoretically two oxidation states are possible. The first, +1, arises by the loss of the single p electron. The resulting helide structure, ns^2, has sufficient stability to give rise to stable ions, eg, Ga^+, In^+, Tl^+. Aluminum has this oxidation state only at elevated temperatures and it is not evident with B, Sc, Y, La.

With the loss of all three valence electrons the +3 oxidation state appears in all the elements of the family. With increasing atomic number the +3 state becomes more electrovalent in character. Boron trichloride is a covalent compound, aluminum chloride is for practical purposes covalent, and gallium(III) chloride has some covalent character. Since a normal octet is not achieved in these compounds an electron deficient structure results. As there are only three electron pairs in the valence shell the electron-pair repulsive forces are weaker, and the molecules become electron-pair *acceptors*. Because of the weaker repulsive forces, these MX_3 molecules give rise to triangular structures with hybrid sp^2 orbitals. The metal occupies the center of the triangle.

By accepting a fourth electron-pair the octet is completed and sp^3 hybrids form. The addends rearrange to give tetrahedral structures with the metal ion in the center of the tetrahedron.

Since the initial compounds, eg, $AlCl_3$, are electron-pair deficient they are Lewis acids. As such they act as catalysts for the Friedel-Crafts synthesis.

Members of this family give rise to an interesting series of double salts, the alums. The common formula is $M^+_2M^{3+}_2(SO_4)_4 \cdot 24H_2O$, where M^+ is a monovalent ion, eg, Na^+, K^+, Rb^+, NH_4^+, Tl^+, and M^{3+} is a trivalent ion, eg, Al^{3+}, Tl^{3+}, Cr^{3+}, Fe^{3+}. The prototype of these double salts is *alum*, $K_2Al_2(SO_4)_4 \cdot 24H_2O$.

Boron

This element appears only in the +3 oxidation state and is a nonmetal. Several oxyacids are known. Metaboric acid, $(HBO_2)_n$, and the metaborate ion do not exist as monomers. Orthoboric acid, $(H_3BO_3)_n$, exists as a hydrogen bonded layered structure, which explains the flaky form in which it is available. Discrete H_3BO_3 molecules exist in the gaseous state and in solution. It is a weak acid, ionizing in solution,

$$H_3BO_3 + 2H_2O \rightleftharpoons H_3O^+ + [B(OH)_4]^-$$

The pH of a $0.1M$ solution is 5.3. In addition there is a tetraborate, available as borax, usually formulated as $Na_2B_4O_7 \cdot 10H_2O$. In water the tetraborate ion reacts as follows,

$$[B_4O_5(OH)_4]^{2-} + 5H_2O \rightleftharpoons 2[B(OH)_3] + 2[B(OH)_4]^-$$

The strong alkalinity of solutions of all borates is due to the reaction,

$$[B(OH)_4]^- \rightleftharpoons [B(OH)_3] + [OH]^-$$

Boric acid is soluble in polyhydroxy compounds, eg, glycerol. In anhydrous media esterification takes place to form "glyceroborate". In aqueous media glyceroboric acid forms, an acid which is valuable in the analytical determination of boric acid.

Since it is a bridge element certain properties of boron resemble those of silicon, its diagonal neighbor in Group IV-A. The boron hydrides and boranes resemble the silanes (page 361). The borohydride ion, $[BH_4]^-$, is commercially available as the sodium salt which is a valuable reducing agent.

Boron and its compounds are toxic, both by ingestion and by absorption through broken or inflamed skin. Numerous fatalities have occurred; especially depressing are those of infants due to the use of dusting powders containing boric acid.

Boric acid and the borates have no germicidal activity and at best are feebly bacteriostatic. On the basis of their toxicity and negligible antiseptic value the use of these compounds is unwarranted.

Boric acid in various dosage forms is employed as a topical anti-infective; in solution it is used as an eye wash. Sodium borate is bacteriostatic and is a frequent ingredient of cold creams, eye washes, and mouth washes. Sodium perborate is an oxidizing type of local anti-infective. Various borate buffers are used in collyria. A common incompatibility in the use of these buffers is the precipitation of insoluble borates from neutral or alkaline buffers. All common metals, except the alkalies, precipitate as insoluble borates.

Boric Acid and Sodium Borate (borax) are cited in NF XV.

Aluminum

Aluminum is the most abundant of the metals and the third most abundant element, being exceeded in natural occurrence only by oxygen and silicon. The metal and its hydroxide are amphoteric but only those compounds in which it acts as a base are pharmaceutically important. As a result of its high charge, small diameter, and electron pair deficiency, the aluminum(III) ion is incapable of independent existence in polar solvents. Due to the very high field strength surrounding this ion, complexation always takes place.

Many insoluble aluminum compounds find use as gastric antacids (page 371). Because of their astringency soluble aluminum salts are used for various skin conditions and in antiperspirants and deodorants (page 371). Kaolin is used as an adsorbent and demulcent, and bentonite is useful as a suspending agent (page 372). In paste form, elemental aluminum is employed topically as a protective (page 321).

There is some concern about chronic aluminum toxicity and its effect on the brain, possibly manifesting itself in the elderly.

Gallium, Indium, and Thallium

These remaining elements of Group III-A are not of interest in pharmacy except for the use of their radioactive isotopes as diagnostic aids, ^{67}Ga, ^{111}In, ^{113}In, and ^{201}Tl (see Chapter 29).

Thallium compounds are among the most toxic and are absorbed from the intestine and through the skin from ointments and creams. Its action is somewhat similar to that of arsenic. Deaths have been recorded from a thallium cosmetic use. Thallium compounds have been used in insecticides, especially ant poisons. Thallium(I) is similar to potassium ion in that TlOH is a strong base and their salts are isomorphous. Thallium(III) is similar in behavior to aluminum(III) and gold(III).

Gallium is interesting because, except for mercury, it has the lowest melting point of the metals (29.75°). It is also unusual for its +2 oxidation state. Since this requires an odd electron it is difficult to explain since gallium(II) compounds are not paramagnetic. It has been postulated that equal numbers of gallium(I) and gallium(III) ions may exist in these compounds to give a formula $M^+[MX_4]^-$. Gallium(III) has properties very similar to iron(III).

Indium is quite similar to both aluminum and gallium. It too, under very special conditions, exists as a divalent chloride.

Elements of Group III-B

Some properties are given in Table XI. These three elements exhibit only the +3 oxidation state and are quite similar. The differences are mostly of degree, dependent on the increasing atomic radius. Since scandium is the smallest, it has the greatest polarizing power and most readily forms complexes of the type K_3ScF_6. Yttrium has properties approximately midway between scandium and lanthanum. This gradation of properties is nicely shown with the three hydroxides: $Sc(OH)_3$ is a weak base, $Y(OH)_3$ is stronger, and $La(OH)_3$ is a very strong base.

Elements of Group IV

The elements of this group are similar in that each has four valence electrons, two of which are s electrons. However, the remaining two valence electrons enter different orbitals to give the structure ns^2np^2 for Group IV-A and $(n-1)d^2ns^2$ for Group IV-B. Because of this there is a strong tendency for all members of the family except carbon and silicon to form "inert pair" ions. Except for the larger atoms many of the compounds are covalent or predominantly covalent. All elements of the family show the +4 oxidation state. Important characteristics of these elements are found in Tables XI and XII.

Table XI—Transition Elements

Element	Group III-B			Group IV-B		
	Scandium	Yttrium	Lanthanum	Titanium	Zirconium	Hafnium
Symbol	Sc	Y	La	Ti	Zr	Hf
Atomic number	21	39	57	22	40	72
Atomic weight	44.96	88.91	138.9	47.90	91.22	178.5
Orbital electrons	[Ar]$3d^14s^2$	[Kr]$4d^15s^2$	[Xe]$5d^16s^2$	[Ar]$3d^24s^2$	[Kr]$4d^25s^2$	[Xe]$4f^{14}5d^26s^2$
Oxidation states	3+	3+	3+	2+,3+,4+	2+,4+	(2+),4+
Atomic radius (Å)	1.51	1.8	1.87	1.36	1.45	1.44
Ionic radii (Å)	0.81(3+)	0.93(3+)	1.15(3+)	1.00(2+)	. . .	. . .
(coordination no 6)				0.75(4+)	0.86(4+)	0.85(4+)
Ionization potential, ev	6.7	6.5	5.6	6.82	6.84	ca 5.5
Electronegativity	1.54	1.53	1.3	. . .	. . .	. . .
% of earth's crust	0.44	0.022	4.5×10^{-4}	0.629	0.028	. . .

Table XII—The Elements of Group IV-A

Element	Carbon	Silicon	Germanium	Tin	Lead
Symbol	C	Si	Ge	Sn	Pb
Atomic number	6	14	32	50	82
Atomic weight	12.01	28.08	72.5$_9$	118.6$_9$	207.2
Orbital electrons	[He]$2s^22p^2$	[Ne]$3s^23p^2$	[Ar]$3d^{10}4s^24p^2$	[Kr]$4d^{10}5s^25p^2$	[Xe]$4f^{14}5d^{10}6s^26p^2$
Oxidation states	4− to 4+	4− to 4+	2+,4+	2+,4+	2+,4+
Atomic radius (Å)	0.77	1.17	1.22	1.41	1.54
Ionic (crystal) radii	2.60(4−)	2.71(4−)	0.87(2+)	0.93(2+)	1.20(2+)
(coordination no 6)	0.30(4+)^a	0.54(4+)	0.67(4+)	0.83(4+)	0.91(4+)
Ionization potential, ev	11.264	8.149	8.09	7.30	7.38
Electronegativity	2.55	1.90	2.01	1.58	1.87
% of earth's crust	2.7×10^{-2}	27.7	7×10^{-4}	6×10^{-4}	1×10^{-3}

^{a} Coordination no 4.

Elements of Group IV-A

Carbon and silicon are usually considered apart from germanium, tin, and lead because of their nonmetallic character and property of catenation. Boron, with which silicon forms a bridge element pair, is quite similar to silicon. The +2 oxidation state is rarely encountered in carbon and silicon. The bonding in carbon is covalent, corresponding silicon bonds have a somewhat greater electrovalent character. Simple carbon compounds are either linear, CO_2, planar triangular, CO_3^{2-}, or tetrahedral, CCl_4. Since the radius of the carbon atom is small, and it lacks d-orbitals to expand its valence shell, carbon never increases its coordination number beyond four. Unlike carbon, because of its available d-orbitals, silicon can achieve sp^3d^2 hybridization and appear in the octahedral configuration, SiF_6^{2-}, with a maximum coordination number of six. Similarly, germanium, tin, and lead have a maximum coordination number of six.

Carbon is exclusively nonmetallic. Metallic properties appear with silicon and germanium and become predominant in tin and lead. The oxides of carbon and silicon are acidic while those of the other elements of the group are amphoteric. The electron configuration, atomic size, electronegativity, etc, of the carbon atom combine to give the chemistry of carbon a uniqueness which is the basis for the classical division of the field of chemistry into inorganic and organic disciplines. Silicon is also unique for the extensive range of complex, insoluble alumino-silicates it forms (page 361).

Carbon

Carbon appears widely distributed in nature, both in the free and combined states. The free element is produced in various forms, eg, coke, lampblack, charcoal. Activated charcoals are prepared from ligneous materials (sometimes pretreated with a dehydrating agent) by carbonization in the absence of air. This is followed by heat and/or chemical treatment to increase surface area and porosity. Activated charcoal is available in two forms, finely powdered (300–350 mesh) for use in liquid media, and coarse, hard, porous particles for gas absorption. The fine form is official in USP XX. It is used as an adsorbent in the treatment of diarrhea.

Carbon dioxide is usually obtained as a by-product from either the production of alcohol by fermentation or by recovery from the stack gases of power plants. Unlike carbon monoxide, its toxicity is not due to interaction with hemoglobin, but through suffocation. Carbon dioxide is an effective respiratory stimulant (page 372), cited in USP XX.

Under appropriate conditions, carbon forms many binary compounds, eg, cyanogen, carbon disulfide, carbon tetrachloride, and numerous carbides. Its important inorganic acids are carbonic, percarbonic (peroxocarbonic), and the pseudobinary hydrocyanic acid, (HCN). All are weak acids and are available primarily in the form of salts.

Sodium bicarbonate and the slightly soluble carbonates or basic carbonates of calcium, magnesium, and aluminum find extensive use as gastric antacids. Potassium bicarbonate is used as a source of potassium ion in electrolyte replenishers. Bismuth subcarbonate is an astringent and protective (page 371). Ammonium carbonate is an effective reflex stimulant (page 371) and expectorant (page 372).

Silicon

Next to oxygen, silicon is the most abundant element on earth. It does not appear free in nature. Silicon forms an inert oxide, silicon dioxide (silica), which occurs abundantly in nature in both amorphous and crystalline states, eg, sand, quartz, opal, siliceous earths.

Siliceous earth (diatomaceous earth, Fuller's earth, Kieselguhr, Celite), and infusorial earth, are the siliceous skeletal remains of diatoms and infusoria. The deposits are in the form of spicules, rods, and stars of silica. Because of their shapes these materials act as excellent, inert, nonadsorbent filter aids. Because of their moderate hardness they are used as mild abrasives. Purified Siliceous Earth is official in NF XV.

Synthetic amorphous silicas are manufactured by two methods. *Silica fume* is prepared by condensation of silica from its vapor phase. *Silica gel* is prepared by hydrolysis of inorganic or organic orthosilicates. Structurally, both forms may be considered condensation polymers of the silicic acids. They are available in various commercial grades, differing in such variables as particle size, degree of hydration, surface type (silanol and/or siloxane), porosity, and hardness. By selection of the product having the desired properties, amorphous silicas find employment as gas adsorbents, desiccants, carriers, fillers, thickeners, and abrasives. Colloidal Silicon Dioxide (fumed form) and Silica Gel (precipitated form) are official in NF XV.

Silicosis is a lung condition resembling chronic tuberculosis, developing after long exposure (seven years or more) to "respirable dust" (silica particles 5 μm or less in mean diameter). Breathing aluminum dust or aluminum oxide dust at regular intervals prevents its development.

Silicon forms numerous silicic acids, eg, metasilicic acid, $[H_2SiO_3]$, orthosilicic acid, $[H_4SiO_4]$, disilicic acid, $[H_6Si_2O_7]$. These and others occur in nature as silicates. Except for the alkali salts, silicates are insoluble in water or acids, but they are readily attacked by hydrofluoric acid forming gaseous silicon tetrafluoride. The alkali silicates do not occur in nature but are prepared by fusion of finely divided silica with the desired alkali base or carbonate.

The "insoluble" silicates have structural arrangements dominated by the large diffuse oxide ion. Since cations of high charge, eg, Si^{4+}, Al^{3+}, are small and compact, they have only a secondary role in determining the structures. Physical properties, eg, density, hardness, refractive index, are almost completely determined by the oxygen "packing" (arrangement).

There are two "close-packed" oxide ion arrangements, cubic and hexagonal. In each the oxygen arranges in identical layers; the difference arises from the placement of the layers with respect to one another. Two types of openings are possible between neighboring spheres. The smaller openings are occupied by small cations, eg, Si^{4+}, resulting in a tetrahedral arrangement of four oxide ions around each cation. The larger openings between adjacent oxide ions are occupied by somewhat larger cations, eg, Li^+, Mg^{2+}, Fe^{3+}. Six oxide ions surround each cation in an octahedral arrangement. The aluminum ion, which is intermediate in size, can occupy either tetrahedral or octahedral spaces. When cations too large to occupy either of the inter-oxide ion spaces, eg, NH_4^+, Na^+, K^+, Ca^{2+}, are present the oxide structure opens in one of two ways. Groups of the oxide ion layers separate to give an overall layered structure with the large cations forming a new layer between. The *clays* have this structure. Or, the oxide ions may spread in a three-dimensional manner to give room-like cavities within the structure. The cavities are occupied by the large cations. Feldspars and zeolites have this latter structure.

A persistent problem preventing early workers from successfully elucidating silicate structures was their failure to recognize that ions of the ideal structure may be substituted to some extent by other ions of the same radius, irrespective of charge. This phenomenon, "isomorphous replacement", is widespread among the silicates. Because of this, empirical formulas, based on analytical data, are meaningless. The illustrative formulas used in the following discussions are "ideal" formulas. Because of isomorphous replacement the actual formula of a given silicate may differ somewhat from the ideal.

Before discussing specific insoluble silicates it must be said that all are chemically inert. The properties which distinguish them and determine their use are structural or related to surface phenomena.

Chain silicates are unidimensional arrangements of silicate tetrahedra sharing two oxygens per tetrahedron; in effect each chain is a macroanion. Since these chains consist of Si—O bonds having 50% covalent character, they are difficult to break. Electrical neutrality is maintained by placing a sufficient number of cations, usually K^+ and/or Ca^{2+}, between the chains. Electrostatic forces being weaker than covalent forces, these crystals cleave readily to give rise to the typical fibrous structure of asbestos, eg, serpentine asbestos, $(HO)_6Mg_6(Si_4O_{11}) \cdot H_2O$. These asbestos chains are useful as filter aids and as insulation. Asbestosis is a pulmonary condition similar to silicosis.

Attapulgite, $Mg_5(Si_8O_{20})(OH)_2 \cdot 8H_2O$, is a double chain structure with rather large open spaces between the chains. These spaces are occupied by water molecules which provide hydrogen bonding to hold the chains together. It has adsorptive properties similar to kaolin.

The layer silicates include talc (talcum, soapstone), the micas, the chlorites (no relationship to ClO_2^-), and the three clay minerals, the montmorillonites (bentonites), kaolins, (kaolinite), and the illites.

Talc, $Mg_3(OH)_2Si_4O_{10}$, is the softest mineral known. There are no cementing cations or molecules between silicate layers; they are held together by van der Waals forces. Consequently the talc layers cleave easily to give the characteristic smooth, unctuous feel. Talc adheres readily to the skin, is chemically inert, and has very low adsorptive powers. It is used in dusting powders as a protective and lubricant, to prevent irritation due to friction. It is also used in medicated dusts and is widely used in cosmetic applications. While there are no problems in its use on intact skin, talc must not be used on broken skin, wounds, or surgical incisions. This precludes its former use as a dusting powder and lubricant for surgical gloves.

Because of its inertness and non-adsorptive character talc is a useful filter aid. Only particles which are passed by a No 80 sieve but retained by a No 100 sieve should be used. Finer particles suspend and are not easily removed by subsequent filtration. Talc is official in USP XX.

In mica, $Al_2[(OH)_2(Si_3O_{10})]K$, and chlorite, $Mg_3[(OH)_2(Si_4O_{10})]$, negatively charged silicate layers are bound together by cations. Thus these silicates cleave readily along the cation layer since the electrostatic forces are weaker than the covalent bonds within the silicate layer. Neither has pharmaceutical applications.

The clays, montmorillonite (Smectite),

$Al_4[(OH)_4(Si_8O_{20})] \cdot 3nH_2O$,

and kaolinite,

$[(OH)_6Al_4][(OH)_2(Si_4O_{10})]$

are layer structures built of alternating layers of aluminum oxide (hydrargillite) and silicate. The montmorillonites have higher $SiO_2:Al_2O_3$ ratios with much isomorphous replacement of aluminum. Magnesium is never present in the kaolins.

The distinguishing feature of the bentonite (montmorillonite) clays is the insertion of up to three distinct layers of hydrogen bridged water molecules between the aluminosilicate layers. Not all water hydrogens are needed to bond the water molecules within their layer; the unused hydrogens bind the layers to each other and to the aluminosilicate layers. These water layers may be removed, one at a time, by heat.

The thickness of the individual crystals decreases in steps as each water layer is removed. By treating with water, the water layers are restored, one at a time, with a return to the original thickness. This may be repeated indefinitely. Because of this phenomenon bentonite clays are known as "swelling clays."

The bentonites have gelling properties which make them useful suspending agents, ion-exchange properties, and detergent properties. Bentonite and Bentonite Magma are official in NF XV.

Kaolins are always found in the form of microcrystals of colloidal dimensions. The properties are somewhat similar to bentonite. They are used as clarifying agents and are good excipients for inorganic salts. They find employment as intestinal adsorbents and protectives. Externally they are used as dusting powders. Kaolin is official in USP XX.

The three dimensional, or lattice silicates have previously been described. In the feldspars, $KAlSi_3O_8$, the most common rock, the large cations, eg, K^+, are trapped in enlarged cavities within the alumino-silicate network. On the other hand, in the zeolites, $CaAl_2Si_4O_{12} \cdot 6H_2O$, and in the synthetic *molecular sieves*, these cavities have connecting openings, or hallways, between one another and to the exterior of the crystal. Thus the cations (and water molecules) in these cavities are free to move about within the crystal and may be exchanged with external cations. These latter silicates are valuable as ion exchangers, desiccants, carriers for catalysts, and for the separation of organic gases, eg, ethylene from ethane. Certain forms of molecular sieves have been tried as antacids. See *Clathrates*, Chapter 14.

Pumice is a porous rock of volcanic origin, usually found in the vitreous state. Being a three dimensionally linked sodium aluminosilicate it is a hard, chemically inert, nonadsorptive material. In the powdered form it is used as a filter medium and dispersing agent. It is found in dental preparations as an abrasive.

Magnesium trisilicate is prepared by precipitation using a soluble silicate and a soluble magnesium salt. Although it has an analytical composition approaching disilicate, it is actually a mixture of magnesium hydroxide, hydrated magnesium oxide and silica gel. The insoluble magnesium compounds are responsible for the antacid action; the silica gel acts as a protective. Magnesium trisilicate is also employed as a suspending agent.

Glass—*Glass* is a generic term used to identify vitreous silicate materials prepared by fusing a base, eg, Na_2CO_3 and $CaCO_3$, with pure silica. On cooling, a clear vitreous mass results. There is no clearly defined melting point; a gradual softening takes place on heating as a result of the somewhat haphazard arrangement of the silicon-oxygen bonds. Certain other cations may be included: manganese dioxide, to hide the blue-green color of the iron usually present in silica, borates, to reduce the coefficient of expansion, potassium ion to give a brown and light-resistant glass, etc.

Since the surface of the glass is an exposed oxide network it can be reactive. On standing in contact with aqueous solutions, alkali will leach from it. This leaching is accelerated by heat, eg, sterilization. The surface of glass also has adsorbing powers, but this can be a problem only in extremely dilute solutions. The compendia usually specify the type of glass container to be used for certain materials and include tests for four types of glass.

Silanes and Siloxanes—The close relationship between carbon and silicon has prompted much interest in the "organic chemistry of silicon." The compounds involved are analogues of carbon compounds or compounds in which silicon functions in place of one or more of the carbon atoms. Simple silanes and their derivatives, such as silane $[SiH_4]$, silanol $[SiH_3OH]$, disiloxane $[H_3SiOSiH_3]$, etc, have long been known. The present interest is in complex compounds that contain both carbon and silicon. The silicones (alkylsiloxanes) are condensation polymers of various types of alkylsilanols and represent a field finding extensive commercial application. Simethicone, USP XX, a polymeric dimethylsiloxane, is employed as an antifoaming agent. It has found use as an antiflatulent in gastric bloating and in postoperative gaseous distention in the GI tract. For further discussion, see Silicones, in Chapter 40.

Germanium

The properties of this element are intermediate to those of silicon and tin. It has no applications in the health sciences. Germanium has remarkable electrical properties which make it valuable in the manufacture of semi-conductors and other microelectronic parts.

Tin

Tin forms compounds in both +2 and +4 oxidation states. The lower oxidation state is somewhat electrostatic but the higher state is largely covalent in character. Both oxides are amphoteric, giving rise to stannate(II) (stannite), $[SnO_2]^{2-}$, and stannate(IV) (stannate), $[SnO_3]^{2-}$, ions.

The only official compound is stannous fluoride [tin(II) fluoride], applied topically as a dental prophylactic. Experimental evidence demonstrates the superiority of this fluoride over other soluble fluorides for this application. The ready susceptibility of tin(II) fluoride to oxidative and hydrolytic decomposition causes problems in the preparation and storage of suitable dosage forms. Various tin dioxide [tin(IV) oxide] preparations have been used externally for their germicidal effect, particularly against staphylococcal organisms often resistant to other germicides.

Lead

This element is the most metallic of the group. However, some residual amphoteric character is present, particularly in the +4 oxidation state. At one time lead compounds found employment in pharmacy and medicine, usually as astringents. Because of its highly toxic nature as a "cumulative poison" it is no longer used. It is readily absorbed in the intestinal tract and broken skin, and deposited in the bone.

Elements of Group IV-B

Because of their minor importance, a detailed treatment is unnecessary. Some important characteristics are given in Table XI. All members of the group occur in nature only in the combined state. The +2 and +4 oxidation states are common to all. All members of the group possess amphoteric properties and their cations readily form complexes.

Titanium

Titanium forms three oxides (TiO, Ti_2O_3, TiO_2) and corresponding binary salts. The soluble salts of divalent and trivalent titanium are violet or red and are powerful reducing agents.

The most important compound is the dioxide, TiO_2, which is official in USP XX. It is used as a solar-ray protective. As such, it is a popular ingredient in various lotions and creams for the prevention of sunburn. This action is the result of its high covering power as a white pigment, a consequence of its high refractive index.

Zirconium and Hafnium

Hafnium occurs in small quantities in zirconium ores. As a consequence, unless highly purified, zirconium compounds include varying percentages of hafnium. Zirconium as the hydrous oxide or carbonate has been used as a lotion or cream for contact dermatitis. The hydrous oxide was also used in deodorant and antiperspirant preparations. However, it has been discovered that zirconium is toxic, and these uses have been discontinued. At present there are no applications of these two elements in the health sciences.

Elements of Group V

The elements of this group have five valence electrons. Two of the electrons occupy s orbitals. The three remaining electrons are in different orbitals in the A and B subgroups, giving the structures ns^2np^3 and $(n-1)d^3ns^2$, respectively.

Elements of Group V-A

This group displays strikingly regular gradations in properties ranging from exclusively nonmetallic nitrogen to almost exclusively metallic bismuth (Table XIII). Oxidation states of +3 and +5 are common to all. Bismuth functions primarily in the +3 state. All members except bismuth also exist in a −3 oxidation state. Hydrides are of the covalent MH_3 type, characterized by an unshared electron pair. This allows these hydrides to form coordinate covalent bonds. The oxides of nitrogen and phosphorus are acidic. Those of arsenic and antimony are amphoteric, but are sufficiently acidic for the elements to be classified as nonmetals. The common oxide of bismuth, Bi_2O_3, is basic; the less important pentoxide is acidic.

Nitrogen

Nitrogen occurs free in the atmosphere (78%) and combined in nitrates and organic compounds. It is a colorless, tasteless, and odorless, inert gas. It is nonflammable and does not support combustion. Due to its stable triple-bond structure, the N_2 molecule shows little reactivity with other elements. The free nitrogen atom is very reactive.

The inertness of nitrogen is the result of the bonding existing in the molecule. There is a σ bond between the atoms, and two π bonds which fuse to form an electron cloud (doughnut) encasing the entire molecule. This electron cloud effectively prevents breaking of the σ bond for reaction with other elements. The cyanide ion and carbon monoxide have electron structures similar to that of the nitrogen molecule and also show an extraordinary stability.

Nitrogen is prepared primarily by the fractional distillation of liquid air. At the temperature of the electric arc it combines with oxygen forming nitrogen(V) oxide, which is converted into nitric acid. In the presence of catalysts and at great pressure and elevated temperature, it combines with hydrogen to form ammonia.

Table XIII—The Elements of Group V-A

Element	Nitrogen	Phosphorus	Arsenic	Antimony	Bismuth
Symbol	N	P	As	Sb	Bi
Atomic number	7	15	33	51	83
Atomic weight	14.01	30.97	74.92	121.7_5	208.98
Orbital electrons	$[He]2s^22p^3$	$[Ne]3s^23p^3$	$[Ar]3d^{10}4s^24p^3$	$[Kr]4d^{10}5s^25p^3$	$[Xe]4f^{14}5d^{10}6s^26p^3$
Oxidation states	3−,1+,3+,5+	3−,3+,5+	3−,3+,5+	3−,3+,5+	3−,3+,5+
Atomic radius (Å)	0.70	1.06	1.21	1.41	1.5
Ionic (crystal) radii (Å)	1.32(3+)	0.58(3+)	0.72(3+)	0.90(3+)	1.17(3+)
(coordination no 6)	0.27(5+)	0.52(5+)	0.60(5+)	0.74(5+)	0.90(5+)
Ionization potential, ev	14.48	11.10	10.5	8.5	8.0
Electronegativity	3.04	2.19	2.18	2.05	2.02
% of earth's crust	4.6×10^{-8}	0.12	5×10^{-4}	10^{-4}	2×10^{-5}

Unlike phosphorus and the other members of the family, nitrogen does not expand its coordination sphere beyond three. The nitric acid of chemistry is the meta acid. There is no ortho acid, hypothetically H_3NO_4. Nitrogen in the +5 state is too small to accommodate four oxygen atoms.

Therapeutically inactive, elemental Nitrogen, NF XV, is employed pharmaceutically as an inert atmosphere in ampules and other containers of substances that would be adversely affected by air. Nitrogen(I) Oxide (nitrous oxide), USP XX, is an inhalatory general anesthetic (page 372). Sodium Nitrite, USP XX, is used as an antidote to cyanide poisoning; it is also a vasodilator but is slower acting than the organic nitrite and nitrate esters commonly used for this purpose. The nitrate ion is frequently used as an anion for medicinally active cations, eg, silver nitrate, thiamine mononitrate.

Nitrite ion is toxic; it reacts with hemoglobin to form methemoglobin. Nitrites are also potentially dangerous since they can form N-nitroso derivatives of amines and amides, which may be carcinogenic. Nitrate ion is reducible to nitrite in the intestine and may cause methemoglobinemia. For the above reasons the use of nitrates and nitrites as food preservatives is being questioned. Various other preservatives are being tried.

Phosphorus

Phosphorus exists in two common allotropic forms, yellow and red. Yellow phosphorus (white phosphorus) has a distinctive, disagreeable, ozone-like odor. On exposure to air, or when heated at about 50°, it ignites spontaneously. It is almost insoluble in water, but is soluble in chloroform, benzene, or carbon disulfide. It is poisonous and on the skin it causes severe, slow to heal burns. Copper(II) sulfate is used as an antidote.

Red phosphorus is a brown to red amorphous powder. It is nonpoisonous and nonflammable in air, except at high temperatures. It is insoluble in any common solvent.

The use of inorganic phosphorus compounds in modern medicine is restricted primarily to the orthophosphates. Tribasic calcium, magnesium, and aluminum phosphates are used as gastric antacids, and the monobasic alkali phosphates are effective urinary acidifiers. Dibasic sodium phosphate is the active ingredient in various saline cathartics and enemas.

Phosphoric Acid, NF XV, is used to form soluble salts of insoluble medicinal bases. The dihydrogen phosphate-monohydrogen phosphate system is a valuable buffer in physiological ranges. Hypophosphorus acid, NF XV, is an antioxidant, used primarily with iodide and iron(II) salts. The radioactive isotope, ^{32}P, is employed therapeutically (Chapter 30).

Phosphorus is essential to plant and animal life. A complex basic calcium phosphate constitutes the main inorganic component of bones and teeth. Dihydrogen phosphate and monohydrogen phosphate ions constitute the ion pair of one of the buffer systems of the blood and body fluids. The phosphate moiety has important roles in the metabolism of various organic materials, eg, carbohydrates.

Arsenic

Inorganic arsenic compounds are rarely employed in modern medicine. There no longer are official compounds; arsenic trioxide and potassium arsenite were the last. They were used as alternatives, tonics, and antileukemics. Sodium arsenate, ^{74}As, has been used as a diagnostic aid.

Arsenic compounds are poisonous. If still in the GI tract, a freshly prepared mixture of iron(III) and magnesium hydroxides is administered orally as an antidote. If already absorbed, dimercaprol by intramuscular injection is effective.

Antimony

Antimony compounds have physiological reactions resembling those of arsenic. The compounds are potentially toxic. Except for Antimony Potassium Tartrate (antimonyl potassium tartrate, tartar emetic), USP XX, antimony compounds are no longer in common medical usage. Antimony potassium tartrate is used in the treatment of schistosomiasis. In the past it was also used as an emetic and expectorant.

Bismuth

With the exception of sodium bismuthate, $[NaBiO_3]$, in which the bismuth functions anionically in the +5 oxidation state, the important bismuth compounds of commerce are the Bi^{3+} variety. The basic salts, bismuth subcarbonate, bismuth subgallate, and bismuth subnitrate, are employed for their astringent, mildly germicidal, and antacid properties. Bismuth Subnitrate and Milk of Bismuth are official in USP XX. Milk of Bismuth owes its antacid properties to the hydroxyl and carbonate ions present. Because of the adherent properties it provides protective action. The small amount of dissolved bismuthyl ion present exerts a mild antiseptic effect.

Hydrogen sulfide, from the breakdown of proteins, reacts with bismuthyl ion to form the insoluble, dark brown, bismuth(III) sulfide. As a result stools appear black. Soluble bismuth compounds are poisonous; intramuscular dimercaprol is an effective antidote.

Elements of Group V-B

Unlike previous transition elements, the valence electron structure of these elements is not identical. Vanadium and tantalum have a $(n-1)d^3ns^2$ structure while niobium has the structure, $(n-1)d^4ns^1$ (Table XIV). The difference has no apparent effect on their chemistry. In addition to the Group V oxidation states, +3 and +5, these elements also appear in a +2 and +4 oxidation state. The −3 oxidation state does not occur. There is a close similarity between niobium and tantalum. Tantalum, because of its size, has a maximum coordination number of eight and the compounds of these elements are colored.

The Group V-B elements are of little pharmaceutical importance as only tantalum metal is employed therapeutically. Since tantalum is unaffected by the body fluids, it is used in sheet form, for the surgical repair of bones. Muscle tissue will attach itself to tantalum as though it were bone.

Table XIV—Transition Elements

	Group V-B			Group VI-B		
Element	Vanadium	Niobium	Tantalum	Chromium	Molybdenum	Tungsten
Symbol	V	Nb	Ta	Cr	Mo	W
Atomic number	23	41	73	24	42	74
Atomic weight	50.94	92.91	180.95	52.00	95.94	183.8_5
Orbital electrons	$[Ar]3d^34s^2$	$[Kr]4d^45s^1$	$[Xe]4f^{14}5d^36s^2$	$[Ar]3d^54s^1$	$[Kr]4d^55s^1$	$[Xe]4f^{14}5d^46s^2$
Oxidation states	2+,3+,4+,5+	2+,3+,4+,5+	2+,3+,4+,5+	2+,3+,4+,6+	2+ . . . 6+	2+ . . . 6+
Atomic radius (Å)	1.22	1.34	1.34	1.18	1.30	1.30
Ionic (crystal) radii (Å) (coordination no 6)	0.40(5+)	0.70(5+)	0.73(5+)	0.76(3+) 0.58(6+)	0.79(4+) 0.73(6+)	0.80(4+) 0.74(6+)
Ionization potential, ev	6.71	6.79	ca 6	6.77	7.38	7.98
Electronegativity	. . .	. . .	1.33	1.66	2.2	2.36
% of earth's crust	0.021	. . .	. . .	2×10^{-2}	ca 5×10^{-4}	ca 1.5×10^{-4}

Elements of Group VI

The members of this group have six valence electrons. Although theoretically a −2 oxidation state is possible for all, −2, and −1, appear only in the subgroup A elements. The common positive oxidation states are +4 and +6; +1 and +2 also exist.

Elements of Group VI-A

There is a very clear gradation of properties in this family (the Chalcogens). Oxygen is nonmetallic in character while polonium is metallic; the other members show both characteristics. Polonium is further distinguished by its natural radioactivity.

The sulfur-selenium-tellurium triad displays especially strong family relationships. Allotropic varieties of each element in the triad are numerous. Although there are quantitative differences, each functions generally in the −2, +4, and +6 oxidation states, forming many analogous compounds. Some of the more important characteristic properties of Group VI-A elements are presented in Table XV.

Oxygen

In free form, oxygen constitutes about one-fifth, by weight, of air. The primeval atmosphere of the earth probably had no oxygen. In combined form, it constitutes about seven-eighths, by weight, of water and important fractional parts of minerals such as $CaCO_3$, Fe_2O_3, etc. The industrial process for preparing oxygen is the fractional distillation of liquid air. When liquid air is allowed to evaporate under controlled conditions, the nitrogen and inert gases escape initially, followed by nearly pure oxygen.

The weighted atomic mass of the mixture of naturally occurring oxygen isotopes was formerly the standard for all chemical atomic weights. This standard has been replaced by the most abundant carbon isotope, ^{12}C. The isotopes of oxygen have been separated and introduced into specific molecules as tracer elements.

Oxygen, USP XX, is employed as a therapeutic gas in the treatment of conditions involving hypoxia. Ozone, O_3, an allotropic form of oxygen, is a powerful oxidizing agent. Ozonized air (air treated to convert some of its oxygen into ozone) is used in various disinfecting and bleaching operations.

Chemically, oxygen is very reactive, combining directly, under appropriate conditions, with all elements except mercury, silver, gold, and members of the platinum family. It is electronegative with respect to all elements except fluorine. The oxides of nonmetallic elements are acidic, while those of metals are basic. The oxides of many elements, eg, antimony and tellurium, are amphoteric. In all, oxygen has the −2 oxidation number.

Hydrogen peroxide and the peroxides are a series of oxygen compounds in which oxygen has an oxidation number of −1. They are valuable oxidizing and reducing agents.

Hydrogen peroxide is prepared by the electrolysis of a concentrated solution of either sulfuric acid or ammonium sulfate. Persulfate, $[S_2O_8{}^{2-}]$, forms in the anode compartment. After electrolysis the anolyte is reacted with water and the hydrogen peroxide formed is separated by distillation under reduced pressure.

Pure concentrated hydrogen peroxide is stable. However, commercial preparations must be stabilized; usually a preservative is added, eg, acetanilid. Traces of mineral acid, eg, phosphoric acid, are often added as the stability increases in acid media.

Hydrogen peroxide is available as the 3%, 6%, 30%, 70%, and 90% solutions. Concentration is also expressed as volume strength, the volume of oxygen gas released from one volume of solution; ten volume is 3%. Hydrogen Peroxide Concentrate, USP XX, is the 30% solution. It is a powerful oxidant and must not be used on the skin, etc. Hydrogen Peroxide

Table XV—The Elements of Group VI-A

Element	Oxygen	Sulfur	Selenium	Tellurium	Polonium
Symbol	O	S	Se	Te	Po
Atomic number	8	16	34	52	84
Atomic weight	16.00	32.06	78.9_6	127.6	(209)
Orbital electrons	$[He]2s^22p^4$	$[Ne]3s^23p^4$	$[Ar]3d^{10}4s^24p^4$	$[Kr]4d^{10}5s^25p^4$	$[Xe]4f^{14}5d^{10}6s^26p^4$
Oxidation states	2−,1−	2−,2+,6+	2−,4+,6+	2−,4+,6+	4+,6+
Atomic radius (Å)	0.66	1.04	1.16	1.37	1.53
Ionic (crystal) radii (Å)					
simple anion	1.26(2−)	1.70(2−)	1.84(2−)	2.07(2−)	1.08(4+)
coordination no 6	. . .	0.43(6+)	0.56(6+)	0.57(6+)	0.81(6+)
Ionization potential, ev	13.61	10.36	9.75	9.0	. . .
Electronegativity	3.44	2.58	2.55	2.1	2.0
% of earth's crust	46.6	0.052	10^{-7}	10^{-7}	10^{-14}

Topical Solution, USP XX, is the 3% solution. It is a mild, fast acting, oxidizing germicide which will destroy most pathogenic bacteria. Hydrogen peroxide, 6%, is the only common bleach mild enough for use on hair.

Hydrogen peroxide is available as a solution in anhydrous glycerine (1.5%) and as urea peroxide, a stable crystalline 1:1 compound, usually in 4–10% solution in anhydrous glycerine. These preparations are preferable to hydrogen peroxide in treatment of oral and ear infections. Zinc peroxide and sodium perborate have been listed in past compendia.

Sulfur

This element exists in several allotropic forms. At room temperature α-sulfur (rhombic sulfur) is the stable form. At the equilibrium point, 96°, β-sulfur (monoclinic sulfur) becomes the stable form. Other allotropes exist. Commercial, Sublimed Sulfur, USP XX, and Precipitated Sulfur, USP XX, are α-sulfur. Precipitated sulfur has a smaller particle size than sublimed; it is therefore more reactive.

As an ointment, precipitated sulfur is used as the scabicide. Sulfur ointments and lotions are used in dermatological applications as keratolytics. Elemental sulfur also has fungicidal action. Sublimed sulfur is used as a cathartic.

Sulfur appears in three series of compounds. The first, based on the −2 oxidation state, gives rise to hydrogen sulfide and the sulfides. The second and third series, based on +4 and +6 oxidation states, give rise to the two sulfur oxides and their acids and salts.

Hydrogen sulfide and soluble sulfides, in solution, react readily with suspended, finely divided, sulfur to give rise to mixtures of polysulfides, S_2^{2-}, S_3^{2-}, S_4^{2-}, S_5^{2-}, usually written S_n^{2-}.

Sulfurated Potash, USP XX, consists largely of potassium polysulfides, sulfate, and thiosulfate. It is prepared by careful heating of a mixture of potassium carbonate and sublimed sulfur. The compound is very soluble in water, giving an alkaline reaction. The polysulfide component is soluble in ethanol. Sulfurated potash is used in the form of lotions, ointments, and aqueous solutions, for the treatment of psoriasis and other chronic skin conditions and has parasiticidal activity.

Sulfurated Lime Topical Solution, USP XX, is prepared by the action of pulverized roll sulfur with hot slaked lime solution. In diluted form the solution is used as a scabicide, and as a keratolytic in the treatment of acnes and other skin conditions.

Both sulfurated potash and sulfurated lime must be stored in tightly sealed containers to prevent reaction with carbon dioxide and oxygen. Both are incompatible with acid.

White Lotion, USP XX, is prepared by adding freshly prepared, filtered, sulfurated potash solution to zinc sulfate solution. The order of mixing is important. It is an astringent and protective.

Selenium Sulfide (and Lotion), USP XX, is employed as a 2.5% suspension in the topical treatment of seborrheic dermatitis (dandruff). Care is essential to prevent introduction into the eyes or mouth. In addition the hands must be thoroughly cleansed after using since selenium is toxic. Cadmium sulfide is also used in the treatment of seborrheic dermatitis. While less irritating, it requires the same precautions as selenium sulfide.

Sulfur Dioxide, NF XV, is usually prepared industrially by burning sulfur. It is the acid anhydride of sulfurous acid and its salts, the sulfites. All are used in pharmaceutical practice as antoxidants and preservatives.

Attempts to crystallize sodium bisulfite yield instead normal sodium sulfite crystals. If the crystallization is carried out under a sulfur dioxide atmosphere crystals of the metabisulfite, $Na_2S_2O_5$, form. On dissolving metabisulfite in water, a solution of bisulfite results:

$$S_2O_5{}^{2-} + H_2O \rightarrow 2HSO_3{}^-$$

Sodium Metabisulfite, NF XV, should be used when sodium bisulfite is specified. It is used as an antoxidant.

Sodium Thiosulfate, USP XX, is prepared from the sulfite by reaction with sulfur. Since the sulfite ion has an unshared electron pair, and elemental sulfur lacks one electron pair of completion of a stable octet, a coordinate covalent bond easily forms, giving the thiosulfate ion. It is used as an antidote for cyanide poisoning. It is a valuable analytical reagent for the determination of iodine.

In the +6 oxidation state sulfur gives rise to sulfuric acid and the sulfates. While not officially cited, sulfuric acid is an important acid. Several sulfates are officially cited but with the exception of sodium sulfate (saline cathartic) all applications are more appropriately ascribed to the cation present, eg, barium sulfate, bleomycin sulfate.

Selenium and Tellurium

In general, selenium and tellurium compounds are analogous to those of sulfur. Observed differences are largely those to be expected in terms of relative atomic size and electronegativity.

While selenium is toxic in large doses, it is an important trace element. It is very slowly absorbed through the skin. Toxicity is usually not a problem if it is applied to small areas of unbroken, unirritated skin. Prolonged contact with the skin results in contact dermatitis. The use of selenium sulfide, the only official compound, has been described in the section on sulfides. Selenomethionine, ^{75}Se, is used in the diagnosis of pancreatic tumors and growths.

Tellurium has no medicinal applications at this time.

Elements of Group VI-B

The elements of this group are metallic in behavior. The lower oxidation state oxides are basic while those of the higher oxidation states are acidic, giving rise to the chromates, molybdates, and tungstates. The cations of high oxidation numbers have a tendency to unite with oxygen to give stable -yl cations, eg, CrO^{2+}, chromyl. These elements show great similarity in behavior to their horizontal neighbors in Groups V-B and VII-B. Some properties are given in Table XIV.

Chromium and molybdenum are essential trace elements. Chromium has a wide margin of safety between amounts usually ingested and those showing adverse effects. The radioactive isotope, ^{51}Cr, is employed as a biological tracer in certain hematological procedures (Chapter 30). There are currently no official compounds of these elements. Their compounds are important in analytical pharmaceutical operations.

Elements of Group VII

The elements of Group VII subdivide into Group VII-A, (Table XVI), members of which have an outer electron configuration ns^2np^5, and Group VII-B, (Table XVII), with the $(n-1)d^5ns^2$ valence electron configuration.

The halogens are nonmetallic in character while the transition elements of the family are metallic. Except for the higher oxidation states of +5 and especially +7 the elements of the subgroups and their compounds are quite dissimilar. While the free halogens are colored almost all of their compounds are not.

Elements of Group VII-A

Examination of the valence electron structure of these elements suggests −1, +1, +3, +5, and +7 as possible oxidation states. Fluorine, the most electronegative element, appears only as the simple fluoride ion (which readily acts as a ligand). Only chlorine forms compounds in all five oxidation states.

The halogen binary compounds may be ionic and/or covalent, depending on electronegativity differences. All halogens unite with hydrogen to form covalent gaseous hydrogen halides. These gases are extremely soluble in water, giving rise to very strong acids, eg, hydrochloric acid. The ionic binary compounds show a displacement series: a halogen of lower atomic weight will displace a halide ion of higher atomic weight,

$$2I^- + Cl_2 \rightarrow 2Cl^- + I_2$$

Thus, of the halogens, fluorine is the strongest oxidizing agent and iodine the weakest. Conversely, iodide is the strongest reducing agent and fluoride the weakest. In fact, the fluoride ion is the most stable of all simple anions.

Chlorine, bromine, and iodine form well-defined oxides,

Table XVI—The Elements of Group VII-A

Element	Fluorine	Chlorine	Bromine	Iodine	Astatine
Symbol	F	Cl	Br	I	At
Atomic number	9	17	35	53	85
Atomic weight	19	35.45	79.90	126.90	(210)
Orbital electrons	$[He]2s^22p^5$	$[Ne]3s^23p^5$	$[Ar]3d^{10}4s^24p^5$	$[Kr]4d^{10}5s^25p^5$	$[Xe]4f^{14}5d^{10}6s^26p^5$
Oxidation states	1−	1−,1+,3+,5+,7+	1−,1+,(3+),5+	1−,1+,(3+),5+,7+	...
Atomic radius (Å)	0.64	0.99	1.14	1.33	...
Ionic (crystal) radii (Å)					
halide anion	1.19	1.67	1.82	2.06	...
coordination no 6	0.022(7+)	0.41(7+)	0.53(7+)	0.67(7+)	0.76(7+)
Ionization potential, ev	17.42	13.01	11.84	10.44	...
Electronegativity	3.98	3.16	2.96	2.66	2.2
% of earth's crust	8×10^{-2}	3×10^{-2}	1.6×10^{-4}	3×10^{-5}	...

Table XVII—Transition Elements

	Group VII-B			Group VIII-First Triad		
Element	Manganese	Technetium	Rhenium	Iron	Cobalt	Nickel
Symbol	Mn	Tc	Re	Fe	Co	Ni
Atomic number	25	43	75	26	27	28
Atomic weight	54.94	(98)	186.2	55.85	58.93	58.71
Orbital electrons	$[Ar]3d^54s^2$	$[Kr]4d^55s^2$	$[Xe]4f^{14}5d^56s^2$	$[Ar]3d^64s^2$	$[Ar]3d^74s^2$	$[Ar]3d^84s^2$
Oxidation states	2+,3+,4+,6+,7+	2+,3+,4+,6+,7+	3+,4+,5+,6+,7+	2+,3+	2+,3+	2+,3+
Atomic radius (Å)	1.17	1.27	1.25	1.17	1.16	1.15
Ionic (crystal) radii (Å)	0.81(2+)	...	0.81(3+)	0.75(2+)	0.79(2+)	0.83(2+)
(coordination no 6)	0.40(6+)	0.56(7+)	0.69(5+)	0.69(3+)	0.69(3+)	0.70(3+)
Ionization potential, ev	7.43	7.23	7.87	7.83	ca 8.5	7.6
Electronegativity	1.55	1.9	1.9	1.85	1.88	1.91
% of earth's crust	0.085	zero(?)	10^{-7}	5	2.3×10^{-3}	8×10^{-3}

oxyacids and their salts, in most of the positive oxidation states. The stability of the higher oxidation states increases with increasing atomic weight. (For nomenclature of these acids and salts see Table I.)

Fluorine

Fluorine is the most reactive of the electronegative elements. With the exception of gold and platinum it attacks all metals at ordinary temperatures. It combines directly with all nonmetals, including the other halogens. Beryllium fluoride is one of the very few fluorides not completely ionized. Fluorine is an essential element and is present in the teeth and bones.

Sodium Fluoride, Stannous Fluoride (Tin(II) Fluoride), Sodium Fluoride and Phosphoric Acid Gel, and Sodium Monofluorophosphate are listed in USP XX. Stannous fluoride is easily oxidized by oxygen of the air to give the tin(IV) ion which is ineffective as a dental prophylactic. For this reason solutions of this salt must be freshly prepared at the time of use. A developing cloudiness of the solution indicates that the oxidation is proceeding since the tin(IV) ion formed is precipitated as the insoluble hydroxide.

Chlorine

Elemental chlorine is a very reactive nonmetallic element. Most common chlorides are water soluble, the main exceptions being $AgCl$, Hg_2Cl_2, and Cu_2Cl_2. A few, eg, $PbCl_2$, are slightly soluble. The oxygenated chlorine compounds are mostly water soluble.

Hydrochloric acid, NF XV, is a pharmaceutical necessity for purposes such as neutralizing, stabilizing, or solubilizing other substances. In diluted form, it is a gastric acidifier but other compounds, more readily amenable to administration, are usually preferred. Sodium, potassium, and calcium chlorides are employed in electrolyte replenishers; the first named is the sole ingredient of physiological salt solution. Ammonium chloride is an expectorant and a systemic acidifying agent. The chloride ion is frequently the carrier of choice for other metal cations such as those of zinc, aluminum, and mercury, but with these the medicinal value is referable to the metal rather than the chloride.

Sodium Hypochlorite Solution, USP XX, is an effective germicide and deodorant because of the oxidizing power of hypochlorous acid. The hypochlorite ion is rapidly reduced by organic matter.

Sodium hypochlorite is prepared by electrolysis of sodium chloride solutions under conditions such that the chlorine formed at the anode reacts with the hydroxyl ion resulting from removal of hydrogen ion as hydrogen gas at the cathode,

$$Cl_2 + 2OH^- \rightarrow ClO^- + H_2O + Cl^-$$

Sodium chloride is always an impurity in the resulting solution. To improve its stability the pH is adjusted to 10 or greater.

Bleaching powder, *calcium hypochlorite*, is one of the most effective and least expensive disinfectants. The product is formed by passing chlorine gas over moist slaked lime. Its composition is variable but hydroxide, hypochlorite, and chloride ions are present in the mixture.

Potassium chlorate is occasionally present in mouth washes, vaginal douches, and other local cleansing preparations; however, its antiseptic value is too weak to be of any value.

Bromine

Bromine is a dark reddish brown, fuming liquid with a suffocating odor. The fumes are highly irritating to the mu-cous membranes and they burn and blister the skin. It attacks most metals and organic tissue. Chemically, bromine resembles chlorine with slight differences referable to the comparative size of the two atoms and their electronegativities.

Bromine is a powerful caustic and germicide but is not employed as such. It is a common chemical reagent. Utmost care should be exercised in handling bromine. All work with bromine should be done under ideal conditions of ventilation. If exposed to bromine, the area should be immediately washed with a solution of sodium bicarbonate and treated with glycerine. Caution—bromine containers should be opened only after they have been thoroughly cooled.

Bromine has no known biological role. In proper dosage the bromide ion provides central depressant action. Sodium, potassium, and ammonium bromides are commonly employed. Excessive continued dosage may elicit a toxic condition, brominism.

Iodine

Except for astatine, iodine is the most metallic of the halogens. Its oxo-salts are very stable while the simple anion is slowly oxidized by the oxygen of the air. When reacting with the other halogens it assumes the cationic role, eg, ICl_3. Many workers consider IOH the hydroxide of iodine. Iodine is an effective antimicrobial.

Iodine solutions include potassium or sodium iodide to enhance the solubility of the iodine by the formation of polyiodide ions. Loss of the element to air is greatly reduced since polyiodide solutions have a lower iodine vapor pressure. Iodine, Potassium Iodide, Sodium Iodide, and various iodine solutions are cited in USP XX, as is Povidone-Iodine. Povidone is a synthetic polymer which has a special affinity for iodine molecules. The advantages of povidone-iodine are reduced volatility of the iodine and a decreased irritation on application. Iodine is also available in the form of cationic and nonionic surface active salts, used as sanitizing agents.

Iodine is essential for proper thyroid functioning and is physiologically utilized either in the elemental form or as potassium or sodium iodide. In proper dosage, iodide ion exerts expectorant action; examples are hydrogen iodide (as hydriodic acid syrup) and potassium iodide. The radioactive isotopes, ^{125}I and ^{131}I have diagnostic and therapeutic applications (Chapter 30).

Elemental iodine is toxic and corn starch and sodium thiosulfate are effective chemical antidotes.

Astatine

Astatine is a synthetic radioactive element. It resembles iodine but is more metallic. It has no pharmaceutical applications.

Pseudohalogens (Halogenoids)

Inorganic anions such as CN^-, CNO^-, CNS^-, N_3^-, and $[Fe(CN)_6]^{3-}$ resemble the halide anions and are known as pseudohalogens. The similarity of the cyanide ion is especially marked; it has properties intermediate to those of the chloride and bromide ions. Similarities include insoluble silver salts soluble in ammonia, preparation of HX by adding concentrated sulfuric acid to the sodium salt, preparation of X_2 by adding MnO_2 and concentrated sulfuric acid to the sodium salt, formation of polyions, etc.

The most striking difference is the very weak acidic character of the pseudohalogen hydrides, eg, the pK_a of HCN is 8.9 while that of HCl is ca -10.

The pseudohalogens have no pharmaceutical applications.

Elements of Group VII-B

The elements of this group are metallic in character. The higher oxides give rise to very stable oxo-salts with the +6 and +7 oxidation states, eg, manganate (MnO_4^{2-}), pertechnetate (TeO_4^-). A summary of important properties appears in Table XVII. Compounds of these elements are colored.

Manganese

Pharmaceutically, manganese is the most important element in this group. Potassium Permanganate, USP XX, is the only official compound. Categorized as a local anti-infective of the oxidizing type, it is also an astringent and a powerful deodorant and cleanser. It is used in the form of dilute (0.01–1%) solutions. As the compound reacts, manganese(IV) oxide precipitates on the skin causing a temporary darkening of the surface. Gastric lavage using dilute permanganate solutions is antidotal for various alkaloids and other toxic substances that have been ingested in small amounts and are readily susceptible to oxidation.

Caution must be exercised to keep permanganate from contact with organic and other easily oxidized compounds either in the dry state or in solution. Dangerous explosions may occur.

Manganese is an essential trace element, being necessary for the activation of a variety of enzymes, eg, pyruvate carboxylase. It is included in mineral supplements, but there are no well-defined deficiency states in man.

Technetium

Technetium (from Greek technetos, meaning artificial) was so named because it was the first element produced artificially. Radioactive technetium, ^{99}Tc, is used diagnostically in various forms (Chapter 30).

Rhenium

Rhenium is a very rare element and finds few technical applications. Alone and in combination with other metals, it has been employed as a catalyst for dehydrogenation.

Elements of Group VIII

This group of elements represents those in which the single electron already present in each of the five d-orbitals is being paired with a second electron of opposite spin. The group consists of three elements (triads) in each of the long rows and fills the space between the elements of Groups VII-B and I-B.

The first triad follows manganese and includes iron, cobalt, and nickel (Table XVII), known as the ferrous metals. They are characterized by their strong ferromagnetism. The second triad follows technetium and includes ruthenium, rhodium, and palladium. The third triad follows rhenium and includes osmium, iridium, and platinum. The elements of these latter two triads are known as the platinum metals. The term *noble*

metals is also used. The platinum metals are characterized by their extreme inertness to chemical reaction.

These elements are definitely metallic and all participate readily in the formation of coordination complexes. The compounds of the first row triad are stable under most conditions while those of the second triad are moderately stable. However, osmium, iridium, and platinum compounds are unstable and easily revert to the free element. All form colored compounds.

None of the elements of the second triad have compounds of medicinal value, but platinum, a member of the third triad, is used in cancer chemotherapy as *cis*-diamminedichloroplatinum(II), Cisplatin.

Elements of the First Triad

The important oxidation states are +2, achieved by the loss of the two s electrons, and +3 in which an additional d electron is lost (Table XVII). The stability of the +2 oxidation state increases from iron to nickel. The free metals and the +2 cations are important reducing agents. The cations have a tendency to form both cationic and anionic complex ions of high stability.

Iron

Iron is widely distributed in nature. It functions in divalent and trivalent states to form iron(II), ferrous, and iron(III), ferric compounds, respectively. Iron(II) compounds are usually green in the hydrated state and white in the anhydrous state. Iron(III) salts are usually yellow to brown in the hydrated state but vary in color when anhydrous. Aqueous solutions of iron(III) salts hydrolyze strongly to give acid solutions. Iron(II) salts undergo slight hydrolysis and are easily oxidized in solution. The behavior of the iron(III) ion is similar to that of aluminum(III).

Iron, in either oxidation state, readily forms soluble coordination complexes with ligands such as phosphate, citrate, tartrate, and amines. Iron does not precipitate from many of these complexes with the usual iron precipitants.

Iron is an essential trace element. It is the important element in the transportation of oxygen by hemoglobin. It functions in various cytochromes, essential oxidative enzymes of the body cells.

Numerous iron(II) and iron(III) compounds, complexes, and solutions have been used as hematinics in the past. However, because of their greater gastrointestinal irritation and poor absorption, iron(III) compounds and preparations are rarely used today. Ferrous Fumarate (and Tablets), Ferrous Gluconate (and Tablets), Ferrous Sulfate (and Oral Solution, Syrup, and Tablets), and Dried Ferrous Sulfate are official in USP XX. Iron Dextran Injection [colloidal iron(III) hydroxide with partially hydrolyzed dextran] and Iron Sorbitex Injection (a complex of iron with sorbitol and citric acid) are cited in USP XX as injectable forms for patients with poor gastrointestinal tolerance or poor absorption of iron. Reduced iron was formerly used as a hematinic. It survives today in the fortification of foods, eg, flour.

Iron(III) compounds are astringent (page 372). Sodium nitroprusside, $Na_2[Fe(CN)_5(NO)] \cdot 2H_2O$, USP XX, is a vasodilator. Iron oxides and hydrous oxides are employed as pigments (page 372).

Cobalt

The important cobalt salts of commerce are those of cobalt(II). Most contain water of hydration and are red in color but when rendered anhydrous they are blue. Because of this color change anhydrous cobalt(II) chloride is included in dehydrating agents for gases to indicate when they are spent.

There is evidence that the presence of traces of cobalt may catalyze the physiological utilization of iron. This has led to the introduction of medicinal specialty products containing iron in association with cobalt designed for use in the treatment of iron deficiency anemias. Cyanocobalamin (vitamin B_{12}), is the only cobalt compound officially cited. The radioactive isotopes, [57]Co and ^{60}Co, are used diagnostically and therapeutically (Chapter 30).

Nickel

The important nickel compounds are in the +2 oxidation state. There are no nickel compounds of medical importance.

Water

Water is omnipresent. About three quarters of the earth's surface is covered with liquid water. Land masses in polar regions are covered with thick sheets of ice. In vapor form, water is an important constituent of the earth's atmosphere. In combined form, water occurs abundantly in many minerals, eg, gypsum ($CaSO_4 . 2H_2O$). In addition, water occurs in all animal and vegetable tissues; it constitutes some 70% of the human body and over 90% of vegetables such as cucumbers and watermelons.

Together with ammonia and hydrogen fluoride, water is distinguished from other covalent hydrides by the strong hydrogen bonds existing between adjacent molecules. Despite the ability of fluoride ion to form stronger hydrogen bonds than oxide, hydrogen bonding reaches its peak in water because two protons are available per molecule. Hydrogen fluoride has only one available proton per molecule and ammonia has only one open site per molecule for hydrogen bonding.

Because of the extensive hydrogen bonding, the physical properties of water are unique among the other hydrides. Most obvious is the existence of water as a liquid under normal conditions. All other covalent hydrides are gases. The heat of fusion and melting point, heat of vaporization and boiling point, specific heat, surface tension, viscosity, and dielectric constant of water are all much higher in absolute value than those of other covalent hydrides. The world as we know it would be impossible without these unusual properties of water.

Water is a chemically stable compound. Even at 2000°K less than 1% is dissociated into its elements. The K_w for water is only 10^{-14}. Despite this relative nonreactivity it acts as a solvent, especially for ionic compounds, as a ligand, as an acid or base, and as an oxidizing or reducing agent. In traces, water is frequently a catalyst. The acid-base properties are discussed later.

Because of its strong permanent dipole, water frequently acts as a ligand in complex substances. Almost all cations form one or more hydrates, divalent cations being more highly hydrated than monovalent because of their stronger electrostatic fields. Having reduced field strengths because of their greater size, large cations, eg, cesium, do not hydrate. Many anions hydrate, eg, $CuSO_4 . 5H_2O$ is actually $[Cu(H_2O)_4][SO_4 . H_2O]$.

Water acts as a solvent for an unusual range of substances. This solvent action results from one or more of its properties, small size, strong permanent dipole, high dielectric constant, and availability of protons for hydrogen bonding.

Natural Waters

Naturally occurring waters contain dissolved minerals indigenous to the region. Such waters are variously described as mineral waters, lithia waters, sulfur waters, etc. Owners of springs or other sources of such waters often claim fanciful therapeutic effects but, in general, these claims have not been substantiated.

Natural waters contain varying amounts of suspended matter, eg, clay, sand, microorganisms, fragments of plants and animals. Commonly they are a very dilute solution (ppm) of calcium, magnesium, iron(III), sodium, and potassium ions having as counter ions, bicarbonate, sulfate, and chloride. The dissolved bicarbonate constitutes *temporary* hardness while sulfate and chloride constitute *permanent* hardness. In addition natural water contains traces of dissolved atmospheric gases, ammonia and metabolic decomposition products. Waters in inhabited areas often include dissolved minerals, eg, nitrate, phosphate, and organic compounds from homes, industry, and farms. Detergents and dissolved traces of insecticides and herbicides are proving especially troublesome. The Environmental Protection Agency (EPA) of the federal government recently established water quality criteria for sixty-four priority pollutants.

Potable Water

This is water that is "fit to drink." Providing potable water is one of the most important functions of modern communities. The overall process involves removal of insoluble matter through appropriate coagulating, settling, and filtering processes; the destruction of pathogenic microorganisms by aeration, chlorination, or other methods; and improvement of palatability through aeration and filtration through charcoal. Activated charcoal also removes some harmful trace impurities, eg, trihalomethanes, not removed or destroyed by previous operations. In regions where water is excessively hard, "softening" is effected by partial removal of dissolved salts by precipitation as carbonates (Ca^{2+} and Mg^{2+}) and hydroxide [iron(III)], by adding lime or ammonia. In order to assure an adequate provision of the essential element fluorine, fluoridation is accomplished by adding sodium fluosilicate. Standards for potable water are issued by the EPA.

In emergencies water may be purified (rendered free of viable microorganisms) by boiling for 15–20 minutes, or by treatment with halazone or iodine.

Purified Water

Purified water is prepared by distillation, ion-exchange (deionized, demineralized), reverse osmosis, or other methods. Potable water, meeting EPA standards, is used in its preparation. The object is the removal of dissolved solids. Ion-exchange and reverse osmosis are particularly effective in removing electrolytes. Distillation is not effective in the removal of weak electrolytes and nonelectrolytes if they are volatile.

Purified water may be rendered sterile and pyrogen-free by repeated distillation.

Primarily because of its solvent powers and physiological inertness, water is an extremely important pharmaceutical agent. It is official in six different monographs: Purified Water, Water for Injection, Bacteriostatic Water for Injection, Sterile Water for Inhalation, Sterile Water for Injection, and Sterile Water for Irrigation.

Heavy Water

The isotopes of hydrogen, unlike those of other elements, have been named, deuterium (two neutrons), and tritium (three neutrons). The presence of three neutrons in tritium results in an unstable nucleus. However, like hydrogen, deuterium is stable and gives rise to deuterium oxide, D_2O. This compound occurs in ordinary water in a few ppm. Because of its greater molecular weight the physical properties of deuterium oxide differ from those of water, eg, bp 101.4°, sp gr 1.10.

Deuterium oxide has no known therapeutic role. It has been used as a research tool in biological and pharmacological investigations. Use of deuterium oxide, for drinking purposes, has caused retardation, or stunted growth in experimental mammals. It is commercially available and finds use as a moderator in nuclear reactors and as a solvent in nuclear magnetic resonance studies.

Acids, Bases, and Buffers

Acids and Bases

Acid-base theories range from the limited classical Arrhenius Theory to the comprehensive theory due to G N Lewis. In between are the Franklin Solvent System of acids and bases and the Brønsted Proton Donor Theory.

Since the body functions with aqueous media and pharmaceuticals are frequently dispensed in aqueous solution, the Brønsted Theory is convenient for use in pharmacy. A molecule or ion which can provide a proton (proton donor) is an acid; one which can accept a proton (proton acceptor) is a base. On accepting a proton, a base becomes an acid; on losing its proton, the acid becomes a base. An acid and its base are related by the presence or absence of a proton, and are known as a "conjugate pair." Neutralization is the transfer of a proton from the acid of one conjugate pair to the base of another conjugate pair. Some conjugate pairs of pharmaceutical interest are given in Table XVIII. It is evident that acids and bases may be cations, neutral molecules, or anions. Some structures may be members of two different conjugate pairs, as an acid in one and as a base in the other.

A strong acid is an acid which loses its proton easily, a weak acid holds its proton tenaciously. The conjugate base of a strong acid is a weak base while that of a weak acid is a strong base. In neutralization the proton goes to the strongest of the bases present. The percent ionization and the ionization constant are measures of the strength of a given acid.

Acids and bases are used in pharmacy for analytical procedures, as buffer systems, and to dissolve insoluble medicinals. To accomplish the latter the insoluble compound must have a functional group capable of acting as a strong base or as an acid. Lidocaine Hydrochloride Injection, USP XX, and Niacin Injection, USP XX, are examples. The former is prepared by reacting lidocaine with hydrochloric acid; the diethylamino group is a stronger base than either the water molecule or the chloride ion. Lidocaine goes into solution as a cation. Niacin Injection is prepared by reacting niacin with either sodium carbonate or sodium hydroxide; the carboxyl group loses its proton to the carbonate or hydroxyl ion and the niacin goes into solution as an anion.

In neutralization, as above, the pharmacist must be cognizant of two requirements which are not important in ordinary chemical neutralizations. The counter-ion being introduced, chloride ion and sodium ion, respectively, in the above examples, must be physiologically compatible with the body fluids. Also, since strong acids or bases are being used, there can be no excess acid or base because of the corrosive nature of these reagents.

Acids and bases are also necessary for the preparation of effervescent mixtures, a medicinal dosage form sometimes used to render a medicinal more palatable for oral administration. Sodium bicarbonate is used as the carbon dioxide source. Solid acids, eg, citric acid, tartaric acid, or sodium dihydrogen phosphate are used, frequently in combination. Reaction rate is very important in these formulations. Sodium bicarbonate must have the correct particle size; if too fine the reaction is too violent, if too coarse the reaction is too slow. To lower the activity of the acid, a normal salt of the acid is included in the mixture as a diluent.

The acids and bases listed in the compendia at present are: Calcium Hydroxide, Calcium Oxide, Potassium Bicarbonate, Potassium Hydroxide, Sodium Bicarbonate, Sodium Carbonate, Sodium Hydroxide, Ammonia Solution, Boric Acid, Hydrochloric Acid and Diluted Hydrochloric Acid, Nitric Acid, Phosphoric Acid and Diluted Phosphoric Acid, and Potassium Dihydrogen Phosphate.

Stability and storage problems of these compounds must be considered. All bases (except $NaHCO_3$) are subject to reaction with carbon dioxide if proper closures are not maintained. Volatile compounds, ammonia and hydrogen chloride, must be tightly sealed at all times, as must hygroscopic compounds such as sodium hydroxide.

Buffers

Buffers are used to maintain the pH of a medicinal at an optimal value. A buffer is a solution of a weak acid and its conjugate base, the base being provided by one of its soluble salts. Refer to Chapter 17 for an extensive discussion of pH and buffers.

Table XVIII—Conjugate Acid-Base Pairs

Acid	Base	Acid	Base
H_2O	OH^-	H_2SO_4	HSO_4^-
H_3O^+	H_2O	HSO_4^-	SO_4^{2-}
NH_4^+	NH_3	H_3PO_4	$H_2PO_4^-$
RNH_3^+	RNH_2	$H_2PO_4^-$	HPO_4^{2-}
HCl	Cl^-	$[Al(H_2O)_6]^{3+}$	$[Al(H_2O)_5(OH)]^{2+}$
H_2CO_3	HCO_3^-	$[Al(H_2O)_5(OH)]^{2+}$	$[Al(H_2O)_4(OH)_2]^+$
HCO_3^-	CO_3^{2-}	$H_3BO_3.H_2O$	$[B(OH)_4]^-$

Physiological Control of pH

Brønsted acids and bases have been used to maintain and adjust the pH of body fluids for many years. By far the greatest interest has been in development of gastric antacids. However, an adequate number of suitable reagents are available for systemic pH adjustments.

Gastric Antacids

The present official magnesium antacids are: Magnesium Hydroxide, Milk of Magnesia, Magnesia Tablets, Magnesia and Alumina Oral Suspension (and Tablets), Magnesium Carbonate, Magnesium Oxide, Magnesium Phosphate, and Magnesium Trisilicate. The official aluminum antacids are: Aluminum Hydroxide Gel, Dried Aluminum Hydroxide Gel (and Tablets), Aluminum Phosphate Gel, Dihydroxyaluminum Aminoacetate (and Magma, and Tablets), Dihydroxyaluminum Sodium Carbonate (and Tablets), and the Alumina and Magnesia preparations already listed. The calcium antacids include: Precipitated Calcium Carbonate (and Tablets), and Tribasic Calcium Phosphate. Miscellaneous official antacids include Milk of Bismuth, Sodium Bicarbonate and Potassium Bicarbonate.

Systemic Alkalizers and Acidifiers

Sodium Bicarbonate and Potassium Bicarbonate, USP XX, are used as systemic alkalizers. Because the bicarbonates are unstable to heat, chemical problems arise in the sterilization of bicarbonate solutions,

$$2HCO_3^- \rightleftharpoons CO_3^{2-} + CO_2 + H_2O.$$

To depress the forward reaction the solution can be saturated with carbon dioxide. To prevent the loss of the gas, which would result in the permanent formation of the strong carbonate base, the ampules used must be tightly sealed before sterilization and made of glass sufficiently strong to withstand the gas pressure developed during sterilization. On cooling the reverse reaction becomes dominant.

Ammonium Chloride, Sodium Biphosphate (dihydrogen phosphate), and Calcium Chloride, USP XX, are employed as systemic acidifiers. Refer to Chapter 41 for a discussion of alkalizers and acidifiers.

Electrolytes and Essential Trace Elements

While the roles and behavior of inorganic elements in these categories are discussed elsewhere in this textbook (Chapter 42) it is instructive to review the physical and chemical properties which make possible their respective roles. Examination of orbital electron structures, ionic radii, oxidation states, etc, as given in Tables VII through XVII, can give valuable clues to their behavior.

The transition elements have incompletely filled 18-electron outer shells and each can exist in several different oxidation states. In most cases the shift between two electron states is relatively easy, eg,

$$Fe^{2+} \rightleftharpoons Fe^{3+} + e^-$$

As a result the transition elements can act as electron *sinks* and are active in those systems involved in oxidation or reduction reactions.

On the other hand an element such as zinc achieves a completely filled outer 18-electron shell on becoming zinc ion.

In the 2+ oxidation state this shell becomes stable. Unlike the tightly held spherical 8-electron shell the 18-electron shell is "mushy" and easily deformed or polarized by external fields. In turn it can cause polarization of other moieties. This ion is not found in redox systems, but rather in systems such as carbonic anhydrase, which aid in the splitting or forming of molecules.

Unlike the incompletely filled shells of the transition elements or the 18-electron shell of the zinc ion, 8-electron shell ions are ordinarily stable and are not easily deformed by external fields. Those 8-electron outer shell ions with a high charge eg, calcium, have intense charge densities in the volume surrounding the ion. This results in strong interactions with the fields of other moieties to form strong permanent associations. However, an 8-electron shell effectively screens the single charge of ions such as sodium. They are therefore chemically inert with very weak interactions with other ions. This explains their simple roles in the body fluids as osmotic regulators, etc.

Topical Agents

Oxidizing Germicides

Hydrogen Peroxide, Sodium Hypochlorite, and Iodine and/or their various solutions are cited in USP XX. The uses of these preparations are discussed in Chapter 64. Hypochlorous acid, the active moiety in sodium hypochlorite solution, owes its germicidal activity to both oxidizing and chlorinating activity.

Precipitating Germicides

Silver Nitrate, Silver Nitrate Ophthalmic Solution and Toughened Silver Nitrate are listed in USP XX, as are Ammoniated Mercury and Yellow Mercuric Oxide (and their ointments). Zinc Acetate, Zinc Chloride, Zinc Sulfate and Zinc Undecylenate are also official. Only two boron compounds are cited; Boric Acid and Sodium Borate. The sole surviving antimony compound is Antimony Potassium Tartrate, USP XX. The applications of these compounds are discussed in Chapter 64.

Astringents

Aluminum ion in solution is an excellent local astringent over wide concentration ranges. It is also mildly antiseptic. Aluminum Chloride (USP XX), was once used in this application, however, the high acidity of its solutions caused problems. The acidity results from ionization of the hexahydrate ion,

$$[Al(H_2O)_6]^{3+} + H_2O \rightleftharpoons [Al(OH)(H_2O)_5]^{2+} + H_3O^+$$

and is about that of acetic acid. Today the mixture of two compounds (aluminum hydroxychloride, aluminum chlorhydrate, aluminum chlorhydrol), obtained by partial neutralization of aluminum chloride is used,

$$[Al(H_2O)_6]^{3+} + OH^- \rightarrow [Al(OH)(H_2O)_5]^{2+} + H_2O$$

$$[Al(OH)(H_2O)_5]^{2+} + OH^- \rightarrow [Al(OH)_2(H_2O)_4]^+ + H_2O$$

The reaction is stopped before complete conversion to the dihydroxy hydrate. The resulting solution (or dried product) retains the excellent astringent (and deodorant) properties of the aluminum ion but the pH of the solutions approximates neutrality (5 to 6). Aluminum Subacetate Topical Solution, (USP XX), is essentially a solution of the above ions prepared from aluminum sulfate using carbonate ion ($CaCO_3$) as the base. Aluminum Sulfate and Alum (USP XX) are also used as astringents. Alum may be either the potassium or ammonium form. It is shaped into "pencils" to be used as styptics.

Iron(III) and aluminum ions are very similar. Iron(III) is astringent, and preparations of ferric salts for such use were formerly recognized. While it is efficient in this capacity its staining property is a major disadvantage. Lime water, a saturated solution of fresh calcium hydroxide, is used as a local astringent. Bismuth subnitrate and the other bismuth sub-salts are used as astringents and protectives.

Protectives

In order to possess good adhering properties protectives must be in very finely powdered form. They must also be relatively inert, insoluble compounds. A wide range of compounds are suitable as protectives. They are usually used externally, but some applications involve the gastrointestinal tract. Some are slightly soluble, eg, ZnO, and give some astringent action; others, eg, kaolin, have adsorbent action.

Zinc Oxide, Calamine (and Calamine Lotion and Phenolated Calamine Lotion), and Zinc Stearate, USP XX, are used for their protective and slightly astringent properties. Calamine is the calcined native zinc oxide ore. The iron oxide impurity gives calamine a flesh color which is cosmetically more appealing. Zinc stearate, a mixture of fatty acid zinc soaps, has an unctuous feel. White Lotion (USP XX), is used for its astringent and protective powers.

Aluminum Paste, USP XX, is prepared by mixing finely powdered aluminum in zinc oxide ointment and is used as a protective.

Magnesium trisilicate, basic aluminum carbonate, and chalk are used as protectives, as are the various insoluble bismuth sub-salts. Talc is used because of its smooth, unctuous feel. Kaolin and bentonite are used as they also have some absorptive properties, titanium dioxide is used as a solar screen.

Inorganic Pigments

The most important innocuous pigments are the iron oxides. They give colors throughout the visible spectrum. Three variables are involved; particle size, oxidation state, and degree of hydration.

Miscellaneous Inorganic Applications

Artificial Atmospheres

Five gases are official: nitrogen, oxygen, helium, carbon dioxide, and nitrogen(I) oxide (nitrous oxide or laughing gas). Nitrogen is used as a diluent for oxygen and may be used as a protective atmosphere for easily oxidized medicinals.

Helium, because of its low density compared to nitrogen, is used to prepare a gaseous mixture composed of 20% oxygen and helium. This air is used to alleviate respiration difficulties. Because of the low solubility of helium in blood the same mixture is used as an atmosphere for those performing under high atmospheric pressures (deep-sea divers, caisson workers). When ordinary air is used, rapid decompression causes bubbles of gaseous nitrogen to form in the blood. The painful, and sometimes fatal, condition known as *bends* results.

Oxygen is used when respiratory problems exist. Ordinarily it is diluted with nitrogen or helium; 100% oxygen should not be used continuously. In hyperbaric oxygen therapy oxygen is breathed inside a tank at up to three atmosphere pressure. While the amount of oxygen carried by the hemoglobin is little affected, the higher oxygen pressure increases the amount of dissolved oxygen in the plasma (Henry's Law).

Nitrogen(I) oxide usually requires 20–25% oxygen during administration. It is used for surgical operations of short duration. Xenon has a general anesthetic action but is too rare for use. Magnesium ion has anesthetic action, however, the anesthetic dose and the toxic dose of magnesium are too close for use as a general anesthetic. Magnesium Sulfate Injection, (USP XX) is used as an anticonvulsant and central depressant.

Carbon Dioxide Absorbers

When, as in general anesthesia, a patient rebreathes air, dangerous levels of carbon dioxide build up. To prevent this carbon dioxide absorbers are used. Soda Lime, USP XX, is prepared by fusing calcium hydroxide with sodium hydroxide and/or potassium hydroxide with sufficient diatomaceous earth to yield a hard, nonfriable product. For Barium Hydroxide Lime, USP XX, barium hydroxide is substituted for the alkali hydroxide. The particles formed must be large enough to allow free passage of air, but small enough to give a large surface area for absorption. The particles must be hard to prevent dust formation with handling. Entrainment of absorber dust in the breathed air could cause serious alkali burns in the respiratory tract. A colored indicator is included in the preparation to indicate when the carbon dioxide capacity is depleted.

Respiratory Stimulants

Carbon dioxide is used as a respiratory stimulant, usually with 5–7% oxygen. Since it is the normal respiratory stimulant it is of no value where the respiratory center is already depressed. Carbon dioxide is also used as an inert gas in the headspace over medicinals in sealed containers.

Ammonium Carbonate (NF XV) is used as a respiratory stimulant. The name is a misnomer; it is a mixture of ammonium bicarbonate and ammonium carbamate. At room temperature it decomposes to ammonia and carbon dioxide, two respiratory stimulants,

$$NH_4HCO_3 + NH_2CO_2NH_4 \rightarrow 3\overline{NH}_3 + 2\overline{CO}_2 + H_2O$$

The substance must be stored in tightly sealed containers.

Aromatic Ammonia Spirit, USP XX, is prepared from ammonium carbonate, strong ammonia solution, various aromatic oils, alcohol, and water. Light resistant containers must be used.

Expectorants

Water vapor is an excellent expectorant, currently considered the best. Ammonium chloride and carbonate, ammonium and potassium iodides, are commonly used expectorants. Hydriodic acid syrup was official at one time. If the iodides are used in solution they must be protected by an antoxidant, eg, sodium thiosulfate.

Laxatives and Enemas

Cathartics are divided into classes according to mode of action. With the exception of sulfur, the inorganic cathartics are saline (osmotic, bulk) laxatives. For laxative action one or both of the ions of the salt must not be absorbed, or be absorbed with difficulty. This sets up an osmotic imbalance in the intestinal tract which the body attempts to correct by secreting water into the intestine. The large volume of fluid in the intestine acts as a mechanical stimulus for peristalsis.

The commonly used salts of the monohydrogen phosphate, monohydrogen tartrate, tartrate, and citrate ions are slowly absorbed, but in laxative doses their osmotic action is rapid and effective. They are swept out of the intestinal tract before appreciable absorption can take place. Sulfate ion is relatively nonabsorbable and is used as either the magnesium or sodium salt (Epsom salt, Glauber's salt). Insoluble laxatives, eg, Milk of Magnesia, must be dissolved in the stomach before they can exert a laxative effect. The soluble magnesium sulfate and citrate of magnesia are widely used as laxatives. However, soluble magnesium salts are frequently not recommended as laxatives because of the danger of absorbing free magnesium ion. Dibasic Sodium Phosphate, Effervescent Sodium Phosphate, Sodium Phosphates Oral Solution, Sodium Citrate Solution, Sodium Citrate and Citric Acid Oral Solution, Sodium Potassium Tartrate, Milk of Magnesia, Sodium Sulfate are officially cited.

Sulfur, when ingested, has an irritant laxative effect. The element is thought to be reduced to hydrogen sulfide by reducing agents present in the intestinal fluid. Hydrogen sulfide is a mild intestinal irritant.

Sodium Phosphates Enema (USP XX), is a mixture of sodium phosphate and sodium biphosphate or sodium phosphate and phosphoric acid in water to give a pH of 5.0–5.8.

Radiopaques

These are compounds capable of interfering with the passage of X-rays. This interference is directly proportional to atomic number. The soft tissues of the body are composed of atoms of very low atomic number, 1, 6, 7, 8, 15, and 16, which do not interfere sufficiently to be discerned. To make the soft tissues, the lumen of organs, and body channels show, high atomic number atoms must be used. Because of the toxicity of these elements the choices are limited. Only two, barium, and iodine, atomic numbers 56 and 53, have proven useful. Barium Sulfate and Barium Sulfate for Suspension, USP XX, are used for studies of the intestinal tract. Iodine is incorporated into organic molecules designed to concentrate in the organ or cavity to be studied, eg, Iopanoic Acid, USP XX, designed for visualization of the gall bladder. Each molecule of the acid has three iodine atoms.

Structural Repairs

Occasionally temporary or permanent replacement of support structures is necessary. The materials used should be chemically inert and insoluble in the body fluids. They must be nontoxic. They must have the strength to withstand any physical stress to which they are subjected. Tantalum has been used as a bone replacement for temporary braces of long bones, and to close openings in the skull. Silver has found similar applications. It reacts slightly with body fluids, but since insoluble silver chloride is the principal product this is not a serious threat. Mercury amalgams of gold and silver are used for dental fillings. Zinc-Eugenol Cement, USP XX, is also used for dental fillings.

Plaster of Paris is used for temporary support structures, especially for broken bones. While the formula, $CaSO_4 \cdot \frac{1}{2}H_2O$, suggests a hemihydrate there is experimental evidence indicating the existence of local gypsum ($CaSO_4 \cdot 2H_2O$) nuclei in anhydrous calcium sulfate.

Plaster of Paris is also used for taking dental impressions. Since it expands slightly on setting it fills all spaces completely to give a true surface replica.

Epilogue

Because of space considerations many less important and older inorganic medicinals have been omitted. The chemistry given is necessarily abbreviated. For further details of basic chemistry and omitted uses and products see Discher.[1] For more thorough discussions of the etiology and treatment involving inorganic substances see the appropriate chapters of this text or of Block et al[4]. For the chemistry and use of many products no longer in general use or entirely abandoned refer to one of the older editions of Soine and Wilson[5].

References

1. Discher CA: *Modern Inorganic Pharmaceutical Chemistry*, John Wiley & Sons, New York, pp 116–126, 1964.
2. Huheey JE: *Inorganic Chemistry*, 2nd ed, Harper and Row, New York, Appendix E, 1978.
3. *Nomenclature of Inorganic Chemistry*, Definitive Rules 1970, 2nd ed., Butterworths, London, 1971. Reprinted in *Pure and Applied Chemistry*, 28: 1, 1971.
4. Block JH, *et al*: *Inorganic Medicinal and Pharmaceutical Chemistry*, Lea & Febiger, Philadelphia 1974.
5. Rogers CH, Soine TO, Wilson CO: *A Textbook of Inorganic Pharmaceutical Chemistry*, Lea & Febiger, Philadelphia (1952).

CHAPTER 24

Organic Pharmaceutical Chemistry

John H Shinkai, PhD

Associate Professor of Pharmaceutical Chemistry, Rutgers University
College of Pharmacy
Piscataway, NJ 08854

Alfonso R Gennaro, PhD

Professor of Chemistry
Philadelphia College of Pharmacy and Science
Philadelphia, PA 19104

It is not the purpose of this text to provide a basic treatment of organic chemistry.[1] Readers are expected to have pursued the usual basic courses in organic chemistry[1] and to be cognizant of the various advanced texts and other readily available works of reference. Accordingly, this chapter is restricted primarily to a listing of the more prominent structural types of organic compounds and to a brief presentation of the various nomenclature systems and of the major chemical classes of official (USP) pharmaceuticals, followed by a discussion on the identification of organic functional groups and the assignment of an approximate acidic, basic, or neutral value. Detailed treatment of the individual pharmaceuticals is provided at other locations in the text (refer to the index).

Types of Organic Compounds

A comprehensive understanding of organic chemistry would be extremely difficult were it not for the fact that the hundreds of thousands of known compounds fall conveniently into a very much smaller number of general types based on molecular structure. Similarities and differences among the physical and chemical properties of the diverse compounds thus become more apparent and understandable, and this is useful both in providing explanations for observed phenomena and in making predictions for possible applications of compounds known and compounds projected for synthesis.

Organic compounds may be classified into types in many ways, the desired intricacy of any particular scheme being dependent on the purpose of performing the classification. Thus, for one purpose it may suffice to construct a single broad class of hydroxy compounds, while for other purposes it is desirable to subdivide this broad class into alcohols and phenols and perhaps even subdivide these further into subclasses of alcohols and phenols. It is appropriate here, for purposes of convenient reference, to list those types of compounds most commonly encountered in the systematic study of organic chemistry and to display their general (type) formulas. The types of compounds which are especially pertinent to pharmacy are treated in greater detail later in the chapter, where examples of official drugs belonging to each class are also provided.

To enhance utility as a reference tool, the listing in Table I is alphabetical rather than by any chemical classification scheme. Prefatorily, the following explanatory notes are provided.

Unless otherwise specified, the formulas shown are for compounds containing only one of the particular functional group involved. Formulas for compounds containing more than one of the same functional group can easily be derived.

Naturally occurring classes of compounds such as carbohydrates, proteins, alkaloids, glycosides, and lipids are not treated as types of compounds in this classification. A separate, more detailed presentation of these is provided in Chapter 25.

Although a few heterocyclic types such as imines (azacyclic), anhydrides of dibasic acids (oxacyclic), lactides (dioxacyclic), etc automatically enter into the listing, it will be observed that parent heterocycles in general (eg, thiophene, pyridine, dioxane, etc) are not included. Heterocycles represented in official drugs are listed later in the chapter.

In type formulas such as in Table I, the symbol R is conventionally employed to denote a hydrocarbon radical. Unless otherwise specified it may be aliphatic, alicyclic, or aromatic, and its valence varies to satisfy the requirements of its attachment to the rest of the molecule. The degree of saturation in R does not enter into the scheme. When a formula contains more than one R, the radicals may be either identical or different. In a few instances, it is possible that even if two monovalent R's are replaceable by a single divalent R the same type of compound is retained; eg, aliphatic ketones (RCOR) and cyclic ketones ($\overline{RCO}$).

The type formulas assume a useful broader meaning if R, instead of being restricted to designate only a *hydrocarbon* radical, is permitted to (1) be a residue from a heterocycle and (2) carry substituent groups. The latter automatically extends the listing to embrace polyfunctional compounds, but it also introduces the complicating feature of order of precedence of functional groups. This matter is discussed later in the chapter.

Unless otherwise specified, the symbol X stands for a member of the halogen family.

In addition to the type formulas, one or more specific examples of each type of compound are also provided, showing how the formulas usually appear in somewhat condensed form and illustrating the manner in which the type names become parts of individual compound names. However, it should be remembered that, although correct, such names are not always the preferred names in modern nomenclature practice.

Only those formulas and structures are depicted which are of pharmaceutical interest.

Nomenclature of Organic Compounds

In the early decades of organic chemistry, newly discovered compounds were commonly provided with names which indicated either the source or some outstanding property of the compound. Thus, marsh gas, wood alcohol, benzoic acid, cadaverine, morphine, chlorophyll, and thousands of other similar names were invented. As more and more compounds were isolated or synthesized, it became apparent, however, that some systematic manner of naming organic compounds in terms of their structure would have to be devised. Early systems of nomenclature, while adequate for the period in which they were invented, soon required modification as the number of known compounds increased. The result has been that the system (or rather the combination of systems) now in use represents an evolution spreading over several decades.

That a truly effective system of nomenclature is bound to be very complex is obvious when one reflects that it must not only discriminate, unequivocally, among the approximately three million compounds already known, but must also allow adequate provision for encompassing new compounds which are being synthesized at a rate of about 75,000 per year. Fundamentally, therefore, such discrimination means that each specific name coined through the system must account

Table I—Types of Organic Compounds

Class	Examples	Class	Examples
Acetals $RC(H \text{ or } R)(OR)_2$ (cf Ketals)	$CH_3CH(OCH_3)_2$ acetaldehyde dimethyl acetal (1,1-dimethoxyethane) $(CH_3)_2C(OC_2H_5)$ acetone diethyl acetal (2,2-diethoxypropane)	Amidines $RC(=NH)NH_2$	$CH_3C(NH)NH_2$ acetamidine
		Amines $RN(H \text{ or } R)(H \text{ or } R)$ RNH_2 types = Amino Compounds	CH_3NH_2 methylamine $(C_2H_5)_2NH$ diethylamine $CH_3N(C_2H_5)C_3H_7$ methylethylpropylamine
Acid Anhydrides 1. Of Monocarboxylic Acids RCOOCOR	$(CH_3CO)_2O$ acetic (acid) anhydride		
2. Of Dicarboxylic Acids $\overline{RCOOCO}$	$\overline{CH_2CH_2COOCO}$ succinic (acid) anhydride	Amino Acids $R(NH_2)COOH$	$CH_2(NH_2)COOH$ aminoacetic acid
Acid Halides (Acyl Halides) RCOX	CH_3COCl acetyl chloride	Ammonium Derivatives $[RH_3N]^+X^-$ where X = OH or a salt anion and any or all H's may be R's. If N is a ring member, specific "ium" nomenclature is em- ployed to denote the heterocycle.	$[(CH_3)_4N]^+I^-$ tetramethylammonium iodide $[(C_2H_5)_2N^+H_2]Cl^-$ diethylammonium chloride (diethylamine hydrochloride) $[\dot{C}H=CHCH=CHCH=N^+-(CH_3)]Br^-$ 1-methyl- pyridinium bromide
Acids (Carboxylic) (other acids are listed under their characteristic names, eg, Sulfonic Acids, Thio Acids, etc) RCOOH	CH_3COOH acetic acid		
		Anilides RCONHR' where NHR' is derived from aniline Note—If NHR' is derived from: toluidine xylidine anisidine phenetidine	$CH_3CONHC_6H_5$ acetanilide Compounds are termed: toluidides xylidides anisidides phenetidides
Acyloins (α-Hydroxy Ketones) RCOCH(OH)R	$CH_3COCH(OH)CH_3$ acetoin $C_6H_5COCH(OH)C_6H_5$ benzoin		
Alcoholates (Alkoxides) ROMetal where R is aliphatic or alicyclic	C_2H_5ONa sodium ethylate sodium ethoxide	Anils (Schiff bases) RCH=NR	$C_6H_5CH=NC_6H_5$ N-Benzylideneaniline
Alcohols ROH where R is aliphatic or alicyclic	C_2H_5OH ethyl alcohol (ethanol) $\overline{CH_2(CH_2)_4}CHOH$ cyclohexyl alcohol (cyclohexanol)	Azides (Acyl Azides) $RCON=N^+=N^-$	$CH_3CON=N^+=N^-$ acetyl azide
Aldehydes RCHO	CH_3CHO acetaldehyde	Azido Compounds $RN=N^+=N^-$	$C_2H_5N=N^+=N^-$ azidoethane
Alkoxides (see Alcoholates)		Azines $R_2C=NN=CR_2$	$(CH_3)_2C=NN=C(CH_3)_2$ acetone azine
Alkylhalosilanes $R(SiH_2)_nX$ where one or more H's may be substituted by addi- tional R's or X's	CH_3SiH_2Cl methylchlorosilane	Azo Compounds RN=NR	$C_6H_5N=NC_6H_5$ azobenzene
Alkylsilanes $R(SiH_2)_nH$ where one or more H's may be substituted by addi- tional R's	CH_3SiH_3 methylsilane $C_2H_5SiH_2SiH_2C_2H_5$ sym-diethyldisilane	Azoxy Compounds RN=N(O)R	$C_6H_5N=N(O)C_6H_5$ azoxybenzene
Alkylsilanols Types here illustrated are limited to derivatives of silane; ie, (mono)-silane, SiH_4. There are similar derivatives of the di-, tri-, etc, silanes. $RSiH_2OH$ $RSiH(OH)_2$ $RSi(OH)_3$ alkylsilanols alkylsilanediols alkylsilanetriols R_2SiHOH $R_2Si(OH)_2$ dialkylsilanols dialkylsilanediols R_3SiOH trialkylsilanols		Benzils (Aromatic α-Diketones) RCOCOR where R is aromatic	p-$CH_3C_6H_4COCOC_6H_4CH_3$-p p,p'-dimethylbenzil
		Benzoins (Aromatic α-Hydroxy Ketones) RCH(OH)COR where R is aromatic	p-$CH_3C_6H_4CH(OH)CO$- $C_6H_4CH_3$-p p,p'-dimethylbenzoin or p-toluoin
		Betaines $R_3N^+(CH_2)_nCOO^-$	$(CH_3)_3N^+CH_2CH_2COO^-$ β-alanine, trimethylbetaine
Alkylsiloxanes Various linear and cyclic types. (see Silicones, page 378). A common linear type consisting of condensation polymers of dialkylsilanediols is shown.	$HO(SiR_2O)_nSiR_2OH$	Borates (see Esters) Carbonates (see Esters) Carbylamines (Isocyanides; Isonitriles) RNC	C_6H_5NC phenyl $\begin{cases} \text{carbylamine,} \\ \text{isocyanide, or} \\ \text{isonitrile} \end{cases}$
Amides $RCONH_2$	CH_3CONH_2 acetamide	Cyanates ROCN	C_6H_5OCN phenyl cyanate

Table I—Continued

Class	Examples	Class	Examples
Cyanides (see Nitriles)		Glycerides	
Cyanohydrins		RCOOCH$_2$CH(OCOR)CH$_2$-	C$_3$H$_5$(C$_2$H$_3$O$_2$)$_3$ or (CH$_3$COO)$_3$-
RC(CN)(OH)(H or R)	CH$_3$C(CN)(OH)CH$_3$	OCOR	C$_3$H$_5$
	acetone cyanohydrin		glyceryl triacetate or triacetin
Diazoamino Compounds (Triazene Derivatives)		Glycols	
RN=NNHR	C$_6$H$_5$N=NNHC$_6$H$_5$	HOCH$_2$(CH$_2$)$_n$CH$_2$OH	CH$_2$(OH)CH$_2$OH
	diazoaminobenzene or	*where n = zero or greater*	ethylene glycol
	1,3-diphenyltriazene		CH$_2$(OH)CH$_2$CH$_2$OH
Diazo Compounds			trimethylene glycol
Type A RNNX	C$_6$H$_5$N=NCl	Guanidino Compounds	
where X = OH or a salt	benzenediazochloride	NH$_2$(C=NH)NHR	NH$_2$(C=NH)NHC$_2$H$_5$
anion			1-ethylguanidine
Type B RN=NOMetal	C$_6$H$_5$N=NONa	Haloalkylsilanes	
(diazoates)	sodium benzenediazoate	XR(SiH$_2$)$_n$H	ClCH$_2$SiH$_3$
Type C C(H or R)(H or R)-	CH$_2$=N$^+$=N$^-$	*where one or more of the H's*	chloromethylsilane
=N$^+$=N$^-$	diazomethane	*in R may be substituted by*	
Diazonium Compounds		*additional X's and one or*	
RN$^+_2$X$^-$	[C$_6$H$_5$N$^+_2$]OH$^-$	*more of silicon hydrogens*	
where X = OH or a salt	benzenediazonium hydroxide	*may be substituted by*	
anion		*additional RX groups*	
Epoxy Compounds		Halohydrins	
CH$_2$(CH$_2$)$_n$CH$_2$O	CH$_2$CH$_2$O	XCH$_2$CH$_2$OH	ClCH$_2$CH$_2$OH
where n = zero or greater	epoxyethane	*where either or both of the*	ethylene chlorohydrin
and any or all H's may		*CH$_2$'s may be CHR or CR$_2$*	
be R's		Hemiacetals	
	CH$_3$CHCH$_2$CH(CH$_3$)O	RC(H or R)(OR)(OH)	CH$_3$CH(OC$_2$H$_5$)OH
	2,4-epoxypentane		acetaldehyde ethyl hemiacetal
Esters (of Carboxylic Acids)			(1-ethoxyethanol)
RCOOR	CH$_3$COOC$_2$H$_5$	Hydrazides	
	ethyl acetate	RCONHNH$_2$	CH$_3$CONHNH$_2$
Esters (of Inorganic Oxy Acids)			acetic acid hydrazide

Esters (of Inorganic Oxy Acids)
The listing here is intentionally limited to esters of the more important oxy acids of nitrogen, phosphorus, sulfur, boron, silicon, and carbon. In each instance, the type formula shown is for the ester which results from the replacement of all acidic H's by R's. Where more than one R is present, acid esters (ie, esters still containing one or more unreplaced H's) are possible.

Class	Type formula	Examples		
			Hydrazines	
			RN(H or R)N(H or R)-	C$_6$H$_5$NHNH$_2$
			(H or R)	phenylhydrazine
			Hydrazones	
Nitrates	RONO$_2$	C$_2$H$_5$NO$_3$, ethyl nitrate	R$_2$(or RH)C=NNH$_2$	(CH$_3$)$_2$C=NNH$_2$
Nitrites	RONO	C$_2$H$_5$ONO, ethyl		acetone hydrazone
		nitrite		C$_6$H$_5$CH=NNH$_2$
(Ortho)phosphates	(RO)$_3$PO	(C$_2$H$_5$)$_3$PO$_4$, ethyl		benzaldehyde hydrazone
		phosphate	Hydrocarbon Halides (Alkyl,	
Metaphosphates	ROPO$_2$	C$_2$H$_5$PO$_3$, ethyl	Alkylene, Alkylidene,	
		metaphosphate	Alkenyl, Aryl, Arylene,	
Pyrophosphates	(RO)$_2$PO—O-	(C$_2$H$_5$)$_4$P$_2$O$_7$, ethyl	etc Halides)	
	—PO(OR)$_2$	pyrophosphate	RX$_n$	CH$_3$Cl
(Ortho)phosphites	P(OR)$_3$	(C$_2$H$_5$)$_3$PO$_3$, ethyl	*where n = valence of R*	methyl chloride (chloromethane)
		phosphite		CH$_2$=CHBr
Hypophosphites	H$_2$P(O)(OR)	C$_2$H$_5$H$_2$PO$_2$, ethyl		vinyl bromide
cf Phosphonic Acids.		hypophosphite		CH$_3$CHCl$_2$
Sulfates	(RO)$_2$SO$_2$	(C$_2$H$_5$)$_2$SO$_4$, ethyl		ethylidene chloride
		sulfate		C$_6$H$_5$I
Sulfites	(RO)$_2$SO	(C$_2$H$_5$)$_2$SO$_3$, ethyl		phenyl iodide (iodobenzene)
		sulfite	Hydroxamic Acids	
Orthoborates	B(OR)$_3$	(C$_2$H$_5$)$_3$BO$_3$, ethyl	RC(=NOH)OH	CH$_3$CH$_2$C(=NOH)OH
		orthoborate		propionohydroxamic acid
Metaborates	ROBO	C$_2$H$_5$BO$_2$, ethyl	Hydroxy Acids	
		metaborate	RCH(OH)COOH	CH$_3$CH(OH)COOH
Orthosilicates	Si(OR)$_4$	(C$_2$H$_5$)$_4$SiO$_4$, ethyl		α-hydroxypropionic acid or
		orthosilicate		lactic acid
Metasilicates	(RO)$_2$SiO	(C$_2$H$_5$)$_2$SiO$_3$, ethyl		
		metasilicate	Hypophosphites (see Esters)	
Orthocarbonates	C(OR)$_4$	(C$_2$H$_5$)$_4$CO$_4$, ethyl	Imides (Carboximides)	
		orthocarbonate	RCON(H or R)CO	CH$_2$CH$_2$CONHCO
Carbonates	(RO)$_2$CO	(C$_2$H$_5$)$_2$CO$_3$, ethyl		succinimide
		carbonate		1,2-ethanedicarboximide
Ethers			Imidic Acids	
ROR		CH$_3$OC$_2$H$_5$	RC(NH)OH	CH$_3$C(=NH)OH
		ethyl methyl ether		acetimidic acid
Fluorophosphates (see Phosphorofluoridates)			Imines	
			R=NH	CH$_3$CH$_2$=NH
				ethylideneimine
				CH$_2$CH$_2$NH
				ethyleneimine

Table I—Continued

Class	Examples	Class	Examples
Iodonium Compounds $[R_2I]^+X^-$ *where X = OH or a salt anion*	$[(C_6H_5)_2I]^+Br^-$ diphenyliodonium bromide	Morpholides $RCON(CH_2)_2OCH_2CH_2$	$CH_3CONCH_2CH_2OCH_2CH_2$ acetomorpholide (4-acetylmorpholine)
Iodoso Compounds RIO	C_6H_5IO iodosobenzene	Nitrates (see Esters) Nitriles (Cyanides; Carbonitriles) RCN	CH_3CH_2CN propionitrile ethyl cyanide ethanecarbonitrile
Iodoxy Compounds RIO_2	$C_6H_5IO_2$ iodoxybenzene		
Isocyanates RNCO	C_6H_5NCO phenyl isocyanate	Nitrites (see Esters) Nitro Compounds RNO_2	CH_3NO_2 nitromethane $C_6H_5NO_2$ nitrobenzene

Isocyanide Dichlorides
    (Imidocarbonyl
    Chlorides)
$RN{=}CCl_2$
	$C_2H_5NCCl_2$
	ethyl isocyanide dichloride
	ethylimidocarbonyl chloride
		Nitroso Compounds
		RNO
			C_6H_5NO
			nitrosobenzene

Isocyanides (see Carbylamines)
Isonitriles (see Carbylamines)
Isothiocyanates
    (Isosulfocyanates;
    Thiocarbimides;
    Mustard Oils)
RNCS
	CH_3NCS
	methyl isothiocyanate, etc.
		Organometallic (Metallo-organic) Compounds
		Note—Restricted here to
		    compounds having a di-
		    rect metal-carbon link-
		    age.
		Commonest types are:
		    MR_v and $R_{(v-1)}MX$
			$(CH_3)_2Zn$
			dimethylzinc

Ketals
$R_2C(OR)_2$
(Commonly treated as
    acetals, qv above)
	$(CH_3)_2C(OC_2H_5)_2$
	acetone diethylketal
	(2,2-diethoxypropane)
		where
		    M = metal functioning
		        with valence v
			$(C_2H_5)_4Pb$
			tetraethyl lead

Ketenes
$RC(H \text{ or } R){=}C{=}O$
	$(CH_3)_2C{=}C{=}O$
	dimethyl ketene
		R = univalent
		    unsubstituted,
		    or, substituted,
		    hydrocarbon
		    radical
			CH_3MgBr
			methylmagnesium bromide

Keto Acids (monobasic) $H(CH_2)_nCO(CH_2)_nCOOH$ *where n = zero or greater and* *any or all H's may be R's.* *May also be polybasic.*	CH_3COCH_2COOH 3-oxobutyric acid or acetoacetic acid $HOOCCH_2COCOOH$ ketosuccinic acid or oxalacetic acid	X = univalent anion	$C_6H_5HgNO_3$ phenylmercuric nitrate Ag_2C_2 silver acetylide
Ketones RCOR *where R's are aliphatic or* *alicyclic. If one or both* *R's are aromatic, com-* *pounds are termed* *Phenones.*	$CH_3COC_2H_5$ ethyl methyl ketone or 2-butanone $C_6H_5COCH_3$ acetophenone	Osazones [Bis(phenylhydrazones)] $(H \text{ or } R)C({=}NNHPh)$- $C({=}NNHPh)(R \text{ or } H)$ *where Ph = phenyl*	$C_6H_5C({=}NNHPh)C({=}NNH$- $Ph)C_6H_5$ benzil osazone [Benzil bis(phenylhydrazone)]
Lactams $\overline{CH_2(CH_2)_nCONH}$ *where n = 2 or more and any* *or all H's may be R's.*	$\overline{CH_2CH_2CH_2CH_2CONH}$ δ-valerolactam (2-piperidone)	Oximes $RC(H \text{ or } R){=}NOH$	$CH_3CH{=}NOH$ acetaldoxime $(CH_3)_2C{=}NOH$ dimethylketoxime (acetone oxime)

Lactides
$\overline{CH_2COOCH_2COO}$
where any or all of the H's
may be R's
	$\overline{CH_3CHCOOCH(CH_3)COO}$
	2-hydroxypropionic acid lactide
	"lactide"
		Oxo Compounds (see Aldehydes,
		    Ketones, Quinones, Keto
		    Acids)	

Lactims as per lactams except $\overline{CH_2(CH_2)_nCONH}$ becomes $\overline{CH_2(CH_2)_nC(OH){=}N}$	$\overline{CH_2CH_2CH_2CH_2C(OH){=}N}$ δ-valerolactim	Ozonides $\overset{O}{RCHOOCHR}$	$\overset{O}{CH_3CHOOCHCH_3}$ 2-butene ozonide
Lactones $\overline{CH_2(CH_2)_nCOO}$ *where n = 2 or more and any* *or all H's may be R's*	$\overline{CH_2CH_2CH_2CH_2COO}$ δ-valerolactone	Peptides (Polypeptides) $NH_2(RCONH)_nRCOOH$	$NH_2(CH_2CONH)_2CH_2COOH$ glycine tripeptides glycyl glycyl glycine
Mercaptans (see Thiols) Mercaptides RSMetal	C_2H_5SNa sodium ethyl mercaptide	Peroxides $ROO(R \text{ or } H)$	$C_2H_5OOC_2H_5$ ethyl peroxide
Mercaptoles $R_2C(SR)_2$	$(CH_3)_2C(SC_2H_5)_2$ acetone diethylmercaptole	Peroxy Acids $RC(O)OOH$	$CH_3C(O)OOH$ peroxyacetic acid

Table I—Continued

Class	Examples	Class	Examples
Phenolates (Phenoxides) ROMetal *where R is aromatic*	C_6H_5ONa sodium phenolate sodium phenoxide		

Phenols
ROH
where R is aromatic — $p\text{-}CH_3C_6H_4OH$ — p-methylphenol (p-cresol)

Phenones (see Ketones)
Phenoxides (see Phenolates)
Phosphates (see Esters)
Phosphites (see Esters)
Phospho Compounds
RPO₂ — $C_6H_5PO_2$ phosphobenzene

Phosphonic Acids
RPO(OH)₂ — $CH_3PO(OH)_2$ methylphosphonic acid or methanephosphonic acid

Phosphorofluoridates (Fluoro-phosphates)
FPO(OR)₂ — $FPO[OCH(CH_3)_2]_2$ diisopropyl phosphorofluoridate diisopropyl fluorophosphate

Phosphorus Compounds (General)
  In addition to the compounds in this listing, phosphorus forms a very large number of types of compounds containing direct linkages between the phosphorus and halogens, cyanogen, nitrogen, and sulfur. Many of these contain also phosphorus-oxygen linkages. For a comprehensive presentation of organic compounds containing phosphorus, see the report entitled *Organic Compounds Containing Phosphorus*, which is available from Chemical Abstracts Service.

Phthaleins, simplest type only
RC(R'OH)₂OCO
where R is o-phenylene, R' is p-phenylene, and either or both may be substituted. — $o\text{-}C_6H_4C(p\text{-}C_6H_4OH)_2OCO$ phenolphthalein

Piperidides
RCON(CH₂)₄CH₂ — $CH_3CONCH_2CH_2CH_2CH_2CH_2$ acetopiperidide (1-acetylpiperidine)

Quaternary Ammonium Compounds
[R₄N]⁺X⁻
where X = OH or a salt anion — $[(CH_3)_4N]^+Cl^-$ tetramethylammonium chloride

Quinones
O=R=O
where R is a quinoid cycle — $p\text{-}O{=}C_6H_4{=}O$ p-benzoquinone

Salts (Metal) — Formulas as per acids except that the acidic H's are replaced by metal equivalent.

Semicarbazones
RC(H or R)=NNHCONH₂ — $(CH_3)_2C{=}NNHCONH_2$ acetone semicarbazone

Silicates (see Esters)
Silicon Compounds (General)
  Because of its position in Group IV of the Periodic Table, it is not surprising that silicon enters freely into organic-type chemical combinations. Like carbon, although to a much lesser extent, silicon forms stable chain compounds containing —SiSi— linkages. Compounds which contain hydrogen as the only other element are termed silanes: eg, SiH_4, silane (silicane, silicomethane); Si_2H_6, disilane (disilicoethane); and Si_3H_8, trisilane. Cyclosilanes, $SiH_2(SiH_2)_nSiH_2$ are also well known. These silicon-hydrogen compounds are analogous to the alkanes and cycloalkanes in the carbon family of compounds. They form various types of derivatives: eg, SiH_3OH, H_2SiO, $HSiOOH$, $HOSiH_2SiH_2OH$, $SiHCl_3$, $H_2Si{=}NH$, $(SiH_3)_2NH$, etc. These formulas are completely analogous to carbon compounds. Silicon also shows a strong tendency to form stable chain compounds containing —SiOSi— linkages; these are the siloxanes: eg, $H_3SiOSiH_3$, disiloxane;

$H_3SiOSiH_2OSiH_3$, trisiloxane; etc. Analogous compounds containing imino instead of oxygen, are also well known. These are the silazanes: eg, $H_3SiNHSiH_3$, disilazane; $H_3SiNHSiH_2$–$NHSiH_3$, trisilazane; etc.
  It will be noted that none of the above types of compounds contain carbon, and in this sense, they are not organic compounds. However, alkyl derivatives of these, which are very numerous, are organic in the same sense as alkyl derivatives of hydrogen compounds of other elements such as nitrogen and sulfur. Since the alkyl groups in the derivatives may also contain substituent functional groups, it is readily apparent that there are a great many types of organic silicon compounds. Only a few of the better known types are included in this listing.

Silylalkanols (Silicoalcohols)
  Alcohols in which one (or more) of the CH hydrogens is replaced by silyl (SiH₃) or substituted silyl groups. In contrast to the silanols compounds of this type contain hydroxyl in true organic combination. — $(C_2H_5)_3SiCH_2CH_2OH$ 2-(triethylsilyl)ethanol
  There are many subtypes.

Sulfamic Acids
RNH(or R₂N)SO₂OH — CH_3NHSO_2OH methanesulfamic acid $(C_2H_5)_2NSO_2OH$ diethylsulfamic acid

Sulfates (see Esters)
Sulfenamides
RSNH₂ — $C_6H_5SNH_2$ benzenesulfenamide

Sulfenic Acids
RSOH — C_6H_5SOH benzenesulfenic acid

Sulfenyl Halides
RSX — C_6H_5SCl benzenesulfenyl chloride

Sulfides (Thio Ethers)
RSR — $(CH_3)_2S$ (di)methyl sulfide (di)methyl thioether

Sulfimides
RCONHSO₂ — $o\text{-}C_6H_4CONHSO_2$ o-benzosulfimide

Sulfinamides
RSONH₂ — $C_6H_5SONH_2$ benzenesulfinamide

Sulfinic Acids
RSOOH — C_6H_5SOOH benzenesulfinic acid

Sulfinyl Halides
RSOX — C_6H_5SOCl benzenesulfinyl chloride

Sulfites (see Esters)
Sulfonamides
RSO₂NH₂ — $C_6H_5SO_2NH_2$ benzenesulfonamide

Sulfones
RSO₂R — $(C_2H_5)_2SO_2$ diethyl sulfone

Sulfonic Acids
RSO₂OH — $C_6H_5SO_2OH$ benzenesulfonic acid

Sulfonium Compounds
[R₃S]⁺X⁻
where X is OH or a salt anion. If S is a ring member, specific "ium" nomenclature is employed to denote the heterocycle. — $[(CH_3)_3S]^+I^-$ trimethylsulfonium iodide

$[CH_2CH_2CH_2CH_2CH_2S^+\text{-}(C_2H_5)]PtCl_6^-$ 1-ethylhexahydrothiapyrylium chloroplatinate

Table I—Continued

Class	Examples	Class	Examples
Sulfonyl Halides RSO$_2$X	C$_6$H$_5$SO$_2$Cl benzenesulfonyl chloride	Thio Ethers (see Sulfides)	
		Thiols (Mercaptans, Acid Sulfides, Hydrosulfides; Sulfhydryl Compounds)	
Sulfoxides RSOR	(C$_2$H$_5$)$_2$SO diethyl sulfoxide	RSH	C$_2$H$_5$SH ethanethiol ethyl $\begin{cases} \text{mercaptan} \\ \text{acid sulfide} \\ \text{hydrosulfide} \end{cases}$
Sultams Analogous to Lactams, qv with —SO$_2$— replacing —CO—.			
Sultones Analogous to Lactones, qv with —SO$_2$— replacing —CO—.		Thiones (Thio Ketones) RCSR	CH$_3$CSCH$_3$ propanethione dimethyl thioketone
Thetins R$_2$S$^+$CH$_2$COO$^-$	(CH$_3$)$_2$S$^+$CH$_2$COO$^-$ S,S-dimethylthetin	Thionium Compounds (see Sulfonium Compounds)	
		Thioureides-Ureides (qv) with the urea oxygen replaced by sulfur.	
Thio Acids 1. Thiolic RCOSH	CH$_3$COSH thioloacetic acid ethanethiolic acid	Ureides, simplest types only acyclic RCONHCONH(H or COR)	CH$_3$CONHCONH$_2$ acetic acid ureide acetylurea
2. Thionic RCSOH	CH$_3$CSOH thionoacetic acid ethanethionic acid	cyclic $\overline{\text{RCONHCONH}}$CO	$\overline{\text{CH}_2\text{CONHCONH}}$CO malonic acid ureide (malonylurea) (barbituric acid)
3. Thionothiolic RCSSH (Dithioic)	CH$_3$CSSH thionothioloacetic acid ethanedithioic acid		
Thio Aldehydes RCHS	CH$_2$CHS thioacetaldehyde	Urethans (Carbamate Esters) NH$_2$COOR	NH$_2$COOC$_2$H$_5$ ethyl urethan (ethyl carbamate)
Thiocyanates (Sulfocyanates; Rhodanates) RSCN	C$_6$H$_5$SCN phenyl thiocyanate, etc.		

for (1) the quantitative elementary composition (molecular formula) and (2) all of the structural features for one, and only one, specific compound.

The IUPAC and CAS Systems of Nomenclature

Of the various comprehensive systems proposed and used to varying extents, the two most widely used and most thoroughly updated through revision and enlargement are those devised by the International Union of Pure and Applied Chemistry (IUPAC) and the Chemical Abstracts Service (CAS). Each of these systems represents an implementation of the rules devised by the IUPAC Commission on the Reform of the Nomenclature of Organic Chemistry, which has been actively and continuously engaged in the subject for several decades. The two systems are identical in most respects. The CAS system intentionally departs from that of IUPAC wherever such departure contributes to the main purpose of Chemical Abstracts, ie, indexing the world's chemical literature. Recognizing the desirability of compatibility of the two systems, however, CAS identifies each such departure and displays the alternative IUPAC treatment.

Because of the difficulty in converting many structural formulas into unique, descriptive names CAS is now assigning a *Registry Number* to every chemical compound (organic and inorganic). Commencing with USP XIX and NF XIV all monographs for pure chemical entities carry the CAS Registry Number, which uniquely identifies every compound. Also, in the same editions of USP and NF "New Chemical Abstracts Names" were assigned. CAS is completely revising the current system (which parallels the IUPAC rules) so that computer searches may be made utilizing nomenclature, rather than topological features, to perform searches for molecular fragments as well as complete molecules.

It is obviously inappropriate and space-prohibitive to include in this text a discussion of the multiplicity of details in either of these two systems. Suffice it to state that, from a structural viewpoint, each system must adequately describe for each compound the following:

Composition and configuration of the carbon skeleton.
Interruptions of the carbon skeleton by heteroatoms.
State of hydrogenation of the skeleton.
Presence and location of substituents, ie, atoms or groups of atoms (radicals) functioning in place of hydrogen.
Features of stereoisomerism.

For the reader desirous of the details of the systems, reference is made to the continuing series of reports issued by the IUPAC Commission on the Nomenclature of Organic Chemistry and to the CAS publication entitled *The Naming and Indexing of Chemical Compounds from Chemical Abstracts*. The latter, which first appeared as an introduction to the Subject Index of Vol 56 of *Chemical Abstracts*, has undergone very extensive revision and enlargement and was concluded by CAS in 1969. The Introduction to the Subject Index of Vol 66 provides a useful summary treatment. Reference is also made to the American Chemical Society publication, *The Ring Index*, for a very detailed systematic presentation of closed-chain systems identified through literature up to 1964.

Because of major changes in nomenclature and indexing procedures, mainly dictated by computerization of nomenclature and two-dimensional structures, each quinquennial index to *Chemical Abstracts* will be accompanied by an *Index Guide* which allow the user to follow the transition between the old and new (or modified) nomenclature.

Three general features common to both systems deserve special comment, *viz*, the employment of trivial names, the order of precedence of functional groups, and permissive ambiguity.

Trivial Names—By a trivial name is meant one which, *per se*, does not rigidly describe a compound in terms of the absolute structure notations embodied in the system, but which has earned worldwide recognition as being specific for that compound. Acetic acid (for ethanoic acid), purine (for 7H-imidazo[4,5-d]pyrimidine), and pregnane (for 10β,13β-dimethyl-17β-ethyl-9α, 14α, 5β, 8β-perhydrocyclopenta[a] phenanthrene) are common examples. Without allowing for the judicious employment of such trivial names, any scheme of nomenclature would be hopelessly complex and of little, if any, practical utility. On the other hand, the wholesale indiscriminate admission of trivial names to a system is equally disastrous. Arriving at a satisfactory compromise between these two extremes obviously requires detailed deliberation, and the compromise position taken by IUPAC has also been adopted by CAS, ie, trivial names admitted by IUPAC are also those admitted by CAS. However, with the advent of computer techniques, long or unwieldy names are handled with relative ease. Thus trivial and systematic names are assuming equal importance since a trivial name index cannot be computer-searched to locate fragments of two-dimensional structures as these fragments are not evident in the name. But with long, systematic names, every portion of a parent molecule, substituent, functional group, etc is apparent in the name and will yield to the computer search.

Precedence Order of Functional Groups—An order of precedence (priority) of functional groups is necessary in order to manage, systematically, polyfunctional compounds. As a simple example, in the absence of a systematic method, the compound $CH_2(NH_2)CH_2CH_2OH$ could be named either as an aminopropanol or as a hydroxypropylamine. But in the order of precedence, hydroxyl is higher than amino and, since the system requires that only the function of highest priority shall be represented by the suffix part of the name, the systematic name becomes 3-amino-1-propanol. The order of precedence of functional groups is clearly prescribed (see Table I of the Introduction to the Subject Index of *Chemical Abstracts*, Vol 66) and is identical in both the IUPAC and CAS systems.

Permissive Ambiguity—Ambiguity (lack of complete structural specificity) is permissive to the extent that it reflects structural features of a compound which either are unknown or have not yet been incorporated into the system. Prohibition of such ambiguity would disallow the cataloging of a very significant percentage of known compounds, especially among those which involve features of stereoisomerism.

Compendial Nomenclature

Lack of adherence to the principles of systematic nomenclature, in both the commercial and academic worlds, has led to a multiplicity in the types of chemical names in actual use. It is not at all unusual to find a specific compound referred to by several different names, each of which is chemically correct. This, of course, creates a very confused state which, if it persists in the indexing literature, often renders searching via nomenclature extremely difficult and, not infrequently, impossible. It is for this reason that, wherever possible, *Chemical Abstracts* translates an author's nonsystematic nomenclature into its CAS equivalent.

Recognizing the advantages of adhering to a standard system of nomenclature, the official compendia (USP and formerly NF) elected to adopt names preferred by CAS. The principle of operation is simply that either the title or one of the subtitles of an official chemical must be the currently preferred CAS name. It is well to observe that the structural relationships established on the basis of principal functional group may automatically hide relationships involving functional groups of lesser priority. Thus, for example, Amphetamine is named as a derivative of phenethylamine, whereas Hydroxyamphetamine becomes a derivative of

phenol; similarly, Sulfamerazine is named as a derivative of sulfanilamide, whereas Phthalylsulfacetamide becomes a derivative of phthalanilic acid. Beginning with USP XIX and NF XIV each monograph carries the "new CAS name" along with the CAS preferred name currently in use.

Chemical Syllables

In addition to whatever numbers, numerical syllables, and individual Greek and English letters are required, systematic chemical names consist of a collection of syllables each of which carries a chemical connotation of some sort. Many, such as chloro-, hydroxy-, methyl-, etc, clearly indicate specific elements or radicals.

Many others, such as andro- (Gr, man), tauro- (Latin, bull), neo- (Gr, new), and pseudo- or ψ (Gr, false), are of no chemical significance from a structural viewpoint, but are often very useful in forming the so-called trivial or common names for complex molecules such as androsterone, taurocholic acid, neoantergan, pseudoglobulin, etc, the correct chemical names for which would often be extremely cumbersome. Because of their lack of structural chemical significance, however, these will not be discussed further here.

The third group of these syllables consists of miscellaneous prefixes and suffixes and is of sufficient importance to warrant abbreviated treatment, because, like those of the first group, these have structural significance and often constitute a necessary part of systematic chemical names. A list of the more commonly encountered ones of this group is provided in Tables II and III. Many of these have multiple meanings, and the definitions given herein represent the commonest sense in which they are used in organic chemistry. Those shown in italics are commonly used in italicized form and/or enclosed in parentheses when used in organic nomenclature. It must also be remembered that the precise meanings shown here do not always apply to trivial names. Thus, for example, the meaning of -ene or of -ylene does not apply to acetylene; similarly, the meaning of -ol does not apply to benzol. Caution must always be exercised in attempting to attach significance to the various parts of such common names.

The systematic treatment of cyclic systems utilizes a generous miscellany of syllables with specific meanings. For listings and explanations of these, consult *The Ring Index*.

Radicals in Organic Chemistry

Through the concept and utilization of radicals, a logical and very helpful classification of the huge number of organic compounds is possible. Furthermore, a knowledge of the chemical properties of the individual radicals commonly makes possible either a prediction or an explanation of the chemical properties of compounds because, in general, the chemical properties of a compound are completely or partly the combined properties of the radicals present in the molecule.

Several hundred different radicals have been recognized, named, and classified. A comprehensive list ordered by both names and formulas is periodically published as part of the *Collective Index* to Chemical Abstracts, as Section IV, *Selection of Index Names for Chemical Substances*, from the Index Guide for Vol 81 of *Chemical Abstracts*.

For purposes of convenient reference, a list of radicals frequently encountered in pharmaceutical chemistry is provided in Table IV. Classification into chemical types has been sacrificed in favor of an alphabetical arrangement. Included in the list are many inorganic radicals which are frequently present in organic combination.

Table II—Prefixes

ald- (or aldo-)	refers to *aldehyde*, as aldoxime and aldohexose
allo-	signifies a *close* (usually isomeric) *relationship*, as allocholesterol (coprostenol) is an isomer of cholesterol
anhydro-	denotes *abstraction of water*, as anhydrohydroxyprogesterone
anti-	equivalent to *trans*, qv, in certain $-\overset{|}{C}=\overset{|}{N}$ geometric isomers, eg, *anti*-benzaldoxime
apo-	usually signifies *formation from the compound* whose name is attached, as apomorphine may be formed (produced) from morphine
ar-	abbreviation for *aromatic*, as aryl
as-	abbreviation for *asymmetric*
bis-	used instead of di-, meaning *two*, before complex expressions, as in bis(*m*-nitrophenyl)-
cis-	refers to that *geometric isomer* in which the two groups are on the *same side*, as *cis*-butenedioic acid, $\overset{\text{CHCOOH}}{\underset{\text{CHCOOH}}{\|}}$
cyclo-	indicates a *cyclic* structure, as cyclopropane
d-	see *dextro-*
D-	signifies a *structural relationship* to D-glyceraldehyde without any reference to direction of optical rotation, as D-glucose
de- (or des-)	denotes *removal of something*, as hydrogen in dehydrocholic acid, and oxygen in desoxyephedrine
Δ (the capital Greek letter *delta*)	used to indicate, or focus attention on, *double bonds*, as in Δ^2-butene [$CH_3CH=CHCH_3$]
dehydro-	see *de-*
desoxy-	see *de-*
dextro- [or *d-* or (+)-]	signifies *dextrorotatory* form, as *d*-glucose
dl- (or *d,l-*)	see *racemic*
E and Z	descriptors used to distinguish stereoisomers differing in the spatial distribution of groups about a doubly-bonded atom pair. *E* signifies that the group of higher priority (by the Cahn–Ingold–Prelog sequence) on one of the atoms and the group of higher priority on the other atom are on opposite sides of the double bond. *Z* signifies that these higher priority groups are on the same side of the double bond. For further discussion, see *J Am Chem Soc. 90:* 509, 1968. Examples:

(*E*)-3-methyl-2-pentenoic acid

(*Z*)-3-methyl-2-pentenoic acid

epi- (or ep-)	connotes a *difference in steric configuration*, as epicholesterol is the 3α-hydroxy epimer of cholesterol; also used to signify a bridge, as in epichlorohydrin and 1,3-epoxybutane.
epoxy-	see *epi-*
gem-	refers to *two groups attached to the same carbon atom*, as the *gem*-dimethyl grouping in 2,2-dimethylpropane and in camphor

hetero-	means *different*, or *not all the same*, as in heterocyclic
hom- (or homo-)	indicates a *homologue* of another compound, as homatropine
hydro- (or hydr-)	refers to *hydrogen*, as hexahydrobenzene and hydracrylic acid
hypo-	signifies a *lower state of oxidation* in relation to another compound, as hypoxanthine
i-	sometimes used instead of iso-
iso- (rarely, *i-*)	denotes an *isomer* of another compound, as isobutane and isopropyl alcohol
levo [or *l-* or (−)-]	signifies *levorotatory* form, as *l*-ephedrine
L-	signifies a *structural relationship* to L-glyceraldehyde without any reference to direction of optical rotation, as L-glucose
m-	see *meta-*
meso-	signifies *optical inactivity due to internal compensation*, as mesotartaric acid
meta- (or *m-*)	indicates the *1,3- positions in benzene*, as in *m*-dihydroxybenzene
n-	abbreviation for *normal*, as *n*-butyl alcohol
N-	refers to *nitrogen*, as in *N*-methylaniline, indicating that the methyl group is attached to the nitrogen.
nor-	indicates a *relationship, usually through alkylation or isomerization*, between the compound whose name carries the prefix and the compound whose name does not. Examples: ephedrine is an *N*-methylated norephedrine; camphane is a trimethylated norcamphane; and leucine (2-amino-4-methylpentanoic acid) is an isomer of the normal form represented by norleucine (2-aminohexanoic acid).
o-	see *ortho-*
ortho- (or *o-*)	signifies the *1,2- positions in benzene*, as in *o*-hydroxybenzoic acid
p-	see *para-*
para- (or *p-*)	signifies the *1,4- positions in benzene*, as in *p*-aminobenzoic acid
per-	signifies *maximum state of substitution or addition*, as in perchloroethane, C_2Cl_6; perchloroethylene, $Cl_2C=CCl_2$; perhydrobenzene, C_6H_{12}. Sometimes used synonymously with peroxy, qv.
poly-	indicates a *union of several* identical molecules or molecular fragments, as in polymers and polysaccharides
R and S	notations used in the Cahn–Ingold–Prelog convention to describe configuration about a chiral center. The system utilizes a set of rules to establish a priority rating for the substituent groups around a center and the rating is then applied to the structure to describe the configuration. Unlike the D-L system, the convention does not involve comparisons with reference compounds. For further discussion, see *J Chem Educ 41 (Mar):* 116, 1964.
racemic [or dl- or (±)-]	signifies *optical inactivity due to equimolecular mixture of* (+)- *and* (−)- *forms*
s-	see *sym-*
S and R	see *R and S*
sec-	abbreviation for *secondary*, as in *sec*-butyl alcohol and *sec*-amines

Table II—Continued

sub-	denotes a *basic salt*, as in aluminum sub-acetate	*trans-* (or *anti-*)	refers to that *geometric isomer* in which the two groups are on *opposite* sides, as *trans*-butenedioic acid,
sym- (or *s-*)	abbreviation for *symmetrical*, as in *sym*-dichloroethane, $ClCH_2CH_2Cl$; specifically signifies the 1,3,5 positions in benzene, as in *sym*-trinitrobenzene		CHCOOH ‖ HOOCCH
syn-	equivalent to *cis*, qv, in certain	tris-	used instead of tri-, meaning *three*, before complex expressions (see *bis-*)
	—C=N │ │	*uns-*	see *unsym-*
	geometric isomers, e.g., *syn*-benzaldoxime	*unsym-* (or *uns-*)	abbreviation for *unsymmetrical*, as in *unsym*-dichloroethane, CH_3CHCl_2; specifically signifies the 1,2,4 positions in benzene, as in *unsym*-trihydroxybenzene
t-	see *tert-*		
tert- (or *t-*)	abbreviation for *tertiary*, as in *tert*-butyl alcohol and *tert*-amines	*v-* *vic-* (or *v-* or *adj-* or *a-*	see *vic-* signifies the *1,2,3 positions in benzene* as *vic*-trimethylbenzene
tetrakis-	used instead of tetra, meaning *four*, before complex expressions (see bis-)	*Z* and *E*	see *E* and *Z*

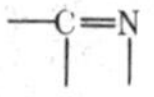

Table III—Suffixes

-al	indicates an *aldehyde*, as methanal, HCHO
-ane	indicates *saturated hydrocarbon or saturated heterocycle* as ethane, androstane, and furane
-ase	characteristic ending for *enzymes*, as zymase, amylase, polypeptidase, etc.
-ate	characteristic ending for *salts and esters of acids* ending in -ic, as acetate, phosphate, etc.
-ene	denotes *one double bond*, as ethene, butadiene, etc. (see also *-ylene*)
-ine	characteristic ending for various *basic nitrogen compounds such as amines and alkaloids*, as histamine, epinephrine, morphine, etc.
-ite	characteristic ending for *salts and esters of acids* ending in -ous, as phosphite, nitrite, etc.
-oic	refers to the *—COOH group*, as in ethanoic, benzoic, etc., acids
-ol	characteristic ending for *alcohols, phenols, naphthols, etc.*, as in ethanol, cyclohexanol, etc.
-one	indicates a *ketone*, as in propanone, acetophenone, etc.
-osan	generic ending for *polysaccharides*, as pentosans, hexosans, etc.
-ose	characteristic *carbohydrate* ending, especially for *sugars*, as dextrose, sucrose, etc.
-oside	generic ending for *glycosides*, as glucoside, rhamnoside, etc.
-oyl	characteristic ending for *acyl* radicals, as ethanoyl (for acetyl), carbamoyl, etc.
-yl	indicates a *radical*, especially a *univalent hydrocarbon radical*, as methyl, phenyl, etc.
-ylene	signifies a *bivalent hydrocarbon radical* with the free bonds on *different* carbon atoms, as in ethylene [—CH_2CH_2—] and o-phenylene

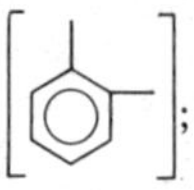

; used also to indicate a *double bond* in olefin hydrocarbons, as in ethylene [CH_2=CH_2]

-ylidene	signifies a *bivalent hydrocarbon radical* with the free bonds on the *same* carbon atom, as in ethylidene [CH_3CH=] and benzylidene 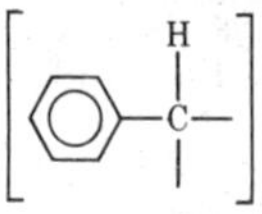

-yne	denotes *one triple bond*, as in ethyne [CH≡CH], ethynyl [CH≡C—], etc.

Chemical Notation Systems

The complexity and cumbersomeness of modern organic chemical nomenclature has encouraged attempts to develop "shorthand expressions" variously referred to as notations, ciphers, codes, and alphamerics which, for certain purposes, would be more convenient to use than the chemical names. Several systems have been proposed;* the only one which survives is that of Wiswesser.[2] In general, these involve assigning chemical meanings to the characters usually available on, or readily adapted to, a standard typewriter keyboard and devising rules for their use in constructing the notations. Final assessment of the overall utility of notations has yet to be made; they are particularly appealing because their brevity (in comparison with descriptive chemical nomenclature as illustrated in Table V) greatly increases storage efficiency in printed indexes and in machine memories. In addition, they automatically avoid the troublesome "trivial name feature" encountered in practical nomenclature. However, they are not pronounceable words and do not eliminate the need for descriptive chemical nomenclature in the written and spoken word.

Several of these notations have been found useful for retrieving compounds on a structural basis from relatively small, usually specialized, files of compounds stored in digital computers in the same notations. The extent to which techniques for accomplishing such retrieval may be usefully applied to a file comprising the universe of chemical compounds is the subject of considerable interest and debate.

Special typewriters have been devised whereby structural formulas may be coded directly on punched tape and also stored in the memory of a digital computer in the form of a matrix which can be searched at any future time on an atom-by-atom basis. This technique permits retrieval of compounds on a highly intimate structural basis which need not involve either nomenclature or the above mentioned notations, but does involve computer programs. Auxiliary devices exist for regenerating the actual structural formulas of retrieved compounds either by actual printout or by display on a cathode-ray tube.

---

* The National Academy of Sciences-National Research Council Publication No 1150 entitled *Survey of Chemical Notation Systems* (1964) provides a comprehensive review of the history of the various systems.

Table IV—Organic Groups and Radicals[a]

acetamido	CH_3CONH-	chloromercuri	$ClHg-$
acetate	CH_3COO- or $C_2H_3O_2{}^-$	cinnamoyl	$C_6H_5CH=CHCO-$
acetonyl	CH_3COCH_2-	cinnamyl	$C_6H_5CH=CHCH_2-$
acetoxy	see *acetate*	citrate	$-OOCCH_2C(OH)(COO-)CH_2COO-$ or
acetyl	CH_3CO-		$C_6H_5O_7{}^{3-}$
acridinyl	$C_{13}H_8N-$ (5 isomers)	cresyl	$CH_3C_6H_4O-$ (3 isomers)
acyl	generic term signifying an acid minus its OH group or groups as *acetyl*, CH_3CO-, and *carbonyl*, $=CO$	cyanato (cyanate)	$N\equiv C-O-$
		cyano (cyanide)	$-CN$
		cyclohexyl	$C_6H_{11}-$
adipoyl	$-CO(CH_2)_4CO-$	cyclopentyl	C_5H_9-
alanyl	$CH_3CH(NH_2)CO-$	cyclopropyl	C_3H_5-
alkoxy	generic term signifying a radical consisting of an alkyl joined to oxygen as *methoxy*, CH_3O-, and *ethoxy*, C_2H_5O-	n-decyl (decyl)	$CH_3(CH_2)_9-$ or $C_{10}H_{21}-$
		dialkylamino	R_2N- wherein R's are *alkyls*
		diazo	$-N=N-$ or $-N(\equiv N)-$
alkyl	generic term signifying a saturated hydrocarbon radical with a valence of one as *methyl*, CH_3-, and *ethyl*, C_2H_5-	diazoamino	$-N=N-NH-$
		diazonium	$N^+(\equiv N)-$
		dimethylamino	$(CH_3)_2N-$
alkylamino	generic term signifying $RNH-$ wherein R is an *alkyl*	dimethylarsino	$(CH_3)_2As-$
		diphenylmethyl	$(C_6H_5)_2CH-$
allyl	$CH_2=CHCH_2-$	dodecyl	$CH_3(CH_2)_{11}-$
amide (amido)	$-CONH_2$, see carbamoyl	epoxy	$-O-$ oxygen united to two different atoms already united in some other way
amidino	$H_2NC(=NH)-$		
amine (amino)	$-NH_2$	ethenyl	see *vinyl*
aminoacetate	H_2NCH_2COO-	ethoxy	C_2H_5O-
aminobenzoate	$H_2NC_6H_4COO-$ (o-, m-, and p-isomers)	ethoxycarbonyl	C_2H_5OCO-
n-amyl (amyl)	see *pentyl*	ethyl	C_2H_5-
tert-amyl	see *tert-pentyl*	ethylamino	C_2H_5NH-
anilino	C_6H_5NH-	ethylene	$-CH_2CH_2-$
anthryl	$C_{14}H_9-$, from anthracene (3 isomers)	ethylenedioxy	$-OCH_2CH_2O-$
aryl	generic term signifying an aromatic hydrocarbon radical as phenyl,	ethylidene	$CH_3CH=$
		ethylthio	CH_3CH_2S-
		ethynyl	$HC\equiv C-$
		fluoro (fluoride)	$F-$
	, o-tolyl , etc	fluorophosphate	see *phosphorofluoridate*
		formamido	$HC(=O)NH-$
auro	$Au-$	formate	$HCOO-$ or $CHO_2{}^-$
azido	$-N=N^+=N^-$	formyl	$-CHO$
azo	$-N=N-$	furfuryl	$OCH=CHCH=CCH_2-$ (two isomers, but used unqualified to refer specifically to the 2-form)
azoxy	$-N(O)=N-$		
benzal	see *benzylidene*		
benzamido	C_6H_5CONH-	furfurylidene	$OCH=CHCH=CCH=$ (two isomers, but used unqualified to refer specifically to the 2-form)
benzenesulfonamido	$C_6H_5SO_2NH-$		
benzenesulfonyl	$C_6H_5SO_2-$		
benzhydryl	see *diphenylmethyl*	furyl	C_4H_3O- (2 isomers)
benzoate	C_6H_5COO- or $C_7H_5O_2{}^-$	glucosyl	$C_6H_{11}O_5-$
benzoyl	C_6H_5CO-		
benzoyloxy (benzoxy)	see *benzoate*	glyceryl	$-CH_2-CH-CH_2-$ or $C_3H_5\equiv$
		glycinate	NH_2CH_2COO-
benzyl	$C_6H_5CH_2-$	glycyl	NH_2CH_2CO-
benzylidene	$C_6H_5CH=$	guanidino	$H_2NC(=NH)NH-$
biphenylyl	$C_6H_5C_6H_4-$ (3 isomers)	n-heptyl (heptyl)	$CH_3(CH_2)_6-$
bisulfate	$HOSO_2O-$ or SO_4H^-	hexadecyl	$CH_3(CH_2)_{15}-$
bisulfide	$-SH$; see *thiol*	hexamethylene	$-CH_2(CH_2)_4CH_2-$
bisulfite	$HOSOO-$ or SO_3H^-	n-hexyl (hexyl)	$CH_3(CH_2)_5-$ or $C_6H_{13}-$
borate (orthoborate)	$B{<}^{O-}_{O-}$ or $BO_3{}^{3-}$	hydrazino	H_2NNH-
		hydrazo	$-NHNH-$
		hydroxy (hydroxyl)	$-OH$
bromo (bromide)	$Br-$	hydroxyamino	$HONH-$
brosyl	*p*-bromobenzenesulfonyl	hydroxyimino	$HON=$
n-butyl (butyl)	$CH_3(CH_2)_3-$	hydroxymethyl (methylol)	$HOCH_2-$
sec-butyl	$CH_3CH_2CH(CH_3)-$		
tert-butyl	$(CH_3)_3C-$	imide	$=NH$, as in succinimide (cyclic)
butyrate (butanoate)	$CH_3CH_2CH_2COO-$ or $C_4H_7O_2{}^-$	imino	$HN=$
		indolyl	C_8H_6N- (several isomers)
cacodyl	see *dimethylarsino*	iodo (iodide)	$I-$
carbamate (carbamoyloxy)	H_2NCOO-	isoamyl	see *isopentyl*
		isobutyl	$(CH_3)_2CHCH_2-$
carbamoyl	H_2NCO-, see amide	isocyanato (isocyanate)	$O=C=N-$
carbethoxy	see *ethoxycarbonyl*		
carbomethoxy	see *methoxycarbonyl*	isocyano (isocyanide)	$-NC$
carbonyl	$=CO$		
carboxyl (carboxy)	$-COOH$	isonitrile	see *isocyano*
cetyl	see *hexadecyl*	isopentyl	$(CH_3)_2CHCH_2CH_2-$
chloro (chloride)	$Cl-$	isopropoxy	$(CH_3)_2CHO-$

Table IV—Continued

isopropyl	$(CH_3)_2CH-$
isothiocyano (isothiocyanato, isothiocyanate)	$S=C=N-$ or NCS^-
keto	see *oxo*
lactate	$CH_3CH(OH)COO-$ or $C_3H_5O_3^-$
malonyl	$-COCH_2CO-$
mandelate	$C_6H_5CH(OH)COO-$
menthyl	$C_{10}H_{19}-$ (several isomers)
mercapto (mercaptan)	$-SH$; see *thiol*
mercuri	$-Hg-$
mesityl	$2,4,6\text{-}(CH_3)_3C_6H_2-$
methenyl	see *methylidene*
methoxy	CH_3O-
methoxycarbonyl	CH_3OCO-
methoxyphenyl	$CH_3OC_6H_4-$ *o-, m-, p-* forms
methyl	CH_3-
methylene	$CH_2=$
methylenedioxy	$-OCH_2O-$
methylidene	$=CH_2$
methylidyne	$HC\equiv$
methylol	see *hydroxymethyl*
methylsulfonyl	CH_3SO_2-
methylthio	CH_3S-
morpholino	$\overline{CH_2CH_2OCH_2CH_2N}-$
naphthyl	$C_{10}H_7-$ (from naphthalene; α and β isomers)
neopentyl	$(CH_3)_3CCH_2-$
nitramino	O_2NNH-
nitrate	$-ONO_2$
nitrile	see *cyano*
nitrilo	$\equiv N$
nitrite	$-ONO$
nitro	$-NO_2$
nitroso	$-NO$
n-nonyl (nonyl)	$CH_3(CH_2)_8-$
n-octyl (octyl)	$CH_3(CH_2)_7-$
oleate	$CH_3(CH_2)_7CH=CH(CH_2)_7COO-$ or $C_{18}H_{33}O_2^-$
oxalate	$-OOCCOO-$ or $C_2O_4^{2-}$
oxalyl	$-COCO-$
oxo	$O=$
oxy	$-O-$ as a connective
palmitate	$CH_3(CH_2)_{14}COO-$ or $C_{16}H_{31}O_2^-$
n-pentyl (pentyl)	$CH_3(CH_2)_3CH_2-$
tert-pentyl	$CH_3CH_2C(CH_3)_2-$ (1,1-dimethylpropyl)
perchlorate	O_3Cl-O- or ClO_4^-
perchloryl	O_3Cl-
peroxy	$-O-O-$
phenethyl	$C_6H_5CH_2CH_2-$
phenoxy	C_6H_5O-
phenyl	C_6H_5-
phenylene	$C_6H_4=$ (*o-, m-* and *p-*isomers)
phenylsulfonyl	see *benzenesulfonyl*
phosphate (orthophosphate)	$O=P{\overset{\displaystyle O}{\underset{\displaystyle O}{\Big\langle}}}O-$ or PO_4^{3-}
phosphino	H_2P-
phospho	$-PO_2$
phosphono	$(HO)_2OP-$
phosphoro	$-PP-$
phosphorofluoridate	$F-{\overset{\displaystyle O}{\underset{\displaystyle O}{\overset{\|}{P}}}}{\Big\langle}^{O-}_{O-}$
phosphoroso	$-PO$
phthalate	$o\text{-}C_6H_4(COO-)_2$
phthalidyl	$o\text{-}\overline{C_6H_4COOCH}-$
phthaloyl	$o\text{-}C_6H_4(CO-)_2$
picrate	$2,4,6\text{-}(NO_2)_3C_6H_2O-$

picryl	$2,4,6\text{-}(NO_2)_3C_6H_2-$
piperidino	$\overline{CH_2CH_2CH_2CH_2CH_2N}-$
piperidyl	2-, 3-, or $4\text{-}C_5H_{10}N-$
pivaloyl	$(CH_3)_3CCO-$
propenyl	$CH_3CH=CH-$
propionate (propanoate)	CH_3CH_2COO- or $C_3H_5O_2^-$
propionyl	CH_3CH_2CO-
propoxy	$CH_3CH_2CH_2O-$
n-propyl (propyl)	$CH_3CH_2CH_2-$
propylene	$CH_3-\overset{\displaystyle \|}{CH}-CH_2-$
pyranyl	C_5H_5O- (3 isomers)
pyrazolidinyl	$C_3H_7N_2-$ (isomers)
pyridyl	C_5H_4N- (3 isomers)
pyrimidinyl (pyrimidyl)	$C_4H_3N_2-$ (3 isomers)
quinolyl	C_9H_6N- (7 isomers)
salicyl	$o\text{-}C_6H_4(OH)CO-$
salicylate	$o\text{-}C_6H_4(OH)COO-$ or $C_7H_5O_3^-$
silyl	$-SiH_3$
stearate	$CH_3(CH_2)_{16}COO-$ or $C_{18}H_{35}O_2^-$
stibo	O_2Sb-
styryl	$C_6H_5CH=CH-$
succinate	$-OOCCH_2CH_2COO-$ or $C_4H_4O_4^{2-}$
succinoyl	$-OCCH_2CH_2CO-$
sulfamoyl	H_2NSO_2-
sulfanilamido	$p\text{-}H_2NC_6H_4SO_2NH-$
sulfanilyl	$p\text{-}H_2NC_6H_4SO_2-$
sulfate	$-OSO_2O-$ or SO_4^{2-}
sulfhydryl	see *thiol*
sulfide	$-S-$; characteristic of thioethers as *ethyl sulfide* (ethyl thioether), $C_2H_5-S-C_2H_5$
sulfinyl	$-SO-$
sulfite	$-OSOO-$ or SO_3^{2-}
sulfo	see *sulfonic acid*
sulfonamido	$-SO_2NH-$
sulfonate	$-SO_2O-$
sulfone	see *sulfonyl*
sulfonic acid	$-SO_2OH$
sulfonyl (sulfone)	$-SO_2-$
sulfoxide	see *sulfinyl*
sulfuryl	see *sulfonyl*
tartrate	$-OOCCH(OH)CH(OH)COO-$ or $C_4H_4O_6^{2-}$
tetradecyl	$CH_3(CH_2)_{12}CH_2-$
tetramethylene	$-CH_2(CH_2)_2CH_2-$
tetrazolyl	CHN_4- (isomers)
thenyl	$C_4H_3SCH_2-$ (2 isomers)
thiazolyl	C_3H_2NS- (3 isomers)
thienyl	C_4H_3S- (2 isomers)
thio	see *sulfide*
thiocarbonyl	$=CS$
thiocyano (thiocyanato, thiocyanate)	$-SCN$
thiol (thiolo, mercapto)	$-SH$
thionyl	see *sulfinyl*
toloxy (tolyloxy)	$CH_3C_6H_4O-$ (*o-, m-,* and *p-*isomers)
toluenesulfonyl	$CH_3C_6H_4SO_2-$ (*o-, m-,* and *p-*forms)
tolyl	$CH_3C_6H_4-$ (*o-, m-,* and *p-*isomers)
tosyl	= *tolylsulfonyl*, qv
trimethylene	$-CH_2CH_2CH_2-$
trityl	$(C_6H_5)_3C-$
ureido	$H_2NCONH-$
valerate (pentanoate)	$CH_3(CH_2)_3COO-$ or $C_5H_9O_2^-$
vinyl	$CH_2=CH-$
xanthenyl (xanthyl)	$C_{13}H_9O-$ (5 isomers)
xenyl	see *biphenylyl*
xylyl	$(CH_3)_2C_6H_3-$ (6 isomers)

---

[a] Anionic radicals have slightly different names than given here when present as ligands. Examples: acetate vs acetato; nitrite vs nitrito; thiol vs thiolo.

Table V—Illustrations of Notation Brevity

Descriptive name (Chemical Abstracts)	Dyson notation	Wiswesser notation
1-chloro-3-methylbutane	C_4C2Ch4	G2Y
p-aminobenzoic acid	B6CXLN4	ZR-DVQ
1-naphthalenemethanol	$B6_2CQ3$	L66J-BLQ

Organic Chemical Literature

The constantly accelerating rate of research and development during the last four decades has created severe literature problems, not only in the areas of basic chemistry but also in the numerous other areas of science and technology where chemical information is primarily applied rather than generated. The history of Chemical Abstracts illustrates the magnitude of this so-called "information explosion." Commencing in 1906, it required 32 years for CA to produce its first million abstracts (1938), but only 17 years for the second million (1955), 8 years for the third million (1963), 6 years for the fourth million (1969), 5 years for the fifth million (1974) and somewhat less than 5 years for the sixth million (1979). By late 1983 the seventh million was surpassed.

Today's volume of chemical literature is so great that many libraries, some even of relatively recent construction, simply do not have enough shelf space to accommodate it and have resorted to microfilming. More important is the fact that selective retrieval of information from the literature has become an extremely arduous task. As a consequence, various industrial, academic, and governmental institutions (several pharmaceutical firms actually pioneered the effort) have developed computerized systems of storage and retrieval of those kinds of chemical information pertinent to their interests. Participating governmental agencies include the Food and Drug Administration, National Library of Medicine, National Science Foundation, US Patent Office, National Aeronautics & Space Administration, and various elements of the Department of Defense. With support from the National Science Foundation, Chemical Abstracts Service has been engaged for several years in computerizing its extensive files and plans to process all of its information via computer in the near future. An experimental computer search system was made available in 1969 which probes connection table representations of structural formulas and furnishes Chemical Abstracts references to compounds contained in a registry numbering in excess of one million compounds and to which compounds are being added at a rate of 5000 per week. Currently, Chemical Abstracts may be searched via its CASIA computerized index file. This service is offered by several vendors and allows very rapid and thorough search of CAS from 1967 to date; the current information is available on computer even before the printed copy reaches the subscriber! Arrangements exist whereby customers may either purchase the magnetic tapes and conduct their own searches or purchase the search service from CAS. The Institute for Scientific Information (ISI) in Philadelphia has also computerized its abstract journal, Index Chemicus, has several million compounds in its registry, and is adding new compounds at a rate of about 150,000 per year. Computer programs are available to customers which provide the capability to search and retrieve on the basis of either structural features via the Wiswesser notation, or properties, applications, and bibliographic information.

The huge continuing flood of published literature has also severely taxed the abilities of abstracting services to keep current. The magnitude of the task is illustrated by Chemical Abstracts experience which shows that the approximate number of papers and patents abstracted annually increased from 50,000 in 1950 to 120,000 in 1959, to 230,000 in 1968, 400,000 in 1973, over half a million in 1978 and approached

750,000 in 1983. The lag between publication of original articles and that of their abstracts has been sufficiently severe to foster the production of various so-called "current awareness tools" and specialty publications such as Index Chemicus and Current Contents of ISI and Chemical Titles, Chemical-Biological Activities (CBAC), Polymer Science and Technology (POST), Basic Journal Abstracts (BJA), and CA Condensates of CAS. These are also computer-based services.

Organic Pharmaceuticals

The contrast between the drugs of today and those of yesterday is a dramatic one in several respects. Only a half-century ago, man relied almost exclusively on nature to produce the organic drugs he needed, and the contributions of pharmacy were confined largely to the preparation of extracts, tinctures, and other dosage forms of the crude drugs and to the isolation of active principles, especially alkaloids and glycosides. Synthetics began to appear at a noticeably accelerated rate in the 1920s, and this is generally attributed to the very large expansion of the American chemical industry fostered by World War I. Many observers view the advent of the sulfa drugs in the early 1930s as marking the beginning of the modern era of synthetic drugs.

The great majority of today's new basic drugs are distinct organic chemical compounds. Most of these are products of synthetic organic chemistry, although some, such as reserpine, ACTH, and most of the antibiotics, are products of natural origin. Even with drugs of the latter group, however, the chemist has played a very important role in devising processes to produce them economically not only in the large quantities required but also in a sufficient state of purity. He has also succeeded in the deliberate chemical alteration of these naturally occurring compounds and produced derivatives which are either more potent or superior in some other respect, e.g., dehydrocholic acid, dihydroergotamine, fluorocorticosteroids, semisynthetic penicillins, methyltestosterone, etc.

Such molecular modification of known pharmacodynamic compounds, both natural and synthetic, constitutes one of the main kinds of research effort in the field of chemotherapy. While it is true that such effort frequently results in cluttering the market with drugs which are not superior to those being imitated, nevertheless a critical review of the results achieved over the past quarter century provides abundant evidence that the effort yields a gratifying percentage of new, highly beneficial drugs (see Chapter 27). Many of the new admissions to the official compendia are of such genesis.

Chemical and Pharmacological Classifications

During the early years of the modern era of synthetic organic pharmaceuticals, it was common practice to classify these new drugs on a chemical basis. This was logical not only because they were fundamentally the products of chemical research but also because the sciences of pharmacology and biochemistry were still in their early stages of development. Indeed, the ever-increasing need for more precise knowledge concerning the efficacy and safety of new drugs has fostered, to a significant degree, the rapid growth of these sciences to their present impressive status, and it will undoubtedly continue to do so in the future. The most comforting result is that these complementary efforts are continuously providing medicine with better tools and knowledge to the end that effective prevention and treatment of human physiological and psychological ills are constantly becoming more and more of a science and less and less of an art.

The guiding hypothesis underlying all efforts to classify organic pharmaceuticals on a chemical basis is simply that some correlation will exist between the chemistry of the compounds and their actions and uses as medicinal agents. Early efforts to discover useful correlations were based largely on gross structural considerations with particular emphasis on the presence and location of chemically active (functional) groups. In more sophisticated form, such efforts continue today, and the net result has been the accumulation of a very large body of knowledge on the broad subject of drug action. This knowledge strengthens materially the belief that the pharmacodynamics of drugs will ultimately be explicable in terms of their chemical characteristics; but it also points indisputably to the fact that a complete understanding of the mechanisms of drug actions is a long way in the future and that it will involve much more information than presently can be visualized from structural formulas and molecular models.

It has become clear that the pharmacological actions of drugs must be viewed as functions of the *total* molecules. For example, all barbituric acids contain the malonylurea fragment, but the relative actions of the different barbiturates vary widely with respect to quantitativeness, onset time, and duration, depending upon substituents at the 1, 3, and 5 positions (Chapter 57). The official sulfa drugs provide another example. The antibacterial portion common to all sulfas is the parent compound sulfanilamide, but chemical alterations at the N^1 and N^4 positions produce derivatives which differ importantly in their actions and chemotherapeutic applications.

Dependence of pharmacological activity on *total* molecular structure is commonly evident with drugs which are polyfunctional from a chemical viewpoint. The sulfa drugs provide a good example of this also; elimination of either the amino or sulfonamido portions, or even a change in their relative positions, results in loss of bacteriostatic activity. Similarly, aspirin loses its analgetic action if either its carboxyl or acetoxy group is completely removed or if the relation of these groups is other than *ortho*.

Similar dependence is common in the area of stereochemistry. Thus, the *trans* form of diethylstilbestrol is estrogenically potent whereas the *cis* form is not. This is reminiscent of the α- and β-forms of estradiol, the latter being about ten times as potent as the former. As an example involving diastereoisomers, one might cite the widely different mydriatic and pressor potencies of ephedrine and pseudoephedrine. Similar differences in physiological activity are also commonly observed between enantiomorphs. Thus, the D- and L-ephedrines differ markedly in mydriatic and pressor potencies; the D-forms of the α-amino acids are vastly inferior to the L-forms as nutrients, and (−)-epinephrine is more than 20 times as potent a sympathomimetic as the (+)-form.

From the preceding discussion, it is clear that difficulties are encountered whenever one attempts to classify organic drugs on a chemical basis and obtain a system which simultaneously separates these drugs on a pharmacologic basis. As will be seen in subsequent parts of this text, drugs that fall into the same chemical category often display, collectively, quite a number of different actions; and conversely, drugs of widely different chemical characteristics frequently provide the same kind of action when used as medicinal agents. Since, from a practical viewpoint, these agents are important because of the actions they provide (irrespective of their chemical composition), their monographs are presented in the subsequent chapters on a pharmacologic basis.

A more extensive treatment of the relationship between molecular structure and biologic activity may be found in Chapter 27.

Heterocycles Present in Official Pharmaceuticals

Many important biochemical compounds and drugs of *natural* origin contain heterocyclic ring structures. Nu-

merous examples occur, e.g., among the carbohydrates, essential amino acids, vitamins, alkaloids, glycosides, antibiotics, etc. The presence of heterocyclic structures in such diverse types of compounds is strongly indicative of the profound effects such structures exert on physiological activity, and recognition of this is abundantly reflected in efforts to find useful *synthetic* drugs. Examples include researches leading to a wide variety of modern drugs such as Chlordiazepoxide (tranquilizer), Methazolamide (carbonic anhydrase inhibitor), Guanethidine (antihypertensive), Stanozolol (anabolic), Dapsone (leprostatic), Cyclophosphamide and Thiotepa (antineoplastics), Hydrochlorothiazide (diuretic and antihypertensive), Imipramine (antidepressant), Lucanthone (antischistosomal), and many others.

As is to be expected, this trend in research finds reflection in the changing character of the contents of official drug compendia. Intensive research in diverse heteroareas continues to yield new medicinal agents, and Table VI is designed to portray the spectrum of heterocycles presently represented in USP and NF drugs. The classification is patterned after that employed in *The Ring Index* and in *Chemical Abstracts*. The rings are presented in the order of increasing complexity. The boldface figures show the total number of atoms in the rings, and the number of boldface figures shows the number of rings present in the systems. As an example, the notation 5, 6 indicates a system composed of two rings, one of which contains five atoms while the other one contains six atoms. The formulas such as C_3NS-C_6 portray the kind and number of atoms present in the ring or rings. Associated with each of these formulas are the graphic formulas and *Ring Index* names[†] of the individual heterocycles, and, *in italics*, one or more examples of official drugs (or the portions of them) containing these heterocycles.

Structures and numbering schemes[‡] are according to *The Ring Index* and thus do not portray any inherent features of stereospecificity.[§] It will be observed that some of the names for the heterocycles are trivial (eg, pyrimidine, nortropane, etc.) while others are rigidly systematic. Trivial names are employed in the table wherever advisable; ie, wherever, through continued use, they have become recognized by chemists (as reflected by *IUPAC* adoption and *Chemical Abstracts* indexing) as denoting the structures to which they refer. In all other instances, systematic names must be used in order to distinguish between the heterocycle of interest and its isomeric forms.

Presentation is exclusively on the basis of the *most complex ring "system"* containing the hetero atom or atoms, the term "system" meaning either a single ring or a combination of rings of the fused, bridged, or spiro types. For example, quinine is presented *only* as a quinoline derivative and *not* also as a pyridine derivative, even though quinoline is a benzopyridine. Similarly, caffeine is presented *only* as a purine derivative and *not* as either a pyrimidine or an imidazole derivative, even though purine is an imidazopyrimidine.

[†] Heterocyclic structures are often actually or theoretically produced by relatively simple chemical operations such as condensation and dehydrogenation on aliphatic structures. Because of this, many authors prefer to name such heterocycles in a manner designed to disclose the relationship to the aliphatics rather than employ *The Ring Index* nomenclature used in this table.

[‡] Extreme caution must be exercised in interpreting position numbers as given in the names of compounds in different texts and works of reference. The situation often arises in which two different numbering schemes, through long continued usage, have become firmly established for a particular ring system; and this leads to different numbers in an otherwise identical pair of names for a given compound. Also, authors of texts frequently indulge in the reprehensible practice of inventing their own pet numbering schemes.

[§] *The Ring Index*, 2nd ed, Am Chem Soc Washington, DC, 1960 and Supplements. Also each annual, quinquennial and decennial index to *Chemical Abstracts*.

Table VI—Heterocycles in Official Drugs

3 C_2N

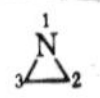

Aziridine (11)[a]
Example: *Thiotepa*

5 CN_4

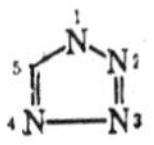

1H-Tetrazole (61)
Examples: *Cefamandole; Cefazolin.*

C_2N_2S

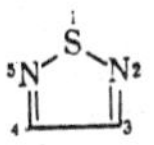

1,2,5-Thiadiazole (89)
Example: *Timolol.*

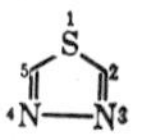

1,3,4-Thiadiazole (90)
Examples: *Acetazolamide; Cefazolin; Sulfamethizole.*

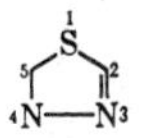

1,3,4-Thiadiazoline (90)
Example: *Methazolamide.*

C_3NO

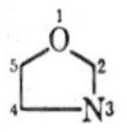

Oxazolidine (119)
Example: *Paramethadione*

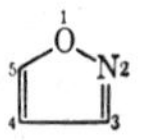

Isoxazole (118)
Examples: *Cloxacillin; Isocarboxazid; Sulfisoxazole.*

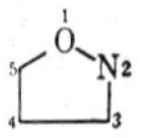

Isoxazolidine (118)
Example: *Cycloserine.*

C_3NS

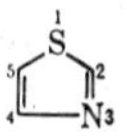

Thiazole (122)
Examples: *Thiabendazole; Thiamine.*

C_3N_2

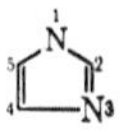

Imidazole (127)
Examples: *Azathioprine; Histamine; Pilocarpine.*

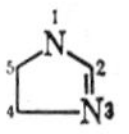

2-Imidazoline (127)
Examples: *Antazoline; Phentolamine.*

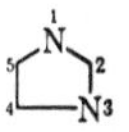

Imidazolidine (127)
Examples: *Hetacillin; Nitrofurantoin; Phenytoin.*

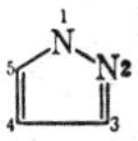

Pyrazole (124)
Example: *Betazole.*

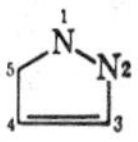

3-Pyrazoline (124)
Example: *Antipyrine.*

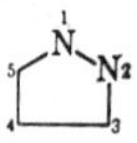

Pyrazolidine (124)
Examples: *Phenylbutazone; Sulfinpyrazone.*

C_4N

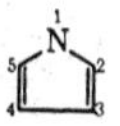

Pyrrole (142)
Example: *Pyrvinium Pamoate.*

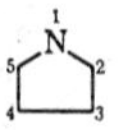

Pyrrolidine (142)
Examples: *Methsuximide; Pyrrobutamine.*

C_4O

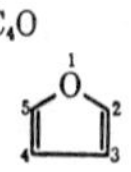

Furan (145)
Examples: *Nitrofurantoin; Nitrofurazone.*

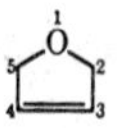

2,5-Dihydrofuran (145)
Examples: *Ascorbic Acid; Digitoxin.*

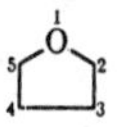

Tetrahydrofuran (145)
Examples: *Polysorbate; Sorbitan; Streptomycin; Sucrose.*

C_4S

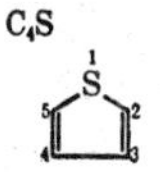

Thiophene (149)
Examples: *Cephaloridine; Methapyrilene.*

6 C_3NOP

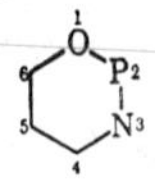

Tetrahydro-2H-1,3,2-oxazaphosphorine (7746)
Example: *Cyclophosphamide.*

C_3O_3

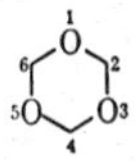

s-Trioxane (222)
Example: *Paraldehyde.*

C_4NO

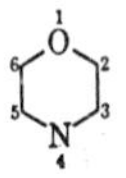

Morpholine (239)
Examples: *Phenmetrazine; Pramoxine; Timolol.*

C_4N_2

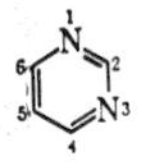

Pyrimidine (249)
Examples: *Pyrimethamine; Sulfadiazine.*

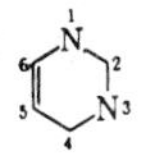

1,2,3,4-Tetrahydropyrimidine (249)
Examples: *Idoxuridine; Propylthiouracil.*

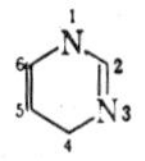

1,4,5,6-tetrahydro form (249)
Example: *Oxyphencyclimine.*

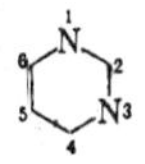

Hexahydropyrimidine (249)
Examples: *All barbituric and thiobarbituric acids; Primidone.*

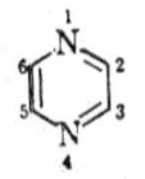

Pyrazine (250)
Example: *Amiloride.*

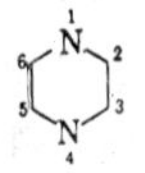

Piperazine; Hexahydropyrazine (250)
Examples: *Chlorcyclizine; Pipobroman; Prochlorperazine.*

C_5N

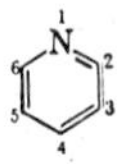

Pyridine (277)
Examples: *Cetylpyridinium Chloride; Niacinamide; Tripelennamine.*

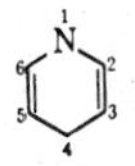

1,4-Dihydropyridine (4H-Pyridine) (277)
Example: *Propyliodone.*

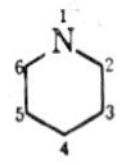

Piperidine; Hexahydropyridine (277)
Examples: *Alphaprodine; Glutethimide; Meperidine.*

C_5O

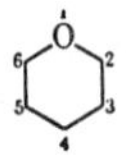

Tetrahydropyran (278)
Examples: *Lactose; Streptomycin.*

7 C_6N

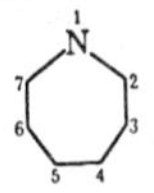

Hexahydroazepine (355)
Example: *Tolazamide.*

8 C_7N

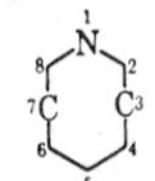

Octahydroazocine (414)
Example: *Guanethidine.*

14 $C_{13}O$

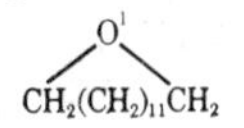

Oxacyclotetradecane (534)
Example: *Erythromycin.*

16 $C_{11}N_5$

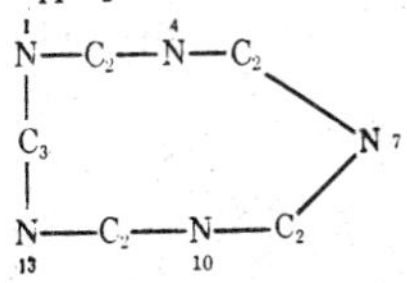

1,4,7,10,13-Pentaazacyclohexadecane
Example: *Viomycin.*

Table VI—Continued

23 $C_{16}N_7$

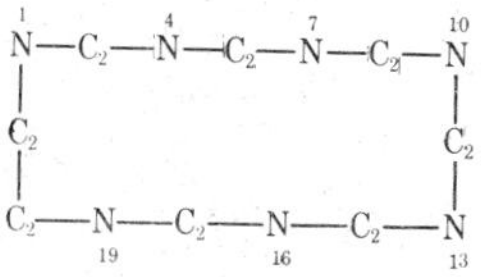

1,4,7,10,13,16,19-Heptaazacyclo-
tricosane (11705)
Examples: *Colistin; Colistimethate
Sodium.*

4,5 C_3N-C_3NS

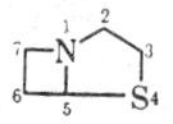

4-Thia-1-azabicyclo[3.2.0]heptane (774)
Example: *Penicillins.*

4,6 C_2HgO-C_6

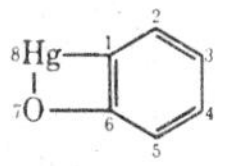

7-Oxa-8-mercurabicyclo[4.2.0]-octa-
1,3,5-triene (796)
Example: *Nitromersol.*

C_3N-C_4NS

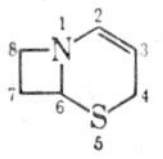

5-Thia-1-azabicyclo[4.2.0]oct-2-ene (11757)
Example: *Cephalothin Sodium.*

5,5 C_4O-C_4O

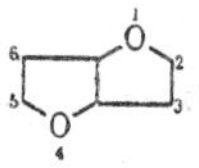

Furo[3,2-*b*]furan, hexahydro form (996)
Example: *Isosorbide Dinitrate.*

5,6 C_2BO_2-C_6

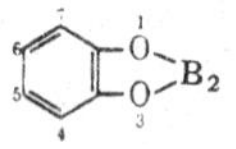

1,3,2-Benzodioxaborole (1040)
Example: *Epinephryl Borate.*

C_3NS-C_6

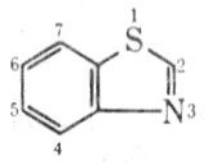

Benzothiazole (1152)
Example: *Ethoxzolamide.*

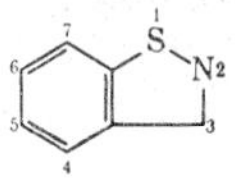

1,2-Benzisothiazole, 2,3-dihydro form (1150)
Example: *Saccharin.*

C_3N_2-C_4N_2

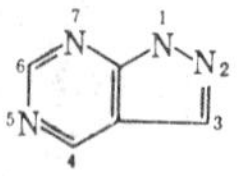

1*H*-Pyrazolo[3,4-*d*]pyrimidine (1174)
Example: *Allopurinol.*

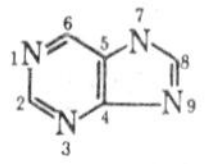

Purine[b] (1179)
Examples: *Azathioprine; Caffeine;
Dimenhydrinate.*

C_3N_2-C_6

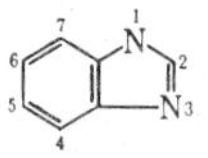

Benzimidazole (1213)
Examples: *Cyanocobalamin; Droperidol; Thiabendazole.*

C_3OS-C_6

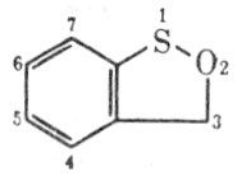

3*H*-2,1-Benzoxathiole (1222)
Example: *Phenolsulfonphthalein.*

C_4N-C_5N

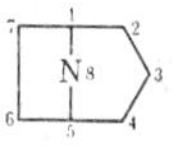

Nortropane (1281)
Examples: *Atropine; Cocaine.*

C_4N-C_6

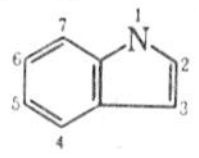

Indole (1286)
Example: *Indomethacin.*

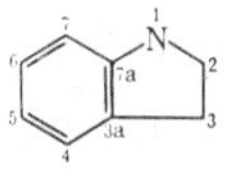

Indoline (1286)
Example: *Indigotindisulfonate Sodium.*

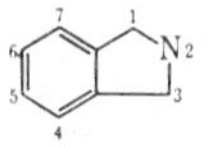

Isoindoline (1290)
Example: *Chlorthalidone.*

C_4O-C_6

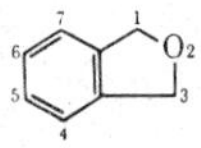

Phthalan (1330)
Examples: *Noscapine; Phenolphthalein.*

6,6 C_3N_2S-C_6

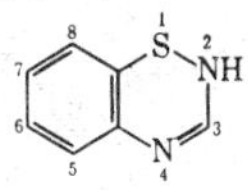

2*H*-1,2,4-Benzothiadiazine (8074)
Examples: *Benzthiazide; Chlorothiazide.*

3,4-dihydro form (8074)
Examples: *Hydrochlorothiazide; Polythiazide.*

C_4N_2-C_4N_2

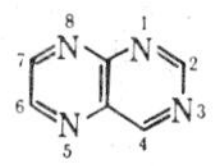

Pteridine (1587)
Examples: *Folic Acid; Methotrexate.*
5,6,7,8-tetrahydro form
Example: *Leucovorin.*

C_4N_2-C_6

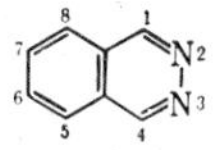

Phthalazine (1628)
Example: *Hydralazine.*

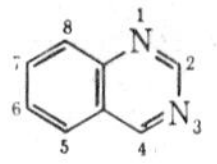

Quinazoline (1626)
Example: *Methaqualone.*

C_5N-C_5N

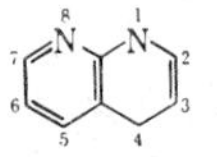

1,8-Naphthyridine, 1,4-dihydro form (1683)
Example: *Nalidixic Acid.*

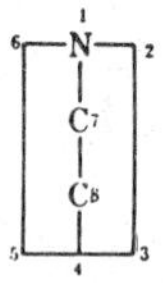

Quinuclidine (1690)
Examples: *Clidinium Bromide; Quinine.*

C_5N-C_6

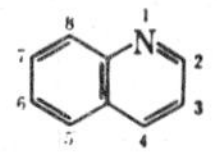

Quinoline (1707)
Examples: *Chloroquine; Pyrvinium
Pamoate; Quinine.*

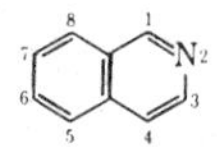

Isoquinoline (1708)
Example: *Papaverine.*
1,2,3,4-tetrahydro form
Example: *Emetine.*

C_5O-C_6

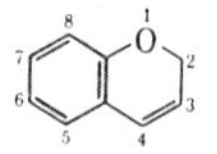

2*H*-1-Benzopyran (1727)
Examples: *Cromolyn Sodium; Dicumarol;
Warfarin.*

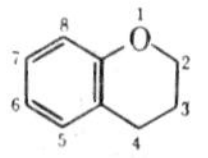

Chroman (Dihydrobenzopyran) (1727)
Example: *Alpha Tocopherol.*

6,7 C_6-C_5N_2

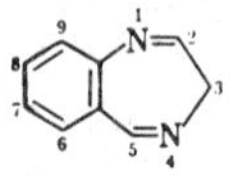

3*H*-1,4-Benzodiazepine (1829)
Example: *Chlordiazepoxide.*

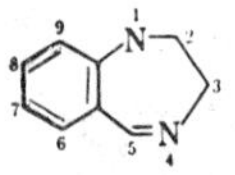

2*H*-1,4-Benzodiazepine, 1,3-dihydro
form (12067)
Examples: *Diazepam; Oxazepam.*

6,36 C_5O-$C_{34}O_2$

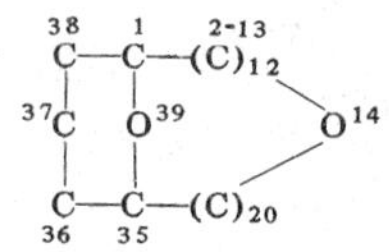

14,39-Dioxabicyclo[33.3.1]nonatriacontane
Example: *Amphotericin.*

3,5,6 C_2O-C_4N-C_5N

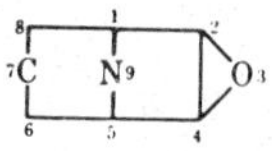

3-Oxa-9-azatricyclo[3.3.1.0^{2,4}]nonane (2072)
Examples: *Methscopolamine Bromide;
Scopolamine.*

Table VI—Continued

3,6,24 C_2O-C_5O-$C_{22}O_2$

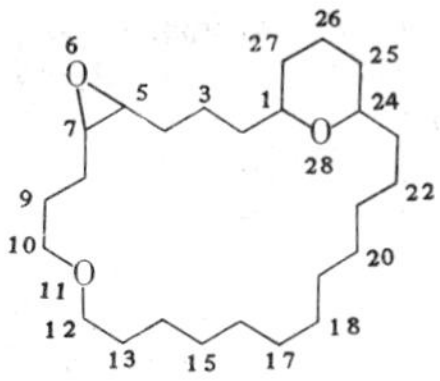

6,11,28-Trioxatricyclo[22.3.1.0^{5,7}]-octacosane
Example: *Natamycin.*

5,5,5 C_3N_2-C_4S-C_4S

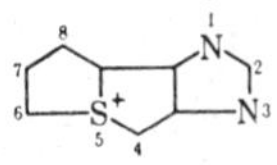

Imidazo[4,5-c]thieno[1,2-a]thiolium, decahydro form (2215)
Example: *Trimethaphan Camsylate.*

5,5,6 C_3NO-C_4N-C_4N_2

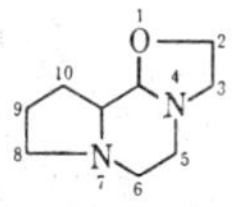

8H-Oxazolo[3,2-a]pyrrolo[2,1-c]-pyrazine, perhydro form (2319)
Example: *Ergotamine.*

C_3N_2-C_4N-C_6

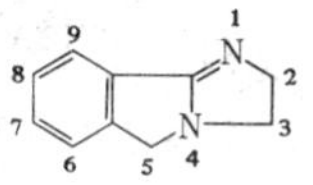

3H-Imidazo[2,1-a]isoindole, 2,5-dihydro form (2384)
Example: *Mazindol.*

C_4N-C_4N-C_6

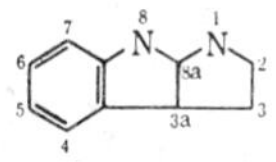

Pyrrolo[2,3-b]indole, 1,2,3,3a,8,8a-hexahydro form (2442)
Example: *Physostigmine.*

5,6,6 C_3O_2-C_4N_2-C_6

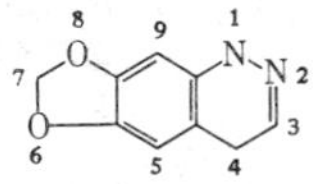

[1,3]-Dioxolo[4,5-g]cinnoline, 1,4-dihydro form (2806)
Example: *Cinoxacin.*

C_3O_2-C_5N-C_6

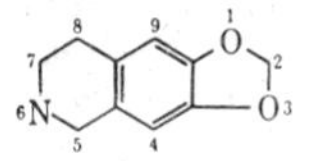

1,3-Dioxolo[4,5-g]isoquinoline, 5,6,7,8-tetrahydro form (2810)
Example: *Noscapine.*

C_4N-C_6-C_6

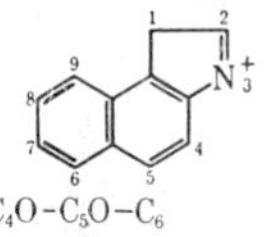

1H-Benz[e]indolium (2933)
Example: *Indocyanine Green.*

C_4O-C_3O-C_6

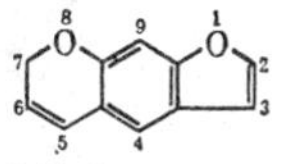

7H-Furo[3,2-g][1]benzopyran (2988)
Examples: *Methoxsalen; Trioxsalen.*

C_4O-C_6-C_6

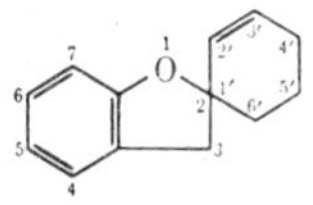

Spiro[benzofuran-2(3H),1'-[2]-cyclohexene] (3028)
Example: *Griseofulvin.*

6,6,6 C_3N_3-C_3N_3-C_3N_3

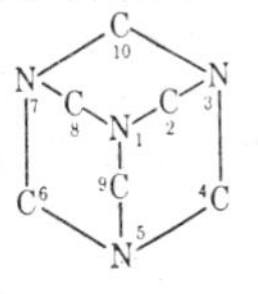

Hexamethylenetetramine (3237)
Example: *Methenamine.*

C_4NO-C_6-C_6

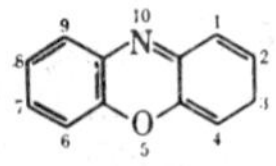

3H-Phenoxazine (3289)
Example: *Dactinomycin.*

C_4NS-C_6-C_6

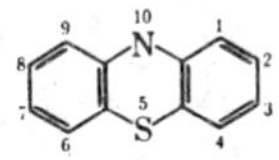

Phenothiazine (3314)
Examples: *Chlorpromazine; Prochlorperazine.*

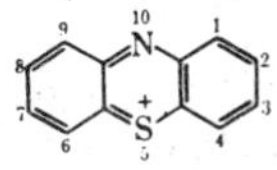

Phenazathionium (3315)
Example: *Methylene Blue.*

C_4O_2-C_5O-C_6

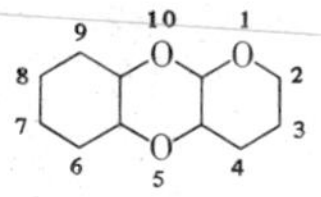

4H-Pyrano[2,3-b][1,4]benzodioxin, decahydro form (12687)
Example: *Spectinomycin.*

C_4N_2-C_4N_2-C_6

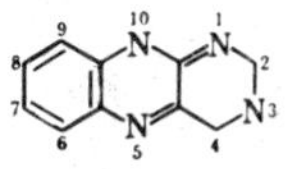

Benzo[g]pteridine, 2,3,4,10-tetrahydro form (3340)
Example: *Riboflavin.*

C_5N-C_5N-C_6

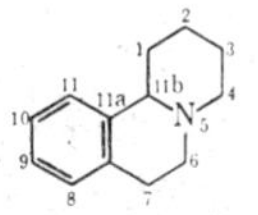

2H-Benzo[a]quinolizine, 1,3,4,6,7,-11b-hexahydro form (3487)
Example: *Emetine.*

C_5N-C_6-C_6

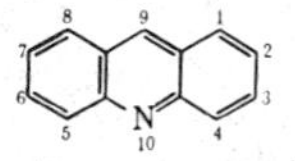

Acridine[b] (3523)
Examples: *Acrisorcin; Quinacrine.*

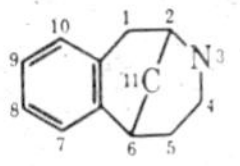

2,6-Methano-3-benzazocine, 1,2,3,4,-5,6-hexahydro form (3535)
Example: *Pentazocine.*

C_5O-C_6-C_6

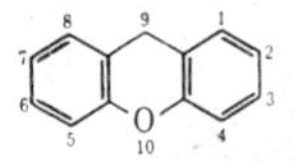

Xanthene[b] (3571)
Examples: *Methantheline; Propantheline.*

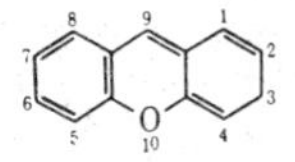

3H-Isoxanthene[b] (3569)
Examples: *Fluorescein Sodium; Rose Bengal Sodium.*

C_5S-C_6-C_6

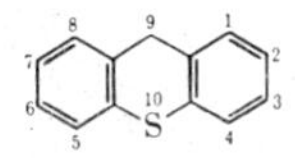

Thioxanthene[b] (3607)
Examples: *Chlorprothixene; Thiothixene.*

6,6,7 C_6-C_6-C_6N

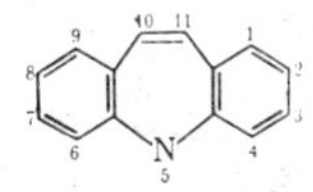

5H-Dibenz[b,f]azepine (3689)
Example: *Carbamazepine.*

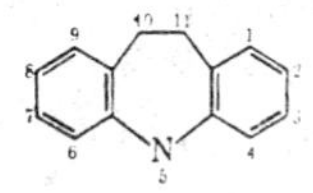

10,11-dihydro form (3689)
Examples: *Desipramine; Imipramine.*

C_6-C_6-C_6O

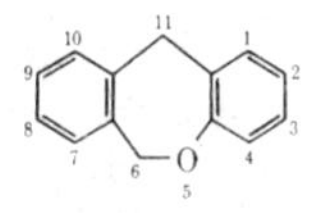

Dibenz[b,e]oxepine, 6,11-dihydro form (3697)
Example: *Doxepin.*

3,5,5,6 C_2N-C_4N-C_4N-C_6

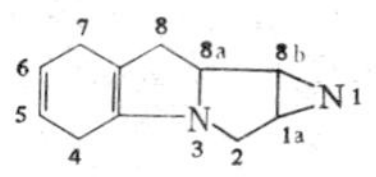

Azirino[2',3':3,4]pyrrolo[1,2-a]indole (12848),1,1a,2,8,8a,8b-hexahydro derivative.
Example: *Mitomycin.*

5,6,6,6 C_4N-C_5N-C_6-C_6

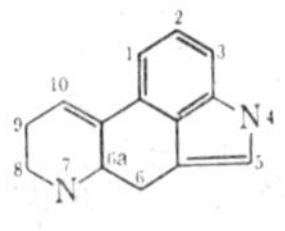

Indolo[4,3-fg]quinoline, 4,6,6a,7,8,9-hexahydro form (4550)
Examples: *Ergonovine; Ergotamine.*

C_5-C_5O-C_6-C_6

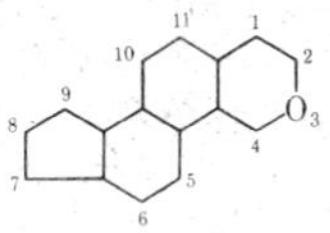

Cyclopenta[5,6]naphtho[1,2-c]pyran, perhydro form (4760)
Example: *Oxandrolone.*

Table VI—Continued

5,6,6,9 $C_4N-C_5N-C_6-C_8N$

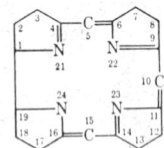

10H-3,7-Methanoazacycloundecino-
[5,4-b]indole, 1,2,4,5,6,7,8,9-octa-
hydro form (13276)
Examples: *Vinblastine; Vincristine.*

5,6,6,24 $C_4O-C_6-C_6-C_{22}NO$

2,7-(Epoxypentadecanimino)naph-
tho[2,1-b]]furan
Example: *Rifampin.*

6,6,6,6 $C_5N-C_6-C_6-C_6$

4H-Dibenzo[de,g]quinoline, 5,6,6a,7-
tetrahydro form (5171)
Example: *Apomorphine.*

2H-10,4a-Iminoethanophenanthrene,[b]
cis-1,3,4,9,10,10a-hexahydro form;
morphinan (5180)
Examples: *Dextromethorphan; Levorphanol.*

5,5,5,5,15 $C_4N-C_4N-C_4N-C_4N-C_{11}N_4$

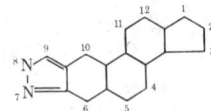

Corrin[b] (5475)
Example: *Cyanocobalamin.*

5,5,6,6,6 $C_3NO-C_5-C_6-C_6-C_6$

1H-Cyclopenta[7,8]phenanthro[3,2-
d]isoxazole, dodecahydro
derivative (11036)
Example: *Danazol.*

5,5,6,6,6 $C_3N_2-C_5-C_6-C_6-C_6$

8H-Cyclopenta[7,8]phenanthro[2,3-c]-
pyrazole, tetradecahydro
derivative (5557)
Example: *Stanozolol.*

$C_4N-C_4N-C_5N-C_6-C_6$

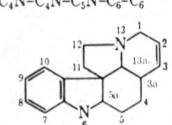

1H-Indolizino[8,1-cd]carbazole,
3a,4,5,5a,6,11,12,13a-octahydro
form (11065)
Examples: *Vinblastine; Vincristine.*

5,6,6,6,6 $C_4N-C_5N-C_5N-C_6-C_6$

Benz[g]indolo[2,3-a]quinolizine,
1,2,3,4,4a,5,7,8,13,13b,14,14a-do-
decahydro form (5874)
Example: *Reserpine.*

$C_4O-C_5N-C_6-C_6-C_6$

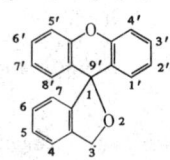

4aH-8,9c-Iminoethanophenanthro-
[4,5-bcd]furan, (5922)
5,7a,8,9-tetrahydro form
Examples: *Codeine; Morphine; Nalorphine.*
5,6,7,7a,8,9-hexahydro form (ring
marked A saturated)
Examples: *Hydrocodone; Hydromorphone.*

$C_4O-C_5O-C_6-C_6-C_6$

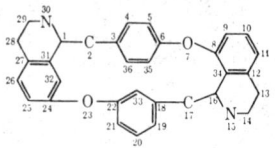

Spiro[phthalan-1,9'-xanthene]
(5935) or Spiro[isobenzofuran-
1(3H),9'[9H]xanthene]
Example: *Fluorescein.*

6,6,6,6,6,6,18 $C_5N-C_5N-C_6-C_6-C_6-C_6-C_{16}O_2$

Octahydro form of Ring Index No
7408.
Examples: *Tubocurarine; Metocurine.*

---

[a] Number in parenthesis is *The Ring Index* number.
[b] Exception to numbering rule.

In a complete presentation of this type, drugs containing two or more *separate* hetero ring systems would appear under each of the systems; eg, quinine would emerge both as a quinoline and quinuclidine derivative.

Wherever possible, only that portion of the official title is used which embraces the heterocycle; eg, thiamine instead of Thiamine Hydrochloride.

Functional Groups and Prediction of Comparative pK Assignments

The understanding of the biological behavior of organic drugs includes the ability to identify the organic functional groups present in the drug and to recognize the chemical and physicochemical properties associated with each group. One fundamental characteristic consists of the acidic and basic properties of organic compounds and their acid-base interactions. This discussion will be limited to a flow sheet (Table VII) approach to the identification of various organic func-

tional groups and to the assignment of approximate acidic, basic, or neutral values. The listing of the *Types of Organic Compounds* (Table I) should be referred to in reviewing the functional groups for the following discussion.

Since the biological environment of a drug is primarily an aqueous solution, the Brønsted-Lowry definition and the quantitative concepts of ionization can be applied to the study of acidic, basic, and amphiprotic drugs. According to the Brønsted-Lowry definition, the strength of an acid depends upon its ability to donate a proton, and the strength of a base depends upon its ability to accept a proton. These strengths can be expressed in terms of the negative log of the acidity constant, pK_a, or of the basicity constant, pK_b. The pK relationship in water between an acid and its conjugate base, or a base and its conjugate acid can be easily established as follows:

$$HA + B \rightleftharpoons A^- + HB^+$$
$$pK_a \quad pK'_b \quad pK_b \quad pK'_a$$

(1)

and $pK_a + pK_b = 14$, $pK'_a + pK'_b = 14$. In the acid-base re-

Table VII—Functional group and pK values on a pK$_b$ 1-14 to pK$_a$ 14-1 plot

pK$_b$				Neutral		pK$_a$	
1	5	10	14	14	10	5	1

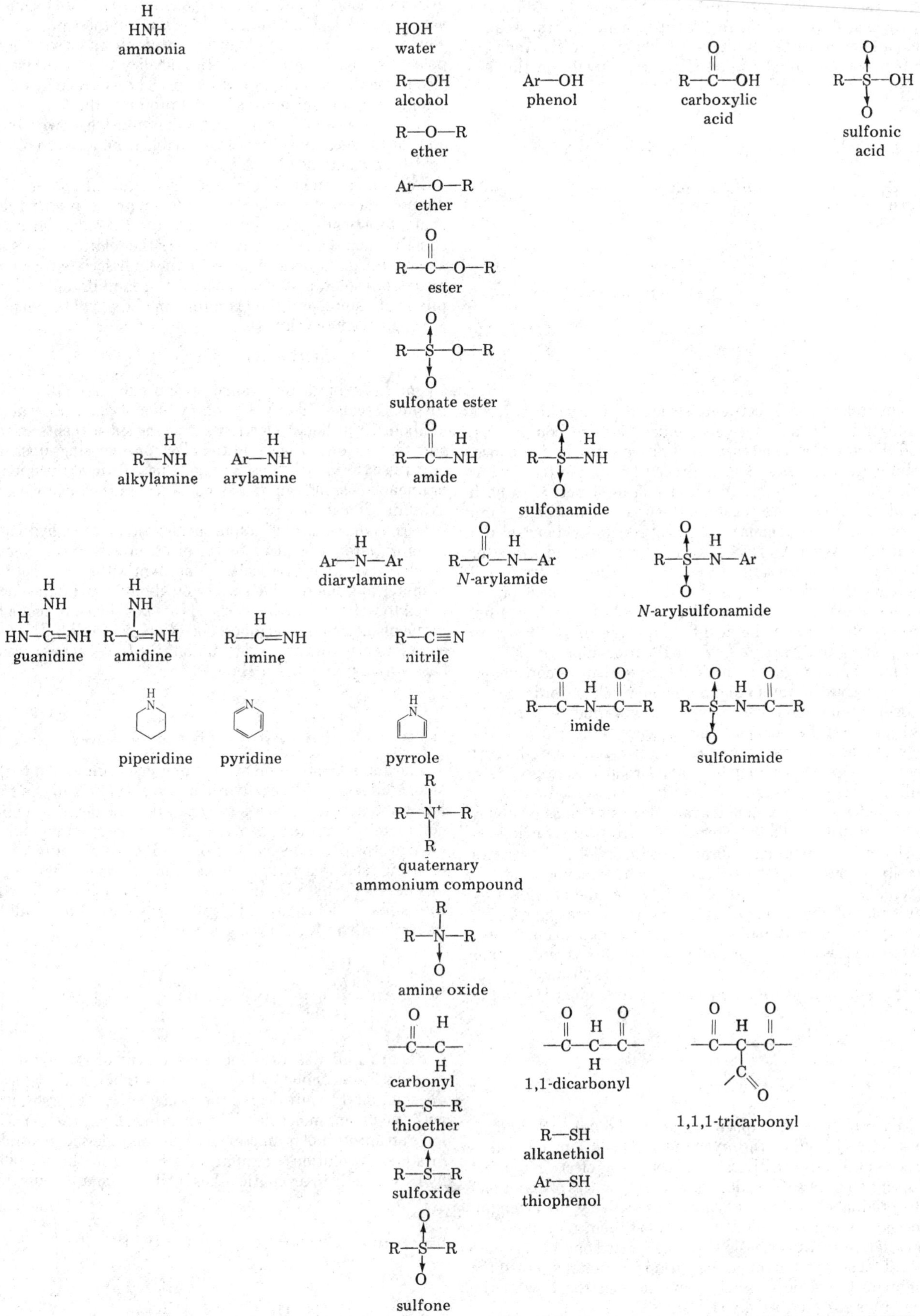

H
HNH
ammonia

HOH
water

R—OH
alcohol

Ar—OH
phenol

R—C(=O)—OH
carboxylic acid

R—S(=O)(=O)—OH
sulfonic acid

R—O—R
ether

Ar—O—R
ether

R—C(=O)—O—R
ester

R—S(=O)(=O)—O—R
sulfonate ester

H
R—NH
alkylamine

H
Ar—NH
arylamine

R—C(=O)—NH—H
amide

R—S(=O)(=O)—NH—H
sulfonamide

H
Ar—N—Ar
diarylamine

R—C(=O)—N(H)—Ar
N-arylamide

R—S(=O)(=O)—N(H)—Ar
N-arylsulfonamide

H
NH
HN—C=NH (with H)
guanidine

H
NH
R—C=NH
amidine

R—C=NH (with H)
imine

R—C≡N
nitrile

O O
R—C—N(H)—C—R
imide

O O
R—S(=O)(=O)—N(H)—C—R
sulfonimide

piperidine

pyridine

pyrrole

R
R—N⁺—R
R
quaternary ammonium compound

R
R—N—R
↓O
amine oxide

O H
—C—C—
H
carbonyl

O O
—C—C—C—
H
1,1-dicarbonyl

O O
—C—C—C—
C
O
1,1,1-tricarbonyl

R—S—R
thioether

R—SH
alkanethiol

O
R—S—R
sulfoxide

Ar—SH
thiophenol

O
R—S—R
O
sulfone

action (Eq 2) between p-aminobenzoic acid(I) and sodium bicarbonate(II), the pK_a values are ~5 (COOH) and ~4 (amine conjugate acid) for I, and for H_2CO_3, pK_{a_1} is ~6 and pK_{a_2} is ~10. This reaction proceeds to the right, since the strongest acid reacts with the strongest base, and the direction of any acid-base reaction favors the formation of the weaker acid and weaker base, or pK_{a_1} = 6 carbonic acid (III) and pK_b = 9 p-aminobenzoate anion (IV), respectively, in this example.

$$H_2N-\text{C}_6H_4-\overset{\overset{\displaystyle O}{\|}}{C}-OH \; + \; {}^-O-\overset{\overset{\displaystyle O}{\|}}{C}-OH \longrightarrow$$

$$\begin{array}{cccc} pK_b & pK_a & pK_{b_1} & pK_{a_2} \\ 10 & 5 & 8 & 10 \\ & (I) & & (II) \end{array}$$

$$HO-\overset{\overset{\displaystyle O}{\|}}{C}-OH \; + \; H_2N-\text{C}_6H_4-\overset{\overset{\displaystyle O}{\|}}{C}-O^-$$

$$\begin{array}{cc} pK_{a_1} & pK_b \\ 6 & 9 \\ (III) & (IV) \end{array}$$

The relationship between structure and acid or base strength has been extensively studied for many compounds, and the results are well correlated with electronic, resonance, orbital hybridization, and hydrogen bonding effects. For example, the *Hammett equation* relates structure to both equilibrium and rate constants for reactions of *meta*- and *para*-substituted (sigma substituent constants) benzene derivatives. With benzoic acid, an electron-withdrawing or electronegative substituent ($+\sigma$) such as the nitro group will increase the acidity (lower the pK_a), while an electron-releasing or electropositive substituent ($-\sigma$) such as the methyl group will decrease the acidity (raise the pK_a). Refer to Chapter 27 on Structure Activity Relationships.

Many of the organic functional groups can be considered as derivatives of water or ammonia in which one or more hydrogen atoms have been replaced by various substituent radicals. For the most part, the influence of the radical on the flow of electrons from the oxygen or nitrogen atom, the first member of periodic Group VI-A and Group V-A, respectively, will determine the resulting acidity, basicity, or neutrality, provided a hydrogen atom is available in situations involving acid ionization. The greater the electron-withdrawing capacity of the substituent radical, the greater will be the relative acidity or lower the relative basicity. Three common radicals often alter the original pK value of water and ammonia by multiples of about five pK units towards increasing relative acidity when substituted into the water or ammonia molecule. These are the aryl, acyl, and alkyl or arylsulfonyl radicals and can be arranged in the following order, using the alkyl radical as the nonelectron-withdrawing group for comparison;

$$R- \; < \; Ar- \; < \; R-\overset{\overset{\displaystyle O}{\|}}{C}- \; < \; R-\overset{\overset{\displaystyle O}{\uparrow}}{\underset{\underset{\displaystyle O}{\downarrow}}{S}}-$$

with the pK altering capacity values of about 0, 5, 10, and 15, respectively. When the aryl or acyl radical is introduced as a second electron withdrawing group, the electronic effect appears to be less than additive, and pK changes of about half the original effect, about 3 and 5, respectively, are often observed. These semiquantitative substituent radical effects on relative acidity or basicity can be plotted on a pK_b 1-14 to pK_a 14-1 scale, with functional group positioning toward the right on the scale favored by greater electron flow of the electrons as described above (Table VII).

Water System

Alcohol, Phenol, Carboxylic Acid, and Sulfonic Acid Sequence—Water can be considered a neutral and strongly hydrogen bonded molecule, and generalizations can be made about how various substituent radicals affect these properties. The replacement of one hydrogen atom in water with nonpolar, electron-releasing aliphatic and alicyclic radicals yields alcohols with a polar hydroxyl group. The alcoholic hydroxyl group does not ionize nor accept a proton in dilute aqueous solution, so alcohols are neutral in the Brønsted-Lowry sense and for the most part indistinguishable from water in dilute acid-base reactions (Table VII).

The replacement of one hydrogen atom in water with nonpolar aromatic radicals results in phenols with their characteristically polar hydroxyl group. In contrast to alkyl substituents, the aryl group increases the relative acidity by about 5 pK units, and compared to the undissociated alcohols in aqueous solution, the phenols exist in equilibrium with the phenolate anion and the oxonium ion (Eq 3). The phenols are slightly more acidic than

$$ArOH + H_2O \rightleftharpoons ArO^- + H_3O^+ \tag{3}$$

alcohols, having a pK_a range of approximately 10 on the pK_b-pK_a scale (Table VII). Many phenols have pK_a values of about 10, although electron-attracting substituents on the ring tend to lower the value and electron-releasing substituents raise the value. The conjugate base form of the phenol or phenolate anion can be assigned a generalized pK_b of 4 and exhibits typical ionic property.

Carboxylic acids and sulfonic acids result when a hydrogen atom in water is replaced by the electron-withdrawing acyl, alkyl or arylsulfonyl radicals. Consistent with the acyl effect of increasing the relative acidity by about 10 pH units compared to water, the carboxylic acids are positioned to the right of the phenols in the neighborhood of pK_a 5 (Table VII). The conjugate base or carboxylate anion (Eq 4) will act as a weak base with a pK_b value of about 9.

$$R-\overset{\overset{\displaystyle O}{\|}}{C}-OH + H_2O \rightleftharpoons R-\overset{\overset{\displaystyle O}{\|}}{C}-O^- + H_3O^+ \tag{4}$$

The aliphatic and aromatic sulfonic acids are similar to the strong mineral acids, eg, hydrochloric acid and sulfuric acid and for practical purposes they can be considered to ionize completely in dilute aqueous solution. The sulfonyl radical changes the pK value by a factor of 15 in the direction of increasing relative acidity, so the sulfonic acids will have a pK of 1 or less (Table VII) and they exhibit ionic behavior in dilute aqueous solution. The sulfonate anion (Eq 5) will be neutral with a pK_b of 14 or greater.

$$R-\overset{\overset{\displaystyle O}{\uparrow}}{\underset{\underset{\displaystyle O}{\downarrow}}{S}}-OH + H_2O \longrightarrow R-\overset{\overset{\displaystyle O}{\uparrow}}{\underset{\underset{\displaystyle O}{\downarrow}}{S}}-O^- + H_3O^+ \tag{5}$$

Ethers and Esters—The replacement of the hydrogen atom in the alcoholic hydroxyl group with aliphatic radicals does not alter to any degree the neutral property associated with the parent molecule. The resulting aliphatic ethers (V) have an aprotic polar functional group, and they act neutrally in aqueous solution. Similar substitution in the phenolic hydroxyl leads to aromatic ethers (VI) which are neutral in

$$\begin{array}{cccc} R-O-R & Ar-O-R & R-\overset{\overset{\displaystyle O}{\|}}{C}-O-R & R-\overset{\overset{\displaystyle O}{\uparrow}}{\underset{\underset{\displaystyle O}{\downarrow}}{S}}-O-R \\ (V) & (VI) & (VII) & (VIII) \end{array}$$

contrast to the weakly acidic parent phenols (pK_a of 10). Likewise, alkyl and aryl replacement of the hydrogen atom of a carboxylic or sulfonic hydroxyl group leads to carboxylate esters (VII) and sulfonate esters (VIII), respectively. The ester functional group is neutral since it no longer has the donor proton essential for acid ionization and complete esters of all of the common acids have aprotic functional groups of varying polarity.

Ammonia System

Alkylamine, Arylamine, Amide, and Sulfonamide Sequence—Hydrogen atom replacement by the four above named substituents of the ammonia molecule yields similar semi-quantitative shifts to the pK values. Ammonia is a strong base with a pK_b of about 5 and an unshared pair of electrons in an sp^3 orbital for reaction with acids and for hydrogen bonding with suitable functional groups. The replacement of one hydrogen atom with electron-releasing aliphatic radicals results in the formation of primary amines and as with the water molecule the pK value changes are minimal. The successive replacement of the second and third hydrogen atom leads to the secondary dialkylamines and tertiary trialkylamines. The additional alkyl groups push electrons toward the nitrogen atom making the unshared electron pair more available for basic reactions. The basicity is also influenced by solvation and steric effects. These differences are not that great except for the stronger pK_b value (about 3) for the low molecular weight secondary amines. So the assignment of a generalized pK_b value of 5 for all aliphatic and alicyclic amines would be rational (Table VII).

The substitution of an aryl group for one hydrogen atom in ammonia leads to arylamines like aniline, an aromatic amine. An aryl group shifts the original pK value by about 5 units, so the arylamines with a pK_b of about 10 are located to the right of the aliphatic amines on the pK_b-pK_a scale (Table VII). And as with the slight basicity differences observed among the primary, secondary and tertiary aliphatic amines, the secondary alkylarylamines and the tertiary dialkylarylamines can be assigned the same weak basic property ascribed to the primary arylamines (pK_b about 10).

The amine salts are conjugate acid forms of various aliphatic, alicyclic, and aromatic amines. The alkylammonium (IX), dialkylammonium (X), and trialkylammonium (XI)

$$
\begin{array}{ccc}
\text{H} & \text{R} & \text{R} \\
| & | & | \\
\text{R}-\overset{+}{\text{N}}-\text{H} & \text{R}-\overset{+}{\text{N}}-\text{H} & \text{R}-\overset{+}{\text{N}}-\text{H} \\
| & | & | \\
\text{H} & \text{H} & \text{R} \\
\text{(IX)} & \text{(X)} & \text{(XI)}
\end{array}
$$

cations, or the aliphatic primary ammonium, secondary ammonium, and tertiary ammonium cations respectively, all have at least one hydrogen attached to the *onium* nitrogen, so they can function as proton donors with a weak acidic strength of about pK_a equal to 9. As expected, the arylammonium (XII), alkylarylammonium (XIII), and dialkylarylammonium (XIV)

$$
\begin{array}{ccc}
\text{H} & \text{R} & \text{R} \\
| & | & | \\
\text{Ar}-\overset{+}{\text{N}}-\text{H} & \text{Ar}-\overset{+}{\text{N}}-\text{H} & \text{Ar}-\overset{+}{\text{N}}-\text{H} \\
| & | & | \\
\text{H} & \text{H} & \text{R} \\
\text{(XII)} & \text{(XIII)} & \text{(XIV)}
\end{array}
$$

cations represent strong conjugate acids with a pK_a of about 4.

The replacement of one hydrogen atom in ammonia by different acid radicals yields various amides. The substitu-

tion by acyl radicals results in the carboxamides or simply, amides. Since the acyl groups change the pK value by a factor of about 10, the conversion from ammonia (pK_b of 5) leads to functional groups with a pK_b of about 14. Hence, amides are neutral molecules (Table VII) and they will not undergo acid-base reactions even with strong mineral acids in dilute aqueous solution. The alkyl and arylsulfonyl radicals alter the pK value by about 15 units, so the resulting sulfonamides will be shifted from the basic ammonia position $pK_b = 5$ to the acidic side on the pK_b-pK_a scale (Table VII). These sulfonamides function as weak acids with a pK_a in the range of about 10, and the conjugate base form or sulfonamidate anion (Eq 6) will act as a fairly strong base with pK_b of about 4.

$$
\underset{\underset{\text{O}}{\parallel}}{\overset{\overset{\text{O}}{\parallel}}{\text{R}-\text{S}-\text{NH}_2}} + \text{H}_2\text{O} \rightleftharpoons \underset{\underset{\text{O}}{\parallel}}{\overset{\overset{\text{O}}{\parallel}}{\text{R}-\text{S}-\text{NH}^-}} + \text{H}_3\text{O}^+ \qquad (6)
$$

Diarylamine, *N*-Arylamide, and *N*-Arylsulfonamide Sequence—The secondary diarylamines are formed by substituting ammonia with two aromatic groups. The influence of the second aryl group in shifting the pK value is less than additive (about 3), so the diarylamines have a pK_b approaching 13. They do not react even with strong mineral acids in dilute aqueous solution. The nitrogen atom in aromatic heterocyclics, such as phenothiazine, 5*H*-dibenz[*b*,*f*]-azepine (Table VI), and the 10,11-dihydro derivative of the latter compound, is equivalent to that in the diarylamines. Thus, these heterocyclics behave as neutral amines in dilute aqueous solution. Likewise, the tertiary triarylamines are neutral compounds, even though they are actually less basic than the diarylamines.

The substitution of an aryl group on the amide or sulfonamide nitrogen has effects similar to the change observed with the primary and secondary arylamines. The *N*-arylamides are relatively more acidic than the neutral amides, but the effect of the aryl group as a second electron-withdrawing function on the nitrogen atom is not sufficient to shift the pK from neutral range. The difference is insignificant in dilute aqueous solution, and the *N*-arylamides can be considered to be neutral compounds (Table VII). The increase in relative acidity is readily discernable with the *N*-arylsulfonamides (Table VII) since they behave as acids with a pK_a of about 7 in contrast to the pK_a of 10 for the unsubstituted sulfonamides. The conjugate base or *N*-arylsulfonamidate anion is a fairly strong base with a pK_b of about 7 (Eq 7).

$$
\underset{\underset{\text{O}}{\parallel}}{\overset{\overset{\text{O}}{\parallel}}{\text{R}-\text{S}-\text{NH}-\text{Ar}}} + \text{H}_2\text{O} \rightleftharpoons \underset{\underset{\text{O}}{\parallel}}{\overset{\overset{\text{O}}{\parallel}}{\text{R}-\text{S}-\overset{-}{\text{N}}-\text{Ar}}} + \text{H}_3\text{O}^+ \qquad (7)
$$

Imide (*N*-Acylamide) and Sulfonimide (*N*-Acylsulfonamide) Sequence—An acyl radical as a second substituent on an amide or sulfonamide nitrogen appears to change the pK value by about 5 units, which is half the 10 pK unit shift observed in monosubstitution situations. Hence, the introduction of an acyl group on the neutral amide nitrogen leads to the weakly acidic imides (pK_a of 10) or *N*-acylamides (Table VII). The imidate anion is a strong base with a pK_b of about 4 (Eq 8).

$$
\underset{\text{O}}{\overset{\text{O}}{\underset{\parallel}{\text{R}-\text{C}}}}-\text{NH}-\underset{\text{O}}{\overset{\text{O}}{\underset{\parallel}{\text{C}}}}-\text{R} + \text{H}_2\text{O} \rightleftharpoons \underset{\text{O}}{\overset{\text{O}}{\underset{\parallel}{\text{R}-\text{C}}}}-\overset{-}{\text{N}}-\underset{\text{O}}{\overset{\text{O}}{\underset{\parallel}{\text{C}}}}-\text{R} + \text{H}_3\text{O}^+ \qquad (8)
$$

Of special interest are the 5,5-disubstituted barbiturates, or cyclic 1,3-diacylureas, consisting of two imide groups sharing a common carbonyl radical for enolization (Eq 9). The barbiturate imide functional group is considerably more acidic, pK_a of 7–8, than the imides of pK_a of 10.

$$\text{(9)}$$

The N-acylsulfonamides, which will be referred to as sulfonimides, are stronger acids than either the unsubstituted sulfonamides or N-arylsulfonamides. Thes sulfonimides are like the carboxylic acids with acidic values in the pK_a range of about 5 (Table VII), and the base form or sulfonimidate anion acts weakly basic with a pK_b of around 9 (Eq 10).

$$\text{(10)}$$

Alkylamine, Imine, and Nitrile Sequence—The conversion of the aliphatic amine carbon-nitrogen single bond into a double or triple bond changes the functional group to an imine and a nitrile, respectively. This change is accompanied by a decrease in relative basicity with increasing order of unsaturation. The unshared pair of electrons on an aliphatic amine (pK_b of 5) occupies an sp^3 orbital. As this electron pair is held more tightly to the nitrogen atom, the electrons become less available for sharing with a proton. The imine unshared electron pair occupying the sp^2 orbital is closer to the nitrogen atom than the sp^3 amine electrons, while the sp orbital unshared electron pair on the nitrile nitrogen is even less available. Hence, the basicity decreases in the order: aliphatic amine > imine > nitrile, or pK_b of 5, 10, and 14 or neutral, respectively, in dilute aqueous solution (Table VII). The conjugate acid of the imine is represented by the strong immonium cation with a pK_a value of 4 (XV).

$$\text{(XV)}$$

Amidine and Guanidine Derivative Sequence—The amidine is the nitrogen isostere of a carboxylic acid and the guanidine derivative that of carbonic acid. Both of these compounds appear to have one imino nitrogen and one or two amide nitrogens. However, they are both very strong bases with resonance of their conjugate acids contributing to the progressive change from the imine (pK_b of 10) and aliphatic amine (pK_b of 5) to the amidine (pK_b of 3) and $pK_b < 1$ for guanidine itself (Table VII). The conjugate acids of these basic compounds are represented by the alkylimmonium, alkylammonium, amidinium, and guanidinium cations. The amidinium cation is a resonance hybrid of two structures (Eq 11) while the guanidinium cation is a hybrid of three (Eq 12). Since resonance stabilizes the guanidinium cation more than the amidinium, the relative order of acidity is alkylimmonium > alkylammonium > amidinium > guanidinium, or pK_a of 4, 9, 11 and $pK_a > 14$ or neutral, respectively.

$$\text{(11)}$$

$$\text{(12)}$$

The heterocyclic 2-imidazoline (Table VI) is a cyclic amidine with similar basicity with a pK_b equal to 3.

Piperidine, Pyridine, and Pyrrole Sequence—There are many heterocyclic amine moieties which appear in the structure of various drugs. The relative basicity of many of

these ring systems can be estimated by considering the nature of the unshared electron pair on the nitrogen atom (Table VII). Piperidine (Table VI) is a saturated heterocycle with an unshared pair of electrons in a sp^3 nitrogen orbital so, like the aliphatic amines, a generalized pK_b value of 5 can be assigned to this molecule even though it exhibits a pK_b value typical of the low molecular weight secondary amines (~3). Pyrrolidine, morpholine, and piperazine (Table VI) are also saturated heterocycles with a pK_b of about 5, although piperazine acts as a diprotic base with the second amine showing a lower basicity in the pK_b range of about 10.

Pyridine (Table VI) is an aromatic compound with an unshared pair of electrons in an sp^2 nitrogen orbital. Like the sp^2 aliphatic imines, pyridine behaves as a weak base with a pK_b on the order of 10. Pyrimidine, quinoline, isoquinoline (Table VI), and other heterocycles with a sp^2 imine-like nitrogen can be assigned the generalized aromatic basicity with a pK_b of 10, although the additional electronegativity of the second nitrogen in pyrimidine reduces that basicity to about $pK_b = 12$. The conjugate acids of these amines are protonated cations with a strong acidic property of pK_a equal to 4.

Pyrrole and indole (Table VI) represent another type of aromatic amine. The nitrogen in pyrrole (XVI) carries an

$$\text{(XVI)}$$

unshared pair of electrons in an sp^2 orbital with three sp^2 orbitals involved in bonding. The unshared pair of electrons, the focus of amine basicity, forms part of the aromatic sextet of electrons in that ring, so this pair of electrons is unavailable for acid-base reactions. Hence, aromatic amines such as pyrrole and indole have a neutral functional group.

Imidazole and pyrazole (Table VI) have aromatic amine properties related to both the pyridine and pyrrole ring systems. The two diazoles have one weakly basic pyridine-like nitrogen with its unshared electron pair in an sp^2 orbital and a neutral pyrrole-like nitrogen with its unavailable electron pair. Hence, they function as monoprotic aromatic amines although imidazole is more basic ($pK_b \sim7$) then pyrazole ($pK_b \sim11$). This basicity enhancement in imidazole may be attributed to its aromatic amidine-like structure.

Quaternary Ammonium Compounds and Amine Oxides—It is important to separate the quaternary ammonium compounds from the primary, secondary, and tertiary ammonium cations. The quaternary ammonium cations, whether tetra-alkylammonium (VII), trialkylarylammonium (XVIII), or N-alkylpyridinium (XIX), no longer have any

| (XVII) | (XVIII) | (XIX) |

hydrogen associated with the ammonium nitrogen, so they have lost their capacity to function as a proton donor. In addition, the ammonium state is indicative of the absence of the unshared pair of electrons. Hence, in the Brønsted-Lowry sense, all quaternary ammonium cations will act neutrally in dilute aqueous solution.

The amine oxides are tertiary amines in which the unshared electron pair is involved in coordinate covalent bonding with an oxygen atom. This functional group, like the quaternary ammonium nitrogen has no proton to donate nor an unshared pair of electrons to accept a proton, so the aliphatic (XX), aromatic (XXI), and heterocyclic (XXII) amine oxides represent neutral molecules.

Table VIII.—Comparison of literature values of pK for drugs with generalized values of pK for functional groups.

Drug Name	Literature[a,c] $pK_a(pK_b)$	Generalized[b,c] $pK_a(pK_b)$	Functional Group
Acetanilid	(13.5)	n	N-arylamide
Benzocaine	(11.2)	(10)	Arylamine
		n	Ester
Chlordiazepoxide	4.8	6	N^2-Arylamidinium cation
Hydrochloride		n	Amide Oxide
Chlorothiazide	6.7	10	Sulfonamide (acidity enhanced by neighboring electronegative groups)
	9.5	10	Second Sulfonamide
		(10)	Aromatic Amine (basicity reduced by neighboring electronegative groups
Dextroamphetamine Sulfate	9.8	9	Alkylammonium cation
Diazepam	(10.7)	(10)	Imine
		n	Amide
Diphenoxylate	(6.9)	(5)	Alicyclic Amine
		n	Ester
		n	Nitrile
Glutethimide	11.8	10	Imide
Histamine	(4.1)	(5)	Alkylamine
	(8.0)	(8)	Aromatic Amidine (imidazole)
Mephenamic Acid	4.3	5	Carboxylic Acid
		n	Diarylamine
Methantheline Bromide		n	Quaternary Ammonium Compound
		n	Ester
		n	Ether
Methylparaben	8.4	10	Phenol
		n	Ester
Nafcillin Sodium	(11.3)	(9)	Carboxylate anion
		n	Amide
		n	Lactam (cyclic amide)
		n	Ether
		n	Thioether
Pentobarbital Sodium	(6)	(6–7)	Barbiturate Imidate anion
Phenobarbital	7.5	7–8	Barbiturate Imide
Phenytoin	(5.7)	(4)	Imidate anion
		n	Amide
Quinine	(5.2)	(5)	Tertiary alicyclic amine
	(10.3)	(10)	Aromatic amine (quinoline)
Sulfamerazine	7.1	7	N-Arylsulfonamide
		(10)	Arylamine
Sulfanilamide	10.4	10	Sulfonamide
		(10)	Arylamine
Tetracycline	3.3	5	1,1,1-Tricarbonyl (acidity enhanced and stabilized in enol state)
	7.7	10	1,1-Dicarbonyl (acidity enhanced and stabilized in enol state)
	9.5	9	Trialkylammonium cation
		n	Amide
		n	Alcohols
		n	Phenol H-bonding with o-carbonyl
Tolazine	10.3	11	Amidinium cation (2-imidazolinium cation)
Tolbutamide	5.3	5	Sulfonimide

[a] Adapted from Appendix B of *Wilson and Gisvold's Textbook of Organic Medicinal and Pharmaceutical Chemistry*, Eighth Edition, Edited by Robert F Doerge, J B Lippincott Co, Philadelphia, PA (1982) pp 841–5.
[b] n = neutral.
[c] If value is in parenthesis it is pK_b.

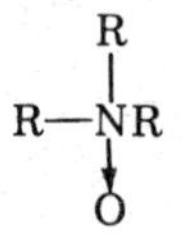

(XX) 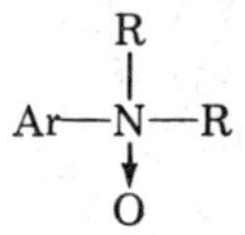   (XXI) 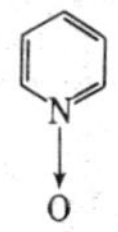   (XXII)

α-Hydrogen Carbonyl System

Carbonyl, 1,1-Dicarbonyl, and 1,1,1-Tricarbonyl System—The aldehydes and ketones are monofunctional representatives of carbonyl-containing compounds. The electron flow in the polar carbonyl group weakens a hydrogen bond on the alpha carbon to promote α-hydrogen ionization. This effect is insignificant in dilute acid-base reactions with monofunctional aldehydes and ketones, so they act neutrally in dilute aqueous solution. As with other systems, the introduction of a second and third electron withdrawing carbonyl group in the proper position increases the relative acidity of the α-hydrogen atom. The functional group with two carbonyls attached to the same carbon atom, such as ethyl acetoacetate, will be referred to as the 1,1-dicarbonyl structure. These 1,1-dicarbonyl structures act as weak acids with a pK_a of about 10. The 1,1-dicarbonyl anion is a strong base, pK_b about 4, stabilized by distribution of the charge among three resonance structures (Eq 13).

$$(13)$$

The proper substitution of a third carbonyl group raises the α-hydrogen acidity into the strong (pK_a value of 5) category; this arrangement will be referred to as the 1,1,1-tricarbonyl structure. The 1,1,1-tricarbonyl anion or enolate anion is a weak base, $pK_b \sim 9$, with the negative charge distributed among four resonance structures. Any additional structural modification of either the 1,1-dicarbonyl or 1,1,1-tricarbonyl structure that is favorable to the enol state will enhance the relative acidity even more.

Hydrogen Sulfide System

Oxygen is a second shell element with $2s$ and $2p$ electrons, while sulfur is a third shell atom with two $3s$ and four $3p$ electrons. Consistent with the higher Group VI-A elements, sulfur exhibits common chemical properties although somewhat different from that of oxygen, the first member of this periodic group. In contrast to the liquid state and neutral acid-base nature of water at room temperature, the isosteric hydrogen sulfide is a gas with low water solubility and acts as a weak diprotic acid with $pK_{a_1} \sim 7$ and $pK_{a_2} \sim 15$.

Alkanethiols and Thiophenols—Several organic functional groups result from the successive alkyl or aryl replacement of the hydrogen atoms in hydrogen sulfide and from the successive oxidation of the disubstituted sulfide. The replacement of one hydrogen with an aliphatic group results in the alkanethiols or thioalcohols with the weakly acidic sulfhydryl functional group. Similarly, the replacement of one hydrogen with an aromatic group yields the comparable weakly acidic thiophenols, not a more acidic compound as might be expected in comparison to the change from a neutral alcohol to a weakly acidic phenol. The thioalcohols and thiophenols can be grouped together as thiols and assigned the generalized weakly acid pK_a value of 10 (Table VII). The thiolate anions, thioalcoholate (XXIII) and

R—S⁻   Ar—S⁻

(XXIII)   (XXIV)

thiophenolate (XXIV), are strong bases with pK_b of 4.

Thioethers, Sulfoxides, and Sulfones—Replacement of the hydrogen atom in thiols with an alkyl or aryl group leads to the formation of thioethers or sulfides. The thioether structure is obviously a neutral functional group. This group appears in such heterocyclic compounds as thiophene, thia-

zole, 4-thia-1-azabicyclo[3.2.0]heptane, and phenothiazine (Table VI).

The oxidation of the thioethers causes the introduction of successive coordinately covalent oxygen atoms. The resulting sulfoxides and sulfones are neither proton donors nor proton acceptors in dilute acid-base reactions, but function as neutral compounds. The presence of the coordinate covalent oxygen and the unshared electron pair about the sulfur atom makes the sulfoxide functional group quite polar, while the two coordinate covalent oxygens are responsible for the polar nature of the sulfone functional group.

Comparison of Experimental and Predicted pK Values

Several drugs will be examined briefly to emphasize the applicability of the generalizations presented in this discussion of pK. Table VIII shows the correlation of the generalized pK values for functional groups with the literature values for various drugs. Considerations of other functional group effects in the drug molecule should explain any appreciable deviation from the generalized pK values.

Since many drugs are acids and bases of varying strength, the degree of their ionization, as determined by the pK of the drug and the pH of the environment, will influence their dissolution, absorption and transportation in the biological system. The Henderson-Hasselbach equation (Eq 14) is useful in determining this effect of the biological pH on the relative ionization of acid and basic drugs.

$$pK_a = pH + \log \frac{[\text{acid}]}{[\text{base}]} \qquad (14)$$

For acidic drugs like tolbutamide with its sulfonimide functional group pK_a of 5, the ratio of drug species at a neutral pH of 7 can be approximated as follows:

$$pK_a = pH + \log \frac{[\text{nonionized sulfonimide}]}{[\text{sulfonimidate anion}]}$$

$$5 = 7 - 2 \text{ or } \frac{[\text{nonionized sulfonimide}]}{[\text{sulfonimidate anion}]} = \frac{1}{100}$$

For basic drugs such as quinine (Table VIII) also at pH of 7, the ratio of drug species of the more basic alicyclic amine with a pK_b of 5 is;

$$pK_a = pH + \log \frac{[\text{cycloalkylammonium cation}]}{[\text{nonionized alicyclic amine}]}$$

$$9 = 7 + 2 \text{ or } \frac{[\text{cycloalkylammonium cation}]}{[\text{nonionized alicyclic amine}]} = \frac{100}{1}$$

From an examination of the data found in Table VIII, the average deviation of the 26 entries is less than 1 pK unit. The maximum variation of 3.3 units between literature and predicted values for chlorthiazide,[15] a variation caused by other influences not built into the simple, convenient system described in this chapter. The level of success demonstrated for this system indicates that it is a valuable way to predict pK values whenever acid-base behavior is a factor in solution phenomena.

References

1. Morrison RT, Boyd RN: *Organic Chemistry*, 4th ed, Allyn & Bacon, Boston, 1983.
2. *Chem Eng News* 33: 2838, 1955.

CHAPTER 25

Natural Products

Vincent S Venturella, PhD

Senior Technical Fellow
Hoffmann-La Roche Inc
340 Kingsland Street
Nutley, NJ 07110

This chapter provides a discussion of the fundamental characteristics of the following, essentially chemical, classes of naturally occurring products.

1. Carbohydrates
2. Glycosides
3. Lipids (Fixed Oils, Fats, Waxes, Sterols, and Phospholipids)
4. Proteins
5. Alkaloids
6. Volatile Oils
7. Plant Exudates (Resins, Oleoresins, Gum Resins, and Balsams)
8. Prostaglandins

Each of the classes enumerated above are either official in the USP, listed in the Food Chemical Codex (FCC), or generally used in pharmacy. Examples are provided at the conclusion of each section. The treatment of all individual monographs is presented at appropriate places elsewhere in the text, the distribution being on a pharmacological basis.

For the location of other classes of natural products, eg, hormones, vitamins, enzymes, antibiotics, etc, consult the general index.

Carbohydrates

Composition

This important class of organic compounds embraces (1) aliphatic polyhydric alcohols in which either the primary alcohol function has been oxidized to aldehyde or the secondary alcohol function has been oxidized to ketone, and (2) condensation polymers of these partially oxidized polyalcohols. The fundamental structural units are thus the aldehyde-alcohols and ketone-alcohols which constitute (1). These are frequently termed *monosaccharides** (sometimes simply *saccharides*) and are subclassified into *aldoses* and *ketoses* according to whether they contain the aldehyde or the ketone group.

The condensation polymers which constitute (2) are sometimes referred to as *saccharide anhydrides;* they are subclassified into *disaccharides, trisaccharides,* etc. according to the number of monosaccharide units present. *Polysaccharides,* on the other hand, contain many monosaccharide units joined in long linear or branched chains. Most polysaccharides contain recurring monosaccharide units of either a single kind or alternating kinds. Polysaccharides have two major biological functions: as storage forms for fuel and as structural elements. The term *polysaccharide* is used differently by different authors, some using it broadly to embrace all of the polymers including the disaccharides, and others restricting it variously so as to exclude the *di-* and sometimes also the *tri-* and *tetra*saccharides. The *di-, tri-,* and up to about the *deca*saccharides are sometimes grouped under the term *oligo*saccharides (*oligo,* of Greek origin, meaning a few).

The term *sugar* is also used with various meanings. It is sometimes employed synonymously with the term carbohydrate. Probably more conventionally, it is used to refer only to those carbohydrates that are soluble and have a sweet taste; and nutritionists frequently restrict it to mean carbohydrates that are physiologically assimilable. The monosaccharides are sometimes termed *simple sugars.*

Classification and Structure

Space permits scarcely more than a statement of the essential features of this complex subject, elucidation of which constitutes a brilliant chapter in organic chemistry.

Monosaccharides have the empirical formula $(CH_2O)_n$, where n = 2 in the case of the aldehydes and 3 in the case of ketones as a minimum. The carbon skeleton of the common monosaccharides is unbranched and each carbon atom, except one, contains a hydroxy group; at the remaining carbon, there is a carbonyl oxygen which, as shall be seen, is often combined in an *acetal* or *ketal* linkage. Thus combining the type of monosaccharide with the number of carbons in the skeletal unit, one can further classify the carbohydrates into being *dioses, trioses, tetroses,* etc, according to the number of carbon atoms they contain and then as aldoses or ketoses depending upon whether or not the main functional carbonyl is an aldehyde or ketone. Thus, in descriptive terminology, xylose is an *aldopentose* (contains the aldehyde function and a total of five carbon atoms); similarly, fructose is a *ketohexose* (contains the ketone function and a total of six carbon atoms).

While the simplest aldose is the diose, glycolaldehyde (Table I), the simplest monosaccharides are the three carbon trioses such as glyceraldehyde and dihydroxyacetone (Table I). Glyceraldehyde is an aldotriose; dihydroxyacetone is a ketotriose. All of the more complex aldoses may be predicted and visualized by inserting additional —(CHOH)— groups in the glycol aldehyde formula, one at a time and always adjacent to the terminal —CH₂OH group, thus passing successively through trioses, tetroses, etc. The same may be said for the series of ketoses insofar as prediction and visualization are concerned, remembering that the addition of each —CH(OH)— group also occurs adjacent to the terminal —CH₂OH group however, and in the simplest ones, the addition is on the down side of the carbonyl carbon. The total scheme for the aldoses and the ketoses is shown in Table I, the intermediate —CH(OH)— groups being represented by horizontal lines drawn to the side to which the OH group is attached. Thus, it will be observed that, starting with the aldotrioses, the insertion of each —CH(OH)— group automatically introduces a chiral center (asymmetric carbon atom), giving rise to an increasing number of stereoisomers. The enantiomorphs of each stereoisomeric pair are distinguished by the *configurational* notations D and L, referring respectively to whether the OH of the last inserted —CH(OH)— is on the right or left of the vertical axis when the formulas are drawn in the *stick* configuration as shown

---

* The syllable "ose" is often used instead of "ide" in saccharide names.

Table I—Monosaccharides*

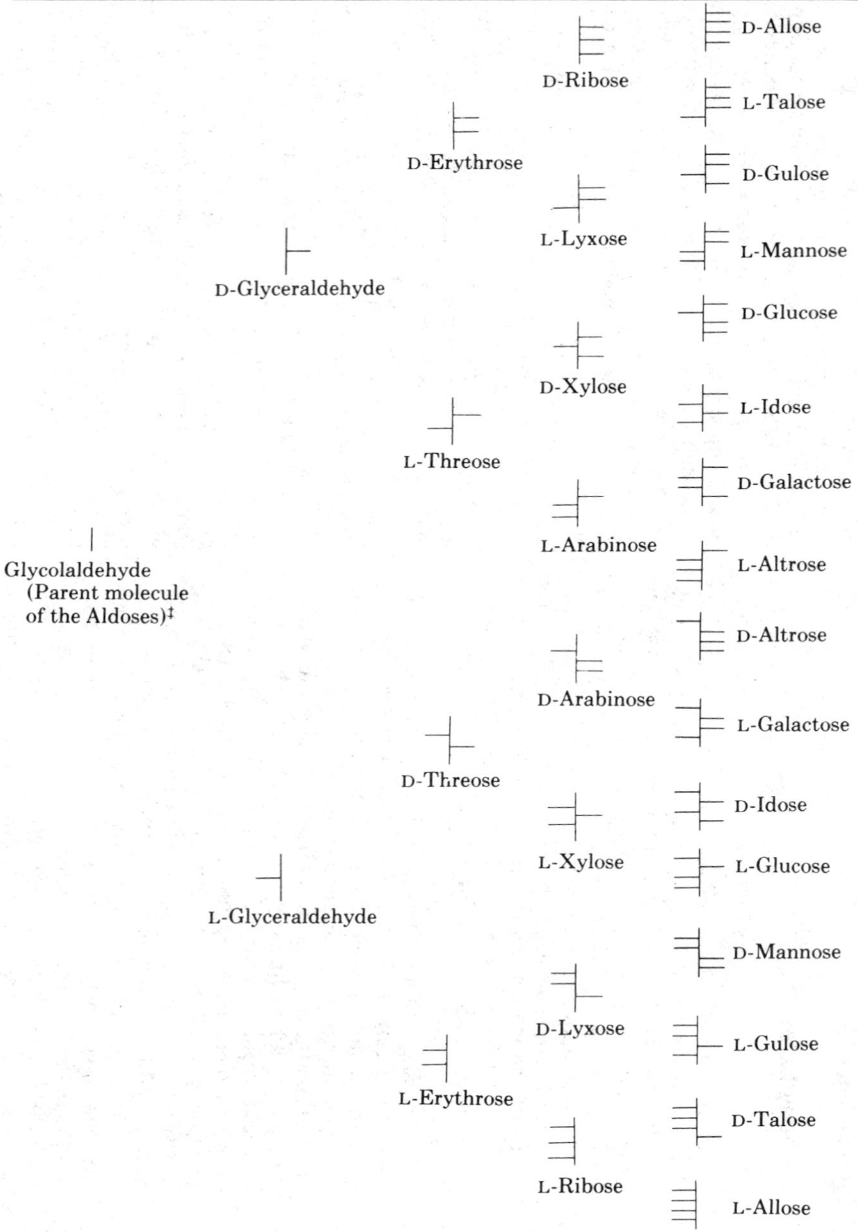

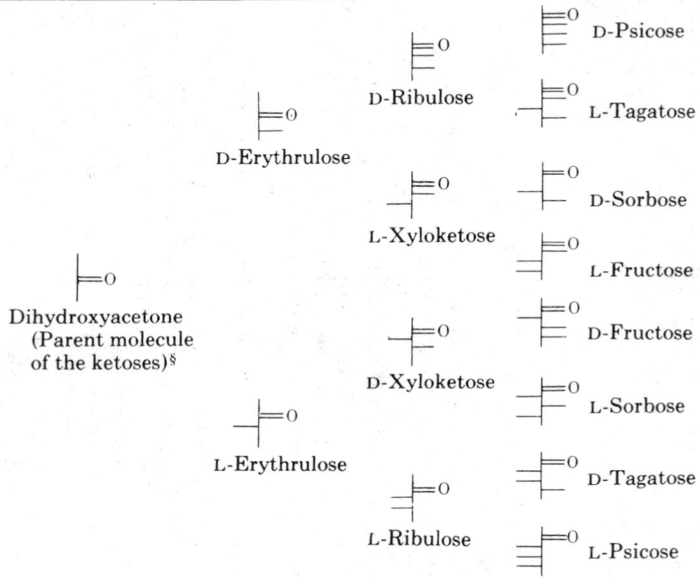

Ketoses†

Triose	Tetroses	Pentoses	Hexoses
			D-Psicose
			L-Tagatose
		D-Ribulose	D-Sorbose
			L-Fructose
	D-Erythrulose	L-Xyloketose	D-Fructose
Dihydroxyacetone (Parent molecule of the ketoses)§			L-Sorbose
		D-Xyloketose	D-Tagatose
	L-Erythrulose		L-Psicose
		L-Ribulose	

Aldoses

Diose	Trioses	Tetroses	Pentoses	Hexoses
			D-Ribose	D-Allose
		D-Erythrose		L-Talose
			L-Lyxose	D-Gulose
		L-Threose		L-Mannose
	D-Glyceraldehyde		D-Xylose	D-Glucose
				L-Idose
			L-Arabinose	D-Galactose
				L-Altrose
			D-Arabinose	D-Altrose
Glycolaldehyde (Parent molecule of the Aldoses)‡		D-Threose		L-Galactose
			L-Xylose	D-Idose
				L-Glucose
			D-Lyxose	D-Mannose
	L-Glyceraldehyde			L-Gulose
		L-Erythrose		D-Talose
			L-Ribose	L-Allose

* Scheme is terminated with hexoses although some higher members are known.

† Scheme is limited to 2-ketohexoses. Other ketoses are not usually treated in carbohydrate chemistry.

‡ In all aldose representations, the vertical line stands for $\begin{matrix} CHO \\ | \\ CH_2OH \end{matrix}$

Thus, for example, the representation $\vert\!-$ for D-Glyceraldehyde actually

portrays H—C—OH ; the representation $-\!\vert$ for L-Threose

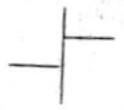

actually portrays H—C—OH , etc.

§ In all ketose representations, the symbol $=\!\!O$ stands for $\begin{matrix} CH_2OH \\ CO \\ CH_2OH \end{matrix}$

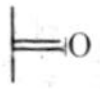

Thus, for example, the representation $=\!\!O$ for D-Erythrulose actually

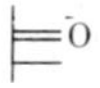

portrays 'H—C—OH ; the representation $=\!\!O$ for L-Xyloketose

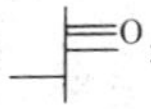

actually portrays H—C—OH ; etc.

in the table. It is important to remember that the D and L notations have nothing to do with direction of optical rotation and also that the actual demonstration of whether a given stereoisomer is D or L is a matter of extensive laboratory experimentation. It should also be noted that the prefixes D and L refer to the asymmetric carbon atom farthest removed from the carbonyl carbon atom.

Two sugars differing only in the configuration around the carbon atom adjacent to the carbonyl group are called epimers of each other. Thus, D-glucose and D-mannose are epimers with respect to carbon atom 2.

The simplest ketose is the triose, dihydroxyacetone. The scheme in Table I depicts the more complex members in the same manner described above for the aldoses.

Cyclic Structures—Measurements of various characteristics (propensity to function as reductants, ability to form acetal derivatives, mutarotation, etc) have demonstrated conclusively that the open-chain formulas shown above do not represent the true structure of at least the higher monosaccharides, the pentoses and hexoses. For example, in aqueous solution, many of the higher monosaccharides behave as if an additional chiral center is present; one more than depicted by the open-chain formulas. Rather, the structures are cyclic and may be looked upon as internal hemiacetals (page 376) formed by condensation of the carbonyl oxygen atom and one of the alcoholic hydroxyls. Although such a reaction can involve any of the hydroxyl groups, theoretical considerations suggest that the γ- and δ-hydroxyl groups are more ideally situated to participate in the cyclization, thus giving rise to furanose (contain the furan ring) and pyranose (contain the pyran ring) structures. Experimental evidence indicates that the aldohexoses, in their normal monosaccharide states, exist largely in the pyranose form.

Thus, for example, the open-chain formula (A) for D-glucose gives way to the corresponding cyclic structures (B):

A B

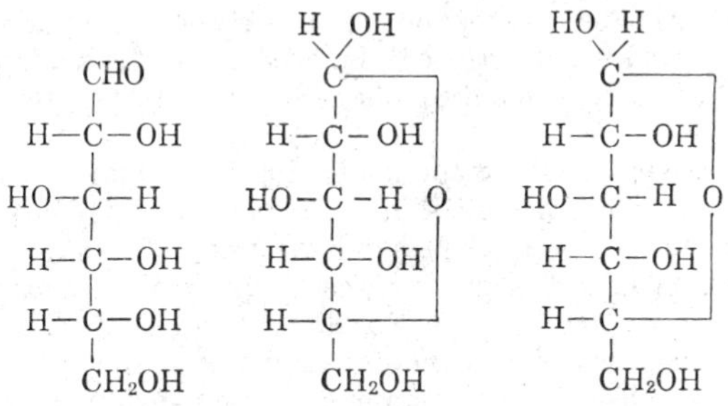

α-form β-form

The two stereoisomeric forms of (B), conventionally distinguished by the alpha and beta type of nomenclature, arise because the cyclization automatically renders the former aldehyde carbon atom asymmetric as previously mentioned. The change or isomerization shown by the Fischer formulas, above, occurs spontaneously in aqueous solution causing the specific rotation to attain a final equilibrium value. This process is termed *mutarotation*. Incidentally, both the α- and β-forms of D-glucose are well known; the D-glucose (dextrose) of commerce is the alpha variety. Isomeric forms of monosaccharides which differ from each other only in configuration of the chiral carbon atom derived from the carbonyl group are *anomers* and the newly formed asymmetric carbon atom is termed the *anomeric* carbon.

The two-dimensional representations of cyclic structures as in (B) have been largely superseded by the Haworth Projection models. In these models, the ring is usually *represented* as planar, the disposition of hydrogen atoms and substituents is portrayed by vertical assignment upward and downward from the ring plane. Haworth structures for some selected hexoses are shown below along with the conventional ring numbering. Note that the edge of the ring nearest the reader is represented by bold lines; thus the plane of the ring is perpendicular to the page. For comparison, both the furanose and pyranose structures are shown for α-D-glucose. Also note that, in the case of sucrose, the stable furan conformation is shown as being dominant for the fructose portion of the molecule.

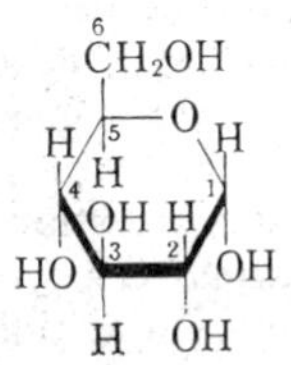

α-D-Glucose
(α-D-Glucopyranose)

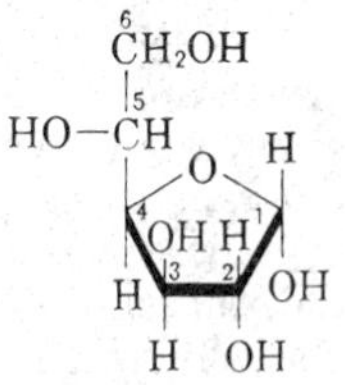

α-D-Glucose
(α-D-Glucofuranose)

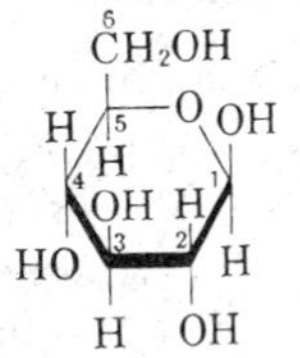

β-D-Glucose
(β-D-Glucopyranose)

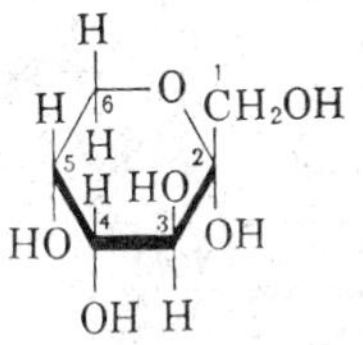

α-D-Fructose
(α-D-Fructopyranose)

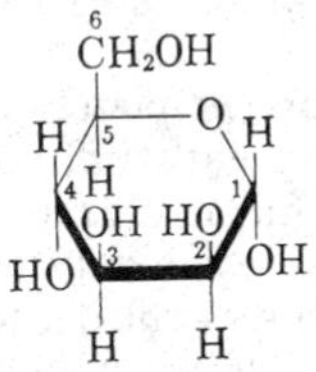

α-D-Mannose
(α-D-Mannopyranose)

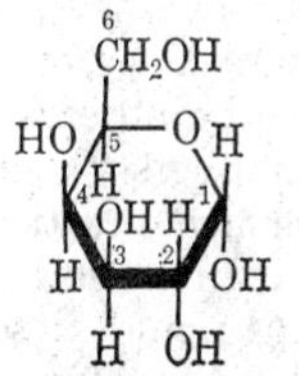

α-D-Galactose
(α-D-Galactopyranose)

The structures and systematic names of the four best-known disaccharides are shown below. It will be observed that the systematic [bracketed] names identify precisely the location of the terminals of the oxygen bridge joining the two monosaccharide residues.

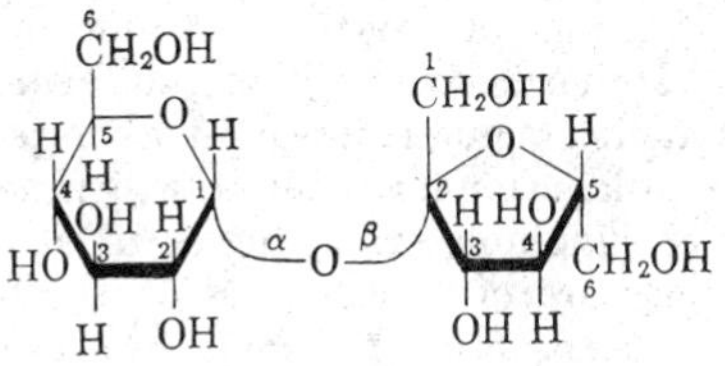

Sucrose
[β-D-Fructofuranosyl-α-D-glucopyranoside]

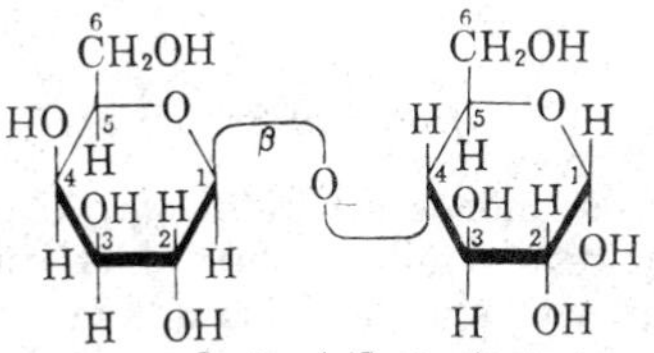

Lactose (α-Lactose)
[4-(*O*-β-D-Galactopyranosyl)-α-D-glucopyranoside]

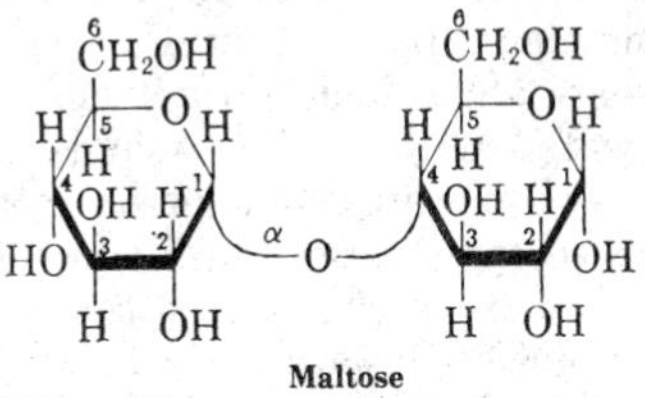

Maltose
[4-(*O*-α-D-Glucopyranosyl)-α-D-glucopyranoside]

Cellobiose

[4-(O-β-D-Glucopyranosyl)-β-D-glucopyranoside]

The Haworth projections are somewhat misleading, however, since they suggest that the five and six-membered furanose and pyranose rings are planar, which is not the actual case. The pyranose rings exist in two conformations, the *chair* form and the *boat* form. The chair form of the pyranose ring, which is relatively rigid and much more stable than the boat form, predominates in aqueous solutions of hexoses. The substituent groups in the chair form are not geometrically and chemically equivalent; they fall into two classes, *axial* and *equatorial*.

Boat   **Chair**

The equatorial hydroxyl groups of pyranoses are more readily esterified than axial groups.

It will also be observed that the completely systematic names are cumbersome and consequently find little use in ordinary chemical practice. Recognizing this, both IUPAC and Chemical Abstracts admit the commonly used trivial names. A pamphlet describing the detailed rules for the systematic nomenclature of carbohydrates and their derivatives is available through Chemical Abstracts Service.

The naturally occurring polysaccharides (eg, the starches, cellulose, glycogen, and inulin), although all classed generally as high-molecular-weight condensation polymers of monosaccharides, vary considerably among themselves in size and structure. Thus, inulin appears to be a relatively small polymer composed of some 30 fructose (fructofuranose) units, whereas cellulose appears to be a relatively large polymer probably containing not less than 1000 glucopyranose units. In some polysaccharides, eg, cellulose, the evidence is strong that the polymers are purely linear; in others; eg, glycogen, a satisfactory explanation for observed experimental data requires that considerable branching occur along the chain. Polysaccharides are often classified on the basis of their monomers; eg, hexosans are polymers of hexoses, and pentosans are polymers of pentoses. Such classification is also frequently rendered specific; eg, cellulose is a glucosan (the hexose unit is D-glucose), and inulin is a fructosan (the hexose unit is D-fructose).

Physical Properties

The common monosaccharides, *viz*, the pentoses and hexoses, are white, crystalline solids which usually melt rather sharply but with simultaneous decomposition. They are readily soluble in water, much less soluble in methanol and ethanol, and relatively insoluble in ether. The common disaccharides, all hexabioses, also display these characteristics. However, the higher polysaccharides—eg, starch, cellulose, and inulin—are amorphous, do not melt sharply, and are much less water-soluble. The soluble, lower-molecular-weight carbohydrates are characterized by a sweet taste, but the relative sweetness varies considerably. This forms the rationale for the use of characteristically similar sugar substitutes which have a lower caloric value on a weight basis. Thus, lactose is only about $\frac{1}{6}$, maltose about $\frac{1}{3}$, and glucose

about $\frac{3}{4}$ as sweet as sucrose; fructose, on the other hand, is about 1.7 times as sweet as sucrose and, therefore is in its own right used as an *artificial* sweetener (of lower caloric value), and is marketed as such.

All carbohydrates are optically active, and their specific rotations serve as one means of differentiation. Many display the phenomenon of *mutarotation*—a continuing change in the value of the rotation until a final fixed value is attained. The classic example is that of α-D-glucose, a freshly prepared aqueous solution of which has an $[\alpha]_D^{20°C}$ of +113°, but which gradually changes to a final value of +52°. This ultimate equilibrium value is derived from the aqueous solution containing about $\frac{1}{3}$ of the α-D-form ($[\alpha]_D^{20} = +112.2°$) and about $\frac{2}{3}$ of the β-D-glucose ($[\alpha]_D^{20} = +18.7°$). Elucidation of this phenomenon constitutes one of the high points in structural carbohydrate chemistry. It has been demonstrated abundantly that such changes in rotation are referable to structural shifts, and that the final value is quantitatively characteristic of the components present in the equilibrium mixture. In the case of glucose, for example, the final rotation value is that to be expected of an equilibrium mixture containing both the α and the β forms of D-glucose. The attainment of the equilibrium state is hastened by acid and by base, hundreds of times more so by the latter. However, hastening the action of the equilibrium should be done with caution and with very dilute solutions of acids and very dilute solutions of weak alkali since acids that are concentrated will yield other compounds such as 5-hydroxymethylfurfural from D-glucose. Additionally, high concentrations of alkali or strong alkali themselves cause D-glucose to form D-fructose and D-mannose through enediol structures in an equilibrium reaction. Rapid equilibration by the addition of base to carbohydrate solutions for equilibration in measuring optical rotation should be done only by the addition of dilute solutions of ammonia.

Chemical Properties

The chemical properties of the carbohydrates are, in general, those to be expected on the basis of their structural features previously described. Treatment here is necessarily limited to a brief mention of the more characteristic reactions.

They behave as compounds having alcohol and carbonyl functions, displaying all of the chemical reactions characteristic of these groups. The aldehyde group of an aldose and the terminal hydroxyl group are each capable of being oxidized to the corresponding mono- or dicarboxylic acid. The carbonyl function can also undergo reduction to the primary or secondary alcohol. Both aldoses and ketoses exhibit the usual addition reactions typical of the carbonyl function.

For identification purposes the carbonyl and adjacent alcohol functions will form phenylhydrazine derivatives known as *osazones*, which give characteristic melting points and exhibit definite crystalline structure. It should be noted that glucose, fructose, and mannose yield the same osazone since the difference in structure and configuration about carbon atoms 1 and 2 are abolished. Also the typical reaction with copper or silver ion, under proper conditions, in which the metal ion is reduced in valence and the carbohydrate is oxidized, is employed to distinguish *reducing* from *nonreducing* sugars.

The hydroxyl groups can be esterified or etherified (a process often used to decrease the polarity and thus increase volatility for identification and separation purposes, especially in gas and liquid chromatography).

All polysaccharides can be hydrolyzed to the simple monosaccharides of which they are composed. Either chemical or enzymatic procedures can be employed with the latter showing much more specificity (in some instances it is possible to hydrolyze only α-linkages, or even cleavage at a specific monosaccharidic linkage in the chain is feasible).

Many microorganisms possess the ability to hydrolyze carbohydrates to simple alcohols, ketones, or acids, usually with the production of carbon dioxide, by the process known as *fermentation*. Ethanol, acetic acid, citric acid, 2-butanone, and butyl alcohol are several of the products derived from sucrose by such a procedure. There are specific microorganisms used in fermentation processes to transform a glucose derivative, L-sorbose, to ascorbic acid (vitamin C), which is actually the γ-lactone of a hexanoic acid having an enediol structure at carbon atoms 2 and 3. This process is quite efficient.

Occurrence

Carbohydrates occur abundantly in nature. Indeed, it has been estimated that more carbohydrate material occurs naturally than all other organic material combined. While they are preponderantly important in the vegetable kingdom, carbohydrates also occur abundantly and play very important biologic roles in the animal world.

Glucose and fructose are the only monosaccharides that occur in the free state to any important extent. They are present in the juices of many ripe fruits. Among the disaccharides, only sucrose (cane or beet sugar) and lactose (milk sugar) occur in important quantities. Prominent, naturally occurring, hexosan polysaccharides include cellulose (the primary structural material in the vegetable world), starch (the primary carbohydrate reserve in the vegetable world), and glycogen, often dubbed animal starch (the primary carbohydrate reserve in the animal world). Pentosan polysaccharides occur abundantly in cereal straws and beans, eg, corn cobs; they are distinguished by the fact that they yield the industrially important furfural upon suitable treatment with sulfuric acid.

Carbohydrate derivatives (chemical combinations with noncarbohydrate substances or carbohydrates slightly altered chemically) occur plentifully in nature. The role of monosaccharide phosphate esters in physiological utilization has already been mentioned. A special class of derivatives, the *glycosides*, are discussed in the next section. Other classes include the *gums*, *pectins*, *mucilages*, *glycoproteins*, and *glycolipids* (*cerebrosides*). Chitin, a condensation polymer of *N*-acetyl-D-glucosamine (contains NH_2 instead of OH in the 2-position), comprises the skeletal material of crabs, lobsters, and insects of the arthropoda class. This same acetylglucosamine is also present in hyaluronic acid, an important constituent of connective tissue. Many bacteria have been shown to elaborate complex carbohydrate materials, and some are known to have immunologic import.

Official Carbohydrates

Examples of official articles in the various classes of carbohydrates follow.

Monosaccharides—Dextrose, and Fructose.

Disaccharides—Lactose, and Sucrose.

Polysaccharides—Dextran (in Iron Dextran), Collagen, Inulin, Starch, and Cotton.

Natural Products (other than the above and which are important because of their carbohydrate or carbohydrate derivative content)— Acacia, Agar, Karaya, Pectin, Plantago Seed, and Tragacanth.

Carbohydrate Derivatives (other than the above)—Alginic Acid, Aurothioglucose, Oxilose Cellacefate, Etlose, Hypromellose 2910, Mellose, Pyroxylin, Sodium Alginate, Carboxymethylcellulose, and Sucrose Octaacetate.

Carbohydrate residues are essential components of glycosides (below) and are frequently present in antibiotics (eg, erythromycin, streptomycin, novobiocin, etc.) and in various other biologically active substances (eg, enzymes, coenzymes, glycoproteins, vitamins, etc.).

Glycosides

Glycosides may be defined broadly as condensation products of sugars with various kinds of organic hydroxy (occasionally thiol) compounds (usually noncarbohydrate in nature), with the added restriction that the OH of the hemiacetal portion of the carbohydrate must participate in the condensation. It is obvious that the polysaccharides are also encompassed in this broad definition. The nonsugar portion is termed an *aglycone* (or *aglycon*), or a *genin*. From a structural viewpoint, the glycosides may be looked upon as internal acetals (see below).

The most characteristic chemical property of the glycosides is their susceptibility to hydrolysis, whereby they yield their sugar and nonsugar moieties. Indeed, it is through identification of the hydrolytic decomposition products that the composition of glycosides is commonly revealed. In general, the hydrolysis is energetically catalyzed by protons and is commonly brought about in the laboratory by digestion with dilute acid.

Acid hydrolysis of the glycosides occurs whether the glycosidic linkage is alpha or beta. However, nature produces many enzymes which also catalyze the hydrolysis; these are often quite specific in their actions. At this point it is instructive to make note of the fact that the naturally occurring enzymes will hydrolyze only the beta glycosides. While one may discuss the specificity of the enzymes that occur naturally with regard to the hydrolysis of the glycosides, it should be noted that there are two enzymes, namely emulsin of almond kernels and myrosin of black mustard seeds, each of which has the ability to hydrolyze a considerable number of glycosides. Glycosides that are derivatives of rhamnose require a special enzyme known as rhamnase for their hydrolysis. The enzymes frequently occur in the same plant along with the glycosides, but usually in different cells. When the structure of the plant is destroyed by grinding or other means, the enzyme contacts the glycoside and soon exerts its hydrolytic action. It is, therefore, necessary to destroy any enzymes that are present before attempting to isolate glycosidal constituents.

Classification—In modern terminology, the glycosides are usually classified according to the identity of their sugar moiety. Thus, in glucosides, the sugar moiety is glucose; in fructosides, it is fructose; in galactosides, it is galactose; etc. In older literature, the term *glucoside* is used in a generic sense and is then synonymous with the modern term *glycoside*.

Classification according to the complexity of the sugar moiety is frequently employed; ie, *monosides* if the sugar is a monosaccharide, *biosides* if a disaccharide, *triosides*, etc. Total classification on the basis of the aglycones, while feasible, is intricate because of the large variety of aglycones; however, with certain classes of glycosides, eg, the cardiotonics, such subclassification is occasionally encountered in the literature.

Occurrence—Glycosides are widely distributed in the plant kingdom. Many fruits and other parts (eg, seeds, barks, and leaves) of plants contain them. The pigments of flowers (anthocyanins) are of glycosidic character. Glycosides of animal origin are relatively rare. The aglycones of the majority of glycosides are of cyclic, and frequently of aromatic, structure. Steroidal aglycones are very common.

Many naturally occurring compounds not usually classed among the glycosides actually contain glycosidic linkages in their structures. Examples include novobiocin and streptomycin among the antibiotics, solanine and various other alkaloids (glucoalkaloids), nucleosides (consist of a purine or pyrimidine base linked with D-ribose or D-2-deoxyribose), etc.

Table II lists a number of common glycosides selected partly on the basis of pharmaceutical interest and partly because they are comprised of a variety of aglycones and sugars.

Structure of Glycosides—Two series of stereoisomeric glycosides are known, the α- and β-glycosides. Taking the methyl-D-glucosides as a simple example, they are represented by the following formulas:

Table II—Selected Glycosides

Names and molecular formulas[a]	Sources[b]	Aglycone (Genin)	Sugar moieties[c]
Amygdalin $C_{20}H_{27}NO_{11}$	Seeds of *Amygdalaceae*, *Drupaceae*, and *Pomaceae*; principally from almonds	D-Mandelonitrile → Benzaldehyde + HCN	Gentiobiose → 2 D-Glucose
Arbutin (Ursin) $C_{12}H_{16}O_7$	Leaves of plants of the *Ericaceae and Rosaceae*	Hydroquinone	D-Glucose
Coniferin (Abietin; Laricin) $C_{16}H_{22}O_8$	Plants of the *Coniferae*, eg, pine, spruce, and fir	Coniferyl alcohol [4-Hydroxy-3-methoxycinnamyl alcohol]	D-Glucose
Cymarin $C_{30}H_{44}O_9$	Various species of *Apocynum*	Strophanthidin (a steroid)	Cymarose (3-Methyldigitoxose)
Daphnin $C_{15}H_{16}O_9$	Barks and flowers of varieties of *Daphne*	7,8-Dihydroxycoumarin	D-Glucose
Digitoxin $C_{41}H_{64}O_{13}$	Leaves of *Digitalis purpurea* and *Digitalis lanata*	Digitoxigenin (a steroid)	3 Digitoxose (Digitoxose is a 2,6-bisdesoxyaldohexose)
Digoxin $C_{41}H_{64}O_{14}$	Leaves of *Digitalis lanata* or *Digitalis orientalis*	Digoxigenin (12-Hydroxydigitoxigenin) (a steroid)	3 Digitoxose
Frangulin $C_{21}H_{20}O_9$	Seeds and barks of various species of *Rhamnus*, especially alder buckthorn	4,5,7-Trihydroxy-2-methylanthraquinone	Rhamnose
Lanatoside A $C_{49}H_{76}O_{19}$	Leaves of *Digitalis lanata*	Digitoxigenin (a steroid)	2 Digitoxose + Acetyldigitoxose + D-Glucose
Lanatoside B $C_{49}H_{76}O_{20}$	Leaves of *Digitalis lanata*	Gitoxigenin (16-Hydroxydigitoxigenin) (a steroid)	2 Digitoxose + Acetyldigitoxose + D-Glucose
Lanatoside C $C_{49}H_{76}O_{20}$	Leaves of *Digitalis lanata*	Digoxigenin (a steroid)	2 Digitoxose + Acetyldigitoxose + D-Glucose
Ouabain (G-Strophanthin) $C_{29}H_{44}O_{12}$	Seeds of *Strophanthus gratus* and several varieties of *Acokanthera*	Ouabagenin (a steroid)	Rhamnose
Phlorizin (Phlorhizin; Phloridzin) $C_{21}H_{24}O_{10}$	Roots and leaves of various plants of the *Rosaceae*	Phloretin [β-(p-Hydroxyphenyl)-2,4,6-trihydroxypropiophenone]	D-Glucose
Prunasin $C_{14}H_{17}NO_6$	Various parts of many *Prunus* plants	D-Mandelonitrile → Benzaldehyde + HCN	D-Glucose
Rutin (Melin, Eldrin, and others) $C_{27}H_{30}O_{16}$	Occurs in many plants Chief source is the buck-wheat plant, *Fagopyrum esculentum*	Quercetin [3,3′,4,′,5,7-Pentahydroxyflavone]	Rutinose → L-Rhamnose + D-Glucose
Salicin $C_{13}H_{18}O_7$	Various *Salix* and *Populus* plants, especially from the bark	Saligenin [o-Hydroxybenzyl alcohol]	D-Glucose
Scillaren A $C_{36}H_{52}O_{13}$	Bulbs of *Urginea maritima*	Scillaridin A (a steroid)	Scillabiose → L-Rhamnose + D-Glucose
Sinigrin (Potassium Myronate) $C_{10}H_{16}KNO_9S_2$	Seeds of *Brassica nigra*, *Brassica juncea*, and other plants of the *Cruciferae*	$CH_2{=}CHCH_2N{=}C(SH)OSO_3K →$ $CH_2{=}CHCH_2NCS + KHSO_4$	D-Glucose
K-Strophanthin-β $C_{36}H_{54}O_{14}$	Seeds of *Strophanthus Kombé*	Strophanthidin (a steroid)	Strophanthobiose → Cymarose + D-Glucose

[a] Shown for the anhydrous forms. As isolated, many glycosides are hydrated.
[b] Typical and well-known, but not exclusive.
[c] Produced on complete hydrolysis or as otherwise indicated.

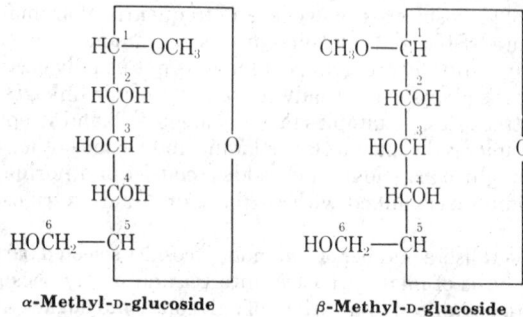

α-Methyl-D-glucoside   β-Methyl-D-glucoside

The glycosidic linkage is formed by dehydration involving a hydroxyl group of the aglycone (methanol here) and the hydroxyl group on the hemiacetal carbon of the sugar, thus forming an acetal type of structure. If the OR (in the above case, OCH_3) group is in the same steric sense as the CH_2OH group on C-5 (for D-family sugars), the glycoside configuration is designated β; if in the opposite steric sense, it is designated as α. For an illustration of how this relationship is reflected in the Haworth-type formulas, see amygdalin, a typical β-glycoside, below. The great majority of naturally occurring glycosides are of the β variety.

The same enzyme is often able to hydrolyze different glycosides, but the α- and β-stereoisomers of the same glycoside are usually not hydrolyzed by the same enzyme. *Emulsin*, for instance, has been found to hydrolyze all β-glycosides and, therefore, those glycosides which are attacked by emulsin are regarded as β-glycosides. Maltase hydrolyzes only α-glycoside.

The sugar in a large number of glycosides is D-glucose, hence the former designation "glucosides," but many important glycosides contain other sugar moieties (see Table II).

The carbohydrate in condensation union with the aglycone is frequently a di- or polysaccharide, eg, amygdalin, digitoxin, and rutin (see Table II). In many instances it is possible, under carefully controlled hydrolysis, to cleave only a portion of the aglycone moiety of the natural (*primary*) glycoside, thus yielding a derived substance which is still glycosidic. Amygdalin, for example, hydrolyzes under the influence of the enzyme amygdalase to yield glucose and prunasin (see Table II). Such derived glycosides are often referred to as *secondary* glycosides.

The synthesis of amygdalin was announced in 1924. It has the structure shown below.

Amygdalin

The glycosidic linkage is considered to be β since it is hydrolyzed by emulsin; therefore, the formula is written as shown above with the linking oxygen on the same side of the plane of the ring as the CH_2OH group on C-5. This compound, like all other glycosides, contains several asymmetric carbon atoms and is optically active. In this instance the aglycone is also optically active due to the asymmetric carbon to which the phenyl, nitrile, hydrogen, and gentiobiose residue are attached. Salicin is another β-glycoside.

Salicin

There are no simple identifying tests for glycosides. The ultimate test involves characterization of the hydrolytic cleavage products. Methods for the detection of glycosides and for their quantitative determination involve the estimation of reducing sugars before and after hydrolysis by boiling with dilute acids, or by the action of enzymes.

Saponins—The saponins are a group of amorphous, colloidal glycosides, which are readily soluble in water and which produce a froth when the aqueous solution is agitated. They are excellent emulsifying agents and the aqueous solutions of some of them, eg, *quillaja* bark, were formerly used as detergents to replace soap. They are acrid in taste and in powder form cause sneezing. Many conform to the general formula $C_nH_{2n-8}O_{10}$.

The aglycones, usually prepared by acid-catalyzed hydrolysis, are usually termed *sapogenins*. Two general types are well known, *viz*, *steroid* as in digitonin and *triterpenoid* as in aesculin.

Much of the research conducted on the saponin-containing plants was motivated by the attempt to discover precursors for cortisone. It would appear that the most outstanding plant steroids for cortisone production are: diosgenin and botogenin from the genus *Dioscorea;* hecogenin, manogenin, and gitogenin from species of *Agave*.

Many of the saponins are markedly toxic. These are called *sapotoxins*. Saponins usually exert a powerful hemolytic action on red blood corpuscles. They have been used as fish poisons.

The saponins are widely distributed in the botanical kingdom. The commercial product *saponin* is prepared from the yucca plant or from Quillaja.

Properties—The greater portion of the known glycosides, when pure, are colorless or white, optically active, and soluble in alcohol or in diluted alcohol. They are extracted from the plant material by water, alcohol, or a mixture of the two. The glycosides occur in the plant in small amounts, and their isolation in a pure state is usually difficult and laborious. The processes used for their production and purification vary according to the nature of the material and the glycoside.

Official Glycosides

Examples of official glycosides are Deslanoside, Digitoxin, Digoxin, and Ouabain.

The physiological actions of many drugs of plant origin are referable to glycosidal constituents. Examples include aloe, cascara, digitalis, gentian, rhubarb, sarsaparilla, senna, squill, strophanthus, taraxacum, viburnum, wild cherry and many others.

Lipids

The lipids, known also as *lipins* or *lipoids*, are the fat and fat-like substances which occur in plants and animals. Like the carbohydrates and proteins, the lipids constitute a very important group of organic substances from the standpoint of physiological utilization. Unlike the carbohydrates and proteins, the lipids comprise a rather heterogeneous group of substances in terms of chemical composition. They are grouped together primarily on the basis of solubility characteristics; in general, they are soluble in the usual fat solvents such as ether and chloroform and are insoluble in water. The lipids may be divided into five classes according to their chemical structure:

1. **Fixed Oils and Fats**—esters of glycerol and fatty acids. An example is olive oil. Fixed oils which are solid at ordinary temperatures are commonly called *fats*. An example is lard.
2. **Waxes**—esters of high-molecular-weight, monohydric alcohols, and high-molecular-weight fatty acids. An example is spermaceti.
3. **Sterols**—alcohols containing the cyclopentanophenanthrene (steroid) nucleus (see page 405). Typical examples include the familiar cholesterol and ergosterol.
4. **Phospholipids (Phosphatides)**—esters consisting of glycerol in combination with fatty acids, phosphoric acid, and certain nitrogenous compounds. Pharmaceutically, the most important members of this group are the lecithins.
5. **Glycolipids (Cerebrosides)**—substances isolated from the brain and from various other sources which on hydrolysis yield fatty acids, galactose, and the nitrogenous compound *sphingosine* (2-amino-4-octadecene-1,3-diol). Examples are phrenosin and kerasin. Because the sugar moiety is usually galactose, the glycolipids are sometimes referred to as galactolipids. At present, the glycolipids have no pharmaceutical applications and will not be further discussed.

Fixed Oils and Fats

Fixed oils and fats are mixtures of glyceryl esters of the so-called high fatty acids, ie, the higher-molecular-weight aliphatic acids, especially palmitic, stearic, and oleic acids. The individual glyceryl esters themselves are frequently referred to as *glycerides*.

The difference in consistency between fixed oils and fats is caused by the relative proportions of liquid and solid glyceryl esters present. Fixed oils contain a relatively high proportion of liquid glycerides (polyunsaturated glycerides), such as glyceryl oleate, whereas fats are relatively rich in solid glycerides (mostly saturated) such as glyceryl stearate. Glycerides of unsaturated fatty acids have lower melting points than those of saturated acids with the same number of carbon atoms. Although most vegetable oils are liquid at room temperature and most animal fats are solids, there are notable exceptions such as cocoa butter (solid) and cod liver oil (liquid).

Fixed oils are to be distinguished sharply from volatile oils.

Physically, the former are nonvolatile under ordinary conditions (hence the name *fixed* oils), in contradistinction to the latter which, as the name implies, are volatile. From the standpoint of composition, the volatile oils differ greatly one from the other; but, as a group, they differ from fixed oils in that they do not contain glyceryl esters. Volatile oils are also known as ethereal oils or essential oils.

Preparation—Most of the fixed oils and fats are obtained by *expression* from the plant or animal tissues in which they occur. Generally the material is first ground and subsequently submitted to hydraulic pressure, and to heat when necessary.

The oils as obtained by the first expression usually are of the highest commercial value, as, for example, olive oil where the first pressings are called *virgin olive oil*, but sometimes the expressed oil from plant tissues is of crude quality and requires subsequent purification, as in the case of cottonseed oil. Fixed oils and fats are frequently bleached by treatment with fuller's earth or similar clays, and subsequent filtration.

Some few oils for technical purposes are not obtained by expression but are extracted from the plant tissues by means of *volatile solvents* which are later recovered. Animal fats and oils are usually separated from the tissues by the process known as *rendering* which consists in heating the tissues until the fat melts and separates mechanically.

Analytical Characteristics—The analytical factors of greatest importance in identifying fixed oils and in judging their quality are the *Iodine Value* (the number of g of iodine monochloride, expressed as iodine, absorbed by 100 g of sample under prescribed conditions); *Saponification Value* (the number of mg of potassium hydroxide required to neutralize the free acids and saponify the esters in 1 g of sample); *Acid Value* (the number of mg of potassium hydroxide required to neutralize the free acids in 1 g of sample); and the refractive index. The specific gravity, color, odor, and congealing point are of little value. Some oils, such as cottonseed oil and sesame oil, are identifiable by specific tests, but the identification of a fixed oil is only inferentially possible as a rule, after taking many physical and chemical factors into account.

Properties—Fixed oils and fats are rather distinctive in their physical properties. They are greasy to the touch and leave a permanent oily stain upon filter paper. They are all lighter than water and insoluble therein, but are soluble in ether, chloroform, and some other water-immiscible solvents. A few of them, such as castor oil, are soluble in alcohol. When purified, they are nearly colorless and of a bland odor and taste with very little distinctiveness. The yellow color of fats is usually due to the presence of carotene, which is one of the provitamins A.

When heated moderately, fats liquefy and oils become less viscous. When heated strongly, they undergo decomposition with the production of acrid, flammable vapors, and when ignited, they burn with a sooty flame. The acidity of an overheated fixed oil or fat is due largely to the formation of *acrolein* (*propenal*).

The property common to all fats and fixed oils is their propensity to undergo hydrolysis to yield glycerol and the fatty acids representative of the fat or oil. Uncatalyzed, the reaction proceeds very slowly; it is therefore commonly accelerated by employing high temperatures and high pressures and by the presence of either acids or alkalies. If alkalies are employed, the liberated acids are automatically converted into their corresponding metallic salts. Since such salts are commonly referred to as soaps, the alkali-catalyzed hydrolysis of fats and fixed oils is frequently referred to as *saponification*. The term is also frequently used to refer to hydrolysis of all kinds of esters, regardless of how accomplished. Many naturally occurring enzymes also catalyze fat and fixed oil hydrolysis. Such enzymes are termed *lipases*. Steapsin of the human pancreatic juice is an important example.

Constituents—Three glycerides, *olein*, *palmitin*, and *stearin*, are common to many fixed oils.

Olein is *glyceryl trioleate* [$C_3H_5(C_{18}H_{33}O_2)_3$], a liquid at ordinary temperature. It is the predominating constituent in expressed almond oil, in lard oil, and in many of the more fluid animal oils and those of vegetable origin. It is separated and purified by cold expression, the other constituents being retained by their lack of fluidity at low temperatures.

Palmitin is *glyceryl tripalmitate* [$C_3H_5(C_{16}H_{31}O_2)_3$]. It is a solid at ordinary temperature (mp 60°). It predominates in palm oil and coconut oil.

Stearin is *glyceryl tristearate* [$C_3H_5(C_{18}H_{35}O_2)_3$]. Its melting point is 71°. It predominates in many of the solid fats and may be separated by expression under controlled temperature conditions, which removes the olein and palmitin.

Olein, and glyceryl esters of other unsaturated acids, may be converted into stearin by *hydrogenation* in the presence of a catalyst such as finely divided nickel. Liquid oils such as cottonseed, soybean, and peanut are often commercially transformed (hardened) by this process into solid fats. The proprietary cooking fat, *Crisco*, is a well-known example. Through partial hydrogenation, the consistency of such hardened oils may be varied between wide limits.

The glycerides in a fixed oil may be *simple* or *mixed*. In simple glycerides, such as olein, palmitin, and stearin, all three fatty acid groups are identical. In the more frequently encountered mixed glycerides more than one fatty acid is present. Because of the many possible combinations in the mixed glycerides, different fats having entirely different physical properties often show the same chemical analysis. The following formula illustrates a mixed glyceride:

$$C_{15}H_{31}COOCH_2 \quad \alpha'$$
$$C_{17}H_{35}COOCH \quad \beta$$
$$C_{17}H_{33}COOCH_2 \quad \alpha$$

α-Oleo-α',β-palmitostearin
(or 1-oleo-3-palmito-2-stearin)

Mono-, di-, and triglycerides, containing, respectively, one, two, or three molecules of fatty acid esterified with one molecule of glycerol, have been prepared synthetically, but only triglycerides occur commonly in nature. The natural fatty acids are nearly all straight-chain and contain an even number of carbon atoms (C_4 to C_{26}).

Of all the fatty acids, stearic, palmitic, and oleic are the most widely distributed. Stearic acid is found mostly in animal fats, but it is occasionally an important constituent in vegetable oils. The saturated fatty acids lower than C_{12} are found in the milk of mammals, although butter fat contains all of the even-numbered fatty acids from C_4 to C_{18} as well as oleic.

Oils and fats, when subjected to pressure at certain temperatures, can be fractionated to some extent into the glycerides composing it. On aging, fixed oils often develop a precipitate of stearin which will reliquefy on warming.

In the days before artificial refrigeration the oils expressed in the summer (at a higher temperature), when the stearin was kept in solution to a greater extent, were found to deposit the stearin much more readily than those oils that were pressed in the winter (at a lower temperature), and "*summer pressed*" and "*winter pressed*" were commercial designations which still persist, although at the present time it is a matter of temperature control at the time of pressing, irrespective of the season.

Drying and Nondrying Oils—Fixed oils are classified into *drying* and *nondrying* oils. The former when exposed to the air undergo oxidation with the formation of a tough hard film. Linseed oil is an example of the class of drying oils which find their greatest use in the manufacture of paints and varnishes.

The nondrying oils when exposed to the air remain sticky to the touch for an indefinite period and therefore cannot be used in paints and varnishes. Olive oil and expressed almond oil are examples of nondrying oils. The drying quality is caused by the presence of unsaturated fatty acids of a distinctive character such as linoleic and linolenic acids.

Uses—Fats and fixed oils contain certain unsaturated fatty acids which are essential foods. Their absence in the human diet has produced eczematous skin conditions, and in experimental animals has resulted in scaly skin, emaciation, necrosis, and premature death. Experimental evidence exists to support the view that fats such as safflower oil which are rich in linoleic acid and possibly other unsaturated acids *may* play an important role in the mobilization and utilization of food cholesterol, provided dietary fat intake is suitably controlled. This is of particular nutritional and medical interest in connection with possibly preventing and correcting the hypercholesterolemia which is commonly observed in atherosclerosis. Certain oils, such as those of peanut and sesame, are used extensively as solvents in the preparation of intramuscular injections. A few oils have medicinal actions in their own right—eg, castor oil as a cathartic, cod liver oil as an antirachitic, and olive oil as an emollient. Chaulmoogra oil was formerly used in the treatment of leprosy.

Salts of several of the fatty acids are fungicidal, such as zinc undecylenate. Other derivatives of glycerides are soaps and various related surface-active compounds which are employed as detergents and germicides.

Waxes

Waxes, like fixed oils and fats, are esters of fatty acids. They differ, however, in that the alcohol represented is *not* glycerol. In place of this trihydric alcohol is found one of the sterols (this page) or one of the higher, even-numbered, monohydric alcohols from C_{16} to C_{36}. Waxes often contain these alcohols and fatty acids (C_{24} to C_{36}) in free state, often as the major component, and some of the waxes obtained from plants also contain paraffin hydrocarbons. The esters in waxes are usually much more resistant to saponification than the glycerides of fats and fixed oils.

Sterols

The sterols are alcohols structurally related to the *steroids*, those naturally occurring compounds, obtained from plants and animals, which contain the partly or completely hydrogenated 17*H*-cyclopenta[*a*]phenanthrene nucleus. In addition to the sterols, the steroids include various other substances, such as compounds of adrenal origin, certain alkaloids, antirachitic vitamins, bile acids, cardiac glycosides, saponins, sex hormones, and toad poisons. The general formula for the basic structure of these compounds may be *represented* as follows. In actual conformation, however, the structure is not planar.

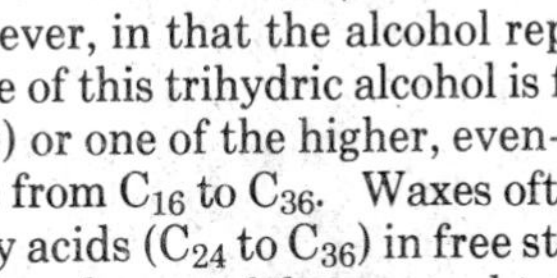

General steroid formula

The rings are conventionally lettered and numbered as indicated. Since usually one or more rings are completely saturated, several centers of asymmetry are present; this, plus restricted rotations due to ring fusions, results in rather complex stereochemical relationships. In the naturally occurring compounds, substitutions in the rings occur most frequently on C-3, C-17 and C-11.

Following the more or less standard convention, the direction of projection from the plane of the ring system of substituting groups located at centers of asymmetry is commonly indicated by use of the letters α and β. An α-substituting group is viewed as projecting beneath the ring plane and is represented by a broken line; a β-substituting group is viewed as projecting above the ring plane and is represented by a solid line. See the examples provided below.

The prefixes *cis* and *trans* are also often employed (but *not* in standardized nomenclature) to distinguish the α- and β-members of a pair of compounds which are otherwise stereochemically identical. However, this requires the selection of a substituting group to serve as a reference point in the steroid molecule, and a "rule" frequently used is that the nearest angular (branching off at a ring fusion) methyl group is so selected. In the case of the sterols, for example, the angular methyl group nearest to the 3-hydroxyl group is the one at C-10 and is represented as having the β-configuration; thus the 3-β-hydroxycholestane becomes *cis*-3-hydroxycholestane, and the 3-α-hydroxycholestane becomes *trans*-3-hydroxycholestane. Most naturally occurring sterols have the 3-hydroxyl group in the β, or *cis*, position. The prefix *epi* is often employed to designate specifically the corresponding epimers in which this OH is α, or *trans;* eg, epicholesterol and epicoprosterol.

Classification of Steroids—Different investigators use slightly different methods of classifying the steroids. One method is to divide them into five classes according to the type of substituent group at carbon 17, ie, group R. A classification commonly used is as follows:

1. *Sterols*—R is an aliphatic side chain. They contain one or more OH groups attached in alicyclic linkage.
2. *Sex Hormones*—C-17 bears a ketonic or hydroxyl group and frequently carried a two-carbon side chain. See page 983.
3. *Cardiac Glycosides*—R is a lactone ring. The glycosides also contain sugars linked through oxygen in other parts of the molecule. Hydrolysis yields this sugar and the *cardiac aglycone*. See page 855.
4. *Bile Acids*—R is a five-carbon side chain terminating in a carboxylic acid group. The bile acids are treated in Chapter 41.
5. *Sapogenins*—R contains an oxacyclic (ethereal) ring system.

Description and Properties—The parent hydrocarbon of natural sterols is cholestane which exists in two forms depending on the configuration of the hydrogen atom at C-5. These are drawn below and labeled with their standard (IUPAC) names and, in parentheses, their trivial names:

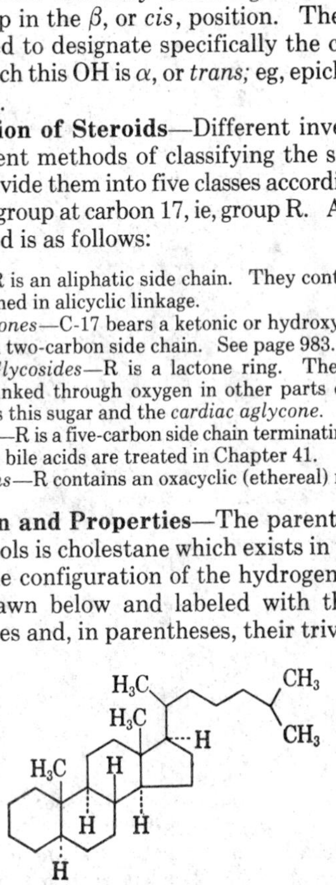

5α-Cholestane
(Cholestane)

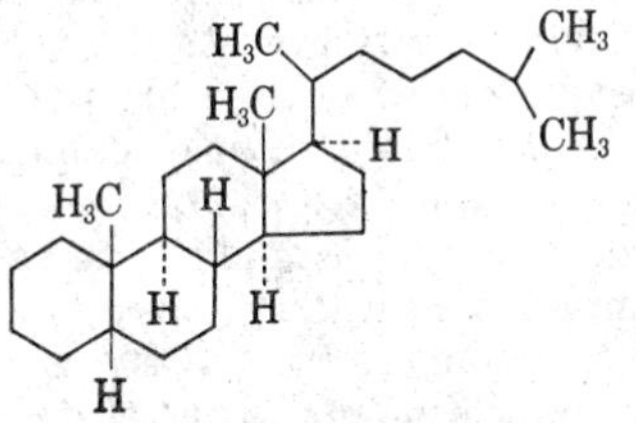

5β-Cholestane
(Coprostane)

The characteristic function of natural sterols is the 3-hydroxyl in *beta* orientation. Thus, 5α-cholestan-3β-ol and 5β-cholestan-3β-ol are commonly looked upon as the parent sterols. Other sterols are often named as derivatives of them although most have commonly accepted trivial names such as cholesterol, ergosterol, stigmasterol, etc. These parent sterols are shown below along with their various names. The two cholesterols are also illustrated. In trivial notation, the prefix *epi-* is employed to denote the unnatural *alpha* orientation of the 3-hydroxyl. Note that in the cholest-5-enols, there is no H at C-5 and thus no α or β accompanies the numeral 5.

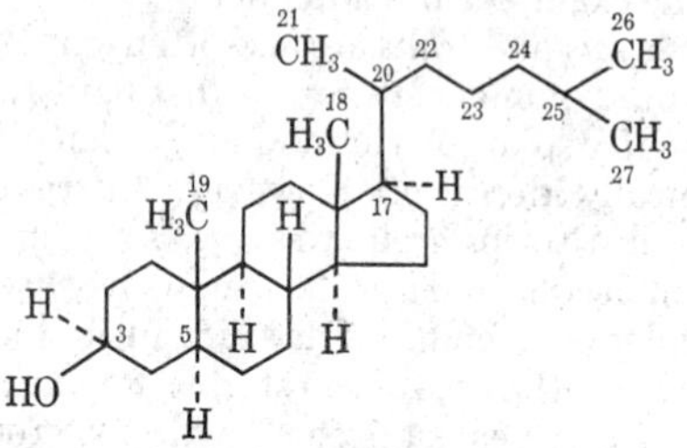

5α-Cholestan-3β-ol
3β-Hydroxy-5α-cholestane
(Cholestanol)

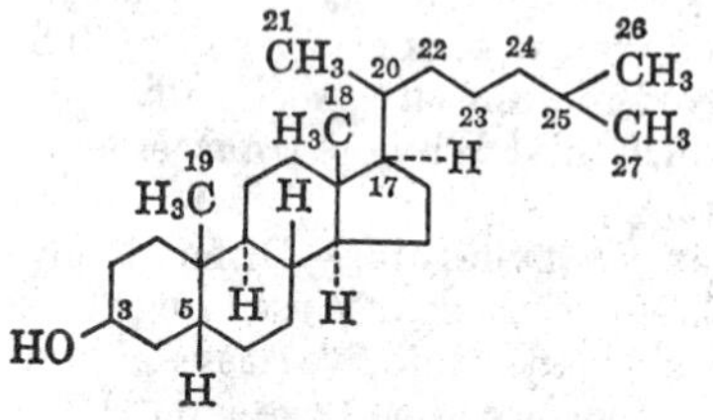

5β-Cholestan-3β-ol
3β-Hydroxy-5β-cholestane
(Coprostanol)

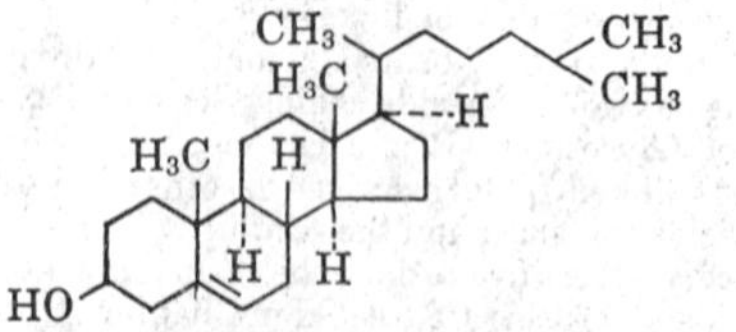

Cholest-5-en-3β-ol
3β-Hydroxycholest-5-ene
(Cholesterol)

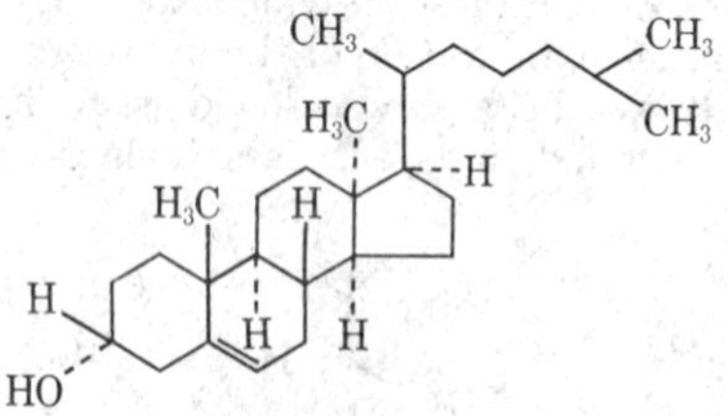

Cholest-5-en-3α-ol
3α-Hydroxycholest-5-ene
(Epicholesterol)

Sterols occur abundantly in nature and often constitute a sizable fraction of the total unsaponifiable portion of lipoidal extractive matter from animal and vegetable tissue.

Several empirical color reactions have been developed which are useful in steroid chemistry for purposes of identification. Most prominently cited are the Salkowski, Liebermann-Burchard, and Rosenheim reactions. For discussion of these, consult reference texts in biochemistry.

The 3β-hydroxysteroids readily form sparingly soluble molecular complexes with the glycoside digitonin. These complexes are commonly referred to as *digitonides*, and they find extensive application in various research operations involving isolation and characterization of the individual steroids.

Several sterols undergo intramolecular rearrangement under the influence of controlled ultraviolet radiation resulting in compounds which display antirachitic (vitamin D) activity. Thus, for example, ergosterol, a mycosterol occurring abundantly in yeast and ergot, is readily converted in good yield to ergocalciferol (vitamin D₂). The structure shown below emphasizes the locus of scission of the cyclic nucleus.

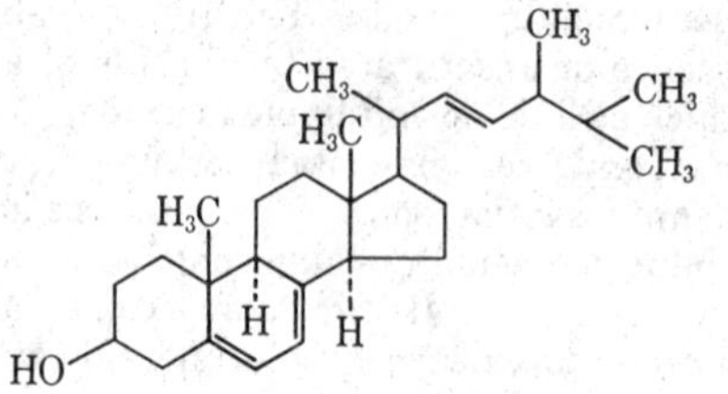

Ergosterol
5,7,22 *E*-Ergostatrien-3β-ol

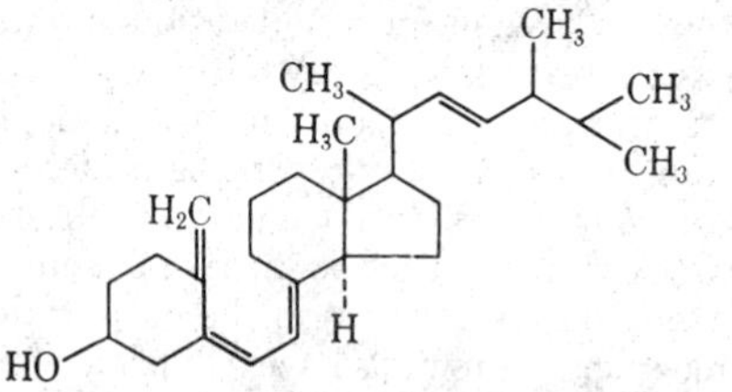

Ergocalciferol (vitamin D₂)
9,10-Seco-5*Z*,7*E*,10(19),22*E*-ergostatetraen-3β-ol

In a similar fashion the natural vitamin D₃ metabolite, 1α,25-dihydroxycholecalciferol (calcitriol) is formed by ultraviolet conversion, hydrolysis, and heat isomerization from 1α,25-diacetoxy-7-dehydrocholesterol. Calcitriol is used for the hypocalcemia associated with chronic renal dialysis.

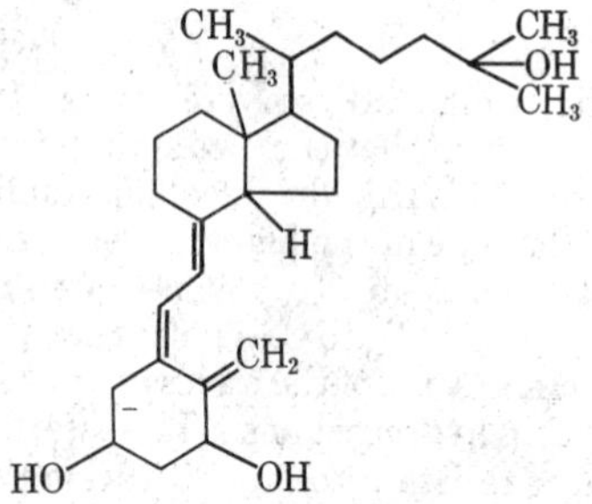

Calcitriol
(1α,2β,5*Z*,7 *E*)-9,10-secocholesta-
5,7,10(19)-triene-1,3,25-triol

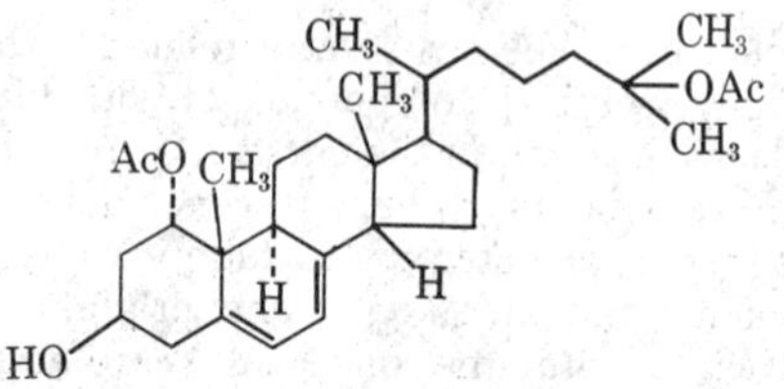

1α,25-diacetoxy-7-dehydrocholesterol

Phospholipids (Phosphatides)

The *phospholipids* (phosphatides) include all lipoidal constituents that contain phosphorus in their molecules. They appear to be essential components of every plant and animal cell, and have been categorized as (1) lecithins, (2) cephalins, and (3) sphingomyelins. The chemical composition in all cases is revealed through quantitative measurement of the products resulting from hydrolysis under various conditions. The only phospholipids with pharmaceutical applications are the lecithins.

The Lecithins—When completely hydrolyzed, each molecule of a lecithin yields two molecules of fatty acid, and one molecule each of glycerol, phosphoric acid, and a basic nitrogenous compound (usually choline).

The fatty acids obtained from lecithins on hydrolysis are usually oleic, palmitic, and stearic. The phosphoric acid may be attached to the glycerol in either an α- or the β-position, forming *α-glycerophosphoric acid* or *β-glycerophosphoric acid*, respectively, and producing the corresponding series of lecithins which are known as α- and β-lecithins. The representations below are in the *zwitterion* (internal salt) form. Each series of lecithins may differ in the fatty acids attached to the glycerol. The naturally occurring lecithins are of the α-variety.

α-Lecithin   *β-Lecithin*

Choline, a very strong base, is a member of the vitamin B complex (page 1014). It functions in the body to prevent accumulation of fat in the liver and also, as the acetylated derivative *acetylcholine*, is released at the parasympathetic nerve endings when these nerves are stimulated and thus controls the transmission of impulses across cholinergic synapses.

Choline

Acetylcholine

Commercially lecithin is obtained by extraction processes from egg yolk, brain tissue, or soybeans. *Ovolecithin* (*vitellin*) from eggs and *vegilecithin* from soybeans as well as purified lecithin from calves brains are used as emulsifiers, antioxidants, and stabilizers in foods and pharmaceutical preparations. Lecithins oxidize readily on exposure to air and, simultaneously, darken in color.

The Cephalins—Cephalins, which are associated with the process of blood clotting, are closely related to lecithin in structure and are known to be essential constituents of various body tissues. They differ from lecithins in that choline is replaced by *cholamine* (ethanolamine), *serine* (page 408), or *meso-inositol* (page 1015).

$HOCH_2CH_2NH_2$ $HOCH_2CH(NH_2)COOH$
Cholamine   Serine

The Sphingomyelins—When completely hydrolyzed, a sphingomyelin yields a fatty acid, phosphoric acid, choline, and a second nitrogenous substance, *sphingosine*, which is the unsaturated amino alcohol, 2-amino-4-octadecene-1,3-diol $[CH_3(CH_2)_{12}CH=CHCH(OH)CH(NH_2)CH_2OH]$. Sphingomyelins are found closely associated with the lecithins and cephalins in the phospholipid fraction of the brain tissue.

Official Lipids

Examples of official articles in the various classes of lipids follow.

Fixed Oils—Castor Oil, Cod Liver Oil, Corn Oil, Cottonseed Oil, Olive Oil, Peanut Oil, and Sesame Oil.

The official Oleovitamin A and D Solution also contains unspecified edible fixed oils. Iodized oil is a synthetic product resulting from the io-dination of vegetable fixed oils containing an oleate radical or other unsaturated fatty acid radicals.

Fats—The only official fat is Cocoa Butter. Cocoa contains from 10 to 22% fat (theobroma oil). Various crude drugs contain significant percentages of fat, but this is incidental and their official status is not a consequence of their fat content. Crude drugs are usually defatted prior to preparing extracts.

Waxes—Carnauba Wax, Cetyl Esters Wax (a synthetic spermaceti), Lanolin, White Wax, and Yellow Wax.

Sterols—The only official sterol is Cholesterol. Ergocalciferol and various other activated sterols are sometimes classed with the sterols although they are actually sterol derivatives (see page 405).

Proteins

Recognition of the universal occurrence of proteins in all forms of animal and vegetable matter and of the intimate roles they play in the fundamental processes of tissue formation, regeneration, and function has won for this class of substances the distinction of being the primary component of all living matter—hence the term protein, of Greek origin, meaning *first*. In sharp contrast with carbohydrates and fats, which are also essential for life and which function primarily as energy sources, proteins vary widely in composition not only from one species to another but also among the various tissues and cellular fluids within a given species. Thus, for example, albumins from different sources vary in composition, and the proteins characteristic of human epithelial tissue, muscle, brain, kidney, and other tissues differ from one another. These differences in composition make for differences in physical and chemical properties which, in turn, are reflected in the diverse biofunctions in which proteins participate.

Occurrence and Isolation

Although proteins are present in all living matter, important differences in distribution are clearly evident. With plants, in which the structural parts are essentially carbohydrate in nature, protein concentration is usually very much higher in the seed than in any of the other plant parts. No similar gross variation is observed in the animal world, but different tissues vary considerably in the approximate percentage of protein they contain; eg, skin, 27; skeletal muscle, 21; brain, 11; adipose tissue, 5.

Insoluble proteins are usually isolated simply by removing contaminating material by means of a suitable array of solvents. Debridement is often facilitated through the appropriate use of enzymes. Soluble proteins are usually obtained first as crude extracts in aqueous solutions from which, after subjecting to dialysis to remove contaminating solutes, the protein is obtained either through precipitation by means of salt solutions or organic solvents or through lyophilization techniques.

As first isolated, proteins are frequently mixtures. Separation into individual components was formerly accomplished only by means of tedious fractional precipitation operations, but is nowadays achieved much more conveniently and completely through chromatographic procedures using ion-exchange resins and various cellulose derivatives.

Composition and Structure

All proteins contain carbon, hydrogen, oxygen, and nitrogen. Sulfur is also generally present, phosphorus frequently, and other elements, eg, iodine, copper, iron, and zinc, occasionally. Nitrogen is the distinguishing element. It constitutes approximately 16% of most proteins and thus leads to the rough factor 6.25 generally employed for converting protein nitrogen found by analysis to protein.

The fundamental structural units of proteins are α-amino acids, about 20 of which (see Table III) participate prominently in protein formation. These building-block molecules contain at least one carboxyl group and one α-amino group,

Table III—Prominent Protein Amino Acids

Neutral Aliphatic

Glycine Gly
  aminoacetic acid

$$CH_2(NH_2)COOH$$

Alanine Ala
  2-aminopropanoic acid

$$CH_3CH(NH_2)COOH$$

Serine Ser
  2-amino-3-hydroxypropanoic acid

$$CH_2(OH)CH(NH_2)COOH$$

Threonine Thr
  2-amino-3-hydroxybutanoic acid

$$CH_3CH(OH)CH(NH_2)COOH$$

Valine Val
  2-amino-3-methylbutanoic acid

$$CH_3CH(CH_3)CH(NH_2)COOH$$

Leucine Leu
  2-amino-4-methylpentanoic acid

$$CH_3CH(CH_3)CH_2CH(NH_2)COOH$$

Isoleucine Ile
  2-amino-3-methylpentanoic acid

$$CH_3CH_2CH(CH_3)CH(NH_2)COOH$$

Neutral Thioaliphatic

Cysteine CySH
  2-amino-3-mercaptopropanoic acid

$$CH_2(SH)CH(NH_2)COOH$$

Cystine CyS-SCy
  3,3′-dithiodi(2-aminopropanoic acid)

$$[-SCH_2CH(NH_2)COOH]_2$$

Methionine Met
  2-amino-4-(methylthio)butanoic acid

$$CH_2(SCH_3)CH_2CH(NH_2)COOH$$

Neutral Aromatic

Phenylalanine Phe
  2-amino-3-phenylpropanoic acid

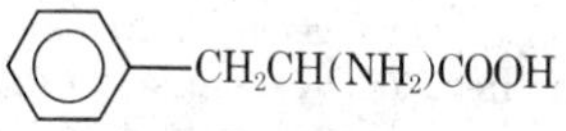

Tyrosine Tyr
  2-amino-3-(*p*-hydroxyphenyl)propanoic acid

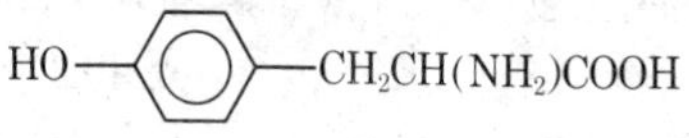

Neutral Heterocyclic

Proline Pro
  2-pyrrolidinecarboxylic acid

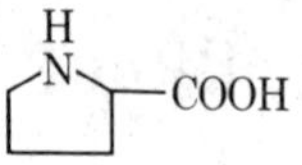

Hydroxyproline Hyp
  4-hydroxy-2-pyrrolidinecarboxylic acid

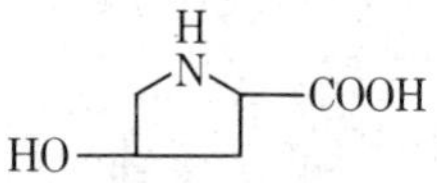

Tryptophan Trp
  α-aminoindole-3-propanoic acid

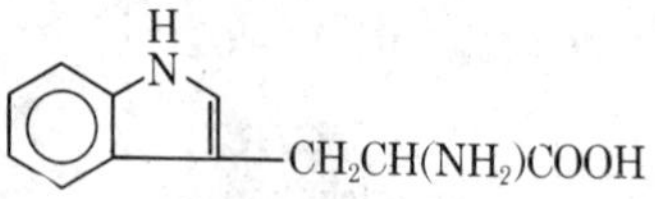

Acidic

Aspartic Acid Asp
  aminosuccinic acid

$$HOOCCH_2CH(NH_2)COOH$$

Glutamic Acid Glu
  2-aminoglutaric acid

$$HOOCCH_2CH_2CH(NH_2)COOH$$

Basic

Histidine His
  α-amino-4-imidazolepropanoic acid

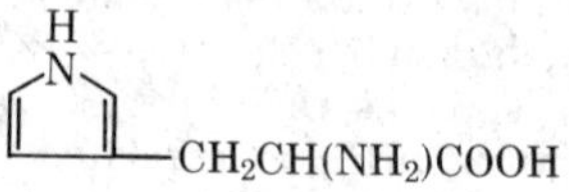

Lysine Lys
  2,6-diaminohexanoic acid

$$CH_2(NH_2)CH_2CH_2CH_2CH(NH_2)COOH$$

Arginine Arg
  2-amino-5-guanidinopentanoic acid

$$NH_2C(=NH)NH-CH_2CH_2CH_2CH(NH_2)COOH$$

but differ in the structure of the remainder of the molecule. All except the simplest one, glycine, are capable of existing in both D and L configurations with respect to their α-carbon but proteins contain only the L-enantiomorphs. The actual protein molecule consists of long-chain polymers which may be looked upon as having resulted from condensation of the amino acids thus producing amide (commonly called peptide) linkages:

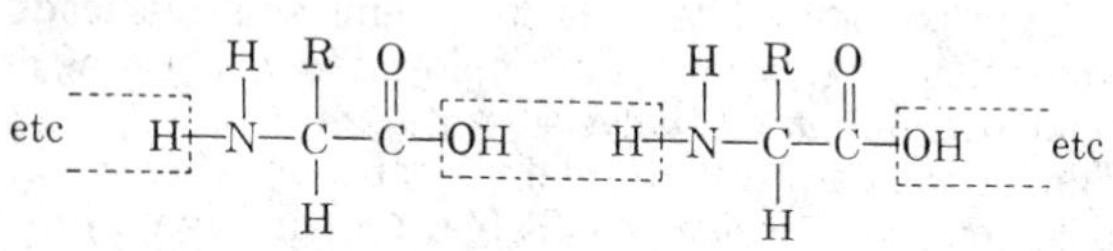

In addition to the twenty standard amino acids given, sev-

eral others of relatively rare occurrence have been isolated from hydrolysates of some specialized types of proteins. All are derivatives of some standard amino acid. Among them is hydroxylysine, the 5-hydroxy derivative of lysine, present in *collagen* (as is hydroxyproline). *Desmosine* and *isodesmosine* occur in the fibrous protein *elastin*. As noted in their structures, *desmosine* and *isodesmosine* can be visualized as formed from four lysine molecules with their side chain moieties joined to form a substituted pyridine ring. Certain muscle proteins have been found to contain several ε-*N*-methylated analogs of *lysine* and *histidine*. *β-Alanine*, *α-aminobutyric acid*, *homocysteine*, *homoserine*, *citrulline*, *ornithine*, *canavinine*, *djenkolic acid*, and *β-cyanoalanine* are some naturally occurring amino acids that are not found in proteins.

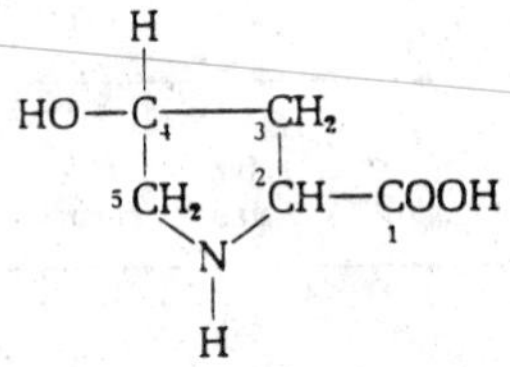

4-Hydroxyproline

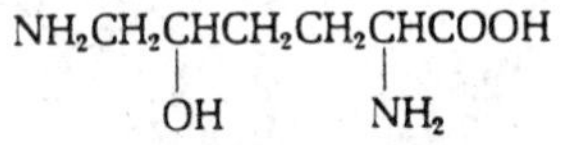

5-Hydroxylysine

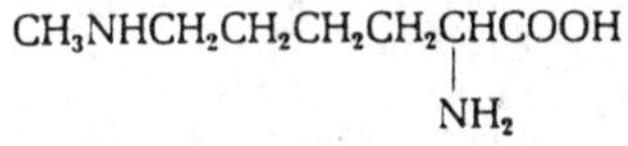

$NH_2CH_2CHCH_2CH_2CHCOOH$
$\quad\quad\quad\ \ OH \quad\quad\quad\ NH_2$

ε-N-Methyllysine

$CH_3NHCH_2CH_2CH_2CH_2CHCOOH$
$\quad\quad\quad\quad\quad\quad\quad\quad\quad NH_2$

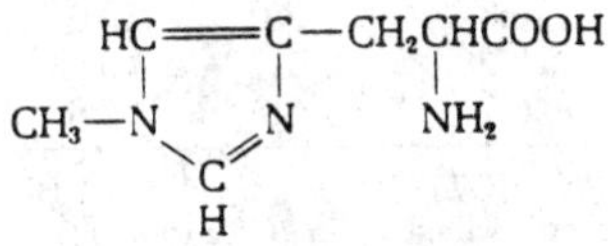

3-Methylhistidine

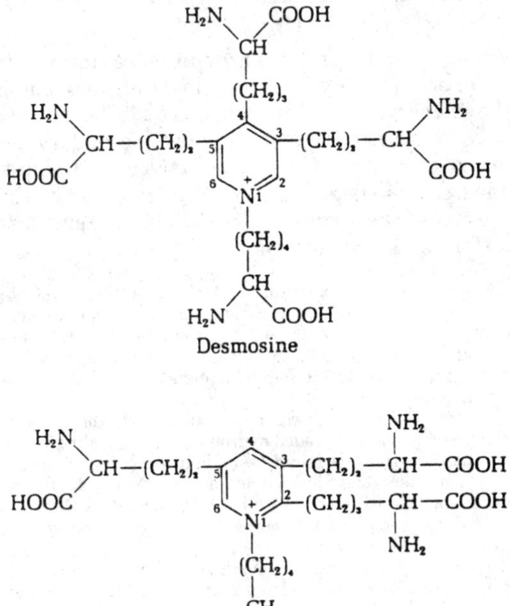

Desmosine

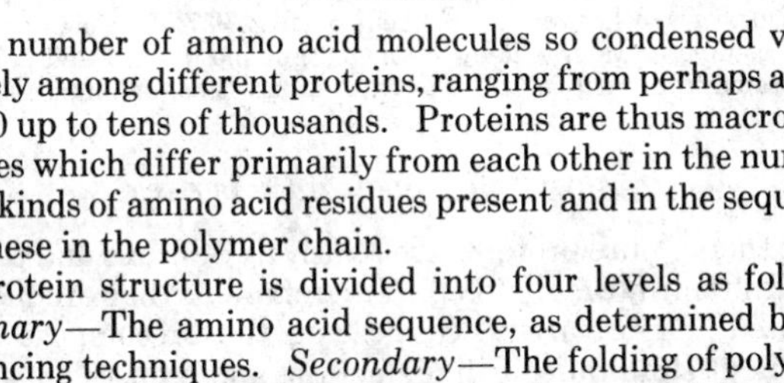

Isodesmosine

The number of amino acid molecules so condensed varies widely among different proteins, ranging from perhaps as few as 30 up to tens of thousands. Proteins are thus macromolecules which differ primarily from each other in the number and kinds of amino acid residues present and in the sequence of these in the polymer chain.

Protein structure is divided into four levels as follows: *Primary*—The amino acid sequence, as determined by sequencing techniques. *Secondary*—The folding of polypeptide chains into coiled structures as determined by X-ray diffraction, optical rotatory dispersion (see Chapter 35) and electron photomicrography. *Tertiary*—The arrangement of chains into specific layers and/or fibers. *Quaternary*—A fourth level of organization where many monomeric units, each displaying primary, secondary and tertiary architecture, associate to form a quaternary structure. Finally, a fifth level is conceivable whereby aggregates of different proteins, each

comprised of the four fundamental structural orders, form macromolecular complexes believed to be involved in fatty acid synthesis and electron transport.

As with other kinds of macromolecules, molecular weights are less meaningful than usual. Determined by various methods, eg, diffusion, sedimentation, viscosity, X-ray analysis, light-scattering, ultracentrifugation, electron microscopy, gel permeation, etc, values for different proteins range from about 10^4 up to about 10^7; and the value found for a given protein often varies with the method used.

Amino Acid Content and Sequence

The two fundamental problems involved in the elucidation of the composition of a protein are (1) quantitative assay of the individual amino acids present and (2) determination of the sequence of all amino acid residues in the chain. Each is a highly specialized field of endeavor. Prior to the advent of modern techniques based on selective adsorption (ion-exchange, paper, thin-layer, high-performance liquid, and gas-liquid chromatography), electrophoresis, countercurrent distribution, and isotope-dilution methods, progress was discouragingly slow. That it is excitingly rapid today is abundantly evident from reports appearing regularly in the literature of biochemistry.

The amino acid composition of various selected proteins is presented in Table IV. In view of the diverse analytical methods employed, slight variations in reported values are expectable and are encountered in the literature. With simple (nonconjugated) proteins, the total mass of the amino acids exceeds the mass of the source protein because of the water which becomes fixed during hydrolytic cleavage of the peptide linkages.

The precise sequence of amino acid residues is now known for a considerable number of proteins among which are insulin, ribonuclease, tobacco mosaic virus, and many of the hemoglobins, the immunoglobulins, and other specialized proteins. A noteworthy example of current progress is the elucidation of the sequence in each of the two identical gamma chains (each contains 146 residues from 18 different amino acids) of the globin in fetal human hemoglobin and the identification of 39 differences in sequence between each of these chains and its analogue in adult human hemoglobin.

Classification

A satisfactory practical classification of proteins on the sole basis of either composition or structure has not been achieved, partly because of their wide diversity and partly because of incomplete knowledge. Classifications in terms of occurrence and function are frequently encountered in the literature but these are designed for special purposes and usually do not embrace the total protein field. A classification having some practical utility has evolved gradually over the years and is presented below. The division into classes is based primarily on solubility, coagulability, conjugation, denaturation, and hydrolysis characteristics.

1. **Simple proteins** are naturally occurring proteins which yield only alpha-amino acids or their derivatives on hydrolysis. They may be of several types and include:

(a) *Albumins*, which are soluble in water and coagulated by heat; eg, ovalbumin in egg white and serum albumin in blood.
(b) *Globulins*, which are insoluble in water but soluble in dilute salt solutions and coagulable by heat; eg, serum globulin in blood.
(c) *Glutelins*, which are insoluble in water or dilute salt solution but soluble in dilute acid and alkali; eg, glutenin in wheat.
(d) *Prolamines*, which are insoluble in neutral solutions but soluble in 80% alcohol; eg, zein in corn and gliadin in wheat.
(e) *Albuminoids*, which are dissolved only by boiling in strong acids; eg, keratins in hair and horny tissue, elastins in tendons and arteries, and collagens in skin and tendons.
(f) *Histones*, which are basic in reaction, soluble in water but insoluble

Table IV—Amino Acid Composition of Selected Proteins[a]

	IUPAC Abbreviation	Gelatins	Milk:* mixed proteins	Casein	Serum albumin*	γ-Globulin	Hemoglobin: horse	Insulin	Clostridium botulinum toxin
Alanine	Ala	9.2	...	3.0	6.2	...	7.4	4.5	3.9
Arginine	Arg	8.8	4.2	4.1	6.0	4.8	3.7	3.1	4.6
Aspartic Acid	Asp	6.3	...	7.1	10.3	8.8	10.6	6.8	20.1
Cystine	CyS-SCy	0.1	1.0	0.3	6.5	3.1	1.0	12.5	0.8
Glutamic Acid	Glu	11.7	21.5	22.4	17.0	11.8	8.2	18.6	15.6
Glycine	Gly	30.5	2.3	2.7	2.0	4.2	5.6	4.3	1.4
Histidine	His	0.7	2.8	3.1	4.0	2.5	8.7	4.9	1.0
Hydroxyproline	Hyp	14.5	...	0	0	0?	0?	0?	...
Isoleucine	Ile	1.9	7.5	6.1	3.0	2.7	0?	2.8	11.9
Leucine	Leu	3.2	11.0	9.2	12.0	9.3	15.2	13.2	10.3
Lysine	Lys	5.1	8.7	8.2	12.7	8.1	8.5	2.5	7.7
Methionine	Met	0.9	3.2	3.4	1.3	1.1	1.0	0	1.1
Phenylalanine	Phe	2.1	5.5	5.0	7.0	4.6	7.7	8.1	1.2
Proline	Pro	16.3	...	11.3	5.1	8.1	8.5	2.5	2.6
Serine	Ser	3.8	4.3	6.3	7.0	11.4	5.8	5.2	4.4
Threonine	Thr	2.2	4.7	4.9	7.1	8.4	4.4	2.1	8.5
Tyrosine	Tyr	0.7	6.0	6.3	5.5	6.8	3.0	13.0	13.5
Tryptophan	Trp	0	1.5	1.2	1.0	2.9	1.7	0	1.9
Valine	Val	3.1	7.0	7.2	6.0	9.7	9.0	7.8	5.3

[a] The data in this table were taken from a more comprehensive table in Hawk, P B, *et al: Practical Physiological Chemistry*, 13th ed, Blakiston, New York, 1954, with the kind permission of the publishers. All values are in g/100 g of protein except those marked * which are in g/16 g total nitrogen.

in dilute ammonia, and difficultly heat-coagulable; eg, thymus histone and hemoglobin.

(g) *Protamines*, which are strongly basic in reaction and soluble in water, dilute acid, and ammonia; eg, salmin and sturin in fish sperm. They precipitate many other proteins.

2. Conjugated proteins are those proteins which are combined in nature with some nonprotein substance. They are classified according to the nature of the prosthetic (nonprotein) group. The classes, which are not mutually exclusive, include:

(a) *Phosphoproteins*—contain a phosphoric acid moiety as the prosthetic group, eg, casein in milk and ovovitellin in egg yolk.
(b) *Nucleoproteins*—the nonprotein portion is a nucleic acid; eg, nuclein in cell nuclei.
(c) *Glycoproteins*—simple proteins united to a carbohydrate group; eg, mucins in vitreous humor and saliva.
(d) *Chromoproteins*—contain a colored prosthetic group; eg, hemoglobin in blood, and flavoproteins.
(e) *Lipoproteins*—proteins in combination with lipid materials such as sterols, fatty acids, lecithin, etc.
(f) *Metalloproteins*—the prosthetic group contains a metal; eg, enzymes such as tyrosinase, arginase, and xanthine oxidase.

3. Derived proteins are substances formed from simple or conjugated proteins by various means such as the action of heat, acids, alkalies, water, enzymes, alcohol, radiant energy, and mechanical shock. They differ in one or more respects from the proteins from which they are formed; and, in general, the extent of this difference, as reflected by changes in various physical and chemical properties, constitutes the basis for the classification described below.

Primary derived proteins are commonly referred to as *denatured proteins*. They differ only slightly from the proteins from which they are derived, probably only in conformation, with the peptide linkages remaining pretty much intact. They are subdivided as follows:

(a) *Proteans*—These are insoluble substances formed during the early stages of the action of water, enzymes, or dilute acid on the original protein. They sometimes result merely from mechanical agitation of a solution of protein. Examples are fibrin from fibrinogen and myosan from myosin.
(b) *Metaproteins*—These are substances formed during the early stages of protein hydrolysis by means of acid or alkali. In general, they are easily soluble in dilute acids and alkalies; this is indicative of some hydrolytic cleavage of the peptide linkages in the original protein. They are insoluble in neutral solvents and, like most natural proteins, are coagulable. Examples are the acid and alkali albuminates.
(c) *Coagulated proteins*—These are insoluble substances formed from proteins usually by the action of heat or alcohol. They may also be pro-

duced from protein solutions by actinic irradiation, by mechanical shock, or by the application of high pressure. Coagulated egg albumin and cooked meat are familiar examples.

Secondary derived proteins are substances formed during the progressive hydrolysis of proteins; thus, in comparison with the primary derived proteins, they differ much more decidedly from their original proteins. Secondary derived proteins cover a very wide range of molecular weights, the weight in each case depending upon the extent of the hydrolytic cleavage of the original protein. They are subclassified into the following broad categories:

(a) *Proteoses*—These constitute the highest molecular weight group and thus represent the least hydrolyzed state of the original protein. They are generally more readily soluble in water than the original protein, and they are of sufficiently reduced complexity as to be noncoagulable by heat. Saturation of their aqueous solutions with ammonium sulfate causes them to precipitate.
(b) *Peptones*—These are lower in molecular weight than the proteoses and thus represent a more degraded hydrolytic state of the original protein. Like the proteoses, they are readily soluble in water and noncoagulable by heat. Due to their lesser molecular complexity, they are not precipitated (salted out) from aqueous solution by saturation with ammonium sulfate. They are precipitated as complexes, however, by phosphotungstic acid.
(c) *Peptides*—These are very small hydrolytic fragments of their original proteins. They contain from 2 to possibly 20 or so amino acids joined via amide linkages, and are commonly subdivided into di-, tri-, etc, peptides according to the number of amino acid residues they contain. Collectively, the higher members are often termed *polypeptides*. Various individual peptides have been isolated from protein hydrolysates. Many have also been synthesized, eg, oxytocin, qv, page 957. The peptides are readily soluble in water. They are noncoagulable by heat and are not precipitated from their solutions by saturation with ammonium sulfate.

Physical and Chemical Properties

In general, pure proteins are relatively odorless and tasteless. In their normal biologic environment, they are highly hydrated. Color varies. On heating, they decompose with or without simultaneous liquefaction, and emit the characteristic odor of singed hair. Since proteins are polyelectrolyte macromolecules with multifunctional groups it is not unlikely that they differ greatly in their physical properties; ie, their solubilities in such solvents as water, salt solutions, monohydric and polyhydric alcohols, and dilute acids and bases, forming colloidal solutions from which heat often precipitates the protein in coagulated form. Precipitation in unaltered form is frequently accomplished, especially at their isoelectric point, by means of salt solutions, eg, sodium chloride and ammonium sulfate, and by diluted ethanol. Many proteins have been obtained in crystalline form but, unlike crystalline substances in general, this is not necessarily evidence of homogeneity since some have been further resolved into two or more components through chromatographic, electrophoretic, and other procedures.

Although the exceptional vulnerability of proteins in general to chemical attack often requires careful control of reaction conditions, nevertheless their chemical characteristics are quite in accord with those to be expected from the functional groups present.

Tests for Proteins and Amino Acids—In addition to the modern chromatographic, electrophoretic, and other procedures mentioned previously, many older test methods still find useful application.

Before dwelling on the older test methods which find useful application, it is worthy of note that current technology is such that high performance liquid chromatographic procedures are becoming more and more useful for the separation and determination of not only the amino acid components themselves but of many of the smaller peptides as well. This is made possible with the advent of post column derivatization techniques with which the peptides and the amino acids are made chromophoric by the use of such fluorescent derivatives as the fluorescamine derivative, the PTH amino acid derivatives, the derivative formed by reaction in the orthophthaldehyde method, and the Dansyl derivative. The advent of these fluorescent and highly sensitive derivatives makes it possible to determine the concentration of individual amino acids and small peptides in mixtures in the *nanomole* and *picomole* range. The hydrolysis of protein yields amino acids which, on treatment with *nitrous acid*, liberate nitrogen. This reaction along with other techniques forms the basis of Van Slyke's nitrogen distribution method which has important uses in clinical chemistry. Amino acids and the free amino groups in proteins react with ninhydrin. The presence of peptide linkages can be shown by means of the *Biuret* test. Numerous color tests are available for individual amino acids, including the *Ehrlich* and *Hopkins-Cole* tests for tryptophan, the *Sakaguchi* test for arginine, the *nitroprusside* test for cystine and cysteine, the *Millon* test for tyrosine, the *xanthoproteic* test for tyrosine and phenylalanine, the *Pauly diazo* test for histidine and tyrosine, and the *basic lead* test for the sulfur-containing acids.

Precipitates are formed with amino acids on the addition of various reagents such as heavy metal salts, and certain acids such as picric, phosphotungstic, trichloroacetic, or sulfosalicylic acids. Simple tests for certain proteins are based on precipitation with heat or acid.

Precursor Functions of Amino Acids

In addition to their role as building blocks of proteins, the amino acids are precursors of many other important biomolecules, including various hormones, vitamins, coenzymes, alkaloids, porphyrins, etc. The aromatic amino acids are particularly versatile as precursors; from them are made many alkaloids, such as morphine, codeine, and papaverine, and a number of hormones. Although hormones are mentioned elsewhere, it should be stated here that with regard to the hormones that are involved in the biotransformation from amino acids, are included such hormones as the thyroid hormone, thyroxine; the plant hormone, indoleacetic acid; and an adrenal hormone, ephinephrine.

Uses for Amino Acids and Proteins

Nutrition—The nutritional value of proteins in our diet involves recognition of the quality as well as the quantity of the protein. Man does not have the ability to synthesize all the amino acids required for normal good health. Those that are required to be supplied by diet are called essential amino acids and include leucine, isoleucine, lysine, methionine, phenylalanine, threonine, tryptophan, and valine. In general it is recommended that an adult should take, in his daily diet, 1.5 g of protein/kg of body weight. Children require about two to three times this amount. Of course this assumes that the protein in the diet has an adequate amount of all essential and nonessential amino acids. Proteins found in eggs, beef, and milk are considered to have the best nutritional value.

Clinical Uses—Adequate protein nutrition requires the intake of sufficient protein to meet daily requirements. This protein must be of the necessary "quality," ie, supply the essential amino acids. Protein deficiency thus may be caused by a reduced intake, or the use of low-quality protein. Obviously, the actual intake of protein may be influenced by factors such as high excretion in conditions of kidney damage or blood loss, or an increased requirement associated with thyrotoxicosis or high fever. Symptoms of deficiency include loss of weight, nutritional edema, and skin changes and are associated with such conditions as nephrosis, sprue, and colitis. Deficiency may result also in a reduced resistance to infection since an adequate protein intake is necessary for the formation of phagocytes, leukocytes, and antibodies. Stress, such as brought on by accidental or surgical trauma, pregnancy, and lactation may also cause a deficiency of amino acids and greater intakes of protein are required in these conditions. The disease kwashiorkor has been shown to respond to adequate supplies of proteins.

For the treatment of protein deficiency several types of products are available. High-protein natural foods should be used where possible. Protein concentrates such as skim milk powder to which may be added casein and lactalbumin are also available. Where the bulk of high-protein foods is undesirable or where the patient is unable to digest whole protein, hydrolysates or mixtures of crystalline amino acids may be indicated (for description, see pages 1027 to 1029).

Official Amino Acids—Those α-amino acids that have official status include alanine, arginine, cysteine, histidine, isoleucine, leucine, lysine, proline, serine, tryptophan, tyrosine, valine, and methionine as racemethionine.

Alkaloids

Sertürner's paper, in 1817, "Morphis, a New Salt-forming Substance, and Meconic Acid, as the Chief Constituents of Opium," opened a new era of discovery in organic plant chemistry. His isolation of the first alkaloid was soon followed by the isolation of narcotine by Robiquet and strychnine by Pelletier and Caventou. These basic compounds were at first called vegetable alkalies, but were later renamed alkaloids, meaning alkali-like. It is of special interest to note that many of the most important alkaloids were discovered by pharmacists.

Alkaloids, as the active principles of many plants, were isolated and announced in rapid succession by various investigators. Various genera of 158 botanical families have yielded compounds with alkaloidal properties. A few are obtained from Cryptogams (flowerless plants), but the majority are extracted from the Phanerogams (flowering plants), most of them being from dicotyledons. The monocotyledons are not excluded since some useful alkaloids are found in species of the *Amaryllidaceae* and *Liliaceae* families. In this connection, it is interesting to note that phytochemists estimate that less than 5% of the known flowering plants have been investigated for possible alkaloid content. Specific alkaloids of complex structures are ordinarily confined to specific plant families (*hyoscyamine*, in *Solanaceae*, *colchicine* in *Liliaceae*). Nicotine, which is found in a number of widely scattered plant families is not an exception to this rule because

Table V—A Partial Classification of Alkaloids

Nucleus	Plant genera	Alkaloids
Benzazulene	Aconitum, Delphinium	Aconitine, delphinine, delsoline
Imidazole	Pilocarpus	Pilocarpine, pilocarpidine, pilosine, *pseudo*pilocarpine, *pseudo*jaborine, *iso*pilocarpine
Indole	Peganum, Psilocybe, Stropharia, Evodia, Corynanthe, Claviceps, Physostigma, Strychnos, Rauwolfia	Brucine, ergonovine, ergotamine, harmine, physostigmine, psilocybin, reserpine, strychnine, yohimbine
Isoquinoline	Hydrastis, Papaver, Corydalis, Berberis, Chondodendron, Ipecacuanha, Sanguinaria	Anhalonine, bebeerine, cephaëline, codeine, corydaline, cotarnine chloride, emetine, erythramine, erythroidine, hydrastine, menispermine, morphine, papaverine, sanguinarine, tubocurarine chloride
Phenylalkylamine	Ephedra, Lophophora	Ephedrine
Purine	Guarana, Cola, Coffea, Thea, Theobroma	Caffeine,[a] theobromine,[a] theophylline[a]
Pyridine	Anabasis, Areca, Conium, Lobelia, Piper, Punica, Ricinus, Nicotiana	Anabasine, aphylline, arecaidine, arecoline, coniine, guvacine, lobeline, nicotine, pelletierine, piperine, ricinine, trigonelline
Quinoline	Cinchona, Cusparia	Cinchonine, cinchonidine, cusparine, ethylhydrocupreine, quinacrine, quinine, quinidine
Quinolizine	Anagyris, Laburnum, Lupinus, Sophora	Anagyrine, cytisine, lupanine, lupinine, matrine, sparteine
Steroidal[b]	Solanum, Veratrum, Lycopersicon, Holarrhena, Schoenocaulon	Cevadine, cevine, conessine, jervine, rubijervine, solanidine, solanine, tomatidine, veratramine, veratridine
Tropane	Erythroxylon, Atropa, Datura, Hyoscyamus, Scopola	Atropine, benzoylecgonine, cocaine, eucatropine, homatropine, hygrine, hyoscyamine, scopolamine

[a] Some authors do not classify these relatively feebly basic compounds as alkaloids.

[b] Various nuclei are represented in this group. In general, they have some resemblance to the steroid (cyclopentanophenanthrene) nucleus.

of the biosynthetic simplicity of its structure. However, the occurrence of ergot alkaloids in the fungus *Claviceps purpurea* and certain *Ipomoea species* (*Convolvulaceae*) is a definite exception and may be attributed to either parallel or conversion evolution of certain complex biochemical pathways.

Notwithstanding the many extremely valuable synthetic medicinal and antibiotic agents that have been added to the list of weapons against disease, the alkaloids still constitute an indispensable and most potent group of substances for the treatment and mitigation of functional disturbances and relief from suffering. It is for this reason that some of the larger pharmaceutical firms maintain continuing programs for the pharmacologic screening of alkaloids, both new and old. Reserpine, much valued today for its antihypertensive and psychotherapeutic actions, emerged from such a program in the 1950s; and an intensive current effort with the *Vinca* (*Catharanthus*) alkaloids has already yielded some oncolytic drugs of value in the treatment of certain types of cancer.

A few alkaloids have been made synthetically and there are also a number of synthetic drugs of an alkaloidal character which do not occur in nature. Distinction should be made between *total synthesis*, in which the end product is the result of chemical processes which employ only materials that can be built up from the elements (carbon, hydrogen, oxygen, etc.), and *partial synthesis* in which the end product is produced from a naturally occurring complex substance which is already closely related structurally to the desired end product (eg, the synthesis of ergonovine from lysergic acid).

In their native environment, alkaloids usually exist in the form of salts, frequently of the simple organic acids such as lactic, malic, tartaric, and citric. Unusual, often distinctive, acids are also encountered, eg, quinic with cinchona and meconic with opium alkaloids. In addition to their basic nitrogen moiety, alkaloids usually contain one or more chemically functional groups. Thus, cocaine contains two ester functions, quinine contains both the secondary alcohol and aromatic methoxy functions, ergonovine contains a substituted amide function, etc. Some alkaloids, eg, solanine and tomatine, actually occur as glycosides.

Perhaps alkaloids should be viewed as products of metabolic experimentation that reflect the intermediary evolutionary stages now obtained by plants. Alkaloid formation might best be described as a metabolic act involving longer or shorter reaction sequences that begin with substances normal and essential in plant metabolism and end with compounds not necessarily serving such a purpose. This process is genetically controlled and, as such, an alkaloid-producing plant is merely a plant in which the additional metabolical reaction has evolved through mutation of one or more genes. Proof that such changes occur regardless of the utility of the element products is given by the thousands of pigments, tannins, polysaccharides, glycosides, volatile oils, and resins to which no essential role in plant metabolism can be ascribed. Therefore, this assumed "metabolic error" will probably be eliminated when plants approach the stage of ultimate adaptation and eliminate all redundant features and processes. They are thus the kind of waste product retained within the organism that produces them. Unlike many substances with which we are familiar, the alkaloids are structurally complex end products of energy requiring reaction sequences.

Classification—Alkaloids may be classified in a variety of ways, eg, according to source, chemical structure, pharmacologic action, etc. Any attempt at comprehensive chemotaxonomic classification is far beyond the scope of concern in this text; for such treatment, consult the continuing encyclopedic work of Manske and Brossi (see *Bibliography*). A partial classification which includes most of the more important pharmaceutical alkaloids is presented in Table V. As in all such condensed classifications, caution must be exercised in interpreting the entries under "Nucleus." Different hydrogenated forms of a given nucleus are often presented in different alkaloids, eg, nicotine contains pyridine whereas piperine contains hexahydropyridine (piperidine). Also, some alkaloids contain more than one nucleus, eg, quinine contains both quinoline and quinuclidine. In many instances, the nucleus shown in the table is merely the best known fragment of the total fused ring system actually present in the alkaloid. Thus, for example, while it is true that each of the ergot alkaloids contains an indole ring in its nucleus, actually the indole is but a fragment of the fused tetracyclic ring system, indolo[4,3-*fg*]quinoline, which constitutes the total nucleus. The complete heteronuclei represented in official alkaloids are included in the display of heterocycles in Table VI, page 387.

Table VI—Classification of Opium Alkaloids

Benzylisoquinoline Group
Codamine [$C_{20}H_{25}NO_4$][d]
Gnoscopine [$C_{22}H_{23}NO_7$][e,b]
Laudanidine [$C_{20}H_{25}NO_4$][d]
dl-Laudanine [$C_{20}H_{25}NO_4$][d]
Laudanosine [$C_{21}H_{27}NO_4$][d]
Narceine [$C_{23}H_{27}NO_8$][a]

Narcotoline [$C_{21}H_{21}NO_7$][e,b]
l-Narcotine [$C_{22}H_{23}NO_7$][e,b]
Oxynarcotine [$C_{22}H_{23}NO_8$][e,b]
Papaverine [$C_{20}H_{21}NO_4$][c]
Xanthaline [$C_{20}H_{19}NO_5$][c]

Cryptopine Group
Cryptopine [$C_{21}H_{23}NO_5$][i]

Protopine [$C_{20}H_{19}NO_5$][f]

Alkaloids of Unknown Structure
Lanthopine [$C_{23}H_{25}NO_4$]
Meconidine [$C_{21}H_{23}NO_4$]

Papaveramine [$C_{21}H_{25}NO_6$]
Rhoeadine [$C_{21}H_{21}NO_6$]

Phenanthrene Group
Codeine [$C_{18}H_{21}NO_3$][h]
Morphine [$C_{17}H_{19}NO_3$][h]
ψ-Morphine [($C_{17}H_{18}NO_3)_2$][h]

Neopine [$C_{18}H_{21}NO_3$][g]

Thebaine [$C_{19}H_{21}NO_3$][f]

Tetrahydroisoquinoline Group
Hydrocotarnine [$C_{12}H_{15}NO_3$][e]

Quinoline Group
Aporeine [$C_{18}H_{17}NO_2$][l]

Derivatives of Natural Alkaloids
Apomorphine[k]
Hydrocodone (dihydro-codeinone)
Hydromorphone (dihydro-morphinone)
Dionine (ethylmorphine)

Heroin (diacetylmorphine)
Metopon (methyldihydro-morphinone)
Nalorphine (N-allylnor-morphine)
Naloxone
Oxymorphone
Oxycodone

---

[a] 2,3-dihydrobenzofuran (coumaran); (1328)
[b] 1,3-dihydroisobenzofuran (phthalan); (1330)
[c] isoquinoline; (1708)
[d] 1,2,3,4-tetrahydroisoquinoline; (1708)
[e] 5,6,7,8-tetrahydro-1,3-dioxolo[4,5-g]isoquinoline; (2810)
[f] 8,9-dihydro-4H-8,9c-iminoethanophenanthro[4,5-bcd]furan; (5922)
[g] 5,6,8,9-tetrahydro-4aH-8,9c-iminoethanophenanthro[4,5-bcd]furan; (5922)
[h] 5,7a,8,9-tetrahydro-4aH-8,9c-iminoethanophenanthro[4,5-bcd]furan; (5922)
[i] 6,7,12,13,14,15-hexahydrobenzo[e]-1,3-dioxolo[4,5-l][2]benzazecine; (4874)
[j] 4,5,6,7,13,14-hexahydrobis[1,3]benzodioxolo[4,5-c:5',6'-g]azecine; (5777)
[k] 4H-dibenzo[de,g]quinoline; (5171)
[l] 6,7,7a,8-tetrahydro-5H-benzo[g]-1,3-benzodioxolo[6,5,4-de]quinoline; (5846)

Properties—The more important characteristic features of alkaloids are the following:

1. In addition to carbon and hydrogen they all contain nitrogen and generally also oxygen. The nitrogen, which is usually contained in whole or in part in the heteronucleus, confers the alkali-like properties to alkaloids.
2. Most of the nonvolatile alkaloids are solid; the volatile ones are mainly liquid and these often contain no oxygen.
3. They are mainly crystallizable, though a few are amorphous. Some, eg, nicotine, are liquid (as the free alkaloid) under ordinary conditions.
4. They are generally white though berberine is yellow and sanguinarine, itself colorless, yields red salts.
5. They are either insoluble or sparingly soluble in water (with a few exceptions, such as colchicine) but soluble in alcohol, chloroform, benzene, some in ether, and a few in petroleum benzin. Their salts behave conversely in the matter of solubility.
6. Most of them are physiologically active, some being extremely poisonous. In the majority of instances they are medicinally important substances of the plants from which they are derived.
7. Alkaloids unite with acids to form substituted ammonium salts. The stability of these salts toward hydrolysis varies with the basic strength of the alkaloid and the nature of the acid used. With the exception of the xanthine group, most common alkaloids have pK values less than 7. The alkaloids are freed from their salts by the addition of alkali.
8. They are precipitated by one or more of the following reagents; with some they form definite chemical compounds which are used for their identification: mercuric-potassium iodide (Mayer's reagent); potassium-cadmium iodide (Marme's reagent); potassium-bismuth iodide (Dragendorff's reagent); phosphomolybdic acid (Sonnenschein's reagent); a solution of iodine with potassium iodide (Wagner's reagent); phosphotungstic acid (Scheibler's reagent); gold chloride; tannic acid; and picric acid.

Identification—Various kinds of tests have been devised to identify known alkaloids. Their effective use, however, usually requires some relevant knowledge of the history of the sample under examination. In general, these tests involve combinations of two or more of the following: melting points of the alkaloid and at least one of its salts or other derivatives, specific rotation, solubility in various solvents, color reactions with specified reagents, and microscopic examination of the crystals obtained by the action of suitable precipitants under controlled conditions.

Closely related alkaloids such as morphine and codeine do not differ sufficiently in their absorption of ultraviolet light to permit differentiation on the basis of their respective spectrograms. However, the infrared spectrum of an alkaloid is individual and if a reference spectrum is available identification can be made with certainty. Modern high resolution NMR techniques make possible even more definitive identification.

Extraction—In a representative type of process the crude milled drug is moistened with an aqueous alkali such as sodium carbonate, sodium bicarbonate or lime—to liberate the alkaloids from their salts—and percolated with benzene, ether, or some other suitable water-immiscible solvent. The solvent layer is extracted with dilute acid to convert the alkaloids into salts and to bring them into the aqueous phase. The free alkaloids, substantially without other plant materials, are precipitated by the addition of alkali and then separated by appropriate means. The operations involved are based on the physical as well as the chemical properties of the alkaloids sought. Purification is usually accomplished by the crystallization of the alkaloidal salts, but distillation and other procedures are also employed.

In some cases, when the alkaloidal content of a drug is low, and large volumes of dilute aqueous solutions are obtained, it is of advantage to adsorb the alkaloids on ion-exchange resins (page 606). If the several alkaloids adsorbed on a resin differ sufficiently in basicity, it may be possible to effect at least a partial separation of the alkaloids in the course of the elution from the resin.

An excellent example of the problems encountered and of some of the modern techniques employed in the separation of a complex mixture of alkaloids is provided by the review[1] of researchers on the *Vinca* alkaloids.

Synthesis—This section briefly presents significant aspects of the very active and diverse roles synthetic organic chemistry has in the alkaloid field.

On the one hand, the total synthesis of a complex alkaloid, eg, strychnine (Chapter 62), even though it has no probable future practical manufacturing importance, is recognized as a monumental achievement; on the other hand, the emergence of what seemed like a simple effective substitute for morphine (methadone) caused a flurry of activity in laboratories throughout the world and resulted in the publication of hundreds of individual chemical research reports and the results of numerous pharmacological investigations. Each type of development will undoubtedly continue to affect the status of alkaloidal drugs.

Total syntheses are usually undertaken with the purely scientific objective of adding to our knowledge. The molecular structure of an alkaloid is deduced from experiments in which (1) the identity of its chemically functional groups is established, and (2) the alkaloid is degraded to simpler fragments. The nature of these functional groups and of the fragments and their own reactions lead to a hypothesis concerning the structure of the original material.* This hypothesis is expressed in the form of a written structural formula or other model, which must adequately explain the chemical and physicochemical properties (spectra, X-ray analysis, nuclear magnetic resonance, etc) of the alkaloid. Final confirmation of the hypothesis can come only from a total synthesis which, step by step, employs unequivocal reactions and at each stage in the buildup produces intermediates of proved structure.

Since the final products usually have several chiral centers, syntheses are further complicated by the requirement that they proceed through stages which will lead to the product with a stereochemical configuration corresponding to that of the natural product. This requirement imposes the need for inventing at appropriate steps stereospecific means for proceeding to the next step or, alternatively, for choosing at a given step, from among a mixture of intermediate products, only the one which is suitable for the further transformations contemplated.

The achievement of a total synthesis is a result of imagination, intellect, and experimental skill. Whether the methods that are used to reach the objective will lend themselves to technological exploitation is usually not germane to the issue. It is, therefore, often very unlikely that total chemical synthesis will compete economically with the processes for deriving the more complex alkaloids from natural sources.[†]

However, the outlook for synthetic analogues of and substitutes for alkaloids is different. Procaine has displaced cocaine to a notable extent; similarly for many uses the synthetic quinolines have replaced quinine, and synthetic morphinan derivatives are replacing some opium alkaloids. From the long-range point of view it appears likely that many of the naturally occurring alkaloids currently in use will eventually be at least partly supplanted by synthetic products.

Using the structural formula of an alkaloid as a prototype, efforts have been made to determine the *pharmacodynamically* important portion of the molecule, that is, the structural arrangement of atoms or groups mostly responsible for the main physiological action of the compound. Once this has been determined (often quite empirically), synthetic variants of the fundamental structure are prepared and tested until a single compound, or family of compounds, is found which offers greatest promise for further pharmacologic study.

The structural resemblance among several alkaloids and their respective analogues or substitutes can be seen from tables presented throughout this chapter.[§] It will also be noted that in some cases large sections of the alkaloidal molecule are not reproduced in the synthetic molecule because they are not fundamentally involved in the physiological effect produced. Very often, also, the complicated stereochemistry of the natural product is not followed in detail in the construction of the synthetic product; morphine has several centers of asymmetry whereas meperidine has only one.

Speculations concerning the *biogenesis* of alkaloids have had fruitful results in increasing our understanding of nature and in stimulating the invention of novel synthetic processes. A biogenetic theory attempts to deduce how the plant, using intermediates known to be present in it, and known conditions of temperature, pH, etc ("physiological conditions"), is able to elaborate a whole group of alkaloids and sometimes several chemical classes of alkaloids. An effort may then be made to reproduce these conditions *in vitro*.

The building blocks of the alkaloids are presumed to be the amino acids and their metabolic degradation products. Formaldehyde sources (eg, glyoxylic and formic acids) are also available, and biological processes of deamination, decarboxylation, and oxidation are operative. How the plant effects the synthesis is best determined by a study of the plant chemistry itself, but *in vitro* experiments often provide strong clues.

Incompatibilities—Most alkaloids are soluble in alcohol and other organic solvents and insoluble in water; they react with acids to form salts which usually are soluble in water and only slightly soluble in alcohol. The addition of a *base*, therefore, to an aqueous solution of an alkaloidal salt, will generally precipitate the free alkaloid. In the same manner, *alkaline salts* such as the *acetates*, *carbonates*, *citrates*, *benzoates*, *salicylates*, and *basic phosphates* of sodium, potassium, and ammonium will precipitate the free alkaloid from such a solution, or, in some instances, will convert it to a less soluble salt.

Iodine and *tannic acid*, sometimes prescribed with alkaloids, form insoluble compounds with most alkaloids. An occasional difficulty arises from the use of a galenical made from a tannin-containing drug. Frequently, a very small amount of alcohol will suffice to prevent these precipitations.

Many of the alkaloids are soluble in liquid petrolatum, while the salts are generally insoluble. Other alkaloids can be rendered soluble in liquid petrolatum by conversion to the oleates.

As a general rule, alkaloids are incompatible with *oxidizing agents*, some undergoing oxidation readily on exposure to air. Various antioxidants such as sodium metabisulfite and sodium sulfite are effective in retarding this deterioration. Oxidation is more rapid in alkaline solution and buffers which maintain the solution at a pH designed to retard it are commonly used. The rate of hydrolysis of ester and glycosidic alkaloids is pH-dependent.

Classification—Alkaloids may be classified in a variety of ways, eg, on a botanical, or chemical, or pharmacological, etc, basis. Various systems are employed depending upon the nature of the primary interests of the various authors. Each system has its advantages and disadvantages, and a realistic appraisal of the present situation points to the firm conclusion that much more needs to be learned about the occurrence, composition, and physiological actions of the alkaloids before a comprehensive classification having maximum practical utility can be produced. The usual chemical classifications take into account the cyclic nuclei and the number, locations, and types of substituent functional groups; and, while it is abundantly evident that these classifications have led to the charting of research paths which have yielded very useful synthetic drugs, nevertheless it is equally clear that the present state of correlation between pharmacologic actions and various features of molecular architecture leaves much to be desired. This has led to a current revival of interest in the various stereochemical aspects of alkaloids in an attempt to resolve the many anomalies, and expectations are high that sufficiently intensive investigation in this area of endeavor will yield useful information.

For the purpose of the abbreviated presentation in this

---

* The review article on *Vinca* alkaloids provides a good illustration of structural elucidation.

[†] It is conceivable that a combination of chemical and biological means (use of enzymes, etc) may in certain cases lead to practical synthesis of alkaloids, but this is not true total synthesis.

[§] Often in the past this resemblance was noted only after the therapeutic effectiveness of a synthetic had been discovered. At the present time more and more alkaloid substitutes are "tailor-made" by design.

chapter, the alkaloids are classified under the following headings.

1. Opium Alkaloids
2. Cinchona Alkaloids
3. Tropane Alkaloids
4. Xanthine Alkaloids
5. Ergot Alkaloids
6. Rauwolfia Alkaloids
7. Veratrum Alkaloids
8. Vinca Alkaloids
9. Miscellaneous Alkaloids

Special attention is called to the fact that the following display is limited strictly to natural alkaloids and derivatives of these which may be produced by effecting relatively simple chemical operations. Deliberately avoided in this section has been any attempt to include synthetic compounds such as (1) meperidine, methadone, and the several synthetic morphinan derivatives which are often included in other texts in the opium group; (2) chloroquine, hydroxychloroquine, and other synthetic antimalarials which are often presented with alkaloids of the cinchona group; (3) eucatropine, procaine, and other synthetics often presented with alkaloids of the tropane group; etc.

Structural Formulas and Nomenclature—The structural formulas for all alkaloids in this text are presented in the style adopted by Chemical Abstracts. This style portrays the alkaloids in what has been termed their "absolute configuration," ie, portrays the stereochemistry of all asymmetric centers, and is employed whenever the stereochemical configuration is definitive and can be expressed unambiguously by the Cahn–Ingold–Prelog sequence convention.

The treatment of alkaloids by Chemical Abstracts frequently abandons the systematic (Ring Index) names in favor of stereospecific trivial names such as aporphine, morphinan, yohimban, etc. It frequently also departs from Ring Index orientation and numbering in favor of schemes more commonly used in the reporting literature. As to be expected, these differences in orientation and numbering are also reflected in differences in nomenclature and thus complicate further literature searches and structural comparisons of compounds. The preferred Chemical Abstracts names for all official alkaloids and alkaloid salts are provided as subtitles to the monograph captions at other locations in the text.

For a detailed discussion of the Chemical Abstracts method of naming, structuring, and indexing alkaloids, see the Introduction to Vol 66 Subject Index and Vol 76 Index Guide to Chemical Abstracts.

Opium Alkaloids

Opium is official as such, and its monograph, along with those on official items containing it, are presented in Chapter 60.

The many alkaloids obtained from the opium poppy, *Papaver somniferum*, are often divided into the following five approximate chemical "groups": (1) *Benzylisoquinoline*, (2) *Phenanthrene*, (3) *Tetrahydroisoquinoline*, (4) *Cryptopine*, and (5) *Alkaloids of Unknown Structure*, and the classification shown in Table VI, giving trivial name, systematic name, and Ring Index designation, is on this basis. An additional group is provided to accommodate the important semisynthetic derivatives of morphine and codeine. The specific heteronuclei present are identified by footnotes; the number in parentheses following the name is the Ring Index (2nd ed) number.

It will be observed that the pharmaceutically important alkaloids displayed in Table VII derive from the so-called benzylisoquinoline and phenanthrene groups.

The parent heterocycle of the phenanthrene group of alkaloids is 4a*H*-8,9*c*-iminoethanophenanthro[4,5-*bcd*]furan. In the hexahydro state characteristic of codeine and morphine, its Ring Index (IUPAC) orientation and numbering are shown below. The specific stereoisomer present in these alkaloids is shown at the right in Chemical Abstracts style which treats

it as a 4,5α-epoxymorphinan and numbers it by the familiar Cahn–Robinson sequence.

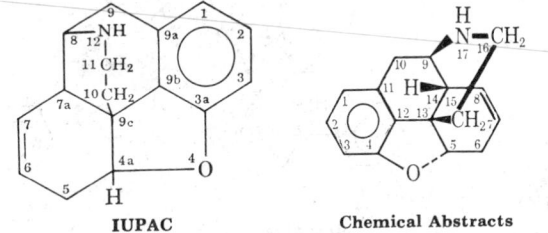

| IUPAC | Chemical Abstracts |

Official Opium Alkaloids and Derivatives

Opium alkaloids and derivatives, official as such and/or as salts, include: Apomorphine, Codeine, Hydrocodone, Hydromorphone, Morphine, Nalorphine, Naloxone, Oxycodone, Oxymorphone, and Papaverine.

Cinchona Alkaloids

There are more than twenty alkaloids obtainable from the bark of various species of *Cinchona* and *Remijia* (*Cuprea*) and many of these are convertible by chemical processes into closely related, useful, synthetic derivatives.

The most important alkaloids of cinchona are the pair of diastereoisomers, *quinine* and *quinidine*, and their 6-demethoxy analogues, *cinchonine* and *cinchonidine*. The structural formulas in Table VIII indicate the close relationships between the various members of this group of alkaloids.

Examination of the formulas of these compounds shows that they all contain a *quinoline* ring attached through a hydroxymethylene group to a *quinuclidine* ring.

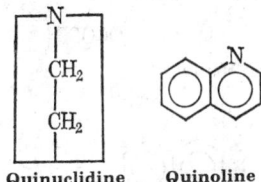

Quinuclidine   Quinoline

By altering the side chains attached to these rings and by esterifying and/or oxidizing the alcohol group, a large number of compounds have been produced and investigated.

Quinine and quinidine both have a *methoxy* group attached to the quinoline ring and a *vinyl* group attached to the quinuclidine ring. Each has the same four centers of asymmetry, but the diastereoisomerism involves only the configurations at the carbinol and 2-quinuclidine carbon atoms. Cinchonine and cinchonidine differ from these two alkaloids in that they do not have a methoxy group on the quinoline ring. Quinidine and cinchonine are dextrorotatory whereas quinine and cinchonidine are levorotatory. *Hydroquinine*, obtained from quinine by reduction with hydrogen and a catalyst, has the same structure as quinine except the vinyl group is reduced to an ethyl group. *Cupreine*, another naturally occurring cinchona alkaloid, has an OH group in place of the methoxy group, and *hydrocupreine* is cupreine with an ethyl group instead of a vinyl group. Thus quinine is the 6-methyl ether of cupreine and hydroquinine is the corresponding ether of hydrocupreine. Quinine was first synthesized in 1944 by Woodward and Doering but the process is too costly for commercial use.

The salts of the alkaloids are typical amine salts. Since there are two nitrogen atoms present in the molecules of the cinchona alkaloids it is possible to form salts containing one or two equivalents of acid, eg, mono- and di-hydrochlorides.

Identification—Quinine and its diastereoisomer, quinidine, are characterized (1) by the blue fluorescence of their solutions in dilute sulfuric or other oxyacids and (2) by the *thalleioquin reaction*. The addition of 2 drops of bromine

Table VII—Opium Alkaloids and Derivatives

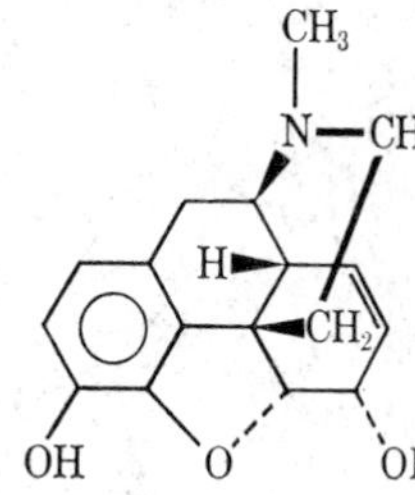

Morphine

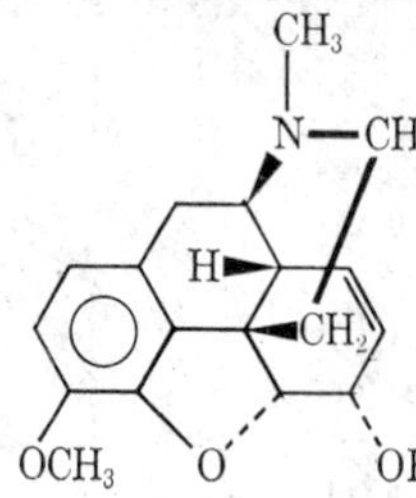

Codeine

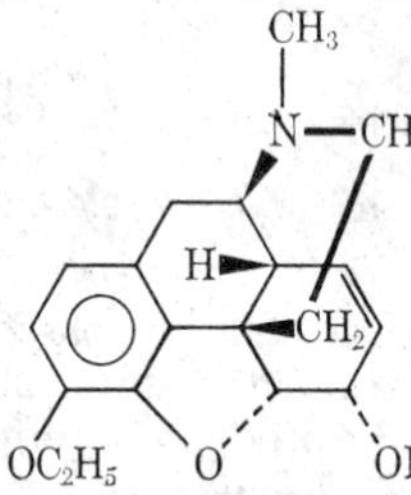

Ethylmorphine

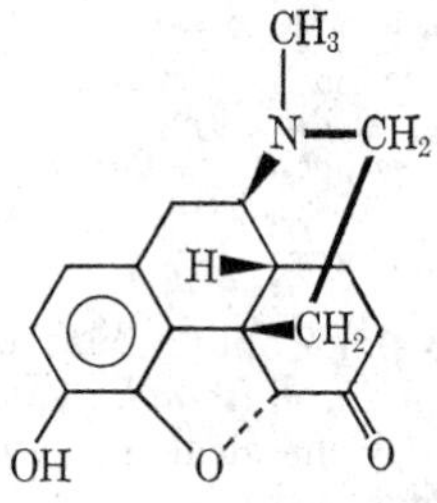

Hydromorphone

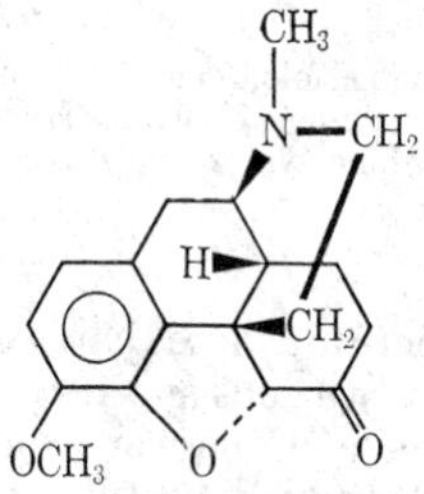

Hydrocodone

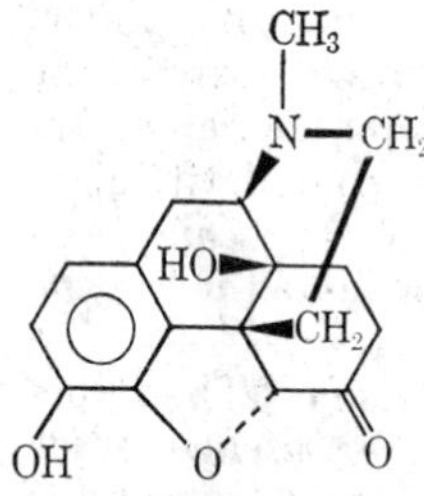

Oxymorphone

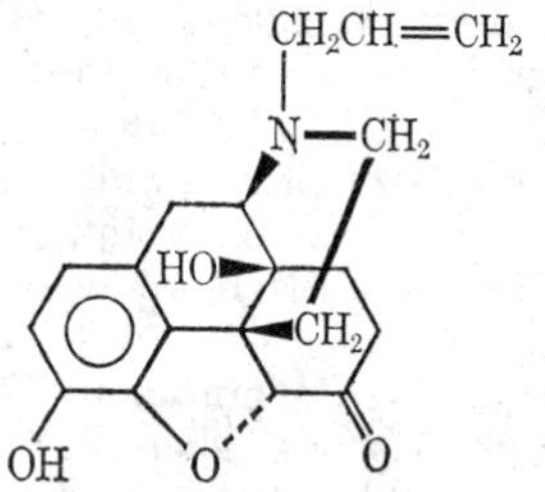

Naloxone

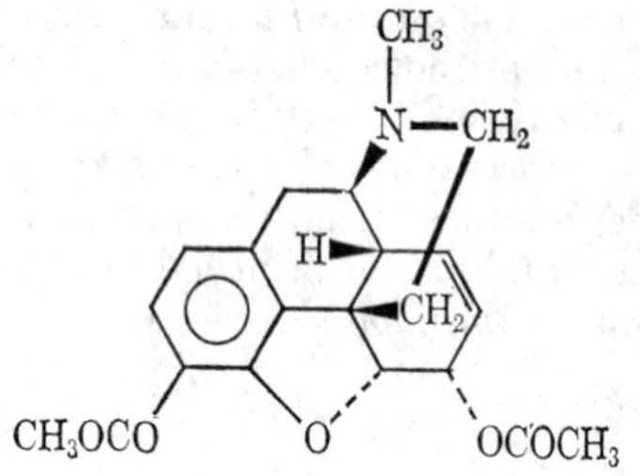

Heroin

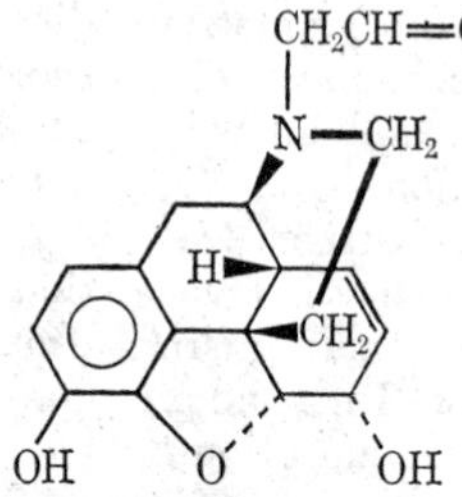

Nalorphine

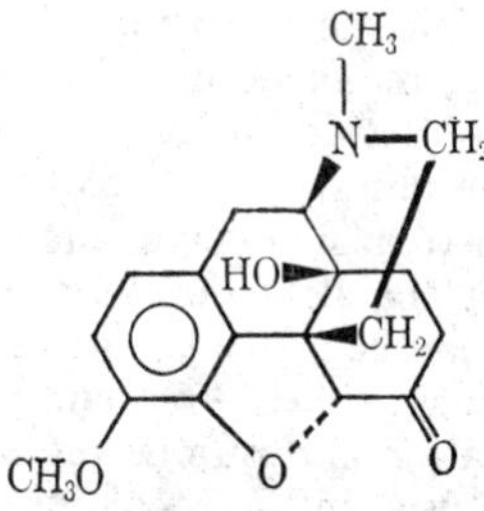

Oxycodone

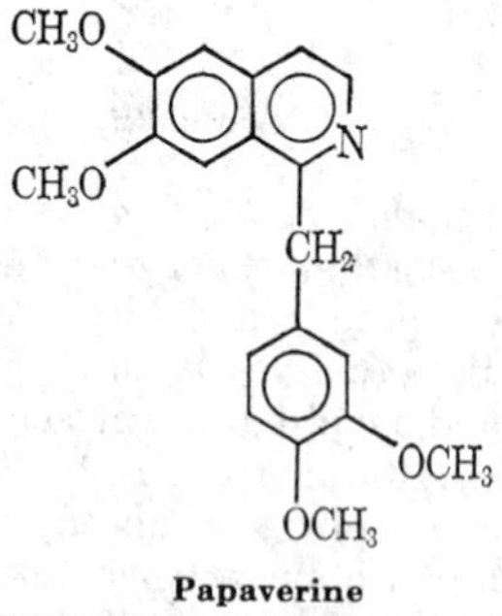

Papaverine

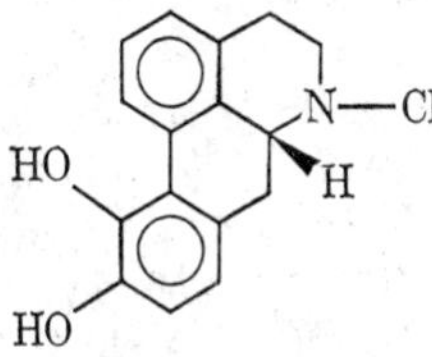

Apomorphine

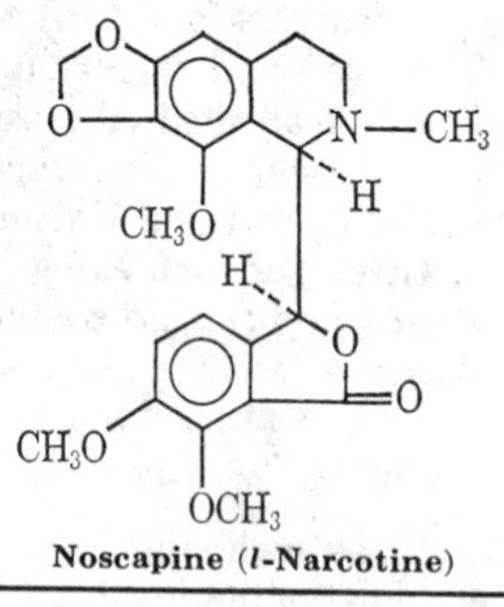

Noscapine (*l*-Narcotine)

TS to 5 mL of a saturated solution of quinine or quinidine or a 1:1000 solution of their salts, followed by 1 mL of ammonia TS produces an emerald green color due to the formation of thalleioquin. They are differentiated by their optical rotations and by their behavior toward alkali tartrate. In neutral or slightly acid solutions quinine is precipitated by this reagent, while quinidine is not. On the other hand, quinidine in moderately dilute solution is precipitated by soluble iodides but quinine is not affected. The same differences are exhibited by cinchonidine and its diastereoisomer cinchonine; the former is levorotatory and, like quinine, it is precipitated by alkali tartrates while cinchonine is unaffected by the reagent and is dextrorotatory.

Cinchona

Cinchona Bark; Peruvian Bark

The dried bark of the stem or of the root of *Cinchona succirubra* Pavon et Klotzsch or its hybrids, known in commerce as Red Cinchona, or of *Cinchona Ledgeriana* (Howard) Moens et Trimen, *Cinchona Calisaya* Weddell or hybrids of these with other species

of *Cinchona*, known in commerce as Calisaya Bark or as Yellow Cinchona (Fam. *Rubiaceae*).

Cinchona yields 5% of the alkaloids of cinchona. The crude drug is no longer official.

History—This drug derives its name from the Countess of Cinchon, who was instrumental in introducing it into European medical practice in 1640. It was also called Jesuit's Bark in recognition of the fact that it was used by the members of this ecclesiastical order in treating fever and ague. Its adoption as a valuable official remedy followed the purchase by Louis XIV, in 1680, of the secret of a proprietary remedy sold by an English apothecary's clerk named Robert Talbor, which contained cinchona as a basis. The romance of Cinchona has been published in various books and is well worth perusal.

Constituents—Other than quinine, quinidine, cinchonine and cinchonidine, 18 other alkaloids have been isolated from cinchona barks. Some of these are found in only one kind of bark, as cupreine, and some are doubtless "split products"—that is, not existing naturally in the bark, but the result of the action of chemical agents upon it.

The acids present in Cinchona are quinic acid (*hexahydro-1,3,4,5-tetrahydroxybenzoic acid*), quinotannic acid, and quinovic acid (*3β-hydroxyurs-12-ene-27,28-dioic acid*). Also present are

Table VIII—Cinchona Alkaloids and Derivatives

Quinine

Quinidine

Cinchonine

Cinchonidine

Hydroquinine

Quinine Ethylcarbonate

Cupreine

Hydrocupreine

Ethylhydrocupreine

α-quinovin (a glycoside), *cinchona-red*, other coloring matter and a volatile oil.

The quinine and total alkaloid content is highest in bark from cultivated cinchona. In bark from the uncultivated plant cinchonine and cinchonidine predominate. Java bark, representing highly cultivated cinchona, contains 7 to 10% of total alkaloids of which about 70% is quinine.

Uses—Little used in modern therapeutics in the US, but is elsewhere employed as a cheap substitute for quinine. It shares the *antimalarial, antipyretic,* and *analgetic* actions of quinine, but the alkaloidal salts are to be preferred to the galenical preparations.

One of the principal difficulties in preserving galenical preparations of cinchona arises from the alteration and precipitation which the cinchotannic acid and its compounds undergo on storage. Glycerin has proved to be very useful by dissolving and holding these in solution, and hence it is present in nearly all of the preparations.

Dose—*Usual,* 1 g.

Official Cinchona Alkaloids

Cinchona alkaloids official as such and/or salts, include: Quinidine and Quinine.

Tropane Alkaloids

The Tropane alkaloids will be considered under two headings: (1) Atropine and Related Alkaloids and (2) Cocaine.

They are grouped together because all are formally derivatives of tropane.

Tropane

Atropine and Related Alkaloids

The alkaloids of the atropine group (Table IX) are closely related chemically. Most of the natural alkaloids are esters of *mandelic acid* or *tropic acid* with *tropine** or *scopine.* For example, atropine is the racemic variety of tropine tropate, hyoscyamine is the levorotatory enantiomorph of the same compound, and scopolamine is scopine tropate. Scopine is epoxytropine, the only difference being the 6,7-oxygen bridge. It is therefore to be expected that these three alkaloids give similar color reactions. Eumydrine is also closely related; it is 8-methylatropinium nitrate, a quaternary ammonium salt. Homatropine is tropine mandelate and Novatropine is 8-methylho-

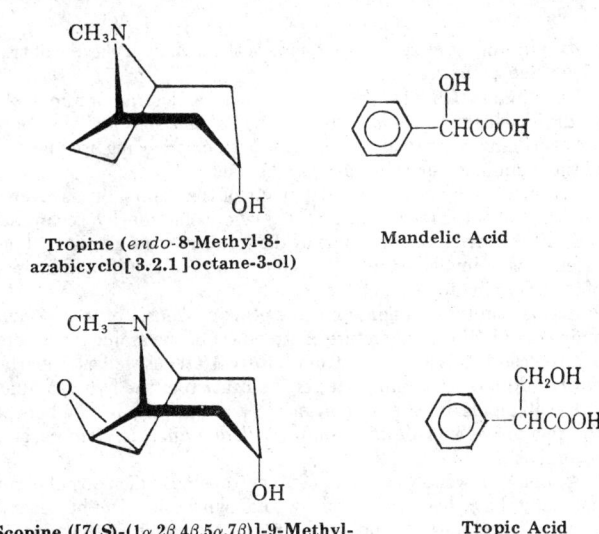

Tropine (*endo*-8-Methyl-8-azabicyclo[3.2.1]octane-3-ol)

Mandelic Acid

Scopine ([7(*S*)-(1α,2β,4β,5α,7β)]-9-Methyl-3-oxa-9-azatricyclo[3.3.1.0²,⁴]nonan-7-ol)

Tropic Acid

* Esters of tropine are called tropeines; eg, tropine mandelate is mandelyltropeine.

Table IX—Atropine and Related Alkaloids and Derivatives

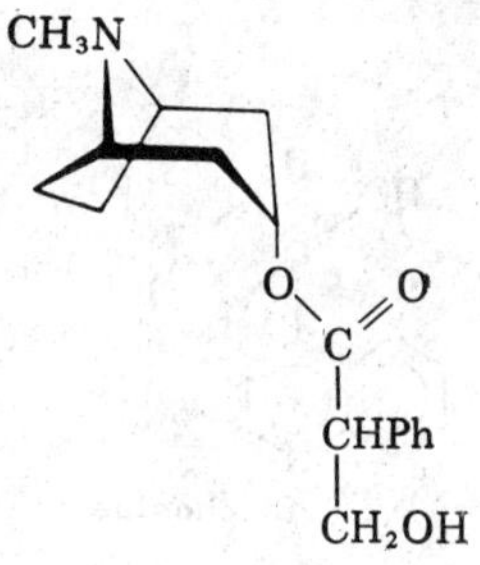

Atropine
(Tropine(±)-Tropate)

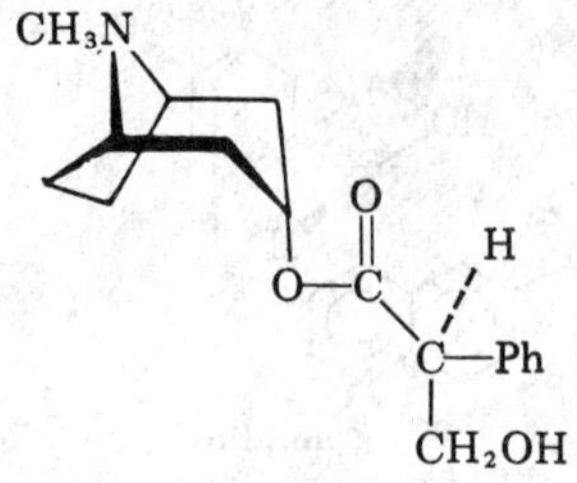

Hyoscyamine
(Tropine(-)-Tropate)

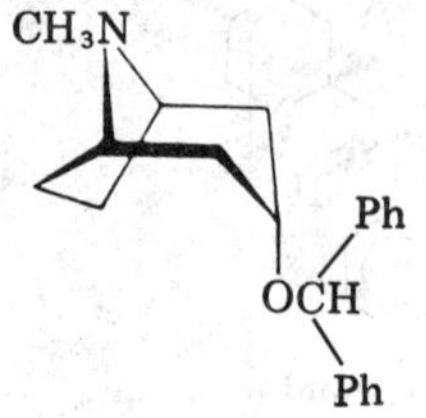

Benztropine

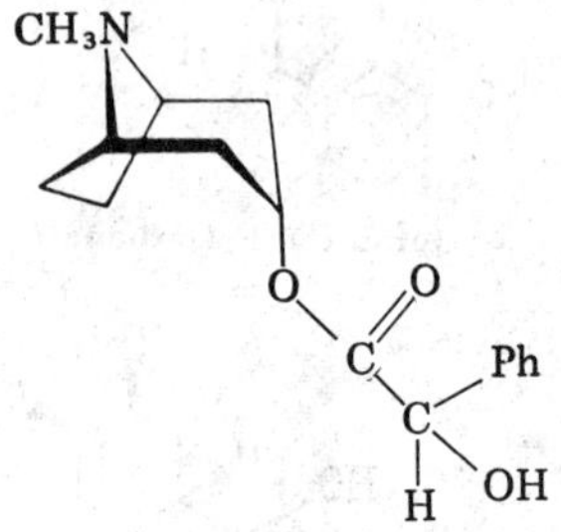

Homatropine

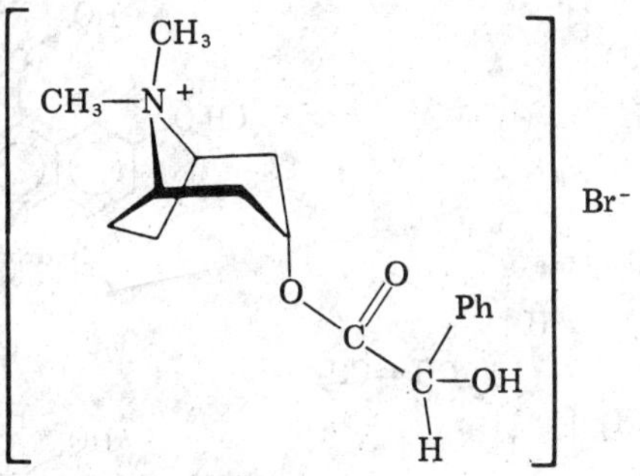

Novatropine
(Homatropine Methylbromide)

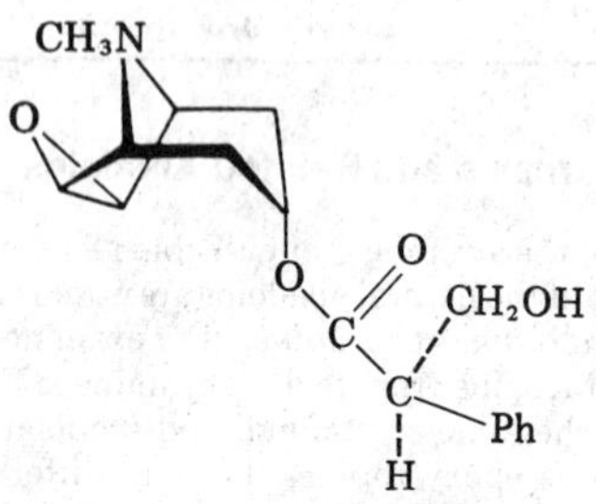

Scopolamine
(6β,7β-Epoxyhyoscyamine)

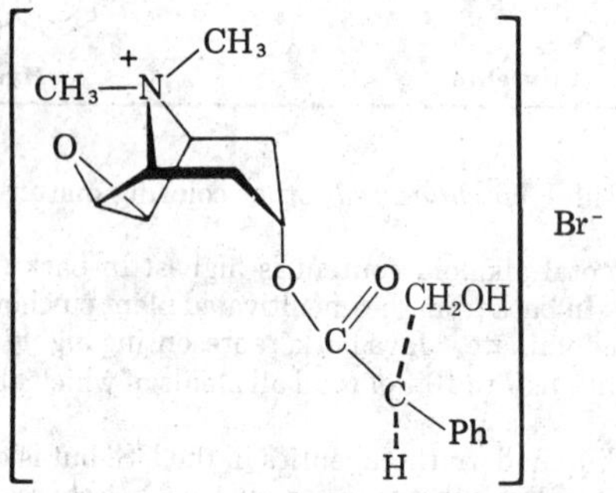

**Methscopolamine
Bromide**

matropinium bromide. Benztropine is the benzhydryl ester of tropine. See Table IX.

Belladonna (Chapter 48), hyoscyamus, and stramonium yield mydriatic alkaloids, characteristic of the *Solanaceae* Family. There are also many other plants of this group which are being used largely in the manufacture of the various alkaloids.

Atropine rarely occurs as such in any of the plants, but is always the product of the racemization of the levo-isomeride, hyoscyamine, which is converted into atropine by the action of weak alkalies. This racemization involves the conversion of the (−)-tropic acid moiety of hyoscyamine to (±)-tropic acid.

In this country stramonium is the principal source of the hyoscyamine used in the manufacture of atropine. Scopolamine (hyoscine) is produced to a large extent from *Datura Metel* as well as from the mother liquors remaining after crystallization of the hyoscyamine. Other alkaloids of lesser importance present in various members of the *Solanaceae* include *atropamine, belladonnine, meteloidine,* and several others.

Atropine, as well as a number of other tropeines which do not occur naturally, have been prepared by total synthesis. Of the several classical syntheses of tropine the most interesting is that due to Robinson[4] in 1917. Variations of this process are employed commercially. Racemic tropic acid has also been synthesized and resolved.

The most characteristic physiological property of the Solanaceous alkaloids is their mydriatic effect (dilation of the pupil of the eye).

This property is the basis for the most sensitive test for their identification. As little as one drop of a 1 in 25,000 solution will cause a distinct dilation of the pupil of a cat's eye.

Cocaine and Related Alkaloids

The cocaine group of tropane alkaloids is distinguished chemically from the atropine group by the presence of an *exo*-carboxyl (or esterified carboxyl) at the 2-position and by the *exo*-configuration (instead of *endo*-) of the 3-ester function. They thus become derivatives of ecgonine ([1R-(*exo,exo*)]-3-hydroxy-8-methyl-8-azabicyclo[3.2.1]octane-2-carboxylic acid) having the general structure:

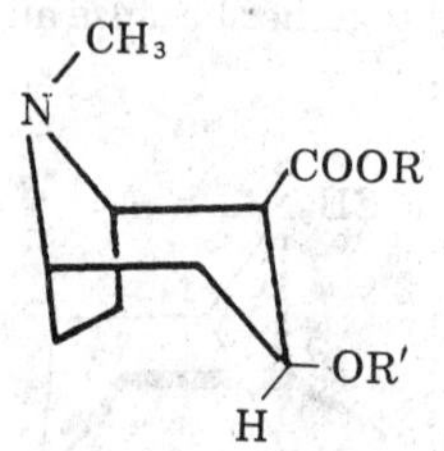

Table X portrays the identities of R and R′ for the common ecgonine derivatives. For further discussion, see *Cocaine*, page 1055.

Table X—Ecgonine Derivatives

R	R'	Name of derivative
H	H	Ecgonine
CH_3	C_6H_5CO-(benzoyl)	Cocaine
H	CH_3	Methylecgonine
H	$C_6H_5CH{=}CHCO$-(cinnamoyl)	Cinnamoylecgonine
H	C_6H_5CO	Benzoylecgonine

Official Tropane Alkaloids and Derivatives

Tropane alkaloids and derivatives, official as such and/or as salts, include: Atropine, Benztropine, Cocaine, Homatropine, Hyoscyamine, Scopolamine, and Methscopolamine.

Xanthine Alkaloids

The purine base alkaloids, better known as the xanthine alkaloids, have three important medicinal agents. These three comprise the bulk of this group. These alkaloids are caffeine, theophylline, and theobromine. These three agents are bases which are all methylated derivatives of 2,6-dioxy-purine (xanthine). The structural relationships of the xanthine alkaloids or purine alkaloids are portrayed in Table XI. The parent molecule of each one is purine. The common practice of portraying the two-dimensional structure in box form is still the one that is used primarily. For example, the xanthine structure can be represented by the following formula:

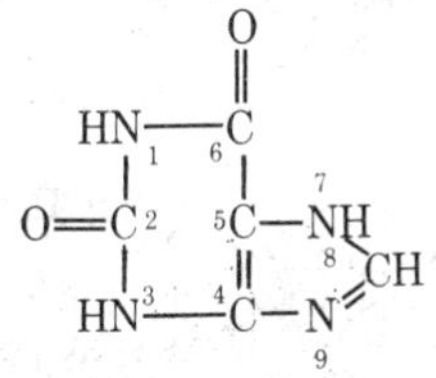

Other bases closely related to purine are *hypoxanthine*, *adenine*, and *guanine*, all of which are normally found in animal tissues. The primary significance of the last two bases is the fact that they are constituents of nucleic acids and nucleoproteins which are found in cell nuclei, and the fact that hypoxanthine is produced in the body during the first stage of adenine oxidation. Subsequent oxidation yields *xanthine*, and finally, *uric acid*. In man the end product of protein metabolism is *urea*. In certain animals the end product is *allantoin*, which is formed by further oxidation of uric acid. The two-dimensional structures of these compounds are illustrated in Table XI. The oxygen-containing compounds are depicted here in keto form but they are often shown in

texts in enol form as illustrated below with xanthine. As noted, the presence of oxygen in several of these structures also causes a slight alteration in the position of unsaturation because of the tautomerization which can occur. The enol forms are often named specifically to reflect the hydroxyl groups, eg, purine-2,6,8-triol or 2,6,8-trioxypurine for uric acid.

Properties—The xanthines are very weak bases, having a pK_b of approximately 13–14. They form salts with the stronger acids which, of course, are readily hydrolyzed. By tautomeric shift of hydrogen from nitrogen to keto oxygen (enolization) a weakly acidic H (pK_a of about 9) is formed on the resulting OH group. Thus xanthine, along with various other oxopurines, and their derivatives form salts with the stronger bases. Having no NH group to participate in enolization, caffeine is an exception.

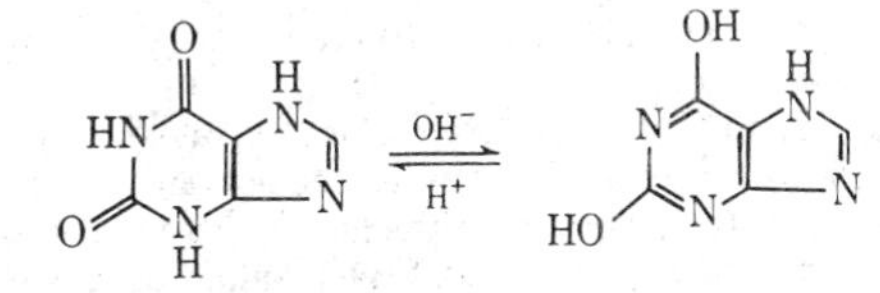

keto structure   enol structure

The xanthines are characterized by the murexide reaction which involves evaporating a nitric acid solution of the test sample to dryness and treating the residue with ammonia whereupon a purplish-red color develops. The color is due to the formation of murexide, an ammonium salt of purpuric acid. Uric acid and various other purine derivatives also respond to the test.

Official Xanthine Alkaloids and Derivatives

Xanthine alkaloids and derivatives, official as such and/or as salts, include: Aminophylline [Theophylline Ethylenediamine Compound (2:1)], Caffeine, and Theophylline.

Ergot Alkaloids

Ergot

Ergot is a morbid growth formed when the fungus *Claviceps purpurea* develops on various plants of the Gramineae (grass) and Cyperaceae (sedge) families such as rye, wheat, oats, barley, and rice. If the infestation of the plant occurs naturally, the resulting ergot is called *natural* ergot; if the infestation is brought about artificially, ie, wholly or partly by man through intention, the resulting ergot is referred to in the trade as *cultivated* ergot. Ergots from different plants vary in composition and they are thus not medicinally equivalent. It is for this reason that rye is stipulated as the source of the official ergot.

Table XI—Xanthine Alkaloids

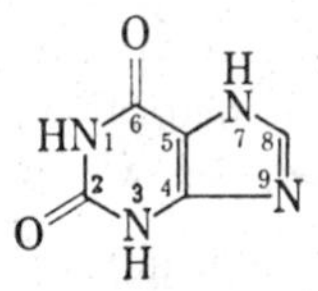

Xanthine
(3,7-Dihydro-1*H*-purine-2,6-dione)

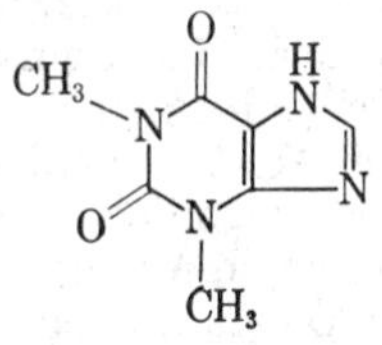

Theophylline
(1,3-Dimethylxanthine)

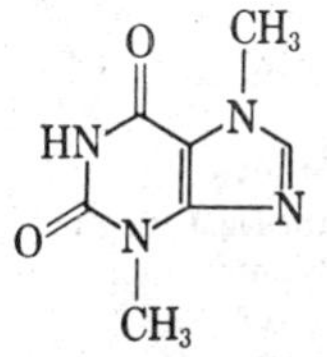

Theobromine
(3,7-Dimethylxanthine)

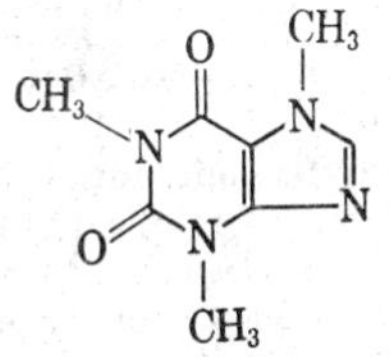

Caffeine
(1,3,7-Trimethylxanthine)

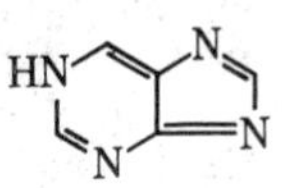

1*H*-Purine

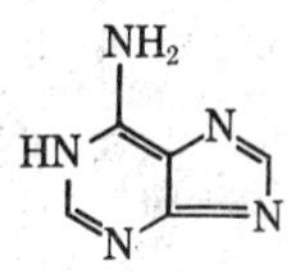

Adenine
(1*H*-Purin-6-amine)

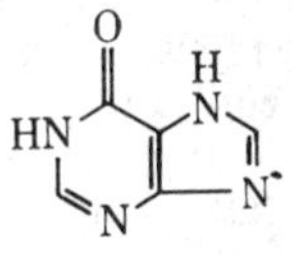

Hypoxanthine
(1,7-Dihydro-6*H*-purine-6-one)

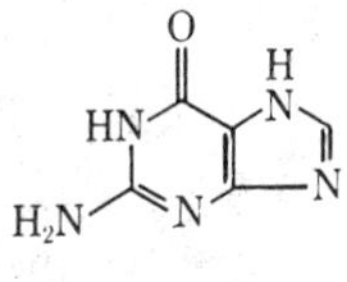

Guanine
(2-Amino-1,7-dihydro-6*H*-purine-6-one)

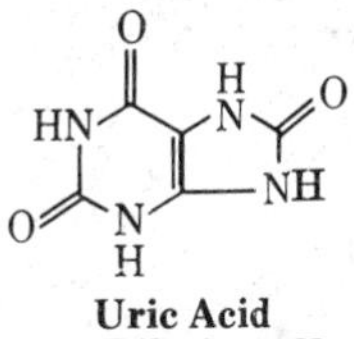

Uric Acid
(7,9-Dihydro-1*H*-purine-2,6,8(3*H*)-trione)

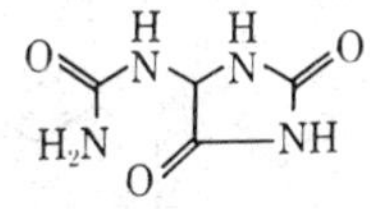

Allantoin
(2,5-Dioxo-4-imidaz-olidinyl)urea

Constituents—Ergot has been referred to as a veritable storehouse of chemicals. In addition to many alkaloids, it contains various carbohydrates, glycerides, sterols (eg, ergosterol and fungisterol), amino acids (eg, histidine, leucine, and tyrosine), amines (eg, histamine and tyramine), quaternary ammonium compounds (eg, choline and betaine), and coloring principles. The lysergic acid group of alkaloids are the important medicinal constituents, and further treatment here is confined to them. They are all substituted amide derivatives of lysergic acid, which is shown below along with the official compounds and the important, but unofficial, diethylamide.

An understanding of the ergot alkaloids requires a knowledge of the isomerism of lysergic acid which exists in two diastereoisomeric forms depending on the spatial configuration of the carboxyl group relative to that of the 5β-hydrogen. In the *normal* lysergic acid (commonly called lysergic acid) this relative configuration is of the *cis* variety (carboxyl in β-configuration); in the *iso*lysergic acid, it is of the *trans* type (carboxyl in α-configuration). Chemical Abstracts treats lysergic and isolysergic acid compounds as derivatives of ergoline which is the 4,6,6aβ,7,8,9,10,10aα-octahydro form of indolo[4,3-*fg*]quinoline, Ring Index No 4550.

Ergot has yielded 12 different, well-defined alkaloids, each of which is an *N*-monosubstituted amide of either the normal or the isolysergic acids. The substituting group on the amide nitrogen is commonly referred to as the *peptide moiety* of the alkaloid because it always contains one or more peptide (amide) linkages.

Ergonovine, simpler by far than any of the other ergot alkaloids, is commercially available both as the natural alkaloid and as a synthetic compound (see page 947). The crude lysergic acid required for the synthesis is readily prepared by subjecting the total ergot alkaloid fraction to alkaline hydrolysis and then acidifying. Lysergic acid itself has been synthesized starting with the commercially available coal tar derivative indole-3-propionic acid but the synthesis is lengthy and the present cost is unfavorable. A microbiologic synthesis utilizing *Claviceps paspali* and suitable for relatively large scale manufacture has been patented.

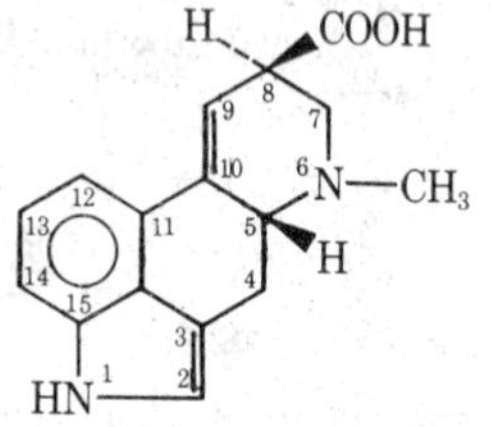

Lysergic Acid
(9,10-Didehydro-6-methylergoline-8β-carboxylic Acid)

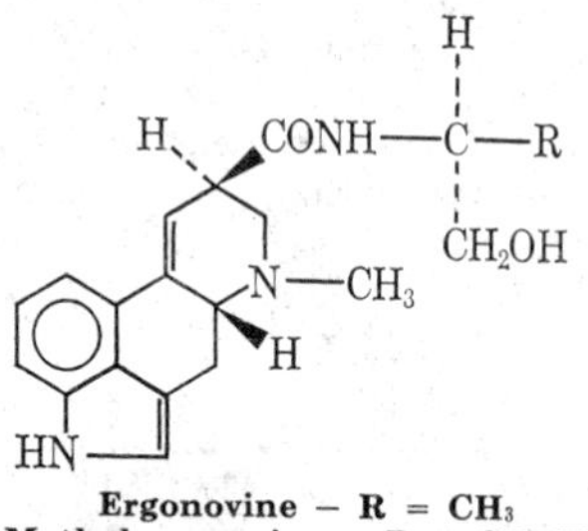

Ergonovine – R = CH₃
Methylergonovine – R = CH₂CH₃

Methylergonovine is not a natural ergot alkaloid. It is synthesized from lysergic acid by the same procedure as that employed for *Ergonovine* (see page 948) except that (+)-2-amino-1-butanol is used to furnish the peptide moiety.

Methysergide, another unnatural alkaloid, is the 1-methyl homologue of methylergonovine.

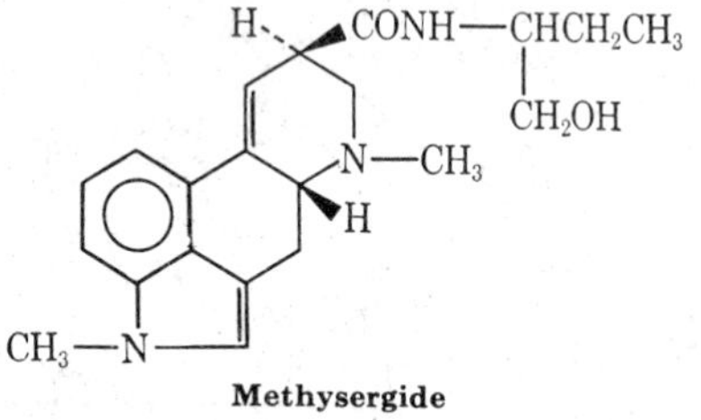

Methysergide

N,N-Diethyl-D-lysergamide, a compound of considerable interest, does not occur in nature. The physiological active isomer is the (+)-enantiomorph of the *N,N*-diethylamide of normal lysergic acid and is commonly referred to as LSD-25 or simply LSD. Methods for its synthesis from lysergic acid have been developed. In normal subjects, LSD elicits a temporary combination of physiological and psychological effects which collectively mimic syndromes characteristic of psychotic states, eg, schizophrenia. LSD has been the subject of intense clinical investigation since the mid-1960s. There are no established therapeutic applications at present, but it has found some application as a diagnostic tool in psychiatry (see page 1098) and as a tool in psychopharmacology. Discovery of the psychotogenic activity of LSD has led to extensive research with various types of lysergic acid derivatives. It has also given rise to serious social problems.

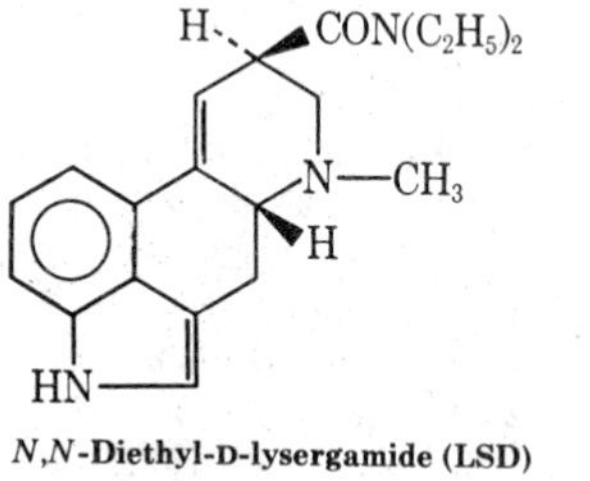

N,N-Diethyl-D-lysergamide (LSD)

Dihydro analogues of lysergic acid and its derivatives form readily by catalytic hydrogenation, the addition occurring at the expense of the 9:10 double bond. Such hydrogenation of the ergot alkaloids results in marked changes in their physiological actions (see *Dihydroergotamine*, page 947). Dihydro-LSD is relatively devoid of psychotogenic action.

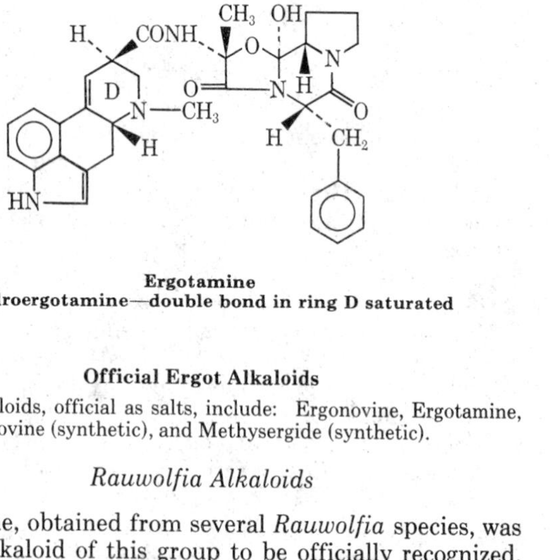

Ergotamine
Dihydroergotamine—double bond in ring D saturated

Official Ergot Alkaloids

Ergot alkaloids, official as salts, include: Ergonovine, Ergotamine, Methylergonovine (synthetic), and Methysergide (synthetic).

Rauwolfia Alkaloids

Reserpine, obtained from several *Rauwolfia* species, was the first alkaloid of this group to be officially recognized. Interest in the remarkable therapeutic properties of these powerful agents became so keen that reserpine alkaloid, injection, and tablets were admitted to the USP XV by Supplement (1959). Rescinnamine soon followed, NF XI (1960), and Syrosingopine gained NF XII recognition (1965). Currently, only reserpine has official status.

The general structure of these three alkaloids is shown below. Chemical Abstracts uses the familiar Barger, Scholz numbering. It will be observed that they are all esters of methyl reserpate, the only difference being in the identity of the acyl group represented in the ester group at locus 18 of the heteronucleus. By the Chemical Abstracts system, methyl reserpate is the methyl ester of 18β-hydroxy-11,17α-dimethoxy-3β,20α-yohimban-16β-carboxylic acid. Yohimban is the 4aβ,13bα,14aα stereoisomer of the 1,2,3,4,4a,5,7,8,-13,13b,14,14a-dodecahydro form of Ring Index No 5874, benz[*g*]indolo[2,3-*a*]quinolizine. Reserpine and Rescinnamine occur naturally; Syrosingopine is synthetic.

Alkaloid	Acyl
Reserpine	3,4,5-trimethoxybenzoyl
Rescinnamine	3,4,5-trimethoxycinnamoyl
Syrosingopine	carbethoxysyringoyl

History—The genus *Rauwolfia*, natural order *Apocynaceae*, contains almost fifty species which grow in tropical and semitropical regions (India, Burma, Ceylon, Java, etc). The genus name honors a German physician and botanist of the 16th century, Leonard Rauwolf, who made a study of medicinal plants in Asia and Africa. The most extensively investigated species at the present time are *R serpentina* Benth, *R canescens* Linn, *R vomitoria* Afzel, and *R heterophylla*, Roem.

In ancient literature mention is made of the use of *Rauwolfia* as a remedy for snake bites and scorpion stings, as a febrifuge, and as a cure for dysentery. The sedative action of the drug was also noted, for it was considered useful in "moon's disease" (lunacy), to induce sleep in children, and in hypochondria.

Despite this long history, very few pharmacological and chemical studies were undertaken on *Rauwolfia* until the Indian investigators Bose and Sen reported successful clinical trials with the drug (1941); the Indian chemists Siddiqui and Siddiqui had isolated the first crystalline alkaloid from the plant in 1931. At present, at least 21 substances have been reported from *R serpentina* alone, which, when assayed as directed, contains not less than 0.15% of reserpine-rescinnamine group alkaloids, calculated as reserpine.

Preparations—*Rauwolfia* preparations (known collectively as Rauwolfia) are available to the pharmaceutical manufacturer in the form of powdered whole root, extracts, selected alkaloidal fractions,* the pure crystalline alkaloids *reserpine* and *rescinnamine*, and the synthetic, *syrosingopine*. For further discussion of the official crude drug, Rauwolfia, see page 908.

Uses—The most prominent actions of the rauwolfia alkaloids are upon the cardiovascular and central nervous systems. They are widely employed as *antihypertensive agents* and as *adjuncts in psychotherapy*.

Veratrum Alkaloids

The veratrum alkaloids are derived from 12 known species of *Veratrum*, the more important of which are *viride*, *album*, *sabadilla*, and *grandiflorum*. The alkaloids may be divided into two groups for which the designations *jerveratrum* and *ceveratrum* have been proposed. Practically all of the alkamines (alkaloids cleaved of ester or glucose moieties) of both groups are polyhydroxylated $C_{27}N$ fused polycyclics which, because they bear some resemblance to the steroid nucleus and also carry the 3β-OH characteristic of natural sterols, are often termed steroidal. In the jerveratrum group, the alkamines contain only 2 or 3 oxygens and the alkaloids consist either of the free alkamine, eg, *jervine* and *rubijervine*, or of the alkamine in D-glucosidic union, eg, *veratrosine*. In the ceveratrum group, the alkamines contain from 7 to 9 oxygens and the alkaloids consist of esters of the alkamines. The

jerveratrum group is devoid of therapeutic activity and further treatment is therefore confined to the ceveratrum group.

Ceveratrum nucleus

The alkamines of the ceveratrum alkaloids are all polyhydroxy derivatives of 4,9-epoxycevane which is shown in the column at the left in Chemical Abstracts orientation and numbering. It is an epoxytrimethyl derivative of a stereospecific hydrogenated form of Ring Index Parent No 11363. Many published papers portray an alternate orientation and numbering.

The relationship among the four alkamines is apparent from the following:

Alkamine	Type of polyol	Location of hydroxyl groups
Veracevine $C_{27}H_{43}NO_8$	heptol	3β,4β,12,14,16β,17,20
Germine $C_{27}H_{43}NO_8$	heptol	3β,4β,7α,14,15α,16β,20
Protoverine $C_{27}H_{43}NO_9$	octol	3β,4β,6α,7α,14,15α,16β,20
Zygadenine $C_{27}H_{43}NO_7$	hexol	3β,4β,14,15α,16β,20

The alkamines can be obtained by subjecting their ester-alkaloids to mild alkaline hydrolysis. In contrast to the ester-alkaloids, the alkamines are relatively devoid of pharmacologic activity.

A partial listing of the ceveratrum alkaloids is presented in Table XII. Listed also are the alkamines along with their loci of esterification and the acids involved. For a complete listing of all veratrum alkaloids (both jerveratrum and ceveratrum groups), consult the Morgan and Barltrop reference.[2] Kupchan and associates have conducted research in-depth on the intimate chemistry of veratrum alkaloids. Under the general title *Veratrum Alkaloids*, their findings have been reported in a lengthy series of papers which, although published in various journals, can be located readily through the *Author Index* to *Chemical Abstracts*.

Uses—Certain veratrum alkaloids and alkaloid mixtures find some use as antihypertensive agents. For further discussion, see *Veratrum Alkaloids*, page 850. The crude drug, Veratrum Viride, was official for many years prior to 1960. Neither it nor any of the veratrum alkaloids is currently official.

Vinca Alkaloids

Pharmacological inquiries during the late 1950s into the purported antihyperglycemic activity of principles contained in the apocynaceous plant, *Vinca rosae* Linn., led to the initial discovery that two of the alkaloidal constituents, vincaleukoblastine and leurosine, possessed certain demonstrable kinds of oncolytic (antitumor) activity. The same inquiries provided evidence of the presence of other alkaloids having similar activity, and pursuit of this lead bore fruit in the later discovery of leurocristine and leurosidine.

The overall result of these discoveries has been that the plant has been the subject, for more than a decade, of one of the most intensive phytochemical studies on record. Upwards of 50 different alkaloids have been demonstrated to be present, and more than half of these are recognized as new

---

* For example, Rauwiloid (*Riker*) and Rautensin (*Dorsey*) contains the fraction known generically as alseroxylon which is claimed to be less toxic over long range administration when compared to other crude Rauwolfia extracts.

chemical compounds. The complete structure has been determined for most of the compounds which have been isolated.

The therapeutic efficacy of vincaleukoblastine and leurocristine has been sufficiently established to accord them official status in the USP in the form of their (1:1) sulfates as antineoplastic agents. The structures of these two closely related alkaloids are portrayed below. The four-ring heterosystem is a stereospecific hydrogenated form of 10H-3,7-methanoazacycloundecino[5,4-b]indole, Ring Index No 13276, and the five-ring system is a similar form of 1H-indolizino[8,1-cd]carbazole, Ring Index No 11065. Leurosine and leurosidine are under clinical investigation.

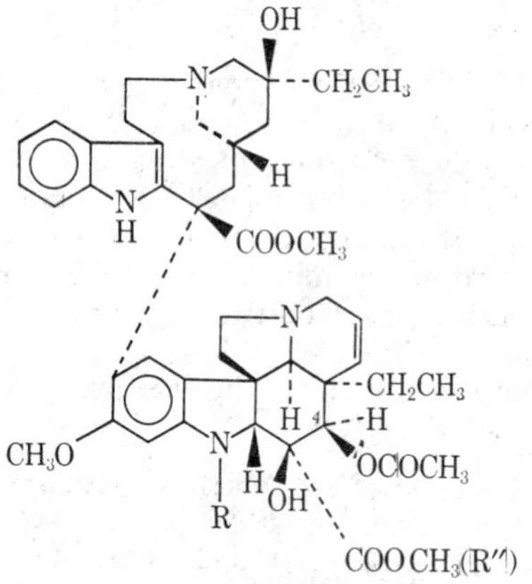

Vinblastine (vincaleukoblastine), R = CH₃
Vincristine (leurocristine), R = CHO
Vinglycinate, R = CH₃, R' = OCOCH₂N(CH₃)₂
Vindesine, R = CH₃, R' = OH, R" = CONH₂

The costliness of vinblastine and vincristine has provided increased interest in producing them synthetically. The five-ring indoline system is known to be available from other natural alkaloid sources, so effort at present is concentrated on synthesizing the four-ring indole system in suitably substituted form for coupling with the indoline moiety. Vinglycinate and vindesine are additions wherein the structure has been synthetically modified.

An excellent review of the accomplishments during the first 7 years of intense research on the Vinca alkaloids with an extensive bibliography is available.[3] For further discussion of the official articles, see the monographs on Vinblastine Sulfate and Vincristine Sulfate at other locations in this text.

Official Vinca Alkaloids

Vinblastine and Vincristine.

Miscellaneous Alkaloids

Several official and unofficial alkaloids, eg, Arecoline, Colchicine, Emetine, Ephedrine, Metocurine Iodide, Physostigmine, Pilocarpine, Tubocurarine, etc, do not fall within the classes of alkaloids presented in this chapter. For locations of discussions of these, consult the general index.

Volatile Oils

Volatile oils, or *essential oils*, are found in various plant organs and tissues. In some countries they are called *olea aetherea*. In some instances they are called *essences*, a name which conflicts with our ordinary use of that word which designates an alcoholic solution of a volatile oil. They usually constitute the savory and odorous principles of the plants in which they exist, and they either pre-exist in the tissues or are produced by the reaction of certain constituents when the tissues are brought into contact with water. Volatile oils are sometimes formed through destructive distillation, as the oils

of tar and of amber, these being occasionally referred to as *pyrolea* or *empyreumatic oils*.

Constituents

In some volatile oils, as thyme, a separation into a solid and a liquid portion occurs on standing in the cold. The solid portion is frequently known by the name *stearoptene*, and the liquid portion is called *eleoptene*. Some of the stearoptenes are of commercial importance (examples: thymol, camphor, menthol).

The following groups of compounds occur in the volatile oils: hydrocarbons, alcohols, acids, esters, aldehydes, ketones, phenols and phenol ethers, lactones, and various nitrogen and sulfur organic compounds.

The hydrocarbons of chief importance are the *terpenes* ($C_{10}H_{16}$) and the *sesquiterpenes* ($C_{15}H_{24}$; literally, "one and one-half terpenes"). The terpenes have the formula C_nH_{2n-4} and can occur theoretically in the following configurations: (1) three double bonds and no cycle, eg, *myrcene* (found in myrcia oil) and *ocimene* (found in the volatile oil from the leaves of *Ocimum gratissimum*); (2) two double bonds and one cycle, eg, *limonene* (of widespread occurrence, but especially in the citrus oils); (3) one double bond and two cycles, eg, either *α-pinene* or *β-pinene* (the first of which is of very widespread occurrence; together, these two terpenes comprise at least 90% of the bulk of turpentine oil); and (4) three cycles. No examples are known of terpenes having the last structure.

Terpenes

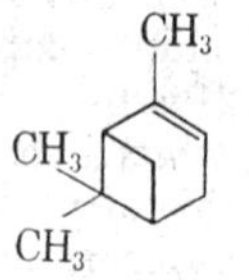

α-Pinene

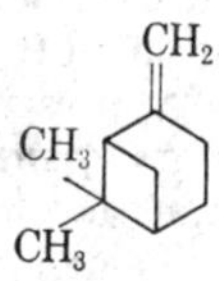

β-Pinene

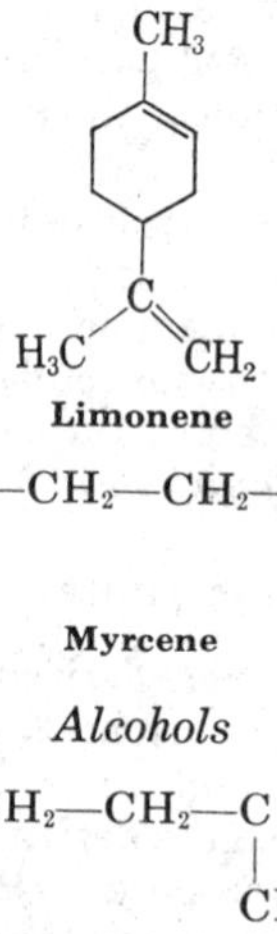

Limonene

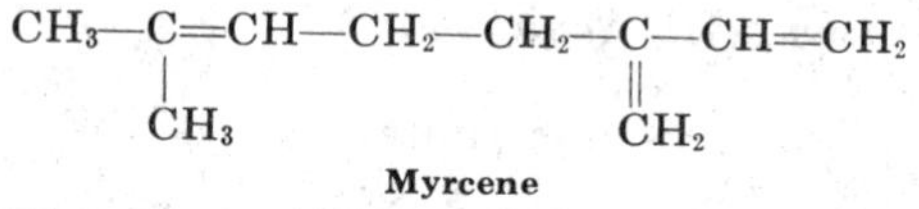

$$CH_3-C=CH-CH_2-CH_2-C-CH=CH_2$$
with CH₃ below first carbon and CH₂ (double bond) below the C

Myrcene

Alcohols

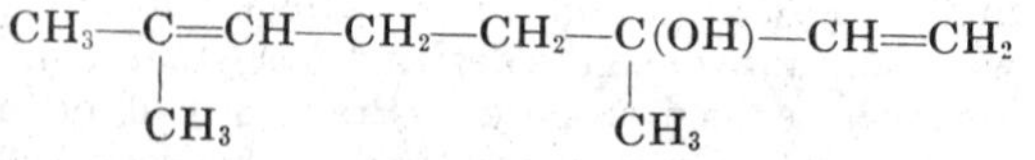

$$CH_3-C=CH-CH_2-CH_2-C(OH)-CH=CH_2$$
with CH₃ groups below

Linalool

$$CH_3-C=CH-CH_2-CH_2-CH-CH_2-CH_2OH$$
with CH₃ groups below

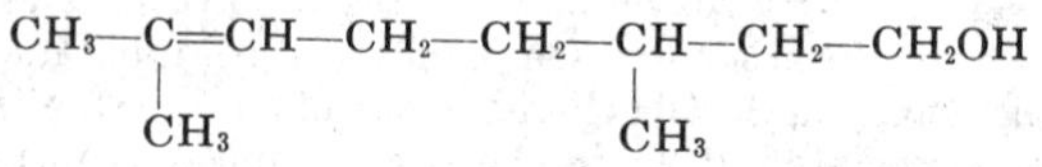

Citronellol

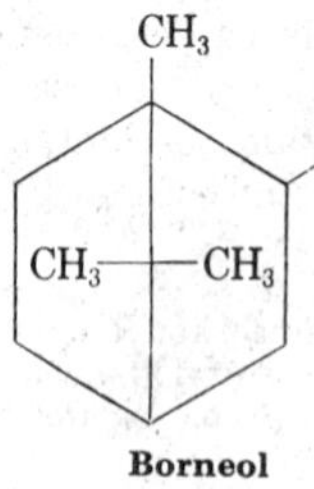

Borneol

Table XII—Composition of Selected Ceveratrum Alkaloids

Alkaloid	Molecular formula	Alkamine	Esterification loci[a]	Acid — Name	Acid — Structure
Cevadine	$C_{32}H_{49}NO_9$	Veracevine[b]	3	*cis*-2-methyl-2-butenoic (angelic)	H_3C H $CH_3C{=}CCOOH$
Germerine	$C_{37}H_{59}NO_{11}$	Germine	3	(+)-2-hydroxy-2-methylbutyric	CH_3 CH_3CH_2CCOOH OH
			7	D-(−)-2-methylbutyric	CH_3 $CH_3CH_2CHCOOH$
Veratridine	$C_{36}H_{51}NO_{11}$	Veracevine[b]	3	3,4-dimethoxybenzoic (veratric)	CH_3O—⬡—$COOH$ OCH_3
Protoveratrine A[c]	$C_{41}H_{63}NO_{14}$	Protoverine	3	(+)-2-hydroxy-2-methylbutyric	CH_3 CH_3CH_2CCOOH OH
			5 and 6	acetic	CH_3COOH
			7	D-(−)-2-methylbutyric	CH_3 $CH_3CH_2CHCOOH$
Protoveratrine B[c]	$C_{41}H_{63}NO_{15}$	Protoverine	3	(+)-*threo*-2,3-dihydroxy-2-methylbutyric	H OH $CH_3{-}C{-}C{-}COOH$ OH CH_3
			5 and 6	as per Protoveratrine A	
			7	as per Protoveratrine A	

[a] Numbering is in the IUPAC-notation described previously for the ceveratrum nucleus.

[b] Formerly thought to be cevine (the 3α-hydroxy analog of veracevine), but subsequent investigation disclosed cevine to be an artifact deduced from failure to recognize a rearrangement which occurred during degradative operations.

[c] Protoveratrines A and B were formerly thought to be only one alkaloid, protoveratrine. See Kloks MV, *et al*: *J Am Chem Soc 74*: 5107, 1952; and Nash HA, Booker RM: *Ibid 75*: 1942, 1953.

The sesquiterpenes have the formula C_nH_{2n-6} and can therefore theoretically occur in an even more varied configuration. Although a number of members of this group of hydrocarbons have been isolated, in many instances the structure is not definitely known. Among those of known structure may be mentioned *zingiberene* (from ginger oil) and *bisabolene* (from Bisabol myrrh oil).

Hydrocarbons other than the terpene types are sometimes present. An example is the saturated hydrocarbon *n*-heptane (C_7H_{16}), which occurs in the volatile oil obtained from the oleoresin of *Pinus Sabiniana* and *P Jeffreyi* and from the fruits of *Pittosporum resiniferum* (the so-called "petroleum nuts" of a tree growing in the Philippines).

The terpenes and sesquiterpenes in general are practically insoluble in water, but soluble in alcohol, ether, chloroform, benzene, petroleum benzin, and the fixed and volatile oils.

Many of the essential oils, however, owe their character and their value to constituents other than hydrocarbons. Among these will be found organic *acids*, such as acetic, benzoic, cinnamic, phenylacetic, etc; *alcohols* like benzyl alcohol, borneol, cinnamyl alcohol, citronellol, geraniol, linalool, menthol, phenylethyl alcohol, terpineol, etc; *aldehydes* such as anisaldehyde, cinnamaldehyde, benzaldehyde, citral, piperonal or heliotropin, salicylaldehyde, vanillin, etc; *ketones* like carvone, camphor, thujone, pulegone, etc; *esters* such as bornyl acetate, methyl salicylate, benzyl benzoate, geranyl acetate, linalyl acetate, etc; *phenols* such as thymol, carvacrol, chavicol, etc; *phenol ethers* like anethol, eugenol, safrol, etc;

and many other more complex compounds, such as coumarin, indole, etc. Many of these products are found in flower oils and are used in the production of synthetic perfumes.

It is beyond the scope of this book to attempt an exhaustive presentation of the chemistry of the numerous constituents occurring in the volatile oils. In the case of those compounds which are official, the structural formulas are given in the respective monographs. In certain other instances, substances such as *carvone, borneol,* and *linalyl acetate* are mentioned in the official text; and since their structures are not provided, a few of the more important of these are given in this article.

Properties

Color—Most of the volatile oils are colorless when pure and fresh, or can be made colorless by redistillation. On exposure to the air they acquire various colors, becoming green, as in oil of wormwood; yellow, as in oil of peppermint; red, as in oil of origanum; brown, as in oil of cinnamon. The blue color of oil of chamomile is an inherent property of the oil even when freshly distilled and is said to be due to the highly unsaturated hydrocarbon *chamazulene* ($C_{15}H_{18}$).

Odor—The odors of volatile oils are extremely variable. It is their most characteristic feature. The odor of an oil is sensibly modified by exposure to the air. Oil of turpentine may be rectified by redistillation in an atmosphere of carbon dioxide, or *in vacuo*, so that it will be almost odorless, or have an agreeable, fragrant odor. A very slight exposure to the air is sufficient, however, to restore the well-known unpleasant odor. Other terpene-containing oils are quickly oxidized and the delicacy and fineness of their flavor and odor seriously impaired. This is especially true of orange and lemon oils.

Taste—The tastes of volatile oils are almost as variable as their odors. Some are sweet, others have a mild, pungent, hot, acrid, caustic, or burning taste.

Density—The specific gravity of official volatile oils also varies (from 0.842 to 1.172). The majority of them are lighter than water.

Optical Activity—This property is used in determining the purity of many oils.

Refractive Index—This property serves as a delicate test for both the identity and purity of oils and fats.

Boiling Range—Owing to the fact that most volatile oils consist of complex mixtures of many types of compounds, the boiling point is of small significance. On heating in a distillation apparatus, the fraction having the lowest boiling point distils first; then the temperature rises until the boiling point of the next higher boiling fraction is reached; and so on.

Aldehydes

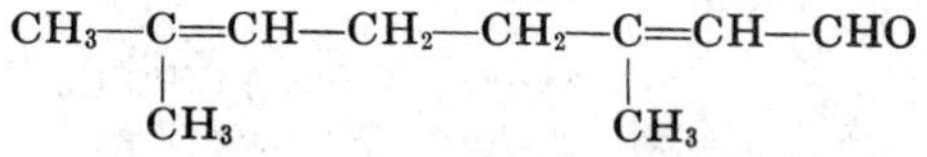

$$CH_3-C=CH-CH_2-CH_2-C=CH-CHO$$

with CH_3 groups below

Citral
(*cis*-**Neral**)
(*trans*-**Geranial**)

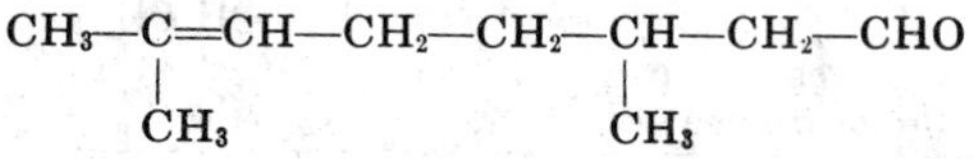

$$CH_3-C=CH-CH_2-CH_2-CH-CH_2-CHO$$

with CH_3 groups below

Citronellal

CHO, OH

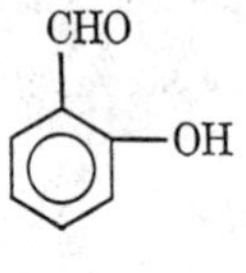

Salicylaldehyde

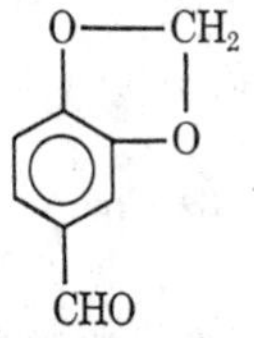

Heliotropin (Piperonal)

Ketones

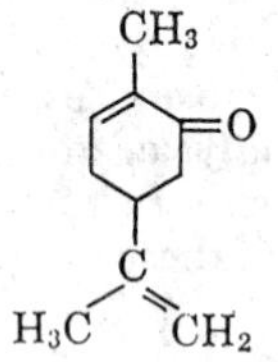

Carvone

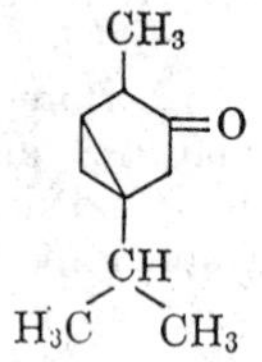

Thujone

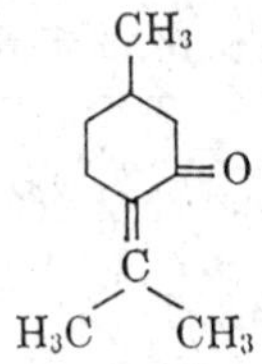

Pulegone

Phenols and Phenol Ethers

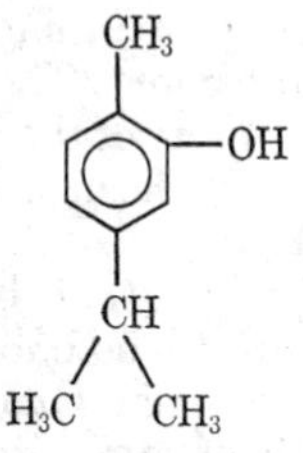

Carvacrol

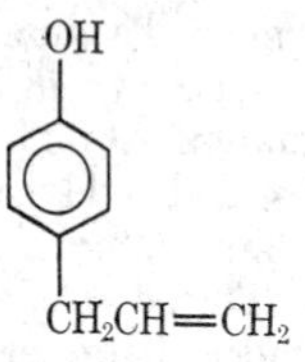

Chavicol

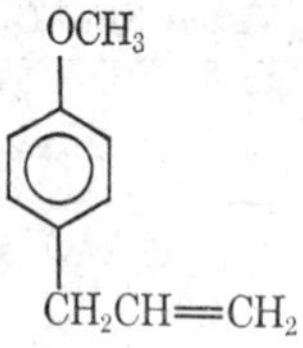

O-Methylchavicol

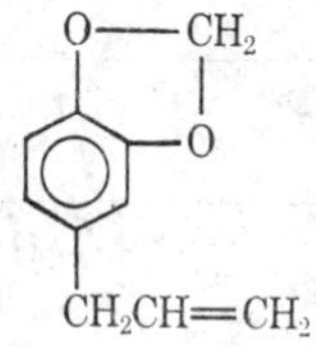

Safrol

Solubilities—Water is a poor solvent for volatile oils, although it acquires a decided odor and flavor when brought in contact with the oil in a finely divided state, as in preparing medicated waters. Alcohol, ether, chloroform, glacial acetic acid, petroleum ether, benzene, and many other organic solvents will dissolve volatile oils. Alcohol is a better solvent for oxygenated oils than for terpenes. Many official oils are required to meet specific solubility tests in 70, 80, or 95% alcohol. Volatile oils freely dissolve fixed oils, fats, resins, camphors, and usually sulfur and phosphorus.

Deterioration—Exposure to light and air impairs the quality and destroys the fragrance of volatile oils. Peroxides frequently develop in oils containing terpenes, and, after extended exposure, the oils thicken and become resinified, or deposit crystalline compounds. The whitening of corks, inserted for a long time in bottles containing certain volatile oils, is due to the bleaching action of the peroxides which are gradually produced during their decomposition. This is true only of oils containing notable amounts of terpenes. Volatile oils should be kept in well-filled, tightly stoppered, amber-colored bottles, in a cool place. A suggestion has been made to replace the air with nitrogen in original packages to prevent oxidation. Storage in tin cans causes pronounced deterioration in odor and the development of color.

Preparation

Volatile oils are generally obtained from plants by the following methods: (1) distillation with steam; (2) distillation *per se;* (3) expression; (4) extraction.

1. Distillation with Steam—This is the method most frequently employed. The general procedure is as follows: Place the substance from which the oil is to be extracted into a still (see RPS-14, pages 184–188), and add enough water to cover it; then distil by a regulated heat into a large condenser. Separate the distilled oil from the water which comes over with it.

**2. Distillation *per se*—By this is meant the distillation of certain bodies without the use of water (*per se*, "by itself"). This is done in the cases of certain oleoresins, copaiba, etc, water not being required in the process, and always being difficult to separate from the distillate.

3. Expression (see Chapter 77)—This method is very limited in its application and generally produces the most fragrant products, because there are very few volatile oils whose aroma is not injuriously affected by the action of heat. The volatile oils of the Citrus family (orange, lemon, bergamot, and lime) are generally obtained by expressing the rind of the fresh fruit. These are usually known as "hand pressed." Three methods are practiced: (1) the sponge process; (2) the écuelle method; and (3) the machine process.

In the *sponge process* the rind is removed from the fruit, and, after dipping in water, is pressed by hand, the oil collecting in a shallow bowl from which it is transferred to a larger container for separation.

In the *écuelle method* the fruit is rolled about in hollow bowls, the walls of which are covered with spikes. The oil cells are punctured and the oil which exudes is collected in the hollow handle.

In the *machine process* either the sponge or the écuelle

processes are adapted to machines which perform the operation on a larger scale.

4. Extraction—Some volatile oils are readily decomposed by distillation, or exist in such minute traces as to make their commercial production impracticable. In such cases the odorous principle may be extracted by some form of solution or absorption. This may be effected by maceration, digestion, percolation with an appropriate immiscible solvent, enfleurage, or extraction with a volatile solvent. For a brief description of these procedures see RPS-15, page 444.

Official Volatile Oils

Volatile oils of the following botanical sources are official: Anise, Caraway, Cinnamon, Clove, Coriander, Eucalyptus, Fennel, Lavender, Lemon, Orange, Orange Flower, Peppermint, Pine Needle, and Spearmint.

Plant Exudates

Plant exudates, for purposes of classification in this textbook, comprise naturally occurring, solid or semisolid, chemically complex mixtures of vegetable origin, such as balsams, gums, oleoresins, and resins. The proportion of their constituents may vary with the climate, season of the year, and other factors. Those plant principles which can be isolated in the pure state and which can be characterized structurally by chemical and physical methods, eg, alkaloids, carbohydrates, glycosides, and vitamins, are considered at other locations under their appropriate headings.

Resins—These are natural or induced solid or semisolid exudations from plants or from insects feeding on plants; they are not to be confused with the large class of so-called synthetic resins prepared by condensation or polymerization of low-molecular-weight organic compounds. They are characterized by being insoluble in water, mostly soluble in alcohol or ether, often uncrystallizable, and softening or melting at a moderate heat. They range in specific gravity from 0.90 to 1.25. Ignited in the air they burn with a smoky flame. They are usually the oxidized terpenes of the volatile oils of plants, and, owing to their insolubility in water, have little taste; they show no uniformity of chemical composition; some of them are acids, and combine with alkalies, forming "soaps" as in the case of common rosin.

A clear distinction must be made between *natural resins* and *prepared resins*. A natural resin is one which occurs as an exudation. The formerly official Mastic is an example. A prepared resin may be made by exhausting a drug, which owes its activity to resinous constituents, with alcohol, pouring the concentrated alcoholic percolate into an excess of water, collecting, washing, and drying the precipitate. Podophyllum Resin (Chap 40) is an example of this class. A prepared resin may also be derived from a natural oleoresin by driving off the volatile oil by heat. Rosin is an example of this class.

Oleoresins—Natural oleoresins are mixtures of volatile oils and resins, generally obtained by incising trunks of trees in which they are found. Turpentine and Copaiba are natural oleoresins formerly recognized by the NF.

A distinction must be made also between the natural and prepared oleoresins. The *prepared oleoresins* are concentrated liquid preparations made by percolating drugs, naturally containing both volatile oil and resin, with an appropriate solvent, ie, acetone, ether, or alcohol, and concentrating the percolate until the solvent has been dissipated. The formerly official Aspidium, Capsicum, and Ginger oleoresins are examples.

Gum Resins—These are natural mixtures of gum and resin, usually obtained as exudations from plants, as the formerly official Myrrh and Gamboge.

Balsams—These are resinous substances containing benzoic or cinnamic acids or their esters, as Tolu Balsam, Peruvian Balsam, etc.

Much faulty nomenclature occurs in the ordinary trade designations for many plant exudates. The word *gum* is frequently the one most misapplied as in *gum thus* for turpentine oleoresin, *gum guaiac* for resin of guaiac, *gum asafetida* for oleo-gum-resin of asafetida. The word *balsam* is also wrongly applied to certain oleoresins, such as Copaiba and Canada Turpentine, neither of which contains any of the constituents characteristic of balsams.

Prostaglandins

In 1933, Swedish Nobel laureate Ulf von Euler, detected the first prostaglandin.[5,6] Independently, he and Maurice Goldblatt, in England, found that one or more substances in human seminal fluid not only stimulated the contraction of a variety of smooth muscles but affected the blood pressure of animals when injected. It was in a paper in 1935 that von Euler suggested the name prostaglandin for the new factor because he found trace amounts of it in prostate gland tissue. The prostaglandins form a class of natural products with diverse and potent biological activities. They are involved in platelet aggregation, blood pressure, GI motility, gastric acid secretion, and *cytoprotection*, pain and inflammation, nerve conduction, fetal development, uterine contraction, thermoregulation and fever production, food intake, vasodilation and vasoconstriction, bronchodilation and bronchoconstriction, and the movement of fluid and electrolytes across membranes. It was not until 1949 that research and knowledge about the prostaglandins started to increase at a fast pace. The natural prostaglandins are unsaturated, hydroxylated fatty acids, all derivatives of the parent compound called prostanoic acid. Indeed, prostaglandins are associated with most mammalian tissues and implicated in an ever-increasing number of physiological systems.

Nomenclature

The parent compound for the prostaglandins is prostanoic acid and nine principal groups or series of modifications are recognized, as listed in Table XIII.

Prostanoic acid

5-Octylcyclopentaneheptanoic acid

The abbreviations in this table are often shortened to the last letter, by dropping the PG prefix.

A subscript following the abbreviation pertains to the prostaglandin depicted in Table XIII or the following modifications:

Subscript 2—Additional double bond at C-5 (Z)

Subscript 3—Two additional double bonds, at C-5 (Z) and C-17 (Z)

Table XIII—Prostaglandins

Abbrev	C=C	>C=O	Substituents –OH	–O–O–	–OOH	–O–
PGA$_1$	10,13E	9	15S	—	—	—
PGB$_1$	8(12),13E	9	15S	—	—	—
PGC$_1$	11,13E	9	15S	—	—	—
PGD$_1$	13E	11	9α,15S	—	—	—
PGE$_1$	13E	9	11α,15S	—	—	—
PGF$_1$	13E	—	9α,11α,15S	—	—	—
PGG$_1$	13E	—	—	9α,11α	15S	—
PGH$_1$	13E	—	15S	9α,11α	—	—
PGR	see PGH series	—	—	—	—	—
PGX	5Z,13E	—	11α,15S	—	—	6,9α

Table XIV—Structures of Representative Prostaglandins

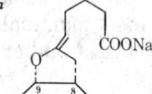

Name	Formula	OH	Double bonds	R_1	R_2	Other
Arbaprostil	$C_{21}H_{34}O_5$	$11\alpha,15\beta$	5–6 cis, 13–14	–OH	$n\text{-}C_4H_9$–	9-oxo, 15α-CH_3–
Carboprost (Prostin/15 M) (Tromethamine* salt and Methyl Ester)	$C_{21}H_{35}O_5$	$9\alpha,11\alpha,15\alpha$	5–6 cis, 13–14	–OH	$n\text{-}C_4H_9$–	15β-CH_3–
Cloprostenol Sodium	$C_{22}H_{28}ClNaO_6$	$9\alpha,11\alpha,15\alpha$	5–6, 13–14	–OH	$m\text{-}ClC_6H_4O$–	—
Dinoprost (Prostin F_2)	$C_{20}H_{34}O_5$	$9\alpha,11\alpha,15\alpha$	5–6, 13–14	–OH	$n\text{-}C_4H_9$–	—
Dinoprostone* (Prostine E_2)	$C_{20}H_{32}O_5$	$9\alpha,15\alpha$	5–6, 13–14	–OH	$n\text{-}C_4H_9$–	9-oxo
Doxaprost	$C_{21}H_{36}O_4$	15β	13–14	–OH	$n\text{-}C_4H_9$–	9-oxo, 15β-CH_3–
Epoprostenol Sodium (Prostacyclin)	$C_{20}H_{31}NaO_5$	$11\alpha,15\alpha$	13–14[a]	–ONa	$n\text{-}C_4H_9$–	15β-CH_3
Fenprostalene	$C_{23}H_{30}O_6$	$9\alpha,11\alpha,15\alpha$	4–5–6 (allene), 13–14	–OCH$_3$	–O–C_6H_5	—
Fluprostenol Sodium	$C_{23}H_{28}F_3NaO_6$	$9\alpha,11\alpha,15\alpha$	5–6, 13–14	–OH	$m\text{-}CF_3C_6H_4O$–	—
Gemeprost	$C_{23}H_{38}O_5$	$11\alpha,15\alpha$	2–3, 13–14	–OCH$_3$	$n\text{-}C_4H_9$–	9-oxo, 16-diCH_3–
Meteneprost	$C_{23}H_{38}O_4$	$11\alpha,15\alpha$	5–6 cis, 13–14	–OH	$n\text{-}C_4H_9$–	9 CH_2=
Prostalene	$C_{22}H_{36}O_5$	$9\alpha,11\alpha,15\alpha$	4–5, 5–6 13–14	–OCH$_3$	$n\text{-}C_4H_9$–	15-methyl
Sulprostone	$C_{23}H_{31}NO_7S$	$11\alpha,15\alpha$	5–6, 13–14	–NHSO$_2$CH$_3$	C_6H_5O–	9-oxo
Tiaprost (tromethamine salt)	$C_{24}H_{39}NO_9S$	$9\alpha,11\alpha,15\alpha$	5–6 cis, 13–14	–OC$_4$H$_{12}$NO$_3$	[thiophene]	—

a [structure with COONa, positions 9 and 8]

* Denotes Official status

The subscripts α or β indicate the configuration at C-9 and the same designation used for the steroids is employed; α is *down* and β is *up*. At C-15 the Cahn-Prelog-Ingold convention defines the chirality and the S configuration (α or dotted line) is found in most natural substances.

Thus, the compound PGF$_{2\alpha}$, or simply, $F_{2\alpha}$ (dinoprost, prostin F$_2$ alpha) is shown below:

PGF$_{2\alpha}$

(5Z,9α,11α,13E,15S)-9,11,15-Trihydroxyprosta-5,13-dien-1-oic acid

The subscript 2 depicting a *trans* (E) configuration at C-13 and *cis* (Z) at C-5, alpha hydroxyl at C-9 and a *cis* (α) diol at C-9 and C-11.

Occurrence

Prostaglandins are known to be widely distributed in mammals. They can be extracted from most animal tissues. The human seminal fluid contains the highest concentration and the greatest number of prostaglandins. Over 31 prostaglandins have been isolated from human seminal fluid.[6] It is present in low concentrations in numerous other organs and fluids, such as in, the iris of the eye, the brain, thymus, the bronchials, the pancreas, the lungs, the human seminal plasma, the ovary, and the uterus. After appropriate stimulation, it was also found that prostaglandins were in the intestines, the adrenal glands, the stomach, the kidneys, the nervous tissues, etc. However, the total prostaglandin production in the adult human is only of the order of 1–2 mg/24 hr. Metabolism occurs by hydroxylation, oxidation, and/or degradation of the carboxylic acid chain. The prostaglandins are perhaps the most versatile, ubiquitous and powerful substances found in humans. Many prostaglandins are characterized both by their multiplicity of effects and their generally short life time.

It has been suggested that the biological activity of the prostaglandin molecule is associated with a right-handed chirality, best visualized as a right-handed wedge in which all the hydrophilic functional groups are oriented to one side and the hydrophobic groups to the other side of the molecule while both ends are hydrophilic.

The Gorgonian, *Plexaura homomalla* (Espers), a Caribbean coral (Florida sea whip) contains from 0.2–1.3% of the 15*R*–PGA$_2$. Although of low biological activity the 15*R* compound easily can be converted chemically to the active 15*S* variety.

Biosynthesis

Prostaglandins are formed from the 20-carbon straight-chain carboxylic acid arachidonic acid, and from closely related fatty acids such as dihomo-γ-linoleic acid. The enzymatic process using vesicular extracts from sheep or bulls yields mainly the E series. Employing lung homogenates as the enzyme source, F_α compounds have been formed by a similar process.

Chemical Synthesis

During the early stages of prostaglandin development, pharmacological studies were the major consumer of the natural materials. The small amounts required were fairly rapidly supplied by biosynthesis. The need to find compounds that more selectively express the diverse effects produced by the prostaglandins and that were more stable to metabolism than was the case with the natural materials led to an overwhelming outburst of synthetic activity in the late 1960s which continues today. The exact number of syntheses is now essentially impossible to determine because of overlapping routes and intermediates from one synthesis to another.

One process known to have industrial importance was developed by Elias J Corey and his group at Harvard University who reported a landmark total synthesis in 1969. This synthesis was particularly notable in several respects. It controls the stereochemistry at every center except C-15, proceeds in excellent yield, and involves an intermediate now known to many as Corey's lactone aldehyde. This intermediate was elaborated to the natural prostaglandins and has been utilized by others for the creation of a host of analogs having modified upper and lower side chains. This route has been refined and modified in varying degrees both by Corey's group and others and appears to be the basis of processes for the preparation of prostaglandins at several pharmaceutical companies. Another industrially important process was developed at Upjohn by Robert C Kelly's group.[6] This process leads to the enone similar to one elaborated in the Corey process and also passes through a core intermediate from which many upper and lower side chain analogs have been prepared. It has been scaled up to produce the equivalent of more than 50 kg per year of $PGF_{2\alpha}$ and has reduced the cost of preparing prostaglandins to less than $1/100$ of that for the biosynthesis.

Activity

The principal pharmacologic activity of the various prostaglandins, where comparative data are available, includes the stimulation of gastrointestinal and reproductive smooth muscle, relaxation and contraction of respiratory smooth muscle, hypotensive activity, inhibition of lipolysis of fatty acids, gastric acid secretion and blood platelet aggregation. Structure-activity relationship for the family of prostaglandin molecules has been only partially characterized and much cross-activity is evident.

Currently, prostaglandins are on the market or are under clinical investigation for potential applications in treating fertility problems, as oxytocic agents, in gastric or cardiovascular therapy, as bronchodilators, and in a variety of uses in animal husbandry. Among the active uses of prostaglandins, for example, is the use of prostacyclin to prevent blood clotting in cardiopulmonary bypass operations.

It was long thought that the mechanism of action of the prostaglandins in anti-ulcer therapy was inhibition of gastric acid secretion. However, a recent study shows that the antiulcer effect may result from both anti-secretory and cytoprotective properties of the prostaglandins.

PGE_1 recently has been introduced for a rare but frequently life-saving application. In certain instances of congenital heart disease, the normal closure of the *ductus arteriosus* is undesirable until corrective surgery has guaranteed the passage of blood to the lungs. Such surgery is more likely to be successful if PGE_1 is infused into the blood of the infant to prevent closure of the ductus until after successful surgery.

Table XIV shows the structures of some representative prostaglandin derivatives currently under investigation.

References

1. Svoboda GH, *et al: J Pharm Sci 51:* 707, 1962.
2. Morgan KJ, Barltrop JA: *Quart Rev (London) 12:* 34, 1958.
3. *J Pharm Sci 51:* 707, 1962.
4. Robinson, R: *J Chem Soc (London):* 762, 1917.
5. *Medical Sci Bulletin*, vol 5, No 5 (Menlo Park, CA) 1982.
6. Nelson NA, *et al: Chem & Eng News*, Aug 16, 1982, pp 30–44.

Bibliography

Briggs MH, ed: *Advances in Steroid Biochemistry and Pharmacology*, Academic, New York, 1970.

Brossi A: *The Alkaloids*, vol 22, Academic, New York, 1983.

Crabbe P, ed: *Prostaglandin Research*, Academic, New York, 1977.

Cuthbert MF, ed: *The Prostaglandins: Pharmacologic and Therapeutic Advances*, Lippincott, Philadelphia, 1973.

Glasby JS: *Encyclopedia of the Alkaloids*, 2 vols, Plenum, New York, 1975.

Guenther E: *The Essential Oils*, 6 vols, Van Nostrand, New York, 1949–1952.

Gunstone F: *An Introduction to the Chemistry and Biochemistry of Fatty Acids and Their Glycerides*, 2nd ed, Chapman & Hall, London, 1968.

Hesse M: *Alkaloid Chemistry*, Wiley-Interscience, New York, 1981.

Honeyman J, Guthrie RD: *An Introduction to the Chemistry of Carbohydrates*, 3rd ed, Clarendon, Oxford, 1968.

Karim SSM, ed: *Prostaglandins: Chemical and Biochemical Aspects*, University Park Press, Baltimore, 1976.

Leach SJ, ed: *Physical Properties and Techniques of Protein Chemistry*, Academic, New York, (Part A) 1969, (Part B) 1970, (Part C) 1973.

Manske RHF: *The Alkaloids*, 17 vols, Academic, New York, 1950–1977.

Manske RHF, Rodrigo RGA: *ibid*, vols 17–20, 1977–1983.

Oesterling TO, *et al: Prostaglandins, J Pharm Sci 61:* 1861, 1972.

Pelletier SW, ed: *Chemistry of the Alkaloids*, Van Nostrand, New York, 1970.

Putnam FW: *The Plasma Proteins*, 3 vols, 2nd ed, Academic, New York, 1975.

Rafauf R: *Handbook of Alkaloids and Alkaloid Containing Plants*, Wiley, New York, 1970.

Shamma M: *The Isoquinoline Alkaloids: Chemistry and Pharmacology*, Academic, New York, 1972.

Sim SK: *Medicinal Plant Alkaloids: An Introduction for Pharmacy Students*, Toronto University Press, Toronto, 1965.

CHAPTER 26

Drug Nomenclature – United States Adopted Names

Mary Celeste Alessandri, MS
Free-Lance Writer
Lisle, IL 60532

Joseph B Jerome, PhD
Secretary Emeritus
United States Adopted Names Council
Chicago, IL 60610

Within recent years advances have been made in many disciplines at such an accelerated rate that the processing of available information has become somewhat of a discipline in its own right. Processing of information includes such subspecialties as collection, collation, abstracting, storage, retrieval, and dissemination.

One area in which it sometimes seems that information has gotten ahead of those seeking it is that involving drugs. The sheer numbers of new potential drug entities that have been researched since the 1950s have made the task of monitoring the literature a formidable one.

If one considers that a given drug may be known by several chemical names, one or more code numbers and/or trivial designations, a formally selected nonproprietary name, and two or three trademarks, plus any variations on these that exist in other countries, it will become apparent that a meaningful nonproprietary nomenclature system is an aid to the efficient use of drug information.

Such a nomenclature system has been developed, and a discussion of its accomplishments and its problems, as well as its history, scope, functions, and operation is the subject of this chapter.

Types of Drug Names

The term "drug nomenclature" indicates several types of names for drugs, each having its own function.

For compounds of known composition, the first name to be applied is generally the *chemical name*. This is a systematically derived name which provides complete and accurate chemical identification. Among the many chemical names which are possible for most compounds, the Chemical Abstracts Index Name, selected by the Chemical Abstracts Service, provides a unique, systematic name which serves as a key to the world's chemical literature. For those substances which are of animal or plant origin, scientific identification of the source is given in terms of technical *biochemical, botanical,* or *zoological names.* Although in either case these designations are scientifically precise, they tend to be very long, unwieldy, and not generally useful to the physician, pharmacist, and others in related fields.

Since chemical names are not suitable for routine use, a potential drug often acquires a *code designation* as a convenient reference for those working with it during laboratory investigations. This kind of nomenclature is generally of two types: (1) a letter and number combination (eg, SH 567) in which the letter(s) generally refers to the laboratory involved and the number is often arbitrarily assigned, and (2) a letter combination (eg, IDU) which is usually derived from portions of the chemical name.

Although code designations are usually considered simply a convenient "shop label" and are generally meant to be discarded when a more appropriate name is selected, many of them find their way into the literature when published reports on early investigative work appear prior to the selection of a nonproprietary name. These code designations must, therefore, be considered as a part of drug nomenclature. Again, however, they cannot be considered acceptable for general usage since, in themselves, they provide no identification of the compound to which they refer. Also, with arbitrarily selected number codes, errors are difficult to detect and, therefore, occur more frequently.

In some instances *trivial names* are assigned (usually by individual researchers working on the drugs) to new compounds during early investigative stages. These are complete names and may be of the type one could loosely call a nonproprietary name. Nomenclature agencies strongly discourage the use of such trivial names, since they are generally coined in a haphazard manner with little concern for the availability (ie, freedom from conflict with established names) of the term used or for the relationship which may exist between the new compound and other drugs previously named.

If a drug has come through the successive research stages and appears to be heading for the market, a *trademark* is assigned; this very often designates not the drug itself, but rather a formulation and its manufacturer.

Trademarks are the legal possessions of their owners and cannot be used in a public sense. Moreover, when a given drug is manufactured by more than one firm, each may market its specific formulation under its own trademark. Trademarks are selected for their brevity, catchiness, and ease of retention or recall. They often fail to indicate the chemical and pharmacological relations that may exist between individual drugs.

Although each type of name mentioned has a specific purpose, none fulfills the need of those in the health professions for a single, simple, informative designation which is freely available for public use. The *nonproprietary name* is intended to fill this specific need. At its best, it is concise, meaningful, and available. The nonproprietary name has also been called a generic name, but this term is inaccurate since each such name is specific for a given compound although the name may possess a structural unit or stem which is common to a related group of drugs. In this discussion the term nonproprietary name is restricted to those names that have been selected through a formal process of adoption carried out between a manufacturer and a nomenclature agency; this artificial restriction will help differentiate such names from the trivial names coined without having been considered by a nomenclature agency.

The USAN Council

In the United States the nomenclature agency responsible for the selection of appropriate nonproprietary names for drugs is the United States Adopted Names (USAN) Council. This expert committee on drug nomenclature is jointly sponsored by the American Medical Association (AMA), the United States Pharmacopeial Convention, and the American Pharmaceutical Association (APhA). Tracing the involvement of these sponsoring agencies in nomenclature selection provides a good history of the practice in this country and is a guide to the evolution of the USAN Council to its present status.

The *United States Pharmacopeia* (USP) has been supplying standards for pharmaceutical preparations since the first edition appeared in 1820. In its concern for the selection of titles for compendium monographs the USP was among the first to recognize the need for a standardized system of drug nomenclature and to take significant action in that direction.

When the APhA began publication of a second compendium, the *National Formulary* (NF), in 1888, this organization also became concerned not only with establishing standards for those drugs admitted to the NF but also with providing nonproprietary names for them.

As the number of new pharmaceutical products increased during this century, the need for providing appropriate nonproprietary names for new compounds became increasingly apparent. This gap was filled, to some extent, by the AMA's Council on Pharmacy and Chemistry (later known as the Council on Drugs).

In 1910 the Council began a nomenclature program to provide names for use in its publications, for those individual drugs that were available under two different trademarks, and in the early 1940s the Council began to require a nonproprietary name for every active compound included in its publications. However, large numbers of drug products were not the subjects of either Council or compendial monographs. These compounds were known by their chemical names, by trivial names or by trademarks selected by the manufacturers.

As drugs, nomenclature, medicine, and pharmacy became more sophisticated, still another need was recognized. Each new drug needed a nonproprietary name selected early in its history; moreover, it was apparent that such names must be systematically selected to assure their appropriateness in the overall nomenclature picture and must be acceptable to the USP, the NF, the AMA, and the manufacturer.

A significant step toward this goal was taken in June, 1961, with the formation of the AMA–USP Nomenclature Committee. Any names adopted by this Committee were deemed automatically acceptable as potential compendia monograph titles, and the term USAN (United States Adopted Name) was coined to designate those drug names so adopted. Although actively participating in the program from its inception, the then publisher of the NF, the APhA, did not become a full sponsor until January, 1964, at which time the name of the group was changed to the USAN Council.

It is advisable here to consider the role of the federal government in nonproprietary nomenclature, both historically and currently.

In 1906 the government legally recognized the significance of the work being done by the USP and the NF by declaring these publications "official" compendia of the US. Since that time monograph titles have had the status of official nonproprietary names.

The 1938 Food, Drug and Cosmetic Act stipulated that "the common or usual name" (the official name or the nonproprietary name established either by the Council on Pharmacy and Chemistry or by use) should be used on the labeling; in the absence of such a name (or until a name attained this status) a chemical name should be used.

The Drug Amendments of 1962 replaced the "common or usual" terminology with the more meaningful requirement that nonproprietary names must be "simple and useful." For the first time the Commissioner of the Food and Drug Administration (FDA) was given the authority (acting for the Secretary of Health, Education and Welfare) to designate an official name if he determined that such action was necessary or desirable.

Although the FDA and the USAN Council had operated in effective liaison for some time, it became clear early in 1967 that a more formal cooperative effort in the development of nonproprietary nomenclature would be of value. This realization resulted in an agreement (effective in June, 1967) between the sponsors of the USAN Council and the FDA: the latter would appoint a member to the USAN Council and agree to accept any name on which the Council is unanimous as the established or official name.

The reorganization agreement reserved the right of the Commissioner of the FDA to select the official name in those instances in which the USAN Council cannot reach unanimous agreement. Also, it should be noted that adoption of USAN as "official names" by the FDA did not follow automatically but was accomplished by publication, subject to public comment, in the *Federal Register*. The USAN Council program remains a privately conducted effort by agencies dedicated to serving the public welfare.

It is emphasized that the adoption of a nonproprietary name does not imply that the article is being offered for either clinical use or investigation; furthermore, its adoption is independent of clinical evaluation or acceptance by the medical profession, by the FDA, or by the USAN Council sponsors of any specific brand(s) of the drug to which the name applies.

The USAN Council, then, under its present organization, is sponsored by the AMA, the APhA, and the USP; it is a five-member group, with one member appointed by each sponsor, one member-at-large who must be approved by all three sponsors, and one member from the FDA.

Council members for 1983 were Lloyd C Miller, PhD; Charles S Kumkumian, PhD; John E Kasik, MD, PhD; John V Bergen, PhD; and Lauren A Woods, MD, PhD. The Council staff, provided by the AMA, is headed by Donald O Schiffman, PhD, Director of the AMA Department of Medical Terminology and Nomenclature. For a number of years Kurt Loening, PhD, of Chemical Abstracts Services, Clarence Van Meter, PhD, John J Hefferren, PhD, and more recently, Dale C Myers have provided expert special services to the USAN Council on essentially every negotiation.

The Council operates primarily through correspondence, with meetings held twice a year to discuss policy matters.

It must be anticipated that, on occasion, difficulties will arise over the adoption or proposed adoption of a particular name. In the majority of such cases, the Council and the interested manufacturer(s) can, in time, work out acceptable solutions. A USAN Review Board has been established as a last resource to handle those situations when the normal procedures fail. The services of this Board have been requested in only four cases (as of May, 1983).

Members of the Review Board for 1983 were Raymond D McMurray, LLB, Chairman*; Durward Dodgen; Harry F Dowling, MD; Joseph B Kirsner, MD; August P Lemberger, PhD; and Joseph V Swintosky, PhD. At the time of any appeal to the Board, representatives of the firms involved in

---

* Deceased 1983.

the specific case can participate in the deliberations but exercise no voting privileges.

The primary functions of the USAN Council are:

1. To negotiate with pharmaceutical manufacturers in the selection of meaningful and distinctive nonproprietary names for new drug entities.
2. To publicize the adopted names, the guiding principles used in devising these names, and the procedures involved in their adoption.
3. To cooperate with other national and international agencies, including the World Health Organization (WHO), in standardizing, as much as possible, the nonproprietary nomenclature for drugs.

Procedure for Selecting a USAN

A proposal for a USAN originates usually from a firm or an individual who has developed a substance of potential therapeutic usefulness to the point where there is a distinct possibility of its being marketed in the US. Occasionally, the initiative is taken by the USAN Council in the form of a request to parties interested in a substance for which a nonproprietary name appears to be lacking.

Proposals are expected to conform to the established Guiding Principles (*vide infra*) and to be reasonably free from conflict with other names, including both trademarks and nonproprietary names. When the initial screening of the proposals suggests that they fail to conform or that they appear to conflict, the USAN Council staff offers suggestions with a view to expediting the selection process.

Each proposal should be accompanied by a statement covering as much as possible of the following information:

1. The chemical structure.
2. The chemical name (preferably the *Chemical Abstracts* index name).
3. Any code designation(s) by which the substance may have been known in the course of its testing and development, particularly if such designations have appeared in the medical or pharmaceutical literature.
4. The source (if it is a product of natural origin) or such other descriptive characteristics as will distinguish it adequately.
5. The kind of pharmacologic activity or therapeutic usefulness claimed for it.
6. Any trademark(s) that may have been applied to it.

This information, supplemented by the results of searches conducted by the staff, is referred to the Council members, whose views then are exchanged until a tentative decision can be submitted to the sponsor for comment. It should be emphasized that although the Council can ascertain the preferred chemical nomenclature for a given structural formula, the Council is not in a position to confirm the structure or the claims for pharmacologic activity.

There is, however, a more important aspect to be considered in the selection of distinctive nonproprietary names. For obvious reasons of safety, names for drugs must be distinctive enough so they do not conflict with other established drug names. The USAN Council takes great care in its screening procedure to limit the possibility of conflict between a name under consideration and any established trademark or nonproprietary name. It is regrettable that it is still rather common industry practice to select trademarks similar to recently assigned USAN; such a practice hinders the selection of new USAN for related drugs and, of course, destroys to some degree such distinctiveness as the USAN possessed at its adoption.

In addition to utilizing the expertise of Council members in this area, the Council staff maintains extensive files on nonproprietary names and, to a lesser extent, on trademarks in use in this country and throughout the world. Moreover, manufacturers are requested to conduct the standard legal searches to help clear names which appear likely to be adopted.

When potential nonproprietary names are proposed they are published in the *Trademark Bulletin* of the Pharmaceutical Manufacturers Association as "Proposed USAN." This informs those who have access to the Bulletin of the Council's intention to adopt the name and serves as an invitation for comments or protests within 30 days following its publication. No disclosure of the name of the manufacturer or of the chemical nature of the substance appears in these Bulletin statements.

Subsequently the same information is referred to Chemical Abstracts Service and to the American National Standards Institute for review of the proposed names as to freedom from conflict with existing names.

The above screening procedures are necessary since nonproprietary names that appear to be rather well established to members of a research group with specialized interests may be unavailable (usually because of conflict with established names) for selection as a USAN; the USAN Council does not desire to adopt as a USAN a designation that would infringe on the valid rights of legally established trademarks or would produce confusion with similar nonproprietary names for compounds that differ significantly in chemical structure and pharmacologic activity.

If the sponsor consents, and in any case if the name and/or nomenclature information has been published elsewhere, the tentatively adopted USAN is then submitted for consideration to several cooperating agencies. These agencies include the WHO, the British Pharmacopoeia Commission, and the French Pharmacopeia Commission, as well as the USP, the NF, and the FDA.

If no significant objections are raised by the cooperating agencies, the USAN Council proceeds toward final adoption. The USAN is then published in the journal, *Clinical Pharmacology and Therapeutics*.

Several drug nomenclature publications, such as the *American Drug Index*, the *Modern Drug Encyclopedia*, and *The Merck Index* give special attention to the USAN.

Despite the efforts to give notice of the proposed adoption of a USAN in the early stages and to exercise care in avoiding conflicts with established names, objections sometimes arise rather late. All valid objections receive conscientious attention from the Council.

Guiding Principles for Coining a USAN

A USAN is a nonproprietary name selected according to the following principles, the primary purpose of which is to assure consistency in the choice of names of maximal usefulness. The principles take into account practical considerations, such as the existence of trademarks, and the fact that the intended uses of the substances for which names are being selected may change. Therefore, the principles are flexible and may be revised in the light of experience.

General Rules

1. A nonproprietary name should be useful primarily to health practitioners, especially physicians, dentists, veterinarians, pharmacists, and nurses.
   a. The principal criterion for judging a name's usefulness is suitability, including safety, for use in the routine processes of ordering, dispensing, and administering drugs throughout the US.
   b. A second criterion is the name's suitability for use in educational programs for students of these health professions.
2. Attributes that contribute to usefulness are simplicity (both brevity and ease of pronunciation) and those qualities that lend euphony and enhance ready recognition and recall. The essential criterion of simplicity is the ease with which the name is used by personnel trained in the above-mentioned professions.
   a. The name for the active moiety of a drug should be a single word, preferably of not more than four syllables.
   b. The name for the active moiety may be modified by a single term, preferably of not more than three syllables, to show a chemical modification (eg, the chemical formation of cortisone acetate from cortisone).
   c. Only under compelling circumstances is a name acceptable with

Table I—Group Relationships: Listing by Syllables[a]	
Syllables	Categories
-actide	.... synthetic corticotropins
-andr-	.... androgens
-arol	.... anticoagulants (dicumarol type)
-azepam	.... tranquilizers (diazepam type)
bol- or -bol-	.... anabolic steroids
-caine	.... local anesthetics
cef-	.... antibiotics (cefazolin type)
-cillin	.... penicillins
-cort-	.... cortisone derivatives
-cycline	.... antibiotics (tetracycline derivatives)
-estr-	.... estrogens
-fibrate	.... antihyperlipidemics (clofibrate type)
-formin	.... guanidine oral hypoglycemics
-gest-	.... progestins
gli-	.... sulfonamide oral hypoglycemics
io-	.... iodine-containing contrast media
-methacin	.... anti-inflammatory substances (indomethacin type)
-mycin	.... antibiotics (*Streptomyces* strains)
nal-	.... narcotic antagonists (normorphine derivatives)
-nidazole	.... antiprotozoal substances (metronidazole type)
-olol	.... anti-adrenergics (β-receptor)
-onide	.... steroids which are acetal derivatives
-orex	.... anorexiants
-orphan	.... narcotic antagonists/agonists related to morphinan
-pramine	.... antidepressants (imipramine type)
-profen	.... anti-inflammatory substances (ibuprofen type)
-prost-	.... prostaglandin derivatives
-relin	.... prehormones or hormone-release modifying agents
sulfa-	.... antimicrobial sulfonamides
-terol	.... bronchodilators (phenethylamine derivatives)
-thiazide	.... diuretics (thiazide derivatives)
-verine	.... spasmolytics having a papaverine-like action

[a] Recommended prefixes and suffixes are of the form gli- and -arol, respectively.

Table II—Group Relationships: Listing by Category	
Categories	Syllables
anabolic steroids	bol- or -bol-
androgens	-andr-
anesthetics, local	-caine
anorexiants	-orex
anti-adrenergics (β-receptor)	-olol
antibiotics (cefazolin type)	cef-
antibiotics (penicillins)	-cillin
antibiotics (*Streptomyces* strains)	-mycin
antibiotics (tetracycline derivatives)	-cycline
anticoagulants (dicumarol type)	-arol
antidepressants (imipramine type)	-pramine
antihyperlipidemics (clofibrate type)	-fibrate
anti-inflammatory substances (ibuprofen type) ..	-profen
anti-inflammatory substances (indomethacin type)	-methacin
antimicrobial sulfonamides	sulfa-
antiprotozoal substances (metronidazole type) ..	-nidazole
bronchodilators (phenethylamine derivatives) ...	-terol
corticotropins, synthetic	-actide
diuretics (thiazide derivatives)	-thiazide
estrogens	-estr-
glucocorticoids (cortisone derivatives)	-cort-
hormone-release modifying agents or prehormones	-relin
hypoglycemics (oral) guanidine	-formin
hypoglycemics (oral) sulfonamide	gli-
iodine-containing contrast media	io-
narcotic antagonists/agonists related to morphinan	-orphan
normorphine derivatives which are narcotic antagonists	nal-
progestins	-gest-
prostaglandin derivatives	-prost-
spasmolytics with papaverine-like action	-verine
steroids which are acetal derivatives	-onide
tranquilizers (diazepam type)	-azepam

more than one modifying term (eg, pharmaceuticals containing radioactive isotopes).

d. Acronyms, initials, condensed words, symbols, and numerals may be acceptable in otherwise appropriate terminology (eg, methyldopa, ibufenac, and dextran 40).

3. A name should reflect pharmacologic, chemical, or other characteristics and relationships of actual practical value to the users.

a. A common syllable or simple word element (a "stem") should be incorporated in the names of all members of a group of drugs when useful common characteristics can thus be indicated (eg, similarity of pharmacologic action) (see Tables I and II). When pharmacologic similarity is found in drugs of distinctly different chemical nature, the stems should differ (eg, reserpine, promazine).

b. Characteristically different terminology is sometimes necessary for specific drugs or groups (eg, insulin I 131, dextran 40).

4. A nonproprietary drug name should be free from conflict with other nonproprietary names or with previously existing trademarks, and should be such that it is neither confusing nor misleading.

5. Preference should be given to the choice of a name of established usage, provided it conforms reasonably well to these principles.

Specific Rules

1. Esters, salts, chelates, and complexes ordinarily require a two-word name to indicate the inactive as well as the active portion.

2. The preferred order for the name of an inorganic salt is cation–anion (eg, sodium bromide). The same order is preferred for well-known salts of simple organic acids (eg, sodium lactate, magnesium citrate, potassium acetate). However, for most organic compounds, the pharmacologically active portion should be named first (eg, oxacillin sodium, codeine phosphate).

3. A name for a salt or ester should in general be derived from the name of the pharmacologically active moiety or corresponding acid (eg, acetic acid, sodium acetate, ethyl acetate). When a non-acid suffix is used, as is customary in the penicillin series, a salt should be named without

modification of the parent acid name (eg, oxacillin, oxacillin sodium). Names for different salts or esters of the same active moiety should differ only in the name of the inactive portion (eg, estradiol enanthate, estradiol undecylenate); exceptions are permissible when both parts of the salt or ester possess pharmacologic activity (eg, aminophylline, prednazate).

4. A name for a quaternary ammonium substance should designate the cation and anion appropriately and separately (eg, octonium bromide, not octonine methylbromide).

5. A name for a complex of two or more components should indicate the composition by means of separate words, the last of which bears the suffix "-*ex*" (eg, bisacodyl tannex).

6. A name for a drug containing a radioactive atom should be constructed in the following pattern: tolpovidone I 131; rose bengal sodium I 131; cyanocobalamin Co 60; potassium bromide Br 82.[1]

7. It is recognized that for some purposes, such as in labeling, in advertising, or in package inserts, the use of standard chemical symbols and abbreviations of certain radicals may be desirable, and such usage is considered acceptable.

8. A name for a substance should not indicate the state of hydration, the morphology, the biologic source (horse, sheep, pig, etc), or the mode of preparation. Such information, however, should be available to the health professions in the literature accompanying the drug.

Preferred Spelling

1. The use of an isolated letter or number, or hyphenation, should be restricted to those groups of substances for which such usage fulfills a clearly demonstrable purpose.

2. To facilitate translation and pronunciation, "f" preferably should be used instead of "ph," "t" instead of "th," and "e" instead of "ae" or "oe." The World Health Organization also recommends that the letters "h" and "y" be avoided as much as possible so that nonproprietary names can be spelled identically in various languages.

3. Syllables such as "methylhydro" and "chlor" preferably should be condensed (eg, to "medro" and "clo").

Preferred Construction

Group relationships in a name preferably should be shown by use of the syllables (stems) listed in Tables I and II; conversely, use of the stem for other than the appropriate group should be avoided. When conflict arises, the stem conveying the most information should be used.

Philosophy of a USAN

An examination of nonproprietary names for drugs currently in use is likely to result in an inaccurate evaluation of present nomenclature activities. Many of these names were coined prior to the adoption of present nomenclature procedures and principles; indeed, many of these names made obvious the need for the action that has been taken by the USAN Council. Existing names, then, reflect a mixture of new and old nomenclature practices.

In many instances poor naming of drugs was due to the early practice of condensing the full chemical name into a chemically oriented nonproprietary name. At the time this practice came into being the chemistry of most drugs was not too complex. With advancing chemical complexity of drug entities, however, nonproprietary names so derived became increasingly long and difficult to spell, pronounce, and remember.

In addition to the problems caused by the complexity of the word itself, chemically derived names have been criticized because they fail to provide useful information to anyone but a scientist involved in drug development. (Although his need is recognized, he has the more scientific and accurate chemical nomenclature to serve his purpose.)

Nonproprietary nomenclature is intended primarily for physicians, pharmacists, and those in related health professions. A physician is not too concerned with the sometimes subtle structural manipulation of molecules which produce a potential new drug. He is more properly concerned with the understanding of the drug's pharmacological and therapeutic properties. Therefore, it must be emphasized again that nonproprietary names should be coined in such a way as to be most useful to, and usable by, their primary users: those in the health professions.

A well-coined nonproprietary name should be distinctive. Repetitious use of chemical prefixes is to be avoided; how many hundreds of drug names begin with di-, meth-, chlor-, oxy-, and phen-? By abandoning strict adherence to chemical antecedents, names can be made not only simpler but more unique.

In order to assign meaningful nonproprietary names to new drug compounds it is necessary to indicate through the name any relationship that exists between the new entity and established drugs. Conversely, inappropriate names suggesting nonexisting relationships are to be avoided. The USAN Council has made use of standardized suffixes, prefixes or stem syllables to apply to particular classes of drugs. The recommended list of these syllables (see Tables I and II) is revised and updated regularly to keep pace with the changing chemical and pharmacologic nature of new drugs.

Again, a random survey of names for drugs currently in use will show a mixture of "old" and "new" nomenclature practices. In fact, such a survey, presented below, should effectively illustrate the principles behind the newer nomenclature approach.

Figure 26-1 presents a pair of compounds named some years ago, meprobamate and carisoprodol, that are related both

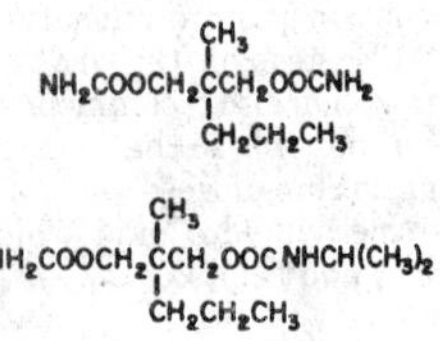

Fig 26-1.   Meprobamate (top) and carisoprodol (bottom) are closely related chemically and pharmacologically; the assigned names, however, do not indicate this relationship.

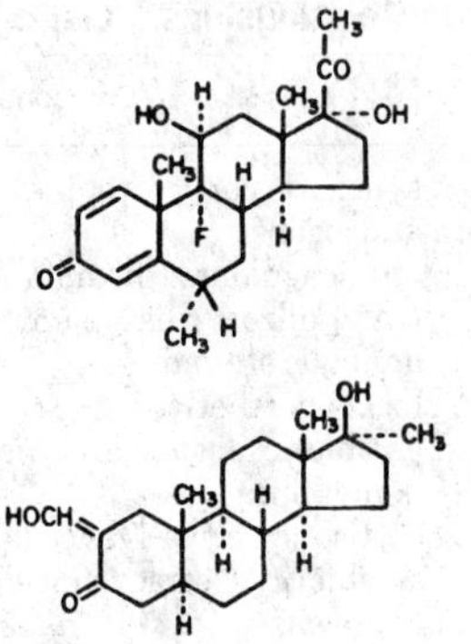

Fig 26-2.   Illustrative of poor practice in nomenclature are the compounds fluorometholone (top) and oxymetholone (bottom). The compounds are not as closely related as the names suggest.

chemically and pharmacologically; despite these similarities, the drugs have dissimilar names.

The opposite situation is illustrated in Fig 26-2; the relationship between fluorometholone and oxymetholone begins and ends with the fact that both compounds are steroids. This class of compounds, however, is so large and so diverse that ring structure alone is hardly sufficient to warrant the use of a common stem (-metholone).

The steroids are, in fact, typical of several large groups of compounds which (within each group) exhibit somewhat similar chemical and pharmacologic properties. Because of diversity within the group, however, it is desirable to establish subseries of names based on the nature of the substituent groups present and on the placement of such substituents. In recent years the USAN Council has increasingly developed this principle, which is typified by the examples in Figs 26-3 and 26-4.

Figure 26-3 depicts a basic glucocorticoid structure (glucocorticoids in themselves being a division of the broader category of steroids) in which the "R" groups indicate the positions at which the principal differences in the subseries occur. There is no common suffix for the entire glucocorticoid series, but the suffixes -olone and -sone are indicative of this series and are used in the stems of the various subseries.

The phenothiazine tranquilizers are a large series of drugs built on the nucleus shown in Fig 26-4. The side chain variations that determine which suffix is to be used are also shown, along with examples of some names in each subseries. Since nuclear substitution has not influenced the selection of the distinguishing suffixes (but on occasion has been used to provide a prefix), the figure neglects nuclear substitution. The suffix -azine is common to each of the five more specific suffixes of the various subseries illustrated and thus helps to exhibit the broad relationship among all these drugs.

The use of common stems to indicate particular classes of drugs is constantly reexamined by the USAN Council. The development of nomenclature for the tetracycline series of

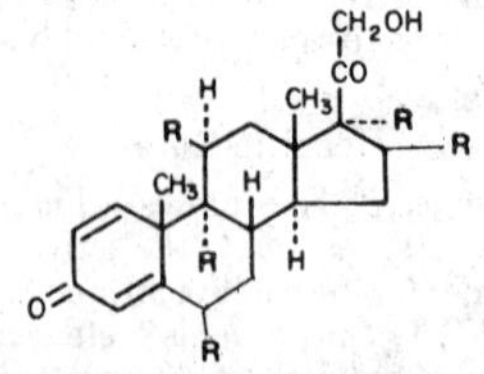

Fig 26-3.   The "R" groups indicate the positions on the glucocorticoid nucleus where the principal variations occur. Such variations give rise to the subseries in which the suffix -olone or -sone is used in the subseries stem—eg, -cinolone (triamcinolone, fluocinolone); -cortolone (clocortolone, flucortolone); -methasone (betamethasone, flumethasone).

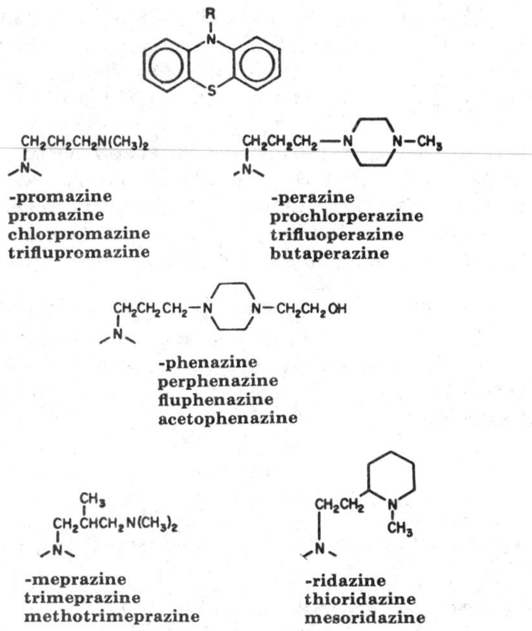

Fig 26-4.   The nucleus of phenothiazine tranquilizers and side-chain variations.

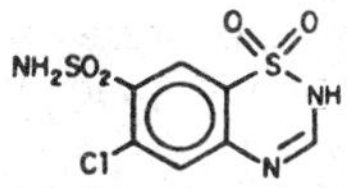

Fig 26-6.   Chlorothiazide; other drugs in this diuretic and antihypertensive series are hydrochlorothiazide, polythiazide, and althiazide.

drugs (see Fig. 26-5) demonstrates the review and revision processes by which the Council's principles are assessed in order to assure their validity in the light of current nomenclature thought.

The first drugs in this series were chlortetracycline and oxytetracycline, both of which can be chemically converted to the parent compound, tetracycline. Further research led to still another variant, demethylchlortetracycline, which, in keeping with the standard practice of the time, was named in strict accordance with its chemical derivation.

The next member of this series to come to negotiation was characterized by a distinctive pyrrolidine group and, following traditional patterns, the name might have become pyrrolidinotetracycline. Instead, the first step was taken toward simplifying names in this series by shortening the prefix and the resulting name became rolitetracycline. The next step was to drop the syllables "tetra" from the suffixes of newer nonproprietary names for drugs in this group thus yielding simpler and more useful designations. Examples of such designations are amicycline, sancycline, and doxycycline.

Although it is a very difficult thing to do, occasionally the need and the opportunity arise to go back and change the poorly coined name of a well-established drug. Such is the case with the above-mentioned drug, demethylchlortetracycline. The name of this compound, which is commercially available as the hydrochloride salt, has been changed to demeclocycline hydrochloride.

Chlorothiazide (Fig 26-6) and the early related compounds which followed it were assigned chemically derived nonproprietary names. The *-thiazide* stem, while chemically oriented, came to have a pharmacologic significance to medical scientists, indicating to them a group of diuretic and antihypertensive drugs. This stem, then, has been retained in the names of all drugs in this group, although excessive dependence on chemical antecedents (as exemplified in the name hydroflumethiazide) has given way to simpler names such as althiazide and polythiazide.

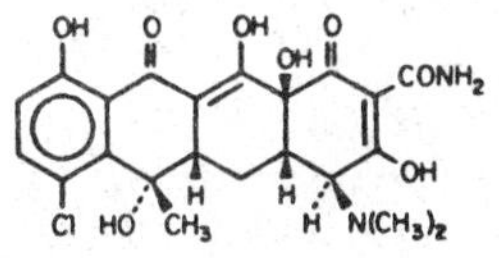

These few examples serve as a guide to the direction of the Council's thought as it seeks to provide appropriate and meaningful nonproprietary names which are, at the same time, relatively simple and useful to members of the medical and related health professions.

International Nonproprietary Names

The USAN Council functions primarily to serve the health professions in the US. However, in an age when drug manufacturers market their products in many countries, when international travel is increasing steadily, and when medical and pharmaceutical literature is read widely around the world, the need for cooperation regarding nomenclature among the major drug-producing countries is clearly evident.

In addition to the USAN Council in the United States, nomenclature agencies exist in Great Britain, France, Italy, Japan, the Nordic countries, and the Union of Soviet Socialist Republics.[2] These agencies operate at varying levels of authority and cooperate with pharmaceutical manufacturers within their areas of jurisdiction in the selection of appropriate nonproprietary names.

The agencies maintain liaison with one another in an effort to secure the wide adoption of the most appropriate designation for each drug. The natural concern of each of these groups is with the drugs that are currently being synthesized, isolated, investigated, produced, or marketed in its own national area. Because such activity for any specific drug rarely, if ever, occurs simultaneously throughout the world, the need for the different agencies to act on a nonproprietary name for a particular drug will vary in time.

The national agencies of the US, Great Britain, and France have set up procedures, with the knowledge and consent of the manufacturers involved, which circulate the names proposed for adoption, along with the pertinent chemical data, to the other agencies with a request that they be reviewed for appropriateness, availability, and the possible existence of another nationally adopted designation for the specific drug. If no valid objection to the proposed name is received, it can be assumed that the name then adopted will receive primary consideration by the other agencies if and when the drug becomes of interest elsewhere.

To prevent the confusion which arises when several nonproprietary names are used for a single drug, either in the same country or in several different countries, the World Health Organization (WHO) has assumed the responsibility of coordinating existing nomenclature efforts at the international level.

Through its Committee on Nonproprietary Names, whose members are drawn primarily from representatives of the national nomenclature agencies, the WHO has developed a procedure and guiding principles for the selection of International Nonproprietary Names (INN). Where national nomenclature agencies exist, they usually act as agents for manufacturers by referring mutually selected designations (usually prior to national adoption) to the WHO with the request that these be considered for selection as international nonproprietary names.

A manufacturer located in a country without a nomenclature agency can direct his request for a nonproprietary name

Fig 26-5.   Chlortetracycline; other names in this series include rolitetracycline, meclocycline, and amicycline.

to the WHO directly or, in some instances, to an existing agency in another country, preferably one in which the pharmaceutical preparation is likely to be marketed.

After the selection of international nonproprietary names, the WHO proposes and, in more favorable cases, recommends to all its member states that such names be adopted at the local level. Formal adoption in accordance with national practice is necessary to provide review of the suitability of the international name for national use and leads to orderly documentation of nomenclature data.

Dissemination of Nomenclature Information

The fact that nonproprietary names for drugs are being selected with ever-increasing thought and skill means little if these names are not brought to the attention of and used by those for whom they are intended. To accomplish this the USAN Council and its sponsors have developed a publication program to disseminate nomenclature information.

The Council publishes a monthly "New Names" column in the *journal, Clinical Pharmacology and Therapeutics*, reprints of which are available on request from the USAN Council staff.

Cumulative compilations of USAN are now included in the book *USAN and the USP Dictionary of Drug Names*, published annually by the United States Pharmacopeial Convention, Inc;[3] each annual edition is cumulative from June 15, 1961, when the USAN program began. This book, alphabetically arranged, also includes current official compendium names, nonproprietary names, brand names, code designations, CAS registry numbers, and a table of molecular formulas and corresponding USAN, in addition to chemical names, graphic formulas, and pharmacologic/therapeutic categories.

Although the advances in drug nomenclature have been significant, the task ahead does not diminish but grows increasingly complex. It remains the aim and hope of the USAN Council to continue to provide an effective service in this field.

References

1. *J Am Med Assoc 218:* 1423, 1971.
2. *International Nonproprietary Names (INN) for Pharmaceutical Substances*, Cumulative List No 6. World Health Organization, Geneva, Switzerland, 1982.
3. *USAN and the USP Dictionary of Drug Names.* United States Pharmacopeial Convention, Inc, Rockville, MD 20852.

CHAPTER 27

Structure-Activity Relationship and Drug Design

Murray Zanger, PhD

Professor of Chemistry
Philadelphia College of Pharmacy and Science
Philadelphia, PA 19104

The seeds of Medicinal Chemistry were planted by the first individual who attempted to use vegetable or mineral preparations for the treatment of disease. Although no one knows when this first occurred, it is well-documented that most ancient cultures utilized a variety of herbal mixtures, teas etc. to treat illness. The active ingredients of some of these concoctions are still found in a modern Pharmacopeia. The Chinese emperor Sheng Nung described a drug for the treatment of malaria in 3000 BC. About the year 1500 Carpensis employed mercury compounds in the treatment of syphilis. Cinchona bark (quinine), to combat malaria, was known in the middle of the 17th century. Nicolaier introduced methenamine, as a urinary antiseptic, about 1895. All of these examples resulted from purely empirical experiences. There was no organized effort to develop better drugs or to study the effects of existing ones under scientific conditions.

Ehrlich, in 1909, with the discovery of arsphenamine (salvarsan) as a treatment for syphilis is credited with being the first to systematically screen compounds for a specific activity. This development along with the concepts of drug activity and drug receptors which he formulated place him among the first of those to whom the title of medicinal chemist could truly be applied.

Following Ehrlich's success, Germany pioneered in drug research. Plasmochin in the year 1924 and Atabrine in 1930 were synthesized as antimalarials. In the late 1930s the sulfonamides began their remarkable career as bacteriostatic agents and about 1940 the first antibiotic, penicillin, was introduced, from England.

It should be noted that most of the medicinal agents mentioned are antibacterial in nature. Because of the protracted efforts of the 19th-century microbiologists, many of the bacterial agents which caused the common, easily diagnosed, human diseases had been identified and could be cultured, studied, and the effect of chemical agents noted. Ehrlich had a target, therefore, for which to fashion his bullet. Such is not the case today, for many human afflictions. Cancer, heart, and mental diseases go unchecked primarily because the causative agent, the "target," has not been defined. In the first quarter of this century pharmacology and chemotherapy were infants, not to mature until World War II provided the impetus. Only in the past 30 years have the biological sciences become sufficiently quantitative so that the more subtle and sophisticated human ailments could be studied and the effects of therapeutic agents evaluated.

Chemotherapy

Chemotherapy is the use of chemical agents in the treatment of disease: a very simple, succinct definition, but extremely difficult to reduce to practice. The problem, in short, is to find a drug or drug combination which can be administered, absorbed, transported to the active site, elicit its desired action and then be metabolized and excreted from the body.

Additionally, unwanted side effects and toxic reactions should be at a minimum. There are several approaches which can be used to achieve these goals. All of them, however, must at present start with an active molecule or type of compound.

Certain organic structures or functional groups are believed to possess or enhance certain biologic activities when incorporated in organic molecules. Table I shows the diversity of activities attributed to the many groups illustrated. It is apparent that the assignment of a specific type of activity to any single functional group is virtually impossible. It is not then possible to construct a medicinal substance by selecting a biologically inert organic substance and appending those functional groups that should impart the desired qualities to the molecule.

The enormity of the problem of drug design begins to become evident. Because of the many biologic activities possessed by a single functional group, the medicinal chemist is confronted with the enigma of nonspecificity. If the drug is not specific it must entertain a degree of toxicity by interference with normal metabolic processes along with the abnormal, disease-causing process. Nonspecificity is only one of a multitude of factors that greatly influence the activity of a drug and because of the large number of variables encountered, it is often surprising that any success is achieved in the attempt to "tailor-make"a drug molecule.

In designing a drug to have a distinctive activity in the treatment of a specific disease, the approaches can be classified broadly as either theoretical or empirical. Historically, the empirical method predates the theoretical by many years and is still the most widely used. For example, it has been shown (Table I) that organic compounds with both amino and ester functions exhibit local anesthetic activity. The chemist may then synthesize several types of molecules possessing these functional groups and the pharmacologist determines the relative activity of each compound. Usually the activities are referred to a standard medicinal agent—a known local anesthetic, in this case.

Or, in generally screening random compounds, the pharmacologist may uncover an interesting biologic activity and communicate his findings to the chemist. Then the chemist utilizes the pharmacologic information to alter his original molecule, providing new compounds for further testing. The pharmacologist, of course, must have previously developed reliable testing procedures.

Other empirical approaches include the random screening of compounds for a variety of pharmacologic activities to uncover "new" active molecules. Often it is a drug metabolite which is the active compound, so studies of the metabolic fate of drugs has also been used as a route to improved drugs. Prontosil forming sulfanilamide, chloral hydrate yielding trichloroethanol, phenacetin going to p-acetamidophenol, oleandomycin yielding the triacetyl derivative (TAO), and zoxazolamine forming chlorzoxazone are several examples of this phenomenon (see Fig 27-1). By identifying, synthesiz-

Table I—Activities Associated with Certain Structural Units[a]

Chemical group	Type structures	Drug example or prototype	Activity
Acetals (see also *Ethers*)	R_2C—O—CH_2CH CH_2NR_2 └─ O ─┘	Glyketal Febrifugine Paraldehyde	Anticholinergic Antimalarial Hypnotic
Acids	RCOOH RCHOHCOOH $RCH(NH_2)COOH$	Propionic acid Chaulmoogric acid Mandelic acid Salicylic acid Salicylates Aspirin Amino acids Thyroxine	Fungistatic Mycobacteriostatic Bacteriostatic Keratolytic Antirheumatic Antipyretic Nutritional Antimitotic Hormonal
Alcohols (see also *Carbohydrates*)	ROH, where R is simple or complex	Benzyl alcohol 3-Pyridinemethanol Ethanol 2-Propanol Vitamins A and E, pyridoxine, thiamine, riboflavin Choline	Local anesthetic Vasodilator Sedative Anticonvulsant Vitamins Transmethylation
Amides (see also *Amidines; Imides; Sulfonamides; Ureides; Semicarbazones; Thioureas*)	RCONHR $ArCONH(CH_2)_nNR_2$ $ArNHCOCH_2NR_2$ heterocyclic-$CONR_2$ Cyclic peptides Cyclic imides Polyfunctional amides	Phenacetin Procainamide Lidocaine Nikethamide LSD ACTH, insulin Oxytocin Polymyxin Barbiturates Idoxuridine Hydantoins Phensuximide Chloramphenicol Halofenate Colchicine Angiotensin Amide	Analgesic Cardiotonic Local anesthetic Analeptic Psychotomimetic Hormonal Antibiotic Hypnotic Antiviral Anticonvulsant Antibiotic Uricosuric Antimitotic Hypertensive
Amidines (see also *Amides; Guanidines*)	$RC(NH_2)$=NH	Phenacine Hydroxystilbamidine	Local anesthetic Trypanocidal
Amines	ArCHOH—CHR—NHR $CH_3(CH_2)_nCH(NH_2)CH_3$ $R_2N(CH_2)_nNR_2$ $R_2CHO(CH_2)_nNR_2$ Carbocyclic-NH_2 Heterocyclic-$NH(CH_2)_nNR_2$ $H_2NArCOOR$ $R_2NCH_2CH_2Cl$ $RN(CH_2CH_2Cl)_2$ RNHCl	Phenethylamine Epinephrine Amphetamine Tuaminoheptane Tripelennamine Diphenhydramine Chlorpheniramine Oxyphencyclimine Methadone Amantadine Primaquine Lucanthone Benzocaine Phenoxybenzamine Nitrogen Mustards Chloramines	Pressor Vasoconstrictor CNS stimulant Vasoconstrictor Antihistamine Antispasmodic Analgesic Antiviral Antimalarial Antischistosomal Local anesthetic Adrenergic block Antineoplastic Antiseptics
Amino alcohols	$ArCHOH(CH_2)_nNR_2$	Acetylcholine Levarterenol Ephedrine Quinine Ethambutol Propranolol	Cholinergic Pressor CNS stimulant Vasoconstrictor Antimalarial Antitubercular agent Antiarrhythmic agent
Amino ethers	R—O—$CH_2CH_2NR_2$	Dimethisoquin Benzodioxanes Phenoxybenzamine Methoxyphenamine Dimenhydrinate Clomiphene	Local anesthetic Antihistamine Sympatholytic Sympathomimetic Antinauseant Ovulation inducing agent

Table I—Continued

Chemical group	Type structures	Drug example or prototype	Activity
Amino ketones	$Ar_2C(COR)(CH_2)_nNR_2$	Methadone	Analgesic
	Cyclic ketone	Tetracyclines	Antibiotic
Ammonium compounds (quaternary)	R_4N^+	Tetraethylammonium	Vasodilator
		Decamethonium	Neuromuscular block
		Hexamethonium	Hypotensive
		Neostigmine	Anticholinesterase
	$R_3\overset{+}{N}CH_2CH_2OCOR$	Methantheline	Anticholinergic
	$ArCH_2\overset{+}{N}(CH_3)_2$—R (long)	Benzethonium	Antiseptic
Carbohydrates (see also *Alcohols*)	$R(CHOH)_nCHO$	ATP	High-energy phosphate
		Lactulose	Cathartic
		Riboflavin	Vitamin
		Streptomycin	Antibiotic
Dyestuffs	Azo dyes	Evans Blue	Diagnostic
	Triphenylmethane type	Gentian Violet	Antibacterial
	Phthaleins	Phenolphthalein	Cathartic
	Pyronine type	Fluorescein	Diagnostic
Enols, enediols	RCOH ‖ RCR and	Ascorbic Acid	Vitamin
	RCOH ‖ RCOH	Tetracycline	Antibiotic
Esters	$RSO_2O(CH_2)_nOSO_2R$	Busulfan	Antineoplastic
	$RONO_2$	Nitroglycerin	Vasodilator
	$H_2NArCOOR$	Benzocaine	Local anesthetic
	$ArCOO(CH_2)_nNR_2$	Procaine	
	Alicyclic aminoester	Cocaine	
		Scopolamine	Cholinergic block
	Heterocyclic aminoester	Meperidine	Analgesic
Ethers (see also *Pyrones*)	R_2O	Ethyl ether	Anesthetic
		Vinyl ether	
	Epoxide	Ethylene oxide	Fumigant
		Scopolamine	Cholinergic block
	Ar—O—R	Codeine	Antitussive
		Mephenesin	Muscle relaxant
		Morphine	Analgesic
		Papaverine	Vasodilator
		Streptomycin	Antibiotic
	Ar—O—Ar	Thyroxine	Hormonal
	$ArOCH_2CH_2NR_2$	Dimethisoquin	Local anesthetic
	$Ar_2CHOCH_2CH_2NR_2$	Diphenhydramine	Antihistamine
Guanidines (see also *Amides; Amidines*)	$RNHC(=NH)NHR$	Streptomycin	Antibiotic
		Guanethidine	Hypotensive
		Cimetidine	Antagonist
Halogen compounds	RCl	Ethyl chloride	Local anesthetic
	CCl_4	Carbon tetrachloride	Anthelmintic
	$CHCl_3$	Chloroform	Anesthetic
	Cl_3CCHO	Chloral	Hypnotic
	Cyclic-Cl	DDT, BHC	Parasiticide
	$HOArCl_n$	Hexachlorophene	Anti-infective
	$RNHCl, RSO_2NHCl$	Halazone	Disinfectant
	Aryl iodinated compounds	Iopanoic acid	Radiopaque
	Fluorinated steroids	Dexamethasone	Glucocorticoids
	Fluorinated heterocycle	Flucytosine	Fungicide
	Fluorinated aromatic side chain	Flufenamic acid	Antiinflammatory
Hydrocarbons		Cyclopropane	Anesthetic
		Ethylene	
Ketones (see also *Pyrones*)	ArCOR	Acetophenone	Sedative
	$Ar(CO)_2$	Diphenadione	Anticoagulant
		Camphor	External analgesic
		Ketonic steroids	Anti-inflammatory, hormonal
	$(HOAr)_2CO$	Dioxybenzone	Ultraviolet screen

Table I—Continued

Chemical group	Type structures	Drug example or prototype	Activity
Lactones (see also *Esters*)		Ascorbic acid	Vitamin
		Dicumarol	Anticoagulant
		Digitoxin	Cardiotonic
		Phenolphthalein	Cathartic
		Pilocarpine	Cholinergic
		Santonin	Anthelmintic
		Tetracyclines	Antibiotic
Mercaptans		Dimercaprol	Chelating agent
		Methimazole	Antithyroid
Mercurials		Thimerosal	Antiseptic
		Meralluride	Diuretic
Nitrile	$RC \equiv N$	Verapamil	Coronary vasodilator
Nitro compounds	$ArNO_2$	Chloramphenicol	Antibiotic
		Nitrofurans	Coccidicidal
			Bactericidal
		Nitrocresols	Weight reducing
Phenols	$ArOH$	Amodiaquine	Antimalarial
		Cresols	Antiseptic
		Estradiol, diethylstilbestrol	Estrogenic
		Guaiacol	Expectorant
		Hexylresorcinol	Anthelmintic
		Hydroxymorphinans	Analgesic
Phosphorus compounds	$R_2N(RO)P(O)NHR$	Cyclophosphamide	Antineoplastic
	$(R_2N)_3P(S)$	Thiotepa	
	$(R_2N)_2P(O)NHCOOR$	Uredepa	
	$R_3\overset{+}{N}(CH_2)_nSP(O)(OR)_2$	Echothiophate	Anticholinesterase
	$F-P(O)(OR)_2$	Isoflurophate	
Pyrones (see also *Ethers; Ketones; Lactones*)		Kojic acid	Antibiotic
		Khellin	Cardiovascular
		Dicumarol	Anticoagulant
		Lucanthone	Schistosomicidal
Quinones (see also *Ketones*)		Emodin	Cathartic
		Vitamin K	Coagulant
		Menadione	
Semicarbazones	$ArCH=NNHCONH_2$	Nitrofurazone	Bacteriostatic
Thiosemicarbazones	$ArCH=NNHCSNH_2$	Thiacetazone	Tuberculostatic
		Methisazone	Antiviral
Silicones	$R_3SiO(R_2SiO)_nSiR_3$	Simethicone	Antiflatulent
Stilbenes	$RArC=CArR$	Hydroxystilbamidine	Trypanocidal
			Fungicidal
		Diethylstilbestrol	Estrogenic
Sulfonamides	H_2NArSO_2NHR	Sulfonamide drugs	Bacteriostatic
		Acetazolamide	Diuretic
	$ArSO_2NHCONHR$	Tolbutamide	Hypoglycemic
Sulfonimides		Saccharin	Sweetening agent
Sulfones	R_2SO_2	Sulfonal	Hypnotic
	Ar_2SO_2	Dapsone	Leprostatic
		Sulfinpyrazone	Uricosuric
Thioureas and Ureides (see also *Thiosemicarbazones*)	$RNHCSNHR'$	Thiouracil	Antithyroidal
		Metiamide	H_2-Antagonist
		α-Naphthylthiourea	Anticoagulant
		Thiobarbiturates	Hypnotic
Ureas	$RNHCONHR'$	Urea	Diuretic
		Diethylcarbamazine	Filaricide
		Suramin	Trypanocidal

Table I—Continued

Chemical group	Type structures	Drug example or prototype	Activity
Ureides (see also *Amides*)	RNHCONHCOR'	Barbiturates	Hypnotic
		Hydantoins	Anticonvulsant
		Theophylline	Diuretic
Urethans (Carbamates) (see also *Amides*)	ROCONH$_2$	Meprobamate	Muscle relaxant
		Ethinamate	Hypnotic
		Novobiocin	Antibiotic
	ROCONR$_2$	Neostigmine	Anticholinesterase
		Trimethadione	Anticonvulsant
	Dithiocarbamates	Disulfiram	Alcoholism
	Metal dithiocarbamates	Thiram	Antifungal

[a] Adapted from a drug prototype listing by Burger.[1]

ing, and pharmacologically testing excreted metabolites, the reactive portion of a molecule often can be ascertained.

Yet another line of research is employed whereby currently used drugs can be improved or modified by altering their absorption, distribution, metabolism and excretion patterns. The concept of *Drug Latentiation* has been promulgated by Harper. It involves the chemical modification of a known biologically active compound to form a new substance, which upon *in vivo* enzymatic attack will liberate the parent compound. Drugs that have been altered in this fashion are also known as *prodrugs*. Several reasons for accomplishing the latentiation process are: to modify duration of action; to modify transportation and distribution of the drug in the body; to reduce toxicity; and to overcome difficulties encountered in pharmaceutical formulation procedures or in the dosage form itself. Typically, this involves conversion of alcohols and thioalcohols either to organic phosphates or esters. Amines may be changed to amides or any active molecule may be transformed into a complex or salt. Aspirin could be considered a prodrug insofar as its activity depends on its salicylic acid moiety. Esterification of the phenolic hydroxyl group greatly reduces the toxicity of salicylic acid.

Another example is the use of stilbestrol phosphate, rather than the free phenol, on the theory that high phosphatase

activity in cancerous tissue will liberate the unesterified drug *in situ*. The phosphate, although possessing a high degree of water solubility, is estrogenically inert. The rate of release of an active drug from the form in which it is transported through the body depends on the steric, electronic, and configurational aspects of the substituent X (Fig 27-2). If the active drug is an ester, as in *a*, *b*, or *d*, the rate of release of the alcohol depends upon the nature of X. That the rate of enzymatic hydrolysis is influenced by electronic factors has been amply demonstrated. Numerous other examples could be cited to substantiate the feasibility of drug latentiation.

Still another approach to drug design has progressed tremendously with the advent of the computer era. If it were possible to evaluate and assess the manner in which all, or at least the important, factors affect the efficacy of a drug and relate these factors to the complex biosystem through which the drug must survive in order to be efficacious, then, perhaps, one could intelligently construct a molecule that would be effective in the treatment of a specific disease state. This goal has never been attained, but enormous gains have been made and it is not improbable that success will be forthcoming in the near future. Later, in this chapter, a more detailed discussion will be given on the use of a mathematical model to correlate chemical with biologic activity.

Two-dimensional structural organic formulas are a very poor means of representing the physical, chemical, or biologic properties of a molecule. Structural formulas merely depict the way the various atoms are strung together to form what is known as a *molecule*. Drugs that are strikingly similar in structure may demonstrate widely differing pharmacologic properties, while two drugs of apparently different structure can exhibit almost identical activity. Reference to Table I easily confirms these facts. There are many factors other than simple structural variation that have an effect on the activity of a drug.

The systematic modification of active molecules, based on

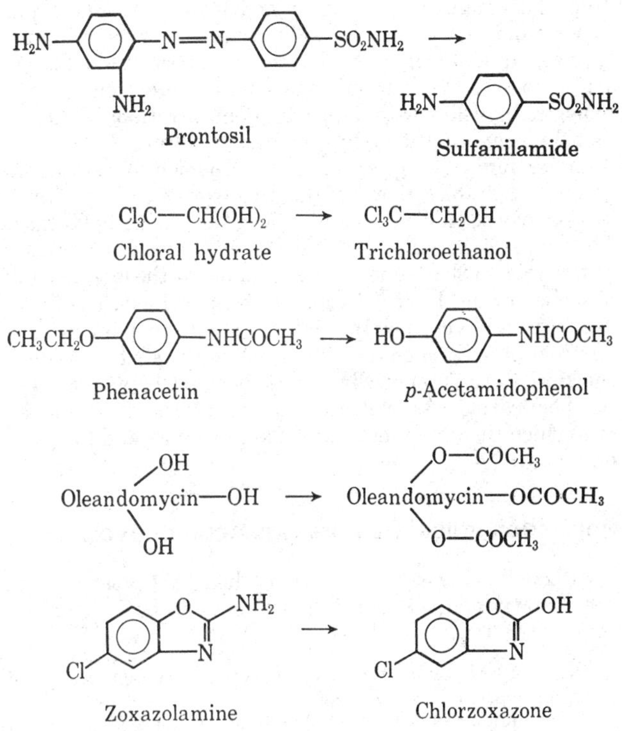

Fig 27-1.

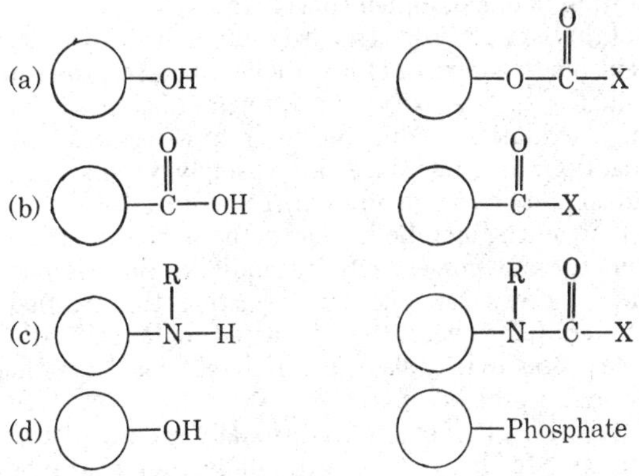

Fig 27-2.

empirical data finds its best expression in the Hansch equation and the Free-Wilson approach to drug design. These and other modern methods will be discussed later in this chapter.

Ideally, theoretical drug design methods should lead to SAR relationships without the need for experimental input. Quantum mechanics may ultimately provide these results but currently, methods based on these calculations are no better or more widely applicable than the empirical modes.

Regardless of how the chemist chooses the method used to modify a structure, the process is complex since many of the factors to be considered are interdependent. In order to more fully appreciate these factors it is important to review the biologic and physicochemical aspects associated with or which have an effect on drug activity.

Biologic Factors

Absorption—Most drugs are administered orally and pass through the stomach, small intestine and colon, from any of which they may be absorbed. During its passage the drug will experience a range of pH starting at about 1.5 in the stomach and reaching the colon whose pH may be as high as 8. Additionally it is subjected to a variety of enzymes and complexing agents, all of which tend to reduce the effective dose of the compound.

In order for the drug to be absorbed (through a lipoid membrane) it should be in the unionized form. The pK_a of the drug and the pH of the absorption site determine (along with lipid solubility) the ease of absorption. Acidic drugs (eg aspirin) are best absorbed from the stomach while basic compounds (quinine) are preferentially absorbed in the colon. Permanently ionized molecules (quaternary ammonium salts) are poorly absorbed from any region of the GI tract.

Finally, the exact mechanism by which a drug is absorbed is unknown. It is not simply the passage of a molecule through a membrane, as in osmosis. Many biochemical reactions occur at the absorption interface, which again influences the survival rate of a drug. That much of the drug does not survive the digestive tract is demonstrated by the fact that in many cases a smaller parenteral dose is required for the same drug than if administered orally.

Transport—The blood is the primary carrier of drugs throughout the body. Independent of the method of administration, the drug must pass through several membranes on its way to the active site. Solubility, degree of ionization, etc, all affect the transport process. Other factors which complicate the transport process are similar to those found above; complexation, protein binding etc. Most drugs move through a membrane by a simple diffusion mechanism (passive transport) while a few compounds which resemble normal body substrates are carried via an "active transport" process. In "active transport," drugs can move against a concentration gradient, that is they can go from a compartment of low concentration to one of higher concentration.

Metabolism—As soon as a drug enters the body it becomes susceptible to a variety of metabolic processes, the purpose of which is to "detoxify" the foreign substance. That is through oxidation, reduction, hydrolysis, esterification, or conjugation the drug is made increasingly water soluble so it can ultimately be excreted from the body.

In fact, a drug metabolite may actually be the active compound or it may possess activity similar to the original compound but after several bio-transformations the modified form is excreted. The liver is the primary site of detoxification but enzyme processes may also occur in the stomach, intestine and other areas in the body.

Metabolic reactions are traditionally separated into two categories. In the first, the drug undergoes what might be termed functional group changes; ring or side chain hydroxylation, nitro-group reduction, aldehyde oxidation, de-alkylation, deamination etc. The second metabolic path is called conjugation, in which the metabolized compound combines with solubilizing groups such as glucuronic acid or glycine to form excretable conjugates.

Because drugs can undergo such a wide variety of chemical changes in the body, the specifics of which are unpredictable, the medicinal chemist must at least be aware of these metabolic processes. At some point in the development of a new drug the molecular structure of the drug may have to be altered in order to change the way in which it is metabolized.

Reactions at Active Sites (see *Antimetabolites*, page 441)—Ehrlich first introduced the concept that a drug must first combine with a *receptor* (active site) in order to be effective. A receptor is considered to be some cellular substance upon which a drug acts to produce its desired (or undesired) effect. It is believed that enzymes are the primary receptors and drug action is a consequence of the influence of the drug on the enzyme. An enzyme system is composed of: a *coenzyme*, usually nonprotein in nature; an *apoenzyme* (the protein portion), which may also enjoin a nonprotein *prosthetic* group; *cofactors*, often inorganic metallic ions; and the *substrate* (that which is acted upon). Exposed on the "active site" may be anionic, cationic, acidic, basic, and neutral sites. Also, the physical shape of the site is such that the contour of the molecule accepted by the receptor must be proper to insure a "fit" (see *Molecular Size and Shape* under *Physicochemical Factors*). Beyond this point little concrete evidence is available to validate the theoretical excursions into the theory of drug action.

Binding and Storage (see Chapter 14)—Mention was made previously of the fact that mucins and proteins bind drugs. That is, some form of molecular adhesion causes the drug to be coupled with protein substances and other macromolecules. If the binding force is strong, the drug may combine quickly with the macromolecule and be thus removed from the transport system, metabolized, and excreted. Besides complexation to macromolecules, storage can also occur by dissolution in the body lipids or chelation by bony tissue, etc. In any case, the location and degree of storage is a factor influencing the potency, toxicity, and duration of action of a drug. For example, the short-acting barbiturates are thought to be bound very rapidly by body tissues and thus the active species is quickly removed from the transport system and its action ceases. Yet suramin sodium has an extremely long biological half-life, with noticeable concentrations occurring months after cessation of dosing with the drug.

Excretion—This process is closely coupled to metabolism and results in the removal of the drug from the body. Elimination may occur via the kidney, liver, skin, lungs, or GI tract. The route of excretion that is utilized is determined largely by the drug—volatile ones (ether, alcohol) via the lungs, poorly absorbed or insoluble substances through the GI tract with the feces, and very few through the skin; the main route of elimination is through the kidney. A thorough discussion of the kidney excretion mechanism is given in Chapter 38. The biochemical aspects relating to the complexity of the biosystem which the drug must survive are intricate and little understood.

Physicochemical Factors (Molecular Level)

Although many individual physicochemical properties have been shown to affect drug activity, they can be divided into three categories:

1. Spatial: Molecular size, stereochemistry, configuration and conformation.
2. Distribution and Binding: Solubility, partition coefficient, pK_a, and surface tension.

3. Structural: Group substitution (isosterism), electronic (inductive and resonance effects), redox potentials and spectroscopic parameters.

Molecular Size and Shape (see also *Metabolite Antagonism*, page 442)—Changing the size or stereochemistry of an active molecule may also alter its physical properties, such as solubility, thus it is not always easy to separate the various physicochemical effects cleanly.

With the above caveat, however, it has been demonstrated in numerous cases that the biological activity of enantiomeric drugs can be vastly different. Using the "lock and key" concept of drug receptors and drawing the analogy of right and left handed gloves, it is easily seen that a "right-handed" drug cannot fit a "left-handed" receptor.

It is postulated that for a drug (or any substrate) to combine effectively with a receptor (usually an enzyme), besides having the proper conformation, an attachment must occur at three separate sites. Thus, what may appear to be a relatively minor defect in the configuration or conformation of a drug, such as the opposite antipode of a stereoisomeric substance, may have appreciable effect on the extent of activity. A typical example is shown in Fig 27-3 for the epinephrine molecule. Thus, there must be a mutual melding of drug and receptor and a mutual adaptation so far as shape and charge distribution are concerned. To further illustrate the point, the antihistamine chlorpheniramine was (and still is) employed for many years before it was discovered that the (+) isomer, dexchlorpheniramine (as the maleate), has about twice the potency of the racemate and a wider margin of safety.

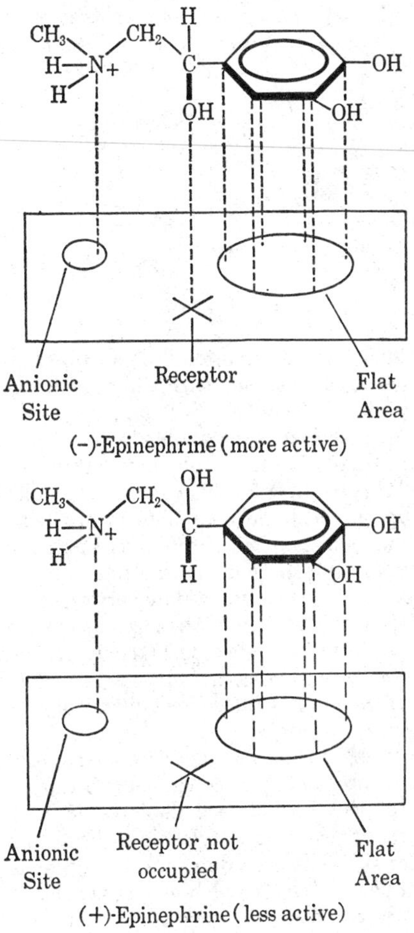

Solubility, Partition Coefficient and pK$_a$— Lipid-soluble drugs usually cross cellular boundaries by dissolving in or interacting with the lipid membranes and diffusing across into the intracellular aqueous phase. Most drugs are weak organic electrolytes, present in equilibrium between two forms, of which only the nonionized form possesses lipid solubility. In general, therefore, water-soluble compounds

$$AH \rightleftharpoons A^- + H^+$$

$$\underset{\text{drug}}{\underset{\text{nonionized}}{}} \quad \underset{\text{drug}}{\underset{\text{ionized}}{}}$$

that are either completely ionized or have lipid-insoluble nonionized forms are poorly absorbed. Quaternary amines and streptomycin are fully ionized and not absorbed to a great extent. At biologic pH values many sulfonamides exist in the nonionic form but are not absorbed well due to lipid insolubility.

Since the solubility of a drug and the partition coefficient between aqueous and lipid phases defines its ability to be absorbed and transported to the active site, these factors must be optimized in the final form of the molecule. Complicating this analysis is the ionization constant (pK$_a$) of the drug. In the calculation of partition coefficient, only that portion of the concentration of the drug in the aqueous phase which is unionized can be considered. With very weak acids or bases, the percent ionization is small but with stronger acids or bases the compound may exist mainly in the ionized form. This results in a greatly reduced effective concentration which in turn will inhibit absorption.

Thus, it should be evident that all of the nuances of molecular structure—interatomic distance, geometric and stereochemical conformation, rigidity and flexibility, and charge distribution—are factors that require attention in the overall consideration of drug design.

The preceding discussion has attempted to illustrate the complexity of the goal of "drug design." Though still largely empirical, the design and development of new drugs is gradually assuming more rational and systematic approaches to the problem. The advent of high speed computers, and their ability to rapidly analyze and correlate enormous amounts of

(−)-Epinephrine (more active)

(+)-Epinephrine (less active)

Fig 27-3.[2]

data is probably the most important tool now available to the medicinal chemist.

Theories and Mechanisms of Drug Action

Theories of drug action address mainly dose/response considerations. That is, why does a given dosage elicit a particular magnitude of response? Why also does drug response peak and then level off? These and other related questions find explanations in various theories of drug action, among them; occupancy theory, rate theory and the induced fit theory.

All of these theories start with the basic concept of a receptor and of how the drug binds to the receptor. Pharmacologists attempt to deal with these questions.

When questions of drug mechanism arise, it is the medicinal chemist who asks them since here it is the basic structures of the drug and the enzyme system it affects which are important. A drug mechanism then, seeks to relate the chemical structure of the active substance with its pharmacologic activity.

Most theories of drug action have evolved from the concept of drug–receptor interactions (see *Reactions at Active Sites*). Receptors are usually thought of as enzymes or other proteins vital to the life process. In a viable biosystem a variety of substrates are known to be metabolized through the intervention of enzyme systems. A large proportion of drugs are believed to act by altering the ability of the substrate to interact with the enzyme or receptor. Without attempting to be comprehensive, extensions of the drug–receptor concept will be discussed which have some experimental verification. The theory of *Metabolite Antagonism* is one that has gained

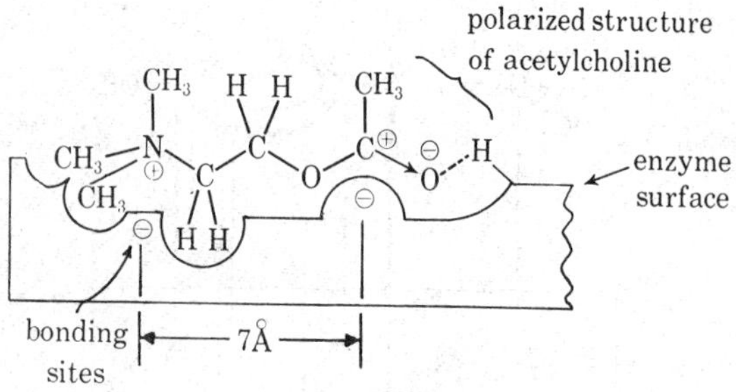

polarized structure
of acetylcholine

enzyme
surface

bonding
sites

|← 7Å →|

Fig 27-4.

PABA   **Sulfanilamide**

$$CH_3—S—CH_2—CH_2—CH—COOH$$
$$\overset{|}{NH_2}$$

Methionine
Fig 27-5.

great currency. An antimetabolite can function in one of several ways; it can complex with a metabolite and thus effectively remove it from the biochemical cycle; in a similar fashion it can inactivate a metabolite by forming a compound with it; and finally it can, through structural or functional group similarity, compete with a metabolite by blocking a site on an enzyme at which the metabolite ordinarily reacts. This latter mechanism, *enzyme inhibition*, has probably been studied by pharmacologists more than any other single mechanism. In its most up-to-date version the theory postulates that on the surface of the enzyme there are sites of particular conformation, spacing, and chemical affinity such that only a molecule that has a shape which mirror-images the enzyme surface and has the correct chemical groups can interact with the enzyme.

The receptor surface of acetylcholinesterase has been studied, and some of the dimensional and functional group properties of this enzyme are depicted in Fig 27-4. By modifying the structure of acetylcholine, the distance between the receptor sites has been determined, and by altering the substituent parts of the acetylcholine molecule, the chemical nature of the receptor sites has been ascertained. Amine (—NH$_2$), sulfhydryl (—SH) and hydroxyl (—OH) are the most common substituents, both on the drug and receptor molecules, through which interactions take place. The spacing, arrangement, and polarity of the binding sites on the receptor surface might be likened to a "lock" and the substrate or drug which interacts with it must fit these sites in order for reaction to occur.

This "lock-and-key" theory would explain, then, why molecules that structurally resemble a metabolite can act pharmacologically by substituting for the metabolite and thus effectively block any further reactions. Two molecules of approximately the same size and shape are called isosteres, and the synthesis of isosteres of known metabolites is one approach to the discovery of new pharmacodynamic agents. Sometimes, however, the chemist is fooled and a synthetic *isostere* (see *Isosterism* under *Molecular Modification*) instead of being antagonistic actually mimics the action of the natural compound. The synthetic vitamins K are good examples of this type of action.

The classic examples of metabolite antagonism by a drug are sulfanilamide and its derivatives. In work carried out by Woods, sulfanilamide was shown to be antagonistic to *p*-aminobenzoic acid (PABA), a biologic precursor of methionine (Fig 27-5). A fascinating feature of these studies was the demonstration that PABA would reverse the effect of sulfanilamide on a bacterial culture, an example of metabolite antagonism in reverse. Since the two compounds are isosteres, it is easy to see why they are mutually antagonistic. Either the metabolite or its antagonist can attach itself to the critical area of the enzyme surface; if the former occurs, the PABA begins its transformation into methionine; if the latter happens, the metabolic process ceases and in the case of bacteria multiplication is inhibited. The degree of inhibition depends on the relative concentrations of the substrate and the inhibitor and has been found to obey the following equa-

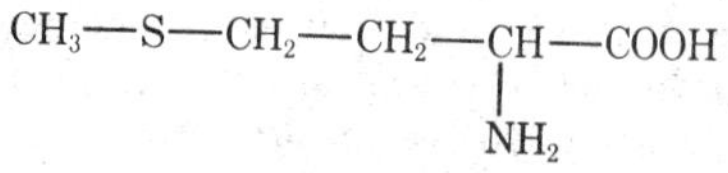

tion:

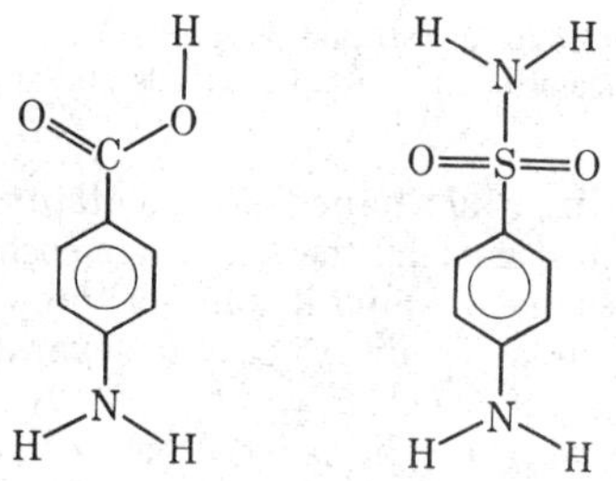

$$K = I/S \times ES/EI$$

where K is the inhibition ratio, I is the inhibitor concentration, S is the substrate concentration, and ES and EI are the enzyme–substrate and enzyme–inhibitor complex concentrations. This expression has been used to determine whether a drug is in fact competing with a substrate for a given site on an enzyme.

Another mode of drug action involves enzyme deactivation without actual competition. Here the drug can react with the enzyme or even the enzyme–substrate complex and in some manner prevent the metabolism of the substrate. The nitrogen mustards and other alkylating agents used for cancer chemotherapy act in this fashion. These drugs are relatively nonspecific enzyme inhibitors that act by forming irreversible bonds with enzyme molecules (Fig 27-6). In doing so they may not necessarily block a particular site but rather many active sites and in this way inactivate the enzyme. Or, by reacting with guanine residues of DNA, to form cross-links, nitrogen mustards can prevent replication and thus arrest cell division.

Another explanation that has been advanced is the *Molecular Perturbation Theory*. It has been well established in recent years that living proteins (enzymes included) assume specific shapes or conformations in an organism. In these conformations certain functional groups are exposed and are spatially related to other groups, thus producing the active sites at which the substrate can attach. Suppose, however, that a noncompetitive drug could bond to an enzyme in such a way as to distort the enzyme surface. The active site would no longer have the same shape or spacings between its bonding groups and the substrate "key" would no longer fit its enzyme "lock." The enzyme, in effect, would have been chemically denatured. Reactions that alter receptor conformation are called *allosteric*. It has been previously mentioned that an antimetabolite can compete with a substrate for an enzyme. Some drugs, however, may act by actual substitution and incorporation into a macromolecule. In this fashion, rather than inactivating an enzyme, they may actually form a new enzyme-like molecule with either no activity or altered activity.

The above discussion has centered largely around mechanisms of drug action involving enzymic processes. Since metabolic pathways are so complex, there are available numerous ways of altering or inhibiting them. Another, albeit poorly understood, aspect of drug action involves the transport of vital ions or metabolites. The movement of molecules either into or out of a cell or across a synapse is an important aspect in the biochemical process. Simple diffusion often is not adequate for the demands of an organism. Thus, there are available other mechanisms of transport that transcend simple diffusion both as to rate and even direction of movement across a membrane. Certain drugs, such as the local anesthetics, appear to act by affecting membrane permeability. Since the structures of these compounds are so dissimilar chemically, it is believed that their action does not involve receptor sites and is probably physicochemical in nature. It also has been demonstrated that sodium, potassium, and calcium ion transport is affected by the administration of various compounds, but how the diffusion rate is changed is not understood. Several tentative explanations of these phenomena have been offered, including membrane depolarization and ion competition, but a really detailed and substantiated mechanism is still forthcoming.

As intimated in the beginning of this section, the mechanisms of drug action remain a fruitful area of investigation. This discussion is merely a brief survey of some of the pathways, which have some experimental basis, through which chemical compounds are assumed to act in a biologic environment. Most of the theories propounded are questioned by certain investigators and among scientists in this field there are all too few areas of general agreement.

Quantitative Drug Design

A long standing goal of workers in the area of quantitative structure-activity relationships (QSAR) has been the development of quantitative methods of determining the activities of a series of compounds. One of the earliest hypotheses which attempted to relate activity to a physicochemical parameter was the Meyer-Overton Narcosis Theory. Working independently, both men in 1901 observed that, for general anesthetics, activity was related to the lipid/water partition coefficient; cyclopropane with a value of 65 was far more effective than nitrous oxide with a coefficient of 2.2.

In the field of theoretical chemistry, Hammett was the first to demonstrate the predictability of the pK_a values of substituted benzoic acids as a function of the various substituents attached to the ring, and their abilities to either donate or withdraw electrons from the carboxyl group. He was then able to extend these results to other reactions and other series of compounds using the same substituent constants he had derived from the benzoic acid series. In his equation,

$$\log k/k_0 = \rho\sigma$$

where k is the rate constant for the reaction of a substituted aromatic compound, k_0 is the rate constant for the unsubstituted aromatic compound, ρ is the reaction constant, and σ is the substituent constant. Later work led to substituent constants in which the electronic effect is separated into inductive and resonance terms and, in the Taft equation, a term E_s is defined as a measure of the steric requirements of a substituent.

In more recent times there have been numerous attempts to correlate mathematically molecular structure with drug activity. Many of these attempts were destined to fail because they grossly oversimplified what we now know as a very complex problem, even more so than "simple" chemical reactivity. Others have had moderate success within narrow limits of drug type, but a universal equation has yet to find expression.

One of the most successful investigators in this field is Hansch, who has derived a general equation based on linear free energy considerations. Inherent in his equation is the ability to incorporate parameters that encompass the full range of known biologic requirements for drug activity. Among these are terms for biologic transport, drug/enzyme binding energies, substituent effects (both electronic and steric), and electron densities of possible active sites on the drug molecule.

The most general form of the Hansch equation is usually written

$$\log 1/C = -a(\log P)^2 + b\log P + \rho\sigma + c$$

Activity is expressed as $1/C$, where C is the concentration of a drug required to elicit a given response. P is the octanol/water partition coefficient and is a measure of the hydrophobic bonding power of the drug. Its magnitude is indicative of the ability of a drug to move through biologic systems. The constant ρ is characteristic of a given molecular type and σ is the Hammett substituent constant which is a measure of the electronic effect on the rate of reaction.

The equation is also expressed

$$\log 1/C = -a\pi^2 + b\pi + \rho\sigma + c$$

where $\pi = \log P_x - \log P_H$, P_x is the partition coefficient of the substituted molecule, and P_H is the partition coefficient of the parent unsubstituted molecule. The particular benefit of the new term π is the observation by Hansch that π values are additive and thus numerous partition coefficients can be calculated without the necessity of synthesizing and measuring P_x of the actual compound. An example was the calculation of P_x values for a series of substituted benzeneboronic acids. The values of π were taken from the known series of substituted benzoic acids and, when added to the $\log P_H$ value for benzeneboronic acid, gave values of $\log P_x$ for the substituted boronic acids (Fig 27-7). When these values were used in a Hansch equation predicting drug penetration into brain tissue, excellent correlation with experimental values was obtained.

Another feature of Hansch's work is his use of the technique of regression analysis. In seeking structure–activity correlation it is often not necessary to include all of the defined parameters in the equation in order to get good results. In effect what has been done is to fit the data to several forms of the equation using the method of least squares. It is then determined which equation is statistically the best. Thus, if good correlation can be obtained by including only π values, it is probable that the electronic effect of substituents is not critical for drug activity in that series. Postulates as to specific drug mechanisms can thus be made when activity dependence, or lack thereof, is found for a given parameter. Further expansions of the equation also permit mechanistic considerations to be formulated. The $\rho\sigma$ term (actually a log k term) can be expanded to include a steric parameter (E_s) or electron density parameters for various parts of a molecule. Thus, if inclusion of a steric substituent constant leads to improved correlation, the steric requirements of the drug/enzyme interaction can be better understood. Several examples are given below for derived equations in which excellent correlation with experimental results is found when one or more parameters are omitted.

For the antibacterial effects on gram-negative bacteria of a series of diguanidines of structure shown in Fig 27-8, the equation

$$\log 1/C = -0.081\pi^2 + 1.483\pi - 1.578$$

predicts quantitative activity very accurately. Substituent effects here are neglected since molecular modification involves only a change in the number of methylene groups.

For the antibacterial activity of substituted phenols of structure of Fig 27-9, the equation

$$\log 1/C = 0.684\log P - 0.921\sigma + 0.268$$

best fits the data. It would seem here that substituents which donate electrons ($-\sigma$ values) would have the highest activity, but in the series studied these compounds have relatively small values of $\log P$ and this offsets much of the substituent effect. Thus, the most active compounds were those that had

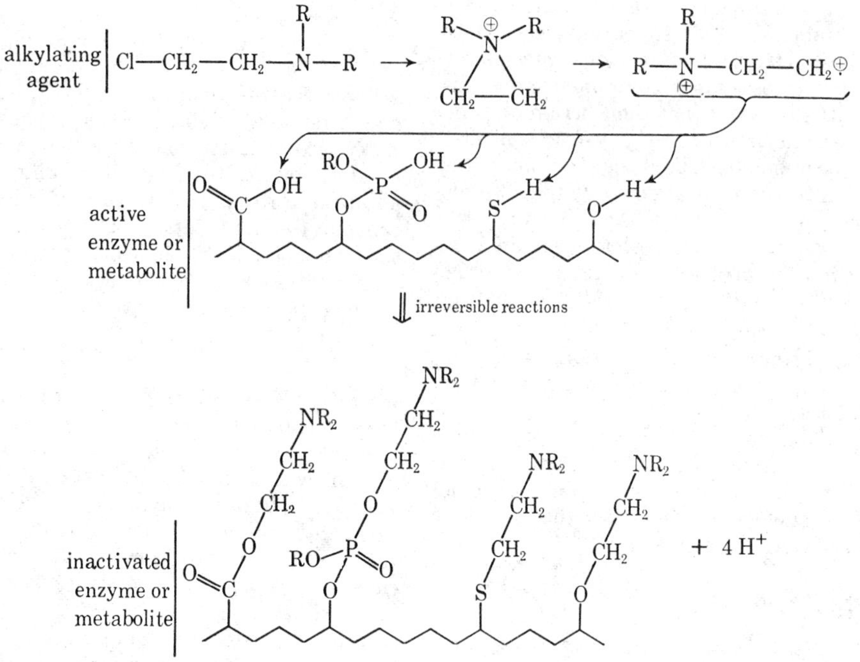

alkylating agent $Cl-CH_2-CH_2-N-R$ →

active enzyme or metabolite

irreversible reactions

inactivated enzyme or metabolite

$+ 4H^+$

Fig 27-6.

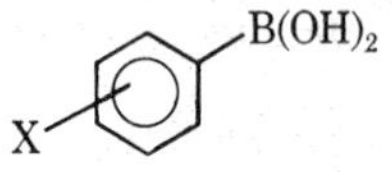

Fig 27-7.

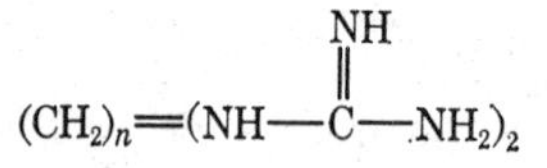

Fig 27-8.

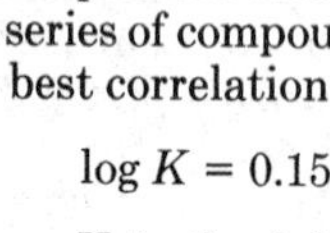

Fig 27-9.

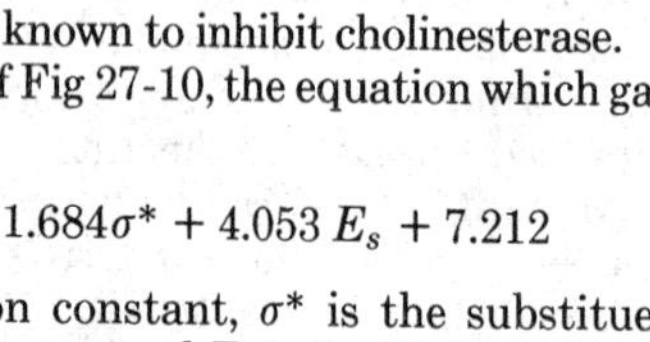

Fig 27-10.

the best balance between partition coefficient and electronic effect.

Phosphonate esters are known to inhibit cholinesterase. In the series of compounds of Fig 27-10, the equation which gave the best correlation was

$$\log K = 0.152\pi - 1.684\sigma^* + 4.053\,E_s + 7.212$$

where K is the inhibition constant, σ^* is the substituent constant for aliphatic systems, and E_s is the Taft steric constant. Here is a series in which steric effect of the substituents plays an important role. The bulkier groups cause a decrease in cholinesterase inhibition.

The above are just a few of the many structure–activity correlations that Hansch has been able to formulate. A study of those equations of best fit can also give us an indication of how to modify a structure in order to affect biologic activity. Thus, in determining the relative sweetness of the derivatives of 2-amino-4-nitrobenzene, electron-releasing groups were found to increase the sweetness. Also, in a study of thyroxine derivatives, it was predicted (and substantiated) that the replacement of iodine by a t-butyl group should lead to a more active molecule. To date, the Hansch equation is the most ambitious attempt to explain drug activity in terms of structural variations. That the equation fails to accurately correlate structure/activity in some systems only indicates that there are still some parameters, perhaps unknown, which should be incorporated.

In designing and identifying the most active drug using the Hansch equation, somewhere between 15 and 25 compounds should be made and tested in order to give a good statistical correlation in fitting the data to an equation. Topliss, using Hansch concepts but eschewing the mathematical and statistical requirements of the equation, devised an operational scheme for drug design.

Initially, the parent compound is synthesized and tested for biological activity. Then, using a table that lists the hydrophobic (π), electronic (σ), and steric (E_s) constants for a large variety of substituents, Topliss chose a substituent with a $+\pi$, $+\sigma$ value and synthesized and tested this compound. The new compound may be either less active, more active, or equally active biologically when compared to the parent compound. Depending on the result, new derivatives would then be prepared in a systematic way such that the electronic, hydrophobic, and steric effects were modified in the direction that leads to increased potency. Using this type of operational approach, the number of compounds that must be synthesized in order to achieve a near maximal biologic response may be decreased to between 8 and 10, a decided advantage.

In the area of theoretical calculations, the last few years have seen a quantum leap, due in large part to the accessibility and increasing sophistication of computers and their attendant software.

Theoretical QSAR calculations can be divided into three areas; quantum mechanics, molecular mechanics and molecular modeling.

Quantum mechanics although the most basic of the QSAR approaches has several drawbacks. The various computer programs which are available under a collection of acronyms (CNDO, MINDO, VRDDO, AB INITIO, etc) provide a range of time vs accuracy results. *Ab initio* calculations, for example, although providing the most accurate results are often impractical for large molecules, while CNDO (complete neglect of differential overlap) which is much faster and more broadly applicable is of necessity less rigorous in its results.

With quantum mechanics, electronic charge distributions, dipole moments, orbital energies, ionization potentials, conformational energies, transition state energies etc can be calculated without requiring empirical data.

Among the results of these methods has been the correlation of the carcinogenic activity of various polycyclic aromatic hydrocarbons vs the electron densities of two regions in the molecules. The antibiotic activities of 3-substituted cephalosporins correlates with the transition state energies (TSE) for the molecules.

The method of molecular mechanics computationally is much faster and less complex but it yields surprisingly good results for conformational energies and other related properties. It gives the medicinal chemist a picture of a molecule in three dimensions.

Molecular modeling is a synthesis of the above theoretical methods with computer graphics. It is now possible to depict a 3-D representation of an enzyme surface (color-coded for electron-rich and electron-deficient areas) and to "on screen" fit various drug structures to the enzyme.

Although the recent manifestations of the above theoretical methods are awesome, they still suffer from obvious deficiencies. Namely, that they ignore parameters of drug activity such as absorption, distribution, steric factors and others previously discussed. Nevertheless, theoretical methods hold a great deal of promise for future results and at present they can offer much in terms of understanding drug/receptor binding at the molecular level.

Somewhere between simplistic physicochemical correlations and the as-yet-unachieved total quantum mechanical description of molecules lies the newly developing area of *molecular topology* or *molecular connectivity*. As was mentioned in the discussion of the mechanisms of drug action, shape is one of the primary aspects of a molecule that determines activity. By defining a molecule as a "graph," an atom as a "vertex," and a bond as an "edge," it becomes possible to describe unambiguously the topology of a molecule. Using these concepts, *connectivity indices* can readily be calculated, and when fit by regression analysis to a suitable equation will often yield excellent structure–activity correlations. Among such correlations that have been determined are those for local anesthetics, enzyme inhibitors, antimicrobial activity, and ether toxicities.

There has been a great deal of other work using statistical methods to define structure–activity relationships. Free and Wilson, and Kopecky among others have been active along lines somewhat similar to the efforts of Hansch. All of these investigators have sought to further the assault on that lofty goal, a quantitative structure–activity relationship of universal application. In summary, there follows a listing of some of the parameters that have been found to correlate with drug activity in specific cases:

solubility, partition coefficients, R_f values
Hammett (substituent) constants
Taft (steric) constants
infrared and ultraviolet data
pK_a values
molecular orbital (MO) electron density calculations
polarographic half-wave potentials
oxidation-reduction potentials
nuclear magnetic resonance chemical shifts
surface activity
dipole moments
electronic polarizability

Drug Design

Literally volumes have been written on the subject of drug design and yet ideal drugs remain to be synthesized. Even aspirin, which might lay claim to the title, cannot be tolerated by certain individuals, and it is also contraindicated by people on anticoagulant drugs and, of course, by patients with ulcers. In spite of the fact that our arsenal of effective drugs is ever expanding and ever improving, the goal is still the ideal drug. One must now consider those aspects of drug action that one seeks to modify by creating new pharmacodynamic agents.

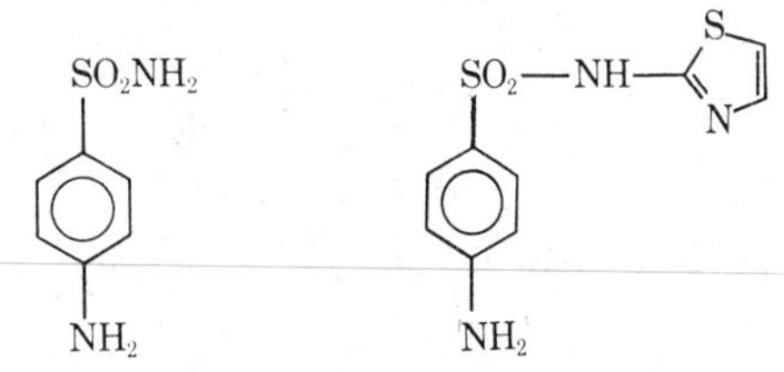

Fig 27-11.

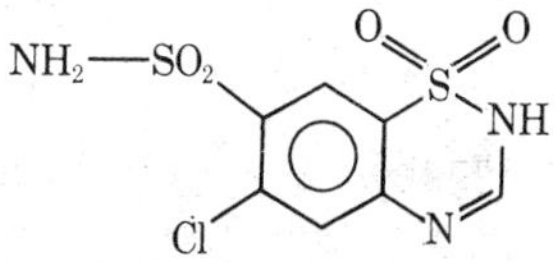

Fig 27-12.

Potency—A known drug may not have a maximal effect at optimum dose. That is, if the therapeutic ratio of a drug or its biologic spectrum is too narrow, a more potent compound should be sought. The first sulfonamide, sulfanilamide, Fig 27-11A, has been supplanted by a host of more effective sulfonamides. By modifying the sulfanilamide structure sulfathiazole (Fig 27-11B) was synthesized, probably the most effective agent (even though the most toxic) in this class of compounds.

Specificity—One of the banes and curses of drug action is its lack of specificity. No drug acts exclusively on one biochemical system and, if a drug is utilized for a specific action, one must often put up with secondary or side effects. If these effects are too deleterious, they may seriously hamper the utility of the drug and may necessitate redesigning the molecular structure to accentuate the positive and eliminate the negative effects. The early antihistamines produced severe drowsiness. Molecular modification has lessened but not eliminated this problem. On the other hand, side effects have often led to new types of drugs. By redesigning the molecule it may be possible to create a new compound in which the secondary effect becomes the primary one. Sulfanilamide exhibited side effects that led to the development of diuretics, exemplified by chlorothiazide (Fig 27-12).

Physiologic Factors—Certain drugs have shown activity *in vitro* and exhibited diminished activity when used *in vivo*. Absorption, distribution, elimination, and detoxification—any of these factors may be the cause. Penicillin G (Fig 27-13), a potent antibiotic, when taken orally is severely degraded by stomach acids. Modification of this structure to Penicillin V (Fig 27-14) led to a compound of comparable potency, identical antibacterial spectrum, but very resistant to acid hydrolysis. In the area of barbiturate sedatives, hexobarbital (Fig 27-15) has a very short onset of action and its action is of short duration. A structural modification gives phenobarbital (Fig 27-16), whose sedative effect may last up to 12 hours.

Ultimately, the medicinal chemist may be able to depict the structure of an as yet unsynthesized molecule, and by making

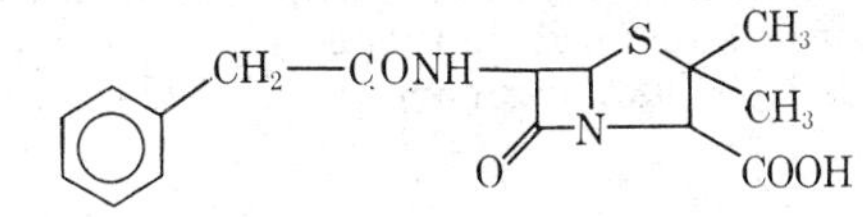

Fig 27-13.

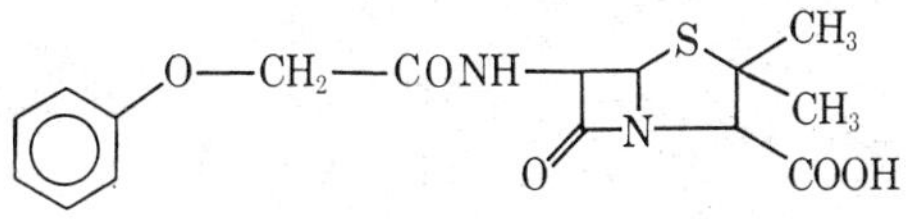

Fig 27-14.

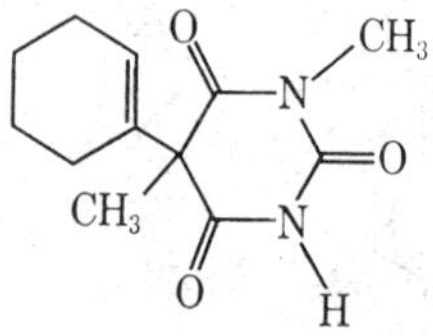

Fig 27-15.

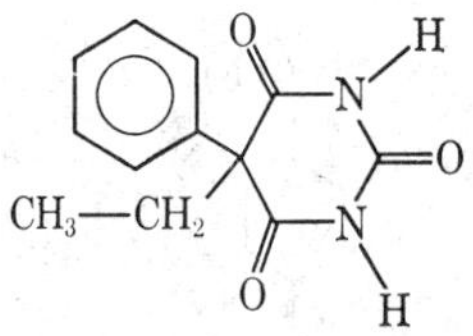

Fig 27-16.

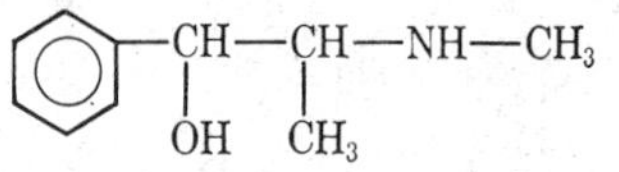

Fig 27-17.

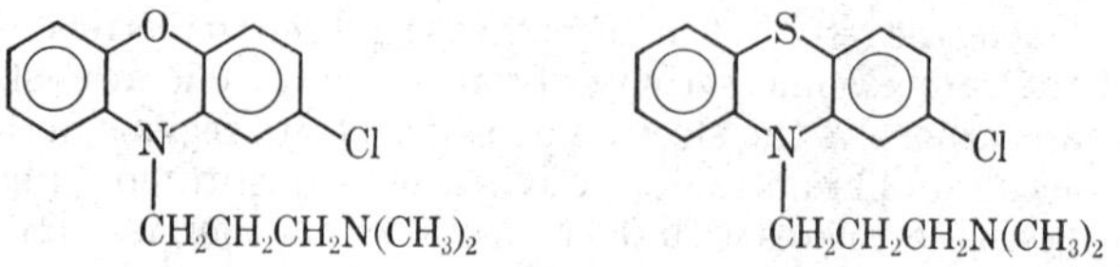

A   B

Fig 27-18.

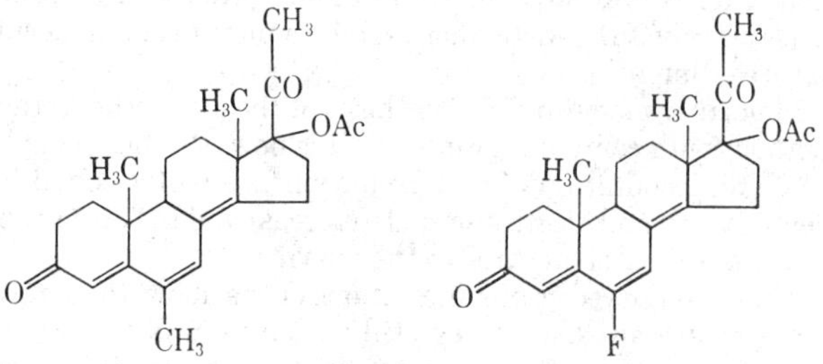

A   B

Fig 27-19.

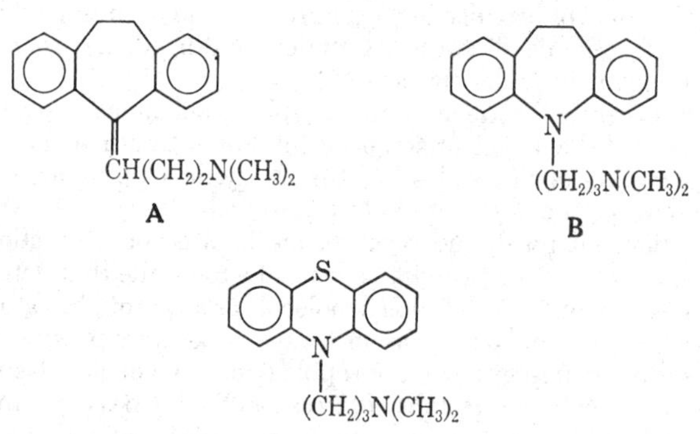

A   B

C

Fig 27-20.

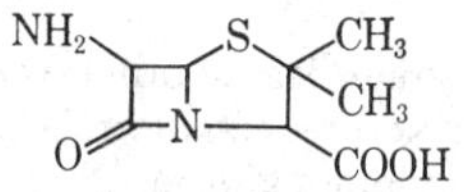

Fig 27-21.

certain *a priori* assumptions, predict both the type and degree of pharmacologic action that the compound will exhibit. There is still a long way to go to attain this goal. In the search for new drugs, the usual approach is to first have in mind some known active compound and then attempt various structural modifications in the hope of either altering or attenuating its known biologic activity. The only alternative to this is a random screening of all organic compounds, across a broad spectrum of possible actions—a monumental and wasteful technique. Molecular modification, too, could verge on the infinite were it not for guidelines that have been established by several generations of investigators.

There are several sources from which we may derive the original structure–activity reference point in our quest for new compounds. Originally, all prototypes came from nature. The adrenergic phenethylamines all derive from ephedrine (Fig 27-17), a naturally occurring compound whose use in medicine goes back some 5000 years. Over the years, however, numerous compounds have been synthesized that exhibit some pharmacologic response. Some were developed from biologic sources, others by exploiting secondary effects of known compounds, and still others by pure luck or serendipity. In any event, we now have a considerable supply of compounds and their modifications that can serve to stimulate and direct our efforts to develop improved drugs (see Table I). The following is a brief description of some of the ways in which an active molecule can be modified to alter and improve its action.

Molecular Modification

Isosterism—When two or more molecules have approximately the same size and shape, they are said to be isosteric. Inherent in this definition are certain qualifications that may or may not apply, depending on how the term is used. The molecules should have the same number and type of bonds and they should be isoelectric. Electron density, resonance energy, and dipole moment should also be similar. In Table II are listed some isosteric equivalents that have been utilized by various chemists.

The following are some examples of isosteres. In the first pair of compounds the oxygen isostere (Fig 27-18A) of chlorpromazine (Fig 27-18B) has only $1/10$ of its tranquilizing activity. In the second pair of compounds the replacement of the CH_3-group in 6-dehydromethylpregnone (Fig 27-19A) with a fluorine atom leads to the more active ovulation inhibitor 6-dehydrofluoropregnone (Fig 27-19B). A final ex-

ample of isosteric replacement shows the evolution of amitriptyline (Fig 27-20A) from imipramine (Fig 27-20B), which in turn derived from promazine (Fig 27-20C). All three drugs have antidepressant and sedative properties even though the heteroatoms of the original phenothiazine (promazine) have evolved into the nonheterocyclic amitriptyline.

Group Substitution—There are two basic ways to modify a drug using group substitution. The first involves changing the type or position of a substituent, usually attached to a ring portion of a molecule. The second method requires that a fundamental portion of the molecule be kept constant while the remainder can be modified quite extensively. The synthetic penicillins typify both types of approach. One of the naturally occurring antibiotics is penicillin G (Fig 27-13). Chemical studies determined that 6-aminopenicillanic acid (6-APA) (Fig 27-21) was the penicillin nucleus and that a

Table II—Isosteric Equivalents

—N=	to	—CH=					—S—	to	—CH=CH—	to	—CH₂—CH₂—	to	—O—
—O—	to	—NH—	to	—CH₂—			—F	to	—H				
—F	to	—OH	to	—NH₂	to	—CH₃	—N—CH₂—	to			—CH=CH—		

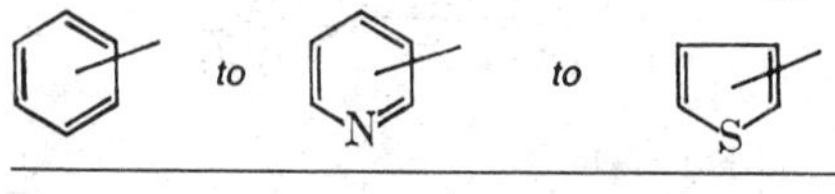

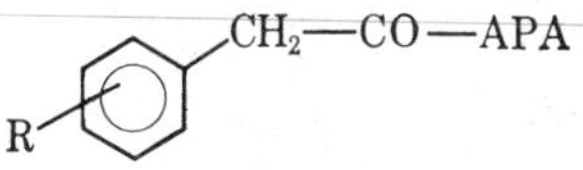

R = *p*-OH, *p*-Cl, *p*-F,
p-Br, *p*-I, *p*-NO$_2$,
p-CH$_3$, *p*-CN,
m-F, *o*-F

Fig 27-22.

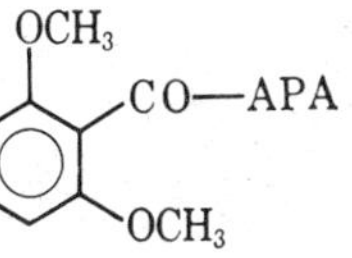

A

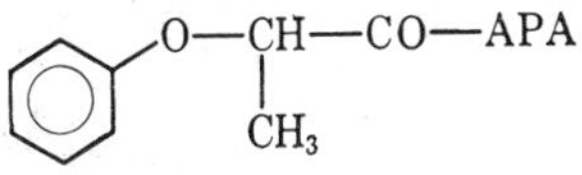

B

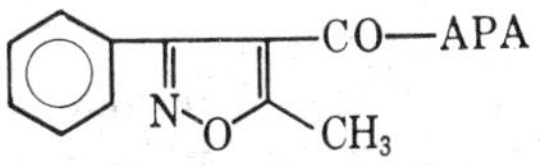

C

Fig 27-23. A: methicillin; B: D(−)phenethicillin; C: oxacillin.

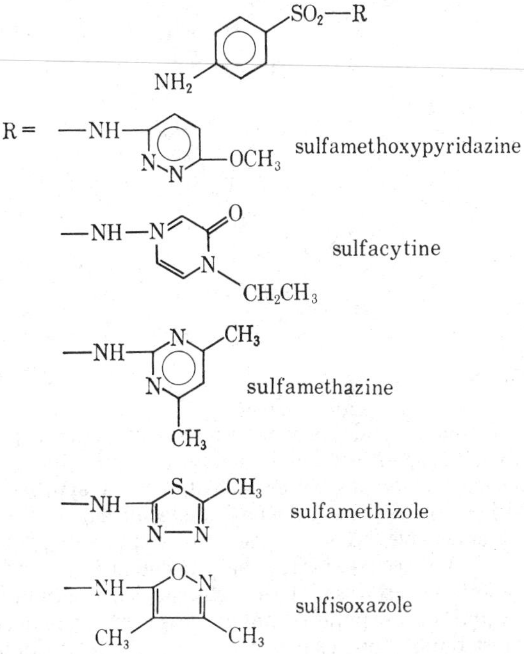

sulfamethoxypyridazine

sulfacytine

sulfamethazine

sulfamethizole

sulfisoxazole

Fig 27-25.

variety of synthetic "penicillins" could be synthesized using this nucleus in combination with a variety of carboxyl-containing compounds. Many semisynthetic penicillins were also made by introducing ring-substituted phenylacetamide precursors into the natural fermentation process. By these means a series of penicillin varieties have been synthesized (Fig 27-22).

In this series the basic penicillin structure has been maintained but a variety of ring substituents have been introduced which by their electronic effects alter both the activity and specificity of the compounds. Synthetic penicillins that are therapeutically useful and those in which the phenylacetyl moiety has been completely changed are pictured in Fig 27-23*A*, *B*, and *C*. These drugs were prepared by acylating 6-APA.

Sometimes nature provides the key to *molecular modification*. Although literally hundreds of semisynthetic penicillins had been prepared and tested, it was thought that the β-lactam-thiazole ring system was essential for antibacterial activity. Attempts at modifying this penicillin "nucleus" had led to loss of activity. In the late 1940s, however, a new antibacterial agent was isolated from a culture and given the generic name *cephalosporin*. When the structure of the cephalosporins was finally elucidated, they were shown to be isomeric with the penicillins. One of the drugs is this class that has since been developed is cephalexin (Fig 27-24*A*). If its structure is compared to that of ampicillin (Fig 27-24*B*), it can be seen that the two are closely related and that what has apparently happened is that the thiazole ring has opened

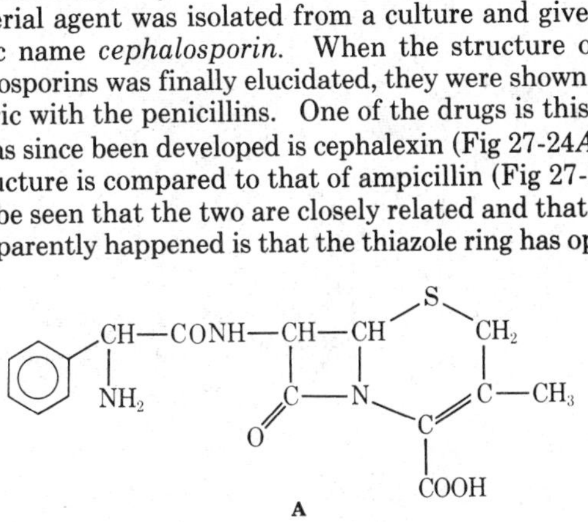

and one of the geminal methyl groups has been incorporated into a newly formed six-membered ring. Recently, chemists have learned to emulate nature and they are able to carry out this very transformation in the laboratory. The cephalosporins are useful because they have a broader antibacterial spectrum and can also be used against certain penicillin resistant strains.

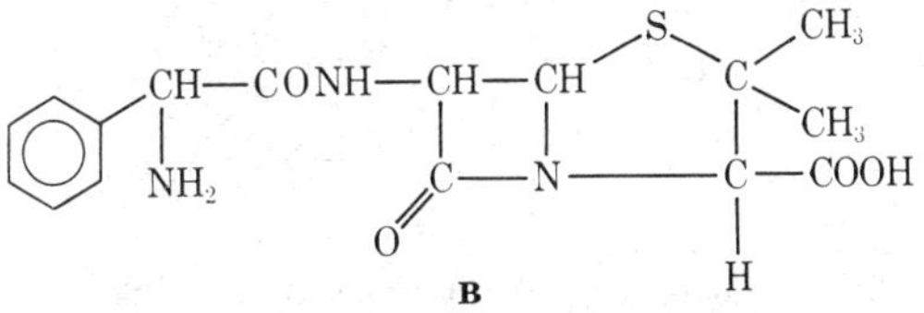

The "nucleus" concept of drug modification is also amply demonstrated by the sulfonamides. With these drugs, the parent compound sulfanilamide is also the nucleus and modification is effected by replacement of the NH$_2$— group by a large variety of heterocyclic amines. Some of the important drugs developed by this technique are shown in Fig 27-25. These few compounds illustrate the variety of heterocyclic amines which have been utilized. Literally thousands of modifications of sulfanilamide have been prepared, only a few of which have become important in medicine.

A final example of group substitution concerns aspirin, one of the oldest and still most useful analgesic, antipyretic, and anti-inflammatory drugs. In all the years of its use (almost 100) none of the molecular modifications of its basic structure proved superior to it. Recently, *diflunisal* (*Dolobid*, MSD), Fig 27-28, has been developed that is claimed to be effective in smaller doses, does not cause gastric distress or bleeding, and still retains the analgesic and anti-inflammatory activity of aspirin. What is unusual in this new drug is the molecular modification of salicylic acid that proved to be so effective—a difluorophenyl ring attached *para* to the phenolic group. If nothing else, this demonstrates that molecular modification of a drug is limited only by chemists' imagination, and that a drug, no matter how well established, can still be improved by this approach.

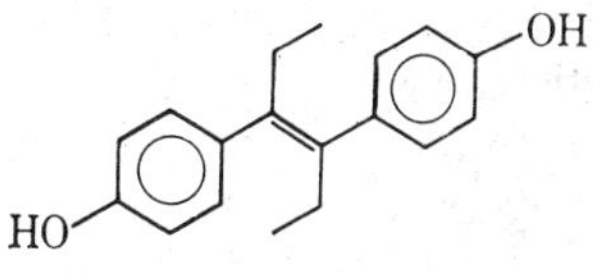

A

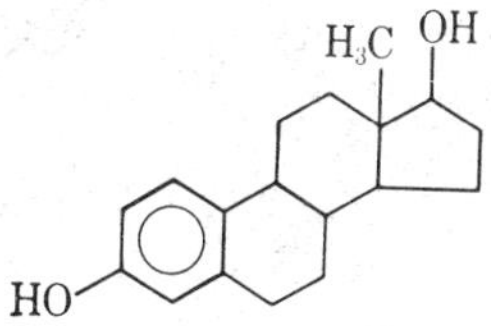

B

Fig 27-24. A: Cephalexin; B: Ampicillin.

A

B

Fig 27-26.

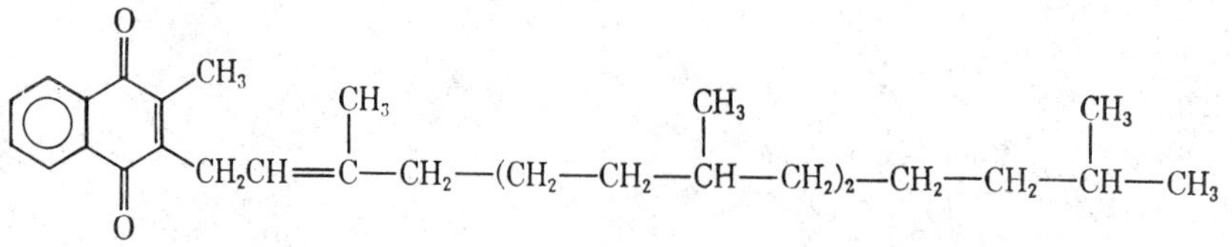

Fig 27-27.   A: vitamin K$_1$.

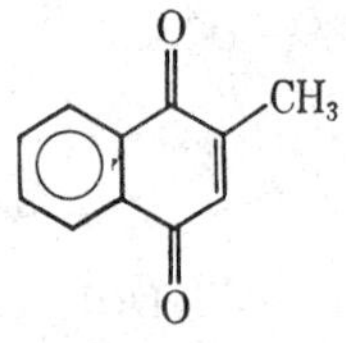

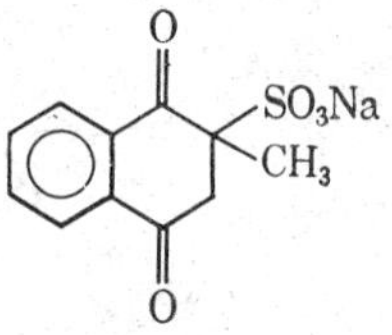

Simplification—Often, when a naturally occurring pharmacodynamic agent has finally had its structure elucidated, the molecule is one of great complexity. Total synthesis or synthetic modifications of the basic molecule may prove difficult or expensive. It is then usually through a long and tedious period of trial and error that the chemist attempts to delineate those portions of the structure which determine the activity and to incorporate them in a less complex molecule. Without a doubt, the most spectacular example of simplification must be diethylstilbestrol (Fig 27-26A). This potent estrogen evolved, via a painstaking synthetic excursion, from estradiol (Fig 27-26B). Unless the structure of diethylstilbestrol is depicted as shown in Fig 27-26A, the simplification is so complete that one could fail to see the similarity that actually exists between the two compounds.

The natural vitamins K are naphthoquinone derivatives bearing a methyl group and a side chain consisting of several isoprene-related units (Fig 27-27A). When it was shown that these compounds were useful in preventing hemorrhage, attempts were made to prepare new drugs of similar activity but less complexity. Menadione (Fig 27-27B), a highly effective drug, resulted by simply removing the isoprene side-chain completely. A further modification led to a water-soluble anticoagulant, menadione sodium bisulfite (Fig 27-27C).

Nowhere has simplification and modification been so thoroughly exploited as in the search for synthetic antimalarials that took place during World War II. Using quinine (Fig 27-29) as the basic molecule, over 14,000 variants were prepared and tested. In the course of this investigation, variation led to variation such that the ultimate active com-

pounds seem remote indeed from the quinuclidine–quinoline composite from which they were derived. Without attempting to describe the synthetic progressions that led to them, the following are representative of the many "quinine inspired" drugs which were developed (Fig 27-30A–D). It is rather discouraging to note that in spite of this vast effort, today still other compounds to combat new drug-resistant malarial parasite strains are being sought.

Isomerism—Molecular modification also can be achieved by preparing compounds that are isomeric with the drug model. These isomers may be of two basic types: positional and steric. Chart I shows examples of some of the different subcategories of isomers that have been utilized in the search for improved drugs.

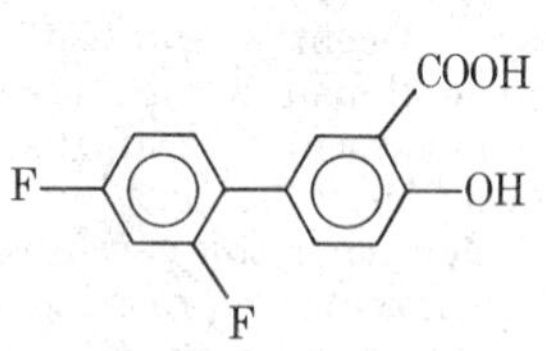

Fig 27-28.   Diflunisal.

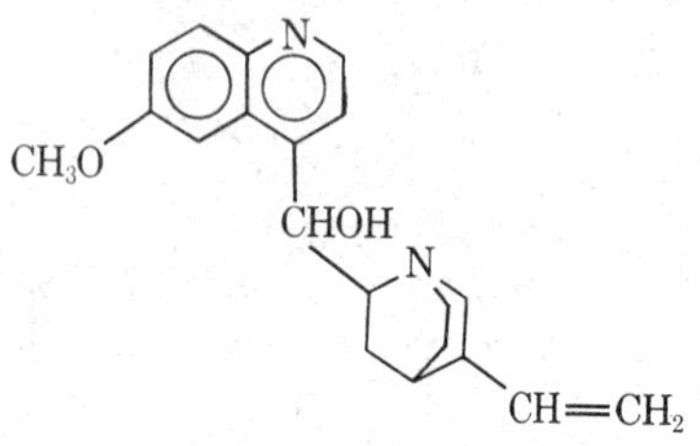

Fig 27-29.

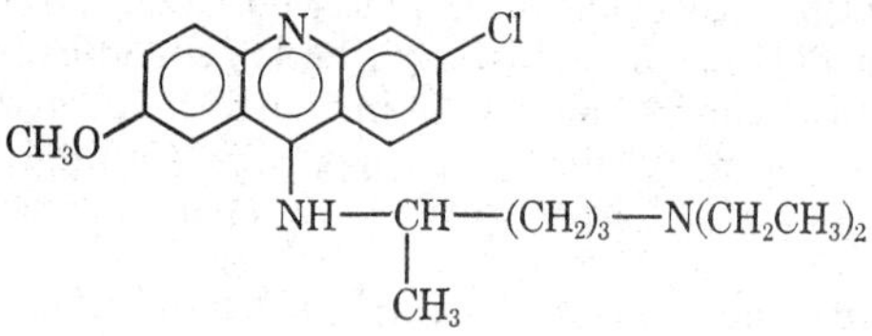

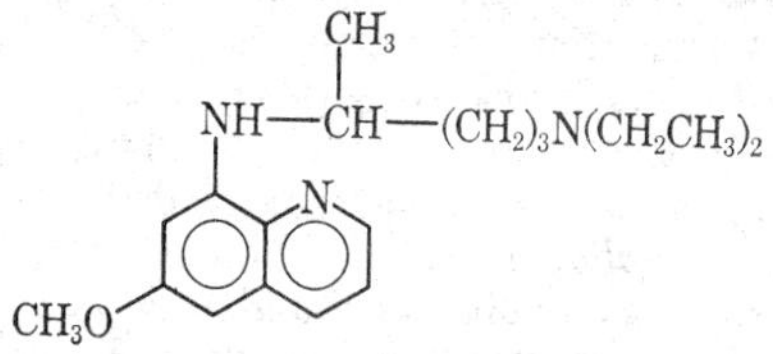

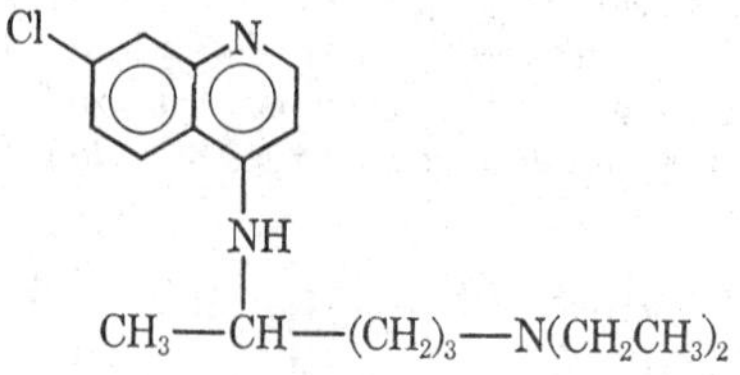

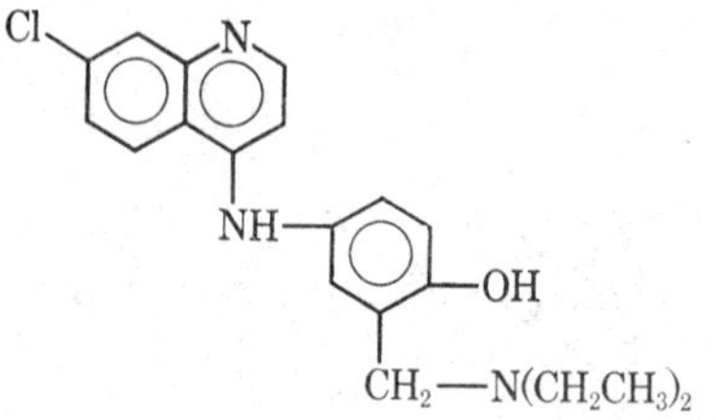

Fig 27-30.   A: quinacrine; B: pamaquine; C: chloroquine; D: camoquine.

Chart I—Structural Modification through Isomer Syntheses

A. Positional isomers

1. Position isomers

A

B

Fig 27-31.

2. Chain isomers

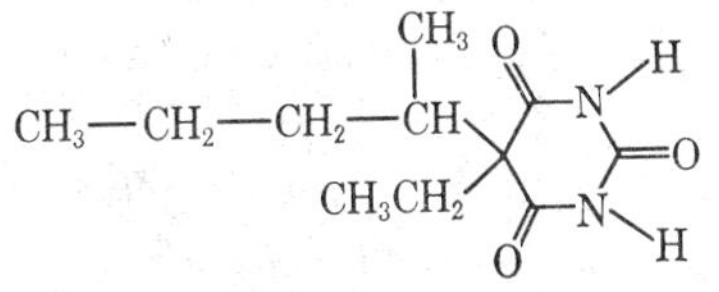

A

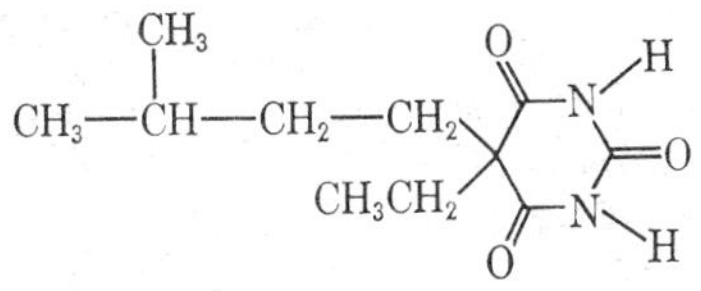

B

Fig 27-32.

3. Functional group isomers

A

B

Fig 27-33.

B. Stereoisomers

1. Geometric isomers

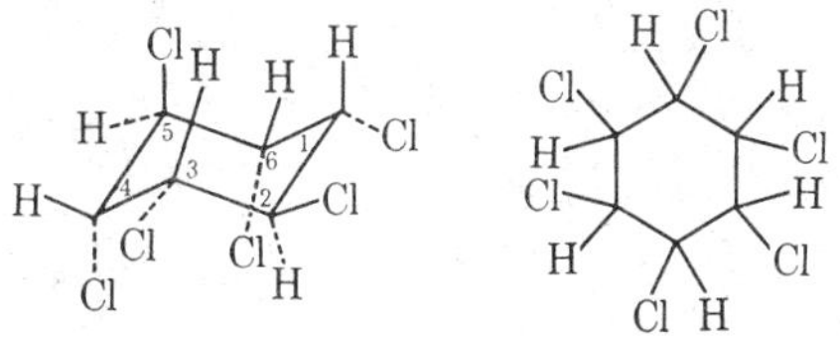

9 stereo-isomers

A

B

Fig 27-34.

2. Enantiomers

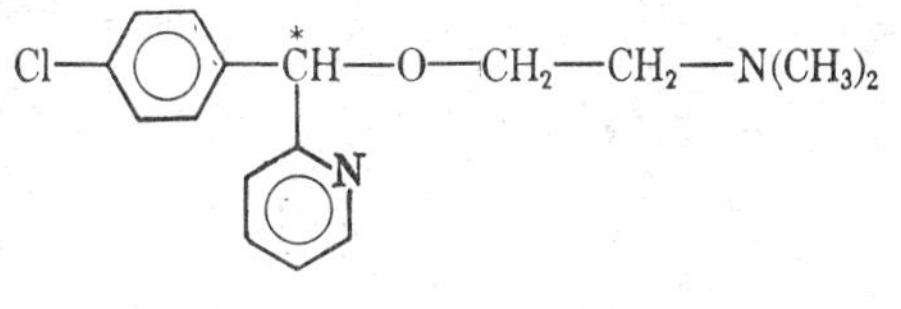

$Cl-\!\!\!\!\langle\bigcirc\rangle\!\!\!-\overset{*}{C}H-O-CH_2-CH_2-N(CH_3)_2$

Fig 27-35.

* = asymmetric carbon atom

Orthoform (Fig 27-31A), a local analgetic, led to Orthoform New (Fig 27-31B), an isomer whose synthesis proved somewhat easier. In the barbiturate family of drugs, pentobarbital (Fig 27-32A) and amobarbital (Fig 27-32B) differ only in the type of 5-carbon side-chain which they bear, but the former has a short duration of action while the latter is of intermediate duration. Betaine ester (Fig 27-33A) and acetylcholine (Fig 27-33B) are isomeric esters with the functional groups reversed. Both are about equal in their cholinergic activity.

Optical isomerism often leads to striking differences in pharmacologic activity. Estradiol (Fig 27-26B) exists in two geometric forms. The *beta*-compound has been shown to be far more active than the *alpha*-isomer. When chlorine is added to benzene, nine benzene hexachloride cis/trans isomers (Fig 27-34B) can be formed. Only one isomer, the *gamma* form (Fig 27-34A), is useful as an insecticide. Since this compound comprises only 10–15% of the reaction product, activity is lessened considerably unless the active isomer is separated. Enantiomerism may produce even more remarkable variations in activity since, to the uninitiated, the isomers are indistinguishable. Carbinoxamine, a potent antihistamine (Fig 27-35) can exist in (+) or (−) forms. Tests have shown that the (−)-isomer (rotoxamine) is more active and exhibits fewer undesirable side effects than its enantiomer. Quinine (Fig 27-29) and quinidine are also enantiomers, the latter being dextrorotatory. Here too, mirror-image isomerism leads to gross differences in activity. Quinidine finds application as a cardiac suppressant while quinine exhibits a broad spectrum of medicinal uses ranging from antipyretic to anesthetic.

Drug design then applies numerous principles, extensive syntheses, comprehensive pharmacologic testing, and the experience and insight to minimize the effort required to evolve a new active molecule. It must be remembered, however, that with all of our background experience and theories, new drugs of superior action and specificity are still discovered infrequently. Were it not for the efforts of countless scientists even these drugs might still not be available.

References

1. Burger A: *J Chem Educ 35:* 142, 1958.
2. Wilson CO, Gisvold O, Doerge, RF: *Textbook of Organic Medicinal and Pharmaceutical Chemistry*, 7th ed, Lippincott, Philadelphia, 1977.

Bibliography

Ariens EJ: *Drug Design*, 6 Vols, Academic Press, New York, 1971–1975.

Ariens EJ: *Physicochemical Aspects of Drug Action*, Pergamon Press, New York, 1968.

Burger A: *Medicinal Chemistry*, 3rd ed, Wiley-Interscience, New York, 1970.

Foye WO: Principles of Medicinal Chemistry, 2nd ed, Lee & Febiger, Philadelphia, 1981.

Gill EW: *Drug Receptor Interactions*, *Progr Med Chem 4:* 39, 1965.

Goldstein A, *et al: Principles of Drug Action*, 2nd ed, Wiley-Interscience, New York, 1974.

Harper NJ: *Drug Latentiation, J Med Chem 12:* 467, 1969.

Kier LB: *Molecular Connectivity in Chemistry and Drug Research*, Academic Press, New York, 1976.

Korolkovas A, *et al: Essentials of Medicinal Chemistry*, Wiley-Interscience, New York, 1976.

Korolkovas A: *Molecular Pharmacology*, Wiley-Interscience, New York, 1970.

Martin YC: Quantitative Drug Design, Marcel Dekker, New York, 1978.

Molecular Modification in Drug Design, Advances in Chemistry Series, No 45, Amer Chem Soc, Washington, 1964.

Roche EB, ed: *Design of Biopharmaceutical Properties Through Prodrugs and Analogs*, Amer Pharm Assoc, Washington, 1976.

Salerni OL: *Natural and Synthetic Organic Medicinal Compounds*, CV Mosby, St Louis, 1976.

Scheuler FW: *Chemobiodynamics and Drug Design*, McGraw-Hill, New York, 1960.

Stuart DM: *Drug Metabolism, Pharm Index 10(9A):* 3, 1968; *ibid. 10(10A):* 4, 1968.

Van Valkenburg W: Symp Chmn: *Biological Correlations-The Hansch Approach*, Amer Chem Soc, Washington, 1972.

PART 4

Radioisotopes in Pharmacy and Medicine

Grafton D Chase, PhD

Professor of Chemistry
Philadelphia College of Pharmacy
and Science
Philadelphia, PA 19104

CHAPTER 28

Fundamentals of Radioisotopes

Grafton D Chase, PhD

Professor of Chemistry
Philadelphia College of Pharmacy and Science
Philadelphia, PA 19104

For years the alchemist sought the secret of *transmutation* without success. Today this nuclear process, which converts one element into another, is commonplace. Yet, our knowledge of nuclear processes is of recent origin. It was not until 1896 that Becquerel observed the fogging of his photographic plates by a uranium salt. His observation aroused the curiosity of the Curies concerning the uranium ore, pitchblende, from which they isolated the elements polonium and radium. Research in the next few years by the Curies, Becquerel, Schmidt, Debierne, and others soon resulted in the discovery and isolation of still other new elements from uranium and thorium ores. These elements, too, were found to fog photographic plates.

It was known that the fogging of photographic plates was caused by some sort of radiation. By 1899 Rutherford concluded that this radiation was of two types, which he called *alpha* and *beta*. The next year P Curie and Villard observed a third, very penetrating, type of radiation which was called *gamma*. The *theory of radioactive disintegration* was proposed by Rutherford and Soddy in 1903. They suggested that atoms of radioactive elements undergo spontaneous emission of alpha and beta particles with the formation of atoms of a new element. These deductions were amazing when one considers the status of atomic knowledge of that day. The *electron*, later found to be physically identical with the beta particle, had been discovered by Thomson in 1897, but the alpha particle was not identified as a positively charged helium nucleus until 1909. That Rutherford and Royds should identify the alpha particle as a helium nucleus in 1909 is also remarkable, for it was not until 1911 that data on alpha particle scattering enabled Rutherford to propose the *nuclear theory*, *viz*, that the positive charge of an atom is concentrated in a centrally located *nucleus* rather than being interspersed with the negatively charged electrons. Two years later Bohr published his theory of atomic structure, based upon Rutherford's nuclear theory and the quantum theory of Planck. The same year (1913) Soddy proposed the name *isotope* (*Greek*, same place), for Aston had just separated two isotopes of neon by fractional diffusion in confirmation of Thomson's discovery of these two forms of neon in 1912.

Rutherford was unquestionably the foremost nuclear scientist of his time. It was he who also observed the first *artificial transmutation* in 1919. This he achieved by bombarding nitrogen with alpha particles, the nitrogen being converted into an isotope of oxygen with a mass of 17. It is regrettable that he should have died in 1937 believing that nuclear power would never be achieved. It was achieved only 5 years later when Fermi built the first nuclear reactor in Chicago.

Constructive research on the nucleus of the atom has not only resulted in the means to harness this tremendous power for the production of electricity and other forms of useful energy but has also provided scientists with more than 1400 different species of atoms. These find innumerable applications in industry, medicine, pharmacy, agriculture, and other disciplines where the atom is used for the benefit of mankind.

Particles and Waves

Elementary Particles—Electrons, protons, and neutrons constitute the basic building blocks of atoms, both stable and radioactive. See Table I. The *electron* is the smallest of these three particles. Its mass, m_e, is 9.1091×10^{-28} g. For simplicity, the mass of the electron, m_e, is used as a unit of mass. Thus, the mass of the proton is 1836 m_e, and that of the neutron is 1838 m_e. Also, for simplicity, the electron is assigned a charge of -1. Thus the charge of the proton is $+1$ and that of the neutron is zero. Although the mass and charge of each of these particles are known with a high degree of accuracy, the size of each is known only approximately. It is in the order of 10^{-13} cm. Size, when applied to such small objects, does not have the customary significance because of inherent uncertainties introduced by the very nature of the measurement to determine size and by the variability of size with velocity.

The *neutrino* is a very unusual particle. Its existence was suggested by Pauli in 1934 and was confirmed by experiment in 1957. It has zero charge and is thought to have zero rest mass. Yet, this particle plays a very important role in beta decay (see page 457).

Particles with mass equal to or less than that of the electron are called *leptons*. Leptons include the electron, positron, and neutrino. Particles found within the nucleus are known as *nucleons* and include the proton and neutron. *Mesons* are those particles with mass greater than that of a lepton but less than that of a nucleon. *Hyperons* have a mass greater than the nucleons. Although mesons and hyperons play an important role in nuclear science, a detailed knowledge of these particles is not essential to an understanding of other topics in this chapter.

Radiation from Radioactive Nuclei—Three types of

Table I—Common Particles of Nature

Particle	Symbol	Charge	Mass[a]
Negatron (Negative beta)	$e^-(\beta^-)$	-1	1
Positron (Positive beta)	$e^+(\beta^+)$	$+1$	1
Proton	p	$+1$	1836
Neutron	n	0	1838
Alpha	α	$+2$	7346
Neutrino	ν	0	0
Gamma ray[b] (a photon)	γ	0	0

[a] Mass is expressed in electron masses.
[b] Although gamma rays are electromagnetic radiation, they do possess particulate properties.

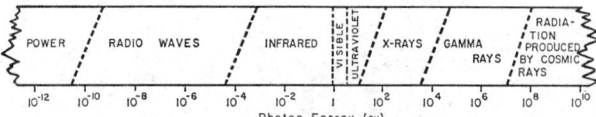

Fig 28-1.   Electromagnetic spectrum.

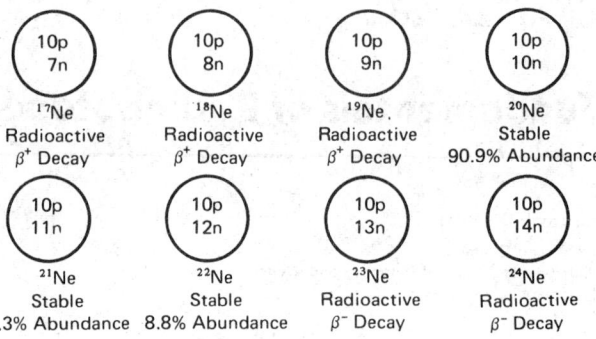

Fig 28-2.   Isotopes of neon.

radiation are most frequently emitted from radioactive nuclei. These are alpha, beta, and gamma radiations.

Alpha particles, which constitute alpha radiation, are compound particles consisting of two protons and two neutrons. Thus, the alpha particle is identical with the helium nucleus; that is, a helium atom less two electrons. As an alpha particle loses energy, its velocity decreases. It then attracts electrons to its *K-shell* and becomes an ordinary helium atom. The *range* of alpha particles in air is about 5 cm, and less than 100 μ in tissue.

Beta radiation is of two types because there are two kinds of electrons, the *negative electron*, or *negatron*, which has been discussed previously, and the *positive electron*, or *positron*. The positron is identical with the negatron in all respects except for its charge of +1 instead of −1. The positron is also known as the *antiparticle* of the electron. When these electrons are emitted from radioactive nuclei, they are called *beta particles*. That is, the two particles β^- and β^+ are the same as e^- and e^+, respectively, except for their origin. Beta particles may have a range of over 10 ft in air and up to about 1 mm in tissue.

Gamma radiation is basically different from alpha and beta radiation. Gamma radiation is electromagnetic, whereas alpha and beta radiation are particulate. Gamma rays are radiated as photons or quanta of energy at a velocity, c, of 3.0 × 10^{-10} cm/sec. Gamma radiation differs from X-rays, ultraviolet rays, visible light, etc, only in wave length (or frequency), as illustrated in Fig 28-1. Gamma rays are the most penetrating of all types of radiation emitted by radioisotopes (except neutrinos) and can easily pass through more than a foot of tissue or several inches of lead.

Atoms and Nuclei

Atomic Structure—A neutral atom consists of a positively charged nucleus (composed of protons and neutrons) with which are associated orbital electrons. The number of orbital electrons is equal to the number of protons in the nucleus, and the number of protons in the nucleus defines the *atomic number*, Z. The *neutron number*, N, is the number of neutrons in the nucleus, and the *mass number*, A, is equal to the sum of the protons and neutrons. Thus, A = Z + N.

The radius of an atom is approximately 10^{-8} cm or 1 Ångstrom unit. The nucleus is roughly 1/100,000 the size of the atom. For example, the radius of the oxygen nucleus is about 3 × 10^{-13} cm, and that of the lead nucleus is about 7 × 10^{-13} cm. To gain some appreciation of the smallness of the nucleus, let us suppose that the oxygen nucleus is magnified until it appears to be the size of a golf ball. The golf ball, similarly magnified, would appear to have a diameter of about 100 million miles, or roughly the distance from the earth to the sun.

Atoms are quite "empty." The nucleus and orbital electrons occupy but a very small fraction of space in matter. Further, most of the mass of matter is concentrated in the nucleus, which has a density of 2.4 × 10^{14} g/cc. For example, 1 cc of the substance of which nuclei are made would weigh over 200 million tons. It is with this very unusual material of the nucleus that we are concerned in nuclear reactions and radioactivity.

Nuclides and Isotopes—In 1912 Thomson developed an analytical process known as "positive ray analysis" by which

he could measure the mass of particles such as atoms. When he attempted to determine the mass of the neon atom, two lines appeared on the screen of his apparatus, indicating two types of neon atoms having masses of 20 and 22, respectively. By use of a process which was the forerunner of mass spectrometry, Thomson demonstrated the existence of nuclei possessing the same number of protons (and, hence, of the same chemical element) but a different number of neutrons (and, hence, of different mass). Soddy later called these *isotopes*.

The atomic number, Z, of neon is 10. From the relationship A = Z + N, we can deduce that the difference between these two forms of neon lies in the number of neutrons, N, in the nucleus.

$$A = 20 = 10 + N \qquad \therefore N = 10$$
$$A = 22 = 10 + N \qquad \therefore N = 12$$

Today at least eight isotopes of neon are known. These are illustrated in Fig 28-2.

Isotopes are species of *nuclides* which possess the same number of protons but a different number of neutrons. That is, isotopes are nuclides of the same chemical element and, therefore, have the same chemical properties but differ in mass. They may also differ in stability. Certain mass numbers may represent stable nuclei, whereas other mass numbers may represent radioactive nuclei. A *nuclide* is any one of the more than about 1400 known species of atoms characterized by the number of protons and the number of neutrons in the nucleus. Nuclides which have the same mass are called *isobars*. Nuclides which possess the same number of neutrons are called *isotones*. Consider the nuclides illustrated in Fig 28-3: ^{1}H, ^{2}H (deuterium), and ^{3}H (tritium) are isotopes; ^{2}He and ^{4}He are isotopes also. On the other hand, ^{3}H and ^{4}He are isobars, and ^{3}H and ^{4}He are isotones.

Nuclear Equations—The nuclear equation expressing the first artificial transmutation observed by Rutherford is expressed by the notation:

$$^{14}_{7}\text{N} + ^{4}_{2}\text{He} \rightarrow ^{1}_{1}\text{H} + ^{17}_{8}\text{O}$$

In this reaction, nitrogen of mass 14 is bombarded with a helium nucleus of mass 4 (ie, an alpha particle) to produce oxygen of mass 17 and a proton. In writing the symbol for a nuclide, the atomic number is written as a subscript preceding the symbol for the element, and the mass number is written as a superscript. Thus the symbol $^{14}_{7}$N describes the nitrogen nucleus whose atomic number, Z, is 7 and whose mass, A, is 14.

It will be noted that nuclear equations must balance. The sum of the masses on the left (14 + 4 = 18) must equal the sum of the masses on the right (1 + 17 = 18). Also, the sum of the atomic numbers on the left (7 + 2 = 9) must equal the sum of the atomic numbers on the right (1 + 8 = 9). This same reaction may also be represented by a "short-hand" notation.

$^{14}N(\alpha,p)^{17}O$

Nuclear Reactions—Nuclear reactions may be either spontaneous or induced. An element which undergoes a spontaneous nuclear reaction is said to be *radioactive*. Such elements are radioactive because the configuration of protons and neutrons in the nucleus produces an unstable structure. During the process of spontaneous decay the ratio of neutrons to protons changes. After one or more decay processes a stable nucleus is formed. Because of its special importance in radiopharmacy and nuclear medicine radioactive decay is discussed in detail in the next section.

Fission is a radioactive process in which a relatively heavy nucleus splits into two new nuclei of nearly equal size with the simultaneous emission of two or three neutrons. Fission may be spontaneous, but normally the reaction is induced by bombardment of the parent nucleus with a neutron,

$$^{235}U + {}^1_0n \rightarrow X + Y + 2.5\ n$$

where X and Y are fission products (new nuclei) with a value of Z between about 30 and 65. Fission reactions may be self-sustaining. For each neutron consumed, an average of 2.5 new neutrons are produced which may initiate the fission of other nuclei. Such a reaction is called a *chain reaction*. If at least one of the 2.5 neutrons produced is used to sustain the reaction, the reaction is said to be *critical*. This is the reaction which occurs in the uranium bomb, as well as in the *atomic reactor*.

Fusion results when two light nuclei are caused to collide with a velocity sufficient to overcome coulombic repulsion, the required velocity representing an enormous amount of energy. This energy must be supplied by high temperatures, ie, millions of degrees. To date such reactions have not been sustained for more than a fraction of a second. When controlled fusion reactions become a reality, the world will be assured of an ample supply of power for many thousands of years. The energy theoretically available from the deuterium found in ordinary water is 150 times greater than would result from burning an equal volume of oil. Deuterons (deuterium nuclei) can react by either of the following processes:

$$^2_1H + {}^2_1H \rightarrow {}^3_2He + {}^1_0n\ (3.2\ MeV)$$

$$^2_1H + {}^2_1H \rightarrow {}^3_1H + {}^1_1H\ (4.0\ MeV)$$

Reactions conducted in a nuclear reactor involve the interaction of nuclei and neutrons. These reactions have special importance as a means for producing radioisotopes. They are discussed in the following section.

Nuclear deexcitation is required when nuclei produced in nuclear reactions are in an *excited state* rather than in the *ground state*. When excited, nucleons occupy high-energy quantum levels. They tend to lose excess energy, returning to the ground quantum state by either of two competing processes—*gamma ray emission* or *internal conversion*. The first process results in emission of one or more gamma rays having energies characteristic of the particular transition involved. Internal conversion results in the emission of an electron from an atomic orbital.

Atomic deexcitation is a process which of necessity must follow any change in the identity of a nucleus. The daughter produced in a radioactive decay process is a different element. Orbital electrons find themselves in excited states and proceed to lose energy either as *fluorescence radiation* or as *Auger electrons* until a stable configuration is achieved.

Radioactive Decay

Statistics—Unstable nuclei which undergo a spontaneous nuclear reaction are said to be radioactive. If a single radioactive atom could be separated for observation, there would

Table II

If the total number of decaying atoms observed is n	There is a 68% chance that the error will be less than $\sigma = \sqrt{n}$	Or a 68% chance that the observed value is in error by no more than $100\ \sigma/n$ %
50	7.07	14.14%
100	10.00	10.00%
500	22.36	4.47%
1000	31.62	3.16%
5000	70.71	1.41%
10000	100.00	1.00%
50000	223.60	0.44%

be no way to predict at which moment decay of its nucleus would occur. If, however, a large number of similar radioactive atoms is considered, it then becomes possible to predict how many will decay within a certain interval of time. This problem can be understood if a comparison is made to the similar situation existing with life insurance. Although the insuring company cannot predict when a particular policy holder will die, the fraction of a large group of policy holders who will die within a given time interval can be predicted. The larger the group considered, the more accurate the prediction can be. Such is the case with nuclei; the greater the number of nuclei considered, the more accurate the measurement of decay rate.

The need to recognize the influence of random decay upon analytical results is extremely important. When radioactivity is measured the value we really want to know is μ, the true count. Since radioactive decay is random, μ cannot be measured. It is expected that replicate measurements of count n_i of the same sample will give a range of values on either side of μ. The best estimate of μ is given by the average

$$\bar{n} = \frac{\sum_i n_i}{N}$$

where N is the number of replicate observations. The precision with which decay rate can be measured is expressed by the standard deviation σ which is a measure of the spread of data on either side of the mean. For radioactive decay an estimate of σ is given by $\sqrt{\bar{n}}$. There is a 68% chance that a particular measurement will fall within the range $\bar{n} \pm \sigma$. About one-third of the observations result in values of n lying outside the range $\bar{n} \pm \sigma$. The significance is illustrated by the statistical analysis in Table II and the normal probability curve depicted (refer to Chapter 10).

Assume that a radioactive sample is decaying at the rate of exactly 500 atoms per minute. If the number of decaying atoms during each of 100 different 1-minute intervals were measured, for 68 of these intervals the data would lie between $500 - \sqrt{500}$ and $500 + \sqrt{500}$ or between 478 and 522. Data for the other 32 per cent of the measurements will fall either below 478 or above 522. Such variations, if truly of a statistical nature, should not be interpreted as indicating faulty equipment, faulty technique, or inaccurately calibrated samples. An increase in counting time to record a greater number of decay processes will result in an increase in counting accuracy.

When radioisotopes are used in analytical procedures the overall error in the measurement is due not only to random decay but also to instrumental error, pipetting, weighing, and other procedural errors. The overall error can be estimated in terms of the sample standard deviation, s, where

$$s = \sqrt{\frac{\sum_i (n_i - \bar{n})^2}{N - 1}}$$

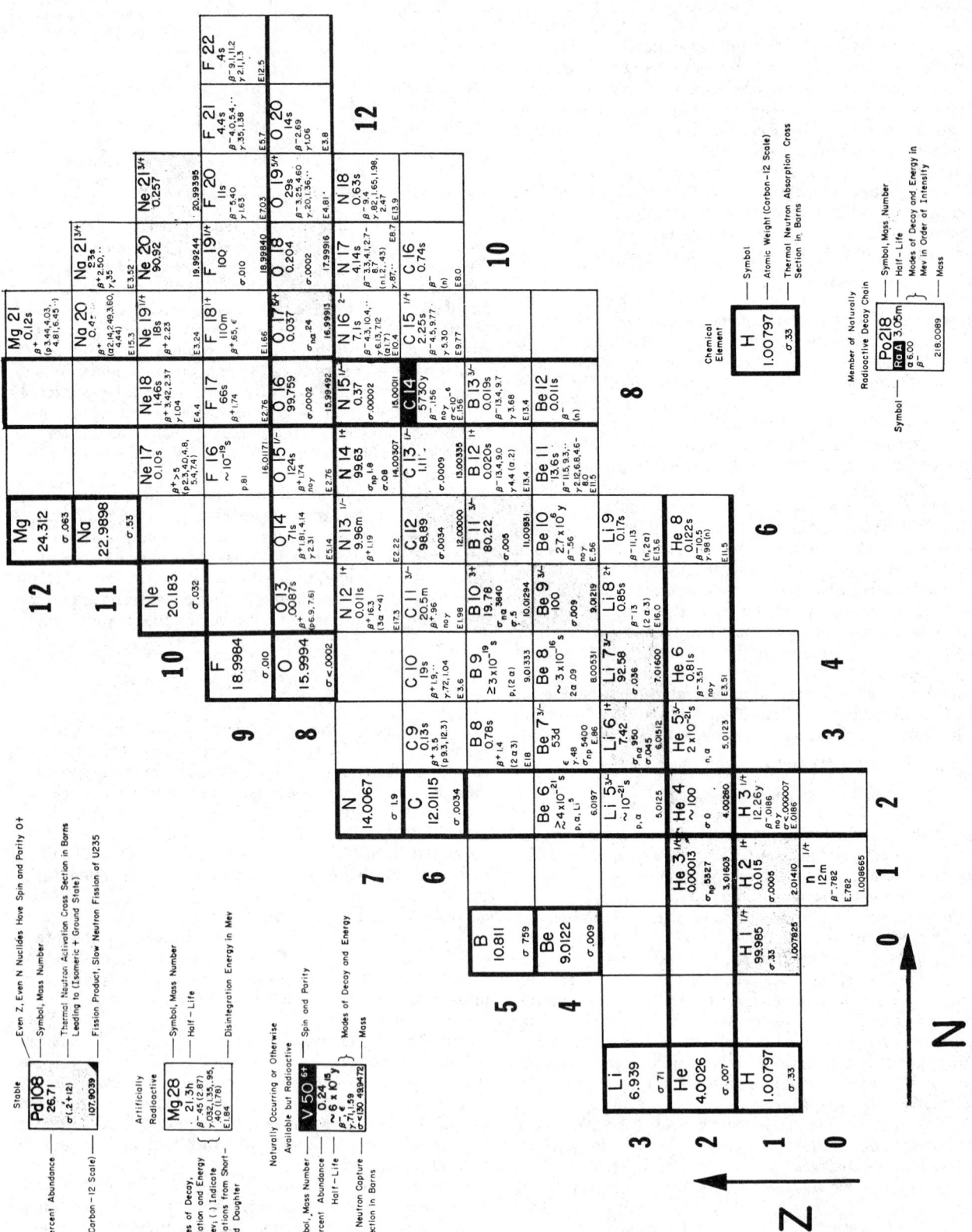

Fig 28-3.   Chart of the nuclides—to mass number 21.   Known nuclides now number about 1400 (courtesy, General Electric).

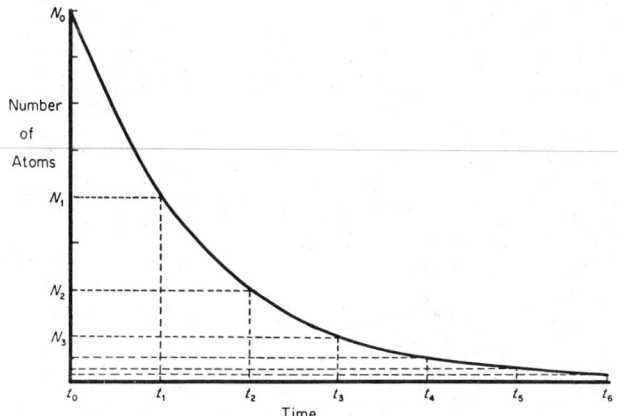

Fig 28-4.   Energy-level diagram for decay of phosphorus-32.

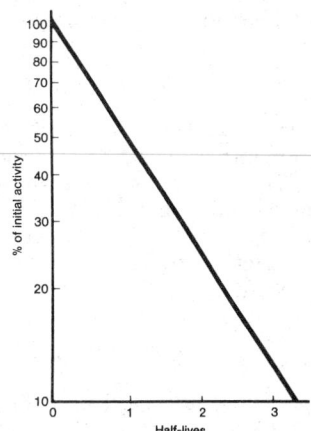

Fig 28-5.   Radioactive decay curve.

If the only source of error is that due to random decay, then the value of s should approach σ as N, the number of observations, approaches infinity.

Kinetics of Decay—*Decay rate* is the time rate at which atoms undergo radioactive disintegration. It is expressed by $-dN/dt$, where $-dN$ is the change in the number of atoms, N, and dt is the change in the time, t. The negative sign merely indicates that the number of atoms is decreasing in time. The rate of decay $(-dN/dt)$ is proportional to the number of atoms, N, present at any time, t. Therefore,

$$-dN/dt = \lambda N$$

where λ is a proportionality constant usually called the *decay constant*. The decay of radioactive atoms is therefore a first-order reaction. Integration of the equation above results in the useful relation

$$\ln \frac{N_t}{N_0} = -\lambda t$$

where N_0 is the number of atoms present at zero time and N_t is the number of atoms present at time t. This relation is sometimes more conveniently used in the exponential form

$$N_i = N_0 e^{-\lambda t}$$

This relation is illustrated graphically in Fig 28-4. The rate of decay, $-dN/dt$, is sometimes called the *activity* and is represented by the symbol, A. Since the activity, A, is proportional to the number of atoms, N, the following useful relations can also be derived.

$$A = \lambda N$$

$$\ln \frac{A_t}{A_0} = -\lambda t \text{ or } A_t = A_0 e^{-\lambda t}$$

or

$$\ln A_t = \ln A_0 - \lambda t$$

The last relationship is illustrated in Fig 28-5.

The *absolute activity* is usually expressed as disintegrations per second (d/s or dps) or disintegrations per minute (d/m or dpm). The *observed activity*, which is less than the absolute activity by a factor equal to the efficiency of the counting system, is expressed in counts per second (c/s or cps) in counts per minute (c/m or cpm).

The *half-life* of a radioactive species is the time required for one-half of a given number of atoms to decay. The half-life, $t_{1/2}$, is related to the disintegration constant, λ, by the equation:

$$t_{1/2} = 0.693/\lambda$$

Consecutive, *sequential* or *series decay* results when a *parent* nuclide A decays to produce a radioactive *daughter*

B which, in turn, decays to C

$$A \xrightarrow{\lambda_A} B \xrightarrow{\lambda_B} C$$

If only atoms of A are present initially, the number of atoms of B present at time t is given by

$$N_B = \frac{\lambda_A}{\lambda_B - \lambda_A} N_{A_0}(e^{-\lambda_A t} - e^{-\lambda_B t})$$

Of particular interest in nuclear medicine are combinations where A has a relatively long half-life and B a short half-life, for example

$$^{99}Mo \xrightarrow{67 \text{ h}} {}^{99m}Tc \xrightarrow{6.0 \text{ h}} {}^{99}Tc$$

After a time equal to many half-lives of the daughter, a state of *secular equilibrium* is said to have been achieved. At this time *in-growth* of the daughter has reached a maximum. This process is utilized in *radioisotope generators* as a source of short-lived isotopes. (See page 458.)

Units of Radioactivity—One g of radium was selected as the unit of radioactivity and was called the *Curie*. It has been extremely difficult to measure the absolute decay rate (dps) of a curie of radium, although the average of many measurements, using a variety of methods, is approximately 3.7×10^{10} dps. In view of these discrepancies, the International Radium Standards Commission has recommended the use of the arbitrary value of exactly 3.7×10^{10} until the third significant figure is agreed upon. Although originally defined in terms of radium, the curie is now used as a standard for the disintegration rate of any radioisotope. For example, 1 curie of carbon-14 means that amount of carbon-14 necessary to provide 3.7×10^{10} disintegrating atoms/sec.

$$1 \text{ millicurie (mCi)} = 10^{-3} \text{ curie}$$

$$1 \text{ microcurie } (\mu Ci) = 10^{-6} \text{ curie}$$

Modes of Radioactive Decay—When it is desired to measure the absolute decay rate of a particular nuclear species, it is necessary to establish its mode of decay in order to determine the relationship of the number of particles or gamma rays emitted to the number of atoms actually undergoing decay. There are several important modes of decay.

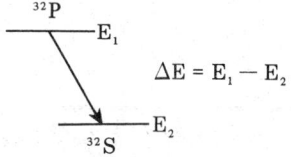

Fig 28-6.   Generalized decay curve.

Alpha decay is illustrated by the decay of polonium-210 to lead-206:

$$^{210}_{84}\text{Po} \rightarrow {}^{4}_{2}\text{He} + {}^{206}_{82}\text{Pb}$$

In this example, the nucleus of lead-206, which contains 82 protons and 124 neutrons, is stable and does not undergo further decay. The majority of nuclides which undergo alpha decay have atomic numbers greater than 82.

There are three types of *beta decay: negatron emission, positron emission*, and *electron capture*. Decay by negatron emission is illustrated by the decay of phosphorus-32 to sulfur-32 (Fig 28-6):

$$^{32}_{15}\text{P} \rightarrow {}^{32}_{16}\text{S} + \beta^- + \nu$$

Note that the atomic number of the *daughter*, sulfur-32, is greater than that of the *parent*, phosphorus-32. In this process a new proton has been produced, but because a neutron has been consumed, there is no change in the mass number. This is explained by the *particle reaction*,

$$^{1}_{0}\text{n} \rightarrow {}^{1}_{1}\text{p} + \text{e}^- + \nu$$

which shows the decay of a neutron into a proton, a negative electron, and a neutrino. Note also the change in the ratio of neutrons to protons as the phosphorus-32 decays to stable sulfur-32.

The beta particles emitted during the decay of a given radioactive species do not all possess the same energy but are emitted with a continuous energy distribution extending from zero to a specific maximum value, E_{max}. That this should be, posed an enigma for some time. The decay of phosphorus-32 of energy E_1 to sulfur-32 of energy E_2 should be associated with the release of energy equal to ΔE, where $\Delta E = E_1 - E_2$ (Fig 28-6). A new particle, the *neutrino*, was postulated to explain the energy change not associated with the beta particle. Thus, the sum of the energies of the beta particle and its associated neutrino is equal to ΔE or E_{max} (Fig 28-7).

If the ratio of neutrons to protons is too *low* for stability, a nucleus may decay by *positron emission* (ie, *positron decay*):

$$^{11}_{6}\text{C} \rightarrow {}^{11}_{5}\text{B} + \beta^+ + \nu$$

In this instance the particle reaction which illustrates the change is

$$^{1}_{1}\text{p} \rightarrow {}^{1}_{0}\text{n} + \text{e}^+ + \nu$$

Again no change in mass number occurs, since the decay of ¹¹C to ¹¹B is accompanied by the change of a proton into a neutron. The energies of the positrons extend from zero to E_{max} in a manner complementary to the energy distribution of negative beta particles since the neutrino is required to account for the balance of the energy.

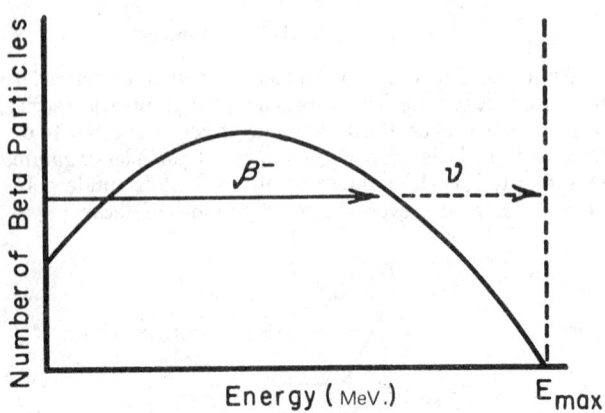

Fig 28-7.   Typical beta spectrum.

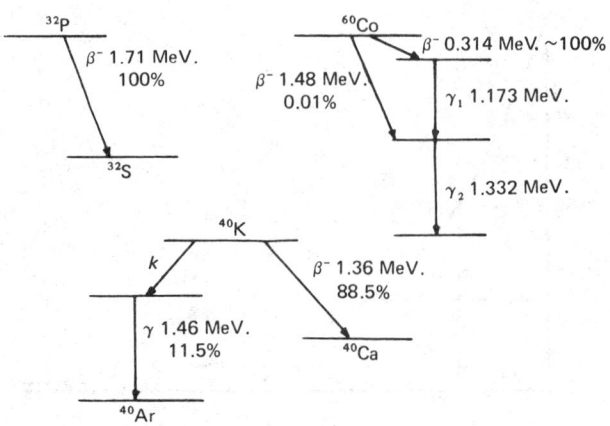

Fig 28-8.   Modes of decay.   Radioactive atoms may decay by any one of numerous processes.   Negatron decay is shown by an arrow slanting to the right, electron or *k*-capture by an arrow slanting to the left, and gamma emission by a vertical arrow.

If insufficient energy is available for positron emission, the neutron–proton ratio is sometimes increased to a stable condition by a process known as *electron capture*. In this process, an orbital electron is captured by the nucleus. An example is the decay of ⁷Be to ⁷Li:

$$^{7}_{4}\text{Be} + \text{e}^-(\text{K}) \rightarrow {}^{7}_{3}\text{Li}$$

The corresponding particle reaction is

$$\text{e}^- + {}^{1}_{1}\text{p} \rightarrow {}^{1}_{0}\text{n}$$

Electron capture has also been called *K-capture* because the electron captured in the process is usually from the K shell. However, the electron may come from the L or M shell instead.

The mode of decay is often represented by an energy-level diagram (see Fig 28-8). Three different modes of decay are illustrated. The first illustrates the simple beta decay of phosphorus-32. In this instance, each decaying atom of ³²P emits one beta particle. Thus, if the number of beta particles is measured, the number of decaying atoms is also known. The decay of an atom of cobalt-60 also results in the emission of a single beta particle but, in addition, two gamma rays are also emitted. Thus, if the decay rate is measured by counting the number of beta particles emitted, a 1:1 ratio exists. If, on the other hand, the decay rate is determined from the number of gamma rays emitted, it must be remembered that the number of decaying atoms is equal to only one-half the number of gamma rays (neglecting a small correction for internal conversion). In the third example, the decay of 113 atoms of ⁴⁰K results in the emission of only 100 beta particles. The other 13 atoms decay by electron capture. Thus, a microcurie of ⁴⁰K does not emit 3.7×10^4 beta particles per second, but only $100/113 \times 3.7 \times 10^4$ beta particles. Fig 28-9 shows similar decay schemes for other nuclides used in medicine.

Units of Radiation and Dosage—Equal quantities (ie, the same number of microcuries or millicuries) of different radioactive species will not produce equal quantities of radiation, nor will equal quantities produce equal doses of radiation. The fundamental reasons for this fact are explained above. Although equal quantities (millicuries) of different radioactive atoms represent equal numbers of atoms decaying per unit of time, the mode of decay must be considered. The number, type, and energy of the radiation emitted are indicated by the decay scheme. These parameters must be known if units of radioactivity are to be related to units of radiation and dosage.

Roentgen—The roentgen is a unit of exposure dose to X-

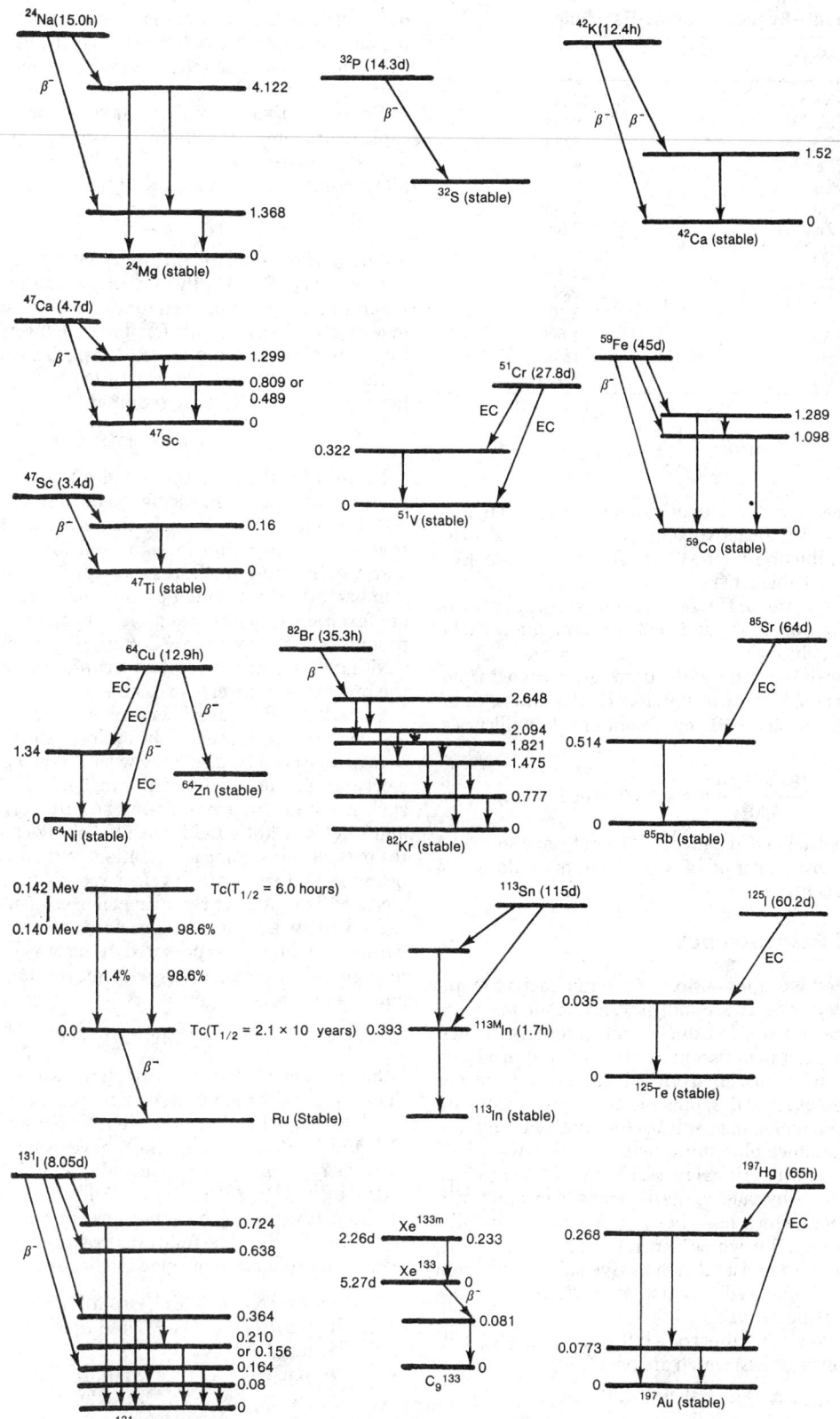

Fig 28-9. Decay schemes for nuclides commonly used in medicine.

or *gamma* radiation. (It is *not* a unit of alpha or beta radiation.) The roentgen is defined as that quantity of X- or gamma radiation which will produce one electrostatic unit of charge in 1 cc of air. While the roentgen is useful for calibrating sources and for measuring the dose in air, the energy dissipated by one roentgen of radiation in air will not be the same as that dissipated in muscle tissue. The *roentgen-equivalent-physical* (*rep*) and the *roentgen-equivalent-man* (*rem*) have been used as units of tissue dose but have now been largely replaced by the *RAD*. The dose is one *RAD* if the energy lost by ionization is 100 ergs/g of tissue.

Units of radioactivity (eg, millicuries) may be related to exposure dose rate (eg, milliroentgens per hour) by the following expression.

Table III—Specific Gamma-Ray Output

Radioisotope	Γ
^{22}Na	12,200
^{24}Na	19,300
^{58}Co	5,600
^{59}Fe	6,500
^{60}Co	12,800
^{64}Cu	1,100
^{65}Zn	3,000
^{86}Rb	500
^{130}I	12,300
^{131}I	2,300
^{192}Ir	5,100
^{198}Au	2,500
^{203}Hg	1,300
^{226}Ra	8,400

$$mr/hr = \frac{\Gamma C}{d^2}$$

C is the number of millicuries of radioactive material, d is the distance to the radioactive source, and values of Γ in milliroentgens/millicurie/hour at 1 cm for several radioisotopes are listed in Table III.

These values of Γ are for the gamma component of the radiation only. For pure alpha and beta emitters, the value of Γ is zero. This includes ^{3}H, ^{14}C, ^{32}P, ^{35}S, ^{45}Ca, and ^{90}Sr.

Suppose we wish to calculate the dose rate received from 10 mg of radium at a distance of 100 cm. By definition, 1 g of radium = 1 curie and, hence, 10 mg of radium = 10 millicuries. Thus,

$$\text{Dose rate} = \frac{(8400)(10)}{100^2} = 8.4 \text{ mr/hr (at 100 cm)}$$

and the dose received at a distance of 100 cm from a source of 10 mg of radium over a period of, say, 10 hours would be 8.4 × 10 = 84 milliroentgens.

Production of Radioisotopes

Pile-Produced Isotopes—Most of the radioactive materials produced today for use in industry, academic research, medicine, etc, are prepared in a nuclear pile (nuclear reactor). In the reactor the uranium fission reaction (p 455) produces a large supply of neutrons. In a critical reactor, one neutron for each uranium atom undergoing fission is used to sustain the reaction. The remaining neutrons (one and one-half) are used either to produce plutonium by interaction with ^{238}U nuclei, are lost from the critical mass, or are used to produce radioactive products by causing the neutrons to interact with specific substances which have been inserted into the pile. The latter process is known as neutron activation. Thus, there are two sources of useful radioactive substances from the pile: (1) those produced as fission products and (2) those produced by neutron activation.

The following reactions illustrate but one of many combinations of fission reactions which are possible.

$$^{238}_{92}\text{U} + ^1_0\text{n} \rightarrow ^{131}_{50}\text{Sn} + ^{106}_{42}\text{Mo} + ^1_0\text{n} + ^1_0\text{n}$$

The ^{131}Sn and the ^{106}Mo are very radioactive and have very short half-lives. They immediately decay by a series of beta decay processes:

$$^{131}_{50}\text{Sn} \rightarrow ^{131}_{51}\text{Sb} \rightarrow ^{131}_{52}\text{Te} \rightarrow ^{131}_{53}\text{I}$$

$$^{106}_{42}\text{Mo} \rightarrow ^{106}_{43}\text{Tc} \rightarrow ^{106}_{44}\text{Ru} \rightarrow ^{106}_{45}\text{Rh}$$

Both ^{131}I and ^{106}Ru are available commercially as fission-produced isotopes. Before use, however, they must be separated chemically from a large number of other fission-pro-

duced radioisotopes. For many of the isotopes produced by fission, separation is too difficult or costly; hence, the majority of radioactive compounds are prepared by neutron activation.

Neutron activation may result either from simple neutron capture or from a transmutation process. For example, radioactive phosphorus (^{32}P) can be prepared from stable phosphorus (^{31}P) by *neutron capture:*

$$^{31}_{15}\text{P} + ^1_0\text{n} \rightarrow ^{32}_{15}\text{P} + \gamma$$

The disadvantage of this method is that the radioactive phosphorus (^{32}P) is highly diluted with stable ^{31}P. ^{32}P of low specific activity can be used for certain purposes, such as the investigation of phosphate fertilizers, but would be less useful for many biological and medical applications.

Radioactive phosphorus can be made by *transmutation* if high specific activities are required.

$$^{32}_{16}\text{S} + ^1_0\text{n} \rightarrow ^{32}_{15}\text{P} + ^1_1\text{p}$$

In this case the radioactive phosphorus can be separated from the unreacted sulfur by chemical procedures. Where ^{32}P is made from ^{31}P such chemical separations are not practical. Transmutation is useful for the preparation of many radioactive nuclides, especially those of low atomic number. As the atomic number increases, "n,γ" reactions are favored over "n,p" reactions. For example, cobalt-60 is produced by the reaction ^{59}Co(n,γ)^{60}Co because the reaction ^{60}Ni(n,p)^{60}Co does not occur with sufficient frequency to make the process commercially feasible.

Cyclotron-Produced Isotopes—Certain radioisotopes are cyclotron-produced. The cyclotron and similar *particle accelerators* can be used only with charged particles such as electrons, protons, deuterons, etc, because the operation of such machines depends upon the interaction of magnetic and/or electrostatic fields with the charge (either + or −) of the particle undergoing acceleration. When the particles have been accelerated to a high velocity, even approaching the velocity of light and representing enormous energies, they are caused to strike a target containing the atoms to be bombarded. Sodium-22 is prepared in this way by the interaction of high-velocity deuterons with magnesium. The nuclear equation is

$$^{24}\text{Mg}(d,\alpha)^{22}\text{Na}$$

Other medically important nuclides which have been produced in a cyclotron by use of high-energy deuterons include ^{11}C, ^{13}N, ^{15}O, ^{18}F, ^{67}Ga, ^{68}Ge, ^{81}Kr, ^{85m}Kr, ^{90}Nd, ^{101m}Rh, ^{111}In, ^{123}I and ^{203}Pb. Those which have been produced using high-energy alpha particles include ^{18}F, ^{43}K, ^{52}Fe, ^{62}Zn, ^{67}Ga, ^{77}Br, ^{81}Rb, ^{87}Y, ^{97}Ru, ^{111}In, ^{123}I, ^{124}I, ^{129}Cs and ^{157}Dy. High-energy protons have been used to produce ^{123}I, ^{127}Xe, ^{201}Pb and ^{203}Pb. The following reactions are typical for the cyclotron production of some medically useful nuclides

^{10}B(d,n)^{11}C	^{18}O(p,n)^{18}F
^{11}B(p,n)^{11}C	^{20}Ne(d,α)^{18}F
^{11}B(d,2n)^{11}C	
^{14}N(p,α)^{11}C	^{66}Zn(d,n)^{67}Ga
	^{68}Zn(p,2n)^{67}Ga
^{10}B(α,n)^{13}N	^{69}Ga(p,2n)^{68}Ge
^{12}C(d,n)^{13}N	
^{16}O(p,α)^{13}N	^{82}Kr(p,2n)^{81}Rb → ^{81}Kr
	^{111}Cd(p,n)^{111}In
^{14}N(d,n)^{15}O	^{112}Cd(p,2n)^{111}In
^{15}N(p,n)^{15}O	
^{16}O(p,pn)^{15}O	^{203}Tl(p,3n)^{201}Pb → ^{201}Tl

Usually a nuclide can be made by more than one reaction. For example, ^{123}I can be prepared either directly or indirectly. Direct reactions include

$$^{123}\text{Te (p,n)}^{123}\text{I}$$
$$^{121}\text{Sb (}^4\text{He,2n)}^{123}\text{I}$$
$$^{122}\text{Te (d,n)}^{123}\text{I}$$
$$^{124}\text{Te (p,2n)}^{123}\text{I}$$

Indirectly, the intermediate ^{123}Xe is prepared which then decays to ^{123}I

$$^{122}\text{Te (}^4\text{He,3n) }^{123}\text{Xe} \rightarrow {}^{123}\text{I}$$
$$^{122}\text{Te (}^3\text{He,2n) }^{123}\text{Xe} \rightarrow {}^{123}\text{I}$$
$$^{123}\text{Te (}^3\text{He,3n) }^{123}\text{Xe} \rightarrow {}^{123}\text{I}$$
$$^{127}\text{I(p,5n)}^{123}\text{Xe} \rightarrow {}^{123}\text{I}$$

Radioisotope Generators—Where clinical tests require that a radioisotope be administered internally, it is advantageous to use an isotope with a short half-life to minimize the radiation dose received by the patient. But it is evident that the shorter the half-life, the greater will be the problem of supply. One answer to this problem is the *radioisotope generator* or *"radioisotopic cow,"* which utilizes the phenomenon of sequential decay. A radioisotope generator or cow (see Fig 28-10) is an ion-exchange column containing a resin or alumina upon which has been adsorbed a long-lived parent nuclide. Radioactive decay of the long-lived parent results in the production of a short-lived radioactive daughter nuclide which is eluted or "milked" from the column by means of an appropriate eluant. Characteristics of a number of parent–daughter systems which have been used in radioisotope generators will be found in Table IV.

The *technetium-99m generator* consists of an alumina column on which molybdenum 99 is adsorbed as ammonium molybdate. Radioactive decay of ^{99}Mo produces ^{99m}Tc which is eluted from the column with sterile, pyrogen-free saline. Upon elution the ^{99m}Tc is in the form of sodium pertechnetate (Na^{99m}TcO$_4$). Elution repeated every 24 hours provides a satisfactory balance between concentration and quantity of eluted ^{99m}Tc. If a high activity of ^{99m}Tc is not required the generator can be eluted more frequently, say every 12 hours, but activity of the ^{99m}Tc will have returned to only about 70% of maximum in that time. A typical elution curve for a ^{99m}Tc generator is shown in Fig 28-11. Normally the generator must be replaced about once a week due to the decay of ^{99}Mo.

In the *indium-113m generator* tin 113 is used as the radioactive parent. The tin 113 is adsorbed on a column of ion-exchange resin from which ^{113m}In is eluted with dilute HCl. Because of the shorter half-life of the daughter (see Table IV) the column can be eluted every 10 to 15 hours.

Table IV—Radioisotope Generators

Parent isotope	Half-life		Daughter isotope	Half-life		Mode of decay
^{68}Ge	250	d	^{68}Ga	68	m	β^+
^{81}Rb	4.7	h	^{81m}Kr	13	s	I.T.
^{82}Sr	25	d	^{82}Rb	1.3	m	β^+
^{87}Y	80	h	^{87m}Sr	2.8	h	I.T.
^{90}Sr	28	y	^{90}Y	64	h	β^-
^{99}Mo	67	h	^{99m}Tc	6.0	h	I.T.
^{109}Cd	453	d	^{109m}Ag	39.2	s	I.T.
^{113}Sn	118	d	^{113m}In	1.7	h	I.T.
^{115}Cd	53.4	h	^{115m}In	4.5	h	I.T.
^{122}Xe	20	h	^{122}I	3.6	m	β^+
^{132}Te	3.2	d	^{132}I	2.3	h	β^-
^{137}Cs	30	y	^{137m}Ba	2.6	m	I.T.
^{144}Ce	285	d	^{144}Pr	17.3	m	β^-
^{178}W	21.5	d	^{178}Ta	9.4	m	β^+
^{191}Os	16	d	^{191m}Ir	4.9	s	I.T.
^{195m}Hg	41	h	^{195m}Au	30.6	s	I.T.

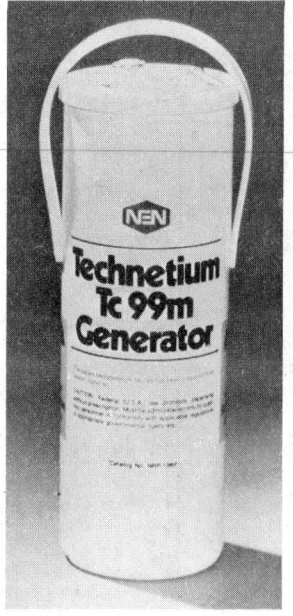
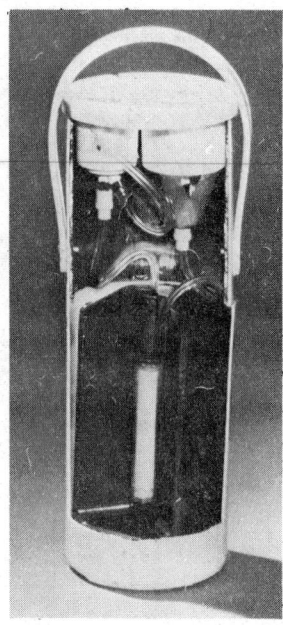

Fig 28-10. Radioisotope generator for production of technetium 99m by elution from molybdenum 99 adsorbed on alumina column. *A:* Outer view. *B:* Cutaway view showing column inside lead shield (courtesy, New England Nuclear).

Natural Radioactivity

The natural radioisotopes include all elements with an atomic number greater than 83, several with atomic numbers of 81 to 83 (isotopes of thallium, lead, and bismuth) and a few isotopes of the lighter elements with atomic numbers less than 81 (^{3}H, ^{14}C, ^{40}K, ^{50}V, ^{87}Rb, ^{115}In, ^{123}Te, ^{138}La, ^{142}Ce, ^{144}Nd, ^{147}Sm, ^{148}Sm, ^{149}Sm, ^{152}Gd, ^{156}Dy, ^{174}Hf, ^{176}Lu, ^{180}Ta, ^{187}Re, and ^{190}Pt).

Some of the heavier radioactive elements disintegrate in a definite known sequence until stable nuclear configurations are achieved. Four such sequences or radioactive series have been established, of which the uranium (or uranium-radium) series is the best known. It commences with uranium-238, passes through a series of decay processes ending with stable radium G (lead-206). Table V shows the uranium series. The mass of each member of this series is given by the expression $4n + 2$ in which n is a whole number. Thus, this relation serves to characterize the uranium-238 series. The actinium series, which has uranium-235 as the parent nuclide, is characterized by the relation $4n + 3$, and the thorium series, which begins with thorium-232 and ends with lead-208, by $4n$. The last series to be discovered, the $4n + 1$ series, is unique in that its members are artificially radioactive. Its initial member is the synthetic element curium-241.

Radium—Ra = 226.02 (At No 88)

History and Occurrence—The word Radium is from the Latin *radius* which means *ray*. Radium was first obtained in 1911 by Mme. Curie and Debierne by electrolysis of a solution of radium chloride.

A salt of radium had been isolated 13 years earlier by M and Mme Curie in 1898 from the ore pitchblende, obtained from North Bohemia. This was an extension of work instituted by Henri Becquerel in 1896. The latter worker, a Frenchman, is credited with the discovery of radioactivity as a result of his work with uranium potassium sulfate which he found to produce blackening of a photographic plate. From several tons of pitchblende Madame Curie extracted a material possessing considerably more activity than uranium. This substance she named *Polonium*, after her native country Poland. During December, 1898, she finally isolated radium from the same ore. Weight for weight it was found to be approximately 2 million times more active than uranium.

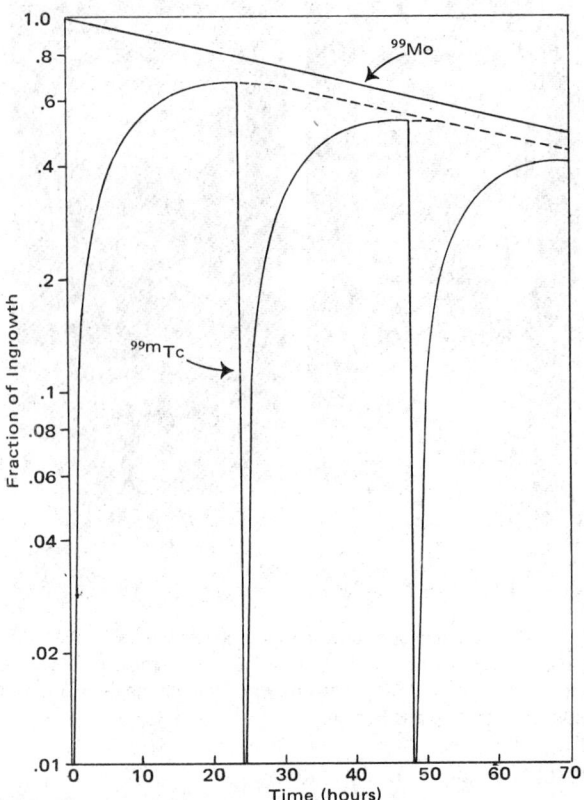

Fig 28-11. Elution curve. The lower solid lines show the theoretical activity of ^{99m}Tc in the generator as a result of ingrowth followed by elution of ^{99m}Tc at 24-hour intervals. If the generator were not eluted, ingrowth would follow the broken line and a secular equilibrium would be established. The upper solid line represents decrease in activity of ^{99}Mo, the parent nuclide, due to radioactive decay.

Today radium is produced primarily from *carnotite* and *pitchblende*. These ores are found chiefly in the Belgian Congo, and in the Great Bear Lake region of Canada. Until 1925 most of the world supply of radium was obtained from the mineral carnotite, which was mined in Colorado and Utah.

Description—A bright, white metal which immediately darkens upon exposure to the air. Its physical constants are given on page 466. It has a valence of 2. Its half-life is 1620 years. 1 g of radium produces 1×10^{-4} ml of radon/day. Radium salts color a flame carmine-red.

Uses—For many years radium enjoyed wide popularity in the medical field as a source of radiation in treating cancer being generally used in the form of radium needles for vaginal application in treat-

Table V—Uranium Disintegration Series

| Old | | Atomic | | |
Name	Element	Wt	No	Half-life
Uranium I	Uranium	238	92	4.51×10^9 y
Uranium X₁	Thorium	234	90	24.1 d
Uranium X₂	Protactinium	234	91	1.18 m
Uranium II	Protactinium	234	91	2.48×10^5 y
Ionium	Thorium	230	90	7.6×10^4 y
Radium	Radium	226	88	1620 y
Radon	Radon	222	86	3.82 d
Radium A	Polonium	218	84	3.05 m
Radium B	Lead	214	82	26.8 m
Radium C	Bismuth	214	83	19.7 m
Radium C′	Polonium	214	84	1.6×10^{-4} sec
Radium C″	Thallium	210	81	1.32 m
Radium D	Lead	210	82	22 y
Radium E	Bismuth	210	83	5.0 d
Radium F	Polonium	210	84	138 d
Radium G	Lead	206	82	stable

ment of cancer of the cervix, and to a lesser degree in the treatment of certain malignant lesions of the oral cavity.

When radium *needles* are used, care must be taken to remove them after the proper dose has been administered. Further, care must be exercised with radium because of the ease with which it is taken up by the circulation and deposited in bone (being in the calcium group, the metabolism is similar thereto). It is interesting that radiation which has the property to *destroy* certain cancers is also capable of *causing* similar growths.

Caution—Radium is an extremely hazardous material and must be handled only by properly protected and adequately trained personnel.

Thorium—Th = 232.04 (At No 90)

History and Occurrence—The name *thorium* was given this element by its discoverer, Berzelius, in honor of the ancient Scandinavian god *Thor*. It occurs in the minerals *thorite* [$ThSiO_4$] and *thorianite*, which contains about 70% of ThO_2 and about 10% of uranium dioxide. Its principal source in the US is *monazite sand* in which it occurs as phosphate to the extent of 3 to 9%.

Description—A white to grayish white metal, having a specific gravity of 11.2 and melting at 1845°. It is scarcely attacked by hydrochloric or nitric acids but is dissolved by nitrohydrochloric acid and converted to sulfate by heating with H_2SO_4.

Thorium is radioactive, yielding a number of disintegration products, the most important of which is *mesothorium*. Due to the fact that thorium has such a high atomic number (90) its insoluble compounds, particularly the oxide or hydroxide, are good absorbers of X-rays. For this reason suspensions of thorium compounds were used to diagnose diseases of the renal pelvis and the urinary tract.

Thorium is tetravalent and its oxide [ThO_2] occurs as the mineral *thoria*. It was used orally or rectally as a contrast medium in roentgenography, and is a constituent in the electron-emitting elements of radio tubes. It was formerly an important constituent of incandescent gas mantles.

Thorium has many properties in common with the alkaline earths as well as with the iron-aluminum group. With potassium sulfate it forms a *thorium alum* which is only very slightly soluble in water.

Uses—All thorium compounds are extremely hazardous if used internally, if not from their chemical toxicity, certainly from the radiation which is emitted. Thorium compounds are retained by the body almost indefinitely. Coupled with the long half-life of thorium, a serious radiation hazard results. Of particular note, thorium dioxide was once employed as a contrast medium in roentgenography, especially for the visualization of blood vessels. It was injected intravenously and produced few immediate toxic effects. However, this agent was retained in the body. Fibrosis of the liver, kidney, spleen, and lymph nodes has been attributed to its persistent radioactivity. The element is now important as a source of fissionable material. Neutron bombardment of thorium-232 yields the fissionable isotope, uranium-233.

Uranium—U = 238.03 (At No 92)

History and Occurrence—*Uranium* was named by its discoverer, Klaproth, in 1789, in honor of the planet *Uranus*. It was first isolated in an elemental state by Peligot, in 1841. The principal sources of uranium and its compounds are the minerals *uranite* and *pitchblende*, found in Czechoslovakia, and *carnotite*, which is potassium uranovanadate. Radioactivity was discovered in 1891 by Becquerel when he observed that uranium salts affected a photographic plate just as did X-rays. In 1898 and 1899 Madame Curie and her husband, Professor Curie, showed that these properties were not due to the presence of uranium but to another substance to which they gave the name radium.

Description—A silvery white and fairly hard metal, but not as hard as steel. Its specific gravity is 18.7, it melts at about 1850°, and it is soluble in the strong mineral acids.

It has two valences, IV and VI, and forms two oxides, the dioxide [UO_2] and the trioxide [UO_3]. The salts derived from tetravalent uranium are termed *uranous;* those containing hexavalent uranium are usually basic salts containing the divalent *uranyl* group, UO_2^{2+}, such as uranyl nitrate, $UO_2(NO_3)_2$. Uranyl salts are often referred to simply as uranium salts; for example, uranyl nitrate is often called simply uranium nitrate.

Uranous salts are green while uranyl salts are yellow with a green fluorescence. Uranyl compounds, except the oxides, phosphate, sulfide, and uranates, are soluble in water.

Uses—Uranyl compounds were used in the manufacture of glass to produce a greenish yellow fluorescent glass known as *uranium glass* or "vaseline" glass. They have also been used for making a black pigment for china painting, and to some extent as intensifiers in photography. Government curtailments and restrictions now prohibit the use of uranium in glass and pottery. The most recent use of uranium metal is in the production of *radioactive isotopes* in the atomic pile.

Instruments for Radiation Measurement

When a radioactive atom decays it emits a particle or electromagnetic radiation or both, depending upon the mode of decay of the nucleus. It is the radiation resulting from the decay of atoms which is detected by the radiation measuring equipment. Various types of radiation detection instruments have been designed, each especially adapted for the detection of a particular type of radiation. If radiation is to be detected with efficiency, the type of radiation must be known and the detector selected accordingly.

It is convenient to separate radiation detectors into two distinct categories: (a) those which depend on collection of ions, and (b) those which depend on collection of photons. On this basis detectors can be classified as follows:

a. Detectors utilizing ion collection
   1. Gas-filled detectors
      Electroscopes
      Ion chambers
      Proportional counters
      Geiger counters
   2. Solid-state detectors
      Barrier-layer detectors
      Lithium-drifted detectors
b. Detectors utilizing photon collection
   1. Sodium iodide scintillation counters
   2. Liquid scintillation counters

Ionization Chambers—Any two conducting surfaces separated by a small distance behave as an electric capacitor. The surfaces may be two flat plates or may consist of a wire mounted inside a hollow metal cylinder. If a potential source is connected between the plates momentarily, the capacitor will be charged. Ionizing radiation passing between the plates will discharge the capacitor. The rate at which discharge occurs is a measure of the radiation intensity. The extent to which discharge has occurred is a measure of the quantity of radiation.

Many types of ionization chambers are available. The classical gold-leaf electroscope is the oldest and best known. Refinements of the electroscope are found in the Landsverk and Lauritsen instruments, and in pocket chambers used for personnel protection. Ion chambers are also useful for routine calibration of isotope shipments, and for calibrating the dose of a radioisotope to be administered to a patient. Ion chambers used for this purpose are sometimes called "dose calibrators." Such an instrument is shown in Fig 28-12. The mode of operation is shown in the simplified diagram (Fig 28-13). A fixed potential is applied to the electrodes of the chamber and the radioactive source to be calibrated is usually placed within the chamber. Current flowing between the electrodes is a function of the degree of ionization occurring in the chamber which, in turn, is a function both of the nature of the radiation emitted by the source and the millicurie strength of the source. The instrument is readily calibrated by use of standard sources. With most instruments a switch permits selection of an appropriate precalibrated meter shunt to compensate for differences in the value of the specific gamma-ray output from one nuclide to another, thereby allowing precalibration for each of several nuclides. In using dose calibrators it is important to remember that samples and

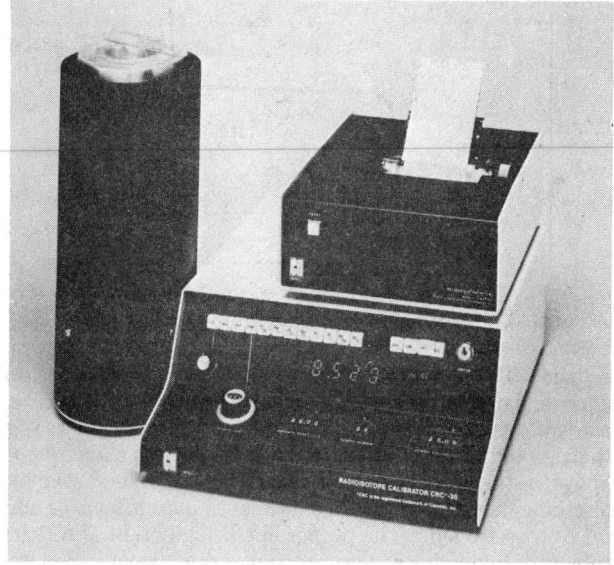

Fig 28-12. Radioisotope calibrator for automatic calibration of patient dose of a radioisotope (courtesy, Capintec, Inc).

standards should be in identical containers to avoid absorption and geometry errors.

Geiger-Müller Counters—The Geiger-Müller counter (Geiger counter or G-M counter) is particularly efficient for the detection of beta particles. It consists of a cylinder of stainless steel, or of glass, silvered on the inner surface, which serves not only as the body of the tube but as the cathode as well. A fine wire, mounted coaxially, is the anode. The space within the cylinder, and hence between the anode and cathode, is filled with a special gas mixture. Radiation passing through the gas causes atoms of gas to ionize. If a potential is maintained between the electrodes, the electrons and the positively charged ions of gas produced by this ionization process are attracted to and collected by the anode and cathode, respectively. The passage of these ions through the Geiger tube constitutes a flow of current. Each particle of radiation causes a brief flow or pulse of current to flow. Each pulse, representing the passage of a particle through the tube, is then recorded by a device such as a scaler to accumulate and indicate the total number of pulses.

To measure the characteristics of a Geiger tube, a radioactive source is placed near the tube. The voltage applied to the tube is then increased by increments, and the observed activity for each voltage setting is recorded and plotted vs the

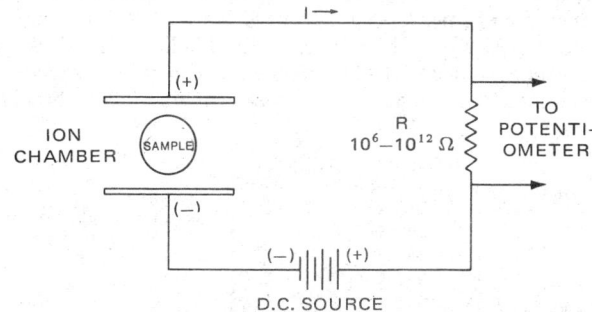

Fig 28-13. Simplified diagram of dose calibrator. Ions produced by radiation from sample migrate to respective electrodes of ion chamber. The resulting current, I, is proportional to extent of radiation and flows through resistor R. The potential produced across resistor R is E = IR, hence the potentiometer reading is proportional to the activity of sample. By adjusting R to compensate for the difference in the value of Γ, the specific gamma ray constant, from nuclide to nuclide, the instrument can be calibrated to read directly in terms of μCi or mCi.

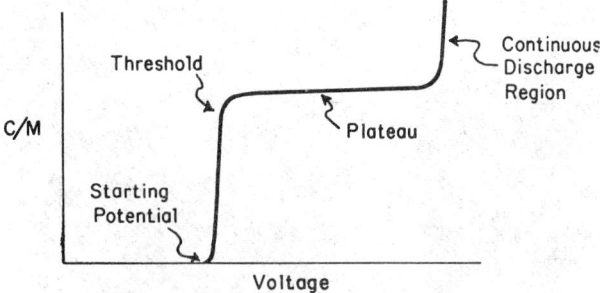

Fig 28-14.   Characteristic curve for Geiger-Müller tube.

voltage. The result is a characteristic plateau curve. Below a particular voltage, the *threshold voltage*, no activity is recorded. At the threshold the observed activity increases sharply and then levels off. The level part of the curve is known as the *plateau*. If the voltage is further increased indiscriminately, the tube will go into *continuous discharge* and may be destroyed. The proper operating potential for the tube is normally in the lower region of the plateau. See Fig 28-14.

Proportional Counters—The basic construction of the proportional counter is similar to that of the Geiger-Müller counter but modified by changing the gas composition and the shape of one or both of the electrodes. An advantage of the proportional counter is its ability to distinguish between alpha and beta particles. If a radioactive source emitting both alpha and beta particles is placed in the chamber, and the voltage applied to the chamber slowly increased, the observed activity in counts per minute will increase. At a certain voltage only alpha particles are detected but at higher voltages both alpha and beta particles are detected by the instrument.

Semiconductor Detectors—Semiconductors or solid-state detectors were first investigated about 1945. Their principal advantage lies in their ability to provide high-energy resolution for alpha, beta, and gamma spectrometry. For charged-particle detection, semiconductor detectors of the *barrier-layer* type are used. They are made by using a combination of N (negative) and P (positive) silicon semiconductors as shown in Fig 28-15. *N silicon* is prepared by adding a minute trace of phosphorus to ultrapure silicon, a process sometimes called *doping*. Phosphorus, having five valence electrons, introduces extra electrons into a lattice of tetravalent silicon atoms. *P silicon* is prepared by doping ultrapure silicon with boron. Since boron has only three valence electrons, the deficit leaves "holes" in the crystal lattice and the semiconductor is known as P silicon. Holes, of course, represent the lack of a negative electron and can therefore be considered as possessing a positive charge. A thin layer of gold deposited on the surface of the P silicon serves as an electrode by means of which a potential can be applied to the detector and at the same time serves as a thin window through

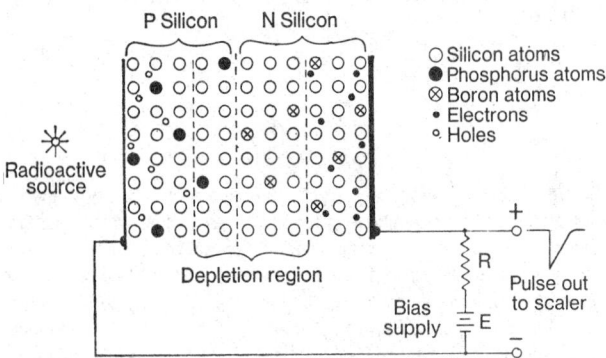

Fig 28-15.   Barrier-layer semiconductor detector.

which radiation is allowed access to the sensitive region of the detector. The opposite electrode, contacting the N silicon, also serves as a physical support for the detector and may be made of aluminum or other suitable metal. An electrical potential called a *bias potential* is now applied to the electrodes. If the positive potential were applied to the gold electrode a current would flow through the device and it would not serve as a radiation detector. Therefore a *reverse bias* is applied. The negative gold electrode attracts the positively charged holes and the positive aluminum electrode attracts the negative electrons. This results in a *depletion region* which is devoid of both electrons and holes. Consequently current ceases to flow. The detector is now said to be in the *quiescent state* since it is dormant or in a state of rest.

When radiation enters the depletion region ionization causes the production of hole-electron pairs. The applied reverse bias sweeps the holes and electrons out of the depletion region. Their migration causes a short burst of current called a *pulse* the amplitude of which is proportional to the energy dissipated by the incident particle in the depletion region. To assure proportionality between the energy of the incident particle and pulse height, the particle must be stopped in the depletion region. A depletion depth of about 60 μm is required for 10 MeV alpha particles while a depletion depth of about 1700 μm is required for 1 MeV beta particles. By increasing the applied reverse bias the depletion depth can be increased.

For gamma rays a much greater depletion depth is required since they are so penetrating. For this purpose lithium-drifted germanium detectors are used. Tetravalent germanium replaces silicon, and lithium, having a single valence electron, is drifted through P-type germanium in order to free a large region of all charge carriers, viz holes, by a process called *compensation*. Although detection efficiency is thereby greatly enhanced it is often necessary to store these detectors at the temperature of liquid nitrogen.

Scintillation Counters—When radiation strikes certain substances known as *phosphors* or *fluors*, a flash of light is produced. One of the oldest and simplest instruments employed for the detection of radiation by this process is the *spinthariscope*. In the spinthariscope flashes of light, produced by the radiation as it strikes a fluorescent screen, are observed by the naked eye. It is possible to measure alpha, beta, gamma, and other types of radiation with scintillation detectors if the detector is suitably modified for the type of radiation to be measured.

Because gamma rays are very penetrating, the phosphor used is a crystal of sodium iodide. The high density of sodium iodide favors the absorption of gamma radiation within the crystal, and this feature, coupled with the ability of the sodium iodide to fluoresce, results in a high gamma detection efficiency. Sodium iodide crystals usually contain about 1% of thallium to enhance the degree of fluorescence. See Fig 28-16.

Gamma radiation passes through a thin light-tight window of aluminum and enters the NaI(Tl) crystal where it produces a small flash of visible light. The crystal is optically coupled to a photomultiplier tube which in turn detects the flash of light and converts it into an electrical impulse. This electrical impulse is then recorded directly by means of a scaler, or pulses may first be amplified and then sorted according to their respective amplitudes before being recorded. This sorting process is accomplished by means of a *pulse-height analyzer* or *pulse-height discriminator*. By the use of such a device it is possible to measure the energy of the gamma rays striking the sodium iodide crystal.

The *liquid scintillation counter*, a modification of the scintillation instrument described previously, is used to measure beta radiation, especially beta radiation of low energy such as that emitted by tritium, carbon-14, and sulfur-35. In

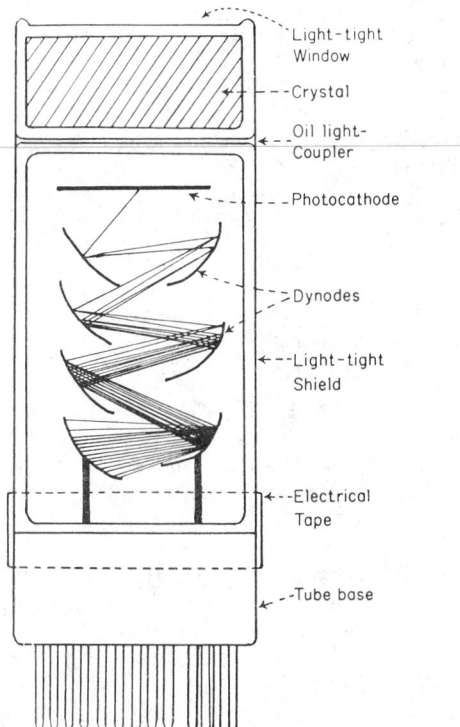

Fig 28-16.   Cross section of a crystal scintillation detector.

place of a solid crystal of sodium iodide one uses a liquid phosphor. A simple liquid scintillator has the following composition.

PPO	(2,5-diphenyloxazole)	3 g
POPOP	(2,2'-paraphenylenebis 5-phenyloxazole)	100 mg
Toluene		1000 mL

The radioactive sample is dissolved or suspended directly in about 10 mL of liquid scintillator in a special vial. The vial containing sample and liquid scintillator is positioned in front of a photomultiplier tube so that each flash of light, produced as a beta particle emitted by the radioactive sample passes through the phosphor, will be detected. Because the beta particle energies in this case are very low, the amplitudes of the corresponding light flashes will also be small, which in turn necessitates a considerable degree of electrical amplification of the pulses. The result is an increase in the number of noise pulses observed. It is common practice, therefore, to reduce the number of noise pulses produced.

The presence of certain chemical substances in a sample interferes with the mechanism for light production in the liquid scintillator. The result is *chemical quenching* (also called thermal quenching). In addition, the presence of color in the sample produces *color quenching* by absorbing light before it reaches the photomultiplier tube. Quenching causes a change in counting efficiency. A quench correction must therefore be applied to all observed count rates.

Accessory Equipment—Various instruments must be used in conjunction with the detectors described above. A *scaler* is the most commonly used device for recording and indicating the total number of impulses produced by Geiger-Müller, proportional, and scintillation counters. A scaler is simply an electronic adding machine. Most scalers also provide a source of high voltage for the operation of the detector, although the high voltage supply may be a separate unit. In addition, an electronic timer or stop-watch must be employed to measure the time during which a given number of pulses is accumulated.

Rate meters are calibrated directly in "counts per minute" or "counts per second"; thus a timer is not required as an ac-

cessory to a rate meter. Rate meters commonly contain a high voltage supply for the operation of the detector. Rate meters, generally, are also equipped with an output jack which enables them to be connected to a recorder. In this way it is possible to record the activity of a sample as a function of time.

Techniques of Radiation Measurement

Relation of Observed Activity to True Activity—The measurement of radiation may be performed with one of two basic objectives in mind; namely, (1) to determine the absolute disintegration rate of a sample or (2) to make only a relative comparison of the activity of one sample with respect to the activity of another. When relative comparisons are made, an accurate knowledge of the absolute disintegration rate is not necessary.

Consider the determination of the absolute disintegration rate, $-dN/dt$. Although it is assumed that absolute activities would normally be determined by methods to be mentioned later, the method of *defined geometry* serves to illustrate the many parameters of measurement which must be considered. Let us suppose the radioactivity of a sample has been measured with a Geiger tube and scaler. The sample was placed, for example, on the second shelf of the sample holder, the scaler was properly adjusted and used, and the count, indicated by the mechanical register and interpolation lights of the scaler, has been recorded. What, now, is the relationship of the activity, A, which has been recorded (in counts per second) to the true activity (disintegrations per second), ie, the absolute disintegration rate, dN/dt?

First, the observed activity or counting rate must be corrected for *coincidence*, which compensates for the dead time or time during which the tube was insensitive to radiation. This results in a corrected counting rate slightly higher than the observed counting rate.

Secondly, the *background* must be subtracted. Not all of the recorded counts are caused by the sample. Some are caused by cosmic radiation, natural radioactivity in the building, etc. All radiation from these outside sources constitutes the background and must be subtracted from the gross count. Application of the coincidence correction and the background correction gives the corrected net count.

The corrected net count of the sample, c/s, may now be related to the absolute disintegration rate of the sample, d/s, by applying a series of geometrical corrections. The general equation for a simple beta-emitting isotope, assuming all radiation entering the sensitive volume of the Geiger tube produces an ionizing event, follows:

$$d/s = \frac{c/s}{G \cdot F_a \cdot F_b \cdot F_d \cdot F_h \cdot F_s \cdot F_w \cdot \epsilon}$$

In this relation, G is the physical geometry factor. It relates the fraction of the beta particles emitted in a direction included by the solid angle formed by the sample and the window of the tube to the total number of beta particles emitted by the sample. F_a is the *forescattering factor* due to air. Beta particles directed initially toward the window of the tube are sometimes deflected by collisions with air molecules and are so deflected that they do not reach the tube. F_b is the *backscattering factor*. Beta particles directed initially away from the Geiger tube toward the planchet holding the sample will interact with the atoms of which the sample support is composed and will be deflected back toward the tube. The extent of backscattering will depend upon the composition of the backing material, ie, the composition of the planchet, as well as the geometrical arrangement of the sample. F_d is the *decay factor* and relates the number of decaying nuclei to the number of particles emitted. F_h is the *sidescattering factor* and corrects for the degree to which beta particles, colliding with the atoms composing the walls of the support holding the sample and Geiger tube, are deflected toward the Geiger tube. The effects of backscattering and sidescattering may be to increase the observed count rate by 100% or more. F_s is the *self-absorption factor*. Just as beta particles may interact with atoms of air before reaching the Geiger tube (*factor* F_a), they may also interact with atoms of the radioactive sample itself. Self-absorption errors are not significant if the radioactive sample is very thin, but if the sample has any thickness whatever, especially if the beta particles are not especially energetic as in the case of carbon-14 and sulfur-35, the self-absorption correction may be considerable, even exceeding that caused by scattering. F_w is the factor for absorption by air and the window of the Geiger tube. Finally, ϵ is the intrinsic efficiency of the detector.

Relative Measurements of Activity—If it is desired to make only a relative comparison of the activities of two or more radioactive samples (of the same radioactive isotope), the procedure is considerably simplified. Fortunately, many of the measurements made of radioactivity fall into this category. Where relative results only are desired, it is necessary to observe one basic precaution. That is, one must reproduce faithfully the exact geometry and counting conditions for all samples, both with respect to the equipment used and to the sample itself. In addition, both the coincidence and background corrections must be employed.

If relative measurements of activity are to be made over a long period of time, it will also be necessary to compensate for changes in instrument efficiency. Changes in the efficiency of a counting system may be brought about in a variety of ways. For example, a change in temperature or pressure may alter the characteristics of the detector. Changes in the line voltage may change the sensitivity of the scaler, as well as the operating point of the detector. Prepared mounts of radioactive samples having long half-lives are used as standards for the measurement of relative efficiency of a counting system so that appropriate corrections can be applied to the observed counting rate. Standards commonly used for this purpose include ^{90}Sr, ^{60}Co, and ^{137}Cs. The activity of this reference standard is measured along with the samples. Changes in the observed activity of the reference standard from day to day are assumed to be caused by changes in instrument efficiency. Thus, all activity data are normalized.

Coincidence Loss—The coincidence loss is the loss of register of events caused by their occurring within a span of time too short to be resolved by an electronic circuit. It is also referred to as the *dead-time loss*, *counting loss*, or *resolving-time loss*. The correction applied is termed the *coincidence correction*. In a Geiger tube, a beta particle entering the sensitive volume initiates a chain of events which requires a finite time (approximately 100 to 300 μsec) to complete. If, during this interval, a second beta particle enters the Geiger tube, it will not be observed, and the result is an error in the observed counting rate. The greater the counting rate, the greater the probability of such a loss, and the greater the counting error. For a dead time of about 300 μsec this loss amounts to $\frac{1}{2}$ of 1% per 1000 counts/min. Thus, if the observed counting rate is 10,000 counts/min the loss is 5% at 20,000 counts/min it is 10%, and at 50,000 counts/min it is 25%. For scintillation detectors resolving time is usually less than one microsecond, allowing measurement of activities as high as 100,000 cpm. Proportional counters also have a relatively short resolving time. Resolving time can be measured by the method of paired sources.

Method of Paired Sources—Two radioactive sources are prepared on identical mounts, each having about the same activity (about 10,000 counts/min). The activity of each source is carefully determined individually and then combined, identical geometry and backscattering being maintained throughout all measurements. The resolving time, T, is then calculated from the relation

$$T = \frac{r_1 + r_2 - r_{1,2}}{2r_1r_2}$$

in which r_1 and r_2 = activities of samples 1 and 2, respectively, and $r_{1,2}$ = activity of the combined samples.

The activity corrected for coincidence may be obtained from the equation

$$R = \frac{r}{1 - rT}$$

in which

R = activity corrected for coincidence
r = uncorrected activity
T = resolving time

Calibration Methods—The calibration of radioactive samples entails the determination of the absolute decay rate, $-dN/dt$, or the determination of the number of radioactive atoms, N. These quantities are related by

$$-dN/dt = \lambda N$$

If two of these terms are known, the third can be calculated. The determination of any two of these terms serves as the basis for all radioactive standardizations. If the decay constant is known or is calculated from a known value of half-life ($\lambda = 0.693/t_{1/2}$), there then remains only one term to be evaluated.

Primary standardization methods are not generally useful as routine calibration procedures in most laboratories, such methods being rather complex and tedious and usually requiring very specialized equipment. It is better, from a practical point of view, to leave primary standardization to laboratories such as those of the National Bureau of Standards. These laboratories, in turn, supply *secondary standards* for distribution to other laboratories throughout the world.

The term "secondary standard" implies a standard which has been calibrated with the use of a primary standard for reference. Secondary standards are available from a number of manufacturers, as well as from the National Bureau of Standards. They are classified as alpha, beta, or gamma standards. Several types are available within each classification. The standard may be prepared from the *same* isotope as the unknown or the standard may be prepared from a *different* isotope than the unknown. *Simulated reference sources* are of the second type. For each classification and type of standard used, attention must be paid to the instrumentation required, the usefulness of the particular standard, and its limitations.

Standards of Same Isotope—When a radioactive standard is prepared from the same isotope as that to be measured, only three simple precautions are required to secure reliable results. These are: (1) readings must be made with the standard in the same position as that at which readings are made on the sample, (2) the sample must be uniformly distributed over approximately the same geometrical area as the standard, and (3) the sample must be supported on a layer of material identical with that supporting the standard, or at least one producing the same backscattering effect. In other words, a relative comparison of the activities is made (see page 465).

Standards of long-lived isotopes (Fig 28-17) are available from a number of manufacturers. The problems of preparation and distribution contingent on a short half-life are, of course, not true of these long-lived standards which may be kept on hand in the laboratory and require only a simple calculation for the determination of their current activity.

Standards of Different Isotope—Short-lived radioactive reference sources are available only periodically and retain a useful amount of activity for only a short time. If it is nec-

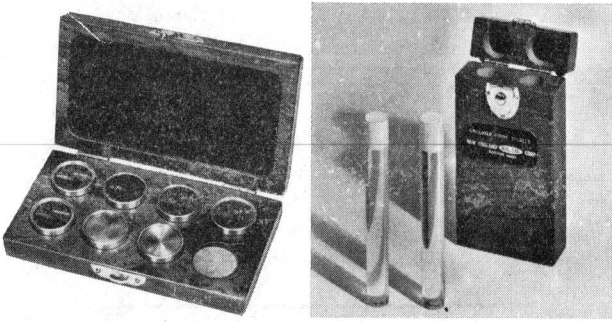

Fig 28-17. Beta and gamma reference sources; *left:* beta; *right:* gamma (courtesy, New England Nuclear).

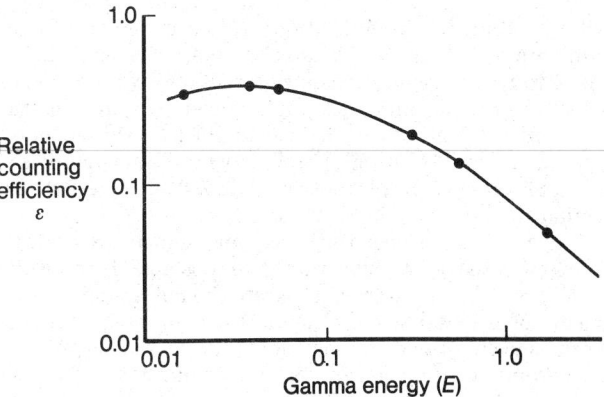

Fig 28-19.   Typical efficiency curve.

essary to calibrate such isotopes at other times, one must resort to the use of standards prepared from long-lived isotopes. These standards will, of course, consist of different nuclear species than the unknowns to be calibrated. When beta radiation is used for calibration the unknown beta sources and the standards should have similar mountings. The beta spectra of the standard and unknown will undoubtedly differ. If the beta energy distributions are not identical, and they will not be, a different degree of absorption by the air and window will occur; hence, the ratio of the radiation detected to that emitted by each source will not be the same, and an error will be introduced into the measurement. A correction for air and window absorption must therefore be applied. To correct for air and window absorption, absorption curves must be plotted for each source using calibrated aluminum absorbers. These absorption curves are then extrapolated to zero absorber thickness.

Calibration by Photopeak Integration—Calibration of a gamma-emitting nuclide can be achieved by comparison to a standard or a set of standards. The area associated with a fixed fraction of the photopeak is determined for each unknown and reference as explained below. These areas are taken as being proportional to radioactivity. Required instrumentation consists of a sodium iodide detector and a multichannel analyzer as described in the section on *Spectrometry*, page 469.

The fixed fraction F of the photopeak taken for comparison, the shaded area in Fig 28-18, is the product of the peak height P and the peak width a measured at $0.606\,P$. That is, $F = aP$. Peaks are assumed to be Gaussian and are therefore most linear at $0.606\,P$. Use of this value simplifies the estimation of a by interpolation of values of activity and channel number.

If the unknown and reference standard are different nuclides the gamma-energy dependence of the detector efficiency must be considered. By use of a series of reference standards of known radioactivity and known gamma energy, a standard curve is constructed relating relative detector efficiency ϵ to gamma energy E. For each reference standard the gamma-ray emission rate, $\gamma = AF_d$, where A is the activity of the source in disintegrations per minute and F_d is the decay

factor (see page 465), is computed. Then

$$\epsilon = \frac{F}{\gamma} = \frac{aP}{AF_d}$$

A typical plot of relative efficiency as a function of gamma energy is shown in Fig 28-19.

To calibrate an unknown source, A is the quantity sought, where

$$A = \frac{aP}{\epsilon F_d} = \frac{F}{\epsilon F_d}$$

It is therefore necessary to measure F from a spectrum using an accurately measured aliquot of the unknown (Fig 28-18), to determine the detector efficiency ϵ from the efficiency curve (Fig 28-19) and to determine the value of F_d by reference to the decay scheme for the nuclide.

Autoradiography—A method of detecting radioactivity that is especially useful in physiological studies of plants and animals is the autoradiographic technique, which may be illustrated by the following example. A radioactive substance is administered to an animal and after sufficient time has elapsed for localization in a given tissue, a bit of that tissue is removed and imbedded in paraffin. Very thin slices are then made with a microtome and these sections are placed in close contact with a photographic emulsion in a darkroom. The radioactive atoms which were collected by the cells in question continue to emit particles which have the same ability to darken a photographic emulsion as does light. Hence, after sufficient exposure time the emulsion is developed and fixed in the routine photographic fashion. By examination under a microscope it is then possible to correlate areas of darkening in the photographic emulsion with cell groups in the tissue and to determine, among other things, the rate at which the radioactive substance was metabolized and also the extent to which it was localized in the tissues studied.

Characterization of Radioactive Substances

Chemical substances are identifiable on the basis of their chemical and physical properties. If a substance is radioactive, it may also be necessary to establish the type or types of radioactive elements present. This may be accomplished by the measurement of certain radiological properties. The properties generally found useful for identification are (1) the half-life of the nuclear species and (2) the type and energy of the radiation emitted.

Half-Life—The most direct approach to the measurement of half-life involves the periodic measurement of the activity of the radioactive substance. An amount of the unknown radioactive material, calculated to give an activity of approximately 10,000 counts per minute, is placed in a planchet or other type of mount in such a way that loss of the sample

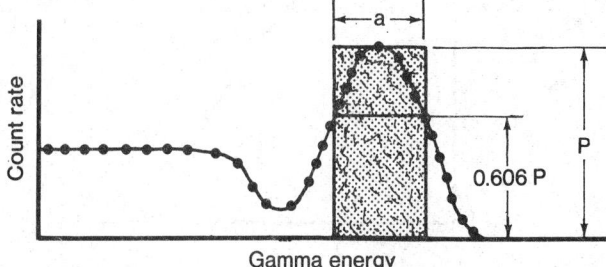

Fig 28-18.   Typical gamma spectrum.

will not occur from volatilization. All measurements of activity are then made on this same sample, special care being taken to reproduce the geometry for all observations of activity. Corrections for background, dead time, and instrument efficiency are applied to the data which are subsequently plotted on semilogarithmic graph paper. If a single nuclear species is present, the plot of these data will be a straight line, similar to that shown in Fig 28-6.

If two or more independently decaying isotopes are present, the slope of the decay curve will not be constant. If this is the case, it may be necessary to separate the nuclear species by means of a suitable radiochemical separation technique. Various techniques which may be employed for this purpose are chromatography, ion exchange, precipitation and coprecipitation techniques, electrodeposition, solvent extraction, distillation, etc. The purpose of separating a mixture of nuclides prior to identification is to simplify the interpretation of data.

Characterization of Radiation

The identification of the type of radiation (ie, alpha, beta, gamma, etc) rests largely upon the interpretation of measurements of the interaction of the radiation with matter or with electric or magnetic fields. For example, the interaction of radiation with a magnetic field will yield a knowledge of the nature of the electrical charge of the radiation. Positively charged alpha particles and positrons are deflected in one direction, negative electrons in the opposite direction, and gamma rays are not influenced at all by a magnetic field.

Range of Radiation—A relatively simple and reliable method for the identification of the most common types of radiation is through the measurement of the range of the radiation. For this purpose, calibrated mica, aluminum, and lead absorbers are used. Absorption of radiation depends upon the *thickness* of the absorbing material and upon the *density* of the absorbing material. Absorbers are therefore calibrated in terms of the product of their thickness (cm) and their density (g/cm³ or mg/cm³), the unit of absorber thickness, therefore, being g/cm² or mg/cm². For radiation range measurements, appropriate absorbers are interposed between the radioactive sample and the detector. The observed relation between activity and absorber thickness is not only characteristic of the type of radiation but can also be utilized to calculate the radiation energy.

Alpha particles are easily absorbed by an absorber thickness of about 5 or 6 mg/cm² or less. An absorber of this thickness is approximately equivalent to one or two sheets of paper. The range of alpha particles, even in air, is only a few centimeters and in aluminum and tissue less than about 100 microns. Calibrated mica absorbers are generally used to determine the range of alpha particles. Alpha radiation is characterized by a sharp decrease in activity as the absorber thickness exceeds a specific value. Because all alpha particles from a given radioactive source are monoenergetic one would anticipate that all alpha particles would have the same range, and this is nearly so. The monoenergetic nature of alpha particles thus accounts for the shape of the absorption curve illustrated in Fig 28-20.

Beta particles are more penetrating than alpha particles, yet, they are less penetrating than gamma radiation. When aluminum absorbers of increasing thickness are interposed between the beta source and the detector, the activity is observed to decrease in a more gradual manner. Whereas alpha particles are monoenergetic, beta particles are not. The less energetic particles are thus stopped by relatively thin absorbers, whereas much thicker absorbers are required to stop the more energetic beta particles. If the logarithm of the observed activity is plotted versus the absorber thickness, a nearly linear relationship is obtained over a portion of the

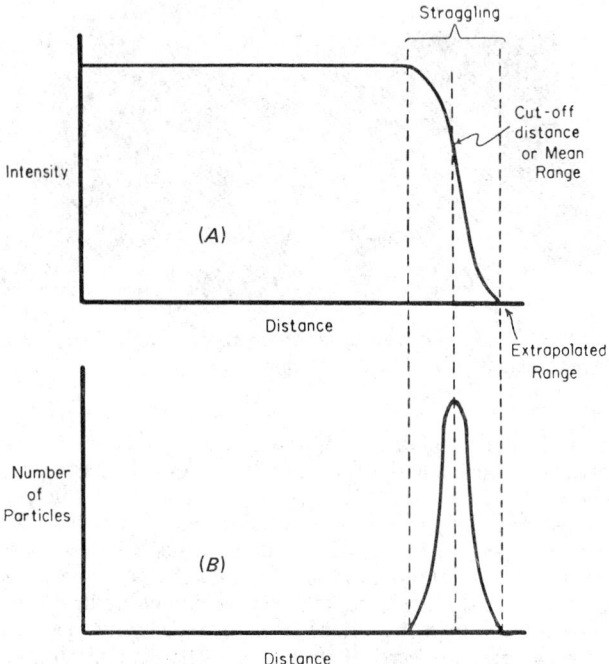

Fig 28-20.   *A:* The relation of alpha-ray intensity to the distance from the source to the detector. *B:* Differential of curve (*A*), which further illustrates the range distribution of alpha particles.

curve. See Fig 28-21. Lack of linearity, though disconcerting, does not prevent the utilization of the slope of such a plot for the identification of a radioactive species. If the curve is assumed to be linear, then

$$A = A_0 e^{-\mu x}$$

or

$$\mu = \frac{2.30 \, (\log A_1 - \log A_2)}{x_1 - x_2}$$

where

μ = absorption coefficient
A_1 = observed activity with an absorber of thickness x_1
A_2 = observed activity with an absorber of thickness x_2

In this case it should be remembered that μ is not a true absorption coefficient since it is not constant over the entire range of data. If, however, an unknown and known are

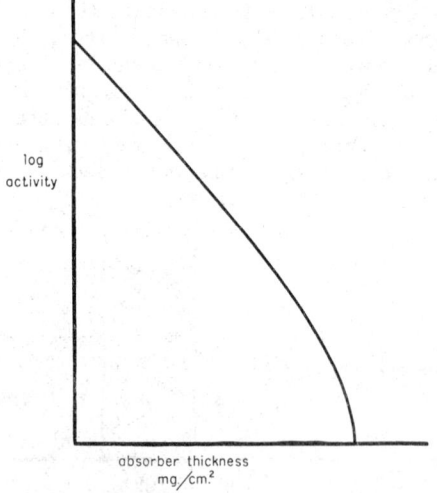

Fig 28-21.   Beta-particle absorption curve.

compared over the same range of absorber thicknesses, the value of this measurement becomes evident.

Gamma radiation is the most penetrating radiation of all. Thus, lead absorbers are most frequently used to study its penetration characteristics, although aluminum absorbers are also useful. The absorption of gamma radiation is essentially logarithmic. That is to say, by analogy with visible light absorption, gamma radiation obeys Beer's law. Thus, the relation

$$\mu = \frac{2.30\,(\log A_1 - \log A_2)}{x_1 - x_2}$$

can be used with less precaution but still not without regard for the effects caused by scattered radiation. Lead shields about the detector and the sample housing also scatter large amounts of radiation, and it is therefore necessary to consider such geometry variables.

Of the several absorption coefficients which have been defined, two are of particular importance here. These are the *linear absorption coefficient* and the *mass absorption coefficient*. If μ is the linear absorption coefficient (units = cm^{-1}), then the mass absorption coefficient (units = cm^2/g or cm^2/mg) is defined by μ/ρ where ρ is the density of the absorber either in g/cm^3 or in mg/cm^3.

Of interest, too, is the half-thickness or half-value-layer (HVL) defined as the thickness of absorber required to reduce the intensity of a beam of gamma radiation to $\frac{1}{2}$ the initial value. The half-thickness, $x_{1/2}$ is related to the linear absorption coefficient

$$x_{1/2} = 0.693/\mu$$

Energy of Radiation—Radiation energy and radiation range are related. Thus, one approach to the determination of radiation energy is to determine the range and then apply the appropriate relation between range and energy. For alpha particles it is found that the energy in MeV is approximately equal, numerically, to the air range of the alpha particles in centimeters. For greater accuracy a graph of the range-energy relation should be consulted.

In the case of beta particles where energy values vary continuously from zero to a particular maximum energy, $E_{\max}$, only the maximum energy is of particular interest and is calculated from the maximum range of the beta particles. Here, the measurement of the maximum range presents a special problem, and special measuring techniques must be used.

Spectrometry—A basic gamma ray spectrometer consists of a scintillation detector (NaI crystal and photomultiplier tube), preamplifier, amplifier, pulse-height analyzer (discriminator), and scaler (or ratemeter and recorder). See Fig 28-22. Its operation depends upon the production of a flash of light in the NaI crystal of the detector, the intensity of which is proportional to the gamma ray energy absorbed in the crystal. The photomultiplier tube, in turn, produces an electric pulse proportional in amplitude to the intensity of the flash of light produced in the crystal and, hence, proportional also to the gamma ray energy. If these pulses are linearly amplified, proportionality is maintained and the pulses become of sufficient amplitude or voltage that they can be sorted electronically according to their voltage. This process is referred to as discrimination or pulse-height analysis. It is thereby possible to measure the number of gamma rays which lie between a particular range of energies (wavelengths or frequencies) and to record this number on a scaler. If, on the other hand, the scaler is replaced by a ratemeter and recorder, and if the pulse height analyzer is made to scan the range of pulse heights at a given rate, it is possible to record a gamma ray spectrum directly. The system described above, using either a scaler or ratemeter, is called a single-channel analyzer (SCA). A typical spectrum prepared by use of such an instrument is shown in Fig 28-23.

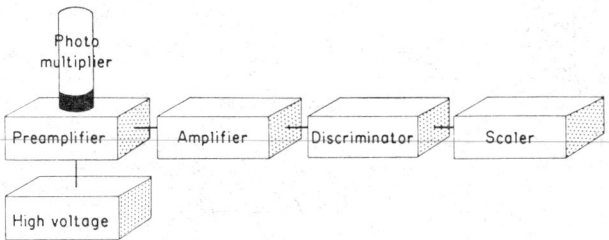

Fig 28-22. Basic gamma ray scintillation spectrometer (courtesy Baird-Atomic, from a handbook, *Scintillation Spectrometry*).

For the identification of short-lived isotopes a multichannel analyzer (MCA) is necessary. One MCA is equivalent to many SCAs since an MCA is capable of registering simultaneously the number of pulses in each of many energy ranges. It is therefore possible to record an entire spectrum in a relatively brief period of time. Since the number of channels is normally given by 2^n, an MCA may typically have 1028 channels and is therefore essentially equivalent to that many SCAs.

With the development of semiconductor detectors spectrometry has taken a giant step forward. Their excellent resolution has eliminated most of the problems related to the overlap of photopeaks. By comparison to the spectra of known nuclides the energies of unknown spectral peaks are readily determined by use of a lithium-drifted germanium Ge(Li) detector coupled to a MCA. The accurate measurement of gamma photopeak energies leads to a ready identification of the particular nuclide.

X-Rays

X-rays were discovered in the fall of 1895 by Wilhelm Konrad Roentgen, Professor of Physics at Würzburg University in Bavaria. Professor Roentgen realized the medical importance of his discovery when, during his investigation, he saw the bones of his hand clearly outlined on a fluorescent screen. After a thorough study of this new phenomenon he telegraphed his findings to the London Medical Society, which was then in session, and the world had its first news of this important discovery.

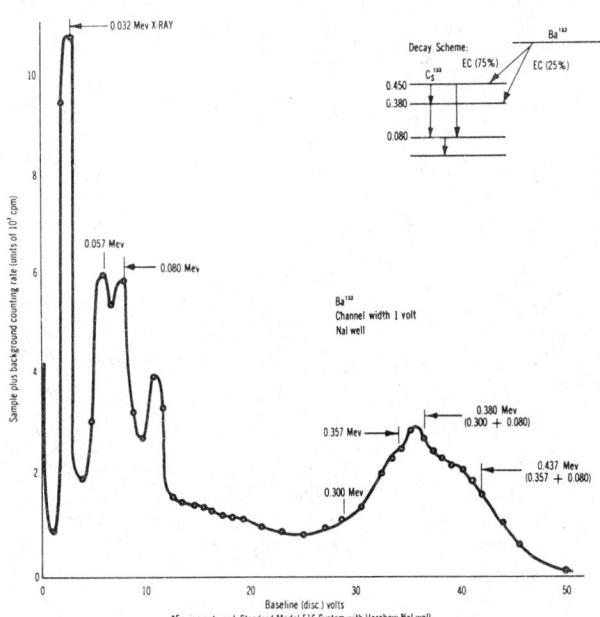

Fig 28-23. Differential gamma-ray spectrum of barium-133 (courtesy, Baird-Atomic, from a handbook, *Scintillation Spectrometry*).

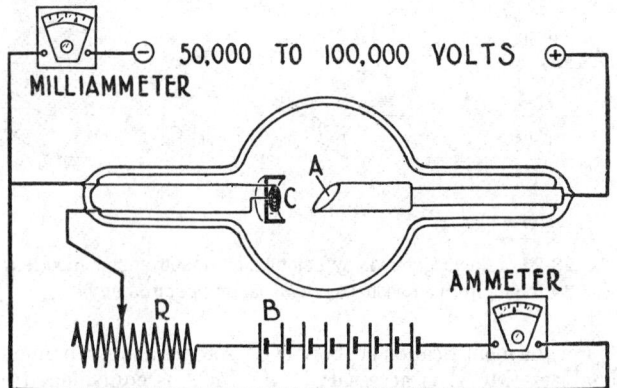

Fig 28-24.   Schematic diagram of an X-ray tube connected in circuit.

Production of X-rays—X-rays are produced by applying a large direct-current voltage across an evacuated tube. The positive terminal of the high voltage is connected to a target which is generally made of some metal with a high melting point such as tungsten or molybdenum, or of a metal with a high coefficient of conductivity of heat, such as copper. The negative terminal is connected to the cathode, which in the modern X-ray tubes consists of a heated filament. It has been found that a heated filament is a copious source of electrons. The electrons are accelerated toward the positively charged target and strike it with a velocity which depends upon the voltage applied across the X-ray tube. The energy, and therefore the velocity, with which the electrons strike the target is given by the following equation:

$$\tfrac{1}{2}mv^2 = Ve$$

$\tfrac{1}{2}mv^2$ is the kinetic energy of the electron, m is its mass, v is its velocity, and e is its charge, while V represents the voltage applied across the X-ray tube (Fig 28-24).

If the applied voltage is above the threshold voltage, and if the accelerated electrons have sufficient energy to penetrate the atoms composing the target of the tube, X-rays are emitted from the target and travel in all directions from it. X-rays are electromagnetic in nature, and therefore behave like visible light waves except that they are much shorter in wavelength. This means they travel with the velocity of light and can be reflected, refracted, polarized, and absorbed as are light waves.

Absorption of X-rays—The penetrating power of X-rays depends on two things; first, the voltage applied across the X-ray tube, and, second, the absorbing ability of the material through which they pass. The higher the voltage across the tube the more penetrating is the X-radiation given off. Very penetrating or deep therapy radiation is produced by applying 100,000 V or more across the tube, while soft, easily absorbed rays are produced by 20,000 V or less. Many hospitals in this country are now using up to 1,000,000 V radiation, and there is a tendency to use even higher voltages in an attempt to concentrate radiation effectively within deeply situated cancers while sparing the overlying normal tissues.

The absorbing ability of a material for X-rays depends upon its atomic weight. It is for this reason that barium in the form of barium sulfate is used as an absorbing material to study the intestinal tract. Iodine-containing compounds and oils also are widely used as "contrast media" in outlining arteries, ureters, kidneys, gall bladder, etc. Both of these materials have a high coefficient of absorption for X-rays because of their high molecular weights. For a given wavelength of X-rays and for a given absorbing material such as lead, for example, the absorption of X-rays by a thickness, t, is determined by the following equation:

$$I = I_0e^{-ut}$$

where I_0 represents the original intensity, I the intensity after passing through a thickness t, e the Naperian base, and u the coefficient of absorption for the material through which it passes.

CHAPTER 29

Medical Applications of Radioisotopes

Grafton D Chase, PhD

Professor of Chemistry
Philadelphia College of Pharmacy and Science
Philadelphia, PA 19104

Radium has the distinction of being the first radioisotope used in medicine, having been employed as early as 1901. This nuclide was the most important medical radioisotope in use up to about 1946 when artificially produced radioisotopes became available in quantity. Since that date, growth in the medical applications of radioisotopes has been very rapid as their usefulness has become more and more apparent in diagnosis, therapy, and medical research and as greater numbers of physicians and other scientific personnel have been trained in their use. Current medical procedures employ more than fifty radioisotopes in a wide variety of chemical and physical forms.

Radioisotopes are used in medicine in two different ways. They may be used (1) as radiation sources or (2) as radioactive tracers. As *radiation sources* their principal role is in therapy. Here, the choice of the isotope for a given application is governed largely by the properties of the radiation required for treatment; type and energy of the radiation and range in tissues are prime considerations. Except in special cases, the chemical properties or chemical form of a given isotope are relatively unimportant.

As a *radioactive tracer* the chemical identity and form of the nuclide are most important since, with but few exceptions, the tracer must be isotopic with the element being traced or must otherwise be capable of being incorporated as a part of a particular molecule. The nature of the radiation emitted by a tracer radioisotope is important primarily from the standpoint of its ease of detection. Radioactive tracers are used in medicine principally for diagnostic purposes.

Therapeutic Applications of Isotopes

For therapy, isotopes are used as radiation sources, not as tracers. These sources may be used either externally or internally. Their use may be summarized as follows:

External sources
   Teletherapy sources—^{60}Co, ^{137}Cs, neutrons, charged particles
   Surface sources—^{90}Sr, ^{32}P
   Extracorporeal irradiation—^{60}Co, ^{90}Sr-^{90}Y, ^{90}Y
Internal sources
   Infusion—^{198}Au, ^{32}P
   Interstitial implant—^{192}Ir, ^{125}I
   Selectively absorbed or concentrated—^{32}P, ^{131}I, ^{90}Y

The therapeutic use of radioisotopes is basically justified by the fact that radioactive material, when present in a tissue or organ in sufficient quantity, will produce emanation capable of destroying existing cells and preventing the formation of new tissue. For this reason isotopic therapy is generally applied only to those diseases in which there exists extensive cellular metabolic malfunction or to those conditions in which an organ or tissue produces physiological harm through overactivity.

External Sources—Where radioisotopes are used as external sources or as sealed sources implanted in a tissue, the dose is terminated by removal of the source. When they are administered internally as an unsealed source, the dose ad-

ministered to the patient, either deliberately in therapy or incidentally in diagnosis, cannot be terminated at will by removal of the source. In therapeutic applications the total dose must be calculated from a knowledge of the effective half-life of the isotope, the type and energy of the radiation emitted, and the concentration of the isotope in the tissue.

Teletherapy units containing kilocurie quantities of ^{60}Co or of ^{137}Cs have been used for many years for the treatment of lesions either postoperatively or where surgical removal of the lesion was not feasible. The monoenergetic nature of gamma rays provides an advantage over high-voltage x-rays which consist of a continuous spectrum of energies in addition to the characteristic energies. On the other hand, radioactive sources have the disadvantage that they cannot be turned off.

Fast neutrons, produced by neutron generators or by nuclear reactors, have received some interest for use in radiation therapy because their relative biological effectiveness surpasses that of X-rays, but their cost, and the lack of detailed knowledge concerning their effects in certain tissues and their penetrability, prevent their more widespread use. Recent research utilizes cyclotrons to generate high-energy, charged particles. Protons, alpha particles, heavy ions such as nitrogen, as well as pi minus mesons, are among the particles that have been considered.

Surface sources for dermatologic and ophthalmologic work consisting of applicators containing pure beta emitters such as ^{32}P and ^{90}Sr have been used. Bladder tumors have been treated by infiltration with ^{32}P. However, results have not created much enthusiasm for these techniques.

Extracorporeal irradiation of blood results in a depletion of lymphocytes thereby producing an alteration in the immunologic response of the individual. X-ray generators were used initially as a source of radiation; later, ^{60}Co sources were used. Attempts have also been made to prevent the rejection of grafts by the use of ^{90}Y so placed that the blood circulating in the graft is irradiated.

Use of *internal sources* for radiotherapy is largely confined to treatment with six different radioisotopes:

1. **Gold Au 198,** introduced as a colloidal gold suspension into a fluid-containing serous cavity, will initially diffuse rapidly throughout the fluid; it will then localize on the surface of the cavity as large aggregates of precipitate. Used in this way, it has found use in the treatment of peritoneal and pleural effusions associated with malignant tumors in those cases in which fluid has accumulated in the abdomen or chest without the presence of large masses or of severe constitutional effects from the tumor. The tumor itself is generally destroyed only superficially or not at all. A side effect of radiation sickness has been noted occasionally.

^{198}Au has also been used experimentally in the treatment of prostate and cervical uterine carcinoma and bladder tumors.

2. **Iridium Ir 192 Seed Ribbons,** consisting of ^{192}Ir seeds spaced at intervals along a nylon ribbon, are used for removable interstitial implant therapy of tumors. The procedure is a surgical one which must be conducted in an operating room.

3. **Sodium Phosphate P 32** may be used in the treatment of polycythemia vera to decrease the rate of formation of the erythrocytes. Since ^{32}P is metabolized in a manner similar to naturally occurring phosphorus, the isotope is readily distributed to all tissues and is concentrated in those tissues where proliferation is most rapid. Thus cancerous tissues con-

centrate the greatest amount of the isotope. A large dose of ^{32}P—1.5 to 5 mCi—will concentrate in the bone marrow but will suppress erythrogenesis only partially. In severe cases of polycythemia a phlebotomy is necessary in conjunction with ^{32}P therapy.

^{32}P may also be utilized in the treatment of chronic granulocytic leukemia. This treatment, however, cannot achieve a cure, but can serve only to alleviate the symptoms of the disease. When ^{32}P is used in conjunction with local x-ray treatment, some phases of the disease may be controlled in the earlier stages.

Radiophosphorus rarely induces a side effect of radiation sickness, but excessive doses can result in serious effects on the hematopoietic system.

4. **Yttrium Y 90** is of special interest because of its 64-hour half-life. It emits a single beta particle with a maximum energy of 2.27 MeV; it emits no gamma radiation. It is readily available by elution of a generator containing ^{90}Sr. The principal disadvantage to the use of ^{90}Y as an internal source lies with the possibility of its contamination by ^{90}Sr leakage from the generator.

^{90}Y has a strong affinity for chelating agents. By controlled manipulation of the chelating agent a significant degree of systemic localization of ^{90}Y has been achieved. Chelation with N-hydroxyethylenediaminetriacetic acid (Ed-ol) will cause ^{90}Y to localize in the bone where it can be made to cause predictable hematologic changes. This chelate has been used to treat leukemia and multiple myeloma.

Chelated with diethylenetriaminepentaacetic acid (DTPA), ^{90}Y has been used for the selective irradiation of lymphatic structures. The method used allows constant levels of radioactivity to be maintained in the body by reinfusion of the patients filtered urine containing the excreted isotope. When reinfusion is interrupted the ^{90}Y-DTPA is rapidly removed from the blood by way of the kidneys. Levels of over 500 mCi of ^{90}Y have been used with this technique.

5. **Sodium Iodide I 131** has several therapeutic applications. In cases of hyperthyroidism, therapeutic doses of ^{131}I will destroy thyroid tissue by means of radiation produced from within the gland. This procedure provides a more desirable mode of therapy than external roentgen-ray treatment since there is less radiation danger to the surrounding tissues. For example, in the treatment of Graves' disease, a thyroid gland that exhibits a 50% uptake at 24 hours averages 2,300–2,400 rads/mCi. The dose to be delivered is generally taken to be 5,000–7,000 rads for this malady. In the case of thyroid cancer the administration of 150 mCi of I-131 will deliver a tumor dose of approximately 25,000 rad, or about five times the absorbed dose that can be achieved through a typical course of external radiation therapy. This course of treatment is especially useful in cases of metastatic thyroid cancer.

To achieve selective absorption of I-131 in the target tissue the radioactive iodine is attached to specific molecules. I-131-labeled m-iodobenzylguanidine (MIGB) is selectively absorbed by the adrenal medullary tissues. Current calculations show that up to 5,000 rads/100 mCi of I-131 MIGB can be delivered to metastases from adrenal medullary carcinoma to brain, skull and axial skeleton. Radioiodinated antibodies and FaB units are also useful. Radioiodinated antibodies, administered in a continuous intravenous drip have been used for the treatment of a malignant melanoma.

^{131}I is used along the same lines in the management of euthyroid cardiac disease including congestive heart failure and angina pectoris. The control of cardiac disease is based on the ability of the isotope to reduce thyroid activity by radiation thyroidectomy, thereby lowering the total metabolic rate of the body and thereby reducing the stress on the heart. Dosage ranges from 10 to 25 mCi, given as a single dose or extended over a period of a few weeks.

Some cases of thyroid carcinoma with metastases may respond to ^{131}I therapy. Dosage must be regulated carefully in treatment of hyperthyroidism since too large a dose may induce hypothyroidism.

6. **Iodine I 125** with a half-life of 60 days and an average photon energy of 28 keV is useful for permanent implants for treatment of deep-seated tumors such as those in the chest which are not surgically resectable. Sufficient ^{125}I to give a dose of about 15,000 RADS is used. About half of this dose is delivered within the first two months.

Diagnostic Applications of Isotopes

For diagnosis, isotopes are used as radioactive tracers and not as radiation sources. If results are to be meaningful the tagged substances must be handled by the body in a manner similar to that of the untagged substance.

When radioisotopes are used for diagnosis, the radiation dose delivered to the patient is maintained at as low a level as possible. This is accomplished through the judicious choice of isotope for the best combination of minimum half-life, minimum retention in the body, and minimum quantity of isotope which will permit its detection and accurate measurement. Accordingly, certain isotopes, such as ^{90}Sr, ^{226}Ra, and many others, are never used as unsealed internal sources

or tracers. In order to reduce the radiation dose to the population there is a trend toward the use of shorter-lived isotopes, when available, for diagnostic purposes. It is for this reason that ^{57}Co and ^{58}Co are often used in place of ^{60}Co, where possible, in diagnostic procedures.

Radioassay Methods in Medicine—Radioisotope studies may be divided into five categories:

1. **Activation Analysis.** An analytical technique capable of detecting and measuring certain elements present in a specimen in relatively low concentration. The sample is exposed to neutrons from a plutonium-beryllium neutron source, a neutron generator or a nuclear reactor. Neutrons are selectively absorbed by those atomic nuclei possessing a large cross section for neutrons. Absorption (or capture) of a neutron usually results in the formation of a radioactive nuclide which is identifiable from the radiation which it emits. The quantity of radiation is related to the quantity of the element present. Na, Cl, Ca, and other elements can be determined quantitatively by this method. One technique uses neutron activation analysis for the determination of protein-bound iodine. The feasibility of using total-body neutron activation analysis has been explored at the Brookhaven National Laboratory where 14 50-Ci Pu-Be neutron sources were used for activation.

2. **Isotope Dilution.** The principles of isotope dilution are discussed in Chapter 28. The clinical application of this technique is illustrated by its use for the measurement of blood volume. The more popular procedure uses radioiodinated human serum albumin injected intravenously; 10 min after injection, a time sufficient to allow adequate mixing of the labeled albumin in the intravascular pool, yet not long enough for metabolic activity or seepage into extravascular pools to occur, a blood sample is withdrawn. The blood volume is calculated from the measured decrease in radioactivity of the injected sample upon its dilution by the blood. Red blood cell volume and plasma volume are related to the blood volume by the peripheral venous hematocrit. RBC volumes can also be determined by the use of cells labeled with ^{51}Cr in the form of sodium chromate.

Radioactive hydrogen, ^{3}H, in the form of tritiated water can be used to determine total body water. Total body potassium, sodium and chloride, usually referred to as "spaces," can be determined by the use of the radioactive isotopes of these elements. In the case of chloride, ^{82}Br is usually used instead of ^{36}Cl because of the long half-life of the latter.

3. **Radiometric Analysis**—Those radioassay methods which require the use of a standard reagent having a known relationship between chemical concentration and radiologic concentration, ie, the radioactivity of a specific radioisotope per unit volume, are called radiometric analyses. For example, a sensitive method for the determination of serum calcium involves the addition of a measured excess of standard ^{14}C-oxalic acid solution to an aliquot of serum. After precipitation of calcium oxalate the radioactivity of the precipitate (or of an aliquot of the supernatant) is determined. This activity is then related to the calcium content of the serum. A variety of similar assays have been developed, including the determination of serum citric acid by use of ^{82}Br.

4. **Competitive Radioassays**—Also known as *saturation analysis*, the basic principle of a competitive radioassay involves competitive reactions in which radioactive substrate (ligand) and nonradioactive substrate, the analyte, P compete with each other for a binding agent Q. The *substrate P* may be a vitamin, hormone, drug, or other substance the concentration of which is to be determined. To perform the assay the same substance must be available with a radioactive tag. This is P*. ^{125}I is the most frequently used tag, with ^{3}H, ^{99m}Tc and ^{57}Co also finding limited use. A constant, known amount of tagged substrate P* is used in all assays. The *binding agent Q* may be an ion-exchange resin, a protein, an antibody or a specific reactor for the particular substrate. The concentration of binding agent used in all assays of a series is also normally held constant. The independent variable is p, the concentration of nonradioactive substrate sought. Its concentration will vary. It can be seen that an increase in the concentration of P will result in an increase in the concentration of nonradioactive bound substrate PQ and a decrease in the concentration of radioactive bound substrate P*Q. The result will be an increase in free tagged substrate P*. Therefore the concentration of substrate P can be determined as some function of any two of the quantities B, F, or T (the bound, free, and total radioactivity, respectively). That is, $p = f(B,F)$, $p = f'(B,T)$ or $p = f''(F,T)$.

$$P^* + Q \rightleftarrows PQ$$
$$P + Q \rightleftarrows P^*Q$$
$$\text{FREE} \qquad \text{BOUND}$$

If the binding between substrate and binder is *nonspecific*, as is the case with certain protein-binding assays, it is frequently necessary to purify the substrate prior to analysis to remove interfering substances. Alternatively, the binding agent can be made more *specific* for the particular substrate. One type of system which shows a very high degree of specificity for a particular substrate is an *immune* system. The assay is known as a *radioimmunoassay (RIA)*, and uses an antigen-antibody reaction.

If the substrate is not already antigenic it is made so by *conjugation* to a protein. Substrates requiring conjugation to a protein to produce antigenicity are known as *haptens*. Rabbits, chickens, goats, and other animals are then injected with antigen to induce the production of antibodies. Usually the antigen is first mixed with an *adjuvant* in order to enhance antibody production. When the antibody level has reached a maximum level, samples of blood are removed from time to time to obtain serum which must then be diluted to produce a suitable antibody concentration for use in the assay. In addition it is necessary to prepare radioactive substrate. If the substrate is a hapten which has been conjugated to a protein, tagging the compound is accomplished readily by iodination with ^{125}I. Sometimes a tritium tag is used instead.

A few specific competitive radioassays do not make use of an immune system. One typical assay is that for vitamin B_{12} in which *intrinsic factor* is used in place of an antibody as a binder. Such a binder is called a *specific reactor*.

In the simplified illustration of a radioimmunoassay described, "ideal" behavior has been assumed. Most radioimmunoassays closely approach this condition. To meet the requirements of ideal behavior the following criteria should be met:

1. The nonradioactive and radioactive antigens, P and P^*, are indistinguishable chemically.
2. Both reactions go to completion. That is, the equilibrium constants are not only equal but are so great they can be considered infinite.
3. Antigen and antibody react in the ratio one-to-one.
4. There are no cross reactions, the antibody being specific only for the single antigen indicated in the reactions.

The purpose of a radioimmunoassay is to determine the concentration p of nonradioactive antigen. To conduct a radioimmunoassay a standard curve must first be constructed where p is plotted as some function of radioactivity. This is known as a dose-response curve. It is constructed using data obtained by use of standard solutions as illustrated in Fig 29-1.

Let the concentration p^* of radioactive antigen added to each of three test tubes be 6 picomoles (pM)/mL. To the first tube (the blank) is added no nonradioactive antigen. To the second tube is added 3 pM/mL and to the third, 12 pM/mL of nonradioactive antigen. Finally, equal amounts of antibody (representing 3 pM of antibody binding sites/mL) are added to each of the three tubes and the content of each tube is well mixed. The tubes are then incubated until the reactions are complete.

Bound and free antigen are now separated by some suitable means and the radioactivity B of bound antigen and the radioactivity F of free antigen are measured for each of the three standards. The total radioactivity, T ($= B + F$), is the sum of the bound and free radioactivities. From Fig 29-1 it can be seen that the data tabulated in Table I are obtained.

The total concentration of antigen C_t ($= C_B + C_F$) is also equal to the sum of the concentrations of radioactive and nonradioactive antigens.

$$C_t = p^* + p$$

Since radioactive and nonradioactive antigen are chemically indistinguishable, they are uniformly distributed in the system. Thus

$$\frac{C_t}{C_B} = \frac{T}{B}$$

By combining these two relationships it follows that

$$p = -p^* + C_B \frac{T}{B}$$

If q is the total concentration of antibody binding sites and q_B is the concentration of bound or occupied binding sites, then, when antigen is in excess, $q = q_B = C_B$ since the reaction is assumed to have gone to completion. Consequently

$$p = -p^* + q \frac{T}{B}$$

By plotting the concentration p of dose antigen (nonradioactive antigen) as a function of the ratio T/B of total to bound radioactivity, a linear re-

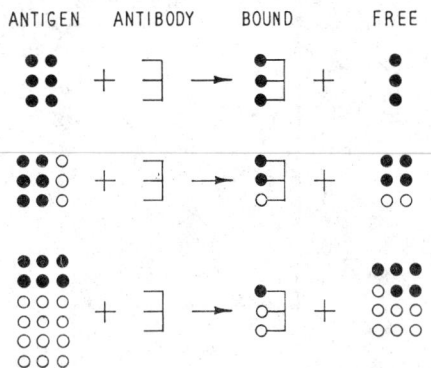

Fig 29-1.   "Ideal" radioimmunoassay.

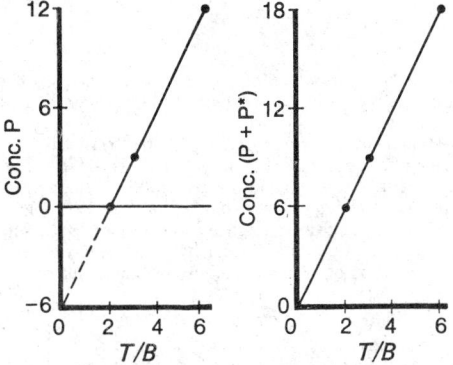

Fig 29-2.   Dose-response curves. The linear relationship illustrated here for an elementary "ideal" radioimmunoassay also holds for most real assays.

lationship is obtained. The y-intercept is $-p^*$ and gives the apparent concentration of radioactive antigen. The slope q gives the concentration of antibody sites. In the assay T/B is the quantity measured and p is the quantity sought. For the example cited

$$p = -6 + 3 \cdot \frac{T}{B}$$

A plot of these data is shown in Fig 29-2.

The usefulness of this method of data reduction lies in its clinical applicability. Radioimmunoassay standard curve data are essentially linearized and can be fit by a linear regression analysis. Suspect data are also readily recognizable.

In a more detailed analysis of competitive assays the equilibrium constant K must be considered. For a single species of binding site the Scatchard equation applies

$$R = \frac{B}{F} = Kq - KC_B$$

Rearrangement shows that

$$C_B = q - \frac{R}{K}$$

The resulting relation is

$$p = -p^* + \left(q - \frac{R}{K} \right) \frac{T}{B}$$

Table I—Data for Simulated Standard RIA Curve

	Concentration of antigen (pM/mL)						Ratios of radioactivities		
Tube no	Radioactive p^*	Nonradioactive p	Total C_t	Bound C_B	Free C_F		F/B	T/B	B/F
1	6	0	6	3	3		1	2	1
2	6	3	9	3	6		2	3	0.5
3	6	12	18	3	15		5	6	0.2

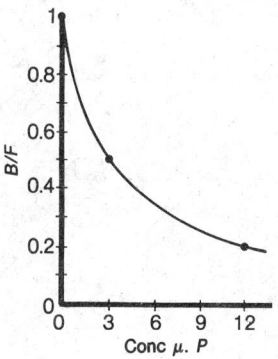

Fig 29-3.   Dose-response curve.   The historical method of plotting B/F vs p is illustrated for an "ideal" radioimmunoassay.   The result is a hyperbola.   The principal disadvantage of this method is the inability to recognize data which are in error.

Here p^* is the true concentration of radioactive antigen. The fit of experimental data is excellent and essentially linear over the clinical range of concentration.

Dose-response curves were originally prepared by plotting the ratio B/F as a function of the concentration of dose antigen p. See Fig 29-3. To improve linearity and to expand the graph in the region of low concentration, the ratio B/F is sometimes plotted as a function of $\log p$ as in Fig 29-4A. Recognizing the advantage of a linear plot of data, especially for rejection of suspect data, a *logit* plot has been used wherein logit Y is plotted as a function of $\ln p$ or $\log p$. According to one definition

$$\text{logit } Y = \ln \frac{Y'}{1 - Y'} \qquad \text{where } Y' = B/B_o$$

where B is the radioactivity of the bound antigen and B_o is the value of B for $p = 0$. For "ideal" conditions a linear plot is obtained as shown in Fig 29-4B. The y-intercept is $\ln p^*$ and the slope is -1 (or -2.303) depending upon whether natural or Naperian logarithms are used. This is expected since it can be shown that

$$\text{logit } Y = \ln p^* - \ln p$$

Although the logit plot is widely used it is not recommended since it is prone to introduce plotting errors.

5. **Immunoradiometric assays (IRMA)**—Immunoradiometric assays utilize a large excess of binder (eg, antibody) so that essentially all of the analyte becomes bound even if the binding constant is not great. In one type of IRMA a radioactively tagged antibody, Q^*, is used. Added to the analyte in large excess, analyte, P, is essentially completely bound.

$$P + Q^* \rightarrow PQ^* \; (+Q^* \text{ excess})$$

The excess of tagged antibody is then removed by use of ligand (analyte) which has been immobilized by bonding to a solid phase, P-sp.

$$Q^* \text{ excess} + P\text{-}sp \rightarrow Q^*P\text{-}sp$$

Radioactivity remaining in solution represents radioactive antibody bound to analyte, PQ^*, and is therefore a measure of analyte concentration in the sample.

In a second, more common type of IRMA known as a "two-site sandwich" assay, analyte, P, is bound to nonradioactive antibody which is

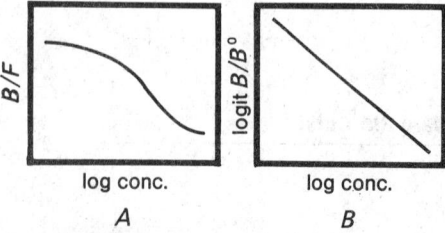

Fig 29-4.   Dose-response curves. A: A semilog plot has been used in an attempt to linearize the data.   This empirical approach represents an improvement over a B/F vs p plot, but falls short of being linear. B: A logit plot is linear for an "ideal" situation as shown here for the plot of "ideal" data.   Its disadvantage is that it is empirical and does not readily explain cases which deviate from linearity.   In addition it cannot be extended to zero concentration of antigen.

bound to a solid phase, Q-sp.

$$P + Q\text{-}sp \rightarrow PQ\text{-}sp \; (+Q\text{-}sp \text{ excess})$$

The amount of analyte bound is then determined by addition of an excess of a second radioactively tagged antibody, Q^*, to the analyte.

$$PQ\text{-}sp + Q^* \rightarrow Q^*PQ\text{-}sp$$

Bound radioactivity is then proportional to the concentration of analyte.

A modification called the "three-site sandwich" assay is similar to the two-site method except that the second antibody, specific for the analyte, is untagged. Bound analyte is then identified and quantitated by addition of a third antibody, radiolabeled anti-gamma globulin, which binds to the second antibody. The advantage of the three-site method is that it uses the same radiolabeled Ig-G to quantify a wide variety of analytes.

6. **Receptor Assays.**—Various receptor systems have been identified in body tissues and organs. These receptor systems are of physiological importance since they act as binders to specific hormones and other compounds having physiological activity. One receptor system of particular clinical importance is the estrogen receptor of breast cancers. It has been observed that breast cancers respond more dramatically to hormone treatment if they contain appreciable numbers of such estrogen receptor sites. Estrogen receptor site assays in breast tumors have therefore become a routine clinical assay.

Receptors may be present either in the cell cytosol or on the cell membrane. At least certain membrane receptors have been shown to be glycoproteins and may have association constants as great as 10^9 to 10^{10} liters/mole.

Receptor assays are similar to competitive binding assays as described above but differ in that it is the binder that is the analyte rather than the ligand. Scatchard analysis is most frequently employed to quantitate the receptor sites and to evaluate their binding constants.

In one type of receptor assay radioactive ligand L^*, specific for the receptor in question, is added to an aliquot of tissue homogenate containing receptor R and the mixture is incubated until an equilibrium condition is achieved.

$$L^* + R \leftrightarrow LR$$

The association constant, K, is given by

$$K = (L^*R)/(L^*)(R)$$

since the ratio of bound-to-free ligand concentration, $(L^*R)/(L^*)f$, is equal to the ratio of bound-to-free radioactivity, B/F, substitution and rearrangement yields

$$B/F = K(R)$$

The total concentration of receptor sites, r, is equal to the sum of free and bound sites, $(R) + (L^*R)$. It follows that $(R) = r - (L^*R)$ and

$$B/F = Kr - K(L^*R)$$

This is one form of the Scatchard equation. This linear form is for a single species of binding site (receptor). By repeating the measurement with a range of concentrations of radiolabeled ligand, L^*, data are obtained to plot B/F as a function of (L^*R), the bound radioactivity. The slope of the resulting curve is $-K$ and the x-intercept is r.

In practice the Scatchard plot is curved concave upward with a long tail to the right. This is due to the presence of nonspecific binding sites. It is customary to take the steepest part of the slope to represent binding to receptor. The slope at the steepest part is used for calculation of the association constant and the intercept of the tangent with the x-axis is taken as the receptor concentration. Another complicating feature sometimes observed is a low-concentration hook resulting from positive cooperativity. The implication of such hooks is that the receptors consist of two interrelated sites, a situation often observed with antibodies.

7. **Functional Radioassays**—Radioassays utilizing radioisotopes as aids in measuring the rate of a biological process are called functional radioassays. They can be divided into three categories:

(a) *Rate of Isotope Transfer.* In these procedures, a labeled substance is injected into one part of the vascular system and the time required for its arrival at another part is determined. This technique has been used widely to determine circulation times, especially in the extremities. ^{24}Na is well suited for this purpose, since it has a short half-life, is a normal body constituent, is not selectively absorbed by any tissue, and is readily detected.

An extension of these methods has been used in the measurement of cardiac output. The passage of a radioisotope through the heart and lungs, following intravenous injection, can be recorded either by assay of serial arterial blood samples or by external counting over the heart. It is important that the radioactive material does not diffuse into the tissues during the studies. Radioiodinated serum albumin has been found most satisfactory; measurements are possible with as little as 25 μCi injected intravenously.

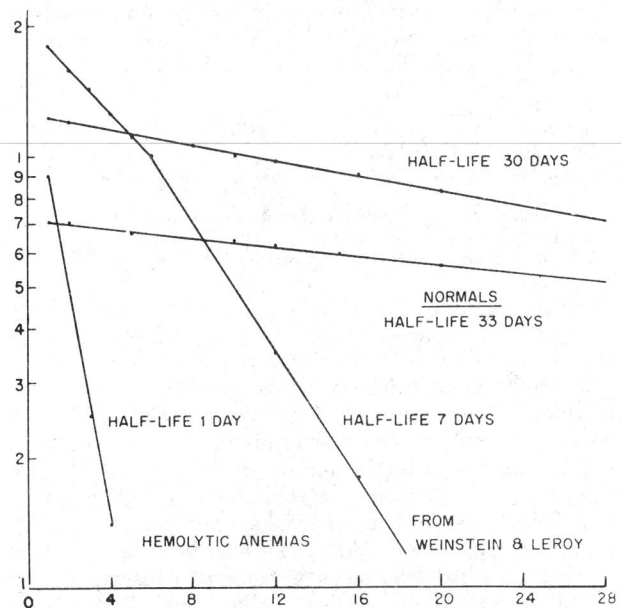

Fig 29-5. Red-cell tagging with ^{51}Cr permits a direct determination of erythrocyte life in anemic patients (courtesy, Picker X-Ray).

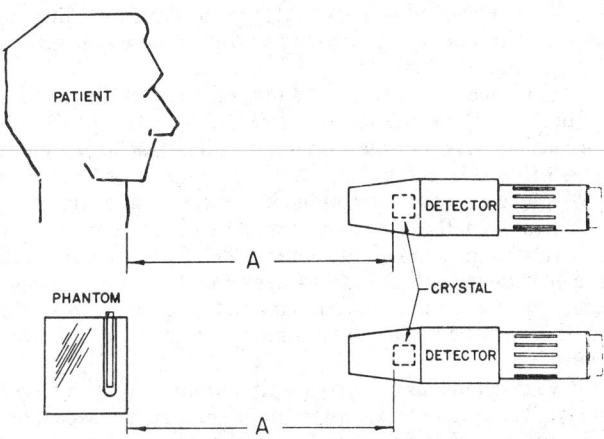

Fig 29-6. In practice, thyroid uptake is measured by intercomparison of the activity of the standard ^{131}I capsules (or source) in a phantom with the activity in the patient's thyroid (courtesy, Picker X-Ray).

(*b*) *Rate of Isotope Disappearance.* The rate at which an isotope disappears from a tissue into which it has been injected is a measure of the circulation in that tissue. This test has been used successfully to determine the extent of circulation in tubed skin grafts in plastic surgery. A small amount of an isotope, eg, radiosodium chloride, is injected directly into the tissue. The disappearance rate of the isotope is measured by means of a counter placed directly over the site of injection.

The RBC destruction mechanism and RBC half-life are measured by means of a disappearance-rate technique. If erythrocytes are labeled *in vitro* with ^{51}Cr and then reinjected, the fate of the tagged cells can be followed by assay of serial blood samples taken every two or three days for at least two weeks. Since the labeled cell group contains cells of all ages, only a mean survival time can be determined for these cells. The rate of decrease in circulating ^{51}Cr is approximately exponential and can thus be characterized by a half-clearance-time. The normal RBC half-life is about 26 days. This study is a valuable aid in the diagnosis of hemolytic anemias. See Fig 29-5.

Gastrointestinal bleeding can be detected and measured by the use of red cells tagged with chromium 51. This procedure can be performed concurrently with the red-cell-survival study mentioned above. Gastrointestinal bleeding will be manifest by the appearance of radioactivity in the stools and, in severe cases, by a decrease in the blood-cell survival time. From quantitative measurements of blood and stool activities, the volume of blood in the stool can be calculated. A loss of up to 2 mL of blood per day is considered normal.

(*c*) *Metabolic Processes and/or Isotope Concentration.* Most of the more familiar radioisotope studies are in this category. The concentration of a particular radioisotope in normal or abnormal tissue or in an organ provides data from which the function of the tissue or the metabolic condition of the organ can be evaluated.

Several studies of thyroid function can be carried out with the aid of radioactive ^{131}I. These studies include: (a) the rate of deposition of iodine in the gland *in vivo;* (b) the total accumulation of iodine in the gland within a specified period of time; and (c) the output of thyroid hormone into which radioactive iodine has been incorporated.

Because the thyroid has such an avidity for iodine, precautions must be taken to prevent exposure to or ingestion of even small amounts of iodine by the patient if valid results are to be obtained. Treatments to be avoided include the external application of iodine, ingestion of iodine-containing medicaments (may influence thyroid uptake for weeks), the use of X-ray contrast media containing organic iodine compounds (these may produce an effect on the thyroid for months), and myelography and bronchography (these may have a permanent effect). The radioiodine thyroid uptake may, in addition, be lowered by such substances as thyroid preparations, antithyroid drugs, thiocyanate and perchlorate,

corticotropin and corticosteroids, phenylbutazone, sulfonamides and *p*-aminosalicylic acid, arsenic, lead, and mercury. Malabsorption syndromes and renal disease will also lower thyroid uptake.

The thyroid gland concentrates inorganic iodide from the blood and converts it to thyroxine, the thyroid hormone, through the action of a peroxidase enzyme. When a thyroid gland is relatively "iodine starved," ie, receiving no more iodine than is found in the normal diet, the administration of a small dose of radioactive iodine results in a portion of the dose being retained by the thyroid while the remainder of the radioactive isotope is excreted in the urine. The amount of radioactive iodine retained by the thyroid is an index of thyroid function.

For *thyroid uptake* the most commonly employed technique involves the oral administration of from 5 to 25 μCi of Na^{131}I followed by measurement of the radioactivity of the thyroid after the elapse of a given time. An identical sample of sodium iodide I 131 is set aside as a standard. After the elapse of, say, 24 hours, the radioactivity of the thyroid is determined with a gamma-sensitive detector and the activity compared to that of the standard when measured under *identical conditions of geometry.* See Fig 29-6.

The radiation emitted from the patient consists of at least three components:

1. Direct radiation from the thyroid—0.36 MeV primaries of ^{131}I plus a small amount of radiation of lower energy.
2. Scattered radiation, resulting especially from Compton interactions of the primary radiation with neck tissue.
3. Radiation from parts of the body other than the thyroid.

Error from the third source is normally small after 24 hours and accounts for only 2 to 3% of the observed radiation. Compton scattering, however, may represent 20 to 30% of the observed radiation. If the *surroundings* of the standard ^{131}I and the thyroid are different, the measurements will be in error as a consequence of the difference in the extent of Compton scattering. A "phantom neck" is sometimes employed with the standard to produce deliberately Compton scattering equivalent to that produced by the patient's neck tissues. It has also been shown that a sheet of lead, 1/32-inch thick, placed in front of the detector, will remove a large percentage of this low-energy scattered radiation while at the same time removing only a small amount of the high-energy direct radiation. A spectrometer may also be used to eliminate scattered radiation through pulse-height analysis.

While the problems of measurement mentioned above result in an increase in the amount of observed radiation, absorption of radiation by the tissues of the neck tends to decrease the observed activity. Absorption errors are difficult to estimate but may generally be reduced in magnitude by using a phantom neck.

The normal range for iodine uptake is about 10 to 40% in 24 hours. Uptakes from 10 to 15% and from 35 to 45% may be considered borderline. An uptake exceeding 50% is highly suggestive of hyperthyroidism while an uptake of less than 15% may usually be interpreted as indicating myxedema.

The use of radioiodine is contraindicated during the second and third trimesters of pregnancy. The fetal thyroid is sufficiently developed at 12 to 14 weeks to pick up iodine from the maternal circulation. Even a tracer dose given to the mother may be sufficient to inhibit or injure the fetal thyroid.

Two mechanisms compete for the iodine circulating in the body: (1) uptake by the thyroid and (2) urinary excretion. The amount of iodine excreted by the kidneys is inversely related to the amount fixed by the thyroid. Urinary excretion may therefore be used as an indirect measure of thyroid function.

An advantage in the use of urinary ^{131}I output over the measure of thyroid uptake rests in the ability to reproduce the counting geometry more accurately. A second advantage is that the patient need not be present when radioactivity measurements are performed. This method has two disadvantages, however, which may introduce serious errors. First, it is necessary to collect a reliable urine specimen; loss of urine will yield low results. Secondly, accuracy of the test is contingent upon normal kidney function.

With a hyperfunctioning thyroid, generally less than 30% of the dose will appear in the urine in 24 hours; with a hypofunctioning gland, over 80% will usually appear. The normal range is approximately 40 to 70%. Theoretically, the iodine uptake plus the urinary excretion should equal about 90% of the dose.

The *thyroid clearance* test measures the rate of clearance of ^{131}I from the plasma. First, a small amount of the isotope is given intravenously, then the rate of uptake over the thyroid gland is measured for 30 min. At the end of this time the urinary excretion of ^{131}I is measured. The iodine collected by the thyroid per min is divided by the average plasma concentration of ^{131}I (μCi/mL) during the elapsed time. The result is thyroid clearance in mL per min. The normal clearance is about 25 mL/min. In hyperthyroidism the value may rise to 250 mL/min while for hypothyroidism the clearance may fall to 2 mL/min.

The *protein-bound iodine conversion ratio* is a measure of thyroid activity. It is the fraction of inorganic iodide converted to thyroid hormone and bound to the plasma proteins in 24 hours.

Assimilated inorganic iodine is concentrated in the thyroid gland where it is converted, in part, to thyroxine. Upon release from the thyroid, the thyroxine is found to be reversibly bound with the serum protein. Treatment of the serum or plasma with trichloroacetic acid (TCA), for example, causes the protein to precipitate. Protein-bound iodine will be found in this precipitate. If, on the other hand, the serum or plasma is passed through a suitable ion-exchange column, inorganic iodine will be retained on the column while the protein-bound fraction passes on through.

The conversion ratio is an expression of the fraction, usually indicated as percent, of radioiodine in the blood that is protein bound to the total iodine present in the serum or plasma at a given time—2, 4, 6, 12, 24 or 72 hours—after administration of the dose.

In humans an oral dose of 50 μCi of Na^{131}I has been found satisfactory for euthyroid patients although only 25 μCi need be used if exophthalmic goiter is indicated and as much as 100 μCi may be required in cases of myxedema.

Current procedures for the determination of the PBI conversion ratio are essentially the same except for the step involving the separation of the protein-bound and the inorganic iodide. The procedure may be outlined as follows:

1. Administration of the dose.
2. Wait for a predetermined period of time.
3. Collection of blood sample.
4. Determination of the activity of an aliquot of the serum or plasma.
5. Separation of the protein fraction from the inorganic fraction.
6. Determination of the activity of the protein fraction.
7. Calculation of the ratio—organic PBI^{131}/total plasma I^{131}.

Normal values are usually in the range of 13 to 42% with hypothyroidism being indicated by values below and hyperthyroidism by values above these limits.

Thyroid activity can be measured by two *in vitro* methods in which ^{131}I in the form of labeled *triiodothyronine* (T-3) is bound to the red cells or to plasma proteins. The first of these is the Hamolsky T-3 RBC uptake which measures the percentage of T-3 absorbed on the surface of the cells. The uptake is increased in hyperthyroidism and decreased in hypothyroidism. Simplified methods have been developed. A Sephadex method determines the capacity of plasma proteins for binding with labeled T-3. A high capacity of plasma proteins indicates hypothyroidism; a low capacity indicates hyperthyroidism. In contrast to *in vivo* studies with ^{131}I, test results with T-3 are but little affected by exogenous iodines or iodides, anxiety, hypertension, congestive heart failure and polycythemia.

The *Schilling Test* is useful for the detection of pernicious anemia and for its differentiation from other macrocytic anemias.

In a normal individual, over 50% of an oral dose of vitamin B$_{12}$ is absorbed through the walls of the gastrointestinal tract. This absorption only occurs in the presence of the intrinsic factor of Castle with which the vitamin must presumably combine in order to pass through the intestinal walls. (The biochemical defect in pernicious anemia is the failure of the gastric mucosa to elaborate intrinsic factor.) By means of ^{60}Co-labeled vitamin B$_{12}$ it has been shown that over half of an oral dose soon appears in the blood. Normally only a small amount of activity appears in the urine, but if a large "flushing" dose (1000 μg) of vitamin B$_{12}$ is given parenterally within an hour after the tagged oral dose, the renal threshold is exceeded and radioactivity is observed in the urine.

In the pernicious anemia patient, there is a deficiency of intrinsic factor which causes poor absorption of the vitamin and most of the ingested B$_{12}$ will therefore be found in the feces. The degree of absorption or of fecal excretion can be measured by the use of labeled vitamin B$_{12}$.

Other anemias, such as those associated with sprue and idiopathic steatorrhea, are also accompanied by a decrease in vitamin B$_{12}$ absorption. They may be differentiated from pernicious anemia through the oral administration of intrinsic factor. A marked increase in vitamin B$_{12}$ absorption results in the pernicious anemia patient but not in the case of sprue and other malabsorption syndromes.

In order to reduce the radiation dose received by the patient, while at the same time improving the available sensitivity of the test, cobalt-57 and cobalt-58 are used instead of cobalt-60 as the radioactive tag for vitamin B$_{12}$ (cyanocobalamin).

If plasma iron is labeled by intravenous injection of Ferrous Citrate Fe 52, Fe 55 or Fe 59, it is possible to obtain a comprehensive evaluation of the *kinetics of iron metabolism*. Among the parameters which can be measured are:

1. Plasma iron clearance half-time
2. Plasma volume
3. Hematocrit
4. Blood volume
5. Red-cell iron incorporation

6. Daily iron clearance (plasma-iron turnover; plasma-iron transport rate)
7. Daily hemoglobin formation
8. % daily hemoglobin replacement

The iron turnover, from the catabolism of hemoglobin, can be estimated in the following way. The average blood volume of a normal adult is about 5000 mL. The hemoglobin content is about 15 g/100 mL of blood or about 750 g/person. Iron represents 0.334% of hemoglobin. The hemoglobin-iron content per person is, therefore, about 2.6 g. If the nominal life of a red cell is 110 to 125 days, then approximately 21 to 24 mg of iron/day is released through the catabolism of red cells. The plasma-iron level is from 2 to 3 mg while the amount of iron excreted amounts to only about 1 mg/day. Hence the plasma-iron turnover rate must be of the order of six to eight times, or more, per day.

^{14}C has been used in many metabolic studies such as those involving cholesterol and steroids. The use of radiocarbon and other radioisotopes for intermediary metabolism studies is for the most part experimental. Limitations on the usefulness of tagging should be considered for accurate measurement.

Oils and fats are composed almost entirely of glycerides—esters of glycerin and fatty acids. Before absorption can occur through the intestinal wall these esters must be hydrolyzed by the action of pancreatic lipase. Following absorption, the fatty acids and glycerin recombine to form neutral triglycerides for distribution throughout the body.

Studies of the *absorption of orally administered radioactive fats and fatty acids* provide useful clinical information in certain disorders of the gastrointestinal tract. Although much of the earlier work was done by measurement of fecal excretion of the labeled fat, more recent studies have shown that the determination of blood levels of radioactivity is an easier and more accurate procedure.

Fats can be labeled with carbon-14 or with iodine, either ^{131}I or ^{125}I. An iodine tag is introduced into the fat molecule by iodination of one of the unsaturated fatty acids, eg, oleic acid. The iodine tag alters the chemical composition of the fat and causes some minor changes in the absorption rate when compared to a carbon-14-labeled fat, but the small difference does not decrease the value of the test as an empiric measure of fat absorption. See Fig 29-7.

The plasma lipid radioiodine level rises over a 6-hour period to about 12% of the administered dose. The normal level is about 8%. In the case of sprue, pancreatitis, etc, the plasma level is much lower. Fecal radioactivity may also be calculated. The normal individual excretes less than 2% of the administered labeled fat in the 48 hours following injection.

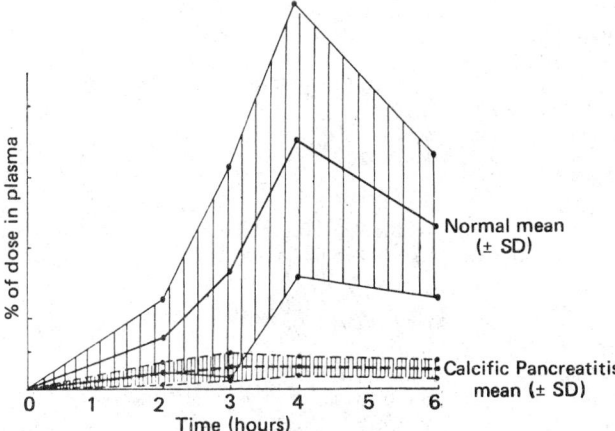

Fig 29-7. The use of triolein (^{131}I) offers a rapid method for the determination of the cause of fat malabsorption (courtesy, Picker X-Ray).

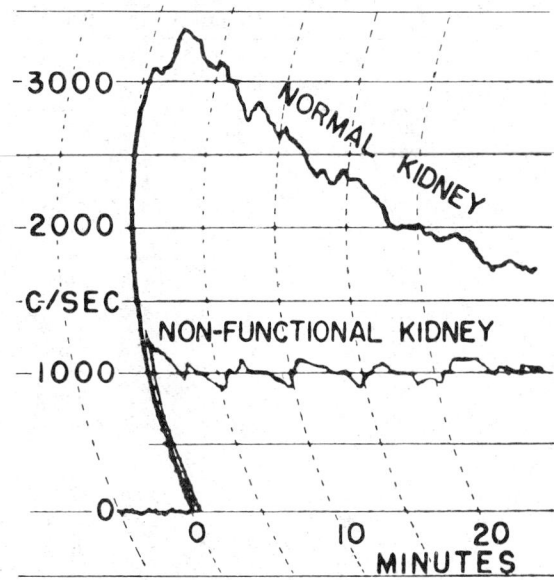

Fig 29-8. Kidney function is studied graphically with *Iodopyracet Injection* which has been labeled with radioactive iodine (courtesy Picker X-Ray).

The rate of gastric emptying and gastrointestinal mobility will influence excretion and absorption patterns. In malabsorption states plasma levels are lower and fecal excretion is increased. Abnormal patterns have been described in individuals with coronary artery disease.

Liver function is measured by intravenous injection of radioiodinated ^{131}I rose bengal and external counting over the area of the liver. Normally radioactivity over the liver reaches a peak 15 to 20 min after injection and falls off gradually as excretion takes place. In liver disease there is a decreased uptake of the dye by the liver. In biliary obstruction the uptake remains normal in the absence of parenchymal involvement, but the excretion rate is diminished. Liver function has also been studied by measurement of the rate of excretion of various labeled radioactive materials such as iodipamide.

In certain types of hemolytic anemias, red cells disappear rapidly from the blood stream, being trapped and eventually destroyed by the spleen. The extent of RBC uptake by the spleen can be determined by tagging the cells *in vitro* with ^{51}Cr, reinjecting them intravenously, counting externally over the spleen and liver and calculating the ratio of spleen:liver radioactivity. A high ratio, associated with decreased RBC survival, may indicate the need for a splenectomy.

The renal function test was introduced by Winter and co-workers in 1956. In their original work they used iodopyracet. However, 10 to 15% of this compound is excreted through the liver. One of the best materials now known is sodium *o*-iodohippurate tagged with either ^{131}I or ^{125}I. This compound was reported to be excreted rapidly and exclusively by the kidney thereby increasing the accuracy of the test and at the same time reducing the time required to perform the test. The isotope is given intravenously and excretion from the renal area is measured externally by means of a pair of radiation detectors. The radioactivity of each kidney is recorded graphically to provide a pattern of the renal function. See Fig 29-8.

^{32}P has been used in attempts to detect and localize gastrointestinal, gastrourinary, pulmonary, and breast tumors, but the results have not been too favorable. ^{32}P has been of value in the detection and delineation of eye tumors. Experiments have been undertaken to localize prostatic metastases and lesions by use of ^{32}P. The isotope is administered

Table II—Properties of Frequently Used Medical Isotopes

Isotope	Radiological half-life		Beta energies[a] (MeV)	Gamma energies (MeV)
^{2}H	stable		. . .	. . .
^{3}H	12.26	years	0.018(100%)	. . .
^{11}C	20.3	min	β^+0.97(99+%)	0.51[b](200%)
^{14}C	5730	years	0.156(100%)	. . .
^{13}N	10.0	min	β^+1.20(100%)	0.51[b](200%)
^{15}O	124	sec	β^+1.70(100%)	0.51(200%)
^{18}F	109.7	min	β^+0.635(97%), EC(3%)	0.51[b](194%)
^{22}Na	2.60	years	β^+0.54(89%), EC(11%)	1.28(100%), 0.51[b]
^{24}Na	15.0	hours	1.39(100%)	1.37(100%), 2.75(10%)
^{32}P	14.3	days	1.71(100%)	. . .
^{35}S	88	days	0.168(100%)	. . .
^{42}K	12.4	hours	3.53(82%), 2.01(18%)	1.52(18%)
^{43}K	22.4	hours	0.82(87%), 0.46(8%)	0.373(85%), 0.619(81%), 0.59(13%)
^{45}Ca	165	days	0.25(100%)	. . .
^{47}Ca-^{47}Sc	4.53	days	0.66(83%), 1.96(17%)	1.31(16%)
(Daughter ^{47}Sc)	3.43	days	0.44(74%), 0.60(26%)	0.16(74%)
^{51}Cr	27.8	days	EC(100%)	0.32(8%)
^{52}Fe	8.2	hours	β^+(56%), EC(44%)	0.165(100%), 0.511(112%)
(Daughter ^{52m}Mn)	21	min	β^+	0.511(193%), 1.434(100%)
^{55}Fe	2.6	years	EC(100%)	. . .
^{59}Fe	45	days	0.46(54%), 0.27(46%)	1.10(57%), 1.29(43%), 0.19(2.8%)
^{57}Co	270	days	EC(100%)	0.122(93%), 0.137(7%)
^{58}Co	71.3	days	β^+0.48(14%), EC(86%)	0.81(100%), 0.51[b]
^{60}Co	5.26	years	0.31(100%)	1.17(100%), 1.33(100%)
^{64}Cu	12.8	hours[5]	EC(43%), 0.57(38%) β^+0.66(19%)	0.51[b]
^{62}Zn	9.3	hours	β^+0.66(18%), EC(82%)	0.51[b]
^{65}Zn	245	days	EC(98.5%), β^+0.325 (1.5%)	1.11(45%), 0.51[b]
^{69m}Zn	13.8	hours		0.439(95%)
^{67}Ga	78	hours	EC	0.093(40%), 0.184(24%), 0.296(22%), 0.388(7%)
^{68}Ga	68.3	min	β^+1.90(88%), EC(12%)	0.51[b](176%), 1.078 (3.5%)
^{74}As	17.9	days	1.36(17%), 0.69(16%), β^+0.90(26%), EC(38%)	0.60(63%), 0.64(16%), 0.51[b]
^{75}Se	120.4	days	EC(100%)	0.265(71%), 0.136(24%), 0.405(14%), 0.077(14%), 0.098(6%), 0.281(5%)
^{75}Br	1.7	hours	β^+(90%), 1.70 (75%) EC(10%)	0.285(75%)
^{77}Br	57	hours	EC(99%), β^+0.34(1%)	0.24(30%), 0.300(67%), 0.52(24%), 0.58(7%), 0.75(2%), 0.82(3%), 1.00(1.3%)
^{82}Br	35.34	hours	0.44(100%)	0.78(87%), 0.55(70%), 0.62(43%), 1.04(30%), 0.70(29%), 1.32(28%), 0.83(26%), 1.48(18%)
^{81m}Kr	13	sec.	IT	0.190(65%)
^{85}Kr	10.76	years	0.67(99+%)	0.052(0.65%)
^{81}Rb	4.7	hours	EC(87%), β^+1.03(13%)	0.51[b](26%)
^{82}Rb	1.3	min	β^+(96%)	0.511(192%), 0.777(9%)
^{86}Rb	18.66	days	1.77(91%), 0.7(9%)	1.08(9%)
^{85}Sr	64	days	EC(100%)	0.514(100%)
^{87m}Sr	2.8	hours	IT	0.388(80%)
^{90}Sr-^{90}Y	28.1	years	0.54(100%)	. . .
(Daughter ^{90}Y)	64.2	hours	2.26(100%)	. . .
^{97}Ru	2.9	days	EC(100%)	0.2154(92%), 0.1091
^{99m}Tc	5.997	hours	. . .	IT0.002(98.6%), 0.140 (98.6%), 0.142(1.4%)
^{111}In	2.8	days	EC	0.173(8%), 0.247(94%)
^{113m}In	100	min		0.393(74%)
^{115m}In	4.50	hours	0.83(5%)	0.335(95%)
^{123m}Te	117	days		0.08846, 0.15900
^{123}I	13.3	hours	EC	0.159(83%)
^{125}I	60	days	EC	0.035(7%), IC(93%)
^{131}I	8.05	days	0.61(87%), 0.33(9%), 0.25(3%)	0.36(80%), 0.64(9%) 0.28(5%), 0.72(3%)

Table II—(Continued)

Isotope	Radiological half-life		Beta energies[a] (MeV)	Gamma energies (MeV)
^{127}Xe	36.4	days	EC	0.203(65%), 0.172(22%), 0.375(20%)
^{133}Xe	5.27	days	0.346(99+%)	0.081(37%)
^{129}Cs	32	hours	EC, no β^+	0.04(2%), 0.28(3%), 0.32(4%), 0.375(48%), 0.416(25%), 0.55(5%)
^{131}Cs	9.70	days	EC, no β^+	Xe, X-rays
^{131}Ba	12	days	EC, no β^+	0.124(28%), 0.216(19%), 0.25(5%), 0.373(13%), 0.496(48%)
^{135m}Ba	28.7	hours		IT, 0.268(16%)
^{153}Sm	47	hours	. . .	0.103(28%), 0.070(5.4%)
^{157}Dy	8.1	hours	EC, no β^+	0.326(91%)
^{169}Yb	32	days	EC	0.063(45%), 0.110(18%), 0.131(11%), 0.177(22%), 0.198(35%), 0.308(10%)
^{178}Ta	2.1	hours	EC	0.328(120%), 0.427(97%), 0.214(75%), 0.093(14%)
^{182}Ta	115	days	1.71(0.3%), 0.216(29%)	0.068(42%), 0.100(14%), 0.152(7%), 0.222(8%), 1.122(34%), 1.189(16%), 1.222(27%), 1.231(13%)
^{192}Ir	74.2	days	0.67(48%), 0.53(41%), 0.26(7%), EC(3.5%)	0.296(29%), 0.31(28%), 0.60(11%), 0.61(7%), 0.48(6%), 0.59(6%)
^{195m}Au	31	sec	IT	0.0567, 0.2615, 0.318
^{198}Au	2.698	days	0.97(99%), 0.28(1%)	0.411(96%), 0.674(1%)
^{197}Hg	64.8	hours	EC(100%)	0.077(19.3%), 0.091 (0.5%)
^{203}Hg	46.9	days	0.21(100%)	0.279(83%), IC(17%)
^{201}Tl	73	hours	EC(100%)	0.167(8%), 0.135(2%)
^{203}Pb	52.1	hours	EC(100%)	0.279(81%), 0.401(5%)
^{226}Ra	1602	years	α4.78(94.3%), α4.59(5.7%)	0.187(4%)
(^{226}Ra daughters)			Many	Many

[a] Unless otherwise specified, the energies given are for negatrons.
[b] Annihilation radiation from positron emission.
Events occurring in less than 1% of the decays have been omitted.

orally and the radioactive uptake by the prostate is determined by means of an internal radiation detector. In the field of brain tumors the isotope may be administered preoperatively and at surgery the marginal limit of the tumor may be delineated by the use of detectors in the brain.

Scanning Techniques—In recent years scanning techniques have developed rapidly and are now among the most useful tools in diagnostic medicine. By means of scanning, tissues and organs can be visualized and such visualization facilitates the detection of abnormalities in their function. In general, a scanning technique consists of (1) administration of a radioactively tagged compound, (2) concentration of the compound in the organ or tissues concerned, and (3) scanning of the region of the organ to prepare a "contour" map of the radioactivity relating the concentration of radioactivity and its physical location. A typical scanner for this purpose is shown in Fig 29-9. A scintillation probe moving evenly and uniformly over the radioactive site detects differences in activity concentrated in the organ. The impulses detected by the probe are amplified and made to modulate a small beam of light which is directed onto a sheet of X-ray film. Since the detector and the light are connected mechanically, visible evidence of the pattern of radiation concentration in the area under examination is produced in the form of a photoscan. Dense regions in the scan, produced by greater exposure to the light, are indicative of regions of high activity. During the recording of the film scan, a mechanical dot scan can also be produced by means of a stylus which transmits the pattern of activity detection to a sheet of electrically sensitive paper.

Variations in activity may be observed throughout the scanning procedure by means of a rate meter and an audio signal. Organs which have been mapped by such techniques with particular success include the lungs, kidneys, thyroid, liver, heart, spleen, bone, and brain.

For detection of the tagged compound to be possible, the radiation emitted by the tagging nuclide must be sufficiently penetrating to pass through tissues so it can reach a detector located outside the body. For this reason, gamma-emitting nuclides must normally be used. (In the interest of minimizing the radiation dose to the patient there should be no alpha component in the radiation and preferably no beta component. In addition, the gamma component should be no "harder" than necessary and the half-lives, both biologic and radiologic, should be as short as convenient.) A list of medically important isotopes and their properties is found in Table II.

One of the first detectors to be used for scanning was the thallium-activated sodium iodide [NaI(Tl)] crystal detector, collimated by means of lead shielding to make it directional. Collimation was improved electronically by means of a pulse-height analyzer adjusted to the photopeak of the tagging nuclide. Problems arising from Compton scattering are thereby largely eliminated. The detector is moved slowly, back and forth, over the area to be scanned. Synchronously, a stylus is moved over a sheet of recording paper. Pulses produced by gamma rays striking the detector are stored electronically. Accumulation of a given number of pulses triggers the stylus causing it to make a mark on the recording

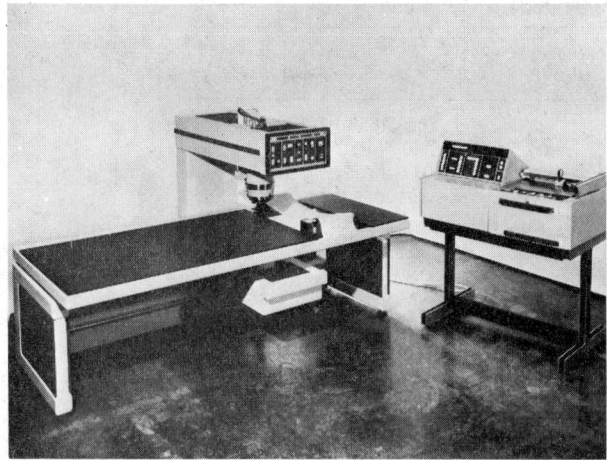

Fig 29-9.   Medical scanner used to visualize tissues and organs in which a diagnostic dose of a radioactively tagged compound has concentrated (courtesy, Picker Corporation).

paper. The greater the radioactivity, the more closely spaced the marks or dots will be. The result is a *dot scan* (Fig 29-10*A*).

Attempts to improve delineation of organs and of "hot" or "cold" spots within organs led to the development of methods by means of which contrast could be increased. One method uses photographic recording. The intensity of a tiny light is modulated by the rate of radiation detection. The light is made to move over a sheet of photographic film synchronously with the motion of the sodium iodide detector over the patient. Development of the film results in the *photoscan*. Contrast can be controlled not only by applying a bias potential to the light bulb but also by appropriate selection of the film. Other methods to improve contrast include low-frequency suppression to reduce background, computer programs, or the simple use of a photocopying process to accent small differ-

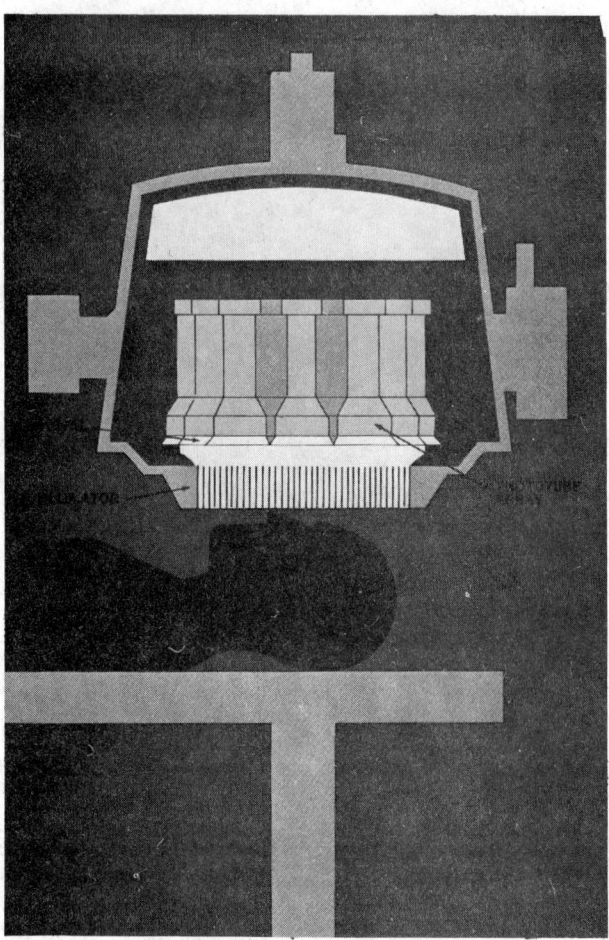

Fig 29-11.   The Anger scintillation camera image detector with multichannel collimator (courtesy, Amersham Searle).

ences in optical density. A typical photoscan is seen in Fig 29-10*C*.

Color scanning represents another approach to improved contrast. In one instrument an eight-color typewriter ribbon is employed, ranging through the spectrum from violet to red. The color region of the ribbon struck by the stylus is selected by the count rate. A dot scan is produced in which "hot" areas are recorded by red dots and the "coolest" areas by violet dots. Quantitative information on the concentration of tagged compound in various regions of the organ is obtained readily from the recording color.

An important disadvantage of single-detector systems, such as those described above, lies in the time required to complete a scan. It is often inconvenient or even impossible for an ill patient to remain immobile long enough to prepare a dot scan or photoscan. A natural solution to this problem is the use of multiple-detector systems. The *Dynapix* is a system in which the detector consists of 10 parallel sodium iodide crystals coupled through light pipes to 10 photomultiplier tubes. The system combines improved detection geometry with data processing and storage. Because data are stored on magnetic tape, worthless scans can be replayed, after resetting controls, to produce useful scans in which the delineation of anatomical details has been optimized.

The *scintillation camera*, also known as the *radiation camera* or *gamma camera*, is a nonscanning device. Several types are available. One consists of a single sodium iodide crystal 11½ inches in diameter which is viewed by an array of 19 photomultiplier tubes. See Fig 29-11. Scintillations produced in the crystal are displayed on an oscilloscope as flashes of light that correspond in position with the original

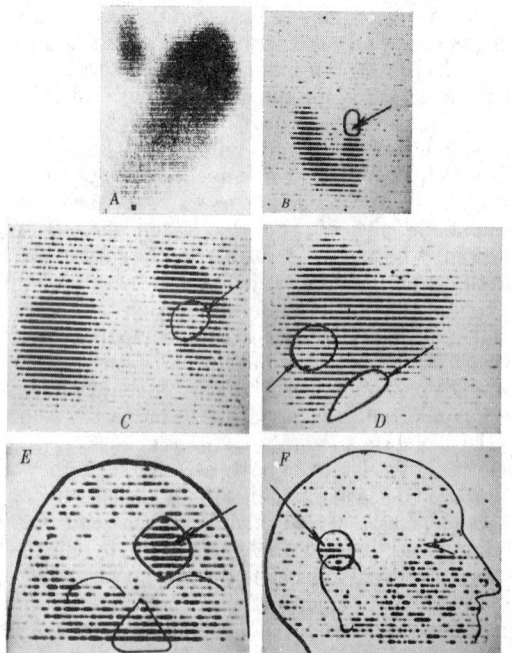

Fig 29-10.   Typical scans.   *A*: Dot scan of thyroid (courtesy, Picker X-Ray); *B*: Photoscan of thyroid; *C*: Photoscan of kidney; *D*: photoscan of liver; *E* and *F*: Photoscans of brain.   Arrows point to malignancies.

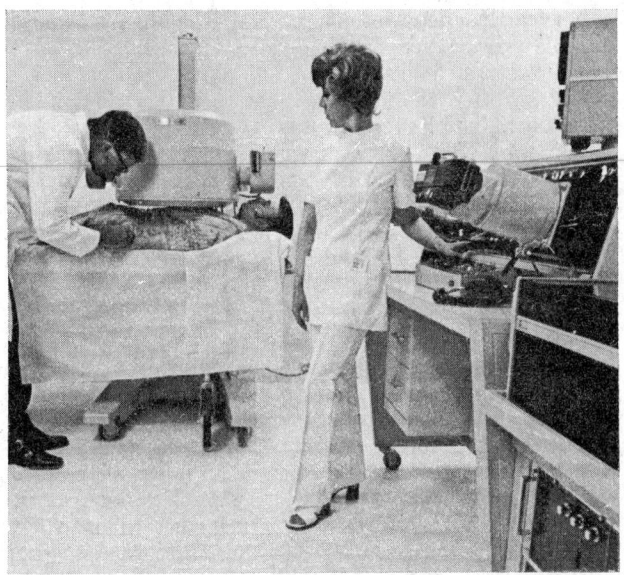

Fig 29-12.   The PHO/Gamma scintillation camera for rapid visualization of the distribution of gamma-emitting radioisotopes within the human body (courtesy, Searle Analytic).

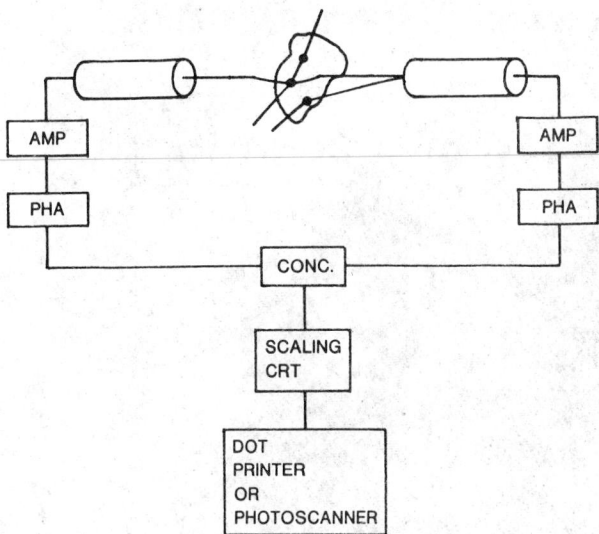

Fig 29-13.   Principle of positron scanning.

image in the scintillation crystal. Images are projected from the radioactive tissue onto the crystal either by pinhole collimation of the radiation or by multichannel collimation. Multichannel collimators consist of a lead block penetrated by a honeycomb-like network of holes. The image appearing on the oscilloscope screen is recorded photographically (see Fig 29-12). The time required to obtain a useful image by means of the scintillation camera is only about $1/10$ that required for scanning.

A second type of scintillation camera is the *Autofluoroscope* in which instead of one large crystal, an array of several hundred crystals is used in combination with multichannel collimation. Each crystal is coupled through light pipes to a rank-and-file system of photocells so that pulses appearing in a particular pair of photocells uniquely identify a particular crystal. Displayed on an oscilloscope, the image can be recorded photographically. Information can also be stored in a magnetic memory for future analysis to optimize contrast. Because scintillation cameras are so fast, dynamic processes can be observed. For example, serial photographs have been prepared showing heart and kidney function.

Digital radiography is a general term for a process in which radiographic images are digitized in order to enhance an area of interest by removal of interfering and uninteresting structures. Clinically significant details can then be more clearly displayed. This is the basis for digital subtraction angiography (DSA). Two types of subtraction techniques have been developed. In the first technique, temporal subtraction, the image obtained before intravenous injection of an iodinated contrast medium is subtracted in a digital computer from the image obtained after injection. The second technique, energy subtraction, is based on the fact that absorption coefficients for X-rays are energy dependent. In energy subtraction, X-ray images obtained using X-rays of different energies are digitized and subtracted. The difference image thus obtained will show some tissues enhanced and others suppressed. To obtain good resolution it is important that the patient be completely immobilized between X-rays.

Positron scintillation scanning or *Positron Emission Tomography* (*PET*) is a technique applicable to the detection of radioisotopes which emit positrons. In tissue, a positron travels only about a millimeter before encountering a negative electron. Their interaction results in the simultaneous emission of two photons, each having an energy of 0.51 MeV, and emitted at an angle of exactly 180° from each other. If two scintillation detectors are placed, one on either side of the tissue in which the isotope is located (Fig 29-13), and the detectors are connected to a coincidence circuit providing an output only when 0.51 MeV gamma rays are detected simultaneously by both, the result is a low background detector, highly specific for the particular isotope used and also giving excellent resolution. The same basic principles applied to a "double" scintillation camera would provide the ultimate in three-dimensional organ imaging. ^{11}C and ^{18}F are among the most frequently used positron-emitting tags.

Computerized Tomography (*CT*)—Tomography is X-ray or gamma-ray photography of a selected plane in the body. In order to reconstruct a picture showing anatomical details clearly it is necessary to process data by computer. Computerized tomography (CT) combines accumulation of radiation data with the advantage of its rapid analysis by computer. CT may operate on the basis of either of two fundamental concepts with regard to the source of radiation: (1) *emission* of radiation from an internally administered radiopharmaceutical and (2) *transmission* of radiation from an external x-ray source. Each type of CT yields distinctly different information. See Figs 29-14 and 29-15.

Emission Computerized Tomography (*ECT*) or *Emission Computerized Axial Tomography* (*ECAT*) utilizes a radioactive pharmaceutical that selectively concentrates in tissues and organs. Radiation data collected by an array of detectors are stored and analyzed by a computer which generates an image or map showing the location and concentration of the radiopharmaceutical in the selected plane of the body. The radiation density in such a *tomograph* depends on the physiological activity of the radiopharmaceutical used.

Transmission or *X-Ray Computerized Tomography* (*TCT*) utilizes an external X-ray source. Transmitted or scattered X-rays are recorded on an array of detectors. When these data are analyzed by computer the image produced depends on the physical density (electron density) of the tissues rather than on the physiological distribution of a radiopharmaceutical. The information thus obtained is therefore substantially different from that obtained by ECT or ECAT.

ECT systems are of two types: (1) *Single Photon Counting* (*SPC*) systems and (2) *Annihilation Coincidence Detection* (*ACD*) systems. SPC systems allow use of any radiopharmaceutical that is generally used for organ imaging with a standard scintillation camera. The SPC system usually uti-

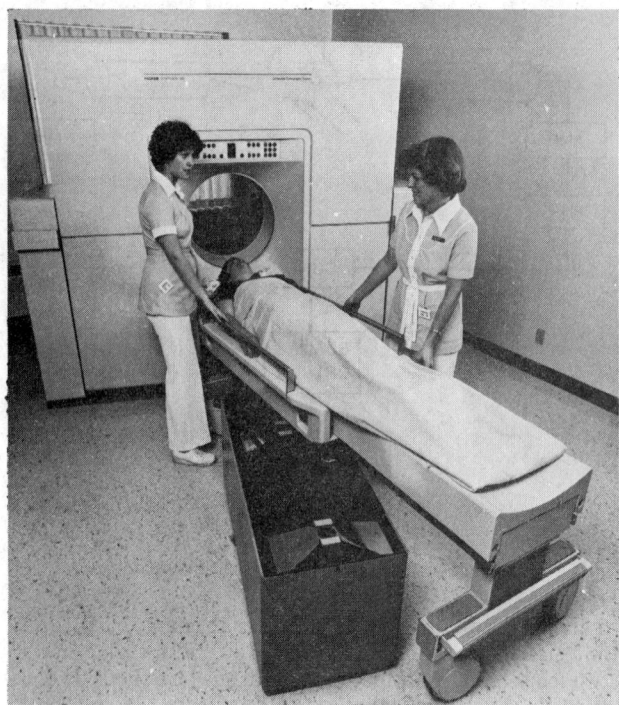

Fig 29-14. A computerized tomography scanner that utilizes 600 stationary detectors and a rotating X-ray tube (courtesy, Picker Corporation).

lizes a scintillation camera mounted on a gantry to allow rotation of the camera about the patient. The position of the camera is synchronized through the computer memory. Through computer reconstruction it is possible to visualize a number of parallel sections with a single scan. Some systems allow visualization of longitudinal as well as transaxial sections by modifying the data processing program.

ACD systems such as the ECAT restrict the choice of nuclide to positron emitters since they utilize annihilation radiation resulting from a positron-negatron interaction but offer the advantage of improved resolution. Opposing detector banks detect the coincident gamma rays. By means of computer analysis of these data a tomographic image is produced representing a map of the location of the positron-emitting radiopharmaceutical.

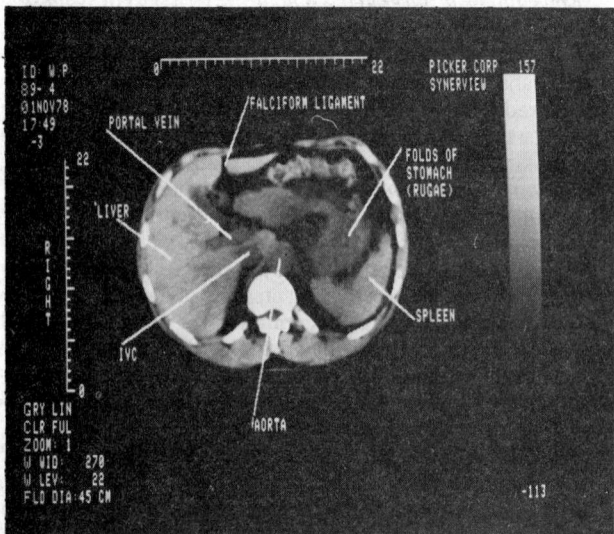

Fig 29-15. A body scan produced with the CT scanner shown in Fig 29-14 (courtesy, Tulane University Medical Center).

Nuclear magnetic resonance (NMR) is one of the most notable of recent advances in diagnostic imaging. NMR reveals structural details not always attainable by other means. NMR also offers the advantage that the patient does not receive any radiation exposure as is the case with computerized tomography (CT). However, NMR provides information which is fundamentally different from that provided by CT. Proton NMR provides essentially a proton or hydrogen map while PET provides a metabolic map and TCT an electron density map. The greatest disadvantage of NMR is that motion of the patient badly degrades images.

Cardiovascular Studies—Thallous Tl 201 Chloride Injection has found extensive use for myocardial imaging and for early detection of infarction. The biological distribution of thallium is similar to that of potassium. On entering the coronary circulation about 85% of the thallium is extracted by the myocardium in a single pass by the potassium-concentrating cell membrane pump and an image of the myocardium can be obtained by use of a gamma camera. In the resulting myocardial scintogram, normal myocardium, having taken up ^{201}Tl, appears "hot" while areas of transient ischemia or of old scar tissue appear "cold." After three or four hours, areas which were originally "cold" due to transient ischemia may appear "hot" while areas of myocardial infarction continue to show up "cold."

Potassium K 42 Chloride and *Potassium K 43 Chloride* have been used similarly to Thallous Tl 201 Chloride, since thallous ions and potassium ions are very similar chemically.

Technetium Tc 99m Sodium Pyrophosphate Injection, while primarily a skeletal-imaging agent, has been used as a cardiac-imaging agent as an adjunct to the diagnosis of acute myocardial infarction. Deposition in the infarcted zone has been explained on the basis of increased Ca^{2+} deposition in such tissues but pyrophosphate seems to be taken up by ischemic tissue as well.

Myocardial perfusion can be used to evaluate the extent of coronary artery disease. Several techniques have been used. The first technique, an invasive approach, consists of a direct intracoronary injection of aggregated albumin or of *albumin microspheres* tagged with ^{99m}Tc or ^{131}I. Gamma-camera images yield information concerning the relative distribution and hence the relative blood flow through the coronary arteries.

A second invasive myocardial perfusion technique consists of injection of inert gas, eg, *Xenon Xe 133*, into the coronary circulation, followed by measurement of the rate of washout from the myocardium. Since the rate of washout is a function of regional coronary blood flow it is possible to quantitate regional myocardial blood from the washout rate.

A third technique for measurement of myocardial perfusion relies on the myocardial distribution of intravenously administered potassium ions (as ^{42}KCl or ^{43}KCl) or of an ion possessing similar chemical properties (in the form of ^{81}RbCl, ^{86}RbCl, ^{129}CsCl, or ^{201}TlCl). The technique differs somewhat from that described above for myocardial infarction. The objective is to identify those areas of the myocardium which are normally perfused under resting conditions, but to which perfusion is not augmented to meet the demands of exercise. Typically a patient receives an injection of *Thallium Tl 201 Chloride* immediately following a treadmill stress test and an image of the heart is recorded. Several days or a week later the administration of Thallium Tl 201 Chloride is repeated under conditions of rest and a second image of the heart is recorded. The images recorded under conditions of stress and rest are then compared.

^{111}*In-oxine* (^{111}In-8-hydroxyquinoline), a lipophilic chelate, has been shown to be an efficient agent for labeling platelets as well as lymphocytes and polymorphs. If blood from a patient is centrifuged at 220 g for 15 minutes the supernatant is platelet-rich plasma. This plasma is removed from the precipitated cells and recentrifuged at 1000 g for 15 minutes, whereupon a platelet-rich precipitate is obtained. After removal of the supernatant, ^{111}In-oxine is added at a pH of 6.5–6.7, and the mixture is incubated for 30 minutes at room temperature to label the platelets. The labeled platelets are then reinjected for studies of platelet kinetics or for *in vitro* detection of phytohemagglutinin and chemotactic substances.

Gallium Ga 67 Citrate, which has been found useful for diagnosis and localization of inflammatory processes, has been used to evaluate myocardial abscesses.

Gated cardiac-imaging or *cine-radionuclide-angiography* (*CRA*) is a new technique which allows the motion of the heart to be visualized in a movie-like manner. After administration of a suitable radiopharmaceutical, eg, ^{99m}Tc-HSA, sequential images of the heart are recorded by use of a scintillation camera. A series of 15 to 30 frames is stored in a computer. Since each frame represents only a fraction of a second it is necessary to accumulate and superimpose data for many cycles in order to obtain clear images. Synchronization of imaging cycles is made possible by use of an EKG-gating device to indicate the beginning of a heart cycle.

Left Ventricular (*LV*) *Function* has been evaluated using a variety of techniques. One important parameter in the evaluation of LV function is the ejection fraction (EF). It is first necessary to measure either the ventricular radioactivity or the ventricular volume during maximum contraction, ie, end-systole (ES) and during maximum volume, ie, end-diastole (ED). The value of EF is then calculated by use of the relationship;

$$EF = \frac{ED - ES}{ED}$$

Several radiopharmaceuticals have been used in these studies, including ^{99m}Tc-DTPA, [113m]In-DTPA, and ^{99m}Tc-HSA. Detection of the radiation has been by use of a single NaI(Tl) gamma counter or with the standard gamma camera. Usually the detector is synchronized to the heart beat by use of an EKG which identifies the times corresponding to ED and ES as in the case of gated cardiac imaging. Methods for the evaluation of LV function may use a "first-pass" or "first-transit" technique wherein data are collected on no more than the first few heart beats following injection of a bolus of the radiopharmaceutical through a cardiac cannula. Alternatively, an "equilibrium" technique may be used, which is essentially an extension of a gated cardiac imaging procedure that includes calculations of ventricular radioactivity or volume, EF, in addition to a sequence of images.

Thyroid Visualization—For many years Sodium Iodide I 131 has been used for thyroid scanning (see Fig 29-10*B*). Through its use one can demonstrate the presence or absence of "hot" or "cold" nodules, which is helpful information in deciding what course of treatment should be followed. Labeling of the thyroid gland is possible with pertechnetate Tc 99m; technetium as [99m]TcO$_4$⁻ has been shown to parallel [131]I⁻ chemistry in many instances. However, metastatic deposits from thyroid carcinoma have not always been readily visible using pertechnetate. Both 4.5-day [124]I and 13.0-hour ^{123}I appear to be especially adaptable to thyroid imaging. Parathyroid tumors have been shown to concentrate selenomethionine Se 75 to a small extent and its use with external scanning has been helpful in some cases for detecting the presence of such a tumor.

Fluorescence scanning of the thyroid utilizes a focused photon source, eg, [241]Am, which emits 60 keV gamma rays, to excite iodine X-rays of the iodine contained in the thyroid. The iodine X-rays are then observed by use of a collimated solid-state detector such as a lithium-drifted silicon or germanium detector. By scanning the thyroid area one is able to obtain a map indicating the distribution of iodine or iodine compounds.

Liver Visualization—A variety of radioactive substances have been used for liver scanning, hepatic function tests, or studies of the reticuloendothelial system. *Rose Bengal Sodium I 131* concentrates in the undifferentiated hepatic cells which are polygonal in shape. Both *Technetium Tc 99m Sulfur Colloid* and *Gold Au 198* are removed from circulation by the Kupffer-cell system, thus concentrating these compounds in the liver. Not only can the general outline of the liver be observed by external scanning but it is also possible to show the presence of nodules (Fig 29-10*D*). Technetium Tc 99m Sulfur Colloid has been used extensively for liver visualization since it combines several advantages over iodine- and gold-tagged compounds; namely, (1) a lower dose is delivered to the patient (^{99m}Tc emits only a 140 keV gamma ray and has a physical half-life of only 6 hours) and (2) increased clarity and resolution of the scan is obtained as the radiation is easily collimated. As a follow-up to Technetium Tc 99m Sulfur Colloid imaging, *Gallium Ga 67 Citrate* studies have been helpful in the detection of hepatoma in patients with cirrhosis and in differentiating cancer and abscess from more benign causes of an abnormal liver scan. Other substances used to test liver function include ortho-^{131}I iodobenzoic acid, *Sodium Iodipamide I 131*, *Technetium Tc 99m Etidronate Sodium*, and *Tc 99m Diethyl-Acetanilido-Iminodiacetate* (Tc 99m Diethyl-IDA).

Colloidal gold Au 198 was the first radioactive material used for reticuloendothelial system (RES) function studies. Recently Technetium Tc 99m Sulfur Colloid has been most frequently used for RES studies. Also used for this purpose are human albumin Tc 99m macroaggregated, ferric hydroxide Tc 99m, indium hydroxide In 113m, stannous oxide Tc 99m, stannous oxide In 113m, sodium phytate Tc 99m, and Tc 99m albumin microspheres.

Gallbladder Visualization—Rose Bengal Sodium I 131 and *Sulfobromophthalein Sodium I 131* were among the first radiopharmaceuticals used to visualize the gallbladder. Later, ^{99m}Tc-Tetracycline, as well as ^{123}I-Rose Bengal and ^{123}I-Bromsulphalein, were introduced for this purpose. Most recent of the compounds showing promise for gallbladder imaging include ^{99m}Tc-Diethyl-Acetanilido-Iminodiacetate and [99m]Tc Pyridoxylideneglutamate.

Pancreatic Scanning—Visualization of the pancreas is complicated by the presence of the liver. *Selenomethionine Se 75* is concentrated by the pancreas but it is also concentrated by the liver, which overlies and obscures it. On the other hand, studies have shown the pancreatic concentration to be 8 to 9 times that of the liver in dogs. It is helpful first to make a liver scan with gold Au 198 several days prior to the pancreatic scan, the pancreas thereby being more readily identified. Another approach utilizes a double-tracer technique. One of the other labeled compounds taken up by the liver is administered simultaneously with selenomethionine Se 75. Then, through pulse-height analysis, it is possible to subtract the contribution from the liver electronically, leaving only the image of the pancreas. Recently, ^{18}F-fluoroamino acids have been tested for pancreatic visualization, and [1-^{11}C]DL-valine has been suggested as a possible pancreas-imaging agent.

Spleen Visualization—A technique for visualization is based on the function of this organ to remove damaged red cells from circulation. If red cells (tagged by means of sodium chromate Cr 51) are heated, they can be converted to spherocytes or spherical fragments without significant release of hemoglobin. These cells are quickly taken up by the spleen allowing it to be identified by scanning. Blood cells tagged with Tc 99m by use of stannous chloride reduction can now be readily prepared. Because the radiation dose to the patient is much less, Tc 99-RBC's are preferred to Cr 51-RBC's.

Other potential radioactively tagged compounds for visualization of the spleen are discussed above under RES studies in the paragraph on liver visualization. Of particular note is the use of Technetium Tc 99m Sulfur Colloid.

Lung Imaging—As early as 1952 colloidal gold Au 198 was used in an attempt to visualize the lungs but variability in particle size of the colloid soon prompted a search for a better scanning agent. Iodinated I 131 Serum Albumin Aggregated was then introduced to visualize the pulmonary vasculature through perfusion lung scanning. The particles of radioactive albumin concentrate selectively in those regions of the lung possessing an adequate blood supply where they are apparently trapped for a short time by the narrow capillaries. The aggregate remains in the lungs long enough to complete a scan. In time they break down to smaller particles and are carried by the blood to the liver where they are phagocytized by the Kupffer cells.

Other compounds which have been used in a similar fashion include ^{51}Cr-labeled albumin aggregate, ^{51}Cr-tagged red cells, ^{203}Hg chlormerodrin and ^{203}Hg-tagged ceramic microspheres but that most frequently used in recent years has been human serum albumin I 131 aggregated. Newer additions to the list of lung-imaging radiopharmaceuticals are human serum albumin Tc 99m and human serum albumin In 133m. HSA Tc 99m microspheres consists of almost perfectly spherical particles of albumin of a very uniform size.

Inhalation lung scans, using the technique of ventilation imaging and employing either a radioaerosol or a radioactive gas, permit bronchial patency evaluation. Some of the radiopharmaceuticals which have been used as aerosols are HSA I 131, sodium rose bengal I 131, iodohippurate sodium I 131, chlormerodrin Hg 197, colloidal gold Au 198, HSA I 125 and HSA Tc 99m. Results are similar to those obtained through the use of perfusion scans. Although one can prepare a lung scan using a radioactive gas by inhalation, gases are usually used to conduct pulmonary function tests such as alveolar clearance. Krypton 85 was one of the first gases to be so used, and ^{127}Xe, ^{133}Xe, and ^{13}N$_2$ are considered to be among the more important gases. Others which have been used or considered include ^{15}O$_2$, ^{11}CO$_2$, CH$_3$^{131}I, ^{15}CO$_2$, ^{15}CO, ^{77}Kr, ^{81m}Kr, ^{85m}Kr, ^{87m}Kr, ^{125}Xe, ^{129m}Xe, ^{131m}Xe, and ^{135}Xe.

Tumor Localization—Diiodofluorescein I 131 was the first radiopharmaceutical to be used for tumor localization. Since then numerous radioactive compounds have been used for cerebral tumor detection (see Fig 29-10*E* and *F*). Iodinated I 131 serum albumin has found extensive use for years, but there are reports that chlormerodrin Hg 203 is faster and gives sharper definition in the scans. Chlormerodrin Hg 197 has replaced the ^{203}Hg compound largely because the dose to the patient is less with the former. Chlormerodrin is also used for kidney scanning. For brain tumor detection a dose of meralluride is usually given first to minimize renal uptake of the labeled chlormerodrin. One of the latest techniques for brain tumor localization employs sodium pertechnetate Tc 99m which is readily available from a "cow." It is the most widely used radiopharmaceutical for this purpose. Atropine is sometimes administered to suppress the uptake of ^{99m}TcO$_4^-$ by mucosa and salivary tissues which would otherwise obscure the frontal area of the brain. Atropine is usually not necessary when chlormerodrin Hg 197, chlormerodrin Hg 203, ^{99m}Tc-diethylenetriaminepentaacetic acid (^{99m}Tc-DTA), ^{113m}In-DTPA, or ^{169}Yb-DTPA are used.

Krypton Kr 85 and *Xenon Xe 133* have been used for the localization of lipomatous tumors. Inert gases have a greater solubility in fatty tissue than in lean. After rebreathing ^{85}Kr or ^{133}Xe in a closed respirometer for about 5 minutes the gas becomes sufficiently incorporated in liposarcomas to permit their visualization.

Gallium 68, being a positron emitter, enables one to use a positron scintillation scanner for localization of areas of ab-

normal uptake. The nuclide is used as ^{68}Ga-EDTA in which form it is superior to ^{64}Cu-EDTA because of its greater instability constant. Human globulin I 124 has also been used for positron scanning.

The use of *gallium citrate Ga 67* to detect soft tissue tumors was first reported in 1969. Carrier-free gallium 67, a cyclotron-produced nuclide, has been useful in the differential diagnosis of liver abnormalities to detect the presence of metastases and cancerous lesions which are not visible roentgenographically. Gallium Ga 67 is primarily useful as an adjunctive test in the evaluation of patients with Hodgkin's disease, histiocytic lymphoma, Burkitt's lymphoma, embryonal cell testicular tumors and in the evaluation of hepatoma, melanoma, and lung carcinoma. The utility of gallium lies in the fact that it is taken up in inflammatory lesions by a combination of direct bacterial incorporation and by neutrophil deposition. Other compounds that have been used for brain scans include sodium arsenate As 74, povidone I 131, and povidone I 125. It has also been found that *Technetium Tc 99m Etidronate Sodium* (^{99m}Tc-HEDP) and other radiopharmaceuticals generally used for bone visualization concentrate in breast tumors. [^{11}C]Carboxyl-labeled 1-aminocyclopentanecarboxylic acid ([^{11}C] ACPC) has also found merit as a tumor-scanning agent, its principal advantage lying in the short half-life of ^{11}C which allows administration of a larger dose, thereby permitting a shorter scanning time.

Kidney Imaging—Kidney scans have been useful for demonstrating both normal and abnormal renal function (see Fig 29-10*C*). Compounds which have been used for this purpose include sodium iodohippurate I 131, sodium iodohippurate I 125, sodium iodohippurate I 123, chlormerodrin Hg 203, and chlormerodrin Hg 197. Generally the advantage of the lower radiation dose obtained using ^{197}Hg is outweighed by the greater resolution available by the use of ^{203}Hg. Renal uptake of chlormerodrin is rapid, thereby permitting scans to be made shortly after administration of the radiopharmaceutical.

Currently the compounds principally used for renal scanning, in addition to sodium iodohippurate I 131, are ^{99m}Tc-iron-ascorbic acid complex and ^{99m}Tc-DTPA. In addition, ^{99m}Tc-tetracycline has been found useful as both a kidney and gallbladder imaging agent. Indications are that this compound behaves similarly to ^{99m}Tc-penicillamine-acetazolamide complex and ^{99m}Tc-caseidin, radiopharmaceuticals which have also been used for renal scanning.

Stannous gluconate Tc 99m is a new promising renal imaging agent providing information on the size and shape of the kidney and allowing delineation of renal lesions and renal vascular disease.

Gallium Ga 67 Citrate and *Technetium Tc 99m Dimethylsuccinate* have been used to follow the response of emphysematous pyelonephritis to antibiotic therapy; the two agents demonstrate a reciprocal relationship to renal uptake as a function of tissue abnormality.

Adrenal Imaging—The imaging of human adrenal glands has been clinically possible since 1971 by use of [^{131}I]19-iodocholesterol, which has been used to identify a number of adrenal disorders, including pheochromocytoma. Uptake of the *iodocholesterol* is increased by ACTH and suppressed by dexamethasone, which has been interpreted to mean that iodocholesterol parallels adrenal steroid production. Therefore an increased uptake of iodocholesterol is generally interpreted to represent hyperfunction of the glands or of an autonomously functioning tumor.

The radiotracer [^{131}I]6β-iodomethyl-19-norcholesterol has a fivefold greater adrenal activity than [^{131}I]19-iodocholesterol, and hence gives better delineation of structure.

Bone and Marrow Imaging—As early as 1942 strontium 89 was observed to accumulate in neoplastic osseous tissue and, in 1948, areas of osteogenesis were demonstrated by the use of gallium 72. Later, calcium 47 was used but its gamma energy (1.31 MeV) requires heavy collimation. Furthermore, it is costly to obtain with a high specific activity. Strontium 85 was then favored as a scanning agent. Its gamma (0.513 MeV) is more readily collimated and, being reactor-produced, it is less costly. In the course of developing suitable bone-scanning agents ^{18}F, ^{87m}Sr, ^{137m}Ba, ^{153}Sm, ^{167}Tm, and ^{171}Er have all been investigated. Recently attention has centered on the use of ^{99m}Tc-labeled polyphosphates, phosphonates and pyrophosphates. Of particular interest are Technetium Tc 99m Etidronate Sodium (^{99m}Tc-hydroxyethylidine diphosphonate, ^{99m}Tc HEDP, or ^{99m}Tc EHDP), Technetium Tc 99m Methylene Diphosphonate (MDP), Technetium Tc 99m Sodium Phosphates (^{99m}Tc Polyphosphate), and Technetium Tc 99m Sodium Pyrophosphate.

Cisternography—This is a technique involving the intraspinal injection—usually lumbar—of a radiopharmaceutical for the purpose of observing the pathway of CSF. After injection of the tracer dose, its distribution is periodically determined by scanning or imaging. Normally the tracer moves up the spinal subarachnoid space or into the basal cisterns, moving toward the brain. Cisternography is useful in the diagnosis of hydrocephalus, intraventricular tumor, subarachnoid hemorrhage, rhinorrhea and other pathologic conditions.

Human serum albumin I 131 has been used extensively for cisternography but human serum albumin Tc 99m is superior because it provides better photon yields. ^{99m}Tc-inulin has been used in a similar manner. Use of ^{169}Yb-DTPA offers the advantage that the longer radiological half life of ^{169}Yb (32 days) and the stability of the ^{169}Yb-DTPA complex allow a strict quality control, a very important feature for a radiopharmaceutical intended for injection in such a critical location.

A comparison of the useful photons per RAD showed ^{111}In to be superior to ^{131}I, ^{99m}Tc, ^{169}Yb and ^{203}Pb. The use of ^{111}In-transferrin, ^{111}In-EDTA, and ^{111}In-DTPA in cisternography has been investigated. The studies show ^{111}In-DTPA to be essentially the ideal radiopharmaceutical for cisternography.

Ophthalmology—^{32}P was first used for the detection of intraocular tumors in 1952. Following injection or oral administration of *Sodium Phosphate P 32*, ocular lesions are detected by comparing the radioactivity observed for one eye versus that observed for the other by placing a small detector directly in contact with the eyeball. For accurate identification it is important that the detector be placed directly over the lesion; a slight error in position can yield incorrect results. This technique is therefore unreliable for posteriorly located lesions.

Chloroquine derivatives, such as ^{125}I-4-(3-dimethylaminopropylamino)-7-iodoquinone, have shown promise in the diagnosis of ocular melanomas. Other radiopharmaceuticals, including ^{82}Rb, ^{125}I-diiodofluorescein and ^{197}Hg-chlormerodrin, have been investigated without success.

Patency of the lacrimal drainage apparatus is evaluated by means of a nuclear dacryocystogram. ^{99m}Tc-pertechnetate in sterile normal saline is placed in the conjunctival sac. Using a gamma camera with a pinhole collimator, a series of scintiphotos are obtained that will indicate if a functional block exists. Radiopharmaceuticals have been used to study the function of the lacrimal gland, and to study aqueous humor dynamics and glaucoma. They have included labeled serum albumin, hippurate, antipyrine, and a number of organic substances labeled with ^{11}C or ^{18}F.

Placental Localization—Diagnosis of bleeding in the third semester of pregnancy is often difficult. The primary conditions to be differentiated are placenta previa and premature separation of the placenta; the treatment may be different.

Sodium chloride Na 24 was first used in the diagnosis but rapid diffusion of the tracer was a severe handicap. In 1957, use of human serum albumin I 131 was reported. It remains in the maternal circulation for a long time and accumulates in the placenta simply because the placenta represents a large pool of blood. Serum albumin Tc 99m replaced the ^{131}I-tagged compound because of its superior ratio of useful photons to the radiation dose delivered. More recently ^{113m}In has been deemed the best tag for placental localization because of its higher energy photons (393 keV compared to 140 keV for ^{99m}Tc). In addition, an interfering image from the bladder is not commonly produced because ^{113m}In is excreted slowly into the urine.

Establishment of a Medical Radioisotope Program

Types of Programs—There are two types of clinical radioisotope programs:

1. Institutional programs sponsored by a medical organization or hospital and carried out under the guidance of a medical isotope committee, and
2. Private medical practice programs.

Among the latter, a distinction may be made between private-practice programs confined primarily to the use of radioactive materials in a private office and private-practice programs where the materials are used within a medical facility. For radiological safety it is advisable that patients receiving a dose of more than 30 microcuries of radioactive material be hospitalized. In most cases physicians have found it desirable to carry out their treatments within a hospital rather than in their private offices. The responsibility still remains with the individual physician, however, the hospital merely providing the facilities.

Personnel—Radioactive compounds used in humans for therapy and diagnosis are radioactive drugs and should be treated as such. The administration of such drugs to humans must be supervised by a physician specially trained in their use. Thus to organize a medical radioisotope program there must be at least one qualified physician. His training must be ample to satisfy the NRC that he can use the radioactive material properly and safely for the particular procedure proposed. Suggested minimum experience requirements for the physician for specific diagnostic and therapeutic procedures have been published by the NRC.

The organization of an isotope committee is highly recommended. Membership on the committee may include physicians, physicists, chemists, pharmacists, business administrators or others as required for the proper functioning of the committee. One member of the isotope committee should be designated as *Health Officer*. His specific responsibility is to see that all radioisotopes are handled with minimum hazard to personnel and that all regulations governing the use of radioisotopes are observed.

Program—One of the first duties of the isotope committee is to outline the radioisotope program for the hospital. Although hospital programs may differ one from the other, they all have certain common problems. Some of the subjects to be considered by the committee are:

Diagnostic or therapeutic procedures to be performed
Facilities and work areas required (treatment room, laboratory, counting areas, etc.)
Instrumentation (selection, cost)
Licensure and reports (NRC, state, city)
Records (licenses, isotopes ordered and received, disposition of isotopes, patients' records, personnel safety records)
Isotopes (procurement, storage, waste disposal)

Facilities and Work Area—An isotope storage area, a laboratory for the manipulation of isotopes and the preparation of prescribed dosage forms, a counting area for calibration of the dose, and a treatment room are among the facilities and work areas which should be considered. With the availability of precalibrated dosage forms of most radiopharmaceuticals, elaborate facilities are not required for many diagnostic procedures. An existing, standard chemical laboratory will normally provide all necessary facilities for the preparation and handling of small amounts of radioactive drugs.

In some hospitals radiopharmaceuticals are dispensed by the hospital pharmacist. Nonradioactive pharmaceuticals have been dispensed by the pharmacist for years. Adding the property of radioactivity to these substances modifies them but does not cause them to be less of a drug than they were before. It therefore seems not only logical but necessary that these products be dispensed by a pharmacist who has taken the initiative to acquire the necessary knowledge and training to work with radioactive pharmaceuticals.

In the selection of the counting area, the location of X-ray equipment and other radiation sources must be considered lest the background in the counting area be erratic or excessively high.

Preparation of Radiopharmaceuticals—Many radiopharmaceuticals in current use require preparation. ^{99m}Tc- and ^{113m}In-cows, for example, which provide valuable, short-lived radioisotopes, complicate procedures for the preparation of radiopharmaceuticals intended for parenteral use since on-site labeling is required. There still remains the need for a sterile, pyrogen-free product for the safety of the patient.

Pyrogens may contaminate parenteral radiopharmaceuticals in many ways. Obvious sources are the solvent or vehicle as well as the solutes used, especially if solutes may have been purified by recrystallization from pyrogen-containing water. Once introduced into a product, pyrogens are essentially impossible to remove. Control of preparation is therefore of utmost importance to ensure a quality product. Glassware must be scrupulously clean. After washing it should be rinsed with pyrogen-free distilled water and heated to 160° for 1 hour.

Adsorption of carrier-free radiopharmaceuticals on the walls of containers can be a problem. Until confidence that adsorption of a particular radiopharmaceutical does not occur, measurement of the radioactivity of the full and "empty" container is recommended to assure delivery of the dose. The use of a carrier may be indicated if such use does not interfere with the intended application of the radiopharmaceutical. In general, reducing the pH of the product or coating the walls of the container with silicone are possible solutions of the problem of adsorption.

Chemicals used in the preparation of radiopharmaceuticals should be of the highest purity obtainable. Trace amounts of impurities may dilute carrier-free substances below the point of acceptability. Chemicals should also be free of pyrogens and are best procured in small bottles rather than the usually more economical large size. It should also be noted that good chemistry laboratory techniques are not always sufficient from the standpoint of radiopharmaceutical formulation.

Water and other vehicles should conform to high standards of purity with regard to pH, sterility, freedom from pyrogens, and dissolved solids. The USP monograph for Water For Injection should be consulted (see Chapter 68).

Additives intended to improve or safeguard the quality of the product (antioxidants, antimicrobial agents, stabilizers, etc.) must be selected carefully because one is usually dealing with an extremely dilute solution of active ingredient in a radiopharmaceutical preparation. Changes too small to be detected chemically can alter the biological behavior of the preparation.

Terminal sterilization of radiopharmaceuticals is usually preferred. This may be accomplished by steam autoclaving; when autoclaving is contraindicated, sterility can be achieved by filtration through a membrane filter, a 0.22-μm filter usually sufficing. Certain products, such as aggregated human serum albumin, cannot be terminally sterilized since the product is heat-labile, and bacterial filters will remove the aggregate. It must be prepared using aseptic techniques from sterile reactants.

Control testing for sterility should be conducted on radiopharmaceutical products prior to use, where half-life and shelf-life permit. Where such testing is not possible prior to use it should be performed after the fact.

Instrumentation—The majority of clinical studies and analyses can be performed with the aid of but a few different types of radiation detection equipment. Of these the scintillation detector will usually be found most useful.

Instruments necessary to carry out a thyroid-uptake study may be considered essential equipment for a clinical radioisotope laboratory. The necessary components of the system are an adjustable gamma scintillation probe attached to a scaler equipped with an elapsed-time clock. With this system the uptake of gamma-emitting isotopes can be measured in any organ of the body. The uptake of ^{131}I by the thyroid and the uptake of ^{51}Cr-labeled red blood cells by the spleen are examples of techniques possible with this basic equipment.

Use of a scintillation counter is greatly enhanced by a pulse-height analyzer. The resulting spectrometer can be "tuned" to a particular isotope. Such a system not only allows the detection of one isotope in the presence of others but also permits the use of a smaller amount of radioactive material in a diagnostic procedure because of the significant reduction in background and the improved statistics resulting therefrom. A further advantage to the use of a spectrometer, again resulting from the possible high selectivity or "tuning" effect, is the resulting discrimination against Compton scattered radiation which could otherwise cause serious errors in the measurements, especially should changes in the counting geometry occur.

For the *in vitro* counting of gamma-emitting isotopes such as those above, a well-type detector will provide detection efficiencies as high as 60% or more. Accordingly, the addition of a well counter to the basic scintillation system or, better, to a scintillation spectrometer system, will provide the necessary instrumentation for performing numerous other diagnostic procedures. Included are blood-volume measurements as well as other isotope-dilution techniques, RBC survival time, test of gastrointestinal bleeding, PBI conversion ratio, triiodothyronine *in vitro* uptake studies, Schilling test, fat absorption, and others.

Measurements to determine the relative concentration of an isotope throughout an organ can be accomplished by means of scintillation scanning. A scintillation scanner such as that described on page 479 permits accurate mapping of radioactivity uptake in such organs as the thyroid, brain, liver, kidneys, spleen, and cardiac blood pool. For the optimum in organ-imaging a gamma camera is recommended.

Licensure and Reports—Until recently all users of radioisotopes in the United States were required to obtain a license for their use from the Atomic Energy Commission, now the Nuclear Regulatory Commission. This is still true in most states. Application for license may be made on forms AEC-313 and AEC-313A which are available from the Nuclear Regulatory Commission, Washington, DC 20545.

Effective March 26, 1962, the Commonwealth of Kentucky assumed certain of the Atomic Energy Commission's regulatory authority in that state. Individuals or organizations desiring to use radioisotopes in Kentucky should contact the State Commissioner of Health, Frankfort, KY. Similar agreements for state regulation have since been made with a number of other states, including Alabama, Arizona, Arkansas, California, Colorado, Florida, Kansas, Louisiana, Mississippi,

Nebraska, New Hampshire, Idaho, New York, North Carolina, Oregon, Tennessee, Texas and Washington.

While the above state programs replace NRC regulations, some states have radiation control programs which supplement those of the NRC. State regulations frequently require registration of radiation sources. Similar registration is desirable with the local municipality, especially with fire and police officials, even though not always required.

Roentgenography

Sources of X-Rays—The most common source of X-rays is the X-ray tube in which electrons, generated at the cathode, are accelerated by means of a high voltage toward the anode. The anode or target is made of tungsten or other high-melting metal. As the accelerated electrons strike target atoms they may interact in different ways. Target atoms may become excited and as they return to the ground state their excess energy is emitted as characteristic X-rays. Other electrons interact with the nuclei of target atoms. Being slowed down in the process their excess kinetic energy is radiated as the continuous X-ray spectrum.

Isotopic X-ray sources are also available. One potential source is ^{125}I. An advantage of an isotopic source is the lack of a continuous spectrum. For example, the radiation from ^{125}I consists of fine discrete energies between 27.2 and 35.4 keV.

Diagnostic Use—In addition to the diagnostic use of X-rays in the examination of broken and carious bones, the teeth, the gums, and the sinuses, there are many other useful applications. X-rays can be used diagnostically in conjunction with materials which have the ability to absorb them strongly. The X-ray-absorbing ability of a material depends on its atomic weight. The higher the atomic weight, the better it will absorb X-rays, all other things being equal. The reason the bones of the body absorb X-rays better than the flesh and muscle is that they are largely composed of calcium, phosphorus, etc, which have higher atomic weights than hydrogen, oxygen, carbon, and nitrogen, which to a large measure are found in the rest of the body.

Therefore, for X-ray diagnostic use, it is desirable to find materials of high atomic number in a form which will have no ill effects on the body. Where liquids are desired, some form of iodine and thorium have proved useful, while the nontoxic forms of barium are used when an emulsion or a suspension is called for. Thorium-containing compounds are no longer considered to be safe for these purposes, however, since they are retained in tissues for years and have been responsible for the formation of cancers and sarcomas. Table III shows a partial list of some of these materials now in common use for X-ray diagnostic purposes.

X-rays can also be used to examine the normal functions of parts or organs of the body. For example, they can be used to "see" the action of the muscle, the joints, the diaphragm,

Table III—Compounds Used in Roentgenography

Part of the Body	Diagnostic Opaques	
Head	Conray	Isopaque
	Hypaque	Reno-M-60
	Hypaque Meglumine	Renographin
Circulatory System	Angio-Conray	Meglumine Diatrizoate
	Cardiografin	Renografin
	Conray	Reno-M-60
	Hypaque-M	Renovist
	Hypaque Sodium	Renovist II
	Isopaque	Vascoray
Digestive System	Barosperse	E-Z-Paque
	Barotrast	E-Z-Paste
	Esophotrast	Sol-O-Pake
	E-Z-Em Barium Enema	Tymtran
Gallbladder and Bile Ducts	Bilopaque Sodium	Oragrafin Sodium
	Cholebrine	Oratrast
	Cholografin Meglumine	Renografin
	Hypaque Sodium	Reno-M-60
	Oragrafin Calcium	Telepaque
Urinary Tract	Conray	Isopaque
	Cysto-Conray	Meglumine Diatrizoate
	Cystografin	Renografin
	Cystotoken	Reno-M-DIP
	Hypaque-Cysto	Reno-M-60
	Hypaque-DIU	Renovist
	Hypaque-M	Renovist II
	Hypaque Meglumine	Vascoray
	Hypaque Sodium	
Obstetrical	Ethiodol	Salpix Contrast Medium
	Hypaque Sodium	
	Hypaque-M	Sinografin
Spinal Cord	Hypaque Meglumine	Reno-M-60
	Renografin	
Joints	Hypaque Meglumine	Reno-M-60
	Renografin	

and the heart. They can also be used diagnostically in the case of pregnancy. Not only is it possible to tell whether or not the fetus is growing and developing properly, but it is possible to tell whether a cephalic or breech delivery is to be expected. X-rays also will clearly show whether the fetus is a singlet, a doublet, or a triplet. Such applications must of course be used with discretion.

Therapeutic Uses—The major use for X-ray therapy is in treatment of *cancer*. Many superficial lesions can be completely cured and for them X-ray therapy is the treatment of choice. However, malignant tumors lying deeper in the body are not regularly cured, though their growth may be halted and they may even regress strikingly, only to return after weeks, months, or years. X-rays are also often used to advantage before the surgical removal of some cancers, particularly of the lower bowel or the uterus, to assist in curing infections which would otherwise complicate healing after surgery. A number of other afflictions are often treated with X-rays. Some controversy exists regarding the advisability of these applications, however, since the possibility of tumor indication years later always exists. It has been shown that the incidence of leukemia (a form of cancer) is higher in radiotherapists than in the population at large.

Dosage—Quite often, as in the treatment of superficial skin cancers, etc, X-ray therapists may deliver between 2000 and 6000 roentgens (see page 458 for definition of roentgen).

It has been found that the intermittent application of fractions of the total ultimate dose produce better therapeutic results with less damage to surrounding normal tissue. Hence, treatment may be prolonged for as long as 3 or 4 weeks with the administration of from 50 to 200 roentgens/day. Ordinarily when doses in this range are employed, changes occur in the skin which are suggestive of ordinary thermal burns. However, these are not burns in the strict sense of the word, and simply indicate that sufficient dosage has been administered. Treatment of these X-ray "reactions" consists simply in keeping the area clean and free from infection, and applying a local anesthetic cream.

Other Applications—In addition to their diagnostic and therapeutic use X-rays have a wide range of applications of interest to the physician, the pharmacist, and the chemist. In the first place X-rays have been used extensively to examine the structure of atoms, molecules, and crystals, and to determine the forces and actions which are going on within the atom, molecule, or crystal. In recent years this method has opened up new frontiers which are of considerable importance and interest to the manufacturing and pharmaceutical chemist. For example, the crystal structures of such simple chemicals as sodium chloride, potassium chloride, and calcium carbonate have long been known, but recently the crystal structures of many complex materials such as insulin, oxalic acid, and glass have been elucidated by X-ray analysis.

Radiopharmaceuticals Used in Medicine

Albumin Microspheres

Tc 99m, In 111, In 113m, Pb 203

Human Albumin Microspheres (HAM); Albumin Microspheres (Human) (*3M*); 3M Brand Instant Microspheres (*3M*); (*Ackerman Nuclear*)

Sterile pyrogen-free spheres of denatured human albumin, usually supplied lyophilized in a special, sterile vial designed to permit rapid and efficient labeling and reconstitution as a suspension.

Preparation—Almost perfect spheres (microspheres) of denatured human albumin of nearly uniform size are prepared by homogenizing 1 mL of 25% human albumin with 100 mL of cottonseed oil. This emulsion is added to an additional 100 mL of heated cottonseed oil, the mixture is stored and maintained at 180° for 10 min, then cooled

in an ice bath, mixed with 200 mL of diethyl ether, and centrifuged. The precipitate, consisting of albumin microspheres, is washed several times with ether, then with alcohol, to remove the oil. The microspheres are suspended in alcohol, filtered through a 14-μm filter, then collected on a 0.22-μm filter, dried, and weighed into vials. The microsphres are tagged with ^{99m}Tc by reducing pertechnetate ^{99m}Tc with combinations of ascorbic acid, $FeCl_2$, and $SnCl_2$. Tagging with ^{111}In or ^{113m}In is accomplished at pH 3 in phosphate, then by adjusting to pH 11 and heating. A ^{203}Pb tag is added by heating at pH 10 with ionic ^{203}Pb.

Uses—Principally for *lung imaging*. The half-life for clearance from the lungs is 14 to 15 hr. Other uses include coronary, urogenital, liver, gastrointestinal, lymphatic, and peripheral circulation.

Note—In making dosage calculations, correct for radioactive decay; for radiological constants, see Table II.

Dose—*Intravenous*, the equivalent of 1 to 4 mCi.

Chromated Cr 51 Albumin Injection

Chromated Cr 51 Serum Albumin; Chromalbin (*Squibb*)

A sterile, pyrogen-free aqueous solution containing 0.5 to 2.5% human albumin in physiological saline. It may contain preservatives and buffers.

Preparation—By incubating ^{51}CrCl$_3$ with human albumin. The unreacted ^{51}Cr is then removed.

Uses—For the *detection* and *quantitation of gastrointestinal protein loss* and *placental localization*. Cr (III) has a strong affinity for plasma proteins without affecting erythrocytes. Conversely, Cr (VI) as Na$_2$^{51}CrO$_4$ binds to erythrocytes without affecting serum protein. These bonds seem to be essentially irreversible.

Note—In making dosage calculations, correct for radioactive decay; for radiological constants, see Table II.

Dose—*Gastrointestinal protein loss*, the equivalent of 30 to 50 μCi; *placental localization*, the equivalent of 30 to 35 μCi.

Iodinated I 125 Albumin Injection

Albumotope ^{125}I (*Squibb*); Risa-125 (*Abbott*); (*Amersham*); Radioiodinated Serum Albumin (Human) (IHSA I-125) (*Mallinckrodt*); Radioiodinated I 125 Serum Albumin (Human) (*Miles*)

A sterile, buffered, isotonic solution prepared to contain not less than 10 mg/mL of radioiodinated normal human albumin, and adjusted to provide not more than 1 mCi/mL of radioactivity. Other forms of radioactivity do not exceed 3% of the total radioactivity.

Preparation—By mild iodination of normal human albumin with ^{125}I to introduce not more than 1 g-atom/g-mol (60,000 g) of albumin. Iodination is usually carried out at 10°, in a slightly alkaline medium, by dropwise addition of very dilute hypochlorite or chloramine-T to a mixture of iodide and the protein. Unbound iodide is removed by an ion-exchange column and the product is sterilized by a Seitz filtration.

Description—Clear, colorless to slightly yellow solution; upon standing the radiation may cause both the albumin and the glass container to darken; pH between 7 and 8.5.

Uses—As *diagnostic aid* in the *determination of total blood* and *plasma volumes*. There are several advantages to the use of ^{125}I as a tag over ^{131}I. The shelf-life of ^{125}I-tagged compounds is greater due to the longer radiological half-life of the isotope and, because ^{125}I emits no beta radiation and its gamma radiation is relatively "soft," the radiation dose is minimal. The resulting decrease in radioautolysis of the tracer compound further increases its shelf-life. Of even greater importance is the decrease in the dose delivered to the patient. Collimation of the radiation is also simpler so it is possible to obtain greater resolution. Shielding problems and the protection of personnel are likewise simplified.

Note—In making dosage calculations, correct for radioactive decay; for radiological constants, see Table II.

Dose—*Intravenous*, the equivalent of 5 to 60 μCi; *usual*, 5 μCi.

Iodinated I 131 Albumin Injection

IHSA-^{131}I; Risa-131 (*Abbott*); Albumotope ^{131}I (*Squibb*); Radioiodinated (I 131) Serum Albumin (*Human*) (*Mallinckrodt*); (*Amersham*); Radioiodinated (I 131) Serum Albumin (*Miles*)

A sterile, buffered, isotonic solution prepared to contain not less than 10 mg/mL of radioiodinated normal human albumin, and adjusted to provide not more than 1 mCi/mL of radioactivity. Other forms of radioactivity do not exceed 3% of the total radioactivity.

Preparation—By mild iodination of normal human albumin with ^{131}I to introduce not more than 1 g-atom/g-mol (60,000 g) of albumin. See *Iodinated I 125 Albumin Injection*.

Description—Clear, colorless to slightly yellow solution; upon standing the radiation may cause both the albumin and the glass container to darken; pH between 7 and 8.5.

Uses—A *diagnostic aid* in the *determination* of *blood or plasma volumes*, *circulation times or cardiac output*, and as an *adjunct* to other diagnostic procedures in the detection and localization of brain tumors, in placental localization and in cisternography. Although available evidence indicates that the immunologic nature of human serum albumin is not altered by radioiodination, it is possible that patients receiving subsequent doses may exhibit allergic reactions.
Note—In making dosage calculations, correct for radioactive decay; for radiological constants, see Table II.
Dose—*Intravenous, blood-volume determination*, the equivalent of 5 to 50 μCi; *usual*, 5 μCi; *placental localization*, 3 to 5 μCi.

Iodinated I 131 Albumin Aggregated Injection

Aggregated Radioiodinated (^{131}I) Albumin (Human); Macroaggregated Albumin I 131; Albumotope-LS (*Squibb*); MAA^{131}I (*Mallinckrodt Nuclear*); Macroscan-131 (*Abbott*)

A sterile, aqueous suspension of normal human albumin that has been iodinated with ^{131}I and denatured to produce aggregates of controlled particle size. The injection contains 0.3 to 3 mg/mL of macroaggregated serum albumin with a specific activity between 0.2 and 1.2 mCi/mg.
Preparation—See *Iodinated I 125 Albumin Injection;* the aggregates are produced by heating under carefully controlled conditions to produce aggregates 10 to 90 μm in size.

Description—Dilute suspension of white to faintly yellow particles which may settle on standing; also, upon standing, the radiation may cause the glass container to darken.

Uses—For the *diagnostic study of the lungs* by radioisotope scanning or organ-imaging techniques. Its principal application is for the diagnosis of pulmonary embolism. Administered intravenously, the fragile clumps of albumin become lodged in the fine pulmonary capillaries where they remain for varying periods of time (a few hours) depending on particle size. Normally fewer than 0.5% of the pulmonary capillaries become blocked so the procedure presents no hazard to the patient through impairment of ventilation. As the aggregates disintegrate they are carried to the liver where they are phagocytized by the Kupffer cells. Prior administration of Lugol's solution minimizes thyroid uptake of released ^{131}I. The biological distribution following injection of mice or rats should indicate a lung uptake to liver uptake ratio of not less than 10:1.
Note—In making dosage calculations, correct for radioactive decay; for radiological constants, see Table II.
Dose—*Intravenous*, the equivalent of 150 to 300 μCi.

Chlormerodrin Hg 197 Injection

Mercury-^{197}*Hg*, [3-[(aminocarbonyl)amino]-2-methoxypropyl]chloro-, Neohydrin-197; (*Mallinckrodt; Squibb; Amersham*)

Chloro(2-methoxy-3-ureidopropyl)mercury-^{197}Hg [10375-56-1] $C_5H_{11}Cl^{197}HgN_2O_2$. *Injection:* A sterile solution containing chlormerodrin in which a portion of the molecules contain radioactive ^{197}Hg in the molecular structure. Other forms of radioactivity do not exceed 5% of the total radioactivity.
Preparation—Allylurea is acetoxymercurated by refluxing with mercuric acetate ^{197}Hg in methanol. Aqueous sodium chloride is then added, whereupon chlormerodrin ^{197}Hg precipitates. ^{197}Hg is obtained by neutron bombardment of enriched ^{196}Hg. A small amount of 24-hour ^{197m}Hg is also formed from ^{196}Hg, as well as a small amount of ^{203}Hg from bombardment of ^{202}Hg. If five days elapse before use of the isotope only about 3% of the ^{197m}Hg will remain.

Description—Clear, colorless solution; pH between 5.5 and 8.5.

Uses—A *diagnostic aid* for *scanning* the *brain* for suspected lesions and the kidneys for anatomical and functional abnormalities. In the brain chlormerodrin concentrates in neoplastic lesions. That which remains in the circulation is rapidly cleared by the kidneys. For brain scans chlormerodrin ^{197}Hg provides several advantages over *Iodinated I 131 Albumin Injection* in that it delivers less than one-half the radiation dose and, because of its rapid clearance from the circulation, a high tumor-to-background activity is achieved in about 4 hours, thereby permitting the scan to be made sooner after administration of the tracer dose. In addition it has a longer shelf-life and, because the radiation is more easily collimated, better resolution is obtained in the scans. A further reduction in radiation dose to the patient is provided through use of chlormerodrin ^{197}Hg.
Note—In making dosage calculations, correct for radioactive decay; for radiological constants, see Table II.
Dose—*Intravenous*, the equivalent of 100 to 150 μCi.

Chlormerodrin Hg 203 Injection

Mercury-^{203}*Hg*, [3-[(aminocarbonyl)amino]-2-methoxypropyl]chloro-, Neohydrin-203; (*Mallinckrodt; Amersham*)

Chloro(2-methoxy-3-ureidopropyl)mercury-^{203}Hg [2042-50-4] $C_5H_{11}Cl^{203}HgN_2O_2$. *Injection:* A sterile solution containing chlormerodrin in which a portion of the molecules contain radioactive ^{203}Hg in the molecular structure. Other forms of radioactivity do not exceed 5% of the total radioactivity.
Preparation—Allylurea is acetoxymercurated by refluxing with mercuric acetate ^{203}Hg in methanol. Aqueous sodium chloride is then added, whereupon chlormerodrin ^{203}Hg precipitates. ^{203}Hg is obtained by neutron bombardment of enriched ^{202}Hg. Small amounts of ^{197}Hg and ^{197m}Hg which are simultaneously formed from ^{196}Hg are allowed to decay before use of the ^{203}Hg.

Description—Clear, colorless solution; pH between 5.5 and 8.5.

Uses—See *Chlormerodrin Hg 197 Injection*.
Note—In making dosage calculations, correct for radioactive decay; for radiological constants, see Table II.
Dose—*Intravenous*, up to a total of the equivalent of 700 μCi; *usual*, the equivalent of 10 μCi/kg.

Chromic Phosphate P 32 Injection

Chromic Phosphate P 32 Suspension; Chromic Phosphate P 32 (*Abbott*); Phosphocol (*Mallinckrodt*)

A sterile suspension of $Cr^{32}PO_4$ [24381-60-0] in a suitable vehicle.
Preparation—By reacting $Na_2H^{32}PO_4$ with chromic nitrate in a saline-carboxymethylcellulose vehicle.

Description—Grayish-green to brownish-green suspension.

Uses—A *neoplastic suppressant* that has given best results for palliative treatment of pleural and peritoneal effusions. For this purpose it has largely replaced *Gold Au 198 Injection*. Because ^{32}P emits no gamma component in its radiation (other than Bremsstrahlung), the hazard to personnel is greatly reduced. In addition, the dose delivered per millicurie during an effective half-life period is about 10 times greater for ^{32}P than for ^{198}Au. Relatively smaller doses of ^{32}P can therefore be used. Since chromic phosphate ^{32}P remains *in situ* on interstitial injection it may be injected directly into a malignancy. It has been investigated for use in the treatment of prostatic carcinoma, urologic tumors, liver metastases, leukemia, and for lymph node irradiation.
Note—In making dosage calculations, correct for radioactive decay; for radiological constants, see Table II.
Dose—*Intravenous, intrapleural effusion*, the equivalent of 6 to 9 mCi; *intraperitoneal*, 10 mCi; *ascites*, 9 to 12 mCi; *leukemia*, 3.5 to 10 mCi.

Cobalt Co 60 and Iridium Ir 192 Sources

Actaloy Wire Sources (*Abbott*); (*Amersham*)

^{60}*Co Sources*—Cobalt rods activated by neutron bombardment and ensheathed in stainless steel. Each rod may contain a radioactivity of up to several thousand curies. Sources possessing a higher activity are obtained by the use of clusters of rods in a suitable support.

^{192}Ir *Sources*—Generally small stainless steel ensheathed seeds measuring approximately 3 mm in length and 0.5 mm in diameter, imbedded in a nylon ribbon, the number and spacing of the seeds depending on the application.

Preparation—^{60}Co *Sources:* By the reaction $^{59}Co + n \rightarrow {}^{60}Co + \gamma$. ^{192}Ir *Sources:* Neutron irradiation of iridium metal by the reaction $^{191}Ir + n \rightarrow {}^{192}Ir + \gamma$. ^{194}Ir produced simultaneously due to the presence of ^{193}Ir in the target will largely decay before use due to its 17.4-hour half-life.

Uses—^{60}Co has replaced radium, which is relatively expensive, for many radiation uses of the latter element. The use of ^{60}Co in alloys rather than the pure metal has increased the physical stability, making quite feasible its incorporation in sealed cells to fit various applicators. The 1.17 and 1.3 MeV gamma radiation is fully the equivalent of radium in biological effectiveness.

^{192}Ir provides a softer radiation, ie, less penetrating; the radioactive source is enclosed in nylon for interstitial use.

Note—In making dosage calculations, correct for radioactive decay; for radiological constants, see Table II.

Dose—^{60}Co *and* ^{192}Ir: *Therapeutic,* up to **7000 rads** in a single or in several doses.

Cyanocobalamin Co 57 Capsules and Solution

Racobalamin-57 (*Abbott*); Rubratope-57 (*Squibb*); Dicopac (*Amersham*); Cyanocobalamin Co 57 Capsules (*Mallinckrodt; Amersham*)

Vitamin B_{12}-^{57}Co [13115-03-2]. Cyanocobalamin (Chapter 53) in which a portion of the molecules contain radioactive ^{57}Co in the molecular structure; specific activity is not less than 0.5 μCi/μg. *Capsules. Solution:* Suitable for oral administration; contains a suitable antimicrobial agent.

Description—*Capsules:* May contain a small amount of solid or solids, or may appear empty. *Solution:* Clear, colorless to pink solution; pH between 4 and 5.5.

Uses—See *Cyanocobalamin Co 60.*
Note—In making dosage calculations, correct for radioactive decay; for radiological constants, see Table II.
Dose—*Schilling test,* usual, the equivalent of **0.5 μCi.**

Cyanocobalamin Co 60 Capsules and Solution

Rubratope-60 (*Squibb*); Racobalamin Co60 (*Abbott*); Cyanocobalamin Co60 Capsules (*Mallinckrodt*)

Vitamin B_{12}-^{60}Co [13422-53-2]. Cyanocobalamin (Chapter 53) in which a portion of the molecules contain radioactive ^{60}Co in the molecular structure; specific activity is not less than 0.5 μCi/μg. *Capsules. Solution:* Suitable for oral administration; contains a suitable antimicrobial agent.

Description—*Capsules:* May contain a small, rectangular solid, or may appear empty. *Solution:* Clear, colorless to pink solution; pH between 4 and 5.5.

Uses—A *diagnostic aid* to study the *absorption* and *deposition* of *vitamin B_{12}* in normal individuals and in patients with megaloblastic anemias. Since the normal human intestine can absorb significant amounts of the usually ingested quantities of vitamin B_{12} only in the presence of the intrinsic factor, radiocyanocobalamin solution is useful in the diagnosis of pernicious anemia, a clinical condition characterized by a marked deficiency or absence of this factor. Three different tests, using the orally administered radioactive substance, have been used for the estimation of intrinsic factor activity: (1) the estimation of the unabsorbed tracer in the stool, (2) the measurement of the radiation emanating from the liver, and (3) the determination of urinary radioactivity following a large parenteral dose of nonradioactive vitamin B_{12}. The first test requires the analysis of total fecal collections for 5 to 10 days; the second necessitates repeated body surface counts using a scintillation counter; and the third directly quantitates, in terms of the administered vitamin B_{12}-^{60}Co, the radioactivity in a 24-hour urine sample. Although the half-life of ^{60}Co is 5.24 years, recent evidence suggests that cyanocobalamin Co 60 solution is subject to decomposition on storage. Therefore, it appears advisable to retest stocks for radiochemical purity at intervals of 1 month or less.

Note—In making dosage calculations, correct for radioactive decay; for radiological constants, see Table II.

Dose—The equivalent of **0.5 to 1 μCi;** *usual,* **0.5 to 2 μg,** containing not more than **1 μCi.**

Ferric Hydroxide In 113m

A sterile nonpyrogenic suspension of ^{113m}In-labeled Fe(OH)$_3$ particles, most of which lie in the range of 20 to 50 μm in diameter.

Preparation—^{113m}In, eluted from a ^{113}Sn-^{113m}In generator with 0.05N HCl, is stirred with FeCl$_3$ solution while titrated with 0.5N NaOH to a pH between 11 and 12. Stirring is continued while 20% gelatin is added to a pH between 7.6 and 8.5 while heating in a boiling water bath. The preparation is then autoclaved. Goodwin, *et al, J Am Med Assoc 206:* 339, 1968.

Uses—A *diagnostic aid* in *lung imaging.*
Note—In making dosage calculations, correct for radioactive decay; for radiological constants, see Table II.
Dose—The equivalent of **0.5 to 2 mCi.**

Ferrous Citrate Fe 59 Injection

Ferrutope (*Mallinckrodt*); Ferrous Citrate Fe 59 (*Abbott*)

A sterile solution of radioactive iron (^{59}Fe) in the ferrous state and complexed with citrate, in Water for Injection [64521-35-3]. It may contain added sodium chloride in an amount to render the solution isotonic, and may contain bacteriostatic agents.

Preparation—By neutron bombardment of iron by the reaction $^{58}Fe(n,\gamma)^{59}Fe$. In the process, ^{55}Fe is also produced by the reaction $^{54}Fe(n,\gamma)^{55}Fe$. If enriched ^{58}Fe is bombarded the resulting ^{59}Fe will be purer.

Description—Clear, slightly yellow solution.

Uses—As a *diagnostic aid* for the evaluation of the *kinetics of iron metabolism.* Among the parameters which can be measured are plasma iron clearance half-time, plasma volume, hematocrit, blood volume, red-cell incorporation (percent utilization), daily iron clearance, daily hemoglobin formation and percent daily hemoglobin replacement. Ferrous citrate is especially useful in that it may be administered directly into the blood stream, where it reacts with the metal-binding globulin normally present in excess, thus avoiding the isolation and *in vitro* tagging of that protein. The rate of disappearance of ^{59}Fe from the blood, the rate of reincorporation into red cells, and the intermediate storage in the reticuloendothelial system may be followed by appropriate gamma-counting techniques.

Note—In making dosage calculations, correct for radioactive decay; for radiological constants, see Table II.
Dose—*Intravenous,* the equivalent of **5 to 10 μCi.**

Ferrous Hydroxide Tc 99m

Technetium-99m Iron Hydroxide (*Diagnostic Isotopes*)

A very fine dispersion of ^{99m}Tc-tagged particles of ferrous hydroxide prepared aseptically to provide a sterile, pyrogen-free product.

Preparation—Typically, by adding 30 mL of sterile, pyrogen-free eluate from a ^{99m}Tc generator to a vial containing 0.5 mL of ferrous sulfate solution equivalent to 2 mg Fe. ^{99m}Tc-Fe(OH)$_2$ is precipitated by adding 0.6 mL of 0.1N NaOH. The pH should be between 7.5 and 10.7. 1 mL of 5% gelatin is added to stabilize the particles and the final pH should be between 7.1 and 8.3.

Description—A very fine dispersion; most of the particles are in the range of 11 to 13 μm; essentially all particles fall within the range of 3 to 50 μm.

Uses—A *diagnostic aid* in *pulmonary scintigraphy.*
Note—In making dosage calculations, correct for radioactive decay; for radiological constants, see Table II.
Dose—*Lung imaging,* the equivalent of **2 to 3 mCi.**

Fibrinogen I 125 Injection

Ibrin (*Amersham*); Radionuclide Labeled (^{125}I) Fibrinogen (Human) Sensor (*Abbott*)

A sterile solution of fibrinogen, suitable for intravenous administration, which has been radioactively labeled with ^{125}I. It is normally supplied as a freeze-dried preparation to be reconstituted by addition of Sterile Water for Injection.

Preparation—Fibrinogen is a very labile protein readily denatured by high temperature (50° or less), and by handling and labeling. One of the more commonly used techniques used for the isolation of fibrinogen is that of Blombäck, which utilizes an alcohol and glycine fractionation of the citrated plasma. Iodination is then accomplished using a modification of one of the standard techniques in which ^{125}I is added in the form of I_2, ICl, or as iodide and subsequently oxidized with chloramine-T, electrolytically or enzymatically. Unreacted iodine is reduced by addition of sodium thiosulfate, and the ^{125}I-fibrinogen is immediately separated from the reaction by-products.

Uses—In the *diagnosis* and *localization* of *deep-vein thrombosis*, the accumulation of ^{125}I-fibrinogen in clots is observable by use of a radiation detector pressed to the surface of the limb. Radiation detectors designed for maximum sensitivity to the 27–35 keV photons emitted by ^{125}I are available for this purpose. Other applications include the detection of renal transplant rejections, tumors, and for the study of fibrinogen turnover.

Note—In making dosage calculations, correct for radioactive decay; for radiological constants, see Table II.

Dose—*Usual*, the equivalent of **100 μCi**.

Gallium Citrate Ga 67 Injection

Gallium-67 Citrate; Neoscan (*Medi-Physics*); Gallium Citrate Ga 67 (*New England Nuclear; Diagnostic Isotopes; Amersham*)

Gallium citrate Ga 67 [41183-64-6]; a sterile, pyrogen-free, isotonic solution.

Preparation—Gallium 67 is produced by proton irradiation of ^{67}Zn-enriched ZnO_2. Reactions are $^{67}Zn(p,n)^{67}Ga$ and $^{68}Zn(p,2n)^{67}Ga$. At the same time ^{66}Ga and ^{65}Ga are formed but they decay rapidly due to their short half-lives. The resulting ^{67}Ga is essentially carrier-free. The expiration date of the product is limited by the 78-hour half-life of ^{67}Ga. ^{67}Ga as the citrate has a biological half-life of 53 days and an effective half-life of 73.5 hours.

Uses—Has been shown to concentrate in tumors of soft tissue and bone. With respect to tumor-to-normal tissue concentration, it is reported to be superior to selenomethionine Se 75, chlormerodrin Hg 203, and human serum albumin I 125. It has been useful for diagnosis of lesions of the lung, breast, maxillary sinuses and liver by using scanning and organ-imaging techniques. A positive ^{67}Ga uptake is a potential indicator of certain malignancies such as lymphomas, bronchogenic carcinoma and Hodgkin's disease. In addition, ^{67}Ga is also useful for placental localization and for the identification of certain inflammatory conditions such as pancreatitis and disc-space infection. The mechanism of ^{67}Ga uptake is unknown.

Note—In making dosage calculations, correct for radioactive decay; for radiological constants, see Table II.

Dose—*Intravenous bolus*, the equivalent of **2.5 mCi**; *scanning*, the equivalent of **2 to 5 mCi**.

Gold Au 198 Injection

Aurcoloid-198 (*Mallinckrodt Nuclear*); Auroscan (*Abbott*); Aureotope (*Squibb*); (*Amersham*)

Gold (^{198}Au) [10043-49-9]. *Injection:* A sterile, colloidal solution of radioactive ^{198}Au stabilized by the addition of gelatin and suitable reducing agents.

Preparation—By neutron activation in a nuclear reactor by the reaction $^{197}Au(n,\gamma)^{198}Au$. The irradiated gold foil is dissolved in aqua regia. A colloidal dispersion is produced by chemical reduction, the pH is adjusted between 4.3 and 7.5, and gelatin is added as a stabilizer.

Description—*Injection:* Distinctly red, colloidal solution; colloidal particle size ranges between 2 and 60 nm; upon standing, the radiation may cause both the injection and the glass container to darken; pH between 4.3 and 7.5.

Uses—A *neoplastic suppressant*. Administration is carried out by allowing a flow of saline from a conventional infusion system to pass through the bottle in which the colloid has been shipped. If the exit needle, leading to the body cavity, is at the bottom of the container, all activity can be transferred with a minimum of exposure to the operators. A silver-coated gold colloid has been studied and found effective, but it does not seem to have met with wide acceptance. Experimentally ^{198}Au has been used for carcinoma of the prostate, carcinoma of the cervix, and tumors of the bladder.

Note—In making dosage calculations, correct for radioactive decay; for radiological constants, see Table II. Do not use the injection if it has changed from the distinctly red color.

Dose—*Antineoplastic, intracavitary injection, the* equivalent of **35 to 150 mCi**; *intravenous, liver scanning*, 1 to 5 **μCi/kg**.

Indium Chlorides In 111

Hydrated indium(3+)-^{111}In chlorides; Indium-111 as Indium Chloride (*Diagnostic Isotopes; Medi-Physics*)

Indium-111 is a cyclotron-produced radioisotope that is available as a mixture of $^{111}InCl_3$ hydrates in 0.05 N HCl.

Indium normally exists in aqueous solution in the 3+ valence state since indium compounds of lower valencies are unstable. For example, indium monochloride and dichloride disproportionate in the presence of water

$$3InCl \rightleftharpoons 2In + InCl_3$$

$$3InCl_2 \rightleftharpoons In + 2InCl_3$$

Indium (3+) ions are colorless and resemble aluminum (3+) ions in many ways. Since the solubility product constant (pK) of $In(OH)_3$ is 33.9, the hydroxide begins to precipitate when the pH is increased to about 3.6. Being amphoteric, indium hydroxide will redissolve in the presence of an excess of strong base.

In aqueous solution it is believed that indium chloride exists as a mixture of the following hydrated chlorides:

$[^{111}In(H_2O)_6]Cl_3$ Hexaaquoindium(3+)-^{111}In trichloride
$[^{111}In(H_2O)_5Cl]Cl_2$ Pentaaquochloroindium(2+)-^{111}In dichloride
$[^{111}In(H_2O)_4Cl_2]Cl$ Tetraaquodichloroindium(1+)-^{111}In chloride
$^{111}In(H_2O)_3Cl_3$ Triaquotrichloroindium-^{111}In

Preparation—A cadmium target is bombarded with 15 MeV deuterons to produce ^{111}In by the reactions $^{110}Cd(d,n)^{111}$In and $^{111}Cd(d,2n)^{111}$In. ^{111}In is then etched from the target with HCl, carrier Fe^{3+} is added, and the ^{111}In is precipitated, along with $Fe(OH)_3$, by adding NH_4OH. The precipitate is separated, dissolved in HCl, and the ferric iron removed by extraction with isopropyl ether.

Uses—^{111}In has been used to tag a variety of compounds. For example, ^{111}In-transferrin, which has been used as a replacement for ^{131}I-HSA; ^{111}In-EDTA and ^{111}In-DTPA, useful for cisternography; ^{111}In-bleomycin, which has been used for tumor localization. ^{111}In-labeled platelets have been used for the noninvasive detection of coronary thrombi. ^{111}In-labeled lymphocytes are useful for monitoring cardiac antirejection therapy and ^{111}In-labeled leucocytes have been used for the diagnosis of upper-abdominal infections, inflammation, and occult sepsis.

Note—In making dosage calculations, correct for radioactive decay; for radiological constants, see Table II.

Dose—For *CSF scan* (*lumbar intrathecal injection*), the equivalent of **0.2 to 1 mCi** of ^{111}In.

Indium Chlorides In 113m Injection

Hydrated indium(3+)-^{113m}In chlorides; Indium (^{113m}In) Chloride Injection; Indium-113m Generator (*New England Nuclear; Commissariat a l'energie Atomique; Amersham*)

A sterile, aqueous solution, suitable for intravenous administration, containing radioactive indium (^{113m}In) in the form of indium chloride. Other chemical forms of radioactivity do not exceed 5% of the total radioactivity.

Preparation—See *Indium Chlorides In 111*, above, for the chemistry of indium. ^{113m}In is formed by radioactive decay of ^{113}Sn and is obtained by "milking" a $^{113}Sn/^{113m}$In generator. The parent nuclide ^{113}Sn is bound to the stationary phase of the generator and indium chloride ^{113m}In is eluted with sterile, pyrogen-free, dilute HCl, using aseptic technique. The generator consists of a glass column containing zirconium oxide, silica gel or other solid support on which the ^{113}Sn is adsorbed. The column should be sterile so that a sterile product will be obtained on elution.

Uses—Indium chloride ^{113m}In has been used for *blood-pool studies*, including visualization of aneurysms, and in *placental scintigraphy*. In the form of various compounds it has also been used for liver, lung, and bone imaging. When administered intravenously at a pH of 4 or less it binds to transferrin, in which form it circulates throughout the vascular system. Because urinary excretion is so low, bladder activity is also low, making ^{113m}In a useful isotope for placental visualization. ^{113m}In-HSA replaces ^{131}I-HSA in various studies. ^{113m}In-colloids, including indium hydroxide ^{113m}In, stannous hydroxide ^{113m}In, ^{113m}In-MAA, indium sulfide ^{113m}In, and rhenium sulfide ^{113m}In have been used for pulmonary scans, liver scans, reticuloendothelial system studies, and placental scanning.

Chelated ^{113m}In-EDTA and ^{113m}In-DTPA have been used for brain scanning, glomerular filtration studies, and renal scanning.

Note—In making dosage calculations, correct for radioactive decay; for radiological constants, see Table II.

Dose—For *placental localization*, the equivalent of **1 mCi**; for *liver* and *spleen scans*, the equivalent of **1 to 3 mCi**.

Indium Hydroxide In 113m Injection

A sterile, aqueous dispersion of indium ^{113m}In hydroxide suitable for intravenous injection.

Preparation—Indium ^{113m}In chloride is obtained by eluting a ^{113}Sn/^{113m}In generator. The resulting sterile eluate is adjusted to a pH of 4 or higher, whereupon indium is converted to the extremely insoluble hydroxide. The particle size of the indium ^{113m}In hydroxide and the stability of the product are controlled by heating and by addition of a stabilizer such as gelatin, mannitol, or PVP and sodium bicarbonate.

Uses—For *liver, spleen* and *bone marrow scintigraphy.*

Note—In making dosage calculations, correct for radioactive decay; for radiological constants, see Table II.

Dose—The equivalent of **3 to 10 mCi**.

Insulin I 125 and I 131

Insulin I 125 (*Mallinckrodt; Amersham*); Imusay-125 (*Abbott*); Insulin I 131 (*Abbott; Mallinckrodt; Amersham*); Imusay-131 (*Abbott*)

Insulin containing a radioactive tag of ^{125}I and ^{131}I, respectively.

Preparation—By mild iodination with high-specific-activity radioactive iodine. Iodination is followed by purification of the product by means of dialysis, ion-exchange, and other processes. It is assumed that the addition of radioactive iodine occurs on available tyrosine moieties.

Uses—For *in vitro assay of circulating insulin,* either free or bound. If prepared for use in humans, these preparations can also be used to study insulin kinetics, including plasma disappearance.

Note—In making dosage calculations, correct for radioactive decay; for radiological constants, see Table II.

Dose—*Insulin* ^{125}I: the equivalent of **1 to 10 μCi**.

Iodohippurate Sodium I 131 Injection

Glycine, *N*-[2-(iodo-^{131}*I*)benzoyl]-, monosodium salt; Hippuran I 131 (*Mallinckrodt*); Hippuran-131 (*Abbott*); Hipputope-131 (*Squibb*); Iodohippurate Sodium I 131 Injection (*CIS Radiopharmaceuticals; Amersham*)

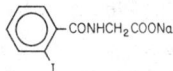

Monosodium *o*-iodo-^{131}I-hippurate [881-17-4] $C_9H_7{}^{131}$INNaO$_3$. *Injection:* A sterile solution containing *o*-iodohippurate sodium in which a portion of the molecules contain radioactive ^{131}I in the molecular structure. Other forms of radioactivity do not exceed 3% of the total radioactivity.

Preparation—*o*-Iodobenzoyl chloride-^{131}I is condensed with glycine with the aid of a dehydrochlorinating agent and the resulting *o*-iodohippuric acid is reacted with NaOH.

Description—Clear, colorless solution; pH between 7 and 8.5.

Uses—The excretion of certain compounds is almost entirely by way of the kidneys. If both kidneys are functioning properly, each should excrete approximately 50% of these compounds or any other substance with a blood concentration in excess of the renal threshold. The performance of the kidneys can be determined by injection of a radioactive compound which is quickly and exclusively excreted by the kidneys. The radioactive tag is selected from those nuclides which emit gamma radiation to permit external detection of the isotope.

The relative concentration of the tagged compound in each kidney can then be measured by means of two identical crystal scintillation detectors, one being positioned over each kidney. Renal malfunction is indicated if the measured activities are unequal.

Note—In making dosage calculations, correct for radioactive decay; for radiological constants, see Table II.

Dose—*Intravenous, renogram,* the equivalent of 1 to **30 μCi**; *scanning,* **200 to 300 μCi**.

Dosage Forms—In such volumes as may be requested by the physician.

Krypton Kr 81m

MPI Krypton Kr 81m Gas Generator (*Medi-Physics*)

Krypton Kr 81m [15678-91-8].

Preparation—Obtained as the decay product of ^{81}Rb, cyclotron-produced by bombardment of ^{79}Br (as sodium bromide) with 30 MeV alpha particles. The reaction is ^{79}Br(α, 2n)^{81}Rb. ^{81}Rb can also be produced using ^{3}He particles by use of the reaction ^{81}Br(^{3}He,3n)^{81}Rb or ^{79}Br(^{3}He,n)^{81}Rb. In a generator ^{81}Rb decays with a 4.7-hour half-life to ^{81m}Kr which in turn decays with a 13-sec half-life to ^{81}Kr emitting a 190-keV gamma ray.

^{81m}Kr gas is obtained by flushing air through a solution of the crude target material. It is filtered to ensure that no ^{81}Rb is carried along mechanically.

A ^{81m}Kr solution can be prepared by eluting a column containing Rb absorbed on zirconium phosphate cation exchanger.

Uses—For *lung function, ventilation,* and *perfusion,* and for *radiocardiology.*

Note—In making dosage calculations, correct for radioactive decay; for radiological constants, see Table II.

Dose—The equivalent of **5 mCi**.

Liothyronine I 125 and I 131

Triiodothyronine I 125 (or 131); ^{125}I-labeled T-3 (or 131); Resomat (*Mallinckrodt; Amersham*); Triomet (*Abbott*)

Liothyronine labeled with either ^{125}I or ^{131}I by mild oxidation. For the structure of liothyronine, see Chapter 52.

Preparation—By exchange of synthetic liothyronine with ^{131}I under carefully controlled conditions. Since such reactions always result in a mixture of products, purification must be effected by column and/or paper strip chromatography.

Uses—For *in vitro* evaluation of *thyroid function.* ^{125}I-labeled T-3, added to an aliquot of the patient's serum, along with a source of secondary binding sites (Sephadex, ion-exchange resin, etc.), will become bound to binding sites on thyroxine-binding proteins (TBP) not occupied by thyroxine. ^{125}I-labeled T-3 not bound to TBP becomes bound to the secondary binding sites in which form it is separated from the serum and measured, thereby providing an estimate of unoccupied binding sites on the TBP.

Note—Due to the high specific activity required, radiation damage can easily take place. This is in part prevented by the use of propylene glycol (50%) as a solvent. Packages should be refrigerated or even frozen during storage, and should not be used longer than 2 weeks.

Note—In making dosage calculations, correct for radioactive decay; for radiological constants, see Table II.

Dose—*Not for internal use.*

Levothyroxine I 125 and I 131

Thyroxine I 125 (*Nuclear Consultants; Amersham*); Thyroxine I 131 (*Abbott; Nuclear Consultants; Amersham*)

L-Thyroxine ($C_{15}H_{13}I_4NO_4$), obtained by synthesis (Chapter 52), tagged with either radioactive ^{125}I [24486-40-6] or ^{131}I [20196-65-0] in the 3′-position.

Uses—To *study the metabolism of endogenous thyroxine,* supplementing other tests of thyroid function. Following administration of a tracer dose, serial blood samples are measured for radioactivity. When data are plotted on semilogarithmic paper the disappearance half-time, calculated from the curve, provides useful information on thyroid function.

Radioactively labeled thyroxine is also used to measure thyroxine-binding protein capacity. When incubated with a small amount of a patient's serum, endogenous and tagged thyroxine will exchange and equilibrate. Separated by electrophoresis, the extent of binding can be determined by measuring the radioactivity of the bound and unbound thyroxine fractions.

Note—In making dosage calculations, correct for radioactive decay; for radiological constants, see Table II.

Oleic Acid I 125 and I 131
Triolein I 125 and I 131

Raoleic Acid-131 (*Abbott*); Raolin-131 (*Abbott*)
Triolein I 125 and I 131 (*Mallinckrodt*)

Oleic acid or triolein that has been iodinated by mild oxidation of ^{125}I or ^{131}I to form iodostearic acid ^{125}I (or ^{131}I) or triiodostearin ^{125}I (or ^{131}I), respectively.

Preparation—Iodinated triolein is prepared by the action of iodine monochloride on the highly purified fat triolein, in a carbon tetrachloride solution. After removal of the solvent, and also all "free iodine," it is diluted with peanut oil to an activity of about 1 mCi/mL. The iodine bond is relatively stable in the digestive tract, but it is liberated as the molecule is metabolized in the blood stream and tissues.

Iodinated oleic acid is prepared in a similar manner and has similar properties.

Uses—As *diagnostic agents* for *measuring fat absorption* in suspected pancreatic disease or other gastrointestinal dysfunction. The use of these agents is based on the fact that the triolein, requiring pancreatic lipase for hydrolysis prior to passage through the gastrointestinal wall, is not absorbed in cases of pancreatitis and cystic fibrosis, while the free acid, not requiring such hydrolysis, is taken up in the normal fashion. The assay for extent of absorption may be made on blood samples taken 2 to 8 hours after administration, or on 24- to 36-hour stool samples.

Note—In making dosage calculations, correct for radioactive decay; for radiological constants, see Table II.

Dose—*Oral* (capsules or oral solution), the equivalent of **25 to 50 μCi.**

Pentetate Indium Disodium In 111 Injection

Indate (2)-^{111}In-, [*N,N*-bis[2-[bis(carboxymethyl)amino]ethyl]-glycinato(5-)]-, disodium; MPI Indium DTPA In III (*Medi-Physics*)

Pentetic Acid

A sterile, aqueous solution of the pentetic acid (diethylenetriaminepentaacetic acid) chelate of indium 111 (^{111}In-DTPA), adjusted to a pH between 7.0 and 7.5, suitable for intravenous administration [60662-14-8]. As supplied, the radioactive concentration is 0.5 mCi/mL at the calibration time; the expiration date is established by the 67.5-hour half-life of ^{111}In.

Preparation—A solution of cyclotron-produced indium chlorides In 111 (see *Indium Chlorides In 111*), at a pH of 3.5 or less to avoid precipitation of indium hydroxide on subsequent chelation, is mixed with pentetic acid to form an indium-111 DTPA chelate. Stability of the chelate is enhanced by adjusting the pH of the solution to between 7.0 and 7.5, corresponding to formation of a trisodium salt of the complex.

Uses—A *diagnostic aid* for studies of *cardiac output*, for *cisternography*, for evaluation of *glomerular filtration*, and in *renal scintigraphy.*

Dose—The equivalent of **0.2 to 1 mCi.**

Pentetate Indium Trisodium In 113m Injection

Sodium salt of pentetic acid In 113m; Diethylenetriaminepentaacetic acid chelate of indium 113m; Indium-113m DTPA; ^{113m}In-DTPA

A sterile, aqueous solution of the pentetic acid chelate of indium 113m, adjusted to a pH between 7.0 and 7.5, suitable for intravenous administration.

Preparation—To a solution of ^{113m}In eluted from a generator with 0.05 *N* HCl (see *Indium Chlorides In 113 m Injection*) is added a solution of pentetic acid containing some ferric ion and HCl; the indium-113m DTPA chelate thus produced is stabilized by adjusting the solution to a pH between 7.0 and 7.5, corresponding to formation of a trisodium salt of the complex. This solution is sterilized.

Uses—A *diagnostic aid* for *brain scanning*, for studies of *glomerular filtration*, and for *kidney imaging.* Indium chelates of DTPA have been used in cisternography to study cerebral spinal fluid circulation; this fluid normally flows from the ventricular system into the subarachnoid space, finally concentrating in the parasagittal area.

Note—In making dosage calculations, correct for radioactive decay; for radiological constants, see Table II.

Dose—The equivalent of **0.5 to 2 mCi.**

Pentetate Ytterbium Trisodium Yb 169 Injection

Sodium salt of pentetic acid Yb 169; Diethylenetriaminepentaacetic acid chelate of ytterbium 169; Yb-169 DTPA; 3M Brand Ytterbium (Yb-169) DTPA (*3M*)

A sterile, aqueous solution of ^{169}Yb-DTPA suitable for oral or intravenous administration.

Preparation—Usually by addition of sterile ytterbium Yb 169 solution to buffered, lyophilized pentetic acid (DTPA) in a sterile ampul.

Uses—For *brain* and *kidney imaging*, and for *cisternographic* diagnosis of *CSF rhinorrhea.*

Note—In making dosage calculations, correct for radioactive decay; for radiological constants, see Table II.

Dose—*Usual*, the equivalent of **1 mCi.**

Potassium Chloride K 42 Injection

Potassium Chloride (^{42}K) Injection (*Amersham*)

A sterile, isotonic solution of Potassium ^{42}K Chloride suitable for intravenous administration.

Preparation—By neutron bombardment of natural potassium in a nuclear reactor, whereby the ^{41}K isotope (present to the extent of 6.9% in natural potassium) undergoes the reaction ^{41}K$(n,\gamma)^{42}$K.

Uses—For *tumor localization* and for studies of *renal blood flow.*

Note—In making dosage calculations, correct for radioactive decay; for radiological constants, see Table II.

Dose—*Intravenous*, the equivalent of **50 to 100 μCi.**

Potassium Chloride K 43 Injection

A sterile, isotonic solution of Potassium ^{43}K Chloride suitable for intravenous administration.

Preparation—By alpha-particle bombardment, using a cyclotron of moderate energy, of a natural argon target by the reaction ^{40}Ar$(\alpha,p)^{43}$K.

Use—For *heart imaging.*

Note—In making dosage calculations, correct for radioactive decay; for radiological constants, see Table II.

Dose—The equivalent of **10 to 50 μCi.**

Rose Bengal Sodium I 131 Injection

Spiro[isobenzofuran-1(3*H*),9'-[9*H*]-xanthene]-3-one, 4,5,6,7-tetrachloro-3',6'-dihydroxy-2',4',5',7'-tetraiodo-, disodium salt, labeled with iodine-131; Robengatope (*Squibb*); Rose Bengal Sodium I 131 Injection (*Mallinckrodt; CIS Radiopharmaceuticals; Amersham*)

Rose Bengal Sodium

4,5,6,7-Tetrachloro-2′,4′,5′-7′-tetraiodofluorescein disodium salt-131I [24916-55-0; 50291-21-9] $C_{20}H_2Cl_4{}^{131}I_4Na_2O_5$. *Injection:* A sterile solution containing rose bengal sodium in which a portion of the molecules contain radioactive 131I in the molecular structure; the injection may contain a suitable buffer. Other forms of radioactivity do not exceed 10% of the total radioactivity.

Preparation—By thermal condensation of tetrachlorophthalic anhydride with 2,4-diiodoresorcinol, and reaction of the resulting phthalein with NaOH. The purified product is labeled by isotope exchange with iodide I 131, which must be first oxidized to iodine. Rose bengal sodium normally contains small amounts of mono-, di-, and tri-iodo compounds as impurities.

Description—Clear, deep-red solution; pH between 7 and 8.5.

Uses—A *diagnostic aid (liver function)*, especially for differential diagnosis of hepatobiliary disease. Following intravenous injection, rose bengal sodium accumulates in the polygonal cells of the liver and is excreted via the biliary system as tetraiodotetrachlorofluorescein; if liver function is impaired excretion occurs via the kidneys.

Note—In making dosage calculations, correct for radioactive decay; for radiological constants, see Table II.

Dose—*Intravenous, usual,* the equivalent of 5 to 25 μCi.

Selenomethionine Se 75 Injection

Butanoic acid, 2-amino-4-(methylseleno-75Se)-, (S)-, L-Selenomethionine-Se 75 (*Amersham*); Selenomethionine-75 (*Diagnostic Isotopes; Mallinckrodt*); Sethotope (*Squibb*); Selenomethionine Se 75 Injection Diagnostic (*CIS Radiopharmaceuticals*)

(S)-2-Amino-4-(methylselenyl-75Se)butyric acid [1187-56-0] $C_5H_{11}NO_2{}^{75}Se$.

A sterile, aqueous solution of L-selenomethionine containing a 75Se radioactive tag. Selenomethionine is the selenium analogue of the naturally occurring amino acid methionine, the sulfur atom of which is replaced by selenium. The general biochemistry of selenomethionine and methionine is therefore quite similar.

Preparation—Extracted from yeast grown on a sulfur-free medium to which trace amounts of sodium selenite, labeled with 75Se, have been added. After hydrolysis of the yeast protein, 75Se-labeled selenomethionine is separated.

Uses—For *scintigraphy of the pancreas and parathyroid glands*. It has also been used to visualize the parotid and prostate glands. Following intravenous administration, selenomethionine Se 75 is localized in organs involved in protein synthesis and is incorporated in newly synthesized proteins. Pancreatic uptake, for example, is related to the synthesis of digestive enzymes in that organ. It has been reported that the blood level of selenomethionine Se 75 reaches a minimum 20 to 45 minutes after intravenous injection, then rises to about three-quarters of the 2-minute level.

Note—In making dosage calculations, correct for radioactive decay; for radiological constants, see Table II.

Dose—The equivalent of 100 to 250 μCi.

Sodium Chloride Na 22 Injection

(Abbott; Amersham)

A sterile, pyrogen-free solution of sodium chloride 22Na [17112-21-9] suitable for injection.

Preparation—Cyclotron-produced by bombarding 24Mg with deuterons. The reaction is $^{24}Mg(d,\alpha)^{22}Na$.

Uses—As an injection for determination of *circulation times, sodium space,* and *total exchangeable sodium.* While use of 24Na has certain advantages over 22Na in medicine, its half-life of only 15 hours creates problems of supply and the usual tracer dose of 22Na is well within the accepted tolerance level. Because 22Na emits positrons it can be detected readily by coincidence counting methods which combine the advantages of low background activity with high resolution.

Note—In making dosage calculations, correct for radioactive decay; for radiological constants, see Table II.

Dose—*Intravenous,* the equivalent of 5 to 10 μCi.

Sodium Chromate Cr 51 Injection

Chromic acid ($H_2{}^{51}CrO_4$), disodium salt; Chromitope Sodium (*Squibb*); Rachromate-51 (*Abbott*); Sodium Chromate Cr 51 Injection (*Mallinckrodt; Amersham*)

Disodium chromate ($Na_2{}^{51}CrO_4$) [10039-53-9]. *Injection:* A sterile solution of radioactive 51Cr processed in the form of sodium chromate in water for injection. For uses where an isotonic solution is required, sodium chloride may be added in appropriate amounts.

The specific activity of the injection is not less than 10 mCi/mg of sodium chromate at the end of the expiration period. Other forms of radioactivity do not exceed 10% of the total radioactivity.

Preparation—By neutron bombardment of enriched 50Cr.

Description—Clear, slightly yellow solution; pH between 7.5 and 8.5.

Uses—A *biological tracer* to measure *circulating red-cell volume, red-cell survival time,* and *whole-blood volume* (red-cell mass and plasma volume). To tag erythrocytes, a sample of the patient's blood or of donor blood is mixed with a solution of $Na_2{}^{51}CrO_4$ and allowed to remain until the isotope diffuses into cells (15 to 60 min). Once inside the cell, the hexavalent anionic chromium ($CrO_4{}^{2-}$) is reduced to the trivalent cationic chromium (Cr^{3+}), which firmly associates with the globin portion of the cell contents. The unbound chromium (in the plasma) is either reduced with ascorbic acid or removed by washing the cells. The treated blood or suspension of cells is then injected into the circulation, time allowed for complete *in vivo* mixing, and samples taken for scintillation counting. Red-cell or whole-blood volume is estimated by the radioisotope dilution method. Normal mean values for whole-blood volume obtained by the isotope method are 65.6 ± 5.96 mg/kg.

Such tagged cells also provide an excellent means of studying red-cell disappearance, as in hemolytic anemias and gastrointestinal bleeding. Platelets may also be labeled, though less effectively. For such purposes, it is essential that the specific activity be high—at least 5 to 15 mCi/mg. Such a solution, prepared by the peroxide oxidation of $CrCl_3$, is essentially colorless.

For greatest tagging efficiency, sterile vials are available containing a special formula ACD solution. The blood and chromate are added directly to these vials wherein tagging takes place.

For those uses where chromic chloride is required, it may be easily secured by the addition of ascorbic acid to the above-mentioned chromate solution.

Sodium radiochromate has not been shown to produce any significant deleterious effects on normal erythrocytes.

The usual dose given below is mixed with 40 or 50 mL of whole blood withdrawn from the patient or from a compatible donor.

Note—In making dosage calculations, correct for radioactive decay; for radiological constants, see Table II.

Dose—*Intravenous,* the equivalent of 15 to 200 μCi; *usual,* 15 to 20 μCi.

Sodium Fluoride F 18 Injection

Sodium Fluoride ($Na^{18}F$); Fluorine 18 Injection (*Medi-Physics*)

A sterile, aqueous solution, suitable for intravenous injection, containing fluoride ion (18F) in sodium chloride injection. Other chemical forms of radioactivity do not exceed 10% of the total radioactivity.

Preparation—Reactor-produced 18F is obtained by neutron bombardment of enriched 6Li in the form of lithium carbonate. The reaction $^6Li(n,\alpha)^3H$ results in the production of energetic tritons (3H or t) which, in turn, react with oxygen according to the reaction $^{16}O(t,n)^{18}F$. The 18F produced in this way is heavily contaminated with tritium, which must be removed before use. When produced in a cyclotron, according to the reaction $^{20}Ne(d,\alpha)^{18}F$, the resulting 18F has a very high specific activity and is much purer than the reactor-produced material.

Use—For *bone imaging, especially to define areas of altered osteogenic activity.*

Note—In making dosage calculations, correct for radioactive decay; for radiological constants, see Table II.

Sodium Iodide I 123

(New England Nuclear; Medi-Physics; Benedict Nuclear)

Sodium iodide (Na[123]I) [41927-88-2]. Radioactive ^{123}I processed in the form of sodium iodide obtained from bombardment of enriched tellurium 124 with protons or enriched tellurium 122 with deuterons or by decay of xenon 123 in such manner that it is carrier-free. Other forms of radioactivity do not exceed 5% of the total radioactivity. *Capsules:* For oral use only. *Solution:* For oral or intravenous administration.

Preparation—[123]I can be produced directly by bombardment of enriched [124]Te with protons or enriched [122]Te with cyclotron-accelerated deuterons from the reaction [122]Te(d,n)[123]I. It is also produced through negatron decay of [123]Xe. One of the best methods for producing [123]Xe is by bombardment of an [127]I target with 50 to 60 MeV protons. The reaction is represented as [127]I$(p,5n)$[123]Xe. After up to three hours of irradiation the iodine target is dissolved in aqueous potassium iodide and helium is flushed through the solution. Water vapor is removed from the helium stream by use of a dry ice-acetone trap and the [123]Xe is collected in a liquid nitrogen trap. Beta decay of the [123]Xe yields [123]I. This method eliminates virtually all radioactive contaminants in the [123]I.

Description—*Capsules:* May contain a small amount of solid or solids, or may appear empty. *Solution:* Clear, colorless; on standing both the solution and the glass container may darken as a result of the effects of the radiation.

Uses—For *diagnostic procedures* in *thyroid function studies* and for other studies utilizing iodinated compounds for *organ imaging*, including the thyroid, liver, lung, and brain. The half-life of 13.2 hours and the radiation characteristics result in a radiation dose far less than that delivered by other iodine isotopes.
Note—*In making dosage calculations, correct for radioactive decay; for radiological constants, see Table II.*
Dose—*Oral,* the equivalent of **10 to 400 μCi;** *intravenous,* **10 to 200 μCi;** for *uptake studies,* **10 to 20 μCi;** for *scanning,* **100 to 400 μCi.**

Sodium Iodide I 125

Iodotope I-125 *(Squibb)*; Sodium Iodide I 125 *(Mallinckrodt; Amersham)*

Sodium iodide (Na[125]I) [24359-64-6]. Radioactive ^{125}I processed in the form of sodium iodide in such manner that it is essentially carrier-free. Other forms of radioactivity do not exceed 5% of the total radioactivity. *Capsules:* For oral use only. *Solution:* For oral or intravenous administration.

Preparation—Reactor reduction by neutron bombardment of xenon gas, represented by the reaction

$$^{124}\text{Xe}(n,\gamma)^{125}\text{Xe} \xrightarrow[18\ \text{hr}]{\text{EC}} {}^{125}\text{I}$$

yields a relatively pure product in large quantities. Xenon, at pressures up to 5000 psi, is irradiated with a high neutron flux for several hours. Irradiation is terminated before large quantities of ^{125}I are produced by decay of the [125]Xe, otherwise the product becomes contaminated with [126]I produced in the reaction [125]I(n,γ)[126]I.

Description—*Capsules:* May contain a small amount of solid or solids, or may appear empty. *Solution:* Clear, colorless; on standing both the solution and the glass container may darken as a result of the effects of the radiation.

Uses—A *diagnostic aid* in determining *thyroid function*. In some applications sodium iodide I 125 is superior to sodium iodide I 131 for organ-imaging because the dose to the patient may be decreased and the organ is often delineated more clearly through improved resolution. Sodium iodide I 125 has been used for thyroid, liver, and brain scans with good results.
Therapeutically ^{125}I has been found useful for treatment of deep-seated tumors such as those in the chest which are not surgically resectable. In such cases, sufficient I 125 to yield a total dose of about 15,000 RADS per year has been found helpful.
Note—*In making dosage calculations, correct for radioactive decay; for radiological constants, see Table II.*
Dose—*Usual diagnostic,* the equivalent of **50 to 100 μCi.**

Sodium Iodide I 131

Iodotope *(Squibb)*; Oriodide-131, Radiocaps-131, Theriodide-131 *(Abbott)*; *(CIS Radiopharmaceuticals; Amersham; Mallinckrodt)*

Sodium iodide (Na[131]I) [7790-26-3]. Radioactive ^{131}I processed in the form of sodium iodide from products of uranium fission or neutron bombardment of tellurium in such manner that it is essentially carrier-free and contains only minute amounts of naturally occurring iodine 127. Other forms of radioactivity do not exceed 5% of the total radioactivity. *Capsules:* For oral use. *Solution:* For oral or intravenous administration.

Preparation—If prepared from the products of uranium fission it is necessary that other radioactive fission products be separated by appropriate chemical techniques. Neutron bombardment of tellurium results in production of ^{131}I through the reactions

$$^{130}\text{Te}(n,\gamma)^{131}\text{Te} \xrightarrow[24.8\ \text{min}]{\beta^-} {}^{131}\text{I}.$$

Description—*Capsules:* May contain a small amount of solid or solids, or may appear empty. *Solution:* Clear, colorless; on standing both the solution and the glass container may darken as a result of the effects of the radiation; pH between 7.5 and 9.0.

Uses—A *diagnostic aid* in determining *thyroid function* and a *neoplastic suppressant.*
Note—*In making dosage calculations, correct for radioactive decay; for radiological constants, see Table II.*
Dose—*Oral* or *intravenous, thyroid function determination,* the equivalent of 5 to 15 μCi; *usual* 5 to 10 μCi; *thyroid inhibitor,* 2 to 10 mCi (2000 to 10,000 μCi) as a single dose or in divided doses 6 to 8 weeks apart; *thyroid scanning,* 30 to 100 μCi.

Sodium Pertechnetate Tc 99m Injection

Pertechnetic acid (H[99m]TcO$_4$), sodium salt
Injection *(Mallinckrodt; Medi-Physics; CIS Radiopharmaceuticals; New England Nuclear)*. Generators *(Abbott; General Radioisotope Products; Mallinckrodt; Squibb; New England Nuclear; Amersham; Union Carbide; IMAJ International)*

Sodium pertechnetate (Na[99m]TcO$_4$) [23288-60-0]. *Injection:* A sterile solution, suitable for intravenous or oral administration, containing radioactive ^{99m}Tc in the form of sodium pertechnetate and sodium chloride to make the solution isotonic. Technetium 99m is formed by decay of molybdenum 99, a radioactive isotope of molybdenum obtained by neutron bombardment of molybdenum 98 or as a product of uranium fission. Other forms of ^{99m}Tc do not exceed 5% of the total radioactivity.

Preparation—Commonly by elution of a generator or "cow" containing [99]Mo (half-life, 67 hours). Decay of [99]Mo results in the buildup of its daughter, ^{99m}Tc, at a rate that permits eluting the generator about once a day.
Generators are usually sterilized by the manufacturer so a sterile, pyrogen-free solution of sodium pertechnetate ^{99m}Tc can be obtained by aseptic elution. Prior to use, the sodium pertechnetate ^{99m}Tc solution should be assayed. [57]Co standards are usually used for this purpose since the 123 keV and 137 keV photopeaks of [57]Co are of nearly the same energy as the 140 keV and 142 keV photopeaks of [99m]Tc.
[99m]Tc is an almost ideal isotope for medical applications. Its half-life is long enough to allow completion of diagnostic procedures using it, yet short enough that the radiation dose to the patient is minimal. Lack of a beta component in the radiation further decreases the dose delivered to the patient. Because greater activities can therefore be used, scanning time can be reduced accordingly. The 140 keV gamma energy is weak enough that good collimation is readily achieved, yet hard enough to penetrate tissue so deep organ-scanning is possible.
The chemistry of technetium is similar to that of other members of Group VIIB, manganese and rhenium. The pertechnetate TcO$_4^-$ resembles iodine in that it is taken up by the thyroid. To reduce thyroid uptake of [99m]Tc a protective dose of potassium perchlorate is often administered.
Uses—Has been used for the *detection and location of cranial lesions, thyroid and salivary gland imaging, placenta localization, and blood pool imaging.* It has also been used to tag many compounds and, in one form or another, has been used to visualize the brain,

liver, kidney, lungs, placenta and other organs and tissues. Erythrocytes have also been labeled with ^{99m}Tc.

Note—In making dosage calculations, correct for radioactive decay; for radiological constants, see Table II.

Dose—*Usual*, the equivalent of 1 to 5 mCi.

Sodium Phosphate P 32 Solution

Phosphoric-^{32}P acid, disodium salt; Radioactive Phosphorus Solution; Phosphotope (*Squibb*); Sodium Phosphate P 32 Injection (*Mallinckrodt; Amersham; Abbott*)

Disodium phosphate-^{32}P [7635-46-3]. *Solution:* A solution, suitable for either oral or intravenous administration, containing radioactive ^{32}P processed in the form of sodium phosphate from the neutron bombardment of elemental sulfur. Inactive sodium phosphate may be added during the process. Other forms of radioactivity are absent.

Preparation—By neutron irradiation of elemental sulfur in an atomic reactor. The ^{32}P, produced by the reaction $^{32}S(n,p)^{32}P$, is leached from the melted sulfur with NaOH solution in the form $Na_3{}^{32}PO_4$. It is then purified chemically as a carrier-free solution of $Na_2H^{32}PO_4$.

Description—Clear, colorless solution; on standing, radiation may cause both the solution and the glass container to darken; pH between 5.0 and 6.0.

Uses—A *neoplastic* and *polycythemic suppressant* and a *diagnostic aid* for the localization of certain ocular tumors.

Note—In making dosage calculations, correct for radioactive decay; for radiological constants, see Table II.

Dose—*Usual*, oral or intravenous, *diagnostic*, the equivalent of 250 μCi to 1 mCi; *therapeutic*, 1 to 7 mCi.

Strontium Sr 85 Injection

Strotope (*Squibb*); Stronscan-85 (*Abbott*); (*Mallinckrodt; Amersham*)

Strontium (^{85}Sr) [13967-73-2]. *Injection:* A sterile solution of ionic radioactive strontium, usually prepared from strontium nitrate [24381-59-7] or strontium chloride [24359-46-4] and suitable for intravenous administration, in water for injection. Sodium chloride may be added to render the solution isotonic.

Preparation—By neutron bombardment of a strontium salt enriched in ^{85}Sr.

Description—Clear, colorless solution; pH between 4 and 7.

Uses—A *diagnostic aid* for scanning bones and bony structures to detect and define lesions and to study bone growth and abnormal formations. The long half-life (64 days) and slow turnover rate for ^{85}Sr are disadvantages since the radiation dose to the bones is necessarily high and repetitive studies are usually not possible.

Note—In making dosage calculations, correct for radioactive decay; for radiological constants, see Table II.

Dose—*Intravenous, usual, adults*, the equivalent of 50 to 100 μCi; *children under 20 years*, 10 to 40 μCi.

Technetium Tc 99m Albumin Injection

CintiChem Technetium 99m HSA Multi-dose Kit (*Union Carbide*); Electrolysis Kit for preparation of ^{99m}Tc-Labeled Human Serum Albumin (*New England Nuclear*); (*Mallinckrodt; Diagnostic Isotopes*)

A sterile, isotonic solution of human albumin in which a portion of the molecules are labeled with ^{99m}Tc. The solution is suitable for intravenous administration.

Preparation—See *Technetium Tc 99m Albumin Aggregated Injection.*

Uses—See *Iodinated I 131 Albumin Injection.*

Note—In making dosage calculations, correct for radioactive decay; for radiological constants, see Table II.

Dose—*Usual*, the equivalent of 3 to 5 mCi.

Technetium Tc 99m Albumin Aggregated Injection

Technetium (^{99m}Tc)-Labeled Macroaggregated Human Serum Albumin Injection; TechneScan MAA (*Mallinckrodt*); Macrotec (*Squibb*); Lung-aggregate Reagent Kit (*Medi-Physics*); MAA Tc 99m Imaging Agent

(*CIS Radiopharmaceuticals*); Pulmolite Technetium Tc 99m Aggregated Albumin Kit (*New England Nuclear*); CintiChem Technetium 99m HSA Multi-dose Kit (*Union Carbide*); (*Ackerman Nuclear; Amersham; Diagnostic Isotopes*); A-N Stannous Aggregated Albumin (*A-N Radiopharmaceuticals*)

A sterile, aqueous suspension of human albumin that has been denatured to produce aggregates of controlled particle size that are labeled with ^{99m}Tc. It is suitable for intravenous administration. It may contain antimicrobial, reducing, chelating, and stabilizing agents, buffers and nonaggregated human albumin. Other forms of radioactivity do not exceed 10% of the total radioactivity.

Preparation—Human albumin, denatured by heating so as to produce aggregates of controlled particle size, may be tagged with ^{99m}Tc by any of several methods which generally involve reducing systems to convert heptavalent Tc as pertechnetate ($TcO_4{}^-$) to a lower oxidation state. Albumin can be tagged by reduction of Tc (VII) with either Sn (II) or Fe (II), alone or in conjunction with ascorbic acid, at an acid pH followed by adjustment to pH 6 with NaOH. Anionic Tc is removed by use of an anion-exchange column. Only pyrogen-free water is used for reagents and the final preparation is sterilized by passage through a microbial filter.

^{99m}Tc-HSA can also be prepared by electrolytic reduction of pertechnetate 99m in the presence of albumin. Sterile ^{99m}Tc freshly eluted from a generator is added to albumin in the presence of dilute HCl and a trace of FeCl$_2$. Reduction of pertechnetate is accomplished by passing a direct current through the solution following which the pH is adjusted by addition of a buffer.

Uses—See *Iodinated I 131 Albumin Injection.* ^{99m}Tc is preferred to ^{131}I as a radioactive tag because of the much smaller radiation dose delivered to the patient. ^{99m}Tc-albumin is a useful radiopharmaceutical for static blood-pool imaging, angiography, dynamic function tests, and visualization of the placenta. The microaggregate is used for liver scanning, the macroaggregate for lung scanning.

Note—In making dosage calculations, correct for radioactive decay; for radiological constants, see Table II.

Dose—*Intravenous, static blood-pool imaging*, the equivalent of 3 to 5 mCi; *angiography*, 10 to 15 mCi; *placental localization*, 1 mCi.

Technetium Tc 99m Etidronate Injection

Phosphonic acid, (1-hydroxyethylidine)bis-, sodium technetium-^{99m} salt; 1-Hydroxyethane-1,1-diphosphonate (EHDP), ^{99m}Tc-labeled; ^{99m}Tc-EHDP; Sodium Etidronate Tc 99m; Tc-99m HEDP (1-hydroxyethylidine diphosphonate); Sodium Diphosphonate (Tin) (*Diagnostic Isotopes*); Osteoscan (*Procter & Gamble*); HEDSPA (*Union Carbide*); MPI Stannous Diphosphonate (*Medi-Physics*); (*Ackerman Nuclear*)

Etidronate Sodium

Sodium technetium-^{99m}Tc (1-hydroxyethylidine)diphosphonate [63951-52-0]. *Injection:* A sterile, clear, colorless solution, suitable for intravenous administration, of radioactive ^{99m}Tc in the form of a chelate of sodium hydroxyethylidinediphosphonate (etidronate sodium). Other forms of radioactivity do not exceed 10% of the total radioactivity.

Preparation—1-(Hydroxyethylidene)diphosphonic acid (etidronic acid) may be prepared by treating acetic acid with PCl$_3$; the disodium salt (HEDSPA) forms when a solution of etidronic acid is adjusted to a pH of 8.5. To the solution of etidronate sodium, stannous chloride and sometimes a stabilizer such as sodium ascorbate are added, and the resulting solution is distributed into vials and lyophilized (alternatively a mixture of dry ingredients may be prepared). The labeled injection is prepared by adding a freshly eluted solution of ^{99m}Tc to a vial and mixing thoroughly.

Uses—A very useful injection for *bone imaging*, since the diphosphonate is more stable than the polyphosphate, and it also has been found superior to ^{18}F bone scans and to roentgen studies; it is frequently more sensitive in detecting metastases to the bone. For this purpose it is considered to be one of the best imaging agents available.

Note—*In making dosage calculations, correct for radioactive decay; for radiological constants, see Table II.*
Dose—*Intravenous*, the equivalent of 5 to 15 mCi.

Technetium Tc 99m Iminodiacetic Acid (IDA) and IDA *N*-Substituted Derivatives

Etifenin, EIDA or diethyl-IDA (*Amersham*); PIPIDA or *p*-isopropyl-IDA (*Diagnostic Isotopes*); HIDA or Hepatobiliary-IDA (*Medi-Physics*); PBIDA of *p*-butyl-IDA (*Syncor*); Hepatolite, Technetium Tc 99m Disofenin Kit, DISIDA or diisopropyl-IDA (*New England Nuclear*); Mebrofenin or 3-bromo-2,4,6-trimethylphenylcarbamoyl-IDA (*Squibb*)

Preparation—Usually in kit form, each vial containing the product in sterile, pyrogen-free, lyophilized form with an appropriate amount of stannous chloride. The solution is reconstituted and the substance tagged by adding sterile, pyrogen-free Sodium Pertechnetate Tc 99m.
Use—Hepatobiliary imaging agents.
Dose—Intravenous: non-jaundiced patient 1–5 mCi, jaundiced patient 3–8 mCi.

Technetium Tc 99m Ferpentate Injection

Renotec, Technetium 99m-Iron Ascorbate-DTPA Kit (*Squibb*)

A sterile, aqueous solution of iron ascorbate pentetic acid that is complexed with ^{99m}Tc. It is suitable for intravenous administration. Other forms of radioactivity do not exceed 10% of the total radioactivity.
Preparation—Usually in kit form, each vial in the kit containing a sterile solution of ferric chloride, N,N-bis[2-[bis(carboxymethyl)amino]ethyl]glycine complex, and ascorbic acid adjusted to a pH of 2 to 4. A sterile solution of sodium pertechnetate ^{99m}Tc, freshly eluted from a generator, is added to the mixture in the vial and, after adjustment of pH with sodium hydroxide, a solution of pentetic acid (diethylenetriaminepentaacetic acid; DTPA; see formula under *Pentetate Indium Disodium In 111 Injection*) is added. The chelate of ^{99m}Tc-iron ascorbate-DTPA is produced on gentle mixing.
Use—For *kidney imaging*.
Note—*In making dosage calculations, correct for radioactive decay; for radiological constants, see Table II.*
Dose—The equivalent of 3 to 5 mCi.

Technetium Tc 99m Pentetate Injection

Diethylenetriaminepentaacetic acid chelate of technetium 99m; Technetium-99m DTPA (Tin); ^{99m}Tc-DTPA; Technetium Tc 99m DTPA (Sn) Kit (*CIS Radiopharmaceuticals; Diagnostic Isotopes; General Radioisotope Products*); (*Cambridge Nuclear; Ackerman Nuclear; Mallinckrodt*); Techneplex (*Squibb; Bio-Dynamics*)

$$\left[Tc^{4+} \begin{array}{c} ^{-}OOCCH_2 \quad CH_2COO^- \ CH_2COO^- \\ NCH_2CH_2NCH_2CH_2 \, N \\ ^{-}OOCCH_2 \qquad\qquad CH_2COO^- \end{array} \right] Na^+$$

A sterile, aqueous solution of the diethylenetriaminepentaacetic acid (pentetic acid; DTPA; see formula under *Pentetate Indium Trisodium In 111 Injection*) chelate of ^{99m}Tc, suitable for intravenous administration [65454-61-7].
Preparation—Usually by addition of sterile pertechnetate ^{99m}Tc saline solution to an aliquot of buffered stock solution of DTPA containing stannous chloride as a reducing agent for pertechnetate. If sterile conditions are maintained no further purification is required. Instant DTPA ^{99m}Tc kits are commercially available which contain vials of lyophilized reagents to prolong shelf-life.
Uses—Although it is thought not to be a true chelate, it does not tend to concentrate in any organ as is the case with pertechnetate 99m, which follows the pathway of iodide. DTPA ^{99m}Tc is uniformly distributed throughout the extracellular space and is rapidly cleared by the kidneys without retention. The compound has been found useful for *brain* and *kidney visualization*, for *vascular dynamic studies* for measurement of *glomerular filtration* and for *lung ventilation* studies.
Note—*In making dosage calculations, correct for radioactive decay; for radiological constants, see Table II.*
Dose—*Intravenous*, for *kidney imaging*, the equivalent of up to 10 mCi; for *brain imaging*, up to 15 mCi.

Technetium Tc 99m Pyrophosphate Injection (Tc-99m PPi)

Tc 99m Pyrophosphate (Sn) Kit (*General Radioisotope Products; Cambridge Nuclear*); TechneScan PYP Kit (*Mallinckrodt*); Stannous Pyrophosphate; Pyrolite (Technetium Tc 99m Pyrophosphate/Trimetaphosphate Kit) (*New England Nuclear*); Phosphotec (Technetium Tc 99m Pyrophosphate-Tin Kit) (*Squibb*); (*CIS Radiopharmaceuticals; Ackerman Nuclear; Diagnostic Isotopes*)

$$NaO\!-\!\overset{\displaystyle O}{\underset{\displaystyle NaO}{P}}\!-\!O\!-\!\overset{\displaystyle O}{\underset{\displaystyle ONa}{P}}\!-\!ONa$$

Sodium Pyrophosphate

A sterile, aqueous solution, suitable for intravenous administration, of pyrophosphate labeled with ^{99m}Tc. It may contain antimicrobial agents, buffers, reducing agents, and stabilizers. Other forms of radioactivity do not exceed 10% of the total radioactivity.
Preparation—Sodium pyrophosphate, mixed with stannous tin, is supplied in kits of single or multiple-dose vials. Each vial contains a measured amount of pyrophosphate and stannous tin as a dry mix or as the residue of a lyophilized solution. The technetium Tc 99m pyrophosphate-tin complex is prepared by adding to the vial sodium pertechnetate Tc 99m injection.
Uses—As a *skeletal imaging agent* it is used to demonstrate regions of altered osteogenesis. For optimal results bone imaging should be performed 2 to 4 hours following administration. As a *cardiac imaging agent* it is used as an adjunct to the diagnosis of acute myocardial infarct; imaging is recommended 45 to 60 minutes postinjection. Under certain conditions technetium ^{99m}Tc pyrophosphate concentrates in muscle tissue. It has been observed to concentrate in contused myocardium, with contused-to-normal ratios of 8 to 41, and in muscle following exercise in patients with McArdle syndrome.
Note—*In making dosage calculations, correct for radioactive decay; for radiological constants, see Table II.*
Dose—For *bone imaging and cardiac imaging*, the equivalent of 10 to 15 mCi administered over a 10- to 20-second period.

Technetium Tc 99m Sulfur Colloid Injection

Collokit (*Abbott*); TechneColl Kit (*Mallinckrodt*); TechneColl (*Medi-Physics*); Tesuloid (*Squibb*); Sulfur Colloid Kit (*New England Nuclear; CIS Radiopharmaceuticals*); TSC Sulfur Colloid Kit (*Union Carbide*); (*Ackerman Nuclear*)

A sterile, colloidal dispersion of sulfur labeled with ^{99m}Tc, suitable for intravenous administration [7704-34-9]. It may contain chelating agents, buffers, and stabilizing agents. Other forms of radioactivity do not exceed 8% of the total radioactivity.

Description—Slightly opalescent, colorless to light-tan colloidal dispersion, pH between 4 and 7.

Uses—A *diagnostic aid* for *liver scanning*. Colloids are phagocytized by the liver. Plasma clearance of ^{99m}Tc sulfur colloid occurs rapidly; the average disappearance half-time is about 2.5 min. Concentration in the liver depends on careful control of the particle size. A test of biological distribution, conducted on mice, should show not less than 80% accumulation in the liver and not more than 5% in the lungs. Other potential uses include the detection of intrapulmonary bleeding and lower GI bleeding, and visualization of the lungs by inhalation of the colloid.
Note—*In making dosage calculations, correct for radioactive decay; for radiological constants, see Table II.*
Dose—*Intravenous*, the equivalent of 1 to 3 mCi.

Technetium Tc 99m Gluceptate Injection

Technetium Stannous Glucoheptonate Agent (*New England Nuclear*); (*Ackerman Nuclear; Mallinckrodt*)

A sterile, aqueous solution, suitable for intravenous administration, of sodium glucoheptonate and stannous chloride that is labeled with ^{99m}Tc; it may contain antimicrobial agents and buffers. Other forms of radioactivity do not exceed 10% of the total radioactivity.
Preparation—Sodium glucoheptonate is available lyophilized in vials with stannous chloride. Addition of freshly eluted pertechnetate

99mTc produces an injection ready for use. The reconstituted injection should be used immediately.

Uses—A *renal imaging agent*, and possibly useful for localization of brain, lung, and gallbladder lesions. Studies have shown that optimal results for both renal and brain imaging are obtained from one to two hours after administration.

Note—In making dosage calculations, correct for radioactive decay; for radiological constants, see Table II.

Dose—The equivalent of 10 to 15 mCi.

Technetium Tc 99m Sodium Methylene Diphosphonate Injection

Technetium Tc 99m Medronate Sodium Kit; Tc-99m MDP (*New England Nuclear; Ackerman Nuclear; Mallinckrodt; Diagnostic Isotopes; Amersham; Union Carbide; Squibb*)

$$NaO-\overset{\overset{O}{\|}}{P}-CH_2-\overset{\overset{O}{\|}}{P}-ONa$$
$$\underset{OH}{}\qquad\underset{OH}{}$$

Sodium Methylene Diphosphonate

Sodium methylene diphosphonate (*sodium medronate*) is supplied as sterile and nonpyrogenic powder, in kits, suitable for reconstitution with sodium pertechnetate Tc 99m.

Uses—On *intravenous* administration, 99mTc-sodium methylene diphosphonate concentrates in areas of altered osteogenesis. It has been shown to be a superior agent for skeletal imaging, compared with other technetium complexes.

Technetium Tc 99m Sodium Phosphates Injection

Sodium Polyphosphate (Tin) (*Diagnostic Isotopes*); (*Ackerman Nuclear*)

$$\left[-O-\overset{\overset{O}{\|}}{P}-\right]_n$$
$$\underset{ONa}{}$$

Sodium Polyphosphate

A sterile, pyrogen-free solution of sodium polyphosphate, a straight-chain dihydrogen sodium phosphate polymer, which has been labeled with 99mTc by addition of 99mTc, freshly eluted from a 99Mo-loaded generator.

Preparation—Sodium polyphosphate is a straight-chain polymer produced by dehydration of NaH_2PO_4. The molecular weight of the polymer used for the preparation of sodium polyphosphate 99mTc should be about 5000. To prepare the 99mTc-labeled compound, commercial kits are available supplying vials each containing lyophilized polyphosphate polymer $-(NaPO_3)_n-$ and stannous chloride. Sodium polyphosphate 99mTc is prepared by adding a sterile, pyrogen-free solution of freshly eluted pertechnetate 99m and shaking. Inclusion of stannous chloride is necessary to ensure reduction of technetium from the heptavalent state ($^{99m}TcO_4^-$) to a lower valence state in which form it chelates to polyphosphate.

Uses—For *bone imaging* and, incidentally, renal imaging.

Note—In making dosage calculations, correct for radioactive decay; for radiological constants, see Table II.

Dose—*Intravenous*, the equivalent of 1 to 4 mCi.

Technetium Tc 99m Sodium Phytate Injection

Sodium Phytate Tc-99m (*Diagnostic Isotopes*); Technetium-99m Stannous Phytate Injection (*New England Nuclear*); (*Ackerman Nuclear*)

A sterile, pyrogen-free solution of sodium phytate prepared by addition of sterile, freshly eluted sodium pertechnetate 99m to a sterile, pyrogen-free mixture of sodium phytate and stannous chloride.

Preparation—Sodium phytate is the sodium salt of inositol hexaphosphate. To prepare the 99mTc-labeled compound, commercial kits are available supplying vials each containing lyophilized sodium phytate and stannous chloride. It is only necessary to add freshly eluted, sterile, pyrogen-free pertechnetate 99mTc solution and mix

to obtain sodium phytate 99mTc. Use of stannous chloride is necessary to reduce Tc (VII) to a lower valence state in which form it will bond to phytate.

Uses—For *liver and spleen imaging*. Over 80% of the activity localizes in the liver and spleen within 30 min following intravenous administration since it is cleared rapidly from the blood by the reticuloendothelial system. This action is believed due to colloid formation, possibly with blood calcium, after administration. The addition of ionic calcium to technetium-99m stannous phytate produces an agent with improved spleenic uptake.

Note—In making dosage calculations, correct for radioactive decay; for radiological constants, see Table II.

Dose—The equivalent of 1 to 8 mCi.

Tetracycline Tc 99m

Tetracycline Kit (*Diagnostic Isotopes*)

A sterile, pyrogen-free solution of tetracycline that has been tagged with 99mTc by addition of freshly eluted sodium pertechnetate 99m to a lyophilized mixture of tetracycline and stannous chloride in a sterile vial.

Preparation—Tetracycline is available in kit forms, each vial containing 20 mg of lyophilized tetracycline and 1 mg of stannous chloride. Addition of 1 to 4 mL of freshly eluted, sterile, pyrogen-free solution of pertechnetate 99mTc, followed by gentle mixing, provides enough tetracycline 99mTc for 1 to 3 scans.

Uses—For *imaging of kidneys* and *gall bladder* which show the greatest concentration of radioactivity. With slightly larger doses, myocardial imaging is also possible.

Note—In making dosage calculations, correct for radioactive decay; for radiological constants, see Table II.

Dose—*Kidney and gall bladder imaging*, the equivalent of 5 to 10 mCi; *myocardial imaging*, 10 to 20 mCi.

Thallium Tl 201 Chloride Injection

Thallous Chloride Tl 201 (*New England Nuclear; Squibb; Mallinckrodt; Medi-Physics*); Thallium-201 Chloride (*Crocker Nuclear Laboratory*, University of California, Davis); (*Diagnostic Isotopes*)

A sterile, isotonic, aqueous solution of 201TlCl suitable for intravenous administration.

Preparation—Thallium is bombarded with protons to produce 201Pb by the reaction $^{203}Tl(p,3n)^{201}Pb$. The lead is complexed and the undesirable thallium target material is removed by ion exchange. The lead isotopes are then affixed to another column from which 201Tl is eluted following its formation by decay of 201Pb.

Uses—In *myocardial perfusion imaging* for diagnosis and localization of myocardial ischemia and infarction. It is an adjunct to angiography. Thallium mimics potassium ions and is taken up by cells of the heart; a decrease in the vitality of the cells is indicated by decreased 201Tl uptake. It has been reported that 201Tl is also useful for thyroid imaging, in particular for the detection of marked goiter and thyroid carcinoma.

Dose—The equivalent of 1 to 1.5 mCi.

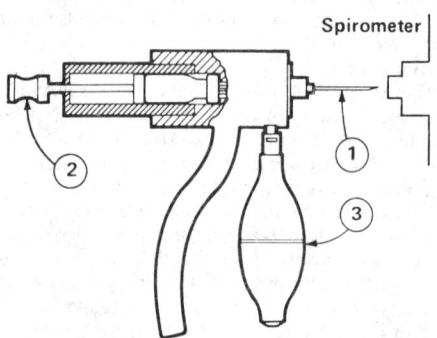

Fig 29-16. Using the Calidose: gas dispensing system. 1: Affix to a spirometer or related breathing apparatus; 2: puncture septum of loaded vial by pushing plunger into dispenser; and 3: immediately squeeze and hold rubber bulb for 5 sec, and then release (courtesy, New England Nuclear).

Xenon Xe 127 Gas

Xenon (^{127}Xe) Gas (*Mallinckrodt*)

Xenon, isotope of mass 127; a gas [13994-19-9]. As produced it contains less than 10% Xenon 129m and less than 10% Xenon 131m; 99% of total radioactivity is as radioxenon.

Preparation—Xenon 127 is produced by proton bombardment of Cesium 133.

Uses—See Xenon Xe 133 Injection.

Dose—Intravenous, cerebral and pulmonary studies, the equivalent of **0.5 to 10 mCi.**

Xenon Xe 133 Injection

Xenon (^{133}Xe) Injection; Xenon-133 (*Diagnostic Isotopes; New England Nuclear; Cambridge Nuclear*); Xeneisol Xe 133 Injection (*Mallinckrodt*); (*Amersham*); MPI Xenon Xe 133 (*Medi-Physics*); (*General Electric*)

Xenon, isotope of mass 133; a gas [14932-42-4]. *Injection:* A sterile, isotonic solution of xenon 133 suitable for intravenous administration. Xenon 133 is a radioactive nuclide prepared from the fission of uranium 235. Other forms of radioactivity do not exceed 10% of the total radioactivity.

Preparation—A product of nuclear fission, xenon 133 can also be prepared by neutron activation according to the reaction $^{132}Xe(n,\gamma)^{133}Xe$. It is available as a gas and, being three times more soluble than oxygen, also as a solution in isotonic saline.

Uses—As a *gas*, for *lung imaging* to detect alveolar blockage. ^{133}Xe can be introduced into a spirometer or breathing apparatus by use of a special assembly illustrated in Fig 29-16. Its biological half-life of approximately 15 min makes it a relatively safe isotope to use. Single-photon tomography of inhaled Xe-133 has been used to map cerebral blood flow.

Dissolve in saline, as a biological tracer for regional blood flow measurements. Injected into a tissue, the rate of clearance is a measure of the regional blood flow. Intravenously, it can be used to measure the potency of the cerebral blood supply, pulmonary functions, etc.

Note—In making dosage calculations, correct for radioactive decay; for radiological constants, see Table II.

Dose—*Intravenous, cerebral,* and *pulmonary studies*, the equivalent of **0.5 to 10 mCi.**

PART 5

Testing and Analysis

Thomas Medwick, PhD

College of Pharmacy
Rutgers—The State University
Busch Campus
New Brunswick, NJ 08903

CHAPTER 30

Analysis of Medicinals

Thomas Medwick, PhD

Professor and Chairman

Karen B Fekety, MS

Research Fellow
Department of Pharmaceutical Chemistry

College of Pharmacy
Rutgers University
Piscataway, NJ 08854

John W Turczan, BS

NMR Spectroscopist
Food and Drug Administration
850 Third Avenue
Brooklyn, NY 11232

Alfonso R Gennaro, PhD

Professor of Chemistry
Philadelphia College of Pharmacy and Science
Philadelphia, PA 19104

From the time of the early apothecaries, who worked with meager equipment in small laboratories, pharmacists have made important contributions in the field of medicinal chemistry, both in discovering or isolating new therapeutic agents and in developing methods for standardizing and controlling medicinals. Today such activity is rarely a function of the prescription laboratory, but in manufacturing laboratories pharmacists often perform physical and chemical analyses either in the course of developing dosage forms of new products or in the control of standard products. In small laboratories the responsibility for performing analyses may be delegated entirely to pharmacist staff members. But whether or not a pharmacist may have occasion to conduct analyses, he or she should at least understand the basic principles involved in the standardization and control of the medicinal agents dispensed.

Analytical Balances

Equipment of a very modest character may be used in the initial stages of the development of an analytical department, and as the need develops and opportunities occur a more complete laboratory can be built up in which work of the most complex type may be performed. The manufacturing pharmacist's first duty, of course, is in the direction of the maintenance of quality and purity in such items of stock as are likely to deviate from the standards, especially those which are apt to change on account of deterioration.

It is assumed that there will be available a balance which is sensitive enough to serve for analytical procedures. These analyses involve the modern methods as well as classical analyses. An analytical balance differs from a high-class prescription balance in the matter of sensitiveness; a satisfactory analytical balance is sensitive to the tenth of a milligram and should never be used for weighing a total load greater than that specified.

The single-pan balance does not require any extra weights and is entirely self-contained. The balance is always under constant load, since to determine the weight of an object, weights are removed from the beam to restore equilibrium. Removal of the weights is accomplished by knobs on the front panel and the amount removed is registered on a dial. Fractions of mass less than 0.1 g are read from a screen on which is focused the image produced by an optical lever. Weighings can be performed with high accuracy very rapidly. As the pan is always under constant load there is little change in sensitivity.

Other types of balances utilize electrical systems; one of these is the electrobalance. It is of the null type (as is the single-pan balance), but the restoring torque is not applied by adding or removing weights but rather by varying a current applied to a coil in a magnetic field, the pointer being attached to the coil. The great advantage of the electromagnetic principle is the freedom from drift or change in sensitivity. The balance can be operated remotely but has a great disadvantage in its low maximum capacity (ca 0.1–1 g). Other electronic analytical balances using load cells are available with capacities of up to 200 g and a readability of ±0.1 mg or ±0.01 mg and have data outputs making them capable of incorporation into automated systems.

Several manufacturers have developed balances which can continuously record variations in weight with time.

Sources of Information

The works of reference needed in an analytical laboratory depend entirely upon the scope of work. For pharmaceutical testing of official substances, the USP is, of course, given primary consideration. Among the indispensable adjuncts of the analyst's library are the latest editions of the following works:

Clarke EGC: *Isolation and Identification of Drugs*, vol 1, 1969, vol 2, 1975.

Connors KA: *Textbook of Pharmaceutical Analysis*, Wiley, New York, 3rd ed, 1982.

Feigl F: *Spot Tests in Organic Analysis*, 7th ed, Elsevier, The Netherlands, 1966.

Florey, K, editor, "Analytical Profiles of Drug Substances," a continuing series starting with Vol 1 1972, Academic Press, New York.

Food Chemicals Codex, 3rd ed, Natl Acad Press, Washington, DC, 1981.

Higuchi T, Brochmann-Hanssen E: *Pharmaceutical Analysis*, Interscience, New York, 1961.

Knevel, AM, Di Gangi, FE and Byrn, SR, "Quantitative Pharmaceutical Chemistry," Waveland Press, Prospect Heights, Illinois, 7th ed, 1983.

Kolthoff IM, *et al*: *Treatise on Analytical Chemistry*, part 1, 12 vols; part 2, 15 vols; part 3, 4 vols (1959–1977).

Merck Index, 10th ed, Merck & Co, Rahway, NJ, 1983.

Ringbom AJ: *Complexation in Analytical Chemistry; Chemical Analysis Series*, vol 16, Interscience, New York, 1963.

Reagent Chemicals, 6th ed, American Chemical Soc, Washington, DC, 1981.

Siggia S: *Quantitative Analysis via Functional Groups*, Wiley, New York, 1963.

Siggia S: *Instrumental Methods of Organic Functional Group Analysis*, Wiley-Interscience, New York, 1972.

Many valuable publications may be obtained from various departments of the US Government.

Specialized Analytical Methods and Equipment

In the following section some important analytical methods used by large manufacturing concerns are discussed. The pharmacist does not as a rule require such sophisticated apparatus as is used for analysis, but should at least be familiar with the type of analyses conducted with each instrument.

A substantial proportion of the medicinal products are still being assayed by the time-honored procedures of gravimetric and titrimetric analysis, although here, too, the use of electronic balances and the recording titrator have considerably improved these classical procedures.

A wide diversity in the types of technique has always been characteristic of assay methods for pharmaceutical products. Simple distillations are very useful in determining the alcohol content of liquids, in the analysis of proteins, and in the determination of certain alkaloids that are volatile in a current of steam. Fractional distillations have for a long time provided suitable methods for the analytical separation of constituents in volatile liquids. An important milestone was reached in the development of a quantitative method for the isolation and measurement of gaseous nitrogen. This procedure has been particularly useful in determining amino acids.

Familiar examples of analytical methods that are purely physical in their nature include those which involve the use of the microscope, the polarimeter, and the refractometer. The identity and relative purity of many substances are often determined by microscopical examination. The polarimeter, which is also referred to as the polariscope, has long been recognized for its usefulness in assaying certain liquids by determining their ability to bend or rotate the plane of polarized light. Both the Abbé and the immersion or dipping types of refractometer are now quite generally used for determining the purity of a substance on the basis of its refractive index.

The determination of the moisture content in various substances involves several types of analytical measurement. These methods include drying in a desiccator or in a heated oven, either under ordinary atmospheric conditions or in vacuum under reduced pressure. An innovation is the "moisture balance" in which the sample pan is directly heated by an infrared lamp, thus eliminating removal of the sample from the balance. Other procedures involve distillation of vegetable drugs with toluene or with benzene, then noting the volume of water that separates in a graduated tube containing the distillate. A more specific and convenient procedure for determining water in many substances is the Karl Fischer titrimetric method. In this procedure, the water is quantitatively measured by titration under anhydrous conditions by the use of a reagent containing iodine, sulfur dioxide, pyridine, and methanol. The end-point may be detected visually, or preferably by the use of the electrometric and automatic titration assembly. Electrical methods for determining water are now being applied to a variety of industrial products, in some cases during continuous processing operations. These are based upon the principle that if a substance is placed between two condenser plates, the capacitance will vary with the dielectric constant of the medium between the plates. Since the dielectric constant of water is greater than that of other substances, the capacitance will vary with the amount of moisture present.

The determination and adjustment of pH or hydrogen ion concentration has become an important function in the control analysis of medicinal products. For a discussion of pH determination see Chapter 34.

Separation techniques, particularly chromatographic methods, are necessary and valuable in the analysis of pharmaceuticals. The partitioning of a solute between two immiscible solvents is used many times to isolate a drug from other components in a mixture. Open column chromatographic methods are likewise used in the separation of a drug from a dosage form matrix or of a drug from a natural biological environment. Separations such as solvent-solvent extraction, open column chromatography, or thin-layer chromatography may be required as a preparatory step when spectrophotometric analysis in the ultraviolet region is to follow. This preliminary treatment introduces specificity by providing for the isolation of the drug from its surroundings prior to its measurement by a relatively non-specific means.

Gas chromatography (GC) and high performance liquid chromatography (HPLC) represent two non-stoichiometric methods that have achieved very great popularity because of their capabilities. In GC, any compound, directly or with derivatization, can be analyzed if it has a perceptible vapor pressure and if a suitable column can be found. The use of various detectors adds another element of selectivity to the procedure. More recently, HPLC has been rapidly developing with the introduction of new pumping methods, more reliable columns and a variety of detectors. But the great attraction of chromatographic techniques to the industrial laboratory is the possibility of automation. The chromatographic procedure and instrumentation may be so designed that the method largely may be automated, involving automated sampling, separations, detection and recording, and finally, calculation and printing of results, leaving only the preparation of drug substance or of dosage form solutions to be done by the analyst. The subject of chromatography is discussed in Chapter 33.

The modern spectrometer which incorporates such features as microprocessor control and diode array detectors has become an especially useful instrument for analysis, since it enables the analyst to seek the answers to his analytical problems with "eyes" that see not only in the visible range, but throughout the electromagnetic spectrum. The analytical possibilities in this direction can be more readily understood when one considers that the ultimate molecules and atoms that make up a material transmit, absorb, and scatter radiation according to their individual natures. Assay methods based upon absorption in the ultraviolet, infrared and visible portions of the spectrum are extensively used. The principles underlying such determinations are discussed in Chapter 34. In some spectrophotometric analytical procedures a colorless substance required to be analyzed is converted to a derivative having color, the intensity of the color being measured in a suitable spectrophotometer and compared with that developed by a known amount of a "reference standard" grade of the same substance.

Other widely used instruments which are quite suitable for routine colorimetric measurements are the colorimeter and the combination nephelocolorimeter which is of considerable value in making quantitative turbidimetric measurements.

Not the least important of spectrometric instruments is the fluorometer, which provides for measurement of fluorescence that may be present in the sample, or, more frequently, may be developed in the sample. This method provides a means of evaluating the potency of many pharmaceutical products, as, for example, those containing thiamine hydrochloride. A solution in which the thiamine has been quantitatively converted into thiochrome is placed in the fluorometer where it is caused to fluoresce on exposure to light. This fluorescence intensity is compared with readings obtained on standard control samples prepared and observed under exactly the same conditions. This comparison serves as a basis on which the potency of the unknown vitamin sample readily can be calculated.

At the opposite end of the electromagnetic spectrum are the infrared radiations. These are heat rays and their utilization marks another important contribution to analytical research.

Table I—Molecular Identification and Analysis[1]

Method	Principal Applications	Molecular Phenomenon	Advantages in Qual Analysis	Advantages in Quant Analysis	Average Spl[2] Desired for Qual Anal	Method Limitations	Sample Limitations
Infrared Spectrometry	Structure determination and identity of organic and inorganic compounds General quant. analysis	Excitation of molecular vibrations by light absorption	Identification of functional groups. Large file of reference spectra available Virtually no sample limitations impurity detection	Widely applicable	3 mg	Medium sensitivity[3] No direct information about size of molecule	Avoid aqueous solutions
Raman Spectroscopy	Structure determination and identity of organic compounds Symmetry of molecular groups in solid state	Excitation of molecular vibrations by light scattering	Identification of functional groups (usually different from those identified by IR) Water solutions	(Special applications)	0.01 mg	Low sensitivity[3] No direct information about size of molecule	Sample must not fluoresce Avoid turbid materials Some restrictions on colored material
Mass Spectrometry	Structure determination and identity of organic compounds Analysis of trace volatiles in non-volatiles	Ionization of molecule, and cracking of molecule into fragment ions	Precision molecular wt (molecular ion) Masses of integral parts of molecule (fragment ions) Very high sensitivity, Impurity detection	High sensitivity Wide applicability to volatile materials	0.1 mg	Dose not detect functional groups directly Comparatively slow	$> \sim 10^{-3}$ Torr vapor pressure at sample inlet temperature
Nuclear Magnetic Resonance	Structure determination and identity of organic compounds Molecular conformation	Reorientation of magnetic nuclei in a magnetic field	Determination of chemical type and number of hydrogen atoms (also ^{11}B, ^{13}C, ^{19}F, ^{31}P) Molecular configuration and conformation impurity determination Applicable to water solutions	Standards not required	10 mg	Medium sensitivity[3] Most useful information only from elements ^{1}H, ^{11}B, ^{13}C, ^{19}F, ^{31}P	Liquid or soluble solid (wide variety of solvent choices)
Ultraviolet and visible spectrometry and colorimetry	Quantitative analysis, esp as end methods in chemical analysis schemes	Excitation of loosely bonded electrons	(Special applications)	High precision High sensitivity Simplicity	0.01 mg	Low specificity; little information on molecular structure	Soluble in UV-transparent solvent (wide variety of choices)
Gas Chromatography	General multi-component quantitative analysis of volatile organics Highly efficient separation technique	Partitioning between vapor phase and substrate	Separates materials for examination by other techniques	Generality—widely applicable to volatile materials Multi-component analyses, High sensitivity in special cases	1 mg	Identifies materials only in special cases Not applicable to materials of low volatility	$> \sim 1$ Torr vapor pressure at sample inlet temperature
Combined Gas chromatography Mass spectrometry	Identification and analysis of trace organic materials	Combines separation efficiency of GC with sensitivity and specificity of mass spec	Applicable to identity of sub-ppm components in mixtures	Specific identification of GC peaks being determined	1 mg	Not applicable to materials of low volatility	>1 Torr vapor pressure at sample inlet temperature
Liquid Chromatography (including ion exchange and thin layer)	Separation techniques for less volatile materials Multi-component quant. analysis	Partitioning between liquid solution and substrate	Separates materials for examination by other techniques	Multi-component analyses of less volatile materials	300 mg	Resolution rather poor compared to other chromatographic methods Method development is time-consuming	(None)
Gel permeation chromatography	Separation on basis of molecular weight Determination of mol wt distribution in polymers	Separation by variation of penetration into cross-linked gel structure	Separates materials for examination by other techniques	Determines molecular weight distribution	500 mg	Requires extensive calibration Time-consuming	Material must be soluble in narrow choice of solvents

Table I—continued

Method	Principal Applications	Molecular Phenomenon	Advantages in Qual Analysis	Advantages in Quant Analysis	Average Spl[2] Desired for Qual Anal	Method Limitations	Sample Limitations
X-ray Diffraction	Identification of crystalline substances, especially inorganic Determination of crystallinity, esp polymers	Diffraction of X-rays from crystal planes	High specificity for crystalline solids, esp inorganics Large file of reference patterns available	Applicable to inorganic crystalline solids	0.1 mg	Limited structural information— essentially a "fingerprint" method	Crystalline solids; partly crystalline polymers
Chemical Reaction Methods (classical analysis)	Variety of specialized quantitative analysis applications	Stoichiometry of chemical reactions	(Special applications)	High precision for assay analyses Absolute calibration	1000 mg	Time-consuming Interferences often a problem	(None)

Notes: (Courtesy of 1966, 1970, 1972, 1979, The Dow Chemical Company)

[1] This table compares only the more widely used techniques, current as of 1979. Methods of identification and analysis of compounds not included in this table can be considered to be specialized techniques.

[2] The amount of sample listed in this column is an estimate of the average minimum sample required. Usually, a larger sample is preferred in order to do the best possible analysis. On the other hand, successful identifications can often be done with much smaller amounts.

[3] "Sensitivity" as used here indicates ability to determine a small amount of one material in the presence of large amounts of other material(s).

Table II—Atomic Identification and Analysis[1]

Method	Principal Applications	Atomic Phenomenon	Advantages in Qual Analysis	Advantages in Quant Analysis	Average[2] Spl Req	Method Limitations	Sample[3] Limitations
Atomic Emission Spectroscopy	General qual. and semi-quant. survey of all metallic elements Trace metal analysis	Light emission from excited electronic states of atoms	General for all metallic elements Simultaneous analysis of all metallic elements	General for all metallic elements High sensitivity in many cases	10 mg	Detects the volatile elements (non-metals) only with difficulty; Calibration required for precision quant analysis	Applicable principally to non-volatile materials
Atomic Absorption Spectroscopy	Precision quant. analysis for a given metal Trace analysis for a given metal	Absorption of atomic resonance line	(Not applicable)	Fast, reliable analysis for a given element High sensitivity in some cases Simplicity	100 mg	Metals analyzed individually, not simultaneously Usually not applicable to non-metallic elements	Element being analyzed must be in a solution (many solvent choices)
X-ray Fluorescence	General qual. and semi-quant. survey of all elements atomic no ≥11 (Na) Precision quant. analysis of elements esp. heavier non-metals (P, S, Cl, Br, I) Trace analysis	Re-emission of X-rays from excited atoms	General for all elements atomic no ≥11 (Na) Minimum sample preparation	General for all elements atomic no ≥14 (Si) High sensitivity in some cases Simplicity; minimum sample preparation	500 mg (non-destructive)	Non sensitive to elements of atomic no <11 (Na) Precision limited by non-uniformity of spl.	Applicable principally to solids and non-volatile liquids
Neutron Activation	Precision quant. analysis of most elements Trace and ultratrace element analysis General qual. analysis of most elements	Counting of radio-active species produced by neutron reactions	Minimum sample preparation	Highest sensitivity for many elements High confidence level Only general instrumental method capable of N, O, and F analysis	100 mg (non-destructive)	Sensitivity varies considerably among elements (but sensitive to amounts <1 μg for most elements) Multi-component analyses present some problems	Applicable to solids and liquids
Chemical Reaction Methods (classical analysis)	Variety of specialized quantitative analysis applications	Stoichiometry of chemical reactions	(Special applications)	High precision for assay analysis Absolute calibration	1000 mg	Time-consuming	(None)

Notes: (Courtesy of 1966, 1970, 1972, 1979, The Dow Chemical Company)

[1] This table compares only the more general techniques, current as of 1979, omitting those which are applicable to only one or a few elements. For each method, the sensitivity and precision with which a given element can be determined can vary considerably. Therefore, this table can be considered only as a very rough guide toward a proper choice for a given analysis.

[2] The amount of sample listed in this column is only a rough index. Sample required will vary enormously depending on whether the problem is identity of a major elemental component, or precision determination of a trace element.

[3] None of these methods handles gases easily and conveniently (although it could be done in special cases). For elemental analysis in gases mass spectrometry is the best general choice.

Infrared spectrometry involves placing the sample in a cell which is traversed by radiation from a hot globar element. The transmitted radiation on passing into the spectrophotometer is dispersed into a spectrum by a prism of sodium chloride, or other salt, or by a diffraction grating. The radiation intensity is sensed by a bolometer, a device capable of detecting exceedingly small changes in temperature, and with the aid of an electronic amplifier, radiation intensity thus measured is recorded by a pen-type recorder. Fourier transform infrared spectrometers are now available (see Chapter 34). An important application of infrared spectrometry in the USP is in the "fingerprinting" of organic compounds, by which means they may be identified.

The spectrograph has long been recognized as a very useful analytical instrument, since it enables the analyst to check the composition of many substances by providing photographic records of their emission spectra. The emission spectrograph is used for identification and for the quantitative measurement of many elements. These include most metals and some nonmetals, such as boron, silicon, and phosphorus. The spectrograph utilizes the principle that elements when vaporized into a high temperature arc or spark discharge emit light in definite wavelengths. This light passes through the narrow slit in the front of the spectrograph and is dispersed by means of a prism or grating. The dispersed light is focused on a recording device, usually a photographic film or plate. When the film is exposed and developed, a series of lines or spectra appear. These lines are images of the slit and correspond to different wavelengths of light. By determining the wavelengths of the lines the various elements present in the sample may be determined by reference to wavelength tables. The sample to be analyzed is placed on a carbon electrode in some suitable manner and becomes one end of the electric discharge. By the use of a densitometer, which measures the relative darkness of the lines, the quantitative evaluation is accomplished. Suitable standards must be prepared for each element to be determined. The elements of an unknown are measured quantitatively by comparing the darkness of its spectral lines with those same lines in the standard. The spectrograph is of special value in determining trace metal contamination in pharmaceutical products. It can be used in conjunction with the heavy metals test to measure the amount of each contaminating metal. The results obtained by trace metal analysis are frequently of considerable value in research and in helping to solve pilot-plant, processing, and control problems.

The flame spectrometer serves a useful purpose in some industrial and hospital laboratories for making routine determinations, particularly of alkali metals and alkaline earth metals. The mass spectrometer and the x-ray spectrometer are among the more sophisticated instruments that are useful as analytical tools.

The recording polarograph provides for rapid qualitative and quantitative analyses by automatic recording of current-voltage curves. In the operation of this instrument reducible ions and organic compounds are reduced at the dropping mercury electrode, yielding polarograms that serve as records of the analysis. The polarogram establishes the identity of the substance by its half-wave potential while the height of the step in the curve is taken as a direct measurement of concentration.

Although the non-stoichiometric methods used in drug analysis are discussed in Chapter 33, *Chromatography*, Chapter 34, *Instrumental Methods of Analysis*, and Chapter 28, *Radioisotopes*, and the stoichiometric analyses are treated in this chapter as they apply to specific drug substances and to specific dosage forms, a tabular summary of analytical methods is provided in Table I which deals with methods useful for molecular qualitative and quantitative analysis and in Table II which deals similarly with methods for atomic systems.

Official Physical and Chemical Assays

There appears to be a misconception on the part of some individuals concerning the assay procedures of the official compendia. A material may well fall within the assay limits stated in the individual monograph for a particular substance, and yet *not* be of suitable quality to conform to the complete specifications indicated for the compound, even though the assay is performed exactly as indicated in the official method. It is essential then to realize that even though a substance meets the purity specifications of an official monograph, as established by a chemical or physical assay procedure, it is *not* of USP quality unless it conforms to *all* of the specifications contained in the monograph for that material. Also, some official substances do not have an assay procedure, as such, listed in the monograph for the basic drug. A quantitative analytical method is not required in such cases since other specifications in the monograph serve to characterize the substance both quantitatively and qualitatively.

In the following sections various aspects of the official drug analyses are considered. The classical titrimetric and gravimetric methods are considered in some detail and, even though the subjects are treated in Chapters 33 and 34, some aspects of instrumental procedures are examined. Then, after a tabulation of indicators and other reagents, some examples of the various classes of analyses are presented, together with an explanation of the chemical principles or other pertinent detail. This list of examples is not complete since a comprehensive tabulation of all official assays is reserved for Table VI, found at the end of this chapter.

Titrimetric Assay Methods

The titrimetric assay procedure is the one most frequently encountered by the pharmaceutical chemist in the standardization of official products. Every titrimetric assay is based on the determination of the volume of a solution of known strength required to complete a chemical reaction with the substance being analyzed. Such a solution is called a *standard solution* or *a volumetric solution* and is commonly referred to by the abbreviation "VS."

Indicators for Determining End Points

It is imperative to avoid the error of using an insufficient amount of a volumetric solution, thus failing to complete a reaction, and it is equally necessary to guard against overstepping a reaction by adding too much of the volumetric solution. To meet this situation a group of chemicals known as *Indicators* is used. These are substances that show when the end point of a reaction has been reached, either by a change in color or by the formation of a precipitate.

Indicator Solutions

Solutions of indicators used for volumetric determinations are referred to as Test Solutions, abbreviated TS, and those used for determination of hydrogen ion concentration are termed pH Indicators.

The indicators used for colorimetric pH determinations are either weakly acid or weakly basic. However, most indicators used for this purpose, such as the phthaleins and sulfonated phthaleins, behave like weak acids.

The usual concentration of the indicator solution is 0.05%. From 0.1 to 0.2 mL of the indicator solution is generally used for 10 mL of the liquid being examined.

Solutions of indicators of the basic type and of the phthaleins are prepared by dissolving them in alcohol. In preparing solutions of indicators containing an acid group, this group must first be neutralized with sodium hydroxide.

Unless otherwise stated each acid-base indicator solution is so adjusted that when 0.15 mL of the indicator solution is added to 25 mL of carbon dioxide-free water, 0.25 mL of 0.02*N* acid or alkali, respectively, will develop the characteristic color changes.

The solutions should be kept in glass-stoppered bottles, and protected from light.

Indicators for Reactions Involving Neutralization

In the USP indicators are used either to indicate the completion of a chemical reaction in volumetric analyses or to indicate the hydrogen ion concentration (pH) of solutions.

Most of the indicators for acid-base titrations and for pH measurement are acidic. They contain a carboxyl, a sulfonic, or a phenolic group. In many instances the same indicator is applicable either to acid-base titrations or to pH measurements, the difference being only in the preparation of the indicator solution. The following are the pH indicators of the Pharmacopeia; in each case Test Solutions (TS) of the following indicators are used.

Bromocresol Green (*Bromocresol Blue: Tetrabromo-m-cresolsulfonphthalein*)—Transition interval: from pH 4.0 to 5.4. Color change: from yellow to blue.

Bromocresol Purple (*Dibromo-o-cresolsulfonphthalein*)—Transition interval: from pH 5.2 to 6.8. Color change: from yellow to purple. This solution and the next two are satisfactory in the titration of weak bases.

Bromophenol Blue (*Tetrabromophenolsulfonphthalein*)—Transition interval: from pH 3.0 to 4.6. Color change: from yellow to blue.

Bromothymol Blue (*Dibromothymolsulfonphthalein*)—Transition interval: from pH 6.0 to 7.6. Color change: from yellow to blue.

Cresol Red (*o-Cresolsulfonphthalein*)—Transition interval: from pH 7.2 to 8.8. Color change: from yellow to red.

Cresol Red–Thymol Blue TS—Transition interval: from pH 7.7 to 9.1. Color change: from yellow to violet.

Malachite Green—The oxalate salt is used. Transition interval: from pH 0.0 to 2.0. Color change: from yellow to green.

Methyl Orange (*Helianthin* or *Tropaeolin D*)—The sodium salt of dimethylaminoazobenzenesulfonic acid or dimethylaminoazobenzene sodium sulfonate. Transition interval: from pH 3.2 to 4.4. Color change: from pink to yellow. Useful in the titration of weak bases.

Methyl Red (*Dimethylaminoazobenzene-o-carboxylic acid; o-carboxybenzeneazodimethylaniline*)—Transition interval: from pH 4.2 to 6.2. Color change: from red to yellow. Useful in the titration of weak bases.

Methyl Red–Methylene Blue TS—Transition interval: from pH 4.8 to 6.2. Color change: from red-violet to green.

Methyl Yellow (*p-Dimethylaminoazobenzene*)—Transition interval: from pH 2.9 to 4.0. Color change: from red to yellow.

Phenolphthalein—Use *Phenolphthalein USP*—Transition interval: from pH 8.0 to 10. Color change: from colorless to red. Useful in the titration of acids with strong bases.

Phenol Red—Use *Phenolsulfonphthalein USP*. Transition interval: from pH 6.8 to 8.2. Color change: from yellow to red.

Quinaldine Red (*5-Dimethylamino-2-styrylethylquinolinium iodide*)—Transition interval: pH 1.4 to 3.2. Color change: from colorless to red.

Thymol Blue (*Thymolsulfonphthalein*)—*Acid*—Transition interval: from pH 1.2 to 2.8. Color change: from red to yellow. *Alkaline*—Transition interval: from pH 8 to 9.2. Color change: from yellow to blue.

Thymolphthalein—Transition interval: from pH 9.3 to 10.5. Color change: from colorless to blue.

Indicators for Reactions Involving Precipitation

Dichlorofluorescein TS.

Eosin Y (Sodium Tetrabromofluorescein) TS.

Ferric Ammonium Sulfate Test Solution—8% in water. This indicator, well-known as *Ferric Alum*, is generally used when titrating with standard ammonium thiocyanate in the presence of silver nitrate. A red color of the ferric thiocyanate complex forms immediately when the silver thiocyanate has been completely precipitated.

Potassium Chromate Test Solution—10% in water. This indicator gives a red precipitate of silver chromate in a neutral or slightly alkaline solution, after silver halides have been completely precipitated by titration with standard silver nitrate.

Sodium Alizarinsulfonate TS.

Tetrabromophenolphthalein TS.

Tetrabromophenolphthalein, Ethyl Ester TS.

Indicators for Nonaqueous Titrations

Azo-violet.

Crystal Violet (TS)—1% in glacial acetic acid.

Malachite Green—Use Malachite Green TS.

Methyl Red—Use Methyl Red TS.

Methyl Violet—Use Methyl Violet TS.

p-**Naphtholbenzein**—4-[α-(4-hydroxy-1-naphthyl)benzylidene]-1-(4*H*)[naphthalenone].

Phenol Red—Use Phenol Red TS.

Quinaldine Red—Use Quinaldine Red TS.

Thymol Blue—Use Thymol Blue TS.

Indicators for Complexometric Titrations

Diphenylamine TS.

Dithizone (*Diphenylthiocarbazone*) **TS.**

Eriochrome Black T—0.05% aqueous solution (should be freshly prepared but can be stabilized).

Hydroxynaphthol Blue.

Murexide (*Acid Ammonium Purpurate*)—Used as a powder; usually mixed with an inert carrier (potassium sulfate) to facilitate handling.

Naphthol Green TS.

1-(2-Pyridylazo)-2-naphthol.

Indicators for Reactions Involving Changes in Valence

2,6-Dichloroquinone-chlorimide (*Dichlorophenolindophenol*)—Usually used as the sodium salt in a solution containing sodium bicarbonate to titrate ascorbic acid dosage forms. In oxidized form it is blue in alkaline and rose-pink in acid solution; when reduced it is colorless.

Dicyanobis(1,10-phenanthroline)iron II Dihydrate—An indicator that reacts similarly to ortho-phenanthroline.

Diphenylamine—Employed in titrations involving potassium dichromate as titrant. In reduced form it is colorless; in a reversible oxidation reaction it produces a brilliant violet diphenylbenzidine derivative.

Iodine—Free iodine serves as its own indicator in assays where it is liberated and determined volumetrically by titration with standard potassium iodate. The end point is the disappearance of the violet color of iodine in chloroform added to the mixture being titrated for the purpose of dissolving and concentrating the iodine.

Methyl Orange—Used as a test solution in titrations with potassium bromate; the color of this external indicator is discharged by excess titrant.

Nitrophenanthroline—An indicator that reacts similarly to ortho-phenanthroline.

Ortho-phenanthroline—Used, in 1.5% concentration in 1.5% ferrous sulfate solution, as an indicator in titrations involving standard ceric sulfate solution. The color changes from red to pale green when the slightest excess of ceric sulfate is added to the oxidized solution.

Oxalic Acid Volumetric Solution—This standard solution is generally used without an indicator since most reactions in which it takes part depend on decolorization of potassium permanganate.

Potassium Permanganate Volumetric Solution—As this highly colored solution is decolorized on being reduced, a separate indicator is not required.

Potassium Thiocyanate—Used in conjunction with ferric chloride volumetric solution, a red compound is produced at the end point.

Starch Iodide Paste Test Solution—Approximately 5% suspension of potato starch in 0.75% potassium iodide with zinc chloride preservative. May be used as an external indicator for titrations with sodium nitrite VS.

Starch iodide paste test solution must show a definite blue streak when a glass rod, dipped in a mixture of 1 mL of tenth-molar sodium nitrite, 500 mL of water, and 10 mL of hydrochloric acid, is streaked on a smear of the paste.

Starch-Potassium Iodide Test Solution—0.5% KI in Starch TS. Must be freshly prepared.

Starch Test Solution—A 0.5% suspension of arrowroot starch in water, freshly prepared. The blue color produced by starch in the presence of free iodine is well known.

Indicator Papers

Strong, white filter paper is treated with hydrochloric acid and washed with water until the washings no longer show an acid reaction to methyl red. It is then treated with ammonia TS and again washed with water, until the washings are no longer alkaline toward phenolphthalein. It is then thoroughly dried.

The dry paper is saturated with the proper strength indicator solution and carefully dried by suspending the paper in a room free from acid or alkali fumes.

The papers so prepared are kept in glass-stoppered bottles, protected from light and moisture.

Lead Acetate Test Paper—Prepared from lead acetate TS.

Litmus Paper, Blue—Usually in the form of strips about 50 mm in length and 6 mm in width.

Litmus Paper, Red—Usually in the form of strips about 50 mm in length and 6 mm in width.

Mercuric Bromide Test Paper—Prepared from alcoholic mercuric bromide TS.

Phenolphthalein Paper—Prepared from a 0.1% solution of phenolphthalein in diluted alcohol.

Potassium Iodate-Starch Paper—Impregnate strips of white filter paper with a solution prepared by mixing a 5% solution of potassium iodate with an equal volume of freshly prepared starch TS.

Starch Iodate Paper—Impregnate strips of white filter paper with a mixture of equal volumes of starch TS and potassium iodate solution (1 in 20).

Starch Iodide Paper—Impregnate strips of white filter paper with a solution of 500 mg of potassium iodide in 100 mL of freshly prepared starch TS.

Turmeric Paper—Impregnate strips of white filter paper with turmeric solution prepared as directed in the USP.

Potentiometric Determination of End Points

The detection of the end point in titrimetric assays by use of colorimetric indicators may sometimes be difficult, especially if the solution being titrated is colored or turbid. In some instances titration to the equivalence or true end point is essential, a requirement that is not conveniently met when an indicator is employed. In such cases the end point may be indicated potentiometrically, most commonly employing the millivolt scale of a pH meter. The potentiometric determination of end points depends upon the fact that in most titrations the potential across two suitable electrodes immersed in the solution being titrated undergoes a sharp change at the true end point (equivalence point), this change corresponding to the point where an indicator undergoes marked change of color. In some titrations neither the change of color nor the change of potential is sharp at the end point, in which case titration to a predetermined voltage or voltage deflection is necessary; since it is generally more convenient to do this potentiometrically, rather than colorimetrically, this electrical method is employed. Suitable electrodes, such as a combination of glass and calomel electrodes, undergo no reaction with the solution being titrated or with the titrant; they serve only as a means of *detecting* the end point.

It may be pointed out here that the change of other electrical properties, such as resistance or the amount of current flowing in a solution being titrated, may be utilized to indicate the end point in a titration. The general term *electrometric titrations* is sometimes applied to such titrations; specific titrations in this category are referred to as *amperometric*, *conductometric*, and *high-frequency* titrations.

*Titrimetric Procedures**

Acid-Base Reactions

Direct Titration of an Acid by Base

In this category a free acid is titrated directly using the method indicated in the monograph to determine the end-point.

Anticoagulant Citrate Dextrose Solution and Anticoagulant Citrate Phosphate Dextrose Solution—for free citric acid (Phth)—for sodium citrate the solution is titrated potentiometrically to pH 1.98.

Boric Acid—The use of glycerin increases the acid strength of the boric acid by formation of a glycero-borate complex according to the equation given here.

$$H_3BO_3 \ + \ 2 \ H-\overset{\displaystyle CH_2OH}{\underset{\displaystyle CH_2OH}{\overset{|}{\underset{|}{C}}}}-OH = H_3O^\oplus \ + \ 2H_2O \ +$$

$$\left[\begin{matrix} CH_2OH & & HOH_2C \\ H-\overset{|}{C}-O & & O-\overset{|}{C}-H \\ & B & \\ H_2\overset{|}{C}-O & & O-\overset{|}{C}H_2 \end{matrix} \right]^{\ominus}$$

Cellulose Acetate Phthalate—phthalyl content.

Dibasic Sodium Phosphate—treatment of the salt with hydrochloric acid forms phosphoric acid and the end point is determined potentiometrically from pH readings. Only one hydrogen of phosphoric acid is titrated in this procedure.

Orange Syrup—citric acid content.

Oxyphenbutazone—even though a phenol, it is sufficiently strong to be titrated directly.

Potassium Phosphate, Monobasic—See *Sodium Phosphate*, below.

Saccharin Calcium—on treatment with mineral acid, free saccharin is liberated, extracted with ether, the solvent removed, and the residual saccharin titrated.

Sodium Phosphates Enema and Oral Solution—The solution is titrated potentiometrically, with standard acid, to two deflection points in the titration curve.

Storax—acid value.

Sulfinpyrazone (and dosage forms)—the sulfonyl group ($-SO_2-$) makes the alpha-hydrogen sufficiently acid so that it may react with base.

Sulfur—sulfur is oxidized to sulfuric acid by the *Oxygen Flask* technique, then titrated. In the *Oxygen Flask* technique the sample is burned in a thick-walled iodine flask in an atmosphere of oxygen, in the presence of an absorbing solution (the nature of which depends on the sample being analyzed). After combustion the flask is shaken to absorb any gaseous product and treated as directed in the specific monograph.

Titration of a Liberated Acid by a Base

Benzaldehyde—See *Lemon Oil*, below.

Cellulose, Oxidized—the sample is shaken with calcium acetate solution, to exchange calcium ion for hydrogen ion of the free carboxyl groups. The liberated hydrogen ion is then titrated with standard base.

Lemon Oil—the aldehydes of the oil react with hydroxylammonium chloride to form the oxime, liberating free hydrochloric acid, which is titrated and the aldehyde content calculated as citral:

$$RCH{=}O + HONH_3Cl = RCH{=}NOH + HCl + H_2O$$

Orange Oil—see *Lemon Oil*, above; results calculated as decanal.

Phenacemide (and Tablets)—the amide is hydrolyzed to phenylacetic acid, extracted with chloroform, evaporated and the free acid titrated.

---

* See Table III for indicator abbreviations.

Table III—Indicators, Color Developing Reagents, Etc. [a]

AAP	4-Aminoantipyrine		MaG	Malachite green, TS
AAPF	4-Aminoantipyrine and potassium ferricyanide		MDB	Metadinitrobenzene
AC	Antimony trichloride		MeB	Methylene blue
ACBD	4-Amino-6-chloro-1,3-benzenedisulfonamide (diazotized)		MeO	Methyl orange
			MeP	Methyl purple, TS
ACT	Ammonium cobaltothiocyanate		MeR	Methyl red, TS
AMDB	Alkaline metadinitrobenzene		MeY	Methyl yellow (p-dimethylaminoazobenzene)
ANB	Alpha-nitroso-beta-naphthol (diazotized)		MP	Molybdophosphotungstate, TS
ANS	1,2,4-Aminonaphtholsulfonic acid		MRB	Methyl red—methylene blue, TS
AP	Alkaline picrate, TS		MV	Methyl violet, TS
AS	Ammonium molybdate and stannous chloride			
AT	Ammonium thiocyanate		Nb	Para-Naphtholbenzein
AV	Azoviolet		NiB	Nile blue hydrochloride
			Np	Nitrophenanthroline, TS
BcB	Bromocresol blue			
BcG	Bromocresol green		ON	Oxidized nitroprusside solution
BcP	Bromocresol purple		ONA	Ortho-Nitroaniline
BF	Basic fuchsin		Op	Ortho-Phenanthroline, TS
BM	Bratton-Marshall reagent; N-(1-naphthyl)-ethylenediamine added to the diazotized solution		PAN	1-(2-Pyridylazo)-2-naphthol
			PBA	Para-Bromoaniline
BnF	Beta-Naphthoquinone sulfonate—formaldehyde		PC	Potassium chromate, TS
BpB	Bromophenol blue		PDA	Para-Dimethylaminoazobenzene
BPy	2,2'-Bipyridine		PDB	Para-Dimethylaminobenzaldehyde
BT	Blue tetrazolium		PdC	Palladium chloride
BtB	Bromothymol blue		PDS	Phenoldisulfonic acid
			PH	Phenylhydrazine hydrochloride
CAN	Ceric ammonium nitrate, TS		Phth	Phenolphthalein
C-S	Cyanogen bromide—sulfanilic acid		Poten	Potentiometric determination of the end point
CR	Cresol red, TS		PR	Phenol red
CRTB	Cresol red—thymol blue, TS		PTB	Phenolphthalein—thymol blue
CrV	Crystal violet, TS		PTC	Potassium thiocyanate
CTA	Chromotropic acid		PyA	Pyridine-acetic anhydride
DCF	Dichlorofluorescein		QR	Quinaldine red
DC	Diphenylcarbazone, TS			
DBP	Dicyanobis(1,10-phenanthroline)iron II dihydrate		R	Reinecke's salt
DBQ	2,6-Dibromoquinone chlorimide		SA	Sulfuric acid in methanol
DcD	2,6-Dichloroquinone chlorimide		SAF	Sodium acetate-potassium ferricyanide
DNP	2,4-Dinitrophenylhydrazine		SAS	Sodium alizarinsulfonate, TS
DP	Diphenylamine, TS		SD	Sudan IV
DT	Dithizone		SN	Sodium nitrite in acid solution
			SNF	Sodium nitroferricyanide, TS
EBT	Eriochrome black T		SaO	Safranin O
EY	Eosin Y, TS		SPI	Starch-potassium iodide, TS, or paper or paste
FAS	Ferric ammonium sulfate, TS		ST	Starch, TS
FC	Ferric chloride, acid, TS			
FCiT	Ferrocitrate reagent		TB	Thymol blue
FCP	Folin-Ciocalteau-Phenol, TS		TBP	Tetrabromophenolphthalein, TS
FEH	Ferric chloride and hydroxylamine		TBPE	Tetrabromophenolphthalein, ethyl ester, TS
FEN	Ferric nitrate		TNP	Trinitrophenol (picric acid)
FET	Ferrous tartrate reagent		TP	Thymolphthalein
			TTC	Triphenyltetrazolium chloride
HDA	Hexanitrodiphenylamine			
HNB	Hydroxynaphthol blue		UV	Ultraviolet radiation
HQ	8-Hydroxyquinoline			
			VS	Vanadyl sulfate
IN	Isoniazid reagent			
IP	Iron-phenol reagent		XyO	Xylenol orange

[a] These are coded in the last column of *Table VI* in this chapter. They are usually employed as solutions, and often are the official Test Solutions (TS).

Polyoxyethylene 50 Stearate (stearic acid)—following saponification, the liberated acid is extracted with hexane, evaporated, and the acid titrated with base.

Sørensen Formol Titration

Meprobamate (and Injection and Oral Suspension)—after hydrolysis of the ester.

Protein Hydrolysate Injection—for alpha-amino nitrogen.

In each case the free amino acid is treated with formaldehyde to form the methylimino or methylol derivative, reducing the basicity of the amino group so that the free carboxyl group may be titrated.

$$RCH(NH_2)COOH + HCHO =$$
$$RCH(NHCH_2OH)COOH \text{ or } RCH(N{=}CH_2)COOH$$

Residual Titration of Excess Base after Interaction with Acid

In this type of assay a measured excess of standard base is added to the prepared sample and the excess titrated with standard acid. Quite often a blank titration is performed, whereby the same volume of base, which was added to the sample, is titrated with standard acid. The difference in the volume of titrant used for the blank and sample is the volume of titrant equivalent to the sample.

Glutaral Concentrate—to a solution of hydroxylamine hydrochloride, neutralized to BpB with triethanolamine, a measured excess of triethanolamine is added, followed by the sample. The HCl liberated in the following reaction combines with triethanolamine and the excess is titrated with standard sulfuric acid. A blank is run on the reagents.

$$OHC(CH_2)_3CHO + 2NH_2OH \cdot HCl =$$
$$HON{=}CH(CH_2)_3CH{=}NOH + 2H_2O + 2HCl$$

Methenamine and Monobasic Sodium Phosphate Tablets—for sodium biphosphate.

All of the phosphates above are assayed by first precipitating ammonium phosphomolybdate from a dilute nitric acid solution of the sample:

$$AlPO_4 + 12(NH_4)_2MoO_4 + 24HNO_3 =$$
$$(NH_4)_3PO_4.12MoO_3 + 21NH_4NO_3 + Al(NO_3)_3 + 12H_2O$$

The precipitated yellow molybdate is filtered, washed free of adhering nitric acid, and dissolved in an excess of standard alkali:

$$(NH_4)_3PO_4.12MoO_3 + 23NaOH = 11Na_2MoO_4 +$$
$$NaNH_4HPO_4 + (NH_4)_2MoO_4 + 11H_2O$$

Excess standard alkali is then titrated with standard acid.
Chloral Hydrate (and Capsules and Syrup).
The chloral-containing compounds are treated with excess standard sodium hydroxide which hydrolyzes the chloral to chloroform and sodium formate. Excess base is titrated with standard acid.

$$CCl_3CHO.H_2O + NaOH = CHCl_3 + HCOONa + H_2O$$

With Chloral Hydrate Syrup a correction must be made for original acidity by a preliminary titration of the sample, with base.
Ethyl Chloride.
For ethyl chloride the halogen is hydrolyzed with excess standard alcoholic alkali and the excess titrated with acid.
Formaldehyde Solution.
The formaldehyde is oxidized to formic acid with peroxide in the presence of excess standard base and the excess titrated.

Direct Titration of Base by Acid

Aminophylline (and Enema, Injection and Tablets)—for ethylenediamine using MeO.
Oxtriphylline—for choline, using MeB.
Potassium Hydroxide—for potassium hydroxide using Phth and for potassium carbonate content using MeO.
Sodium Citrate and Citric Acid Solution—For citric acid by titration to a phenolphthalein end point.
Theophylline Olamine (and Solution)—for monoethanolamine using MeO.
Thiotepa—sodium thiosulfate reacts with each ethyleneimine group to liberate one equivalent of alkali, which is titrated with standard acid.

$$—N\big\langle\begin{smallmatrix}CH_2\\|\\CH_2\end{smallmatrix} + Na_2S_2O_3 + H_2O =$$
$$—NHCH_2CH_2S_2O_3Na + NaOH$$

Tromethamine (and for Injection)—for tromethamine using BcP.

Titration of Volatile Bases after Distillation

Compounds in this category are usually hydrolyzed by boiling with strong alkali and the ammonia or amines formed are distilled into excess standard acid or into a saturated boric acid solution. In either case, the excess standard acid is titrated with standard base, or the ammonia-boric acid complex titrated with acid, methyl red being the indicator for either method. If the nitrogen content only is determined, the Kjeldahl procedure is used.

Calcium Pantothenate—nitrogen content by Kjeldahl method.
Glucagon—nitrogen content by Kjeldahl method.
Ichthammol (and Ointment)—for ammonia; make alkaline and distil into excess standard acid.
Neostigmine Methylsulfate—dimethylamine distilled.
Pyrazinamide—amide hydrolyzed and ammonia distilled.

Titration of Metal Salts with Acid

Caffeine and Sodium Benzoate Injection—the caffeine is extracted with chloroform, ether is added to the residual aqueous solution and the mixture titrated with acid, shaking vigorously. As free benzoic acid is liberated by titration with hydrochloric acid it is immediately extracted into the ether phase. As the end point is exceeded, excess titrant causes the indicator (MeO) to change.

Residual Titration of Excess Acid after Interaction with Base

For this category a basic substance is treated with a measured excess of standard acid and the excess acid titrated with standard base.

Ammonia Spirit, Aromatic—for the total ammonia assay, the sample is boiled with excess standard acid and the excess titrated with sodium

hydroxide. The ammonium carbonate is converted into an equivalent amount of sodium carbonate.
Magnesium Trisilicate—for magnesium oxide (MeO).
Zinc Undecylenate—excess standard sulfuric acid is boiled with the salt, the liberated undecylenic acid extracted with hexane and the aqueous phase titrated with standard base (MeO).

Residual Titration of Excess Acid following Liberation of a Base by a Stronger Base

Assays of this kind are also applied to extractions made of vegetable drugs containing alkaloidal principles and to the pharmaceutical preparations obtained from them.

All of the assays are based on the principle that relatively weak organic bases are readily displaced from their salts by a stronger base, such as sodium hydroxide, sodium carbonate, or ammonium hydroxide. The last compound is more generally employed to liberate alkaloids from their salts. The liberated free bases are then extracted into an organic solvent (ether or chloroform) and the separated organic phase evaporated.

Titration of Carbonate Residues from Ignited Salts

In general the ignition of an alkali metal salt of a carboxylic acid forms sodium carbonate, carbon dioxide, and water as exemplified by sodium citrate:

$$2Na_3C_6H_5O_7 + 9O_2 = 3Na_2CO_3 + 9CO_2 + 5H_2O$$

Excess standard acid is added to the ignition residue and the residue titrated with base. The volume of standard acid consumed is multiplied by the appropriate conversion factor to determine the amount of alkali salt in the sample taken.

Magnesium Citrate Oral Solution—for citric acid (Phth), after precipitation of calcium citrate and ignition of the filtered salt.
Ringer's Injection, Lactated—for sodium lactate (MeO).

Residual Titration Involving Saponification of an Ester

In general, esters are determined by a saponification procedure of boiling the sample in excess standard alcoholic alkali, which acts as a mutual solvent. The excess alkali is determined with standard acid. A blank is usually run on the same volume of alkali used for the saponification procedure.

Oxandrolone—the ester is present in lactone form.
Peppermint Oil—for total menthol content. The free menthol is first acetylated with acetic anhydride to form the ester, menthyl acetate. After purification, to remove excess acetic acid and water, the ester is subjected to the saponification procedure.
Polysorbates—saponification value.
Polyvinyl Alcohol—saponification and hydrolysis values.
Storax—saponification value.
Tolu Balsam—saponification value.

Residual Titration following an Acylation Reaction

The general method involves the treatment of an alcohol with an acylating reagent, usually acetic anhydride or phthalic anhydride in pyridine. Any excess anhydride remaining after the esterification reaction is converted to the free acid with water, and the acid titrated with standard base. A blank is usually run employing all the reagents except the sample. The difference in titer between the blank and the sample is the volume of base equivalent to the alcohol content of the sample taken.

Polyethylene Glycol—for average molecular weight, using phthalic anhydride in pyridine.

Residual Titration following the Hydrolysis of Alkoxyl Groups

A previously neutralized sample is saponified with excess standard base and the excess determined in the usual manner.

Pectin—for methoxyl groups (galacturonic acid).

Precipitation Reactions

Titration of Liberated Nitric Acid

In assays of this type silver nitrate reacts with the substance being assayed, to form an insoluble silver derivative, simultaneously releasing an equivalent amount of nitric acid which is titrated with standard alkali.

Ethinamate—an acetylenic hydrogen reacts with silver nitrate.
Oxtriphylline—for theophylline. The solution from the choline assay is treated with silver nitrate and the above method followed.

Direct Titration of a Theophylline–Silver Complex

The theophylline-silver complex is separated by filtration, dissolved in nitric acid and the liberated silver ion titrated with thiocyanate (FAS indicator).

Aminophylline Suppositories—for theophylline.

Residual Titration of a Theophylline–Silver Complex

The insoluble silver complex is precipitated from an ammoniacal solution of the sample by warming with excess standard silver nitrate. After filtration, the excess silver ion is determined in the filtrate by titration with thiocyanate (FAS indicator).

Aminophylline (and Injection and Tablets)—for theophylline.
Dimenhydrinate—for 8-chlorotheophylline.
Theophylline Olamine (and Enema)—for theophylline.

Direct Titration of Halogen

These assays may involve the conversion of organic halogen to halide ion (if covalently bound), before titration. Silver nitrate is the titrant in all cases.

The following are titrated without previous treatment:

Anticoagulant Heparin Solution and Heparin Lock Flush Solution—for NaCl.

The following require hydrolysis with alkali:

Melphalan
Methyclothiazide—although two chlorine atoms occur in the molecule only the benzylic halogen is sufficiently active to be hydrolyzed and then titrated with silver nitrate.
Pipobroman

The following require refluxing with zinc and alkali to liberate the halogen:

Diatrizoate Meglumine (and Injection)
Diatrizoate Meglumine and Diatrizoate Sodium Injection—the assay gives both compounds and a correction is made for Diatrizoate Meglumine
Diatrizoate Sodium (and Injection and Solution)
Diatrizoic Acid
Iocetamic Acid and Tablets
Iodipamide
Iodipamide Meglumine Injection
Iopanoic Acid
Iothalamate Meglumine Injection
Iothalamate Meglumine and Iothalamate Sodium Injection
Iothalamate Sodium Injection
Iothalamic Acid
Ipodate Calcium and for Oral Suspension
Ipodate Sodium and Capsules
Methiodal Sodium and Injection

Residual Titration of Halogen

Excess standard silver nitrate is added to a solution of the prepared sample containing ionic halogen. The excess silver nitrate is then titrated with standard ammonium thiocyanate. This method is known as the Volhard procedure. Nitrobenzene is added, in the titration involving silver chloride, to prevent its interaction with thiocyanate. Ferric Alum (FAS) is the usual indicator. Quite often the ionic halogen must be liberated from an organic compound.

Chlorobutanol—after hydrolysis with base.
Mannitol and Sodium Chloride Injection—for sodium chloride.
Sodium Chloride and Dextrose Tablets—for sodium chloride.

Titration with Thiocyanate

Silver ion or mercury (II) ion is titrated with thiocyanate. With silver, insoluble silver thiocyanate is formed; with mercury (II) un-ionized mercuric thiocyanate is produced. Ferric alum (FAS) is the usual indicator.

Benzoylpas Calcium—p-benzamidosalicylic acid is precipitated as the silver salt with excess standard silver nitrate and the excess titrated with thiocyanate.
Nitromersol (and Solution and Tincture)—the sample is digested with sulfuric acid and peroxide, and oxidized with permanganate to form mercuric ion.
Phenylmercuric Acetate and Phenylmercuric Nitrate—both are decomposed with formic acid to release mercury, which is scavenged with zinc metal and then dissolved in nitric acid.

Titration with Thorium (IV)

Sodium Monofluorophosphate—The sample, acidified with sulfuric acid, is distilled and the fluoride-containing distillate is titrated with thorium nitrate solution, using sodium alizarinsulfonate indicator. Insoluble thorium tetrafluoride is formed in the acid solution, and when all the fluoride ion is precipitated the pink-red thorium salt of the indicator is produced.

Redox Reactions

Titrations Involving Direct Oxidation with Ceric Sulfate

Ceric sulfate is of value in titrating iron(II) salts in mixtures that contain excipients or diluents which have a reducing action on permanganate, but have no effect on ceric sulfate. The equation which applies is:

$$2FeSO_4 + 2Ce(SO_4)_2 = Fe_2(SO_4)_3 + Ce_2(SO_4)_3$$

Ferrous Fumarate—prior to titration with ceric sulfate, stannous chloride is added to insure that all the iron is in the reduced state; excess tin is removed by precipitation with mercuric ion.
Homatropine Hydrobromide—following hydrolysis with base, the mandelic acid thereby liberated is oxidized by the titrant.
Menadione (and Tablets)—the quinone groups are reduced with zinc and acid to hydroquinone and then reoxidized with the titrant.
Menadione Sodium Bisulfite Injection—menadione released by treatment with alkali is determined as stated above.

Direct Titration with Potassium Permanganate

The sample is directly oxidized by the permanganate titrant. No indicator is required, as a slight excess of permanganate imparts a distinct pink color indicating the end point.

Cherry Juice—for malic acid, which is converted to an equivalent amount of calcium maleate, the calcium of which is precipitated as calcium oxalate and determined as stated above.
Hydrogen Peroxide Concentrate (and Topical Solution).

Titration Utilizing Ferric Alum and Permanganate

In this reaction category an excess of ferric ammonium sulfate is added to the sample, which reduces the ferric iron to iron (II), and the latter is titrated with permanganate.

Titanium Dioxide—the sample is dissolved by heating with sulfuric acid and ammonium sulfate, the titanium (IV) is reduced to titanium (III) with zinc amalgam, ferric alum is added to reoxidize the titanium with simultaneous formation of an equivalent amount of ferrous ion which is titrated with permanganate.

Residual Titration Utilizing Oxalic Acid and Permanganate

Potassium Permanganate (and Tablets for Solution)—an excess of standard oxalic acid is reacted with a warm, acidified solution of the sample; the excess oxalic acid is then titrated with permanganate.
Sodium Nitrite—the nitrite is first oxidized to nitrate with an excess of standard permanganate, the unreacted permanganate is reduced with an excess of oxalic acid, which is titrated with more standard permanganate. The reason for using an excess of permanganate in the first step is to prevent loss of nitrous acid on acidifying the sodium nitrite, and the addition of an excess of oxalic acid is to insure reduction of permanganate to manganous ion rather than an intermediate of higher valence.

Dichlorophenol-Indophenol Titration

Ascorbic Acid may be quantitatively oxidized by titration with dichlorophenol-indophenol volumetric solution, which also serves as its own indicator. During the titration the blue color of the dichlorophenol-indophenol solution is discharged by the reducing action of the ascorbic acid; when the end point is reached a permanent reddish color is imparted by the slightest excess of titrant. The reaction is explained as follows:

2,6-dichlorophenolindophenol
(blue in alkaline—
red in acid solution)

reduced indicator
(colorless)

Sodium Tetraphenylboron Titration

Quaternary ammonium salts are capable of forming chloroform-soluble compounds with bromophenol blue as indicated below:

bromophenol   quaternary   chloroform-
blue   salt   soluble product

The product is extracted from alkaline solutions into chloroform. Titration with sodium tetraphenylboron removes the quaternary salt from the product, discharging the color from the chloroform layer. In this assay the quaternary salt and bromophenol blue, in a mixture of chloroform and water, is titrated with the sodium tetraphenylboron solution.

Assays Involving Diphasic Amine–Surfactant Titration

Cetylpyridinium Chloride Lozenges—see A, below.
Dicyclomine Hydrochloride Dosage Forms—see A, below.
Docusate Calcium—see B, below (TBA).
Docusate Sodium—see B, below (TBA).
Methylbenzethonium Chloride Dosage Forms—see A, below.

A. In this type of assay the amine salt is dissolved in chloroform, indicator added and the mixture shaken. The indicator dissolves in the organic phase. Titration of this two-phase system (with adequate shaking) with a surfactant solution, such as sodium lauryl sulfate, produces a water-soluble complex between amine and surfactant. As the end point is exceeded the excess surfactant reacts with the basic dye (in the organic layer) and the indicator color changes from pale yellow to red(MeY), blue(BpB) or pink(SaO). Standardization of the titrant is effected using a pure sample of the substance being assayed as the standard.
B. In this modification the surfactant is the substance being assayed and is added to the chloroform–water–indicator mixture. The titration is now performed utilizing a solution of a quaternary amine (cetalkonium chloride–CAC or tetrabutylammonium iodide–TBA) and the end point is reached when the color *disappears* from the chloroform layer.

Direct Titration with Titanium Trichloride

These titrations depend upon the reduction of the colored sample and subsequent discharge of the color at the end-point.

Residual Titration with Titanium Trichloride

The sample is heated with excess standard titanium trichloride, in an inert atmosphere. Excess reagent is determined by titration with ferric ammonium sulfate; thiocyanate ion, as the indicator, gives the familiar red end point.

Titration of Iodine Liberated from Potassium Iodide

Assays in this category involve addition of the substance being assayed to an acidified solution of potassium iodide as exemplified by the equation with cupric sulfate:

$$2CuSO_4 + 4KI = 2CuI + I_2 + 2K_2SO_4$$

The liberated iodine is titrated with thiosulfate, starch being employed as the indicator:

$$I_2 + 2Na_2S_2O_3 = 2NaI + Na_2S_4O_6$$

In many cases the sample requires an initial special treatment.

Dextrothyroxine Sodium—see A, below.
Dextrothyroxine Sodium Tablets—see B, below.
Ethiodized Oil Injection—see A, below.
Ethylcellulose—for ethoxyl, by the Zeisel alkoxy procedure.
Ferric Oxide—as for Ferrous Fumarate Tablets, replacing nitric acid with hydrochloric acid.
Ferrous Fumarate Tablets—the sample is decomposed with nitric and perchloric acids. Addition of KI to the iron(III) solution causes reduction of the iron and liberation of free iodine, which is titrated with thiosulfate.
Iodoquinol (and Tablets)—see A, below.
Iophendylate and Injection—treatment with sodium biphenyl in toluene liberates iodide ion which is extracted into dilute phosphoric acid. Addition of hypochlorite then liberates free iodine.

Methylcellulose Ophthalmic Solution and Oral Solution—methoxyl; see *Ethylcellulose*, above.
Phenindione—Bromine halogenates the carbon alpha to both carbonyl groups, the excess bromine is destroyed, KI added, which reacts with the active alpha halogen to liberate iodine.
Propyliodone (and Dosage Forms)—see A, below.
Selenium Sulfide (and Lotion)—after treatment with fuming nitric acid to form selenous acid. Potassium iodide then reduces the selenium, liberating iodine.

$$H_2SeO_3 + 4KI + 4H^+ = Se + 2I_2 + 4K^+ + 3H_2O$$

Thyroglobulin (and Tablets)—see B, below.
Thyroid (and Tablets)—see B, below.

A. Substances in this category are initially decomposed using the *Oxygen Flask Combustion Method*, and the sample is treated with bromine, etc, as directed for B, below.
B. The sample is fused with potassium carbonate, acidified, and oxidized with bromine to form iodate and bromide ions. The solution is boiled to expel bromine; phenol or formic acid is added to scavenge any remaining halogen; then KI is added and the iodate ion liberates free iodine which is titrated.

Titrations with Potassium Iodate

When potassium iodate solution is titrated into an acidified solution of an alkali metal iodide, free iodine is liberated according to the following equation:

$$5KI + KIO_3 + 6HCl = 6KCl + 3I_2 + 3H_2O$$

When this step of the reaction is complete, and if a sufficiently high concentration of hydrochloric acid is present, the liberated iodine is converted into iodine monochloride, as is shown by:

$$KIO_3 + 2I_2 + 6HCl = KCl + 5ICl + 3H_2O$$

combining both reactions:

$$KIO_3 + 2KI + 6HCl = 3KCl + 3ICl + 3H_2O$$

The end point of this titration is the disappearance of the iodine color from a few mL of chloroform added to serve as an indicator.

Benzalkonium Chloride (and Solution)—each equivalent of the quaternary chloride yields one equivalent of iodide ion, which is titrated according to the above reaction.
Hydralazine Hydrochloride Injection and Tablets—the hydrazino group of hydralazine is oxidized by potassium iodate to nitrogen and is replaced by a hydroxyl group on the phthalazine ring in accordance with the following equation:

hydralazine

$$+ KIO_3 + 2HCl =$$

1-phthalazinol

$$KCl + ICl +$$ $$+ N_2 + 2H_2O$$

Iodine Topical Solution—for sodium iodide; free iodine is first reduced by titration with arsenite.
Iodine Solution Strong—for potassium iodide; as for *Iodine Solution*.
Iodine Tincture, Strong Iodine Tincture—for sodium iodide; as for *Iodine Solution*.
Stannous Fluoride—for tin(II); in HCl solution, KI is added and iodide is converted to iodine, which is titrated with iodate.

Reaction of KI with Excess Periodate

Diatrizoate Meglumine and Diatrizoate Sodium Solution—the meglumine (*N*-methylglucamine) component of the diatrizoate adduct consumes four moles of periodate on oxidation, forming four moles of iodate. On addition of an excess of KI both iodate and periodate oxidize iodide to iodine, but iodate forms six equivalents while periodate yields eight equivalents of iodine. The difference in the thiosulfate titer of the blank (only periodate) and the sample (iodate plus periodate) is the thiosulfate equivalent of the iodine deficiency resulting from oxidation of the sample. As each mole of periodate consumed is equivalent to two gram-atoms of iodine, the equivalent weight of diatrizoate meglumine is one-eighth the formula weight.

Mannitol (and Injection)—an acidified solution of the prepared sample is heated with periodate and acid, oxidizing the mannitol as follows:

$$C_6H_{14}O_6 + 5HIO_4 = 2HCHO + 4HCOOH + 5HIO_3 + H_2O$$

The excess periodate and the iodate formed in the reaction react with KI to liberate iodine:

$$HIO_3 + HIO_4 + 12HI = 7I_2 + 7H_2O$$

A blank is performed and the difference in the volumes of thiosulfate titrant is equivalent to the mannitol in the sample.

Mannitol and Sodium Chloride Injection—for mannitol, as above.

Direct Titration of Iodine with Thiosulfate

No preliminary preparation of the sample is necessary, as the iodine is present in the free state.

Povidone–Iodine—for available iodine.

Residual Titration of Iodine following Dichromate Precipitation

These assays are based on the insolubility of the dichromate precipitated from an aqueous solution of the sample on the addition of excess standard potassium dichromate. After removal of the precipitate the excess dichromate in the filtrate is determined by adding excess KI, which liberates free iodine and is titrated with thiosulfate.

$$Cr_2O_7{}^{2-} + 14H^+ + 6I^- = 3I_2 + 2Cr^{3+} + 7H_2O$$

Residual Titration of Excess Standard Iodine

A sample of the assay material is oxidized or converted to a periodide or iodine substitution product with standard iodine and the excess iodine determined by titration with thiosulfate.

Racemethionine (and dosage forms)—being a thioether, the methionine, in a phosphate buffer, is treated with excess standard iodine, which oxidizes the ether to the sulfoxide and the excess iodine is titrated with thiosulfate.

$$CH_3SCH_2CH_2CH(NH_2)COOH + I_2 + 3H_2O =$$
$$CH_3SOCH_2CH_2CH(NH_2)COOH + 2I^- + 2H_3O^+$$

Phenelzine Sulfate (and Tablets)—the hydrazine is oxidized by iodine as is indicated by the equation

$$C_6H_5CH_2NHNH_2.H_2SO_4 + 2I_2 + 5NaHCO_3 =$$
$$C_6H_5CH_2I + 3NaI + Na_2SO_4 + 5CO_2 + 5H_2O + N_2$$

Iodimetric Determination of Phenols

In these assays a bromophenol derivative is precipitated by adding a bromine (potassium bromate-potassium bromide) volumetric solution to a solution of the sample and acidifying to release free bromine, according to the reaction:

$$5KBr + KBrO_3 + 6HCl = 6KCl + 3Br_2 + 3H_2O$$

The free bromine immediately reacts with the phenolic substance according to the following equation, using phenol as an example:

$$C_6H_5OH + 3Br_2 = C_6H_2Br_3OH + 3HBr$$

Potassium iodide is then added and the excess bromine liberates free iodine:

$$2KI + Br_2 = 2KBr + I_2$$

and it is titrated with thiosulfate. A blank is run on the same quantity of reagents, omitting the sample.

Direct Titration with Standard Iodine

The sample is titrated directly, starch TS usually being employed as the indicator.

Ascorbic Acid—a direct titration. If ascorbic acid is present in a multiple vitamin preparation, the dichlorophenol-indophenol procedure is employed.

Carbarsone (and Dosage Forms)—the sample is first subjected to an acid digestion and reduction of arsenic to the trivalent form. The resulting arsenite is then titrated:

$$Na_2HAsO_3 + I_2 + H_2O = Na_2HAsO_4 + 2HI$$

Added sodium carbonate reacts with the HI formed to prevent reversal of the reaction.

Echothiophate Iodide (and for Ophthalmic Solution)—the ester is first hydrolyzed with pH 12 buffer to yield the free mercaptan, which is then oxidized, by titration with iodine, to the disulfide. Any free mercaptan in the original sample is corrected for by a preliminary titration. The following equations apply:

$$[(C_2H_5O)_2(PO)—S—CH_2CH_2N(CH_3)_3]^+I^- + H_2O =$$

Echothiophate

$$[HSCH_2CH_2N(CH_3)_3]^+I^- + (C_2H_5O)_2(PO)OH$$

$$2[HSCH_2CH_2N(CH_3)_3]^+I^- + I_2 =$$

mercaptan

$$2[—SCH_2CH_2N(CH_3)_3{}^+]I^- + 2HI$$

Sulfur Dioxide—on absorption in sodium hydroxide bisulfite ion is produced and then titrated with iodine.

Residual Titration of Excess Thiosulfate with Iodine

Mechlorethamine Hydrochloride and Mechlorethamine Hydrochloride for Injection—thiosulfate reacts with the active chlorine atoms according to the equation

$$CH_3N(CH_2CH_2Cl)_2.HCl + NaHCO_3 + 2Na_2S_2O_3 =$$
$$CH_3N(CH_2CH_2S_2O_3Na)_2 + 3NaCl + CO_2 + H_2O$$

Direct Titration of Iodine with Arsenite

Free or liberated iodine is titrated with a standard sodium arsenite solution.

Iodine Topical Solution—for iodine.
Iodine Solution, Strong—for free iodine.
Iodine Tincture and Strong Iodine Tincture—for free iodine.

Direct Titration with Ferric Chloride

Articles in this category are titrated with ferric chloride using thiocyanate indicator.

Direct Titration with Standard Bromine

Thymol—a warm solution of the sample is titrated to produce a bromo-derivative, analogous to the determination of phenols. However, an excess is not employed, since methyl orange whose color is bleached as the equivalence point is exceeded is used as an indicator.

Direct Titration with Potassium Ferricyanide

Methyprylon (and Capsules and Tablets)—in this assay ferricyanide oxidizes the diketopiperidine ring effecting loss of 2 atoms of hydrogen; 2 moles of ferricyanide are consumed per mole of methyprylon. The end-point is determined potentiometrically.

methyprylon   **dehydro derivative**

Titrations Involving Sodium Nitrite Solution

Most compounds in this group, being primary aromatic amines or derivatives which may be converted to such amines, are capable of undergoing quantitative diazotization of the amino group substituted on the aromatic ring, as illustrated by the following equation utilizing p-aminobenzoic acid.

$$H_2NC_6H_4COOH + NaNO_2 + 2HCl =$$
$$ClN_2C_6H_4COOH + NaCl + 2H_2O$$

The titration with sodium nitrite is performed potentiometrically in a solution containing crushed ice, to prevent decomposition of the diazonium salt, or until a drop of the titrated solution produces an immediate blue color with starch iodide paste used as an external indicator.

Sulfonamides in which the reactive amino group is acylated must first be hydrolyzed to release the free amine form of the sulfonamide prior to diazotization.

Table IV—Systems for Nonaqueous Titrations

Type of Solvent	Acidic (for titration of bases and their salts)	Relatively Neutral (for differential titration of bases)	Basic (for titration of acids)	Relatively Neutral (for differential titration of acids)
Solvent[1]	Glacial Acetic Acid Acetic Anhydride Formic Acid Propionic Acid Sulfuryl Chloride	Acetonitrile Alcohols Chloroform Benzene Chlorobenzene Ethyl Acetate Dioxane	Dimethylformamide n-Butylamine Pyridine Ethylenediamine Morpholine	Acetone Acetonitrile Methyl Ethyl Ketone Methyl Isobutyl Ketone tert-Butyl Alcohol
Indicator	Crystal Violet Quinaldine Red p-Naphtholbenzein Alphazurine 2-G Malachite green	Methyl Red Methyl Orange p-Naphtholbenzein	Thymol Blue Thymolphthalein Azo Violet o-Nitroaniline p-Hydroxyazobenzene	Azo Violet Bromothymol Blue p-Hydroxyazobenzene Thymol Blue
Electrodes	Glass-calomel Glass-silver–silver chloride Mercury–mercuric acetate	Glass-calomel Calomel-silver–silver chloride	Antimony-calomel Antimony-glass Antimony-antimony[2] Platinum-calomel Glass-calomel	Antimony-calomel Glass-calomel Glass-platinum[2]

[1] Relatively neutral solvents of low dielectric constant such as benzene, chloroform, or dioxane may be used in conjunction with any acidic or basic solvent in order to increase the sensitivity of the titration end-points.
[2] In titrant.

Primaquine Phosphate (and Tablets)—this substance contains a secondary amino group and nitrosation rather than diazotization occurs, the $=NH$ group being converted to $=N—NO$ (N-nitroso).
Procaine and Tetracaine Hydrochlorides and Levonordefrin Injection—for procaine and tetracaine, after removal as the thiocyanate.
Trisulfapyrimidines Oral Suspension (and Tablets)—assay for total sulfapyrimidines.

Complexation Reactions

Direct with Ethylenediaminetetraacetic Acid (EDTA)

EDTA complexes with many polyvalent metals to form an undissociated chelate. A buffered solution of the sample is titrated with EDTA (as the disodium salt). The indicator used is a dye which forms a weak chelate with the assay material. At the end point the color changes when the indicator–metal complex can no longer exist.

Alumina and Magnesia Oral Suspension (and Tablets)—for magnesium hydroxide, using ammonium hydroxide and ammonium chloride buffer (EBT).
Calcium Pantothenate (and Tablets)—calcium content.
Calcium Pantothenate, Racemic—calcium content.
Edetate Calcium Disodium (and Injection)—mercury (II) nitrate is the titrant.
Edetate Disodium (and Injection)—primary standard calcium carbonate, after suitable preparation, is titrated with a solution of the *Assay Preparation.*
Edetic Acid—calcium carbonate (primary standard) is titrated with a solution of the *Assay Preparation.*
Magaldrate (and Oral Suspension and Tablets)—for magnesium oxide.
Magnesia and Alumina Oral Suspension (and Tablets)—for magnesium Oxide.
Ringer's Injection and Irrigation—calcium content.
Ringer's Injection, Lactated—calcium content.

Residual Titration Involving EDTA

To assay for aluminum in many combinations containing both magnesium and aluminum a residual method is employed. Excess EDTA is added to a suitably buffered sample and the excess determined by titration with standard zinc sulfate solution. By use of proper buffers and masking agents (weak complexing materials) it is often possible to determine mixtures of calcium and aluminum, calcium and magnesium, or zinc and aluminum without preliminary separation.

Alumina and Magnesia Oral Suspension (and Tablets)—for aluminum oxide (DC).
Aluminum Acetate Topical Solution—for aluminum oxide (DC).
Aluminum Subacetate Topical Solution—for aluminum oxide (DC).
Magaldrate (and Oral Suspension and Tablets)—for aluminum oxide (DC).
Magnesia and Alumina Oral Suspension (and Tablets)—for aluminum oxide (DC).

Miscellaneous Complexometric Methods

Penicillamine (and Capsules)—direct titration with mercury (II) acetate; penicillamine is an excellent complexing agent and readily combines with mercury. As the end point is passed, excess titrant forms the violet mercury–diphenylcarbazone.

Acid-Base Reactions in Nonaqueous Solvents

Titrimetric methods employing nonaqueous solvents are extensively used for the assay of certain materials which cannot be easily titrated in aqueous systems. Water is a leveling solvent and many weak acids or bases do not give a sufficiently sharp break in the titration curve to evidence a distinct end point. However, in a nonaqueous solvent, such as glacial acetic acid, weak organic bases and their salts can be titrated with an acetic acid solution of perchloric acid. While the strongest acid available in aqueous medium is the oxonium ion, H_3O^+, in acetic acid the proton of perchloric acid forms the acetacidium ion, $CH_3C(OH)_2^+$.

$$CH_3COOH + HClO_4 = CH_3C(OH)_2^+ + ClO_4^-$$

The reaction between acetacidium ion and an amine (a weak base) is illustrated by the following equation, forming the ammonium ion and acetic acid.

$$CH_3C(OH)_2^+ + RNH_2 = CH_3COOH + RNH_3^+$$

No difficulty is experienced in the titration of amine salts other than salts of halogen acids. In the latter case mercury (II) acetate is added to form undissociated mercury (II) halide, thus preventing interference by the halogen acid which would be liberated in its absence (Pifer-Wollish method).

Weak organic acids, such as carboxylic acids, phenols, barbiturates, sulfonamides or enols may also be titrated in nonaqueous medium using a strong base. These include the sodium or lithium salts of methanol or ethanol and the reaction is of the ordinary neutralization type, as illustrated below for an organic acid with sodium ethoxide.

$$RCOOH + C_2H_5ONa = RCOONa + C_2H_5OH$$

In both types of titration, acid or base, the end point may be determined with indicators or potentiometrically as depicted in the accompanying chart (Table IV) taken from the USP.

Titration of Basic Substances

Dimenhydrinate—for diphenhydramine (poten).

Diphenoxylate Hydrochloride and Atropine Sulfate Oral Solution and Tablets—for diphenoxylate hydrochloride.

Isobucaine Hydrochloride and Epinephrine Injection—for isobucaine.

Mepivacaine Hydrochloride and Levonordefrin Injection—for mepivacaine.

Potassium Acetate—titration of a salt of a carboxylic acid.

Potassium Sorbate—see *Potassium Acetate*.

Titration of Acidic Substances

A strong base is used to titrate very weak acids. Special precautions must be employed to exclude atmospheric carbon dioxide, which interferes with the titration. The titrants used frequently are indicated.

Titrants employed:

1—Lithium methoxide solution.
2—Sodium methoxide solution.
3—Tetrabutylammonium hydroxide solution.
4—Tributylethylammonium hydroxide solution.

Gravimetric Methods

In gravimetric methods of analysis the assay results are generally obtained either by determining the weight of a substance in the sample, or the weight of some other substance derived from the sample, the equivalent weight of which serves as the basis for calculating the result. Separation of the substance ultimately weighed is frequently accomplished by purely physical methods. On the other hand, there are many instances in which it is necessary to utilize a chemical reaction in order to convert the substance to a corresponding amount of some other substance which can be separated, purified, and weighed. The various types of official gravimetric assays may be conveniently grouped into the following categories.

Weighing the Active Ingredient after Separation

The active principle is separated, dried, and weighed.

Caffeine and Sodium Benzoate Injection—for caffeine, after solution of the sodium benzoate in water.

Collodion—pyroxylin is precipitated by water, dried, and weighed.

Estrone Injection—an elaborate purification procedure is involved whereby the estrone is converted to a water-soluble derivative using trimethylacethydrazide ammonium chloride (Girard's reagent for carbonyl compounds); the aqueous extract contains only ketonic material as the reagent reacts only with carbonyl compounds. The aqueous extract is then decomposed with acid to regenerate estrone, which is extracted into chloroform, the solvent removed, and the residue weighed.

Zinc-Eugenol Cement—for rosin by loss in weight after chloroform extraction.

Weighing of the Residue after Ignition of the Sample

Aluminum Monostearate—as aluminum oxide.

Silica Gel—see *Silicon Dioxide, Colloidal*.

Silicon Dioxide, Colloidal—silica is determined by difference; the sample is weighed before and after treatment with hydrofluoric acid, which converts silica into the volatile silicon tetrafluoride. The difference in weight represents the silica content of the sample.

Zinc-Eugenol Cement—for total zinc, as the oxide.

Zinc Oxide and Salicylic Acid Paste—for total zinc, as the oxide.

Precipitation and Weighing of a Derivative of the Active Ingredient

Anticoagulant Citrate Phosphate Dextrose Solution—for dextrose a precipitate of Cu_2O, from reaction with Fehling's solution, is weighed.

Barium Sulfate—the sample is fused with sodium carbonate, forming barium carbonate which is dissolved in acid and the barium precipitated as the chromate and weighed.

Camphor Spirit—for camphor as the 2,4-dinitrophenylhydrazone.

Ichthammol (and Ointment)—for total sulfur as barium sulfate after oxidation with nitric acid and perchlorate (see *Sulfur Ointment*).

Lanolin Alcohols—the cholesterol content is determined by precipitation as digitonide.

Magnesium Citrate Solution—for MgO as the 8-hydroxyquinolate.

Parachlorophenol, Camphorated—for *para*-chlorophenol: silver chloride is precipitated after release of chloride by oxidation with hot permanganate. For camphor: as the 2,4-dinitrophenylhydrazone.

Potash, Sulfurated—for sulfur by treatment with copper (II) sulfate to precipitate copper (II) sulfide, which is ignited to oxide and weighed.

Sorbitan Esters—the sample is saponified, the fatty acid separated from the acidified aqueous solution and weighed. The aqueous phase is concentrated, extracted with ethanol, the extract concentrated to yield the *polyols*, which are weighed.

Sulfur Ointment—the sample is oxidized with nitric acid to convert sulfur to sulfate, which is precipitated and weighed as barium sulfate.

Spectrometric Methods

Photometric analysis depends upon the measurement of the amount of light absorbed by a solution (*spectrophotometry*), or by a suspension (*turbidimetry*), or the amount of light scattered by a suspension (*nephelometry*), or the intensity of the light emitted by an element when subjected to high temperatures (*flame photometry*). The measurement of light in the visible region (*colorimetry*) may be accomplished using a colorimeter or spectrophotometer or less accurately by visual comparison with color standards. See Chapter 34 for a more detailed treatment.

Radiant energy waves that are of importance to spectrophotometry range from 200 to 400 nm in the ultraviolet, from 400 to 750 nm in the visible range, and from 750 to 25,000 nm in the near infrared and infrared regions. The relatively large number of spectrometric assays that are now described in the official compendia testifies to the widespread development and general acceptance of the analytical methods that belong in this category.

Visible Absorption (Colorimetry) Assays

If an absorption spectrometric analysis is specified in the USP-NF, a formula is provided to ensure accuracy in the calculation of the analytical result. In most cases, a numerical constant is found in the formula and may be deduced as follows.

Since Beer's Law holds for both the analyte (A) and standard (S) solutions, Eqs 1 and 2 may be written.

$$A_A = abc_A \qquad (1)$$

$$A_S = abc_S \qquad (2)$$

where A_A is the absorbance of the analyte solution whose concentration is C_A; A_S is the absorbance of the standard solution whose concentration is C_S; a is the absorptivity of the drug substance and b is the path length or cell thickness. If cells of the same thickness are used, Eq 1 may be divided by Eq 2 and the resulting expression solved for C_A to give Eq 3.

$$C_A = \frac{A_A}{A_S} C_S \qquad (3)$$

In order for a solution to have a proper concentration such that the absorbance may be in the range of the spectrometer, an initial analyte sample, large enough to minimize weighing errors, is chosen and the initial solution is then carried through a series of dilutions to produce the final desired solution concentration. Since the final analytical measurement should be related back to the original analyte sample, W_A in mg, Eq 4 may be written to indicate the total volume, V_A in liters, of solution of concentration C_A, in mg per liter, that would result if the entire quantity, W_A, were diluted directly.

$$W_A = V_A C_A \qquad (4)$$

Eq 4 may be solved for C_A and substituted into Eq 3 to yield Eq 5. Thus, the constant V_A is the numerical constant that is found in spectrophotometric analyses and represents the total volume of solution of concentration C_S that could be made from the entire initial analyte sample, W_A.

$$W_A = V_A \frac{A_A}{A_S} C_S \qquad (5)$$

Under this heading, are considered those assays that depend on the development of color or upon the color of the substance being assayed. The absorbances are accordingly measured at wavelengths that are within the visible range of the spectrum. These colorimetric assays generally consist of adding a reagent to the assay preparation or to the substance being tested, in order to produce a color which is compared with that of a standard preparation that has been prepared simultaneously and contains approximately an equal quantity of a reference standard. When the absorbance of a frequently assayed substance has been found to conform to Beer's law over a reasonable range of concentration, it is considered permissible to utilize a standard curve, prepared with the respective reference standard, for interpolation of the data obtained with the assay preparation.

In some instances characteristic colors are developed in *flame photometers* by subjecting an inorganic element or its compound in solution to an intensely hot flame. The intensity of the colors (radiations) is compared photoelectrically in a suitable spectrometer with standard solutions containing the same element.

The various models of available spectrometers are suitable for making these colorimetric measurements. Photoelectric colorimeters of the filter type, in which the light absorption is measured by sensitive photoelectric cells, are also largely used for making these determinations and several of them are commercially available.

Dye-Complex Method

Quaternary salts and many amines are capable of forming chloroform-soluble complexes with indicators, such as bromophenol blue. The usual procedure is to shake a mixture of the assay preparation, chloroform, and a buffer containing the indicator. The dye-complex partitions into the organic layer, which is separated, filtered to remove any adhering aqueous phase and the absorbance determined.

Colorimetry Involving a Chromogenic Reagent

If a three-digit number followed by a letter code is given, this indicates the analytical wavelength and color-developing reagent employed.

Anticoagulant Citrate Phosphate Dextrose Solution—for monobasic sodium phosphate; 660, ANS: for sodium citrate; 425, PyA.

Carbachol Ophthalmic Solution—hypochlorite is employed to form the *N*-chloroamide and this derivative with KI forms free iodine which reacts with starch TS, 590.

Cobalamin Concentrate—see *Cobalamin Assay—Radiotracer Method*, USP XX; 361 and 550.

Ergotamine Tartrate and Caffeine Suppositories (and Tablets)—for ergotamine; 515, PDB.

Ethynodiol Diacetate and Ethinyl Estradiol Tablets—for ethinyl estradiol; 536, SA.

Isobucaine Hydrochloride and Epinephrine Injection—for epinephrine; 530, FCiT.

Isoproterenol Hydrochloride and Phenylephrine Bitartrate Inhalation Aerosol—for isoproterenol hydrochloride; 530, FCiT; for phenylephrine bitartrate; 495, HgSO₄, SN.

Mepivacaine Hydrochloride and Levonordefrin Injection—for levonordefrin; 530, FCiT.

Meprobamate Tablets—as for *Carbachol Ophthalmic Solution*, but omitting starch; 358.

Meprylcaine Hydrochloride and Epinephrine Injection—for epinephrine; 530, FCiT.

Methenamine and Monobasic Sodium Phosphate Tablets—for methenamine; 570, CTA.

Norethindrone Acetate and Ethinyl Estradiol Tablets—for ethinyl estradiol; 536, H₂SO₄.

Norgestrel and Ethinyl Estradiol Tablets—for ethinyl estradiol; 536, H₂SO₄.

Procaine and Phenylephrine Hydrochlorides Injection—for phenylephrine; 500, AAP.

Procaine and Tetracaine Hydrochlorides and Levonordefrin Injection—for levonordefrin; 530, FCiT.

Procaine and Propoxycaine Hydrochlorides and Levonordefrin Injection—for levonordefrin; 530, FCiT.

Propoxycaine and Procaine Hydrochlorides and Norepinephrine Bitartrate Injection—for norepinephrine; 530, FCiT.

Propoxyphene Napsylate and Aspirin Tablets—for aspirin; 530, FEN.

Reserpine, Hydralazine Hydrochloride and Hydrochlorothiazide Tablets—for reserpine; 390, SN: for hydralazine hydrochloride; 510, FAS-Op.

Stannous Fluoride—for fluoride; 590; a zirconium-dye lake is bleached by fluoride ion.

Terpin Hydrate and Dextromethorphan Hydrobromide Elixir—for dextromethorphan; 420, BcG.

Spectrometric Assays in the Ultraviolet

Spectrometric assays in which the absorbances are directly measured in the ultraviolet range are described in official monographs.

Applied to solutions, spectrometry is more specific than colorimetry because the absorption depends upon wavelength in a complicated manner that is generally characteristic of the chemical composition of the absorbing substance. Measurement of absorption at several wavelengths may permit identification of the solute as well as the determination of its concentration. Tests of this kind are made usually on solutions, rarely on pure liquids or solids.

Solvents used for dilution usually require special purification which is often exacting and different from the requirements for other uses. Some

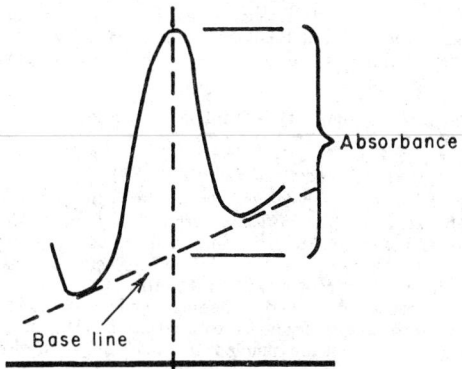

Fig 30-1.   Illustration of base-line technique.

assays direct that blank runs be made on the solvent and reagents used to obtain a correction for their inherent absorbances.

Spectrometers used in official assays must be carefully calibrated with the aid of standard glasses or standard solutions.[1]

Reference Standards—In practically all cases a Reference Standard is used in conjunction with the sample under assay. The standard preparation is prepared and observed in the same manner as the test specimen. The purpose of this specification is to avoid errors due to wavelength or slit-width variation among various spectrophotometers, as well as to avoid errors arising from differences in transmittance and placement of cells.

Infrared Assays

The quantitative estimation of compounds by infrared methods is quite similar to the techniques employed in the ultraviolet and visible regions. However, due to the difficulties involved in measuring the absolute absorbance at a particular absorbance maximum, the "baseline" technique is often utilized. In this method a synthetic "baseline" is constructed between the minima at the sides of the absorption maximum and a vertical line, intersecting the peak of the maximum, is erected perpendicular to the abscissa. The length of the vertical line, measured from the intersection of the synthetic base line and the peak of the absorption maximum is used as the absorbance in quantitative calculations, as illustrated in Fig 30-1.

For a further discussion of the theory involved in infrared absorption, see Chapter 34.

Assays Involving Flame Photometry

This method deals with the emission of energy of a particular wavelength when a dilute solution of a metallic ion is sprayed into a colorless flame. The intensity of the emitted radiation is determined by a suitable spectrometer and compared to standards. Sodium, at 588 nm, and potassium, at 766 nm, are determined by this technique for the official substances indicated below.

Potassium Citrate and Citric Acid Tablets for Oral Solution—for potassium.

Ringer's Injections and Irrigation—for potassium and sodium.

Fluorometric Assay Methods

Riboflavin in official vitamin preparations is quantitatively assayed by measuring its degree of fluorescence in ultraviolet light. Thiamine is also assayed by a fluorometric method, the principal difference from the riboflavin assay being that thiamine is first oxidized to thiochrome, the fluorescence of which is quantitatively measured in isobutyl alcohol solution. The intensity of fluorescence is measured at right angles to the incident monochromatic radiation in an instrument known as a fluorometer, or in certain spectrometers equipped with the required accessories. Quantitative evaluation of the fluorescence data is achieved through comparison with similar data obtained with solutions containing known amounts of reference standard thiamine hydrochloride.

Multivitamin preparations are assayed also for riboflavin and thiamine by this procedure.

Atomic Absorption Analysis

This technique is similar to flame photometry except that the photometer determines the decrease in intensity of a beam of energy passed through a flame in which the metallic ion under test is sprayed. The incident radiation is generated by a lamp, the cathode of which is fabricated from the same metal as the ions of the solution being assayed. See Chapter 34 for a detailed discussion.

Nuclear Magnetic Resonance Methods

With NF XIV, a new spectrometric technique for the assay of organic pharmaceuticals was employed. Since this technique is an absorptive process, the area under the resonance peak is related to the concentration of that substance. The methods are similar to IR or UV techniques, and an *internal* standard is often employed. See Chapter 34 for further discussion.

Amyl Nitrite (and Inhalant)—benzyl benzoate internal standard.

Polarographic Analysis

Quantitative polarographic methods of analysis are specified for several official substances. The *diffusion current* (i_d) is proportional to the concentration of the electro-active species under test while the *half-wave potential* ($E_{1/2}$) is characteristic of the kind of electro-active species and is independent of concentration. In the official assay methods the diffusion current of a sample and a reference standard solution is measured under identical conditions and the concentration of the sample is calculated from the ratio of the sample to reference standard diffusion currents.

A complete review of the theory of polarography can be found in Chapter 34.

Miscellaneous Methods

Gasometric Assay Methods

Gasometric methods of analysis depend upon the measurement of the volume of a gas liberated under the conditions that are described in the assay, or of the decrease in volume of a gas when a suitable reagent is used to remove one of the gases present. These determinations are usually conducted in a gas buret or nitrometer, which is provided with a two-way stopcock and a two-way outlet and is properly connected with a balancing tube.

Carbon Dioxide—the sample is absorbed in 50% potassium hydroxide and the volume of residual gas measured, as for *Ethylene*, below.
Cyclopropane—the sample is absorbed by concentrated sulfuric acid and the residual volume measured, as for *Ethylene*.
Nitrogen—the gas sample is exposed to the action of an ammoniacal copper solution, which removes oxygen. The residual gas volume is nitrogen.
Oxygen—same method as for *Nitrogen*, but the residual volume is a measure of the impurities present.

Assays Involving Volumetric Measurements

Assays that depend on the separation and measurement of oily or aqueous immiscible layers are considered here. In general, these volumetric measurements are made possible as the result of processes that involve solvent separations, steam distillations, or chemical changes, in which an important constituent of the official substance (ie, volatile oil), such as an aldehyde, a ketone, or a phenol, is purposely converted to a water-soluble substance. In the latter case, the volume of residual oil is measured and the assay result is then determined by difference.

Caraway Oil—the ketone, carvone, is converted into a water-soluble bisulfite addition compound and the residual oily volume measured.
Cinnamon—for volatile oil content; by steam distillation and measurement of the volume of insoluble oily layer in the distillate.
Cinnamon Oil—for aldehydes; as for *Caraway Oil*.
Clove Oil—for phenolic substances; the phenols are converted into water-soluble phenolates by potassium hydroxide and the residual, insoluble oil volume measured.
Orange Spirit, Compound—for mixed oils; as for *Peppermint Spirit*.
Peppermint Spirit—for mixed oils; the oils are separated in a Babcock bottle after first mixing and centrifuging with kerosene and an acidified, saturated calcium chloride solution. A correction in the measured volume is made for the kerosene used.
Spearmint Oil—for carvone, as for *Caraway Oil*.
Tetrachloroethylene Capsules—the sample is distilled with glycerin in a toluene moisture apparatus and volume of the lower layer of the distillate measured.

Assays Depending on Measurement of Optical Rotation

Many organic substances, or their solutions, have the property of rotating the plane of polarized light either to the right or to the left and this property is referred to as the optical activity, or optical rotation, of that substance. Measurement of this rotatory power serves as the basis for determining the purity, as well as the identity, of a number of official substances since the optical activity is a function of their chemical constitution, as well as their concentration. When the rotation is to the right the dissolved substance is said to be dextrorotatory, while levorotatory substances are those which rotate the plane of polarized light to the left. The extent of observed rotation is measured and expressed in terms of degrees and the instrument used in making these measurements is called a polariscope or polarimeter.

The term *optical rotation* when used in the official monographs refers to *angular rotation* and this represents the number of degrees a substance, or its solution, under specified conditions of wavelength of the polarized light, concentration, temperature, and length of the tube, will rotate the plane of polarization.

The *specific rotation*, [α], of a liquid is defined as the angular rotation in degrees through which the plane of polarization of polarized monochromatic light is rotated by passage through 1 decimeter (100 mm) of the liquid, calculated on the basis of a specific gravity of 1. In the case of solutions of an optically active substance the specific rotation is calculated on the basis of a concentration of 1 g solute in 1 mL of solution.

For calculating the specific rotatory power of an optically active liquid substance, or the solution of an optically active solid, the following formulas apply generally:

$$For\ liquid\ substances,\ [\alpha]_{\text{D}}^{t} = \frac{a}{ld}$$

$$For\ solutions,\ [\alpha]_{\text{D}}^{t} = \frac{100a}{lpd}$$

$$or\ [\alpha]_{\text{D}}^{t} = \frac{100a}{lc}$$

a = the observed rotation in degrees of the liquid at a temperature t, using a sodium light;
l = the length of the tube in decimeters;
d = the specific gravity of the liquid or solution at the temperature of observation;
p = the concentration of the solution expressed as the number of g of active substance in 100 g of solution;
c = the concentration of the solution expressed as the number of g of active substance in 100 mL of solution.
t = temperature of measurement.
D = D line of sodium (light source).

Anticoagulant Citrate Dextrose Solution—for dextrose.
Dextrose and Sodium Chloride Injection—for dextrose.
Diatrizoate Meglumine and Diatrizoate Sodium Injection—for diatrizoate meglumine.
Epinephrine Inhalation, Injection, Nasal Solution—rotation of the triacetyl derivative.
Epinephryl Bitartrate Ophthalmic Solution—as for *Epinephrine Nasal Solution*.
Iothalamate Meglumine and Iothalamate Sodium Injection—for iothalamate meglumine.
Sodium Chloride and Dextrose Tablets—for dextrose.
Sterile Epinephrine Oil Suspension.

Specific Gravity

Many substances are mixtures of several compounds and can have varied composition. A simple assay procedure will not establish the purity or efficacy of such a material and, therefore, they are quite often characterized by physical methods, one of which may be specific gravity.

Assays Involving Measurement of Radioactivity

In this type of assay, the radioactivity of a sample and of a calibrated radioactive standard are determined at the same time and under identical geometric conditions, as outlined in *Radioisotopes in Pharmacy and Medicine*, Chapter 28.

The radiochemical purity of many official radioactive substances is determined by first chromatographing the substance on a paper strip and determining the radioactive distribution on the developed chromatogram.

The Assay of Enzyme-Containing Substances

The official enzymatic assays depend on the ability of enzymes to catalyze reactions of a certain type under the conditions that are described in the assay. These enzymes that bring about the conversion of starch into water-soluble sugars are known as diastatic enzymes. Other official enzyme-containing substances are those that digest proteins and peptides, changing them into peptones and eventually amino acids. These are called proteolytic enzymes. A third type of enzyme encountered in the official assays is the one which causes or prevents the coagulation of serum. In all of these assays the enzymatic activity of the sample is determined by comparison with that of a reference standard.

Chymotrypsin—a dilute hydrochloride solution of the sample is incubated with buffered *N*-acetyl-L-tyrosine ethyl ester in a spectrometer cell with the instrument set at 237 nm. The change in absorbance with respect to time is noted. One Chymotrypsin Unit is the activity causing a change in absorbance of 0.0075/min under the conditions of the assay.
Heparin Sodium (and Injection, Anticoagulant Heparin Solution, and Lock Flush Solution)—the anticoagulant activity of heparin sodium

is determined by its ability to inhibit the clotting of sheep plasma *in vitro*. Assay preparations are compared to a reference standard and calculation of potency is based on determinations of the extent of clotting which has occurred 1 hour after addition of heparin and calcium chloride to samples of citrated plasma.

Hyaluronidase (and for Injection)—Hyaluronidase activity is assayed on the basis of the ability of preparations of the enzyme to decrease the turbidity of colloidal suspensions of a substrate consisting of potassium hyaluronate and protein *in vitro*. Assay preparations are compared to a reference standard and calculation of potency is based on measurements of the absorbance of solutions containing hyaluronidase, potassium hyaluronate, hydrolyzed gelatin, phosphate buffer, and serum.

Pancreatin—the *starch digestive power* (amylase activity) is determined on a prepared sample by testing its quantitative ability to hydrolyze starch to the extent that no blue or reddish color develops upon the addition of iodine. The *casein digestive power* (protease activity) is determined by placing a suitably prepared casein solution in each of two tubes. To one tube is added a solution of Pancreatin and to the other tube is added a similar amount of Pancreatin Reference Standard. Both mixtures are diluted and incubated at 40° for 1 hour. The addition of alcoholic acetic acid solution produces no more haze in the tube containing Pancreatin than in that containing the Reference Standard, indicating that the proteolytic activity of the former is at least as great as that of the latter. The *fat digestive power* (lipase activity) is determined on an olive oil substrate by titration of liberated fatty acid with base. The activity is determined from a standard curve in *mean acidity released* per minute.

Protamine Sulfate (and Injection and for Injection)—the activity of Protamine Sulfate Injection is assayed on the basis of its ability to nullify the anticoagulant action of sodium heparin *in vitro*. Varying concentrations of sodium heparin are added to a series of test tubes containing uniform amounts of citrated sheep plasma, calcium chloride-thromboplastin solution, and Protamine Sulfate Injection. Calculation of potency is based on that amount of heparin sodium which results in a clotting time most nearly approaching the clotting time observed in the control tube.

Sutilains (and Ointment)—using a casein substrate and a tyrosine reference standard, the amount of tyrosine cleared per unit time, measuring the absorbance at 275 nm, is related to the enzyme activity.

Trypsin—the method is similar to that used for *Chymotrypsin*; *N*-benzoyl-L-arginine ethyl ester hydrochloride is the substrate measured at a wavelength of 253 nm. One Trypsin Unit is the activity causing a change in absorbance of 0.003/min under the conditions of the assay.

Proximate Assays

At one time the extensive use of vegetable drugs, extracts and other galenicals in pharmacy required that the analyst be concerned with a great many *proximate assays*. Currently, due to the majority of more specific, well-defined medicinals, usually of synthetic origin, in common use, the proximate assay is required to a much lesser degree. By proximate assay is meant the determination of the amount of any organic constituent which may be present in any vegetable drug or plant to which its value or therapeutic activity is attributed. The separations are dependent mainly on the use of a variety of solvents selected after elaborate and painstaking research. Acid and alkali solutions, chloroform, ether, alcohol and many other organic solvents play an important role in proximate assays.

Although largely associated with the alkaloidal content of vegetable drugs, proximate assays also include the determination of alcohol-soluble, ether-soluble or water-soluble constituents of various drugs by solvent extraction.

The officially described proximate assays that involve weighing the dried residue obtained upon evaporating a complete solvent extraction of the drug are listed as follows:

Official Standards

Aloe	Not less than 50% of water-soluble extractive
Benzoin	Not less than 75% of alcohol-soluble extractive from Sumatra Benzoin and not less than 90% of alcohol-soluble extractive from Siam Benzoin
Cocoa	Not less than 10% nor more than 22% of nonvolatile ether-soluble extractive
Podophyllum	Not less than 5% of Podophyllum resin by alcohol–chloroform extraction
Vanilla	Not less than 12% of diluted alcohol-soluble extractive

Alkaloidal Drug Assays

Alkaloidal assays present the most important application of proximate assay methods with which the pharmaceutical chemist has to deal. Quantitative experiments must necessarily be done with great care and in conducting proximate assays of alkaloidal drugs particular attention must be paid to all details. The alkaloidal substances to be separated are organic chemical compounds which are difficult to extract from the drug.

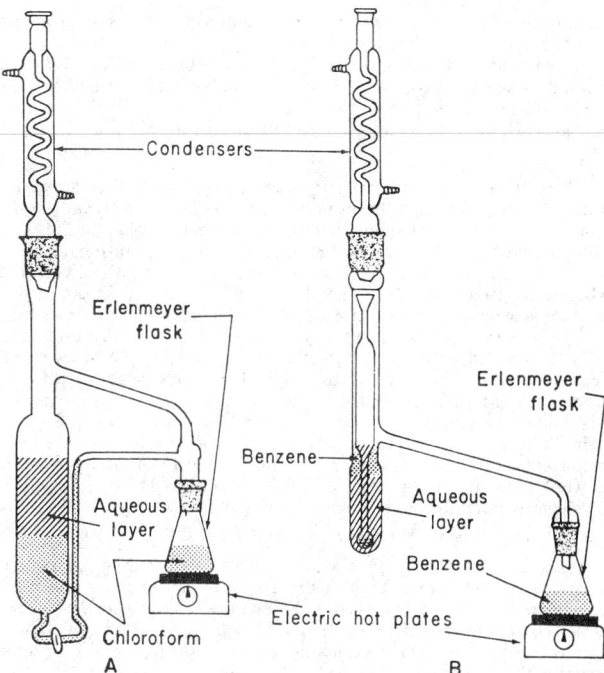

Fig 30-2. Automatic extraction apparatus for alkaloids.

They are present in comparatively small quantities and in many cases are easily destroyed by improper manipulation.

These assays are conducted largely through the use of immiscible solvents, such as chloroform, ether, amyl alcohol, etc, except where the properties of the alkaloid sought necessitate a special method, as for morphine in opium. Advantage is taken of the fact that the free alkaloids are practically insoluble in water (except colchicine, ephedrine, sparteine, nicotine, and a few others), whereas they are very soluble in one or more of the immiscible solvents such as chloroform, ether, etc. The salts of the alkaloids behave in the reverse manner, being practically insoluble in the immiscible solvents and soluble in water. There are several exceptions, such as the salts of caffeine, theobromine, colchicine, etc, which bases are feebly basic and the salts of which hydrolyze readily with the liberation of the free alkaloid.

Three general steps are required for the separation and estimation of alkaloids in vegetable drugs:

1. Extraction of the drug.
2. Subsequent separation and purification of the alkaloid.
3. Determination of the amount of alkaloid obtained, either by gravimetric or titrimetric means.

Extraction of the Crude Drug

After reduction to proper fineness by grinding, the drug may be "defatted" by extraction with petroleum benzin, or directly treated with a solvent to extract the active constituent. Depending on the alkaloid present the drug is treated in one of the following methods:

1. Extraction with an organic solvent, after addition of ammonia to insure the complete liberation of the basic alkaloid (belladonna and ipecac).
2. Extraction with water (morphine in opium).
3. Extraction with acidulated water, if the alkaloid is present as such or in the form of weakly combined organic salts.

The extraction procedure is usually accomplished by use of separatory funnels (separators) with mechanical agitation or in a Soxhlet extraction apparatus.

The assay processes for extracts, fluidextracts, tinctures and powdered extracts of an alkaloidal drug are in general similar to those described for the crude drug. *Powdered and pilular extracts* are usually liquefied by the use of an appropriate solvent and then extracted directly. *Fluidextracts* are often diluted with water and *tinctures* are concentrated to a small volume by means of a preliminary evaporation. After the mixture is made alkaline it is extracted, directly, with the most suitable solvent.

Automatic Extraction Apparatus—The need for an automatic extraction apparatus for use in the assay of alkaloidal galenicals prompted the design of an improved apparatus. The simple type is easily constructed, requires only a small amount of solvent and practically no attention, and gives a clear extraction in one operation.

In the simple type of apparatus (Fig 30-2) the same jacket, condenser, and boiling flask are used for light and heavy solvent. For light solvents the funnel tube containing very small openings at its lower end, is used in the jacket, as shown in *B*. For heavy solvents, as shown in *A*, the wide tube open at both ends is used. The manner in which the extractors function is shown by the illustrations.

In both cases the extracting solvent is continuously returned to the boiling flask and reused. In A, the chloroform returns to the boiling flask under the bottom and around the inner jacket, whereas in B, the non-aqueous layer is always on top and is returned by overflow.

Separation and Purification of the Alkaloid

The extract of the crude drug or galenical usually contains impurities which may interfere with the ultimate method of assay: especially in the case of extraction with immiscible solvents, whereby oils, tannins and soluble coloring matter can obscure the end point in a titration or add to the weight of a gravimetric method. For these reasons purification of the alkaloidal extract is accomplished by: crystallization, as in the case of morphine in opium; removal of associated alkaloids by chemical methods; or by use of immiscible solvents. This latter method is most often employed and involves repeated extraction of the alkaloid from aqueous and organic solvent. For example, the original organic solvent extract containing the basic alkaloid is shaken with dilute acid, thus transferring the alkaloid to the aqueous layer due to the formation of the more polar acid salt. The aqueous acid layer is then made basic with ammonia (or a stronger base if required) and again extracted into an immiscible organic solvent as the free base. This process is repeated until the alkaloid is sufficiently pure for the final assay.

Estimation of the Alkaloid

Final determination of the alkaloid is accomplished either by a quantitative gravimetric or volumetric procedure, the latter being preferred. In the gravimetric method all, or a definite fraction (aliquot), of the solution containing the extract is evaporated to dryness in a tared container, the increase in weight of the container representing the weight (or some fraction thereof) of the alkaloid in the sample.

In the volumetric method the solvent is carefully evaporated to a small volume and an excess of standard acid plus a small amount of alcohol is added and the evaporation continued. The residual titration method is used since the acid, by converting the alkaloid(s) to salt(s), prevent loss of some alkaloids that are fairly volatile in the form of the free base.

Miscellaneous Assay Methods or Functional Tests

Barium Hydroxide Lime—the weight of carbon dioxide absorbed under specified conditions of rate of gas flow and time is determined.

Charcoal, Activated—the adsorptive power with respect to alkaloids (strychnine) and dyes (methylene blue) is determined by measuring the amount (if any) of unadsorbed material.

Mecamylamine Hydrochloride—phase solubility analysis is applied to 50- to 250-mg portions of sample by equilibration with isopropyl alcohol and determination of the solution concentrations of the portions. From a plot of these concentrations vs the system concentrations the purity of the sample may be calculated (see *Phase Solubility Analysis* in Chapter 16).

Soda Lime—see *Barium Hydroxide Lime*, above.

Sodium Alginate—the carbon dioxide liberated when the sample is heated with hydrochloric acid in a special apparatus for assay of alginates is drawn into an excess of standard base and the excess titrated with acid.

Biological Assays

Substances in this category may not need to be assayed by a chemical or physical method. If a biological assay is required, information con-cerning it may be found in Chapter 31. Many of these substances require batch certification by either the Food and Drug Administration or the National Institutes of Health.

Multivitamin Dosage Forms

The analysis of vitamins in a mixture of vitamins may be different from the procedures used when the individual vitamins are alone. The following methods are used in multivitamin mixtures.

Vitamin A—spectrometric measurements at 310, 325 and 334 nm.
Vitamin D—HPLC method.
Vitamin C—dichlorophenol-indophenol titration.
Calcium pantothenate—microbiological method.
Cyanocobalamin—microbiological method.
Folic Acid—spectrometric measurement at 550 nm.
Niacinamide—reaction with cyanogen bromide and then reaction of the product with sulfanilic acid to produce a colored derivative whose color intensity is measured at 450 nm.
Pyridoxine—reaction with 2,6-dichloroquinonechloroimide to produce a colored compound whose color intensity is measured at 650 nm.
Riboflavin—permanganate is added to oxidize interferences after which the riboflavin fluorescence is measured at 530 nm.
Thiamine—reaction with alkaline potassium ferricyanide produces thiochrome whose fluorescence is measured at 435 nm.
α-Tocopherol—reaction with iron (III) and 2,2'-bipyridine produces a color whose intensity is measured at 520 nm.
Decavitamin Capsules and Tablets.
Hexavitamin Capsules and Tablets.

Fixed Oils and Waxes

The fixed oils (corn, cottonseed, olive, etc) and waxes are largely composed of mixtures of fatty acid esters and it is possible that each component has a relatively wide concentration limit without sacrificing the quality of the oil. It is for this reason that a single-substance assay is of little value and many parameters are necessary to stipulate the quality of the oil. Some of the many kinds of tests performed on the materials in this category are: saponification value, acid number, acetyl value, iodine number, specific gravity, melting range of fatty acids, etc.

Penicillin Class Antibiotic Assays

Iodometric Assay

Treatment of penicillins with alkali or penicillinase causes the β-lactam to open yielding a derivative with an acidic and an amine function (eg, penicillin yields penicilloic acid). The derivative consumes iodine whereas the initial intact penicillin antibiotic does not. This behavior forms the basis for the Iodometric Assay.

Hydroxylamine (Hydroxamic Acid) Assay

When penicillins are reacted with hydroxylamine, the β-lactam is opened and a hydroxamic acid derivative forms. The derivative reacts with iron III to produce a color whose intensity is used as a measure of the penicillins. This method is specific since the β-lactam must be intact in order for the hydroxamic acid derivative to form.

Reference

1. *Standards for Checking the Calibration of Spectrophotometers* (200–1000 mμ), Letter Circular LC-1017, Jan, 1955, National Bureau of Standards, Washington, DC 20234.

Table V—Classification Used for Official Assays

I. TITRIMETRIC METHODS
  A. Acid-Base Reactions
    1. Direct Titrations
      a. Titration of an acid by a base
        i. Titration of a liberated acid
        ii. Sorenson—Formol titration
        iii. Nonaqueous titration
      b. Titration of a base by an acid
        i. Titration of metal salts
        ii. Nonaqueous titration
        iii. Nonaqueous titration—Pifer-Wollish Reagent
      c. Kjeldahl Determination
    2. Residual Titrations
      a. Titration of excess acid by a base
        i. After distillation of a volatile base
        ii. After addition to carbonate residues
        iii. After acylation reactions
        iv. Nonaqueous titration
      b. Titration of excess base by an acid
        i. After saponification of an ester
        ii. After hydrolysis of an alkoxyl group
        iii. After distillation of a volatile base
  B. Precipitation Reactions
    1. Direct Titrations
      a. With silver nitrate
      b. With thiocyanate
        i. Of theophylline—silver compound
        ii. Of halogen
        iii. Of mercury
      c. Of a halogen with mercuric ion
      d. Of a halogen with thorium (IV)
      e. Of liberated nitric acid
      f. Of thiol with mercuric ion
    2. Residual Titrations
      a. With thiocyanate
        i. Of theophylline—silver compound
        ii. Of silver

Table V—continued

C. Redox Reactions
  1. Direct Titrations
     a. Involving ceric sulfate or ceric ammonium nitrate
     b. Involving potassium permanganate
        i. Utilizing ferric alum and potassium permanganate
     c. Involving dichlorophenol-indophenol
     d. Involving potassium dichromate
     e. Involving ferrous ammonium sulfate
     f. Involving titanium trichloride
     g. Involving ferric chloride
     h. Involving standard bromine
     i. Involving potassium ferricyanide
     j. Involving sodium nitrite
     k. With iodine
     l. Involving iodine and thiosulfate
        i. Iodimetric determination of phenols
        ii. Titration of iodine liberated from potassium iodide
        iii. Reaction of potassium iodide with excess periodate
     m. Of iodine with arsenite
     n. Involving potassium iodate
  2. Residual Titrations
     a. Of excess standard iodine
        i. Titration of iodine following dichromate reaction
     b. Of excess thiosulfate with iodine
     c. Of generated iodine with thiosulfate
     d. Of residual titanium with iron (III)
     e. Of residual oxalic acid by potassium permanganate
     f. Of residual iodine by sodium thiosulfate
D. Complexation Reactions
  1. Direct Titrations
     a. With EDTA
     b. With miscellaneous titrant
  2. Residual Titrations
     a. With EDTA
     b. With metal ion
E. Large Anion Reagent and Large Cation Reagent Reactions
  1. Titration with sodium tetraphenylboron
  2. Titration with sodium lauryl sulfate
  3. Titration with tetra-n-butyl ammonium iodide
  4. Titration with dioctyl sodium sulfosuccinate

II. GRAVIMETRIC METHODS
  A. Weighing Drug After Separation
  B. Weighing a Derivative After Separation
  C. Weighing a Residue After Ignition
III. SPECTROMETRIC METHODS
  A. Visible Absorption (Colorimetry)
     1. Steroid
     2. Dye—Complex
     3. Direct
     4. Derivative formed
  B. Ultraviolet (UV) Absorption
     1. Direct
     2. Derivative formed
     3. Amphetamine

C. Infrared (IR) Absorption
  1. Direct
  2. Derivative formed
D. Flame Photometric Emission
E. Fluorimetric Emission
  1. Native fluorescence
  2. Fluorescent derivative formed
F. Atomic Absorption (AA)
  1. Flame
  2. Furnace used
G. Nuclear Magnetic Resonance (NMR) Absorption
  1. Absolute method
  2. Relative method

IV. ELECTROCHEMICAL METHODS
  A. Voltammetry
     1. Polarography
     2. Differential pulse polarography
     3. Use of electrodes other than DME
  B. Potentiometry
     1. Ion-selective electrodes

V. CHROMATOGRAPHIC METHODS
  A. Gas Chromatography (GC)
     1. Direct assay
     2. Derivative formed
  B. High Performance Liquid Chromatography (HPLC)
     1. Direct assay
        a. Normal phase
        b. Reverse phase
     2. Derivative formed
        a. Normal phase
        b. Reverse phase
  C. Thin-Layer Chromatography (TLC)
     1. Mobile Phase
        a. Normal
        b. Reverse

VI. MISCELLANEOUS METHODS
  A. Gasometric Assay
  B. Assays Involving Liquid Volume Measurements
  C. Assays Involving Optical Rotation
     1. Direct
     2. Derivative formed for assay
  D. Assays Involving Specific Gravity
  E. Assays of Radioactivity
  F. Enzyme Assay
  G. Proximate Assay
     1. Alkaloid assay
  H. Biological Assay
  I. Miscellaneous
     1. Fixed oils and waxes
  J. Distillation
  K. Functional Test
  L. Vitamin Assays
  M. Phase Solubility
  N. Antibiotic Assays
     1. Microbial
     2. Iodometric
     3. Hydroxylamine

Classification of Official Assays

For the purpose of this chapter the official chemical, physicochemical and physical assay methods have been classified according to the outline, presented as Table V, "Classification Used for Official Assays." The first two classes are stoichiometric analyses, the next three are modern or non-stoichiometric analyses whereas the last class encompasses miscellaneous methods, many older procedures together with some more modern ones.

Table VI presents a classification of the assay for the majority of official drugs. In column 1 the drug substance or dosage form is listed; column 2 gives the Assay Category whose interpretation may be taken from Table V; column 3 gives the analytical wave-length for Spectrometric Analyses (Class III) in nm for visible and ultraviolet regions and in μm for the infrared and also gives the detector type that is used for Chromatographic Methods (Class V). For example, for GC methods, FID-P represents a flame ionization detector—temperature programmed mode, whereas TC-I means thermal conductivity detector—isothermal mode. For HPLC, UV-280 means a UV detector used at 280 nm, RI indicates refractive index, and EC electrochemical detectors. Finally, column 4 lists the indicator employed in titration procedures or the internal standard, where used, for the chromatographic procedures and for the quantitative NMR analyses.

Table VI—Assay Index of Official USP-NF Drugs According to the Classes of Table V

Drug	Assay category	Analytical wavelength and/or detector	Indicator or internal standard
Acacia	None		
Syrup	None		
Acetaminophen	IIIB1	244	
Capsules	IIIB1	249	
for Effervescent Oral Solution	IIIB1	243	
Elixir	IIIB1	249	
Oral Suspension	IIIA4	430	
Tablets	IIIB1	249	
and Aspirin Tablets	VB1b	UV-280	benzoic acid
Acetazolamide	IIC1	7.38	
Tablets	IVA1		
Acetazolamide Sodium Sterile	IIIB1	265	
Acetic Acid	IA1a		Phth
Diluted	IA1a		Phth
Glacial	IA1a		Phth
Irrigation	IA1a		Phth
Otic Solution	IA1aiii		TB
Acetohexamide	IIIB1	247	
Tablets	VA1	FID-P	CrV
Acetone	IA1bii		
Acetophenazine Maleate Tablets	IIIB1	278	Phth
Acetylcholine Chloride for Ophthalmic	IA2b	RI	
Solution	VB1b		
Acetylcysteine Solution	VB1b	UV-214	(±)-phenylalanine
and Isoproternol Hydrochloride Inhalation	VB1b	UV-214	(±)-phenylalanine
Solution	VB1b	UV-214, 280	(±)-phenylalanine, acetaminophen
Acrisorcin	IA1bii		
Cream	IIIA3	400	Poten
Agar	None		
Alanine	IA1bii		
Albumin Human	None		
Alcohol	None		
Dehydrated	None		
Dehydrated Injection	None		Poten
Diluted	IIIA2, IA2bi		
Rubbing	VIJ, VIC		
and Dextrose Injection	IA1aiii	410	Phth
Alginic Acid	IIIB1		
Allopurinol	None		
Tablets	IIIB1	250	Poten
Almond Oil	None		
Aloe	VIG		
Alphaprodine Hydrochloride	IA1biii		CrV
Injection	IA1bii		MeR
Alum	ID2a		DT
Alumina and Magnesia Oral	ID2a, ID1a		DT, EBT

Drug	Assay category	Analytical wavelength and/or detector	Indicator or internal standard
Aminosalicylic Acid	VB1b	UV-254	sulfanilamide and acetaminophen
Tablets	VB1b	UV-254	sulfanilamide and acetaminophen
Amitriptyline Hydrochloride	IA1bii		CrV
Injection	IIIB1	265	
Tablets	IIIB1	265	
Strong Ammonia Solution	IA2a		MeR
Aromatic Ammonia Spirit	IA2a, IA1b		MeR, MeO
Ammonium Carbonate	IA2a		MeO
Ammonium Chloride	IB2a		
Injection	IA1c		FAS
Tablets	IA1c		FAS
Ammonium Phosphate	IA1b		FAS
Amobarbital	IA1aiii		Poten
Elixir	VA1	FID-I	TB
Tablets	VA1	FID-I	
Amobarbital Sodium	IIA	239	
Capsules	IIIB1		barbital
Sterile	IIA		barbital
Amodiaquine	IIIB1	342	SPI
Amodiaquine Hydrochloride	IIIB1	342	SPI
Tablets	IIIB1	342	SPI
Amoxicillin	VIN2		SPI
Capsules	VIN2		SPI
for Oral Suspension	VIN2		SPI
Tablets	VIN2		SPI
Amphetamine Sulfate	IIIB3	257, 280	SPI
Tablets	IIIB3	257, 280	
Amphotericin B	VIN1		
Cream	VIN1		
Injection	VIN1		
Lotion	VIN1		
Ointment	VIN1		
Ampicillin	VIN2		
Capsules	VIN2		
for Oral Suspension	VIN2		
Sterile	VIN2		
Sterile for Suspension	VIN2		
Tablets	VIN2		
Sterile Sodium	VIN2		
and Probenecid Capsules	VIN2, IIIB1	257	
and Probenecid for Oral Suspension	VIN2, IIIB1	257	
Amprolium	IIIA4		
Oral Solution	IIIA4	520	
Soluble Powder	IIIA4	520	
Amyl Nitrite	IIIG1	520	
Inhalant	IIIG1		
Amylene Hydrate	VA1	TC-I	
Anethole	None		
Anileridine	IA1bii		benzyl benzoate
Injection	IIIA4		benzyl benzoate
Anileridine Hydrochloride	IA1biii	560	CrV

Name	Code	λ	Note
Suspension	ID2a, ID1a		DT, EBT
Tablets	ID2a, ID1a, ID1a		DT, EBT, HNB
Alumina, Magnesia and Calcium Carbonate Oral Suspension	ID2a, ID1a, ID1a		DT, EBT, HNB
Tablets	ID2a, ID1a		DT, EBT
Alumina and Magnesium Trisilicate Oral Suspension	ID2a, IA2b		DT, Phth
Aluminum Acetate Topical Solution	ID2a		DT
Aluminum Chloride	ID2a		DT
Aluminum Hydroxide Gel	ID2a		DT
Dried	ID2a		DT
Dried Tablets	IIC		Phth
Aluminum Monostearate	IA2b		DT, Phth
Aluminum Phosphate Gel	ID2a, IA2b		DT
Aluminum Subacetate Topical Solution	ID2a		Poten
Aluminum Sulfate	IA1bii		Poten
Amantadine Hydrochloride Capsules	IA1bii		Poten
Syrup	IA1bii		CrV
Ambenonium Chloride Tablets	IA1bii		BpB
Amcinonide	ID1b	UV-254	dibutyl phthalate
Cream	VB1b	UV-254	CrV
Ointment	VB1b	UV-254	CrV
Amikacin	None		Poten
Injection	IA1bii		Poten
Amiloride Hydrochloride Tablets	VB1b	UV-286	CrV
and Hydrochlorothiazide Tablets	VB1b	UV-286	Poten
Aminobenzoate Potassium Capsules	IC1j	270	Poten
for Oral Solution	IIIB1		Poten
Tablets	IIIB1	270	Poten
Aminobenzoate Sodium	IC1j		salicylic acid
Aminobenzoic Acid Gel	IC1j		Poten
Topical Solution	VB1b		CrV
Aminocaproic Acid Injection	IC1j		CrV
Syrup	IA1bii		CrV
Tablets	IA1bii		Poten
Aminoglutethimide Tablets	IA1bii	242	Poten
Aminohippurate Sodium Injection	IA1bii		Poten
Aminohippuric Acid	IIIB1		FAS
Aminophylline	IC1j		FAS
Enema	IC1j		FAS
Injection	IB1bi	270	FAS
Suppositories	IIIB1		Poten
Tablets	IB1bi		Poten
Aminosalicylate Calcium Capsules	IB1bi		Poten
Tablets	IB1bi		Poten
Aminosalicylate Potassium Tablets	IC1j		
Aminosalicylate Sodium	VB1b	UV-254	sulfanilamide and acetaminophen
Tablets	VB1b	UV-254	sulfanilamide and acetaminophen
Tablets	IIIA4	560	Poten
Anise Oil	None		
Antazoline Phosphate	IA1bii	UV-365	
Anthralin	VB1b		anthracene
Ointment	IIIA3	354, 432	Poten, Phth
Anticoagulant Citrate Dextrose Solution	IA1b, IA1a, VIc1		
Anticoagulant Citrate Phosphate Dextrose Solution	IIIA4, IA1a, IIB	425, 660	Phth
Anticoagulant Heparin Solution	VIF, IB1a		PC
Anticoagulant Sodium Citrate Solution	IA1bii		Poten
Cryoprecipitated Antihemophilic Factor	None		
Antimony Potassium Tartrate	IC1k		ST
Antipyrine	IC1l		ST
Antivenin (Latrodectus mactans)	None		
Apomorphine Hydrochloride Tablets	IA1bii		CrV
Arginine	IA2a		MeR
Arginine Hydrochloride Injection	IA1bii		Poten
Aromatic Elixir	IA1bii		Poten
Ascorbic Acid	IIIA4	520	ST
Injection	None		
Oral Solution	IC1k		
Tablets	IC1c		
Ascorbyl Palmitate	IC1c		
Aspirin	IC1c		Phth
Capsules	IC1k	280	
Suppositories	IA2b	280	
Tablets	IIIB1	UV-280	
Atropine	VB1b		CrV
Atropine Sulfate Injection	IA1bii	TC-I	Poten
Ophthalmic Ointment	IA1bii	TC-I	homatropine hydrobromide
Ophthalmic Solution	VA1	TC-I	homatropine hydrobromide
Tablets	VA1	TC-I	homatropine hydrobromide
Aurothioglucose Sterile Suspension	VA1		homatropine hydrobromide
Azatadine Maleate	VA1		homatropine hydrobromide
Azathioprine	IIC		CrV
Tablets	IIC		TB
Azathioprine Sodium for Injection	IA1bii		
Sterile Azlocillin Sodium	IA1aii		
Bacampicillin Hydrochloride for Oral Suspension	IVA1	480	
Tablets	IVA1		
Bacitracin	VIN3		
Ointment	VIN2		
Ophthalmic Ointment	VIN2		SPI
Sterile	VIN2		SPI
Zinc	None		SPI
Zinc Ointment	VIN1		
Sterile Zinc	None		
Zinc and Polymixin B Ointment	None		

Table VI—continued

Drug	Assay category	Analytical wavelength and/or detector	Indicator or internal standard
Bacitracin Zinc and Polymixin B Ophthalmic Ointment	None		
Adhesive Bandage	None		
Gauze Bandage	None		
Barium Hydroxide Lime	VIK		
Barium Sulfate	IIB		
for Suspension	IIB		
BCG Vaccine	None		
Beclomethasone Dipropionate	VB1b	UV-254	testosterone propionate
Belladonna Extract	VA1	TC-I	homatropine hydrobromide
Tablets	VA1	TC-I	homatropine hydrobromide
Belladonna Leaf	VA1	TC-I	homatropine hydrobromide
Tincture	VA1	TC-I	homatropine hydrobromide
Bendroflumethiazide	IA1aiii		AV
Tablets	VB1b	UV-270	
Benoxinate Hydrochloride	IA1bii		Poten
Ophthalmic Solution	IIIB1	308	
Bentonite	None		
Magma	None		
Benzaldehyde	IA1ai		BpB
Compound Elixir	None		
Benzalkonium Chloride	IC1n		BpB
Solution	IC1n		SPI
Benzestrol	IIIA4	750	
Tablets	IIIA4	750	BpB
Benzethonium Chloride	IE1		
Tincture	IIB		
Topical Solution	IE1		Poten
Benzocaine	IC1j		Poten
Cream	IC1j		Poten
Ointment	IC1j		Poten
Otic Solution	IC1j		Poten
Topical Aerosol	IC1j		
Topical Solution	IC1j		Phth
Benzoic Acid	IA1a	311, 275	
and Salicylic Acid Ointment	IIIB1		
Benzoin	VIG		
Compound Tincture	None		
Benzonatate	IA2bi		Btb
Capsules	IIIA4	500	
Hydrous Benzoyl Peroxide	IC1lii		
Gel	VB1b	UV-254	ethyl benzoate
Lotion	VB1b	UV-254	ethyl benzoate
Benzoylpas Calcium	IB2a		Poten
Tablets	IIIB1	274	
Benzthiazide	IIIB1	283	
Tablets	IIIB1	295	
Benztropine Mesylate	IA1bii		MeR
Injection	VB1b	UV-259	
Tablets	VB1b	UV-259	
Blood Grouping Serums	None		
Blood Grouping Serums Anti D, Anti C, Anti E, Anti c, Anti e	None		
Leukocyte Typing Serum	None		
Blood Group Specific Substances A, B and AB	None		
Red Blood Cells	None		
Whole Blood	None		
Boric Acid	IA1a		Phth
Botulism Antitoxin	None		
Bromocriptine Mesylate	IA1bii	UV-300	Poten
Tablets	VB1b		
Bromodiphenhydramine Hydrochloride	IA1bii		CrV
Capsules	IA2a		MeR
Elixir	IA2a		MeR
Brompheniramine Maleate	IA1bii		CrV
Elixir	IA1bii		CrV
Injection	IIIB1	262	dibutyl phthalate
Tablets	IIIB1	264	CrV
Bupivacaine and Epinephrine Injection	VB1b	UV-263	dibutyl phthalate
Bupivacaine Hydrochloride	IA1bii		Phth
Injection	VB1b	UV-263	Phth
Busulfan	IA1ai		
Tablets	IA1ai		
Butabarbital Sodium	IIIB1	240	
Capsules	VA1	FID-I	secobarbital
Elixir	VA1	FID-I	secobarbital
Tablets	VA1	FID-I	secobarbital
Butacaine Sulfate	IC1j		SPI
Topical Solution	IIIB1	280	Poten
Butalbital	IB1a		SPI
Butamben	IC1j		CrV
Butane	VA1	TC-I	
Butorphanol Tartrate	IA1bii	UV-280	propylparaben
Injection	VB1b	FID-I	4-tert-butylphenol
Butylated Hydroxyanisole	VA1		BtB
Butylated Hydroxytoluene	None		
Butylparaben	IA2b		Poten
Caffeine	IA1bii		MeO
and Sodium Benzoate Injection	IIA, IA1b		MeO
Calamine	IA2a		
Lotion	None		
Phenolated Lotion	None		
Calcifediol	VB1a	UV-254	testosterone
Capsules	VB1a	UV-254	testosterone
Calcium Carbonate, Precipitated	ID1a		HNB
Calcium Carbonate and Magnesia Tablets	ID1a		HNB
Calcium Carbonate, Magnesia, and Magnesium Carbonates Tablets	ID1a		HNB, EBT
Calcium Gluceptate	ID1a		HNB, EBT
Calcium Gluceptate Injection	ID1a		HNB
Calcium Gluconate	ID1a		HNB

Name	Code	No.	Note
Benzyl Alcohol	None		
Benzyl Benzoate	IA2bi		Phth
Lotion	IA2bi		Phth
Benzylpenicilloyl Polylysine	IIIB2		
Concentrate		282	
Injection	IIIB2	282	
Bephenium Hydroxynaphthoate	IA1bii	420	CrV
for Oral Suspension			
Beta Carotene	IIIA2	455	
Capsules	IIIA3	452	
Betaine Hydrochloride	IIIA4		CrV
Betamethasone	IA1biii	UV-254	propylparaben
Cream	VB1b	UV-254	propylparaben
Syrup	VB1b	525	
Tablets	IIIA1	525	
Betamethasone Acetate	IIIA1	239	
Betamethasone Benzoate	IIIB1	UV-254	betamethasone dipropionate
Gel	VB1b	364	
Betamethasone Dipropionate	IIIB2	UV-254, 240	beclomethasone dipropionate
Topical Aerosol	VB1b	UV-254, 240	beclomethasone dipropionate
Cream	VB1b	UV-254, 240	beclomethasone dipropionate
Lotion	VB1b	UV-254, 240	beclomethasone dipropionate
Ointment	VB1b	UV-254, 240	beclomethasone dipropionate
Betamethasone Sodium Phosphate	VB1b	UV-254	beclomethasone dipropionate
Sterile	VB1b		butylparaben
and Betamethasone Acetate			
Suspension	IIIB1, IIIA1	241, 525	
Betamethasone Valerate	VB1b	UV-254, 240	beclomethasone dipropionate
Topical Aerosol	VB1b	UV-254, 240	beclomethasone dipropionate
Cream	VB1b	UV-254, 240	beclomethasone dipropionate
Lotion	VB1b	UV-254, 240	beclomethasone dipropionate
Ointment	VB1b	UV-254, 240	beclomethasone dipropionate
Betazole Hydrochloride	IIB		
Injection	IIB		
Bethanechol Chloride	IA1bii		
Injection	IIB		CrV
Tablets	IIB		
Biperiden	IA1bii		
Biperiden Hydrochloride	IA1bii	408	CrV
Tablets	IIIA2	408	CrV
Biperiden Lactate Injection	IIIA2		
Bisacodyl	IA1bii		Nb
Suppositories	IIIB1	263	
Tablets	IIIB1	263	
Milk of Bismuth	IIC		XyO
Bismuth Subnitrate	ID1a		
Sterile Bleomycin Sulfate	VIN1		
Anti-A Blood Grouping Serum	None		
Anti-B Blood Grouping Serum	None		

Name	Code	No.	Note
Injection	ID1a		HNB
Tablets	ID1a		HNB
Calcium Hydroxide	ID1a		HNB
Topical Solution	IA1b		Phth
Calcium Lactate	ID1a		HNB
Tablets	ID1a		HNB
Calcium Levulinate	ID1a		HNB
Injection	VIH		
Calcium Pantothenate	VIH		
Tablets	None		
Racemic	ID1a		HNB
Dibasic Calcium Phosphate	ID1a		HNB
Tablets	ID1a		HNB
Tribasic Calcium Phosphate	ID1a, IIC		HNB
Calcium Saccharate	ID1a		HNB
Calcium Silicate	ID1a		HNB
Calcium Stearate	None		
Calcium Sulfate	IIB		
Camphor	None		
Spirit	None		
Candicidin	None		
Ointment	None		
Sterile Capreomycin Sulfate	VIB		
Caramel	IA1biii		
Caraway	IIIA4		
Oil	IIIA4		
Carbachol	IIIB1	590	CrV
Intraocular Solution	IIIB1	590	
Ophthalmic Solution	IC1lii	285	
Carbamazepine	IC1k	285	
Tablets	IC1k		
Carbamide Peroxide Solution	VIN1		
Carbarsone	VIC1		ST
Capsules	VB1b		ST
Sterile Carbenicillin Disodium	VB1b		ST
Carbenicillin Indanyl Sodium	IA1bii	UV-280	
Carbidopa	IA1bii	UV-280	
and Levodopa Tablets	IA1bii		
Carbinoxamine Maleate	None		CrV
Elixir	IA1a		CrV
Tablets	VIA		CrV
Carbol-Fuchsin Topical Solution	VB2b		
Carbomer 934P	VB2b		Poten
Carbon Dioxide	None		
Carboprost Tromethamine	IA1bii	UV-254	
Injection	IA1bii	UV-254	
Carboxymethylcellulose Calcium	None		guaifenesin
Carboxymethylcellulose Sodium	None		guaifenesin
Paste	None		Poten
Tablets	IIIA4		Poten
12	IIIA4		Poten
Cardamom Oil	IIIA4		
Seed	None		
Compound Tincture	None		
Carphenazine Maleate	IIIA4	485	
Oral Solution	IIIA4	485	
Tablets	IIIA4	485	
Carrageenan	None		
Cascara Sagrada	IIIA4	515	
Extract	IIIA4	515	
Fluidextract	None		

Table VI—continued

Drug	Assay category	Analytical wavelength and/or detector	Indicator or internal standard
Cascara Sagrada	None		
Aromatic Fluidextract	IIIA4	515	
Tablets	None		
Castor Oil	None		
Aromatic	None		
Capsules	None		
Emulsion	VA1	FID-I	bis(2-ethylhexyl)-phthalate
Hydrogenated	None		
Cefaclor	VIN3	480	
Capsules	VIN3	480	
for Oral Suspension	VIN3	480	
Cefadroxil	VIN3	480	
Capsules	VIN3	480	
for Oral Suspension	VIN3	480	
Tablets	VIN3	480	
Cefamandole Nafate, Sterile	IVA1		
for Injection	IVA1		
Sterile Cefamandole Sodium	IVA1		
Sterile Cefazolin Sodium	VIN1		
Sterile Cefoperazone Sodium	VB1b	UV-254	
Sterile Cefotaxime Sodium	VIN3	480	
Sterile Cefoxitin Sodium	VIN3	480	
Microcrystalline Cellulose and Carboxymethylcellulose Sodium	IC1e		Poten
	IA1bii		
Oxidized Cellulose	IA1a		Phth
Regenerated	IA2b		Phth
Cellulose Acetate	None		
Cellulose Acetate Phthalate	None		
Powdered Cellulose	IC1e		
Cephacetrile Sodium	VIN3	480	
for Injection	VIN3	480	
Cephalexin	VIN1		
Capsules	VIN1		
for Oral Suspension	VIN1		
Tablets	VIN1		
Cephaloglycine	VIN1		
Capsules	VIN1		
Sterile Cephaloridine	VIN1		
Sterile Cephalothin Sodium	VIN1		
for Injection	VIN3	480	
Injection	VIN1		
Sterile Cephapirin Sodium	VIN1		
Cephradine	VIN1		
Capsules	VIN1		
for Oral Suspension	VIN1		
Tablets	VIN3	480	
Sterile	VA1	FID-I	
for Oral Suspension	VA1	FID-I	
Cetostearyl Alcohol	None		
Cetyl Alcohol	IE1		BpB
Cetyl Esters Wax	IE2		MeY
Cetylpyridinium Chloride			
Lozenges			

Drug	Assay category	Analytical wavelength and/or detector	Indicator or internal standard
Ophthalmic Ointment	VIN1		
Sterile	VIN1	UV-254	2,7-naphthalenediol
Chlorthalidone	VB1b	UV-254	2,7-naphthalenediol
Tablets	VB1b	282	
Chlorzoxazone	IIIB1	282	
Tablets	IIIB1	UV-280	phenacetin
and Acetaminophen Capsules	VB1b	UV-280	phenacetin
and Acetaminophen Tablets	VB1b	UV-254	
Cholecalciferol	VB1a		
Cholera Vaccine	None		
Cholesterol	None		
Cholestyramine Resin	None		
Cholestyramine for Oral Suspension	IIIB2	318	
Sodium Chromate Cr51 Injection	IIIB1, VIE	370	
Chromic Chloride	IC1iii	357.9	ST
Injection	IIIF1		
Chymotrypsin	VIF		
for Ophthalmic Suspension	VIF		
Cinnamon	VIB		
Oil	VIB		
Cinoxacin	VB1b	UV-254	sulfanilic acid
Capsules	IIIB1	352	Phth
Cinoxate	IA2b		
Lotion	IIIB1	308	Phth
Citric Acid	IA1a		Poten
Chloroprocaine Hydrochloride	IA1biii	278	
Injection	IIIB1		
Chloroquine	IA1bii	343	CrV
Chloroquine Hydrochloride	IIIB1		
Injection	IIIB1	343	
Chloroquine Phosphate	IIIB1	343	
Tablets	VB1b	UV-254	
Chlorothiazide	IIIB1	292	
Oral Suspension	IVA1		
Tablets	IVA1		
Chlorothiazide Sodium for Injection	IIIB1		
Chlorotrianisene	IB2aii	292	FAS
Capsules	IIIB1		
Chlorpheniramine Maleate	IA1bii	310	CrV
Injection	IIIB1	264	
Syrup	IIIB1	264	
Tablets	IIIB1	264	
Chlorphenoxamine Hydrochloride	IA1biii		
Tablets	IIIB1	258	Poten
Clemastine Fumarate	IA1bii		
Tablets	VB1b	UV-220	
Clidinium Bromide	IA1biii		
Capsules	IIIA2	410	Poten
Clindamycin Hydrochloride	VA1	FID-I	cholestane
Clindamycin Palmitate	VA1	FID-I	cholestane
Hydrochloride for Oral Solution	VA1	FID-I	cholesteryl benzoate
Clindamycin Phosphate	VA2	FID-I	cholesteryl benzoate
Injection	VA2	FID-I	hexacosane
		FID-I	hexacosane

Name	Method	Wavelength	Note
Topical Solution	IE1		BpB
Activated Charcoal	None		
Cherry Juice	IC1b		
Cherry Syrup	None		
Chloral Hydrate	IA2b		
Capsules	IA2b		
Syrup	IA1a		
Chlorambucil	VB1b		
Tablets	VIN1	UV-254	propylparaben
Chloramphenicol	VIN1		
Capsules	VIN1		
Cream	VIN1		
Injection	VIN1		
Oral Solution	VIN1		
Ophthalmic Ointment	VIN1		
Ophthalmic Solution	VIN1		
for Ophthalmic Solution	VIN1		
Otic Solution	VIN1		
Sterile	VIN1		
Tablets	VIN1		
and Hydrocortisone Acetate for Ophthalmic Suspension	VIN1, VB1b	UV-254	fluoxymesterone
and Polymixin B Sulfate Ophthalmic Ointment	VIN1		
Polymixin B Sulfate and Hydrocortisone Acetate Ophthalmic Ointment	VIN1, VB1b	UV-254	fluoxymesterone
and Prednisone Ophthalmic Ointment	VIN1, VB1b	UV-254	
Chloramphenicol Palmitate	VB1b	UV-280	
Oral Suspension	VB1b	UV-280	
Sterile Chloramphenicol Sodium Succinate	IIIB1	278, 276	
Chlorcyclizine Hydrochloride	IA1biii		
Chlordiazepoxide	VB1b	UV-254	
Tablets	VB1b	UV-254	Poten
and Amitriptyline Hydrochloride Tablets	VB1b	UV-254	
Chlordiazepoxide Hydrochloride	VB1b	UV-254	
Capsules	IIIB1	245	
Sterile	IA1biii		
Chloroazodin	IC1		CrV
Chlorobutanol	IC1		ST
Chloroform	IB2aii		ST
Chlorpromazine	None		FAS
Suppositories	IA1bii	254, 277	
Chlorpromazine Hydrochloride	IIIB1	254, 277	CrV
Injection	IA1bii	254, 277	
Syrup	IIIB1	254, 277	Poten
Tablets	IIIB1	254, 277	
Chlorpropamide	IIIB1	232	
Tablets	IIIB1	232	MeR
Chlorprothixene	IA1bii	324	
Injection	IIIB1	324	
Oral Suspension	IIIB1	324	
Tablets	IIIB1	324	
Chlortetracycline Hydrochloride	VIN1		
Capsules	VIN1		
Ointment	VIN1		

Name	Method	Wavelength	Note
Sterile	VA2	FID-I	hexacosane
Topical Solution	VA2	FID-I	hexacosane
Clocortolone Pivalate Cream	IIIA4	405	
Clofibrate	IIIA4	390	
Capsules	IIIB1	226	
Clomiphene Citrate	IIIB1	226	
Tablets	IA1bii	232.5	CrV
Clonazepam	IIIB1		NiB
Tablets	IA1bii	UV-254	o-dichlorobenzene
Clonidine Hydrochloride	VB2b		Poten
Tablets	IA1bii	UV-220	Nb
and Chlorthalidone Tablets	VB1b	UV-220	MeY
Clotrimazole	IA1bii		MeY
Cream	IE2		MeY
Topical Solution	IE2		
Vaginal Tablets	IE2		
Clove Oil	VIB		
Cloxacillin Sodium	VIN1		
Capsules	VIN1		
for Oral Solution	VIN1		
Coal Tar	None		
Ointment	None		
Topical Solution	None		
Cobalamin Concentrate	IIIB1, IIIA4	361, 550	
Cyanocobalamin Co 57 Capsules	VIE		
Oral Solution	VIE		
Cyanocobalamin Co 60 Capsules	VIE		
Oral Solution	VIE		
Cocaine	IA1bii		CrV
Cocaine Hydrochloride	IA1bii		QR
Tablets for Topical Solution	IA2a		MeR
Coccidioidin	None		Poten
Cocoa Butter	VIG		
Butter	None		sulfanilamide
Syrup	None		sulfanilamide
Cod Liver Oil	None		sulfanilamide
Codeine	VIL		sulfanilamide
Codeine Phosphate	IA2a		MeR
Injection	IA1bii	350	Poten
Tablets	IA1b		MeR
Codeine Sulfate	IA1b		MeR
Tablets	IA1bii		Poten
Colchicine	IA2a	350	MeR
Injection	IA1bii		Poten
Tablets	IIIB1		
Cold Cream	IIIB1		
Sterile Colistimethate Sodium	None		
Colistin Sulfate	VIN1		
for Oral Suspension	VIN1		
and Neomycin Sulfate and Hydrocortisone Acetate Otic Suspension	VIN1, IIIA4	410	
Collodion	IIA		
Flexible	None		
Coriander Oil	None		
Corn Oil	None		
Corticotropin	VIH		
Injection for Injection	VIH		
Repository Injection	None		

Table VI—continued

Drug	Assay category	Analytical wavelength and/or detector	Indicator or internal standard
Corticotropin Sterile Zinc Hydroxide Suspension	VIH		
Cortisone Acetate	VB1b	UV-254	fluorometholone
Sterile Suspension	VB1b	UV-254	fluorometholone
Tablets	VB1b	UV-254	fluorometholone
Purified Cotton	None		
Cottonseed Oil	None		
Cresol	IIIB1	326	
Cromolyn Sodium for Inhalation	IIIB1	326	
Cromitamiton	IIIB1	242	
Cream	VB1b	UV-254	butyl benzoate
Croscarmellose Sodium	None		
Crospovidone	None		
Cupric Chloride	IC1lii		
Injection	IC1lii	324.8	ST
Cupric Sulfate	IIIF1		
Injection	IIIF1	324.8	ST
Cyanocobalamin	IIIB1	361	SPI
Injection	IIIB1	361	SPI
Cyclacillin	VIN2		CrV
Tablets	VIN2		
Cyclizine	IA1bii		Poten
Cyclizine Hydrochloride	IA1bii	264	
Tablets	IIIB1	264	
Cyclizine Lactate Injection	IIC1	14.2	Poten
Cyclobenzaprine Hydrochloride	IA1bii	290	
Tablets	IIIB1	290	CrV
Cyclomethycaine Sulfate	IA1bii		
Cream	IIIB1	261	
Jelly	IIIB1	261	
Ointment	IIIB1	261	
Suppositories	IA1bii	261	
Cyclopentamine Hydrochloride	IA2a		CrV
Cyclopentolate Hydrochloride	IA1bii		MeR
Ophthalmic Solution	IIIA4	500	CrV
Cyclophosphamide			ethylparaben
for Injection	VB1b	UV-195	ethylparaben
Tablets	VB1b	UV-195	ethylparaben
Cyclopropane	VIA		
Cycloserine	VIN1		
Capsules	VIN1		
Cyclothiazide	IA1aiii	271	ONA
Tablets	IIIB1		
Cycrimine Hydrochloride	IIIA2	405	CrV
Tablets	IA1biii		
Cyproheptadine Hydrochloride	IIIB1		CrV
Syrup	IIIB1	286	
Tablets	IC1lii	286	
Cysteine Hydrochloride	IVA1		
Injection	IIIB1	285	ST
Cytarabine			
Sterile	IIIB1	285	
Ophthalmic Solution	IIIA1	525	
Dexbrompheniramine Maleate	IA1bii		CrV
Dexchlorpheniramine Maleate	IA1bii		CrV
Syrup	IIIB1	264	
Tablets	IIIB1	264	
Dexpanthenol	IA2aiv		CrV
Preparation	IA2aiv		CrV
Dextrates	None		
Dextroamphetamine Phosphate	IIIB3	257, 280	
Tablets	IIIB3	257, 280	
Dextroamphetamine Sulfate	IA1bii		Poten
Capsules	VB1b	UV-254	
Elixir	IIIB1	257, 280	
Tablets	IIIB1	257	
Dextromethorphan	IA1bii		CrV
Dextromethorphan Hydrobromide	IA1biii		CrV
Syrup	IIIB1	278	
Dextrose	None		
Excipient	None		
Injection	VIC1		DCF
and Sodium Chloride Injection	VIC1, IB1a		
Dextrothyroxine Sodium	IC1lii		ST
Tablets	IC1lii		ST
Diacetylated Monoglycerides	None		
Diatrizoate Meglumine	IB1a		TBP
Injection	VIC1, IB1a		TBP
and Diatrizoate Sodium Injection	IC1lii, IB1a		TBP
and Diatrizoate Sodium Solution	IB1a		ST, TBP
Diatrizoate Sodium	IB1a		TBP
Injection	IB1a		TBP
Solution	IB1a		TBP
Diatrizoic Acid	IA1bii		Poten
Diazepam	VB1b	UV-254	sulfanilamide
Capsules	VB1b	UV-254	tolualdehyde
Injection	VB1b	UV-254	ethylparaben
Tablets	IA1aiii		TP
Diazoxide	IIIB1	280	
Capsules	IIIB1	280	
Injection	VB1b	UV-254	
Oral Suspension	IA1bii		hydrochlorothiazide
Dibucaine	IIIB1	247	CrV
Cream	IIIB1	247	
Ointment	IIIB1	320	
Suppositories	IA1bii		
Dibucaine Hydrochloride	IIIB1	247	CrV
Injection	None		
Dichlorofluoromethane	None		
Dichlorotetrafluoroethane	VB1b	UV-280	
Dichlorphenamide	IVA1		
Tablets	VIN1		
Dicloxacillin Sodium	VIN1		
Capsules	VIN1		
Sterile	VIN1		
for Oral Suspension	VIN1		

Table VI—continued

Drug	Assay category	Analytical wavelength and/or detector	Indicator or internal standard
Dimethisoquin Hydrochloride	IIIB1	328, 360	
Lotion	IIIB1	328, 360	
Ointment	IIIB1	328, 360	
Dimethyl Sulfoxide	None		
Irrigation	VA1	FID-P	
Dioxybenzone	IIIB1	325	
and Oxybenzone Cream	IIIB1	325	
Diperodon	IA1bii	235, 300	
Ointment	IIIB1	325	CrV
Diphemanil Methylsulfate	IIIB1	412	
Tablets	IIIA2	412	
Diphenadione	IIIB1	289	
Tablets	IIIB1	289	
Diphenhydramine Hydrochloride	IIIB1	258	
Capsules	IA1biii	258	CrV
Elixir	IIIB1	258	
Injection	IIIB1	258	
Diphenoxylate Hydrochloride and Atropine Sulfate Oral Solution	IA1biii, VA1	FID-I	Poten, homatropine hydrobromide
and Atropine Sulfate Tablets	IA1biii, VA1	FID-I	Poten, homatropine hydrobromide
Diphenylpyraline Hydrochloride	IA1biii	258	CrV
Tablets	IIIB1	258	
Diphtheria Antitoxin	None		
Diphtheria Toxin for Schick Test	None		
Diphtheria Toxoid Adsorbed	None		
Diphtheria and Tetanus Toxoids Adsorbed	None		
and Pertussis Vaccine Adsorbed	None		
and Pertussis Vaccine Adsorbed	None		
Dipyridamole	IA1bii		Poten
Tablets	VB1b	UV-288	
Disopyramide Phosphate	IA1bii	268	Poten
Capsules	IIIB1		
Disulfiram	IC2c		
Tablets	IC2c		
Dobutamine Hydrochloride	VA2	FID-I	n-triacontane
for Injection	VA2	FID-I	n-triacontane
Docusate Calcium	IC2c		BpB
Capsules	IIIA2	545	BpB
Docusate Potassium	IE3	RI	BpB
Capsules	VB1b		
Docusate Sodium	IE3	RI	BpB
Capsules	VB1b		
Solution	IE3		p-toluenesulfonic acid
Syrup	VB1b	UV-214	p-toluenesulfonic acid
Tablets	VB1b	UV-214	BpB
Dopamine Hydrochloride	IIIA2	UV-280	Poten
Injection	IA1biii	UV-280, RI	
Doxapram Hydrochloride	VB1b		CrV cholesterol
Injection	IA1biii	FID-I	
and Dextrose Injection	VA1	FID-I	chlorpheniramine maleate
Doxepin Hydrochloride	VA1	FID-I	

Drug	Assay category	Analytical wavelength and/or detector	Indicator or internal standard
Epinephrine Bitartrate	IA1bii	530	CrV
Inhalation Aerosol	IIIA4		
for Ophthalmic Solution	VIC2		
Ophthalmic Solution	VIC2		
Epinephryl Borate Ophthalmic Solution	VIC2		phenol
Equilin	VB1b	UV-280	
Ergocalciferol	VB1a	UV-254	
Capsules	VB1a	UV-254	
Oral Solution	VIL		
Tablets	VB1b	UV-280	
Ergoloid Mesylates Oral Solution	VB1b	UV-280	
Tablets	VIL		
Ergonovine Maleate	VB1b	550	
Injection	VB1b	UV-312	
Tablets	IIIA4	UV-312	
Ergotamine Tartrate	IIIA4	546	CrV
Inhalation Aerosol	IA1bii	545	
Injection	VB1b	545	
Tablets	IIIA4	550	
and Caffeine Suppositories	IIIA4	276, 545	
and Caffeine Tablets	IIIA4, IIIB1	276, 545	
Eriodictyon	None		
Fluid extract			
Erythrityl Tetranitrate, Diluted	IIIA4	405	
Erythromycin	IIIA4	405	
Capsules	VIN1		
Ointment	VIN1		
Ophthalmic Ointment	VIN1		
Tablets	VIN1		
Topical Solution	VIN1		
Erythromycin Estolate	VIN1		
Capsules	VIN1		
Oral Suspension	VIN1		
Tablets	VIN1		
Erythromycin Ethylsuccinate	VIN1		
Injection	VIN1		
Sterile	VIN1		
for Oral Suspension	VIN1		
Oral Suspension	VIN1		
Tablets	VIN1		
and Sulfisoxazole acetyl for Oral Suspension	VIN1, VB1b	UV-254	
Sterile Erythromycin Gluceptate	VIN1		
Erythromycin Lactobionate for Injection	VIN1		
Erythromycin Stearate	VIN1		
for Oral Suspension	VIN1		
Tablets	VIN1		
Erythrosine Sodium	None		
Topical Solution	IIIA3	530	benzanilide

Capsules	IIB1		
Oral Solution	IIB1	292	
Doxorubicin Hydrochloride	VB1b	292	
for Injection	VB1b	UV-254	
Doxycycline	VIN1		
for Oral Suspension	VIN1		
Doxycycline Calcium Oral	VIN1		
Suspension	VIN1		
Doxycycline Hyclate	VIN1		
Capsules	VIN1		
for Injection	VIN1		
Sterile	VIN1		
Tablets	VIN1		
Doxylamine Succinate	IA1bii		
Syrup	IIB1		
Tablets	IIB1		
Dromostanolone Propionate	VA1	262	cholesterol
Droperidol	VA1	262	cholesterol
Injection	FID-I		Nb
Droperidol	FID-I		
Injection	IIB1	246	CrV
Absorbable Dusting Powder	IA1bii	246	
Dyclonine Hydrochloride	IIB1		
Gel	IA1biii		
Topical Solution	VB1b		EBT
Dydrogesterone	VB1b	UV-254	CrV
Tablets	IIA4	285	
Dyphylline	IIA4	420	SD
Injection	IA1bii		
Tablets	VB1b	UV-254	
Edetic Acid	VB1b	UV-254	
Edetate Disodium	ID1a		
Injection	ID1a		
Edetate Calcium Disodium	ID1b		DC
Injection	ID1b		DC
for Ophthalmic Solution	IC1k		HNB
Echothiophate Iodide	IC1k		HNB
Edetate Disodium	IC1k		HNB
Injection	IA2a	Poten	CrV
Edetate Calcium Disodium	IA2a	Poten	
Injection	VA1	273	CrV
Emetine Hydrochloride	IA1biii		MeR
Injection	IIB1		CrV
Edrophonium Chloride	IIB1, 2		MeR
Injection	IIB2		
Enflurane	IA1bii		
Ephedrine	IIB2	242	MeR
Ephedrine	IA1bii	242	CrV
Ephedrine Hydrochloride	IIB2	242	MeR
Ephedrine Sulfate	IA1bii	242	
Capsules	IIB2	242	
Injection	IIB2		MeR
Nasal Solution	IA1bii		
Syrup	IIB2		
Tablets	IIB2	240, 242	
Epinephrine and Phenobarbital Capsules	IIB1, 2	242	CrV
Epinephrine	IIB2	242	
Inhalation	VIC2		
Inhalation Aerosol	IIB1		
Injection	VIC2	EC	dopamine hydrochloride
Nasal Solution	VB1b		
Ophthalmic Solution	VIC2	280	
Sterile Oil Suspension	VIC2		MeR

Soluble Tablets	IIIA3	530	dotriacontane
Estradiol	VA2	FID-I	dotriacontane
Pellets	VA2	520	dotriacontane
Sterile Suspension	IIIA4	FID-I	
Estradiol Benzoate	VA2	520	testosterone benzoate
Injection	IIIA4	230	testosterone benzoate
Estradiol Cypionate	IIB1	UV-280	
Injection	VB1b	UV-280	
Estradiol Valerate	IIA4	281	CrV
Injection	IIB1	300	CrV
Estriol	VB1b	281	
Conjugated Estrogens	IIA4	635, 515	
Tablets	IIA	635, 515	Progesterone
Esterified Estrogens	VA1	635, 515	
Tablets	VB1b	UV-280	
Estrone	IIA4	UV-280	
Injection	IIA4	241	ST
Sterile Suspension	IIA4	450	CrV
Estropipate	IA1bii		CrV
Tablets	IVA1	660	
Vaginal Cream	IIB1	660	MRB
Ethacrynate Sodium for Injection	IIB1		MRB
Ethacrynic Acid	IIA4		
Tablets	IA1bii		
Ethambutol Hydrochloride	IA1biii		MRB
Tablets	IC2c		
Ethamivan	IVA1	5, 80	
Injection	IA1ai		
Ethionamide	None		
Tablets	IA1ai		
Ethchlorvynol	IIB1	290	ST
Capsules	IA1aii	290	
Ether	IIB1		
Ethinamate	IC1i	538	MeO
Capsules	IC1ii	538	
Ethosuximide	IA1aiii	254, 277	AV
Capsules	None		AV
Ethopropazine Hydrochloride	IA2b		
Tablets	IA2b		
Ethoxzolamide	IIB1	299	Phth
Tablets	IIB1	299	Phth
Ethyl Acetate	IA1aii		
Ethyl Chloride	IA1aii		
Ethyl Oleate	IIB1		
Ethyl Vanillin	IA1b		
Ethylcellulose	IC1lii		
Ethylenediamine	IA1b		
Ethylnorepinephrine Hydrochloride	IA1biii	402	BrB
Injection	IIA4		CrV
Ethylparaben	IA2b		
Ethynodiol Diacetate and Ethinyl Estradiol Tablets	VB1a	RI	
Ethinyl Estradiol and Mestranol Tablets	IIIB1, IIIA4	236, 536	
Etidronate Disodium	VB1b	F-505	XyO
Eucalyptus Oil	ID1b		
Eucatropine Hydrochloride	None		
Ophthalmic Solution	IA2a		
	IIB2	242	MeR

Table VI—continued

Drug	Assay category	Analytical wavelength and/or detector	Indicator or internal standard
Eugenol	None		
Evans Blue	IIIA3	610	
Injection	IIIA3		
Factor IX Complex	None		
Fennel Oil	None		
Fenoprofen Calcium	VA2	FID-I	docosane
Capsules	VA2	FID-I	diphenamid
Tablets	VA2	FID-I	diphenamid
Fentanyl Citrate	IA1bii		Nb
Injection	VA1	FID-I	papaverine hydrochloride
Ferric Oxide, Red	IC1iii		
Yellow	IC1iii		ST
Ferrous Fumarate	IC1a		ST
Tablets	IC1a		Op
Ferrous Gluconate	IC1iii		ST
Capsules	IC1a	522	Op
Elixir	IIIA4		Op
Tablets	IC1a		Op
Ferrous Sulfate	IIIA4	522	Op
Oral Solution	IC1a		Op
Syrup	IC1a		Op
Tablets	IC1a		Op
Dried	IC1a		Op
Floxuridine	IA1aiii		Op
Sterile	IIIB1		Poten
Flucytosine	IA1bii		Poten
Capsules	IIIB1	268	
Tablets	IIIA1		
Fludrocortisone Acetate	IIIA1	285	
Tablets	VB1b	525	norethindrone
Flumethasone Pivalate	IIIA1	520	norethindrone
Cream	IIIB2	390	
Flunisolide	VB1b		
Nasal Solution	VB1b	UV-254	norethindrone
Fluocinolone Acetonide	VB1b	UV-254	
Cream	VB1b	UV-254	norethindrone
Ointment	VB1b	UV-254	norethindrone
Topical Solution	IIIA1	UV-254	norethindrone
Fluocinonide	VB1b	525	norethindrone
Cream	VB1b	UV-254	norethindrone
Gel	VB1b	UV-254	norethindrone
Ointment	VB1b	UV-254	norethindrone
Fluorescein	IIE1	515	
Injection	IIE1	515	
Fluorescein Sodium	IIE1	515	
Ophthalmic Strips	VB1b	515	
Fluorometholone	VB1b	UV-254	fluoxymesterone
Cream	VB1b	UV-254	
Ophthalmic Suspension	IA1aiii		
Fluorouracil	VB1b		
Cream	IIIB1	266	TB
Injection	IIIB1	266	
Topical Solution	IIIB1	266	

Drug	Assay category	Analytical wavelength and/or detector	Indicator or internal standard
Otic Solution	IIIB1, IIIA4	266, 544	
Suppositories	None		
Glyceryl Monostearate	VA2	FID-I	hexadecyl hexadecanoate
Glycine	IA1bii		CrV
Irrigation	IA1aii		hexadecanoate
Glycobiarsol	ICIj		Phth, TB
Tablets	ICIj		SPI
Glycopyrrolate	ICIj		SPI
Injection	IA1bii		CrV
Tablets	IIIA2	410	
Glycyrrhiza	IIIA2	410	
Pure Extract	None		
Fluid Extract	None		
Gold Au 198 Injection	VIE		
Gold Sodium Thiomalate	IIC		
Injection	IIC		
Chorionic Gonadotropin	VIH		
for Injection	VIH		
Gramicidin	VIN1		
Green Soap	None		
Tincture	None		
Griseofulvin	VA1	FID-I	tetraphenylcyclopentadienone
Capsules	VA1	FID-I	tetraphenylcyclopentadienone
Oral Suspension	VA1	FID-I	tetraphenylcyclopentadienone
Tablets	VA1	FID-I	tetraphenylcyclopentadienone
Ultramicrosize Tablets	VA1	FID-I	tetraphenylcyclopentadienone
Guaifenesin	IIIB2	276	tetraphenylcyclopentadienone
Capsules	VA1	FID-I	tetraphenylcyclopentadienone
Syrup	VA1	FID-I	dextromethorphan hydrobromide
Tablets	VA1	FID-I	dextromethorphan hydrobromide
Guanethidine Monosulfate	IIIA4	500	dextromethorphan hydrobromide
Tablets	IIIA4	412	
Guanethidine Sulfate	IIIA4	500	
Tablets	IIIA4	500	
Guar Gum	None		
Gutta Percha	None		
Halazone	ICIlii		
for Solution	ICIlii		
Haloperidol	IA1bii		
Injection	IIIB1	245	ST
Oral Solution	IIIB1	245	ST
Tablets	IIIB1	245	Nb
Haloprogin	IC1n		
Cream	IIIB1	298, 320	
Halothane	None		

Name	Code	No.	Ref.
Fluoxymesterone			
Tablets	VB1b	UV-254	
Fluphenazine Enanthate			
Injection	IA1bii	UV-254	
Fluphenazine Hydrochloride			
Elixir	IA1biii		
Injection	IIIA4	485	
Oral Solution	IIIA4	485	
Tablets	IIIA4	485	
Flurandrenolide			
Cream	VB1b	485	
Lotion	VB1b	485	
Tape	VB1b	485	
Flurazepam Hydrochloride			
Capsules	IA1biii	UV-240	
Flurothyl	VIC1		
Folic Acid			
Injection	VA1	TC-P	Poten
Tablets	VB1b	UV-254	
Formaldehyde Solution	VIL		
Fructose			
Injection	IA2b	239	
Fumaric Acid	VIC1		
Basic Fuchsin	VIC1, IB1a		
and Sodium Chloride Injection	None		
Absorbent Gauze	None		
Petrolatum Gauze	None		
Gelatin	None		
Gallium Citrate Ga 67 Injection	IA1a	367	Phth
Gallamine Triethiodide			
Injection	VIE	416	BpB
Gemfibrozil			
Capsules	IIIB1	271	
Tablets	IIIB1	271	
Absorbable Sponge	VB1b	UV-276	
Absorbable Film	None	UV-276	
Gentamicin Sulfate			
Cream	VIN1		
Injection	VIN1		
Ointment	VIN1		
Ophthalmic Ointment	VIN1		
Sterile	VIN1		
Ophthalmic Solution	VIN1		
Gentian Violet			
Cream	VIN1		Cr-V
Topical Solution	IIIA3	435	Cr-V
Pharmaceutical Glaze	IC2d		FAS
Glucagon	IIA		
for Injection	None		
Glucose	VIH		
Liquid Glucose	None		
Glutaral Concentrate	IA1b		
Disinfectant Solution	IIIB1	257	
Glutethimide			
Capsules	IIIB1	257	ST
Tablets	IIIB1	257	ST
Glycerin			
Ophthalmic Solution	IC1liii		ST
Oral Solution	IC1m		ST

Name	Code	No.	Ref.
Helium	VA1	TC-I	PC
Heparin Lock Flush Solution	VIH, IB1a		
Heparin Sodium	VIH		
Injection	VIH		
Injection	None		
Hepatitis B Immune Globulin	None		
Hepatitis B Virus Vaccine Inactivated	None		
Hetacillin	VIN1		
Hetacillin for Oral Suspension	VIN1	299	Poten
Tablets	VIN1		
Hetacillin Potassium	VIN1		
Capsules	VIN1		
Sterile	VIN1		
Hexachlorophene	IA1a		
Cleansing Emulsion	IIIB1	240	
Liquid Soap	IIIB1	232	TB
Hexafluorenium Bromide	IA1biii	275	Poten
Injection	IIIB1		
Hexavitamin Capsules	VIL		
Tablets	VIL		
Hexobarbital	IA1aiii	242	
Tablets	IIIB1		
Hexylcaine Hydrochloride	VB1b	UV-254	
Injection	IIIB1	UV-254	
Topical Solution			
Hexylresorcinol	IC2c		
Pills	IC2c		
Histamine Phosphate	IA1a	460	Poten
Injection	IIIA4		
Histidine	IA1biii		
Histoplasmin	None		Np
Homatropine Hydrobromide	IC1a	273	
Ophthalmic Solution	IIIB2		
Homatropine Methylbromide	IA1biii		
Tablets	IIIA4	525	Cr-V
Hyaluronidase Injection	VIF		
for Injection	IIIA4		
Hydralazine Hydrochloride	IA1a		
Injection	IA1a		
Tablets	IC1n		
Hydrochloric Acid	IC1n		
Diluted	IA1bii		
Hydrochlorothiazide	IIIB1		
Tablets	IA1biii		
Hydrocodone Bitartrate	VB1b		
Tablets	VB1b	UV-254	
Hydrocortisone			
Cream	VB1b	525	
Enema	IIIA1	UV-254	
Gel	VB1b	525	
Lotion	VB1b	UV-254	prednisone
Ointment	VB1b	525	prednisone
Sterile Suspension	IIIA1	UV-254	prednisone
Tablets	VB1b	525	
Hydrocortisone Acetate			
Cream	VB1b	UV-254	fluoxymesterone
Lotion	VB1b	UV-254	fluoxymesterone
Ointment	IIIA1	UV-254	fluoxymesterone
Ophthalmic Ointment	IIIA1	525	fluoxymesterone
Ophthalmic Suspension	IIIA1	525	
Sterile Suspension	IIIA1	525	

Table VI—continued

Drug	Assay category	Analytical wavelength and/or detector	Indicator or internal standard
Hydrocortisone Cypionate			
Oral Suspension	VB1b	UV-254	medroxyprogesterone acetate
Hydrocortisone Hemisuccinate	VB1b	UV-254	medroxyprogesterone acetate
Hydrocortisone Sodium Phosphate			
Injection	VB1b	239	fluorometholone
Hydrocortisone Sodium Succinate			
for Injection	IIIA1	525	
Hydrocortisone Valerate			
Cream	VB1b	UV-254	fluorometholone
Topical Solution	IIIB1	273	ethyl benzoate
Hydroflumethiazide			
Tablets	IIIB1	273	
Hydrogen Peroxide Concentrate			
Topical Solution	IC1b		
Hydromorphone Hydrochloride	IC1b		
Injection	IA1biii		CrV
Tablets	IIIA4	440	
Hydroquinone			
Cream	IC1a	440	
Topical Solution	IIIB1	293	DP
Hydroxocobalamin Injection	VB1b	UV-280	
Hydroxyamphetamine	IIIB2	361	
Hydrobromide	IA1biii	361	CrV
Hydroxychloroquine Sulfate			
Tablets	IIIB1	343	
Hydroxyethyl Cellulose	None	343	
Hydroxyprogesterone Caproate			
Injection	IIIB1	240	
	IIIB2	380	ST
Hydroxypropyl Cellulose	IA1biii		
Hydroxypropyl Methylcellulose	IC1I	UV-230	
1828	VA2	TC-I	toluene
2208	VA2	TC-I	toluene
2908	VA2	TC-I	toluene
2910	VA2	TC-I	toluene
Ophthalmic Solution	IIIA4	635	
Phthalate 220731	None		Poten
Phthalate 220824	None		Poten
Hydroxystilbamidine Isethionate			
Sterile	IC1h		ST
Hydroxyurea			
Capsules	IC2b		ST
Hydroxyzine Hydrochloride			
Injection	IC2b		QR
Syrup	IA1biii	UV-230	tetracaine hydrochloride
Tablets	VB1b	UV-232	
Hydroxyzine Pamoate			
Capsules	VB1b	UV-232	
Oral Suspension	VB1b	UV-254	
Hyoscyamine			
Tablets	VA1	UV-232	
		TC-I	CrV; homatropine hydrobromide

Drug	Assay category	Analytical wavelength and/or detector	Indicator or internal standard
Meglumine Injection	IB1a		TBPE
Iodochlorhydroxyquin	VA1		pyrene
Cream	VA1		pyrene
Ointment	VA1		pyrene
Compound Powder	IIIB1	267	
Iodoquinol	IIB		
Tablets	IC1Iii		ST
Iopanoic Acid	IC1Iii		ST
Tablets	IB1a		ST
Iophendylate	IA1a		TB
Injection	IC1Iii		TBP
Iothalamate Meglumine Injection and Iothalamate Sodium Injection	IC1Iii		TB
Iothalamate Sodium Injection	IC1Iii		ST
Iothalamic Acid	VIC1, IB1a		ST
Ipecac	IB1a		ST
Powdered	IB1a		Poten
Syrup	IB1a		Poten
Ipodate Calcium for Oral Suspension	IB1a		
Ipodate Sodium	IB1a		
Capsules	IB1a		
Ferrous Citrate Fe59 Injection	VIE		EY
Iron Dextran Injection	IIIA4	510	EY
Iron Sorbitex Injection	IIIA4	510	EY
Iso-Alcoholic Elixir	None		EY
Isobucaine Hydrochloride and Epinephrine Injection	IA1bii, IIIA4	530	MeR
Isobutane	VA1		MeR
Isocarboxazid	ICIj		MeR
Tablets	ICIj		Poten
Isoetharine Hydrochloride	IIIA4		Poten
Inhalation	VB1b		
Isoetharine Mesylate	VB1b		
Inhalation Aerosol	None		
Isoflurane	VA1		
Isoflurophate	VA1		
Ophthalmic Ointment	IA1bii		
Isoleucine	VA1	420	
Isoniazid	ICIj		
Injection	ICIj		
Syrup	ICIj		
Tablets	ICIj		
Isopropamide Iodide	IA1bii		
Tablets	IIIB1		
Isopropyl Alcohol	IA1bii	280, 258	CrV
Rubbing	VA1	TC-I	MeR
Azeotropic	VID	UV-278	
Isopropyl Myristate	VA1	UV-278	cyclohexanone
Isopropyl Palmitate	VA1	UV-254	cyclohexane
Isoproterenol Hydrochloride	None	UV-254	cyclohexane
	VA1	TC-P	Poten
	VB1b	UV-278	Poten
		FID-I	Poten
		FID-I	Poten
		FID-P	Poten
		FID-P	CrV
		UV-278	

Name	Code	No.	Reagent
Hyoscyamine Hydrobromide	IA1bii		CrV
Hyoscyamine Sulfate	VA1		Poten
Elixir	VA1		homatropine hydrobromide
Injection	VA1	TC-I	homatropine hydrobromide
Oral Solution	VA1	TC-I	homatropine hydrobromide
Tablets	VA1	TC-I	homatropine hydrobromide
Hypophosphorous Acid	IA1a		
Ibuprofen	VA1	FID-I	n-nonadecane
Tablets	VA1	FID-I	n-nonadecane
Ichthammol	IA1a		
Idoxuridine	IA2a		homatropine hydrobromide
Ointment	IA2a, IIB		homatropine hydrobromide
Ophthalmic Ointment	IA1aiii		homatropine hydrobromide
Ophthalmic Solution	IIB1		Phth
Imidurea	None	320, 283	MeR
Imipramine Hydrochloride	IA1bii	320, 283	TB
Injection	IIB1	250	
Tablets	IIB1	250	
Indigotindisulfonate Sodium	IIB1	610	
Injection	IIA3	610	
Indium In 111 Pentetate Injection	IIIA3		
Indium Chlorides In 113m Injection	VIE		
Indocyanine Green	VIE	785	
Sterile	IIIA3	785	
Indomethacin	VB1b	UV-254	CrV
Capsules	IIB1	318	
Influenza Virus Vaccine	None		
Insulin	VIH		
Injection	VIH		
Globin Zinc Injection	VIH		
Isophane Suspension	VIH		
Zinc Suspension	VIH		
Extended Zinc Suspension	VIH		
Prompt Zinc Suspension	VIH		
Protamine Zinc Suspension	VIH		
Inulin	None		
and Sodium Chloride Injection	IIIA4, IB1a	435	
Iocetamic Acid	IB1a	435	DCF
Tablets	IB1a		Poten
Iodine	IB1a		
Topical Solution	IC1l		ST
Strong Solution	IC1l		ST
Tincture	IC1m, n		ST
Strong Tincture	IC1m, n		ST
Sodium Iodide I123 Capsules	IC1m, n		ST
Iodinated I125 Albumin Injection	VIE		
Sodium Iodide I125 Capsules	VIE		
Iodinated I131 Albumin Injection	VIE		
Sodium Iodide I131	VIE		
Aggregated	VIE		
Iodohippurate Sodium I131	VIE		
Injection	VIE		
Rose Bengal Sodium I131 Injection	IIIA3, VIE	550	
Sodium Iodide I131 Capsules	VIE		
Iodipamide	IB1a		TBPE

Name	Code	No.	Reagent
Inhalation Aerosol	IIIA4	530	norepinephrine hydrochloride
Inhalation	VB1b	UV-278	
Injection	VB1b	UV-280	
Tablets and Phenylephrine Bitartrate	VB1b	530	triethyleneglycol
Inhalation Aerosol	IIIA4	495, 530	triethyleneglycol
Isoproterenol Sulfate	VB1b	UV-278	
Inhalation Aerosol	IIIA4	530	
Inhalation Solution	VB1b	UV-278	
Isosorbide Concentrate	VA1	TC-I	Poten
Oral Solution	VB1b	TC-I	Poten
Inhalation Aerosol	IVA1		Poten
Tablets	VA1		
Isosorbide Dinitrate, Diluted	IIB1		
Isoxsuprine Hydrochloride	IIB1	269, 300	
Injection	IVA1	275	CrV
Tablets	VA1	275	CrV
Juniper Tar	None		
Kanamycin Sulfate	VIN1		
Capsules	VIN1		
Injection	VIN1		
Sterile	VIN1		
Kaolin	IIB1		
Ketoconazole	IA1bii	269	Phth
Injection	IIB1		
Ketamine Hydrochloride	None		
Injection	IA2b		
Krypton Kr 81m	None		
Lactic Acid	VIE		
Lactose	VIF		
Lactulose Concentrate	VIF		
Syrup	None		
Lanolin	IIB		Phth
Alcohols	None		
Anhydrous	None		
Lavender Oil	IA2b		
Lecithin	None		
Lemon Oil	IA2a		
Leucine	IIIB1	284	Poten
Leucovorin Calcium	IIIB1	284	Poten
Injection	IIB1		
Levallorphan Tartrate	IIIA2	420	Poten
Injection	IA1bii		
Levodopa	IA1bii	280	
Capsules	IIB1	280	
Tablets	IA1bii		
Levonordefrin	IA1bii		
Levopropoxyphene Napsylate	IA1bii		
Capsules	VA1		
Oral Suspension	IA1bii	FID-I	CrV
Levorphanol Tartrate	VA1	FID-I	CrV
Injection	IA2a	UV-225	n-tricosane
Tablets	IA2a	UV-225	n-tricosane
Levothyroxin Sodium	VB1b		
Tablets	IA2a		
Lidocaine	IA1bii		BcG
Topical Aerosol	IA2a		CrV
Ointment	IA2a		Poten
Oral Topical Solution	IA1bii		CrV
Lidocaine Hydrochloride	VB1b		CrV
Injection	IA1bii		MeR
Jelly	IA2a	UV-246	Poten

Table VI—continued

Drug	Assay category	Analytical wavelength and/or detector	Indicator or internal standard
Lidocaine Hydrochloride			
Topical Solution	IA2a		Poten
Sterile	IA1biii		CrV
and Dextrose Injection	VB1b, VIC1	UV-261	
and Epinephrine Bitartrate Injection	VB1b	UV-254, EC	norepinephrine bitartrate
and Epinephrine Injection	VB1b	UV-261, EC	norepinephrine bitartrate
Lime	None		
Sulfurated Topical Solution	ID1a		HNB
Lincomycin Hydrochloride	VA2	FID-I	n-dotriacontane
Capsules	VA2	FID-I	n-dotriacontane
Injection	VA2	FID-I	n-dotriacontane
Sterile	VA2	FID-I	n-dotriacontane
Syrup	VA2	FID-I	n-dotriacontane
Lindane	IB2aii		FAS
Cream	VA1		methylene chloride
Lotion	VA1		methylene chloride
Shampoo	VA1		methylene chloride
Liothyronine Sodium	VB1b	UV-225	
Tablets	VB1b	UV-225	
Liotrix Tablets	IA2a	225	MeO
Lithium Carbonate	IIIB1		MeO
Capsules	IIID	671	
Tablets	IIID	671	
Lithium Citrate	IIID	671	
Syrup	IIID	671	
Lithium Hydroxide	IIID	671	
Loperamide Hydrochloride	IIIA4		Phth
Capsules	IA1b	410	Nb
Lymphogranuloma Venereum Antigen	VB1b		
Lysine Acetate	IIIA4		
Lysine Hydrochloride	None		
Lypressin Nasal Solution	IA1bii		
Mafenide Acetate	IA1biii	267	
Cream	VIH	267	
Magaldrate	IIIB1		EBT, DT
Oral Suspension	IIIB1		EBT, DT
Tablets	IIIB1		EBT, DT
Milk of Magnesia	IIIF1		EBT, DT
Magnesia Tablets	IA2a		EBT
Magnesia and Alumina Oral Suspension	ID1a, IIIF1	309, 285	EBT, DT
Tablets	ID1a, ID2b		EBT, DT
Magnesium Aluminum Silicate	IIIF1	589	EBT
Magnesium Carbonate and Sodium Bicarbonate for Oral Suspension	IA2a		MeO
Magnesium Chloride	ID1a, ID2b		EBT
Magnesium Citrate Oral Solution	ID1a, ID2b		EBT
Magnesium Gluconate	ID1a, ID2b		EBT
Tablets	ID1a		EBT
Magnesium Hydroxide	ID1a		Phth
Magnesium Oxide	ID1a, IIB		MeR
Magnesium Phosphate	ID1a, ID2b		MeO / Phth

Drug	Assay category	Analytical wavelength and/or detector	Indicator or internal standard
Menthol	None		Poten
Mepenzolate Bromide	IA1biii		
Syrup	IIIA4	620	CrV
Tablets	IIIA4	620	CrV
Meperidine Hydrochloride	IA1biii		CrV
Injection	IIIB1		
Syrup	IIIB1		
Tablets	IIIB1		
Mephentermine Sulfate	IA		
Injection	IA1biii		
Tablets	IIIB1		
Mephenytoin	IA1biii		
Tablets	IIIB1		
Mephobarbital	IIIB1		
Tablets	IIIB1	257	TP
Mepivacaine Hydrochloride	IA1aiii	257	TP
Injection	IA1biii		
and Levonordefrin Injection	IA1biii, IIIA4		
Meprednisone	IIIB1	530	MeR
Tablets	IIIA1	238	MeR
Meprobamate	IIIA1	525	
Injection	IA1ai		Phth
Oral Suspension	IA1ai		Phth
Tablets	IA1ai		Phth
Meprylcaine Hydrochloride and Epinephrine Injection	IIIB2	358	
Mercaptomerin Sodium	IA2a		
Injection	IA2a, IIIA4	530	MeR
Mercaptopurine	IIB	530	MeR
Injection	IIB		
Tablets	IA1aiii		
Ammoniated Mercury	IIIB1	325	TB
Ointment	IA1bi		MeR
Chlormerodrin Hg 197 Injection	IIB		
203 Injection	VIE		
Mesoridazine Besylate	IIB		Poten
Injection	IA1bii	262	
Oral Solution	IIIB1	267	
Tablets	IIIB1	267	
Mestranol	IIIB1	547	
Metaraminol Bitartrate	IIIA4		CrV
Injection	IA1bii		
Methacholine Chloride	IIIA4		
Methacycline Hydrochloride	IA1bii	UV-264	Phth
Methacrylic Acid Copolymer	VB1b		
Methadone Hydrochloride	IA1a		Phth
Capsules	IA1biii		
Oral Solution	VIN1		
Oral Concentrate	VIN1		
Oral Suspension	VIN1		
Injection	VIN1		
Tablets	IA1a		
Methamphetamine Hydrochloride	IA1biii		CrV
Injection	IA1bii		procaine
Tablets	VA1	UV-280	procaine
Methandriol	VB1b	UV-254	pyrilamine maleate
Methandrostenolone	IIIB1	FID-I	procaine
Tablets	IIIB1	UV-254	benzhydrol
Methantheline Bromide	IIIB1	245	CrV
Sterile	IA1bii		CrV
Tablets	IA1biii		CrV

Name	Code	No.	Method
Magnesium Salicylate Tablets	IIB1	296	MeO
Magnesium Silicate	IIB1	296	EBT
Magnesium Stearate	IA2a, IIC		EBT
Magnesium Sulfate	ID1a		EBT
Magnesium Sulfate Injection	ID1a		MeO
Magnesium Trisilicate	ID1a		Phth
Malic Acid	IA2a		EBT
Manganese Chloride Injection	IA1a		
Manganese Sulfate	ID1a		
Manganese Sulfate Injection	IIF1		
Mannitol	ID1a	279	EBT
Mannitol Injection	IIF1		
Mannitol and Sodium Chloride Injection	IC1liii		
Maprotiline Hydrochloride Tablets	IC1liii, IB2aii	273, 300	CrV amitriptyline hydrochloride
Mazindol Tablets	IA1bii	279	
Measles Virus Vaccine Live	VB1b	UV-254	
Measles and Mumps Virus Vaccine Live	None		
Measles, Mumps and Rubella Virus Vaccine Live	None		
Mebendazole	None		
Mebendazole Tablets	IA1bii	247	Poten
Mecamylamine Hydrochloride Tablets	VIM		MeR
Mechlorethamine Hydrochloride for Injection	IA2a		ST
Meclizine Hydrochloride	IC2b		ST
Meclizine Hydrochloride Tablets	IC2b		Poten
Meclocycline Sulfosalicylate Cream	IA1bii	UV-340	Poten
Meclofenamate Sodium Capsules	VB1b	UV-340	Phth
Medroxyprogesterone Acetate Sterile Suspension	VB1a	UV-254	progesterone
Medroxyprogesterone Acetate Tablets	VB1a	UV-254	progesterone
Medrysone Ophthalmic Suspension	VB1a	242	progesterone
Megestrol Acetate	IIB1	242	propylparaben
Megestrol Acetate Tablets	IIB1	242	propylparaben
Meglumine	IIB1	UV-280	MeR
Melphalan	IA1a	UV-280	Poten
Melphalan Tablets	IIB1		Poten
Menadiol Sodium Diphosphate	IIB1		Poten
Menadiol Sodium Diphosphate Injection	IC1a	UV-254	Poten
Menadione	IC1a		Poten
Menadione Injection	IC1a		Poten
Menadione Tablets	IIIA4	635	Op
Menadione Sodium Bisulfite Injection	IC1a	250	Op
Meningococcal Polysaccharide Vaccine	IB1a		Op
Group A	None		
Group B	None		
Group C	None		
Menotropins for Injection	VIH		

Name	Code	No.	Method
Methapyrilene Fumarate Tablets	IA1bii		CrV
Methapyrilene Fumarate Syrup	IIB1		Poten
Methapyrilene Hydrochloride	IA1bii	313	
Methaqualone Capsules	IIB1	313	
Methaqualone Injection	IIB1	313	Poten
Methaqualone Tablets	IA1bii		
Methaqualone Hydrochloride	IIB1		CrV
Methaqualone Hydrochloride Capsules	IA1bii		
Metharbital	IA1bii		CrV
Metharbital Tablets	IIB1		
Methazolamide	IIB1	252, 275	MeR
Methazolamide Tablets	IIB1	460	
Methdilazine	IVA1	244	
Methdilazine Tablets	IIIB1	288	
Methdilazine Hydrochloride	IIIB1	235	
Methdilazine Hydrochloride Syrup	IIIA4	235	
Methdilazine Hydrochloride Tablets	IIIA4		
Methenamine	IA2a	570	MeR
Methenamine Elixir	IIIA4	570	
Methenamine Tablets	IIIA4	570	
Methenamine and Monobasic Sodium Phosphate Tablets	IIIA4, IA2a		Phth
Methenamine Hippurate	IA1a		CrV
Methenamine Mandelate	IA1a		TP
Methenamine Mandelate for Oral Suspension	IB1a		Poten
Methenamine Mandelate Tablets	IB1a		Poten
Methenamine Mandelate Oral Suspension	IB1a		Poten
Methicillin Sodium for Injection	VIN1		
Methimazole	IA1a		BtB
Methimazole Tablets	IA1a		BtB
Methiodal Sodium	IB1a		TBPE
Methiodal Sodium Injection	IB1a		TBPE
Methionine	IA1bii	274	Poten
Methionine Injection	IIB1	UV-274	
Methocarbamol	VB1b	UV-274	caffeine
Methocarbamol Injection	VB1b	5, 93	caffeine
Methocarbamol Tablets	VB1b	247	
Methohexital Sodium for Injection	IIC1	247	
Methotrexate	IIB1	UV-302	
Methotrexate Injection	VB1b	UV-302	
Methotrexate Tablets	VB1b	UV-302	Phth
Methotrexate Sodium for Injection	IA1bii		
Methotrimeprazine	IIA2	274	CrV
Methotrimeprazine Injection	IA1bii	300	MeR
Methoxamine Hydrochloride	IA1a	300	
Methoxamine Hydrochloride Injection	IA2a	TC-I	CrV
Methoxsalen	IIIB1		
Methoxsalen Capsules	IIB1	415	
Methoxsalen Topical Solution	IIB1		
Methoxyflurane	VA1		
Methoxyphenamine Hydrochloride	IA1bii	300	benzphetamine hydrochloride
Methoxyphenamine Hydrochloride Tablets	VB1b	300	benzphetamine hydrochloride
Methscopolamine Bromide	IIIA2	420	MV benzphetamine hydrochloride
Methscopolamine Bromide Injection	VB1b	UV-254	
Methscopolamine Bromide Tablets	VB1b		
Methsuximide	IIIB1	247	
Methsuximide Capsules	VB1b	247	EY
Methyclothiazide	IB1a		

Table VI—continued

Drug	Assay category	Analytical wavelength and/or detector	Indicator or internal standard
Methyclothiazide Tablets	IIIB1		
Methyl Alcohol	VA1	FID-I	
Methyl Isobutyl Ketone	None		
Methyl Salicylate	IA2b	268	Phth
Methylbenzethonium Chloride	IC1n		
Lotion	IE4		SaO
Ointment	IE4		SaO
Powder	IE4		SaO
Methylcellulose	VA2		
Ophthalmic Solution	IC1lii	TC-I	toluene
Oral Solution	IC1lii		ST
Tablets	IC1lii		ST
Methyldopa	IIA		
Oral Suspension	IC1lii		
Tablets	IA1bii		
Methyldopa and Hydrochlorothiazide Tablets	IIA4, VB1b	520, UV-270	CrV
Methyldopate Hydrochloride Injection	IIIB1	UV-280	
Methylene Blue Injection	VB1b	663	Nb
Methylene Chloride	VA1	TC-I	
Methylergonovine Maleate Injection	IIA3	555	
Tablets	IIA3	555	
Methylparaben	VA1	283	
Methylphenidate Hydrochloride Tablets	IIA4	405	BtB
Methylprednisolone	IA1bii	UV-254	prednisone
Injection	VB1b	UV-264	prednisone
Tablets	VB1b	UV-254	prednisone
Methylprednisolone Acetate Cream	IIIA1	525	prednisone
for Enema	VB1b	UV-254	prednisone
Sterile Suspension	VB1b		fluorometholone
Methylprednisolone Hemisuccinate	IIIA1	525	fluorometholone
Methylprednisolone Sodium Succinate for Injection	VB1a	525	fluorometholone
Methyltestosterone Capsules	IIA4	241	
Tablets	IA1bii	241	
Methylthiouracil Tablets	IA1aiii	241	TB
Methyprylon Capsules	IIB1		Poten
Tablets	IIB1		Poten
Methysergide Maleate Tablets	IIB1		CrV
Metocurine Iodide Injection	IIB1	322	Poten
Metoprolol Tartrate Tablets	IA1bii	UV-254	oxprenolol hydrochloride
Metronidazole Injection	VB1b	UV-320	MaG
Tablets	IA1bii		
Metyrapone	IIIB1	260	Poten

Drug	Assay category	Analytical wavelength and/or detector	Indicator or internal standard
Ophthalmic Ointment	VIN1		
Oral Solution	VIN1		
Sterile Tablets	VIN1		
and Bacitracin Ointment	VIN1		
and Bacitracin Zinc Ointment	VIN1	525	
Phosphate Cream	VIN1, IIIA1		
and Dexamethasone Sodium Phosphate Ointment	VIN1, IIIA1	525	
and Dexamethasone Sodium Phosphate Ophthalmic Solution	VIN1, IIIA1	525	
and Fluocinolone Acetonide Cream	VIN1, VB1b	UV-238	
and Fluorometholone Ointment	VIN1, VB1b	UV-254	fluoxymesterone
and Flurandrenolide Cream	VIN1, VB1b	UV-240	
and Flurandrenolide Ointment	VIN1, VB1b	UV-240	
and Gramicidin Ointment	VIN1		
and Hydrocortisone Cream	VIN1, VB1b	UV-254	
and Hydrocortisone Ointment	VIN1, VB1b	UV-254	
and Hydrocortisone Acetate Cream	VIN1, VB1b	UV-254	
and Hydrocortisone Acetate Ointment	VIN1, VB1b	UV-254	
and Methylprednisolone Acetate Ophthalmic Suspension	VIN1, IIIA1	525	fluoxymesterone
Neomycin and Polymyxin B Sulfates Solution for Irrigation	VIN1		
Ophthalmic Ointment	VIN1		
Ophthalmic Solution	VIN1		
and Bacitracin Ointment	VIN1		
and Bacitracin Ophthalmic Ointment	VIN1		
and Bacitracin Zinc and Hydrocortisone Acetate Ointment	VIN1, VB1b	UV-254	fluoxymesterone
Bacitracin and Hydrocortisone Acetate Ointment	VIN1, VB1b	UV-254	fluoxymesterone
Bacitracin Zinc and Hydrocortisone Acetate Ophthalmic Ointment	VIN1		
and Bacitracin Zinc Ointment	VIN1		
and Bacitracin Zinc Ophthalmic Ointment	VIN1		
and Bacitracin Zinc Powder	VIN1		
and Bacitracin Zinc Topical Aerosol	VIN1		
Bacitracin Zinc and Hydrocortisone Ophthalmic Ointment	VIN1, VB1b	UV-254	fluoxymesterone
Bacitracin Zinc and Hydrocortisone Ophthalmic Ointment	VIN1, VB1b	UV-254	fluoxymesterone

Name	Classification	Ref	Notes
Tablets	IIIA4	450	
Metyrosine	IIIA4	450	
Tartrate Injection	IA1bii		
Capsules	IIIB1	274	
Sterile Mezlocillin Sodium	VIN3	280	
Miconazole	IIIA4	540	Nb
Injection	IA1bii		
Mineral Oil	None		
Emulsion	None		
Light	None		
Minocycline Hydrochloride	VIN1		
Capsules	VIN1		
Sterile	VIN1		
Oral Suspension	VIN1		
Tablets	VIN1		
Mitomycin	VIN1	268	
for Injection	VIN1		
Mitotane	IIIB1	268	
Tablets	IIIB1		
Mono and Di-Acetylated	None		
Monoglycerides	None		
Mono and Di Glycerides	VA1	FID-I	
Monoethanolamine	IA1b	FID-I	Poten
Monosodium Glutamate	IA1bii		BcG, MeR
Monothioglycerol	IC1k		Poten
Morphine Sulfate	IA1aiii		ST
Injection	IIIB1	285	PR
Morrhuate Sodium Injection	IA2a		
Moxalactam Disodium for Injection	VB1b	UV-254	MeO
Mumps Skin Test Antigen	None		
Mumps Virus Vaccine Live	None		
Nafcillin Sodium	None		
Capsules	VIN1		
for Injection	VIN1		
for Oral Solution	VIN1		
Sterile	VIN1		
Tablets	VIN1		
Nalidixic Acid	IA1aii		TP
Oral Suspension	IIIB1	258	
Tablets	IIIB1	258	
Nalorphine Hydrochloride	IIIB1	285	
Injection	IIIB1	285	
Naloxone Hydrochloride	IA1biii	285	
Injection	VA1	FID-I	MV papaverine
Nandrolone Decanoate	IIB1	239	
Injection	IIB2	380	
Nandrolone Phenpropionate	IIB1	239	
Injection	IIB2	380	
Naphazoline Hydrochloride	IIB1		
Nasal Solution	IIB1	280	MeR
Ophthalmic Solution	IIB1	280	
Naproxen	IA1a		
Naproxen Sodium	IIB1		
Tablets	IA1bii	332	Phth
Natamycin	IIIB1	332	Nb
Ophthalmic Suspension	VIN1		
Neomycin Sulfate	VIN1		
Cream	VIN1		
Ointment	VIN1		

Name	Classification	Ref	Notes
Suspension	VIN1, VB1b	UV-254	
and Dexamethasone Ophthalmic	VIN1		
Ointment	VIN1, VB1b	UV-254	
and Dexamethasone Ophthalmic	VIN1		
Suspension	VIN1		
and Gramicidin Cream	VIN1, VB1b	UV-254	
and Gramicidin Ophthalmic	VIN1, VB1b	UV-254	
Solution			
and Hydrocortisone Ophthalmic	VIN1, IIIA1	525	
Suspension			
and Hydrocortisone Otic Solution	VIN1, VB1b	525	
and Hydrocortisone	VIN1, VB1b	525	
Suspension			
Neomycin Sulfate and Prednisolone	VIN1, IIIA1	525	
Acetate Ophthalmic			
Suspension			
Ointment			
Ophthalmic Ointment			
Neomycin Sulfate and Prednisolone	VIN1, IIIA1		fluoxymesterone
Sodium Phosphate Ophthalmic			
Ointment			
Neomycin Sulfate and	VIN1, VB1b	UV-254	
Triamcinolone Acetonide			
Ophthalmic Ointment			
Neostigmine Bromide	IA1biii	420	CrV
Tablets	IIIA2		
Neostigmine Methylsulfate	IA1c	420	MeP
Injection	IIIA2		
Netilmicin Sulfate	VIN1		
Injection	VIN1		
Niacin	IIIB1	262	
Injection	IIIA4	450	
Tablets	IIIA4	450	
Niacinamide	IIIB1	262	
Injection	IIIA4	450	
Tablets	IIIA4	450	
Nifedipine	IIIB1	350	
Capsules	IIIB1	340	
Nitric Acid	IA1a		
Nitrofurantoin	IVA1	375	
Oral Suspension	IVA1	375	
Tablets	IVA1	375	
Nitrofurazone	IIIB1	375	
Cream	IIIB1	375	
Ointment	IIIB1	375	
Topical Solution	VA1	375	
Nitrogen	IIIB1		
Nitroglycerin Tablets	IIIA4	410, 600	
Nitromersol	IB1biii	TC-I	FAS
Nitrous Oxide	IB1biii		FAS
Tincture	VA1	TC-I	FAS
Nonoxynol 10	None		
Norepinephrine Bitartrate	IA1a		
Injection	IA1biii	UV-278	CrV
Norethindrone	VB1b, VIC1	240	MeR
Tablets	IIIB1	380	
and Ethinyl Estradiol Tablets	IIIB2, IIIE22	375, 556	
and Mestranol Tablets	IIIB2, IIIE2	249, 568	
Norethindrone Acetate	IIIB1	240	
Tablets	IIIB1	240	

Table VI—continued

Drug	Assay category	Analytical wavelength and/or detector	Indicator or internal standard
Norethindrone Acetate and Ethinyl Estradiol Tablets	IIIB1, IIIA4	240, 536	
Norethindrone and Ethinyl Estradiol Tablets	IIIB1	240	
Norethynodrel and Ethinyl Estradiol Tablets	IIIB1	241	
Norgestrel Tablets	IIIB1	380	
Norgestrel and Ethinyl Estradiol Tablets	IIIB2	241, 536	
Nortriptyline Hydrochloride Capsules	IIIB1, IIIA4		Poten
Oral Solution	IA1bii	239	
Noscapine	IIIB1	239	
Novobiocin Cream	VIN1		
Novobiocin Calcium Oral Suspension	VIN1		CrV
Novobiocin Sodium Capsules	VIN1		
Nutmeg Oil	None		
Nystatin Cream	VIN1		
Lotion	VIN1		
Ointment	VIN1		
Topical Powder	VIN1		
Oral Suspension	VIN1		
for Oral Suspension	VIN1		
Tablets	VIN1		
Vaginal Suppositories	VIN1		
Vaginal Tablets	VIN1		
Neomycin Sulfate, Gramicidin and Iodochlorhydroxyquin Ointment	VIN1, IIIA4	650	
Neomycin Sulfate, Gramicidin and Triamcinolone Acetonide Ointment	VIN1, VB1b	UV-254	fluoxymesterone
Neomycin Sulfate, Gramicidin and Triamcinolone Acetonide Cream	VIN1, VB1b		fluoxymesterone
Octoxynol 9	None		
Hydrophilic Ointment	None		
Oleic Acid	VIL		
Oleovitamin A and D Capsules	VIL	285	Poten
Oleyl Alcohol	None		
Olive Oil	None		
Opium Powdered	IIIB1	285	
Tincture	IIIB1	285	
Orange Flower Oil Water	None		
Orange Oil	IA2a		
Sweet Orange Peel Tincture	VIB		
Compound Orange Spirit	None		
Orange Syrup	None		
Orphenadrine Citrate	IA1bii		
Injection	IA1a	410	Phth
Ouabain	IIIA4	495	
Injection	IIIA4	495	CrV
Oxacillin Sodium	VIN1		

Drug	Assay category	Analytical wavelength and/or detector	Indicator or internal standard
Parachlorophenol Camphorated	IC2c, IIB, IIB	FID-I	ST
Paraffin	None		
Paraldehyde	None	FID-I	1-decanol
Sterile	None	FID-I	cyclohexanol
Paramethadione	None	FID-I	cyclohexanol
Capsules	VA1		
Oral Solution	VA1		
Paramethasone Acetate Tablets	IIIB1	242	
Paregoric	IIIB1	6.04	
Pargyline Hydrochloride Tablets	IIIC1		Phth
Parathyroid Injection	VIH	285	benzophenone
Paromomycin Sulfate Capsules	IA1bii	UV-262	Poten
Syrup	VB1b		
Peanut Oil	None		
Pectin	None		
Penicillamine Capsules	IA2b, IA1a		Phth
Tablets	ID1b		DC
Penicillin G Benzathine Oral Suspension	ID1b		DC
Sterile Suspension	ID1b		DC
Tablets	VIN2		SPI
Penicillin G Potassium and Penicillin G Suspension Tablets	VIN2		SPI
Penicillin G Potassium Capsules	VIN2		SPI
for Injection	VIN2		SPI
for Oral Solution	VIN2		SPI
Sterile	VIN2		SPI
Tablets	VIN2		SPI
Tablets for Oral Solution	VIN2		SPI
Penicillin G Procaine, Sterile Suspension	VIN2		SPI
for Suspension	VIN2		SPI
with Aluminum Stearate Suspension	VIN2		SPI
Penicillin G Sodium for Injection Sterile	VIN2		SPI
Penicillin V for Oral Suspension	VIN2		SPI
Tablets	VIN2		SPI
Penicillin V Benzathine Oral Suspension	VIN2		SPI
Penicillin V Hydrabamine Oral Suspension	VIN2		SPI
Tablets	VIN2		SPI
Penicillin V Potassium for Oral Solution	VIN2		SPI
Tablets	VIN2		SPI
Pentaerythritol Tetranitrate Tablets	IIIA4	409	SPI

Table VI—continued

Drug	Assay category	Analytical wavelength and/or detector	Indicator or internal standard
Phenoxybenzamine Hydrochloride Capsules	IA1biii		
Phenprocoumon Tablets	IIIB1	275	Poten
Phensuximide Capsules	IA1a	311	Poten
Oral Suspension	IIIB1	258	
Phentermine Hydrochloride Capsules	IIIB1	258	
Tablets	VB1b	UV-254	MRB
Phentolamine Hydrochloride Capsules	IA1biii	UV-254	Poten
Tablets	VB1b		
Phentolamine Mesylate for Injection	IIIA4	410	Poten
Phenylalanine	IA1aiii	410	Poten
Phenylbutazone Capsules	IIIB1	264	Poten
Tablets	IA1aiii	264	Poten
Phenylephrine Hydrochloride Injection	IC2c	271	ST
Nasal Jelly	IIIB1	UV-280	AV
Nasal Solution	VB1b	271	AV
Ophthalmic Solution	IIIB1	271	CrV
Phenylethyl Alcohol	None	271	
Phenylmercuric Acetate	IIIB1		FAS
Phenylmercuric Nitrate	IB1b		FAS
Phenylpropanolamine Hydrochloride	IIIB1		CrV
Phenytoin	IA1biii		
Oral Suspension	IA1aii		
Tablets	IA1aiii		
Phenytoin Sodium Extended Capsules	IIA	UV-254	
Injection	VB1b		
Prompt Capsules	IIA		
Injection	IIA		
Sterile	VIE		
Chromic Phosphate P32 Suspension	VIE		
Sodium Phosphate P32 Solution	IIA		
Phosphoric Acid Diluted	IIA		
Phthalsulfathiazole	ICIj		TP
Tablets	ICIj		TP
Physostigmine	IA1bii	246	Poten
Physostigmine Salicylate Injection	IIIB1		Poten
Ophthalmic Solution	IIIB1		Poten
Physostigmine Sulfate Ophthalmic Ointment	IA1bii	305	Poten
Phytonadione Injection	IIIB1	248	Poten
Tablets	VB1b		Poten
Pilocarpine Ocular System	VB1b		
Pilocarpine Hydrochloride Ophthalmic Solution	IIIB1	215	Poten
	IA1biii	UV-254	
	IIIB1		
	VB1a	UV-220	CrV

Drug	Assay category	Analytical wavelength and/or detector	Indicator or internal standard
and Potassium Chloride for Effervescent Oral Solution	IB1a	766.5	FAS
and Potassium Chloride Effervescent Tablets for Oral Solution	IB2aii, IIIF1	766.5	FAS
	IB2ai, IIIF1	766.5	
Potassium Chloride	IB1a		Poten
Extended Release Capsules	IIIF1	766.5	
Extended Release Tablets	IIIF1	766.5	
Elixir	IIIF1	766.5	
Injection	IIIF1	766.5	
Oral Solution	IIIF1	766.5	
for Oral Solution in Dextrose Injection	VIC1, IB1a	766.5	DCF, CrV
Potassium Citrate and Citric Acid Oral Solution	IIIF1	766.5	Poten, Phth
	IID, IA1a	766.5	
Potassium Gluconate Elixir	IIIF1	766	Poten
Tablets	IIIF1	766.5	Poten
Potassium Guaiacolsulfonate	IIIF1	766.5	Poten
Potassium Hydroxide	IIIB1	279	Phth, MeO
Potassium Iodide Oral Solution	IA1b		Poten
Tablets	IB1a		Poten
Potassium Metaphosphate	IB1a		Poten
Potassium Permanganate	IB1a		Phth
Tablets for Topical Solution	IA2a		
Monobasic Potassium Phosphate	IA2b		
Dibasic Potassium Phosphate	IC2e		
Potassium Phosphates Injection	IC2e		
Potassium Sodium Tartrate	IA1a		MeB
Potassium Sorbate	IA1a, b	279	CrV
Povidone	IA2aii		
Povidone-Iodine	IA1bii		
Ointment	None		
Topical Aerosol Solution	IC1I		
Topical Cleansing Solution	IC1I		
Topical Solution	IC1I		
Pralidoxime Chloride	IC1I	336	
Sterile	IC1I	336	
Tablets	IC1I	336	
Pramoxine Hydrochloride Cream	IIIB1		
Jelly	IIIB1		
Prazepam Capsules	IA1biii		
Tablets	IIIB1		
Prazosin Hydrochloride Capsules	VB1b	286	CrV
Prednisolone Cream	VB1b	UV-254	CrV
Tablets	IA1biii	UV-254	CrV
Prednisolone Acetate Sterile Suspension	IIIB1	UV-254	Poten
Prednisolone Hemisuccinate	IIIB1	410	Poten
Prednisolone Sodium Phosphate	VB1b	UV-254	Poten
	VB1b	525	Poten
	IIIA4	525	
	IIIA1	243	betamethasone
	IIIA1	241	betamethasone

Name	Code	No.	Ref.
Pilocarpine Nitrate			
Injection	IA1bii		
Ophthalmic Solution	VB1a	UV-220	Poten
Pine Needle Oil	IA2b		Phth
Pine Tar	None		
Sterile Piperacillin Sodium	VB1b	UV-254	CrV
Piperacetazine			
Tablets	IA1bii		
Piperazine	IIIB1	283	
Tablets	IA1bii		
Piperazine Citrate			
Syrup	IA1bii		Poten
Tablets	IIB		CrV
Piperazine Phosphate			
Tablets	IIB		
Piperidolate Hydrochloride			
Tablets	IA1bii		
Pipobroman			
Tablets	IA1bii		
Posterior Pituitary Injection	IA1bii		
Plague Vaccine	IB1a		
Plantago Seed	None		
Plasma Protein Fraction	None		
Platelet Concentrate	None		
Plicamycin	None		
Plicamycin for Injection	None		
Podophyllum	IB1a		
Podophyllum Resin	VB1b	UV-278	
Podophyllum Resin Topical Solution	VB1b	UV-278	
Polacrilin Potassium	VIG	UV-278	
Poldine Methylsulfate	VIG		
Tablets	IIID	766	
Poliovirus Vaccine Inactivated	IA2b		
Poliovirus Vaccine Inactivated Live Oral	IIIB2	257	CR
Poloxalkol / Poloxamer	None		
Polycarbophil	None		
Polyethylene Glycol	None		
Ointment	None		
Polymixin B Sulfate	VIN1		
Sterile	VIN1		
Polymixin B Sulfate and Hydrocortisone Otic Solution	VIN1, VB1b	UV-254	
Sterile Otic Solution	VIN1		
Polyoxyl 10 Oleyl Ether	None		
Polyoxyl 20 Cetostearyl Ether	None		
Polyoxyl 35 Castor Oil	None		
Polyoxyl 40 Hydrogenated Castor Oil	None		
Polyoxyl 40 Stearate	None		
Polypropylene Glycol	None		
Polysorbate 20	None		
Polysorbate 40	None		
Polysorbate 60	None		
Polysorbate 80	None		
Polythiazide	IIIB1	268	
Tablets	IIIB1	268	
Polyvinyl Alcohol	IIB		
Sulfurated Potash	None		
Potassium Acetate			
Injection	IA1bii	766.5	CrV
Potassium Bicarbonate Effervescent Tablets for Oral Solution	IIF1	766.5	MeO
	IA1b		
	IIIF1		

Name	Code	No.	Ref.
Injection	IIIB1	241	
Ophthalmic Solution	IIIB1	241	
Prednisolone Sodium Succinate for Injection	IIIA1	525	
Prednisolone Tebutate Sterile Suspension	VB1a	254	procaine hydrochloride
Prednisone Tablets	IIIB1	UV-254	procaine hydrochloride
Prednisone Oral Suspension	VB1a	UV-254	procaine hydrochloride
Prednisone Tablets	VB1a	UV-254	procaine hydrochloride
Primaquine Phosphate Tablets	IA1bii	244, 350	acetanilide
Prilocaine Hydrochloride Injection	VB1b	UV-254	acetanilide
Primidone	IC1j		CrV
Oral Suspension	IC1j	257	Phth
Tablets	IIIB1	257	androsterone
Probenecid Tablets	VA1	257	Poten
Probenecid and Colchicine Tablets	IIIB1	FID-I	Poten
Procainamide Hydrochloride	IIIB1	257	
Capsules	VB1b	UV-254	Poten
Procaine Hydrochloride			
Injection	VB1b	UV-254	Poten
Procaine Hydrochloride Injection	IC1j	530	SPI
Procaine and Epinephrine Injection	IC1j	280	Poten
Procaine and Phenylephrine Hydrochloride Injection	IC1j	272, 500	procaine hydrochloride
Tetracaine Hydrochloride and Levonordefrin Injection	IC1j, IIIA4	280	procaine hydrochloride
Procarbazine Hydrochloride Capsules	IIIB1, IIIA4	UV-254	procaine hydrochloride
Prochlorperazine	IA1a		Poten
Suppositories	IA1bii	254, 278	
Prochlorperazine Edisylate Injection	IA1a	254, 278	CrV
Oral Solution	VB1b	254, 278	CrV
Syrup	IIIB1	254, 278	
Prochlorperazine Maleate Tablets	IIIB1	254, 278	Poten
Procyclidine Hydrochloride Tablets	IIIB1	405	
Progesterone Injection	IA1bii	241	Poten
Progesterone Intrauterine Contraceptive System	IA1bii	UV-254	
Progesterone Injection	IIA2	241	
Proline	IA1bii	UV-254	methyltestosterone
Promazine Hydrochloride Injection	IIIB1	254, 278	
Oral Solution	IIIB1	254, 278	methyltestosterone
Syrup	IIIB1	301	
Tablets	VB1b	301	UV-254
Promethazine Hydrochloride Injection	IA1bii	301	
Syrup	IIIB1	301	
Tablets	IVA1	405	
Propane	IA1a	254, 278	CrV
Propantheline Bromide	IIIB1	298	
	IIIB1	298	
	IIIB1	304	
	VA1	TC-I	Poten
	IA1biii		

Table VI—continued

Drug	Assay category	Analytical wavelength and/or detector	Indicator or internal standard
Propantheline Bromide	IA1biii		
Sterile	IA1biii		Poten
Tablets	IA1biii		Poten
Proparacaine Hydrochloride			
Ophthalmic Solution	IIB1		CrV
Propiomazine Hydrochloride	IA1bii	310	
Injection	IIIA4	465	
Propionic Acid	IIIA4	465	
Propoxycaine Hydrochloride	IA1a		
Propoxyphene Hydrochloride	IC1j		SPI
Injection	IIIB1, IIIA4	272, 296, 530	Phth
Procaine Hydrochloride and Levonordefrin Injection	IIIB1, IIIA4	272, 296, 530	
Procaine Hydrochloride and Norepinephrine Bitartrate Injection	IA1bii		CrV
Propoxyphene Hydrochloride Capsules	IIIB1, VA1	FID-I	n-tricosane
and Acetaminophen Tablets	IIIA4, VA1	249, FID-I	n-tricosane
Aspirin and Caffeine Capsules	IIIA4, VA1	530, FID-I	n-tricosane
and APC Capsules	IA1bii	530, FID-I	n-tricosane
Propoxyphene Napsylate	IIIA4, VA1	FID-I	CrV
Oral Suspension	VA1	FID-I	n-tricosane
Tablets	VA1	FID-I	n-tricosane
and Acetaminophen Tablets	VA1, 2	FID-I	n-tricosane
Propranolol Hydrochloride and Aspirin Tablets	VA1, IIIA4	FID-I, 530	n-tricosane, n-tetradecane
Propranolol Hydrochloride	IA1biii		
Injection	IIIB1	FID-I	n-tricosane
Tablets	IIIB1		Poten
Propyl Gallate	IIIB1	293	Phth
Propylene Carbonate	IA1b	293	
Propylene Glycol	VA1	273	
Diacetate	IA1b	TC-P	Phth
Monostearate	None		
Propylhexedrine	IA1b		MeR
Inhalant	IA2a		MeR
Propyliodone	IC1l		ST
Sterile Oil Suspension	IC1l		
Propylparaben	IA2b	274	
Propylthiouracil	IA1ai		
Tablets	IIIB1		
Protamine Sulfate	VIH		
Injection	VIH		
for Injection	None		
Protein Hydrolysate Injection	VIH		
Protriptyline Hydrochloride	IIIB1	292	CrV
Tablets	IA1biii		
Pseudoephedrine Hydrochloride	IA1biii	UV-254	
Syrup	IA1biii	UV-254	
Tablets	VB1b		
Psyllium Husk	VB1b		
Pumice	None		
Pyrantel Pamoate	None		
Oral Suspension	IIIB1	311	
Pyrazinamide	IIIB1	311	
Tablets	IA1c	268	MeR
	IIIB1		

Drug	Assay category	Analytical wavelength and/or detector	Indicator or internal standard
Rocky Mountain Spotted Fever Vaccine	None		
Rolitetracycline, Sterile for Injection	VIN1		
Ritodrine Hydrochloride	VIN1		
Injection	VB1b	UV-254	Phth
Tablets	VB1b	UV-254	Phth
Rose Oil	VB1b	UV-254	Phth
Rose Water Ointment	None		
Stronger	None		
Rosin	None		
Rubella Virus Vaccine Live	None		
and Mumps	None		
Saccharin	None		Phth
Saccharin Calcium	IA1a		Phth
Saccharin Sodium	IA1ai		Phth
Salicylic Acid	IA1ai		
Tablets	IA1a	UV-257	
Oral Solution	IA1a	269	
Collodion	IIIB1		
Gel	IA1a		BtB
Plaster	IA1a		Phth
Topical Foam	IC2c		ST
Schick Test Control	VB1b		
Scopolamine Hydrobromide	None	UV-280	benzoic acid
Injection	IA1biii		CrV
Ophthalmic Ointment	VA1	TC-I	homatropine
Ophthalmic Solution	VA1	TC-I	homatropine hydrobromide
Tablets	VA1	TC-I	homatropine hydrobromide
Secobarbital	VA1	TC-I	homatropine hydrobromide
Elixir	IA1aii		homatropine hydrobromide
Secobarbital Sodium	VA1	TC-I	homatropine hydrobromide
Capsules	IIB	FID-I	TB
Injection	VA1	FID-I	butabarbital
Sterile	IIIB1	FID-I	butabarbital
and Amobarbital Sodium	IIB		
Capsules	VA1	TC-I	aprobarbital
Selenomethionine Se 75 Injection	VIE		
Selenium Sulfide	IC1lii	505	
Lotion	IC1lii	505	
Senna	None		
Fluidextract	None		
Syrup	None		
Sennosides A and B	IIIE2	260	
Tablets	IA1bii		
Serine	IIIE2		
Sesame Oil	None		
Shellac	None		
Silica Gel	IIC		ST
Purified Siliceous Earth	None		ST
Colloidal Silicon Dioxide	IIC		Poten

Name	Category	λ (nm) / value	Method
Pyridostigmine Bromide Injection	IA1bii	269	QR
Syrup	IIB1	415	
Tablets	IIIA2	269	
Pyridoxine Hydrochloride Injection	IIIB1	269	
Injection	IA1biii		
Tablets	VIL		
Pyrilamine Maleate Injection	VIL		
Tablets	IA1bii	312	CrV
Pyrimethamine Tablets	IIB1	273	QR
Pyroxylin	IIIB1		
Pyrobutamine Phosphate	None		
Oral Suspension	IA1bii	505	CrV
Tablets	IIIA3	505	
Pyrvinium Pamoate Oral Suspension	IIIA3	505	
Tablets	IIIA3	505	
Quinacrine Hydrochloride Tablets	IIIA3	425	Poten
Injection	IA1bii	538	
Quinestrol Tablets	IIIA3		
Capsules	IA1bii		
Oral Suspension	IIIA4		
Tablets	VB1b	UV-281	
Quinethazone Tablets	IA1aii	UV-281	Poten
Quinidine Gluconate Injection	IIIC1	7.45	Nb
Tablets	IIIC1	UV-235	
Quinidine Sulfate Injection	VB2b	UV-235	Nb
Capsules	VB2b		
Tablets	IA1bii		
Quinine Sulfate Capsules	VB2b	UV-235	
Oral Suspension	VB2b	UV-235	
Tablets	IA1bii	249	
Rabies Immune Globulin	VB2b	UV-235	
Vaccine	IIB1		
Racemethionine	VB2b		
Capsules	None		
Tablets	IC2f	390	ST
Rauwolfia Serpentia	IC2f	390	ST
Powdered	IC2f	390	ST
Tablets	IIIA4	390	
Purified Rayon	IIIA4	390	
Reserpine	IIIA4	390	
Elixir	None	390	
Injection	IIIA4	390	
Tablets	IIIA4		
Hydralazine Hydrochloride and Hydrochlorothiazide Tablets	IIIA4	271, 390	
	IIIA4	390, 271, 510	ST
Resorcinol	IIIA4, IIIB1		
Compound Ointment and Sulfur Lotion	IC2c		
Resorcinol	None		
Riboflavin	IC1k, VB1b	UV-280	ST, caffeine
Monoacetate	None		
Injection	IIIE1	530	
Tablets	IIIE1	530	
5'-Phosphate Sodium	IIIE1	530	
Rifampin	IIIE1	530	
Capsules	IIIE1	530	
Ringer's Injection	VIN1		
and Isoniazid Capsules	VIN1		
Lactated, Injection	VIN1, IC1h	766	Poten
Irrigation	IC1a, IIID, IB1a	766	HNB, DCF
	IC1a, IIID, IB1a, IA2a	766	HNB, DCF, MeR
	IC1a, IIID, IB1a	766	HNB, DCF

Name	Category	λ (nm) / value	Method
Silver Nitrate Ophthalmic Solution	IB1b	7.9	FAS
Toughened	IB1b	7.9	FAS
	IB1b	7.9	FAS
Simethicone Emulsion	IIIC1		Nb
Oral Suspension	IIIC1		Phth
Tablets	IIIC1		ST
Sisomicin Sulfate Injection	IIIC1		CrV
Smallpox Vaccine	VIN1		CrV
Soda Lime	VIN1		
Sodium Acetate Injection	None		
Solution	None		
Sodium Alginate	IA1bii		MeO
Sodium Ascorbate	IA1bii		MeO
Sodium Benzoate	IIID		MeO
Sodium Bicarbonate Injection	IIID		MeO
Oral Powder	IA2b		MeO
Tablets	IC1k		MeR
Sodium Borate	IA1bii		MeR
Sodium Carbonate	IC1n		
Sodium Chloride Inhalation	IA1b		DCF
Injection	IA1b		DCF
Bacteriostatic Injection	IA1b		DCF
Irrigation	IA1b		DCF
Ophthalmic Solution	IA1b		DCF
Tablets	IA1b		FAS
Tablets for Solution and Dextrose Tablets	IB1a		FAS
Sodium Citrate and Citric Acid Oral Solution	IB1a		FAS
Sodium Dehydroacetate	IB1a		FAS
Sodium Fluoride Oral Solution	IB1a		Poten
Tablets	IB1a		Nb
and Phosphoric Acid Gel and Phosphoric Acid Topical Solution	IB2aii		
Sodium Formaldehyde Sulfoxylate	IB2aii		ST
Sodium Hydroxide	IB2aii		Phth
Sodium Hypochlorite Solution	IB2aii, VIC1		ST
Sodium Iodide Solution	IIID, IA1a		
Sodium Lactate Injection	IA1bii		ST
Solution	IA1bii		SAS
Sodium Lauryl Sulfate	ID1b		
Sodium Metabisulfite	IVB1		CrV
Sodium Monofluorophosphate	IVB1		Poten
Sodium Nitrite	IVB1		
Injection	IC1k	589	Poten
Sodium Nitroprusside Sterile	IA1b		
Monobasic Sodium Phosphate	IC1lii		Phth
Dibasic Sodium Phosphate	IC1n		Poten
Effervescent	IC1n		Poten
Sodium Phosphates Enema Injection	IA1bii		None
Oral Solution	IA1bii		Poten
	None		Poten
	IC2a		
	ID1b		
	IC2e		
	IC2e		
	IB1a		
	IVA1		
	IVA1		
	IB1a		
	IA1b		
	IA2a		
	IA1b		
	IA2b		
	IA1a, b		
	IA2b		

Table VI—continued

Drug	Assay category	Analytical wavelength and/or detector	Indicator or internal standard
Sodium Polystyrene Sulfonate	None		
Sodium Propionate	IA1bii		
Sodium Salicylate	IA1b		
Tablets	IA1b		
Sodium Starch Glycolate	IA1bii	FID-I	
Sodium Stearate	VA2		
Sodium Sulfate	IIB		CrV
Injection	IIB		CrV
Sodium Thiosulfate	IC1k		BpB
Injection	IC1k		Poten
Sorbic Acid	IA1a		ST
Tablets	IA1a		ST
Sorbitan Monolaurate	IIA, IIA		
Monooleate	IIA, IIA		
Monopalmitate	IIA, IIA		
Monostearate	IIA, IIA		
Sorbitol	VA2		Phth
Solution	VA2		
Soybean Oil	None		
Spearmint	VIB		
Oil	VA2	FID-I	
Sterile Spectinomycin	VA2	FID-I	
Hydrochloride	VB1b	FID-I	triphenylantimony
Spironolactone	VB1b	UV-254	
Tablets	VB1b	UV-254	
Squalene	None	590	
Stannous Fluoride	IC1n, IIIA4		ST
Stanzolol	IA1bii		CrV
Tablets	IIIB1	235	
Starch	None		
Pregelatinized	None		
Glycerite	None		
Topical	None		
Glycerite	None		
Stearic Acid	VA2		
Purified	VA2	FID-I	methyl nonadecanoate
Stearyl Alcohol	VA1	FID-I	methyl nonadecanoate
Storax	None	FID-I	
Streptomycin Sulfate Injection	VIN1		
Sterile	VIN1		
Succinylcholine Chloride	VIN1	UV-214	
Injection	VB1b	UV-214	
Sterile	VB1b	UV-214	
Sucrose	None		
Octaacetate	IA2b		Phth
Compressible Sugar	VIC1		
Confectioner's Sugar	None		
Sulfabenzamide	IA1aiii		TB
Sulfacetamide	IC1j		Poten
Sulfacetamide Sodium	IC1j		Poten
Ophthalmic Ointment	IC1j		Poten
Ophthalmic Solution	IIIA4		
Sulfadiazine	VB1b	545	
Tablets	IC1j	UV-254	
Sulfadiazine Sodium	VB1b	UV-254	
Injection	IC1j		Poten
Sulfadoxine	IC1j		Poten
Gluceptate Injection	VIF	550	Poten
Medronate Injection	VIF	550	
Oxidronate Injection	VIF		
Pentetate Injection	VIF		
Pyrophosphate Injection	VIF		
(Pyro- and trimeta-) Phosphates Injection	VIF		
Sulfur Colloid Injection	VIF		
Terbutaline Sulfate	IA1bii		
Injection	IA1bii		
Tablets	IIIA4		
Terpin Hydrate	VA1	FID-I	
Elixir	VA1	FID-I	biphenyl
and Codeine Elixir	VA1	FID-I	biphenyl
and Dextromethorphan Hydrobromide Elixir	VA1, IIIA2	FID-I, 420	biphenyl, N-phenylcarbazole dodecyl alcohol
Testolactone	IIIA4	415	
Sterile Suspension	IIIA4	415	
Tablets	IIIA4	415	
Testosterone	IIIA4	415	
Pellets	IIIB1	241	
Sterile Suspension	IIIB1	241	
Testosterone Cypionate	IIIA4	241	
Injection	IIIA4	380	cholesteryl caprylate
Testosterone Enanthate	IIIA4	380	cholesteryl caprylate
Injection	IIIA4	380	
Testosterone Propionate	IIIA4	380	
Injection	IIIA4	380	
Tablet	VB1b	UV-254	propylparaben
Tetanus Antitoxin	None		
Immune Globulin	None		
Toxoid	None		
Toxoid Adsorbed	None		
Toxoid Adsorbed and Diphtheria Toxoids Adsorbed for Adult Use	None		
Tetracaine	IC1j		
Ointment	IIIB1		
Ophthalmic Ointment	IIIB1		
and Menthol Ointment	VA1, IIIB1		
Tetracaine Hydrochloride	IIIB1	241	
Cream	IC1j	241	
Injection	IIIB1	380	
Ophthalmic Solution	IIIB1	380	
Topical Solution	VIB		
Sterile	None		
Tetrachloroethylene	IIIB1	310	SPI
Capsules	IIIB1	310	1-decanol
Tetracycline	VIN1	FID-I, 310	Poten
Oral Suspension	VIN1	310	
for Oral Suspension	VIN1	310	
and Amphotericin B Capsules	VIN1	310	
and Amphotericin B Oral Suspension	VIN1	310	
Tetracycline Hydrochloride	VIN1		

and Pyrimethamine Tablets	VB1b	UV-254	phenacetin
Sulfamerazine Tablets	IC1j		SPI
Sulfamethazine Tablets	IC1j		phenacetin
Sulfamethizole Tablets	IC1j		Poten
Sulfamethizole Oral Suspension	IC1j		Poten
Sulfamethoxazole Tablets	IC1j		Poten
Sulfamethoxazole Oral Suspension	IC1j		Poten
Sulfamethoxazole and Trimethoprim Oral Suspension	IC1j		Poten
Sulfamethoxazole and Trimethoprim Tablets	IC1j		Poten
Sulfapyridine Tablets	VB1b	UV-254	phenacetin
Sulfasalazine Tablets	IC1j	359	Poten
Sulfathiazole Tablets	IC1j	359	Poten
Sulfacetamide and Sulfabenzamide Vaginal Cream	IIIB1		sulfapyridine
Sulfabenzamide and Sulfacetamide and Sulfabenzamide Vaginal Tablets	IIIB1	UV-280	sulfapyridine
Sulfabenzamide Vaginal	VB1b		phenacetin
Sulfinpyrazone Capsules	IA1a	UV-254	Phth
Sulfinpyrazone Tablets	IA1a		Phth
Sulfisoxazole Tablets	IIIB1	260	TB
Sulfisoxazole Acetyl Oral Suspension	IA1aiii		TB
Sulfisoxazole Diolamine Injection	IA1aiii		Poten
Sulfisoxazole Ophthalmic Ointment	IC1j		TB
Ophthalmic Solution	IC1j		TB
Sulfobromophthalein Sodium Injection	IA1aiii	540	TB
Sulfoxone Sodium Tablets	IA1aii	580	
Injection	IA4	580	
Sulfur, Precipitated Ointment	IIA4	535	
Sublimed	IIB	535	
Sulfur Dioxide	IA1a	535	
Sulfuric Acid	IIIA4		
Sulindac Tablets	IIIA3	UV-332	Phth
Sutilains Ointment	IIIA4		ST
Absorbable Surgical Suture	IA1aii		MeO
Nonabsorbable	IA1a		Poten
Syrup	IA1a		AV
Talbutal Tablets	IIIB1	241	
Talc	IC1k		
Tamoxifen Citrate Tablets	IA1a	UV-254	Poten
Tannic Acid	IA1a		Phth
Adhesive Tape	VB1a		
Technetium Tc 99m Albumin Aggregated Injection	VIF		
Etidronate Injection	VIF		
Ferpentetate Injection	VIF		

Capsules for Injection	VIN1		QR
Ophthalmic Ointment	VIN1		
Ophthalmic Solution	VIN1		
Sterile	VIN1		
for Topical Solution	VIN1		
Ophthalmic Suspension	VIN1		
Tablets	VIN1		
and Nystatin Capsules	VIN1		
Tetracycline Phosphate Complex Capsules	VIN1		
for Injection	VIN1		
Sterile	VIN1		
Tetrahydrozoline Hydrochloride Nasal Solution	IA1bii	570	BtB
Ophthalmic Solution	IIIA4	415	
Thallous Chloride Tl 201 Injection	IIIA2		
Theophylline Capsules	VIE	UV-254	FAS
Tablets	IA1ai		FAS
Oral Suspension	VB1b	UV-241	FAS
Elixir	IB2ai		FAS
Theophylline and Guaifenesin Capsules	VB1b		CrV
Theophylline Sodium Glycinate Elixir	IB2ai	302	
Tablets	IB2ai	365	
Theophylline Olamine	IB2ai	365	
Enema	IB2ai	365	
Theophylline, Ephedrine Hydrochloride and Phenobarbital Tablets	VB1b	365	caffeine
Thiabendazole Tablets	IA1bii		
Oral Suspension	IB2ai		
Thiamine Hydrochloride Elixir	IIIE2	365	
Injection	IIIE2	365	
Tablets	IIIE2	365	
Thiamine Mononitrate	IIE2	365	
Thiamylal Sodium for Injection	IA	263	Poten
Thiethylperazine Malate Injection	IA1bii	263	CrV
Thiethylperazine Maleate Suppositories	IA1bii	263	
Tablets	IA1bii	263	
Thimerosal	IIE2		
Topical Aerosol	IIF1	254	
Topical Solution	IIF1	254	
Tincture	IIF1	254	
Thioguanine Tablets	IIB1	254	
Thiopental Sodium for Injection	IIB1	254	
Thioridazine Oral Suspension	IIB1	263	
Thioridazine Tablets	IIB1	263	
Thioridazine Hydrochloride Oral Solution	IA1bii	304	Poten
Thiotepa for Injection	IA1bii	348	Phth
Thiothixene Capsules	IIB1	348	Poten
Thiothixene Hydrochloride Injection	IIC1	10,75	
for Injection	IIB1	265	
Oral Solution	IIB1	265	

Table VI—continued

Drug	Assay category	Analytical wavelength and/or detector	Indicator or internal standard	Drug	Assay category	Analytical wavelength and/or detector	Indicator or internal standard
Thonzonium Bromide	IA1biii		CrV	and Pseudoephedrine Hydrochloride Tablets	VB1b	UV-254	
Threonine	IA1bii		Poten	Trisulfapyrimidines Oral Suspension	VB1b	UV-254	BcP
Thrombin	None			Tablets	VB1b		BcP
Thymol	IC1h		MeO	Suspension			CrV
Thyroglobulin	IC1lii		ST	Trolamine	IA1bii		MeR
Tablets	IC1lii		ST	Troleandomycin	VIN1		MeR
Thyroid	IC1lii		ST	Capsules	VIN1		MeR
Tablets	IC1lii		ST	Oral Suspension	VIN1		MeR
Sterile Ticarcillin Disodium	VIN1			Tromethamine	IA1b		
Timolol Maleate	IA1bii			for Injection	IA1b		
Ophthalmic Solution	IIIB1			Tropicamide	IA1bii		
Tablets	VB1b	294	Poten	Ophthalmic Solution	IIIB1	253	
and Hydrochlorothiazide Tablets	VB1b	UV-295	Poten	Crystallized Trypsin for Inhalation Aerosol	VIF		
Titanium Dioxide	IC1bi			Tryptophan	VIF		
Tobramycin	VIN1			Tuaminoheptane	IA1bii		
Ophthalmic Ointment	VIN1			Inhalant	IA1a		
Ophthalmic Solution	VIN1			Tuaminoheptane Sulfate	IA1a		
Tobramycin Sulfate Injection	VIN1			Nasal Solution	IA1bii		
Tolazamide	VB1a	UV-254	tolbutamide	Tuberculin	IA2ai		
Tablets	VB1a	UV-254	tolbutamide	Tubocurarine Chloride	IA2ai		
Tolazoline Hydrochloride	IA1bii		Poten	Injection	None		
Injection	IIIA4	565		Tyloxapol	VIH		
Tablets	VB1a	565		Typhoid Vaccine	VIH		
Tolbutamide	VB1a	UV-254	tolazamide	Typhus Vaccine	None		
Tablets	VB1a	UV-254	tolazamide	Tyropanoate Sodium	None		
Tolbutamide Sodium	IIIB1	263		Capsules	IB1a	237	TBPE
Sterile	VB1a		Poten	Tyrosine	IB1a		
Tolmetin Sodium	IA1bii	322	Poten	Tyrothricin	IA1bii		
Capsules	IIIB1	322		Undecylenic Acid	VIN1		Poten
Tablets	IIIB1			Compound Ointment	VIN1		
Tolnaftate	IIIB1	258	progesterone	Uracil Mustard	IIIB1		
Topical Aerosol Powder	IIIB1	258	progesterone	Capsules	IA1a		Poten
Cream	IIIB1	258	progesterone	Urea	IIIF1, VA2	214, FID-1	Phth tridecanoic acid
Gel	IIIB1	258		Sterile	IIIA4	466	
Powder	IIIB1			Vaccinia Immune Globulin	IIIB1	256	MRB
Topical Solution	VB1b	UV-254		Valine	IA1c		
Tolu Balsam	IIIB1			Vancomycin Hydrochloride	IA1a		
Tincture	None			for Oral Solution	None		
Tragacanth	None			Sterile	None		Poten
Tranylcypromine Sulfate	IA1bii			Vanilla	IA1bii		
Tablets	IIIB1.	271	TB	Tincture	VIN1		
Tretinoin	IA1aiii			Vanillin	VIN1	308	
Cream	IIIB1	358		Varicella-Zoster Immune Globulin	VIG		
Gel	IIIB1	365		Vasopressin Injection	None		
Topical Solution	IIIB1	352		Hydrogenated Vegetable Oil	IIIB1		
Triacetin	IA2bi		Phth	Vidarabine Concentrate for Injection	None		
Triamcinolone	IIIB1			Ophthalmic Ointment	None		
Tablets	VB1b	UV-254	hydrocortisone methylparaben	Sterile	VIH		
Triamcinolone Acetonide	VB1b	UV-254	fluoxymesterone	Vinblastine Sulfate	None		
Topical Aerosol	VB1b	UV-254	fluoxymesterone	Sterile	IIIB1	267	
Cream	VB1b	UV-254	fluoxymesterone	Vincristine Sulfate	IIIB1	UV-254	
Lotion	VB1b	UV-254	fluoxymesterone	Sterile	VB1b	UV-297	
Ointment	VB1b	UV-254	fluoxymesterone				
Dental Paste	VB1b	UV-254	fluoxymesterone				

Name	Category	Ref.	Method
Sterile Suspension	IIB1	238	UV-254
Triamcinolone Diacetate	IIIB1	525	
Sterile Suspension	IIIA1	525	
Syrup	IIIA1	525	UV-254
Triamcinolone Hexacetonide	VB1b	525	UV-254
Sterile Suspension	VB1b		UV-254
Triamterene	IA1bii	357.5	Poten
Capsules	IIB1	357.5	
Trichlormethiazide	IA1aiii		PR
Tablets	IIB1	267	Phth
Trichloroacetic Acid	IIB1		Phth
Trichloromonofluoromethane	IA1a		PR
Trichlorates Oral Solution	None		
Tridihexethyl Chloride	IIB1	766	
Tablets	IIA2	408	TB
Injection	IIB1	408	Phth
Trifluoperazine Hydrochloride	IA1biii		
Injection	IA1bii	255	CrV
Syrup	IIB1	255	
Tablets	IIB1	255	
Trifluopromazine	IIB1	255	
Oral Suspension	IA1bii	255	CrV
Trifluopromazine Hydrochloride	IA1biii	255	
Injection	IIB1	255	CrV
Tablets	IIB1	255	
Trihexyphenidyl Hydrochloride	IIB1	766	n-tricosane
Elixir	VA1	766.5	n-tricosane
Tablets	VA1	766.5	n-tricosane
Trikates Oral Solution	IIF1		CrV
Trimeprazine Tartrate	IA1bii	251	
Syrup	IIB1	251	CrV
Tablets	IIB1	251	
Trimethadione	IIB1	255	CrV
Capsules	VA1	255	1-decanol cyclohexanol
Oral Solution	VA1	255	cyclohexanol
Tablets	IIB1	258	cyclohexanol
Trimethaphan Camsylate	IIA2	420	Poten
Injection	IA1bii		
Trimethobenzamide Hydrochloride	IA1biii	258	Poten
Capsules	VA1	258	
Injection	VA1		
Trimethoprim	IIB1	258	Poten
Tablets	IIB1	252	
Trioxsalen	IIB1	252	
Tablets	IIB1	252	
Tripelennamine Citrate	IIB1		CrV
Elixir	IA1bii	313	
Tripelennamine Hydrochloride	IIB1	313	CrV
Tablets	IA1biii	313	
Triprolidine Hydrochloride	IIB1		Poten
Syrup	IA1bii		
Tablets	VB1b		
and Pseudoephedrine Hydrochloride Syrup	VB1b		

Name	Category	Ref.	Method
fluoxymesterone for Injection	VB1b	UV-297	hexadecyl hexadecanoate
Vinyl Ether	None		hexadecyl hexadecanoate
Sterile Viomycin Sulfate	VIN1		hexadecyl hexadecanoate
Vitamin A	VIL		
Capsules	VIL		
Vitamin E	VA1	FID-I	
Preparation	VA1	FID-I	
Capsules	VA1	FID-I	
Warfarin Potassium	IIIB1	308	TB
Tablets	IIIB1	307	MeO
Warfarin Sodium	IIIB1	308	EBT
for Injection	IIIB1	307	EBT
Tablets	IIIB1		EBT
Water for Injection	None		
Bacteriostatic for Injection	None		
Sterile for Injection	None		
Sterile for Irrigation	None		
Purified	None		
Wax	None		
Carnauba	None		
Emulsifying	None		
Microcrystalline	None		
White	None		
Yellow	None		
White Lotion	None		
Xanthan Gum	None		
Xenon Xe 133	IA2b		Phth
Injection	VIE		
Xylometazoline Hydrochloride	VIE		
Nasal Solution	IA1bii	565	Nb
Xylose	IIIA4	565	
Yellow Fever Vaccine	None	520	
Ytterbium Yb 169 Pentetate	None		
Injection	VIE		
Zinc Acetate	VIE		
Zinc Chloride	ID1a		EBT
Injection	ID1a		EBT
Zinc-Eugenol Cement	ID1a		
Zinc Gelatin	IIA, C	213.8	
Impregnated Gauze	IIF1		
Zinc Oxide	None		
Paste	ID1a		
Ointment	IA1aiii, IIC		
and Salicylic Acid Paste	IIC		
Zinc Stearate	ID1a		TB
Zinc Sulfate	ID1a		MeO
Injection	ID1a		EBT
Ophthalmic Solution	IIF1	213.8	
Zinc Undecylenate	ID1a		PAN
Zonepirac Sodium	IA2a		MeO
Tablets	IA1bii	328	Poten
	IIIB1		

CHAPTER 31

Biological Testing

G Victor Rossi, PhD
Professor of Pharmacology
Philadelphia College of Pharmacy and Science
Philadelphia, PA 19104

Biological testing includes the quantitative assay of drugs by biological methods as well as the application of qualitative biological tests. Such testing utilizes intact animals, animal preparations, isolated living tissues, or microorganisms.

The majority of currently available therapeutic agents are assayed by quantitative chemical or physical analyses. There remains, however, a limited number of useful drugs which cannot be assayed satisfactorily by chemical or physical means. Such drugs, which are primarily of natural origin, are assayed by biological methods. Biological standardization procedures are generally less precise, more time-consuming, and more expensive to conduct than chemical assays; therefore, they are generally reserved for use mainly:

1. If the chemical identity of the active principle has not been fully elucidated.
2. If no adequate chemical assay has been devised for the active principle, although its chemical structure has been established, e.g., insulin.
3. If the drug is composed of a complex mixture of substances of varying structure and activity, eg, digitalis, posterior pituitary.
4. If purification of the crude drug, sufficient for the performance of a chemical assay, is not possible or practical, eg, the separation of vitamin D from certain irradiated oils.
5. If the chemical assay is not a valid indication of biological activity, due, for example, to lack of differentiation between active and inactive isomers.

There are several situations in which factors such as specificity, sensitivity, or practicality dictate the use of a biological rather than a chemical assay procedure.

A chemical assay quantitatively determines the amount of a specific compound or structural moiety present in a given sample. On the basis of the established concentration, an assumption is made relative to the biological activity of the sample. In contrast, a biological assay measures the actual biological activity of a given sample, which may represent the algebraic sum of the interaction of numerous chemical and physical-chemical factors. For example, the data obtained from a chemical assay may not provide information concerning the contribution to the net biological activity of trace amounts of substances which do not influence the chemical analysis. Such substances may produce qualitative variations in biological activity which may be responsible for unexpected side-effects or toxic reactions. Furthermore, the augmentatory or inhibitory influence of variations in the physical state of the active principle is not reflected in the results of a chemical assay. The safety, efficacy, and dependability of dosage of drugs are contingent upon standardization, and biological assays must be employed in some instances even though the chemical identities of the active principles in the preparation may be known.

Animals

As animals are an important "unknown" factor in most biological assays the need for their proper selection and adequate care thereafter is self-evident. Most laboratories seek a reliable source of animals which can supply their needs from colonies maintained for this purpose. In any one test it is desirable to use animals of only one strain. Actually bioassayists may adopt a specified strain for all work of a particular type. In this manner experience is gained as to the normal variation that is to be expected. For some assays a specific sex must be employed, eg, estrogenic tests; in other assays either sex may be used but the effect that sex may play in the response should not be overlooked. The male rat, for instance, has a faster growth rate than the female; therefore indiscriminate use of both males and females in a rat growth test should be avoided. Differences in the response of sexes may extend into other categories, eg, response toward toxic materials.

Bioassay Procedures

Bioassays are conducted by determining the amount of a preparation of unknown potency required to produce a definite effect on suitable test animals or organs under standard conditions.

Reference Standards—To minimize the source of error resulting from animal variation, standard reference preparations are used in certain bioassay procedures. The principle of the standard consists of testing successively the unknown and standard preparations on two groups of similar animals, or in some cases (eg, epinephrine, posterior pituitary) on the same animal or organ. The amount of the unknown preparation required to produce an effect equal to that produced by a certain amount of the standard will be inversely proportional to their relative potencies. The potency of the unknown can therefore be expressed as a percentage of that of the standard.

In some assays it is necessary to adopt precise methods of calculating potency based upon observations of relative but not necessarily equal effects. Likewise, methods of computation have been devised to determine the statistical reliability of the results. These procedures are discussed in Chapter 10. The section on General Tests in the USP also presents a detailed consideration of factors germane to the Design and Analysis of Biological Assays.

Reference standards, for use in assays in which they are required, are available as a service from USP-NF Reference Standards, 12601 Twinbrook Pkwy., Rockville, MD 20852. They are standardized in terms of such corresponding International Standards as may exist.

Disadvantages of Bioassays—Biological assays leave much to be desired in several respects. Although some are extremely sensitive in detecting small differences in concentration, their quantitative accuracy usually falls considerably below that obtainable with most chemical analyses. The techniques and interpretations involved can often vary with different operators in spite of the rigid requirements specified by the official publications, and hence there is a considerable subjective element present. Furthermore, the effect which the drug is measured in the test animals is often not that which the drug is intended to produce in treating patients. The importance of this discrepancy was formerly minimized, but recent studies have shown that when several active principles are present in a crude drug, those producing the maximal therapeutic effect are not necessarily the ones chiefly responsible for the action measured in the assay. As a result, samples found to be of equal strength by assay may show different potencies when employed clinically. An example of this situation is found in the discussion on digitalis.

Classification of Bioassay Procedures—Bioassays are classified in three groups according to whether the effect produced is all or none (as death), graded (as rise in blood pressure), or is characterized by developing in a measured period of time (as the curative response to thiamine). It should be noted that in all three types, with few exceptions, the calculations of potency are based on the sizes of doses necessary to produce approximately equal effects and not on the intensities of the responses. Furthermore, *the results derived from all are quantitative* in that the potency of the unknown is expressed in terms of the standard.

Animal Assays

In the following section biological assay procedures involving the use of intact animals, animal preparations, or isolated, surviving, animal tissues or organs are considered. The presentation is restricted largely to the general principles and basic experimental approaches involved in each of several representative types of biological assay methods. For complete details of the official procedures the reader is directed to the corresponding official compendium monographs.

Digitaloid Drugs

The digitaloid group of drugs includes Digitalis (the dried leaf of *Digitalis purpurea*), which is used medicinally as the powdered material in the form of capsules or tablets. These products of natural origin contain, in addition to the cardioactive glycosides *digitoxin* and *gitoxin*, a saponin-like glycoside, termed *digitonin*, largely devoid of the cardiac effects of Digitalis, and a complex mixture of constituents including digitoflavin, digitophyllin, lipids, carbohydrates, and other nonspecific plant components. Although the cardioactive glycosides are similar in chemical structure and pharmacodynamic activity, they differ markedly in milligram potency, efficiency of gastrointestinal absorption, speed of onset, and duration of action. Furthermore, there is considerable variation among different lots of crude drug in respect to the total active glycoside content and the relative concentration of each active principle.

It is apparent that *chemical* assay procedures, such as the determination of total glycosides or total aglycones, cannot adequately measure the pharmacodynamic activity of the crude drug or galenical preparation of Digitalis. Such drugs, composed of a complex mixture of substances of varying structure and activity, must be subjected to a *biological* assay.

The biological assay of Digitalis is based on determination of the amount of test material required to cause death due to cardiac arrest in the anesthetized pigeon, relative to the amount of a reference standard preparation required to produce the same effect.

As a rule, it is desirable that the parameters of a biological assay simulate, as closely as practicable, the conditions generally associated with clinical usage of the drug in question. In this respect the currently employed biological assay procedure for Digitalis has several disadvantages and limitations. For example, the preparation to be assayed is given by fractional, intermittent, intravenous injection, whereas in the treatment of patients with cardiac disorders digitaloid drugs are most often administered orally. The assay procedure does not, therefore, take into consideration variations in clinical effectiveness among different members of this medicinal group which may be attributable to differences in the rate and completeness of absorption from the gastrointestinal tract. Furthermore, the calculation of potency is based on the amount of drug required to produce death of the test animal due to cardiac arrest. Thus the end-point of the assay cor-

responds to a toxic rather than a therapeutically desirable event. However, it may be claimed that the toxic effects of Digitalis on the heart constitute extensions of the cardiodynamic changes which are beneficial in certain cardiac disorders. Because of the limitations of the pigeon method many attempts have been made to develop more satisfactory bioassay procedures. None of the alternatives devised to date has any impelling advantage over the current official method.

Separation and identification of the active principles of crude drugs having characteristic digitalis-like effects on the heart has resulted in the availability of a single relatively pure cardiotonic glycoside. These additional members of the digitaloid group of drugs include Acetyldigitoxin, Deslanoside, Digoxin, and Lanatoside C (all of which are derived from *Digitalis lanata*), Digitoxin (a glycosidal constituent of both *Digitalis lanata* and *Digitalis purpurea*), and Ouabain (a glycoside obtained from the seeds of *Strophanthus gratus*). Preparations containing these glycosides are assayed quantitatively by spectrometric methods described in Chapter 30. Chemical assay procedures enable precise determination of the amount of glycoside present in a particular dosage formulation. However, it must be emphasized that the response to digitaloid drugs varies considerably among cardiac patients. A "clinical assay" must, therefore, be performed with each patient regardless of whether the digitaloid preparation being used was standardized on the basis of a chemical or biological assay procedure.

Biological assay by the pigeon method is specified for the following official preparations: *Digitalis, Powdered Digitalis, Digitalis Capsules,* and *Digitalis Tablets.*

Insulin

Insulin is a hormone secreted by *beta* cells of the islet tissue of the pancreas. Structurally, insulin is composed of two polypeptide chains (A and B) having a total molecular weight of approximately 6000. The A chain, comprising 21 amino acids, is linked by two disulfide (—S—S—) bridges to the B chain, composed of 30 amino acids. Although there are some variations in the amino acid sequence and immunological specificity of insulins isolated from different animal species, they have fundamentally similar biological activities.

Since the isolation of insulin by Banting and Best in 1922, the hormone has constituted the keystone of the therapeutic control of diabetes mellitus. Most of the insulin used for medicinal purposes is prepared by extraction of the pancreas obtained from domestic animals. Biosynthetic human insulin (BHI) has recently been developed through recombinant DNA technology; it is probable that, in the near future, BHI will largely replace purified animal insulins.

Accurate standardization of insulin preparations is essential inasmuch as discrepancies in the order of 10% from the required dose may result in severe adverse reactions in the diabetic patient. Inadequate insulin replacement therapy may be associated with the appearance of any of the characteristic symptoms of diabetes mellitus including ketoacidosis and diabetic coma; overdosage may result in marked hypoglycemic reactions.

Insulin Zinc Suspension, Extended Insulin Zinc Suspension, and *Prompt Insulin Zinc Suspension* are not subject to biological assay, whereas *Insulin, Insulin Injection, Isophane Insulin Suspension, Protamine Zinc Insulin Suspension*, and *Globin Zinc Insulin Injection* are standardized on the basis of biological assay. Briefly the assay is based on a comparison between the potencies of the unknown and the standard preparation in lowering the blood sugar level of intact rabbits following subcutaneous injection.

In addition to the quantitative bioassay procedures a qualitative identification test, which also depends on hypoglycemic activity, is described for these preparations. The test is performed by demonstrating that the convulsions induced in rabbits by subcutaneous injection of high doses of the preparation are relieved by the intravenous injection of dextrose solution (refer to the section on *Identification Tests*, in the pertinent USP/NF monographs).

Insulin preparations are subject to the regulations of the Federal Food, Drug and Cosmetic Act, which requires certification by the Food and Drug Administration (FDA) of each lot marketed. Many of the tests and criteria employed by the FDA follow closely those specified by the official compendia. In addition to the biological assays, certain chemical and bacteriological tests must be performed to meet the requirements for certification by the FDA. The Act (particularly Section 506) and regulations thereunder should be consulted for specific details concerning the steps that must be followed in obtaining such certification.

Insulin Injection is available as solutions containing 40, 100, and 500 USP Insulin Units per mL. Globin Zinc Insulin Injection and Protamine and Protamine Zinc Insulin Suspensions provide either 40, or 100 units/mL. A variation of not more than 5% from the labeled potency is permitted.

Glucagon

Glucagon is a polypeptide hormone secreted by the *alpha* cells of the pancreatic islets of Langerhans. Glucagon stimulates the adenylate cyclase–cyclic AMP system in the liver, which leads to the activation of phosphorylase, the rate-limiting enzyme in the conversion of glycogen to glucose. This hormone is obtained commercially from the pancreas glands of domestic animals used for food by man. Glucagon for Injection USP is a mixture of the hydrochlorides of glucagon with one or more suitable dry diluents.

Parenteral administration of glucagon in persons with adequate hepatic glycogen stores elicits a prompt elevation of the blood-sugar level. This reaction constitutes the basis of the primary therapeutic indication (ie, termination of hypoglycemic coma) and biological assay of Glucagon for Injection.

The bioassay of Glucagon for Injection fundamentally involves comparison of the blood-sugar elevation induced in healthy, fasted, anesthetized cats by intravenous injection of alternating doses of suitable dilutions of the test sample and USP Glucagon Reference Standard. Specific procedures relating to preparation of assay dilutions of test sample and reference standard, sequence of injection and blood sampling, and calculation of potency are detailed in the USP.

Parathyroid

The parathyroid hormone plays an important physiological role in the regulation of calcium metabolism. The hormone consists of a linear peptide of 84 amino acids with no cross-linking. The renal and skeletal activity apparently resides in the 34 amino acids at the amino terminal end of the chain.

The only official parathyroid preparation, *Parathyroid Injection*, is prepared from an aqueous extract of the parathyroid glands of domestic animals. Biological assay of this material is based on its hypercalcemic activity. Parathyroid Injection possesses a potency of not less than 100 USP Parathyroid Units/mL. By definition, 100 units produces an average rise in the serum calcium of normal dogs of 1 mg/100 mL within 16 to 18 hours after subcutaneous administration.

Posterior Pituitary

Extracts of the posterior lobe of the neurohypophysis when injected into responsive animals may exert a variety of pharmacodynamic effects including a rise in blood pressure, contraction of uterine smooth muscle (oxytocic effect), an increased renal tubular reabsorption of water (antidiuresis), and milk-ejection (galactokinesis) in the lactating mammary gland. Although there is no conclusive agreement on the number of different hormones elaborated by the neurohypophysis, two distinct active principles have been separated from extracts of this structure. These are *oxytocin* which possesses primarily oxytocic and galactokinetic activities, and *vasopressin*, which exhibits predominantly pressor and antidiuretic activities. Both of these principles are octapeptides; the amino acid sequences of these fractions obtained from several animal species have been determined and corresponding octapeptide amides have been synthesized.

Posterior Pituitary (powder) and Posterior Pituitary Injection, which are prepared from the posterior lobe of the pituitary gland of domestic animals, contain oxytocic and vasopressor principles in varying amounts.

Each mg of Posterior Pituitary possesses an oxytocic activity equivalent to 1 USP Posterior Pituitary Unit,* the permissible lower limit of assayed potency being 0.85 Unit/mg.

Although the standardization of Posterior Pituitary is based on *oxytocin* content, the major therapeutic use of this preparation (i.e., control of diabetes insipidus) depends primarily on the *vasopressin* (antidiuretic hormone) content.

Each mL of Posterior Pituitary Injection possesses an oxytocic activity equivalent to 10 USP Posterior Pituitary Units (permissible range, 8.5 to 12 Units), and not less than 5 Units of vasopressin. Since the separate fractions (oxytocin and vasopressin) are available in purified form, Posterior Pituitary Injection, which represents a mixture of the active principles, is used relatively infrequently.

Oxytocin Injection possesses, in each mL, an oxytocic activity equivalent to 10 USP Posterior Pituitary Units (permissible range of assayed potency is 8.5 to 12 Units). Oxytocin Injection is subject to a maximum allowable limit of pressor activity, corresponding to not more than 0.01 USP Posterior Pituitary Unit for each USP Unit of oxytocic activity found in the assay.

Each mL of Vasopressin Injection possesses a pressor activity equivalent to 20 USP Posterior Pituitary Units, the permissible lower and upper limits being 17 and 24 Units, respectively. The oxytocic activity of Vasopressin Injection may not exceed that which corresponds to 1.2 USP Posterior Pituitary Units for each 20 USP Units of pressor activity found in the assay.

The oxytocic activity of Posterior Pituitary and Posterior Pituitary Injection was formerly assayed on the basis of contractions induced in the isolated guinea pig uterus. Although unrelated to the therapeutic objective of oxytocic agents, the transient decrease in blood pressure elicited in the anesthe-

---

* One USP Posterior Pituitary Unit represents the potency of 0.5 mg of USP Posterior Pituitary Reference Standard.

tized chicken by intravenous injection of posterior pituitary extracts provides a criterion for biological assay which is more reproducible, convenient, and specific for oxytocin. The *Chicken Vasodepressor Method* constitutes the current assay for the primary biological activity of Posterior Pituitary, Posterior Pituitary Injection, and Oxytocin Injection. However, due to interference with the vasodepressor assay by a predominance of pressor substances, the small but permissible amount of oxytocic activity in Vasopressin Injection is determined on the basis of the *Guinea-Pig Uterus Method.* The potency of Vasopressin Injection is standardized on the basis of the *Rat Vasopressor Method.* Briefly the assay involves measurement of the blood-pressure elevation produced by intravenous injection of the hormone preparation in anesthetized male rats previously treated with phenoxybenzamine (Dibenzyline—SKF). Replacement therapy in the treatment of diabetes insipidus constitutes the major use of Vasopressin (Injection and Tannate). Since pressor and antidiuretic activities are properties of the same molecule, potency may be determined on the basis of blood-pressure elevating (i.e., vasopressor) activity, although the inappropriately named *vasopressin* is no longer recommended for use as a *pressor* agent. The small but permissible limit of pressor activity in Oxytocin Injection is determined also by the *Rat Vasopressor Method.*

Corticotropin

Corticotropin Injection is a sterile preparation of the principle or principles derived from the anterior lobe of the pituitary of mammals used for food by man, which exert a tropic influence on the adrenal cortex.

Corticotropin acts on the cortex of the adrenal gland to stimulate the secretion of adrenocortical steroid hormones, predominantly hydrocortisone. Secretory activity is reflected by a reduction in the concentration of ascorbic acid in the adrenal gland. The USP biological assay is essentially that devised by Sayers and his associates[3] and is based on the extent of depletion of ascorbic acid in the adrenal glands of the hypophysectomized rat.

Corticotropin Injection labeled for intramuscular or subcutaneous administration is biologically assayed by a method involving *subcutaneous* injection into the test animal. The procedure for the assay of the potency of Corticotropin Injection labeled for intravenous administration only is similar to the above except that the preparation is injected *intravenously* into the test animal. Corticotropin Injection may be labeled for administration either subcutaneously or intramuscularly or intravenously provided the ratio of the observed potency by *subcutaneous* assay and that by *intravenous* assay is not less than 0.80 and not more than 1.25.

Repository Corticotropin Injection is corticotropin in a solution of partially hydrolyzed gelatin. The gelatin menstruum retards the absorption of corticotropin at the site of intramuscular injection thereby prolonging the period of therapeutic effectiveness. The biological assay of Repository Corticotropin Injection is identical with that specified in the *subcutaneous* method for Corticotropin Injection.

Sterile Corticotropin Zinc Hydroxide Suspension represents corticotropin adsorbed on a suspension of zinc hydroxide. Following intramuscular administration, the absorption of the preparation is delayed in comparison to Corticotropin Injection. In preparation for biological assay, sufficient 0.1 N hydrochloric acid is added to Sterile Corticotropin Zinc Hydroxide Suspension to effect complete solution. Using this solution, the assay is identical with that specified in the *subcutaneous* method under Corticotropin Injection.

The official compendium specifies an upper limit on the permissible vasopressor activity of Corticotropin Injection and Repository Corticotropin Injection; the *Rat Vasopressor*

Method, described in the section on *Vasopressin Injection,* is employed for determination of this activity.

Tubocurarine Chloride Injection

Tubocurarine, typical of the *curariform drugs,* is a valuable adjuvant to general anesthesia because of the muscular relaxation it produces by depression of transmission at the neuromuscular junction. Since doses slightly in excess of the desired amount can result in respiratory paralysis, its accurate assay is of extreme importance. The alkaloid has been isolated in pure form and can be assayed chemically in this state. However, similar substances of variable pharmacological potency are often present and consequently a biological assay is necessary. Biological assay of the skeletal-muscle-paralyzing activity of Tubocurarine Chloride Injection is based on the amount required to produce temporary paralysis of the neck muscles, or "head drop," when administered by fractional, intermittent intravenous injection into unanesthetized rabbits. The activity of Tubocurarine Chloride Injection is compared with that of USP Tubocurarine Chloride Reference Standard.

The assay for Metocurine Iodide and Metocurine Iodide Injection is similar to that outlined for Tubocurarine Chloride Injection, except that the standard solution for the former assay is prepared from Metocurine Iodide Reference Standard.

Chorionic Gonadotropin

Chorionic gonadotropin is a gonad-stimulating principle, of placental origin, prepared from the urine of pregnant women. The biological activity of chorionic gonadotropin is essentially identical to that of the luteinizing hormone (interstitial cell-stimulating hormone) of the anterior pituitary. Chorionic gonadotropin is used in sequence with menotropins (human menopausal gonadotropins) in the treatment of infertility in women in whom anovulation is due apparently to low or absent endogenous gonadotropins. Follicular growth and maturation are promoted by initial treatment with menotropins, following which chorionic gonadotropin is administered to induce ovulation by simulating the normal preovulatory surge of luteinizing hormone. Chorionic gonadotropin is also used in the treatment of cryptorchism in cases in which there is no apparent anatomical obstruction to descent of the testis. Combined therapy with this hormone and menotropins may promote spermatogenesis in patients with hypogonadotropic eunuchoidism. Diagnostically, chorionic gonadotropin is used to evaluate Leydig cell responsiveness.

Chorionic Gonadotropin for Injection is a sterile, dry mixture of chorionic gonadotropin with suitable diluents and buffers. Biological assay of the preparation is based on the increase in weight of the uterus excised from young female rats sacrificed 2 days after the last of 3 daily subcutaneous injections of dilutions of the test sample. The response is compared to that obtained in a series of animals similarly treated with USP Chorionic Gonadotropin Reference Standard. The uterotrophic effect is dependent upon elaboration of ovarian hormones in response to the gonad-stimulating activity of chorionic gonadotropin. Chorionic Gonadotropin for Injection is satisfactory if it contains not less than 80% and not more than 125% of the potency stated on the label. It is also necessary to ascertain, biologically, that Chorionic Gonadotropin for Injection meets the requirements of the estrogenic activity test. This is accomplished by examination of vaginal smears taken from ovariectomized rats on each of three successive days following subcutaneous injection of 0.25 mL. of chorionic gonadotropin test solution twice daily (morning and afternoon) for 2 days. The requirements of the test are met if the cellular elements in the smears consist of leukocytes and a few nucleated epithelial cells, but no cornified epithelial cells.

Heparin

Heparin is a mucopolysaccharide composed of repeating units of glucuronic acid or iduronic acid and sulfated glucosamine; it is a relatively strong acid which readily forms water-soluble salts, eg, heparin sodium. Heparin inhibits blood clotting both *in vitro* and *in vivo*; the anticoagulant effect is evident immediately upon the mixing of heparin with blood. A major factor in heparin anticoagulation is neutralization of thrombin and other serine protease clotting factors. The antithrombin activity of heparin requires an alpha-globulin cofactor.

Heparin used medicinally is extracted from the lungs, intestinal mucosa or other suitable tissues of domestic mammals used for food by man. Heparin Sodium is biologically assayed on the basis of its ability to prevent the clotting of sheep plasma under standardized conditions, as compared with the activity of USP Heparin Sodium Reference Standard. The official compendium requires that Heparin Sodium Units contain not less than 120 USP Heparin Units when derived from lungs and not less than 140 Units when derived from other tissues, and not less than 90% nor more than 110% of the potency stated on the label.

The potency of commercial preparations of heparin sodium ranges from 140 to 190 units/mg. Inasmuch as 100 mg of heparin sodium may represent between 12,000 and 19,000 units of activity, depending on the preparation dispensed, the dosage of heparin should be expressed in units rather than in milligrams.

Summary Table

Major aspects of the biological assay procedures for several official compounds are summarized in Table I.

Vitamins

Chemical or spectrometric assay procedures are specified for all preparations of vitamin A, vitamin B₁ (thiamine), and vitamin D. A biological assay for determination of vitamin D activity of Cod Liver Oil, Nondestearinated Cod Liver Oil, Oleovitamin A and D, and descriptions of formerly official biological assay methods for vitamins A and B₁ will be found in RPS-13, pp. 1600–1604.

Protamine Sulfate

Protamine sulfate is a purified mixture of simple protein principles obtained from the sperm or testes of suitable species of fish. The positively charged protein reacts with negatively charged heparin to form an inactive complex. Protamine Sulfate Injection, administered intravenously, serves as a specific and effective antidote if severe hemorrhage develops during heparin therapy.

Protamine sulfate is assayed biologically on the basis of its ability to neutralize the anticoagulant activity of heparin sodium in sheep plasma under standardized conditions. Each mg of protamine sulfate neutralizes not less than 80 USP Units of heparin activity derived from lung tissue or not less than 100 USP Units of heparin activity derived from intestinal mucosa. Protamine Sulfate Injection contains not less than 90% and not more than 120% of the labeled amount of protamine sulfate.

Table I—Summary of Biological Assay Procedures

Compendial article	Activity assayed	Animal employed	Route of administration of test material	End point of assay	Unitage	Additional biological tests required
Digitalis	Cardiac (cardiotonic) action	Pigeon	IV infusion	Cardiac arrest (death)	100 mg is equivalent to not less than 1 USP Digitalis Unit	—
Insulin injection	Hypoglycemic	Rabbit	SC injection	Reduction of blood glucose level	1 mL is equivalent to 40, 100 or 500 USP Insulin Units (potency not less than 95% and not more than 105% of that stated on the label)	Identification (convulsions following SC injection in fasting rabbits; relieved by IV dextrose)
Globin zinc insulin injection	Assay procedure and biological identifica-tion test as described for Insulin Injection	—	—	—	1 mL is equivalent to 40 or 100 USP Insulin Units	—
Isophane insulin suspension						
Protamine zinc insulin suspension						
Glucagon for injection	Hyperglycemic	Cat (injected IP with dextrose 16 hr prior to assay)	IV injection	Elevation of blood glucose level	—	—
Parathyroid injection	Hypercalcemic	Dog	SC injection	Elevation of serum calcium level	1 mL is equivalent to not less than 100 USP Parathyroid Units	—

Table I—(continued)

Compendial article	Activity assayed	Animal employed	Route of administration of test material	End point of assay	Unitage	Additional biological tests required
Oxytocin injection	Vasodepressor activity in anesthetized chickens as an index of oxytocic activity	Chicken	IV injection	Intermittent	Reduction of arterial blood pressure	1 mL possesses USP Posterior Pituitary Units equivalent to 10	Pressor activity—oxytocin injection must not contain excessive vasopressor activity as determined by elevation of arterial blood pressure following IV injection of the test sample in phenoxybenzamine pretreated rats
Vasopressin injection	Vasopressor	Rat (pretreated with phenoxybenzamine)	IV injection	Intermittent	Elevation of arterial blood pressure	1 mL possesses a pressor activity equivalent to 20 USP Posterior Pituitary Units	Oxytocic activity—vasopressin injection must not contain excessive oxytocic activity as determined by contraction of uterine smooth muscle isolated from the guinea pig
Posterior pituitary injection	Vasodepressor and Vasopressor	—	—	—	1 mL possesses USP Posterior Pituitary activity equivalent to 10 Units of oxytocic activity and not less than 5 Units of vasopressin activity	Refer to assays for Oxytocin Injection and Vasopressin Injection	
Corticotropin injection Sterile corticotropin injection Repository corticotropin injection Sterile corticotropin zinc hydroxide suspension	Adrenal cortical stimulation	Hypophy-sectomized rat	SC injection	Reduction of ascorbic acid content of adrenal glands	—	Vasopressin activity—corticotropin injection must not contain excessive vasopressor activity as determined by elevation of arterial blood pressure following IV injection of the test sample in phenoxybenzamine-pretreated rats (this test is not required with Sterile Corticotropin Zinc Hydroxide Suspension)
Tubocurarine chloride injection	Skeletal muscle relaxant	Rabbit	IV injection	Intermittent	Head-drop (paralysis of skeletal musculature of neck)	—	—
Metocurine iodide injection	Skeletal muscle relaxant	Rabbit	IV injection	Intermittent	Head-drop (paralysis of skeletal musculature of neck)	—	—

As previously noted in this chapter, *biological assay* refers to measurement of the relative potency or activity of compounds by determining the amount required to produce a stipulated effect on a suitable test animal or organ under standard conditions. The experimental animals mentioned in specific test procedures described in the previous section include mice, rats, guinea pigs, rabbits, cats, dogs, and pigeons. In its broadest sense, however, a biological assay may involve observations or measurements of effects obtained in any form of living matter, plant or animal. The term *microbial* (contraction of microbiological) *assay* designates a type of biological assay, specifically, a biological assay performed with microorganisms, eg, bacteria, yeasts, and molds.

The principles involved in microbial assays are in general those which apply to assays utilizing higher forms of plant or animal life. One notable difference involves the relative size of the experimental population. In a typical bioassay procedure the response of each individual test animal is noted and the results obtained with a series of animals are subjected to statistical analysis to calculate mean activity, standard error, etc. In a typical microbial assay each evaluation is performed with a culture of microorganisms and the measurement represents the average response of an extremely large population of test organisms. In the case of most bioassays a linear relationship exists between the *log dose* and the response, whereas in most microbial assays there is a linear relationship between the *dose* and the response (within certain limits). The importance of this relationship in the evaluation of microbial assays is considered in Chapter 10.

Vitamins

Microbiological procedures are available for the assay of Calcium Pantothenate, Niacinamide, and Vitamin B₁₂ activity.

Microbial Assays

Table I—(continued)

Compendial article	Activity assayed	Animal employed	Route of administration of test material	End point of assay	Unitage	Additional biological tests required
Chorionic gonadotropin for injection	Chorionic gonadotropin	Gonad-stimulating	Female rat	SC injection daily for 3 days	Increase in weight of uterus	1 mg is equivalent to not less than 1500 USP Chorionic Gonadotropin Units	Estrogenic activity—chorionic gonadotropin must not contain excessive estrogenic activity as determined by cytological examination of vaginal smears taken from ovariectomized rats injected SC with the test sample Pyrogen Safety (determined by minimal toxicity in mice injected IV with 1000 USP Chorionic Gonadotropin Units)
Heparin sodium injection	Heparin sodium	Anticoagulant	Sheep	*In vitro* addition of heparin sodium to blood plasma	Inhibition of clot formation	1 mg is equivalent to not less than 120 USP Heparin Units when derived from lungs and not less than 140 USP Heparin Units when derived from other tissues (e.g., intestinal mucosa)	Pyrogen
Protamine sulfate for injection Protamine sulfate injection	Heparin neutralization	Sheep	*In vitro* addition of protamine sulfate to blood plasma containing known amounts of heparin	Reduction of clotting time of heparinized plasma	1 mg neutralizes not less than 80 USP Units of heparin activity from lung tissue or not less than 100 USP Units of heparin derived from intestinal mucosa	Pyrogen
Cod liver oil Nondestearinated cod liver oil	Antirachitic (vitamin D)	Rachitic rat	Oral feeding (one-half of total dose on day 1; one-half on day 3 or day 4)	Calcification of rachitic metaphysis of radius and tibia	1 g contains not less than 2.125 µg (85 USP Units) of vitamin D	1 g also contains not less than 255 µg (850 USP Units) of vitamin A (assayed by a spectrophotometric method)

of Cyanocobalamin Co 57 Solution and Capsules, and Cyanocobalamin Co 60 Solution and Capsules.

A fundamental requirement in a microbial assay for the activity of a vitamin or amino acid (factor) is the inability of the test organism to synthesize the factor being assayed. Furthermore, the test organism must require the factor in question for normal growth, and should be sensitive to very small amounts of the required factor. For such microbial assays special media are prepared which are nutritionally complete in all respects except for the factor under study. Control tubes containing the suitable media inoculated with the test species exhibit no, or only minimal, growth. If the basic requirements specified above are satisfied, the growth response of the test organism is, within limits, proportional to the amount of factor added to the medium.

The extent of the growth response may be determined either turbidimetrically, spectrophotometrically, or by titration of the acid produced. The turbidity of the culture is proportional to the amount of microbial growth; the development of acidity also reflects quantitatively the growth response. Sufficient levels of reference standard are included to enable construction of a curve of response for each assay. The activity of an assay dilution is determined by interpolation from the standard curve.

Niacin or Niacinamide

The techniques and procedures used in the microbiological assay for niacin are common to many of the microbiological methods and a description of the niacin method will serve to give the pattern generally employed.

The Microorganism—In the case of niacin there has been adequate demonstration that the assay organisms employed metabolize only the forms of niacin that are available to the animal. The fact that some organisms are more limited than the animal in their ability to utilize niacin derivatives serves as a basis for differentiating such compounds in biological materials. For example, *Lactobacillus plantarum* is able to utilize, in addition to the free niacin, niacinamide, nicotinuric acid, cozymase, and niacinamide nucleoside.

Although a number of microorganisms require niacin for their metabolic processes, and are unable to synthesize it for themselves, the acid-forming organism *L. plantarum* is most widely used for assay purposes. It is nonpathogenic, easy to culture, and is affected to only a limited degree by stimulatory or inhibitory substances normally found in foods or pharmaceutical preparations containing niacin. It may be grown on a simple stab-culture medium containing gelatin, yeast extract, and glucose, and is cultured for use in the assay tubes by direct transfer to the liquid medium consisting of the basal assay medium containing an optimum amount of added niacin.

One important advantage of microbiological procedures is that only a minute quantity of a vitamin is needed to give a measurable response. For example, the range of niacin added to the series of standard tubes is 0.05 to 0.5 μg/tube. Thus the niacin content of extremely small amounts of biological materials may be readily measured. Modifications utilizing microanalytical apparatus, and a lower range of vitamin additions have been described for blood and tissue analysis.

The Test Solution—The first step in the assay procedure is the preparation of the test solution of the material to be assayed. If the sample is a dry or semisolid material, the niacin is extracted by heating the sample in a measured volume of dilute H_2SO_4 in an autoclave for 30 min. Liquid preparations are autoclaved 30 min after addition of the H_2SO_4 to give a concentration of one-normal. Although niacin is soluble in water, certain precursors, found particularly in cereals, are unavailable to the test organism unless hydrolyzed. Either acid or alkali is equally effective for the extraction but acid is preferred, owing to the possibility of hydrolysis of trigonelline in alkaline solution. Preparation of the test solution is completed by neutralizing with strong NaOH solution, then diluting to a volume that contains 0.1 μg of niacin per mL. Further purification of the test solution is not ordinarily important since *L. plantarum* is relatively unaffected by substances that inhibit or stimulate other test organisms.

The Medium—The basal medium employed in a niacin assay is simple to prepare and with properly treated casein hydrolysate is otherwise nutritionally complete. A medium suitable for use in the amino acids is prepared by replacement of the casein hydrolysate with an amino acid mixture, omitting in each instance the acid under assay. Both dehydrated complete media and dehydrated casein hydrolysates are available commercially and appear to be entirely satisfactory for assay purposes.

Details of the microbial assay procedure for niacin (including preparation of standard niacin solution, spectrophotometric determination of cell density, and calculation of the niacin content of the test samples) are given in the official compendium.

Calcium Pantothenate

In the assay of Calcium Pantothenate, the turbidimetric procedure is followed, using *Lactobacillus plantarum*.

Vitamin B12 Activity

Determination of vitamin B_{12} activity requires special treatment of the material to be assayed in order that the vitamin may be made available to the test organism, which, in this case, is a culture of *Lactobacillus leichmannii*. The basal medium used is quite complex, being prepared as a mixture in solution, of a great variety of essential nutritional components. To one set of tubes containing this medium are added measured amounts of the material to be assayed, and to a corresponding second set are added measured amounts of the Standard Cyanocobalamin Solution. The tubes are inoculated with a small amount of culture of the test organism and then incubated. The extent of growth which has occurred is measured by determining light transmittance by means of a spectrophotometer. A concentration-response curve is drawn by plotting the transmittance for each level of the Standard Cyanocobalamin Solution against the concentrations in the respective tubes in terms of nanograms. The amount of vitamin B_{12} contained in the test solution is determined by proper interpolation of the observed values on the standard curve.

Antibiotics

The term antibiotic, as used in the official compendia, designates a medicinal preparation containing a significant quantity of a chemical substance that is produced by a microorganism or artificially by synthesis and that has the capacity to inhibit or destroy microorganisms in dilute solution. Under the terms of the Federal Food, Drug and Cosmetic Act of 1938, as amended by Public Law 87-781, all antibiotics intended for use in man are subject to production and testing controls under federal supervision, including batch certification prior to distribution. For the purposes of administering the certification program, standards of potency and purity for antibiotics are established by the Food and Drug Administration in the form of regulations published from time to time in the *Federal Register*. Since all recognized antibiotics are subject to the provisions of the regulations, the latter determine the official standards. The federal regulations governing all aspects of antibiotic testing are extremely detailed and subject to periodic amendment; they should be consulted with regard to prescribed methods for the assay of individual antibiotics and their preparations.

In evaluation of the potency of antibiotic substances the measured effect is inhibition of the "growth" of a suitable strain of microorganisms, ie, prevention of the multiplication of the test organisms. The procedures employed in microbial assay of antibiotics may be divided into two broad classifications: the *Cylinder-Plate Method* and the *Turbidimetric Method.*

Cylinder-Plate Method

The Cylinder-Plate (Cup) Assay of antibiotic potency is based on measurement of the diameter of zones of microbial growth inhibition surrounding cylinders (cups) containing various dilutions of test compound, which are placed on the surface of a solid nutrient medium previously inoculated with a culture of a suitable organism. Inhibition produced by the test compound is compared with that produced by known concentrations of a Reference Standard.

Turbidimetric Method

The Turbidimetric Assay of antibiotic potency is based on inhibition of microbial growth as indicated by measurement of the turbidity (transmittance) of suspensions of a suitable microorganism in a fluid medium to which have been added graded amounts of the test compound. Changes in transmittance produced by the test compound are compared with those produced by known concentrations of reference material.

In the context of *bioassay*, a biological test has as its objective the qualitative determination of a specific characteristic of a biological product or of the container in which it is supplied (eg, transfusion assemblies). These tests are designed to determine with a high degree of certainty the absence or presence of a type of activity (antibacterial activity, pressor activity, etc), or quality (nonantigenicity, toxicity, etc), or constituent (depressor substances, pyrogen, etc). Animals are employed in some tests and microorganisms in others.

Biological Tests

Summary Table

An outline of compendial articles subject to identification, activity or toxicity tests of a biological nature is presented in Table II.

References

1. *Federal Register 32:* 3270-3282, 1967.
2. *Guide for the Care and Use of Laboratory Animals* (DHEW Publ No (NIH) 78-23), DHEW, Washington, DC, 1978.
3. Sayers MA: *Endocrinol 42:* 379, 1948.

Table II—Summary of Biological Test Procedures[a]

Compendial article	Activity tested	Animal or test system employed	Route of administration of test material	End point of test procedure
Iron dextran injection	Absorption of iron compound	Rabbit	IM	No heavy black deposit of unabsorbed iron 7 days after injection
Antiseptics, disinfectants, fungicides, germicides	Kills or prevents growth of pathogenic or nonpathogenic organisms	Microbial cultures	Microbial	Absence of microbial growth
Diphtheria toxoid, tetanus toxoid and combinations with pertussis vaccine	Antigenicity	Guinea pig	SC	Not less than 80% survival (for at least 10 days) of immunized animals injected with test doses of toxin
Protein hydrolysate injection	Nutritional completeness	Rat	PO	Weight gain while maintained on test product and nitrogen deficient diet
Parenteral forms of various antibiotics	Depressor activity	Cat	IV	Arterial blood pressure not depressed more than by 0.1 µg/kg histamine
Atropine	Mydriatic	Cat	Ocular instillation	Pupil dilation
Isofluorophate ophthalmic ointment and solution	Miotic	Cat	Ocular instillation	Pupil constriction
Insulin products	Hypoglycemic convulsions	Rabbit	SC	Convulsions relieved by IV dextrose
Technetium TC99m-containing compounds	Distribution of radioactivity	Rats or mice	IV	Residual radioactivity in specified tissues
Diphtheria toxoid, tetanus toxoid	Toxin poisoning	Guinea pig	SC	No symptoms of toxin poisoning within 21 days
Parenteral solutions	Pyrogens/bacterial endotoxins	Rabbits	IV	Rectal temperature increase not more then 0.6°C
Elastomeric closures, plastic containers, transfusion assemblies	Systemic toxicity of incubate	Mouse	IP, IV	No toxic reaction within 48 hours
	Intracutaneous toxicity of incubate	Rabbit	Intracutaneous	No irritation
	Implantation toxicity of designated material	Rabbit	Aseptic implant	No reaction

[a] These tests are described in detail in the USP/NF and the Official Supplements

CHAPTER 32

Clinical Analysis

Robert D Smyth, PhD
Vice President, Research Support

Lorraine Evans, DS, H(ASCP)
Clinical Pathology
Bristol-Myers Company
Syracuse, NY 13221

Characterization and quantitation of the various components of blood, urine, and other body fluids are the primary functions of the clinical laboratory. The major divisions of clinical analysis are clinical biochemistry, hematology, blood-bank technology, histopathology, immunology, and microbiology. Accurate diagnosis of disease and determination of a potential therapeutic regimen are frequently based on the laboratory analysis of blood, urine, feces, gastric secretions, or cerebrospinal fluid. Modern medical practice is tending toward greater reliance on laboratory results as definitive measures of pathologic or normal states.

The pharmacist should familiarize himself with the basic principles involved in sample collection, analysis and diagnostic significance of the various clinical parameters. The role of the pharmacist in community health necessitates his comprehension of the methodology and diagnostic value of clinical laboratory procedures. The influence of various drugs and drug interactions on these parameters must be considered in both the clinical and drug-abuse situation.

Hematology

Determination of the morphologic, physiologic, and biochemical properties of peripheral blood and the blood-forming organs (hematopoietic system) is a function of the hematology laboratory. The functional categories of hematology are (1) analysis of cellular elements, and specific biochemical and physiological parameters of peripheral blood and the hematopoietic system; (2) blood-coagulation analysis; and (3) blood-bank technology.

Peripheral blood is a biphasic liquid tissue system of cellular elements suspended in a liquid plasma phase. The cellular phase comprises about 45% of the blood volume and contains erythrocytes (red blood cells, RBC), leukocytes (white blood cells, WBC), and thrombocytes (platelets). The plasma phase is primarily water (90-92%) and protein (7%).

Hematologic analysis of blood is primarily concerned with enumeration and differentiation of the various cellular elements. Analysis of the hematopoietic system (eg, bone marrow and lymphoid tissue) determines the status of blood-cell precursors in these tissues. Determinations of specific biochemical (hemoglobin) and physiologic (blood or plasma volume) parameters are performed in a complete evaluation of the erythron system (blood and marrow RBC and their precursors). The normal hematologic values in the adult are presented in Table I.

Erythrocytes and Hemoglobin—The erythrocytic system is composed of the mature erythrocytes in peripheral blood and their precursors in bone marrow. The precursors of

The author acknowledges the assistance of Dr Joseph P Usavage of Rorer Group Ltd, in the preparation of the Microbiology section and Dr Alfred H Free of the Ames Co for the Urinalysis section.

erythrocytes, as found in the erythropoietic system (red bone marrow), are classified as to the degree of nucleation and characteristics of cytoplasmic constituents. The sequence of erythrocyte formation in bone marrow, based on gradual denucleation of the cell, generation of the chromatin structure, and changes in nucleolar structure and cytoplasmic constituents, is as follows: pronormoblast → basophilic normoblast → polychromatic normoblast → orthochromatic normoblast → polychromatophilic erythrocyte → erythrocyte.

The first four types are nucleated and are normally seen only in bone marrow. In normal erythrocyte formation these immature bone marrow cells are designated as *normoblastic* or *normocytic*. In pernicious anemia and related conditions, these immature cells become abnormally large and are designated *megaloblastic* or *megalocytic*. In iron-deficiency anemia, these cells become abnormally small and are designated *microblastic* or *microcytic*—of the iron-deficiency type. Normal blood contains 0.5 to 1.5% of circulating erythrocytes as reticulocytes. These cells contain a fine network of basophilic reticulum that is demonstrable on staining with a vital dye such as brilliant cresyl blue. The number of these cells

Table I—Normal Hematological Values in Man

	Normal value	Normal range of values
Erythrocytes (cu mm × 10^6)		
Male	5.4	4.6-6.2
Female	4.8	4.2-5.6
Reticulocytes (cu mm × 10^3)	50	10-100
Hemoglobin (g%)		
Male	16.0	14.0-18.0
Female	14.0	12.0-16.0
Hematocrit (%)		
Male	47.0	40.0-54.0
Female	42.0	37.0-47.0
Mean corpuscular volume (μm^3)	87	82-92
Mean corpuscular hemoglobin (pg)	29	27-31
Mean corpuscular hemoglobin concentration (%)	34	32-36
Mean corpuscular diameter (μm)	7.3	6.7-7.7
Leukocytes (cu mm × 10^3)	7.0	5.0-10.0
Leukocyte differential (%)		
Neutrophils	63	57-67
Eosinophils	1	1-3
Basophils	1	0-1
Lymphocytes	30	25-33
Monocytes	5	3-7
Platelets (cu mm × 10^5)	3.0	1.4-6.0
Erythrocyte sedimentation rate (Wintrobe), (mm/hr)		
Male	4	0-9
Female	10	0-20

in the blood is a measure of effective erythropoiesis. High circulating-reticulocyte values are an index of erythropoietic activity and are found in the first few days of life, after hemorrhage, and after treatment of iron or vitamin B_{12} deficiency anemias.

The normal *erythrocyte* (normocyte) is a flexible, elastic, biconcave, enucleated structure with a mean diameter of 7.3 μm and a thickness in the range of 2.2 μm. The chemical constituents of the red blood cell include water (63%), lipids (0.5%), glucose (0.8%), minerals (0.7%), nonhemoglobin protein (0.9%), methemoglobin (0.5%), and hemoglobin (33.6%). The primary function of the erythrocyte is transport of oxygen and carbon dioxide. The red cell membrane, a dynamic, semipermeable component of the cell, is associated with energy metabolism in the maintenance of the permeability characteristics of the cell to various cations (Na^+, K^+) and anions (Cl^-, HCO_3^-). The stroma of insoluble material which remains after red-cell disruption (hemolysis) constitutes 2–5% of the wet cell weight; it is primarily protein (40–60%) and lipid (10–12%). The membrane includes stromatin (a fibrous or structural protein) and mucopolysaccharides associated with A, B, and O blood-group substances. The lipid fractions include phosphatides (lecithin, cephalin), cholesterol, cholesterol esters, neutral fats, cerebrosides, and sialic acid glycoproteins.

Erythrocytes may be enumerated by either visual or electronic procedures. In the visual procedures, a measured quantity of blood is diluted with a fluid which is isotonic with blood and which will prevent its coagulation. The diluted blood is then placed in a counting chamber (hemocytometer) and the number of cells in a circumscribed area is enumerated microscopically. Hayem's solution (sodium sulfate, 2.5 g; sodium chloride, 0.25 g; mercuric chloride, 0.25 g; distilled water, 100 mL), Toison's fluid (sodium sulfate, 8 g; sodium chloride, 1 g; methyl violet, 0.025 g; glycerin, 30 mL; distilled water, 180 mL), or 0.9% sodium chloride are used as diluting fluids. The overall error of this method is about 8%.

A greater degree of accuracy and reproducibility can be achieved by erythrocyte enumeration in an electronic counting apparatus; eg, Coulter Counter or Ortho cell counters. The Coulter method (Fig 32-1A) determines the number and size of particles suspended in an electrically conductive liquid. The blood cells traverse a small aperture and displaces its own volume in diluent as to produce a change in resistance between electrodes; the magnitude of the voltage pulse is proportional to cell volume, and the resultant pulses are then amplified, scaled, and automatically counted.

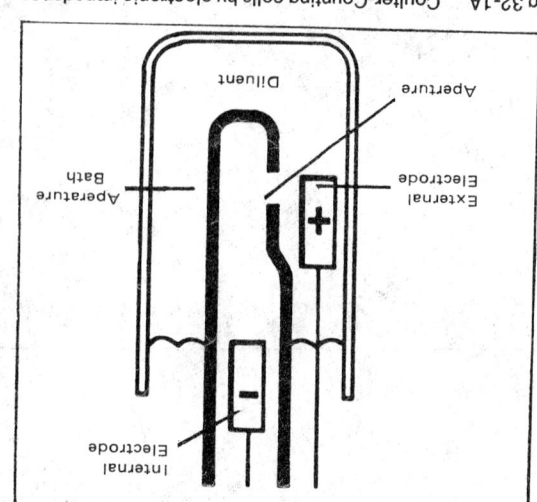

Fig 32-1A. Coulter-Counting cells by electronic impedance (Coulter Electronics, Inc).

The *hematocrit value* is also a measure of the erythrocyte portion of blood. A sample of blood containing anticoagulant is placed in a graduated hematocrit capillary tube, centrifuged, and the volume ratio of packed red cells to total blood volume (hematocrit) determined. The centrifuged sample in the hematocrit tube appears as a red layer of packed erythrocytes over which is found an off-white layer of packed leukocytes and platelets, and a supernatant plasma phase. The hematocrit value is an index of both the number and size of the red cells.

Hemoglobin, a conjugated hemoprotein with an approximate molecular weight of 67,000, contains basic proteins, the globins, and ferroprotoporphyrin, or heme. It is essentially a tetramer, consisting of four peptide chains, to each of which is bound a heme group. Heme, which constitutes about 4% of the weight of the molecule, consists of a divalent iron atom in the center of a pyrrole-porphyrin structure. Four distinct polypeptide chains (α, β, γ, δ) can be incorporated into hemoglobin. Normal adult hemoglobin is HbA = $\alpha_2\beta_2$. Fetal hemoglobin contains 2α and 2γ chains and is designated HbF = $\alpha_2\gamma_2$.

Differences in the structural sequences of amino acids in the peptide portion of the hemoglobin molecules are genetically controlled and are responsible for different types of hemoglobin. Based on characteristic mobility of the hemoglobin, in an electric field (electrophoresis) on starch, paper, cellulose acetate, agar, or acrylamide gel media, many hemoglobin types have been recognized (see Chapter 33). Only types P, F, and A_1-A_4 are considered normal. Sickle-cell anemia and β-thalassemia are hemolytic anemias associated with abnormal hemoglobins (ie, Type S in sickle-cell anemia and abnormal production of β chain in β-thalassemia). In homozygous HbS *disease* sickling of the red cells is due to the low solubility of the abnormal hemoglobin in its reduced state, with the production of semicrystalline bodies (tactoids), which distort and elongate the cells. In the sickle-cell trait (heterozygous), the blood smear shows no sickle cells. In the

In the Ortho ELT-8 technique (Fig 32-1B), the principles of laser flow cytometry are used to count cells. Hydrodynamic focusing and laminar flow are combined in the system to count a large number of individual cells. Light focused by a helium-neon laser is scattered by the cells as they pass through the flow channel. The scattered light is monitored by a photoelectric sensor and transfers the electrical pulses which are processed by the systems circuitry. In addition to increased speed of counting, the overall error of the electronic procedures is reduced to about 1%.

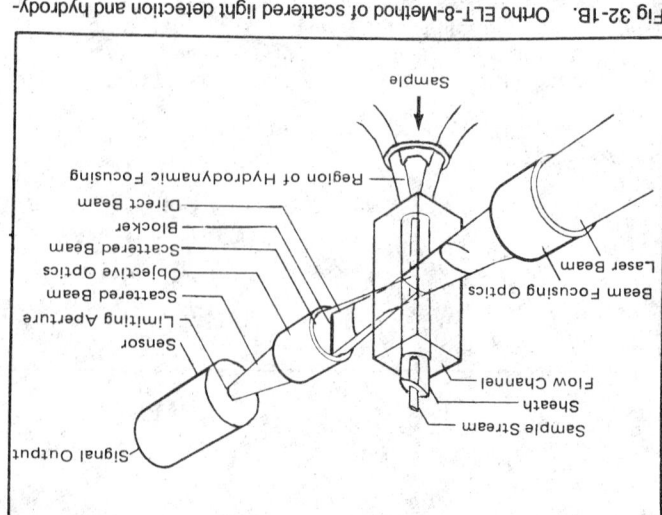

Fig 32-1B. Ortho ELT-8—Method of scattered light detection and hydrodynamic focusing for cell counting (From Clinical Instrument Systems, Oct 1980).

homozygous condition, HbS accounts for nearly all of the hemoglobin with small amounts of HbF. In the heterozygous, HbS constitutes 50% or less of the hemoglobin, with the balance as HbA.

The detection of sickle-cell disease is performed by microscopic observation of the induction of red-cell sickling in the presence of a reducing agent such as sodium metabisulfite or by quantitative determination of urea-dispersible turbidity induced by dithionite following reduction of HbS to deoxy-HbS in RBC lysates. The microscopic procedure will only detect homozygotes, whereas HbAS and HbS and its structural variant HbC-Harlem are both detected in the urea-dithionite technique. Commercial qualitative test kits are available for detecting sickle cell trait and anemia by solubility determinations. All hemoglobins positive to dithionite test must be electrophorized (cellulose acetate, citrate agar or starch gel) to differentiate HbS from HbC and thalassemia traits.

The *hemoglobin* concentration is measured spectrophotometrically after lysis of whole blood and conversion of hemoglobin to hematin, oxyhemoglobin, or cyanmethemoglobin. The addition of strong base (NaOH) to pH 10 converts oxyhemoglobin, carboxyhemoglobin, and methemoglobin to hematin, which can be estimated photometrically. Weaker bases (Na_2CO_3 or NH_4OH) convert hemoglobin to oxyhemoglobin for analysis.

Total hemoglobin is also measured by conversion to cyanmethemoglobin utilizing alkaline sodium cyanide-potassium ferricyanide reagent. Hemoglobin standards certified by the Clinical Standards Committee of the College of American Pathologists are used in the above procedures, and all results are expressed as "g hemoglobin per 100 mL blood."

In the normal state, the oxygen consumption of the RBC is low and it is involved in the conversion of hemoglobin to oxidized (Fe^{3+}) methemoglobin (HbM) which cannot bind oxygen. The normal balance of HbM (<0.5%) is maintained by two enzyme systems—NADH and NADPH methemoglobin reductases. An inherited deficiency of the RBC enzyme, *glucose 6-phosphate dehydrogenase* (G-6-PD) will decrease the rate of reduction of glutathione and methemoglobin, make the cell more vulnerable to oxidative attack and result in susceptibility to drug-induced or nonspherocytic hemolytic anemia. G-6-PD deficiency is found predominantly in Mediterranean peoples, Southeast Asians, Africans, and American negroes. The enzyme can be quantitated spectrophotometrically or by fluorophelometry by measuring the rate of reduction of nicotinamide adenine dinucleotide phosphate (NADP) in the presence of G-6-PD. Presumptive screening tests based on reduced glutathione (GSH) content of blood before and after incubation with acetylphenylhydrazine are also used.

Erythrocyte count, hemoglobin content, and hematocrit value are used to determine various blood indices in the diagnosis and treatment of anemia. These measurements are:

$$\textit{Mean corpuscular volume } \{MCV\ (\mu m^3)\} = \frac{\text{Hematocrit (\%)} \times 10}{\text{Erythrocyte count (millions/cu mm)}}$$

$$\textit{Mean corpuscular hemoglobin } \{MCH\ (pg)\} = \frac{\text{Hemoglobin (g/100 mL)} \times 10}{\text{Erythrocyte count (millions/cu mm)}}$$

$$\textit{Mean corpuscular hemoglobin concentration } \{MCHC(\%)\} = \frac{\text{Hemoglobin (g/100 mL)} \times 100}{\text{Hematocrit (\%)}}$$

An additional parameter used to characterize red cell variation is the red cell distribution width (RDW) determined on the Coulter S-Plus II. The RDW is directly calculated by the standard deviation and coefficient of variation from a red cell histogram on the S-Plus II. The difference in cell size may be used to monitor patients with pernicious anemia and hemorrhagic anemia.

Anemias are classified as to red cell volume and hemoglobin concentration. *Macrocytic* (large cell: MCV > 94), *normocytic* (normal cell: MCV, 82-92), or *microcytic* (small cell: MCV < 80) are the classifications according to cell volume. Cellular hemoglobin concentration categorizes the cells as to *hyperchromic* (MCHC > 38), *normochromic* (MCHC = 32-36), or *hypochromic* (MCHC < 30). Examples of anemias:

I. Hypochromic microcytic—erythroid normoblastic anemia in bone marrow
  A. Iron Deficiency—low hemoglobin (Hbg) and RBC. Low serum iron, High total iron binding capacity, absent hemosiderin.
    1. Dietary—low iron intake
    2. Intestinal problems—decreased iron absorption
    3. Pregnancy, infants—increased iron requirements
    4. Iron loss—due to chronic hemorrhage, parasitic infections, GI tract lesions, excess menstrual bleeding.
  B. Hereditary Sideroblastic Anemia—defect in the heme synthesis, an inability to utilize ingested iron.
  C. Thalassemia—genetic abnormality which produces normal to increased HbF and/or HbA_2.

II. Normochromic Normocytic
  A. Hemolytic Anemias—increased destruction of erythrocytes
    1. Autoimmune hemolytic
    2. Cold agglutinin hemolytic
    3. Mechanical destruction of RBC's
    4. Paroxysmal Nocturnal hemoglobinuria
    5. Lymphomas and Hodgkin's disease
    6. Infections
  B. Hemoglobinopathies—abnormalities in structure of alpha or beta chains of hemoglobin molecule. Normoblastic erythroidhyperplasia in bone marrow.
    1. Sickle cell anemia
    2. Hemolysis
    3. Hemoglobin CC
  C. Acute Hemorrhage
  D. Other Anemias
    1. Aplastic Anemia, Leukemia, Malignancy
    2. Renal failure and drug related anemias caused by chloramphenicol and antineoplastic drugs.

III. Normochromic Macrocytic—due to deficiency of vitamin B_{12} or folate. Bone marrow is hypercellular with increased erythroid precursors.
    1. Pernicious Anemia
    2. Sideroblastic Anemia
    3. Sprue—total iron binding capacity is decreased; hemosiderin increased in the bone marrow.
    4. Pregnancy

Determinations of the suspension stability of whole blood and erythrocyte fragility are useful adjuncts in the diagnosis of various diseases. The *erythrocyte sedimentation rate* (ESR) is an estimate of the suspension stability of red cells in plasma; it is related to the number and size of the red cells and to the relative concentration of plasma proteins, especially fibrinogen and the α- and β-globulins. This test is performed by determining the rate of sedimentation of blood cells in a standard tube. Normal blood ESR is 0–15 mm/hour. Increases are an indication of active but obscure disease processes such as tuberculosis and ankylosing spondylitis. ESR is affected by anemia and does not respond linearly with changes in asymmetrical macromolecules such as fibrinogen and globins. The *zeta sedimentation ratio* (ZSR) technique overcomes these disadvantages. It is based on a measure of the closeness with which RBC will approach each other after standardized cycles of dispersion and compaction. The *erythrocyte fragility test* is based on resistance of cells to hemolysis in decreasing concentrations of hypotonic saline. Increased osmotic fragility of the red cells is associated with various types of spherocytosis and acquired hemolytic anemia; increased resistance has been observed in thalassemia, sickle-cell anemia, and hypochromic anemia. The test can be performed manually by colorimetric estimation of hemoglobin released by hypotonic cell rupture or automatically in an instrument which continually records the increase in light transmittance through a suspension of red cells in a continuously decreasing salt gradient during dialysis.

LEUKOCYTES—Mature leukocytes (white blood cells, WBC) in peripheral blood and their precursors in bone and lymphoid tissue comprise the leukocytic system. Various types of leukocytes are found in normal blood. Differentiation of the lymphocytic, monocytic, and granulocytic leukocyte types is based on cell size, color, chromatin structure, and cytoplasm constituents.

The primary function of leukocytes is the development of the various defensive and reparative processes in inflammatory and immune response mechanisms. Migration of leukocytes to the site of inflammation is associated with the release or activation of various biochemical substances (5-hydroxytryptamine, histamine, complement, immunoglobulins, prostaglandins, lysosomal enzymes). The tissue histiocyte or monocyte (macrophage) can also engulf and destroy foreign particles by the process of endocytosis, and certain leukocyte types by phagocytosis.

The chemical composition of the leukocyte includes water (82%), nucleoprotein, phospholipids, and trace minerals. Enzyme content, glycogen, and histamine levels vary in the different types of white cells. Deficiency in enzymes associated with glycolytic metabolism (hexokinase) and increases in phosphomonoester hydrolases (alkaline phosphatase) have been observed in leukocytes of certain leukemia patients.

The precursors of granulocytic leukocytes are found in bone marrow and are classified according to degree of cytoplasmic granulation, dye-affinity of the granules and shape of the nucleus (Schilling, Arneth, or Cooke-Ponder Classification). As undifferentiated cells (myeloblasts) mature (promyelocyte → myelocyte → metamyelocyte → band leukocyte → segmented leukocyte), metachromatic granules appear in the cytoplasm (granulocytes). All segmented leukocytes are motile, a requirement for participation in the inflammatory or phagocytic processes.

In the mature *basophilic* and *eosinophilic leukocytes*, these granules develop an affinity for a basic or acidic dye, respectively; those cells containing granules which do not stain are called *neutrophils*. In peripheral blood, the mature granulocytic cells are designated *polymorphonuclear leukocytes—neutrophilic, eosinophilic, or basophilic*.

The other types of white cells normally observed in peripheral blood have no granules and are classified as to size and shape into the *monocyte* and *lymphocyte*, which are formed in lymphoid tissue. The small lymphocyte is thymic-derived and is found in the circulation and the germinal centers of lymphoid tissue. The origin of the large lymphocyte is a gut-associated lymphoid stem cell which can further differentiate into the immunoglobulin-producing plasmacyte. The interaction of thymic (T) and bone marrow (B) lymphocytes is the basis for the development and maintenance of humoral and cellular immune mechanisms.

Leukocytes are enumerated by procedures similar to those utilized for erythrocytes. In the visual procedures, the blood is diluted with a fluid (3% v/v acetic acid) which lyses the red cells, and total leukocyte count is determined microscopically. Eosinophils may also be differentially analyzed by use of a diluting fluid which renders the red cells nonrefractile and invisible, and lyses the base-labile leukocytes, leaving the base-stable eosinophils intact. A suitable diluting fluid for this purpose is Pilot's Fluid (propylene glycol, 50 mL; distilled water, 40 mL; 1% phloxine, 10 mL; 10% sodium carbonate, 1 mL; and heparin sodium, 100 units). Electronic counting procedures are similar to those used for erythrocytes with the added advantage of speed, accuracy, and reproducibility.

The normal adult leukocyte value is 5,000 to 10,000 cells/cu mm. Values greater than 10,000 (*leukocytosis*) are encountered in the newborn infant, young children, after violent exercise, convulsive seizures of epilepsy, leukemia, and cancer. Values of less than 5,000 (*leukopenia*) are observed in certain microbial infections (eg, typhoid fever, measles, malaria, overwhelming septicemia), cirrhosis of the liver, pernicious anemia, radiation injury, and replacement of marrow by malignant tissue.

A *differential count of the leukocytes* will provide information as to the relative numbers of each type. A thin film of blood is prepared on a microscope slide stained with a polychromatic preparation such as the Leishman, Wright, or Giemsa stain, and analyzed microscopically. Wright's stain contains polychromed methylene blue and eosin dyes; the erythrocytes are stained pink; the nuclei of the leukocytes, purplish-blue; neutrophilic granules, violet-pink; eosinophilic granules, red; basophilic granules, blue; and platelets, blue. The recent introduction of automated systems for differential white cell counts will significantly reduce the errors inherent with the subjective nature of the visual counting procedure. Differentiation of the various cell types can be made on the basis of cytochemistry and staining properties of enzymes specific for a single cell type. The granules of neutrophils and eosinophils are stained by their action on 4-chloro-1-naphthol to form a colored quinone in the presence of a peroxide and further differentiated by the optimum pH for peroxidase activity between these two cell types. The monocytic lipase is used as a specific marker by reaction of basic fuchsin with α-naphthol liberated by lipase on α-naphthylbutyrate substrate. The lymphocytes are not stained in this procedure, but are measured by electronic sizing.

Automated differential WBC counts have also been obtained in systems which count large populations of cells by simultaneous measurement of two optical properties (axial light loss and/or narrow-angle scatter and/or multiple-wavelength fluorescence). Laser light is also utilized to differentiate cell size, granularity, and volume of cells. The collected light measured by forward versus right angle scatter is converted to a histogram giving the percent of lymphocytes, monocytes and granulocytes. Another system involves computer processing of two-dimensional images of the various cell types using an automatic scanning microscope.

Polymorphonuclear neutrophilic leukocytes (neutrophils, "polys") normally comprise 62% (50-67%) of the total leukocyte count. These cells are irregular in shape (10-15 μm in diameter) and usually contain a multilobated nucleus with fine, lightly stained cytoplasmic granules. An immature or juvenile form of neutrophil, with a band-shaped nonsegmented nucleus constitutes 3-5% of peripheral blood leukocytes. Increases in the relative percentage of these cells (neutrophilia) is observed in acute microbial infections (eg, meningitis, smallpox, poliomyelitis), metabolic disorders (diabetic acidosis, gout), drug intoxication (digitalis, epinephrine), vaccination, coronary thrombosis, and malignant neoplasms.

Polymorphonuclear eosinophilic leukocytes (eosinophils) normally comprise about 1-3% of total circulating white blood cells. In appearance they are similar to the neutrophil with the exception of large, red-stained cytoplasmic granules. Eosinophilia has been observed in certain skin diseases (psoriasis, eczema), parasitic infestations (pork round worm—trichinosis), certain hypersensitivity reactions, scarlet fever, and pernicious anemia. Charcot-Leyden crystals, which are found in bronchial secretions from asthmatics, are derived from nucleoprotein disintegration products of eosinophils.

Polymorphonuclear basophilic leukocytes (basophils) possess large cytoplasmic granules which stain a deep blue. These cells, which are primarily sources of blood heparin and histamine constitute less than 1.0% of the leukocytes. Basophilic leukocytosis is seen in chronic myelocytic leukemia, hemolytic anemia, and Hodgkin's disease. Basophilic leukopenia occurs following radiation or therapy with glucocorticoids.

Lymphocytes have a cell diameter from 7–10 μm (small) to 10–18 μm (large). They have a round, or slightly indented, deeply stained nucleus and normally comprise 25–33% of the leukocytes. Lymphocytosis is seen in infectious mononucleosis, lymphocytic leukemia, rickets, and in most conditions associated with neutrophilic leukopenia (neutropenia).

Monocytes constitute 3–7% of the leukocytes. They are larger (12–20 μm) than the other leukocytes and possess an abundant, pale, bluish-violet-stained cytoplasm with a fine, reticulated chromatin structure in the nucleus. The monocytes (macrophages) phagocytize bacteria, parasitic protozoa, foreign particles, and even erythrocytes. Monocytosis is seen in certain microbial infections (tuberculosis, typhus, malaria), Hodgkin's disease, and monocytic leukemia.

Drug therapy frequently causes neutrophil dysfunction which can be characterized by decreased number of mature neutrophils or a defect in cellular function. This results in the inability of the body to defend itself against infection. Drugs such as nitrogen mustard and chloramphenicol degenerate bone marrow stem cells and DNA synthesis is impaired by antimetabolites such as methotrexate and flurouracil. Depolymerization of DNA is caused by procarbazine and alkylating agents. Mitosis is inhibited by colchicine and vinca alkaloids. The following outline lists drugs which cause granulocytopenia.[2]

Nonchemotherapeutic rifampin fistocetin benzene nitrous oxide ethanol	**Phenothiazides** chlorpromazine mepazine methotrimeprazine prochlorperazine thoridizine
Antithyroid carbimazole methimazole thiouracil	**Antibiotics** chloramphenicol carbenicillin griseofulvin isoniazid novobiocin
Diuretics acetazolamide chlorthalidone chlorothiazide hydrochlorothiazide ethacrynic acid mercurials	**Cardiovascular** diazoxide procainamide methyl dopa quinidine propranolol
Antihistamines ethylenediamine thenalidine metaphenylene pyribenzamine	

As qualitative and quantitative changes in leukocytes in peripheral blood and their precursors in bone marrow and lymphatic tissue are associated with the various types of *leukemia*, this disease has been classified on the basis of the predominating type of leukocyte, ie, myelocytic (granulocytic), lymphocytic, monocytic, plasmacytic. Leukemia may be either acute or chronic and involve replacement of bone marrow elements by malignant cells, infiltration of the reticuloendothelial system, anemia, thrombocytopenia and hemorrhage. Leukemia is usually associated with an elevated WBC count and increase in the specific cell and its precursors in peripheral blood, but in certain instances there is an aleukemic blood picture with no evidence of leukocytosis. Leukocytes are more immature ("blast"-type cells) in acute leukemia than those encountered in the chronic type.

In many diseases of the hematopoietic system, it is necessary to examine the bone marrow to determine the rates of formation, maturation, and release of blood cells into peripheral circulation. Using a puncture biopsy needle, samples of *bone marrow* may be obtained from the sternum, iliac crest, or proximal end of the tibia. Smears of marrow are then prepared, stained (Wright's stain or specialized histopathological procedure), and examined microscopically. The ratio of myeloid leukocyte to nucleated red cells in bone marrow, the presence of abnormal (*nonmyeloid*) cells, the number of platelet precursors (*megakaryocytes*), signs of cell maturation arrest, and the presence of focal lesions are important factors in the diagnosis of various disease states.

Systemic lupus erythematosus (LE) is a disease characterized by numerous clinical and pathological manifestations associated with various organs. Although the disease chiefly affects the lymphatic system, the cardiac, renal, and articular systems are also involved. The diagnosis of this disease is based on the presence of a LE-cell factor in the gammaglobulin fraction of blood in the diseased state. This factor dissolves the nuclei of leukocytes by depolymerization of deoxyribonucleic acid to form the LE-body. If serum from patients with LE is incubated with white cells, the "polys" will engulf the liberated LE-body and form the typical LE-cell with a characteristic progressive loss of nuclear detail. These antibodies to nucleoprotein can also be detected by immunological techniques. In the double antibody technique, the test serum containing antibodies to nuclear protein is incubated with a rat kidney slice (antigen). The second antibody is a fluorescein-labeled goat antihuman immunoglobulin (IgG) which combines with the human IgG bound to the antigen site in a positive test. The fluorescence is estimated by immunomicroscopy. Normal light microscopy can be used if the goat-antihuman IgG is labeled with peroxidase.

Thrombocytes—The primary functions of *thrombocytes* (blood platelets) are the maintenance of hemostasis (arrest of blood flow from a vessel) and blood coagulation (clot formation). Platelets are oval to spherical in shape and have a mean diameter of 2–4 μm. They originate from an immature cell (*megakaryocyte*) in bone marrow and ranges of 140,000–450,000/cu mm have been reported in normal blood.

Adhesiveness, aggregation, and agglutination are the principal physical properties of platelets responsible for hemostasis and coagulation reactions. Chemically, they contain protein (60%), lipid (15%), and carbohydrate (8.5%). Their content of serotonin, epinephrine and norepinephrine aids in promoting constriction at the site of injury. Release of "platelet thromboplastin," a cephalin-type phosphatide, and ADP are important in blood coagulation.

As at the present time, there is no satisfactory manual method for accurate enumeration of blood platelets. The size and physical properties of the platelet seriously deter the development of accurate and reproducible methodology. Indirect methods of analysis are based on the proportion of platelets to erythrocytes in a stained blood smear. Blood samples obtained directly from the fingertip puncture are diluted with an anticoagulant fluid which will simultaneously stain the platelets. The ratio of platelets to red cells is then determined microscopically and the number calculated from the predetermined red cell count (normal 3–8 platelets/100 RBC). In the direct procedures, a sample of blood is obtained by venipuncture, placed in a siliconized tube, diluted, and subsequently analyzed by counting the platelets in a microscopic counting chamber using conventional or phase microscopy apparatus. Suitable diluting fluids are the Rees-Ecker Fluid (sodium citrate, 3.8 g; formaldehyde, 0.22 mL; brilliant cresyl blue, 0.05 g; water, qs 100 mL) or Brecker Fluid (1% ammonium oxalate). Automated procedures for platelet counting have increased the accuracy to ±5 to 10%. Blood is collected in a special anticoagulant, diluted and centrifuged at specified speeds to obtain a "platelet-rich" supernatant fluid, which is then counted in an automated counting apparatus similar to those used for RBC counting.

Methods for counting platelets in whole blood include electronic impedence instruments and laser-optical counters utilizing hydrodynamic focusing.[3] These new hematology multi-parameter analyzers provide greater accuracy, precision, and increased rate of analysis performed on a small volume of blood. The automated instruments provide precise platelet measurements for monitoring chemotherapy-induced thrombocytopenia and transfusion therapy.

Persistent increases in platelet count (*thrombocythemia* or *plasthrenemia*) have been observed in chronic myelocytic leukemia, polycythemia, megakaryocytic hyperplasia, and splenic atrophy. Acute or temporary increases in platelet values (*thrombocytosis*) are seen in trauma and asphyxiation. *Thrombocytopenia* or a decrease in platelets to values less than 60,000/cu mm occurs in various purpuras or hemorrhagic states (idiopathic or symptomatic thrombocytopenic purpura). Inherited platelet defects include Glanzmann's thrombasthenia which is characterized by prolonged bleeding time and poor clot retraction while Bernard-Soulier Syndrome and Von Willebrand's disease demonstrates defective platelet adhesiveness. Defects in the release reaction includes "Storage Pool Deficiency" and "Aspirin-like" syndrome. Leukemia, extensive burns, splenic disorders, and agents such as quinidine, sulfonamides, hydrochlorothiazide, diuretics, antiepileptics, and neuropharmacological agents have been implicated in the etiology of symptomatic thrombocytopenia. Decreases in platelet count are also accompanied by morphologic changes in the size, shape, and cytoplasmic granulation of these cells and changes in adhesiveness and normal function in hemostasis and coagulation.

Studies on *platelet aggregation* have been of significant value in the study of platelet abnormalities and their role in disease states. The rate and extent of the aggregation and clotting response to adrenaline, ADP, collagen and thrombin have been measured by observing changes in optical density of platelet-rich plasma on addition of these agents or other test substances. Low amounts of ADP give reversible aggregation, while a biphasic aggregation pattern occurs with intermediate concentrations of ADP or with epinephrine. The second phase is the release of the platelets endogenous ADP. High concentrations of ADP result in an irreversible aggregation. Aspirin acts as an inhibitor of the intrinsic platelet and the collagen reaction.

Reticulocytes—In normal peripheral blood 0.5–1.5% of the erythrocytes possess a fine reticulum in the cytoplasm. In blood smears prepared with Wright's, Giemsa, and other Romanowsky methods, basophilic stippling of the erythrocytes occurs in lead poisoning (*plumbism*). This is not to be confused with the basophilic staining of the reticulocyte which can only be seen when wet cells are stained by supravital procedures (mixture of dyes with wet blood prior to preparation of air-dried blood smear). The observed granular filaments or reticulum of this immature erythrocyte are a result of endoplasmic coagulation by lipophilic dyes used in the supravital procedures. *Reticulocytes* are enumerated by supravital staining of fresh blood with an anticoagulant-dye solution.

The usual method of expression is:

$$\% \text{ Retics} = \frac{\text{No reticulocytes}/1000\ \text{RBC}}{10}$$

The "corrected" reticulocyte count is calculated for a more meaningful clinical approach in the degree of anemia by expressing the percentage of reticulocytes per mm^3 of whole blood.

$$\text{corrected reticulocyte count} = \text{reticulocyte count} \times \frac{\text{(Patient's Hematocrit)}}{\text{(Normal Hematocrit)}}$$

In indirect counting methods a thin film of the blood-dye mixture is prepared on a microscope slide, counterstained with Wright's stain, and the reticulocytes enumerated in proportion to a predetermined erythrocyte count. In direct procedures, reticulocytes are enumerated in wet films without counterstaining. Suitable dyes are brilliant cresyl blue, methylene blue and Janus green. These methods are subject to high counting error.

An increase in the number of reticulocytes is an index of accelerated hematopoiesis and is observed in acute hemorrhage or adequate therapeutic management of iron-deficiency or pernicious anemia. In cases of chronic blood loss or bone-marrow depression a decrease in reticulocytes is seen.

Blood Volume and Erythropoietic Mechanisms—The mean red cell mass in normal males is 2095 ± 384 mL (30 mL/kg), the average plasma volume is 2766 ± 459 mL (40 mL/kg) and the total blood volume 4861 ± 795 mL (70 mL/kg). The specific determination of *red cell mass* is accurately estimated by tagging erythrocytes with ^{51}Cr *in vitro* or ^{59}Fe *in vivo*. These isotopes are incorporated into the β-polypeptide (Cr) or porphyrin (Fe) of hemoglobin in the RBC and subsequent isotope dilution in blood after injection of tagged erythrocytes is used for calculation of red cell mass. In hemolytic anemia there is also a decrease in the normal life span (108–120 days) of the erythrocyte as indicated by a decreased survival time of ^{51}Cr-tagged red cells in blood (refer to Chapter 29).

Plasma volume is estimated by measurement of hemodilution of IV injected ^{125}I or ^{131}I human serum albumin. The activity of labeled albumin steadily decreases after injection due to loss of albumin to the extravascular space. Estimates of zero-time radioactivity levels can be made by extrapolation of a typical first-order blood level decay curve. Dyes (Evans Blue) and other isotopes are less satisfactory for accurate assessment of plasma volume. The *total blood volume* is equal to the red cell mass and plasma volume.

Chronic expansion of the red cell mass is seen in primary and secondary polycythemia associated with erythrocytosis due to hypoxia, tumors, and renal disease. In these conditions, there is an increased hemoglobin and hematocrit and absolute increase in red cell mass. In relative polycythemia, the high hematocrit is due to contraction of the plasma volume. *Chronic expansion of the blood volume* with a resultant decrease in hematocrit value and, in some cases, a "hemodilution" anemia, is seen in cardiac failure, normal pregnancy, hepatic cirrhosis, splenomegaly and arteriovenous fistula.

The metabolic defect in *pernicious anemia*, characterized by inadequate gastrointestinal absorption of vitamin B$_{12}$, is readily diagnosed by monitoring urinary radioactivity following oral administration of cyanocobalamin-^{57}Co with and without intrinsic factor. The percent recovery of the isotope in normal patients is 3–25% and in pernicious anemia 0–2.5%.

^{51}Cr-tagged erythrocytes are also used in studying the effects of various compounds, such as the nonsteroidal anti-inflammatory drugs, on *gastrointestinal (GI) bleeding*. The patient's blood cells are tagged with ^{51}Cr and the agent under test is administered. If GI bleeding occurs, there is an increase in ^{51}Cr content of fecal samples as a result of blood loss into the lumen of the GI tract.

Measurement of the absorption of radioactive iron (^{59}Fe), its tissue distribution (liver, spleen, precordium and sacral bone marrow), plasma elimination and urinary excretion establish various *ferrokinetic parameters*. Iron is absorbed to the greatest extent as the ferrous salt in the upper small intestine. Absorption is decreased in iron overload, decreased erythropoiesis and various malignant, inflammatory or infectious diseases. Iron is transported in plasma bound to transferrin—a specific iron-binding protein. Alterations in plasma iron and iron-binding capacity are seen in pregnancy, thalassemia major and iron deficiency (hypochromic) anemia. Iron is stored in the liver, bone marrow, skeletal muscle and spleen as ferritin and hemosiderin. The daily turnover of iron is about 35 mg, primarily from an "erythropoietic labile pool" in bone marrow. *Hemosiderosis* is simply an increase in iron storage, whereas *hemochromatosis* denotes increased iron storage with associated tissue damage. Both of these states can result from oral or parenteral medicinal/transfusion iron overload. Iron excretion is limited and occurs by desquamation of iron-containing cells from bowel, skin and urinary tract. Iron-deficiency anemia is a symptom and not a disease. Treatment is based on evaluation of ferrokinetic parameters, correction of hemoglobin and tissue-iron deficiency and recognition of the underlying cause (eg, chronic blood loss).

Blood Coagulation—*Hemostasis*, the arrest of blood flow from a vessel, is regulated by extravascular (muscle, skin, and subcutaneous tissue), vascular (blood vessels), and intravascular (platelet adhesion, clot retraction and blood-coagulation) mechanisms. The following discussion will be limited to those processes related to the blood-coagulation mechanism. When blood is allowed to clot, the free-flowing liquid is converted into a firm cell clot surrounded by serum. If an anticoagulant is added to blood, coagulation does not occur and the blood cells are suspended in a liquid phase—plasma. The clotting mechanism involves three stages: (1) formation of plasma *thromboplastin*, (2) conversion of *prothrombin to thrombin*, and (3) conversion of *fibrinogen to fibrin*.

The International Committee on Nomenclature of Blood Clotting Factors has numerically designated the blood-coagulation factors (Table II). Fibrinogen and Factors V and VIII are absent in normal blood serum as a result of the clotting process. The absorption characteristics of certain blood-coagulation factors on calcium phosphate or barium sulfate are used in the differential analysis of specific factors. Interaction of coagulation factors may be initiated through either the intrinsic or extrinsic pathways. In the intrinsic system all the factors are present in the blood, while the extrinsic system is activated by the release of tissue thromboplastin. The figure below shows the activities of both pathways to form a stabilized fibrin clot.

In Stage 1 of the coagulation process, the contact of injured tissue with blood results in the activation of Factor XII, which reacts with calcium, PTA, PTC, and Factors III, V, and X to yield intrinsic or blood thromboplastin. This stage is normally completed in 3–5 min. Extrinsic or tissue thromboplastin is formed rapidly (<12 sec) in various tissues in the body such as lung and brain in the presence of calcium and Factors V, VII, and X. In Stage 2, thromboplastin catalyzes the conversion of prothrombin to thrombin (8–15 sec) in the presence of Factors V, VII, X, and calcium. In Stage 3, the thrombin rapidly converts fibrinogen into fibrin. The fibrin then forms a network of fibers which traps red cells and thus forms the blood clot. Although the exact nature of the enzymatic sequences in the coagulation process is not clear, it is definitely a biological amplification process starting from the small reaction of tissue contact to rapid conversion of fibrinogen to fibrin.

Blood contains natural inhibitors of coagulation such as antithrombin, heparin, and antithromboplastin which can prevent a particular reaction in the coagulation sequence. The dissolution of blood clots occurs by action of blood proteolytic enzyme—plasmin or fibrinolysin. Plasmin is formed from its precursor, plasminogen, after activation by tissue and body fluids or substances of bacterial origin (streptokinase).

The routine tests performed in the coagulation laboratory are indices of vascular function (vascular phase and platelet adhesion) or intrinsic clotting mechanisms. Determinations of *bleeding time* and *capillary fragility* provide estimates of vascular factors. In the Ivy method for determination of *capillary bleeding time*, a blood-pressure cuff is placed on the forearm and inflated to 40 mm Hg; a puncture wound is made and the time required for bleeding to stop is noted. The normal bleeding time, as determined by this method is 1–9 min. Dextran, pantothenyl alcohol, and derivatives and streptokinase-streptodornase may cause a prolonged bleeding time. The *Simplate II* (General Diagnostics Division of the Warner Lambert Company) is a standardized, disposable, springloaded bleeding time device for platelet function testing. It uses 2 blades that are released automatically to produce 2 uniform incisions 6 mm long X 1 mm deep, making the procedure reliable and reproducible.

The *capillary fragility* or *tourniquet* test is based on the incidence of petechiae (small red marks) formation produced by an inflated blood-pressure cuff over a 5-min period. Normally, a few tiny petechiae may appear. The most common cause of abnormalities in vascular function and platelet adhesion tests is thrombocytopenia.

Table II—Blood-Coagulation Factors

Factor	Synonym
I	Fibrinogen
II	Prothrombin
III	Thromboplastin (tissue)
IV	Calcium
V	Labile factor, proaccelerin, Ac globulin
VI	Accelerin
VII	Stable factor, proconvertin, serum prothrombin conversion accelerator (SPCA)
VIII	Antihemophilic globulin (AHG)
IX	Christmas factor, plasma thromboplastin component (PTC)
X	Stuart-Prower factor
XI	Plasma thromboplastin antecedent (PTA)
XII	Hageman factor
XIII	Fibrin-stabilizing factor (FSF)

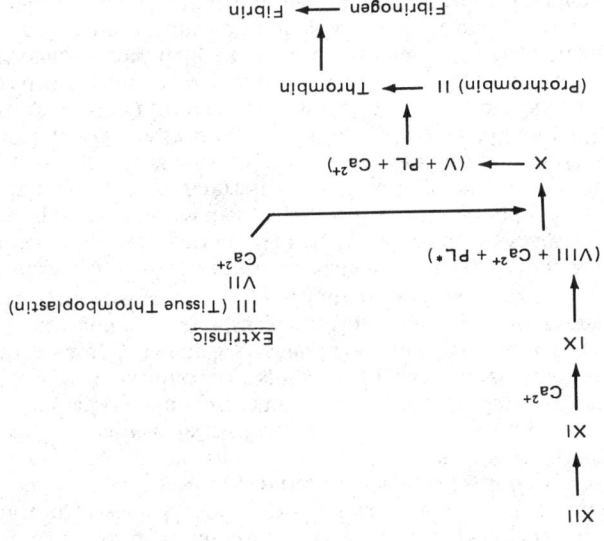

Analysis of the intrinsic coagulation mechanism is concerned with determination of levels of the specific clotting factors in whole blood. In preliminary studies of a suspected hemorrhagic disorder, determinations of coagulation time, clot retraction, platelet count, bleeding time, and capillary fragility are usually performed.

In the Lee-White procedure, the coagulation time of whole blood is determined in regular or siliconed tubes. Normal values are 8.5–15 min in glass and 19–60 min in siliconed tubes. Anticoagulants and tetracyclines may cause increased times while corticosteroids and epinephrine cause decreased values. Siliconization of glassware prevents platelet aggregation and thus delays coagulation. The samples used in the analysis and coagulation time are then inspected at 0.5, 1, 2, 4, and 24 hours after clotting to determine the time required for various phases of clot retraction. The tubes are also observed for evidence of clot lysis or dissolution. The clot will normally start to retract in 30 min, completely retract within 24 hours, and will show no evidence of lysis over a 72-hour period. Prolonged coagulation times are associated with hemophilia, hypofibrinogenemia, and Factor IX deficiency. Abnormalities in any of the above tests indicate the requirements for further coagulation studies.

The *prothrombin time test* is a measure of the levels of all coagulation factors, except III, IV, and VII, and is an index of the capacity of plasma to form thrombin. In the "One Stage" test, the plasma sample is mixed with calcium chloride and tissue thromboplastin, and the time required for fibrin-clot formation is determined. Results are compared with a normal plasma control, and the prothrombin time is reported either in seconds or as percent prothrombin calculated from a standard activity curve. Correction studies using normal serum, adsorbed normal plasma or whole normal plasma added to test serum indicate deficiencies of Factors VII and X, Factor V and Factor II, respectively. If none of these additives shorten the prothrombin time, a circulating anticoagulant problem can be suspected.

A modification (*prothrombin-proconvertin procedure*) of this technique using a 1:10 dilution of both patient and control plasma in the presence of prothrombin-free plasma as a source of Factors I and V, is a more sensitive index of specific deficiencies in prothrombin, Factor VII, IX, and X.

Owren's *thrombotest*, as performed on whole blood, is sensitive to changes in both extravascular and intravascular clotting mechanisms, including Factor IX. The dosage of anticoagulant drugs, such as dicumarol, is adjusted in accordance with prothrombin time determinations; patients are usually maintained within a therapeutic range of 20–40% prothrombin activity (normal range, 80–130%). Reduced prothrombin levels, with prolonged prothrombin times, are observed in vitamin K deficiency, hemorrhagic disease of the newborn, excessive anticoagulant therapy, liver, and biliary disease. The interaction of other drugs with anticoagulants may cause increased prothrombin times. Drugs such as salicylates, phenylbutazone, oxyphenbutazone, indomethacin, and some sulfonamides increase the amount of active anticoagulant activity. Other drugs decrease the amount of vitamin K produced by gut bacteria which include chloramphenicol, kanamycin, neomycin, streptomycin, and sulfonamides.

The *prothrombin consumption test* is an index of the efficiency of conversion of prothrombin to thrombin in the coagulation process. The blood sample is allowed to clot under standardized conditions and then the quantity of prothrombin complex removed in the serum is determined in the presence of extrinsic fibrinogen. At least 80% of the prothrombin is normally consumed. Reduced consumption of prothrombin (<80%) is observed in coagulation deficiencies (hemophilia) related to thromboplastin generation.

Other types of coagulation tests detect deficiencies in the *thromboplastin generation mechanism*. The *thromboplastin generation time test* (TGT) provides a means of detecting specific deficiencies of Factors V, VIII, IX, X, XI, or XII. In the initial phase of this procedure the clotting time of the patient's adsorbed plasma is determined in the presence of a standardized platelet factor reagent, calcium chloride, plasma substrate reagent (Factors I, II, and V), and the patient's serum. If the clotting time is abnormal (>16 sec), further tests are performed with the patient's plasma or serum. Adsorption of the plasma sample on barium sulfate removes Factors II, VII, IX, and X and facilitates differentiation of a Factor IX–X from V–VIII deficiency in the thromboplastin generation mechanism. Thromboplastin generation is reduced in hemophilia and thrombocytopenia.

The *activated partial thromboplastin time test* (PTT) is based on the observation that hemophilic plasma has a normal clotting time in the presence of a complete thromboplastin (extrinsic-saline extract of brain tissue), as used in prothrombin determinations, but will give a markedly prolonged clotting time with an incomplete thromboplastin (cephalin). Cephalin is a thromboplastic, ether-soluble phospholipid factor with platelet-like activity. In this test the clotting time of the patient's plasma is determined in the presence of calcium chloride and activated cephalin. This test is used primarily to detect deficiencies in Stage 1 of the coagulation mechanism and is rather sensitive to changes in Factors VIII and IX, as seen in classical hemophilia, and Factor IX deficiency (Hemophilia B or Christmas Disease).

In Stage 3 of the coagulation process, the presence of adequate levels of fibrinogen and thrombin is critical. *Fibrinogen levels* are analyzed semiquantitatively by determining the clotting time of a diluted plasma sample in the presence of extrinsic thromboplastin. This test is basically independent of prothrombin levels. Fibrinogen concentrations of 125 mg% or greater are adequate; deficiencies (hypofibrinogenemia) have been observed in liver disease, carcinomatosis, and in certain complications of pregnancy.

Increased levels of *fibrinogen degradation products* (FDP) have been demonstrated in serum due to primary activation of the fibrinolytic system (pathological fibrinolysis) or by secondary activation following increased blood clotting (disseminated intravascular coagulation). Fibrinogen (mw 3.4×10^5) is sequentially degraded to fragments X, Y, D and E with molecular weights 2.7, 1.65, 0.85 and 0.55×10^5, respectively. Fragments X and Y are more potent anticoagulants than fragments D and E and are responsible for hemorrhagic states in defibrination. Complexes between fibrin monomer, fragment X and other FDP interfere with thromboplastin generation and platelet formation. FDP can be measured by immunological techniques involving latex agglutination of particles sensitized with specific antibodies to FDP or by an hemagglutination inhibition test. The normal level of serum FDP is $4.9 \pm 2.8 \ \mu g/mL$. Increased levels are seen in acute myocardial infarction, menstruation, complications of pregnancy, hypoxic newborns, malignancy and renal disease.

Deficiencies in the clotting mechanisms can usually be partially and temporarily corrected by transfusion of normal blood or plasma. When this fails, the presence of circulating *anticoagulants* (antithrombin, antithromboplastins, heparin) must be considered. Circulating anticoagulants are detected by determining the effect of normal plasma on the clotting time (*recalcification time*) of the patient's oxalated plasma in the presence of calcium chloride. If the addition of the normal plasma does not shorten the prolonged recalcification time, a circulating anticoagulant state can be reported.

Since the end point of all coagulation tests is the conversion of fibrinogen to fibrin, it is vital that the analyst rigidly standardize his concepts of fibrin formation in visual recording procedures. The use of mechanical instrumentation in the detection of clot formation has significantly increased the standardization, accuracy, and reproducibility of coagulation procedures. These instruments measure and record the process of fibrin formation via increased turbidity (coagulogram or photometric clot detection) or changes in electrical conductance in the reaction mixtures. As well as performing routine laboratory tests simultaneously or sequentially, updated systems can run Fibrinogen and Factor assays achieving rapid throughput and accuracy. New performance features are available with many of the automated coagulation instruments. These include monitoring temperature zones, digital displays of the individual clotting times, automatic dilutions or patients samples, and programmable parameters for testing flexibility.

Hemophilia is a classic deficiency of AHG, Christmas disease of PTC, and Hageman trait of Factor XII. Hereditary or acquired deficiencies of Factors II, V, VII, X and XI are also associated with disease states. The process of blood coagulation, analysis of coagulation factors, and interpretation of results comprise a highly complex system. The coagulation laboratory and the physician function together in the diagnosis and treatment of coagulation-deficiency diseases.

Blood-Bank Technology

Blood-bank technology in the modern laboratory is part of the blood-transfusion service. As whole blood for transfusion and its components are biologically active therapeutic substances, a complete analysis of their chemical and biologic characteristics is vital to the assurance of successful therapeutic effects. The transfusion service is responsible for:

1. Reception and examination of the donor.
2. Collection, processing, and storage of the blood.
3. Typing of recipient and donor for ABO and Rh blood-group factors.
4. Compatibility (crossmatching) testing before transfusion.
5. Issuance of blood for transfusion and extracorporeal circulation.
6. Evaluation of transfusion complications.
7. Performance of special serologic tests pertinent to blood groups and other factors.

In this section a discussion of pertinent factors related to the various phases of the transfusion service will be presented.

Reception and Examination of the Donor—A complete registry[4] of prospective donors should be maintained, with specific reference to age, sex, weight, address, occupation, and telephone number. Computerized blood banking has increased the efficiency of this service. Donors should preferably be between the ages of 21 and 60 and should weigh no less than 110 lb. The donor may be rejected on the basis of previous or active incidence of certain microbial diseases (recurrent malaria, syphilis, infectious or homologous serum hepatitis, tuberculosis), bleeding abnormalities, convulsions, allergic syndromes, skin or heart diseases, diabetes, alcohol or drug addiction, pregnancy, cancer, recent immunization with live vaccine product, acquired immune deficiency syndrome (AIDS), or blood pressure abnormalities (acceptable blood pressure: between 100/50 and 200/100; pulse rate: 60 to 120/min.).

A period of at least 8 weeks should have elapsed since blood was withdrawn and the blood hemoglobin level should be 12.5–13.5 g% or greater. Serum bilirubin and transaminase levels should also be evaluated in donors with previous incidence of jaundice.

Collecting, Processing, and Storage of the Blood—A tourniquet is applied to the arm of the donor to occlude the venous return, the skin area is sterilized, and the blood is collected by venipuncture (phlebotomy). NIH Formula A or B [ACD(Acid–Citrate–Dextrose) or ACD-phosphate] so-

lutions are used as anticoagulants in the sterile blood-collecting containers. Evacuated containers may be of regular or siliconed glass; collapsible plastic containers offer many advantages in donation, blood-banking, and transfusion procedures.

The preservation of the red cells in blood is improved by complete removal of trapped air in the blood collection apparatus, rapid cooling after collection, and storage at 4°. Properly collected whole blood is usually stable for 21 days at 1°–6°. Deterioration of whole blood is related to increased cellular fragility (increased plasma K^+) and decreased glucose utilization. Blood which is used for correction of any bleeding tendency or clotting defect should be as fresh as possible. Leukocytes, platelets and Factors V and VIII deteriorate in stored plasma or whole blood.

ABO Blood-Group Classification[5]—Human red cells can be classified into various groups or types on the basis of reactivity of certain blood factors (*agglutinogens*) located on the erythrocyte membrane. The Landsteiner system (Table III) for the four blood groups is based on the presence or absence of either A or B agglutinogen on the cell surface (Group A, B, AB, or O, respectively).

Serum does not contain the antibody (*agglutinin*-IgM type) for the antigen present in an individual's own red cells, but does contain the isoagglutinin (eg, anti-B in blood group A) due to exposure, early in life, to bacterial and plant antigens similar in structure to the A-B antigens. The clumping or agglutination of the red cells by reaction of agglutinogen with agglutinin is utilized in blood-grouping techniques. In certain instances hemolysin antibodies, present in serum containing anti-A or anti-B agglutinins, cause the disruption of cells and release of hemoglobin (hemolysis).

Human blood cells are grouped by two separate reactions: cellular or "front" grouping and serum or "reverse" grouping. The blood group is ordinarily determined by testing an individual's red cells with standardized anti-A or anti-B serum (certified by Div. of Biological Standards, NIH). Confirmation of the blood group (reverse typing) is accomplished by analysis of an individual's agglutinin titer. In this procedure the individual's serum is heated at 56° for 10 min to destroy hemolysins, and then mixed with known subgroup A_1 or B_1 human red (Rh negative) cells in the agglutination test. These two tests should be in agreement prior to release of blood for transfusion.

Although human blood cells of Group B react uniformly with Anti-B serum, Group A and AB cells show a wide range of reactivity with Anti-A or Anti-A_1B serum. Blood group A may be further categorized into Subgroups A_1, A_{int}, A_2, A_3, A_0, and A_x on the basis of the reaction with absorbed Anti-A, Anti-A_1-lectin, anti-H-lectin, Anti-$A_{1,2}$ and Anti-AB serum and the presence of anti-A_1 in the serum. Certain Group O individuals possess anti-H in their serum and are further subcategorized into the Bombay or O_h phenotype. Tests for A, B, and H in saliva can establish the genotype of an individual, ie, A and H in saliva of blood group A, B and H in B,

Table III—Blood-Group Systems

Blood group	Agglutinogen in cell	Agglutinin in serum	Reaction[a] with anti-A serum	Reaction[a] with anti-B serum	Frequency (%) in caucasians
A	A	Anti-B	+	−	41
B	B	Anti-A-A_1	−	+	10
AB	AB	None	+	+	4
O	None	Anti-A and B	−	−	45

[a] Agglutination.

As the human blood cell contains many antigens with rather complex biochemical and immunochemical properties, the blood factors have been further classified into various sub-systems. The Kell (K), Lutheran (Lu), Lewis (Le), Duffy (Fy), Kidd (Jk), Sutter (Js), Diego (Di), and P blood-factor systems are based on the detection of a specific antigen on or within the red cell by means of antibody (*isohem-agglutinin*) reactions with specific antisera or panels of re-agent red cells. Some of these factors (e.g., Kidd, Kell, and Lewis) have been involved in transfusion reactions.

The Rh-Hr System and Antihuman Globulin Test—
The presence or absence of Rh_0 *antigen* in human blood is of prime importance in transfusion reactions, paternity disputes, and isosensitization phenomena. There are eight blood Rh phenotypes which are determined by their reaction with three specific serum agglutinins (Anti-Rh_0, Anti-rh', and Anti-rh''): rh, rh', rh'', rh'rh'', Rh_0, Rh_0', Rh_0'', Rh_0''. The rh groups do not contain the Rh_0 factor on the cell surface and are des-ignated "Rh negative." The terminology of the Wiener sys-tem (Rh, rh) is comparable to the Fisher-Race (CDE) as fol-lows: rh"(C), Rh_0(D), rh"(E). The Rosenfield system uses numerical classification: RHI = Rh_0.

The absence of the Rh antigen in about 15% of the popu-lation does not preclude the presence of other factors; the use of specific antisera (Anti-hr' and Anti-hr'') has demonstrated the existence of the Hr factors (Hr_0, hr', hr''). For example, the Rh-negative cell (rh') possesses rh''hr'Hr_0. The antigen Rh_0(D) is the most potent immunogen of all the Rh antigens.

The Rh antibodies are either *saline agglutinins* (complete) or "*blocking*" *antibodies* (incomplete). The latter are of the IgG type. They are used in Rh testing procedures and are produced more commonly, and in higher titer in the human isosensitization or autoantibody reactions. They will not agglutinate saline suspensions of normal Rh-positive red cells except in the presence of a high concentration of albumin, serum, or conglutinin (AB serum with albumin) at a temper-ature of 35-37°.

In routine Rh testing procedures, a sample of blood (oxa-lated or heparinized) or a suspension of cells in serum or al-bumin is mixed with Anti-Rh_0 serum on a slide or in a tube at 37-47°. The presence of clumping indicates that the blood possesses Rh_0 antigen. Confirmation of an Rh-negative test may be performed by retesting with Anti-rh''Rh_0'h'' serum.

In Rh testing procedures, red cells from patients with ac-quired hemolytic anemia are partially coated with human autoantibody, and cells from erythroblastic infants are coated with maternal antibody globulins and may be falsely clumped by Rh typing serum containing a high protein concentration, or may appear to be Rh-positive in the saline cell suspension test. Demonstration of anti-Rh_0(D) in an eluate from these antibody-coated cells can help to establish true Rh type.

Anti-Rh antibodies are not normally present in human serum. Such antibodies may be acquired via isosensitization. The transfusion of Rh-positive blood to an Rh-negative re-cipient, or transfer of cells of Rh-positive fetus through the placental barrier to the Rh-negative mother will result in formation of antibodies to Rh agglutinogens not present in the cells of the recipient or mother, respectively.

Hemolytic blood-transfusion reactions and hemolytic dis-ease of the newborn (erythroblastosis fetalis) involve iso-sensitization phenomena usually related to the Rh_0 antigen. Hr and ABO antigens can also be responsible for hemolytic disease of the newborn. If an expectant mother is Rh-nega-tive and the father is Rh-positive, the Rh genotype of the fa-ther should be determined. If the father is homozygous, the erythrocytes will contain a pair of Rh_0 factors and the off-spring will inherit the Rh_0 factor; if he is heterozygous, one Rh_0 and one Hr_0 factor will be present and his offspring may or may not inherit the factor.

If the fetus is Rh-positive, the mother may be sensitized to the Rh antigen and in subsequent pregnancies the develop-ment of high titers of Anti-Rh_0 antibodies will result in he-molytic disease of the fetus. These antibodies enter the fetal circulation via the placental barrier, coat the red cells of the fetus, and cause excessive erythrocyte destruction, hyper-bilirubinemia and associated potential for brain damage, hydrops fetalis (edema), and congenital anemia of the new-born. This Rh disease can now be avoided by proper thera-peutic use of Rh_0(D) Human Immune Globulin (Rho-GAM, *Ortho*) to prevent the postpartum formation of active anti-bodies in the Rh_0(D) negative, Du negative mother who has delivered an Rh_0(D) positive or Du positive infant.

The *Coombs' antiglobulin test* is a method of detecting the blocking-type antibodies, globulins and complement which are attached to red cell antigens in isosensitization phe-nomena.

In the "direct" test procedure, a saline suspension of washed red cells is mixed with anti-human gamma globulin antiserum and agglutination is indicative of the combination of human antibody with antigen on the red cell, eg, maternal incomplete isoantibody on infant's red cells in hemolytic disease of the newborn.

An "indirect" procedure is utilized to demonstrate the presence of blocking antibody in the serum of pregnant Rh-negative women and in transfusion reactions. In this proce-dure the patient's serum is incubated with a suspension of Group O Rh-positive red cells; the cells are washed and then antihuman globulin antiserum is added to detect the coating of the red cells with antibody globulin from the patient's serum by agglutination phenomena. If agglutination occurs in the first part of the procedure, a saline agglutinin is also present. Anticomplement sera (anti-nongamma-globulin antiserum) are used to detect reactions involving anti-JK.

The Du allele is a clinically important variant of the Rh_0 factor and usually associated with rh'(C) and rh''(E). These individuals are considered Rh-positive, and the red cells fail to react with anti-Rh_0 in the saline tube method but reacts with incomplete anti-Rh_0(D) by other slide or tube techniques. Rh-negative donors should be tested for Du factor. If posi-tive, their blood must only be given to Rh-positive recipi-ents.

Drug Related Problems—Hematologic abnormalities may be caused by the administration of drugs which can cause a positive direct antiglobulin test and immune hemolytic anemia eg, cephalothin, cephaloridine (*Keflin*), methyldopa (*Aldomet*), penicillin, L-dopa, quinidine, phenacetin and in-sulin.

Compatibility Testing—Cross-matching procedures are designed to detect incompatibilities in the blood of donors and recipient. The test is designed to prevent transfusion reaction and assure maximum benefit to the patient. Although erro-neous ABO grouping will usually result in an incompatible cross match, no such protection exists in the Rh system. An incorrectly-typed Rh-positive donor can result in pri-mary immunization to Rh_0(D) antigen if transfused to a Rh-negative recipient. For each transfusion, a *major* and *minor cross match* should be performed.

In the *major cross match*, (1) a saline suspension of the donor's cells is mixed with the recipient's serum, and (2) the donor's cells are suspended in recipient's serum or in serum with added albumin. The saline cross match is an additional check on the ABO typing and may detect incompatibilities caused by antibodies to M, N, S, P and Lu subgroups. The high protein or albumin cross match can demonstrate anti-bodies in the Rh system. The presence of agglutination or hemolysis indicates incompatibility. The *minor cross match*

Techniques of Analysis

This section will describe the principles of the procedures used in the analyses of various substances in blood, plasma, or urine. Examples of the significance of such tests in clinical diagnosis will be presented. A complete description of the physiologic and pharmacologic aspects of these blood constituents can be found in publications listed in the Bibliography.

Instrumentation—The development of instrumentation has accelerated many advances and much progress in clinical chemistry. An excellent review of the principles and applications in clinical chemistry of automation, atomic-absorption spectroscopy, ultraviolet and visible spectrophotometry, fluorimetry, phosphorimetry, infrared and Raman spectroscopy, microwave and radiowave spectroscopy and nucleonics was prepared by Broughton and Dawson.[7] Quality control techniques are a vital part of any clinical laboratory. Standard reference materials,[8,9] standardization of quantities and units[10] and continual evaluation of precision and accuracy of various determinations[11] are incorporated into procedures of all reliable clinical laboratories. The manufacture of certified standards and reagents and the certification of clinical chemists and clinical laboratories are under the supervision of either FDA, NIH, Pharmaceutical Manufacturers Association (PMA), American Association of Clinical Chemists or the College of American Pathologists.

Interaction of Drugs with Clinical Laboratory Tests—Drugs may interfere with the interpretation of laboratory tests by three mechanisms: (I) chemical or biochemical interference due to reaction of a drug or its metabolite in biological fluids with test reagents in analytical procedures, (II) pharmacological interference due to normal drug-induced alterations in various physiological parameters, and (III) toxicological interference as a consequence of the toxicity of a drug.

Examples of class I interference include false positive urine glucose results due to the reducing properties of drugs or metabolites such as ascorbic acid, p-aminosalicylic acid, tetracycline, cephalordine, and levodopa, which are excreted in urine. Spironolactone therapy will result in an elevation of certain urinary ketosteroids through cross-reaction of the drug in the analytical procedure.

Examples of class II interference include the decrease in serum-potassium levels in patients receiving thiazide diuretics, the alteration in serum uric acid with probenecid therapy and the elevation in various plasma proteins and thyroid function tests with estrogen-progesterone combinations. Drug-drug interaction can also result in changes in these parameters. Guanethidine enhances the effect of coumarin anticoagulants. Barbiturates induce hepatic microsomal enzyme synthesis, subsequently increase the metabolism and decrease the therapeutic effect of drugs, such as warfarin, even after barbiturate therapy is terminated.

Examples of class III interference include changes in liver and kidney function tests and hematological parameters (anemia, agranulocytosis, and leukopenia) due to drug-induced toxicity and positive LE and ANA tests due to a "lupus-like" syndrome induced by hydralazine.

It is beyond the scope of this chapter to include a complete listing of drug interactions in laboratory tests. The reader is referred to an annual, readily available, computerized review of the effect of normal therapeutic drug doses, as well as overdoses, on clinical laboratory tests[12] and to other review articles.[13]

Blood

Collection of Blood and Preparation for Chemical Analysis—Using aseptic technique, a blood sample is ob-

includes the donor's serum and the recipient's cells, and is useful as a check of the ABO typing and indication of the possibility of transfusion reactions caused by rare antigen on recipient's cells or uncommon antibodies directed against an antigen in the serum of the donor. The minor cross match has been replaced in many instances with screening of the donor's serum against a panel or pool of red cells of known antigenicity.

The *indirect antihuman globulin* procedure must also be performed with recipient's serum and donor's cells with and without albumin (major side) and may be tested with the donor's serum and recipient's cells (minor side). The use of proteolytic enzymes (bromelain) enhances the agglutination of red cells by low-titer or weakly reacting Rh-Hr antibodies, probably by removing sialic acid residues on the RBC surface. The red cells used in the indirect Coombs test are treated with the enzyme prior to absorption of antibodies and addition of antiglobulin reagent.

The usual cross-matching techniques involve (1) a room temperature or 30° procedure, preferably with the addition of albumin; (2) a high-protein procedure; and (3) an antiglobulin procedure.

The presence of nonspecific *autoantibodies, cold agglutinins,* and *bacteriogenic agglutination* sometimes complicates the cross-matching procedure. If the recipient's serum reacts more strongly with his own cells than with the donor's, then autoantibodies should be suspected. Cold agglutinins will usually agglutinate all blood, regardless of type, at low temperatures, but will not react at 37°. Agglutination as a result of bacterial contamination of blood is called panagglutination.

Hepatitis Testing—Post-transfusion hepatitis is associated with the transmission of virus-like particles referred to as *Australia or serum hepatitis antigen or the hepatitis antigen (HAA)*. All donor blood must be tested for associated antigen (HAA). Agar gel diffusion (AGD), counterelectrophoresis (CEP), complement fixation (CF), and rheophoresis procedures can be used.[25] The rheophoresis procedure uses a modified gel diffusion technique for detection of HAA by precipitin-type reaction with HAA antibody. It offers the sensitivity of CEP and CF procedures with the simplicity of the AGD procedure. Other tests for HAA are based on radioimmunoassay (RIA) technique for detection of antigen by hemagglutination (HA) or HA-inhibition for the presence of HAA antibody. In the RIA (radioimmunoassay) technique, donor's serum is added to a test tube coated with HAA antibody (solid RIA). If the serum contains HAA, it will bind to the antibody. ^{125}I-HAA is then added to the tube. If the antibody binding site is previously occupied with HAA from donor's serum, then ^{125}I-HAA will not bind and determination of ^{125}I bound vs. free is an index of HAA content of the donor's serum.

Issuance of Blood and Evaluation of Transfusion Reactions—Whole blood, red cell or leukocyte suspensions, plasma, platelet-rich plasma, platelet concentrates, leukocyte-poor blood, AHF, factor IX complex, plasma protein fractions, and RhoGAM are products of the transfusion service.[6] Transfusion reactions are related to antibody phenomena or transmission of disease. The hemolytic reaction resulting from transfusion of incompatible cells is the most serious problem. Transfusion of microbially contaminated blood can result in a pyrogenic reaction or transmission of infectious diseases, such as malaria, syphilis or hepatitis. Allergic reactions (urticaria, asthmatic seizures), circulatory overload, embolic complications (blood clot or air emboli) may also be encountered. Leukocyte and platelet antibodies may develop in repeat transfusions and in transplantation patients. The transfusion service is an integral unit in the evaluation of such complications.

tained by venipuncture and usually placed in evacuated glass tubes. The choice of anticoagulant, type of specimen, stability of test component and use of preservatives depends on the type of analysis requested and the specific analytical procedure involved. If serum is desired, the blood sample is allowed to clot and the serum is separated by centrifugation. When whole blood or plasma is to be used in the analysis, an anticoagulant is added to the collecting tube.

The following concentrations of specific anticoagulants are routinely used per 10 mL blood: lithium, potassium or sodium oxalate (15–25 mg); sodium citrate (40–60 mg); heparin sodium (2 mg); disodium or tripotassium ethylenediamine-tetraacetate (EDTA-Na₂), 10–30 mg) or ACD-Formula B solution (1.0 mL).

Heparin prevents blood coagulation by inhibiting thrombin-catalyzed conversion of fibrinogen to fibrin. The other anticoagulants either precipitate blood calcium or convert ionized calcium into a nonionized (chelated) form which cannot function in the coagulation reaction. Heparin and EDTA do not significantly alter the cellular elements of blood. Sodium fluoride and thymol are used as preservatives or enzyme inhibitors to prevent deterioration of various substances in the blood sample, eg, glucose → lactic acid. Preservatives and anticoagulants can interfere with some enzyme tests. Serum is usually used for these procedures.

The separation of plasma or serum, and chemical analysis, are usually performed as soon as possible after collection of the sample. The addition of polystyrene granules to the blood sample prior to centrifugation facilitates the isolation of serum or plasma. Hemolysis interferes with analytical procedures for bilirubin, albumin, nonprotein nitrogens, pH, phosphorus, potassium and various enzymes. The serum should also be observed for presence of lipemia. Changes in the ratio of CO_2, chloride, and electrolytes in cells and plasma, glycolytic conversion of glucose to lactic acid, hydrolysis of ester phosphate to free inorganic phosphate, bacterial conversion of urea to ammonia, and conversion of pyruvate to lactate are examples of changes that can occur in contaminated, improperly preserved, or unrefrigerated blood specimens.

The first stage in many of the chemical determinations is the removal of blood protein and preparation of protein-free blood filtrate. The protein is precipitated with tungstic acid, trichloroacetic acid, zinc hydroxide, or organic solvents such as alcohol and acetone, and then filtered or centrifuged to remove the protein coagulum. Tungstic acid precipitation is performed by mixing 1 volume of blood with 9 volumes of stabilized tungstic acid reagent. The filtrate obtained in this procedure should be in the pH range 3.0–5.1 to assure adequate removal of proteins (<2 mg% in filtrate).

The Somogyi filtrate is prepared by mixing 1 volume of blood with 5 volumes of water, 2 volumes of 5% zinc sulfate and 2 volumes of 0.3 N barium hydroxide. The barium sulfate is precipitated and the zinc hydroxide, formed in the reaction, precipitates the blood protein. Trichloroacetic acid (10%), in a ratio of 9:1 with blood, yields greater volumes of filtrate due to a more complete formation of protein aggregates.

Blood Glucose—Methods for the determination of blood glucose are based on the utilization of glucose as a reducing agent and on the enzymatic oxidation of glucose to gluconic acid. In the Folin-Wu technique, glucose is determined in a protein-free blood filtrate by reduction of alkaline cupric sulfate and subsequent reaction with phosphomolybdic or arsenomolybdic acid reagent to form a blue complex which can be estimated colorimetrically. The Nelson-Somogyi method uses a protein-free blood filtrate prepared with zinc hydroxide to remove most of the interfering reducing substances.

The presence of a terminal aldehyde in the glucose molecule is the basis of a colorimetric determination with phenolic hydroxyl reagents (phenol in aqueous methyl salicylate or phosphorylated 1,3-dihydroxybenzene) in the presence of strong sulfuric acid and heat.

The o-toluidine procedure is a color reaction specific for hexoses—glucose, mannose, and galactose. Since aldohexoses other than glucose are normally present in very small concentrations, results obtained by this method approach the true value of glucose. o-Toluidine is condensed with glucose in glacial acetic acid to yield a green chromogen by formation of an equilibrium mixture of a glycosylamine and Schiff base.

In the preceding techniques, interfering substances such as lactose, galactose, and glutathione are measured and the value is reported in the nonspecific term "sugar." Enzymatic determination with glucose oxidase is the only test specific for blood glucose. Blood glucose is converted to gluconic acid and hydrogen peroxide by glucose oxidase; the peroxide is then estimated by iodimetric procedures or by oxidation of a chromogen (o-dianisidine or 2,2'-azino[diethylbenzothiazol-inesulfonic acid]) in the presence of peroxidase to form a colored product.

Another enzymatic procedure utilizes the hexokinase-catalyzed conversion of glucose to glucose 6-phosphate (G-6-P), and then to 6-phosphogluconate and NADPH in the presence of NADP and G-6-P dehydrogenase. The NADPH thus formed is equivalent to the amount of glucose present and is estimated spectrophotometrically at 340 or 366 nm.

Normal fasting blood-sugar values for adults are 80–120 mg/100 mL; true glucose is 65–100 mg/100 mL. When the blood-sugar values exceeds 120 (hyperglycemia), diabetes mellitus should be suspected and can be confirmed by evidence of diminished carbohydrate tolerance. The effect of ingested carbohydrate on blood sugar can be determined by the glucose tolerance test; 100 g of glucose (1.75 g/kg) in water or a flavored beverage, is administered orally and glucose determinations are performed on blood and urine samples at hourly intervals for 3 hr. Values above 160 at 1 hr and 110 at 2 hr in blood samples are abnormal. The renal threshold for sugar is 180–200 mg/100 mL of blood, and, therefore, sugar should not appear in the urine of normal subjects in the tolerance test.

Hyperglycemia and decreased glucose tolerance are seen in diabetes mellitus (to 500 mg/100 mL), and hyperactivity of the adrenals, pituitary, and thyroid glands. Hypoglycemia, with a blood-sugar value of <60 mg/100 mL and increased glucose tolerance, is encountered in insulin overdose, glucagon deficiencies, and hypoactivity of various endocrine glands. Intravenous glucose tolerance studies are used in order to circumvent defective absorption of glucose in the gastrointestinal tract, eg, steatorrhea.

Monitoring hemoglobin A_{1c} is another way to follow patients with hyperglycemia. Hemoglobin A_{1c} is more specific for diagnosing diabetes but less sensitive than the glucose tolerance test.[14] Normally hemoglobin A_{1c} accounts for 3% to 6% of the total hemoglobin while in diabetics it is 6% to 12%. The concentration of Hgb A_{1c} in the blood reflects the patients carbohydrate status over a period of time, providing a marker for hyperglycemia. Pancreatic function tests include studies on IV and oral glucose, glucagon and tolbutamide tolerance. The beta cells of pancreatic islet tissue secrete insulin and the alpha cells secrete glucagon, a substance antagonistic to insulin and having a hyperglycemic effect induced by its glycogenolytic action. In glucagon tolerance studies the effect of parenteral administration of glucagon on blood-sugar values is useful in the diagnosis of pancreatic and hepatic function. Insulin and tolbutamide tolerance studies are used in the diagnosis of endocrine disorders, differentiation of insulin-resistant diabetics, and determination of functional hypoglycemia and islet-cell tumors.

Galactosemia, the presence of galactose (>4.5 mg%) in blood, is usually due to an inborn error of galactose metaboism. Congenital deficiencies in galactokinase or galactose 1-phosphate uridyl transferase result in inadequate galactose metabolism with accumulation of galactose 1-phosphate in the liver. Oral administration of galactose in galactosemia leads to a decrease in blood glucose and to increasing concentrations of galactose in urine and blood. Galactose is measured by estimation of NADH liberated in the conversion of galactose to galactonolactone in the presence of NAD and galactose dehydrogenase. Deficiencies in intestinal disaccharidases such as lactase will preclude efficient conversion of lactose to galactose and glucose, and oral administration of lactose will cause no increase in blood galactose and usually produce diarrhea. Galactose-loading studies are useful in the diagnosis of toxic or inflammatory conditions of the liver. In hepatic cirrhosis, there is a decrease in galactose metabolizing capacity of liver due to inhibition of hepatic diphosphogalactose-4-epimerase.

Lactic acid is a product of glucose metabolism; it is converted into pyruvic acid and NADH by lactic dehydrogenase (LDH) in the presence of NAD. Blood lactic acid is estimated by reaction with LDH to form pyruvate and NADH; the NADH level is determined spectrophotometrically at 340 nm and is a function of lactic acid concentration. It is elevated (>20 mg/100 mL) following exercise, anesthesia, and certain types of acidosis. The *blood lactate/pyruvate* ratio should be calculated in order to determine the presence of excess lactic acid in blood in acidosis, thiamine deficiency, and decompensated heart disease.

Blood *pyruvic acid* is determined by the reverse procedure; ie, conversion of pyruvate to lactate in the presence of LDH and NADH. Normal blood pyruvic acid ranges from 0.6–1.3 mg/100 mL, by chemical methods and 0.3 to 0.7 mg/100 mL by enzymic procedures.

Nonprotein Nitrogen Compounds—*Nonprotein nitrogen (NPN)* refers to all nitrogen-containing compounds in biologic fluids exclusive of protein. This includes nitrogen from amino acids, low-molecular-weight peptides, urea, nucleotides, uric acid, creatinine, creatine, and ammonia. Blood NPN is usually determined by digestion of a protein-free blood filtrate with sulfuric acid in the presence of a catalyst (SeO_2) to convert nitrogen to ammonium sulfate (Kjeldahl digestion); the excess acid is then neutralized and ammonia determined by Nesslerization or reaction with alkaline hypochlorite.

The normal blood NPN is 25–45 mg/100 mL (48% urea N, 14% amino acid N, 4% creatine N, 1% creatinine N, 3.0% uric acid N, and 30% residual N). In renal damage, NPN is elevated to values ranging from 60–500 mg/100 mL (*azotemia*). As variations in NPN mainly reflect alterations in blood urea nitrogen (BUN), urea determinations are more sensitive and preferred as a guide to kidney function.

The primary pathway of nitrogen metabolism in man is the synthesis of urea from ammonia in the liver and then rapid renal excretion of urea. In renal disease (nephritis), the excretion of urea is diminished and blood NPN and BUN are increased. In BUN procedures, *urea* is enzymatically converted to ammonia by urease; the ammonia is then determined by Nesslerization, reaction with phenol-alkaline hypochlorite, aeration into standard acid and subsequent titration, or reaction with salicylate-nitroprusside reagent at pH 12.0 in the presence of alkaline dichloroisocyanurate to form a green chromogen which can be estimated colorimetrically. The ammonia can also be estimated by spectrophotometric determination of NAD produced in conversion to ammonia and α-ketoglutarate to glutamate by NADH-L-glutamate dehydrogenase. Direct chemical determinations of urea are based on reaction with 2,3-butanedione in an acid medium (Fearon reaction).

BUN (normal = 5–25 mg/100 mL) is increased in chronic and acute nephritis, metallic poisoning, and cardiac failure;

reduced levels occur in rapid dehydration or following diuresis. In severe liver damage due to diminished urea formation, an increase in blood ammonia and decrease in BUN are observed. Urine urea output (6–17 g/day) is an index of *glomerular filtration rate (GFR)* and kidney function. Increased dietary protein and gastrointestinal hemorrhage will increase urine urea. Decreases in urea excretion involve either tubular reabsorption or secretion defects.

The *nitrogen balance* represents the balance between nitrogen input or produced (N_{in}) and nitrogen excreted (N_{out}); in normal individuals $N_{in} = N_{out}$. N_{out} is regulated by renal GFR; in renal disease GFR is decreased, $N_{in} > N_{out}$ and BUN is increased. The rate of urinary excretion of parenterally administered dyes (phenolsulfonphthalein), inulin sodium, *p*-aminohippurate, and mannitol are sensitive indices of GFR in renal clearance studies.

Creatine (methylguanidoacetic acid) and *creatinine* (creatine anhydride) are involved in the physiology of muscle contraction. Creatine phosphate is an intracellular source of high-energy phosphate bonds via the reaction of ATP and creatine kinase. Creatinine is the waste product of creatine metabolism and is the normally excreted compound. Serum creatinine is determined by reaction with alkaline picrate to form a red chromogen. These values usually represent 20–30% non-creatinine-interfering substances. Absolute determinations can be made by absorption of creatinine from protein-free blood filtrates on aluminum silicate prior to the final determination. Creatine is determined after hydrolytic conversion to creatinine with boiling aqueous picric or hydrochloric acid.

Renal clearance of endogenous creatinine is related to GFR and is normally 1–2 g/day (creatinine coefficient = 20–26 mg/kg/24 hours). Normal serum creatinine is 1–2 mg/100 mL; creatine 0.2–1.0 mg/100 mL. Higher values (5 mg/100 mL) indicate glomerular damage or cardiac insufficiency.

Uric acid is a catabolite of purine metabolism as derived from nucleic acids or nucleotide cofactors. Direct methods for determination of uric acid involve reaction with alkaline phosphotungstic acid to form a "tungsten blue," which is estimated colorimetrically. In another method, alcoholic NaOH is added to a protein-free filtrate to eliminate interfering reducing substances (ascorbic acid, glutathione) prior to reduction of uric acid with acid copper chelate to form a cupric chromogen complex.

In indirect procedures, uric acid is hydrolyzed by the enzyme uricase; the decrease in absorbance at 290–293 nm is a function of initial concentrations of uric acid. The normal blood value is 1.5–6.0 mg/100 mL. It is elevated in renal disease, in gout due to increased metabolic pools of uric acid, and in leukemia as a result of increased turnover of cellular nucleoprotein.

Amino acid determinations in blood are performed by conventional colorimetric ninhydrin techniques or reaction with alkaline β-naphthoquinone-4-sulfonate. Normal plasma values range from 3.9–7.8 mg/100 mL. A variety of metabolic disorders may be detected by analysis of increased levels of specific amino acids in urine or blood. Total urine amino acids are determined by formol titration; formaldehyde reacts with basic amino groups and thus permits subsequent titration of the acidic groups of the amino acids. Daily excretion of amino acid nitrogen ranges from 100–400 mg, constituting 1–2% of total urine nitrogen.

Identification and quantitation of specific amino acids in blood and urine are accomplished by paper, thin-layer (TLC), column and ion-exchange chromatographic and electrophoretic separation of electrolytically desalted blood or urine samples. See Chapter 33, *Chromatography.* Abnormal amino acid metabolism (*aminoacidopathies*) usually results in the presence of abnormal quantities of specific amino acids in the urine (aminoaciduria).

The aminoacidurias are divided into two main groups: 1. *Primary overflow aminoaciduria* in which blood amino acids are elevated [phenylketonuria (PKU), maple syrup urine disease (MSUD), tyrosinosis, and alkaptonuria]; 2. Aminoacidurias characterized by elevated amino acid urine levels with normal blood levels (*transport diseases* with a defect in the kidney tubule—eg, cystinuria—and "no threshold" aminoaciduria in which the kidney has no mechanism for reabsorbing the amino acid involved—eg, homocystinuria).

PKU, a disease characterized by mental deficiency, is associated with the presence of phenylpyruvic acid in the urine and elevated serum phenylalanine levels due to an hereditary (autosomal recessive) deficiency of hepatic phenylalanine hydroxylase which converts phenylalanine to tyrosine. The availability of treatment through dietary intake is predicated upon early detection. Many states have passed legislation for mass screening for PKU in all infants. The Guthrie test is performed by placing filter paper discs impregnated with serum or blood on the surface of an agar culture medium containing β-(2-thienyl)alanine at a concentration sufficient to inhibit the growth of a *B subtilis* organism. *Phenylalanine* will reverse this inhibition and the Bacterial Inhibition Assay (BIA) is a direct measure of this amino acid. Serum phenylalanine determinations can also be performed by estimating the fluorescence of a complex with ninhydrin and copper in the presence of L-leucyl-L-alanine.

MSUD is characterized by the odor of the urine and is rapidly fatal to infants. It is associated with a deficiency in the oxidative decarboxylation of α-keto acids leading to an accumulation of both the keto acids and amino acids in the blood and urine (valine, leucine, isoleucine). TLC and BIA assays can be used to detect MSUD.

Alkaptonuria is a rare, hereditary disease in which homogentisic acid cannot be further metabolized due to a lack of homogentisic acid oxidase. This causes homogentisic aciduria, ochronosis, and arthritis.

In *Hartnup disease,* indole and tryptophane appear in the urine due to defective renal and intestinal absorption of tryptophane. Tryptophane is an intermediary metabolite in the synthesis of serotonin (5-hydroxytryptamine) and 5-hydroxyindole acetic acid (HIAA). Excessive production of *serotonin* and the presence of its HIAA metabolite in urine are associated with metastatic carcinoid tumors. HIAA is measured after removal of interfering keto acids with dinitrophenylhydrazine, extraction, and estimation with nitrosonaphthol reagent.

Routine screening tests for congenital metabolic defects and the substance under test in the newborn include PKU (phenylalanine), MSUD (leucine), tyrosinemia (tyrosine), homocystinuria (methionine), histidemia (histidine), valinemia (valine), galactosemia (galactose or galactose uridyl transferase), orotic aciduria (orotidine-1-phosphate decarboxylase), argininosuccinuria (argininosuccinic lyase), hereditary angioneurotic edema (C_1-esterase inhibitor), and sickle-cell disease (hemoglobin S).

The analyses for these substances are based on BIA, metabolite bacterial inhibition assay (MIA), enzyme auxotraph bacterial assay (ENZ-Aux), fluorescent spot tests or TLC and electrophoresis.

Proteins—The *plasma proteins* (albumins, globulins, and fibrinogen) are involved in nutrition, electrolyte and acid-base balance, transport mechanisms, coagulation, immunity, and enzymatic action. *Total plasma proteins* may be determined by Kjeldahl, Nesslerization, specific ion pair (bromcresol green dye plus albumin), or biuret procedures. The last technique is based on the reaction of —CONH— groups joined by carbon or nitrogen linkages in protein with alkaline copper sulfate to yield the biuret complex which can be estimated colorimetrically. Total protein can also be estimated by specific gravity, refractometric or UV spectrometric methods. These

methods are subject to large errors in the presence of a pathology involving increased glucose, lipid, urea, or abnormal protein concentrations.

The *albumin-globulin (A/G) ratio* is determined by the biuret method after precipitation of the globulins with a sodium sulfate-sulfite reagent. The normal range is 5.5–8.0 g% total protein with an A/G ratio of 1.4–2.4. Changes in total protein and A/G ratio occur in kidney and liver disease, multiple myeloma, rheumatoid arthritis, dehydration, hemorrhage, and GI bleeding. Gastrointestinal albumin loss, as seen in GI bleeding, ulcerative colitis, sprue and enteritis, can be detected by monitoring fecal radioactivity after IV injection of ^{51}Cr-human serum albumin.

The physiochemical properties of the plasma proteins—molecular weight (68,000–300,000) and isoelectric point (pH of minimum solubility and ionic neutrality)—provide the basis for the electrophoretic separation of plasma proteins (Fig 32-2). The plasma sample is spotted on a paper or cellulose acetate strip, or in a polyacrylamide gel ("disc" or gel electrophoresis) at pH 8.6. At this pH the proteins are electroanionic and, under the influence of electric current, will migrate to the anode at a rate dependent on their isoelectric point and, in the case of cellulose acetate or gel electrophoresis, their molecular size. The strips are then stained with a protein dye (bromophenol blue, Amidoschwarz, or Ponceau S), and the concentrations of the various proteins are estimated by densitometric scanning.

The normal ranges for the major proteins are (in g%): albumin 3.8–5.0; total globulin 2.0–3.9; α_1-globulin 0.1–0.5; α_2-globulin 0.5–0.9; β-globulin 0.5–1.2; γ-globulin 0.7–1.6.

Ordinary electrophoresis does not identify the subgroups of *immunoglobulins,* IgA, IgM, IgG, and IgE. This is accomplished by immunoelectrophoresis, a process involving electrophoresis and immunodiffusion. The sample is electrophorized in an agar gel (zone electrophoresis) and then antiserum to the specific Ig or to total globulins is placed in a trough aligned parallel to the axis of the original electrophoresis. The serum proteins and antisera diffuse toward each other and form precipitin (antigen-antibody complex) lines. Ordinary cellulose acetate or gel electrophoresis will permit the recognition of diffuse polyclonal elevation of serum immunoglobulins seen in chronic infections, isolated M-protein peaks of macroglobulinemia and multiple myeloma and absent gamma component in a hypogammaglobulinemia or agammaglobulinemia. Immunoelectrophoresis will indicate specific Ig abnormalities, or by noting the presence of any

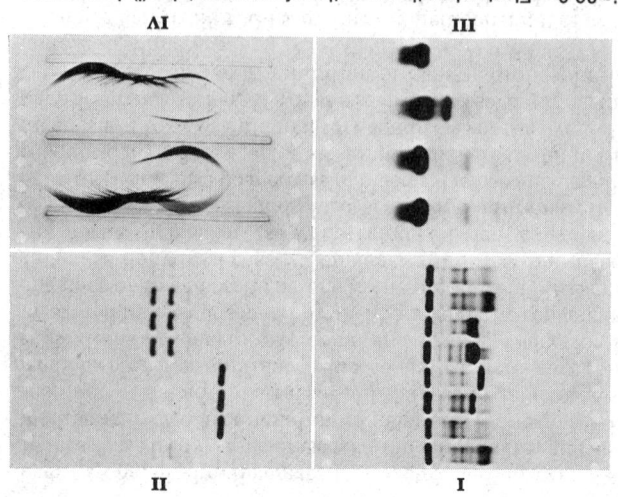

Fig 32-2. Electrophoretic separation of serum proteins (I), isoenzymes (II), hemoglobins (III), and immunoelectrophoresis of plasma protein (IV) (courtesy, Spinco).

Nephelometric techniques detect immunological constituents by measuring the light-scattering properties of various antibody-antigen complexes in a test solution. The Hyland system measures the amount of laser beam deflection at an angle by employing a photomultiplier tube which is sensitive in the red region of the spectrum. Results are calculated by an electronic screening system and read in percent relative light scatter on a digital readout.

Radial immunodiffusion is a simple process which can be also used for quantitation of IgA, IgM and IgG.[15] It is performed by incorporating the antibody in an agar gel and then introducing the antigen or test sera into wells punched in the agar. The antigen diffuses radially out of the well into the surrounding gel media and a visible precipitin line forms where antigen and antibody have reacted. Quantitation of IgA, IgM and IgG aids in the diagnosis and differentiation of collagen diseases, chronic infections and liver disease. IgE is best quantitated by immunoelectrophoresis or RIA (see section on Immunology for basis and principles of RIA).

displacement, bowing, or broadening of the precipitin band will aid in the diagnosis of the paraimmunoglobulin monoclonal diseases such as multiple myeloma, macroglobulinemia or chronic lymphatic leukemia.

Enzymes—Enzymes are proteins whose biologic function is the catalysis of chemical reactions in living systems. Enzymes combine with the substances on which they act (substrate) to form an intermediate enzyme-substrate complex which is then converted to a reaction product and liberated enzyme, which continues its catalytic function. Enzymes are highly specific; a few enzymes exhibit absolute specificity and will catalyze only one particular reaction, while other enzymes will be specific for a particular type of chemical bond, functional group, or stereoisomeric structure.

Most serum enzymes of clinical significance are intracellular in origin and are elevated in hyperactivity disease, malignancy, or injury to cardiac, hepatic, pancreatic, muscle, bone tissue. As the specific tissue involved will determine the type of enzyme that will be elevated, such determinations are valuable diagnostic tools in the differentiation of various pathologic states.

Enzymes are named and classified according to the type of reaction that they catalyze, and to their substrate specificities. Enzyme activity is usually expressed in International Units (IU) where one unit (U) is that amount of enzyme which will catalyze the transformation of 1 μmole of substrate/min at definite temperature, pH and substrate concentration conditions. Refer to Chapter 54 for a more complete discussion of enzymes.

Transferases are enzymes that catalyze the transfer of amino or phosphate groups from one compound to another. Aspartate aminotransferase (AST) and alanine aminotransferase (ALT) are important in clinical diagnosis. These enzymes catalyze the transfer of the amino group from glutamic acid to keto acids (oxaloacetic or pyruvic) to form aspartic and α-ketoglutaric acids with AST (aspartate aminotransferase) and alanine and α-ketoglutaric acid with ALT (alanine aminotransferase).

Colorimetric methods of determination are based on estimation of reaction products (oxaloacetic or pyruvic acid) with dinitrophenylhydrazine, or substrate (α-ketoglutaric acid) by coupling with 6-benzamido-4-methoxy-m-toluidine diazonium chloride.

Spectrophotometric methods of analysis are based on the reaction of the product pyruvate with lactic dehydrogenase and NADH, or of oxaloacetate with malic dehydrogenase and NADH. The rate of NADH utilization is measured by decrease in absorbance at 340 or 360 nm and is directly proportional to transaminase activity.

Normal AST and ALT levels are <40 mU/mL. AST is present in large amounts in liver, cardiac, and skeletal muscle,

whereas ALT is primarily found in liver tissue. AST is elevated in myocardial infarction and Duchenne muscular dystrophy; AST and ALT are increased in liver disease, acute toxic or viral hepatitis, infectious mononucleosis, obstructive jaundice, and hepatic cirrhosis.

Creatine Kinase (CK) is a transferase found in muscle and brain tissue. It catalyzes the transfer of phosphate groups from creatine phosphate to adenosine diphosphate (ADP) to form adenosine triphosphate (ATP). Activated CK activity is measured by following the increase of ATP in the creatinine phosphate-ADP reaction in the presence of glutathione or cysteine thiol activators. The ATP can be measured by fluorimetric determination of light emitted by luciferinase conversion of luciferin to adenyl-oxyluciferin in the presence of ATP. Normal serum levels are <50 mU/mL. It is elevated in myocardial infarction and Duchenne muscular dystrophy, but remains at normal levels in liver disease.

Ornithine transcarbamylase (OTC) in serum is the only enzyme of the urea cycle which has been used in the clinical investigation of liver disease. It catalyzes the conversion of ornithine to citrulline. The normal serum value is 0–0.4 mU/mL.

Oxidoreductases or *dehydrogenases* are enzymes that catalyze hydrogen transfer in cellular oxidation processes. *Lactic* (LDH), *α-hydroxybutyric* (HBDH), *malic* (MDH), *glutamic* (GLDH), *isocitric* (ICDH), *and sorbitol* (SDH) *dehydrogenases* are of diagnostic importance in myocardial and liver disease.

LDH catalyzes the reversible conversion of pyruvic to lactic acid in the presence of NADH. The activity may be estimated colorimetrically by formation of the pyruvic acid hydrazone with 2,4-dinitrophenylhydrazine; spectrophotometric or fluorimetric estimation of NADH in this reaction is also used to estimate enzyme activity. The normal serum LDH value is <200 mU/mL (pyruvate → lactate) and <50 mU/mL (lactate → pyruvate). LDH is increased to a much greater extent and for a more prolonged period than AST or CK in myocardial infarction; it is also increased to varying degrees in certain types of hepatic disease, disseminated malignancies, pernicious anemia, and muscular dystrophy.

Recent advances in protein chemistry and technical methodology have led to fractionation of enzymes, previously thought to be homogeneous, into heterogeneous moieties. These multiple molecular forms of enzymes (*isoenzymes*) have similar substrate specificity but different biophysical properties. LDH, MDH, CK, phosphatases, and leucine aminopeptidase exist in isoenzyme forms.

Serum contains five LDH isoenzymes, each a tetramer composed of one or two monomers. LDH 1 and 2 are found in preponderance in heart, kidney, and RBC; whereas liver and skeletal muscle largely contain LDH 4 and 5. Intermediate forms prevail in lymphatic tissues and many malignancies. Fractionation of LDH isoenzymes is important in the differential diagnosis of cardiac, muscle and liver disease. Fractionation can be accomplished with DEAE-cellulose chromatography, electrophoresis, sulfite or urea inhibition of specific isoenzymes, thermal stability, and substrate concentration requirements.

HBDH reduces α-ketobutyric acid to α-hydroxybutyric acid in the presence of NADH; estimation of the α-keto acid via hydrazone formation or NADH is the basis of activity measurements. The normal serum HBD level is <140 mU/mL; it is elevated in myocardial infarction. LDH-1 is high in HBDH activity. The ratio of total LDH/HBDH is often used in place of LDH isoenzyme determination. Ratios >0.8 are seen in myocardial infarction, and <0.6 in acute liver damage.

MDH and *SDH*, in the presence of NAD, catalyze the conversion of malate or sorbitol to oxaloacetate or fructose, respectively. They are of diagnostic value in myocardial infaction (MDH >48 mU/mL) and acute liver injury (SDH >96 mU/mL).

ICDH oxidizes isocitrate, in the presence of NADP or NAD, to α-ketoglutarate; it is elevated (>5.0 mU/mL) in acute hepatitis.

Hydrolases are enzymes that catalyze the addition of the elements of water across the bond which is cleaved. *Amylases, lipases, phosphatases, 5'-nucleotidase, γ-glutamyl-transpeptidase,* and *leucine aminopeptidase* are specific examples of clinically important hydrolases.

Salivary and pancreatic *amylases* hydrolyze the substrate starch to maltose and dextrins. Amylase activity can be measured by procedures based on the loss in certain properties of starch as it is hydrolyzed (*amyloclastic*), or generation of reducing substances (*saccharogenic*). The amyloclastic methods utilize the decrease in viscosity and turbidity of hydrolyzed water-soluble starch substrates, or the reaction of starch with iodine as the method of estimation. A recent procedure utilizes the colorimetric determination of water-soluble dye-dextrin fragments released by amylolytic hydrolysis of a cross-linked, water-insoluble, dye-starch polymer. The saccharogenic methods determine the reaction products (reducing sugars) by previously described methodology. The normal serum level is 140 mU/mL; elevations are noted in acute pancreatitis, acute abdominal conditions (perforated peptic ulcer, common bile-duct obstruction), and salivary gland disease.

Lipases catalyze the conversion of triglycerides to glycerol and fatty acids. Clinical determinations are based on titrimetric analysis of fatty acids liberated from an emulsified olive oil substrate, or fluorimetric estimation of fluorescein liberated from a fluorescein fatty acid ester substrate. Serum lipase is increased in pancreatic carcinoma.

Phosphatases catalyze the hydrolysis of orthophosphoric acid esters and are classified according to pH of optimal activity into alkaline or acid phosphatases. Activity (alkaline, pH 8–10; acid, pH 4–6) is measured with phenyl phosphate, glycerophosphate, *p*-nitrophenyl phosphate, or thymol-phthalein monophosphate substrates. With the latter two chromogenic substrates, the amount of *p*-nitrophenol or thymolphthalein liberated by phosphatase hydrolysis is estimated colorimetrically in an alkaline medium. With glycerophosphate or phenyl phosphate substrate, the liberated phosphorus is determined by molybdenum blue formation with phosphomolybdic-phosphotungstic acids; phenol may also be estimated with 4-aminoantipyrine or Folin-Ciocalteau reagent.

Acid phosphatase activity may be differentiated by the use of inhibitors in the assay mixture; formaldehyde has no effect on acid phosphatase of prostatic origin, but it inhibits other acid phosphatases, while tartrate is a selective inhibitor of the prostatic enzyme.

Normal values for *alkaline phosphatase* activity depend on the substrate used; elevations in osteomalacia and in bone tumors depend on the degree of osteolytic or osteoblastic activity. The enzyme (isoenzyme) is also elevated in obstructive jaundice, bone and liver disease. *Acid phosphatase* is of a primary diagnostic value in metastatic carcinoma of the prostate.

The enzyme *5'-nucleotidase* is an alkaline phosphomonoesterase that hydrolyzes nucleotides with a phosphate radical attached to the 5'-position of the pentose (eg, adenosine monophosphate). The normal serum value is 17 mU/mL; it is elevated in hepatic disease.

Leucine aminopeptidase (LAP) is an exopeptidase which hydrolyzes the peptide bond adjacent to a free amino group. It liberates amino acids from the *N*-terminal group of proteins and polypeptides in which the free amino group is a L-leucine residue. Activity is determined by spectrophotometric estimation following hydrolysis of the amide bond of a leucin-

amide substrate at 238 nm. Clinical estimations are usually performed on synthetic substrates, and since there is no correlation between cleavage of leucinamide and these substrates, the LAP-like activity is designated *leucine arylamidase.* A fluorometric determination of naphthylamine liberated from a leucyl-β-naphthylamide substrate or colorimetric determination of *p*-nitroaniline liberated from leucine-*p*-nitranilide substrate has also been utilized. The normal value is 8–22 mU/mL; it is elevated in the last trimester of pregnancy, hepato-biliary disease, and pancreatic carcinoma.

Serum *γ-glutamyl transpeptidase* (γGT) is increased in diseases of the liver, bile ducts and pancreas. Together with alkaline phosphatases, LAP and 5'-nucleotidase, γGT is usually tested in the group of cholestasis-indicating enzymes. The assay is based on hydrolysis of γ-glutamyl-*p*-nitranilide.

Serum lysozyme (muramidase) activity is increased in certain types of leukemia. Serum arginase, an enzyme which hydrolyzes arginine to ornithine and urea, and serum guanase are sensitive indicators of hepatic necrosis.

Lyases are enzymes which split C—C bonds without group transfer. *Aldolase* is a glycolic lyase which catalyzes the reversible splitting of fructose 1,6-diphosphate to form dihydroxyacetone phosphate and glyceraldehyde 3-phosphate. In estimation of activity, the triose phosphate reaction products are hydrolyzed with alkali and the resultant trioses are reacted with 2,4-dinitrophenylhydrazine to form chromogenic hydrazones for colorimetric analysis. A spectrophotometric estimation is made by coupling the aldolase reaction products with a dehydrogenase acting on one of the triose phosphates and measuring concomitant changes in NADH. The normal value is <8 mU/mL; it is elevated in muscular dystrophy, polymyositis, and acute hepatitis.

The significance of serum enzyme changes in hepatitis is seen in Fig 32-3A and enzyme activity following myocardial infarction in Fig 32-3B.

Lipids—The major classes of blood lipids are: *fatty acids, cholesterol, triglycerides, phospholipids, and lipoproteins.* Hyperlipidemia is not a single aberration and there are a number of different hyperlipidemic states. Lipid-profile tests include measurements of cholesterol, triglyceride, phospholipids, and determination of lipoprotein phenotypes.

Cholesterol, a sterol molecule, is an essential substance in steroid hormone synthesis by the adrenal cortex and bile acid production in the liver. It exists in blood as the free sterol and as cholesterol esters of fatty acids.

In the determination of *total cholesterol,* the serum is extracted with an alcohol-ether mixture and the cholesterol estimated colorimetrically after reaction with acetic anhydride-sulfuric acid reagent (Liebermann-Burchard reaction). Precipitation of free cholesterol with digitonin will differentiate free from esterified cholesterol. Chromatographic separation of cholesterol from its esters on alumina, silicic acid, or magnesium silicate columns with organic solvents has also been used.

Gas chromatographic procedures have resulted in separation and quantitation of cholesterol, its metabolites, and precursors; this is a type of partition chromatography in which a volatilized sample is partitioned between a liquid stationary phase and a mobile gas phase. The normal adult total serum cholesterol level is 150–270 mg/100 mL; it is increased in hyperlipidemia and specifically in hyper-β-lipoproteinemia, nephrosis, diabetes mellitus, and myxedema, and decreased in hyperthyroidism and hepatic disease. Free cholesterol comprises 20–40% and the ester fraction 60–80% of the total serum cholesterol.

Phospholipids are "compound" or "heterolipids" which contain phosphorus, a nitrogen base and a long-chain fatty acid. Lecithin (phosphatidylcholines) and cephalin (phosphatidylethanolamine or serine) are the principal plasma from the oral cavity of the newborn is an accurate assessment of fetal maturity and the respiratory distress syndrome. Changes in phospholipid biosynthesis during gestation reflect the aging of the fetal lung, as the L/S ratio normally increases.

Tay-Sachs disease is a lipid storage disease in which the central nervous system degenerates because of the progressive intraneuronal accumulation of excess amounts of the sphingolipid ganglioside GM_2. The accumulation of the lipid ganglioside GM_2 in Tay-Sachs disease has been shown to be caused by a lack of the enzyme hexosaminidase A. Therefore, measurement of serum, WBC or amniotic fluid *hexosaminidase A* is important in evaluating carriers and in diagnosing Tay-Sachs disease in the fetus.

Both hexosaminidase A (heat-labile) and hexosaminidase B (heat-stable) can catalyze the conversion of 4-methylumbelliferyl-N-acetylgalactosamine (a synthetic substrate) to N-acetylgalactosamine and 4-methylumbelliferone. The cleavage product, 4-methylumbelliferone, fluoresces under ultraviolet radiation and the intensity of the fluorescence is a measure of the activity of the enzyme. In noncarriers, 50 to 75% of the total hexosaminidase activity is heat-labile (hexosaminidase A), and in carriers 20 to 45% of the total hexosaminidase activity is heat-labile.

The blood fatty acids occur in esterified (EFA) and nonesterified (NEFA) forms. *Triglyceride* determinations are of value in differentiating the hyperlipidemic states, ie, essential (diet-induced) hypertriglyceridemia from familial hypercholesterolemia with or without triglyceridemia. After preliminary separation from phospholipids, triglycerides are most often determined in terms of their glycerol moiety. The glycerol released by saponification is oxidized to formaldehyde and the latter determined by fluorimetric or colorimetric procedures. Triglycerides can also be determined by coupling the glycerol liberated from lipase/α-chymotrypsin treatment of serum with a glycerol kinase-pyruvate kinase-LDH system, and spectrophotometric estimation of NADH. Normal triglyceride levels are 110-140 mg/100 mL. An increase in triglycerides will produce a milky appearance in serum (lipemic). EFA analyses are also based on the reaction of alkaline hydroxylamine with esters of fatty acids to form hydroxamic acids which produce a red color with ferric chloride.

Gas chromatographic procedures have been used to quantitate the various *fatty acids;* ie, palmitic, stearic, oleic, linoleic, and linolenic acids. Mono-, di-, and triglycerides can also be separated into classes and quantitated by column or thin-layer chromatography, and infrared spectroscopy. The total fatty acids of plasma range from 200-450 mg/100 mL in the fasting state; they are derived from glycerides, cholesterol esters and phospholipids.

All the lipids in plasma circulate in combination with protein. The free fatty acids are bound to albumin and the lipids aggregate with other proteins to form *lipoproteins.* Electrophoresis and ultracentrifugation are the principal methods used to separate and identify lipoprotein families. *Chylomicrons* (S_f <400) *pre-β-lipoproteins* (S_f 20-400), *β-lipoproteins* (S_f <400), and *α-lipoproteins* (S_f 0-20), and are the 4 major classes in order of increasing density and migration on cellulose acetate electrophoresis. *Chylomicrons* are representative primarily of dietary or exogenous triglycerides, pre-β-lipoproteins of endogenous glycerides, β-lipoproteins of cholesterol and its esters, and α-lipoproteins of cholesterol and phospholipids. Abnormal lipoproteins that may appear in plasma include: floating β-lipoprotein, lipoprotein X and complexes of normal lipoproteins with IgA and IgG myeloma proteins (autoimmune hyperlipoproteinemia). Age, sex, diet, fasting, posture changes, and trauma can alter the lipid profile.

The lipoprotein classes are usually separated by paper, agarose or cellulose acetate electrophoresis. The strips are stained with fat-soluble dyes (Sudan Black or Oil Red O) and

phospholipids, which normally comprise one-third of total plasma lipids. They are usually bound to lipoproteins. These serum lipids are extracted into an alcohol-ether mixture, digested with sulfuric acid-hydrogen peroxide, and the liberated phosphorus determined by colorimetric techniques. The normal lipid phosphorus is 6-11 mg/100 mL; about one-half is lecithin. The average ratio of cholesterol to lipid phosphorus when cholesterol is normal is 21. Phospholipid changes are usually associated with cholesterol changes and are of interest in coronary artery and liver diseases and the hyperlipoproteinemias.

Sphingolipids differ from lecithin and cephalin. They are phosphate esters of sphingosine bound to choline or ethanolamine and are primarily found in brain tissue (eg, sphingomyelin, galactolipin). The ratio of lecithin to sphingomyelin (L/S) in amniotic fluid or resuscitated amniotic fluid

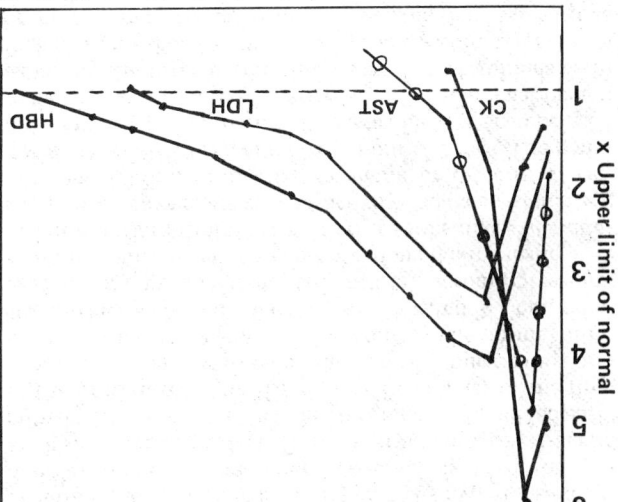

Fig 32-3B. Serum enzymes following myocardial infarction, AST, CK, LDH, and HBD are compared.

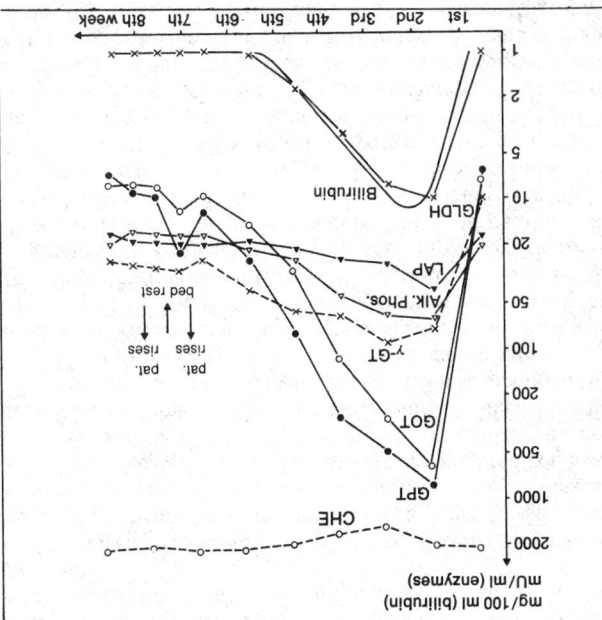

Fig 32-3A. Typical course of alterations in serum enzyme activity in acute viral hepatitis (courtesy, Schmidt E, Schmidt FW Med Welt 21: 805, 1970).

quantitated by densiometric scanning. Primary hyperlipoproteinemias are classified into normal and five abnormal types based on cholesterol and triglyceride levels and lipoprotein analysis. Hyperchylomicronemia (Type I), hyper-β-lipoproteinemia (Type II), broad β-band (Type III), hyper-pre-β-lipoproteinemia (Type IV), and hyper-pre-β-lipoproteinemia and chylomicronemia (Type V) are the major classes. Carbohydrate and fat-tolerance studies, post-heparin lipase activity and clinical symptomatology are also integrated into diagnosis of the various subclasses. The presence or predisposition to coronary artery disease and other disease states is associated with the various types.[16]

Steroids and Other Hormones—The steroids possess a common structure, the perhydrocyclopentanophenanthrene nucleus. This group includes cholesterol, bile acids, androgens, and the adrenocortical, adrenomedullary, estrogenic and progestational hormones.

Androsterone, dehydroepiandrosterone, etiocholan-3α-ol-17-one, 11-ketoandrosterone, 11-ketoetiocholanolone, 11β-hydroxyandrosterone and 11β-hydroxyetiocholanolone are the principal urinary *17-ketosteroids (17KS)*. These androgenic hormones are derived from the adrenal and, in males, testicular function. The principal urinary steroid metabolites in this group of androgens are found both in the free form, and as conjugates of glucuronides, sulfates, or acetates. Their determination in urine involves acid hydrolysis of the conjugates, extraction with organic solvent, reaction with alkaline *m*-dinitrobenzene (Zimmerman reaction), and colorimetric estimation of the chromogen. The individual 17KS can be separated by TLC prior to analysis to obtain further information on the individual steroids. The normal adult urine values are: male, 9–24 mg/day; female, 5–17 mg/day. Decreased excretion is seen in hypoactive disease of the pituitary, gonads, and adrenals. Increased excretion is seen in hyperplasia, cancer or tumors of the adrenals.

Testosterone is the most potent androgen in blood. Measurement of urinary or serum testosterone is useful in distinguishing normal and hypogonadal males and in treating hirsutism in the female. This hormone is determined by gas chromatography, competitive protein-binding, isotope dilution or RIA procedures. Normal serum testosterone is 0.2–1.1 µg/100 mL in the male and <0.1 µg/100 mL in the female.

The natural *estrogenic hormones* are estradiol, estrone and estriol, produced in gonads, adrenals and placenta. The relative amounts of the three estrogens rise and fall concomitantly during the menstrual cycle. Maternal urinary total estrogen excretion, especially estriol, is an indirect index of the integrity and viability of the feto-placental unit. Analysis involves acid or glucuronidase-arylsulfatase hydrolysis of the conjugates, removal of urinary glucose if present, extraction and colorimetric or fluorimetric analysis. In the determination, after acid hydrolysis and ether extraction of the urine, the estrogens are methylated with dimethyl sulfate and chromatographically separated prior to reaction with phenolsulfuric acid to yield a red chromogen for colorimetric analysis. The normal estrogen output is 4–60 µg/24 hours in the female and up to 25 µg in the male. Estrogen deficiency can be related to ovarian failure and pituitary deficiency.

Progesterone is a progestational hormone which is secreted by the corpus luteum of the ovary and also by the adrenal cortex. Serum progesterone determination is of value in detection of ovulation and is a measure of the secretory activity of the placenta during pregnancy. Progesterone is determined in serum by RIA, double-isotope derivatization, gas liquid chromatography or competitive protein binding techniques. Normal menstrual cycle serum progesterone levels vary between 0 and 1.6 µg/100 mL.

Pregnanediol is the principal metabolite of progesterone. Urinary determination of pregnanediol excretion is an indirect index of progesterone levels, but is subject to variation due to individual differences in hepatic metabolism of this hormone and is not representative of total endogenous progesterone production.

Adrenal cortex steroids include glucocorticoids, androgens, estrogens, progesterone, and mineralocorticoids. Glucocorticoids can be determined as plasma cortisol (plasma *17-OH corticosteroids*), urinary free (unconjugated cortisol) or total urinary *17-OH corticosteroids*. The latter are determined in urine as *17-ketogenic steroids (17KGS)*. The 17KS in urine are reduced with borohydride to alcohols; the 17-OH steroids are oxidized with sodium bismuthate or periodate to 17KS and quantitated by the alkaline dinitrobenzene method. The 17-OH steroids can be quantitated directly by the phenylhydrazine-sulfuric acid reaction after hydrolysis of glucuronide conjugates and chromatographic purification. The 17-OH steroid analysis only determines compounds with the dihydroxyacetone side chain, such as tetrahydrocortisol or tetrahydrocortisone; the 17KGS analysis includes the 17-OH-corticosteroids with the dihydroxyacetone side chain and the pregnanetriol type of compound. Normal 17KGS daily urinary excretion is 5–23 mg in the male and 3–15 mg in the female. They are significantly reduced in myxedema and adrenal or anterior pituitary insufficiency. Plasma cortisol is usually measured by fluorimetric or gas chromatography procedures.

Aldosterone is the most active member of the mineralocorticoid group. Determination of urinary aldosterone is of value in differentiating benign essential hypertension from primary aldosteronism (Conn's syndrome) which is caused by an adrenal adenoma and is accompanied by hypertension. A double-isotope derivatization technique is used for this analysis. Urinary aldosterone is acetylated with ^{3}H-acetic anhydride; aldosterone-^{14}C-diacetate standard is added early in the procedure. The ^{3}H/^{14}C specific activity of the final product is measured after chromatographic purification and is a direct measurement of aldosterone. The normal aldosterone levels of about 10 µg/day are elevated in Conn's disease and are usually associated with low serum potassium, sodium retention and low concentration alkaline urine.

The anterior pituitary secretes three substances (*gonadotropins*) which regulate gonadal activity: *follicle-stimulating hormone (FSH), luteinizing hormone or interstitial cell hormone (ICSH, LH)*, and *luteotropin (LTH)*. The gonadotropins are glycoproteins. Bioassay methods can be used to determine gonadotrophic activity. After fractionation and isolation, the urine extract is assayed in test animals as to follicular growth of the ovaries in hypophysectomized animals or increase in testicular, ovarian or uterine weight in various animal models. RIA techniques have been developed for these gonadotropins and represent the most sensitive and precise measurement method.

Analysis of serum or urinary *placental lactogen (HPL)* and *chorionic gonadotropin (HCG)*, a placental-derived protein hormone, is useful in the diagnosis of threatened abortion, hydatiform mole and choriocarcinoma. HCG, pregnanediol and progesterone, and total and fractionated estrogens are useful in testing for pregnancy. HCG and HPL are readily measured by RIA and low values are seen in threatened abortion and intrauterine fetal death.

The increase in HCG in serum or urine of the pregnant female is the basis of a routine *pregnancy test*. Test components consist of an antigen in the form of HCG latex particles and an HCG antiserum. When antiserum is mixed with urine containing a detectable level of HCG, it is neutralized and no agglutination of latex-antigen particles occur (*agglutination inhibition test*). Commercial application of the HCG assay gives laboratories a rapid accurate pregnancy test by taking advantage of monoclonal antibody specificity and sensitivity. A monoclonal slide procedure on urine, Duoclon (*Organon Diagnostics*), uses two different monoclonal antibodies, one against HCG and one against the HCGβ subunit for maximum specificity. Agglutination indicates a positive test with a sensitivity level of 500 mIU HCG/mL, detecting pregnancy a few days after conception.

Human growth hormone and *insulin* are proteins which are of diagnostic value in growth-rate studies and diabetes. They are best quantitated by RIA.

Epinephrine and *norepinephrine* are biologically active catecholamines derived from the adrenal medulla and sympathetic nerve endings. Catecholamines are measured in blood and urine after fractionation on alumina or ion-exchange columns, oxidation at pH 3.5 or 6.0, and subsequent fluorimetric analysis. Urine catecholamines are increased to >350 μg/24 hours in adrenal medullary tissue tumors (pheochromocytoma). The normal plasma level is 2.1–6.5 μg/L, with about 80% as norepinephrine.

Vanillylmandelic acid (VMA) is the urine metabolite of these two catecholamines. Its quantity in urine reflects the endogenous secretion of catecholamines. VMA can be determined colorimetrically, after extraction of the urine with ethyl acetate, and diazotization with *p*-nitroaniline and ethanolamine in the presence of carbonate ion. VMA can also be measured spectrophotometrically following periodate oxidation to vanillin and solvent extraction. The normal output is 0–12 mg/24 hours.

Homovanillic acid (HVA) is not a metabolite of epinephrine or norepinephrine, but is produced from a common precursor, dopamine. Elevated HVA excretion is diagnostic in cases of neuroblastoma.

The biosynthesis of *serotonin* (5-hydroxytryptamine) and urinary excretion of its metabolite, 5-hydroxyindoleacetic acid (5-HIAA) are increased in argentaffine tumors. These tumors have a very large capacity to metabolize tryptophane stores to serotonin. Urinary 5-HIAA increases from 1–7 mg/24 hours to as much as 1 g/24 hours in this type of tumor.

Bilirubin, a tetrapyrrole which is derived from senescent red cell degradation, normally occurs in low concentration in the blood. In bile it is present as the water-soluble conjugated acyldiglucuronide. In blood, bilirubin is tightly bound to plasma albumin. The reduction of bilirubin in the intestine yields urobilinogen which is, in turn, oxidized to a brown pigment—urobilin.

Serum bilirubin is determined by coupling with diazotized sulfanilic acid to form azobilirubin for colorimetric analysis. The *direct or conjugated bilirubin* test is performed in aqueous media; the *indirect or free bilirubin* analysis is performed in methanol or caffeine-sodium benzoate solution. Normal values in serum are: direct, 0–0.3 mg/100 mL; total, 0–1.5 mg/100 mL.

Clinical jaundice is a yellowing of the tissues associated with hyperbilirubinemia; in hemolytic disease of the newborn due to Rh and ABO incompatibilities, indirect serum bilirubin is elevated, whereas acute hepatitis results in increases in the direct type.

Electrolytes—The normal plasma electrolyte level is 154 mEq/L of cations and 154 mEq/L of anions. The osmotic effects of chloride, bicarbonate, sodium, and potassium are important in the maintenance of normal muscle contraction and water distribution between cells, plasma, and interstitial fluid.

Flame photometry, atomic absorption spectroscopy, neutron-activation analysis, X-ray fluorescence, ion-specific electrodes and colorimetric techniques are used in the identification, and determination of cations or anions in biological fluids. Advances in technology have developed multi-phase systems capable of measuring not only sodium and potassium but also chloride, carbon dioxide, and calcium simultaneously.

Sodium and *potassium* serum concentrations are readily measured by flame photometry or highly sensitive and specific atomic-absorption spectroscopy. The latter technique is similar to emission-flame photometry, except that it measures energy as it is absorbed by atoms rather than as it is emitted by atoms. Both techniques are based on the characteristic absorption or emission wavelengths of the cations. Ion-specific glass electrodes are also used for Na+ and K+ determinations eliminating the use of a flame or combustible gas and can be performed on whole blood, plasma, or serum.

Chloride levels in serum or urine are determined by titration with acid mercuric nitrate solution in the presence of s-diphenylcarbazone indicator. They also may be determined potentiometrically with a silver-silver chloride pH electrode assembly. The normal serum values are 135–155 mEq Na/L, 3.9–5.6 mEq K/L, and 95–106 mEq Cl/L; urine levels are 150–197 mEq Na/day, 20–64 mEq K/day, and 180–270 mEq Cl/day.

Serum sodium, potassium, chloride and bicarbonate determinations are useful indicators in adrenal cortical insufficiency, renal and cardiac failure, anuria, dehydration, alimentary tract diseases associated with diarrhea and vomiting, and increased renal electrolyte excretion (diuretic therapy). The determination of excess *chloride* (>50 mEq/L) in the perspiration of patients with pancreatic *cystic fibrosis* is an accurate diagnostic tool. Perspiration is stimulated by placing the patient's hand in a plastic bag for 15–20 min or, preferably, by an iontophoresis technique in which pilocarpine nitrate ions are transported through small areas of the skin to produce local perspiration. The chloride content may be quantitated with silver nitrate–potassium chromate-impregnated papers or with selective ion electrodes.

Bicarbonate, phosphates, sodium, potassium, and chloride concentrations are related to maintenance of acid-base balance in the body. The pH of the blood reflects the state of the acid-base balance and is mathematically related to HCO₃⁻ concentration and partial pressure of CO₂ (pCO₂) in blood by the Henderson-Hasselbalch equation.

$$pH = 6.1 + \log \frac{[HCO_3^-]}{[H_2CO_3]}$$

Blood pH, as measured electrometrically, has a normal range of 7.36–7.40 for venous samples and 7.38–7.42 for arterial samples. The *pCO₂ level* in blood is determined by measuring the pH of the blood at three different pCO₂ concentrations—one native to the blood and the other two obtained by equilibration with gas mixtures of known pCO₂. Blood bicarbonate levels also may be determined by measuring the amount of acid neutralized by plasma or serum and pCO₂ calculated by the above equation. The relationship between pCO₂ and carbonic acid concentration is:

$$[H_2CO_3] = 0.03 \times pCO_2 \qquad \frac{mM \ per \ L.}{mm \ Hg}$$

The role of oxygen and hemoglobin in respiration has been discussed previously. Measurements of blood pH and CO₂ content are used in differentiating respiratory acidosis (low pH, high CO₂) from metabolic acidosis (low pH, low CO₂). *Blood oxygen* (pO₂) and *percent oxygen saturation* are measured by a polarographic method; the blood sample is placed in a chamber and separated from a combined platinum and silver-silver chloride electrode by a polypropylene membrane. By diffusion through the membrane, equilibrium is established between the pO₂ of the blood and a film of solution in contact with the electrode. A current, which is proportional to blood pO₂, is generated after application of a polarizing voltage.

Calcium and phosphorus are important minerals in the processes of bone calcification, nerve irritability, muscle contraction, and blood coagulation. Calcium is present in plasma as an ultrafilterable (ionic and nonionic) form, and a electrolytes, blood acid-base balance, routine urinalysis, and the clearance of administered compounds in the urine. Most *clearance studies* are performed with substances that are not resorbed or secreted by the renal tubules: inulin, mannitol, sodium *p*-aminohippurate, or ^{125}I-iothalamate sodium (sodium 5-acetamido-2,4,6-triiodo-*N*-methylisophthalamate). These substances are administered intravenously and the rate of urine clearance and glomerular filtration is estimated by analysis of the urine. The excretory capacity of the renal tubular epithelium can be determined by measuring the clearance rate of phenolsulfonphthalein (PSP). The dye is injected IV and the rate of its clearance in urine is determined. PSP is loosely bound to serum albumin and is rapidly removed from the blood by the renal tubules.

Sodium iodohippurate (^{125}I), which is almost completely extracted from the blood on a single passage through the kidney, has also been used in renal function studies; a *reno-gram* or isotopic scan of both kidneys is performed. The test provides data on renal tubular secretion, renal vascular competence and renal evacuation and is primarily useful as a comparison of individual kidney function. It is important to note that 50% of kidney function can be compromised without any significant change in the routine renal function parameters.

Thyroid function tests usually measure the circulating levels of the thyroid hormones, and not the end-organ effect. The thyroid gland converts inorganic iodide to *thyroxine* (T_4) and *triiodothyronine* (T_3). T_3 and T_4 are stored in the colloid part of the gland as part of the thyroglobulin molecule. Hypothalamic *thyrotropin-releasing hormone* (TRH) mediates the release of the pituitary thyrotropin (*thyroid-stimulating hormone, TSH*). Excess levels of circulating T_4 depress and low levels of T_4 increase TSH release. TSH stimulates proteolytic degradation of thyroglobulin to release T_4 and T_3, and increases organification of iodine. T_4 accounts for 90% of secreted thyroid hormones and exists in blood bound to *thyroxine-binding globulin* (*TBG*) or *thyroxine-binding prealbumin* (*TBPA*) or to albumin. T_3 is not protein-bound and has 5–10 times the biological potency of T_4 on a weight basis. Therefore, T_4 represents the major part of protein-bound iodine (PBI). The level of *free thyroxine* (FT_4), the active fraction in blood, is regulated by T_4 and T_3 release and the levels of binding proteins in blood and tissues.

The uptake of orally administered Na ^{131}I preparations by the thyroid gland can be estimated by isotopic scanning of the gland 24 hr after ^{131}I administration and is an index of glandular function (hyperactive, >50% uptake; hypoactive, <15%).

PBI determinations are based on precipitation of protein-bound thyroxine, removal of inorganic iodine by basic- or anion-exchange chromatography, alkaline incineration to convert thyroxine to inorganic iodide, and finally, quantitation of iodide by reaction with arsenous acid and ceric ammonium sulfate. PBI is a good estimate of total circulating hormonal iodine. The normal range is 4–8 µg/100 mL serum.

T_4 can be determined by column chromatography in which the T_4 is separated and isolated by ion-exchange chromatography, and then analyzed colorimetrically. Non-isotope thyroid assays have been developed using fluorescence polarization methods for T_4 and free thyroxin index. In the competitive protein-binding assay for T_4, serum T_4 competes with ^{125}I-T_4 for binding sites on a known amount of TBG. The ratio of bound to free ^{125}I-T_4 is determined by adsorption of ^{125}I-T_4 not bound to TBG on an anion-exchange resin embedded in a polyurethane sponge or a porous dextran gel, and is a direct index of T_4 levels. The presence of mercurials, inorganic iodide, or iodinated radiographic compounds in serum will interfere with the T_4 column and PBI procedures. The competitive binding procedure will be affected by the presence of highly protein-bound drugs or changes in TBG

protein-bound fraction. Blood phosphorus consists of inorganic phosphorus, organic phosphate ester (G-6-P, ATP), and phospholipids.

Serum and urine calcium levels are routinely determined by titration with EDTA or EGTA using a fluorescent calcein or calcichrome indicator. Other methods are based on colorimetric analysis of calcium-methylthymol blue complex in the presence of 8-quinolinol to prevent interference by magnesium. Bis-(*o*-hydroxyphenylimino)ethane forms a colored complex with calcium and in the presence of polyvinylpyrrolidone, to inhibit phosphate interference, is a sensitive and specific method for calcium. Calcium is best determined by atomic-absorption spectroscopy. As with all cations, calcium can be determined by emission- or absorption-flame photometry.

Inorganic phosphorus levels are determined by reaction with acid molybdate reagent to form phosphomolybdic acid which, in turn, is reduced with aminonaphtholsulfonic acid or *p*-dimethylaminophenol sulfate to give a blue complex which is estimated colorimetrically. Normal serum levels are: 2.5–4.5 mg P/100 mL, 9–11 mg Ca/100 mL.

Calcium levels are decreased and phosphorus increased in hyperparathyroidism; an opposite effect is seen in hyperparativity of this gland. In rickets and osteomalacia, the concentrations of both elements are decreased.

Copper, magnesium, zinc, and iron are trace elements in blood. They are readily quantitated by flame photometric, colorimetric or atomic-absorption techniques.

Organ Function Tests—Analyses of various blood or urine constituents, determination of metabolic excretion rates of exogenous compounds or endogenous metabolites, and effect of exogenous stimuli on these parameters are utilized for evaluation of *in situ* activity and function of various organs. Organ function studies are performed in diseases associated with the liver, kidney, parathyroid, thyroid, and pituitary gland, gastrointestinal tract, pancreas, adrenals and gonads. The principles and significance of the analysis used in such evaluations have also been described in other sections of this chapter.

Tests for *hepatic function* are based on bilirubin metabolism and excretion, carbohydrate metabolism (galactose tolerance test), plasma-protein changes (cephalin flocculation test and A/G ratio), abnormal fat metabolism, detoxification mechanisms (hippuric acid synthesis), excretion of injected substances [bromosulfophthalein (BSP)], prothrombin formation and previously discussed enzyme levels.

Diseases of the liver are due to cellular alterations (hepatocellular) or obstructions to the flow of bile (obstructive jaundice). Hepatocellular liver disease can be of the chronic (postnecrotic cirrhosis, carcinoma) or acute (viral hepatitis, alcoholism, toxin- and chemical-induced) types.

The *cephalin flocculation test* is based on the flocculation of cephalin-emulsified cholesterol by γ-globulin. In normal serum an albumin-like protein will inhibit this reaction; in hepatic diseases, which produce abnormal γ-globulin or reduced albumin levels, the flocculation will occur.

The *detoxification mechanisms of the liver* can be evaluated by intravenous administration of sodium benzoate and estimation of the benzoic acid metabolite, hippuric acid, in the urine. In hepatoparenchymal disease, a reduced capacity of the liver to form hippuric acid by conjugation of glycine and benzoic acid is observed.

The ability of the liver to excrete an injected dye is determined in the *BSP test*; the serum is analyzed for dye concentration at a suitable time interval after IV administration of 2–5 mg BSP/kg. Radioiodinated (^{131}I) Rose Bengal Sodium dye has also been used in dye-excretion studies with isotopic estimation of urine dye levels.

Kidney function tests are based on the determination of blood nonprotein nitrogen (urea, uric acid and creatinine),

Table IV—Reference Values[a]

Electrolytes

Calcium	9.0–10.6 mg/dL	2.25–2.65 mmol/L
Chloride		98–109 mmol/L
CO_2 content		23–30 mmol/L
Magnesium	1.2–2.4 mEq/L	0.6–1.2 mmol/L
Phosphorus	2.5–5.0 mg/dL	0.81–1.62 mmol/L
Potassium		3.7–5.3 mmol/L
Sodium		138–146 mmol/L

Metabolites

Bilirubin	0.1–1.2 mg/dL	1.7–20.5 µmol/L
Cholesterol	150–250 mg/dL	3.9–6.5 mmol/L
Creatinine	0.7–1.5 mg/dL (adults)	62–123 µmol/L
Glucose	60–95 mg/dL	3.33–5.28 mmol/L
Iron	50–165 µg/dL	9.0–29.5 µmol/L
Triglycerides	20–180 mg/dL	0.22–1.98 mmol/L
Urea nitrogen (BUN)	8–26 mg/dL	2.9–9.3 mmol/L
Uric acid	2.5–7.0 mg/dL	0.15–0,41 mmol/L

Proteins and enzymes

Alanine aminotransferase	(ALT, SGPT)	5–40 U/L at 37°
Albumin	3.5–5.0 g/dL	35–50 g/L
Alkaline phosphatase	35–120 U/L at 37° (adults)	50–400 U/L at 37° (children)
Amylase	60–180 Somogyi Units	110–330 U/L
Aspartate aminotransferase	(AST, SGOT)	8–40 U/L at 37°
Carcinoembryonic antigen (CEA)	<2.5 ng/mL	<2.5 µg/L
Creatine kinase (CK)		10–180 U/L at 37°
Glutamyl transferase (GGT)		5–40 U/L at 37°
Lactate dehydrogenase (LDH)	60–220 U/L at 37°	(lactate → pyruvate)
Total protein	6.0–8.0 g/dL	60–80 g/L

Hormones

Cortisol in plasma	7–20 µg/dL (at 8:00 AM)	3–13 µg/dL (at 4:00 PM)
	(200–550 mmol/L)	(80–360 mmol/L)
Cortisol (FREE) in urine	20–90 µg/24 hours	55–248 nmol/24 hours
Follicle-stimulating hormone (FSH)	Adult males	Adult Females
	2–15 mIU/mL	Follicular phase 3–15 mIU/mL
		Ovulatory spike 10–50 mIU/mL
		Luteal Phase 3–15 mIU/mL
		Postmenopause 30–200 mIU/mL
17-Hydroxycortico-steroids in urine	3–10 mg/24 hours	
17-Ketosteroids in urine	5–15 mg/24 hours	(adult females)
	8–20 mg/24 hours	(adult males)
	0.1–3.0 mg/24 hours	(prepubertal children)
Luteinizing hormone (LH)	Adult males	Adult females
	5–25 mIU/mL	Follicular phase 5–30 mIU/mL
		Ovulatory spike 50–150 mIU/mL
		Luteal phase 5–40 mIU/mL
		Postmenopause 30–200 mIU/mL
Metanephrine in urine	<1.3 mg/24 hours	
Prolactin	1–20 ng/mL (males)	1–25 ng/mL (females)
	(1–20 µg/L)	(1–25 µg/L)
Thyroxine (Ty)	5.5–12.5 g/dL (adults)	7.8–16.0 µg/dL (newborns)
	(72–163 nmol/L)	(101–208 nmol/L)
Vanillylmandelic acid (VMA) in urine	<6.8 mg/24 hours	

[a] Serum specimens unless otherwise indicated.[17]

levels in serum. The normal range of serum T_4 is 2.9–6.4 µg/100 mL by column and 3.0–7.0 µg/100 mL by binding assay. T_4 and PBI are increased in hyperthyroidism and early stages of hepatitis. T_4 and PBI are decreased in hypothyroidism and nephrosis.

FT_4 is also determined in a competitive protein-binding assay in which $^{125}IT_4$ and serum are incubated, and then dialysed to determine the percent dialyzable $^{125}I\text{-}T_4$. FT_4 analysis is used in suspected abnormalities in protein-binding globulins. T_4 binding capacity of serum TBG, albumin and prealbumin can be determined after electrophoretic separation of these proteins.

T_3 analysis is determined by the resin uptake test. The uptake of $^{125}I\text{-}T_3$ by a resin is determined in the presence of the test serum. In hyperthyroidism, the primary TBG-binding sites are saturated and $^{125}I\text{-}T_3$ is taken up by the resin. The resin uptake is decreased in hypothyroidism, and most of $^{125}I\text{-}T_3$ is bound to TBG in serum. A *free thyroxine index* can be obtained by multiplying T_3 (resin) × T_4 (competitive binding) × 0.01. This product deviates from normal in the same direction as T_3 and T_4 in hyperthyroidism and hypothyroidism. This product is stable during euthyroidism in spite of changes in binding proteins, eg, a euthyroid patient on phenytoin therapy will show a decreased TBG and T_4 and increased T_3, but (T_4 × T_3) is normal. The indication of hyper- or hypothyroidism in the presence of abnormal amounts of TBG is observed in the (T_4 × T_3) product.

The determination of *TSH* by RIA appears to be the most useful test in discriminating patients with primary hyperthyroidism from the euthyroidism or hypothyroidism secondary to pituitary disease. Serum TSH is increased in the primary disease state.

The *PBI conversion ratio* is an estimate of the rate of conversion of inorganic iodide to PBI. Radioiodide-(^{131}I) is administered to the subject; after 24 hours, a sample of blood is obtained and the ^{131}I to PB^{131}I is estimated by radiochromatographic procedures with ion-exchange resins (normal conversion, 13–42%).

Adrenocortical function is evaluated by estimation of serum or urinary 17-ketosteroids and 17-hydroxycorticosteroids (17-OH-CS) (androgen and corticosteroid metabolism), serum electrolytes (aldosterone metabolism) and blood adrenocorticotrophic hormone (ACTH) levels in the basal state, after stimulation with IM or IV ACTH, or after adrenal inhibition with dexamethasone. In the normal individual, ACTH will increase plasma cortisol and urine 17-OH-CS, and dexamethasone will suppress plasma cortisol. Metapirone, an inhibitor of 11β-hydroxylase, will cause selective secretion of compound S (11-deoxycortisol) by the adrenals in place of cortisol. Compound S will not inhibit the adrenal-pituitary feedback mechanism, the pituitary will secrete more ACTH, and the adrenal will secrete more compound S. Determination of urinary 17-OH-CS or tetrahydro-compound S (THS) following metapirone administration is a good index of the functional integrity of the pituitary-adrenal axis; patients with virilizing adrenal hyperplasia excrete excessive THS due to a 11β-hydroxylase defect.

Common chemistry reference values are listed in Table IV.[17]

Automated Analysis—Automation of analytical techniques used in blood and urine chemistry, hematology, blood typing and immunology has increased the productivity and accuracy of the clinical laboratory.[18] *Computerization* of the automated analytical system has also increased rapidity of reporting test results, reduced clerical error, and provided a unified and updated report of the laboratory tests for each patient.

In the SMA-12 (or SMA-20) Autoanalyzer (*Technicon*), a continuously-operating, multiple-channel proportioning pump moves the samples, diluents, and reagent streams. Air bubbles segment the flowing streams of samples and reagents, which may then flow through dialyzers to remove interfering substances, move them into chambers preset at desired temperatures, and, finally, into detection devices (colorimeters, fluorometers, flame photometers, spectrophotometers). A serum standard is run simultaneously with the samples. The results can be read directly from a recorder or can be coupled into a digital computer output. Sequential multiple analyses in the SMA-12 are accomplished by distributing the sample to 12 different analytical streams, so that all 12 analyses are in progress at the same time. The *SMA-12 profile* usually determines calcium, inorganic phosphorus, glucose, BUN, uric acid, cholesterol, total protein, albumin, total bilirubin, alkaline phosphatase, LDH and AST. The Mark X (*Hycel*), Ektachom 400 (*Kodak*), ACA, (*Dupont*) and DSA-560 (*Beckman*) are also used in automated clinical laboratory techniques.

The rapid growth of more sophisticated chemistry analyzers increase the capacity of any clinical laboratory and is associated with small specimen requirements incorporating batch analysis, profiles, and stat capabilities. In addition to routine chemistry testing, the systems test for enzymes, immunoassay, therapeutic drug tests, coagulation (fibrinogen, antithrombin III, plasminogen) and electrolytes. Techniques eliminating liquid requirements of other reagent systems are available from *Kodak* and *Ames* utilizing dry reagents. The reagents are impregnated in pads on a strip or slide and read by a reflectance photometer.

Automated hematology and simultaneous determination of RBC, WBC, hemoglobin and hematocrit, MCV, MCH, and MCHC can be performed on the SMA-7A (*Technicon*) Analyzer. The automated Technicon Hemalog system will provide data of SMA-7A and CCV (conductivity cell volume), prothrombin time, partial thromboplastin time and platelet count. *Automated leukocyte differential* was previously discussed in the *Hematology* section.

Urine

The formation of urine and its excretion are critical physiological activities of the body which provide a mechanism for the maintenance of a constant internal environment for all cells, tissues and organs. This internal ecology of the body is well recognized and is known as homeostasis. Inasmuch as the urine reflects what is occurring within the body, it offers a fluid which is an important source of information that is most useful as an aid in the definition of states of health and disease. More specifically, the kidney, by means of urine formation, (1) regulates the body water, (2) excretes metabolic waste products, many of which are of a nitrogenous nature, (3) excretes toxic substances of both endogenous and exogenous origin, (4) regulates the electrolyte equilibrium of the body by either excreting or retaining each specific ion, (5) maintains the delicate balance of pH within the body by ex-

Table V—Normal Constituents of Urine

Constituent	g/day	Constituent	g/day
Water	1400	Amino acids	2.1
Total solids	60	Purine bases	0.01
Urea	30	Phenols	0.03
Uric acid	0.4	Proteins (total)	0.025
Hippuric acid	0.9	Chloride (as NaCl)	12
Creatinine	1.2	Sodium	5
Indican	0.01	Potassium	2
Citric acid	0.8	Calcium	0.2
Lactic acid	0.2	Magnesium	0.15
Oxalic acid	0.03	Sulfur (total)	1.0
Nicotinic acid	0.00025	Phosphate as P	1.1
Allantoin	0.04	Ammonia	0.7

cretion of excess acid or excess base and, (6) provides an important route for the elimination of pharmaceutical agents and their break-down products from the body. Normal urine contains several thousand compounds most of which occur in minute quantities. Table V identifies some of the constituents of normal urine which are of particular significance.

Urine is quite widely studied as a means of identifying abnormalities associated with disease. The importance of such study is emphasized by the fact that the number of tests carried out on urine far exceeds those made on all other body fluids combined. Urine not only is of importance in providing information relating to kidney disease, but it may provide information relative to many other body activities. Information from urine studies is of diagnostic value in functional diseases of the kidney, liver, pancreas, blood, bone, muscle and the urinary, gastrointestinal and cardiovascular systems. Urine studies provide vital clinical information on electrolyte and water balance, acid-base equilibrium, intermediary metabolism, inborn errors of metabolism, drug abuse, intoxication, pregnancy and hormone balance. Most of these parameters have been discussed in previous sections and this section will be devoted to routine urinalysis.

It is important to recognize that urine test information, like all other laboratory data, helps provide a picture of the whole body, but any single result requires interpretation to be most meaningful. It should also be recognized that negative results can be essentially as useful as positive results in a great many instances. The ready availability of urine is an advantage that makes it practical as a material for monitoring the course of treatment of disease as well as for its recognition and definition.

Most urine examinations include observations with regard to the majority of the following—color, odor, turbidity, pH, protein, glucose (or reducing substances), ketone bodies (acetone), occult blood, bilirubin, urobilinogen, bacteria (culture or chemical tests), specific gravity, and microscopic examination of sediment, including erythrocytes, leukocytes, casts, epithelial cells, crystals, bacteria, parasites, and exfoliative cytology. A *"routine" urinalysis* varies in different institutions but ordinarily involves the inclusion of the majority of the above tests. Urine for laboratory study should be collected in clean containers—preferably into a disposable unit (polystyrene tube) with a capacity of 15 mL which can be used for collecting, transporting, centrifuging and testing. Refrigeration is desirable for any specimen which is not tested within 1 to 2 hours. If urine is to be transported through the mails or is to be held for significant time intervals at room temperature, it is desirable to add a urine preservative (formalin, methenamine, thymol, toluene) which will interfere with microbial growth in the specimen. Several proprietary urine preservative tablets are available. If urine is allowed to stand at room temperature, bacteria will grow in the specimen and cause degradation of many urine constituents.

Frequently, the bacteria decompose urea into ammonium carbonate with a resulting increase in the alkalinity of the specimen. Formed elements, particularly casts and red blood cells, disintegrate in alkaline solution.

The majority of urine tests are done on random specimens but, in certain instances, it is necessary to have a 24-hour specimen for certain specialized analyses. For urine sugar testing in diabetes detection, it is desirable to utilize a postprandial urine specimen (ie, after a meal). For protein tests, chemical or culture tests for bacteriuria, the first morning specimen is preferred. Most laboratories utilize commercially-available, standardized, reagent-impregnated strips ("dipstrips") or tablets (*Ames*) for routine urinalysis. The specific test procedures with these reagents will be discussed.

Instrumentation in Urinalysis—Automated urine testing systems, semi-automated reagent strip readers and a system which performs the complete urinalysis procedure have been developed. The strip reader is a reflectance photometer which measures urine pH, protein, glucose, ketones, blood, bilirubin, nitrate, and urobilinogen. The IRIS AIM (*International Remote Imaging Systems*) measures urine specific gravity by refractometry, urine sediment by staining and classifies analytes, controlled fluid dynamics, video microscopy with an image processor, a chemistry system to read a standard dipstick by reflectance photometry and color and appearance. These systems achieve standard results for routine urinalysis and increase accuracy and precision.

Volume—The normal volume of urine excreted during a 24-hour period is usually in the range of 1000–1500 mL. It is possible for a healthy person to modify the volume either by severe fluid restriction or by ingestion of excessive quantities of fluid. In certain disorders there is a change in urine volume. Urine volume increases are identified as polyuria and are encountered in diabetes mellitus, diabetes insipidus and in certain stages of chronic renal disease. Urine volume is increased during diuretic therapy and with the ingestion or injection of large volumes of fluid. A decrease in urine volume usually occurs in dehydration, water restriction and in acute or terminal renal disease. Extensive water loss from severe diarrhea or vomiting causes oliguria or decreased urine volume. Acute renal failure precipitated by shocks, poisons or transfusion reaction may result in a complete absence of urine excretion or anuria. In the majority of instances urine study does not require volume measurements, but these are quite critical in severely ill persons where oliguria or anuria is present.

Specific Gravity-Osmolality—The urine density or specific gravity is related to the amount of solids excreted in a given volume of urine. In the majority of instances in healthy persons the specific gravity varies between 1.010 and 1.030 and is related to dietary habits of fluid and food ingestion and secondarily to the loss of fluid by other routes such as by extensive sweating. The measurement of urine density or specific gravity is a part of "routine urinalysis," and as such provides information with regard to water and solids turnover in the body. The specific gravity information alone is not nearly so important as it may be in conjunction with other observations. Thus, if dehydration is suspected a specific gravity in the mid-range of 1.015 would cast a doubt about dehydration unless there was a concurrent renal dysfunction.

The kidney possesses a remarkable ability to either form a concentrated urine or a very dilute urine ranging from a specific gravity of 1.001 to 1.032. This concentrating or diluting capacity is diminished in cases where there is a loss of renal function. In fact one of the sensitive tests for measuring renal function involves so-called dilution-concentration tests where fluid is administered or withheld, and the specific gravity of the urine is measured. With serious loss of renal function, the kidney cannot excrete a urine in excess of 1.020 even with marked fluid restriction. In advanced renal disease the specific gravity of the urine may become "fixed" or constant in the range of 1.010 to 1.012 with all urine being of this specific gravity regardless of whether there is overhydration or dehydration.

Specific gravity is readily measured by means of a special hydrometer, which is called a urinometer. There is a correlation between the density of urine and its refractive index, and a special refractometer has been designed which gives readings in specific gravity units on a single drop of urine.

Certain abnormal constituents of urine, such as glucose or protein, when present in high concentrations, will cause significant increases in specific gravity. Certain X-ray contrast media when excreted in the urine will also cause marked increases in specific gravity.

Urine specific gravity is only an indirect index of solute concentration, ie, 1 mole of urea will produce a lower specific gravity than 1 mole of glucose. Osmolality is a direct measure of the molal concentration of solutes in solution regardless of their molecular weight, ie, 1 mole of NaCl dissociates into 1 mole of chloride ion and 1 mole of sodium ion. Osmolality is determined in a direct-reading osmometer by comparing the freezing point of urine with that of a standard sodium chloride solution.

The kidneys normally excrete 800 to 1400 mOsm/kg (an osmol is that weight of any substance when dissolved in water depresses the freezing point 1.86°) of solutes per day. Man concentrates urine and eliminates the daily solute load at a maximum volume of 1200 mOsm/kg water. Urine osmolality is an inverse function of urine volume in the normal catabolic state. Urine volume is regulated by the antidiuretic hormone (ADH) and sodium excretion by the hormone aldosterone. Increased osmolality of body fluids stimulates, and increased dilution inhibits release of ADH. The major determinant of body fluid osmolality is sodium. Sodium conservation is mediated through the renin-angiotensin-aldosterone axis. Determinations of plasma and urine sodium, and osmolality and urinary volume are of diagnostic value in Addison's disease, vasomotor nephropathy (acute tubular necrosis), inapparent volume depletion, incomplete urinary tract obstruction and hepatorenal disease.

pH (Reaction)—Freshly voided urine usually has a slightly acid reaction. The normal pH range is 5 to 8, and essentially this is also the abnormal pH range. The kidneys, by reason of excreting a urine of variable pH, provide a regulatory mechanism for the body to get rid of excess acid or alkaline waste products. Since the normal pH range and the abnormal pH range are comparable, the measurement of pH alone provides minimal information, but when utilized in conjunction with other information, it is a very useful urinary parameter. In conditions of acidosis, the urine is quite acid and in conditions of alkalosis, the urine pH is above 7. When metabolic or respiratory acidosis is suspected, an alkaline urine pH result almost eliminates the possibility of acidosis. Conversely, if respiratory or metabolic alkalosis is suspected, the excretion of an acid urine indicates that alkalosis is likely not present. *Dip-and-read* tests are widely used for pH testing, but pH meter measurements are less commonly utilized. In certain situations involving kidney stone susceptibility, it is quite important to maintain a narrow range of urinary pH. For example, in cystinuria an alkaline pH is maintained to keep the cystine solubilized and to avoid as much as possible the crystallization of cystine into renal calculi. Maintenance of urinary pH is also important for optimum results in certain types of drug therapy.

Color—Urine normally has a yellow color, mostly due to urochrome; the color varies from a pale straw to a dark amber shade. Darker specimens usually have a high specific gravity. Occasionally either normal or abnormal urine may show a color different from yellow. Bilirubin may cause fresh urine to be dark in color. In addition, urine which is allowed to stand darkens because of the oxidation of urobilinogen to urobilin. Red, reddish-brown or "smoky" urine is usually due to the presence of hemoglobin (hemoglobinuria), myoglobin (myoglobinuria) or red blood cells (hematuria). Porphyria is an uncommon cause of red coloration. Black urine can be caused by melanin, which may occur in the urine of patients with far advanced malignant melanoma. An inborn error of metabolism, alkaptonuria, is characterized by the urinary excretion of homogentisic acid which causes the urine to turn dark brown or black on standing. Many of the unusual colors occasionally found in urine are derived from exogenous sources, including both foods and drugs. Among these are the red color caused by beets, particularly in infants, the golden yellow or orange-red color of metabolites of pyridium-like drugs or azo drugs and the green or blue color from methylene blue.

Odor—Normal, freshly voided urine has a faint aromatic and characteristic odor, which is more intense in concentrated specimens. If the urine is allowed to stand, the odor becomes strongly ammoniacal and unpleasant because of bacterial destruction of urea. Freshly voided urine having a foul odor indicates severe infection. A sweet, fruity odor may be due to ketones.

Appearance—Freshly voided urine is usually clear. On standing a precipitate may form which usually consists of amorphous urates if the urine is acid or calcium and magnesium phosphates if the urine is alkaline. The formation of precipitate is more likely to occur if the urine is refrigerated. Most specimens will become clear again if they are warmed gently to room temperature. Large quantities of mucus, cells, leukocytes, or bacteria may cause cloudiness. Protein does not usually cause cloudiness.

Protein—A small amount of protein is present in the urine obtained from healthy subjects although the quantity is not sufficient to give a positive reaction with the tests commonly used for the recognition of protein in urine. The majority of the 25 to 50 mg of protein that is excreted daily is microprotein (low-molecular-weight polypeptide), which has properties quite different than those of albumin and globulin, which are the principal proteins of the blood serum. Albumin and globulins do occur in the normal urine in minute concentrations. Plasma proteins, hemoglobin, abnormal Bence-Jones protein and proteins (nucleo-, phospho- and glyco-proteins) derived from leukocytes and mucus may be present in urine in nephritis, nephrosis, lesions of the urinary tract, GI dehydration and renal congestion. Abnormal amounts of protein in the urine may be recognized by precipitation tests or by colorimetric tests. The precipitation depends on the heat coagulation of the protein or on the chemical precipitation of the protein. Most popular of the heat-precipitation tests is the heat-and-acetic acid test in which a tube of urine is heated to boiling after the addition of a drop or two of acetic acid. Sulfosalicylic acid is commonly employed in chemical precipitation tests and in this test equal quantities of 3% sulfosalicylic acid and urine are mixed in a test tube and the mixture is examined for turbidity indicative of precipitated protein. Colorimetric tests for proteins involve *dip-and-read* type of systems and are based on the *protein error* of indicators. Certain indicators have a point of color change which is different in the presence of protein as compared to the same system in the absence of protein. Thus, by buffering the indicator tetrabromophenol blue on this dip-strip at a specific pH, it is possible to have a yellow color in the absence of protein and a green or blue color in the presence of protein. This test Albustix (*Ames*), not only indicates the presence or absence of protein in the urine, but can also be made to indicate the approximate amount of protein. Strongly alkaline or

fermented urines will give false-positive results. The sensitivity of the colorimetric method is such that quantities of 10 to 20 mg of albumin per 100 mL of urine are recognized with confidence.

A positive test for protein in the urine may have any one of several meanings, and it is only when this information is related to other observations that it has optimum value. Proteinuria may be benign and appear following strenuous exercise or simply as a result of standing (orthostatic proteinuria). Protein frequently occurs in the urine during pregnancy and in some instances this is benign, but in other cases it is indicative of renal complications. Transient proteinuria may occur following severe infections, high fever, exposure to cold and in congestive heart failure. Proteinuria may be an early and sensitive indicator of renal disease and may indicate an abnormality prior to other signs and symptoms of renal impairment in the glomerulus or tubules. In the majority of instances there is not a correlation between the amount of protein in the urine and the severity of the renal disease. Patients with severe nephrosis may lose up to 25 g of protein per day. Such a marked loss of protein causes a decrease in plasma protein concentration with an accompanying edema. In both chronic and acute glomerulonephritis there is protein in the urine. Tumors of the kidney and renal infection will usually have an accompanying proteinuria. Bence-Jones protein is a unique protein which occurs in the urine of about 50% of patients with multiple myeloma. It has the unusual property of precipitating between 50 and 60° and dissolving at higher temperatures.

Glucose (Reducing Substances)—Glucose normally occurs in urine in such low concentration that it escapes detection by the usual testing methods. The urine of untreated or poorly controlled diabetic patients characteristically contains easily detectable amounts of glucose. A positive test for glucose in urine usually suggests hyperglycemia and the diagnosis of diabetes mellitus; further studies such as the glucose tolerance test to confirm the diagnosis are indicated. Glycosuria may also occur when the renal tubules fail to reabsorb glucose normally, and glucose appears in the urine despite normal blood glucose levels in contrast to true diabetes. Glucose is the sugar almost always found in urine; however, lactose, galactose, levulose, sucrose, and pentoses may be encountered. These other sugars are identified by paper chromatography, selective fermentation, polaroscopy, special chemical tests or the formation of their osazones. Other reducing substances occur in urine and may cause falsely positive reducing reactions for glucose. Examples are ascorbic acid, glucuronides, many drugs, homogentisic acid and the preservatives formalin and chloroform. The traditional method for glucose in urine (Benedict's test) relies on the reduction of cupric ions in alkaline solution to reddish-orange insoluble cuprous oxide. The copper is totally reduced by large amounts of glucose and results in a brick-red sediment with no remaining blue color. Lesser concentrations form green to rust colored solutions with some red sediment. A modification of this test, Clinitest (*Ames*), is available in tablet form. The tablet contains copper sulfate, anhydrous sodium hydroxide, citric acid and sodium carbonate. When added to dilute urine, the tablet dissolves and generates enough heat and effervescence to yield results comparable with the Benedict test. A specific but extremely simple enzyme test for glucose is available (Tes-Tape (*Lilly*), Clinistix (*Ames*), and Multistix (*Ames*)). Reagent strips are impregnated with glucose oxidase, peroxidase and orthotolidine. When dipped into a solution of glucose, oxidation occurs and hydrogen peroxide is formed which oxidizes orthotolidine to a blue color. This test is more sensitive than Clinitest, but is not as reliable for estimating the concentration of glucose. The enzymatic test is specific and thus useful in determining whether or not a reducing substance is glucose. Diastix (*Ames*) is a specific urine glucose test utilizing glucose oxidase which also indicates the quantity of glucose present.

Ketone Bodies—The ketone bodies acetone, acetoacetic acid and beta-hydroxybutyric acid are present in the urine when fats are incompletely metabolized. Ketonuria is most commonly seen in poorly controlled diabetes and indicates ketonemia and diabetic acidosis. Other causes for ketonuria are starvation, fever, protracted vomiting, and Von Gierke's disease. Ketonuria also occurs following anesthesia. Acetoacetic acid and acetone produce a distinctive purple color when treated with a mixture of sodium nitroprusside, ammonium sulfate and concentrated ammonium hydroxide. A similar reagent is available in tablet form (Acetest, *Ames*). A drop of urine is placed on the tablet; if ketones are present, a lavender to deep purple color develops in 30 sec. The color intensity indicates the concentration of ketones. The reagent strip Ketostix (*Ames*), used as a *dip-and-read* test on urine or serum, contains the same reagents, which are available on Multistix (*Ames*) and other multiple reagents as well. These tests will detect 5 to 10 mg of acetoacetic acid per 100 mL of urine.

Phenylpyruvic Acid—Phenylketonuria (or PKU) is an inborn error of metabolism in which the normal conversion of phenylalanine to tyrosine in the body does not occur and there is a build-up of phenylalanine concentration in the blood. This metabolic disorder causes mental retardation. A portion of the phenylalanine is excreted by the kidneys into the urine and in the process is converted to phenylpyruvic acid (or phenylketone). If this genetic disorder is discovered soon after birth, it is possible to place the infant on a diet very low in phenylalanine-containing proteins and thus minimize the phenylalanine build-up in the body, averting the serious mental retardation which is ordinarily seen in the untreated PKU patient.

Recognition of PKU can be made by the use of a test for phenylpyruvic acid using a dip-and-read reagent composition containing ferric ions. This test, Phenistix (*Ames*), can be used on urine from all newborn babies. A positive reaction gives a green color, whereas a normal infant urine gives a pale ivory or yellow color to the strip. PKU can also be recognized by the employment of a chemical or microbiological test for elevated phenylalanine in serum, as discussed in the section on *Amino Acids*.

Bilirubin—Bilirubin is found in the urine of patients with hepatitis or obstructive jaundice but not patients with hemolytic jaundice. Tests for bilirubin and urobilinogen combine to give excellent information in the differential diagnosis of jaundice. Tests for bilirubin are of two kinds; oxidation tests form a green color of biliverdin from bilirubin usually using ferric chloride as the oxidative reagent, and diazotization tests form colored compounds when bilirubin reacts with diazonium salts in strongly acid medium. Most oxidation tests adsorb the bilirubin onto barium sulfate or similar material before the addition of Fouchet's reagent. The tablet test Ictotest (*Ames*) is the most sensitive diazo test and it uses an absorption mat to concentrate the bilirubin from 5 drops of urine. A reagent tablet is added to the moist spot on the mat and two drops of water are added to dissolve the effervescent reagent and wash some of it off the tablet onto the mat where the reaction takes place. A blue or purple color on the mat around the tablet in 30 sec indicates the presence of bilirubin. In addition, a *dip-and-read* test composition also based on the diazo reaction has been incorporated into the multiple urinalysis reagent strips, Bili-Labstix and Multistix (*Ames*). It is less sensitive than the tablet test, but its convenience allows it to be used in routine urinalysis quite readily. An incidence of approximately 0.1% positives on health screening population groups, 0.2% on clinic patients and 0.9% on hospitalized patients has been reported.

Urobilinogen—Bilirubin in the bile is reduced to urobil-inogen by bacteria in the lower intestine. A portion of the urobilinogen is reabsorbed from the intestine into the blood. A portion of this urobilinogen is excreted into the urine by the kidney and the balance is re-excreted via the bile into the intestine. Although the quantity of urobilinogen in the urine is quite small, it is an important indicator of liver function and red-blood-cell catabolism. If there is an obstruction to bile flow such as occurs in obstructive jaundice, the amount of urobilinogen formed and reabsorbed into the blood and excreted in the urine is decreased. With impairment of liver function, the excretion of urobilinogen in the bile is decreased, the blood concentration increases and there is a corresponding increase in urinary urobilinogen excretion. Actually, the increase in urinary urobilinogen is one of the most sensitive tests for impaired liver function and this test may indicate an abnormality when all other tests of liver function remain unchanged from normal. In hemolytic diseases where there is an increased rate of hemoglobin breakdown, the amount of bilirubin formation is increased with a corresponding increase in urobilinogen formation and excretion in the urine. The concentration of urobilinogen in urine can be established by the use of a *dip-and-read* test which utilizes the interaction of urobilinogen and p-dimethylaminobenzaldehyde (Urobilistix, *Ames*).

Hematuria, Hemoglobinuria, and Myoglobinuria—Hematuria refers to a condition in which intact red blood cells appear in the urine. This condition is indicative of a specific defect in the microscopic functional unit (the nephron) of the kidney or it may be indicative of bleeding in the kidney, the ureter, the bladder or the urethra. In the female, there may be variable numbers of red blood cells in the urine during menstruation.

Hemoglobinuria is a condition in which free hemoglobin is present in the urine without red blood cells. This may be caused by intravascular hemolysis as a result of a transfusion reaction or by poisoning or by toxins. The free hemoglobin in the plasma is excreted by the kidney into the urine. In some situations actual total hemolysis of the red cells occurs after they have entered the urine. This occurs particularly with alkaline urines. Myoglobin is the red respiratory pigment of muscle. This pigment is quite comparable to hemoglobin in its composition and chemical reactions. Myoglobin may be liberated from muscle cells in certain types of injury and in such cases will circulate in the plasma and will be excreted in the urine. There are also certain genetic muscle disorders in which myoglobin is lost from the muscles and appears in the plasma and subsequently in the urine.

Chemical tests for red cells, free hemoglobin and myoglobin are based on the peroxidase-like activity of hemoglobin or myoglobin. When a chromogen mixture such as orthotolidine and peroxide is exposed to this peroxidase activity it will rapidly interact to generate an intense blue color. A *dip-and-read* solid state system is available which is called Hemastix (*Ames*). This specific composition utilizes cumene hydroperoxide as the peroxide. The same *dip-and-read* test for occult blood is incorporated as a component part of multiple urine *dip-and-read* tests, eg, Multistix (*Ames*).

Microscopic Examination—Ordinarily, urine contains a number of formed elements or solid structures of microscopic dimensions. These are readily studied by centrifuging 10 to 15 mL of urine, pouring off the supernatant and resuspending the sediment in the drop or so of urine which remains in the tube. This suspension of sediment is placed on a microscope slide and viewed with a low-power magnification of the microscope. Specific structures can be studied with higher magnification. The urinary sediments can be classified into unorganized (chemical substances) and organized (cells and casts) constituents.

In an alkaline urine, amorphous or crystalline ammonium-magnesium phosphates, calcium carbonate or oxalate crystals, and ammonium urate may occur normally. Amorphous or crystalline urates, uric acid, and calcium oxalates are normally seen in acid urines. The presence of tyrosine, leucine, or cystine crystals is associated with various diseases. Chemical crystals are identified by solubility in acid and/or alkali, colorimetric reactions, and crystalline structure.

The urine sediment ordinarily contains residues of epithelial cells, crystals and an occasional red blood cell or white blood cell. Increased numbers of erythrocytes are seen where there is bleeding into the urinary tract. If the red cells are formed into a red cell cast, it is suggestive that bleeding has occurred at the glomerular level. An increased number of leukocytes is suggestive of infection and inflammation of the kidney. Casts are microscopic concretions which have the form of a tubule. These structures have a matrix of precipitated protein and depending on their appearance may be identified as hyaline casts, granular casts, waxy casts, and red cell casts. Renal failure casts are larger and are associated with severe necrosis of the kidney.

Numerous crystals, mucus fibers, bacteria, yeast cells, spermatozoa, and parasites (*Trichomonas vaginalis*) may be indentified in the urine sediment. The majority of these crystals do not have any unusual significance but in certain disorders may be indicative of crystal deposits in kidney tissue or predisposition to formation of calculi.

Tissue cells can be recognized in urine sediment. This provides an excellent means of detection and diagnosis of cancer of the lower urinary tract when the sediment is fixed in alcohol and stained by the Papanicolaou procedure. Exfoliative cytology of urine may be applied as a routine to all urology patients. In one large clinic the number of positive cases found among urology patients was almost 5 percent, which is much higher return of positive results than is obtained with routine staining of cervical smears.

Bacteria—Freshly voided specimens of urine ordinarily contain a few microorganisms, which primarily represent bacteria picked up from the external genitalia. There are fewer contaminating organisms in a *clean-catch* specimen which involves extensive washing of the external genitalia prior to collection of the specimen. A specimen collected at the mid-point of urination or a "mid-stream" specimen ordinarily has more organisms than a clean-catch specimen, but fewer than a so-called random specimen. When there is an infection of the kidney or urinary tract, the number of organisms in the urine is markedly increased. Ordinarily, if the urine contains 100,000 or more organisms per mL, the result strongly suggests the presence of an active infection. Infection of the urinary tract with accompanying bacteriuria is relatively common in young girls and in women. Quite often the condition is asymptomatic and is only recognized as a result of study of the urine. If bacteriuria is not treated, it may lead to serious renal injury.

If there is a very large number of bacteria in the urine, the specimen may actually be turbid. This can be recognized by gross visual inspection of the urine. Bacteriuria can also be recognized by microscopic examination of the urine sediment particularly if there is a large number of organisms present. The most widely employed procedure for recognizing bacteria involves plating a specimen of diluted urine on a culture plate and then counting the number of colonies after the plate has been incubated. A more convenient approach to this same measurement involves the use of a microscope slide which is coated with nutrient agar. Such a slide when dipped in a urine specimen and then incubated will indicate the presence or absence of bacteriuria and also the approximate count.

Methods to determine the presence of significant numbers of bacteria in urine samples are available on various automated systems.[19] The Bac-T-Screen (*Marion Laboratories*) system is a dispensing and filtering system used with a straining process to detect the presence of bacteria on special filter cards by noting the color change on the card. Analysis on the Abbott MS-2 performed by photometric monitoring of bacterial growth changing the light transmitted in a broth culture over a period of time. A decrease in the light transmission due to turbidity or color identifies a positive specimen. The Lumac Biocounter M2010 measures bacterial adenosine triphosphate (ATP) in urine by the bioluminescence produced in a luciferin-luciferase system. Once these rapid techniques are performed to determine which specimen have increased bacteria, then further identification and sensitivity testing are performed. Chemical tests for the metabolic activity of bacteria have been utilized in studying bacteriuria. The most popular chemical test is that for nitrite. Ordinarily, all urine specimens contain nitrate, but do not contain nitrite. If *E coli* or certain other organisms are present in sufficient numbers they will reduce the nitrate to nitrite.

Calculi—Knowledge of the composition of renal and bladder calculi ("stones") is essential in the planning of the therapeutic regimen in such diseases. Mixed calcium phosphate and oxalate stones usually occur over the entire urine pH range. Uric acid, cystine and calcium hydrogen phosphate calculi are generally associated with acid urines, while magnesium ammonium phosphate calculi usually occur in alkaline urine. Hyperexcretion of one of the calculi components, pH, renal blockage, and the presence of foreign objects in the urinary tract are the most probable causal factors in the formation of renal calculi. Calcium oxalate stones are the most common type. The chemical content of the stones is established by routine qualitative analysis for calcium, magnesium, ammonium, phosphate, carbonate, oxalate, uric acid and cystine. Subsequent confirmation by optical crystallography, X-ray diffraction, and infrared spectroscopy is also utilized in characterization of the physical properties of the calculi.

Feces

Normal feces consists of undigested food remnants, products of digestion, bacteria, and secretions of the gastrointestinal tract. *Macroscopic*, *chemical*, and *microscopic* determinations are routinely performed. The normal quantity of feces is about 200 g/day. The brown color is due to the reduction of bilirubin to urobilinogen and then to uribilin (stercobilin); bilirubin is not normally present in feces, but porphyrins and biliverdin (a component of meconium) is excreted during the first days of life. Bilirubin can be detected by tests previously described for bile pigments.

Color changes in the stool can be a result of dietary intake or diagnostic for biliary obstruction, and gastrointestinal bleeding.[20] Patients with steatorrhea and malabsorption may show a yellow bulky stool containing fat and gas. The feces is clay colored when bile is prevented from entering the gut. A red or black stool can occur when excessive doses of anticoagulants, phenylbutazone, or salicylates are taken, producing bleeding in the gastrointestinal tract. Substances which interfere with the coloration of the stool include antacids (whitish or speckling), bismuth salts (black), iron salts (black), pyridium (orange), senna (yellow to brown), and tetracyclines (red).

Fecal urobilinogen can be determined colorimetrically by reduction of urobilin to urobilinogen with alkaline ferrous sulfate, and then reaction with acidified *p*-dimethylaminobenzaldehyde (Ehrlich's reagent). Fecal urobilinogen is increased from a normal range of 40–280 mg daily to 400–1400 mg in hemolytic jaundice (dark brown stool), and is decreased in obstructive jaundice (clay-colored stool).

Porphyrins and porphyrinogens do not arise from hemoglobin catabolism, such as bilirubin, but are by-products of the synthesis of heme. Increases in fecal and urinary elimination of coproporphyrin, uroporphyrin and protoporphyrin are valuable diagnostic aids in distinguishing the various hepatic and erythropoietic porphyrias. Fecal coproporphyrins (CP) and coproporphyrinogens (CPP) are determined after extraction, conversion of CPP to CP by iodine, and triple-point spectrophotometric estimation at 380, 401 and 430 nm to correct for interfering substances (also see *Urinalysis* section).

Fecal occult blood is readily detected by the *o*-tolidine, benzidine, guaiac or diphenylamine tests; this is valid only if the patient has been on a meat-free diet for 3 days. Guaiac and diphenylamine are preferred due to the carcinogenic potential of other two chemicals.

The Hemoccult test kit (*SmithKline Diagnostics*) uses an impregnated guaiac paper slide for detecting occult blood, which is a useful screening test for colon cancer. Two slides are prepared each day for three days from different parts of the same stool while the patient is on a meat free high bulk diet. Interfering substances include aspirin, because it can produce bleeding and Vitamin C which interferes with the oxidation reaction of the test. If bleeding occurs high in the GI tract, the blood is digested and converted to acid hematin; 50 mL of blood in the feces will cause melena (black stool). Bleeding from the lower GI tract is apparent from red streaking of stools. The use of ^{51}Cr-tagged erythrocytes has been used to quantitate and locate the source of gastrointestinal bleeding. The subject's red cells are mixed with an isotonic ^{51}Cr solution and then reinjected intravenously. If bleeding occurs, the ^{51}Cr-isotope content of the feces will be increased. Location of the hemorrhagic area can also be approximated by an isotopic scan of the abdominal area.

The presence of excessive quantities of *mucus* is usually indicative of dysentery, colitis, or other inflammatory processes in the intestinal mucosa. Strongly alkaline or acidic reaction in the feces is indicative of excessive quantities of protein or carbohydrate in the diet, respectively.

Quantitative determination of *fecal nitrogen* is useful in analysis of pancreatic function. In pancreatic disease, increases in fecal nitrogen will occur as a result of decreased secretion of pancreatic proteolytic enzymes. The normal individual will excrete 4–13% of ingested nitrogen in the feces; in chronic pancreatitis, 9–30%. Fecal nitrogen can be determined by the Kjeldahl digestion procedure.

Fecal fat is present in the form of triglycerides of fatty acids (neutral fat), free fatty acids (FFA), and soaps. Fat determinations are based on the solubility of neutral fat and FFA in ether; the soaps are insoluble in ether and have to be acid hydrolyzed to their respective FFA prior to extraction. Neutral fat will liberate FFA only on alkaline hydrolysis. The FFA, isolated from the above fractionations, are then determined by titrimetric, colorimetric, or gas chromatographic procedures.

Determinations of blood, urine, and fecal ^{125}I after oral administration of an iodinated glyceryl trioleate or ^{125}I-oleic acid preparation is an index of both *pancreatic, biliary and intestinal absorptive function* and correlates with *fecal fat excretion*. The bile must emulsify the ^{125}I-triglyceride prior to enzymatic hydrolysis by pancreatic lipase to yield FFA-^{125}I which is subsequently absorbed and metabolized. An increased amount of ^{125}I in the feces is associated with pancreatic diseases (cystic fibrosis with achylia), obstructive jaundice, malabsorption disease (sprue, celiac disease) and steatorrhea. The latter entity can be differentiated as to a pancreatic lipase or intestinal absorptive defect. In the "absorptive" disease, increased excretion of ^{125}I is seen after administration of ^{125}I-triolein or oleic acid. In the pancreatic defect, adequate absorption of ^{125}I oleic acid occurs but fecal ^{125}I is increased after the triolein meal.

A *microscopic examination* of emulsified feces includes analysis for the presence of crystals, food residues, body cells, bacteria, and parasites. Crystals of triple phosphate, calcium oxalate, fat and cholesterol, starch granules, vegetable fibers and neutral fat globules are normally present. Octahedral needle-shaped crystals (Charcot-Leyden crystals) are present in parasitic infestation and mucous colitis. Excessive quantities of fat or starch are seen in malabsorption disease.

Adult, larval, or ova phases of parasites may be encountered in the feces. The most common parasitic infestations are caused by *cestodes* (tapeworms), *trematodes* (flukes), *nematodes* (roundworms), and *protozoa* (amoeba). (See *Microbiology* section.)

Toxicology

Determination of drug or chemical concentrations in biological fluids is an important aspect in the diagnosis and treatment of the toxic syndrome induced by various agents in acute or chronic drug abuse situations or in chemical poisoning.

Barbiturates, glutethimide, methaqualone, chlordiazepoxide, diazepam, diphenhydramine, ethchlorvynol, morphine, phenothiazines, and salicylates are encountered in drug abuse situations. Preliminary screening of serum or urine samples for drug substances is accomplished by TLC procedures. Analysis of serum or urine levels of intact drug or its metabolites is usually performed by extraction of the sample with an organic solvent, separation by gas-liquid (GLC), or high performance liquid (HPLC) chromatography, and quantitation by spectrophotometric, fluorometric, or electrochemical techniques. The interpretation of the serum concentration data in relation to clinical significance and toxicology must not be limited to numbers. In acute drug overdosage, the time of drug ingestion, time of blood or urine sampling and severity of clinical symptoms or time of death must be interpreted in reference to data on the absorption, tissue distribution, metabolism and elimination of the drug and its metabolites. The specificity of the chemical assay as to interference from other drugs or metabolites of the parent drug must be considered. The extent of absorption of many drug substances is not directly related to the dose when large amounts of drug are ingested in comparison to the therapeutic dose. The tissue distribution and metabolic rates can be affected by large drug overdoses in which renal or hepatic failure is encountered. The plasma elimination rate can also be affected and it is important to recognize the change in elimination kinetics and to be aware of the nature of plasma elimination as defined by a mono-, bi- or poly-exponential elimination curve. The drug overdose usually involves several drug substances and the chemical, metabolic and pharmacological aspects of drug interaction must be considered.

The methodology for analysis of drugs in biological fluids or tissues can be found in the books listed in the *Bibliography*. Analysis for serum *barbiturate* levels will be described in this section as a specific example of the analytical methodology. Serum is extracted at pH 6.5 with chloroform; the chloroform extract is washed with pH 7.0 phosphate buffer and extracted with 0.45N NaOH. The UV spectrum of the alkaline aqueous layer is determined at pH 13 and 10.5. The UV spectra are characteristic and distinguish barbiturates, N-methylbarbituric acids and thiobarbiturates. The barbiturates can also be detected by acidifying the alkaline layer, extracting with chloroform and spotting this organic extract on a silica-gel TLC plate. Sequential spraying of the plate with $KMnO_4$, $HgSO_4$, and diphenylcarbazone will show R_f values and color reactions typical of the various barbiturates. Blood barbiturates can be determined more accurately by a GLC procedure in which the retention times are used to identify the specific barbiturates. The degree of severity of clinical symptoms has been correlated with blood barbiturate levels. Comatose, areflexic signs are observed at 5.0 mg% amobarbital, 2.0 mg% pentobarbital, 8.0 mg% phenobarbital and 1.5 mg% secobarbital.

Opiates, amphetamines, barbiturates and methadone can be rapidly detected by "*homogenous*" *enzyme assay.*[21] In this procedure, addition of drug antibodies to a conjugate of drug and lysozyme results in inhibition of lysozyme activity. Addition of free drug to this reaction mixture increases the enzyme activity in proportion to the amount of free drug added. The sensitivity of this type of assay is 0.1 μg/mL of amphetamine and barbiturates, 0.5 μg/mL of methadone, 0.3 μg/mL of opiates and 1.0 μg/mL of benzoylecgonine, a cocaine metabolite. This assay is applicable to large drug-screening programs.

Electron-spin-labeling techniques can also be employed on large-scale drug screening programs. In this procedure, known amounts of drug antibodies are mixed with drug labeled with a stable nitroxide radical (spin-label) and with the specimen to be analyzed. Due to competition for antibody between spin-labeled drug and drug in the specimen, the spin-labeled drug becomes detached from the antibody and can be detected by electron-spin resonance spectroscopy. This procedure is 1000 times more sensitive than TLC.

Blood-alcohol levels may be determined by aeration, distillation, gas chromatography, or specific enzymatic analysis with alcohol dehydrogenase. In the chemical techniques the blood sample is either oxidized or distilled into a dichromate-sulfuric acid mixture; the excess dichromate is then determined by titration with potassium iodide or methyl orange-ferrous sulfate solutions or by colorimetric analysis. The gas-chromatographic and enzyme procedures are specific for ethanol, whereas the chemical techniques are influenced by other volatile or oxidizable substances in the blood. The enzymatic method is based on the reaction of ethanol and NAD in the presence of alcohol dehydrogenase to form acetaldehyde and NADH; the acetaldehyde is removed with semicarbazide and the NADH formed in the reaction is estimated spectrophotometrically at 340 nm. Ethanol levels of >0.10% are indicative of intoxication and apparent psychomotor disturbance. Levels of 0.40–0.50% are associated with medullary and diencephalic disturbances such as tremors, coma, respiratory depression, peripheral collapse, and death.

Specific analysis of heavy metals is best performed by atomic-absorption spectroscopy. Analyses for arsenic, beryllium, bismuth, copper, iron, lead, lithium, mercury, nickel, thallium, and zinc are frequently encountered in the toxicology laboratory. *Blood lead* is determined by forming a lead-dithiocarbamate chelate in the presence of ammonium pyrrolidinedithiocarbamate and extraction of the chelate into methyl isobutyl ketone for subsequent atomic absorption analysis. A lead concentration of >60 μg/mL in children usually reflects significant absorption and accumulation of lead and is interpreted as an indicator of lead toxicity (plumbism).

Increased lead exposure will result in a decrease in delta-*aminolevulinic acid (ALA)* conversion to porphobilinogen by ALA-dehydrase in heme synthesis. ALA blood levels will increase to the point that ALA is excreted in the urine. Determination of urinary ALA is performed by removing urine porphobilinogen and urea by ion-exchange chromatography, reaction of ALA with *p*-dimethylaminobenzaldehyde and colorimetric determination of the chromogen. Urinary ALA levels >2.5 mg/100 mL are unacceptable in children and industrial lead workers. Urinary ALA levels are not as sensitive an indicator of lead toxicity as blood lead, but can be used to monitor prophylactic treatment procedures.

Cholinesterase determinations are of value in the diagnosis of suspected cases of organophosphate or carbamate pesticide poisoning. Two types of cholinesterase are found in tissues. True cholinesterase is found in RBC and nerve tissue and exhibits a specificity for acetylcholine substrate. Pseudocholinesterase is found in plasma and has a greater affinity for hydrolyzing butyrylcholine and other esters. The organophosphate and carbamate insecticides inhibit both enzymes. The activity of the plasma enzyme is inhibited more rapidly than the RBC cholinesterase, and recovers more rapidly due to synthesis of new enzyme by the liver. The recovery of the erythrocyte enzyme is slow and is governed by red cell turnover rate. Cholinesterase activity is usually determined by measuring changes in pH after incubation of plasma or RBC lysates with acetylcholine. The normal range of this enzyme is 4.5–10.9 (plasma), 3.4–5.7 (whole blood) and 6–10.5 (RBC) units/mL.

Gastric Analysis

The chief constituents of gastric juice are hydrochloric acid, gastric proteases (pepsin and gastricsin), hematopoietic factor (intrinsic factor and vitamin B_{12} binders), gastric hormones, and mucosubstances (aminopolysaccharides, mucopolyuronides, mucoids and mucoproteins). Tests for *gastric function*[22] are usually performed on gastric juice samples collected by direct intubation into the stomach. The fasting content (normal, <100 mL) of the stomach is removed and gastric secretion is collected in the basal state, or after stimulation by the oral administration of caffeine-benzoate or alcohol, or parenteral administration of histamine, insulin, or the hormone pentagastrin. Samples are collected by continuous aspiration and analyzed for acidity and gastric protease activity at various time intervals. The extent of recovery of total juice can be estimated by oral nonabsorbable indicators (polyethylene glycol-^{14}C, phenol red and ^{125}I-HSA) instilled into the stomach prior to the aspiration. The recovery and specific concentration of these indicators in gastric juice is an index of gastric secretory volume, completeness of collection and gastric emptying rate.

Gastric juice is a heterogeneous mixture of clear juice and flocculent, clear mucus. The *color* of the juice should be noted as to the appearance of blood, bile and excessive quantities of mucus. *Acidity* can be determined by simple pH measurement and conversion to mEq H$^+$ or by titration of centrifuged gastric juice to pH 3.5, 4.5 and 7.4, the respective end points for free acid (HCl), protease activity and physiological neutrality. The *basal acid output* is about 1 mEq/hour in normal subjects and 2–4 mEq/hour in duodenal ulcer patients. The *peak acid output (PAO)* after histamine stimulation is 10–20 mEq/hour in normals and 40–50 mEq/hour in duodenal ulcer; PAO following pentagastric stimulation is similar to histamine. Gastric acid secretion is decreased in atrophic gastritis, gastric carcinoma and certain types of gastric ulcer. Hypersecretion is seen in duodenal ulcer, Zollinger-Ellison (Z.E.) syndrome and hyperparathyroidism.

In situ measurements of pH may be made with a *Heidelberg capsule apparatus.* In this technique the subject swallows a small pH-sensitive capsule (transmitter); radiowaves are transmitted from the capsule to a sensing device (receiver), and the signals are recorded as a function of pH. The normal pH of the stomach is 1.2–1.8.

Tubeless gastric acidity analysis is performed by oral administration of Diagnex Blue (*Squibb*), a carbacrylic ion-exchange resin reacted with azure blue dye. The hydrogen ions in the gastric juice exchange with the dye on the resin; the dye is absorbed and then excreted in the urine. The dye concentration in the urine is a function of gastric acidity. The normal value is >0.6 mg dye in the urine 2 hr after administration.

The principal gastric proteases are *pepsin and gastricsin;* pepsinogen is a precursor which is converted to active pepsin by free HCl and by an autocatalytic process. *Total gastric protease activity* is determined on hemoglobin or radioiodinated human serum albumin (RISA) substrates at pH 1.8–3.1 (RISA-^{125}I); protease activity on hemoglobin will liberate tyrosine which can be estimated spectrophotometrically at 280 nm; with RISA, liberated tyrosine-^{125}I, as estimated by isotopic procedures, is an index of proteolytic activity.

Pepsin activity can be distinguished from the total protease activity by estimation of the 3,5-diiodotyrosine liberated from *N*-acetyl-L-phenylalanyl-3,5-diiodotyrosine substrate at pH 2.1. Pepsin will react on this substrate, gastricsin will not. Normal gastric juice protease activity ranges from 200–1200 μg total protease activity/mL and 50–300 μg pepsin/mL. The presence of bile, blood, saliva, or excess mucus in the sample will decrease both acidity and gastric protease activity.

Gastrin, cholecystokinin, secretin and pancreozymin are gastrointestinal hormones.[26] The role of gastrin and its interaction with other gastrointestinal hormones in the etiology and proliferation of ulcer disease is of recent interest. Accurate RIA techniques have been developed for gastrin and secretin-6-tyrosine due to the availability of pure synthetic polypeptide. Biological assays based on the effect of these substances on gastric, pancreatic and biliary secretion have also been utilized.

Gastrin is found in various species in two forms, G-I and G-II. The only difference is in sulfation of the 12-tyrosyl residue in G-II of the heptadecapeptide amides. Gastrin is found primarily in the gastrin-producing cells (G-cells) of the antral mucosa. The C terminal tetrapeptide represents the biologically active part of the molecule. Gastrin infusion will stimulate secretion of gastric acid, pepsin and intrinsic factor. It has a slight secretin-like effect and a powerful pancreozymin-like effect on pancreatic secretion. Gastrin also stimulates bile flow. Instillation of HCl into the stomach will inhibit gastrin release; protein and meal stimulation will increase serum gastrin.

RIA of serum gastrin is of diagnostic value in ZE syndrome, pernicious anemia and duodenal ulcer. Basal serum gastrin levels in the normal individual are 20–30 μg/mL and increase about 2-fold after a protein meal stimulus. Basal serum gastrin levels in duodenal ulcer are normal or slightly elevated, but increase 4- to 5-fold after a protein meal stimulus. Basal serum gastrin levels are elevated in ZE to 500–4000 pg/mL due to the presence of a gastrin-producing tumor. The ZE patient is uniquely sensitive to IV calcium stimulation which will increase both gastric acid secretion and serum gastrin in this syndrome. Basal serum gastrin levels are also elevated in gastric hyposecretion as seen in pernicious anemia and Type A gastritis, and in chronic renal failure due to decreased metabolic turnover of gastrin in the kidney.

The RIA of serum gastrin is based on competition of gastrin in test sample with ^{125}I-gastrin for gastrin antibody binding sites. The antibodies used in this procedure are usually cospecific for gastrin I and II. However, they detect all forms of circulating gastrin, ie, Big-Big Gastrin (G-39), Big Gastrin (mw 7000; G-33), gastrin heptadecapeptide (G-17, mw 2200), G-13 and G-8 (mini-gastrin). The Big components can be converted to gastrin by trypsin hydrolysis. The significance of changes in the ratio of the circulating gastrins is not known, but it has been suggested that G-39 and G-33 predominate in the basal state and cleave to G-17 which is the major serum form after a protein meal.

Other Body Fluids

Physical, chemical, and microscopic examination of cerebrospinal fluid, synovial fluid, human milk, transudates, and exudates are also performed by the clinical laboratory. The principles of the various determinations are similar to those described for blood and urine.

Microbiology

Clinical medical microbiology is a science which is concerned with the isolation and identification of disease-producing microorganisms, ie, bacteria, fungi (including yeast), viruses, rickettsia, and parasites. The techniques employed in the isolation and identification of the suspect organism(s) involve the propagation on suitable primary culture media, selective isolation on special culture media, use of suitable living host material (mouse, embryonated egg, tissue culture, etc.), determination of morphologic and, where applicable, staining characteristics of the organism, and confirmation by biochemical and/or immunochemical analysis. Suitable animal inoculation, where applicable, may be employed to determine pathogenicity. Site, timing, technique (aseptic), instrumentation, and transportation of clinical specimens (blood, urine, feces, cerebrospinal fluid, etc) are prime variables involved in the final differentiation and confirmation process.

Rapid manual enzymatic and immunologic test kits have been introduced to identify pathogens for cerebrospinal fluid analysis. The latex agglutination test coats a specific antibody onto latex particles and when an antigen is present, the latex particles are visible.[23] In the coagglutination test, the specific antibody is bound to protein A on the surface of a staphylococcal cell and the presence of antigen produces agglutination.[23]

Staphylococcus aureus (*Micrococcus pyogenes* var *aureus*) is a Gram-positive coccus frequently found on normal human skin and mucous membranes and frequently associated with abscesses, septicemia, endocarditis, and osteomyelitis. Some strains elaborate an exotoxin capable of causing food poisoning. Primary isolation is on blood-agar and in thioglycollate broth. With feces and other heavily contaminated specimens, phenylethyl alcohol agar and/or mannitol-salt agar should be inoculated to suppress growth of other bacteria. Identification of pathogenic staphylococci is based on colonial (pigmentation) and microscopic morphology (grape-like clusters), positive catalase production, positive coagulase production (staphylocoagulase-plasma clotting factor), and positive mannitol fermentation.

Streptococcus pyogenes is another Gram-positive coccus frequently associated with tonsillitis or pharyngitis, erysipelas, pyoderma and endocarditis. Neopeptone agar containing 5% defibrinated sheep blood is preferred for primary isolation and to demonstrate characteristic hemolysin production by observing zone of clear (beta) hemolysis around the colonies on blood agar. Streptococcal groups are identified by precipitin tests with group-specific antisera for A, B, C, D, F, and G. Streptex (*Wellcome Diagnostics*) uses a latex agglutination system for identifying the Lancefield group of streptococci. Other groups are not usually associated with human clinical materials.

Neisseria gonorrheae is a Gram-negative diplococcus associated with the venereal disease gonorrhea. Identification is based on the primary isolation of the gonococcus from urethral exudates on chocolate agar or Thayer-Martin (TM) medium. Microscopic observation of Gram-negative intracellular diplococci resembling the gonococcus constitutes a presumptive positive diagnosis of gonorrhea. Confirmation of the oxidase enzyme activity of the gonococci is performed by reaction with *p*-dimethylaminoaniline which turns oxidase-positive colonies black. A positive oxidase test by Gram-negative diplococci isolated on TM medium constitutes a presumptively positive test for *N gonorrheae*. Final identification as *N gonorrheae* rests on typical sugar fermentation or specific (fluorescent antibody) staining.

Neisseria meningitidis is the primary cause of bacterial meningitis and of septicemia. Primary isolation is based on culturing of a specimen (blood, spinal fluid, or nasopharyngeal secretions) on a Mueller-Hinton medium or chocolate agar containing vancomycin-colistimethate-nystatin antibiotic mixture. Confirmation of the isolate by biochemical reactions (positive oxidase, positive catalase, etc) and serologic agglutination with group-specific (A, B, and C) antiserum is used in the differentiation. Young cultures of groups A and C may show capsular swelling (Quellung reaction) in the presence of specific antiserum.

The enteric bacilli (*Enterobacteriaceae*) are Gram-negative, nonsporulating rods associated with dysentery (*Shigella sp*), typhoid fever (*Salmonella typhi*), urinary tract and tissue infections (*Escherichia coli*, *Proteus sp*, and *Pseudomonas sp*), and pulmonary infections (*Klebsiella sp*). Primary isolation of enteric bacilli is on selective and differential infusion agar such as MacConkey and eosin-methylene blue (EMB), and enrichment media such as selenite broth and tetrathionate broth. Primary isolation of *Salmonella sp.* is on Leifson's deoxycholate citrate agar (LDC) or *Salmonella-shigella* agar (SS); whereas if *Salmonella typhi* is suspected, brilliant green agar (BG) and bismuth sulfite agar (BS) may be used and would constitute a presumptively positive diagnosis of *S typhi*.

Confirmation and identification of enteric bacilli may be performed by serological tests and biochemical reactions: H_2S production (triple sugar iron agar), indole production, acetylmethylcarbinol production, citrate utilization, urease, lysine and arginine decarboxylase and phenylalanine deaminase activity. Enterotube (*Roche Diagnostics*) employs conventional media to perform eleven standard biochemical tests which can be inoculated simultaneously in one compartmented tube, with a single bacterial colony. Serological identification of *Salmonella* and *Shigella sp.* is based on the agglutination of antigens that fall into three categories; "K" capsular (*Klebsiella sp* and *Shigella sp*), "O" (*Salmonella sp*, *Arizona sp*, *E coli*, *Shigella sp*, etc) and "H" flagellar (*Salmonella sp*).

Other Gram-negative rods of medical importance are the hemophilic bacilli (*Bordetella pertussis*, whooping cough and *Hemophilus influenzae*, bacterial meningitis), the hemorrhagic bacilli (*Pasteurella pestis*, bubonic plague, and *P tularensis*, tularemia), and pyrogenic bacillus (*Brucella melitensis*, undulant fever).

Spore-forming Gram-positive rods of medical importance belong to the genus *Clostridium*, which are associated with tetanus (*Cl tetani*), gas gangrene (*Cl perfringens* or *welchii*) and botulism (*Cl botulinum*). The isolation of these organisms requires anaerobic conditions. Once the strain to be identified is obtained in pure culture by single-colony selection, its morphological characteristics are noted and then grown in a variety of definitive media to determine catalase activity, hydrogen peroxide decomposition, and fermentation or hydrolysis of carbohydrates and organic acids. Analysis of fermentation products (gas chromatography) is also used for identification of pathogenic anaerobic *Clostridia*. The major clostridial exotoxin type can be determined by typing with specific antitoxin sera. A Gram-positive, aerobic, spore-former of medical importance is *Bacillus anthracis*, responsible for anthrax, a disease of animals transmissible to man.

The mycobacteria are acid-fast bacilli associated with tuberculosis in man (*Mycobacterium tuberculosis*), in cattle (*Mycobacterium bovis*), and with leprosy (*Mycobacterium leprae*). Tubercle bacilli in man are isolated from sputum cultured on a tubed or bottled egg medium (Lowenstein-Jensen) following enzymatic digestion and concentration of the specimens. A provisional diagnosis of tuberculosis is usually made by demonstrating acid-fast bacilli microscopically, X-ray diagnosis, and a positive tuberculin skin test.

Other weakly and partially acid-fast bacilli of medical importance are members of the *Actinomycetales*, *Nocardia*

asteroides, and *Nocardia brasiliensis*, which are responsible for severe pulmonary infections, and cutaneous and subcutaneous abscesses.

Bacteriophages (phages) are a special group of viruses that are hosted by bacteria. Any given phage is highly host-specific and when in contact with its host, lysis of the host occurs (phage-typing). They are primarily used as epidemiological tools in subtyping strains of *E coli*, staphylococci, *Salmonella sp*, that are presumed to be related epidemiologically. Phages also furnish ideal material for studying host-parasite relationships and virus multiplication.

Medically important fungal diseases include the superficial mycoses, ie, fungal invasion is restricted to the outermost layers of the skin or to the hair shafts, (*Microsporum audouini*, ringworm of the scalp, *Trichophyton sp*, athlete's foot, and *Epidermophyton floccosum*, *Tinea pedis*) and the systemic pathogenic fungi (*Blastomyces dermatitidis*, *Coccidioides immitis*, *Histoplasma capsulatum*, *Candida albicans*). Diagnosis of the causative agent is based on the isolation of organisms on Sabouraud's dextrose agar or trypticase soy agar with or without cycloheximide and chloramphenicol to suppress growth of saprophytic fungi and bacteria, macroscopic examination of morphological characteristics, and microscopic examination using KOH or lactophenol cotton-blue stain. Biochemical reactions are usually limited to *Candida sp*. Immunologic reactions include skin tests, where applicable, agglutination tests, such as latex particle agglutination for histoplasmosis, and tube precipitin and complement-fixation tests.

An *antimicrobial susceptibility test* is a determination of the least amount of an antimicrobial chemotherapeutic agent that will inhibit the growth of a microorganism *in vitro*, using a tube dilution method, agar cup or disc diffusion method. The test may function as an aid in the selection of a chemotherapeutic agent by the physician. Also the concentration of antimicrobial agents in body fluids may be determined by biological assay with an organism of known susceptibility for the specific agent.

The laboratory diagnosis of *viral infections* is based upon (1) examination of infected tissues for pathognomonic changes or for the presence of viral material; (2) isolation and identification of the viral agent; (3) demonstration of a significant increase in antibody titer to a given virus during the course of the illness; (4) detection of viral antigens in lesions—using fluorescein-labeled antibodies; and (5) electron microscopic examination of vesicular fluids or tissue extracts. Blood is used for serological tests, seldom for virus isolation. Acute and convalescent-phase blood specimens must be examined in parallel to determine whether or not antibodies have appeared or increased in titer during the course of the disease. Some examples of human viral infections are: respiratory infections (Adenovirus group), diseases of the nervous system, ie, polio and coxsackie viruses of the picornavirus group, smallpox (poxvirus group), measles (paramyxovirus group), chicken pox (herpesvirus group), and influenza (myxovirus group).

Members of *Mycoplasmatacea* pleuropneumonia-like organisms (PPLO) are of a range of size similar to the larger viruses. They are highly pleomorphic because they lack a rigid cell wall, they can reproduce in cell-free media, and they do not revert to or from bacterial parental forms as the L-forms. Specimens (sputum, bronchial secretions, urinary sediment, etc) for the primary isolation of mycoplasmas (*M pneumoniae*, *M hominis*, etc) should be cultured on agar media containing peptone, serum, ascitic fluid, whole blood, or egg yolk. Species identification may be by growth inhibition on agar medium containing type-specific rabbit antisera. Antigenic variants or subspecies may be detected by immunodiffusion. Various PPLO are pathogenic, parasitic, or saprophytic. Mycoplasmas have a predilection for mucous membranes and are associated with primary atypical pneumonia and bronchitis.

Clinical parasitology is a science which is concerned with the parasitic protozoa (amoeba), the helminths (cestodes, tapeworms; trematodes, flukes; nematodes, roundworms) and the arthropods. The identification of protozoan ova is based on detailed microscopic morphology (nuclei, etc) using wet mounts (saline or iodine) or stained preparations (iron hematoxylin, etc) obtained from fecal specimens (fresh or preserved with polyvinyl alcohol), which are concentrated by sedimentation, centrifugation, or flotation techniques. Trophozoite and/or cystic stages may be detected in fecal specimens associated with intestinal protozoa as in amoebic dysentery caused by *Entamoeba histolytica*.

Commonly encountered helminths are *Necator americanus* (hookworm), *Trichuris trichiura* (whipworm), and *Enterobius vermicularis* (pinworm); they are identified by characteristic ova. Characterization of tapeworm segments (proglottids), or head (scolex) in a fecal specimen will differentiate *Taenia saginata* (beef tapeworm) from *Taenia solium* (pork tapeworm). Eggs of *T solium* and *T saginata* cannot be differentiated on a morphological basis.

Adult flukes oviposit a characteristic egg which may reach the urine, sputum or feces. *Schistosoma japonicum* eggs have a small, indistinct spine; *S mansoni*, a distinct, large lateral spine; and *S haematobium*, a distinct terminal spine.

Arthropoda constitute the largest of the animal phyla which are characterized by a segmented body with the segments usually grouped in two or three distinct body regions, by a chitinous exoskeleton, by several pairs of jointed appendages, and by characteristic internal organs. Most arthropods can be preserved in 70% alcohol. Arthropods are of medical importance since they can infest man and cause mechanical trauma or produce hypersensitivity from repeated exposure (*Cimex lectularius*, the bedbug), or by toxin injection (*Latrodectus mactans*, the black widow spider), by skin invasion (*Sarcoptes scabiei*, the itch mite), and by transmitting disease (*Anopheles* mosquitoes, malaria), and *Yersinia pestis* in fleas (plague).

Serodiagnosis of parasitic diseases includes the following immunodiagnostic tests: complement-fixation (trichinosis); precipitin test (schistosomiasis); bentonite flocculation (ascariasis); hemagglutination (echinococcosis); latex agglutination (trichinosis); cholesterol flocculation (schistosomiasis); fluorescent antibody (malaria); and methylene blue dye test (toxoplasmosis).

Immunochemistry

Clinical immunopathology[24] includes *general immunology* (immunofluorescence, immunodiffusion, immunoelectrophoresis and agglutination tests), *radioimmunoassay* (RIA-hormones, vitamins, drugs, immunoglobulins), *tissue typing* (histocompatibility tests in organ transplants), *cellular immunology*, *cancer immunology*, and *immunohematology*. Examples of each of these disciplines are discussed in this section and other parts of this chapter.

The ELISA, *enzyme-linked immunosorbent assay*, detects antibodies by an indirect technique using enzyme-linked antibodies to label antigenic substances in tissue or body fluid. The antigen is attached to a solid matrix and reacts with a specimen that may contain a complimentary antibody. The antihuman globulin which is conjugated with the enzyme is added and the antigen reacts with the bound antibody of the patient. By adding the substrate molecule the enzyme is detected. This system has been used to identify antibodies to viruses, parasites, bacterial products, and quantitation of some drugs. *Antibody response* is a complex process involving the lymphoid cell system response to foreign stimulus

or antigen. Hematopoietic cells in the fetal yolk sac, liver or marrow develop into lymphoid stem cells, which in turn, differentiate into T-lymphocytes of thymic origin and B-lymphocytes of bone marrow origin. The T-cells further differentiate into lymphoblasts which are responsible for *cell-mediated cellular immunity* (graft vs host reaction, tissue transplant rejection, tuberculin skin testing, *delayed-type hypersensitivity*). B-cells differentiate into plasma cells which are responsible for humoral immunity which is mediated by circulating serum immunoglobulins (*immediate-type hypersensitivity*). Macrophages can cooperate in presentation of antigen to the T or B lymphoblasts. Cooperation between T and B cells, immunological memory, development of immune tolerance to antigens and genetic control of the immune response are integral properties of the immune system and are related to development of immune deficiency and autoimmune disease.

Identification and determination of *immunoglobulins* (IgG, IgM, IgA) by radial immunodiffusion and immunoelectrophoresis have been discussed in the *Protein* section of this chapter. *IgM* (γM) is the earliest antibody found in the primary immune response and falls rapidly after the onset of IgG antibody synthesis. *IgG* (γG) is the major class of antibody in both the primary and secondary immune response. IgG can cross the placenta to provide the early forms of antibody protection for the newborn. IgG and IgM can participate in complement fixation reaction. *IgA* (γA) is found predominantly in saliva and secretions of the gastrointestinal and respiratory tracts. In contrast to IgM and IgG, only a small portion of total IgA is found in blood. IgA functions in protection against pathogens that enter the host through the respiratory or gastrointestinal tract. *IgD* (γD) is found in trace quantities in sera and its function is unknown. *IgE* (γE) is probably the most important antibody in acute hypersensitivity or allergic reactions. Reaction of mast cell- or basophil-bound IgE with antigen initiates release of histamine, slow-reacting substance (SRS), serotonin and bradykinin and the subsequent allergic response. IgE is best quantitated by RIA. Mean serum levels (mg%) in healthy adults are IgG 1200 ± 500, IgA 210 ± 140, IgM 140 ± 70, IgD 3, IgE <0.1.

Heterophile antibodies are agglutinins which are capable of reacting with antigens that are entirely unrelated to those which stimulate their production. These antibodies, which occur in the serum of patients with infectious mononucleosis or serum sickness, will agglutinate formalized horse erythrocytes. In order to distinguish the specific *heterophile agglutinins of infectious mononucleosis*, the serum sample is mixed with guinea-pig kidney tissue or beef erythrocyte stromata; the infectious mononucleosis antibody will be absorbed and inactivated by the beef cells but not by the kidney tissue, and subsequent agglutination of horse erythrocytes will occur only in the kidney-tissue system. This test is used to detect infectious mononucleosis even prior to clinical symptoms. The heterophile titer has no relation to the course or severity of the disease.

Two protein constituents of human plasma, *rheumatoid factor* (RF) and *C-reactive protein* (CRP) are of value in the differential diagnosis of rheumatoid diseases. CRP is a protein present in the serum of patients in the acute stages of bacterial and viral infections, collagen diseases, and other inflammatory processes. The presence of this antigen in serum is detected by agglutination of polystyrene latex particles sensitized with specific CRP antibody globulin. In the management of rheumatic fever, decreases in CRP blood levels are used to measure the effectiveness of therapy.

Rheumatoid arthritis is characterized by the presence of a reactive group of macroglobulins known as RF in blood and synovial fluid. RF is a protein of the IgM globulin fraction and is regarded as an autoantibody against antigenic determinants of IgG. Analysis of RF is based on agglutination procedures employing polystyrene latex particles coated with a layer of adsorbed human gamma globulin. The RF-antibody reaction causes a visible agglutination of the inert latex particles. CRP is not elevated in rheumatoid arthritis.

β-Hemolytic streptococci, the causative agent in rheumatic fever, produce streptolysin O and S, streptokinase, hyaluronidase, desoxyribonuclease, and NADase in the body. Growth of streptococci in tissue with elaboration of these proteins serves as the antigenic stimulus to evoke the production of specific antibodies (eg, *antistreptolysin-O, ASO*). The quantitation of the antibody titer to these enzymes is an index of the strength of the antigenic stimulus and the extent of the streptococcal infection. These antibodies can be detected by latex agglutination (ASO) or tests dependent on inhibition of enzyme action by the antibody (anti-hyaluronidase inhibition of hyaluronic acid depolymerization by hyaluronidase).

The laboratory diagnosis of *syphilis* (treponemal disease) and evaluation of chemotherapeutic approach is based on serological tests. Demonstration of an antibody-like substance, *reagin*, or of true antitreponemal antibody in the serum of infected individuals is accomplished by complement fixation or flocculation tests for reagin, or immunofluorescent techniques for treponemal antibody.

In the *complement fixation* tests (Kolmer CF), reagin reacts with a complex phosphatidic acid antigen (cardiolipin) and complement; the complement is bound and will not lyse hemolysin-sensitized red cells which were added in the second phase of the test. In normal serum the reagin-cardiolipin complex is not formed and the complement is free to react with hemolysin and lyse the erythrocytes.

Flocculation tests for determination of syphilis use a cardiolipin-lecithin-cholesterol antigen which clumps in the presence of serum reagin occurring in nontreponemal diseases and syphilis (*Venereal Disease Research Laboratory—VDRL Test; rapid plasma reagin—RPR test*).

Treponemal antibody can be detected also by reaction of the patient's serum with treponemal antigen and subsequent confirmation with fluorescein-labeled antihuman globulin as an indicator of primary antigen-antibody reaction (*fluorescent treponemal antibody-FTA test*). The patient's serum can be treated with an extract of treponemes prior to the FTA test to remove interfering antibodies and eliminate biological false-positives (FTA-Abs Test). False positives occur in related treponematosis such as yaws, pinta and bejel. Increased reagin titers also occur in malaria, leprosy, infectious mononucleosis, chronic rheumatoid arthritis or systemic lupus erythematosus and in patients on hydralazine therapy.

Febrile antibodies are present in the serum of patients with certain bacterial or rickettsial infections (spotted, typhus, or Q fever). In typhus disease the patient's serum contains a febrile antibody which will agglutinate a suspension of *Proteus OX-19* bacteria (Weil-Felix Reaction). *Salmonella* O-H, *Pasteurella tularensis*, and *Brucella abortus* antigens are used in febrile antibody tests for diagnosis of typhoid or paratyphoid fever, tularemia, and brucellosis, respectively.

Toxoplasmosis is a major cause of birth defects. An expectant mother may become infected with oocysts in uncooked meat or from cat fur and infect the fetus transplacentally. Toxoplasmosis testing is based on detecting serum antibody by a hemagglutination procedure. Red cells sensitized by exposure to toxoplasmosis antigen are agglutinated by the specific antibody.

Radioimmunoassay (RIA)[25,27] has been mentioned in various sections of this chapter as an analytical tool in the measurement of hormones, immunoglobulins, drugs, and steroids. The basic principle of RIA is:

$$Ag^* + Ag + Ab \leftrightharpoons Ag^*Ab + AgAb + Ag^* + Ag$$

RIA is not to be confused with the *specific reactor assay* using labeled antigen and nonantibody protein receptors which is used for vitamin B_{12}, T^4, T^3 and cortisol assays.

All procedures are based on the observation that radiolabeled antigens (Ag*) compete with nonlabeled antigen (Ag) for binding sites on specific antibody (Ab) in the formation of antigen-antibody complexes (Ag*Ab, AgAb). When increasing amounts of Ag are added to the assay, the binding sites of Ab are progressively saturated and the antibody can bind less Ag*. Therefore, the ratio of bound to free Ag* (B/F) or % Ag* bound is a direct index of the concentration of Ag in the assay.

The requirements for RIA are (1) preparation and characterization of Ag, (2) radiolabeling of Ag, (3) preparation of specific Ab, and (4) development of the assay system and methods to separate free (Ag, Ag*) from antibody bound (AgAb, Ag*Ab) antigen.

Antigens can be prepared from natural tissue sources or preferably synthesized. ^3H, ^{14}C or ^{125}I-labeled antigens are routinely used in the assay. The biological and immunochemical activity of the antigen must not be altered in the tagging procedure, and the specific activity of Ag* must be extremely high so that tracer quantities can be used in the assay. Tritium labeling and iodination (^{125}I) produce the highest specific activity, but also increase susceptibility of Ag* to internal degradation and self-radiolysis, in contrast to ^{14}C. In many instances, the original antigen cannot be iodinated, but can be chemically altered in such a way as to retain full antigenic cross-reactivity in RIA, eg, cyclic AMP, has no tyrosyl or histidyl residue for iodination; ^{125}I-succinylcyclic AMP-tyrosine methyl ester retains full cross-reactivity with antibodies to cyclic AMP and is used in the assay.

Hormones, steroids and drug substances are *haptens*. They do not produce antibody response when injected by themselves, but will produce antibodies specific for the hapten when injected as a hapten-protein carrier conjugate. Gastrin (hapten) is coupled to albumin (protein-carrier) by treatment with carbodiimides (CCD) which couple functional carboxyl, amino, alcohol, phosphate or thiol groups. Morphine must be converted to the 3-O-carboxymethyl derivative prior to CCD coupling with albumin to provide a functional coupling group in the hapten. The hapten-conjugate is usually emulsified in a mineral oil preparation of killed *Mycobacterium* (Complete Freunds Adjuvant) and injected intradermally in rabbits or guinea pigs on several occasions. The serum antibody must have both high specificity and affinity for the antigens.

The *assay system* contains Ag*, sample containing endogenous Ag or a standard Ag, and antibody, at specified pH (6.5–8.5). After incubation at 5–37° for anywhere from 1 hour to several days, free and antibody-bound antigen must be separated. This is accomplished by *double antibody technique, solid-phase RIA, resin techniques* or *salt or solvent precipitation*. In the double antibody technique, antiglobulin (Ab′) serum is added to the assay system after incubation. Ab-Ag* and Ab-Ag complexes are antibody-globulin antigen complexes. The antiglobulin will react to form insoluble Ab′-Ab-Ag* and Ab′-Ab-Ag complexes which can be removed by centrifugation. The free Ag*, Ag is in the supernate.

The solid phase RIA is performed by coating tubes with Ab. Ag and Ag* react, compete and bind with Ab on the wall of tube. Unreacted Ag and Ag* is separated by decanting and rinsing the tube. Ab can also be covalently bound with isothiocyanate to dextran gel particles. Ag and Ag* will compete and bind with Ab on particles. Bound antigen can then be separated from free antigen by centrifugation.

RIA has been applied to analysis of hormones (ACTH, angiotensin I, II, gastrin, HCG, FSH, GH, glucagon, HLH, HPL, insulin, thyroxine), steroid hormones (aldosterone, androstenedione, glucocorticoids, testosterone, estrones, progesterone), drug substances (digoxin, digitoxin, amphetamines, barbiturates, morphine, LSD, ouabain), endogenous substances (cyclic AMP, cyclic GMP, prostaglandins, immunoglobulins, hepatitis antigen and carcinoembryonic antigen—CEA). Examples of the specific assays are discussed in other sections.

CEA and AFP (α-1-fetoprotein) are proteins found in fetal tissue. CEA analysis was first proposed as a specific test for early detection of bowel cancer. Although the test does not have absolute specificity for this disease, it may prove of value as a diagnostic aid and therapy monitor. CEA can be detected by RIA. Serum levels >2.5 ng CEA/mL are found in 60–70% of patients with adenocarcinoma of the colon; positive levels are also found in lower percentages in carcinomas of the pancreas, stomach, liver, breast, endometrium, ovary, kidney, and bronchus and in other conditions such as gastrointestinal polyps, colitis, diverticulitis and cirrhosis. CEA appears to be primarily associated with tumors of entodermally derived epithelial tissue. The similarity between CEA and cell surface glycoproteins and sialic acids has stimulated considerable research interest in a new approach to cancer chemotherapy.

The study of *tissue transplantation antigens* is an important factor in studies on tissue and organ transplants. ABO blood group antigens are involved in survival of skin and renal grafts. Because of the presence of natural occurring anti- A and B, avoidance of ABO incompatibility is important in clinical grafting. The *HL-A antigens* are found on tissue and on the white cells. There is one major histocompatibility locus comprising a number of alleles or linked genes, on a single chromosome segment. Each allele controls four to five groups of major transplantation antigens. These HL-A isoantigens affect the survival of allogenic tissue grafts and organ transplants. HL-A antigens can be typed by a leukoagglutination method in which the patient's or donor's white cells are reacted with specific HL-A antisera. HL-A typing can also be performed by a cytotoxicity test in which lymphocytes are mixed with antisera and complement. The antibody can destroy the lymphocytes if a corresponding antigen is present on the cell surface.

References

1. *Detection of Fibrinogen Degradation Products*, Wellcome Res Labs England, 1973.
2. Christensen RL, Triplett DA: "Neutrophil Dysfunction: Quantitative and Qualitative Disorders," *Laboratory Medicine*, Vol 13, No 11: 666–672, November 1982.
3. Bollinger P, Brailas CD, Drewinko B: "Evaluation of Whole-Blood Platelet Analyzers," *Laboratory Medicine, 14*, 492–502, 1983.
4. *Central File for Rare Donors*, Am Assoc Blood Banks, Milwaukee.
5. *ABO and Rh Systems*, Ortho Diagnostics, Raritan, NJ, 1969.
6. *Fed Reg 37FR17419*, Aug 26, 1972.
7. Broughton PMG, Dawson JB: *Advan Clin Chem 15:* 288, 1972.
8. Mears T, Young D: *Am J Clin Pathol 50:* 411, 1968.
9. Meinke W: *Anal Chem 43:* 28A, 1971.
10. Dybaker R: *Std Methods Clin Chem 6:* 223, 1970.
11. Flokstra JH, Soda JA: *Am J Med Sci 254:* 429, 1967.
12. Young DS, *et al: Clin Chem 21:* 1D–423D, 1975.
13. Constantino NV, Kabat HF: *Am J Hosp Pharm 30:* 24–71, 1973.
14. Peterson CM: "What We Are Learning From Glycosylated Hemoglobin," *Diagnostic Medicine*, 73–83 July/August: 1980.
15. *Radial Immunodiffusion and Immunoelectrophoreses for Qualitation and Quantitation of Immunoglobulins* (DHEW Publ. HSM-72-8102), USD-HEW, Washington, DC, 1972.
16. *Bull WHO 43:* 891, 1970.
17. Statland BE: *Clinical Decision Levels For Lab Tests*, Medical Economics Company Inc., Oradell, NJ, 1983.
18. White W, *et al: Practical Automation for the Clinical Laboratory*, Mosby, St. Louis, 1972.
19. Szilagyi G, Aning V, Karmen A: "Comparative Study of Two Methods for Rapid Detection of Clinically Significant Bacteriuria," *J Clinical Laboratory Automation*, 3, 117–122, 1983.
20. Bradley GM: "Fecal Analysis," *Diagnostic Medicine*, 63–74 March/April, 1980.
21. Rubenstein K, *et al: Biochem Biophys Res Comm 47:* 846, 1972.
22. Baron J: *Scand J Gastroenterol 5:* 9, 1970.
23. Kuhn PJ: "Microbiology Gears Up For Prospective Payment," *MLO* 108–116, September 1983.
24. Feldman M, Nossal GJ: *Quart Rev Biol 47:* 269, 1972.
25. Berson S, Yalow R: *Gastroenterol 62:* 1061, 1972.
26. Jorpes J, Mott V: *Secretin, CCK, Pancreozymin and Gastrin*, Springer Verlag, New York, 1973.
27. Skelley DS, *et al: Clin Chem 19:* 146, 1973.

Bibliography

Wintrobe M: *Clinical Hematology*, 6th ed, Lea & Febiger, Philadelphia, 1967.
Lynch MJ: *Medical Laboratory Technology*, 2nd ed, Saunders, Philadelphia, 1969.
Faulkner W, King J: *Manual Clinical Laboratory Procedures*, Chemical Rubber Co, Cleveland, 1970.
Faulkner W, *et al: Handbook Clinical Laboratory Data*, Chemical Rubber Co., Cleveland.
Roth K, Saunders A: *Evaluation of Methods for White Cell Identification and Counting-Advances in Automated Analysis*, Technicon International Congress, 1970.
Dacie J, Lewis S: *Practical Hematology*, 3rd ed, Churchill, London, 1963.
Frankel S, Reitman S, eds: *Clinical Laboratory Methods and Diagnosis*, 6th ed, Mosby, St. Louis, 1963.
Wintrobe MM: *Laboratory Medicine-Hematology*, 2nd ed, Mosby, St. Louis, 1962.
Manual of Blood Coagulation Technics, 2nd ed, Warner-Chilcott, Morris Plains, NJ, 1966.
Detection of Fibrinogen Degradation Products, Wellcome Res Labs, England, 1973.
A Manual of Methods for the Coagulation Laboratory, BD & Co, Rutherford, NJ, 1965.
Technical Methods and Procedures of the American Association of Blood Banks, Am Assoc Blood Banks, Chicago, 1962.
Standards for Blood Transfusion Service, 4th ed, Am Assoc Blood Banks, Chicago, 1963.
Griffiths JJ, Elliott J: *Blood Bank Procedures*, Dade Reagents, Miami, 1967.
Chromatography in Mass Screening for Disorders of Amino Acid Metabolism, Hyland, Los Angeles, 1966.
Rosalki S, Wilkinson J: *Diagnostic Enzymology*, Dade Reagents, Miami, 1966.
Wilkinson J: *Introduction to Diagnostic Enzymology*, Edward Arnold, Ltd., London, 1962.
Davidsohn I, Henry J: *Todd-Sanford Clinical Diagnosis by Laboratory Methods*, 15th ed, Saunders, Philadelphia, 1974.
Peron FG, Caldwell BV: *Immunologic Methods in Steroid Determination*, Appleton-Century, New York, 1970.
Winsten S, Dalal F: *Clinical Laboratory Procedures for Nonroutine Problems*, Chemical Rubber Co., Cleveland, 1972.
Specialized Diagnostic Laboratory Tests, Bioscience Labs., Van Nuys, CA, 1971.
Kark RM, *et al: A Primer of Urinalysis*, 2nd ed, Harper & Row, New York, 1963.
Sunderman FW, Sunderman FW, Jr: *Laboratory Diagnosis of Renal Diseases*, Warren H Green, Inc, St. Louis, 1970.
Faust E, Russell P: *Clinical Parasitology*, 7th ed, Lea & Febiger, Philadelphia, 1964.
Sunshine I: *Manual of Analytical Toxicology*, Chemical Rubber Co., Cleveland, 1972.
Clarke, E: *Isolation and Identification of Drugs*, vols 1 and 2, Pharmaceutical Press, London, 1969, 1975.
Blair JE, *et al: Manual of Clinical Microbiology*, Williams & Wilkins, Baltimore, 1970.
Edwards PR, Ewing WH: *Identification of Enterobacteriaceae*, 3rd ed, Burgess, Minneapolis, 1972.
Holdeman LV, Moore WEC: *Anaerobe Laboratory Manual*, 2nd ed, VPI Anaerobe Lab, Blacksburg, VA, 1973.
Connant NF, *et al: Manual of Clinical Mycology*, 3rd ed, Saunders, Philadelphia, 1971.
Bach F, Good R: *Clinical Immunobiology*, Academic, New York, 1972.
Clinical RIA. *Lab Management:* May 1973.
Manual of tissue typing techniques. *Natl Inst All Infect Dis Bull:* 1972.

Directory of Rare Analysis. *Clin Chem 23:* 323–446, 1977.

Doucet LD, *Medical Technology Review*, JB Lippincott Company, Philadelphia, 1981.

Hansten Philip D, *Drug Interactions*, 3rd ed, Lea & Febiger, Philadelphia, 1975.

Kaplan A, Szabo LL, *Clinical Chemistry: Interpretation and Techniques*, 2nd ed, Lea & Febiger, Philadelphia, 1983.

Miller SE, Weller JM, *Textbook of Clinical Pathology*, 8th ed, Williams & Wilkins, Baltimore, 1971.

Peacock J, Tomar R, *Manual of Laboratory Immunology*, Lea & Febiger, Philadelphia, 1980.

Pertinent Reference Journals

Advan Clin Chem	*J Clin Lab Automation*
Am J Clin Pathol	*Diagn Med*
Am Clin Prod Rev	*J Lab Clin Med*
Am J Hosp Pharm	*Lab Medicine*
Am J Med Technol	*Lab Notes Med Diag*
Anal Chem	*Med Lab Obs*
BioTechniques	*Med Lab Tech*
Clin Chem	*Scand J Clin Lab Invest*
Clin Chim Acta	*Std Methods Clin Chem*

CHAPTER 33

Chromatography

Leonard C Bailey, PhD

Associate Professor of Pharmaceutical Chemistry
Rutgers University College of Pharmacy
Piscataway, NJ 08854

Modern pharmaceutical formulations are complex mixtures including, in addition to one or more medicinally active ingredients, a number of inert materials such as diluents, disintegrants, colors, and flavors. In order to ensure quality and stability of the final product, the pharmaceutical analyst must be able to separate these mixtures into individual components prior to quantitative analysis. Moreover, comparison of the relative efficacy of different dosage forms of the same drug entity requires the analysis of the active ingredient in biological matrices, eg, blood, urine, and tissue. Among the most powerful techniques available to the analyst for the resolution of these mixtures are a group of highly, efficient methods collectively called *chromatography*. Because this technique is so intimately involved in all aspects of pharmaceutical research and development, the pharmacist should possess a working knowledge of chromatographic principles and techniques. Although electrophoresis is fundamentally different than chromatography, a short discussion of this important separation technique is provided at the end of this chapter.

Chromatography comprises a group of methods for separating molecular mixtures that depend on the differential affinities of the solutes between two immiscible phases. One of the phases is a fixed bed of large surface area while the other is fluid which moves through, or over the surface of, the fixed phase. The components of the mixture must be of molecular dimensions which requires that they be in solution or in the vapor state. The relative affinity of the solutes for each of the phases must be reversible to ensure that mass transfer occurs during the chromatographic separation.

The fixed phase is called the *stationary phase*, and the other is termed the *mobile phase*. The stationary phase may be a porous or finely divided solid, or a liquid that has been coated in a thin layer on an inert supporting material. It is necessary that the stationary phase particles be as small as possible in order to provide a large surface area so that sorption and desorption of the solutes will occur frequently. The mobile phase may be a pure liquid or a mixture of solutions (eg buffers) or it may be a gas (pure or a homogeneous mixture).

Chromatographic methods can be classified according to the nature of the stationary and mobile phases. If the stationary phase is a solid, the process is called *adsorption chromatography*, whereas if the stationary phase is a liquid, it is termed *partition chromatography*. The difference between adsorption and partition chromatography can be ascribed to the nature of the forces which influence the distribution of the solutes between the two phases.

In adsorption chromatography, the mobile phase containing the dissolved solutes passes over the surface of the stationary phase. Retention of the components and their consequent separation depends on the ability of the atoms on the surface to remove the solutes from the mobile phase and adsorb them temporarily by means of electrostatic forces. If the mobile phase is a liquid, the process is called *liquid-solid chroma-*

tography (*LSC*) but when the mobile phase is a gas, the method is called *gas-solid chromatography* (*GSC*).

In partition chromatography, an inert solid material, such as silica gel or diatomaceous earth, serves to support a thin layer of liquid which is the effective stationary phase. As the mobile phase containing the solutes passes in close proximity to this liquid phase, retention and separation occur due to the relative solubility of the analytes in the two fluids as determined by their partition coefficients. If the mobile phase is a liquid, this type of partition chromatography is called *liquid-liquid chromatography* (*LLC*) and if the mobile phase is a gas the process is termed *gas-liquid chromatography* (*GLC*).

Two other modes of chromatography in which the stationary phase is a solid are classified differently from LSC and GSC because of the unique nature of their separation processes. These are *ion-exchange chromatography* and *size-exclusion chromatography*.

In *ion-exchange chromatography* the stationary phase consists of a polymeric matrix onto the surface of which ionic functional groups, eg, carboxylic acids or quaternary amines, have been chemically bonded. As the mobile phase passes over this surface, ionic solutes are retained by forming electrostatic chemical bonds with the functional groups. The mobile phases used in ion-exchange chromatography are always liquid.

In *size-exclusion chromatography*, the stationary phase is a polymeric substance containing numerous pores of molecular dimensions. Solutes whose molecular size is sufficiently small leave the mobile phase to diffuse into the pores. Larger molecules which will not fit into the pores remain in the mobile phase and are not retained. This method is most suited to the separation of mixtures in which the solutes vary considerably in molecular size. The mobile phase in size-exclusion chromatography may be either liquid or gaseous.

The classifications given above for the various types of chromatography can be deceptive in their simplicity. Except in isolated cases, pure adsorption or partition chromatography rarely occur. The ultimate success of a chromatographic separation depends on the ability of the analyst to recognize the limitations of the methods and adjust his experiments accordingly.

The Chromatographic Process

In order to appreciate the theory and applications of chromatography, it is worthwhile to consider the events taking place in an ideal chromatograph. Conceptually, chromatography may be considered as being similar to the processes occurring in fractional distillation or sequential solvent extraction. In distillation, mixtures of liquids are separated by a series of steps involving vaporization and subsequent condensation. Each step involves an equilibrium between a vapor enriched in the more volatile component and a liquid condensate of the same composition. Each single equilibra-

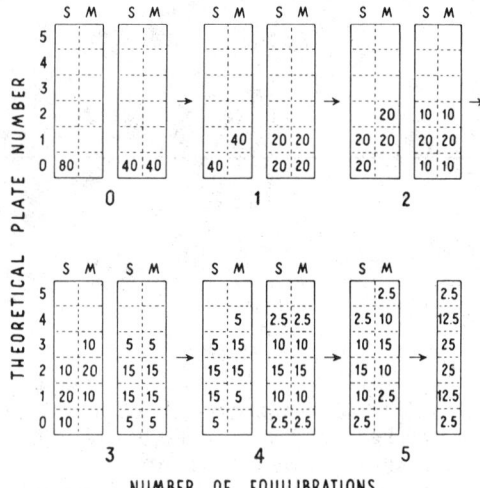

NUMBER OF EQUILIBRATIONS

Fig 33-1. Chromatography depicted as a discontinuous equilibrium process. For purposes of illustration the stationary (S) and mobile (M) phases are shown separately. The mobile phase migrates up the paper strip causing a solute with a partition coefficient of unity to successively equilibrate between the two phases.

tion between the phases is termed a *theoretical plate* and the length of the column required for one equilibration is called the *height equivalent to a theoretical plate* or *HETP*. The nomenclature has been adopted by chromatographers to describe the equivalent transfer of solute between the mobile and stationary phases.

In solvent extraction, a solute, commonly dissolved in an aqueous vehicle, is partially transferred in one step into an immiscible solvent. The amount of solute transferred is determined by its partition coefficient which is the ratio of its concentration (in reality, activity) in the nonaqueous and aqueous phases, respectively. After the first step, the layers are separated, fresh solvent is brought in contact with the aqueous phase and, as a result, a new equilibrium based on the partition coefficient is established and more solute is transferred to the nonaqueous phase. Each of these extraction steps is equivalent to one theoretical plate and is analogous to the solute transfer process occurring in a chromatographic system.

With the aid of Fig 33-1, these concepts can be applied to the visualization of the passage of a solute through a chromatographic system containing six theoretical plates. The process is started by applying 80 μg of a solute with a partition coefficient of unity to the area of the first theoretical plate. As mobile phase is brought in contact with the stationary phase, the solute distributes itself equally into each phase according to its partition coefficient. Next, the mobile phase is allowed to flow so that it carries its dissolved solute into the area of the next theoretical plate. Now, the solute retained on the stationary phase in the first plate partitions equally into fresh mobile phase while the solute in the mobile phase of the second plate distributes itself into the stationary phase. If the process is continued through the remainder of the plates, an equilibrium is established such that equal amounts of solute are present in the mobile and stationary phases.

If the flow is stopped after the last equilibration and the total amount of solute in each plate is plotted as a function of plate number (as in Fig 33-2a), it can be seen that the graph assumes the approximate shape of a Gaussian distribution. This shape is characteristic of an elution distribution and from it some inferences about chromatographic behavior can be drawn.

First, as a solute moves through a chromatographic system, it is subject to a phenomenon called *band-broadening*. Even though the entire mass of solute is introduced into one theo-

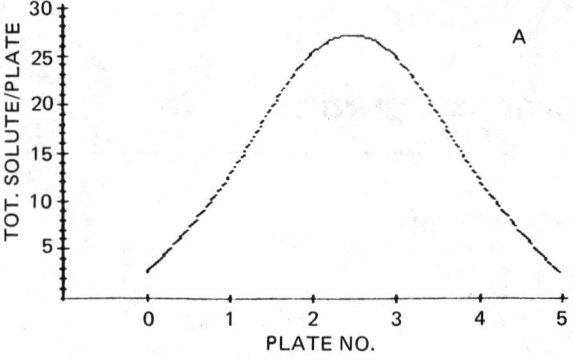

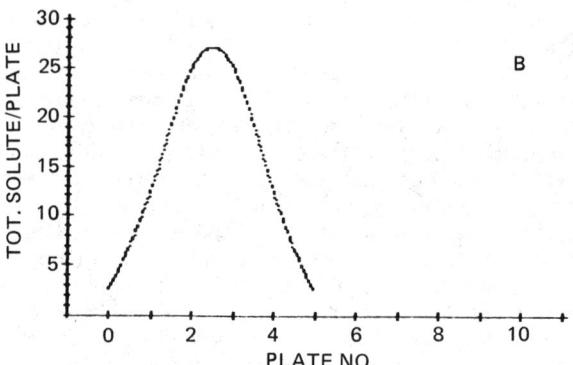

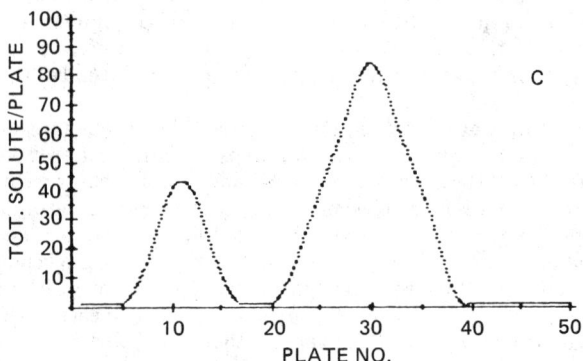

Fig 33-2. Effect on peak shape of the number of theoretical plates in a chromatographic system. A. Typical Gaussian curve produced by an eluting solute. B. Compression of the curve as the plate height is reduced. C. Separation of solute bands as the number of plates is increased.

retical plate, it soon becomes distributed over a broader area of the system. However, the large majority is concentrated at the center of the band as predicted by the Gaussian distribution. If the system is altered (by changing the mobile or stationary phases, or both) so that more theoretical plates are present, the HETP is reduced and the band becomes narrower (as in Fig 33-2b). This increases the efficiency of the system and so it has become common to compare the efficiencies of different chromatographic processes by stating N, the number of theoretical plates, or the respective HETP's.

Second, the separation of a mixture of compounds can only be achieved if their bands can be made to move at different rates through the system so that eventually they do not overlap. This is possible only if the partition coefficients of the solutes are appreciably different. This condition can be demonstrated by carrying out the idealized elution procedure as before except for assuming that the partition coefficient of the second solute is 3. By using the same stepwise scheme as in Fig 33-1, it can be shown that after six equilibrations the greater mass of the second solute will be concentrated in the second plate whereas the first solute is predominantly in the third and fourth plates. As more and more plates are introduced, the bands become narrower and no longer overlap. This results in an elution pattern similar to the one in Fig 33-2c, in which each solute is concentrated in a different area of the column and complete separation is achieved.

Although the example presented above is sufficient to give a understanding of the basic processes occurring in chromatography, it should be realized that actual chromatograms may depart significantly from this ideal state since the process is not a discontinuous one as described above. Rather, the mobile phase is moving at a more or less constant rate over the stationary phase. If the rate of solute transfer from one phase to the other is not much faster than the linear velocity of the mobile phase, equilibrium will not be attained at each plate. This results in broadening of the band to a size greater than would be predicted by the ideal treatment and subsequent loss of separation. In more severe cases, this may result in peaks which are *asymmetric (skewed; tailed)*. The efficiency and sensitivity of the method is reduced and its potential for quantitative analysis is lessened.

Techniques of Column Development

As stated previously, chromatographic processes are classified according to the physical states of the mobile and stationary phases, ie, whether they are gaseous, liquid, or solid. Each of these techniques may be further classified depending on the method of mobile phase development into *frontal analysis, displacement analysis, and elution analysis.*

Frontal Analysis—Frontal analysis was one of the earliest methods of chromatography. From 1898 to 1903, DT Day and his associates separated crude oil samples on large columns of limestone and powdered Fuller's earth. By percolating the crude oil through these columns, they found that the mixture could be separated into aliphatic hydrocarbons followed by aromatic hydrocarbons and nitrogen and sulfur compounds of increasing complexity.

In frontal analysis, a large volume of a sample mixture is allowed to flow continuously through a chromatographic column. The most weakly retained component of the mixture emerges alone from the column first (as in Fig 33-3). After a period of time during which the first component elutes continually at a constant rate, a sharp front appears indicating the appearance of the next most weakly retained compound. This now elutes as a mixture with the first component. The appearance of the next front indicates the emergence of the

third most weakly retained compound in a mixture with the first two. This process continues until the effluent has the same composition as the sample being introduced into the column. After this point, no further separation can occur.

Because only the component which elutes first can be obtained in a pure state, frontal analysis has never been used extensively. However, recent research has indicated that it may be useful for the analysis of complex mixtures which cannot be resolved by other means. If the first derivative of the frontal chromatogram is taken, the resulting graph resembles exactly a normal elution pattern (as in Fig 33-2c). The point of maximum height of the peak for each component corresponds to the inflection point of each rising front. The flat portions of the frontal chromatogram, since they are constant, give derivatives of zero and thus form the baseline. The computations of the derivatives can be done easily by a computer.

Displacement Analysis—In displacement analysis, the sample mixture, dissolved in a small volume of solvent, is introduced onto the column as a narrow band at the top. The mobile phase, containing a *displacing agent*, is then allowed to pass through the column. The displacing agent is a substance which is more strongly retained by the stationary phase than any of the components of the sample mixture and it therefore forces them off the surface of the stationary phase into the mobile phase. As each of the displaced solutes move through the column in the mobile phase, it in turn acts as a displacing agent for less strongly retained compounds. The final result is that the solute that is least firmly bound is eluted first, followed in order by those more tightly bound and finally by the displacing agent. A displacement chromatogram is illustrated in Fig 33-4. The pattern is similar to that obtained with frontal analysis except that the trailing edge of each solute zone does not extend back through the length of the column.

Although displacement analysis is not used in quantitative studies, it has two potential advantages. First, it is possible to isolate in a pure state at least a portion of each of the compounds eluting from the column. Second, in the course of the separation process the sample is concentrated instead of being diluted as usually occurs in chromatographic analyses.

Elution Analysis—Elution analysis is the most frequently used technique of chromatographic development. Credit for the initial discovery of this method is usually accorded to Michael Tswett, a Russian botanist working at the University of Warsaw, who used it to separate leaf pigments, such as chlorophyll. Instead of percolating a large volume of sample solution through the column, he applied a small amount of a petroleum ether extract to the top of a calcium carbonate column. He then *developed* the column with pure solvent and was able to separate the extract into seven colored bands.

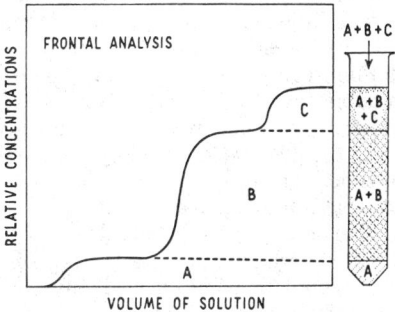

Fig 33-3. Frontal analysis for determining the number of components in a mixture. A solution containing a mixture of the Solutes A, B, and C is percolated through the adsorption column at the right. A is least strongly adsorbed and appears first in the effluent solution. This is followed by a mixture of A + B and finally A + B + C. The elution diagram illustrates the increasing concentration of solutes in the effluent.

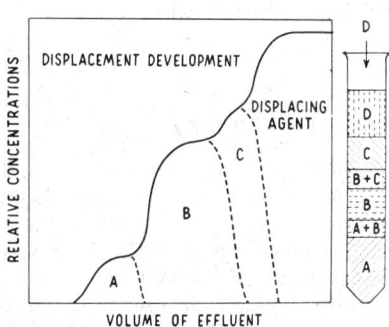

Fig 33-4. Displacement development for determining number, nature, and concentration of solutes. A sample containing Solutes A + B + C is applied to the top of an adsorption column. The chromatogram is developed with a solvent containing a displacing agent (D) which is more strongly adsorbed on the column than either A, B, or C.

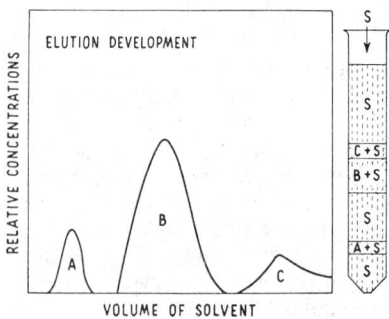

Fig 33-5.   Elution development for separating components of a mixture.   A sample containing Solutes A + B + C is applied to the top of an absorption column, and the chromatogram developed by percolating pure solvent (S) through the column.   The component separate as they pass down the column and are collected separately in the effluent.

He is also credited with coining the terms *chromatography* (color-writing) to describe the process and *chromatogram* to describe the developed column.

As indicated above, elution analysis is carried out by introducing the sample in as small a volume as possible onto the head of the column.   The mobile phase is then allowed to flow through the system.   The components with larger partition coefficients will be retarded in their passage through the system and will "elute" later.   A typical elution chromatogram is shown in Fig 33-5.   The advantages of elution chromatography are that each component of a separated mixture can be isolated in a relatively pure state contaminated only by mobile phase and that the method can be readily used for quantitative analysis.   If the strength of the mobile phase is not changed during the course of the development of the chromatogram, the technique is called *isocratic elution analysis.*

A widely used modification of elution analysis, which is capable of overcoming the difficulties of long elution times and poor resolution of complex mixtures, is called *gradient elution analysis*.   In this adaptation, two eluting solvents, one *weak* and one *strong*, are used to develop the chromatogram.   The *weak* solvent has a lower affinity for the solutes whereas the *strong* solvent has a higher affinity.   The elution begins using only the weak solvent and as the development progresses, the strong solvent is gradually mixed in until the final mobile phase has a composition approaching that of the strong solvent.   The mixing is done in a specially designed chamber at the top of the column.   The result is that the composition and strength of the mobile phase change constantly during the analysis.   Weakly retained solutes are eluted first by the weak solvent, and strongly retained solutes, which would not elute at all with the weak solvent or which would have undesirably long retention times, are eluted by the increasingly stronger mobile phase.

Theory of Chromatography

Two theoretical approaches have been developed to describe the processes involved in the passage of solutes through a chromatographic system.   The first of these, the *plate theory*, based on the work of AJP Martin and RLM Synge[1], considers the chromatographic system as a series of discrete layers of theoretical plates.   At each of these, equilibration of the solute between the mobile and stationary phases occurs.   Movement of the solute is considered as a series of stepwise transfers from plate to plate.   The second, or *rate theory*, discussed in the book by Giddings, considers the dynamics of the solute particle as it passes through the void spaces between the stationary phase particles in the system as well as its ki-

netics as it is transferred to and from the stationary phase. Aspects of both of these theories will be presented in the discussion following in order to exemplify the basic principles underlying the chromatographic process and introduce the experimental parameters necessary for the understanding and interpretation of chromatograms.

Chromatographic systems achieve their ability to separate mixtures of chemicals by selectively retarding the passage of some compounds through the stationary phase while permitting others to move more freely.   Therefore, the chromatogram may be evaluated qualitatively by determining the R_f, or *retardation factor*, for each of the eluted substances. The R_f is a measure of the fraction of its total elution time that any compound spends in the mobile phase.   Since the solute particle proceeds down the column only when it is in the mobile phase, the R_f is directly related to the fraction of the total amount of solute that is in the mobile phase, and it can be expressed as:

$$R_f = \frac{V_M C_M}{V_M C_M + V_S C_S}$$

where V_M is the volume of the mobile phase, and V_S is the effective volume of the stationary phase, ie, the volume available for interaction with the solutes.   The variables C_M and C_S indicate the concentrations of the solute in the respective phases at any time.   By dividing each term of the fraction by C_M, this can be simplified to:

$$R_f = \frac{V_M}{V_M + K V_S}$$

where K, the partition coefficient, equals C_S/C_M, the ratio of the solute concentration in the stationary phase to that in the mobile phase, and is an equilibrium constant that indicates the differential affinity of the solute for the two phases.   It can be seen from this expression that a component with a large partition coefficient, that is, one which is strongly attracted to the stationary phase, will have a small R_f and a long elution time since only a small fraction of its total mass will be in the mobile phase at any time.   By dividing each term of the fraction by V_M, an alternate expression results:

$$R_f = \frac{1}{1 + k'}$$

where the *capacity factor, $k' = K V_S/V_M$.*   The capacity factor, which is normally constant for small samples, is a parameter that expresses the ability of a particular solute to interact with a chromatographic system.   Since the volumes of the stationary and mobile phases are constant for any chromatographic experiment, k' is directly proportional to the partition coefficient.   Therefore, the larger the value of k', the more the sample is retarded.

Both the retardation factor and the capacity factor may be used for qualitative identification of a solute or for developing strategies for improving separations.   In terms of parameters easily obtainable from the chromatogram, the R_f is defined as the ratio of the distance from the origin traveled by the solute band to the distance traveled by the mobile phase in a particular time.   The R_f is most conveniently used in *complete chromatography*, eg, paper and thin-layer chromatography, which occurs when the mobile phase is allowed to develop to a predetermined point in the system and is then stopped.   Solutes will then have moved only a fraction of the distance traveled by the mobile phase.   In *continuous chromatography*, as exemplified by the gas and liquid column techniques, mobile phase development is permitted to continue indefinitely until the solutes elute from the end of the stationary phase.   Measurement of the capacity factor, described below, is more useful in the latter cases.

The time which elapses from the start of the chromatogram to the elution maximum of the solute is called the *retention time*, t_R, and it is a function of the length of the column and the rate of travel of the solute.   The rate of travel is determined by the expression:

$$RATE = \mu \, R_f$$

where μ is the linear velocity of the mobile phase, usually expressed in cm/sec.   Thus

$$t_R = \frac{Length}{Rate} = \frac{L}{\mu}\,(1 + k') = t_0(1 + k')$$

where t_0 is the time for the elution of a solute that is not retained by the chromatographic system.   From this, a convenient expression for the experimental determination of the capacity factor can be formulated:

$$k' = \frac{(t_R - t_0)}{t_0}$$

The values of k' should ideally be between one and ten, i.e., solutes should be retained from two to eleven times as long as the unretained compound.   Values of k' greater than ten result in longer retention times and broad peaks, while values less than one lead to poor separation.

Another parameter used to describe the retardation of a solute is the *retention volume*, V_R, which is equal to the volume of mobile phase required to elute a compound from the system.   Therefore, the retention volume is equal to the product of the retention time and the flow rate of the mobile phase, $t_R F$, or $t_0(1 + k')F$.   Since $t_0 F$ is equal to the volume of mobile phase in the system (V_M, or the *void volume*), the retention volume can be expressed as:

$$V_R = V_M(1 + k') = V_M + K\,V_S$$

Therefore, the retention volume of a solute depends on the relative volumes of the two phases and on the partition coefficient.   Since the phase volumes are identical for each solute in a mixture, the most important influence on retention arises from the partition coefficient.   A large partition coefficient results in long retention since the solute spends more time in the stationary phase.

Retention time and retention volume frequently vary slightly from run to run due to small changes in operating parameters such as temperature and flow rate.   In order to minimize the errors caused by these variations, retention time and/or volume are frequently measured with respect to another peak in the chromatogram rather than from the origin.   Since the peak of interest and the reference peak are affected similarly by the changes in experimental conditions, the retention measurements are more accurate.   In these cases, the parameters are termed *relative retention time*, *RRT*, and *relative retention volume*, *RRV*.

As was mentioned previously, the elution pattern of an ideal chromatographic peak is a curve whose shape is Gaussian.   Thus, it can be described by parameters derived from the Normal statistical distribution, ie, the standard deviation, σ, and the variance, σ.[2]   It can be seen clearly by reference to Fig 33-6 that the peak width at any point can be expressed as a multiple of the standard deviation.   The inflection points are located at one standard deviation on either side of the mean at a level which is 60.7% of the overall height of the peak.   The width at this point is therefore 2σ.   If tangents to the peak are drawn through the inflection points and extended to the baseline, the width at the base, W_B, is 4σ.   The width at half the height is 2.354σ (W_H).

Two further characteristics of the peak are the height and area.   The area is equal to the integral of the equation representing the curve from the point where it leaves the baseline to the point where it returns and is proportional to the amount or concentration of the solute.   The height is measured at the maximum and therefore corresponds to the greatest concentration in the zone.   It is at the point of maximum height that retention times and volumes are measured.

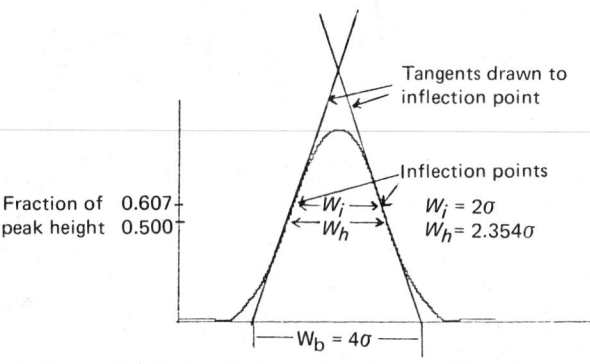

Fig 33-6.   Distribution characteristics of a typical Gaussian peak.

Two parameters commonly used for estimating the effectiveness of a chromatographic system are N, the number of theoretical plates, and H, the Height Equivalent to a Theoretical Plate (HETP), which is defined as L/N where L is the length of the column.   Since the width and standard deviation of a peak can vary depending on experimental conditions, a better indicator of the sharpness of a peak is its *relative standard deviation* (RSD), σ/t_R.   In practice, N is defined in terms of the reciprocal of the RSD by the expression $N = (t_R/\sigma)^2$.   Since it would be difficult to determine σ for each peak, the relationships given above ($W_B = 4\sigma$, $W_H = 2.354\sigma$) can be substituted to arrive at the equations

$$N = 16(t_R/W_B)^2 \text{ and } N = 5.545(t_R/W_H)^2$$

which are readily evaluated from the chromatogram.   Although these are mathematically equivalent expressions, the former is used more frequently.   However, the latter is particularly useful for non-ideal peaks of unsymmetrical shape and possibly skewed or tailed, since the asymmetry is less pronounced at the half-height.   At any particular retention time a system with a greater number of theoretical plates will produce a narrower peak and will therefore be capable of separating more complex mixtures.

Chromatographic systems are available in which N is 50,000/meter or better.   These values are established with selected test compounds, and the analyst should be aware that such levels will not be obtained with every sample.   Because of intrinsic differences in the affinities of different compounds for the stationary phase, every solute will have a unique value for N in a particular system.

The procedures discussed above enable the chromatographer to derive from the experimental data a number of parameters which characterize the retention behavior of individual compounds in a system.   However, the greatest utility of chromatography lies in its ability to separate mixtures of solutes so that a number of individual substances may be quantitated or isolated in a pure state.

To develop strategies for accomplishing these objectives, consideration must be given to parameters which describe the interrelationships of both the retention and peak shape variables for more than one peak.   The most significant of these parameters are *separation*, which is concerned with the relative positions of the band centers, and *resolution*, which describes the overlap of the leading and trailing edges of successive peaks.   These are illustrated in Fig 33-7.   In Fig 33-7a, a chromatogram with poor separation and resolution indicates the presence of two peaks, but is useful neither for quantitation nor for isolation of either substance.   In Fig 33-7b, adequate separation has been achieved, but resolution remains poor because of overlap of the trailing edge of peak 1 and the leading edge of peak 2.   In Fig 33-7c, the separation

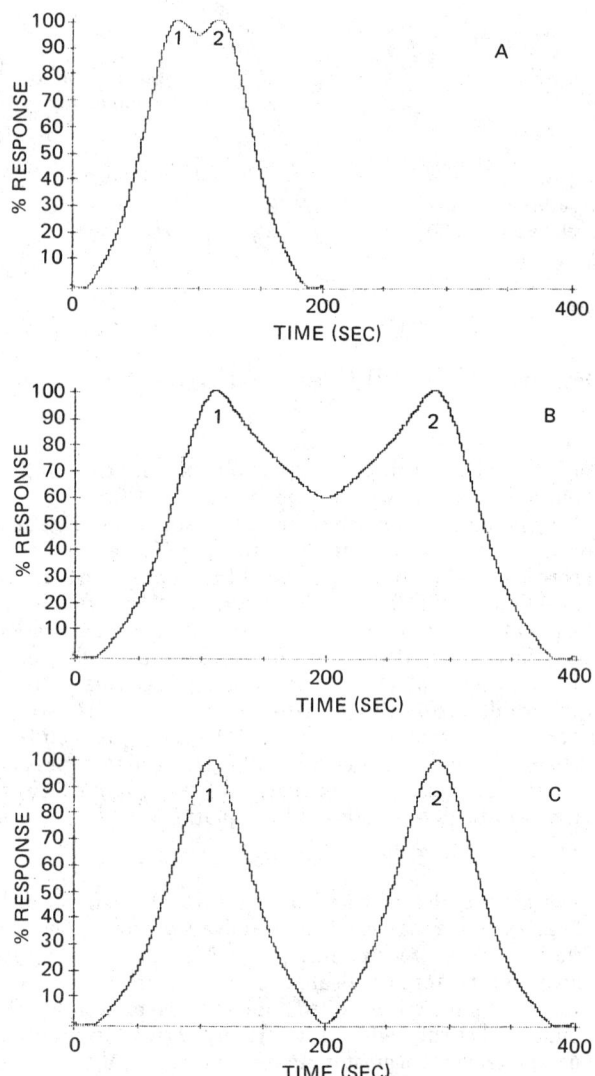

Fig 33-7. Effect of changes in separation and resolution on the elution pattern of adjacent peaks. A. The band centers are poorly separated and resolution is poor. B. Separation has been increased but band overlap remains, causing poor resolution. C. Peak separation is the same as in Fig 33-7B but overlap is reduced, giving good resolution.

has remained constant while resolution has been optimized to lessen band overlap, resulting in an ideal chromatogram.

In order to achieve adequate separation of two adjacent peaks it is necessary to adjust the experimental variables so that the band centers or peak maxima elute at significantly different points on the chromatogram. As previously indicated, this requires that the partition coefficients of the two solutes be sufficiently different, so that one substance is more strongly retained than the other. Therefore, α, the *separation factor* or *selectivity factor*, may be defined as K_2/K_1, that is, the ratio of the partition coefficient of the solute producing the second band to that of the solute producing the first. Since k', the capacity factor, is directly proportional to K, the separation factor may also be stated as the ratio of the respective k' values, ie k_2'/k_1'. From an experimental viewpoint, this is more useful, since k' can be more easily determined from peak retention parameters than K. Therefore, the separation factor is usually stated in terms of the adjusted retention times or volumes as:

$$\alpha = \frac{(t_r)_2 - t_0}{(t_r)_1 - t_0} = \frac{(V_R)_2 - V_M}{(V_R)_1 - V_M}$$

Since it is based on Relative Retention Times and Relative Retention Volumes, the separation factor is also termed the *relative retention*. In addition to being useful in optimizing chromatographic separation, α also has value in qualitative analysis by chromatography. If, under identical experimental conditions, an unknown compound has the same relative retention as a known substance, the identity of the unknown substance can be inferred. However, more positive identification, with greater confidence, requires that the same relative retention for the test sample be exhibited in two *different* chromatographic systems.

As shown in Fig 33-7b, it is possible to attain adequate separation of the peak maxima and yet fail to have a useful chromatogram because of overlap of the adjacent portions of the two peaks. In this case the partition coefficients of the two compounds are sufficiently different to effect separation but the efficiency of the chromatographic system in terms of the number of theoretical plates is low. For the purpose of comparison, the *resolution* between two adjacent peaks can be defined as the distance between the band centers divided by the average peak width:

$$R_S = \frac{2(t_{R2} - t_{R1})}{W_1 + W_2}$$

where the peak widths at the baseline are measured by drawing tangents through the inflection points and are therefore taken as four times the standard deviation. For two adjacent peaks of equal size, when $R_S = 1.00$ there will be a 4% contamination of each component by the other due to overlap. At $R_S = 1.25$, the overlap will be 2%, and at $R_S = 1.50$ it will be 0.3%. The calculation of resolution is especially useful when chromatography is being used to isolate pure compounds, since it gives the chromatographer an indication of where to start and end collection of the peak in order to achieve the desired purity. A more detailed discussion of resolution, especially in those cases where the adjacent peaks are not equal in size and shape, can be found in the text by Snyder and Kirkland.

Techniques of Chromatography

The four basic modes of chromatography—adsorption, partition, ion-exchange, and size-exclusion—can be applied to the analysis of pharmaceutical systems through the use of a number of techniques which differ from each other according to the nature of the stationary and mobile phases and the apparatus used to perform the chromatography. While it may be possible to analyze a sample using more than one of these methods, the choice of a particular technique depends on a number of factors, including the complexity of the sample, the chemical and physical properties of the compounds to be separated, the resolution required, the ease and speed of the technique and its ability to be automated, the availability and cost of the equipment, and the need to isolate the separated analytes.

If the materials are volatile and stable in the gas phase, gas chromatography may be the technique of choice since it is simple to perform, rapid, and capable of high resolution. If it is necessary to isolate eluted compounds in quantity, then liquid partition or thin-layer chromatography may be a more advantageous choice. Gas chromatographic columns cannot handle large quantities of material and it is difficult to retrieve the eluants from the hot effluent gases. If the substances are of high molecular weight, such as proteins, triglycerides, or polymers, liquid chromatography using the size-exclusion mode is necessary to achieve separation. For compounds which are ionized in solution, eg amino acids, the ion-exchange mode of liquid chromatography is particularly useful. Highly polar or hydrophilic compounds of intermediate molecular weight, such as sugars, can be separated by partition techniques involving paper or column chromatography. Substances which are nonionizable, hydrophobic, or nonpolar are amenable to separation by liquid adsorption methods. The following sections provide a discussion of the various techniques available to the chromatographer, including the modes applicable to each technique, the apparatus required, and applications to specific separations.

Gas Chromatography

In 1941, in their paper on partition chromatography which outlined the plate theory, Martin and Synge[1] proposed the technique of gas chromatography with the following statement:

"The mobile phase need not be a liquid but may be a vapour . . . Very refined separations of volatile substances should therefore be possible in a column in which a permanent gas is made to flow over gel impregnated with a non-volatile solvent in which the substances to be separated approximately obey Raoult's Law."

In the subsequent ten years, no one followed up on this suggestion, so Martin returned to it himself and with AT James developed the first separations using gas chromatography.[2] Once the validity and utility of the method had been demonstrated, other workers quickly adopted it and gas chromatography became more rapidly and broadly applied to scientific research than any other analytical technique developed before that time. Tens of thousands of papers have been published using it as the analytical technique and thousands of instruments are in use in laboratories throughout the world.

Gas chromatographic methodology is divided into two classes depending only on the nature of the stationary phase, since the mobile phase is always a gas. These are *gas-solid chromatography (GSC)*, in which the stationary phase is a solid adsorptive material and solute particles are removed from the mobile phase by electrostatic forces, and *gas-liquid chromatography (GLC)*, in which the stationary phase is a thin layer of liquid, usually as a coating on the surface of an inert particle. In this method solute molecules are retained in the liquid phase based on their partition coefficients between it and the gaseous mobile phase.

Theory—In the mid 1950's, a group of Dutch chemical engineers began a study of the processes which caused band-broadening in chromatography. They derived an expression, commonly called the van Deemter equation, relating the height equivalent to a theoretical plate (HETP) to a number of experimental parameters, including the diameter of stationary phase particles, the diffusion coefficients of the solute in the stationary and mobile phases, and the flow rate of the mobile phase. For descriptive purposes, the original complicated equation is frequently given in the simplified form:

$$\text{HETP} = A + B/\mu + C\mu$$

where μ is the linear velocity, in cm/sec, of the mobile phase, and A, B, and C are coefficients which describe the various diffusion processes occurring in the chromatography which lead to band broadening.

The coefficient A is called the *eddy diffusion* or *multiple-path coefficient* and is concerned with the different paths traveled by the molecules of a particular solute during their passage through the column. The particles of the stationary phase, whether irregularly or spherically shaped, are packed as tightly as possible and the solute molecules must pass around them in order to proceed along the column. Because of the large number of possible paths, some molecules of the same kind will reach the end of the column before others. On the average, however, most molecules travel paths of approximately the same length and the greatest mass of solute is concentrated near the band center. Faster molecules are

found in the leading edge of the peak, and slower ones form the trailing edge. The net effect of this distribution is band broadening. Eddy diffusion effects can be reduced by using small, uniformly packed particles.

The coefficient B in the van Deemter equation is termed the *coefficient of longitudinal diffusion*. Since the concentration of solute is lower at the edges of the band than in the center, a gradient exists and, during the travel of the band through the column, solute is continually diffusing through the mobile phase away from the center of the band. This phenomenon occurs at both the leading and trailing edges of the peak and contributes further to band broadening. Since the equation predicts that the contribution to the HETP of this term is inversely proportional to the mobile phase velocity, the effect is more pronounced at low flow rates. Diffusion effects are more severe in gas chromatography than in liquid chromatography since diffusion coefficients are several orders of magnitude higher in a gas. The contribution of longitudinal diffusion to band broadening can be lessened by proper adjustment of flow rate and by increasing the viscosity of the mobile phase.

The third term of the van Deemter equation, the *coefficient of mass transfer*, C, is concerned with the transfer of the solute between the two phases. Since the mobile phase is moving rapidly, equilibrium between the two phases may not be attained. Therefore, some solute molecules in the mobile phase are not transferred to the stationary phase quickly enough, and, as a result, are carried ahead of the center of the band. Those in the stationary phase are retained too long, and hence lag behind. In contrast to longitudinal diffusion, the contribution to the plate height of this term is directly proportional to flow rate, so that in order to minimize the overall effect, a compromise in flow rate is necessary. Mass transfer effects may also be lessened by using small particles with a very thin coating of stationary phase so that the area in contact with the mobile phase is maximized while diffusion deep into the stationary phase is reduced.

In Fig 33-8 a graph of the simplified form of the van Deemter equation is shown as well as the contributions of each of the terms throughout a range of flow rates. A distinct minimum corresponding to a narrow range of flow velocities can be seen. Although this ideal curve may not be achieved in practice, it is possible to optimize a gas chromatographic analysis by running the test compound at various flow rates, determining the respective values for HETP, and plotting the van Deemter curve. In this manner the HETP for any solute under a particular set of experimental conditions can be minimized. For a more detailed treatment of the applicability of the van Deemter equation to both gas and liquid chromatography, the excellent review by Hawkes[3] is recommended.

Basic Instrumentation—The essential components of a gas chromatograph are the same whether the instrument is an inexpensive student grade apparatus or a research instrument costing thousands of dollars. The basic components are shown in the block diagram in Fig 33-9. The *carrier gas*, which serves as the mobile phase, is supplied in steel tanks under high pressure. In order to reduce the pressure to a level compatible with the requirements of the instrument, a suitable two-stage diaphragm-controlled pressure regulator is fitted to the tank. The carrier gas, now at a pressure of approximately 40–80 psi, passes into a flow controller which allows the operator to adjust the flow rate to the desired operating level (usually 50–100 mL/min) before the carrier gas moves into the instrument proper, which is contained within an oven capable of maintaining a constant temperature ranging from ambient to as high as 400°. The next component in the line of flow is the sample injection port. This is a small chamber, usually separately heated to a temperature slightly above that of the column, in which the analytical

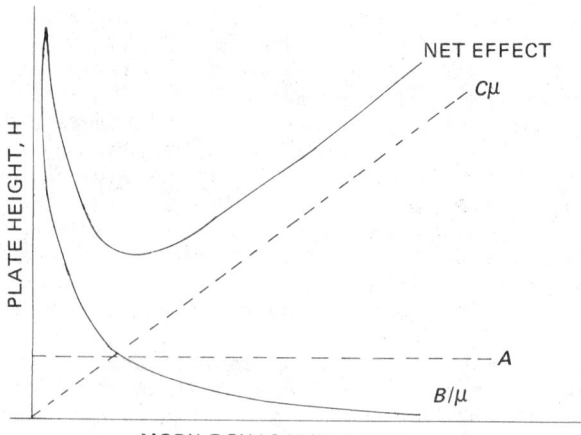

Fig 33-8. Graph of the simplified form of the van Deemter equation showing the contribution of each of the terms throughout a range of flow rates.

sample is made to vaporize rapidly before entering the column. The sample is introduced into the flowing gas stream through a self-sealing rubber or silicone *septum* using a microliter syringe. The sample may be injected into the chamber directly on the beginning of the column to minimize diffusion due to turbulence. Samples may be pure liquids, solids dissolved in liquid solvents, or gases. The gaseous mixture next enters the column which is a tube, usually glass or stainless steel, from 1–3 m long and with an internal diameter of from 2–5 mm. The column may be straight, coiled, or U-shaped.

The interior of the column is filled with either a solid adsorbent material for GSC or, in the case of GLC, a packing of inert, solid particles whose surface is coated with a thin layer of liquid. Based on their electrostatic attraction for the surface of the solid or their partition coefficients between the two fluids, the solutes are retained temporarily by the stationary phase. As the carrier gas continues to flow, the retained molecules diffuse back into the mobile phase.

At the end of the column, each of the separated solutes ex-

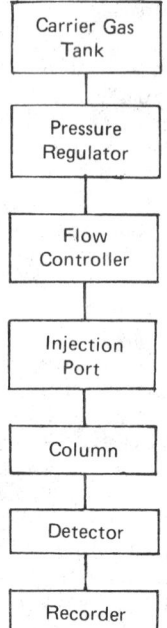

Fig 33-9. Block diagram of a gas chromatograph showing the essential components of the system.

ists as a binary mixture with carrier gas and moves into the detector, which may also be heated to a level slightly higher than that of the column to prevent condensation of the solutes. The detector is a device which converts some physical property of the solute, eg thermal conductivity, ionizability, electron-capturing ability, into an electrical signal which is proportional to the amount of solute in the carrier gas. This is amplified electronically and fed to a suitable recorder which produces a graphic record of the level of the signal versus time. The output may also be sent simultaneously to a computer for storage.

Carrier Gas—Since it is the mobile phase, the choice of the carrier gas is crucial to the success of the chromatography. In theory any gas may be used, but, for practical reasons, usually helium or nitrogen and occasionally hydrogen or argon are employed. One of the most important considerations is the purity of the gas, since a contaminated carrier gas will cause a drifting or elevated baseline or it may deposit its impurities on the column. This in effect changes the nature of the stationary phase, thereby altering the partition coefficients and results in a progressive degradation of the column. Although carrier gases are typically from 99.99 to 99.9999% pure when purchased they may be contaminated with small amounts of hydrocarbons and water, which may be removed by a filter trap inserted in the gas stream prior to the injection port.

In addition, it is essential that the carrier gas be inert with respect to the sample components, the column packing materials, and the components of the instrument. This quality is especially important in GSC, since a reactive gas would compete with the solute molecules for binding sites on the column. The viscosity is also important since low viscosity gases such as hydrogen and helium allow higher flow rates to be maintained, while a gas with relatively high viscosity, such as nitrogen, may be useful in lessening longitudinal diffusion of the solutes and thereby reducing band broadening.

One of the chief disadvantages of gas chromatography is that the choice of mobile phases is so limited that the analyst can affect resolution and separation only by changing the stationary phase. A fairly large inventory of columns with different stationary phases must be maintained and time is lost cooling the instrument, fitting a new column, and returning to operating temperature.

Stationary Phase—The interior of a GC column contains either an uncoated solid material for GSC or an inert *solid support* coated with a thin layer of *liquid phase* for GLC. The particles of the packing material are small (80 to 120 mesh) in order to minimize *void volume* (total volume of interstitial space between particles) while at the same time providing a large surface area for interaction with the solutes.

In GSC, the adsorbents most frequently used are activated charcoal, silica gel, alumina, and glass beads. For the analysis of low molecular weight compounds, such as water and alcohols, a group of porous polymers made from styrene and divinylbenzene are available. These are manufactured in such a way that their porosity is carefully controlled, and their separation ability is achieved by a combination of adsorption and size exclusion.

For GLC, the most commonly used solid support material is diatomaceous earth which is treated with acid and base to remove impurities and then calcined to activate the surface. Nonporous supports such as glass microbeads have also been used. The liquid phase is uniformly coated on the surface of the solid support usually at levels of 1–5% by weight. For the separation of compounds which are only slightly retained, amounts as high as 40% have been used. The liquid must be chemically stable, have a low vapor pressure at operating temperatures and have specific solvent properties toward the compounds to be analyzed.

In the thirty years since the introduction of gas chromatography, hundreds of substances have been tried as stationary phases including such materials as stopcock grease and ordinary household laundry detergent. Most of these have fallen into disuse since they could not be purified or standardized and reproducible results could not be obtained from batch to batch. Today, there are in common use about fifteen or twenty highly purified liquid phases which differ from each other in their overall polarity and their specific selectivity for particular functional groups on the solute molecules. Most of these are based on silicone polymers with substituents such as phenyl, cyano, and trifluoropropyl introduced in order to affect polarity and selectivity. Ethylene glycol polymers are also frequently used, mainly for the separation of polar compounds, eg, alcohols and amines. In the case of the nonpolar liquid phases, the elution of a mixture of solutes occurs in order of increasing molecular weight, since the larger the compound the more nonpolar it is likely to be and the more strongly it will be retained. As the polarity of the liquid phase is increased, elution order will be based more on the relative polarities of the solutes, with the most polar substances being more strongly retained.

Several methods have been developed in order to facilitate the choice of the most efficient stationary phase for a particular analysis. The Retention Index system of Kovats, a measure of the relative retention of a compound with respect to a series of n-alkanes, was formulated in order to catalog the relative polarities of the liquid phases. If the retention of the compound is determined on a polar and a nonpolar column, the difference in relative retention is a measure of the column polarity. Subsequently, Rohrschneider and then McReynolds developed more efficient methods for predicting the selectivity of liquid phases. The method of McReynolds[4] is the one most frequently used and suppliers of chromatographic materials will indicate the McReynolds constants for each of the liquid phases offered in their catalogs. These constants are based on the difference in retention of a series of test compounds between a standard column with the stationary phase of 20% squalane and a column containing the liquid phase whose selectivity is to be determined. The test compounds—benzene, 1-butanol, 2-pentanone, nitropropane, and pyridine—were chosen because each has a different functional group to interact with the stationary phase. A high McReynold's number indicates a strong interaction of that liquid phase with the particular functional group. By consulting the McReynold's numbers for various liquid phases, the chromatographer is able to make a more logical selection of the optimum stationary phase.

Column Design—For the great majority of GC applications, the column is a stainless steel or glass tube which is 1–3 m in length and has an inner diameter of 2 to 4.6 mm. It is attached at either end to the injection port and the detector using compression fittings to achieve a gas-tight seal. Since the shape of the column has no effect on the chromatographic process, it is designed to conform to the dimensions of the oven. Shorter columns may be straight or U-shaped but longer ones are usually coiled into a spiral.

In addition to stainless steel, various other metals have been used for the fabrication of columns, including copper and aluminum. These latter two have the advantage of being less expensive than stainless steel and being more flexible so that columns may be easily made and bent to shape in the laboratory. However, they are less durable and their surfaces are more reactive so that unstable solutes are more likely to degrade in copper and aluminum columns than in steel.

For certain compounds, notably steroids, which are highly susceptible to degradation and molecular rearrangement on hot metal surfaces, glass columns are widely employed since their surfaces are relatively inert. The disadvantages of glass are that it is difficult to get a gas-tight seal at the injector and

detector connections and they are brittle enough to break under limited stress. A recent development, which promises to overcome the negative aspects of stainless steel or glass, is the use of nickel tubing for column fabrication. The surface of nickel is claimed to be as inert as glass while it has the strength and durability of steel.

Because of the relatively low viscosity of the mobile phase in gas chromatography, the contribution of solute diffusion to band-broadening can be substantial. In an effort to reduce the volume within which the solute can diffuse, narrow-diameter columns are frequently used. A small increase in efficiency has been achieved by using tubing with an inner diameter of about 1 mm. However, the greatest increase in efficiency has occurred with the use of *capillary columns*. These are tubes of glass or highly purified fused silica with internal diameters of 0.2 to 0.5 mm and lengths of up to 300 meters. The liquid phase is contained within these columns in either of two ways. In *wall-coated open tubular (WCOT)* columns the stationary phase is deposited as an extremely thin layer directly on the inner surface of the tube, while in *support-coated open tubular (SCOT)* columns the inner surface of the tube is coated with a layer of inert support and the liquid phase is coated onto this. Because of the irregularity of the support particles, the surface area of the SCOT column is larger, and more stationary phase is therefore available to interact with the solutes. Another method which has been used to increase the available surface of the liquid phase is to bond it chemically to the wall of the capillary column. This is advantageous since it prevents *bleeding* or loss of the liquid phase due to its volatility at elevated temperatures.

Because of the extremely low void volume in a capillary column, the ratio of V_S to V_M is high in comparison to a larger diameter column. This results in much higher efficiencies and columns of several hundred thousand theoretical plates have been described. The disadvantage of capillary columns is that they have low capacities, so injections must be made through a *splitter* which diverts more than 95% of the sample away from the column. The method is also not useful when it is desirable to collect the eluted solutes.

Operating Conditions—Most chromatographic analyses are done in the *isothermal* mode in which the temperature of the instrument is maintained constant throughout the run. However, this method is frequently unsatisfactory for complex mixtures, when both volatile and comparatively nonvolatile solutes are present. If for these mixtures the column is operated at a high temperature the low-boiling solutes will be eluted rapidly but not resolved while the less volatile substances may be satisfactorily separated. At a lower operating temperature all substances may be resolved but the retention time for the less volatile compounds will be excessively long and the peaks may be so broad as to be undetectable.

In order to obviate these problems, the technique of *temperature-programming* may be used. In this method the temperature of the column is raised at a preset rate beginning at the time of injection of the sample. The programming rate may be constant during the run or, in more sophisticated instruments, periods of isothermal operation may be interspersed between temperature rises. The result of temperature programming is a chromatogram with evenly spaced peaks having good heights resulting in an overall saving of time. The initial temperature should be chosen in order to minimize the retention time for the least retained solute while the final temperature must be sufficient to elute the least volatile compound in a reasonable time without exceeding the operating limits of the liquid phase.

An alternative method for complex mixtures involves the use of *flow-programming*, in which the velocity of the mobile phase is varied during the run. This has the advantage of not exposing solutes and stationary phases to high temperatures. However, it has not gained wide usage since special equipment is required and flow changes have a lesser effect on retention time than temperature changes.

In either the isothermal or temperature programmed modes, some of the liquid phase is constantly volatilizing and entering the detector causing drift of the baseline. In isothermal runs, this is constant and can be compensated for by adjusting the detector, but when the temperature is programmed the drift increases continually and can be a problem, especially when high detector sensitivity is required. This effect can be compensated for by using a liquid phase with lower volatility or by using a dual column system in which the sample is injected into one column while the other acts as a baseline monitor. The output signal of the second column can be subtracted electronically from that of the first thereby cancelling the effect of the drifting baseline.

Detectors—Much of the overall progress in gas chromatography has resulted from the development of detectors which are sensitive to amounts of solute in the sub-microgram range and which have responses rapid enough to prevent band-broadening. These are grouped into two general classifications, *mass flow rate* detectors, which are sensitive to the rate of flow of the solute through the detector, and *concentration sensitive* detectors, which respond to the concentration of solute in the mobile phase in the detector.

The *Thermal Conductivity Detector* (*TCD*), also called the *Hot Wire Detector* (*HWD*) *or katharometer* is widely used because it is a universal detector, that is, it responds to all solutes. In this device a coil of fine wire, usually made of a tungsten–rhenium alloy, resides in a small chamber into which the column effluent flows. In practice most TC detectors consist of a matched pair of wires, one of which is placed in the gas stream before it enters the column, while the other is at the end of the column. An electrical potential is placed across the wire filaments and they heat up due to their resistance. The resistance of the filament is a function of its temperature. When only carrier gas is flowing through the chamber, the filaments maintain a steady temperature which is determined by the thermal conductivity of the gas, but when a binary mixture of solute and carrier gas emerges from the column, the mixture has a different thermal conductivity and heat is conducted from the sample filament at a greater or lesser rate. This changes the resistance of the wire and the change in resistance or current is a measure of the concentration of the solute in the detector.

The thermal conductivities of hydrogen and helium are as much as ten times higher than those of most organic compounds, so even a small amount of solute will cause a large change in the output of the detector. Nitrogen, however, has a conductivity close to that of most organic compounds so that sensitivity is lower with this carrier gas and, in fact, it is possible to obtain negative peaks. TC detectors are simple, inexpensive, and nondestructive to the sample. They are relatively insensitive, however, in comparison to other detectors and are not useful for analyses requiring detection of low levels of solutes eg, drugs in biological fluids.

The *Flame Ionization Detector* (*FID*) is the most frequently used detector in GC since it is highly sensitive, able to detect microgram quantities of solutes, being as well an almost universal detector. It responds well to most organic compounds but is insensitive to water and most inorganic substances. In this device, hydrogen and air or oxygen are introduced into the column effluent stream. The mixture is ignited and, as a result of the energy of the flame, electrons are stripped from the solutes and ions are formed. These charged particles migrate to a pair of oppositely charged electrodes in the chamber and cause a small electrical current to flow. The current, which is amplified to produce a useful signal, is proportional to the rate of flow of solute through the detector. In addition to their exceptional sensitivity, flame ionization detectors are useful because of their large *linear dynamic*

range. They will respond in a linear manner to amounts of solute which differ in concentration by several orders of magnitude.

Other highly sensitive detectors are available but their response is limited to compounds containing certain specific functional groups, such as nitrogen, phosphorus, and the halogens. This property of selectivity can be very useful, however, since even if the chromatographic separation is not optimal an interfering solute will not be detected unless it contains the functional group for which the detector is specific. Thus, they impart a second level of selectivity to the procedure.

The *Electron Capture Detector* (*ECD*) is one of the most sensitive of detectors, being able to respond to nanogram, or even picogram quantities of materials having functional groups which possess high electron affinity, such as the halogens or nitro groups. In this device, a radioactive source, usually ^{63}Ni, emits beta particles which interact with the carrier gas molecules to form positive ions and electrons. These, in turn, migrate to oppositely charged electrodes in the detector chamber to produce a *standing current.* When a detectable solute elutes from the column, it is able to "capture" some portion of the electrons, thereby lowering the standing current. This decrease in the current is detected electronically and is proportional to the amount of solute.

The ECD is extremely sensitive to low levels of halogenated compounds, eg pesticides. However, its linear response range is narrow and it is very susceptible to permanent saturation if it is exposed to too high a concentration of a halogenated compound.

The *Alkali Flame Ionization Detector* (*AFID*), also called the *Thermionic Specific Detector* (*TSD*), is a modified form of the FID which shows increased response to compounds containing nitrogen and phosphorus. It consists of a standard FID with a crystal of a solid alkali metal compound, such as rubidium bromide or potassium chloride, suspended in the area above the flame. The mechanism of action is not fully understood, but its sensitivity for nitrogen and phosphorus containing compounds is 10^3–10^4 times greater than for other organic compounds. It, too, has important applications in pesticide residue analysis.

Another modification of the FID which has increased selectivity for sulfur and phosphorus containing compounds is the *Flame Photometric Detector* (*FPD*). The eluted compounds are first burned in the usual FID flame, from which the products of the pyrolysis then pass to another flame where sulfur and phosphorus atoms are excited to a higher energy state and subsequently detected by emission spectroscopy. The sensitivity of this device to S and P is about 10^5 times greater than that for carbon compounds.

There are a number of other detectors which are available for use in gas chromatography, but which are used less frequently since they do not offer any advantages over the devices currently employed. These include detectors whose operating principles are based on coulometry, conductivity, and photoionization.

Special Techniques—It is not unusual in the practice of gas chromatography to encounter samples which cannot be analyzed satisfactorily no matter what combination of mobile and stationary phases are used. For example, petroleum fractions contain tars and other high-boiling hydrocarbons which chromatograph with difficulty, if at all. In addition, many drugs which contain carboxylic acid or primary amine functional groups are volatile enough to chromatograph but will give badly tailed peaks due to nonideal interactions of the functional groups with the stationary phase. However, for research and quality control purposes, the pharmaceutical and chemical industries require that these substances be analyzed and, to overcome the problem posed by these compounds, special techniques, such as *pyrolysis* and *derivatization* have been developed.

Pyrolysis gas chromatography is used frequently for the analysis of very high molecular weight compounds eg, crude oil fractions, rubber vial closures, and packaging materials. In this technique, the high molecular weight substances are decomposed to lighter and more volatile compounds by controlled heating in a furnace, which may be external to the gas chromatograph or an integral part of the instrument. The resulting lighter compounds will then be chromatographed as usual, frequently using capillary columns.

Since the nature of the decomposition products rarely is known with any certainty, the chromatogram which is produced represents a "fingerprint" of the original sample. If the time and temperature of pyrolysis are carefully controlled, the method is reproducible and is valuable for checking raw materials from different suppliers to determine if the source or the chemical composition have changed over a period of time.

A number of compounds, such as steroids, do not chromatograph well because they are not sufficiently volatile or they decompose at the higher temperatures needed for successful GC. Others, eg, fatty acids, yield poorly shaped peaks. It is frequently possible to obviate these problems and obtain good chromatograms by forming derivatives of these substances. Many of the procedures used to produce derivatives in these cases are the same as those used in qualitative organic analysis, eg acylation of alcohols, formation of oximes and hydrazones of carbonyls, and esterification of fatty acids. However, for gas chromatography, a different class of derivatizing reagents called *silylating agents* has been used most often. These agents are intended to react with compounds containing labile protons such as alcohols, amines, carboxylic acids, and thiols to produce the corresponding ethers, silyl amines, esters, and thioethers. Because of the reduced polarity, the derivatives have greater volatility and stability than the original compounds. A number of derivatizing agents have been used, the most common of which are trimethylchlorosilane, hexamethyldisilazane, and *N,O*-bistrimethylsilylacetamide. The byproducts of the reactions are very volatile and elute very rapidly so they do not interfere with the chromatography.

Other than being useful as derivatizing agents, silylating compounds are also used to deactivate solid supports and the surfaces of glass columns. In these applications, they react readily with the silanol groups on the silica surface, thereby blocking polar sites which would interfere with the separation process.

Qualitative Analysis—Although gas chromatography is primarily used as a quantitative technique, it is also valuable in the qualitative analysis of unknown substances. This may be accomplished in either of two ways: by comparing the retention parameters of the unknown with known compounds or by trapping the effluents as they leave the column and subjecting them to classical chemical or spectroscopic identification procedures.

In terms of parameters derived from the chromatogram, the retention or relative retention times or their corresponding volumes are useful indicators of identity when compared with the same parameters for a known compound. The related variables, the capacity factor k', and the separation factor, α, may also be used. If the unknown compound is suspected of being a member of a homologous series and sufficient known members of the series are available, plots of log t_R vs carbon number or log t_R on a polar column vs log t_R on a nonpolar column will give a straight line for homologs.

It is also possible to identify solutes after GC by collecting individual fractions as they elute from the column. This can be done manually or automatically using a fraction collector which is activated by the signal from the detector. In this manner, the entire procedure can be automated and carried out unattended over an extended period of time in order to ensure that adequate amounts are collected for subsequent analysis. Since the effluents are gases at high temperatures, collection is done by passing the eluate through a solvent which is subsequently evaporated or by collecting in chilled tubes. Because the FID is a destructive detector, these procedures are most frequently accomplished using the thermal conductivity detector or by employing parallel columns with one attached to a detector and the other to the collecting device.

After the fractions have been collected and the solvents, if any, removed, the substances may be identified by standard qualitative chemical reactions or by spectrometric techniques. Specialized gas chromatographs are available in which the effluent can be made to pass through an ultraviolet or infrared spectrometer after it leaves the column. Fractions from the beginning, middle, and end of the peaks may be scanned to determine if more than one substance is co-eluting in a single peak.

Probably the most sensitive and useful qualitative analyses can be made by combining a gas chromatograph with a mass spectrometer. Using a suitable separator to remove the carrier gas allows direct introduction of the solute into the ionization chamber of the mass spectrometer after it exits the column. This technique has the advantage of extremely high sensitivity (10^{-12}–10^{-15} g) so that usually only one injection of the unknown is required. The GC-MS technique is also useful for quantitative analysis by using selective ion monitoring.

Quantitative Analysis—In addition to providing rapid and efficient separations of complex mixtures and qualitative information about the eluted substances, gas chromatography can also furnish the analyst with accurate and precise quantitative data.

The parameter which is proportional to the concentration of a compound in the GC effluent is the area under the elution peak, which is the integral of the elution curve from the point where it leaves the baseline to the point where it returns. Using computerized techniques, this integral can be determined exactly, but since this requires specialized dedicated equipment, a number of manual integration methods are employed. These are based on the assumption that the shape of the peak is Gaussian and while they do not yield the true peak area, the results obtained are proportional to it and may be used with equal confidence. Some of these methods are:

1. *Triangulation*—Tangents to the inflection points of the peak are drawn from the baseline to the point where they meet above the peak. The third side of the triangle is drawn along the baseline, and the area is determined by multiplying the base width by half the height. The resulting value is equal to 96% of the actual area of the Gaussian peak.

2. *Height times width at half height*—The baseline portions of the chromatogram before and after the peak are joined with a straight line. The height is measured from this base and multiplied by the width at half height. The result is equal to 84% of the true area.

3. *Height*—If the conditions of temperature and flow rate are rigorously controlled, the peak height produced by a given quantity of solute will be constant from run to run. It may therefore be used directly as an estimate of the area.

4. *Cutting and Weighing*—In this method, the peaks are cut out with a scissors and weighed on an analytical balance. Although this is very tedious, it is more precise than any of the previous three procedures. If peaks are extremely narrow the peak may be traced onto aluminum or lead foil of uniform thickness, prior to cutting, in order to increase the amount weighed.

5. *Computer Integration*—The computer, or integrator,

converts the analog voltage produced by the detector into a digitized quantity and computes the results. This is by far the most precise method, as well as being applicable to peaks whose shape is not ideally Gaussian, but it requires expensive, elaborate equipment.

Once the relative areas of the peaks in the chromatogram have been determined, this data which is proportional to the concentration of each of the species, must be used to determine exact concentrations. This is accomplished in one of three ways:

1. *Area Normalization*—The assumption is made that each substance in the injected mixture produces a separate peak in the chromatogram. The weight of the material in any peak is found by determining the ratio of its peak area to the sum of the total areas of all the peaks and multiplying this by the total weight of solute in the amount injected. This method is used infrequently since the initial assumption is not usually valid.

2. *External Standardization*—A pure reference standard material corresponding to the substance to be determined is dissolved in a solvent at a known concentration. Exactly measured quantities of this solution, eg 1, 2, 3, 4, and 5 μL, are successively injected. The areas of each of the peaks produced are plotted *vs* the mass of solute injected and a calibration curve is produced. Next, the unknown solution is injected, the area of the peak determined and the concentration found by interpolation. This method is very accurate but it is necessary that the analyst be skilled in the use of microliter syringes, since the volumes injected must be known exactly. It is also assumed that instrument parameters remain constant for the period during which the samples are introduced; an assumption not always valid.

3. *Internal Standardization*—To obviate the difficulty of introducing precisely measured quantities into the GC, the internal standard method may be used. This procedure requires two standards, the analytical standard, being a pure sample of the compound to be analyzed and the other an *internal standard*. This is normally a substance which elutes at a position near the substance being analyzed and is well resolved ($R_S > 1.25$) but which cannot be converted to the analyte under the conditions of the analysis. A series of solutions is prepared containing varying amounts of the analytical standard and constant amounts of the internal standard. These are chromatographed and a calibration curve is determined by plotting the ratio of the areas of the two peaks *vs* the ratios of their concentrations. The unknown is then dissolved in a suitable solvent, the same amount of internal standard is added, and the mixture is chromatographed. The ratio of the areas is calculated and, by interpolation on the calibration curve, the amount of the unknown is determined. This method is the most frequently used technique for quantitative analysis by GC since it is not necessary to know the exact amount of solution injected. Any other inaccuracies are compensated for by using the ratios of the responses.

Liquid Chromatography

Although Michael Tswett, in 1906, published a comprehensive paper on liquid chromatography in which he clearly explained the nature of the process and his appreciation of its potential, the method was not widely adopted until many years later. In 1941, Martin and Synge, who had been unsuccessful in using countercurrent extraction for the separation of amino acids in wool samples, developed a liquid chromatographic process in which they used a packed column containing water-saturated silica gel and a mobile phase of butanol–chloroform. They perfected the experimental techniques and explained the theoretical aspects of the procedure so thoroughly that they were awarded the Nobel Prize

in 1952 for this work. Since that time, liquid chromatography has become one of the most versatile techniques available to the analyst because of its simplicity and capacity for high resolution separations. Separations may be developed based on such diverse characteristics as the polarity of the solutes, their ionic nature, their molecular weight, their partitioning ability, or their ability to form affinity complexes.

The term liquid chromatography is used today to refer to those methods in which the separation takes place within a packed column. The packing material is the stationary phase and may be a solid with adsorptive capabilities or an inert support coated with a liquid phase. A liquid mobile phase is used as the eluant. Although thin layer chromatography and paper chromatography use a liquid mobile phase and a solid stationary phase, they differ in that the separations take place on a planar surface rather than in a column.

The process of liquid chromatography can be performed using either of two methods. In the first, the classical procedure developed by Tswett, called *open-column chromatography*, the mobile phase is allowed to flow through the packed column under the influence of gravity or, at most, low pressure, eg, 50–100 psi. In the second the mobile phase is forced through the packed column under high pressure. This method is called *high performance liquid chromatography (HPLC)*, due to the extremely high efficiencies (as many as 50,000 plates per meter) attainable or *high pressure liquid chromatography*, because of the high pressures (1000–3000 psi) required. In HPLC, particle diameter is typically 10 μm or less, and as a result columns are packed more tightly and develop high back pressures which necessitate pumping the mobile phase through the column.

Whether HPLC or open column methods are used, the mode of separation is primarily dependent on the nature of the stationary phase. Five modes are available: adsorption, partition, ion-exchange, size exclusion, and affinity. Each of these will be discussed in detail.

Adsorption Chromatography—In this mode of liquid chromatography, as in gas-solid chromatography, solutes are retained as a result of the ability of the stationary phase to bond them temporarily to its active surface. The forces involved are usually relatively weak and are effective only over short distances. These include van der Waals and London forces, dipole and induced dipole interactions with polar groups on the active surface, charge transfer forces, and hydrogen bonding. With this type of binding, termed *physical adsorption*, the energy required to break the bonds is small and the mobile phase, through its ability to dissolve and displace the solutes, can effectively counteract these attractive forces. Therefore, an efficient chromatographic process can occur based on the competition between dissolution of the solute in the mobile phase and binding at the surface of the stationary phase. However, when stronger chemical bonds form between solutes and the adsorbent, as in the process of *chemisorption*, the mobile phase is not able to provide sufficient energy to desorb the solutes. In this case, equilibrium between the two phases is not reached, and solutes are irreversibly adsorbed or give unsatisfactory, tailed elution peaks.

Some of the most common of the large variety of substances which have been used as adsorbents are shown in Table I. In addition to adsorptivity, surface area, particle size, and surface activity are of primary importance in determining the utility of a potential adsorbent. A large surface area is necessary to provide effective contact between the two phases and ensure frequent exchange of the solute. Although areas of 5–200 m^2/g are quoted by suppliers of adsorbents, these values may be lower than the actual effective surface area, since the methods of measurement used do not accurately account for the porous nature of the adsorbent particles or the true shape of the solute molecules. Particle size is important, not only

Table I—Adsorbents Used in Column Chromatography

Sucrose	(weakest)
Starch	
Inulin	
Talc	
Calcium carbonate	
Calcium phosphate	
Magnesia	
Silica gel	
Magnesium silicate	
Alumina	
Charcoal	(strongest)

as an indicator of surface area, but also because it determines the resistance of the packed column to solvent flow. While very small particles may provide a large area for solute interaction, they may pack so tightly that a reasonable flow rate cannot be achieved without using high pressure techniques with a consequent loss in sample capacity. Particles in the range of 75–150 μm in diameter are a useful compromise providing a large surface area with good permeability. Surface activity refers to the energy of the active site of the adsorbent and may vary depending on the nature of the substance and on the amount of water adsorbed. In order to provide a reproducible surface it is common practice to activate an adsorbent by heating it to expel most of the water and then deactivate it to a desired level by exposure to a climate of known humidity, returning a known quantity of moisture to the adsorbent.

Among the commonly used adsorbents, silica gel and alumina have surfaces rich in hydroxyl groups and oxygen atoms and they thus interact strongly with polar solutes. Charcoal, activated at 1000° to make it nonreactive to polar compounds, has a very porous surface which slows down the adsorption-desorption process and makes it more prone to chemisorption. Separations on charcoal are based mainly on molecular weight, with larger compounds being retained more strongly. Magnesium silicate has an acid surface characteristic of the insoluble silicates and is similar to alumina in adsorptive properties.

Table II lists a number of the solvents most commonly used in liquid-solid chromatography cataloged in a standard order, ie, according to their relative energy of adsorption per unit

Table II—Characteristics of Solvents Used in Chromatography

Solvent	Eluotropic value, E^0	Dielectric constant	Solubility parameter
Heptane	0.00	1.92	7.4
Hexane	0.01	1.88	7.3
Isooctane	0.01	1.94	7.0
Cyclohexane	0.04	2.02	8.2
Carbon tetrachloride	0.18	2.24	8.6
Toluene	0.29	2.38	8.9
Benzene	0.32	2.27	9.2
Ethyl ether	0.38	4.33	7.4
Chloroform	0.40	4.81	9.1
Methylene chloride	0.42	8.93	9.6
Tetrahydrofuran	0.45	7.58	9.1
Acetone	0.56	20.7	9.4
Dioxane	0.56	2.25	9.8
Ethyl acetate	0.58	6.02	8.6
Acetonitrile	0.65	37.50	11.8
Pyridine	0.71	12.30	10.4
1-Propanol	0.82	20.33	10.2
Ethanol	0.88	24.30	11.2
Methanol	0.95	32.70	12.9
Acetic acid	large	6.15	12.4
Water	large	78.54	21.0

surface area on alumina. A listing such as this is called an *eluotropic series*, and although the relative energies of adsorption differ slightly on other surfaces, the choice of solvents is usually made according to this series. An exception to this is made in the case of charcoal, however, because of its tendency to adsorb nonpolar substances, the order of solvent strength is reversed. The solvent used for a particular separation must be chosen with regard to the properties of the solutes as well as the stationary phase. For example, if a group of very polar compounds is to be separated using silica gel, the solvent must be polar enough to overcome the strong attraction between the solutes and the surface or very large retention times will result. If a mixture of less polar solutes is to be analyzed, a weaker solvent must be used to permit a longer residence time on the column and more equilibrations between the phases. For a more detailed discussion of the methods used to correlate solute structure with retention time using adsorption chromatography the text by Snyder is recommended.

Partition Chromatography—In this mode of liquid chromatography, mixtures of solutes are separated according to the relative tendencies of their components to partition between a mobile phase and a stationary phase consisting of a layer of liquid coated onto the surface of a solid support. The liquid is present as an extremely thin layer so that equilibration between the phases may be attained rapidly by minimizing the diffusion of the solutes into the stationary phase. The surface of the solid support is frequently treated, eg, by silylation, in order to eliminate adsorptive effects.

Although it has been used for many successful analyses, liquid-liquid partition chromatography was until relatively recently an inconvenient method to use experimentally. The liquid phase had to be coated onto the solid support by evaporation of a solution or by injecting it onto the column with the mobile phase flowing. In either case, it was difficult to obtain stationary phases which were stable and reproducible. In addition, the choice of mobile phase was necessarily restricted to those in which the liquid coating had limited solubility. For example, if a polyethylene glycol was to be used to provide a very polar stationary phase, a mobile phase of hexane or some other hydrocarbon of very low polarity had to be used. Even so, the liquid stationary phase would be slowly but continually stripped from the column thereby changing the characteristics of the separation. In order to prevent stripping, either the mobile phase was saturated with the liquid phase material or a precolumn containing a high concentration of the liquid phase coated on a solid support was inserted into the system before the analytical column. In either case, the nature of the mobile phase was changed and partition coefficients became less favorable.

Recently the problems presented by unstable stationary phases have been solved by the development of *bonded-phase chromatography*, in which liquid phase is permanently bonded chemically to the surface of the solid support. Silica gel, with its high surface population of hydroxyl groups, provides an excellent medium onto which various substances can be bonded using appropriately substituted silylating agents. For example, octadecyldimethylsilyl chloride reacts with silica gel to form a stable, non-polar stationary phase called ODS (octadecylsilyl). Because of steric effects, not all of the hydroxyl groups of the silica gel are derivatized by the ODS reagent, so the remainder are then reacted with trimethylsilyl chloride in a process called *capping* to reduce adsorption effects. Bonded phases are advantageous in that they can be made reproducibly from batch to batch and the surface does not change during the chromatography. They have the disadvantages of being expensive and of being effective only over the pH range within which the backbone of silica gel is stable, usually pH 2–7. Compared to the inconveniences of the former method, however, these disadvantages are not very restrictive, and the use and development of new bonded phases is an active area in current research, especially with respect to HPLC.

Partition chromatography may be conducted in either of two ways: *normal* or *reversed phase*. In the normal phase mode the stationary phase is a polar substance, such as polyethylene glycol, and the mobile phase is nonpolar, eg, hexane. Under these circumstances polar compounds are preferentially retarded and nonpolar substances elute more quickly. In reversed phase chromatography the stationary phase in nonpolar, eg, ODS, and the mobile phase is polar, usually a mixture of water, methanol, and/or acetonitrile. Nonpolar compounds are retained more strongly by this system, while polar solutes elute first. Reversed phase separations are the most frequently used methods in HPLC.

Because of the efficiency and availability of reversed phase materials, especially the ODS or C-18 type, attempts have been made to use them to separate mixtures of ionic compounds, eg, amino acids. Normally these compounds would not be retained in a reversed phase packing, since they are too polar to partition appreciably onto the stationary phase. Several techniques, all of which involve altering the mobile phase, have been developed to permit successful chromatography of ionic compounds using these stationary phases. These methods are called *ion-suppression chromatography*, *ion-pairing chromatography*, and *"soap" chromatography*.

Ion suppression is used for substances such as weak acids ($pK_a > 2$) and weak bases ($pK_a < 8$), which are partly ionized at the neutral pH values characteristic of the usual mobile phases. For example, a carboxylic acid with $pK_a = 5$ will, at pH = 7, be present in both ionized and unionized with the anionic carboxylate predominating by a ratio of 100 to 1. In order to enhance the retention of the anion in a reversed phase system, the pH of the mobile phase can be adjusted to a value low enough to suppress the ionization of the acid, eg, pH < 3. This causes the free acid to predominate and since it is much less polar than the anion it will be able to partition into the stationary phase.

For stronger acids or bases which remain ionized throughout the pH range (2–7) where silica is stable, ion-pairing chromatography is the technique of choice. In this method a reagent which dissociates to give ions opposite in charge to those of the solutes is added to the mobile phase. Although the mechanism of action has not yet been fully understood, the added ions may interact with the charged solutes in two ways. First, they may combine directly with the charged solutes to form ion pairs which are nonpolar and will partition more readily into the stationary phase. Alternatively, the nonpolar end of the ion-pairing reagent may itself partition into the stationary phase, leaving its polar end extending from the surface into the mobile phase, where it acts as an ion exchanger. In either case, the retention of ionic solutes in the reversed phase materials is increased. Examples of ion-pairing reagents are heptanesulfonic acid, used for cationic species, such as protonated amines, and tetra-*n*-butylammonium hydroxide, which pairs with anionic substances.

The third method, "soap" chromatography, is actually a form of ion-pairing in which the added reagent is a detergent or soap. Examples are sodium lauryl sulfate for cations and cetyltrimethylammonium chloride for anions. Soap chromatography is especially useful for the separation of proteins, since the soap not only neutralizes the charge on the molecule but also affects the conformation of the protein to allow it to interact more favorably with the stationary phase. The practical aspects of ion-pair chromatography are discussed in more detail by Gloor and Johnson.[5]

Another special technique which can be used with partition chromatography is *metal ion complexation*. In this process, a small quantity of a metal ion, eg, Ag^+, is added to the mobile phase in the chromatography of olefinic compounds. The ionic silver interacts with the double bonds, forming charge transfer complexes and altering the partitioning behavior of the olefinic solute. This technique is useful for separating mixtures of compounds which differ in the extent and placement of the unsaturation.

Ion Exchange Chromatography—Although ion-pairing techniques have proved useful in many cases for the separation of mixtures of ionic substances, the usual method for the analysis of these compounds is *ion-exchange chromatography*. This method provides a greater degree of selectivity due to the larger number of combinations of mobile and stationary phases which can be employed. It is especially useful for inorganic cations, amino acids, and similar groups of closely related compounds.

The stationary phase materials used to effect these separations are called *ion exchangers*, and they comprise a group of natural or synthetic organic or inorganic polymers which are capable of reversibly removing ions from a solution, while at the same time replacing them with ions of equivalent charge. At all times during this exchange process the principle of electroneutrality must be obeyed both in the ion exchanger and the solution. An ion exchanger contains *fixed ions*, which are permanently incorporated into its insoluble skeleton, and loosely bound *counter ions* which are opposite in charge to the fixed ions and are capable of being exchanged when charged species are adsorbed from solution. If the counter ions are positively charged, the material is called a *cation exchanger*; if they are negative it is an *anion exchanger*.

The inorganic polymers used in this type of chromatography are aluminosilicates which have lattice, or cage-like, structures. Because of the preponderance of oxygen atoms in the polymer it is negatively charged and the counter ions, usually calcium or sodium, are positive. Therefore, they are cation exchangers. The naturally occurring members of this group are called *zeolites*, while the synthetic ones, which were developed to provide standardized structures with constant pore sizes, are called *molecular sieves*. Because of their low capacities for ion exchange, these inorganic substances are used primarily for the size separation of small molecules.

The most frequently used ion exchange materials are organic copolymers made from styrene (vinylbenzene) and divinylbenzene (DVB). The styrene polymerizes to give long twisted chains of carbon atoms, with a benzene ring at every other carbon. Divinylbenzene is added to cross-link these chains and give a three-dimensional bead-like structure. Commercially available ion exchange resins are identified according to their percent cross-linking, as ×2, ×4, ×6, etc, corresponding to the initial percentage of DVB in the reaction mixture. Since the styrene-DVB copolymers have no intrinsic ion exchanging properties of their own and act only as a skeleton, charged functional groups must be added. Reaction with chlorosulfonic acid places a sulfonic acid group on each of the non-linked benzene rings, yielding a *strong cation exchanger*, ie, one in which the counter ions can be removed easily from the fixed ions. If methacrylic acid is used in the polymerization in place of styrene, the resulting copolymer has carboxylic acid groups attached to the skeleton and functions as a *weak cation exchanger*, that is, one in which the counter ions do not dissociate at low pH. *Strong anion exchange* resins can be made from the same skeleton by introducing quaternary amine functional groups, while weak anion exchangers use polyamines as the ionizable groups.

Many other substances are used both as the skeletal components and the functional groups for ion exchange. Carbohydrate polymers, such as dextran and cellulose, when used as the insoluble matrix change the selectivity of a resin. For example, solute ions with attached polyaromatic groups, such as the anthraquinonesulfonic acids, do not chromatograph well on polystyrene-based ion exchangers, since they associate too strongly with the benzene rings of the resin. On a cellulose based exchanger, however, separation is possible since the mechanism is limited entirely to the ion exchange process. Silica gel is also used as a support matrix for preparing ion exchangers, especially in HPLC, where strength of the particle is important, as it must not be crushed by the high operating pressure of the system.

Other functional groups used frequently are diethylaminoethyl (DEAE) and triethylaminoethyl (TEAE), both of which are anion exchangers, and carboxymethyl (CM), which is used in cation exchange resins. Attached to matrices of cellulose or dextran, these substances have been widely employed for the separation of proteins and peptides.

The mechanism of action in this mode of chromatography depends on the replacement of the counter ions of the resin by the ionic species being separated. This can be illustrated by the procedure used for purifying water by passing it through a mixed-bed resin. Using sodium chloride as a typical contaminant, the mechanism is:

(1) $RESIN—SO_3H + Na^+ = RESIN—SO_3Na + H^+$

(2) $RESIN—N(CH_3)_3OH + Cl^-$
$$= RESIN—N(CH_3)_3Cl + OH^-.$$

Water of the exceptionally high purity needed for making mobile phases for HPLC is prepared by an ion exchange column, followed by passage through a charcoal adsorption column to remove nonionizable organic compounds and microfiltration to exclude particulate matter and bacteria.

Ion exchange materials achieve retention and separation efficiency because of their selectivity, that is, their ability to exchange one ion in preference to the counter ion. The exchanged ion binds to the resin and, among a group of solute ions, the ones retained most tightly are those which form the strongest bonds with the fixed ions. For a mixture of solute ions which differ in charge, the more highly charged species are preferentially retained. Thus, on a sulfonic acid resin, aluminum is bound more strongly than calcium, and calcium more strongly than sodium. The binding of negatively charged species to strong anion exchange resins follows the same trend. Among substances of the same charge, retention is related to the size of the hydrated ions, with smaller ions being held more tightly. Since the smaller elements in the periodic table bind more molecules of water, their hydrated ions are larger, and therefore for the alkali metals the order of retention is $Cs^+ > Rb^+ > K^+ > Na^+ > Li^+$. Another parameter which affects retention is the nature of the substituents attached to the charged portion of the solute species. Polystyrene resins exhibit preference for ions containing aromatic groups over aliphatic groups because, in addition to binding due to the electrostatic forces of ion exchange, the aromatic groups of the solute interact directly with the skeleton of the resin.

Ion exchange chromatograms may be developed either by displacement or by elution methods. In the former case, an ion which is more strongly retained than any of the solute ions displaces them from the resin, and a continuous series of bands results (see Fig 33-4). In elution development, the eluting agent is an ion for which the resin has less selectivity than it has for the solute ions. Transfer of the solute ions to and from the resin depends on their exchange equilibria with the eluting ion. The resulting chromatogram consists of a series of separate Gaussian peaks, as in Fig 33-5.

Mobile phases used in ion exchange chromatography are usually aqueous salt solutions which may be buffered to a desired pH or adjusted to a constant ionic strength. Choice of the mobile phase depends on a knowledge of the selectivity of the resin for the solute ions and the influence of solution equilibria due to pH or complexation. Mixed aqueous-or-

ganic or organic solvents may be used if the stationary phase is not altered. Gradient elution is used for difficult separations.

Chromatofocusing, first described in 1978 by Sluyterman,[6] is a special method of ion exchange chromatography which is of great utility in the separation of mixtures of proteins. In this case a buffer, adjusted to a specific pH, is added to an anion exchange column previously adjusted to a different pH. As the buffers mix, a pH gradient is formed along the length of the column, ranging from the initial pH at the far end to that of the added buffer at the beginning. If the pH at the start of the column is lower than the isoelectric point of the protein to be analyzed it will carry a positive charge and will not interact with the anion exchanger. Instead, it will migrate along the column to a point where the pH is just greater than the isoelectric point, at which time it will acquire a negative charge and bind to the resin. Thus, a group of proteins will arrange themselves on the column in order of their isoelectric points. As the pH gradient moves down the column, the proteins will migrate downward, so as to remain negatively charged, until each elutes from the column at its isoelectric point. Fractionation of complex mixtures of proteins is therefore possible using this method of separation.

Size Exclusion Chromatography—*Size exclusion chromatography*, also called *gel chromatography*, is a relatively new technique used to separate groups of solutes based on their effective size in solution. The stationary phases used to attain these separations are polymers which have been cross-linked to yield an open network with numerous pores of consistent size. The degree of cross-linking is carefully controlled to yield a series of gels having different pore sizes and fractionation ranges. When a mobile phase containing a mixture of solutes of various sizes is passed through a column of these materials, molecules which are too large to fit within the pores are "excluded" and remain completely in the mobile phase. They are, therefore, eluted rapidly near the void volume. Molecules of smaller size are free to diffuse in and out of the pores so that, in effect, their path through the column is longer, and they will elute later, as is depicted in Fig 33-10. The extent of retention depends on the size of the included molecules relative to the size of the pores. Thus, the smallest molecules will enter all of the pores, while molecules of intermediate size, because of the velocity of the mobile phase, will not have sufficient time to diffuse into all of the pores into which they would fit normally, and therefore will be retained less effectively. The result is a chromatogram which consists of an initial peak containing all of the totally excluded substances, followed by a group of peaks representing all of the substances which have been partially retained and separated, and finally another single peak caused by all of the totally included solutes.

The stationary phases used in this mode of partition chromatography are of two types. First, the soft gels, are usually made from cross-linked carbohydrates, such as dextran (*Sephadex*), agarose (*Sepharose*), or polyacrylamide (*Bio-*

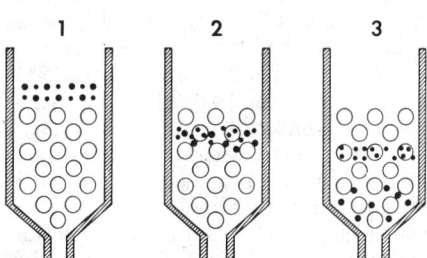

Fig 33-10.   Size exclusion chromatography. Small soluble molecules (•) penetrate the pores of the gel (O) and are retarded. Macromolecules (●) are excluded from the gel matrix and elute first.

Table III—Stationary and Mobile Phases Used in TLC

Technique	Stationary phases	Mobile phases
Adsorption	Silica gel Alumina Charcoal Polyamide	Nonpolar or polar organic solvents Polar organics
Partition	Cellulose Silica gel	Mixed aqueous, organic solvents
Reversed phase partition	ODS silica gel Coated silica Acetylated cellulose	Mixed aqueous, polar solvents
Ion exchange	Ion exchange resins DEAE- and CM- cellulose	Buffered aqueous solutions
Size exclusion	Dextran gels	Aqueous buffers

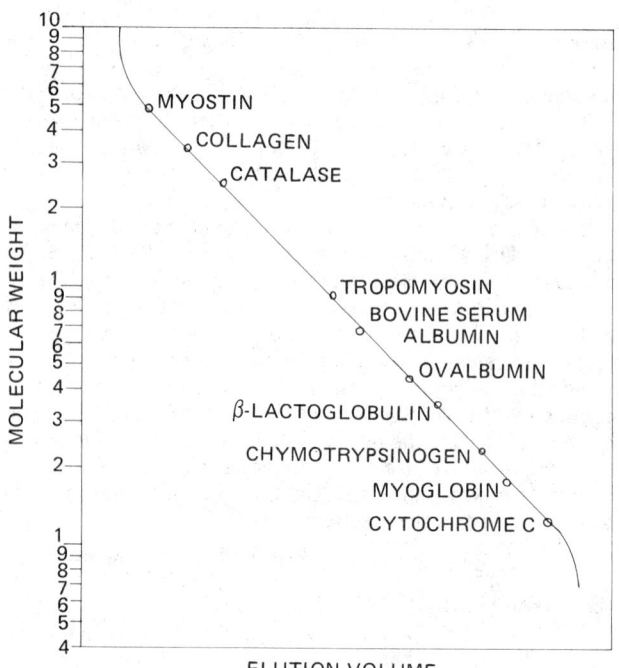

Fig 33-11.   Typical size exclusion calibration curve of elution volume, V_E, vs $log\ M$ for a series of protein standards.

Gel); the use of which was first described by Porath and Flodin.[7]   These are very hydrophilic, and before the column can be packed, they must be mixed with the mobile phase until they have *imbibed* enough liquid to become completely swollen.   Once the column has been packed, the composition of the mobile phase cannot be altered, since this would change the amount of imbibed solvent, resulting in shrinking of the bed, or in further swelling, which may burst the column. These gels are used with mobile phases which are primarily aqueous, and the technique is called *gel filtration*.   Because of the low structural strength of the soft gels they cannot be used under high pressure.   Size exclusion media made from silica gel with controlled pore sizes have been developed for HPLC; they do not deform under pressure and can be used with aqueous or nonaqueous mobile phases.

The second type of stationary phase, the *semi-rigid* or *rigid gels*, consist of materials such as cross-linked polystyrene, controlled-porosity glass beads, and alkylated dextran.   These can be used for the separation of organic-soluble polymers using nonaqueous mobile phases, such as chloroform, acetone, pyridine, or tetrahydrofuran.   This technique is called *gel permeation*, and was first described in 1964 by JC Moore.[8]

Ideally, the only separation mechanism occurring in size exclusion chromatography is that which depends on the diffusion of the solutes into and out of the pores.   However, depending on the nature of the solute and the stationary phase, other retention mechanisms such as ion exchange, hydrophobic partitioning, and hydrogen bonding may have an effect on certain solutes.   These can result in long retention times, irreversible adsorption, or loss of activity in biological molecules.   Such difficulties can be minimized by changing ionic strength or pH of the mobile phase to reduce charge effects, or by using additives, such as detergents, which modify the shape and charge of biological molecules.

Size exclusion chromatography is used most often in procedures involving large biological molecules, such as proteins, nucleic acids, and polysaccharides, which are not chromatographed well by other techniques.   Among the procedures for which these gels are useful are desalting, concentration, molecular weight determination, and fractionation.

Desalting is frequently necessary for the purification of biochemicals which have been separated from tissue using techniques involving buffers and precipitating reagents.   In this procedure, a gel with a fairly low exclusion limit, ie, equivalent to a molecular weight of 1000–2000, is used.   Because of the great differences in molecular weight between the biologial molecules and the contaminating salts, short columns and high flow rates may be used.   The macromolecules will

be eluted in the void volume with little dilution, while the salts are retained on the column.

Concentration of dilute solutions of large molecules may be achieved with gels whose exclusion limit is less than the molecular weight of the substances involved.   The solution is mixed with a small quantity of dry gel which will absorb ten to twenty times its weight in water.   Some salts and small molecules are taken up also, leaving the macromolecules in a solution of almost unchanged pH and ionic strength but significantly decreased volume.

Perhaps the greatest value of size exclusion chromatography is for the fractionation and molecular weight determination of macro-molecules.   It has been found that since the size of a molecule is approximately proportional to its molecular weight, M, the elution volume, V_E, can be expressed by the formula

$$V_E = a + b\ log\ M$$

where a and b are constants dependent on the mobile and stationary phases.   To determine the molecular weight of a substance, the system must be calibrated by using an extremely large molecule, such as blue dextran, to establish the void volume of the system, and a substance such as deuterium oxide or sucrose to determine the retention time for a totally included solute.   A series of standard proteins or polymers is then used to calibrate the region between these limits.   A typical calibration curve of V_E vs $log\ M$ for a series of protein standards is shown in Fig 33-11.   Once the elution volume of the unknown compound is determined, the molecular weight can be estimated by interpolation.

Affinity Chromatography—In situations where very specific separations are desired, *affinity chromatography*, a highly specialized form of adsorption chromatography may be employed.   This technique makes use of a specific ligand, which has been immobilized by being chemically bound to an insoluble matrix, to reversibly adsorb a single molecular species from a mixture of solutes.   This method differs from other modes of chromatography already discussed in that, rather than attempting to separate a mixture of solutes for qualitative or quantitative analysis, it is concerned only with removing a single species from the mixture. It achieves its greatest utility as a highly specific purification technique for biological molecules.

Affinity chromatography owes its high degree of specificity to the nature of the binding forces between the ligand and the substance to be purified. Many biological molecules, as a result of their unique structure and conformation, form strong, non-covalent bonds to related compounds, as a drug would to a cellular receptor. Examples of this are found in the association of enzymes with coenzymes, antigens with antibodies, lectins with carbohydrates, and polynucleotides with nucleic acids. If either member of the above mentioned pairs is permanently bonded to a chromatographic matrix, it will be able to remove the other from solution without interacting at all with any other solute in the mixture. Since the ligand-target molecule binding is reversible, a suitable mobile phase can be passed through the column to dissociate the pair and elute the purified substance. A recent example of the utility of this technique involves the purification of interferon A for structural studies and clinical trials.[9] The interferon is synthesized by cells of the bacterium *E coli* which contain recombinant DNA carrying the gene for human interferon. An extract of the *E coli* cells containing the interferon along with the thousands of other proteins synthesized by the bacterium was chromatographed using an affinity column in which a monoclonal antibody to the interferon protein had been attached to inert beads. The interferon bound to the surface and after all of the other proteins had been washed through the column, a weakly acidic mobile phase was used to elute it in sufficient purity to permit crystallization.

The principle of enzyme-substrate interaction has also been applied to purification of enzymes that do not interact specifically with insoluble porous materials. Instead of a substrate being used, a competitive inhibitor of the enzyme (a ligand) is covalently bound directly to a porous stationary phase. Sepharose, a water-insoluble spherical form of an agarose gel, is used widely. It displays little nonspecific adsorption of proteins, has good flow properties, contains many functional groups for ligand derivatization, and has sufficiently high porosity to permit the entrance and exit of large macromolecules (molecular weight $> 1 \times 10^6$). The agarose matrix is activated by reaction with cyanogen bromide and is subsequently bound covalently to the amino groups of a ligand. Competitive inhibitors are used as ligands rather than substrates since the enzyme would act on and be released from a substrate.

Binding the inhibitor directly to the matrix of Sepharose results in the necessity to use a rather potent inhibitor (inhibition constant, $K_I < 10^{-5} M$) as the ligand. Under these conditions binding of the enzyme is more difficult because of steric hindrance. The interposition of lengthy hydrocarbon "spacer arms" between the matrix and the ligand makes the inhibitor more accessible to the enzyme. The arm thereby promotes better enzyme binding and results in a higher capacity adsorbent that yields better separations. Hydrocarbon arms can be attached to Sepharose using the cyanogen bromide procedure or the agarose matrix may be purchased with various hydrocarbon arms already attached. Agaroses with aminoalkyl, carboxyl, aminophenyl, sulfhydryl, and other groups substituted are available for coupling with ligands which have amino, carboxyl, imidazole, etc. functional groups. For example, an inhibitor with a carboxyl function may be coupled with aminoalkyl agarose by a simple water-soluble carbodiimide method. The resulting adsorbent has the following type arms with ligands (R) attached:

$$\text{agarose}-NH(CH_2)_3-NH(CH_2)_3NHCOR$$

The coupling must not, of course, totally destroy the inhibitory nature of the ligand. However, even if some potency is lost,

ie, the K_I increases from $1 \times 10^{-6} M$ to $1 \times 10^{-4} M$, the affinity may still be great enough to adsorb the enzyme because the ligand is not hindered by the agarose matrix. The addition of hydrocarbon arms permits the use of competitive inhibitors with K_I values as high as $1 \times 10^{-3} M$.

A number of different and highly specific adsorbents also have been devised for the separation of nucleic acids. These utilize hydrogen-bonding or salt linkages as the adsorptive forces. It was first demonstrated that DNA and RNA could be resolved from each other and also subfractionated on columns when methylated serum albumin was adsorbed onto diatomaceous earth. About the same time several investigators prepared modified celluloses to which purines, pyrimidines, and synthetic and naturally occurring nucleic acids were either adsorbed or covalently bound. Nucleic acids are adsorbed onto the column by the formation of hydrogen bonds with the base or nucleic acid attached to the column packing. Development is achieved by gradient elution utilizing a changing salt concentration. This technique can produce highly specific fractionations based on bonding between complimentary sequences in amino acids.

Experimental Factors and Instrumentation

Classical Column Chromatography—The experimental setup for performing this type of chromatography is relatively simple. The column into which the stationary phase is packed consists of a glass or Teflon tube 10–50 mm in diameter and 5–100 cm in length although much longer columns have been used for difficult separations and preparative work. The bottom of the column is fitted with a stopcock or another type of flow restrictor in order to provide control over the flow rate of the mobile phase. The packing material is supported inside the column by means of a fritted glass disc or a piece of glass wool.

The packing may be introduced into the column either as a dry powder or as a slurry in the mobile phase. In either case, it is essential that the bed be formed evenly with no air bubbles or channels to disrupt the flow of the mobile phase. If it is packed dry, the stationary phase is introduced in small quantities and allowed to settle with the aid of gentle tapping or vibrating on the outside of the column. If a slurry packing technique is used, the stopcock is left open to allow the solvent to flow through the solid material and solvent is added as necessary to prevent the column from going dry, while tapping is used to dispel air bubbles. When the bed has reached the desired height, the stopcock is closed and a layer of mobile phase left at the top of the bed. In slurry packing, positive pressure or vacuum or a tamping rod may be used to ensure that the material is firmly packed.

The sample is placed on the top of the column in either of two ways. It may be mixed with a small portion of the stationary phase which is then packed as before or it may be dissolved in mobile phase and deposited on the packing after the mobile phase has been allowed to run a slight distance into the stationary phase. More mobile phase is then added and the stopcock is opened to allow flow to begin. The chromatogram may then be developed by allowing the solvent to flow from a reservoir under the force of gravity or, since this method gives variable flow rates due to changes in pressure or temperature, by introducing it under low pressure using a peristaltic pump. The effluent from the column is collected in fractions as a function of time or volume and the eluates tested for the presence of the various solutes.

High Performance Liquid Chromatography—Because of the relatively high pressures necessary to perform this type of chromatography, a more elaborate experimental setup is required. Figure 33-12 shows the block diagram of a complete HPLC apparatus. As will be detailed below, all of these

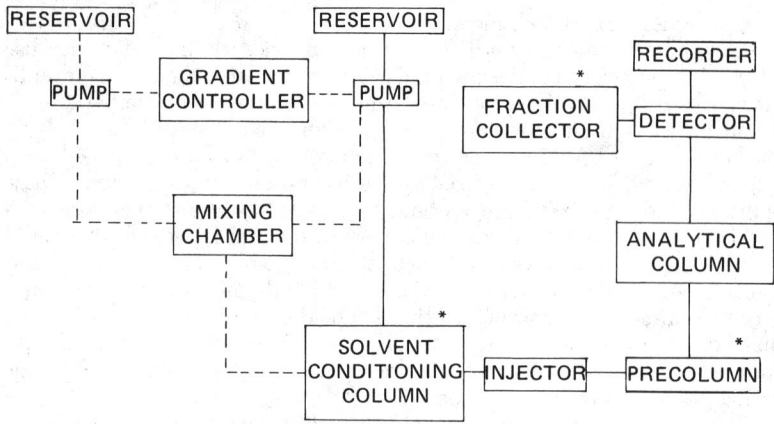

Fig 33-12.   Block diagram of a complete HPLC. The items connected by dashed lines are necessary only for gradient elution.   Those marked with an asterisk are optional for both gradient and isocratic analysis.

components are not necessary to achieve successful analyses. The parts connected by dashed lines are used only in gradient elution and the starred components are optional in either the gradient or isocratic modes.

The *solvent reservoirs* are glass or stainless steel containers capable of holding up to a liter of mobile phase which may consist of pure organic solvents or aqueous solutions of salts or buffers.   The substances used to prepare these mixtures should be of the highest purity available since contaminants will be eventually deposited on the column and disrupt the chromatography.   The mobile phases are also degassed using vacuum or sonication to eliminate outgassing in the pump or detector and then they are filtered to remove particulate matter which may clog the system.

Since the particles which are used to pack HPLC columns are small enough to prevent solvent flow by gravity, pumps which develop pressures up to 5000 psi are needed to force the mobile phase though the column.   Two types are available; mechanical, which deliver at a constant flow rate and pneumatic, which produce a constant pressure.   Of the mechanical pumps, the most frequently used is the reciprocating piston type in which a motor-driven cam drives a sapphire plunger into a small liquid-end chamber to force out the solvent. Check valves control the flow of solvent into and out of the liquid-end and prevent backflow.   Since the flow pulses every time the plunger moves in and out, the pressure variations may cause an unstable baseline and these pumps are usually equipped with a pulse damping device.   They may have two liquid chambers arranged in such a manner that, while one is filling, the other is delivering.   The pneumatic pumps may be either the gas-displacement type which uses direct pressure from a highly compressed gas to force solvent out of a tube, or the pneumatic amplifier type in which compressed gas at a lower pressure impinges on the large end of a piston to force the smaller end to deliver the liquid.   The amplification of the original gas pressure is proportional to the ratio of the areas of the two ends of the piston.   The pneumatic pumps have the advantage of pulseless operation.

If gradient analysis is necessary to achieve a particular separation, the most common way of forming the gradient is to include a second reservoir and pump and a *gradient controller*.   This is an electronic device which synchronizes the operation of the two pumps to provide a mobile phase mixture of the desired concentration.   For example, if a 50–50 mixture of the solvents in the two reservoirs is desired at an overall flow rate of 1.0 mL/min, the controller will adjust the rate of delivery of each pump to 0.5 mL/min.   The individual solvents are then combined in the *mixing chamber* and delivered to the chromatograph.   The controllers are able to provide linear, convex, concave, or step gradients, thereby yielding a solvent mixture of constantly increasing strength to enable the resolution of complex mixtures.

The next component, a *solvent conditioning column*, is used only under special circumstances.   Most HPLC column packing materials are prepared from silica gel which will dissolve slowly in solvents whose pH values are below 2 or above 7.   This results in a shrinkage of the packing material giving rise to void spaces in which separated solutes remix or are diluted, thereby leading to a loss of resolution.   Therefore, to minimize this occurrence and to protect the expensive silica-based packing materials, a small column (5–10 cm) packed with HPLC grade silica gel is inserted into the liquid stream after the pump.   The material in this column is preferentially dissolved, saturating the mobile phase and preserving the analytical column.   Although there is some slight dissolution of the silica even in the pH range of 2–7, conditioning columns need not always be used and may be a disadvantage if fractions are collected with the object of recovering the solutes, since silica is difficult to remove from the solute.

The solute mixture is introduced into the chromatograph by means of a suitable *injection device*.   Septum injectors are available, in which the sample solution is injected through a self-sealing rubber or Teflon disc using a microliter syringe. This may be done while the mobile phase is flowing or while it has been temporarily stopped.   Although these devices are inexpensive and easy to use, it is difficult to achieve reproducible injections and to automate their operation.   Therefore, sample introduction is done mainly by using a rotary valve-and-loop injector.   This consists of a stainless steel and Teflon block which has been drilled to provide two alternate paths for solvent flow each selectable by a rotating valve. When the valve is in the "fill" position, the solvent flows through one path directly onto the column.   In the other path there is a fixed-volume (20–1000 μL) loop of narrow-bore stainless steel tubing which is filled with the sample solution using a syringe or suction.   When the valve is moved to the "inject" position, the mobile phase path is diverted through the loop and washes its contents onto the column.   The results obtained are very reproducible and the injector can be automated by using a solenoid to change the valve position.

The next component in the instrument, called a *pre-column*, is optional and may be used for either of two reasons. When stationary phases consist of a thin layer of a liquid coated on a solid support, the liquid slowly dissolves in the mobile phase causing a degradation of resolution.   In this case, the pre-column will contain solid support coated with a higher percent of liquid phase than the analytical column in order to saturate the mobile phase and retard dissolution.   Since most stationary phases used currently in HPLC are permanently bonded and not subject to dissolution, the pre-column is mainly used to protect the main column by trapping particulate matter and retaining substances which would be irreversibly adsorbed on the analytical column.   In this case it is usually called a *guard column*.   The guard column is packed with a stationary phase chemically identical to that in the main column, except that its particle size is larger so that it will not restrict the flow. The larger material is relatively inexpensive and easy to pack so the contents of the guard column can be changed frequently. Because of its short length (2–10 cm), it does not usually affect the separation.

The *analytical column*, in which the actual separation takes place, is a stainless steel tube, usually 25 cm in length, with an internal diameter of 2 to 4.6 mm. It is packed with the stationary phase in one of two ways. For materials of larger particle size (> 30 μm) the dry packing is introduced in small amounts through a funnel while the outside of the column is vibrated or tapped to ensure settling of the material into a firm bed. For the more commonly used stationary phases with particle sizes less than 10 μm, the packing is slurried in a solvent or solvent mixture approximately equal in density to it and then forced into the column under pressures of up to 6000 psi. This method is superior to dry packing since it gives a tighter, more uniform bed.

The materials used to pack the column are of two types, *superficially porous* or, *pellicular*, and *totally porous*. The pellicular substances consist of a layer of porous stationary phase coated on a solid core, usually a glass bead. Solute molecules can penetrate the surface layer but not the solid support. Because of the size of the core, the particles are relatively large (37–50 μm) and they are less efficient than the smaller particles which are totally porous. Pellicular packing materials are mainly used as the support in conditioning, pre- and guard columns. The totally porous materials are microparticulate and are available in sizes of 3, 5, 10, and 20 μm with the particle size distribution closely controlled so that they will give a uniform bed when packed. They have a very high surface area to interact with the solutes and their average pore diameter of about 80 Å permits most substances to diffuse into the pores. Materials with larger pore sizes are available for molecules like proteins which are trapped in the ordinary packings and elute poorly or not at all.

Silica gel is the material most frequently employed for microparticulate column packings. It may be used as such for adsorption chromatography, but more often liquid phases for partition chromatography are bonded chemically to its surface. These include alkyl groups with chain lengths of 1, 2, 8 or 18 (ODS) carbons, cyanopropyl groups, and ion exchangers. Packings are also available with chiral stationary phases for the separation of optical isomers.

A satisfactory general purpose detector similar to the FID used in gas chromatography has not yet been developed for HPLC. However, a number of sensitive and specific detection systems based on the spectrometric, refractometric, and electrochemical properties of the solutes are employed. The most frequently used instrument is an ultraviolet-visible spectrometer which has been fitted with a flow cell of very small volume (8 μL). The simplest of these are fixed at one wavelength, usually 254 nm, since most aromatic organic compounds absorb strongly at or near this wavelength and the low pressure mercury lamps used as light sources have a strong emission line at this point. Fixed wavelength models are also available at 280 nm, where the aromatic amino acids of proteins and peptides absorb, or at 214 nm, where isolated double bonds such as the carbonyl group absorb. The fixed wavelength detectors have the advantages of low cost and high sensitivity, being able to detect some compounds at low nanogram range. Sensitivity can sometimes be increased by using a variable wavelength detector since it can be set to the exact point of maximum absorptivity for the solute. More elaborate models are also found which can scan the entire UV spectrum repeatedly during the elution of a peak to determine if more than one substance is co-eluting.

A much more sensitive but less broadly applicable detector is the fluorescense spectrometer. Sensitivities in the picogram range can be attained with those compounds which fluoresce naturally or can be made to do so by derivatization. The less expensive models of these instruments are filter fluorimeters while the more sensitive ones use a prism or grating to provide monochromatic excitation and emission radiation.

The most generally applicable detector available for use in HPLC is the differential refractometer, which is capable of measuring refractive index changes of 10^{-4}–10^{-5} RI units. Although this detector reacts to almost all organic and inorganic compounds, it is not as sensitive as a spectrometer. In addition, changes in ambient temperature cause severe drift and it cannot be used with gradient elution since in both cases differences in the RI are attributable to the solvent and not the solution.

Detectors based on electrochemical measurements such as amperometry, coulometry, polarography, and photoconductivity are used for readily oxidizable or reducible compounds such as the catecholamines.

Derivatization—Derivatization procedures are used in HPLC for a number of reasons, among which are: (a) to allow chromatography of compounds which could not otherwise be detected by the instruments currently available eg, aliphatic amines, alcohols, and carboxylic acids; (b) to improve resolution by adding a functional group which enhances the interaction of the solutes with the stationary phase eg, esterification of acids; and (c) to improve the sensitivity of the method eg, formation of fluorescent derivatives of amino acids.

Most of the derivatization reactions commonly used involve adding a substituted phenyl group to enhance detectability at 254 nm. These include the formation of p-bromophenacyl esters of alcohols, p-nitrobenzyl esters of carboxylic acids, and p-nitrobenzyl oximes of carbonyls. Fluorescent derivatives (fluorescamine adducts of primary amines) are especially useful since they not only increase the sensitivity greatly but they also allow selective detection of derivatizable compounds in the presence of co-eluting substances which do not react with the reagent.

Derivatization may be done before the sample is introduced onto the column or after it has been eluted. Pre-column reactions provide a functional group which may enhance the separation of the solutes as well as their detectability eg, the formation of phthalaldehyde derivatives of amino acids.[10] Post-column derivatization allows the separation of the solutes based on their own functionalities but introduces a reagent into the column effluent before it reaches the detector in order to increase the sensitivity. Special items of equipment are available which have the capability of adding reagent, heating the reaction mixture, and providing a time delay to allow quantitative derivatization to occur before introducing the sample into the detector.

Qualitative and Quantitative Analysis—The methods used for qualitative and quantitative analysis in HPLC are the same as those used in gas chromatography and the interested reader should consult that section for the relevant information.

Recent Developments in HPLC

Microbore Chromatography—A recent development in HPLC, *microbore chromatography* combines extremely high efficiencies with speed and economy of operation. The columns used in this technique are narrow bore (1 mm or less) fused silica or glass lined stainless steel. The tubes may be coated with liquid phase or packed with microparticulate stationary phases of the same types used in ordinary HPLC. Special equipment is necessary for operation in this mode, including pumps which can deliver accurate volumes at flow rates of less than 100 μL per minute, injectors which introduce samples of less than 1 μL, and detector flow cells with volumes of less than 1 μL.

The chief advantage of this method lies in the efficiency of the columns, with HETPs of less than 20 μm having been reported. In addition, columns can be connected in series to achieve additive increases in efficiency, a procedure which is not possible with ordinary HPLC columns. Other advantages include significant savings in solvents, since flow rates lower than 50 μL per minute are required, and finally the possibility of direct coupling to a mass spectrometer. The major disadvantage is a result of the low solute capacity of the columns, which makes preparative work impractical. The method seems ideal for the pharmaceutical quality control laboratory, where large numbers of samples must be analyzed in the shortest possible time and at low cost.

Supercritical Fluid Chromatography—This technique is based on the use as a mobile phase of a *supercritical fluid*, that is, one which is held at conditions of temperature and pressure such that it has viscosity and diffusivity values midway between those of its gaseous and liquid states. The usual HPLC columns and packing materials are used, but modifications must be made to the pumps, injectors, and detectors to allow operation at supercritical conditions.

The advantages of this method are high column efficiencies, short analysis times, and the ability to program the temperature or pressure to improve the separation. The most commonly used mobile phase, carbon dioxide, has the desirable qualities of being inexpensive, non-toxic, and non-flammable. Although successful separations have been reported, this technique is still experimental and needs more development before being used routinely.

Thin Layer Chromatography

Thin layer chromatography (TLC) is a method of analysis in which the stationary phase, a finely divided solid, is spread as a thin layer on a rigid supporting plate and the mobile phase, a liquid, is allowed to migrate across the surface of the plate. It differs from the techniques previously discussed in that the separation does not take place in a closed column, but rather on a planar surface and the mobile phase does not flow under the influence of gravity or high pressure, but is drawn across the plate by capillary action. Although separation efficiencies equivalent to those obtained with gas or high pressure liquid chromatography cannot be obtained by this method, it has the advantages of speed, versatility, and simplicity. No dedicated, expensive equipment is needed to perform separations by TLC and the analyst can modify the experimental conditions easily and quickly. It is used for such diverse purposes as trial runs to test stationary and mobile phases for liquid chromatography, monitoring the progress of synthetic reactions, clinical diagnosis, and monitoring of drug abuse.

Like liquid chromatography, TLC was not widely accepted at the time when its utility and simplicity were first demonstrated. The earliest definitive work in this field, done in 1938 by Izmailov and Schraiber[11] at the Ukranian Institute for Experimental Pharmacy, involved the analysis of plant material for alkaloids using thin layers of alumina on microscope slides. Despite the success of this and subsequent work, widespread acceptance of the technique was not achieved until the late 1950s, when Stahl,[12] who had been working in the area for a number of years, publicized the method and developed a kit of basic equipment which was made commercially available. Since then TLC has remained an important tool for both qualitative and quantitative analyses.

A wide variety of stationary phases are available in size ranges suitable for use in TLC. Since the mechanism of this method is essentially the same as that of liquid column chromatography, the only distinction being that the separation

takes place on a flat surface, the same modes used in liquid chromatography—adsorption, partition, ion exchange, and size exclusion—are available for thin layer separations. These processes are listed in Table III, along with some of the more commonly used mobile and stationary phases.

Silica gel, the most frequently used stationary phase, is employed as such for adsorption TLC and modified for reversed phase separations by coating with a thin layer of a nonpolar substance, such as silicone oil, or by binding a nonpolar functional group to it, eg, octadecylsilyl (ODS). The surface of silica is acidic due to the presence of many silanol hydroxyl groups and it is therefore best suited to the analysis of acidic compounds. It is also preferable for polar compounds, such as amino acids and sugars. Alumina (aluminum oxide) has a basic surface and is chosen over silica gel for the separation of basic and weakly polar compounds. Polyamide (nylon) is a long chain polymer, which, because it has many free amide and carboxyl groups on its surface, is an adsorbent with strong hydrogen bonding abilities. It will readily bond phenols, carboxylic acids, quinones, and nitro compounds, all of which require polar solvents such as methanol and dimethylformamide to displace them. Less active and less frequently used sorbents are calcium phosphate, calcium carbonate, and diatomaceous earth.

Cellulose, a polysaccharide, has numerous neutral hydroxyl groups on its surface and can adsorb water or polar solvents by hydrogen bonding, making it useful for partition TLC. The surface coverage of water on cellulose or silica gel can be controlled by drying the plates in an oven and then storing them in a controlled humidity chamber.

Reversed phase TLC is performed on plates coated with the same material as is packed in HPLC columns. This makes it a highly efficient technique and especially useful for trial runs on solvent systems for HPLC analysis. Although it is much less effective and convenient, reversed phase TLC can be done using silica gel, diatomaceous earth, or cellulose coated with nonpolar liquids, such as silicone oils or long chain hydrocarbons.

The stationary phases used in ion exchange and size exclusion TLC are also identical to those used in liquid chromatography. They must, however, be in a finely divided state so as to prevent band spreading. Because dextran must be swollen with solvent to be effective, TLC plates coated with size exclusion gels are stored "wet." Capillary action through these gels is slow, and development takes ten to twenty times longer than comparable analyses performed using liquid chromatography.

In order to ensure that the stationary phase adheres firmly to the backing plate and does not flake off during the development, binders such as calcium sulfate (gypsum), starch, or carbomethylcellulose are added to the adsorbent. Since these substances are not totally inert, it is likely that they influence the chromatography, and the analyst must take this into account when developing a separation. Commercially available plates of the same type, eg, silica gel, may contain different kinds and quantities of binders and therefore a separation successfully achieved on plates from one supplier may not work on those of another.

The solvents used as mobile phases in TLC are identical to those used in liquid chromatography, and can be chosen using the eluotropic series shown in Table II. They must be of high purity, since additives, such as ethanol in chloroform or antioxidants in ethers, can affect the separation and must be removed or their effects determined. Changes in the viscosity of the solvent due to impurities will alter its rate of travel since the more viscous the solvent, the more slowly it is drawn up the plate. If possible, it is preferable to use a single solvent to develop the chromatogram, rather than a multicomponent mixture, because solvents are preferentially adsorbed by the stationary phase and, as the mixture moves up the plate, the composition of the mobile phase is always changing. Compounds which travel a greater distance up the plate will therefore be exposed to a different mobile phase than those which are strongly retained. If a mixture must be used, the components should be measured carefully so that subsequent experiments will be reproducible and the solvents should also be volatile so they can be evaporated from the plate after the development is completed.

Selection of the optimum solvent or mixture for use as the mobile phase depends also on the nature of the solutes and stationary phase and is largely empirical. A useful procedure for initial trials is to run two separate plates, one using a very polar solvent, eg, ethanol, and the other employing a nonpolar liquid, such as hexane. After observing which type of mobile phase moves the solutes from the origin and determining their k' or R_f values, the solvent may be modified to increase selectivity and resolution in a number of ways. The polarity may be altered by adding other solvents chosen by consulting tables of strength or dielectric constant. Substances with functional groups similar to those of the solutes, such as ethers, alcohols, or carboxyls may be added to increase the R_f value by promoting solubility in the mobile phase. Acids or bases (acetic acid or ammonia) may be added to affect the charges on the solutes to prevent tailing.

An alternate procedure which has a sound theoretical basis involves the use of the Hildebrand solubility parameters of the solvents. The solubility parameter (δ) is related to the heat of vaporization of the liquid and indicates the selectivity of the solvent according to its ability to interact with solutes by dispersion or London forces, by dipole interactions, or as a proton donor or acceptor. The solubility parameter of a mixture depends on the values of δ for the individual solvents and on their volume fractions:

$$\delta_{MIXTURE} = \delta_A \phi_A + \delta_B \phi_B + \ldots$$

where ϕ_A and ϕ_B are the volume fractions of solvents A and B, respectively. This approach is useful for changing the selectivity of a solvent without changing its overall strength. For example, if a preliminary separation of solutes using a mixture of heptane:ethyl acetate (80:20) yielded good R_f values but unacceptable resolution, the analyst may wish to try a modifier more selective than ethyl acetate, such as acetone or ethanol. Using the formula above, the solubility parameter of the heptane-ethyl acetate mixture is calculated to be 7.6. The mixture of heptane and acetone which yields an identical δ value may be determined by

$$\delta_{MIXTURE} = \delta_{HEPTANE} \cdot X + \delta_{ACETONE}(1 - X)$$

where X is the volume fraction of heptane. The result of this calculation and a similar one for ethanol indicates that a mixture of 90:10 heptane:acetone or 95:5 heptane:ethanol has the same solvent strength as 80:20 heptane:ethyl acetate, though they differ significantly in selectivity.

Preparation of Plates—One of the greatest advantages of TLC is that the experimental set-up is simple and the chromatographer therefore can prepare plates quickly and easily in the laboratory. Although the coatings may not be as reproducible as those on plates from commercial suppliers, the procedure is less expensive and the opportunity is present to make stationary phases expressly modified for a particular separation.

The simplest method for producing an acceptable TLC plate is to dip a microscope slide into a slurry of stationary phase suspended in a volatile solvent, such as chloroform. The solvent is then removed by air drying or in an oven, and the plates can be used directly. Although it takes some practice to achieve a uniform, reproducible coating and the plates are small, development time is very short, and this method is used extensively for monitoring the progress of a

synthetic reaction or evaluating solvents as mobile phases for a particular separation.

Larger plates with dimensions of 5 × 20 cm or 20 × 20 cm are necessary to attain the greater efficiency required for more difficult separations. These are usually made of glass, but plastic, stainless steel, or aluminum backings are also used. The material must be scrupulously cleaned to prevent interaction of the solutes with contaminants on the backing.

In order to reduce band broadening, the stationary phase should consist of small particles of uniform size, so as to provide a large area for interaction and a small void volume. The particles are mixed with water or an organic solvent to form a slurry, a suitable binding agent is added and fluorescent indicators, such as zinc silicate, may be included to aid in detection of the solutes after the development. The slurry can be coated onto the plates in either of two ways. In the first, a spreading trough similar to the one first developed by Stahl is filled with the mixture and drawn across the plates, depositing a uniform layer of gel, the thickness of which is determined by an adjusting device. In the second method two or three layers of tape are placed on the edges of the plate, slurry is poured into the outlined area, and levelled off with a stirring rod. Either of these methods produces satisfactory plates but the first is preferred as it is both faster and more convenient.

Instead of coating a plate with one sorbent, two different substances may be applied simultaneously, so that the layer is made of a gradient mixture of both. For example, silica gel and alumina can be used to prepare a pH gradient across the width of the plates. This may yield separations which would otherwise be impossible.

The thickness of the layer of stationary phase is important to the success of the chromatography, since excessively thick layers allow the solutes to diffuse laterally, and, as in liquid column chromatography, band broadening results. Layers from 0.1 to 2 mm in depth are used most often, with thinner ones (250 μm) being most suitable for precise separations and thicker coatings for preparative work, due to their greater solute capacity.

Commercially available plates may differ in a number of ways from those extemporaneously prepared. They may be coated with lanes of stationary phase separated by uncoated dividers to prevent spreading and overlap of adjacent bands. They may also contain a preadsorbent area at the bottom of the plate, consisting of a 2 to 3 cm layer of an inert material, such as diatomaceous earth, running the width of the plate, which does not interact with the solutes. When the mobile phase moves across this area, it will concentrate the solutes in a narrow band, which it then transfers to the adsorbent. This makes sample applications easier and lessens band broadening.

Sample Application and Development—After the plates have been dried and conditioned, if necessary, in a controlled humidity chamber, the samples, which may range from a few μg to mg dissolved in 10 to 1000 μL of a volatile solvent, are spotted usually with a capillary tube or a microliter syringe. Samples may be applied as spots or as thin streaks, but it is essential that all of the solvent be evaporated between repeated applications and the area of sample application be kept as small as possible, since the bands will broaden as they travel up the plate. Such care is not necessary when using plates with a preadsorbent area, since the solvent will compress the applied solute into a narrow streak before depositing it on the plate.

For ascending development of the thin layer chromatogram, the plate is placed in a rectangular jar which contains developing solvent to a depth of about 0.5 cm. The atmosphere of the jar should be completely saturated with the mobile phase before development; a process usually performed by lining the jar with a piece of filter paper which has been wet with mobile phase. Instead of this arrangement, a sandwich chamber may be used, in which a second glass plate is clamped tightly against the TLC plate, the edges sealed with gaskets, and the assembly placed in a tray containing mobile phase and allowed to develop. Since the free space inside the chamber is very small, the problem of saturation is minimized. The solvent is allowed to move up the plate until it has travelled a distance of about 15 cm from the point of application of the sample, on a 20 cm plate. The plate is then removed from the tank, the mobile phase front is marked by scratching the surface, and the solvent is evaporated in an oven or, if the sample is heat labile, in the air.

In order to increase resolution, the techniques of *multiple development* and *two dimensional development* have been used. In the former, the plate after being dried, is returned to the chamber and redeveloped in the same direction, using the same mobile phase. The process may be repeated as many times as is necessary to ensure effective separation. This technique is useful for increasing the R_f values of compounds which move only a short distance from the origin, since they are exposed to solvent travel for a longer time period than faster eluting substances. In two dimensional TLC the sample is applied as a small spot in the lower left corner of the plate, about 2.5 cm from each edge. After the plate has been developed in the usual manner, it is dried, rotated ninety degrees counterclockwise, and placed in another chamber with a different developing solvent. The separated spots produced by the first elution are now located at the origin of the second. This method is especially useful for complicated mixtures containing many components or groups of substances with different functionalities, because selectivity effects of the mobile phases can be exploited more efficiently using two solvents. Two dimensional TLC is also helpful in determining if degradation of any of the solutes takes place during the chromatography. If the plate is developed in the usual two dimensional manner, except that the same mobile phase is used in both directions, all of the spots from the original sample should lie on a diagonal line running from the point of initial application to the opposite corner. Those spots not on the diagonal were not components of the original sample, and should be assumed to be degradation products.

Detection Methods—Once the chromatogram has been developed, the solute spots must be made visible in order to determine their R_f values. If the substances are highly colored, eg, dye pigments, there is no difficulty in visual detection. Most organic compounds, however, especially those of biological origin, do not absorb visible light and special methods must be used for their detection. These methods should be very sensitive since it is often necessary to detect sub-microgram quantities of material as, for example, in the analysis of drugs and their metabolites in biological fluids.

The most routinely used method of detection is examination of the plate under an ultraviolet light to detect fluorescence, using light sources which have their maximum emission lines at 254 or 365 nm. The longer wavelength is especially useful for inducing fluorescence in susceptible compounds, while the shorter wavelength is used to detect substances which absorb in that region of the ultraviolet spectrum. *Fluorescence quenching* is a particularly useful technique for detection of compounds which absorb at 254 nm. In this process a substance which will fluoresce at the given wavelength (zinc silicate) but which will not affect the separation is added to the stationary phase before the plates are prepared. After development, when the plate is irradiated at 254 nm, the entire surface will fluoresce except in those places where a compound which absorbs at this wavelength is located. The background fluorescence is thus quenched, and the absorbing compounds are visible as dark spots on a bright surface.

Many specific and nonspecific methods have been developed for detecting compounds on TLC plates using chemical

Table IV—Commonly Used Derivatizing Agents

Compound Class	Reagent	Color Produced
General	Iodine vapor	Brown
General	Sulfuric acid (50%)	Black
Acids	Bromcresol green	Yellow
Aldehydes and ketones	2,4-Dinitrophenylhy-drazine	Yellow-red
Amines and amino acids	Ninhydrin	Fluorescent
Alkaloids	Mercuric nitrate	Yellow to brown
Barbiturates	Diphenylcarbazone	Purple
Carbohydrates	Aniline phthalate	Gray-black
Lipids	Bromthymol blue	Light green
Steroids	Antimony trichloride	Various

reactions. The two most frequently employed nonspecific methods involve the use of iodine vapor and charring of organic compounds. Iodine vapor is employed for the detection of organic compounds by placing the plate in a chamber containing some iodine crystals, which sublime to produce an atmosphere saturated by their vapor. Iodine associates with practically all organic compounds, especially with unsaturated or aromatic compounds forming charge-transfer complexes. In any case the solutes will become visible as brown spots. The spots must be marked as soon as the plate is removed from the chamber, since the association between the iodine and the compound is usually weak, and the color will quickly disappear. Caution should be observed since iodine vapor is very toxic, but the method is fast, broad in its application, and non-destructive as the iodine will evaporate off the plate or can be removed by warming.

Charring is a very widely employed technique for the detection of carbon containing compounds, since it is effective for almost all organic compounds. The process involves spraying the plate with sulfuric acid, usually as a 50% (v/v) mixture with methanol, and then heating it in an oven at 110° for ten to thirty minutes. The organic compounds are destroyed by the acid and a dark deposit of carbon (charcoal) remains at the spot. Though this method is effective for most organic solutes, it is destructive, and hence cannot be used if the compounds are to be removed from the plates. It is also not applicable in those cases where a carbon based stationary phase, such as cellulose or dextran, is used, since the entire surface is then degraded.

The more specific methods of detection involve spraying the plates with reagents designed to react with specific functional groups to produce visible derivatives. These reactions may produce products of three types: (a) those which are directly detected in visible light (2,4-dinitrophenylhydrazones of carbonyls), (b) those which absorb ultraviolet light and quench fluorescence (benzoate esters of alcohols), (c) those which fluoresce directly (phthalaldehyde derivatives of amino acids). Some of the more common derivatizing reagents, and the classes of compounds with which they react, are shown in Table IV.

The incorporation of radioactive elements, such as ^{14}C or ^3H, into the solutes provides another convenient method of detection, since special instruments are available which will scan a TLC strip and produce a chart recording similar to that obtained in gas chromatography. Alternatively, adjacent sections may be scraped from the plates and counted in a scintillation counter. Also, the plate may be clamped to a piece of X-ray film, which then becomes exposed in the areas containing radioactivity, producing an *autoradiograph*. These radioactive detection methods are used extensively in metabolic studies of new drug entities, where radio-labelled drug is administered to animals and their urine is collected, extracted, and chromatographed to isolate and identify metabolites.

Qualitative Analysis—In thin layer chromatography, qualitative correlations of unknown compounds with standards is accomplished primarily by comparing the value of the R_f, which is the distance from the origin to the point of maximum intensity in the spot divided by the total distance of solvent travel. Because TLC is a technique of complete chromatography, the solutes never travel the full length of the stationary phase, and therefore all R_f values are less then one. Moreover, because fewer theoretical plates are involved than in a continuous chromatogram, the R_f values are not as reliable as retention times obtained by gas or liquid chromatography.

Greater confidence can be obtained in a qualitative identification by combining the knowledge of the R_f with a specific detection reaction. If an unknown has an R_f and color identical to that of a standard, their equivalence can be assumed with a high level of confidence if the total number of unknown possibilities is limited to a relative few. This method is used with great success in monitoring drugs of abuse in the urine of addicts undergoing treatment. More than twenty narcotic and stimulant drugs can be detected in a single sample using a combination of R_f and the various colors produced by overspraying with different reagents.[13]

Quantitative Analysis—Quantitation may be performed either while the solute is still on the plate or after it has been removed. The solute can be isolated from the plate in a number of ways. Using descending development, the mobile phase can be allowed to run continuously until the compound of interest is eluted from the end of the plate. This is rarely done and is hard to control due to the rigidity of the plate. Alternatively, the area of adsorbent containing the substance can be removed from the plate by scraping or by aspirating it into a Pasteur pipet. The compound is then eluted from the adsorbent using a suitable solvent and the solid stationary phase is removed by centrifugation or filtration. The solute may then be identified or quantitated by the usual spectrometric or chromatographic methods.

In those cases in which the solute band cannot be seen except by chemical reaction, an underivatized solute may be obtained by running portions of the same sample in adjacent lanes or a sample in one lane and a standard in the next. After development the sample lane is masked with a piece of glass and the remainder of the plate is sprayed with developing reagent to determine the location of the desired spot. The other lane is uncovered and the adsorbent removed in the area adjacent to the visualized solute.

Since the bonding between the solutes and adsorbents is frequently quite strong, complete removal from the stationary phase is often not achieved. Therefore, quantitative analysis of the substance while it is still on the plate is more reliable. Manual methods such as comparing the spot sizes and intensities between unknown and standard using a template or tracing the spot outline on paper and weighing it have been used but they are tedious and give high levels of variability. An automated method called *spectrodensitometry* is much more convenient, and is capable of yielding quantitation in the submicrogram range. In this method, the plate is placed on a movable stage which is driven by a motor so that the lane of interest passes under a beam of light. The wavelength of the light is one which is absorbed by the compounds on the plate and it is selected using a monochromator. The change in the intensity of the beam which results from its interaction with the samples is measured as transmittance by a detector placed below the plate or as reflectance by a detector on the same side of the plate as the incident beam. The results are recorded and presented on a chart as a series of Gaussian peaks which can be integrated and quantitated. The accuracy and precision of this technique may be optimized by adding a suitable internal standard in the chromatogram. Spectrodensitometric measurements may be made on substances which are colored or absorb UV, those which have been charred, those which quench fluorescence, and even on photographs or X-ray films. A more detailed discussion of the quantitative aspects of densitometry can be found in the paper by Touchstone.[14]

Paper Chromatography

Although successful paper chromatographic separations of dyes, salts, and other substances had been reported as far back as the middle of the 19th century, the method was not widely used until 1944 when AJP Martin and his coworkers rediscovered and developed it just as they had done for liquid partition and gas chromatography. Consden, Gordon, and Martin[15] not only optimized the experimental procedure, they also developed the theory of the separation process and formulated equations to describe the factors influencing the technique. Their work led to an appreciation of the method and its subsequent widespread application.

In this type of chromatography the stationary phase ordinarily consists of a sheet of filter paper with controlled texture and thickness. Since the paper is made from cellulose, a highly hydroxylated polysaccharide, it has a great affinity for water and other polar solvents. The tightly bound water is the actual stationary phase and, as a mobile phase passes over the surface of the paper, the solutes distribute themselves between the bound layer of water and the mobile phase solvent. Therefore, the mechanism that predominates is liquid-liquid or partition chromatography although adsorption to the cellulose surface may also occur. Papers especially impregnated to permit ion exchange and reversed phase chromatography are also available.

Stationary Phase—The paper used in this method is especially prepared from cotton fibers and highly purified so as to be about 99% alpha-cellulose which consists of polymers of glucose with molecular weights above 50,000. The chains of cellulose are bound together by hydrogen bonds in two different types of cross-linking. In some areas the fibers are held tightly enough to be highly structured and almost crystalline giving the paper its strength. A looser association of the polymer chains in the rest of the surface yields an almost amorphous structure with a porous surface which can absorb water molecules and swell. About 6% of the weight of the cellulose consists of water molecules permanently bound to the sugar hydroxyl groups, while another 10 to 20%, depending on humidity, are held more loosely. Because of the potential variability of the water content of the paper, moisture must be carefully controlled in its manufacture, storage and use in order to achieve reproducible results. Some of the more important chromatographic papers and their characteristics are shown in Table V.

Another variable introduced in the manufacture of the paper concerns the orientation of the fibers in the direction of motion of the machines which form it. Since the mobile phase travels across the paper by capillary action, the physical orientation of the channels is important in determining the rate of movement and, as a result, the flow is greater in the direction of the fiber orientation (*grain*) and slower perpendicular to it. In addition, there is a distance effect resulting in a slower flow as the distance from the origin increases.

Some of the hydroxyl groups of the glucose molecules can be oxidized to aldehydes, ketones, or carboxylic acids, due to the processes used during manufacture. This results in the possibility of adsorption or ion exchange occurring in addition to partition. However, the extent of such occurrences is small and in most cases they do not contribute significantly to the chromatographic separation. Modified cellulose papers with a higher carboxyl content or attached ion exchange functional groups (diethylaminoethyl, DEAE or carboxymethylcellulose, CM) are available for the separation of cations, amines, and

Table V—Types and Properties of Common Chromatographic Papers

Paper	Thickness mm	Water ascent[a]	Development time[b]	Character-istics
Whatman				
No. 1	0.16	140–220	15–16	Standard paper
No. 3MM	0.31	140–180	11	Preparative
No. 4	0.19	70–100	9	Fast
No. 31ET	0.50	60–120	4	Very fast
No. 54	0.17	60–120	6	Washed, fast
Schleicher & Schuell				
2040a	0.18	90–140	7	Fast
2043b (MGI)	0.23	220–260	15	Standard paper
2045b (GI)	0.16	300–400	45	Slow
2071	0.67	274–290	23	Preparative

[a] Time in minutes for water to ascend 30 cm up the paper.
[b] In hours, for the system: 1-butanol : acetic acid : water (4 : 1 : 5).

amino acids. For hydrophobic substances, cellulose ester papers or those impregnated with mineral oil or silicone oil are used with polar organic solvents. Glass fiber paper (Whatman GF/A) has been used, the main advantage being that it is not affected by reagents which are too corrosive for cellulose.

Mobile Phase—The solvents used for paper chromatographic analysis are similar to those employed in other forms of partition chromatography. However, since the surface of the paper binds solutes strongly, mobile phases tend to be more polar than those used in thin layer chromatography. Mixtures of alcohols, such as butyl or isopropyl, and water are commonly employed with ammonia or acetic acid added to control the charge on the solutes and reduce tailing.

Many organic substances are insoluble in water but soluble in polar organic solvents. For these compounds, paper impregnated with 20 to 40% formamide in ethanol is used. In most cases, chloroform (for hydrophilic substances), benzene (for substances of medium polarity), cyclohexane (for hydrophobic substances), or a mixture of these solvents is used as the mobile phase. The advantages of these solvents are good separating ability and relatively short developing times, ranging from one to four hours.

Sample Preparation and Application—Drugs are frequently applied to the paper in solution in volatile solvents, such as ethanol, acetone, or chloroform, in quantities of 0.1 to 1000 μg, depending on the sensitivity of the detection method and the purpose of the analysis. In the determination of pharmaceutical or biological materials in which test substances occur at low concentrations, an extraction step must generally be employed, since substances like proteins, lipids, and inorganic ions may have undesirable effects when present in large amounts, and must therefore be removed before the sample is applied to the paper. It is often advantageous to chromatograph derivatives when the original compounds are volatile, in order to enhance separation and identification.

Samples are applied at an origin which is located approximately 7 to 9 cm from the upper edge of the paper for descending development, 3 to 5 cm from the lower edge in ascending development, and on a circle with a radius of 1 to 3 cm for radial development. The optimum size of the spot varies from 3 to 8 mm in diameter and adjacent spots should be 2 to 3 cm apart. Samples are applied with capillary pipets or microliter syringes, using multiple applications for large sample volumes, and drying each spot between applications.

Development of the Chromatogram—The development of a paper chromatogram takes place in a glass or glass lined stainless steel chamber of a size commensurate with the dimensions of the paper. This may range from a test tube for a small strip to a large cabinet or jar able to contain papers

almost two feet long. The chamber must be kept sealed and saturated with the mobile phase solvents. If the mobile phase is a mixture (eg, butanol-water) the two reagents are mutually saturated by shaking in a separatory funnel, the layers separated, and the butanol layer is transferred to the mobile phase reservoir in the chamber. The aqueous layer is then poured into a second container and placed in the chamber, the chamber is sealed, and the vapors of the two solvents are allowed to come to equilibrium. The paper is spotted and placed in the chamber, but not yet allowed to contact the mobile phase, and the cellulose is permitted to equilibrate with the vapors.

The chromatogram is developed by allowing the mobile phase to travel over the surface of the paper in one of a number of ways—*ascending, descending, radial, linear horizontal,* or *spiral.* In the ascending mode the paper may be suspended by clips from the top of the tank or rolled into a cylinder and stapled in place. The end of the paper nearest to the sample spot is dipped into the mobile phase at the bottom of the tank and the mobile phase is drawn up the paper by capillary action. In the descending mode, the mobile phase is contained in a trough or Petri dish, which is supported in place at the top of the chamber by small shelves attached to the glass wall, or by a steel framework. The sample bearing end of the paper is placed in the solvent trough, and is held in place with a glass rod. The solvent runs over the edge of the trough, and is drawn down the paper by capillary action. In ascending chromatography the paper must be looped over a glass rod (anti-siphon rod) placed several cm above the trough or solvent flow will be erratic due to siphoning.

A simple apparatus for radial development may be constructed from two pie plates slightly smaller in diameter than the paper circle containing the sample. One of the plates is inverted over the other, with the paper secured between them. The mobile phase is placed in the bottom plate, and is carried up to the paper by a wick. The solvent then disperses radially from the point of contact, and the paper is removed from the chamber when the solvent front nears the edge of the plate.

The linear horizontal and spiral methods are used far less frequently than the previous techniques. In the linear horizontal mode a flat tray is used as the developing chamber, with the filter paper strips or sheets resting in a glass rack. Horizontal development trays occupy less space than the chambers already described permitting bench area to be utilized more efficiently. In the spiral mode the paper is rolled up in a Teflon sheet and one end is held in a solvent trough by a glass rod. This permits a long (19 inch) strip of paper to be developed in a small chamber.

Once the solvent has reached a point near the end of the paper the chromatography is stopped by removing the sheet from the chamber and allowing the solvent to evaporate. The spots are then made visible by methods similar to those employed in TLC, with the exception of charring, which is not useful because of the cellulose paper.

Qualitative analysis is also accomplished in the same manner as in TLC. The R_f values are determined and compared with standards, as are the results of specific derivatization reactions. Areas of the paper containing the compound of interest may be cut out and treated with a solvent to elute the substances. In descending chromatography, spots may be eluted off the paper and collected in small containers at the bottom of the chamber.

Quantitative analysis may be accomplished by comparing spot size and intensity with standards developed under identical conditions, by densitometry, or by subjecting the material to standard spectrometric methods after eluting it off the paper.

Electrophoresis

Electrophoresis is the migration of charged molecules under the influence of an electrical field. When run in the absence of a stabilizing medium the technique is termed *free boundary* or *moving boundary electrophoresis*. This method yields information on isoelectric points and mobility of compounds and requires some theoretical considerations for interpretation. Several problems are associated with the technique, including stabilization of ion boundaries, boundary anomalies, and the need for specialized equipment.

Zone electrophoresis is performed on a stabilizing medium which eliminates problems associated with the free boundary technique. Many types of stabilizing media are available including paper, agar or polyacrylamide gels, and starch blocks. The name *electrochromatography* has been used for this process because, like chromatography, a narrow zone of solute is applied to a support and migration is influenced by adsorptive or steric exclusion properties of the support. However, chromatography and electrophoresis are two fundamentally different processes; consequently, the term electrochromatography must be considered a misnomer. Electrophoresis is discussed at this point because some of the techniques are similar to chromatographic techniques with which they are readily combined.

One of the simplest procedures in electrophoresis involves spotting a mixture of solutes in the middle of a paper strip, moistening the paper with some electrolyte, and placing it between two sheets of glass. The ends of the paper strip extending beyond the glass plates are immersed in beakers of the electrolyte. A potential of approximately 5 v/cm of paper length is placed on this system, from a direct current source. Electrophoresis is allowed to continue for a period of several hours. Usually, sufficient movement occurs in that time to obtain good separations, but longer periods are sometimes required.

Many other supporting media have been used for electrophoretic separations. *Cellulose acetate* strips, which are widely used in clinical laboratories, produce excellent separations of 7 to 9 protein fractions in a few hours. This material is exceedingly fine and homogeneous, and little "tailing" is encountered due to negligible adsorption. It is especially useful for separating α_1-globulins from albumin and provides a good background for staining glycoproteins (see Chapter 32).

Electrophoresis in compact gels also has been used for the separation of protein fractions, depending at least in part on molecular sieving effects to achieve fractionation. *Starch gels* have been particularly valuable in this respect. *Agar gels* and *polyacrylamide gels* also are being used. The latter has been applied to "disc electrophoresis," where the protein fractions in the gel column are so sharply defined that they appear as thin discs after staining.

Migration of particles in a electrophoretic system depends on properties of the particles as well as the laboratory system. Based on Stoke's Law, the mobility of a particle, μ, may be calculated from Eq 1,

$$\mu = \frac{Q}{6\pi rn} \qquad (1)$$

where Q is the charge on the particle in esu, μ is in cm^2/volt-sec, r is the particle radius in cm and n is the viscosity of the medium in poises.

For ions and peptides with a molecular weight of at least 5000 that do not obey Stokes Law, Eq (2) is valid,

$$\mu = \frac{Q}{A\pi r^2 n} \qquad (2)$$

where A has a value that ranges from 4 to 6 and is related to the particle shape.

Solution conditions are important variables. The solution pH determines the nature of species. For example, an acidic pH would favor protonation of basic centers of a protein resulting in a positively charged molecule whereas an alkaline pH leads to loss of protons from the protein producing a negatively charged molecule. It is not desirable to choose a pH such that the protein is at its isoelectric point and exists as the uncharged zwitterion, a species not mobile in the imposed electrical field. Electrophoretic mobility decreases with the supporting electrolyte ionic strength. Generally, the ionic strengths employed in electrophoresis range from 0.01 to 0.10. Temperature of the solution is important because the solution viscosity varies with temperature and the mobility increases with temperature. Since heat is generated during the electrophoretic process, this must be provided for in apparatus design and in experimental conditions.

The phenomenon of electroendosmosis arises since the solution itself migrates in an electrical field. This migration, which results from surface charges on the apparatus walls, is usually increased when a gel is added in order to stabilize the electrolyte and prevent the mixing of separated zones because of thermal gradients or diffusion. The stabilizing media used in zone electrophoresis develop a negative charge which causes the electrolyte and all zones, even the neutral compounds, to be carried to the cathode. Electroendosmosis effects are large with agar gels but small with polyacrylamide gels.

When no stabilizing medium is present or when a very porous system is used, the separations of species is related to the charge to size ratios as is seen in Eq 1. If stabilizing media are present, interaction of the species undergoing separation with molecules of the media introduce another consideration into the process.

Molecular sieving may be effective in electrophoresis. For example, the pore sizes in polyacrylamide may be varied by the synthesis procedure used in preparing the polymer. Gradient pore gels are available to produce a molecular sieving which permits migration as far as the lattice allows. Molecular size may be determined in this manner, under non-denaturing conditions.

Under some conditions, inclusion of a detergent in both the polyacrylamide gels and the protein samples allows the electrophoretic separation based on molecular size to be directly proportional to molecular weight. Electrophoresis in gel media can also be used for preparative purposes.

Enzymatic and immunological methods also have been used to detect proteins following electrophoresis in gels. Immunochemical methods add an additional dimension to protein identification. Following electrophoresis in an agar gel backed with a microscope slide, antibody is placed into a trough cut parallel to the direction of electrophoresis. Antibody and electrophoretically separated antigens diffuse toward each other resulting in precipitin arcs where antigen-antibody complexes form. This technique has been referred to as *immunoelectrophoresis*.

Polyacrylamide gels also have been used successfully for the fractionation of DNA and RNA. The technique yields separations which are superior to those obtained by zone centrifugation through sucrose density gradients; thus, the time of analysis is greatly reduced. Larger columns of starch, cellulose, and silica gel are suitable for preparative work, yielding highly purified fractions in sufficient quantity for chemical analysis.

A recent modification of electrophoretic technique called *isoelectric focusing* is rapidly becoming an important tool for the separation of ampholytes, especially proteins. All proteins have an isoelectric point, pI, which is the pH value when the molecule has no net charge. When electrophoresis is run in a solution buffered at a constant pH, proteins having a net charge will migrate toward the opposite electrode as long as the current flows. The use of a pH gradient across the supporting medium causes each protein to migrate to an area of specific pH. Proteins are focused at the point in the gradient where they carry no net charge, i.e., the pI of the protein equals the pH of the gradient, thus resulting in sharp, well-defined protein bands.

References

1. Martin AJP, Synge RLM: *Biochem J 35:* 1358, 1941.
2. Martin AJP, James AT: *Biochem J 50:* 679, 1952.
3. Hawkes SJ: *J Chem Ed 60:* 393, 1983.
4. McReynolds WO: *J Chromat Sci 8:* 685, 1970.
5. Gloor, Johnson: *J Chromat Sci 15:* 413, 1977.
6. Sluyterman LA, Elgersma O: *J Chromat 150:* 17, 1978.
7. Porath J, Flodin P: *Nature 183:* 1657, 1959.
8. Moore JC: *J Polymer Sci Part A, 2:* 835, 1964.
9. Pestka S: *Scientific American 249(2):* 36, 1983.
10. Jones BN, Paabo S, Stein S: *J Liq Chromat 4:* 565, 1981.
11. Izmailov NA, Schraiber MS: *Farmatsiya 3:* 1, 1938.
12. Stahl E: *Chemiker Ztg 82:* 323, 1958.
13. TLC Toxicology System, Bulletin No 502, Whatman Inc, Clifton, NJ.
14. Touchstone JC, Levin SS, Murawec T: *Anal Chem 43:* 858, 1971.
15. Consden R, Gordon AH, Martin AJP: *Biochem J 38:* 224, 1944.

Bibliography

Dilts RV: *Analytical Chemistry*, Van Nostrand, New York, 1974.
Advances in Chromatography (a series), Marcel Dekker, New York.
Frei RW, Lawrence JF: *Chemical Derivatization in Analytical Chemistry*, vol 1: Chromatography, Plenum, New York, 1981.
Fried G, Sherma J: *Thin Layer Chromatography*, Marcel Dekker, New York, 1982.
Snyder LR, Kirkland JJ: *Introduction to Modern Liquid Chromatography*, 2nd ed, Wiley & Sons, New York, 1979.
Sherma J, Zweig G: *Paper Chromatography*, Academic, New York, 1971.
Snyder LR: *Principles of Adsorption Chromatography* (vol 3 of Giddings JC, Keller RA, eds: *Chromatographic Science Series*), Marcel Dekker, New York, 1968.
Giddings JC: *Dynamics of Chromatography*, Part I, Marcel Dekker, New York, 1965.
Miller JM: *Separation Methods in Chemical Analysis*, Wiley, New York, 1975.
Touchstone JT, Dobbins MR: *Practice of Thin Layer Chromatography*, Wiley, New York, 1978.
Grob RL, ed: *Modern Practice of Gas Chromatography*, Wiley-Interscience, New York, 1977.
Reed E, ed: *Assay of Drugs and Other Trace Compounds in Biological Fluids*, vol 5, *Methodological Developments in Biochemistry*, Elsevier/North-Holland, Amsterdam, 1976.
Deyl Z, ed: *Electrophoresis—a survey of techniques and applications*, vol 18, *Journal of Chromatography Library*, Elsevier, New York, 1979.

Acknowledgment

The author wishes to acknowledge with gratitude the editorial, computational, and secretarial assistance of Leonard C Bailey, Jr.

CHAPTER 34

Instrumental Methods of Analysis

Hamed M Abdou, PhD

Director of Product Quality Control
ER Squibb & Sons, Inc
New Brunswick, NJ 08903

The recent advances in instrumental methods of analysis have helped to establish this rather new technique, as the mainstream of the analytical laboratory. The conventional wet chemical methods gradually became obsolete or played a minor role in the analytical discipline.

Also, one of the major scientific achievements during the last few years was the introduction of the computer. The invention of the ubiquitous microchip in the mid-seventies and the overwhelming spread of microelectronics created a new revolution in the analytical laboratory, the proportions of which we still cannot fully foresee. The microcomputer, in one form or another has become an integral part of almost every analytical instrument. From the analytical balance to the most sophisticated mass spectrometer, it controls the operating parameters, acquiring the data and manipulating it as well as managing its storage and retrieval. Large separate computers with terminals at many locations can perform several functions, such as sample preparation and instrument control in addition to data acquisition and laboratory management.

It should be noted however, that the ultra sophistication of analytical instruments of today, combined with the immense controlling power of the microcomputer, is creating a new challenge for the analytical chemist. The ability to handle infinitesimal amounts of samples with such high accuracy and precision is changing our traditional concept of the analytical process. Therefore, it is essential today to realize that chemical analysis should only be applied to the problems that the sample represents rather than the sample itself.

Hence, the analytical chemist is increasingly required to understand the system under observation as well as the sophisticated measurement device in use.

This chapter includes three major sections of analytical disciplines: (1) spectrometric methods, (2) electrometric methods, and (3) thermometric methods. Chromatographic methods of analysis are discussed separately in Chapter 33 and radiochemical measurement in Chapter 30. The discussion in this chapter is, in general, a survey of many analytical techniques. For a full discussion of any particular topic the reader is referred to the bibliography supplied at the end of this chapter.

Under *spectrometric methods*, instruments based on the absorption or emission of electromagnetic (EM) radiation as a result of its interaction with matter are described and their applications explored. These include, X-ray, ultraviolet (UV), visible, infrared (IR), nuclear magnetic resonance (NMR), atomic absorption (AA), mass spectroscopy (MS), fluorescence, and light scattering techniques.

Under *electrometric methods*, the electrochemical behavior of matter characterized by measuring different electrical quantities, such as voltage, current, resistance, etc., is discussed. These include potentiometry, polarography, amperometry, and voltammetry.

Under *thermometric methods*, the thermodynamic changes brought about by raising the temperature of the sample under study are monitored. These methods include thermogravimetry (TGA), differential thermal analysis (DTA) and differential scanning calorimetry (DSC).

Spectrometric Methods

A study of the theory and applications of spectrometric methods of analysis necessitates a brief understanding of electromagnetic (EM) theory. The old Newtonian views regarding the corpuscular nature of light were abandoned during the nineteenth century as they could not explain many observed wave properties such as interference, diffraction, and refraction. The concept of the electromagnetic field was first expressed by Maxwell in 1860. His equations theorized the existence of waves that travel through electromagnetic fields and whose properties are identical to those of light. The oscillation of an electron gives rise to EM radiation. As is illustrated in Fig 34-1, at each point in the direction of the beam, the electric field and magnetic field, represented by two vectors, are perpendicular to each other. The wavelength, λ, is defined as the distance between successive maxima or minima, and is expressed in nanometers (nm) or 10^{-9} meters, formerly Angstroms (Å), (one Å $= 10^{-8}$ cm). The frequency in cycles per second (cps or Hz) is denoted by ν. The frequency is related to λ by $\nu = c/\lambda$, where c is the velocity of light in vacuum. The time required for the completion of 1 cycle

is designated by τ, which is related to ν by $\tau = 1/\nu$. The reciprocal of wavelength, $1/\lambda$, is referred to as wave number, $\bar{\nu}$, expressed in reciprocal centimeters, cm^{-1}. The wave number is employed particularly in describing the position of peak maxima for IR spectra.

Initially, the assignment of wave properties to EM radiation did not seem to encounter any difficulty as both light and waves share identical properties. Both are forms of energy,

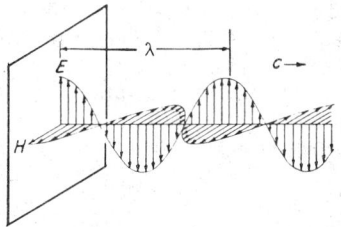

Fig 34-1. A plane-polarized electromagnetic radiation. *E:* electric vector; *H:* magnetic vector.

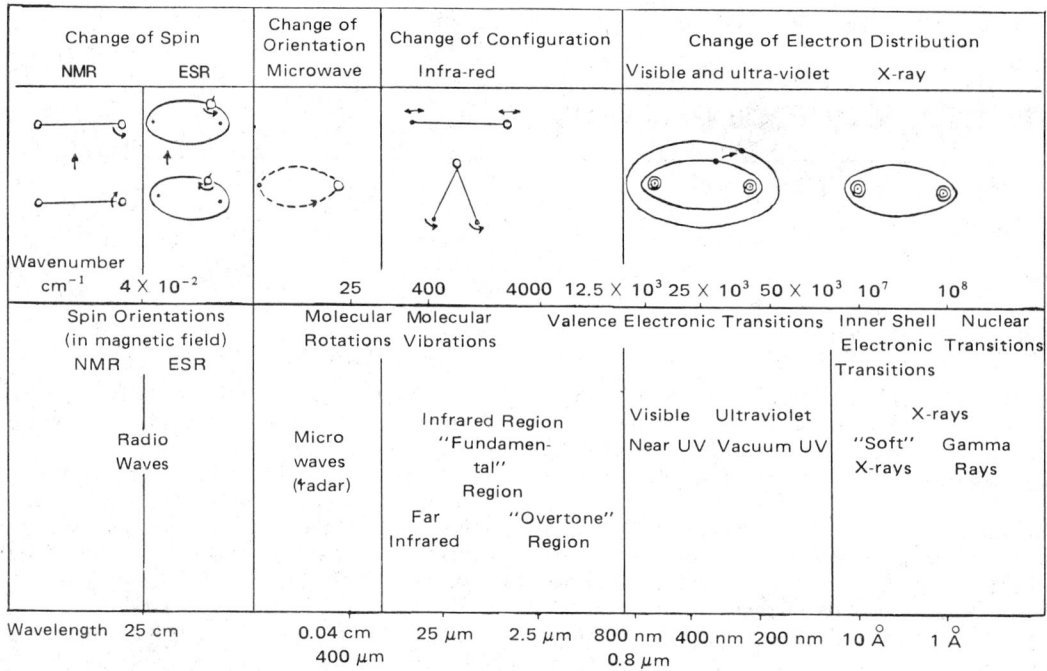

Fig 34-2.　A schematic diagram of the electromagnetic spectrum.

and have intensity (amplitude), wavelength, and frequency or velocity. Maxwell, therefore, was believed to have settled the corpuscular vs wave question for all time. However, only a few years later (1881–1889), Michelson and Morley proved experimentally the apparent absence of any medium capable of sustaining the electromagnetic oscillations. Planck, in 1900, formulated his concept of quantum restriction. He stated that oscillating atoms of a hot body can have only energies that are integral multiples of $h\nu$. In other words, the energy of an oscillator is discontinuous and any change in the energy can occur only by a jump between two energy states. Planck showed that the energy in a photon of light is related to wave frequency by the expression $E = h\nu = hc/\lambda$, where h is Planck's constant, 6.6256×10^{-27} ergs/sec. In 1903, Einstein conducted his experiments on the photoelectric effect of light. He concluded that electrons are emitted from the surface of a specific metal upon its illumination with light of a relatively low wavelength such as blue light. Red light, irrespective of its intensity, fails to eject an electron from a similar metal. These findings by Michelson and Morley, Planck, Einstein, and others could not be explained by Maxwell's assigned wave properties. Considering these facts, a reliance on the dual nature of light, behaving both like a wave and a particle, seemed to be indispensable for resolving many physicochemical phenomena.

Interaction between Molecules and EM Radiation— The presence of radiation of a particular frequency is necessary, but is not always sufficient, to induce a change in the energy level of a molecule. Quantum restrictions specify certain conditions for the interaction of radiation with a molecule. On many occasions energy is absorbed only if the radiation frequency corresponds to the components of the molecular frequency. This is referred to as resonance absorption.

The position of maximum absorption, λ_{max}, for a molecule in a particular region of the spectrum is a function of the total structure of the molecule with a transition energy corresponding to a given wavelength. The intensity of the absorption maximum, ϵ_{max}, is a function of the probability of EM radiation–molecule interaction and polarity of the excited state. At room temperature a molecule is normally in its lowest energy state; ie, the ground state. The transition be-

tween E_1 and E_2, two energy states or levels of a molecule, occurs by the interaction of EM radiation with a molecule. The difference between E_1 and E_2 is designated by ΔE, whose frequency of radiation is expressed as $\Delta E = h\nu$ ergs.

Very high energies ($>10^8$ cm^{-1}) disturb and cause changes in the nucleus of the atom that is independent of its environment. Less energy however, causes a change in the electronic distribution around the nucleus.

Regions of the Spectrum

The whole range of EM radiation is divided arbitrarily into a number of regions. Interaction between a molecule and various kinds of EM radiation gives rise to a change in the electronic energy and/or kinetic energy of the molecule. In most cases, the energy absorbed is quickly converted to vibrational, rotational, and translational energy. However, in particular cases emission occurs either immediately as in *fluorescence*, or after a short time as in *phosphorescence*. As will be seen later, these specific changes in the energy of a molecule result in the generation of a characteristic spectrum that can be utilized by the pharmaceutical chemist for both structural elucidation and quantitative determination. Fig 34-2 depicts a wavelength and frequency scale for the different regions of the EM radiation spectrum.

A theoretical and practical description of various types of spectroscopy of primary interest in the pharmaceutical sciences is given in the following sections. An arbitrary order has been adopted in organizing this chapter, beginning with the instrumental methods using the highest frequency EM radiation (X-ray) and proceeding toward the lowest frequency (microwave, NMR). The length of discussion of each topic is based on the extent of the applicability of the method in pharmaceutical analysis.

X-Ray Methods

The shortest wavelength section of EM radiations wherein the energy change of the involved atoms is reversible lies between 1–10 Å and is known as the X-ray region. When a sample is irradiated with photons in this region, electrons in the inner shell of the atoms will be displaced. As electrons

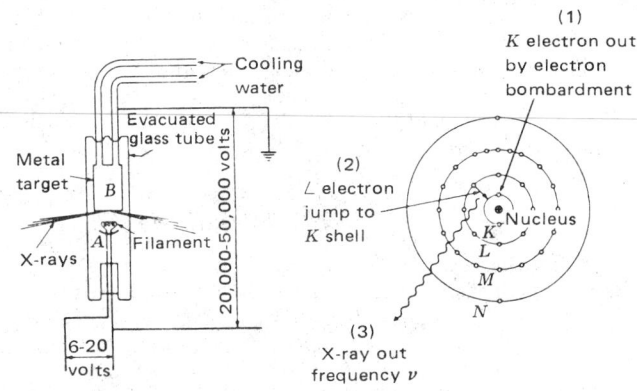

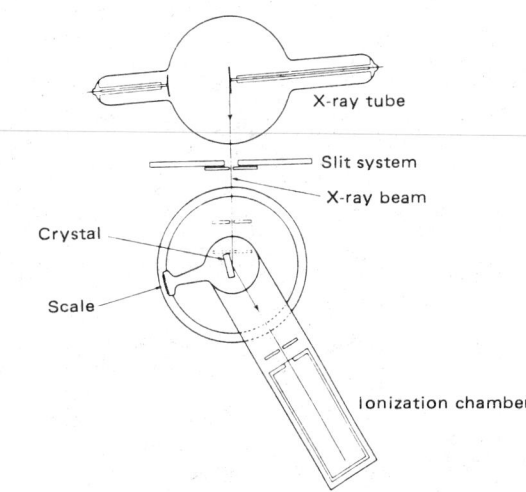

Fig 34-3.   The production of X-rays. (Reproduced from RL Murray, *Introduction to Nuclear Engineering*, Prentice-Hall, 1961).

return to their normal states in the atoms, X-rays will be emitted with frequencies that are dependent only on the atom, not on the state of the chemical binding: this X-ray emission line (including fluorescence) could therefore only be utilized for the quantitative estimation and qualitative identification of elements present in the sample. A second type of emission of X-radiation, a continuous spectrum, results from the transfer of the kinetic energy of the impinging electrons to the atoms of the target. Since not all electrons lose all their energy and some are less decelerated, a distribution of energy or a spectrum occurs. It should be noted that the characteristic sharp lines of the X-ray emission are superimposed on the continuous distribution. The generation of the X-ray spectrum is caused by the expulsion of an electron from one of the lower quantum levels of the atom. This vacancy is filled by an electron from one of the upper shells, which results in the emission of a photon possessing energy identical to that which was lost by the original electron; ie, $\Delta E = E_1 - E_2$, where E_1 and E_2 are the initial and final energy of the electron, respectively. If the vacancy produced in the K shell is filled with an electron from the L shell, the radiation is called $K\alpha$; if it is filled with an electron from the M shell, $K\beta$. Fig 34-3 shows the production of X-rays, Fig 34-4 is a diagram of an X-ray spectrometer and Fig 34-5 depicts the peaks for molybdenum.

The frequency of the emitted radiation is given by;

$$\nu = Z^2 \frac{2\pi^2 me^4}{h^3}\left(\frac{1}{N_1^2} - \frac{1}{N_2^2}\right) \qquad (1)$$

where Z is the atomic number of the atom, m and e are the mass and charge of the electron, h is Planck's constant, and N_1 and N_2 are 1 and 2 for K and L shell, respectively.

An X-ray tube consists of an evacuated tube containing a heated cathode and an anode (target). The emitted electrons are accelerated to the target by imposing a high voltage across the electrodes. Usual X-ray methods for obtaining a characteristic spectrum of a substance are made by using the sample as an anode or affixing the specimen on the target anode. The detector is most often the energy dispersive spectrometer (EDS) with a liquid nitrogen cooled Si(Li) detector at its heart. Two X-ray methods are described: powder diffraction and emission spectrometry (including fluorescence).

X-Ray Diffraction

In 1912, Max von Laue pointed out that if the wavelength of EM radiation became as small as the distance between atoms in the crystals, a diffraction pattern should result. Later it was found that the X-ray region has the right wavelength and a definite diffraction pattern was obtained for

Fig 34-4.   Bragg x-ray spectrometer. (Reproduced from WJ Moore, *Physical Chemistry*, 3rd Ed, Prentice-Hall, Inc, Englewood, NJ, 1962.)

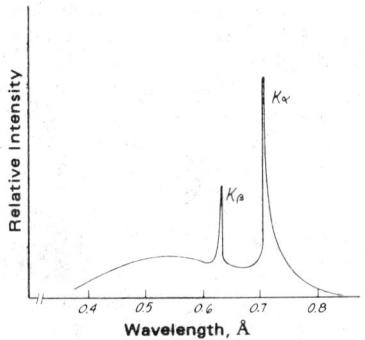

Fig 34-5.   The X-ray emission spectrum of molybdenum.

$CuSO_4$ crystals. In essence, the crystal diffracts X-rays similar to a diffraction grating, whose plane diffracts ordinary light. The three-dimensional crystal functions like a series of plane gratings stacked one above the other. The wavelength of the X-rays, λ, is related to the angle of incidence, θ, and the interatomic distance, d, by Bragg's equation;

$$n\lambda = 2d \sin \theta \qquad (2)$$

where n is the order of the diffraction, 1, 2, 3, . . .

For a single crystal the diffracted X-rays consist of a few lines; with powder, due to a random distribution of crystals, the diffraction pattern consists of a series of concentric cones with a common apex on the sample. The atoms in a crystal possess the power of diffracting the X-ray beam. Each substance scatters the beam in a particular diffracting pattern, producing a *fingerprint* for each atomic crystal or molecule (Fig 34-6).

If an unknown powder sample is to be identified, its diffraction pattern may be compared with those of known substances or its d values calculated from the diffraction diagram and compared with the d values of known compounds.

If the diffraction pattern of a single crystal is to be determined, the crystal is mounted on a thin glass capillary and the capillary is fastened to a brass pin. Metal samples are machined into an appropriate shape whereas plastics are prepared in a desirable shape by extrusion. A substance in powder form can be ground finely and transformed into a small rod using collodion as a binder or held in a specific device with an open cup. Single crystal X-ray diffraction is one of the most frequently used techniques for the study of molecular structure and configurations in the crystal.

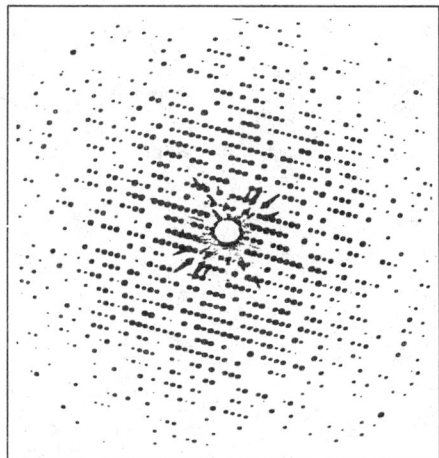

Fig 34-6. X-ray diffraction pattern from a crystal of sperm whale myoglobin, using a Buerger precession camera. (Reproduced from WJ Moore).

Powder X-ray diffraction analysis is employed for characterization of crystalline structure. It has been utilized to determine the existence of polymorphic forms of many substances, such as carbon in graphite or in diamond and drugs. The method also is used to distinguish between various oxides such as FeO and Fe_2O_3 and to aid in the identification of Levopropoxyphene Napsylate, Flurandrenolide, etc. The X-ray diffraction method is applied also in polymer chemistry to determine the degree of orientation of the fibers.

New pulsed X-ray sources have short beam durations with high intensity outputs which are appropriate for flash X-ray radiographs of rapid events. They also have some diffraction applications. Other techniques such as diffraction topography, double-crystal diffractometry, interferometry, strain measurements and texture analysis are very important techniques today for the study of crystal perfection, structure defect, grain structure and orientation. The analysis of diffraction data ranges from the use of simple calculations to very involved computations using mini-computers. Due to its complexity, there are separate computation packages available for single-crystal structure analysis and for powder diffraction analysis.

X-Ray Emission Spectrometry

X-ray spectrometric analysis gives qualitative and quantitative data about the elements in a sample. The intensity of the X-rays emitted by a given element as the target depends on the wavelength. There is a broad continuous emission (white X-radiation) and superimposed upon this are sharp line emissions characteristic of the target material. The study of these characteristic X-ray spectra provides a considerable insight into the atomic structure of the sample.

X-Ray Fluorescence

As a K electron is expelled, either by bombardment with high-energy electrons or by absorption of X-ray, it is replaced by an L or M electron. Emission of energy of a wavelength longer than the excited wavelength is known as fluorescence radiation. In X-ray fluorescence, the sample is a secondary target and is irradiated by a beam produced by bombarding a primary target with high-energy electrons. The sample is rotated to insure uniformity of exposure. The emitted fluorescence lines, which are characteristic of a given substance, are collimated and directed onto the surface of the analyzing crystal. The analyzing crystal consists of a flat, single crystal

plate. The reflected radiation is directed through an exit slit to the detector, where the X-ray energy is transformed into electrical impulses. X-ray fluorescence is applicable to the quantitative determination of elements, especially those for which no other reliable "wet" analytical methods exist such as niobium and the rare earths. The method is also complementary to emission spectrometry.

Electron Probe Microanalysis (EPMA)

Traditional X-ray emission has not proven to be very useful for microanalysis. The current availability of low-cost microcomputers however, has led to the emergence of a new class of techniques that have X-ray spectrometry as their dominant partner and are very useful for the qualitative and quantitative determination of an extremely small number of atoms of a specific contaminant in complex matrices, (sensitivity $\simeq$ $10^{-7}\%$ of the sample). These techniques are collectively known as electron probe microanalysis (EPMA) or analytical electron microscopy (AEM) and are currently experiencing widespread growth in surface analysis as they only scan the first few angstroms in thickness of the sample surface. EPMA in general is concerned with the measurement of core-electron binding energies. When a molecule is bombarded with high energy electron beams some electrons are elastically bounced off when they approach the sample and these have little analytical information to offer. Others are absorbed by the sample and exhibit what is known as inelastic bouncing; this latter phenomenon is the basis of the information about the structure of the sample surface that EPMA techniques offer. Two types of X-ray high vacuum spectrometers could be employed. The first and the most common is the energy dispersive spectrometer (EDS) and the second is the wavelength dispersive spectrometer (WDS).

Auger Electron Spectrometry (AES)

This technique differs from other EPMA methods in the depth of analysis utilized, which depends on the atomic number of the sample. While traditional X-ray emission penetrates between 1000–4000 Å deep, AES penetration extends only about 20 Å, a very shallow depth and therefore it is effective for the elemental analysis of the surface of a film and layers of metallurgical samples. It is not suitable for a glass or polymer however, as it destroys these materials. AES utilizes a sample size of only 0.2 μL or small area of 100 Å and can detect all elements except hydrogen.

X-ray Photoelectron Spectroscopy or Electron Spectroscopy (ESCA)

When a molecule or atom is bombarded with an X-ray of sufficient energy, all electrons whose binding energies are less than the energy of the exciting X-ray are ejected. The kinetic energies of these photoelectrons are then measured by an electron analyzer. The advantage of ESCA is that it is the most sensitive technique to determine the chemical shifts observed in the core-electron binding energies. These binding energies are affected by the valence electrons and therefore by the chemical state of the sample. Since chemical shifts are observed for every element in the periodic table except hydrogen, ESCA is very valuable and more versatile than NMR from the perspective of elemental sensitivity. Due to this sensitivity and its excellent quantitative ability, ESCA currently enjoys a phenomenal growth as an analytical technique.

Ion Scattering Spectroscopy (ISS), and Secondary Ion Mass Spectrometry (SIMS)

These ion techniques can also sample about 20 Å or less of the surface. Unlike AES, both ISS and SIMS techniques do not destroy the sample but they require a larger sample size. In SIMS, the plasma generated by primary ions produces a secondary ion beam that is characteristic of each element. SIMS can detect less than 1 ppm and in some cases 1 ppb of certain elements such as Cu, Cr, and Ba on the sample surface. It is the only EPMA technique that can detect and quantitate hydrogen on the surface of a sample. The only limitation of SIMS is its prohibitive cost ($\simeq \$1$ million).

Absorption Spectrometry

Absorption spectrometry is the measurement of the selective absorption by atoms, molecules, or ions of electromagnetic radiation having a definite and narrow wavelength range, approximating monochromatic energy. Absorption spectrometry encompasses the wavelength regions: ultraviolet (200–380 nm), visible (380–780 nm), near-infrared (780 nm–2.5 μm), and infrared (2.5 μm–40 μm). The region between 10 nm to 200 nm, known as the far UV or vacuum UV (as it requires the complete absence of air due to its interference) has minimal application in pharmaceutical analysis. Atomic absorption spectrometry involves the measurement of radiation absorbed by the unexcited atoms of a chemical substance that have been aspirated into a flame or other high energy sources.

Theory—When electromagnetic radiation travels through a medium containing atoms, molecules, or ions, a number of events may take place. 1) The intensity of the emergent energy is identical to the intensity of the incident energy. This indicates that no absorption of radiation has occurred. 2) Reflection, refraction and/or scattering may occur. 3) The intensity of the emergent energy is less than that of the incident energy. This indicates that some absorption has taken place (absorption spectrometry). As a result of this absorption, the species in solution are activated from their lowest energy state (ground state) to higher energy states (excited states). For absorption to occur, the energy of the exciting radiation must match the quantized energy difference between the ground state and one of the excited states of the species. In atomic absorption, excitation occurs only through electronic transition. In visible and ultraviolet spectrometry, radiation energy can excite only the outermost or valence electrons. Accompanying the electronic excitation (E_e) is a change in vibrational energy (E_v) and rotational energy (E_r) of the molecule. For polyatomic molecules, vibrational and rotational transitions can occur in addition to electronic excitation. As a result, the molecular spectrum consists of closely spaced absorption bands instead of the sharp lines as in atomic absorption. Pure vibrational and some rotational transitions can be achieved by infrared radiation. The lifetime of the excited state is brief (10^{-8}–10^{-9} sec), its existence being terminated by any of several *relaxation* processes. The most common relaxation is through the production of heat, which may cause a slight increase in the temperature of the medium. Another form of relaxation occurs as the decomposition of the excited state into new species (photochemical reactions) according to the following equation;

$$M + h\nu \rightarrow M^* \text{ (excited state)}$$

$$M^* \rightarrow M + \text{heat}$$

$$M^* \rightarrow M' \text{ (new species)}$$

Alternatively, relaxation may result in emission of radiation at specific wavelengths characteristic of the excited species (emission spectroscopy), or in emission of radiation at longer wavelengths than the incident beam, immediately (fluorescence) or after a short time (phosphorescence).

Ultraviolet and Visible Absorption Spectrometry

As mentioned previously, UV and visible absorption bands are due to electronic transitions in the region 200 nm–780 nm. In case of organic molecules, the electronic transitions could be ascribed to the σ, π, or an n electron transition from the ground state to an excited state (σ^* & π^*). Since the σ electron is involved firmly in the construction of a single bond, its transition requires much more energy (usually in far UV) than the n electron (nonbonding electrons) or less tightly bonded π electrons.

There are four types of absorption bands that occur due to the electronic transition of a molecule:

R-Bands: $n \rightarrow \pi^*$, in compounds with C=O or NO_2 groups $\epsilon_{max} < 100$

K-Bands: $\pi \rightarrow \pi^*$, in conjugated systems $\epsilon_{max} > 10,000$

B-Bands (benzenoid bands): due to aromatic and heteroaromatic systems, $\epsilon_{max} < 2000$

E-Bands (ethylenic bands): in aromatic systems, ϵ_{max} 2,000 to 14,000

Beer's Law—If incident light with wavelength λ and intensity I_0 impinges on a solution with concentration, c, and pathlength, l, of 1 cm, the radiant energy of the light is diminished in an exponential fashion. Thus, if a given concentration of a substance absorbs 50% of the incident radiation, doubling the concentration will not absorb 100% but rather 75% of the light. The thickness of the sample or pathlength has a similar effect on the absorption. Mathematically, the radiation-concentration and radiation-pathlength relation can be expressed by the following equations;

$$\frac{dI}{dc} = -k_1 I \quad \text{and} \quad \frac{dI}{dl} = -k_2 I \qquad (3)$$

Integration of the equations in Eq. 3 gives;

$$\int_I^{I_0} \frac{dI}{I} = -k_1 \int_0^c dc \quad \text{and} \quad \int_I^{I_0} \frac{dI}{I} = -k_2 \int_0^C dc \qquad (4)$$

Evaluation of the integrals between limits, combining the two formulae, and incorporating the value 2.303 (for transforming the natural log into a log of base 10) in the constant provides the more familiar equation used in spectrometry;

$$\log (I_0/I) = \epsilon cl \qquad (5)$$

where I_0 is the intensity of the incident energy, I is the intensity of the emergent energy, c is the concentration, l is the thickness of the absorber (in cm), and ϵ is the molar absorptivity (formerly expressed as molar extinction coefficient) for concentration in moles/L.

If the concentration is expressed in grams/L, absorptivity is designated by a instead of ϵ. The term $\log I_0/I$ or $\log (1/T)$ is referred to as absorbance, A (formerly stated as optical density or extinction); T is Transmittance or I/I_0. $E_{1cm}^{1\%}$, which is encountered less frequently in the literature, represents a concentration of 1% w/v and a 1-cm cell thickness and is primarily used in the investigation of those substances of unknown or undetermined molecular weight (usually impure natural products).

A typical UV absorption spectrum, shown in Fig 34-7, is the result of plotting wavelength vs absorptivity. The wavelength corresponding to maximum absorptivity, ϵ_{max} is denoted by λ_{max}.

UV Terminology—A few of the most generally employed terms in absorption spectrometry follow;

Chromophore—A moiety of a molecule responsible for selective absorption of radiation in a given range.

Auxochrome—A chemical group which does not give rise to an absorption band by itself, but upon being attached to a chromophore alters both the position and intensity of the peak.

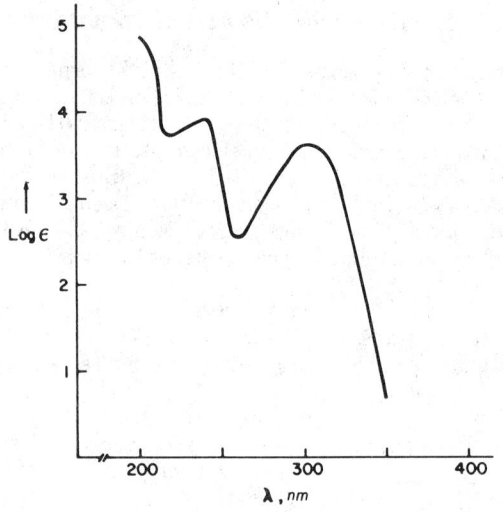

Fig 34-7.   The UV absorption spectrum of salicylic acid.

Bathochromic Shift—A shift of the peak position (λ_{max}) to a higher wavelength due to the effect of a substituent or solvent (red shift).

Hypsochromic Shift—A shift of λ_{max} to lower wavelength (blue shift).

Hyperchromic and Hypochromic Effect—These terms refer to an increase and decrease in absorptivity, respectively.

Quantitative Applications of UV and Visible Spectrophotometry—One of the major uses of UV and visible spectrometry is for quantitative measurements. An unknown concentration of a known compound, if it conforms to Beer's Law, can be determined by using Eq 5. A representative calibration curve, shown in Fig 34-8 is constructed by plotting absorbance (A) vs concentration.

Analytical Procedure—Samples for UV absorption can be examined in the form of a vapor or a solution. Both polar and nonpolar solvents can be employed for preparing an analytical sample. The cutoff point of a solvent, however, should be recognized. A cutoff point is the wavelength at which the absorbance of a solvent approaches unity, using water as a reference. The cutoff points for many solvents can be found in the literature and in solvent charts supplied by several suppliers of solvents.

A thorough understanding of the limitations of Beer's law must be taken into consideration. Some of these are of such a fundamental nature that they constitute a real limitation of the law; they are due to the fact that the law does not take into consideration the effects of pH, temperature, wavelength, or solute-solvent and solute-solute interactions, eg, association (intermolecular hydrogen bonding), dissociation, chemical reaction, etc. Due to these limitations, the law usually applies only to dilute solutions, where these interactions are insig-

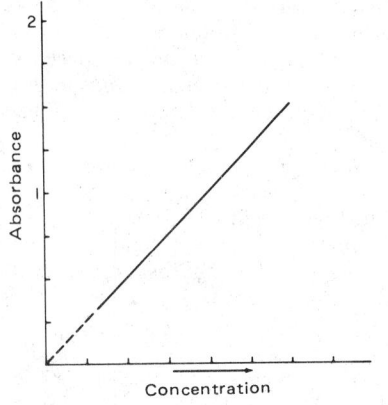

Fig 34-8.   A representative Beer's law plot.

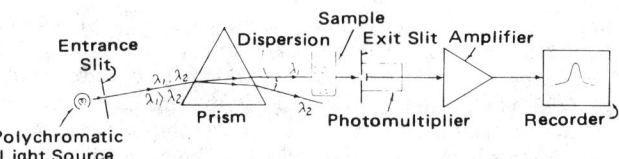

Fig 34-9.   A classical UV-visible spectrometer. (Newer instruments use grating instead of prisms.)

nificant. Another limitation to the Beer's law is due to the inability of most instruments to provide monochromatic radiation.

Instrumentation—A simplified diagram of a UV-visible spectrometer is presented in Fig 34-9 and its major components are described below.

Radiation Source—The source for the UV range is usually a high-pressure hydrogen (or deuterium) discharge lamp, which covers a range of 200 to 375 nm. A xenon arc or a mercury vapor lamp provides a more intense radiation. The source employed for the visible range is a 6- or 12-V tungsten lamp.

Monochromator—The primary function of a monochromator is the dispersion of polychromatic energy by means of a prism or grating. The desired monochromatic ray, whose position is determined by the angular position of the prism or grating, is directed toward the sample compartment.

Sample Compartment—This is the section where monochromatic energy encounters the sample. In a double-beam instrument, this compartment contains a beam-chopping device or a beam-switching assembly which allows the beam to pass alternatively through the sample and reference cells (about 35 times/sec). This allows the sample-reference relationship to remain unaffected by slight changes in the source or optics of the instrument.

Detector—The detector is usually a photomultiplier tube. As depicted in Fig 34-10, the cathode consists of a surface coated with a light-sensitive layer. When energy strikes the layer, it emits electrons. A series of electrodes called dynodes, which are also coated with a energy-sensitive layer, are connected by a voltage-dividing network of resistors. The electrons are attracted from the cathode to dynode 1, from dynode 1 to 2, etc, each impinging quantum thus producing an avalanche of about 10^6 electrons. The collection of electrons on the anode creates a few milliamperes of current which can be measured as voltage across a resistor.

The output from the detector is amplified and observed on a meter, a recorder, or a cathode ray tube. Some spectrometers are manually operated, while others are equipped for automatic and continuous recordings. Spectrometers employing the latest technology can be interfaced with a digital computer through an analog to digital converter for the direct determination of difference spectra of analytes as well as for the storage of reference spectra.

New Spectrometric Techniques

In the last few years, there has been significant progress in the use of holographic gratings and microprocessor control in

Fig 34-10.   The circuit of a photomultiplier.

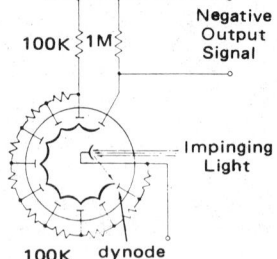

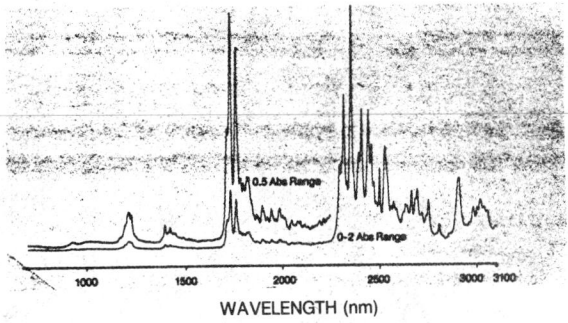

Fig 34-11.   NIR absorption spectrum of cyclohexane.
(Reproduced from Varian Publication (VIA)).

WAVELENGTH (nm)

the design of modern spectrometers. Recent models feature automatic control of all operating parameters such as wavelength selection and calibration, baseline correction, programmed scanning, first-, second-, third- and fourth-derivative spectra, light emitting diode (LED) readouts of absorbance or concentration in addition to screen monitoring and hard-copy printouts.

Also, because of the advent of stable microelectronics, in addition to the wide availability of microprocessor controlled and fully automated spectrometers, new interest is rising in all of the UV-visible absorption techniques that normally require substantial instrument control and data manipulation. These include simultaneous multicomponent analysis, reaction rate determinations and dual-wavelength derivatives. Also, there is a significant increase in the use of *Difference Spectrometry* as a means for increasing sensitivity, improving detection limits, and decreasing noise as compared to conventional absorption spectrometry.

Other new high-sensitivity spectrometric techniques have recently gained wide attention, especially in trace analysis application and determination of solvent spectra.

These new techniques include:

1. Laser-absorption intracavity techniques based on the dye-laser oscillating mechanism, which is capable of measuring absorbances in the 5×10^{-6} range and is more suitable for aqueous systems.
2. Wavelength modulation (peak-sensing method) suitable for measuring two different samples simultaneously as well as double derivation of reflectivity, with a sensitivity of up to 1 $\times 10^{-7}$ g.
3. Colorimetric methods for the measurement of energy absorbed by the solution utilizing laser sources. These methods have a range of detection between 1×10^{-7}–8×10^{-8} g and they include thermocouple colorimetry, photoacoustic colorimetry and thermal lens techniques. Both photoacoustic and thermal lens methods suffer great loss of sensitivity in aqueous media.
4. Photon counting and diode array detectors.

Near Infrared Spectrometry (NIR)

NIR, or the overtone region, comprises the spectral region from 800 nm to 2.5 μm. It is concerned with low energy electronic transitions in molecular species that are associated with stretching and bending vibrations of mostly hydrogenic groups, eg, CH, NH, OH. Discussion of these different modes of vibration and the underlying theory are presented later under Infrared Spectrometry. Actually, the NIR technique is midway between the UV visible and Infrared where it enjoys the excellent quantitative abilities of the former and the wide qualitative properties of the latter. Table 34-1 lists the absorption bands of the hydrogenic groups common to various organic compounds. The spectrum of cyclohexane may be seen in Fig 34-11. NIR also has important applications in organic chemistry where it has been used in the study of metal

complexes and rare earth and transition metal compounds. It is widely used in the determination of water content in different materials utilizing the —OH overtones bands at 1400–1500 nm and combination bands at 2000 nm. Other studies include water-protein binding and interaction, determination of water in pharmaceutical formulations and crystal structural studies of hemo proteins. Most NIR instruments are UV-visible spectrometers with an extended long wavelength range. Solid state lead sulfide detectors are commonly used for photodetection. The light source is usually the tungsten-halogen lamp generally utilized for the visible region. The technique for analysis and sample handling is similar to the UV-visible region, where sample cells (0.1–10 cm pathlength) can be used. Carbon tetrachloride is commonly the solvent of choice in NIR; however, water is useful for measurements below 1400 nm. A recent introduction of instrumentation in this field is the Varian Model 2300 UV-VIS-NIR spectrometer and the Perkin-Elmer PE 330 which offers the NIR capability together with such features as touch key-selection of analytical parameters, eg, wavelength, scanning and attenuation, microprocessor-controlled operation, CRT display of results and optimal minitape cassette memory for method storage. Dedicated NIR instruments such as the Technicon Infranalyzer are currently available. This will significantly help the acceleration of research in this long-neglected spectral region.

Infrared Spectrometry (IR)

The range of EM radiation between 0.8 μm to 500 μm is referred to as infrared (IR) radiation. Development of a commercial IR instrument did not begin until the late 1940s. At present the IR spectrometer is one of the instruments most frequently employed in the characterization of organic molecules. Unlike the UV-visible spectral plots, the IR spectrum is usually represented with percent transmittance rather than

Table I—Near Infrared Bands

Hydrogenic Group	Absorption Wavelength (nm)
—CH$_3$	900, 1150, 1700, 2300
=CH$_2$	850, 1120, 1640, 2200
≡CH	1550, 3050
—CH (aromatic)	850, 1300, 1700, 2450
—CH (aldehyde)	970, 2080
—NH$_2$	1020, 1500, 2000, 2900
=NH	1020, 1550, 3010
—OH (alcohol)	920, 1420, 2050, 2750
—OH (acid)	980, 1430, 2120, 2830
—OH (peracid)	2950
—OH (water)	1400, 1900, 2680
—FH	2620
—SH	2000

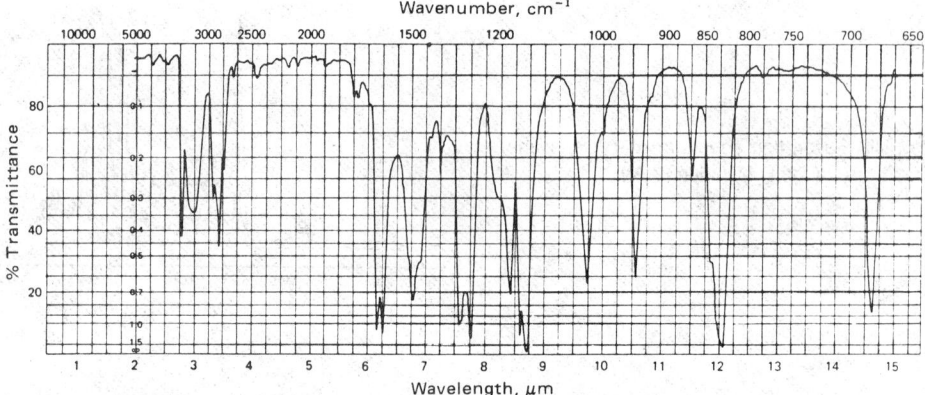

Fig 34-12.   Infrared absorption spectrum of 3,5-dimethylphenol.   (Reproduced from Skoog, DA and West, DM, *Principles of Instrumental Analysis*, Holt, Rinehart and Winston 1971).

absorbance as the ordinate.   Also, it is customary to use the unit of reciprocal centimeter (cm^{-1}) or the wave number for the abscissa rather than the wavelength.   This is because of the direct proportionality between the wave number and the energy as well as the frequency of the radiation; the frequency can, in turn, be directly related to molecular vibrational frequencies.   An example of an IR spectrum is shown in Fig 34-12.   The most commonly used region of the IR spectrum in pharmaceutical chemistry is the region between 2.5 μm (4000 cm^{-1}) to 16 μm (625 cm^{-1}).

Near Infrared (NIR) or the overtone region refers to the region from 780 nm (12,500 cm^{-1}) to 2.5 μm (4000 cm^{-1}); the Far Infrared (FIR) or the rotational region is between 400 and 20 cm^{-1}.

Theory—In order for IR radiation to be absorbed by a molecule, two criteria must be met: (1) the molecule should possess a vibrational or rotational frequency identical to that of the impinging EM radiation, and (2) a net change in the magnitude or direction of the dipole moment should occur as a result of radiation-molecule interaction.   When IR radiation impinges upon a molecule at the proper frequency, the vibration and/or rotation of the molecule is altered.   If the frequency of the impinging EM radiation matches a natural vibrational frequence of the molecule, a net transfer of energy occurs that creates a greater amplitude of vibration and, as a result, absorption of radiation occurs.

The longest wavelength (lowest energy) of IR radiation that induces a change in the vibratory motion of a molecule gives rise to an absorption band known as the *fundamental band*. There is only one fundamental band in a diatomic molecule, although multiples of the band frequency (ν), known as overtones, can occur as 2ν, 3ν, etc.

Rotation of unsymmetric molecules around their centers of mass results in a periodic dipole change which interacts with the incident EM radiation causing a higher frequency of the molecular rotation and absorption of radiation occurs.   The energy required to cause a change in rotational levels only is very small (<100 cm^{-1}) and comprises the Far IR region. Absorption by gases in this region appears as discrete, well defined lines.   However, because of the intramolecular collisions and interactions in liquids and solids, broadening of the absorption lines occurs and usually appears as a continuum. The Far IR region which is experimentally difficult to study has little application in pharmaceutical chemistry and will not be discussed further.

Since absorption of IR radiation alters both vibrational and rotational characteristics of a molecule, absorption bands are not defined lines but are bands which are centered upon one frequency.   Since the total kinetic energy is a combination of translational, rotational, and vibrational energies of a molecule

(ie, $E_t = E_{tr} + E_r + E_v$), a polyatomic molecule consisting of n atoms will have 3n degrees of freedom of motion.   The possible fundamental vibrational modes of a molecule can be calculated by subtracting 3 for translational energy and 3 for rotational energy (2, if the molecule is linear).   This gives a total of 3n-6 possible vibrational modes.   The theoretical number of fundamental absorption bands, however, is not observed due to such factors as weak absorptivity, coalescence of several closely located bands, and lack of required change in dipole moment.   Since the 2–16 μm region normally employed for IR investigation covers both fundamental and *overtone* regions, the total number of absorption bands in an IR spectrum may greatly exceed the theoretical number.

The atomic stretching vibration can be approximated mechanically by Hooke's law, $F = -kx$, where F is the restoring force, k is the proportionality or the force constant (dyne/cm) and x is the displacement distance.   For a diatomic molecule with atoms of masses m_1 and m_2, the frequency of fundamental vibration is expressed by;

$$\nu = \frac{1}{2\pi} \sqrt{\frac{k}{\mu}} \qquad (6)$$

or in terms of wave number by;

$$\bar{\nu} = \frac{1}{2\pi c} \sqrt{\frac{k}{\mu}} \qquad (7)$$

where μ is known as the reduced mass, defined by;

$$\mu = \frac{m_1 m_2}{m_1 + m_2} \qquad (8)$$

Application of the equation for the C—H stretching frequency with $k = 5 \times 10^5$ dynes/cm, $m_1 = 19.8 \times 10^{-24}$ g, and $m_2 = 1.64 \times 10^{-24}$ g gives the value 3040 cm^{-1} (slightly higher than the observed value, 2950 cm^{-1}, which is caused by neglect of the environmental effect).   The vibrational modes of a CH_2 group are depicted in Fig 34-13.   It should be observed that more energy is required for the stretching vibration than for the bending vibration.

The position of the absorption bands is determined by the symmetry of a molecule, the masses of atoms, the force constants of the chemical bonds, and the interaction of vibrations (Fermi interactions).   Hydrogen bonding affects the position of the bands by shifting the frequency of the stretching vibration to a lower frequency and that of the bending vibration to a higher frequency.

Characterization of Molecules—There are two major applications of IR spectrometry in the characterization of various molecules: (1) determination of the identity of a compound by means of spectral comparison with that of an authentic sample and (2) verification of the presence of

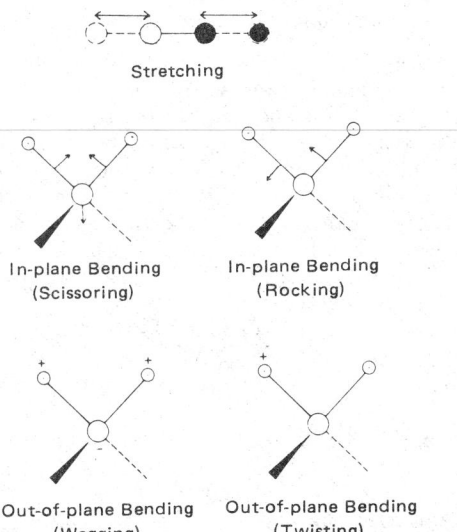

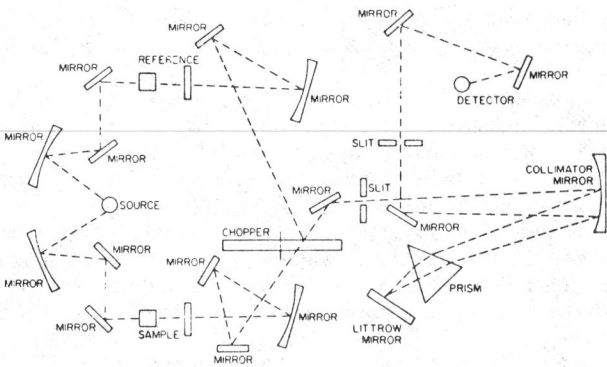

Fig 34-14. The optical system of a classical IR spectrometer. (Newer instruments use gratings instead of prisms).

Fig 34-13. Types of molecular vibrations. + indicates motion from plane of page toward reader, − indicates motion from plane of page away from reader. (Reproduced from Skoog and West).

functional groups in an unknown molecule. The latter aspect is quite important in the structural elucidation of synthetic organic compounds or substances isolated from natural sources.

The position of the absorption bands due to stretching and in-plane bending vibrations of the functional groups such as C=O, C—H, N—H, O—H, etc, are somewhat independent of the influence of the neighboring groups in the molecule. These bands usually occur at 4000–1300 cm⁻¹. The position of the bands below 1300 cm⁻¹ is markedly influenced by neighboring groups in the molecule. The portion of the spectrum from 1300–400 cm⁻¹ is referred to as the "fingerprint" region.

Extensive charts and tables of the characteristic group absorption frequencies for common organic functional groups can be found in many of the texts listed in the *Bibliography*. Several catalogs of reference spectra have been published, the most voluminous of which is that of the Sadtler Research Laboratories, currently in excess of 70,000 spectra. Only a brief treatment of structure–absorption frequency correlation can be given here.

C—H stretching and bending vibrations occur at 3300–2800 cm⁻¹. Each particular type of hydrocarbon has its own characteristic band position, eg, saturated acyclic and cyclic hydrocarbons have stretching $\bar{v}$ at 2960–2850 cm⁻¹ and in-plane bending $\bar{v}$ at 1470–1360 cm⁻¹, unsaturated olefinic C—H stretching at 3090–3000 cm⁻¹ and unsaturated acetylenic C—H stretching $\bar{v}$ at 3300–3270 cm⁻¹, aromatic C—H stretching $\bar{v}$ at 3100–3000 cm⁻¹, and the out-of-plane bending is at 900–650 cm⁻¹. The most characteristic band for aromatic compounds, however, is at 1610–1590 cm⁻¹ (due to aromatic skeletal vibration).

O—H Vibration—Stretching at 3700–3350 cm⁻¹, depending on the extent of hydrogen bonding.

C—O Vibration—Stretching at 1280–1000 cm⁻¹, depending on whether it is an alcohol, phenol, ester, ether, etc.

C=O Vibration—Stretching at 1950–1640 cm⁻¹. These bands are quite intense and very conspicuous. Hydrogen bondings, field effect and conjugation affect the position.

N—H Vibration—Stretching at 3500–3300 cm⁻¹, hydrogen bonding at lower frequency. Bands for N⁺H₃, N⁺H₂ and N⁺H occur at about 3200, 2700 and 2000 cm⁻¹, respectively.

C—N Vibration—Stretching of aliphatic compounds at 1210 cm⁻¹ and for aromatic at 1250–1350 cm⁻¹. For C≡N,

a band occurs at 1680–1640 cm⁻¹ and for C≡N at 2250 cm⁻¹.

Quantitative IR—Although IR spectrometry is generally employed for qualitative identification, rather limited use of its quantitative aspects is being made. Because of the uniqueness of its spectra, quantitative methods may not require prior separation of the analyte from excipients. The Beer's law, as discussed under UV-Visible spectrometry is also applicable to IR spectrometry. The sensitivity of IR analysis, however, is poor, only 0.01 to 0.001 of the sensitivity of UV, and therefore it has only a few applications in quantitative analysis.

Instrumentation—A brief description of the major components of an IR spectrometer is given below, and an IR instrument is illustrated in Fig 34-14.

Radiation Source—Generally, IR radiation is obtained by electrically heating a Nernst glower (a mixture of oxides of zirconium, yttrium, and thorium) or a globar unit (a small rod of silicon carbide).

Monochromator—The most commonly used prism materials for dispersion of IR radiation are:
1. NaCl with a refractive index of 1.5442. This provides good dispersion at 2000–650 cm⁻¹, but poor dispersion beyond 2000 cm⁻¹.
2. KBr, with a refractive index of 1.53, disperses at 1600–370 cm⁻¹.
3. CsBr, with a refractive index of 1.69, disperses at 1000–250 cm⁻¹.

In recent years grating systems have been employed more widely than the prism, primarily because of their high resolving power.

Detector—The thermocouple and bolometer are two types of detectors which are used in IR spectrometry, the former being employed to a greater extent. A bolometer is comprised of a resistance element in a bridge circuit. A change in the resistance upon heating causes an unbalance signal which can be amplified and recorded.

As seen in Fig 34-14, the source beam is reflected by mirrors to form the sample and reference beam. After passing through the sample and reference, the beams are chopped by a mirror which serves to focus each beam alternately onto the entrance slit of the monochromator. If the sample absorbs part of the radiation, the intensity of the two beams will be unequal. This inequality results in the development of an out of balance signal in the detector. After amplification and rectification, the signal is relayed to a comb or wedge to drive the reference beam attenuator to reduce the intensity of the reference beam. As the difference between the two beams becomes zero, the out of balance signal also becomes zero. The pen of a recorder, which is connected to the attenuator, will perform the function of plotting the absorption coordinates on a paper chart. The speed of the chart is a function of frequency, and the resulting tracing of % transmission vs frequency is known as an IR spectrum.

Preparation of the Sample—Samples for IR determination can be prepared in the form of a gas, liquid, or solid. Liquid samples are prepared "neat" (pure form) or in solution using a liquid cell. Carbon tetrachloride and carbon disulfide are two commonly used solvents. With solutions, the solvent alone should be placed in the path of the reference beam in order to cancel absorption due to the solvent. This method is particularly useful in the study of various types of hydrogen bonding.

Solid samples are prepared either as a KBr disc or in the form of a dispersion in mineral oil. A KBr disc of a sample is prepared by grinding the sample with KBr powder, placing the mixture between a punch and die, and applying a pressure of about 50,000 psi.

A mineral oil dispersion of a sample is usually placed between two sodium chloride windows. This method possesses an inherent disadvantage in that the C—H absorption bands in the sample will be masked by those of the oil.

Fourier Transform Infrared Spectrometry (FT-IR)

The wide availability of high powered microcomputers at reasonable cost has helped popularize the applications of transform spectroscopy in general and Fourier transform in particular to several branches of spectrometry. These include IR, NMR, and MS. FT-IR, however, has been one of the first techniques developed and today is the instrumentation of preference over dispersive IR for handling ever smaller and more complex samples. Superior sensitivity and resolution, absolute wavelength accuracy and higher precision of measurements are some of the reasons behind the rapid growth of FT-IR.

Basically, the technique is a coupling of a Michelson interferometer with a sensitive infrared detector. However, because of the enormous amount of data generated, a microcomputer is essential for data handling. In Michelson's interferometer, there is no monochromator and radiation of many frequencies passes through the sample. The source radiation is split between a fixed mirror and a movable one. The two reflected beams are then combined either constructively or destructively at the beam splitter, depending on the position of the movable mirror. As the path difference between the two beams is altered and because only the nonabsorbed frequencies reach the detector, the signal pattern becomes the sample interferogram. For monochromatic radiation, the amplitude of the signal is a cosine function of the mirror position. For polychromatic radiation, the signal is a summation of all the constructive reinforcement or destructive interferences of each wavelength interacting with every other wavelength and results in a unique interferogram for each particular sample. In order to handle the complex mathematical treatment needed for calculations, it was found that the cosine Fourier transform can relate the intensity of the interferogram as a function of the mirror travel, $I(x)$ (Eq 9) and the intensity of the frequency $I(\nu)$ (Eq 10) of the IR radiation;

$$I(x) = \int_{-\infty}^{\infty} I(\nu) \cos(2\pi\nu x)\, d\nu \qquad (9)$$

and after calculating (using a computer) the inverse transforms;

$$I(\nu) = \int_{-\infty}^{\infty} I(x) \cos(2\pi\nu x)\, dx \qquad (10)$$

by which the interferogram could be related back to the IR spectrum.

Modern FT-IR spectrometers such as Nicolet FT-IR, MX or DX systems and Perkin-Elmer FT-IR model 1500 provide full spectra that can be monitored continuously on a CRT screen while scanning. Standard software packages include spectral subtraction, baseline correction, integration, peak picking, multicomponent and factor analysis, quantitative analysis and spectral library searching. The use of a new mercury cadmium telluride (MCT) detector and diffuse reflectance accessory are recent features that enhances the instrument's sensitivity.

Advantages and Limitations of FT-IR

The speed and high sensitivity of FT-IR, which makes it ideal for microanalysis, arise from two factors. First the utilization of what is known as the multiplex or the Fellgett advantage where a very high signal-to-noise ratio exists due to the fact that the sample and, hence, the detector is affected by all frequencies at one time. Secondly the fact that the radiation power throughput of the interferometer is significantly larger than for the dispersive instrument (about 40 times). These advantages of FT-IR make it the technique of choice for coupling the qualitative power of IR to such separation techniques, as gas and liquid chromatography (GC-FT-IR & LC-FT-IR). The limitation of FT-IR however, lies in its high cost.

Nuclear Magnetic Resonance Spectrometry (NMR)

In 1921, AH Compton suggested that an electron can possess an intrinsic angular momentum or "spin" and thus act as a tiny magnet. In 1925, Wolfgang Pauli suggested that similarly, the nuclei of certain atoms could also have the property of spinning or rotating around their axis. The spinning of these charged particles, ie the circulation of charge, generates a magnetic moment along the axis of spin, or creates a nuclear dipole, so that these nuclei act like tiny bar magnets. As a consequence, when these nuclei are exposed to an external magnetic field, their energies are split into two or more quantized levels. The reason, according to quantum mechanics, is that the spinning, charged particles must align themselves either *with* the external magnetic field (more stable, lower energy level, ground state) or *against* it (less stable, higher energy level, excited state). Transitions among the different energy levels can only be brought about if EM radiation of the current frequency is absorbed and the tiny bar magnet is "flipped" to the less stable excited state (alignment against the field).

The experimental verification of these theoretical concepts, however, was not an easy task. It took about 21 years until two scientists, Block from Stanford and Purcell from Harvard, working independently, were able to demonstrate the absorption of radiation in the radio frequency portion of the EM spectrum as a consequence of energy level transitions by nuclei exposed to a strong external magnetic field. The radio frequency radiation ranges from 0.1–100 MHz or 3000–3m wavelength.

Although NMR is a general term that can apply to any of several atoms, unless otherwise specified it usually refers to proton (or ^{1}H) NMR, a technique that grew to be most vital for structural elucidation of organic molecules. Most of the discussion in this chapter will relate to proton magnetic resonance, since it is the most commonly used version.

Theory—As discussed above, the angular momentum of the spinning charge is expressed by a spin quantum number, I (in units of $h/2\pi$, where h is Planck's constant). The I value for isotopes may vary by integral values 1, 2, 3, . . . , or half-integral values $\frac{1}{2}, \frac{3}{2}, . . . \frac{9}{2}$. An I value equal to zero indicates no spin. The spin number of isotopes can be determined by observing the following rules:

1. Nuclei with an even number of protons and neutrons have a spin number of zero, or no spin (eg, ^{4}He, ^{12}C, ^{16}O).
2. Nuclei with an odd number of protons and neutrons have an integral spin of 1, 2, 3, . . . (eg, ^{2}H, ^{14}N, ^{10}B).
3. Nuclei with an odd mass number have a half-integral spin of $\frac{1}{2}, \frac{3}{2}$, . . . $\frac{9}{2}$; either an odd number of protons and even number of neutrons (eg, ^{1}H, ^{19}F, ^{31}P) or an even number of protons and odd number of neutrons (eg, ^{13}C).

The nuclei of an isotope ($I > 0$) placed in a magnetic field will assume a number of orientations equal to $(2I + 1)$. Since I for the proton is $\frac{1}{2}$, there will exist 2 orientations or spin

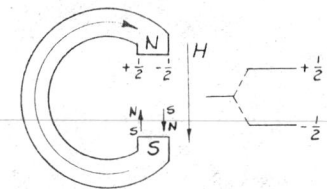

Fig 34-15.   Orientation of nuclear magnets in an external magnetic field.

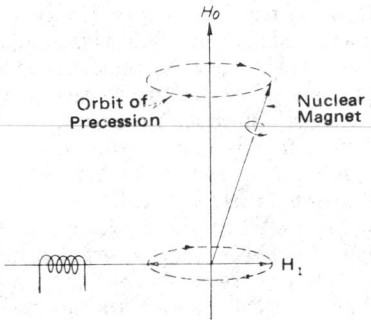

Fig 34-16.   The spinning and precessing of a nuclear magnet in an external magnetic field.

states: (1) a low-energy state, wherein the nuclei are in alignment with the external magnetic field (parallel orientation, N pole of nucleus near S pole of magnet) and (2) a high-energy state, wherein the nuclei are in alignment against the external magnetic field (antiparallel orientation, S pole near S pole) (see Fig 34-15). The separation of the energy levels is a function of the nuclear magnetic moment, μ, and the external magnetic field strength, H_0, and inversely proportional to the spin quantum number, I, according to the formula;

$$E = \frac{\mu H_0}{I} \tag{11}$$

As shown in Fig 34-16, the spin axis of the nucleus precesses about the axis parallel to the field direction. If H_0 is increased, the precessional frequency of the nucleus increases proportionally. The angular velocity, ω_0, of the precessing nucleus is expressed as;

$$\omega_0 = \gamma H_0 \tag{12}$$

where γ is the magnetogyric ratio (a nuclear constant). The flipping from one energy state to another can occur by absorption or transmission of radiation according to the formula;

$$\nu = \frac{\gamma H_0}{2\pi} \tag{13}$$

where ν is the radio frequency (rf), corresponding to the precessional frequency of the nucleus, which causes nuclear transition from a low-energy to a high-energy state. Restated, if the rotating magnetic vector of rf equal to ω_0 is introduced perpendicular to H_0, the system will be attuned; ie, the frequency of the precessing nucleus and inserted frequency will be in resonance.

Combining Eqs 12 and 13 gives;

$$\omega_0 = 2\pi\nu \tag{14}$$

If H_0 is 14,092 gauss, an external frequency of 60 mHz (a weak magnetic field H_1) is required to induce "flipping" of protons. The direction of the rotating magnetic field, H_1, is perpendicular to the direction of H_0. When resonance occurs, the nuclei flip over (revert to alternate energy states). This results in an induced voltage in a receiving coil placed at a right angle to both H_0 and H_1.

In practice the rf oscillator is maintained at a constant frequency and H_0 is swept over a narrow range (usually of the order of a few milligauss).

Population of nuclei in each energy level is given by;

$$N_{\text{upper}}/N_{\text{lower}} = e^{-\Delta E/kT} \tag{15}$$

where k is the Boltzmann constant (1.38×10^{-16} erg degree^{-1}). In the case of proton nuclear spin, $\Delta E = 5 \times 10^{-19}$ erg in a 15,000 gauss field at a temperature of $T = 300°$K, $N_{\text{upper}}/N_{\text{lower}} \approx e^{-5 \times 10^{-19}/4.2 \times 10^{-14}}$ or $1-1.2 \times 10^{-5}$ for such nuclei. It is this excess that is responsible for the observed absorption of radiation. Since the excess of nuclei is very slight, it is important that too large an amount of energy not be introduced into the system. If this occurs, all of the excess nuclei are in the excited state and the intensity of the absorption

signal may decrease or even vanish. This is the phenomenon of saturation, a situation to be avoided if the quantitative nature of energy absorption by nuclei is to be preserved. Therefore, the required condition for nuclear resonance is the maintenance of excess nuclei in the lower energy level. This is accomplished by a process known as relaxation, mechanisms by which a nucleus returns from the higher to the lower energy state.

Two types of relaxations are operative: spin–spin relaxation and spin–lattice relaxation. Spin–spin (transverse) relaxation involves the mutual exchange of energy between two proximal precessing nuclei. This type of relaxation does not contribute to the maintenance of an excess lower state spin population, but it decreases the lifetime of the excited state nucleus, which affects spectral linewidth.

Spin–lattice (longitudinal) relaxation involves a transfer of the nuclear energy, as a result of transition to a lower state, to the energy of the lattice components. The term lattice refers to the framework of molecules in a system in any physical state. Translational, rotational, and vibrational energies of the molecules are the components of a lattice. Owing to the magnetic properties of these various types of energies, the lattice contains a variety of magnetic fields whose proper alignment with a precessing nucleus can cause transition to a lower state. The energy thus released increases the translational, vibrational, and rotational energies. There is no net change of energy in the system. This process is responsible for maintaining the small excess nuclei in the lower energy level.

Both spin–spin and spin–lattice relaxations are responsible for spectral line width. The line width is inversely proportional to the lifetime of nuclei in the excited state. In solids or viscous liquids, restriction of molecular motion does not allow frequent occurrence of proper magnetic orientation, resulting in a long spin–lattice relaxation time. This condition, however, creates a proper orientation of nuclei so that the mutual exchange of energy becomes quite facile, thus shortening spin–spin relaxation time, which in turn results in the broadening of the spectral line.

Interpretation of Spectra—The value of NMR spectra in qualitative determinations arises from the nature of the proton resonances. Depending on the nature of the immediate molecular environment, protons will resonate at characteristic frequencies, allowing protons in different environments to be differentiated. The interaction of protons gives rise to the phenomenon of splitting, a behavior that makes an NMR spectrum complex. In order to be able to interpret such a spectrum correctly, it is essential to understand the following terms which are unique to NMR.

Shielding Effect—The frequence of resonance in an NMR spectrum depends on the magnetic environment of the protons in a molecule. This concept can be elaborated by considering the phenomenon that, when placed in an external magnetic field, electrons in an atom or molecule will circulate.

The circulating electrons create a new magnetic field which opposes the external magnetic field, thus reducing its effect on the nucleus. This is known as the shielding effect, and its magnitude is determined by the density of the electrons around the nucleus. Since the electron density around each proton is a function of its environment, protons surrounded by different substituent groups will experience an unequal effect of the external magnetic field.

Chemical Shift—When the frequency of the rotating magnetic field, H_1, whose plane is perpendicular to H_0, becomes equal to the precessional frequency of the nucleus, energy will be absorbed and nuclear transitions will occur and an NMR spectrum is obtained. Therefore, the NMR spectrum is a plot of resonant absorption frequencies (or magnetic field strength) vs an arbitrary intensity scale. The area under each peak (when properly evaluated, as will be discussed later) is proportional to the number of protons in the environment producing such a peak or combination of peaks. Tetramethylsilane (TMS) is used as a reference standard since all of the protons are equivalent; thus, only one resonant peak is observed and it occurs at a point farther "up-field" from most other proton resonances. All other proton resonances are referred to TMS (arbitrarily assigned a value of zero) and are measured from the TMS value using a concept known as a *chemical shift* (distance from the TMS value, measured in ppm—see below). Since the chemical shift is a function of the magnetic field strength, its value will vary if instruments with different rf magnetic fields are employed for measurement (eg, 60, 100, and 400 mHz). To make the chemical shift expression independent of field strength, a chemical shift symbol, δ, in dimensionless units of parts per million (ppm) is used;

$$\delta = H_S - H_{TMS}/H_1 \times 10^6 \qquad (16)$$

where H_S and H_{TMS} are the field strengths (in Hz) corresponding to resonance for the sample and reference, respectively. H_1 is the frequency of the rf signal used. The designation τ (where $\tau = 10 - \delta$) is also used to designate chemical shift.

It should be emphasized at this point that although the electronegativities of atoms proximal to protons are a contributory factor in determining chemical shift values, the position of the resonance peak is influenced also by several other structural features. A classic example is the peak for acetylinic protons at 2.35 ppm which is more shielded than the olefinic proton at 4.60 ppm. This apparent anomaly can be explained by considering the *diamagnetic anisotropy* effect; ie, the orientation of the chemical bond in a magnetic field. In Fig 34-17A, the lines of force, induced by circulating π electrons of the acetylenic C≡C bond, shield the proton. In contrast, the induced magnetic field deshields an aldehyde proton (Fig 34-17B).

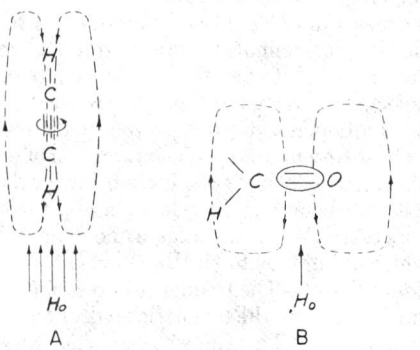

Fig 34-17.   **The electron-induced magnetic lines of force.**   *A:* Shielded acetylenic proton; *B:* deshielded aldehyde proton.

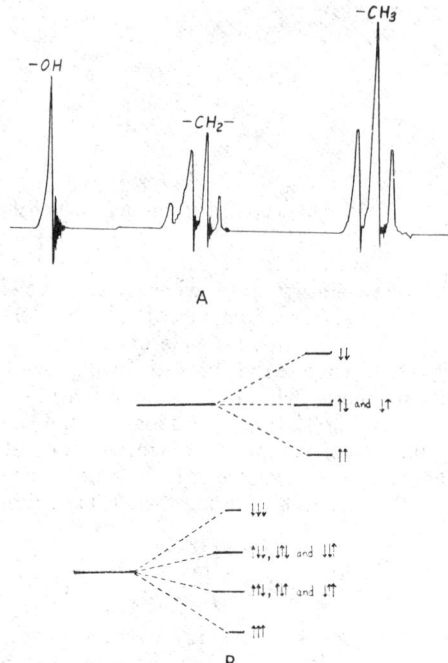

Fig 34-18.   *A:* A high-resolution NMR spectrum of ethanol; *B:* spin–spin splitting presentation of proximal CH_3 and CH_2.

Spin–Spin Coupling—Fig 34-18A depicts the NMR spectrum of ethanol as determined by a high resolution instrument. Instead of observing three distinct peaks indicative of the methyl (CH_3—), methylene (—CH_2—), and hydroxyl (—OH) protons, with peak areas in the relation 3:2:1, several peaks are noted in each area. Each peak representative of certain types of protons has been *split* by coupling with adjacent protons. The concept of spin–spin coupling can be visualized by considering the effect of one proton on a neighboring proton connected by not more than three bonds (conjugated systems excepted). The splitting occurs because of the tendency of the electron to pair its spin with that of the nearest proton. For a simple explanation of spin–spin splitting, consider a molecule with nonequivalent protons, H_1 and H_2, in a magnetic field. If the nucleus H_1 is in an antiparallel position, the field experienced by H_2 becomes augmented, corresponding to a higher precessional frequency. The resonance line for H_2 occurs at a lower field if H_1 is absent. An opposite effect is observed if the nucleus H_1 has the parallel position. A similar effect is exerted on H_1 by H_2. The combination of these effects thus gives rise to two doublets.

Fig 34-18B illustrates the probable nuclear arrangement of the —CH_2— and —CH_3 groups of ethanol. The multiplicity caused by the effect of one group on a neighboring group is given by the formula $2nI + 1$, where n is the number of equivalent nuclei of spin I. In the case of protons with $I = \frac{1}{2}$, the formula can simply be written as $n + 1$. In Fig 34-18A the CH_2 group in ethanol consists of four peaks with intensities of 1:3:3:1; the CH_3 group has three peaks with intensities of 1:2:1. The ratio of the total area of CH_2 to that of CH_3 is 2:3.

The distance between multiplets is referred to as the coupling constant, J, expressed in Hz and the letter J is subscripted (eg, J_{AB}-see below) to denote the protons or atoms involved in coupling. For protons, the J value rarely exceeds 20 Hz. The separation of two resonance lines, $\Delta\nu$, is expressed in Hz. Unlike chemical shift, the J value is independent of the strength of the applied magnetic field, H_0, and its magnitude is a function of the extent of coupling between two nuclei. Chemically equivalent protons also undergo spin–spin coupling but the transitions are forbidden and not observed.

Qualitative Measurement of NMR Spectra—The use of NMR for qualitative analysis involves several properties of the spectrum. First, the chemical shift establishes the general nature of the proton. Then the multiplicity of the proton resonance indicates the nature of the proton environment and the interaction of protons. For the simplest cases, the first-order spectra follow idealized rules and may be interpreted directly. More complex spectra may prove to be too complex for noncomputer assisted interpretation, and in these cases qualitative analysis may be established by use of reference standard materials. The magnitude of the resonance intensity of a proton singlet or multiplet is directly proportional to the number of protons. Thus, if the area of the singlets or multiplets in a spectrum is integrated, it is possible to assign relative values to the areas and determine the number of protons that a particular multiplet represents. This information simplifies interpretation of spectra and the identification of compounds.

Instrumentation—The NMR spectrometers available commercially are of either the continuous wave (CW) or Fourier transform (FT) type and vary as to magnetic field strength and, accordingly, the resonance frequency imposed by the radio frequency oscillator. The FT instrument systems that permit signal enhancement are particularly useful when weak resonance signals are encountered, as in the case of ^{13}C, an isotope present in nature only to the extent of 1.11%, or in those cases when very dilute samples of strongly absorbing nuclei are studied.

The available spectrometers have different radio frequency oscillators, eg, 60 MHz, 100 MHz, 200 MHz or 400 MHz. This variation makes it convenient to express field strength in a manner independent of oscillator frequency. Fig 34-19 depicts a 60-mHz NMR CW instrument, consisting of the following major parts:

Magnet—Either a permanent magnet or electromagnet can be employed in NMR to supply H_0. Currently, superconducting magnets cooled in liquid helium are being used in instruments with high magnetic fields. Since chemical shift is a function of magnetic field strength, greater dispersion is achieved at a higher magnetic field strength. In practice, the field is varied over a very small range (about a few milligauss) with the aid of a sweep coil. If a sawtooth voltage is employed to change the field of the large magnet and the same sawtooth is used as an x axis driving voltage, the signal can be observed on a recorder or an oscilloscope.

Radiofrequency Oscillator (Transmitter)—This rf field is provided by a transmitter coil whose magnetic vector component moves in a plane perpendicular to the direction of H_0. The field induces nuclear transitions when its frequency equals ω_0.

Radiofrequency Receiver (Detector)—The flipping of nuclei as a result of rf insertion induces a voltage in the receiving coil, whose axis is at a right angle to the axis of the transmitter coil and H_0.

Oscilloscope and Recorder (Display Device)—The voltage from the receiving coil is amplified and observed in an oscilloscope or a recorder. The peaks of an NMR spectrum are the result of plotting intensity vs frequency of resonance (field strength).

Preparation of the Sample—A sample for NMR spectral determination should be dissolved in a solvent devoid of protons or in which the protons have been replaced by deuterium, such as: CCl_4, $CDCl_3$, D_2O, $SO(CD_3)_2$, $CO(CD_3)_2$, CF_3COOD, etc. The choice of solvent depends on the nature of the substance and obviously, the solute and solvent must not interact.

Usually, 30–70 mg of the compound under investigation is dissolved in about 0.2 mL of the solvent in an NMR tube. A small amount of TMS is added for reference. Due to the insolubility of TMS in some solvents, such as water, an external TMS standard is often used. This is done either by placing a sealed TMS-containing capillary tube inside the NMR tube or by marking the reference point, just prior to determining the spectrum of a sample, with a TMS solution in CCl_4 or $CDCl_3$.

Spin-Spin Decoupling

Spin-Spin Decoupling (double irradiation or double resonance) is a useful technique for simplifying NMR spectra in order to find the relative positions of protons in a molecule or for locating a masked absorption. All protons can be decoupled as long as they are more than 20 Hz apart at 100 MHz. In spin-spin decoupling, the nucleus is essentially irradiated with a strong radio frequency signal at its resonance frequency, while scanning other nuclei to detect which ones are affected by decoupling from the irradiated nucleus. Decoupling has been usually applied to ^{14}N, ^{31}P, or ^{19}F because of the large difference from proton resonance. Internuclear double resonance (INDOR) is another technique which is used to examine coupling between two nuclei of very different relative sensitivities such as ^1H and ^{15}N.

Shift Reagents—These are ions in the rare earth (Lanthanide) series coordinated to organic ligands such as tris-(6,6,7,7,8,8,8-heptafluoro-2, 2-dimethyl-3, 5-octanedionato)-europium, Eu(fod)$_3$. The addition of these reagents helps to spread out the NMR absorption patterns without increasing the strength of the applied magnetic field. This occurs due to a significant magnification of the chemical shift differences of nonequivalent protons.

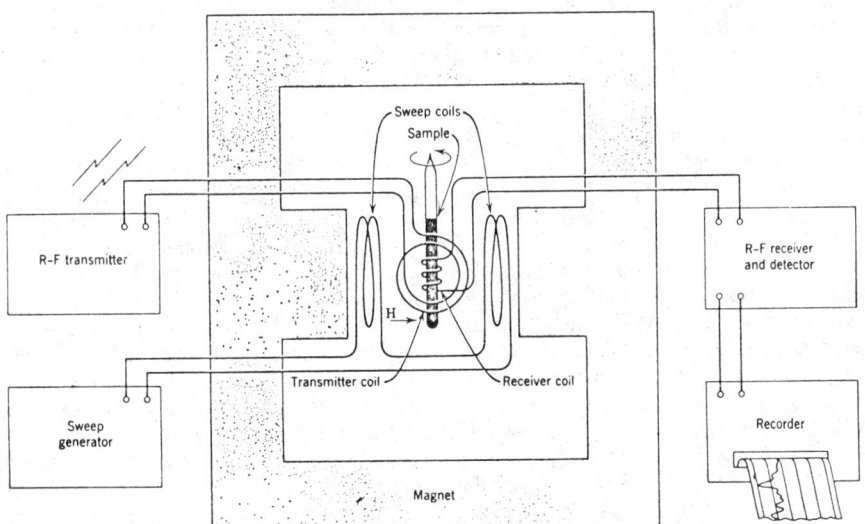

Fig 34-19.   A basic NMR instrument (courtesy, Varian).

Quantitative Applications of NMR—The ability to integrate areas under the resonance peaks in NMR spectra has quantitative applications. Two methods can be employed for quantitative measurements. First is the relative method where the integral areas from two different proton types within the same molecule are compared. The second method is the absolute method where a known quantity of an organic compound is in the same solution with a known quantity of internal standard. An internal standard is a pure organic compound with a structure such that the integral for the area of the resonance peak(s) of a single kind of proton may be used as an absolute measure of the protons. The integral area for one kind of analyte protons may be compared with the integral area for the internal standard protons and quantitative analysis accomplished.

Several factors must be considered when selecting a particular resonance peak or cluster of resonance peaks for quantitative measurement. First, the analytical moiety that gives rise to the resonance peak(s) should be stable under analytical conditions. Second, the strongest resonance peak or multiplet should be chosen to obtain the most sensitive measurement. Third, the internal standard should be a compound that possesses a strong resonance signal, preferably a singlet, in the proximity of the peak of interest.

Some of the limitations of quantitative NMR are the cost of the instrument and, in the case of CW instruments, lack of sensitivity. Also, complexity of the sample may give rise to peak overlap. Another major problem arises from the very small excess nuclei in the lower energy state which can lead to the saturation problem. However, by controlling the relaxation time for the species, the power of the source and the scanning rate, this problem can be minimized. The characterization of chemical or biological samples by multidimensional data followed by appropriate data analysis provides a means for the quantitative classification of new samples.

Isotopes NMR—As discussed under the theory section, several other isotopes possess magnetic moments and, thus, can be studied by the magnetic resonance technique. The most important nuclei studied so far are the following.

^{13}C NMR—This is the most exceedingly interesting nucleus for which an increasing amount of work has been reported recently. [13]C has a nuclear spin of $\frac{1}{2}$ which can usually be studied at a frequency of 10.705 MHz at a field of 10 kilogauss. However, due to the very low natural abundance of this isotope (1.1% compared to ^{12}C), its resonance has only 1.6% the sensitivity of ^{1}H NMR. Another difficulty with ^{13}C NMR is that its relaxation time is significantly longer than [1]H. Because of these problems, ^{13}C requires relatively larger samples and sophisticated instrumentation where pulsed FT-NMR could be applied and computer analysis is used for data manipulation and spectra interpretation. It should be pointed out that the basic rules for interpretation of ^{13}C spectra are essentially similar to proton NMR since the spin number for ^{13}C is the same as for [1]H ($\frac{1}{2}$). However, the coupling constants for [13]C-^{1}H are large (100–250 Hz) and thus interpretation of the ^{13}C spectra is usually difficult because of the overlapping [13]C-^{1}H multiplets. Recent studies showed that the complicated ^{13}C spectra could be simplified by completely decoupling the ^{13}C nuclei from all the ^{1}H nuclei using a spin-spin decoupling technique (double resonance). Recently, the development of superconducting magnets, together with Fourier transform techniques and advanced computer technology has helped ^{13}C NMR to develop into one of the most important techniques in structure elucidation.

^{19}F NMR—Fluorine-19 has a spin quantum number of $\frac{1}{2}$ and its resonance frequency is about 56.5 MHz at 14,000 gauss (as compared with 60.0 MHz for ^{1}H). Therefore, ^{19}F can be investigated with a slightly modified proton NMR spectrometer. Although ^{19}F absorption was found to be also sensitive to its molecular environment, the structural correlations of the fluorine shift are few by comparison to proton NMR.

^{31}P NMR—Phosphorous-31, has a spin quantum number of $\frac{1}{2}$ and its resonance frequency at 14,000 gauss is 24.3 MHz. It exhibits sharp peaks with chemical shifts extending over a range of 700 ppm. Recently the use of ^{31}P NMR as a direct, noninvasive measurement of several kinetic studies in biological systems has opened a new and exciting field for this technique. Employing an Mg-ATP thermometer, measurements with small surface coils have been used to observe phosphorous metabolism of perfused hearts within localized regions in order to assess the altered regional metabolism resulting from myocardial infarction and response to drug treatment. Also ^{31}P NMR of free Mg-ion, Mg-ATP, and Mg-ADP in intact Ehrlich ascites tumor cells has been reported.

High Resolution NMR and its Analytical Applications—The development of new, pulse and multiple pulse NMR techniques has made the study of the NMR of low abundance and/or low sensitivity nuclei almost a conventional technique. Today, these high resolution NMR techniques constitute a major role in the study of molecular structure and conformation, kinetics and biochemical studies. The ubiquitous distribution of hydrogen in the human body and the nature of FT NMR techniques have made it possible to apply absorption of NMR radiation by hydrogen to the development of a non-invasive imaging technique for the human body. The technique is based on the fact that the detected EM signal is unique in intensity and duration to each type of tissue in the body. Through computerized data acquisition, the NMR signal is displayed as a vivid cross sectional images of the specific organ under study. The new technique avoids the harmful effects of the ionizing radiation caused by the current prevailing technique, Computerized Axial Tomography (CAT) scanning, as well as the pain and danger associated with the necessary injections of contrast agents. The technique, still in its infancy, has also proven to be a far superior and effective diagnostic tool. Recent reports have shown an accuracy of 100% in identifying multiple sclerosis lesions, as compared to the present success rate of 5–35% for the CAT scan. It can also reveal the damage from a stroke buried deep beneath the skull and differentiates between the gray and the white matter of the brain. The potential of the new technique is astounding as it promises to reveal not only the cellular structure of the body, but its *in vivo* chemistry as well.

Pulsed Fourier Transform NMR (Pulsed FT-NMR)—Since its introduction in the late nineteen sixties by Ernst and Anderson, Pulsed FT-NMR has been the major force behind the significant achievements in high resolution NMR and in solid-state NMR. In the traditional continuous wave method, a frequency/field sweep is applied to the sample and each magnetic resonance line has to be recorded sequentially. In Pulsed FT-NMR, the sample is irradiated with a high powered pulse of radio frequency energy. The transient response or signal, which results in the time domain (known as free induction decay or "FID") is stored in a computerized data acquisition system where it undergoes Fourier transformation to generate the usual frequency-domain spectrum. Therefore, in FT-NMR the data of all resonance lines over a specific region is gathered and processed simultaneously. This great time saving is of extreme importance in understanding the high sensitivity of FT-NMR. Also its ability to handle natural low-abundance nuclei, such as ^{13}C, where consecutive scanning and averaging over long periods of time is necessary for resolution enhancement, is an obvious advantage. Pulsed FT-NMR can be performed either as a single radio frequency pulse sequence followed by the acquisition of the FID or in a multiple pulsed mode where a series of carefully timed radio frequency pulses is applied to the sample prior to the acquisition of the FID in order to measure

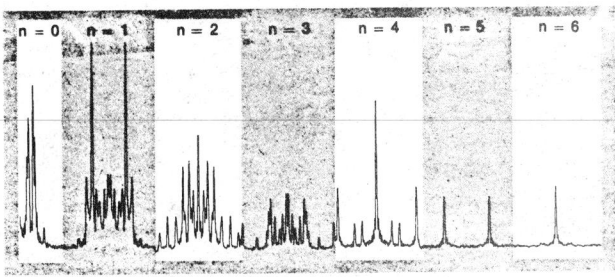

Fig 34-20A.   Oriented benzene spectrum in quantum NMR simplification of the spectra by using higher quantum numbers (Baum, RM, *Chem and Eng News*, Jan 1983, pp 30–31).

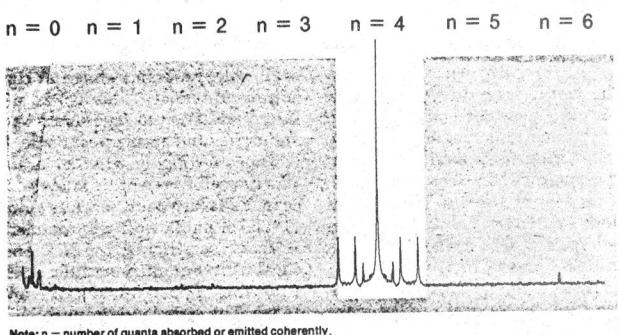

Note: n = number of quanta absorbed or emitted coherently.

Fig 34-20B.   Quantum NMR oriented benzene spectrum using selective, four-quantum excitation.   (Baum, RM).

the spin-lattice relaxation time (T_1) and the spin-spin relaxation time (T_2). The important applications of multiple pulse techniques include:

(1) *Two-Dimensional NMR* (2D-NMR) where data are collected as a function of two independent time domains, followed by double Fourier transformation. The spectrum has two frequency axes and one intensity axis. 2D-NMR is very useful in simplifying very complex conventional spectra;

(2) *Insensitive Nucleus Enhancement by Polarization Transfer* (INEPT), which is especially applicable for sensitivity enhancement in the study of relatively insensitive multinuclei resonance such as ^{15}N, ^{17}O, etc;

(3) *Incredible Natural Abundance Double Quantum Transition Experiment* (INADEQUATE) which is of unique value in providing detailed C—C bonding information by observing the natural abundance ^{13}C—^{13}C scalar (spin-spin) couplings;

(4) *Multiple Quantum Technique* (MQ-NMR), a technique developed by Pines where several quanta of energy are absorbed or emitted, and several spins flip simultaneously. A multiple-quantum transition occurs when several separate transitions occur coherently. MQ-NMR is generating new excitement in the study of the orientation of molecules in space when coupling between proton spins produces a large number of lines in the NMR spectrum. The higher the quantum number, the more simplified is the spectrum (see Fig 34-20 for Benzene).

Solid-State NMR—Conventional NMR spectra of solids consists largely of broad peaks that are caused by a high proton dipolar (H_D) and quadrupolar (H_Q) nuclear spin Hamiltonians (in liquids both H_D and H_Q vanish and only chemical shift (H_{CS}) and scalar coupling terms (H_J) contribute). Lately newer techniques have been introduced to deal with the broadening problem: (a) magic angle sample spinning (MASS), where the sample spins rapidly about an axis inclined at the magic angle of 54° 44′ of H_O; (b) multiple pulse techniques, which significantly narrow the lines; (c) magnetic

dilution. ^{13}C satisfies this condition for being magnetically dilute; hybrid experiments of all three techniques have also been applied with great success.

Electron Spin Resonance (ESR)

According to Bohr's nuclear theory, the atomic spectra of alkali metals should have a single spectral line corresponding to the unpaired valence electron. Careful examination, however, showed that the spectra have two closely spaced lines. In 1925, W Pauli suggested that the doublet could be explained only if the electron exists in two distinct states of angular momentum, an idea first introduced in 1921, by H Compton, who hypothesized that the electron may have an intrinsic magnetic momentum or a spin which makes it act as a tiny magnet. A new quantum number for spin "s" with values $\pm\frac{1}{2}$ was then added to the other 3 quantum numbers of the electron n, l and m. Therefore, the intrinsic angular momentum of the electron may have the value of $\frac{1}{2}(h/2\pi)$ or $-\frac{1}{2}(h/2\pi)$. The angular momentum of the electron is almost 1000 times larger than that of the proton and, therefore, the energy differences between its magnetic quantum levels are much larger than for the nucleus corresponding to about 10,000–80,000 MHz, which falls in the microwave region of the EM radiation spectrum.

ESR spectrometry depends on the splitting of the electron's magnetic energy levels upon subjecting it to an external magnetic field. Only unpaired electrons, contained in an ion, a molecule or an atom can exhibit ESR. Compounds such as transitional-metal ions and their complexes, free radicals and molecules with triplet-state electrons have successfully been studied by ESR spectrometry.

The basic principles of ESR are very similar to NMR spectrometry. Instruments consist of a power source that produces radiation at a constant frequency of approximately

9500 MHz and the peaks are obtained by varying the field. A 3500 gauss electromagnet is usually employed with sweep coils that allow for field variation within a narrow range. The sample is contained in a microwave cavity within the field of the magnet.

ESR spectrometry has not yet enjoyed the popular acclaim and analytical importance accorded to NMR. This may be in part due to its high initial set-up costs but more importantly because of the fact that most molecules fail to exhibit an ESR spectrum since they contain an even number of electrons. In certain cases, however, ESR has proven to be of prime value in providing unique analytical information, such as in the detection and identification of free radicals. Other recent applications include polymer characterization and metal ion-complexes studies.

Emission Spectrometry, Flame Photometry, and Atomic Absorption

The study of atomic spectra is probably the most basic scientific phenomenon that has captured the curiosity and the imagination of physicists, astronomists and chemists since the sixteenth century. The information gained from the intensive and unrelenting pursuit to establish its fundamental theories, was a major factor behind the development of our modern physical and chemical sciences.

Theory—When gaseous ions or an aerosol form of metals and some nonmetallic elements are heated to a high temperature, the kinetic energy of the atoms or molecules is increased. A collisions occurring at such elevated energy incur a high probability of transforming the kinetic energy into excitation energy. The electronically excited species are unstable and, if no chemical reaction occur after 10^{-4} to 10^{-7} sec, the energy is lost by emission of EM radiation in the UV and visible region, with wavelengths that are characteristic of the species under investigation.

Commonly employed methods of excitation are flame, AC arc, DC arc, and AC spark. Flame provides low-energy excitation and is used for easily activated substances; it has been used more recently with great success in Inductively Coupled Plasmas (ICP) where a high temperature argon torch is used to excite most atoms. Electrical excitation by discharge is also very effective in volatilizing and exciting samples and a temperature range of 4000–8000°K is attainable by this method. An AC spark provides excitation energies greater than the arc and is produced by application of a high voltage (10–50 kV) across the electrodes. Excitation also can be achieved with an optical ruby laser.

Emission Spectrometry

Instrumentation—The optical system of a typical emission spectrograph is shown in Fig 34-21. A diffraction grating can be used in place of a prism for radiation dispersion.

Analytical Procedure—For the qualitative analysis of metallic samples, the metal usually is fabricated into the electrodes. If quantitative analysis is desired, the sample is prepared in the form of a powder or solution and introduced onto pure graphite or copper electrodes mounted vertically. The lower electrode contains a small depression in the tip for powder samples. A solution may be placed on the electrode

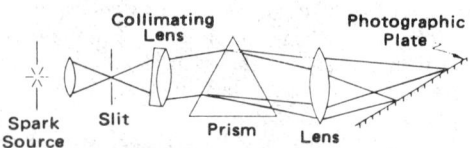

Fig 34-21.   A simplified optical diagram of an emission spectrophotometer.

and evaporated; the residue then yields an emission spectrum. A densitometer is used to identify unknowns by comparing the lines at various wavelengths with the lines in the previously photographed spectra of known metals. Iron is a valuable internal standard.

The major application of emission spectrometry is in the qualitative detection of all metals and most of the nonmetallic elements. Detection limits lie in the ppm or ppb range. Quantitative application, which used to be limited, has grown very rapidly lately, especially with the introduction of inductively-coupled plasma techniques and laser sources. Currently, emission spectrometry provides an excellent rapid technique for the simultaneous or sequential quantitative determination of up to 30 elements.

Flame Photometry (Flame Emission Spectrometry)

Flame photometry employs an emission-measuring device and utilizes a gas–air flame (1100–1300°) for excitation. The detection is limited to group IA and IIA metals of the periodic table which have a low-lying electronic level. Sodium is the most active in the series with a detection limit of 0.0002 ppm and beryllium is the least active with a detection limit of 25 ppm. The detection limit of a few elements is listed in Table II.

Instrumentation—A flame photometer is composed of the following parts:

The Flame Source—This part consists of pressure regulators and flow meters for the fuel, atomizer, and burner. The burner has inlets for fuel and oxygen or air. In order to insure constant emission, a major requirement of the flame is the maintenance of a steady state. The quality of the burner is important in attaining a proper spectrum.

The Optical System—The optical system is identical to that of the atomic absorption spectrometer. In recent years instruments have been designed to combine both flame photometry and atomic absorption spectrometry. In flame photometric measurement, a chopping device, located between the flame and the monochromator, is employed to provide an AC signal at the detector. The chopping of the signal is stopped when the instrument is being used for absorption purposes. Other parts of the instrument are identical to those required for atomic absorption spectrometry.

Analytical Procedure—Samples are dissolved in a solvent and introduced into the burner via an atomizer. Standard solutions used for analysis should be similar to the sample solution since variables such as viscosity and temperature affect the nature of atomization, thus the degree of excitation. In clinical laboratories the quantitative measurement of sodium, potassium, and calcium in biological samples is made by means of flame photometers.

Plasma Emission—Conventional atomization methods, such as combustion flame, furnaces and electric arcs, are usually adequate for most of the traditional applications of atomic emission spectroscopy. These techniques however, have several limitations, the most important of which are the instability of the atomization source, the possibility of chemical interaction such as metal oxide formation, the re-

Table II—The Detection Limits of Some Elements Using Flame Photometry [a]

Element	Wavelength, nm	Detection limit, ppm
Barium	553.6	1.3
Calcium	422.7	0.003
Cesium	852.1	0.1
Lithium	670.8	0.002
Magnesium	285.2	0.2
Potassium	766.5	0.001
Sodium	589.3	0.0002

[a] Courtesy, Beckman.

quirement of a relatively large size sample, low sensitivity, and finally, the inability to conduct simultaneous or sequential multielemental analyses. In order to overcome these limitations, new techniques called plasma emission spectroscopy have been developed. A plasma is a partially ionized gas, usually a mixture of the sample vapor and a support gas. The plasma is electrically generated and once formed, larger electric power can be transferred to it, raising its temperature to 9000°K. Such a high temperature provides the analyst with a rich and stable source of atoms that act as a reservoir of free and highly excited atoms. The other advantages of plasma include a wide linear dynamic range, excellent sensitivity, high accuracy and good precision. Also its suitability for simultaneous multielemental determinations at the ng/mL level has made it the method of choice for the analysis of trace constituents in samples of very limited volume. Although there have been different types of plasma emission sources, the most popular sources that have gained wide application are the Direct-Current Argon plasma and the Inductively Coupled Plasma.

Direct-Current Argon Plasma (D/C Argon Plasma)—The main advantage of DC Argon plasma is its excellent stability even in the presence of solvents, organics and high acid or alkali concentrations. It usually consists of two carbon anodes, between which the plasma jet is formed, and a tungsten cathode. It requires about 1 kw of power and once ignited can be sustained by a low voltage. The plasma can sustain a temperature as high as 10,000°K. Samples are introduced in an aerosol form, and their emission spectra are observed in a region isolated from the main plasma core; a procedure by which the sensitivity is greatly enhanced. Multielemental sequential analysis can be easily achieved with much lower detectable limits than with conventional flame emission. The DC Argon plasma also has a special advantage in the determination of trace amounts of arsenic and other nonmetallic elements. One limitation, however, is its unsuitability for automation, since the plasma supporting electrodes have to be replaced or reshaped after about 2 hours of operation.

Inductively Coupled Argon Plasma "ICP"—The main difference between ICP and DC plasmas is that the ICP derives its sustaining power by induction from a high frequency magnetic field. The pioneering work of Reed in the early nineteen sixties laid the basis for ICP as an exciting new technique that can be used for the simultaneous determination of all of the periodic table elements with a lower limit of detectability in the ppb range.

ICP (see Fig 34-22) simply consists of a quartz tube (2.5 cm diameter) placed inside a coil that is connected to a high frequency generator (4–50 MHz range) with output levels of 2.5 kW. Because argon is a nonconductor, a seed of electrons (from a Tesla discharge coil) is first introduced before turning on the power. Argon is fed into the quartz tube and is ionized by the magnetic field produced by the induction coil. The seed electrons interact with the magnetic field and gain in intensity enough to ionize the gas flow and an eddy current, induced by the magnetic field, flows in circular closed paths around the discharge tube. After complete ionization, a coned flame plasma is formed at the tip of the torch.

Because there is no electrode contact in ICP (cf DC plasma), the excitation and emission zones are separated from each other. This, besides the inert environment and the high temperature achieved, allows complete ionization of the sample with minimum chemical interference and a high signal-to-noise ratio of the sample's emission. These excellent conditions are the main reasons for the extreme sensitivity of ICP, typically in the ppb range.

Therefore, ICP offers the threefold potential of ultra-trace determinations on a multielement basis, utilizing a very small sample size (microliter or microgram level), in any type of

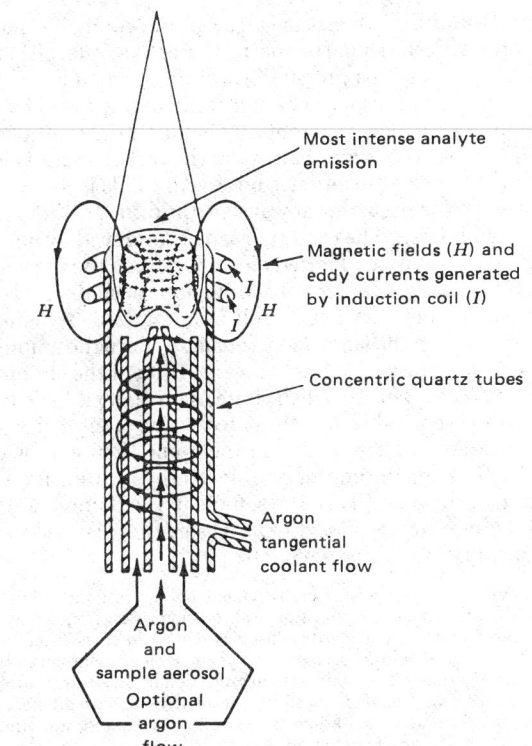

Fig 34-22.   Schematic diagram of an argon ICP. (Reproduced from Willard, HH, Merritt, LL, Dean, JA and Settle, PA, *Instrumental Methods of Analysis*, 6th Edition, D VanNostrand Co, NY, 1981).

matrix. ICP is also very amenable to complete automation and the simultaneous determinations of a vast array of both metals and metalloids.

Atomic Absorption Spectrometry (AA)

As early as 1860 Kirchhoff described the basic principles of atomic absorption spectra. It was not until 1955, however, that the theoretical background for its analytical applications were demonstrated by Walsh and by Alkemade and Milatz. The simplicity of this technique makes it an attractive tool for the analysis of many elements. At present, many chemical and clinical laboratories use this method for the quantitative determination of most of the elements in multivitamin and mineral formulations, drugs, and biological fluids.

Theory—In AA spectrometry, the elements are transformed into the atomic vapor form by drawing an aerosol of the sample solution into an open flame. A fraction or most of the freed atoms are then excited by exposure to a suitable source of radiation. The radiation absorbed by the unexcited atoms is related to the sample concentration. In this sense, AA could then be envisaged as the inverse of emission spectrometry, where the radiation emitted by the thermally excited atoms is related to concentration. It should be emphasized that usually the fraction of atoms excited by heat (via a flame or an electric arc) is relatively small for most elements. Also the atomic absorption of any element is generally at its resonance line, ie, a narrow range of wavelengths, usually in the UV or visible region of the spectrum, corresponding to the electronic transition between the lowest excited state and the ground state.

Factors Affecting Atomic Absorption Spectra—*Solvents*—In general, an organic solvent enhances the absorption signal, and therefore, it may alter the absorption intensity.

Anions—These can bond strongly with metals and tend to reduce the signal intensity. EDTA chelation could eliminate such effect.

Metal Binding—Sometimes, the presence of one metal interferes with the signal of another. For example, either Si or Al interferes with a proper absorption signal of Sr if both are present in a solution. The signal can be improved by the addition of La which preferentially binds the interferants.

Ionization—If a large quantity of the test element is ionized, a very weak absorption is observed. This is due to the ionic absorption occurring at wavelengths different from that of the atomic one. The condition can be improved by adding a large excess of easily ionized elements; eg, in the measurement of Ca, a large amount of sodium ion is usually added.

Emission from the flame itself is minimized by using a chopper between the lamp and the flame. Since the amplifier is designed to amplify only an ac signal (that of the chopping frequency) the intensity of light from the hollow cathode tube can be observed and recorded. A reduction of intensity due to the presence of the sample in the flame then will be detected. The magnitude of the decrease in intensity is a function of the quantity of the sample in the flame.

Instrumentation—An atomic absorption spectrometer consists of the following elements:

Source—Single-element or multielement hollow cathode tubes are generally employed as sources in atomic absorption. Less frequently, the bright continuum of a xenon arc has been used as a source. The cathode of the hollow cathode tube is comprised of an element identical to that under investigation in the flame. Upon excitation by an electric current, metal atoms are sputtered off. Collision of these atoms with an inert gas such as argon induces excitation of the metal atoms and subsequent emission of characteristic radiation.

Burner—The quality of the burner, the type of fuel, and the ratio of fuel to oxidant are the most important factors which affect the result of analysis by an atomic absorption instrument. The burner can be compared to a sampling cell in a spectrometer. The following characteristics are desirable in a burner: stability sensitivity, freedom from memory, freedom from background, linearity, and lack of self-emission. Either oxyacetylene or nitrous oxide-acetylene flames are employed in the burner. The latter mixture has the advantage of providing a hot flame with lower explosion hazard.

Monochromator, Phototube, and Amplifier—These parts are identical to those employed in visible spectrometry. The monochromator, however, should be able to pass the resonance line and filter out others. A large bandpass causes the absorbance curve to bend. Most of the elements are determined at slitwidths corresponding to bandpasses of 7–40 Å; in atomic absorption a 10 Å wavelength accuracy is sufficient.

Analytical Procedure—It is desirable to dissolve the sample in an organic solvent and for higher sensitivity the strongest absorption line must be chosen. In general, the resonance line resulting from the lowest excited state is usually the line exhibiting the strongest absorption. The instruction manual of each instrument suggests the choice of the line and the sampling technique.

New Atomization Techniques in AA Spectrometry—While flame atomic absorption is still widely used for the routine determination of more than 60 elements with new records of detection limits, lately there has been a considerable interest in the utilization of other atomization techniques. These include the mercury cold vapor atomic absorption, hydride generation techniques especially for As and Se, and an electrothermal atomization method. Recent research has concentrated on the latter technique as a new powerful tool for the study of trace amounts of lead in different matrices.

Fluorescence Spectrometry (Fluorometry)

When certain chemical substances are electronically excited by the absorption of UV or visible radiation, they emit light at a longer wavelength. This phenomenon is called "Luminescence" and depending on the life span of the excited species, two different processes could be distinguished. The first is fluorescence, where the luminescence stops within 10^{-8}–10^{-4} sec after the source of excitation is removed, and the second is phosphorescence, where the luminescence continues for a slightly longer period of time ($\simeq 10^{-4}$–10 sec).

Theory—Upon absorption of visible or UV radiation by a molecule (usually $\pi \rightarrow \pi^*$ transition), the electron from S_0 (singlet ground state) is promoted to S_1 or S_2 (singlet excited states). The excited species, may return to the ground state by dissipation of energy through collision or by vibrational relaxation of the excited state. The vibrationally relaxed species can return to the ground state with the emission of radiation with a wavelength longer than that which originally was absorbed. This radiation is referred to as fluorescence. Fig 34-23 illustrates different electron spin states.

There is also a nonradiative process in which the excited state gives off energy and proceeds to a lower energy (triplet) state T, by a decay process. A return from T to S_0 gives off a long-lived radiation, which is called phosphorescence. The absorption and emission of radiation is specific for a particular molecule. Fig 34-24 is an energy level diagram that summarizes the electronic processes.

In order for a molecule to fluoresce, an absorbing molecular structure is required. Fluorescence may be expected to occur generally with molecules containing a highly conjugated system. At least one electron-donating group such as NH_2 or OH should be a part of the conjugated system. Electron withdrawing groups such as COOH or NO_2 diminish, and in some cases prevent, fluorescence. Fluorescence is enhanced as the rigidity of the molecule increases; ie, a reduction in the internal vibration of the molecule.

In case of dilute atomic vapors, resonance fluorescence occur (at the same wavelength as the excitation), however, in more complex organic compounds in addition to the resonance radiation, emission of radiation at longer wavelength occurs (Stokes' shift).

The position and intensity of the fluorescence bands are affected by pH. The quantum yield, ϕ, of fluorescence is lower than unity due to a "quenching" process; ie, not all of the excited molecules return to the ground state by emitting fluorescence radiation. Energy may be lost by bond dissociation and deactivation.

Fluorescence spectrometry offers detection limits lower than those of absorption spectrometry. A quantity of 1.1 $\mu g/L$ can be measured and linearity can be maintained up to 10,000 $\mu g/L$. The method is applicable in the quantitative determination of fluorescing substances.

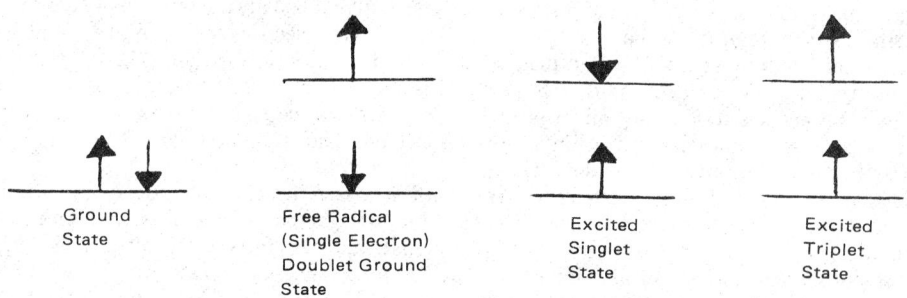

Ground State   Free Radical (Single Electron) Doublet Ground State   Excited Singlet State   Excited Triplet State

Fig 34-23.   Illustration of the different electron spin states.

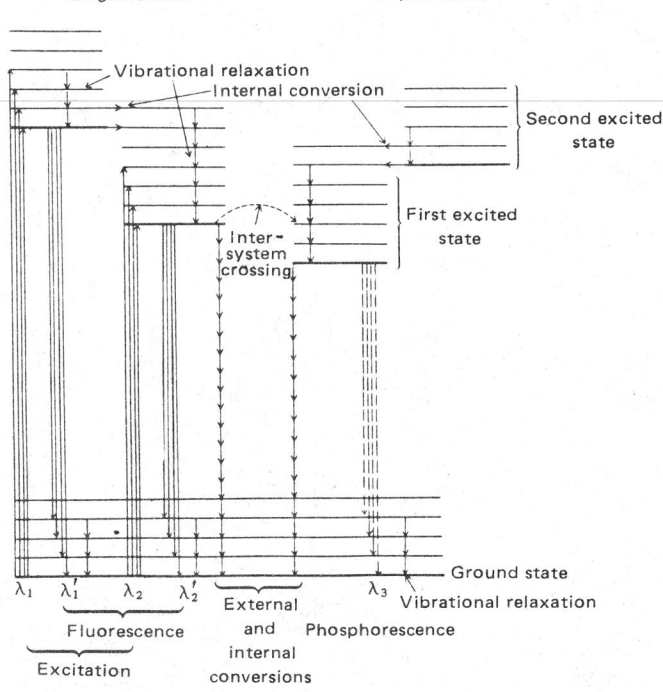

Singlet states   Triplet states

Vibrational relaxation
Internal conversion
Second excited
state

First excited
state

Inter-
system
crossing

Ground state
Vibrational relaxation

λ_1 λ_1' λ_2 λ_2' λ_3

Fluorescence   External   Phosphorescence
and
Excitation   internal
conversions
(quenching)

Fig 34-24.   Energy level diagram for a photoluminescent system. (Reproduced from Skoog and West).

Instrumentation—The source of irradiation of the sample is a mercury-discharge lamp or xenon lamp. Selection of the exciting wavelength can be accomplished by means of a filter; this type is called a filter fluorometer. In a true fluorescence spectrometer two monochromators usually are employed, one for the excitation source and the other for analyzing fluorescence emission. If the fluorescence spectrum is strong, the excitation spectrum can be determined by placing the desired solution in the instrument and evaluating the fluorescence while varying the wavelength of the exciting light. The detector is a photomultiplier tube whose output is connected to a meter, a digital display, or a recorder. The preparation of the sample is similar to that for UV.

Application—Fluorescence spectrometry has the greatest inherent sensitivity of all spectrophotometric techniques. Concentrations as low as $10^{-7}M$ can be accurately and precisely measured. It also has a high selectivity, which makes it useful in the analysis of trace amounts of drugs and metabolites in biological fluids. Fluorescence, however, is less widely used than other absorption techniques due to the relatively limited number of organic compounds in which fluorescence can be induced.

Lately, because of computer enhanced techniques, new areas are being investigated such as Derivative Fluorescence Spectroscopy. In addition, fluorescence has proven to be of great value in HPLC where either natural or induced fluorescence can significantly lower the limit of detection. Furthermore, pre- and post-column derivatization with such compounds as o-phthalaldehyde are becoming increasingly common.

Nonabsorptive Interaction of Matter with EM Radiation

The phenomenon of nonabsorptive interaction of matter with EM radiation is applied in such analytical procedures as light-scattering photometry, refractive index, and polarimetry. These interactions are not quantized, except for Raman spectroscopy, and therefore are considered to be nonspecific. However, each compound possesses its own characteristic interaction. The differentiation of stereoisomers with a polarimeter, the quantitative analysis of various substances with a refractometer, and the determination of the molecular weight of macromolecules by light-scattering are examples of this type of instrumental analysis.

Light-Scattering Spectrometry

As in reflection and refraction, the scattering of radiation results when it passes through a transparent medium in which particles of a second phase are suspended. In order for EM radiation to be scattered by particles, two criteria should be met: (1) the dimensions of particles should be equal to or smaller than the incident wavelengths and (2) the dispersing medium should have a refractive index different from that of the particles.

Particles of 1–10,000 Å scatter EM in the UV and visible regions. If a beam of light is allowed to illuminate a colloidal suspension in a test tube, a pencil of light will be observed in the tube, due to the light-scattering phenomenon. This is known as the *Tyndall effect* and is an indication of the presence of suspended particles. The simplest kind of scattering is that observed by small, spherical, and optically isotropic particles and is known as *Rayleigh scattering*.

Turbidimetry, nephelometry, and Raman spectroscopy are analytical techniques that are based on the light scattering phenomenon. However, only Raman spectroscopy will be discussed here.

Raman Spectrometry

In 1928, CV Raman, an Indian physicist, noted that under certain conditions, when an intense monochromatic light is scattered by molecules, the wavelength of a fraction of the scattered radiation is different from that of the incident beam. Fig 34-25A is a diagram of the various types of scattering of radiation. This shift (called the Raman effect) was found to be related to the chemical structure of the sample, and, therefore, offered a new technique for structural elucidation and, in some cases, quantitative determination of several organic and inorganic compounds, in a way similar to IR spectroscopy. Raman spectra, however, arise under certain con-

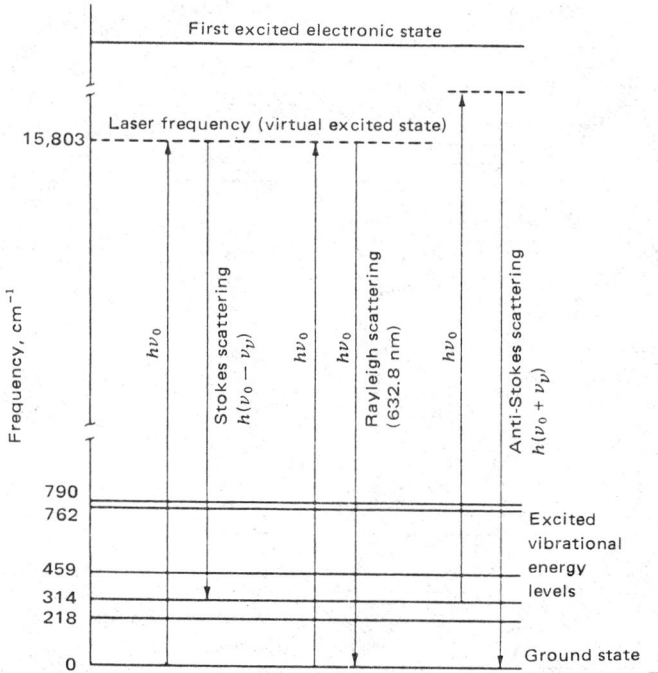

Fig 34-25A. Energy interchange involved in rayleigh and raman scattering (CCl_4 Molecule, Source is a He-Ne Laser). (Reproduced from Skoog and West).

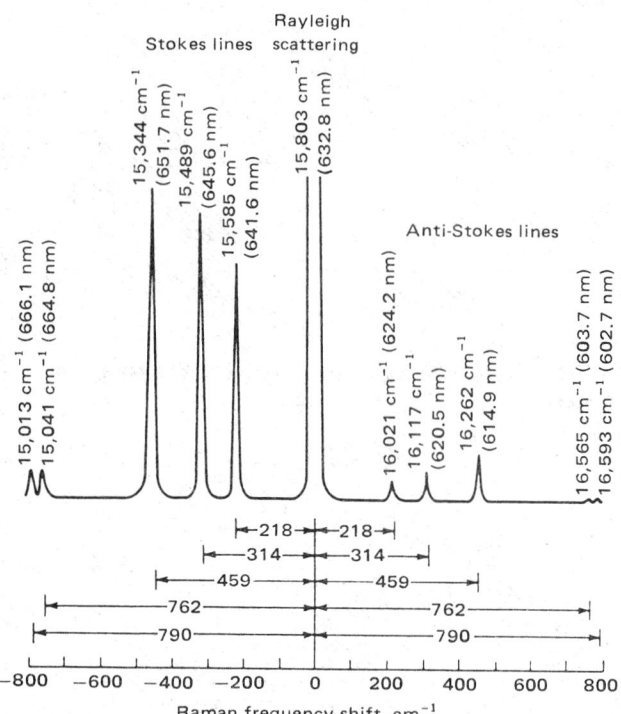

Fig 34-25B. Raman Spectrum of CCl_4 Obtained with a He-Ne Laser. (Reproduced from Skoog and West).

ditions that are entirely different from IR. For example, molecules have to undergo a change in their polarizability as they vibrate under quantum conditions, but do not have to have a dipole moment as in IR. Therefore, vibrations that are inactive in the infrared, may be active in the Raman, such as in the homonuclear diatomic molecules. Also Raman spectra, unlike IR, can be used to study aqueous media. The main limitation of Raman spectroscopy however, is that it is a weak effect, with low sensitivity and high vulnerability to many interferences. Meticulous sample preparation is required, as any dust contamination would cause Tyndall scattering. Lately, laser sources, usually a helium-neon laser, have been employed to provide an intense, coherent, monochromatic beam, and this has improved the sensitivity significantly and raised new interest in the technique. Fig 34-25B is the Raman spectrum of carbon tetrachloride.

Polarimetry

The fundamental principle of polarimetric analysis is based on the existence of optical activity in a substance; ie, the ability of a material to rotate plane-polarized light.

Polarimetry is applicable to the determination of the molecular structure of substances which do not have a rotation–reflection symmetry axis (*vide infra*). Determination of the sugar content of foodstuffs is an example of the quantitative application of polarimetry.

Modern polarimeters are capable of measuring optical rotation at more than just the traditional D-line of sodium. Some instruments measure optical rotation discretely at a number of different wavelengths. When the optical rotation is measured continuously as a function of wavelength, the technique known as Optical Rotatory Dispersion (ORD) results. ORD has found some use in structural studies.

Mass Spectrometry (MS)

The phenomenon of deflection of ions in electric or magnetic fields was first proposed by Wien in 1898. Using this

principle, Thompson in 1912 and Aston in 1919 performed some experimental work on the identification and quantification of isotopes. A mass spectrometer for general use, however, did not become available until the mid-1930s.

In MS, the sample, usually in the vapor form, is bombarded by an electron beam converting it into a gaseous ionic state, consisting of the parent ion and several ionic fragments of the original molecule, using different magnetic focusing techniques. The ions are then separated according to their mass/charge ratio (m/e) (the majority of ions are singly charged). The mass spectrum·records the amounts of different kinds of ions formed under specific conditions plotted against the m/e ratio. The spectrum is characteristic for every compound and, therefore, can provide valuable information about its chemical structure and, in most cases, a very accurate measurement of its molecular weight.

MS is a very sensitive, highly selective and quantitative analytical technique. Sample size is usually in the mg to the nanogram range and fragmentation patterns are highly reproducible even for multicomponent mixtures. The main limitations of MS are its relatively high cost, its need for extensive computerization of data analysis, its requirement of highly skilled analysts for the proper operation and maintenance of the mass spectrometer as well as for the successful interpretation of the mass spectral data. The recent quantum leaps in computer technology, however, have made the overcoming of these limitations an attainable task and today MS data is becoming an almost routine adjunct to the IR and NMR spectra.

Theory and Instrumentation—The theoretical and instrumental aspects of mass spectrometry are somewhat intermingled and it is appropriate, therefore, to discuss them together.

The principle of mass spectrometry consists of the (1) generation of positive (or in some techniques, negative) ions (primarily from organic molecules), (2) separation of these ions according to their mass (and charge), and (3) collection of ions and recording the quantity of each species. Molecules

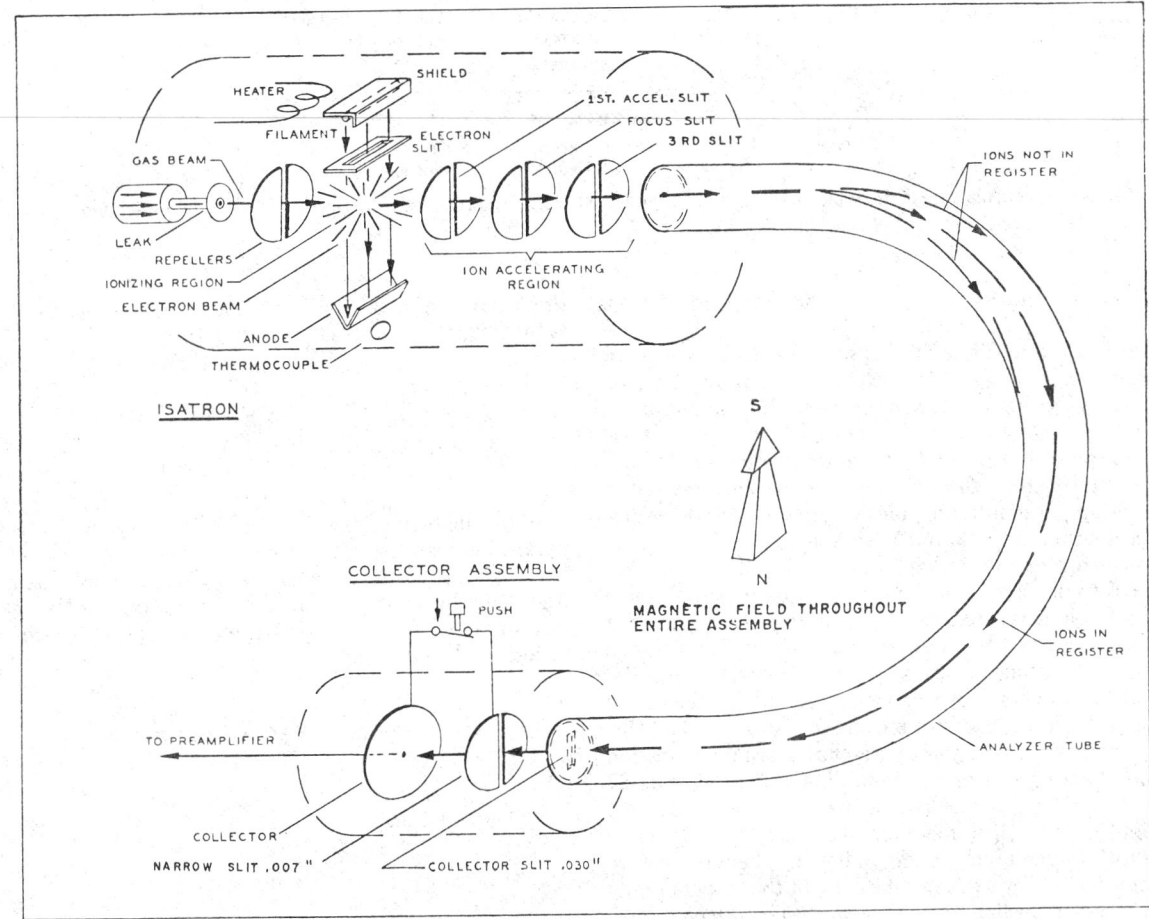

Fig 34-26.   The CEC Model 21-103C mass spectrometer.

up to a mass of 500 can be analyzed by single-focusing (magnetic-focusing) instruments. The double-focusing instruments, in which a combination of electrostatic and magnetic fields has been employed, provide a higher resolution. An accurate molecular weight (to six significant figures) can be obtained by the latter instrument. A typical magnetic focusing mass spectrometer is shown in Fig 34-26. The following sequence provides the analytical procedure common to most mass spectrometric measurements.

Introduction of Sample and Ion Production—A gas sample is introduced from a gas bulb into a small glass manifold. A known volume is passed into a reservoir where the pressure is about 10^{-2} torr. Liquids are introduced by a micropipet or by injection through a silicone rubber dam using a hypodermic syringe and needle. Due to the vacuum in the reservoir, the liquid is drawn in as a vapor.

Solid samples are ordinarily volatilized by heating and a vapor pressure of 10^{-2} torr is necessary, while a sample is still below its decomposition temperature, in order to introduce sufficient sample into the ionization chamber. In recently developed instruments, the sample can be heated in high vacuum in the proximity of the electron beam. A compound must be stable at a temperature at which its vapor pressure is about 10^{-7} torr. Special handling techniques are required for compounds exhibiting thermal instability. The sample in the vapor form enters the ion-producing chamber via a small orifice, known as *molecular leak*.

The sample vapor can be transformed into ions by various means; the electron bombardment of the vapor is the most widely used. The ionization chamber, where the neutral molecules from the molecular leak enter, is maintained at a pressure of 10^{-6} torr. A hot, carbonized, tungsten filament provides electrons which are drawn off by a pair of positively charged slits and directed on the vaporized sample molecules. The collision of electrons with molecules produces both negative and positive ions. The electric field can be varied from 6 to 100 eV and *parent ions* and fragments with various mass numbers are produced in this potential range.

The positive parent ions and fragment ions are accelerated toward the analyzing tube by one positively charged repeller slit, placed after the molecular leak, and two negatively charged slits located between the electron beam and the entrance to the analyzer tube. The ions can be accelerated up to 150,000 miles/sec by applying voltages ranging from 400 to 4000 V across the two accelerating slits. The potential energy, eV, of an accelerated ion will be equal to its kinetic energy; ie, $eV = \frac{1}{2}mv^2$, where m is the mass of the ion of charge e and velocity v in terms of the accelerating voltage V.

The Analyzer Tube—This tube which guides the ions to the collector is located between two magnetic poles and is maintained at a pressure of 10^{-7} to 10^{-8} torr. The path of the ions is shown in Fig 34-26. Varying the current in the electromagnet increases or decreases the force imposed upon the ions; thereby, each ion beam is brought into focus at the exit slit.

Ion Collector—The ion beam, upon passing through the exit slit of the analyzer tube, carries a current of 10^{-18} to 10^{-10} amp. This current is amplified by an electrometer prior to recording.

Recorder—Five separate galvanometers can be used to record simultaneously the peaks for fragment ions and the parent ion. The relative galvanometer sensitivity ratios are 1:3:10:30:100. This procedure, however, requires extensive data manipulation as all peaks have to be counted, measured and then normalized before any interpretation is possible. This consumes time and effort and because of this, electronic data handling has become increasingly employed.

Computerized Data Processing—Digitized electrical data from the ion collector is fed into a computer memory where it can be further processed and simultaneously matched with a host of possibly identical spectra stored in the computer. This allows rapid accumulation, manipulation and interpretation of the mass spectra. Cathode ray tubes (CRT) are usually connected to the computer central processing unit (CPU) in order to give a real time display of the mass spectrum.

Resolution Enhancement—Resolution in mass spectrometry is defined as the mass divided by the difference between closely related mass numbers; ie, $M/\Delta M$. For example, to differentiate between O_2 of mass 31.9898 and S of mass 31.9721, a resolution of 1800 is necessary. A mass spectrometer can be considered high resolution if it can separate two ions differing in mass by at least one part in 10,000–15,000;

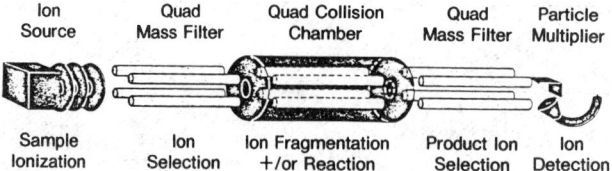

Fig 34-27.   Conceptual diagram of the triple quadrupole mass spectrometer. (Reproduced from Borman Stuart, *Instrumentation in Analytical Chemistry*, Vol 2, Amer Chem Soc, Washington, DC, 1982).

ie, can separate an ion of mass 500.00 from one of mass 499.95.

Quadrupole and Time of Flight Mass Analyzers—In addition to the double-focusing technique to improve the mass resolution, two techniques recently have been introduced. In the Quadrupole Mass Analyzer, four electric poles (a quadrupole) replace the magnetic field application procedure. The ions entering from the top, travel with a constant velocity in a direction parallel to the poles (Z direction) and acquire stable oscillation in the X and Y directions. This is usually accomplished by applying a dc voltage as well as radio frequency (rf) to the poles. Only one m/e ratio can pass through the quadrupole mass analyzer and be detected for a given rf potential and rf frequency. Therefore, a very rapid sweep can be performed by varying the rf frequency while rf and DC potentials are constant or vice versa. An advantage of the quadrupole is that it does not require focusing slits and this results in higher sensitivity as the resolution is only a function of the number of cycles an ion spends in the field. Fig 34-27 is a diagram of a triple quadrupole mass spectrometer.

In Time of Flight Spectrometers, the ions of different mass are given the same kinetic energy allowing them to acquire different velocities, and have a time of flight that depends only on their mass; ie, the lighter the ions, the faster they can travel through the field-free region. Hence, the original beam of ions tends to separate into several layers of ions depending on their mass which bombarded the cathode of the ion-detector sequentially, and their transit time is calculated. Because a complete mass spectrum can be repeated 20,000 times in one second, the Time of Flight instrument is extremely useful in kinetic studies of fast reactions or in GC-MS, where the effluent peak of the gas chromatograph could be scanned simultaneously on-line.

Chemical Ionization Mass Spectrometry (CI/MS)—For certain compounds, the negative ion spectrum is significantly more intense than that of the positive ion. For these compounds, a new technique called Chemical Ionization/Mass Spectrometry (Bimolecular) has been introduced where both the negative and positive ions are subjected to an appropriate potential and thereby are alternately pulsed from the chemical ionization source through a quadrupole analyzer to a separate electron multiplier. To collect the negative ions, a positive potential is applied to the first dynode of the multiplier. Because of its high sensitivity and unique spectra, CI (Bimolecular) has become an equal competitor to the traditional electron impact (unimolecular, field ionization) technique. Actually, several mass spectrometers today have both ionization modes available in the same instrument.

In the CI mode, a reagent gas is introduced into the ionization chamber to form the new molecular ions that can be separated on the basis of the m/e ratio. The major advantage of the CI technique is that less fragmentation occurs and the mass spectrum is usually much simpler to interpret.

Mass Spectra and Molecular Structure—With the low-energy electron beams in the order of 8–14 eV it is possible to observe only the molecular ion (parent ion). Unlike other analytical methods, mass spectrometry gives an exact molecular weight. The mass spectrum of toluene shows a peak at $m/e = 92$ (m/e is the mass to charge ratio; for the parent ion

this value is also the molecular weight), which is developed according to the process;

$$\left[\begin{array}{c}\text{CH}_3\end{array}\right] \xrightarrow{e} \left[\begin{array}{c}\text{CH}_3\end{array}\right]^+ + e \qquad (33)$$

With a high-energy electron beam, in the order of 70 eV, the parent ion disintegrates, due to the removal of several electrons, giving positively charged and uncharged fragments. Adopting the symbolism for the transfer of a single electron by a single-headed arrow, two typical examples for fragmentation can be given by;

$$R\!\!\frown\!\!CH_2\!\!\frown\!\!NH_2 \longrightarrow R^{\cdot} + CH_2\!\!=\!\!\overset{+}{N}H_2$$

(34)

$$\underset{77}{}\underset{105}{}\underset{121}{}\underset{135}{}\underset{176}{}$$

The mass spectrum of a compound, therefore, is a display of masses of molecular fragments together with the mass of the parent ion vs the relative abundance of each species as depicted by the peak heights.

The graphic form of the mass spectrum of toluene and its tabular presentation is depicted in Fig 34-28. The most intense mass peak is referred to as the *base peak* and is assigned an arbitrary value of 100; the other peaks are normalized relative to the base peak. Since the ratios of fragment abundance for a given compound remains constant, a mass spectrum (like an IR spectrum) becomes a "fingerprint" for each molecule.

The isotope abundance of atoms such as Cl, Br, S, and Si leads to the detection of these elements by mass spectrometry. For example, the ratio of ^{35}Cl to ^{37}Cl is 100 to 32.5.

For compounds of the general formula $C_w H_x N_y O_z$, contribution from the heavy isotopes can be calculated by;

$$100\,\frac{P+1}{P} = 1.11w + 0.015x + 0.37y + 0.037z \qquad (28)$$

and;

$$100\,\frac{P+2}{P} =$$

$$0.0002wx + 0.004wy + 0.006w(w-1) + 0.20z \qquad (29)$$

where P is the monoisotopic peak (parent peak; equivalent to the nominal molecular weight value) and $P+1$ and $P+2$ are the monoisotopic mass number plus one and two mass numbers, respectively. The relative isotope abundance of the heavy isotopes of each element determines the height of the

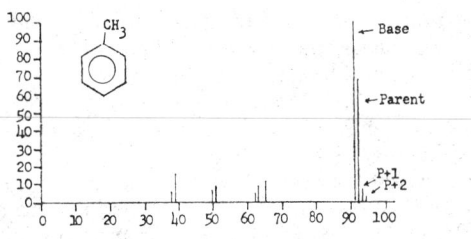

m/e	% of base peak	m/e	% of P
38	4.4	92 (P)	100
39	16	93 (P + 1)	7.37
45	3.9	94 (P + 2)	0.29
50	6.3		
51	9.1		
62	4.1		
63	8.6		
65	11		
91	100 (Base)		
92	68 (Parent)		
93	5.3 (P + 1)		
94	0.21 (P + 2)		

Fig 34-28.   Relative abundance of various fragments shown in mass spectrogram of toluene.

$P + 1$ and $P + 2$ peaks.   By consulting special tables of abundance factors for the $P + 1$ and $P + 2$ peaks, it is possible to determine an exact molecular formula from mass spectral data.

The following example represents the use of isotopic contribution in structural elucidation.

A compound with a mass spectrum of $P = 110$ (100%), $P + 1 = 111$ (5.5%), and $P + 2 = 112$ (0.3%) could be sorted out of the following molecular formulas with the molecular weight of 110:

Formula	$P + 1$	$P + 2$
$C_3H_2N_4O$	4.84	0.30
$C_4H_2N_2O_2$	5.20	0.51
$C_4H_4N_3O$	5.57	0.33
$C_4H_6N_4$	5.94	0.15
$C_5H_2O_3$	5.55	0.73
$C_5H_4NO_2$	5.93	0.55

The data reveal that the molecular formula of the compound is $C_4H_4N_3O$.

The fragmentation patterns of a few representative chemical classes are illustrated below.   More detailed information can be obtained by consulting reference books on mass spectrometry.

Several empirical rules of molecular fragmentation are listed below:

1.   Cyclic compounds show an intense parent peak and a peak at the mass number of the ring.
2.   Saturated cyclic compounds lose side-chains at the α-carbon.   The peaks resulting from the loss of two atoms from the ring is more intense than the peaks from the loss of one atom.
3.   In cyclic compounds containing a double bond next to the side-chain, cleavage occurs at the bond β to the ring.
4.   In olefins, cleavage occurs β to the double bond.
5.   In compounds with heteroatoms, cleavage occurs at the bond β to the heteroatom.
6.   In hydrocarbon molecules, the ease of cleavage is in the following order: tertiary > secondary > primary.   The positive charge remains on the branched fragment.
7.   In carbonyl-containing compounds, cleavage occurs at this group, the positive charge remaining on the fragment containing;

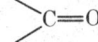

Molecular fragmentation may occur by one or a combina-

tion of the following processes: simple fission, simple rearrangement, complex fission, and complex rearrangement.

New Techniques in Mass Spectrometry

Mass Spectrometry has traditionally served as an excellent tool for the elucidation of elemental and isotopic composition of organic compounds that are volatile or may be made volatile after simple derivatization reaction.   However, the recent dramatic improvements in instrumentation capabilities combined with the vigorous growth in computer technology, at affordable costs, have propelled a new host of applications that have significantly increased the analytical potential of MS.   Nonvolatile substances such as polar compounds with high molecular weights, solid-state mixtures, the gas phase of ionic or radical species, and transition states of chemical processes can be analyzed with these new techniques.

Mass Spectrometry/Mass Spectrometry (MS/MS)—In this technique, sequential mass analyzers are used to both separate and identify ions in a single instrument.   The first analyzer generates several "parent ions" from the sample that are separated based on their m/e ratios.   Some of these ions are then selected for further fragmentation to form "daughter ions" that can be mass-analyzed.   There are several methods for the secondary fragmentation, but the most common procedure is allowing the parent ion to collide with a neutral target gas.   An MS/MS spectrometer consists of the sample ionization source (usually dual CI/EI), two analyzers separated by a reaction region and finally the detector.   The analyzers can be of the sector type (electric or magnetic), quadrupole mass filters or hybrids of both the sector and quadrupole.   In triple quadrupole instruments, the first quadrupole serves as a mass filter for ion selection, then an RF-only quadrupole that can be pressurized with a collision gas is utilized for ion fragmentation and/or reaction.   A second quadrupole mass filter is used for product ion-selection.   The main advantage of MS/MS is in the direct analysis of mixtures due to its large mass range (up to 12,000), high resolution, and extreme sensitivity.

Fourier Transform Mass Spectrometry (FTMS)—This method is based on the old Ion Cyclotron Resonance (ICR) mass spectrometry.   In FTMS, the analyzers are temporally rather than physically separate.   This kind of separation of the ion formation, excitation and detection allows very short scanning time.   FTMS essentially makes use of the Fellgett (a multiplex) advantage common to all Fourier spectroscopies, where the noise is detector and not source limited.   This is generally achieved by the simultaneous observation of the signals from all excited ions in the time domain, rather than the space domain, followed by Fourier transformation of the data to yield a frequency domain that can be assigned mass values according to their known relationship in order to provide the familiar mass spectrum.   Experimentally this involves obtaining the entire spectrum in a single measurement which requires a massive computer memory in order to accommodate the huge amount of data instantaneously.   The major advantages of FTMS are its high-resolution measurements, its high speed of scanning, and its extreme accuracy in mass measurements.   This makes it ideal for coupling to high performance (capillary) gas chromatography, chemical ionization measurements and MS/MS techniques.   It also proved to be a powerful tool for the study of the kinetics of gas-phase ionic reactions and ion chemistry.

Soft Ionization Techniques in Mass Spectrometry— These techniques allow the ionization of molecules directly from the solid state and are used, mainly, for nonvolatile substances of high molecular weights.   The main concept is to allow the sample to be distributed over a large surface area in order to greatly reduce the intramolecular forces between the molecules and thus make the evaporation process more dependent on the interactions of the sample-surface forces rather than the sample-sample forces that prevail during the regular sample heating processes. Early techniques included the "In-beam" or "direct CI exposure," where the sample is coated on a surface of a probe that can be placed inside the source as close to the ionization area as possible. The sample is rapidly heated to enhance the evaporation of the intact neutral compounds without pyrolysis. These early inert probe techniques have mostly been replaced by new active desorption emitters such as Field Desorption methods (FD), Plasma Desorption (PD) and Laser Desorption. Those techniques are suitable for intermediate molecular weight, heat labile or polar compounds. The most recent technique, however, is "Fast Atom Bombardment" (FAB) mass spec-trometry, and is revolutionizing the analysis of underivatized polar molecules in the mass range of 1000–6000, such as carbohydrates, peptides and glycopeptides.

Secondary Ion Mass Spectrometry (SIMS)—This technique has been previously discussed under X-ray Analytical Techniques.

Mass Spectrometry—Hyphenated Techniques—Recently MS has been successfully coupled to both gas chromatography (GC/MS) and liquid chromatography (HPLC/MS). Essentially, MS is employed as a detector for mass and a means of molecular structure determination of the effluents compounds. It has also been used for the qualitative assay of trace amounts of compounds in biological fluids and in environmental analysis.

Electrometric Methods

Chemical analyses in which electrical current, voltage, or resistance is involved are known as electrochemical methods. To facilitate discussion of this topic, some fundamental concepts of electrical and electrochemical phenomena should be reviewed.

Although the electrical waves associated with the generation of power and lighting equipment are classified under EM radiation, their interaction with matter differs from the relatively high-frequency optical waves such as UV and visible. The signals from the former travel in metal but those from the latter travel in space.

The following are a few commonly employed units in electricity:

Coulomb (Q)—The coulomb is a quantity of electricity. One electron has a charge of 1.602×10^{-19} Q. One Q can deposit 0.0011180 g of silver.

Faraday (F)—The Faraday is 96,489 Q, the charge carried by an equivalent weight.

Ampere (I)—The ampere is the unit of electric current. A rate of flow of 1 Q/sec is designated as 1 ampere.

Ohm (Ω)—The ohm is the electrical resistance of a uniform column of mercury at 0° with a mass of 14.4521 g, a length of 106.300 cm, and uniform cross section.

Volt (V)—The volt is the potential difference required to produce a current of 1 amp through a resistance of 1 ohm. The symbol for potential is E. Volt is equal to the product of current and resistance ($E = $ IR).

Watt (W)—The watt is the unit of power; work performed at a rate of 1 joule/sec. It is equal to the product of current and voltage.

For a proper understanding of electrochemical methods, it is appropriate to describe a few pertinent components and terms.

Electrodes—Metal or carbon conductors immersed in electrolytes are known as electrodes. A negative electrode (cathode) is the supplier of electrons in a chemical cell. A collector of positive ions in a gas-filled tube is also known as an electrode (anode). Electrodes are also discussed under *Potentiometry*. Gases, liquids and solutions which are capable of conducting current depositing materials at the electrodes, or dissolving the electrodes are known as electrolytes.

The standard electrode potential ($E°$) is the potential of the electrode immersed in a solution of its ions at unit activity ($a = 1$). All the electrode potentials are referred to the hydrogen electrode set at $E°_{Pt, H_2, H^+} = 0$.

When a cell is operating reversibly, the electrical work (ΔG) obtained per g-atom is the maximum work given by;

$$\Delta G = -nFE \qquad (41)$$

where G is the free energy, n is the valence change, F is a Faraday (96,489 coulombs), and E is the voltage or electromotive force (EMF) of the cell.

Electrical Cell—An electrical cell is an electrical circuit which consists of two electrodes and a solution of electrolyte(s). One electrode functions as an electron acceptor and the other as an electron donor. There are two general types of electrochemical cells:

1. A galvanic cell is one in which the chemical energy is converted into electrical energy by spontaneous chemical reaction. The current, which occurs as a result of an oxidation–reduction reaction, usually continues as long as all the components are available.

2. An electrolytic cell is one in which chemical reactions occur as a result of an applied potential whether the cell is galvanic or electrolytic. The electrode at which chemical reduction occurs is called "cathode," and that at which oxidation occurs is called "anode." Some electrochemical cells have the electrodes sharing the same electrolyte solution (cells without liquid functions). On the other hand, if each electrode has to have its own electrolyte solution, it becomes inperative to separate the two electrolytes (cells with liquid functions). In many cases, a simple fritted glass plate can serve as a liquid junction. In other cases, however, a "Salt Bridge" is used as a separator. This can take the form of a U-shaped tube containing a saturated solution of potassium chloride (double liquid-junction cell).

Electrochemical methods display a reasonable degree of sensitivity and accuracy. The apparatus is often very simple, modestly priced, rugged and requires little training to operate. Also, in some cases, a very small amount of sample is needed with some procedural preparations. In pharmaceutical analysis, however, the main limitation of electrochemical procedures is that generally they are not stability-indicating methods, and in many cases, they are subject to matrix interferences and require complex clean-up procedures.

In electrochemical analysis, four basic parameters are involved: current, resistance (or conductance), voltage and time. Each parameter has been utilized alone or in combination with others for analytical purposes. Most of the analytical techniques can be classified under three major categories:

1. *Potentiometry* involves determination of the EMF of chemical cells. In these methods (nonpolarized), an equilibrium or steady state is maintained and the electrode potential is related to the concentration by the Nernst equation.

2. *Voltammetry* involves the application of an external potential to the system in order to carry out various electrochemical analyses (limited electrolysis). In these methods no equilibrium exists, therefore, they may be called transient or dynamic (polarized) in nature.

3. *Other Electrochemical Methods* include those procedures during which exhaustive electrolysis takes place such as coulometry and electrogravimetry or during which conductance is measured.

Potentiometry

Potentiometric methods of analysis consist of the measurement of the EMF of chemical cells.

The EMF of a cell is the sum of three potentials:

$$E_{cell} = E_{ref} + E_{ind} + E_{jcn} \qquad (42)$$

where the subscripts denote *reference*, *indicator*, and *junction* potentials, respectively. E_{jcn} is the potential at the liquid junction which is constant. Since the E_{ref} is known, the indicator electrode then can provide information about the concentration of a species involved in electron exchange. An inert electrode, such as platinum, immersed in a solution of an oxidation-reduction system, provides or accepts electrons and indicates the ratio of oxidized to reduced species. A general expression of this phenomenon is given by the Nernst equation:

$$E = E^0 - \frac{0.0591}{n} \log [A_{red}/A_{oxid}] \qquad (43)$$

where A is the activity of oxidized or reduced species.

A chemical cell consists of a reference electrode half-cell and an indicator electrode half-cell.

Potentiometric methods encompass two types of electrochemical analysis. The first is the direct measurement of the potential of an indicator electrode with respect to a reference electrode, from which the calculation of the activity (or concentration) of the ion of interest can be achieved. The second category called "Potentimetric Titrations" involves the measurement of the changes in the EMF of the cell brought about by adding a titrant, ie, the monitoring of the potential serves only to locate the equivalence point for a titration.

Reference Electrodes—These have to be reversible, easily reproducible with no need for special assembly, with a small temperature coefficient and reasonable stability with time. The most widely used reference electrodes are the so-called electrodes of the-second-kind, which consist of either a mercury-calomel electrode or a silver-silver chloride electrode:

$$Hg\,|\,Hg_2Cl_2(s),\ KCl\ soln$$

or;

$$Ag\,|\,AgCl(s),\ HCl\ soln.$$

For the calomel electrode the connection to the test solution is made through a saturated solution of KCl, whereas the electric connection is by a platinum wire that is in contact with the mercury. The half-cell reaction is given by;

$$2Hg + 2Cl^- = Hg_2Cl_2 + 2e^- \tag{44}$$

Indicator Electrodes

a. *Noble Metals Electrodes.* These are widely used as indicator electrodes. For example, platinum is used for the Fe^{2+}–Fe^{3+} or H_2–H^+ potentiometric system.

b. *Electrodes of The-First-Kind.* These are a metal in contact with its own ions; example, Zn/Zn^{2+} electrode. They are limited to metals below hydrogen in the electromotive series, and are only partially ion selective.

c. *Electrodes of The-Second-Kind.* These consist of the metal part covered by a layer of one of its slightly soluble salts and immersed in an acid or a salt solution with the same anion. They include:

1. *Oxides Electrodes*—These are responsive to H^+ and are employed in nonaqueous acid-base titrations. Examples are Sb–Sb_2O_3 and Hg–Hg_2O electrodes.

2. *Specific-Ion Electrodes*—These are the most widely used indicator electrodes today. Due to their selectivity, they offer a simple, sensitive, and accurate method for direct potentiometry. Their selectivity is brought about by the use of a membrane, a special crystal or any other suitable discriminating element that allows a selective ion-exchange at the boundary of the solution membrane. In general, they are composed of an insoluble membrane or layer as the sensitive element, an inside electrolyte solution and an internal reference electrode. The difference in potential develops between the inner and the outer surfaces of the membrane. One of their advantages, is that they also allow the measurement of an anion of a slightly soluble salt. Ion-selective electrodes (membrane electrodes) include the glass electrodes, liquid membrane electrodes, crystalline solid-state membrane electrodes, precipitate-impregnated silicone rubber layers and enzymes or other reactive substances in gel-layer electrodes.

Glass-Membrane Electrodes

Hydrogen-ion-sensitive glass electrodes—This electrode is for the determination of H^+ concentration in aqueous solutions. The silicate network of the membrane absorbs water and alkali metal ions and becomes hydrated. An exchange of ions from solution to surface and vice versa occurs

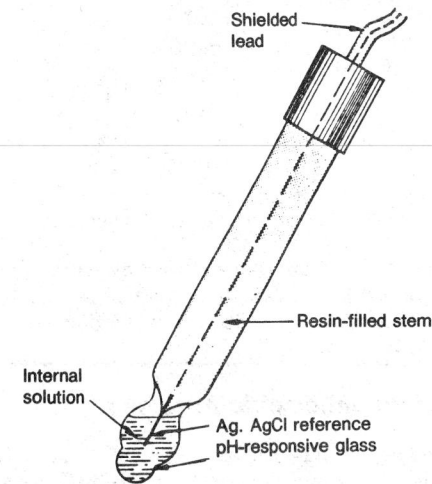

Fig 34-29.   Representative pH electrode. (Reproduced from Strobel, H, *Chemical Instrumentation*, 2nd Edition, 1973, Addison-Wesley Publishing Co, Inc, Reading, MA).

on a limited scale. The inner and outer glass surfaces assume potentials which depend on the solution with which they are in contact. The glass-electrode potential varies only with the pH of the external solution. The membrane of the electrode has a high resistance; ie, 5–1000 megohms at 25°. Considering this, the current drawn from this cell must be kept smaller than 10^{-11} amp if an error greater than 1 mV is to be avoided (10^{-11} amp $\times$ 100 megohms = 1 mV). A representative glass electrode is shown in Fig 34-29.

Metal-ion-sensitive glass electrodes (Specific-ion Electrodes)—One of the limitations of the glass membrane electrode is that at very low H^+ concentration (pH >9) it responds not only to H^+ ion but also to the alkali metal ions, this is known as the "alkaline error." Studies were first directed to a glass composition that minimizes this effect. Later, however, it became clear that if this "alkaline error" could be significantly potentiated, new glass electrodes that are selectively sensitive to an alkali ion could be introduced. It was demonstrated that Al_2O_3 or B_2O_3 in glass leads to such an effect, and the development of membranes that are selective for cations other than hydrogen has been growing fast. These metal-ion-sensitive glass electrodes have been constructed by replacing part of the silica in the glass structure with oxides of aluminum or boron. This type of glass electrode responds to univalent cations other than H^+, but not to polyvalent cations. Some of these electrodes are particularly sensitive to Na^+, Ag^+, and other cations.

Liquid Membrane Electrodes—These are based on the use of an immiscible ion-exchange organic liquid that has an ability to selectively bond with the ion of interest. The potential that is generated across the interface between the membrane and the aqueous solution to be analyzed is related to the specific ion concentration. Therefore, these electrodes can be used for the direct potentiometric determination of several polyvalent cations as well as certain anions.

Precipitate and Solid-State Electrodes—It is known that the sensitivity of the glass electrode is due to anionic sites on its surface that have special affinity for certain cations. Solid-state electrodes consist of sparingly soluble compounds or crystals that have surface cationic sites and, therefore, have a special affinity for anions. These electrodes are usually used for the determination of Cl^-, Br^-, I^-, sulfates and phosphates. They are insensitive to cations.

Measurement of the Cell EMF—This measurement is done potentiometrically by the null-balance method. The diagram of a simple potentiometric circuit is depicted in Fig 34-30.

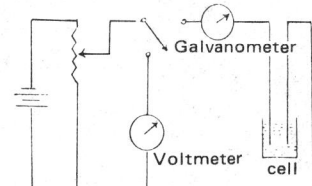

Fig 34-30.   A simplified potentiometer circuit.

It should be pointed out that all direct measurements using specific ion electrodes indicate the activity of the electro-active species in solution and not its concentration (see Nernst equation, Eq 43).

Classes of Potentiometric Analyses

Measurement of pH—Determination of the activity of H^+ is done either (1) potentiometrically or (2) by direct reading with a pH meter. For the potentiometric measurements, the apparatus consists of a potentiometer whose sensitivity has been increased by electronic amplification of the unbalanced current. The second type is a circuit designed to give meter-needle deflection as a function of pH. This is essentially an electronic vacuum tube voltmeter (VTVM) with a high-input resistance.

Acid–Base Titration—An acid–base titration curve can be obtained by using a pH meter with a recorder (or manually

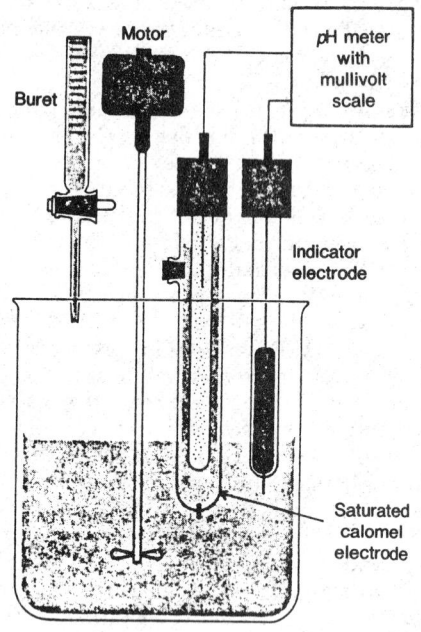

Fig 34-31A.   Apparatus for a potentiometric titration.

plotting points). In an aqueous system, in order to obtain proper curves with well-resolved end points, the acid or base to be titrated should be stronger than water, and the concentration prepared for titration should be higher than the hydrogen or hydroxyl concentration of water. If the EMF (E) obtained during the titration is plotted against volume (v) of the titrant, the end-point is the inflection point, or the steepest slope. The apparatus necessary for potentiometric titration is shown in Fig 34-31A.

Precipitation and Complexation—An ion may be determined by a potentiometric precipitation or complexation titration. This method requires an indicator electrode that can detect one of the ions precisely or that the reaction be accompanied by a change in electrochemical potential. To arrive at an exact equivalence point, the salt formed during the titration should have a low solubility or the complex should demonstrate high stability. Examples of precipitation titrations are the formation of insoluble or undissociated salts of Ag^+ and Hg^+ with Cl^-, Br^-, I^-, CN^-, and CNS^-. Fig 34-31B shows three means of plotting potentiometric data in order to determine the end point.

Complexation titration by potentiometry has been employed for quantification of ions such as Cu^{2+}. Ethylenediaminetetraacetic acid (EDTA) in the form of its disodium salt is the most widely used complexing agent. An indicator electrode that is sensitive either to the pH or to the metal ion is employed for detection of the end-point;

$$M^{2+} + H_2(EDTA)^{2-} = M(EDTA)^{2-} + 2H^+ \qquad (45)$$

Titrations in Nonaqueous Systems—Many organic acids and bases are too weak to be titrated in aqueous solvents. As is discussed in Chapter 17 and Chapter 30 (see analyses utilizing nonaqueous solvents), water is a leveling solvent, hydroxide ion being the strongest base and hydrogen ion the strongest acid which can be titrated. Any substance which is a weaker base or acid than water cannot be effectively titrated in an aqueous medium.

There are three general types of solvents:

1. Amphiprotic solvents, which have both acidic and basic properties. Examples: water, the lower alcohols, and acetic acid.
2. Aprotic solvents, which possess no acidic or basic properties. Due to their low dielectric constant, they have a low ionizing potential. Examples: hydrocarbons and carbon tetrachloride.
3. Basic solvents, which have no acidic properties. Examples: amines, ketones, and ethers.

The acidic strengths of various solute molecules vary as a function of the dielectric constant of the solvent. Generally, a nonaqueous potentiometric titration is unsuitable in solvents with a dielectric constant less than 5. A decrease in the dielectric constant of a solvent increases the acidic strength of a positively charged acid, such as NH_4^+, but lowers that of a negatively charged acid, such as the hydrogen succinate ion. For the titration of weak bases, a solvent with a low basic

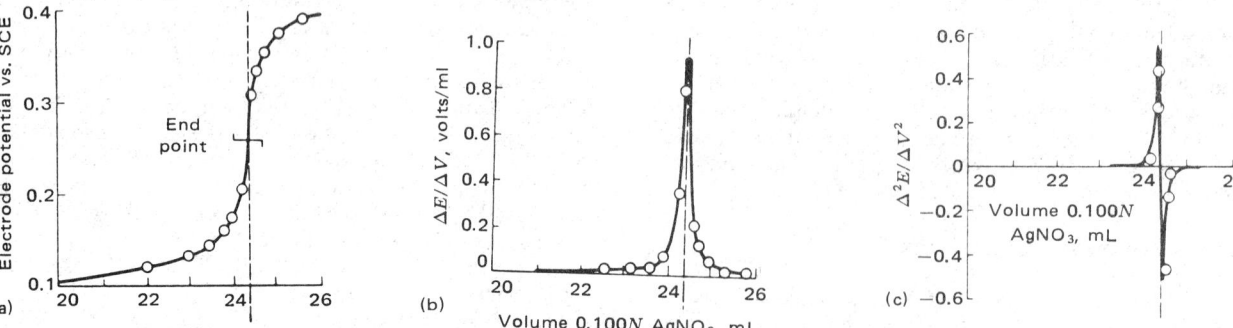

Fig 34-31B.   (a) Potentiometric titration curve for 2.433 meq of Cl^- with 0.100N AgNO$_3$; **(b)** First derivative curve; **(c)** Second derivative curve. (Reproduced from Skoog and West).

strength such as acetic acid is suitable; likewise, for weak acids, solvents with moderate basic strength are desirable. In the former case the titrant is usually perchloric acid in dioxane or acetic acid; in the latter case, sodium ethoxide in toluene–methanol or quaternary ammonium hydroxides in isopropanol.

Oxidation–Reduction Reactions—An inert electrode, such as platinum, which is unaffected by oxidizing agents, is used in redox titrations. A calomel electrode can be used as a reference electrode. The electrode generates a potential proportional to the logarithm of the activity ratio of the two oxidation states of the reactant or titrant. Titration of iron II with cerium IV is an example. The electrode potential changes gradually during the major portion of the titration. As the equivalence point approaches, the activity ratio changes rapidly.

Voltammetry

Voltammetry includes all electroanalytical techniques which involve the application of an external potential on the system and utilize the current-potential relationship arising at a polarizable microelectrode to calculate the concentration of the electroactive species. Two major types of electrochemical analysis based on voltammetric principles are:

   1. Polarography and amperometry, in which a very small fraction of the test solution is involved in the analysis. These methods can be used both for quantitative and qualitative analysis.

Both aqueous and nonaqueous solvents are employed in voltammetry. The analysis is primarily for inorganic substances, but a number of organic compounds have been analyzed, especially in detecting eluting compounds in liquid chromatography.

Polarography—In 1922, J Heyrovsky, a Czechoslovakian chemist, noted that the current passing between a polarizable, dropping mercury electrode (DME) and a nonpolarizable current-carrying electrode, when a certain potential is applied, is related to the concentration of one of the electroactive species in solution. Soon after, Heyrovsky realized that this phenomenon could serve as the basis for an elegant, sensitive and selective quantitative analytical technique for the determination of virtually all elements in one form or another. At this time, instrumental methods of analysis were a rarity, and the dominant techniques were the traditional volumetric and gravimetric methods. Polarography then, offered a new and exciting analytical tool that allowed for the first time, the measurements of concentrations at the submillimolar level without heroic efforts. However, the classical DC polarography never gained the widespread use in the analytical laboratory due, mainly, to three reasons: first, the wave-forms are usually not sharply defined which makes the data difficult to calculate; second, unless ideal conditions exist, the technique is vulnerable to several interferences due to nonfaradic currents which are not diffusion controlled; and third, efforts were futile in trying to apply the technique to nonaqueous organic solutions. Fortunately, most of these problems have been recently overcome, and modern polarographic methods such as differential pulse polarography and anodic stripping voltammetry are enjoying a rapid and wide growth in the analytical field.

Theory and Instrumentation—Polarographic analysis is based on the current-voltage curves arising in a cell consisting of a dropping mercury electrode (DME) or a microelectrode and a nonpolarizable current-carrying electrode in an unstirred solution. Substances in a concentration range of 10^{-5} to 10^{-2} M can be analyzed, both qualitatively and quantitatively, provided they can undergo cathodic reduction or anodic oxidation.

Polarography provides (1) a limiting electrolysis current that is proportional to the concentration of a given compound

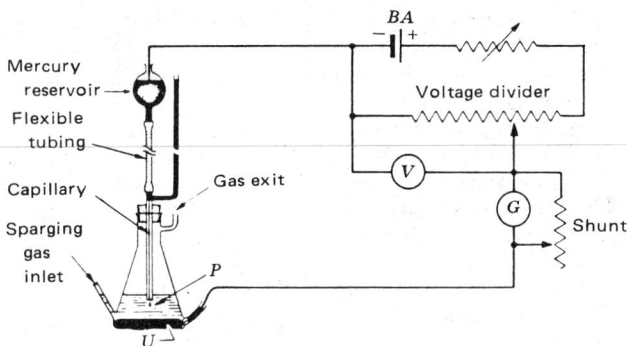

Fig 34-32.   Schematic diagram of a simple polarographic apparatus. P, dropping mercury electrode; U, unpolarizable mercury pool electrode; G, galvanometer; V, voltmeter.   (Reproduced from Strobel).

and (2) a half-wave potential, which is characteristic of an individual species. Fig 34-32 shows the simple circuit of a polarograph. The voltage applied across the electrodes may be increased gradually and the resulting electrolysis current measured with a galvanometer. The plot of EMF (voltage) vs current (μ amp) provides the curve shown in Fig 34-33. Until the decomposition potential is reached, there will be only a minor increase in current. The decomposition potential is a function of E° of the reaction and the concentration of the ions involved. At this point there will be a sharp rise in the current. A further voltage increase will cause the curve to level off. The sharp increase in current, called the diffusion current (i_d), is due to the diffusion of the ions to the electrode whereupon the ions are plated out. This plating causes the concentration at the solution-mercury interface to be lowered and results in a concentration gradient being established which causes ions to diffuse from the body of the solution into the interface at a rate proportional to the concentration difference. The current-voltage curve levels off when complete concentration–polarization occurs; ie, the diffusion rate becomes constant and proportional to the ion concentration in the body of the solution.

A mixture of two ions, Cd^{2+} and Zn^{2+}, with standard oxidation potentials of +0.4 and +0.76, respectively, gives the polarogram shown in Fig 34-33. The diffusion current for Zn^{2+} is the difference between the total diffusion current and that for Cd^{2+}.

In addition to the diffusion current, ions attracted to the DME by electric forces also create some current, referred to as *migration current*. The limiting current is therefore the sum of a migration current and the diffusion current. Current in an electrolytic cell is carried by all the ions present, irrespective of their participation in electrode reaction; therefore, if an inert electrolyte such as KCl (which at the low potentials employed in the polarography of Zn^{2+} or Cd^{2+} is neither oxidized nor reduced) is added in excess to the solution, the mi-

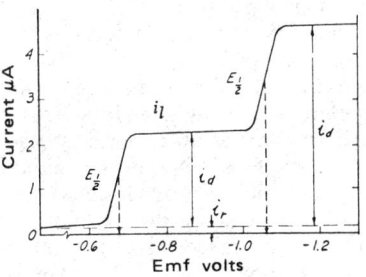

Fig 34-33.   The polarogram of a solution containing Cd^{2+} and Zn^{2+}. D_p: decomposition potential; $E_{1/2}$: half-wave potential; i_r: residual current; i_d: diffusion current; i_l: limiting current.

gration current will be carried almost entirely by the KCl ions. The limiting current observed then will be the diffusion current for the ions under investigation. The KCl is called the supporting electrolyte.

Another type of current that occurs in polarography is residual current. Even with inert ions, it is observed that an increase in voltage gives rise to a small but observable current. This is due to charges acquired by the DME on application of higher voltages. In polarography, compensation is allowed for this residual current.

The diffusion current obtained with the DME is given by Ilkovic's equation:

$$i_d = 607nD^{1/2}m^{2/3}t^{1/6}C \qquad (46)$$

where i_d is the average current in μ amp during the life of the drop, n is the number of Faradays of electricity required/mole of the electroactive species, D is the diffusion coefficient of the reducible or oxidizable substance in $cm^2\ sec^{-1}$, m is the rate of flow of Hg from the DME capillary in mg sec^{-1}, C is the concentration of electroactive solute in moles/L, and t is the drop time in sec (an optimum drop time is 2–5 sec). The equation is simplified by keeping all the factors except C constant:

$$i_d = k_cC \qquad (47)$$

Plotting i_d vs C will give a straight line.

Half-Wave Potential—As shown in Fig 34-33, the half-wave potential ($E_{1/2}$) is an oxidation or reduction potential at the current mid-point of a polarographic curve. A half-wave potential is characteristic of an electrolyzable species, is independent of concentration, and is related to the standard electrode potentials (E° values). The half-wave potential of a compound, however, is related to the form in which an oxidizable or reducible molecule exists. For example, it can be shifted by varying the pH of a solution. Two compounds, whose half-wave potentials overlap at a given pH, can possibly be resolved by varying the pH or adding a complexing agent. For example, in acid solutions the half-wave potential of tin and antimony are −0.47 V and 0.20 V, respectively, but in alkaline solutions they are −1.1 V and 1.8 V. Therefore, the latter condition is preferred in determining these ions in a mixture.

Electrodes—In polarography the indicator or polarizable electrode is most often a DME which is for reduction reactions. In some cases, a platinum electrode (stationary or rotating) is used for oxidation reactions. The curves provided by these reactions are known as cathodic and anodic waves, respectively. By convention, diffusion currents are designated as follows: reduction, positive; oxidation, negative. The advantages of the DME are that it provides a smooth renewable surface and the diffusion currents obtained are reproducible. However, it has the disadvantage in that at a small positive potential anodic dissociation occurs. Therefore, platinum is preferred. Precision obtainable with a platinum electrode is about ±5%. For a reference electrode, a saturated calomel electrode is used.

Both manual and recording polarographs are available, of which the recording type is the most widely used.

Oxygen Waves—The dissolved oxygen in any solution to be analyzed polarographically often interferes with accurate determinations and therefore its removal by deaeration before the analysis is essential (usually by ultrasonification, vacuum or purging with nitrogen). Oxygen interference is due to two equal oxygen waves, the first is produced by its reduction to hydrogen peroxide and the second is by the further reduction of the hydrogen peroxide to water. On the other hand, these reductive reactions and their well defined waves could also, if desired, serve as the basis for the polarographic measurement of dissolved oxygen in aqueous solutions.

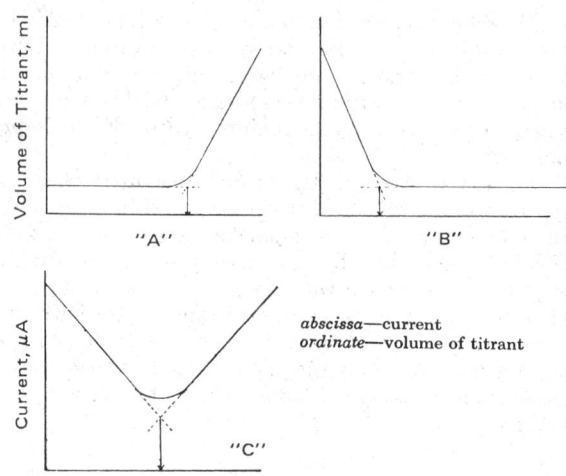

Fig 34-34.   Titration of A: SO_4^{2-} with Pb^{2+}; B: Pb^{2+} with SO_4^{2-}; C: Pb^{2+} with $Cr_2O_7^{2-}$.

Amperometry—This method is based on the principle of polarography, with the exception that the voltage is maintained constant during a titration procedure. Substances which cannot be analyzed polarographically, due to the absence of a diffusion current, can be determined amperometrically by using a titrant which yields a diffusion current. Figs 34-34A, B, and C illustrate typical amperometric titration curves. The equivalence point is the intersection of the two extrapolated straight lines whose slopes are a function of the diffusion current. In contrast to a polarographic measurement, in which several ions in a mixture can be determined, the amperometric titration involves determinations of a single substance only. The substance and its half-wave potential must be known prior to titration. A change in volume during the titration is usually minimized by selecting a titrant five to ten times more concentrated than the material to be analyzed. The best potential for the microelectrode is chosen by referring to the half-wave potentials of the sample and titrant. The applied voltage is located on the plateau of the electrolysis wave.

As shown in Fig 34-34A, the titration of SO_4^{2-} with Pb^{2+} is carried out at a potential more negative than −0.46 V (Pb^{2+} + 2e → Pb, −0.46 V half-wave potential). As sulfate ions are removed and Pb^{2+} concentration is increased, the diffusion current increases. The opposite is true if Pb^{2+} is to be titrated with SO_4^{2-}. In the titration of Pb^{2+} with sodium or potassium dichromate at −1.2 V, when the equivalence point is passed, the excess $Cr_2O_7^{2-}$ gives an increase in the diffusion current.

In amperometric titrations (as in polarography) an inert electrolyte must be added to eliminate the effect of migration current and, prior to titrating, nitrogen is bubbled through the solution to remove dissolved oxygen. The titrations are performed in an H-shaped cell. Either a DME or a rotating platinum electrode can be used with a saturated calomel electrode (SCE) as the reference electrode.

The amperometric procedure is applied to the measurement of ions which cannot be evaluated potentiometrically. For example, no suitable electrode is available to determine sulfate anion potentiometrically. Amperometrically, however, excellent results are obtained. A similar application is utilized in the determination of fluoride ion with thorium or lanthanum nitrate, and in titrations involving reagents such as iodine and bromine (as bromate). However, the greatest use of the amperometric end-point is for titrations where a slightly soluble precipitate is formed.

Amperometric Titrations Utilizing Two Indicator Electrodes—When a reversible redox reaction is present in the system, the amperometric method can be modified to use two polarized microelectrodes (usually of platinum) immersed in the well stirred titration cell. The current starts flowing when a small potential is applied between the two electrodes. This current can be monitored as a function of the volume of the titrant until the end-point, when the current drops to zero or close to zero. The technique used to be called the "Dead-stop end-point."

Modern Voltammetric Analytical Techniques—Classical or DC polarography only refers to electrochemical analysis utilizing the dropping mercury electrode under a constant DC potential. Because of the limitations inherent in this technique, several modifications have been introduced that helped to generate a new renaissance in polarographic and voltammetric methods of analysis that features much higher sensitivity and better selectivity. The new procedures do not utilize the standard dropping mercury electrode.

Derivative Polarography—In this modification, the current/voltage curves are differentiated in order to obtain a peak-shaped response that can be easily and accurately measured in place of the traditional sigmoid polarographic waves that are hard to interpret. These differential methods usually employ the potentiostatic capabilities of a working electrode potential that are based on a three electrode system. In addition to two working electrodes, the third electrode is a reference electrode of constant potential that draws no current.

Single-Sweep Polarography (Oscillographic Polarography)—In this technique, a voltage range between 0.3–0.5 V is scanned or swept linearly during the last two to three seconds of the life of a mercury drop. An oscilloscope is used to monitor this rapid scan on a polarogram that is quite different from that obtained in regular polarography (see Fig 34-35). An advantage of this technique is its better sensitivity due mainly to a lower residual current and higher "summit" currents. Another advantage is its easy and more accurate measurement due to the peak-shaped response.

Pulse Polarography—One of the major difficulties in DC polarography is the interference by the non-Faradaic capacitance current that flows across the interface. In the early 1950's, while experimenting with square-wave polarography, G Barker discovered that a sudden change in the applied potential causes the capacitance current to decay almost to zero before the Faradaic (redox) current is observed. A small, fixed-height potential pulse ($\simeq$50 msec duration) is superimposed at regular intervals of about one second against the linearly increasing DC potential normally associated with classical polarography. The pulse is usually applied near the end of the life of the mercury drop and is synchronized with its maximum growth. Two pulse techniques are common. In the "normal or integral pulse" procedure, square waves of successively increasing amplitude are applied to consecutive mercury drops from the dropping mercury electrode at a constant pressure. The polarograms are similar in shape to DC polarography with a greatly reduced capacitance component. This allows about six times the sensitivity of classical polarography. In the "differential pulse" methods, pulses of equal amplitude are applied on a linear potential ramp. The current is sampled twice, just before the pulse application and at the end of the pulse. These currents are stored on a memory capacitance, and the difference is plotted vs the potential yielding peak-shaped polarograms. Differential pulse methods have less sensitivity than the normal pulse method, but they display greatly enhanced detection limits because of better resolution of the half-wave potential. One of the major advantages of the pulse technique is its suitability for the analysis of organic compounds and several irreversible electrochemical systems.

AC Polarography—A small amplitude, low frequency periodic potential (usually a sinusoidal wave) is superimposed

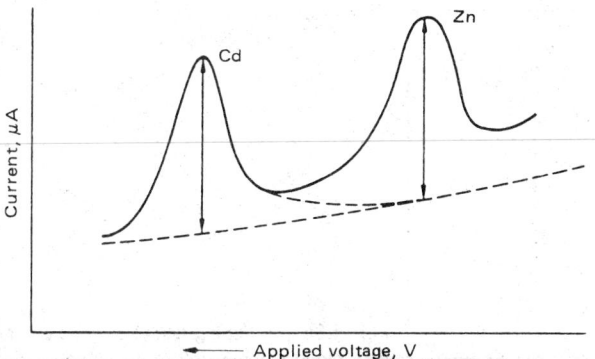

Fig 34-35.   Single sweep polarogram.   Baseline (dashed) gives current in supporting electrolyte alone as a blank.   (Reproduced from Strobel).

against the slow linear DC voltage. The instrumentation employed, utilizes electronic circuitry that only allows the measurement of the alternating components of the total current flowing into the working electrode (eliminating the DC component). This in effect allows the monitoring of the difference in current that flows between the minimum and the maximum applied potential during the modulation period. Therefore, the polarogram is a peak-shaped response with its maximum height at the half-wave potential. In AC polarography, the capacitance current can be separated from the Faradaic current by a simple phase-sensitive lock-in amplifier.

Cyclic Voltammetry (Fast Linear Sweep)—In this technique, the normal, slow DC sweep employed in classical polarography is substituted with a fast sweep of about 100 mV/sec and higher, applied to a stationary electrode in a diffusion-controlled system. The technique is very fast, is more sensitive than classical polarography and can supply information about the reversibility of the reaction as well as its kinetics. It also does not require the highly sophisticated instruments usually associated with pulse polarography. For identification purposes, cyclic voltammetry monitors four properties of a redox system, *viz* the peak potential, wave slope, reversibility and the effect of changing the supporting electrolyte.

Chronopotentiometry—In this technique, the change in the potential of a working electrode is monitored as a function of time while a constant current is passed through the solution under study (electrolysis). The transition time is a measure of the rate at which the species at the electrodes is reduced up to a point where it can no longer sustain the required current. Although chronopotentiometry is not a voltammetric technique in the real sense, it like polarography, depends on a diffusion-controlled phenomenon. It is usually employed to study electrodes processes. It requires a higher concentration due to its relatively low sensitivity.

Voltammetric Stripping Analysis—The stripping analysis technique has been the fastest growing voltammetric application in recent years. The main reasons for its wide popularity are the high degree of sensitivity by means of which concentrations below parts per billion can be easily measured with inexpensive instrumentation. Also, its suitability for simultaneous multielemental analysis is an attractive feature that other polarographic techniques lack. While the technique itself is a bulk procedure, where the whole solution is subjected to the electrolytic process as in a coulometric determination, it usually uses a mercury microelectrode which is subjected to a single-sweep voltage scan, and, therefore, it is usually classified as a voltammetric method. The stripping concept consists of two basic steps; the first is the deposition or the concentration step, where the desired electroactive species are deposited anodically or cathodically through a long

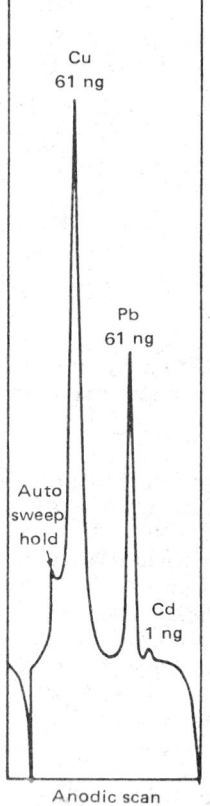

Auto sweep hold

Anodic scan

Fig 34-36.   Stripping analysis, anodic scan of a blood sample (0.2 mL). Experimental data: Plating time, 30 min; plating potential, −1.0 V; sweep rate, 60 mV/sec; chart speed, 12.7 cm/min; current range, 200 μA full scale; anodic stripping time, 16 sec. (Reproduced from Willard, Merritt, Dean & Settle).

electrolysis stage ($\simeq$20–40 minutes), and the second is the stripping step, where the deposited elements are stripped from the microelectrode through a reversed electrolysis process, usually a linear-potential sweep, such as the one used in single sweep polarography. The resulting current/voltage polarograms are then recorded. The anodic scan of a blood sample that was analyzed for metals (Cu, Pb, Cd) is seen as Fig 34-36. Unlike polarography, the working electrode is stationary, usually a hanging mercury electrode (a thin mercury film on nickel or platinum) or other solid electrodes such as platinum or gold in anodic stripping voltammetry (ASV) or a glassy carbon electrode in cathodic stripping voltammetry (CSV). The solid electrodes, however, have several disadvantages. Their performance depends on their past history and is affected by oxide film formation. In ASV, the electroactive elements of interest are first reduced (or concentrated) at the working electrode under fixed conditions of diffusion and electrode surface area. The stripping process (or oxidation step) is carried out by linear anodic scan, usually 2–5 mV sec^{-1}. Usually very little capacitive current exists during stripping and, therefore, the Faradaic current is very high and, hence, the extreme sensitivity of this technique. In CSV, the electroactive species is deposited as an insoluble layer with varying potential depending on the concentration of the element to be determined. Stripping is carried out through a reversed electrolysis process following the anodic pre-electrolysis step. The stripping voltammograms show peak shaped responses for the electroactive species, their heights or areas are used for quantitative purposes and their potential for identification in a way similar to the half-wave potentials in polarography.

Differential Pulse Stripping Voltammetry (DPSV)—In this technique, relatively large amplitude (50–100 mV) pulses are periodically superimposed on a slow, linear potential range of about 5 mV sec^{-1} for short periods of time. As discussed before, this allows a great enhancement in the Faradaic current due to the fast decay of the capacitive current. The current is measured just before the pulse application and again

at the end of the pulse. The difference between these two currents is amplified and displayed on a recorder. The hanging mercury drop electrode is the working electrode of choice in DPSV.

Fast Fourier Transform Data Acquisition (FFT) for Electrochemical Relaxation Measurements (ERM)—The on-line FFT data acquisition and processing procedure, familiar in spectroscopic analysis such as NMR & IR, has been applied to electrochemical techniques with great success, especially in polarographic and voltammetric analyses. This is because most of the techniques are actually relaxation measurements of an electrochemical cell, initially at approximate equilibrium, and then observations are made of a time-varying response to an applied electrical perturbation. Also, the wide availability of relatively inexpensive computers with high memory capacity that can handle the complex Fourier transforms, convolutions and deconvolutions helped make FFT quite affordable. Actually, many scientists believe that within a few years FFT data treatments will be used in all chemical applications as often as our familiar logarithmic transforms, due to its unprecedented speed and precision in data acquisition and processing.

Coulometry—Coulometry involves exhaustive electrolysis and requires currents larger than those employed in polarography plus an unpolarized working electrode. Either constant current or constant voltage techniques can be employed and elaborate electronic regulating devices are commercially available.

In coulometry it is possible to generate a reactant or titrant in situ, therefore, unstable reagents may be employed in the analytical procedure.

The quantity of the reactant formed is proportional to Q, the number of coulombs when the current is constant;

$$Q = it \qquad (48)$$

where i is the current and t is the time of electrolysis. One Faraday of electricity is 96,487 Q, which causes chemical changes in mw/n g-ions, where n is the number of electrons. If the current is maintained constant, the weight of the reactant can be calculated by;

$$\frac{it}{96,487} = \frac{\text{weight of } x}{\text{equivalent weight of } x} \qquad (49)$$

There are two important factors to be considered in coulometric analysis: (1) the substance of interest must be electrolyzed completely and (2) the exact time at which the reaction is completed must be determined.

In the electrical generation of the analytical reagent, three points must be observed: (1) the working electrode must remain inert during analysis—eg, due to the tendency of halide to react with platinum giving PtX_6^{2-}, platinum cannot be employed as an anode when a halide is present, (2) oxygen should be removed, and (3) interference occurring as a result of participation of electrons in the electrolysis of another substance, such as a solvent, must be eliminated. In order to avoid the involvement of the solvent or impurities during an analysis, a constant-current procedure is used for the electrical generation of the reactant. The use of an excess quantity of the inactive form of a reagent (titrant) provides a proper control of the electrode voltage. For example, in the titration of Fe^{2+}, a large excess of Ce^{3+} is added. On passage of current, Ce^{4+} is easily generated at the working electrode (anode) and Fe^{2+} is oxidized;

$$Ce^{4+} + Fe^{2+} \rightarrow Fe^{3+} + Ce^{3+} \qquad (50)$$

Generation of Ce^{4+} ceases at the end-point.

Analytical Procedure and Instrumentation—A constant-current coulometer is the most widely used instrument. A power supply provides a constant current for the cell.

Usually a current of less than 250 mA is employed and the time of electrolysis varies from about 10 to 200 sec. An accurate electric timer starts or stops the electrolysis by controlling a switch. The end-point can be detected potentiometrically, amperometrically, or with an absorption photometric detector. If the potentiometer is set at a predetermined voltage, the imbalance observed during the analysis will be decreased so that at the end-point the galvanometer deflection will show zero. Silver or platinum are the most generally employed electrodes.

Electric Conductance Methods—Electric conductivity of a solution under a given potential is a function of the nature of the solute and its concentration. The current is conducted by the ions that migrate under the influence of an electric field. Conductance in *mho* units is $1/R$, where R is the resistance in ohms. Specific conductance, κ, is the reciprocal of the resistance of a 1-cm cube of liquid and is defined by;

$$\kappa = \frac{1}{R}\frac{d}{A} \tag{52}$$

where A is the area of the electrodes and d is the distance between the electrodes. In a cell with electrodes of 1-cm² area and a 1 cm separation, equivalent conductance, Λ, is

$$\Lambda = (1000/C_s)\kappa \tag{53}$$

where C_s is the concentration of the solution in moles per liter.

The equivalent conductance of a solution increases on dilution due to an increase in ionic mobility and, in the case of a weak electrolyte, also to an increase in the degree of dissociation. The degree of dissociation of a weak electrolyte, α, is given by;

$$\alpha = \Lambda/\Lambda_o \tag{54}$$

where Λ_o is the equivalent conductance at infinite dilution. Λ_o, which is also denoted by Λ_∞, is the summation of the conductances of the cations and anions.

The dissociation constant of weak electrolytes, K_a at an initial concentration of C_s, can be calculated by;

$$K_a = \alpha^2 C_s/(1 - \alpha) \tag{55}$$

Spectroelectrochemistry—Spectroelectrochemistry is a hybrid analytical technique that combines electrochemistry with a suitable optical measuring device. In general, redox reactions are initiated at the electrodes and simultaneously the electrolysis solution is monitored by spectrometry to study the nature of the newly electro-generated ions. The most common spectrometric techniques are UV or IR, where the light beams are directed at a transparent electrode and its nearby analytical solution. Internal reflectance spectrometry also has been utilized as well as Raman spectrometry. Spectroelectrochemistry has been applied mostly to specific redox reactions of organic, inorganic and complex biological systems.

Thermal Methods of Analysis

Thermal analysis is a technique in which a physical property of a substance is monitored as a function of controlled temperature increase. Modern thermal analytical methods can measure weight loss on heating, melting points, heat and energy of transitions and changes in form, in dimensions or in the viscoelastic properties of the substance. They find wide applications in material characterization, purity of medicinal substances, study of relative heat stabilities and dynamic properties of new compounds, as well as in crystallography, chemical kinetics and generation of phase diagrams.

Theory

Most thermodynamic events are accompanied by a loss of heat or require addition of heat from an external source in order to proceed. The event may be a phase transition, loss of a volatile component or a chemical reaction. Each of these occurrences can be followed thermodynamically by noting either change of temperature of the sample under study or energy changes of the sample with respect to time. If the sample loses a volatile substance by evaporation, sublimation or chemical conversion to a gas, it is also possible to follow the course of events by noting weight loss with respect to time, as the temperature of the sample is increased at a constant rate.

The general laws of thermodynamics, specifically those governing calorimetry, serve as the basis for understanding the theoretical concepts involved in the different thermal analytical methods of analysis. Refer to Chapter 15 for these fundamental relationships. For equilibrium transitions, where $\Delta G = 0$ the heat of transition ΔH_n is related to the entropy of transition ΔS_n by the following equation.

$$\Delta S_n = \frac{\Delta H_n}{T_n} \tag{57}$$

Modern instruments for thermal methods of analysis are based on these parameters; mass, temperature and heat flow.

Table III illustrates the use of these functions and typical data outputs.

Thermogravimetry (Thermogravimetric Analysis, TGA)

TGA is perhaps the simplest form of thermal analysis and utilizes a *thermobalance* as the analytical instrument. The apparatus may be no more than a modified single pan analytical balance provided with a digital electronic output so that a plot of weight change (y axis) can be made with respect to time or temperature. An infrared lamp may be the source of heat to irradiate the balance pan. Many modifications of such a device are used to determine the moisture content of tablet granulations, hydrated substances, etc. Much more sophisticated instruments are also commercially available which include temperature programming and the use of a variety of beam, spring, cantilever or torsion balances to determine changes in weight of the sample. Since the atmosphere surrounding the heated sample may influence (retard or hasten) decomposition, provision is often made to control the atmosphere by addition of inert gases (nitrogen, helium), or reactive gases (oxygen, hydrogen, etc). The result of a thermogravimetric evaluation of calcium oxalate monohydrate may be seen in Fig 34-37.

Recently several types of thermogravimetric devices have been coupled to a gas chromatograph or mass spectrometer so that the effluent products of decomposition can thus be characterized.

Differential Thermal Analysis (DTA)

In this technique a sample and a thermally inert reference material are heated (or cooled) linearly with the aid of a programming device, and the temperature difference between the sample and the reference is measured as a function of the temperature applied. Because, during transition, the sample may either absorb or evolve heat, the difference in the tem-

Table III—Typical Curves Produced in Thermal Gravimetry Analysis (TGA), Differential Thermal Analysis (DTA), and Differential Scanning Calorimetry (DSC)

Technique	Parameter measured	Instrument employed	Typical curve
Thermogravimetry (TG)	Mass	Thermobalance	
Differential thermal analysis (DTA)	$T_s - T_r (\Delta T)$	DTA apparatus	
Differential scanning calorimetry (DSC)	Heat flow, dH/dt	Calorimeter	

perature between the sample and the standard is equivalent to the temperature of transition and can indicate if the transition is endothermic or exothermic. Usually ΔT is plotted against the temperature, T, or as a function of time (t). A block diagram of a typical differential thermal analyzer is depicted in Fig 34-38 and a schematic diagram of a modern DTA instrument is illustrated in Fig 34-39. DTA data is probably the most accurate of all thermal techniques, because the thermocouple is inserted into the sample; however, only the temperature of transition and not the amount of heat can be measured from a DTA curve, as the area under the peak is not proportional to the amount of energy transferred into or out of the sample.

Differential Scanning Calorimetry (DSC)

Another technique, very closely related to TGA, is DSC which differs only that the sample and reference containers are not contiguous, but are heated separately by individual coils that are heated (or cooled) at the same rate. Platinum resistance thermometers monitor the temperature of the sample and reference holders and electronically maintain the temperature of the two holders constant.

If a thermodynamic event occurs which is either endothermic or exothermic, the power requirements for the coils maintaining a constant temperature will differ. This power

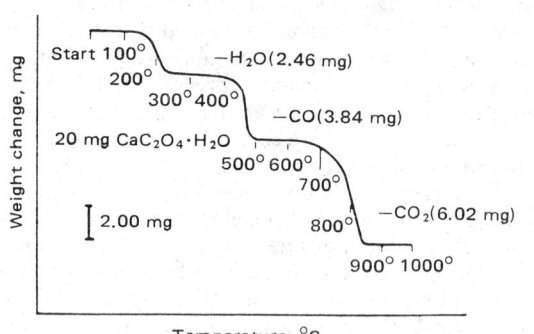

Fig 34-37. Thermogravimetric evaluation of calcium oxalate monohydrate, heating rate 6°/min. (Reproduced from Strobel.)

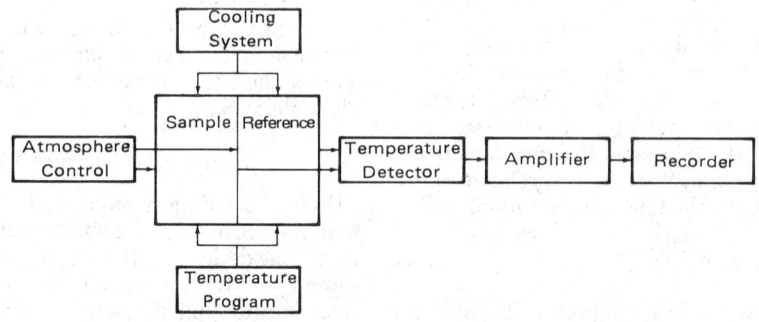

Fig 34-38. Block diagram of differential thermal analyzer.

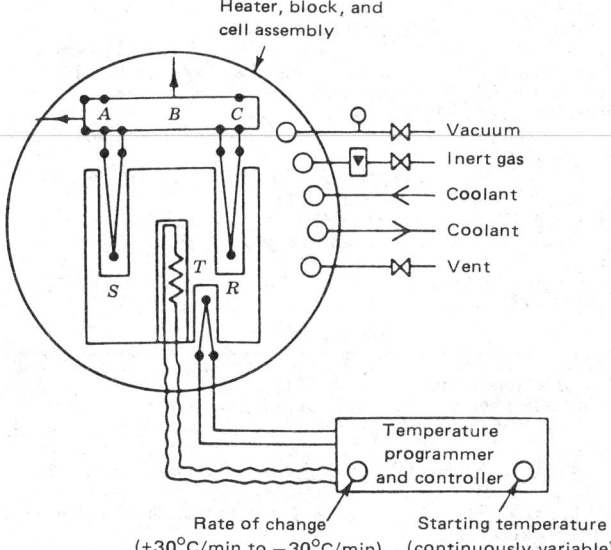

Heater, block, and
cell assembly

Vacuum
Inert gas
Coolant
Coolant
Vent

Temperature
programmer
and controller

Rate of change
(+30°C/min to −30°C/min)

Starting temperature
(continuously variable)

Fig 34-39   Schematic diagram of the Du Pont differential thermal analysis apparatus. (Reproduced from Willard, Merritt, Dean & Settle).

difference (ΔP) is plotted as a function of the temperature recorded by the programming device.

Unlike DTA, in DSC the amount of heat put into the system is exactly equivalent to the amount of heat absorbed or liberated during a specific transition (transition energy).

Thermomechanical Analysis (TMA)

This technique is useful for the measurements of changes in shape, volume or dimensions, penetration characteristics and viscoelastic properties of different materials as a function of controlled temperature elevation. The sample is usually contained in a small tube that is connected through a quartz probe to a differential transformer. Any movement in the sample upon heating is monitored by the displacement of the transformer. Modifications in the sample stage and probe enable the measurements of other sample characteristics, such as tensile strength, volume expansion, penetration, elasticity, etc.

Bibliography

Instrumental Methods of Analysis, General

Ewing GW: *Instrumental Methods of Chemical Analysis*, 4th ed, McGraw-Hill, New York, 1975.
Mann CK, *et al: Instrumental Analysis*, Harper-Row, New York, 1974.
Strobel HA: *Chemical Instrumentation*, 2nd ed, Addison-Wesley, Reading, MA, 1973.
Willard HH, *et al: Instrumental Methods of Analysis*, 5th ed, Van Nostrand, New York, 1974.
Skoog DA, and West DM: *Principles of Instrumental Analysis*, Holt, Rinehart and Winston, Inc, 1971.
Moore WJ: *Physical Chemistry*, 3rd Edition, Prentice-Hall, Inc, Englewood Cliffs, NJ, 1962.
Pharmaceutical Analysis, Modern Methods, Part A, Edited by JW Munson, Marcel Dekker, Inc, NY, 1981.
Analytical Chemistry, Fundamental Reviews, April 1982, American Chemical Society, Washington, DC.
Instrumentation in Analytical Chemistry, Vol 2, Edited by SA Borman, 1982, American Chemical Society, Washington, DC.

X-Ray Spectrometry

Bertin EP: *Principles and Practice of X-Ray Spectrometric Analysis*, 2nd ed, Plenum, New York, 1975.
Birks L: *X-Ray Spectrochemical Analysis*, 2nd ed, Interscience, New York, 1969.
Liebhafsky H, *et al: X-Rays, Electrons and Analytical Chemistry: Spectrochemical Analysis with X-Ray*, Wiley, New York, 1972.

Nuffield EW: *X-Ray Diffraction Methods*, Wiley, New York, 1966.
Nyburg SC: *X-Ray Analysis of Organic Structures*, Academic, New York, 1961.
Johnson Q, Mitchell AC, Smith IP: *Rev Sci Instr 51*, 741–749, 1980.
Tanner BK: *X-ray Diffraction Topography;* Pergamon: Oxford, England, 1976, p 188.
Attard AE, Lee HC: *J Chem Ed 56*, 650, 1979.
Gabe EJ, Lee FI: *Acta Crystallogr Sect A*, (Denmark) *A37*, 1981 (Supp).
Mallony CL, Snyder RL: *Adv X-ray Anal 22*, 121–131, 1978.

Ultraviolet and Visible Spectrometry

Braude EA: in *Determination of Organic Structures by Physical Methods*, Academic, New York, Chap 4, 131–194, 1955.
Duncan ABF, Matsen FA: in Weissberger A, ed: *Technique of Organic Chemistry*, vol IX, 2nd ed, Interscience, New York, 581–706, 1968–1970.
Hershenson HM: *Ultraviolet and Visible Absorption Spectra, Index*, 1930–1963, 6 vols, Academic Press, New York, 1966.
Jaffe HH, Orchin M: *Theory and Applications of Ultraviolet Spectroscopy*, Wiley, New York, 1962.
Lang L: *Absorption Spectra in the Ultraviolet and Visible Region*, vols 1–17, Academic, New York, 1961–1973.
Scott AI: *Interpretation of the Ultraviolet Spectra of Natural Products*, Pergamon, New York, 1964.
Organic Electronic Spectral Data, vols I–VII, Interscience, New York, 1960–1971 (covers literature from 1946 to 1967).
ASTM Index to Ultraviolet and Visible Spectra, ASTM Tech. Publ. 357, ASTM, Philadelphia, 1963.
Harris TD: *Analytical Chemistry, 54*, 741A, 1982.
Montegu B, Langier A, Fournier J: *J Phys E, 12*, 1153–1158, 1979.

Near IR Spectroscopy

Abu-Shumays A: *Varian Instruments Literatures* (VIA).
Kermit BW: *Near Infrared Spectrophotometry*, Appl Spect Rev 2, 1, 1968.

Infrared Spectrometry

Bellamy LJ: *The Infrared Spectra of Complex Molecules*, 3rd ed, Wiley, New York, 1975.
Dyer JR: *Organic Spectral Problems*, Prentice-Hall, Englewood Cliffs, NJ, 1972.
Hershenson HM: *Infrared Absorption Spectra, Index*, 1947–1954, 2 vol, Academic Press, 1965.
Lang L, ed: *Absorption Spectra in the Infrared Region*, vols I and II, Butterworths, London, 1974 and 1976.
Martin AE: *Infrared Instrumentation and Techniques*, Elsevier, New York, 1966.
Nyquist RA, Kegel RO: *Infrared Spectra of Inorganic Compounds*, Academic Press, New York, 1971.
Catalog of Infrared Spectra, Sadtler Research Labs., Philadelphia.
Silverstein RM, *et al: Spectrometric Identification of Organic Compounds*, 3rd ed, Wiley, New York, 1974.
Szymanski HA, Erickson RE: *Infrared Band Handbook*, rev ed, Plenum, New York, 1970 (Suppls 1 and 2 cover the 200–600 cm⁻¹ region).
Vornhederand PF, Brabbs WJ: *Anal Chem 42*, 1454, 1970.
Marshall A: *Fourier, Hadamard, and Hilbert Transforms in Chemistry*, Plenum Press, NY, 1982.
Hurley WJ: *J Chem Educ 43*, 236, 1966.
Low MJD: *J Chem Educ 47*, A163, A255, and A415, 1970.
Colthup NB, Daly LH and Wiberly SE: *Introduction to Infrared and Raman Spectroscopy*, Academic Press, NY, 2nd Ed, (1975), pp 111, 112.
Silverstein RM, Bassler GC, and Morrill TC: *Spectrometric Identification of Organic Compounds*, 3rd Edition, John Wiley and Sons, Inc, NY, 1974, p 194.

Nuclear Magnetic Resonance

Bible RH, Jr: *Interpretation of NMR Spectra*, Plenum New York, 1965.
Bible RH, Jr: *Guide to the Empirical Method: A Workbook*, Plenum, New York, 1967.
Hershenson HM: *Nuclear Magnetic Resonance and Electron Spin Resonance Index*, 1958–1963, Academic, New York, 1965.
Jackman LM, Sternhell S: *Applications of Nuclear Magnetic Resonance Spectroscopy in Organic Chemistry*, 2nd ed, Pergamon, New York, 1969.
Nuclear Magnetic Resonance Spectra, Sadtler Res Labs, Philadelphia.
High Resolution NMR Spectra Catalogue, vols 1 and 2, Varian Associates, Palo Alto, CA, 1962–1963.
Sadtler Guide to NMR Spectra of Polymers, Sadtler Res Labs, Philadelphia, 1973.
Simons WW, Zanger M: *Sadtler Guide to NMR Spectra*, Sadtler Res Labs, Philadelphia, 1972.

Szymanski HA, Yellin RE: *NMR Band Handbook*, Plenum, NY, 1968.

Stothers JB: *Carbon-13 NMR Spectroscopy*, Academic Press, New York, 1972.

Johnson LF, Jankowski WC: *Catalog of Carbon-13 NMR Spectra*, Wiley, New York, 1972.

Nunnally RL, Bottomley PA: *Science, 211*, 177–180, 1981.

Norton RD: *Bull Magn Reson, 3*, 29–48, 1980.

Farrar TC, Becker ED: *Pulse and Fourier Transform NMR*, Academic Press, New York, 1971.

Shaw D: *Fourier Transform NMR Spectroscopy*, Elsevier, New York, 1976.

Baum RM: *C&EN*, Jan 1983, (pp 30–31).

Paudler WW: *Nuclear Magnetic Resonance*, Allyn and Bacon, Boston, MA, 1971.

Emsley JW, Feeney T, and Sutcliffe LH: *High Resolution NMR Spectroscopy*, Vol I and II, Pergamon Press, NY, 1967.

ESR

Gordy W: *Theory and Applications of Electron Spin Resonance*, Wiley, NY, 1980.

Bertini I, Drago RS: *ESR and NMR of Paramagnetic Species in Biological and Related Systems*, Kluwer Boston, Inc, Hingham, MA, 1980.

Woodward AE, Bovey FA, Eds: *Polymer Characterization by ESR and NMR*, American Chemical Society, Washington, DC, 1980.

Emission Spectrometry, Flame Photometry, and Atomic Absorption Spectrometry

Ahrens LH, Taylor SR: *Spectrochemical Analysis*, 2nd ed, Addison-Wesley, Reading, MA, 1961.

Brode WR: *Chemical Spectroscopy*, 2nd ed, Wiley, New York, 1943.

Elwell WT, Gidley JAF: *Atomic Absorption Spectrophotometry*, 2nd rev ed, Pergamon, New York, 1966.

Mavrodineanu R, ed: *Analytical Flame Spectroscopy*, Springer-Verlag, Berlin, 1971.

Meggers WF, *et al: Tables of Spectral-Line Intensities*, Parts I and II. Natl Bur Std (US) Monograph 32, USGPO, Washington, DC, 1961–1962 (Corliess CH, rev ed, 1967).

Walsh A: *Spectrochim Acta*, 7, 108, (1955).

Alkemade CTJ and Milatz JMW: *Appl Sci Research, B4*, 289, 1955, J Opt Soc Amer, *45*, 583, 1955.

Van Loon JC: *Analytical Atomic Absorption Spectroscopy, Selected Methods*, Academic Press, NY, 1980.

Pinta M: *Atomic Absorption Spectrometry*, Vol 2, Application to Chemical Analysis, 2nd Ed, Masson: Paris, 1980.

Godden RG, Thomerson DR: *Analyst* (London) *105*, 1137, 1980.

Dedina J, Rubeska I: *Spectrochim Acta*, Part B, *35B*, 119, 1980.

Styris DL, Kaye JH: *Spectrochim Acta*, Part B, *36B*, 41, 1981.

Willard H, Merritt L, Dean J, Settle F: *Instrumental Methods of Analysis*, 6th Edition, D Van Nostrand Company, NY, 1981.

Read TB: *J Appl Phys, 32*, 821, 2534, 1961.

Reed TB: *Int Sci Technol*, 142, (June 1962).

Fluorescence and Phosphorescence Spectrometry

Guilbault GC: *Fluorescence: Theory, Instrumentation and Practice*, Dekker, NY, 1967.

Hercules DM, ed: *Fluorescence and Phosphorescence Analysis: Principles and Applications*, Interscience, NY, 1966.

Udenfriend S: *Fluorescence Assay in Biology and Medicine*, Academic, NY, 1962.

Light Scattering, Refractometry, and Polarimetry

Batsanov SS: *Refractometry and Chemical Structure II*, Consultant Bureau Enterprises, NY, 1961.

Crabbe P: *ORD and CD in Chemistry and Biochemistry*, Academic, NY, 1972.

Djerassi C: *Optical Rotatory Dispersion*, McGraw-Hill, NY, 1960.

Stacey K: *Light-Scattering in Physical Chemistry*, Butterworths, London, 1956.

Weissberger A, ed: *Physical Methods in Organic Chemistry*, vol 1, 3rd ed, Interscience, NY, Part II, 1960.

Mass Spectrometry

Beynon JH, *et al: The Mass Spectra of Organic Molecules*, Elsevier, NY, 1968.

Budzikiewicz H, *et al: Interpretation of Mass Spectra of Organic Compounds*, Holden-Day, San Francisco, 1964.

Budzikiewicz H, *et al: Structure Elucidation of Natural Products by Mass Spectrometry*, vols I and II, Holden-Day, San Francisco, 1964.

Silverstein RM, Bassler GC: *Spectrometric Identification of Organic Compounds*, 3rd ed, Wiley, NY, 1974.

Catalog of Mass Spectra Data, Am Petrol Inst Res Pro 44, Carnegie Inst Technol, Pittsburgh.

Index of Mass Spectral Data, ASTM Spec Tech Publ 356, ASTM, Philadelphia, 1963.

Busch K, Cooks R: *Analytical Chemistry, 55*, 38A, 1983.

Comisarow M, Marshall A: *Chem Phys Lett, 25*, 282–283, 1974; 26, 489–490, 1975.

Comisarow M, Marshall A: *Can J Chem, 52*, 1997–99, 1974.

Fellgett P: *J Phys Radium*, 1958, 19 (187–91).

Electrochemistry

Brezina M, Zuman P: *Polarography in Medicine, Biochemistry, and Pharmacy*, Interscience, Wiley, New York, 1958.

Hills GJ: *Polarography*, vols I and II, Interscience, New York, 1966.

Latimer WM: *Oxidation Potential*, 2nd ed, Prentice-Hall, Englewood Cliffs, NJ, 1956.

Meites L: *Polarographic Techniques*, 2nd ed, Interscience, New York, 1965.

Milner GW, Phillips G: *Coulometry in Analytical Chemistry*, Pergamon, New York, 1968.

Stock JT: *Amperometric Titration*, Wiley, New York, 1965.

Pinta M: *Modern Methods for Trace Element Analysis*, Ann Arbor Science Publishers, Ann Arbor, MI, (1978).

Bond AM: *Modern Polarographic Methods in Analytical Chemistry*, Marcel Dekker, New York, 1980.

Meites I: *Polarographic Techniques*, Interscience, New York, 1965.

Vydra F, Stulik K, Julakova E: *Electrochemical Stripping Analysis*, Halstead Press-Wiley, New York, 1973.

Brainina KZ: *Stripping Voltammetry in Chemical Analysis*, Halstead Press-Wiley, New York, 1974.

Sadana R: *Anal Chem, 55*, 304–307, 1983.

Schenidman F, Lewis M, Jarved I: *American Laboratory*, June 1982, pp 47–54.

Winograd N and Kuwana T: *Electroanalytical Chemistry*, Vol 7, AJ Bard, Ed, Marcel Dekker, New York, 1974.

McIntyre JDE: *Advances in Electrochemistry and Electrochemical Engineering*, Vol 9, RH Muller, Ed, Wiley-Interscience, New York, 1973.

Thermal Analysis

Schwenker RF, Garn PD: *Thermal Analysis*, 2 vols, Academic, New York, 1969.

Smothers WJ, Chiang MS: *Differential Thermal Analysis*, Chemical Publishing, New York, 1958.

Wendlandt WW: *Thermal Methods of Analysis*, 2nd ed, vol 19 of Chemical Analysis, Wiley, New York, 1974.

Wunderlich B: *The Impact of Computers on Thermal Analysis*, American Laboratory, June 1982, p 28–44.

Mackenzie RC: *Differential Thermal Analysis*, (Vol 1&2), Academic Press, New York, 1970–1972.

Kambe H, and Garn PD: *Thermal Analysis, Comparative Studies on Materials*, Wiley, New York, 1974.

Daniels T: *Thermal Analysis*, John Wiley & Sons, New York, 1973.

Liptay G: *Atlas of Thermoanalytical Curves*, Vol 1–5, Heyden & Sons, Ltd, London, 1976.

The author would like to express his deepest gratitude to Dr AR Gennaro, the previous author of this chapter and present chairman of Remington's Editorial Board for his input and valuable recommendations which were extremely helpful in completing this work in its present format. The author is also indebted to Dr T Medwick, College of Pharmacy, Rutgers University, Dr E Gusmano, Dr C Papastephanou, Dr GL Hassert, Dr G Brewer and Dr J Kirschbaum of ER Squibb and Sons Inc for their many contributions to the proofreading of the manuscript. I wish also to thank Ms C Mathews for her patience and professional expertise in typing and preparing the manuscript, and finally my wife Faye and my daughter Nyier for their unwavering support and sacrifices that were imposed during the writing of this chapter.

CHAPTER 35

Dissolution

Hamed M Abdou, PhD

Director of Product Quality Control
E R Squibb & Sons, Inc
Georges Rd, New Brunswick, NJ 08903

Dissolution is the process by which a solid solute of only fair solubility characteristics enters into solution. The earliest reference to dissolution is probably an article by Noyes and Whitney in 1897, about "The Rate of Solution of Solid Substances in Their Own Solution." The authors suggested that the rate of dissolution of solid substances is determined by the rate of diffusion of a very thin layer of saturated solution that forms instantaneously around the solid particle. Noyes and Whitney developed the mathematical relationship that correlates the dissolution rate to the solubility gradient of the solid. Their equation is still the basic formula upon which most of the modern mathematical treatments of the dissolution phenomenon revolve. Noyes and Whitney's work however, as well as most of the work which has been conducted during the first part of this century, was concentrated on the study of the physicochemical aspects of dissolution as applied to chemical substances. Most important of these studies were the application of Fick's law of diffusion to the Noyes and Whitney equation by Nernst and Brunner in 1904 and the development of the famous cubic root law of dissolution by Hixson and Crowell in 1931.

At the middle of the century, emphasis started to shift to the examination of the effects of dissolution behavior of drugs on the biological activity of pharmaceutical dosage forms. One of the earliest studies with this purpose in mind was conducted by J Edwards in 1951 on aspirin tablets. Based on his findings, Edwards reported that "because of its poor solubility, the analgesic action of aspirin tablets would be controlled by its dissolution rate within the stomach and the intestine." No *in vivo* studies, however, were conducted by Edwards to support his postulate. About eight years later, Shenoy *et al* proved the validity of Edward's suggestion of the *in vitro/in vivo* correlation by demonstrating a direct relationship between the bioavailability of amphetamine from sustained release tablets and its *in vitro* dissolution rate. Other studies, especially those reported by Nelson, Levy and Hays, confirmed beyond doubt, the significant effect of the dissolution behavior of drugs on their pharmacological activities. Because of the novelty and importance of these findings, dissolution testing began to emerge as a dominant topic within both the pharmaceutical academia and the drug industry. In the late sixties biopharmaceutics were established as an important discipline in the pharmaceutical sciences and dissolution testing became a mandatory USP requirement for several dosage forms. Dissolution, however, is still far from being understood perfectly. In spite of the reported success of several *in vitro/in vivo* correlation studies, dissolution is not a predictor of therapeutic efficiency. Rather, it is a qualitative tool which can provide valuable information about the biological availability of a drug as well as batch to batch consistency. Another area of difficulty is the fact that the accuracy and precision of the testing procedure is dependent to a large extent on the strict observance of so many subtle parameters and detailed operational controls.

In spite of these shortcomings, dissolution is considered today as one of the most important quality control tests performed on pharmaceutical dosage forms.

Theory of Dissolution

Diffusion Layer Model (Film Theory)

In 1897, Noyes and Whitney studied the dissolution rate of benzoic acid and lead chloride, two practically insoluble substances, by rotating a cylinder of each compound in water at a constant rate and sampling the solution for analysis at specific time intervals. In order to examine their data quantitatively, Noyes and Whitney developed an equation based on Fick's second law, to describe the dissolution phenomenon;

$$\frac{dc}{dt} = K(c_s - c_t) \tag{1}$$

where,

dc/dt = dissolution rate of the drug
K = the proportionality constant
c_s = the saturation concentration (maximum solubility)
c_t = concentration at time t
$c_s - c_t$ = concentration gradient

The proportionality constant K is also called the dissolution constant and the equation has been shown to obey first order kinetics (Fig 1).

In their experiments, Noyes and Whitney maintained a constant surface area by using sticks of the insoluble substance. However, because such a condition is not always applicable, Brunner and Tolloczko modified Eq 1 to incorporate the surface area, S, as a separate variable.

$$\frac{dc}{dt} = k_1 S(c_s - c_t) \tag{2}$$

In order to explain the mechanism of dissolution, Nernst in 1904 proposed the film model theory. Under the influence of no reactive or chemical forces, a solid particle immersed in a liquid, undergoes two consecutive steps; first is the solution of the solid at the interface, forming a thin stagnant layer or film, h, around the particle; and second, is the diffusion from this layer at the boundary to the bulk of the fluid. The first step, solution, is almost instantaneous, the second, diffusion, is much slower and therefore, is the rate limiting step (see Fig 2).

In the same year, Brunner was investigating factors other than surface area that affect the dissolution process in order to determine the fundamental components of the proportionality constant in Eq 1. By utilizing Fick's first law of diffusion and Nernst's newly proposed film theory, Brunner expanded Eq 2 to include the diffusion coefficient, D, the thickness of the stagnant diffusion layer, h, and the volume of the dissolution medium, v, producing Eq 3.

$$\frac{dc}{dt} = k_2 \frac{DS}{vh}(c_s - c_t) \tag{3}$$

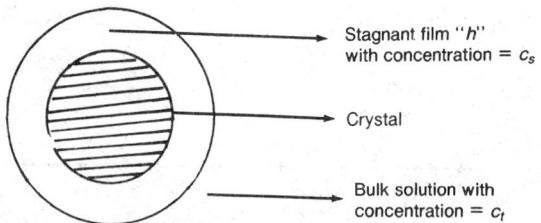

Fig 35-1. Diffusion layer model (film theory).

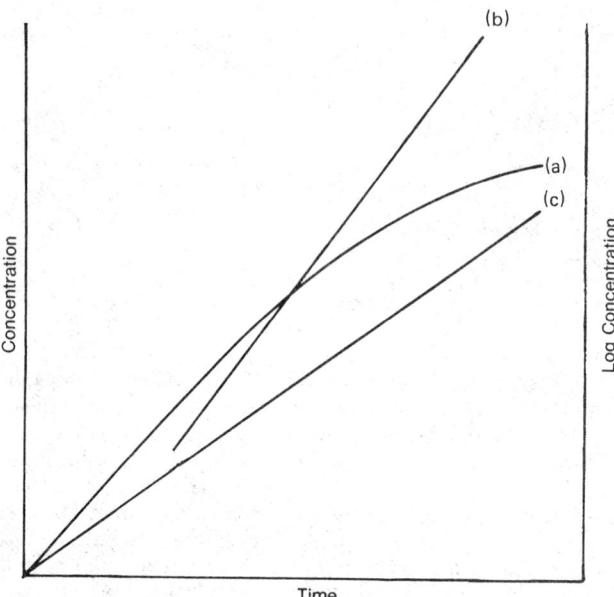

Fig 35-2. First-order kinetic plot. (A) Linear (dissolution rate under non-sink condition). (B) Semi-log (dissolution rate under non-sink condition). (C) Linear (dissolution rate under sink condition).

The proportionality constant k_2 is known as the intrinsic dissolution rate constant and is characteristic of each chemical compound.

Sink Condition

The term *sink* condition originated from a fact long known by pharmacologists that the drug concentration on both sides of the epithelial layer of the intestinal wall approaches equilibrium in a short time, and that the gastrointestinal tract acts as a *natural sink*; ie, the drug is instantaneously absorbed the moment it dissolves. Therefore, under *in vivo* conditions, there is no concentration buildup and hence the retarding effect of the concentration gradient on the dissolution rate, as predicted by Eq 1, does not occur.

In order to simulate the *in vivo* sink condition, *in vitro* dissolution testing is usually conducted using either a large volume of dissolution medium or a mechanism by which the dissolution medium is constantly replenished with fresh solvent at a specified rate so that the concentration of the solute never reaches more than 10–15% of its maximum solubility. If such a parameter is maintained, the dissolution testing is said to be conducted under *sink* conditions, ie, under no influence of the concentration gradient. This could be seen from the following mathematical treatment.

Assuming that $c_s \gg c_t$, Eq 3 becomes,

$$\frac{dc}{dt} = k_2 \frac{DS}{vh} c_s \tag{4}$$

As c_s and D are constants for each specific chemical substance, therefore they could be incorporated in k_2 and Eq 4 becomes,

$$\frac{dc}{dt} = k_3 \frac{S}{vh} \tag{5}$$

If the volume of the dissolution medium and the surface area are kept constant during the duration of the dissolution test, then

$$\frac{dc}{dt} = K \tag{6}$$

Eq 6 predicts a constant dissolution rate under sink condition and represents a zero order kinetic process, ie, the concentration of the drug increases linearly with time. Eq 6 is also believed to approximate the *in vivo* condition where the dissolution rate of sparingly soluble drugs plays a fundamental role in determining their bioavailability. Figure 2 presents plots of data that would be expected under sink and non-sink conditions.

Hixson and Crowell Cubic Root Law for Dissolution

In Eq 2, the surface area was considered constant for the duration of the dissolution test. Although this could be achieved by using a nondisintegrating disk of the chemical substance, a technique usually employed for the determination of the intrinsic dissolution rate, the same could not be

maintained for a dissolving crystal or a regular solid dosage form where complete disintegration is a priority. Therefore, in order to develop a dissolution equation that is based on a changing surface area, Hixson and Crowell modified Eq 2 to represent the rate of appearance of the solute in the solution by multiplying each side of the equation by v (volume), letting $k_2 v = K$;

$$\frac{dW}{dt} = KS(c_s - c_t) \tag{7}$$

where W is the weight of solute in solution.

They also assumed that $S = kw^{2/3}$, where k is a constant containing the shape factor and the density of the particle, and w is the weight of undissolved particles at time t,

$$\frac{dW}{dt} = K(kw^{2/3})(c_s - c_t) \tag{8}$$

After multiple mathematical treatments involving the application of Fick's first law and integration under the condition that w is equal to w_o, the initial weight of the particle at time zero, Eq 9 results,

$$w_o^{1/3} - w^{1/3} = K^1 t \tag{9}$$

Eq 9 is called the Hixson and Crowell's "Cubic Root Law" for dissolution.

Theoretical Concepts for the Release of a Drug from Dosage Forms

In determining the dissolution rate of drugs from solid dosage forms under standardized conditions, one has to consider several physicochemical processes in addition to those previously discussed under dissolution of pure chemical substances. These include the wetting characteristics of the solid dosage forms, the penetration ability of the dissolution medium into the dosage forms, the swelling process, disintegration and deaggregation. Wagner proposed the following scheme for the processes involved in the dissolution of solid dosage forms.

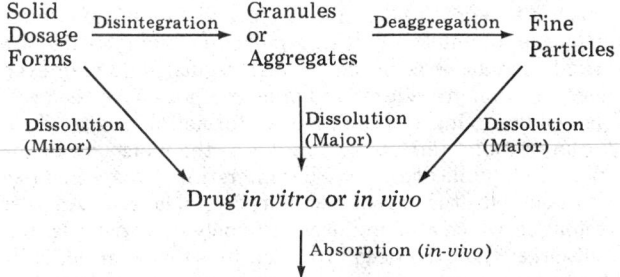

Drug in Blood and Other Fluids and Tissues

Carstensen explained that the wetting of the dosage solid surface controls the liquid access to the solid surface and, many times, is the limiting factor in the dissolution process. The speed of wetting is directly dependent upon the surface tension at the interface (interfacial tension) and upon the contact angle, θ, between the solid surface and the liquid. Generally, a contact angle of more than 90° indicates poor wettability. Incorporation of a surfactant, either in the formulation or in the dissolution medium, lowers the contact angle and enhances dissolution. Also, the presence of air in the dissolution medium causes the air bubbles to be entrapped in the tablet pores and act as a barrier at the interface. For capsules, the gelatin shell is extremely hydrophilic, and, therefore, no problems in wettability exist for the dosage itself (although it may exist for the powders inside).

After the solid dosage form disintegrates into granules or aggregates, penetration characteristics play a prime role in the deaggregation process. Hydrophobic lubricants, such as talc and magnesium stearate, commonly employed in tablet and capsule formulations, slow the penetration rate and, hence, the deaggregation process. A large pore size facilitates penetration, but if it is too large it may inhibit penetration by decreasing the internal strain caused by the swelling of the disintegrant.

After deaggregation and dislodgement occur, the drug particles become exposed to the dissolution medium and dissolution proceeds as previously discussed under the Film Theory. Fig 3 graphically presents the model proposed by Carstensen.

Correlation Between Disintegration and Dissolution

The close correlation between disintegration and dissolution has been studied by many investigators. Both processes exhibit "S"-shaped curves and a probit or a weibul function were suggested to explain the data. In general, however, disintegration has proved to be a poor indicator of bioavailability because of the turbulent agitation maintained during the test. Several other factors such as solubility, particle size, and crystalline structure, among others, have been found to affect seriously the dissolution of the drug substance but have no relevance to distintegration.

Factors Affecting the Rate of Dissolution

Factors that affect the dissolution rate of drug dosage forms can be classified under three main categories as delineated below.

1.   Factors Relating to the Physiochemical Properties of the Drug

The physicochemical properties of the drug substance play a prime role in controlling its dissolution from the dosage form. The modified Noyes and Whitney equation as expressed in Eq 3 shows that the aqueous solubility of the drug is the major

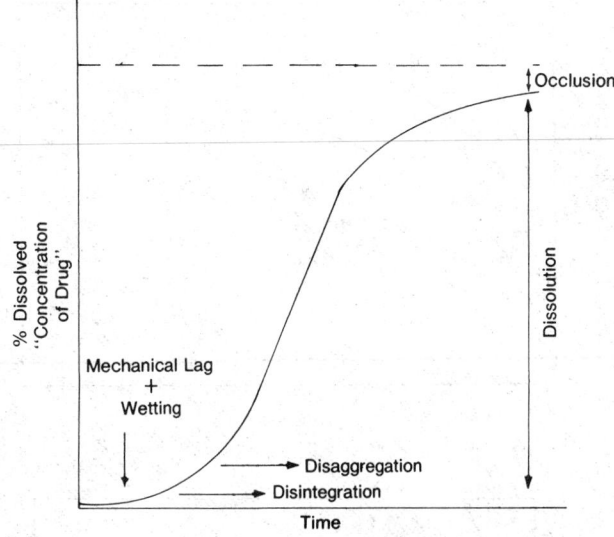

Fig 35-3.   The S-shaped dissolution curve of solid dosage forms. (Cartensen, J: Procedures of the Second Wisconsin Update Conference, "Dissolution—State of the Art 1982," October 25–27, 1982.

factor which determines its dissolution rate. Actually, some studies showed that drug solubility data could be used as a rough predictor of the possibility of any future problems with bioavailability, a factor that should be taken into consideration in the formulation design.

Other factors that affect dissolution rate include particle size; crystalline state, such as polymorphism and state of hydration, solvation, complexation, as well as surfactants and other reactive additives (acids, bases, buffers, etc). Other physical properties such as density, viscosity, and wettability contribute to the general dissolution problems of flocculation, flotation and agglomeration. Adsorption characteristics of the drug have also been found to have a significant effect on the dissolution of certain drugs.

Effect of Particle Size on Dissolution Rate

Eq 3 shows a direct relationship between the surface area of the drug and its dissolution rate. Since the surface area increases with decreasing particle size, higher dissolution rates may be achieved through reduction of the particle size. This effect has been highlighted by the superior dissolution rate observed after *micronization* of certain sparingly soluble drugs as opposed to the regularly milled form. Micronization increases the surface area exposed to the dissolution medium and, hence, improves the rate of dissolution. Several investigations have demonstrated an increased absorption rate for griseofulvin after micronization. Similar effects have been reported for chloramphenicol, tetracycline salts, sulfadiazine, and norethisterone acetate. In the case of chloramphenicol, studies showed that formulations containing smaller particles (50–200 μm) were absorbed faster than formulations containing larger particles (400–800 μm). Fig 4 presents the effect of particle size differences on the dissolution rate of phenacetin and phenobarbital.

It should be recognized, however, that the mere increase in the surface area of the drug does not always guarantee an equivalent increase in dissolution rate. Rather, it is the increase in the *effective* surface area, or the area exposed to the dissolution medium, and not the absolute surface area, that is directly proportional to the dissolution rate.

Physical properties of the drug particles other than size also affect indirectly the effective surface area by modifying the shear rate of the fresh solvent that comes in contact with the solid. These properties include the particle shape and the density.

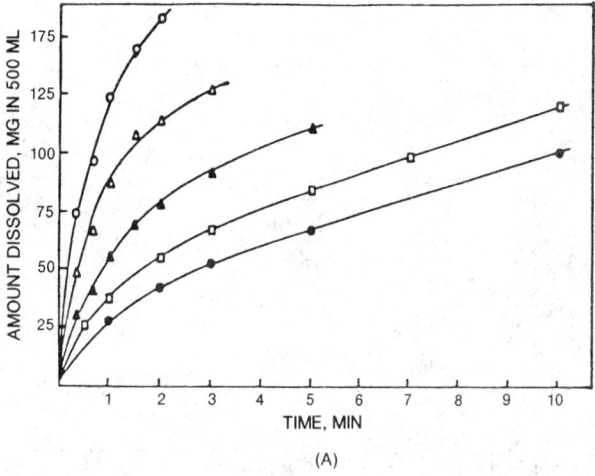

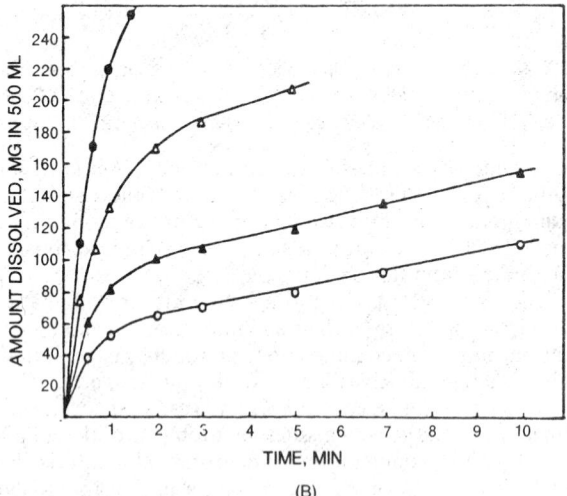

Fig 35-4.   Effect of particle size on the dissolution rate of drugs from solid dosage forms.   (Reproduced from P Finholt, "Dissolution Technology," p 108, published by the Industrial Pharmaceutical Technology Section of the Academy of Pharmaceutical Science, 1974, Editors, L Leeson and J Cartensen.)

(A) *Key:*   (Phenacetin) ○ particle size: 0.11–0.15 mm; △ particle size: 0.15–0.21 mm; ▲ particle size: 0.21–0.30 mm; □ particle size: 0.30–0.50 mm; ● particle size: 0.50–0.71 mm.   (B) *Key:* Phenobarbital ● particle size: 0.07–0.15 mm; △ particle size: 0.15–0.25 mm; ▲ particle size: 0.25–0.42 mm; ○ particle size: 0.42–0.71 mm.

Effect of Particle Size on Solubility

Another mechanism by which the reduction in particle size improves dissolution is through the enhancement of the drug solubility (c_s).   It should be pointed out that Eq 3 has an inherent limitation in assuming that c_s is independent of the particle size.   Actually c_s and the surface area can be correlated by the Ostwald-Freundlich equation.

$$ln\ S = \frac{2M\gamma}{\rho RT} \cdot \frac{1}{r} = \frac{\alpha}{r} \tag{10}$$

where M is the molecular weight, ρ is the density, γ is the interfacial tension or surface free energy of the solid, r is the radius of the particle, and T is the temperature.

From Eq 10 we have

$$S = S_\infty \cdot e^{\alpha/r} \tag{11}$$

The equation shows that the solubility is inversely proportional to particle radius.   Therefore, S could be viewed as the solubility of the micro particles and S_∞ as the solubility of the macro particles.   However, it is obvious that the particle radius has to be reduced to a micro level before it can effect a change in solubility.   This extreme reduction in particle size usually cannot be achieved through regular milling or even micronization procedures and other methods have been recommended.   One of these involves formation of a *solid-solution* or *molecular dispersion* where the molecules of the sparingly soluble drug are either interstitially dispersed in a water-soluble drug or replaced in its crystal lattice.   Another technique, which also produces extremely small particles but still larger than the ones produced by solid solution, is by dispersion of the drug into a soluble carrier such as polyvinylpyrrolidone (PVP) solution.   These techniques are usually employed for the enhancement of dissolution rate of insoluble drugs.

Effect of the Crystalline State of the Drug on Dissolution Rate

The solid phase characteristics of drugs, such as amorphicity, crystallinity, state of hydration and polymorphic structure have been shown to have a significant influence on the dissolution rate.   Mullins and Macek showed that the amorphous form of novobiocin has a greater solubility and higher dissolution rate than the crystalline form.   Blood level studies confirmed such findings where administration of the amorphous form yielded about 3–4 times the concentration compared to the administration of the crystalline form.   Similar differences were demonstrated for griseofulvin, phenobarbital, cortisone acetate, and chloramphenicol.

2.   Factors Relating to the Solid Dosage Form

The effects of various formulations and manufacturing processing factors on the rate of dissolution and the bioavailability of the active ingredients from tablets and capsules have been well documented by several investigators since the early sixties.   Although the magnitude and significance of these effects must be determined individually for each tablet or capsule product, the following discussion of earlier and current findings can certainly serve as a guideline for the pharmaceutical scientist, especially during the initial stages of formulation design and product development.

Effect of Formulation Factors on Tablet Dissolution Rate

It has been shown that the dissolution rate of a pure drug can be altered significantly when mixed with various adjuncts during the manufacturing process of solid dosage forms.   These adjuncts are added to satisfy certain pharmaceutical functions such as diluents (fillers), dyes, binders, granulating agents, disintegrants, and lubricants.   Generically identical tablet and capsule products, manufactured by different pharmaceutical houses, were found to exhibit significant differences in dissolution rates for their active ingredients.   In certain cases, several studies showed that poor tablet and capsule formulations have been shown to cause a marked decrease in bioavailability and impairment of the clinical response.   Such findings during the sixties, especially in the case of digoxin and tolbutamide tablets, as well as chloramphenicol and tetracycline HCl (all lifesaving drugs), were the main triggering factors that compelled drug regulatory agencies and compendial authorities to institute the dissolution test as a legal requirement for most solid dosage forms.

Diluents and Disintegrants

Levy, in 1963, studied the effect of starch, the most commonly used diluent, on the rate of dissolution of salicylic acid tablets manufactured by the dry, double compression process (Fig 5).   Increasing the starch content from 5 to 20% resulted in a dramatic increase in the dissolution rate (almost 3 fold).

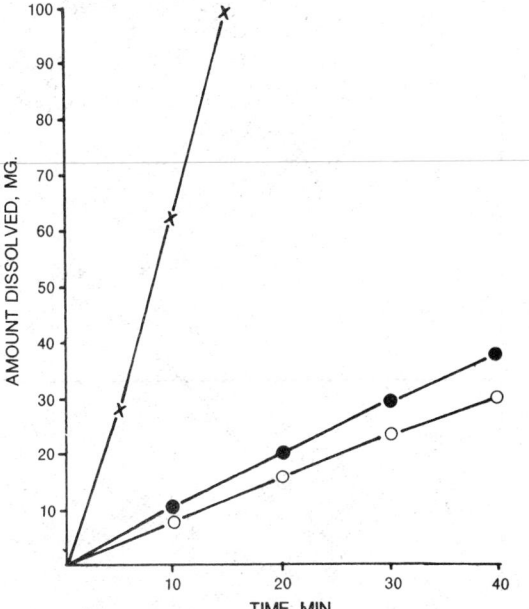

Fig 35-5.   Effect of starch content on dissolution rate.   [Reproduced from Levy, G, *et al*, J Pharm Sci: *52*, 1050, 1963.]
Key: O, 5%; ●, 10%; ×, 20% starch in granules.

This was attributed to better and more thorough disintegration.   Later, however, Finholt suggested that the hydrophobic drug crystals acquire a surface layer of fine starch particles that impart a hydrophilic property to the granular formulation and thereby increases the effective surface area and hence the dissolution rate.

Binders and Granulating Agents

Differences in binders used for tolbutamide tablets resulted in variable dissolution characteristics and differences in the hypoglycemic effects observed clinically.   Wet granulation, in general, has been shown to improve dissolution rates of poorly soluble drugs by imparting hydrophilic properties to the surface of the granules.   Solvang and Finholt showed that phenobarbital tablets granulated with gelatin solution dissolved much faster in human gastric juice than those prepared with sodium carboxymethylcellulose or polyethylene glycol 6000 as a binder.   They suggested that gelatin imparts hydrophilic characteristics to the hydrophobic drug surface, whereas polyethylene glycol forms a complex with poor solubility and sodium carboxymethylcellulose is converted to its less soluble acid form in low pH gastric juice (Fig 6).

Lubricants

Levy and Gumtow investigated the effects of different types of lubricants on the dissolution rate of salicylic acid tablets. They found that magnesium stearate, a hydrophobic lubricant, tends to retard the dissolution rate of salicylic acid tablets, while a water-soluble surface-active lubricant, sodium lauryl sulfate, enhanced the dissolution rate significantly (Fig 7).   Investigating the mechanism of retardation they suggested that hydrophobic lubricants, such as magnesium stearate, aluminum stearate, stearic acid, and talc, decrease the effective drug-solvent interfacial area by changing the surface characteristics of the tablets which results in reducing its wettability, prolonging its disintegration time, and decreasing the area of the interface between the active ingredient and solvent.   The enhancing effect of sodium lauryl sulfate, on the other hand, was suggested to be due, in part, to an increase in the microenvironment pH surrounding the sparingly soluble weak acid and to increased wetting and better solvent

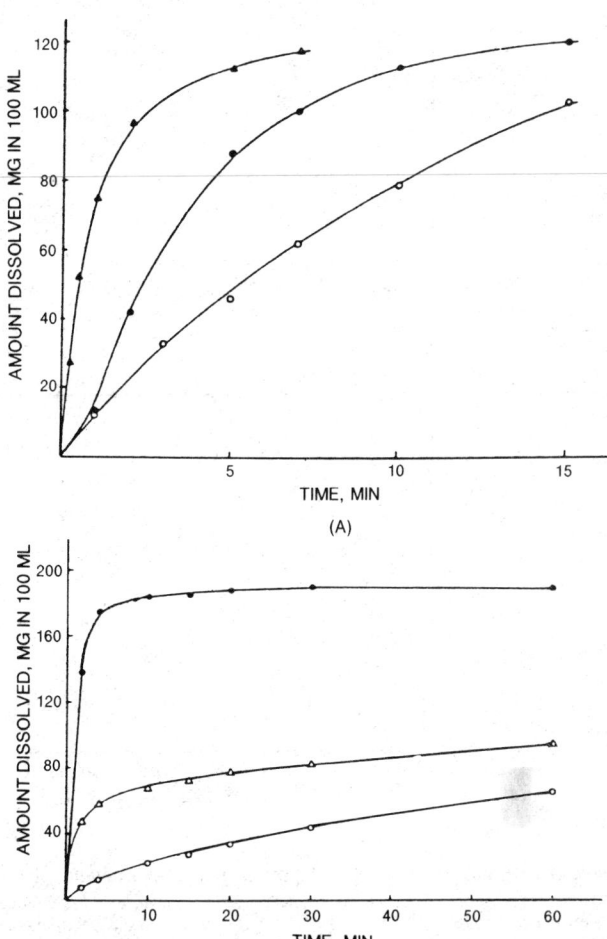

(A)

(B)

Fig 35-6.   Effect of binders and granulating agents on dissolution rate of tablets.   [Reproduced from Solvang and Finholt, J Pharm Sci: *59*, 50, 51, 1970.]

(A) Rate of dissolution of phenacetin from powder, granules, and tablets in diluted gastric juice (surface tension 42.7 dynes cm.$^{-1}$, pH 1.85). *Key:* O, phenacetin powder; ▲, phenacetin granules; ●, phenacetin tablets.   (B) Dissolution rate of Phenobarbital Tablets in Diluted Gastric Juice (surface tension 39.4 dynes cm^{-1}, pH 1.50). *Key:* ● Gelatin Binder, △ CMC, O Polyethylene glycol 6000.

penetration into the tablets and granules as a result of lowering the interfacial tension between the solid surface and the solvent.   The fact that sodium lauryl sulfate is a water-soluble lubricant was not considered a factor in improving the dissolution rate of the tablet, since sodium stearate, another water-soluble lubricant, was found to have a retarding effect on the dissolution rate.

Effects of the Processing Factors on Dissolution Rates of Tablets

The many processing factors used in tablet manufacturing greatly influence the dissolution rates of the active ingredients. The method of granulation, the size, density, moisture content and age of the granules, as well as the compression force utilized in the tableting process, all contribute to the dissolution-rate characteristics of the final product.

Method of Granulation

Studies have shown that the granulation process, in general, enhances the dissolution rate of poorly soluble drugs.   The use of fillers and diluents, such as starch, spray-dried lactose and microcrystalline cellulose, tend to increase the hydrophilicity of the active ingredients and improve their dissolu-

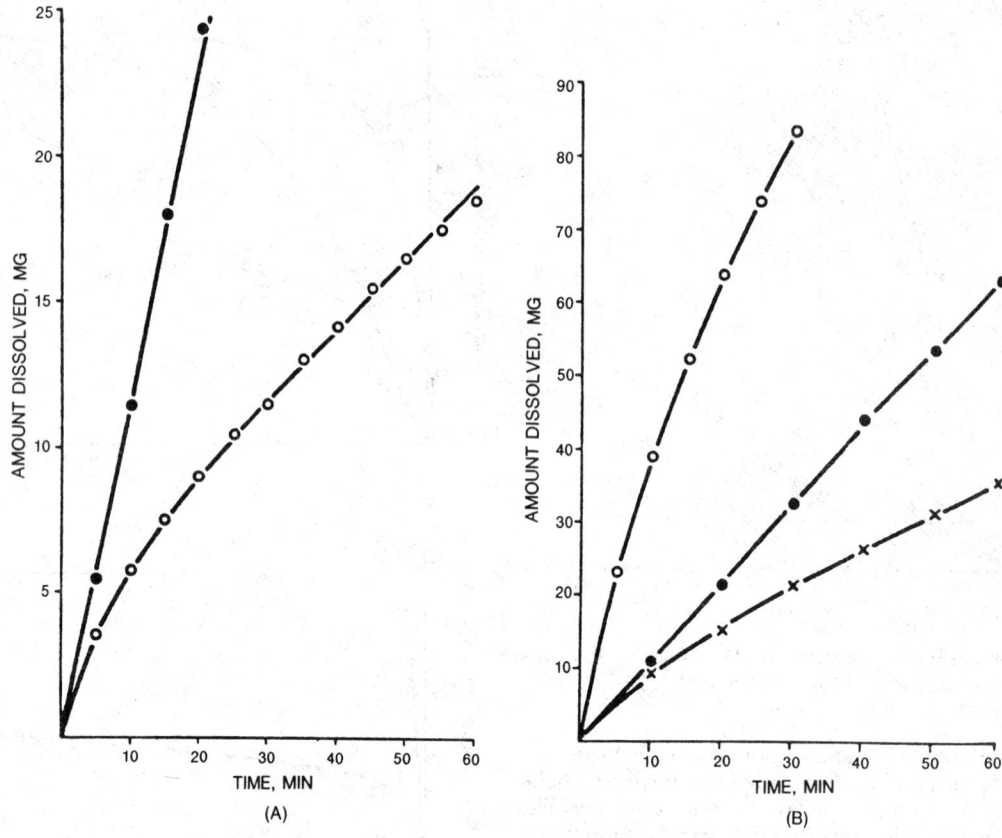

Fig 35-7. Effect of lubricant on the dissolution rate of tablets. [Reproduced from Levy and Gumtow, J Pharm Sci: *52*, 1140, 1963.]
(A) Effect of magnesium stearate on dissolution rate of salicylic acid from rotating disks made from fine salicylic acid powder. *Key:* O, 3% magnesium stearate; ●, no lubricant added. (B) Effect of lubricant on dissolution rate of salicylic acid contained in compressed tablets (formula A). *Key:* ✕, 3% magnesium stearate; ●, no lubricant; O, 3% sodium lauryl sulfate.

tion characteristics. In this regard, the wet granulation procedure was traditionally considered as a superior method compared to the dry or double compression procedure. With the advent of newer tabletting machines and materials, however, it became more evident that the careful formulation and proper mixing sequence and time of adding the several

ingredients are the main criteria that affect the dissolution characteristics of the tablets and not the method of granulation per se. Fig 8 shows the effect of different granulation methods on the dissolution rate of tablets.

Effects of Compression Force on Dissolution Rate

In his early studies of the physics of tablet compression, Higuchi (1953), pointed to the great influence of the compressional force employed in the tabletting process on the apparent density, porosity, hardness, disintegration time, and average primary particle size of compressed tablets. There is always a competing relationship between the enhancing effect due to the increase in surface area through the crushing effect and the inhibiting effect due to the increase in particle bonding that causes an increase in density and hardness and, consequently, a decrease in solvent penetrability. The high compression also may inhibit the wettability of the tablet due to the formation of a firmer and more effective sealing layer by the lubricant under the high pressure and temperature that usually accompanies a strong compressive force (Fig 9).

The curve profile of the compressive force of the tablet versus dissolution rate can take one of several shapes, as is observed in Fig 10.

Modified-Release Dosage Forms

Since the early fifties, pharmaceutical preparations with controlled-release characteristics have been introduced with the purpose of optimizing the bioavailability through the modulation of the time course of the drug concentration in the blood. Such designed control is intended to complement the pharmacological activity of the medicament in order to achieve better selectivity and/or longer duration of action.

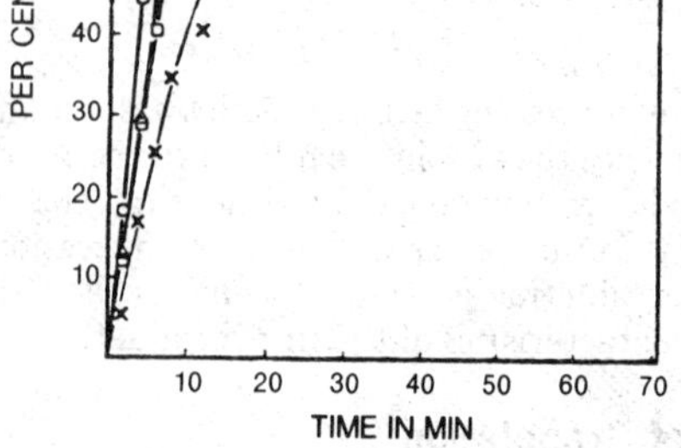

Fig 35-8. Effect of manufacturing process on the dissolution rate of tablets. [Reproduced from Marlowe and Shangraw, J Pharm Sci: *56*, 500, 1967.]

Key: B₁ Direct compression with spray dried lactose, B₂ Wet granulation with ethylcellulose and lactose, B₃ Acacia mucilage and lactose, B₄ Starch paste and lactose.

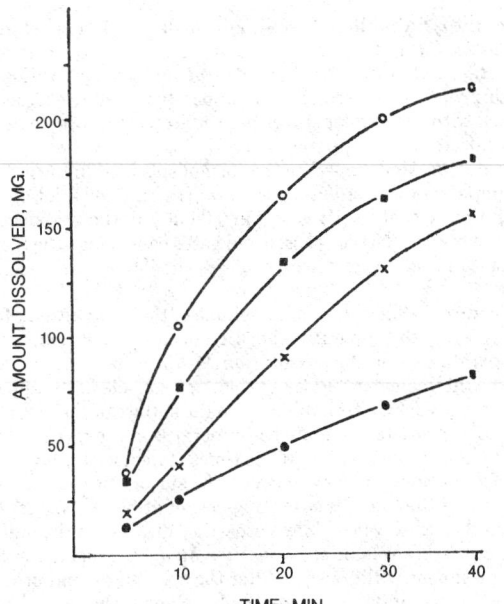

Fig 35-9. Effect of precompression pressure on the dissolution rate of tablets. [Reproduced from Levy, et al, J Pharm Sci: *52*, 1050, 1963.]

Key: Effect of precompression pressure on dissolution rate of salicylic acid contained in compressed tablets. *Key:* ●, 715 Kg.; ✕, 1430 Kg.; ■ 2860 Kg.; ○, 5730 Kg. pressure per cm.² (Average of five tablets each, formula D.)

This adds an extra dimension to the traditional functions of the dosage form being a mere vehicle for drug storage, portability and administration.

Modified-release dosage forms is a relatively new term used by the compendia to describe those dosage forms for which the drug-release characteristics vs time and/or conditions at the site of dissolution are chosen to accomplish therapeutic or convenience objectives not offered by conventional dosage forms such as solutions, ointments or compressed tablets and capsules. For the present, two types of modified-release dosage forms have been proposed in the *Pharmacopeial Forum.*

Delayed-Release Dosage Forms are defined as those that release a drug (or drugs) at any time other than promptly after administration. Enteric coated products are an example of such dosage forms. The proposed USP limit for the enteric coated tablets requires that the tablets survive a one-hour acid treatment in the disintegration apparatus (no disks) and, if they pass this step, they must show 75% dissolution in 45 minutes in pH 6.8 buffer.

Extended Release Dosage Forms (popularly known as timed-release or sustained-release) are defined as those that allow at least a two-fold reduction in dosing frequency as compared to the drug presented in a conventional form, eg, a solution or a prompt drug-releasing conventional solid dosage form.

Dissolution Apparatus Design

As the concept of dissolution developed in importance during the last two decades, the methods and techniques

utilized in the *in vitro* procedure have evolved considerably from a simple, rudimentary apparatus that can be built from everyday laboratory tools to a highly sophisticated, microprocessor-controlled and fully automated instrument. The various dissolution apparatuses and techniques are usually classified according to their associated hydrodynamics.

Three general categories are recognized: the first covers the beaker methods, the second includes the open flow-through compartment systems and the third is based on the "dialysis" concept.

The design of the apparatus affects the dissolution results through a number of factors. These include the geometry and structure of the container, the type and intensity of agitation as well as the composition and volume of the dissolution medium. These factors, in turn, affect the abrasion rate of the intact solid dosage form on the particles, the dispersion of the disintegrated particles, the homogeneity of the dissolution fluid and finally the reproducibility of the system from run to run.

Beaker Methods

These include all closed-compartment systems with a forced convection mixing mechanism, where a relatively large volume of the dissolution medium (200–2000 mL) is contained in a beaker or a flask and agitation is performed by some type of a stirring, rotating or oscillating mechanism.

All the three official apparatuses described in USP XX/NF XV belong to this category.

The following text and Fig 11 are the official specifications and descriptions of these apparatuses as reported by the compendia.

Apparatus 1—The assembly[1] consists of the following: a covered, 1000-mL vessel made of glass or other inert, transparent material[2]; a variable-speed drive; and a cylindrical basket. The vessels are immersed in a suitable water bath of any convenient size that permits holding the temperature at 37 ± 0.5° during the test and keeping the bath fluid in constant, smooth motion. No part of the assembly, including the environment in which the assembly is placed, contributes significant motion, agitation, or vibration beyond that due to the smoothly rotating stirring element. Apparatus that permits observation of the specimen and stirring element during the test is preferable. The vessel is cylindrical, with a spherical bottom. It is 16 cm to 17.5 cm high, its inside diameter is 10.0 cm to 10.5 cm, and its nominal capacity is 1000 mL. Its sides are flanged near the top. A fitted cover may be used to retard evaporation.[3] The shaft is positioned so that its axis is not more than 0.2 cm at any point from the vertical axis of the vessel. A speed-regulating device is used that allows the shaft rotation speed to be selected and maintained at the rate specified in the individual monograph, within ±4%.

The metallic shaft is 6 mm to 10.5 mm in diameter, and rotates smoothly and without significant wobble. The basket consists of two

---

[1] A suitable vessel is available commercially as Kimble Glass No 33730, from laboratory supply houses, or as Elanco Products Division No EQ-1900, from Eli Lilly and Co, PO Box 1750, Indianapolis, IN 46206. A suitable basket is available commercially from Hanson Research Corp, PO Box 35, Northridge, CA 91324, and from Van-Kel Industries, PO Box 311, Chatham, NJ 07928.
[2] The materials should not sorb, react, or interfere with the specimen being tested.
[3] If a cover is used, it provides sufficient openings to allow ready insertion of the thermometer and withdrawal of specimens.

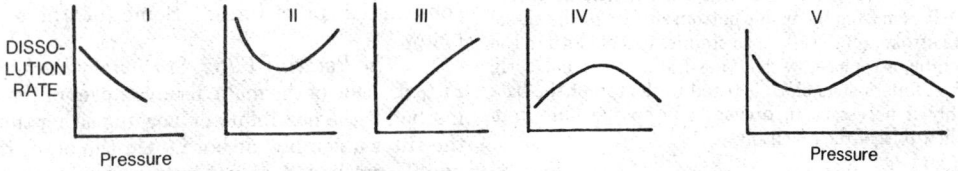

Fig 35-10. Different types of relations between compressional force of tablets and dissolution rate. (Reproduced from P Finholt, *loc cit*, pp 134, 135).

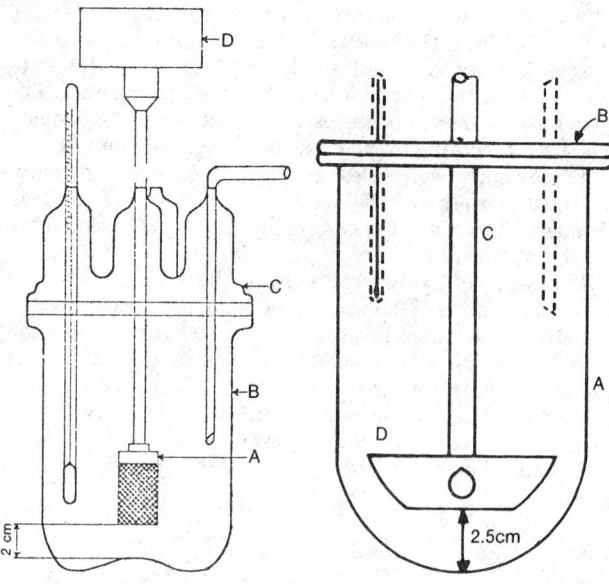

Fig 35-11. Official dissolution apparatus.

Apparatus 1: A—rotating basket assembly; B—container for dissolution fluid; C—4-hole cover for container; D—varying speed stirring motor.

Apparatus 2: A—container for dissolution fluid; B—3-hole cover for container; C—stirring shaft attached to varying speed motor D—stirring blade (paddle) held in horizontal position.

parts, one of which, the top, is attached to the shaft. It is of solid metal except for a 2-mm vent, and it is fitted with three spring clips that allow removal of the lower part to admit the test specimen, and that firmly hold the lower part of the basket concentric to the axis of the vessel during rotation. The detachable part of the basket is fabricated of welded-seam, stainless-steel cloth, formed into a cylinder 3.66 cm high and 2.5 cm in diameter, with a narrow rim of sheet metal around the top. Shaft and basket components are fabricated of stainless steel, usually type 316. Unless otherwise specified in the monograph, use 40-mesh cloth. A basket having a gold coating 0.0001 inch (2.5 μm) thick may be used for tests carried out in dilute acid media. The dosage unit is placed in a dry basket at the beginning of each test. The basket is lowered into position before the rotation is started. The distance between the inside bottom of the vessel and the basket is maintained at 2.5 ± 0.2 cm during the test.

Apparatus 2—Use the assembly from *Apparatus 1*, except that a paddle formed from a blade and a shaft is used as the stirring element.[4] The shaft, 10 ± 0.5 mm in diameter, is positioned so that its axis is not more than 0.2 cm at any point from the vertical axis of the vessel, and rotates smoothly without significant wobble. The stirring blade, 3.0 mm to 5.0 mm thick, forms a section of a circle having a diameter of 83 mm, and is subtended by parallel chords of 42 ± 1 mm and 75 ± 1 mm. The blade passes through the diameter of the shaft so that the bottom of the blade is flush with the bottom of the shaft, and the blade is positioned horizontally at the end of the rotating shaft so that the 42-mm edge is nearest the lowest inner surface of the vessel. The distance of 2.5 ± 0.2 cm between the blade and the inside bottom of the vessel is maintained during the test. The metallic blade and shaft comprise a single entity that may be coated with a suitable fluorocarbon polymer. The dosage unit is allowed to sink to the bottom of the vessel before rotation of the blade is started. A small, loose piece of nonreactive material such as wire or glass helix may be attached to dosage units that would otherwise float.

Apparatus 3—Use the apparatus described under *Disintegration* ⟨701⟩, with these exceptions: (a) the disks are not used; (b) the apparatus is adjusted so that the bottom of the basket-rack assembly descends to 1.0 ± 0.1 cm from the inside bottom surface of the vessel on the downward stroke; (c) the 10-mesh stainless-steel cloth in the basket-rack assembly is replaced with 40-mesh stainless-steel cloth; and (d) 40-mesh stainless-steel cloth is fitted to the top of the basket-rack assembly if necessary to prevent any dosage unit from floating out of the tubes of the assembly.

---

[4] A suitable paddle is available commercially from Hanson Research Corp and from Van-Kel Industries.

Apparatus Suitability Test—Individually test 1 tablet of the *USP Dissolution Calibrator, Disintegrating Type* and 1 tablet of *USP Dissolution Calibrator, Non-disintegrating Type*, according to the operating conditions specified. The apparatus is suitable if the results obtained with each tablet are within the stated acceptable range for that calibrator in the apparatus tested.

Dissolution Medium—Use the solvent specified in the individual monograph. If the *Dissolution Medium* is a buffered solution, adjust the solution so that its pH is within 0.05 unit of the pH specified in the monograph. [NOTE—Dissolved gases can change the results of the test. In such cases, dissolved gases should be removed prior to testing.]

Procedure—Place the stated volume of the *Dissolution Medium* in the vessel of the apparatus specified in the monograph, assemble the apparatus, warm the *Dissolution Medium* to 37 ± 0.5°, and remove the thermometer. Place 1 tablet or 1 capsule in the apparatus, taking care to exclude air bubbles from the surface of the dosage-form unit, and immediately operate the apparatus at the rate specified in the individual monograph. At the times stated, withdraw the specimens from a zone midway between the surface of the *Dissolution Medium* and the top of the rotating basket or blade, not less than 1 cm from the vessel wall. Unless otherwise directed in the individual monograph, add a volume of *Dissolution Medium* equal to the volume of the specimens withdrawn. Filter the specimens, and proceed as directed in the individual monograph. Repeat the test with additional dosage-form units.

Interpretation—Unless otherwise specified in the individual monograph, the requirements are met if the quantities of active ingredient dissolved from the units tested conform to the accompanying acceptance table. Continue testing through the three stages unless the results conform at either S_1 or S_2. The quantity, Q, is the amount of dissolved active ingredient specified in the individual monograph, expressed as a percentage of the labeled content; both the 5% and 15% values in the acceptance table are percentages of the labeled content so that these values Q are in the same terms.

USP Dissolution Acceptance Criteria

Stage	Number Tested	Acceptance Criteria
S_1	6	Each unit is not less than $Q + 5\%$.
S_2	6	Average of 12 units $(S_1 + S_2)$ is equal to or greater than Q, and no unit is less than $Q - 15\%$.
S_3	12	Average of 24 units $(S_1 + S_2 + S_3)$ is equal to or greater than Q, and not more than 2 units are less than $Q - 15\%$.

USP Calibrators

Although precise geometry of the dissolution apparatus and strict tolerance limits in its design and operational specifications are the best guarantee of reproducible and meaningful dissolution results, the USP recommends the use of two types of calibrators, disintegrating (prednisone) and nondisintegrating (salicyclic acid) tablets, as a regular performance check for both the rotating basket and paddle methods. The tablets are available from the USP headquarters in Rockville, MD, and come with complete instructions for the allowable dissolution limits of each type of tablet.

Nonofficial Methods

Although probably more than one hundred different dissolution methods have appeared in the literature, only a few have maintained their popularity after the introduction of the compendial procedures. Some of these are described below.

1. *The Rotating Filter/Stationary Basket Method (Spin Filter)*. One of the main disadvantages of the rotating basket method is the possibility of clogging either the basket screen, the filter assembly, or both. On the other hand, while the paddle method does not suffer from such a problem, the possibility of floating tablets and/or particles, as well as nonreproducible tablet locations at the bottom of the flask

constitute distinct deficiencies. Shah *et al* designed a system that virtually eliminates most of the problems associated with the compendial procedures (Fig 12). It consists of a magnetically driven rotating filter assembly and a 12-mesh wirecloth basket in which the dosage form is placed. The sample is withdrawn through the spinning filter for analysis. The system provides uniform, mild, laminar and nonturbulent agitation that is essential for reproducible results. It also ensures a representative sample of the bulk fluid with minimum abrasion to the solid dosage form. Because of the wide mesh screen used for the basket and the constantly spinning filter, no possibility of clogging exists in the system. It has been criticized, however, because of its complexity and the long time needed for setting up and cleaning.

2. *Rotating Bottle Method for Sustained Release Formulations.* This is probably the oldest dissolution apparatus originally developed during the late fifties for the determination of the dissolution rate of sustained release formulations. Newer versions have been in use; one of them was suggested in NF XIII, but has never been considered as an official method. The system consists of 12 small bottles (15 × 3 cm), attached to a horizontal shaft which rotates at a slow speed of 6–50 rpm. The whole assembly is placed in a constant temperature water bath. Each bottle contains 60 mL of dissolution fluid which is decanted through a 40 mesh screen after each sampling period and is replaced by fresh fluid. Usually five fluids of different pH are utilized: pH 1.2 for 1 hour, pH 2.5 for 1 hour, pH 4.5 for 1.5 hours, pH 7.0 for 1.5 hours and, finally, pH 7.5 for 2 hours for a total dissolution time of 7 hours.

Although a considerable data base has been generated using the rotating bottle method, most of the new sustained release formulations are tested by the compendial methods.

Open Flow-Through Dissolution Systems

In the beaker methods discussed above, (also known as closed compartment methods) a forced convection type of agitation is generated in a relatively large vessel through a stirring, rotating, or oscillating mechanism. In open flow-through methods (also known as open compartment methods), the dosage form is contained in a small vertical glass column with built-in filter through which a continuous flow of the dissolution medium is circulated upward at a specific rate from an outside reservoir using a peristaltic or centrifugal pump. The dissolution fluid is usually collected in a separate reservoir as it leaves the dissolution cell and thereby the dosage form is continuously exposed to fresh solvent (noncumulative mode), and a perfect sink condition is maintained. On the other hand, if a sink condition could easily be met using a limited volume of dissolution medium, the circulating fluid can be routed back to the original reservoir (cumulative mode).

The open flow methods have several advantages over the beaker methods. Because the apparatus utilizes no stirring mechanism, the dosage form and drug particles are continuously exposed to a homogeneous, nonturbulent laminar flow that can be precisely controlled. All the problems of wobbling, shaft eccentricity, verticity, vibration, stirrer position, etc, simply do not exist. Also, the turbulent solvent flow associated with stirring mechanisms imparts variable degrees of physical abrasion of the solids but is avoided here.

Langenbucher's system consists of a cone-shaped dissolution cell with a filter attached to the top (Fig 13A and B). The solvent is circulated from the bottom of the cone in which glass beads are placed to help maintain a laminar flow. Although a pulsating pump was first used to minimize filter clogging, it was later shown that pulsation affects the dissolution rate significantly, and a centrifugal pump is preferred.

The open flow-through system, however, has its own dis-

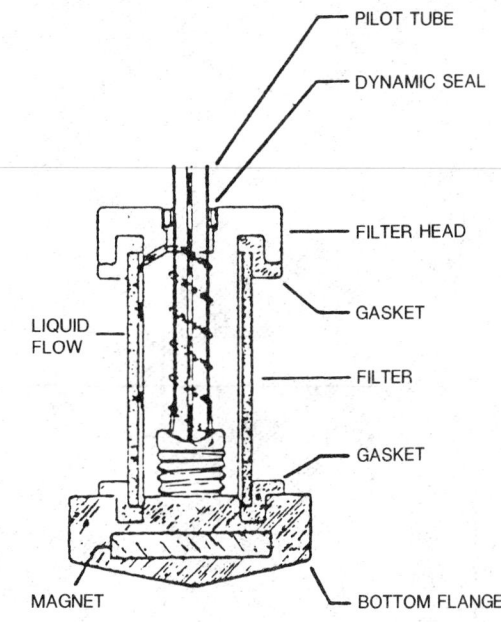

CROSS SECTION

Fig 35-12.   The rotating filter assembly.   [Reproduced from Shah, *et al*, J Pharm Sci: *62*, 671, 1973.]

advantages, the most important of which is the tendency of the filter to clog because of the unidirectional flow. Pressure tends to build near the end of the run and, in many cases, it is necessary to have built-in pressure transducers and a feedback mechanism to increase the pressure gradually in order to keep the flow rate constant. Another limitation, which should be pointed out, is the "pump" effect. Different types of pumps, such as the peristaltic and centrifugal varieties, have been shown to give different dissolution results.

A variation of the flow-through concept, is a closed column-type system which was introduced by Abdou *et al*. The system is a combination of a miniaturized rotating basket with a closed flow-through apparatus to keep the concentration of the drug at an acceptable range for quantitative determination (Fig 14A). The system is semiautomated in conjunction with an HPLC and is used for the determination of the dissolution rate of 0.1 mg fludrocortisone acetate tablets (Fig 14B).

Automation in Dissolution Testing

Due to the large amount of testing required in determining the dissolution rate of drugs, automation of the process seemed almost a necessity and not simply a convenience to the analyst. Also, because of the modular nature of the dissolution apparatus, automation can be easily accomplished in different ways and by various techniques.

At present, however, the set up of the apparatus, media preparation and introduction of the dosage forms mostly are done manually. The rest of the process including the withdrawal of the sample, maintenance of a certain pH or of sink conditions, assay performance and data acquisition and calculations are, in most cases, fully automated. The automation process not only saves money, time, and effort on the part of the analyst but more significantly it improves the overall reliability and enhances the reproducibility of testing procedures. Several approaches have been tried for the automation of dissolution such as those recommended by Shroeter and Wagner, Bayer and Smith, Cioffi *et al* and Abdou *et al*. Details of these systems could be found in the indexed literature at the end of this chapter. Several commercial companies have also introduced semi and fully automated dissolution

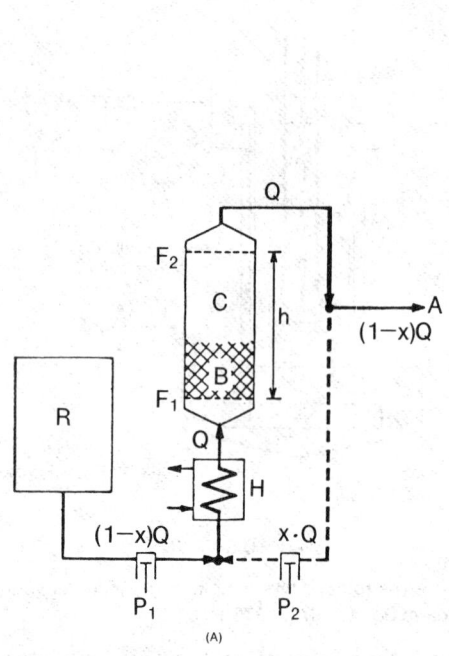

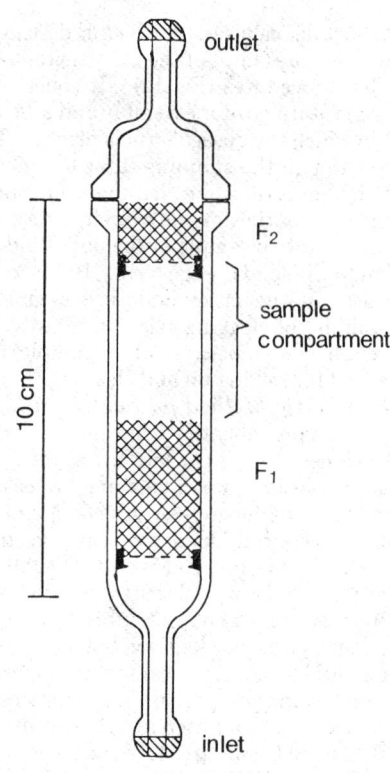

Fig 35-13.   Column-type dissolution method (open flow-through system by Langenbucher).   [Reproduced from Langenbucher, F, J Pharm Sci: *58*, 1265, 1969.]

(A) Sketch of the column dissolution apparatus (schematic).   *Key:* B, particle bed: C, cell: F_1, F_2, screens: H, heat exchanger; h, height of cell: P_1, P_2, volumetric pumps; R, liquid reservoir; x, circulation factor; Q, xQ, (1-x) Q, volumetric flow rates.   (B) Specifications for the 4-cm.^{2} dissolution cell (drawn to scale).   Inner cell diameter 22.6 mm.   Height of sample compartment 40 mm. F_1: stainless steel sieve with 30-mm. bed of glass beads 1 mm. in diameter. F_2: 40 mesh stainless steel sieve with glass beads.

systems.   Most important of these are Hanson Research Corporation's Dissolution System, Northridge, Calif.   (Dissoette and Dissograph apparatuses), Technicon, Tarrytown, NY (Sasdra apparatus) and Applied Analytical, Wilmington, NC.

Effects of Test Parameters on Dissolution Rate

Agitation

The relationship between intensity of agitation and the rate of dissolution varies considerably according to the type of agitation used, the degree of laminar and turbulent flow in the system, the shape and design of the stirrer, and the physico-chemical properties of the solid (Fig 15).   When a stirring device is used, such as the basket, paddle, rotating filter, etc, the speed of agitation generates a flow that continuously changes the liquid/solid interface between the solvent and the drug in a way similar to the flow rate in the flow-through dissolution apparatus.   In order to prevent turbulence and sustain a reproducible laminar flow, which is essential for obtaining reliable results, either the speed of agitation or the flow rate, depending on the type of apparatus employed, should be maintained at a relatively low level.

Polli reviewed the literature concerning the effect of agitation on the rate of heterogeneous reactions and many of these studies have led to the empirical relationship between the rate of dissolution and the intensity of agitation.

$$K = a(N)^b \qquad (12)$$

where N is the speed of agitation, K is the dissolution rate, and a and b are constants.   If the dissolution process is diffusion controlled, the value of b should be 1 or close to 1 in accordance with the Nernst-Brunner film theory, which states that the film thickness is inversely proportional to the stirring speed.   However, if the dissolution process is purely controlled by an interfacial reaction, the stirring speed would have no influence on dissolution and b should approach zero.   If both processes are involved (such as dissolution of weak acids in buffer solution), the value of b should fall between 0 and 1.   Also, as the nature of the flow changes from laminar to turbulent and the distance from the interface increases, the value of b would also vary according to the type of agitation utilized.   Other factors that affect the correlation between agitation and dissolution rate include the density of the solid phase, the size and characteristics of the solid, the stirrer, the dissolution vessel and the heat of solution of the solute.

Temperature

Since drug solubility is temperature dependent, its careful control during the dissolution process is very important and should be maintained within 0.5°.   Generally, a temperature of 37° is always maintained during dissolution determinations.   The effect of temperature variations of the dissolution medium depends mainly on the temperature/solubility curves of the drug and excipients in the formulation (Fig 16).   For a dissolved molecule, the diffusion coefficient, D, is dependent upon the temperature T according to the Stokes equation.

$$D = kT/(6\pi \eta r) \qquad (13)$$

where k is the Boltzmann constant and $6\pi \eta r$ is the Stokes force for a spherical molecule (η is the viscosity in cgs or poise units and r is the radius of the molecule).

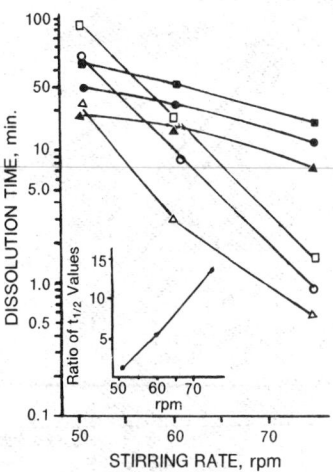

Fig 35-15. Effect of agitation on dissolution rate. [Reproduced from Levy, *et al*, J Pharm Sci: *56*, 1365, 1967.]
1980, (a); and Nogami, H, Chem Pharm Bull: *17*, 499, 1969, (b).]
Dissolution rate of aspirin from type A (open symbols) and type B (solid symbols) tablets as a function of stirring rate. Triangles, $t_{1/3}$, circles, $t_{1/2}$, squares, $t_{2/3}$. Inset: ratio of $t_{1/3}$, type B: type A tablets, as a function of stirring rate.

studies show a specific need for the acidic solution in order to generate meaningful dissolution data. Another approach for avoiding the deleterious effects of hydrochloric acid is to replace it with acidic buffers, such as sodium acid phosphate, to maintain the required low pH.

Surface Tension of the Dissolution Medium

Surface tension has been shown to have a significant effect on the dissolution rate of drugs and their release rate from solid dosage forms. Surfactants and wetting agents lower the contact angle and thereby improve the penetration process of the matrix by the dissolution medium. Measurable enhancement in the dissolution rate of salicyclic acid from an inert matrix was reported by Singh *et al* when the contact angle, θ was lowered from 92° (water) to 31° (using 0.01% dioctyl sodium sulfosuccinate Fig 17A). The surface tension was also correspondingly lowered from 60 to 31 dynes/cm. The same findings were obtained in benzocaine studies when polysorbate 80 was used as the surface active agent (Fig 17B).

Other studies conducted on conventional tablet formulations and capsules also showed significant enhancement in the dissolution rate of poorly soluble drugs when surfactants were added to the dissolution medium, even at a level below the critical micelle concentration, probably by reducing the interfacial tension. Low levels of surfactants were recommended to be included in the dissolution medium as this seemed to give a better correlation between the *in vitro* data and *in vivo* condition. Finholt and Solvang compared the dissolution behavior of phenacetin and phenobarbital tablets in human gastric juice to that in dilute hydrochloric acid with and without various amounts of polysorbate 80 in the dissolution medium. The data showed that both pH and surface tension have significant influences on the dissolution kinetics of the drug studies. For example, they found that not only was the dissolution rate much faster in diluted gastric juice, but that it increased with decreasing particle size, whereas the opposite was the case when 0.1N HCl was used.

Viscosity of the Medium

In the case of diffusion-controlled dissolution processes, it would be expected that the dissolution rate decreases with an increase in viscosity. In the case of interfacial controlled dissolution processes however, viscosity should have very little

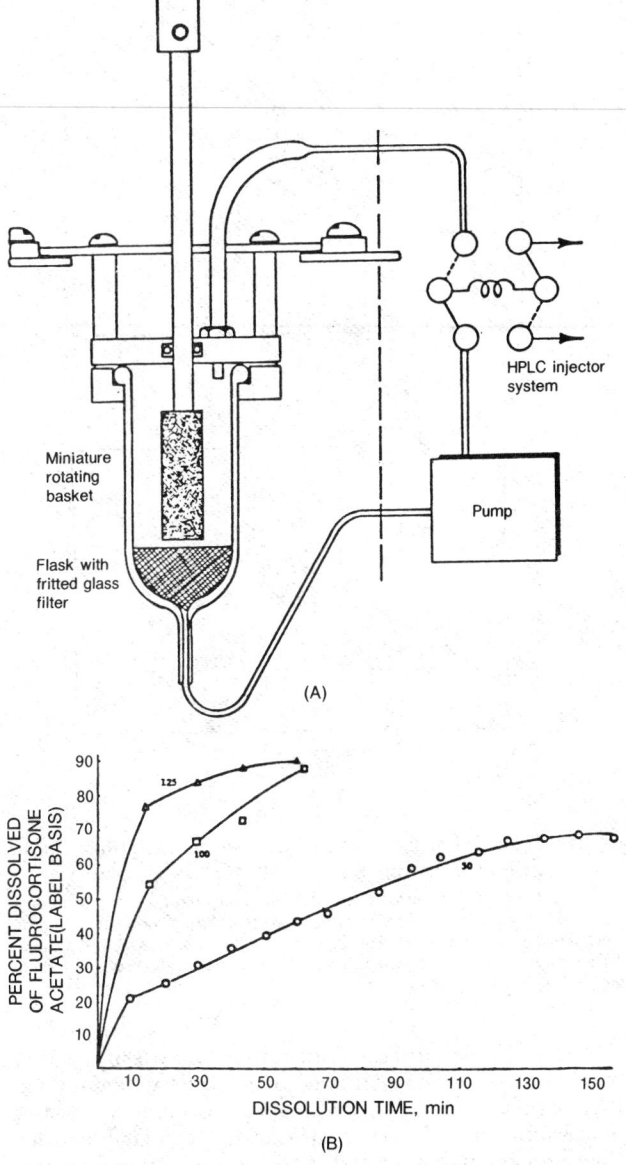

Fig 35-14. Apparatus for the determination of the dissolution rate of dosages with extremely small amounts of active ingredients. [Reproduced from Abdou, *et al*, J Pharm Sci: *67*, 1397, 1978.]
(A) Miniaturized USP basket apparatus, combined with a flow-through mechanism. (B) Comparison between the dissolution rate of fludrocortisone acetate at different rotation speeds. Each point is an average of six tablets of the same lot. *Key:* O, 50 rpm; □, 100 rpm; and △, 125 rpm.

Dissolution Medium

The selection of the proper fluid for dissolution testing depends largely on the solubility of the drug, as well as mere economics and practical reasons.

pH of the Dissolution Medium

Great emphasis and effort was first placed on simulating *in vivo* conditions, especially pH, surface tension, viscosity, and sink condition. Most of the early studies were conducted in 0.1N HCl or buffered solutions with a pH close to that of the gastric juice (pH ~1.2). The acidic solution tends to disintegrate the tablets slightly faster than water and thereby it may enhance the dissolution rate by increasing the effective surface area. However, because of the corroding action of the acid fumes on the dissolution equipment, currently it is a general practice to use distilled water unless investigative

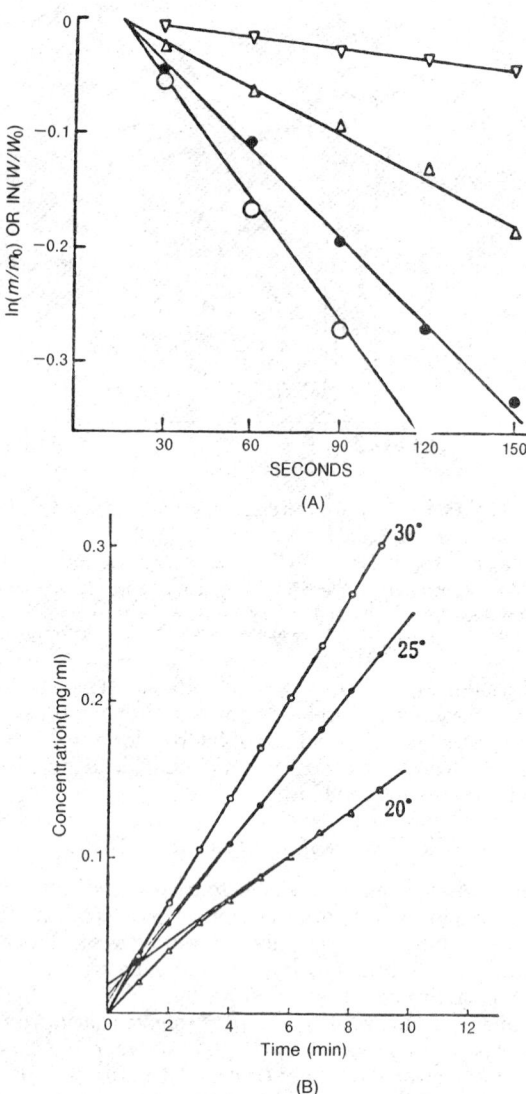

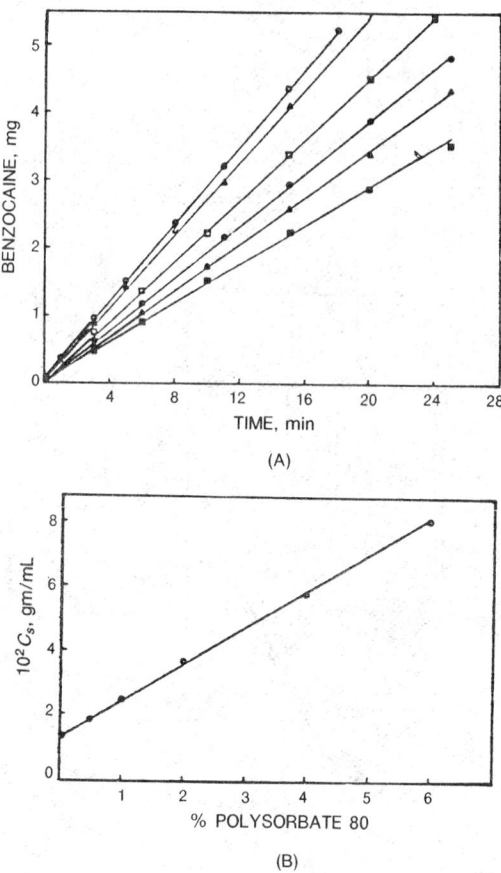

Fig 35-17. Effect of surfactants on dissolution rate. [Reproduced from Singh, P et al, J Pharm Sci: *57*, 959, 1968.]

(A) Dissolution data for benzocaine in different concentrations of polysorbate 80 using the propeller-driven stirrer apparatus at a stirring speed of 150 r.p.m. *Key:* Polysorbate conc.—O, 6%; △, 4%; □, 2%; ●, 1%; ▲, 0.5%; ■, 0%.
(B) Solubilization data for benzocaine in different concentrations of polysorbate 80.

Fig 35-16. Effect of temperature on dissolution and disintegration rates of tablets. [Reproduced from Carstensen, *et al*, J Pharm Sci: *89*, 291, 1980, (a); and Nogami, H, Chem Pharm Bull, *17*, 499, 1969, (b).]
(A) Dissolution and disintegration curves according to Eqs. 1 and 2 for position II of the USP basket. *Key:* ▽, dissolution at 10°; △, dissolution at 20°; ●, dissolution at 30°; and O, disintegration at 5°. (B) Dissolution of Phenobarbital Anhydrate at Various Temperatures under 300 rpm.

effect. The Stokes-Einstein equation describes the diffusion coefficient D as a function of viscosity (Refer to Chapt 21 and 22).

Braun and Parrott showed that the dissolution rate of benzoic acid is inversely proportional to the viscosity of the dissolution medium utilizing various concentrations of sucrose and methylcellulose solutions (Fig 18).

Dissolution of Suspensions

Although most dissolution studies during the last two decades have concentrated on tablets and capsules, some studies have pointed to the importance of the dissolution characteristics of drugs administered in suspension. This is hardly surprising as suspensions are similar to the disintegrated form of tablets and capsules and, if dissolution has become a priority for these formulations, it is logical to extend its concept to suspensions. Indeed, several studies have shown that the absorption of several poorly soluble drugs administered in suspension formulations is dissolution-rate limited.

Such *in vivo/in vitro* correlation studies have confirmed the importance and the viability of dissolution rate determinations of suspensions as a discriminative test for rapid screening of new formulations and to control lot-to-lot variability within the same manufacturer and between different commercial manufacturers. In general, most of the dissolution apparatuses that have been described for tablets and capsules could easily be utilized for suspensions. The USP Apparatus II (Paddle) has been used frequently at a rotation speed between 25–50 rpm. However, the rotating filter apparatus by Shah, with the basket removed, has gained wide acceptance for suspensions since it provides mild laminar liquid agitation and it also functions as an *in situ* nonclogging filter. Sufficient volume of the dissolution medium should be used to maintain sink condition (about 900–1000 mL) and a temperature of 37° should be maintained. Rotation speeds of up to 300 rpm have also been used on occasion.

Dissolution of Topical Dosage Forms (Creams, Ointments and Gels)

Drug-release studies from gels, creams and ointments are becoming an important step both during the developmental stages of new formulations and as a routine quality control test for assuring the uniformity of the finished product. Also these studies often can provide useful information on some physicochemical parameters involved in the *in vivo* percutaneous absorption, such as the diffusion coefficient and the solubility of the drug in the specific vehicle utilized.

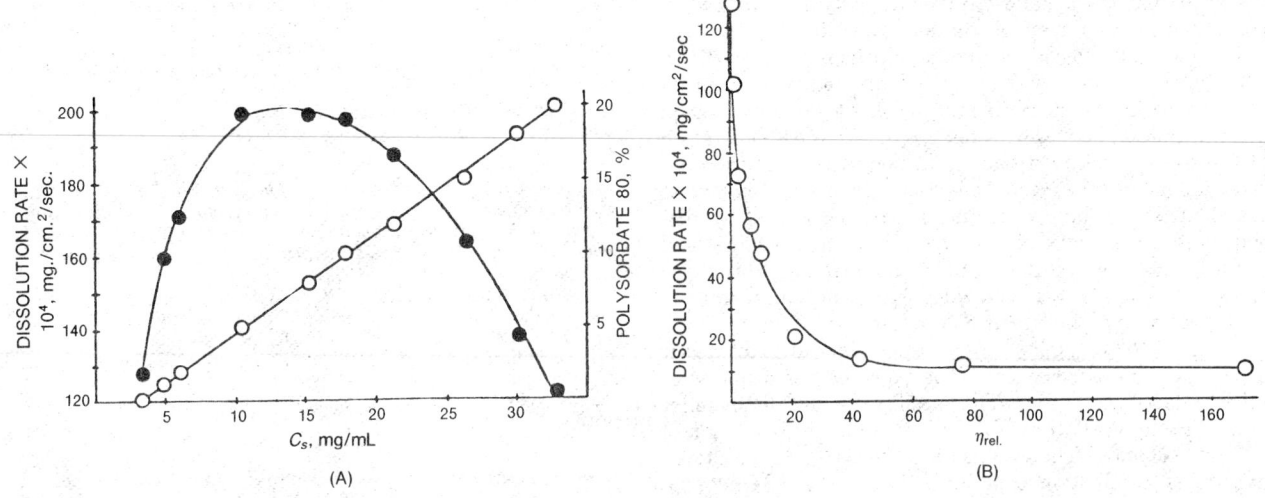

Fig 35-18.   Effect of viscosity on dissolution rate.   [Reproduced from Braun and Parrott, J Pharm Sci: *61*, 175, 1972.]
(A) Relationship of total solubility (C_s) of benzoic acid at 25° to dissolution rate and concentration of polysorbate 80.   *Key:* ●, rate; and ○, concentration.   (B) Relationship of viscosity to dissolution rate of benzoic acid in aqueous methylcellulose solutions at 25°.

Although many investigators have conducted drug release rate studies from topical dosage forms, it appears that no single apparatus or procedure has yet emerged as the most favored, or to be widely accepted as a quasi-standard for others in the field.   In reviewing the literature, however, it appears that two general techniques have been commonly employed.   In the first, the sample is placed in direct contact with the receptor phase which acts as an aqueous sink, and the second utilizes various types of barriers to isolate the donor phase from the receiving medium.   The barrier could be a dialysis membrane, a filter membrane, a membrane of animal origin or a polymer membrane.

Dissolution of Suppositories

Although most of the early work on suppositories has been concerned with their physical characteristics such as softening and liquefaction ranges, homogeneity, smoothness and neutrality, several reports appeared in the early literature pointing to the direct correlation between their efficacy and the release characteristics of the active ingredients.   It has been reported that fatty bases, such as the popular cocoa butter, tend to release hydrophobic drugs that are highly soluble in the oily base very slowly but that emulsification of the fatty base significantly improved the drug-release rate.   Incorporation of surface active agents was found to dramatically improve the release rate of water soluble drugs from the fatty suppository base.

Although many investigators have conducted extensive research on the release of drugs from suppositories, no single method or apparatus design has yet emerged as the standard procedure for the pharmaceutical laboratory.   Most of the methods for the determination of the dissolution rate of suppositories are based on the dialysis technique where the suppository is placed in a dialyzing bag made of special membrane or cellophane material.   The bag is placed in a beaker or wide mouth bottle containing a known volume of distilled water and the concentration of drug outside of the bag is measured as a function of time.

A slight variation of the basket method of the USP dissolution apparatus I has been used.   Hanson Research Corporation markets a basket apparatus for suppository dissolution testing.   Hanson's modified basket uses slots instead of mesh to provide a porosity of about 52%.   The use of such a basket avoids the blocking of the mesh opening of the regular USP basket when oil-based suppositories are used.   The system also has the advantage of being capable of testing supposito-

ries that float or have such low specific gravity that it interferes with the flow dynamics in the paddle method.

Developing a New Dissolution Method

Dissolution data, based on a discriminating and well thought dissolution test is of tremendous value in the selection of the proper formulation.   The dissolution test can also serve as a routine control mechanism to assure the uniformity of regular production batches.   One of the first decisions to be made in the process of developing a new dissolution method is the choice of the apparatus.   There are three types of apparatuses in the compendia and several others are in current use by pharmaceutical companies, universities, and regulatory agencies.   Apparatuses differ, in great respect, with regard to the shape and geometry of the dissolution vessel, the type and intensity of agitation, the position of the dosage form, the dispersion of particles, the volume of the dissolution medium, the ability to change the solvent at a certain rate to maintain sink conditions, and the reproducibility of the system.   Wagner cautioned that the inherent variability in the dissolution method should be less than the inherent variability that can be tolerated in the product.   He also recommended that the apparatus must be scientifically realistic, be economically sound, and have the ability to provide an effective hydrodynamic condition.

In deciding on which apparatus is to be utilized for testing, it should be emphasized that its features should allow for a convenient and reproducible mechanism for introducing the dosage form at a fixed position in the dissolution medium with minimal hydrodynamic disruption.   The temperature of the dissolution medium should be rigorously maintained with minimum vibration and no localized overheated spots.

The dissolution apparatus should also allow for the maintenance of sink conditions by allowing for continuous exchange of the dissolution fluid with fresh solvent.   The apparatus should also provide for the testing of various types of dosage forms with a convenient and reproducible sampling technique that results in a minimum disruption of the dosage form dissolving bed or the hydrodynamic condition of the dissolution medium.   Automatic filtration mechanisms that are inserted in the dissolution fluid are preferred, as they avoid the removal of insoluble drug powder.   Simple and rapid analytical methods should be utilized, as many drugs tend to degrade rapidly in dilute aqueous solutions.

In reviewing the above criteria for a sound dissolution apparatus, it could easily be recognized that the compendial dissolution methods I and II do not actually fair badly when compared to other available dissolution systems.

In general, if the compendial apparatus is to be used, 900 mL of distilled water with an agitation speed of 100 rpm for the rotating basket and 50 rpm for the paddle method is a good starting point. However, a check to determine if deaeration of the water is necessary has to be conducted. If such parameters prove to be inadequate, a slightly higher stirring rate may be tried. If not successful, the composition of the dissolution medium could be changed. Dilute hydrochloric acid or buffer systems of different pH could be used. In the case of enteric coated or sustained-release preparations, media pH change may be required during the test.

In regard to the quality control aspect, it is advisable to set dissolution guidelines close to the expected performance of the selected formulation. The specification usually includes both DT_{50} and DT_{85} or DT_{85} (DT_x = time for dissolution of 50% or 85%) only. The specifications, however, can be altered as further production experience is obtained. Once the specification is finalized, any batch which does not comply should be completely reviewed to find the cause of its poor dissolution.

A knowledge of the dissolution rate of poorly soluble drug substances (intrinisic dissolution rate, $K = kD/h$ from Eq 3), is very useful in predicting whether their biological absorption is dissolution limited or not. Such information is essential during the early stages of formulation of a new drug dosage form as it can point to a future bioavailability problem. Depending on how slow the intrinsic dissolution rate is, the formulator may choose to improve it by micronization, complex formation, derivatization, or any of the other techniques generally utilized for enhancing the dissolution rate of insoluble drugs. The information is also very useful for improving existing formulations that have exhibited bioavailability problems.

For the determination of the intrinsic dissolution rate, most investigators compress the pure powdered drug under extremely high pressure in the absence of any additives. The resulting nondisintegrating disk is then transferred to any of the previously discussed dissolution apparatuses. Because of the nondisintegrating characteristic of the disk, the surface area is essentially constant during the entire duration of the test. This facilitates the calculation and interpretation of the results. Usually the modified form of Noyes and Whitney equation, previously discussed is utilized as the basis for calculation.

Also, the effects of the various formulation factors as well as the key processing factors such as the compression force, mixing time and in-process storage conditions have to be determined. This will provide information on how critically these important variables have to be controlled during routine production.

Furthermore, appropriate stability studies should be conducted to establish what changes take place, if any, in the dissolution characteristics of the selected formulation after it has been held in stability storage for a reasonable period of time. Accelerated conditions (stress studies) could also be utilized for the same purpose. After the dissolution pattern of the selected formulation has been established, an *in vivo* study may be conducted to establish *in vitro/in vivo* correlation. It is advisable that these studies be conducted on humans and not on animals, since man will be the final vehicle for drug dissolution.

Bibliography

1. Leeson, LJ and Carstensen, TJ: *Dissolution Technology*, The Industrial Pharmaceutical Technology Section of the Academy of Pharmaceutical Science, 2215 Constitution Ave, NW, Washington, DC, 20037, 1974.
2. Procedures of the Second Wisconsin Update Conference, *Dissolution—State of the Art 1982*, Extension Services in Pharmacy, University of Wisconsin—Extension, 425 N Charter Street, Madison, WI 53206.
3. Hanson, WA: *Handbook of Dissolution Testing*, Pharmaceutical Technology Publication, 320 North A Street, Springfield, Oregon, 97477, 1982.
4. Crank, J: *The Mathematics of Diffusion*, New York: Oxford University Press, 1956.

References

1. Noyes, AA and Whitney, WR: J Am Chem Soc, 19, 930, (1897).
2. Nelson, KG and Miller, KW: *Principles of Drug Dissolution and Absorption Related to Bioavailability*, a chapter in Blanchard, J, Sawchuk, RJ, and Brodic, BB, *Principles and Perspectives in Drug Bioavailability*, S-Karger, Basel, (1979).
3. Wurster, DE and Taylor, PW: ibid, 54, 670, (1965).
4. Wagner, J and Pernarowski, M: *Biopharmaceutics and Relevant Pharmacokinetics*, Hamilton, Il, Drug Intelligence Publications, (1971).
5. Gibaldi, M and Perrier, D: *Pharmacokinetics*, Dekker, New York, NY, pp 270, 281, (1974).
6. Wagner, JG: Drug Intelligence and Clinical Pharmacy, 4, 137, (1970).

General

Leeson, Lewis J and Carstensen, Thuro J: *Dissolution Technology*, The Industrial Pharmaceutical Technology Section of the Academy of Pharmaceutical Science, 2215 Constitution Ave, NW, Washington, DC, 20037, 1974.

Particle Size

1. Levy, G: Amer J Pharm, 135, 78, (1963).
2. Kornblum, S and Hirsohorn, J: ibid, 60, 445, (1971).

Crystalline State of the Drug

1. Poole, J: Current Therapeutic Research, 10, 292, (1968).
2. Aguiar, A, Kre, J, Kinkel, A and Samyn, J: ibid, 56, 847, (1967).

Formulation and Processing Factors for Tablet Formulations

1. Levy, G, Antlkowiak, J, Proknal, J, and White, D: J Pharm Sci, 52, 1047, (1963).
2. Marlowe, E and Shangraw, R: J Pharm Sci, 56, 498, (1967).
3. Chowhan, Z, Yang, I, Amaro, A and Chi, L: J Pharm Sci, 71, 1371 (1982).

Factors Relating to the Dissolution Apparatus and Test Parameters

1. Pernarowski, N: *Dissolution Technology* by L Leeson and J Carstensen, Industrial Pharm Tech Section, Academy of Pharm Sci, Washington, DC (1974).
2. Stavchansky, S: *Dissolution—State of the Art 1982*, Procedures of the Second Wisconsin Update Conference, Extension Services in Pharmacy.
3. Hanson, W: *Handbook of Dissolution Testing*, Pharm Tech Publications, Springfield, Oregon, pp 88–89.
4. Langenbucher, F: Pharm Acta Helv, 49, 187, (1974).
5. Abdou, H, Ast, T, and Cioffi, F: ibid, 67, 1397, (1978).

Intrinsic Dissolution Rate

1. Tingstad, J, Gropper, E, Lachman, L, and Shami, E: ibid, 62, 293, (1973).
2. Cartensen, J and Musa, M: ibid, 61, 223, (1972).

Effect of Dissolution Medium
Effect of pH and Surface Tension

1. Singh, P, Desai, S, Simonelli, A and Higuchi, W: J Pharm Sci, 57, 217 (1968).
2. Felmeister, A: J Pharm Sci, 61, 151 (1972).
3. Solvang, S and Finholt, P: ibid, 59, 49 (1970).

Automation in Dissolution Testing

1. Beyer, W, and Smith, E: ibid, 60, 1556, (1971).
2. Shah, A, Poet, C, and Ochs, J: ibid, 62, 671, (1973).
3. Cioffi, F, Abdou, H, and Warren, A: ibid, 65, 1236, (1976).
4. Abdou, H, Ast, T, and Cioffi, F: ibid, 67, 1397, (1978).

Effects of Agitation on Dissolution Rate

1. Levy, G, Leonard, J, Procknal, J: ibid, 56, 1365, (1967).

Modified Release Dosage Forms

Pharmacopeial Forum, May–June 1983, pp 2991–3000.

Effect of Temperature

Carstensen, J, Kothari, R, Prasad, V and Sheridan, J: ibid, 69, 290 (1980).

Effect of Viscosity

Braun, R, and Parrott, E, J Pharm Sci, 61, 175 (1972).

Developing a New Dissolution Method

1. Wagner, G: *Biopharmaceutics and Relevant Pharmacokinetics*, Drug Intelligence Publications, Hamilton, Ill, 1971, p 110.
2. Sarapu, A and Clark, L: J Pharm Sci, 69, 129, (1980).

PART 6

Pharmaceutical and Medicinal Agents

Stewart C Harvey, PhD

Professor of Pharmacology
The University of Utah
Medical Center
School of Medicine
Department of Pharmacology
Salt Lake City, UT 84132

Ewart A Swinyard, PhD

Professor Emeritus of Pharmacology
College of Pharmacy and
School of Medicine
University of Utah
Salt Lake City, UT 84112

Alfonso R Gennaro, PhD

Professor of Chemistry
Philadelphia College of Pharmacy
and Science
Philadelphia, PA 19104

CHAPTER 36

Diseases: Manifestations and Pathophysiology

John A Bosso, Pharm D

Associate Professor of Clinical Pharmacy and Adjunct Associate Professor of Pediatrics
College of Pharmacy and School of Medicine, University of Utah
Salt Lake City, UT 84112

Steven J Padula, MD

Instructor, Department of Medicine
University of Connecticut Health Center
Farmington, CT 06032

James W Freston, MD, PhD

Professor and Chairman
Department of Medicine
University of Connecticut Health Center
Farmington, CT 06032

This chapter provides a brief overview of certain basic information about some major diseases, the objective being to prepare students and practitioners of pharmacy for more effective service as drug information specialists and consultants on drug therapy.

Included in this presentation are signs and symptoms of the diseases, also their pathophysiology, etiology, and epidemiology; some discussion of relevant physiology, biochemistry, anatomy, and pathology serves to provide a better understanding of the diseases. Some diseases are discussed more extensively than others; many are not discussed at all. This uneven treatment is the result of variables such as state of knowledge, frequency of disease, applicability of drug therapy, and space constraints. For additional information the reader should refer to textbooks of medicine or to textbooks of basic science disciplines for amplification of introductory material provided here.

The use of some medical jargon is deliberate. The reader may struggle with some unfamiliar terms, even as the pharmacist does in working in the clinical environment. It is intended that such exposure here may facilitate communication with other members of the health team.

Infectious Diseases

Urinary Tract Infections

Urinary tract infections (UTIs) include: pyelonephritis, cystitis, prostatitis and urethritis, and are infections of the kidneys, bladder, prostate gland and urethra, respectively. Each of these infections may be asymptomatic but each has characteristic signs and symptoms. The infections may be acute or chronic.

Normal Anatomy and Physiology—The urinary tract is a closed system for drainage of urine from kidneys to bladder and eventually to the outside via the urethra. Under normal circumstances the entire urinary tract except for the anterior urethra is sterile. Various defense mechanisms prevent infection in the urinary tract. The outward flow of urine serves to wash out organisms. This is probably the most important defensive mechanism and can clear 99% of organisms experimentally inoculated into the bladder. The urine itself has certain characteristics that discourage bacterial growth. These include an acidic pH (5.5), as bacteria prefer a more alkaline medium, pH = 6 to 8; low osmolarity, usually below that required for optimal bacterial growth; and the presence of urea and weak organic acids. The urinary-tract anatomy prevents retrograde flow of urine. Valves at the ureterovesicular junction prevent reflux of urine from bladder into ureters and perhaps the kidneys. Females have a shorter urethra than males (4 cm vs 12 cm) which contributes to the much higher incidence of urinary tract infections in women. Also, the urethra in women is easily colonized by organisms from the vagina or rectum because of their close proximity. Prostatic secretions are probably antibacterial. The kidney is particularly susceptible to infection due to the hypertonic state of the papillae and medulla. This leads to impairment of leukocyte migration, complement activity and phagocytosis; plus the development of spheroplasts or protoplasts by bacteria which make them less susceptible to antibiotics.

Epidemiology—The incidence of urinary tract infections depends on the age, sex, sexual activity and underlying diseases in the population. Women have a 20% risk of a UTI during their lifetime; 5% during the first 10 years, 4% during childbearing years, 4 to 8% during pregnancy and 2 to 10% after 50 years of age. Celibate women have a 0.4 to 1.6% incidence of urinary tract infection. In infancy, the rate of UTIs in males, usually associated with a structural anomaly, exceeds that of females. Men under 50 years old rarely have UTIs. In patients with underlying disease, the incidence of UTIs is 20% for diabetes mellitus, 14% for hypertension, 85% for hydronephrosis and nephrolithiasis and greater than 50% for long term indwelling urinary catheters. Twenty-five percent of pregnant women with asymptomatic bacteriuria go on to develop acute pyelonephritis.

Etiology—Most UTIs are caused by gram-negative organisms that normally inhabit the large intestine. *Escherichia coli* account for 85% of first urinary tract infections. Other organisms, including *Klebsiella*, *Enterobacter*, *Proteus*, and *Pseudomonas*, are less commonly seen. Instrumentation of the urinary tract is a predisposing factor for development of a UTI caused by *Proteus* or *Pseudomonas*. Urethritis may be caused by *Neisseria gonococcus*, *chlamydia* and vaginal organisms.

Pathophysiology—Most urinary tract infections are caused by bacteria that ascend the urinary tract through the entrance to the urethra. This ascent is easier in the shorter urethra of females. The anterior urethra is normally colonized by bacteria from the large intestine in females. The trauma to the male urethra that occurs during sexual intercourse can result in the entrance of bacteria into the bladder. Instrumentation of the lower urinary tract frequently results in infection. Bacteriuria commonly occurs within 24 to 48 hours after the placement of an indwelling urinary catheter.

Normally the flow of urine would wash out any bacteria that enter the bladder. However, certain conditions interfere with this flow and therefore predispose the individual to the development of UTIs. Tumors, stones, strictures, bladder diverticulum, anatomical abnormalities and prostatic hypertrophy may impede flow of urine. These conditions, as well as a neurogenic bladder, may also prevent complete emptying of the bladder so that bacteria remain in the residual urine and continue to multiply. Conditions that allow retrograde flow of urine increase the incidence of UTIs. In vesicoureteral reflux, urine from the bladder is forced up the ureters and perhaps into the renal parenchyma by increased pressure in the bladder, as occurs in voiding. Urethrovesicle reflux may bring urine back into the bladder after being contaminated by the bacteria in the urethra during coughing, sneezing, or laughing. In pregnancy the urine flow is partially obstructed by the enlarged uterus and the dilated ureters and decreased peristaltic activity of the bladder allow reflux.

Rarely, urinary tract infections may be caused by the hematogenous spread of bacteria from other sites. This usually involves seeding of the kidney by staphylococcus.

Signs and Symptoms—Urethritis is accompanied by symptoms related to micturition, including urgency and dysuria. Cystitis is characterized by symptoms of frequency, urgency, dysuria and perhaps pain or pressure in the lower abdomen. Systemic signs or symptoms are uncommon with cystitis. Acute pyelonephritis is manifested by symptoms which develop over a few hours to two days, including aching pain in the lumbar region (flank pain), fever to 39°C, shaking chills, nausea, vomiting and local symptoms of urgency and dysuria. On physical examination, there may be tenderness over the kidney in the area of the costovertebral angle.

The urinalysis in a UTI may show bacteria, leukocytes, red blood cells and epithelial debris. The presence of white blood-cell casts is indicative of pyelonephritis.

The diagnosis of a UTI is usually based on the presence and quantitation of bacteria in the urine. The culture is taken from a midstream, clean-voided, urine specimen. If fewer than 1000 bacterial colonies/mL of urine are cultured, significant infection is not present as the bacteria are probably contaminants from the urethra or perineal areas. If between 10^3 and 10^4 organisms/mL of urine are cultured, then the culture cannot be interpreted and should be repeated. If there are more than 10^5 organisms/mL of urine, then the diagnosis of a UTI will be correct in 80% of the cases. If three urine specimens result in the growth of greater than 10^5 organisms/mL, then there is a 95% chance that the patient has a UTI. Less than 10^5 organisms/mL may grow on culture although the patient has a UTI when the pH of the urine is less than 5, when bacteriostatic medication is present or if the organism multiplies slowly. When urine is obtained from the bladder, ureters or renal pelvis by sterile technique, the presence of any number of bacteria indicates a UTI. An intravenous pyelogram (IVP) will usually show evidence of pyelonephritis if this disease is present.

The extent of the diagnostic workup of a patient with a UTI depends on whether it is the first infection, the age and sex of the patient and the presence of underlying disease. Male children should receive a complete evaluation to rule out anatomical abnormalities. A female in the childbearing years may be diagnosed on the basis of urinalysis and gram stain of the urine if this is the first infection. Cultures are obtained in other situations. Recurrent UTIs require a complete diagnostic workup.

In patients with acute urinary tract infections, the symptoms may resolve with or without therapy. Acute pyelonephritis may resolve spontaneously or recur over many years. Patients without underlying disease usually do not have continuing asymptomatic bacteriuria. However, in patients with obstruction or anatomical abnormalities, the eradication of the organism is difficult. Recurrent urinary tract infections are often caused by the same organisms.

Chronic pyelonephritis is a chronic interstitial nephritis resulting from bacterial infection. Hypertension, anemia and, on occasion, renal failure may result. Proteinuria is usually absent. Patients with chronic pyelonephritis may do well for many years.

Sexually Transmitted Disease (STD)

Sexually transmitted disease refers to a disease acquired through sexual activity. There are many diseases in this category and STD refers to no specific one; therefore, the term is confusing.

Gonorrhea (GC) is an extremely common disease that is transmitted by sexual activity. The incidence of gonorrhea in the US today is such that it may be the most common bacterial infection.

Etiology—Gonorrhea is caused by the nonmobile, nonspore-forming gram-negative diplococcus, *Neisseria gonorrhea*. This organism requires precise conditions for growth. It dies quickly on a dry swab, survives only briefly on a moist towel and does not grow at room temperature. Culture of the organism requires a special enriched medium that contains antibiotics to suppress growth of other organisms and an atmosphere containing 3–10% carbon dioxide. Certain strains of *N. gonorrhea* are resistant to penicillin. There are no nonhuman reservoirs of gonorrhea.

Epidemiology—Gonorrhea has reached epidemic proportions in the US and the incidence of infections has been rising exponentially over the past few years. Incidence in the US is about one million cases annually. The reason for the increased incidence relates primarily to the spread of the disease by infected people who are asymptomatic or who have been inadequately treated. In the US there is little emphasis on tracing and treating contacts, as there is in European countries which are not experiencing the same epidemic of gonorrhea. The incidence and prevalence of gonorrhea relate to age, sex, race, socioeconomic status and marital status. These factors correlate with sexual activity, the motivation to seek medical attention and accessibility to health care.

Pathophysiology—Gonococci are inoculated onto mucous membranes by an infected person. The hallmark of GC is copious, yellow pus. Common sites of inoculation are the pharynx, urethra, cervix, and anus. The incubation period for gonorrhea is 3 to 5 days. Once inoculated in the genital tract, the infection may ascend, particularly in the female. Epididymitis and prostatis are rare. In the female, the gonococcus does not survive well in the uterus but infects the fallopian tubes in about 15% of cases. This may cause scarring and later sterility. About 1–3% of affected adults develop gonococcemia, two-thirds of these are females. Distant sites of infection include the joints, the meninges and the heart valves.

Signs and Symptoms—Clinical manifestations of gonorrhea depend on the site and duration of infection and whether there has been local or systemic spread.

A profuse, purulent, yellow urethral discharge associated with dysuria and frequency develops in 90–95% of infected males. If untreated, the urethritis will resolve in 8 weeks. Anorectal and pharyngeal gonococcal infections are common among homosexual men. Anorectal infections are usually asymptomatic but may produce anorectal burning or pruritus, tenesmus, and a bloody mucopurulent rectal discharge. These symptoms may subside without treatment. Pharyngeal infections may produce an exudative tonsilitis but are most commonly asymptomatic.

Only 5–10% of infected females develop symptoms, which include dysuria, frequency, increased vaginal discharge, abnormal menstrual bleeding, and anorectal discomfort. The symptoms of urethritis may be confused with a urinary tract infection, and the increased vaginal discharge may be attributed to vaginitis. Both of these other diseases may occur concomitantly with GC. Pelvic inflammatory disease may occur and is manifested by lower abdominal tenderness and pain, and perhaps fever, chills, nausea, vomiting and leukocytosis. Physical examination reveals signs of pelvic peritonitis.

Gonococcemia may be the first sign of infection and includes fever, polyarthralgias and papular, petechial, pustular, hemorrhagic or necrotic skin lesions that are usually located on the distal extremities. The joint infection is a tenosynovitis or a septic arthritis of a single large joint or of several joints. The signs and symptoms of gonococcemia may not precede onset of arthritis. The synovial fluid is purulent, and joint destruction occurs very rapidly without proper treatment.

Diagnosis of gonorrhea in a male is made on a gram stain of the urethral discharge by the presence of gram-negative diplococci within leukocytes. If gram-negative diplococci are seen but are extracellular, a culture is required for diagnosis. The diagnosis of gonorrhea in females can only be made by culture. The anal canal and pharynx should also be cultured in women and homosexual men. Blood cultures are unlikely to be positive for gonococcus 48 hours after the onset of gonococcemia. Joint cultures are unlikely to be positive for gonococcus later in the course of the arthritis.

Syphilis is a chronic systemic infection that is seen in three stages which progress over many years. In untreated syphilis, degeneration occurs in the central nervous and cardiovascular systems.

Etiology—Syphilis is caused by the spirochete *Treponema pallidum*, a spiral-shaped organism that is not seen under an ordinary light microscope but can be visualized using the dark-field technique. The organisms have not been cultured because their growth requirements are so precise. The only naturally occurring host for *T pallidum* is man.

Epidemiology—The incidence of syphilis has remained the same over the last few years. The incidences of tertiary and congenital syphilis have been declining since 1943. As with other venereal diseases, syphilis is more common among indigent nonwhites living in urban areas and in homosexuals.

Pathophysiology—Nearly all cases of syphilis are acquired by sexual contact with infectious lesions. Syphilis may be rarely acquired by non-sexual personal contact, contact with contaminated fomites, following blood transfusions and *in utero*. The spirochete penetrates intact mucous membranes or abraded skin and enters the lymphatics and blood within a few hours. The average incubation time for syphilis is 21 days; however, it ranges from 10 to 90 days depending on the size of the inoculum. Primary syphilis is manifested by a single, usually raised and indurated lesion which appears at the site of inoculation. This lesion is known as a chancre and heals spontaneously in 2 to 6 weeks. The chancre is an infectious lesion. Secondary syphilis appears approximately 6 weeks after the chancre has healed and is manifested by a symmetrical maculopapular rash and non-tender generalized lymphadenopathy. The rash subsides in 2 to 6 weeks and the patient enters the latent stage, which is detectable only by serologic testing. About 25% of untreated patients have one or more recurrences of the rash during the first 2 to 4 years. About one-third of untreated patients develop tertiary syphilis, which may be manifested by the presence of gummas in any part of the body, or degeneration of the central nervous or cardiovascular systems.

Signs and Symptoms—The chancre begins as a papule which rapidly becomes eroded and forms an ulcer. The chancre is most commonly found on the external genitalia or the anal canal but can be found anywhere. It is painless if located on the genitals. The chancre is accompanied by painless lymphadenopathy. Atypical primary lesions may also occur.

Secondary syphilis is characterized by appearance of nonpruritic red or pink macules on the trunk and proximal extremities. In about 1–2 months, red papular lesions also appear that may progress to pustular or necrotic lesions. The lesions are widespread and may involve the palms, soles, face and scalp. The papules may scale but vesicles are not seen. In warm, moist areas of the body the papular lesions enlarge, erode and produce moist pink or gray-white lesions known as condyloma lata. The lesions may also occur on mucous membranes as painless erosions. Fever, anorexia, weight loss, malaise and headache may accompany the rash.

Latent syphilis is detected only by positive serologic tests. The blood is intermittently infectious and pregnant women may infect the fetus *in utero*. This condition may persist throughout life or tertiary syphilis may develop. Spontaneous cures probably do not occur.

Tertiary syphilis may involve the central nervous system in one of three ways and is seen in 4 to 6.5% of patients. Meningovascular syphilis may occur 5 to 10 years after the primary infection and involves inflammation of the pia and the arachnoid. There may be either focal or widespread symptoms. General paresis reflects widespread parenchymal damage to the brain and results in changes in personality, changes in affect, hyperactive reflexes, a small irregular pupil which accommodates but does not react to light, changes in sensorium including illusions, delusions and hallucinations, changes in intellect including decreased recent memory, impaired orientation, judgment and insight, and an inability to perform simple calculations and difficulty with speech. General paresis is seen about 20 years after infection. Tabes dorsalis is due to demyelinization of the posterior columns, dorsal roots and dorsal-root ganglia of the spinal cord. Signs and symptoms include ataxia, wide-based gait, foot-slap, paresthesias, bladder disturbances, impotence and loss of position, deep pain, and temperature sensations. Trophic degeneration of joints, and ulcers of the feet may develop as a result of loss of pain sensation. Tabes dorsalis occurs 25 to 30 years after infection.

Endarteritis obliterans of the small blood vessels that supply blood to the walls of large blood vessels results in medial necrosis and loss of elastic tissue. This occurs primarily in the ascending and transverse arch of the aorta. The result is aortitis, aortic regurgitation, saccular aneurysm and coronary artery stenosis. Only 10% of patients with cardiovascular syphilis are symptomatic, while lesions are found in 50% of affected individuals at autopsy. Cardiovascular syphilis appears 10 to 40 years after infection.

Genital Herpes, also known as herpes genitalis is the second most common sexually transmitted disease in this country. It occurs in acute (primary) and recurrent forms.

Etiology—The vast majority of cases of genital herpes are caused by Herpes Simplex Virus type 2 (HSV-2). A very small number may be caused by Herpes Simplex Virus type 1 (HSV-1) or a concurrent infection with both types. HSV is a DNA virus and is identified through cultures and serologic testing for antibodies to the virus.

Epidemiology—Genital herpes has reached epidemic proportions in this country and the rate of occurrence seems to be increasing. The peak incidence is during the sexually active years although all age groups are affected. Herpes infections occur in all socio-economic groups. Recurrent episodes may be more frequent than primary ones.

Pathophysiology—Genital herpes is contracted through sexual contact with an individual who has an active infection. After the primary infec-

tion, the virus resides in the local neural ganglia and periodically descends to the skin to cause lesions. The causes of reactivation from this latent stage have not been clearly identified. It is often difficult to identify primary cases of herpes genitalis as many cases are asymptomatic. Recurrent episodes generally are shorter in duration, less severe, and less likely to be associated with systemic involvement than are primary cases.

Signs and Symptoms—A prodromal stage usually precedes the appearance of skin lesions. Symptoms during this phase may include pain, tingling sensations or itching. Usually within 24 hours lesions appear, which initially are papular and rapidly progress through vesicular, ulcer and crusting stages in an otherwise asymptomatic patient. Systemic involvement may occur in neonates and immunocompromised patients.

A typical primary episode lasts two to three weeks while recurrent cases are much shorter (five to ten days). Recurrent disease is more likely to occur in patients with a more severe initial episode, a prior recurrence, history of sexually transmitted disease, younger age, and immunosuppression. While lesions are often limited to the genitals and perineal area, they may also occur on the thighs and buttocks.

The diagnosis of herpes genitalis is made through history and physical exam as well as culture and serologic techniques.

Respiratory Tract Infections

Respiratory tract infections are the most common of acute illnesses. Etiologic agents include viruses, bacteria, mycoplasma and on unusual occasions other organisms. Lower respiratory tract infections usually indicate an impairment of host defenses.

Normal Anatomy and Physiology—A number of organisms normally colonize the nasopharynx. Most of these organisms are not pathogenic and will return if eradicated by antibiotics. The normal flora may inhibit growth of pathogenic organisms. Potential pathogens often colonize the upper respiratory tract. These organisms will not often result in infection to the individual but may be the source of disease in others when transmitted, (eg, meningococcus). Transient colonizers may become infectious in some individuals. Anaerobic organisms constitute 90% of the normal flora of the upper respiratory tract. Also, normal flora usually do not extend below the larynx; the remainder of the respiratory tract is sterile in healthy people.

The lungs are protected by several defense mechanisms. The lining of the respiratory tract is composed of sticky surfaces on which particles adhere. Particles larger than 5 μm are usually efficiently filtered and do not reach the alveoli. The lungs also have mechanisms to remove particles which reach the bronchi or alveoli. Coughing and sneezing are natural defenses for removing particles. Ciliated epithelial cells line the lower respiratory tract. Mucus secretion by goblet cells helps trap particles and suspend them for transport by the cilia. This mucociliary transport system is the most important means for clearing particles. Macrophages located in alveoli can engulf particles. Secretory IgA helps with immunologic clearance. If a particle cannot be removed or destroyed within the lung, a granuloma forms around it to wall it off.

Environmental factors such as air pollution, cigarette smoking, drugs such as alcohol and anesthetics, and other disease states such as congestive heart failure and leukemia can suppress the normal defensive mechanisms of the lung.

Approximately 95% of upper respiratory tract infections are due to *viruses*.

Etiology—More than 150 serotypes, representing 12 groups of viruses, have been associated with URIs. Rhinoviruses cause 40% of respiratory illness, adenoviruses cause 2 to 10%, with the remainder being caused by respiratory syncytial virus, coronavirus, and influenza viruses.

Epidemiology—URIs follow seasonal variation, with the incidence being highest in winter and lowest in summer. This type of virus infection is transmitted mainly through the coughing and sneezing of infectious aerosolized droplets, but transmission also occurs through contamination of hands and objects by nasal secretions and saliva. Infection depends on the size of the inoculum and the response of the host.

Pathophysiology—Respiratory viruses cause mucosal denuding and consequent decreased lung defense mechanisms. This predisposes to serious bacterial infections, although this superinfection occurs in only a minority of patients.

Signs and Symptoms—The signs and symptoms of a viral URI are familiar and are known as the "common cold." These include a coryzal syndrome characterized by nasal stuffiness and discharge, sneezing, moderate sore throat, and mild constitutional symptoms. Fever may or may not be present. Children may develop bronchitis, bronchiolitis and pneumonia with rhinoviruses. Both children and adults may develop lower respiratory infection with adenovirus, respiratory syncitial virus, and influenza viruses.

Streptococcal infections are important because of the seriousness of the acute illness as well as the late complications which are not infective but are immunologically mediated. Acute respiratory tract infections include streptococcal pharyngitis, scarlet fever, and pneumonia. The late complications include acute rheumatic fever, rheumatic heart disease, and acute glomerulonephritis.

Epidemiology—Streptococcal infections occur throughout the population. Respiratory streptococcal infections are more common during the colder months. Scarlet fever is usually a disease of children between 6 months and 10 years of age. Infants less than 3 months old rarely have streptococcal infections. Streptococcal pharyngitis occurs commonly among children and young adults. As many as 20% of the population are asymptomatic carriers of group A streptococcus. A streptococcal URI may be spread by inhalation of respiratory secretions. Epidemics of streptococcal URIs occur.

Etiology—Streptococci are gram-positive cocci that tend to form chains. Three groups have been identified by their ability to hemolyze red cells in culture media by the enzymes streptolysin O and S. Alpha streptococcus, or viridans, beta hemolytic streptococcus, and gamma-nonhemolytic streptococcus are the three groups. There are 13 serologic types of streptococci designated by the letters A to O. Most URIs are caused by Group A streptococci. The late complications of rheumatic fever and glomerulonephritis have only been attributed to Group A streptococci.

Pathophysiology—Streptococci are inhaled into the nasopharynx and are normally cleared by defense mechanisms or become transient colonizers. The size of the inoculum, the virulence of the organism, the presence of type-specific immunity and the defense mechanisms of the host determine if an infection is to occur. Type-specific immunity lasts for years.

Signs and Symptoms—Streptococcal infections present a variable clinical syndrome and as many as 40% of individuals may be asymptomatic. The incubation period usually lasts 3 to 5 days. The onset is acute and the illness includes fever, chills, headache, sore throat, anorexia, malaise, and in children nausea and vomiting. Symptoms reach a maximum in 1–2 days. The sore throat is worsened by swallowing, hoarseness is present, and nasal stuffiness, nasal discharge and a nonproductive cough may occur. Earache is common. Scarlet fever is streptococcal pharyngitis followed by a rash with circumoral pallor.

Patients with streptococcal pharyngitis may be mildly to moderately ill, with fever to 40°C, tachycardia, and a diffusely red posterior pharynx and soft palate. The uvula is edematous. Characteristically, there is an exudate on the tonsils which may be scraped off without bleeding. The nasal discharge is thick, mucopurulent and may contain blood.

The clinical course of a streptococcal URI is short with the fever resolving in 3–4 days or 5–9 days in adults and children respectively. Exfoliation of the epithelium begins as the rash fades.

A positive throat culture for beta-hemolytic streptococci in the setting of the characteristic history, signs and symptoms makes the diagnosis of streptococcal pharyngitis.

Pneumonia is an infection in the alveoli that only occurs when impairment of host defenses allows the organism access to alveoli and the infectious process cannot be contained. Pneumonias occur in individuals with underlying diseases such as congestive heart failure, lung cancer, chronic bronchitis, asthma, etc.; those who are immunologically compromised, such as the elderly, patients with leukemia or lymphoma, patients being treated with cancer chemotherapy, corticosteroids or immunosuppressive agents, in cigarette smokers and alcoholics or in individuals who recently had a viral pneumonia or general anesthesia. Pneumococcus (*Streptococcus pneumoniae*) accounts for 60% of community acquired pneumonias severe enough to require hospitalization. Other organisms include *Hemophilus influenzae*, *Staphylococcus*, *Klebsiella*, and *Pseudomonas*. This discussion will focus only on pneumococcal pneumonia.

Etiology—*Streptococcus pneumoniae* is a gram-positive encapsulated coccus that usually grows in pairs; hence the name diplococcus. There are 85 serotypes of pneumococcus that are pathogenic for man. Capsular forms 1 through 8 account for 60% of infections.

Epidemiology—Approximately 5–60% of the population are asymptomatic carriers of the pneumococcus, depending on the season. The infection is more prevalent in winter and spring. Pneumococcal pneumonia accounts for approximately 10% of admissions to acute medical wards. Incidence of the disease is highest among males 30 to 50 years old with chronic bronchitis and/or emphysema. The incidence of pneumococcal pneumonia has changed little although the mortality has greatly decreased with the advent of antibiotics.

Pathophysiology—Pneumococcal infections of the nasopharynx or pharynx do not occur. Impairment of normal defense mechanisms of the lungs allows pneumonia to occur. Pneumococci are aspirated into the lung and usually lodge in the right-lower, right-middle or left-lower lobe, where they multiply rapidly. The response to the multiplying organisms involves transudation of fluid into the alveoli which becomes a growth medium for the organism and a mode for local spread to other alveoli, segments, lobules, lobes, and pleura. Polymorphonuclear leukocytes come in to phagocytize the bacteria. Macrophages appear later to clean up the fibrin and debris. Antibodies against the pneumococcus enhance phagocytosis and cause organisms to agglutinate and adhere to the alveolar wall, thus slowing spread of the infection. Bacteremia is usually transient. Complications include infections of the meninges, joints, peritoneum, and pleural and pericardial spaces.

Signs and Symptoms—The clinical course of pneumococcal pneumonia is classic. The pneumonia may be preceded by a URI syndrome by a few days. The onset is abrupt and patients may state the hour of onset. In 80% of patients there is a sudden shaking chill and a rapid rise in temperature with tachycardia and tachypnea. In 75% of patients pleuritic chest pain and a productive cough develop. The sputum is mucoid and pink or rusty in color. Dyspnea is a common complaint. The patient will appear acutely ill but will not complain of nausea, headache or malaise. If untreated the signs and symptoms last for 7 to 10 days. Then there is diaphoresis, a sudden drop in temperature and dramatic improvement. Circulatory collapse and heart failure are common in fatal cases.

On physical examination, breath sounds are decreased and rales and rhonchi are present. The chest radiograph shows a homogeneous density in the affected areas. There is a leukocytosis with 70 to 90% of the WBC being mature or immature polymorphonuclear leukocytes, the "shift to the left." Blood culture is positive in only 20–30% of cases. Gram-stain of the sputum shows many PMNs and gram-positive cocci usually in pairs.

Poor prognostic signs include leukopenia, bacteremia, multilobar involvement, infection outside the lungs, underlying systemic disease, and circulatory collapse. The fatality rate in pneumococcal pneumonia is about 5% despite appropriate treatment.

Respiratory Tract Infections Due to Mycoplasma— Mycoplasma, which has been called pleuropneumonia-like organisms (PPLO), do not have a cell wall, reproduce by fission, and grow outside of cells. *Mycoplasma pneumoniae* causes asymptomatic infections, upper respiratory infections and pneumonia. Mycoplasma pneumonia is also called atypical pneumonia, Eaton's agent pneumonia, and cold agglutinin positive pneumonia.

Epidemiology—The infection, which is spread by inhalation of respiratory secretions, is characterized by occurrence among many family members or in large numbers of people living in crowded environments such as military bases and college dormitories. Mycoplasma infections are common among children and young adults and rarely occur in individuals over 40 years old. *Mycoplasma pneumoniae* accounts for 15–20% of all pneumonias. Mycoplasma infections are more common in the winter.

Etiology—Mycoplasmas are unique organisms of extremely small size. Instead of a cell wall, mycoplasmas are surrounded by a unit membrane. Mycoplasmas cause the production of specific cold-reacting antibodies (IgM) and are resistant to penicillin. Mycoplasmas may frequently be found as normal flora in the upper respiratory tract. It takes 2 to 4 weeks to culture mycoplasma.

Signs and Symptoms—The incubation period for mycoplasma varies from 9 to 12 days. The disease begins as a URI that progresses to bronchitis and pneumonia in 3 to 10% of cases. A nonproductive cough is the most characteristic symptom. In cases of pneumonia, the cough may become productive of blood-tinged sputum later in the course. Headache, general malaise, muscle aches, nasal congestion, and sore throat are common. Usually 40% of household members have the same symptoms.

The clinical course of the disease is variable. Fever may persist for two weeks in untreated cases. Abnormalities in the chest radiograph last for 7 to 10 days or longer in treated cases and 3 weeks in untreated cases. The pneumonia is usually multilobar and may be bilateral. Lower lobes are more commonly involved than upper lobes. The infiltrate is less dense than in bacterial pneumonia and often is of an interstitial pattern. The physical findings on chest examination usually are much less striking than the severity of disease noted on the chest radiograph.

Complications are rare even without treatment.

The diagnosis is based on the history and clinical picture plus the chest radiograph. There is a minimal increase in WBC count without a "shift to the left." Lymphocytosis with atypical forms may be present. Cold agglutinins are positive in 50% of the cases after the second week of the illness. Monocytes may be seen in the sputum.

Tuberculosis (TB)

Tuberculosis is a bacterial infection that has greatly decreased in prevalence in the US. Although TB can involve many organs, pulmonary TB is the most common. Bovine tuberculosis has essentially been eradicated.

Etiology—*Mycobacterium tuberculosis* is a rod-shaped organism that requires high oxygen tension for optimum growth and produces no toxins or enzymes. The organism has unique staining properties due to the lipid content of the cell wall. Carbol-fuchsin stain does not wash off with acid, hence the name "acid fast." The bacilli can be cultured.

Epidemiology—Since the beginning of the 20th century the incidence of TB has been declining in the US. In 1980 about 28,000 new cases were reported. There is evidence that the rate of decline has stopped, possibly due to the recent immigration to the United States of large numbers of refugees from Southeast Asia. In any case, the majority of people with TB today have either healed or dormant TB. Tuberculosis is no longer a leading cause of death. The declining mortality and morbidity due to TB is related to an increased standard of living with better nutrition and less crowded living conditions, as well as antituberculosis therapy.

Tubercle bacilli are aerosolized as droplets during coughing by a person with cavitary disease. The fresh droplets, which are 1 to 5 μm in diameter, reach the alveoli and establish an infection in a susceptible host. The infectiousness of a patient is related to the severity of the disease, the number of bacilli in the lesion and the closeness and length of the contact. An infected person is considered no longer contagious after about 2 weeks of appropriate chemotherapy. Transmission is also blocked by exposure of the air to UV light and adequate ventilation.

Pathophysiology—Tubercle bacilli are inhaled and deposited in peripheral alveoli throughout the lung. Before the infection can be contained by a local cellular response, the bacilli are drained to lymph nodes in the hilum and then disseminated throughout the body by the bloodstream.

Sites that are seeded by bacilli include the apices of the lungs, the kidney, the growing ends of bones, and other areas of high oxygen tension. Cellular immunity involving lymphocytes, macrophages and giant cells develops in several weeks. Once cellular immunity develops the reaction forms granulomas at the sites of infection and in time caseous necrosis may develop in these granulomas. During caseation, cytotoxic material is released from T lymphocytes which destroys the bacilli as well as the surrounding tissue. The sites then heal by resolution, fibrosis and calcification. In some cases the immunity is inadequate and overwhelming infection develops. The healed lesions still contain viable tubercle bacilli. These may remain dormant for the life of the individual. In 10% of cases, these lesions develop into clinical disease sometime after the initial infection. Reactivation usually occurs under circumstances of decreased immunity as in malnutrition, underlying disease, old age, or treatment with corticosteroids.

Signs and Symptoms—The initial infection or primary TB usually does not produce many signs or symptoms. The incubation period is 4 to 8 weeks. Mild fever and malaise may occur as tuberculin hypersensitivity develops. In some cases, especially in a child less than 3 years old or in elderly people, an overwhelming infection may result from the primary infection.

Pulmonary tuberculosis usually occurs after a period of dormancy in a previously infected individual. The onset is insidious. The patient may be asymptomatic with a routine chest radiograph leading to the diagnosis. Fever to 40°C may occur in the late afternoon or evening. Night sweats are common. General malaise, fatigue, irritability and weight loss may occur. A cough, particularly early in the morning and productive of green or yellow sputum that may be blood streaked is common. When cavitation occurs highly infectious material is spilled into the bronchi for expectoration. The blood in the sputum is usually from ulceration of the bronchial mucosa and this bleeding will subside. Massive hemorrhage can occur if a pulmonary artery in a tuberculous cavity ruptures. Death may occur from exsanguination or obstruction of airflow.

Spread of pulmonary tuberculosis into the pleura results in pleuritic

chest pain and the formation of a pleural effusion as part of the inflammatory reaction. The presence of a large effusion may compromise lung function and result in the complaint of dyspnea. Tuberculosis can also spread from the lung or the lymph nodes into the pericardium where the same inflammatory process occurs. An acute pericardial effusion may cause cardiac tamponade. Later, the inflamed pericardium may scar down, calcify and become restrictive to motion, be heard as a friction rub and present as congestive heart failure.

During the dissemination phase, bacilli are seeded in the kidney, bone, adrenals and meninges. At each site the same inflammatory process occurs with caseation and liquefaction. If the infection cannot be contained, local spread may occur. Tuberculosis in the kidney may result in infection of the rest of the genitourinary tract and present as cystitis, epididymitis or prostatitis. Gross or microscopic hematuria is seen on urinalysis. Although pyuria is present the urine is "sterile" by routine culture. An intravenous pyelogram will show characteristic lesions in the kidney. In females, tuberculosis of the fallopian tubes and uterus may result in abdominal pain, vaginal discharge, sterility or ectopic pregnancy. Tuberculosis of the bone occurs most commonly in childhood. Spondylitis may result in localized back pain or compression of the spinal cord. Tuberculosis of the adrenal glands may cause total destruction of the glands and result in Addison's disease. Tuberculous meningitis is also seen. Signs and symptoms include headache, restlessness, irritability, nausea, vomiting and stiffness of the neck. A change in mentation may be the only sign of the disease.

Miliary tuberculosis is a massive dissemination of tubercle bacilli throughout the body. Lesions are found, in addition to the previously mentioned sites, in the liver, spleen, bone marrow and other organs which do not have a high oxygen tension. The signs and symptoms are nonspecific and include dyspnea, weight loss, weakness, fever, night sweats and gastrointestinal disturbances. Death is certain unless appropriate treatment is promptly instituted. Diagnosis is based on a biopsy of the liver or bone marrow showing caseating granulomas.

The diagnosis of tuberculosis rests on the use of a skin test with tuberculin which is the protein fraction of the tubercle bacilli. Active versus dormant disease, however, cannot be separated by this test. Sensitized lymphocytes accumulate at the site of intradermal injection of tuberculin. Five tuberculin units are injected and the skin test is read 48 to 72 hours. A positive test is greater than 10 mm of induration. False negative tests occur in 15 to 20% of patients with clinical tuberculosis. The skin test does not become positive until the development of cellular immunity. In patients with a decreased number of lymphocytes, an overwhelming infection, a pleural effusion or a fever, the skin test may be falsely negative and tests for anergy should also be given. The chest radiograph is also essential to the diagnosis of tuberculosis. It shows multinodular infiltrates with or without cavitation in one or both upper lobes. Acid-fast bacilli may be seen on an appropriately stained smear of sputum from a patient with tuberculosis. Sputum may also be cultured for the organisms.

Viral Hepatitis

Acute viral hepatitis is a systemic infection affecting predominantly, but not exclusively, the liver. Various viruses can cause acute hepatitis but Type A, Type B, and Type non-A, non-B are the most common. Cases of hepatitis A (HA) and B (HB) generally differ in their incubation period, mode of transmission and sequelae. Precise differentiation, however, depends on the presence of distinct serological markers. Type non-A, non-B hepatitis (HNANB) resembles HB clinically but is serologically distinct.

Etiology—HAV is an RNA virus while HBV is a DNA virus. Little is known of the nucleic acid composition of NANB virus(es).

Epidemiology—HA is transmitted almost exclusively by the fecal-oral route. Children and young adults are most commonly infected with HA, which often occurs in epidemics in crowded medical facilities such as state institutions for the mentally retarded. Good hygiene, particularly washing hands, decreases the transmission of HA. Type B virus is transmitted parenterally, transcutaneously, orally, and sexually. The risk of post-transfusion HB has nearly been eliminated by screening donors. HNANV is transmitted primarily by transfusion of blood products containing the agent.

Pathology—The liver injury caused by all three viruses includes panlobular infiltration with small lymphocytes or monocytes, hepatic cell degenerative swelling, ballooning and perhaps necrosis, hyperplasia of Kupffer cells and variable degrees of cholestasis without fatty infiltration. In uncomplicated cases the reticulum framework is maintained and orderly regeneration of hepatic cells occurs. In severe cases liver-cell necrosis is extensive, the reticulum framework is destroyed, and fibrosis between liver lobules occurs. This is called subacute hepatic necrosis. In massive hepatic necrosis, a small shrunken liver is found at autopsy.

Pathophysiology—In HB the liver cell replicates the virus and the virus or its fragments are incorporated into liver-cell membranes. Humoral antibodies, IgG and IgM, are formed against the viruses. Antibodies attack the "foreign" plasma membranes. Cellular immunity is involved in the liver damage. Circulating immune complexes and complement activation are responsible for the systemic manifestations seen in hepatitis. Thus the consequences of HB are largely due to the immune response to the infection rather than to the cytotoxicity of the virus. The pathophysiology of the other forms of viral hepatitis is less well understood.

Signs and Symptoms—Classically HA has a short incubation period of 15 to 45 days and an acute onset; HB has a long incubation period, 45 to 160 days, and an insidious onset. HA is a mild disease with complete recovery and the carrier state does not develop. HB may be a severe disease with a poor prognosis, can progress to chronic hepatitis and a carrier state may develop. HNANB resembles HB.

The prodromal symptoms vary and may include anorexia, nausea, vomiting, changes in the senses of smell and taste, fatigue, malaise, arthralgias, myalgias, headache, photophobia, pharyngitis, cough, coryza and fever. The symptoms usually occur 1 to 2 weeks before the onset of jaundice. Dark urine and clay-colored stools may occur 1 to 5 days before the jaundice. During the icteric phase, the liver is enlarged and tender and there may be right upper quadrant pain. Splenomegaly and cervical lymphadenopathy may also occur. The symptoms subside during the recovery phase but laboratory abnormalities remain. The recovery phase lasts from 2 to 12 weeks, being longer in HB. Laboratory recovery occurs in 3 to 4 months.

Several liver-cell enzymes, including serum aminotransferases, increase during the prodromal phase of acute viral hepatitis. The degree of the rise does not correlate with the severity of the disease. The liver-cell enzymes peak with the onset of jaundice. Jaundice is visible in the skin and sclera when the serum bilirubin level exceeds 2.5 mg/100 mL.

Serological markers are used to distinguish between the three types of viral hepatitis. In HA the onset of symptoms is accompanied by a sharp rise in IgM anti-HAV and a gradual but lasting rise in IgG anti-HAV. HB is characterized by several antigens derived from the virus and antibodies to the antigens. The antigens include surface and core antigen as well as an enigmatic e antigen, which appears to be derived from the core of the virus. The surface antigen, HBsAg, rises sharply before clinical or biochemical abnormalities occur. Antibody to core, HBcAb, and e antigen, HbeAg, appear in the serum in close proximity to the clinical and biochemical abnormalities. In uncomplicated cases HbsAg and HbeAg are "cleared" within about four to six months and the antigens are supplanted in serum by their respective antibodies. The diagnosis of acute HB is made definitely by demonstrating the occurrence of HbsAg, HbcAb and HbeAg in serum. Often, however, a presumptive diagnosis is based on the history, physical findings, biochemical abnormalities (eg, elevated serum bilirubin and aminotransferases) and the presence of HbsAg in serum. There are no serological markers for HNANB; the diagnosis usually is made on the basis of compatible clinical features and the absence of serological markers of acute HA and HB.

Nearly all patients with HA and the majority of patients with HB and HNANB recover without sequelae. Poor prognostic signs include the presence of subacute hepatic necrosis, a serum bilirubin level of greater than 20 mg/100 mL that persists, and an elevated prothrombin time indicating extensive hepatocellular damage. Elderly patients or patients with underlying disease may have a more severe form of hepatitis. The mortality rate is 0.1% and 1 to 2% for HA and HB hepatitis respectively.

Chronic hepatitis occurs as a complication of HB in 5 to 10% of patients and 30% of patients with HNANB. About 0.1 to 1.0% of patients with HB develop a carrier state of HbsAg. Such individuals usually are asymptomatic and non-infectious but they have an increased risk of developing hepatocellular carcinoma.

Delta agent is a recently-discovered incomplete RNA virus that causes hepatitis only in patients who are persistently HbsAg positive.

Infectious Diarrhea

Normal Physiology—The gastrointestinal tract has a number of normal defense mechanisms that prevent infections. The stomach normally is sterile because the acidity destroys most organisms. In situations where the pH of the stomach is increased, the number of pathogens required for the establishment of an infection is significantly decreased. The remainder of the gastrointestinal tract has a normal bacterial flora which inhibits the growth of other organisms. The normal flora of the large intestine is composed predominantly of anaerobes. Some species of the normal flora produce short-chain fatty acids or antibiotics such as clostin which prevent the growth of pathogens. Other members of the normal flora decrease the growth of pathogens by competing with them for nutrients. Antibiotics that suppress normal flora predispose to bacterial infection. The gastrointestinal tract is lined by cells which produce mucus. This mucus forms a barrier to bacterial invasion of the gut wall. Locally produced IgA and antibodies produced elsewhere, such as IgG, enhance phagocytosis of bacteria within the GI tract. Motility of the gastrointestinal tract moves organisms out and thus prevents infections. Diarrhea increases transit and rids the body of organisms. Antimotility agents interfere with this defense.

Diarrhea is defined as an increase in numbers of stools per day and/or an increase in stool volume. Acute diarrhea is sudden in onset, lasts for less than 2 weeks and is usually caused by an infectious agent. Chronic diarrhea is of longer duration and is usually due to noninfectious gastrointestinal disease.

Etiology—Diarrhea may be caused by bacterial toxins, bacterial organisms, viruses, or parasites. Diarrhea need not be caused by a pathogen but may be due to changes in normal flora or by normal colonic flora reaching the small intestine. Bacteria commonly causing diarrhea by the production of toxins include enterotoxigenic *Escherichia coli*, *Staphylococcus*, *Clostridium perfringens*, and *Clostridium difficile*. Bacterial diarrhea is caused by *Shigella*, *Salmonella*, *Campylobacter jejuni* and *Yersinia enterocolitica* in the US and *Vibrio cholera* in other countries. Reovirus-like agent (Norwalk agent), Echo, and coxsackie viruses commonly cause diarrhea while influenza viruses do not. Parasites include *Entamoeba histolytica* and *Giardia lamblia*.

Epidemiology—The transmission of the causative agent is via the fecal-oral route in most cases. Contaminated objects, food and water may transmit the agent.

Pathology—Viral diarrhea may cause villous shortening in the small intestine, an increase in the number of crypt cells and widening of the lamina propria. Diarrhea caused by bacterial invasion results in hyperemia, leukocyte infiltration, and frank ulceration of the bowel wall. *Entamoeba histolytica* produces an inflammatory colitis similar to ulcerative colitis except for the presence of the parasite and larger, flask-shaped ulcers of the colonic mucosa.

Pathophysiology—Bacteria may cause diarrhea via enterotoxin induced hypersecretion or invasion of the gut wall by the bacteria. Enterotoxins stimulate adenyl cyclase in the mucosal cells of the intestine which results in massive secretion of fluid and electrolytes into the bowel lumen. Mucosal integrity is preserved and absorption is normal. In bacterial invasion, the damage to the mucosa results in defective absorption. *Giardia* probably produces diarrhea by the same mechanism since invasion of the small bowel occurs. *C difficile* causes pseudomembranous colitis (antibiotic-associated colitis).

Signs and Symptoms—Systemic symptoms including fever, headache, anorexia, vomiting, malaise and myalgias may accompany diarrhea regardless of the etiology except when toxins are ingested.

Twelve to 24 hours after eating food contaminated by *Clostridium perfringens* or *Staphylococcus*, diarrhea with abdominal pain, cramps, and nausea, but no vomiting or systemic symptoms occurs. The diarrhea contains no pus or blood. Recovery occurs in 12 to 24 hours.

In diarrhea in which organisms invade the mucosa, such as *Shigella* or *Salmonella*, systemic symptoms occur along with lower abdominal cramps, tenesmus, and rectal urgency. Pus and erythrocytes or gross blood are found in the stool. *Shigella* causes an explosive diarrhea and fever. The disease is usually self-limited with the fever subsiding in four days and the diarrhea subsiding in one week. *Shigella* also produces a neurotoxin that may cause seizures in children. *Salmonella* produces a less acute clinical picture.

Enterotoxigenic *E coli*, frequently the causative agent in "turista" or "traveler's diarrhea" may produce mild or severe symptoms. The incubation period is 24 to 48 hours and the diarrhea lasts for 2 to 7 days. The stools contain no blood and few white blood cells.

Viral diarrhea is usually accompanied by nausea and vomiting and other systemic symptoms. The diarrhea is usually mild, recovery occurs in 48 hours but malabsorption due to lactase deficiency may persist for several weeks. No red blood cells or white blood cells are seen in examination of the stool.

The prognosis of acute infectious diarrhea is usually excellent when treated with adequate fluid replacement. Complications are rare except in infants or extremely debilitated patients who are unable to tolerate the dehydration. Pseudomembranous colitis usually responds promptly to discontinuation of the causative antibiotic, although some cases require treatment with an antibiotic directed at *C. difficile.*

Central Nervous System Infection

Meningitis and encephalitis are medical emergencies requiring rapid diagnosis and specific therapy. While meningitis involves only the leptomeninges, encephalitis involves the brain tissue itself and may also involve the meninges.

Etiology—Meningitis is often caused by bacteria; the most common pathogens in most age groups being *Streptococcus pneumoniae, Haemophilus influenzae,* and *Neisseria meningitis.* In the neonatal age period, *Escherichia coli* and group B streptococci are common. Viruses such as enteroviruses and mumps virus also cause meningitis. Fungal meningitis occurs predominantly in immunocompromised patients. Encephalitis is usually caused by viruses such as mumps and herpes viruses.

Epidemiology—The peak incidence of meningitis is during the winter months and is often associated with respiratory tract infections. The majority of cases occur in children less than four years of age especially in infants between three and 18 months of age. Between 30,000 and 40,000 cases occur each year.

Pathophysiology—Infection of the subarachnoid space results in inflammation of the leptomeninges and the cerebrospinal fluid (CSF). Pus may also accumulate. Such inflammation may result in disruption of the natural flow of CSF leading to hydrocephalus. In association with the presence of bacteria or other microorganisms and inflammation, CSF levels of glucose, protein and lactic acid may be altered. In encephalitis, the brain matter itself is involved. While the mode of infection in meningitis and encephalitis is usually through the hematogenous route, meningitis and brain abscesses may occur via direct extension of infection, often secondary to trauma.

Signs and Symptoms—Systemic manifestations of central nervous system infection include such features as fever, irritability and somnolence. A single seizure prior to diagnosis is not uncommon. Nuchal rigidity and headache are often present. The definitive diagnosis of meningitis usually depends on analysis of CSF obtained through lumbar puncture. In classical bacterial meningitis, CSF glucose is decreased, protein is increased, and white blood cells (predominantly polymorphonuclear cells) and bacteria are present. These findings are quite variable in viral and fungal meningitis, however. While such findings may also be present with encephalitis, these patients often have more severe central nervous system dysfunction with symptoms such as coma and paresis. A culture of brain material obtained through biopsy is often necessary to clearly identify the etiologic agent in encephalitis.

Infective Endocarditis

Infective endocarditis is an infection of the heart valves or the endocardial lining of the heart wall. The etiologic agent is most commonly bacterial but may be fungal. Based on the clinical course the endocarditis is said to be either acute or subacute (duration greater than 6 wks).

Epidemiology/Etiology—Acute endocarditis is caused by virulent organisms which infect a normal valve. Subacute endocarditis, on the other hand, is usually caused by relatively avirulent, less invasive organisms affecting an abnormally structured valve. The structural abnormality may be acquired or congenital.

The bacteria of acute endocarditis include such organisms as *S aureus*

(most frequent), *S pneumoniae,* group A streptococcus, *N gonorrhoeae,* salmonella, other members of the *Enterobacteriaceae,* and *P aeruginosa.* It is important to note, however, that these agents sometimes are associated with a subacute course.

Bacterial species usually associated with subacute endocarditis are members of the indigenous flora. The most common organisms include "viridans" streptococci, enterococci, nonhemolytic streptococci, non-group A beta-hemolytic streptococci, microaerophilic streptococci, and anerobic streptococci. These agents are commonly found in the oral cavity and in the gastrointestinal and genitourinary tracts.

Approximately 10% of cases are "culture-negative" endocarditis. These are clinically consistent with endocarditis but repeated blood cultures fail to grow organisms. The most common causes of culture-negative endocarditis include previous antibiotic usage, infection with species with fastidious growth requirements, and endocarditis of the tricuspid and pulmonic valves with relatively avirulent organisms.

The relatively recent increase in incidence of "*S. aureus*" endocarditis with involvement of the valves of the right side of the heart is correlated with the widespread use of intravenous drug abuse. Fungal and gram-negative endocarditis also occur more frequently in this setting. Hospitalized patients who receive intravenous fluids and hyperalimentation for prolonged periods also are at increased risk.

A new infectious disease has attended the advent of prosthetic valve replacement surgery. Endocarditis arising on a prosthetic valve is divided into early (clinically apparent within 60 days of surgery) and late infection. Early prosthetic valve endocarditis usually is a result of contamination during surgery; the organisms are those of acute bacterial endocarditis. Late prosthetic valve endocarditis is caused by transient bacteremia with organisms of the indigenous flora.

Pathophysiology—In subacute endocarditis the congenital or acquired abnormal valve causes flow disturbances which injure the endocardial lining of the heart valves or wall. This area of injury becomes a focus of thrombus formation which is seeded with bacteria during transient periods of bacteremia. Bacteremia with indigenous flora can be caused by dental work or manipulation of either the gastrointestinal or genitourinary tracts with endoscopes, catheters and surgical instruments. Acute endocarditis results from direct attack of normal valves by aggressive organisms which can destroy valves rapidly.

Endocarditis is associated with injury to many organs. The pathophysiology involves emboli (both septic and sterile) from the heart focus and immune complexes. In the setting of chronic infection with continued stimulation of the immune system, immune complexes of antibody and antigen form and deposit in various organs, thereby initiating a potentially harmful inflammatory response. Some manifestations of emboli and immune complex deposition are described in the following section.

Signs and Symptoms—Subacute endocarditis often begins with non-specific constitutional complaints. Fever, sweats, anorexia, malaise, myalgias, and arthralgias are prominent. These symptoms often persist and the patient may receive several courses of antibiotics, a practice which interferes with correct diagnosis.

A previous heart murmur may change or a new murmur occurs. Petechia may appear in the conjunctive, mucosal surfaces, or skin. Linear subungual splinter hemorrhages are a feature of this disease as are peculiar lesions on the hands and finger tips (Janeway lesions and Osler's nodes). In acute endocarditis skin pustules occur. Arthritis and osteomyelitis, splenomegaly, and retinal lesions may develop. Renal manifestations (flank pain; hematuria) may be secondary to renal infarction by emboli or immune complex-mediated glomerulonephritis. Pulmonary infiltrates caused by septic emboli may occur with right-sided endocarditis. Cardiac conduction defects or congestive heart failure may develop as the infection erodes into the conduction system or chordae tendineae, respectively. Stroke, seizures, or meningitis are more commonly seen in patient with acute bacterial endocarditis and are embolic in origin.

Laboratory tests usually reveal a leukocytosis, anemia, elevated erythrocyte sedimentation rate, rheumatoid factor (seen in subacute endocarditis), and circulating immune complexes. Hematuria, proteinuria, and even azotemia may be seen. The sustained bacteremia is evident by the positive blood cultures.

Pulmonary

Normal Physiology

Respiration involves all the processes in the transfer of oxygen from the air to the mitochondria of cells and of carbon dioxide from the cells back to the air. Four major steps are involved in respiration: (1) ventilation, (2) alveolar diffusion, (3) transport, and (4) tissue diffusion.

Ventilation is the functioning of the lungs to move air in and out to maintain the appropriate concentrations of oxygen and carbon dioxide in the alveoli. The process of ventilation requires proper functioning of the respiratory center in the medulla, the peripheral nerves to the muscles, the muscles such as the diaphragm, the intercostals, the abdominals and others, and the lungs themselves. Spirometry is a technique that is used to measure the ventilatory functioning of the lungs.

For purposes of measuring lung function, the lung is arbitrarily divided into various volumes and capacities. Tidal Volume (TV) is the amount of air moved in and out of the lung during a normal breath. The amount of air remaining in the lungs after a maximal exhalation is called the Residual Volume (RV). The level to which the lung volumes return after a normal breath is called the Functional Residual Capacity (FRC). If one takes a maximal inspiration, filling the lungs with as much air (or gases) as possible, one then reaches the Total Lung Capacity (TLC). The Vital Capacity (VC) is the maximum amount of air which can be exhaled following a maximal inspiration. The VC represents the ability of the subject to change the size of the thoracic cavity or the bellows function of the lung. Age, sex, size, and disease may affect the vital capacity. When the vital capacity is forcibly exhaled, the measurement is called the Forced Vital Capacity (FVC). The rate of exhaling the FVC is measured at time intervals, ie, Forced Expiratory Volume in one second (FEV_1), FEV_2, etc. The volume exhaled during the timed interval may be expressed as percentage of the vital capacity (FEV_1/FVC). This value is useful in assessing the severity of obstructive airway disease. The measurement of the airflow during the middle 50% of the Vital Capacity is relatively independent of patient effort and is useful in determining the mechanical properties of the lung. This is called the Forced Expiratory Flow from 25% to 75% of the VC, ($FEV_{25-75\%}$). This measurement is the most sensitive spirometric measurement for the detection of early obstructive lung disease.

Each breath contains a portion of air which does not come in contact with a gas exchanging membrane, such as the air in the large conducting airways. This is called dead space. The larger the dead space, the smaller the proportion of each breath which reaches a gas exchanging membrane and this affects the alveolar and arterial content of oxygen (O_2) and carbon dioxide (CO_2). In a steady state, the amount of CO_2 eliminated from the lung per minute is equal to the amount of CO_2 produced by the body. Since the partial pressure of CO_2 in the artery (P_{aCO_2}) is almost equal to the partial pressure of CO_2 in the alveoli (P_{ACO_2}), the measurement of P_{aCO_2} assesses the adequacy of alveolar ventilation. An elevated P_{aCO_2} means alveolar hypoventilation and a decreased P_{aCO_2} means alveolar hyperventilation.

Alveolar Diffusion—Gases are exchanged across the alveolar-pulmonary capillary membranes. The ability for this diffusion to occur depends on (1) the surface area of the alveoli, (2) the gradient between the partial pressures of gases in the alveoli and those in the blood, (3) the condition of the membranes, and (4) the amount of hemoglobin in the red blood cells. When a person breathes 100% oxygen, the gradient between the partial pressure of O_2 in the alveoli and that in the blood is so great the oxygen is transferred at a very rapid rate into the blood regardless of any decreases in surface area, changes in the condition of the membranes or decreases in hemoglobin concentration. Under normal circumstances, the partial pressure of oxygen in the arteries (P_{aO_2}) approximates the partial pressure of oxygen in the alveolus (P_{AO_2}). The difference in these measurements, the alveolar-arterial oxygen gradient ($P_{(A-a)O_2}$) is a measurement of the efficiency of the lungs in transferring oxygen into the blood. A normal $P_{(A-a)O_2}$ is 10–15 mg Hg in young people. This value increases with age.

Transport in the Blood—The maximum amount of oxygen that the blood can carry is called oxygen capacity and is determined by the amount of hemoglobin in the blood. One gram of hemoglobin can carry 1.39 mL of oxygen. The presence of hemoglobin increases the oxygen-carrying capacity of the blood by 30- to 100-fold. Normally 97% of the oxygen is carried bound to hemoglobin. The actual amount of oxygen carried, which is usually less than the oxygen capacity, is the oxygen content. The oxyhemoglobin saturation (S_{aO_2}) is the O_2 content divided into O_2-carrying capacity × 100 and is expressed as a percent. The oxygen content can be calculated from the oxygen saturation and the hemoglobin content. This measurement rather than the arterial partial pressure of oxygen (P_{aO_2}) is more indicative of tissue oxygenation. A patient with normal lungs but with an extremely low hemoglobin would have a normal P_{aO_2} because the amount of O_2 dissolved in the plasma would be normal but the blood would actually be carrying little O_2 to the tissues because of the decreased carrying capacity. Also, the oxygen-carrying capacity of hemoglobin may be affected by physiologic conditions that change the pH or temperature of the blood.

Pathophysiology of Hypoxemia

Hypoxemia refers to decreased amounts of oxygen in the arterial blood. There are five general mechanisms for the development of hypoxemia.

Low Inspired Oxygen Tension—This is not a disease but is the result of the person breathing air that has less than the normal amount of oxygen. Such conditions exist at high altitudes and in some deep mines where methane may replace oxygen. As long as the lungs are normal, the $P_{(A-a)O_2}$ will be normal. Ventilation remains normal or may be increased so the elimination of CO_2 is normal or increased.

Primary Hypoventilation—This condition occurs when the lungs no longer move air in and out to maintain appropriate concentrations of gases. The lungs themselves may or may not be normal. Primary hypoventilation may be caused by abnormalities in (a) the respiratory center, (b) the

peripheral nerves to the muscles, (c) the muscles of respiration, or (d) the chest wall. If the lungs are normal, the $P_{(A-a)O_2}$ will be essentially normal but the P_{aCO_2} will be increased indicating inadequate alveolar ventilation. Drugs suppressing the ventilation centers are probably the most common cause of primary hypoventilation.

Mismatching of Ventilation to Perfusion ($\dot{V}/\dot{Q}$ abnormalities)—If each alveolus were perfused with the appropriate amount of blood for maximum gas exchange, the ventilation-to-perfusion ratio would equal one. Normally in the erect position, there is excess ventilation to perfusion in the apices of the lung and excess perfusion to ventilation at the lung bases. At the apex $\dot{V}/\dot{Q} = 3$ and at the bases $\dot{V}/\dot{Q} = 0.6$. In normal individuals the overall $\dot{V}/\dot{Q} = 0.8$. Airflow obstruction decreases ventilation while perfusion remains unchanged. In this situation the $\dot{V}/\dot{Q}$ ratio is less than normal. If blood flow to an area is restricted while ventilation remains normal, the $\dot{V}/\dot{Q}$ ratio is very high. When no ventilation is present but perfusion is normal, $\dot{V}/\dot{Q} = 0$, this is defined as a true shunt. When there is no perfusion but ventilation is normal, $\dot{V}/\dot{Q} = \infty$, this is defined as dead space. High $\dot{V}/\dot{Q}$ ratios do not decrease the P_{aO_2} as ventilation is more than adequate to supply O_2 to the capillaries which have decreased blood flow. However, low $\dot{V}/\dot{Q}$ ratios do cause hypoxemia as ventilation is inadequate to oxygenate the relatively increased blood flow to that area. $\dot{V}/\dot{Q}$ mismatching, which is the most common cause of hypoxemia, may be corrected by allowing the patient to breathe 100% oxygen for 10 to 15 minutes. This is because the alveolar P_{O_2} is raised by replacing nitrogen (which is normally 79% of the gas in the alveolus) with oxygen. Also $\dot{V}/\dot{Q}$ mismatching results in an increased $P_{(A-a)O_2}$. Low $\dot{V}/\dot{Q}$ ratios which occur normally at the lung bases, probably account for much of the normal $P_{(A-a)O_2}$. Chronic bronchitis, emphysema, asthma, and many other lung diseases cause hypoxemia by affecting ventilation and lowering the $\dot{V}/\dot{Q}$ ratios in many areas of the lung.

True Right-to-Left Shunting—This occurs when venous blood goes from the right heart through the pulmonary circulation without contacting a gas-exchanging surface (ventilated alveolus). Such a situation exists in pulmonary arteriovenous malformations where the pulmonary capillaries are bypassed, in the adult respiratory distress syndrome, in atelectasis where alveoli are airless and in pneumonia and pulmonary edema where the air in the alveoli is replaced by fluid. Since the blood is not in contact with a alveolar membrane which can exchange oxygen, breathing 100% oxygen will not correct the hypoxemia due to right to left shunting.

Diffusion Defects—Diffusion defects are caused by thickened alveolar membranes. This is not a cause of significant hypoxemia in a resting patient but probably does play a role during exercise. Breathing 100% oxygen may increase the gradient across the alveolar membrane sufficiently to overcome a diffusion defect.

Airflow Obstructive Disease

Obstructive disorders, the commonest diseases of the lungs, are characterized by an increase in airway resistance. Alterations in resistance may be acute or chronic, reversible or irreversible.

Chronic bronchitis is a disease associated with excessive tracheobronchial mucus production sufficient to cause daily cough with expectoration of sputum for at least 3 months per year for two consecutive years. Chronic bronchitis is a clinical diagnosis which is made after other pulmonary diseases are excluded. Emphysema is defined as distention of the airspaces distal to the terminal bronchioles with destruction of the alveolar septa. The diagnosis of emphysema is based on anatomical alterations and is frequently made at autopsy. However, the entity can be considered to be present on the basis of certain physiologic studies. These two diseases, although distinct processes, are often present simultaneously in patients.

Etiology—The etiology of these diseases has not been clearly delineated although a variety of host and environmental factors have been implicated. Air pollution has been incriminated in the etiology of both chronic bronchitis and emphysema. Also, people who work in occupations associated with dusts and noxious gases have a higher incidence of chronic bronchitis. Respiratory infections with viruses, mycoplasma and bacteria may play a role in the development of chronic bronchitis. Cigarette smoking correlates with the prevalence and severity of chronic bronchitis and emphysema. These diseases are currently more commonly seen in males over 35 years old although the incidence in females is increasing, paralleling the increase in cigarette smoking by women. The hereditary deficiency of the enzyme alpha-1-antitrypsin is associated with the development of severe emphysema relatively early in life in both men and women.

Pathology—Chronic bronchitis is associated with hyperplasia and hypertrophy of the mucus-producing glands in the large airways. In the small airways, there is goblet-cell hyperplasia, mucosal and submucosal inflammation and edema, peribronchial fibrosis, and intraluminal mucus plugs. Ciliated cells are lost. Emphysema is classified according to the pattern of involvement distal to the terminal bronchioles. Centrilobular or centroacinar emphysema involves the respiratory bronchioles. Panacinar emphysema involves the respiratory bronchioles, the alveolar ducts, the alveoli and their blood supply. Both forms of emphysema often occur in a single patient although one form may predominate.

Pathophysiology—Both chronic bronchitis and emphysema can exist without clinically significant airflow obstruction. However, using sophisticated pulmonary function testing, early disease can be detected in young smokers. Both diseases result in narrowing of the airways with increased airway resistance and decreased Forced Expiratory Flow rates. Due to the altered pressure-airflow relationships, the work of breathing is increased in chronic bronchitis and emphysema. In both diseases, the Total Lung Capacity (TLC) and residual lung volume are increased. The hypoxemia results from ventilation to perfusion mismatching. The P_{aCO_2} may be normal, be decreased because of hyperventilation or be elevated in severe disease or during an acute exacerbation. The chronic hypoxia leads to pulmonary vascular constriction and pulmonary artery hypertension. The chronic increased afterload on the right heart ultimately leads to right heart failure (cor pulmonale). Other sequelae of severe hypoxemia include polycythemia and alteration of the patient's mental status.

Signs and Symptoms—Dyspnea on exertion and functional disability result from severe airway obstruction with its increased work of breathing.

Predominant Emphysema—These patients have a long history of exertional dyspnea with little cough or sputum production. The typical patient is thin, uses accessory muscles to breathe, is tachypneic, with prolonged expiration through pursed lips, frequently leans forward when sitting, has a hyperresonant percussion note and has diminished breath sounds by auscultation. The chest radiograph reveals low and flattened diaphragms and signs of hyperinflation. The clinical course is progressive severe dyspnea for which little can be done. Resting blood gases become abnormal late in the course of the disease.

Predominant Bronchitis Along with Emphysema—The typical patient has an impressive history of cough and sputum production for many years. Acute exacerbations increase in frequency, duration and severity over the years. After each episode the patient's baseline status may have deteriorated slightly. The presenting complaints may include cough, sputum production, exertional dyspnea or peripheral edema secondary to right heart failure. This patient is usually overweight, cyanotic and only slightly tachypneic. On auscultation coarse rhonchi and wheezes may be heard throughout the lung fields. Arterial blood gas analysis reveals hypoxia and hypercapnia. The Vital Capacity is normal or only slightly decreased while the Forced Expiratory Flow rates are low. These patients develop emphysema with the resultant symptoms. A patient with chronic bronchitis may experience many episodes of acute respiratory failure usually precipitated by a respiratory tract infection.

Reversible Airway Obstruction

Bronchial asthma is defined as a disease characterized by increased responsiveness of the trachea, bronchi, and bronchioles to various stimuli and manifested by widespread narrowing of the airways that changes in severity either spontaneously or as a result of therapy.

Etiology and Epidemiology—Asthma affects at least 2% of the population. About one-half of the cases develop before age ten and another third develop before age forty. Childhood asthma occurs in males predominantly (2:1) but after age thirty there is no sex difference.

Because of the diversity of the disease, the classification of asthma is difficult. Allergic or extrinsic asthma is usually found in individuals with a history or a family history of atopy or allergic diseases such as rhinitis, urticaria, and eczema. Allergic asthma, which accounts for 25% of the cases, tends to be seasonable and occurs more commonly in children and young adults. Nonseasonal allergic asthma may be due to antigens such as animal dander, molds, and dust. In another group of patients, ingestion of aspirin or nonsteroidal anti-inflammatory agents may aggravate the asthma. Asthma may also occur during times of heavy air pollution, on exposure to a variety of compounds involved in industry; during physical exercise or emotional upset; during bronchitis or bronchiolitis due to infections; and as a result of congestive heart failure or pulmonary embolism or with treatment with certain drugs such as cholinergic agents or beta adrenergic blockers. Asthma that occurs without an identifiable cause is labeled intrinsic or idiosyncratic.

Pathology—The hallmarks of acute asthma are overdistention of the lungs, gelatinous plugs in the bronchioles, hypertrophy of the bronchial smooth muscle, mucosal edema, denudation of the surface epithelium, pronounced thickening of the basement membranes and eosinophilic infiltration of the bronchial wall. Emphysematous changes are usually absent.

Pathophysiology—In those with allergic asthma, bronchoconstriction and alterations in bronchial secretions are the result of an immediate hypersensitivity reaction. In this response the interaction of antigen and antibody, particularly IgE, causes the release of chemical mediators from sensitized mast cells in the lungs. The mediators include histamine, slow-reacting substance of anaphylaxis (SRS-A—now known to be a form of leukotriene) platelet-activating factor (PAF), eosinophil chemotactic factor of anaphylaxis (ECF-A) and neutrophil chemotactic factor of anaphylaxis (NCF-A). Secondary mediators include prostaglandins and bradykinin. These mediators constrict bronchial smooth muscle and increase vascular permeability.

Adenyl cyclase catalyzes the formation of the cyclic nucleotide, cyclic 3′,5′-adenosine monophosphate (cyclic-AMP), from adenosine triphosphate (ATP). Cyclic-AMP is an intracellular mediator that inhibits the release of the chemical mediators. An increase in the concentration of cyclic-AMP causes relaxation of bronchial smooth muscle. It is thought that bronchoconstriction in asthmatics might result from a defect in cyclic-AMP as a result of non-responsiveness to endogenous catecholamines. Catecholamines stimulate adenyl cyclase to increase the intracellular concentration of cyclic-AMP.

A second cyclic nucleotide, cyclic 3′,5′-guanosine monophosphate (cyclic-GMP), opposes the action of cyclic-AMP. Actions that are facilitated by cyclic-AMP are suppressed by cyclic-GMP and vice versa. Cyclic-GMP promotes the release of bronchoconstricting substances from mast cells. Guanyl cyclase catalyzes the synthesis of cyclic-GMP in response to stimulation by acetylcholine. Anticholinergics such as atropine block the action of acetylcholine and prevent the release of mediators.

Signs and Symptoms—Symptoms include dyspnea, chest tightness, cough, and wheezing. All patients with asthma do not wheeze and may have only dyspnea and/or cough. The symptoms are episodic and frequently occur at night. In asthma the contraction of bronchial smooth muscle and the presence of mucosal edema and thick tenacious mucus result in airflow obstruction. Hypoxemia is present during an acute severe attack. Blood gas analysis usually shows decreased P_{aCO_2} and respiratory alkalosis. Normal or elevated levels of carbon dioxide during an acute episode should be viewed as impending respiratory failure. Clinical signs and symptoms are unreliable for judging tissue oxygenation. When severe symptoms persist for days or weeks the condition is known as status asthmaticus. Sputum and blood eosinophilia are helpful but not specific for asthma. The chest radiograph shows hyperinflation and is not diagnostic.

Restrictive Lung Disease

This is a general term applied to a wide spectrum of diseases with a decrease in total lung capacity. In advanced cases, other lung volume components are also reduced. Most patients with restrictive lung diseases have intrinsic structural and functional abnormalities of the lung which cause a stiff lung. Stiffness of the lungs is defined by a decrease in lung compliance, or change in lung volume per unit change in pressure. A minority of patients have normal lungs but have reduced lung volumes because of abnormalities of the chest wall, pleura, or abdomen.

Pathology—Although some restrictive lung diseases have unique pathology many have similar non-specific end-stage changes. Such changes may include pulmonary fibrosis of the alveolar septa, peribronchiolar fibrosis, mononuclear inflammatory cell infiltrate, smooth muscle proliferation within the interstitium, metaplasia of the alveolar lining cells sometimes leading to carcinoma, and vascular obliteration with pulmonary hypertension.

Etiology—Restrictive lung disease may be acute or chronic. An example of an acute, reversible restrictive lung disease is pulmonary edema. The diverse group of chronic diseases may be classified as those whose etiology is known, eg, asbestosis, hypersensitivity pneumonitis, drug or toxin induced, those associated with a well-defined systemic illness, eg, sarcoid, collagen vascular diseases; or those whose cause is unknown but have distinctive pathology, eg, pulmonary aveolar proteinosis, desquamative interstitial pneumonitis (DIP).

Signs and Symptoms—The hallmark of all restrictive lung diseases is a sensation of shortness of breath, or dyspnea. This results from the increased work of breathing caused by stiff lungs. In addition, air flow resistance is increased because patients breathe at low lung volumes which allows small airways to close. Tachypnea and a non-productive cough are common findings. Although fine rales may be heard, auscultatory findings are usually minimal compared to the degree of pathologic changes. Patients with extensive fibrosis may experience recurrent pneumothorax. Pulmonary hypertension advancing to cor pulmonale may be seen as a late sequela. This complication is caused by obliteration of the pulmonary vascular bed.

The chest X-ray in restrictive lung diseases may show decreased lung volumes and increased interstitial markings (reticular-nodular pattern). Arterial blood gases often reveal hypoxemia and hypocapnia.

Abnormalities on physiologic testing include an increased aveolar-arterial oxygen gradient and a decreased diffusion capacity.

Adult Respiratory Distress Syndrome (ARDS)

ARDS is a common cause of acute respiratory failure in a hospitalized patient. Its hallmark is damage to the pulmonary capillaries and alveolar epithelium leading to increased permeability and acute pulmonary edema. The etiology of this syndrome is multiple and includes shock, infection, near drowning, drug and toxin exposure, acute pancreatitis and aspiration pneumonia. Despite the wide spectrum of diseases which may lead to ARDS, in all cases there is a similar clinical picture. Acute respiratory failure is accompanied by a diffuse infiltrate on chest X-ray and physiologic disturbances of restrictive lung disease. On pathology there is edema, hemorrhage, hyaline membranes, inflammatory cells, and fibrosis.

Deep Venous Thrombosis and Pulmonary Embolism

Both deep venous thrombosis (DVT) and pulmonary embolism (PE) are significant causes of mortality and morbidity. The most important factor for decreasing morbidity and mortality is prevention of DVT.

Normal Anatomy and Physiology—Veins are thin-walled vessels composed mainly of collagen with some smooth muscle and little elastic tissue. They normally contain a large proportion of the circulating blood but at significantly lower pressures than arteries. The venous system of the lower extremities is composed of the deep, superficial, and communicating veins.

Blood return from lower extremities depends on the contraction of skeletal muscles, especially in the calves. Retrograde flow of blood in the veins is prevented by valves. These valves are present in venules as small as 0.08 mm in diameter and their number decreases in the proximal veins. The valves are composed of elastic and collagen tissue and operate passively in response to pressure changes.

The lung has two arterial blood supplies. The pulmonary artery exits from the right ventricle, immediately divides into the right and left branches, and carries deoxygenated blood from the systemic venous system to the lungs for gas exchange. The bronchial arteries branch off the aorta and carry oxygenated blood to the supporting tissue of the lung.

Normally clots do not form within the vascular system. The smooth endothelial surface of the blood vessels and a negatively charged protein layer on the endothelial surface that repels platelets are probably the most important factors in preventing clot formation. Two factors prevent excessive clotting. Approximately 85% of the thrombin formed is adsorbed to the fibrin threads, which prevents spread of the thrombin. The remaining thrombin is inactivated in 20 minutes by combining with antithrombin III.

Plasma normally contains a protein called plasminogen which when activated forms plasmin. Plasmin is a proteolytic enzyme which digests fibrin, fibrinogen, prothrombin, and Factors V, VIII, and XII. The process that activates plasminogen is poorly understood. Plasminogen is incorporated in all blood clots and is involved in dissolution of intravascular clots.

Etiology—A number of conditions and situations have been associated with increased risk of DVT and/or PE. These include prolonged bed rest, immobilization, cancers (particularly adenocarcinomas of the pancreas, lungs, or prostate), polycythemia vera, congestive heart failure, administration of estrogens, the postpartum state, orthopedic injuries, major surgery, trauma, chemical irritations, and infections. Approximately 85% of pulmonary embolic episodes are caused by DVT.

Epidemiology—It is difficult to estimate the incidence of DVT. The incidence of PE has been estimated as high as 630,000 cases per year and as the cause of 200,000 deaths per year in the US. On autopsy, PE is found in 10% of deaths in general hospitals, 25% of deaths in nursing homes, and as many as 50% of deaths due to CHF. The risk of DVT and PE is markedly increased in individuals over 40 years old. It is postulated that the diagnosis of PE is frequently missed in elderly chronically ill patients.

Pathophysiology—Three factors were described over 100 years ago by Virchow as necessary for venous thrombosis: stasis, hypercoagulability, and vessel wall factors. Increased platelet adhesiveness and aggregation may also be involved.

The veins have a propensity for development of stasis. The edges of the valves cause turbulent blood flow with eddy formation and stasis. The areas adjacent to the valves and the junctions of tributaries are also areas of stasis. Dilated veins (varicose veins) or previously damaged veins may have sluggish flow and incomponent valves. Lack of pumping of the blood in the veins by skeletal muscle contraction or compression of the veins by the muscle mass may explain the increased risk of DVT during bedrest or immobilization, and part of the increased risk during surgery. In polycythemia vera the blood is viscous and prone to stasis. Congestive heart failure may also increase the stasis of blood in the lower limbs. The stasis may allow the activation of factors as well as inhibit the dilution or removal of activated factors.

Various risk factors for DVT and PE are associated with hypercoagulable states. Cancers are thought to increase production of Factors V, VIII, IX and XI; release tissue thromboplastin from necrotic tumor and decrease the efficiency of the fibrinolytic system. Trauma and surgery may increase plasma concentration of fibrinogen and procoagulants, increase platelet adhesiveness, and decrease fibrinolysis. Administration of estrogens increases the production of Factors I, II, VIII, IX and X, increases platelet adhesiveness and decreases the activity of antithrombin III. Estrogens also cause venous dilatation which promotes stasis.

Increasing age predisposes individuals to thrombosis because of increased stasis caused by venous dilatation, malfunction of venous valves, decreased skeletal muscle mass, decreased physical activity and decreased cardiac output. Hypercoagulation may be caused by increased Factor VIII activity and decreased antithrombin III.

If the vessel wall is disrupted, collagen is exposed and/or tissue thromboplastin is released. The intrinsic coagulation system is activated by the exposed collagen; the extrinsic system by the tissue thromboplastin. Platelets adhere to the exposed collagen, aggregate to form a platelet plug and release platelet Factor III. Platelet Factor III is similar to tissue thromboplastin in that it initiates the extrinsic coagulation system. Platelet Factor III can also activate Factors VIII, IX, XI, and XII. The end product of coagulation is the thrombus, which is composed of fibrin and trapped serum and blood cells. The clot itself initiates a vicious cycle which promotes more clotting. The clot extends until it reaches an area of faster flowing blood.

The most feared form of DVT involves the iliofemoral veins as thrombi here are most likely to result in large emboli to the lungs and severe vascular injury to the limb.

When a embolus lodges in a pulmonary artery, the area is being ventilated but not perfused. The area is now dead space. The alveoli transiently constrict due to hypocapnia. Surfactant is lost and atelectasis develops in 24 to 48 hours. Hypoxemia usually develops. In massive PE pulmonary hypertension may result and lead to acute right heart failure. Infarction of the lung may or may not occur depending on the size of the embolus and the dual pulmonary blood flow. Many PEs are quickly dissolved by the fibrinolytic system. Recanalization may occur in a week. Some vessels however remain totally occluded with the resultant loss of lung function.

Signs and Symptoms—DVT may present as swelling of the calf or thigh with edema of the lower extremity. The area over the thrombosis may be tender, warm and erythematous. The thrombosed vein may be felt as a hard cord. Physical maneuvers of the limb or walking may worsen the pain. However, no signs or symptoms are present in many cases of DVT. More than 50% of patients with signs and symptoms normally attributed to DVT do not have it. The diagnosis of DVT is made conclusively by phlebography. Other causes of the signs and symptoms include pulled muscles, nonthrombotic inflammation of varicose veins, trauma, cramps, and a ruptured Baker's cyst. DVT can lead to PE, the postphlebitic syndrome (edema, pain, increased pigmentation, eczema, induration, and ulceration), or recurrence of DVT.

The signs and symptoms of PE depend on the size of the embolus and the presence of infarction. The classic presentation of PE is the sudden onset of dyspnea. If infarction occurs, pleuritic chest pain and hemoptysis may also be present. Hypoxemia and an increased alveolar-arterial oxygen gradient may be seen. Physical examination may or may not demonstrate the signs and symptoms of DVT. Rales, local wheezes and a pleuritic friction rub may be heard on auscultation. Tachycardia and tachypnea are seen. Signs of acute right-heart failure can be seen in massive PE. However, the physical examination may be completely normal. Laboratory examination is not diagnostic. The chest radiograph is often normal but may show a pleural effusion and/or infiltrate and/or changes in size or disappearance of blood vessels. A ventilation perfusion scan may give presumptive evidence for the diagnosis of PE. The test is associated with false negatives if the area involved is small or false positives if other lung diseases are present. Pulmonary arteriography is the most accurate method used to diagnose a PE.

Cystic Fibrosis

Cystic fibrosis is a disease with diverse clinical manifestations characterized by abnormal exocrine gland secretions. Although cystic fibrosis presents in childhood, with improved methods of detection in mild cases and better treatment more adults are now followed for this disease.

Etiology and Epidemiology—Cystic fibrosis is an autosomal recessive disease. It affects both sexes equally and occurs predominantly in caucasians. In the past cystic fibrosis was considered a fatal disease of childhood. With better techniques for earlier detection and improved methods of treatment the mean life expectancy has been raised to near 20 years of age. There is as yet no reliable test to identify those heterozygous for the disease.

Pathogenesis—The basic chemical defect in the abnormally thick mucus secreted has not been determined. Although a number of abnormalities (low water content, altered metabolism of glycoproteins) have been described, no consistent feature has been documented. A circulating factor which is toxic to cilia has been postulated but not documented.

Signs and Symptoms—The initial manifestation may be intestinal obstruction in the newborn secondary to abnormally thick meconium. Early in life pulmonary complications develop. Thick tenacious mucus results in bronchial obstruction with subsequent atelectasis and infection. The initial bacterial pathogens including *S. aureus* are later replaced by *P. aeruginosa* and other gram-negative organisms. Death in cystic fibrosis is usually due to overwhelming pulmonary infection and respiratory failure. With longer survivals cor pulmonale and recurrent hemoptysis are seen more frequently.

Pancreatic insufficiency develops in approximately 80% of patients and causes malabsorption characterized by steatorrhea and deficiencies of vitamin B_{12} and the fat soluble vitamins. Some patients experience recurrent bouts of pancreatitis. Biliary cirrhosis develops in approximately 10% of patients. The incidence of gallstones is increased. Most male patients are sterile secondary to a structural defect in the reproductive organs. Secondary sex characteristics are normal. The fertility rate among females is approximately one-fifth that of a control population. The reason for this is probably the increased viscosity of the cervical mucus and the possible presence of a cervical plug.

The most accurate diagnostic test is the sweat test. There is usually a three-to-fivefold increase in the concentration of sodium and chloride in the sweat of patients with cystic fibrosis. The level of sweat electrolytes does not correlate with severity of disease. The sweat test is a difficult test to perform correctly and must be obtained in a reliable, experienced laboratory.

Heart Disease

Atherosclerosis

Atherosclerosis is the single most important cause of mortality in the US because it is involved in the development of ischemic heart disease and cerebrovascular disease.

Normal Anatomy and Physiology—Arterial walls have three layers, the intima, media and adventitia. The intima is composed of endothelial cells; the media of smooth muscle cells and the adventitia of collagen, elastic fibers, fibroblasts and some smooth cells.

Arteries are not inert conduits. They are metabolically complex structures which maintain smooth muscle tension and carry out numerous endothelial cell functions, including local inhibition of blood clotting and maintenance of cellular integrity. During the lifetime of the individual, arteries withstand tremendous physical forces. Areas of particular stress, friction and turbulence include bifurcations and openings of branch arteries.

Epidemiology—In all populations studied, early changes of atherosclerosis have been seen in young individuals who died of unrelated causes. Mortality and morbidity from atherosclerotic disease is more common in men than premenopausal women. After menopause, the differences decrease. The incidence of atherosclerotic disease is also different in different nationalities. The mortality from atherosclerotic disease in North Americans and Scots is twice that of Swedes. The incidence is low in Japan and in native Africans. Incidence of atherosclerotic disease in immigrants to the United States is similar to that of native Americans rather than to age-matched individuals who did not immigrate. Primary relatives of individuals who become symptomatic from atherosclerotic disease before 50 years of age are likely to develop symptomatic atherosclerotic disease at an earlier age.

Etiology—The etiology of atherosclerosis is unknown. However, clinical and epidemiologic studies of atherosclerosis suggest that many factors accelerate the disease process, regardless of the underlying pathologic events. The two most important risk factors are advancing age and male sex. For the male aged 35 to 65 other significant factors include plasma cholesterol level, arterial blood pressure, and cigarette smoking. These risk factors also probably apply to postmenopausal women.

Other risk factors associated with a high incidence of atherosclerotic disease include diet, diabetes mellitus, lack of physical activity, obesity, competitive aggressive personality (Type A) and heredity. These factors may not be independent of the others already listed.

Pathology—Atherosclerosis is a patchy thickening and hardening of arterial walls that is characterized in the early stages by streaks of cholesterol and other lipids ("fatty streaks") and later by atheromas. The lesions initially involve the intima and progress to involve the media.

Pathophysiology—The mechanism for the development of atherosclerosis is poorly understood. Lesion development is thought to be accelerated by the increased stress associated with increased blood pressure and turbulent flow. The actual initiating event in the intima is unknown but minute tears in this layer occur and may be important. Platelet aggregation is important in the development of the atheroma as are changes in endothelial permeability and fibrin deposition.

These changes may induce smooth muscle proliferation in the intima with subsequent lipid accumulation. Another theory advocates lipid deposition as the inciting and most important event. Later, fibrosis, calcification, hemorrhage, ulceration and thrombosis develop causing eventual rupture or further lumen narrowing causing tissue blood flow to be critically reduced.

The lipids in the blood are cholesterol and triglycerides, which are carried in combination with phospholipids and proteins, and are called lipoproteins. Acceleration of atherosclerosis is principally correlated with elevations of the LDL fraction (low density lipoprotein) which is rich in cholesterol and poor in triglycerides. Elevation of the HDL fraction (high density lipoprotein) actually has been shown to have a protective effect against atherosclerosis development. This may result from the HDL function of transporting cholesterol from peripheral tissues to its site of metabolism in the liver.

Signs and Symptoms—The signs and symptoms of atherosclerotic disease depend on the location and degree of impairment of blood flow to an organ. Atherosclerotic disease presents as sudden death (probably due to a ventricular arrhythmia), angina pectoris, myocardial infarction, cerebrovascular accident, dissecting aneurysm, thrombosis of a major vessel, ischemic renal disease, intermittent claudication or peripheral vascular disease. Only those which are not discussed elsewhere will be discussed here. Intermittent claudication is pain in the legs which is precipitated by exercise and relieved by rest. Other signs and symptoms of peripheral vascular disease include pain in the legs at night when gravity is not helping blood perfusion, atrophy and weakness of leg muscles, loss of pulses in the feet, loss of hair on the feet and legs, neuropathy, extreme sensitivity to cold, and eventually dry gangrene. Atherosclerosis of the mesenteric vessels may cause abdominal pain which is precipitated by eating (abdominal angina) and weight loss, diarrhea and steatorrhea. Thrombosis of these vessels will cause bowel infarction. The diagnosis of atherosclerotic disease is usually based on signs and symptoms of reduced organ perfusion. Noninvasive studies and angiography are often helpful in defining the sites of vessel narrowing.

Coronary Artery Disease (CAD)

Coronary artery disease (CAD) is also referred to as *ischemic heart disease* (IHD); an imbalance between myocardial oxygen supply and demand which is most commonly caused by coronary artery atherosclerotic disease. Other causes of decreased oxygen delivery to the myocardium include: embolism, coronary ostial stenosis in tertiary syphilis and coronary artery spasm. Also, a decrease in oxygen-carrying capacity of the blood may be due to anemia, carboxyhemoglobinemia and hypoxemia from lung disease. Perfusion of the myocardium is decreased in hypotension. Myocardial oxygen demand is increased with exertion and in myocardial hypertrophy and thyrotoxicosis. In the majority of cases of CAD atherosclerosis is the underlying disorder.

Normal Anatomy—The myocardium is supplied by arteries from the aorta. The right coronary artery supplies the right atrium, right ventricle, left atrium, posterior septum, AV node and, in greater than 50% of individuals, the SA node. The left coronary artery branches into two arteries. The circumflex supplies the anterolateral, lateral, posteriolateral, inferior lateral and inferior wall of the left ventricle, left atrium and, in about 45% of individuals, the SA node. The left anterior descending supplies the anterior, anterolateral and apical left ventricular wall, the septum and the right ventricle adjacent to the septum.

Normal Physiology—Under normal resting conditions, the myocardium extracts about 70% of the available oxygen from the coronary blood flow. This is in contrast to resting skeletal muscle which extracts only 25% of available oxygen. Unlike skeletal muscle, the myocardium is capable of anaerobic metabolism for only a short time and cannot incur an oxygen debt. Increased myocardial oxygen demand must be met by increased coronary blood flow. The myocardium normally receives 5% of cardiac output. The normal heart can increase coronary blood flow by five-fold by increasing cardiac output. Blood flow to the myocardium occurs almost exclusively during diastole. Local tissue hypoxia results in potent vasodilatation and may increase coronary blood flow. Local tissue factors are more important than neuronal factors in regulating vasodilatation.

Oxygen consumption by the myocardium is determined by (a) systolic wall tension, (b) fraction of the cardiac cycle time spent in systole and (c) myocardial contractility. The systolic wall tension (t) is determined by the systolic ventricular pressure (P) and the radius (r) of the ventricular cavity, according to the Law of Laplace: $P = t/r^4$. The greater the cavity size, the greater the tension necessary to generate the pressure. The ventricular systolic pressure is determined by the aortic diastolic pressure (afterload). The fraction of time spent in systole is determined by heart rate and ejection time. The myocardial contractility is determined by the rate the muscle contracts. The oxygen demand of the myocardium is determined by the amount of work the muscle must perform.

Pathology—Most of the atherosclerotic lesions occur in the proximal portion of the coronary arteries as this is not a small vessel disease. Lesions in the left anterior descending artery are usually within 3 cm of the bifurcation of the left main coronary artery. Lesions in the right coronary artery usually occur within 6 to 8 cm of the ostium. A lesion which occludes less than 50% of the lumen of the vessel usually does not produce symptoms.

Pathophysiology—As the lumen of the vessels begins to narrow blood flow is decreased. Vessels distal to the obstruction dilate to maintain flow, presumably in response to hypoxia. When the obstruction reaches a critical size, the distal vessels become permanently dilated. Oxygen supply can only be increased at this point by increasing cardiac output which also increases oxygen demand.

Ischemia causes changes in the biochemical, electrical and mechanical properties of the heart. The myocardium normally oxidizes glucose and free fatty acids completely to carbon dioxide and water. In ischemia, lactate, pyruvate, and other metabolic products accumulate in the myocardium. Ischemia also alters the electrical properties of the heart; repolarization particularly is affected. Electrical instability results and arrhythmias may occur. Ischemia causes decreased contractility transiently and necrosis causes irreversible loss of contractility. Ischemia may cause asymmetry and asynchrony of ventricular contraction.

The location of the lesion is important because this determines the size and location of the ischemia. The presence of collateral vessels may prevent the development of permanent injury. Unfortunately, the only known stimulus for collateral vessel formation is ischemia. A sudden decrease in lumen size as with thrombosis or hemorrhage is a catastrophic event as collateral vessels have not yet formed and therefore cannot provide an alternative source of oxygen. There is a group of people in whom coronary artery spasm plays a role in ischemic heart disease with or without fixed atherosclerotic lesions. The mechanism of the production of pain by the ischemia is unknown.

Angina pectoris is classified according to its frequency, severity and precipitating event. Unstable angina describes a syndrome of attacks of recent onset or of increasing frequency, severity or duration, or occurring with less exercise or at rest. Myocardial infarction and arrhythmias are more likely to develop during periods of unstable angina. Stable angina describes a clinical picture of similar attacks. Noc-

turnal angina occurs during sleep and may be associated with either dreams and rapid eye movement (REM) sleep or increased venous return in a patient with congestive failure. Prinzmetal angina is atypical angina. It occurs at rest, is associated with ventricular arrhythmias and is thought to be due to coronary artery spasm.

Signs and Symptoms—CAD may present as ventricular arrhythmias or myocardial infarction, which will be discussed below. The other manifestation of CAD is angina pectoris which is a clinical syndrome that results from transient myocardial ischemia but with no evidence of permanent damage.

The patient with angina pectoris usually describes the chest discomfort as heaviness, pressure, tightness or squeezing. The patient usually will not use the word "pain" and may ascribe his symptoms to indigestion. The substernal discomfort may radiate to the left arm, throat, jaw, shoulder, back or abdomen. The discomfort typically is precipitated by exercise, and also but less often by eating, emotional upset, exposure to cold, and cigarette smoking. It is relieved by rest. The episodes usually last longer than one minute and not longer than 30 minutes.

The physical examination of these patients is normal between attacks. The diagnosis of angina is made from the history. Early evidence of ischemia on EKG stress testing is inversion of T waves and depression of the S-T segment. Angiography and a therapeutic response to nitroglycerin may be helpful in establishing the diagnosis. Other causes of chest pain such as other forms of heart disease, gastrointestinal and musculoskeletal disease must be considered in the differential diagnosis.

Ischemic heart disease is the leading cause of death among males over 35 years old in the US and accounts for one-third of male deaths before age 65. The chief prognostic factors are the state of left ventricular function and the extent of the atherosclerotic disease. Yearly mortality for patients with normal ventricular function and atherosclerotic disease of the 3 coronary vessels is 11%; with 2 vessel disease mortality is 8% and with single vessel disease mortality is 2%.

Myocardial Infarction (MI)

Myocardial infarction may be totally asymptomatic, can be fatal or cause a variety of complications.

Pathology—The coronary blood vessels may or may not show thrombosis and it is controversial whether thrombosis is the cause or the result of a myocardial infarction. Myocardial infarction is death of myocardial tissue. Most infarctions involve the endocardial layer. If the area of necrosis exceeds 3 cm in diameter, the infarct is likely to be transmural. Twenty-four hours after the infarction occurs the myocardial fibers show clumping, coagulation and interstitial edema. By the fourth day the area is necrotic and shows fatty change and phagocytosis of fibers by neutrophils. Between the fourth and tenth days the area shows distinct fatty change, may contain hemorrhage and is maximally soft. By the tenth day vascularized scar tissue begins to replace the infarct. The infarction has completely healed by the sixth to eighth week.

Signs and Symptoms—Chest pain is usually the presenting complaint. It is described as severe, excruciating, deep, heavy, squeezing or crushing. No precipitating cause for the pain may be identified. The pain is similar to the pain of angina pectoris but is more severe, lasts longer and is not relieved by rest or sublingual nitroglycerin. The pain may wax and wane. In 25% of patients, the substernal pain radiates to the arms; the pain may also radiate to the jaw, neck, abdomen and back. Weakness, diaphoresis, nausea, vomiting, light-headedness, marked anxiety, and a sense of doom accompany the pain. The patient attempts in vain to find a comfortable position. Myocardial infarction may be asymptomatic in 15–20% of patients. Elderly persons may complain of dyspnea rather than pain. Other presentations of myocardial infarction include syncope, confusion, arrhythmias and hypotension. Greater than 50% of the deaths following MI occur within the first 24 hours and are due to arrhythmias.

Physical examination typically discloses an anxious patient who is sweating and has cool extremities. Auscultation of the heart may reveal decreased heart sounds, S_3, S_4 or the murmur of mitral regurgitation. Temperature may be elevated to 38°C.

Laboratory examination may reveal an increased white blood count to 15,000/mm³. Enzymes released from damaged myocardial cells are used to diagnose myocardial infarction. The serum concentrations of these enzymes follow a characteristic pattern with creatine phosphokinase (CPK) and serum glutamic oxaloacetic transaminase (SGOT) rising and falling quickly while lactic acid dehydrogenase (LDH) rises later and remains elevated longer. CPK is found in skeletal muscle and brain as well as in myocardium. An intramuscular injection can elevate the serum CPK two-to three-fold. SGOT is also found in skeletal muscle, in red blood cells and liver. LDH is a ubiquitous tissue enzyme. Isoenzymes for CPK and LDH identify the enzymes of myocardial origin and are helpful in diagnosis. It is often difficult to correlate enzyme elevation with size of the infarct.

The EKG initially shows T-wave inversion and S-T segment depression, nonspecific signs of ischemia. When the infarct is transmural Q-waves appear. Infarction may also cause decreased voltage in the precordial leads.

Complications of Myocardial Infarction—Arrhythmias are the most common cause of deaths in the early stages of MI. Ventricular arrhythmias are the most ominous and ventricular fibrillation is the most common fatal arrhythmia. Coronary care units which prevent or aggressively treat arrhythmias have decreased mortality due to this complication.

Cardiac failure is now the primary cause of death in hospitalized patients with MI. If greater than 40% of the myocardium is destroyed, the prognosis is poor.

Mitral regurgitation may occur as a result of rupture or dysfunction of the papillary muscles. This may decrease cardiac output and contribute to cardiac failure.

Thromboembolism contributes to the cause of death in 25% of cases. Mural thrombosis may develop on the endocardium of the left ventricle. Embolization of this thrombus may cause strokes or a new MI. Deep venous thrombosis may develop in the legs and embolize to the lungs (pulmonary embolism).

Rupture of the infarct may occur during the first week when the infarct is maximally soft. The blood pressure falls rapidly and the patient loses consciousness. The EKG may not change immediately. Cardiac tamponade occurs as the pericardium fills with blood. This complication is almost always fatal. The septum may rupture leading to left-to-right shunting. A pansystolic murmur is heard and cardiac output decreases.

Ventricular aneurysm occurs when the scar of the ventricular wall balloons outward while the remaining myocardium contracts. Because this portion of the wall has lost contractility, cardiac output decreases and congestive heart failure may develop. Systemic embolism may arise from a mural thrombus in the aneurysm. Arrhythmias are common with ventricular aneurysms.

Pericarditis may develop 2 to 3 days after the infarction. Pericardial pain is usually sharp, knife-like, substernal, may radiate to the neck and shoulders, is relieved by leaning forward, and is worsened by deep breathing. A pericardial friction rub may be heard. The pericarditis usually resolves with the healing of the infarct. However, organization may occur with the development of adhesions. Dressler's syndrome is pericarditis that develops from 1 to 6 weeks after an MI. The patient develops a fever and complains of pleuritic and pericardial pain. The syndrome is thought to be due to an autoimmune pericarditis, pleuritis and pneumonitis.

Heart Failure

Heart failure is defined as an inability of the heart to pump blood at a rate sufficient to meet the metabolic demands of the tissues. The inability to pump blood can be due to various abnormalities in the myocardium. When the heart pumps blood at an insufficient rate, salt and water are retained by the kidneys and fluid accumulates in interstitial spaces. Thus the term congestive heart failure is usually used. However, not all types of fluid overload or congestion are due to heart failure. Other causes of fluid overload include nephrotic syndrome, renal failure, liver disease, and starvation. Heart failure may develop acutely or chronically and may be mild to severe. Severe heart failure is synonymous with cardiogenic shock.

Normal Physiology—The functioning of the heart as a pump depends upon: the number of functioning muscle fibers; the length of muscle fiber at the onset of contraction which is determined by the end diastolic volume (EDV), or what is referred to as *preload*, and the intrinsic myocardial activity or the contractile state. Cardiac output (CO) is determined by the heart rate and the stroke volume. The normal stroke volume (SV) is 70 mL and the normal end systolic volume is 5–60 mL. SV is described by the equation: end diastolic volume minus end systolic volume.

The heart contracts in two phases. In the isovolumic phase the length of the fiber remains constant while the tension increases. When the left ventricular pressure reaches 80 mm Hg the ejection phase occurs, during which contraction occurs as the fibers shorten. Heart rate determines filling time for the ventricles which in turn determines cardiac output. Between 50 to 180 beats/minute, cardiac output remains stable. The afterload or the resistance against which the heart works influences cardiac output—the higher the resistance the lower the CO.

Normally the heart will pump out the blood that flows into it so that cardiac output is equal to venous return which is controlled by the tissues. Cardiac output can be increased within certain limits by automatic stimulation, hypertrophy of the heart muscle, and an increase in blood volume. The heart has tremendous reserve capacity and can increase CO by increasing both heart rate and stroke volume.

The Frank-Starling principle describes the relationship between the cardiac output and the length of the fibers at the end of diastole. Increased contractility results from sympathetic stimulation and decreased contractility indicates a failing heart. This relationship shows that for a given end diastolic pressure, the ventricles receive and eject a higher stroke volume when contractility is increased and a lower stroke volume when contractility is decreased. The Frank-Starling law of the heart describes the ability of the heart to adapt to changing amounts of inflowing blood. Within physiologic limits, the more the chamber is filled the greater the quantity of blood that will be pumped. If the muscle fibers are stretched by volume, the muscle contracts with greater force; thereby increasing CO. The amount of actin that overlaps myosin determines the force of contraction. There is an optimal muscle fiber length at which the greatest surface area of actin-myosin overlap occurs.

Etiology—Processes that cause the heart to fail are those that increase the work of the heart, usually over many years, or that damage the myocardial fibers. As a result, cardiac output decreases. The most common cause of left ventricular failure is systemic hypertension. Stenotic valvular disease leads to failure. An incompetent heart valve eventually leads to failure. Congenital defects may result in increased cardiac work. Cardiomyopathies, atherosclerotic coronary disease and myocardial infarction damage muscle fibers and impair contractility. Tachyarrhythmias and atrial-ventricular dissociation result in less filling of the ventricles, and ventricular arrhythmias decrease contractility. Pericarditis may impair ventricular filling or contraction. The most common cause of right-heart failure is left-heart failure. Pulmonary embolism may precipitate acute right ventricular failure. Cor pulmonale is right-heart failure due to pulmonary hypertension which can occur as a complication of hypoxemia from lung disease.

Increased metabolic demands or decreased oxygen-carrying capacity of the blood may exceed cardiac reserve. Causes of high-output heart failure (see below) include hyperthyroidism, anemia, A-V fistulas, pregnancy, infections (particularly pulmonary infection) and beriberi.

Pathophysiology—The majority of cases of CHF are due to low-output failure as occurs in hypertension, atherosclerotic heart disease or valvular disease. In certain cases of heart failure, the cardiac output is greater than normal and is known as high-output failure. This is due to the metabolic demands of the tissue being greatly increased or the oxygen-carrying capacity of the blood being greatly decreased. Hyperthyroidism and pregnancy are causes of increased metabolic demands of the tissues. Anemia, arteriovenous fistulas and hypoxemia are examples of decreased oxygen content of the blood. Another cause of high-output failure which is exceedingly rare is beriberi or chronic thiamine deficiency, which increases venous return to the heart.

Compensatory Mechanisms of Low Cardiac Output—When cardiac output falls, reflexes occur immediately. The baroreceptors sense the decreased arterial pressure and increase sympathetic tone while decreasing parasympathetic tone. This increases the force of contraction of the heart, increases heart rate, raises mean systemic arterial pressure, and increases venous return. These reflexes are maximal at 30 seconds after a drop in arterial pressure.

Redistribution of blood flow occurs resulting in maintenance of blood flow to the myocardium and brain. Blood flow to the skin and skeletal muscle are greatly decreased by norepinephrine-induced vasoconstriction. Blood flow is also decreased to the kidney in CHF.

Decreased cardiac output reduces the glomerular filtration rate because of both decreased renal blood flow and sympathetic vasoconstriction of afferent renal arterioles. Blood flow within the kidney is redistributed by the vasoconstriction to the medulla at the expense of the cortex. Renin production by the juxtaglomerular apparatus is increased in response to decreased blood flow or sodium transport. Renin cleaves angiotensinogen to angiotensin I which is converted by angiotensin converting enzyme (ACE) to angiotensin II. This end substance is a potent peripheral vessel constrictor and stimulator of aldosterone secretion by the adrenal cortex. Aldosterone promotes the retention of sodium and water by the distal convoluted renal tubule, causes expansion of the blood volume and accumulation of fluid in interstitial spaces. Serum sodium remains normal or is decreased although total body sodium is increased.

Increased blood volume and increased systemic blood pressure increase venous return to the heart. Eventually the heart can no longer keep pace with the increased venous return. In mild heart failure, the increased fluid volume helps to increase cardiac output by applying some stretch to the myocardial fibers. In severe heart failure, the amount of fluid overload becomes so great that the fibers are stretched beyond the limits of efficient contraction and the fibers descend to a lower Frank-Starling curve. A greater end diastolic pressure is necessary to maintain CO on this lower curve. The increase in left ventricular end diastolic pressure (LVEDP) is transmitted as increased hydrostatic pressure to the pulmonary veins, capillaries and arteries. Eventually the increased pressure in the pulmonary arteries causes the right ventricle to fail. Increased right ventricular end diastolic pressure translates into increased hydrostatic pressure in the systemic veins and capillaries.

Edema Formation—Most of the fluid accumulation in interstitial spaces results from increases in hydrostatic pressures. The colloidal pressure of the blood that holds fluid in the vascular compartment is about 25 to 30 mm Hg. When the hydrostatic pressure in the capillaries exceeds 25 mm Hg, fluid is pushed into the interstitial spaces. Congestive heart failure involves fluid retention in both the intra and extravascular space. When LVEDP exceeds 28 mm Hg, the pressure transmitted to the pulmonary capillaries causes pulmonary edema. Oxygen does not diffuse efficiently in alveoli filled with edema fluid so hypoxemia results. Fluid retention also results in distention of the venous reservoirs in the liver and spleen.

Many of the symptoms of CHF are due to fluid overload. Dyspnea develops due to hypoxemia but also due to the decreased compliance of the lungs due to the accumulation of fluid. The decreased compliance increases the work of breathing and the oxygen required for breathing. Dyspnea may occur during the night because of the normal decrease in respiratory drive that occurs during sleep may result in severe hypoxemia. Also sympathetic stimulation is decreased during sleep so cardiac output may decrease even further. Gravity normally causes the edema to pool in the limbs or the bases of the lung. When a recumbent position is assumed, the fluid may be redistributed throughout the lung resulting in hypoxemia, or return to the vascular compartment and increase venous return, which may compromise cardiac output even further. Cyanosis develops because of increased levels of reduced hemoglobin. Central nervous system symptoms occur because of decreased oxygen delivery to the brain. Hemoptysis occurs because of rupture of engorged pulmonary capillaries. Anorexia, nausea and vomiting occur due to congestion of the liver and digestive tract. Stasis and peripheral edema of the lower extremities predispose to venous thrombosis and skin ulceration.

Signs and Symptoms—Patients with left ventricular CHF most commonly complain of a sensation of shortness of breath (dyspnea). Initially the dyspnea is present only on exertion (DOE) but the amount of activity necessary to precipitate dyspnea progressively lessens until the patient is dyspneic at rest. Orthopnea is the sensation of breathlessness that occurs in the recumbent position and may be relieved by elevating the head on several pillows or by sitting. Paroxysmal nocturnal dyspnea (PND) is severe dyspnea occurring at night that awakens the patient with a sensation of smothering. PND is usually accompanied by coughing and/or wheezing. The patient may produce frothy pink sputum.

Patients with left-sided CHF also may experience fatigue, weakness and alterations in mental status such as confusion, difficulty in concentrating, impaired memory, headache, insomnia, and anxiety.

Physical examination of the patient with left heart failure reveals a person who may have lost considerable body mass. The patient may be unable to lie flat during the examination. The pulse may be weak although the blood pressure remains normal until very late in the course. The extremities will be pale and cool. Cyanosis of the lips and nailbeds may be present. Examination of the heart reveals tachycardia and S_3 gallop. Moist crepitant inspiratory rales over the lung bases in moderately severe CHF and over the entire lung fields in pulmonary edema are heard. Chest radiograph shows the enlarged heart and signs of pulmonary venous congestion.

Patients with right ventricular failure complain of weight gain and the accumulation of fluid. A 10% gain in body weight may occur before pitting edema occurs. In ambulatory patients the edema is symmetrical in the ankles and legs. Since gravity influences the distribution of the edema, the buttocks and sacrum may be edematous in bedfast patients. Anasarca is massive body fluid overload including generalized edema, ascites and pleural effusions. As fluids accumulate in the pleural cavity, the patient may develop dyspnea. Patients experience an increased girth as fluid accumulates in the peritoneal cavity. The liver may become enlarged and tender and result in right upper quadrant pain. Anorexia, nausea and abdominal fullness occur. The patient becomes jaundiced as impairment of liver function becomes severe.

Physical examination of the patient with severe right-sided heart failure will reveal pleural effusions, ascites, jugular venous distention, hepatomegaly, splenomegaly and pitting edema. Urine volume will be decreased and pre-renal azotemia may be present.

Valvular Heart Disease

Valvular heart disease occurs when the heart valves become damaged and no longer open or close properly. If fibrous scar tissue forms or calcium deposits on the valve, the valve becomes stenotic and no longer opens easily. If the valve leaflets shrink or do not oppose each other properly when closing due to scarring or are destroyed by infection, the valve no longer is competent and blood flows in a retrograde fashion. A single valve may be both stenotic and incompetent. More than one valve may be involved. The consequences of valvular disease include congestive heart failure, arrhythmias and systemic emboli. The hallmark of valvular disease is a murmur—a noise representing turbulence of blood flow across the valve.

Normal Anatomy and Physiology—The valves between the atria and the ventricles, tricuspid on the right side and mitral on the left side, are large and normally offer little resistance to flow. The semilunar valves, the aortic and pulmonic are smaller. The atrioventricular valves are supported by chordae tendineae but the semilunar valves are not. The valves open and close passively in response to pressure gradients.

The opening and closing of the valves cause the heart sounds. The first sound ("lub") occurs at the beginning of systole and represents the closure of the mitral and tricuspid valves. The second sound ("dub") is heard at the beginning of diastole and signals closure of the aortic and pulmonic valves. In normal individuals the second sound may be split because the aortic and pulmonic valves do not close simultaneously. The loudness of the heart sounds is proportional to the rate of change of pressure across the valves. A loud first sound is heard with rapid systole and increased force of contraction. A loud second sound indicates a rapid increase in pressure as in systemic and pulmonary hypertension. A third heart sound (S_3) is caused by blood flowing into the ventricles, particularly in the dilated ventricles of CHF. A fourth heart sound (S_4) emanates from the atria contracting forcefully and is heard in conditions of decreased compliance of the ventricles as in hypertensive heart disease.

Etiology—Most valvular lesions are due to rheumatic fever: 40% of mitral stenosis (MS), 50% of mitral insufficiency (MI), and 80% of aortic insufficiency (AI). MS is rarely a congenital lesion while (MI) may be. Two-thirds of patients with MS are female while most patients with pure MI or aortic stenosis (AS) and three-fourths of patients with pure AI are male. Subacute bacterial endocarditis may damage the valves, usually the mitral or aortic valve. The aortic valve may become stenotic due to idiopathic calcification thought to be due to the "wear and tear" of aging. Congenital bicuspid aortic valves cause AS and AI. In patients with rheumatic heart disease (RHD) 40% have mitral disease alone, 40% have both mitral and aortic disease and 10 to 15% have aortic disease alone. Pulmonic valve involvement in RHD is uncommon. Mitral insufficiency may occur when the chordae tendineae or papillary muscles are damaged by atherosclerotic heart disease or a myocardial infarction. A large dilated chamber can lead to regurgitation through its entrance valve.

Pathology—In acute rheumatic fever the valve leaflets become swollen and thickened and small beadlike nodules develop along the valve closure lines and on the chordae. These nodules are composed of fibrin, platelets and white blood cells. The inflammation may subside with the acute attack or develop into a subacute or chronic process. The inflammation leads to erosion of the endothelial surface and deposition of collagen by fibroblasts. The fibrous scarring during organization leaves a permanently thickened, distorted, rigid valve. Contraction of the scar results in shortening of the leaflets and distortion of the architecture of the valve. The edges of the deformed valve fail to fit together during closure causing valvular incompetency. The chordae may also be involved in scarring and shortening. Fibrous adhesions may occur across the cusp edges. Irregular fibrous thickening and scarring are also associated with calcification. Adhesions and calcification increase the rigidity of the valve and cause stenosis. Stenosis and the uneven surface are associated with increased turbulence of flow across the valve.

Mitral Stenosis (MS). *Pathophysiology*—The normal opening of the mitral valve is 4 to 6 cm^2 in adults. Symptoms of MS occur when the area is reduced to 1.5 cm^2. If the valve is stenotic, greater pressures are required to pump the blood from the left atrium to the left ventricle. Normally the systolic pressure in the left atrium is 12 mm Hg. A valve opening of less than 1 cm^2 requires a pressure of 25 mm Hg in the left atrium to pump the blood into the left ventricle. The elevated atrial pressure is transmitted back into the pulmonary veins, capillaries and arteries. Pulmonary arteries develop medial hypertrophy and intimal thickening which leads to high resistance and pulmonary hypertension. Alveolar fibrosis may also occur. When the pressure in the pulmonary vessels exceeds the osmotic pressure of blood, pulmonary edema develops although the patient does not have left ventricular failure and left ventricular end diastolic pressure is normal. Eventually the right heart fails.

Left ventricular output may be normal or decreased. The flow across the valve depends on heart rate as well as size of the opening. Increasing heart rate decreases the time available for flow across the mitral valve.

Signs and Symptoms—Two decades usually elapse between the initial attack of rheumatic fever and the development of the signs and symptoms of MS. Most patients become symptomatic during the fourth decade of life. Once the symptoms occur the prognosis is poor with death occurring in 2 to 5 years unless the valve is replaced or corrected. The symptoms begin with dyspnea and cough during extreme exertion, but over the years the amount of exercise necessary to produce symptoms decreases until dyspnea occurs at rest. Orthopnea and paroxysmal nocturnal dyspnea may occur. With long standing MS, atrial arrhythmias are common. Chronic atrial fibrillation is a poor prognostic sign.

Extensive fibrosis of the alveolar walls and pulmonary capillary thickening lead to decreased vital capacity, total lung capacity, maximum breathing capacity and oxygen uptake. $\dot{V}/\dot{Q}$ mismatching occurs. Decreased compliance of the lung increases the work of breathing and increases the sensation of breathlessness. Hemoptysis results from rupture of small vessels in the bronchioles.

Patients with MS, particularly those with atrial fibrillation, are likely to embolize thrombi from the left atrium to the brain, kidneys, spleen or extremities.

The physical examination of patients with MS often discloses cyanosis of the lips and nails, and signs of right heart failure. The first heart sound is accentuated. The opening snap of the mitral valve may be heard. A low pitched rumbling diastolic murmur is characteristic of mitral stenosis. Chest radiograph shows an enlarged left atrium, pulmonary arteries and right ventricle as well as markings of increased pulmonary venous pressure. EKG shows signs of left atrial enlargement and may disclose an atrial arrhythmia.

Mitral Insufficiency (MI). *Pathophysiology*—Blood now flows from the left ventricle in two directions: into the aorta and back into the left atrium. Early in the disease cardiac output is maintained, first by more complete emptying of the left ventricle. Later, as left ventricular function deteriorates, left-end diastolic volume is increased. Finally, left-end diastolic pressure is increased but cardiac output eventually decreases.

Signs and Symptoms—The patients present with symptoms of decreased cardiac output such as fatigue, dyspnea, weakness, and perhaps cachexia. Palpitations due to atrial arrhythmias may be felt. If pulmonary vascular resistance is increased, right heart failure results. If pulmonary pressures are high the patient may complain of orthopnea, DOE and PND. The symptoms of MI are less episodic than those of MS.

Physical examination discloses a loud holosystolic murmur that may radiate to the axilla. The EKG reveals evidence of left ventricular and/or right ventricular hypertrophy, left atrial enlargement and in chronic cases, atrial fibrillation. Chest X-ray may show extreme left atrial enlargement and left ventricular enlargement. Calcifications of the mitral valve may be seen on chest radiograph. The clinical course of MI generally is more prolonged than that of MS.

Aortic Stenosis. *Pathophysiology*—Aortic stenosis causes obstruction to the flow of blood from the left ventricle. Cardiac output is maintained by the generation of increased pressures by the left ventricle. The left ventricle responds to this situation by developing concentric hypertrophy without dilatation if the obstruction develops gradually. The diameter of the normal aortic orifice is 3–3.5 cm^2 and a reduction to 0.5–1.0 cm^2 is critical.

The patient initially develops symptoms during exercise because cardiac output cannot be increased to meet the oxygen demands of exercise. Later, as the left ventricle begins to fail, cardiac output cannot be maintained at rest.

Signs and Symptoms—Aortic stenosis may exist for years before symptoms develop. The onset of symptoms for rheumatic aortic stenosis is usually in the fourth or fifth decade. The characteristic symptoms are fatigue, exertional dyspnea, angina, and syncope. The syncope is usually exertional and occurs when cardiac output cannot be increased. Reduced cerebral blood flow may cause syncope. An arrhythmia may also result in decreased cardiac output and syncope. Very late in the course of the disease the patient has the signs and symptoms of left ventricular failure and finally in the preterminal phase signs and symptoms of right heart failure.

When aortic stenosis occurs with mitral stenosis, less blood fills the left ventricle so less of a pressure gradient develops across the aortic valve. The left ventricle does not hypertrophy as much and less angina occurs. When aortic stenosis occurs with mitral stenosis, the patient has more of the signs and symptoms of mitral stenosis.

On physical examination of the patient with aortic stenosis, an opening snap may be heard as well as closure of the aortic valve if the valve is not calcified. The pulmonary valve may close before the aortic valve resulting in paradoxical splitting of the second heart sound. A S$_3$ gallop may be

heard indicating left ventricular hypertrophy and increased LVEDP. A systolic ejection murmur which begins after the first heart sound, increases in intensity reaching a peak in the middle of the ejection period and decreases in intensity until closure of the aortic valve is heard. The ejection murmur is thus referred to as diamond-shaped.

Once the patient has become symptomatic the prognosis is poor with an 80% mortality at 4 years. Congestive heart failure accounts for mortality in up to two-thirds of the patients and its onset suggests an average prognosis of 1½ years. Ten to 20% of the patients die from an arrhythmia.

Aortic Insufficiency. *Pathophysiology*—In aortic insufficiency a fraction of the stroke volume flows retrograde into the left ventricle so that cardiac output decreases. To compensate for the decrease in cardiac output, left ventricular end diastolic volume increases to allow for greater stroke volume. The left ventricle dilates to accommodate the increased end diastolic volume. Eventually left ventricular function fails and cardiac output decreases. The enormous left ventricular dilatation stretches the mitral ring and causes malalignment of the papillary muscle-chordae tendinae apparatus inducing MI. In later stages, pressure increases in the left atrium, pulmonary vessels and right ventricle.

Signs and Symptoms—A patient who develops AI is usually asymptomatic for 10 to 20 years. The first symptom is an uncomfortable awareness of the heart beat particularly in the supine position or during exertion or emotional upset. Next exertional dyspnea develops as a sign of decreased cardiac reserve. Later signs of left ventricular failure appear. The patient may complain of chest pain that is due to pounding of the chest wall. Typical or atypical angina may develop, may be prolonged and does not respond to nitroglycerin. Finally signs and symptoms of systemic fluid overload and right heart failure appear. The cause of death may be pulmonary edema. Syncope is rare.

Physical examination of patients with AI reveals an increased systolic pressure and decreased diastolic pressure with a wide pulse pressure. A diastolic high-pitched blowing decrescendo murmur is heard. The murmur becomes louder and longer as the AI worsens. EKG shows left ventricular hypertrophy. Chest radiograph shows left ventricular enlargement and dilatation of the ascending aorta.

The prognosis in decompensated AI is poor. Surgical correction is necessary before left ventricular deterioration occurs.

Tricuspid Stenosis. *Pathophysiology*—Tricuspid stenosis presents an obstruction to outflow of the right atria and results in an increased end diastolic pressure in the right atrium. The increased right atrial pressure causes backup of blood and congestion in the systemic circulation. Cardiac output decreases because of decreased return to the left atrium.

Signs and Symptoms—The patient presents with the signs and symptoms of right heart failure. A diastolic murmur is characteristic of tricuspid stenosis.

Tricuspid Insufficiency. *Pathophysiology*—The flow of blood from the right ventricle flows back into the right atrium leading to enlargement of the right atrium and increased right atrial pressure. The increased right atrial pressure leads to systemic venous congestion.

Signs and Symptoms—The patient with advanced tricuspid insufficiency exhibits the signs of right heart failure and decreased cardiac output. A blowing holosystolic murmur is heard in tricuspid insufficiency. Atrial fibrillation may be present.

Disorders of Cardiac Rhythm (Electrophysiology)

Arrhythmias or dysrhythmias are irregularities in the heart beat that result from disturbances in the rate or conduction of the impulse. Certain arrhythmias occur in the absence of any detectable disease of the heart. Other arrhythmias occur characteristically in certain diseases of the heart or with toxic amounts of drugs. Predisposing factors for the development of an arrhythmia include ischemic heart disease, congestive heart failure, hypoxemia, electrolyte imbalance, acidosis and treatment with certain drugs such as sympathomimetics or cardiac glycosides. The treatment of an arrhythmia may be difficult unless all predisposing factors are corrected.

Normal Physiology—The conduction of an impulse through the myocardium proceeds in an orderly fashion so that the atria and the ventricles each contract as a unit and the atria fill the ventricles. Thirty percent of the blood is added to the ventricles by atria contraction which increases ventricular effectiveness by 40 to 50%. The heart rate is normally controlled by the SA node, which fires at 60 to 100 beats/minute. The SA node and all other pacemaker cells have a decreasing potential at rest until threshold is reached. The electrophysiology of the pacemaker dictate that the faster pacemaker controls the heart rate: SA node 60 to 100/min.; AV node 40–60/min; ventricular pacemaker 20–40 min.

An impulse is conducted from the SA node through the atria to the AV node. Atrial depolarization is the P wave of the EKG. The AV node slows the impulse so that the atria may contract to fill the ventricles. The impulse then proceeds down the common bundle of His, the bundle branches and into the Purkinje fibers. The QRS complex of the EKG is ventricular depolarization and the T wave is ventricular repolarization.

The slope of cellular depolarization is the major factor in controlling rate. Depolarization is accomplished by a rapid influx of sodium—Phase 0. The change in membrane potential allows an influx of calcium ions which are responsible for contraction. Potassium is pumped rapidly from the cells.

Repolarization (Phase 3) to restore the membrane to its potential of −80 mv is accomplished by the rapid efflux of sodium and the rapid influx of potassium. Phase 4 represents slow spontaneous depolarization which allows threshold potential to be reached.

Pathophysiology—Many arrhythmias result from a decrease or increase in automaticity in myocardial tissue. Increased automaticity may result from (1) more rapid rate of depolarization, (2) a more negative threshold potential, (3) a less negative resting potential, or (4) a combination of these alterations. A decreased automaticity results from the opposite situations. Conduction disturbances, particularly slowing or failure of propagation, may also cause arrhythmias. Conduction disturbances are caused electrophysiologically by low resting potential, a slowly rising action potential and delayed recovery from depolarization.

Many paroxysmal tachyarrhythmias are due to reentrant phenomena, ie, a circus movement, in which an impulse is continually propagated in a circuit of excitable tissue. Such circuits may exist because of structural abnormalities, such as a bypass tract, or because of functional abnormalities of diseased heart tissue. When a critically timed impulse comes to two potential pathways with different refractory periods, it may be blocked down one pathway but conducted down the second. The impulse can then be conducted up the initially refractory pathway in a retrograde direction and back down the second pathway thus setting up the circus movement.

Arrhythmias may have various or no effects on the individual. Significant changes in the heart rate may impair cardiac output. In bradycardia, cardiac output is not increased during conditions of increased demand such as exercise, infection or stress. In tachycardia the synchrony of atrial-ventricular contraction may be lost or the time for ventricular filling may be decreased so that cardiac output is decreased.

Heart rate is a determinant of myocardial oxygen consumption. Coronary artery blood flow to the ventricles occurs only in diastole. Tachycardia increases cardiac oxygen demand while decreasing supply.

Ventricular contraction is not as efficient during tachycardia and myocardial function is depressed by long periods of tachycardia for unknown reasons.

Pathophysiology and Signs and Symptoms of Common Arrhythmias—*Sinus bradycardia* is a heart rate of less than 60 beats per minute with the impulse originating in the sinus node. Sinus bradycardia occurs in individuals who are in excellent physical condition, have increased intracerebral pressure, have hypothyroidism or in patients with SA node dysfunction due to degenerative or ischemic heart disease.

Sinus arrest refers to total cessation of sinus node activity. This may occur because of complete sinoatrial block (interference of conduction between sinus node and atrium) or loss of automaticity. There is a prolonged pause between 2 P waves on the EKG. Etiology of sinus arrest include excessive vagal stimulation, ischemic heart disease and digitalis toxicity.

Sinus arrhythmia is usually not a dysrhythmia but a normal change in heart rate (less than 10% variation in length of adjacent sinus cycles) that occurs with respiration. Heart rate increases during inspiration and decreases during expiration.

Sinus tachycardia is a heart rate of greater than 100 beats per minute with the impulse originating in the sinus node. Usually sinus tachycardia is less than 140 beats/minute. The etiologies of sinus tachycardia include: anxiety, fever, anemia, blood loss, thyrotoxicosis, pregnancy, pheochromocytoma, hypoxemia and electrolyte disturbances.

Premature atrial contractions (PACs) are ectopic atrial beats. Usually PACs are of little significance although they may precede a more serious atrial arrhythmia. The rhythm with PACs is usually irregular. The P wave is abnormal in PACs or may be hidden in the T wave. A PAC may be confused with a premature ventricular contraction. The etiology of PACs is related to stimulation by nicotine, caffeine or sympathomimetics or the deranged electrophysiology of a failing atria.

Paroxysmal atrial (supraventricular) tachycardia (PAT) is a sudden attack of atrial tachycardia that is sustained by reentry. The heart beat is regular and 140 to 250 beats/minute. This is a benign arrhythmia unless the rate is very rapid. PAT occurs in young people with no obvious cardiac disease and the precipitating event is usually emotional upset, trauma, fatigue, indigestion, stimulant drugs or alcohol ingestion. The patient may become very anxious because of prominent palpitations. PAT may end abruptly, spontaneously or be terminated by carotid massage or medications. The prognosis for PAT is excellent unless the rapid rate results in CHF, angina or myocardial infarction.

Atrial flutter is a regular rhythm with an atrial rate of 250 to 350, usually 300 beats per minute. The ventricular rate is 75 to 150 beats per minute reflecting AV block. The rhythm is sustained by reentry. The EKG shows sawtooth flutter waves instead of P waves. Atrial flutter occurs in patients with ischemic heart disease, mitral stenosis, thyrotoxicosis, atrial septal defect and hypoxemia due to chronic lung disease.

Atrial fibrillation is an arrhythmia in which the atria do not contract. The atrial rate is 400 to 600 and the ventricular rate is 80 to 180. The ventricular rate, which is slower than the atrial rate because of AV block, is usually rapid and irregularly irregular. The EKG shows fibrillating undulations instead of P waves. Because the atria do not contract, cardiac output is decreased and the signs and symptoms of congestive heart failure may be seen. Blood stagnates in the fibrillating atria and thrombi may form that embolize to either the lungs or the systemic circulation. The patient may also complain of palpitations due to the irregular rhythm. Paroxysmal atrial fibrillation may precede the onset of permanent atrial fibrillation in patients with mitral stenosis, constrictive pericarditis, ischemic heart disease, CHF, and thyrotoxicosis. Atrial fibrillation may occur in digitalis intoxication.

Premature ventricular contractions (PVCs) are beats that originate in an ectopic ventricular pacemaker. No P waves precede the QRS complex which appears widened and bizarre. PVCs are a benign arrhythmia when they occur in young people without underlying heart disease. The precipitating factors in these individuals include the consumption of caffeine, nicotine or alcohol, emotional stress, and reflexes from the GI tract. PVCs may be a more serious arrhythmia when the frequency increases, they occur in pairs or runs, occur near the T wave, or originate from multiple foci. In these cases, the arrhythmia may precede ventricular tachycardia or ventricular fibrillation. PVCs are associated with ischemic heart disease, myocardial infarction and digitalis intoxication.

Ventricular tachycardia is an arrhythmia with a rate of 150 to 250 and a regular rhythm. The rhythm is originating from an ectopic ventricular pacemaker by a reentrant mechanism. The P wave is independent of the QRS complex (A-V dissociation). Cardiac output is markedly decreased and the patient is usually unconscious if the arrhythmia is sustained. Ventricular fibrillation may originate from ventricular tachycardia. The most common cause of ventricular tachycardia is an acute myocardial infarction. Other causes include ischemic heart disease and digitalis and Type I antiarrhythmic drug toxicity. Ventricular tachycardia rarely occurs in a healthy individual.

Ventricular fibrillation is an irregular chaotic rhythm that is associated with no cardiac output and death if the arrhythmia is prolonged. The EKG is chaotic and does not reveal discernible wave forms. Treatment involves immediate DC electroshock.

Abnormalities of Conduction

Normally the AV node delays the impulse from the atria. In pathologic conditions, the impulse may be abnormally delayed or blocked completely.

First-degree (1°) heart block is an arrhythmia that usually requires no treatment. In 1° heart block the delay of atrial impulses by the AV node is prolonged (PR interval is greater than 0.20 seconds). Each atrial impulse is conducted through the AV node and results in a ventricular impulse. First-degree heart block can result from any inflammatory or degenerative disease of the heart, ischemic heart disease, and multiple medications. In healthy persons, an increase in vagal tone may result in first degree-heart block.

Second-degree heart block is an arrhythmia where the atrial rate is greater than the ventricular rate. *Mobitz Type I* (Wenckebach) is a progressive lengthening of the PR interval until an atrial impulse is not conducted by the AV node and the corresponding ventricular beat does not occur. The dropped ventricular beat may occur after every 6 to 8 atrial beats or after every second beat, 2:1 block. The block may disappear during exercise or with a decrease in vagal stimulation. The atrial rate is regular while the ventricular rate is irregular. Mobitz Type I block is caused by ischemic heart disease, disease which involves the AV node, and increases in vagal tone. The arrhythmia requires no treatment unless cardiac output is impaired.

Mobitz Type II is a more serious block of the lower AV node–His bundle complex that may progress to complete heart block. The EKG shows a normal or increased PR interval that remains constant. QRS complexes may be dropped after the P wave on a 2:1, 3:1, 4:1 or irregular basis. Mobitz Type II block occurs after a myocardial infarction, in myocarditis and in sclerosing diseases of the myocardium.

Complete or third-degree (3°) heart block involves a normal P wave that is unrelated to QRS complexes. The atrial impulse is completely blocked from conducting into the ventricles and the CO is maintained by the ventricles' own pacemakers. Third-degree heart block is caused by digitalis toxicity, a myocardial infarction, and degeneration of the conduction tissue. The prognosis for 3° heart block depends on whether the patient is symptomatic and the exact site of the block. Treatment is by pacemaker insertion.

Syncopal episodes due to complete atrioventricular heart block with resultant decreased CO is known as the *Stokes-Adams-Morgagni syndrome.*

Hypertension

Hypertension means abnormally elevated blood pressure. It may refer to increased pressure in any blood vessel, such as pulmonary or portal hypertension. However, it usually refers to an elevated systemic arterial blood pressure. Hypertension is not a disease but is a physical finding. Hypertension is often defined as a diastolic pressure of greater than 90 mm Hg because at this value the frequency of complications due to hypertension rises significantly. Systolic hypertension may also occur. Increased cardiovascular complications are also associated with elevated systolic blood pressure.

Normal Physiology—Blood pressure is determined by cardiac output and peripheral resistance ($BP = CO \times PR$). Cardiac output is determined by stroke volume and heart rate ($CO = SV \times HR$). Peripheral resistance is proportional to the fourth power of the internal radius of the blood vessels, according to the law of Laplace ($P = t/r^4$). Therefore, variations in the internal lumen of blood vessels profoundly affect the blood pressure. Blood pressure varies throughout the day in any individual and is affected by physical activity, emotional upset, and other factors.

Epidemiology—Approximately 10 to 20% of the population in the United States has hypertension. The incidence of hypertension depends on age, race, and gender. For example, Blacks at any age have twice the incidence of hypertension as Caucasians. Hypertension is slightly more common in males than in females.

Etiology—Between 5 and 20% of cases of hypertension have an identifiable cause, and these are called secondary hypertension. Causes of secondary hypertension include renal disease, endocrine disorders, and coarctation of the aorta, which will be discussed below. The remaining 80 to 95% of the cases of hypertension have no known cause and are called idiopathic, primary, or essential. The etiology of essential hypertension is probably multifactorial and may involve a number of abnormalities in physiologic regulatory systems. The pressure receptors in the cardiovascular system, ie, baroreceptors, may become reset at a higher pressure in response to chronic stress, overactivity of the sympathetic nervous system or heredity. The kidneys may retain too much salt and water in response to altered reflexes which tend to maintain abnormal intravascular fluid volumes. Statistical evidence correlates the incidence of hypertension with the quantity of dietary sodium. Some individuals with essential hypertension have elevated serum levels of renin.

Systolic hypertension occurs in situations of increased cardiac output such as anemia, fever, beriberi, aortic valve insufficiency, arteriovenous fistulas, and thyrotoxicosis. Systolic hypertension also occurs in elderly individuals with stiff, noncompliant blood vessels, ie, atherosclerosis.

Pathophysiology—Hypertension is a major risk factor for atherosclerosis and cardiovascular complications such as CHF, MI, and angina pectoris (see previous discussions). Sustained hypertension results in damage in the target organs: the eyes, brain, heart, and kidneys.

Damage to the eyes has been classified by Keith-Wagener-Barker. Grades I and II retinopathy correlate well with duration of hypertension, while Grades III and IV correspond to severity. The classes are cumulative.

Grade I: AV narrowing with mild depression of the venule by the crossing arteriole.
Grade II: greater AV narrowing and nicking of the venule by the crossing arteriole (AV nicking).
Grade III: arteriolar spasm, hemorrhages, exudates, tapering and disappearance of the venule under the arteriole.
Grade IV: all other findings, plus papilledema.

Hypertensive retinopathy leads to visual disturbances.

Damage to the brain results from cerebral edema, thrombosis and hemorrhage (see discussion of strokes). Strokes are 12 times more common in hypertensive patients. The stroke may be small and result in focal signs or a large fatal cerebral hemorrhage.

The heart compensates for the increased work imposed by the increased afterload with left ventricular hypertrophy. Eventually left ventricular function deteriorates, the chamber dilates, and left ventricular failure occurs (see previous discussion of heart failure). Mortality from hypertensive congestive heart failure is 50% in 5 years. Hypertension accelerates coronary atherosclerotic heart disease and increases myocardial oxygen consumption. Angina pectoris and myocardial infarction are more common in hypertensive patients (see previous discussion of CAD).

Hypertension causes fibrin deposition in the glomeruli and muscular hypertrophy of afferent arterioles. Severe hypertension causes intimal hypertrophy and fibrinoid necrosis in the afferent arterioles. Malignant hypertension accelerates damage to the kidney. Eventually renal failure occurs (see discussion of chronic failure below).

Signs and Symptoms—Hypertension *per se* causes no signs or symptoms unless the BP is very high. The signs and symptoms of essential hypertension are secondary to target organ damage. For example, retinopathy causes scotomas, blurred vision, and finally blindness. Brain damage may cause such symptoms as dizziness, light-headedness, vertigo, tinnitus, syncope, lethargy, confusion, increased neuromuscular irritability, convulsions, and coma. Damage to the heart results in angina pectoris or the signs and symptoms of CHF or MI. The signs and symptoms of chronic renal failure are described later.

Elevated blood pressure may be an incidental finding during routine physical examination. The diagnosis of hypertension is based on documentation of increased blood pressure on several independent readings, unless target organ damage is already present. The adequate treatment of hypertension reduces its mortality and morbidity.

Secondary Hypertension—This presently accounts for only 5 to 20% of the cases. It may be cured if the underlying disorder is successfully treated.

Renal vascular hypertension is mediated by the renin-angiotensin system. Renal blood flow is decreased by renal artery stenosis secondary to fibromuscular dysplasia or atherosclerosis. The renal artery lesion may be either unilateral or bilateral. The decreased renal blood flow is sensed by the juxtaglomerular apparatus which secretes renin. Renin cleaves angiotensinogen to angiotensin I (a decapeptide). Converting enzyme in the pulmonary circulation converts angiotensin I to angiotensin II. Angiotensin II (an octapeptide) constricts blood vessels and stimulates aldosterone production. Aldosterone stimulates the retention of sodium and water by the distal convoluted tubule and the excretion of potassium.

Renal parenchymal disease is also associated with hypertension; the mechanism is not well understood. The decreased clearance of sodium and water that occurs in renal failure results in volume expansion which contributes to hypertension.

Endocrine disorders cause hypertension usually by the production of hormone by tumors of endocrine glands. Hypertension is seen in Cushing's syndrome, primary hyperaldosteronism and hyperparathyroidism (see later discussion of these disorders). A very rare cause of hypertension is a tumor of the adrenal gland known as pheochromocytoma, which secretes excessive quantities of norepinephrine and epinephrine. Elevations of blood pressure are often episodic. Accompanying symptoms of excessive catecholamines include acute pounding headache, tachycardia, and sweating. Administration of oral contraceptives can cause hypertension that occurs in greater than 5% of users. Estrogens increase hepatic synthesis of renin substrate and angiotensin I. The hypertension reverts to normal when the oral contraceptives are discontinued.

Coarctation of the aorta is a congenital malformation of the aorta resulting in a narrow area in the aorta, usually in the arch. Alterations in hemodynamics lead to a decreased renal blood flow which activates the renin-angiotensin system.

Rheumatology

Normal Physiology

Joints allow movement of one bone upon another. The ends of the bones are covered with hyaline cartilage and diarthrodial joints are covered by collagenous tissue called the joint capsule. The synovial membrane lines the joint space side of the joint capsule. The synovial membrane is a relatively acellular, highly vascular, delicate membrane which secretes the synovial fluid. The cartilage, which is avascular, derives its nutrition from the synovial fluid. Various inflammatory diseases, trauma and degeneration may involve the joint.

Rheumatoid Arthritis

Rheumatoid arthritis (RA) is a chronic systemic illness manifested primarily by inflammatory arthritis involving small peripheral joints symmetrically. The disease also may affect the cardiovascular, hematologic and pulmonary systems and the eye.

Etiology—The etiology of RA is unknown. Many infectious organisms have been postulated to be the etiologic agents. Histocompatibility typing has recently proven that a predisposition for the disease is inherited. Unknown environmental factors may play a role in the development of RA.

Epidemiology—Approximately 4½ million people in the United States have RA. The onset is most common in the third and fourth decades but may affect all age groups, including children. Women develop the disease more commonly than men by a ratio of 3:1.

Pathology—The disease is characterized by inflammation of the synovium. Infiltration of lymphocytes, monocytes, and polymorphonuclear leukocytes occurs with edema, vascular congestion, and fibrin deposition. As a result of chronic inflammation, the synovium thickens, forms large villi and is referred to as a pannus. The pannus erodes the underlying cartilage and bone. The degree of functional joint disability correlates with the destruction of the cartilage. The joint space is reduced and even eliminated as the cartilage is destroyed. The joint may become ankylosed or fixed as fibrous or bony connections develop between the bones. The inflammatory process and the destruction of normal joint anatomy results in weakening of tendons, ligaments, and other supporting structures. This leads to instability and partial dislocation (subluxation) of the joint. Tendons may rupture due to inflammation of the tendon sheath.

Rheumatoid nodules, characteristic of RA, are most commonly found in subcutaneous tissue over pressure points such as the elbows, extensor surface of the forearms, and the occiput. However, they may also be found in the lung, heart or vocal cords. An area of necrosis and cellular debris forms the center of the nodule. This is surrounded by several layers of palisading large monocytes. Severe RA may also be complicated by vasculitis involving multiple organs.

Pathophysiology—Antibodies against immunoglobulin G (IgG) are found in the serum and synovial fluid of most patients with RA. The antibodies are of the IgM, IgG, and IgA classes of immunoglobulins and are called rheumatoid factors. Chronic antigenic stimulation is thought to stimulate production of these antibodies. The exact role of rheumatoid factors in the development of RA has not been demonstrated. However, immunologic mechanisms do appear to play a role in the pathogenesis of RA. Immune complexes of immunoglobulins, rheumatoid factor and complement generate vasoactive and chemotactic substances in the joint. Lysosomal enzymes, which cause tissue injury, are released after phagocytic cells ingest the immune complexes. Immunoglobulins and complement are also found in the vascular lesions and immunoglobulins may contribute to the development of the systemic manifestations of RA.

Signs and Symptoms—The onset of RA is usually insidious. Fatigue, weakness, joint stiffness, arthralgias, and myalgias may precede signs of joint inflammation. The joints gradually become tender, red, swollen, hot, and painful. Joint stiffness, particularly after a prolonged period of rest, ("gelling") is a major complaint of patients with RA. The joints most commonly involved include some of those in the hands (proximal interphalangeal and metacarpophalangeal joints) and feet (metatarsophalangeal joints), shoulders, knees, elbows, ankles, and wrists; the cervical spine, hips and tempomandibular joints may also become involved. RA tends to affect joints symmetrically.

The hypertrophied synovium of involved joints may be palpated. Muscle weakness and atrophy often parallel the severity of the joint disease. Range of motion, especially extension, becomes limited. Flexion contractures and ankylosis develop as the disease progresses. Swan-neck, boutonniere and cockup toes are terms used to describe the deformities of the hands and feet. Ulnar deviation of the fingers can occur.

Duration of morning stiffness, which is usually measured in hours, may be used to monitor disease activity. Other indicators include grip strength, time required to walk a certain distance, number and clinical assessment of joints involved and radiographs demonstrating erosion of bone, loss of joint space and soft tissue swelling of inflammation.

Rheumatoid arthritis is a systemic disease involving multiple organ systems besides the joints. The rheumatoid nodules are found in 20% of RA patients. Less than 5% of the patients have the vasculitis which may result in peripheral neuropathy, nail-fold thrombi, digital gangrene and leg ulcers. The most common ocular manifestation is keratoconjunctivitis sicca (Sjögren's syndrome); episcleritis may also occur. In the lungs, interstitial fibrosis, rheumatoid nodules and pleural effusions are seen. Inflammation of the pericardium may cause pericarditis and cardiac tamponade. Rheumatoid nodules on the heart valves may lead to murmurs, and nodules in the heart muscle cause electrical conduction disturbances.

Patients with severe arthritis may develop Felty's syndrome—RA, splenomegaly and leukopenia.

A mild to moderate anemia that is normochromic or hypochromic is found in patients with RA. The severity of the anemia parallels the activity of the disease. In these patients serum iron is low but total iron-binding capacity is normal. The defect is thought to be in iron utilization in hemoglobin synthesis. (See anemia of chronic disease.)

Other abnormal laboratory tests include a rapid erythrocyte sedimentation rate which may be used to monitor disease activity. The latex aggregation test for IgM rheumatoid factor is positive in 85 to 90% of patients. However, other diseases of chronic inflammation are also associated with a positive rheumatoid factor test. Antinuclear antibodies and lupus erythematosus (LE) cells may be present. The serum complement level is usually normal or elevated. Analysis of the synovial fluid, while not diagnostic, typically shows neutrophils (10,000 to 50,000/mm³), decreased levels of complement, presence of fibrinogen, and decreased levels of glucose.

The highly variable clinical course of RA makes prognosis difficult in individual patients. Spontaneous remissions and exacerbations are characteristic. Remissions occur most frequently in the early stages of the disease. As many as 35% of patients may experience a complete remission with little or no joint deformity. Approximately 50% of patients have a chronically progressive course over many years with development of varying degrees of joint damage. A smaller group, 10 to 15%, have a relentless destructive course that results in severe deformities and crippling. The unpredictable course of RA also makes evaluation of therapy particularly difficult and contributes to the quackery seen in this field.

The diagnosis of RA is based on the clinical picture of symmetrical inflammatory arthritis usually involving small joints, characteristic radiograph changes and a positive rheumatoid factor test. Other causes of inflammatory arthritis: Reiter's syndrome, psoriatic arthritis, systemic lupus erythematosus, and arthritis associated with inflammatory bowel disease, must be excluded. The arthritis associated with rheumatic fever and viral infections, such as rubella and hepatitis B, may mimic RA. Initially, degenerative joint disease is easily distinguished from RA although both diseases may occur simultaneously.

Degenerative Joint Disease

DJD, also known as *osteoarthritis* and *hypertrophic arthritis*, is characterized by loss of joint cartilage and hypertrophy of bone. Stress and wear and tear probably contribute to the loss of cartilage in some patients.

Etiology and Epidemiology—Approximately 40 million Americans have radiographic evidence of DJD but many have no symptoms attributable to the disease. The prevalence of DJD increases with age, 85% of people 70 years old or older have characteristic radiographic changes. Epidemiologic evidence indicates that heavy use of a joint, so-called "wear and tear," may play a role in initiating the degeneration of cartilage. In younger persons, degenerative changes occur when the cartilage has been damaged by infection, acute trauma, excessive use, or congenital deformities. The precise mechanisms of cartilage loss in DJD are unknown.

Pathology—Histologically, degenerative changes are seen in cartilage as progressive loss of metachromasia, which is evidence of proteoglycan loss. Chondrocytes increase in number and form clusters. The surface of the cartilage loosens and flakes off; and fissures form as deeper layers become involved. The cartilage may be lost completely. The bone at joint margins responds by osteophyte formation and hypertrophy. The subchondral bone which has lost the covering cartilage becomes dense, smooth, and glistening (eburnation). Cystic areas may develop below the joint surface. Inflammation of the synovium and joint capsule is usually mild.

Pathophysiology—Collagen fibers and proteoglycans give normal cartilage the properties of compressibility and elasticity. The proteoglycan molecules bind large numbers of water molecules which are released when the cartilage is compressed and are regained when the force is removed. The proteoglycan molecules do not bind water properly in DJD because the molecule is smaller and the composition is altered.

In normal adult cartilage, chrondrocytes do not synthesize DNA or divide but in DJD chrondrocytes perform both of these processes. The chrondrocytes are continuously rebuilding the cartilage matrix in DJD. The amount of hydrolases is increased in DJD. As the disease progresses, the destruction exceeds the rate of repair, resulting in a net loss of cartilage. Cartilage laid down during the rebuilding process of DJD is of the type normally found in tendons and skin but not in bone. Simultaneously, the subchondral bone sclerosis and marginal bone overgrowths (spurs) develop.

Degenerative joint disease may be either primary or secondary. No predisposing cause can be identified in primary DJD. In secondary DJD the underlying abnormality or cause is found and the onset is usually several decades earlier in life. Causes of secondary DJD include infection, trauma, fractures, unusual use, damage by inflammation as in RA and congenital abnormalities. In addition, acromegaly, alcaptonuria, hemochromatosis, and chrondrocalcinosis are predisposing factors for secondary DJD.

Signs and Symptoms—Pain in the joints particularly with motion or weight bearing is characteristic of DJD. The pain is usually described as aching. Joint stiffness occurs after rest and quickly subsides after resuming movement. The duration of morning stiffness is measured in minutes rather than hours as in RA.

Examination of the joints reveals decreased range of motion, local tenderness, bony enlargement but usually no heat or erythema. Joint involvement in primary DJD is symmetrical. DJD commonly involves the distal interphalangeal (DIP) joints, in contrast to RA. Bony enlargement of the DIP joints is called Heberden's nodes. Involvement of the PIP joints is known as Bouchard's nodes. Metacarpophalangeal joints, wrists, elbows, and shoulders are infrequently involved in DJD unless occupational trauma predisposes the development. DJD involves the spine and may cause compression of spinal nerve roots by the bony spurs which can lead to a variety of complaints. DJD of the hip may be the most disabling form of the disease.

There are no laboratory abnormalities characteristic of DJD. The diagnosis is based on radiographic changes of joint space narrowing and bony spur formation and the signs and symptoms of the patient. The clinical course of DJD usually is progressive.

Crystal-Induced Arthritis

Several distinct diseases are characterized by crystal deposition in and about joint spaces. The deposition can lead to acute inflammation of the joint. Gout is a disorder of sodium urate deposition whereas pseudogout is characterized by deposition of calcium pyrophosphate dehydrate crystals. Recently arthritis has been attributed to hydroxyapatite deposition.

Gout is a disorder typified by hyperuricemia with recurrent attacks of acute arthritis and tophaceous deposits of sodium urate. Primary causes of gout are defects in the metabolism of purines to uric acid or a specific decrease in renal clearance of uric acid. Secondary gout results from other disorders which result in hyperuricemia.

Epidemiology—Contrary to folklore, gout is not related to socioeconomic class. Few individuals with gout consume excessive quantities of purine-containing foods. Primary gout is a disease of the adult male. Only 5% of cases occur in females and these are usually in the postmenopausal group. Secondary gout accounts for only 5–10% of all cases. Primary gout may be inherited. The mode of inheritance may be autosomal dominant, autosomal recessive, or sex-linked depending on the metabolic abnormality responsible for the hyperuricemia. Diabetes mellitus, obesity, hypertension coronary and cerebral atherosclerosis and hypertriglyceridemia all occur more frequently among gouty patients for unknown reasons.

Pathophysiology—The rates of production and elimination of uric acid determine the amount of uric acid in the body. Exogenous (dietary) and endogenous purines are oxidized to uric acid. Of the uric acid eliminated, the kidney excretes two-thirds and the gastrointestinal tract excretes the remainder. The two most important processes in the development of hyperuricemia are abnormalities of endogenous purine production and of uric acid excretion by the kidney. The majority of patients with gout have a defect of uric acid clearance through the kidney. Specific enzyme abnormalities which have been identified include: decreased hypoxanthine-guanine phosphoribosyltransferase and increased PP-ribose-P synthetase, which result in the over-production of uric acid.

Uric acid is filtered by glomeruli, but 98% of the filtered amount is reabsorbed by the tubules. The majority of the uric acid excreted (80–85%) is actively secreted into the urine by the renal tubules. The exact reason for undersecretion of uric acid by the tubules is unknown. Metabolic acidosis or increased acid load as occurs in chronic renal failure, after a prolonged fast or with ethanol ingestion, inhibits the secretion of uric acid.

Hyperuricemia is defined statistically as a serum uric acid level of above 7.5 mg per 100 mL for males and a serum uric acid level of above 6.6 mg per 100 mL for females using the automated colorimetric method of determination. The risk of developing gout correlates with the serum uric acid level. Gout is rare in patients with uric acid levels of less than 7 mg per 100 mL, whereas 83% of patients with a uric acid level greater than 9 mg per 100 mL develop gout. Although the exact reason for the sudden attack of gout in a hyperuricemic patient is unknown, acute attacks may be precipitated by acute fluctuations in serum uric acid level, trauma or acute decreases in uric acid secretion. The likelihood of developing gout increases with age.

Pathology—The pathognomonic lesion of gout is the tophus which is a sodium urate deposit surrounded by inflammatory and foreign-body reaction. The water-soluble crystals are anisotropic (negatively birefringent) when viewed under a polarized light microscope. Sodium urate is deposited in cartilage, epiphyseal bone, periarticular structures and kidneys. Common sites for tophi include the earlobe, the olecranon and patellar bursas and tendons. Urate deposits in the joints result in cartilage degeneration, synovial proliferation and pannus formation, destruction of subchondral bone, proliferation of marginal bone and fibrous or bony ankylosis.

Sodium urate crystals are found in the medulla of the kidney with interstitial inflammatory or vascular reaction. The interstitial inflammation which may be acute or chronic results in tubular damage. Vascular reaction includes arterial and arteriolar sclerosis.

Signs and Symptoms—Primary gout has three manifestations: asymptomatic hyperuricemia, acute gouty arthritis which recurs after asymptomatic intervals and chronic gouty arthritis. Many patients with hyperuricemia never develop gouty arthritis, urolithiasis or renal damage.

Acute Gouty Arthritis—The onset of the attack is abrupt and usually involves the great toe, although the instep, ankle or knee may be involved. The pain is intense or excruciating. Fever may be present. The initial attack usually subsides in a few days to a few weeks and recovery is complete.

The interval following the initial attack may be from a few weeks to many years. Later the attacks become more frequent, may involve more joints, and are more severe.

The acute attack begins with sodium urate crystallization from the supersaturated synovial fluid. The crystals activate complement and Hageman factor; chemotactic and vasoactive substances are produced; leukocytes accumulate and phagocytize the crystals which in turn destroys the leukocytes releasing their lysosomal enzymes. The enzymes attack and destroy cartilage.

Chronic Gouty Arthritis—Without treatment and after many years visible tophi develop, permanent joint destruction occurs, and symptoms become chronic. The tophi are relatively painless. However, there is progressive stiffness and persistent aching of affected joints. Destruction of joints and large tophi may lead to grotesque deformities and crippling. The tophi may ulcerate and extrude the chalky sodium urate. Eventually acute attacks occur less frequently and lessen in severity.

Urolithiasis—Patients with gout have an increased incidence of renal stones with 20% of patients with normal uric acid excretion and 40% of patients with elevated uric acid excretion developing stones; 84% of the stones are composed of uric acid which is only slightly water-soluble. Development of urolithiasis may precede the acute attack of gout. A predisposing factor to urate renal stone formation is the excretion of a more acidic urine.

Secondary Gout—Acquired hyperuricemia occurs in patients with polycythemia vera, secondary polycythemia, leukemia, lymphoma, multiple myeloma, chronic hemolytic anemia and after radiation or chemotherapy for a variety of cancers. Both overproduction and under-secretion of uric acid play a role in the development of secondary gout. Serum and urinary levels of uric acid tend to be higher than in primary gout. Drugs that interfere with secretion of uric acid, such as the thiazide diuretics, may also cause secondary gout. Chronic renal disease may cause hyperuricemia but gouty arthritis is not usually seen. Patients who have had lead intoxication develop gout.

The acute attack is diagnosed by the presence of needle-like crystals, birefringent under polarized light in leukocytes from the synovial fluid. Chronic gouty arthritis may be confirmed by chemical analysis of tophaceous material. Pseudogout must be excluded.

Calcium pyrophosphate dihydrate (CPPD) deposition disease—CPPD is characterized by chondrocalcinosis and acute attacks of pseudogout. The prevalence of CPPD increases with age. Associations with other diseases such as hemochromatosis, hyperparathyroidism, ochronosis, Wilson's disease, and hypothyroidism have been demonstrated. Pseudogout describes acute inflammatory arthritis in which positively birefringent rhomboid crystals of CPPD are identified on synovial fluid analysis. By far the most commonly involved joint is the knee. Between attacks the joint may be entirely asymptomatic or show changes of osteoarthritis. Radiographic evidence of calcinosis in cartilage and other joint related structures is usually found.

Hydroxyapatite crystals have been described recently in the synovial fluid of acutely inflamed joints. They are not resolvable by light microscopy and require electron microscopic or microanalytic techniques for identification. The knee and shoulder are most commonly involved.

Systemic Lupus Erythematosus

Systemic lupus erythematosis (SLE) is a multisystem disease of unknown etiology which predominately affects young women but can affect men and women of all ages. It is often viewed as the prototypic autoimmune disease in which antibodies are formed against one's own tissues.

Etiology—Although many potential etiologies, eg, viral infections have been proposed none have been clearly substantiated. A small percentage of patients given procainamide or hydralazine have developed a syndrome which mimics SLE.

Pathophysiology—Antibodies are formed against one's own DNA. These autoantibodies bind the antigen (DNA) and complement, forming immune complexes which when deposited in various organs cause injury.

Signs and Symptoms—SLE patients may manifest non-specific constitutional symptoms such as fever, malaise, anorexia, weight loss, arthralgias or myalgias. Specific signs may include photosensitive rashes, "butterfly" malar rash, scarring "discoid" rash, alopecia, mucosal ulcerations, arthritis, serositis, vasculitis, cerebritis, and glomerulonephritis. Laboratory abnormalities may include leukopenia, hemolytic anemia, thrombocytopenia, false positive serologic test for syphilis, abnormal urinary sediment and proteinuria, antinuclear antibodies (ANA) and antibodies against double-stranded DNA, and hypocomplementemia.

Scleroderma

This is a disease of unknown etiology and pathogenesis which is characterized by increased fibrous tissue disposition and obliteration of small vessels in many organ systems. The skin of the face, hands and feet typically becomes swollen and then firm, thickened and leathery in appearance. Patients may also manifest one or more of a collection of findings referred to collectively as "CREST" (*c*alcinosis, *R*aynaud's phenomenon, *e*sophageal involvement, *s*clerodactyly, and *t*elangiectasis). The most feared complication of this disease is malignant hypertension with rapid onset of renal failure.

Polymyositis and Dermatomyositis

Polymyositis and dermatomyositis (when there is associated skin involvement) are diseases in which there is inflammation primarily of skeletal muscles. The myositis is characterized by both degenerating and regenerating muscle fibers and a mononuclear cell infiltrate. Proximal muscle weakness dominates the clinical picture. Some patients also have an associated malignancy or another rheumatic disease. Diagnosis is based on compatible signs and symptoms, increased muscle enzyme levels in the serum, abnormal electromyogram, and muscle biopsy.

Vasculitis

Vasculitis is a term used to describe inflammatory changes of blood vessels which can lead to necrosis, thrombosis and obliteration of the involved vessels. Vasculitis can be a manifestation of an underlying systemic disease or constitute the primary process of a collection of disease entities. Understanding of the vasculitides has been hampered by the lack of a universally accepted and clear classification system. Classifications have been based on clinical, histopathologic, and etiologic considerations. A major obstacle to classification is the fact that vasculitis represents a spectrum of disease and most individual cases do not fit precisely into a well-defined category. Selected aspects of several of the vasculitides will be described briefly.

Since vasculitis can involve all organs a multitude of clinical expressions is seen. Many patients have constitutional complaints such as fever, malaise, anorexia, weight loss, myalgias and arthralgias. Other features include glomerulonephritis, ischemic heart disease, peripheral neuropathy (mononeuritis multiplex) or central nervous system involvement, pulmonary infiltrates or effusions, ischemic bowel disease and rash. Laboratory tests usually suggest a nonspecific inflammatory reaction (eg, elevated erythrocyte sedimentation rate). Diagnosis is based on the clinical presentation in conjunction with biopsy and angiographic results.

Polyarteritis nodosa primary involves medium size vessels and is characterized at an early stage by infiltration of the vessels with polymorphonuclear leucocytes. In a majority of cases the etiology is unknown but a few patients have hepatitis B antigenemia. The vessel injury may be mediated through deposition of immune complexes of hepatitis B antigen, antibody, and complement with resultant damage by neutrophils drawn to the lesions by chemotaxis.

Hypersensitivity angititis is a small vessel vasculitis predominantly involving the skin. It appears to be a manifestation of an allergic reaction to an exogenous (drug, infection) or endogeneous (tumor) antigen. The histopathology is described as "leukocytoclastic angitis," which is vasculitis with neutrophils and their nuclear dust, extravasated red blood cells, and fibrinoid necrosis of the vessel wall. This type of vasculitis also occurs with the other collagen vascular diseases such as systemic lupus erythematosus, rheumatoid arthritis, and dermatomyositis.

Wegener's granulomatosis is a disease characterized by granulomatous vasculitis of the upper (sinusitis, nasal ulcerations, otitis media) and lower (cavitary and nodular infiltrates) respiratory tracts, glomerulonephritis, and a variable degree of small vessel involvement.

Giant cell arteritis (also called temporal arteritis, cranial arteritis) is characterized by segmental involvement of large vessels (primarily branches of the carotid artery) with a mononuclear infiltrate including giant cells and destruction of the internal elastic lamina. This disease primarily affects older patients (greater than 50 years of age). It is often accompanied by symptoms of polymyalgia rheumatica which include achiness and stiffness of the proximal muscles of the shoulders and pelvis. The most dreaded complication of giant cell arteritis is sudden blindness due to ischemic optic neuritis.

Neurology

Epilepsy

Epilepsy is a chronic disorder of cerebral functions that is characterized by recurrent seizures. The seizures have a definite onset and ending and usually last less than ten minutes.

Epidemiology—Approximately 1% of the population suffers from epilepsy with two to four million people in the US being affected. The age of onset is characteristic for particular types of epilepsy. For example, "petit mal" seizures usually begin in childhood. Approximately one in 15 children will have a seizure in the first seven years of life.

Etiology—Many diseases may cause one or several seizures. These are not epilepsy. Diseases involving the central nervous system such as brain tumors, cerebral vascular accidents, meningitis, lipid storage diseases, and cerebral injuries may cause epilepsy. In many cases the cause of the epilepsy is unknown and the condition is referred to as idiopathic.

Pathology—Various lesions in the brain such as gliosis and abnormal vascularization have been associated with epilepsy in some patients and not in others. It is not always possible to diagnose an epileptogenic lesion when the clinical information indicates focal seizures.

Pathophysiology—The convulsion results from sudden excessive disorderly neuronal discharges in an apparently normal or a diseased cortex. The mechanisms and reasons for the discharge are not well understood. One theory is that a group of diencephalic nerves normally exerts a constant restraining influence on cortical neurons preventing excessive discharge. In epilepsy the neurons are deafferented, supersensitive, and susceptible to activation or depolarization by a variety of stimuli. Another theory states that there is a decreased amount of gamma-aminobutyric acid (GABA) which is one of the inhibitory transmitters in the brain. A lower seizure threshold may also be genetically determined.

The excessive disorderly neuronal discharge involving the entire brain immediately results in loss of consciousness, disturbances in sensation and/or convulsive movements. A focal brain lesion may cause generalized convulsions exclusively.

Signs and Symptoms—The signs and symptoms of epilepsy depend on the type. Seizures may generally be classified as generalized or partial. Generalized convulsions which involve the entire cerebral cortex are the most frequent. "Grand mal" seizures are a type of generalized convulsion which is characterized by a sudden loss of consciousness, a cry, falling, tonic then clonic movements of the muscles and incontinence of sphincters. After the motor activity ceases, the patient may be unconscious for as long as 30 minutes. On awakening, the patient may complain of a headache. Other generalized convulsions may consist of clonic rhythmic jerking or tonic spasms without a typical sequence.

"Petit mal," also known as absence seizures, is a generalized convulsion characterized by loss of consciousness for a few seconds. The patient has a blank facial expression and may blink the eyelids or jerk the arm.

Partial seizures start on one side of the brain but may become generalized. Focal epilepsy originates from a certain area within the brain and the signs and symptoms may be attributed to that area. A structural abnormality may be identified in that site. Focal epilepsy is also called partial epilepsy with either elementary or complex symptomatology. "Jacksonian epilepsy" is a type of partial seizure which begins with twitching of the fingers of one hand, the face or one foot. The movement then spreads to other muscles on the same side of the body. It may become generalized.

"Psychomotor" epilepsy is a partial seizure with complex symptomatology. It is often associated with a lesion in the temporal lobe. The patient acts as though he were conscious, although he is amnestic. The patient may continue with activity or perform tasks but may not be able to respond to questions or commands. The seizure is often preceded by an aura which consists of sensations or experiences often recognized by the patient as a warning of an impending seizure. Motor activity due to the seizure is chewing, lip smacking, and tonic spasms of the extremities. This type of seizure may last for hours.

Somatic sensory epilepsy may be focal or marching and originates in the parietal lobe. The patient complains of numbness, tingling, crawling or other sensations that involve the lips, fingers and toes. Other types of somatic sensory seizures involve visual hallucinations of moving lights or colors.

The diagnosis of epilepsy is based on the clinical history and the electroencephalogram. The EEG is characteristically abnormal during a seizure but may be normal between seizures. The cerebral spinal fluid, skull X-rays, CT scans of the head and arteriogram are normal, unless there is a primary neurologic disease as the cause of the epilepsy. The frequency of seizures varies from one per year to many per day. Mental deterioration is not caused by epilepsy.

Parkinsonism

Parkinsonism, also called paralysis agitans, is a disorder of the extrapyramidal system that was originally described in 1817. James Parkinson described a tremor which occurs at rest, decreased muscle power, lip flexion and festination, but sparing the senses and intellect.

Etiology—The cause of parkinsonism is unknown. Many of the persons who survived the pandemic of von Economo encephalitis in 1918 and 1922 developed parkinsonism 20 to 30 years later. Psychoactive drugs such as the phenothiazines and butyrophenones can cause a syndrome similar to parkinsonism. An identical but reversible disorder may be caused by infections, tumors and certain chemicals and drugs. The term Parkinson's disease is reserved for paralysis agitans of unknown cause.

Epidemiology—Parkinsonism usually occurs in middle or late life between 50 and 70 years, though it is rarely seen in young people. There is a 2% risk of being affected by this disease and 200,000 to 300,000 are presently affected in this country.

Pathology—The melanin is lost from nerve cells in the brainstem, particularly in the substantia nigra, usually accompanied by some loss of nerve cells and reactive gliosis.

Pathophysiology—The basal ganglia normally control postural tone and provide the background adjustments for intentional movements. The dopaminergic pathway from the caudate nucleus to the thalamus inhibits the inhibition of voluntary movement. This pathway is opposed by the cholinergic pathway, which is excitatory for the inhibition of voluntary movement. The cholinergic pathway in the caudate nucleus is inhibited by a dopaminergic pathway from the substantia nigra. The loss of inhibition and the unbalance of opposing pathways result in the movement difficulties of parkinsonism. The origin of the tremor is less clear. Decreased dopamine is found in the substantia nigra, caudate nucleus and putamen in parkinsonism.

Signs and Symptoms—The signs and symptoms of parkinsonism are characteristic. The typical tremor occurs at rest and lessens with voluntary movement. The tremor may involve the hands, legs, lips, tongue and eyelids when the eyes are closed. In the early stages of the disease, the tremor is unilateral but becomes bilateral later in the course. The tremor occurs at a frequency of 4 to 8 cycles per second. The hand tremor is described as "pill rolling."

In the early stage of the disease, there is bradykinesia as all movement is slowed. Later, the patient has particularly difficulty initiating movement. Finally, there is absence of movement or akinesia. The spontaneous movements of posture change, such as arm swinging while walking, disappear. The face becomes expressionless and is known as mask-like facies. The voice becomes monotonous. The posture is stooped. Because the patient cannot make reflex adjustments to the posture changes of walking, "he walks with quick shuffling steps at an accelerating pace, as if attempting to catch up with his center of gravity." Passive movement of the extremities elicits "cog wheel" motion because both flexors and extensors are contracted.

Anxiety and tension aggravate the symptoms. The patient with parkinsonism may also have seborrhea and excessive sweating and salivation.

Eventually the patient is incapacitated by the rigidity and the tremor disappears. The clinical course is one of gradual progression of the disease. In five years, 25% of patients are disabled; in 15 years, 80% are disabled. Dementia occurs very late in the course of the disease but often occurs earlier than in persons not affected by parkinsonism.

Stroke Syndromes

A stroke is a process involving one or more blood vessels in the brain, which results in the sudden and dramatic development of a focal neurologic deficit. The deficit reflects the location and size of brain injury. Three separate entities are recognized: transient ischemic attacks (TIA), progressing stroke and completed stroke. While TIAs are transient, progressing and completed strokes are not.

Etiology—The vast majority of strokes are caused by atherosclerotic disease of the cerebral arteries. Embolism from the heart or from ulcerated atherosclerotic plaques in the carotid arteries also causes strokes. Cerebral hemorrhages are most often due to hypertension but may also be due to the rupture of an aneurysm. Less frequent causes of strokes include trauma, excessive anticoagulation and inflammatory diseases of cerebral blood vessels.

Normal Physiology—The effects of the blood vessel occlusion relate to the location and the availability of collateral or anastomotic blood flow. The circle of Willis provides collateral circulation and is protective of the brain. Infarction will be prevented by these collaterals if the lesion is proximal. Retrograde flow from the external carotid may prevent damage when the internal carotid is occluded. Collaterals for the vertebral artery exist. Anastomoses may prevent or lessen damage if the lesion is distal to the circle of Willis.

Pathophysiology—Atherosclerosis occurs in the arteries of the brain as elsewhere in the body (see discussion of atherosclerosis). A thrombotic stroke results when a thrombus develops on an atherosclerotic plaque, the lumen of the vessel is narrowed or may be completely occluded, and collaterals are insufficient to preserve function. Extension of the thrombus may block collateral blood flow.

Cerebral embolism most commonly originates from a thrombus in the heart which is in atrial fibrillation. Other sources of embolic strokes are mural thrombi that occur after myocardial infarction and pieces of intraarterial thrombi. The emboli usually become lodged at bifurcations. Emboli cause hemorrhagic infarction.

Intracranial hemorrhage is the third most frequent cause of stroke. Intracranial hemorrhage is most commonly due to hypertension, rupture of saccular aneurysm and bleeding disorders. Cerebral hemorrhages due to hypertension involve a penetrating artery and occur within the brain tissue. Adjacent tissue is compressed and displaced by the mass of blood.

Saccular aneurysms or berries are thin-walled blisters protruding from the arteries of the circle of Willis or major branches of the circle at bifurcations. Developmental defects in the media of the arteries cause the aneurysms, which are composed of intima and adventitia. The defect in the wall structure is congential, but enlargement and eventual rupture occur during later life, reaching a peak at 35 to 65 years of age. In 20% of the cases there is more than one aneurysm. Rupture of the aneurysm results in bleeding into the subarachnoid space and occasionally into the brain as well.

Signs and Symptoms—The location of the lesion determines the nature of the deficit. Lesions in the carotid system result in unilateral signs of hemiplegia, hemihypoesthesia, hemianopsia, aphasia and agnosia. Lesions in the basilar system result in bilateral signs, motor and sensory deficit, brainstem deficit and variable cranial nerve abnormalities. Cerebellar infarction results in severe dizziness, nausea, vomiting, ataxia, and nystagmus.

In 80% of cases of thrombotic stroke a TIA has occurred previously. A TIA due to temporary or partial occlusion of all or part of the carotid-middle cerebral artery system may consist of hemiplegia, hemiparesthesia, monocular blindness, or other focal signs, depending on the area of brain affected. A TIA due to temporary or partial occlusion of the vertebral-basilar system consists of dizziness, diplopia, numbness, impaired vision, and dysarthria. A TIA usually lasts for about 10 minutes but may last for a few seconds up to 12 hours. Between the TIAs the patient may have no neurologic deficit. A bruit may be heard over the carotid arteries if they are severely atherosclerotic.

A thrombotic stroke begins suddenly but may progress over several days. Parts of the body may become involved in a stepwise fashion. A completed stroke is defined as 18 to 24 hours without progression for the carotid system and 72 hours without progression for the vertebral-basilar system.

Prognosis in a thrombotic stroke is difficult to predict. Comatose patients have a poor prognosis. Improvement generally occurs as functions are taken over by other parts of the brain or when edema surrounding an infarct subsides. If improvement has not begun by the second week, prognosis is poor. Any deficit that remains at the end of 6 months is likely to be permanent.

Embolic strokes develop the most rapidly and are fully developed within minutes. No warning symptoms precede an embolic stroke. Focal deficits such as motor aphasia, receptive aphasia or a sensorimotor paralysis may occur. The ultimate prognosis depends upon the correction of the underlying disease.

Cerebral hemorrhage due to hypertension occurs without warning and evolves over hours. It occurs more commonly and at a younger age in Blacks. The signs and symptoms depend on the site and size of the hemorrhage. Hemorrhage is most common in the putamen, where it causes hemiplegia, hemisensory loss and homonymous visual loss and aphasia when the lesion is on the dominant side. Severe headache and vomiting occur at the onset. Eighty-five percent of patients with cerebral hemorrhages due to hypertension do not survive the first eight hours.

Rupture of a saccular aneurysm may present with sudden unconsciousness with or without preceding excruciating headache. There are no lateralizing neurologic signs when the blood is confined to the subarachnoid space. The hemorrhage tends to recur if surgical correction is unsuccessful. Prognosis is poor if the patient is comatose; however, if the patient awakes, recovery is likely.

Headache

The three major types of headaches are migraine, cluster, and muscle contraction headaches. Migraine headaches may be subdivided into classic and common types. Muscle contraction headaches are the most common type.

Pathogenesis and Pathophysiology—Classic migraine headaches occur in three stages. The symptoms of each are described below and are related to an initial vasocontriction and subsequent vasodilatation of the blood vessels of the head. The initial vasoconstriction which is also called the prodrome is quickly followed by vasodilatation. The common migraine headache does not include a prodromal phase. A release of serotonin and histamine by mast cells is thought to play a role in migraine headaches. Females experience migraine headaches more often than males. Eighty percent of all migraine headaches are the common type. Several so-called trigger factors have been associated with migraine headaches. These include psychological factors (eg, stress), certain foods (eg, those containing tyramine), hormones (eg, oral contraceptives), and others. As the name implies, cluster headaches occur in closely-spaced groups. They are rare compared to migraine headaches, and their pathophysiology is unclear. Muscle contraction headaches, the most common type, are caused by contraction of muscles in the neck and head.

Signs and Symptoms—The first stage of classic migraine headaches consists chiefly of visual disturbances. These include blurred or cloudy vision, scotomas, and/or flashes of light Vertigo, chills, tremors, unilateral numbness, aphasia, photophobia or pallor may also occur. In the second stage, the patient experiences a severe, throbbing headache which initially is unilateral. Nausea, vomiting, diarrhea, chills, tremors and perspiration may also occur at this time. The third stage is a recovery phase. The pain decreases markedly but the head is tender and exhaustion is present. The common migraine headache includes no prodromal stage (stage I) but the actual headache may last longer (more than two hours) than with classic migraine. Cluster headaches are usually unilateral and nonthrobbing. The patient experiences excruciating pain lasting 20 to 90 minutes. Muscle contraction headaches may cause intermittant, recurrent or constant pain. Patients may describe scalp soreness with pain on combing their hair, bandlike pain or tightness and pressure.

Neuromuscular Disease

Guillain-Barre Syndrome

Etiology—The cause of most cases of Guillain-Barre Syndrome or acute idiopathic polyneuritis is unknown, although a number of cases were reported in association with the swine flu vaccination program of the 1970s.

Pathophysiology—Pathologic changes observed in patients who die of Guillain-Barre syndrome include perivascular lymphocytic infiltrates usually associated wth demyelination of the affected nerves. Infiltrates may also occur in the liver, spleen, lymph nodes and heart. Although the pathogenesis is unclear, the syndrome may involve a cell-mediated immunologic reaction directed at peripheral nerves.

Signs and Symptoms—The principal symptom is muscle weakness of both proximal and distal limbs. The weakness may advance to muscles of the trunk. While loss of sensation is unusual, paresthesias often occur. Affected patients are afebrile but sometimes have elevations of white blood cells in the cerebrospinal fluid along with increased protein. In severe cases the respiratory system may be affected, requiring respiratory assistance. Death is rare and complete recovery occurs in the majority of cases.

Myasthenia Gravis

Myasthenia gravis is a disease characterized by muscle fatigability and weakness most prominently affecting the muscles of the eye and cranium.

Incidence and Epidemiology—The incidence of myasthenia gravis is 1 in 20,000 in the general population. All age groups are affected with females predominating in the 20 to 40 year age group.

Etiology and Pathophysiology—While the underlying cause of myasthenia gravis remains a mystery, the physiologic defect has been clarified. Although it was thought for many years that this disorder resulted from impaired production of acetylcholine, it is now known that, there is instead of reduction in number and effectiveness of acetylcholine receptors at the neuromuscular junction. It is believed that this reduction is secondary to an autoimmune mechanism but the source of the immune stimulation remains to be identified. In experimental models, massive phagocytic infiltration of motor end plates with large areas of postsynaptic membrane destruction and associated decrease in acetylcholine receptors is observed. This process results in the denervation of muscle fibers.

Signs and Symptoms—The typical clinical presentation includes drooping eyelids, aphasia, and the inability to perform usually simple muscular functions. Early in the disease only a few muscles are affected in many patients. Neuromuscular fatigue is a cardinal sign when patients are unable to sustain or repeat muscular movements.

Electromyelography is a useful diagnostic technique, and shows a rapid decline in the amplitude of muscle action potentials with repetitive muscle contraction. Other tests used in diagnosis include the regional curare test and the use of anticholinesterase agents. Antibodies to acetylcholine receptors can be demonstrated in 90% of patients.

Multiple Sclerosis

A number of neurologic disorders are characterized by the degeneration of the myelin sheath of nerve fibers. Of these, only multiple sclerosis will be discussed. Other diseases falling into this classification include acute disseminated encephalomyelitis (postvaccinal and postinfectious encephalomyelitis) and acute necrotizing hemorrhagic encephalomyelitis.

Normal Physiology—Many of the nerve fibers of the body are covered with a layer of lipid material called myelin. This myeline sheath is interrupted at intervals by spaces termed nodes of Ranvier. Myelinated nerves are found in great number in cranial and spinal processes and in the white matter of the brain and spinal cord. The myelin sheath influences the rate of nerve impulse conduction with transmission being more rapid in myelinated nerve fibers.

Etiology and Epidemiology—The etiology of multiple sclerosis is unclear although several epidemiologic factors may offer some clues. This disease is rare between the equator and latitudes 30 to 35° north and south. It occurs more frequently with increasing latitude. Multiple sclerosis is more common in some families suggesting simultaneous exposure to some etiologic agent or perhaps a hereditary factor. These factors suggest to some an infectious etiology with a resultant autoimmune response.

Pathophysiology—The pathologic lesions vary in size and appearance but always include or reflect demylinization. While brain matter is not affected, involvement of the spinal cord and the optic nerves is frequent. The associated pathophysiologic change is a decrease in speed of nerve impulse conduction. Symptoms worsen with age, reflecting the ongoing nature of the disease.

Signs and Symptoms—While most patients present with evidence of spinal cord or brainstem involvement, about 40% present with only optic neuritis. The former presentation may include paresthesias, numbness, or weakness in an asymmetrical distribution. Diplopia, nystagmus, and cerebellar ataxia may also occur. The latter presentation may include partial or complete blindness in one or both eyes, scotomas or pain with eye movement. This disease progresses with time with interspersed exacerbations and may eventually result in quadraplegia and coma. The usual patient survives 20 or more years from the time of the initial diagnosis.

Dementia

Dementia is a generic term referring to a syndrome of decreasing memory and intellectual function. The clinical course of the disorder is extremely variable and the causes are probably multiple.

Pathophysiology—Many types of dementia involve structural disease of the cerebrum and diencephalon. A degeneration and loss of nerve cells with secondary changes in the cerebral white matter are often observed. These changes may occur in one or many parts of the brain. While the underlying etiology is often undetectable, dementia with its various lesions may be due to identifiable disorders such as chronic hydrocephalus, syphilis, and certain virus infections.

Signs and Symptoms—The initial presentation of dementia is quite variable. Symptoms include irritability, lack of interest, distractibility, unclear thinking, loss of memory, and wide mood swings. As the disorder progresses, incontinence, aphasia and speech disorders often develop. Eventually, the patient becomes unable to care for himself and apparently has no interest in doing so. The course of dementia is variable with progression occurring over months or years. It should be stressed that dementia may be due to a wide variety of disorders, many of which are treatable. Therefore, a detailed diagnostic effort is warranted.

Dermatology

Normal Anatomy and Physiology

The skin is the largest organ in the body. The functions of the skin include sensation, temperature control, prevention of water loss or penetration, synthesis of vitamin D and protection from organisms and irritants. The skin is composed of three layers: the epidermis, the dermis and the hypodermis or subcutaneous tissue. The outer layer of the epidermis is the stratum corneum or horny layer. The cells of the stratum corneum are fully keratinized and are without nuclei or granules. In the process of keratinization the cells from the basal layer migrate upward, flatten, lose water and fill with keratin. This process normally requires 28 days from formation of a daughter cell (through mitotic division of a cell in the basal layer of the epidermis) until that cell is shed at the surface of the stratum corneum. The cells of the stratum corneum are normally shed invisibly as scales.

The dermis is composed of connective tissue in which are found blood vessels, lymphatics, nerves, arrectores pilorum muscles, fibroblasts, mast cells and dermal appendages—hair follicles, sebaceous glands and sweat glands. The elastin and collagen embedded in mucopolysaccharide give the skin its elasticity. Blood vessels in the papillae of the dermis bring nutrients to the avascular epidermis. Sebaceous glands are attached to hair follicles and produce sebum which lubricates the skin and may help prevent water loss. Sebum also has some antiseptic and antifungal properties. Hairs are specialized keratinous structures. Nails are a modified type of keratin.

The subcutaneous tissues are composed of connective tissue and fat.

Certain microorganisms may be found on the skin as normal flora. Other microorganisms may transiently colonize the skin.

Acne Vulgaris

Acne vulgaris is a common disease which primarily affects teenagers and which has as the characteristic lesions the open comedo (blackhead) and closed comedo. The majority of patients have only mild acne and never consult a physician although they may spend large sums of money on over-the-counter acne aids. In severe forms acne may lead to extensive scarring. Even the milder forms cause considerable psychological distress for the patients.

Epidemiology and Etiology—Almost everyone has some acne during the adolescent years. Acne may continue in some people until 30 to 40 years of age or appear postmenopausally in women. Administration of certain drugs, such as corticosteroids, halogens, androgens, lithium, and anticonvulsants, may result in acne. Acne may also be associated with certain occupations in which tars, oil, and chlorinated hydrocarbons come in contact with the skin. The application of certain cosmetics including moisturizers has been associated with acne.

The etiology of acne is multifactorial. Heredity plays a role. Androgenic stimulation of sebum production by the sebaceous glands at puberty is the main event in the production of acne. Bacteria present on the surface of the skin are also involved in the etiology of acne. These include *Proprionibacterium acnes*. There is no scientific evidence that diet commonly plays a role in the development of acne so restrictive diets are usually unnecessary. Anxiety, fatigue, heat and humidity probably do aggravate acne.

Pathology—The characteristic lesions in acne are the open comedo and closed comedo which are due to sebaceous glands that have become plugged with sebum and keratin debris. The black color is the result of oxidation of pigment granules in shed cells in the plug. When the epidermis covers the opening of the sebaceous gland so that oxidation cannot occur, the lesion is known as a whitehead. Comedones are not inflamed. When they become inflamed the other lesions of acne are formed; papules, pustules, and nodular-cystic lesions. Acne most commonly occurs on the oily areas of the skin, primarily the face, ears, neck and upper trunk. Healed acne may result in atropic, pitted, or hypertrophic scars.

Pathophysiology—Androgens cause sebaceous glands to mature and to produce large quantities of sebum. Both males and females produce androgens. The sebaceous glands respond to very low levels of androgens. Obstruction of flow of sebum from the sebaceous gland to the surface of the skin results in a comedo. Increased amounts of sebum, increased viscosity of sebum, and keratin debris contribute to the obstruction. Chronic obstruction of the sebaceous gland leads to follicular dilatation (enlarged pores). Sebum is composed of triglycerides, waxes, cholesterol, squalene and minute amounts of free fatty acids. Normally sebum is not inflammatory. However, bacterial flora in the follicle hydrolyze the triglycerides to free fatty acids, which are extremely irritating and initiate the inflammatory process. In addition, *P acnes* releases chemotactic factors which enhance the inflammatory process. The inflamed follicle may rupture and spread the process to the adjacent dermis, causing increased inflammation via a foreign body reaction.

Signs and Symptoms—The comedones and other lesions, including scars, are the physical abnormalities of acne. The course is usually chronic throughout adolescence until hormonal balance is achieved, usually in the early 20s. Occasional flares are common during the course. The objective of treatment is to clear the lesions, prevent scarring, and minimize psychological distress.

Psoriasis

Psoriasis is a chronic disease characterized by epidermal hyperplasia and a greatly accelerated rate of epidermal turnover. The lesions are characteristically red, slightly raised and scaly. Although psoriasis is usually a minor disorder, generalized forms and systemic manifestations also occur.

Epidemiology—Approximately 1 to 3% of individuals in the US have some form of psoriasis. A higher incidence occurs in Northern European countries, while the disease does not appear in some races. Males and females are equally affected. Peak incidence occurs in early and middle adulthood but psoriasis may occur at any time during life.

Etiology—The etiology of psoriasis is unknown. Heredity is thought to play a role in transmission being autosomal dominant with incomplete penetrance or multifactorial. Frequently, the first lesions of psoriasis are associated with previous injury to the site, which is known as the Koebner phenomenon. Environmental factors such as decreased humidity may aggravate psoriasis.

Pathology—The histopathological changes of psoriasis include parakeratosis (retention of nuclei in cells in the keratin layer) layered with neutrophiles, hyperkeratosis (increased thickness of the keratin layer), hypogranulosis (loss of the granular layer), elongation of the epidermal rete ridges, pustules with surrounding intercellular edema (spongiform pustules), and papillomatosis (increased height of the dermal papillary pegs) with thinning of the suprapapillary epidermis. There is an inflammatory infiltrate in the upper dermis and proliferation of small blood vessels in the papillae (vascular ectasia). Mitotic figures are seen in the bottom three cell layers of the epidermis rather than just in the basal layer.

Pathophysiology—The characteristic change is the markedly shortened rate of turnover of the epidermal cells. Instead of the normal 28 days from cell division in the basal layers until the cell is shed from the stratum corneum, in psoriasis it takes only 3 to 4 days for this to occur. The mechanism for this and the other signs and symptoms of psoriasis is not understood at this time.

Signs and Symptoms—The lesions of psoriasis are discrete or confluent erythematous plaques and papules covered with white or silvery scales. The lesions are characteristically found on the extensor surfaces such as the elbows and knees and the back and scalp. However, any area of skin can be involved. Nails are commonly involved with pitting and ridging while mucous membranes are rarely involved. The lesions may be localized or generalized and are usually asymptomatic but may cause discomfort usually from burning and itching. Auspitz sign is characteristic (punctate bleeding that occurs when psoriatic scales are removed). The onset of psoriasis is usually insidious although it may be explosive. The clinical course of psoriasis is chronic and recurring with periods of remission. Spontaneous cures rarely occur. Most cases of psoriasis are only cosmetically disfiguring. Some forms such as psoriatic erythroderma and pustular psoriasis may be life-threatening. Although pustular psoriasis looks like an infection, the lesions are sterile. A form of arthritis that closely resembles rheumatoid arthritis but affects the distal joints is associated with psoriasis in some cases. There are no characteristic laboratory abnormalities of psoriasis.

Allergic Skin Diseases

Allergic skin diseases may be caused by a variety of antigens and may be manifested in a variety of ways. These reactions may be classified according to time from exposure to onset in the sensitized individual. Immediate reactions occur within 1 to 60 minutes of exposure to the antigen and are manifested by generalized pruritus and urticaria. IgE is the mediator of immediate reactions. These reactions are the most dangerous as they may be associated with laryngeal edema and/or anaphylaxis. Accelerated reactions occur within 1 to 72 hours of contact with the antigen and are also manifested by generalized urticaria and pruritus. An exanthematic eruption is rarely seen with this type of reaction. A late reaction may occur from 3 to 21 days after exposure to the antigen and may be manifested by urticaria. The urticaria in this case may subside even though the exposure to the antigen is not terminated because of the development of IgG and IgA blocking antibodies. The most common form of the late reaction is the exanthematic eruption. The eruption may not begin until the exposure to the antigen is discontinued and may last from 2 weeks to 4 months. As the exanthem fades, there is usually scaling. Late reactions are mediated by IgM. Chronic reactions continue longer than 6 weeks. Usually the antigen cannot be identified in chronic reactions.

Urticaria or hives is a skin reaction characterized by wheal formation and is a member of the atopy complex which indicates a hereditary allergic background.

Epidemiology and Etiology—Approximately 15 to 20% of the population will experience at least one episode of urticaria. Young adults are most frequently afflicted by the acute form. The chronic form, lasting longer than 6 weeks, is usually seen in patients over 35 years old. Individuals with urticaria or their family members are likely to be allergic to a number of antigens and to also suffer from seasonal rhinitis, asthma and atopic dermatitis. In the acute form the antigen can usually be identified but no mechanism is known for 70% of the chronic cases of urticaria. Urticaria is also seen in association with parasitic infections, systemic lupus erythematosus, bacterial infections and occult malignancy. Exposure to physical agents such as cold, heat, UV light or mechanical pressure may precipitate urticaria in some individuals.

Pathophysiology—Urticaria may develop as a result of several different processes although all involve liberation of histamine from mast cells in the dermis. Systemic exposure to an antigen may result in formation of IgE antibodies toward that antigen. The antibodies are fixed to mast cells in the dermis and lungs and to circulating basophils. The interaction of antigen and antibody results in liberation of histamine and other mediators (prostaglandin E and kinins). These substances cause arteriolar dilatation and increased capillary permeability in the skin. Histamine is quickly degraded in tissues so urticaria seldom lasts for more than 48 hours. A degranulated mast cell is refractory to further stimulation until histamine granules reform.

Other antibodies may be involved in the liberation of histamine and mediator substances from mast cells. IgG and IgM may be formed against antigens. These antibodies, when they interact with antigens, may activate the complement cascade which results in histamine release. Cold and solar urticaria are mediated by antibodies (IgE) that are only active at decreased temperature or upon exposure to light.

Histamine may be released from mast cells by nonimmunologic mechanisms. Certain chemicals stimulate mast cells directly to liberate histamine. These chemicals include drugs such as morphine, codeine, and dextrans, crayfish toxin, and snake venom. Direct physical pressure may cause release of histamine from mast cells.

Signs and Symptoms—The lesions are well circumscribed discrete wheals with erythematous raised serpiginous borders and blanched centers. The lesions, which involve only the superficial layer of the skin, may be scattered, localized or may coalesce. The patient will complain of intense pruritus or burning. Urticaria alone is seldom life-threatening but it may indicate a future anaphylactic reaction. Skin testing is usually of little value in these individuals in that they are allergic to numerous antigens. The acute form usually lasts less than 6 weeks. The chronic form may last for years but does not last forever.

Atopic Dermatitis (Eczema)—Eczema is a skin disease which is also a member of the atopy complex. Atopic dermatitis is characterized by itching. The appearance and distribution of the lesions depends on the age of onset.

Etiology—The etiology of atopic dermatitis is unknown. Seventy percent of the patients with atopic dermatitis have a family history of atopy and 50% also have either hayfever or asthma. Atopic dermatitis can occur at all ages and usually remits when the patient is in the mid 20s. Irritants, excessive bathing, wide temperature variation, low humidity and nervous tension may aggravate atopic dermatitis.

Pathology—Pathologic changes in atopic dermatitis are those of nonspecific dermatitis. Epidermal vesicles due to intercellular edema, parakeratosis, acanthosis and an inflammatory infiltrate of the epidermis and dermis are seen in acute atopic dermatitis. In the chronic form, hyperkeratosis, parakeratosis, acanthosis and a lymphocytic infiltrate of the thickened upper dermis are seen.

Pathophysiology—The mechanisms for the development of atopic dermatitis are not understood. Various immunologic theories have been postulated to explain the development of atopic dermatitis but no one theory explains all cases. Some patients with atopic dermatitis have elevated levels of IgE and perhaps elevated levels of IgG and IgM. Atopic dermatitis also occurs commonly in immune deficient individuals and may be due to an impairment of delayed hypersensitivity or impaired phagocytosis. Depressed IgA has also been reported in atopic patients.

Signs and Symptoms—Infant type atopic dermatitis (infantile eczema) begins during the first few months of life, perhaps as a reaction to food, although this is controversial. The eruption is generalized, acutely inflamed, vesicular, and spreads rapidly. The scalp, face, trunk, extremities and diaper area are involved. There is considerable oozing and crusting associated with the lesions along with intense pruritus. The skin may become secondarily infected. The child usually outgrows the disease spontaneously at 2 to 3 years of age.

The childhood type of atopic dermatitis may be a recurrence of infant type or may be the first appearance of the disease. In contrast to the vesicles and oozing of the infant type, these lesions are dried, lichenified plaques and patches. The lesions are also more localized in the childhood type and are found on the flexor surfaces and the face, neck, feet, genitalia and scalp. Again there is intense pruritus. The disease may clear or persist into adulthood.

In the adult type of atopic dermatitis, the lesions consist of chronic lichenified patches which are intensely pruritic and may be hyperpigmented. Commonly flexures and the creases of the neck and eyelids are involved as well as the same areas as in the childhood type. The clinical course of atopic dermatitis is chronic and is characterized by spontaneous exacerbations and remissions. Eventually the disease fades.

Allergic Contact Dermatitis—An extremely common skin disease caused by direct contact with the substance and the development of delayed hypersensitivity. Primary irritant contact dermatitis is caused by contact with noxious agents such as acids or corrosives. The inflammatory skin reaction that results from such a contact occurs in all individuals exposed to these agents and does not involve the development of hypersensitivity.

Epidemiology—Many patients with dermatological problems have allergic contact dermatitis. This disease affects any age group and is equally common in both sexes.

Etiology—Substances capable of forming a stable bond with cutaneous proteins and being transported to a lymph node are allergens for contact dermatitis. These include Rhus (poison ivy and poison oak), ragweed, fruits and vegetables, solvents, low molecular weight polymers, metals, particularly nickel, household detergents and cleaning agents and waxes.

Pathology—The changes of a spongiotic (intercellular edema) dermatitis are seen.

Pathophysiology—The chemical group binds to skin protein and is transported to the lymph nodes. Cellular proliferation occurs in the paracortical area of the lymph nodes. Small lymphocytes become sensitized to the antigen within 7 to 10 days of the first exposure. The sensitized lymphocytes react with the antigen and release soluble chemotactic factors which attract other lymphocytes and macrophages into the area. Also, the sensitized lymphocytes release migratory inhibitory factors which inhibit the movement of macrophages and other cells away from the area. Lysosomal enzymes released from the macrophages result in skin destruction. On subsequent exposures, reaction will occur within 24 to 48 hours of exposure.

Signs and Symptoms—The distribution of the lesions in contact dermatitis is characteristic: the rash occurs where the allergen came in contact with the skin. The scalp is rarely involved. The lesions begin as intense, relatively well-limited areas of erythema that are soon associated with edema. Papules and vesicles form, with subsequent oozing and weeping. Sometimes the lesions are bullous. The erythema lessens and is replaced with crusting and scaling. Pruritus in varying degrees of severity is always present. If contact with the allergen is eliminated, healing occurs in 1 to 3 weeks. With chronic exposure, a chronic contact dermatitis may develop with thickening, fissuring, scaling, and hyperpigmentation of the area. Vesiculation is minimal in the chronic form. Intense itching and burning may result in excoriation and secondary infection. The disease will recur if there is another contact with the allergen or the acute form may persist. Diagnosis may be made via patch testing, although the patient may react to a variety of allergens including some which s/he is not allergic to.

Photoallergic Reactions—Uncommon delayed hypersensitivity reactions that require three factors: light, skin, and an allergen. Distribution is limited to the areas exposed to light. Photoallergic reactions must be distinguished from the more common phototoxic reaction, which occurs when a photosensitizing substance ingested or applied externally, plus minimal exposure to sunlight or artificial lighting, results in an exaggerated sunburn in 6 to 18 hours. No immunologic mechanisms are involved in phototoxic reactions which can occur with the first exposure to the substance. Pigment is protective in the phototoxic reaction and tanning results as the reaction subsides.

Epidemiology and Etiology—Photoallergic reactions are rare but occur predominantly in males (7:1) and in the age group of 40 to 60 years old. Pigment and dark skin are not protective for this reaction. Numerous drugs, chemicals and cosmetics can cause both phototoxic and photoallergic reactions.

Pathophysiology—The energy of light depends on the wavelength in the electromagnetic spectrum. A molecule when exposed to light may dissipate the absorbed energy as heat or may undergo one of numerous photochemical reactions including chemical bond formation. The chemical and the cutaneous protein are the antigen for the development of delayed hypersensitivity.

Signs and Symptoms—A photoallergic reaction occurs as an urticarial or eczematous eruption in the areas of sun exposure. The initial eruption will not be seen until 7 to 10 days after the first exposure but occurs within 24 to 48 hours on subsequent exposures. No tanning occurs as the reaction subsides. The reaction may recur with each reexposure. Diagnosis may be made by photo-patch testing.

Adverse Reactions to Drugs as Manifested by the Skin

Adverse reactions to drugs as manifested by the skin are among the most common adverse reactions to drugs. The significance of these reactions varies from minor to life-threatening. Nonallergic drug reactions of the skin include alopecia, purpura, secondary infections, and phototoxic reactions. Allergic reactions include urticaria, the rash seen with serum sickness, allergic contact dermatitis, and photoallergic reactions as already discussed. In addition, several less common but potentially more serious reactions may occur.

Exfoliative Dermatitis (Erythroderma Syndrome)—A potentially fatal complication that may occur as a result of an extension of another dermatitis.

Etiology—Exfoliative dermatitis is seen with generalized spreading of a drug reaction, psoriasis, contact dermatitis, seborrheic dermatitis, atopic dermatitis and in association with leukemia or lymphoma.

Pathophysiology—The pathophysiology is entirely unknown.

Signs and Symptoms—There is a generalized erythematous eruption with scaling involving all the skin surface. In extensive exfoliative dermatitis the metabolic demand is such that the patient develops negative nitrogen balance, edema, hypoalbuminemia and loses muscle mass. Serious water and electrolyte imbalance can result from the greatly increased loss of water through the skin. The course is determined by the cause and complications. The erythroderma syndrome in patients with malignancy persists. If psoriasis, atopic dermatitis, or other skin diseases cause the exfoliative dermatitis, improvement occurs over 8 to 10 months. Prognosis is better if the etiologic factor can be removed. Approximately 30% of patients with exfoliative dermatitis die.

Erythema Multiforme—A characteristic skin reaction that occurs as a result of a systemic allergic reaction to various agents. The syndrome may include only a few typical skin lesions or become a severe toxic illness known as Stevens-Johnson syndrome.

Etiology—Infectious agents including herpes virus and *Mycoplasma pneumoniae*, drugs including penicillin, aspirin, anticonvulsants and sulfonamides, and malignancy may cause erythema multiforme.

Pathology—Histopathologically, the changes seen are those of a spongiotic dermatitis with epidermal necrosis, ballooning, and vacuolar alteration. An associated superficial perivasculitis and interface lymphohistiocytic infiltrate is present.

Pathophysiology—Erythema multiforme is probably antigen-antibody mediated.

Signs and Symptoms—The lesions of erythema multiforme may be papules, macules, urticarial, vesicles or bullae. The type of lesion may change as the disease progresses. The lesions are symmetrical in distribution and are most commonly found on extensor surfaces, the backs and palms of hands, and the tops and soles of feet. Both mucous membranes and skin are involved in the severe form. The lesions begin as a bright redness that extends peripherally as the center pales, becomes indurated, and may contain the bullae. The lesions are called target lesions because of their appearance, are characteristic of erythema multiforme but do not always occur in the disease. In Stevens-Johnson syndrome the skin, conjunctiva, and mucous membranes are involved. This reaction includes toxemia, prostration, high fever, cough, and inflammation of the lungs. The disease usually resolves within a few weeks after the inciting agent is removed although the severe form may be fatal.

Skin Infections

Impetigo—A common superficial bacterial infection of the skin that may arise from normal skin or as a secondary infection of dermatitis, intertrigo, infestations, other infections or trauma.

Etiology and Epidemiology—The causative organisms are beta-hemolytic streptococci and coagulase-positive staphylococci. In secondary forms, gram-negative organisms may also be found. Impetigo may occur at any age but is most common in children. The lesions may be autoinoculable and are somewhat contagious.

Signs and Symptoms—Impetigo begins as a macule that progresses to a vesicle covering about 2 to 3 cm^2 in area. The vesicle, which is located just below the stratum corneum, becomes a pustule filled with polymorphonuclear leukocytes. The pustule ruptures and may spread the bacteria to the adjacent skin. The lesion is now denuded and seeps. The seropurulent fluid quickly dries, forming the characteristic friable honey-colored crust of impetigo.

Mycotic Infections

Dermatophytoses (also known as ringworm) are mycotic infections of the skin that involve the epidermis, nails and hair. The diseases differ as to causative organism, area affected, mode of transmission, and response to therapy.

Tinea capitis usually occurs in prepuberal children and may occur in epidemics in schools or institutions. The lesions are found on the scalp and appear as scaly, crusted patches with the hair broken off close to the scalp. Inflammation and deeper lesions may occur and may result in scarring alopecia. The fungus is of the *microsporum* species.

Tinea corporis is classic ringworm. The lesions occur anywhere on the glabrous skin of the body. A papule begins and spreads centrifugally as a scaly red rim with central clearing. The border of the lesions may contain vesicles. The causative organisms are of the *microsporum* and *trichophyton* species.

Tinea cruris is more commonly known as "jock itch." The lesions begin as a scaly red eruption of the groin and inner thighs which is symmetrical. Chronic lesions are more brown in color. The lesions have specific margins and the margins are more inflamed than the center. Severe pruritus accompanies the eruption. The fungus belongs to either *epidermophyton* or *trichophyton* species. Heat and humidity are aggravating factors for the development of *Tinea cruris*. This condition must be distinguished from a similar eruption that is caused by another fungus, *Candida albicans*.

Tinea pedis or athlete's foot is perhaps the most common of the dermatophytoses. Darkness, heat and humidity predispose an individual to the development of this infection. *Trichophyton mentagrophytes* cause an inflammatory eruption with vesicles and weeping. *Trichophyton rubrum* causes a dry scaly eruption.

Tinea unguium is a fungal infection of the nails, most commonly the toe nails. The nails become yellow in color, brittle, thickened and raised by the underlying debris. Infections of the nails are difficult to eradicate.

Endocrine

Endocrine glands are organs that secrete substances known as hormones directly into the blood. The major endocrine glands are the anterior pituitary, posterior pituitary, thyroid, adrenals, parathyroids, and ovaries or testes. The anterior pituitary gland controls the function of the other glands with the exception of the parathyroids and posterior pituitary. The pituitary is controlled by the hypothalamus and the central nervous system. Hormones regulate metabolism. Endocrine disorders arise when there is an excess or a deficiency of a hormone(s). The majority of patients with endocrine dysfunction can be successfully treated.

The Hypothalamus

The hypothalamus is responsible for the integration of the central nervous system and the endocrine system and is particularly related to the physiologic response to stress.

Normal Physiology—The hypothalamus controls the pituitary gland. Neurosecretory cells in the hypothalamus synthesize and release small molecular-weight peptides into the pituitary portal veins. These are called releasing/inhibiting hormones because they stimulate or inhibit the release of a corresponding trophic hormone by the anterior pituitary gland. Thyrotropin-releasing hormone (TRH), lutenizing hormone-releasing hormone (LHRH), and gonadotropin-releasing hormone (GNRH) have been identified and characterized. Corticotropin-releasing factor (CRF), growth-hormone-releasing factor (GRF) and prolactin-releasing hormone are thought to exist but they have not been characterized. TRH also stimulates the release of prolactin and a prolactin-inhibiting factor (PIF) which may be dopamine inhibits the release of prolactin. Somatostatin is growth-hormone release-inhibiting hormone which also has other physiologic effects such as depressing pancreatic glucagon and insulin secretion.

Antidiuretic hormone (ADH), also known as vasopressin, is secreted by the hypothalamus and stored in the posterior pituitary. It is released when the baroreceptors in the aorta and carotids sense a decreased blood pressure, the volume receptors in the left atrium sense a decreased volume, or the osmoreceptors in the supraoptic nucleus sense an increased serum osmolarity. The other posterior pituitary hormone, oxytocin, stimulates contraction of the uterus during childbirth and the ejection of milk from the breast.

The secretory cells of the anterior pituitary and other endocrine glands are responsive to the feedback effects of circulating hormone levels. High hormone levels inhibit the releasing mechanism and low hormone levels stimulate the releasing process. Autonomy is a state in which feedback control of the gland is lost and the hormone is secreted in excess regardless of the hormone level. Hormone secretion normally follows a diurnal pattern over 24 hours, being highest in the morning.

Destruction of the hypothalamus would lead to a deficiency of the releasing/inhibiting hormones. A clinical picture resembling panhypopituitarism would result but prolactin levels would be increased resulting in galactorrhea.

Anterior Pituitary Disorders

The pituitary gland is located at the base of the brain in the sella turcica. The anterior lobe contains agranular, chromophobic, eosinophilic and basophilic cells.

Normal Physiology—The anterior pituitary gland secretes trophic hormones in response to stimulation by releasing hormones from the hypothalamus. These anterior pituitary hormones include adrenocorticotropin (ACTH), thyroid-stimulating hormone (TSH), and gonadotropins, follicle-stimulating hormone (FSH) and luteinizing hormone (LH). The anterior pituitary also secretes growth hormone (GH) and prolactin. Melanocyte-stimulating hormone (MSH) does not exist in humans.

Adrenocorticotropin regulates the production of cortisol, aldosterone and sex hormones by the adrenal glands. ACTH, however, is not the major regulator of aldosterone production and functions in this regard for only short periods of stress.

Thyrotropin stimulates the uptake of iodine by the thyroid gland and the synthesis and release of thyroid hormones.

Gonadotropins are two hormones produced in both the male and female but with different functions in each sex. FSH stimulates the growth of graafian follicle and the production of estrogen in the female and promotes spermatogenesis in the male. LH stimulates ovulation and luteinization of the mature follicle in the female and androgen production in the male. The normal cyclic pattern of estrogen and progesterone production and inhibition via feedback mechanisms is responsible for the menstrual period.

Growth hormone has no single target gland but affects physiologic processes in general. The main function of growth hormone is to promote the growth before puberty. Metabolic functions of growth hormone include anabolism, decreased lipid synthesis and antagonism of the effects of insulin. Growth hormone is released in response to hypoglycemia and stimulates gluconeogenesis in the liver while inhibiting the uptake of glucose by peripheral tissue. Removal of growth hormone after puberty causes no known clinical problems.

Prolactin stimulates the secretion of milk from the breast after delivery. The functions of prolactin at other times in the female and in the male are unknown.

Pathophysiology—Tumors develop in the anterior pituitary which cause increased production of TSH, ACTH, GH and prolactin. Only a few tumors that produce increased amounts of gonadotropins have been identified. A tumor that secretes excess TSH is a rare cause of hyperthyroidism. A basophilic tumor may secrete excess ACTH and result in Cushing's disease (vide infra). Growth hormone secreting tumors cause gigantism or acromegaly. If the tumor occurs before puberty and closure of the epiphyseal plate, gigantism with generalized overgrowth of the skeleton and soft tissue occurs. After puberty, a GH secreting tumor causes acromegaly which is characterized by overgrowth of bone and cartilage in the distal parts of the body such as the face, head, hands and feet. Acromegaly is also associated with early osteoarthritis, psychological disturbances, glucose intolerance and hypertension. Prolactin secreting tumors usually are chromophobe adenomas and cause galactorrhea and amenorrhea.

The anterior pituitary may be destroyed by a nonsecreting tumor, usually a chromophobe adenoma. Sheehan's syndrome is destruction of the pituitary due to hypotension during delivery. The clinical manifestations of panhypopituitarism depends on whether the destruction occurs pre or post puberty. Prepuberal destruction results in stunted growth and lack of sexual development. Postpuberal destruction results in gonadal, thyroid and adrenal insufficiency.

Signs and Symptoms—Pituitary tumors cause headaches, loss of temporal visual fields, bilateral hemianopsia, loss of visual acuity and blindness. The other signs and symptoms relate to the excess of lack of hormone(s).

Posterior Pituitary Disorders

The posterior pituitary secretes ADH and oxytocin.

Normal Physiology—ADH secretion is regulated by reflexes reaching the hypothalamus via the vagus nerve. ADH is a vasoconstrictor and conserves total body water. The action of ADH on the kidney is to promote the reabsorption of water in the collecting tubules and thus to concentrate urine. ADH maintains serum osmolarity within a very narrow range despite wide variations in fluid and salt intake. ADH release may be also controlled by the autonomic nervous system.

Diabetes Insipidus—A disorder due to decreased production of ADH. Tumors may compress the posterior pituitary or it may be removed surgically. Nephrogenic diabetes insipidus occurs when the kidney tubules are not responsive to the action of ADH.

Signs and Symptoms—The hallmark of diabetes insipidus is polyuria with excessive thirst and polydipsia. In severe forms the urine volume is 16 to 24 liters per day. Micturition may be required every half hour, day and night. Urine osmolarity is low and urine specific gravity is less than 1.005. If intake does not equal output, the patient may become severely dehydrated.

Syndrome of Inappropriate ADH Secretion—Caused by continual release of ADH regardless of plasma osmolarity. Diseases of the lung including TB and oat-cell carcinoma, CNS trauma or disease and drugs such as chlorpropamide, vincristine, carbamazepine, etc., cause inappropriate ADH release.

Signs and Symptoms—Ingested fluids are retained so volume expansion and dilutional hyponatremia occur. The patient complains of weight gain, weakness, lethargy, and mental confusion. The serum sodium is low, as is plasma osmolarity and the urine is concentrated.

Thyroid Disorders

The thyroid gland, which is located in the anterior neck, secretes thyroid hormones which control a number of metabolic processes.

Normal Physiology—TRH from the hypothalamus stimulates the anterior pituitary to secrete TSH. TSH regulates thyroid hormone synthesis and secretion. The thyroid gland actively takes up iodine so that iodine is 500 times more concentrated in the gland than the rest of the body. Iodide peroxidase oxidizes the iodine. Organic iodination forms monoiodotyrosine and diiodotyrosine. Coupling of these two molecules results in triiodothyronine (T3) or thyroxine (T4). The hormones are stored in the gland bound to thyroglobulin and are released following proteolysis. Both T3 and T4 enter the cells but T3 is three times more potent than T4 in stimulating metabolic processes. About 30 percent of T4 is converted to T3 in the blood. Both T3 and T4 circulate in the blood bound to plasma proteins such as thyroxine-binding globulin (TBG), T4 binding prealbumin and albumin. Disorders that affect serum proteins can affect the amount of bound T3 or T4 but not the metabolic status of the patient.

Actions of thyroid hormone include maintenance of body temperature and weight, control of skin texture, stimulation of protein catabolism, stimulation of myocardial contractility, increased metabolism of cholesterol and proper functioning of the central nervous system. At the tissue level the actions of thyroid hormone are synergistic with those of epinephrine.

Hypothyroidism—A state of deficient thyroid hormone production. Cretinism is hypothyroidism which begins at birth and results in developmental abnormalities and severe mental retardation. Myxedema is severe hypothyroidism with the accumulation of hydrophilic mucopolysaccharides in the dermis.

Etiology—Various mechanisms may cause hypothyroidism. An inherited defect in thyroid synthesis may occur. The diet may be deficient in iodine. The pituitary may no longer produce TSH, as well as other hormones such as ACTH and gonadotropins. Antibodies against the thyroid gland may destroy it. The treatment of hyperthyroidism by either surgery or radioactive iodide usually results in hypothyroidism.

Signs and Symptoms—The cretin is constipated and somnolent and has a hoarse cry and feeding problems. The child does not develop normally. Physical abnormalities include short stature, coarse features, protruding tongue, broad flat nose, widely set eyes, a protuberant abdomen and an umbilical hernia. The child is mentally retarded.

Hypothyroidism in adults is insidious in onset. Complaints include cold intolerance, lethargy, constipation, menorrhagia, slowing of intellectual and motor activity, a modest weight gain, dry hair that falls out, dry skin, stiff aching muscles and a deep hoarse voice. Patients with myxedema have a dull expressionless face, sparse hair, periorbital puffiness, a large tongue, and pale, cool, rough, doughy skin. Coma is a poor prognostic sign.

Physical examination of patients with hypothyroidism is remarkable for the skin changes, bradycardia and prolonged relaxation phase of deep tendon reflexes. Goiter is caused by hyperplasia of the thyroid gland due to excessive stimulation by TSH in conditions where there is a defect in thyroid hormone synthesis. In primary hypothyroidism the serum concentrations of T3 and T4 are reduced and TSH level is increased. In secondary hypothyroidism serum T3, T4, and TSH are reduced.

Hyperthyroidism—A state of excess thyroid hormone production. A goiter may become autonomous and toxic after many years. A single adenoma of the thyroid whose function is independent of TSH may occur. Very rarely carcinoma of the thyroid may cause hyperthyroidism.

Graves' Disease is hyperthyroidism with diffuse goiter, ophthalmopathy and dermopathy. All three features are not necessary for the diagnosis, and the course of each may be independent.

Etiology and Epidemiology—The etiology of Graves' disease is unknown but there is a familial predisposition. The disease has a female: male ratio 7:1 and usually occurs in the third or fourth decade of life.

Pathophysiology—The mechanism of the development of Graves' disease is unknown. Long-acting thyroid stimulator (LATS) is an IgG immunoglobulin found in about 50% of patients with Graves' disease. The antigen that stimulates production of LATS has not yet been identified.

Pathology—The thyroid gland shows diffuse hyperplasia and hypertrophy with lymphocytic infiltration. The orbit and orbital muscles have an inflammatory infiltrate of lymphocytes and plasma cells. The dermis is thickened and infiltrated by lymphocytes and hydrophilic mucopolysaccharides over the tibia.

Signs and Symptoms—The patient with Graves' disease may complain of a goiter, a fine tremor particularly when the fingers are spread, increased nervousness, emotional instability, increased sweating, heat intolerance, weight loss, palpitations, loss of strength, weakness, increased appetite, hyperdefecation, nausea, vomiting, dyspnea, and amenorrhea. Physical examination reveals wasting of muscles, sinus tachycardia, atrial arrhythmias and perhaps congestive heart failure. The skin is warm, moist, and velvety and the hair fine and silky. The goiter is usually diffuse and a bruit may be heard over the gland.

The patient may also complain of decreased lacrimation, eye redness, and a sensation of sand in the eyes. The ocular signs include the characteristic stare and frightened facies, infrequent blinking, lid lag, failure of convergence and failure to wrinkle the brow on upward gaze. Varying degrees of ophthalmoplegia occurs as does proptosis. Corneal ulceration may occur as a complication. The exophthalmos is usually bilateral.

Adrenal Disorders

The adrenal glands produce three principal hormones. Disorders may involve an excess or a deficiency of any one or a combination of the hormones. The disorders may be primary, in the adrenal gland, or secondary, due to a problem outside the adrenal gland.

Normal Physiology—The adrenal glands synthesize glucocorticoids, mineralocorticoids, and adrenal androgens from cholesterol. The principal glucocorticoid is cortisol, which is secreted in a diurnal cycle. Aldosterone is the principal mineralocorticoid. Dehydroepiandrosterone, which is metabolized to testosterone, is the principal adrenal androgen.

The hypothalamus and anterior pituitary gland control the adrenal gland by CRF and ACTH respectively. The secretion of CRF and ACTH is controlled by the plasma level of free cortisol, stress and the sleep-wake cycle. The peak ACTH level occurs just before arising and the trough occurs just before retiring. The cycle of ACTH secretion conforms to the sleep-wake cycle. Stress increases ACTH release. Within minutes of ACTH release, glucocorticoid concentration in the blood rises. ACTH is only a minor stimulus for aldosterone secretion. The renin-angiotensin system is the most potent stimulus for aldosterone production.

Glucocorticoids regulate the metabolism of carbohydrates, proteins, lipids and nucleic acids. Glucocorticoids increase protein breakdown and nitrogen excretion. They mobilize amino acids from proteins in peripheral

supporting structures such as bone, skin, muscle and connective tissue and decrease protein synthesis in these areas. Glucagon is secreted in response to the increased serum amino acid level and stimulates gluconeogenesis. Glucocorticoids increase hepatic glycogen content and decrease the peripheral utilization of glucose, an anti-insulin effect. Certain hepatic enzymes are induced by glucocorticoids. Glucocorticoids inhibit the synthesis of nucleic acids in most tissues but not the liver. They enhance the activity of cellular lipase and cause fatty acid mobilization. Under the influence of these steroids, abdominal and interscapular fat accumulates.

Glucocorticoids have anti-inflammatory actions by a variety of mechanisms that are not well understood. They may alter the ability of an antigen-antibody complex to cross cell membranes to reach receptor sites. They may limit the number of white blood cells that migrate to the area of inflammation and stabilize lysosomal membranes. The leakage of fluid and proteins from capillaries is decreased by glucocorticoids. Cellular mediated immunity is impaired by glucocorticoids but antibody production is not.

Glucocorticosteroids have a major role in maintaining blood pressure. They increase glomerular filtration rate and increase sodium reabsorption in exchange for potassium.

The major mineralocorticoid is aldosterone. Aldosterone is the most important agent in controlling extracellular fluid volume and potassium concentration. Volume is regulated by the promotion of sodium reabsorption in the distal convoluted tubule in exchange for potassium. Water passively follows the sodium. Sodium is also exchanged for hydrogen ion. Angiotensin II, which is formed by renin in response to a perceived decreased blood volume, stimulates the production of aldosterone. ACTH also stimulates aldosterone production. Increased serum potassium level stimulates the production of aldosterone independently of the other two stimuli.

Adrenal androgens are produced in response to ACTH and not gonadotropins. Androgens cause development of secondary sexual characteristics in the male and increase protein synthesis in both sexes.

Cushing's Syndrome—Caused by increased production of cortisol by the adrenal gland.

Etiology—Cushing's disease is the result of increased cortisol production due to bilateral adrenal hyperplasia often caused by an ACTH producing tumor of the pituitary gland which acts independently of feedback mechanisms. Nonendocrine tumors, such as bronchogenic carcinoma, bronchial adenoma, and pancreatic carcinoma secrete an ACTH-like peptide that causes Cushing's syndrome. Cushing's syndrome may also result from adrenal adenomas or adrenal carcinomas.

Epidemiology—Cushing's syndrome is seen more commonly in females 30 to 40 years of age.

Signs and Symptoms—The syndrome was originally characterized by truncal obesity, hypertension, weakness and fatigability, hirsutism, amenorrhea, purple abdominal striae, edema and osteoporosis. Approximately 80% of patients have the first four signs and symptoms.

The signs and symptoms of Cushing's syndrome are secondary to the excess cortisol. Increased cortisol levels promote the deposition of adipose tissue in the face (the moon facies), in the interscapular area (the buffalo hump) and in the mesenteric bed (the truncal obesity). The obesity is modest; not extreme. Mobilization of protein from peripheral supporting tissue results in muscle weakness, fatigability, osteoporosis, striae, ecchymoses and easy bruising. Because of increased hepatic gluconeogenesis and insulin resistance, glucose intolerance or diabetes mellitus occurs. Hypertension is almost always present. Marked emotional changes from irritability, emotional instability and euphoria to severe depression and psychosis occur. Amenorrhea, acne, and hirsutism are seen in females. Acne is seen in both sexes.

Laboratory tests reveal a mild neutrophilic leukocytosis with eosinopenia, normal serum sodium, hypokalemia, metabolic alkalosis and increased serum glucose with intermittent glucosuria. Radiographs show generalized osteoporosis, particularly of the spine and pelvis, and perhaps compression fractures of the vertebrae.

The diagnosis of Cushing's syndrome is based on elevated serum levels of cortisol. Patients with a pituitary tumor producing ACTH will have decreased morning cortisol levels after 4 mg dexamethasone at midnight. Patients with a nonendocrine tumor producing ACTH do not have a marked fall in morning cortisol level with dexamethasone suppression. Patients with an adrenal tumor have increased serum cortisol but decreased serum ACTH.

Primary Hyperaldosteronism—Due to excessive production of aldosterone by an adrenal tumor.

Etiology—Conn's syndrome is primary hyperaldosteronism due to an adrenal adenoma. This disease occurs twice as frequently in females than males and usually between the ages of 30 to 50 years. Rarely adrenal carcinoma or bilateral cortical nodular hyperplasia causes primary hyperaldosteronism. Secondary hyperaldosteronism occurs in states of overstimulation of the renin-angiotensin system such as in renal vascular hypertension or the edema formation of hepatic cirrhosis, nephrotic syndrome or congestive heart failure.

Signs and Symptoms—The hallmarks of hyperaldosteronism are hypokalemia, hypertension and volume expansion. The hypokalemia leads to muscle weakness and fatigue, particularly in the legs, and EKG changes. Hypokalemia may predispose to the development of pyelonephritis. The patients complain of polyuria and polydipsia.

Adrenal Virilism—The excessive production of adrenal androgens.

Etiology—Congenital enzyme defects lead to the syndrome of adrenal hyperplasia. Tumors which produce excess ACTH also increase adrenal androgen production.

Pathophysiology—The enzyme defect is most commonly C-21 hydroxylase deficiency which prevents the formation of cortisol so the feedback mechanism does not inhibit ACTH production with resultant overproduction of androgens.

Signs and Symptoms—The syndrome which occurs at birth causes ambiguous external genitalia in females and premature virilization of males. In the adult female hirsutism, acne, temporal baldness, deepening of the voice, decrease in breast size, atrophy of the uterus, amenorrhea and enlargement of the clitoris occur.

Primary Adrenal Insufficiency—A disease originally described by Addison which has a poor prognosis if untreated.

Etiology—The adrenal glands are destroyed. Approximately 90% of the glands must be destroyed before clinical manifestations occur. Chronic granulomatous infections such as tuberculosis or fungal infection or acute infections such as meningococcemia can cause the destruction. Most cases of *Addison's disease* are due to idiopathic atrophy of the adrenal glands which may be immunologically mediated and have a genetic predisposition.

Signs and Symptoms—Addison's disease presents as progressive fatigability, weakness, anorexia, nausea, vomiting, weight loss, increased skin and mucosal pigmentation, and hypotension. Other symptoms include those due to hypoglycemia and abdominal pain, diarrhea, constipation, salt craving and syncope. The most prominent symptom is fatigue. The hyperpigmentation is brown, tan or bronze in both exposed and nonexposed areas and particularly over pressure points or in skin creases.

Secondary Adrenal Insufficiency—An ACTH deficiency caused by pituitary destruction or pituitary atrophy secondary to prolonged administration of exogenous corticosteroids. The patient has the same signs and symptoms as the patient with Addison's disease but not the hyperpigmentation. ACTH deficiency due to pituitary destruction usually occurs along with other hormone deficiencies.

Adrenal Crisis—A state of acute adrenal insufficiency.

Etiology—Stress, surgery, trauma, or infection may precipitate acute adrenal insufficiency in a patient who has been chronically adrenally insufficient. Adrenal hemorrhage due to septicemia or anticoagulants or rapid withdrawal of exogenous steroids may precipitate an adrenal crisis.

Signs and Symptoms—The signs and symptoms of chronic adrenal insufficiency become severe and intractable. The nausea, vomiting and abdominal pain are difficult to control and contribute to the dehydration. Somnolence is profound. The blood pressure is low and the patient may die of hypovolemic shock.

Diabetes Mellitus

Diabetes mellitus is a disorder of glucose metabolism that results from a relative an absolute (Type I) or a relative (Type II) lack of insulin and of complications that include accelerated atherosclerosis and microangiopathy. The interrelationship between the glucose intolerance and the vascular disease has not been clearly defined.

Epidemiology—Diabetes mellitus is a disease that occurs worldwide with about 4.2 million diabetics in the US. The incidence of diabetes is higher in relatives of diabetics, people older than 45 years and those who are currently or were obese. The incidence of diabetes is increasing because female diabetics are now able to have children.

Etiology—One form of diabetes is inherited although the mode of inheritance has not been worked out. Diabetes also occurs spontaneously in patients without a positive family history. Destruction of the pancreas by chronic pancreatitis, hemochromatosis or carcinoma results in diabetes. Other endocrine disorders, such as Cushing's syndrome, hyperpituitarism and hyperthyroidism, are associated with diabetes. Glucose intolerance occurs during pregnancy or times of excessive stress and with the administration of glucocorticosteroids, thiazides and oral contraceptives.

Pathology—The beta cells of the pancreas are decreased in number or degranulated in diabetes. The reduction in number of beta cells corresponds to the lack of insulin. In Type I diabetes there are no beta cells; in adult onset diabetes only about one-half of the beta cells are present. In some cases the beta cells are infiltrated with lymphocytes, suggesting an autoimmune mechanism for diabetes. The atherosclerosis that occurs in diabetes is the same as the atherosclerosis previously discussed but it occurs as frequently in females as males and at an earlier age. The microangiopathy consists of a thickened basement membrane in capillaries due to the deposition of glycoprotein. In the kidney, nodular glomerulosclerosis (Kimmelstiel-Wilson's) is seen, which is the deposition of glycoprotein in ball-like masses in the mesangial regions of the capillary tufts. Diffuse glomerulosclerosis, which is the deposition of glycoprotein in the mesangium, is also seen, as well as tubular basement membrane thickening. The hallmark of diabetic retinopathy is the formation of microaneurysms. Proliferative retinopathy, the formation of new blood vessels around the optic disk, occurs with long standing diabetes. Repeated hemorrhages cause scar formation that may lead to retinal detachment. The changes of hypertensive retinopathy are also seen in diabetics with hypertension.

Pathophysiology—The lack of insulin results in a peripheral underutilization and a hepatic overproduction of glucose which results in hyperglycemia. Insulin facilitates the entry of glucose into cells of adipose tissue and muscle, stimulates fat synthesis in cells and stimulates protein synthesis. The lack of glucose in muscle cells leads to glycogenolysis and the release of amino acids for gluconeogenesis. Lack of insulin and glucose in adipose tissue leads to impaired triglyceride synthesis and release of free fatty acids. The liver metabolizes free fatty acids to ketones which are used by muscles for energy to a limited extent. Lack of insulin also results in hepatic overproduction of glucose from glycogenolysis and gluconeogenesis. Another hormone, glucagon, is increased in diabetes. Glucagon effects oppose insulin physiologically.

Hyperglycemia results in glucosuria when the serum level of glucose exceeds the renal threshold for reabsorption of glucose. The osmotic diuresis results in polyuria and polydipsia and may result in dehydration. Excess ketones are also excreted in the urine, as strong acids. This results in urinary loss of bicarbonate and potassium and dehydration.

Normally insulin is only released in response to a glucose load such as a meal. Serum insulin levels rise within 15 to 20 minutes after eating. Patients with juvenile onset diabetes do not produce insulin. Those with adult onset diabetes produce too little insulin too late to prevent hyperglycemia. Obese people have hypertrophied adipose cells which, because of their size, are less sensitive to the action of insulin.

The vascular complications of diabetes mellitus have been related to the hyperglycemia. It is postulated that glycoprotein is deposited in the capillaries when glucose levels are elevated. Formation of cataracts and neuropathy are thought to occur because glucose is metabolized to sorbitol by aldose reductase in hyperglycemia. The sorbitol causes osmotic swelling and damage. Diabetic patients are predisposed to infections because phagocytes do not function properly and have impaired killing action in the presence of hyperglycemia.

Signs and Symptoms—Onset of Type I diabetes is sudden and characterized by polyuria, polydipsia, polyphagia, weight loss, decreased muscle strength, irritability and perhaps a return of bed wetting. The presentation may be ketoacidosis. About one-third of these patients have a remission shortly after the onset of the diabetes. The remission may last for weeks to one year and the patient does not require insulin during this time. After the remission, Type I diabetics require insulin for the remainder of their lifetime. Usually juvenile onset diabetics are very sensitive to the effects of insulin and physical activity. Their course is marked by both hypoglycemia and ketoacidosis. The prognosis for juvenile onset diabetes is death within 20 to 30 years of the onset of the disease.

The clinical presentation of adult onset diabetes may be the insidious onset of weight loss, nocturia, vascular complications, decreased or blurred vision, fatigue, anemia, or signs and symptoms of neuropathy. The disease may be diagnosed from an elevated glucose level without any symptoms. Type II diabetics are usually not prone to ketoacidosis. The majority of Type II diabetics respond to weight loss.

The diagnosis of diabetes mellitus is based on the documentation of elevated fasting blood sugar, elevated blood glucose two hours postprandially or an abnormal glucose tolerance test. The accuracy of a glucose tolerance test is influenced by diet, physical activity, age, underlying diseases and drugs.

Complications of Diabetes Mellitus

Ketoacidosis occurs in diabetic patients who develop high levels of glucose and ketones plus metabolic acidosis. The usual cause is lack of compliance with insulin therapy but ketoacidosis may be the first episode for an undiagnosed diabetic or a manifestation of an infection. The signs and symptoms of ketoacidosis include nausea, vomiting, abdominal pain and air hunger (Kussmaul breathing—heavy labored breathing as a compensatory mechanism to the decreased pH). The dehydration may be severe. Oliguria and hypotension may be present. Hyperglycemia, decreased bicarbonate, hypokalemia, azotemia and acidosis are seen on laboratory evaluation.

Hyperglycemic hyperosmolar nonketotic coma occurs in patients with Type II diabetes. The patients are usually elderly and have some renal impairment. Neurological manifestations are preceded by polyuria and polydipsia. The osmotic diuresis results in loss of large amounts of free water so serum sodium is increased. The patient presents with hyperpyrexia, hypotension, tachycardia, hyperventilation and the signs of dehydration. Hyperreflexia, mild disorientation, confusion, seizures or coma reflect the intracellular dehydration of the central nervous system. Laboratory examination is remarkable for increased serum osmolarity, hyperglycemia without ketosis, hypernatremia and normal pH.

Retinopathy occurs in the majority of diabetics after 20 years of the disease. Venous dilatation, the formation of microaneurysms and small hemorrhages into the macula occur but do not interfere with vision. Hemorrhages into the vitreous cause temporary blindness. Retinal detachment occurs due to repeated hemorrhages and scar formation. Secondary hemorrhagic glaucoma occurs in proliferative retinopathy. Diabetes is the second leading cause of blindness. Cataracts are also associated with diabetes.

Neuropathy results from the sorbitol pathway or from ischemia because of the vascular disease. Diabetic neuropathy most frequently involves the peripheral nerves but can involve any nerve. Manifestations of diabetic neuropathy include sexual dysfunction in the male, gastric atony, nocturnal diarrhea, fecal incontinence, orthostatic hypotension, neurogenic bladder, paresthesias and loss of sensation.

Diabetic ulcers and gangrene result from either the neuropathy, the vascular disease, or both. The painless foot is more prone to injury. The ischemic foot is less likely to heal. The patient usually has a history of intermittent claudication, nocturnal leg pain and cramps, loss of hair and muscle atrophy. Both feet or legs usually become involved.

Nephropathy occurs with diabetes of 15 years or more duration, and usually occurs along with the other complications. The first sign of diabetic nephropathy is mild proteinuria. Later the nephrotic syndrome may appear and renal function deteriorates or progressive renal failure occurs without the nephrotic syndrome. Diabetic nephropathy may cause hypertension. Urinary tract infections and pyelonephritis are more common in the diabetic and may contribute to the renal failure. Renal failure is the cause of death in the majority of diabetics.

Accelerated Atherosclerosis—Diabetics have an increased incidence and severity of coronary atherosclerotic heart disease. (See previous discussion.)

Disorders of Calcium Metabolism

Disorders of calcium metabolism may relate to dysfunction of the parathyroid glands or to vitamin D deficiency.

Normal Physiology—Calcium and phosphate homeostasis is maintained by parathyroid hormone (PTH), vitamin D and calcitonin. The normal serum calcium varies only slightly for an individual. Dietary vitamin D or that produced in the skin by sunlight is inactive. The molecule is hydroxylated at the 25-position by the liver and at the 1-position by the kidney to form the active 1,25-dihydroxycholecalciferol. Parathyroid hormone is necessary for the hydroxylation in the kidney. Parathyroid hormone and vitamin D work together and are synergistic. Their action is to stimulate gastrointestinal absorption of calcium, bone resorption of calcium, and kidney reabsorption of calcium. The actions of vitamin D and parathyroid hormone are opposed by calcitonin. Parathyroid hormone promotes the excretion of phosphate by the kidney.

Vitamin D promotes phosphate absorption from the gastrointestinal tract.

Primary Hyperparathyroidism—An overproduction of PTH with increased serum calcium and decreased serum phosphate.

Etiology—Most cases of primary hyperparathyroidism are caused by benign adenomas of one parathyroid gland. Some cases are caused by chief cell hyperplasia in all four parathyroid glands. A few cases are caused by carcinoma of the parathyroids. Pseudohyperparathyroidism is caused by nonendocrine neoplasms, without metastases to the bone, which secrete a PTH-like peptide.

Signs and Symptoms—The majority of patients with primary hyperparathyroidism are asymptomatic and the diagnosis is discovered after routine screening demonstrates elevated serum calcium.

Some patients present with recurrent nephrolithiasis that leads to urinary-tract obstruction, recurrent urinary-tract infections, a predisposition to pyelonephritis and chronic renal failure. The stones are usually either calcium oxalate or calcium phosphate. Nephrocalcinosis or deposition of calcium in the renal parenchyma can also occur as a result of hyperparathyroidism. Nephrocalcinosis may lead to chronic renal failure.

The effect of increased levels of PTH on the bone results in decreased number of trabeculae, increased osteoclasts, and replacement of normal bone by fibrous tissue which is known as osteitis fibrosa cystica. The hands and skull are most commonly affected. Radiographs show phalangeal resorption.

Increased serum calcium can result in mental status changes from mild personality disturbances to severe psychotic disorders, obtundation and coma. Proximal muscle weakness, easy fatigability and muscle atrophy are caused by increased serum calcium. Patients with hyperparathyroidism have a high incidence of duodenal ulcers which may be related to the increased serum calcium.

Other causes of hypercalcemia, such as osteolytic metastases from various malignancies, prostaglandins from various cancers without metastases to the bone, vitamin D intoxication, milk-alkali syndrome, and prolonged immobilization must be excluded. The serum level of PTH is not elevated in these situations.

Secondary Hyperparathyroidism—Occurs in situations in which serum calcium falls and the parathyroids are intact. Chronic renal failure causes secondary hyperparathyroidism. Thus osteitis fibrosa cystica is a part of the bone disease of chronic renal failure. The serum calcium level is normal although the serum phosphate and PTH levels are high.

Hypoparathyroidism—Production of PTH is decreased. Pseudohypoparathyroidism is a resistance of the renal tubules to the action of PTH. Serum calcium is low and serum phosphate is high.

Etiology—Hypoparathyroidism is most commonly caused by the surgical removal or damage to the glands. A congenital absence of PTH occurs rarely. Pseudohypoparathyroidism is an X-linked inherited disorder.

Signs and Symptoms—The hypocalcemia causes neuromuscular irritability which is manifested by tingling and numbness around the lips and of the hands and feet. Tetany and convulsions are the most serious manifestations of hypocalcemia.

The patient with pseudohypoparathyroidism is of short stature and has short metacarpals and metatarsals. The serum PTH level is high. In addition to the signs and symptoms of hypocalcemia, these patients have resorption of bone and soft tissue calcifications as in primary hyperparathyroidism.

Osteomalacia and Rickets—Due to defective mineralization of the normal bone matrix. Osteomalacia refers to the disorder which occurs after the bones have ceased growing; rickets refers to the disorder in growing bones.

Etiology—The defect is a deficiency of vitamin D. Vitamin D deficiency may result from consumption of a deficient diet, inadequate exposure to the sun, intestinal malabsorption of vitamin D (a fat-soluble vitamin), chronic acidosis, renal tubular defects, and therapy with anticonvulsants.

Pathophysiology—A precise concentration of calcium and phosphate is required for mineralization of bone matrix. A deficiency of vitamin D results in decreased absorption of calcium and phosphate from the gastrointestinal tract. The hypocalcemia stimulates the production of PTH which increases calcium resorption from the bone and phosphate excretion by the kidneys. Mineralization cannot occur because of the decreased calcium and decreased phosphate.

Signs and Symptoms—A child with rickets has skeletal deformities, an increased susceptibility to bone fractures, muscular weakness, hypotonia, delayed dental eruption, defects in the enamel of the teeth and, in severe cases, tetany. Adults with osteomalacia have skeletal pain, bone tenderness, muscular weakness and fractures of the bones with minimal trauma.

Osteoporosis—Not a disorder of calcium metabolism. The amount of calcium in the bone is normal in osteoporosis but the amount of bone is decreased. Osteoporosis occurs with aging as bone resorption exceeds bone formation. Osteoporosis occurs in the spine leading to back pain, and collapse of vertebrae and deformity of the spine. Long bones and hips are also susceptible to osteoporosis with subsequent ease of fracture.

The Hyperlipoproteinemias

The hyperlipoproteinemias result from disturbances in the synthesis or degradation of lipoproteins. The morbidity and mortality associated with this family of disease result from the ability of abnormally high lipoprotein levels to cause atherosclerosis and pancreatitis. Primary lipoproteinemias are due to disorders in lipoprotein metabolism and have a genetic basis while secondary hyperlipoproteinemias occur because of a concurrent disease such as diabetes mellitus and hypothyroidism. As a complete discussion of all hyperlipoproteinemias is not possible here, only two of the more common primary types, familial hypercholesterolemia and familial hypertriglyceridemia, will be presented.

Normal Physiology—The physiologic role of the lipoproteins is to transport lipids (ie, triglycerides and cholesterol esters) through plasma. Lipoproteins are comprised of triglycerides, cholesterol, phospholipids, and protein (apoprotein). Various lipoproteins differ in the quantity of these components and thus density and size. Lipids are transported in the body by lipoproteins through exogenous and endogenous pathways. In the exogenous pathway, dietary lipids are incorporated with lipoproteins into chylomicrons which are transported to adipose and muscle tissue where the triglycerides are removed. The remainder of the chylomicron, or remnant particle, is transported to the liver for further metabolism. The endogenous pathway has its base in the liver, where carbohydrates are converted to triglycerides. The liver secretes these triglycerides into the blood as very low density lipoproteins (VLDL). These particles are handled in much the same way as chylomicrons except that after removal

of the triglycerides by adipose tissue, a further transformation occurs. Most of the protein is removed, yielding low density lipoprotein (LDL) which is chiefly composed of cholesterol. These LDL particles supply cholesterol for various uses, including cell membrane composition and glucocorticoid synthesis. In addition, some LDL particles are degraded by the reticuloendothelial system. As the cells of this system turn over, cholesterol is released to form high density lipoprotein (HDL) which is then transferred to VLDL and thus to LDL, forming a cycle.

Familial Hypercholesterolemia—This common hyperlipoproteinemia affects approximately 1 in 500 individuals in the general population.

Pathophysiology—The defects occurring with this disorder are an inability to bind and/or transport LDL into cells for subsequent catabolism. Thus plasma LDL are elevated. More is taken up by the reticuloendothelial system resulting in accumulations in various locations in the body. These accumulations are called xanthomas. LDL also infiltrates the walls of blood vessels, ultimately resulting in artherosclerosis.

Signs and Symptoms—Patients with familial hypercholesterolemia have high LDL blood levels from birth and throughout life. The chief manifestation is myocardial infarction which results from coronary atherosclerosis. Myocardial infarctions may occur in this population as early as the third decade of life, and by 60 years of age 85% have experienced one. This complication occurs earlier in males than females. Xanthomas, a common sign of this disorder, increase in frequency with age. They tend to occur in tendons and the eyelids. With the homozygous form of this disease, xanthomas may also form in the skin over the knees, elbows, and buttocks as well as between fingers. A diagnosis of familial hypercholesterolemia is suggested by high plasma cholesterol (or LDL) in the face of normal triglyceride levels.

Familial Hypertriglyceridemia—This disease involves elevated blood levels of VLDL with resultant hypertriglyceridemia.

Pathophysiology—The underlying defect is unclear although it may be in VLDL catabolism. The incidence of diabetes mellitus and obesity is higher in this patient population and both contribute to the hypertriglyceridemia.

Signs and Symptoms—These patients usually exhibit hyperglycemia, hyperinsulinism and obesity in addition to hypertriglyceridemia. Such findings are usually not manifested until after puberty. As with familial hypercholesterolemia, atherosclerosis is frequent and may lead to myocardial infarction. Unlike hypercholesterolemia, xanthomas are not common. In addition to the inherent complications of diabetes and obesity, both contribute to the hypertriglyceridemia and thus to the artherosclerosis. The diagnosis of familial hypertriglyceridemia is suggested by the finding of elevated plasma triglycerides with normal cholesterol levels. Some patients have elevated chylomicron levels in addition to the increased VLDL.

Gastroenterology

Disease of the Esophagus

Diseases of the esophagus are mainly related to failure of the organ to transport swallowed material from the mouth to the stomach or to failure to prevent the retrograde flow of gastrointestinal contents into the esophagus. Dysphagia is the sensation of swallowed material sticking in the esophagus. Odynophagia is painful swallowing. Heartburn is a pain that usually begins in the upper epigastrium and migrates upward substernally.

Normal Physiology—The esophagus is not simply a hollow conduit through which swallowed material passes from the mouth to the stomach. Rather, it is an organ of unique structure and function. The superior sphincter separates the pharynx and the esophagus and prevents air from entering the alimentary tract during inspiration. A lower esophageal sphincter (LES) separates the stomach from the esophagus and prevents gastric contents from entering the esophagus. The propulsive force of the upper one-fourth of the esophagus is provided by striated voluntary muscle. Swallowing initiates the opening of both esophageal sphincters and a primary peristaltic wave, which propels the bolus down the esophagus. Secondary peristalsis differs from primary peristalsis in that it is not initiated by swallowing but by the bolus itself. Secondary peristalsis

may occur in response to reflux of material from the stomach into the esophagus. Tertiary contractions of the esophagus are uncoordinated, nonpropulsive muscle contractions which serve no known purpose. They may occur spontaneously or in response to swallowing. Tertiary contractions occur in normal people, particularly the elderly. In some cases, however, tertiary contractions interfere with esophageal function and cause symptoms.

Regulation of esophageal motor function is poorly understood but probably is under parasympathetic and hormonal control. Denervation of the esophagus abolishes primary and secondary peristalsis. The LES pressure is increased by cholinergic stimulation, muscurinic agents, gastrin and several other gastrointestinal hormones. LES pressure is reduced by ganglionic stimulants, dopamine, secretin, cholecystokinin and other hormones. However, the role of gastrin and other gastrointestinal hormones in regulating LES pressure under normal conditions is unclear.

Reflux and Esophagitis—The movement of gastric contents into the esophagus with resultant inflammation of the esophagus.

Pathophysiology—An incompetent LES allows reflux of gastric contents into the lower esophagus. The normal LES pressure is about 20 mm Hg. Pressures below 10 mm Hg usually are associated with reflux esophagitis. Reflux of either gastric acid or bile can cause esophagitis.

In some cases the major abnormality is the failure of secondary peristalsis to clear quickly and completely refluxed material from the esophagus. Chronic reflux esophagitis is characterized by inflammation, thickening of the basal layer of epithelial cell and in severe cases, ulceration and stricture formation. Rarely, the inflamed squamous epithelium may be replaced by an aberrant epithelium that resembles that of the stomach or intestine (Barrett's esophagus). This abnormal epithelium is predisposed to develop adenocarcinoma.

Signs and Symptoms—Heartburn is the hallmark of gastroesophageal reflux. This burning epigastric or retrosternal pain usually moves upward and occurs after eating. Heartburn may be accompanied by an acid taste ("water brash"). Overeating, lying down after eating, bending over and straining may precipitate heartburn. Standing up, drinking anything or taking antacids will relieve the pain. Severe heartburn may mimic angina or myocardial infarction and radiate to the jaw or arms. Dysphagia may occur with chronic reflux esophagitis due to esophageal spasm or stricture.

The diagnosis of reflux and esophagitis depends on demonstrating that reflux occurs and that the reflux causes the symptoms. Reflux of barium from the stomach may be demonstrated radiographically but this is an insensitive test unless ulceration and/or stricture are also demonstrated. Esophagoscopy with biopsy usually reveals esophageal inflammation. The most sensitive diagnostic procedure is to measure LES pressure and esophageal pH using a tube.

Hiatal Hernia—The protrusion of a portion of the stomach into the chest through the diaphragm. Hiatal hernia is a common disorder, occurring in 40 to 50% of the population. In contrast to previous belief, hiatal hernia is usually asymptomatic and rarely causes gastroesophageal reflux.

Achalasia—A motor disorder of the esophagus of unknown etiology that causes dysphagia.

Pathophysiology—The cholinergic innervation of the esophagus is impaired due to a loss of the myenteric plexuses. The pressure in the LES is increased and the LES relaxes by less than 50% with swallowing. Primary and secondary peristaltic waves are absent or infrequent and of low amplitude. The contractions are mainly of the tertiary type. The esophagus above the LES becomes progressively dilated.

Signs and Symptoms—The disorder presents as progressive dysphagia to solids and liquids. The dysphagia may be accompanied by the pain of esophageal spasm. Weight loss occurs. The patient may have massive regurgitation when a supine position is assumed. Aspiration is possible.

Radiographs establish the diagnosis by showing a tortuous dilated esophagus without peristalsis and a narrow LES that fails to dilate. The condition is treated by mechanical dilatation or surgery.

Diffuse Esophageal Spasm—A motor disorder of the esophagus characterized by frequent and severe tertiary contractions.

Pathophysiology—Diffuse esophageal spasm occurs predominantly in elderly patients. Neuromuscular disorders can cause diffuse esophageal spasm as can disorders that irritate the esophagus such as gastroesophageal reflux. The LES is normal and typically relaxes by greater than 50 percent.

Signs and Symptoms—Diffuse esophageal spasm presents as severe retrosternal pain with or without dysphagia to liquids and solids. Symptoms occur intermittently. The spasm may be precipitated by cold drinks or by eating while emotionally upset.

The diagnosis is made by barium swallow or by pressure measurements in the esophageal lumen.

Dysphagia—May be a diagnostic sign. Dysphagia to solids and liquids is indicative of a motor disorder of the esophagus such as diffuse esophageal spasm. Dysphagia to solids but not liquids is characteristic of a mechanical obstruction such as cancer or stricture. In these cases, dysphagia to liquids occurs only after the esophageal lumen is severely narrowed.

Peptic Ulcer Disease

Peptic ulcer disease is a chronic relapsing disorder characterized by deep ulceration in the stomach or duodenum or both. It is the most common disease of the upper gastrointestinal system and affects approximately one in 10 persons during a lifetime.

Normal Physiology—The parietal cells in the fundus of the stomach secrete hydrochloric acid throughout the day in response to neurogenic and hormonal stimuli. Basal acid secretion is mediated by the vagus nerve and follows a circadian rhythm, being highest at 8:00–12:00 pm, and accounts for about 30% of daily acid secretion. Acid secreted in response to meals is quantitatively more important. The cephalic phase of meal-related acid secretion is stimulated by the sight, smell, taste or even thought of food. The vagus nerve mediates this phase and stimulates the parietal cells to secrete acid and the G-cells of the antrum to release gastrin. Gastrin is liberated into the portal vein and returns to the parietal cells via the systemic circulation. Gastrin is the most potent stimulator of acid secretion. The gastric phase is mediated largely by gastrin which is released in response to food, particularly protein derivatives, and possibly to antral distention. The role of various mediators in stimulating the parietal cell to secrete acid is unclear. One theory holds that histamine is the common mediator for both gastrin and acetylcholine. Gastrin and possibly acetylcholine appear to stimulate paracrine cells in the gastric mucosa to release histamine, which stimulates histamine-H2 receptors on parietal cells. Another theory proposes that histamine, gastrin and acetylcholine are independent mediators for the stimulation of acid secretion. Acid secretion is partially inhibited by an intragastric pH of 3.0 or less, an effect that appears to be due to inhibition of gastrin release caused by somatostatin. Somatostatin is present in the gastric antrum. The intestinal phase of gastric acid secretion is one of inhibition. The passage of peptides and acid into the duodenum causes release of various hormones which inhibit gastric acid secretion. Candidate hormones include enterogastrone, secretin, and gastrointestinal inhibitory peptide (GIP).

A coating of mucus helps protect the gastric mucosa from acid injury. Certain substances, such as bile, aspirin, ethanol, and other drugs, can alter the integrity of the gastric mucus barrier. This allows diffusion of HCl back into the mucosal cells, a process which causes cellular injury and possibly gastric ulceration.

Duodenal Ulcer—The most common of the peptic diseases, accounting for about 80% of ulcerations of the upper gastrointestinal tract.

Epidemiology—Males between the ages of 20 and 50 years are most commonly affected. The male to female ratio was about 7:1 but has narrowed considerably to about 2:1, largely due to an increased incidence in women. Women after menopause have the same risk as men. Cigarette smoking increases the risk.

Pathology—The depth of the crater varies but the submucosa is always penetrated and the ulcer usually erodes the muscle layer. The ulcer is surrounded by edema and hyperemia. The ulcer base is composed of fibrin, necrotic debris, granulation tissue, and inflammatory reaction. Healed ulcers have a scar. Most duodenal ulcers are located within 3 cm of the pylorus on either the anterior or posterior wall.

Pathophysiology—The pathogenesis of duodenal ulcers is multifactorial. Duodenal ulcers never occur in the absence of gastric acid. However, only about 50% of patients with the disease secrete excessive quantities of acid. This hypersecretion may be due to an increased parietal cell mass, excessive gastrin release during meals, enhanced sensitivity to gastrin or to other factors. Some patients have an increased rate of gastric emptying of acid. Genetic factors clearly predispose to development of duodenal ulcers. Neuropsychiatric factors are now thought to be of less importance. The notion that patients with duodenal ulcer disease are hard-driving, ambitious, "over-achievers" is false; the disease occurs as often in socially disadvantaged manual laborers. Duodenal ulcer disease occurs more frequently in patients with hyperparathyroidism, emphysema, alcoholic cirrhosis and rheumatoid arthritis.

Signs and Symptoms—Duodenal ulcer disease is characterized by remissions and exacerbations. Curiously, relapse often occurs during spring and autumn. Relapses in 50 to 90% of patients within a year of the first attack. It is not yet possible to predict who will relapse but cigarette smoking increases the risk.

The classical symptom of duodenal ulcer is a steady, gnawing or burning pain in the mid-epigastrium which is relieved by ingestion of food or antacids. The pain begins about 2 hours after a meal, may awaken the patient between midnight and 3:00 a.m. but almost never is present before breakfast. The patient often gains weight because eating relieves the pain. Approximately 20% of patients have no pain. Their disease may be expressed by hemorrhage.

Physical examination is within normal limits except occasionally for mild tenderness in the mid-epigastrium. Laboratory examination may show iron deficiency anemia. Radiographs usually show the ulcer crater or distortion of the duodenum due to spasm or scarring.

Endoscopy is the most accurate means of diagnosis but usually is unnecessary.

Complications of duodenal ulcer disease account for approximately 7,000 deaths per year in the United States. The ulcer may perforate into the peritoneal cavity resulting in peritonitis and sepsis. It may penetrate directly into the pancreas, causing pancreatitis. Hemorrhage is the most common complication and may be massive. Inflammation and edema or scarring may narrow the pyloric channel causing obstruction. These complications usually are indications for surgery.

Gastric Ulcer—Less common than duodenal ulcer as a clinical diagnosis.

Epidemiology—Gastric ulcers occur with equal frequency in men and women. The average age of onset of gastric ulcer is between 40 and 55 years.

Pathology—Gastric ulcers appear grossly as punched-out craters, usually with smooth but heaped up margins and a fibrin base. All layers of the wall may be involved. Most gastric ulcers are found in the antrum or at the antral-fundal junction. Approximately 20% of patients have or have had duodenal ulcers.

Pathophysiology—Benign gastric ulcers also do not occur in the absence of acid. However, as a group, patients with gastric ulcers secrete less acid than do normal people. Postulations regarding the pathogenesis include gastric hypomotility, abnormalities in mucosa blood flow and alterations in the gastric barrier which allow the back diffusion of hydrogen ions into the mucosa. Cigarette smoking and aspirin ingestion increase the risk of developing gastric ulcer disease.

Signs and Symptoms—The classic pain-food-relief cycle of duodenal ulcer may also be present with gastric ulcer but usually is less clearly defined. The pain of gastric ulcer often is described as burning or gnawing and is less localized than duodenal ulcer pain. The pain from gastric ulcer rarely occurs at night. The course is chronic with relapses and remissions. The complications are the same as those of duodenal ulcer disease. It is extremely doubtful that gastric ulcer causes cancer. However, gastric cancer may ulcerate and masquerade as benign gastric ulcer disease. The discovery of a crater in the stomach therefore requires evaluation for cancer.

Diarrhea and Constipation

There are no precise and agreed upon definitions for either diarrhea or constipation. Changes in bowel habits must be defined within the context of usual bowel habits for an individual patient.

Normal Physiology—The function of the colon is to reabsorb water and electrolytes and to store feces.

Constipation generally denotes the infrequent or difficult evacuation of feces.

Etiology—Constipation is a symptom which accompanies a variety of medical disorders including hypothyroidism, hyperparathyroidism and other hypercalcemic states, tuberculosis, urinary tract disease, lead poisoning, congestive heart failure, psychosis, major depression, parkinsonism, a recent myocardial infarction, and diabetes. The ingestion of various inorganic ions, aluminum and calcium, can cause constipation.

The sudden occurrence of constipation in a previously normal individual suggests a problem of innervation or muscular function of the intestine or associated reflexes and accessory muscles. These abnormalities may be caused by severe infections, acute mesenteric circulatory events, renal colic, CNS infection or damage, or drug ingestion.

Constipation may be a major complaint in the irritable bowel syndrome, a common functional disorder related to anxiety. Other gastrointestinal disorders such as diverticulosis, toxic megacolon, tumors of the intestine and painful anal lesions may present as constipation. The most common causes of constipation include inadequate intake of dietary fiber, changes in daily routine such as travel and decreased physical activity.

Pathophysiology—Normal defecation requires a complex interaction of nervous reflexes, smooth and skeletal muscle contraction, and voluntary initiation. Peristaltic contractions occur over only short distances to advance material through the gastrointestinal tract. Massive contractions in the colon move material over longer distances. The massive contractions occur reflexly in association with eating and gastric emptying. Segmental contractions of circular muscles also influence bulk flow through the intestine. These contractions occur most frequently in the proximal small bowel. The law of Laplace describes the important relationship between the tension in the muscle walls, the radius of the bowel lumen and the pressure in the lumen ($P = t/r^4$). The tension of the muscle walls is largely a function of smooth muscle contractions. Increased muscle contraction, particularly in the colon, increases intraluminal

pressure and retards forward fecal movement. This increases the contact time for the absorption of water from the fecal mass and may lead to constipation. A reduced luminal diameter because of a low fiber diet may also increase intraluminal pressure..

A defecation reflex is initiated by distention of the muscles of the rectum. The abdominal and pelvic floor muscles contract during defecation. Weak muscles in these areas impair defecation. Squatting improves the performance of these muscles. If the impulse for defecation is voluntarily suppressed, the external and sphincter contracts and the sigmoid colon relaxes allowing the fecal mass to return to the lower portion of the colon. Repeated or prolonged suppression of the defecatory reflex can lead to constipation.

Signs and Symptoms—The only agreed-upon signs and symptoms of constipation are infrequent or difficult evacuation of feces and perhaps weight gain in severe cases. It is doubtful if constipation *per se* actually causes the nonspecific symptoms ascribed to it, such as indigestion, anorexia, flatulence, lower abdominal pain, malaise and headache. The concept of autointoxication due to the absorption of toxins from feces is a myth except in patients with portal systemic encephalopathy in which absorbed ammonia contributes to the syndrome.

Diarrhea is regarded as increased frequency or increased fluid content of bowel movements.

Etiology—Various infectious agents such as *Shigella*, *Salmonella*, enteropathogenic *E. coli*, viruses and parasites may cause diarrhea (see previous discussion). Diarrhea may also be associated with a variety of gastrointestinal diseases including chronic inflammatory bowel diseases, malabsorption, etc. Many other medical disorders may also be associated with diarrhea.

Pathophysiology—The classification of diarrhea by pathogenesis is more meaningful than listing diseases that cause diarrhea.

Osmotic diarrhea is caused by the accumulation of nonabsorbable solutes in the gastrointestinal tract. These solutes inhibit the reabsorption of water and electrolytes and cause water to move into the gut from the plasma. This type of diarrhea is seen in lactase deficiency and the dumping syndrome.

Secretory diarrhea is caused by the secretion of water and electrolytes into the gut by the intestinal epithelial cells. The secretion of bicarbonate, chloride and water is mediated by stimulation of adenyl cyclase which increases intracellular cyclic-AMP. This is a proposed mechanism for the diarrhea of cholera, toxigenic *E. coli*, bile-acid irritation of the colon and some diarrheogenic islet cell tumors of the pancreas.

Anatomical derangement can cause diarrhea by decreasing the surface area available for absorption. Sprue results in a loss of villi and substantial reduction in intestinal surface area. Surgical resection of the bowel and intestinal by-pass operations cause diarrhea largely by reducing surface area.

Abnormal intestinal motility may cause diarrhea but the mechanism(s) is unclear. Decreased gastrointestinal transit encourages overgrowth of bacteria which in turn can result in steatorrhea by interfering with bile acid metabolism. The bacteria may also form laxating hydroxy fatty acids. Decreased smooth muscle contractions in the gastrointestinal tract removes the resistance to forward flow and permits rapid transport of contents through the bowel without allowing time for the absorption of water and electrolytes. Vagotomy, diabetic neuropathy, other neurologic disorders and the irritable bowel syndrome are examples of conditions which cause diarrhea by altering intestinal motility.

Exudative diarrhea is due to the outpouring of cells, colloid and even whole blood from an inflamed or ulcerated bowel. Ulcerative colitis, amebiasis and shigellosis are examples of this type of diarrhea.

Signs and Symptoms—Acute diarrhea usually lasts for 48 to 72 hours and resolves spontaneously. Chronic diarrhea lasts for months to years. Blood in the stool is associated with infection with invasive organisms, inflammatory bowel disease or cancer of the GI tract. Pus in the stool suggests infection or inflammatory bowel disease. Greasy, bulky, foul-smelling stools are characteristic of steatorrhea. Mucus in the stool and diarrhea alternating with constipation are characteristic of the irritable bowel syndrome. Nocturnal diarrhea occurs with diabetic neuropathy. The diarrhea may be accompanied by other signs and symptoms characteristic of the underlying disorder. Dehydration and electrolyte imbalance may result from severe diarrhea particularly in infants or elderly patients.

Inflammatory Bowel Disease

This is a group of disorders characterized by chronic diarrhea and stools containing blood and pus. The most common of these diseases are ulcerative colitis and Crohn's disease.

Ulcerative Colitis (UC)—A chronic inflammatory bowel

disease of unknown etiology in which the inflammation begins in the rectal mucosa and progresses proximally.

Epidemiology—Ulcerative colitis occurs predominantly in adults 25 to 40 years of age. It is more common in females, Caucasians, Jews, and in those who reside in urban settings. UC is rare in Africa and Asia and American Indians are rarely affected. The incidence of UC appears to be rising.

Pathology—The inflammation in UC is confined to the mucosa and submucosa. It begins in the rectum and spreads uniformly and continuously up the colon. During acute phases, neutrophils and eosinophils are seen in the crypts. In the chronic phase, lymphocytes and plasma cells are the predominant cells. The crypts become irregular and may contain abscesses at the bases. The mucosa is hyperemic and friable. The ulcerations usually are too small to be seen with the naked eye. Hyperplastic overgrowth of regenerating mucosa results in the formation of pseudopolyps. The rectum is involved in 95% of cases. Two-thirds of the patients have only rectal and left colonic involvement. One-third of patients have pancolitis. In severe chronic cases goblet cells are replaced by non-mucus producing cells. In toxic megacolon, areas of mucosa become necrotic and perforation of the grossly dilated thin-walled colon may occur.

Pathophysiology—The inciting event for the inflammation has not been identified. Most likely an autoimmune mechanism is involved rather than infection or psychologic factors. The inflammation results in the inability of the colon to absorb water and electrolytes and disturbs colonic motility. These disturbances together with exudation of colloid and blood cause diarrhea. The inflammation may result in systemic toxicity. The ulceration and bleeding result in iron-deficiency anemia, the anemia of chronic diseases and hypoalbuminemia.

Signs and Symptoms—Bloody diarrhea is the hallmark of UC. The stool also contains pus. The number of stools may be as many as 30 per day although stool volume is a more accurate index of the severity and extent of the disease. The diarrhea may be accompanied by abdominal cramps, tenesmus and fever. Weight loss is common.

Laboratory data are nonspecific and show anemia, increased white blood-cell count, decreased albumin and electrolyte disturbances, particularly hypokalemia.

Sigmoidoscopy reveals mucosal granularity, friability and an exudate containing pus and blood. Pseudopolyps may be present. Barium enema typically reveals irregularity of the rectal margins, loss of haustral markings and shortening of the colon. In toxic megacolon the colon is grossly dilated and without evidence of motility.

The clinical course of UC is variable. A few patients have a spontaneous remission for 10 to 15 years after the initial acute attack. Most have an intermittent course with near normal health between attacks. Some patients have a chronic unremitting course with continuous diarrhea and systemic symptoms until the colon is removed surgically.

Complications—The inflamed bowel wall can perforate, resulting in peritonitis. Toxic megacolon results when the chronically inflamed thin-walled colon loses motility and rapidly dilates. Antimotility drugs, cathartics, or enemas may precipitate toxic megacolon or it may occur spontaneously in patients with severe pancolitis. Toxic megacolon has a poor prognosis: the mortality is from 25 to 40%.

The risk of adenocarcinoma of the colon is greatly increased in patients with UC involving more than the rectum. The risk is increased in pancolitis and in individuals with a family history of colon cancer. The risk of developing colon cancer is seven to 8% after 10 years of UC and 23% after 20 years of the disease. The mortality of colon cancer in patients with UC is greater than 50%.

UC is accompanied by a number of extracolonic manifestations whose course generally parallels that of the colitis. Most of these subside with colectomy. The extracolonic manifestations include erythema nodosum, pyoderma gangrenosum, uveitis, iritis, episcleritis, arthritis and a variety of liver and biliary tract disorders.

Crohn's Disease—A granulomatous disease of the large and small intestine. When confined to the small bowel, it usually is called regional enteritis.

Epidemiology—Crohn's disease is less common than UC. However, it is also more common in Jews and is uncommon in nonwhites. The peak incidence is between 15 and 35 years of age. Both sexes are affected equally. The incidence is rising for unknown reasons.

Etiology—The etiology is unknown but genetic factors appear to be involved and recent evidence implicates a transmissive agent.

Pathology—Chronic inflammation may involve all layers of the intestinal wall and even adjacent mesentery and lymph nodes. The bowel wall becomes thickened and the lumen is narrowed. Stenosis may occur in any part of the small bowel but usually occurs in the terminal ileum. The mucosa eventually becomes ulcerated and the submucosa thickened. Noncaseating granulomas with multinucleated giant cells are found in 25 to 75% of cases. Fistulas, adhesions and abscesses occur. The disease is patchy with normal areas between involved areas. The terminal ileum is the most common site of involvement. One-third to one-half of patients have both large and small bowel involvement.

Pathophysiology—Inflammation impairs the absorptive ability of both the small and large intestine and the thickened bowel disturbs motility. Bleeding is not as severe as in UC because much of the inflammation is below the mucosa, particularly early in the disease process. Fistulas form because the inflammation is transmural. The thickening and shortening of the bowel result in stenosis and strictures. Peritonitis or sepsis occurs frequently.

Signs and Symptoms—The presentation may be acute or insidious. The acute onset presents with right lower quadrant (RLQ) pain, fever, and leukocytosis. Most of these patients recover without sequelae. An insidious onset is more common and is characterized by diarrhea and abdominal pain. Fatigue, weight loss, anorexia and nausea may also occur. The pain is the most prominent feature and is described as steady, crampy or colicky. The diarrhea is of moderate severity and does not contain gross blood.

Laboratory data are nonspecific and show evidence of inflammation. Physical examination is remarkable for RLQ tenderness and mass. Radiographs may show loss of mucosal detail, rigidity, stenosis, strictures, fistulas, and the segmental distribution of involvement.

Several of the complications of Crohn's disease differ from those of UC. Intestinal obstruction occurs in 20 to 30% of patients. Fistula formation is common. Rectal fissures, perirectal abscesses and rectal fistulas are very common. Extracolonic manifestations are similar to those of UC but do not occur as frequently. Patients with ileal disease have an increased incidence of cholesterol gallstones, presumably due to interruption of the enterohepatic circulation of bile acids.

The clinical course of Crohn's disease is variable. Most patients develop one or more complications. A colectomy is not necessarily curative in Crohn's disease of the colon.

Malabsorption

Normal Physiology—Complex foods are broken down to simple molecules by the process of digestion. Acid and pepsin begin the process in the stomach. The enzymes from the pancreas, mainly trypsin, amylase and lipase, continue the process in the upper small intestine. Carbohydrates are absorbed as monosaccharides and disaccharides; protein as amino acids and small peptides, and lipids as fatty acids and monoglycerides. Molecules are absorbed by active transport, passive diffusion and facilitated diffusion. The proximal intestine is the major site of absorption for iron, calcium, water-soluble vitamins and fats. Sugars are absorbed mostly in the duodenum and jejunum. Amino acids and peptides are absorbed largely in the mid-intestine. The terminal ileum is the site of bile acid and vitamin B_{12} absorption. The colon absorbs practically only water and electrolytes.

Carbohydrate Absorption: Starches are split to disaccharides by salivary and pancreatic enzymes. Disaccharides cannot be absorbed and are hydrolyzed to absorbable monosaccharides by disaccharidases in the brush border of the microvilli of the intestine. Monosaccharides such as galactose and glucose are absorbed by active transport; sugars enter the intestinal cell coupled to sodium.

Protein and Amino Acid Absorption: Pepsin digests some protein in the stomach. Pancreatic enzymes (trypsin, chymotrypsin, and carboxypeptidase) digest proteins in the small intestine. Tri- and dipeptidases in the microvilli continue the breakdown of peptides. Dipeptides and amino acids are absorbed along with a small quantity of protein.

Fat Absorption: Long-chain triglycerides are ingested in the diet. Bile acids emulsify the water-insoluble lipids in the small intestine, thereby greatly increasing their surface area and enhancing the activity of pancreatic lipase. In the lipolytic phase, lipase splits the triglycerides into monoglycerides and fatty acids. The effect of lipase, is significantly enhanced by colipase, a protein in pancreatic juice which holds lipase at the surface of the triglyceride droplet. In the micellar phase, fatty acids and monoglycerides are surrounded by bile acids to form mixed micelles. In the mucosal phase, the mixed micelles are not absorbed but the lipid contents are. Lipids are absorbed by diffusion. In the mucosa, long-chain fatty acids (ie, containing C-16 to C-18 fatty acids) are reesterified intracellularly and formed into chylomicrons with lipoproteins, phospholipid and cholesterol. The chylomicrons are secreted by the mucosal cell into the lymphatics. Medium-chain fatty acids (less than 12 carbons) are absorbed directly into the portal venous system and bound to albumin.

Etiology and Pathophysiology of Fat Malabsorption—Disorders which decrease the ability of the pancreas to excrete lipase result in malabsorption of fat. Pancreatic exocrine insufficiency results in the most severe cases of lipid malabsorption. Chronic pancreatitis due to alcoholism and cystic fibrosis are the most common causes of chronic pancreatic exocrine insufficiency. Pancreatic carcinoma may also cause malabsorption if the pancreatic duct is occluded.

A deficiency in bile acids causes a decrease in the activity of lipase. Disorders in which bile acid secretion is impaired contribute to a lipolytic phase defect. Bile acids are synthesized in the liver from cholesterol, secreted into hepatic bile, stored in the gallbladder and delivered to the small intestine. Bile acids are reabsorbed by the terminal ileum. (See discussion of bile acids under gallbladder disease.) Any disorder which decreases the synthesis, secretion or reabsorption of bile acids can result in fat malabsorption by impairing emulsification and micelle formation. A sufficient amount of bile acids is not synthesized in severe liver disease. Intrahepatic cholestasis and occlusion of bile ducts prevent the delivery of bile acids to the intestine. Inflammatory disorders of the terminal ileum and ileal resection decrease reabsorption of bile acids. Bacterial overgrowth in the small intestine causes deconjugation and dehydroxylation of bile acids which may then precipitate and fail to be reabsorbed.

Inflammatory or infiltrative diseases of the small intestine impair the function of the mucosal cells in fat absorption or reduce surface area. These disorders also usually decrease bile acid reabsorption. Disorders of the lymphatics can prevent the delivery of chylomicrons to the circulation.

Malabsorption leads to weight loss. If bile acids are not absorbed by the terminal ileum, they irritate the colon and increase the secretion of water and electrolytes into the lumen, causing diarrhea. The malabsorption of fat-soluble vitamins results in multiple deficiencies. Vitamin K deficiency causes impaired blood coagulation. Vitamin A deficiency causes night blindness. Vitamin D deficiency along with the malabsorption of protein and calcium results in osteomalacia. Malabsorption of protein results in edema formation. The malabsorption of iron, folate and vitamin B_{12} causes anemia.

Signs and Symptoms—The hallmark of fat malabsorption is steatorrhea, which is fat-laden, bulky, yellowish, malodorous diarrhea. The patient may also complain of abdominal distention and bloating. Weight loss ensues. Bleeding tendency or night blindness may be present. Bone pain and pathologic fractures result from osteomalacia. The signs and symptoms of iron, folate or vitamin B_{12} deficiency anemia may be present.

Lactase Deficiency—The absence of the enzyme in the brush border of the microvilli that splits lactose to glucose and galactose.

Etiology—The deficiency is probably inherited. During adolescence or early adulthood the enzyme disappears. These individuals were able to tolerate milk during childhood. This is not an allergic or hypersensitivity reaction to milk proteins. Lactase deficiency occurs in inflammatory bowel diseases and commonly occurs temporarily after an episode of acute infectious diarrhea.

Epidemiology—Lactase deficiency is more common in certain races. The incidence in Caucasians in the US is 10 to 20%. The incidence among American Negros, Africans and Asians is 60 to 90% and the incidence among Jews and American Indians is 60 to 70%.

Pathophysiology—The absorption of water from the intestine is inhibited by the osmotic effect of the lactose retained in the bowel lumen. This results in osmotic diarrhea. Bacteria in the colon digest the lactose, producing gas and small carbohydrate fragments.

Signs and Symptoms—The patient complains of bloating, cramping abdominal pain, flatulence and diarrhea after the ingestion of milk or certain milk products. The amount of milk that is necessary may vary from one to four glasses.

Liver Disease

The liver performs a vast array of metabolic functions. This organ is responsible for most of the synthetic and detoxification processes in the body. The liver is involved in the metabolism of proteins, lipids and carbohydrates. Amino acids are synthesized by the liver to tissue and plasma proteins, mainly albumin. It synthesizes nonessential amino acids and all of the coagulation factors except factor VIII. The liver also synthesizes triglycerides, cholesterol and lipoproteins. Glucose is stored in the liver as glycogen and gluconeogenesis takes place there as well. The liver conjugates bilirubin, a product of hemoglobin metabolism, converting it to a more polar form so that it can be excreted in bile and to a lesser extent in urine. The liver detoxifies and excretes many other endogenous compounds as well as lipid-soluble exogenous substances by utilizing a number of enzyme systems. Conjugation, reduction, oxidation, hydroxylation and deamination are examples of biotransformation reactions occurring in the liver that result in detoxification and excretion of various compounds.

The liver differs from most other organs in that it has two blood supplies. The veins from the gastrointestinal tract and spleen drain into the portal vein which perfuses the liver. The liver is also perfused by blood from the hepatic artery. Blood from both sources mixes and flows through the sinusoids adjacent to the liver cells. Approximately one-fourth of cardiac output normally flows through the liver at a given time. Most of the oxygen requirements of the liver are met by portal blood.

The liver responds to injury in a limited number of ways. Liver cells may undergo necrosis, accumulate fat or exhibit other degeneration. Inflammation may occur throughout the liver or be confined to certain areas, especially portal tracts. Granulomas occasionally form in response to liver injury. Massive necrosis or sustained inflammation and possibly fatty change trigger fibrogenesis which may in turn cause hepatic scarring. The liver possesses a remarkable capacity to regenerate itself if the agent causing the injury is removed. However, if significant scarring has already occurred, the regeneration does not result in restoration of normal liver architecture.

Cirrhosis—A nonspecific term which indicates that the liver is diffusely fibrotic and contains nodules of regenerating liver cells. The architecture is distorted and the vascular bed is contracted. There is a net loss of hepatocytes and the function of the remaining cells is compromised. The condition is irreversible. Because of the numerous functions provided by the liver, patients with cirrhosis are metabolically bankrupt.

Etiology—Various toxins and infectious agents can cause cirrhosis. In some cases, especially those with end-stage disease, it may be difficult to identify the etiology.

The most common form in the US is Laennec's cirrhosis which is due to the chronic consumption of ethanol. The quantity of alcohol consumption required to cause cirrhosis is uncertain but a pint of whiskey or 160 grams of ethanol in any form daily for five to 10 years is sufficient in most cases. Smaller daily doses over longer periods may also cause cirrhosis in some people. Contrary to popular belief, a nutritious diet does not prevent Laennec's cirrhosis.

Postnecrotic cirrhosis may follow infection with Type B hepatitis or the exposure to certain toxins including drugs. Biliary cirrhosis, which is due to chronic impairment of bile excretion, may be either a primary or a secondary condition. Primary biliary cirrhosis is an idiopathic disorder which begins with destruction of intrahepatic bile ductules; cirrhosis is a late development. Secondary biliary cirrhosis is due to chronic obstruction of the common bile duct by gallstones or stricture. A rare cause of cirrhosis is hemochromatosis and is due to iron overload in the liver. Although there is a genetic basis for the iron overload, concomitant liver injury by alcohol is commonly involved.

Pathology—Laennec's cirrhosis is characterized by diffuse fine scarring, hepatocyte necrosis and regeneration in micronodules. Weblike septa or connective tissue divide the hepatic lobules. Inflammation and bile stasis is minimal. Fatty infiltration is present if the patient is currently drinking. The degree of cell necrosis eventually exceeds the degree of regeneration and the liver shrinks in size.

Postnecrotic cirrhosis is characterized by massive loss of liver cells with the development of broad bands of scar tissue. Regenerating hepatocytes form large nodules (macronodules).

Primary biliary cirrhosis is a diffuse necrotizing and chronic inflammatory process around the portal triads with destruction of ductal and portal duct cells. Bile ducts eventually disappear entirely. Secondary biliary cirrhosis is characterized by expansion of portal tracts by edema, fibrosis, and acute inflammatory cells. The fibrosis extends between portal tracts. There is extensive proliferation of bile ducts and bile stasis in hepatocytes and canaliculi.

Pathophysiology—The consequences of cirrhosis are due to portal hypertension and to the loss of hepatocyte function.

Portal hypertension results from increased intrahepatic resistance to blood flow. The increased resistance is caused largely by the fibrosis and expanding regenerative nodules, both of which compress sinusoids and hepatic venules. As portal hypertension progresses, collateral vessels open and deliver blood to the vena cava without passing through the liver. The collateral veins around the rectum form hemorrhoids. Collateral blood flow through gastroesophageal veins causes these veins to dilate (esophageal varices). Periumbilical or abdominal wall collateral veins form the "caput medusa." Since blood is unable to flow through the liver, splenic blood flow increases and the spleen enlarges. Abnormal sequestration and destruction of blood cells occurs in the enlarged, congested spleen, a condition known as hypersplenism. Since blood from the gastrointestinal tract is shunted around the liver in portal hypertension, various toxic products of digestion are not removed by the liver and enter the systemic circulation (see portal systemic encephalopathy below).

Ascites is the accumulation of fluid in the abdominal cavity. The formation of ascites in cirrhosis is a complex process that requires the interaction of several factors. Portal hypertension increases hydrostatic pressure in the portal veins and forces fluid from the veins. Hypoalbuminemia, due to reduced hepatic albumin synthesis, decreases the oncotic pressure that holds fluid within the blood vessels. Hyperaldosteronism causes increased renal sodium and water retention. The fluid retained is driven into the abdominal cavity by the imbalanced hydrostatic and oncotic pressures. The hyperaldosteronism is caused by increased stimulation of aldosterone production by the renin-angiotensin system due to decreased blood flow near the juxtaglomerulosa and by decreased aldosterone metabolism by the liver. There is also movement of lymphatic fluid from the liver across the liver capsule into the abdominal cavity. The exudation is caused by increased intrahepatic vascular resistance.

Portal systemic encephalopathy (PSE) is a complex syndrome of disturbed sensorium and abnormal neurological signs. The symptoms may be acute or chronic. PSE is largely due to failure of hepatocytes to extract and detoxify various neurotoxins because of mesenteric blood bypassing the liver and flowing directly into the systemic circulation and also because of severe hepatocyte dysfunction. Nitrogenous products, particularly ammonia, are not removed by the liver and reach the brain in high concentrations. Ammonia is not the only product involved in PSE. Other substances such as short-chain fatty acids, indoles, and false neurotransmitters such as octopamine also appear to be important. The damaged liver may no longer be producing substances that are necessary for normal brain function.

Decreased catabolism of estrogens results in loss of secondary sexual characteristics and feminization in the male as well as other signs, such as palmar erythema and spider angiomas in both sexes.

Signs and Symptoms—As liver function is lost there is a gradual onset of weakness and fatigue, anorexia, jaundice, edema, and increasing abdominal girth. The signs of PSE usually appear late. The first notable change is often a change in sleep pattern such that the patient sleeps during the day rather than at night. The patient becomes apathetic, forgetful, and confused. Personality changes include irritability and euphoria. Behavior is inappropriate and social graces are lost. Stupor and coma eventually ensue. Neurologic signs are multiple and include asterixis or flapping tremor of the hands (liver flap) when the wrists are extended, inability to draw a star or write legibly, slurred speech, muscular rigidity and hyperreflexia. The electroencephalogram shows nonspecific changes of metabolic encephalopathy.

Gynecomastia, testicular atrophy and loss of body hair occur in the male. Females may have menstrual irregularity or amenorrhea. Spider angiomas and palmar erythema may be noted.

Laboratory abnormalities in end-stage cirrhosis are multiple and include hyperbilirubinemia, decreased serum albumin, prolonged PT and PTT, increased serum ammonia, glucose intolerance, hyponatremia and hypokalemia. Pancytopenia may be present if portal hypertension is severe and the spleen is enlarged.

Primary biliary cirrhosis usually presents with intense pruritus; later dark urine, pale stools, steatorrhea, xanthelasmas, and xanthomas appear. Laboratory data include a markedly increased alkaline phosphatase and a variable increase of serum bilirubin and cholesterol. Antibodies to mitochondria usually are present in the serum. Eventually, the signs and symptoms of end-stage cirrhosis occur.

Laennec's cirrhosis has a poor prognosis. The signs and symptoms of liver failure may become acutely worse during a drinking binge. Mortality is 60% in 3 to 5 years if the patient continues to drink. The fatal event is usually hepatic coma precipitated by bleeding esophageal varices. The prognosis in symptomatic primary biliary cirrhosis is poor with death occurring within 5 to 10 years of the onset of the symptoms. However, the advent of multiple chemical tests from a single blood sample has detected many patients with asymptomic primary biliary cirrhosis by the finding of a greatly elevated alkaline phosphatase. Such patients have not yet been found to have decreased longevity. Secondary biliary cirrhosis may be improved by removal of the obstruction. The prognosis of postnecrotic cirrhosis is variable but longevity is generally longer than it is in patients with Laennec's cirrhosis who continue to drink alcohol.

Gallbladder

The gallbladder stores and concentrates bile and is the usual location of gallstones.

Normal Physiology—The gallbladder fills passively with bile secreted by the liver. The filling process is facilitated by the closing of the sphincter of Oddi between meals which enables pressures within the biliary tree to rise. The gallbladder is not an inert sac. The gallbladder epithelium concentrates bile 10–20-fold by absorbing water. The water absorption occurs passively, mostly in response to active transport of sodium and

chloride. The intact gallbladder epithelium is relatively impermeable to the organic constituents of bile. The gallbladder contracts and empties its concentrated bile in response to cholecystokinin release from the duodenal mucosa during a meal. Branches of the vagus nerve innervate the gallbladder but neuronal stimulation is relatively unimportant in gallbladder emptying.

Bile is a unique fluid. It is an aqueous medium in which large quantities of lipid are dissolved. Bile contains sodium, chloride, potassium, calcium and traces of other electrolytes. Several organic compounds, such as cholesterol, lecithin, bile acids, and bilirubin, are also found in bile. Cholesterol is highly insoluble in water. It is dissolved in bile by incorporation in mixed micelles. These macroaggregates are composed largely of detergent bile acids and lecithin, which together solubilize cholesterol. There is a limit to the quantity of cholesterol that can be dissolved in micelles; the limit is determined by the relative amounts of bile acids, lecithin, and cholesterol. If the quantity of cholesterol exceeds the required quantity of bile acids or lecithin or both, cholesterol will precipitate.

Bile acids are synthesized from cholesterol in liver cells. The primary bile acids, cholic acid and chenodeoxycholic acid, are conjugated in the liver, excreted into the bile and eventually reach the small intestine where they participate in the digestion and absorption of lipids. The terminal ileum actively absorbs approximately 90% of bile acids which are returned to the liver via the portal circulation. This enterohepatic circulation of bile acid maintains constancy of the bile acid pool. The liver synthesizes bile acids to replace the small quantity that is lost in the stool. The bile acid pool undergoes enterohepatic recirculation two to three times with each meal.

Gallstones (Cholelithiasis)—Gallstones are common and constitute the major cause of acute and chronic cholecystitis. In the US most gallstones consist largely of cholesterol. Some consist largely of bilirubin pigment and are more commonly found in patients with hemolytic anemia.

Epidemiology—Approximately 12 million women and 4 million men in the United States have gallstones. Seventy percent of American Indian women of certain tribal origin have gallstones by the age of 30. The incidence of gallstones is increased in individuals who are diabetic, obese, elderly, multiparous, or cirrhotic. The incidence also rises in those who have chronic hemolysis, are being treated with estrogens or clofibrate, or have undergone resection of the terminal ileum.

Pathophysiology—The pathogenesis of cholesterol gallstone formation has been clarified. Failure of cholesterol solubilization leads to precipitation and potentially to a gallstone. Normal people may secrete lithogenic bile (supersaturated with cholesterol) during fasting when bile acid secretion is minimal but all people obviously do not develop gallstones. Nevertheless, certain defects have been identified in patients with cholesterol gallstones. Lean people with gallstones tend to have reduced biliary secretion of bile acids and phospholipid. Obese individuals secrete excessive quantities of cholesterol into bile. Some individuals have a contracted bile acid pool because their bile acid loss exceeds the maximum rate of liver synthesis of bile acids. For example resection or chronic inflammatory disease of the ileum may cause the net loss of bile acids as may the chronic ingestion of the binding resin, cholestyramine.

Once a crystal is formed as a result of cholesterol precipitation from bile, the crystal may grow or several crystals may aggregate. This phase of gallstone formation is poorly understood but appears to involve the entrapment of crystals by gallbladder mucus and the process may be fostered by impaired gallbladder emptying.

Information regarding pigment stone formation is scarce. Many patients have increased bilirubin production as a result of chronic hemolysis. Thus the liver conjugates and excretes increased quantities of bilirubin. Beta-glucuronidase in bile may deconjugate bilirubin, making it less soluble in bile and possibly fostering precipitation.

Gallstones cause morbidity by irritating the gallbladder mucosa directly (cholecystitis) or by impacting in the cystic duct. They may also pass into and obstruct the common duct. Rarely a gallstone erodes through the gallbladder wall and through adjacent bowel. The stone may then obstruct the ileum (gallstone ileus).

Signs and Symptoms—About 50% of patients with gallstones are asymptomatic. The characteristic symptom is epigastric pain that may lateralize to the right side and radiate to the tip of the right scapula. The pain is a severe, aching sensation that is not influenced by body position. The pain begins suddenly, grows in intensity, and disappears rather abruptly. The duration of pain is variable but usually is about two to six hours. Nausea and vomiting may accompany the pain. Jaundice may appear in several days if the stones remain in the common bile duct. Fever and chills often occur with acute cholelithiasis because of infection in the biliary tree. Sepsis may occur. The signs and symptoms of flatulence, bloating and fatty food intolerance frequently attributed to gallbladder disease are not characteristic of gallbladder disease and are more likely to be due to irritable bowel syndrome.

Physical examination in the acute case reveals tenderness, muscle guarding and rigidity over the area of the gallbladder. A mass is rarely palpable. Serum levels of alkaline phosphatase and bilirubin may be increased; WBC count is elevated in infection. Ultrasound or oral cholecystography discloses gallstones in about 95% of cases.

Pancreas

This organ is a vital participant in the digestive process and in glucose metabolism. Diseases of the pancreas are usually expressed as pain or as pancreatic endocrine or exocrine insufficiency.

Normal Physiology—The pancreas is a retroperitoneal organ with both endocrine and exocrine functions. Pancreatic exocrine secretion is under hormonal and neuronal control. Secretin is released by duodenal cells when the pH of the duodenum falls below 4.5. Cholecystokinin (CCK) is released when long-chain fatty acids and amino acids reach the duodenum. Secretin stimulates the secretion of bicarbonate and water by the ductular epithelial cells of the pancreas. CCK and the vagus nerve stimulate the secretion of pancreatic enzymes from the pancreatic acinar cells. The bicarbonate in pancreatic juices neutralizes the HCl from the stomach, providing optimal pH for pancreatic enzyme function.

The proteolytic enzymes of the pancreas are secreted as inactive precursors or zymogens. Another enzyme, enterokinase, is released by the mucosal cells of the duodenum in the presence of bile acids. This enzyme converts trypsinogen to trypsin. Trypsin activates trypsinogen and other zymogens. Trypsin, chymotrypsin and procarboxypeptidase hydrolyze the peptide bonds in proteins. The pancreas also secretes amylase which cleaves polysaccharides to di- or monosaccharides, lipase which hydrolyzes the ester linkages of triglycerides to form fatty acids and monoglycerides, and phospholipase which hydrolyzes phospholipids to fatty acids. The exocrine reserve of the pancreas is large. As much as 90% of the gland must be destroyed before maldigestion occurs.

Etiology—Acute pancreatitis is usually caused by alcoholism, biliary tract disease, or trauma. Rare causes include hyperlipidemia and hypercalcemia. Some cases are idiopathic. Chronic pancreatitis is usually due to alcoholism or cystic fibrosis.

Pathophysiology—Pancreatic enzymes become active in the pancreas and digest the pancreas and surrounding tissue. The initiating event is not clearly understood. The flow of pancreatic enzymes may become blocked within the pancreas or in the duct. The enzymes become activated during the stasis. Some abnormality may cause the reflux of bile and/or activated pancreatic enzymes from the duodenum back into the pancreas. Toxins, particularly alcohol, may result in inflammation of the acinar cells in the pancreas.

Once the process of autodigestion has begun it comes self-perpetuating. The inflammation may be mild or progress to severe hemorrhagic necrosis. Kinins and other vasoactive substances are released into the circulation which cause hypotension. The destruction of the pancreas and enzyme attack on surrounding tissue has been likened to a burn: tremendous amounts of fluid are lost into the peritoneal cavity causing ascites and hypotension. Peritonitis can occur. During fat necrosis calcium is deposited in the form of soaps. This can lead to hypocalcemia and tetany. Because of prolonged hypotension, acute tubular necrosis occurs. Adult respiratory distress syndrome and disseminated intravascular coagulation are among the numerous other complications.

Chronic destruction of the pancreas leads to steatorrhea. Glucose intolerance or diabetes mellitus also occurs. The risk of pancreatic cancer is increased in patients with chronic pancreatitis.

Signs and Symptoms—Acute pancreatitis presents as severe pain in the upper abdomen. The pain is described as a steady, boring pain that radiates to the back or chest. Nausea, vomiting, abdominal distention and fever may accompany the pain. Shock may be the presenting manifestation or an early sequelae.

Physical examination reveals a distressed patient who may be near shock. There is tenderness and voluntary guarding in the upper abdomen. Bowel sounds may be absent. Radiographs of the abdomen may show calcification in chronic pancreatitis. Laboratory examination typically reveals an elevated WBC count, signs of hemoconcentration and increased serum and urinary amylase levels. Serum calcium may be decreased.

The clinical course in acute pancreatitis may be resolution of the edema in a few days, a prolonged illness due to pancreatic necrosis and secondary infection or sudden death from cardiovascular collapse. Chronic pancreatitis may begin as an acute attack and follow a course of recurrent mild attacks. A persistent form of chronic pancreatitis occurs which is unremitting.

Hematology

Normal Physiology-Hematopoiesis

Blood is an organ that performs many functions. It is the transport system for the body. Oxygen, glucose, amino acids, and fats are transported to cells for metabolism. Waste products of metabolism are transported to organs for excretion. The functions of organs and tissues are regulated by hormones transported by blood. Blood cells and proteins are responsible for host defenses against infection and cancer. Blood also has the self-preserving function of hemostasis or clot formation.

In the embryo, the yolk sac is the blood-forming organ until about three months of gestation. The liver and spleen then become the blood-forming organs. These organs do not normally continue to form blood cells after birth. The bone marrow becomes a hematopoietic organ at six months of gestation and continues so after birth. An adult has active bone marrow in the axial skeleton whereas hematopoiesis during childhood occurs in the long boxes. With age the bone marrow in the long bones becomes progressively replaced by fat. In disease states where the need for red blood cells (RBCs) is greatly increased, bone marrow may revert to the infant pattern, increasing RBC production five- to eight-fold. When this compensatory mechanism is also exceeded, the spleen and liver may assume hematopoietic functions. The fetus makes hemoglobin F which carries oxygen more efficiently at low oxygen tensions. At birth hemoglobin F is largely replaced by hemoglobin A although production of hemoglobin F continues throughout life, especially in certain diseases. The fetus has a high RBC count which falls at birth since the increased number of RBCs is no longer needed.

Blood cells follow certain principles of maturation. Bone-marrow stem cells are pluripotential and can become a RBC, WBC, or platelet. During maturation the size of a blood cell decreases. Young cells are capable of protein synthesis while mature cells, except lymphocytes and macrophages, are not. The nucleus in a young cell is large and contains loose fine chromatin. A mature cell has a small nucleus without nucleoli and with dense chromatin. Each blood cell has specific inclusions related to the function of the cell. The number and amount of specific inclusions increases with the age of the cell.

The reticulocyte is the next to last step of maturation. The nucleus is absent in the reticulocyte but some RNA and ribosomes are still present. These are absent in mature RBCs. Reticulocytes are seen in the peripheral circulation and normally comprise 1% of the RBCs. A normal RBC has a life span of 120 days. The production of red blood cells is stimulated by erythropoietin which is synthesized, in part, in the kidney in response to hypoxia. Androgens also increase RBC production probably through their effect on erythropoietin.

The synthesis of hemoglobin requires the heme (porphyrin) pathway, the absorption, transport, and utilization of iron and globin synthesis. These pathways are complex and subject to a number of defects. After the destruction of a RBC by the spleen and liver, all of the components are conserved and recycled.

The granulocytes have the primary function of phagocytosis. Bacteria are prepared for phagocytosis by coating with opsonins, which are primarily antibodies and complement. The specific inclusions in the granulocyte are the lysosomes, which contain digestive enzymes. The band is the youngest granulocyte that is seen normally in the peripheral circulation. The mature polymorphonuclear leukocyte or "seg" has an intravascular life span of 6 to 8 hours. One-half of the WBCs in the periphery are found in the circulation while the other one-half are marginated along the endothelial surfaces of blood vessels. Stress, epinephrine and other stimuli can cause demargination of the WBCs and effectively double the white blood cell count without changing the differential count. In bacterial infections increased numbers of bands are seen in the circulation. This is known as a "shift to the left."

Platelets are very small packets of granules and cytoplasm that function in hemostasis. The megakaryocyte is the precursor cell to the platelet and buds to shed hundreds of platelets. The life span of a platelet is 8 to 10 days.

Lymphocytes are cells of the immune system, which are produced in the bone marrow, thymus, spleen, and lymph nodes. The B-lymphocytes produce antibodies to specific or nonspecific antigens. The T-lymphocytes function in delayed hypersensitivity as well as augmenting or suppressing a variety of immune reactions.

Anemia

Anemia is a clinical state, not a disease, which is characterized by a decreased red cell mass and corresponding reduction in oxygen-carrying capacity of the blood. The hematocrit, or percent volume of packed red cells, hemoglobin, and red-blood-cell count are measured to assess anemia.

Pathophysiology—In a normal state, RBC production equals RBC cell destruction. Anemia may result from decreased production due to a deficiency of components such as iron or co-enzymes, as in vitamin B_{12} and folic-acid deficiency. Anemia also results when RBC production does not respond appropriately to decreased red-blood-cell mass, as in anemia of chronic disease and anemia associated with endocrine disorders. Anemia due to decreased production is seen when the bone marrow no longer produces RBCs, as in myelophthisis, which is a replacement of the bone marrow by cancer cells or granulomas; or aplastic anemia, a state of bone-marrow failure. A measure of decreased RBC production is a decreased reticulocyte count.

Anemia may also result from increased destruction of RBCs. Defective RBCs are destroyed more quickly than normal RBCs. Abnormalities in the red cell membrane, hemoglobin or enzymes may decrease the life span of a RBC. Increases in indirect bilirubin, urobilinogen and reticulocyte count indicate increased destruction of red blood cells.

Some anemias have features of both decreased production and increased destruction of RBCs.

Anemias may also be classified according to cell size and shape. Normocytic anemia is few RBCs but the cell size is normal. Microcytic anemia is a decrease in number and size of RBCs. Macrocytic anemia is a decreased number of RBCs but the RBCs are larger than normal. Hypochromic anemias are those with less than the normal amount of hemoglobin.

Signs and Symptoms of Anemia—The signs and symptoms of anemia are nonspecific. The patient frequently complains of tiredness, weakness, dyspnea on exertion, and easy fatigability. Females complain of menstrual problems, including amenorrhea, irregularity, increased frequency or increased flow. With long-standing anemia, pallor develops which may be detected in the conjunctiva, nailbeds or the creases of the palms. A functional systolic heart murmur may be heard in anemia. If the hemoglobin falls below 8 grams/100 mL, the O_2-carrying capacity of blood is critically decreased and compensatory mechanisms to prevent tissue hypoxia develop. Tachycardia, increased cardiac output, selective vasodilation and redistribution of blood flow occur. Patients with underlying atherosclerotic heart disease may develop angina or CHF.

Iron-Deficiency Anemia—This is an example of an anemia of decreased production due to lack of a component. The cells are typically microcytic hypochromic and have a slightly decreased life span.

Normal Physiology—The average adult consumes approximately 10–20 mg of iron per day in the diet, of which 10 to 20% is absorbed. The iron is absorbed as heme molecules in the stomach or as ferrous ion in the duodenum. Iron absorption can be increased when iron is needed. Iron is conserved and reused. There is no mode for iron excretion. Loss is via desquamated cells from the skin and the gastrointestinal tract. The normal male loses 1 mg per day in this fashion. Menstruating females lose an additional 0.5 to 1 mg iron per day or an average of 17 mg of iron per period.

Most of the iron in the body is found in hemoglobin. Myoglobin and certain enzymes also contain iron. A small amount of iron is found in the serum bound to a transport protein, transferrin. Transferrin is normally only 20 to 45% saturated with iron. Iron is stored in the bone marrow, liver, and spleen as ferritin and hemosiderin. Males store about 1 gram of iron, premenopausal women have only 100 to 400 mg stored. The amount of stored iron determines the ability to meet increased requirements. The average pregnancy requires an additional 700 mg of iron. Children require an additional 1.5 mg iron per day for growth. The loss of 1 mL of blood constitutes the loss of 0.5 mg of iron.

Etiology—Diet inadequate in iron is no longer a problem except in socioeconomically deprived situations. Increased demand of childhood growth, pregnancy or menstruation is the most common etiology for iron deficiency. Occasionally iron deficiency is due to increased demand and decreased absorption of iron in patients with gastrectomy or steatorrhea. Iron absorption may be decreased because of complex formation with phosphates or tannates. The most common cause of iron deficiency in adult males and in women who no longer menstruate is chronic loss of blood. The gastrointestinal tract is the most common site for this blood loss. Diseases such as peptic ulcer, hookworms, gastritis from alcohol or aspirin, hemorrhoids, and gastrointestinal cancer can cause chronic blood loss. Five to 10 mL of blood may be lost each day via the GI tract without the patient noticing it.

Signs and Symptoms of Iron-Deficiency Anemia—The majority of patients with iron-deficiency anemia are asymptomatic. Symptoms correlate with severity of the anemia. Iron deficiency may lead to abnormalities in the epithelial tissue which are seen as a sore or atrophic tongue, sore mouth, angular stomatitis, and thinning or spooning of the nails.

Examination of the peripheral blood usually reveals a microcytic, hypochromic anemia. Calculations of the mean corpuscular volume and mean corpuscular hemoglobin concentration are correspondingly decreased. White blood cells and platelets are normal. Serum iron is decreased and total iron-binding capacity is increased. A saturation index of less than 10% is strongly suggestive of iron deficiency. Serum ferritin is decreased. Bone marrow examination reveals red cell hyperplasia and the absence of iron stores.

Megaloblastic Anemia—This is a disorder of red blood-cell maturation due to impaired DNA synthesis and nuclear maturation. Cytoplasmic maturation is normal. The most common causes of megaloblastic anemia are deficiencies of vitamin B_{12} and folic acid.

Normal Physiology—Vitamin B_{12} cannot be synthesized by man. Dietary sources are animal products and the MDR is 2.5 μg. Ingested vitamin B_{12} forms a complex with intrinsic factor, a glycoprotein produced by the parietal cells of the stomach; the complex is resistant to digestion. The mucosal brush border of the distal ileum contains receptors for absorption of the intrinsic factor–vitamin B_{12} complex. Vitamin B_{12} is transported to the bone marrow and liver where it is stored. An average adult has a 3- to 6-year supply of vitamin B_{12} stored.

Folic acid or pteroylmonoglutamic acid also cannot be synthesized by man. Dietary sources are fresh fruits and vegetables and are susceptible to destruction by cooking. The dietary forms of folic acid are conjugates of polyglutamic acid and require the action of conjugases in the intestinal lumen for conversion to the mono- or diglutamates for efficient absorption in the proximal jejunum. The MDR for folic acid is 50 μg but this may increase in times of rapid growth or pregnancy. Approximately 5 to 10 mg of folic acid is stored in the liver and bone marrow. The active form is tetrahydrofolinic acid.

Vitamin B_{12} and folic acid are involved in the transfer of methyl groups in DNA synthesis. Vitamin B_{12} is required for conversion of deoxyuridylate to deoxythymidylate. Folic acid as tetrahydrofolinic acid is required for two steps in purine synthesis and for conversion of homocysteine to methionine and uridylate to thymidylate.

Pernicious Anemia—This is megaloblastic anemia with achlorhydria and, in some cases, neurologic abnormalities.

Etiology—Heredity plays a role in the development of pernicious anemia as 13% of patients have relatives with pernicious anemia.

Epidemiology—Pernicious anemia is the most common cause of vitamin B_{12} deficiency in the United States. The disease is uncommon in Blacks, Orientals, and Southern Europeans. Both sexes are equally affected. The average age of onset of pernicious anemia is 60 years.

Pathophysiology—It is characterized by lack of intrinsic factor secretion and atrophy of the gastric mucosa. It is currently thought to be caused by an autoimmune reaction against gastric parietal cells. Autoantibodies against parietal cells and intrinsic factor are found in these patients although the cause and effect relationship between these antibodies and pernicious anemia is unclear.

Other causes of vitamin B_{12} deficiency include total gastrectomy, stomach damage due to corrosives, intestinal malabsorption due to inflammatory disease, resection of the ileum and competition for vitamin B_{12} by bacterial overgrowth or the fish tapeworm.

Signs and Symptoms of Megaloblastic Anemia—The nonspecific signs and symptoms of anemia occur. Because of defects in epithelial cells a red, sore, glazed tongue is seen. The neurologic abnormalities consist of numbness, tingling, and loss of vibratory sense in the extremities, loss of position sense, loss of fine coordination, spasticity, irritability, memory loss and mild depression. The GI complaints include anorexia and significant weight loss. Examination of the blood shows oval macrocytes. The red blood cells may be bizarrely shaped (poikilocytosis) and of different sizes (anisocytosis). The reticulocyte count is decreased. The nuclei of the neutrophils have five or more lobes (hypersegmented) and there may be a mild to moderate neutropenia and thrombocytopenia with the platelets, also bizarre in appearance. The bone marrow shows megaloblasts, erythroid hyperplasia, abnormal mitoses in the red cell series, large leukocytes with bizarrely shaped nuclei and decreased numbers of megakaryocytes.

Folic-Acid Deficiency Anemia—A megaloblastic anemia due to folic-acid deficiency that may be confused with vitamin B$_{12}$ deficiency anemia.

Etiology—Most cases of folic-acid deficiency anemia are due to an inadequate diet. Folic-acid deficiency is seen frequently in alcoholics. A dietary deficiency may also be combined with increased demand, as in pregnancy, hemolytic anemia, hemoglobinopathies, myelofibrosis and other conditions. Malabsorption of folic acid occurs in inflammatory small bowel diseases. Certain drugs such as methotrexate, pyrimethamine, triamterene, pentamidine, and trimethoprim inhibit conversion of folic acid to its biologically active form. Oral contraceptives, barbiturates, phenytoin and ethanol inhibit conversion of dietary folic acid to the absorbable monoglutamate.

Signs and Symptoms—In addition to the other signs and symptoms of anemia, the patient with folic acid deficiency may appear wasted. Diarrhea is a prominent complaint. No neurologic deficits are attributed to folic acid deficiency.

Anemia of Chronic Disease—This is seen in association with a number of chronic inflammatory or infectious diseases.

Pathophysiology—The problem in anemia of chronic disease involves a defect which prevents transport of iron from storage depots. The bone marrow does not increase red blood cell production although anemia is present.

Signs and Symptoms—The anemia is usually normocytic normochromic but may be microcytic normochromic or even hypochromic. The serum iron is low and the total iron binding capacity is normal or low. The saturation index is greater than 10%. The serum ferritin level is normal to increased. Increased amounts of iron are stored in the bone marrow reticuloendothelial system.

Anemia of Renal Failure—An anemia, usually severe, that is multifactorial in origin.

Pathophysiology—The anemia of renal failure may be due to iron deficiency because blood is lost from the gastrointestinal and genitourinary tracts in uremia. A hemolytic anemia occurs possibly because of toxins in the blood. Bone marrow is suppressed by the accumulation of toxins. The kidneys are the source of erythropoietin and production of erythropoietin is decreased in chronic renal failure.

Signs and Symptoms—Anemia of renal failure is usually severe with hematocrit values of 15 to 30%. However, patients are not as symptomatic as the severity of the anemia would suggest. The anemia is normochromic normocytic unless iron deficiency is also present.

Hemolytic Anemia

This involves the destruction of RBCs in the blood stream or by macrophages in the liver and spleen.

Etiology—Hemolysis may be caused by a variety of factors. Excessive external trauma, such as marching or jogging or excessive internal trauma such as occurs with a cardiac valve prosthesis may cause hemolysis. Toxins from the venom of a cobra snake, the brown recluse spider and *Clostridium welchii* cause hemolysis. Infections of the RBCs with malaria and bacteremia due to pneumococcus, staphylococcus and *E coli* cause hemolysis. Antibodies may develop toward RBCs as a result of sensitization, exposure to drugs, infections or spontaneously. The RBCs may be made defectively because of an inherited error in metabolic enzyme systems.

Autoimmune Hemolytic Anemia

Characterized by development of IgG or IgM antibodies against the patient's own RBCs.

Etiology and Epidemiology—The disease can occur at any age and may be idiopathic or occur in association with another immune disorder such as lymphoma, chronic lymphocytic leukemia or systemic lupus erythematosus.

Signs and Symptoms—The anemia is mild to severe. The reticulocyte count is increased. Spherocytes are seen on the peripheral blood smear. Bilirubin is increased. Thrombocytopenia may occur. The course is variable but may end in fatal massive hemolysis. The direct Coombs' test is positive. A direct Coombs' test detects IgG, IgM, or C$_3$ coating the circulating RBCs by specific antisera which cause agglutination.

Drug-Induced Immune Hemolytic Anemia

Three types may occur. Methyldopa induces an autoimmune hemolytic anemia identical to the idiopathic form. The antibody is an IgG against the Rh antigen. The direct Coombs' test is positive. There is intravascular hemolysis. Penicillin and cephalosporins produce an hemolytic anemia by serving as a hapten. The hapten forms a complex with the RBC and antibodies are produced against the drug-red blood cell complex. The hemolysis is extravascular. The direct Coombs' test is positive. Quinine and quinidine cause hemolysis by the "innocent bystander" mechanism. The drug forms a complex with plasma proteins and IgG and IgM antibodies form against the drug-protein complex. The antibody-drug-plasma protein complex settles on the RBC and fixes complement. C$_3$ remains attached to the RBC. The direct Coombs' test is positive. Intravascular hemolysis occurs. Hemoglobin appears in the urine and acute tubular necrosis may result.

Hemolytic Anemia Due to Hexose Monophosphate Shunt Defects

Glucose metabolism via the hexose monophosphate shunt increases several times when the RBC is exposed to oxidants. The shunt generates glutathione to protect the sulfhydryl group of the hemoglobin from oxidation. Oxidized hemoglobin precipitates in RBCs, forming Heinz bodies. The spleen removes RBCs with Heinz bodies from the circulation. The most common defect in the hexose monophosphate shunt is a hypofunction of glucose 6-phosphodehydrogenase (G-6-PD) of which there are more than 100 variants. The G-6-PD gene is located on the X chromosome (sex-linked trait).

Epidemiology—The two most clinically significant forms of G-6-PD deficiency occur in Blacks who originated in Central Africa, and in Eastern Mediterraneans, particularly Sephardic Jews.

Pathophysiology—Some patients with G-6-PD deficiency are only symptomatic when the RBCs are subject to the stress of infections or oxidants including drugs such as sulfonamides, antimalarials, nitrofurantoins, etc. Heterozygous women have two populations of cells, one with normal enzyme concentration and one deficient.

Signs and Symptoms—Within a few hours of infection or exposure to a drug, the patient has acute hemolysis. Generally the older RBCs are deficient in G-6-PD and are destroyed. Therefore, the hemolysis is self-limited even if the exposure to the oxidant continues. The Mediterranean form is characterized by more severe hemolysis. The patient has a decreased hematocrit, increased level of unconjugated bilirubin and hemoglobinuria. A test for G-6-PD will be falsely negative if done shortly after a hemolytic crisis.

Sickle-Cell Anemia

The most common congenital hemolytic anemia. It is due to the substitution of valine for glutamic acid on the β-chain of hemoglobin, which results in hemoglobin S (HbS).

Etiology—The disorder is inherited according to Mendelian genetics, so that one-fourth of off-spring from heterozygous parents are homozygous, one-fourth are normal and one-half are heterozygous.

Epidemiology—Approximately 8% of Black Americans are heterozygous or carry the sickle-cell trait. The disease or homozygous form is seen in 0.15% of Black American children.

Pathophysiology—A red blood cell must be able to withstand distortion of shape in order to traverse the microcapillary circulation. A RBC which contains HbS changes from a biconcave disc to an elongated crescent-shaped (sickle) cell on deoxygenation. The HbS forms fibers consisting of stable helical polymers. The sickled cells obstruct capillary blood flow, resulting in tissue hypoxia, further deoxygenation of RBCs and further sickle formation. A small area of ischemia may become a large area of infarction as the process continues. Formation of sickle cells is initially a reversible process but with time RBC membrane damage occurs and the sickle formation becomes irreversible. Patients who are homozygous also have 2 to 20% hemoglobin F, which prevents polymerization of hemoglobin S. RBCs with a high concentration of hemoglobin F do not irreversibly sickle. Any condition that causes hypoxia or dehydration of RBCs increases sickle-cell formation. HbS has decreased affinity for oxygen so the oxygen content of the blood is decreased. Sickled cells are removed from the circulation by the spleen and have an average life span of 15 days. Because of the increased erythropoiesis, folic acid deficiency may develop and worsen the anemia.

Signs and Symptoms. Individuals with the sickle-cell trait, but not the disease, do not usually have significant clinical problems. Severe hypoxia is necessary to cause a sickle-cell crisis in these individuals. A person who is homozygous for sickle-cell anemia develops symptoms at about 6 months of age when much of the hemoglobin F has been replaced. Initial symptoms may be impairment of growth and development, and failure to thrive. Later a severe hemolytic anemia develops.

The mortality and morbidity of sickle cell anemia is related to recurrent episodes of vascular occlusion. A crisis is an episode of sickle-cell formation resulting in severe pain in the chest, abdomen, joints, or other sites. The frequency of the crises varies. A crisis may be precipitated by an infection, or exposure to cold resulting in vasospasm or conditions that lead to dehydration. Many times the crisis is mistaken for an "acute abdomen" and the patient is taken to surgery. Chronic organ damage results from recurrent crises. Lung function is decreased because of recurrent pulmonary infarcts. CHF results from the chronic severe anemia, hypoxemia, and pulmonary hypertension. Gallstones develop because of increased bilirubin turnover. Hepatic infarcts may become hepatic abscesses and if enough liver tissue is infarcted, liver function decreases. The hypertonic, hypoxic, acidotic renal medulla is most susceptible to infarction. After repeated infarctions the ability to concentrate urine is lost. Papillary necrosis also occurs. Prolonged hematuria may result in iron deficiency anemia. Osteomyelitis may develop in bony infarcts. Aseptic necrosis of the femur occurs. Retinal infarcts, vitreous hemorrhage and retinal detachment occur. Chronic skin ulcers are seen on lower extremities. Cerebral vascular occlusion can result in stroke, seizures, or coma. With repeated splenic infarcts, splenic function becomes impaired so susceptibility to infection, particularly pneumococcal, increases.

Blood Dyscrasias

Blood dyscrasias is a term used to indicate a general disorder of the blood. The most common blood dyscrasias include aplastic anemia, agranulocytosis and thrombocytopenia. Many drugs and chemicals have been cited as the causative agents in blood dyscrasias.

Aplastic Anemia—This term is actually a misnomer. A more accurate description is pancytopenia resulting from damaged pluripotent stem cells. It is characterized by an acellular or hypocellular bone marrow.

Etiology—A number of drugs and chemicals have been associated with production of aplastic anemia, including benzene, chloramphenicol, phenylbutazone, gold, and cancer chemotherapeutic agents. Radiation, infectious hepatitis, and other diseases may also be associated with aplastic anemia. Approximately one-half of the cases of aplastic anemia have no identifiable cause.

Signs and Symptoms—The patient complains of progressive weakness and fatigue, mild bleeding from mucous membranes, ecchymoses, and petechiae. The usual signs of infection are not present even though an infection exists. Signs and symptoms of anemia are present. Examination of the blood reveals a severe normochromic, normocytic anemia with no reticulocytes. The white-blood-cell count is low and is comprised mostly of lymphocytes. There is no increase in bilirubin unless liver disease is also present.

Agranulocytosis—Is characterized by a marked reduction or disappearance of neutrophilic granulocytes in the peripheral blood. Severe neutropenia is defined as less than 500 polymorphonuclear leukocytes/mm^3. The incidence of infection directly correlates with the number of PMNs.

Etiology—Various drugs may cause agranulocytosis, including cancer chemotherapeutic agents, thiouracils, phenothiazines, sulfonamides, thiazides, etc.

Pathophysiology—Several mechanisms lead to a decreased number of circulating PMNs. Drugs used in cancer chemotherapy as well as radiation will predictably decrease the production of PMNs. This interference with production is usually reversible when the agent is discontinued, unless precursor cells in the bone marrow have been destroyed. Other drugs decrease production of PMNs in an unpredictable fashion and by an unknown mechanism. These drugs include the phenothiazines, sulfonamides and thiouracils. The decrease in PMNs occurs about 20 days after initiation of therapy with the drug. When the drug is withdrawn the WBC count returns to normal. In some cases the drug may be readministered without problems. Neutropenia may result from increased destruction of PMNs. In severe infections the rate of PMN utilization may exceed the rate of production. Aminopyrine is the prototype for drug-induced granulocytopenia via the "innocent bystander" mechanism. The drug serves as a hapten with plasma proteins and antibodies are formed against the drug-protein complex. The antibody-drug-protein complex settles on the granulocyte and fixes complement. The WBC is removed from the circulation by the spleen. Initially, with increased destruction, production increases but eventually the bone marrow is not able to keep pace.

Signs and Symptoms—The patient may have fever, chills, severe prostration, severe sore throat and oral ulcers. There is no accumulation of pus at the sites of infection.

Thrombocytopenia—A dyscrasia characterized by a platelet count of less than 100,000/mm^3. Spontaneous bleeding occurs when the platelet count is less than 20,000/mm^3.

Pathophysiology—A number of drugs, such as cancer chemotherapeutic agents, gold, ethanol, thiazides, and sulfonamides, can decrease production of platelets. Other drugs act as haptens and induce formation of antibodies against the drug-platelet complex. These include quinidine, quinine, analgesics, antibiotics, sedatives, and sulfonamides. Drugs that cause folate deficiency or aplastic anemia also cause thrombocytopenia.

Signs and Symptoms—The patient complains of petechiae, purpura and ecchymoses over the back, upper chest and limbs and of mucosal bleeding. Blood-filled bullae are found in the mouth. Bleeding may occur from any mucosal surface. Spontaneous bleeding may occur which may last for several days. The most serious site of bleeding is into the brain. Bleeding time is prolonged.

Disorders of Hemostasis

Clotting disorders may result from a defect in any of the steps of coagulation. They may be mild or severe. The coagulation defect may be inherited or acquired.

Normal Physiology—When a blood vessel is cut two events occur to prevent blood loss: (1) platelet plug formation, and (2) blood coagulation. Platelets adhere to the injured vessel surfaces and also aggregate to each other. During adherence and aggregation, platelets assume bizarre shapes with many protruding processes or pseudopods that overlap. The next step in hemostasis is blood coagulation. Either the intrinsic or extrinsic coagulation pathway is activated by the surfaces of the injured vessel or by substances liberated by the traumatized tissue or platelets. This process is complete within less than 10 minutes. The clot is composed of a fibrin meshwork with entrapped blood cells, platelets, and serum. The final step in hemostasis is clot retraction, which expresses the serum from the clot and physically draws the torn edges of the blood vessels together. Clot retraction occurs within one hour. Clots which form in repairing an injured blood vessel are later replaced by scar tissue. Other clots dissolve.

Bleeding Disorders Due to Platelet Defects

Thrombocytopenia may be an adverse reaction to a drug, a congenital defect, an acquired defect or occur in association with other diseases.

Etiology and Pathophysiology—A congenital defect of production can cause thrombocytopenia. A decreased production of platelets occurs when the bone marrow is replaced by fibrous tissue or cancer cells. Vitamin B_{12} and folate deficiency can lead to defective maturation of platelets. In massive splenomegaly, 80% of the platelets are sequestered by the spleen. Increased destruction of platelets is usually antibody-mediated and occurs in systemic lupus erythematosus, chronic lymphocytic leukemia, and Evan's syndrome (thrombocytopenia with autoimmune hemolytic anemia). Congenital defects in platelet adherence, aggregation or ADP release occur. Abnormal platelet function occurs in uremia and liver diseases.

Idiopathic Thrombocytopenic Purpura—This usually occurs in young women. An acute idiopathic thrombocytopenic purpura may occur in children following a URI.

Pathophysiology—IgG which sensitizes platelets for sequestration by the spleen or liver develops so that platelet life span is shortened.

Signs and Symptoms—Consists of purpura over the limbs, upper chest and back, and mucosal bleeding. Onset is sudden. No adenopathy, fever, or malaise is associated with the bleeding. The bone marrow shows a normal or increased number of megakaryocytes. The platelet count is low. The bleeding time is prolonged.

Hemophilia A—This is due to an inherited deficiency of factor VIII activity.

Epidemiology—Hemophilia A is a sex-linked recessive trait that occurs in one in 10,000 people and is the most common genetic coagulopathy. Males and homozygous females have the disease.

Pathophysiology—Factor VIII is a large glycoprotein found in trace amounts in normal plasma. It has three components: clot promoting or antihemophiliac factor activity, antigen, and the von Willebrand factor. Von Willebrand factor is needed for normal platelet function. The defect in hemophilia A is a deficiency of clot promoting activity. The defect may be in the activity of factor VIII rather than the amount.

Signs and Symptoms—In severe hemophilia bleeding is often spontaneous, whereas in milder cases excessive bleeding may occur only after injury or surgery. The severity of the bleeding depends on the degree of Factor VIII deficiency. Spontaneous bleeding occurs into joints and muscles. Recurrent hemarthroses are characteristic of the disease and result in permanent joint damage and deformity. Bleeding into the urogenital or gastrointestinal tracts also occurs. Hemorrhage may occur into any organ and may be fatal. Patients with severe hemophilia do not have a normal life span.

Tests of platelet function, bleeding time, and platelet count are normal. The prothrombin time is normal but the partial thromboplastin time is prolonged.

Vitamin K Deficiency—This results in deficiencies of factors II, VII, IX, and X. Vitamin K is a fat-soluble vitamin found in leafy green vegetables. Stores of vitamin K are limited and deficiency develops in one to three weeks if intake is stopped.

Etiology—Vitamin K deficiency is multifactorial in etiology and involves decreased absorption due to decreased bile acids, impaired intestinal absorption due to inflammatory bowel disease, and changes or decreases in gut flora which synthesize vitamin K.

Signs and Symptoms—The signs and symptoms due to vitamin K deficiency are those signs and symptoms of bleeding seen in other coagulopathies. The prothrombin time and partial thromboplastin time are prolonged.

Liver disease results in coagulopathy due to decreased synthesis of all factors except Factor VIII. Also removal by the liver of proteases or enzymes that inactivate the clotting factors is decreased causing a consumption coagulopathy. The signs and symptoms of the coagulopathy due to liver disease are similar to those of other coagulopathies. The prothrombin time, thrombin time and partial thromboplastin time are prolonged. In addition, hemostasis is further impaired by thrombocytopenia and platelet dysfunction.

Glomerulonephritis

Glomerulonephritis, also known as Bright's disease, is an immunologically mediated inflammation of the glomeruli which involves both kidneys symmetrically. Glomerulonephritis (GN) must be differentiated from interstitial nephritis, which is inflammation of the connective tissue between the glomeruli.

Etiology—The antigen that initiates the immune reaction may be either endogenous or exogenous. Examples of endogenous antigens include glomerular basement membrane (Goodpasture's syndrome) and DNA (systemic lupus erythematosus). Exogenous antigens include group A streptococcus, serum from other species, drugs and possibly viruses.

Epidemiology—Glomerulonephritis is the leading cause of chronic renal failure. Lupus nephritis occurs in two-thirds of patients with the disease.

Pathology—In acute GN, such as post-streptococcal, the glomeruli are swollen, infiltrated with PMNs and there is proliferation of endothelial and epithelial glomerular cells. In severe cases epithelial crescents form in Bowman's capsule. In immune complex GN granular, nodular or "lumpy bumpy" deposits of immunoglobulin are found in the glomeruli. In antiglomerular basement membrane nephritis, antibodies are seen in a linear pattern along the glomerulus.

The pathologic classification of chronic GN includes membranoproliferative, membranous, focal or diffuse proliferative and rapidly progressive GN. A description of the histopathologic features of these forms of GN is beyond the scope of this chapter.

Pathophysiology—All cases of GN are the result of immune reactions. Nearly 95% of the cases involve formation of antibodies against circulating extrarenal antigens. These antibodies are usually IgG and also circulate in the blood. Antigen-antibody complexes are formed when a critical ratio of antibody to antigen is reached in the blood. The complexes become trapped in the glomeruli during filtration, hence the name immune complex glomerulonephritis. The process actually is more complex than simple trapping and involves dysfunction of the mesangial cells, the reticuloendothelial cells in the glomeruli that normally remove foreign materials. The antigen-antibody complexes in the glomeruli activate the complement cascade via the classic or alternate pathways. Activation of complement also activates Factor XII and the clotting system which leads to the deposition of fibrin. Factor XII also activates the kinin system which causes release of chemotactic factors and substances that increase permeability of blood vessels. The inflammatory reaction with the release of lysosomal enzymes damages the glomeruli. Fibrosis ensues.

The remaining 5% of cases of GN are due to development of antibodies against glomerular basement membrane. These antibodies are also active against alveolar basement membrane. The inflammatory reaction is responsible for the damage to the glomeruli and alveoli.

Signs and Symptoms—The hallmarks of GN are gross or microscopic hematuria (RBCs in the urine), proteinuria, and facial, periorbital and pedal edema. These latter two signs are also part of the nephrotic syndrome and will be discussed below. Glomerulonephritis may also be associated with hypertension, fatigue, anorexia, and congestive symptoms such as orthopnea and dyspnea on exertion. The urine may also contain red-blood-cell casts, white blood cells, granular or hyaline casts, and epithelial debris. Chronic GN eventually leads to the signs and symptoms of chronic renal failure.

The onset of acute post-streptococcal glomerulonephritis is manifested typically by oliguria, "coke-colored" or "smoky" urine, bilateral steady flank pain, and malaise. The edema develops in a few days unless fluid is restricted.

The prognosis of acute post-streptococcal GN is excellent in children: 90% recover completely, although the urinary signs may persist for a year. The prognosis for chronic GN is also variable. Some forms progress slowly while others deteriorate rapidly to chronic renal failure.

Nephrotic Syndrome

The nephrotic syndrome is not a disease but a constellation of abnormalities which occur when the glomerular capillary wall becomes permeable to protein.

Normal Physiology—Only small quantities of protein are filtered by normal glomeruli, a situation largely explained by the barriers to protein filtration and the nature of the proteins. The normal glomerular capillary wall is almost impermeable to protein. The endothelium is not a barrier but the glomerular basement membrane prevents filtration of large proteins and blood cells. The podocytes of the epithelium that cover the glomeruli prevent filtration of smaller proteins. The negative charge on the podocytes repels protein molecules. Thus only proteins with a molecular weight of less than 40,000 may be filtered normally by the glomeruli and the tubules reabsorb these proteins so that insignificant quantities of protein appear in the urine.

Etiology—The nephrotic syndrome may be caused by any glomerular disease that involves the basement membrane and/or the epithelial cell foot processes and allows leakage of protein. The most common cause of nephrotic syndrome is lipoid nephrosis. Other causes include glomerulonephritis, diabetes mellitus, amyloidosis, renal-vein thrombosis, collagen vascular diseases, and nephrotoxins such as mercury, gold, bismuth, anticonvulsant drugs, and penicillamine. Tubular disorders may cause mild to moderate proteinuria but do not cause nephrotic syndrome unless a glomerular disease is also present.

Pathophysiology—Large quantities of protein, mainly albumin, are lost in the urine in nephrotic syndrome. In adults the proteinuria is usually 3 to 4 grams per day but may be as high as 30 to 40 grams per day. Albumin synthesis by the liver can keep pace with a 3-gram per day loss if dietary protein intake is adequate. When the loss exceeds the synthetic capacity of the liver, hypoalbuminemia occurs. Hypoalbuminemia results in a decreased oncotic pressure within blood vessels. Decreased oncotic pressure drives fluid from the capillaries into tissues resulting in edema. Loss of vascular fluid volume causes hypotension. The kidneys respond to the fall in blood pressure and volume by retaining sodium and water via the renin-angiotensin system. Up to 20 liters of water may be retained in a futile attempt to restore blood volume as the retained water simply becomes more edema fluid. Proteinuria leads to cast formation in the tubules. These may be seen as hyaline, granular or waxy casts.

Hyperlipidemia occurs in nephrotic syndrome for unknown reasons. Triglycerides, cholesterol and phospholipids increase. Lipiduria also occurs.

Signs and Symptoms—The classical signs and symptoms of nephrotic syndrome are proteinuria (greater than 3.5 gm/m^2/day), hypoalbuminemia, and edema. The edema may be dependent and occur in the feet and ankles, or accumulate in compliant periorbital and facial tissue. The edema occasionally involves the entire body, a condition known as anasarca. The hyperlipidemia and lipiduria may or may not be present and are not essential for the diagnosis. Complications of nephrotic syndrome include hypotension and possibly shock, congestive heart failure, protein malnutrition, and a predisposition to thrombosis.

The prognosis of nephrotic syndrome is related to the prognosis of the underlying cause. However, nephrotic syndrome due to any cause may be fatal if fluid overload is not corrected.

Renal Failure

Renal failure is the inability of the kidney to perform its usual physiologic functions and maintain homeostasis. Renal failure may be classified as acute, subacute or chronic, depending on the time course of events.

Normal Physiology—The kidneys perform many functions. The fluid volume and serum osmolality are maintained by regulation of both sodium and water excretion. The pH of body fluids is maintained within very narrow limits, normally pH = 7.40 ± 0.2. Numerous waste products are excreted by the kidneys.

The normal range for renal function is extremely wide because intake of salt, water and protein varies widely. The normal glomerular filtration rate (GFR) is 125 mL/min and decreases with increasing age. The kidney can excrete 20% of the glomerular filtrate if blood volume is expanded, which means that water intake could be as high as 35 L/day. The obligatory osmolar load requires a urine output of 400 to 500 mL/day. The kidney can excrete as much as 500 mEq of sodium per day or maintain sodium balance if intake of sodium is limited to 5 mEq per day. The kidneys normally excrete 50 to 80 mEq of potassium per day but this figure cannot be reduced even if potassium intake is severely restricted. A person ingesting 70 grams of protein forms 40 to 60 mEq of acid per day. The range of pH compatible with life is 6.9 to 7.6 but the normal range is much narrower. One half of the acid is excreted as titratable acid: Na$_2$HPO$_4$ + H$_2$CO$_3$ → NaH$_2$PO$_4$ + NaHCO$_3$. The other half is excreted by ammonia formation: 2NH$_3$ + Na$_2$SO$_4$ + 2H$_2$CO$_3$ → (NH$_4$)$_2$SO$_4$ + 2NaHCO$_3$. Filtered bicarbonate is completely reabsorbed.

The kidneys are responsible for excreting other waste products. Approximately 20% of filtered phosphate is excreted in the urine. A diet of 80 grams of protein per day results in the formation of 30 grams of urea, which is excreted. The blood level of urea (blood urea nitrogen, BUN) is normally maintained below 20 mg %. The kidneys also excrete uric acid, magnesium, calcium, and other substances to maintain homeostasis.

The kidneys have several endocrine or metabolic functions. They produce erythropoietin, which regulates the red blood cell mass. Renin, which regulates blood pressure and sodium and water balance, is produced by the kidneys. The kidneys degrade gastrin and possibly parathyroid hormone. The kidneys also participate in vitamin D metabolism and thus calcium homeostasis by converting a derivative of vitamin D, 25-hydroxycholecalciferol, to the biologically active form, 1,25-dihydroxycholecalciferol.

Acute Renal Failure—This is most commonly due to acute tubular necrosis (ATN) but may also be due to pre-renal causes and to obstruction of the ureters, bladder or urethra. All excretory renal function is lost within a few days.

Etiology—ATN is most commonly due to ischemia or toxins. Any event which leads to shock and intense vasoconstriction within the renal

vascular bed may lead to ATN. Hemorrhage, hypotension during anesthesia, burns, sepsis, crush injuries, massive intravascular hemolysis, heart surgery requiring extracorporeal oxygenation, and childbirth may cause ATN. Toxins alone or combined with ischemia may cause ATN. These include bichloride of mercury, carbon tetrachloride, ethylene glycol, methanol, myoglobin from crush injuries, and hemoglobin from intravascular hemolysis. Some cases of ATN have no identifiable cause.

Pathology—Ischemia causes patchy necrosis of the tubular epithelial cells and basement membrane. Other areas of the tubule may appear normal. Toxins cause diffuse necrosis of the tubular endothelial cells but do not injure the basement membrane. The glomeruli are spared in ATN unless the injury is severe and prolonged. The lesions are reversible if the patient survives.

Pathophysiology—Immediately after the injury renal blood flow may be reduced by as much as 50% by arteriolar constriction. The fluid filtered by the glomeruli leaks back into the interstitium through the damaged tubules. The subsequent edema of the interstitium increases the hydrostatic pressure, which further decreases renal blood flow and causes the tubules to collapse. Casts of degenerating epithelial cells block urine flow in the tubules and cause further increases in interstitial fluid. The kidneys can no longer maintain homeostasis by the excretion of sodium, water and waste products.

Signs and Symptoms—Oliguria (urine volume of less than 40 mL/day) usually is the first sign of ATN but does not appear until several days after the injury. The urine formed is essentially glomerular filtrate which also contains protein and RBCs. The sodium concentration of the urine is fixed at about 50 mEq/L. Oliguria may not occur but the urine volume may be fixed at 800 to 1200 mL/day. The BUN begins to rise and the pH falls. If fluid therapy is not managed appropriately, hyponatremia and edema develop. Hyperkalemia occurs. The patient complains of nausea and lethargy. Death may occur within a few days because of acidosis and/or hyperkalemia.

During the second week, nausea, somnolence, weakness, and thirst ensue. The BUN continues to rise and the acidosis, edema, hyponatremia, and hyperkalemia worsen. Complications are common during this phase. Pulmonary edema, congestive heart failure and hypertension may develop because of fluid overload. Hyperkalemia may cause cardiac arrhythmias. Metabolic encephalopathy, particularly due to hyponatremia and hypocalcemia, results in neurologic deterioration, convulsions and coma. Anemia due to decreased RBC production, increased RBC destruction and dilution appears in the second week. A nosocomial infection is the most common cause of death in this phase.

During the recovery phase urine volume increases daily. The BUN may continue to rise until urine volume has exceeded 1000 mL per day for several days. Polyuria (urine volume of greater than 3000 mL/day) may develop. Weight loss is rapid as the edema resolves. Since the tubules may not yet be able to conserve water, sodium or potassium, dehydration, hyponatremia and hypokalemia may develop. The diuresis may continue for 1 to 3 weeks. The GFR may never return to normal but the signs and symptoms of renal failure resolve.

Chronic Renal Failure—A loss of kidney function that occurs over a number of years. Azotemia is the accumulation of nitrogenous waste products in the blood which may or may not be caused by renal failure. Uremia is the syndrome of signs and symptoms that is caused by CRF when renal function is less than 10% of normal. CRF is the fourth leading cause of death in the US.

Etiology—Many diseases can destroy renal parenchymal tissue and result in CRF. These include chronic glomerulonephritis, hypertension, diabetes mellitus, polycystic kidney disease, analgesic nephropathy, nephrocalcinosis, chronic pyelonephritis, obstructive uropathy, and interstitial nephritis. In certain patients, more than one disease may have caused the CRF. In some cases it is not possible to establish the cause.

Pathophysiology—CRF develops because the number of functioning nephrons decreases below that necessary to maintain homeostasis. Renal failure and uremia occur when 90 to 95% of the nephrons are destroyed. As renal function deteriorates, hypertrophy occurs in the remaining nephrons, and the amount of solute and water excreted per nephron may increase. Compensatory mechanisms eventually are overwhelmed by even the normal daily intake of water, sodium, potassium, acid and nitrogen. Uremia ensues.

The earliest renal impairment is loss of ability to concentrate urine. This is partially due to the increased solute load per nephron. The patient must then increase water intake to prevent dehydration. The diurnal pattern of water excretion is reversed.

In some forms of renal failure salt wasting occurs early because the kidneys are unable to conserve sodium even when sodium intake is restricted. The osmotic diuresis of the solute load causes an obligatory sodium loss. Hyponatremia and dehydration may occur·and worsen renal failure by reducing the GFR. Salt wasting eventually ceases and the kidneys are then unable to excrete dietary sodium. The sodium and water retention results in edema, congestive heart failure and hypertension.

The serum potassium is normal during the early stages of renal failure. The renin-angiotensin-induced production of aldosterone stimulates potassium excretion and the osmotic diuresis further enhances potassium excretion. Eventually the urine volume may fall below 500 mL/day and serum potassium will begin to rise. Acidosis worsens the hyperkalemia by causing the movement of potassium out of cells.

As renal function deteriorates, ability to form ammonia and therefore excrete hydrogen is impaired. Ability to reabsorb filtered bicarbonate is also impaired. Acidosis ensues.

The percentage of phosphate excreted decreases as the GFR declines. The increased serum phosphate level and other factors described below cause a drop in the serum calcium level. Hypocalcemia stimulates the production of parathyroid hormone which increases renal excretion of phosphate and resorption of calcium from bones. When the GFR reaches less than 20 mL/min, the increased serum PTH level is no longer effective in increasing phosphate excretion.

Hypocalcemia is due to other factors besides the increased serum phosphate. Hypoalbuminemia reduces the quantity of carrier proteins for calcium. Absorption of calcium from the gastrointestinal tract is impaired because of lack of the active metabolite of vitamin D. The ionized fraction of serum calcium is decreased because ions such as sulfate, phosphate, and citrate bind the calcium. The serum concentrations of calcium and phosphate may exceed the solubility of calcium phosphate, which is then deposited in skin, conjunctiva, blood vessels, and joints.

Magnesium levels do not usually rise until the GFR is below 30 mL/min. Uric acid levels usually do not rise above 10 mg % and gouty arthritis is rare.

Urea is not excreted in CRF and the BUN rises. The magnitude of the rise correlates poorly with the symptoms of uremia except for the gastrointestinal symptoms. Increased quantities of urea are excreted into the intestinal lumen, presumably contributing to irritation and ulceration. Urea precipitates in the pericardial sac and causes pericarditis. A uremic pneumonitis which appears as a butterfly pattern on the chest radiograph may occur.

Other presumably toxic substances accumulate in uremia. These include indoles, phenols, amino acids, organic acids, and derivatives of guanidine. The accumulation of carotene-like pigments results in sallow skin color.

A normochromic normocytic anemia parallels the severity of the azotemia. The pathogenesis of the anemia is complex. Decreased RBC production occurs because of bone-marrow suppression by toxins, erythropoietin deficiency and iron deficiency due to chronic GI blood loss. Decreased RBC survival occurs probably because of toxins. The anemia of chronic disease is also found in these patients (see previous discussion).

A bleeding tendency is caused by platelet dysfunction. The accumulation of guanidinosuccinic acid may be responsible for loss of platelet adhesiveness and aggregation.

Osteomalacia occurs in part because vitamin D is not converted to the active metabolite.

Hypertension is exacerbated by increased renin production. Peptic ulcer disease may be caused by the lack of degradation of gastrin.

A peripheral demyelinating neuropathy, mostly in the legs, results in decreased nerve conduction and loss of motor and sensory function.

Renal-failure patients are predisposed to infections because of poor nutrition, pulmonary edema, lack of physical activity, vascular insufficiency, and the number of venipunctures required during treatment. Repeated transfusions increase the risk of viral hepatitis.

Signs and Symptoms—The onset of renal failure is insidious. The first signs may be polyuria or nocturia or both. As renal function deteriorates, the signs and symptoms relate to the organ systems involved.

Fluid accumulation produces the signs and symptoms of edema, congestive heart failure, and hypertension. Hyponatremia causes inability to concentrate the urine, drowsiness, lethargy, psychotic disturbances, stupor, and coma. Hyperkalemia may cause cardiac arrhythmias. Acidosis contributes to nausea, fatigue, malaise, and dyspnea and causes Kussmaul respiration. Hypocalcemia may result in tremor, muscle twitchings, muscle cramps, and convulsions. The increased PTH level leads to the erosive and cystic changes and bone pain of osteitis fibrosa cystica. Calcium deposition in the skin contributes to severe itching, in the eyes to conjunctivitis, in the blood vessels to gangrene, and in the joints to pain. Hypermagnesemia results in bladder retention, drowsiness, muscle weakness, and coma.

The ammonia formation from urea in the gastrointestinal tract contributes to the unpleasant taste, anorexia, nausea, vomiting, and hiccoughs. The pericarditis may cause pain and be detected by

hearing a friction rub. The pneumonitis may cause dyspnea and hypoxemia. Urea in sweat precipitates on the skin and is known as "uremic frost." This may contribute to the itching.

The signs and symptoms of anemia are seen when the hematocrit falls below 15 to 20%. Patients with renal failure experience ecchymoses, epistaxis, and oozing of blood from mucous membranes due to coagulation abnormalities.

The neuropathy results in numbness, tingling, muscular weakness and on occasion paralysis.

The signs and symptoms of uremia progressively worsen. Renal failure is fatal unless the patient is treated by hemo- or peritoneal dialysis or receives a renal transplant.

Acid-Base and Fluid and Electrolyte Disturbances

Acid-base and fluid and electrolyte disturbances can be caused by a wide variety of diseases including the kidney disorders previously discussed in this section. They may also be caused by gastrointestinal (eg, severe diarrhea), pulmonary (eg, chronic obstructive lung disease), or metabolic (eg, diabetes) disorders. The defects observed with these diseases have been described in earlier sections of this chapter.

Normal Physiology—A number of mechanisms act to maintain normal plasma pH (7.35–7.45). One such mechanism is the chemical buffering by extra- and intracellular buffer systems. These include hemoglobin, plasma proteins, and the carbonic acid-bicarbonate buffer system. Hydrogen ions (H^+) migrate into or out of cells in exchange for potassium (K^+) to maintain electrical neutrality. The respiratory system contributes through the exchange of carbon dioxide (an acid). Lastly, the kidneys help to maintain normal pH through the elimination or conservation of H^+ and bicarbonate (HCO_3^-). Each of these mechanisms act to maintain a constant HCO_3:CO_2 ratio of approximately 20:1. As long as this ratio is maintained, the pH will be 7.4 (see Chapter 17).

The human body is largely comprised of water. Fifty to sixty percent of total body weight is water. Body water is distributed between the intracellular space (intracellular fluid or ICF) and the extracellular space (extracellular fluid or ECF). Two-thirds of all body water is contained in the ICF and the remaining $1/3$ in the ECF. The ECF is further divided into intravascular fluid (IVF) and interstitial fluid (ISF) containing $1/4$ and $3/4$, respectively. Electrolytes are unequally divided between ICF and ECF. Potassium is the major ICF cation and phosphate, sulfate, and organic ions are the ICF anions. Sodium is the major ECF cation and chloride and bicarbonate are the ECF anions. Although water moves readily in and out of cells, electrolytes do not, often requiring active transport. While electrolyte concentrations vary between the ICF and ECF, osmolarity is equal.

Water homeostasis is regulated by the interrelationships between water intake, kidney function, and water loss through the lungs, skin and gastrointestinal tract. A decrease in ECF volume or an increase in osmotic pressure of plasma both stimulate water intake. The kidneys act to preserve water homeostasis through their relationship to antidiuretic hormone (ADH) which was discussed in the endocrine section. ADH release is under the control of both osmotic and volume factors. Increased osmotic pressure or decreased ECF volume stimulate increased ADH production and secretion. The glomeruli of the kidney filter all blood delivered to them. Thus the glomerular filtration rate (GFR) is normally 125 mL/min. The GFR is affected by renal blood flow, hydrostatic pressure in Bowman's space and plasma protein concentration. Essentially everything in the plasma, except protein, is filtered. The kidney tubules both resorb and secrete solutes via active transport and passive diffusion. Almost all water (90%) and electrolytes initially filtered are reabsorbed by active transport in the tubules and Henle's loop. Ammonia and urea are secreted into the filtrate.

Pathophysiology—Acid-base disorders may be divided into respiratory acidosis and alkalosis and metabolic acidosis and alkalosis. Respiratory acidosis is associated with disorders that cause an impairment of gas exchange and thus CO_2 retention. Arterial blood gases (ABG's) show a decreased pH, elevated pCO_2 (dissolved CO_2 gas) and elevated bicarbonate. Respiratory alkalosis is caused by conditions that result in hyperventilation with an abnormally large loss of CO_2. ABG's reflect an increased pH and decreased pCO_2 and HCO_3^-. Metabolic acidosis occurs secondary to either the addition of acid or a loss of bicarbonate. Acids may be endogenous, as in the case of diabetic ketoacidosis or exogenous, as in the case of methanol ingestion. Bicarbonate may be lost through diarrhea or through the kidney as in renal tubular acidosis. ABG's show low pH, HCO_3 and PCO_2. Calculation of the anion gap [(Na^+)—(Cl^-+HCO_3^-)] is helpful in determining whether metabolic acidosis is due to addition of acid or loss of HCO_3^-. The normal anion gap is 10 to 12 mEq/L and is elevated when acidosis is due to addition of acid. Metabolic alkalosis is usually due to the loss of acid (H^+) but may occasionally occur with excessive HCO_3^- ingestion. It is characterized by elevated pH and HCO_3^-.

Once one of the above conditions occurs, the body compensates with another. For example, in cases of metabolic acidosis, the body compensates with increased respiratory activity thus removing CO_2 and thereby increasing pH.

The causes of fluid and electrolyte imbalances are many. Such derangements may be interrelated, occurring together, or may occur independently. Fluid losses occur with such gastrointestinal disorders as vomiting and diarrhea. In such cases, electrolytes are lost with the water. In others, the losses of electrolytes and water are not proportional resulting in hypo- or hyperosmolarity. In the various renal disorders, a number of fluid and electrolyte shifts are common. In nephrotic syndrome, large volumes of fluid are lost due to lack of reabsorption. In acute renal failure, large shifts of water are often involved. This water is not necessarily lost from the body but may be lost from the vascular compartment, frequently in the form of edema. In addition to the fluid shifts, electrolyte disturbances ensue. Secondary to decreased renal blood flow and thus, decreased glomerular filtration rate, the renin-angiotensin system is activated causing further fluid retention. The specifics of renal disease associated fluid and electrolyte disturbances have been described in greater detail earlier in this section.

Signs and Symptoms—Signs of dehydration include decreased skin turgor, dry mucous membranes, lack of tearing, hypotension and cloudy sensorium. Excessive hypovolemia can result in shock. Fluid excess may be manifested by edema, hypertension or ultimately congestive heart failure. Of all electrolyte disturbances, only one of the more serious, that involving K^+, will be discussed here. Others have been discussed in previous sections. Signs of hyperkalemia include muscle weakness and cardiac dysrhythmias. Severe hyperkalemia results in cardiac standstill. Hypokalemia may also be reflected as muscle weakness. Abdominal distress may occur from impaired intestinal smooth muscle mobility. Abdominal distention and depressed deep tendon reflexes may be evident. Cardiac rhythm disturbances also occur with hypokalemia.

The measurement of ABG's, plasma electrolytes, urine output and electrolytes, and blood pressure are all helpful in assessing a patient with acid-base or fluid and electrolyte disorders.

Bibliography

1. Petersdorf RG, *et al.*, eds: *Harrison's Principles of Internal Medicine*, 10th ed, McGraw-Hill, New York, 1983.
2. Sleisenger MH, Fordtran JS, eds: *Gastrointestinal Disease*, 3rd ed, Saunders, Philadelphia, 1983.
3. Hurst JW, ed: *The Heart*, 5th ed, McGraw-Hill, New York, 1982.
4. Hoeprich FP, ed: *Infectious Diseases*, 3rd ed, Harper and Row, Hagerstown, MD, 1983.
5. Gilman AG, Goodman LS, Gilman A, eds: *The Pharmacologic Basis of Therapeutics*, 6th ed, Macmillan, New York, 1980.
6. Fishman AP, ed: *Pulmonary Diseases and Disorders*, McGraw-Hill, New York, 1980.

CHAPTER 37

Drug Absorption, Action, and Disposition

Stewart C Harvey, PhD
Professor of Pharmacology
School of Medicine, University of Utah
Salt Lake City, UT 84132

Although drugs differ widely in their pharmacodynamic effects and clinical application, in penetrance, absorption, and usual route of administration, in distribution among the body tissues, and in disposition and mode of termination of action, there are certain general principles that help explain these differences. These principles have both pharmaceutic and therapeutic implications. They facilitate an understanding of both the features that are common to a class of drugs and the differentia among the members of that class.

In order for a drug to act it must be absorbed, transported to the appropriate tissue or organ, penetrate to the responding subcellular structure, and elicit a response or alter ongoing processes. The drug may be simultaneously or sequentially distributed to a number of tissues, bound or stored, metabolized to inactive or active products, or excreted. The history of a drug in the body is summarized in Fig 37-1. Each of the processes or events depicted relates importantly to therapeutic and toxic effects of a drug and to the mode of administration, and drug design must take each into account. Since the effect elicited by a drug is its *raison d'etre*, *drug action* and *effect* will be discussed first in the text that follows, even though they are preceded by other events.

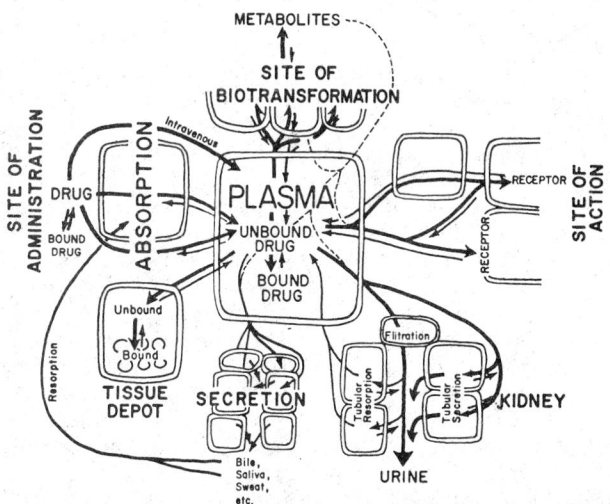

Fig 37-1. The absorption, distribution, action, and elimination of a drug (arrows represent drug movement). Intravenous administration is the only process whereby a drug may enter a compartment without passing through a biological membrane. Note that drugs excreted in bile and saliva may be resorbed.

Drug Action and Effect

The word *drug* imposes an action–effect context within which the properties of a substance are described. The description must of necessity include the pertinent properties of the recipient of the drug. Thus, when a drug is defined as an analgesic, it is implied that the recipient reacts in a certain way, called pain,* to a noxious stimulus. Both because the pertinent properties are locked into the complex and somewhat imprecise biological context and because the types of possible response are many, descriptions of the properties of drugs tend to emphasize the qualitative features of the effects they elicit. Thus a drug may be described as having analgesic, vasodepressor, convulsant, antibacterial, etc, properties. The specific effect (or use) categories into which the many drugs may be placed are the subject of Chapters 40 through 67 and will not be elaborated upon in this chapter. However, the description of a drug does not end with the enumeration of the responses it may elicit. There are certain intrinsic properties of the drug–recipient system that can be described in quantitative terms and which are essential to the full description of the drug and to the validation of the drug for specific uses. Under *Definitions and Concepts*, below, certain general terms are defined in qualitative language; under *Dose–Effect Relationships* the foundation is laid for an appreciation of some of the quantitative aspects of pharmacodynamics.

Definitions and Concepts

In the field of pharmacology, the vocabulary that is unique to the discipline is relatively small, and the general vocabulary is that of the biological sciences and chemistry. Nevertheless, there are a few definitions that are important to the proper understanding of pharmacology. It is necessary to differentiate among action, effect, selectivity, dose, potency, and efficacy.

Action vs Effect—The *effect* of a drug is an *alteration of function* of the structure or process upon which the drug acts. It is common to use the term action as a synonym for effect. However, action precedes effect. *Action* is the *alteration of condition* that brings about the effect.

The final effect of a drug may be far removed from its site of action. For example, the diuresis subsequent to the ingestion of ethanol does not result from an action on the kidney but instead from a depression of activity in the supraopticohypophyseal region of the hypothalamus, which regulates the release of antidiuretic hormone from the posterior pituitary gland. The alteration of supraopticohypophyseal function is, of course, also an effect of the drug, as is each subsequent change in the chain of events leading to diuresis. The action of ethanol was exerted only at the initial step, each subsequent effect being then the action to a following step.

Multiple Effects—No known drug is capable of exerting a single effect, although a number are known that appear to have a single mechanism of action. Multiple effects may

---

* Sophisticated studies indicate that pain is not simply the *perception* of a certain kind of stimulus but rather a *reaction* to the perception of a variety of kinds of stimuli or stimulus patterns.

derive from a single mechanism of action. For example, the inhibition of acetylcholinesterase by physostigmine will elicit an effect at every site where acetylcholine is produced, is potentially active, and is hydrolyzed by cholinesterase. Thus physostigmine elicits a constellation of effects.

A drug can also cause multiple effects at several different sites by a single action at only one site, providing that the function initially altered at the site of action ramifies to control other functions at distant sites. Thus a drug that suppresses steroid synthesis in the liver may not only lower serum cholesterol, impair nerve myelination and function, and alter the condition of the skin (as a consequence of cholesterol deficiency) but also may affect digestive functions (because of a deficiency in bile acids) and alter adrenocortical and sexual hormonal balance.

Although a single action can give rise to multiple effects, most drugs exert multiple actions. The various actions may be related, as, for example, the sympathomimetic effects of metaraminol that accrue to its structural similarity to norepinephrine and its ability partially to suppress sympathetic responses because it occupies the catecholamine storage pools in lieu of norepinephrine; or the actions may be unrelated, as with the actions of morphine to interfere with the release of acetylcholine from certain autonomic nerves, to block some actions of 5-hydroxytryptamine (serotonin), and to release histamine. Many drugs bring about immunologic (allergic or hypersensitivity) responses that bear no relation to the other pharmacodynamic actions of the drug.

Selectivity—Despite the potential most drugs have for eliciting multiple effects, one effect is generally more readily elicitable than another. This differential responsiveness is called *selectivity*. It is usually considered to be a property of the drug, but it is also a property of the constitution and biodynamics of the recipient subject or patient.

Selectivity may come about in several ways. The subcellular structure (receptor) with which a drug combines to initiate one response may have a higher affinity for the drug than that for some other action; atropine, for example, has a much higher affinity for muscarinic receptors (page 876) that subserve the function of sweating than it does for the nicotinic receptors (page 876) that subserve voluntary neuromuscular transmission, so that suppression of sweating can be achieved with only a tiny fraction of the dose necessary to cause paralysis of the skeletal muscles. A drug may be distributed unevenly, so that it reaches a higher concentration at one site than generally throughout the tissues; chloroquine is much more effective against hepatic than intestinal (colonic) amebiasis because it reaches a many times higher concentration in the liver than in the wall of the colon. An affected function may be much more critical to or have less reserve in one organ than in another, so that a drug will be predisposed to elicit an effect at the more critical site; some inhibitors of dopa decarboxylase (which is also 5-hydroxytryptophan decarboxylase) depress the synthesis of histamine more than that of either norepinephrine or 5-hydroxytryptamine (serotonin), even though histidine decarboxylase is less sensitive to the drug, simply because histidine decarboxylase is the only step and hence is rate-limiting in the biosynthesis of histamine. Dopa decarboxylase is not rate-limiting in the synthesis of either norepinephrine or 5-hydroxytryptamine until the enzyme is nearly completely inhibited. Another example of the determination of selectivity by the critical balance of the affected function is that of the mercurial diuretic drugs. An inhibition of only 1% in the tubular resorption of glomerular filtrate will usually double urine flow, since 99% of the glomerular filtrate is normally resorbed; aside from the question of the possible concentration of diuretics in the urine, a drug-induced reduction of 1% in sulfhydryl enzyme activity in tissues other than the kidney is not usually accompanied by an observable change in function. Selectivity also can be determined by the pattern of distribution of destructive or activating enzymes among the tissues and by other factors.

Dose—Even the uninitiated person knows that the *dose* of a drug is the amount administered. However, the appropriate dose of a drug is not some unvarying quantity, a fact sometimes overlooked by pharmacists, official committees, and physicians, and the practice of pharmacy is entrapped in a system of fixed-dose formulations, so that fine adjustments in dosage are often difficult to achieve. Fortunately, there is usually a rather wide latitude allowable in dosages. It is obvious that the size of the recipient individual should have a bearing upon the dose, and the physician may elect to administer the drug on a body-weight basis rather than as a fixed dose. Usually, however, a fixed dose is given to all adults, unless the adult is exceptionally large or small. The dose for infants and children is often determined by one of several formulas which take into account age or weight, depending on the age group of the child and the type of action exerted by the drug. Infants are relatively more sensitive to many drugs, often because enzyme systems which destroy the drugs may not be fully developed in the infant.

The nutritional condition of the patient, the mental outlook, the presence of pain or discomfort, the severity of the condition being treated, the presence of secondary disease or pathology, genetic, and many other factors affect the dose of a drug necessary to achieve a given therapeutic response or to cause an untoward effect (Chapter 69). Even two apparently well-matched normal persons may require widely different doses for the same intensity of effect. Furthermore, a drug is not always employed for the same effect and hence not in the same dose. For example, the dose of a progestin necessary for an oral contraceptive effect is considerably different from that necessary to prevent spontaneous abortion, and a dose of an estrogen for the treatment of the menopause is much too small for the treatment of prostatic carcinoma.

From the above it is evident that the wise physician knows that *the dose of a drug is "enough"* (ie, no rigid quantity but rather that which is necessary and can be tolerated) and individualizes his regimen accordingly. The wise pharmacist will also appreciate this dictum and recognize that official or manufacturer's recommended doses are sometimes quite narrowly defined and may be very wide of the mark. They should serve only as a useful guide rather than as an imperative.

Potency and Efficacy—The *potency* of a drug is the reciprocal of dose. Thus it will have the units of persons/unit weight of drug or body weight/unit weight of drug, etc. Potency generally has little utility other than to provide a means of comparing the relative activities of drugs in a series, in which case *relative potency*, relative to some prototype member of the series, is a parameter commonly used among pharmacologists and in the pharmaceutical industry.

Whether a given drug is more potent than another has little bearing on its clinical usefulness, provided that the potency is not so low that the size of the dose is physically unmanageable or the cost of treatment is higher than with an equivalent drug. If a drug is less potent but more selective, then it is the one to be preferred. Promotional arguments in favor of a more potent drug are thus irrelevant to the important considerations that should govern the choice of a drug. However, it sometimes occurs that drugs of the same class differ in the maximum intensity of effect; that is, some drugs of the class may be less efficacious than others, irrespective of how large a dose is used.

Efficacy connotes the property of a drug to achieve the desired response, and *maximum efficacy* denotes the maximum achievable effect. Even huge doses of codeine often cannot achieve the relief from severe pain that relatively small doses of morphine can; thus codeine is said to have a lower maximum efficacy than morphine. Efficacy is one of the primary determinants of the choice of a drug.

Dose–Effect Relationships

The importance of knowing how changes in the intensity of response to a drug vary with the dose is virtually self-evident. Both the physician, who prescribes or administers a drug, and the manufacturer, who must package the drug in appropriate dose sizes, must translate such knowledge into everyday practice. Theoretical or molecular pharmacologists also study such relationships in inquiries into mechanism of action and receptor theory (see page 718). It is necessary to define two types of relationship: (1) the dose–intensity relationship—ie, the manner in which the intensity of effect in the individual recipient relates to dose—and (2) dose–frequency relationship—ie, the manner in which the number of responders among a population of recipients relates to dose.

Dose–Intensity of Effect Relationships—Whether the intensity of effect is determined *in vivo* (eg, the blood-pressure response to epinephrine in the human patient) or *in vitro* (eg, the response of the isolated guinea pig ileum to histamine), the dose–intensity of effect (often called dose-effect) curve usually has a characteristic shape, namely a curve that closely resembles one quadrant of a rectangular hyperbola.

In the dose–intensity curve depicted in Fig 37-2, the curve appears to intercept the *x* axis at 0 only because the lower doses are quite small on the scale of the abscissa, the smallest dose being 1.5×10^{-3} µg. Actually, the *x* intercept has a positive value, since a finite dose of drug is required to bring about a response, this lowest effective dose being known as the *threshold dose*. Statistics and chemical kinetics predict that the curve should approach the *y* axis asymptotically. However, if the intensity of the measured variable does not start from zero, the curve may possibly have a positive *y* intercept (or negative *x* intercept), especially if the ongoing basal activity before the drug is given is closely related to that induced by the drug.

In practice, instead of an asymptote to the *y* axis, dose–intensity curves nearly always show an upward concave foot at the origin of the curve, so that the curve has a lopsided sigmoid shape. At high doses the curve approaches an asymptote which is parallel to the *x* axis, and the value of the asymptote establishes the maximum possible response to the drug, or *maximum efficacy*. However, experimental data in

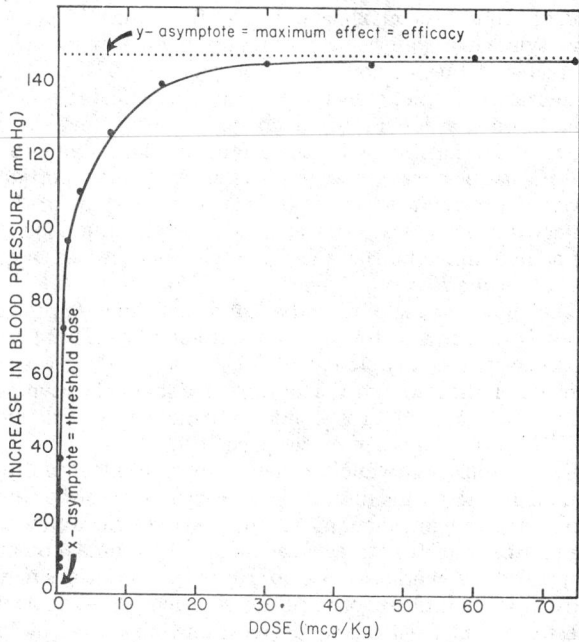

Fig 37-2.   The relationship of the intensity of the blood-pressure response of the cat to the intravenous dose of levarterenol.

the regions of the asymptotes are generally too erratic to permit an exact definition of the curve at the very low and very high doses. The example shown represents an unusually good set of data.

Because the dose range may be 100 or 1000 fold from the lowest to the highest dose, it has become the practice to plot dose–intensity curves on a logarithmic scale of abscissa; ie, to plot the log of dose vs the intensity of effect. Fig 37-3 is such a semilogarithmic plot of the same data as in Fig 37-2. In the figure the intensity of effect is plotted both in absolute units (at the left) or in relative units, as percent (at the right).

Although no new information is created by a semilogarithmic representation, the curve is stretched out in such a way as to facilitate the inspection of the data; the comparison of results from multiple observations and the testing of different drugs is also rendered easier. In the example shown, the curve is essentially what is called a *sigmoid curve* and is nearly symmetrical about the point which represents an intensity

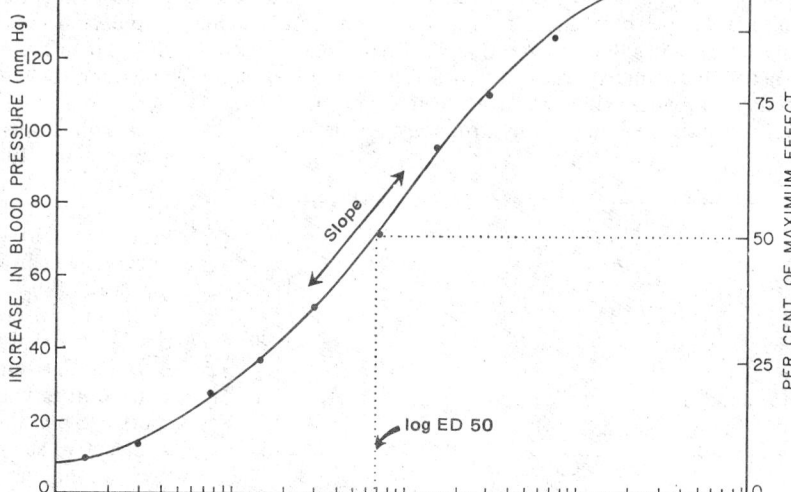

Fig 37-3.   The relationship of the intensity of the blood-pressure response of the cat to the log of the intravenous dose of levarterenol.

equal to 50% of the maximal effect, ie, about the mid-point. The symmetry follows from the rectangular hyperbolic character of the previous Cartesian plot (Fig 37-2). The semilogarithmic plot reveals better the dose–effect relationships in the low-dose range, which are lost in the steep slope of the Cartesian plot. Furthermore, the data about the mid-point are almost a straight line; the nearly linear portion covers approximately 50% of the curve. The slope of the "linear" portion of the curve, or, more correctly, the slope at the point of inflection, has theoretical significance (see *Drug Receptors and Receptor Theory*, page 718).

The upper portion of the curve approaches an asymptote, which is the same as that in the Cartesian plot. If the response system is completely at rest before the drug is administered, the lower portion of the curve should be asymptotic to the x axis. Both asymptotes and the symmetry derive from the law of mass action (see page 719).

Dose–intensity curves often deviate from the ideal configuration illustrated and discussed above. Usually, the deviate curve remains sigmoid but not extended symmetrically about the mid-point of the "linear" segment. Occasionally other shapes occur, sometimes quite bizarre ones. Deviations may derive from multiple actions that converge upon the same final effector system, from varying degrees of metabolic alteration of the drug at different doses, from modulation of the response by feedback systems, from nonlinearity in the relationship between action and effect, or from other causes.

It is frequently necessary to identify the dose which elicits a given intensity of effect. The intensity of effect that is generally designated is the 50% of maximum intensity. The corresponding dose is called the *50% effective dose*, or *individual ED50* (see Fig 37-3). The use of the adjective *individual* distinguishes the ED50 based upon the intensity of effect from the median effective dose, also abbreviated ED50, determined from frequency of response data in a population (see *Dose–Frequency Relationships*, this page).

Drugs that elicit the same quality of effect may be graphically compared. In Fig 37-4, five hypothetical drugs are compared. Drugs *A*, *B*, *C*, and *E* can all achieve the same maximum effect, which suggests that the same effector system may be common to all. *D* may possibly be working through the same effector system, but there are no *a priori* reasons to think this is so. Only *A* and *B* have parallel curves and common slopes. Common slopes are consistent with but in no way prove, the idea that *A* and *B* not only act through the same effector system but also by the same mechanism. Although drug–receptor theory (see *Drug Receptors and Receptor Theory*, page 718) requires that the curves of identical mechanism have equal slopes, examples of exceptions are known. Furthermore, mass-law statistics require that all simple drug-receptor interactions generate the same slope; only when slopes depart from this universal slope in accordance with distinctive characteristics of the response system do slopes provide evidence of specific mechanisms.

The relative potency of any drug may be obtained by di-

viding the ED50 of the standard or prototype drug by that of the drug in question. Any level of effect other than 50% may be used, but it should be recognized that when the slopes are not parallel, the relative potency depends upon the intensity of effect chosen. Thus the potency of *A* relative to *C* (in Fig 37-4) calculated from the ED50 will be smaller than that calculated from the ED25.

The low maximum intensity inducible by *D* poses even more complications in the determination of relative potency than do the unequal slopes of the other drugs. If its dose–intensity curve is plotted in terms of percent of its own maximum effect, its relative inefficacy is obscured, and the limitations of relative potency at the ED50 level will not be evident. This dilemma simply underscores the fact that drugs can better be compared from their entire dose–intensity curves than from a single derived number like ED50 or relative potency.

Drugs that elicit multiple effects will generate a dose–intensity curve for each effect. Even though the various effects may be qualitatively different, the several curves may be plotted together on a common scale of abscissa, and the intensity may be expressed in terms of percent of maximum effect; thus all curves can share a common scale of ordinates in addition to common abscissa. Separate scales of ordinates could be employed, but would make it harder to compare data.

The selectivity of a drug can be determined by noting what percent of maximum of one effect can be achieved before a second effect occurs. As with relative potency, selectivity may be expressed in terms of the ratio between the ED50 for one effect to that for another effect, or a ratio at some other intensity of effect. Similarly to relative potency, difficulties follow from nonparallelism. In such instances, selectivity expressed in dose ratios varies from one intensity level to another.

When the dose–intensity curves for a number of subjects are compared, it is found that they vary considerably from individual to individual in many respects: threshold dose, mid-point, maximum intensity, etc, and sometimes even slope. By averaging the intensities of the effect at each dose, an average dose–intensity curve can be constructed.

Average dose–intensity curves enjoy a limited application in comparing drugs. A single line expressing an average response has little value in predicting individual responses unless it is accompanied by some expression of the range of the effect at the various doses. This may be done by indicating the standard error of the response at each dose. Occasionally, a simple scatter diagram is plotted in lieu of an average curve and statistical parameters (see Fig 10-2, page 106). An average dose–intensity curve may also be constructed from a population in which different individuals receive different doses; if sufficiently large populations are employed, the average curves determined by the two methods will approximate each other.

It is obvious that the determination of such average curves from a population sufficiently large to be statistically meaningful requires a great deal of work. Retrospective clinical data occasionally are treated in this way, but prospective studies are infrequently designed in advance to yield average curves. The usual practice in comparing drugs is to employ a quantal (all-or-none) end point and to plot the frequency or cumulative frequency of response over the dose range, as discussed below.

Dose–Frequency of Response Relationships—When an end point is truly all-or-none, such as death, it is an easy matter to plot the number of responding individuals (eg, dead subjects) at each dose of drug or intoxicant. Many other responses that vary in intensity can be treated as all-or-none if simply the presence or absence of a response (eg, cough or no cough, convulsion or no convulsion, etc) is recorded,

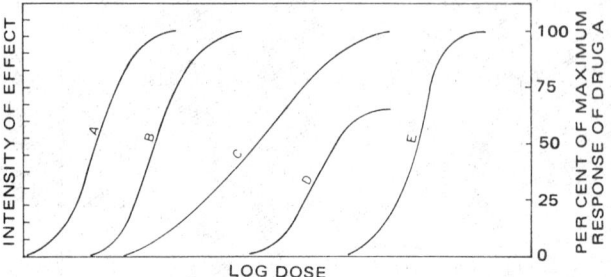

Fig 37-4.   Log dose–intensity of effect curves of five different hypothetical drugs (see text for explanation).

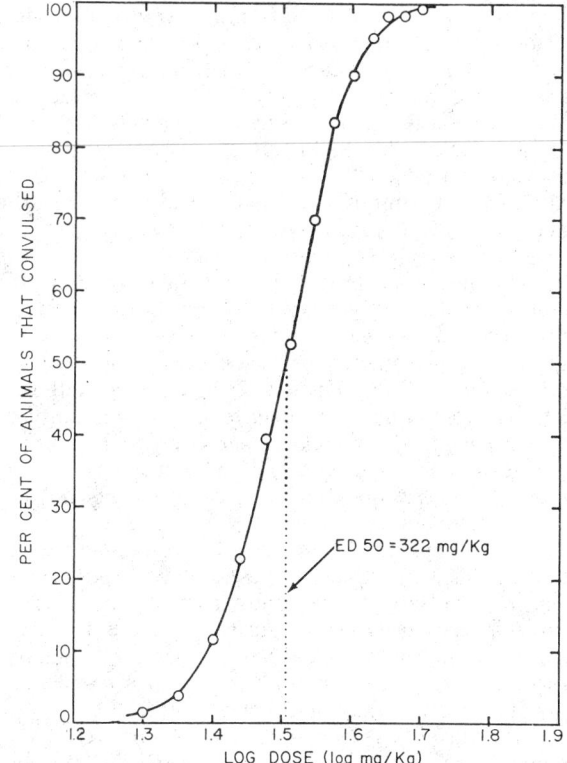

Fig 37-5.   The relationship of the number of responders in a population of mice to the dose of pentylenetetrazol (courtesy, Drs DG McQuarry and EG Fingl, University of Utah).

without regard to the intensity of the response when it occurs.

When the response grades from the basal or control state in a less abrupt manner (eg, tachycardia, miosis, rate of gastric secretion, etc) it may be necessary to designate arbitrarily some particular intensity of effect as the end point. If the end point is taken as an increase in heart rate of 20 beats/min, then all individuals whose tachycardia is less than 20/min would be recorded as nonresponders, while all those with 20 or above would be recorded as responders. When the percent of responders in the population is plotted against the dose, a characteristic dose–response curve, more properly called a *dose–cumulative frequency* or *dose–percent* curve, is generated. Such a curve is, in fact, a cumulative frequency–distribution curve, the percent of responders at a given dose being the frequency of response.

Dose–cumulative frequency curves are generally of the same geometric shape as dose–intensity curves (namely, sigmoid) when frequency is plotted against log dose (see Fig 37-5). The tendency of the cumulated frequency of response (ie, percent) to be linearly proportional to the log of the dose in the middle of the dose range is called the *Weber–Fechner law*, although it is not invariable, as a true natural law should be. In many instances, the cumulative frequency is simply proportional to dose rather than log dose. The Weber–Fechner law applies to either dose–intensity or dose–cumulative frequency data. The similarity between dose–frequency and dose–intensity curves may be more than fortuitous, since the intensity of response will usually have an approximately linear relationship to the percent of responding *units* (smooth muscle cells, nerve fibers, etc) and hence is also a type of cumulative frequency of response. These are the same kind of statistics that govern the law of mass action.

If only the increase in the number of responders with each new dose is plotted, instead of the cumulative percent of responders, a bell-shaped curve is obtained. This curve is the first derivative of the dose–cumulative frequency curve and is a *frequency–distribution* curve (see Chapter 10). The distribution will be symmetrical—ie, *normal* or Gaussian (see Fig 10-6, page 109)—only if the dose–cumulative frequency curve is symmetrically hyperbolic. Because most dose–cumulative frequency curves are more nearly symmetrical when plotted semilogarithmically (ie, as log dose), dose–cumulative frequency curves are usually *log-normal*.

Since the dose–intensity and dose–cumulative frequency curves are basically similar in shape, it follows that the curves have similar defining characteristics, such as ED50, maximum effect (maximum efficacy), and slope. In dose–cumulative frequency data, the ED50 (*median effective dose*) is the dose to which 50% of the population responds (see Fig 37-5). If the frequency distribution is normal, the ED50 is both the arithmetic mean and median dose and is represented by the mid-point on the curve; if the distribution is log-normal, the ED50 is the median dose but not the arithmetic mean dose. The efficacy is the cumulative frequency summed over all doses; it is usually but not always 100%. The slope is characteristic of both the drug and test population. Even two drugs of identical mechanism may give rise to different slopes in dose–percent curves, whereas in dose–intensity curves the slopes are the same.

Statistical parameters (such as standard deviation)—in addition to ED50, maximum cumulative frequency (efficacy), the slope—characterize dose-cumulative frequency relationships (see Chapter 10).

There are several formulations for dose–cumulative frequency curves, some of which are employed only to define the linear segment of a curve and to determine the statistical parameters of this segment. For the statistical treatment of dose–frequency data, see Chapter 10. One simple mathematical expression of the entire log-symmetrical sigmoid curve is

$$\log \text{dose} = K + f \log \left(\frac{\% \text{ response}}{100\% - \text{response}} \right) \qquad (1)$$

where percent response may be either the percent of maximum intensity or the percent of a population responding. The equation is thus basically the same for both log normal dose–intensity and log normal dose–percent relationships. K is a constant that is characteristic of the mid-point of the curve, or ED50, and $1/f$ is characteristically related to the slope of the linear segment, which, in turn is closely related to the standard deviation of the derivative log normal frequency distribution curve.

The comparison of dose–percent relationships among drugs is subject to the pitfalls indicated for dose–intensity comparisons (see page 715), namely, that when the slopes of the curves are not the same (ie, the dose–percent curves are not parallel), it is necessary to state at which level of response a potency ratio is calculated. As with dose–intensity data, potencies are generally calculated from the ED50, but potency ratios may be calculated for any arbitrary percent response. The expression of selectivity is likewise subject to similar qualifications, inasmuch as the dose–percent curves for the several effects are usually nonparallel.

The term *therapeutic index* is used to designate a quantitative statement of the selectivity of a drug when a therapeutic and an untoward effect are being compared. If the untoward effect is designated as T (for toxic) and the therapeutic effect as E, the therapeutic index may be defined as TD50/ED50 or a similar ratio at some other arbitrary levels of response. The TD and the ED are not required to express the same percent of response; some clinicians use the ratio TD1/ED99 or TD5/ED95, based on the rationale that if the untoward effect is serious, it is important to use a most severe therapeutic index in passing judgment upon the drug. Unfortunately, therapeutic indices are known in man for only a few drugs.

There will be a different therapeutic index for each untoward effect that a drug may elicit, and, if there is more than one therapeutic effect, a family of therapeutic indices for each therapeutic effect. However, in clinical practice, it is customary to distinguish among the various toxicities by indicating the percent incidence of a given side effect.

Variations in Response and Responsiveness—From the above discussion of dose–frequency relationships and Chapter 10, it is obvious that in a normal population of persons there may be quite a large difference in the dose required to elicit a given response in the least-responsive member of the population and that to elicit the response in the most-responsive member. The difference will ordinarily be a function of the slope of the dose–percent curve, or, in statistical terms, of the standard deviation. If the standard deviation is large, the extremes of responsiveness of responders are likewise large.

In a normal population 95.46% of the population responds to doses within two standard deviations from the ED50 and 99.73% within three standard deviations. In log normal populations the same distribution applies when standard deviation is expressed as log dose.

In the population represented in Fig 37-5, 2.25% of the population (two standard deviations from the median) would require a dose more than 1.4 times the ED50; an equally small percent would respond to 0.7 the ED50. The physician who is unfamiliar with statistics is apt to consider the 2.25% at either extreme as abnormal reactors. The statistician will argue that these 4.5% are within the normal population and that only those who respond well outside of the normal population, at least three standard deviations from the median, deserve to be called abnormal.

Irrespective of whether the physician's or the statistician's criteria of abnormality obtain, the term *hyporeactive* applies to those individuals who require abnormally high doses and *hyperreactive* to those who require abnormally low doses. The terms *hyporesponsive* and *hyperresponsive* may also be used. It is incorrect to use the terms hyposensitive and hypersensitive in this context; *hypersensitivity* denotes an allergic response to a drug and should not be used to refer to hyperreactivity. The term *supersensitivity* correctly applies to hyperreactivity that results from denervation of the effector organ; it is often more definitively called denervation supersensitivity. Sometimes hyporeactivity is the result of an immunochemical deactivation of the drug, or *immunity*. Hyporeactivity should be distinguished from an increased

dose requirement that results from a severe pathological condition. Severe pain requires large doses of analgesics, but the patient is not a hyporeactor; what has changed is the baseline from which the end-point quantum is measured. The responsiveness of a patient to certain drugs sometimes may be determined by the history of previous exposure to appropriate drugs.

Tolerance is a diminution in responsiveness as use of the drug continues. The consequence of tolerance is an increase in the dose requirement. It may be due to an increase in the rate of elimination of drug, as discussed elsewhere in this chapter, to reflex or other compensatory homeostatic adjustments, to a decrease in the number of receptors or in the number of enzyme molecules or other coupling proteins in the effector sequence, to exhaustion of the effector system or depletion of mediators, to the development of immunity, or to other mechanisms. Tolerance may be gradual, requiring many doses and days to months to develop, or acute, requiring only the first or a few doses and only minutes to hours to develop. Acute tolerance is called *tachyphylaxis*.

Drug resistance is the decrease in responsiveness of microorganisms, neoplasms, or pests to chemotherapeutic agents, antineoplastics, or pesticides, respectively. It is not tolerance in the sense that the sensitivity of the individual microorganism or cancer cell decreases; rather it is the survival of normally unresponsive cells which then pass the genetic factors of resistance on to their progeny.

Patients who fail to respond to a drug are called *refractory*. Refractoriness may result from tolerance or resistance, but it may also result from the progression of pathological states that negate the response or render the response incapable of surmounting an overwhelming pathology. Rarely, it may result from a poorly developed receptor or response system.

Sometimes a drug evokes an unusual response that is *qualitatively* different from the expected response. Such an unexpected response is called a *meta-reaction*. A not uncommon meta-reaction is a central nervous stimulant rather than depressant effect of phenobarbital, especially in women. Certain pathological states and pain sometimes favor meta-reactivity. Responses that are different in infants or the aged than in young and middle-aged people are not meta-reactions if the response is usual in the age group. The term *idiosyncrasy* also denotes meta-reactivity, but the word has been so abused that it is recommended that it be dropped. Although hypersensitivity may cause unusual effects, it is not included in meta-reactivity.

Drug Receptors and Receptor Theory

Most drugs act by combining with some key substance in the biological milieu that has an important regulatory function in the target organ or tissue. This biological partner of the drug goes by the name of *receptive substance* or *drug receptor*. The receptive substance is mostly considered to be a cellular constituent, although in a few instances it may be extracellular, as the cholinesterases are, in part. The receptive substance is thought of as having a special chemical affinity and structural requirements for the drug. Drugs such as emollients, which have a physical rather than chemical basis for their action, obviously do not act upon receptors. Drugs, such as demulcents and astringents, which act in a nonselective or nonspecific chemical way are also not considered to act upon receptors, since the candidate receptors have neither sharp chemical nor biological definition. Even antacids, which react with the extremely well-defined hydronium ion, cannot be said to have a receptor, since the reactive proton has no permanent biological residence.

Because of early preoccupation with physical theories of action and the classical and illogical dichotomy of chemical and physical molecular interaction, there is a reluctance to admit receptors for drugs such as local anesthetics, general anesthetics, certain electrolytes, etc, which are not generally accepted to combine with cellular or organelle membrane constituents. The word receptor is used often inconsistently and intuitively. However, the term is a legitimate symbol for that biological structure with which a drug interacts to initiate a response. The fact that we are ignorant of the identities of most receptors does not detract from but rather increases the importance of the term and general concept.

Once a receptor is identified, it is frequently no longer thought of as a receptor, although such identification may afford the basis of profound advances in receptor theory. Since the effects of anticholinesterases are only indirectly derived from inhibition of cholinesterase and no drugs are known that stimulate the enzyme, it may be argued that it is not a receptor. Nevertheless, it is probable that a number of drugs ultimately will be revealed to act indirectly through the inhibition of such modulator enzymes, and it is important for the theoretician to develop models based upon such indirect interrelations.

Enzymes, of course, readily suggest themselves as candidates for receptors. However, there is more to cellular function than enzymes. Receptors may be membrane or intracellular constituents that govern the spatial orientation of enzymes, compartmentalization of the cytoplasm, contractile or compliant properties of subcellular structures, or permeability and electrical properties of membranes. For nearly every cellular constituent there can be imagined a possible way for a drug to affect its function; therefore, few cellular constituents can be dismissed *a priori* as possible receptors. The nicotinic receptor appears to be a membrane constituent that regulates the "gates" of certain ionic channels through the membrane. The beta adrenoreceptor appears to be a membrane constituent which modulates the closely proximate enzyme, adenylate cyclase.

Occupation and Other Theories

Drug-receptor interactions are governed by the law of mass action, a concept initiated by Langley in 1878. However, most chemical applications of mass law are concerned with the rate at which reagents disappear or products are formed, whereas receptor theory usually concerns itself with the fraction of the receptors combined with a drug, similar to theories of adsorption. The usual concept is that only when the receptor is actually occupied by the drug is its function transformed in such a way as to elicit a response. This concept has become known as the *occupation theory*. The earliest clear statement of its assumptions and formulations is often credited to Clark in 1926, but both Langley and Hill made important contributions to the theory in the first two decades of this century.

In all receptor theories, the terms agonist, partial agonist, and antagonist are employed. An *agonist* is a drug that combines with a receptor to initiate a response.

In the classical occupation theory, two attributes of the drug are required: (1) *affinity*, a measure of the equilibrium constant of the drug-receptor interaction and (2) *intrinsic activity*, or *efficacy* (not to be confused with efficacy as maximum effect), a measure of the ability of the drug to induce a positive change in the function of the receptor.

A *partial agonist* is a drug that can elicit some but not a maximal effect and which antagonizes an agonist. In the occupation theory it would be a drug with a favorable affinity but a low intrinsic activity.

A *competitive antagonist* is a drug that occupies a significant proportion of the receptors and thereby preempts them from reacting maximally with an agonist. In the occupation theory the prerequisite property is affinity without intrinsic activity.

A *noncompetitive antagonist* may react with the receptor in such a way as not to prevent agonist–receptor combination but to prevent the combination from initiating a response, or it may act to inhibit some subsequent event in the chain of action–effect–action–effect that leads to the final overt response.

The mathematical formulation of the receptor theories derives directly from the law of mass action and chemical kinetics. Certain assumptions are required to simplify calculations. The key assumption is that the intensity of effect is a direct linear function of the proportion of receptors occupied. The correctness of this assumption is most improbable on the basis of theoretical considerations, but empirically it appears to be a close enough approximation to be useful. A second assumption upon which formulations are based is that

the drug-receptor interaction is at equilibrium. Another common assumption is that the number of molecules of receptor is negligibly small compared to that of the drug. This assumption is undoubtedly true in most instances, and departures from this situation greatly complicate the mathematical expression of drug-receptor interactions.

The first clearly stated mathematical formulation of drug–receptor kinetics was that of Clark.[1] In his equation,

$$Kx^n = \frac{y}{100 - y} \qquad (2)$$

where K is the affinity constant, x is the concentration of drug, n is the molecularity of the reaction, and y is the percent of maximum response. Clark assumed that y was a linear function of the percent of receptors occupied by the drug, so that y could also symbolize the percent of receptors occupied. When the equation is rearranged to solve for y,

$$y = \frac{100Kx^n}{1 + Kx^n} \qquad (3)$$

A Cartesian plot of this equation is identical in form to that shown in Fig 37-2. When y is plotted against log x instead of x, the usual sigmoid curve is obtained. Thus it may be seen that the dose–intensity curve derives from mass action equilibrium kinetics, which in turn derive from the statistical nature of molecular interaction. The fact that dose–intensity and dose–percent curves have the same shape shows that they both involve the same kind of statistics.

If Eq 2 is put into log form,

$$\log K + n \log x = \log \frac{y}{100 - y} \qquad (4)$$

a plot of log $y/100 - y$ against log x will then yield a straight line with a slope of n; n is theoretically the number of molecules of drug which react with each molecule of receptor. At present, there are no known examples in which more than one molecule of agonist combines with a single receptor, hence n should be equal to 1, universally. Nevertheless, n often deviates from 1; deviations occur because of cooperative interactions among receptors (*cooperativity*), *spare receptors* (see below), amplifications in the response system ("*cascades*"), receptor coupling to more than one sequence (eg, to both adenylate cyclase and calcium channels, etc), and other reasons. In these departures from $n = 1$, the slope becomes a characteristic of the mechanism of action and response system.

The probability that a molecule of drug will react with a receptor is a function of the concentration of both drug and receptor. The concentration of receptor molecules cannot be manipulated like the concentration of a drug. But as each molecule of drug combines with a receptor, the population of free receptors is diminished accordingly. If the drug is a competitive antagonist, it will diminish the probability of an agonist–receptor combination in direct proportion to the percent of receptor molecules preempted by the antagonist. Consequently, the intensity of effect will be diminished. However, the probability of agonist–receptor interaction can be increased by increasing the concentration of agonist, and the intensity of effect can be restored by appropriately larger doses of agonist. Addition of more antagonist will again diminish the response, which can, again, be overcome or *surmounted* by more agonist.

Clark showed empirically and by theory that as long as the ratio of antagonist to agonist was constant, the concentration of the competitive drugs could be varied over an enormous range without changing the magnitude of the response (see Fig 37-6). Since the presence of competitive antagonist only diminishes the probability of agonist–receptor combination at a given concentration of agonist and does not alter the molecularity of the reaction, it also follows that the effect of

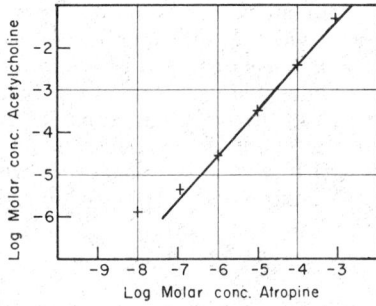

Fig 37-6. Direct proportionality of the dose of agonist (acetylcholine) to the dose of antagonist (atropine) necessary to cause a constant degree of inhibition (50%) of the response of the frog heart (courtesy, adaptation, Clark[1]).

the competitive antagonist is to shift the dose–intensity curve to the right in proportion to the amount of antagonist present; neither shape nor slope of the curve is changed (see Fig 37-7). Both Figs 37-6 and 37-7 are from Clark's original paper on competitive antagonism.[1]

Many refinements of the Clark formula have been made, but they will not be treated here; details and citations of relevant literature can be found in references 2–6 and among various works on receptors cited in the Bibliography. Several refinements are introduced to facilitate studies of competitive inhibition. The introduction of the concept of intrinsic activity[3] and efficacy[4] required appropriate changes in mathematical treatment.

Another important concept has been added to the occupation theory, namely the concept of *spare receptors*. Clark assumed the maximal response to occur only when the receptors were completely occupied, which does not account for the possibility that the maximum response might be limited by some step in the action–effect sequence subsequent to receptor occupation. Work with isotopically labelled agonists and antagonists and with dose–effect kinetics has shown that the maximal effect is sometimes achieved when only a small fraction of the receptors are yet occupied. The mathematical treatment of this phenomenon has enabled theorists to explain several puzzling observations that previously appeared to contradict drug–receptor theory.

The classical occupation theory fails to explain several phenomena satisfactorily, and it is unable to generate a real-

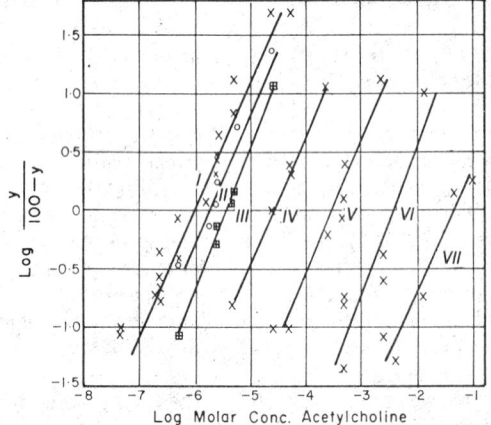

Fig 37-7. Effect of an antagonist to shift the log dose–intensity curve to the right without altering the slope. The effector is the isolated heart. *I:* no atropine; *II:* atropine, $10^{-8}M$; *III:* 10^{-7}; *IV:* 10^{-6}; *V:* 10^{-5}; *VI:* 10^{-4}; *VII:* 10^{-3}. *Y:* % of maximum intensity of response; the function $\log y/(100-y)$ converts the log dose–intensity relationship to a straight line (courtesy, adaptation, Clark[1]).

istic model of intrinsic activity and partial agonism. A rate theory, in which the intensity of response is proportional to the rate of drug–receptor interaction instead of occupation, was proposed to explain some of the phenomena that occupation theory could not, but the rate theory was unable to provide a realistic mechanistic model of response generation, and it had other serious limitations as well.

The phenomena that neither the classical occupation nor rate theory could explain can be explained by various theories in which the receptor can exist in at least two conformational states, one of which is the active one; the drug can react with one or more conformers. In a *two-state* model[7]

$$R \rightleftharpoons R^*,$$

where R is the inactive and R^* is the active conformer. The agonist combines mainly with R^*, the partial agonist can combine with both R and R^*, and the antagonist can combine with R, the equilibrium being shifted according to the extent of occupation of R and R^*. Other variations of occupation theory treat the receptor as an aggregate of subunits which interact cooperatively (see Ref 8).

The Nature of Receptor Groups and Models of Receptors

A *receptor group* is that portion of the receptor molecule with which an agonist acts and which is vital to the function of the receptor. Studies of receptor group composition and configuration are too complex for the purposes of this text; consequently, only a brief sketch will be made here to orient casually the reader to the nature of the approach.

From the chemical configuration and reactivity of agonists and antagonists certain deductions can be made about the structure of a receptor group. For example, all highly active agonists of muscarinic receptors are cations at physiological pH. This suggests that the receptor group contains an anionic group and that the force of attraction is electrostatic, at least in part, which agrees with thermodynamic data. That van der Waals forces (especially Heitler-London fluctuation forces) may also make an important contribution to binding is suggested by the requirement for *N*-methyl groups and by the low but definite activity of the nonionizable quaternary carbon analogue of acetylcholine, 3,3-dimethylbutyl acetate. This establishes a requirement for an auxiliary structure close to the anionic site. Studies of the contribution to activity of ester and carbonyl oxygen among analogues of acetylcholine, of intramolecular distances, and of the stereospecificity of various isomers and conformers have indicated a partial cationic (proton donor) site between 2.5 and 4 Å and a region of high electronic density (electron donor) between 5 and 7 Å from the anionic site. This is similar to the way in which the active site of acetylcholinesterase was mapped (see text, page 442, and Fig 27-4).

The structure–activity relationships among competitive inhibitors must also be consistent with any model of a receptor. However, binding sites additional to the receptor group can be involved, and results are frequently more difficult to interpret than those with agonists. Nevertheless, studies with antagonists have made a substantial contribution to receptor group analysis. There is considerable interest in antagonists that combine irreversibly with the receptor, since such drugs offer a way of marking (affinity labeling) the receptor for isolation and for identification of the receptor group.

Since receptors for autonomic agonists appear to be embedded in the cell membrane, they have been difficult to isolate without inactivation. Several laboratories have succeeded in isolating proteins, the chemical properties of which are consistent with those expected of the nicotinic receptor. Receptors for steroid hormones have been easier to isolate, and some have been relatively well characterized. The student interested in further details of drug–receptor interactions and the nature of receptors should peruse Refs 9–17 and the various works on receptors cited in the bibliography.

Up and Down Regulation—In many receptor-effector systems, if there is a paucity of agonist, the system will respond by increasing the responsiveness, by increasing the number of receptors on the effector membrane or number of coupling proteins or enzymes in the effector system. This is known as *up-regulation*. In adrenergic systems, sympathetic denervation has been shown to increase the number of postsynaptic β-adrenoreceptors at some junctions and the availability of nucleotide-binding protein units and/or adenylate cyclase molecules at others. Hyperthyroid activity also increases the number of β-adrenoreceptors in heart muscle, which explains the excessive heart rate. Prolonged blockade of receptors by antagonists may also cause up-regulation. The abrupt discontinuation of treatment, such that drug levels fall faster than re-regulation, may be followed by excessive activity, as, for example, pernicious tachycardia and angina pectoris from abrupt withdrawal of propranolol.

Excessive agonism will lead to a decrease in the number of receptors or in stimulus-response coupling. This one cause of tachyphylaxis or tolerance, such as occurs to the bronchodilator effects of β-adrenoreceptor agonists. Abrupt withdrawal may result in poor residual function or in rebound effects, depending upon the type of effect caused by the agonist.

Mechanism of Drug Action

Any metabolic or physiological function provides a potential mechanism of action of a drug. The term *mechanism of action* has been employed in a number of ways. In the past it was often the habit to confuse the site or locus of action with the mechanism of action. For example, the mechanism of the hypotensive action of tetraethylammonium ion was originally described as that of ganglionic blockade, which did nothing more than identify the anatomical structure upon which the drug acted. In a general sense, this was a partial elucidation of the mechanism of action, if mechanism is used in the mechanical sense of the entire linkage between the input and output of a machine. However, there has been a gradual narrowing of the definition of mechanism of action to be restricted to only the first event in the action–effect sequence, that is, only to the alteration of receptor function by the drug. In this sense the mechanism of action of tetraethylammonium is more appropriately defined as that of competition with acetylcholine for nicotine cholinergic receptors on the postsynaptic ganglion cell membrane, even though the alteration in receptor function is not defined. The ultimate mechanism of action is known for only a few drugs.

It is customary to speak of a drug as a stimulant or a depressant, of the action as being excitatory or inhibitory, etc. Such terms describe only the effect and not the action, and they have no bearing upon whether the drug augments receptor function or diminishes it. In biological systems positive and negative modulation and feedback occur at every level, the organ as well as the subcellular. Thus an agonist to a negative modulator may be able to bring about the same effect as an antagonist to a positive modulator. It is possible for an antagonist or inhibitor to elicit an excitatory effect. An example is the convulsant action of strychnine, which results from its antagonism of glycine, an important mediator of postsynaptic inhibition in the central nervous system. Conversely, it is possible for an agonist to elicit an inhibitory effect. An example is the reflex bradycardia that results from the stimulant action of veratrum alkaloids on chemoreceptors in the left ventricle.

Because of the central role *enzymes play* in cellular function, it is not surprising that thinking about the mechanism of action of drugs has focused largely upon enzymes. Agonist drugs conceivably could serve as substrates, cofactors, or activators. At the present time, no drug is definitely known to exert its action as a substrate or as a cofactor, exclusive of vitamins and known nutrients. However, at least three classes of drugs are known and several are suspected to work through the activation of enzymes.

The most notable example of enzyme activation is that of epinephrine and similar β-adrenoreceptor agonists, which activate adenyl cyclase to increase the production of 3′,5′-cyclic adenylic acid (cyclic AMP; CAMP). The metabolic and cardiac effects of catecholamines are attributable in part to the increment in cyclic AMP. One modulator of adenyl cyclase is the β-adrenergic receptor. The β-adrenoreceptor is coupled to adenylate cyclase through a regulatory protein that binds GDP and GTP. When GDP is present, the agonist-receptor complex is associated with the regulatory protein. GTP causes transfer of the regulatory protein to adenylate cyclase and dissociation of the β-adrenoreceptor. Glucagon also owes its hyperglycemic action to activation of hepatic adenylate cyclase. There is thus the interesting phenomenon of one enzyme, adenyl cyclase, being activated by two chemically unrelated drugs. Since β-adrenergic blocking agents do not antagonize glucagon, it is obvious that glucagon works upon a different receptor than does epinephrine.

CAMP activates protein kinases that increase the activity of phosphorylase, actomyosin, the sequestration of calcium by the sarcoplasmic reticulum, and calcium channels. Thus a brief activation of the β-adrenoreceptor sets in motion a cascade of events that greatly amplify the signal.

Other important enzymes coupled to receptors are guanylate cyclase and phospholipases A and C, which are involved with membrane fluidity and calcium channels, respectively.

Many drugs are inhibitors of enzymes. When the drug is a *competitive inhibitor* of a natural endogenous substrate of the enzyme, it is called an *antimetabolite* (see also page 442). Examples of antimetabolites are sulfonamides, which compete with para-aminobenzoic acid and thus interfere with its incorporation into dihydrofolic acid, and methotrexate, which competes with folic acid for dihydrofolate reductase and thus interferes with the formation of folinic acid. It might seem that anticholinesterases are also antimetabolites, although they are never placed into that classification. The reason is that the products of cholinesterase–acetylcholine interaction do not subserve important metabolic functions, as do folic and folinic acids, so that the organism is not deprived of an important metabolite by the action of the cholinesterase inhibitors.

Some drugs are competitive inhibitors of enzyme systems whose natural function appears not to produce useful metabolites but to rid the body of foreign substances. Inhibitors of the hepatic microsomes and probenecid fall into this category; the hepatic microsomes do perform a few biotransformations on endogenous substrates, but the renal tubular anion transport system does not appear to be required to eliminate any important endogenous substances.

Since neither the hepatic microsomes nor the tubular anion transport system seems to be involved in response systems, inhibitors of these enzyme systems are antagonists without corresponding agonists. Indeed, even natural endogenous substrates of enzymes are rarely considered to be agonists.

Noncompetitive enzyme inhibitors among drugs are also known. Examples are cyanide, fluoride, disulfiram, and cardiac glycosides. When enzyme inhibition brings about a positive response—eg, the cholinergic effects of the anti-cholinesterases or the effects of diazoxide consequent to inhibition of phosphodiesterase—the drug appears to be an agonist. Yet there can be no competitive antagonist to such an inhibitor, since the competitor to the drug is more substrate, to which the effect of the drug is actually attributable.

Acetylcholine increases the permeability of the subsynaptic membrane to cations and the heart muscle membrane to potassium. The mechanism is generally thought to involve a change in conformation of a membrane constituent so that pore size or permeability constant is affected. Other autonomic agonists are also known to alter the permeability to ions, in part through activation of adenyl cyclase, guanyl cyclase, phospholipase-c, or other enzymes. Many drugs and toxins, among them local anesthetics, some sedative–hypnotics, general anesthetics, and tetrodotoxin, act through *alterations in the structural and physical properties of membranes.* To the extent that some of such substances may disperse themselves generally throughout the lipid phase of the membrane rather than to combine with special chemical entities, no definite receptors for such drugs can be said to exist.

The mechanism of action of certain drugs, especially autonomic drugs, is often stated to be *mimicry* of a natural neurohumor or hormone. Thus methacholine mimics acetylcholine as an agonist. This does not define the mechanism of action, unless the mechanism of action of the natural substance is known.

Mimicry usually occurs because of a structural similarity between the natural substance and the mimetic drug. Mimicry in agonist functions is easy to demonstrate, but the site of action may not always be mimicry of the natural agonist at its receptor but rather at its storage site to *release* the natural agonist.

Examples of mimetics that act by release of the natural mediator are sympathomimetics such as *d*-amphetamine, mephentermine, ephedrine (in part), tyramine, and others, which are now known to act by displacing norepinephrine from storage sites within the adrenergic neuron. Many of such indirectly acting sympathomimetics lack a direct action on the adrenergic receptor, although some, like ephedrine, act both upon the receptor and the storage complex. Another mimetic by a release mechanism is carbachol, which promotes the presynaptic discharge of acetylcholine.

In these examples there is a close structural similarity between the mimetic and the released mediator. In the case of many releasers of histamine (such as tubocurarine, polymyxin, or morphine) no close chemical relationship exists between the releaser and the released. In such instances release has been explained by activation of receptors on the mast-cell membrane which promote exocytosis of the histamine-containing granules, by an influx of calcium, and activation of microtubules, all of which may be involved in moving the granules out of the mast cell.

Structural similarity may also aid mimicry by promoting chemical combination with an enzyme of destruction or some other means of disposition. For example, metaraminol, amphetamine, etc *inhibit membrane transport* into the neuron and hence inhibit the neuronal recapture of released norepinephrine. Consequently, the extraneuronal concentration of norepinephrine in the nearby region of the receptors does not drop as rapidly as in the absence of the mimetic, and the action of the mediator is sustained.

Some inhibitors of the enzymes of the destruction of mediators are structurally similar enough to the mediator to have some agonist action. This is true of neostigmine, which has a direct stimulant action on nicotinic receptors in addition to its anticholinesterase action. In contrast, the anticholinesterase physostigmine has some antagonist actions on cholinergic receptors and also an effect to interfere with acetylcholine synthesis.

The above multiple actions come about because all the structures that interact with a small molecule mediator (the receptor, synthesizing enzyme, destructive enzyme, storage molecule, membrane transport carrier) must have some common structural features and affinities. A drug that reacts with one of these molecules has a distinct probability of interacting with another.

The recognition of the critical role of *ions* in the function of membranes, the excitability of cells, and the activity of many enzymes has generated a renewed interest in ions in the mechanism of action of certain drugs. The inorganic ions, some of which are used as drugs, lend themselves automatically to a discussion of ionic mechanisms. The repair of electrolyte deficiencies by replacement therapy warrants no further comment here. Some nonphysiological ions act as imperfect impersonators of physiological ions; lithium partly substitutes for sodium, bromide for chloride and thiocyanate for iodide, and each may owe its pharmacological action, in part, to a sluggish mobility through membrane channels, through which their sister ions normally pass readily when traffic is not impeded by "slowly moving vehicles." Iodide has an effect to increase the penetrance of drugs into caseous and necrotic areas, to aid in the resolution of gummatous lesions, to reduce the viscosity of mucous secretions, and other odd effects; it is thought to do so by increasing the hydration of collagen and mucoproteins by a poorly understood mechanism. The transition and heavy metals have in common the ability to form complexes with a variety of physiologically active substances, particularly the active centers of many enzymes. *Chelation* and other *complexation* are the mechanisms of action of several drugs used to treat heavy metal intoxication, diseases that involve abnormal body burdens or plasma levels of heavy metals, and hypercalcemia. Chelates and chelation are discussed in more detail on pages 187 and 188.

There is much interest in the effects of drugs on ion movements. Cardiac glycosides are known to inhibit an ATPase involved in the membrane transport of sodium and several other substances, which indirectly causes an increase in intracellular calcium content. In part, the mechanisms of action of local anesthetics, quinidine, and various other drugs are also speculated to involve calcium movements. More recently, there has appeared a whole new class of drugs, the calcium channel blockers.

Concomitant with the development of molecular biology was the appreciation that drugs act through *nuclear* and *extranuclear genetic mechanisms.* Nitrogen mustards have long been known to interfere with the replication of DNA. Streptomycin, kanamycin, neomycin, and gentamicin cause misreading by the ribosomes of the code incorporated into messenger RNA; tetracyclines, erythromycin, and chloramphenicol inhibit the synthesis of protein at the ribosomes; and chloroquine, novobiocin, and colchicine inhibit DNA polymerase. Other drugs induce the the production of enzymes; aldosterone appears to act by inducing the synthesis of the enzyme, membrane ATPase, necessary to sodium transport. Many drugs induce one or more of the hepatic and extrahepatic cytochrome P-450 enzymes.

A number of drugs have simple mechanisms that do not involve an action at the cellular level. Examples are bulk and saline cathartics, osmotic diuretics, and cholestyramine. Although such drugs usually do not generate much excitement among pharmacologists, they do serve to remind us of the many avenues through which mechanism of action may be expressed. Throughout the various chapters of Part 6 specific mechanisms of action may be mentioned.

Absorption, Distribution, and Excretion

No matter by which route a drug is administered it must pass through several to many biological membranes during the processes of absorption, distribution, biotransformation, and elimination. Since membranes are traversed in all of these events, the subject of this section will begin with a brief description of biological membranes and membrane processes and the relationship of the physiochemical properties of a drug molecule to penetrance and transport.

Structure and Properties of Membranes

The concept that a membrane surrounds each cell arose shortly after the cellular nature of tissue was discovered. The biological and physiochemical properties of cells seemed in accord with this view. In the past, from time to time the actual existence of the membrane has been questioned by brilliant men, and ingenious explanations have been advanced to explain cellular integrity and the osmotic and electrophysiological properties of cells. Microchemical, X-ray diffraction, electron microscopic, nuclear magnetic resonance, electron spin resonance, and other investigations have proved both the existence and nature of the plasma, mitochondrial, nuclear and other cell membranes. The description of the plasma membrane that follows is somewhat oversimplified, but it will suffice to provide a background for an understanding of penetrance into and through membranes.

Structure and Composition—The cell membrane has been described as a "mayonnaise sandwich," in which a bimolecular layer of lipid material is entrained between two parallel monomolecular layers of protein. However, the protein does not make continuous layers, like the bread in a sandwich, but rather is sporadically scattered over the surfaces, like icebergs; like icebergs, much of the protein is below the surface. In Fig 37-8 the lipid layers are represented as a somewhat orderly, closely packed lamellar array of phospholipid molecules associated tail-to-tail, each "tail" being an alkyl chain or steroid group and the "heads" being polar groups, including the glycerate moieties, with their polar ether and carbonyl oxygens and phosphate with attached polar groups. In reality the lamellar portion is probably not so orderly, since its composition is quite complex. Chains of fatty acids of different degrees of saturation and cholesterol cannot array themselves in simple parallel arrangements. Furthermore, the polar heads will assume a number of orientations depending upon the substances and groups involved. Moreover, the lamellar portion is penetrated by large globular proteins, the interior of which, however, like the lipid layers, has a high hydrophobicity, and some fibrous proteins.

The plasma membrane appears to be asymmetrical. The lipid composition varies from cell type to cell type and perhaps from site to site on the same membrane. There are, for example, differences between the membrane of the endoplasmic reticulum and the plasma membrane, even though the membranes are coextensive. Where membranes are double, the inner and outer layers may differ considerably; the inner and outer membranes of mitochondria have been shown to have strikingly different compositions and properties. Some authorities have expressed doubt as to the existence of the protein layers in biological membranes, although the evidence is preponderantly in favor of at least an outer glycoprotein coat. Sugar moieties are also attached to the outer proteins; these sugar moieties are important to cellular and immunological recognition and adhesion and have other functions as well.

The cell membrane appears to be perforated by water-filled pores of various sizes, varying from about 4–10 Å, being predominantly around 7 Å. Probably all major ion channels are through the large globular proteins that traverse the membrane. Through these pores pass inorganic ions and small organic molecules. Since sodium ions are more hydrated than potassium and chloride ions, they are larger and do not pass as freely through the pores as potassium and chloride. The vascular endothelium appears to have pores at least as large as 40 Å, but these seem to be interstitial passages rather than transmembrane pores. Lipid molecules small enough to pass through the pores may do so, but they have a higher probability of entering into the lipid layer, from where they will equilibrate chemically with the interior of the cell. From work on monolayers, some workers contend that it is not necessary to postulate pores to explain the permeability to water and small water-soluble molecules.

Stratum Corneum—Although the stratum corneum is not a membrane in the same sense as a cell membrane, it offers a barrier to diffusion, which is of significance in the topical application of drugs. The stratum corneum consists of several layers of dead keratinized cutaneous epithelial cells enmeshed in a matrix of keratin fibers and bound together with cementing desmosomes and penetrating tonofibrils of keratin. Varying amounts of lipids and fatty acids from dying cells, sebum, and sweat are contained among the dead squamous cells. Immediately beneath the layer of dead cells and above the viable epidermal epithelial cells is a layer of keratohyaline granules and various water-soluble substances, such as alpha-amino acids, purines, monosaccharides, and urea.

Both the upper and lower layers of the stratum corneum are involved in the cutaneous barrier to penetration. It is barrier to penetration from the surface is in the upper layers for water-soluble substances and the lower layers for lipid-soluble substances, and the barrier to the outward movement of water is in the lowest layer of the stratum corneum.

Membrane Potentials—Across the cell membrane there exists an electrical potential, always negative on the inside and positive on the outside. If a cell did not have special membrane electrolyte transport processes, its membrane potential would be mainly the result of the Donnan equilibrium (see Chapter 14) consequent to the semipermeability of the membrane. Such potentials generally lie between 2 and 5 mv.

A cell with a membrane across which diffusible electrolyte distribution is purely passive would be expected to have a high internal concentration of sodium, such as is true for the erythrocytes of some species. However, the interior of most cells is high in potassium and low in sodium, as depicted in Fig 37-8. This unequal distribution of cations attests to special electrolyte transport processes and to differential permeabilities of diffusible ions, so that the membrane potential is higher than that which would result from a purely passive Donnan distribution. In nerve and skeletal or cardiac muscle the membrane potential ranges upwards to about 90 mv. The electrical gradient is on the order of 50,000 v/cm, because of the extreme thinness of the membrane. Obviously, such an intense potential gradient will strongly influence the transmembrane passages of charged drug molecules.

Diffusion and Transport

Transport is the movement of a drug from one place to another within the body. The drug may diffuse freely in uncombined form with a kinetic energy appropriate to its thermal environment, or it may move in combination with extracellular or cellular constituents, sometimes in connection with energy-yielding processes that allow the molecule or complex to overcome barriers to simple diffusion.

Simple Nonionic Diffusion and Passive Transport—

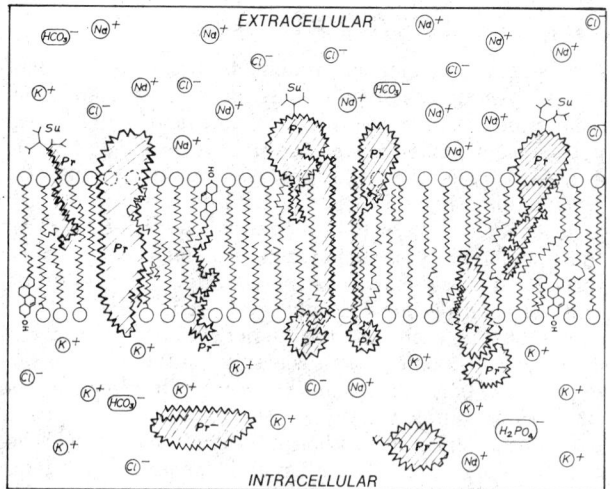

Fig 37-8. Simplified cross section of a cell membrane (components are not to scale). The lipid interior of the lamellar portion of the membrane consists of various phospholipids, fatty acids, cholesterol (c), and other steroids. Ions are indicated in order to illustrate differences in size relative to the channel. *Pr:* protein; *Su:* sugar.

Molecules in solution move in a purely random fashion, providing they are not charged and moving in an electrical gradient. Such random movement is called *diffusion*, and if the molecule is uncharged it is called *nonionic diffusion*.

In a population of drug molecules, the probability that during unit time any drug molecule will move across a boundary is directly proportional to the number of molecules adjoining that boundary and therefore to the drug concentration. Except at dilutions so extreme that only a few molecules are present, the actual rate of movement (molecules/unit time) is directly proportional to the probability and therefore to the concentration. Once molecules have passed through the boundary to the opposite side, their random motion may cause some to return and others to continue to move further away from the boundary. The rate of return is likewise proportional to the concentration on the opposite side of the boundary. It follows that, although molecules are moving in both directions, there will be a net movement from the region of higher to that of lower concentration and that the net transfer will be proportional to the concentration differential. If the boundary is a membrane, which has both substance and dimension, the rate of movement is also directly proportional to the permeability and inversely proportional to the thickness. These factors combine into Fick's Law of Diffusion,

$$\frac{dQ}{dt} = \frac{\overline{D}A(C_1 - C_2)}{x} \tag{5}$$

where Q is the net quantity of drug transferred across the membrane, t is time, C_1 is the concentration on one side and C_2 on the other, x is the thickness of the membrane, A is the area, and $\overline{D}$ is the diffusion coefficient, related to permeability. The equation is more nearly correct if chemical activities are used instead of concentrations. Since a biological membrane is patchy, with pores of different sizes and probably with varying thickness and composition, both $\overline{D}$ and x probably vary from spot to spot. Nevertheless, some mean values can be assumed.

It is customary to combine the membrane factors into a single constant, called a permeability constant or coefficient, P, so that $P = \overline{D}/x$, A in Eq 5 having unit value. The rate of net transport (diffusion) across the membrane then becomes

$$\frac{dQ}{dt} = P(C_1 - C_2) \tag{6}$$

As diffusion continues, C_1 approaches C_2, and the net rate, dQ/dt, approaches zero in exponential fashion characteristic of a first-order process. Equilibrium is defined as that state in which $C_1 = C_2$. The equilibrium is, of course, dynamic, with equal numbers of molecules being transported in each direction during unit time. If water is also moving through the membrane, it may either facilitate the movement of drug or impede it, according to the relative directions of movement of water and drug; this effect of water movement is called *solvent drag*.

Ionic or Electrochemical Diffusion—If a drug is ionized, the transport properties are modified. The probability of penetrating the membrane is still a function of concentration, but it is also a function of the potential difference or electrical gradient across the membrane. A cationic drug molecule will be repelled from the positive charge on the outside of the membrane, and only those molecules with a high kinetic energy will pass through the ion barrier. If the cation is polyvalent, it may not penetrate at all.

Once inside the membrane, a cation will be simultaneously attracted to the negative charge on the intracellular surface of the membrane and repelled by the outer surface; it is said to be moving along the *electrical gradient*. If it is also moving from a higher towards a lower concentration, it is said to be moving along its *electrochemical gradient*, the electrochemical gradient being the sum of the influences of the electrical field and the concentration differential across the membrane.

Once inside the cell, cations will tend to be kept inside by the attractive negative charge on the interior of the cell, and the intracellular concentration of drug will increase until, by sheer numbers of accumulated drug particles, the outward diffusion or mass escape rate equals the inward transport rate, and electrochemical equilibrium is said to have occurred. At electrochemical equilibrium at body temperature (37°C), ionized drug molecules will be distributed according to the Nernst equation,

$$\pm\log\frac{C_o}{C_i} = \frac{ZE}{61} \tag{7}$$

where C_o is the molar extracellular and C_i the intracellular concentration, Z is the number of charges per molecule, and E is the membrane potential in millivolts. Log C_o/C_i is positive when the molecule is negatively charged and negative when the molecule is positively charged.

Facilitated Diffusion—Sometimes a substance moves more rapidly through a biological membrane than can be accounted for by the process of simple diffusion. This accelerated movement is termed *facilitated diffusion*. It is thought to be due to the presence of a special molecule, called a *carrier*, within the membrane, with which carrier the transported substance combines. There is considered to be a greater permeability to the carrier–drug complex than to the drug alone, so that the transport rate is enhanced. After the complex traverses the membrane it dissociates. The carrier must either return to the original side of the membrane to be reused or be constantly produced on one side and eliminated on the other in order for the carrier process to be continuous. Many characteristics of facilitated diffusion formerly attributed to ion carriers can be explained by ion exchange. Although facilitated diffusion resembles active transport, below, in its dependence upon a continuous source of energy, it differs in that facilitated diffusion will only transport a molecule along its electrochemical gradient.

Active Transport—Active transport may be defined as energy-dependent movement of a substance through a biological membrane against an electrochemical gradient. It is characterized by the following:

1. The substance is transported from a region of lower to one of higher electrochemical activity.

2. Metabolic poisons interfere with transport.

3. The transport rate approaches an asymptote (ie, saturates) as concentration increases.

4. The transport system usually shows a requirement for specific chemical structures.

5. Closely related chemicals are competitive for the transport system.

Many drugs are secreted from the renal tubules into urine, from liver cells into bile or from the cerebrospinal fluid into blood by active transport, but the role of active transport of drugs in the distribution into most body compartments and tissues is less well known. Active transport is required for the penetrance of a number of sympathomimetics into neural tissue.

Pinocytosis and Exocytosis—Many, perhaps all, cells are capable of a type of phagocytosis called *pinocytosis*. The cell membrane has been observed to invaginate into a saccular structure containing extracellular materials and then pinch off the saccule at the membrane, so that the saccule remains as a vesicle or vacuole within the interior of the cell. Since metabolic activity is required and since an extracellular substance may be transported against an electrochemical gradient, pinocytosis shows some of the same characteristics as active transport. However, pinocytosis is relatively slow and inefficient compared to most active transport, except in gastrointestinal absorption, in which pinocytosis is of considerable importance.

It is not known to what extent pinocytosis contributes to the transport of most drugs, but many macromolecules and even larger particles can be absorbed by the gut. Pinocytosis probably explains the oral efficacy of the Sabin polio vaccine. Some drugs themselves affect pinocytosis; for example, adrenal glucocorticoids markedly inhibit the process in macrophages and other cells involved in inflammation.

Exocytosis is more or less the reverse of pinocytosis. Granules, vacuoles or other organelles within the cell move to the cell membrane, fuse with it, and extrude their contents into the interstitial space.

Physicochemical Factors in Penetrance

Drugs and other substances may traverse the membrane primarily either through the pores or by dissociation into the membrane lipids and subsequent diffusion from the membrane into the cytosol or other fluid on the far side of the membrane. The physicochemical prerequisites are different according to which route is taken. To pass through the pores the "diameter" of the molecule must be smaller than the pore, but the molecule can be longer than the pore diameter. The probability that a long, thin molecule will be oriented properly is low, unless there is also bulk flow, and the transmembrane passage of large molecules is slow.

Water-soluble molecules with low lipid solubility are usually thought to pass through the membrane mainly via the pores and to a small extent by pinocytosis, but recent work with lipid monolayers suggests that small water-soluble molecules may also be able to pass readily through the lipid, and the necessity of postulating the existence of pores has been questioned. Nevertheless, experimental data on penetrance overwhelmingly favor the concept of passage of water-soluble lipid-insoluble substances through pores. If there is a membrane carrier or active transport system, a low solubility of the drug in membrane lipids is no impediment to penetration, since the drug-carrier complex is assumed to have an appropriate solubility, and energy from an active transport system enables the drug to penetrate the energy barrier "imposed by the lipids." Actually, the lipids are not an important energy barrier; rather the barrier is the force of attraction of the solvent water for its dipolar to polar solute, so that it is difficult for the solute to leave the water and enter the lipid.

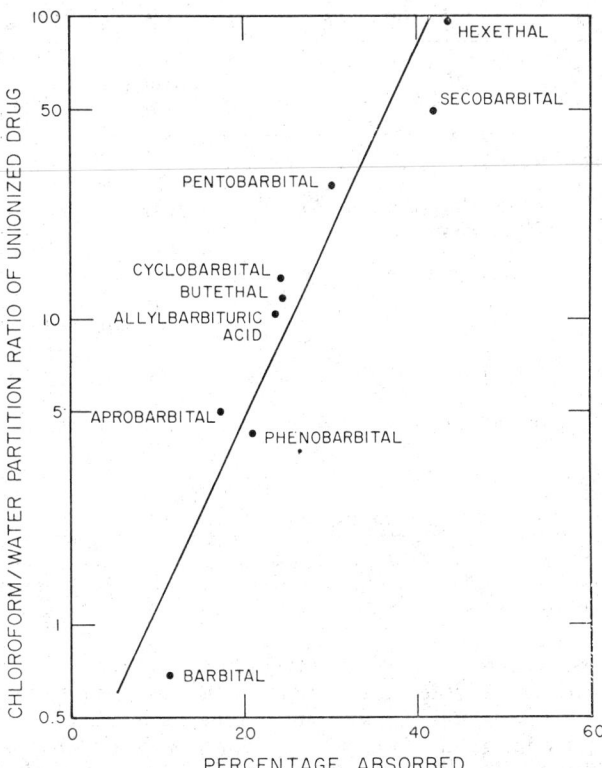

Fig 37-9. The relationship of absorption of the unionized forms of drugs from the colon of the rat to the chloroform:water partition coefficient (courtesy, Schanker[18]).

Drugs with a high solubility in the membrane lipids, of course, pass easily through the membrane. Even when their dimensions are small enough to permit passage through pores, lipid-soluble drugs primarily pass through the membrane lipids, not only because chemical partition favors the lipid phase but because the surface area occupied by pores is only a small fraction of the total membrane area.

Lipid Solubility and Partition Coefficients—As early as 1902 Overton investigated the importance of lipid solubility to the penetrance and absorption of drugs. Eventually it was recognized that more important than lipid solubility was the lipid–water distribution coefficient; that is to say, a high lipid solubility does not favor penetrance unless the water solubility is low enough that the drug is not entrained in the aqueous phase.

In Fig 37-9 is illustrated the relationship between the chloroform–water partition coefficient and the colonic absorption of barbiturates. Chloroform is probably not the optimal lipid solvent for such a study, and natural lipids from nerve or other tissues have been shown to be superior in the few instances in which they have been employed. Nevertheless, the correlation shown in the figure is a convincing one.

When the water solubility of a substance is so low that a significant concentration in water or extracellular fluid cannot be achieved, absorption may be negligible in spite of a favorable partition coefficient. Hence mineral oil, petrolatum, etc. are virtually unabsorbed. The optimal partition coefficient for permeation of the skin appears to be lower than that for the permeation of the cell membrane, being perhaps as low as one.

Dipolarity, Polarity, and Nonionic Diffusion—The partition coefficient of a drug depends upon the polarity and the size of the molecule. Drugs with a high dipole moment, even though un-ionized, have a low lipid solubility and hence

Table I—Rates of Entry of Drugs in CSF and the Degrees of Ionization of Drugs at pH 7.4[19]

Drug	% binding to plasma protein	pK_a[a]	% unionized at pH 7.4	Permeability constant $(P\ min^{-1}) \pm$ S.E.
Drugs mainly ionized at pH 7.4				
5-Sulfosalicylic acid	22	(strong)	0	<0.0001
N'-Methylnicotinamide	<10	(strong)	0	0.0005 ± 0.00006
5-Nitrosalicylic acid	42	2.3	0.001	0.001 ± 0.0001
Salicylic acid	40	3.0	0.004	0.006 ± 0.0004
Mecamylamine	20	11.2	0.016	0.021 ± 0.0016
Quinine	76	8.4	9.09	0.078 ± 0.0061
Drugs mainly unionized at pH 7.4				
Barbital	<2	7.5	55.7	0.026 ± 0.0022
Thiopental	75	7.6	61.3	0.50 ± 0.051
Pentobarbital	40	8.1	83.4	0.17 ± 0.014
Aminopyrine	20	5.0	99.6	0.25 ± 0.020
Aniline	15	4.6	99.8	0.40 ± 0.042
Sulfaguanidine	6	>10.0[b]	>99.8	0.003 ± 0.0002
Antipyrine	8	1.4	>99.9	0.12 ± 0.013
N-Acetyl-4-aminoantipyrine	<3	0.5	>99.9	0.012 ± 0.0010

[a] The dissociation constant of both acids and bases is expressed as a pK_a—a negative logarithm of the acidic dissociation constant.

[b] Sulfaguanidine has a very weakly acidic group (pK_a > 10) and two very weakly basic groups (pK_a 2.75 and 0.5). Consequently, the compound is almost completely undissociated at pH 7.4.

poor penetrance. An example of a highly dipolar substance with a low partition coefficient and which does not penetrate into cells is sulfisoxazole. Sulfadiazine is somewhat less dipolar, has a chloroform–water partition coefficient ten times that of sulfisoxazole, and readily penetrates cells. Ionization not only greatly diminishes lipid solubility but may also impede passage through charged membranes (see *Ionic Diffusion*, page 724).

It is often stated that ionized molecules do not penetrate membranes, except for ions of small diameter. This is not necessarily true, because of the presence of membrane carriers for some ions, which carriers may effectively shield or neutralize the charge (ion-pair formation). The renal tubular transport systems, which transport such obligate ions as tetraethylammonium, probably form ion-pairs. Furthermore, if an ionized molecule has a large nonpolar moiety such that an appreciable lipid solubility is imparted to the molecule in spite of the charge, the drug may penetrate, although usually at a slow rate. For example, various morphinan derivatives are passively absorbed from the stomach even though they are completely ionized at the pH of gastric fluid. Nevertheless, when a drug is a weak acid or base, the unionized form with a favorable partition coefficient passes through a biological membrane so much more readily than the ionized form that, for all practical purposes, only the unionized form is said to pass through the membrane. This has become known as the *principle of nonionic diffusion*.

This principle is the reason that only the concentrations of the unionized form of the barbiturates are plotted in Fig 37-9.

For the purpose of further illustrating the principle, Table I is provided. In the table the permeability constants for penetrance into the cerebral spinal fluid of rats are higher for unionized drugs than for ionized ones. The apparent exceptions—barbital, sulfaguanidine, and acetylaminoantipyrine—may be explained by the dipolarity of the unionized molecules. With barbital, the two lipophilic ethyl groups are too small to compensate for the considerable dipolarity of the unionized barbituric acid ring; it may be also seen that barbital is appreciably ionized, which contributes to the relatively small permeability constant. Sulfaguanidine and acetylaminoantipyrine are both very polar molecules. Mecamylamine might also be considered an exception, since it shows a modest permeability even though strongly ionized; there is no dipolarity in mecamylamine elsewhere than the amino group.

Absorption of Drugs

Absorption is the process of movement of a drug from the site of application into the extracellular compartment of the body. Inasmuch as there is a great similarity among the various membranes that a drug may pass through in order to gain access to the extracellular fluid, it might be expected that the particular site of application (or *route*) would make little difference to the successful absorption of the drug. In actual fact, it makes a great deal of difference; many factors other than the structure and composition of the membrane determine the ease with which a drug is absorbed. These factors are discussed in the following sections, along with an account of the ways that drug formulations may be manipulated to alter the ability of a drug to be readily absorbed.

Routes of Administration

Drugs may be administered by many different routes. The various routes include oral, rectal, sublingual or buccal, parenteral, inhalation, topical, etc. The choice of a route depends upon both convenience and necessity.

Oral Route—This is obviously the most convenient route for access to the systemic circulation, providing that various factors do no militate against this route. Oral administration does not always give rise to sufficiently high plasma concentrations to be effective; some drugs are absorbed unpredictably or erratically; patients occasionally have an absorption malfunction. Drugs may not be given by mouth to patients with gastrointestinal intolerance, or who are in preparation for anesthesia, or who have had gastrointestinal surgery. Oral administration is also precluded in coma.

Rectal Route—Drugs that are ordinarily administered by the oral route usually can be administered by injection or by the alternative *lower enteral* route, through the anal portal into the rectum or lower intestine. With regard to the latter, *rectal suppositories* or *retention enemas* were formerly used quite frequently, but their popularity has abated somewhat,

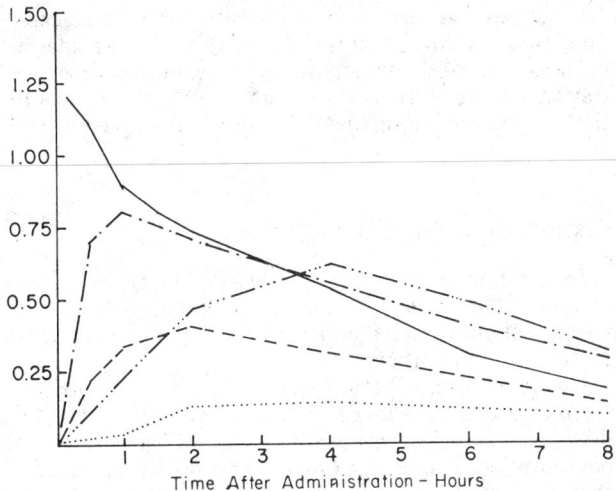

Fig 37-10.   Blood concentration in mg/100 ml of theophylline (ordinates) following administration to humans of aminophylline in the amounts and by the routes indicated. Doses: per 70 kg. Theophylline-ethylenediamine by various routes: —— *intravenous, 0.5 g; –*·–·–*retention enema, 0.5 g;* ——···——···—— *oral tablets-Pl., 0.5 g;* ---*oral tablets-Pl., 0.3 g;* ···· *rectal suppository, 0.5 g* (courtesy, Truitt, et al[20] adapted).

owing to improvements in parenteral preparations. Nevertheless, they continue to be valid and sometimes very important ways of administering a drug, especially in pediatrics and geriatrics. In Fig 37-10 the availability of a drug by retention enema may be compared with that by the intravenous route and by oral and rectal suppository administration. It is apparent that the retention enema may be a very satisfactory means of administration but that rectal suppositories may be inadequate where rapid absorption and high plasma levels are required. The illustration is not intended to lead the reader to the conclusion that a retention enema will always give more prompt and higher blood levels than the oral route, for converse findings for the same drug have been reported,[21] but rather to show that the retention enema may offer a useful substitute for the oral route.

Sublingual or Buccal Route—Even though an adequate plasma concentration eventually may be achievable by the oral route, it may rise much too slowly for use in some situations where a rapid response is desired. In such situations parenteral therapy is usually indicated. However, the patients with angina pectoris may get quite prompt relief from an acute attack by the *sublingual* or *buccal* administration of nitroglycerin, so that parenteral administration may be avoided. When only small amounts of drugs are required to gain access to the blood, the buccal route may be very satisfactory, providing the physicochemical prerequisites for absorption by this route are present in the drug and dosage form. Only a few drugs may be given successfully by this route.

Parenteral Routes—These routes by definition include any route other than the oral–gastrointestinal (enteral) tract, but in common medical usage the term excludes topical administration and includes only various hypodermic routes. Parenteral administration includes the intravenous, intramuscular, and subcutaneous routes. Parenteral routes may be employed whenever enteral routes are contraindicated (see above) or inadequate.

The *intravenous* route may be preferred on occasion, even when a drug may be well absorbed by the oral route. There is no delay imposed by absorption before the administered drug reaches the circulation, and blood levels rise virtually as rapidly as the time necessary to empty the syringe or infusion bottle. Consequently, the intravenous route is the preferred route when an emergency calls for an immediate response.

In addition to the rapid rise in plasma concentration of drug, another advantage of intravenous administration is the greater predictability of the peak plasma concentration, which with some drugs can be calculated with a fair degree of precision. Smaller doses are generally required by the intravenous than by other routes, but this usually affords no advantage, inasmuch as the sterile injectable dose form costs more than enteric preparations, and the requirements for medical or paramedical supervision of administration may also add to the cost and inconvenience.

Because of the rapidity with which drug enters the circulation, dangerous side effects to the drug may occur which are often not extant by other routes. The principal untoward effect is a depression of cardiovascular function, which is often called *drug shock*. Consequently, some drugs must be given quite slowly to avoid vasculotoxic concentrations of drug in the plasma. Acute serious allergic responses are also more likely to occur by the intravenous route than by other routes.

Many drugs are too irritant to be given by the oral, intramuscular, or subcutaneous route, and must of necessity be given intravenously. However, such drugs may also cause damage to the veins (phlebitis) or, if extravasated, cause necrosis (slough) around the injection site. Consequently, such irritant drugs may be greatly diluted in isotonic solutions of saline, dextrose, or other media and given by slow infusion, providing that the slower rate of delivery does not negate the purpose of the administration in emergency situations.

Absorption by the *intramuscular* route is relatively fast, and this parenteral route may be used where an immediate effect is not required but a prompt effect is desirable. Intramuscular deposition may also be made of certain repository preparations, rapid absorption not being desired. Absorption from an intramuscular depot is more predictable and uniform than from a subcutaneous site.

Irritation around the injection site is a frequent accompaniment of intramuscular injection, depending upon the drug and other ingredients. Because of the dangers of accidental intravenous injection, medical supervision is generally required. Sterilization is necessary.

In *subcutaneous* administration the drug is injected into the alveolar connective tissue just below the skin. Absorption is slower than by the intramuscular route but nevertheless may be prompt with many drugs. Oftentimes, however, absorption by this route may be no faster than by the oral route. Therefore, when a fairly prompt response is desired, with some drugs the subcutaneous route may not offer much advantage over the oral route, unless for some reason the drug cannot be given orally.

The slower rate of absorption by the subcutaneous route is usually the reason why the route is chosen, and the drugs given by this route are usually those in which it is desired to spread the action out over a number of hours, in order to avoid either too intense a response, too short a response, or frequent injections. Examples of drugs given by this route are insulin and sodium heparin, neither of which is absorbed orally and both of which should be absorbed slowly over many hours. In the treatment of asthma, epinephrine is usually given subcutaneously to avoid the dangers of rapid absorption and consequent dangerous cardiovascular effects. Many repository preparations, including tablets or pellets, are given subcutaneously. As with other parenteral routes, irritation may occur. Sterile preparations are also required. However, medical supervision is not always required, and self-administration by this route is customary with certain drugs, such as insulin.

Intradermal injections, in which the drug is injected into rather than below the dermis is rarely employed, except in certain diagnostic and test procedures, such as screening for allergic or local irritant responses.

Occasionally, even by the intravenous route it is not possible, practical, or safe to achieve plasma concentrations high enough so that an adequate amount of drug penetrates into special compartments, such as the cerebrospinal fluid, or various cavities, such as the pleural cavity. The brain is especially difficult to penetrate with water-soluble drugs. The name *blood-brain barrier* is applied to the impediment to penetration. When drugs do penetrate, they are often secreted back into the blood very rapidly, so that adequate levels of drugs in the cerebrospinal fluid may be difficult to achieve. Consequently *intrathecal** or *intraventricular* administration may be indicated.

Body cavities such as the pleural cavity are normally wetted by a small amount of effusate which is in diffusion equilibrium with the blood and hence is accessible to drugs. However, infections and inflammations may cause the cavity to fill with serofibrinous exudate which is too large to be in rapid diffusion equilibrium with the blood. *Intracavitary* administration may thus be required. It is extremely important that sterile and nonirritating preparations be used for intrathecal or intracavitary administration.

Inhalation Route—Inhalation may be employed for delivering gaseous or volatile substances into the systemic circulation, as with most general anesthetics. Absorption is virtually as rapid as the drug can be delivered into the alveoli of the lungs, since the alveolar and vascular epithelial membranes are quite permeable, blood flow is abundant, and there is a very large surface for absorption.

Aerosols of nonvolatile substances may also be administered by inhalation, but the route is infrequently used for delivery into the systemic circulation, because of various factors that contribute to erratic or difficult-to-achieve blood levels. Whether or not an aerosol reaches and is retained in pulmonary alveoli depends critically upon particle size: particles greater than 1 μm in diameter tend to settle in the bronchioles and bronchi, whereas particles less than 0.5 μm fail to settle and are mainly exhaled. Aerosols are mostly employed when the purpose of administration is an action of the drug upon the respiratory tract itself. An example of a drug commonly given as an aerosol is isoproterenol, which is employed to relax the bronchioles in asthma.

Topical Route—Topical administration is employed to deliver a drug at or immediately beneath the point of application. Although occasionally enough drug is absorbed into the systemic circulation to cause systemic effects, absorption is too erratic for the topical route to be used for systemic therapy. Recent work with aprotic solvent vehicles such as dimethyl sulfoxide (DMSO) has, however, renewed interest in topical administration for systemic effects. A large number of topical medicaments are applied to the skin, although topical drugs are also applied to the eye, nose and throat, ear, vagina, etc.

In man, percutaneous absorption probably occurs mainly from the surface. Absorption through the hair follicles occurs, but the follicles in man occupy too small a portion of the total integument to be of primary importance. Absorption through sweat and sebaceous glands generally appears to be minor. When the medicament is rubbed on vigorously, the amount of the preparation that is forced into the hair follicles and glands is increased. Rubbing also forces some material through the stratum corneum without molecular dispersion and diffusion through the barrier. Rather large particles of substances such as sulfur have been demonstrated to pass intact through the stratum corneum. When the skin is diseased or abraded, the cutaneous barrier may be disrupted or

---

* Intrathecal administration denotes administration into the cerebrospinal fluid at any level of the cerebrospinal axis, including injection into the cerebral ventricles, which is the most common mode of intrathecal administration.

defective, so that percutaneous absorption may be increased. Since much of a drug that is absorbed through the epidermis diffuses into the circulation without reaching a high concentration in some portions of the dermis, systemic administration may be preferred in lieu of or in addition to topical administration.

Factors That Affect Absorption

In addition to the physicochemical properties of drug molecules and biological membranes, various factors affect the rate of absorption and determine, in part, the choice of route of administration.

Concentration—It is self-evident that the concentration, or, more exactly, the thermodynamic activity, of a drug in a drug preparation will have an important bearing upon the rate of absorption, since the rate of diffusion of a drug away from the site of administration is directly proportional to the concentration. Thus a 2% solution of lidocaine will induce local anesthesia more rapidly than a 0.2% solution. However, drugs administered in solid form are not necessarily absorbed at the maximal rate (see *Physical State of Formulation and Dissolution Rate* below).

After oral administration the concentration of drugs in the gut is a function of the dose, but the relationship is not necessarily linear. Drugs with a low aqueous solubility (eg, digitoxin) quickly saturate the gastrointestinal fluids, so that the rate of absorption tends to reach a limit as the dose is increased. The peptizing and solubilizing effects of bile and other constituents of the gastrointestinal contents assist in increasing the rate of absorption but are in themselves somewhat erratic. Furthermore, many drugs affect the rates of gastric, biliary, and small intestinal secretion, which causes further deviations from a linear relationship between concentration and dose.

Drugs that are administered subcutaneously or intramuscularly also may not always show a direct linear relationship between the rate of absorption and the concentration of drug in the applied solution, because osmotic effects may cause dilution or concentration of the drug, if the movement of water or electrolytes is different from that of the drug. Whenever possible, drugs for hypodermic injection are prepared as isotonic solutions. Some drugs affect the local blood flow and capillary permeability, so that at the site of injection there may be a complex relationship of concentration achieved to the concentration administered.

Physical State of Formulation and Dissolution Rate—The rate of absorption of a drug may be greatly affected by the rate at which the drug is made available to the biological fluid at the site of administration. The intrinsic physicochemical properties, such as solubility and the thermodynamics of dissolution, are only part of the factors which affect the rate of dissolution of a drug from a solid form. Other factors include not only the unavoidable interactions among the various ingredients in a given formulation but also deliberate interventions to facilitate dispersion (eg, comminution, Chapter 76, and dissolution, Chapter 35) or retard it (eg, coatings, Chapter 91, and slow release formulations, Chapter 92). There are also factors that affect the rate of delivery from liquid forms. For example, a drug in a highly viscous vehicle is more slowly absorbed from the vehicle than a drug in a vehicle of low viscosity; in oil-in-water emulsions, the rate depends upon the partition coefficient. These manipulations are the subject of biopharmaceutics (see Chapter 92).

Area of Absorbing Surface—The area of absorbing surface is an important determinant of the rate of absorption. To the extent that the therapist must work with the absorbing surfaces available in the body, the absorbing surface is not subject to manipulation. However, the extent to which the existing surfaces may be utilized is subject to variation. In those rare instances in which percutaneous absorption is intended for systemic administration, the entire skin is available.

Subsequent to subcutaneous or intramuscular injections, the site of application may be massaged in order to spread the injected fluid from a compact mass to a well-dispersed deposit. Alternatively, the dose may be divided into multiple small injections, although this recourse is generally undesirable.

The different areas for absorption afforded by the various routes account, in part, for differences in the rates of absorption by those routes. The large alveolar surface of the lungs allows for extremely rapid absorption of gases, vapors, and properly aerosolized solutions; with some drugs the rate of absorption may be nearly as fast as intravenous injection. In the gut the small intestine is the site of the fastest, and hence most, absorption because of the small lumen and highly developed villi and microvilli; the stomach has a relatively small surface area, so that even most weak acids are predominately absorbed in the small intestine despite a pH partition factor that should favor absorption from the stomach (see *The pH Partition Principle*, page 731).

Vascularity and Blood Flow—Although the thermal velocity of a freely diffusible average drug molecule is on the order of meters per second, in solution the rate at which it will diffuse away from a reference point will be much slower; collisions with water and/or other molecules, which causes a random motion, and the forces of attraction between the drug and water or other molecules slow the net mean velocity.

The time taken to traverse a given distance is a function of the square of the distance; on the average it would take about $1/_{100}$ sec for a net outward movement of 1 μm, 1 sec for 10 μm, 100 sec for 100 μm, etc. In a highly vascular tissue, such as skeletal muscle, in which there may be more than 1000 capillaries/sq mm of cross section, a drug molecule would not have to travel more than a few microns, hence less than a second on the average, to reach a capillary from a point of injection.

Once the drug reaches the blood, diffusion is not important to transport, and the rate of blood flow determines the movement. The velocity of blood flow in a capillary is about 1 mm/sec, which is 100 times faster than the mean net velocity of drug molecules 1 mm away from their injection site. The velocity of blood flow is even faster in the larger vessels. Less than a minute is required to distribute drug molecules from the capillaries at the injection site to the rest of the body.

From the above discussion it follows that absorption is most rapid in the vascular tissues. Drugs are absorbed more rapidly from intramuscular sites than from less vascular subcutaneous sites, etc. Despite the small absorbing surface for buccal or sublingual absorption, the high vascularity of the buccal, gingival, and sublingual surfaces favors an unexpectedly high rate of absorption. Because of hyperemia, absorption will be faster from inflamed than from normal areas, unless the presence of edema lengthens the mean distance between capillaries and thus negates the effects of hypermia on absorption.

Vasoconstriction may have a profound effect upon the rate of absorption. When a local effect of a drug is desired, as in local anesthesia, absorption away from the infiltered site may be greatly impeded by vasoconstrictors included in the preparation. Unwanted vasoconstriction sometimes may cause serious problems. For example, in World War II many wounded soldiers were given subcutaneous morphine without evident effect. As a result, injections were sometimes repeated more than once. When the patient was removed to the field hospital, toxic effects would suddenly occur. The explanation is that cold-induced vasoconstriction occurred in the field; when the patient was warmed in the hospital,

vasodilation would result and the victim would be flooded with drug. Shock also contributes to the effect, since during shock the blood flow is diminished, and there may also be a superimposed vasoconstriction; repair of the shock condition then facilitates absorption.

Molecules too large to pass through the capillary endothelium will of necessity enter the systemic circulation through the lymph. Thus the lymph flow may be important to the absorption of a few drugs.

Movement—A number of factors combine so that movement at the site of injection increases the rate of absorption. In the intestine, segmental movements and peristalsis aid in dividing and dispersing the drug mass. The continual mixing of the chyme helps keep the concentration maximal at the mucosal surface. The pressures developed during segmentation and peristalsis may also favor a small amount of filtration. Movement at the site of hypodermic injection also favors absorption, since it tends to force the injected material through the tissue, increasing the surface area of drug mass and decreasing the mean distance to the capillaries. Movement also increases the flow of blood and lymph. The selection of a site for intramuscular injection may be determined by the amount of expected movement, according to whether the preparation is intended as a fast-acting or a repository preparation.

Gastric Motility and Emptying—The motility of the stomach is more important to the rate at which an orally administered drug is passed on to the small intestine than it is to the rate of absorption from the stomach itself, since for various reasons, noted above, absorption from the stomach is usually of minor importance.

The average emptying time of the unloaded stomach is about 40 min, and the half-time is around 10 min, though it varies according to its contents, reflex and psychological factors, the action of certain autonomic drugs, or disease. The effect of food to delay absorption is due in part to its action to prolong emptying time. The emptying time causes a delay in the absorption of drug, which may be unfavorable or favorable according to what is desired. In the case of therapy with antacids, gastric emptying is a nuisance, since it removes the antacid from the stomach where it is needed.

Solubility and Binding—The dissolution of drugs of low solubility is generally a slow process. Indeed, low solubility is the result of a low rate of departure of drug molecules from the undispersed phase. Furthermore, since the concentration around the drug mass is low, the concentration gradient from the site of deposition to the plasma is small, and the rate of diffusion is low, accordingly.

When it is desired that a drug have a prolonged action but not a high plasma concentration, a derivative of low solubility is often sought. The "insoluble" estolates and other esters of several steroids have durations of action of weeks because of the slow rates of absorption from the sites of injection. Insoluble salts or complexes of acidic or basic drugs are also employed as repository preparations; for example, the procaine salt of penicillin G has a low solubility and is used in a slow release form of the antibiotic.

The solubility of certain macromolecules is critically dependent on the ionization of substituent groups. When they are amphiprotic, they are least soluble at their isoelectric pH. Insulin is normally soluble at the pH of the extracellular fluid; but by combining insulin with the right proportion of a basic protein, such as protamine, the isoelectric pH can be made to be approximately 7.4, and the complex can be used as a low-solubility prolonged-action drug. For more details, see Chapter 92.

Some drugs may bind with natural substances at or near the site of application. The strongly ionized mucopolysaccharides in connective tissue, ground substance, and mucous secretions of the gut are retardants to the absorption of a number of drugs, especially large cationic or polycationic molecules. In the gut, the binding is the least at low pH, which should favor absorption of large cations from the stomach; however, absorption from the stomach is slow (see above), so that the absorption of large cations mainly occurs in the upper duodenum where the pH is still relatively low. Pharmacologically inactive quaternary ammonium compounds are sometimes included in an oral preparation of a quaternary ammonium drug for the purpose of saturating the binding sites of mucin and other mucopolysaccharides and thereby enhancing the absorption of drug.

In addition to mucopolysaccharides in mucous secretions, food in the gastrointestinal track binds many drugs and slows absorption. Antacids, especially aluminum hydroxide plus other basic aluminum compounds and magnesium trisilicate, bind amine and ammonium drugs and interfere with absorption.

Donnan Effect—The presence of a charged macromolecule on one side of a semipermeable membrane (impermeable to the macromolecule) will alter the concentration of permeant ionized particles according to the Donnan equilibrium (page 732). Accordingly, drug molecules of the same charge as the macromolecule will be constrained to the opposite side of the membrane. The presence of appropriately charged macromolecules not only will influence the distribution of drug ions in accordance with the Donnan equation but will increase the rate of transfer of the drug across the membrane, because of mutual ionic repulsion. This effect is sometimes used to facilitate the absorption of ionizable drugs from the gastrointestinal tract. The Donnan effect also operates to retard the absorption of drug ions of opposite charge; however, the mutual electrostatic attraction of a macromolecule and drug ion generally results in actual binding, which is more important than the Donnan effect.

Vehicles and Absorption Adjuvants—Drugs that are to be applied topically to the skin and mucous membranes are often dissolved in vehicles that are thought to enhance the penetrance. For a long time it was thought that oleaginous vehicles promoted the absorption of lipid-soluble drugs. However, the role and effect of the vehicle has proven to be quite complex. In the skin at least five factors are involved:

1. The effect of the vehicle to alter the hydration of the keratin in the barrier layer.
2. The effect of the vehicle to promote or prevent the collection of sweat at the surface of the skin.
3. The partition coefficient of the drug in a vehicle–water system.
4. The permeability of the skin to the undissolved drug.
5. The permeability of the skin to the vehicle.

The effect of the vehicle to aid in the access of the drug to the hair follicles and sebaceous glands may also be involved, although in man the follicles and glands are probably ordinarily of minor importance to absorption.

A layer of oleaginous material over the skin prevents the evaporation of water, so that the stratum corneum may become macerated and more permeable to drugs. In dermatology it is even sometimes the practice to wrap the site of application with Saran wrap or some other waterproof material for the purpose of increasing the maceration of the stratum corneum. However, the layer of perspiration that forms under an occlusive vehicle may itself become a barrier to the movement of lipid-soluble drugs from the vehicle to the skin, but it may facilitate the movement of water-soluble

drugs. Conversely, polyethylene glycol vehicles remove the perspiration and dehydrate the barrier, which decreases the permeability to drugs; such vehicles remove the aqueous medium through which water-soluble drugs may pass down into the stratum corneum but at the same time facilitate the transfer of lipid-soluble drugs from the vehicle to the skin.

Even in the absence of a vehicle it is not clear what physicochemical properties of a drug favor cutaneous penetration, high lipid-solubility being a prerequisite according to some authorities and an ether–water partition coefficient of approximately 1 according to others. Yet the penetrances of ethanol and dibromomethane are nearly equal, and other such enigmas exist. It is not surprising, then, that the effects of vehicles are not altogether predictable.

A general statement might be made that if a drug is quite soluble in a poorly absorbed vehicle, the vehicle will retard the movement of the drug into the skin. For example, salicylic acid is 100 times as permeant when absorbed from water than from polyethylene glycol, and pentanol is 5 times as permeant from water as from olive oil. Yet ethanol penetrates 5 times faster from olive oil than from either water or ethanol, all of which denies the trustworthiness of generalizations about vehicles.

In recent years there has been much interest in certain highly dielectric aprotic solvents, especially dimethyl sulfoxide (DMSO). Such substances generally prove to be excellent solvents for both water- and lipid-soluble compounds and for some compounds not soluble in either water or lipid solvents. The extraordinary solvent properties are probably due to a high polarizability and van der Waals bonding capacity, a high degree of polarization (dipole moment), and a lack of association through hydrogen bonding. As a vehicle, DMSO greatly facilitates the permeation of the skin and other biological membranes by numerous drugs, even including such large molecules as insulin. The mechanism is not understood. Such vehicles have a potential for many important uses, but they are at present only experimental, pending further investigations on toxicity.

From time to time a claim is made that a new ingredient of a tablet or elixir enhances the absorption of a drug, and a comparison of plasma levels of the old and new preparations seems to support the claim. Upon further investigation, however, it may be revealed that the new so-called absorption adjuvant is replacing an ingredient that previously bound the drug or delayed its absorption; thus the new "adjuvant" is not an adjuvant but rather it is only a nondeterrent.

Other Factors—A number of other less-well-defined factors affect the absorption of drugs, some of which may operate, in part, through factors already cited above. Disease or injury has a considerable effect upon absorption. For example, debridement of the stratum corneum increases the permeability to topical agents, meningitis increases the permeability of the blood–brain barrier, biliary insufficiency decreases the absorption of lipid-soluble substances from the intestine, acid–base disturbances can affect the absorption of weak acids or bases, etc. Certain drugs, such as ouabain, that affect active transport processes may interfere with the absorption of certain other drugs. The condition of the ground substance, or "intracellular cement" probably bears on the absorption of certain types of molecules. Hyaluronidase, which depolymerizes the mucopolysaccharide ground substance, can be demonstrated to facilitate the absorption of some, but not all, drugs from subcutaneous sites.

Drug Disposition

The term *drug disposition* is used here to include all processes which tend to lower the plasma concentration of drug, as opposed to drug absorption, which elevates the plasma level. Consequently, the distribution of drugs to the various tissues will be considered under Disposition. Some authors use the term disposition synonymously with elimination, that is, to include only those processes which decrease the amount of drug in the body. In the present context, disposition comprises three categories of processes: distribution, biotransformation, and excretion.

Distribution, Biotransformation, and Excretion

The term *distribution* is self-explanatory. It denotes the partitioning of a drug among the numerous locations where a drug may be contained within the body. *Biotransformations* are the alterations in the chemical structure of a drug that are imposed upon it by the life processes. *Excretion* is, in a sense, the converse of absorption, namely, the transportation of the drug or its products out of the body. The term applies whether or not special organs of excretion are involved.

Distribution

The body may be considered to comprise a number of compartments: enteric (gastrointestinal), plasma, interstitial, cerebrospinal fluid, bile, glandular secretions, urine, storage vesicles, cytoplasm or intracellular space, etc. Some of these "compartments," such as urine and secretions, are open-ended, but since their contents relate to those in the closed compartments, they must also be included.

At first thought it may seem that if a drug were passively distributed (ie, by simple diffusion) and the plasma concentration could be maintained at a steady level, the concentration of a drug in the water in all compartments ought to become equal. It is true that some substances, such as ethanol and antipyrine, are distributed nearly equally throughout the body water, but they are more the exception than the rule. Such substances are mainly small, uncharged, nondissociable, highly water-soluble molecules.

The condition of small size and high water solubility allows for passage through the pores without the necessity of carrier or active transport. Small size also places a limit on van der Waals binding energy and configurational complementariness, so that binding to proteins in plasma or cells is slight. The presence of a charge on a drug molecule makes for unequal distribution across charged membranes, in accordance with the Donnan distribution. Dissociability causes unequal distribution when there is a pH differential between compartment, as discussed under *The pH Partition Principle* (see below). Thus, even if a drug is distributed passively, its distribution may be uneven throughout the body. When active transport into or a rapid metabolic destruction occurs within some compartments, uneven distribution is also inevitable.

The pH Partition Principle—An important consequence of nonionic diffusion is that a difference in pH between two compartments will have an important influence upon the partitioning of a weakly acidic or basic drug between those compartments. The partition is such that the unionized form of the drug has the same concentration in both compartments, since it is the form that is freely diffusible; the ionized form in each compartment will have the concentration that is determined by the pH in that compartment, the pK, and the concentration of the unionized form. The governing effect of pH and pK on the partition is known as the *pH partition principle*.

To illustrate the principle, consider the partition of salicylic acid between the gastric juice and the interior of a gastric mucosal cell. Assume the pH of the gastric juice to be 1.0,

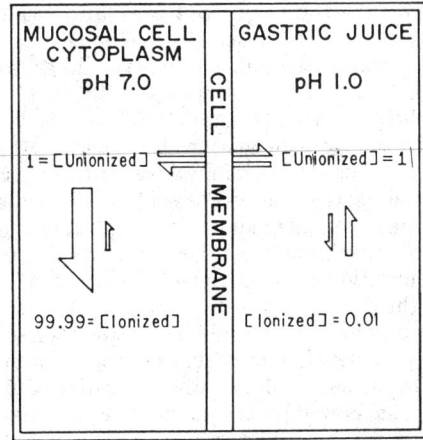

Fig 37-11. Hypothetical partition of salicylic acid between gastric juice and the cytoplasm of a gastric mucosal cell. It is assumed that the ionized form cannot pass through the cell membrane. The intragastric concentration of salicylic acid is arbitrarily arranged to provide unit concentration of the unionized form. *Bracketed values:* concentration; *arrows:* relative size depicts the direction in which dissociation-association is favored at equilibrium.

which it occasionally becomes. The pK$_a$ of salicylic acid is 3.0 (Martin[22] provides one source of pK values of drugs). With the Henderson–Hasselbalch equation (see page 244) it may be calculated that the drug is only 1% ionized at pH 1.0.* The intracellular pH of most cells is about 7.0. Assuming the pH of the mucosal cell to be the same, it may be calculated that salicylic acid will be 99.99% ionized within the cells. Since the concentration of the unionized form is theoretically the same in both gastric juice and mucosal cells, it follows that the total concentration of the drug (ionized + unionized) within the mucosal cell will be 10,000 times than in gastric juice. This is illustrated in Fig 37-11. Such a relatively high intracellular concentration can have important osmotic and toxicologic consequences.

Had the drug been a weak base instead of an acid, the high concentration would have been in the gastric juice. In the small intestine, where the pH may range from 7.5 to 8.1, the partition of a weak acid or base will be the reverse of that in the stomach, but the concentration differential will be less, because the pH differential from lumen to mucosal cells, etc., will be less. The reversal of partition as the drug moves from the stomach to the small intestine accounts for the phenomenon that some drugs may be absorbed from one gastrointestinal segment and returned to another. The weak base, atropine, is absorbed from the small intestine, but because of pH partition it is "secreted" into the gastric juice.

The pH partition of drugs has never been demonstrated to be as marked as that illustrated in Fig 37-11 and in the text. Not only do many drug ions probably pass through the pores of the membrane to a significant extent, but some may also pass through the lipid phase, as explained above for the morphinans and mecamylamine. Furthermore, ion-pair formation in carrier transport also bypasses nonionic diffusion. All processes that tend toward an equal distribution of drugs across membranes and among compartments will cause further deviations from theoretical predictions of pH partition.

---

* The relationship of ionization and partition to pH and pK has been formulated in several different ways, but the student may calculate the concentrations from simple mass law equations. More sophisticated calculations and reviews of this subject are available.[18,23-28]

Electrochemical and Donnan Distribution—A drug ion may be passively distributed across a membrane in accordance with the membrane potential, the charge on the drug ion, and the Donnan effect. The relationship of the membrane potential to the passive distribution of ions is quantitatively expressed by the Nernst equation (Eq 7, page 724) and has already been discussed. Barring active transport, pH partition, and binding, the drug will be said to be distributed according to the electrical gradient or to its "equilibrium" potential. If the membrane potential is 90 mv, the concentration of a univalent cation will be 30 times as high within the cell as without; if the drug cation is divalent, the ratio will be 890. The distribution of anions would be just the reverse. If the membrane potential is but 9 mv, the ratio for a univalent cation will be only 1.4 and for a divalent cation only 2.0. It can thus be seen how important membrane potential may be to the distribution of ionized drugs.

It was pointed out under *Membrane Potentials*, page 723, that large potentials derive from active transport of ions but that small potentials may result from Donnan distribution. Donnan membrane theory is discussed in Chapter 14. According to the theory, the ratio of the intracellular/extracellular concentration of a permeant univalent anion is equal to the ratio of extracellular/intracellular concentration of a permeant univalent cation. A more general mathematical expression that includes ions of any valence is

$$\left(\frac{A_i}{A_e}\right)^{1/Z_a} = \left(\frac{C_e}{C_i}\right)^{1/Z_c} = r \qquad (8)$$

where A_i is the intracellular and A_e the extracellular concentration of anion, Z_c is the valence of cation, Z_a is the valence of anion, C_i is the intracellular and C_e the extracellular concentration of cation, and r is the Donnan factor. The value of r depends upon the average molecular weight and valence of the macromolecules (mostly protein) within the cell, and the intracellular and extracellular volumes. Since the macromolecules within the cell are negatively charged, the cation concentration will be higher within the cell, that is, $C_i > C_e$. Since a Donnan distribution results in a membrane potential, the distribution of drug ion will also be in keeping with the membrane potential.

The Donnan distribution also applies to the distribution of a charged drug between the plasma and interstitial compartment, because of the presence of anionic proteins in the plasma. Eq 8 applies by changing the subscript i to p, for plasma, and e to i, for interstitial. The Donnan factor, r, for plasma–interstitial space partition is about 1.05:1.

Binding and Storage—Drugs are frequently bound to plasma proteins (especially albumin), interstitial substances, intracellular constituents, and bone and cartilage. If binding is extensive and firm, it will have a considerable impact upon the distribution, excretion, and sojourn of the drug in the body. Obviously, a drug that is bound to a protein or any other macromolecule will not pass through the membrane in the bound form; only the unbound form can negotiate among the various compartments.

The partition among compartments is determined by the binding capacity and binding constant in each compartment. As long as the binding capacity exceeds the quantity of drug in the compartment, the following equation generally applies:

$$\log D_b = \log K + a \log D_f \qquad (9)$$

where D_b is the concentration of bound drug, D_f is the concentration of free drug, and a and K are constants characteristic of the drug and binding macromolecule. The equation is that of a Freundlich isotherm. As the binding capacity is approached, the relationship no longer holds. For a nondissociable drug at equilibrium, D_f will be the same in all com-

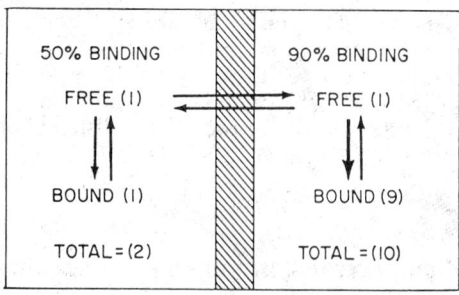

Fig 37-12. Distribution of a drug between two compartments between which the degrees of binding to protein differ. The percent of binding is indicated. Only the unbound drug can pass through the membrane. *Bracketed values:* concentration (courtesy, Schanker[24]).

municating compartments, so that it would be possible to calculate the partition if K and a are known for each compartment. Except for plasma, the values of a and K are generally unknown, but the percent bound is often known. From the percent bound the partition can also be calculated, as in Fig 37-12. However, the logarithmic relationships shown in Eq 9 serve as a reminder that the percent bound changes with the concentration, so that the partition will vary with the dose. If the drug is a weak acid or base, the unionized free form negotiates among the compartments, but the ionized form is often the more firmly bound, and calculations must take into account the dissociation constant and the different a's and K's of the ionized and unionized forms.

It is commonly misbelieved that binding in the plasma interferes with the activity of a drug and the intracellular binding in a responsive cell increases activity or toxicity. Both binding in plasma and in the tissues decreases the concentration of free drug; but this is easily remedied by adjusting the dose to give a sufficient concentration for pharmacological activity. The distribution and activity of the free form is not affected by binding. The principal effect of binding is to increase the initial dose requirement for drug and to create a reservoir of drug from which the drug may be withdrawn as the free form is excreted or metabolized. However, if the binding is extremely firm and release is slow, the rate of release may not be enough to sustain the free form at a sufficient level for pharmacological activity; in such instances the bound drug cannot be considered a reserve.

The effect of binding upon the sojourn of a drug may be considerable. For example, quinacrine, which may be concentrated in the liver to as much as several thousand times the concentration in plasma, may remain in the body for months. Some iodine-containing radiopaque diagnostic agents are strongly bound to plasma protein and may remain in the plasma for as long as 2 years. In pathological conditions, such as nephrosis, diabetes, and cirrhosis, in which plasma protein levels may be decreased, the plasma protein binding, loading dose, and duration of action may all be decreased.

If a drug is bound to a functional macromolecule, binding may relate to pharmacological activity and toxicity, provided that the binding is at a critical center of the macromolecule. The binding by nucleic acids of certain antimalarials, such as quinacrine, undoubtedly contributes to the parasiticidal actions as well as to toxicity.

Most drugs are bound to proteins by relatively weak forces, such as van der Waals (London, Keesom, or Debye) forces, or hydrogen or ionic bonds. Consequently, binding constants are generally small and binding is usually readily reversible. The larger the molecule, the greater the van der Waals bonding, so that large drug molecules are more likely to be strongly bound than are small ones.

Just as shape and the nature of functional groups is important to drug–receptor combination, so they also are to

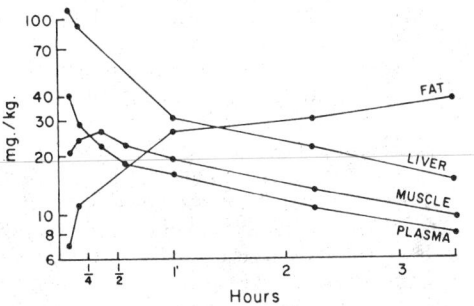

Fig 37-13. Predisposition of thiopental for fat. 25 mg/kg was given to a dog. After a brief sojourn of thiopental in the more vascular tissues, it gradually transfers to fat, where the lipid-soluble drug dissolves in fat droplets (courtesy, Brodie and Hogben[25]).

binding. Drugs of similar shape and/or chemical affinities may bind at the same sites on a binding protein and hence compete with one another. For example, phenylbutazone displaces warfarin from human plasma albumin, which may cause an increase in the anticoagulant effect of warfarin. Some drugs may also displace protein-bound endogenous constituents. For example, sulfisoxazole displaces bilirubin from plasma proteins; in infants with kernicterus the freed bilirubin floods the central nervous system and causes sometimes fatal toxicity.

According to the lipid–water coefficient, a drug may be taken up into fat. The ratio of concentration in fat to that in plasma will not be the same as the partition coefficient because of the content of water and of non-lipids in adipose tissue and because electrolytes and other solutes alter the dielectric constant and hence solubilities from those of pure water. Lipoproteins and even nonpolar substituents on plasma proteins also take up lipid-soluble molecules, so that solubility in plasma can be considerably higher than that in water. The relatively high solubility of ether in plasma makes plasma a pool for ether, the filling of which delays the onset of anesthesia. However, ether and other volatile anesthetics are gradually taken up into the adipose tissue, which acts as a store of the anesthetic. The longer the anesthetic is administered, the greater the store and the longer it takes for anesthesia to terminate when inhalation has been discontinued.

Another notable substance that it readily taken up into fat is thiopental. Even though there is a high solubility of this barbiturate in fat, the low rate of blood flow in fat limits the rate of uptake. Because the blood flow in the brain is very high, thiopental rapidly enters brain tissue. However, it soon equilibrates with the other tissues, and the brain concentration falls as that in the other tissues (eg, muscle, liver) increases. Gradually, however, the fat accumulates the drug at the expense of other compartments. The gradual entry of thiopental into fat at the expense of plasma, muscle, or liver is illustrated in Fig 37-13.

Nonequilibrium and Redistribution—Thus far the distribution of drugs has been mainly discussed as though equilibrium or steady state conditions exist after a drug is absorbed and distributed. However, since most drugs are administered at intervals and the body content of drug rises and falls with absorption and destruction-excretion, neither a true equilibrium among the body compartments nor a steady state exists.

The term equilibrium is misleadingly used to describe the conditions that exist when the plasma concentration and the concentration in a tissue are equal, as exemplified at the point of intersection of the curves for plasma and muscle or plasma and fat in Fig 37-13. But such "equilibrium" with fat occurs much later than "equilibrium" with muscle, so that no true equilibrium really exists among all the compartments. Fur-

thermore, the cross-over point for plasma and any one tissue is not necessarily an equilibrium point, because the rates of ingress and egress from the tissue are not necessarily equal when the internal and external concentrations are equal, since there are numerous factors that make for unequal distribution (pH partition, Donnan effect, electrochemical distribution, active transport, binding, etc).

A study of Fig 37-13 shows that the distribution of thiopental continually changed during the $3\frac{1}{2}$ hr of observation. At the end of the period, the content in fat was still increasing while that in each of the other compartments was decreasing. This time-dependent shift in partition is called *redistribution*. Eventually, the content in fat would have reached a peak, which peak would represent as nearly a true equilibrium point as could be achieved in the dynamic situation where metabolic destruction and a slight amount of excretion of the drug was taking place. Once the concentration in the fat had reached its peak, its content would have declined in parallel with that in the other tissues, and the partition among the compartments would have remained essentially constant. Redistribution, then, takes place only until the concentration in the slowest filling compartment reaches its peak, so long as the kinetics of elimination are constant.

An index of distribution known as the *volume of distribution* (amount of drug in the body divided by plasma concentration) is of considerable usefulness in pharmacokinetics but is of limited value in defining the way in which a drug is partitioned in the body. Volume of distribution is discussed on page 756.

The word *space* is often used synonymously with volume of distribution. It is especially employed when the distributed substance has a volume of distribution that is essentially identical to a physical real space or body compartment. *N*-Acetyl-4-aminoantipyrine is distributed evenly throughout the total body water and is not bound to proteins or other tissue constituents. Thus the acetylaminoantipyrine space or volume of distribution coincides with that of total body water. Inulin, sucrose, sulfate, and a number of other substances are essentially confined to extracellular water, so that an inulin space, for example, measures the extracellular fluid volume. Evans blue is confined to the plasma, so that the Evans blue space is the plasma volume. Such space measurements with standard space indicators are a necessary part of studies on the distribution of drugs, since it is desirable to compare the volume of distribution to a drug to the standard spaces.

Biotransformations

Most drugs are acted upon by enzymes in the body and converted to metabolic derivatives called metabolites. The process of conversion is called biotransformation. Metabolites are usually more polar and less lipid-soluble than the parent drug because of the introduction of oxygen into the molecule, hydrolysis to yield more highly polar groups, or conjugation with a highly polar substance. As a consequence, metabolites often show less penetrance into tissues and less renal tubular resorption than the parent drug, in accordance with the principle of the low penetrance of polar and high penetrance of lipid-soluble substances. For similar reasons, metabolites are usually less active than the parent drug, often inactive; even if they are appreciably active, they are generally more rapidly excreted. Therefore, the usual net effect of biotransformation may be said to be one of *inactivation* or *detoxication*.

There are, however, numerous examples in which biotransformation does not result in inactivation. Table III (page 758) lists a number of drugs that generate active metabolites; in a few instances activity derives entirely from the metabolite.

There are also examples in which the parent drug has no activity of its own but is converted to an active metabolite. Parathion, malathion, and certain other anticholinesterases require metabolic activation, inactive chloroguanide is converted to an active triazine derivative, phenylbutazone is hydroxylated to the antirheumatic hydroxyphenylbutazone, inactive pentavalent arsenicals are reduced to their active trivalent metabolites, and there are other examples of an activating biotransformation.

When a delayed or prolonged response to a drug is desired or an unpleasant taste or local reaction is to be avoided, it is a common pharmaceutical practice to prepare an inactive or nonoffending precursor, such that the active form may be generated in the body. This practice has been termed *drug latentiation*. Chloramphenicol palmitate, dichloralphenazone, and the estolates of various steroid hormones are examples of deliberately latentiated drugs. Because inactive metabolites do not always result from biotransformation, the term detoxication should not be used as a synonym for biotransformation.

Biotransformations take place principally in the liver, although the kidney, skeletal muscle, intestine, or even plasma may be important sites of the enzymatic attack of some drugs. Since plasma lacks the enzymes and structures required for electron transport, biotransformations in plasma are mostly hydrolytic.

Endoplasmic Reticulum and Microsomal System—Biotransformations in the liver mainly occur in *smooth endoplasmic reticulum*. The endoplasmic reticulum is a tubular system which courses through the interior of the cell but also appears to communicate with the interstitial space, and its membrane is continuous with the cell membrane. Some of the reticulum is lined with ribonucleoprotein particles, called ribosomes, which are engaged in protein synthesis; this is the *rough* endoplasmic reticulum. Although the smooth endoplasmic reticulum lacks such a granular appearance, it is heavily invested with numerous enzymes which biotransform many drugs and some endogenous substances.

When a broken cell homogenate of the liver is prepared, the reticulum becomes fragmented, and the fragments form vesicular structures called *microsomes*. Although the microsomes are artifacts, it is the practice to refer to the *microsomal drug metabolizing system* rather than to the smooth endoplasmic reticulum.

The microsomal system is peculiar in that both oxidations and reductions usually require the reducing cofactor NADPH (TPNH). This is because microsomal oxidations proceed by way of the introduction of oxygen rather than by dehydrogenation, and NADPH is essential to reduce one of the atoms of O_2. The drug first binds to an oxidized cytochrome P-450. The drug-cytochrome complex is then reduced by NADPH-cytochrome reductase; the reduced complex then combines with O_2, after which the metabolite is released and oxidized cytochrome P-450 is regenerated. Cytochrome P-450 is a generic term that includes at least six, and probably more, separate enzymes[29].

Some of the enzymes of the microsomal system are quite easily *induced;* that is, a substrate of the enzyme may considerably increase the activity of that enzyme by increasing the biosynthesis of that enzyme. An increase in the amount of smooth endoplasmic reticulum is also sometimes demonstrated concomitantly with enzyme induction.

Treatment of an experimental subject with phenobarbital will greatly increase the rate of metabolism of phenobarbital, which necessitates larger and more frequent doses of the drug in order to maintain a constant sedative effect. Moreover, phenobarbital may induce an increased metabolism of some other but not all barbiturates as well as some unrelated drugs, such as strychnine and warfarin. Oddly, warfarin does not readily induce its own biotransformation. At the present time, both self-induction and cross-induction appear capricious and unpredictable.

Induction may create therapeutic problems. For example, the use of phenobarbital during treatment with warfarin increases the dose requirement for warfarin. If the physician is unaware of this interaction and fails to increase the dose, the patient may suffer a thrombotic episode. If the dose of warfarin has been increased and the phenobarbital is then discontinued, the rate of metabolism of warfarin may drop to its previous level, so that the patient is overdosed, with hemorrhagic consequences. Some drugs inhibit rather than induce the microsomal system, which reduces the dose requirement and may lead to toxicity. Cimetidine is an example of a drug that inhibits the hepatic metabolism of a number of other drugs.

The activity of the microsomal system is affected by many factors other than the presence of drugs. Age, sex, nutritional states, pathological conditions, body temperature, and genetic factors are among the influences that have been identified. Age, particularly, has received considerable attention. Infants have a poorly developed microsomal system, which accounts for the low dose requirement for morphine and also explains the high toxicity of chloramphenicol in infants.

The activity and selectivity of the microsomal system varies greatly from species to species, so that care must be exercised in extrapolating experimental findings in laboratory animals to man.

Types of Biotransformations—Biotransformations may be *degradative*, wherein the drug molecule is diminished to a smaller structure, or *synthetic*, wherein one or more atoms or groups may be added to the molecule. Very few drugs are degraded completely. However, it is more useful to categorize biotransformations with respect to "metabolic" (nonconjugative) biotransformations and conjugative biotransformations. The former is called phase I and the latter phase II. In phase I pharmacodynamic activity may be lost, however, active and chemically reactive intermediates may also be generated. The polarity of the molecule may or may not be increased sufficiently to increase excretion markedly. In phase II, metabolites from phase I may be conjugated, and sometimes the original drug may be conjugated, thus bypassing phase I. Phase II generates metabolites of high polarity which are readily excreted.

Biotransformations may be placed into five categories: (1) oxidation, (2) reduction, (3) hydrolysis, (4) conjugation, and (5) miscellaneous. Oxidation, reduction and hydrolysis comprise phase I. Conjugation comprises phase II. Most of the miscellaneous belong in phase I.

Oxidation—Oxidation is more common than any other type of biotransformation. Oxidations that occur primarily in the liver microsomal system include side-chain hydroxylation, aromatic hydroxylation, deamination (which is oxidative and results in the intermediate formation of RCHO), N-, O-, and S-dealkylation (which probably involves hydroxylation of the alkyl group followed by oxidation to the aldehyde), and sulfoxide formation. N-Demethylation involves a different system from N-dealkylation of higher radicals.

Oxidations that occur elsewhere than the microsomes are generally dehydrogenations followed by the addition of oxygen or water. Examples are the oxidation of alcohols by alcohol dehydrogenase, the oxidation of aldehyde by aldehyde dehydrogenase, and the deamination of monoamines by monoamine oxidase and diamines by diamine oxidase. The oxidation of purines like caffeine and theophylline is also extramicrosomal.

Reduction—Reductions are relatively uncommon. They mainly occur in liver microsomes, but they occasionally take place in other tissues. Examples are the reduction of nitro and nitroso groups (as in chloramphenicol, nitroglycerin, and organic nitrites), of the azo group (as in prontosil), and of certain aldehydes to the corresponding alcohols (as with the deaminated serotonin metabolite, 5-hydroxytryptophal, to 5-hydroxytryptophol).

Hydrolysis—Hydrolysis is a common biotransformation among esters and amides. Esterases are located in many structures besides the microsomes. For example, cholinesterases are found in plasma, erythrocytes, liver, nerve terminals, junctional interstices, and postjunctional structures, and procaine esterases are found in plasma. Various phosphatases and sulfatases are also widely distributed in tissues and plasma, although few drugs are appropriate substrates. The hydrolytic deamidation of meperidine occurs primarily in the hepatic microsomes.

Conjugation—A large number of drugs or their metabolites are conjugated. Conjugation is the biosynthetic process of combining a chemical compound with a highly polar and water-soluble natural substance to yield a water-soluble, usually inactive, product. Conjugations generally involve either esterification, amidation, mixed anhydride formation, hemiacetal formation, or etherization.

Glucuronic acid is the most frequent partner to the drug in conjugation. Actually, the drug reacts with uridine diphosphoglucuronic acid rather than with simple glucuronic acid. The drug or drug metabolite combines at the number 1 carbon (aldehyde end) and not at the carboxyl end of glucuronic acid. The hydroxyl group of an alcohol or a phenol attacks the number 1 carbon of the pyran ring to replace uridine diphosphate. The product is a hemiacetyl-like derivative. Since the product is not an ester, the term *glucuronide* is appropriate. Rarely, thiols and amines may form analogous glucuronides.

Carboxyl compounds form esters, appropriately called *glucuronates*, in replacing the uridine diphosphate. *Sulfuric acid* is also a frequent conjugant, especially with phenols and to a lesser extent with simple alcohols. The sulfurated product is called an *ethereal sulfate*. Occasionally sulfuric acid conjugates with aromatic amines to form *sulfamates*. *Phosphoric acid* also conjugates with phenols and aromatic amines. The conjugation of benzoic acid with glycine to yield hippuric acid is a classical example of an *amidation* conjugative process. Cysteine may take the place of glycine, through the intermediation of glutathione, to yield mercapturic acids with certain aromatic acids.

Amidations with amino acids are less frequent than *acetylation*, partly because few drugs are carboxylic compounds. Aromatic amines and occasionally aliphatic amines or heterocyclic nitrogen are frequently acetylated. Acetyl-CoA is the biological reagent rather than acetic acid itself. Unlike most other conjugates, the acetylate (amide) is usually less water-soluble than the parent compound. The acetylation of the para-amino group of the sulfonamides is a prime example of this type of conjugation.

Although most conjugations occur in the liver, the microsomal system is not involved. Some conjugations occur in the kidney or in other tissues.

Miscellaneous—Many amines, especially derivatives of β-phenylethylamine and heterocyclic compounds, are methylated in the body. The products are usually biologically active, sometimes more so than the parent compound. *N-Methylation* may occur in the cell sap of the liver and elsewhere, especially in chromaffin tissue in the case of phenylethylamines.

Phenolic compounds may be *O*-methylated. *O-Methylation* is the principal route of biotransformation of catecholamines such as epinephrine and norepinephrine, the methyl group being introduced on the meta hydroxy substituent. Both *N*- and *O*-methylation require *S*-methyladenosyl cysteine.

Desulfuration, in which oxygen may replace sulfur, takes place in the liver. Thiopental is in part converted to pentobarbital by desulfuration, and parathion is transformed to paraoxon.

Dehalogenation of certain insecticides and various halogenated hydrocarbons may take place, principally in the liver but not in the microsomes.

Excretion

Some drugs are not biotransformed in the body. Others may be biotransformed, but their products still remain to be eliminated. It follows that excretion is involved in the elimination of all drugs and/or their metabolites. Although the kidney is the most important organ of excretion, some substances are excreted in bile, sweat, saliva, gastric juice, or from the lungs.

Renal Excretion—The excretory unit of the kidney is called the *nephron* (Fig 37-14). There are several million nephrons in the human kidney. The nephron is essentially a filter funnel, called *Bowman's capsule*, with a long stem, called a *renal tubule*. It is also now recognized that the collecting duct is functionally a part of the nephron. The *blood vessels* that invest the capsule and the tubule are also an essential part of the nephron.

Bowman's capsule is packed with a tuft of branching interconnected capillaries (*glomerular tuft*), which provide a large surface area of capillary endothelium ("filter paper") through which fluid and small molecules may filter into the capsule and begin passage down the tubule. The glomerular tuft together with Bowman's capsule constitute the *glomerulus*. The glomerular capillary endothelium and the sup-

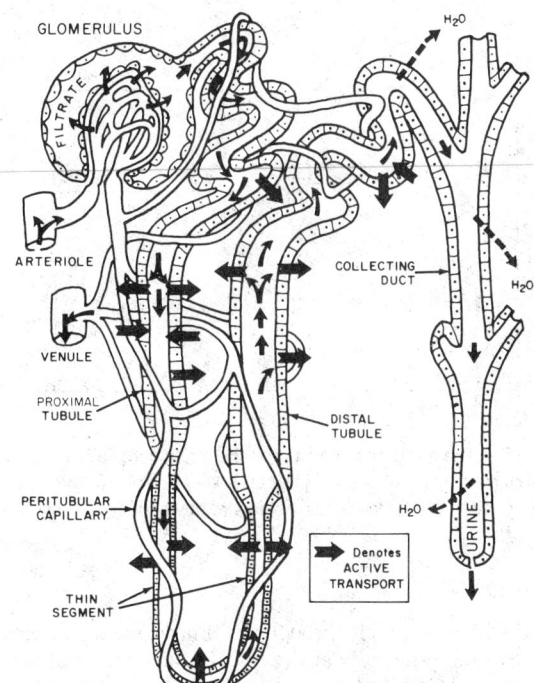

Fig 37-14. Diagram of a mammalian nephron. Note how the lower loops of the postglomerular capillaries course downward and double back along with the tubule. This allows countercurrent distribution to maintain hyperosmolar urine within the thin segment.

porting layer of Bowman's capsule have channels ranging upwards to 40 Å. Consequently, all unbound crystalloid solutes in plasma and even a little albumin pass into the glomerular filtrate.

The postglomerular vessels which lie close to the tubules are critically important to renal function in that substances resorbed from the filtrate by the tubule are returned to the blood along these vessels. The tubule is not straight but rather first makes a number of convolutions (called a *proximal convoluted tubule*), then courses down and back up a long loop (called the *loop of Henle*), makes more convolutions (the *distal convoluted tubule*), and finally joins the collecting duct. The loop of Henle is divided into a *proximal (descending) tubule*, a thin segment, and a *distal (ascending) tubule*.

As the glomerular filtrate passes through the proximal tubule, some solute may be resorbed (*tubular resorption*) through the tubular epithelium and returned to the blood. Resorption occurs in part by passive diffusion and in part by active transport, especially with sodium and glucose. Chloride follows sodium obligatorily.

In the proximal region, the tubule is quite permeable to water, so that resorbed solutes are accompanied by enough water to keep the resorbate isotonic. Consequently, although the filtrate becomes diminished in volume by approximately 80% in the proximal tubule, it is not concentrated.

Some *acidification* occurs in the proximal tubule as the result of carbonic anhydrase activity in the tubule cells and the diffusion of hydronium ions into the lumen. In the lumen the hydronium ion reacts with bicarbonate ion, which is converted to resorbable nonionic CO_2.

There is also active transport of organic cations and anions into the lumen (*tubular secretion*), each by a separate system. These active transport systems are extremely important in the excretion of a number of drugs; for example, penicillin G is rapidly secreted by the anion transport system and tetraethylammonium by the cation transport system. Probenecid is an inhibitor of anion secretion and hence decreases the rate of loss of penicillin from the body.

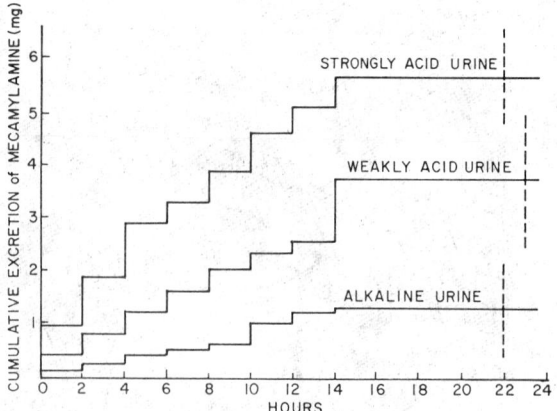

Fig 37-15. The effect of urinary pH on the mean cumulative excretion in man of mecamylamine during the first day after oral administration of 10 mg. *Vertical broken lines:* standard deviation (courtesy, Milne, *et al*[30]).

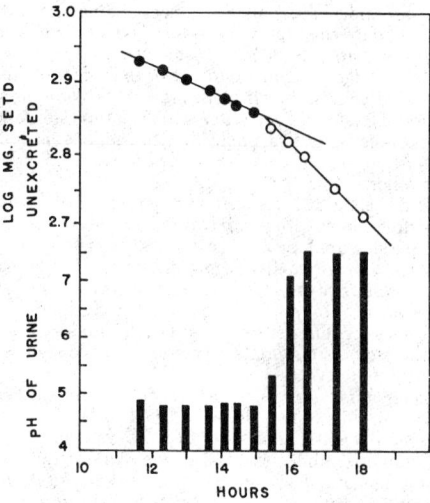

Fig 37-16. The effect of urinary pH on the excretion of sulfaethidole in a human subject after oral administration of 2 g. *Bars* (lower half): urinary pH; *circles* (open and closed, top): log of the amount of drug remaining in the body; *negative slopes* (of lines defined by the circles): a function of the rate constant of excretion. Note the abrupt increase in rate when the urinary pH is changed from acidic to neutral or slightly alkaline (courtesy, Kostenbauder, *et al*[31]).

As the filtrate travels through the thin segment it becomes concentrated, especially at the bottom, as a result of active resorption and a countercurrent distribution effect enabled by the recurrent and parallel arrangement of the ascending segment, the parallel orientation of the collecting duct, and the similar recurrent geometry of the associated capillaries.

In the thick segment of the ascending loop of Henle, both sodium and chloride are transported actively.

In the distal tubule sodium resorption occurs partly in *exchange* for potassium (*potassium secretion*) and for hydronium ions. Adrenal mineralocorticoids promote distal tubular sodium resorption and potassium and hydronium secretion. *Ammonia secretion* also occurs, so that the urine may be either acidified or alkalinized, according to acid–base and electrolyte requirements.

Water is resorbed selectively from the distal end of the distal convoluted tubule and the collecting ducts; water resorption is under the control of the antidiuretic hormone.

Drugs may also be resorbed in the distal tubule; the pH of the urine there is extremely important in determining the rate of resorption, in accordance with the principle of nonionic diffusion and pH partition. The pH of the tubular fluid also affects the tubular secretion of drugs.

As an example of the importance of urine pH, in humans the secondary amine, mecamylamine, is excreted more than four times faster when the urine pH is less than 5.5 than when it is above 7.5; Fig 37-15 illustrates the effect of urine pH on the excretion of this amine. The effect of urine pH on the excretion of a weak acid, sulfaethidole (for structure, see page 1109, RPS-15), is shown in Fig 37-16.

The urine pH and hence drug excretion may fluctuate widely according to the diet, exercise, drugs, time of day, and other factors. Obviously, the excretion of weak acids and bases can be partly controlled with acidifying or alkalinizing salts, such as NH_4Cl or $NaHCO_3$, respectively. Comparative studies on potency and efficacy in man have demonstrated the importance of controlling urinary pH. Urine pH is important only when the drug in question is a weak acid or base of which a significant fraction is excreted. The plasma levels will change inversely to the excretory rate. For example, it has been shown clinically with quinidine that alkalinization of the urine not only decreases the urine concentration but increases the plasma concentration and toxicity.

The collecting duct also resorbs sodium and water, secretes potassium, acidifies, and concentrates the urine. Antidiuretic hormone (ADH) controls the permeability to water of both the collecting duct and the distal tubule.

Renal clearance and the kinetics of renal elimination are discussed in Chapter 38 (page 746).

Biliary Excretion and Fecal Elimination—Many drugs are secreted into the bile and thence pass into the intestine. A drug that is passed into the intestine via the bile may be reabsorbed and not lost from the body. This cycle of biliary secretion and intestinal resorption is called *enterohepatic circulation*. Examples of drugs enterohepatically circulated are morphine and the penicillins. The biliary secretory systems greatly resemble those of the kidney tubules. The enterohepatic system may provide a considerable reservoir for a drug.

If a drug is not completely absorbed from the intestine, the unabsorbed fraction will be eliminated in the feces. An unabsorbable drug that is secreted into the bile will likewise be eliminated in the feces. Such fecal elimination is also called *fecal excretion*. Only rarely are drugs secreted into the intestine through the succus entericus (intestinal secretions), although a number of amines are secreted into gastric juice.

Alveolar Excretion—The large alveolar area and high blood flow make the lungs ideal for the excretion of appropriate substances. Only volatile liquids or gases are eliminated from the lungs. Gaseous and volatile anesthetics are essentially completely eliminated by this route. Only a small amount of ethanol is eliminated by the lungs, but the concentration in the alveolar air is so constantly related to the blood alcohol concentration that the analysis of expired air is acceptable for legal purposes. The high aqueous solubility and relatively low vapor pressure of ethanol at body temperature account for the retention of most of the substance in the blood. Carbon dioxide from those drugs that are partly degraded to CO_2 also is excreted in the lungs.

Pharmacokinetics

Pharmacokinetics is the science that treats of the rate of absorption, extent of absorption, rates of distribution among body compartments, rate of elimination, and related phenomena. Because of its importance, two chapters, *Basic Pharmacokinetics* (page 741) and *Principles of Clinical Pharmacokinetics* (page 762), have been devoted to the subject.

Drug Interaction and Combination

It is frequent that a patient may receive more than one drug concurrently. Case records show that surgical patients commonly receive more than 10 and sometimes as many as 30 drugs and that the patient is often under the influence of several drugs at once, sometimes unnecessarily. Multiple-drug administration is also common to patients hospitalized for infections and for many other disorders. Furthermore, a patient may be suffering from more than one unrelated disorder which demands simultaneous treatment with two or more drugs. In such instances interactions are unsolicited and often unexpected.

In addition to the administration of drugs concurrently for their independent and unrelated effects, drugs are sometimes administered concurrently deliberately to make use of expected interactions.

Types of Interaction and Reasons for Combination Therapy

A drug may affect the response to another drug in a quantitative way. On the one hand, the intensity of either the therapeutic effect or side effect may be augmented or suppressed. On the other hand, a qualitatively different effect may be brought out. The mechanisms of such interactions are many and are not always understood. A drug may not necessarily affect either the quality or initial intensity of effect of another drug but may cause significant to profound changes in the duration of action. The nature of this type of interaction is generally fairly well understood, although it may not yet have been ascertained for any particular drug combination. The deliberate use of combined interacting drugs is most valid when the mechanism of the interaction is understood and the combined effects are both quantifiable and predictable. The rationales of drug combination and the principles involved are discussed below.

Combinations to Increase Intensity of Response or Efficacy—Sometimes the basis for the action of one drug to increase the intensity of response to another is well understood, but often the reason for a positive interaction is obscure. A terminology has grown up that is frequently not enlightening as to mechanisms and principles but also which is somewhat confusing.

Drugs that elicit the same quality of effect and are mutually interactive are called *homergic*, regardless of whether there is anything in common between the separate response systems. Thus the looseness of the term admits a pressor response consequent to an increase in cardiac output to be homergic with one resulting from arteriolar constriction, even though there is not one common responsive element, the blood pressure itself being but a passive indicator. However, homergic drugs usually have in common at least part of a response system. Thus both norepinephrine and pitressin stimulate some of the same vascular smooth muscle, even though they do not excite the same receptors.

Two homergic drugs can be agonists of the same receptor, so that the entire response system is common to both. Such drugs are called *homodynamic*. As discussed under *Drug Receptors and Receptor Theory* (page 718), homodynamic drugs will generate dose–intensity of effect curves with parallel slopes but not necessarily with identical maxima or efficacies, if one of the drugs is a partial agonist.

From mass law kinetics and dose–effect data of the separate drugs it is possible to predict the combined effects of two agonists to the same receptor. If both drugs are full agonists, theory predicts that an *EDx* of Drug *A* added to an *EDy* of Drug *B* should elicit the same effect as that of an *EDy* of Drug *A* added to an *EDx* of Drug *B*. An example is shown in Fig

37-17. Dose–percent data with homodynamic drugs can be treated in the same way.[33]

Drugs whose combined effects fit the above conditions are called *additive*. If the response to the combination exceeds the expected value for additivity, the drugs are considered to be *supra-additive*. Purely homodynamic drugs do not show supra-additivity; however, if one drug in the pair has an additional action to affect the concentration or penetrance of the other or to prime the response system in some way, two agonists to the same receptor may exhibit supra-additivity. Two homergic drugs are *infra-additive* if their combined effect is less than expected from additivity. As with supra-additivity, infra-additivity must involve an action elsewhere than on a common receptor.

Two drugs are said to be *summative* if a dose of drug that elicits response x added to a dose of another drug that elicits response y gives the combined response $x + y$. Very little significance can usually be attached to summation. Unless the dose–intensity curve of each drug is linear rather than log-linear, summation cannot be predicted from the two curves. When summation does occur with the usual clinical doses of two drugs, it almost never occurs over the entire dose range; indeed, if the dose of each of the two drugs is greater than an ED50, summation is theoretically impossible unless it is possible to increase the maximal response. At best, summation is an infrequent clinical finding limited to one or two doses.

Two drugs are said to be *heterergic* if the drugs do not cause responses of the same quality. When heterergy is positive, ie, the response to one drug is enhanced by the other, *synergism* is said to occur. The word has often been used to describe any positive interaction, but it should be used only to describe a positive interaction between heterergic drugs. The term *potentiation* has been used synonymously with synergism, but misuse of the term has led to the recommendation that the term be dropped. Synergism is often the result of an effect to interfere with the elimination of a drug and thus to increase the concentration; synergism may also result from an effect on penetrance or upon the responsivity of the effector system. Examples of a synergistic effect in which responsivity is enhanced are the action of adrenalcorticoids to enhance the vasoconstrictor response to epinephrine and the increase of

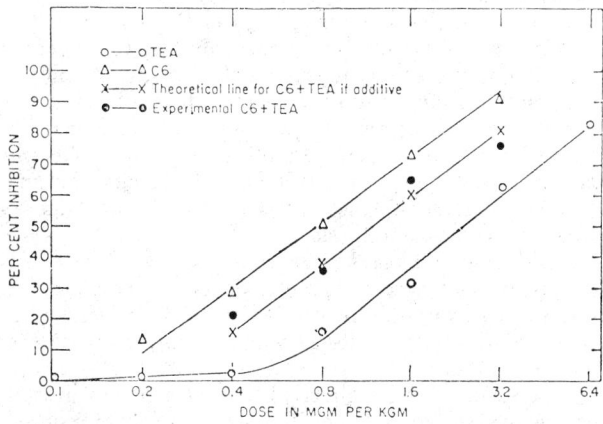

Fig 36-17. Additive inhibitory effects of tetraethylammonium (TEA) and hexamethonium (C6) on the superior cervical ganglion of the cat. The theoretical line for additivity was calculated on the basis that an increment of TEA added to an EDx of C6 should have the same effect as if it were added to an EDx of TEA. When TEA and C6 were administered together, an equal amount of each was given. The dose is the sum of the doses of the two components (courtesy, Harvey[32]).

epinephrine-induced hyperglycemia consequent to impairment by theophylline of the enzymatic destruction of the cyclic-AMP which mediates the response.

In clinical practice two homodynamic drugs are rarely coadministered for the purpose of increasing the response, since a sufficient dose of either drug should be able to achieve the same effect as a combination of the two. Most clinical combinations with positively interacting drugs are with heterergic drugs.

Combinations to Decrease Individual Doses and Toxicity—When homodynamic drugs are coadministered, it is usually for the purpose of decreasing toxicity. If the toxicities of two homodynamic drug are infra-additive, the toxicity of combined partial doses of the two drugs will often be less than with full doses of either drug. This principle is valid for trisulfapyrimidines mixture (see page 1176).

Combinations to Attack a Disease Complex at Different Points—With many diseases more than one organ or tissue may be affected or events at more than one locus may bear upon the ultimate perturbation. For example, in duodenal ulcer, psychic factors appear to increase activity in the vagus nerve which modulates gastric secretion, so that it was rational to explore the effects of sedatives, ganglionic blocking drugs, antimuscarinic drugs, and antacids, singly and in combination. In heart failure the decrement in renal plasma flow and changes in aldosterone levels promote the retention of salt and water, so that diuretics and digitalis are usually employed concomitantly. Pain, anxiety, and agitation or depression are frequent accompaniments of various pathologic processes, so that it is to be expected that analgesics, tranquilizers, sedatives or antidepressives will frequently be given at the same time, along with other drugs intended to correct the specific pathology.

Combinations to Antagonize Untoward Actions—The side effects of a number of drugs can be prevented or suppressed by other drugs. An antagonist may compete with the drug at the receptor that initiates the side effect, depress the side-effector system at a point other than the receptor, or stimulate an opposing system.

Antagonism at the receptor is *competitive antagonism* if the antagonist attaches at the same receptor group as the agonist (see page 719). Antagonism at a different receptor group or inhibition elsewhere in the response system is *noncompetitive antagonism*. Both competitive and noncompetitive antagonism are classified as *pharmacological antagonism*. The stimulation of an opposing system is *physiological antagonism*.

Clinical examples of pharmacological antagonism are the use of atropine to suppress the muscarinic effects of excess acetylcholine consequent to the use of neostigmine and the use of antihistaminics to prevent the effects of histamine liberated by tubocurarine. Examples of physiological antagonism are the use of amphetamine to correct partially the sedation caused by anticonvulsant doses of phenobarbital and the administration of ephedrine to correct hypotension resulting from spinal anesthesia.

Combinations That Affect Elimination—Only a few drugs are presently used purposefully to elevate or to prolong plasma levels by interfering with elimination, although continued interest in such drugs will probably increase the number.

Probenecid, which has already been mentioned to antagonize the renal secretion of penicillin, was originally introduced for this purpose. However, the inexpensiveness of penicillin G, repository preparations of penicillin G, and oral preparations (which obviate the need for injection) make it less imperative to retard the excretion of penicillin. The low non-allergenic toxicity of penicillin permits very large doses to be given without concern for the high plasma concentrations that result, which also means that there is little necessity for increasing the biological half-life of the drug. Consequently, probenecid routinely is not used much today in combination with penicillin.

The use of vasoconstrictors to increase the sojourn of local anesthetics at the site of infiltration continues, but few other clinical examples of the deliberate use of one drug to interfere with either the distribution or elimination of another can be cited. Nevertheless, the subject of the effect of one drug on the elimination of another has become immensely active. Innumerable drugs affect the fate of others, and the therapist must be aware of such interactions.

Drugs that induce cytochrome P-450s enhance the elimination of drugs that are metabolized by the liver microsomes. There would be very little point ordinarily to solicit combinations that would shorten the duration of action or lower plasma levels unless it were to reduce an overdosage. However, since such combinations are unwittingly or unavoidably used, this type of interaction is of great clinical importance.

Combinations to Alter Absorption—In the section on *Vehicles and Absorption Adjuvants* (page 730) it was mentioned that certain substances facilitate the absorption of others. The use of such absorption adjuvants is generally included under the subject of formulation rather than under drug combination. Although drugs which increase blood flow, motility, etc have an effect to increase the rate of absorption, the use of such drugs has so far not proven to be very practical. When it is desired to slow the absorption of drugs, various physical or physicochemical means prove to be more effective and less troublesome than drug combinations.

Fixed Combinations of Drugs

Concomitant treatment with two or more drugs is frequently unnecessary, and it generally immeasurably complicates therapy and the evaluation of response and toxicity. Nevertheless, it is often warranted, even essential, and cannot be condemned categorically. However, with fixed-dose or fixed-ratio combinations, in which the drugs are together in the same preparation, have certain disadvantages, except for a few rare instances like trisulfapyrimidines.

The disadvantages are as follows: patients differ in their responsivity or sensitivity to drugs, and adjustments in dosage or dose-interval may be necessary. If adjustment of only one component of the mixture is required, it is undesirable that the schedule of the second component be obligatorily adjusted, as it is in a fixed combination. According to which way the dose is adjusted, either toxicity or loss of the therapeutic effect may result. Furthermore, when adverse effects to either component occur, both drugs must be discontinued. The fixed combination denies the physician flexible control of therapy. Especially when one component in a mixture is superfluous yet potentially toxic, as is often the case, the promotion of fixed combinations is reprehensible. However, the separate administration of drugs used in combination often complicates treatment for the patient, who, in an outpatient situation and sometimes in the hospital, may not take all of his medication or who may take it at inappropriate intervals. The resulting consequences may be worse than those of fixed combinations in certain instances. Consequently, a summary dismissal of fixed combinations is unwarranted. Rather, the fundamentals of pharmacokinetics and clinical experience must be brought together with biopharmaceutics to analyze present combinations and to predict possible new allowable combinations.

Dangers in Multiple-Drug Therapy

Some objections to fixed-dose combinations were stated above. Also the unanticipated effects of drug combinations have been touched upon, particularly with respect to effects upon elimination. But it should be made clear that more is at stake than simply the biological half-life of a drug. On page 733 was given an example of the grave clinical consequences of the effect of phenobarbital to enhance the biotransformation of warfarin. Other examples of dangerous interactions, such as the effect of several antidepressants greatly to synergize catecholamines, may be cited. Even some antibiotics antagonize each other and increase mortality.

In addition to the obvious pitfalls posed by the interactions themselves, the use of multiple-drug therapy fosters careless diagnosis and a false sense of security in the number of drugs employed. Multiple-drug therapy should never be employed without a convincing indication that each drug is beneficial beyond the possible detriments or without proof that a therapeutically equivocal combination is definitely harmless. Finally, the expense to the patient warrants consideration.

References

1. Clark AJ: *J Physiol (London) 61:* 547, 1926.
2. Waud DR: *Pharmacol Rev 20:* 49, 1968.
3. Ariens EJ, ed: *Molecular Pharmacology,* vol 1, Academic, New York, 176–193, 1964.
4. Stephenson RP: *Brit J Pharmacol 11:* 379, 1956.
5. McKay DJ: *J Pharm Pharmacol 18:* 201, 1966.
6. Furchgott RF: *Ann Rev Pharmacol 4:* 21, 1964.
7. Rang HP: *Brit J Pharmacol 48:* 475, 1973.
8. Colquhoun D: The relation between classical and cooperative models for drug action. In Rang HP, ed: *Drug Receptors:* University Park, Baltimore, 1973.
9. Cuatracasas P, Greaves MF, eds: *Receptors and Recognition,* Halsted, New York, 1976.
10. Danielli JF, *et al,* eds: *Fundamental Concepts in Drug-Receptor Interactions,* Academic, New York, 1970.
11. DeRobertis E: *Synaptic Receptors, Isolation and Biology,* Dekker, New York, 1975.
12. DeRobertis E, Schacht J, eds: *Neurochemistry of Cholinergic Receptors,* Raven, New York, 1974.
13. Porter R, O'Connor M, eds: *Molecular Properties of Drug Receptors,* Churchill, London, 1970.
14. Robson JM, Stacey RS: Drug-Receptor Theories. In *Recent Advances in Pharmacology,* Little, Brown, Boston, 1968. Chapter 4.
15. Triggle DJ, *et al,* eds: *Cholinergic Ligand Interactions,* Academic, New York, 1971.
16. Triggle DJ: *Neurotransmitter-Receptor Interactions,* Academic, London, 1971.
17. Rang HP, ed: *Drug Receptors,* University Park, Baltimore, 1973.
18. Schanker LS: *Advan Drug Res 1:* 71, 1964.
19. Brodie BB, *et al: J Pharmacol Exp Ther 130:* 20, 1960.
20. Truitt EB, *et al: J Pharmacol Exp Ther 100:* 309, 1950.
21. Lillehei JP: *J Am Med Assoc 205:* 531, 1968.
22. Martin AN, *et al: Physical Pharmacy,* 2nd ed, Lea & Febiger, Philadelphia, 247, 253, 1969.
23. Jacobs MH: *Cold Spring Harbor Symp Quant Biol 8:* 30, 1940.
24. Schanker LS: *Pharmacol Rev 14:* 501, 1961.
25. Brodie BB, Hogben CA: *J Pharm Pharmacol 9:* 345, 1957.
26. Hogben CA: *Proc Fed Am Soc Exp Biol 19:* 864, 1960.
27. Albert A: *Pharmacol Rev 4:* 136, 1952.
28. Ariens EJ, *et al:* In Ariens, EJ, ed. *Molecular Pharmacology,* vol 1, Academic, New York, 7–52, 1964.
29. Lu AYH, West SB: *Pharmacol Rev, 31:* 277, 1980.
30. Milne MD, *et al: Clin Sci 16:* 599, 1957.
31. Kostenbauder HB, *et al: J Pharm Sci 51:* 1084, 1962.
32. Harvey SC: *Arch Intern Pharmacodyn 114:* 232, 1958.
33. Weaver LC, *et al: J Pharmacol Exp Ther 113:* 359, 1955.

Bibliography

Albert A: *Selective Toxicity,* 6th ed, Chapman and Hall, London, 1979.

Albert A: *The Selectivity of Drugs,* Chapman and Hall, London, 1975.

Ariens EJ, ed: *Drug Design,* vols 1 and 2, Academic, New York, 1971.

Ariens EJ, ed: *Drug Design,* vol 5, Academic, New York, 1975.

Ariens EJ, ed: *Molecular Pharmacology,* vol 1, Academic, New York, 1964.

Ariens EJ, ed: *Physico-Chemical Aspects of Drug Action,* Pergamon, London, 1968.

Barlow RB: *Quantitative Aspects of Chemical Pharmacology,* University Park, Baltimore, 1980.

Berridge MJ: Receptors and Calcium Signalling, *TIPS 1982:* 419.

Binns TB, ed: *Absorption and Distribution of Drugs,* Livingston, London, 1964.

Boeynaems JM, Dumont JE, eds: *Outlines of Receptor Theory,* Elsevier/North Holland, Amsterdam, 1980.

Brodie BB, Hogben CA: Some physicochemical factors in drug action, *J Pharm Pharmacol 9:* 345, 1957.

Capaldi RA, ed: *Membrane Proteins and their Interaction with Lipids,* Dekker, New York, 1977.

Cuatracassas P, Greaves MF, eds: *Receptors and Recognition,* Halsted, New York, 1976.

DeRobertis E: *Synaptic Receptors, Isolation and Biology,* Dekker, New York, 1975.

Featherstone RM, ed: *A Guide to Molecular Pharmacology,* Parts I and II, Dekker, New York, 1973.

Finean JB, Michell RH, eds: *Membrane Structure,* Elsevier/North Holland, Amsterdam, 1981.

Fink BR, ed: Molecular mechanisms of anesthesia. *Progr Anesthesiol 1:* 1–652, 1975.

Goldstein A: The interactions of drugs and plasma proteins. *Pharmacol Rev 1:* 102, 1949.

Goldstein A, *et al: Principles of Drug Action,* 3rd ed, Wiley, New York, 1985.

Gregoriadis G, *et al: Targeting of Drugs,* Plenum, New York, 1982.

Hartiala H: Metabolism of hormones, drugs, and other substances in the gut. *Physiol Rev 53:* 496, 1973.

Hogben CAM, Lindgren P, eds: *Drugs and Membranes,* Macmillan, New York, 1963.

Jakoby WB, *et al: Metabolic Basis of Detoxification,* Academic, New York, 1982.

Jenner P, Testa B, eds: *Concepts in Drug Metabolism,* Part A, Dekker, New York, 1980.

Jenner P, Testa B, eds: *Concepts in Drug Metabolism,* Part B, Dekker, New York, 1981.

Kotyk A, Janáček K, eds: *Membrane Transport,* vol 9, of *Biomembranes,* Plenum, New York, 1977.

Kreuzer F, Slegers JFG, eds: *Passive Permeability of Cell Membranes,* Plenum, New York, 1972.

Kunos G, ed: *Adrenoreceptors and Catecholamine Action,* Part A, Wiley Interscience, New York, 1981.

Lamble JW, ed: *Towards Understanding Receptors,* Elsevier/North Holland, Amsterdam, 1981.

Lamble JW, ed: *More About Receptors,* Elsevier/North Holland, Amsterdam, 1982.

Lefkowitz RJ, ed: *Receptor Regulation,* Chapman and Hall, London, 1981.

Lefkowitz RJ, *et al:* Mechanism of Hormone-Receptor-Effector Coupling: The B-Adrenergic Receptor and Adenylate Cyclase, *Proc Fed Am Socs Exptl Biol 41:* 2664, 1982.

Levine RR: *Pharmacology: Drug Actions and Reactions,* 2nd ed, Little, Brown, New York, 1978.

Levine RR, Pelikan EW: Mechanisms of drug absorption and excretion. Passage of drugs out and into the gastrointestinal tract. *Ann Rev Pharmacol 4:* 69, 1964.

Levitzki A: Activation and Inhibition of Adenylate Cyclase by Hormones: Mechanistic Aspects, *TIS 1982:* 203.

Martonosi AN: *Membranes and Transport,* Plenum, New York, 1982.

Meyer UA: Role of Genetic Factors in the Rational Use of Drugs, Chapter 18 in, Melmon KL, Morrelli, HF, eds: *Clinical Pharmacology,* 2nd ed, Macmillan, New York, 1978.

Milne MD: Nonionic diffusion and excretion of weak acids and bases. *Am J Med 24:* 709, 1958.

Nebert DW, *et al:* Genetic Mechanisms Controlling the Induction of Polysubstrate Monooxygenase (P-450) Activities, in *Ann Rev Pharmacol Toxicol 21:* 431, 1981.

Park DV, Smith RL, eds: *Drug Metabolism—From Microbes to Man,* Taylor & Francis, London, 1977.

O'Brien RD, ed: *The Receptors,* vol 1. *General Principles and Procedures,* Plenum, New York, 1979.

Rang HP, ed: *Drug Receptors,* University Park, Baltimore, 1973.

Roberts GCK: *Drug Action at the Molecular Level,* University Park, Baltimore, 1977.

Sandler M, ed: *Enzyme Inhibitors as Drugs,* University Park, Baltimore, 1980.

Schanker LS: Passage of drugs across body membranes. *Pharmacol Rev 14:* 501, 1961.

Schanker LS: Physiological transport of drugs. *Advan Drug Res 1:* 71, 1964.

Seeman P: The membrane actions of anesthetics and tranquilizers. *Pharmacol Rev 24:* 583–655, 1972.

Smythes JR, Bradley RJ, eds: *Receptors in Pharmacology,* Dekker, New York, 1978.

Stenlake JB: *The Chemical Basis of Drug Action,* Athlone, London, 1979.

Symposium (various authors; Anton AH, Solomon HM, eds): *Drug-Protein Binding. Ann NY Acad Sci 226:* 1–362, 1973.

Triggle DJ: *Neurotransmitter-Receptor Interactions*, Academic, New York, 1971.

Usdin E, *et al: Neuroreceptors*, Wiley & Sons, Chichester, 1981.

Van Rossum JM, ed: *Kinetic of Drug Action*, Springer-Verlag, Berlin, 1977.

Vesell E: Pharmacogenetics. *Biochem Pharmacol 24:* 445, 1975.

Vesell ES: The influence of host factors on drug response. I. Ethnic background, *Rational Drug Ther 13*, no 8: 1, 1979.

Weissman G, Claiborne R, eds: *Cell Membranes: Biochemistry, Cell Biology and Pathology*, HP Publishing, New York, 1975.

Yamamura HI, *et al*, eds: *Neurotransmitter-Receptor Binding*, Raven, New York, 1978.

CHAPTER 38

Basic Pharmacokinetics

Stewart C Harvey, PhD
Professor of Pharmacology

and C Dean Withrow, PhD
Associate Professor of Pharmacology
School of Medicine, University of Utah
Salt Lake City, UT 84132

Pharmacokinetics is the discipline that treats of the rates of movement of a drug or its metabolites into the body, among its many compartments, and out of the body, and also which treats of the rates of biotransformations of the drug and its metabolites. As in chemistry, it primarily involves following the rate of change in concentration in the appropriate compartment(s), most often in the extracellular fluid (plasma) and/or urine. However, pharmacokinetics is by no means limited to observations on concentration; rates of movement of a drug can be followed by isotopes or other means. The application of pharmacokinetics to drug formulation and treatment regimens is also within the scope of this title. The application to treatment regimens and other clinical uses of pharmacokinetics are treated in Chapter 39, *Principles of Clinical Pharmacokinetics.*

Orders of Processes

The order of any process is determined by the probability that the appropriate unit events will occur in a given population within a given time. Processes may be zero order, first order, second order, etc, depending upon the number of variables that determine the probability. In pharmacokinetics, only zero-order and first-order processes are important, the latter being of overwhelming importance; consequently, only the kinetics of these two processes will be treated in this chapter.

First-Order Processes

When activity is random within a population of a single species, the probability that a given event will occur is directly proportional to the size of the population. For example, the probability that some atom in a population of radionuclides will disintegrate in any instant is directly proportional to the number of radionuclide atoms in the current as well as the original population. Similarly, the number of molecules of drug that diffuse across a given boundary, for example, the vascular endothelium, per unit time will be directly proportional to the number of molecules near the boundary, which, in turn, is proportional to the concentration. This is the basis of Fick's Law of Diffusion (page 724). Any process in which the rate of change in a population is directly proportional to the population is known as a *first-order* process. In such a process, the time-dependent change in concentration is defined by the equation

$$C = C_0 e^{-kt} \qquad \text{[units of wt} \cdot \text{vol}^{-1} \text{ or molar, etc]} \qquad (1)$$

where C is the concentration at time t, C_0 is the initial concentration (time zero), t is time, e is the natural (Naperian) log base, and k is a proportionality constant known as the rate constant. (For a derivation of Eq 1, see page 249.) In a diffusion process, the magnitude of k is determined by the temperature, mobility, permeability, and other factors. The numerical value of k will also depend upon the time units (min vs hr, etc) chosen.

Eq 1 predicts that as t approaches infinity, C approaches zero, which would be true for irreversible processes like radioactive decay, diffusion into infinite space, some exentropic SN_1 chemical decompositions, and certain enzymatic reactions. However, in a confining space, diffusion and many chemical reactions reach an equilibrium state in which C approaches a finite asymptote as t approaches infinity. Fig 38-1 illustrates a simple situation in which the asymptote is nec-

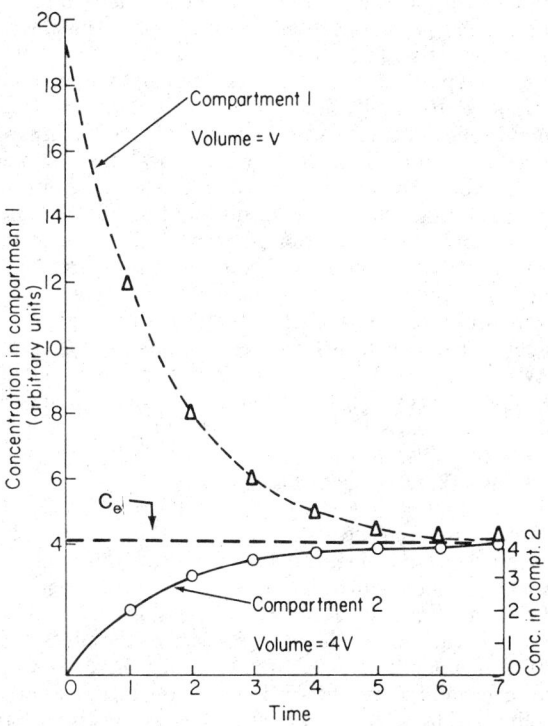

Fig 38-1. Idealized diffusion kinetics of a hypothetical drug that equilibrates between two compartments. Transfer is from Compartment 1 into Compartment 2. The equilibrium concentration is ⅕ of that initially in Compartment 1, because the final volume of distribution is 5 times that of Compartment 1.

essarily finite. To satisfy the conditions of this closed system, $(C_0 - C_e)$ must be substituted for C_0 in Eq 1, C_e being the equilibrium concentration.

In Eq 1, the algebraic sign of k is usually negative, which indicates a diminishing concentration with time. However, in Fig 38-1 the concentration in compartment 2 rises logarithmically with time; nevertheless, k is negative, since the rate diminishes exponentially with time. The equation for the logarithmically rising concentration in compartment 2 will take the form of Eq 4 (page 743), in which C_e would be used in lieu of C_p^{∞}.

Eq 1 can be written in the log form,

$$\log C = \log C_0 - 0.434kt \qquad \text{[no units]} \qquad (2)$$

The coefficient 0.434 results from the conversion of the natural log base, e, to log base 10 ($0.434 = 1/2.303$). The equation determines that a plot of $\log C$ against t will be rectilinear (bottom of Fig 19-1, page 249) with a slope of $-0.434k$ and an ordinate-intercept of C_0. For pharmacokinetics, this is a useful type of plot, because, in the straight line form, back extrapolation to estimate C_0 is easier and more accurate than from a curve, and k can also be determined without the need for computation.

Rate Constants and Half-Life—Since first-order processes are characterized by exponential or logarithmic kinetics, it follows that a constant fraction of the present or instantaneous population (eg, concentration) changes per unit time,

that fraction being equal to $0.434k$; k has the units of t^{-1}. Another way of expressing the rate of change is that of half-time (or especially *half-life*, if the population is decreasing), with the notation $t_{1/2}$. The half-time is the time that it takes the population to decrease (or increase) by 50% of the total possible change. By setting C equal to $\frac{1}{2}C_0$ in either Eqs 1 or 2 and solving for t (which is $t_{1/2}$ under these constraints),

$$t_{1/2} = \frac{0.693}{k} \qquad \text{[units of time]} \qquad (3)$$

Zero-Order Processes

When an enzyme or transport system is saturated, the activity cannot be further increased by increases in the concentration of substrate. Consequently, the rate remains constant so long as the concentration of substrate is in excess of the saturating concentration. In this situation, the rate is independent of the concentration. The kinetics are described as being of *zero-order*, and it is customary to speak of the process as being a zero-order process; however, as the process continues, the concentration will eventually fall to subsaturation levels, and the kinetics will change, usually to first-order kinetics, so that it is more appropriate to speak of the initial kinetics and not the process as being zero-order.

Pharmacokinetic Models

The plasma, cerebrospinal fluid, interstitial space, glandular or renal tubular lumina, gall bladder, etc, and each cell are all compartments which a drug may or may not enter or leave with different rate constants. In addition, binding to protein or other sequestration (such as in granules or vacuoles) within or without cells is also governed by characteristic rate processes. Consequently, it is to be expected that the kinetics of absorption, distribution and elimination would be very complex and perhaps beyond analysis and mathematical description. Fortunately, the rates of distribution among the various tissues and myriad cells generally are not greatly dispersed, so that the kinetics behave as though the drug were being distributed among one, two, or at the most, a few compartments. Like the volume of distribution (page 743), a compartment is fictive or virtual and may be difficult to define in precise anatomical terms. Therefore, a compartment is defined mainly by its pharmacokinetic parameters. The mathematical treatment of the kinetics and the pertinent parameters are based upon hypothetical models which assume one, two, or more functional compartments arrayed in parallel or serially, etc, according to the model and with certain other assumed constraints.

Open One-Compartment Model

In this model, the body is assumed to behave as though it were a single compartment, that is, as though there were no barriers to movement of drug within the total body space and the final equilibrium distribution is attained instantaneously. In practice, the model adequately describes the pharmacokinetic behavior of a drug if the final equilibrium distribution is attained rapidly in comparison to the rates of absorption and elimination. The term *open* indicates that input and output (from any and all routes of administration and elimination, respectively) are unidirectional and that the one compartment (ie, body) is not within a confined space and hence does not come into chemical equilibrium with its external environment. In simple diagram, such an open one-

compartment model is depicted in Fig 38-2. In the diagram, the compartment represents the entire body (excluding the lumina of the gastrointestinal tract, urinary tract, pulmonary alveoli, etc, which communicate with the open environment). V_d is the *volume of distribution* (see page 743, below). However, V_d is not necessarily that of the body or even total body water; as noted on page 743, the volume of distribution, V_d, is a fictive one considered to be equal to fD/C_p (where f is the fraction absorbed, D is the dose, and C_p is the plasma concentration), in which it is hypothetically assumed that the concentration is the same throughout the volume and is equal to the plasma concentration. In reality, concentration is not homogeneous throughout, but this cannot be determined from C_p alone (which simply averages all inputs and outputs); as long as distribution equilibrium is rapidly achieved, the kinetics as perceived through blood or urine concentrations are the same whether distribution is homogeneous or heterogeneous.

In order to derive formulae to describe time-related changes in C_p, it is convenient to consider absorption and elimination separately, as though each were occurring in the absence of

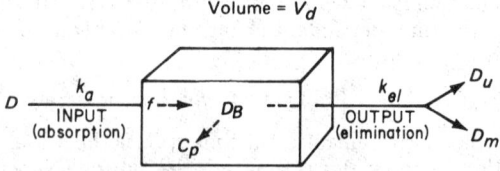

Fig 38-2. Diagram of the open one-compartment pharmacokinetic model. An amount of drug, D_B, is absorbed from the administered dose, D, with a rate constant of k_a into a compartment with volume V_d and is distributed instantaneously to reach a plasma concentration C_p. V_d is obtained by dividing D_B by C_p. D_B = dose D times f, the fraction absorbed. Drug is eliminated from the compartment with a rate constant k_{el}. D_u is the amount excreted into urine, feces, expired air, sweat, milk, etc.; D_m is the amount of drug metabolized.

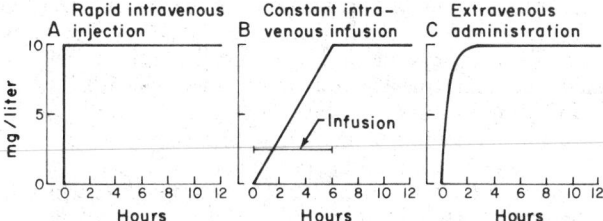

Fig 38-3.   Time-concentration curves for injection (A), infusion (B), and extravenous (C) administration of drug in the one-compartment model. The volume of the compartment is 100 L ($V_d = 100$ L); the amount of drug administered in each instance is 1,000 mg. Drug elimination has been set to zero, so that the time-concentration curve for each model of administration can be examined without the complication of simultaneous elimination (courtesy, Bigger[1], adapted).

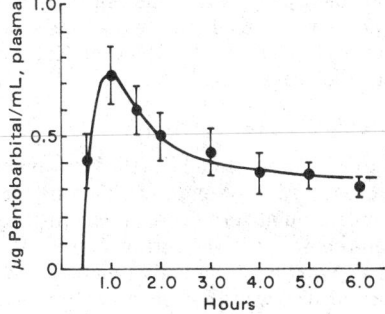

Fig 38-4.   The time course of pentobarbital in the blood of a fasting human subject following the oral administration of 50 mg. The figure shows a lag-time of about 20 min, approximately the emptying time of the fasting stomach (courtesy, Dittert[2]).

the other, then to add them algebraically to determine the total integral kinetics.

Absorption—If a drug is administered intravenously by single rapid injection, absorption is by-passed. The time for such injections is usually so short compared to other pharmacokinetic processes that it is customary to consider the peak plasma concentration and equilibrium distribution to occur instantaneously in one-compartment systems. This is depicted in panel A of Fig 38-3. In the model for the figure, there is no elimination, and C_p remains constant once injection is accomplished. With constant intravenous infusion (panel B) C_p rises rectilinearly so long as infusion continues at a constant rate. With other routes of administration, absorption also usually manifests first-order kinetics, since most drugs are absorbed by simple diffusion. Thus the drug disappears exponentially from the site of administration (as from compartment 1 in Fig 38-1). The equation for the concentration of drug in the plasma after a single extravascular dose of drug, assuming no elimination takes place, is

$$C_p = C_p^\infty - C_p^\infty e^{-k_a t} \qquad \text{[units: wt} \cdot \text{vol}^{-1}, \text{etc]} \qquad (4)$$

where C_p is the concentration at time t, C_p^∞ is the final concentration at "infinite" time, and k_a is the absorption rate constant. Absorption is characterized by a half-time equal to $0.693/k_a$. Bimolecular absorption processes, such as facilitated diffusion or active transport, also often show first-order kinetics, especially at drug concentrations well below those at which the carrier system will become saturated. At saturation, the kinetics become zero-order. Even the rate of dissolution of a drug approximates a first-order process, provided that the drug is readily soluble and diffuses rapidly. If the solubility and diffusibility are low, it will approximate a zero-order process as long as there is saturation around the solid phase. Some sustained-release dosage forms are designed to release drugs at a constant rate (zero-order) over long periods of time.

Absorption by the oral route rarely conforms to simple first-order kinetics. A drug is absorbed at different rates from the stomach and the three segments of the intestine, partly simultaneously and partly sequentially. Absorption from the stomach is usually quite slow compared to that from the small intestine, and it is sometimes so slow that a significant amount of drug appears in the blood only after the stomach contents are emptied. Thus there may be a *lag*, that is, the curve describing the time-dependent rise in C_p does not pass through the origin. An example of lag in the absorption of pentobarbital is shown in Fig 38-4. Enteric-coated or other delayed-release dosage forms also cause lag. The mathematical formulation of lag will be deferred to the next section in connection with Eq 27. Other factors that complicate oral absorption are binding to gastrointestinal contents, changes in intraluminal pH, gastric emptying time, intestinal motility,

biliary secretion, mucosal blood flow, and sustained-release or other complex or insoluble dose-forms. Some changes in gastrointestinal conditions during the course of absorption are part of diurnal rhythms or are caused by the drug itself, which make it impossible to establish a steady basal state for description; others may result from emotionality, ingestion of foodstuffs, water, other drugs, etc, and can be adequately controlled for scientific purposes but may greatly vary in practical circumstances. Absorption by other routes is also subject to variability. Factors affecting absorption are enumerated on page 728. Some drugs that are completely absorbed in normal patients may not be absorbed in persons with abnormal gastrointestinal function, as the result of genetic, pathological or surgical factors. Many drugs are not completely absorbed even when gastrointestinal function is optimal. Absorption can be limited by the physical state of the drug and by other substances in the dosage form. The amount of drug absorbed into the body (D_B) is related to the dose as follows:

$$D_B = fD \qquad \text{[units: wt]} \qquad (5)$$

where D_B is the amount absorbed (drug in the body), f is the fraction absorbed, and D is the dose administered. The property of a drug to be absorbed from its dosage form is known as *bioavailability*, and f is the bioavailability factor. The bioavailability factor is often determined by comparison of the area under the concentration curve (AUC) of a given dose of drug given orally with that of the same dose given intravenously (see page 753).

Distribution—In the open one-compartment model, the body is treated as though it were a single compartment in which absorbed drug is mixed instantaneously and homogeneously. Clearly, the assumption of instantaneous equilibrium establishes only an ideal mathematical boundary condition to facilitate pharmacokinetic calculations. At best, no drug could be equilibrated in less than one circulation time, and no drug has been shown to distribute so rapidly. However, for practical purposes, a few minutes distribution time is negligible compared to absorption and elimination times. Only small, water-soluble drugs which are completely confined to the extracellular space equilibrate rapidly enough to meet the requirements of the ideal one-compartment model, but, for clinical purposes, the one-compartment model is adequate to describe the pharmacokinetics of a large number of drugs.

Volume of Distribution and Distribution Coefficient—The hypothetical volume within which a drug is distributed is known as the *volume of distribution*, V_d. It may be calculated by dividing the amount of drug in the body, D_B, by the plasma concentration, C_p, where C_p is the concentration in plasma. It is important to note that C_p is the total concentration, of unbound plus bound drug. Under real conditions, D_B and C_p vary with time, and computation must be made in such a way as to eliminate the time variable. One such way is to extrapolate C_p to zero time (eg, see Figs 38-6 and 38-8), in which case

$$V_d = f D/C_p, \quad (6)$$

where D is the dose administered, f is the bioavailability factor (fraction that reaches the systemic circulation), and C_p is the plasma concentration at zero time, determined by extrapolation. When the drug is given intravenously, $D_B = D$.

Of course, V_d will vary with body weight, so that it needs to be normalized in a way that allows comparisons among individuals of different body weights. Therefore, the *distribution coefficient*,* Δ', is more serviceable;

$$\Delta' = V_d/BW, \quad (7)$$

where BW is body weight. Units are usually mL/g or L/kg, and care must be taken to employ the appropriate units of weight, concentration, and volume in Eqs 6 and 7.

Although V_d and Δ' are derived as though the concentration were equal to C_p throughout the volume, concentration is, in fact, almost never homogeneous, and consequently V_d and Δ' are only imaginary (fictive, virtual) volumes. Factors that make for inhomogeneous distribution are: binding to proteins, dissolution into body lipids, pH partition, active transport, electrochemical and Donnan distributions, etc. Even if C_p (free) rather than C_p (total) were to be used to calculate V_d, V_d would not represent a real space, because of these manifold factors that cause uneven distribution. Consequently, the principal utility of V_d or Δ' is not so much in permitting an estimation of where the drug is distributed but rather as a measure of the reservoir from which a drug is being delivered and/or cleared (see page 745 and Table II, page 747). However, with appropriate considerations, V_d or Δ' may also serve to indicate the general ability of a drug to penetrate membranes, dissolve in fat or bind extensively to extravascular macromolecules.

Highly polar, poorly penetrant drugs tend to be confined mostly to the extracellular space; if they are little bound to plasma proteins, they will have Δ's of about 0.3 mL/g, less if there is significant binding to plasma proteins. The lower limit to Δ' is about 0.04 mL/g, which is approximately equal to the plasma volume. Ethanol and antipyrine are distributed throughout body water and are not bound or concentrated; consequently, their Δ's are approximately 0.7 mL/g, the Δ' of body water. Lipid-soluble drugs that are negligibly bound to plasma protein have Δ's that usually range from about 0.7 to 3–4 mL/g, depending upon water-lipid distribution coefficients. Some drugs that strongly bind to nucleo-proteins have Δ's that exceed 1000. However, many drugs combine penetrance, lipid solubility and protein binding in such proportions to make it difficult to interpret the meaning of Δ' without ancillary information.

Since, by definition, V_d varies reciprocally with C_p, it is essential to recognize that binding to plasma proteins, by increasing C_p, will decrease V_d. Despite this, plasma protein binding has no *real* effect on extravascular distribution. Since it is only the free form that moves among the spaces and tissues, it follows that alterations in plasma protein binding alone will not alter the extravascular (indeed, extraplasma) distribution. Only the calculated, fictive quantity, Δ', is affected. For example, nafcillin has a Δ' of 0.29 mL/g and is 90% bound to plasma proteins. Were there no protein binding, Δ' would equal 2.9 mL/g, a volume sufficiently larger than that of water to suggest considerable extravascular binding. However, it is not the masking of the degree of extravascular distribution that is the source of difficulty when there is sig-

* Δ' is not to be confused with water-lipid distribution coefficients.

nificant binding to plasma proteins, but rather it is the fact that the extent of protein binding is not always constant. Both the quantity and binding properties (affinity and capacity) of human plasma proteins can vary in health, disease, and the presence of other drugs (see pages 192 and 732). If the degree of binding of nafcillin to plasma proteins were to change to 50% as the result of hypoalbuminuria, Δ' would become nearly 0.48 mL/g. The Δ' of ampicillin, which is bound only to the extent of 18%, would not be so greatly affected. A further complication of binding to plasma proteins is occasioned when the degree of binding, and hence the magnitude of Δ', is dose dependent. There are a number of known examples in which Δ' varies with the dose.

Elimination—Once a drug is absorbed, it is transported by the blood to the tissues, among which it is distributed, metabolized and/or excreted, all of which processes lower the plasma concentration of the drug. Each separate process ordinarily has first-order kinetics, and the overall change in plasma concentration is described by the linear combination (or algebraic addition) of the separate equations. In the one-compartment model, the kinetics of distribution are ignored, since distribution occurs so rapidly that distribution occurs before any practical blood-sampling or repetitive dosing occurs. Thus, after intravascular administration the plasma concentration, C_p, will fall exponentially according to Eq 1. Such an exponential elimination of theophylline, given intravenously, is shown in Fig 38-5. According to Eq 2, if the data of Fig 38-5 are plotted semilogarithmically, as in Fig 38-6, a straight line should result. Several derived data can be obtained from such a plot. Extrapolation to zero time (ie, the y intercept) gives C_p^0, the theoretical plasma concentration at time zero. It is a theoretical concentration, because neither injection nor distribution is actually instantaneous. Nevertheless, C_p^0 is a very practical figure. For example, from it may be derived the volume of distribution, V_d, simply by dividing the dose, D, by C_p^0 (see page 743). In the figure, C_p^0 = 0.0115 mg/mL, so that V_d is 43.5 L, or about 89% of the volume of total body water in a 70 kg adult. The plasma half-time, $t_{1/2}$, can be determined directly from the graph or from the elimination rate constant, k_{el}, by means of Eq 3. (Conversely, k_{el} could be derived from $t_{1/2}$, determined visually from a graph.) When determining k_{el} from the slope, it must be kept in mind that the log of the concentration must be used rather than the antilog that is plotted on the log-scaled ordinate in the figure. In natural logarithms, the slope (ln C_{p1} − ln C_{p2})/($t_2 - t_1$) is equal to k_{el}; in decilogarithms, the slope (log C_{p1} − log C_{p2})/($t_2 - t_1$) is equal to $0.434 k_{el}$. From the figure, k_{el} is found to be 0.22 hr^{-1}, ie, during each hour the plasma concentration decreases by 22% of the concentration

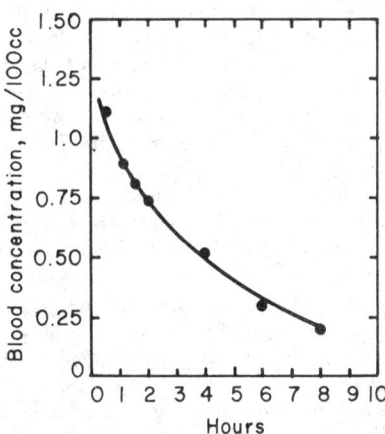

Fig 38-5. Elimination curve of average blood levels of theophylline in 11 human subjects after intravenous administration of 0.5 g aminophylline per 70 kg to each (courtesy, data, Truitt *et al*[3]).

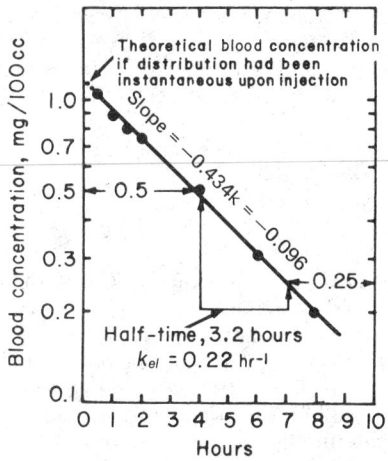

Fig 38-6. Semilog plot of the elimination curve in Fig 38-5. Note the log scale of the ordinate.

at the beginning of the hour. The elimination half-time, $t_{1/2}$, is equal to 0.693/0.22, or 3.2 hr.

Within the group of 11 subjects in the above study, there were considerable differences in k_{el} or $t_{1/2}$ among the members. One cannot overemphasize the caveat not to take too literally the average half-life data found in various tables or other literature but rather to assume a considerable probability that the half-life in a given patient may depart considerably from that average value. The half-lives of some drugs vary over a wide range even in normal individuals. The half-life of amitriptyline, a drug with a complex metabolic and excretory elimination, varies nearly tenfold; even the half-life of penicillin, a drug with a simple excretory elimination, varies twofold. In persons with hepatic or renal failure, the published mean half-life data may not even be in a range applicable to such persons.

The half-time may vary widely from species to species; for example, in man, the half-life of sulfaethidole is about 8 hr, whereas in cattle it is less than 2 hr. Half-lives also vary considerably even among congeneric drugs, as may be seen with the sulfonamides shown in Table I.

The biological half-life must not be confused with the time for the response to decline by 50%, since dose, the requirement for a threshold concentration, latency of response, and other factors may cause a nonparallelism between blood concentration and intensity of response. In fact, because the relationship between effect and plasma concentration is usually logarithmic, effect tends to decline in a linear, not loglinear fashion.

In Fig 38-2, the rate constant for elimination is designated k_{el}, without reference to the mode or route of elimination. However, k_{el} may be a compound constant equal to the sum of the rate constants that define the various simultaneous (ie, parallel) contributory processes, such as biotransformation, renal excretion, biliary secretion, etc. Thus the compound or overall constant is $K = k_1 + k_2 + k_3 \ldots k_n$, where $k_1, k_2 \ldots k_n$ are the rate constants of the separate contributory processes. Consider the case in which a drug is simultaneously biotransformed and excreted unchanged in the urine. The

Table I—The Approximate Biologic Half-Life in Man of Several Sulfonamides[4]

Drug	$t_{1/2}$ (hr)
Sulfamethylthiadiazole	2
Sulfaethidole	8
Sulfisoxazole	8
Sulfamethoxypyridazine	34

initial concentration, C_p^0, will therefore be diminished by both $C_p^0 e^{-k_m t}$ and $C_p^0 e^{-k_u t}$, where m designates metabolism and u renal excretion. In some notations, k_u is designated k_r, k_{10}, k_3 or k_e. Eq 2 adapted for the two processes becomes

$$\log C_p = \log C_p^0 - 0.434 k_m t - 0.434 k_u t$$
$$= \log C_p^0 - 0.434(k_m + k_u)t \quad \text{[no units]} \quad (8)$$

Thus $k_m + k_u$ combine to make a single constant, which is the overall elimination rate constant. In order to identify it as a compound, or overall, constant it is sometimes designated as K, rather than k_{el}.

Clearance and Routes of Elimination—The half-life of a drug is a useful pharmacokinetic parameter. Since half-life is expressed in units of time, it is an easily understood, concise indication of the rate of disappearance or accumulation of a drug. Further, it is used to estimate the time necessary to attain a new steady state whenever a steady state is altered by a change in the factors determining dose regimen, namely, drug dose, bioavailability, the dose interval, rate of elimination, and volume of distribution (see page 743). However, the elimination half-life of a drug is a complex function of drug distribution, biotransformation, and elimination. A more direct expression of the rate of drug elimination is drug clearance.

Clearance is the rate of removal of a drug or other substance from the body, expressed as the *in vivo* volume equivalent of the substance being removed per unit time. In order to illustrate the concept, assume that drug D is being eliminated from the body at a rate of 0.1% per minute. The absolute amount of drug that was eliminated would therefore be equal to 0.1% D_B per minute. Since D_B is distributed as though it were in a volume V_d (volume of distribution, page 756), one can calculate the fictive volume equivalent of the amount of drug lost per minute, which in this instance would be 0.1% V_d/min. Since the relative rate of loss, 0.1%/min or 0.001/min is, in fact, k_{el}, it may be seen that

$$Cl_t = k_{el} \times V_d \quad \text{[vol/unit time]} \quad (9)$$

where Cl_t is total body clearance. It is usually expressed in units of mL/min. It must be emphasized that clearance is a hypothetical or fictive quantity, since the body rarely clears a drug completely from a specific volume of body fluid. Only when elimination is flow-limited is the blood that passes through the eliminating organs(s) totally cleared, so that the effluent blood is essentially devoid of drug; in such an instance the clearance approximates the rate of blood-flow. If the concentration in the effluent blood were to be only 0.5 of the affluent blood, then the clearance would be said to be 0.5 that of the blood flow.

Although clearance is the dV/dt equivalent of dD_B/dt or the volume equivalent of the drug lost per unit time, the hypothetical volume cannot be regarded as having also been eliminated. Just as the depleted effluent blood from the eliminating organ is returned to the systemic circulation to mix with all the blood and as drug is redistributed and re-equilibrated among the vascular and extravascular components of V_d, the fictive volume that is "cleared" remains a part of V_d, so that the only change that is effected is one in concentration, of which C_p is the index. Since V_d and k_{el} are both constant, it follows that Cl_t is also constant.

The concept of clearance can be applied to the whole body or to specific organs. The former application is a convenient way to indicate overall drug elimination; the latter application is used to indicate the contribution of a specific organ to drug disappearance.

Total Systemic (Whole Body) Clearance—Total body clearance is the sum of all of separate clearances that contribute to drug elimination, ie, $Cl_{tot} = Cl_{metab} + Cl_{renal}$, etc. It is essential that k_{el} be expressed in the same time units as are used in clearance (usually min). In Eq 9, dividing by 60 converts k_{el} in hr^{-1} to min^{-1}, so that clearance can be expressed in mL/min. Whole body clearance in a one-compartment system is also equal to dose divided by the area under the curve:

$$Cl_{tot} = D/AUC_0 \quad [\text{mL} \cdot \text{min}^{-1}] \quad (10)$$

where AUC_0 is the area under the curve. AUC is discussed on page 753. The determination of Cl_{tot} in the two-compartment system is discussed on page 756.

Renal Excretion and Clearance—The principles of renal excretion and clearance have been used for approximately 50 years as tools for studying renal physiology and pathology and hence were early adapted to pharmacokinetics. Consequently, renal clearance of drugs is a classic illustration of the general subject of clearance. As discussed in Chapter 37, all drugs are filtered in the glomerulus and some are also secreted into the urine by renal tubular cells; there is also resorption of drugs from the tubular luminal fluid back into the blood as the fluid passes along the tubule. Glomerular filtration is the passage through the glomerular vascular endothelium of the plasma fluid and all solutes therein small enough to pass through the pores, that is, it is the filtration of water and all micromolecular solutes. Thus it is independent of the presence of drug and is a function of the filtration pressure (which relates to blood pressure) and the mean transit time across the glomerular capillaries. The rate of filtration is known as the *glomerular filtration rate, GFR*, and it has the units of vol/min (usually mL/min). In turn, the transit time is determined by the rate of flow of blood through the glomeruli; this rate of blood flow is known as the *renal plasma flow*, designated *RPF*. Since only a fraction of the plasma is filtered during passage through the glomerulus, it is useful to designate this fraction as the filtration fraction, *FF*, where $FF = GFR/RPF$. The average renal *plasma* (not blood) flow in the adult human male is approximately 600–700 mL/min, and the glomerular filtration rate is approximately 100–125 mL/min (of which 99% of the water is resorbed and returned to the blood); thus the filtration fraction is approximately 0.2.

Under basal conditions, the *GFR* is roughly constant in time. Therefore, the only major variable that determines the rate of filtration of free drug is the concentration of drug in the plasma. Thus

$$F = C_{pf} \cdot GFR \quad [\text{units: mL} \cdot \text{min}^{-1}] \quad (11)$$

where F is the filtration rate of the drug, usually in units of mg/min and C_{pf} is the amount of *free* drug in the plasma. If the drug is unbound, $C_{pf} = C_p$. If the drug is bound to plasma protein, then

$$F = [C_p(1 - p)] \cdot GFR \quad [\text{mL} \cdot \text{min}^{-1}] \quad (12)$$

where p is the fraction bound to plasma protein.

The *GFR* may be determined by the steady-state rate of excretion of any non-bound chemical substance that is not subsequently secreted and/or resorbed by the renal tubules, so that the amount of substance which appears in the urine is all of that which was filtered and no more. Two such substances are *creatinine* and *inulin*. With creatinine, the endogenous plasma levels are nearly constant, and thus creatinine lends itself readily to the determination of *GFR*. Either inulin or creatinine may be given by constant intravenous infusion. Usually, creatinine is used. However, it is not customary to express the glomerular filtration rate of creatinine or of drugs as *F*, in terms of mg/min, but rather in terms of *clearance*. As discussed above, clearance is a hypothetical volume of plasma which, if completely cleared of its content of drug in unit time, would be equivalent to the amount of drug that disappears in unit time. In the instance of filtration, it is easy to visualize clearance as that volume filtered per min,

since the filtered volume is actually physically separated from the blood. Thus the *creatinine clearance*, or *GFR*, is equal to the total amount of creatinine found in the urine (equal to urine concentration times urine volume) divided by the plasma concentration.

The general concept of clearance can be applied to the kidney according to the equation

$$Cl_{ren} = \frac{\overline{C}_u V}{\overline{C}_p t} \quad [\text{mL} \cdot \text{min}^{-1}] \quad (13)$$

where Cl_{ren} is renal clearance, $\overline{C}_u$ is mean concentration during time t of drug in the urine in mg/mL, V is urine volume in mL generated in time t (min) and $\overline{C}_p$ is the mean concentration (during time t) of drug in the plasma in mg/mL; the units are thus mL/min. This equation obtains whether the drug is "cleared" by filtration or by tubular secretion and whether or not tubular resorption occurs. If the drug is protein-bound, the formula becomes

$$Cl_{ren(corr)} = \frac{\overline{C}_u V}{\overline{C}_p t(1 - p)} \quad [\text{mL/min}] \quad (14)$$

where $Cl_{ren(corr)}$ is the corrected renal clearance.

The ratio between Cl_{ren} and Cl_{creat}, Cl_{ren}/Cl_{creat} (or Cl_{ren}/Cl_{inulin}), is known as the *clearance ratio*. If the drug is protein-bound and the *corrected clearance* is used, the ratio $Cl_{ren(corr)}/Cl_{creat}$ is known as the *excretion ratio*.

If an unbound drug is only filtered and not resorbed, the excretion ratio will be 1 and the clearance about 125 mL/min; if the drug is subsequently resorbed, the excretion ratio will be less than 1 and the clearance will lie between 125 and 1 mL/min, the values depending on the degree of resorption. A clearance of 1 mL/min suggests distribution and elimination like those of water. If there is tubular secretion (plus obligatory filtration), the excretion ratio may exceed 1, and the clearance could be as high as 600–700 mL/min, depending upon the extent of tubular secretion and resorption. *Para-aminohippuric acid* (PAH) is not bound to plasma protein, is not tubularly resorbed, and is secreted so fast by the renal tubules that the plasma passing through the kidney is 90% cleared of PAH. Thus Cl_{PAH} is equal to 0.90 *RPF*. This is called the effective renal plasma flow, *ERPF*. The excretion ratio of PAH is about 5 to 6. The almost total clearance of a drug from the blood as it passes through an organ is known as *total clearance*.

Eq 9 can be rearranged so that

$$\frac{\overline{C}_u}{t} = \frac{\overline{C}_p Cl_{ren}}{v} \quad [\text{wt} \cdot \text{vol}^{-1} \cdot \text{min}^{-1}] \quad (15)$$

Thus it may be seen that the concentration of drug in newly formed urine is directly proportional to the plasma concentration. Since moment-to-moment the plasma concentration falls exponentially during time t, it follows that the instantaneous urine concentration in the collecting ducts likewise must fall exponentially and hence the rate of fall can be expressed by a first-order rate constant, k_u. This constant relates to renal clearance as follows:

$$k_u = \frac{Cl_{ren}}{V_d} \quad [\text{min}^{-1}] \quad (16)$$

The excretory rate constant may be simple, as with a drug like creatinine, or compound, as with a drug that is tubularly secreted and/or resorbed.

The overall renal elimination constant, k_r, is defined by

$$k_r = k_g + k_{ts} - k_{tr} \quad [\text{min}^{-1}] \quad (17)$$

where k_g is the constant for glomerular filtration, k_{ts} for tubular secretion, and k_{tr} for tubular resorption. Although k_r might be thought to be the same as k_u on page 745, in practice it is not, because clearance data are obtained from time-averaged concentrations and cannot provide instantaneous rates.

Table II—Hypothetical Half-Lives of Drugs of Differing Volumes of Distribution and Clearances

Drug No.	Distribution	V_d, liters	Renal Disposition	Clearance mL/min	Half-Life
1	Total body water	50	Filtered and resorbed with water	1	24 days
2	Total body water	50	Filtered, no resorption	125	4.67 hr
3	Total body water	50	Tubular secretion, total clearance	700	50 min
4	Extracellular water	15	Tubular secretion, total clearance	700	15 min
5	Strongly bound in tissues	50,000	Filtered and resorbed with water	1	66 years
6	Strongly bound in tissues	50,000	Tubular secretion, total clearance	700	35 days

However, creatinine-derived k_r is close to the instantaneous k_u at the midpoint of the collection period.

By combining Eqs 3 and 16 and assuming that there is no other route of elimination

$$t_{1/2} = 0.693 \frac{V_d}{Cl_{ren}} \quad [\text{time}] \quad (18)$$

The units of time must be the same for both $t_{1/2}$ and Cl_{ren}. The equation enables the calculation of some thought-provoking information about the biological half-lives of non-metabolized drugs of different excretion profiles and volumes of distribution. Approximate hypothetical half-lives of drugs of different volumes of distribution and renal clearance are shown in Table II. The drugs are assumed to be eliminated only by renal excretion. A volume of distribution of 50 L is that of total body water, 15 L is that of extracellular water, and 50,000 L is that of a drug strongly bound in the tissues. Because of biotransformations, few drugs have half-lives longer than a year. However, a few radioopaque iodine-containing diagnostic agents are so tightly bound that their half-lives exceed a year. At the other extreme, a half-life of 15 min by renal elimination is uncommon, because few drugs that are totally cleared have volumes of distribution as small as that of extracellular water. However, the half-life of penicillin G is about 30 min.

Although data from collected urine cannot provide instantaneous rates, it does allow the calculation of the plasma half-life. The instantaneous excretion rate, dD_u/dt (where D_u is the amount in urine), is directly proportional to the body burden, D_B, such that

$$dD_u/dt = k_u D_B \quad [\text{wt} \cdot \text{min}^{-1}] \quad (19)$$

But D_B is falling exponentially with a rate constant k, so that $D_B = D_B^0 e^{-kt}$; therefore, $dA/dt = k_u D_B^0 e^{-kt}$. It follows that the slope of a plot of the log of the excretion rate versus time will have a slope of $-0.434k$, analogous to Eq 2 (adapted to total content rather than concentration). The y intercept of such a plot is $\log k_{el} - D_B^0$, where D_B^0 is the amount of drug in the body at zero time. (For a derivation, see ref 9, pp 6–7). However, data on excretion rates require renal catheterization and are subject to considerable error. An alternative, usually more accurate, method of estimating k from urine concentration is to employ the cumulative amount excreted. In this method

$$D_u = \frac{D_B k_u}{k}(1 - e^{-kt}) \quad [\text{wt}] \quad (20)$$

Since k_u/k expresses the proportion of D_B being transferred to the urine, $D_B^0 k_u/k$ represents the total amount of drug excreted, or D_u^∞, where ∞ designates infinite time. Eq 20 in log form, with the above substitution and transposition, becomes

$$\log(D_u^\infty - D_u) = \log D_B^0 \frac{k_u}{k} - 0.434kt$$
$$= \log D_u^\infty - 0.434kt \quad [\text{no units}] \quad (21)$$

The slope of the plot against time is also $-0.434k$. The

equation applies if drug is administered intravascularly. This is known as the sigma minus method (sigma for the integral D_u^∞ and minus for the $-D_u$). Urine needs to be collected for only 3 or 4 half-lives in order for the semilog plot to yield a reliable slope and $t_{1/2}$. The method is especially useful when plasma concentrations are low.

Hepatic Clearance—The concept of hepatic clearance is like that of renal clearance, and hepatic clearance is likewise a hypothetical volume of blood per min imagined to be totally cleared of drug during passage through the liver. Unlike renal clearance, the input is both portal venous and hepatic arterial blood and the output is both hepatic venous blood and bile, rather than arterial blood and urine, respectively. Portal venous blood and bile cannot be readily sampled, so that the concepts involved in hepatic clearance serve better to provide a model for understanding the role of the liver in pharmacokinetics than a clinical methodology for its direct measurement.

Although the mathematical treatment of hepatic clearance has been developed for steady-state conditions, rather than for exponentially falling drug concentrations in the inputs and outputs to the liver, the subject is appropriate at this place, in conjunction with other clearances.

The *hepatic clearance*, Cl_H, can be defined by the equation

$$Cl_H = HBF\left(\frac{C_{ap} - C_v}{C_{ap}}\right) = HBF \cdot E \quad [\text{mL} \cdot \text{min}^{-1}] \quad (22)$$

where HBF is the total hepatic blood flow, C_{ap} the hypothetical mean of mixed hepatic arterial and portal venous concentrations, and C_v is the hepatic venous concentration. The ratio, $(C_{ap} - C_v)/C_{ap}$, is the *extraction ratio, E*. Unlike glomerular filtration, there is an upper limit to the absolute quantity of drug that can be cleared and hence to the extraction ratio. Extraction is flow-limited only so long as the biotransforming enzyme system is not approaching saturation. The maximal clearance in the presence of normal blood flow has been called the *total intrinsic clearance, Cl_{intr}*. The extraction ratio expressed in terms of Cl_{intr} is

$$E = \frac{Cl_{intr}}{HBF + Cl_{intr}} \quad [\text{no units}] \quad (23)$$

which may be substituted into Eq 21, to yield

$$Cl_H = HBF\left(\frac{Cl_{intr}}{HBF + Cl_{intr}}\right) = HBF \cdot E \quad [\text{mL} \cdot \text{min}^{-1}] \quad (24)$$

The intrinsic clearance becomes

$$Cl_{intr} = \frac{HBF \cdot E}{1 - E} \quad [\text{mL} \cdot \text{min}^{-1}] \quad (25)$$

Cl_{intr} is thus somewhat analogous to V_{max}/K_m in enzyme kinetics.

Eqs 22 through 25 emphasize that hepatic clearance and extraction are functions both of hepatic blood flow and the capacity of hepatic enzymes to biotransform (or secrete into bile) the drug that is delivered. In order to appreciate the relative dependencies on Cl_{intr} and HBF, various assumed values may be substituted into the equations. What will be found is that the larger the Cl_{intr}, the more Cl_H tends to be flow-limited (ie, dependent on the rate of delivery of blood), whereas when Cl_{intr} is small, Cl_H is metabolism-limited. At constant blood flow with a drug in which elimination is predominately hepatic, when intrinsic clearance and hence extraction ratios are small, a significant change in intrinsic clearance will be accompanied by a significant change in $t_{1/2}$; when intrinsic clearance is high, a significant change may be accompanied by a small, often insignificant change in $t_{1/2}$ but a significant decrease in bioavailability. In the latter instance, $t_{1/2}$ is determined mostly by the fraction of the cardiac output that passes through the liver. Figures illustrating these features and an excellent discussion of hepatic clearance of the model may be found in ref 5, as may be a treatment of the effect of binding of drug to plasma protein. Binding to plasma protein limits clearance when intrinsic clearance is low but not when it is high.

Although the determination of Cl_{intr} is too involved for routine investigative purposes, it may be estimated according to the equation

$$Cl_{intr} = \frac{\left(1 - \dfrac{D_{un}}{fD}\right)D}{AUC_0} \qquad [\text{mL} \cdot \text{min}^{-1}] \qquad (26)$$

where D_{un} is the total quantity of drug excreted unchanged, f is the fraction absorbed, D is the dose administered, and AUC_0 is the total area under the blood concentration-time curve after intravenous administration. The meaning of AUC will be discussed later (page 753).

Some drugs may be used to illustrate some of the points emphasized by the model. For example, at blood concentrations of ethanol above 0.02–0.04%, the hepatic alcohol dehydrogenase system is saturated, and hence hepatic blood flow will have little effect on Cl_H of ethanol above the concentration indicated. This implies that liver disease or injury will not much affect the rate that ethanol is cleared from the blood, a fact of some forensic importance. The hepatic biotransformations of pentobarbital and phenytoin are relatively slow, that is, Cl_{intr} are low; consequently, the induction of hepatic cytochrome P450 will increase Cl_H, almost in proportion to the degree of induction, and the $t_{1/2}$ will be shortened accordingly. The hepatic biotransformation of lidocaine is extremely rapid, that is, the Cl_{intr} is very high, so that Cl_H is limited by delivery. This means that by the oral route, in which all of the absorbed drug obligatorily passes through the liver, only very small amounts will survive the pass through the liver into the systemic circulation. This nearly total clearance as the drug passes through the liver into the rest of the body is known as the *first-pass effect*. The clinical significance of the first-pass effect is discussed in Chapter 39. The flow-limitation in the hepatic metabolism of lidocaine also means that in congestive heart failure or shock, in which hepatic blood flow is diminished, the rate of biotransformation will decrease and $t_{1/2}$ will increase.

Biliary secretion contributes to hepatic clearance and hence is included in the above pharmacokinetic considerations. However, drugs that are excreted intact or in a form from which the drug can be sequestered in the intestines and subsequently resorbed may have complex pharmacokinetics if the rate of biliary secretion is an appreciable fraction of the hepatic clearance and if the enterohepatic reservoir is large.

Other Routes and Clearances—The kidney and liver are usually the major organs in the elimination of drugs, and all other routes combined often contribute negligibly. However, with the volatile anesthetics, pulmonary clearance is the major route, and pulmonary clearance becomes dominant; pulmonary clearance of gases is completely flow-limited. With some

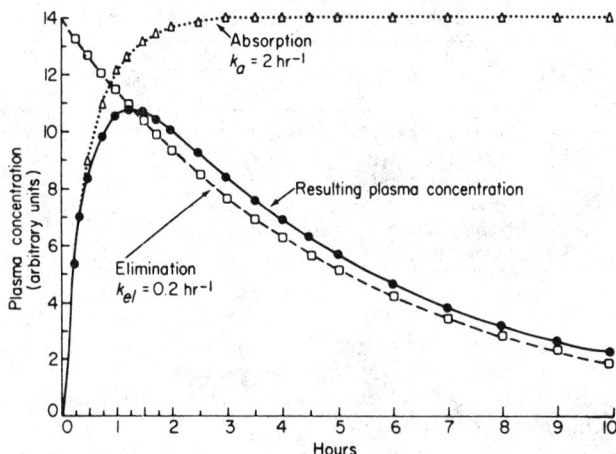

Fig 38-7. Time course of the plasma concentration of a hypothetical drug with simple first-order absorption and elimination kinetics. The rate constants are shown in the figure. The half-time for elimination is 3.47 hr.

drugs, mammary secretion is appreciable, and the presence of drug in milk may present hazards to nursing children; however, pharmacokinetics in the mother is not usually affected by lactation. Salivary secretion is too small to affect systemic pharmacokinetics, but the concentration of drug in saliva usually parallels that in plasma, so that it is possible to follow systemic pharmacokinetics by sampling saliva.

Absorption Plus Elimination—The kinetics of absorption and disposition must now be put together to define the time-related curve which describes the plasma concentration of a drug. The curve is determined by the algebraic sum of all processes involved in absorption, distribution, and elimination. Since disposition (distribution plus elimination) begins as soon as the drug enters the blood stream, the plasma concentration reflects all these processes from the outset.

The time course of the plasma concentration of a drug in a one-compartment body can be obtained by combining algebraically Eqs 1 and 4, with appropriate rate constants, and substituting fD/V_d for C_p^∞. When the equations for absorption and elimination are thus combined,

$$C_p = \frac{fDk_a}{V_d(k_a + k_{el})}(e^{-k_{el}t} - e^{-k_a t}) \qquad [\text{wt} \cdot \text{vol}^{-1}] \quad (27)$$

where f is the fraction absorbed, D is the dose, etc.

This equation simplifies to

$$C_p = C_p^0 e^{-k_{el}t} - C_p^0 e^{-k_a t} \qquad [\text{wt} \cdot \text{vol}^{-1}] \qquad (28)$$

where C_p^0 and the C_p^∞ of Eq 4 are the same, since they both represent all of dose, D, distributed in V_d. If there is a lag, the t-factor in the exponents of e should be $t - t_1$, where t_1 is the lag time. Fig 38-7 shows a plot of the plasma concentration for each of absorption and elimination separately and when the two are combined.

In Fig 38-7 the parameters of absorption and elimination were assumed, in order to construct the figure. In practice, drug concentration-time data are obtained empirically, and the parameters are obtained from a semilog plot of the data, as in Fig 38-8. The rising phase of the plot is not loglinear, since that which is added by absorption is being diminished by elimination. Only after absorption is complete does the plot become loglinear, since now there is no opposing process at work against the monoexponential decline in concentration. The time at which absorption is essentially complete is called the *absorption time* and is detected as that time at which the plot becomes loglinear. However, prior to the absorption time, the concentration at the site of deposition becomes equal to that in plasma. This is called the *equilibrium time*. It is

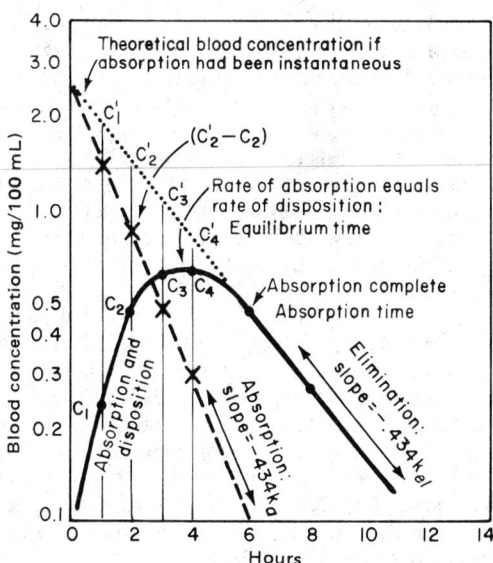

Fig 38-8. Kinetics of absorption and disposition of theophylline in the human subject after oral administration of 0.5 g of aminophylline per 70 kg. Blood concentration is plotted on a log scale (courtesy, data, Truitt et al[3]).

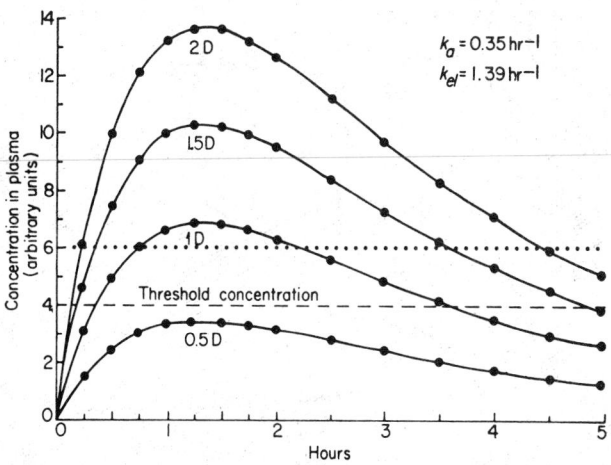

Fig 38-9. The effect of the size of the dose of a drug on the peak concentration, time of peak concentration, and duration of action. The data are calculated from a one-compartment model.

also the *peak-time* for plasma concentration. Because of the interplay of physicochemical and active transport factors that affect the distribution of a drug, true chemical equilibrium is not necessarily reached at the pharmacokinetic equilibrium point. The loglinear line described by the elimination phase, when back-extrapolated to the y-axis, yields a theoretical C_p^0, just as with intravascular injection, and $V_{d(extrap)}$ can be calculated accordingly. Furthermore, the slope of the loglinear elimination segment of the semilog plot is equal to $-0.434k_{el}$, as with intravascular injection. The absorption rate constant, k_a, can also be obtained from the plot, if the empirical curve is subtracted from the back-extrapolated elimination line. This is done by subtracting the real values for C_p (C_1, C_2, etc) at various times during the absorption phase from the extrapolated values for C_p, designated C', on the back-extrapolated elimination line. It must be remembered that the antilog and not the log of C must be used if log C is plotted in cartesian coordinates. This method of dissecting a compound function into its separate components is known as the *method of residuals*, or "*back-feathering.*" The back-feathered "absorption" line is the dashed line; its slope is negative, as though it were being seen from the site of administration.

The *peak concentration*, *time of peak concentration*, and *duration of action* are affected by various factors, some of which are discussed below.

Peak Concentration—That the peak concentration should vary with the dose is self-evident; according to Eq 27, it is directly proportional to the dose (assuming that absorption and elimination are first order processes). Fig 38-9 shows how peak concentration varies directly with dose. Note that the time of peak concentration is the same for all doses; this independence of peak time from dose also approximately obtains in all multicompartment systems. Departures from the generalization occur especially when the rate of absorption or elimination is different at high than at low concentration, ie, when it is dose-dependent (see page 759).

Time of Peak Concentration—The time of peak concentration must not be confused with the time of peak effect. Effect often lags behind plasma concentration, sometimes because the tissue concentration at the point of action has not yet reached its peak and sometimes because a response may have a considerable latency. The latency of effect of reserpine or phenytoin (in its anticonvulsant effect) is measured in hours

to days. Occasionally, the time of peak effect may precede the time of peak concentration because of a reflex or other compensatory process which limits effect before the concentration becomes maximal. This is often true with oral ethanol or ephedrine. Both the peak concentration and time of peak concentration are considerably affected by the rate constants for absorption and elimination. In Fig 38-10, the effect of differences in absorption rate is shown; the higher the absorption rate, the higher the peak concentration and the earlier the time of peak concentration. Fig 38-11 shows the effect of differences in rate of elimination; the higher the elimination rate the lower the peak concentration but the earlier the time of peak concentration. The two effects of absorption rate and elimination rate can be treated as a single phenomenon, if the ratio of k_a/k_{el} is considered rather than the separate rate constants (Fig 38-12).

The effects illustrated in Figs 38-10 to 38-12 have certain clinical implications:

1. *Differences in the rate of absorption are of more significance for slowly than for rapidly absorbed drugs.* In Fig 38-10, the blood levels achieved when $k_a = 2$ hr^{-1} are not greatly different than when $k_a = 20$ hr^{-1}, but the difference in the level when $k_a = 0.5$ is considerably different

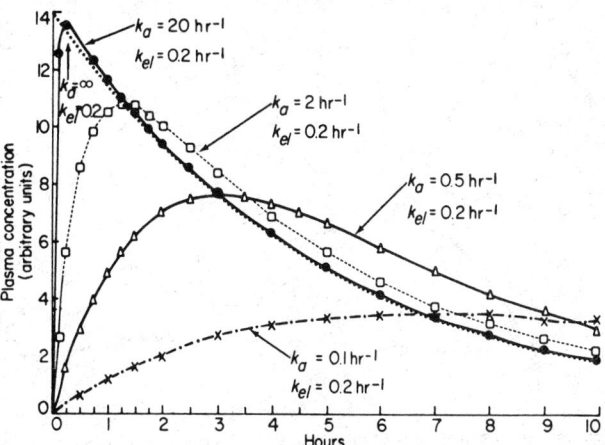

Fig 38-10. The effect of differences in the rate of absorption of drugs on the peak concentration, time of peak concentration, and sojourn in the body. The rate of elimination is the same for all curves. The dotted line ($k_a = \infty$) is approximately what the concentration curve would be, had the drug been given intravenously. The data were calculated from a one-compartment model.

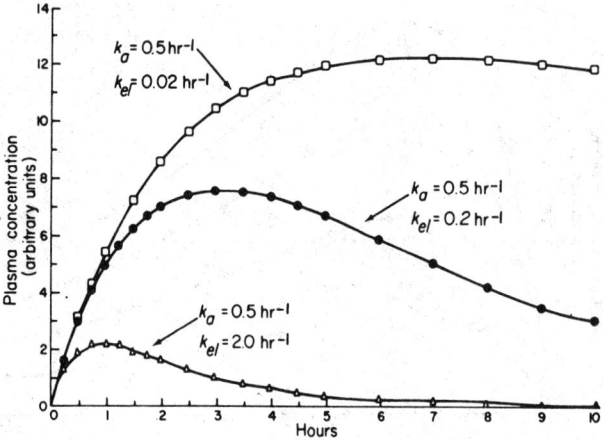

Fig 38-11.   The effect of differences in the rate of elimination of drugs on the peak concentration, time of peak concentration, and sojourn in the body.   The rate of absorption is the same for all curves.   The data were calculated from a one-compartment model.

from that when $k_a = 0.1$, even though in the latter the rate difference was less than in the former comparison.   It is thus apparent that differences in the release rates among different products of the same drug, or in gastrointestinal motility, blood flow, etc, may be important, depending upon k_a/k_{el}.   This point has an especial relevance to sustained-release and depot formulations.   With a number of drugs, especially among the anorectic drugs, the dose with a sustained-release form is often approximately the same as that of a rapid-release form; thus the former has a long duration in the body but yields low blood levels when used in a single dose.   Except with the initial dose, the differences are of lesser importance in a multiple-dose regimen.   Small differences in the rate of absorption of rapidly absorbed drugs are usually of minor significance.

2.   *When the rate of absorption is fast relative to that of elimination, differences in the rate of elimination do not greatly affect the peak concentration consequent to a single dose* (compare top two curves of Fig 38-12).   Thus in such instances, the peak concentration is relatively insensitive to normal variations in the rate of elimination.   Consequently, with such a drug, the size of the initial dose in a multiple-dose regimen often may not need to be diminished in the presence of renal or hepatic impairment; however, subsequent doses require adjustment.

3.   *A change in the time of peak concentration or of peak effect is usually an indication of a change in one of or both k_a and k_{el}.*

Duration of Action—The duration of action of a drug is related to its pharmacokinetics in a rather complicated way.

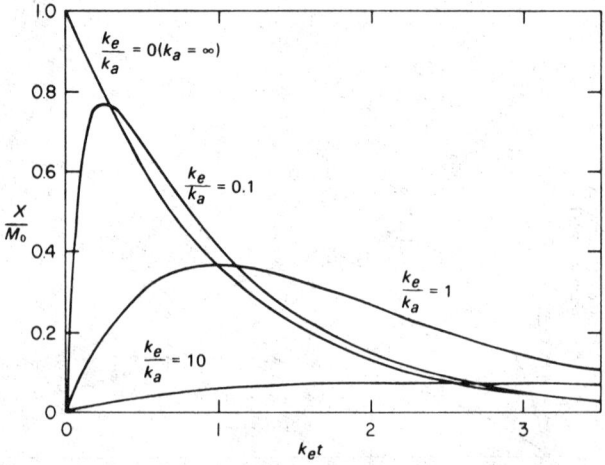

Fig 38-12.   The effect of differences in the ratio, k_{el}/k_a (k_e/k_a in diagram), on the peak concentration, time of peak concentration, and sojourn in the body.   The ordinate, X/M_0, actually represent the fraction of a dose that is in the body, but they are directly proportional to concentration and thus serve to represent concentration.   The abscissa can be converted to time by dividing by k_e, the elimination rate constant (courtesy, Goldstein *et al*[6]).

It is usually shorter than the sojourn of the drug in the body, because a threshold, or minimal effective, concentration must be reached before the effect occurs (see Fig 38-9), and the effect usually ceases when the plasma concentration falls below the threshold level.   In a one-compartment system, duration of action tends to be proportional to log dose.   In a two-compartment system it tends to be proportional to log dose only when the site of action is in the central compartment and the effective concentrations (minimum to maximum) are entirely within the concentrations found during the elimination phase.   In Fig 38-9, the duration of action is 3.25 hours with dose D, 4.6 hours with $1.5\ D$, and 5.4 hours with $2\ D$; were the threshold at 6 (dotted line), instead of 4, (dashed line), the respective durations would have been 1.5, 3.25, and 4.25 hours.   Although the example in which the threshold is 6 provides that the duration of action would be disproportionately prolonged as the dose is increased, the contrary is seen when the threshold is 4.   Consequently, *increasing the dosage is usually not a feasible way of increasing the duration of action*, and toxic concentrations are often reached more predictably than duration is prolonged.

With a few drugs, there is no mathematically definable relationship between duration of action and persistence of the plasma concentration.   With reserpine, for example, the effect outlasts the sojourn of the drug, because of the depletion of a slowly replaceable biological mediator.*

Multiple-Dose Administration—*Multiple-dose administration* is the administration of a succession of doses at intervals such that the drug does not completely leave the body in each interval between doses.   The usual procedure in a multiple-dose regimen is to administer a drug repetitively with a constant dose interval, designated τ, with both dose and τ chosen so as to maintain the plasma concentration in the therapeutic range.   Some features of such repetitive dosing may be seen from the construction reproduced in Fig 38-13.

Accumulation and Plateau Principle—If the novice reader will make his own construction it will greatly aid his understanding of the subject.   In the construction, the amount of drug in the body (D_B) is plotted against time.   Dose, D, is given repetitively, intravenously, at intervals such that $\tau = t_{1/2}$, in order to facilitate the construction.   The first dose is given at 0τ; since it is given intravenously, the amount in the body rises to $1\ D_B$ essentially instantaneously.   Immediately, D_B falls exponentially with the first-order kinetics of Eq 1, except that whole-body content, rather than C_p is plotted.   Since $\tau = t_{1/2}$, at τ, $D_B = \frac{1}{2}D$, when the next dose, D, is added, it brings the body content up to $D + \frac{1}{2}D$.   During each dose interval, D_B falls exponentially to one-half the previous post-injection peak.   As D_B rises after each administration, the rate (*not* the rate constant) of elimination rises proportionately, until eventually the amount eliminated during τ essentially equals the amount injected.   The maximum and minimum values of D_B, $D_{B(max)}$ and $D_{B(min)}$, during τ, approach respective asymptotes, shown on the graph.   As $t \rightarrow \infty$, $D_{B(max)} \rightarrow 2D$ and $D_{B(min)} \rightarrow D$.   Thus, although D_B fluctuates between $D_{B(max)}$ and $D_{B(min)}$, once the asymptotes are closely approximated, D_B can be thought of as having reached a qualified *steady-state* condition, and the pharmacokinetics are sometimes called steady-state pharmacokinetics. D_b is also said to have reached a *plateau*.   It is important to note that the rate at which the plateau is reached is exactly the same rate at which drug is eliminated from the body after a single dose.   Thus the exponentially falling line for the elimination of D given at 0τ (had no further doses been

---

* Careful studies show that trace amounts of reserpine in the body outlast the effect, and the duration of action may be related to these trace amounts.   These residual amounts, however, are much smaller than are required to initiate the catecholamine-depleting action.

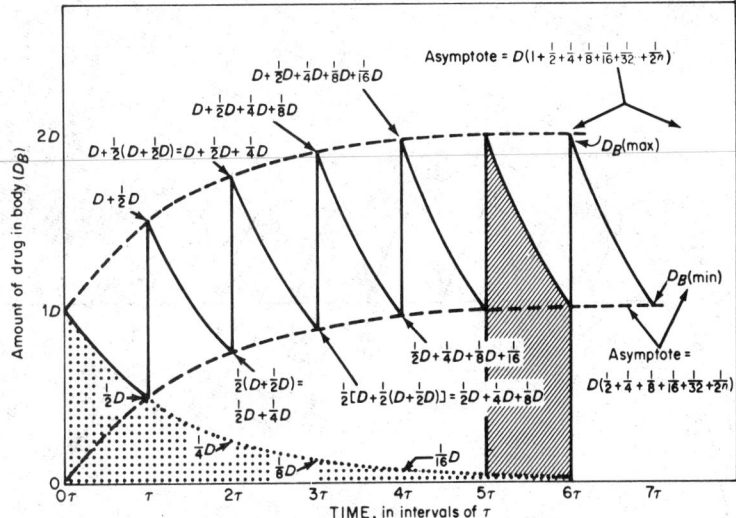

Fig 38-13. The accumulation of drug in the body during a regime of multiple dosing. Dose, D, is administered intravenously at intervals (τ) equal to the half-life ($t_{1/2}$). Thus after each dose, the amount in the body, D_B, has decreased to half the previous peak amount at the time each dose is administered. When the cumulated amount in the body after injection reaches $2D$, the body content will fluctuate from $2D$ to $1D$ during each dose interval thereafter. Approximately 5 half-lives are required before this leveling off (plateau) of the body content occurs. The stippled area is the area under the elimination curve of a single injection if no second dose had been given. The cross-hatched area is the area under the curve during a single dose interval. The two areas are equal.

given) is the mirror image of the line connecting the sequential $D_{B(max)}s$. The principle that *when the rate of absorption is fast compared to the rate of elimination ($k_a > 5k_{el}$) the rate at which the multiple-dose steady state is approached is determined only by k_{el}* is known as the *plateau principle.* This is the fundamental feature of one-compartment multiple-dose kinetics. It obtains irrespective of the value of τ. However, the plateau concentrations do depend upon τ (see below).

In Fig 38-13, drug was administered intravenously, so that no time-dependent absorption had to be considered. When absorption is involved, the $C_{p(max)}$ is not as high as with intravascular administration, is blunted, and occurs with a latency after administration that is determined by k_a/k_{el}, just as in single dose administration. The appearance of the C_p-time curve with multiple dose administration is shown in Fig 38-14. The value of C_p at any time during multiple-dose administration can be calculated according to Eq 29:

$$C_p = \frac{fk_a}{V_d(k_{el} - k_a)}\left[\left(D^* e^{-nk_{el}\tau} + D \cdot \frac{1 - e^{-nk_a\tau}}{1 - e^{-k_a}}\right)\right.$$
$$\left. - \left(D^* e^{-nk_{el}\tau} + D \cdot \frac{1 - e^{-nk_{el}\tau}}{1 - e^{-k_{el}\tau}}\right)\right] \quad [wt \cdot vol^{-1}] \quad (29)$$

where n is the nth dose, τ is the dose-interval, t is the time since the last dose, D is the maintenance dose, D^* is the initial or loading dose (see below), and f is the fraction absorbed (bioavailability factor). With this equation, C_p, rather than D_B, is calculated; however, it will be recalled that $C_p^0 = D/V_d$, and similarly, $C_p = D_B/V_d$, so that the equation is easily modified to calculate either C_p or D_B, and the same principles obtain in either form.

It is important to know how many half-lives must transpire before the plateau is approached closely enough to be considered complete for practical purposes. $D_{B(min)}$ is approximately 93% complete at 4τ and 97% at 5τ; $D_{B(max)}$ is 97% at 4τ and 98.5% at 5τ. Thus it may be stated that, for practical purposes, the plateau state is approximately reached in five half-lives, provided $k_a > 5k_{el}$. This is another form of the *plateau principle. The principle applies whenever the steady state conditions are perturbed; that is, 5 half-times will be required to reach a new plateau, whether the plasma*

concentration is rising or falling to a new plateau (see Fig 38-14).

Maximum and Minimum Concentrations—During multiple dosing, $C_{p(max)}$ and $C_{p(min)}$ are described by Eqs 30 and 31:

$$C_{p(max)n} = \frac{C_p^0 (1 - e^{-nk_{el}t_a})}{1 - e^{-k_{el}\tau}} \quad [wt \cdot vol^{-1}] \quad (30)$$

$$C_{p(min)n} = \frac{C_p^0 (1 - e^{-nk_{el}\tau})}{1 - e^{-k_{el}\tau}} \quad [wt \cdot vol^{-1}] \quad (31)$$

where n is the nth dose, C_p^0 is the concentration that would have occurred from instantaneous absorption and distribution (obtained by extrapolation of the elimination curve to zero time), and t_a is the absorption time. During the plateau state, $1 - e^{nk_{el}\tau}$ becomes $e^{-k_{el}\tau}$, and $C_{p(max)}$ and $C_{p(min)}$ are designated C_{max}^{ss} and C_{min}^{ss}, respectively. The equation is valid only

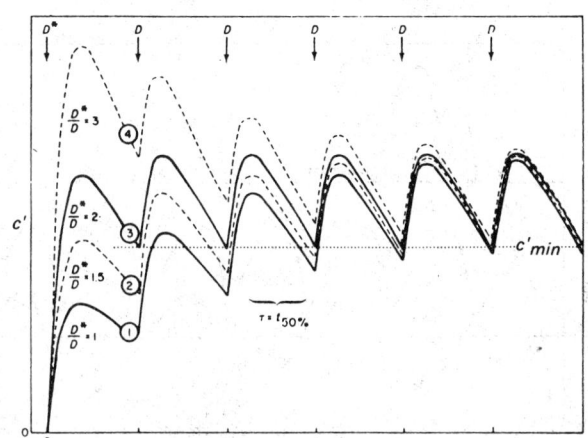

Fig 38-14. Time course of the plasma concentration of a drug administered according to a multiple-dose schedule. C' (ordinate): concentration; t (abscissa): time; D^*: initial dose; D: maintenance dose; τ: dose-interval (equal to $t_{1/2}$ in this illustration); C'_{min}: minimum concentration after each dose (same as $C_{p(min)}$ in text) (courtesy, Krüger-Thiemer[7]).

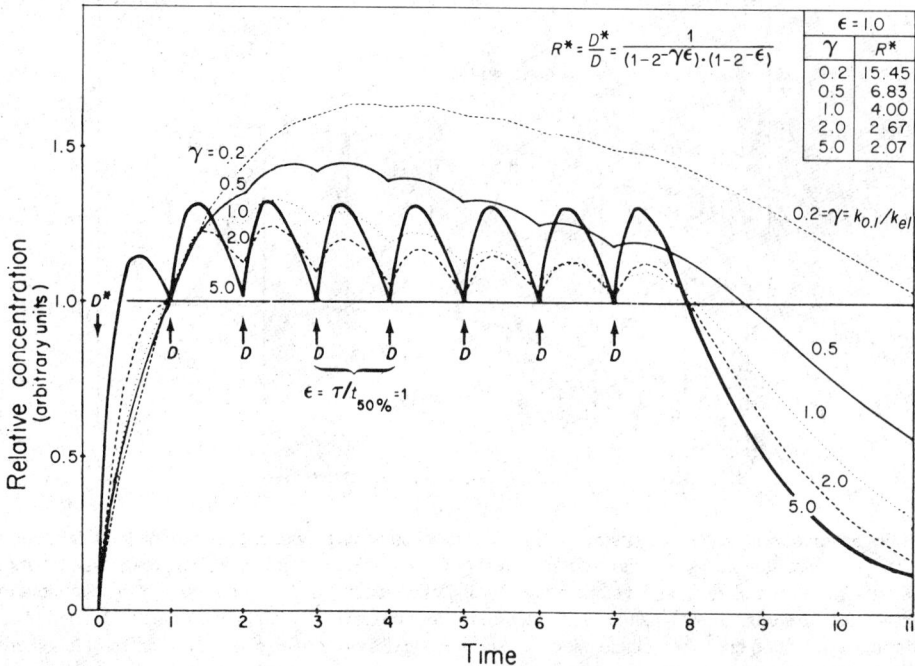

Fig 38-15. The effect of differences in k_a/k_{el} (k_{01}/k_{el} in diagram) on the plasma concentration of five different drugs administered in a multiple dose regimen. In the figure, $\gamma = k_a k_{el}$. D^* was determined from the dose ratio R^*, calculated according to the formula in the upper right. In the original figure, the ordinate was expressed in terms of relative quantity in the body, but the principle and relative fluctuations are the same. The value of 1 corresponds to steady state $C_{p(min)}$ for a drug with $\gamma = 5$, when $\tau = t_{1/2}$. τ is the dose-interval. Time is in multiples of the half-lives (courtesy, Krüger-Thiemer[7], adapted).

when $k_a > 5k_{el}$. It can be seen that $C_{p(max)}$ is determined by both k_a and k_{el} (k_a shows itself only indirectly, in t_a) and $C_{p(min)}$ by k_{el}. The greatest difference between $C_{p(max)}$ and $C_{p(min)}$ occurs when the drug is given intravenously; when $\tau = t_{1/2}$, after intravenous injection, $C_{p(max)}/C_{p(min)}$ is theoretically equal to 2. With extravascular administration, the ratio is always less than that with intravenous administration, the ratio being determined by k_a/k_{el}. As k_a/k_{el} decreases, $C_{p(max)}/C_{p(min)}$ decreases; this effect is illustrated in Fig 38-15.

Average Concentration and Body Content—The average concentration during the plateau state is described by the equation

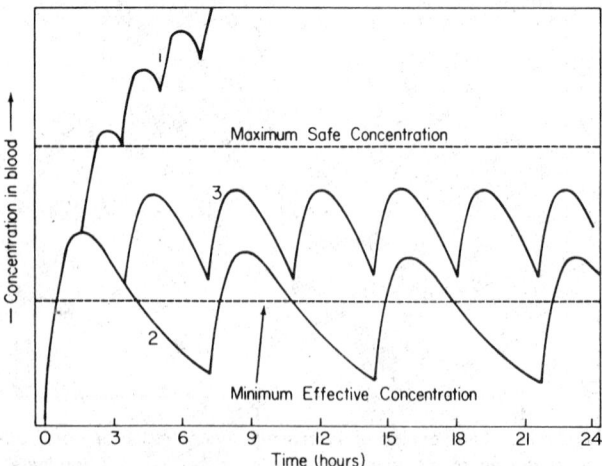

Fig 38-16. The effect of the dose interval on the time course of the plasma concentration of a drug administered in a multiple-dose regimen. $D^* = 4$, $D = 3$, and $k_a/k_{el} = 3$. The dose interval is 1.7 hr in Curve 1, 7.7 hr in Curve 2, and 3.8 hr in Curve 3 (courtesy Notari[8]).

$$C_{p(ave)} = \frac{fD}{V_d k_{el} \tau} = \frac{1.44\, t_{1/2} fD}{V_d \tau} \qquad [\text{wt} \cdot \text{vol}^{-1}] \qquad (32)$$

The coefficient 1.44 is the reciprocal of 0.693 in Eq 3. $C_{p(ave)}$ is a time-averaged concentration and is therefore really a mean concentration. Since $C_p = D_B/V_d$, it follows that

$$D_{B(ave)} = \frac{fD}{k_{el} \tau} = \frac{1.44\, t_{1/2} fD}{\tau} \qquad [\text{wt}] \qquad (33)$$

It is self-evident that the plasma concentration or amount of drug in the body is directly proportional to the fraction of drug absorbed (f, bioavailability factor). The appearance of f in these equations and Eq 29, however, serves to remind us that a change from one drug product to another with a different bioavailability, f', will be accompanied by changes in $C_{p(ave)}$ and $D_{B(ave)}$ as well as in the maxima and minima. The equations also reemphasize that a change in $t_{1/2}$ (or k_{el}) will affect $C_{p(ave)}$ and $D_{B(ave)}$, all other factors being held constant. Since k_{el} and f (and sometimes V_d in relation to weight) vary from patient to patient, the dosage of certain drugs will always need to be ascertained with laboratory assistance and acumen. The effects of changes in τ are discussed below.

Importance of Dose-Interval—The ratio $C_{p(max)}/C_{p(min)}$ depends on the dose-interval, τ. If the interval is increased and the dose is unchanged, $C_{p(max)}$, $C_{p(min)}$, and $C_{p(ave)}$ all decrease, but $C_{p(max)}/C_{p(min)}$ is increased. If τ is decreased, then $C_{p(max)}$, $C_{p(min)}$, and $C_{p(ave)}$ increase, but $C_{p(max)}/C_{p(min)}$ is decreased. This is shown in Fig 38-16. To avoid a change in $C_{p(ave)}$ consequent to a change in τ, the dose may be appropriately changed, in accordance with Eqs 31 and 32. Nevertheless, the wider fluctuations between $C_{p(max)}$ and $C_{p(min)}$ when τ is lengthened cannot be avoided simply by adjusting the dose (see Fig 38-17, broken lines). If $C_{p(min)}$, rather than $C_{p(ave)}$, is held constant, the fluctuations become even larger (Fig 38-17, solid lines), and the hazard of the concentration reaching the toxic range is increased. Conversely, *the greater the number of divided doses, the smaller*

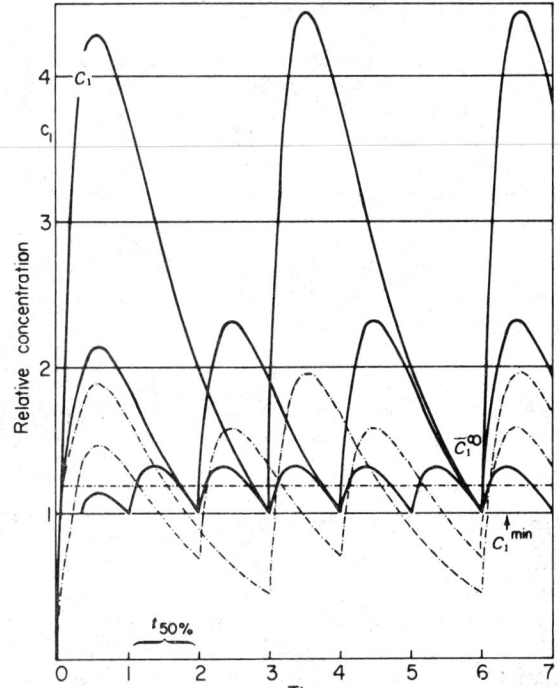

Fig 38-17.   Fluctuations in the plasma concentration of a drug when the dose interval is changed but the dose is altered to maintain the same minimal (solid lines) or average (broken lines) concentration during maintenance. C_1^{min} is the minimal concentration (corresponding to $C_{p(min)}$ in the text), and $\overline{C}_1^\infty$ is the average concentration during maintenance (corresponding to $C_{p(ave)}$ in the text). The initial dose was calculated according to the formula in Fig 38-15. Time is in multiples of the half-life (courtesy, Krüger-Thiemer[7], adapted).

the fluctuations in plasma concentration. With drugs with a narrow therapeutic range, it is usually inadvisable to dose at intervals longer than $t_{1/2}$. With digitoxin, τ is much smaller than $t_{1/2}$, and the fluctuations in plasma concentration are consequently less than 10%. However, with drugs with a high therapeutic index and which do not require a steady plasma concentration for an adequate therapeutic action, dose intervals much larger than $t_{1/2}$ may be conveniently used. Penicillin G is such a drug, for which it is more convenient to give large doses at 4-hour intervals, or longer, than at 30- to 60-min intervals ($t_{1/2}$ = 30 to 60 min).

Cumulation Ratio and Persistence Factor—From the above, it is evident that the drug cumulated in the body during the repetitive administration approaches different amounts (asymptotes) in the plateau state according to the magnitude of τ in relation to $t_{1/2}$ (or k_{el}). The dose-interval must be a convenient interval that not only is easy for the patient or medical and paramedical personnel to keep track of but also one which does not subject the patient to an annoying or difficult number of doses per day. Furthermore, $t_{1/2}$ varies from patient to patient. Consequently, it is rare when $\tau = t_{1/2}$, although it is sometimes close enough that the difference is inconsequential. Therefore, it is important to be able to estimate the extent of cumulation with any dose interval in any patient. This can be done with information derived from a single dose, by means of the *accumulation factor*, r_a.

$$r_a = \frac{1}{1 - e^{-k_{el}\tau}} \qquad \text{[no units]} \qquad (34)$$

The component factor, $e^{-k_{el}\tau}$, is the persistence factor, r, which is the fraction by which C_p or D_B falls during the dose interval. When the plateau, or steady state, is reached, the cumulated plasma concentration or body content will be larger

than that from the first dose by a factor known as the *cumulation ratio*, (or *drug amount ratio*), R_c:

$$R_c = \frac{1}{k_{el}\tau} = \frac{1.44\, t_{1/2}}{\tau} = \frac{\overline{C}_\tau^{ss}}{\overline{C}_0^\infty} \left(\text{or } \frac{\overline{D}_{B\tau}^{ss}}{\overline{D}_{B0}^\infty}\right) \quad \text{[no units]} \quad (35)$$

where $\overline{C}_\tau^{ss}$ is the mean concentration during one dosage interval during the steady state and $\overline{C}_0^\infty$ is the mean concentration from $t = 0$ to $t = \infty$ after a single dose; $\overline{D}_{B\tau}^{ss}$ and $\overline{D}_{B0}^\infty$ are the corresponding respective body contents. Since both $\overline{C}_0^\infty$ and $\overline{C}_\tau^{ss}$ can be estimated from the area under the curve (AUC), it is appropriate to discuss AUC further.

Area Under Curve (AUC)—The area under the monoexponentially falling, single-dose plasma concentration-time curve is the integral of the differential form of Eq. 1, from $t = 0$ to $t = \infty$:

$$AUC^{0\to\infty} = \overline{C}^{0\to\infty} = \int_0^\infty C\, dt$$

$$= \int_0^\infty C_p^{0} e^{-k_{el}t} dt = \frac{C_p^0}{k_{el}} \qquad \text{[wt} \cdot \text{vol}^{-1} \cdot \text{time]} \quad (36)$$

Although its units are concentration times time, its value is equal to the time-averaged concentration, and hence is called the *average concentration* $\overline{C}_0^\infty$, although it is more appropriately a *log mean* concentration. If the amount of drug in the body is used, instead of plasma concentration, then the AUC is equal to the *time-averaged body content*. The average body content, could, of course, be calculated from $\overline{C}_0^\infty$ by multiplying by V_d.

Even when two or more exponential processes act additively on the plasma concentration (or body content), as in absorption plus elimination, the $AUC^{0\to\infty}$ equals $\overline{C}_p^{0\to\infty}$ (or $D_B^{0\to\infty}$). The interested student may verify this by integrating any of Eqs 27–29. In the two-compartment system (see below), $AUC^{0\to\infty}$ for a plasma concentration-time curve correctly equals $\overline{C}_p^{0\to\infty}$; however, $D_B^{0\to\infty}$ cannot be calculated from $\overline{C}_p^{0\to\infty}$, because the plasma concentration differs from the average body concentration.

Since $AUC^{0\to\infty} = C_p^0/k_{el}$ in the one-compartment system, it is obvious that AUC does not provide any new information that cannot otherwise be obtained, as by back-extrapolation or regression analysis. Nevertheless, AUC is frequently used in lieu of C_p^0/k_{el}. For example, in the determination of the bioavailability factor, f, the $AUC^{0\to\infty}$ after *extra*vascular administration ($AUC_{ev}^{0\to\infty}$) divided by the AUC after *intra*vascular administration ($AUC_{iv}^{0\to\infty}$) is equal to f.

$AUC^{0\to\infty}$ is not the only AUC that may be used in pharmacokinetics. The AUC during different time intervals under supposedly steady state conditions could be employed to detect time- or concentration-related changes in or clearance (eg, see Eqs 10 and 26). During the plateau, or steady state, the AUC during one dose interval (AUC^{ss}) is of especial interest. $AUC^{0\to\infty}$ requires many samples and a long time over which samples are taken, which is an inconvenience to the subject or patient. AUC^{ss} can provide the same derived information with fewer samples and less time. This is because $AUC^{ss} = AUC^{0\to\infty}$. Thus, in Fig 38-13, the stippled area, which is $AUC^{0\to\infty}$, would be exactly equal to the cross-hatched area, AUC^{ss}, except for the negligible stippled area that remains during $5\tau - 6\tau$. At $t = \infty$, the two areas would be identical. In this comparison of AUCs, the identical areas do not mean that $C_p^{0\to\infty}$ is identical to $\overline{C}_p^{ss}$, but it does enable AUC^{ss} to be used to calculate values of single dose parameters and vice-versa.

Constant Infusion and Sustained Release—A constant infusion or sustained release of a drug may be regarded as a series of minidoses given at infinitely short dose intervals. When infusion is intravascular, the plasma concentration will rise in logarithmic fashion with the same time course and cumulation factor as with multiple dosing, that is, with a rate

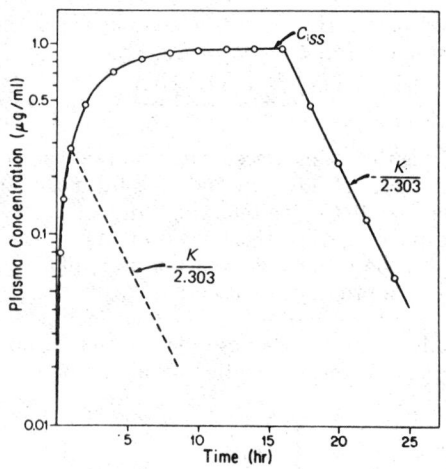

Fig 38-18. Semilogarithmic plot of plasma concentration during and after cessation of a constant intravenous infusion of a drug in a one-compartment system. Whether infusion is stopped prior to the attainment of a plateau or after, the plasma concentration will fall loglinearly with a slope of $-0.434k_{el}$. In the figure, K is k_{el} and $1/2.303$ = 0.434. C_{ss} is the steady-state concentration, C_p^{ss}(courtesy, Gibaldi and Perrier[9]).

constant of k_{el}. Thus, the plateau principle applies equally to constant infusion and multiple dosing. After discontinuation of infusion, the plasma concentration falls exponentially with a rate constant, k_{el}, in accordance with Eq 1. These principles are illustrated in Fig 38-18.

The steady-state plasma concentration, C_p^{ss}, is equal to the infusion rate divided by the whole body clearance:

$$C_p^{ss} = \frac{R^0}{Cl_{tot}} = \frac{R^0}{V_d k_{el}} \qquad [\text{wt} \cdot \text{vol}^{-1}] \qquad (37)$$

where R^0 is the infusion rate. V_d must be expressed in the same volume units as R^0; Cl_{tot} and R^0 must be in the same time units as k_{el}.

With sustained-release dosage forms in which the release is approximately constant for long periods of time, the pharmacokinetics are like those of constant infusion.

Loading and Maintenance—In Fig 38-13, $D_{B(max)} \to 2D$; consequently, had $2D$ been given for the first dose and D thereafter, the plateau condition would have been reached immediately. This illustrates the *principle of loading*. The same effect of loading is shown by curve 3 in Fig 38-14; in both these figures, $\tau = t_{1/2}$. The initial dose is called the *loading dose*, D^*, and each subsequent dose is called the *maintenance dose*, D. Since it takes about 5 half-lives to reach the plateau state, it is very important to use a loading dose with drugs that have long half-lives or in situations in which it is desirable that the optimal therapeutic concentration be reached rapidly.

The loading dose, D^*, should approximate the amount of drug in the body which will be contained during maintenance (ie, the plateau state). The optimal oral loading dose, D^*, may be calculated as follows:

$$D_0^* = \frac{D}{(1 - e^{-k_a \tau})(1 - e^{-k_{el} \tau})} \qquad [\text{wt}] \qquad (37)$$

where D is the maintenance dose. The equation correctly applies only when $k_a > 3k_{el}$; Fig 38-15 shows the inadequacy of the loading dose formula when k_a/k_{el} is small. D_0^* is also equal to D/R_c. The time course of the plasma concentration after different loading doses is shown in Fig 38-14. When D^* = $2D$, the plateau maintenance concentration is closely approximated when $\tau = t_{1/2}$ but is smaller than 2 when $\tau < t_{1/2}$ and greater when $\tau > t_{1/2}$.

In Fig 38-14, it should be noted that if the loading dose is not optimal, either too low or too high, the plateau state is

approached with the same time course as when no loading dose is given.

When a constant intravenous infusion is used, the principle of loading also applies, because the plateau principle applies; loading may be accomplished with one or more rapid intravenous doses, called boluses or slugs, or by an initial period of rapid infusion to bring the plasma concentration to the maintenance level. The loading dose can be calculated from the infusion rate and half-time, as

$$D_0^* = \frac{R_0 t_{1/2}}{0.434 \log 2} \qquad [\text{wt}] \qquad (39)$$

or from the steady state concentration,

$$D_0^* = C_p^{ss} V_d \qquad [\text{wt}] \qquad (40)$$

D_0^* is equal to the body content at steady state. Eq 40 applies equally well to multiple dosing, except that V_d^{ss} should be employed.

Open Two-Compartment Model

The one-compartment model adequately describes the pharmacokinetics of many drugs. However, with an even larger number of drugs, after intravenous administration, the decline in plasma concentration is not monoexponential but rather manifests two or more monoexponential components which are discernible in the semilogarithmic plot of C_p vs. time. The most common is a decline which manifests two components; the open two-compartment model most adequately describes such pharmacokinetics. Other models having more compartments or other complexities will be briefly mentioned later.

Description of the Model—In the open two-compartment model, the body is considered to comprise two compartments in dynamic equilibrium, as depicted in Fig 38-19. The compartment into which the drug is directly absorbed and from which the drug is eliminated is called compartment 1, or the *central compartment*. The blood is a part of this compartment, is the transporting and distributing medium, and is the medium actually sampled for chemical and phar-

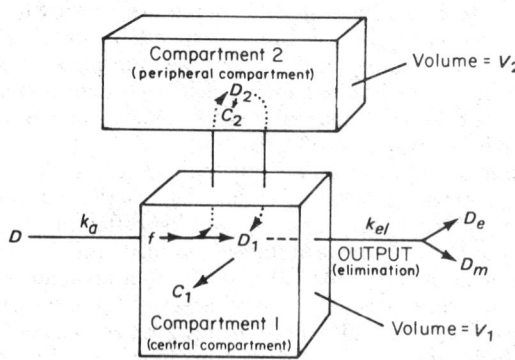

Fig 38-19. Diagram of open two-compartment pharmacokinetic model. An amount of drug, fD, is absorbed from the administered dose, D, with a first-order rate constant of k_a into compartment 1 of volume V_1. Some of the absorbed drug enters compartment 2 with a first-order rate constant of k_{12} and is returned into compartment 1 with a first-order rate constant of k_{21}. D_1 is the amount of drug in compartment 1 and D_2 in compartment 2; C_1 and C_2 are the respective concentrations in compartments 1 and 2 ($C_1 = C_p$). Drug is eliminated from compartment 1 with a first-order rate constant, k_{el}, which, however, is obscured by the lag in transfer of drug from compartment 2 to compartment 1. D_u is the amount excreted into urine, feces, expired air, sweat, milk, etc; D_m is the amount of drug metabolized. The relative volumes of V_1 and V_2 may vary greatly, V_1 sometimes being the larger and other times the smaller.

macokinetic analysis; consequently, compartment 1 is sometimes misleadingly called the blood or plasma compartment, even though the erythrocytes or plasma proteins may sometimes behave kinetically as though they were part of compartment 2. In the simple two-compartment model, compartment 2 is closed and communicates with the environment only through the central compartment, being, as it were, peripheral to the events of absorption and elimination; consequently, it is called the *peripheral compartment*. It is also sometimes called the tissue compartment, which is misleading, since usually some tissues, or certain cell types within otherwise peripheral tissues, may be kinetically in compartment 1. It is important to reiterate that the compartments are fictive and are defined by the kinetic behavior of the drug within the body and not necessarily by identifiable anatomical entities. To avoid confusion and to enable a simple numerical designation of model components and distribution rate constants by number, the terms compartment 1 and compartment 2 will be used hereinafter.

The movement of drug between compartments is defined by characteristic first-order rate constants. The subscript indicates the direction of movement; thus k_{12} (subscript one-two, not twelve) indicates movement from compartment 1 to compartment 2 and k_{21} the reverse direction. The constants k_a and k_{el} are entirely analogous to the like-designated respective absorption and elimination rate constants of the one-compartment model. However, k_{el} is not directly observed from the decline in plasma concentrations, since both the characteristic overall rate of the elimination processes and the rates of diffusion into and recruitment from compartment 2 combine to control the rate of decline in plasma concentration (see below). Once an infinitesimal amount of drug is absorbed, all processes occur simultaneously, that is, in parallel. Nevertheless, since the various processes have different time constants, one process will run its course to a practical end earlier than another, and events may be thought of as occurring sequentially, with overlap, in the order absorption, distribution and elimination. As long as $k_a > (k_{12} + k_{21})/k_{21} > k_{el}$, the terminal phase will be a steady decline in concentration (see Fig 38-20), during which the distribution ratio, C_1/C_2, will be constant.

Absorption—Absorption does not differ from that in the open one-compartment model and does not require further description. However, the determination of absorption characteristics from the log plasma concentration-time curves is complicated by the distribution phase, and the method of residuals (page 749) entails the resolution of three, rather than two components (see below).

Distribution and Elimination—After the intravascular administration of a drug which obeys two-compartment kinetics, the plasma concentration falls in a complex two-process fashion, but in an arithmetic plot the two components may not always be evident to the eye. When concentration-time data are plotted semilogarithmically, however, the separate processes of distribution and elimination are easily identified by the method of residuals (back-feathering, page 749 and Fig 38-8), if the rate of distribution significantly exceeds that of elimination. In Fig 38-20, such a resolution has been made for the drug pralidoxime. In the figure, it may be seen that after 2 hr the curve assumes a loglinear character. The assumption is made that the distribution phase is essentially complete and a pseudoequilibrium has been reached between the two compartments. Therefore, the late loglinear segment of the line, with the slope -0.434β, represents the elimination phase. If this line is subtracted from the curve, the distribution phase is the residual line. In order to do this, the loglinear segment is back-extrapolated. From this extrapolated line are obtained the antilogs to be subtracted from the temporally corresponding antilogs on the unresolved, original curve. The respective differences, or residuals, are then

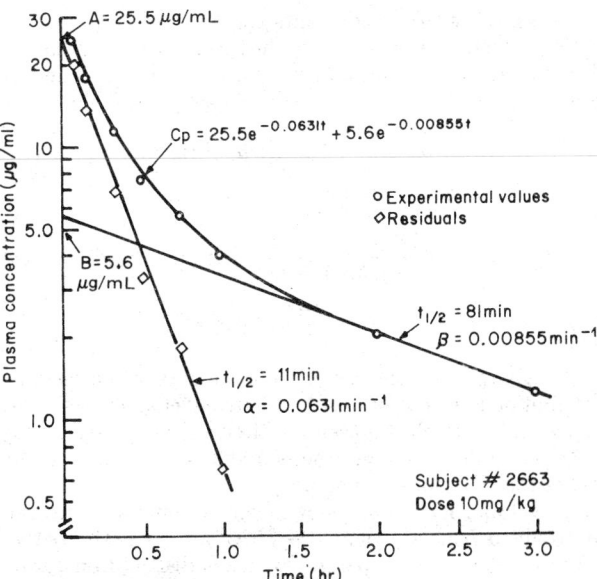

Fig 38-20. Resolution of the plasma concentration curve for pralidoxime after intravenous administration into its distribution and elimination components. Note that plasma concentration is plotted on a logarithmic scale. The time constant for the elimination phase is determined from the slope, -0.434β; it is a hybrid constant and β is not the same as k_{el} (see text). Likewise, the time constant for distribution, α, is obtained from the slope, -0.434α, of the distribution line; α is also a hybrid constant (courtesy, Gibaldi and Perrier[9]).

plotted semilogarithmically to reveal the loglinear line that represents distribution only. From the loglinear properties of the separate but algebraically additive lines representing the two processes of distribution and elimination it may be inferred that the equation for the original compound curve was

$$C_1 = Ae^{-\alpha t} + Be^{-\beta t} \qquad [\text{wt} \cdot \text{vol}^{-1}] \qquad (41)$$

where C_1 is the concentration of drug in compartment 1 (the central compartment), α and β are first-order rate constants for the distribution and elimination phases, respectively, and A and B are fictive plasma concentrations to be discussed on page 756. The constant β describes the late rate of disappearance of drug from compartment 1 but is not the same as k_{el} (see below). It is the rate constant from which the biological half-life is calculated in a two-compartment system ($t_{1/2} = 0.693/\beta$).

Hybrid and Prime Kinetic Parameters—In Fig 38-20, the slope of the late, slower elimination line is -0.434β, where β is a first-order time constant for elimination. However, β is not determined only by the rate capacities of the irreversible elimination processes but also by the rates at which drug is transferred out of and back into compartment 1. Therefore, β is a compound, or hybrid, rate constant. It is equal to the fraction of drug in the central compartment, f^*, in the post-distributive ("elimination") phase times the elimination constant, k_{el}, for the central compartment. Thus

$$\beta = f^* k_{el} \qquad [\text{time}^{-1}] \qquad (42)$$

Alpha, α, is a hybrid constant that combines k_{21}, k_{el}, and β:

$$\alpha = \frac{k_{21} k_{el}}{\beta} \qquad [\text{time}^{-1}] \qquad (43)$$

Interestingly, the equation for α does not include k_{12}, although f^* does depend upon $(k_{12} + k_{21})/k_{21}$. The sum of α and β can be entirely expressed in terms of prime constants:

$$\alpha + \beta = k_{12} + k_{21} + k_{el} \qquad [\text{time}^{-1}] \qquad (44)$$

However, these prime constants cannot be determined directly, and must be derived from the hybrid constants that are obtainable from graphical or regression analysis. The formulae are

$$k_{el} = \frac{A + B}{\dfrac{A}{\alpha} + \dfrac{B}{\beta}} \quad [\text{time}^{-1}] \tag{45}$$

$$k_{12} = \frac{AB\,(\beta - \alpha)^2}{(A + B)(A\beta + B\alpha)} \quad [\text{time}^{-1}] \text{ and} \tag{46}$$

$$k_{21} = \frac{A\beta + B\alpha}{A + B} \quad [\text{time}^{-1}] \tag{47}$$

where A and B are the zero-time intercepts of the residual distribution line and the postdistributive ("elimination") line, respectively. Each represents a fictive concentration that describes a limit when the other variable is set to zero (ie, the other process is non-existent).

The volume of compartment 1 (central compartment) can be obtained from C_p^0 (ie, $V_1 = fD/C_p^0$). From the fictive concentration, B, the apparent volume of distribution during the postdistributive phase, can be calculated, since $A + B = C_p^0$. From $A - B$ may be obtained the value of compartment 2. (Volumes of distribution are discussed below.) C_p^0 can be more accurately determined by summing the two loglinear extrapolates than from the extrapolation of the unresolved curve. A and B are also hybrid coefficients, since the value of B depends upon all of k_{21}, k_{12} and k_{el}.

Volumes of Distribution—The volume of distribution, V_d, of a drug is a useful pharmacokinetic parameter that relates C_p to D_B (see page 744). Even though it is fictive, it not only provides some insight into distribution but also it importantly relates to the rate of clearance of drug from plasma, and changes in pathological conditions reveal changes in the physiological-biochemical conditions. By means of the distribution coefficient, Δ', data from one patient may be applied to others of different body weights (see page 744).

In the open two-compartment system, the determination of V_d is complicated by the slow attainment of distribution "equilibrium" (ie, steady state) between two compartments, and the volume of distribution is continually changing during the distribution phase. It is especially important to know V_d during the postdistribution phase (in which case V_d only applies during postdistribution times) or to estimate V_d by methods that cancel the distributive factors.

The most theoretically accurate method for estimating V_d is known as the *steady-state* method, of which there are three variations. In this, the ideal procedure is to give a continuous intravenous infusion until the steady state (ie, plateau) is reached. During the steady state, the amount of drug in the peripheral compartment (compartment 2) is constant. Under these conditions

$$V_d^{ss} = \frac{k_{12} + k_{21}}{k_{21}} \cdot V_1 \quad [\text{vol}] \tag{48}$$

Note that V_d^{ss} is independent of k_{el} and β. There are, however, several disadvantages to this approach, the principal ones being that for most drugs the steady state is reached only after prolonged infusion, since 5 or more half-lives will often require days of infusion, and that V_1, k_{12}, k_{21} and β need to be determined. This can be done by discontinuing infusion and resolving the curve of the declining plasma concentration into its component parts. Fortunately, the same information can be obtained from the mean plasma concentration during one dose interval at steady state, $\overline{C}^{ss}$. In this,

$$V_d^{ss} = \frac{fD(k_{12} + k_{21})}{\overline{C}^{ss}k_{21}k_{el}\tau} \quad [\text{vol}] \tag{49}$$

where k_{el} is the rate of elimination from the central compartment. Provided that elimination occurs only from the central compartment, Eqs 48 and 49 are valid for any n-compartment model. This method has the same disadvantage as the infusion method in that dosing must be continued to the steady state, which, however, with repetitive dosing is more comfortable and less expensive than continuous infusion. An advantage is that extravascular routes may be employed and that only one dose-interval need be sampled, thus making the determination of V_d^{ss} applicable to drugs with long half-lives.

V_d^{ss} can also be determined from areas under the curve (AUC) during and after constant intravenous infusion:

$$V_d^{ss} = \frac{D_\Sigma \cdot AUC_{t(ss)}}{\overline{C}^{ss} \cdot AUC^{0 \to \infty}} \quad [\text{vol}] \tag{50}$$

where $t(ss)$ is the time to reach steady state, D_Σ is the cumulated dose at $t(ss)$, $AUC_{t(ss)}$ is the area under the plasma concentration-time curve from $t = 0$ to $t = t(ss)$, and $AUC^{0 \to \infty}$ is the total area under the curve from $t = 0$ to $t = \infty$, providing that the infusion is stopped at the achievement of steady state or that the AUC during any overrun into the plateau state be eliminated from the determination of $AUC^{0 \to \infty}$. The method has the advantage that the determination of k_{12}, k_{21}, k_{el}, or V_1 are not necessary.

A second method of determining V_d is that in which V_d is calculated from V_1, k_{el}, and β:

$$V_{d(\beta)} = \frac{V_1 k_{el}}{\beta} \quad [\text{vol}] \tag{51}$$

The designation $V_{d(\beta)}$ indicates the method of calculation. The rationale for the method is the valid assumption that plasma and tissue concentrations decline in parallel during the postdistributive phase, so that the distribution ratio, which will be equal to Δ', is constant after the distributive phase has come to completion. The method has been shown to yield the same values for V_d as one based on area:

$$V_{d(area)} = \frac{fD}{AUC^{0 \to \infty}} = \frac{fD}{(A/\alpha + B/\beta)\beta} = V_{d(\beta)} \quad [\text{vol}] \tag{52}$$

The method is independent of the route of administration, so long as the fraction absorbed, f, is used.

On page 755, on which the parameters derived from curves such as that in Fig 38-20 were discussed, it was pointed out that the zero-time extrapolates A and B were fictive concentrations from which apparent volumes of distribution could be obtained. The extrapolate β gives a volume known as $V_{d(extrap)}$:

$$V_{d(extrap)} = \frac{D}{B} \quad [\text{vol}] \tag{53}$$

The method does not take into account the effect of process k_{21} to limit the size of the peripheral compartment and hence tends to overestimate D_B, except at zero time. However, it has the advantage of rapid determination.

$V_{d(area)}$ is the most correct value of V_d to apply to the postdistribution phase. $V_{d(ss)}$ is correct for constant infusion at steady state but otherwise underestimates D_B.

Clearance—The definition and concept of clearance can be found on page 745. The definition of clearance applies whether the elimination occurs in a one- or multi-compartment system, hence clearance is model-independent. However, mathematical identities of clearance do depend on the model. In the open two-compartment model, β and $V_{d(area)}$ are applicable in the calculation of total body clearance:

$$Cl_{tot} = \beta V_{d(area)} \quad [\text{usually mL} \cdot \text{min}^{-1}] \tag{54}$$

Since it is customary to express clearance in units of mL/min, β must be expressed in min and $V_{d(area)}$ in mL. An analogous formula is based on the condition of the model that elimination occurs only from the central compartment, so that the applicable volume and elimination rate constant are used:

$$Cl_{tot} = k_{el}V_1 \qquad [\mathrm{mL \cdot min^{-1}}] \qquad (55)$$

Cl_{tot} can also be expressed in terms of α, A, β, B and D:

$$Cl_{tot} = \frac{D}{A/\alpha + B/\beta} \qquad [\mathrm{mL \cdot min^{-1}}] \qquad (56)$$

Absorption Plus Distribution and Elimination—After extravascular administration in a two-compartment system, there are three first-order processes occurring simultaneously: absorption, distribution, and elimination. These processes all add algebraically, as follows:

$$C_p = Ae^{-\alpha t} + Be^{-\beta t} - C_p^0 e^{-k_a t} \qquad [\mathrm{wt \cdot vol^{-1}}] \qquad (57)$$

They can be resolved by various methods, of which the easiest is the method of residuals already illustrated in Figs 38-8 and 38-20. However, in a two-compartment system, the first residual line is a compound line (absorption + distribution) and must be further resolved into its two component lines. Fig 38-21 is an example of the method of residuals applied to two-compartment data. The first step is the subtraction of the late postdistribution (elimination) line (with slope -0.434 β) from the curve, which leaves a two-component residual curve. This residual curve has a late, postabsorptive loglinear segment of slope $-0.434\ \alpha$. If the absorption segment of the curve of residuals is subtracted from the extrapolated α-line, a loglinear second residual line with a slope of $-0.434k_a$ will be generated. The extrapolated intercepts A and B have the meanings previously discussed. The zero-time intercept of the absorption residual line is equal to C_p^0 and hence theoretically equals $A + B$. Kinetic parameters other than α, A, β, and B are calculated by means of Eqs 42 and 43. The absorption parameters for other routes of absorption can be similarly determined, except with certain sustained-release dosage forms, which release approximately at a steady rate over long periods of time.

In the example illustrated by Fig 38-21, only two or three points each could be used for establishing the loglinear segments of the residual distribution and absorption lines, which therefore may be in considerable error. This indicates the importance of taking frequent enough samples, especially during the absorption and distribution phases, to provide reliable kinetic data.

Multiple-Dose Administration—Equations 29–31, which describe various aspects of the fluctuating plasma concentrations in the one-compartment system, are complex. It may be appreciated that the additional complexities conferred by two compartments renders the analogous equations intricate and difficult to follow for the non-specialist. However, one-compartment equations modified in minor ways apply to two-compartment systems with reasonable accuracy, when the distribution phase after one dose is approximately complete before the next dose is administered. Under these conditions, β may be substituted for k_{el} and $V_{d(area)}$ for V_d, to adapt one-compartment equations to two-compartment systems for rough approximations of the two-compartment parameters and plasma concentrations. Thus

$$\overline{C}^{ss} = \frac{fD}{\beta V_{d(area)}\tau} \qquad [\mathrm{wt \cdot vol^{-1}}] \qquad (58)$$

Adaptation of one-compartment equations for accumulation ratios and loading dose also usually give values that satisfactorily approximate those calculated with more rigorous equations. The respective adapted equations are

$$R_c = \frac{1}{1 - e^{-\beta\tau}} \qquad [\text{no units}] \quad \text{and} \qquad (59)$$

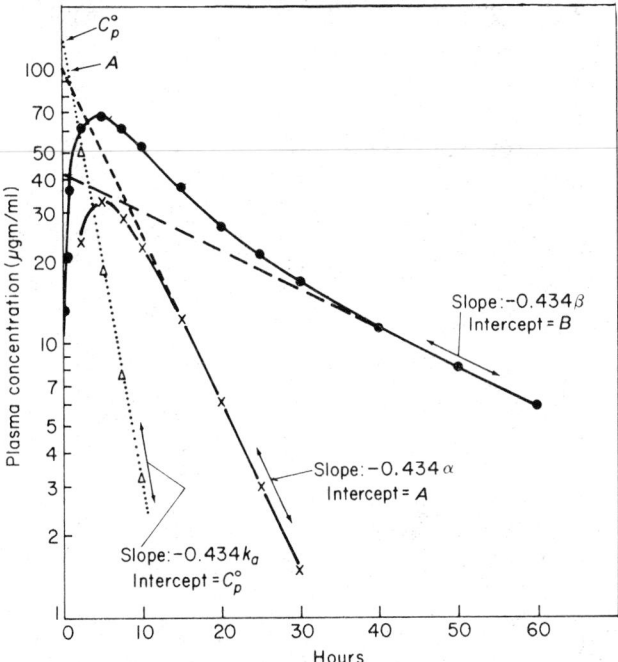

Fig 38-21. Resolution of absorption, distribution, and elimination components of a concentration-time curve of a drug with two-compartment kinetics. The solid curve is a semilogarithmic plot of plasma concentrations. The method of residuals was used to resolve the component lines. The postdistribution, or elimination, line of slope -0.434β (— —) was subtracted from the concentration-time curve. The difference, or residual line (X—X) retained the absorption and distribution components. The loglinear segment of this line represents the postabsorption ("distribution") line, of slope -0.434α. A second residual line representing the absorption phase was obtained by subtracting the absorptive segment (first four points) of the first residual curve (X—X) from the extrapolated α line of slope -0.434α (----) to give the residual absorption line of slope $-0.434k_a$ (·····). The zero-time intercepts of the extrapolated lines defined by k_a (·····), α (----), and β (— —) are C_p^0, A and B, respectively (courtesy, data, Gibaldi and Perrier[10]).

$$D_0^* = R_c D \qquad [\text{wt}] \qquad (60)$$

where R_c, D_0^*, and D are the accumulation ratio, optimal loading dose, and maintenance dose, respectively.

The rate at which the steady state is attained depends almost entirely on β. The plateau principle essentially applies, and approximately 5 half-lives, based on β, are required to reach the "steady state." Essentially all precepts emanating from the one-compartment plateau principle are applicable if two-compartment β is used in place of one-compartment k_{el}.

Nonconformities and Miscellany

Fallibility of Assumptions—General pharmacokinetic concepts are applicable to many drugs without significant modification. Implicit in these concepts are certain assumptions which, however, do not apply to all drugs or drug recipients. Some of the basic assumptions are that the pharmacological effect is elicited by the drug administered (and which is being assayed in the blood), that the pharmacokinetic parameters remain constant with both time and dose, and that the peak effect occurs when the concentration is at its peak at the site of action, that binding and sequestration follow first-order kinetics, and, in short, that the models chosen for kinetic analysis are correct. When these

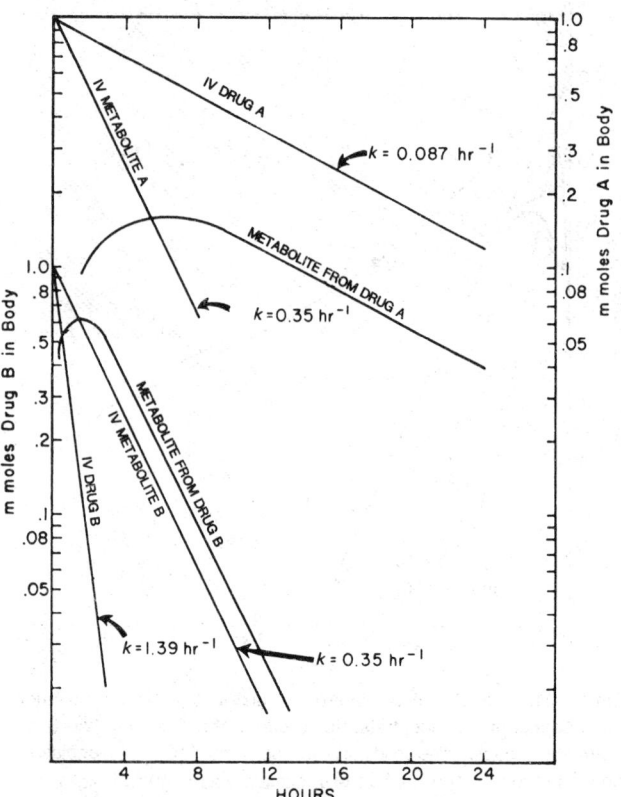

Fig 38-22. Computer plot of the relationship of the amount of drug metabolite in the body to the amount of drug in the body at different relative rates of disposition of drug and metabolite. With Drug A, the metabolite is eliminated at a much faster rate than the parent drug. Curve "IV Metabolite A": the blood concentration when the metabolite is given intravenously; curve "Metabolite from Drug A": the concentration of metabolite actually biotransformed from Drug A. With Drug B the metabolite is eliminated at a much slower rate than the parent drug (courtesy, combined replot of two figures, Martin[11]).

Table III—Some Drugs With Pharmacologically Active Metabolites

Parent Drug	Active Metabolite(s)
Acetohexamide	Hydroxyhexamide
Allopurinol	Alloxanthine
Aldophosphoramide	Phosphoramide mustard
Amitriptyline	Nortriptyline
Chloral Hydrate	Trichloroethanol
Chlordiazepoxide	Desmethylchlordiazepoxide, Demoxepam
Codeine	Morphine
Dacarbazine	5-Aminoamidazole-4-carboxamide
Diazepam	Desmethyldiazepam
Digitoxin	Digoxin
Flurazepam	Desalkylflurazepam
Fluorouracil	Fluorodeoxyuridine phosphate
Glutethimide	4-Hydroxyglutethimide
Imipramine	Desipramine
Lidocaine	Glycinexylidide
Meperidine	Normeperidine
Mephobarbital	Phenobarbital
Methyldopa	α-Methylepinephrine, α-methylnorepinephrine
Methamphetamine	Amphetamine
Phenacetin	Acetaminophen
Phenylbutazone	Oxyphenbutazone
Prednisone	Prednisolone
Primidone	Phenobarbital
Propoxyphene	Norpropoxyphene
Procainamide	N-Acetylprocainamide
Propranolol	4-Hydroxypropranolol
Spironolactone	Canrenone, Canrenoate
Sulfasalazine	Sulfapyridine
Tamoxiphen	4-Hydroxytamoxiphen
Trimethadione (TMO)	Dimethadione (DMO)

assumptions are not valid, significant clinical consequences accrue, and theoretical and/or empirical modification of the models may be necessary. Therefore, it is worthwhile to examine some departures from the more common or commonly assumed behavior and some miscellaneous pharmacokinetic considerations not stressed elsewhere in this chapter.

Active Metabolites and Latentiation—Some drugs are biotransformed to a metabolite that has a pharmacological action like that of the parent drug. With these, the pharmacokinetics of each of parent drug and its metabolite may or may not be simple and easy to define, but the combined pharmacodynamic (and sometimes pharmacokinetic) action may rise and fall in a complex way because of the different time courses, distributions and routes of elimination of the two active molecules. For example, the anticonvulsant trimethadione (TMO) is un-ionized at body pH, is little excreted and has a V_d of about 600 mL/kg and a half-life of about 4 hr, whereas its anticonvulsant metabolite, dimethadione, is a weak acid, is excreted and excretion is affected by urine pH, has a V_d of 400 mL/kg and a half-life of about 10 days. It is obvious that a study of the pharmacokinetics of TMO alone would be of little value in predicting a therapeutic regimen and precautions.

Two or more active metabolites may greatly increase the complexity. There are a few drugs in which it is only the metabolite, not the parent drug, that is active; with these, the relationship of pharmacokinetics to pharmacodynamics is simpler, provided that it is the metabolite that is followed. It is sometimes deliberately the practice to prepare a drug that

is inactive with the intention that the drug be converted to an active metabolite once it is in the tissues. This practice is known as *latentiation*. Latentiation may be used when it is desired to slow down the rate of delivery of drug to the tissues, a kind of systemic sustained release, as it were, or when the active metabolite is locally toxic at the site of administration. Some drugs which generate active metabolites are shown in Table III. Not shown are drugs the metabolites of which have no therapeutic activity but which have toxic or other pharmacodynamic activity.

The amount of a metabolite of a drug in the body at any one time depends upon both the rate of transformation of the drug to metabolite and the rate of disposition of the metabolite. The body content of metabolite will continue to rise as long as the content of precursor is high enough that the rate of biotransformation to metabolite exceeds the rate of elimination of the metabolite. When the concentration of drug or precursor falls to a level below which there is no longer a net gain in content of metabolite, the metabolite concentration will fall.

The kinetics of the fall in concentration depends upon which rate is faster, the elimination of drug precursor or the elimination of metabolite. If that of the drug is faster, the content of metabolite will rise above that of the drug, and drug will soon disappear. This eventually leaves the content of cumulated metabolite to decline according to the kinetics of its own disposition.

In Fig 38-22, drug B illustrates the rate-limiting effect of the disposition of a metabolite. When the rate constant for the elimination of the drug or precursor is slower than that of the metabolite, as with drug A in Fig 38-22, the content of metabolite never reaches that of the drug and it eventually declines according to the kinetics of biotransformation of the drug. That is, the content of metabolite is mainly that which is being produced moment-to-moment. The figure is adapted from a plot of data from a computer analysis of a multivariable model.

The kinetics of the generation and elimination of a metabolite relative to those of its drug precursor are important when the metabolite is either toxic or therapeutically active. In the latter instance the kinetics are the kinetics of latentiation. Where the metabolite is toxic, a pattern such as in A would be less likely to generate toxic concentrations as in B.

When the disposition of the drug precursor involves more than one process or when there is more than one metabolite, the kinetics are necessarily more complex than in the illustrations presented above.

Other Pharmacokinetic Models—Apparent kinetic nonconformities may result when the system does not obey the simple open one- or two-compartment models. In the two-compartment model discussed in this chapter, elimination took place from the central compartment; however, other two-compartment models in which elimination takes place partly or entirely in the peripheral compartment are more appropriate with some drugs. Even absorption appears to be into a peripheral compartment with some drugs. In addition to alternate two-compartment models, three- or multi-compartment models are occasionally required to account for the pharmacokinetic behavior of certain drugs. In the common *three-compartment* model, the central compartment communicates with two peripheral compartments (which are not interconnected), one called the *shallow compartment* and the other the *deep compartment*. Distribution into the shallow compartment is faster than into the deep compartment.

Many drugs that are described as having one- or two-compartment kinetics actually have more complicated kinetics. There is no drug that displays true one-compartment kinetics, since distribution is never instantaneous. With any drug, sampling within the first minute to half hour will show one or more distribution phases.

Nonlinearities—Nonlinearity is a term applied to all nonconformities in which a semilogarithmic plot of plasma concentration-time data cannot be completely resolved into loglinear components, that is, into first-order processes. There may be various causes, such as capacity-limited elimination (ie, saturation of elimination system), capacity-limited absorption or transport, changes in protein binding, changes in pH at the site of absorption, changes in blood flow to the site of absorption and/or elimination, low or erratic dissolution or release rates from dosage forms, low solubility of the drug, drug-induced or other change in body temperature, etc. Some apparent nonlinearities are the result of fitting straight lines to nonlinear data under the assumption that deviations are experimental error.

Protein Binding—The binding of a drug to protein or other macromolecules can affect the pharmacokinetics, the magnitude of the effect being dependent on the fraction of the drug that is bound, the fraction of the binding sites that are occupied by the drug, and the rates of association and dissociation. If only a small fraction of drug is bound, the kinetic consequences may be minor or negligible, even if binding is very tight. The effect of the binding of a large fraction of drug depends somewhat upon whether the drug is bound tightly or loosely; if the rate of dissociation is quite rapid in comparison to the rate of delivery to sites of distribution and elimination or in comparison to the intrinsic rate of elimination, the kinetic consequences may also be minor. The greatest consequences accrue to binding with high capacity and slow dissociation.

It cannot be overemphasized that in the analysis of plasma the total concentration of drug, that is both free and bound drug, is determined. However, it is only the free drug that can

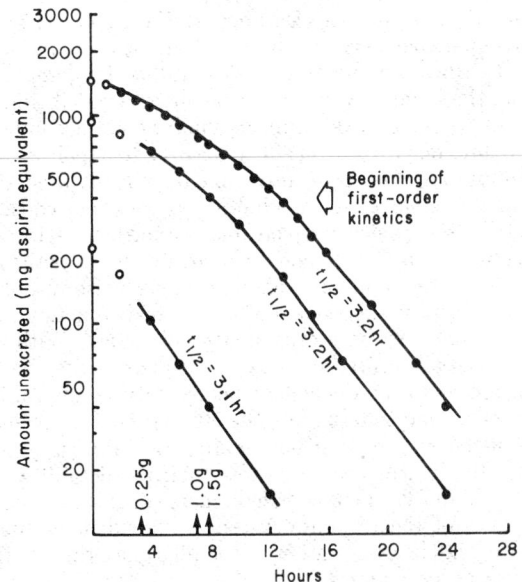

Fig 38-23. Dose-dependent elimination of salicylate in a normal 22-year-old male. Doses taken were 0.25, 1.0 and 1.5 g aspirin, respectively. Vertical arrows on the time axis indicate the time necessary to eliminate 50 per cent of the dose. Stated half-times ($t_{1/2}$) are for straight-line portion of curves where elimination rate is first-order. However, during the early hours after the larger doses, the slope at any time (tangent to the curve) is flatter, hence $t_{c1/2}$ is longer, than during the first-order phase (courtesy, Gibaldi and Perrier[9], modified from Levy[12]).

move across cell membranes, and equilibrium or steady state conditions are established only through the movement of free drug. Therefore, total drug concentrations are defective indicators of a true kinetic situation unless a correction is made for the extent of protein binding. Without such corrections, errors can be serious. Binding to plasma protein has a profound effect not only on V_d but also on apparent renal filtration fraction and clearance, as may be seen in Eqs 12 and 14. If the plasma concentration were not corrected for binding, Cl_{ren} would be in error by a factor of $1/(1 - p)$, where p is the fraction bound; however, when excretion is mainly by active tubular transport, protein binding often has a negligible effect on renal clearance. Similarly, when intrinsic hepatic clearance is low, protein binding greatly affects the clearance, the effect being to decrease clearance.

The binding of a drug to plasma proteins retards the rate of distribution and delays the attainment of equilibrium or steady-state conditions. It is as though the transport of some molecules of drug across a membrane has to wait until these molecules dissociate and are free to diffuse.

When the amount of a drug bound to plasma proteins does not approach saturation, that is, the binding capacity of the proteins, the fraction of drug bound is approximately constant over a therapeutic dose range. However, when the amount exceeds about 50% of the saturation value, the percent of drug bound may vary considerably with dose, which will give rise to dose-dependent kinetics (see below). Under the condition of near-saturation, changes in the protein content of the blood will also make large differences in the percent bound and hence in the various pharmacokinetic parameters. Certain pathological conditions, such as uremia, some congestive heart failure, starvation, etc, may be accompanied by hypoproteinemia and albumin with altered binding properties and hence abnormal pharmacokinetics.

Time-Dependent Kinetics—A drug with low to intermediate intrinsic clearance and which induces an increase in the activity of its own biotransforming enzyme system will decrease $t_{1/2}$ and increase clearance, and, if its kinetics show two-compartment kinetics, its V_d. Since such an induction requires time, usually several dose intervals of repetitive dosing, the kinetics vary with time and are called time-dependent. Allosteric (or feedback) inhibition by accumulated metabolites of a drug or an effect of a drug to impair its route or elimination will also cause time-dependent (and dose-dependent) changes in the kinetics. Drugs that cause the depletion of some slowly repleteable intermediary factor, such as the depletion of norepinephrine by reserpine or the irreversible inhibition of acetylcholinesterase by isoflurophate, will manifest time-dependent effects on body function which do not correlate with the drug pharmacokinetics. With some drugs, especially central nervous system depressants, the drug effect recruits time-dependent homeostatic counteradjustments that tend to terminate the effect prematurely and to increase the dose requirement for effect (ie, causes tolerance), so that the pharmacokinetics lose their predictability with time. Similarly, drug-induced changes in the receptor properties of the response system will tend to produce a time-dependent dissociation of the pharmacokinetics from the pharmacodynamics.

Dose-Dependent Kinetics—With some drugs, the pharmacokinetics are different with high than with low doses. Such changes may be due to the saturation of a biotransforming enzyme or excretory transport system, to toxic impairment of the organ of excretion at high doses, to differences in intercompartment permeability and V_d at high and low doses, to drug-induced changes in blood flow and hence in distribution and clearance, to saturation of protein binding sites or the recruitment of new binding sites at high doses, etc. In those instances in which the elimination route is saturated (also called capacity-limited), it is evident that the half-life will increase, as can be seen in Fig 38-23. The cause of the dose-dependent increase in $t_{1/2}$ at the higher doses is the saturation of the enzyme systems that form salicyluric acid and carboxybenzoxyglucuronide. It is usual to speak of the kinetics during the saturation phase as being zero-order, but they are not truly zero-order. The saturated system manifests zero-order kinetics, but alternative routes of elimination, such as through salicyl glucuronide and glomerular filtration and renal tubular secretion, etc, still manifest first-order kinetics, so that elimination is a mixture of zero- and first-order processes. In any event, since elimination is no longer completely a first-order process in the saturation phase, there is no overall elimination rate constant and hence no constant half-life. During repetitive dosing with the large doses, the new $\overline{C}^{ss}$ will be determined by both the zero-order and first-order elimination processes, as well as the dose; but the time required to reach the new plateau will be determined only by the remaining first-order processes; since the first-order overall elimination constant, K, has been diminished, the time-to-plateau will be increased accordingly.

Examples of important drugs which show dose-dependent kinetics are aspirin, phenylbutazone, probenecid, levodopa, phenytoin, and dicumarol. Ethanol obeys essentially zero-order elimination kinetics at blood concentrations above 0.02–0.04%, which is a fact of considerable importance in court cases involving ethanol. The clinical significance of dose-dependent kinetics will be discussed further in Chapter 39.

Kinetics in the Evaluation of Drugs and Drug Products

The utility of pharmacokinetics to the devising of appropriate dosage regimens is obvious. Kinetic studies are also important to the study of the influence of inhibitors of elimination, such as that of probenecid on the excretion of penicillin, and the effect of one drug on the disposition of another.

Plasma or tissue concentrations and their kinetics are not only valid but essential in comparing the bioavailability of drug products in which the excipients, adjuvants, etc, may vary but the active ingredients are the same. Such data are critical to a proper appraisal of the practice of prescribing drugs by proprietary names.

Kinetics are also employed to compare different drugs, but the meaning of such comparisons is often obscure, and claims of therapeutic superiority based upon kinetics must be accepted cautiously. The kinetics of disposition are important to a comparison of drugs in a class in which toxic effects are frequent; it is often desirable to use a drug with a short biological half-life, so that a toxic episode may be quickly terminated upon discontinuation of medication. Furthermore, it is valid to compare among drugs the fluctuations in plasma concentration consequent to multiple-dose administration, provided, of course, that for the class of drugs in question the extent of fluctuation has an important bearing on efficacy or toxicity. In the case of penicillin, fluctuations in blood level have very little effect on either efficacy or toxicity.

A comparison of peak or mean blood levels achieved by equal doses of different drugs is not entirely meaningless. It is true that the dose of a drug may be adjusted to compensate for a difference in potency from some reference drug, but it is often difficult for the physician to alter the dose except in multiples of the unit dose provided by the manufacturer. Partly because of the inertia of precedence and habit and partly because it is easier for the physician to memorize doses as a group, closely related drugs whose potencies differ only moderately may all be available in the same dose. Thus tetracyclines are available as "250's" or "500's", even though they are not equipotent, sulfonamides as 1 g, etc. It is therefore valid for the physician to choose the drug whose unit dose yields a blood level closest to the optimum. Unfortunately, many physicians do not have the prerequisite knowledge for such a choice and hence may be susceptible to misleading promotional arguments about the superiority of one product over another. Some of these points will be elaborated in the following chapter on *Clinical Pharmacokinetics*.

References

1. Bigger JT: *Am J Med 58:* 479, 1975.
2. Dittert LW: *Drug Intel Clin Pharm 8:* 222, 1974.
3. Truitt EB Jr, *et al: J Pharmacol Exp Ther 100:* 309. 1950.
4. Swintosky JV: *Proc Am Assoc Coll Pharm Teacher's Seminar 13:* 140, 1961.
5. Wilkinson GR, Shand DG: *Clin Pharmacol Ther 18:* 377, 1975.
6. Goldstein A, *et al: Principles of Drug Action* 2nd ed, Wiley and Sons, New York, 1974, p 334.
7. Krüger-Thiemer E. In Ariens EJ ed: *Physico-chemical Aspects of Drug Actions*, Vol 7, Pergamon, London, 1968, pp 63–113.
8. Notari RE: *Biopharmaceutics and Pharmacokinetics* 2nd ed, Dekker, New York, 1975, p 170.
9. Gibaldi M, Perrier D: *Pharmacokinetics*, Dekker, New York, 1975, pp 30, 54.
10. *Ibid*, pp 290–292.
11. Martin BK: *Brit J Pharmacol Chemother 31:* 420, 1967.
12. Levy G: *J Pharm Sci 54:* 959, 1965.

Supplementary Reading

Baggot JD: *Principles of Drug Disposition in Domestic Animals.* WB Saunders, Philadelphia, 1977.

Clark, B and Smith DA: *An Introduction to Pharmacokinetics.* Blackwell Scientific Publications, Oxford, 1981.

Creasy WA: *Drug Disposition in Humans.* Oxford University Press, New York, 1979.

Curry SH: *Drug Disposition and Pharmacokinetics*, 3rd edn. Blackwell Scientific Publications, Oxford, 1980.

Fingl E: Absorption, Distribution and Elimination: Practical Pharmacokinetics. In *Antiepileptic Drugs:* Woodbury DM, Penry JK and Schmidt RP, eds. Raven Press, New York, 1972, p 7.

Gibaldi M: *Biopharmaceutics and Clinical Pharmacokinetics*, 2nd edn. Lea & Febiger, Philadelphia, 1977.

Gibaldi M and Perrier D: *Pharmacokinetics*, Marcel Dekker, Inc., New York, 1975.

Goldstein A, Aronow L and Kalman SM: *Principles of Drug Action*, 2nd edn, John Wiley and Sons, New York, 1974, p 301.

Greenblatt DJ and Koch-Weser J: Clinical Pharmacokinetics. *New Eng J Med*, *293:* 702, 964, 1975.

Levine RR: Pharmacology. *Drug Actions and Reactions*, 3rd edn, Little, Brown and Company, Boston, 1983.

Niazi S: *Textbook of Biopharmaceutics and Clinical Pharmacokinetics.* Appleton-Century-Crofts, New York, 1979.

Notari RE: *Biopharmaceutics and Pharmacokinetics:* An Introduction. 3rd edn. Marcel Dekker, Inc., New York, 1980.

Ritschel WA: *Handbook of Basic Pharmacokinetics.* Drug Intelligence Publications, Inc., Hamilton, Ill., 1976.

Rowland M: Drug Administration and Regimens. In, *Clinical Pharmacology. Basic Principles in Therapeutics.* 2nd edn. Melmon KL and Morelli HF, eds. Macmillan Publishing Co., Inc., New York, 1978.

Wagner JG: *Biopharmaceutics and Relevant Pharmacokinetics.* Drug Intelligence Publications, Inc., Hamilton, Ill., 1971.

CHAPTER 39

Clinical Pharmacokinetics

Douglas E Rollins, MD, PhD

Associate Professor of Medicine and Pharmacology
School of Medicine and College of Pharmacy
University of Utah
Salt Lake City, UT 84112

In Chapter 37 the basic principles of pharmacokinetics were presented. Clinical pharmacokinetics is the discipline in which basic pharmacokinetic principles are applied to the development of rational dosage regimens. In the present chapter the concepts of pharmacokinetics are placed into perspective with the development of individualized drug dosage regimens. The clinical significance of the processes of drug absorption, distribution and elimination and influence of disease states on these processes are emphasized. Examples will be given of the ways pharmacokinetic principles can be applied in the calculation and adjustment of dosage regimens designed to fit the pharmacokinetic and pharmacodynamic properties of drugs and specific disease states that alter drug disposition. The principles of therapeutic drug monitoring and the rational use of this clinical science in the management of patients are also topics discussed in this chapter.

An individualized dosage regimen for a patient involves a decision about the dose or amount of drug to be administered, the interval between doses, the route of administration, and patient factors that may change during the course of drug administration. The latter implies that there is a plan for monitoring the therapeutic and adverse effects of the drug. Decisions about drug dose, dosage intervals and route of administration are based on clinical knowledge of the disease being treated, the efficacy of the drug in treating the disease and the absorption, distribution and elimination of the drug.

Absorption

Drugs are administered by a variety of routes including intravenous, intramuscular, inhalation, oral, rectal, vaginal and topical application to the skin. The choice of the route by which a drug is administered is dependent on the many patient- and drug-related factors discussed in Chapter 37. In practical terms, the important considerations in this choice include the systemic availability of a particular dosage form, the rate and extent of drug absorption, and patient convenience.

Oral Route—The oral route of drug administration is most frequently chosen because of ease of administration and patient acceptance. However, the number of variables involved in the absorption of drugs from the stomach and small intestine make the oral route of administration quite complex. Plasma concentration-time curves will reflect some of these complexities. One of these is the relative rates of absorption of different preparations of the same drug. This is illustrated in Fig 39-1. In the figure, A represents a simple, rapidly absorbed preparation of a drug. Preparation B is a more slowly absorbed derivative of the same base. The bioavailabilities of A and B are identical. Preparation C is the same compound as B, but in a dosage form that is only 50% as bioavailable as B. Preparation A is rapidly absorbed (ie, k_a for preparation A is greater than for preparations B or C) and the peak level

is in the therapeutic plasma concentration range. The advantage of such a preparation is that a pharmacodynamic response can be expected to occur quickly, provided the response is related to plasma concentration. To appreciate the clinical relevance of the situation, consider preparation A to be quinidine sulfate, an antiarrhythmic drug. For quinidine sulfate, the absorption rate constant (k_a) is large in relation to the elimination rate constant (k_{el}), and the peak concentration usually occurs in 1–2 hours. The rapid absorption is important in clinical situations in which some degree of urgency exists. It may be desirable in the initiation of therapy of ominous ventricular premature contractions to use a preparation with the characteristics of quinidine sulfate. The half-life of quinidine is 4–6 hours, so that frequent doses (every 4 hours) are necessary to maintain effective blood concentrations of the drug. The short half-life can be an advantage, since steady-state concentrations of quinidine are achieved within twenty-four hours (plateau principle). Therefore, one can decide within a day whether quinidine will be useful in suppressing the ventricular premature contractions. However, the fact that a dose must be administered every 4–6 hours to maintain therapeutic plasma concentrations is somewhat of a disadvantage in that it is inconvenient and may result in noncompliance. Preparation B, with its slower rate of absorption, reaches a lower peak concentration at a considerably later time even though given in the same dose. There are clinical consequences of this. For example, if preparation B were the sustained-release form of quinidine gluconate, it

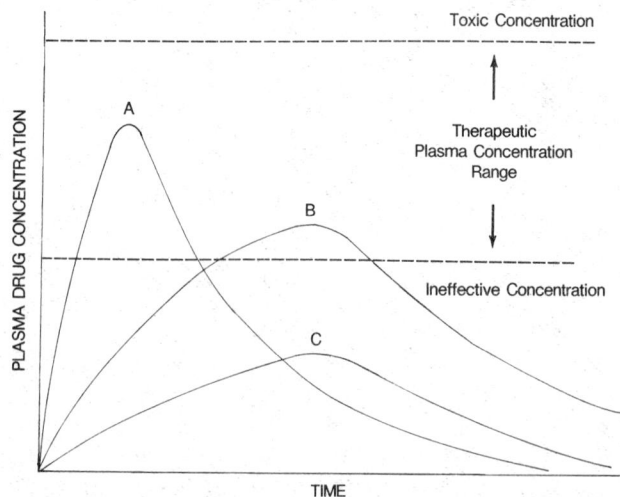

Fig 39-1. Plasma drug concentration-time curves of three preparations of the same drug. Preparation A is rapidly and completely absorbed. Preparation B is not absorbed as rapidly as A but is 100% available. Preparation C has the same time-to-peak concentration as B but is only 50% as available (Courtesy, adaptation, Benet[1]).

would be less desirable than quinidine sulfate for the initiation of drug therapy where a rapid therapeutic response is needed. Because of its prolonged absorption, this preparation is commonly administered every 8–12 hours. This is so because the slower rate of absorption enables the dose to be increased commensurate with a longer dose-interval without peak concentrations that rise into the toxic range. When treating a patient in which a rapid (but not immediate) effect is required (as with asymptomatic ventricular premature contractions), it is advisable that a dosage form that is rapidly and completely absorbed be used to initiate therapy. Once the drug is shown to be effective in a particular patient, the dosage form can be changed to one with characteristics similar to B, so that less frequent dosing is required and patient compliance is improved. The preparation represented by C *in the same dose* as A or B is probably not an acceptable way to administer this drug. The total amount of drug C that is absorbed in only half of that of B (area-under-the-plasma concentrations-time curve, AUC, for C is half of AUC for B). Thus, it would require twice the dose to attain blood levels equivalent to A or B.

Treatment of asthma with theophylline is an example in which a rapidly absorbed dosage form is used to initiate therapy and a prolonged-release dosage form is used for maintenance therapy. When a patient presents with an acute asthma attack or worsening bronchitis that requires bronchodilator therapy, it is advisable to use the theophylline-ethylenediamine complex (aminophylline). This dosage form can be administered either intravenously or orally. The former route of administration should be used to initiate treatment in the acute asthmatic patient who requires prompt therapy, so that neither a delay in achieving therapeutic plasma concentrations nor bioavailability are factors in the initial therapeutic response. Following the administration of a loading dose (see discussion on loading dose in section on *Distribution*, page 765), the drug should be given by continuous intravenous infusion until the acute symptoms have subsided, which may take 24 to 72 hours. In the patient with less severe symptoms, aminophylline can be administered orally four times a day. Once the patient's condition has improved and an effective dose of theophylline has been established, then it may be possible to switch the patient to a prolonged-release formulation for maintenance therapy. The absorption and bioavailability of Theodur and Sustaire, two sustained-release theophylline preparations, permit 12-hour dosing intervals; Slo-Phyllin Gyocaps should be given every eight hours. The total daily dose of theophylline that was required during intravenous aminophylline administration is divided into smaller oral doses given at intervals appropriate for the characteristic of the preparation or dosage form used. It is important to keep in mind that the absorption and plasma-time curve characteristics for these preparations usually have been established in healthy volunteers or asthmatic patients without other illnesses. Patients who eliminate theophylline rapidly (ie, smokers) may have increased dose requirements, and the dose interval may have to be shortened to avoid recurrent asthmatic symptoms between doses.

Prolonged-release dosage forms have the additional advantage that fluctuations in blood levels of the drug will be less than with rapidly absorbed dosage forms. There is evidence for some drugs that the reduction in rapidly changing blood levels may improve efficacy and decrease adverse effects. For example, the dose of fentanyl or ketamine required to maintain anesthesia was reduced by nearly 50% when the drugs were given by continuous infusion rather than by intermittent bolus.[2] This reduced dosage also resulted in more rapid recovery with less prolonged sedation. These findings suggest that a reduction of fluctuation in the plasma concentrations will reduce total dosage requirement. If such a reduction in

Table I—Drugs that Exhibit First-Pass Metabolism

Acetylsalicylic acid	Metoprolol
Alprenolol	Morphine
Amitriptyline	Nitroglycerin
Desipramine	Nortriptyline
Dopamine	Pentazocine
Imipramine	Prazosin
Isoproterenol	Propoxyphene
Lidocaine	Propranolol
Meperidine	Salicylamide

plasma concentration fluctuation also applies to oral prolonged-release dosage forms, it would provide a distinct advantage for their use.

Bioavailability of a particular drug product, by any route of administration, can be determined by comparison of the area under the concentration curve (AUC) of a drug given by the route of interest with that of the same dose given intravenously (see Chapter 37). In the case of an orally administered drug, it is the ratio of the AUC after an oral dose to the AUC after an intravenous dose. Decreased bioavailability of an oral drug may be due to poor gastrointestinal absorption of the drug because the drug does not go completely into solution, because it is degraded in the gastrointestinal lumen, or because it does not pass across the intestinal mucosa. Furthermore, in order to reach the general circulation, drugs taken orally must pass through the wall of the gastrointestinal tract and then to the liver via the portal vein. Thus, drug metabolism may occur in the gut wall or in the liver and severely limit the delivery of parent drug to the general circulation. If the extraction of drug by the liver is efficient, oral administration results in low bioavailability and sometimes limited pharmacologic effect. This is commonly referred to as *first-pass metabolism*. Table I lists some of the drugs known to exhibit first-pass metabolism. Because their extraction is high and their rate of metabolism great, the rate-limiting step in the clearance of drugs in Table I is liver blood flow. The metabolism of these drugs can be referred to as *flow-limited*. The clinical significance of changes in liver blood flow on drug bioavailability will be discussed under the section on *Drug Therapy in Hepatic Disease*.

Different dosage forms of the same drug may have different systemic bioavailabilities. The ratio of the AUC for one dosage form to that of another dosage form is termed the *relative bioavailability*. A drug usually has the highest bioavailability if administered orally an an aqueous solution; finely comminuted drugs in suspension follow closely. However, as a drug is packed into hard gelatin capsules or compacted into tablets, its bioavailability decreases. Furthermore, a drug in one dosage form made by one manufacturer may have a different bioavailability from that of another manufacturer. With drugs in which bioavailability varies significantly from product to product, if one product initially has been efficacious, it is advisable to continue with that product. If for economical or other reasons the product must be changed to that manufactured by a different company, it is wise to observe the patient carefully for a possible change in clinical response indicative of a change in bioavailability. Products designed for prolonged-release sometimes have a low bioavailability. However, this may not be a problem during maintenance therapy as long as therapeutic serum concentrations are consistently achieved.

The presence of food in the stomach or intestine can have a profound influence on the rate and extent (bioavailability) of drug absorption. Initial absorption studies for a new drug are commonly performed in healthy volunteers in a fasting condition. Therefore, the effect that food may have on drug absorption may not be known when a drug is introduced into the market. Unfortunately, food-drug interactions are not consistent, and the presence of food may enhance or diminish the absorption of drugs. The most common type of interaction occurs when a food constituent binds the drug and the food-drug complex cannot pass through the gut wall. For example, complexation of tetracycline antibiotics may occur when these drugs are administered with dairy products or with antacids containing aluminum, calcium, or magnesium. The presence of a large meal in the stomach will delay gastric emptying. If a drug that is absorbed in the intestine is ingested with a large meal, the delay in gastric emptying may result in a delay in absorption of the drug. However, the presence of food in the stomach has also been shown to *increase* absorption of some drugs. For example, the bioavailabilities of the β-adrenergic blocking drugs, propranolol and metoprolol, are enhanced by the presence of food.[3] Therefore, because of the difficulty in predicting the absorption pattern of a drug in the presence of food, it is usually advisable to administer drugs when the stomach is empty. An exception to this advice is with drugs which cause gastrointestinal irritation and nausea. These drugs must be given with food to prevent these side effects. It is recommended that such drugs *always* be taken with food to compensate for the differences in absorption that might occur if they were given one time with food and another time without food.

Water taken concomitantly with certain drugs may increase bioavailability. The administration of aspirin, erythromycin stearate, amoxicillin or theophylline with 250 mL of water results in greater bioavailability than if the same drugs are ingested with only 25 mL of water.[4] It is probable that the increased amount of water enhances the amount of drug absorbed by improving drug dissolution as well as by hastening gastric emptying.

Diseases that affect the structure and function of the gastrointestinal tract are also capable of altering the absorption of drugs after oral administration. However, no consistent pattern develops; rather, there appears to be a complex relationship between the effect of the disease on stomach and intestinal functions and the absorption of the drug in question. For example, diseases such as diabetes mellitus or chronic renal failure, diseases that delay gastric emptying, will markedly delay the absorption and onset of effect of drugs that must reach the small intestine before they are absorbed. This has been a problem with the use of phenytoin in patients with chronic renal failure. Celiac disease and Crohn's disease, two diseases that alter the intestinal epithelium, have been studied in detail.[5] In these diseases, absorption of some drugs is greatly affected, but there is no consistent pattern of altered drug absorption.

When a drug is to be administered orally to a patient with altered gastrointestinal motility, diseases of the stomach and small or large intestine, previous stomach or intestinal surgery, or gastrointestinal infection, there is a considerable probability that drug absorption characteristics in these patients will differ from those in healthy volunteers. This may result in a change in the time of peak blood level or the extent of absorption. It is advisable to observe such patients closely for clinical effect during initial drug administration and during chronic dosing in order to assess the influence of alterations in absorption and to correct dosing regimens accordingly. The monitoring of drug blood concentrations may be beneficial in adjusting dose.

Non-Oral Routes—Drugs are administered by a variety of non-oral routes. These include: subcutaneous, intramuscular, intravenous, inhalation, percutaneous, rectal, buccal, sublingual, vaginal, intra-arterial and intrathecal. In the cases of inhalation, topical application to the skin or mucous membranes, rectal, vaginal, intra-arterial or intrathecal administration, the route is often chosen to ensure that drugs reach a specific site with a minimum of systemic absorption.

The rationale is that the maximum concentration of drug will be at the site of action so that side effects will be lessened. Nevertheless, if large doses are administered by these routes, enough drug may reach the general circulation to produce side effects. Therefore, the dose and preparation should be such that limited quantities of drug reach the systemic circulation. The beta-adrenergic agonists, metaproterenol and albuterol, when administered by inhalation produce bronchodilatation at doses that avoid serious systemic side effects. Similarly, the corticosteroid, beclomethasone, can also be administered by this route for the management of chronic asthma. Low doses of beclomethasone by inhalation are without the serious systemic side effects of oral steroids. However, as the dose is increased beyond two inhalations four times a day, for an average daily dose of 400 µg, there is a greater incidence of side effects, including adrenal suppression.

The *topical* administration of drugs is rapidly becoming an important route of drug administration of systemic drugs. Previously used only for the application of drugs for local effects in diseases of the skin, it is now being explored as a means of administering drugs for their systemic effects. Nitroglycerin is commonly applied to the skin in the form of an ointment or transdermal patches; it is rapidly absorbed and provides sustained blood levels. Sublingual nitroglycerin is also employed to produce therapeutic blood levels; it produces a maximal effect on anginal pain within 3 to 5 mins but lasts only 20 to 60 min. In contrast, nitroglycerin ointment provides peak blood concentrations in about one hour and the effect on anginal pain may last for several hours. The sublingual tablets should be used to suppress acute angina attacks, whereas nitroglycerin ointment or transdermal patches may be useful to prevent recurrence of episodes of angina for prolonged periods, such as during the night. Whether or not the continuous administration of nitrates by this route will result in the development of tolerance is not clear at this time. There are several other drugs, such as those used to treat hypertension, for which percutaneous administration is being investigated as a means of attaining sustained plasma levels.

Close *intra-arterial* administration of drugs is used to get drugs directly to a target site or organ in high concentration. After it has passed through the target region it is distributed in the entire blood volume, which reduces the systemic levels of the drug and the consequent side effects. One example of this mode of drug administration is the use of cytotoxic drugs for the treatment of primary or metastatic tumors of liver. The infusion of drugs into the hepatic artery exposes the tumor to higher drug concentrations than can be tolerated with intravenous administration. If the drug is efficiently extracted by liver, the exposure of sensitive tissues such as bone marrow and gastrointestinal epithelium to the drug will be decreased. For example, after hepatic artery infusion of floxuridine (FUDR) hepatic vein concentrations are 2 to 6 times higher than comparable drug concentrations following intravenous infusion yet systemic blood concentrations are 75% less. Thus, the therapeutic index of FUDR in the treatment of liver cancer is considerably increased by hepatic arterial infusion. This type of selective drug administration may be beneficial with other drugs that have low therapeutic indices.

Intrathecal injection is used to deliver drugs to the brain in sufficient concentration to produce an effect but at the same time to reduce the incidence or severity of systemic side effects. The intrathecal administration of the cancer chemotherapeutic agent, methotrexate, is frequently employed in the management of leukemic involvement of the central nervous system. The epidural administration of morphine, which produces long-lasting (6–30 hrs) analgesia with minimal side effects, is proving to be of benefit in the management of chronic pain.

Distribution

Once a drug is absorbed into the general circulation, it distributes into various tissues and body fluids. The nature and extent of this distribution depends on several factors such as the extent of drug binding to plasma or tissue proteins, blood flow to selected areas of the body, and lipid-solubility of the drug and consequently its ability to permeate membranes. In clinical practice, concern about drug distribution often arises regarding the penetration of an antibiotic into the central nervous system, into abscesses at any location, into bone for the treatment of osteomyelitis, and into specific body fluids such as synovial fluid. In most cases, the distribution of a drug within the body is determined by the nature of the drug. However, distribution occasionally is altered by the disease process for which it is being used. For example, in healthy individuals, the concentration of penicillin in the nervous system is much less than in serum. However, in patients with inflamed meninges, as in bacterial meningitis, large daily parenteral doses of penicillin can result in bactericidal concentrations in the cerebrospinal fluid. Thus, pneumococcal and meningococcal meningitis can be treated effectively with intravenous penicillin. Increased penetration into the brain in these diseases occurs because the inflamed meninges are more permeable to the penicillin. Also, active transport of penicillin out of the cerebrospinal fluid back into plasma may be impaired in meningitis, thus causing an increase in penicillin concentration in the brain.

In Chapter 38 the term *volume of distribution* (V_d) was introduced. Despite the fact that the V_d of a drug is a very important pharmacokinetic term, it is important to recall that knowing the V_d of a drug does not necessarily indicate how or where a drug is distributed within the body. The abstract nature of the volume of distribution is illustrated with a drug such as the tricyclic antidepressant, amitriptyline. The V_d for amitriptyline is 20 L/kg, which represents a total V_d of 1400 L in a 70 kg man. This large volume of distribution indicates that the amount of drug in the plasma is small in relation to the amount in extravascular compartments and implies that tissue concentrations of the drug are probably very large. Since the volume of total body water in a 70 kg man is less than 70 L, a V_d of 1400 L also illustrates that V_d does not represent a real volume. Drugs with a large volume of distribution are usually extensively distributed to tissues where they are commonly bound to tissue constituents such as DNA or other macromolecules, or dissolved in lipids, whereas drugs that are extensively bound to *plasma* proteins will have smaller V_ds.

One situation in which knowledge of the size of the volume of distribution is useful clinically is in the management of the patient with a severe drug overdose. If a drug such as amitriptyline has a large volume of distribution, it is likely that after an overdose neither hemodialysis nor hemoperfusion will be an effective way of lowering the total body concentration of the drug. Dialysis may lower the plasma drug concentration temporarily, but there will be redistribution from tissues into plasma soon after the dialysis is stopped.

Knowledge of the V_d is also important in determining the loading dose of a drug. This is the dose of a drug administered initially to bring the plasma concentration to a level anticipated during maintenance. An example will illustrate how the V_d is used to determine the loading dose of theophylline. The V_d of theophylline is approximately 0.5 L/kg, and a commonly desired plasma concentration is 10 μg/mL (10 mg/L). Equation 6, page 744, shows that

$$V_d = \frac{fD}{C_p},$$

where f is the bioavailability factor or the faction of drug administered that reaches the systemic circulation, D is the dose of drug administered, and C is the plasma concentration desired. Since the f for theophylline is 0.96 it can be considered to be 1. Thus,

$$0.5 \text{ L/kg} = \frac{1 \cdot D}{10 \text{ mg/L}},$$

and

$$D = 5 \text{ mg/kg} = 350 \text{ mg/70 kg}.$$

This dose, administered as a 30-minute intravenous infusion, an oral solution, or as an uncoated, rapidly dissolving tablet, will result in a peak plasma theophylline concentration of approximately 10 mg/L in patients who have not recently received theophylline.

The V_d is usually considered to be a constant parameter of a drug, so that the loading dose is independent of subsequent changes in drug elimination produced by disease. For example, the loading dose of gentamicin in a patient with severe renal failure will usually not be different from that in a patient with normal renal function. Therefore, therapy can be started with the conventional loading dose without knowing the actual status of renal function. The severity of renal failure as measured by creatinine clearance (see below) will nevertheless have to be determined prior to calculation of the maintenance dose. There are some clinical situations, however in which V_ds of various drugs may be altered so that the loading dose may have to be appropriately altered. The volume of distribution of a drug may be affected by a variety of factors such as protein binding, disease states, body habitus, and age. As a rule, the effect of changes in protein binding on V_d are important only for drugs which are bound 90% or greater to plasma proteins. Propranolol provides an example in which in patients with chronic liver disease V_d is significantly increased because plasma protein binding is decreased. This occurs because a greater fraction of unbound drug has access to tissue. The V_d of digoxin in patients with severe congestive heart failure is usually decreased from that in patients with normal cardiac output. Consequently, the loading dose of digoxin is reduced in these patients. Severe dehydration and sepsis result in contraction of the extracellular space and a consequent decrease in the V_d of drugs that are largely confined to this physiological space.

The degree of obesity may also affect the volume of distribution of some drugs. The relative volume of distribution (Δ'; V_d/kg) of water-soluble, lipid-insoluble drugs varies inversely with percent body fat; Δ' of lipid-soluble, water-insoluble drugs varies directly with body fat. Even in extremely obese patients the increase in body weight may not be accompanied by an increase in V_d for water-soluble drugs, such as aminoglycoside antibiotics, which will not distribute into fat tissue. Calculation of the loading dose of these antibiotics in obese patients illustrates this problem. If actual body weight rather than the ideal body weight or lean body mass is used to calculate a loading dose of an aminoglycoside, elevated peak concentrations may occur in obese patients. Nevertheless, an excessive loading dose is preferable to the risk of possible subtherapeutic concentrations from a miscalculated adjusted dose in a seriously ill patient. Calculations of maintenance dosing should be made with ideal body weight to avoid consistently elevated peak plasma concentrations. In the first year of life, infants are known to have a larger extracellular space per unit of body weight than adults so that the Δ' of some drugs is also greater. This has been shown to be true for ampicillin, ticarcillin and amikacin. Changes in V_d occur frequently in elderly patients as the result of changes in lean body mass. A linear increase in Δ' with increasing age has been demonstrated to occur with diazepam.

It should be kept in mind that the V_d for a particular drug in an individual patient may change during therapy. An example might occur when a severely dehydrated patient is treated with intravenous fluids. Unfortunately, there are no accurate means by which the V_d of a particular drug can be determined in an individual patient without first administering the drug in question. Therefore, in situations where one suspects that the V_d may be altered, it is important to monitor blood concentrations of drug or clinical response to ensure that therapeutic and neither toxic nor inadequate plasma concentrations are being achieved. This is particularly true during initial cumulative drug administration or when a loading dose is being given.

Protein Binding—Pharmacologic effect is closely related to the free concentration of drug at its site of action. However, all drugs are bound to some extent to plasma and/or tissue proteins, and the free drug concentration may often represent only a fraction of the amount of drug in the body. For most drugs the total drug concentration is measured in plasma and related to an observed therapeutic effect. Thus, recommended therapeutic concentrations are commonly expressed as the total drug concentration in plasma, simply because total drug concentration is much easier to assay than free drug concentration. If something occurs that perturbs the protein binding of drug, then either more or less may be free in plasma (and thus free at the site of action) and "standard" therapeutic drug concentration guidelines no longer apply. This situation is made more complex because changes in protein binding may alter elimination as well as distribution. There is definitely a need to understand the therapeutic consequences of alterations in drug-protein binding in order to individualize drug therapy.

The major factors that affect drug-protein binding include: the types of proteins available for binding, the binding affinities and capacities, and the presence of competing substances, such as endogenous substances and other drugs. Albumin is the major protein in serum, and drug binding to albumin has consequently been studied in detail. Drug binding to alpha$_1$-acid glycoprotein and lipoprotein has also been shown to be of clinical significance for certain drugs. There are little data on the ability of other plasma proteins to bind most drugs.

For the purpose of discussing protein binding, drugs can be classified as either acidic or basic (Table II). Acidic drugs commonly bind to plasma albumin, and concomitantly-administered acidic drugs may displace one another from their binding sites. Basic drugs may bind to either albumin or alpha$_1$-acid glycoprotein. If a drug is displaced from its binding protein by another drug or by a disease process, the concentration of free drug in plasma (and at the receptor site) will temporarily increase, an effect which may then temporarily increase the pharmacologic response. The clinical impact of displacement depends on the total amount of drug in the body that is bound, the extent of displacement, whether the drug is also tissue-bound, the V_d, and whether the drug is a high-clearance or low-clearance drug. High-clearance drugs are those with an extraction ratio (see below) of close to 1, so that the extraction is usually insensitive to the extent of protein binding. A low-clearance drug, on the other hand, has a lower extraction ratio, and the clearance of the drug may be very sensitive to protein binding. Warfarin is an example of a low-clearance drug for which the clearance has been shown to vary with the fraction of unbound drug. Thus, after warfarin has been displaced from protein binding sites, $C_{p(\text{free})}$ increases and clearance increases. The increased metabolism will result in the elimination of excess $C_{p(\text{free})}$ and restore the original free drug levels. Nevertheless, the initial release of bound drug may cause temporary depletion of clotting factors and consequent bleeding.

The effects of protein displacement are usually of clinical significance only when binding exceeds 85–90%. Let us consider a drug which is 98% bound to plasma proteins. A displacement of 2% potentially will increase free drug concentration by 100%. However, this does not necessarily mean that free drug concentration in plasma will actually increase by 100%, because free drug usually quickly distributes into tissues. After redistribution, the actual increase in free drug concentration in plasma depends on the V_d. If V_d is large, the increase in plasma concentration may be minimal; if V_d is small, the concentration at the receptor site may significantly rise and elicit an increase in intensity of drug action. To make matters more complex, a decrease in protein binding can also directly increase the V_d by decreasing the total concentration in plasma, from which V_d is calculated.

Diseases can alter drug-protein binding by decreasing the amount of protein available for binding and by inhibiting drug binding. Table III lists some conditions that increase or decrease plasma proteins. Hypoalbuminemia and elevated alpha$_1$-acid glycoprotein have been shown to have the most dramatic effect on drug-protein binding. A normal concentration of serum albumin is 4 gm/dL, and a concentration of 2 gm/dL would be considered severe hypoalbuminemia. The effect of hypoalbuminemia on drug-protein binding has the greatest impact if 90% or greater of the drug is bound, if the number of binding sites on albumin are limited, and if the drug has a low V_d. It has been shown that a change in plasma albumin concentration from 3.5 down to 2.3 gm/dL causes protein binding of phenytoin to change from 90% to 80.8%.[8] The reduced protein binding results in an inversely proportional increase in total plasma clearance, so that in steady-state the unbound drug concentration remains unchanged. Thus, it is probably unnecessary to alter the total daily dose. However, the decrease in total plasma drug concentration poses a potential problem for the interpretation of routine plasma concentrations. This problem is discussed in further detail in the section on *Drug Therapy in Renal Disease*.

Table II—Drugs Bound to Plasma Proteins Greater than Ninety Percent

Basic Drugs	Acidic Drugs
Amitriptyline	Acetylsalicylic acid
Chlorpromazine	Penicillin
Desipramine	Phenylbutazone
Diazepam	Phenytoin
Imipramine	Probenecid
Lidocaine	Sulfinpyrazone
Nortriptyline	Tolbutamide
Propranolol	Warfarin
Quinidine	

Table III—Conditions Capable of Altering Plasma Proteins

	Albumin	Alpha$_1$-Acid Glycoprotein
Decreased plasma protein	Burns	Nephrotic syndrome
	Chronic liver disease	
	Cystic fibrosis	
	Protein-losing enteropathy	
	Nephrotic syndrome	
	Pregnancy	
	Chronic renal failure	
	Trauma	
Increased plasma protein	Hypothyroidism	Celiac disease
		Crohn's disease
		Myocardial infarction
		Renal failure
		Rheumatoid arthritis
		Trauma

Diseases can also affect the affinity of drugs for albumin. The best known example occurs in chronic renal failure, in which accumulated endogenous compounds that are not significantly removed by dialysis displace acidic drugs from albumin binding sites. In disorders or situations in which free fatty acid levels are increased, acidic drugs are displaced from albumin binding sites. Quantitatively, when the free fatty acid/albumin ratio exceeds 3.5, binding of acidic drugs is usually significantly reduced.[9]

Elimination

The elimination of drugs from the body usually occurs either by excretion into the urine or by biotransformation to metabolites that are eliminated in the urine or feces. The mechanisms whereby the kidneys and liver eliminate drugs and the pharmacokinetic principles behind these processes were presented in Chapters 37 and 38, respectively. In this section, emphasis will be placed on the practical application of these principles toward the development of individualized dosage regimens.

When drugs are approved by the Food and Drug Administration, their elimination has been studied in detail usually only in healthy volunteers. Nevertheless, there is often enough information available to make rational decisions about the individualization of drug doses in patients who might have impaired elimination. The most important information is whether the drug is eliminated unchanged in the urine or biotransformed in the liver. For a drug the major route of elimination of which is renal it is necessary to know if it is excreted by tubular secretion or glomerular filtration or by a combination of secretion and filtration. For a drug the elimination of which is by the liver it is necessary to know: 1) if the biotransformation is primarily by a phase I (oxidation) reaction or a phase II (conjugation) reaction; 2) if the metabolite(s) is/are pharmacologically active; and 3) if the drug exhibits first-pass metabolism. With the knowledge of these facts about each drug, one can determine whether or not it is necessary to adjust the dosage regimen in a patient with kidney or liver impairment.

As indicated in Chapter 38, drug clearance is a more direct expression of elimination than is half-life. This is mentioned here only to remind the reader to be cautious about equating impaired renal or hepatic function with a change in drug half-life. If a decrease in the renal elimination of a drug is accompanied by an increase in half-life, it is necessary to know this to adjust the dosage regimen. However, the elimination half-life of a drug is a complex function of elimination and the volume of distribution, and it is possible to have a change in V_d in patients with renal or hepatic impairment such that there is no alteration in half-life. Furthermore, it is possible to have a drug with a high total body clearance yet a long half-life. This seeming contradiction occurs when drugs with a very high clearance also have a large V_d. One class of drugs that displays this contradiction is the tricyclic antidepressants; the members have rapid clearances of about 1500 mL/min as the result of hepatic metabolism, but their plasma elimination half-life may be as long as 20 hours. Because of their large V_d (1000 − 2000 liters) and rapid redistribution between tissues and plasma, drug cleared from the plasma is almost completely replaced by drug from the peripheral compartment. As already mentioned, this is important to remember when deciding about the use of extracorporeal (hemodialysis or hemoperfusion) systems to remove drugs from the body of an overdosed patient. For a drug with a half-life of 20 hours it might appear that an extracorporeal system would enhance drug elimination. However, clearance of the tricyclic antidepressants by dialysis is small compared to normal hepatic clearance. If the drug also has a large V_d then redistribution would likely keep the plasma levels elevated and hemodialysis

or hemoperfusion would have to be continued for an unusually long time to enhance significantly the removal of drug from the body.

Renal Excretion—Unchanged drug or drug metabolites can be eliminated from the body by way of the kidneys, as mentioned above. Drug excretion by this route takes place either as a result of filtration through the glomerulus or by tubular secretion, or both. A knowledge of how a drug is excreted can be useful in predicting the effect that renal disease will have on its elimination. Drugs that are excreted by tubular secretion can generally be divided into organic acids, such as penicillin and probenecid, and organic bases such as cimetidine. As indicated in Chapter 37, the organic acids and bases are secreted by separate transport systems. Among the organic acids there is competition in transport such that the coadministration of two such drugs can result in decreased elimination and elevated blood concentrations of each. Sometimes this competition can be used to advantage, as in the case of the administration of probenecid in combination with penicillin in the treatment of gonorrhea. The result is that the clearance of penicillin is reduced and the plasma penicillin concentrations remain high for a prolonged period of time; the combination is more effective than penicillin alone. Since the therapeutic index of penicillin is high, such interactions are useful. However, if probenecid is administered with the cytotoxic drug, methotrexate, the secretion of the latter drug is impaired and significant toxicity may occur. When tubular secretion is high, plasma protein binding does not usually affect active secretion by the proximal tubule.

Most drugs are excreted by the kidney via filtration across the glomerular membrane. Glomerular filtration is a passive, nonsaturable process. Because of the small size of the pores of the glomerular membrane, only free drug in plasma can be filtered; consequently, drugs that are bound to plasma proteins are poorly filtered. Displacement from proteins can actually increase the amount of drug filtered in the glomerulus and hence eliminated in the urine.

The glomerular clearance of drugs is directly proportional to the glomerular filtration rate (GFR). It follows that a decrease in GFR will result in a proportional decrease in the rate of glomerular elimination of a drug. Thus, measurement of the GFR can be very helpful in the individualization of dose regimens in patients with impaired renal function. The GFR is generally estimated by measuring the clearance of either inulin or creatinine. Inulin must be infused intravenously, whereas creatinine, a product of muscle metabolism, is released *in vivo* at a relatively constant rate, thus obviating the need for constant intravenous infusion. Urinary creatinine excretion usually exceeds the amount filtered by about 10% because of a small amount of renal tubular secretion of creatinine. However, because determination of GFR by creatinine clearance is inexpensive and easy to do, and because the difference between inulin and creatinine clearance is not *clinically* significant, creatinine clearance is commonly used to estimate GFR. It is very important to realize that the creatinine clearance is an accurate estimate of GFR only if renal function is stable. If renal function is decreasing, serum creatinine concentrations will be increasing and it may take several days to reach a new steady-state. Until a new steady-state is reached, the GFR cannot be accurately estimated from serum creatinine concentrations, and serum creatinine should not be used to calculate an individualized dose of a drug. Although creatinine clearance only measures the GFR, it is frequently used in the determination of the dose regimens of drugs that are eliminated both by filtration and by tubular secretion. Unfortunately, there is no simple test to measure tubular secretion. Therefore, dosage adjustment based on creatinine clearance may not be appropriate for patients receiving drugs that are actively secreted by the renal tubules.[10]

The effect of changes in urine pH and urine flow on drug excretion have already been discussed in Chapter 37. In routine drug therapy, these parameters are not considered to be of great importance. However, alkalinization of urine to pH 8 by the administration of sodium bicarbonate is routinely used to treat overdoses of phenobarbital and salicylates, since ionization of these weak acids reduces their reabsorption and increases their elimination.

Drug Therapy In Renal Disease—Drug administration to patients with impaired renal function is complicated by their associated medical problems, by the number of drugs they receive and by the alterations in drug disposition and elimination that occur. In renal disease, the protein binding of acidic or neutral but not basic drugs in plasma is usually altered. Some of the reasons to explain changes in protein binding include: 1) hypoalbuminemia that occurs as a result of protein loss in the urine, 2) competition for protein binding sites with small acidic molecules that accumulate in uremia, 3) changes in the conformation of albumin that results in decreased affinity for binding sites, and 4) the accumulation of drug metabolites that might displace parent drug from proteins. Whichever the cause for changes in binding, the clinical importance of changes in plasma binding and/or protein concentration is that care must be used to interpret plasma drug concentrations. Measured drug concentrations in plasma are usually reported as total drug, that is, bound plus free drug. For example, therapeutic plasma concentrations of phenytoin in persons with normal plasma protein content are 10–20 mg/L, of which only 1–2 mg/L represents free drug. In patients with renal failure, the *free* phenytoin concentration is unchanged, whereas the *total* drug concentration falls to 5–10 mg/L, because of changes in protein concentration. The clinician might, therefore, be mislead into thinking that an increase in dose was necessary to increase the plasma concentration. In fact, because the free phenytoin levels are unchanged in patients with renal disease a dosage adjustment is not warranted. The renal elimination of metabolites can also be affected by impaired renal function.

The uremic state has been shown to have an effect on the biotransformation of many drugs. However, effects of uremia on drug metabolism are often inconsistent and not predictable, and the clinical significance of such effects are usually not known. The clinical importance of the reduced elimination of drug metabolites is better understood. Table III in Chapter 38 lists active drug *metabolites*, many which are eliminated by the kidneys. Procainamide is acetylated in the liver to *N*-acetylprocainamide, which has cardiac effects similar to those of the parent drug. This metabolite is eliminated by the kidneys, and its plasma concentration is increased in patients with impaired renal function. Patients with renal failure who are treated with procainamide should be observed closely for signs of clinical procainamide toxicity, and plasma concentrations of both procainamide and N-acetylprocainamide should be monitored.

Dosage adjustment of drugs in patients with renal impairment should be based on a knowledge of the pharmacokinetic parameters of the drug and, when indicated, on monitoring of plasma drug concentration. The aim of individualizing dosing regimens in patients with impaired elimination (renal or hepatic) is to maintain an average plasma concentration ($C_{p(ave)}$) similar to that of patients with normal elimination and thus to avoid unnecessary toxicity or loss of efficacy. In equation 31 in Chapter 38 it can be seen that $C_{p(ave)}$ is a direct function of dose (D) and bioavailability (f) and an inverse function of the dosing interval (τ) and clearance ($V_{d} \cdot k_{el}$). In the patient with impaired elimination or decreased clearance, $C_{p(ave)}$ will increase until a new plateau is reached (plateau principle). If clearance is markedly impaired or if the therapeutic index of the drug is small, toxicity may occur. It is apparent from the same equation that either an appropriate

decrease in dose or increase in the dosing interval will offset a decrease in elimination, and a $C_{p(ave)}$ can be attained that is similar to that of a nonimpaired patient.

In the patient with renal impairment, individualization of drug therapy requires knowledge of the degree of impairment and the effect of that degree of impairment on drug elimination in order to choose a proper dose or dosing interval to achieve a desired $C_{p(ave)}$. As discussed above, the endogenous creatinine clearance is usually the most practical index of glomerular filtration rate and it is widely used (with the limitations indicated) to determine the degree of renal impairment in a patient with renal disease. Translation of the degree of impairment into a dosage regimen is not simple. In the literature there are a variety of nomograms and equations available that aid in calculation of dosing regimens in patients with renal impairment. Each has its proponents and opponents and each is based on a set of assumptions that provide limitations to its use. None take into account all of the complexities discussed above. Therefore, a nomogram or an equation used to determine a dose of a drug to be given to a patient with renal impairment must be used only as a guideline and, when possible, should be used along with monitoring of plasma drug concentration, when indicated, and careful clinical observation to ensure optimal therapy.

Drug clearance in patients with renal insufficiency (Cl_{ri}) can be estimated from the relationship of the creatinine clearance in the renally-impaired patient, the creatinine clearance of normal persons and the clearance of drug by renal and nonrenal clearance mechanisms according to the equation

$$Cl_{ri} = Cl_{renal} \times \frac{Cl_{creat\ impaired}}{Cl_{creat\ normal}} + Cl_{nonrenal}, \qquad (1)$$

where Cl_{renal} = normal renal clearance, $Cl_{creat\ impaired}$ = the creatinine clearance in the patient, $Cl_{creat\ normal}$ = the creatinine clearance in normal persons and $Cl_{nonrenal}$ = nonrenal clearance. The renal and nonrenal clearances may not be available. Therefore, in this situation, to determine a proper dosage regimen, one must rely on pharmacokinetic information that is available in the literature. The elimination rate constants, k_{el}, in normal patients and in patients with complete anuria are frequently available in the literature. The values for these constants for many drugs have been listed in Table IV. Dettli[11] has derived a nomogram in which these elimination rate constants and the creatinine clearance can be used to determine an individualized dosage regimen for patients with decreased renal function. This nomogram is reproduced in Fig 39-2.

An example of how this nomogram can be applied is as follows: the ratio $k_{el(anephric)}/k_{el(normal)}$ is the fraction of the usual dose of a drug to be administered when there is anuria. When this ratio is entered on the left ordinate of the nomogram in Figure 39-2 and connected by a line to the upper right hand corner, the dose fraction is described for a range of creatinine clearances from 0 to 100 mL/min (100 mL/min is that of a normal 70 kg person). A line is then drawn vertically from the patient's creatinine clearance on the abscissa to the dose fraction line. From this point of intersection, a second line is drawn horizontally to the left ordinate of the nomogram. The point of intersection on the left ordinate is the dose fraction for that particular drug corresponding to the compromised creatinine clearance.

Insofar as the maintenance dose is concerned, the dosage regimen in the patient in renal failure can be modified by adjusting either the dose or the dosing interval according to the calculated dose fraction. The maintenance dose can be adjusted by multiplying the normal dose by the dose fraction as follows:

$$D_{ri} = D \cdot \text{Dose Fraction}, \qquad (2)$$

Table IV—Drug Elimination Rate Constants in Normal and Anephric Patients

Drug	Normal k_{el} (hr^{-1})	Anephric k_{el} (hr^{-1})
Alpha-methyldopa	0.17	0.03
Amikacin	0.40	0.04
Amoxicillin	0.70	0.10
Amphotericin B	0.04	0.02
Ampicillin	0.70	0.10
Carbenicillin	0.60	0.05
Cefazolin	0.40	0.04
Cephacetrile	0.70	0.03
Cephalexin	1.00	0.03
Cephalothin	1.40	0.04
Cephaloridine	0.50	0.03
Chloramphenicol	0.30	0.20
Chlorpropamide	0.02	0.008
Chlortetracycline	0.10	0.10
Clindamycin	0.47	0.10
Cloxacillin	1.40	0.35
Colistimethate	0.20	0.04
Digitoxin	0.004	0.003
Digoxin	0.017	0.006
Doxycycline	0.03	0.03
Erythromycin	0.50	0.14
Ethambutol	0.58	0.09
Fluorocytosine	0.24	0.01
Gentamicin	0.30	0.01
Isoniazid		
(fast acetylators)	0.60	0.20
(slow acetylators)	0.20	0.08
Kanamycin	0.40	0.01
Lidocaine	0.40	0.36
Lincomycin	0.15	0.06
Methicillin	1.40	0.17
Minocycline	0.05	0.03
Nafcillin	1.20	0.48
Oxacillin	1.40	0.35
Oxytetracycline	0.08	0.02
Penicillin G	1.40	0.05
Polymyxin B	0.16	0.02
Procainamide	0.22	0.01
Propranolol	0.20	0.16
Quinidine	0.07	0.06
Rifampin	0.25	0.25
Streptomycin	0.27	0.01
Sulfadiazine	0.08	0.03
Sulfamethoxazole	0.70	0.70
Tetracycline	0.08	0.01
Ticarcillin	0.60	0.06
Tobramycin	0.36	0.01
Trimethoprim	0.60	0.02
Vancomycin	0.12	0.003

where D_{ri} is the dose in renal insufficiency, D is the usual dose in normal persons, and dose fraction is the value determined from the nomogram as described above. The dosing interval, τ, can be adjusted by dividing by the dose fraction as follows:

$$\tau_{ri} = \tau/\text{Dose Fraction}, \qquad (3)$$

where τ_{ri} is the dose interval in renal insufficiency. An example of an adjustment in a gentamicin dosage regimen for a patient with an impaired creatinine clearance of 35 mL/min is as follows: the usual gentamicin dosage regimen in a patient with normal renal function is a loading dose of 80 mg followed by 80 mg every 8 hours. From Table IV it can be seen that

$$k_{el(anephric)}/k_{el(normal)} = 0.01/0.30 = 0.03.$$

When 0.03 is entered on the left ordinate of the nomogram and a line is extended to the upper right corner, the dose-fraction line for gentamicin is described. From a creatinine clearance

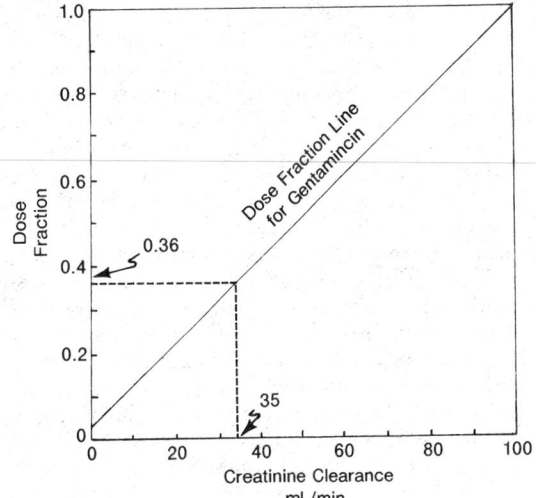

Fig 39-2. Nomogram used to determine the fraction of a dose that should be administered to a patient with a particular creatinine clearance. An example is given for a patient with a creatinine clearance of 35 mL/min and a ratio of $k_{el(anephric)}/k_{el(normal)}$ of 0.03. The dose fraction in this case is determined to be 0.36. This dose fraction is then used to adjust the dose or dosing interval for a patient with that degree of renal impairment. (Courtesy, adaptation, Dettli[11]).

of 35 mL/min on the abscissa a line is drawn vertically to the gentamicin dose-fraction line. From this point of intersection a corresponding point on the left ordinate of the nomogram is a dose-fraction of 0.36. The dosing interval can then be adjusted as follows:

$$\tau_{ri} = \tau/\text{Dose Fraction}$$

$$= 8 \text{ hours}/0.36$$

$$= 22.2 \text{ hours.}$$

Thus, in a patient with such an impaired renal function, a once-a-day dose of 80 mg is likely to maintain therapeutic plasma concentrations. The maintenance dose for gentamicin in this patient could also be adjusted using equation 2 as follows:

$$D_{ri} = D \cdot \text{Dose Fraction}$$

$$= 80 \text{ mg} \cdot 0.36$$

$$= 28.8 \text{ mg.}$$

Thus, 29 mg administered every eight hours would provide therapeutic plasma concentrations in this patient. The decision to adjust the dose or the dosing interval should also be individualized. Fluctuations in plasma concentration of gentamicin will be less if the dosing interval is lengthened to 24 hours. However, there may be a therapeutic reason to have peak plasma concentrations occur three times a day rather than only once. As mentioned above, this or any other nomogram or calculation for dosage adjustment is only an approximation. Once the dosage adjustment has been made, careful clinical observation and, when indicated, monitoring of plasma concentrations are warranted. Since the loading dose depends primarily on V_d, a change in only k_{el} does not necessitate a change in the loading dose.

Drug Therapy in Hepatic Disease—The biotransformation of drugs is discussed extensively in Chapter 37. Although many organs are involved in drug biotransformation, the liver is the most important. One might therefore assume that all patients with liver disease would demonstrate a predictable decline in drug elimination by the liver. This is not the case. There are several factors that complicate the management of drug therapy in patients with liver disease.

First, there are no routinely-performed laboratory tests that predict the effect of liver disease on drug metabolism. Unlike the correlation between creatinine clearance and renal clearance of drugs, there is not a good correlation between the commonly available tests of liver function and drug clearance by the liver. In fact, there are many biotransformed drugs the elimination rates of which are unaffected by liver disease. Second, drug elimination by the liver may be affected by several factors including liver blood flow, protein binding and volume of distribution, in addition to drug-metabolizing capacity. Third, liver disease is not a single well-defined entity but comprises a number of various structural and functional alterations. These include inflammation and necrosis, which generally alter only liver cell function and hence drug metabolizing activity; cirrhosis, which may impair both liver cell function and liver blood flow; cholestasis, which may impair both biotransformation and biliary elimination; and neoplasia, which may both impair cell function and decrease blood flow.

The discussion of biotransformation in Chapter 37 indicates that the process of hepatic elimination of drugs is complex, involving many different types of chemical reactions. While this is true, for practical purposes it is most important to know whether a drug is metabolized by an oxidation (Phase I) or conjugation (Phase II) reaction. The specific type of chemical reaction is of less clinical importance. Many drugs are biotransformed first by an oxidation reaction and the resulting metabolite is then conjugated to facilitate urinary excretion. In these cases it is the oxidation reaction that is probably most important. The clinical significance of knowing the general reactions involved in the metabolism of drugs is related to administration of such drugs in the patient with hepatic impairment. It is generally accepted that liver disorders that affect hepatocyte cell function will impair drug oxidation long before drug conjugation is altered. A specific example occurs within the benzodiazepine class of drugs. On the one hand, chlordiazepoxide and diazepam are metabolized initially by oxidation reactions that have been demonstrated to be impaired in patients with alcoholic cirrhosis.[7,12] Accordingly, the elimination of these drugs is decreased, and elevated blood levels may result during chronic therapy. On the other hand, oxazepam and lorazepam undergo only conjugation with glucuronic acid prior to being eliminated in the urine. Glucuronidation does not appear to be affected in clinically stable alcoholic cirrhosis, and the elimination of these drugs is no different than in healthy volunteers.[13,14] From a pharmacokinetic point of view, oxazepam and lorazepam are more rational choices than diazepam or chlordiazepoxide for use in patients with alcoholic cirrhosis.

Most studies of drug elimination in patients with liver disease have been performed in patients with either acute viral hepatitis or alcoholic liver disease. One should be careful about extrapolating these data to patients with other types of liver disease, such as chronic forms of hepatitis, neoplasias of the liver or cholestasis. Furthermore, one must not extrapolate studies of the metabolism of one drug in patients with liver disease to another drug, even though the metabolic reactions appear to be similar. There is a multiplicity of subpopulations of cytochrome P-450 enzymes. One drug may be metabolized by one of these subpopulations, while another drug is metabolized by another enzyme. For this reason, there is often poor correlation between the oxidations of two drugs.

Hepatic disease can also produce changes in serum proteins and in liver blood flow which can influence the elimination of drugs. Because the liver is the site of synthesis of serum proteins, patients with severe chronic liver disease frequently have decreased protein binding of drugs. In addition, there may be decreased protein binding as a result of qualitative changes in serum proteins. Liver blood flow is dominated by

the portal venous system that drains the mesenteric veins. Thus, all drugs absorbed from the oral route pass through the liver via the portal vein. In certain types of liver disease, most commonly alcoholic cirrhosis, there is shunting of the portal circulation away from functioning hepatocytes. This leads to increased pressures within the portal system and shunting of drugs away from the drug-metabolizing enzymes.

One method of classifying drugs by the characteristics of hepatic elimination is to divide them into those with a high hepatic extraction ratio and those with a low hepatic extraction ratio. As described in equation 21 of Chapter 38, the hepatic extraction ratio is defined as

$$ E = \frac{C_{ap} - C_v}{C_{ap}}, $$

where C_{ap} is the hypothetical mean of mixed hepatic arterial and portal venous drug concentrations, and C_v is the hepatic venous drug concentration. The hepatic clearance, Cl_H, of a drug is determined by its extraction ratio as follows:

$$ Cl_H = HBF{\cdot}E, $$

where HBF is total hepatic blood flow. The classification of drugs according to their hepatic extraction ratios is shown in Table V. Hepatic blood flow is usually the rate-limiting factor in the hepatic clearance of drugs with high extraction ratios, and the metabolism of such drugs are considered to be *flow-limited* metabolism. These drugs demonstrate first-pass metabolism in that after oral administration a major portion of the drug does not reach the systemic circulation. Their bioavailability is low and their metabolism is sensitive to anything that alters hepatic blood flow. Thus, for example, the elimination of lidocaine can be substantially decreased in patients with congestive heart failure, which usually causes a reduction in hepatic blood flow. In patients with cirrhosis and portal hypertension, the shunting of blood away from functioning hepatocytes has the greatest impact on drugs with a high hepatic extraction ratio. In patients with portal hypertension, the bioavailability of drugs with a high extraction ratio may be significantly increased, so that toxic blood levels may result. At the present time there is no routine laboratory test that will predict this effect in an individual patient. Rather, it is advisable to start with a low dose of drug and increase the dose slowly to achieve the desired response.

The rate of metabolism for drugs with a low extraction ratio is dependent on the concentration of drug at the hepatic enzyme site, which is proportional to the free concentration of drug in plasma. Consequently, drugs in this class can be further divided into those in which hepatic elimination is either sensitive or insensitive to protein binding. Drugs the hepatic elimination of which is distinctly sensitive to protein

Table V—Classification of Drugs According to Their Hepatic Extraction Ratios

Drugs with an Extraction Radio Greater than 0.5

Lidocaine	Nortriptyline
Propranolol	Morphine
Pethedine	Labetalol
Pentazocine	Verapamil
Propoxyphene	Metoprolol

Drugs with an Extraction Ratio Less than 0.5

Binding-Sensitive	*Binding-Insensitive*
Phenytoin	Theophylline
Diazepam	Acetaminophen
Tolbutamide	Hexobarbital
Warfarin	Chloramphenicol
Chlorpromazine	
Digitoxin	
Quinidine	

binding are generally 80–99+% bound, whereas drugs the hepatic elimination of which is clearly insensitive to protein binding are less than 30% bound. Conditions that affect plasma protein binding can have a significant effect on the hepatic clearance of binding-sensitive drug but usually not a binding-insensitive drug.

Although much is known about the hepatic metabolism of drugs and the factors that can affect their hepatic elimination, the use of drugs in patients with potential altered hepatic clearance is still empirical in that there are no specific guidelines relating the severity of hepatic disease and drug elimination. To a great extent this is due to the multiplicity of drug metabolizing enzymes, and it is unlikely that a single or simple battery of laboratory tests will suffice to predict the hepatic elimination of all drugs. Applying the known facts about liver disease along with the knowledge of drug elimination by the liver will usually permit a rational use of drugs in patients with disorders of the liver.

Therapeutic Drug Monitoring

Rational drug therapy requires individualization of the dosage regimen for a particular patient. In many instances this can be done by *monitoring the clinical response* to drug therapy. For example, if a patient with hypertension is not responding to therapy and there is no reason to suspect poor compliance, then it may be appropriate to increase the dose until the patient's blood pressure is under control. Whenever a drug is administered, well-defined therapeutic end points should be a preferred part of the management plan. Observation of the clinical response or monitoring a reliable laboratory test may be easy with certain classes of drugs such as antihypertensives, oral hypoglycemics, oral anticoagulants, analgesics or drugs used to lower serum uric acid or serum lipids. For other drugs, the definition of a therapeutic end point may not be clear or the onset of toxicity may occur at dosages only slightly above therapeutic concentrations. For some of these drugs one should monitor the serum drug concentration and thus determine if the dose administered to an individual patient is achieving therapeutic concentrations.

The following are several criteria and typical examples that should be considered before measured drug serum concentrations are of clinical value.

1. *The drug must have a reversible action.* An example of drugs with irreversible action would be the alkylating agents which exert a lasting effect after a single dose. At the present time there seems to be little need for routinely monitoring the plasma concentration of these drugs.
2. *The development of tolerance at the receptor site should not occur.* A therapeutic concentration range for morphine is not rational, since the dose requirements may increase with use.
3. *The pharmacokinetic properties of the drug are taken into account in the blood sampling schedule.* If sampling is performed in a maintenance regimen, steady-state should have been achieved prior to sampling. Steady-state may occur 4–5 half-lives after the initiation of therapy if a loading dose is not administered. Changes in drug half-life produced by disease must be taken into accounts. For drugs with a short half-life, peak (1 or 2 hours after dosing) and trough (pre-dosing) determinations are advisable. The distribution phase should be complete before drug concentrations are measured.
4. *The presence of active metabolites should be taken into consideration.* The serum concentrations of the N-acetylprocainamide metabolite of procainamide should be considered when assessing antiarrhythmic activity after administering procainamide. This is particularly true in patients with renal failure who may eliminate the metabolite slowly.
5. *The analytical method must be sensitive enough to measure accurately the expected serum concentrations and selective enough to be certain that interfering substances will not influence the results.*

6. *The data must be evaluated in the context of sound clinical judgment.* Treat the patient, not the serum drug concentration. An example is the patient who is taking digoxin and develops a low plasma potassium. Hypokalemia makes the myocardium more sensitive to the rhythm disorders produced by digoxin. Thus, the patient with a normal serum digoxin concentration may experience drug-induced cardiotoxicity if hypokalemia is also present.

Therapeutic drug monitoring requires as much clinical skill as does titration of an oral anticoagulant dose by monitoring the prothrombin time. A basic assumption in this principle is that free drug at the *active site* is in equilibrium with total drug in plasma or serum. This has been shown probably to be true for many drugs. Furthermore, for these drugs, optimum therapeutic effects and minimal toxicity is observed when the serum drug concentration lies within an empirically-determined therapeutic plasma concentration range. However, there is overlap between the therapeutic and subtherapeutic serum drug concentrations. Therefore, therapeutic drug monitoring should be considered as an aid to, not a substitute for, careful clinical observation in the management of drug therapy.

The purpose of this section is to provide some guidelines to follow for therapeutic drug monitoring, and some of the salient features of the drugs being monitored. Table VI contains a list of drugs commonly monitored and the serum concentrations thought to represent the therapeutic range.

Interpretation of plasma drug concentrations clearly requires a broad knowledge of clinical pharmacokinetics. Recently several sources of pharmacokinetic data have become available. The Sixth Edition of Goodman and Gilman contains an Appendix of Pharmacokinetic Data developed by Benet and Sheiner.[15] (The Seventh Edition will contain an updated version of this Appendix.) Included are excellent compilations of availability, urinary excretion, protein binding, clearance, volume of distribution, half-life and therapeutic and toxic concentrations for most of the currently used drugs. Data are accompanied by references so that the original work can be documented. Another useful reference is the book by Gerson.[16] Included are chapters on the major drug classes with detailed discussions of the commonly used drugs.

Table VII provides important pharmacokinetic information for commonly monitored drugs. A sound knowledge of the clinical pharmacokinetics of each drug, a critical use of plasma drug concentrations as described above, and a thorough

Table VI—Therapeutic Ranges for Drugs

Amikacin	Trough	4–8	mg/L
	Peak	20–30	mg/L
Carbamazepine		4–8	mg/L
Digoxin		0.8–2	μg/L
Disopyramide		2–5	mg/L
Ethosuximide		40–100	mg/L
Gentamicin	Trough	0.5–2	mg/L
	Peak	5–10	mg/L
Lidocaine		1.2–5	mg/L
Phenobarbital		15–40	mg/L
Phenytoin		10–20	mg/L
Primidone (see phenobarbital)		5–12	mg/L
Procainamide		4–10	mg/L
N-Acetylprocainamide		10–30	mg/L[a]
Quinidine		1.5–4.5	mg/L
Theophylline		10–20	mg/L
Tobramycin	Trough	0.5–2	mg/L
	Peak	4–10	mg/L
Valproic Acid		50–100	mg/L

[a] Total of procainamide and N-acetylprocainamide.

Table VII—Pharmacokinetic Parameters of Commonly Monitored Drugs

Drug	Volume of Distribution (L/kg)	Protein Binding (%)	Oral Availability (%)	Route of Elimination	Half-Life		Dose Adjustment Required	
					Normal	Anephric	Renal Failure	Liver Failure
Amikacin	0.25	<5	Parenteral only	Renal	3 hr	2–4 days	Yes	No
Carbamazepine	0.8–1.4	75	70	Hepatic—epoxide metabolite is active	10–26 hr	—	No	No
Digoxin	5.1–7.4	20–40	50–93	Renal	33–51 hr	3.6 days	Yes	No
Disopyramide	0.5	50–80	80–85	Renal and Hepatic	6–10	45	Yes	No
Ethosuximide	0.62	Negligible	100	Hepatic	60 hr adults 30 hr children	—	No	No
Gentamicin	0.25	<5	Parenteral only	Renal	2 hr	2–3 days	Yes	No
Lidocaine	1.6	60	Parenteral only	Hepatic—metabolites are active	1.5 hr	—	No	Yes
Phenobarbital	1.0	46	80–100	Hepatic primarily	3–4 days	—	No	Yes
Phenytoin	0.6	90	90	Hepatic	10–30 hr concentration dependent	—	No	Only in severe cases
Primidone	0.6	14	Complete	Hepatic—phenobarbital and phenyl-ethylmalonyl-amide (PEMA) are active metabolites	3–12 hr 29–36 hr metabolites	—	No	No
Procainamide	2.2	15	75–95	Renal and Hepatic N-acetylprocainamide is active	2.5–4.5 hr	10–15 hr	Yes	No
Quinidine	0.5	60–80	70–95	Hepatic—metabolite active	11–7 hr	—	No	No
Theophylline	0.3–0.6	55	Complete	Hepatic	3–9 hr	—	No	Yes
Tobramycin	0.25	<5	Parenteral only	Renal	2 hr	2–4 days	Yes	No
Valproic acid	0.2	90	70–100	Hepatic	10–15 hr	—	No	Yes, use with caution

clinical evaluation of the patient will provide the data required for the development of rational drug therapy.

References

1. Benet LZ: Input factors are determinants of drug activity: Route, dose, dosage regimen and the drug delivery system. In McMahon FG, ed: *Principles and Techniques of Human Research and Therapeutics:* Futura Publishing, Mount Kisco, New York, 1974.
2. White PF: Use of continuous infusion versus intermittent bolus administration of fentanyl or ketamine during outpatient anesthesia, *Anesthiology 59:* 294, 1983.
3. Melander A *et al*: Enhancement of the bioavailability of pro-pranolol and metoprolol by food, *Clin Pharmacol Ther 22:* 108, 1979.
4. Welling PG: Drug bioavailability and its clinical significance. In Bridges JW and Chasseavel LF, ed: *Progress in Drug Metabolism 4:* John Wiley & Sons, New York, 1980.
5. Welling PG: Effects of gastrointestinal disease on drug absorption. In Benet LZ et al ed: *Pharmacokinetic Basis for Drug Treatment:* Raven Press, New York, 1984.
6. Ensminger WD *et al*: A clinical pharmacological evaluation of hepatic arterial infusions of 5-fluoro-2'-dioxyuridine and 5-fluorouracil *Cancer Research 38:* 3784, 1978.
7. Klotz U *et al*: The effect of age and liver disease on the disposition and elimination of diazepam in adult man, *J Clin Invest 55:* 347, 1975.
8. Gugler R *et al*: Pharmacokinetics of drugs in patients with ne-phrotic syndrome, *J Clin Invest 55:* 1182, 1975.
9. Spector AA *et al*: Influence of free fatty acid concentration on drug binding to plasma albumin, *Ann NY Acad Sci 226L* 247, 1973.
10. Hori R *et al*: Ampicillin and cephalexin in renal insufficiency, *Clin Pharmacol and Therap 34:* 792, 1983.
11. Dettli L: Drug dosage in renal disease. *Clin Pharmacokinet 1:* 126, 1976.
12. Roberts RK *et al*: Effects of age and parenchymal liver disease on the disposition and elimination of chlordiazepoxide (Librium), *Gastroenterol 75:* 479, 1978.
13. Kraus JW *et al*: The effects of aging and liver disease on the disposition of lorazepam in man, *Clin Pharmacol Ther 24:* 411, 1978.
14. Shull HJ *et al*: Normal disposition of oxazepam in acute viral hepatitis and cirrhosis, *Ann Intern Med 84:* 420, 1976.
15. Benet LZ and Sheiner LB: Design and optimization of dosage regimens; pharmacokinetic data. In Gilman et al, eds: *The Pharmacological Basis of Therapeutics:* Macmillan, New York, 1980.
16. Gerson B: *Essentials of Therapeutic Drug Monitoring*, Igaku-Shoin, New York, 1983.

CHAPTER 40

Topical Drugs

Stewart C Harvey, PhD

Professor of Pharmacology
College of Medicine, University of Utah
Salt Lake City, UT 84132

A large number of chemical agents may be applied to the skin and mucous membranes for their local effects. Many of these, such as antibiotics, antiseptics, corticosteroids, antineoplastics, and local anesthetics, belong to distinct pharmacological classes treated elsewhere in this text, and will not be discussed in this chapter. The remainder comprise a heterogeneous group of agents which, by exclusion, are mostly nonselective in action.

Those locally acting agents that have limited chemical and pharmacologic activity generally have a *physical* basis of action. Included in this group are protectives, adsorbents, demulcents, emollients, and cleansing agents. The relative inertness of many of these substances renders them of value as vehicles and excipients. Consequently, many in this group are also pharmaceutical necessities and may be treated in Chapter 68.

Those locally acting agents that have general *chemical* reactivity include most astringents, irritants, rubefacients, vesicants, sclerosing agents, caustics, escharotics, many keratolytic (desquamating) agents, and a miscellaneous group of dermatologics including hypopigmenting and antipruritic agents.

Although the skin and mucous membranes differ considerably in structure and function, they are similar in penetrability (to chemical agents) and in their response to certain physical and pharmacological stimuli. Thus, many of the agents found in this chapter may be applied to both types of surfaces. Nevertheless, it is obvious that many agents, for which there is either contraindication or no rationale for their application to the mucous membranes, may be applied only to the skin.

In its broadest pharmacologic sense a protective is any agent that isolates the exposed surface (skin or mucous membrane) from harmful or annoying stimuli. In common practice only those substances that protect by mechanical or other physical means are considered to be protectives, although the surface action of adsorbents and demulcents cannot be divorced from their chemical properties. Protectives such as demulcents and emollients are customarily placed in separate categories; that practice is followed here.

The abridged category of protectives mainly comprises the dusting powders, adsorbents, mechanical protective agents, and plasters.

Protectives and Adsorbents

Dusting Powders

Certain relatively indifferent (inert and insoluble) substances are used to cover and protect epithelial surfaces, ulcers, and wounds. Usually these substances are very finely subdivided. They generally absorb moisture and therefore also act as cutaneous desiccants. The absorption of skin moisture decreases friction and also discourages certain bacterial growth.

The water-absorbent powders should not be administered to wet, raw surfaces because of the formation of cakes and adherent crusts. Starch and other carbohydrate powders may not only become doughy but they may also ferment. Consequently, such powders often contain an antiseptic. Most impalpable powders are to some extent absorptive. Whether absorption of substances other than water contributes to the protection of the skin is uncertain; however, absorption of fatty acids and other constituents of perspiration, along with cutaneous drying, contributes to a deodorant action of the powders. It is generally held that the adsorptive capacity is important to the gastrointestinal protective action of chemically inert powders taken internally.

The chemically inert dusting powders are not entirely biologically inert, despite the name. When entrained in pores or wounds or left upon parietal surfaces, certain of the dusting powders, eg, talc, may cause irritation, granulomas, fibrosis, or adhesions. Even without direct irritation or obstruction of the perspiration, dust can be troublesome.

Several of the dusting powders are incorporated into ointments, creams, and lotions.

Bentonite—page 1297.
Boric Acid—page 1310.
Calcium Carbonate, Precipitated—page 794.
Talc—page 1319.
Titanium Dioxide—page 790.
Zinc Oxide—page 779.

Zinc Stearate

Octadecanoic acid, zinc salt

Zinc stearate [557-05-1]. A compound of zinc with a mixture of solid organic acids obtained from fats, and consists chiefly of variable proportions of zinc stearate and zinc palmitate. It contains the equivalent of 12.5–14.0% of ZnO(81.38).

Preparation—An aqueous solution of zinc sulfate is added to a sodium stearate solution and the precipitate is washed with water until free of sulfate and dried.

Description—Fine, white, bulky powder, free from grittiness with a faint characteristic color. It is neutral to moistened litmus paper.

Solubility—Insoluble in water, alcohol, or ether but is soluble in benzene.

Uses—In *water-repellent* ointments and as a *dusting powder* in dermatologic practice for its desiccating, astringent, and *protective* effect. It has been removed from baby dusting powders, owing to accidental, fatal inhalations.

Mechanical and Chemical Protectives

Several materials may be administered to the skin to form an adherent, continuous coat which may be either flexible or semirigid, depending upon the substances and the manner in which they are applied. Such materials may serve three purposes: (1) to provide occlusive protection from the external environment, (2) to provide mechanical support, and (3) to serve as vehicles for various medicaments.

The two principal classes of mechanical protectives are the collodions and plasters. Neither is used to much extent today. This is because there is increasing recognition of the beneficial effects of air in maintaining a normally balanced cutaneous bacterial flora of low pathogenicity. Also, the mechanical protectives may of themselves be somewhat irritating because of interference with normal water transport through the skin caused by certain oleaginous and resinous ingredients, especially in plasters. It is also recognized that rubber in adhesive plaster may induce eczema. The cerates may be employed similarly to the plasters. Bandages, dressings, and casts also afford mechanical protection and support (see Chapter 105 for additional information). A brief discussion of plasters is included in Chapter 88.

A number of insoluble and relatively inert powders remain essentially unchanged chemically in the gastrointestinal tract. If the particles possess surface properties that favor their clinging to the gastrointestinal mucosa, and especially if they split up into tabular shapes, they offer mechanical protection against abrasion and may even offer slight protection against toxins and chemical irritants. Many such protectives also are adsorbents (charcoal, bismuth compounds, kaolin) or astringents (zinc and bismuth compounds). They are discussed under those categories.

Aluminum Hydroxide Gel—page 793.

Collodion

Contains not less than 5.0%, by weight, of pyroxylin.

Pyroxylin	40 g
Ether	750 mL
Alcohol	250 mL
To make about	1000 mL

Add the alcohol and the ether to the pyroxylin contained in a suitable container, and stopper the container well. Shake the mixture occasionally until the pyroxylin is dissolved.

Description—Clear, or slightly opalescent, viscous liquid. It is colorless, or slightly yellowish, and has the odor of ether. Specific gravity between 0.765 and 0.775.
Alcohol Content—22 to 26% of C_2H_5OH.

Uses—Chiefly to seal small wounds or for the preparation of medicated collodions.
Caution—Collodion is highly flammable.

Flexible Collodion [Collodium Flexile]—See *RPS 16*, page 717. See also *Salicylic Acid Collodion* (page 785).

Absorbable Gelatin Film

Gelfilm (*Upjohn*)

A sterile, nonantigenic, water-insoluble, gelatin film obtained from a specially prepared gelatin-formaldehyde solution by drying on plates at constant temperature and humidity with subsequent sterilization by dry heat at 146° to 149°C for 12 hours.

Description—Light amber, transparent, pliable film that becomes rubbery when moistened.
Solubility—Insoluble in water; it assumes a rubbery consistency after being in water for a few minutes.

Uses—Both as a *mechanical protective* and as a *temporary supportive structure* and *replacement matrix* in *surgical repair of defects in membranes*, such as the dura mater and the pleura. When emplaced between damaged or operated structures, it prevents adhesions. When moistened, the film becomes pliable and plastic, so that it can be fitted to the appropriate surface. Absorption requires 1 to 6 months. Absorbable gelatin film is also a component of stomadhesive, to be placed around an ostomy.

Dose—Applied in the form of sheets, previously soaked in isotonic sodium chloride solution and cut to the desired shape. The film blanks are 100 × 125 × 0.16 mm in size.

Zinc Gelatin

Zinc Gelatin Boot; Unna's Boot; Unna's Paste

Zinc Oxide	100 g
Gelatin	150 g
Glycerin	400 g
Purified Water	350 g
To make about	1000 g

Gradually add the gelatin to the cold purified water, with constant stirring, allow the mixture to stand for 10 min, and then heat on a steam bath until the gelatin dissolves. Add the zinc oxide, which previously has been rubbed to a smooth paste with the glycerin, and stir carefully until a smooth jelly result.

Uses—Melted and applied in the molten state between layers of bandage to act as a *protective* and to support varicosities and similar lesions of the lower limbs. After a period of about 2 weeks the dressing is removed by soaking with warm water.
Dose—*External*, as an occlusive boot.
Dosage Forms—Impregnated Gauze, in 10-yd lengths in following widths: 2¼, 2½, 3, and 4 inch; impregnated with white or pink paste (the latter colored with a small amount of ferric oxide).

Kaolin—page 811.

Lanolin—page 1304.

Lanolin, Anhydrous—page 1303.

Mineral Oil—page 805.

Mineral Oil Emulsion—page 805.

Mineral Oil, Light—page 1315.

Olive Oil—page 1310.

Peanut Oil—page 1295.

Petrolatum—page 1302.

Other Mechanical and Chemical Protectives

Petrolatum Gauze [Petrolated Gauze]—Absorbent gauze saturated with white petrolatum. The weight of the petrolatum is 70–80% of the weight of the Gauze. It is sterile. *Preparation:* Add, under aseptic conditions, molten, sterile, white petrolatum to dry, sterile, absorbent gauze, previously cut to size, in the ratio of 60 g of petrolatum to each 20 g of gauze. *Uses:* A *protective* dressing; also as packing material for postoperative plugs, packs, rolls, and tampons, and as a wick or drain or wrap-around for tubing. It is claimed that there is no danger of tissue maceration and that no growth of granulation tissue through the Gauze occurs.

Dimethicone [Poly(dimethylsiloxane; poly[oxy(dimethylsilylene)] [9006-65-9] $(C_2H_6OSi)_n$]—A water-repellent silicone oil consisting essentially of dimethyl siloxane polymers of the 200 series of fluids (see *Silicones*, below). It is a water-white, viscous, oil-like liquid; immiscible with water and alcohol; miscible with chloroform and ether. *Uses:* Has skin-adherent and water-repellent properties. It is both a protective and an emollient, for which its FDA classification is category I. Applied to the skin, it forms a *protective* film that provides a barrier to ordinary soap and water and water-soluble irritants. The film may last several hours if the skin is exposed mainly to aqueous media. The film provides a less effective barrier to synthetic detergents and lipid-soluble materials, such as organic solvents. Dimethicone should not be applied except in contact dermatoses and dermatoses aggravated by substances that can be repelled by the silicone. It is useful in preventing irritation from ammonia produced by the urine of infants, but it may exacerbate preexisting irritation. The occlusive protection by the silicone is detrimental to inflamed, traumatized, abraded, or excoriated skin and to lesions requiring free drainage. However, applied adjacent to such lesions, it offers protection against irritating discharges and maceration. Dimethicone is itself nearly harmless, and does not sensitize skin but it does cause temporary irritation to the eyes. It may be incorporated into ointments, creams, and gels. *Dose:* Apply uniformly with rubbing 3 or 4 times for the first day or two, then twice daily. *Dosage Forms:* Aerosol; Cream; Ointment: 20 and 30%. All concentrations from 1 to 30% are approved.

Silicones (*polyorganosiloxanes*)—These are organosilicon polymers containing chains of alternating oxygen and silicon atoms with substituent organic groups, frequently methyl or phenyl, attached to each silicon atom.

Preparation: These polymers may be prepared synthetically by condensing alkylated or arylated *silanols.* Disubstituted *silanediols* [$R_2Si(OH)_2$] form linear polymers having the general formula:

$$HO-\underset{\underset{R}{|}}{\overset{\overset{R}{|}}{Si}}-O-\left[\underset{\underset{R}{|}}{\overset{\overset{R}{|}}{Si}}-O\right]_n-\underset{\underset{R}{|}}{\overset{\overset{R}{|}}{Si}}-OH$$

Cross-linked polymers result from condensation of mixtures of substituted silanediols and monosubstituted *silanetriols* [$RSi(OH)_3$]; represented by the following partial formula where R is a hydrocarbon radical:

$$\left[\begin{array}{c}\overset{\overset{R}{|}}{}\quad\overset{\overset{R}{|}}{}\quad\overset{\overset{R}{|}}{}\\-O-Si-O-Si-O-Si-O-\\ \underset{\underset{R}{|}}{}\quad\underset{\underset{O}{|}}{}\quad\underset{\underset{R}{|}}{}\\ \overset{R}{|}\quad\quad\overset{R}{|}\\ -O-Si-O-Si-O-Si-O-\\ \underset{R}{|}\quad\underset{R}{|}\quad\underset{R}{|}\end{array}\right]_n$$

One method of preparation involves interaction of silicon tetrachloride with appropriate Grignard reagents to yield alkylated or arylated dichlorosilanes. After hydrolysis to the corresponding substituted silanols, dehydration procedures are used to effect condensation polymerization. The overall reaction, as it involves a disubstituted silanediol, may be represented as:

$$SiCl_4 \xrightarrow{RMgX} R_2SiCl_2 \xrightarrow{HOH} R_2Si(OH)_2 \xrightarrow{-HOH} HO[Si(R)_2O]_nH$$

Silicon Tetrachloride	Disubstituted Dichlorosilane	Disubstituted Silanediol	Silicone Linear Polymer

Properties: Silicones with a wide range of properties may be produced by varying the substituent R and the degree of cross-linking. Physically, silicones vary from mobile liquids through viscous liquids and semisolids to solids. Viscosities range from 0.65 to 1,000,000 centistokes. In general, they display high- and low-temperature stability. They are odorless, tasteless, relatively inert chemically and physiologically, water-repellent, and possess antifoam characteristics. Unmodified silicones are generally insoluble in water; because of this the liquids are often termed *silicone oils;* however, a water-soluble sodium salt of a simple silicone, chemically *sodium methyl siliconate* [$CH_3Si(OH)_2ONa$] has been marketed.

Uses: Preparations containing silicones have various dermatological uses (see *Dimethicone*) and are used as ingredients of bases for ointments and liniments. In the form of inhalation sprays, silicone preparations have been employed in the treatment of pulmonary edema involving frothing of fluid in the upper respiratory tract. They are also used orally as antiflatulent or gastric defoaming agents (see *Simethicone*, page 814). A silicone *bouncing putty* has found acceptance for use as a physical agent in treatment of conditions requiring finger exercise. The water-repellent properties of the silicones have found considerable use in a great variety of applications where complete drainage of aqueous fluids from surfaces is desirable.

Silicones are virtually nonirritating; consequently, silicone rubbers are used in various indwelling catheters, tubes, etc., and in some types of prostheses. Liquid silicones are used also to fill in hypoplastic body areas for cosmetic purposes, although they tend to relocate because of flow under gravity and motion.

In addition to uses involving antifoaming, water-repellent, and nonirritating characteristics, silicones are employed also to prevent sticking of one object to another and are then commonly referred to as release agents. Examples of such employment include release of rubber and plastics from molds, food from metal, ice from the wings of aircraft, and capsules and tablets from molds and dyes in which they are fabricated.

Silicone rubbers are used to encapsulate steroid hormones and other drugs intended for chronic use, in order to retard absorption and effect a repository action lasting in some instances for as long as a year. Continuing developments in this field offer interesting possibilities.

Zinc Carbonate—$CO_3Zn(125.38)$. *Description*—White rhombohedroids. *Solubility*—10 ppm in water at 15°; soluble in dilute acids, alkalies, and solutions of ammonium salts. *Uses:* Zinc carbonate is used both for its lubricity and as a drying agent. As a skin protectant it falls into FDA Category I. It is included in commercial topical burn and sunburn products and extemporary protectants. *Dose:* 0.2 to 2%.

Demulcents

Demulcents are protective agents that are employed primarily to alleviate irritation (*demulcere*—to smooth down), particularly of mucous membranes or abraded tissues. They are also often applied to the skin. They are generally applied to the surface in viscid sticky preparations that cover the area readily. The local action of chemical, mechanical, or bacterial irritants is thereby diminished, and pain, reflexes, spasm, or catarrh are attenuated. They also prevent drying of the affected surface. The demulcents may be applied to the skin in the form of lotions, cataplasms or wet dressing, to the gastrointestinal tract in the form of demulcent liquors or enemas, and to the throat in the form of pastilles, lozenges, or gargles. Demulcents are also included in artificial tears and in wetting agents for contact lenses. When demulcents are applied as solid material (as in lozenges or powders), the liquid is provided by secreted or exuded fluids. Demulcents are frequently medicated. In such instances the demulcent may be an adjuvant, a corrective, or a pharmaceutical necessity. Many of the demulcents are also laxatives (page 799) and are used as such, or they are used with laxatives or antacids for their demulcent and lubricating action.

A variety of chemical substances possess demulcent properties. Among these are mucilages, gums, dextrins, starches, certain sugars, and polymeric polyhydric glycols. Mucus in itself is a natural demulcent. Certain silicates that form silicic acid on exposure to air or to gastric juice, and glycerin, although it is of low molecular weight and has relatively low binding power, are frequently placed among the demulcents. Also the colloidal hydrous oxides, hydroxides, and basic salts of several metals are claimed to be demulcent, but acceptable clinical proof of the claim has not been provided.

The hydrophilic colloidal properties of most of the demulcents make them valuable emulsifiers and suspending agents in water-soluble ointments and suspensions. They also retard the absorption of many injections and thus may be employed in sundry depot preparations. Many of the demulcents mask the flavor of medicaments by means of at least three physical phenomena: (1) They apparently coat the taste receptors and render them less sensitive; (2) they incorporate many organic solutes into micelles and thereby diminish the free concentration of such solutes; and (3) they coat the surfaces of many particles in suspension. Because of the adhesiveness of the demulcents, they are widely employed as binding agents in tablets, lozenges, and similar dosage forms. Consequently, certain demulcents will be discussed in Chapter 68.

Acacia—page 1296.

Benzoin

Gum Benjamin; Benzoe

The balsamic resin obtained from *Styrax benzoin* Dryander or *Styrax paralleloneurus* Perkins, known in commerce as Sumatra

Benzoin, or from *Styrax tonkinensis* (Pierre) Craib ex Hartwich, or other species of the Section *Anthostyrax* of the genus *Styrax*, known in commerce as Siam Benzoin (Fam *Styraceae*).

Sumatra benzoin yields not less than 75.0% of alcohol-soluble extractive, and Siam benzoin yields not less than 90.0% of alcohol-soluble extractive.

Constituents—Siam benzoin contains about 68% of crystalline *coniferyl benzoate* [$C_{17}H_{16}O_4$]; up to 10% of an amorphous form of this compound is also present. Some *coniferyl alcohol* (*m-methoxy-p-hydroxycinnamyl alcohol*, mp 73–74°) occurs in the free state as well. Other compounds that have been isolated are *benzoic acid* 11.7%, *d-siaresinolic acid* 6%, *cinnamyl benzoate* 2.3%, and *vanillin* 0.3%.

Sumatra benzoin has been reported to contain benzoic and cinnamic acid esters of the alcohol *benzoresinol* and probably also of coniferyl alcohol, free *benzoic* and *cinnamic acids*, *styrene*, 2 to 3% of *cinnamyl cinnamate* (also called *styracin*), 1% of *phenylpropyl cinnamate*, 1% of *vanillin*, a trace of *benzaldehyde*, a little *benzyl cinnamate*, and the alcohol *d-sumaresinol* [$C_{30}H_{48}O_4$].

Description—*Sumatra Benzoin:* Blocks or lumps of varying size made up of compacted tears, with a reddish brown, reddish gray, or grayish brown resinous mass. *Siam Benzoin:* Compressed pebble-like tears of varying size and shape. Both varieties are yellowish to rusty brown externally, milky white on fracture; hard and brittle at ordinary temperatures but softened by heat; aromatic and balsamic odor; taste aromatic and slightly acrid.

Uses—A *protective* application for irritations of the skin. When mixed with glycerin and water, the tincture may be applied locally for *cutaneous ulcers*, *bedsores*, *cracked nipples*, and *fissures* of the lips and anus. For throat and bronchial inflammation, the tincture may be administered on sugar. The tincture and compound tincture are sometimes used in boiling water as steam inhalants for their *expectorant* and *soothing action* in acute laryngitis and croup. In combination with zinc oxide, it is used in baby ointments.

Compound Benzoin Tincture [Balsamum Equitis Sancti Victoris, Balsamum Commendatoris, Balsamum Catholicum, Balsamum Traumaticum, Balsamum Vulnerarium, Balsamum Persicum, Balsamum Suecium, Balsamum Friari, Balsamum Vervaini, Guttae Nader, Guttae Jesuitarium, Tinctura Balsamica, Balsam of the Holy Victorius Knight, Commander's Balsam, Friar's Balsam, Turlington's Drops, Persian Balsam, Swedish Balsam, Vervain Balsam, Turlington's Balsam of Life, Balsam de Maltha, Ward's Balsam, Jerusalem Balsam, Saint Victor's Balsam, Wade's Drops, Wound Elixir, and Balsamic Tincture]—*Preparation:* With Benzoin (in moderately coarse powder, 100 g), Aloe (in moderately coarse powder, 20 g), Storax (80 g), and Tolu Balsam (40 g), prepare a tincture (1000 mL) by Process M (page 1516), using alcohol as the menstruum. *History:* This popular preparation has had more different Latin titles and synonyms since its origin in the 15th or 16th century than any other official preparation. Many of these are significant of its uses or its originators, introducers, or patrons, for it has figured as a nostrum as well as in the pharmacopeias of the past 300 years. *Alcohol Content:* 74 to 80% of C_2H_5OH. *Uses:* Especially valuable in acute *laryngitis*, also in croup, when added to hot water and the vapor inhaled. By adding a teaspoonful of the tincture to boiling water in an inhaler, and inhaling the vapor, very effective results may be obtained. See Chapter 104. Also administered, on sugar, for throat and bronchial inflammation and as a local application, when mixed with glycerin and water, for *ulcers*,

bedsores, *cracked nipples*, and *fissures* of the lips and anus. *Dose:* *Topically*, as required.

Carbomer Methylcellulose—page 1297.

Gelatin—page 1297.

Glycerin—page 1308.

Glycerin Suppositories—page 802.

Glycyrrhiza—page 1286.

Hydroxypropyl Cellulose—page 1298.

Hydroxypropyl Methylcellulose—page 1298.

Hydroxyethyl Cellulose—page 1297.

Hydroxypropyl Methylcellulose Ophthalmic Solution

A sterile solution of hydroxypropyl methylcellulose, of a grade containing 19.0–30.0% methoxy and 4.0–12.0% hydroxypropoxy groups; may contain antimicrobial, buffering, and stabilizing agents.

Uses—A wetting solution for contact lenses. The demulcent action of hydroxypropyl methylcellulose decreases the irritant effect of the lens on the cornea. It also imparts viscous properties to the wetting solution, which assists the lens in staying in place. The demulcent effect also finds application in ophthalmic decongestants. "Artificial tear" formulations containing hydroxypropyl methylcellulose may be used when lacrimation is inadequate. One or 2 drops of the ophthalmic solution may be applied topically to the conjunctiva 3 or 4 times a day.

Dosage Forms—0.5, 0.8, 1, and 2.5% solutions.

Methylcellulose—page 1298.

Methylcellulose Ophthalmic Solution

A sterile solution of methylcellulose; may contain antimicrobial, buffering, and stabilizing agents. Used for the same purposes, and in the same manner, as *Hydroxypropyl Methylcellulose Ophthalmic Solution*, above.

Dosage Forms—0.25, 0.5, and 1%.

Pectin—page 811.

Polyvinyl Alcohol—page 1299.

Polyvinyl Alcohol Ophthalmic Solution

A sterile solution of polyvinyl alcohol, which may contain antimicrobial, buffering, and stabilizing agents and other demulcent substances.

Uses—A wetting solution for contact lenses. The polyvinyl alcohol has a demulcent action that helps protect the eye from irritation by the contact lens. It is also used in "artificial tears" employed when there is insufficient lacrimation. It is applied to the conjunctiva, 1 or 2 drops 3 or 4 times a day or as needed.

Dosage Forms—1, 1.4, 2, 3, and 4% solutions.

Emollients

Emollients are bland, fatty or oleaginous substances which may be applied locally, particularly to the skin, and also to mucous membranes or abraded tissues. Water-soluble irritants, air, and air-borne bacteria are excluded by an emollient layer. The skin is also rendered softer (*emollier*—to soften) and more pliable through penetration of the emollient into the surface layers, through the slight congestion induced by rubbing and massage upon application, and especially through mechanical interference with both sensible and insensible water loss.

Emollients have certain disadvantages. It is now recognized that retention of perspiration below the emollient and exclusion of air render conditions favorable to the growth of anaerobic bacteria. Furthermore, the rubbing during application aids in the spreading of cutaneous bacteria. Con-

sequently, use of emollients to cover burns and abrasions is diminishing. The liquid emollients may be used for mild catharsis (page 800) and for protection against gastrointestinal corrosives; however, castor oil is hydrolyzed in the gut to the irritating ricinoleic acid and hence is employed as an emollient only externally. Orally administered liquid emollients may be aspirated into the trachea and lungs, especially in infants and in the debilitated, and thus induce "oil aspiration pneumonia." This condition may also be induced by emollient nose drops.

The chief use of emollient substances is to provide vehicles for lipid-soluble drugs (as in ointments and liniments), hence many of them are described among the pharmaceutical necessities (Chapter 68). It is widely but incorrectly held that such vehicles facilitate the transport through the skin of their active ingredients. On the contrary, when the oil:water partition coefficient is greater than 1.0, the penetration is retarded, and the emollient vehicle prolongs the action of the active ingredient. Emollient substances also are commonly employed in both cleansing and antiphlogistic creams and lotions. Compound ointment bases, creams, and other medicated applications are treated elsewhere in this book (Chapter 87). Only the simple emollients and important compounded ointments that are used frequently for their emollient actions are listed below.

Castor Oil—page 801.
Castor Oil, Sulfated—page 1303.
Cocoa Butter—page 1312.
Coconut Oil—page 1309.
Cold Cream—page 1307.
Corn Oil—page 1295.

Cottonseed Oil—page 1295.
Ointment, Hydrophilic—page 1304.
Rose Water Ointment—page 1304.
Sesame Oil—page 1295.
Theobroma Oil—page 1312.
White Ointment—page 1301.
Yellow Ointment—page 1301.

Other Emollients

Myristyl Alcohol [Tetradecyl Alcohol [112-72-1] $CH_3(CH_2)_{12}$-CH_2OH]—White crystalline alcohol; specific gravity 0.824; melts at 30°. Insoluble in water soluble in ether; slightly soluble in alcohol. *Use:* Emollient in cold creams.

Shark Liver Oil—The oil extracted from the livers of the *soupfin shark, Galeorhinus zyopterus* or *Hypoprion brevirostris*, both of which are rich in vitamins A and D. *Uses:* An emollient and protectant, the FDA classification of which is Category I. It is used in burn and sunburn ointments. *Dose:* Usually 3%.

Astringents and Antiperspirants

Astringents are locally applied protein precipitants which have such a low cell penetrability that the action is essentially limited to the cell surface and the interstitial spaces. The permeability of the cell membrane is reduced, but the cells remain viable. The astringent action is accompanied by contraction and wrinkling of the tissue and by blanching. The cement substance of the capillary endothelium is hardened, so that pathological transcapillary movement of plasma protein is inhibited and local edema, inflammation and exudation are thereby reduced. Mucus or other secretions may also be reduced, so that the affected area becomes drier.

Astringents are used therapeutically to arrest hemorrhage by coagulating the blood (*styptic* action, page 831) and to check diarrhea, reduce inflammation of mucous membranes, promote healing, toughen the skin, or decrease sweating. The *antiperspirant* effect is the result both of the closure of the sweat ducts by protein precipitation to form a plug and peritubular irritation that promotes an increase in inward pressure on the tubule. Astringents also possess some *deodorant* properties by virtue of interaction with odorous fatty acids liberated or produced by action of bacteria on lipids in sweat, and by an action suppressing bacterial growth, partly because of a decrease in pH.

Many astringents are irritants or caustics in moderate to high concentrations. Consequently, strict attention must be paid to the appropriate concentration. Most astringents are also antiseptics, hence many of them are discussed in Chapter 64.

The principal astringents are (1) the salts of aluminum, zinc, manganese, iron, and bismuth, (2) certain other salts that contain these metals (such as permanganates) and (3) tannins, or related polyphenolic compounds. Acids, alcohols, phenols, and other substances that precipitate proteins may be astringent in the appropriate amount or concentration; however, such substances generally are not employed for their astringent effects, because they readily penetrate cells and promote tissue damage. Strongly hypertonic solutions dry the affected tissues and are thus often but wrongly called astringents, unless protein precipitation also occurs.

Alcohol—page 1159.

Alum

Sulfuric acid, aluminum potassium salt (2:1:1), dodecahydrate; Sulfuric acid, aluminum ammonium salt (2:1:1), dodecahydrate; Alumen; Alumen Purificatum; Purified Alum

Aluminum ammonium sulfate (1:1:2) dodecahydrate [7784-26-1]; anhydrous [7784-25-0] (237.14); or aluminum potassium sulfate (1:1:2) dodecahydrate [7784-24-9]; anhydrous [10043-67-1] (258.19).

The label of the container must indicate whether the salt is Ammonium Alum [$AlNH_4(SO_4)_2.12H_2O$ = 453.32] or Potassium Alum [$AlK(SO_4)_2.12H_2O$ = 474.38].

Preparation—Alum is prepared from the mineral *bauxite* (a hydrated aluminum oxide) and sulfuric acid, with the addition of ammonium or potassium sulfate for the respective alums. Ammonium alum is prevalent on the market because of its lower cost.

Description—Large, colorless crystals, crystalline fragments, or a white powder. It is odorless and has a sweetish, strongly astringent taste. Its solutions are acid to litmus.

Solubility—1 g ammonium alum is soluble in 7 mL water, and 1 g potassium alum is soluble in 7.5 mL water. Both are soluble in about 0.3 mL boiling water but they are insoluble in alcohol. Alum is freely but slowly soluble in glycerin.

Incompatibilities—When alum is dispensed in powders with *phenol, salicylates*, or *tannic acid*, gray or green colors may be developed due to traces of iron in the Alum. A partial liberation of its water of crystallization permits it to act as an acid toward *sodium bicarbonate*, thus liberating carbon dioxide. Ammonia is liberated simultaneously from ammonium alum. *Alkali hydroxides and carbonates, borax*, and *lime water* precipitate aluminum hydroxide from solutions of alum. The alums possess the incompatibilities of the water-soluble sulfates.

Uses—A powerful *astringent* in acidic solutions. It is slightly antiseptic, probably due to bacteriostasis through liberation of acid on hydrolysis. Alum is sometimes used as a local *styptic*, and is frequently employed in making astringent lotions and douches. It is used especially by athletes to toughen the skin. As an astringent it is used in concentrations of 0.5 to 5%. Some vulvovaginal cleansing and deodorant preparations contain alum.

Styptic pencils are made by fusing Potassium Alum, usually with the addition of some potassium nitrate, and pouring into suitable molds.

Caution—Do not confuse *styptic* pencils with *caustic* pencils (page 784); the latter contain *silver nitrate*.

Dose—*Topical*, as a 0.5 to 5% solution.

Aluminum Acetate Topical Solution

Acetic acid, aluminum salt; Liquor Burowii, Burow's Solution

$$Al(OCOCH_3)_3$$

Yields, from each 100 mL, 1.20–1.45 g of aluminum oxide [Al_2O_3 = 101.96], and 4.24–5.12 g of acetic acid [$C_2H_4O_2$ = 60.05], corresponding to 4.8–5.8 g of aluminum acetate [139-12-8] $C_6H_9AlO_6$ (204.12). It may be stabilized by the addition of not more than 0.6% of boric acid.

Caution—This solution should not be confused with Aluminum Subacetate Topical Solution which is a stronger preparation.

Note—Dispense only clear Aluminum Acetate Solution.

Description—Clear, colorless liquid having a faint acetous odor, and a sweetish, astringent taste. Specific gravity about 1.022; pH 3.6–4.4.

Uses—As an astringent dressing or as an astringent mouth wash and gargle. Aluminum acetate is included in preparations to treat athlete's foot, dermatidides, diaper rash, dry skin, poison ivy poisoning and inflammation of the external ear.

Dose—*Topical*, to skin, as a wet dressing containing a 1:10 to 1:40 dilution of the solution.

Aluminum Chloride

Aluminum chloride, hexahydrate

Aluminum chloride hexahydrate [7784-13-6] $AlCl_3.6H_2O$ (241.43); *anhydrous* [7446-70-0] (133.34).

Preparation—By heating aluminum in chlorine gas, then dissolving the product in water and crystallizing; or by dissolving freshly precipitated aluminum hydroxide in hydrochloric acid and concentrating to permit crystallization.

Description—White or yellowish white, crystalline powder; deliquescent; sweet, astringent taste; solutions are acid to litmus.

Solubility—1 g in about 0.9 mL water, 4 mL alcohol; soluble in glycerin.

Uses—Extensively employed on the skin as an astringent and anhidrotic; it is included in some proprietary preparations formulated for this purpose. It is used especially in the treatment of soggy athlete's foot, to promote drying and hence to enhance the efficacy of specific antifungal drugs. For ordinary antiperspirant use the basic salt *aluminum chlorohydroxide*, $Al_2Cl(OH)_5$, is preferable as it is less irritating and causes less deterioration of clothing than does aluminum chloride. Aluminum chloride may have a special use in the treatment of *hyperhidrosis of the palms, soles, or axillae*, for which a 20% solution in absolute ethanol is used. In the presence of water, aluminum chloride hydrolyzes to aluminum chlorohydroxide and hydrochloric acid, which can cause irritation, especially in fissures, and discomfort and also deterioration of clothing. Concentrations below 15% cause a low incidence of irritation. Consequently, it is essential that the area to be treated is completely dry before application. To protect bedclothes, the treated area is sometimes covered with plastic wrap, but such occlusion of the axillae may result in boils or furuncles. Aluminum chloride should not be applied to the axillae immediately after shaving or used where the skin is irritated or broken. Concentrations above 15% are used as caustics.

Dose—*Topical*, to skin, as **6.25** to **30**% solution. The 20% alcoholic solution may be applied on two successive days and twice a week thereafter, except that it may be applied twice daily for athlete's foot.

Aluminum Chlorohydrates

The hydrate of aluminum chloride hydroxide [1327-41-9] $Al_2Cl(OH)_5$].

Uses—Aluminum chlorohydrates mainly are employed in antiperspirant products, for which they have been rated safe and effective in concentrations of 25% (as anhydride) or less. Since solutions or suspensions of chlorohydrates are less acidic than those of aluminum chloride, they cause a lower incidence of irritation to the skin.

Dose—*Topical*, to the axilla, as a 2.5 to 25% ointment, solution, or suspension.

Aluminum Subacetate Topical Solution

Aluminum, hydroxybis (acetato-O)-

Hydroxybis(acetato)aluminum [142-03-0] $Al(OH)(OCOCH_3)_2$. The solution yields, from each 100 mL, 2.30–2.60 g of aluminum oxide [Al_2O_3 = 101.96], and 5.43–6.13 g of acetic acid [$C_2H_4O_2$ = 60.05]. It may be stabilized by the addition of not more than 0.9% of boric acid.

Description—Clear, colorless, or faintly yellow liquid, having an acetous odor. It gradually becomes turbid on standing, due to separation of a more basic salt. Heat accelerates precipitation. It is acid to litmus.

Uses—For external use as an *antiseptic* and *astringent* in the treatment of acute vesicular or exudative eczema and other dermatoses. It is also used to make Aluminum Acetate Solution.

Dose—*Topical*, to the skin or mucous membranes, as a wet dressing containing a 1:20 to 1:40 dilution of the Solution.

Aluminum Sulfate

Sulfuric acid, aluminum salt (3:2), hydrate; Cake Alum; Patent Alum; Pearl Alum; Pickle Alum; "Papermaker's Alum"

Aluminum sulfate (2:3) hydrate [17927-65-0] $Al_2(SO_4)_3.xH_2O$; anhydrous [10043-01-3] (342.14).

Preparation—By reacting freshly precipitated aluminum hydroxide with an appropriate quantity of sulfuric acid. The resulting solution is evaporated and allowed to crystallize.

Description—White crystalline powder, shining plates, or crystalline fragments. It is stable in air. It is odorless and has a sweet, mildly astringent taste. The aqueous solution (1 in 20) is acid and has a pH not less than 2.9.

Solubility—1 g in about 1 mL water; insoluble in alcohol.

Uses—A powerful *astringent*, acting much like alum. It is widely used as a *local antiperspirant* and is the effective ingredient in some commercial antiperspirant products. Solutions are usually buffered with sodium aluminum lactate to make them less irritating. Aluminum Sulfate is used for water purification in the "alum flocculation" process. Aluminum Sulfate is a *pharmaceutical necessity* for *Aluminum Subacetate Solution*.

Dose—*Topical*, to the skin, as an 8% solution.

Bismuth Subcarbonate—page 797.

Bismuth Subnitrate—page 794.

Calamine

Iron oxide (Fe_2O_3), mixt. with zinc oxide; Prepared Calamine; Lapis Calaminaria; Artificial Calamine

Calamine [8011-96-9]; contains, after ignition, not less than 98.0% ZnO (81.38).

Preparation—By thoroughly mixing zinc oxide with sufficient ferric oxide (usually 0.5 to 1%) to obtain a product of the desired color.

Calamine was originally obtained by roasting a native zinc carbonate, then known as *calamine;* hence the name. This name is also applied by mineralogists to a native form of zinc silicate, which is not suitable for making medicinal calamine.

Description—Pink powder, all of which passes through a No 100 standard mesh sieve. It is odorless and almost tasteless.

Solubility—Insoluble in water, but dissolves almost completely in mineral acids.

Uses—Similar to those of zinc oxide, being employed chiefly as an *astringent* and in *protective* and soothing ointments and lotions for *sunburn, ivy poisoning*, etc. It is often prescribed by dermatologists to give opacity and a flesh-like color to lotions or ointments.

Dose—*Topical*, to the skin, in various concentrations in lotions and ointments.

Calamine Lotion [Lotio Calaminae]—*Preparation:* Dilute bentonite magma (250 mL) with an equal volume of calcium hydroxide solution. Mix calamine (80 g) and zinc oxide (80 g) intimately with glycerin (20 mL) and about 100 mL of the diluted magma, triturating until a smooth, uniform paste is formed. Gradually incorporate the remainder of the diluted magma. Finally add calcium hydroxide solution (qs) to make 1000 mL, and shake well. If a more viscous consistency in the Lotion is desired, the quantity of bentonite magma may be increased to not more than 400 mL. *Note: Shake thoroughly before dispensing.*

Phenolated Calamine Lotion [Lotio Calaminae Composita; Compound Calamine Lotion]—*Preparation:* Mix liquefied phenol (10 mL) and calamine lotion (990 mL) to make 1000 mL. Commercial preparations also contain 8.4% isopropyl alcohol and have various other modifications. See *Calamine. Note: Shake thoroughly before dispensing.*

Ferric Chloride Tincture—RPS-13, page 491.

Glutaral—page 1160.

Potassium Permanganate—page 1168.

Resorcinol—RPS-16, page 1107.

Silver Nitrate—page 1165.

White Lotion

Lotio Alba; Lotio Sulfurata

Zinc Sulfate	**40 g**
Sulfurated Potash	**40 g**
Purified Water, a sufficient quantity,	
To make	1000 mL

Dissolve zinc sulfate and sulfurated potash separately, each in 450 mL purified water, and filter each solution. Add slowly the sulfurated potash solution to the zinc sulfate solution with constant stirring. Then add the required amount of purified water, and mix.

Note—Prepare freshly and shake thoroughly before dispensing. For further discussion see *Sulfurated Potash* (page 1318).

Uses—An *astringent, protective,* and mild antimicrobial preparation. The astringency is attributable to the zinc ion. The thiosulfates and polysulfides in sulfurated potash exert antibacterial and antifungal actions (see *Sodium Thiosulfate*, RPS-16, page 1176). White lotion is used in the treatment of acne vulgaris.

Dose—*Topical*, to the skin, as required.

Zinc Chloride

Zinc chloride [7646-85-7] $ZnCl_2$ (136.29).

Preparation—By reacting metallic zinc or zinc oxide with hydrochloric acid and evaporating the solution to dryness.

Description—White, or nearly white, odorless, crystalline powder, or as porcelain-like masses, or in moulded pencils. It is very deliquescent. The aqueous solution (1 in 10) is acid to litmus.

Solubility—1 g in 0.5 mL water, about 1.5 mL alcohol, and about 2 mL glycerin. Its solution in water or alcohol is usually slightly turbid, but the turbidity disappears on addition of a small quantity of HCl.

Incompatibilities—Soluble zinc salts are precipitated as zinc hydroxide by alkali hydroxides, including ammonium hydroxide; the precipitate is soluble in an excess of either the fixed or the ammonium hydroxide. *Carbonates, phosphates, oxalates, arsenates,* and *tannin* cause precipitation. The precipitation with sodium borate can be prevented by addition of an amount of glycerin equal in weight to the sodium borate. In weak aqueous solutions, zinc chloride has a tendency to form the insoluble basic salt by hydrolysis and about one-half its weight of ammonium chloride has been used for the purpose of stabilization. Zinc chloride is very *deliquescent*. It has the incompatibilities of chlorides, being precipitated by *silver* and *lead salts*.

Uses—In high concentrations, it is caustic, and has been used as a caustic agent to treat corns, calluses, and warts. In low concentrations it is astringent and mildly antibacterial. It is used in vaginal douches to suppress trichomonal and hemophilus infections. Although it is used in mouthwashes, the contact time is too short, and only an astringent and not antibacterial action results. It also is used to desensitize teeth, but care is required, since it is irritating to the mucous membranes.

Dose—*Topical*, to the teeth, as a **10%** solution; to skin and mucous membranes for astringency and antimicrobial actions, as a **0.2 to 2%** solution; as a caustic, in pencils or as a 30% solution in ethanol.

Zinc Oxide

Flowers of Zinc; Zinc White; Pompholyx; Nihil Album; Lana Philosophica

Zinc oxide [1314-13-2] ZnO (81.38).

Preparation—By heating zinc carbonate at a low red heat until the carbon dioxide and water are expelled.

Description—Very fine, odorless, amorphous, white or yellowish white powder, free from gritty particles. It gradually absorbs carbon dioxide from the air. When strongly heated it assumes a yellow color which disappears on cooling. Its suspension in water is practically neutral.

Solubility—Insoluble in water and alcohol but is soluble in dilute acids, solutions of the alkali hydroxides, and ammonium carbonate solution.

Incompatibilities—Reacts slowly with fatty acids in *oils* and *fats* to produce lumpy masses of zinc oleate, stearate, etc. *Vanishing creams* tend to dry out and crumble. Whenever permissible, it is advisable to levigate it to a smooth paste with a little mineral oil before incorporation into an ointment.

Uses—Has a mild *astringent, protective,* and *antiseptic* action. In the form of its various official ointments and pastes it is widely employed in the treatment of dry skin and such skin disorders and infections as *acne vulgaris, prickly heat, insect stings and bites, ivy poisoning, diaper rash, dandruff, seborrhea, eczema, impetigo, ringworm, psoriasis, varicose ulcers, pruritus.* It is contained in some sunscreens. It is included in some vulvovaginal deodorant preparations and in preparations for the treatment of hemorrhoids. It is also used in dental cements and temporary fillings.

Dose—*Topical*, as a **15 to 25%** lotion, ointment, or paste.

Zinc Phenolsulfonate—RPS-13, page 1252.

Zinc Pyrithione—page 1168.

Zinc Sulfate—page 1165.

Zinc Undecylenate—page 1231.

Other Astringents and Antiperspirants

Aluminum Zirconium Chlorhydrate—*Uses:* Used mainly in antiperspirant products. Because of the propensity of the zirconium to elicit allergic reactions and sarcoid-like granulomas, the compound is not included in aerosols, because of possible pulmonary complications if inhaled. *Dose:* To the axilla, in a concentration not to exceed 20% (as anhydride).

Tannic Acid [Gallotannic Acid; Tannin; Digallic Acid] [1401-55-4]—A tannin usually obtained from nutgalls, the excrescences produced on the young twigs of *Quercus infectoria* Olivier, and allied species of *Quercus* Linné (Fam *Fagaceae*). *Description:* Yellowish white to light brown amorphous powder, glistening scales, or spongy masses; usually odorless with a strong astringent taste; gradually darkens on exposure to air and light. *Solubility:* 1 g in about 0.35 mL water, 1 mL warm glycerin; very soluble in alcohol; practically insoluble in chloroform, ether. *Incompatibilities:* Solutions of tannic acid gradually darken on exposure to air and light through oxidation of phenolic groups to quinoid structures. Tannic acid is incompatible with most enzymes, gums, salts of many metals, and many other substances.

Uses: Tannic acid is used in the treatment of minor burns, for which it is applied as a 5% jelly. It promotes the formation of a firm eschar that helps protect the burned tissue from infection, preserving body fluids, and adding to the comfort of the patient. A disadvantage of tannic acid is that it is not an active germicide. It is also absorbed from denuded surfaces and may cause serious systemic toxicity, particularly liver damage. Furthermore, it causes necrosis of viable tissue in the burned area. It has lost favor as an astringent in the treatment of major burns and is now little used for that purpose.

An ointment or spray of tannic acid has been used in the treatment of bed sores, weeping ulcers, ingrown toenails, and ivy poisoning. In high concentrations, it is used to treat corns, calluses, and warts. For the treatment of athlete's foot it has been placed in Category II. Tannic acid is included in one product for the treatment of toothache, canker, and cold sores.

The tannic acid in tea accounts for the use of strong tea as an internal antidote, presumably for the dual purpose of precipitating toxic alkaloids and hardening the surface of the gastrointestinal mucosa and its mucous layer.

Zinc Acetate [Acetic acid, zinc salt, dihydrate [5970-45-6] $C_4H_6O_4Zn.2H_2O$ (219.50)]—*Preparation:* One method reacts zinc oxide with acetic acid. *Description:* White crystals or granules, having a slight acetous odor and an astringent taste; slightly efflorescent; pH (1 in 20 solution) between 6.0 and 8.0. *Solubility:* Freely soluble in water and boiling alcohol; slightly soluble in alcohol. *Uses:* An *astringent* in low concentrations and an irritant at high concentrations. It also has mild *antibacterial* actions similar to those of *Zinc Sulfate* (page 1165). Zinc acetate is used for treating minor cuts and burns. When applied to cuts, it exerts a *styptic* action. After oral ingestion, it causes emesis, and it is sometimes employed as an *emetic*. It is also a pharmaceutical necessity for zinc-eugenol dental cement for temporary fillings. *Dose: Topical*, **0.2 to 2%**.

Zinc Caprylate [Zinc octanoate (351.79)]—Lustrous scales. Sparingly soluble in boiling water; moderately soluble in boiling alcohol. *Uses:* Zinc caprylate is used in the treatment of athlete's foot. The astringency of the zinc decreases inflammation and wetness. The caprylate has a weak antifungal action. *Dose:* As a 5% ointment.

Zinc Ricinoleate [Zinc [R-(Z)]-12-hydroxy-9-octadecenoate ($C_{18}H_{33}O_3$)$_2$Zn (660.24). *Uses:* Used only as a deodorant for ostomies.

Zirconium Oxide [Zirconium Dioxide; Zirconic Anhydride, Zirconia; ZrO_2 (123.22)]—White powder or crystals. Insoluble in water; soluble in acids. *Uses:* Has weak astringent and adsorptive activity, for which it is employed in topical preparations for treating rhus dermatitis (ivy and oak poisoning). However, it is not only poorly effective for this purpose but it also can cause allergic reactions that may give rise to sarcoid-like granulomas. Consequently, its use should be condemned. Zirconium salts also are subject to the same criticisms.

Irritants, Rubefacients, and Vesicants

The *irritants* are drugs that act locally on the skin and mucous membranes to induce hyperemia, inflammation and, when the action is severe, vesication. Agents that induce only hyperemia are known as *rubefacients*. Rubefaction is accompanied by a feeling of comfort, warmth, and sometimes itching and hyperesthesia. Appropriately low concentrations of directly applied or inhaled vapors of volatile aromatic irritants, such as camphor or menthol, induce a sensation of coolness rather than of warmth. When the irritation is more severe, plasma escapes from the damaged capillaries and forms blisters (vesicles). Agents that induce blisters are known as *vesicants*. Most rubefacients also may be vesicants in higher concentrations. Certain irritants may be relatively selective for various tissues or cell types, so that hypersecretion of the surface, seborrheic abscesses, paresthesia or other effects may be noted in the absence of appreciable hyperemia.

Irritants have been used empirically for many centuries, probably even prehistorically. They may be employed for counterirritation, the mechanism of which is poorly understood. A moderate to severe pain may be obscured by a milder pain arising from areas of irritation appropriately placed to induce reflex stimulation of certain organs or systems, especially respiratory. Sensory and visible effects of irritation sometimes give the patient assurance that he is receiving effective medication. Taken internally, many irritants exert either an emetic or laxative action. Irritant laxatives are listed on page 800. A few irritants, especially cantharides, on absorption into the blood stream irritate the urogenital tract and consequently have been dangerously employed as *aphrodisiacs*. Certain irritants also possess a healing action on wounds, possibly the result of local stimulation. Many condiments are irritants. In high concentrations, many irritants are corrosive.

Alcohol—page 1159.

Alcohol, Rubbing—page 1160.

Ammonia Spirit, Aromatic—page 1507.

Anthralin

1,8,9-Anthracenetriol; Dithranol;
Dioxyanthranol; Cignolin; Anthra-Derm (*Dermik*); Lasan (*Stiefel*)

1,8-Dihydroxyanthranol [480-22-8] $C_{14}H_{10}O_3$ (226.23).

Preparation—Anthraquinone is sulfonated to the 1,8-disulfonic acid, which is isolated from the reaction mixture and then heated with a calcium hydroxide-calcium chloride mixture to form 1,8-dihydroxy-9,10-anthraquinone, which is reduced with tin and HCl to anthralin.

Description—Yellowish brown, crystalline powder; odorless and tasteless; melts between 175° and 181°.

Solubility—Insoluble in water; slightly soluble in alcohol; soluble in chloroform; slightly soluble in ether.

Uses—Although anthralin has long been considered to be an irritant, its principal therapeutic action is the reduction of epidermal DNA synthesis and mitotic activity. It is used in the treatment of *psoriasis*, *eczema*, and other *chronic dermatoses*. It is usually used in combination with ultraviolet light and a daily coal tar "bath." To avoid harmful irritation, medicaments containing anthralin should not be used on the face, scalp, genitalia, or intertriginous skin areas; they should not be applied to blistered, raw, or oozing areas of the skin, and should be kept from the eyes, since they may cause severe conjunctivitis, keratitis, or corneal opacity. Renal irritation, casts, and albuminuria may result from systemically absorbed anthralin. The

hands should be washed immediately after applying medication. A reversible slight discoloration of the skin may occur.

Dose—*Topical*, to the skin, as a 0.1 to 1% ointment. The concentration should be low initially and increased only as necessary.

Dosage Forms—Ointment: 0.1, 0.25, 0.5, and 1%.

Benzoin Tincture, Compound—page 776.

Camphor

Bicyclo [2.2.1] heptane-2-one, 1,7,7-trimethyl-, 2-Camphanone;
Gum Camphor; Laurel Camphor

2-Bornanone [76-22-2] $C_{10}H_{16}O$ (152.24). A ketone obtained from *Cinnamomum camphora* (Linné) Nees et Ebermaier (Fam *Lauraceae*) (Natural Camphor) or produced synthetically (Synthetic Camphor).

Preparation—Natural crude camphor may be obtained by steam distilling chips of the camphor tree; the crude camphor so obtained is purified, usually by sublimation.

One method of producing synthetic camphor starts with *pinene* [$C_{10}H_{16}$], a hydrocarbon obtained from turpentine oil. The pinene is saturated with hydrogen chloride at 0° forming bornyl chloride [$C_{10}H_{17}Cl$]. On heating the bornyl chloride with sodium acetate and glacial acetic acid it is converted into isobornyl acetate, which is subsequently hydrolyzed to isobornyl alcohol [$C_{10}H_{17}OH$] and oxidized with chromic acid to camphor.

Synthetic camphor resembles natural camphor in most of its properties except that it is a racemic mixture and therefore lacks optical activity.

When camphor is mixed in approximately molecular proportions with chloral hydrate, menthol, phenol, or thymol, liquefaction ensues; such mixtures are known as *eutectic mixtures* (see page 180).

Description—Colorless or white crystals, granules, or crystalline masses; or as colorless to white, translucent, tough masses. It has a penetrating, characteristic odor, a pungent, aromatic taste, and is readily pulverizable in the presence of a little alcohol, ether, or chloroform. Specific gravity about 0.99. It melts between 174° and 179° and slowly volatilizes at ordinary temperature and in steam.

Solubility—1 g in about 800 mL water, 1 mL alcohol, about 0.5 mL chloroform, and 1 mL ether; freely soluble in carbon disulfide, solvent hexane, and fixed and volatile oils.

Incompatibilities—Forms a liquid or a soft mass when rubbed with *chloral hydrate, hydroquinone, menthol, phenol, phenyl salicylate, resorcinol, salicylic acid, thymol*, and other substances. It is precipitated from its alcoholic solution by the addition of water. It is precipitated from camphor water by the addition of soluble salts.

Uses—Locally, weakly *analgesic*, mildly *analgesic* (*antipruritic*), and *rubefacient* when rubbed on the skin. The spirit is applied locally to allay itching caused by insect stings. It is also used as a counterirritant in humans for *inflamed joints*, *sprains*, and *rheumatic* and other *inflammatory* conditions such as colds in the throat and chest. Although the patient may feel improved, the inflammation is not affected. However, reflexly induced local vasoconstriction may mediate a mild nasopharyngeal decongestant effect.

When taken internally in small amounts it produces a feeling of warmth and comfort in the gastrointestinal tract, and was therefore formerly much used as a *carminative*. Systemically, camphor is a reflexly active *circulatory* and *respiratory stimulant*. However, its use as a stimulant is obsolete. It also possesses a slight *expectorant* action.

Concentrations above 11% are not safe. Toxicity consists of nausea and vomiting, headache, feeling of warmth, confusion, delirium, convulsions, coma, and respiratory arrest.

Camphor is a pharmaceutical necessity for *Flexible Collodion* and *Camphorated Opium Tincture*.

Dose—*Topical*, to skin, as a **0.1** to **3**% lotion or ointment, or **10**% tincture (spirit), no more than 3 to 4 times a day. For topical analgesia, concentrations of 0.1 to 3% are used; for counterirritation, 3 to 11%.

Camphor Spirit is an alcohol solution containing, in each 100 mL, about 10 g $C_{10}H_{16}O$.

Coal Tar

Pix Carbonis; Prepared Coal Tar BP; Pix Lithanthracis; Gas Tar

The tar obtained as a by-product during the destructive distillation of bituminous coal.

Description—Nearly black, viscous liquid, heavier than water, with a characteristic naphthalene-like odor and a sharp burning taste. On ignition it burns with a reddish, luminous, and very sooty flame, leaving not more than 2% of residue.

Solubility—Only slightly soluble in water, to which it imparts its characteristic odor and taste and a faintly alkaline reaction; partially dissolved by alcohol, acetone, methanol, solvent hexane, carbon disulfide, chloroform, or ether; to the extent of about 95% by benzene, and entirely by nitrobenzene with the exception of a small amount of suspended matter.

Uses—A *local irritant* used in the treatment of *chronic skin diseases*. Like anthralin, its primary action is to decrease the epidermal synthesis of DNA and hence to suppress hyperplasia.

Occasionally, coal tar may cause rash, burning sensation, or other manifestations of excessive irritation or sensitization. Since photosensitization may occur, the treated area should be protected from sunlight. Coal tar should be kept away from the eyes and from raw, weeping, or blistered surfaces. Temporary discoloration of the skin may occur.

Dose—*Topical*, to the skin, in a **1%** ointment or shampoo or **20%** solution, 2 or 3 times a day. Nonofficial ointments may contain much higher than 1% coal tar. Emulsions for the bath contain 50%.

Creosote—RPS-15, page 1102.

Eucalyptol—page 1291.

Eucalyptus Oil—page 1286.

Green Soap—page 786.

Green Soap Tincture—page 786.

Histamine Phosphate—page 1125.

Ichthammol

Ammonium Ichthosulfonate; Sulfonated Bitumen; Ictiol; Ichthymall (*Mallinckrodt*), Ichthyol (*Stiefel*)

Ichthammol [8029-68-3]. It is obtained by the destructive distillation of certain bituminous schists, sulfonating the distillate, and neutralizing the product with ammonia.

Ichthammol yields not less than 2.5% of NH_3 (ammonia) and not less than 10% of total S (sulfur).

Constituents—Ichthammol belongs to a class of preparations containing as essential constituents salts or compounds of a mixture of acids designated by the group name *sulfoichthyolic acid*, formed by sulfonation of the oil obtained in the destructive distillation of certain bituminous shales. Sulfoichthyolic acid is characterized by a high sulfur content, the sulfur existing largely in the form of sulfonates, sulfones, and sulfides.

Description and Properties—Reddish brown to brownish black, viscous fluid, with a strong, characteristic, empyreumatic odor.

Solubility—Miscible with water, glycerin, and fixed oils or fats, but is partially soluble in alcohol or ether.

Incompatibilities—Becomes granular in the presence of *acids* or under the influence of *heat*. In solution, it is precipitated by acids and *acid salts* as a dark, sticky mass. *Alkalies* liberate ammonia. Many *metallic salts* cause precipitation.

Uses—A mildly astringent irritant and local antibacterial agent with moderate emollient and demulcent properties. It is used alone or in combination with other antiseptics for the treatment of skin disorders such as *insect stings and bites*, *erysipelas*, *psoriasis*, and *lupus erythematosus*, and to produce healing in *chronic inflammations*. It is also used to treat *inflammation* and *boils* in the external ear canal. Medical opinion is divided as to whether this agent is useful. In higher concentrations, irritation is frequent, and rashes may develop. It should be kept away from the eyes and other sensitive surfaces. It has been reported to cause hyperepithelialization, an action that would be counterproductive in the treatment of psoriasis.

Dose—*Topical*, to the skin or external ear canal, as a **10%** ointment.

Menthol

Cyclohexanol, 5-methyl-2-(1-methylethyl)-, Peppermint Camphor

p-Menthan-3-ol [1490-04-6] $C_{10}H_{20}O$ (156.27). An alcohol obtained from diverse mint oils or prepared synthetically. Menthol may be levorotatory [(−)-Menthol] from natural or synthetic sources, or racemic [(±)-Menthol].

Preparation—Peppermint oil owes its odor chiefly to menthol, which is obtained from it by fractional distillation and allowing the proper fraction to crystallize, or by chromatographic processes.

Among numerous methods of synthesis of an optically inactive menthol, the most popular involves the catalytic hydrogenation of thymol (obtained from natural sources or synthesized from m-cresol or cresylic acid).

The difficulty in the synthesis of (−)-menthol arises from the fact that menthol contains three asymmetric carbon atoms, and there are thus eight stereoisomers, designated as (−)- and (+)-menthol, (−)- and (+)-isomenthol, (−)- and (+)-neomenthol, and (−)- and (+)-neoisomenthol. To obtain a product meeting USP requirements, it is necessary to separate (−)-menthol from its stereoisomers, for which purpose fractional crystallization, distillation under reduced pressure, or esterification may be used. The other stereoisomers differ from the official (−)-menthol in physical properties and possibly to some extent in pharmacological action.

Description—Colorless, hexagonal, usually needle-like crystals, or fused masses, or a crystalline powder, with a pleasant, peppermint-like odor. (−)-Menthol melts between 41° and 44°, and (±)-Menthol congeals at 27° to 28°.

Solubility—Very soluble in alcohol, chloroform, ether; freely soluble in glacial acetic acid, mineral oil, and in fixed and volatile oils; slightly soluble in water.

Identification—When mixed with about an equal weight of camphor, chloral hydrate, phenol, or thymol, Menthol forms a "eutectic" mixture liquefying at room temperature.

Incompatibilities—Produces a liquid or soft mass when triturated with *camphor, phenol, chloral hydrate, resorcinol, thymol*, and numerous other substances.

Labeling—The label on the container indicates whether the Menthol is levorotatory or racemic.

Uses—In low concentrations, menthol selectively stimulates the sensory nerve endings for cold and hence causes a sensation of coolness. Some local analgesic effects also accompany this effect. Higher concentrations not only stimulate sensory endings for heat and other pain, but also may cause some irritation. Consequently, there may first be a sensation of coolness then a slight prickly and burning sensation.

The local analgesia and the sensation of coolness are employed in the treatment of insect bites and stings, itching (antipruretic effect), minor burns and sunburn, hemorrhoids, toothache, cankers, cold sores, and sore throat. The local analgesic effect also is the probable basis of the antitussive use, although the value of menthol as an antitussive remains unproved. Care must be taken to avoid the inhalation of irritant concentrations. In ophthalmology, the mild analgesia and cooling sensation appear to relieve scleral and conjunctival irritation, but it has the disadvantage of masking the sense of a foreign body on the eye or in the conjunctival sack. In the treatment of colds and allergic coryza and rhinorrhea, a nasal spray or the inhalation of menthol not only appears to exert a local analgesia but also to cause decongestion, possibly through local vasoconstriction. The contribution of a placebo effect to some of these effects cannot be discounted.

Menthol is incorporated into irritant products used to treat acne vulgaris, dandruff, seborrhea, calluses, corns, warts, and athlete's foot and in vaginal preparations to lessen the sense of irritation.

Whatever effects the rubbing of menthol-containing ointment on the chest have to relieve pulmonary congestion in colds and allergy are attributable to counterirritation and placebo effects. Menthol is also contained in counterirritants for the treatment of muscle aches.

Dose—*Topical*, to the skin, as a **0.1 to 2%** lotion or ointment; to the throat, as a 0.08 to 0.12% lozenge. *Inhalation*, **15 mL** of 1% liquid or **10 mL** of 2% ointment per quart of water, to be dispensed by steam inhalation.

Methyl Salicylate—page 1287.

Resorcinol—RPS-16, page 1107.

Resorcinol Ointment, Compound—RPS-16, page 1107.

Resorcinol Monoacetate—RPS-16, page 1107.

Storax—page 1318.

Tolu Balsam—page 1290.

Turpentine Oil, Rectified—RPS-16, page 808.

Other Irritants, Rubefacients, and Vesicants

Cantharidin [(3aα,4β,7β,7aα-Hexahydro-3a,7a-dimethyl-4,7-epoxy-isobenzofuran-1,3-dione[56-25-7] $C_{10}H_{12}O_4$ (186.21)]—The active principle of *Cantharides*. *Description and Solubility:* White platelets soluble 1 g in 40 mL acetone, 65 mL chloroform, 560 mL ether, 150 mL ethyl acetate; also soluble in oils. *Uses:* Cantharidin produces intradermal vesiculation. It is used to remove warts, particularly the periungual type. It is applied under an occlusive bandage. The vesicle eventually breaks, becomes encrusted and falls off in one to two weeks. *Dose:* Topical, to the wart, as a 0.7% solution.

Capsicum—The dried ripe fruit of *capsicum frutescens* L, *Solonaceae*, which contains less than 1% of capsaicin [(*E*)-*N*-[4-Hydroxy-3-methoxyphenyl)methyl]-8-methyl-6-nonaneamide[404-86-4] $C_{18}H_{27}NO_3$ (305.40)], which is the active ingredient. *Uses:* The active ingredients of capsicum are mildly irritant, causing erythemia and a feeling of warmth without vesication. Capsicum preparations are used as counterirritants. *Dose:* The equivalent of 0.025 to 0.25% of capsicum applied to the skin no more than 3 or 4 times a day.

Juniper Tar [Cade Oil]—The empyreumatic volatile oil obtained from the woody portions of *Juniperus oxycedrus* Linné (Fam *Pinaceae*). *Description:* Dark brown, clear, thick liquid, having a tarry odor and a faintly aromatic, bitter taste. *Solubility:* Very slightly soluble in water; 1 volume dissolves in 9 volumes of alcohol; dissolves in 3 volumes of ether, leaving a slight, flocculent residue; miscible with chloroform.

Uses: A mildly irritant oil that is employed as a topical antipruritic in several chronic dermatologic disorders, such as *psoriasis*, *atopic dermatitis*, *pruritus*, *eczema*, and *seborrhea*. Since it is irritant to the conjunctiva and also may cause chemosis of the cornea, care should be taken to keep the tar out of the eyes. Systemic absorption may result in renal damage. *Dose: Topical*, as 1 to 5% ointment applied once a day; it is also used as a 4% shampoo or 34% bath.

Methyl Nicotinate [Methyl 3-pyridinecarboxylate, Midalgan; $C_7H_7NO_2$ (137.13)]—*Description and Solubility:* Low melting, white crystals; soluble in water, alcohol and benzene. *Uses:* A vasodilator and mild irritant used for counterirritation. Erythema and cutaneous warming occur at the site of application. It does not cause vesication in therapeutic concentrations. *Dose:* Topical, to the skin, as a 0.25 to 1.0% solution no more than 3 or 4 times a day.

Peruvian Balsam [Peru Balsam; Balsam of Peru; Indian Balsam; Black Balsam]—Obtained from *Myroxylon pereirae* (Royle) Klotzsch (Fam. *Leguminosae*). *Constituents:* Contains from 60 to 64% of a volatile oil termed *cinnamein* and from 20 to 28% of *resin*. Cinnamein is a mixture of compounds, among which the following have been identified: The esters *benzyl benzoate, benzyl cinnamate, cinnamyl cinnamate (styracin)*, and the alcohol *peruviol* (considered by some to be identical with the sesquiterpene alcohol *nerolidol*, $C_{15}H_{26}O$) as ester, free *cinnamic acid*; about 0.05% of *vanillin*; and a trace of *coumarin*. The resin consists of benzoic and cinnamic acid. *Description and Solubility:* Dark brown, viscid liquid. It is transparent and appears reddish brown in thin layers, has an aggreable odor resembling vanilla, a bitter, acrid taste, with a persistent after-taste, and is free from stringiness or stickiness. It does not harden on exposure to air. Specific gravity 1.150 to 1.170. Nearly insoluble in water, but soluble in alcohol, chloroform, and glacial acetic acid, with not more than an opalescence; only partly soluble in ether and solvent hexane. *Uses: A local irritant and vulnerary*. It is a valuable dressing to promote growth of epithelial cells in the treatment of *indolent ulcers*, *wounds* and certain *skin diseases*, eg, scabies. In combination with dimethicone, it is used in the treatment of decubitus ulcer, intertrigo, and diaper rash. It is an ingredient in suppositories used in the treatment of hemorrhoids and anal pruritus. Allergic reactions to Peruvian balsam occasionally occur. Ointments containing both Peruvian balsam and sulfur present a problem in compounding, since the resinous part of the balsam tends to separate. This difficulty may be overcome by mixing the balsam with an equal amount of castor oil, prior to incorporating it into the base; or alternatively, by mixing it with solid petroxolin. *Dose: Topical*, to skin as required, usually in ointment or in alcohol solution.

Pine Tar [Pix Pini; Pix Liquida; Tar]—The product obtained by the destructive distillation of the wood of *Pinus palustris* Miller, or of other species of *Pinus* Linné (Fam *Pinaceae*). *Preparation:* Tar is usually obtained as a by-product in the manufacture of charcoal or acetic acid from wood. It is a complex mixture of phenolic bodies for the most part insoluble in water. Among these are *cresol, phlorol, guaiacol, pyrocatechol, caerulignol*, and *pyrogallol* ethers. Traces of *phenol* and *cresols* are also present as well as hydrocarbons of the paraffin and benzene series. *Description:* Very viscid, blackish brown liquid. It is translucent in thin layers, but becomes granular and opaque with age. It has an empyreumatic, terebinthinate odor, a sharp, empyreumatic taste, and is more dense than water. Its solution is acid to litmus. *Solubility:* Miscible with alcohol, ether, chloroform, glacial acetic acid, and with fixed and volatile oils. It is slightly soluble in water, the solution being pale yellowish to yellowish brown. *Uses:* Externally as a mild *irritant* and *local antibacterial* agent in chronic *skin diseases*, especially eczema and psoriasis. The volatile constituents of tar are claimed to be *expectorant* but their efficacy is unproven; tar inhalations were formerly used for this purpose.

Sclerosing Agents

A number of irritant drugs are sufficiently active to damage cells but are not sufficiently active to destroy large numbers of cells at the site of application. Such agents promote fibrosis and are used to strengthen supporting structures and to close inguinal rings, etc. The intimal surface of blood vessels may break down under attack by such agents and thus initiate thrombosis, which may be an undesirable side effect. This action is the basis of the use of sclerosing agents in the reduction of varicose veins and hemorrhoids. Sclerosing agents are generally regarded as obsolete. They can be harmful when improperly used and sometimes even when used with caution.

Sclerosing Agents

Morrhuate Sodium Injection—A sterile solution of the sodium salts of the fatty acids of cod liver oil. It contains 50 mg of sodium morrhuate/mL. A suitable antimicrobial agent, not to exceed 0.5%, and ethyl or benzyl alcohol, not to exceed 3%, may be added. *Note: Sodium Morrhuate Injection may show a separation of solid matter on standing. Do not use the material if such solid does not dissolve completely upon warming. Preparation:* By heating cod liver oil with alcoholic sodium hydroxide until completely saponified. After dilution with water the al-

cohol is removed by distillation. Dilute H_2SO_4 is then added to the aqueous solution, and the liberated organic acids are separated or preferably extracted with a suitable immiscible solvent such as ether. Just sufficient aqueous NaOH is then added to neutralize the acids. About 20 mg of benzyl alcohol/mL of the Injection is usually added to lessen the pain of injection. *Uses:* Formerly widely used as a *sclerosing* and *fibrosing agent* for obliterating *varicose veins*. Irritants of this type have also been employed for closure of hernial rings, fibrosing of uncomplicated hemorrhoids, the removal of condylomata acuminata, and in other conditions where the ultimate objective is production of fibrous tissue. *Dose: Intravenous*, by special injection, 0.5 to 5 mL of a 5% injection to a localized area; *usual*, 1 mL. *Dosage Forms:* 2 and 5 mL.

Sodium Tetradecyl Sulfate [7-Ethyl-2-methyl-4-undecanol hydrogen sulfate sodium salt [139-88-8] $C_{14}H_{29}NaO_4S$ (316.43); STS; Sotradecol Sodium (*Elkins-Sinn*)]—*Preparation:* One method reacts the corresponding alcohol with $ClSO_3H$ and neutralizes the resulting hydrogen sulfate ester with Na_2CO_3. *Description and Solubility:* A white, waxy, odorless solid. Soluble in water, alcohol, and ether. *Uses:* A *sclerosing agent* similar in action to sodium morrhuate. It was formerly widely used as a buffered solution in the *obliteration of varicose veins and internal hemorrhoids*. For such purposes, the solution is injected directly into the vein. Injection outside of the vein may cause sloughing. For this reason, the substance is not used to close inguinal rings. The principal untoward effect is pain immediately upon injection, although brief, mild anaphylactoid and idiosyncratic responses rarely occur. Because the substance is an anionic surface-active agent, it is also used as a wetting agent to promote spreading of certain topical antiseptics. *Dose:* By injection directly into the target vein, as a 1 or 3% solution, depending on the size of the vein. The volume then to be injected at any one site varies from 0.2 to 2.0 mL, depending on the concentration and the number of previous injections at the site, the larger volumes being given only after several previous injections. No more than 10 mL of the 3% solution or 6 mL of the 5% solution should be given at any one sitting. The interval between injections varies from 5 to 7 days. *Dosage Form:* Injection: 1 and 3% in 2-mL ampuols.

Caustics and Escharotics

Any topical agent that causes destruction of tissues at the site of application is a *caustic* (or corrosive).

Caustics may be used to induce desquamation of cornified epithelium ("keratolytic" action) and are therefore used. to destroy warts, condylomata, keratoses, certain moles, and hyperplastic tissues.

If the agent also precipitates the proteins of the cell and the inflammation exudate, there is formed a scab (or eschar), which is later organized into a scar; such an agent is an *escharotic* (or cauterizant). Most, but not all, caustics are also escharotic. Furthermore, certain caustics, especially the alkalies, redissolve precipitated proteins, partly by hydrolysis, so that no scab or only a soft scab forms; such agents penetrate deeply and are generally unsuitable for therapeutic use. Escharotics are sometimes employed to seal cutaneous and aphthous ulcers, wounds, etc. Since most escharotics are bactericidal, it was formerly thought that chemical cauterization effected sterilization; however, sterilization is not always achieved, especially by those agents which remain bound to the protein precipitate. The growth of certain bacteria may even be favored by the chemically induced necrosis and by the protection of the scab.

Acetic Acid, Glacial—page 1158.

Alum—page 777.

Aluminum Chloride—page 778.

Gentian Violet—page 1167.

Phenol—page 1315.

Podophyllum

Mandrake; May Apple

The dried rhizome and roots of *Podophyllum peltatum* Linné (Fam. *Berberidaceae*); it yields not less than 5% of podophyllum resin.

Constituents—From 3 to 6% of resin along with up to 1% of quercetin and podophyllotoxin and peltatin glucosides. At least sixteen different compounds have been isolated and characterized. The aglycone *podophyllotoxin* [$C_{22}H_{22}O_8$] is the lactone of 1-hydroxy-2 - (hydroxymethyl) - 6,7 -methylenedioxy -4- (3′,4′,5′-trimethoxyphenyl)-1,2,3,4-tetrahydronaphthalene-3-carboxylic acid. Hydrolytic rupture of the lactone ring yields *podophyllic acid* [$C_{22}H_{24}O_9$], the 2,3-*trans* form of which is *podophyllinic acid* while the 2,3-*cis* form is *picropodophyllinic acid.*

Although podophyllotoxin has been demonstrated to possess marked caustic, cathartic, and toxic properties, it is believed that not it, but an amorphous *resin*, called *podophylloresin*, is the chief cathartic principle of the drug. However, podophyllotoxin is safer and will probably ultimately replace the crude preparations.

Uses—The chief therapeutic use in humans is as a *caustic* for removal of *warts, calluses, fibroids, condyloma acuminatum,* and *papillomas* or as a source of the more effective resin. It is not selective enough against skin cancer to be safely used. It was formerly used as a *cathartic*. Its actions differ from those of most caustics in that action is neither direct nor immediate; rather, cell division is arrested and other cellular processes are impaired, which leads eventually to the disruption of the cells and erosion of the tissue. In appropriate concentration, normal tissue is spared.

Dose and Dosage Forms—Topical, to the affected area, as a 5 or 25% tincture or liquid containing various other ingredients. See *Podophyllum Resin* and *Podophyllum Resin Topical Solution*, below.

Podophyllum Resin [Podophylin] is the powdered mixture of resins removed from podophyllum by percolation with alcohol and subsequent precipitation from the concentrated percolate on addition to acidified water. *Description:* An amorphous powder, varying in color from light brown to greenish yellow, turning darker when subjected to a temperature exceeding 25° or when exposed to light. It has a slight, peculiar, faintly bitter taste. *Solubility:* Dissolves in alcohol with only a slight opalescence; its alcohol solution is acid to litmus paper; only partially soluble in ether and in chloroform. *Caution—Podophyllum Resin is highly irritating to the eye and to mucous membranes in general. Uses:* See *Podophyllum* (above). The resin is superior to the crude podophyllum. The resin is also an unpredictable and frequently toxic irritant cathartic; consequently, its cathartic use is mainly restricted to animals. *Dose: Topical,* as a 12 to 25% dispersion in compound benzoin tincture or as a solution in ethanol once a week. It is commonly suspended in mineral oil, 25% for warts and 1–12% for papillomata of the bladder. Solutions in ethanol (20%) have also been employed in the treatment of warts.

Podophyllum Resin Topical Solution is prepared by mixing 25 g of the alcohol-soluble extractive of podophyllum resin in alcohol and 10 g of the alcohol-soluble extractive of benzoin in alcohol and diluting with alcohol to make 100 mL. *Caution—This solution is highly irritating to the eye and to mucous membranes in general. Care must be exercised when applying the drug so that the adjacent area is not affected. Use:* As topical application to certain papillomas, 1 to 5 times a day.

Potassium Hydroxide

Caustic Potash; Lye; Potash Lye

Potassium hydroxide [1310-58-3] contains not less than 85.0% of total alkali, calculated as KOH (56.11), including not more than 3.5% of K_2CO_3 (138.21).

Caution—Exercise great care in handling Potassium Hydroxide, as it rapidly destroys tissues. Do not handle it with bare hands.

Preparation—By electrolysis of a solution of potassium chloride in a diaphragm cell that does not allow liberated chlorine to react with the potassium hydroxide.

Potassium hydroxide, known commercially as *caustic potash*, is prepared in the form of sticks, pellets, flakes, or fused masses. Sticks or pellets are made by evaporating a solution of potassium hydroxide to a fluid of oily consistency and then pouring the hot liquid into suitable molds in which it solidifies.

Description—White, or nearly white, fused masses, small pellets, flakes, sticks, and other forms. It is hard and brittle and shows a crystalline fracture. Exposed to air it rapidly absorbs carbon dioxide and moisture, and deliquesces. It melts at about 360–380°. When dissolved in water or alcohol, or when its solution is treated with an acid much heat is generated. Solutions of potassium hydroxide, even when highly diluted, are strongly alkaline.

Solubility—1 g in 1 mL water, 3 mL alcohol, and 2.5 mL glycerin at 25°. It is very soluble in boiling alcohol.

Incompatibilities—Bases react with *acids* to form salts, liberate alkaloids from aqueous solutions of *alkaloidal salts*, and promote various hydrolysis reactions such as the decomposition of *chloral hydrate* into chloroform and a formate or the breakdown of *salol* into phenol and a salicylate.

Only the alkali hydroxides are appreciably soluble in water. Nearly all common *metals* will be precipitated as hydroxides when solutions of their salts are added to solutions of the alkali hydroxides. Certain hydroxides, however, notably those of aluminum, zinc, arsenic, and lead, will dissolve in excess of sodium or potassium hydroxide.

Uses—A *caustic*, principally in veterinary practice. The end of a stick of potassium hydroxide may be inserted into a section of rubber tubing, or wrapped several times with tin foil, to avoid cauterizing the fingers of the operator. It is used also as a *pharmaceutical necessity* in several pharmacopeial preparations.

Salicylic Acid—page 785.

Silver Nitrate—page 1165.

Toughened Silver Nitrate

Molded Silver Nitrate; Fused Silver Nitrate; Silver Nitrate Pencils; Caustic Stick or Pencil; Lunar Caustic

Contains not less than 94.5% of silver nitrate [7761-88-8] $AgNO_3$ (169.87), the remainder consisting of silver chloride (AgCl).

Preparation—By fusing silver nitrate with addition of HCl to produce a small amount of silver chloride, which has the effect of toughening the fused mass and making the sticks less brittle, and casting in silver molds.

Description—White, crystalline masses, generally molded as pencils or cones; breaks with a fibrous fracture; becomes gray or grayish black on exposure to light; its solution is neutral to litmus.

Solubility—Soluble in water to the extent of its nitrate content (there is always a residue of silver chloride); partially soluble in alcohol; slightly soluble in ether.

Uses—In the cauterization of wounds and for the removal of warts and other abnormal epithelium, granulation tissues, etc. Silver nitrate is toughened to lessen the danger of breakage when applied inside the oral cavity. It is usually provided in pencil-shaped applicators that may be sharpened. Death has resulted more than once through the careless use of silver nitrate cones in cauterizing the throat, the cone having slipped and then swallowed by the patient. Other caustics are generally preferred.

Dose—*Topical*, to the skin, after the tip is dipped in water.

Small wooden sticks, dipped in fused toughened silver nitrate, sufficient for one application, are sometimes used, as are 3- or 6-inch wooden sticks on which is fused a mixture of 75% silver nitrate and 25% potassium nitrate. See *Medicated Pencils* (RPP XII, page 428).

Trichloroacetic Acid

Acetic acid, trichloro-,

$$CCl_3COOH$$

Trichloroacetic acid [76-03-9] or $C_2HCl_3O_2$ (163.39).

Preparation—This acid is usually made by oxidizing chloral hydrate with fuming nitric acid.

Description—Colorless, deliquescent crystals having a slight, characteristic odor. Melts at about 58° and boils at 196°–197°.

Solubility—1 g in about 0.1 mL water; soluble in alcohol and ether.

Uses—Precipitates proteins, and it is used as a *caustic* on the skin or mucous membranes to destroy local lesions and for treatment of various dermatologic diseases. Its chief use is to destroy ordinary warts and juvenile flat warts. It is extensively employed as a precipitant of protein in the chemical analysis of body fluids and tissue extracts, also as a decalcifier and fixative in microscopy.

Caution—*Trichloroacetic Acid is highly corrosive to the skin.*

Dose—*Topical*, to the skin, as a 15 to 100% w/v solution, carefully applied with a cotton-tipped applicator or glass rod. Concentrations above 50% are not recommended.

Zinc Chloride—page 779.

Other Caustics and Escharotics

Dichloroacetic Acid [Dichloroacetic acid $C_2H_2Cl_2O_2$ (128.95)]—Pungent liquid miscible with water, alcohol, and ether. *Uses:* See *Trichloroacetic Acid.*

Ferric Subsulfate [Monsel's Solution; the molecular formula approximates $Fe_4O(SO_4)_5$]—*Preparation:* By the action of hot sulfuric and nitric acids on ferrous sulfate (*US Dispensatory*, 25th ed, page 574). *Uses:* Used mainly as a hemostatic in minor surgical procedures. The chemical coagulates tissue and blood proteins at the site of application, the coagulum closing the bleeding vessels. Electrocautery at the same site may cause the precipitation of elemental iron and insoluble iron compounds with a resulting cosmetic disfigurement ("tatoo"). *Dose:* Topical, to the site, as a solution containing 21% iron.

Nitric Acid—Contains 67–71% HNO_3. It is a fuming liquid, very caustic, and has a characteristic, highly irritating odor. It boils at 120° C; specific gravity about 1.41. It is miscible with water. *Uses:* As a cauterizing agent for the immediate sterilization of dangerously infected wounds, such as the bite from a rabid animal; it does not penetrate too deeply and forms a firm eschar.

Keratolytics (Desquamating Agents)

The epidermis consists of layers of flat cells, called *stratified squamous epithelial cells*. They are bound together by desmosomes and penetrating tonofibrils, both of which largely consist of keratin. The outer layer of the epidermis, the cornified epithelium or stratum corneum, is made up of the collapsed ghosts of the squamous cells and, as such, is principally a tight network of keratin and lipoprotein. Certain fungi, especially the dermatophytes, utilize keratin and therefore reside in the stratum corneum in those places where the degree of hydration and the pH are sufficiently high. One way such mycoses may be suppressed is that of removal of the stratum corneum, a process that is called *desquamation*. Certain chemical substances, especially among phenols and sulfhydryl compounds, loosen the keratin and thus facilitate desquamation. These substances are called *keratolytics*. Aqueous maceration of the stratum corneum also favors desquamation. In addition to the treatment of epidermophytosis, keratolytics are used to thin hyperkeratotic areas. Most keratolytics are irritant. Irritants also can cause desquamation by causing damage to and swelling of the basal cells.

Hydrous Benzoyl Peroxide

Peroxide, dibenzoyl; Epi-Clear (*Squibb*); Oxy-5 (*USV*); Persadox (*Owen*); Panoxyl (*Steifel*); Vanoxide (*Dermik*)

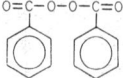

Benzoyl peroxide [94-36-0] $C_{14}H_{10}O_4$ (242.23); contains 65–82% of benzoyl peroxide; also contains about 26% of water for the purpose of reducing flammability and shock sensitivity.

Preparation—Benzoyl chloride is reacted with a cold solution of sodium peroxide.

Description—White, granular powder, having a characteristic odor.

Solubility—Sparingly soluble in water and alcohol; soluble in acetone, chloroform, and ether.

Caution—It may explode at temperatures higher than 60° or cause fires in the presence of reducing substances. Store it in the original container, treated to reduce static charges. Do not transfer it to metal or glass containers fitted with friction tops. Do not return unused material to its original container, but destroy it by treatment with NaOH solution (1 in 10) until addition of a crystal of KI results in no release of free iodine.

Uses—Possesses mild antibacterial properties, especially against anaerobic bacteria. It is also mildly irritant, and it exerts moderate keratolytic and antiseborrheic actions. Its principal use is in the treatment of *acne vulgaris* and *acne rosaceae*, but it is also used in the treatment of athlete's foot.

Benzoyl peroxide causes stinging or burning sensations for a brief time after application; with continued use these effects mostly disappear. After 1 or 2 weeks of use there may be a sudden excess dryness of the skin and peeling. The drug must be kept away from the eyes, and from inflamed, denuded or highly sensitive skin, such as the circumoral areas and neck, and the skin of children. It should not be used in conjunction with harsh abrasive skin cleansers. Benzoyl peroxide can cause contact dermatitis. It can bleach hair and fabrics.

Dose—*Topical*, as a **5** to **10**% cream, gel, or lotion, initially applied once a day, then 2 to 4 times a day.

Dosage Forms—Cream: 5 and 10%; Gel: 5 and 10%; Lotion: 5 and 10%.

Fluorouracil—page 1149.

Resorcinol—RPS-16, page 1107.

Resorcinol Ointment, Compound—RPS-16, page 1107.

Salicylic Acid

Benzoic acid, 2-hydroxy-, *o*-Hydroxybenzoic Acid

Salicylic acid [69-72-7] $C_7H_6O_3$ (138.12).

Preparation—Mostly by the Kolbe-Schmidt process in which CO_2 is reacted with sodium phenolate under pressure at about 130° to form sodium salicylate followed by treatment with mineral acid.

Description—White, fine, needle-like crystals or as a fluffy, white, crystalline powder. Synthetic salicylic acid is white and odorless. It has a sweetish, afterward acrid, taste, is stable in the air, and melts between 158° and 161°.

Solubility—1 g in 460 mL water, 3 mL alcohol, 45 mL chloroform, 3 mL ether, 135 mL benzene, and about 15 mL boiling water.

Uses—Salicylic acid is used *externally* on the skin, where it exerts a slight *antiseptic* action and considerable *keratolytic* action. The latter property makes it a beneficial agent in the local treatment of certain forms of *eczematoid dermatitis*. It is also included in products for the treatment of *psoriasis*, for which the FDA classification is Category I. Tissue cells swell, soften, and ultimately desquamate. Salicylic Acid Plaster is often used for this purpose. Salicylic acid is especially useful in the treatment of *tinea pedis* (athlete's foot) and *tinea capitis* (ringworm of the scalp), since the fungus grows and thrives in the stratum corneum. Keratolysis both removes the infected horny layer and aids in penetration by antifungal drugs. It is usually combined with benzoic acid in an ointment long known as Whitfield's Ointment. It is also commonly combined with zinc oxide, with sulfur, or with sulfur and coal tar. Salicylic acid is incorporated into preparations for the treatment of acne, dandruff, and insect bites and stings and into soaps and vaginal douches, but efficacy remains to be established. In high concentrations it is *caustic* and may be used to remove *corns*, *calluses*, *warts*, and other growths.

Continuous application of salicylic acid to the skin can cause dermatitis. Systemic toxicity resulting from application to large areas of the skin has been reported. It is not employed internally as an analgesic because of its local irritating effect on the gastrointestinal tract.

Dose—*Topical*, to the skin, for *keratolysis*, as a 2 to 10% collodion, 6% gel, 3 to 10% ointment, or 3.5% soap; as a *caustic*, a 20% collodion, 25 to 60% ointment, or 40% plaster.

Salicylic Acid Collodion is prepared by dissolving 100 g of salicylic acid in about 750 mL of flexible collodion and then adding sufficient flexible collodion to make the product measure 1000 mL, mixing well.

Salicylic Acid Plaster is a uniform mixture of salicylic acid in a suitable base, spread on paper, cotton cloth, or other suitable backing material.

Sulfur, Precipitated—page 1240.

Sulfurated Lime Solution—RPS-16, page 1187.

Tretinoin

Retinoic acid; Retin-A (*Ortho*)

all *trans*-Retinoic acid [302-79-4] $C_{20}H_{28}O_2$ (300.44).

Preparation—By oxidation of vitamin A aldehyde which may be obtained by oxidation of vitamin A. *Biochem J 90:* 569, 1964.

Description—Yellow to light-orange crystals or crystalline powder with the odor of ensilage. It should be stored in cold and protected from light and air. It melts between 176 and 181°.

Solubility—Insoluble in water; slightly soluble in alcohol; slightly soluble in chloroform; 1 g in 10 mL boiling benzene.

Uses—Tretinoin is retinoic acid, or so-called *vitamin A acid*, which is formed when the aldehyde group of retinene (retinal) is oxidized to a carboxyl group. It is not known whether retinoic acid has a physiological function, but some authorities consider it to be the form of vitamin A that acts in the skin. This view is supported by the fact that retinol and retinal have very little action on the skin but large systemic doses of vitamin A evoke prominent dermatologic changes.

Topical tretinoin causes inflammation, thickening of the epidermis (acanthosis), and local intercellular edema, which leads to some separation of the epidermal cells. The stratum corneum loosens, and exfoliation may occur. High concentrations can cause vesiculation. These actions are used in the treatment of *acne vulgaris*. The loosened horny layer makes it easier for the comedo to rise up and discharge, and the inflammatory response mobilizes white cells which attack the bacteria in the follicle. In the early stages of treatment, the sudden surfacing of obscured preexisting comedones makes it appear that the acne has been exacerbated, but the new comedones do not coalesce into cysts or nodules, and scarring does not occur. The exaggerated stage may last for as long as 6 weeks, after which improvement comes rapidly. Shortly after discontinuation of treatment, relapses readily occur. Deep cystic nodular acne (acne conglobata) or severe cases are usually not improved by tretinoin.

Various hyperkeratotic conditions are reported to respond to tretinoin, responses being sometimes exceptionally dramatic. *Solar keratosis, ichthyosis, keratosis palmaris* and *plantaris*, and other hyperplastic dermatoses have been successfully treated with the drug.

Tretinoin is an antioxidant and free radical scavenger. There is some evidence not only that topical applications may provide some protection from actinic and other radiation effects on the skin, including cancer, but that internally it may be protective against carcinogenesis from radiation and carcinogens. Systemically, it does not cause the toxic effects of large doses of vitamin A.

In concentrations of 0.05 to 0.1%, tretinoin causes a transient feeling of warmth or mild stinging, and erythema follows. Peeling of the skin may occur. Irritation and peeling are more marked when the concentration exceeds 0.1%. When peeling, crusting, or blistering occurs, medication should be withheld until the skin recovers, or the concentration should be reduced. The drug should not be applied around the eyes, nose, or angles of the mouth, because the mucosae are much more sensitive than the skin to the irritant effects. Tretinoin also may cause severe irritation on eczematous skin. It should not be applied along with or closely following other irritants or keratolytic drugs. Exposure to sunlight should be avoided if possible. Both hypo- and hyperpigmentation have been reported, but the conditions appear to be reversible and temporary.

Dose—*Topical*, *usual*, to the skin, **0.01 to 0.1%**, once a day at bedtime.

Dosage Forms—Cream: 0.05 and 0.1%; Gel: 0.01 and 0.025%; Swabs: 0.05%; Topical Solution: 0.05%.

Trichloroacetic Acid—page 784.

Zinc Oxide Paste with Salicylic Acid—RPS-16, page 723.

Other Keratolytics

Urea [Carbamide [57-13-6] $CO(NH_2)_2$ (60.06)]—A product of protein metabolism; prepared by hydrolysis of cyanamide or from carbon dioxide by ammonolysis. Colorless to white crystals or white, crystalline powder; almost odorless but may develop a slight odor of ammonia in presence of moisture; melts between 132° and 135°. 1 g dissolves in 1.5 mL water, 10 mL alcohol; practically insoluble in chloroform, ether. *Uses:* Urea is a protein denaturant that promotes hydration of keratin and mild keratolysis in dry and hyperkeratotic skin. It is used topically in the treatment of psoriasis, ichthyosis, atopic dermatitis, and other dry, scaly conditions. It was once used in the treatment of wounds and ulcers. Systemically, in doses in excess of the renal tubular maximum for resorption, it acts as an osmotic diuretic, and is sometimes used in the treatment of cerebral edema, to reduce intraocular pressure and vitreous volume and to increase urinary excretion in patients with inappropriate secretion of antidiuretic hormone. It is given by amniocentesis to cause abortion. *Dose:* Topical, as 2 to 30% cream or lotion. *Intravenous*, 1 to 1.5 g/kg in adults and 0.5 to 1.5 g/kg in children, administered as a 30% solution containing 5 or 10% dextrose, at a rate of no greater than 4 mL/min. *Intraamniotic*, 135 to 200 mL of a 40 to 50% solution containing 5% dextrose.

Cleansing Preparations

The skin may be cleansed with detergents, solvents, or abrasives, singly or in combination. Among the detergents, the soaps have enjoyed the greatest official status, more through custom than through especial merit. The nonsoap detergents became important not only as household hand cleansers but also in dermatologic and surgical practice as well. However, because many nonsoap detergents do not decompose in sewage disposal plants, there has been a return to real soap. Some of the antiseptic "soaps" still contain synthetic detergents. Soap interferes with the action of many antiseptics, which is one reason synthetic detergents are often used in antiseptic cleansing preparations. However, synthetic detergents also interact with some antiseptics. Anionic nonsoap skin detergents rarely sensitize and thus are prescribed when the user is allergic to soap.

Ordinary soaps tend to be alkaline, with pH ranging from 9.5 to 10.5. Superfatted soaps have a pH in the lower end of the range. Synthetic detergents usually have a pH of 7.5 or less.

Shampoos are liquid soaps or detergents used to clean the hair and scalp. Both soaps and shampoos are often used as vehicles for dermatologic agents.

It is commonly but erroneously believed that soap has an antiseptic action. The promotion of either soap or synthetic detergents alone for the control of acne is unwarranted; antiseptic substances must be added to the cleansing material or be used separately. Quantitative studies of the cutaneous flora before and after cleansing with soap or with other anionic detergents show a negligible antiseptic effect. However, the removal of loose epidermis lessens the likelihood that cutaneous bacteria will be transferred from the skin to other structures. Certain cationic detergents employed in dermatology are antiseptic. Detergents are treated under *Surface-Active Agents* (page 267).

The choice of organic solvents to cleanse the skin depends largely upon the nature of the material to be removed. In medical practice ethanol and isopropanol are the most frequently employed organic solvents. Cleansing creams act both as solvents and as detergents.

Alcohol—page 1159.

Alcohol, Rubbing—page 1160.

Benzalkonium Chloride—page 1159.

Green Soap

Sapo Mollis Medicinalis; Soft Soap; Medicinal Soft Soap USP XVI

A potassium soap made by the saponification of suitable vegetable oils, excluding coconut oil and palm kernel oil, without the removal of glycerin. Green soap may be prepared as follows:

The Vegetable Oil	380	g
Oleic Acid	20	g
Potassium Hydroxide (total alkali 85%)	91.7	g
Glycerin	50	mL
Purified Water, a sufficient quantity,		
To make about	1000	g

Mix the oil and oleic acid, and heat the mixture to about 80°. Dissolve the potassium hydroxide in a mixture of the glycerin and 100 mL of purified water, and add the solution, while it is still hot, to the hot oil. Stir the mixture vigorously until emulsified, then heat while continuing the stirring until the mixture is homogeneous and a test portion will dissolve to give a clear solution in hot water. Add sufficient hot purified water to make the product weight 1000 g, continuing the stirring until the soap is homogeneous.

Note—The vegetable oil to be used in the formula given above may be corn, cottonseed, linseed, olive, soybean, or a similar oil which has a saponification value not greater than 205 and an iodine value not less than 80. These specifications limit the degree of saturation (iodine value) and the average molecular weight of the fatty acids present in the oil (saponification value). Iodine values less than 80 indicate that the oils are not sufficiently unsaturated and are likely to produce a soap which is too hard. Saponification values above 205 indicate molecular weights which are too low. The lower fatty acids produce soaps which are too irritating for this product. For these reasons *coconut* and *palm kernel oils* are excluded. Since glycerin is added only to accelerate the saponification, it may be omitted if desired.

The quantity of potassium hydroxide given in the formula is based on an alkalinity equivalent to 85% KOH. If the potassium hydroxide is of any other strength, a proportionately larger or smaller quantity should be taken. The oleic acid is added to form an emulsion nucleus which aids in dispersion of the fixed oil, thus aiding in its saponification. A slight excess of alkali is desirable to promote detergency.

A variety of soft soap prepared from green, colored oils, such as green olive oil, or artificially colored, is known as "Green Soap." The official soap is not green in color. It has been demonstrated that the green color adds nothing to the therapeutic value and linseed oil soap has long been used with satisfaction. On a large scale the soap may be prepared without the addition of alcohol or glycerin, heat and concentrated alkali producing saponification. It should contain a little free alkali, but too much must be avoided. The amount is limited by official standards.

Description—A soft, unctuous, yellowish white to brownish or greenish yellow, transparent to translucent mass, with a slight, characteristic odor, often suggesting the oil from which it was prepared, and an alkaline taste. Its solution (1 in 20) is alkaline to bromothymol blue TS.

Incompatibilities—Incompatible with *acids*, which liberate the free fatty acids, and with many *metallic salts*, which form insoluble soaps.

Uses—Green soap has three major uses as a *detergent* applied *topically* on the skin:

1. *The preoperative preparation of operative sites*—For this purpose there is required a soap that is a good fat emulsifier that contains just enough reserve alkalinity to make it quickly effective in the removal of sebaceous secretions from the skin. The soap must contain such proportions of unsaturated fatty acids that it is soluble in and lathers with water and is not too easily affected by hard water. The fatty acids must not be of such low molecular weight that they are irritating to the skin, yet the amount of free alkali must be enough to give prompt detergent activity without at the same time having the powerful caustic effect of free alkali upon the skin. The germicidal efficacy of Green Soap is negligible. In *Green Soap Tincture* it is the ethanol that is antiseptic.

2. *The cleansing of the skin and hair in dermatological conditions*—Green soap is used when it is necessary to remove greasy substances or greasy preparations that have been added for therapeutic reasons, to produce a clean area where other medicinal agents may be used, or to remove irritating discharges. It is prescribed by dermatologists for use as a shampoo when commercial shampoos are suspected of causing allergic rash and other untoward effects.

3. *The cleansing of the surgical operator and assistants*—The soap for this use likewise must have excellent detergent power, must be fairly resistant to hard water, and must be equally free from irritating effects of fatty acids or alkalies upon the surgeon's hands. Germicidal detergents, generally containing hexachlorophene, iodophors, or chlorhexidine have considerably replaced Green soap in the surgical scrub.

Coconut and *palm oil soaps* are excellent detergents and they are much less easily affected by hard water than are those soaps that are employed in the official preparation, but they are irritating to the skin and therefore excluded.

4. *The decontamination of the skin*—This soap is widely used in the emergency decontamination of the skin when the contaminant is a hydrocarbon or other lipid-soluble substance.

Green Soap Tincture is locally irritating.

Dose—*Topical*, to the skin, usually as of *Green Soap Tincture* (below).

Green Soap Tincture [Linimentum Saponis Mollis Medicinalis; Soft Soap Liniment; Medicinal Soft Soap Liniment USP XVI; Tinctura Saponis Viridis]—*Preparation:* Mix lavender oil (20 mL) with alcohol (300 mL), dissolve in this the green soap (650 g) by stirring or by agitation, set the solution aside for 24 hours, filter through paper, and add alcohol (qs) to make 1000 mL. *Alcohol Content:* 28 to 32% (v/v) C₂H₅OH. *Dose: Topical*, to skin.

Hexachlorophene Cleansing Emulsion—page 1161.
Isopropyl Rubbing Alcohol—page 1162.

Soap, Hard—RPS-15, page 1269.
Sodium Lauryl Sulfate—page 1299.

Miscellaneous Dermatologics

Gargles, nasal washes, douches, enemata, etc., generally contain as basic ingredients substances described under other categories in this chapter. These preparations are described under *Aqueous Solutions*, page 1494. *Antiphlogistics* include alcohol and several creams and lotions that cool by evaporation. Many antiphlogistic preparations also contain an astringent and a local anesthetic or camphor or menthol. Commonly employed *antipruritics* also depend largely upon local anesthetics and the soothing effect of cooling, although emollients or demulcents may be included, especially depending upon the etiology of the pruritus. The antipruritic properties of phenol preparations largely derive from superficial local anesthesia. *Vulnerary* and *epithelizing* properties are attributed to numerous irritants and to several dyes; however, few reliable data exist to support most claims to vulnerary action. *Sunscreens* contain aromatic compounds, like aminobenzoic acid, which efficiently absorb the harmful ultraviolet rays from the incident sunlight and transmit mainly the less harmful wavelengths, or titanium dioxide, which reflects sunlight from the surface of application. Ultraviolet light in the spectral range of 290–320 nm causes suntan and sunburn; therefore, a sunscreen to prevent tan or burn should have a high molar absorptivity in this range. However, *photosensitization* (ie, the photoactivation of chemicals to make them toxic or allergenic) may occur with wavelengths as high as 500 nm; consequently, to protect recipients of certain drugs (tetracyclines, sulfonamides, erythromycin, promazine, chlorpromazine, promethazine, psoralens), sunscreens with a broader absorption spectrum are required. An adequate broad spectrum is usually achieved with combinations of sunscreens (eg, dioxybenzone and oxybenzone). *Melanizers* are substances that promote the pigmentation of the skin. Most melanizers produce their effect by sensitizing the skin to ultraviolet light,* so that the effect is principally the same as if the subject had been exposed for a long time to the sun. *Skin bleaches,* or *demelanizers,* mostly contain either ammoniated mercury or hydroquinone derivatives. *Hair bleaches* generally contain peroxides. There is a large variety of depilatories on the market. Many of them are sulfhydryl compounds, especially thioglycollates, which reduce the disulfide bonds of keratin, thus softening the hair to the point where it can be separated easily from the epidermis. Some of the same compounds are used in lower concentrations in hairwaving preparations. *Antiperspirants* have been included among the astringents.

Aminobenzoic Acid

Benzoic acid, 4-amino-, PABA

p-Aminobenzoic acid [150-13-0] $C_7H_7NO_2$ (137.14).
Preparation—*p*-Nitrotoluene is oxidized with permanganate to *p*-nitrobenzoic acid and the nitro group is then reduced to amino with iron and hydrochloric acid.

---

* This action is termed a *photodynamic action.* The term has been used loosely to include all instances of enhanced sensitivity to light, but in strict definition it is confined to photosensitization in which the participation of oxygen is required. In the photodynamic process, light of wavelengths too long to be ordinarily effective may be utilized, so that the activating spectrum may be shifted toward longer wavelengths.

Description—White or slightly yellow, odorless crystals or crystalline powder; melts between 186° and 189°. Discolors on exposure to air or light.
Solubility—Slightly soluble in water and chloroform; freely soluble in alcohol and solutions of alkali hydroxides and carbonates; sparingly soluble in ether.

Uses—A *sunscreen.* It absorbs ultraviolet light of wavelengths in the region of 280 to 320 nm; its molar absorptivity at 288.5 nm is 18,300. However, it does not absorb throughout the near ultraviolet range, so that drug-related photosensitivity and phototoxicity may not be prevented by aminobenzoic acid, but in combination with benzophenone it does protect against some drug-induced phototoxicities. Nevertheless, in the 280–320 nm range, it has the highest protection index of current sunscreen agents.
For animal species that do not use preformed folic acid, which contains the *p*-aminobenzoyl moiety, aminobenzoic acid is a B-vitamin. However, man does not use aminobenzoic acid, and its promotion in vitamin preparations preys on the ignorance of the consumer. Aminobenzoic acid or its potassium salt is promoted as an agent that softens or regresses fibrotic tissue in Peyronie's disease, scleroderma, dermatomyositis, morphea and pemphigus. It has also been claimed to be useful in treating disseminated lupus erythematosus and lymphoblastoma cutis, but it is no longer promoted for such uses. The claims for the antifibrotic actions are poorly substantiated, and the actions and uses are not mentioned in major works on pharmacology and therapeutics. Aminobenzoic acid does have a legitimate use in combination with salicylates in the treatment of rheumatic fever; it retards the conjugation of salicylic acid and hence prolongs the action of the salicylates.
Topical aminobenzoic acid is rarely allergenic to recipients but phototoxicity and photoallergenicity occur.
Dose—*Topical,* as a sunscreen, 4 to 15% in solutions, lotions, creams, ointments, and lipsticks. *Oral,* in combination with salicylates, **600 mg** 4 to 6 times a day.
Dosage Forms—Cream: 4%; Gel: 5%; Solution: 5%.

Cetyl Alcohol—page 1304.

Dioxybenzone

Methanone, (2-hydroxy-4-methoxyphenyl)(2-hydroxyphenyl)-,
Cyasorb UV 24 (*American Cyanamid*); Solaquin (*Elder*)

2,2′-Dihydroxy-4-methoxybenzophenone [131-53-3] $C_{14}H_{12}O_4$ (244.25).
Preparation—By a Friedel-Crafts reaction in which *o*-methoxybenzoyl chloride is added gradually to a mixture of 1,3-dimethoxybenzene, chlorobenzene, and aluminum chloride. The reaction conditions are such that both methoxy groups ortho to the carbonyl bridge in the initial condensation product are demethylated. US Pat 2,853,521.

Description—Off-white to yellow powder; congeals not lower than 68°.
Solubility—Practically insoluble in water; freely soluble in alcohol and toluene.

Uses—A *sunscreen* of intermediate molar absorptivity (11,950 at 282 nm), but it absorbs throughout the ultraviolet spectrum and hence affords protection not only against sunburn but also against the photodynamic, photosensitizing, and phototoxic effects of drugs. At present, dioxybenzone is marketed in combination with the closely related *Oxybenzone* (page 788).
Dose—*Topical,* as a **3%** lotion.
Dosage Forms—Dioxybenzone and Oxybenzone Cream: 3% of each ingredient.

Hydrogen Peroxide Solution—page 1167.

Hydroquinone

1,4-Benzenediol; *p*-Dihydroxybenzene; Hydroquinol; Quinol; Tecquinol; Eldoquin, Eldopaque (*Elder*)

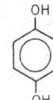

Hydroquinone [123-31-9] $C_6H_6O_2$ (110.11).

Preparation—Various processes are employed. One involves reacting a sulfuric acid solution of aniline with manganese dioxide and reducing the resulting *p*-benzoquinone with sodium bisulfite.

Description—Fine, white needles; darkens on exposure to air; melts between 172 and 174°.

Solubility—1 g in about 17 mL water, 4 mL alcohol, 51 mL chloroform, and 16.5 mL ether.

Uses—A *hypopigmenting* agent employed percutaneously to lighten localized areas of hyperpigmented skin, such as skin blemishes, lentigo, melasma, chloasma, freckles, etc. Its action is only temporary, so that it is necessary to repeat the application at frequent intervals. It is a mild irritant, and erythema or rash may develop, which requires discontinuation of the drug. It should not be used near the eyes or in open cuts. It is contraindicated in the presence of sunburn, miliaria, or irritated skin. Hydroquinone is not to be used in children.

Dose—*Topical*, to the skin, as a **2 to 4%** cream, lotion, or ointment to the affected area once or twice daily.

Dosage Forms—Cream: 2%; Lotion: 2%; Ointment: 2 and 4%.

Hydroxyurea—page 1155.

Isotretinoin

13-*cis*-Retinoic Acid; Accutane (*Hoffmann-LaRoche*)

3,7-Dimethyl-9-(2,6,6-trimethyl-1-cyclohexen-1-yl)-2-*cis*-4-*trans*-6-*trans*-8-*trans*-nonatetraenoic acid [4759-48-2] $C_{20}H_{28}O_2$ (300.44). Differs from tretinoin (vitamin A) only in the configuration of the unsaturation at the α and β carbon atoms, which is *cis* rather than *trans*.

Uses—Although isotretinoin is not a topical drug, it is a dermatological agent and hence is described here. Its primary action is to decrease the production of sebum, which lends itself to the treatment of severe *modular* and *cystic acne* (acne conglobata). The size of the sebaceous gland is decreased and there is a change in the morphology and secretory capacity of the cells (dedifferentiation). Complete clearing of lesions is seen in about 90% of cases. A single course of treatment usually brings about long-lasting, sometimes permanent, remissions.

Isotretinoin also appears to diminish hyperkeratosis and has been reported to be effective in lamellar ichthyosis, Darier's disease, pityriasis rubra pilaris, and keratocanthoma.

Adverse effects include facial dermatitis, fragile skin, thinning and drying of the hair, reversible cheilitis, and dry skin, mouth, eyes and conjunctivitis in 25 to 80% of recipients. Peeling of the palms and soles and sensitivity to sunburn occur in about 5% of users. Urethral inflammation also frequently occurs. Joint pains and exacerbation of rheumatoid arthritis has also been reported to occur in about 16% of patients. Sedimentation rate, serum triglyceride concentration, and serum levels of alanine and aspartate transaminases transiently occur in about 25% of users. In spite of the relatively high incidence of side effects, treatment rarely has to be discontinued.

After oral administration, peak blood concentrations occur within 1 to 4 hr. The compound is oxidized to 4-hydroxy-13-*cis*-retinoic acid, which is then glucuronidated and is secreted into the bile. The elimination half-life is 11 to 39 (mean 20) hr.

Dose—*Oral, adult*, **1 to 2 mg/kg** a day in two divided doses for 15 to 20 weeks. If the cyst count has not been reduced by more than 70%, a second course of treatment may be given after a wait of two months. Persons over 70 kg of body weight or who have severe chest and back involvement usually require doses at the high end of the range.

Mercury, Ammoniated—page 1167.

Methoxsalen

7*H*-Furo [3,2-*g*][1]benzopyran-7-one, 9-methoxy-, Ammoidin; 9-Methoxypsoralen; Xanthotoxin; Meloxine (*Upjohn*); Oxsoralen (*Elder*)

9-Methoxy-7*H*-furo[3,2-*g*][1]benzopyran-7-one; 8-methoxypsoralen [298-81-7] $C_{12}H_8O_4$ (216.19).

Preparation—Occurs naturally in *Psorales coryfolia*, *Ammi majus*, *Ruta chalepensis*, and various other plants. It may be synthesized by methods described in *J Am Chem Soc 79:* 3491, 1957, and US Pat 2,889,337.

Description—White to cream-colored, odorless, fluffy, needle-like crystals; melts between 143° and 148°.

Solubility—Practically insoluble in cold water, sparingly soluble in boiling water, and freely soluble in chloroform. Soluble in boiling alcohol, acetone, and acetic acid. Soluble in aqueous alkalies with ring cleavage; reconstitution occurs on neutralization.

Uses—A psoralen melanizer. It increases the photodynamic pigmentation of skin; it does not induce pigmentation in the absence of ultraviolet light. It is used in the treatment of *vitiligo*. Severe sunburning can occur with topical application; it is customary to protect the surrounding skin with a sunscreen. After oral administration gastrointestinal upset and central nervous toxicities, such as vertigo and excitement, also occur. Consequently, the drug should be used orally only under medical supervision.

Dose—*Topical*, as a 1% lotion. *Oral*, adults and children over 12 years of age, **20 mg** once a day 2 to 4 hr before exposure to ultraviolet light.

Dosage Forms—Capsules: 10 mg; Lotion: 1%.

Monobenzone

Phenol, 4-(phenylmethoxy)-, Monobenzyl Ether of Hydroquinone; Benoquin (*Elder*)

p-(Benzyloxy)phenol [103-16-2] $C_{13}H_{12}O_2$ (200.24).

Preparation—Prepared in various ways. One method involves condensing sodium *p*-nitrophenolate with benzyl chloride to produce benzyl *p*-nitrophenyl ether followed by (1) reduction of nitro to amino, (2) diazotization of amino, and (3) hydrolytic decomposition of the diazonium compound to the corresponding phenol.

Description—White, odorless, crystalline powder possessing very little taste. Melts between 117° and 120°.

Solubility—1 g in >10,000 mL water, 14.5 mL alcohol, 29 mL chloroform, 14 mL ether.

Uses—A *depigmenting agent* or *demelanizer*. It acts by interfering with the formation of melanin, which is the principal cutaneous pigment. It is used in the treatment of *lentigo*, *severe freckling*, and other types of *hyperpigmentation*. It is not effective against pigmented moles or malignant melanoma. Its pigment-decreasing action is somewhat erratic. Irritation of varying degrees occurs in a considerable number of patients.

Dose—*Topical*, to the skin, as a **20%** ointment 1 or 2 times daily.

Dosage Forms—Ointment: 20%.

Oxybenzone

Methanone, (2-hydroxy-4-methoxyphenyl)phenyl-, Spectra-Sorb UV9 (*American Cyanamid*)

2-Hydroxy-4-methoxybenzophenone [131-57-7] $C_{14}H_{12}O_3$ (228.25).

Preparation—Benzoic acid is condensed with resorcinol monomethyl ether by heating in the presence of $ZnCl_2$, polyphosphoric acid (103% H_3PO_4 equivalent), and PCl_3. US Pat 3,073,866.

Description—White to off-white powder; congeals not lower than 62°.

Solubility—Practically insoluble in water; freely soluble in alcohol and toluene.

Uses—A *sunscreen*. It has a high molar absorptivity (20,381 at 290 nm), and it absorbs in both the long and short ultraviolet spectrum. Therefore, it serves not only to prevent sunburn but also to protect against the photodynamic, photosensitizing, and phototoxic effects of various drugs. Contact with the eyes should be avoided. At present, oxybenzone is marketed only in combination with other sunscreens.

Dose—*Topical*, as a **5%** cream, **0.5%** lipstick, and **2 or 3%** lotion in combination with other sunscreens.

Ringer's Irrigation—RPS-16, page 762.
Sodium Bicarbonate—page 796.

Sodium Borate

Sodium Tetraborate; Sodium Pyroborate; Sodium Biborate

Borax [1303-96-4] $Na_2B_4O_7.10H_2O$ (381.37); anhydrous [1330-43-4] $Na_2B_4O_7$ (201.22).

Preparation—Found in immense quantities in California as a crystalline deposit. The earth, which is strongly impregnated with borax, is lixiviated; the solution is evaporated and crystallized.

Calcium borate, or *cotton balls*, also occurs in the borax deposits of California, and sodium borate is obtained from it by double decomposition with sodium carbonate.

Description—Colorless, transparent crystals, or a white, crystalline powder. It is odorless. The crystals are often coated with white powder due to efflorescence. Its solution is alkaline to litmus and to phenolphthalein; pH about 9.5.

Solubility—1 g in 16 mL water, 1 mL glycerin, and 1 mL boiling water; insoluble in alcohol.

Incompatibilities—Precipitates many *metals* as insoluble borates. In aqueous solution it is alkaline and precipitates *aluminum salts* as aluminum hydroxide, *iron salts* as a basic borate and ferric hydroxide, and *zinc sulfate* as zinc borate and a basic salt. *Alkaloids* are precipitated from solutions of their salts. Approximately equal weights of *glycerin* and boric acid react to produce a decidedly acid derivative generally called glyceroboric acid. Thus the addition of glycerin to a mixture containing sodium borate overcomes incompatibilities arising from an alkaline reaction.

Uses—Saturated solution of sodium borate has limited usefulness as an *antipruritic* for the skin. Solutions are also sometimes used as a mouth wash in the treatment of *stomatitis* and *gingivitis* (see *Boric Acid*, page 1310); the low concentrations used and short contact times preclude an antimicrobial action. Sodium borate should not be administered internally. Chronic intoxication has occurred from the use of borate-containing mouthwashes.

Pharmaceutically, it is frequently used in small quantities in some ointments, in hand lotions, vaginal douches, eyewashes, acne products, preparations for athlete's foot, and in cosmetics. In these, it has a questionable efficacy except, perhaps, as a buffer. It forms a soap that serves as an emulsifying agent in the preparation of the ointment. It is a frequent ingredient in eye lotions, but is incompatible with zinc sulfate, since insoluble zinc borate is formed. As a pharmaceutical necessity, it is used as an alkalizing agent and as a buffer for alkaline solutions.

Sodium Fluoride

Sodium fluoride [7681-49-4] NaF (41.99).

Preparation—By interaction of hydrofluoric acid (40% HF) with an equivalent quantity of NaOH or Na_2CO_3.

Description—White, odorless powder.
Solubility—1 g in 25 mL water; insoluble in alcohol.

Uses—A *dental caries prophylactic*. Fluoridation of municipal water supplies is considered a safe and practical public health measure, a concentration of about 1 ppm of fluoride in the water supply resulting in a 50 to 65% reduction in the incidence of dental caries in permanent teeth. Ingested fluoride is effective only while teeth are being formed. The fluoride is incorporated into tooth salts as fluo-

roapatite. Excessive intake during development of teeth may cause mottling; hence, mottling of newly erupted teeth is an indication to reduce fluoride intake. Where drinking water contains less than 0.7 ppm of fluoride, dietary supplements for children with unerupted teeth may provide some future protection.

Topical application results in changes only in the outer layers of enamel or exposed dentin. In children, repeated application of a 2% solution of sodium fluoride to cleaned teeth results in a 16 to 49% reduction of dental caries; adult teeth are protected to a lesser extent by topical fluoride.

In experimental trials, orally administered sodium fluoride produced new bone formation in some patients with osteoporosis, especially when calcium and vitamin D were concomitantly administered to facilitate mineralization of the new bone. However, the bone may become brittle.

Fluoride removes calcium from tissues and also poisons certain enzymes. Oral doses may cause nausea and vomiting, which usualy can be prevented by taking the substance with food. Solutions and gels for topical applications should not be swallowed.

Dose—*Topical*, to the teeth, as a **0.02 to 2%** solution, **0.5%** gel or **0.22 to 2.3%** paste. *Oral*, 1.5 to **3 ppm** of sodium fluoride (equivalent to 0.7 to 1.3 ppm of fluoride ion) in drinking water; as a supplement, when the drinking water contains less than 0.2 ppm of fluoride ion, **1.1 mg** of sodium fluoride once a day for children under 3 yr of age and **2.2 mg** for those over 3 yr, and when the drinking water contains 0.2 to 0.6 ppm of fluoride ion, **550 μg** of sodium fluoride once a day for children under 3 yr of age and **1.1 mg** for those over 3 yr. The fluoride ion equivalents of 550 μg, 1.1 mg, and 2.2 mg of sodium fluoride are 250 μg, 500 μg, and 1 mg, respectively. For *osteoporosis*, **50 mg**/day. *Caution: Sodium fluoride is poisonous.*

Dosage Forms—Solution: 1.1, 3.3, 5.5, and 20 mg/mL; Tablets: 1.1 and 2.2 mg. Sodium Fluoride and Orthophosphoric Acid: Gel and Solution, each containing 1.23% fluoride ion and 1% phosphoric acid.

Sodium Monofluorophosphate

Phosphorofluoridic acid, sodium salt

$FPO(ONa)_2$

Disodium phosphorofluoridate [10163-15-2] (143.95).

Preparation—Substantially pure sodium monofluorophosphate is produced by fusing a mixture of sodium metaphosphate and sodium fluoride, in stoichiometric proportion, in a closed vessel from which moist air is excluded.

Description—White to slightly gray, odorless powder.
Solubility—Freely soluble in water.

Uses—Like sodium fluoride, above, sodium monofluorophosphate promotes the replacement of the hydroxyapatite by fluoroapatite in the tooth salts and hence is used as a *dental prophylactic* against dental caries. It has the advantage over sodium fluoride in that the teeth do not require special preparation before application, it is effective when included in dentifrices, and that in dentifrices there is no hazard with respect to local toxicity to the gingivae or systemic intoxication from ingestion.

Dose—*Topical*, to the teeth, in dentifrice containing 0.76% of sodium monofluorophosphate.

Stannous Fluoride

Tin Difluoride; Fluoristan

Tin fluoride (SnF_2) [7783-47-3] (156.69); contains not less than 71.2% Sn^{2+} (stannous tin), and about 24% F (fluoride).

Preparation—Stannous oxide is dissolved in 40% HF and the solution is evaporated out of contact with air.

Description—White, crystalline powder with a bitter, salty taste. Melts at about 213°.
Solubility—Freely soluble in water; practically insoluble in alcohol, ether, and chloroform.

Uses—Alters the composition and crystalline structure of the hydroxyapatite-like salts that make up the bulk of enamel, especially, and dentin, so that the tooth material is more resistant to acidic erosion and dental caries (decay). The substance is applied only topically, so that the tooth substance is only affected in the superficial layers, and stannous fluoride must be applied periodically. It is most effective when applied to the tooth surface after the teeth have been cleaned thoroughly by a dentist. However, there is good evidence that even when incorporated into tooth pastes the drug has a retardant effect on the development of dental caries.

Dose—*Topical*, to the teeth, generally as **0.1%** gel or 8% (2% fluoride) solution.

Dosage Forms—Capsules (for solution): 0.4, 0.65, and 0.8 g; Concentrate: 30%; Gel: 0.1%.

Titanium Dioxide

Titanic Anhydride; A-Fil (*Cooper*)

Titanium oxide (TiO$_2$) [13463-67-7] TiO$_2$ (79.90).

Preparation—By adding ammonia or an alkali carbonate to a solution of titanyl sulfate (TiOSO$_4$). Titanic acid [Ti(OH)$_4$ or TiO(OH)$_2$] is precipitated and, after filtration and washing, is dried and ignited.

Description—White, amorphous, tasteless, odorless, infusible powder. Density about 4. Its suspension in water (1 in 10) is neutral to litmus.

Solubility—Insoluble in water, HCl, HNO$_3$, and dilute H$_2$SO$_4$.

Uses—Titanium dioxide powder has a very high reflectance at visible and ultraviolet wavelengths, and hence it serves as an excellent white pigment. In ointments or lotions it reflects a very high proportion of incident sunlight and hence protects the skin from sunburn and hence serves as a *sunblock*. It is also used in cosmetics and as a dusting powder. Topically, it is devoid of toxicity.

Dose—*Topical*, as 12 to 25% cream, lotion or ointment as required.

Trioxsalen

7*H*-Furo[3,2-*g*][1]benzopyran-7-one, 2,5,9-trimethyl-, 6-Hydroxy-β,2,7-trimethyl-5-benzofuranacrylic Acid δ-Lactone; Trisoralen (*Elder*)

2,5,9-Trimethyl-7*H*-furo[3,2-*g*][1]benzopyran-7-one [3902-71-4] C$_{14}$H$_{12}$O$_3$ (228.25).

Caution: Avoid contact with the skin.

Preparation—2-Methylresorcinol is cyclized with ethyl acetoacetate with the aid of sulfuric acid to 7-hydroxy-4,8-dimethylcoumarin (I). Treatment with allyl bromide in the presence of potassium carbonate transforms I into the 7-allyloxy compound which, on reacting with acetic anhydride in the presence of *N,N*-diethylaniline and anhydrous sodium acetate, rearranges and esterifies to give the 7-acetoxy-6-allyl compound (II). Bromination of II followed by reaction with sodium methoxide yields trioxsalen. US Pat 3,201,421.

Description—White to off-white, odorless, tasteless crystalline solid; stable in light, air, and heat; melts at about 230°.

Solubility—1 g in 1150 mL alcohol, 84 mL chloroform, and 43 mL methylenedichloride; practically insoluble in water.

Uses—Although trioxsalen is not a topical drug, it closely relates to other drugs in this section. It facilitates the action of near ultraviolet light to induce melanin (skin pigment) formation. It is used to cause repigmentation in idiopathic *vitiligo* and to enhance pigmentation to *increase tolerance to sunlight* or for *cosmetic purposes*. The increased tolerance to sunlight does not occur until enhanced pigmentation has occurred, and the user must be cautioned that severe sunburning with less than normal exposure can occur early during the course of treatment. The increase in dermal pigment occurs gradually over a period of several days of repeated exposure. Care must be taken to protect the eyes and lips during treatment. The manufacturer's recommended schedule of exposure should be used except at high altitudes, where exposure times should be appropriately reduced.

Trioxsalen is contraindicated in persons with photosensitizing diseases, such as infectious leukoderma, porphyria, or lupus erythe-matosus and when photosensitizing drugs are being given. The drug may sometimes cause gastric irritation and emesis. Children under 12 should not take the drug.

Dose—*Oral*, adults and children over 12 yr of age, **5** to **10 mg** 2 hours before exposure to sunlight. For the treatment of vitiligo the exposure should be repeated once daily for 4 days, and subsequent exposures should be determined according to the results of the initial 4 days. For the enhancement of pigmentation, treatment should not exceed 2 weeks, and the total accumulated dose in any one treatment course should not exceed 140 mg. Persons who show side effects of the drug should take only 5 mg; the duration of use will be necessarily prolonged over that in persons taking the usual dose of 10 mg.

Dosage Forms—Tablets: 5 mg.

Urea—page 935.

Other Miscellaneous Topical Drugs

Allantoin [5-Ureidohydantoin [97-59-6]; C$_4$H$_6$N$_4$O$_3$ (158.12)]—Prepared by oxidation of uric acid; colorless crystals melting at 238°; 1 g dissolves in 190 mL water and 500 mL alcohol; nearly insoluble in ether. *Uses:* In World War I it was noticed that maggot-infested wounds seemed to heal better than uninfested wounds, an effect attributed to allantoin produced by maggots. Used topically as a vulnerary to stimulate tissue repair in suppurating wounds, resistant ulcers, acne, seborrhea, cold sores, hemorrhoids, and various dermatologic infections and psoriasis. Frequently combined with astringents, keratolytics, coal tar, antiseptics, and antifungal drugs. The silver salt has been used in the topical treatment of extensive burns. *Dose: Topical,* 0.2 to 2% in creams, lotions, or shampoos and 0.3 to 0.5% in ointments for hemorrhoids.

Aluminum Chlorhydroxyallantoinate—*Uses:* This substance combines the astringent properties of aluminum ion with the vulnerary property of allantoin. It is used to treat acne vulgaris and hemorrhoids. *Dose:* Topical, 0.2%, as a powder, cleanser, or medical pad.

Cinoxate [2-Ethoxyethyl *p*-methoxycinnamate [104-28-9]; C$_{14}$H$_{18}$O$_4$ (250.29)]—A viscous liquid that may have a slightly yellow tinge; boils at about 185°; practically insoluble in water; miscible with alcohols. *Uses:* A *sunscreen* with relatively high molar absorptivity (19,400 at 306 nm) but not absorbing well throughout the entire offending range of ultraviolet light. Consequently, it is used principally in preparations intended to promote tanning rather than to protect against photosensitivity and phototoxicity. *Dose: Topical,* 1.75 to 4% in creams, gels, or lotions.

Dextranomer [Dextran 2,3-dihydroxypropyl-2-hydroxy-1,3-propanediyl ether [56087-11-7] Dextran polymer; Debrisan (*Pharmacia*)]—Small, dry beads of a three-dimensional dextran polymer; highly hygroscopic; 1 g absorbs about 4 g water. *Uses:* For drying, cleansing, and debridement of exudative *venous stasis ulcers, infected wounds,* and *burns;* it is not useful for cleansing nonexudative wounds or lesions. The beads not only absorb water but also proteins, including fibrin/fibrinogen degradation products, and thus prevent encrustation. The beads are poured into the cleansed wound, which is circumscribed with petroleum jelly, and a compress is taped in place to retain the material. Changes may be made up to 3 or 4 times a day, as needed. The beads must be removed before skin grafting is attempted. Care must be taken to prevent cross-contamination from patient to patient. On the floor the beads are slippery and thus hazardous.

Digalloyl Trioleate—A sunscreen used topically as a 3.5% cream or 2.5% lipstick.

Dihydroxyacetone [1,3-Dihydroxydimethyl ketone; C$_3$H$_6$O$_3$ (90.08)]—The ketone resulting from oxidation of the secondary alcohol group of glycerin. A crystalline powder; fairly hygroscopic; characteristic odor and sweet taste. The normal form is the dimer, slowly soluble in 1 part of water and 15 parts of alcohol; the monomer formed in solution is very soluble in water, alcohol, ether. *Uses:* Interacts with keratin in the stratum corneum to form a dark pigment that simulates the appearance of a suntan. It is incorporated in several sunscreen preparations. Since the sunscreen component is usually present in a concentration lower than optimal, such preparations may not provide protection to photosensitive persons.

Glyceryl *p*-Aminobenzoate [1,2,3-Propanetriol 1-(4-aminobenzoate); C$_{10}$H$_{13}$NO$_4$ (211.21)]—Prepared by esterification of aminobenzoic acid with glycerin. A waxy semisolid or syrup; insoluble in water, oils, and fats; soluble in ethanol, isopropanol, and propylene glycol. *Uses:* A sunscreen with relatively high molar absorptivity (17,197 at 295 nm) but a limited spectrum, therefore used primarily to promote tanning rather than to protect sensitive persons. *Dose: Topical,* 3% in lotions.

Homosalate [3,3,5-Trimethylcyclohexyl salicylate [118-56-9]; homomenthyl salicylate; C$_{16}$H$_{22}$O$_3$ (262.36); ing. of Coppertone (*Plough*); Filtrosol "A" (*Norda*); Heliophan (*Greeff*)]—*Uses:* A liquid with relatively low molar absorptivity (6,720 at 310 nm) and limited absorption in the near-ultraviolet range, so that it is used mainly to promote tanning. Photosensitive persons may not be protected from burns and phototoxicity. *Dose: Topical,* 4 to 10% in creams, lotions, or oils.

Methyl Anthranilate [Methyl 2-aminobenzoate; C$_8$H$_9$NO$_2$

(151.16)]—A constituent of several essential oils; also obtained by esterifying anthranilic acid with methyl alcohol. A crystalline substance; melts at 25°; slightly soluble in water; freely soluble in alcohol and ether. *Uses:* A sunscreen, with the lowest molar absorptivity of all sunscreens (941 at 315 nm); also, it does not absorb throughout the near-ultraviolet range and therefore is used in combination with other sunscreens or light-protectives. It is also used as a perfume in ointments and cosmetics. *Dose: Topical,* 5% in creams, lotions, or ointments.

Octyldimethylaminobenzoate—*Uses:* A sunscreen of moderate molar absorptivity. As with aminobenzoic acid, the UV absorption spectrum is relatively narrow, so that the compound does not protect against phototoxicity. *Dose:* Topical, to the skin as a 1.4% to 8% cream, lotion, or oil.

Padimate O 2-Ethylhexyl 4-(dimethylamino)benzoate [14779-78-3] $C_{14}H_{21}NO_2$ (235.33); Escalol (*Van Dyk*)—*Uses:* A sunscreen of moderate molar absorptivity but relatively narrow UV absorption spectrum characteristic of other aminobenzoic acid derivatives. *Dose*, topical, to the skin as a 1.4 to 8% cream, foam, lotion, or stick.

Red Petrolatum—*Uses:* Owing to its opacity, it is used in sunblock creams, ointments, and sticks. Concentrations range from 30 to 100%.

CHAPTER 41

Gastrointestinal Drugs

Ewart A Swinyard, PhD, DSc (Hon)

Professor Emeritus of Pharmacology
College of Pharmacy and School of Medicine
University of Utah
Salt Lake City, UT 84112

Drugs appropriate for this chapter include antacids, H_2-receptor antagonists, digestants, laxatives, emetics, antiemetics, adsorbents, and some miscellaneous agents which act on the gastrointestinal tract. The latter group includes such diverse agents as cholestyramine resin, diphenoxylate hydrochloride, simethicone, and sucralfate. A number of other drugs not included in this chapter are often administered for their effect on the gastrointestinal tract. Opium and morphine are frequently used to treat diarrhea and to relieve severe abdominal pain; antispasmodics such as papaverine and the parasympatholytic agents are used to suppress gastric acid secretion and to treat gastrointestinal spasm; cholinergics and posterior pituitary are occasionally used to increase the peristaltic activity of the gastrointestinal tract and to allay distention; and the anthelmintics, amebicides, and certain sulfonamides are used in the treatment of infections of the gastrointestinal tract.

Gastric Antacids

Gastric antacids are drugs which on ingestion react with the hydrochloric acid of the gastric contents to lower the acidity. They are prescribed by physicians for the symptomatic relief of hyperactivity associated with the diagnosis of *peptic ulcer*, *gastritis*, *peptic esophagitis*, and *gastric hyperacidity* and *hiatal hernia*. Unfortunately, they are used by the laity for a large variety of symptoms. Indiscriminate use of these agents, as encouraged by the communications media, is to be condemned since such use may lead to severe *uncompensated alkalosis*, a condition which is frequently unrecognized despite its high incidence.

In order for a product to be labeled an "antacid," according to the FDA Antacid Panel it must consist of one or more approved (active) ingredients. Each active ingredient must contribute at least 25% of the total acid-neutralizing capacity of the product. The finished product must contain at least 5 mEq/dose unit of neutralizing capacity and raise the pH of gastric secretions to 3.5 or greater within 10 minutes. This ruling does not apply to an antacid ingredient specifically added as a corrective to prevent a laxative or constipating effect or to adjunctive ingredients, such as simethicone, demulcents, or antipeptic agents. It is clear, therefore, that no more than four active antacid ingredients can be combined in any one product and that this ruling (see *Federal Register 39*, (108): 19862–19877, 1974) eliminates many marginal and/or ineffective products which have been promoted to the public.

Antacid products are required by law to carry certain warnings on the label or package inserts: products causing either constipation (aluminum-containing agents) or laxation (magnesium-containing agents) in 5% or more individuals taking the maximum dose must carry appropriate warnings; those which contain 50 mEq of magnesium or 25 mEq of potassium in the usual daily dose must indicate they are not to be used by patients with kidney disease; antacids which contain 5 mEq of sodium in the maximum daily dose must state they are contraindicated in patients on a sodium-restricted diet; and those containing more than 5 grams of lactose must warn individuals allergic to milk or milk products against their use. The pharmacist should be familiar with these warnings and counsel individuals using these products accordingly.

The goal of antacid therapy is to reduce the concentration and the total load of acid in gastric juice. This is not difficult to do. For example, one can neutralize 50% of the acid in a given amount of gastric juice with a pH of 1.3 by raising the pH to 1.6, 90% by raising the pH to 2.3, and 99% by raising the pH to 3.3. Antacids also have the ability to irreversibly inactivate pepsin if the gastric contents are brought to a pH above 6. The ultimate goal of therapy is to bring the gastric contents to a pH between 3.5 and 5, but it is difficult to maintain the desired pH because antacids tend to increase the activity of secreting gastric cells, and their effects are temporary and disappear when medication is discontinued. Furthermore, acid is usually secreted in greater amounts in the duodenal ulcer patient than in the normal individual.

Several factors must be considered when selecting an antacid product. *The patient:* The choice among various products is markedly reduced if the patient has impaired renal function, edema, high blood pressure, is allergic to milk or milk products or must take certain prescription drugs (see below). *Systemic vs nonsystemic:* A *systemic* antacid, such as sodium bicarbonate, is soluble, readily absorbed, and capable of producing systemic electrolyte disturbances and the symptoms of alkalosis. This imposes upon the kidney the burden of electrolyte readjustment. *Nonsystemic* antacids, such as calcium carbonate or basic aluminum substances, form compounds that are not appreciably absorbed and thus do not exert any systemic effect. It is generally agreed that when intensive antacid therapy is indicated only nonsystemic agents should be employed in order to avoid the potential danger of alkalosis induced by systemic antacids. *Neutralizing capacity:* Antacids differ enormously in their ability to neutralize gastric secretions. For example, 5 mL of aluminum hydroxide suspension (Amphojel) will neutralize 6.5 mEq of acid in 60 minutes, whereas a similar volume of aluminum hydroxide–magnesium hydroxide suspension (Delcid) will neutralize 42 mEq in the same period of time. *Dose:* It is generally agreed that 50 mEq per hour of *available* antacid is required to neutralize continuously the gastric contents of 90% of patients with duodenal ulcer. Based on the neutralizing capacity given above, this would require a dose of 6 mL of Delcid or 39 mL of Amphojel. *Dose interval:* An ideal antacid should be rapid in onset and provide a continuous buffering action. Antacids with a rapid onset include magnesium hydroxide, magnesium oxide, and calcium carbonate; those with an intermediate onset, magaldrate and magnesium carbonate; and those with a slow onset, magnesium trisilicate and the aluminum compounds. The duration of buffering action is largely determined by when the antacid is administered; if administered while food is in the stomach the buffering action will last for 2 hours. An additional dose 3 hours after meals will extend the buffering time by one hour. Therefore, the ideal dose interval is *one and three hours after meals and at bedtime*. *Cost:* It should be obvious that when cost to the patient is a factor, the decision should be based on neutralizing capacity per dose unit rather than cost per dosage unit.

Both the physical and chemical nature of antacids suggest a high potential for drug interaction by absorption and by alterations of the gastric pH. Calcium, aluminum, and magnesium decrease the gastric absorption of *tetracyclines*. Aluminum hydroxide decreases the absorption of *digoxin*, *isoniazid, phenytoin, corticosteroids, quinidine*, and *warfarin*. Antacids may also impair the absorption of oral *anticholinergics, phenothiazines*, and *oral iron* products. *Systemic antacids* may accelerate the excretion of *acidic drugs* (*salicylates*) and *inhibit* the urinary excretion of *basic drugs* (*amphetamines, quinidine*, etc). Since the effect of antacid therapy on the absorption of many drugs has not been studied, it seems advisable to administer other drugs at least one-half to one hour before antacid ingestion in order to assure consistent absorption and effect. Long-term use of antacids should be avoided when other drugs are taken, unless antacid use is clinically indicated and is of proven benefit.

The excess use of any antacid may produce adverse side effects. Sodium bicarbonate may produce *sodium overload* and *systemic alkalosis*. Magnesium preparations may induce *diarrhea* and are dangerous in patients with renal failure. Calcium carbonate can result in *hypercalcemia, renal impairment*, and *stimulation of gastric secretion*. Aluminum hydroxide may lead to *phosphate depletion* and, subsequently, *muscle weakness, bone resorption*, and *hypercalciuria*. Many antacid preparations contain large amounts of sodium, and, consequently, are contraindicated in patients with *hypertensive* and/or *cardiac disease*.

Aluminum Hydroxide Gel

Colloidal Aluminum Hydroxide; Amphojel (*Wyeth*); Alu-Tab (*Riker*)

Aluminum Hydroxide [21645-51-2] Al(OH)$_3$ (78.00); a suspension each 100 g of which contains the equivalent of 3.6–4.4 g of aluminum oxide [Al$_2$O$_3$ = 101.96], in the form of aluminum hydroxide and hydrated oxide.

It may contain peppermint oil, glycerin, sorbitol, sucrose, saccharin, or other suitable flavors, and it may contain suitable antimicrobial agents.

Preparation—One process for the preparation of this type of aluminum hydroxide is as follows:

Dissolve 1000 g of Na$_2$CO$_3$.10H$_2$O in 400 mL of hot water and filter. Dissolve 800 g of ammonium alum in 2000 mL of hot water and filter into the carbonate solution with constant stirring. Then add 4000 mL of hot water and remove all gas. Dilute to 80,000 mL with cold water. Collect and wash the precipitate and suspend it in 2000 mL of purified water flavored with 0.01% peppermint oil and preserve with 0.1% of sodium benzoate. Homogenize the resulting gel.

The principal property desired is a very fine particle size to achieve large surface and thus maximum adsorption capacity.

Description—White, viscous suspension, from which small amounts of water may separate on standing; translucent in thin layers; affects both red and blue litmus paper slightly but is not reddened by phenolphthalein.

Incompatibilities—The use of Aluminum Hydroxide Gel and similar materials to reduce the gastrointestinal problem accompanying use of tetracycline antibiotics has resulted in complexation and decreased absorption of the antibiotic.

Uses—Primarily as an antacid in the management of *peptic ulcer, gastritis, peptic esophagitis, gastric hyperacidity*, and *hiatal hernia*. It is also used as a skin protectant and mild astringent. Contrary to popular views, the compound is not an adsorbent, but reacts chemically to neutralize the gastric contents. It is a relatively weak antacid and does not elevate gastric pH sufficiently to inhibit pepsin activity.

Aluminum hydroxide does not have significant demulcent properties. Although aluminum hydroxide is a nonsystemic antacid and the fraction absorbed is very small, significant amounts are absorbed in patients with renal failure. Aluminum hydroxide is excreted as the phosphate. This provides the basis not only for the occasional use of aluminum hydroxide for the treatment of *phosphate nephrolithiasis*, but also is the cause of the phosphate depletion syndrome sometimes observed after chronic administration. Aluminum hydroxide has been used for *intestinal toxemia*, but more effective agents are available. The major advantage of aluminum hydroxide is that no systemic alkalosis is produced. Aluminum compounds decrease the absorption of certain drugs, such as the tetracycline antibiotics. It also interferes with the defoaming action of simethicone. These compounds are also constipating.

Dose—5 to 30 mL up to 12 times daily; *usual, adult, oral suspension:* **10 mL** 5 to 6 times a day between meals and at bedtime. *Tablets:* two 300-mg or one 600-mg 5 or 6 times daily between meals and at bedtime.

Other Dose Information—One 600-mg tablet or 10 mL of suspension will neutralize 18 and 13 mEq, respectively, of acid in 60 minutes.

Dosage Forms—Capsules 475 mg; Oral Suspension, 600 mg/5 mL; Dried, Tablets: 300 and 600 mg; Tablets (Chewable), 487.5 mg.

Dried Aluminum Hydroxide Gel yields not less than 50.0% of aluminum oxide [Al$_2$O$_3$ = 101.96]. *Preparation:* Aluminum hydroxide, prepared as described under *Aluminum Hydroxide Gel*, is dried at a low temperature until it has the required amount of Al$_2$O$_3$. *Description:* White, odorless, tasteless, amorphous powder. The filtrate from the aqueous suspension (1 in 25) is neutral to litmus. *Solubility:* Insoluble in water and alcohol; soluble in diluted mineral acids and solutions of fixed alkali hydroxides. *Dose:* The equivalent of 300 mg to 5 g of aluminum hydroxide daily; *usual*, the equivalent of 300 mg of aluminum hydroxide, 4 to 6 times a day.

Alumina and Magnesia Oral Suspension

Aludrox (*Wyeth*); Creamalin (*Winthrop*); Kolantyl (*Merrell-National*); Maalox (*Rorer*); WinGel (*Winthrop*)

Uses—A popular *antacid* mixture that combines the slowly acting aluminum hydroxide with the rapidly acting magnesium hydroxide. The various products described herein contain from 3.0 to 6.5% aluminum hydroxide and 1.5 to 4.0% magnesium hydroxide. The aluminum hydroxide is not only an effective antacid, but it is used to counteract the laxative effect of the magnesium hydroxide. The doses employed are usually capable of neutralizing continuously 40 to 50 mEq of gastric acid for 60 minutes. Combinations of this type are contraindicated in patients on antibiotic (tetracycline) medication.

Dose—*Usual, adult, oral,* **5 to 20 mL,** as indicated in the product literature, one hour after each meal and at bedtime.

Other Dose Information—Neutralizing capacity in mEq and sodium content (mg) per 5 mL: Aludrox, 14 (1.5); Creamalin, 12 (2.3); Kolantyl, 10.5 (2.6); Maalox, 13.5 (2.5); and WinGel, 10.2 (2).

Dosage Forms—Suspension containing indicated mg of aluminum hydroxide and magnesium hydroxide, respectively, in each 5 mL: Aludrox, 307 and 103; Creamalin, 320 and 75; Kolantyl, 150 and 150; and WinGel, 180 and 160.

Alumina and Magnesia Tablets

Aludrox (*Wyeth*); Creamalin (*Winthrop*); Kolantyl (*Merrell-National*); Maalox and Maalox 2 (*Rorer*); WinGel (*Winthrop*)

Uses—An *antacid* combination. The various products described herein contain from 180 to 248 mg of aluminum hydroxide and 75 to 170 mg of magnesium hydroxide per dosage unit. See *Alumina and Magnesia Oral Suspension*.

Dose—*Usual, adult, oral,* 1 to 4 **tablets** (or wafers), as indicated in product literature, one hour after each meal and at bedtime.

Other Dose Information—Neutralizing capacity in mEq and sodium content (mg) per dosage unit: Aludrox, 11.5 (1.6); Creamalin, 12.8 (<41); Kolantyl (wafer), 10 (0); Maalox, 11.5 (0.8); Maalox 2, 18 (1.8); WinGel, 12.3 (<1.7).

Dosage Forms—Tablets containing indicated mg of aluminum hydroxide and magnesium hydroxide in each tablet: Aludrox, 233 and 83; Creamalin, 248 and 75; Kolantyl (wafer), 180 and 170; Maalox, 200 and 200; Maalox 2, 400 and 400; and WinGel, 180 and 160.

Alumina, Magnesia, and Simethicone Oral Suspension

Gelusil and Gelusil II (*Warner*); Maalox Plus (*Rorer*); Mylanta and
Mylanta II (*Stuart*)

Uses—An *antacid* mixture that combines the slowly acting aluminum hydroxide and the rapidly acting magnesium hydroxide with the antifoaming agent simethicone. The various products described herein contain approximately equal parts of aluminum hydroxide and magnesium hydroxide with 0.4 to 0.6% simethicone. The aluminum hydroxide is used to counteract the laxative effect of magnesium hydroxide. The doses employed are usually capable of neutralizing continuously 40 to 50 mEq of gastric acid for 60 minutes. Combinations containing aluminum hydroxide are contraindicated in patients on antibiotic (tetracycline) therapy.

Dose—*Usual, adult, oral,* **5 to 10 mL,** as indicated in the product literature, one hour after each meal and at bedtime.

Other Dose Information—Neutralizing capacity in mEq and sodium content (mg) per 5 mL: Gelusil, 12 (1); Gelusil II, 24 (2); Maalox Plus, 13.5 (2.5); Mylanta, 12.7 (3.8); and Mylanta II, 25.4 (8).

Dosage Forms—Suspension containing indicated mg of aluminum hydroxide, magnesium hydroxide, and simethicone, respectively, in each 5 mL: Gelusil, 200, 200 and 25; Gelusil II, 400, 400 and 30; Maalox Plus, 225, 200 and 25; Mylanta, 200, 200 and 20; and Mylanta II, 400, 400 and 30.

Bismuth Subnitrate

Basic Bismuth Nitrate; Bismuth Oxynitrate; Spanish White; Bismuth
Paint; Bismuthyl Nitrate

Bismuth hydroxide nitrate oxide [1304-85-4] $Bi_5O(OH)_9(NO_3)_4$ (1461.99); a basic salt which, dried at 105° for 2 hours, yields upon ignition not less than 79% of Bi_2O_3 (465.96).

Preparation—A solution of bismuth nitrate is added to boiling water to produce the subnitrate by hydrolysis.

Description—White, slightly hygroscopic powder; suspension in distilled water is faintly acid to litmus (pH about 5).

Solubility—Practically insoluble in water and organic solvents; dissolves readily in an excess of hydrochloric or nitric acid.

Incompatibilities—Slowly hydrolyzed in *water* with liberation of nitric acid; thus it possesses the incompatibilities of the acid. *Reducing agents* darken it with the production of metallic bismuth.

Uses—A *pharmaceutical necessity* in the preparation of milk of bismuth. It is also used as an *astringent, adsorbent,* and *protective.* However, its value as a protective is questionable. Fatalities have been reported from oral use of bismuth subnitrate, especially in infants suffering from severe infectious diarrheas, due to formation of nitrite ion. This agent, like other insoluble bismuth salts, is used topically in lotions and ointments.

Dose—*Usual,* **5 mL.**

Bismuth Subsalicylate

Basic Bismuth Salicylate; Pepto-Bismol (*Norwich Eaton*)

[14882-18-19] $C_7H_5BiO_4$ (362.11).

Solubility—Practically insoluble in water or alcohol; soluble in alkali; decomposed by hot water.

Uses—Bismuth subsalicylate is the principal ingredient in a popular OTC product employed for *indigestion, nausea,* and *diarrhea.* As an antidiarrheal agent it shows good activity vs *salmonella,* but less activity vs *E Coli.* As an anti-ulcer drug, gastroscopic studies show little effective coating of the mucosa; nevertheless, it seems to increase the rate of healing of peptic ulcers. Since this agent is a salicylate, it may cause ringing of the ears if taken with aspirin. Bismuth subsalicylate may cause a temporary darkening of the stool and tongue.

Dose—*Usual, adult, oral,* two tablespoonfuls of the liquid or 2 tablets every ½ to 1 hour as needed to a maximum of 8 doses. *Children* (10–14 years), 4 teaspoonfuls; *children* (6 to 10 years), 2 teaspoonfuls or 1 tablet; *children* (3 to 6 years), 1 teaspoonful or ½ tablet.

Dosage Form—Liquid: 262 mg/15 mL (tablespoonful). Tablets: 300 mg.

Precipitated Calcium Carbonate

Carbonic acid, calcium salt (1:1); Creta Praecipitata; Precipitated
Chalk; Precipitated Carbonate of Lime

Calcium carbonate (1:1) [471-34-1] $CaCO_3$ (100.09).

Preparation—By double decomposition of calcium chloride and sodium carbonate in aqueous solution. Its density and fineness are governed by the concentration of the solutions; heavy and light forms are available on the market.

Description—Fine, white, microcrystalline powder, without odor or taste, and stable in air; aqueous suspension is practically neutral to litmus.

Solubility—Practically insoluble in water (its solubility in water is increased by the presence of any ammonium salt and by the presence of carbon dioxide; alkali hydroxide reduces its solubility); insoluble in alcohol; dissolves with effervescence in dilute acetic, hydrochloric, and nitric acids.

Uses—A rapidly-acting *antacid.* Calcium carbonate is classified as a "nonsystemic" *antacid* in that it does not tend to cause a systemic alkalosis. However, long-term therapy with large doses taken with milk or other sources of phosphate will cause renal pathology (milk-alkali syndrome) and some systemic alkalosis. The salt reacts with hydrochloric acid in the stomach to form calcium chloride which is largely (90%) converted to insoluble calcium salts in the intestinal tract. A variable proportion of the calcium (7 to 19%) is absorbed, probably in proportion to the amount of acid neutralized. Increased urinary calcium also favors calcific renal stones. Calcium salts by mouth are apt to be constipating. For this reason, calcium and magnesium antacids are often alternated in therapy or given in fixed combination.

Large doses of calcium carbonate (above 2 g) increase gastric secretion for a period of time that considerably outlasts the elevation of pH. Presumably this results from a local action in the intestine to cause gastrin release. A dose of only 0.5 g of calcium carbonate (the amount found in most antacids) may increase acid secretion in patients with and without duodenal ulcer. For this reason, it may seem that the stimulation of acid secretion is counterproductive; however, continuous neutralization with any antacid may cause maximal gastric secretion, so that the hypersecretion effect of large doses of calcium carbonate is of significance only when the dose-intervals are too large.

Theoretical and clinical considerations indicate that a dose of 2.5 g/hour (45 mEq) should effectively and continuously neutralize the acid of 90% of duodenal ulcer patients. However, the recommended 4- to 6-hour interval is much too long for maximum efficacy; the emptying time of the otherwise empty stomach is 30 to 40 min. For many years, the standard dose of calcium carbonate used by authorities was 4 g every hour. For OTC products, the usual dose is 1 to 2 g as needed (up to 160 mEq/day).

Precipitated calcium carbonate is also employed in dentifrices and is a pharmaceutical necessity for *Aluminum Subacetate Solution* and antacid oral suspension dosage forms.

Dose—1 to **10 g** daily; *usual,* **1 g** 4 to 6 times a day.

Other Dose Information—Two 420-mg tablets or 5 mL of suspension (Titralac) will neutralize 15 and 19 mEq, respectively, of acid in 60 minutes.

Dosage Forms—Suspension: (*Titralac;* Riker); Tablets: 420, 600 mg and 1 g.

Calcium Hydroxide Solution—page 1310.

Calcium Phosphate, Dibasic—page 834.

Calcium Phosphate, Tribasic—RPS-16, page 774.

Dihydroxyaluminum Sodium Carbonate

Aluminum, [carbonato(1-)-*O*]dihydroxy, monosodium salt; Rolaids
(*Warner Lambert*)

Sodium (*T*-4)-[carbonato(2-)-*O,O'*]dihydroxyaluminate (1-) [16482-55-6] $NaAl(OH)_2CO_3$ (144.00); contains the equivalent of 34.8–38.2% of Al_2O_3 (aluminum oxide).

Preparation—Aluminum isopropoxide is reacted with a basic solution of sodium bicarbonate. US Pat 2,783,179.

Description—Fine, white powder that is odorless and tasteless; stable in light, slightly hygroscopic at room temperature, and dehydrates and loses CO_2 above 100°.

Solubility—Practically insoluble in water; dissolves in dilute mineral acids.

Uses—A single molecule which combines the antacid properties of aluminum hydroxide and sodium bicarbonate. Hence, it is a partial systemic *antacid*. It has a rapid onset of action as gastric acid reacts with the sodium carbonate portion of the molecule; this is followed by a sustained, but less intense, antacid action due to the generated aluminum hydroxide. Since each tablet contains 53 mg of sodium, it is contraindicated in patients on a sodium-restricted diet.

Dose—*Usual*, **300** to **600 mg** as required. *Other dose information*—each tablet (334 mg) neutralizes approximately 7.5 mEq of acid in 60 minutes.

Dosage Form—Tablets: (chewable), 334 mg.

Magaldrate

Aluminum magnesium hydroxide; Riopan and Riopan Plus (*Ayerst*)

$$AlMg_2(OH)_7.H_2O$$

[1317-26-6] (212.66); contains the equivalent of 29–40% of MgO (magnesium oxide), and the equivalent of 18–26% of Al_2O_3 (aluminum oxide).

Preparation—By precipitation using aqueous solutions of sodium or potassium aluminate and a magnesium salt under controlled conditions of concentration and temperature. The precipitated product is collected by filtration, washed to remove soluble by-products, and dried. US Pat 2,923,660. The formulas shown above have been suggested although the substance is also described as an indefinite mixture of magnesium and aluminum hydroxides.

Description—White, odorless, crystalline powder.

Solubility—Insoluble in water and alcohol; soluble in dilute solutions of mineral acids.

Uses—A chemical combination of magnesium and aluminum hydroxides used as an *antacid*. It is said to have a rapid action, uniform buffering action, high acid-consuming capacity, no alkalinization or acid rebound, and a very low sodium content. It is indicated for the relief of *heartburn*, *sour stomach*, and/or *acid indigestion*. It is also used for the symptomatic relief of *hyperacidity* associated with the diagnosis of *peptic ulcer*, *gastritis*, *peptic esophagitis*, *gastric hyperacidity*, and *hiatal hernia*. It is somewhat more effective as an antacid than aluminum hydroxide. Magaldrate disturbs neither electrolyte balance nor bowel function. It should not be used in patients taking any form of tetracycline. It is also available in combination with simethicone.

Dose—*Usual*, **480** to **960 mg** of magaldrate as required, preferably taken between meals and at bedtime.

Other Dose Information—Each tablet (480 mg) or 5 mL of suspension (400 mg) neutralizes 13.5 mEq of acid in 60 minutes and contains 0.65 mg of sodium.

Dosage Forms—Oral Suspension: 480 mg/5 mL (Riopan); 480 mg and 20 mg simethicone/5 mL (Riopan Plus). Chewable Tablets: 480 mg (Riopan); 480 mg and 20 mg simethicone (Riopan Plus). Swallow Tablets: 480 mg (Riopan).

Magnesia and Alumina Oral Suspension

Maalox Therapeutic (*Rorer*); Delcid (*Merrell-Dow*); Aludrox Suspension (*Wyeth*)

Uses—An *antacid* composed of magnesium hydroxide (103 mg, Aludrox; 300 mg, Maalox; 665 mg, Delcid) and aluminum hydroxide (307 mg Aludrox; 600 mg, Maalox and Delcid) in each 5 mL of suspension. The aluminum hydroxide counteracts the laxative effect of the magnesium hydroxide. This preparation tends to decrease the absorption of tetracyclines and some other drugs (*see* introduction to this section).

Dose—*Usual*, *adult*, *oral*, **5 mL** one hour after each meal and at bedtime.

Other Dose Information—Neutralizing capacity in mEq and sodium content (mg) per 5 mL: Delcid, 42 (<15); Aludrox, 14 (1.15); Maalox, 28.3 (0.8).

Dosage Form—Suspension.

Magnesium Carbonate

Carbonic acid, magnesium salt, basic or Carbonic acid, magnesium salt (1:1), hydrate; Light Magnesium Carbonate; Heavy Magnesium Carbonate

Magnesium carbonate, basic [39409-82-0] *or* magnesium carbonate (1:1) hydrate [23389-33-5]; *anhydrous* [546-93-0] (84.31); contains the equivalent of 40–43.5% of MgO (magnesium oxide).

Medicinal magnesium carbonate is available in *light* and *heavy* forms; the light, which is 2 to $2\frac{1}{2}$ times as bulky as the heavy, is the most commonly used.

Preparation—Largely from *dolomite* [$MgCO_3.CaCO_3$] by first calcining it, suspending the calcined product in water and saturating with CO_2 under pressure. Some lime also dissolves as calcium bicarbonate, but when the temperature, after the treatment with carbon dioxide, is raised, nearly all of the dissolved lime precipitates as the insoluble carbonate. The filtered solution is then heated to the boiling temperature whereupon the magnesium bicarbonate loses CO_2 and H_2O and magnesium carbonate precipitates. This process generally yields the light carbonate.

The heavy carbonate is generally produced by precipitating a hot, concentrated solution of magnesium chloride or sulfate with a solution of sodium carbonate.

Description—Light, white, friable masses, or a bulky, white powder; odorless, but readily absorbs odors; stable in air.

Solubility—Practically insoluble in water, to which however, it imparts an alkaline reaction, but it is appreciably soluble in water containing carbon dioxide; insoluble in alcohol; dissolved by dilute acids with effervescence.

Uses—An *antacid* and *cathartic* with pharmacologic properties similar to magnesium oxide. It differs from the latter, however, in that carbon dioxide is liberated during neutralization. As an antacid, it is relatively weak; its neutralizing capacity *in vitro* is 20 mEq per g, only a fraction of which is available for neutralization *in vivo*. Its rate of reaction is considerably slower than that of calcium carbonate. It is usually alternated with calcium carbonate to overcome the constipating action of the latter salt.

Dose—*Usual*, **500 mg** to **2 g** 4 times a day.

Magnesia, Alumina, and Calcium Carbonate

Camalox (*Rorer*)

Uses—An antacid containing magnesium hydroxide (200 mg), aluminum hydroxide (225 mg), and calcium carbonate (250 mg) per dose unit. It is contraindicated in patients on antibiotic (tetracycline) medication.

Dose—*Usual*, *adult*, *oral*, **10** to **20 mL** of the suspension or two to four tablets one-half to one hour after each meal and at bedtime.

Other Dose Information—Neutralizing capacity in mEq and sodium content (mg) per 5 mL of suspension or one tablet: 18 (2.5) and 18 (1.5), respectively.

Dosage Forms—Suspension and Tablets.

Magnesium Hydroxide

Magnesium hydroxide [1309-42-8] $Mg(OH)_2$ (58.32).

Preparation—By precipitation using aqueous solutions of magnesium chloride or sulfate and sodium hydroxide. US Pat 3,127,241. A method for preparing it in various particle sizes is described in US Pat 3,232,708.

Description—White, very fine, bulky powder; slowly absorbs carbon dioxide on exposure to air.

Solubility—Practically insoluble in water and in alcohol; dissolves in dilute acids.

Uses—The same as *Magnesium Oxide*.

Dose—*Usual*, *antacid*, **300** to **600 mg**; *cathartic*, **2** to **4 g**.

Dosage Forms—Tablets: 300 mg.

Milk of Magnesia [Magnesium Hydroxide Mixture; Cream of Magnesia; Magnesia Magma; MOM] is a suspension of magnesium hydroxide, each 100 g of which contains 7–8.5% of $Mg(OH)_2$ (58.32). It may contain 0.1% of citric acid, and may contain not more than 0.05% of a volatile oil or a blend of volatile oils, suitable for flavoring purposes. *Note*—Citric acid may be added to minimize the interaction of glass containers and this preparation. No formula is now included in the USP as there are various satisfactory methods of preparation and any one of these may be used if the finished product conforms to the official specifications. *Description:* White, opaque, more or less viscous suspension from which varying proportions of water usually separate on standing; pH about 10; absorbs carbon dioxide from the air; alkaline to litmus and phenolphthalein. *Incompatibilities:* The fact is occasionally overlooked that milk of magnesia has an alkaline reaction and possesses the incompatibilities typical of such a reaction. Thus, *alkaloids* are liberated from solutions of their salts. *Uses:* A nonsystemic gastric *antacid* and mild *cathartic.* Each mL of milk of magnesia is capable of neutralizing approximately 2.7 mEq of acid. When used routinely as an antacid, the cathartic effect may be minimized by the occasional use of calcium carbonate. It should be used with caution in patients with kidney disease, since 5 to 10% can be absorbed. Prolonged use may result in kidney stones. *Dose:* 5 to 50 mL/daily; *usual antacid,* 5 mL/4 times a day; *usual, cathartic,* 15 to 30 mL.

Magnesium Oxide

Magnesia; Light Magnesia; Calcined Magnesia; Heavy Magnesium Oxide; Heavy Magnesia; Heavy Calcined Magnesia; Magnesia Usta

Magnesium oxide [1309-48-4] MgO (40.30).

Preparation—Light or heavy magnesium carbonate is exposed to red heat whereupon carbon dioxide and water are expelled, and light or heavy magnesium oxide is left. The density of the oxide is also influenced by the calcining temperature, higher temperatures yielding more compact forms.

Description—Very bulky, white powder known as light magnesium oxide or as a relatively dense, white powder known as heavy magnesium oxide. Readily absorbs moisture and carbon dioxide when exposed to air.

Solubility—Practically insoluble in water to which, however, it imparts an alkaline reaction; insoluble in alcohol; soluble in dilute acids.

Uses—An effective, fairly long-acting, nonsystemic *gastric antacid.* Since in water it is converted to the hydroxide, its biological properties are the same as the hydroxide. Consequently, it does not neutralize gastric contents excessively and does not liberate carbon dioxide. It is sometimes employed as a *cathartic.* Either the light or heavy form may be employed.

Light magnesia is preferable to the heavy for administration in liquids because, being a finer powder, it suspends more readily.

Dose—**250 mg** to **4 g** daily; *usual,* **250 mg** 4 times a day.

Other Dose Information—One g has a neutralizing capacity of 50 mEq of acid; however, only 8 to 20 mEq react with gastric acid in 30 minutes.

Magnesium Phosphate

Phosphoric acid, magnesium (2:3), pentahydrate; Tribasic Magnesium Phosphate

Magnesium phosphate (3:2) pentahydrate [10233-87-1] Mg$_3$(PO$_4$)$_2$.5H$_2$O (352.93); *anhydrous* [7757-87-1] (262.86).

Preparation—By precipitation using aqueous solutions of tribasic sodium phosphate and magnesium sulfate or chloride.

Description—White, odorless, and tasteless powder.

Solubility—Almost insoluble in water; readily soluble in diluted mineral acids.

Uses—An *antacid* used like *Tribasic Calcium Phosphate* (RPS-16, page 774). It neutralizes the excess acid of the stomach but produces no excess alkalinization of the system. It has a mild laxative action.

Dose—*Usual,* 1 g.

Magnesium Trisilicate

Silicic acid (H$_4$Si$_3$O$_8$), magnesium salt (1:2), hydrate; Hydrated Magnesium Silicate

Magnesium silicate hydrate [39365-87-2] 2MgO.3SiO$_2$.xH$_2$O; *anhydrous* [14987-04-3] (260.86); a compound of magnesium oxide and silicon dioxide with varying proportions of water. It contains not less than 20% of magnesium oxide [MgO = 40.30] and not less than 45% of silicon dioxide [SiO$_2$ = 60.08].

Preparation—By precipitating a solution of sodium silicate of the proper composition [Na$_4$Si$_3$O$_8$, or having a ratio of Na$_2$O to SiO$_2$ = 1:1.5] with a solution of magnesium chloride or sulfate.

Description—Fine, white, odorless, tasteless powder, free from grittiness; its suspension is neutral or only slightly alkaline to litmus.

Solubility—Insoluble in water and in alcohol; readily decomposed by mineral acids with the liberation of silicic acid.

Uses—A nonsystemic *antacid* and *adsorbent.* As an antacid, it has slow onset of action and is relatively weak; as a single entity it can not meet current pH requirements for nonprescription antacids. Approximately 5% of the magnesium and 7% of the silicate may be absorbed. Therefore, a number of cases of siliceous nephrolith have been reported following chronic use. Large doses may cause diarrhea due to the action of the soluble magnesium salts on the enteric tract. It is available only in combination with other antacids.

Dose—1 to 16 g daily; *usual,* 1 g 4 times a day.

Dosage Forms—Tablets: 500 mg.

Sodium Bicarbonate

Carbonic acid monosodium salt; Baking Soda; Sodium Acid Carbonate

Monosodium carbonate [144-55-8] NaHCO$_3$ (84.01).

Preparation—May be produced by the ammonia-soda process, or *Solvay Process,* as it is usually called. In this process carbon dioxide is passed into a solution of common salt in ammonia water, sodium bicarbonate is precipitated, and ammonium chloride, being much more soluble, remains in solution. The ammonium chloride solution is heated with lime whereby the ammonia is regenerated and returned to the process.

Description—White, crystalline powder; odorless and has a saline and slightly alkaline taste; solutions, when freshly prepared with cold water without shaking, are alkaline to litmus paper; alkalinity increases as the solutions stand, are agitated, or heated; stable in dry air, but slowly decomposes in moist air.

Solubility—1 g in 12 mL water; with hot water it is converted into carbonate; insoluble in alcohol.

Uses—Widely employed as a gastric *antacid,* especially by the laity, despite its many disadvantages. Sodium bicarbonate reacts with hydrochloric acid to produce carbon dioxide, thus giving rise to epigastric distress. Although the onset of action is rapid, the duration of action is short. Sodium bicarbonate is readily absorbed and prolonged therapy with large doses will produce systemic alkalosis. Moreover, chronic therapy along with milk or calcium may precipitate the milk-alkali syndrome. Also, even moderate amounts may expand plasma volume, increase blood pressure, and lead to edema. Therefore, it may be hazardous in patients with renal insufficiency, hypertension, or cardiac failure.

In the treatment of *systemic acidosis,* sodium bicarbonate is specific in that the salt is composed of the two ions essential to correct this condition.

Sodium bicarbonate is used locally on the skin in the form of a moist paste or a solution. In this form, it is an effective *antipruritic.* The salt is also an ingredient of many effervescent mixtures, alkaline solutions, douches, etc.

Dose—**300 mg** to **16 g** daily; *usual,* **300 mg** to 2 g 1 to 4 times a day.

Other Dose Information—The maximum daily intake is 200 mEq of bicarbonate in patients under 60 years of age and 100 mEq in those over 60. Each g will neutralize 12 mEq of gastric acid in 60 minutes.

Dosage Forms—Injection: 1%/20 mL, 1.4 and 5%/500 mL, 7.5%/50 mL, 8.4%/40 mL; Tablets: 325, 487.5, 520, and 650 mg.

Other Gastric Antacids

Aluminum Carbonate, Basic [Basaljel (*Wyeth*)] is an aqueous suspension of an aluminum hydroxide carbonate prepared by the interaction of soluble aluminum salts and soluble carbonates. It contains the equivalent of 5.1% of Al$_2$O$_3$ and not less than 2.4% of CO$_2$. *Description:* White, creamy, thixotropic gel having a pH of 6.6 to 7; if not kept in tightly closed containers, it gradually loses CO$_2$. *Uses:* To control gastric hyperacidity and as an adjunct in the treatment of peptic ulcer. It is also used in the management of nephrolithiasis when the stones are composed of phosphate salts. The drug has a tendency to produce constipation which can easily be controlled with a mild laxative. *Dose: Antacid,* adult oral, 2 capsules or tablets, 10 mL of regular suspension (in water or fruit juice) or 5 mL of extra strength suspension as often as every 2 hours, up to 12 times a day. *Prevention of phosphate stones,* capsules or tablets: 2 to 6, 1 hour after meals and at bedtime. Suspension: 10 to 30 mL or extra strength suspension 5 to 15 mL, 1 hour after each meal and at bedtime. In the management of phosphatic urinary calculi, larger doses (30 mL 4 times daily) are used to combine with phosphate in the intestine and decrease phosphate absorption.

Other Dose Information: 5 mL of the suspension or 1 swallow tablet will neutralize 14 mEq of acid in 60 minutes; this volume of suspension also contains 15 mg of sodium. Five mL of extra strength suspension or 1 capsule will neutralize 11 and 13 mEq of acid in 60 minutes.

Bismuth Subcarbonate [Bismuth subcarbonate [5892-10-4] approximately $(BiO)_2CO_3 \cdot \frac{1}{2}H_2O$ (518.98); a basic salt, which yields on ignition not less than 90% of Bi_2O_3 (465.96).] *Preparation:* To a solution of bismuth nitrate is added, with constant stirring, an excess of an approximately 20% solution of sodium carbonate and allowed to stand for some time. After filtering and washing the precipitate until the washings are neutral, the subcarbonate is dried at about 50°. *Description:* White, or pale yellowish white, odorless, and tasteless powder; stable in air, but slowly affected by light. *Solubility:* Practically insoluble in water and alcohol; dissolved by excess of nitric and hydrochloric acids with copious effervescence, forming the corresponding salts. *Uses:* A very *weak antacid;* bismuth compounds are incapable of increasing the gastric pH above 2. It is used internally as an *astringent* and *adsorbent.* It is also used topically as a *protective* in lotions and ointments. Bismuth subcarbonate is given in the dose of 1 to 4 g every 2 to 4 hours in the treatment of *enteritis, diarrhea, dysentery,* and *ulcerative colitis. Dose: Topical,* in lotions and ointments. *Other Dose Information:* The oral range is 1 to 4 g, *usual,* 1 g 4 times a day.

Milk of Bismuth [Bismuth Magma; Bismuth Cream] Bismuth hydroxide and bismuth carbonate in suspension in water; yields 5.2–5.8% (w/w) of Bi_2O_3 (bismuth trioxide = 465.96). Refer to RPS-16, page 736 for a preparation recipe from bismuth subnitrate, nitric acid, ammonium carbonate, and ammonia. *Description:* Thick, white, opaque suspension which separates upon standing; odorless and almost tasteless. *Solubility:* Miscible with water and alcohol. *Uses:* An *astringent* and *antacid.* It is used either alone or in combination with paregoric in the management of *diarrhea* and intestinal inflammation. Its weak antacid properties render it unsuitable for use in the management of peptic ulcer. *Dose: Usual,* 5 mL.

Dihydroxyaluminum Aminoacetate [Basic Aluminum Glycinate [41354-48-7] $C_2H_6AlNO_4 \cdot xH_2O$; anhydrous [13682-92-3] (135.06)] Yields 35.5–38.5% of Al_2O_3 [aluminum oxide = 101.96]; may contain small amounts of aluminum oxide and of aminoacetic acid. *Preparation:* By precipitation on adding a solution of aluminum isopropoxide in propanol to an aqueous solution of glycine. *Description:* White, odorless powder having a faintly sweet taste; pH (1 in 25 aqueous suspension) between 6.5 and 7.5. *Solubility:* Insoluble in water; dissolves in dilute mineral acids and in solutions of fixed alkalies. *Uses:* A relatively weak *antacid.* Its actions are almost identical with those of the aluminum hydroxide gel preparations, and it has the same advantages and disadvantages. The drug may be employed as a constituent of almost any regimen to control *hyperacidity ie, gastritis, gastric hyperacidity, peptic esophagitis,* and *hiatal hernia.* Substitution of another form of antacid therapy may occasionally be necessary to alleviate the constipation which may occur after prolonged use of any of the aluminum preparations. This drug is contraindicated for patients taking any form of tetracycline; it markedly decreases the absorption of the antibiotic. *Dose:* 500 mg to 2 g; *usual,* 500 mg to 1 g 4 times a day. *Other Dose Information:* Each tablet (500 mg) neutralizes approximately 7 mEq of acid in 60 minutes. *Dosage Forms:* Magma: 500 mg/5 mL; Tablets: 500 mg.

H₂-Receptor Antagonists

Histamine contracts many smooth muscles, such as those of the bronchi and gut, but markedly relaxes others including those of the small blood vessels. It is also a potent stimulus to gastric acid production and elicits various other exocrine secretions. Although these actions dominate the overall response of the drug, it also induces edema formation and stimulation of the sensory nerve endings. Some of these actions, such as bronchoconstriction and contraction of the gut, are mediated by one type of receptor, the H_1 receptors (Ash and Shild, *Br J Pharmacol 27:* 427–439, 1966) which are readily blocked by the classical antihistamines (see chapter 61). Other effects most importantly gastric acid secretion, involve the H_2 receptors and are susceptible to inhibition by histamine H_2-receptor blocking drugs (Black, *et al, Nature, 236:* 385–390, 1972). Still other effects of histamine, such as hypotension resulting from vascular hypotension, are mediated by both H_1 and H_2 receptors and are blocked by a combination of both H_1- and H_2-receptor inhibitors.

The H_2-receptor antagonists were the result of the intentional modification of the histamine structure and deliberate search for a chemically related substance that would act as a competitive inhibitor of the H_2 receptors. Burimamide, the first agent discovered with substantial antagonistic activity

against histamine, was only effective intravenously. This success, however, stimulated the development of another substance, metiamide, which is an effective inhibitor of gastric secretion after either oral or intravenous administration. This agent was abandoned because it produced agranulocytosis, an effect presumably related to a thiourea group in the molecule. Cimetidine, approved for clinical use August 1977 by the Food and Drug Administration, contains a substituted imidazole ring like that in histamine. After five years of clinical experience in 25 million patients, cimetidine is considered the prototype drug for ulcer therapy. In June 1983 another H_2 receptor antagonist, ranitidine, was approved by the FDA for use in the management of duodenal ulcer and hypersecretory states. Ranitidine contains a substituted furan ring rather than the imidazole ring common to cimetidine and histamine. These two agents, as well as other H_2-receptor antagonists under clinical trial, are presented in this section.

Cimetidine

Guanidine, N''-cyano-N-methyl-N'-[2-[[(5-methyl-1H-imidazol-4-yl)-methyl]thio]ethyl]-; Tagamet (*Smith Kline & French*)

2-Cyano-1-methyl-3-[2-[[(5-methylimidazol-4-yl)methyl]thio]-ethyl]guanidine [51481-61-9] $C_{10}H_{16}N_6S$ (252.34).

Preparation—Methods of synthesis of analogs of histamine capable of functioning as H_2-receptor antagonists, of the type of cimetidine, are described in German Pats 2,344,779 and 2,344,833 (see *CA 80:* 146167h, 146168j, 1974). In one of these methods a substituted guanidine, such as $CH_3NHC(:NCN)SCH_3$, is refluxed with a histamine-related imidazole, as $NH_2CH_2CH_2SCH_2Z$ (in which Z is a methylimidazole), in methyl cyanide to produce the product $N\!\!\equiv\!\!CHNH(CH_3)C\!\!=\!\!CHCH_2CH_2SCH_2Z$.

Description—White to off-white, crystalline powder; unpleasant odor; melting range 141°–143°; pK_a 6.8.

Solubility—1 g in about 200 mL water, 18 mL alcohol, 1000 mL chloroform; insoluble in ether.

Uses—Cimetidine is used for the treatment of endoscopically or radiologically confirmed duodenal ulcers. It is also used in the treatment of pathological hypersecretory conditions such as Zollinger-Ellison syndrome, systemic mastocytosis, and multiple endocrine adenomas. Although total gastrectomy has been considered the treatment of choice for Zollinger-Ellison syndrome, clinical studies now suggest cimetidine may be preferred because of the lesser risks. Cimetidine has also been used with some success in the short-term treatment of gastric ulcers. Preliminary studies also suggest that this agent may be effective in stress ulcers, peptic esophagitis, and upper gastrointestinal bleeding. The relative value of cimetidine in these latter disorders as compared with conventional therapy remains to be established.

Cimetidine has a pK_a of 6.8 and cimetidine hydrochloride has a pK_a of 7.11. Cimetidine competitively inhibits the action of histamine on the H_2 receptors of parietal cells, reducing gastric acid output and concentration. This reduction occurs under basal conditions as well as when gastric acid secretion is stimulated by food, insulin, betazole, histamine, pentagastrin, and caffeine. The oral administration of 300 mg of cimetidine reduces basal gastric acid output by 100% for at least 2 hours and by 90% throughout the 4 hour study in fasting duodenal ulcer patients. The gastric pH in all subjects was increased to 5 or greater for at least $2\frac{1}{2}$ hours. A 300 mg dose of cimetidine inhibited nocturnal basal secretion in fasting duodenal ulcer patients by 100% for at least one hour and by 89% over a 7-hour period. Gastric pH was increased to 5.0 or greater for 3 or 4 hours. Administered orally after a standard meal, 300 mg of cimetidine inhibited gastric secretion in duodenal ulcer patients by 50% during the first hour and by 75% during the subsequent 2 hours.

Cimetidine is rapidly and well absorbed after oral administration. A small portion of the drug is metabolized on its first pass through the liver; the average bioavailability is 70% when compared to intravenous injection; 19% is bound to serum proteins; volume distribution is 1.5 L/kg; 48% is excreted unchanged; elimination half-life ranges from 2 to 3 hours; mean serum concentration is 500 ng/mL; and mean peak blood level is 1440 ng/mL.

Cimetidine has been reported to reduce hepatic metabolism of drugs that are metabolized primarily by cytochrome P450, thereby delaying elimination and increasing blood levels of these drugs. Therefore, cimetidine should be used with caution in patients on *warfarin-type anticoagulants*, *phenytoin*, *beta-adrenergic blocking agents*, *lidocaine*, and *theophylline*; cimetidine reduces the hepatic metabolism of these substances, delays their elimination, and increases their blood levels. The half-life of benzodiazepines is increased in patients also taking cimetidine. A *decrease* in serum digoxin may occur in patients taking both *digoxin* and cimetidine.

Adverse reactions are usually mild and transient; diarrhea, muscular pain, dizziness, and rash have been reported in a few patients. A few cases of headache, ranging from mild to severe, have been reported. Reversible arthralgia and myalgia, and exacerbation of joint symptoms in patients with pre-existing arthritis are observed on rare occasions. Mild gynecomastia has been reported in about 4% of patients with hypersecretory conditions; in all others the incidence was about 0.3 to 1%. A few cases of reversible confusional states in elderly or severely ill patients have been observed. Small increases in plasma creatinine, serum transaminase, and interstitial nephritis have also been reported; all of these cleared when the drug was withdrawn. The safe use of cimetidine in pregnant women or nursing mothers has not been established. A report of gastric cancer observed in several patients receiving cimetidine has prompted ongoing studies to determine if any cause-effect relationship exists.

Dose—*Usual, adult, oral*, **300 mg** 4 times daily with meals and at bedtime; *Dose range*, **1.2** to **2.4 g** daily. *Usual, adult, intravenous* (as the hydrochloride) **300 mg** administered in 20 mL of 0.9% sodium chloride solution or **300 mg** 100 mL of 5% dextrose by intermittent infusion. Although commonly used with antacids, cimetidine should be administered between doses of the antacid to avoid possible inhibition of cimetidine absorption.

Dosage Forms—Injection (as the hydrochloride): 150 mg/mL; Liquid, 300 mg/5 mL. Tablets: 200 and 300 mg.

Cinnamon—page 1285.

Cinnamon, Ceylon—page 1285.

Cinnamon Oil—page 1285.

Coriander Oil—page 1286.

Ranitidine

1,1-Ethenediamine, *N*-[2-[[[5-[(dimethylamino)methyl]-2-furanyl]-methyl]thio]ethyl]-*N*′-methyl-2-nitro-, Zantac (*Glaxo*)

[66357-35-5] $C_{13}H_{22}N_4O_3S$ (314.40).
Preparation—See US Pat 4,128,658.

Description—White solid melting about 70°.

Uses—Ranitidine, a substituted furan derivative, is an H_2-receptor antagonist indicated for the short-term treatment of *duodenal ulcer* and the management of *hypersecretory conditions*, such as *Zollinger-Ellison Syndrome* and *systemic mastocytosis*. The pharmacokinetic profile of ranitidine is similar to that for cimetidine. Neither product is long acting and they have similar half-lives. Oral absorption appears to be variable and decreased if given concurrently with antacids; bioavailability after an oral dose of 150 mg is approximately 50% (range 40 to 88%); 15% is bound to plasma protein; volume distribution 1.4 L/kg; 30% of the administered dose is excreted unchanged; elimination half-life ranges from 2.5 to 3.0 hours; serum concentrations vary from 36 to 94 ng/mL; and mean peak blood levels are 440 to 545 ng/mL. Ranitidine is not inherently long acting and it lacks a predictable dose/response relationship. For example, 75, 100, and 150 mg of ranitidine inhibits nocturnal gastric acid output by 95, 96, and 92%, respectively. Although the limited clinical experience suggests that ranitidine may interact with only a limited

number of other drugs, interactions with warfarin, benzodiazepines, fentanyl, metaprolol, nefedipine, and acetaminophen have been reported. Likewise, few adverse reactions have been encountered; headache, malaise, dizziness, constipation, nausea, abdominal pain, and rash have been observed most frequently. Decreased white blood cell and platelet count have also been reported. Increases (up to 5 times the upper limit of normal) in serum transaminase and gammaglutamyl transpeptidase have been noted. Rare cases of hepatitis have also been reported. In normal volunteers, SGPT were increased at least twice the pretreatment levels in 6 of 12 subjects given 100 mg 4 times a day intravenously for 7 days and in 4 of 24 subjects given 50 mg 4 times daily intravenously for 5 days. This dose-related effect suggests that ranitidine is potentially hepatotoxic. With respect to use in pregnancy and lactation, studies in rats and rabbits have revealed no evidence of impaired fertility or harm to the fetus. Nevertheless, it should not be used in pregnancy unless needed. Ranitidine is secreted in milk; therefore, it should not be used in nursing mothers unless absolutely necessary. Overall, ranitidine appears to have a profile of action similar to cimetidine. However, an accurate comparative assessment cannot be made until ranitidine has been used in many more ulcer patients.

Dose—*Usual, adult, oral, duodenal ulcer:* **150 mg** twice daily. *Hypersecretory conditions* (such as Zollinger-Ellison Syndrome): **150 mg** twice daily. *Impaired renal function:* **150 mg** every 12 to 24 hours.

Dosage Forms—Tablets: 150 mg.

Other H_2-Receptor Antagonists

Oxmetidine Hydrochloride [5-(1,3-Benzodioxol-5-ylmethyl)-2-[[2-[[5-methyl-1*H*-imidazol-4-yl)methyl]thio]ethyl]amino]-4(1*H*)-pyrimidinone hydrochloride [63204-23-9] $C_{19}H_{21}N_5O_3S.2HCl$ (472.39)]. A histamine H_2-receptor antagonist currently under clinical trial for use in duodenal ulcer and various gastric hypersecretory disorders. Oxmetidine appears to have a pharmacological profile similar to that for cimetidine and ranitidine.

Digestants

Digestants are drugs which promote the process of digestion in the gastrointestinal tract. They have limited usefulness in the treatment of conditions characterized by a deficiency of one or more of the specific substances essential for the digestion of foodstuffs in the alimentary canal. Thus, in a general way, they may be classified as drugs used for replacement therapy in deficiency states. The digestants commonly employed are the *choleretics* (bile, bile acids, bile salts) and hydrochloric acid.

Although bile is composed of a variety of substances, only the bile salts (salts of the native bile acids, page 779) are therapeutically important. When given by mouth the bile salts are absorbed from the intestine and reexcreted by the liver in the bile, thus entering the same cyclic process as endogenous bile salts. They are of value in promoting the absorption of fats and fat-soluble vitamins (see Chapter 53) from the intestinal tract when the normal biliary output is either reduced or absent.

Hydrochloric acid exerts several physiological functions in the gastrointestinal tract. It converts pepsinogen to active pepsin, renders gastric contents relatively sterile, plays a role in the normal emptying of the stomach, aids in the secretion of intestinal and pancreatic juices, and, finally, is essential for the absorption of certain inorganic salts. Gastric hydrochloric acid secretion is deficient in 10 to 15% of the general population. This condition is commonly called *hypochlorhydria*. *Achlorhydria* is frequently associated with gastritis, gastric carcinoma, pernicious anemia, etc. It may also be present in individuals with no demonstrable gastric lesion. Symptoms usually attributed to achlorhydria include vague epigastric distress, belching, abdominal distention, coated tongue, nausea, vomiting, and diarrhea. Hydrochloric acid or its substitutes are effective in relieving such deficiency symptoms in a significant number of individuals.

Bile, Bile Acids, and Bile Salts

The bile, a viscid, bitter, alkaline (pH 7.8), fluid, isotonic with the blood and yellowish brown to a golden yellow in color, is excreted by adults at the rate of 500 to 1100 mL in 24 hours. The principal organic constituents are bile acids (as salts), bile pigments, cholesterol, lecithin, mucin, neutral fats, nucleoproteins, and phosphatides. The principal inorganic constituents are sodium, calcium, copper, iron, magnesium, potassium, bicarbonate, phosphate, and sulfate.

The bile acids, present as the sodium salts of a mixture of acids, are divided into two groups: (1) the *glycocholic acids* and (2) the *taurocholic acids*. The first group consists of the various cholic acids combined through peptide linkages at their COOH groups with the amino acid *glycine* [H_2NCH_2COOH] and the second group consists of the cholic acids combined in a similar manner with *taurine* [$H_2NCH_2CH_2SO_3H$].

The predominant cholic acids represented in bile are cholic, desoxycholic, and lithocholic. The structural relationships among these and their parent molecule, 5β-cholanic acid, are shown below. The essentially synthetic dehydrocholic acid is included for comparison.

The composition of bile varies considerably with the species of animal; the glycocholates predominate in human bile whereas the reverse is true of the bile of carnivora. The bile salts can be isolated as stable crystals soluble in water. The free bile acids can be obtained; they are only slightly soluble in water. These acids combine with the fatty acids in varying proportions, depending on the size of the aliphatic acid molecule, by means of secondary valence forces to form *choleic acids*. The latter are responsible for emulsifying, dispersing, and thus promoting the absorption of fats, cholesterol, and the oil-soluble vitamins.

Dehydrocholic Acid

Cholan-24-oic acid, 3,7,12-trioxo-, (5β)-, Cholan-DH (*Pennwalt*); Decholin (*Miles*); Delabil (*Breon*)

3,7,12-Trioxo-5β-cholan-24-oic acid [81-23-2] $C_{24}H_{34}O_5$ (402.53). Dehydrocholic acid for parenteral use melts between 237° and 242°.

Preparation—Has been isolated in minute quantities from cow's bile. It is readily prepared from cholic acid, the main steroid constituent of ox bile, by oxidation with chromic acid in acetic and sulfuric acid solution.

Description—White, fluffy, odorless, bitter powder; melting range 231° to 242°, with a range of not more than 3° for a given sample; the higher the melting temperature, the greater the purity.

Solubility—Practically insoluble in water; slightly soluble in ether; 1 g in about 100 mL alcohol and about 35 mL chloroform; soluble in solutions of alkali hydroxides and carbonates.

Uses—A semisynthetic cholate that evokes bile secretions of a low specific gravity (hydrocholeretic drug). It is used as a *laxative* for the temporary relief of constipation. Frequent use may result in dependence on laxatives. It has also been used to wash out fragments of gallstones and to flush the biliary tree. The sodium salt has been used to determine arm-to-tongue circulation time (see page 798). However, safer agents for this purpose are available (calcium gluconate). It enhances the absorption of lipids and lipid-soluble vitamins.

Dose—*Usual, adult, oral, laxative,* **250** to **500 mg** 2 to 4 times a day.

Dosage Forms—Tablets: 250 mg.

Glutamic Acid Hydrochloride

Acidulin (*Lilly*); Muriamic (*Merrell-Dow*)

L-Glutamic acid hydrochloride [138-15-8] $C_5H_9NO_4 \cdot HCl$ (183.59).

Preparation—Glutamic acid, usually obtained from gluten, casein, or other proteins by acid hydrolysis, is reacted with HCl.

Description—White crystalline powder; solution is acid to litmus.

Solubility—1 g in about 3 mL water; almost insoluble in alcohol and ether.

Uses—Administered orally to counterbalance a deficiency of hydrochloric acid in the gastric juice, and to inhibit the growth of putrefactive microorganisms in ingested food. A deficiency of hydrochloric acid is often associated with pernicious anemia, gastric carcinoma, congenital achlorhydria, and allergy. Since it is administered in capsules, dental enamel is not exposed to the acid. It is less effective than free hydrochloric acid in lowering gastric pH. One 340-mg capsule contains approximately 1.8 mEq of hydrochloric acid.

Dose—*Usual,* 1 to 3 capsules (**340** to **1020 mg**) 3 times daily before meals.

Dosage Form—Capsules: 340 mg.

Diluted Hydrochloric Acid

Diluted hydrochloric acid [7647-01-0]; contains, in each 100 mL, 9.5–10.5 g of HCl (36.46).

Hydrochloric Acid	226 mL
Purified Water, a sufficient quantity,	
To make	1000 mL
Mix the ingredients	

Description—Colorless, odorless liquid, strongly acid to litmus; specific gravity about 1.05 at 25°.

Uses—In the treatment of *gastric achlorhydria* and *hypochlorhydria*. Hydrochloric acid is often given in conjunction with iron therapy in the treatment of *hypochromic anemia*. In the treatment of pernicious anemia, it is also prescribed, if the accompanying achlorhydria gives rise to intestinal symptoms. See also *Glutamic Acid Hydrochloride*.

Dose—*Usual,* **5 mL,** well diluted in water.

Other Dose Information—The recommended dose may vary from 1 to 10 mL since there is no unanimity of opinion among physicians as to what constitutes an adequate dose. The acid should be diluted with 25 to 50 volumes of water or fruit juice and sipped through a glass tube to prevent a solvent reaction upon the dental enamel. It is usually taken during or after meals.

Malt Extract—page 1300.

Pancreatin—page 1037.

Resorcinol—RPS-16, page 1107.

Laxatives

Laxatives are drugs that affect fecal consistency, accelerate the passage of feces through the colon, and facilitate elimination of feces from the rectum. Consequently, they are used to ease the pain of elimination in patients with anorectal disorders, such as thrombosed hemorrhoids, and fissures, perianal abscesses, or other inflammatory rectal conditions. They are also used to minimize the hazardous excessive blood pressure which may occur with excessive straining during defecation, especially in patients with diseases of the cerebral or coronary arterial vessels. Appropriate agents may also be used to relieve acute constipation during pregnancy or the puerperal period, in geriatric patients whose abdominal and perineal muscles have become atrophied or whose rectal reflex has been lost or blunted, in children with acquired or congenital megacolon, to prepare the bowel prior to surgery or radiologic, proctoscopic, or colonoscopic procedures, to provide a fresh stool for parasitologic examination, to facilitate excretion of various parasites and the vermifuge after anthelmintic therapy, and to eliminate drug and food poisons from the gastrointestinal tract.

Chronic constipation, not of organic origin, may be effectively treated with diet and exercise. This is especially true for cases involving a low-fiber diet and habitual use of laxatives. A low-fiber diet produces a low-bulk stool, and habitual use of laxatives weakens bowel muscle tone. Dietary fiber is that part of a whole grain, vegetables, fruits, and nuts that resists digestion in the gastrointestinal tract. Such fiber has a significant effect on bowel habits; it holds water, stools tend to be softer and bulkier, and fecal material passes through the colon more rapidly. Moreover, it is believed that an increase in dietary fiber can lessen the incidence of constipation and provide symptomatic relief in cases of colonic diverticulitis. Exercise in any form improves muscle tone, but that which involves the abdominal muscles is the most useful in improving intestinal muscle tone. Daily exercise and an increase in the fiber content of the diet should prove effective in the relief of most cases of constipation.

Patients who use laxatives should be reminded of the following points: Laxatives are not for long-term use; if they are not effective after one week, a physician should be consulted. Laxative products which contain more than 15 mEq (345 mg) of sodium, more than 25 mEq (975 mg) of potassium, or more than 50 mEq (600 mg) of magnesium in the maximum daily dose should not be used if kidney disease is present. Phenophthalein preparations should be discontinued if a skin rash appears. Saline laxatives should not be given orally to children under 6 or rectally to infants under 2 years; mineral oil should not be given to children under 6 years of age. To be effective, enemas and suppositories must be administered properly. *The use of laxatives to relieve gastrointestinal symptoms of unknown cause cannot be too emphatically condemned.*

Although occasional use of a laxative is relatively harmless, depletion of fluids and electrolytes can result from their chronic use. Dioctyl sodium sulfosuccinate should not be used with mineral oil. Mineral oil should be given at bedtime in order to minimize its interference with the absorption of fat-soluble vitamins in the diet. In addition, aspiration of mineral oil may result in chronic pneumonitis; consequently, it is contraindicated in patients with disorders of gastric or esophageal emptying. Even the soft bulk-forming laxatives have been reported to cause enteric obstruction in an occasional patient with inflammatory or neoplastic strictures of the gut.

Traditionally, laxatives are divided into five groups: *stimulant laxatives, saline laxatives, bulk-forming laxatives, lubricant laxatives,* and *fecal softeners.* It should be emphasized, however, that this classification is merely for convenience, since it does not relate to mechanisms responsible for either increasing fecal water excretion or altering intestinal fluid movement. Ricinoleic acid (the active ingredient of castor oil) and bisacodyl, two stimulant laxatives, can convert net fluid and electrolyte absorption to net fluid accumulation, alter mucosal permeability, induce changes in intestinal motility, and occasionally produce mucosal damage. It has been proposed that the laxative action of magnesium, the classical cation among saline laxatives, is mediated through the release of endogenous cholecystokinin-pancreozymin, a hormone which promotes the accumulation of fluid and electrolyte within the intestine. The demonstration that bran changes the composition of fecal bile acids suggests that the mechanism of bulk-forming laxatives may require clarification. Until these and other possible mechanisms of action have been established, classification based on the pathophysiological mechanisms by which laxatives alter fluid and electrolyte movement can not be developed.

Stimulant Laxatives

The *stimulant laxatives* act on the intestinal tract to increase its motor activity. The more commonly employed agents are the anthraquinone laxatives, *cascara sagrada* and *senna;* the diphenylmethane derivatives, *phenolphthalein* and *bisacodyl;* and *castor oil.*

The *anthraquinone-containing laxatives*, such as cascara, senna, and danthron, are widely used. The active glycosides are absorbed in the small intestine, circulated through the portal system and into the general circulation, and excreted in the bile, urine, saliva, colonic mucosa, and in the milk of lactating women. These glycosides stimulate Auerbach's plexus to increase peristalsis. These agents usually act in 6 to 12 hours after ingestion. The *diphenylmethane derivatives,* such as phenolphthalein, and bisacodyl, have similar pharmacological actions; they stimulate sensory nerves in the colonic mucosa to initiate reflex peristalsis. Phenolphthalein is usually active within 6 to 8 hours after administration; bisacodyl results in a smooth, formed stool within 6 to 10 hours after oral administration and 15 to 60 minutes after rectal administration. *Castor oil* is classified as a stimulant laxative because lipolysis in the small intestine liberates ricinoleic acid, a short-chain fatty acid which stimulates peristalsis and inhibits the absorption of water and electrolyte from the small intestine. *Glycerin,* in the form of suppositories, promotes defecation by stimulating the rectal mucosa; it also acts to lubricate and soften inspissated fecal material. The stimulant laxatives have many characteristics in common; they increase peristalsis, cause griping and intestinal cramps, increase mucous secretion, and increase fluidity of the stool. Intensity of effect is related to dosage, but effective doses vary markedly from one individual to another.

Bisacodyl

Phenol, 4,4'-(2-pyridinylmethylene)bis-, diacetate (ester); Dulcolax (*Boehringer-Ingelheim*); Theralax (*Beecham*)

4,4'-(2-Pyridylmethylene)diphenol diacetate (ester) [603-50-9] $C_{22}H_{19}NO_4$ (361.40).

Caution—Avoid inhalation and contact with the eyes, skin, and mucous membranes.

Preparation—2-Pyridinecarboxaldehyde is condensed with phenol with the aid of a suitable dehydrant such as sulfuric acid and the resulting 4,4'-(2-pyridyl)diphenol is esterified by treatment with acetic anhydride and anhydrous sodium acetate. US Pat 2,764,590.

Description—White to off-white, crystalline powder in which particles having a longest diameter smaller than 50 μm predominate; melts between 131° and 135°.

Solubility—1 g in >10,000 mL water, 210 mL alcohol, 2.5 mL chloroform, 275 mL ether.

Uses—A contact laxative which acts directly on the colonic mucosa to increase peristalsis throughout the large intestine. It is administered either orally or rectally for constipation and for evacuation of the bowel prior to surgery, proctoscopy, or radiologic examination.

It is usually effective overnight or within 6 hours. Bisacodyl provides satisfactory cleansing of the bowel, obviating the need for an enema. Side effects are usually limited to abdominal cramps. Continued use of the suppository may cause rectal irritation. There are no contraindications to the use of bisacodyl, except for an acute surgical abdomen.

Dose—*Oral*, 10 to 30 mg; *usual, oral* and *rectal*, **10 mg**; *usual, pediatric, rectal,* **8 mg/m²**, or 5 to 10 mg; *oral*, **0.3 mg/kg** or **8 mg/ m²**.

Other Dose Information: Do not chew or break tablet coating. Do not take within 1 hour after ingestion of antacids or milk.

Dosage Forms—Suppositories: 10 mg; Tablets, Enteric Coated: 5 mg.

Cascara Sagrada

Sacred Bark; Chittem; Dogwood; Bear-berry; Bitter Bark

The dried bark of *Rhamnus purshiana* De Candolle (Fam *Rhamnaceae*).

Note—Cascara Sagrada should be collected at least 1 year prior to use.

Constituents—The following active principles have been reported: *Aloe-emodin* (1,8-dihydroxy-3-hydroxymethylanthraquinone), *chrysophanic acid* (1,8-dihydroxy-3-methylanthraquinone), *isoemodin* (3,5,8-trihydroxy-2-methylanthraquinone), *methylhydrocotoin* (2,4,6-trimethoxybenzophenone), and *purshianin*, a glycoside forming red-brown crystals, melting at 237°. Cascara also contains several resins, one of which is very bitter and gives a bright-red color with potassium hydroxide solution.

Uses—A widely used *cathartic*. Its precise mechanism of action is unknown. It has very little action on the small intestine, but promotes peristalsis in the large intestine. Of its several preparations, the fluidextract or aromatic fluidextract is perhaps the most effective. The action of cascara is mild and is unaccompanied by discomfort or griping. Indeed, it is the least griping of the emodin cathartics. A therapeutic dose causes a single evacuation of the bowel in approximately 8 hours. The stool may be solid or semifluid. Prolonged ingestion frequently results in a benign melanotic pigmentation of the rectal mucosa which may regress after cascara sagrada is discontinued. It should not be given to lactating mothers, since it is excreted in breast milk.

*Note—*When ground cascara sagrada is moistened and mixed with magnesium or calcium hydroxide the drug loses its intensely bitter taste, the acid constituents being neutralized and apparently rendered insoluble. Such treatment seems to lessen its activity.

Cascara Sagrada Extract [Cascara Dry Extract; Powered Cascara Sagrada Extract; Rhamnus Purshiana Extract]—1 g of cascara sagrada extract represents 3 g of cascara sagrada. *Preparation:* Mix cascara sagrada in coarse powder (900 g), with boiling water (4000 mL), and macerate the mixture during 3 hours. Then transfer it to a percolator, allow it to drain, and exhaust it by percolation, using boiling water as the menstruum and collecting about 5000 mL of percolate. Evaporate the percolate to dryness, reduce the extract to a fine powder, and add sufficient starch, dried at 100°, to make the product weigh 300 g. Mix the powders thoroughly and pass the extract through a fine sieve. *Dose: Usual*, 300 mg.

Cascara Sagrada Fluidextract [Cascara Liquid Extract; Rhamnus Purshiana Fluidextract]—*Preparation:* With cascara sagrada (in very coarse powder, 1000 g), prepare a fluidextract by Process D (page 1516). Evaporate the percolate until it measures 800 mL, and when it is cold, gradually add 200 mL of alcohol and, if necessary, sufficient water to make the product measure 1000 mL. Mix thoroughly. *Alcohol Content:* 18 to 20%. *Uses:* A mild and effective *cathartic*, especially valuable because it does not produce habitual or after constipation. Its usefulness is limited because of its intensely bitter taste. See *Cascara sagrada. Dose: Usual*, 1 mL.

Cascara Tablets are prepared from cascara sagrada extract. *Dose: Usual*, 300 mg of cascara sagrada extract.

Aromatic Cascara Fluidextract [Aromatic Rhamnus Purshiana Fluidextract; Elixir of Cascara Sagrada]—*Preparation:* Mix cascara sagrada (in very coarse powder, 1000 g) with magnesium oxide (120 g), moisten it uniformly with boiling water (2000 mL), and set it aside in a shallow container for 48 hours, stirring it occasionally. Pack it in a percolator, and percolate with boiling water until the drug is exhausted. Evaporate the percolate, at a temperature not exceeding 100°, to 750 mL, and at once dissolve in it pure glycyrrhiza extract (40 g). When the liquid has cooled, add alcohol (200 mL), in which saccharin (2 g), methyl salicylate (0.1 mL), anise oil (0.65 mL), and coriander oil (0.15 mL) have been dissolved, and finally add water (qs) to make 1000 mL, mix. *Alcohol Content:* 18 to 20%. *Uses:* This mild and effective cathartic is the most frequently employed form of cascara sagrada. The treatment with magnesium oxide (hydroxide in the presence of water) precipitates the acidic constituents and makes the preparation more palatable, particularly in the presence of the aromatic flavoring agents employed. The cathartic activity is also lessened. *Dose:* 5 to 15 mL daily; *usual*, 5 mL.

Castor Oil

The fixed oil obtained from the seed of *Ricinus communis* Linné (Fam *Euphorbiaceae*).

Preparation—By cold expression and subsequent clarification of the oil by heat. It consists chiefly of glycerides of ricinoleic and isoricinoleic acids. The purgative action has been attributed to hydrolysis of ricinolein in the intestine, ricinoleic acid being produced. The seeds contain two principles, *ricin*, a very poisonous albumin (150 mg toxic *per os*), and *ricinine*, a poisonous base (1,2-dihydro-4-methoxy-1-methyl-2-oxonicotinonitrile). Because of the presence of these toxic substances, the seeds are definitely poisonous.

Description—Pale yellowish or almost colorless, transparent, viscid liquid with a faint, mild odor, and a bland followed by a slightly acrid and usually nauseating taste; specific gravity between 0.945 and 0.965.

Solubility—Soluble in alcohol; miscible with dehydrated alcohol, glacial acetic acid, chloroform, and ether.

Uses—Externally as an *emollient*, internally as a *laxative*. The oil is bland and soothing to the skin. When administered orally it produces one or more copious stools within 2 to 6 hours after ingestion. It is frequently used to empty the gastrointestinal tract of gas and feces prior to proctoscopy or X-ray studies of the gastrointestinal tract. It should not be used in the therapy of acute constipation. Chronic use is not recommended, since absorption of nutrients may be reduced.

Dose—**15 to 60 mL** daily; *usual* **15 mL.**

Other Dose Information—No harm results if this dose is exceeded inasmuch as the cathartic action of the first portion of the oil sweeps the remaining oil through the intestinal tract.

Aromatic Castor Oil—*Preparation:* Dissolve cinnamon oil (3 mL), clove oil (1 mL), saccharin (0.5 g), and vanillin (1 g) in alcohol (30 mL), add castor oil (qs), and mix thoroughly to make 1000 mL. *Alcohol Content:* 2 to 3%. *Uses:* A *cathartic*. The aromatics assist in its administration by masking the disagreeable taste of the castor oil. *Dose: Usual*, 15 mL.

Danthron

9,10-Anthracenedione, 1,8-dihydroxy-, Chrysazin; Dorbane (*Riker*); Istizin (*Winthrop*); Modane (*Adria*)

1,8-Dihydroxyanthraquinone [117-10-2] $C_{14}H_8O_4$ (240.21).

Preparation—From anthraquinone as described in the synthesis of anthralin, page 780. Its chemical structure closely resembles the anthraquinone derivatives which exist in glycosidic combination in cascara sagrada and the other irritant glycoside cathartics.

Description—Orange-colored crystalline powder; begins to sublime at about 75° and melts between 190° and 197°.

Solubility—1 g in >10,000 mL water, 2100 mL alcohol, 50 mL chloroform, 650 mL ether.

Uses—An anthraquinone derivative with the same mechanism of action as other drugs in this group. It is a *laxative* which produces a soft or semisolid stool in 6 to 8 hours. Prolonged administration may result in temporary brownish staining of the mucosa (melanosis coli). The drug also appears in the milk of nursing mothers and may cause catharsis in the nursing infant. Danthron is eliminated in the urine and imparts a pinkish color to alkaline urine. It has not gained wide acceptance in clinical medicine, but is used mainly in veterinary medicine.

Dose—*Usual, oral, adult,* **37.5** to **150 mg** with or one hour after evening meal. *Children 6 to 12 years of age,* one-half adult dose.

Dosage Forms—Tablets: 37.5 and 75 mg; Liquid: 75 mg/10 mL.

Glycerin Suppositories

Glycerin	91 g
Sodium Stearate	9 g
Purified Water	5 g
To make about	100 g

Heat the glycerin in a suitable container to about 120°. Dissolve the sodium stearate, with gentle stirring, in the heated glycerin. Then add the purified water, mix, and immediately pour the hot mixture into a suitable mold, which, if made of metal, previously has been heated and is used while hot. Cool the suppositories completely before removal.

Note—If preferred, the sodium stearate for glycerin suppositories may be prepared during the making of the suppositories by the direct reaction between stearic acid and sodium bicarbonate, sodium carbonate, or sodium hydroxide, these being taken in correct proportion.

Uses—Occasionally used as a laxative, especially in infants and children. Fecal evacuation usually occurs within 15 to 30 minutes after insertion. They act by stimulating the rectal mucosa and by softening inspissated fecal material. They may also be used to reestablish habit time.

Dose—*Usual, adult, rectal,* **3 g.** *Children, under 6 years of age,* 1 to **1.5 g.**

Dosage Forms—Suppositories: 1.5 and 3 g.

Phenolphthalein

1(3*H*)-Isobenzofuranone, 3,3-bis(4-hydroxyphenyl)-, (*Various Mfrs*)

3,3-Bis(*p*-hydroxyphenyl)phthalide   [77-09-8] $C_{20}H_{14}O_4$ (318.33).

Preparation—A mixture of phenol, phthalic anhydride, and sulfuric acid is heated at 120° for 10 to 12 hours. The product is extracted with boiling water, the residue dissolved in dilute NaOH solution, filtered, and precipitated with acid.

Description—White or faintly yellowish white, crystalline powder; odorless and stable in air; melts no lower than 258°.

Solubility—Practically insoluble in water; 1 g in about 15 mL alcohol and about 100 mL ether.

Uses—One of the most widely used of the *cathartic* drugs, being the basis of many proprietary laxatives. Classified as an irritant cathartic, although the precise mechanism of action is unknown. When taken orally, it is thought to be dissolved by the intestinal juices and bile and to stimulate the intestinal musculature, chiefly that of the colon. It acts within 4 to 8 hours after ingestion. In susceptible individuals, phenolphthalein may cause allergic reactions, including Stevens-Johnson syndrome, and lupus erythematosus; the skin lesions may persist for months after discontinuing the drug. Deaths have been attributed to allergy to this drug. It should also be remembered that phenolphthalein colors an alkaline urine red, and small portions may appear in the urine after oral ingestion. It is also used as an indicator in volumetric analysis.

Dose—*Usual, adult, oral,* **60 mg;** *pediatric, oral,* 15 to 30 mg.
Dosage Forms—Tablets: 60 and 120 mg.

Senna

Senna Leaf; Senna Leaves

The dried leaflet of *Cassia acutifolia* Delile, known in commerce as Alexandria Senna, or of *Cassia angustifolia* Vahl, known in commerce as Tinnevelly Senna (Fam *Leguminosae*).

Constituents—The principal cathartic constituents are reported to be: *aloe-emodin* and *rhein* and their glycoside derivatives; *sennaemodin* and an emodin glycoside; *chrysophanic acid (chrysophanol); cathartic acid* (formerly believed to be the chief purgative principle); *cathartomannite,* and *sennanigrin.* Also present are *sennacrol, sennarhamnetin, kaempferol* [$C_{15}H_{10}O_6$], its glycoside *kaempferin,* and a small amount of an essential oil. When senna leaves are macerated in strong alcohol, the principles which produce

griping and give odor and taste are said to be eluted while the purgative properties are unaffected. Water and diluted alcohol are good solvents for its active principles.

Uses—An active *laxative* causing a single thorough evacuation of the bowels within 6 to 12 hours after administration. Its action is usually accompanied by considerable griping. Although it is an anthraquinone-type laxative, *melanosis coli* has not been reported to occur after continued use. Senna preparations may impart a yellowish-brown color to acid urine and a reddish color to alkaline urine.

Dose—*Usual,* **2 g.**

Senna Fluidextract—*Preparation:* With senna (in coarse powder 1000 g), prepare a fluidextract by Process A (page 1516) using a mixture of 1 volume of alcohol and 2 volumes of water as the menstruum. Macerate the drug for 24 hours, then percolate at a moderate rate, and reserve the first 800 mL of percolate. *Alcohol Content:* 23 to 27%. *Uses:* A *laxative,* frequently producing griping when used alone. It is chiefly used to make other preparations. *Dose: Usual,* 2 mL.

Senna Syrup—*Preparation:* Mix coriander oil (5 mL) with senna fluidextract (250 mL), and gradually add purified water (330 mL). Allow the mixture to stand for 24 hours in a cool place, with occasional agitation, then filter, and pass enough purified water through the filter to obtain 580 mL of filtrate. Dissolve the sucrose (635 g) in this liquid, and add sufficient purified water to make the product measure 1000 mL. Mix well and strain. *Alcohol Content:* 5 to 7%. *Uses:* A *laxative,* frequently in combination with other drugs. *Dose: Usual,* 8 mL.

Sennosides A and B

Glysennid (*Dorsey; Sandoz*)

A natural complex of anthraquinone glycosides found in senna, isolated from *Cassia angustifolia* as calcium salts; contains 55–65% of the calcium salts.

Description—Brownish powder; pH (mixture, 1 g/10 mL water) between 6.3 and 7.3.

Uses—A *laxative.* Evacuation of the bowels occurs 8 to 10 hours after oral administration.

Dose—*Usual, adult,* and *children over 10 years of age,* 12 to 24 mg daily. *Children, 6 to 10 years of age,* 12 mg.

Dosage Form—Tablets: 12 mg of Sennosides A and B.

Other Stimulant Laxatives

Aloe—The dried latex of leaves of *Aloe barbadensis* Miller (*Aloe vera* "Linné"), known in commerce as Curaçao Aloe, or of *Aloe ferox* Miller and hybrids of this species with *Aloe africana* Miller and *Aloe spicata* Baker, known in commerce as Cape Aloe (Fam *Liliaceae*); yields not less than 50% of water-soluble extractive. The active principles are pentosides, including *aloin* (barbaloin, socaloin, or capaloin), *beta-barbaloin,* and *iso-barbaloin.* Uses: Aloe is still employed as a cathartic in a few old, irrational mixtures. The active principles yield on hydrolysis in the intestine anthraquinone derivatives that are responsible for the cathartic action. The action of aloe is accompanied by intestinal griping and pelvic vascular congestion, the latter property having given to aloe the undeserved classification of emmenagogue. The laxative action of aloe occurs 8 to 12 hours after ingestion. Use of aloe as a cathartic is irrational and should be abandoned. Aloe is also an ingredient of *Compound Benzoin Tincture,* which gives it official status as a pharmaceutic aid.

Casanthranol [Peristim Forte (*Mead-Johnson*); ing of Peri-Colace (*Mead-Johnson*)]—A purified mixture of the anthranol glycosides extracted from cascara sagrada. *Uses:* One of the anthraquinone-containing stimulant laxatives; reported to be 10 times as potent as cascara sagrada. In most patients a semisoft stool is produced in 8 to 12 hours. Casanthranol is an ingredient in numerous proprietary laxative preparations. Adverse reactions reported are abdominal cramping, diarrhea, nausea, and rectal bleeding in a patient with ulcerative colitis. *Dose: Usual,* 90 mg at bedtime; 180 mg may be required in laxative-dependent patients. *Dosage Form:* Capsules: 90 mg.

Saline Laxatives

A number of magnesium salts as well as other sulfates, phosphates, and tartrates are used as *saline laxatives.* These cations and anions are not absorbed, or at most only slightly absorbed, from the gastrointestinal tract. Consequently, when given orally in hypertonic solutions, they draw water from the tissues into the intestine, increase peristalsis, and induce a profuse, watery stool. This *traditional explanation* for the mechanism of action of *saline laxatives* has been questioned. Indeed, several studies indicate that different mechanisms, independent of osmotic effect, are responsible for the laxative properties of these salts. It has been shown that magnesium stimulates release of endogenous cholecystokinin-pancreozymin, a hormone which causes the accumulation of fluid and electrolytes within the human small intestine. The laxative action of magnesium-containing salts, therefore, may result from their ability to diminish the net absorption of fluid and electrolytes.

Although the choice of saline laxative is usually based on cost and palatability, there are situations in which the injudicious use of a saline laxative results in serious effects. As much as 20% of the magnesium ion may be absorbed after oral administration of a magnesium salt. If renal function is normal, the absorbed ion is excreted so rapidly that no change in the blood level of the ion can be detected. In patients with impaired renal function, however, toxic concentrations of the ion can accumulate. Laxatives that contain sodium are contraindicated in individuals with edema and congestive heart disease. Chronic use of saline laxatives may also result in excessive dehydration. Other contraindications will be mentioned in the respective monographs.

Magnesium Carbonate—RPS-16, page 738.

Magnesium Citrate Oral Solution

1,2,3-Propanetricarboxylic acid, hydroxy-, magnesium salt (2:3); Citrate of Magnesia, "Citrate"

Magnesium citrate (3:2) [3344-18-1] $C_{12}H_{10}Mg_3O_{14}$ (451.12); contains, in each 100 mL, not less than 7.59 g of $C_6H_8O_7$ (anhydrous citric acid) and an amount of magnesium citrate corresponding to 1.55–1.9 g of MgO (magnesium oxide).

Magnesium Carbonate	15 g
Anhydrous Citric Acid	27.4 g
Syrup	60 mL
Talc	5 g
Lemon Oil	0.1 mL
Potassium Bicarbonate	2.5 g
Purified Water, a sufficient quantity,	
To make	350 mL

Note—An amount (30 g) of citric acid containing 1 molecule of water of hydration, equivalent to 27.4 g of anhydrous citric acid, may be used in the above formula.

Dissolve the anhydrous citric acid in 150 mL of hot purified water in a suitable dish, add slowly the magnesium carbonate, previously mixed with 100 mL of purified water, and stir until it is dissolved. Then add the syrup, heat the mixed liquids to the boiling point, immediately add the lemon oil, previously triturated with the talc, and filter the mixture, while hot, into a strong bottle (previously rinsed with boiling purified water) of suitable capacity. Add enough boiled purified water to make the product measure 350 mL. Stopper the bottle with purified cotton, allow to cool, add the potassium bicarbonate, and immediately stopper the bottle securely. Lastly, shake the solution occasionally until the potassium bicarbonate is dissolved, cap the bottle, and sterilize or pasteurize the solution.

Note—In this process the 2.5 g of potassium bicarbonate may be replaced by 2.1 g of sodium bicarbonate, preferably in tablet form. The solution may be further carbonated by the use of CO_2, under pressure. Carbon dioxide alone, instead of the potassium or sodium bicarbonates, should not be used, as the citrates formed from the latter have a desired therapeutic effect.

The stability of magnesium citrate solution may be improved by pasteurizing or sterilizing the solution. For solutions not intended to be pasteurized or sterilized, stability may be improved by employing 30 g of citric acid and a quantity of magnesium carbonate equivalent to 6.0 g of MgO for each 350 mL of solution. The excess is necessary in order to form carbon dioxide when the bicarbonate is added, thus adding to the flavor due to carbonation and to the therapeutic effectiveness through the formation of alkali citrates.

In this connection it should be noted that official magnesium carbonate contains the equivalent of 40.0 to 43.5% of MgO, corresponding to from 6.0 to 6.47 g of MgO from the 15 g of the carbonate.

Solutions containing amounts of magnesium oxide approaching the lower official limit are more stable than those containing higher percentages. Precipitation on standing is increased by the presence of sucrose and carbon dioxide and decreased by sterilization of the finished product.

Description—Colorless to slightly yellow, clear effervescent liquid having a sweet, acidulous taste and a lemon flavor.

Uses—A pleasant *saline laxative.*
Dose—*Usual*, 200 mL.

Magnesium Oxide—page 796.

Magnesium Sulfate

Sulfuric acid magnesium salt (1:1), heptahydrate; Bitter Salts; Epsom Salts

Magnesium sulfate (1:1) heptahydrate [10034-99-8] $MgSO_4.7H_2O$ (246.47); *anhydrous* [7487-88-8] (120.36).

Preparation—Magnesium sulfate can be prepared by neutralizing sulfuric acid with magnesium carbonate or oxide, but it may also be obtained directly from natural sources. In the form of double salt with alkali metals it occurs abundantly in several mines, and these comprise a large source of the salt. It is also produced in large quantities from the magnesium salts occurring in the brines used for extraction of bromine. The "liquors" after the removal of bromine are treated with calcium hydroxide, thus precipitating magnesium as the hydroxide. Sulfur dioxide and air are passed into an aqueous suspension of the magnesium hydroxide, yielding magnesium sulfate:

$$Mg(OH)_2 + SO_2 + \tfrac{1}{2}O_2 \rightarrow MgSO_4 + H_2O$$

Description—Small, colorless crystals, usually needlelike, and has a cooling, saline, and bitter taste; effloresces in warm, dry air; at 100° it loses 5 molecules of its water; aqueous solution is neutral to litmus.

Solubility—1 g in 0.8 mL water, 0.5 mL boiling water, 1 mL glycerin; sparingly soluble in alcohol.

Incompatibilities—Addition of *alcohol* may cause a precipitation of magnesium sulfate from an aqueous solution. *Alkali hydroxides* form insoluble magnesium hydroxide, *alkali carbonates* form a basic carbonate, and the *salicylates* form a basic salicylate. *Arsenates, phosphates,* and *tartrates* may cause precipitation of the corresponding magnesium salts. *Sulfates* are precipitated by lead, barium, strontium, and calcium.

Uses—An effective and widely employed *saline laxative.* The laxative action probably results from two factors: (1) magnesium sulfate is not absorbed from the intestinal tract, and thus retains sufficient water within the lumen of the bowel to make an isotonic solution, and (2) the magnesium ion stimulates the release of cholecystokinin-pancreozymin which causes an accumulation of fluid and electrolytes within the small intestine (*see* Introduction this section). It is the increased bulk which promotes the motor activity of the bowel. If dissolved in iced water, its nauseous taste is not so perceptible as when water at ordinary temperature is used; it may be still further disguised by the use of orange juice.

A cold, wet compress of saturated magnesium sulfate solution in water has been employed in the treatment of such skin disorders as erysipelas. Hot concentrated, aqueous solutions of magnesium sulfate (about 1 lb/pint of water) are sometimes used in the treatment of deep-seated infections; cloths are saturated and applied while hot. The action is much like that of a poultice.

For parenteral anticonvulsant use see *Magnesium Sulfate Injection,* page 1078.

Dose—2 to 30 g daily; *usual*, 15 g.

Potassium Sodium Tartrate

Butanedioic acid, 2,3-dihydroxy-, [R-(R^*,R^*)]-, monopotassium monosodium salt, tetrahydrate; Rochelle Salt; Seignette Salt; Sodium Potassium Tartrate

```
       COOK
        |
   H—C—OH
        |              · 4H₂O
  HO—C—H
        |
       COONa
```

Monopotassium monosodium tartrate tetrahydrate [6381-59-5] $C_4H_4KNaO_6.4H_2O$ (282.22); *anhydrous* [304-59-6] (210.16).

Preparation—By neutralizing potassium bitartrate with sodium carbonate.

Description—Colorless crystals, or a white, crystalline powder, having a cooling saline taste; effloresces slightly in warm, dry air; the crystals are often coated with a white powder; aqueous solution is alkaline to litmus paper, but is not reddened by phenolphthalein.

Solubility—1 g in 1 mL water; practically insoluble in alcohol.

Incompatibilities—*Acids* cause a precipitation of potassium bitartrate. *Magnesium sulfate* and *calcium* salts produce a precipitate. The tartrates are weak reducing agents.

Uses—A *saline laxative.*
Dose—*Usual,* **10 g.**

Sodium Phosphate

Phosphoric acid, disodium salt, heptahydrate; Dibasic Sodium Phosphate; Disodium Orthophosphate; Disodium Hydrogen Phosphate; Secondary Sodium Phosphate

Disodium phosphate heptahydrate [7782-85-6] $Na_2HPO_4.7H_2O$ (268.07); *anhydrous* [7558-79-4] (141.96).

Preparation—From *bone phosphate* or *bone ash*, obtained by heating bones to whiteness, which consists chiefly of tribasic calcium phosphate. The mineral *phosphorite*, which is a tribasic calcium phosphate, is also used. The finely ground phosphatic material is digested with sulfuric acid, the mixture is then leached with hot water, neutralized with sodium carbonate, and the sodium phosphate crystallized from the filtrate.

Description—Colorless, or white, granular salt; effloresces in warm, dry air; solutions are alkaline to litmus and phenolphthalein (pH about 9.5).

Solubility—1 g in 4 mL water; very slightly soluble in alcohol.

Uses—One of the most palatable of the *saline laxatives*. It is also used in the form of the oral solution (see below) as an *antihypercalcemic.*

Caution—This phosphate should not be confused with tribasic sodium phosphate which is very alkaline and has a caustic action.

Dose—4 to 8 g; *usual,* **4 g.**

Dried Sodium Phosphate [Exsiccated Sodium Phosphate]—*Description:* White powder which readily absorbs moisture. *Solubility:* 1 g in about 8 mL water; insoluble in alcohol. *Uses:* A *saline laxative.* It is used chiefly in the form of Effervescent Sodium Phosphate for which purpose it should be dried before use, otherwise it will be variable in its water content. It rapidly absorbs as much as 15 to 20% of water if exposed to a moist atmosphere. *Dose:* 2 to 4 g.

Effervescent Sodium Phosphate—*Preparation:* Powder citric acid (monohydrate crystals, 162 g), mix it intimately with dried sodium phosphate (dried and powdered, 200 g) and tartaric acid (in dry powder, 252 g), and thoroughly incorporate sodium bicarbonate (in dry powder, 477 g) to make about 1000 g. Place the mixed powders on a plate of glass or in a suitable dish in an oven previously heated to between 93° and 104°. Manipulate the mixture carefully, with a spatula which is acid-resistant, and when it has become moist rub it through a No 6 tinned-iron sieve. Dry the granules at a temperature not exceeding 54°, and immediately transfer the salt to suitable containers and seal them tightly. *Note:* The proportions of tartaric acid and citric acid may be varied if desired, but their combined acidity must be equivalent to the acidity indicated in the official formula. *Uses:* One of the most pleasant of the *saline laxatives*, being an effervescent mixture which combines the cathartic action of the phosphate and tartrate ions. *Dose:* 10 to 20 g.

Sodium Phosphate Oral Solution contains, in each 100 mL, the equivalent of 71–79 g of $Na_2HPO_4.7H_2O$. *Preparation:* Add sodium phosphate (755 g), citric acid monohydrate (130 g), and glycerin (150 mL) to purified water (150 mL), and digest on a steam bath until solution is effected. Filter, and pass sufficient purified water through the filter to make the product measure 1000 mL. *Note:* 400 g of dried sodium phosphate may be used in place of the 755 g of sodium phosphate specified in the formula. If this alternative is followed, the 150 mL of purified water specified in the direction should be increased to 500 mL. *Description:* Clear, colorless liquid, of a thick, syrupy consistency, practically odorless, and with a cooling, saline taste; specific gravity about 1.39 at 25°; acid to litmus and produces effervescence with sodium carbonate. *Uses:* This Solution, which corresponds to 0.75 g of the official hydrated salt in each mL, furnishes a convenient form for the administration of a *saline laxative* and *antihypercalcemic.* The citric acid is added to prevent the salt from crystallizing, and the glycerin assists in its preparation, especially in preventing the development of microorganisms. *Dose: Usual,* 10 mL (one usual dose contains about 7.5 g).

Sodium Phosphate and Sodium Biphosphate Enema

Sodium Phosphates Enema; Fleet Enema (*Fleet*)

Uses—A *laxative* administered as an enema. It should not be used in the presence of abdominal pain, nausea, or vomiting.

Dose—*Usual, rectal,* **120 mL.** *Usual, pediatric, rectal,* dosage not established in children under 2 years of age; over 2 years of age, **60 mL.**

Dosage Forms—Enema: 6% sodium phosphate and 16% sodium biphosphate.

Sodium Phosphate and Sodium Biphosphate Oral Solution

Sodium Phosphates Oral Solution; Fleet Phospho-Soda (*Fleet*)

Uses—An orally administered saline *laxative.* It is usually effective overnight or within 1 hour if taken before meals. It should not be used in patients with abdominal pain, nausea, or vomiting.

Dose—*Usual, oral,* **2.5 to 20 mL;** mix with ½ glass water and then follow with a glass full of water; *usual, pediatric, oral,* **2.5 to 5 mL** for children 5 to 10 years of age; **5 to 10 mL** for children over 10 years of age.

Dosage Forms—Solution: 18% sodium phosphate and 48% sodium biphosphate.

Sodium Sulfate

Sulfuric acid disodium salt, decahydrate; Glauber's Salt

Disodium sulfate decahydrate [7727-73-3] $Na_2SO_4.10H_2O$ (322.19); *anhydrous* [7757-82-6] (142.04).

Preparation—Largely as a by-product in the manufacture of hydrochloric acid from sodium chloride and sulfuric acid. Also occurs in various minerals, mineral springs, and salt brines.

Description—Large, colorless, odorless, transparent crystals or a granular powder; effloresces rapidly in air; liquefies in its water of hydration at about 33°; at 100° it loses all of its water of hydration; solutions are neutral to litmus.

Solubility—1 g in 1.5 mL water; soluble in glycerin; insoluble in alcohol.

Uses—Orally, an effective *saline laxative.* An isotonic (3.89%) solution of sodium sulfate decahydrate, administered intravenously, is used as an *antihypercalcemic.*

Dose—As *laxative, usual, adult, oral,* **15 g.** As *antihypercalcemic,* by *intravenous infusion,* **1 to 4 L** of isotonic solution (containing **3.89%** of $Na_2SO_4.10H_2O$) over a period of 9 to 15 hr.

Other Saline Laxatives

Potassium Bitartrate [Cream of Tartar; Acid Potassium Tartrate; $C_4H_5KO_6$ (188.18)]—*Preparation:* By purifying *argol* or *tartar*, a substance deposited in wine casks during the fermentation of grape juice, which substance consists of about 80% potassium bitartrate. *Description* and *Solubility:* Colorless or slightly opaque crystals, or as a white, crystalline powder having a pleasant, acid taste; saturated solution is acid to litmus. 1 g dissolves in 165 mL water, 8820 mL alcohol, or 16 mL boiling water. *Incompatibilities:* Because it contains an acidic hydrogen, it can react with alkaline substances. Its slight solubility sometimes causes difficulty in liquid mixtures. *Uses:* Occasionally as a *laxative.* It is largely used in baking powders and in the manufacture of hard candies. *Dose: Usual,* 2 g.

Potassium Phosphate [Dibasic Potassium Phosphate; Dipotassium Hydrogen Phosphate; K_2HPO_4 (174.18)]—*Preparation:* By reacting potassium carbonate or potassium hydroxide with phosphoric acid. *Description* and *Solubility:* Colorless or white granules or powder; deliquescent when exposed to moist air; solutions are alkaline to phenolphthalein TS. 1 g dissolves in 3 mL water; very slightly soluble in alcohol. *Uses:* Same as *Sodium Phosphate* (page 803) and is also an official reagent. *Dose: Usual,* 4 g.

Bulk-Forming Laxatives

The bulk-forming laxatives include a wide range of natural and semisynthetic polysaccharides and cellular derivatives that are only partially digested. The undigested portions are hydrophilic and swell in the presence of water to form a viscous solution or gel. The increased intraluminal pressure reflexly stimulates peristalsis, diminishes colonic transit time, and produces a soft gelatinous stool. Other mechanisms may also be involved. For example, bile-salt metabolism may be altered and a laxative action may reflect a choleretic effect.

Bulk-forming laxatives usually exert a laxative effect in 12 to 24 hours but may require as much as 3 days. Each dose of laxative should be taken with a full glass of water. These drugs interact and combine with other drugs, such as salicylates, digitalis, etc. Consequently, they should not, as a general rule, be taken with other drugs.

Carboxymethylcellulose Sodium—page 1297.

Methylcellulose—page 1297.

Plantago Seed

Psyllium Seed; Plantain Seed

The cleaned, dried, ripe seed of *Plantago psyllium* Linné, or of *Plantago indica* Linné ((*Plantago arenaria* Waldstein et Kitaibel), known in commerce as Spanish or French Psyllium Seed; or of *Plantago ovata* Forskal, known in commerce as Blond Psyllium or Indian Plantago Seed (Fam *Plantaginaceae*).

Uses—By virtue of its indigestibility and mucilaginous character, it acts as a mild *laxative*. It is contraindicated in patients with intestinal obstruction.

Dose—4 to 15 g; *usual*, **7.5 g**.

Polycarbophil—page 812.

Other Bulk-Forming Laxatives

Plantago Ovata Coating—A cream-colored to brown, granular powder; practically odorless and tasteless. It consists principally of the separated outer mucilaginous layers of plantago ovata seeds (blond psyllium). *Uses*: For correction of simple constipation of functional or nervous origin due to lack of sufficient bulk in the stool. *Dose*: Oral, 5 to 10 g 3 times daily in a glass of water or milk.

Psyllium Hydrophilic Muciloid [Metamucil (*Searle*) and others]—A white to cream-colored, slightly granular powder with little or no odor, and a slightly acid taste. It consists of the mucilaginous portion (outer epidermis) of blond psyllium seeds. *Uses*: A bulk-forming laxative. *Dose*: Oral, 4 to 7 g 1 to 3 times daily in a glass of liquid, followed by another glass of liquid.

Sterculia Gum [Gum Karaya]—The dried gummy exudate from *Sterculia urens* Roxburgh or other species of *Sterculia* Linné (Fam *Sterculiaceae*) or from species of *Cochlospermum* Kunth (Fam *Bixaceae*). *Uses*: An indigestible laxative that swells when moistened. It is also used as an ostomy appliance "glue."

Lubricant Laxatives

The *lubricant laxatives* (mineral oil and vegetable oils) lubricate the intestinal tract, soften the fecal contents, and facilitate the passage of feces. The many untoward effects induced by mineral oil, such as *aspiration oil pneumonitis* and *lipoid avitaminosis A*, suggest that habitual use be avoided.

Cottonseed Oil—page 1295.

Mineral Oil

Liquid Paraffin; Liquid Petrolatum; White Mineral Oil; Heavy Liquid Petrolatum

A mixture of liquid hydrocarbons obtained from petroleum. It may contain a suitable stabilizer.

Preparation—After removing the lighter hydrocarbons from petroleum by distillation the residue is again subjected to distillation at a temperature between 330° and 390° and the distillate treated first with H_2SO_4, then with NaOH, and afterward decolorized by filtering through bone black, animal charcoal, or fuller's earth. The purified product is again chilled, to remove paraffin, and redistilled at a temperature above 330°. In some instances the H_2SO_4 treatment is omitted.

Description—Colorless, transparent, oily liquid, free or nearly free from fluorescence; tasteless and odorless when cold and develops not more than a faint odor of petroleum when heated; specific gravity between 0.860 and 0.905; kinematic viscosity not less than 38.1 centistokes at 37.8°.

Solubility—Insoluble in water or alcohol; miscible with most fixed oils, but not with castor oil; soluble in volatile oils.

Uses—A vehicle formerly used for drugs to be applied to the nasal mucous membranes, and internally as a *laxative*. It is now recognized that neither of these procedures is as benign as once supposed. A small portion of mineral oil may be aspirated into the lungs after topical application to nasal mucous membranes and may cause "lipid" pneumonia.

When taken internally, mineral oil, by virtue of its ability to soften fecal contents and retard the absorption of water, is a mild laxative. It is probably harmless in occasional laxative doses, but if taken continuously in large amounts it may impair appetite, reduce somewhat the absorption of fat-soluble vitamins, and possibly be absorbed to an extent sufficient to cause recognizable changes in the liver and mesenteric lymph nodes.

Dose—*Adult*, oral, **15 to 45 mL** once a day. *Children over 6 years of age*, **10 to 15 mL**.

Dosage Forms—Emulsion (see below).

Mineral Oil Emulsion [Liquid Petrolatum Emulsion; Liquid Paraffin Emulsion]—*Preparation*: Mix mineral oil (500 mL) with acacia (in very fine powder, 125 g) in a dry mortar, add purified water (250 mL) all at once, and emulsify the mixture. Then add, in divided portions, triturating after each addition, a mixture of syrup (100 mL), purified water (50 mL), and vanillin (40 mg), dissolved in alcohol (60 mL). Finally add sufficient purified water to make the product measure 1000 mL, and mix well. *Note*: In preparing mineral oil emulsion, other methods of emulsification may be used and the quantity of acacia may be reduced or it may be replaced by agar, gelatin, tragacanth, or mixtures of any of these emulsifying agents, provided the resulting emulsion is similar in viscosity and appearance to the emulsion made by the formula given. The vanillin may be replaced by not more than 1% of any other official flavoring substance or mixture of official flavoring substances. Sixty mL of sweet orange peel tincture, or 2 g of benzoic acid may be used as a preservative in place of the alcohol. Heavy mineral oil should be used in preparing this emulsion as that variety is preferable for internal administration and is less likely to cause "leakage." *Alcohol Content*: When present, 4 to 6%. *Uses*: A palatable form of liquid petrolatum for administration as an intestinal lubricant and laxative. *Dose*: Usual, 30 mL.

Light Mineral Oil—page 1315.

Olive Oil—page 1301.

Fecal Softeners

The fecal softeners represent the most recent approach to the management of constipation and fecal impaction. Substances included in this category are "surface-acting" or "wetting" agents which are nonabsorbable, and relatively nontoxic. Their action is attributed to their surface-active property; by lowering surface tension they permit the intestinal fluids to penetrate the fecal mass more readily, and thus produce soft, easily passed stools. However, agents such as dioctyl sodium sulfosuccinate have been shown to increase mucosal cyclic AMP and alter ion transport in a manner similar to the bile acids. Thus, cyclic AMP-mediated active anion secretion may account for the increased accumulation of luminal fluid. The relative importance of these two mechanisms remains to be determined.

Docusate Calcium

Butanedioic acid, sulfo-, 1,4-bis(2-ethylhexyl) ester, calcium salt; Bis(2-ethylhexyl) *S*-Calcium Sulfosuccinate; Dioctyl Calcium Sulfosuccinate; Surfak (*Hoechst-Roussel*)

[128-49-4] $C_{40}H_{74}CaO_{14}S_2$ (883.22).

Preparation—*Docusate Sodium* (page 806) is dissolved in isopropanol and reacted with a methanolic solution of calcium chloride. US Pat 3,035,973.

Description—White, amorphous solid having the characteristic odor of octyl alcohol; free of the odor of other solvents.

Solubility—1 g in 3300 mL water, <1 mL alcohol, <1 mL chloroform, <1 mL ether.

Uses—A *fecal-softening* agent useful in *preventing constipation* or in patients where laxative therapy is undesirable or contraindicated. It does not cause peristaltic stimulation and, therefore, may be used in patients in whom cathartic medication is contraindicated. Except for occasional mild, transitory cramping pains, dioctyl calcium sulfosuccinate is free from side effects and contraindications. It is also used as an emulsifying, wetting, and dispersing agent for external preparations.

Dose—*Usual, adult, oral,* **240 mg.** *Children,* and *adults with minimal needs,* **50 mg** 1 to 3 times a day.

Dosage Forms—Capsules: 50 and 240 mg.

Docusate Sodium

Butanedioic acid, sulfo-, 1,4-bis(2-ethylhexyl) ester, sodium salt; Dioctyl Sodium Sulfosuccinate; Aerosol OT Dry (*Am Cyanamid*); Colace (*Mead-Johnson*); DioMedicone (*Medicone*); Doxinate (*Hoescht-Roussel*)

$$
\begin{array}{l}
\mathrm{C_2H_5} \\
| \\
\mathrm{COOCH_2CH(CH_2)_3CH_3} \\
| \\
\mathrm{CH_2} \\
| \\
\mathrm{CH-SO_3Na} \\
| \\
\mathrm{COOCH_2CH(CH_2)_3CH_3} \\
| \\
\mathrm{C_2H_5}
\end{array}
$$

Sodium 1,4-bis(2-ethylhexyl) sulfosuccinate [577-11-7] $C_{20}H_{37}NaO_7S$ (444.56).

Preparation—Several patents have been issued covering the preparation of this compound. In general, maleic anhydride is treated with 2-ethylhexanol to produce the so-called dioctyl maleate which is then reacted with sodium bisulfite under conditions conducive to saturation of the olefinic bond with simultaneous rearrangement of the bisulfite to the sulfonate structure.

Description—White, wax-like, plastic solid with a characteristic odor suggestive of octyl alcohol; usually available in the form of pellets.

Solubility—1 g slowly in about 70 mL water; freely soluble in alcohol and glycerin.

Uses—A surface-active agent used internally in the management of constipation and fecal impaction. It is used to soften the stools in impaction associated with megacolon, anal fissures, and postoperative anal atresia. It is also useful for constipation in geriatric, pediatric, and obstetric patients. However, 1 or 2 days of treatment may be necessary before an effect is observed. Although its action is attributed to its "detergent" or "wetting" properties, it does increase mucosal cyclic AMP in a manner similar to bile acids. As a pharmaceutic aid, it is used as an emulsifying, wetting, and dispersing agent in formulations for external use.

Dose—50 to **500 mg** daily; *usual,* **100 mg** 2 or 3 times a day.

Other Dose Information—For infants and children the dose is 10 to 20 mg daily.

Dosage Forms—Capsules: 50, 60, 100, 120, 240, 250, and 300 mg. Solution: 10 mg/mL; Syrup: 20 and 150 mg/5 mL; Tablets: 50, 100, and 300 mg.

Emetics

An *emetic* is a drug which induces vomiting. Although vomiting is primarily a respiratory function, the final result of this act is to evacuate the stomach. Therefore, the *emetics* are considered here with the gastrointestinal drugs. Such drugs may act directly by stimulation of the *chemoreceptor trigger zone* located in the area postrema of the medulla oblongata, (eg, apomorphine, morphine, hydrogenated ergot alkaloids, and digitalis glycosides) or they may act reflexly by irritant action on the gastrointestinal tract (eg, copper sulfate, mustard, sodium chloride, and zinc sulfate). They may also produce stimulation of the nodose ganglion of the vagus (eg, veratrum) or excitation of receptors in the heart, in the central nervous system rostral to the brain stem, and in other organs. The clinical value of emetics has been lessened by the stomach tube, a safer and more efficient tool for emptying the stomach.

Emetics should not be used in patients who are unconscious, semicomatose, or in whom coma is imminently expected, as well as those with significant central nervous system depression or shock. Also, they should not be used in patients with severe heart disease, tuberculosis, hernia, or advanced pregnancy. They are also contraindicated in debilitated patients and in poisoning caused by corrosive or petroleum products.

Apomorphine Hydrochloride

4*H*-Dibenzo[*de,g*]quinoline-10,11-diol, 5,6,6a,7-tetrahydro-6-methyl-, hydrochloride, hemihydrate (*R*)-,

6aβ-Aporphine-10,11-diol hydrochloride hemihydrate [41372-20-7] $C_{17}H_{17}NO_2 \cdot HCl \cdot \frac{1}{2}H_2O$ (312.80); *anhydrous* [314-19-2] (303.79). For the structure, see page 416.

Preparation—By heating morphine in a closed tube with a great excess of HCl for 2 or 3 hours at a temperature of 140° to 150°. The elements of one mole of H_2O are abstracted from the morphine, resulting in a change in the molecular structure. On cooling, crude apomorphine hydrochloride crystallizes.

Description—Minute, white or grayish white, glistening crystals or white powder; gradually acquires a green color on exposure to light and air; odorless; solutions are neutral to litmus.

Solubility—1 g in about 50 mL water and about 50 mL alcohol; 1 g in about 20 mL water at 80°; very slightly soluble in chloroform and in ether.

Uses—An *expectorant* in doses of 1 mg and a powerful *emetic* in doses of 5 mg. It should be employed with caution because in certain conditions (depression of the nervous system from poisons or overdoses of hypnotics) apomorphine may fail to cause emesis and will then cause further depression of the central nervous system. A narcotic antagonist (levallorphan, 0.02 mg/kg; nalorphine, 0.1 mg/kg; or preferably, naloxone, 0.01 mg/kg) may be used to terminate the vomiting and to alleviate the depression. Collapse, coma, and even death have occurred from the injudicious use of this powerful alkaloid. If vomiting does not occur from the first dose, a second should not be given. It is better to administer a gastric tube and lavage the stomach than to employ emetic drugs. Apomorphine is classified as a *Schedule II* drug under the *Controlled Substances Act.*

Dose—*Usual, subcutaneous,* **5 mg.**

Dosage Forms—Tablets (hypodermic): 6 mg.

Emetine Hydrochloride—page 1229.

Ipecac—page 868.

Sodium Chloride—page 835.

Zinc Sulfate—page 1165.

Antiemetics

The *nausea-vomiting complex* is one of the most frequent symptoms of disease. It is often induced by certain drugs and occurs after operations and radiation therapy, during pregnancy, in gastrointestinal carcinoma, and as the result of certain types of motion in hypersensitive persons. Often it is mild and self-limiting; at times, it is very disturbing. A number of drugs which block this action, the *antiemetics* (*antinauseants*), are therapeutically effective. Useful agents are found among the sedatives, antihistamines, and ataraxics. Of these, the phenothiazine derivatives appear to be the most potent and the only drugs known to depress directly the *chemoreceptor trigger zone* (see this page). Others may act either locally, on the cerebral cortex, or on the vestibular apparatus. Since the mechanism of action of many antiemetic agents is not fully understood, the selection of drug continues to be largely based on empirical reasons.

Antiemetics fall mainly into five groups:

1. *Sedatives and hypnotics* (barbiturates), which depress stimuli arising in the cerebral cortex or vomiting center.

2. *Anticholinergic agents* (scopolamine), which act largely to reduce excitability in the labyrinth and depress conduction in the vestibular pathways.

3. *Antihistamines* (dimenhydrinate and many others), which act upon the vestibular apparatus and are especially useful in motion sickness.

4. *Phenothiazines*, which act upon the chemoreceptor trigger zone, the vomiting center, or both.

5. *Miscellaneous agents* (diphenidol, trimethobenzamide, benzquinamide, etc) which act either upon the aural vestibular apparatus or upon the chemoreceptor trigger zone.

Centrally acting antiemetics, such as trimethobenzamide, prochlorperazine and similar agents, should not be used for the treatment of uncomplicated vomiting in children; their use should be restricted to prolonged vomiting of known etiology. There are three reasons for this caution: (1) there has been some suspicion that centrally acting antiemetics may contribute, in combination with viral illnesses, to the development of Reye's syndrome, a potentially fatal acute childhood encephalopathy; (2) the extrapyramidal symptoms which may occur secondary to these agents may be confused with the central nervous system signs of an undiagnosed primary disease responsible for the vomiting, eg, Reye's syndrome or other encephalopathy; and (3) it has been suspected that drugs with hepatotoxic potential may unfavorably alter the course of Reye's syndrome. Such drugs, including large doses of salicylates and acetaminophen, should therefore be avoided in children whose signs and symptoms (vomiting) could represent Reye's syndrome.

The phenothiazine antiemetics are capable of potentiating central nervous system depressants (eg, anesthetics, opiates, alcohol, etc) as well as atropine and phosphorus-containing insecticides. Phenothiazines may also reverse the pressor effect of epinephrine.

Adverse reactions include the following: *Sedatives and hypnotics*, drowsiness to stupor; *anticholinergic agents*, drowsiness, excitement or hallucinations, dryness of the mouth, mydriasis, blurred vision, and urinary retention; *antihistamines*, drowsiness, dizziness, blurred vision, dryness of the mouth, urinary retention; *phenothiazines (aliphatic)*, drowsiness, orthostatic hypotension, ocular changes, and anticholinergic effects; *phenothiazines (piperazine)*, extrapyramidal reactions (dystonia, akathisia, parkinsonian syndrome, dysarthria), hypersensitivity reactions, amenorrhea, reversal of epinephrine pressor effect, enhancement of CNS depressant drugs, gynecomastia, lactation, hyperglycemia, hypoglycemia, and glycosuria. Since drowsiness is common to most of these agents, patients should be cautioned not to drive or operate hazardous machinery while on these drugs.

Persistent vomiting results in loss of hydrochloric acid, alkalosis, and dehydration which, in turn, may precipitate further vomiting. Hence electrolyte therapy may be necessary after vomiting has been present for some time (see pages 821 and 832).

Benzquinamide Hydrochloride

2H-Benzo[a]quinolizine-3-carboxamide, 2-(acetyloxy)-N,N-diethyl-1,3,4,6,7,11b-hexahydro-9,10-dimethoxy-, monohydrochloride; Emet-con (*Roerig*)

N,N-Diethyl-1,3,4,6,7,11b-hexahydro-2-hydroxy-9,10-dimethoxy-2H-benzo[a]quinolizine-3-carboxamide acetate (ester) monohydrochloride [30046-34-5] $C_{22}H_{32}N_2O_5$.HCl (440.97).

Preparation—See US Pat 3,053,845.

Description—White or pale yellow, crystalline powder; melts between 222° and 230°; light-sensitive; stable in solution between pH 2 and 4; pK_a 5.9.

Solubility—1 g in 12.5 mL water, 43 mL alcohol.

Uses—A benzoquinolizine derivative, chemically unrelated to the phenothiazines, with antiemetic, antihistaminic, mild anticholinergic, and sedative properties. It is indicated for *prevention* and *treatment* of *nausea* and *vomiting* associated with anesthesia and surgery; contraindicated in patients with demonstrated hypersensitivity to the drug. It should not be used either in pregnant women or in children. The onset of antiemetic activity occurs within 15 min; 5 to 10% of an administered dose is excreted unchanged in the urine and the remainder metabolized by the liver. The plasma half-life is about 40 min; 58% of the drug is bound to plasma protein. Drowsiness appears to be the most common adverse effect. Other adverse reactions reported are as follows: *autonomic nervous system*—dry mouth, shivering, sweating, hiccups, flushing, salivation, blurred vision; *cardiovascular system*—hypertension, hypotension, dizziness, atrial fibrillation, premature atrial and ventricular contractions; *central nervous system*—drowsiness, insomnia, restlessness, headache, excitement, nervousness; *gastrointestinal system*—anorexia, nausea; *musculoskeletal system*—twitching, shaking, tremors, weakness; *other systems*—fatigue, chills, increased temperature.

Dose—*Usual, intramuscular,* **50 mg** repeated in 1 hour, with subsequent doses every 3 or 4 hours as necessary. *Intravenous,* 25 mg slowly as a single dose.

Dosage Form—Injection: 50 mg, to be reconstituted with 2.2 mL sterile water.

Chlorpromazine—page 1087.

Cyclizine

Piperazine, 1-(diphenylmethyl)-4-methyl-, Marezine (*Burroughs-Wellcome*)

1-(Diphenylmethyl)-4-methylpiperazine [82-92-8] $C_{18}H_{22}N_2$ (266.39).

Preparation—Benzhydryl chloride is condensed with N-carbethoxypiperazine and the carbethoxy group is split off by heating with potassium hydroxide. The N-benzhydrylpiperazine thus formed is isolated from the reaction product and methylated at the N^4-position by treatment with formic acid and formaldehyde to give cyclizine.

Description—White, or creamy white, crystalline, practically odorless powder; melts at about 106°; pH (saturated solution) between 7.6 and 8.6.

Solubility—Soluble in alcohol and chloroform; slightly soluble in water.

Uses—Antihistamine used as the hydrochloride and the lactate in the prevention and treatment of *motion sickness* (nausea, vomiting, and vertigo). It is also used for the control of postoperative nausea and vomiting. The antiemetic activity appears within 30 min and, after the indicated dose, persists for 4 to 6 hrs. Cyclizine also has anticholinergic properties and reduces the sensitivity of the labyrinthine apparatus. The exact mechanism of action is unknown. Because of its anticholinergic properties, it should be used with great caution in patients with glaucoma, obstructive disease of the gastrointestinal or urinary tract, and in elderly males with possible prostatic hypertrophy. The drug should not be used in women during pregnancy and those likely to become pregnant unless specifically directed by the physician. Large doses may cause drowsiness and dryness of the mouth. See introduction (in this section).

Dose—See *Cyclizine Hydrochloride* and *Cyclizine Lactate Injection.*

Cyclizine Hydrochloride

Piperazine, 1-(diphenylmethyl)-4-methyl-, monohydrochloride, Marezine Hydrochloride (*Burroughs-Wellcome*)

1-(Diphenylmethyl)-4-methylpiperazine monohydrochloride [303-25-3] $C_{18}H_{22}N_2$.HCl (302.85). For the structure of the base, see *Cyclizine.*

Preparation—The purified base may be converted conveniently into the hydrochloride by passing hydrogen chloride into a solution of the base in an appropriate organic solvent. For the preparation of the base, see *Cyclizine.*

Description—White, crystalline powder or small colorless crystals; odorless or nearly so and has a bitter taste; melts indistinctly and with decomposition at about 285°.

Solubility—1 g in about 115 mL water, 115 mL alcohol, and 75 mL of chloroform; insoluble in ether.

Uses—See *Cyclizine*.

Dose—*Usual, adult, oral*, **50 to 200 mg** daily; for motion sickness, **50 mg** ½ hour before departure and **50 mg** every 4 to 6 hours if required, not to exceed 4 tablets/day. *Children*, 6 to 10 years of age, ½ the above dose.

Dosage Forms—Tablets: 50 mg.

Cyclizine Lactate Injection

Piperazine, 1-(diphenylmethyl)-4-methyl-, mono(2-hydroxypropanoate); Marezine Injection (*Burroughs-Wellcome*)

1-(Diphenylmethyl)-4-methylpiperazine monolactate [5897-19-8] $C_{18}H_{22}N_2.C_3H_6O_3$ (356.46). For the structure of the base, see *Cyclizine*.

Preparation—Cyclizine base is reacted with an equimolar quantity of lactic acid. For the preparation of the base, see *Cyclizine*.

Description—pH between 5 and 6.

Dose—*Usual, adult, intramuscular*, **50 mg** every 4 to 6 hours as necessary. *Children*, 6 to 10 years of age, ½ the adult dose; under 6 years of age, ¼ the adult dose.

Dosage Form—Injection: 50 mg/mL.

Dimenhydrinate

1*H*-Purine-2,6-dione, 8-chloro-3,7-dihydro-1,3-dimethyl-, compd. with 2-(diphenylmethoxy)-*N*,*N*-dimethylethanamine (1:1); Dramamine (*Searle*); (*Various Mfrs*)

8-Chlorotheophylline, compound with 2-(diphenylmethoxy)-*N*,*N*-dimethylethylamine (1:1) [523-87-5] $C_{17}H_{21}NO.C_7H_7ClN_4O_2$ (469.97); contains 53–55.5% of diphenylhydramine ($C_{17}H_{21}NO$), and 44–47% of 8-chlorotheophylline ($C_7H_7ClN_4O_2$).

Preparation—By interaction of diphenhydramine, a base, with 8-chlorotheophylline, an acid, in isopropyl alcohol.

Description—White, crystalline, odorless powder; melts between 102° and 107°.

Solubility—Slightly soluble in water; freely soluble in alcohol and in chloroform; sparingly soluble in ether.

Uses—An *antihistaminic* compound which is a combination of diphenhydramine (Benadryl, *Parke-Davis*) and 8-chlorotheophylline. The latter contributes little, if anything, to its action as an antiemetic or an antihistaminic agent. It is chiefly employed as an *antinauseant* in *motion sickness* (*air-*, *train-*, *sea-sickness*, etc). It has also been used with success in the management of the vertigo associated with Ménière's syndrome, radiation sickness, and vestibular dysfunction resulting from streptomycin therapy. Mild sedation commonly attends its use. See page 1128.

Dose—25 to 600 mg daily; *usual, adult, oral*, **50 to 100 mg** every 4 hours. *Children 8 to 12 years of age, orally or rectally*, **25 to 50 mg** 2 or 3 times daily.

Dosage Forms—Injection: 50 mg/mL; Liquid: 12.5 mg/4 mL; Tablets: 50 mg.

Diphenhydramine Hydrochloride—page 1128.

Diphenidol

1-Piperidinebutanol, α,α-diphenyl-, Vontrol (*Smith Kline & French*)

α,α-Diphenyl-1-piperidinebutanol [972-02-1] $C_{21}H_{27}NO$ (309.45).

Preparation—Piperidine is reacted with 1-bromo-3-chloropropane in benzene with the aid of trimethylamine and the resulting 1-(3-chloropropyl)piperidine is converted to a Grignard reagent and reacted with benzophenone in tetrahydrofuran. Hydrolysis of the Grignard reaction complex yields crude diphenidol which may be purified by recrystallization from isopropanol. US Pat 2,898,340.

Description—White, crystalline powder that is odorless and has a slightly bitter taste; stable in light and air; melts between 103° and 107°.

Solubility—Freely soluble in chloroform, ether; sparingly soluble in alcohol; insoluble in water.

Uses—An antiemetic agent for the control of peripheral (labyrinthine) vertigo and associated nausea and vomiting as seen in Meniere's disease middle- and inner-ear surgery. It is also used to control nausea and vomiting in post operative states, malignant neoplasms, and labyrinthine disturbances. Experimentally, it has been shown to exhibit weak parasympatholytic actions, but to lack significant sedative, tranquilizing, or antihistaminic properties. *Its use should be restricted to patients under close medical supervision, since auditory and visual hallucinations, disorientation, and confusion have been reported.* Other untoward effects such as drowsiness, dry mouth, dizziness, skin rash, heartburn, headache, nausea, blurred vision, malaise, etc have been infrequent and minor in nature. Since diphenidol does possess parasympatholytic properties, it should be used cautiously in patients with glaucoma, prostatic hypertrophy, peptic ulcer, pyloric or duodenal obstruction, or cardiospasm. Animal experiments have revealed no evidence of teratogenic effects. Nevertheless, it is not recommended for use in the nausea and vomiting of pregnancy, since its safe use in this condition has not been established.

Dose—*Usual, adult, oral*, **25 to 50 mg** every 4 hours. *Children* (50 to 100 lbs) **25 mg** every 4 hours. Not recommended for use in infants under 6 months of age or 25 lbs.

Dosage Forms—Tablets: 25 mg.

Diphenidol Hydrochloride

1-Piperidinebutanol, α,α-diphenyl-, hydrochloride; Vontrol Hydrochloride (*Smith Kline & French*)

α,α-Diphenyl-1-piperidinebutanol hydrochloride [3254-89-5] $C_{21}H_{27}NO.HCl$ (345.91). For the structure of the base, see *Diphenidol*.

Preparation—*Diphenidol* is dissolved in a suitable solvent and reacted with hydrogen chloride.

Uses and **Dose**—See *Diphenidol*.

Dosage Forms—Tablets: 25 mg.

Fluphenazine Hydrochloride—page 1087.

Meclizine Hydrochloride

Piperazine, 1-[(4-chlorophenyl)phenylmethyl]-4-[(3-methylphenyl)-methyl]-, dihydrochloride, monohydrate; Antivert (*Roerig*); Bonine (*Pfizer*)

1 - (*p* - Chloro - α - phenylbenzyl) - 4 - (*m* - methylbenzyl)piperazine dihydrochloride [31884-77-2] $C_{25}H_{27}ClN_2.2HCl.H_2O$ (481.89); *anhydrous* [1104-22-9] (463.88).

Preparation—Meclizine is formed by condensing *N*-(*m*-methylbenzyl)piperazine with *p*-chlorobenzhydryl chloride in the presence of triethylamine. The purified base is dissolved in a suitable solvent and converted to the dihydrochloride by a stream of hydrogen chloride.

Description—White or slightly yellowish, crystalline powder; slight odor; tasteless; melts between 217° and 224°, with decomposition.

Solubility—Practically insoluble in water and ether; freely soluble in chloroform; slightly soluble in alcohol.

Uses—A long-acting antihistaminic agent effective in the prevention or treatment of *nausea*, *vomiting* and *dizziness* associated with *motion sickness.* It is also used in *vertigo* associated with diseases affecting the vestibular system. The antiemetic activity starts within 60 min and lasts for 12 to 24 hours. Like other antihistamines, it may cause drowsiness and other side actions, such as blurred vision, dryness of the mouth and fatigue. The action of a single dose persists for 9 to 24 hours. Use of the drug in pregnancy or in women who may become pregnant is contraindicated. See page 806.

Dose—*Usual, adult, oral,* **25** to **50 mg** 1 hour prior to embarkation for protection against motion sickness. The dose may be repeated every 24 hours for the duration of the trip.

Dosage Forms—Tablets: 25 mg. Chewable Tablets: 25 mg.

Pheniramine Maleate—page 1131.

Metoclopramide Hydrochloride

Benzamide, 4-amino-5-chloro-*N*-[2-(diethylamino)ethyl]-2-methoxy-, monohydrochloride, monohydrate; Reglan (*Robbins*)

4-Amino-5-chloro-*N*-[2-(diethylamino)ethyl]-*o*-anisamide, monohydrochloride, monohydrate [54143-57-6] $C_{14}H_{22}ClN_3O_2 \cdot HCl \cdot H_2O$.

Preparation—See *Arch Pharm 313:* 297, 1980.

Description—White crystals melting about 185° with decomposition.

Solubility—Soluble 1 g in about 0.7 mL of water, 3 mL of alcohol, or 55 mL of chloroform. A 10% aqueous solution has a pH of about 5.5.

Uses—Metoclopramide (methoxychloroprocainamide) is used for the prophylaxis of *vomiting* associated with *cisplatin* and other *cancer chemotherapy;* relief of symptoms associated with *acute* and *recurrent diabetic gastric ptosis;* facilitation of *small bowel intubation* in adults and children in whom the tube does not pass the pylorus with conventional maneuvers; and the *promotion of gastric emptying and intestinal transit of barium* in cases where delayed emptying interferes with radiological examination of the stomach and small intestine. In addition to its ability to stimulate the gut, it also has cholinergic properties, apparently sensitizing intestinal smooth muscle to the action of acetylcholine rather than acting directly on cholinergic receptors. In addition, it is a potent dopamine antagonist.

Metoclopramide is rapidly absorbed, single oral dose peak plasma concentrations are reached within 40 to 120 minutes, and plasma half-life is about 4 hours. Approximately 75% of the orally administered drug is excreted in the urine. Pharmacological activity appears within 1 to 3 minutes following intravenous administration and 10 to 15 minutes following intramuscular injection; pharmacological effects persist for 1 to 2 hours.

Common adverse effects include somnolence, nervousness and dystonic reactions. Parkinsonism and tardive dyskinesia have also been observed; increased pituitary prolactin release, galactorrhea, and menstrual disorders have been reported. Metoclopramide should not be used in epileptics or patients receiving other drugs which are likely to cause extrapyramidal reactions, since the frequency and severity of seizure or extrapyramidal reactions may be increased.

Dose—*Prevention of cisplatin-induced emesis:* **1** or **2 mg/kg** diluted in 50 mL of a large volume parenteral solution; infuse slowly over a period of not less than 15 minutes, 30 minutes before beginning cisplatin every 2 hours for 2 doses, then every 3 hours for 3 doses. *Diabetic gastroparesis:* **10 mg** orally, 30 minutes before each meal and at bedtime for 2 to 8 weeks. *Direct intravenous injection: adults* **10 mg (2 mL),** *children (6 to 14 years)* **2.5** to **5 mg,** and *children under 6 years,* **0.1 mg/kg** injected slowly over a period of 1 to 2 minutes.

Dosage Forms—Injection: 5 mg/mL in 2 and 10 mL ampuls. Syrup: 5 mg/5 mL. Tablets: 10 mg.

Prochlorperazine

10*H*-Phenothiazine, 2-chloro-10-[3-(4-methyl-1-piperazinyl)propyl]-, Compazine (*Smith Kline & French*)

2 - Chloro - 10 - [3 - (4 - methyl - 1 - piperazinyl)propyl]phenothiazine [58-38-8] $C_{20}H_{24}ClN_3S$ (373.94).

Preparation—A toluene solution of 1-(3-chloropropyl)-4-methylpiperazine and 2-chlorophenothiazine is refluxed with sodamide for several hours. After filtering and distilling off the toluene, the prochlorperazine is obtained by short-path distillation under high vacuum.

Description—Clear, pale yellow, viscous liquid; sensitive to light.

Solubility—Very slightly soluble in water; freely soluble in alcohol, chloroform, and ether.

Uses—A piperazine-type phenothiazine with actions, uses, and limitations similar to those of *Prochlorperazine Maleate.* However, prochlorperazine, as the base, is administered rectally.

Dose—*Usual, rectal, children,* **2.5** to **10 mg** daily, according to weight, in divided doses; *adults,* **25 mg** 2 times daily.

Other Dose Information—The *child's rectal* dose should not exceed 7.5, 10, and 15 mg daily for a 20 to 29-lb, 30 to 39-lb, and 40 to 58-lb child, respectively. It is not recommended for children weighing less than 20 lb.

Dosage Forms—Suppositories: 2.5, 5, and 25 mg.

Prochlorperazine Edisylate

10*H*-Phenothiazine, 2-chloro-10-[3-(4-methyl-1-piperazinyl)propyl]-, 1,2-ethanedisulfonate (1:1); Prochlorperazine Ethanedisulfonate; Compazine (*Smith Kline & French*)

2-Chloro-10-[3-(4-methyl-1-piperazinyl)propyl]phenothiazine 1,2-ethanedisulfonate (1:1) [1257-78-9] $C_{20}H_{24}ClN_3S \cdot C_2H_6O_6S_2$ (564.13).

For the structure of the base, see *Prochlorperazine.*

Preparation—*Prochlorperazine* is dissolved in a suitable solvent and treated with an equimolar portion of 1,2-ethanedisulfonic acid. The salt precipitates.

Description—White to very light yellow, odorless, crystalline powder; solutions are acid to litmus.

Solubility—1 g in about 2 mL water and about 1500 mL alcohol; insoluble in ether and chloroform.

Uses—Same actions and uses as prochlorperazine maleate except that it may be administered intramuscularly as well as orally. Parenteral therapy is usually reserved for the treatment of severe nausea and vomiting, for the immediate control of acutely disturbed psychotics or for patients who cannot or will not take oral medication. It should not be used in children with uncomplicated vomiting of unknown etiology. See *Prochlorperazine Maleate.*

Dose (as base equivalent)—*Adult, oral, antiemetic,* **5** to **10 mg** 3 or 4 times daily as required; *tranquilizer,* **5** to **35 mg** 3 or 4 times daily. *Usual range of oral dose,* **5** to **150 mg** daily. *Intramuscular* or *intravenous, antiemetic,* **5** to **10 mg** 6 to 8 times daily as required; *tranquilizer,* **10** to **20 mg** 4 to 6 times daily as required. *Usual range of parenteral dose,* as antiemetic, **5** to **40 mg** daily; as tranquilizer, **10** to **200 mg** daily.

Other Dose Information—No more than 40 mg of base equivalent should be injected in any 24-hour period unless the patient is hospitalized and under adequate observation. For acutely disturbed patients, the usual dose is 20 to 40 mg intramuscularly at intervals of 1 to 6 hours.

Dosage Forms (base equivalent)—Injection: 5 mg/mL; Syrup: 5 mg/5 mL; Concentrate (for institutional use): 10 mg/mL.

Prochlorperazine Maleate

10*H*-Phenothiazine, 2-chloro-10-[3-(4-methyl-1-piperazinyl)propyl]-, (*Z*)-2-butenedioate (1:2); Compazine (*Smith Kline & French*)

2 - Chloro - 10 - [3 - (4 - methyl - 1 - piperazinyl)propyl]phenothiazine maleate (1:2) [84-02-6] $C_{20}H_{24}ClN_3S \cdot 2C_4H_4O_4$ (606.09).

For the structure of the base, see *Prochlorperazine.*

Preparation—By the method described for *Prochlorperazine Edisylate* except that maleic acid is employed instead of ethanedisulfonic acid and it is employed in double equimolar quantity in relation to the prochlorperazine base.

Description—White or pale yellow, practically odorless, crystalline powder; saturated solution is acid to litmus.

Solubility—Practically insoluble in water and alcohol; slightly soluble in warm chloroform.

Uses—An *antiemetic, antipsychotic,* and *tranquilizing agent.* It is an effective *antiemetic* in the control of mild or severe nausea and vomiting due to a variety of causes, such as early pregnancy, anesthesia and surgery, and radiation therapy. It should not be used in children with uncomplicated vomiting of unknown etiology (*see* page 806). The drug is also an *effective antipsychotic* and is used in severe psychiatric disorders such as schizophrenia, mania, involutional psychoses, degenerative conditions, and senile and toxic psychoses. Beneficial results ascribed to its action include, among others, reduction in psychomotor agitation and excitement, diminished aggressiveness and destructiveness, mitigation of hallucinations and delusions and a general calming effect. As a *tranquilizing agent,* it is possibly effective in mild mental disorders in which anxiety, tension, and agitation predominate.

Adverse reactions may include *drowsiness, dizziness, amenorrhea, skin reactions, hypotension, cholestatic jaundice, neuromuscular (extrapyramidal) reactions, motor restlessness, dystonias, pseudoparkinsonism, persistent tardive dyskinesia,* and *contact dermatitis.* Children with acute infections (chickenpox, CNS infections, measles, gastroenteritis) or dehydration are more susceptible to neuromuscular reactions, particularly dystonias; such patients should be kept under close supervision. This agent may mask signs of overdosage of toxic drugs or obscure diagnosis of conditions such as intestinal obstruction or brain tumor. Adverse drug reactions can be minimized by periodically evaluating the dosage employed by patients on long-term therapy.

Dose (as base equivalent)—*Adult, oral, antiemetic,* **5** to **10 mg** 3 or 4 times daily as required; *tranquilizer,* **5** to **35 mg** 3 or 4 times daily, the initial low dose being increased gradually until the desired response is obtained, for which 50 to 150 mg daily is usually required.

Dosage Forms (base equivalent)—Tablets: 5, 10, and 25 mg; Sustained Release Capsules: 10, 15, 30, and 75 mg.

Scopolamine Hydrobromide—page 917.

Thiethylperazine Malate

10*H*-Phenothiazine, 2-(ethylthio)-10-[3-(4-methyl-1-piperazinyl)-propyl]-, 2-hydroxy-1,4-butanedioate (1:2); Torecan (*Boehringer-Ingelheim*)

2-(Ethylthio)-10-[3-(4-methyl-1-piperazinyl)propyl]phenothiazine malate (1:2) [52239-63-1] $C_{22}H_{29}N_3S_2.2C_4H_6O_5$ (533.71).

Preparation—*Thiethylperazine* is reacted with a double equimolar quantity of malic acid.

Description—White to faintly yellow crystalline powder; not more than a slight odor; pH (freshly prepared 1 in 100 solution) between 2.8 and 3.8.

Solubility—1 g in 40 mL water, 90 mL alcohol, 525 mL chloroform, 3400 mL ether.

Uses—See *Thiethylperazine Maleate.* Because of its solubility, this salt is used to prepare the injection.

Dose—*Intramuscular, usual,* **10** to **30 mg** daily.

Dosage Form—Injection: 10 mg/2 mL.

Thiethylperazine Maleate

10*H*-Phenothiazine, 2-(ethylthio)-10-[3-(4-methyl-1-piperazinyl)-propyl]-, (*Z*)-1,4-butenedioate (1:2); Torecan (*Boehringer-Ingelheim*)

2-(Ethylthio)-10-[3-(4-methyl-1-piperazinyl)propyl]phenothiazine

maleate (1:2) [1179-69-7] $C_{22}H_{29}N_3S_2.2C_4H_4O_4$ (631.76). For the structure of the base refer to *Thiethylpyrazine malate.*

Preparation—Thiethylperazine is prepared by reacting 2-(ethylthio)phenothiazine with 1-(3-chloropropyl)-4-methylpiperazine in the presence of sodamide or another dehydrochlorinating agent. The base is dissolved in a suitable solvent and reacted with a double molar quantity of maleic acid to produce the official salt. The starting phenothiazine compound may be prepared by condensing phenothiazine with ethanethiol, and the piperazine compound similarly from methylpiperazine and trimethylene chloride. US Pat 3,336,197.

Description—Faintly yellowish, fine, crystalline, voluminous powder; odorless or has a very slight odor and is bitter to the taste; melts at about 183°, with decomposition; pH (1 in 1000 solution, warmed) between 2.8 and 3.8.

Solubility—1 g in 1700 mL water, 530 mL alcohol, >10,000 mL chloroform, >10,000 mL ether.

Uses—A phenothiazine antiemetic *effective* in the relief of *nausea and vomiting* from various causes. It is also *possibly effective* for the management of *vertigo.* It should not be used in pregnancy or children under 12 years of age. Other contraindications and side effects are the same as those for other phenothiazines (see Page 1084). The malate salt (above) is used to prepare the injection.

Dose—*Usual, adult, oral,* **10** to **30 mg** daily.

Other Dose Information—The usual intramuscular and rectal dose is 10 to 30 mg/day.

Dosage Forms—Suppositories: 10 mg; Tablets: 10 mg.

Trimethobenzamide Hydrochloride

Benzamide, *N*-[[4-[2-(dimethylamino)ethoxy]phenyl]methyl]-3,4,5-trimethoxy-, monohydrochloride; Tigan (*Beecham*)

N-[*p*-[2-(Dimethylamino)ethoxy]benzyl]-3,4,5-trimethoxybenzamide monohydrochloride [554-92-7] $C_{21}H_{28}N_2O_5.HCl$ (424.92).

Preparation—4-[2-(Dimethylamino)ethoxy]benzylamine is condensed with 3,4,5-trimethoxybenzoyl chloride by refluxing in an inert solvent. The resulting trimethoxybenzamide may be converted to the hydrochloride by dissolving it in a suitable solvent and treating with HCl. The starting amine may be prepared in various ways, eg, by condensing sodium *p*-aminomethylphenoxide with 2-chloro-*N,N*-dimethylethylamine.

Description—White crystalline powder; slight phenolic odor; melts between 186° and 190°.

Solubility—1 g in 2 mL water, 59 mL alcohol, 67 mL chloroform, 720 mL ether.

Uses—A dimethylaminoethanol derivative indicated for the control of *nausea* and *vomiting.* Its antiemetic potency is about one-tenth that of chlorpromazine when given subcutaneously and ¼ that of the latter when given orally. Minor side effects which have been reported include drowsiness, vertigo, diarrhea, and local irritation. In patients with acute febrile illness, encephalitides, gastroenteritis, dehydration, and electrolyte imbalance (especially in children and the elderly and debilitated) CNS reactions such as opisthotonos, convulsions, coma, and extrapyramidal symptoms, have been reported, but it is not certain that these effects were in all cases due to use of the drug. Therefore, caution should be exercised when trimethobenzamide hydrochloride is used in these conditions (*see* page 806). The use of the injectable form of the drug in children, the suppositories in premature or newborn infants, and the use of the drug in patients hypersensitive to it are contraindicated. Also, suppositories should not be used in patients known to be sensitive to benzocaine or similar types of local anesthetics.

Dose—*Usual, adult, oral,* **250 mg** 3 or 5 times daily; *rectal* or *intramuscular,* **200 mg** 3 or 4 times daily. Children (30 to 90 lbs), *oral* or *rectal,* **100** to **200 mg** 3 or 4 times daily. *Intramuscular* not recommended for use in children.

Dosage Forms—Capsules: 100 and 250 mg; Injection: 100 mg/mL in 2-mL ampuls and 20-mL vials; Suppositories: 100 and 200 mg.

Adsorbents

Adsorbents are chemically inert powders that have the ability to adsorb gases, toxins, and bacteria. The fine state of subdivision of these inert powders confers high adsorptive capacity upon them. However, in the complex milieu of the gastrointestinal secretions, physical (van der Waals) adsorbents are more likely to be selective for surface-active substances such as bile salts than for bacterial toxins and other noxious substances. Consequently, only certain materials that possess chemical adsorptive properties lend themselves effectively to gastrointestinal detoxification and to the adsorption of gases resulting from abnormal intestinal fermentation. Such substances are kaolin, which is employed supposedly to adsorb bacterial toxins in diarrhea, dysentery, and chronic ulcerative colitis, and activated charcoal, which is employed to adsorb organic intoxicants especially, and gastrointestinal gases. It is doubtful that either is an effective adsorbent in the lower gastrointestinal tract since passage through the upper tract saturates and deactivates the agent; however, the effectiveness of these agents in bulk in entraining and dispersing bacterial aggregates may contribute to beneficial effects in the lower bowel.

Many of the nonsystemic antacids may serve as internal protectives and adsorbents, especially after regeneration in the alkaline small intestine. Magnesium trisilicate is claimed to exert a protective action also in the stomach by virtue of released silicic acid, which acts more as a demulcent than as a solid protective. *Antacids* are commonly combined with kaolin or other adsorbents.

Bismuth Subcarbonate—page 797.

Bismuth Subnitrate—page 794.

Activated Charcoal

Medicinal Charcoal

The residue from the destructive distillation of various organic materials, treated to increase its adsorptive power.

Preparation—Under the name *Carbo Ligni* or *Wood Charcoal* there was formerly used a product made by burning wood out of contact with air, the residue obtained consisting of nearly pure carbon. Charcoal made by this process was variable in its adsorptive powers, frequently being entirely devoid of such properties. It was found that the adsorptive powers of charcoal could be tremendously increased by treating it with various substances such as steam, air, carbon dioxide, oxygen, zinc chloride, sulfuric acid, or phosphoric acid, or a combination of some of these substances, at temperatures ranging from 500° to 900°. This treatment is referred to as activation, the activating agent presumably removing substances previously adsorbed on the charcoal and, in some instances at least, breaking down the granules of carbon into smaller ones having a greater total surface area. It has been estimated that 1 mL of charcoal, finely divided, possesses a total surface of approximately 1000 m^2.

In addition to wood many other substances are used as sources of charcoal, such substances including sucrose, lactose, rice starch, coconut pericarp, bone, blood, various industrial wastes, etc. As many different activated charcoals are available for various purposes, one should be certain to use only the medicinal variety for medicinal purposes.

Description—Fine, black, odorless, and tasteless powder, free from gritty matter.

Solubility—Insoluble in water or the other known solvents.

Uses—The most valuable single agent as an emergency *antidote* in many forms of poisoning because of its adsorptive powers. Indeed, except for mineral acids, alkalies, and substances insoluble in aqueous acidic solution, such as tolbutamide, it is the emergency treatment of choice for virtually all drugs and chemicals. Unfortunately, adsorption is not a specific action, thus nutrients and enzymes, as well as noxious substances, are adsorbed. Therefore, it has no recognized therapeutic value in dyspepsia, diarrhea, and dysentery.

Industrially it is used in large quantities in chemical and pharmaceutical manufacturing as a decolorizer.

Activated charcoal is marketed under the names of *Nuchar*, *Darco*, and *Norit*, less pure forms used for decoloration of solutions during manufacturing processes. See *Clarification and Decoloration* (Chapter 78).

Dose—5 to **50 g**; *usual, adult, oral,* **50 g**; *children, oral,* **25 g**.

Other Dose Information—Generally, charcoal is underutilized and given in insufficient doses; it should be given in a ratio of at least 10:1 of charcoal to estimated dose of toxin. Charcoal should not be administered simultaneously with ipecac, since it binds ipecac.

Kaolin

Light Kaolin; White Bole; China Clay

A native hydrated aluminum silicate, powdered, and freed from gritty particles by elutriation.

Preparation—Kaolin is widely distributed in nature. Most kaolin deposits, however, are frequently contaminated with ferric oxide (hence the red color of ordinary clay) and some other impurities, such as calcium carbonate, magnesium carbonate, etc. To render such kaolin suitable for pharmaceutical use it has to be purified by treatment with hydrochloric acid or sulfuric acid, or both, then washed well with water.

Kaolin of a high degree of purity, directly suitable for pharmaceutical use without acid purification, has been mined in the state of Georgia. England has large deposits of a fine grade of kaolin. The kaolin from these deposits is freed of coarse particles by elutriation or by screening. Kaolin is essentially a colloid, and the *colloid kaolin* on the market differs only from ordinary kaolin in that it contains a larger percentage of fine particles and it is prepared by special screening.

The BP also recognizes a native *Heavy Kaolin* (*Kaolinum Ponderosum*) for use in poultices. The Light Kaolin BP (Kaolin) is prepared from the heavy variety by elutriation.

Description—Soft, white, or yellowish white powder, or lumps; characteristic earthy or clay-like taste and, when moistened with water, it becomes darker and develops a pronounced clay-like odor.

Solubility—Insoluble in water, in cold diluted acids, and in solutions of the alkali hydroxides.

Uses—Either alone or as *Kaolin Mixture with Pectin* (see page 812) it is used medicinally as an *adsorbent*. It is of value chiefly in the treatment of *diarrhea* caused by agents capable of being adsorbed, as, for example, the diarrhea of food poisoning or dysentery. Kaolin has also been used in the treatment of chronic ulcerative colitis, but it is doubtful whether any adsorptive capacity is retained by the time the preparation reaches the colon. Externally kaolin has some use as a poultice, dusting powder, and an ingredient of toilet powders.

It has been used as a clarifying and decolorizing medium and as a filtering medium, but it must never be used as a filtering agent for liquids containing alkaloids, as it has been shown that it adsorbs alkaloids, often separating them completely from the liquids filtered. Sometimes employed as a tablet diluent, kaolin must never be used in tablets containing cardiac glycosides, alkaloids, estrogens, etc which may be adsorbed by kaolin.

Dose—It is usually given suspended in water in the dose of from **50 to 100 g**, at 3-hour intervals.

Magnesium Trisilicate—page 796.

Pectin

A purified carbohydrate product obtained from the dilute acid extract of the inner portion of the rind of citrus fruits or from apple pomace. It consists chiefly of partially methoxylated polygalacturonic acids.

Pectin yields not less than 6.7% of methoxy groups and not less than 74.0% of $C_6H_{10}O_7$ (galacturonic acid), calculated on the dried basis.

Pectin may be standardized to the convenient "150 jelly grade" by addition of dextrose or other sugars, and it may contain sodium citrate or other buffer salts. Such pectin is not suitable for medicinal use.

Description—Coarse or fine powder, yellowish white in color, almost odorless, and with a mucilaginous taste.

Solubility—Almost completely soluble in 20 parts of water at 25°, forming a viscous, opalescent, colloidal solution which flows readily and is acid to litmus; insoluble in alcohol or in diluted alcohol, and in other organic solvents; dissolves in water more readily if first moistened with alcohol, glycerin, or simple syrup, or if first mixed with 3 or more parts of sucrose.

Incompatibilities—Precipitated from solution by an excess of *alcohol*. *Metals*, particularly the heavy metals, form insoluble derivatives. In the presence of *alkalies*, pectin undergoes progressive hydrolysis resulting in a demethylation followed by a splitting of the glycosidic linkages of the galacturonic acid units. *In cold acid solution* it is more stable; prolonged heating of such a solution causes hydrolysis. Liquefaction of pectin pastes may be due to a hydrolysis which accompanies growth of certain types of *mold*.

Uses—A *protective* of value in the treatment of *diarrhea* in infants and children. The unchanged molecules of the polygalacturonic acids may have an *adsorbent* action in the intestine. As a *pharmaceutic aid*, it is used as an *emulsifying* and *thickening* agent.

Polycarbophil

Acrylic Acid-Divinyl Glycol Copolymer

Polycarbophil [9003-97-8]; polyacrylic acid cross-linked with divinyl glycol.

Preparation—Acrylic acid and divinyl glycol (1,5-hexadiene-3,4-diol) are copolymerized in a hot salt slurry using azobis[methyl-propionitrile] as the initiator. US Pat 3,202,577.

Description—White to creamy white granules, having a slight, characteristic, esterlike odor; contains a maximum of 1.5% water.

Solubility—Swells but is insoluble in water; insoluble in most organic solvents.

Uses—A pharmacologically inert substance which has the capacity to bind free fecal water. Hence, it is used in diarrheal disorders to decrease the fluidity or looseness of stools. Orally administered, polycarbophil exerts its most marked hydrosorptive action only on reaching the slightly acid or alkaline medium of the small intestine and colon. Polycarbophil is also used as a bulk-forming laxative. This hydrophilic polyacrylic resin is indigestible, nonabsorbable, and binds more water than other laxatives of this type. Polycarbophil is reported to have no effect on digestive enzymes, and that it is metabolically inactive. The only adverse effect noted is a sense of fullness and bloating in some patients; this can be minimized by giving smaller doses at shorter intervals.

Dose—*Usual, adult, oral,* **4 to 6 g,** divided into 4 doses, daily. *Children 6 to 12 years of age,* **1.5 to 3 g;** *2 to 5 years of age,* **1 to 1.5 g;** *under 2 years of age,* **0.5 to 1 g.**

Other Adsorbents

Kaolin Mixture with Pectin [(Various Mfrs)]—*Preparation:* Mix kaolin (200 g) with purified water (500 mL). Triturate pectin (10 g), powdered tragacanth (5 g), and sodium saccharin (1 g) with glycerin (20 mL) and add to this, with constant stirring, benzoic acid (2 g) dissolved in boiling purified water (300 mL). Allow the mixture to stand until it cools to room temperature and all the pectin is dissolved. Add peppermint oil (0.75 mL) and the kaolin-water mixture, mix thoroughly, and finally add sufficient purified water to make 1000 mL. In order to obtain a product with suitable consistency when larger amounts are prepared, the quantity of tragacanth and, if necessary, the quantity of pectin may be altered. However, if the proportion of pectin in the form is altered by more than 10%, the pectin content of the preparation must be clearly stated on the label. *Uses:* An *adsorbent demulcent.* See *Kaolin* (page 811). *Dose: Usual,* 30 mL as needed.

Miscellaneous Gastrointestinal Drugs

Several drugs with diverse actions on the gastrointestinal tract are included in this section. They range from the empirical carminative *peppermint spirit* to the novel gallstone dissolution agent chenodiol, and the well established *diphenoxylate hydrochloride–atropine sulfate* antidiarrheal combination. Carminatives are substances which were at one time used to relieve gaseous distention of the stomach or intestines. Many carminative volatile oils are used as flavoring agents (*see* Chapter 68 and the cross-references listed below).

Anise Oil—page 1285.
Camphor—page 780.
Camphor Spirit—page 781.

Caraway—page 1285.
Caraway Oil—page 1285.
Cardamom Oil—page 1285.
Cardamom Seed—page 1285.
Cardamom Tincture, Compound—page 1294.

Chenodiol

Cholan-24-oic acid, 3,7-dihydroxy-, (3α,5β,7α)-, Chenix (*Rowell*)

[474-25-9] $C_{24}H_{40}O_4$ (392.58).

Preparation—A naturally occurring bile acid in most vertebrates as the glycine or taurine conjugate. It is usually prepared from cholic acid (*J Amer Chem Soc 72:* 5530, 1950 and *J Org Chem 24:* 1367, 1959).

Description—White needles melting about 120°; $[\alpha]_D^{20}$ + 11.5° (dioxane).

Solubility—Practically insoluble in water and hydrocarbon solvents; freely soluble in alcohol or acetone.

Uses—An alternative to surgery for the treatment of symptomatic radiolucent cholesterol gallstones in patients with well-functioning gallbladders. Approximately 20 million people in this country have gallstones; about 1 million new cases appear each year. Some 80% of gallstones are composed of cholesterol or are mixed stones that contain 50% cholesterol. Cholesterol crystals form in bile when its capacity to solubilize cholesterol is exceeded (Sedaghat and Grundy, *New Engl J Med: 302,* 1274, 1980). Neither the mechanism involved in the aggregation of cholesterol crystals into stones nor the mechanism by which chenodiol dissolves gallstones is known. It is known, however, that chenodiol suppresses the hepatic synthesis of cholesterol and decreases biliary cholesterol secretion.

Chenodiol, a naturally occurring human bile acid, is well absorbed from the small intestine, taken up by the liver, conjugated, and then secreted in the bile. Since first pass hepatic clearance accounts for 60 to 80% of the drug, the body pool of chenodiol resides mainly in the enterohepatic circulation; serum and urinary bile acid levels are not significantly altered. At steady state a portion of the drug (approximately the daily dose) reaches the colon where it is converted by bacterial action to lithocholic acid. About 80% of the lithocholic acid is excreted in the feces; the remainder is absorbed and conjugated in the liver.

Clinical studies indicate that stones dissolved completely in 13.5 to 27% of patients taking 750 mg and 15 mg/kg, respectively, of chenodiol for two years; stones were partially dissolved in an additional 27% of patients taking 750 mg/day (*Ann Intern Med: 95,* 257, 1981; *Dig Dis Sci:* 28, 545, 1983). After treatment was stopped, the stones formed again in 50% of patients within 5 years.

Potential drug interactions include decreased absorption when given with cholestyramine, colestipol, and antacids. Estrogens, oral contraceptives, clofibrate and other drugs that increase cholesterol secretion may counteract the effectiveness of chenodiol. A possible carcinogenic effect was observed in rats given 40 to 65 times the maximum recommended human dose for 2 years.

Adverse effects appear to include an increase in serum SGOT levels and an increase in low density lipoprotein cholesterol concentrations. About 40% of patients on 750 mg/day developed diarrhea; this subsided when dosage was reduced. Other less frequent adverse effects include urgency, cramps, heartburn, constipation, nausea and vomiting, anorexia, epigastric distress, dyspepsia, flatulence and abdominal pain. The safety and effectiveness in pregnant women, nursing mothers, and children have not been established.

Dose—*Usual, adult, oral,* **13 to 16 mg/kg/day,** divided into 2 doses; start with 250 mg twice daily for two weeks and increase by one tablet each week until the recommended dosage is reached or intolerance develops.

Dosage Form—Tablets: 250 mg.

Chlorobutanol—page 1278.
Chloroform—page 1312.

Cholestyramine Resin

Cuemid *(MSD)*; Questran *(Mead-Johnson)*

Cholestyramine [11041-12-6]; a strongly basic anion-exchange resin in the chloride form, consisting of styrene-divinylbenzene copolymer with quaternary ammonium functional groups. Each g exchanges 1.8–2.2 g of sodium glycocholate, calculated on the dried basis.

Preparation—Polystyrene trimethylbenzylammonium chloride is copolymerized through cross-linkage with divinylbenzene.

Description—White to buff-colored, hygroscopic, fine powder; odorless or has not more than a slight amine-like odor; pH between 4 and 6, in a slurry (1 in 100).

Solubility—Slightly soluble in water and alcohol; insoluble in chloroform, and ether.

Uses—An ion-exchange resin with an affinity for bile salts indicated as adjunctive therapy to diet in the management of patients with elevated cholesterol levels due to primary type II hyperlipoproteinemia. *It has not been established, however, whether drug-induced lowering of serum cholesterol, or other lipid levels has a detrimental, a beneficial, or no effect on the morbidity due to atherosclerosis or coronary heart disease.* It is also used for the relief of pruritus associated with bile stasis which occurs in biliary cirrhosis and with various forms of partial obstructive jaundice. It is contraindicated in hypersensitive patients and in patients with complete biliary obstruction. The safe use of cholestyramine resin during pregnancy has not been established. Chronic use may be associated with constipation, fecal impaction, and a tendency to increased bleeding; hyperchloremic acidosis may also occur. Cholestyramine may bind other drugs given concurrently. For example, it may interfere with fat absorption and thus prevent absorption of fat-soluble vitamins such as A, D, and K. Reduced absorption of folic acid, phenylbutazone, warfarin, chlorothiazide, tetracycline, phenobarbital, thyroid, and thyroxine has also been reported. The resin should not be taken in the dry form; it should always be mixed with water or other fluids before ingesting.

Dose—10 to **24 g** daily; *usual,* **4 g** 3 times a day. Dosage in infants and children has not been established.

Dosage Form—for Oral Suspension: Powder: 4 g of anhydrous cholestyramine in 9 g of powder.

Dexpanthenol

Butanamide, 2,4-dihydroxy-*N*-(3-hydroxypropyl)-3,3-dimethyl-, *(R)*-, Ilopan *(Adria)*; Panthoderm *(USV)*

$$HOCH_2-\overset{CH_3}{\underset{CH_3}{\overset{|}{C}}}-\overset{OH}{\underset{H}{\overset{|}{C}}}-CONHCH_2CH_2CH_2OH$$

D(+)-2,4-Dihydroxy-*N*-(3-hydroxypropyl)-3,3- dimethylbutyramide. *d*-Pantothenyl alcohol [81-13-0] $C_9H_{19}NO_4$ (205.25).

Preparation—By combination of propanolamine with the lactone of D-2,4-dihydroxy-3,3-dimethylbutyric acid through ring rupture. US Pat 2,413,077.

Description—Viscous, somewhat hygroscopic liquid with a slightly bitter taste.

Solubility—Freely soluble in water and alcohol; slightly soluble in ether.

Uses—This alcohol analogue of D-pantothenic acid is said to increase the amount of coenzyme A available for the synthesis of acetylcholine. The increased formation of acetylcholine is thought to increase peristalsis and intestinal tone. Hence, dexpanthenol has been proposed for *prophylactic use* immediately after major abdominal surgery to minimize the possibility of *paralytic ileus.* It is also recommended for *intestinal atony causing abdominal distention;* postoperative or postpartum *retention of flatus;* or postoperative *delay in* the resumption of *intestinal motility.* Dexpanthenol should not be injected directly into a vein and it should not be administered within one hour of succinylcholine. Rare instances of allergic reactions of unknown cause have been observed in patients receiving this drug and other drugs such as antibiotics, narcotics, or barbiturates. Adverse effects observed in one or more patients include itching,

tingling, difficulty in breathing, dermatitis, urticaria, slight hypotension, intestinal colic, vomiting, and diarrhea. Dexpanthenol prolongs bleeding time and, hence, is contraindicated in hemophilia. It should not be used in combination with parasympathomimetic drugs.

Dose—*Usual, adult, intramuscular,* **250** or **500** mg repeated in 2 hours and then every 6 hours for the prevention of gastrointestinal atony and distention.

Dosage Form—Injection: 250 mg/mL.

Diphenoxylate Hydrochloride

4-Piperidinecarboxylic acid, 1-(3-cyano-3,3-diphenylpropyl)-4-phenyl-, ethyl ester, monohydrochloride; ing of Lomotil *(Searle)*

Ethyl 1-(3-cyano-3,3-diphenylpropyl)-4-phenylisonipecotate monohydrochloride [3810-80-8] $C_{30}H_{32}N_2O_2$·HCl (489.06).

Preparation—Ethyl 4-phenylisonipecotate (prepared as described under *Meperidine Hydrochloride* (page 1108) except omitting the final step of *N*-methylation), is condensed with 2,2-diphenyl-4-bromobutyronitrile by refluxing in toluene using either an excess of the ester or another suitable dehydrobrominating agent. US Pat 2,898,340.

Description—White, odorless, crystalline powder; pH (saturated solution) about 3.3; melts between 220° and 226°.

Solubility—Sparingly soluble in alcohol and acetone; slightly soluble in water and isopropyl alcohol; freely soluble in chloroform; practically insoluble in ether and solvent hexane.

Uses—Diphenoxylate, a synthetic congener of meperidine, inhibits excessive gastrointestinal propulsion by slowing intestinal motility. It is *effective as adjunctive therapy* in the management of *diarrhea*, for which purpose it has been used in the treatment of diarrhea associated with gastroenteritis, irritable bowel, functional hypermotility, regional enteritis, acute infections, ulcerative colitis, food poisoning, and side effects of some drugs. It is also useful in the control of *intestinal transit time* in patients with *ileostomies* and *colostomies.*

In high dosage (40 to 60 mg) diphenoxylate can produce morphine-like euphoria and prevent withdrawal symptoms in narcotic addicts, but in the recommended dosage range for antidiarrheal therapy no evidence for addiction liability has been reported. The available dosage forms contain a subtherapeutic dose of 0.025 mg of atropine sulfate and a 2.5-mg dose of diphenoxylate hydrochloride. The atropine sulfate decreases gastrointestinal motility after accumulative dosage and also discourages usage of excessive amounts, thereby minimizing abuse. The combination is listed in *Schedule V* under the *Controlled Substances Act. Caution:* This combination *(Lomotil)* is *not* an innocuous drug and dosage recommendations should be strictly adhered to, especially in children.

Side effects are usually minor and include nausea, sedation, dizziness, vomiting, pruritus, skin eruption, insomnia, and abdominal cramps. Numbness of the extremities, headache, blurring of vision, swelling of gums, and general malaise have also been reported. The drug is contraindicated in patients with cirrhosis or advanced liver disease, and in children under 2 years of age. It should be used with caution in patients on barbiturates, tranquilizers, and alcohol, because the activity of these drugs may be potentiated by diphenoxylate. Concurrent use with monoamine oxidase inhibitors may, in theory, precipitate a hypertensive crisis.

Dose—**5** to **30 mg**/day; *usual, adult, oral,* **5 mg** 4 times a day. Lomotil is contraindicated in children under 2 years of age; in children 2 to 12 years of age the liquid form should be used; *2 to 5 years*, **4 mL (2 mg)** 3 times daily; *5 to 8 years of age*, **4 mL (2 mg)** 4 times daily; and *8 to 12 years of age*, **4 mL (2 mg)** 5 times daily.

Dosage Forms—Diphenoxylate Hydrochloride and Atropine Sulfate Solution *(Lomotil*, Searle): 2.5 mg of diphenoxylate hydrochloride and 0.025 mg (25 µg) of atropine sulfate/5 mL; Diphenoxylate Hydrochloride and Atropine Sulfate Tablets: 2.5 mg of diphenoxylate hydrochloride and 0.025 mg of atropine sulfate.

Ether—page 1041.
Fennel Oil—page 1286.

Lactulose

D-Fructose, 4-O-β-D-galactopyranosyl-, Cephulac (*Merrell*)

4-O-β-D-Galactopyranosyl-D-fructofuranose [4618-18-2] $C_{12}H_{22}O_{11}$ (342.30).

Preparation—Lactulose (a disaccharide containing one molecule of galactose and one molecule of fructose) may be prepared by epimerization of lactose (a disaccharide containing one molecule of galactose and one molecule of glucose) in a lime water medium. *J Am Chem Soc 52*: 2101, 1930.

Description—White powder; melts at about 169°; levorotatory; reduces Fehling's solution; yields galactose and fructose on acid hydrolysis. The commercially available syrup is a pale yellow to yellow, viscous, sweet liquid; each 15 mL contains 10 g of lactulose (and less than 2.2 g galactose, less than 1.2 g lactose, and 1.2 g or less of other sugars).

Solubility—Very soluble in water; very slightly soluble in alcohol.

Uses—Lactulose (syrup) is used to reduce blood ammonia levels in patients with portal-systemic encephalopathy, thereby generally reducing the degree of the affliction and improving the patients' mental state and EEG patterns, although not altering the course of the underlying liver disease. The action of lactulose, which is poorly absorbed after oral administration, depends on its breakdown by saccharolytic bacteria in the colon to carbon dioxide, lactic acid, and small amounts of acetic and formic acids, which acidify the contents of the colon. This acidification results in retention of ammonia in the colon (as ammonium ion) and diffusion of ammonia from blood into the colon. The laxative action of lactulose and/or its metabolites then expels the trapped ammonium ions from the colon. Therapy with lactulose is reported to reduce blood-ammonia levels by 25 to 50%, and to effect a favorable clinical response in about 75% of patients.

Lactulose may produce gaseous distention with flatulence or belching and abdominal discomfort such as cramping in about 20% of patients. Excessive dosage may produce diarrhea. Nausea and vomiting have been reported infrequently.

Lactulose syrup contains some monosaccharides (see under *Preparation*, above) and should be used with caution in diabetics. Concomitant use of neomycin with lactulose may result in elimination of colonic bacteria by neomycin that are essential for the required degradation of lactulose and thus prevent acidification of the colon. Other laxatives should not be used especially during the initial phase of therapy because loose stools may falsely suggest that lactulose dosage is adequate. Lactulose does not alter the course of the underlying liver disease, for which other therapy may be required. The safety of lactulose syrup during pregnancy and the effect on the mother and fetus have not been evaluated.

Dose—*Oral, usual*, **30** to **45 mL** of syrup (**20** to **30 g** of lactulose) 3 or 4 times daily; dosage may be adjusted every day or two to produce 2 or 3 soft stools daily.

Dosage Form—Syrup, each 15 mL containing 10 g of lactulose.

Loperamide Hydrochloride

1-Piperidinebutanamide, 4-(4-chlorophenyl)-4-hydroxy-*N,N*-dimethyl-α,α-diphenyl-, monohydrochloride; Imodium (*Ortho*)

4-(*p*-Chlorophenyl) - 4 - hydroxy - *N,N*-dimethyl-α,α-diphenyl-1-piperidinebutyramide monohydrochloride [34552-83-5] $C_{29}H_{33}ClN_2O_2 \cdot HCl$ (513.51).

Preparation—4-Bromo-2,2-diphenylbutyric acid is converted in a series of reactions to dimethyl(tetrahydro-3,3-diphenyl-2-furylidene)ammonium bromide, which is reacted with *p*-chlorophenyl-4-piperidinol to produce loperamide. US Pat 3,714,159; *J Med Chem 16:* 782, 1973.

Description—White to faintly yellow, amorphous or microcrystalline powder; melts at about 222°.

Solubility—Slightly soluble in water; soluble in alcohol.

Uses—A synthetic agent used for the control and symptomatic relief of *acute nonspecific diarrhea* and *chronic diarrhea* associated with inflammatory bowel disease. It is also used for *reducing the volume of discharge* from ileostomies. Plasma levels are highest 5 hours after oral administration. The elimination half-life is 10.8 hours with a range of 9.1 to 14.4 hours. Unchanged drug remains below 2 nanograms/mL after the intake of a 2-mg capsule. Most of the drug is excreted in the feces. The safe use of this agent during pregnancy, by nursing mothers, infants and children has not been established. Adverse effects are minimal and usually self-limiting. The following patient complaints have been reported: abdominal pain, constipation, drowsiness, dizziness, dry mouth, nausea and vomiting, and tiredness. Hypersensitivity reactions have been reported. Loperamide should be discontinued if abdominal distention occurs or if other untoward symptoms develop in patients with ulcerative colitis. Loperamide is listed in *Schedule V* under the *Controlled Substances Act*.

Dose—*Usual, adult, oral,* **4 mg** initially followed by **2 mg** after each unformed stool until diarrhea is controlled. Daily dosage should not exceed 16 mg. Clinical improvement is usually observed within 48 hours.

Dosage Form—Capsules: 2 mg.

Peppermint Spirit

Essence of Peppermint

Contains, in each 100 mL, 9–11 mL of peppermint oil.

Peppermint Oil	**100 mL**
Peppermint, in coarse powder	**10 g**
Alcohol, a sufficient quantity,	
To make	$\overline{\text{1000 mL}}$

Macerate the peppermint leaves, freed as much as possible from stems and coarsely powdered, for 1 hour in 500 mL of purified water, and then strongly express them. Add the moist, macerated leaves to 900 mL of alcohol, and allow the mixture to stand for 6 hours with frequent agitation. Filter, and to the filtrate add the oil and sufficient alcohol to make the product measure 1000 mL.

The maceration of the peppermint leaves with water is for the purpose of removing brownish-colored pigments. If this processing were not performed, the finished product would not possess a brilliant green color since the undesirable pigments are also soluble in alcohol. On the other hand, the maceration with water does not remove chlorophyll.

Alcohol Content—79 to 85%.

Uses—A *carminative* in *flatulence* and *nausea*.

Dose—*Usual*, **1 mL** 3 times a day.

Peppermint Water—page 1288.

Pimenta Oil—page 1292.

Simethicone

Mylicon (*Stuart*); Silain (*Robins*)

Simethicone [8050-81-5]; a mixture of fully methylated linear siloxane polymers containing repeating units of the formula $[-(CH_3)_2SiO]_n$, stabilized with trimethylsiloxy end-blocking units of the formula $[(CH_3)_3SiO-]$, and silicon dioxide.

Description—Translucent, gray, viscous fluid; specific gravity between 0.964 and 0.984; refractive index between 1.400 and 1.410; viscosity (25 ± 0.1°) not less than 300 centistokes.

Uses—An agent with antifoaming and water-repellent properties used as adjunctive therapy in conditions in which gas is a problem, such as *postoperative gaseous distention, air swallowing, functional* *dyspepsia, peptic ulcer, spastic* or *irritable colon* and *diverticulitis.* It is also used in antacid combinations to defoam gastric juice, in order to decrease the tendency to gastroesophageal reflux; however, it does *not* decrease the antacid requirement. It is thought to be physiologically inert and devoid of toxicity. However, definitive clinical usefulness remains to be established.

Dose—*Usual, adult, oral,* Tablets: **40** to **80 mg** 4 times daily after each meal and at bedtime. Chew tablets thoroughly. Drops: **40 mg** 4 times daily after meals and at bedtime.

Dosage Forms—Drops: 40 mg/0.6 mL; Tablets: 40, 50, and 80 mg.

Spearmint Oil—page 1290.

Sucralfate

α-D-Glucopyranoside, β-D-fructofuranosyl-, octakis(hydrogen sulfate), aluminum complex; Carafate (*Marion*)

$(R$ is $SO_3[Al_2(OH)_x(H_2O)_y])$

Sucrose octakis(hydrogen sulfate) aluminum complex [54182-58-0] $C_{12}H_mAl_{16}O_nS_8$ (*m* and *n* are approximately 54 and 75 respectively giving an average molecular weight of about 2086 daltons).

Preparation—See US Pat 3,432,489.

Description—White powder; pK_a between 0.43 and 1.19.
Solubility—Practically insoluble water; soluble in fixed alkali or acids.

Uses—For the short-term (up to 8 weeks) treatment of duodenal ulcer. Antacids may be prescribed as needed for pain relief. Sucralfate is absorbed minimally from the gastrointestinal tract. The mechanism by which sucralfate accelerates healing of duodenal ulcer remains to be fully defined. It is thought that sucralfate forms an ulcer-adherent complex with proteinaceous exudate at the ulcer site; this complex covers the ulcer site and protects it against further attack by acid, pepsin, and bile salts. Sucralfate has negligible acid neutralizing properties; therefore, its anti-ulcer effects cannot be attributed to neutralization of gastric acid. There are no known contraindications. Nevertheless, it should not be used during pregnancy or in nursing mothers unless clearly needed. Since sucralfate is an aluminum salt of a sulfated disaccharide, it may prevent absorption of tetracycline. Adverse effects occur in approximately 5% of patients; constipation is most common (2.2%). Other adverse effects include diarrhea, nausea, gastric discomfort, indigestion, dry mouth, rash, pruritus, back pain, dizziness, sleepiness, and vertigo.

Dose—*Usual, adult, oral for duodenal ulcer*, **1 g** 4 times a day on an empty stomach (1 hour before each meal and at bedtime).

Dosage Form—Tablets: 1 g.

Other Miscellaneous Gastrointestinal Drugs

Ursodeoxycholic Acid [3α,7β-Dihydroxy-5β-cholan-24-oic acid [128-13-2] $C_{24}H_{40}O_4$, 392.58]. A white crystalline powder melting about 200°; practically insoluble in water; freely soluble in alcohol; slightly soluble in chloroform; very slightly soluble in ether. For the isolation see *J Biochem (Japan) 185:* 151, 1929. *Uses:* Ursodeoxycholic acid, the 7-beta-hydroxy epimer of chenodiol (chenodeoxycholic acid) is used to dissolve gallstones. Clinical results obtained in Europe indicate that it rarely induces hepatic abnormalities and that it is much less likely to induce diarrhea (*Dig Dis Sci: 27,* 737, 1982; *Ann Intern Med 97:* 351, 1982). See Chenodiol (page 812).

CHAPTER 42

Blood, Fluids, Electrolytes, and Hematologic Drugs

Stewart C Harvey

Professor of Pharmacology
School of Medicine, University of Utah
Salt Lake City, UT 84132

Blood is a unique tissue. As a tissue, it can be withdrawn from the body, and an extensive array of its parts can be separated for use in therapy. As a circulating body fluid, blood serves a vital set of physiologic functions. A large number of drugs exert useful specific actions directed at maintaining or restoring these functions.

This chapter is organized as follows:

Whole Blood and Blood Components. The term blood components has been used increasingly to designate the parts of blood which are separated and dispensed in blood centers and blood banks.

Drugs, or *biologicals obtained by fractionation of human plasma*, are sometimes called *blood constituents* or *blood derivatives*. The presentation is organized according to functional uses of these drugs.

Plasma Expanders and Intravenous Fluids, which include plasma protein biologicals, dextran, and balanced electrolyte solutions.

Antibodies and Isoagglutinins. These are purely of blood origin.

Agents Affecting Coagulation of Blood.
Electrolytes.
Hematologic Drugs which affect the production of blood and its parts.
Miscellaneous Drugs.

The reader is referred to Chapter 32 for a basic discussion of hematology and blood banking technology.

The responsibility for promulgating and administering federal regulations applicable to blood and blood products is that of the Food and Drug Administration, Bureau of Biologics. The applicable regulations are found in the *Code of Federal Regulations*, *21 CFR 273.3*. Standards are also set by the American Association of Blood Banks and the World Health Organization.

Whole Blood and Blood Components

The blood is both an important regulator and a mirror of the proper functioning of body cells. Although it does not come into direct contact with cells other than the vascular endothelium, the interstitial fluid and lymph so resemble plasma, except that they are nearly devoid of protein, that plasma may be thought of as the culture medium of the tissue cells. Consequently, its electrolyte and organic composition is of the utmost importance. Plasma is the vehicle for the transport of most nutrients to, and many wastes from, the tissues. Plasma transports drugs, often in combined, or bound, form; plasma is therefore an important factor in determining the effectiveness of drugs (Chapter 37). The proteins in plasma are importantly involved in the regulation of the hydration of the tissues by virtue of osmosis resulting from the impermeability of the vascular endothelium to most of the protein. Some of the plasma proteins are intimately involved in the clotting of blood and therefore in its conservation. The erythrocytes are especially involved with oxygen and carbon dioxide transport. Leukocytes play major roles in the defense against infection, and platelets exert a variety of important functions in hemostasis and response to injury.

Uses for Blood and Blood Components—The many physiologic functions of blood derive from the specific roles of its many parts; in addition to the formed elements there are more than 70 discrete proteins in the plasma. When whole blood has been lost, as by hemorrhage, whole blood is required for replacement. However, the use of whole blood to overcome a deficiency of a single part constitutes a dissipation of the other useful parts. In the majority of instances, the administration of a single component in concentrated form elicits a far better response than the administration of that component in whole blood. Furthermore, by using the specific parts of the blood, the supply of blood can be used more economically; the net result is utilization of the components of a single donation for several purposes.

The number of products now available is increasing but is still short of the number of known parts of blood. For example, the red cells can be made available for treatment of anemia, the albumin for treatment of shock, the immune globulins for the prophylaxis of certain infectious diseases, granulocytes for granulocytopenia, and platelets for thrombocytopenia. These and other important available blood components are discussed in the following sections.

In the US, the collection, processing, preservation, and distribution of blood and its separated components are carried out by a wide variety of enterprises. For the purpose of this discussion, however, what is important is where and how blood and its components are made available for the use of patients and the public at large. The main channels for dispensing blood services and blood products are as follows:

1. Blood centers and blood banks provide a wide array of services which reach the patient on prescription usually through a hospital blood bank or transfusion service. The major services include the provision of whole blood, separated red cells, platelets, granulocytes, cryoprecipitated Factor VIII, single donor plasma and fresh frozen plasma. These are usually referred to as blood and blood components. They are distinguished by the fact that they are prepared locally in the blood center and are dispensed in the form of individual units identified by donor.

2. The pharmaceutical manufacturer and the pharmacy. This applies to the products of plasma fractionation, which are prepared by pharmaceutical manufacturers from large lots of pooled human plasma and are therefore subject to biologic control regulations separate from those applying to simple units of blood and its components.

3. Public health agencies and large blood centers, which may dispense directly to physicians or even to individual patients under certain circumstances.

Transmission of Infection—The use of blood and its components is accompanied by some risk of transmission of serum hepatitis cytomegalovirus, AIDS, Epstein-Barr virus, herpes simplex, infectious mononucleosis, syphillis, malaria, Chaga's disease, etc. This risk is different depending on which part of the blood is used, and also on how it was prepared. In the case of units of whole blood and blood components prepared and distributed by blood banks and blood centers, the degree of risk depends on the ability to detect the infectious agent in donor blood. Rapid progress is being made in this area. However, it will be probably some time, if ever, before the risk will reach zero; ie, before the absolute safety of donor blood can be assured. Still, the risk may be diminished or indeed eliminated by suitable processing treatments. Thus, immune globulin prepared by the ethanol-water fractionation procedure is free of virus even without specific viricidal treatment. *Human Albumin* carries no risk of virus transmission, as a result of heating the solution to 60°C for 10 hours. Therefore, it is likely that any product which can be heated at 60°C for 10 hours will have a greatly diminished, if not zero, risk of viral transmission. Unfortunately, very few products can withstand such rigorous treatment, and other means have been sought to inactivate viruses, but with less than complete success. These include irradiation with ultraviolet light, or with cathode rays, and chemical treatment with various substances such as β-propiolactone. None of these methods, as presently used, can be relied on to inactivate completely all viruses that might be present, although they diminish the risk associated with use of the material. In short, except for certain products such as albumin and immune globulin which are known to be free of virus, most blood derivatives must be assumed to involve a risk of virus transmission, and this risk must be weighed against the medical consequences of withholding the product.

Whole Blood

Blood may be collected for human use only from persons who are certified by a physician as being free of transmissible disease, as far as can be determined from the donor's personal history and physical examination, etc. Unfortunately, in mass donations (bloodmobiles, etc) these tend to be hasty and limited. The usual amount drawn is 500 mL. The blood is collected into an anticoagulant solution. A sample of blood is collected at the time of bleeding and subjected to serologic and virologic tests.

The use of the anticoagulant mixtures known as CPD and CPDA-1 (see pages 828–9) extends the useful life of the red cells with the result that, following storage under proper conditions, the blood can be used with safety for a period of 3 weeks after collection. The addition of adenine to CPD solution increases the shelf life by another 2 weeks, thus enabling a useful storage time of 35 days. Use of these solutions has greatly extended the flexibility of hospital and community blood banks.

If whole blood is used, it is carefully handled and stored in the cold without further processing or testing, except for occasional observation to detect evidence of hemolysis or contamination.

Whole Blood

Blood that has been drawn from suitable human donors under rigid aseptic precautions. It contains citrate ion (acid citrate dextrose or citrate phosphate dextrose or citrate phosphate dextrose with adenine) or heparin as an anticoagulant. Preparations are designated CPD Whole Bood, CPDA-1 Whole Blood or Heparinized Whole Blood according to the anticoagulant used. Whole blood from which one or more components has/have been removed is designated Modified Whole Blood (page 819).

Description—Deep red, opaque liquid from which the corpuscles readily settle on standing for 24 to 48 hours, leaving a clear, yellowish or pinkish supernatant layer. If the blood has been drawn soon after the donor has eaten, it may, on standing, acquire a layer of fatlike material near its surface. A deep pink or red color in the plasma, or a purplish tint at the surface of the cell portion, usually indicates that the blood is unsatisfactory for use.

Uses—Whole blood is the natural replenisher for lost blood and hence is indicated when there has been hemorrhage or traumatic blood loss of over 20% of the blood volume. When the blood loss is small, it is not essential that all of the lost blood be replaced, except in persons with high oxygen demand (thyrotoxicosis, beri-beri, etc.) or in anemia. Consequently some practitioners may replace only part of the lost blood and make up the remainder of the deficit with a saline, hetastarch, or dextran solution. In hemorrhagic shock, some medical opinion holds that the entire volume deficit should not be repaired by whole blood alone because of erythrocyte aggregation and sludging, and a dextran is also sometimes added concomitantly, not only to suppress erythrocyte aggregation but also platelet aggregation, since intravascular clotting is sometimes a complication. Adverse effects of whole blood include reactions from improperly matched blood, passive transfer of allergies, serum hepatitis and other infections, volume overload in improperly monitored administration, and increased viscosity of the circulating blood. Stored whole blood is nearly devoid of platelets and may also be deficient in factors V and VII, so that clotting and coagulation defects may occur after massive transfusions.

Dose—*Intravenous, infusion*, as needed to replenish blood volume; *usual* **1 unit**, repeated as necessary. The dose is based on the estimated blood loss, laboratory determination of need, or central venous pressure. One unit is 450 ± 45 mL of whole blood to which 63 mL of CPD or CPDA-1 solution has been added. Units must be administered through a 170 μm filter.

Dosage Forms—Between 468 and 558 mL.

Blood Components

Blood collection agencies—blood centers and blood banks—provide an array of blood services to areas they serve. These include providing whole blood and several blood components prepared in the center from fresh donor blood. Blood components are made from single units of blood without opening or breaking the sterility of the plastic bag system in which the blood was originally collected. These components are thus individualized with respect to donor; if greater amounts are required than those available from one donor, multiple units are used. In addition to whole blood, components commonly available are CPD or CPDA-1 red blood cells, frozen red blood cells, saline-washed red blood cells, leukocyte-free red blood cells, granulocyte concentrate platelet concentrate, cryoprecipitated antihemophilic factor (page 819), fresh frozen plasma, and liquid plasma.

Single-Donor Plasma

Human Plasma

The liquid portion of a single unit of CPD- or CPDA-1-whole blood, the separation of which was accomplished within the expiration time of the whole blood. It is stored at 1 to 6°; it may be stored for 5 days beyond the dating period of the whole blood from which it was separated (26 and 40 days if from CPD- or CPDA-1-whole blood, respectively). ABO compatibility is that of the donor whole blood. One unit is 220 to 250 mL.

Description—A straw-colored transparent fluid which may sometimes exhibit a slight opalescence.

Uses—Used mostly for *volume replenishment* in the treatment of *shock*, especially after severe burns, in which plasma protein loss is considerable. It is occasionally used as a source of the stable coagulation factors II, VII, IX, and X, and thus can be used to treat hemophilia B. ABO compatibility is desirable but is not a prerequisite to use.

Dose—*Intravenous infusion*, variable dose, depending upon the magnitude of the volume deficit or requirement for stable coagulation factors and upon the clinical response. When the plasma is ABO-incompatible with the blood of the recipient and a volume deficit is large, the physician may elect to repair only part of the deficit with plasma and the remainder with another plasma expander.

Single-Donor Plasma Fresh Frozen

Human Plasma, Fresh Frozen; Antihemophilic Plasma

Single-donor human plasma frozen within 6 hr of collection and stored at a temperature of −20° or lower (preferably below −30°). The frozen plasma shall not be stored beyond 12 mo. As a source of coagulation factors, the expiration time of thawed fresh frozen plasma is 24 hr; as a volume replenisher, the expiration time is that of Single-Donor Plasma. ABO compatibility is that of the donor whole blood. One unit is 200 to 250 mL.

Description—The frozen plasma is light yellow to deep cream in color. When viewed microscopically, a reticulated structure without evidence of fusion may be seen.

Uses—The labile coagulation factors V and XIII are preserved in fresh frozen plasma, so that this preparation is especially indicated for the treatment of *multiple coagulation factor deficiencies*, such as that which occurs in cases of massive transfusion with stored blood, after heparinization in disseminated intravascular coagulation, or in lover disease and for *hemophilia*. The preparation also may be used as *Single-Donor Plasma* (above), although such use is unnecessarily expensive. It is the plasma of choice in patients with thrombotic throbocytopenic purpura. It is also of value in patients with deficiencies of immunoglobulin and/or complement. Serum hepatitis virus is not killed by freezing.

Dose—*Intravenous infusion*, variable dose, depending upon the magnitude and type of coagulation factor deficit and the clinical response or upon the volume deficit and response.

Platelet Concentrate

Platelets taken from plasma obtained by whole blood collection, by plasmapheresis, or by plateletpheresis, from a single suitable human donor of whole blood; or from a plasmapheresis donor; or from a plateletpheresis donor. One unit of platelet concentrate consists of not less than 5.5×10^{10} platelets suspended in a specified volume of the original plasma. (See USP for collection procedure.)

Preserved platelets can be successfully reinfused into recipients suffering from platelet deficiency. Platelets obtained by plateletpheresis must be used within 24 hr of collection, because the open system allows bacterial contamination. It is now possible to store platelets for up to 120 hr, and it is likely methods to preserve them for a longer period will be devised in the near future.

Uses—Platelets are used to arrest or prevent bleeding resulting from thrombocytopenia or thrombopathia. In platelet deficiency consequent to disseminated intravascular coagulation and thrombocytopenic purpura (in which a type of intravascular coagulation occurs) the platelets must be coadministered with heparin. When thrombocytopenia is caused by immune destruction, administration of platelets is mostly futile because of rapid destruction of the added platelets. Likewise, in drug-induced thrombocytopenia, the effects of the platelets are mostly voided unless the drug is discontinued, preferably in advance. Platelets can be used in the priming of extracorporeal circuits, but they may be subjected to faster destruction in the circuit than endogenous platelets. The half-life of platelets is about 1 to 2 days.

Dose—*Intravenous*, usually **1 unit,** which will increase the platelet count in an an average adult by about 35,000 per μL in a 70-kg recipient without platelet antibodies, splenomegaly, sepsis, or coagulopathy. Units must be administered through a 170 μm filter.

Dosage Form—1 Unit (which contains approximately 10^{11} platelets).

Red Blood Cells

Packed Human Blood Cells USP XVIII; Human Red Blood Cells; Red Cell Concentrate.

Red cells of whole human blood, separated from plasma by centrifuging or subsidence during the dating period of the blood from which it is derived but not later than 21 days after the blood is drawn; if acid citrate dextrose adenine solution has been used as anticoagulant, such preparation may be made within 35 days therefrom. The expiration dates are valid only if the hematocrit does not exceed 80%. Preparations are designated CPD Red Cells, CPDA-1 Red Cells or Heparinized Red Cells according to the anticoagulant used.

Description—Dark red when packed and may show a slight creamy layer on the surface and a small supernatant layer of yellow or opalescent plasma. Resuspended human blood cells is a dark red fluid.

Uses—A *blood replenisher* in any condition in which the primary deficiency in the blood is that of the erythrocytes. Thus they are used in the emergency treatment of a number of the anemias wh. h formerly were treated with whole blood transfusions. They may also be returned to the donor by autologous transfusion after plasmapheresis or apheresis of other components. Human blood cells are not suitable alone as a replacement fluid in hemorrhage, but they may be employed in cases where chronic blood loss is not too great to decrease appreciably the plasma volume and plasma protein content. Each unit of concentrate is preferrably mixed with 50 to 100 mL of 0.9% NaCl injection to decrease the viscosity. Lactated Ringer injection is contraindicated because it provides enough calcium to initiate coagulation; dextrose injection is contraindicated because it causes hemolysis. The half-life is about 4 weeks, but varies considerably according to the recipient.

Dose—*Usual, intravenous infusion,* as needed to replenish red cells or to prime extracorporeal circuits, etc., the equivalent of **1 Unit** (500 mL) of whole blood, repeated as necessary. One unit in a 70-kg recipient increases the hematocrit about 3%.

Dosage Form—The red-cell equivalent of 1 Unit (about 500 mL) of human blood.

Red Blood Cells Frozen

Red Blood Cells (Human) Frozen; Red Cells Fresh Frozen

A preparation in which human red cells are suspended in a glycerol solution and frozen at temperatures ranging from −80° to −120°. There are two types of preparation: one in which a low concentration of glycerol and rapid freezing are used, and the other in which a high concentration of glycerol and slow freezing are used. Such cells can be kept frozen for periods of 2 years or more without deterioration. Before use the suspension is thawed and the glycerol medium is replaced with a physiologic solution. At this stage the preparation is designated Deglycerolized Red Cell Concentrate.

Uses—By freezing erythrocytes immediately or shortly after withdrawal, both ATP and 2,3-diphosphoglyceric acid (2,3-DPG) are better preserved than in the classical preparation and storage methods, and frozen erythrocytes have better oxygen-transport capacity. Therefore they are especially suited for use in newborn and premature infants, and in older patients with excessive oxygen demands. Because of their single-donor origin they are especially used for autologous transfusions. They are also used when there is a rare blood requirement, in elective gynecologic and cardiac surgery, hemodialysis, and kidney transplantation. They are essentially free of irregular antibodies and plasma proteins. Since there are few surviving leukocytes, the risk of graft vs host response is diminished. The freeze-thaw procedure removes senescent erythrocytes, thus leaving a younger population of cells with a longer survival time in the recipient. The post-thaw washing procedure greatly decreases the risk of serum hepatitis and pyrogenic reactions to debris from leukocytes and platelets. The preparation may be used in lieu of washed red cells in patients who continue to have febrile reactions and in patients with paroxysmal nocturnal hemoglobinuria. Frozen red cells are very expensive.

Dose and **Dosage Form**—See the corresponding paragraphs under *Red Blood Cells* (above).

Other Whole Blood and Blood Components

Granulocyte Concentrate—A single-donor concentrate of leukocytes obtained either by separation from sedimented whole blood or by pheresis with a continuous or intermittent flow centrifuge. The granulocytes (and entrained lymphocytes) are resuspended in the plasma of the recipient. The component should be used within 24 hr of collection. *Uses:* Heterologously in patients with severe leukopenia, usually that which results from cancer chemotherapy or other adverse drug reactions. *Dose:* That which is necessary to bring the granulocyte count above 500/μL. It is difficult to administer more than 10% of the normal daily output of granulocytes.

Lymphocytes, Frozen—A single-donor frozen concentrate of lymphocytes obtained by differential sedimentation from whole blood or from the removal of lymph from the thoracic duct. The cells are cooled at a rate of 3.5°/min. DMSO is added to a 5% concentration when the temperature reaches 0°. Reconstitution requires careful thawing and repeated wash-out of DMSO. Viable cells are quantified from the uptake of radiothymidine into phytohemagglutinin-stimulated suspensions. *Uses:* Used investigationally in the treatment of neoplastic diseases, as exchange replacement for lymphocytes pheresed from the blood of patients afflicted with certain thymocyte-mediated auto-immune disorders, and as a diagnostic agent in specialized in-vitro assessments of immune function.

Single-Donor Plasma, Freeze-Dried [Human Plasma Freeze-Dried]—Single-donor plasma that has been cryodessicated. If Fresh Frozen Plasma is the source of the cryodessicate, the plasma may be designated as an Antihemophilic Plasma. The expiration time of the reconstituted plasma is that of Single-Donor Plasma. *Uses and Dose:* If the dessicate is made from *Fresh Frozen Plasma*, see the monograph (page 818); if made from Frozen Plasma, see *Single-Donor Plasma* (page 817).

Single-Donor Plasma Frozen [Human Plasma Frozen]—Single-donor plasma that has been frozen within the expiration time of the liquid plasma but longer than 6 hr after removal from the donor. The expiration time of the thawed plasma is that of *Single Donor Plasma. Uses and Dose:* See *Single-Donor Plasma*, page 817.

Red Blood Cells, Leukocytes Removed [Red Cell Concentrate, Leukocyte-poor]—A single-donor red cell concentrate which contains less than 25% of the original leukocytes. The expiration time is that of *Red Blood Cells* (page 818) and is determined by the type of anticoagulant used. The hematocrit usually ranges from 0.7 to 0.8. *Uses:* Mostly for autologous transfusion in leukemic individuals in whom a reduction in circulating leukocytes is imperative. May be used in heterologous erythrocyte replenishment if the original donor blood was normal (ie, donor blood served as a source of therapeutic leukocytes). Because the preparation has fewer pyrogenic leukocyte fragments than does Red Blood Cells, febrile reactions are less severe and less frequent. *Dose:* See *Red Blood Cells* (page 818).

Red Blood Cells, Saline Washed [Red Cell Concentrate, Washed]—A single-donor red cell concentrate in which most of the plasma, leukocytes and platelets have been removed by one or more washes with an isotonic saline solution. The hematocrit usually lies between 0.7 and 0.8. *Uses:* Washing may be employed for five purposes: 1) to remove adverse components in specific disorders (eg, lymphocytes and/or immune globulins in certain autoimmune disorders, Rh factors in alloimmunity, anticoagulation factors in certain bleeding disorders, thyroid hormone in thyroid storm, etc); in such instances, the erythrocytes are to be reinfused into the donor. 2) To reduce the risk of blood-transmissable infections (not malaria); the erythrocytes are intended for heterologous transfusion. 3) To remove citrate from citrated blood when the volume to be transfused is large and the intended recipient has a liver dysfunction in which citrate cannot be tolerated. 4) To decrease the intensity of heterologous transfusion reactions in emergency situations in which out-of-group (non-matched) blood must be used. 5) To decrease the incidence and severity of febrile transfusion reaction caused by fragments of leukocytes and platelets.

Whole Blood, Modified—Single donor whole blood from which one or more non-erythrocyte components has/have been removed. Components and plasma may be removed either by sedimentation methods or by continuous separation devices; after selective separation, the plasma is reunited with the erythrocytes. The expiration time is that of *Red Blood Cells* (page 818). *Uses:* The uses are determined, in part, by the health of both the donor and recipient and the reason for removal of the component(s). If the reason for component-pheresis is to remove an adverse component, such as leukocytes in a leukemia or lymphocytes in an autoimmune disorder, the modified whole blood is returned autologously to the donor. If, instead, the donor is healthy and pheresis is conducted to provide a heterologous source of the component(s) for therapeutic purposes, the residual modified whole blood may be used for the same purposes as *Whole Blood* (page 817), provided that the volume to be transfused is small enough so as not to cause by dilution a clinically-significant deficit of the corresponding component(s) in the recipient.

Plasma Expanders and Intravenous Fluids

Protein and Colloid Solutions

Hemorrhage and shock result in loss of blood volume, which, if carried beyond a certain critical point, leads to circulatory failure. Replacement of the plasma proteins, or injection of a substance having similar osmotic properties, will restore the blood volume at least temporarily, so that circulation of oxygen to the tissues may be maintained. Many substances have been employed for this purpose: *whole blood*, which in certain situations is ideal but which is not always immediately available; *plasma*, which is extremely effective but is unstable in the liquid form, relatively cumbersome in the dry form, involves injection of salt and water, which are in some cases undesirable, and, finally, cannot readily be rendered free of pathogenic viruses; and *serum albumin*, the protein in the plasma which functions to control blood volume.

Physiologically, the most clearly established role of albumin appears to be its water-retaining (osmotic) capacity. It is due chiefly to plasma albumin that the water of the plasma, instead of diffusing into the tissues, is retained in the blood stream, maintaining the volume of blood which is necessary for effective cardiac output, and circulation. Albumin, although it comprises less than 60% of the plasma proteins, by virtue of having the lowest molecular weight of these proteins contributes 80% of their osmotic effect. Another highly important property of albumin is its capacity to bind various chemical substances, including numerous ions and drugs.

Methods have been devised for preparing human plasma albumin more than 99% pure. Unlike most plasma proteins, it is extraordinarily stable. It does not require desiccation or continuous refrigeration, and therefore can be kept on hand as a 25% sterile solution, ready for instant use. Separation of the albumin leaves the remaining plasma proteins as by-products. It is possible to derive many specific pharmaceutical agents from one blood donation, enabling more efficient use of a given quantity of blood.

Albumin Human

Normal Serum Albumin (Human); Albumisol (*Merck Sharp & Dohme*); Albuspan (*Parke-Davis*)

Human albumin is a sterile, nonpyrogenic preparation of serum albumin obtained by fractionating blood, plasma, serum, or placentas from healthy human donors and tested for absence of hepatitis B surface antigen, made by a process ensuring safety for intravenous use. Not less than 96% of the total protein is albumin. It is a solution containing in each 100 mL either 25 g of serum albumin osmotically equivalent to 500 mL of normal human plasma, or 20 g equivalent to 400 mL, or 5 g equivalent to 100 mL, or 4 g equivalent to 80 mL of normal human plasma. It contains no added antimicrobial agent, but may contain sodium acetyltryptophanate, with or without sodium caprylate, as a stabilizing agent. It has a sodium content of not less than 130 mEq per L and not more than 160 mEq per L. It meets the requirements of tests for limit of heme, for heat stability, and for pH. Solutions are heated in final containers at 60° for 10 hours to kill any pathogenic organisms that may be present. The storage temperature is indicated on the label. The solution is not to be used if it is turbid or there is a sediment.

Description—Moderately viscous, clear, brownish fluid; practically odorless; may develop a slight granular or flaky deposit during storage. When dried, has a slight yellow to deep cream color.

Uses—In the treatment of *shock* or *hemorrhage* albumin serves as an emergency agent for restoration of blood volume. It is especially indicated when blood loss exceeds 20% of blood volume. If albumin is administered in hypertonic concentrations, it will abstract water from interstitial and intracellular fluids and increase blood volume by an amount more than the volume administered; in isotonic concentration it will expand blood volume only by an amount equal to the volume added. Each gram of albumin holds about 18 mL of water in the blood stream. Because its action depends on the availability of tissue water, hypertonic albumin should not be used in severely dehydrated patients without simultaneous administration of saline or glucose solutions. It has been used in protein replacement therapy where serum protein levels are low due to excessive loss, as in extensive burns and nephrosis, certain skin diseases, and other conditions, or due to inadequate formation of proteins because of nutritional disturbances, cirrhosis, or other causes. However, the value of albumin in the therapy of chronic nephritis or cirrhosis is less impressive than in acute hypoalbuminemia. Hyperoncotic albumin solutions may be used to cause transient diuresis in edematous patients or in those undergoing renal dialysis. It is also used in the treatment of hyperbilirubinemia and erythroblastosis fetalis to increase the binding capacity for bilirubin.

Low salt content and the high stability of the single protein component present make "salt-poor" albumin the agent of choice in certain types of protein replacement therapy, bearing in mind the following limitations: Albumin does not in any sense replace red cells and therefore should not be used in hemorrhagic shock except as an emergency remedy. It lacks the other proteins contained in plasma, hence is not an adequate agent for treatment of deficiencies of specific plasma proteins (eg, fibrinogen, prothrombin) such as occur in acute hepatitis or burns. It does not replace lost fluids, and therefore must be given with ample quantities of crystalloid solution when used in dehydrated patients, as noted above. Human albumin is not completely free of the risk of serum hepatitis. Chills, fever, urticaria, and perturbations of respiration and blood pressure sometimes occur. Albumin is contraindicated in congestive heart failure. Large doses should not be given in severe anemia, low cardiac reserve and in the absence of hypoalbuminuria.

Dose—*Intravenous*, for *replacement* or *plasma extension*, volumes equivalent to **25 to 125 g** (not to exceed 250 g) of albumin daily, depending on the need. The 5% solution may be infused directly and the 25% solution infused as a mixture of 20 mL of 25% albumin diluted to 100 mL with an isotonic solution, the infusion rate being maintained at 2 to 4 mL/min. When the 25% solution is infused directly, the rate should not exceed 1 mL/min. In *burns*, initially **500 mL** of 5% or **100 mL** of **25%** solution along with an electrolyte solution. Children, for *hyperbilirubinemia* and *erythroblastosis* fetalis, **1 g/kg** of body weight is given with each exchange transfusion; for nonemergency use, **6.25 to 12.5 g.**

Dosage Forms—Injection: 5 and 25%; foreign products of 4 and 20% albumin are also approved for use in the US.

Antihemophilic Factor—page 825.

Fibrinogen—page 825.

Plasma Protein Fraction

Plasma Protein Fraction (Human); (*Hyland*)

A sterile solution of selected proteins derived from the blood plasma of adult human donors. It contains 4.5–5.5 g of protein/100 mL, of which about 83–90% is albumin, and the remainder is alpha and beta globulins. It contains no antimicrobial agent but may contain suitable stabilizers.

Preparation—By a process similar to that by which albumin is made. The product resembles plasma from which certain unstable globulins have been removed, including gamma globulin and certain lipoproteins. The solution is treated by heating at 60° for 10 hours to reduce the risk of virus transmission. The solution is isotonic with normal plasma and is isotonic with respect to diffusible ions, the major ions being sodium and chloride.

Description—Transparent, nearly colorless or slightly brownish liquid; nearly odorless; may develop a slight, granular or flaky deposit during storage.

Uses—Like albumin, plasma protein fraction is indicated as a substitute for plasma in treating nonhemorrhagic *shock*. It is also a convenient source of protein for intravenous nutrition. Because it does not contain any clotting factors, it is not a substitute for fresh plasma in treating hemorrhagic states. The plasma half-life is about 27 days.

Untoward effects are uncommon; they include nausea, vomiting and increased salivation. Care must be exercised to prevent circulatory overload, especially in nonhypovolemic patients. Solutions of this fraction should not be mixed with other intravenous fluids, either in the bottle or in the tubing.

Dose—*Intravenous infusion, adults, shock*, **250 mL** of **5%** solution at a rate of 5 to 8 mL/min; *burns*, initially **500 mL** to 1 **L**; *hypoproteinemia*, 1 to **1.5 L/day.** *Infants* and *small children*, 22 to **33 mL** of 5% solution/**kg** of body weight at a rate not exceeding 8 mL/min.

Dosage Forms—Solution: 5%, in 50, 250, and 500-mL containers.

Plasma Extenders (Volume Expanders)

Much effort has been expended in the search for nontoxic substances, not of human origin, which might be used in an emergency to restore blood volume. It should be emphasized that these substances are in no sense substitutes for plasma; following their emergency use, plasma or blood must be replaced as rapidly as possible. Some substitutes, however, have favorable actions on the rheology of blood and on platelet adhesiveness, hence they may sometimes be administered along with blood or plasma just for these effects. Furthermore, in some kinds of hypovolemic shock, the plasma is not really lost from the vascular tree but is sequestered in various vascular beds. In these situations, it is not necessary to give plasma, because repair of the fictive volume deficit with a plasma extender will mobilize some of the plasma back into the circulation. Even plasma proteins lost into interstitial spaces return by way of the lymph. In hypovolemia from dehydration or adrenal insufficiency, appropriate electrolyte or dextrose solutions are indicated.

Volume expansion (plasma extension) is not clearly indicated unless the pulmonary arterial wedge pressure (PAW), an approximation of the pulmonary venous pressure, is below 12 torr. It is advisable to give a test injection (about 200 mL) of isotonic saline or dextran solution. If the PAW rises only slightly but cardiac output more substantially, further plasma extension is indicated; if PAW rises sharply but cardiac output does not, plasma extension is redundant, and treatment must be directed toward improving cardiac function. In volume expansion, the end point is usually 16 torr (rarely 18 torr), and further expansion will tend to cause pulmonary edema.

Volume expanders are also used to prime extracorporeal circuits.

Albumin—page 819.

Dextran 40

Gentran 40 (*Travenol*); LMD (*Abbott*); Rheomacrodex (*Pharmacia*); Rheotran (*Pharmachem*)

Dextran [9004-54-0] $(C_6H_{10}O_5)_n$; a polymer of glucose, with an average mol wt of about 40,000 in which the glucosidic linkages are predominantly of the $\alpha(1 \rightarrow 6)$ type.

Preparation—Sucrose is subjected to the action of the bacterium *Leuconostoc mesenteroides* B 512, and the crude, high-molecular-weight dextran thus formed is hydrolyzed and fractionated to an average molecular weight of about 40,000 as measured by light-scattering techniques. US Pat 2,644,815.

Description—White, amorphous powder that is odorless and tasteless; its 10% solution in 5% dextrose in water darkens slightly over a long storage period as with other dextrose-containing solutions; darkening is accelerated by increased ambient temperatures.

Solubility—Freely soluble in water; soluble in dimethyl sulfoxide; insoluble in alcohol, and ether.

Uses—As an isotonic solution to prime pumps or improve flow in surgery requiring *cardiopulmonary bypass*. It has the property of lowering the viscosity of blood and improving flow; in part the improvement in flow is the result of hemodilution. For this reason, 10% of dextran 40 in isotonic saline solution or 5% dextrose is superior to dextran 40 in whole blood. Dextrans decrease platelet adhesiveness. This property is used for *prophylaxis of thrombosis and thromboembolism during and after surgery* and occasionally to decrease coagulopathies in the shock-lung syndrome. Otherwise, Dextran 40 is seldom used in shock, because of the short duration in the body (2 to 4 hr) and also because of frequent adverse effects.

The size of the molecule is such that the polysaccharide is filtered in the glomeruli more rapidly than larger macromolecules, such as dextran 75. As the filtrate is concentrated in the renal tubules, it may sometimes become too viscid to flow, and renal damage can ensue. For this reason many surgeons prefer to prime their bypass with other solutions. Renal failure, severe congestive heart failure, severe coagulation disorders, hypervolemia, hypersensitivity, and severe dehydration contraindicate use of this substance. Dextran 40 can cause allergic reactions. Dextran 40 interferes with the cross-matching of blood, especially when enzyme methods are used. It also interferes with some tests of renal and hepatic function and with assays for blood sugar in which acid-hydrolysis is used.

Dose—As a primer for extracorporeal circuits, **500 mL to 1 L**, depending on volume requirement. *Intravenous infusion*, for *hypovolemia*, **10 mL/kg** of 10% solution in isotonic sodium chloride or dextrose solution, not to exceed 20 mL/kg of body weight a day on the first day and 10 mL/kg/day thereafter; for *prophylaxis* of thrombosis or thromboembolism, **500 mL to 1 L** prior to surgery, then 500 mL a day for the next 2 or more days, according to the persistence of the risk. *Children*, proportioned to the adult dose according to body weight or surface, not to exceed 20 mL/kg a day.

Dosage Forms—Injection: 10% in 5% dextrose solution, 500 mL; 10% in 0.9% sodium chloride solution, 500 mL.

Dextran 70

Dextran 70 (*American McGaw*); Hyskon, Macrodex (*Pharmacia*)

Dextran [9004-54-0] $(C_6H_{10}O_5)_n$; a polymer of glucose with an average mol wt of about 70,000, in which the glucosidic linkages are predominantly of the $\alpha(1 \rightarrow 6)$ type. For the structural formula see *Dextran 40*.

Preparation—As described for *Dextran 40* except that the hydrolysis and fractionation are adjusted to yield a product of average mol wt of about 70,000.

Description—A fine, white, amorphous powder that is odorless and tasteless. It is stable in light and is very hygroscopic. Commercial grades usually contain about 5% water.

Solubility—Freely soluble in hot water, dimethyl sulfoxide; insoluble in alcohol, ether.

Uses—A plasma expander for the prevention or treatment of *hypovolemic shock*. The macromolecule is contained within the plasma and hence retains fluid in the vascular bed by osmosis. Hypertonic solutions cause the dehydration of tissues, the abstracted water being added to the plasma. For this reason it is useful in the treatment of *toxemia of pregnancy* and *nephrosis*. Although dextran 70 solution is inferior to plasma, it has the advantage that refrigeration is not required or that the solution does not have to be prepared immediately before use. Thus, it may be kept ready for use in emergency vehicles, field kits, etc. It is also less expensive than plasma. Like plasma, it is inferior to whole blood as replacement when hypovolemia is due to hemorrhage. When hypoproteinemia exists, it should not be used in place of plasma. Dextran 70 decreases platelet adhesiveness and hence increases clotting time. In some cases this may be a disadvantage, although hemorrhage occurs mainly in the presence of clotting disorders. In some types of shock the effect on platelet adhesiveness is an advantage, because shock-induced coagulopathies will be attenuated. The anticoagulant effect of dextran 70 can be clinically useful; it has been shown to be equal to dicumarol in *preventing thrombosis* after femoral neck fractures and major pelvic surgery. A dextran 70 solution is also used to distend the uterus for hysteroscopy and to irrigate the cavity.

A small part of dextran 70, corresponding to the low-molecular-weight molecules, is excreted during the first 1 or 2 days. The remainder is taken up by the reticuloendothelial system and is later metabolized, which requires approximately 10 days.

Side effects of dextran 70 include mainly allergic reactions (hives, angioedema, bronchospasm, and anaphylaxis). The substance may interfere with cross-matching of blood if unsuitable dilutions of erythrocytes and serum are used. The drug is contraindicated when there is hypersensitivity, severe coagulation disorders, severe congestive heart failure, and hypervolemia.

Dose—*Intravenous*, *adult*, **250 to 1500 mL**, not to exceed 20 mL/kg, in the first day; *usual*, **500 to 1000 mL** of a 6% solution in isotonic saline, 5% dextrose or 10% invert sugar solution. The rate

of infusion is usually 20 to 40 mL/min but may be accelerated if hypovolemia is severe. For *nephrosis* or *toxemia of pregnancy*, **500 mL** of a **10%** solution in 5% dextrose or 10% invert sugar may be given at a rate of about 60 mL/hour. *Children*, proportioned to the adult dose according to body weight or surface, not to exceed 10 mg/kg/day. *Intrauterine*, to be administered by canula with a pressure of about 100 torr and maintained at a pressure of less than 150 torr during examination.

Dosage Forms—Injection: 6% in 5% dextrose solution, 500 mL; 6% in 0.9% sodium chloride solution, 500 mL; Solution: 32% in 10% dextrose solution.

Dextran 75

Dextran 75 (*Abbott*)

Chemistry, **Preparation, Description, Solubility**—See *Dextran 70* (above); read 75,000 in place of 70,000.

Uses and **Dose**—See *Dextran 70*, above. Dextran 75 is not used as an aid to hysteroscopy.

Dosage Forms—Injection: 6% in 5% dextrose solution. 500 mL; 6% in 0.9% sodium chloride solution, 500 mL.

Hetastarch

Uses—A 6% hetastarch solution is osmotically equivalent to 5% albumin solution. In the blood, it abstracts some water from interstitial and intracellular fluids, thus expanding the blood volume somewhat in excess of the volume infused. The expansion persists for 1 to $1\frac{1}{2}$ days. Hetastarch is used in the prevention and treatment of *hypovolemic shock*. It is also used as a suspension medium for leukapheresis.

Hetastarch does not cause the coagulation abnormalities that does dextran nor does it interfere with the cross-matching of blood. There is general but not complete agreement that it is less likely than dextran to cause anaphylaxis and other allergic manifestations (fever, chills, urticaria, pruritis). The incidence of anaphylactoid reactions is stated to be less than 0.1%.

Elimination has complex kinetics, mainly because of heterogeneity in molecular size and linkage. About 40% is eliminated in 1 day, 64% in 8 days, 90% in 41 days, and 100% in 48 days. Larger molecules are taken up by the reticuloendothelial system and degraded by amylase. Smaller molecules are excreted in the urine.

Dose—*Intravenous infusion*, *adults*, for *hypovolemia*, *intially* **500 mL to 1 L** repeated as needed up to 3 or 4 L/day in severe hypovolemia. The rate of infusion depends upon the hemodynamic indices, but ranges up to 20 mL/kg/hr. For *leukapheresis*, **250 to 700 mL** in a 1:8 ratio with venous whole blood.

Single-Donor Plasma—page 818.

Electrolyte Solutions

Ringer's Injection

Isotonic Solution of Three Chlorides

A sterile solution of sodium chloride (8.6 g), potassium chloride (0.30 g), and calcium chloride (0.33 g) in one liter of solution prepared with Water for Injection. It contains approximately 147.5 mEq of sodium, 4.0 mEq of potassium, 4.5 mEq of calcium, and 156 mEq of chloride ion per liter; antimicrobial agents are not present.

Description—Colorless, odorless solution having a salty taste; pH between 5.0 and 7.5.

Uses—Theoretically superior to Sodium Chloride Injection as a *fluid and electrolyte replenisher* in that it supplies the three important cations of the extracellular fluid. However, in actual practice, the addition of potassium and calcium increases only slightly the therapeutic value of an isotonic sodium chloride solution. Neither potassium nor calcium is present in sufficient concentration to render Ringer's injection useful for the repair of deficits of these ions. Further, while administration of large volumes of Ringer's injection would result in minimal distortion of the cation composition of the extracellular fluid, like *Sodium Chloride Injection*, it would alter acid–base balance. Ringer's injection is frequently used to prime pumps for cardiopulmonary bypass in heart surgery. It may also be applied topically for purposes of irrigation.

Dose—*Intravenous infusion*, **500** to **1000 mL**. However, the dose may be larger or smaller, according to the size and clinical condition of the patient.

Dosage Forms—Injection: 250, 500 and 1000 mL.

Lactated Ringer's Injection

Hartmann's Solution

A sterile solution of calcium chloride, potassium chloride, sodium chloride, and sodium lactate in water for injection. It contains no antimicrobial agents. The calcium, potassium, and sodium contents are approximately 2.7, 4, and 130 mEq/liter, respectively.

Description—pH between 6.0 and 7.5.

Uses and **Dose**—See *Ringer's Injection*. Except for the concentration of lactate and absence of bicarbonate, the composition of lactated Ringer's injection closely approximates that of the extracellular fluids. It is employed as a *fluid and electrolyte replenisher*. The lactate ultimately metabolizes to bicarbonate and thus has an alkalinizing effect in the body; in persons with normal cellular oxidative activity, this requires 1 to 2 hr to be fully effective. Lactated Ringer's injection is inappropriate in the treatment of lactic acidosis. The absence of bicarbonate from the solution stabilizes the calcium, which sometimes tends to precipitate as calcium carbonate from heated solutions which contain bicarbonate.

Dose—*Intravenous infusion*, **500** to **1000 mL**. However, the dose may be larger or smaller, according to the size and clinical condition of the patient. Do not administer with blood. Pediatric dosage can be determined from an analysis of the acid–base status of the young patient.

Dosage Forms—Injection: 250, 500, and 1000 mL.

Sodium Chloride—page 835.

Miscellaneous Intravenous Fluids

Dextrose Injection

Injection of Glucose

A sterile solution of dextrose in water for injection. It contains 95–105% of the labeled amount of $C_6H_{12}O_6.H_2O$. It contains no antimicrobial agents.

Preparation—Undoubtedly represents one of the most extensively used injections, especially in hospital practice. The strength of the solution may vary from 5%, which is generally considered satisfactory as an isotonic solution, to 10, 20, 25, and 50%. Usually the 5% solution is used in hospitals. Quantities which are administered may vary from 100 mL to 1000 mL or more. With such large amounts being administered, a hospital will require considerable quantities of this solution daily, and many short-cuts have been developed for its manufacture. It is general practice to prepare concentrated solutions and then to dilute these with water for injection, thus saving an immense amount of labor and time, particularly in the filtration operation.

Care should be exercised in the selection of dextrose, since the sugar itself may be a source of pyrogens, and extreme care must be observed throughout the preparation of the dextrose injections to prevent contamination, for the conditions are practically ideal for the development of bacteria and therefore pyrogens.

Weaker solutions may be sterilized in an autoclave without producing any change in color, but with the more concentrated solutions there is greater possibility of producing a slight change in color on sterilization with high temperatures. Consequently, sterilization by filtration is often resorted to in these cases.

The pH of dextrose solutions is lowered on heating. Nevertheless, buffers are seldom added directly to the solution during its preparation since this is often the cause of discoloration and the buffer capacity diminishes after the solution stands for a period of time. Where buffers are desired, they should be dispensed separately so that the physician may add the buffer extemporaneously when the prep-

aration is to be administered. Dextrose solutions should be tested for mold.

Note—Antimicrobial agents are prohibited since such large quantities of dextrose are administered at one time that excessive doses of the antimicrobial agent would thus be given.

Description—Clear, colorless solution having a pH between 3.5 and 6.5, determined on a portion of injection diluted with water, if necessary, to a concentration of not more than 5% of dextrose.

Uses—Dextrose provides a readily metabolizable nutrient. During periods of inanition, intravenous injection of isotonic solution of dextrose *provides both fluid and carbohydrate*. One liter of 5% solution provides about 170 calories. A 20 to 50% solution may be infused into a high-flow vein as a source of calories in total parenteral nutrition. A 50% solution is given in insulin or suspected insulin-coma. Twenty to 50% solution with or without insulin is used in hyperkalemia, to move potassium intracellularly. Body protein is spared and starvation ketosis and acidosis are prevented. Dextrose injection is also employed for parenteral fluid therapy when it is desired to supply water unaccompanied by electrolyte. In the body, the dextrose is slowly converted to glycogen or metabolized, thus leaving the water component of the injection without an osmotic component; the final result is the same as if water were given, but without the hemolysis that accompanies intravenous infusions of water. The injection also provides a suitable *vehicle for the slow intravenous infusion* of numerous drugs.

Dextrose is usually administered intravenously as a 5% solution which is isoosmotic with body fluids. Subcutaneous injection of dextrose solution is less desirable since such solutions are irritating and can cause local necrosis. In addition, such solutions cause temporary sequestration of extracellular electrolyte in the subcutaneous depot, and anuria, oliguria, and circulatory collapse can result. If the subcutaneous route is to be employed, *Dextrose and Sodium Chloride Injection* should be used.

When administered rapidly intravenously, hypertonic solutions of dextrose cause cellular dehydration which may be of benefit in the treatment of *cerebral edema*, *shock*, and *circulatory collapse*. However, dextrose and sodium chloride injection is preferred. Hypertonic solutions of dextrose are also administered intravenously to initiate *osmotic diuresis*. Dextrose in the glomerular filtrate in excess of that which can be reabsorbed by the renal tubule causes excretion of an osmotic equivalent of water. Additional quantities of extracellular electrolyte also escape renal tubular reabsorption during the osmotic diuresis.

Dose—*Intravenous*, variable, as determined by the use, clinical condition, and size of the individual. For 5% dextrose solution, the dose frequently ranges from 500 to 1000 mL. The maximum rate of infusion that will not cause glycosuria is 0.5 g/kg/hr; about 95% is retained when the rate is 0.8 g/kg/hr. The usual diuretic dose is 50 mL of 50% solution. For emergency treatment of suspected insulin coma, 50 mL of 50% solution.

Dosage Forms—Injection: 2.5, 5, 10, 20, 40, 50, 60, and 70%, in various volumes. Solutions of 2.5 to 10% are for nonelectrolyte and caloric replacement; 20 to 50% are for caloric provision with minimal hydration; 50% is for use in insulin hypoglycemia; 40 to 70% solutions are for mixing with other solutions for parenteral alimentation.

Dextrose and Sodium Chloride Injection

Sodium Chloride and Dextrose Injection

A sterile solution of dextrose and sodium chloride in water for injection. It contains 95–105% of the labeled amount of $C_6H_{12}O_6.H_2O$ and of NaCl. It contains no antimicrobial agents.

Preparation—This preparation may represent a highly concentrated solution for use as a sclerosing agent, or much weaker solutions to be used in a manner similar to the use of 5 or 10% dextrose solution. This may be a mixture of equal parts of isotonic sodium chloride solution and isotonic dextrose solution, or it may represent 5% of dextrose in isotonic sodium chloride solution. Both of these should be prepared according to the suggestions given for the preparation of *Dextrose Injection*.

Description—Clear, colorless solution having a pH between 3.5 and 6.5, determined on a portion of injection diluted with water, if necessary, to a concentration of not more than 5% of dextrose.

Uses—To provide dextrose as a nutrient (see above) in a medium that does not hydrate the tissues, or it may be employed as a source of isotonic sodium chloride, or both. When hypertonic solutions of dextrose are employed in cerebral edema or in hydrated states, isotonic sodium chloride in the injection prevents a delayed rebound hydration. Since dextrose, alone, cannot safely be given by the subcutaneous route (see *Dextrose Injection*, above), dextrose and sodium chloride injection is the preferred preparation.

Dose—*Intravenous*, variable, as determined by the use, clinical condition, and size of the patient. It frequently ranges from 500 to 1000 mL.

Dosage Forms—Various percentages of each ingredient, ranging from 2.5% dextrose:0.45% NaCl to 25% dextrose:0.9% NaCl, in various sizes.

Fructose Injection—page 1029.

Fructose and Sodium Chloride Injection—page 1029.

Protein Hydrolysate Injection—page 1029.

Other Plasma Extenders and Intravenous Fluids

Miscellaneous Parenteral Fluids—There are numerous commercially available parenteral fluids, some of which differ only slightly and others considerably from one or more of those described in the foregoing sections. Excellent summary tables of the composition, names, and manufacturers of these products may be found in *AMA Drug Evaluations* and *Drug Facts and Comparisons* (listed under *Parenteral Nutrients*). *AMA Drug Evaluations* also provides a useful table of peritoneal dialysis solutions.

Antibodies and Isoagglutinins

Human plasma contains antibodies of various types, which are almost entirely concentrated in Fractions II and III. Some of these occur naturally, others arise as a result of infection or are stimulated by artificial immunization.

The serum of all human beings contains antibodies (agglutinins or isoagglutinins) which react with those principal blood group factors (agglutinogens) which the individual does *not* possess.

Thus, for example, 45% of the population of the US possesses the blood group O factor in their red cells, and agglutinins against the A and B factors in the plasma. Should the whole blood or cells of a Group A individual be injected into a Group O patient, the anti-A agglutinins of the patient will clump the cells received, and will usually destroy (lyse) them, causing a serious reaction in many cases, even if the volume of cells injected is as little as 50 mL. The importance of establishing the blood group of anyone either giving or receiving whole blood is therefore obvious. This is done by mixing a specimen of the cells of the subject with the serum of a selected individual whose group is known; for example, if the cells of an untyped donor are clumped by the serum of a known Group B subject, but not by the serum of a known Group A subject, the donor evidently belongs to Group A. In practice, anti-A isoagglutinins obtained from selected group B subjects, and anti-B isoagglutinins from similarly selected Group A subjects, have for years provided highly effective reagents for identification of the blood groups. It has been demonstrated that administration of small quantities of the specific blood group substances A or B (which can be obtained from red blood cells or, in larger quantities, from other animal tissues) to individuals having the corresponding isoagglutinins will induce a tremendous rise in titer of the agglutinin. In this fashion, extremely potent blood grouping sera have been prepared in ample quantities. It is also possible to produce blood grouping sera as a by-product of ethanol fractionation of plasma.

Blood Group Factors

Factors present	Blood groups (cells) Frequency in population	Isoagglutinins (plasma)
O	45%	Anti-A and Anti-B
A	41%	Anti-B
B	10%	Anti-A
AB	4%	None

In practice (see Chapter 32), it is customary not only to determine the blood group of a donor and recipient of a blood transfusion, but to "cross match" the cells of the donor with the serum of the patient and *vice versa*, so as to detect any otherwise unpredictable incompatibility in the bloods of the two individuals. This extra precaution is invaluable, not only for the purpose indicated but also as a final check against mistaken identity of the specimens. Numerous other precautions are involved in correct blood grouping, so that it has become a highly specialized technique, which should only be performed by a qualified technician.

The Rh Factor—A much rarer antibody occurs in a small proportion of individuals as a result of injection of so-called "Rh-positive blood," or absorption of such blood across the placenta during pregnancy in gravid females. This "Rh factor" actually consists of at least nine different factors, any one or several of which may be present in the red cells of a given individual. Isoagglutinins reacting with these factors do not occur normally in humans, but appear only as a result of accidental "immunization" of an individual with a type of Rh factor which he or she does not possess. Actually, the blood of about 85% of Western Europeans or Americans contains one or two of the commonest of these factors, which also are the most potent as antigens. Therefore in general practice it is customary and quite permissible to classify individuals simply as either "Rh-positive" or "Rh-negative." The technique of Rh typing is essentially like that of blood grouping.

Like anti-A and anti-B blood grouping serum, the principal source for Rh typing serum is the blood of human donors who, by chance or intention, have become hyperimmunized to one of the Rh factors. One of the commonest sources is the blood of Rh-negative women who have borne several Rh-positive infants, absorbed their Rh factor, and thereby have become sensitized. Another source is Rh-negative individuals who have been transfused with Rh-positive blood. Injection of small amounts of Rh substance in the latter individuals will induce very high antibody titers, rendering them suitable donors of hyperimmune serum for typing purposes. The danger of mismatched transfusion in such individuals is actually decreased, since they become extremely easy to identify.

Blood Grouping and Typing Serums

Blood-Group Specific Substances A, B, and AB

A sterile, isotonic solution of the polysaccharide-amino acid complexes that are capable of reducing the titer of the anti-A and the anti-B isoagglutinins of group O blood. The blood-group specific substance A is prepared from hog gastric mucin and the blood-group specific substances B and AB are prepared from the glandular portion of horse gastric mucosa. Blood Group Specific Substances A, B, and AB contains no preservative.

Description—Clear solution, which may have a slight odor due to the preservative; pH between 6.0 and 6.8.

Uses—Added to group O blood as a *neutralizer of isoagglutinins* and hence it makes the blood reasonably safe for transfusions into patients whose blood is of another group. It may also be used to condition plasma. However, conditioned plasma which contains immune anti-A and anti-B agglutinins may cause reactions. Furthermore, it must not be forgotten that blood from group O donors that have previously received conditioned group O blood may contain A and B isohemagglutinins. Such blood is dangerous to use in universal donation unless it is conditioned with blood group specific substances A and B.

Dose—*Intravenous*, one transfusion unit in approximately **500 mL** of group O blood.

Anti-A Blood Grouping Serum

Derived from high-titered serums of humans, with or without stimulation by the injection of group-specific red cells or substances. It agglutinates human red cells containing A antigens; ie, blood groups A and AB (including subgroups A_1, A_2, A_3, A_1B, and A_2B). It may contain a suitable antibacterial preservative.

Description—Clear or slightly opalescent fluid unless artificially colored, when it has a blue or blue-green color. The dried product is light yellow to deep cream color, unless artificially colored as indicated for liquid serum, and is microscopically of a honeycomb-like structure.

Use—As a diagnostic agent.

Anti-B Blood Grouping Serum

Derived from high-titered serums of humans, with or without stimulation by the injection of group-specific red cells or substances. It agglutinates human red cells containing B antigens; ie, blood groups B and AB (including subgroups A_1B and A_2B). It may contain a suitable antibacterial preservative.

Description—Clear or slightly opalescent fluid unless artificially colored when it has a yellow color. The dried product is light yellow to deep cream color, unless artificially colored as indicated for liquid serum and is microscopically of a honeycomb-like structure.

Use—As a diagnostic agent.

Anti-Rh Blood Grouping Serums

Blood Grouping Serums Anti-D, Anti-C, Anti-E, Anti-c, Anti-e

Derived from the blood of humans who have developed specific Rh antibodies. Anti-Rh Blood Grouping Serums are free from agglutinins for A or B antigens and from alloantibodies other than those for which claims are made in the labeling. They may contain suitable antimicrobial agents.

Two varieties of Anti-Rh Grouping Serums are recognized: ie, (1) complete ("saline-agglutinating") serums, which specifically agglutinate human red blood cells in saline TS, and (2) incomplete ("blocking") serums, which agglutinate human red blood cells only in a medium containing protein or other macromolecular substances, which may be furnished in an accompanying diluent. Complete serums commonly are designated "for saline tube test," and the incomplete serums are designated "For slide or modified (rapid) tube test." In liquid form, the latter contain, as additives, the required micromolecular substances.

The left-hand column of the accompanying table lists the designations of the most commonly used anti-Rh blood grouping serums, and the right-hand column lists the blood factor(s) with which each serum specifically reacts. The designations used in an alternative system of nomenclature are indicated parenthetically.

Uses—As diagnostic agents.

Immune Globulins

Adult blood contains antibodies specific for various infectious agents to which the individual has built up a resistance. In pooled normal plasma used for fractionation some of these are in high enough concentration to have a protective action.

Serum	Antigen(s) Reacting
Anti-D (Anti-Rh_0)	D (Rh_0)
Anti-C (Anti-rh')	C (rh')
Anti-E (Anti-rh'')	E (rh'')
Anti-CD (Anti-Rh_0')	D (Rh_0), C (rh')
Anti-DE (Anti-Rh_0'')	D (Rh_0), E (rh'')
Anti-CDE (Anti-Rh_0''')	D (Rh_0), C (rh'), E (rh'')
Anti-c (Anti-hr')	c (hr')
Anti-e (Anti-hr'')	e (hr'')

This is usually true of measles and poliomyelitis antibodies. Antibodies from adult plasma will protect against the disease if given after exposure. In certain other conditions, it is possible to select individuals with already detectable antibody levels and by injection of an appropriate vaccine to raise their antibody level to very high titers, much as was described for blood grouping and Rh typing sera above. This practice has been most employed in the production of pertussis hyperimmune globulin for the treatment or prophylaxis of whooping cough.

During the fractionation of plasma, most of the antibodies are concentrated into a single fraction (Fraction II); electrophoretically the proteins in this fraction are characterized as gamma globulins. Isolated immune globulins, dispensed as a 16% solution, represent a concentration of most antibodies approximately 25 times greater than in plasma. As a result, they have been found useful in the prophylaxis of certain infectious diseases, including measles, infectious hepatitis (not to be confused with serum hepatitis), and poliomyelitis. The usefulness derives from the immunity conferred by the *added* antibody. However, since the added antibody is slowly metabolized and therefore disappears, the immunity is passive, and lasts only as long as the concentration of antibody is above an effective level, usually from one to two months. Thereafter, the recipient once again becomes susceptible to infection. Alternatively, and particularly when exposure to infection can be ascertained with reasonable accuracy, as in measles, a modifying dose of antibodies may be administered. While failing to prevent active infection, the added antibody lessens the severity of the disease and the patient responds to the infection by producing antibodies of his own. This production of antibodies persists for long periods thereafter, thus conferring long-lasting immunity.

Immune globulin is administered intramuscularly; it cannot be used intravenously. Reactions are uncommon and when they do occur are chiefly local and usually mild. Another source of gamma globulin is the blood from normal human placentas. Application of the methods of processing immune globulin from human blood, however, has made possible the preparation of a similar globulin from placentas.

Immune Globulin—page 1391.

Rh_0 (D) Immune Globulin—page 1391.

Immune Sera

Various biological products obtained from the blood of humans or animals and used for their prophylactic or therapeutic effects, eg, antitoxins, immune sera, and immune globulin, are discussed in Chapter 74.

Agents Affecting Coagulation of the Blood

The clotting of blood is a very important process (see Chapter 32). It depends on the existence of a complex system of reactions involving plasma proteins, platelets, tissue factors, and calcium ion. This system is normally in a state of balance. However, if a factor is missing, as is the case in hemophilia, a hemorrhagic tendency exists which can lead to major hemorrhage under certain circumstances. In hemophilia, the defect is congenital. Other defects, often transient, may arise as the result of disease or malnutrition. Under certain circumstances, the reverse situation is encountered. Hypercoagulability—an abnormal tendency for the blood to clot—can be very serious, leading to thrombosis.

Various agents are available with which to achieve at least partial control over this system.

Blood Clotting Proteins

Although it should technically be possible to prepare therapeutically useful concentrates of several clotting factors, only a few are presently marketed.

Antihemophilic Factor

Actif VIII (*Merieux*); Factorate (*Armour*); Hemofil (*Hyland*); Humafac (*Parke-Davis*); Koāte (*Cutter*); Profilate (*Alpha*)

A sterile, freeze-dried concentrate of human antihemophilic factor prepared from the Factor VIII-rich cryoprotein fraction of human venous plasma.

Preparation—Precipitated by glycine from a solution of AHF-rich first precipitate from pooled normal human plasma. After treatment to lower the content of glycine and inactive proteins, a solution of the active fraction is sterilized by filtration, aseptically filled into final containers, dried aseptically from the frozen state, stoppered under vacuum, and assayed for AHF content.

Description—White or grayish, to yellow, amorphous substance dried from the frozen state; colorless or opalescent when reconstituted with the diluent provided.

Uses—The coagulation defect in classical hemophilia (hemophilia A) is predominately a deficit of the coagulation factor VIII, called antihemophilic factor (AHF). In severe hemorrhage in the patient with hemophilia A, it is used as a cryoprecipitate or concentrate, or in fresh plasma or whole blood, as required to *terminate hemorrhage* or to prevent hemorrhage in surgery or consequent to various procedures in which bleeding may occur. The concentrate is generally preferred to plasma or whole blood since the AHF titers of blood and plasma are quite variable, but in von Willebrand's disease the cryoprecipitate (below) is more effective. The preparation is poorly effective in hemophilia B. The preparation is also used as a *source of fibrinogen*. AHF has a distribution half-life of 4 to 8 hr, and an elimination half-life of 12 to 15 hr. The preparation is not entirely free of possible contamination by serum and other hepatitis virus. Traces of ABO isohemoagglutinins are present, so that large doses may sometimes cause severe hemolysis. Mild allergic reactions are frequent. Occasionally there may be chills, fever, erythema, urticaria, bronchospasm, headache, lethargy, somnolence, and backache. The concentrate is more expensive than the cryoprecipitate.

Dose—*Intravenous*, from **5 Units/kg** of body weight once a day to **25 Units/kg** every 8 to 12 hr, depending on severity of hemorrhage and its location, or whether use is for prophylaxis. To raise plasma concentration of AHF by 10% of the normal content, 4 to 5 Units/kg are usually required. The following levels of normal are desirable: for *hemarthrosis*, 20 to 30%, except 50% if severe; *hemorrhage into CNS*, or *peritoneal* or *pleural spaces*, 50%; overt bleeding, 20 to 40% for 3 or 4 days; *bleeding from massive wounds*, 40% until wounds are healed; *muscle hemorrhage adjacent to vital structures*, 20 to 30% with tapering over 6 days; *surgery*, 30 to 60%, beginning 1 day prior and continuing 10 days after; *general prophylaxis*, 10 to 15%. Appropriate laboratory tests are necessary to ascertain the adequacy of dosage.

Dosage Forms—Vials containing 80, 125, 175, 225, 250, 275, 325, 375, 700, and 1000 Units; also available in many other quantities, the amount of which is shown on the label only.

Cryoprecipitated Antihemophilic Factor

A sterile, frozen concentrate of antihemophilic factor prepared from the Factor VIII-rich cryoprotein fraction of a single unit of human venous plasma obtained from whole blood or by plasmapheresis. It can be kept for 1 year at −18° or below, and is thawed at a temperature not to exceed 37° just before use.

Uses and **Dose**—See *Antihemophilic Factor* (above). The cryoprecipitated form is used when an autologous replacement is necessary. Also, cryopreservation maintains the potency better than liquid preservation. The cryoprecipitate contains other factors, including one that improves the bleeding time in patients with von Willebrand's disease. This factor is not present in marketed preparations of antihemophilic factor, and the cryoprecipitated preparation or fresh frozen plasma should be used, instead. Since the cryoprecipitate is type-specific, it may be cross-matched to the patient's blood to avoid hemolysis.

Factor IX Complex

Konȳne (*Cutter*); Profilnine (*Alpha*); Proplex (*Hyland*)

A preparation of pooled human plasma protein fraction containing clotting factors II, VII, IX, and X. The preparation is standardized in terms of Factor IX; the activity is not less than 0.7 and is usually 1 unit/mg of protein.

Preparation—See US Pat 3,717,708.

Description—White powder with a slight odor; fairly stable in light and air but unstable in heat. After reconstitution solutions are stable up to 12 hr at room temperature; they should, however, be prepared only immediately before use.

Solubility—Soluble in water.

Uses—Principally as a source of Factor IX for treatment of hemophilia B, a form of hemophilia separate and distinct from the more prevalent hemophilia A, or classic Factor VIII-deficient hemophilia. It can also be used in the treatment of congenital deficiencies of the other vitamin-K dependent coagulation factors, namely, factors II, VII, and X. Because some preparations of the product have been found to cause post-transfusion hepatitis, caution is indicated and physicians should weigh the risks against expected benefits.

Factor IX manifests two-compartment pharmacokinetics, with a distribution half-life of 3–6 hr, and a terminal half-life of 22–41 hr.

Dose—*Intravenous*, the dose is determined according to previous evaluation of the patient, the circumstances, and the response. In Factor IX-deficient patients, 1 unit/kg will cause an average increment of Factor IX of 1% of normal; in Factor VII-deficient patients, 2 units/kg will cause an increase in Factor VII of about 4%. Presurgically, it is advisable to achieve 60% of normal initially, although a maintenance of 20% is minimally sufficient. Maintenance should continue for 8 days. Prophylactically, for ambulatory patients with a Factor IX deficiency in normal circumstances, 500 units/week.

Dosage Form—Vials containing approximately 500 or 1000 Factor IX units, equivalent to Factor IX activity of 500 or 500 mL, respectively of normal plasma. The actual number of units is indicated on the label. Products differ in the volume of sterile water to be added for reconstitution.

Other Blood Clotting Proteins

Anti-Inhibitor Coagulant Complex [Autoplex]—A cryodesiccated complex of activated and precursor clotting factors and factors of the kinin generating system which is prepared from pooled human plasma. It is standardized by its ability to restore normal clotting time to Factor VIII-deficient plasma. One correctional unit will correct the clotting time to 35 sec in the ellagic acid-APTT test. The complex is reconstituted with sterile water for injection. There should be no more than 2 units/mL of heparin and 0.02 M citrate after reconstitution. *Uses:* As an alternative treatment for hemorrhagic diathesis in patients with titers of factor VIII inhibitors above 5 Bethesda units/mL only after the failure of conventional treatment. It is contraindicted when signs of fibrinolysis or disseminated intravascular coagulation are extant. It may cause transient hypofibrogenemia in children, so that fibrinogen levels should be monitored in young patients. Headache, flushing, tachycardia and hypotension may result from too rapid infusion. It is not free of the risk of serum hepatitis. *Dose: Intravenous*, initially 25 to 100 units/kg, to be adjusted according to APTT 30 min after the end of infusion. The infusion rate should not exceed 10 mL/min. *Dosage Form:* Powder, in 30-mL vials.

Anticoagulants

Anticoagulants are substances or drugs which delay coagulation of blood. They are of three general types.

1. *Calcium Sequestering Agents*—Calcium is essential to several steps in the clotting process; hence, its removal prevents clotting. The calcium-sequestering agents tie up calcium and other divalent cations; these agents are employed only in withdrawn blood. They thus find their most common use in anticoagulant solutions used by blood banks. These substances act rapidly, and their effect can be overcome rapidly by adding back or otherwise restoring calcium to normal. Thus citrate-containing blood is in effect recalcified on transfusion back into the blood stream.

2. *Heparin and Heparin Substitutes*—These agents combine with antithrombin III; the complex then interacts with certain activated clotting factors, namely, factors IX, X, XI, and XII, to prevent the conversion of prothrombin to thrombin; in high concentrations the complex interacts with thrombin and inhibits its effects to promote conversion of fibrinogen to fibrin. They inhibit the aggregation of platelets. They are fast-acting drugs. Heparin has the advantage of being a naturally occurring substance.

3. *Prothrombopenic Anticoagulants (Oral Anticoagulants)*—In this group dicumarol provides the prototype of action but not necessarily of structure. Prothrombopenic anticoagulants competitively inhibit vitamin K in the hepatic production of prothrombin (Factor II), the plasma content of prothrombin is thus reduced and coagulation of the blood impaired. These drugs also suppress formation of Factors VII, IX, and X, although the effect on prothrombin is the predominant one. Drugs in this category are slow-acting because their effect is directed at inhibition of protein synthesis and there is a latency determined by the long half-life (ca 60 hr) of prothrombin. By the same token, their action is overcome only slowly by Vitamin K.

The heparin and prothrombopenic anticoagulants are generally not employed for the same purpose, since chronic medication with heparin is expensive and entails the nuisance of parenteral administration. Rather, they may be complementary, heparin being employed acutely or initially, and prothrombopenic anticoagulants being employed for longer term therapy.

The enzymes urokinase and streptokinase are not true anticoagulants, although their effects to increase the fibrinolytic activity of blood have the effect of retarding red thrombus formation. They are described in Chapter 54.

Prothrombopenic Anticoagulants

Dicumarol

2*H*-1-Benzopyran-2-one], 3,3'-methylenebis[4-hydroxy-, Biscumarol; Bishydroxycoumarin; Dicoumarol; (*Various Mfrs*)

3,3'-Methylenebis[4-hydroxycoumarin]   [66-76-2] $C_{19}H_{12}O_6$ (336.30).

Preparation—Methyl acetylsalicylate is stirred with sodium thus effecting ring closure through demethanolation to form the sodium derivative of 4-hydroxycoumarin. Treatment with HCl liberates the 4-hydroxycoumarin, which readily forms bishydroxycoumarin on heating with formaldehyde and water.

Description—White or creamy white, crystalline powder, with a faint, pleasant odor and a slightly bitter taste; melts at about 290°.

Solubility—Practically insoluble in water, alcohol, and ether; slightly soluble in chloroform; readily soluble in solutions of fixed alkali hydroxides.

Uses—A *prothrombopenic anticoagulant*. It depresses hepatic production of prothrombin, probably by competing with vitamin K, both for transportation into liver cells and at the major site of vitamin-K dependent synthesis of clotting factors; the resultant lowering of the blood level of prothrombin renders the blood less coagulable. The plasma levels of VII, IX, and X are also depressed; indeed, in some persons the major effect of dicumarol is upon these factors. Plasma levels of factor VII are the first to fall, since factor VII has a

half-life of about 6 hr; the half-lives of factors IX, X, and II (prothrombin) are 20, 40, and 60 hr, respectively.

Dicumarol has advantages over heparin (see page 828) for ambulatory and prolonged anticoagulant therapy in that it is *orally effective*, has a longer duration of action (2 to 7 days; plasma half-life, about 8.2 hr at low doses, but up to 30 hr at high doses) and is considerably less expensive; it is unsuitable for short-term or emergency therapy in that the maximal effect of a full initial dose does not occur for 48 to 96 hours after administration, which reflects both the long half-life of prothrombin and the slow onset of the steady state. During the period of onset of action, heparin may be given. Dicumarol or one of its congeners is employed for long-term therapy to a much greater extent than heparin; however, the necessity for frequent prothrombin tests, which are more difficult to determine than clotting time, restricts the use of dicumarol to physicians having access to properly equipped laboratories and trained personnel. Dicumarol may be used in the treatment of the following: *pulmonary embolism*, to prevent further embolism; primary acute and postoperative *thrombophlebitis* and *traumatic injuries to blood vessels*, to forestall *venous thrombosis* and to prevent *thromboemboli;* sudden *arterial occlusion from thrombosis or embolism;* prophylaxis of *postoperative venous thrombosis or embolism; vascular surgery*. In the absence of specific contraindications, it is frequently used routinely in acute *coronary thrombosis* with myocardial infarction. It is also advocated in the treatment of chronic diseases that predispose to thrombi or emboli such as congestive heart failure, persistent phlebitis migrans, recurrent thrombophlebitis, recurrent coronary thrombosis and atrial fibrillation; however, the exact status of such long-term therapy is undetermined.

The aim of treatment is to maintain the blood prothrombin activity at a level of 15 to 25% of normal.

With the recommended dosage, the incidence of hemorrhage is 2 to 4%, and strict laboratory control is mandatory to prevent hemorrhagic diatheses. Bleeding is most common from the mucous membranes, skin, gastrointestinal tract, and urogenital tract and uterus. Stools should be monitored for occult blood loss and urine for hematuria. Hemorrhage can be arrested by vitamin K (which has a latency), fresh frozen plasma, whole blood, or factor IX concentrate (which contains prothrombin along with other vitamin K-dependent coagulation factors).

Other side effects include anorexia, nausea, vomiting, and diarrhea. Rarely there may be hypersensitivity reactions, such as purpura, alopecia, urticaria, necrosis of the skin and breast, and purple coloration of the toes.

Dicumarol is sensitive to interaction with other drugs and to the nutrition and other status of the patient, all of which may lead to unpredictable results. Therefore, whenever a patient on dicumarol is subjected to a new drug regimen or an old drug is withdrawn, it is essential that the patient's prothrombin time be monitored and the dosage of dicumarol be adjusted if necessary.

Drug interactions occur in various ways. Mechanisms of antagonism and offending drugs are as follows (*underscores* indicate the most important clinical interactions): Interference with absorption: *griseofulvin*, *cholestyramine*, clofibrate. Stimulation of synthesis of clotting factors: *vitamin K*, glucocorticoids, estrogens. Induction of hepatic enzymes: *barbiturates, ethchlorvynol, glutethimide, carbamazepine, griseofulvin*, meprobamate, phenytoin, *rifampin*.

Mechanisms of increasing the response to dicumarol, and the offending drugs are as follows: Displacement from plasma protein: *chloral hydrate* (as the trichloroacetate metabolite), *clofibrate*, diazoxide, ethacrynic acid, *mefenamic acid*, nalidixic acid, *phenylbutazone* and *hydroxyphenylbutazone*, long-acting sulfonamides. Inhibition of hepatic metabolism: *chloramphenicol*, *clofibrate*, oral hypoglycemics, *cimetidine*, *disulfiram*, allopurinol, disulfiram, mercaptopurine, methylphenidate, nortriptyline. Decrease in availability of vitamin K: *anabolic steroids, broad-spectrum antibiotics, clofibrate, cholestyramine, mineral oil*, D-thyroxine. Inhibition of synthesis of clotting factors: acetaminophen, *anabolic steroids, glucagon*, mercaptopurine, *quinidine, salicylates*. Increased catabolism of clotting factors: *anabolic steroids*, D-thyroxine. Increased binding affinity to receptor enzyme: D-thyroxine. Additivity of anticoagulant effects: *heparin, salicylates*, quinidine.

Dicumarol is contraindicated if laboratory facilities are unavailable for determining prothrombin levels, and vitamin K, fresh blood or plasma are not available. It is also contraindicated in any person with hemorrhagic tendencies, blood dyscrasias, peptic ulcer, ulcerative colitis, colitis, diverticulitis, subacute bacterial endocarditis, recent operations on the CNS, regional or lumbar block anesthesia, and severe renal or liver disease. Not only is it contraindicated in threatened abortion, but it should be withheld in pregnancy, since hemorrhage in the fetus can occur, and embryonic chondroplasia punctata has been attributed to use of the related drug warfarin. Patients with congestive heart failure are more sensitive to dicumarol than persons with normal cardiac function.

Dose—*Oral, adults,* **200 to 300 mg** on the first day, for loading; *maintenance,* ranges from **25 to 200 mg** a day, according to prothrombin time.

Dosage Forms—Capsules: 25 and 50 mg; Tablets: 25, 50, and 100 mg.

Phenindione

1*H*-Indene-1,3(2*H*)-dione, 2-phenyl-, Hedulin (*Merrell Dow*)

2-Phenyl-1,3-indandione [83-12-5] $C_{15}H_{10}O_2$ (222.24).

Preparation—Phthalide is condensed with benzaldehyde with the aid of sodium alcoholate.

Description—Creamy white to pale yellow crystals or crystalline powder; almost odorless; melts between 148° and 151°.

Solubility—Very slightly soluble in water; slightly soluble in alcohol and ether; freely soluble in chloroform.

Uses—A *prothrombopenic anticoagulant* with the same actions and uses as *Dicumarol.* It has a more rapid onset of action, namely, 18 to 24 hours. The effect lasts for 1 to 2 days after medication is discontinued. As with all short-acting prothrombopenic drugs, its actions are erratic, and its short duration of action is of little therapeutic advantage.

The untoward effects of phenindione include jaundice, hepatitis, nephropathy, with albuminuria and massive edema, severe exfoliative dermatitis, leukocytosis, leukopenia, and rarely agranulocytosis. The drug frequently imparts a red or orange color to the urine, which the patient may confuse with hematuria; therefore, the patient should be forewarned. The urinary discoloration may mask an important sign of impending hemorrhagic diathesis. For this reason, more serious hemorrhagic episodes occur with this drug than with any other prothrombopenic drug. The hemorrhagic complications and drug interactions are those of *Dicumarol.*

Dose—*Oral, adults,* **300 mg** the first day, **200 mg** the second day, and **100 mg** on subsequent days until the prothrombin time, determined daily, shows a desirable response; thereafter the daily dose is adjusted downward until the prothrombin time stabilizes at the desired level. *Maintenance,* ranges from **50 to 150 mg** a day, in two divided doses.

Dosage Forms—Tablets: 50 mg.

Phenprocoumon

2*H*-1-Benzopyran-2-one, 4-hydroxy-3-(1-phenylpropyl)-, Liquamar (*Organon*)

3-(α-Ethylbenzyl)-4-hydroxycoumarin [435-97-2] $C_{18}H_{16}O_3$ (280.32).

Preparation—Diethyl (α-ethylbenzyl)malonate is reacted with acetylsalicylic acid chloride by heating with a suspension of powdered sodium in dry benzene. The resulting diethyl (*o*-acetoxybenzoyl)(α-ethylbenzyl)malonate is dissolved in absolute ether and treated with sodium methylate whereby ethyl acetate is split off with concomitant cyclization to the coumarin derivative, 3-carbethoxy-3-(α-ethylbenzyl)-4-oxodihydrocoumarin. This is saponified and decarboxylated by heating with aqueous sodium hydroxide, following

which acidification with H_2SO_4 liberates phenprocoumon. Recrystallization is from 80% ethanol. US Pat. 2,701,804.

Description—Fine, white, crystalline powder that is odorless or has a slight odor; melts between 177° and 181°.

Solubility—Practically insoluble in water; soluble in chloroform, and solutions of alkali hydroxides.

Uses—A *prothrombopenic anticoagulant* with actions and uses similar to those of *Dicumarol.* Its onset of action is 48 to 72 hours, and its duration of action may be as long as 7 days. Like other drugs of this class, the effective dose and duration of action are affected by a number of factors, including dietary intake and enteric bacterial synthesis of vitamin K, and concurrent drugs which affect the hepatic "microsomal" drug metabolizing system. The hemorrhagic complications and drug interactions are those of *Dicumarol.*

Overdose of the drug may cause hemorrhagic diathesis; phytonadione (vitamin K_1) can be used to antagonize the overdose, but there is a long delay before prothrombin levels return to a safe range. The drug may cause diarrhea, or other mild gastrointestinal disturbances, such as anorexia, nausea, and vomiting, and dermatitis. Leukopenia, urticaria, erythema, or hemorrhagic infarction of the skin and digits may occur.

Dose—*Oral, adults,* **24 mg** the first day, followed by **0.75 to 6 mg** a day, as determined by the prothrombin levels.

Dosage Form—Tablets: 3 mg.

Warfarin Potassium

2*H*-1-Benzopyran-2-one, 4-hydroxy-3-(3-oxo-1-phenylbutyl)-, potassium salt; Athrombin-K (*Purdue-Frederick*)

3-(α-Acetonylbenzyl)-4-hydroxycoumarin potassium salt [2610-86-8] $C_{19}H_{15}KO_4$ (346.42).

Preparation—Warfarin (see *Warfarin Sodium*) is reacted with an equimolar portion of KOH.

Description—White, odorless, crystalline powder, having a slightly bitter taste; discolored by light; pH (1 in 100 solution) between 7.2 and 8.3.

Solubility—1 g in 1.5 mL water, 1.9 mL alcohol, >10,000 mL chloroform, >10,000 mL ether.

Uses—See *Warfarin Sodium.* The potassium salt has the same uses as the sodium salt.

Dose—*Oral, intramuscular* or *intravenous,* **10 to 15 mg** the 1st day followed by a daily *maintenance* dose of **2 to 10 mg,** according to prothrombin time.

Dosage Forms—Tablets: 5 mg.

Warfarin Sodium

2*H*-1-Benzopyran-2-one, 4-hydroxy-3-(3-oxo-1-phenylbutyl)-, sodium salt; Coumadin (*Endo*); Panwarfin (*Abbott*)

3-(α-Acetonylbenzyl)-4-hydroxycoumarin sodium salt [129-06-6] $C_{19}H_{15}NaO_4$ (330.31); an amorphous solid or a crystalline clathrate. The clathrate consists principally of sodium warfarin, isopropyl alcohol, and water, the molecular proportions of which vary between 8:4:0 and 8:2:2. Refer to the previous monograph for the structure of the warfarin moiety.

Preparation—By addition of 4-hydroxycoumarin to benzalacetone under the catalytic influence of a mildly basic substance such as ammonia or piperidine. The reaction is a typical Michael "condensation." Conversion to the sodium salt is effected by reacting purified warfarin with an equimolar portion of dilute NaOH solution at room temperature.

Description—White, odorless, amorphous or crystalline powder, having a slightly bitter taste; discolored by light; pH (1 in 100 solution) between 7.2 and 8.3.

Solubility—Very soluble in water, freely soluble in alcohol, and very slightly soluble in chloroform and ether.

Uses—A *prothrombopenic anticoagulant* (see *Dicumarol*). Although it is usually administered orally, its chief distinction from other prothrombopenic drugs is the fact that it is water-soluble and may be administered intravenously. By the intravenous route its onset of action is 12 to 18 hours and its duration is 5 to 6 days. The plasma half-life is 41 to 57 hours, except about 27 hours in alcoholics and probably even less in persons using phenobarbital or other hepatic microsomal enzyme inducers.

The hemorrhagic complications and drug interactions are those of *Dicumarol*.

Dose—*Oral, intramuscular,* or *intravenous, adults,* **10 to 15 mg** the first day, followed by a daily *maintenance* dose of **2 to 10 mg,** according to the prothrombin time.

Dosage Forms—for Injection: 50 mg; Tablets: 2, 2.5, 5, 7.5, and 10 mg.

Other Prothrombopenic Anticoagulants

Anisindione [2-*p*-(Methoxyphenyl)-1,3-indandione [117-37-3] $C_{16}H_{12}O_3$ (252.27); Miradon (*Schering-Plough*)]—Prepared by rearrangement of 3-(*p*-methoxybenzylidene)phthalide (US Pat 2,899,359). White or off-white, crystalline powder; practically insoluble in water. *Uses:* A prothrombopenic anticoagulant with actions and uses similar to those of *Dicumarol*. Its onset of action is 24 to 72 hr, and duration of action is ordinarily 3 to 5 days. The effective dose and duration of action are affected by factors including dietary intake, bacterial synthesis of vitamin K, and concurrently administered drugs that affect the hepatic microsomal drug-metabolizing system. Untoward effects include hemorrhagic diathesis resulting from overdosage, also dermatitis. Overdoses can be antagonized with phytonadione (vitamin K_1) but there is a long delay before prothrombin levels return to a safe range. If fever or dermatitis appear the drug should be discontinued because of the possible danger of blood dyscrasias. Anisindione may cause some orange discoloration of urine that may obscure onset of hematuria, an important sign of impending hemorrhage; the color disappears on acidification. Hemorrhagic complications and drug interactions are as for *Dicumarol*. *Dose: Oral, adults,* 300 mg the first day, 200 mg the second day, and 100 mg the third day; for maintenance, 25 to 250 mg a day. *Dosage Form:* Tablets: 50 mg.

Nonprothrombopenic Anticoagulants

Anticoagulant Citrate Phosphate Dextrose Solution

CPD Solution

A sterile solution of citric acid ($C_6H_8O_7$), sodium citrate ($C_6H_5Na_3O_7.2H_2O$), sodium biphosphate ($NaH_2PO_4.H_2O$), and dextrose ($C_6H_{12}O_6.H_2O$) in water for injection. It contains no antimicrobial agents.

Citric Acid (anhydrous)	**3.0 g**
Sodium Citrate (dihydrate)	**26.3 g**
Sodium Biphosphate (monohydrate; $NaH_2PO_4.H_2O$)	**2.22 g**
Dextrose (monohydrate)	**25.5 g**
Water for Injection, a sufficient quantity, To make	**1000 mL**

Dissolve the ingredients, and mix. Filter the solution until clear, place immediately in suitable containers, and sterilize.

If desired, 3.27 g of monohydrated citric acid may be used instead of the indicated amount of anhydrous citric acid; 23.1 g of anhydrous sodium citrate may be used instead of the indicated amount of dihydrated sodium citrate; 1.93 g of anhydrous sodium biphosphate may be used instead of the indicated amount of monohydrated sodium biphosphate; and 23.2 g of anhydrous dextrose may be used instead of the indicated amount of monohydrated dextrose.

Description—Clear, colorless, odorless liquid; pH between 5.0 and 6.0.

Uses—Citrate ion chelates calcium thus making calcium unavailable to the coagulation system. Citric acid, sodium citrate, and sodium biphosphate are in the proper proportions to buffer the solution at the optimal pH for the storage of blood and its components. Dextrose provides a substrate for glycolysis and increases both storage and post-transfusion lives of blood cells. The expiration time of whole blood with CPD solution is 21 days. The 2,3-diphosphorglycerate (2,3-DPG) content of erythrocytes stored in CPD solution is 120% of the original content at 7 and 40% at 21 days. The preservation helps keep the oxygen affinity of hemoglobin low so that it can yield its

oxygen readily to the tissues. Consequently, CPD is the preferred anticoagulant for blood to be used for exchange transfusion.

The sodium concentration is 284 mEq/L, and 17.8 mEq are thus added to each unit of whole blood.

Application—In the proportion of 14 mL of solution for each 100 mL of whole blood.

Size Available—63 mL in a blood-collecting container.

Anticoagulant Citrate Phosphate Dextrose Adenine Solution

CPDA-1 Solution; CPD-Adenine Solution (*Travenol*)

Uses—The addition of adenine to CPD solution increases the storage life of blood by 40%, that is, blood can now be stored for 35 days. However, CPDA-1 solution does not preserve 2,3-diphosphoglycerate as well as does CPD solution; there is 97% of the initial content at 7 days but only 10% at 21 days. Therefore, CPDA-1 whole blood should not be used in exchange transfusion.

Application—In the proportion of 14 mL of solution for each 100 mL of whole blood.

Heparin Sodium

Heparin; Lipo-Hepin (*Riker*); Liquaemin Sodium (*Organon*); Panheprin (*Abbott*)

A mixture of active glycosaminoglycans, having the property of prolonging the clotting time of blood. It is usually obtained from the lungs, intestinal mucosa, or other suitable tissues of domestic mammals used for food by man. Potency: not less than 120 (when derived from lungs) and not less than 140 (when derived from other tissues) USP Heparin Units*/mg.

Preparation—Heparin is the body's natural anticoagulant, taking part in the physiological function of maintaining the fluidity of the blood. It is produced by the mast cells of Ehrlich, which are clustered in the perivascular connective tissue of the walls of major blood vessels and capillaries. Heparin is a polysulfuric ester of mucoitin. The molecular skeleton is constructed from acetylated glucosamine and glucuronic acid. The disaccharide unit is similar to that in *mucoitin sulfuric acid* and *hyaluronic acid*. Protein-free samples of heparin contain about 10% of sulfur present as ester sulfates. Original preparations of heparin contain mixtures consisting of mucoitin disulfuric and trisulfuric acids. The anticoagulant action is greater in preparations with the highest sulfuric content. Heparin in the final, therapeutic form is supplied in a solution made from the sodium salt, but in the steps of its purification the barium salts of heparin are prepared. Heparin, being a mixture of the several sulfuric esters, is not entirely homogeneous, and there is debate as to whether a truly crystalline or homogeneous preparation has been or ever can be prepared.

Description—White or pale-colored amorphous powder: odorless, or nearly so; hygroscopic. A 1% solution has a pH of 5.0 to 7.5. It will not dialyze through a parchment membrane, and only slightly through a collodion membrane. Heparin is resistant to all kinds of chemical agents; it gives an insoluble precipitate with protamine and with toluidine blue; and interference with the sulfuric groups reduces its anticoagulant activity. Heparin has a very low osmotic pressure in respect to its high degree of ionization. In contrast to the effect of oxalate, heparin has no osmotic influence on red blood cells. Heparin may be stored for long periods without loss of activity.

Solubility—1 g in 20 mL of water; soluble in alcohol, acetone, and glacial acetic acid.

Uses—The anticoagulant actions of heparin are described on page 826. In addition to these actions, heparin releases lipoprotein lipase from the vascular endothelium, which has the effect of clearing chylomicrons and very-low-density lipoproteins from blood; only low doses are needed for this action. Heparin also has anti-inflammatory and antiallergy actions through its effects on the Hageman factor (XIIa), kallikreins, and other enzymes that have active groups containing or act on substrates with lysine and/or arginine moieties.

Heparin is employed clinically in conditions in which a rapid reduction in the coagulability of the blood is desired. It is often employed to initiate prolonged anticoagulant therapy in order to cover

---

* *Note*—USP Heparin Units are consistently established on the basis of the USP assay, independently of International Units, and the respective units are not equivalent.

the latent period of onset of action of dicumarol-type anticoagulants. Heparin is also used in lieu of dicumarol-type drugs in prolonged therapy when laboratory facilities are unavailable for determination of prothrombin time. Some of the primary clinical applications are nonfatal *pulmonary embolism*, primary and postoperative *thrombophlebitis*, sudden *arterial occlusion* from thrombosis or embolism, prophylaxis of postoperative *venous thrombosis* or embolism, and after *vascular surgery*. For these purposes, low doses given subcutaneously are popular; however, recent reports indicate that blood levels are erratic and monitoring is advisable. It is indicated for treatment of *diffuse intravascular coagulation* (consumptive coagulopathy) and *immune thrombocytopenia* (in which vasculitis causes coagulopathy and consumption of platelets). It is sometimes given during and after conversion of atrial fibrillation to prevent thrombosis from emboli and mural thrombi. It is advocated by some for immediate therapy of *coronary occlusion*, but its status in that condition is still controversial after nearly four decades of use. It appears to decrease mortality in women but not in men. However, heparin does protect against venous thrombosis resulting from stasis during coronary care. The indications for prolonged therapy with heparin are the same as with prothrombopenic anticoagulants (see *Dicumarol*), but usually heparin is used only during the early stages of treatment when the disorder is acute and to keep blood clotting suppressed until oral anticoagulants can be given and take effect. Heparin also has special uses, such as prevention of clotting of blood samples, to *prevent clotting* during blood transfusions, to prevent clotting during *extracorporeal hemodialysis* and during *cardiopulmonary bypass*, and for the heparin tolerance test. It is used in low concentrations in solutions for flushing intravenous catheters for intermittent injections; the residual heparin in the catheter keeps clots from occluding the catheter orifice. It is also used to prevent pleural and peritoneal *adhesions*. Sometimes heparin is used as an adjuvant to antineoplastic therapy to suppress formation of a fibrin network through which the neoplasm can spread.

Hemorrhage is the principal toxic effect, usually the result of overdosage; protamine, with which heparin combines, may be employed for immediate control of hyperheparinemia. Heparin must be administered cautiously when oral anticoagulants are in use because of the enhanced risk of hemorrhage; it also interferes with laboratory tests for the effect of oral anticoagulants. The risk of hemorrhage is also increased by salicylates, dipyridamole, glyceryl guaiacolate, and other inhibitors of platelet adhesiveness. Certain amine or ammonium compounds, especially bifunctional ones, interact directly with heparin and thus decrease the circulating levels in the blood; cimetidine, various antihistamines, quinine and quinidine are examples. Even tetracyclines supposedly interact. Polymyxins and colistins are known to interact during simultaneous infusion but have not been reported to interact when administered separately. Heparin favors hematomas fromn various intramuscular injections.

Hypersensitivity and other adverse side effects may occur. Manifestations include bronchospasm (dyspnea, tightness in chest, wheezing), skin rash, urticaria, pruritis, chills, fever, vasospasm (chest pain, pain in extremities, priapism), neuropathy with paresthesias, and hair loss.

Heparin is inactive orally and must be administered parenterally. Its plasma half-life is 1.3 to 1.6 hours.

Dose—Dosage should be determined by laboratory tests of coagulability of blood during the course of therapy in each patient and not by a rigid regimen. Usually, a coagulation time 2.5 to 3 or a partial prothombin time (PPT) 1.5 to 2.5 times normal is desired. The following doses only provide an approximate guide to dosage. Doses are in USP units. *Intravenous, adults, therapeutic, initially* **10,000 Units** followed by **5,000** to **10,000 Units** every 4 to 6 hr or **100 Units/kg** every 4 hr; *children, initially* **50 Units per kg** of body weight (or 1667 Units per m² of body surface) followed by **100 Units per kg** (or 3333 Units per m²) every 4 hr. *Intravenous infusion, adults,* initially **35** to **70 Units/kg** or **5000 Units** rapidly followed by **20,000** to **40,000 Units** (in 1 L isotonic sodium chloride) per 24 hr; *children,* initially **50 Units/kg** rapidly followed by **100 Units/kg** every 4 hr or **20,000 Units/m²** every 24 hr. *Deep subcutaneous* ("intrafat"), *adults, therapeutic, initially* **10,000** to **20,000 Units** followed by **8,000** to **10,000 Units** every 8 hr or **15,000** to **20,000 Units** every 12 hr; for *low-dose prophylaxis,* initially **5,000 Units** 2 hr prior to surgery, repeated at 8- to 12-hr intervals for 7 days or until the patient is fully ambulatory, whichevery is the longer. For *blood transfusion* or *extracorporeal circuits,* **400** to **600 Units per 100 mL** of whole blood. For laboratory *blood samples,* **70** to **150 Units per**

10 to 20 mL. For *filling* and *flushing intravenous catheters,* as an isotonic saline solution containing **10** or **100 Units/mL.**

Dosage Forms—Injection: 10, 100, 1000, 2500, 5000, 7500, 10,000, 15,000, 20,000, and 40,000 Units per mL.

Sodium Citrate

1,2,3-Propanetricarboxylic acid, 2-hydroxy-, trisodium salt

$$CH_2(COONa)C(OH)(COONa)CH_2COONa$$

Trisodium citrate [68-04-2] $C_6H_5Na_3O_7$ (258.07) or trisodium citrate dihydrate [6132-04-3] (294.10).

Preparation—Usually by adding sodium carbonate to a solution of citric acid until effervescence ceases, evaporating, and granulating the product.

Description—Colorless crystals, or a white, crystalline powder; a cooling, saline taste; stable in air; the aqueous solution is slightly alkaline to litmus but should not be reddened by phenolphthalein.

Solubility—1 g in 1.5 mL water at 25° and in 0.6 mL boiling water; insoluble in alcohol.

Uses—The most important use of sodium citrate is as an *anticoagulant* for blood or plasma that is to be fractionated or for blood that is to be stored. The anticoagulant effect is due to conversion of ionized calcium in the blood to a citrato-calcium chelate. Sodium citrate is an ingredient of *Anticoagulant Citrate Dextrose Solution, Anticoagulant Citrate Phosphate Dextrose Solution,* and *Sodium Citrate and Citric Acid Solution.*

Sodium citrate is also used as an *expectorant* and systemic and urine *alkalinizer.* Saline expectorants are especially useful when it is desired to liquefy thick, tenacious sputum. In the body sodium citrate is oxidized to bicarbonate and excreted in urine; thus, when given orally it is useful in acidosis, to overcome excessive urinary acidity and to assist in the dissolution of uric acid nephroliths.

Sodium citrate is a chelating agent and thus increases *urinary excretion* of *calcium* and *lead*; it has been employed in hypercalcemia and to facilitate elimination of lead in poisoning due to the latter. As a *pharmaceutic aid,* sodium citrate may be used to prevent darkening when iron is included in preparations containing tannin.

Dose—*Usual, expectorant,* 1 to 2 **g,** well diluted with water, every 2 hr; for *metabolic acidosis,* 1 to 4 **g** 4 times a day. Since sodium citrate is not used alone as an anticoagulant, there is no statement of application or dosage forms here.

Anticoagulant Sodium Citrate Solution

A sterile 4% solution of sodium citrate $[C_6H_5Na_3O_7.2H_2O$ (294.10)] in water for injection. It contains no antimicrobial agents.

Sodium Citrate (dihydrate)	**40 g**
Water for Injection, a sufficient quantity,	
To make	$\overline{1000\ mL}$

Note—Anhydrous sodium citrate (35.1 g) may be used instead of the dihydrate.

Dissolve the sodium citrate in sufficient water for injection to make 1000 mL, and filter until clear. Place the solution in suitable containers, and sterilize.

Description—Clear, colorless solution possessing a slightly saline taste; pH between 6.4 and 7.5.

Uses—Prevents clotting of blood by forming an undissociated calcium citrate chelate. The solution also prevents either crenation or swelling of the cells. The sterile solution is employed for preparation of blood for fractionation, for banked blood for transfusion, and for preparation of citrated human plasma.

Application—10 mL per 100 mL of whole blood or plasma.

Edetate Disodium—page 838.

Other Nonprothrombopenic Anticoagulants

Heparin Calcium [Calciparine [9005-49-6]]—A creamy white powder obtained from the lungs or mucosa of cattle, sheep, or pigs. Refer to heparin sodium, page 828. *Uses and Dose: See Heparin Sodium,* page 828. The calcium salt is used in low doses to prevent postoperative thromboembolism. The claim that it causes fewer and less severe hemorrhagic disturbances has not been supported by controlled clinical trials. The calcium salt is especially indicated when it is desirable to restrict sodium intake. *Dosage Forms:* Injection: 5,000, 12,500, and 20,000 units/mL.

Potassium Oxalate [$K_2C_2O_4.H_2O$]—The oxalate anion of potassium oxalate combines with calcium ions to form the very insoluble calcium oxalate. Thus when it is added to withdrawn (shed) blood it acts as an anticoagulant, for which purpose it may be employed in clinical laboratory procedures. It may also be used as a reagent in the determination of serum or other calcium by the permanganate method, the washed precipitated calcium oxalate being redissolved in acid and the oxalate anion make this permanganate. The reducing properties of the oxalate titrated with substance useful as a cleaning and bleaching agent, especially for straw. Care must be exercised in its storage and use because it is highly toxic.

Sodium Oxalate [$Na_2C_2O_4$]—The actions and uses of sodium oxalate are virtually identical to those of *Potassium Oxalate*, above.

Antiplatelet Drugs

Platelets play a key role in hemostasis and thrombus formation. Platelets adhere to thrombin, collagen, immunologicaly sensitized surfaces, and various other substances. At the site of vascular injury, collagen is exposed thus causing platelet adhesion and the release of ADP, prostaglandins PGG_2 and PGH_2, TXA_2, and other substances. The growing platelet aggregate becomes a "white thrombus" which may plug a small vascular break or grow sufficiently large to cause vascular occlusion. In a blood clot, adhesion to thrombin causes an aggregate known as the "white head" of a red thrombus, which by a self-regenerating process (since ADP and TXA_2 cause further aggregation) enlarges the thrombus. Serotonin, PGG_2, PGH_2, TXA_2 and PDGF cause local vasospasm, which helps arrest bleeding from ruptured capillaries.

Vascular endothelium generates prostacycline (PGI_2). PGI_2 suppresses platelet adherence and aggregation and thus is a protective substance that helps limit the progression of a white thrombus beyond the point of injury. PGI_2 is also a potent vasodilator.

Platelets adhering to the wall of a blood vessel promote atherogenesis. PDGF causes local smooth muscle cells to increase cholesterol synthesis, bind low-density lipoprotein (LDL), increase the rate of cell replication, and to change into the foam cells characteristic of an atheroma. Platelets are also crucial to the process of thrombotic vascular occlusion once an athheroma has ruptured.

So-called antiplatelet drugs may suppress platelet adherence and aggregation and extend platelet viability by acting directly on mechanisms within the platelet (true antiplatelet activity) or indirectly to decrease the availability of nonplatelet-derived agonists that promote aggregation. The greatest publicity has been of inhibitors of prostaglandin and thromboxane synthesis, especially of *aspirin* (page 1112). Aspirin irreversibly inhibits (by acetylation) the cyclooxygenase system that generates prostaglandins, prostacycline and TXA_2. The effect to decrease TXA_2 decreases platelet aggregation, but this is at first counterbalanced by a decrease in PGI_2. However, vascular endothelial cells continue to synthesize cyclooxygenase, whereas anuclear platelets do not. Therefore, within a few hours after the administration of aspirin, PGI_2 synthesis returns to normal but TXA_2 synthesis does not. This has led to the dogma that "low dose" (once-a-day) aspirin is more effective than continuous aspirin treatment. Other nonsteroidal antiinflammatory drugs (NSAID), such as other salicylates, hydroxychloroquin, indomethacin, etc are not irreversible inhibitors of cyclooxygenase and are not as effective as antiplatelet drugs. *Sulfinpryrazone* (page 1115) is a weak inhibitor of cyclooxygenase and may possibly have another mechanism of action. Aspirin also has an action to suppress secretion of ADP-containing dense granules from platelets, which also contributes to antiplatelet activity.

Other drugs work in other ways. *Dipyridamole* (page 854) inhibits platelet phosphodiesterase thus increasing cyclic AMP levels, which suppresses dense-granule secretion. *Calcium channel blockers* (page 861) decrease intraplatelet calcium concentration and hence also suppress dense-granule secretion. *β-Adrenergic blockers* (page 902) prevent β-receptor operation of calcium channels. α-Blockers prevent α-agonist-induced dense-granule secretion. *Anagrelide* suppresses platelet response to all stimuli; its mechanism may be that of inhibiting a distinct pool of cAMP phosphodiesterase. *Ticlopidine* blocks the effects of secreted ADP. Other inhibitors of platelet function are dextrans 70 and 75 (page 821), glyceryl guaiacolate (very active), penicillin, tricyclic antidepressants, glucocorticoids, clofibrate, pyridinol carbamate, PGE_1, glucagon, antiserotonin drugs, certain antihistamines, caffeine, theophyllin pentoxifyllin, general anesthetics, and ethanol in high concentration.

No clinical use of antiplatelet drugs is without some controversy. Furthermore, efficacy, when it is reported, seems mainly to be in men and almost negligible in women. In general, except for dextrans 70 and 75, antiplatelet drugs have not been found effective alone in preventing or limiting venous thrombosis and pulmonary embolism, but they probably improve the response to oral anticoagulants; in such a combination, aspirin increases the incidence and severity of gastrointestinal hemorrhage whereas dipyridamole does not. Antiplatelet-anticoagulant drug combinations appear to be superior to oral anticoagulants alone in preventing thombosis from prosthetic heart valves and other foreign surfaces. After hip surgery, aspirin alone (in men), aspirin-dipyridamole, and hydroxychloroquin have been reported to be of value in preventing venous thrombosis and pulmonary embolism. Sulfinpyrazone decreases the incidence of systemic embolism in rheumatic mitral valve stenosis.

Aspirin is approved in the US for the prevention of certain platelet-fibrin embolic vascular occlusions (in men only); namely, transient ischemic attacks (reduced by 50%), amaurosis fugax, and strokes. Completed strokes are not affected. In elderly men, sulfinpyrazone appears to be more effective than aspirin. Occlusive microvascular disorders in the fingers are resolved in 2 to 3 days after treatment using aspirin and further prevented. Microvascular occlusion after organ transplants also appear to be diminished by aspirin. Aspirin and dipyridamole prevent vascular occlusion after coronary-artery bypass operations.

There is much interest in the reputed ability of antiplatelet drugs to decrease the rate of myocardial reinfarction. In a controversial study, sulfinpyrazone was reported to reduce the rate by 50%. The efficacies of aspirin and clofibrate have been reported to be somewhat less. In men with unstable angina, aspirin decreases the *de novo* infarction rate. Aspirin and sulfinpyrazone also decrease the incidence of sudden death, presumably by ventricular fibrillation, in the early period (hours to a few weeks) after myocardial infarction. Platelets may not be involved, and an effect to decrease prostaglandin-modulated release of norepinephrine has been postulated.

Anticoagulant Antagonists

Anticoagulant therapy carries the risk of serious hemorrhage, so that there may be need to arrest the anticoagulant action. Prothrombopenic anticoagulants, as expected from their mode of action, are antagonized by vitamin K or its synthetic substitutes. Not all vitamin K preparations are equally effective, vitamin K_1 (phytonadione) being superior and menadione inferior. The efficacy of vitamin K preparations also varies according to the anticoagulant, but all agents of the dicumarol group may be antagonized by an appropriate dose of vitamin K_1. The antagonism is not manifested immediately, since normal coagulation is obtained only after the liver has had time to replenish the prothrombin and prothrombinogen. High doses of vitamin K_1 can antagonize oral anticoagulants despite their continuing inhibition at their site of action, because high doses can activate a second latent enzyme not significantly productive with ordinary concentrations of vitamin K and which enzyme is not inhibited by the anticoagulants. Heparin is antagonized by various amines, ammonium compounds, and basic proteins, which precipitate the polysulfate. Circulating heparinoid substances in the blood can also be assayed with such substances.

Menadiol Sodium Diphosphate—page 1010.

Menadione—page 1011.

Menadione Sodium Bisulfite—page 1011.

Phytonadione—page 1011.

Protamine Sulfate

A purified mixture of simple protein principles obtained from the sperm or testes of suitable species of fish, which has the property of neutralizing heparin. Each mg neutralizes not less than 80 USP Units of heparin activity derived from lung tissue and not less than 100 USP Units of heparin activity derived from intestinal mucosa.

Preparation—Frozen ripe salmon testes are ground, water-washed, centrifuged, and dehydrated by means of solvents and vacuum drying. The dried material is then extracted with 10% H_2SO_4 and, after filtering, a protamine sulfate-rich fraction is precipitated from the filtrate with cold alcohol. After collecting, this fraction is dissolved in hot water, and the protamine sulfate separates as an oil upon cooling. This protamine-rich oil is dissolved in hot water and fractionated again with cold alcohol. After collecting, this fraction is dehydrated by means of solvents and vacuum drying.

Description—Fine, white or faintly colored, amorphous or crystalline, hygroscopic powder.

Solubility—Sparingly soluble in water.

Uses—A *heparin antagonist*. Because it is a strongly basic macromolecule, it combines avidly with heparin, which is a polyanionic macromolecule. Protamine combines with heparin in an approximate 1:1 ratio by weight regardless of the source of heparin; since the potency of heparin from different sources varies, the dose of protamine based on USP unitage also varies. It is injected slowly intravenously after suitably diluting with physiological salt solution, to counteract the effect of *overmedication with heparin*. The duration of the effect is about 2 hours.

Untoward effects are uncommon. They include abrupt hypotension, dyspnea, bradycardia, flushing, and a feeling of warmth. An overdose can itself exert an anticoagulant effect.

Dose—*Intravenous*, *adults* and *children*, **1 mg** for each 90 Units of heparin from lung or 115 units of heparin from intestinal mucosa, to be injected slowly over a span of 1 to 3 min; no more than 50 mg should be given in any 10-min period. In calculating the dose, the disappearance of heparin from the blood should be taken into account. Since the half-life of heparin is 1.3 to 1.6 hr, a dose of protamine sulfate given 1.5 hr after a single dose of heparin would be based on 50% of the dose of heparin. However, during steady-state heparin treatment, the dose of protamine sulfate required may be even greater than that estimated from the last dose of heparin, especially if the protamine dose comes shortly after the heparin. Therefore, laboratory checks on coagulation of blood are important in determining adequacy of dosage.

Dosage Forms—Injection: 10 mg/mL; for Injection: 50 mg.

Fibrinolysin Inhibitors

Aminocaproic Acid

"Epsilon" Aminocaproic Acid; Amicar (*Lederle*)

$$H_2C(CH_2)_3CH_2COOH$$
$$\underset{NH_2}{|}$$

6-Aminohexanoic acid [60-32-2] $C_6H_{13}NO_2$ (131.17).

Preparation—The lactam group of the commercially available caprolactam (hexahydro-2*H*-azepin-2-one) is cleaved at the C-N linkage by heating an aqueous solution with calcium hydroxide. The calcium aminocaproate thus formed is reacted with sulfuric acid to free the official acid and precipitate the calcium. Various other methods of preparation are also available.

Description—Fine, white, crystalline powder that is odorless, or nearly so, and tasteless, stable in light and air; melts at about 205°.

Solubility—1 g in 3 mL water; slightly soluble in alcohol; practically insoluble in chloroform and ether.

Uses—A competitive inhibitor of activators of profibrinolysin and, to a lesser extent, of fibrinolysin. As a consequence, it suppresses the formation of fibrinolysin, an enzyme which destroys fibrinogen, fibrin, and other clotting components. For vascular integrity a low rate of fibrin deposition is normal; excessive fibrinolysis leads to hemorrhage. Aminocaproic acid is used in the treatment of *procedures or disorders in which fibrinolysis is enhanced*, such as cardiac bypass, postcaval shunt, major thoracic surgery, prostatic postoperative hematuria and also nonsurgical hematuria, leukemia, metastatic prostatic carcinoma, cirrhosis and other hepatic diseases, eclampsia, intrauterine fetal death, amniotic fluid embolism, and abruptio placentae. Aminocaproate has been reported to be of use in angioedema and subarachnoid hemorrhage. The drug is of no value in hemorrhage due to thrombocytopenia, hyperheparinemia, or other coagulation defects, or to vascular disruption.

Aminocaproic acid may cause itching, erythema, skin rash, diuresis, heartburn, nausea, and diarrhea. It also has an antiadrenergic effect similar to guanethidine, so that nasal stuffiness, conjunctival suffusion, and hypotension may occur. The drug may enhance thrombotic processes by suppression of reactive fibrinolysis, which tends to limit clot formation and to favor clot resolution. Therefore, aminocaproate should not be given unless there is unequivocal evidence that disseminated intravascular clotting is not the cause of elevated fibrinolytic activity. The drug is teratogenic in animals and hence should not be used in humans in the first two trimesters of pregnancy and in the third trimester only if its use is imperative.

Aminocaproic acid is excreted by the kidney; in the presence of renal disease the dose should be reduced.

Dose—*Intravenous infusion*, *adults*, for *peripheral acute hemorrhage*, **4 to 5 g** during 1 hr followed by **1 g/hr** for 8 hr or until an adequate response occurs, up to 30 g/day; *children*, **100 mg/kg** (or 3 g/m² of body surface) in 1 hr followed by **33.3 mg/kg/hr**, not to exceed 18 g/m²/day. *Intravenous infusion* or *bolus*, *adults*, for *subarachnoid hemorrhage*, 1 to **1.5 g/hr**. *Oral*, *adults*, for *peripheral acute hemorrhage*, *initially* **5 g** followed by 1 or **1.25 g/hr** for 8 hr or until an adequate response occurs; *children*, same as intravenous dose.

Dosage Forms—Injection: 250 mg/mL; Syrup: 250 mg/mL; Tablets: 500 mg.

Other Fibrinolytic Inhibitors

Tranexamic Acid [*trans*-4-(Aminomethyl)cyclohexanecarboxylic acid [1197-18-8] $C_8H_{15}NO_2$ (157.21)]—Preparation of tranexamic acid is described in *J Org Chem* 24: 115, 1959, and in US Pat 3,499,925. Crystals; 1 g dissolves in about 6 mL of water; very slightly soluble in alcohol, ether. *Uses*: Tranexamic acid resembles aminocaproic acid in decreasing the activity of the fibrinolysin system, in part by inhibiting plasminogen; it has the same potential uses. Its most interesting use has been in the treatment of malignant ovarian tumors, to promote formation of a fibrin capsule to wall off and inhibit growth of the tumor. It also causes regression of ascites secondary to carcinoma. In these uses heparin was given concomitantly to prevent intravascular coagulation. *Dose*: Oral, *adult*, 4 to 6 g a day in divided doses.

Hemostatics and Styptics

Many substances not especially related to the clotting mechanism are capable of promoting clotting. Upon contact with most surfaces, platelets disintegrate, thereby liberating a thromboplastin. Spongy and gauzy materials, which provide a large surface area, are thus used to arrest bleeding; absorbable sponges may be left permanently at the site of bleeding. Fibrin, fibrinogen, and thrombin are also potent hemostatics (see page 832). Astringents (see Chapter 40) also initiate clotting by precipitating proteins and by labilizing platelets; ferric salts are mostly employed as styptics.

Alum—page 777.

Cellulose, Oxidized—page 1873.

Desmopressin—page 958.

Fibrinogen—RPS-16, page 765.

Absorbable Gelatin Sponge

Gelfoam (*Upjohn*)

Gelatin in the form of a sterile, absorbable, water-insoluble sponge.

Description—Light, nearly white, nonelastic, tough, porous, hydrophilic solid; 10-mm cube weighing approximately 9 mg will take up approximately 45 times its weight of well-agitated oxalated whole blood; it is stable in dry heat at 150° for 4 hours.

Solubility—Insoluble in water, but absorbable in body fluids; completely digested by a solution of pepsin.

Uses and **Application**—A *hemostatic* and *coagulant* used to control bleeding. It is moistened with sterile sodium chloride solution or thrombin solution and may then be left in place following closure of a surgical incision. It is absorbed in from 4 to 6 weeks.

Application Forms—Prostatectomy Cones; Dental Packs; Sterile Packs; Sterile Sponges; Sterile Compressed Sponges.

Thrombin

Thrombin, Sterile (*Upjohn*); Thrombin, Topical (*Parke-Davis*)

A sterile protein substance prepared from prothrombin of bovine origin through interaction with added thromboplastin in the presence of calcium. It is capable, without the addition of other substances, of causing the clotting of whole blood, plasma, or a solution of fibrinogen. It may contain a suitable antibacterial agent.

Note: Solutions of thrombin should be used within a few hours after preparation, and are not to be injected.

Description—White or grayish, amorphous substance dried from the frozen state.

Uses—Concentrated thrombin has an extraordinarily potent hemostatic or clotting effect on blood. Its powerful coagulant action is employed in coagulating fibrinogen solution. It is also useful for local application to *cuts* or *injuries*. In surgery and in emergency, it is useful for local application in the control of minor oozing. For more extensive or inaccessible *hemorrhage*, a matrix must be applied to hold the thrombin in place and provide a structure for clot formation. Such a matrix is provided by various products, including fibrin foam, gelatin sponge, etc. It is ineffective in arterial bleeding. It is used orally to arrest gastrointestinal bleeding.

Dose—*Topical*, as a powder or as a solution containing 100 to 2000 NIH units/mL in 0.9% sodium chloride solution or sterile water. In gastrointestinal hemorrhage it may be administered in phosphate buffer after aspiration of the gastric contents, or in milk after a supposedly buffering quantity of milk (1 to 2 oz! which will hardly affect the pH); 10,000 to 20,000 units suspended in 2 oz of buffer or milk and ingested, 3 times a day for 4 or 5 days.

Dosage Forms—Powder: 1000, 5000, 10,000, and 20,000 units.

Zinc Acetate—page 779.

Other Hemostatics and Styptics

Carbazochrome Salicylate [Adrenosem Salicylate (*Beecham*)]—An adrenochrome monosemicarbazone (3-hydroxy-1-methyl-5,6-indolinedione-5-semicarbazone) sodium salicylate complex [25512-32-7] $C_{10}H_{12}N_4O_3 \cdot C_7H_5NaO_3$ (396.35) occurring as an orange-red powder; soluble in water. *Uses:* Proposed for systemic control of capillary bleeding of various types. Its clinical usefulness for this purpose is scientifically unjustified. Stinging may occur at the site of injection. *Dose: Intramuscular, adults* and *children over 12 yr of age*, preoperatively for prophylaxis, 10 mg the night before surgery and 10 mg with the on-call medication; postoperatively, 5 mg every 2 hr if patient has been premedicated as above or 10 mg otherwise; *children under 12 yr*, 5 mg the night before, 5 mg on-call, and 5 mg every 2 hr thereafter. *Oral*, same as intramuscular, except used only for postoperative medication.

Collagen, Microfibrillar [Avitene]—A preparation of animal origin of the polypeptide substance occurring as the main constituent of skin, connective tissue, and the organic substance of bones. *Uses:* Platelets naturally adhere to collagen and are stimulated to release substances that promote further aggregation. Microfibrillar collagen is used to arrest bleeding, especially during surgery. It usually stops capillary bleeding in 1 min, "brisk" bleeding in 4 to 5 min, and oozing from bone in 5 to 10 min. The collagen is absorbed in less than 84 days. It may cause mild, chronic inflammation at the site of application, probably as the result of slight contamination by bovine albumin. It does not interfere with regeneration of bone. Spillage on nonbleeding surfaces should be avoided because it may cause adhesions. *Application:* 1 g per 50 cm² of previously dried surface. Handle with forceps, as it is adhesive. *Dosage Forms:* Fibrous: 1 and 5 g; Web: 70 × 70 × 1 mm and 70 × 35 × 1 mm sterile blister packs.

Gelatin Powder, Absorbable—Sterile gelatin powder is used to arrest bleeding or weeping from chronic leg ulcers, decubitus ulcers, or other oozing lesions. It is also used to stimulate formation of granulation tissue in open sores or wounds. In nonsterile form it is used to arrest gastrointestinal hemorrhage. *Dose: Topical*, as powder, covered with a dressing and left in place for 7 days, at which time loose (not adherent) gelatin is removed and replaced by fresh powder. *Oral*, initially 10 g mixed with 2 oz of milk followed by 50 mL of thrombin solution (5 units/mL) at 2-hr intervals during the first 3 or 4 days, then 5 g per dose thereafter.

Negatol [Negatan (*Savage*)]—A relatively high molecular weight copolymer of formaldehyde and metacresol sulfonic acid. There are 6 components. Soluble in water. Acidic, a 5% solution having pH = 1. *Uses:* Combines with various proteins. In the vagina it coagulates cervical mucous, which tends to arrest bleeding from capillaries and small arterioles. Used as a styptic to control bleeding from the vagina, cervix and vulva. It is irritant to the eyes, mucous membranes and abraded skin. It may cause burning, erythema and desquamation; treatment is lavage. Local hypersensitivity sometimes occurs. It soils and attacks clothing so that a perineal pad should be worn. *Dose: Topical*, initially as a 4.5% solution (1:10 dilution), to be increased if necessary. *Dosage Form:* Solution: 45%.

Electrolytes and Systemic Buffers

The concentration of several of the electrolytes in the plasma is critical for proper functioning of cells, especially those of the excitable tissues. The proper balance of the several ions is complex; it depends not only on the concentration in the extracellular fluid (of which plasma is one compartment) but also on the intracellular concentration, the ratio across the cell membrane being an essential factor, and on the ratio of one ion type to another. Thus, plasma electrolyte concentrations provide only a crude clue to the electrolyte status of the patient, and balance or other ancillary studies are often necessary to determine the true electrolyte needs. Certain electrolytes, for example calcium and phosphate, serve also as structural elements in hard tissues (bone, teeth, etc.) and may be employed for that purpose.

Several of the phosphates described in this section are often used not to add an electrolyte but rather to remove calcium from blood in hypercalcemia and to prevent and even dissolve calcific kidney stones.

Calcium Chloride

Calcium chloride, dihydrate [10035-04-8] $CaCl_2 \cdot 2H_2O$ (147.02); *anhydrous* [10043-52-4] (110.99).

Preparation—By saturating HCl with chalk or marble, then adding calcium hydroxide to alkalinity and boiling, which precipitates magnesium, iron, and other metals. After filtering, the filtrate is neutralized with HCl and evaporated until it contains about 24% of water.

Description—White, hard, odorless fragments or granules; deliquescent.

Solubility—1 g in 0.7 mL water; 4 mL alcohol.

Uses—Calcium chloride provides calcium ions in the treatment of hypocalcemic tetany. For this purpose, 5 to 20 mL of 5% solution is given by slow intravenous injection. It is also given during exchange transfusions, in order to repair the calcium deficit in citrated blood; calcium gluceptate is preferred for this use. Calcium chloride is also *antispasmodic* to smooth muscle and is effective in relieving the abdominal pain and diarrhea of *intestinal tuberculosis* and *lead colic;* for this purpose it is given orally, a neutral salt being preferred. It stimulates cardiac automaticity and contractility and is used in *cardiac resuscitation.*

Calcium chloride is a specific antidote in cases of *magnesium poisoning.* It is also used in the treatment of *hyperkalemia,* since it antagonizes the cardiac effects of potassium.

As an *electrolyte replenisher* calcium chloride is a pharmaceutical necessity for *Ringer's Injection, Lactated Ringer's Injection,* and *Ringer's Solution.*

Side effects result from too rapid injection; these include vasodilation and a burning sensation in the skin. Overdosage can cause hypercalcemia. Because of the danger of overdosage, calcium chloride is contraindicated in renal insufficiency, even if hypocalcemia exists. It should be given cautiously to the digitalized patient, and the electrocardiogram should be monitored. Extravasation can cause tissue necrosis.

Other calcium salts are preferred to calcium chloride.

Dose (as dihydrate)—*Intravenous, adults,* **6.8 to 13.6 mEq** (500 mg to 1 g) at a rate not to exceed 0.5 to 1 mL of 10% solution/min, repeated at intervals of 1 to 3 days, if necessary; *children* (rarely), **1.02 mEq** (75 mg) per kg of body weight (or 27.2 mEq or 2 g per m^2 of body surface) as a solution containing 2.72 mEq/100 mL (2%) 4 times a day. *Intracardiac* (into ventricle), **200 to 800 mg.**

Dosage Forms (as dihydrate)—Injection: 50 and 100 mg/mL.

Calcium Gluceptate

D-*glycero*-D-*gulo*-Heptonic acid, calcium salt (2:1); Calcium
Gluceptate (*Lilly; Abbott*)

$$\left[HOCH_2-\overset{H}{\underset{OH}{C}}-\overset{H}{\underset{OH}{C}}-\overset{OH}{\underset{H}{C}}-\overset{H}{\underset{OH}{C}}-\overset{H}{C}-COO- \right]_2 Ca$$

Calcium D-*glycero*-D-*gulo*-heptonate (1:2) [17140-60-2] $C_{14}H_{26}CaO_{16}$ (490.43); *hydrate* [56348-83-5] (508.45).

Preparation—From sodium glucoheptonate, US Pat 3,033,900.

Uses—To provide calcium ions when rapid availability is required. The clinical conditions in which calcium is required are stated under *Calcium Chloride.* Calcium gluceptate is even less irritating than *Calcium Gluconate,* so that it is preferred when intramuscular administration is required, as in neonatal tetany. Many authorities also prefer the gluceptate to the gluconate for intravenous injection, but, once symptoms are controlled, maintenance is usually achieved with calcium gluconate given by intravenous infusion. The duration of action after intravenous administration is 2 to 3 hours and after intramuscular injection, 1 to 4 hours.

After rapid intravenous injection there may be tingling sensations and a chalky taste. The effects of overdoses, precautions, and drug interactions are those of *Calcium Chloride.* Mild local reactions may occur at the site of injection, but abscesses apparently do not occur.

Dose (calcium equivalent)—*Intravenous, adults,* **4.5 to 18 mEq** (90 to 360 mg) to be given at a rate not to exceed 0.23 mEq/min (0.26 mL/min of a solution containing 0.9 mEq/mL or 18 mg of calcium/mL); more may be given, if necessary to control symptoms; *neonates,* in exchange transfusion, **0.45 mEq** (9 mg) after each 100 mL of blood exchanged. *Intramuscular, adults* and *children,* **1.8 to 4.5 mEq** (36 to 90 mg) into the buttocks or lateral thigh; *infants,* **1.8 to 4.5 mEq** (36 to 90 mg) into several sites in the lateral aspect of the thigh.

Dosage Form (calcium equivalent)—Injection: 4.5 mEq (90 mg)/5 mL. (4.5 mEq of calcium is equivalent to 90 mg of calcium or 1.1 g of calcium gluceptate monohydrate.)

Calcium Gluconate

D-Gluconic acid, calcium salt (2:1); (*Various Mfrs*)

$$\left[HOCH_2-\overset{H}{\underset{OH}{C}}-\overset{H}{\underset{OH}{C}}-\overset{OH}{\underset{H}{C}}-\overset{H}{\underset{OH}{C}}-COO- \right]_2 Ca$$

Calcium gluconate (1:2) [299-28-5] $C_{12}H_{22}CaO_{14}$ (430.38).

Preparation—D-Glucose is oxidized to gluconic acid in the presence of calcium carbonate. The oxidation may be effected by certain molds, eg, *Aspergillus niger,* or by bromine.

Description—White, crystalline granules or powder, without odor or taste. It is stable in air and does not lose its water on drying without undergoing decomposition. Its solutions are neutral to litmus paper. It is decomposed by dilute mineral acids into gluconic acid and the calcium salt of the mineral acid used.

Solubility—1 g slowly in about 30 mL water and about 5 mL boiling water; insoluble in alcohol and many other organic solvents.

Uses—A source of calcium ion in the treatment of *hypocalcemic tetany* or *hyperkalemia.* It is less irritating than calcium chloride and may be given orally or by intramuscular or intravenous injection. However, intramuscular injection may cause abscesses. Calcium gluconate is usually considered to be the calcium salt of choice for intravenous use.

Dose—*Intravenous, adults,* usually **2.25 to 9 mEq** (1 g), to be injected at a rate not to exceed 0.23 mEq/min (0.5 mL of 10% solution/min), at intervals of 1.5 hr to 3 days, if necessary; as little as 4.5 mEq/week may be sometimes sufficient and as much as 67.5 mEq/day necessary; *children,* usually **0.575 mEq** (125 mg) per kg or 13.8 mEq (3 g) per m^2 of body surface, given in diluted form over a period of no less than 20 min, 4 times a day. *Oral, adults,* **2.25 to 4.5 mEq** (500 mg to 1 g) 3 or more times a day; *children,* **0.575 mEq** (125 mg)/kg or **13.8 mEq** (3 g) per m^2 3 or more times a day.

Dosage Forms—Injection: 0.45 mEq (0.1 g)/mL; Powder: 120 g and 1 lb. Tablets: 1.25, 3, and 4.5 mEq (500, 650, and 1000 mg).

Calcium Lactate

Propanoic acid, 2-hydroxy-, calcium salt (2:1), hydrate

$$\left[\overset{CH_3 CHCOO-}{\underset{OH}{}} \right]_2 Ca \cdot x H_2O$$

Calcium lactate (1:2) hydrate [41372-22-9] $C_6H_{10}CaO_6.xH_2O$; *anhydrous* [814-80-2] (218.22); *pentahydrate* (308.30).

Preparation—By fermenting hydrolyzed starch with a suitable mold in the presence of calcium carbonate, and purifying until the product meets USP purity requirements. It is also obtained, now in decreasing quantities, by fermentation of the mother liquors resulting from the production of milk sugar.

Description—White, almost odorless powder or granules, somewhat efflorescent; it becomes anhydrous at 120°. Aqueous solutions are prone to become moldy.

Solubility—1 g in about 20 mL water; practically insoluble in alcohol.

Uses—An excellent source of calcium ion in the oral treatment of *calcium deficiency.* It causes less gastrointestinal irritation than does calcium chloride.

Dose (as pentahydrate)—*Oral, adults,* **2.11 to 33.8 mEq** (325 mg to 5.2 g) 3 times a day with meals; children, **1.14 mEq** (175 mg)/**kg** body weight or **19.4 mEq** (or 3 g)/m^2 of body surface up to 4 times a day.

Dosage Forms (as pentahydrate)—Powder: 1 lb; Tablets: 325 and 650 mg (2.11 and 4.22 mEq).

Calcium Levulinate

Pentanoic acid, 4-oxo-, calcium salt (2:1), dihydrate; (*Various Mfrs*)

$$\left[CH_3COCH_2CH_2COO- \right]_2 Ca \cdot 2H_2O$$

Calcium levulinate (1:2) dihydrate [5743-49-7] $C_{10}H_{14}CaO_6.2H_2O$ (306.33); *anhydrous* [591-64-0] (270.30).

Preparation—From levulinic acid and calcium carbonate. The acid may be obtained from crude cellulose and as a by-product in manufacture of furfural. *Ind Eng Chem 48:* 1331, 1956.

Description—White, crystalline or amorphous powder having a faint odor suggestive of burnt sugar; bitter, salty taste.

Solubility—Freely soluble in water, slightly soluble in alcohol; insoluble in ether and chloroform.

Uses—Calcium levulinate is much like *Calcium Glucepteate* in that it is less irritating than calcium gluconate. The side effects are also essentially the same. The effects of overdoses, precautions, and drug interactions are those of *Calcium Chloride*.

Dose (as dihydrate)—*Intravenous*, *adults*, **1 g** (6.5 mEq) once a day; *children*, **0.2** to **0.5 g** (1.3 to 3.25 mEq) once a day.

Dosage Form (as dihydrate)—Injection: 100 mg (0.65 mEq)/mL.

Dibasic Calcium Phosphate

Phosphoric acid, calcium salt (1:1); Dicalcium Orthophosphate;
(*Various Mfrs*)

Calcium phosphate (1:1) anhydrous [7757-93-9] $CaHPO_4$ (136.06); *dihydrate* [7789-77-7] (172.09).

Preparation—A phosphate mineral, eg, *apatite*, or preferably ignited animal bone, is decomposed with H_2SO_4, resulting in the production of phosphoric acid and calcium sulfate. After filtering off the calcium sulfate, the proper quantity of calcium hydroxide is added to form dibasic calcium phosphate.

It may also be prepared from animal bones as described under the preparation of *Tribasic Calcium Phosphate*, using only sufficient calcium hydroxide to form the dibasic salt.

Description—White, odorless, tasteless powder; stable in air; aqueous suspension is neutral to litmus.

Solubility—Practically insoluble in water; readily soluble in diluted hydrochloric and nitric acids; insoluble in alcohol.

Uses—An excellent *source of calcium* and *phosphorus* during pregnancy, lactation, or mild to moderate *hypocalcemia* characterized by a low degree of tetany. Because of the phosphate content, it is contraindicated in hypoparathyroidism. If the tetany is severe, intravenous calcium medication is administered. See *Calcium Chloride*, *Calcium Gluconate*, *Calcium Glucepteate*, or *Calcium Levulinate*.

Dose (as dihydrate)—*Oral*, *adults*, **500 mg** to **1.5 g** (5.8 to 17.4 mEq) 2 or 3 times a day with meals; *children*, **125 mg** (1.45 mEq)/**kg** of body weight up to 4 times a day. The calcium is better absorbed if taken in small doses at frequent intervals.

Dosage Form (as dihydrate)—Powder: 1 lb; Tablets: 500 mg (5.8 mEq).

Magnesium Sulfate Injection—page 1078.

Potassium Chloride

Potassium chloride [7447-40-7] KCl (74.55).

Preparation—Occurs in sea water and in many mineral springs. Formerly it was largely imported from Germany where it is mined at Stassfurt, occurring there as *carnallite* [$KCl.MgCl_2.6H_2O$] and as *sylvite* [KCl]. It is now obtained from the Searles Lake deposit in the Mojäve Desert of southern California and from deposits of carnallite and sylvite in New Mexico and Texas. Another source of potassium chloride is the Dead Sea, where considerable quantities are found as dissolved carnallite. This double salt, in aqueous solution, is treated with live steam, the two separate salts form, and the less soluble salt, potassium chloride, crystallizes out as the solution cools. In the laboratory it may be prepared from potassium carbonate or bicarbonate and HCl.

Description—Colorless, elongated, prismatic, or cubical crystals, or as a white granular powder; odorless, has a saline taste, and is stable in air; pH (aqueous solution) about 7.

Solubility—1 g in 2.8 mL water at 25° and about 2 mL boiling water; insoluble in alcohol.

Uses—The salt most frequently employed when the action of potassium cation is desired. It is used when *hypokalemia* or *hypochloremic alkalosis* exists, as after prolonged diarrhea or vomiting or consequent to adrenal steroid therapy or treatment with certain diuretics, especially the thiazides. It is also used when it is desired to elevate normal plasma potassium levels, as in the treatment of digitalis intoxication. It may be used as a diuretic. Potassium chloride is also of value for the relief of the symptoms of *hypokalemic periodic paralysis*, a rare disease characterized by recurrent attacks of muscular weakness. Potassium salts have also been found to relieve the symptoms of *Ménière's disease*. Potassium chloride is an ingredient of *Lactated Potassic Saline Injection*, *Ringer's Solution*, *Lactated Ringer's Injection*, and *Ringer's Injection*.

Potassium chloride is irritant to the gastrointestinal tract: oral preparations may cause nausea, vomiting, epigastric distress, abdominal discomfort, and diarrhea. High local concentrations in the gastrointestinal tract can lead to ulceration. Esophageal ulceration may occur if there is dysphagia and gastric ulceration, especially if gastric emptying is delayed. Enteric coating lessens the incidence of such side effects but favors development of small bowel lesions, especially when thiazides are concurrently used. Potassium chloride in a wax matrix has been promoted as a safe form, but esophageal, gastric, and small bowel ulcerations nevertheless occasionally occur. It is best to avoid solid forms; if they are used, they should be taken with one or more full glasses of water. Overdoses may cause paresthesias, generalized weakness, flaccid paralysis, listlessness, vertigo, mental confusion, hypotension, cardiac arrhythmias, and heart block. Death may ensue. Signs of toxicity may occur even with apparently normal blood levels; consequently the signs must be frequently monitored, and ambulatory patients must be apprised of premonitory symptoms. Most patients can be managed adequately and more safely with foods high in potassium and low in sodium (fruits, especially dried, and cereals).

Potassium chloride must be administered cautiously in the presence of heart or renal disease. It is contraindicated in untreated Addison's disease, heat cramps, adynamia episodica hereditaria, acute dehydration, and hyperkalemia from any cause.

Dose—*Oral*, *adults*, **20** to **40 mEq** (1.44 to 2.98 g) a day to *prevent depletion* and **40** to **100 mEq** (2.98 to 7.55 g) a day for *replacement*, in 3 or 4 divided doses; *children*, **1** to **3 mEq** (75 to 225 mg)/**per kg** (or 15 to 40 mEq/m² of body surface) per day in several divided doses. Doses may be higher or lower, as indicated by serum potassium levels. The oral solution should be diluted, such that each 20 mEq is contained in at least 90 mL of water or juice. Enteric-coated and wax-matrix tablets and extend-release capsules are not recommended for children; however, effervescent tablets can be used. *Intravenous infusion*, *adults*, when plasma potassium is above 2.5 mEq/L, at a rate not to exceed **10 mEq** (750 mg)/*hour* and a total dose not to exceed **200 mEq**/*day*; when plasma potassium is less than 2 mEq/L and the clinical condition is serious, **40 mEq** (3 g)/*hour* may be given, up to a total daily dose of **400 mEq**. For the slower rate of infusion, a 30 mEq/L (0.25%) solution is recommended, and for the faster rate of infusion, 60 mEq/L (0.5%). *Children*, **up to 3 mEq/kg** (or 40 mEq/m² of body surface) per day; volume of solution should be proportional to body size.

Dosage Forms—Extended-Release Capsules: 8 mEq (600 mg); Injection: 0.67, 1, 1.5, 2, 3, and 3.2 mEq/mL; Oral Powder (for oral solution): 15, 20, and 25 mEq/packet; Oral Solution: 0.67, 1.34, 2, and 2.66 mEq/mL (5, 10, 15, and 20%, respectively); Effervescent Tablets: 20, 25, and 50 mEq; Enteric-Coated Tablets: 4, and 13.4 mEq (325, and 1000 mg, respectively); Wax-Matrix Tablets: and 8 and 10 mEq (600 and 750 mg, respectively).

Dibasic Potassium Phosphate

Potassium phosphate dibasic [7758-11-4] K_2HPO_4 (174.18).

Preparation—By partial neutralization of phosphoric acid with potassium hydroxide or carbonate.

Description—A hygroscopic granular powder. A 5% aqueous solution has a pH of about 8.5.

Solubility—Very soluble in water.

Uses—In the body, $HPO_4{}^{2-}$ anion interacts with calcium ion in a way that favors the deposition of both calcium and phosphate in bone salts and in other tissue depots. Some of the phosphate is also converted to pyrophosphate, which is a chelator of calcium, the calcium-pyrophosphate complex being excreted in the urine. Furthermore, high plasma phosphate levels decrease calcitriol levels and thus decrease absorption of calcium. Thus $KHPO_4$ causes all of redistribution from plasma to tissue, decorporation and diminished incorporation of calcium. Its principal use is in the treatment of *hypercalcemia*. It is not used alone as a source of phosphate in phosphate deficiency. It is a component of *Potassium Phosphates* (page 837), *Potassium and Sodium Phosphates* (page 837) and *Dibasic Potassium and Sodium Phosphates* (page 837). It is also a reagent and pharmaceutical necessity for various buffers and parenteral fluids. It is no longer used as a laxative; it may cause diarrhea by the oral route. See *Monobasic Potassium Phosphate* (below) for other adverse effects.

Dose—*Oral, adults*, for *hypercalcemia*. **8 to 16 mmol** (250 to 500 mg of P) 4 times a day, after meals and at bedtime.

Dosage Forms—Tablets: extemporaneous.

Monobasic Potassium Phosphate

Potassium phosphate monobasic [7778-77-0] K₂HPO₄ (136.09).

Preparation—See the dibasic salt, above.

Solubility—One gram dissolves in about 5 mL of water. A 5% aqueous solution has a pH of about 5.

Uses—See *Dibasic Potassium Phosphate* (above) for actions to decrease calcium absorption, depress calcium levels in plasma, and enhance calcium excretion as pyrophosphate complex. The dibasic salt is likewise used to treat *hypercalcemia*. It is also used to treat *nephrolithiasis* when the stones are calcific. In this, the decrease in free calcium excretion into the urine decreases stone formation and acidification of the urine (H₂PO₄⁻ causes *acidosis*) and free pyrophosphate ion favor dissolution of stones. KH₂PO₄ is a component of *Potassium Phosphates* (page 837), *Monobasic Potassium and Sodium Phosphates* (page 837), *Potassium and Sodium Phosphates* (page 837), *Potassium and Sodium Phosphates* (page 837), *Potassium and Sodium Phosphates*) (page 837), and a pharmaceutical necessity for various parenteral fluids and buffers.

Adverse effects are diarrhea by the oral route (it is poorly absorbed orally and acts as an osmotic cathartic), hypocalcemia (paresthesias, confusion, weakness, muscle cramps, dyspnea, irregular heartbeat) when employed vigorously in nonhypercalcemic patients, and the passing of loosened kidney stones.

Dose—*Oral, adults*, for *hypercalcemia*, **8 to 16 mmol** (250 to 500 mg of P) 4 times a day, with meals and at bedtime; for *urolithiasis*, **7.4 mmol** (1 g of salt; 228 mg of P) 4 times a day, with meals and at bedtime. Because of the acidity, the dose must be diluted with 180 to 240 mL of water.

Dosage Form—Tablets: 3.7 mmol (500 mg of salt; 124 mg P).

Ringer's Injection—page 822.

Lactated Ringer's Injection—page 822.

Sodium Bicarbonate—page 796.

Sodium Chloride

Salt; Table Salt; Rock Salt; Sea Salt

Sodium chloride [7647-14-5] NaCl (58.44). It contains no added substance.

Preparation—Common salt is widely distributed over the world, and may be obtained by mining, as rock salt, by evaporating a purified solution of saline deposits, or by evaporating sea water, and purifying afterward. If free from contaminating salts, it is not hygroscopic.

Description—Colorless, cubic crystals, or a white crystalline powder; odorless and has a saline taste; the solution is practically neutral. A 23% solution in water freezes at −20°.

Solubility—1 g in 2.8 mL water, 10 mL glycerin, 2.7 mL boiling water; slightly soluble in alcohol.

Uses—Solutions of sodium chloride more closely approximate the composition of the extracellular fluid of the body than solutions of any other single salt. For example, more than 90% of the cation of the extracellular fluid is sodium, more than 60% of the anion is chloride. Furthermore, a 0.9% solution of sodium chloride has approximately the same osmotic pressure as body fluids, ie, is isotonic with body fluids. Thus, an isotonic sodium chloride solution (injection) can be injected without affecting the osmotic pressure of the body fluids and without causing any appreciable distortion in chemical composition. An isotonic solution of sodium chloride is therefore the choice as a vehicle for many drugs which have to be administered parenterally. Sodium Chloride 0.9% Injection is widely used as a substitute for plasma in *volume expansion*, most practitioners preferring it to a dextran because it not only is free of allergenicity but also increases the flow of lymph. The solution has the added advantage of being nonirritating to tissue. Isotonic solutions of sodium chloride may be used as an enema or applied topically to intact or exposed tissues for purposes of irrigation, to keep tissues moist or to keep a cavity flushed, as in irrigation of the urinary bladder; for this purpose 0.45 or 0.9% *Sodium Chloride Irrigation* is used. The irrigation is sterile but not pyrogen-free and should not be injected parenterally. Hypertonic solutions (2 or 5%) may be applied to the cornea, to diminish corneal edema in inflammation or chemosis. Hypertonic solutions (20%) are also injected into the amniotic fluid to cause abortion; since accidental intravenous injection can cause shock, pneumonia, fever, and other adverse effects, this procedure should be performed only if an intensive care unit is available.

Sodium chloride injection is also used as an *electrolyte replenisher* for maintenance or replacement of deficits of extracellular fluid. Since the solution is potentially capable of producing metabolic acidosis (by diluting bicarbonate ion) and does not supply all major cations of the extracellular fluid, other solutions, such as lactated Ringer's injection, may be preferred if large volumes of fluids are to be administered. Other solutions of appropriate composition must also be employed if the composition of the extracellular fluid is markedly distorted. Sterile, pyrogen-free solutions are administered, usually intravenously. In persons who are unable to take fluids by mouth, a hypotonic sodium chloride injection (0.45%) may be used as a source of water, but hypotonic balanced electrolyte solutions with dextrose are usually preferred. In patients in which a salt deficit exists disproportionately to dehydration, a hypertonic sodium chloride injection (3 or 5%) may be used, preferably in conjunction with sodium bicarbonate.

Sodium chloride is administered orally for the prevention of *heat cramps* (miner's cramps, low-sodium syndrome) caused by the depletion of sodium salts through copious perspiration. It is common to use tablets, but a beverage containing only 0.5% of sodium chloride will prevent development of the symptoms. This salt is also given in adrenal cortical insufficiency (*Addison's Disease*) where it decreases the requirement for adrenal cortical extract. It is also used in the treatment of hypercalcemia, to increase glomerular filtration and consequent excretion of calcium.

Common salt is used as a preservative; 6% or more prevents the growth of *Cl. botulinum* and other pathogens.

Overdosage may cause pulmonary edema, generalized edema, hypernatremia (characterized by diarrhea, muscle twitching, hyperreactivity, confusion, stupor, convulsions or coma), and occasionally cellular dehydration. Sodium chloride must be used cautiously in patients with cardiac or renal impairment or hypoproteinemia.

Dose—*Oral*, **17.1 to 34.2 mEq** (1 to 2 g) 3 times a day. *Intravenous infusion*, variable, according to the weight of the patient, clinical situation, the plasma electrolyte concentration, and the intake-output balance, but usually about 1 L of 0.9% injection (154 mEq), except when the plasma is hypotonic, in which case a 3 to 5% injection may be given at a rate not to exceed 100 mL/hr. *Topically*, usually as **0.9%** solution, but 0.45 or 0.9% for bladder irrigation and 2 or 5% with added oncotic substances for corneal turgescense. *Rectal*, as *enema*, **0.9%** solution. *Intraamniotic*, **200 to 250 mL** of 20% sterile solution.

Dosage Forms—Injection (0.9%): 100, 150, 250, 500, and 1000 mL; Injection (0.45%): 100, 500, and 1000 mL; Injection (3%): 500 mL; Injection (5%), 500 mL; Injection (20%): 250 mL; Injection for Admixtures (0.9%): 50, 100, 400 mEq; Injection for Diluents (0.9%): 5, 10, 20, 30, 50, and 100 mL; Irrigation (0.9%): 250, 500, 1500, 2000 and 3000 mL; Irrigation (0.45%): 1000 and 2000 mL; Ophthalmic Solution: 2 or 5%; Tablets: 450, 455, 600, 650 mg, and 1 and 2.25 g; Enteric-Coated Tablets: 1 g; Sustained-Release Tablets, 600 mg; various tablets containing NaCl in combination with dextrose, CaCO₃, Ca₃(PO₄)₂, MgCO₃ or KCl.

Sodium Lactate Injection

Propanoic acid, 2-hydroxy-, monosodium salt

CH₃CH(OH)COONa

Monosodium lactate [72-17-3] C₃H₅NaO₃ (112.06); a sterile solution of lactic acid (C₃H₆O₃) in water for injection prepared with the aid of NaOH.

Note—Sterilize sodium lactate injection preferably by steam under pressure.

Preparation—A weighed quantity of lactic acid, sufficient to yield the desired amount of sodium lactate, is diluted with water for injection. A volume of assayed concentrated NaOH solution, equivalent to the quantity of lactic acid, is added and the mixture gently boiled until all the lactic anhydride also has been converted into sodium lactate. After quickly cooling, the solution is diluted with water for injection to the proper volume, promptly filtered if necessary, ampuled, and sterilized.

Description—pH, diluted if necessary to about 0.16 M (20 mg/mL), between 6.0 and 7.3.

Uses—Sodium lactate is employed as a substitute for sodium bicarbonate in solutions for *parenteral fluid* and *electrolyte therapy*. Since lactate ion is generally rapidly metabolized in the body, sodium lactate is a potential source of fixed cation for correction of metabolic *acidosis*. However, in shock, severe liver disease, and various other hyperlactic acidemic states lactate oxidation is impaired, and the compound is contraindicated. In persons with normal cellular oxidative capacity, lactate will be converted to bicarbonate in 1 to 2 hr. An advantage of sodium lactate over sodium bicarbonate is that its solutions may be sterilized by boiling. Sodium lactate is also used to accelerate the heart in hypopotassemia.

Dose—*Intravenous infusion, adults*, **500 to 1000 mL** of **0.167 M** solution (equivalent to 140 to 180 mL of 5% $NaHCO_3$ solution), the dose varying according to the clinical condition of the patient, the laboratory evaluation, and the response. It is given at a rate no faster than 300 mL/hr. For antagonizing the cardiac effects of hypopotassemia, 100 mL of 1 molar solution is given in 2 to 5 min, after which infusion is continued at a rate of 2 to 5 mL/min until the desired effect is achieved.

Dosage Forms—0.167 M solution in 150-, 150-, and 1000-mL containers; 2.5 M solution in 20-mL containers; 4 M solution in 500- and 1000-mL containers.

Dibasic Sodium Phosphate—page 804.

Monobasic Sodium Phosphate

Phosphoric acid, monosodium salt, monohydrate; Sodium Acid Phosphate; Sodium Dihydrogen Phosphate; Monosodium Orthophosphate; Monobasic Sodium Phosphate
Monosodium phosphate monohydrate [10049-21-5] $NaH_2PO_4.H_2O$ (137.99); *anhydrous* [7558-80-7] (119.98).

Preparation—By adding phosphoric acid to a hot concentrated solution of disodium phosphate until the liquid ceases to give a precipitate with barium chloride. The solution is then concentrated to the crystallization point.

Description—Colorless crystals or a white, crystalline powder; odorless and slightly deliquescent; solutions are acid to litmus and effervesce with sodium carbonate.

Solubility—Freely soluble in water; practically insoluble in alcohol.

Incompatibilities—Since sodium biphosphate is an acid salt, it is incompatible with *carbonate* and *alkalies* in general. In solution with *methenamine* it causes a slow evolution of formaldehyde.

Uses—The actions, therapeutic uses, and adverse effects are those of *Monobasic Potassium Phosphate* (page 1316). In addition, it is used as a source of phosphorus in *hypophosphatemia* and *nutrition*. It is a pharmaceutical necessity for *Sodium Phosphates Injection* (below). Sodium *Phosphates Oral Solution* (page 804), *Monobasic Potassium and Sodium Phosphates* (page 837), and *Potassium and Sodium Phosphates* (page 837), various parenteral and topical solutions, enemas, and buffers. Additional adverse effects are those of sodium (hypertension, edema in heart failure, ascites in hepatic dysfunction, etc).

Dose—*Oral, adults, hypercalcemia*, 8 to **16 mmol** (250 to 500 mg of P) 4 times a day, after meals and at bedtime.

Sodium Phosphates Injection

The usually available injection contains 276 mg (2 millimoles) of monobasic sodium phosphate ($NaH_2PO_4.H_2O$) and 142 mg (1 millimole) of dibasic sodium phosphate (Na_2HPO_4) per mL, equivalent to a total of 93 mg (3 millimoles) of phosphorus.

Uses—Sodium phosphates injection may be used as a source of phosphorus for *replacement* in phosphorus-depleted patients. It can also be used to treat *hypercalcemia*, since elevated plasma levels of phosphate promote deposition of calcium in bone salts and also loss in urine. The injection should be diluted before use and should be infused slowly to avoid phosphate intoxication. The patient should be monitored for serum levels of calcium, phosphorus, and sodium, and for renal function at frequent intervals. Concurrent administration with thiazides may cause renal damage. Each mL of the injection described above represents 92 mg (4 mEq) of sodium, which should be taken into consideration in use of the injection in patients on sodium restriction.

Dose (phosphorus equivalent)—*Intravenous infusion, adults, usual*, for *replacement*, **10 to 15 mmol** (310 to 465 mg of phosphorus) once a day; for *hypercalcemia*, **100 mmol** (3.1 g of phosphorus) per day as needed; infusion should be slow, over a period of 6 to 8 hr.

Tromethamine

1,3-Propanediol, 2-amino-2-(hydroxymethyl)-, Tham-E (*Abbott*)

$$
\begin{array}{c}
CH_2OH \\
| \\
HOCH_2CCH_2OH \\
| \\
NH_2
\end{array}
$$

2-Amino-2-(hydroxymethyl)-1,3-propanediol [77-86-1] $C_4H_{11}NO_3$ (121.14).

Preparation—Nitromethane is additively reacted with formaldehyde to yield tris(hydroxymethyl)nitromethane, and the nitro compound is then hydrogenated with the aid of Raney nickel. US Pat 2,174,242.

Description—White, crystalline powder with a slight, characteristic odor and a faint, sweet, soapy taste; stable in light and air; melts between 168° and 172°; pH (1 in 20 solution) between 10.0 and 11.5.

Solubility—1 g in 1.8 mL water, 46 mL alcohol, >10,000 mL chloroform.

Uses—A weak amine base with a pK_b of 7.8 at body temperature. This is close to plasma pH (7.4), so that the compound is well suited to the preparation of a buffer mixture for controlling extracellular pH. Furthermore, at pH 7.4 it is 30% un-ionized and hence it gradually penetrates cells, where it may also buffer the intracellular contents. Tromethamine can react with any proton donor, and the notion that it reacts primarily with carbonic acid or carbon dioxide is erroneous. By removing protons from hydronium ions, ionization of carbonic acid is shifted so as to decrease pCO_2 and to increase bicarbonate. The excess bicarbonate is then gradually excreted in the kidney. This is an especially useful way to manage excessively high pCO_2 in *respiratory acidosis* (respiratory distress syndrome, asphyxia neonatorum, status asthmaticus, chronic respiratory insufficiency, drug intoxication, etc), in which pulmonary ventilation is inadequate. However, tromethamine is equally useful in the management of *metabolic acidosis* (drug intoxications, cardiac surgery, diabetic acidosis, etc), especially when the intracellular pH is low, since it readily penetrates cells. It is used to prevent acidosis in cardiac bypass surgery, and it may be used in conjunction with other drugs in the treatment of cardiac arrest. Ionized tromethamine is excreted by the kidney, so that the effect is that of excretion of hydrogen ions. Elimination of the drug from the body is entirely by renal excretion. Excretion of tromethammonium ion is accompanied by osmotic diuresis, since clinical doses of the drug considerably add to the osmolarity of the glomerular filtrate. The drug should be used cautiously in renal disease. Tromethamine is also used to buffer blood for transfusions, and it may be added to ACD blood as a buffer for storage purposes.

The principal untoward effects are related to its buffering action, namely that overdoses may cause alkalosis; respiration may be depressed because of the decrease in pCO_2 and increase in pH in plasma. Also, it is locally irritant because of its alkalinity, and a slough may develop at a site of extravasation, and venospasm and thrombosis may also occur. The fact that about 70% remains in extracellular space means that a sufficient amount of water must be given to prevent hyperosmolarity and hence to avoid tissue dehydration and the hemodynamic consequences of an increased blood volume. Plasma hyperosmolarity, in general, causes hepatic and renal damage, and tromethamine is no exception. The hemorrhagic liver necrosis seen frequently in newborn infants treated with the drug may possibly have another origin, perhaps related to the route of administration (umbilical vein). The drug also causes hyperkalemia, hypoglycemia, and may depress the respiratory center, especially in neonates and premature infants.

Dose—*Intravenous*, variable, depending upon the cause of acidosis and the degree of acid-base distortion. The preferred dose is calculated by the formula; mL (of 0.3 M) = body weight in kg × base deficit in mEq/L × 1.1. It is frequently given in a single dose of **2.5 mEq** (300 mg)/**kg** given over a period of not less than 1 hour. Doses of up to **4.1**

mEq (500 mg)/**kg** may be required depending upon the severity and progression of the acidosis.

Dosage Forms—Injection: 0.3 M solution in 500 mL (18 g).

Other Electrolytes

Calcium Glucobionate [(4-O-β-D-Galactopyrosyl-D-gluconato-O^1)-(D-gluconato-O^1) calcium monohydrate, Neo-Calglucon (*Sandoz*) [12569-38-9] $C_{18}H_{32}CaO_{19}.H_2O$ (610.53)]. *Uses:* As a source of calcium, more as a dietary supplement than for the treatment of hypocalcemia. *Dose:* Oral, 5.9 to 17.8 mEq (115 to 345 mg of Ca) 3 times a day with meals. *Dosage Form:* Syrup: 5.9 mEq (115 mg Ca)/5 mL.

Potassium Acetate [127-08-2] $C_2H_3KO_2$ (98.14). *Preparation*—Potassium bicarbonate or carbonate is reacted with acetic acid, previously diluted with water, and the solution is evaporated to dryness. *Description and Solubility:* Colorless, monoclinic crystals or a white, crystalline powder, rapidly deliquescing in moist air; has a saline and slightly alkaline taste; its aqueous solution is alkaline to litmus paper, but does not affect phenolphthalein TS. Soluble 1 g in about 0.5 mL of water, about 3 mL alcohol. *Uses:* Therapeutically as a systemic and urinary *alkalinizer*, and for the effects of the *potassium ion*. The value of potassium acetate in hypokalemia is limited, since the condition is frequently associated with a hypochloremic alkalosis. Consequently, potassium chloride is usually preferred in hypokalemia. Acetate anion is metabolized to bicarbonate. When used orally as an alkalinizer the salt should be liberally diluted with water or fruit juice to avoid gastric distress. Indiscriminate use of potassium acetate or other potassium salts may produce toxic manifestations of hyperkalemia (see *Potassium Chloride*, below). *Dose: Intravenous infusion, adults*, for *hypokalemia*, when plasma potassium is above 2.5 mEq/L, up to 200 mEq per day, given in a concentration of no more than 40 mEq/L at a rate of no more than 10 mEq/hr; when plasma potassium is less than 2.0 mEq/L, up to 400 mEq per day at a rate of no more than 40 mEq/hr; *children*, up to 3 mEq/kg (or 40 mEq/m² of body surface) a day; the volume of fluid should be varied in proportion to body size. *Oral*, **1 g** up to 4 times daily, in solution. *Dosage Forms:* Injection: (not available commercially) 2, 2.5, 3, and 4 mEq/mL are convenient concentrations.

Potassium Gluconate Kaon (*Warren-Teed*) [299-27-4] $C_6H_{11}KO_7$ (234.25). *Preparation:* Glucose may be oxidized to gluconic acid by various processes, eg, electrolytic oxidation of an alkaline solution, reaction with hypobromites, or by fermentation using *Aspergillus niger* or other microorganisms. Neutralization with potassium hydroxide provides the salt. *Description and Solubility:* White to yellowish white, crystalline powder or granules; odorless and has a slightly bitter taste; stable in air; solutions are slightly alkaline to litmus. Soluble 1 g in 3 mL water; practically insoluble in dehydrated alcohol, ether, and chloroform. *Uses:* A source of potassium for management of hypokalemic states, such as occur consequent to adrenocorticosteroid therapy or use of thiazide diuretics, or for deliberate production of hyperkalemia, as for treatment of digitalis intoxication. The gluconate anion supposedly makes the compound better tolerated in the gastrointestinal tract than is potassium chloride. It is also claimed that the potassium of the gluconate is absorbed high in the gastrointestinal tract, above the location where mucosal lesions sometimes occur in combined thiazide–potassium therapy, whereas other salts are not so quickly absorbed. Such faulty suppositions and claims ignore the unavoidable chemical fact that irrespective of the salt used, potassium is completely dissociable and hence is unaffected in its irritant actions and absorption by the anion in the compnound. Sugar-coated potassium gluconate tablets dissolve at a higher level than do enteric-coated tablets of potassium chloride but, by this very fact, are free to cause the irritation for which the chloride tablet was coated. The fact that potassium gluconate may cause nausea, vomiting, diarrhea, and abdominal discomfort shows that the gluconate has no advantage over nonenteric-coated potassium chloride tablets. A full glass of water taken with either greatly reduces the irritant effects of either salt. Hypochloremia is a frequent accompaniment of hypokalemia; in such instances the chloride is definitely preferred. Furthermore, since gluconate metabolizes to bicarbonate, it contributes to alkalosis, which may also be present in hypokalemia. Only in a hypokalemic, hyperchloremic acidosis (as in renal failure, dehydration, and occasional diabetic acidosis) is the drug rational; however, clinical experience indicates no obvious superiority over KCl. The use and toxicity of and contraindications to potassium gluconate are the same as those for *Potassium Chloride*. *Dose: Oral, adults*, 5 to 20 mEq (2.34 to 4.68 g) 2 to 4 times a day, after meals. As the elixir, the dose should be diluted with a glass of water or fruit juice; *children*, 2 to 3 mEq/kg (or 20 to 40 mEq/m² of body surface) per day as the elixir in several divided doses well diluted in water or juice. The tablets are not recommended.

Potassium Mixtures—A number of potassium-containing products are mixtures of: KCl and $KHCO_3$; KCl $KHCO_3$ and K_2CO_3; KCl, $KHCO_3$ and citric acid; KCl $KHCO_3$ and potassium citrate; $KHCO_3$ and citric acid; KCl and potassium gluconate; $KHCO_3$, potassium citrate and potassium acetate; and potassium citrate and potassium gluconate. Those that combine $KHCO_3$ with citric acid are effervescent; some effervescent preparations contain betaine · HCl or lysine · HCl in lieu of or in addition to citric acid. Those that are not constituted for effervescence are intended for their alkalinizing effects in addition to their effects to repair

potassium deficits. $KHCO_3$ and K_2CO_3 are directly alkalotic; potassium acetate, citrate and gluconate all metabolize to $KHCO_3$. Since hypokalemia is usually accompanied by *alkalosis*, there are few situations in which an alkalinizing source of potassium is rational. Examples in which hypokalemia and acidosis co-exist are renal failure, dehydration and sometimes diabetic acidosis. Even in these, clinical experience is that KCl alone seems to be as useful as the combinations.

Potassium Phosphates—A mixture of monobasic and dibasic potassium phosphate in the ratio described under each category below: *Uses:* For actions, uses and adverse effects see *Dibasic Potassium Phosphate* (page 834) and *Monobasic Potassium Phosphate* (page 835). Mainly used for *hypercalcemia* and *hypophosphatemia*. *Dose: Oral, adults*, for *hypercalcemia* 8 or 16 mmol (150 to 500 mg of P), 4 times a day, after meals and at bedtime; *children*, for *hypophosphatamia*, 6.4 mmol (200 mg of P) 4 times a day, after meals and at bedtime; when Capsules for Oral Solution are used, they must be dissolved in at least 10 mL/mmol of phosphate. *Intravenous, adults*, for *hypercalcemia*, 100 mmol (3.1 g of P) infused over 6 to 8 hr once a day; for *hypophosphatemia*, 10 mmol (310 mg of P)/day; *children over 4 yr* of age, for *hypophosphatemia*, 1.5 to 2 mmol (46 to 62 mg of P)/day. *Dosage Forms:* Injection: 3 M (93 g of P, 224 g KH_2PO_4 and 236 g of K_2HPO_4 per L); Capsules for Oral Solution: 8 mmol (250 mg of P); for Oral Solution: 71 g of powder to be constituted with 3.785 L of water (1 gal) to make 8 mmol (250 mg of P)/75 mL of solution.

Dibasic Potassium and Sodium Phosphates—A mixture of dibasic potassium and dibasic sodium phosphates. *Uses:* See *Dibasic Potassium Phosphate* (page 834) and *Sodium Phosphate* (page 836). The mixture is advantageous in that it lessens the risk of sodium or potassium overload from a single-entity preparation. Used mainly for *hypercalcemia* and *hypophosphatemia*. *Dose: Oral, adults*, 8 to 16 mmol (250 to 500 mg of P) with 240 mL (8 fl oz) of water 4 times a day; for *hypophosphatemia*, 11 mmol (346 mg of P) with 240 mL (8 fl oz) of water 4 times a day. *Dosage Form:* 5.5 mmol (173 mg of P).

Monobasic Potassium and Sodium Phosphates—A mixture of monobasic potassium and monobasic sodium phosphates. *Uses:* See *Monobasic Potassium Phosphate* (page 835), and *Monobasic Sodium Phosphate* (page 836). The combination is used to treat both hypercalcemia and hypophosphatemia. The combination is advantageous in that it lessens the likelihood of excessive intake of either sodium or potassium from that of the single entity components. *Dose: Oral, adults*, for *hypercalcemia*, 8 to 16 mmol (250 to 500 mg of P) 4 times a day, after meals and at bedtime; for *hypophosphatemia*, 8 mmol (150 mg of P) 4 times a day, after meals and at bedtime; *children over 4 yr* of age for *hypophosphatemia*, 6.4 mmol (200 mg of P) 4 times a day, after meals and at bedtime. When Capsules for Oral Solution are used, at least 10 mL/mmole must be used. *Dosage Forms:* Capsules for Oral Solution: 8 mmol (250 mg of P); Oral Solution: 8 mmol (250 mg of P)/75 mL.

Potassium and Sodium Phosphates—A mixture of the mono- and dibasic potassium and sodium phosphates. *Uses:* See *Dibasic Potassium Phosphate* (page 834), *Monobasic Sodium Phosphate* (page 836), *Dibasic Sodium Phosphate* (page 804). The mixture is advantageous in that it lessens the risk of sodium or potassium overload from a single-entity preparation. It is used mainly for *hypercalcemia* and *hypophosphatemia*. *Dose: Oral, adults*, 8 mmol (250 mg of P) for *hypophosphatemia* and 8 to 16 mmol (250 to 500 mg of P) 4 times a day, after meals and at bedtime; *children*, over 4 yr of age for *hypophosphatemia*, 6.4 mmol (200 mg of P) 4 times a day, after meals and at bedtime; Capsules for Oral Solution should be dissolved in no less than 10 mL of water/1 mmol of PO_4. *Dosage Forms:* Capsules for Solution: 8 mmol (250 mg of P); for Oral Solution: 64 g of concentrate powder, to be reconstituted in 3.875 L (1 gal) of water; each 75 mL will contain 8 mmol of PO_4 (250 mg of P).

Sodium Acetate [Sodium acetate trihydrate [6131-90-4] C_2H_3Na-$O_2.3H_2O$ (136.08); anhydrous [127-09-3] (82.03)]—*Preparation:* By neutralization of acetic acid with sodium carbonate. *Description:* Colorless, transparent crystals, or granular, crystalline powder; slightly bitter, saline taste; effloresces in warm, dry air; the trihydrate liquefies at about 60°. *Solubility:* 1 g dissolves in 0.8 mL water, 19 mL alcohol. *Uses:* The acetate ion is rapidly and completely metabolized in the body; consequently administration of sodium acetate is eventually equivalent to giving sodium bicarbonate. Solutions of sodium acetate are stable and readily sterilized, and this salt has been used for parenteral therapy of metabolic acidosis. It may also be used to alkalinize the urine. It is a pharmaceutic necessity used in solutions for hemodialysis and peritoneal dialysis. *Dose: Usual*, 1 to 2 g, but more or less may be given, depending on the size of the patient and the clinical condition.

Sodium Citrate and Citric Acid Solution—A solution of sodium citrate and citric acid in purified water. It contains, in each mL, 95–105 mg of sodium citrate dihydrate ($C_6H_5Na_3O_7.2H_2O$), and 57–63 mg of anhydrous citric acid ($C_6H_8O_7$). It may contain preservatives and flavoring agents. *Uses:* A *systemic* and *urinary alkalinizer*. In the body the citrate is metabolized to bicarbonate, so that the effect is that of a dose of bicarbonate. The citric acid is metabolized to carbon dioxide and water and thus has only a transient effect on the systemic acid-base status; its function is as a temporary buffer component. Citrate can mobilize calcium from the bones and increase its renal excretion; this, along with the elevated urine pH, may predispose to urolithiasis. *Dose: Oral, adults,* usually 10 to 30 mL 4 times a day, but as much as 150 mL may be given per day; *children,* 5 to 15 mL 4 times a day. Each 10 mL of solution should be diluted with a fluid ounce of water for adults and 2 fluid ounces for children. The first three doses are to be given after meals and the fourth at bedtime.

Cation Complexing Agents

The monovalent cations do not form strong complexes with sequestering agents; thus, hyperkalemia and hypernatremia cannot be treated by simple chemical means. However, the divalent and polyvalent cations do form complexes easily and can be removed from the plasma; thus, hypercalcemia is a frequent target for complexing agents. It is generally difficult to complex magnesium in the presence of calcium; however, disorders of magnesium metabolism are rare. The complexing agents may also be employed for removing certain foreign toxic cations from the body.

Deferoxamine Mesylate

Butanediamide, *N'*-[5-[[4-[[5-(acetylhydroxyamino)pentyl]amino]-1,4-dioxobutyl]hydroxyamino]pentyl]-*N*-(5-aminopentyl)-*N*-hydroxy-, monomethanesulfonate; Desferal Mesylate (*Ciba*)

$$H_2N(CH_2)_5NC(CH_2)_2CNH(CH_2)_5NC(CH_2)_2CNH(CH_2)_5NCCH_3 \cdot CH_3SO_3H$$

N-[5-{3-[(5-Aminopentyl)hydroxycarbamoyl]propionamido}pentyl] - 3 - {[5 - (*N* - hydroxyacetamido)pentyl]carbamoyl}propionohydroxamic acid monomethanesulfonate (salt) [138-14-7] $C_{25}H_{48}N_6O_8 \cdot CH_4O_3S$ (656.79).

Preparation—Isolated from cultures of *Streptomyces pilosus* by the method of Bickel, *et al* (*Helv Chim Acta 43:* 2118, 1960) or synthesized by the method of Prelog and Walser (*Helv Chim Acta 45:* 631, 1962).

Description—White crystals; reconstituted solutions are stable for 2 weeks at room temperature.
Solubility—Freely soluble in water.

Uses—A chelating agent that is specific for iron. It is used for the *treatment of severe iron intoxication,* iron overload resulting from hemolysis (from drugs, thalassemia, sickle-cell anemia, frequent blood transfusion, etc) or *iron storage disease.* Stoichiometrically, 100 mg of deferoxamine sequesters 8.5 mg of ferric iron. Although it does not appreciably bind ferrous ion, it has nevertheless proven useful in the treatment of intoxication by ferrous as well as by ferric salts, probably partly because some of the toxicity of ferrous salts is due to ferric ion resulting from oxidation of the divalent ion and partly because complexation of the ferric ion favors further oxidation of ferrous ion and so promotes a diminution in the content of the divalent form. The drug is not absorbed orally and must be given parenterally. By intermittent or continuous subcutaneous infusion the drug is 2 to 3 times more effective than by intramuscular or intravenous injection; this can be achieved in ambulatory patients with an automatic syringe strapped to the waist. Ascorbic acid, 1 g twice a day, also greatly increases the efficacy of deferoxamine.

Pain and induration may occur at the site of an intramuscular injection. Other untoward effects include erythema, flushing, diarrhea, blurring of vision, abdominal discomfort, muscular spasms in the legs, itching, tachycardia, and fever. In long-term therapy, various allergic reactions, including anaphylaxis, have been reported. Because of the side effects, deferoxamine should not be used to treat mild iron intoxication. The drug is contraindicated in severe renal impairment. The iron chelate (ferrioxamine) is excreted by the kidney and imparts a reddish color to the urine.

Dose—*Intravenous* or *intramuscular, adults,* in *acute intoxication,* initially **1 g** (500 mg twice at 4-hr interval), then **0.5 g** every 4 to 12 hr, not to exceed 6 g/day; in *chronic iron overload,* **0.5 to 1 g** a day; in chronic iron overload, if blood is to be infused, 2 g must be administered for each unit of blood. Intravenous infusion is reserved only for iron-intoxicated patients in a state of cardiovascular collapse. The rate of intravenous infusion must not exceed 15 mg/kg/hr. *Subcutaneous,* by *infusion,* **1 to 2 g** a day. *Intramuscular* or *intravenous, children,* **50 mg/kg** every 6 hr, the rate of infusion not to exceed 15

mg/kg/hr and the dose and total daily dose not to exceed 2 g and 6 g, respectively.
Dosage Form—for Injection: 500 mg to be constituted to 2 mL.

Dimercaprol—page 1224.
Edetate Calcium Disodium—page 1225.

Edetate Disodium

Glycine, *N,N'*-1,2-ethanediylbis[*N*-(carboxymethyl)-, disodium salt, dihydrate; Disotate; Endrate (*Abbott*); Sodium Versenate (*Riker*)

$$(HOOCCH_2)_2NCH_2CH_2N(CH_2COONa)_2 \cdot 2H_2O$$

Disodium (ethylenedinitrilo)tetraacetate dihydrate [6381-92-6] $C_{10}H_{14}N_2Na_2O_8 \cdot 2H_2O$ (372.24); *anhydrous* [139-33-3] (336.21).

Preparation—(Ethylenedinitrilo)tetraacetic acid (edetic acid, page 1260) is dissolved in a hot solution containing two equivalents of NaOH and the disodium salt is allowed to crystallize.

Description—White, crystalline powder.
Solubility—Soluble in water; pH (1 in 20 solution) between 4.0 and 6.0.

Uses—Since it readily chelates calcium, edetate disodium may be employed to remove free calcium ions from solution; thus it may be used as an *anticoagulant* in the same manner as sodium citrate. Intravenously, it temporarily *lowers plasma calcium* concentration, but the effect is too brief to be of value in the treatment of hypercalcemia, but constant infusion can yield a more sustained effect. It is employed occasionally to *terminate* abruptly *the effects of injected calcium* and to antagonize digitalis toxicity or suppress *tachyarrhythmias.* The drug is not effective in the treatment of arteriosclerosis, since calcium is more easily mobilized from bone. Edetate disodium can also dissolve precipitated calcium salts.

Edetate disodium may cause nausea, vomiting, diarrhea, transient circumoral paresthesias, numbness, headache, and a transient hypotension. Too rapid an injection can cause death. Fever, anemia, exfoliative dermatitis, and other toxic effects on skin and mucous membranes occasionally occur. Intravenous edetate disodium sometimes has a nephrotoxic action. Overdosage can result in damage to the reticuloendothelial system. Prolonged infusion may cause zinc deficiency. It is contraindicated in patients with impaired renal function with severe azotemia, and it should be used cautiously in the presence of liver impairment.

Dose—Depends on the use and the amount of calcium to be sequestered; 1 g chelates 0.12 g of calcium. *Usual, intravenous infusion, adults* **50 mg/kg,** up to a maximum of 3 g/day. The drug is usually employed as a 3% solution in isotonic saline or glucose. It is given by slow intravenous drip such that 3 or more hours are required to accomplish the infusion. Five consecutive daily doses may be given, after which there should be a rest of 2 days before resuming treatment; no more than a total of 15 doses should be given. For *children,* the recommended daily dose is **40 mg/kg** to be infused over a period of no less than 3 hr; the maximum daily dose is 70 mg/kg.
Dosage Forms—Injection: 3 g/15 and 20 mL.

Penicillamine—page 1225.

Sodium Polystyrene Sulfonate

Benzene, ethenyl-, homopolymer, sulfonated, sodium salt; Kayexalate (*Breon*)

Styrene polymer sulfonated, sodium salt; a cation-exchange resin prepared in the sodium form. Each g exchanges (2.8–3.5 mEq) of potassium.

Description—Golden brown, fine powder that is odorless and tasteless.
Solubility—Insoluble in water.

Uses—An ion-exchange resin used for the treatment of hyperkalemia resulting from acute renal failure. The resin is given orally by a stomach tube or as a high retention enema. The sodium moiety of the resin is in part replaced by potassium which is subsequently eliminated from the body when the resin is excreted in the feces or in the enema. The potassium-removing capacity of the resin is approximately ⅓ of that possible when measured under conditions in which potassium is the only cation present. The resin should be an adjunct to other therapeutic measures, such as restriction of electrolyte intake, control of acidosis, and high caloric diet. Untoward effects include anorexia, nausea, vomiting, and constipation. Constipation and fecal impaction can be minimized by the administration of 70% sorbitol solution every 2 hours as needed to produce watery stools. Serum potassium levels should be determined daily in order to avoid hypokalemia.

The resin may cause gastric irritation, nausea, vomiting, and occasional diarrhea. Especially in elderly patients, large doses may cause fecal impaction. Since the resin can sequester calcium and magnesium, hypocalcemia or hypomagnesemia or related effects may occur, and mineral metabolism should be monitored during prolonged treatment. The drug should be used with caution in patients with actual or impending cardiac failure; the absorption of the released (exchanged) sodium may be hazardous in such patients. Sodium polystyrene sulfonate may also exaggerate the effects of digitalis.

Dose—*Oral, adults,* **15 g** 1 to 4 times a day. Each dose should be suspended in 20 to 100 mL of water or syrup. By *enema,* **25 to 100 g** in 150 to 200 mL of water, 5% dextrose solution, or 2% hydroxy methylcellulose solution as retention enema once or twice a day; a cleansing enema should follow. Duration of treatment depends on clinical condition and response, and it may be as short as 3 days; it is discontinued when plasma potassium reaches 4 to 5 mEq/L. *Oral* or *rectal, children,* **1 g** of resin for every mEq of potassium that is to be removed. One level teaspoonful contains approximately 3.5 g.

Dosage Form—Powder: jars containing 1 lb. *Note:* Each gram of sodium polystyrene sulfonate contains 4.1 mEq (94 mg) of sodium.

Other Cation Complexing Agents

Sodium Cellulose Phosphate [Calcibind (*Mission*)]. An insoluble, non-absorbable ion exchange resin with a great affinity for calcium ions described in US Pat 2,759,924. It is a white to cream colored powder which must be stored in tightly closed containers to minimize hydrolysis during storage. *Uses:* Exchanges sodium for calcium and other polyvalent cations. By the oral route it decreases the amount of calcium absorbed from the diet, supposedly without altering calcium balance. It is used to treat a type of absorptive hypercaluria which occurs even on low-calcium diets. The effectiveness in suppressing nephrolith formation ranges from nil to much according to various reports. During treatment, hyperoxaluria and hypermagnesemia occur, both of which favor certain kinds of kidney stones. The drug is unpalatable and may also cause gastrointestinal discomfort. Acute arthralgias from drug-induced hyperparathyroidism have been reported. Every 15 g contains 25 to 50 mEq of sodium. *Dose: Oral, adults,* 5 g 3 times a day (with meals) when urine calcium output exceeds 300 mg/day and 20 g/day in 3 divided doses when calcium output falls to less than 150 mg/day. *Dosage Form:* 2.5 g.

Hematologic Drugs

Hematopoietics

Hematopoietics are *antianemics* that aid in production of red and white blood cells; *hematinics* are *antianemics* that increase the hemoglobin content of blood through erythropoiesis or through an increase in hemoglobin content of erythrocytes. The hematinic to be employed is critically dependent upon the nature of the anemia. The hypochromic anemias are nearly all iron-deficiency anemias in character and are treated with iron preparations. Occasionally, other accessory factors are indicated in the treatment of the hypochromic anemias. As long as 6 months of treatment may be required to restore the body stores of iron and correct various anemias. For example, the anemia of nurslings may require copper to facilitate the mobilization of iron from the gut and tissues. Ascorbic acid occasionally helps promote the antianemic action of iron. When given with iron salts, it promotes the absorption of iron, in part by reducing the less well absorbed ferric ion to the better absorbed ferrous ion or maintaining the ferrous state of administered ferrous salts, and in part by forming an absorbable complexonate with iron. However, ascorbic acid appears to have an additional but obscure role in hematopoiesis. Ascorbic acid is included in a number of iron-containing products. Cobalt and molybdenum probably also play a role in hematopoiesis, but deficiency syndromes in man are unknown, and the inclusion of these metals in hematinic preparations is irrational. The use of cobalt may even be dangerous. Although copper is known to have a hematopoietic function, a deficiency in man severe enough to impair erythropoiesis has never been demonstrated (see page 1032). The macrocytic anemias all respond to cyanocobalamin, but the route of administration and accessory factors are critically dependent upon the particular anemia. In tropical sprue, the absorption of folic acid is impaired to a greater extent than that of vitamin B_{12}, so that folic acid usually elicits the greater hematopoietic response. For reasons stated elsewhere (below and on page 1014), the promiscuous use of folic and folinic acids should be condemned. In pyridoxine deficiency, protoporphyrin synthesis and hence erythropoiesis are impaired, and pyridoxine restores normal erythropoiesis.

Iron and Iron Compounds

Iron is used in medicine in the following forms: (1) inorganic and simple organic ferrous compounds (ferrous sulfate, etc) and (2) complex ferrous compounds.

Complex (nonionic) iron compounds do not respond to the ordinary tests for ferrous or ferric ions because the iron in them is part of a complex radical. The stabilities of these complex radicals differ widely. Some are converted to simple ionic iron by action of dilute acids while others resist treatment with strong acids or with alkalies. The complex iron compounds occurring naturally in animal and vegetable tissues (termed food irons) belong generally to the more resistant class, while the complex iron compounds produced artificially are as a rule decomposed rather readily. There is, however, no sharp line of distinction between the natural complex iron compounds and those products artificially produced, nor is there any good evidence that they differ in therapeutic action.

Uses—The principal use of iron is in the treatment of *hypochromic, iron-deficiency anemias*, that is, in anemias characterized by a deficiency of hemoglobin. The two most common causes of such anemias are nutritional (deficient intake, especially in infancy, in childhood, at puberty, during pregnancy, and late in menstrual life or at the menopause), and chronic blood loss (especially bleeding peptic ulcer, carcinoma of the colon or stomach, bleeding from the urinary tract, or excessive loss of blood during menstruation). Iron therapy is of no particular value in other forms of anemia, such as pernicious anemia, unless the patient has entered an iron-deficiency stage of his disease.

Complex iron compounds are generally less prone to produce gastric distress than the simple ferrous compounds; they are also less efficiently utilized physiologically. Indeed, in some complexes the iron may be so effectively chelated as to escape utilization altogether.

A difference exists between the different iron preparations in their local irritant and astringent action, which is absent in most of the complex iron compounds; for this reason the less astringent and less irritant ferrous salts are used rather than ferric salts. The irritation occurs mostly in the stomach and upper duodenum, where the pH is low. It can exacerbate peptic ulcer, regional enteritis, ulcerative colitis, and other gastrointestinal disorders. Enteric coatings allow the preparation to pass into the more alkaline portions of the gut before release occurs. However, the absorption of iron from enteric-coated preparations is less than in uncoated ones, especially in persons with bowel hypermotility. In steatorrhea or in persons with partial gastrectomy, iron preparations are often poorly absorbed. Antacids also diminish absorption. Constipation consequent to local actions of iron may be countered by cathartics, properly individualized. Suitable diet (especially liver, kidney, and meat) is sometimes more effective than the iron preparations, presumably by the co-operation of other factors.

All of the iron preparations are capable of causing severe intoxication in overdoses, especially in children. Iron preparations are a common cause of lethal intoxication in children.

Ascorbic Acid—pages 1012 and 1021.

Ferrous Fumarate

2-Butenedioic acid, (*E*)-, iron(2+) salt; (*Various Mfrs*)

Iron(2+) fumarate [141-01-5] $C_4H_2FeO_4$ (169.90).

Preparation—Ferrous sulfate and sodium fumarate are metathesized in hot aqueous solution whereupon the sparingly soluble, anhydrous ferrous fumarate precipitates.

Description—Reddish orange to red-brown, odorless powder; may contain soft lumps that produce a yellow streak when crushed.

Solubility—Slightly soluble in water; very slightly soluble in alcohol; its solubility in dilute HCl is limited by the separation of insoluble free fumaric acid.

Uses—In the clinical management of *iron-deficiency anemias*. Its efficacy is about the same as that of ferrous sulfate, but the untoward effects are somewhat less severe. The drug may sometimes be employed without difficulty in patients who cannot tolerate other preparations of iron. When side effects occur, they include anorexia, nausea, vomiting, cramping, and constipation or diarrhea. Like other iron preparations, ferrous fumarate may exacerbate gastrointestinal diseases, especially ulcerative ones. The effects generally subside as therapy is continued. The untoward effects are minimized if the dose is taken shortly after eating.

Dose—*Oral, adults*, **200 mg**, once a day for *prophylaxis* and 3 times a day for *treatment*, except **300 mg**/day for prophylaxis and 3 times a day for treatment with extended-release tablets; *children*, usually as the oral suspension, **3 mg/kg** once a day for prophylaxis and 3 times a day for treatment. For treatment, doses may be gradually doubled, if necessary.

Dosage Forms—Oral Suspension: 100 mg (33 mg Fe)/100 mL, 45 mg (15 mg Fe)/0.6 mL; Tablets: 195, 200, 300, 324, 325 mg (64, 66, 99, 106, 107 mg Fe, respectively); Chewable Tablets: 100 mg (33 mg Fe); Extended-Release Tablets: 324 mg (106 mg Fe).

Ferrous Gluconate

D-Gluconic acid, iron(2+) salt (2:1), dihydrate; (*Various Mfrs*)

Iron(2+) gluconate (1:2) dihydrate [12389-15-0] $C_{12}H_{22}FeO_{14}$.$2H_2O$ (482.17); *anhydrous* [299-29-6] (446.14).

Preparation—By metathesis between hot solutions of calcium gluconate and ferrous sulfate whereby ferrous gluconate and insoluble calcium sulfate are formed. The mixture is filtered while hot to minimize the solubility of calcium sulfate and the filtrate is evaporated to crystallization.

It may also be produced by heating freshly prepared ferrous carbonate with the proper quantity of gluconic acid in aqueous solution.

Description—Fine, yellowish gray or pale greenish yellow powder, or granules, with a slight burnt-sugar-like odor. It is affected by light and the ferrous iron slowly oxidizes to ferric on exposure to air. Its aqueous solution is acid to litmus. The color of the solutions depends on pH; they are light yellow at pH 2, brown at pH 4.5, and green at pH 7. The iron rapidly oxidizes at higher pH.

Solubility—1 g in about 5 mL water with slight heating; practically insoluble in alcohol; it forms supersaturated solutions which are stable for a period of time; its solubility is increased by addition of citric acid or the citrate iron.

Uses—A *hematinic*, similar to other ferrous salts. Its side effects and toxicity are those of all iron compounds; it is claimed that it causes fewer side effects than ferrous sulfate (see *Iron and Iron Compounds* in the introduction in this section). The elixir can cause staining of teeth if taken undiluted.

Dose—*Oral, adults*, **320** or **325 mg** once a day for *prophylaxis* and 4 times a day for *treatment*, except **435** mg once a day for prophylaxis and twice a day for treatment with extended-release capsules; *children, under 2 yr* of age, to be individualized; *2 yr* of age *and over*, **8 mg/kg** once a day for *prophylaxis* and **16 mg/kg** 3 times a day for treatment. Adult doses may be doubled gradually, if necessary.

Dosage Forms—Capsules: 325 and 435 mg (38 and 50 mg Fe); Elixir: 300 and 325 mg (35 and 38 mg Fe)/5 mL; Tablets: 320 and 325 mg (37 and 38 mg Fe).

Ferrous Sulfate

Sulfuric acid, iron(2+) salt (1:1), heptahydrate; Ferri Sulfas; Feosol (*Various Mfrs*)

Iron(2+) sulfate (1:1) heptahydrate [7782-63-0] $FeSO_4.7H_2O$ (278.01); *anhydrous* [7720-78-7] (151.90).

Note—Do not use Ferrous Sulfate that is coated with brownish yellow basic ferric sulfate.

Preparation—By dissolving iron in diluted H_2SO_4. The resulting solution is filtered and concentrated, if necessary, to the point of crystallization of ferrous sulfate. Commercially, scrap iron is used in the process.

Description—Pale, bluish green crystals or granules. It is odorless, has a saline, styptic taste, and effloresces in dry air, becoming white. Oxidizes readily in moist air to form brownish yellow basic ferric sulfate. The solution (1 in 10) is acid to litmus; pH about 3.7.

Solubility—1 g in 1.5 mL water and 0.5 mL boiling water; insoluble in alcohol.

Uses—Ferrous sulfate is one of the most commonly employed *hematinic* preparations used in iron-deficiency anemias (see *Iron and Iron Compounds* in the introduction in this section). The drug is most commonly dispensed as tablets, coated for protection from air and moisture. The salt is sometimes mixed with glucose or lactose to protect it from oxidation.

The adverse effects of ferrous sulfate are those of iron compounds in general, but they are rarely severe when the salt is taken in therapeutic doses; however, relatively small overdoses can cause serious intoxication in infants and children. The oral solution can cause staining of teeth if used undiluted.

About 20% of ferrous sulfate is absorbed when taken orally. Timed-release and enteric-coated preparations tend to be more erratically absorbed and are not recommended. Magnesium and aluminum hydroxides, present in some preparations, make the iron unavailable for absorption.

Dose—*Oral, adults* **300 mg** once a day for *prophylaxis* and *initially* 2 times a day, gradually increased to 4 times a day, if necessary, for *treatment; children*, usually as liquid, **5 mg/kg** a day for *prophylaxis* and **10 mg/kg** 3 times a day for treatment.

Dosage Forms—Capsules: 190 mg (60 mg Fe); Extended-Release Capsules: 150, 167 (exsiccated), 225, 250, and 390 mg (30, 50, 45, 50, and 78 mg of Fe, respectively); Liquids: 75 mg (15 mg Fe)/0.6 mL, 125 mg (25 mg Fe)/1 mL, 195 mg (38 mg Fe)/4 mL, 90 and 220 mg (18 and 44 mg Fe)/5 mL; Tablets: 190 (exsiccated), 195, 200 (exsiccated), 300 and 325 mg (60, 39, 65, 60 and 65 mg Fe, respectively); Extended-Release Tablets: 525 mg (105 mg Fe).

Other Iron Compounds

Iron Dextran [Imferon (*Merrell Dow*) [9004-66-4]]. A sterile, colloidal solution of ferric hydroxide in complex with partially hydrolyzed dextran of low molecular weight, in water for injection. It may contain not more than 0.5% of phenol as a preservative. *Preparation:* To an aqueous solution of partially depolymerized dextran (intrinsic viscosity 0.04 to 0.07) is added a solution of alkali and a solution of a ferric salt. The mixture is heated, then cooled to room temperature and clarified by centrifugation, and the solution is dialyzed against running water. After concentrating to the required iron content, the solution is filtered, ampuled, and sterilized by autoclaving. It is a dark brown, slightly viscous liquid; pH 5.2 to 6. *Uses:* Because iron is strongly chelated by dextran, it is not locally irritating on intramuscular injection. Absorption is rapid from an intramuscular site. Thus the drug is used for intramuscular injection in patients with iron-deficiency anemias in whom oral therapy cannot be tolerated or does not evoke a therapeutic response. If the drug is administered to persons not in an iron-deficiency state, hemosiderosis may occur. Absorption is very slow from a subcutaneous site and a brown stain occurs that may remain for 1 to 2 years. Consequently, in injecting the drug, care must be taken to prevent leakage under the skin. Injections are given deeply into the upper-outer quadrant of the buttock by a special technique called a Z-track injection, which diminishes leakage to subcutaneous sites. In the human the lymphatic system is well developed and the dose of the complex is relatively low, so that the danger of malignancy, such as occurs in some animals, is very slight. However, it can cause fibrosis at the site of injection. Allergic reactions, even anaphylaxis, have occurred. Consequently, a test of 0.5 mL of the injection should be given prior to therapeutic administration. Headache, fever, nausea, vomiting, parenthesias, and regional lymphadenopathy are relatively common side effects. Hypotension, reactivation of quiescent arthritis, leukocytosis with fever, and sterile abscesses at an intramuscular injection site may occur. Phlebitis occasionally occurs after intravenous administration. *Dose: Intramuscular, adults,* daily dose in

$$\text{mg Fe} = 0.3 \times \text{wt in lb} \left(\frac{100 - \text{Hb in g\%} \times 100}{14.8.} \right)$$

To convert to mL of injection, divide by 50. The daily dose should not exceed 25 mg Fe for infants under 10 lb. 50 mg Fe for 10 to 20 lb, or 100 mg Fe for persons under 110 lb. *Intravenous,* up to 50 mg Fe may be given slowly (less than 1 mL/min) once a day. *Intravenous infusion* (not approved in US), the calculated dose is placed in 200 to 250 mL of isosotonic sodium chloride; if a test dose of 25 mg infused over 5 min evokes no adverse effect, the infusion is completed over 1 to 2 hr. *Dosage Form:* 50 mg/mL in 2, 5 and 10 mL vials.

Iron Polysaccharide—*Uses:* For the treatment of iron-deficiency anemias. The complex is less astringent than ferrous salts and hence is more palatable in oral suspension. *Dose: Oral, adults,* the equivalent of 50 mg Fe once a day for *prophylaxis* and twice a day, gradually doubled, if necessary, for *treatment; children,* the equivalent of 1.5 mg Fe/kg/day, for *prophylaxis* only. *Dosage Forms:* Capsules: 125 mg Fe; Elixir: 200 mg Fe/5 mL; tablets: 50 mg Fe.

Agents for Macrocytic Anemias

The macrocytic anemias are characterized by the presence of large erythrocytes. They include *pernicious anemia*, the *anemia* of *sprue, macrocytic tropical anemia, fish tapeworm anemia, achrestic anemia*, and anemias resulting from gastric carcinoma and resection or disease of the intestinal tract. In all of these, insufficient intake or absorption of *cyanocobalamin* (vitamin B_{12}) is the cause of the disorder, the vitamin being essential to normal hematopoiesis and to the integrity of the central nervous system. Early work on pernicious anemia had established the need for a dietary factor, called the *extrinsic factor*, and a gastric and upper duodenal secretory factor, called the *intrinsic factor*. It is now well established that cyanocobalamin is the extrinsic factor; the vitamin is also the *antianemia principle* of liver. The intrinsic factor is essential to the proper absorption of vitamin B_{12}. The intrinsic factor is absent in pernicious anemia; in this disease the secretion of hydrochloric acid and pepsin is also diminished or absent. Before the advent of cyanocobalamin, various liver preparations were employed as sources of extrinsic factor and stomach preparations as sources of the intrinsic factor. Since orally administered liver was not reliable because it did not provide the intrinsic factor, it was necessary to administer a stomach preparation at the same time or to administer the liver parenterally. Today, the preparation of choice is cyanocobalamin, which is cheaper and which causes

less discomfort at the site of injection than liver. Oral cyanocobalamin, of course, like liver, optimally requires a source of intrinsic factor.

For the patient with uncomplicated pernicious anemia in relapse, the initial dose of cyanocobalamin is 30 μg daily, parenterally, or every other day for 5 to 10 doses, followed by 15 to 30 μg once or twice weekly until the blood picture is normal. For maintenance; 40 to 60 μg every 2 weeks or 80 to 100 μg once a month is usually adequate. If there is demonstrable neurological damage, it may be necessary to administer 1000 μg weekly for several months before switching to the maintenance schedule. Therapy must be maintained for life, since the basic deficiency in gastrointestinal physiology remains. Nevertheless, the patient may be kept in good health and may lead a fairly normal life.

Despite the superiority of cyanocobalamin, liver and stomach preparations are still available. The ingestion of 200 to 400 g of whole liver may be irregularly effective in inducing a remission in pernicious anemia. Concentrates for oral administration are made from such amounts of liver, but concentration results in some loss of activity. Extracts suitable for parenteral administration may be prepared from 10 to 15 g of liver. Similar effects may be produced by the ingestion of 30 to 40 g of desiccated stomach; however, the combinations of stomach and liver are required for optimal oral therapy. Liver preparations for injection may be assayed microbiologically, employing *Lactobacillus leichmannii* ATCC 7830, the assay being expressed in terms of vitamin B_{12}. However, since oral preparations are rarely effective, owing to the absence of the intrinsic factor, assay must be made in the human pernicious anemia patient in relapse, and the assay is expressed in terms of oral units. This reflects the ridiculousness of using archaic and irregularly effective preparations when the active ingredient, vitamin B_{12} or cyanocobalamin, or derivatives, is readily available and is more easily and safely administered.

Megaloblastic anemia of infancy, megaloblastic anemia of pregnancy, achrestic anemia, and nutritional macrocytic anemia generally respond better to liver preparations than they do to cyanocobalamin, and deficiencies in *folic* and *folinic acid* intake or metabolism are implicated; thus, either of these two acids may evoke a dramatic response in such anemias. Ascorbic acid also may occasionally confer additional benefits. The metabolic functions of folic or folinic acid and vitamin B_{12} converge in certain respects. Thus, folic or folinic acid may induce a remission in the blood pathology in pernicious anemia, but it will not revert or delay the progression of the epithelial and neurological pathology, which may develop insidiously and emerge explosively and irreversibly. Therefore, folic or folinic acid therapy of pernicious anemia is to be condemned. *Equally offensive and irresponsible is the inclusion of these acids in liver or multivitamin-hematinic preparations* because, in allaying the blood pathology of undiagnosed pernicious anemia, they prevent detection of the disease until the neurological pathology has advanced to a dangerous state. Unfortified liver preparations also may contain enough folic acid to constitute the same danger. *In general, a hematinic should be employed only upon accurate diagnosis of the anemia and upon specific indication.* Multiple preparations are to be avoided. For descriptions of cyanocobalamin, hydroxocobalamin, and folic acid, see Chapter 52.

Antihematopoietic Drugs

Polycythemia and erythrocytosis are conditions in which there is an increase in the number of circulating erythrocytes. The cause is usually the result of a deficient oxygenation of the arterial blood, and either condition may be corrected by management of the underlying primary disorder. However, in *polycythemia rubra vera* the condition is primary, and therapy is thus directed at the erythrocytes, either by their removal by venesection, their destruction by phenylhydrazines, or the suppression of their formation by antihematopoietic drugs or by X-irradiation. Several of the antineoplastic drugs such as the nitrogen mustards, the antifolic acids, ar-

senicals, and radiophosphate may be employed. The *leukemias* result from excessive leukocytic hematopoietic activity of a neoplastic nature; either the bone marrow (myelogenous or granulocytic leukemia) or lymphatic tissue (lymphocytic leukemia) may be involved. In myelogenous leukemia there may be anemia because the erythropoietic cells are crowded out by leukopoietic cells. Drugs used in the therapy of the leukemias and polycythemia are treated in Chapter 63.

Miscellaneous Drugs That Affect Blood

Hemin

Ferrate(2-), chloro[7,12-diethenyl-3,8,13,17-tetramethyl-21*H*,23*H*-porphine-2,18-dipropanoato(4-)-N^{21},N^{22},N^{23},N^{24}]-, dihydrogen-, (*SP*-5-13)

Chlorohemin[16009-13-5] $C_{34}H_{32}ClFeN_4O_4$ (651.96).

Preparation—Usually from hemoglobin by treatment with a hot saline acetic acid solution. *Org Syn Coll Vol III*, 442(1955).

Description—Polychromatic chrystals (usually brownish to blue) which do not melt under 300°.
Solubility—Freely soluble in dilute base through conversion to *hematin* by replacement of the chlorine atom by hydroxyl. Sparingly soluble in alcohol; insoluble in water.

Uses—Hemin inhibits the biosynthesis of porphyrin in juvenile erythrocytes and hence also indirectly decreases the rate of formation of porphyrins. It is used to ameliorate symptoms in *intermittent porphyria*, *porphyria variegata*, and hereditary *coproporphyria*. In some but not all patients pain, tachycardia, hypertension, mild to moderate neurological impairment and abnormal mentation are abated. Neurological improvement is sometimes delayed weeks to months after treatment. Remissions are not permanent.

Hemin is contraindicated in hypersensitivity to hemin and in porphyria cutanea tarda. Excessive doses may cause renal failure. Phlebitis may occur in the injected vein. Coagulopathy has been reported.

Hemin is partially converted to bilirubin and partially excreted into the bile intact. Bilirubin metabolites and urobilinogen appear in the urine.

Dose—*Intravenous infusion* into large high-flow vein, **1 to 4 mg/kg** over a 10- to 15-min period once a day for 3 to 14 days. In severe cases, the dose may be repeated at 12-hr intervals, not to exceed 6 mg/kg/day.

Dosage Form—Powder for injection: 313 mg to be reconstituted to 43 mL with sterile water (makes 7 mg/mL).

Methylene Blue

Phenothiazin-5-ium, 3,7-bis(dimethylamino)-, chloride, trihydrate; Methylthionine Chloride; Aniline Violet

C I Basic Blue 9 trihydrate [7220-79-3] $C_{16}H_{18}ClN_3S.3H_2O$ (373.90); *anhydrous* [61-73-4] (319.85).

Preparation—By treating a solution of *N*,*N*-dimethyl-*p*-phenylenediamine and *N*,*N*-dimethylaniline hydrochlorides with H_2S and $FeCl_3$ or another suitable oxidizing agent.

Description—Dark green crystals or a crystalline powder, having a bronze-like luster; odorless or having a slight odor; stable in air; solutions have a deep blue color.
Solubility—1 g in 25 mL water, 65 mL alcohol; soluble in chloroform.

Uses—Readily reduced to leukomethylene blue, which, in turn, is readily reoxidized to methylene blue. Thus, it is useful as a reversible *oxidation–reduction* indicator. Its principal therapeutic

use, in the *treatment of methemoglobinemia*, stems from this chemical property. Methylene blue acts as an electron-acceptor in the transfer of electrons from reduced pyridine nucleotides (NADPH and NATPH) to methemoglobin, thus facilitating reduction of ferric to ferrous iron. Glucose 6-phosphate dehydrogenase is required; if this enzyme is absent, as it is in certain hemolysis-prone individuals, the drug is ineffective. If the dose of methylene blue is high, the oxidation potential favors the formation of methemoglobin from hemoglobin. This effect is used in the *treatment of cyanide poisoning*. The methemoglobin so formed complexes cyanide, which tends to spare the cytochrome system. However, other drugs are superior.

Methylene blue was formerly employed as a urinary antibacterial agent, but this use is now obsolete. An outgrowth of this use is the belief that the drug is effective in the treatment of urolithiasis. Although a slight effect to retard crystal formation *in vitro* has been reported, no clinical benefits have been proven, and expert opinion holds the dye to be ineffective. Its use as an analgetic, antipyretic, and parasiticide has likewise been abandoned. The dye is used as a bacteriologic stain.

Methylene blue colors urine and feces green and the skin blue. It may cause bladder irritation, nausea, vomiting and diarrhea. Large doses may cause vertigo, headache, confusion, sweating methemoglobinemia (paradoxical) and chest and abdominal pains. It can cause hemolysis in persons with glucose-6-phosphate dehydrogenase-deficient erythrocytes.

Dose—*Oral*, for chronic *idiopathic methemoglobinemia*, **65 to 130 mg** 3 times a day, in conjunction with large doses of ascorbic acid; for *urolithiasis* (but see comments above), **65 mg** 2 or 3 times a day. *Intravenous*, for *drug-induced* or *toxic methemoglobinemia*, **1 to 2 mg/kg**, and for *cyanide poisoning*, **500 mg** (50 mL of 1% solution).

Dosage Forms—Injection: 10 mg/1 mL and 100 mg/10 mL; Tablets: 65 mg.

Sodium Nitrite

Nitrous acid, sodium salt

Sodium nitrite [7632-00-0] $NaNO_2$ (69.00).
Preparation—By various methods, as by reduction of sodium nitrate with lead, a sulfite, or sulfur dioxide, or by absorption of NO obtained from catalytic oxidation of ammonia in sodium carbonate solution.

Description—White to slightly yellow, granular powder or white or nearly white, opaque, fused masses or sticks; deliquescent in air. Solutions are alkaline to litmus.
Solubility—1 g in 1.5 mL water; sparingly soluble in alcohol.

Uses—The principal use of sodium nitrite is for treatment of *cyanide poisoning*, based on its causing methemoglobinemia. In cyanide poisoning, sodium nitrite is injected intravenously in very large doses to produce methemoglobin, which combines with the highly lethal cyanide and renders it temporarily inactive as cyanmethemoglobin. Sodium thiosulfate (RPS-16, page 1176) is then injected intravenously to form the nontoxic thiocyanate. Nitrite ion relaxes smooth muscle, so that sodium nitrite causes hypotension. Solutions of sodium nitrite are unstable and should be prepared directly before use.

Dose—*Intravenous*, *adult*, **10 mL** of 3% solution, given at a rate of 2.5 to 5 mL/min; *pediatric*, **0.2 mL** of 3% solution **per kg** of body weight (or 6 to 8 mL/m² of body surface), not to exceed 10 mL.

CHAPTER 43

Cardiovascular Drugs

Stewart C Harvey, PhD
Professor of Pharmacology

C Dean Withrow, PhD
Associate Professor of Pharmacology

School of Medicine, University of Utah
Salt Lake City, UT 84132

Any drug that affects the heart or blood vessels, directly or indirectly, is a cardiovascular drug, although the term generally connotes only those drugs which are used for their cardiovascular actions. Many such drugs exist. Nearly every autonomic drug has clinically applicable cardiovascular actions. *Sympathomimetics* (see Chapter 45) may be used to elevate blood pressure, stimulate the heart, slow the heart reflexly, etc., depending on the particular agents and the clinical conditions. *α-Adrenergic blocking drugs* (see Chapter 47) may be used in vasospastic conditions, in the diagnosis and management of pheochromocytoma, and rarely in malignant and toxemic hypertensive crises. β-Adrenergic blocking drugs (Chapter 47) are employed in the treatment of essential hypertension, portal hypertension, angina pecdisorders. The anticholinesterase, edrophonium (page 899), is used in the diagnosis and treatment of paroxysmal atrial is used in the diagnosis and treatment of paroxysmal atrial tachycardia. Atropine and other *antimuscarinic drugs* (see Chapter 48) may be used to block the cardiac vagus nerve in Adams-Stokes syndrome and certain other bradycardias. The *ganglionic blocking agents* are treated in this chapter. Most of the *antihypertensive agents* can be considered autonomic drugs. A large number of drugs other than the autonomic agents have useful cardiovascular actions. *Digitalis* and its allies, the *coronary* and *peripheral dilators*, and the *antidysrhythmic agents* are included below. *Parenteral fluids* (see Chapter 42), which may be used in the treatment of shock, *diuretics* (see Chapter 50), which are adjuvants in the treatment of heart failure and hypertension, are discussed elsewhere, as are numerous miscellaneous drugs.

Antihypertensive and Hypotensive Drugs

Antihypertensive drugs are used in the treatment of hypertension, although certain ones (eg, ganglionic blocking drugs) enjoy scattered uses in other therapeutic, diagnostic, and surgical procedures. Some are used as hypotensive drugs in nonhypertensive patients. The predominant types of diastolic hypertension are primary (essential, idiopathic) and secondary hypertension. Malignant hypertension is a severe, progressive phase of primary hypertension. Unfortunately, there is no specific therapy for primary hypertension, and individual cases vary widely in response to various drugs.

Many studies in the past have led to the belief that diastolic hypertension is not a disorder of sympathetic function, except, perhaps, that there may be an involvement of the sympathetic nervous system in the early stages of the disease. However, evidence today suggests that there may be, after all, a sympathetic factor, at least in some types of hypertension formerly classified as diastolic or essential hypertension. It has long been thought that there is a component of sympathetic involvement in malignant hypertension, which differentiated it from essential hypertension. Where a sympathetic neural

influence exists, it seems to be not so much one directly on blood vessels but rather one on the renin-producing system in the kidney. Irrespective of whether there is an abnormal sympathetic neural factor involved, removal of the normal sympathetic nervous support of vascular tone and cardiac output usually decreases blood pressure in the hypertensive person and favors a retardation of the progression of the disease.

In recent years there has been considerable controversy regarding the role of the renin-angiotensin system (see page 849) in the pathogenesis of essential hypertension and in the antihypertensive actions of various drugs. Clinical studies alone indicate that the renin-angiotensin system is involved in less than one third of cases of essential hypertension, but the effects of converting-enzyme inhibitors and antagonists of angiotensin indicate that the renin-angiotensin system is involved in at least 70% of cases of essential hypertension. It is possible that the effect of sundry antihypertensive drugs to decrease plasma renin activity contributes importantly to their efficacy.

The therapy of diastolic hypertension has been in flux since 1958 because of the large number of agents introduced since then. The finding that the diuretic chlorothiazide (see page 938) not only is mildly antihypertensive but also greatly potentiates the antihypertensive effects of other drugs initiated a revolution in the medical management of hypertension. Closely following chlorothiazide came reserpine and guanethidine, (see page 908), and later alpha-methyldopa, certain monoamine oxidase inhibitors (see Chapter 59), mebutamate (see the index) and various experimental drugs that necessitated revisions in concepts and approach.

At the present time in the US expert opinion holds that in young persons, a diastolic blood pressure over 90 torr is an indication for treatment and in persons over 35 years of age, 95 torr. Long-term studies have unequivocally proven that treatment both decreases morbidity and prolongs life expectancy. Usually, the first drug to be used is a thiazide diuretic, but it now appears that therapy may just as well be initiated with prazosin or other drugs. Propranolol, captopril and "mini-dose" guanethidine have also been used as single agents in early hypertension. If no single drug is effective alone, then two are used in combination. In mild hypertension, the first drugs to be added to a thiazide are α_1-adrenergic blockers, β-blockers, centrally-acting antihypertensives or calcium entry blockers. In moderate hypertension, hydralazine or converting enzyme inhibitors are added. Severe hypertension is popularly treated with guanethidine or minoxidil, in combination with a diuretic. Since β-adrenergic blockers and converting enzyme inhibitors decrease angiotensin II levels, they are indicated whenever renin levels are high and possibly even when they are normal. β-Blockers are also commonly combined with vasodilators, such as hydralazine, to prevent reflex tachycardia and stimulation of renin secretion. Hydralazine is likely to be replaced by α_1-blockers, less toxic vasodilators and converting enzyme inhibitors. Diuretics and the related diazoxide and sodium nitroprusside, captopril, guanethidine or hydralazine, and to a lesser extent alkaloids and trimethaphan are employed in the treatment of hypertensive crises, such as eclampsia.

It is difficult to anticipate how and when treatment of hypertension will stabilize. It seems likely that converting enzyme inhibitors, renin inhibitors, angiotensin II antagonists, calcium channel blockers, and α_1-blockers will dominate the field; the diuretics will become secondary agents; there will be a marked decline in use of guanethidine, reserpine, methyldopa, and clonidine; hydralazine will be used mainly for ventricular unloading; and the presently minor agents will disappear from use.

Saluretics

It has long been known that certain hypertensive persons have abnormal salt metabolism, and epidemiologic and endemiologic studies have established a relationship between sodium intake and blood pressure. In the essential and malignant hypertensive individual with an expanded blood volume and high sodium burden, the rationale for use of saluretic drugs is almost self-evident. However, saluretic drugs even have been found to lower blood pressure of persons with essential hypertension who have small extracellular fluid volumes. It is widely held that the vascular smooth muscles in such persons have a high intracellular sodium content. When thiazide saluretics are given, the fall in blood pressure in the first week or two correlates with saluresis and the decrement in extracellular fluid volume (hence in venous return, stroke output, and systolic blood pressure); in this phase, heart rate is accelerated and peripheral resistance is increased. The antihypertensive action passes into a phase in which the extracellular volume and heart rate return toward normal and peripheral resistance falls. Not all saluretics are alike in this effect, which suggests that something more than saluresis is involved. For example, high-ceiling saluretics never lower the vascular resistance, and blood pressure is lowered only because cardiac output is decreased. Spironolactone is a useful antihypertensive agent only when aldosterone or 18-hydroxycorticosterone levels are high.

Homeostatic mechanisms increase plasma renin activity 2 to 8 times, which counterproductively increase plasma levels of the potent endogenous vasoconstrictor, angiotensin. Drugs that inhibit renin secretion are thus rational agents to combine with diuretics.

At present, thiazide-like saluretics are usually the first drugs to be used in the treatment of essential hypertension, usually being used alone in mild essential hypertension; other drugs are added in moderate and severe essential hypertensions. Thiazides are also correctives for the counterproductive salt and water retention that occurs as side effects to most other antihypertensive drugs. High-ceiling diuretics are inappropriate for general use and should be withheld for use only in hypertensive emergencies in which salt and water have accumulated or in combinations with drugs in which salt and water retention are especially severe (eg, methyldopa, minoxidil, hydralazine).

For the pharmacology of specific saluretics, see Chapter 50.

Peripheral Antiadrenergic Drugs

Irrespective of whether there is a sympathetic component in the perpetuation of essential or malignant hypertension, a reduction of whatever sympathetic activity exists can effect a lowering of blood pressure four ways. (1) A decrease in sympathetically (α_1-receptor)-mediated arteriolar constric-

tion will decrease systemic peripheral resistance. (2) A decrease in sympathetically (α_1-receptor)-mediated venous tone will increase venous capacitance and decrease venous return and hence cardiac output. However, this effect tends not to be sustained in the long run because of compensation by fluid retention. (3) A decrease in sympathetically (β_1-receptor)-mediated support of cardiac contractility and heart rate will decrease cardiac output. (4) A decrease in sympathetically (β_1-receptor)-modulated secretion of renin by the juxtaglomerular apparatus of the kidney will decrease the plasma levels of angiotensin II, a potent vasoconstrictor and sensitizer to sympathetic nervous activity and stimulant of the secretion of aldosterone, an antisaluretic hormone.

Drugs such as reserpine and guanethidine, which act on adrenergic nerve terminals to deplete norepinephrine or prevent release of norepinephrine, potentially are antihypertensive by all four ways, although their actions are not exerted evenly throughout the sympathetic nervous system, and the heart may be affected more than the vessels, etc. Alpha-adrenoreceptor blocking drugs, such as phenoxybenzamine and phentolamine, have antihypertensive actions, but reflex cardiac stimulation and increased renin secretion limit their efficacy. However, both phenoxybenzamine and phentolamine are important antihypertensives in the treatment of pheochromocytoma. By a unique selectivity for only α_1-receptors, prazosin causes less of such counterproductive homeostatic adjustments and hence is more efficacious. Beta-adrenoreceptor blocking drugs, such as propranolol, act to decrease cardiac output and renin secretion. However, they reflexly increase sympathetic activity and hence peripheral vascular resistance. Nevertheless, they are not only effective alone but are also important adjuncts to vasodilator drugs, which cause reflex sympathetic cardiac stimulation and increased renin secretion, and to diuretics, which increase renin secretion. β-Blocking drugs also have actions at the adrenergic nerve terminals to decrease norepinephrine release. Newer drugs, such as labetolol, with both α- and β-adrenoreceptor blocking activity may possibly considerably change the treatment of essential hypertension, since blockade of one type of receptor cannot result in counteractive reflex activation of the other.

The following important antihypertensive α- and β-adrenoreceptor-blocking and drugs that act on the adrenergic nerve terminals and neuroeffectors are described in Chapter 47, *Adrenergic Blocking Drugs:* Atenolol, Guanethidine, Labetolol, Nadolol, Metoprolol, Phenoxybenzamine, Phentolamine, Pindolol, Propranolol, Reserpine, and Timolol.

Prazosin Hydrochloride

Piperazine, 1-(4-amino-6,7-dimethoxy-2-quinazolinyl)-4-(2-furanylcarbonyl)-, monohydrochloride; Minipress (*Pfizer*)

1-(4-Amino-6,7-dimethoxy-2-quinazolinyl)-4-(2-furoyl)piperazine monohydrochloride [19237-84-4] $C_{19}H_{21}N_5O_4 \cdot HCl$ (419.87).

Preparation—Synthesis of prazosin and other hypotensive 2,4-diaminoquinazolines, starting with 2,4-dichloro-6,7-dimethoxyquinazoline, is described in British Pat 1,156,973, corresponding to US Pat 3,511,836.

Description—White, crystalline powder; pK_a 6.5 (in 1:1 water-ethanol solution).

Solubility—Slightly soluble in water; very slightly soluble in alcohol.

Uses—Prazosin lowers blood pressure by blocking α_1-adrenoreceptors that subserve vasoconstrictor functions. It differs from other α-blocking agents in that it does not block α_2-adrenoreceptors on the adrenergic nerve terminals, which receptors serve a negative feedback function to limit the release of norepinephrine. Nondiscriminatory α-blocking drugs block these receptors and thus cause an excessive continuing release of norepinephrine, which in the heart gives rise to often intolerable tachycardia and palpitation, and in the juxtaglomerular apparatus in the kidney to elevated plasma renin activity. Prazosin is unique in avoiding this neurotransmitter overflow and hence causes less reflex cardiac stimulation and increased plasma renin activity than do other α-blocking drugs. It is also unique in being the first non-diuretic drug, since chlorothiazide was introduced as an antihypertensive drug, to be accepted as a drug that can be used alone, without the ritualistic, obligatory foundation of a concomitant saluretic drug.

Prazosin can often be used alone in the treatment of *mild to moderate essential hypertension* and *with other drugs in severe hypertension*. Used alone, it is effective in 40 to 75% of patients, and, in combination, in about 80%. In these, the peripheral resistance is decreased because of α-blockade of sympathetic stimulation to the arterioles. Venous capacitance is increased, also because of α-blockade, but this plays a minor role in the antihypertensive actions, except with the first few doses. Because of the relative selectivity for the vascular resistance and cardiac impedance, prazosin is useful to *decrease cardiac overload* and hence increase cardiac output in severe acute congestive heart failure and cardiogenic shock; with mild to moderate doses, the slight effect on capacitance does not decrease venous return ("preload") sufficiently to compromise cardiac output, but large doses will decrease preload, even in the supine position.

The most common side effect of prazosin is palpitation (15%), even though this is much less than occurs with other α-adrenoreceptor blocking drugs and vasodilators. Dizziness occurs in about 10% of patients, headache in 8% of recipients; nasal stuffiness is also a frequent complaint. With small to moderate doses, postural hypotension (from α-blockade of reflex stimulation of capacitance veins) during maintenance is usually only slight to moderate, but during initiation of treatment, or when dosage is abruptly increased, a severe postural hypotension, sometimes with syncope, occurs in about 1% of patients; therefore, treatment must begin slowly and dose increments should be made gradually; with large doses, severe postural hypotension is frequent. Diuretics increase the incidence and severity of the postural hypotension. Other side effects include dry mouth, lassitude (7%), urinary incontinence, drowsiness (8%), nausea (5%), impotence, blurred vision, sweating, psychic depression, and polyarthralgia. Fluid retention frequently occurs but is usually sufficiently limited that the drug can often be given without the coadministration of a saluretic. Plasma renin levels may increase little, if at all, and do not correlate with fluid retention. Renal blood flow and filtration fraction are very little affected. Rashes and pruritus have been reported. The safety of prazosin in pregnancy has not been established. Not only do saluretics favor orthostatic hypotension and syncope, but various vasodilators, such as nitroglycerin, do also.

Prazosin is completely absorbed by the oral route; the absorption time is 1.7 to 4.55 hr. About 97% in plasma is bound to proteins. The volume of distribution is about 1.7 mL/g. Prazosin is mainly eliminated by metabolism in the liver. The β-half-life is 3 to 4 hr, but the antihypertensive effect outlasts the plasma levels, the duration of action being about 10 hr.

Dose (base equivalent)—*Oral, adult*, initially **0.5 to 1 mg** 3 times a day, to be gradually increased in increments of only 1 mg a day to a maximum of 20 mg a day; very little further effect is usually achieved above 20 mg a day, but a few patients may show increased response up to 40 mg a day. When a diuretic or another antihypertensive drug is added, the dose of prazosin should be decreased to 1 or 2 mg 3 times a day, to be followed by gradual increases in dosage, if necessary.

Dosage Forms (base equivalent)—Capsules: 1, 2, and 5 mg.

Other Peripheral Antiadrenergic Drugs

Trimazosin Hydrochloride—[4-(4-Amino-6,7,8-trimethoxy-2-quinazolinyl)-1-piperazinecarboxylic acid, 2-hydroxy-2-methylpropyl ester, monohydrochloride, monohydrate [53746-46-6] $C_{20}H_{29}N_5O_6 \cdot HCl \cdot H_2O$ (489.96)]—White crystals melting about 170° with decomposition. *Uses:* Trimazosin is closely related to prazosin (above) and closely resembles it in pharmacological actions. Vasodilatation is probably by α_1-adrenergic blockade. Heart rate is increased only reflexly by a few beats/min. Renin secretion and extracellular fluid volume are not affected. The first-dose postural hypotension characteristic of prazosin is mostly absent. It is used to treat essential hypertension and for ventricular unloading in heart failure. *Dose: Oral, initially* 50 mg 3 times a day, to be gradually increased at 2-wk intervals, if necessary, up to as much as 900 mg/day.

Centrally Acting Antihypertensive Drugs

Several drugs act directly or indirectly on the vasomotor center and/or in the spinal cord to decrease sympathetic outflow to the blood vessels. Most of them also depress the cardioaccelerator center. Less is known about central inhibition of outflow to the juxtaglomerular apparatus, but the clinically significant drugs of this class all decrease plasma renin activity. Only clonidine, guanabenz, methyldopa, and methyldopate are described in this section. The various sedative and antianxiety drugs have never been shown to have antihypertensive actions, although it might seem that a salutary effect on the progression of the reactive stage of early essential hypertension should accrue to their use. Nevertheless, the pharmaceutical industry has convinced a large proportion of the medical profession that sedatives are important adjuvants to antihypertensive treatment, and it is common to prescribe an "antianxiety" drug (phenobarbital or a benzodiazepine) along with antihypertensive drugs.

Clonidine Hydrochloride

2-(2,6-Dichlorophenylamino)-2-imidazoline hydrochloride;
Catapres (*Boehringer Ingelheim*)

2-(2,6-Dichloroanilino)-2-imidazoline monohydrochloride [4205-91-8] $C_9H_9Cl_2N_3 \cdot HCl$ (266.56).

Preparation—For information concerning the synthesis of clonidine see US Pat 3,202,660.

Description—White to off-white, odorless, bitter-tasting, crystalline powder; stable in light, air, and heat; does not exhibit polymorphism; melts about 300° with decomposition; pK_a 8.2.

Solubility—1 g in about 13 mL water (20°), about 25 mL alcohol, and about 5000 mL chloroform.

Uses—An antihypertensive drug used in the treatment of moderate *primary* (essential) *hypertension*. It is also used in the treatment of *postmenopausal vasomotor instability*, *dysmenorrhea*, and in the prophylaxis of *migraine headache*. It suppresses opiate withdrawal symptoms and is an investigational drug in the management of opiate addiction. The antihypertensive actions are in part a central action: a decrease in sympathetic activity causes vasodilation, bradycardia, and a decrease in renin release from the kidney; an increase in vagal activity also causes bradycardia. The central actions, in part, appear to be the result of a stimulant action on α_2-adrenergic receptors in the vasomotor and cardioinhibitory centers, and in the spinal cord on preganglionic sympathetic neurons. Clonidine also appears to have a peripheral action to reduce release of norepinephrine from sympathetic nerves; it stimulates α_2-adrenergic receptors on the sympathetic nerve terminals, which stimulation feeds back negatively to suppress release of the mediator.

In moderate doses clonidine causes sedation in about 65% of patients, dry mouth in about 50%, and mild to moderate orthostatic hypotension in about 25%. Salt and water retention occur in the first few days of treatment but usually do not persist. Impotence, constipation, depression, and nightmares also occur in an appreciable proportion of recipients. Various side effects secondary to too-marked reductions in blood pressure can occur, as with most antihypertensive drugs. Tolerance sometimes occurs. After prolonged treatment, clonidine potentiates the pressor actions of sympathomimetics and angiotensin, and antagonizes the depressor actions of isoproterenol. Serious rebound hypertension may occur if the drug is discontinued abruptly. Tricyclic antidepressants antagonize the antihypertensive actions of clonidine. In combination with methyldopa, excessive sedation occurs.

Clonidine is readily absorbed by the oral route, with an absorption time of 2 to 4 hr. It is excreted mostly unchanged into the urine. The half-life is 6 to 23 hr (av 13). The duration of action is 6 to 10 hr.

Dose—*Oral, adults,* for *mild* to *moderate* essential *hypertension,* initially **0.1 mg** twice a day, followed by gradual adjustments in increments of 0.1 to 0.2 mg a day until the desired effect occurs; *main-*

tenance doses usually range from **0.2** to **0.8 mg** a day; *severe hypertension*, initially **0.2 mg** then **0.1 mg** every hr until the blood pressure is controlled or 0.7 mg have been given; for *vasomotor instability*, **25** to **75 μg** (0.025 to 0.075 mg) twice a day; for severe *dysmenorrhea*, **25 μg** (0.025 mg) twice a day 2 weeks before and during menses; for *migraine*, **25 μg** 2 to 4 times a day to **50 μg** 3 times a day.

Dosage Forms—Tablets: 0.1, 0.2 mg and 0.3.

Methyldopa

L-Tyrosine, 3-hydroxy-α-methyl-, sesquihydrate; Alpha-methyldopa; Aldomet (*Merck Sharp & Dohme*)

L-3-(3,4-Dihydroxyphenyl)-2-methylalanine   [41372-08-1] $C_{10}H_{13}NO_4.1\frac{1}{2}H_2O$ (238.24); *anhydrous* [555-30-6] (211.22).

Preparation—The product of the reaction of 3,4-dimethoxy-phenylacetonitrile with sodium ethoxide is hydrolyzed with acid to give 3,4-dimethoxyphenylacetone. This is reacted with ammonium carbonate and potassium cyanide to form a substituted hydantoin intermediate which, on alkaline hydrolysis, yields racemic methyldopa. The acetylated form of this racemate is resolved using (−)-α-methylbenzylamine. The isolated acetylated (−)-methyldopate salt is deacetylated with base and treated with mineral acid to liberate (−)-methyldopa. US Pat 2,868,818.

Description—White to yellowish white, odorless, fine powder, which may contain friable lumps. It is almost tasteless and relatively stable in both light and air. It melts above 290° with decomposition.

Solubility—Sparingly soluble in water; very soluble in diluted hydrochloric acid; slightly soluble in alcohol; practically insoluble in ether.

Uses—Methyldopa is employed as an *antihypertensive* in the treatment of moderate to severe essential hypertension, including malignant hypertension: the antihypertensive effect is greater than that of oral reserpine but somewhat less than that of guanethidine. It has a slight effect on cardiac output and heart rate. Renal blood flow remains nearly normal in patients without previous renal damage. The degree of orthostatic hypotension is considerably less than with guanethidine, which is an advantage. Its action is erratic, and one third of treated patients may not respond to the drug. Tolerance sometimes develops in up to a third of initially responsive patients; it is largely the result of retention of salt and water, and may be overcome by increasing the dose of concomitant diuretic drug. Methyldopa has some usefulness in the treatment of *pheochromocytoma* and *carcinoid tumor*. It acts to inhibit dopa decarboxylase (which is also 5-hydroxytryptophan decarboxylase) and thus to suppress biosynthesis of norepinephrine, epinephrine, and 5-hydroxytryptamine (serotonin) in chromaffin and argentochromaffin cells; norepinephrine synthesis in adrenergic neurons is not affected by therapeutic doses, since decarboxylation is not the rate-limiting step there.

In the brain, methyldopa appears to induce release of norepinephrine from storage sites in noradrenergic neurons and to interfere with release in response to stimuli, probably through the action of the decarboxylated metabolites of methyldopa—methyldopamine and methylnorepinephrine. These metabolites displace norepinephrine from storage sites and are themselves released as "false transmitters" by nervous impulses in the adrenergic nerves. The metabolite α-methylepinephrine has potent α_2-agonist activity and probably acts to decrease blood pressure in the same way as does clonidine. The effects accumulatively result in failure of effective transmission. In the vasomotor center the result is a decrease in sympathetic vasomotor outflow, which decreases blood pressure and lowers plasma renin activity. The action of methyldopa begins in about 2 hr, becomes maximal in 6 to 8 hr, and lasts 18 to 24 hr. Methyldopa also depletes tissue 5-hydroxytryptamine by interference with tryptophan decarboxylase.

The most prominent side effect of methyldopa is somnolence; tolerance to the sedative effects usually occurs in a few days to a few weeks. Side effects consequent to blockade of sympathetic nerves include occasional orthostatic hypotension with vertigo, nausea, weakness and headache, bradycardia, nasal stuffiness, diarrhea, and impotence. Other side effects include frequent dry mouth, maculopapular skin rashes, decreased libido in males, breast enlargement, and paresthesias. Like reserpine, it may cause edema and rarely psychic depression and nightmares, parkinsonism, arthralgia, and

myalgia. Lactation and breast engorgement occur rarely. Depression of liver function characterized by fever and malaise and occasionally jaundice may occur. The direct Coombs test may be positive in about 20% of recipients. Rarely, a lupus erythematosus-like syndrome, granulocytopenia, or thrombocytopenia occurs. Methyldopa is contraindicated in the presence of active liver disease and in persons known to be sensitive to the drug.

About 50% of methyldopa is absorbed by the oral route. Most of the drug is excreted unchanged, but some is conjugated to the *O*-sulfate. Most of the drug is excreted before distribution is complete. The plasma concentration falls with an α-phase half-life of about 1.7 hr; however, in renal failure only 50% is excreted during the distribution phase ($t_{1/2}$ = 3.5 hr), and accumulation can occur.

Dose—*Oral, adults*, **250 mg** every 8 or 12 hr during the first 2 days then, if necessary, upward adjustments are made at intervals no shorter than 2 days, up to a total daily dose of 2 g; while occasional patients have responded to higher doses (maximum of 3 g daily) it is recommended that if 2 g is insufficient, another antihypertensive drug be added to the regimen rather than to increase the dose. *Children*, initially **10 mg/kg** of body weight a day in 2 to 4 divided doses, or 100 mg/m² of body surface every 8 hr, to be adjusted, as necessary, at 2- to 4-day intervals; the maximum *maintenance* dose is 65 mg/kg or 2 g/m², up to a maximum total of 3 g a day.

Dosage Forms—Tablets: 125, 250, and 500 mg.

Methyldopate Hydrochloride

L-Tyrosine, 3-hydroxy-α-methyl-, ethyl ester, hydrochloride; Aldomet Ester Hydrochloride (*Merck Sharp & Dohme*)

L-3-(3,4-Dihydroxyphenyl)-2-methylalanine ethyl ester hydrochloride [5208-79-4] $C_{12}H_{17}NO_4.HCl$ (275.73).

Preparation—By converting methyldopa to its ethyl ester and passing hydrogen chloride into a solution of the ester in a suitable organic solvent.

Description—White or practically white crystalline powder which is odorless or practically odorless and has a bitter taste. It is relatively stable both in light and air. It melts at about 160°. pH (1 in 100 solution) between 3.0 and 5.0.

Solubility—Freely soluble in water, alcohol, and methanol; slightly soluble in chloroform; practically insoluble in ether.

Uses—The actions and uses are the same as those of *Methyldopa*. The ester is employed for intravenous use in hypertensive crises or in patients who are unable to take antihypertensive drugs by mouth. In the body the ethyl group is removed by hydrolysis to yield methyldopa. The onset of action by the intravenous route is 4 to 6 hours, whereas that by the oral route may be 1 to 2 days. The duration of action is 10 to 16 hours.

Dose—*Intravenous infusion, adults*, **250 to 500 mg** in 100 mL of 5% dextrose injection over a period of 30 to 60 min every 6 hr, if needed; single doses of as much as 3 g have been given, but syncope is more likely with such large doses, especially in arteriosclerotic patients: *children*, **5 to 10 mg/kg** of body weight (150 to 300 mg/m² of body surface) every 6 hr if necessary.

Dosage Form—Injection: 250 mg/5 mL.

Other Centrally Acting Antihypertensive Drugs

Guanabenz Acetate [[(2,6-Dichlorobenzylidene)amino]guanidine acetate [23256-50-0] $C_8H_8Cl_2N_4.C_2H_4O_2$ (291.14)]—*Uses:* Guanabenz depresses the vasomotor and cardioaccelerator centers and thus decreases the sympathetic outflow to the arterioles and heart. It appears to act as an α_2-adrenergic agonist at presynaptic nerve terminals in the CNS, thus decreasing release of neurotransmitter. Guanabenz also has peripheral adrenergic neuron-blocking actions. It is effective in mild to moderately severe essential hypertension. Although it is usually effective alone, efficacy is enhanced by saluretics. It is as effective as methyldopa, but the incidence of side effects may be greater. The duration of action is 12 to 24 hr. It causes a mild, usually insignificant, postural or exercise hypotension. Dry mouth, sedation and occasional anxiety, depression, insomnia and cardiac dysrhythmias occur. It does not interfere with ejaculation or cause diarrhea, hepatitis, or immune disorders. Withdrawal hypertension occurs after large doses. *Dose: Oral*, initially 8 mg in 1 or 2 divided doses, to be gradually increased to 64 mg/day, if necessary.

Guanfacine Hydrochloride—[*N*-(Aminoiminomethyl)-2,6-dichlorobenzeneacetamide hydrochloride [29110-48-3] $C_9H_2Cl_2N_3O.HCl$

(282.56)]—White needles melting about 215°. *Uses:* Guanfacine is an α_2-agonist which acts in the vasomotor center and the bulbospinal tract to decrease sympathetic outflow to the blood vessels and to a lesser extent, to the heart. It is thus like clonidine (page 845) and guanabenz. However, its effects last longer. It is used (usually along with a saluretic) mostly to treat mild to *moderate hypertension*, but it is also effective in *toxemia of pregnancy* and may ultimately prove to be useful in hypertensive emergencies. Tolerance is common in the absence of a saluretic. Adverse effects are mainly those of clonidine (page 845). Withdrawal hypertension may occur 2 to 7 days after discontinuation of treatment. Elimination is by both hepatic metabolism and renal excretion, the former being the more important; dosage is said not to require adjustments in renal failure. The elimination half-life is 14 to 17 hr. *Dose:* Oral, *adults*, initially 0.5 mg twice a day, to be gradually increased as needed; maintenance doses usually lie between 1 and 3 mg/day.

Antihypertensive Direct Vasodilators

Direct vasodilators act by several mechanisms, such as inhibition of cyclic nucleotide phosphodiesterase, adenosine mimicry, impairment of calcium and sodium influx in vascular smooth muscle, and unknown mechanisms. Their usefulness in the ambulatory treatment of hypertension depends a great deal on the selectivity of the drug for the resistance blood vessels, namely, the arterioles, which causes a lowering of blood pressure. If the capacitance veins are also dilated, venous return to the heart, and hence cardiovascular adjustments to posture and exercise, is impaired, and the patient may experience postural and exercise hypotensions, sometimes to the point of syncope. A slight degree of interference with venous return is usually considered to be desirable, especially in the treatment of severe hypertension, because it enables a greater lowering of blood pressure than does arteriolar dilatation alone. Direct vasodilators invariably cause reflex palpitation and tachycardia and also increases in plasma renin activity, all of which tend to counter the hypotensive action; the cardiac effects give rise to patient discomfort. Therefore, it is advisable to combine the vasodilators with β-blocking drugs to antagonize these effects. In addition to the ultimate edema-causing sequelae to increased renin secretion, the lowering of blood pressure may decrease both pressure natriuresis and renal blood flow. This decrease promotes sodium and water retention, which, in turn, may decrease the antihypertensive effects of the drug; therefore, it is rational to use saluretics in combination with vasodilators.

Diazoxide

2*H*-1,2,4-Benzothiadiazine, 7-chloro-3-methyl-, 1,1-dioxide; Hyperstat (*Schering*)

7-Chloro-3-methyl-2*H*-1,2,4-benzothiadiazine 1,1-dioxide [364-98-7] $C_8H_7ClN_2O_2S$ (230.67).

Preparation—One method reacts 2,4-dichloronitrobenzene with benzyl mercaptan and KOH and the 2-(benzylthio) group thus introduced is converted to —SO_2Cl with chlorine and aqueous acetic acid and thence to —SO_2NH_2 by reaction with NH_3. After reducing the NO_2 to NH_2 with Fe and NH_4Cl, cyclization is effected by condensation with ethyl orthoacetate. *Science 133:* 2067, 1961. US Pats. 2,986,573 and 3,345,365.

Description—White to cream-white crystals or crystalline powder; odorless; melts at about 330°.
Solubility—Practically insoluble to sparingly soluble in water.

Uses—Diazoxide exerts prominent vasodepressor actions, especially by the intravenous route. In therapeutic doses, vasodepression is primarily the result of arteriolar dilatation, so that orthostatic hypotension is usually minimal. However, some venous dilatation does occur, which at times is sufficient to cause orthostatic hypotension. The smooth muscle-relaxing effects result from both phosphodiesterase inhibition and interference with calcium activation of the contractile system. Diazoxide is used as a hypotensive drug in *acute hypertensive crises*. Its side effects preclude its use in the chronic management of essential hypertension, but it may be used to initiate treatment in order to control blood pressure until the oral antihypertensives can be used.

Although diazoxide is a benzothiazide, it is not a diuretic but instead actually causes salt and water retention and consequent gain in weight. This action sometimes precipitates congestive heart failure, especially if renal function is impaired. It also causes hyperglycemia, which is usually more prominent by the oral route because the absorbed drug must all pass through the liver, where phosphodiesterase inhibition promotes glycogenolysis. Occasionally it is necessary to administer oral hypoglycemics or insulin to suppress the hyperglycemia. Oral diazoxide is sometimes employed in the treatment of hypoglycemia, especially the leucine-sensitive type in children. Other side effects include nausea, vomiting, and other gastrointestinal upsets, burning sensations along the vein of injection (because of the high pH of solutions), mild tachycardia, substernal pain, occasional orthostatic hypotension, transient hyperuricemia, headache, and drowsiness. Overdosage by the intravenous route can cause shock. With chronic use, hirsutism, hyperosmolar nonketotic coma, dermatoses, neutropenia, thrombocytopenia, and eosinophilia may occur.

Diazoxide is contraindicated in toxemia of pregnancy unless other antihypertensives have failed; its effect on the fetus is unknown; also, it relaxes uterine smooth muscle and may interfere with impending delivery. Diazoxide should be used in diabetics only when blood glucose is closely monitored. Blood glucose also should be determined in all persons receiving multiple injections. It should be used cautiously in persons with coronary or cerebral insufficiency and patients with impaired renal function. However, it may be safer to use in renal hypertensive crises than other antihypertensives. The drug is contraindicated if hypersensitivity to thiazides exists. Thiazide diuretics and other antihypertensive drugs increase the response to diazoxide, even when they fail to lower blood pressure themselves. Some authorities administer furosemide along with diazoxide, in order to prevent salt and water retention. Diazoxide displaces dicumarol-type anticoagulants from plasma proteins, which can lead to a hemorrhagic diathesis.

Diazoxide is well absorbed orally. It is about 90% protein-bound, but rapid intravenous injection permits distribution to smooth muscle before it is bound to protein. Thus a greater and longer-lasting fall in blood pressure accrues to faster rates of injection. It is of interest that the drug persists in blood longer than the hypotensive effect; the plasma half-life is 10 to 31 hr in persons with normal renal function, but the hypotensive effect lasts only 2 to 15 hr. Different populations may eliminate the drug differently, some mostly by renal excretion and others mostly by biotransformation.

Dose—*Intravenous, adults*, for *hypertensive emergencies*, initially up to **150 mg** (or 1 to 3 mg/kg), repeated in 5 to 15 min, if necessary, with dose adjusted according to response, then every 4 to 24 hr until the blood pressure is under control and an oral antihypertensive drug can be substituted; *children, initially* 1 to **3 mg/kg** (or 30 to 90 mg/m^2 of body surface), repeated as for adults. *Oral, adults*, for *hypoglycemia, initially* 3 to **8 mg/kg/day** in 2 or 3 evenly divided doses (no more than 15 mg/kg/day); *children, initially* **3.3 mg/kg** every 8 hr, adjusted according to response, then 8 to **15 mg/kg/day** in 2 or 3 evenly divided doses.

Dosage Forms—Capsules: 50 and 100 mg; Injection: 300 mg/20 mL; Oral Suspension: 50 mg/mL.

Hydralazine Hydrochloride

Phthalazine, 1-hydrazino-, monohydrochloride; Apresoline (*Ciba*)

1-Hydrazinophthalazine monohydrochloride [304-20-1] $C_8H_8N_4$·HCl (196.64).

Preparation—Phthalazone is converted to 1-chlorophthalazine by treatment with phosphorus oxychloride, condensed with hydrazine hydrate to form hydralazine, and neutralized with HCl to produce the hydrochloride.

Description—White to off-white, crystalline powder; melts in the range of 270° to 280°, with decomposition.

Solubility—1 g in 25 mL water, 500 mL alcohol; very slightly soluble in ether.

Uses—Hydralazine is a vasodilator of unknown mechanism of action. It is one of the few drugs that causes substantial vasodilatation in the kidney, and it increases renal plasma flow even when the blood pressure drops considerably. Vasodilatation is also pronounced in the splanchnic, cerebral, and coronary vascular beds; it exerts only slight vasodilator actions in skin and skeletal muscle. The veins participate very little in the effect, so that postural hypotension is negligible. As the result of the fall in blood pressure, reflex tachycardia, palpitations, and increases in plasma renin activity occur, although the renin activity sometimes decreases in long-term treatment. Hydralazine may be used in the treatment of *essential, early malignant hypertension* and *hypertensive emergencies*, virtually always in conjunction with other antihypertensive drugs; however, mainly because of its side effects, it is generally not used until other safer therapy has failed. Because it increases renal blood flow, it is often used to treat *toxemia of pregnancy*. It is also sometimes used in *acute congestive heart failure* or *after myocardial infarction* because it decreases cardiac afterload with very little effect on preload, so that cardiac output is improved.

The principal serious toxic effects of hydralazine hydrochloride are syndromes resembling rheumatoid arthritis or lupus erythematosus, appearance of which necessitates withdrawal of the drug. Most patient complaints are of tachycardia and palpitations. These effects are counterproductive in that they tend to limit the fall in blood pressure. Furthermore, they may precipitate attacks of angina pectoris. β-Adrenergic blocking drugs prevent these effects and also the reflex rise in plasma renin levels and hence increases the antihypertensive response. Other frequent side effects include tachycardia and palpitation (sometimes causing anginal pain), dizziness, headache and cardiomegaly. Paresthesias, anxiety, nausea, vomiting, malaise, disorientation, depression, edema, nasal congestion, lacrimation, red eyes, rash, giant urticaria, drug fever, agranulocytosis, leukocytosis, and anemia also occasionally occur. It sometimes causes a lupus-like syndrome. Even when the plasma renin activity is suppressed, a counterproductive sodium and water retention occurs; saluretics suppress the effect and improve the antihypertensive effects.

Hydralazine is absorbed by the oral route; food enhances the bioavailability. Elimination is by both ring hydroxylation and *N*-acetylation, and only 10% of hydralazine is excreted unchanged. The half-life is 1.5 to 8 hr; the difference between slow and fast acetylators is usually minor. Hydralazine accumulates in fat in vascular smooth muscle, where it has a life longer than in plasma.

Dose—*Oral, adults*, initially **5 to 10 mg** 4 times a day for 2 to 4 days, then **25 mg** 4 times a day for the rest of the week; the dose may be increased to **200 mg** a day in 2 to 4 divided doses thereafter; the daily dose should not exceed 200 mg, but in preeclampsia the total daily dose may be as high as 400 mg, reached by *daily* increments of 40 to 50 mg until the desired effect is achieved; *children*, initially **0.75 mg/kg** of body weight (or 25 mg/m² of body surface) daily, divided into 4 doses. *Intramuscular* or *intravenous, adults*, **10 to 20 mg,** increased to **40 mg** if necessary, repeated as necessary; *children*, **1.7 to 3.5 mg/kg** of body weight (or 50 to 100 mg/m² of body surface) daily, divided into 4 to 6 doses.

Dosage Forms—Injection: 20 mg/mL; Tablets: 10, 25, 50, and 100 mg.

Minoxidil

2,4-Pyrimidinediamine, 6-(1-piperidinyl)-, 3-oxide; Loniten (*Upjohn*)

2,4-Diamino-6-piperidinopyrimidine 3-oxide [38304-91-5] $C_9H_{15}N_5O$ (209.25).

Preparation—Described in US Pat. 3,461,461.

Description—White to off-white, crystalline powder.

Solubility—1 g in about 500 mL water; soluble in alcohol; practically insoluble in chloroform.

Uses—Minoxidil dilates arterioles by an undetermined mechanism and lowers the total peripheral vascular resistance and hence the blood pressure. The maximum achievable decrease in mean blood pressure is usually at least 35 torr in most hypertensive patients. Dilatation of capacitance veins is only slight to moderate and sympathetic vascular reflexes are unimpaired, so that postural and exercise hypotensions are usually minimal. Reflex tachycardia and palpitations occur, but they are less than that expected from the fall in blood pressure, which suggests cardioaccelerator-suppressant actions not yet elucidated; nevertheless, a β-adrenoreceptor blocking drug may need to be coadministered to suppress reflex cardiac stimulation. Renal plasma flow and glomerular filtration rate are very little affected, which implies a substantial renal vasodilatation. Plasma renin activity may be elevated as the result of reflex sympathetic activity or diminished by an unknown mechanism. Irrespective of the plasma renin activity, salt and water retention occur sufficiently to cause considerable tolerance to the antihypertensive effects, and saluretics, even occasionally high-ceiling diuretics, are necessary to restore the antihypertensive effects. In appropriate dosage, minoxidil can be used to treat all types of hypertension, although most experience has been in the treatment of *moderate* to *severe essential hypertension*. It is often effective in hypertensions refractory to all other therapy. It is also useful in *hypertensive emergencies* and for *ventricular unloading*, the effect being mainly to decrease afterload.

Adverse effects include fluid retention, cardiac stimulation, and mild postural hypotension, anginal attacks (from both cardiac stimulation and decreased coronary perfusion pressure), moderate but usually reversible hypertrichosis with increased pigmentation in about 70% of patients, and rare pulmonary hypertension (controversial), pericardial effusion, and breast tenderness. A slight anemia (7% decrease in RBC, in part the result of hemodilution) and small increase in alkaline phosphatase and 6% increase in plasma creatinine and BUN transiently occur. No teratogenic effects have thus far been observed, but it is wise to avoid the drug during pregnancy. It should also probably be withheld within a month after a myocardial infarction.

Minoxidil is absorbed by the oral route. It is concentrated in vascular tissue. Metabolism in the liver accounts for about 90% of elimination, and no modification of dose is required in renal failure or hemodialysis. The apparent half-life of about 4 hr appears to be a distribution parameter; the β-half-life is about 24 hr. The duration of action is 1 to 3 days.

Dose—*Oral, adult*, and *children over 12 years of age*, initially **5 mg** a day, with dose adjustments at 3-day intervals, if necessary, usually up to 20 to 40 mg and no more than 100 mg a day; *children under 12 years*, *initially* **0.2 mg/kg** of body weight a day, to be gradually increased at 3-day intervals, usually up to 0.25 to 1 mg/kg and no more than 50 mg a day. In severe hypertension in which a rapid reduction in blood pressure is desired, dose adjustments can be made at 6-hr intervals, if the patient is carefully monitored.

Dosage Forms—Tablets: 2.5 and 10 mg.

Nifedipine—page 862.

Nitroprusside Sodium

Ferrate(2-), pentakis(cyano-*C*)nitrosyl-, disodium, (*OC*-6-22)-dihydrate; Sodium Nitroferricyanide; Nipride (*Roche*); Nitropress (*Abbott*)

Disodium pentacyanonitrosylferrate(2-) dihydrate [13755-38-9] $Na_2[Fe(CN)_5NO].2H_2O$ (297.95); *anhydrous* [14402-89-2] (261.92).

Preparation—Potassium ferrocyanide is dissolved in 50% HNO_3 and the solution is boiled for about an hour. After cooling and filtering to remove potassium nitrate, the solution is neutralized with Na_2CO_3, and evaporated to crystallization.

Description—Reddish brown, practically odorless, crystals or powder.

Solubility—1 g in about 2.5 mL water; slightly soluble in alcohol.

Uses—Sodium nitroprusside is a directly acting peripheral vasodilator presumably because of an effect to shut down receptor-operated calcium transport. Its actions on arterioles decrease the total systemic vascular resistance, which is the main cause of the fall in blood pressure it evokes. It has a lesser action on capacitance veins so that, with usual doses, venous return is insignificantly impaired in the recumbent position; however, in the upright position there is considerable orthostatic hypotension. Cardiac output is increased in the recumbent and decreased in the upright position. Heart rate is invariably increased reflexly. There is a variable effect on renal plasma flow and glomerular filtration rate, but it is usually increased in the recumbent position. Plasma renin activity is increased.

Nitroprusside is given by continuous intravenous infusion for treatment of *hypertensive emergencies* and for *ventricular unloading* in acute congestive heart failure and after myocardial infarction; its predilection for the arterioles enables it to reduce selectively the cardiac afterload. It is also used for controlled hypotension during surgery. Owing to an extremely brief duration of action, the drug must be given intravenously. Since there is a very narrow therapeutic range, the rate of infusion and the blood pressure must be monitored continuously at first and then at intervals of 5 min throughout the course of the infusion. For this reason, the drug is usually employed only in desperation.

Overdosage can cause hypertensive instead of hypotensive effects. Other adverse effects are tachycardia (in part reflex, hence unavoidable), nausea, retching, vomiting, transient restlessness, agitation, tremors, and muscular twitching. Dyspnea, cyanosis, mydriasis, and cardiovascular collapse have occurred as the result of too marked a fall in blood pressure.

The fate of nitroprusside anion is unknown. Since it does not produce methemoglobinemia in adults, it can be presumed that the rate of release of nitrite ion is quite slow. A trace of cyanide ion is formed, but it is far too little to cause cyanide intoxication. However, it is possible that the hypertensive phase of action and part of the tachycardia is from the stimulation of the carotid chemoreceptors by cyanide. Cyanide is converted to thiocyanate by the enzyme rhodanase; infants lack this enzyme, so that the drug should not be used in neonates and probably also not in the treatment of toxemia of pregnancy.

Dose (as the dihydrate)—*Intravenous*, by slow infusion, *adults*, *initially* **0.5 μg/kg** of body weight per minute of a solution containing 50 mg dissolved in 500 to 1000 mL of 5% dextrose injection, adjusted in 0.5 μg-increments, as needed, up to a limit of 10 μg/kg/min or a total dose of 3.5 mg/kg in brief infusions; *children*, **1.4 μg/kg/min,** adjusted slowly, if necessary. A fresh solution should be prepared immediately before use.

Dosage Form—Powder for preparation of injection: 50 mg.

Ganglionic Blocking Agents

The ganglionic blocking agents act by competing with acetylcholine for the cholinergic receptors of the autonomic postganglionic neurons. Like acetylcholine, most of these agents are quaternary ammonium agents, although a few amines also possess ganglionic blocking properties. Since the ganglia of both the sympathetic and parasympathetic nervous systems are cholinergic, these drugs interrupt the outflow through both systems; thus, it is not possible to achieve a therapeutic block of autonomic outflow to a given locus without a number of undesirable but unavoidable side effects resulting from the blockade of other autonomic nerves. Blockade of sympathetic outflow to the blood vessels causes hypotension and increased blood flow (with a pink, warm skin). Blockade of sympathetics to the heart may cause slowing, but the parasympathetic outflow is also blocked, so that acceleration can result in persons with predominantly parasympathetic tone. Orthostatic hypotension results from blockade of reflex adjustments to posture. Blockade of parasympathetic outflow results in dry mouth, mydriasis, cycloplegia (loss of ocular accommodation), diminished gastrointestinal motility, and urinary retention.

Ganglionic blocking drugs are erratically absorbed after oral administration, but some are well enough absorbed to be given by mouth. They are all secreted into the urine by the cation transport system, but some are filtered more than secreted.

The ganglionic blocking agents are used mostly for their interruption of the sympathetic outflow in *hypertension*, *vasospastic disorders*, and *peripheral vascular disease*, thus lowering the blood pressure and increasing the peripheral blood flow. This is not to imply, however, that increased sympathetic activity occurs in all disorders for which these agents are used; rather, a reduction in even normal sympathetic tone is conducive to symptomatic improvement. In *arterial embolism, herpes zoster, acute thrombophlebitis, acrocyanosis, trench foot, immersion foot, reflex dystrophy,* and *Raynaud's disease* sympathetic hyperactivity may occur at some point in the disease; in essential and malignant hypertensions, diabetic gangrene, thromboangiitis obliterans, and arteriosclerosis obliterans there is no evidence of significant sympathetic hyperactivity.

The ganglionic blocking agents should be used cautiously when other hypotensive, antihypertensive or anesthetic drugs are concomitantly used, because the hypotension may be exaggerated to such an extent that blood flow through the brain, heart, or kidney may be jeopardized. Overdose of the ganglionic blocking drug alone can have this effect. Because compensatory cardiovascular reflexes are suppressed by the ganglionic blocking drugs, pressor drugs given during ganglionic blockade may elicit dangerously enhanced responses.

Ganglionic blocking drugs are contraindicated when there is pyloric stenosis, cerebral arteriosclerosis, coronary insufficiency, recent myocardial infarction, or glaucoma. They should be used cautiously in elderly patients and in patients with renal insufficiency.

Mecamylamine Hydrochloride

N,2,3,3-Tetramethyl-2-norbornanamine hydrochloride [826-39-1]

$C_{11}H_{21}N.HCl$ (203.75); Inversine (*Merck Sharp & Dohme*). Prepared from camphene (see RPS-15, page 781). White, crystalline powder; freely soluble in water.

Uses—Mecamylamine differs from most other ganglionic blocking agents in that it is not a quaternary ammonium compound; it is poorly ionized in the small intestine and thus is readily and completely absorbed. Consequently its actions are more predictable than those of most other ganglionic blocking agents, and it is also more potent by the oral route. Its nonionic form permits it to pass into the central nervous system, so that occasional bizarre central disturbances may result. It has a low renal clearance and hence a longer duration of action than most ganglionic agents.

Like the ganglionic blocking agents in general, mecamylamine may produce a variety of unpleasant unavoidable side effects that result from the interruption of both sympathetic and parasympathetic outflow. Orthostatic hypotension, blurring of vision, dry mouth, diarrhea followed by constipation, occasional paralytic ileus, nausea and vomiting, urinary retention, fatigue, sedation and impotence are among these general side effects. Tremor and delusions or hallucinations may occur; these actions are not shared by the quaternary ammonium ganglionic blocking agents.

Dose—*Oral, adults,* **2.5** to **25 mg** daily; *usual, initial,* **2.5 mg** 2 times a day, increased by **2.5-mg** increments at intervals of not less than 2 days as required, *maintenance*, **7.5 mg** 3 times a day.

Dosage Forms—Tablets: 2.5 and 10 mg.

Drugs Affecting Renin-Angiotensin System

Renin is a protease that acts on the plasma α_2-globulin substrate, angiotensinogen, to yield the decapeptide, angiotensin I. Angiotensin I is hydrolyzed by a *"converting enzyme"* to yield the octapeptide, angiotensin II. Angiotensin II may lose one aminoacid residue to yield angiotensin III. Angiotensins II and III are destroyed by carboxypeptidases.

Angiotensin I is inactive in the cardiovascular system, although it may have some effect to contract the renal glomerular mesangium. Angiotensin II has several cardiovascular-renal actions: 1) It stimulates the zona glomerulosa of the adrenal cortex to secrete aldosterone. Aldosterone causes the renal retention of sodium (and hence of water) and the loss of potassium. The extracellular fluid volume and body burden of sodium are thus increased, which promotes an increase in blood pressure in many persons and to edema in congestive heart failure. 2) It is a very potent vasoconstrictor, which contributes to an elevation of blood pressure in most persons and to reduced cardiac output (from increased afterload) in congestive heart failure. 3) It facilitates transmission in sympathetic ganglia, increases the release of norepinephrine at adrenergic nerve terminals, and increases the response of blood vessels and the heart to norepinephrine, thus amplifying sympathetic factors in the maintenance of elevated blood pressure. 4) It stimulates the release of ADH (vasopressin) from the neurohypophysis and thirst receptors, thus adding to volume and vasopressor factors in some conditions of hypertension and in congestive heart failure. Angiotensin II is also a putative neurotransmitter in the CNS. Angiotensin III also stimulates the adrenal secretion of aldosterone.

The most important site of the angiotensin converting enzyme (CE) is in the lung, but CE is found in the kidney, CNS and elsewhere. A form of CE circulates in the plasma. The enzyme also doubles as kininase II. Therefore, inhibition of CE not only decreases the amount of the vasoconstrictor, angiotension II, but increases the amount of the vasodilator kinins. At one time it was thought that much of the antihypertensive effects of CE inhibitors was attributable to kinins, but careful studies have discounted this involvement. Furthermore, kinins probably do not account for rashes caused by captopril, as is commonly thought.

Converting enzyme inhibitors are used to treat *hypertension*, especially when plasma renin activity (PRA) is high, although they are somewhat antihypertensive even when PRA is not elevated. They are also used in *refractory congestive heart failure*, to unload the ventricle and to suppress the renin angiotensin factor in edema formation.

There is one available competitive antagonist of angiotension II, *saralasin*, but it has a very brief half-life and is not orally effective. Long-acting, orally effective antagonists are under investigation. There are also promising investigational inhibitors of renin. Some of these may be introduced before the next edition of this book.

Captopril

L-Proline, 1-[(2S)-3-mercapto-2-methyl-1-oxopropyl]-, Capoten (*Squibb*)

[62571-86-2] $C_9H_{15}NO_3S$ (217.28)
Preparation—See *Science 196*: 441, 1977.

Description—White crystals melting about 88° which resolidify and melt again at about 105°. $pK_1 = 3.7$, $pK_2 = 9.8$.
Solubility—Freely soluble in water, alcohol, or chloroform.

Uses—Captopril is an orally effective converting enzyme inhibitor which is a triumph of drug design. For the uses, see the general statement (above). It is most effective in renal and malignant hypertensions.

Rashes (erythematous, morbilliform, macropapular, edematous, urticarial) occur during the first 4 weeks of treatment in about 10% of recipients. Approximately 7 to 10% of these manifest eosinophilia and antinuclear antibody, so that the rashes may have an immune origin. Eruptions do not occur until the dose exceeds 600 mg/day; they will sometimes disappear even with continued treatment. Approximately 7% of recipients may have chest pain, vertigo or syncope (especially in salt-depleted patients), swelling of the hands, feet or mouth (angioedema), and tachycardia and/or dysrhythmia. Sore throat (with severe neutropenia) and chills and fever occur in about 0.3%. Neutropenia is "dose-related" and occurs within 10 to 30 days of treatment; it persists for about 2 weeks after discontinuation; granulocyte counts are mandatory. Captopril increases blood urea nitrogen, creatinine, and liver enzymes in some patients. It may cause false positive tests for urinary acetone. Since captopril decreases aldosterone levels, drugs or situations that cause hyperkalemia, hyponatremia or hypoveolemia may interact adversely.

Dose—*Oral, adult, initially* **25 mg** 3 times a day to be increased after 2 weeks to 50 mg 3 times a day, if necessary; up to 150 mg 3 times a day may be given; *children, initially* **360 μg** (0.36 mg)/**kg,** to be increased, if necessary, by 360 μg/kg at 8- to 24-hr intervals up to the optimal dose.
Dosage Forms—Tablets: 25, 50 and 100 mg.

Other Drugs Affecting Renin-Angiotensin System

Enalapril Maleate [(S)-1-[N-[1-(Ethoxycarbonyl)-3-phenylpropyl]L-alanyl]-L-proline (Z)-2-butenedioate (1:1) [76095-16-4] $C_{20}H_{28}N_2O_5 \cdot C_4H_4O_4$ (492.52)]. A white to off-white powder melting about 144°: The pH of a 1% aqueous solution is about 2.6. *Uses:* Enalapril is a converting enzyme inhibitor used in the treatment of *hypertension*. It lowers blood pressure irrespective of whether plasma renin activity is high or low, and lowering of blood pressure does not correlate well with suppression of plasma converting enzyme activity. Unlike captopril, enalapril does not increase left ventricular performance, even though cardiac impedance is lowered, possibly because norepinephrine-release by sympathetic nerves is decreased. The advantage of enalapril over captopril is the absence of hematologic and dermatologic adverse effects. In fact, captopril-induced rashes resolve after enalapril is substituted. *Dose* (Not firmly established): *Oral, adults, initially* 5 mg twice a day, to be increased to 10 mg twice a day if necessary; no greater effect is achieved with higher doses.
Saralasin Acetate [1-(N-Methylglycine)-5-L-valine-8-L-alanine-angiotensin acetate [39698-78-7] $C_{42}H_{65}N_{13}O_{10} \cdot xC_2H_4O_2 \cdot xH_2O$ (912.06-base) Sarenin (*Norwich-Eaton*)] Fluffy white powder melting

about 255°. Soluble in water, aqueous alcohol and dextrose solutions. *Uses:* Saralasin is a competitive antagonist of angiotensin II. It also has some partial agonist activity, particularly in low-renin, high-sodium hypertensive patients, who seem to have altered angiotensin receptors. Saralasin is used as a diagnostic drug to indicate the extent of involvement of the renin-angiotensin system in the maintenance of hypertension. After a transient rise in blood pressure, a fall during infusion indicates "angiotensinogenic" hypertension. There are some false positives, of unknown cause. False negatives mostly occur among patients with a high sodium load. For these reasons, the manufacturer recommends sodium depletion with furosemide before the test. However, this introduces an artifact in that furosemide itself considerably increases plasma renin activity and angiotensin II levels, thus guaranteeing a more favorable situation for a positive response. Dietary sodium restriction may be a more acceptable procedure, although it also tends to increase plasma renin activity. Newer angiotension II antagonists without partial agonist activity will correct this fault of saralasin. Adverse effects are headache, light headedness, malaise, nausea, and discomfort at the injection site. Pressor responses, when they occur, are sometimes severe. In pheochromocytoma, hypertensive crises may be evoked, especially in patients who respond with marked vasodepression. Twelve to 13 hr after discontinuation of treatment, there is sometimes a rebound hypertension. Saralasin is rapidly destroyed by proteolysis, the half-life being about 3 min. Consequently, it is not orally effective and must be given by continuous intravenous infusion. Newer analogs that are stable in the GI tract and body will permit not only oral testing of outpatients but also will provide drugs for antihypertensive treatment. *Dose: Intravenous, infusion, adults, initially* 0.5 μg/kg/min, to be increased at 10-min intervals, if necessary, to 5, then 10, then 20 μg/kg/min. If a pressor response occurs, the infusion time should not exceed 8 min.

Miscellaneous Antihypertensives and Hypotensives

A large number of substances are capable of lowering the blood pressure, at least briefly. Few of these, however, are employed for their hypotensive action. Examples of drugs with prominent hypotensive actions that are rarely used for such actions are histamine, parasympathomimetics, azapetine, and tolazoline; however, they may be used to increase peripheral blood flow.

Veratrum Alkaloids

Cryptenamine Acetates [Unitensen Aqueous (*Mallinckrodt*)] is the acetate salts of a mixture of alkaloids derived from an extract of *Veratrum viride*. White to tan, amorphous powder that is odorless, stable in aqueous solution, and melts over a wide range. Very soluble in water and alcohol. *Uses:* Cryptenamine lowers the blood pressure and slows the heart by stimulating sensory receptors in the left ventricle and in the lung. There may also be minor contributions to the cardiovascular effects by reflexes arising elsewhere and by central actions. Somewhat higher doses, occasionally reached in man, depress respiration, also by a combination of reflex stimulation and central inhibition. Cryptenamine acetates are employed only in selected cases of hypertensive encephalopathy, preeclampsia, and eclampsia, for which they are obsolete. They are given only by the intravenous or intramuscular routes; the hypotensive effect is prompt and lasts 3 to 6 hours. The range between the therapeutic and the toxic dose is quite narrow; in patients, the veratrum alkaloids frequently cause epigastric and substernal burning, unpleasant taste, salivation, sweating, hiccough, nausea and vomiting, and other lesser side effects. Overdosage can cause severe hypotension and cardiovascular collapse. Atropine and ephedrine can counteract the bradycardia and hypotension, respectively. The physician must select his therapeutic regimen carefully and adjust the dosage to the patient's needs and response. Dosage schedules are complex and must continually be readjusted; tolerance may also develop. For each individual preparation it is advisable to consult the manufacturer's recommendations. *Dose: Intravenous,* 1 mg diluted with 20 mL of isotonic dextrose solution, to be infused at the rate of 1 mL/min and to be repeated as needed; *intramuscular, initial,* 1 mg at hourly intervals until the hypertension is controlled, then at 3- to 6-hour intervals; 0.2-mg increments may be necessary.
Cryptenamine Tannates [Unitensen (*Mallinckrodt*)] is the tannate salts of a mixture of alkaloids derived from an extract of *Veratrum viride*. Tan, amorphous powder that is odorless, stable in light and air, and melts over a wide range. Soluble in alcohol; very slightly soluble in water. *Uses:* See *Cryptenamine Acetates* (above). The tannates are given only by the oral route and are preferred only in the absence of a hypertensive crisis. *Dose: Oral, initial,* 2 mg twice daily. Increments may be made at weekly intervals, if necessary, by increasing the number of daily doses rather than the size of the individual dose.

Pargyline Hydrochloride

N-Methyl-N-2-propynylbenzylamine hydrochloride [306-07-0] $C_{11}H_{13}N \cdot HCl$ (195.69); Eutonyl (*Abbott*). Prepared by interaction of 2-propynyl bromide and N-methylbenzylamine. White, crystalline powder; very soluble in water. *Uses:* An inhibitor of monoamine oxidase.

It has a weak *antihypertensive* action. It does not appreciably lower the blood pressure of hypertensive patients when they are recumbent, but only when they are standing. Thus it causes only an orthostatic hypotension and has little demonstrable peripheral action or influence on the disease process. The mechanism of its action is unknown; it appears to promote the exchange of the weak sympathomimetic, octopamine, for norepinephrine in the adrenergic terminals. Pargyline has been claimed to have a euphoriant or antidepressant action, but controlled clinical observation has not shown the effect to be significant. Untoward effects of the pargyline are vertigo, weakness, and syncope (the result of orthostatic hypotension), nausea and vomiting, constipation, dry mouth, sweating, headache, hyperexcitability, nervousness, insomnia, nightmares, impotence, and difficulty in ejaculation, arthralgia, increased appetite, fluid retention, rash, drug fever (rare), thrombocytopenia, and extrapyramidal disorders of movement. It potentiates dangerously the effects of narcotics, anesthetics and sedatives (including alcohol), psychomotor stimulants, sympathomimetics, antihistaminics, and hypotensives. Because it inhibits monoamine oxidase, which normally destroys tyramine and other pressor amines in foods, hypertensive crises sometimes occur on eating certain cheeses and also drinking certain red wines. It may cause emergence of concealed psychoses. Thus both physician and patient are required to be on continuous alert. *Dose: Initially* 10 to 25 mg once a day, then increase the dose by 10 mg once a week until the desired response is obtained. If used in combination with other antihypertensives, or in elderly or sympathectomized patients, the initial dose is preferably 10 mg and the maintenance dose should not exceed 25 mg a day.

Peripheral Vasodilators

Peripheral vasodilators are substances which dilate the arterioles and increase blood flow in the numerous systemic vascular beds, especially in the extremities. To the pharmacologist, the word *peripheral* may indicate that the action is directly on the arterioles, but to the clinician the word merely indicates the site of the final effect. Thus, centrally acting, reflexly acting, or ganglionic blocking drugs that reduce sympathetic tone to the periphery are peripheral vasodilators, clinically speaking; consequently, all of the hypotensives listed in the previous section may be considered to be peripheral dilators. Some sympathomimetics with prominent beta-receptor stimulant actions are employed for their peripheral vasodilator effects. The adrenergic blocking drugs are also used to improve flow through specific peripheral vascular beds.

Peripheral vasodilators are employed in the treatment of vasospastic disorders such as *Raynaud's disease, causalgias* and *reflex dystrophy*, vasospasm associated with *arterial embolism* and *thrombophlebitis, immersion foot, trench foot, herpes zoster, decubitus ulcers*, and degenerative arterial diseases such as *thromboangiitis obliterans, arteriosclerosis obliterans, acrocyanosis*, and *diabetic gangrene*. However, there is a great deal of justifiable skepticism about the value of peripheral vasodilators in most uses, since vasospastic ischemia is usually self-limiting because of autoregulatory factors that counteract the spasms. An organic obstruction cannot be corrected for by vasodilatation, since the obstruction is the principal resistance in the line. However, vasodilatation may (or may not) improve circulation in the ischemic area through collateral vessels.

Isoxsuprine Hydrochloride—page 892.

Niacin—pages 1015 and 1024.

Nitrates and Nitrites (see **Coronary Drugs**)—pages 852 to 854.

Nylidrin Hydrochloride—page 892.

Phentolamine—page 906.

Tolazoline Hydrochloride

1*H*-Imidazole, 4,5-dihydro-2-(phenylmethyl)-, monohydrochloride; Priscoline (*Ciba-Geigy*); (*Various Mfrs*)

2-Benzyl-2-imidazoline monohydrochloride [59-97-2] $C_{10}H_{12}N_2.HCl$ (196.68).

Preparation—Benzyl cyanide and ethylenediamine are heated together in the presence of carbon disulfide, whereby hydrogen sulfide and ammonia are liberated, and tolazoline is formed. After purification by distillation, the base is converted to the hydrochloride with hydrogen chloride.

Description—White or creamy white, crystalline powder; its solutions are slightly acid to litmus; melts between 172° and 176°.

Solubility—Freely soluble in water and alcohol.

Uses—A vasodilator with weak alpha-adrenergic blocking activity. Its clinical usefulness rests on the vasodilator properties, and adrenergic blockade is not established with therapeutic doses. It has a sympathomimetic effect to stimulate the heart, so that blood pressure is sometimes moderately elevated, despite vasodilation. It has a histamine-like effect to stimulate gastric secretion and an acetylcholine-like effect to increase gastrointestinal motility. It also causes mydriasis by a sympathomimetic action.

Tolazoline is of some use in the treatment of *vasospastic disorders*, such as the early stages of *Raynaud's disease, frostbite, endarteritis, causalgia, acrocyanosis*, and the vasospastic components of *embolism* and *phlebitis*. It is not useful in the treatment of occlusive vascular diseases such as thromboangiitis obliterans, phlebothrombosis, coronary occlusion, or cerebral vascular accidents.

Side effects include flushing, tingling, formication, nausea, vomiting, diarrhea, abdominal pain, gastric hyperacidity, pilomotor stimulation, palpitation, tachycardia and mydriasis. The drug is contraindicated when there is a history of angina pectoris or peptic ulcer.

Dose—*Intramuscular, intravenous*, or *subcutaneous, adults, initially* **25 mg** slowly, to test responsiveness, then up to **50 to 75 mg** twice a day to 2 or 3 times a week.

Dosage Forms—Injection: 25 mg/mL.

Trimethaphan Camsylate

Thieno[1′,2′:1,2]thieno[3,4-*d*]imidazol-5-ium, decahydro-2-oxo-1,3-bis-(phenylmethyl)-, salt with (+)-7,7-dimethyl-2-oxobicyclo[2.2.1]-heptane-1-methanesulfonic acid (1:1);
Arfonad (*Hoffman-LaRoche*)

(+)-1,3-Dibenzyldecahydro-2-oxoimidazo[4,5-*c*]-thieno[1,2-*a*]-thiolium 2-oxo-10-bornanesulfonate (1:1) [68-91-7] $C_{32}H_{40}N_2O_5S_2$ (596.80).

Preparation—Trimethaphan bromide, prepared from an intermediate produced in the synthesis of biotin, is metathesized with silver *d*-camphor-10-sulfonate; the silver bromide is removed by filtration and trimethaphan camsylate is obtained by evaporating the filtrate.

Description—White crystals or crystalline powder; melts in the range of 230° to 235°, with decomposition.

Solubility—Freely soluble in water, alcohol, chloroform; insoluble in ether.

Uses—Trimethaphan is usually classified as a ganglionic blocking agent, but it only moderately blocks ganglia in the therapeutic dose range; rather, its hypotensive effects result from a direct peripheral vasodilator action. It has an extremely brief duration of action. Thus the hypotension induced is subject to moment-to-moment control simply by varying the rate of intravenous infusion. It is sometimes used in the treatment of *hypertensive emergencies*, but other drugs are usually preferred. It has been used in *acute congestive heart failure* and after a myocardial infarction to relieve pulmonary congestion, but other drugs have more favorable actions; the action of trimethaphan is mainly dilatation of capacitance veins and consequent reduction in venous return to the right side of the heart, and the consequence is a decrease in cardiac output at a time when there is already a critical deficit in output. Trimethaphan is occasionally used for *induction of brief hypotension*, as for surgical procedures to reduce an otherwise bloody field or for certain diagnostic procedures.

Adverse effects are mostly the result of ganglionic blockade. They necessitate a reduction in dosage. They are anorexia, nausea, vomiting, constipation and possibility of paralytic ileus, mydriasis, cycloplegia and possibility of glaucomatous attack, dry mouth, anginal pain, tachycardia, postural hypotension, and urinary retention. Trimethaphan causes release of histamine, so that it must be used with caution in allergic and asthmatic persons.

Dose—*Slow intravenous infusion, adults,* for *hypertensive emergency, initially* **0.5 to 1 mg/min** then **1 to 15 mg/min** for *maintenance,* according to blood pressure; for *controlled hypotension,* initially **3 to 4 mg/min** then **0.2 to 6 mg/min,** according to response; *children, initially* **0.1 mg/min,** adjusted according to response.

Dosage Form—Injection: 250 mg/10 mL, to be diluted to 500 mL before use.

Other Peripheral Vasodilators

Cyclandelate [3,3,5-Trimethylcyclohexyl mandelate [456-59-7] $C_{17}H_{24}O_3$ (276.36); Cyclospasmol (*Ives*)]—Prepared by esterification of mandelic acid with 3,3,5-trimethylcyclohexanol. Crystals, melting at about 52°; insoluble in water. *Uses:* An antispasmodic drug with actions similar to those of papaverine. It relaxes vascular smooth muscle and erratically increases blood flow. It is *"possibly effective"* in the treatment of thrombophlebitis, Raynaud's disease, nocturnal leg cramps, and favorable cases of cerebral ischemia. It is considered an obsolete drug. Side effects include flushing and tingling, vertigo, nausea, heartburn, eructation, colic, headache, sweating, and hypotension. *Dose: Oral, adults,* initially 1.2 to 1.6 g a day in divided doses followed by 400 to 800 mg a day in 2 to 4 divided doses.

Ethaverine [Tetraethyl homologue of papaverine [486-47-5] $C_{24}H_{29}NO_4$ (395.48); Neopavrin (*Savage*)]—A synthetic homologue of papaverine in which ethoxy groups replace the four methoxy groups of papaverine. *Uses:* The same as for papaverine (see *Papaverine Hydrochloride,* below). *Dose: Oral, adults,* usually 100 mg 3 times a day, but 200 mg per dose may be given in nonresponsive cases; in sustained-release form, 150 mg every 12 hr.

Nicotinyl Alcohol [3-Pyridinemethanol [100-55-0] $C_4H_4NCH_2OH$ (109.12); Roniacol (*Roche*)]—Prepared by catalytic hydrogenation of 3-pyridinecarboxaldehyde. A colorless, somewhat hygroscopic liquid; freely soluble in water. *Uses:* In the body, nicotinyl alcohol is converted to nicotinic acid, and it is believed that the pharmacologic properties of the alcohol are mediated through the acid, although it has not been proven that the vasodilator and antihyperlipidemic actions of nicotinic acid (not shared by nicotinamide) are not mediated by nicotinyl alcohol. Given in very large oral doses, it is a peripheral vasodilator and causes flushing of the skin in the blush area and a feeling of warmth and tingling. It is "possibly effective" in the treatment of vasospastic disorders, such as Raynaud's disease, acrocyanosis, varicose ulcers, decubital ulcers, Meniere's syndrome, vertigo and chilblains. However, no sound clinical studies have established that the usual doses effect any beneficial action in these diseases. Even more dubious are scattered claims of effectiveness in the treatment of obliterative vascular diseases. However, the drug has an undisputed efficacy in lowering plasma beta-lipoproteins (and cholesterol) and very-low-density lipoproteins; it is mainly used to treat familial hypercholesterolemia (not approved). Duration of action is brief except when given in sustained-release form (as the tartrate salt). Side effects include flushing on the face and neck, tingling, mild swelling of extremities, nausea, vomiting, and rarely, syncope. For adverse effects in antihyperlipidemic therapy, see *Niacin* (page 1024). *Dose: Oral, adults,* for vasodilatation, 50 or 100 mg 3 times a day, except 150 to 300 mg at morning and night with sustained-release forms; for *antihyperlipidemic* therapy, 1.8 to 7.4 g a day in divided doses.

Papaverine Hydrochloride [6,7-Dimethoxy-1-veratrylisoquinoline hydrochloride [61-25-6] $C_{20}H_{21}NO_4$.HCl (375.85)]—An alkaloid of opium that may be obtained from opium after separation of morphine, or prepared synthetically, as by a procedure of 10 to 12 major steps from vanillin. Papaverine hydrochloride occurs as white crystals or a white, crystalline powder, melting at about 220°, with decomposition. 1 g dissolves in 30 mL water, 120 mL alcohol; soluble in chloroform; practically insoluble in ether. *Uses:* A nonselective *smooth muscle relaxant,* although with therapeutic doses different organs are affected to varying degrees. It is most effective in hypertonic conditions. It is also a rather feeble central analgetic and local anesthetic. Its toxicity is low, and neither tolerance nor habituation has been reported. It has been used in various spasmodic conditions of smooth muscles, especially in all kinds of gastric and intestinal spasms, in biliary colic, ureteral colic, and in bronchial spasms, angina pectoris, cardiac dysrhythmias, and other disorders, but *authoritative opinion holds it to be ineffective and obsolete for these purposes.* Perhaps the chief use is in *peripheral arterial* or *pulmonary embolism,* in which many pulmonary specialists hold it to be of value. Its action is to dilate the arteries and allow collateral blood supply to reach the obstructed region. For this purpose it is given intravenously. It may be of short-term

value in *Meniere's disease.* In normal subjects, papaverine dilates cerebral vessels moderately. Consequently it is used to treat cerebral ischemia, although its vasodilator effect on diseased cerebral vessels is less marked. Although large doses can suppress extrasystoles, they also depress A-V and intraventricular conduction and hence replace one arrhythmia with an often more serious one. Adverse effects include drowsiness, weakness, diplopia, constipation, jaundice, and irritation at the injection site. It decreases the efficacy of levodopa. The plasma half-life of papaverine is 0.5 to 2 hr. *Dose: Oral, adults,* as tablets, 75 to 300 mg 3 to 5 times a day; as timed-release capsules or tablets, from 150 to 200 mg every 12 hr to 150 mg every 8 hr to 300 mg every 12 hr. *Intraarterial,* 40 mg over 1 to 2 min. *Intramuscular* or *intravenous,* 30 to 120 mg every 3 hr. *Intravenous* (only in urgent situations), 100 mg, slowly over a period of 2 min, every 3 hr.

Coronary Drugs

Most vasoactive substances dilate the coronary vessels, even though their peripheral effects may be that of constriction. Thus, sympathomimetics, which are peripheral vasoconstrictors, dilate the coronary beds by autoregulatory mechanisms. But, a useful coronary *vasodilator* should have minimal effects on the blood pressure and should not increase cardiac work. Thus, most autonomic agents, hypotensives and peripheral vasodilators do not fall in this class. The principal coronary dilators are smooth muscle relaxants in general and may be employed as spasmolytics in certain instances. However, coronary dilatation makes a minimal contribution to the antianginal effects, since the diseased coronary arteries are usually incapable of dilating. Rather, arterial dilation, which reduces arterial impedance, and venous dilation, which reduces venous return and hence stroke volume, combine to reduce cardiac work and thus give relief.

Propranolol and other β-adrenoreceptor blocking drugs increase exercise tolerance in angina because they improve the flow to the vulnerable subendocardium by slowing the heart and increasing diastolic time, during which subendocardial perfusion mainly occurs. It is also widely believed that β-block decreases myocardial oxygen utilization; sympathetically increased heart work has a slightly higher oxygen cost than that effected through the Starling mechanism. Therefore, β-blockade forces the heart to select the more energy-efficient mechanism to increase the work demanded by exercise.

At present much attention is being given to the prevention or eradication of coronary atherosclerosis. Many claims of the efficacy of polyunsaturated fats and certain dietary factors in the reduction of atherosclerosis have been made, but no claim has yet been widely accepted by authorities in the field. Antiplatelet drugs, such as aspirin and sulfinpyrazone, are under intense investigation as prophylactics, with the rationale that thrombosis subsequent to rupture of the atheromatous plaque may be prevented or, alternatively, that white thrombus formation and release of a transforming factor precedes the atheromatous development. Preliminary data strongly suggest a prophylactic efficacy in men but not in women.

Amyl Nitrite

Mixture of nitrous acid, 2-methylbutyl ester, and nitrous acid, 3-methylbutyl ester

A mixture of nitrite esters of 3-methyl-1-butanol and 2-methyl-1-butanol [8017-89-8] $C_5H_{11}NO_2$ (117.15).

Preparation—A good grade of commercial amyl alcohol (isoamyl alcohol) boiling above 125° is esterified with nitrous acid. The acid is generated in contact with the alcohol from sodium nitrite and dilute H_2SO_4.

Description—Clear, yellowish liquid with an ethereal, fruity odor and pungent, aromatic taste; boils at about 96° but is volatile even at low temperatures and is flammable; slowly decomposes on exposure to air and light; moisture accelerates decomposition; specific gravity between 0.870 and 0.876.

Solubility—Practically insoluble in water; miscible with alcohol, chloroform, and ether.

Uses—Amyl nitrite, being exceedingly volatile, can be inhaled to obtain the therapeutic effects of nitrite ion in the body rapidly. In practice however, amyl nitrite is employed rarely in the treatment of attacks of *angina pectoris* but somewhat more frequently for the relief of *biliary* or *renal colic*. The actions are those of *Nitroglycerin* (page 854), except that amyl nitrite causes more reflex arteriolar constriction. An unusual but at times life-saving use for amyl nitrite is in the emergency treatment of *cyanide poisoning*, where nitrites are given to produce methemoglobin, which temporarily inactivates the toxic cyanide ion by combining with it to form cyanmethemoglobin. For this purpose, sodium nitrite is employed intravenously, but amyl nitrite may be inhaled while the solution of sodium nitrite is being prepared. It is administered by crushing a glass *perle of amyl nitrite* in a handkerchief and inhaling the liquid which volatilizes, or by dropping a small quantity on a handkerchief and inhaling the vapor. It has become a drug of abuse. Abuse may cause methemoglobinemia, hemolytic anemia and immunologic disorders.

Caution—Amyl Nitrite is very flammable. Do not use where it may be ignited.

Dose—By *inhalation*, **0.18** to **0.3 mL** as required.

Dosage Forms—Inhalant: 0.18 and 0.3 mL.

Erythrityl Tetranitrate

1,2,3,4-Butanetetrol, tetranitrate, ($R*,S*$)-, Tetranitrol; Cardilate (*Burroughs Wellcome*)

$$CH_2ONO_2$$
$$H---C---ONO_2$$
$$H---C---ONO_2$$
$$CH_2ONO_2$$

Erythritol tetranitrate [7297-25-8] $C_4H_6N_4O_{12}$ (302.11); a dry mixture with lactose or other suitable inert excipients, to permit safe handling and compliance with federal ICC regulations pertaining to interstate shipment.

Caution: Undiluted erythrityl tetranitrate is a powerful explosive, and proper precautions must be taken in handling. It can be exploded by percussion or by excessive heat. Only extremely small quantities should be isolated.

Preparation—Erythritol is reacted with nitric acid in the presence of sulfuric acid under controlled temperature.

Description—White powder having a slight odor of nitric oxides and a bitter taste; unstable in light and heat.

Solubility—Undiluted erythrityl tetranitrate is soluble in acetone and alcohol; practically insoluble in water.

Uses—A *vasodilator* similar in action to other organic nitrates. By the sublingual route, it has a relatively long duration of action (about 2 hr) within its class. By the oral route, the duration is longer but quite variable. Its principal use is in the prophylaxis of *angina pectoris* in *acute* situations in which an attack can be anticipated. Medical authorities do not consider it useful as a chronic routine prophylactic because of development of a prominent tolerance. In fact, it has been shown to be not as good as a placebo. Sensitivity can be restored by a 1- to 2-week rest. As with nitroglycerin and other organic nitrates, its peripheral effects to decrease venous return and arterial impedance and not coronary vasodilation account for the improved exercise tolerance in anginal patients.

Untoward effects include tachycardia, headache, flushing, dizziness, syncope, and nausea; tolerance to these effects often develops. It should be given cautiously to patients with glaucoma.

The bioavailability by the oral route is unpredictable because of differences among individuals and also from time-to-time as the result of variations in hepatic metabolism during absorption. Phenobarbital increases the metabolism.

Dose—*Oral, adults*, initially, **10 mg** of erythrityl tetranitrate 4 times a day, gradually increased to 20 mg, if necessary, not to exceed 100 mg/day; *sublingual, adults*, **5** to **10 mg** 3 or 4 times a day, with adjustments as needed. The interval between increments of dosage should not be shorter than 2 days. Despite the fact that "round-the-clock" regimes are common, they run counter to authoritative medical opinion regarding proper use of so-called long-acting organonitrates, namely, that they should be administered only in advance of anticipated situations known to cause anginal pain. Steady use causes tolerance and loss of effectiveness; to break tolerance the drug must be discontinued for more than a week, during which time other organonitrates cannot be used.

Dosage Forms—Sustained-Release Capsules: 30, 45, and 60 mg; Tablets: 10, 20 and 40 mg; Sustained-Release Tablets: 80 mg.

Isosorbide Dinitrate

D-Glucitol, 1,4:3,6-dianhydro-, dinitrate; Isordil (*Ives*); Sorbitrate (*Stuart*); Sorquad (*Reid-Provident*)

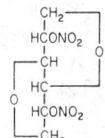

1,4:3,6-Dianhydro-D-glucitol dinitrate [87-33-2] $C_6H_8N_2O_8$ (236.14).

Preparation—An aqueous syrup of 1,4:3,6-dianhydro-D-glucitol is slowly added to a cooled mixture of HNO_3 and H_2SO_4. After standing a few minutes the mixture is poured into cold water and the precipitated product is collected and recrystallized from ethanol.

Description—*Diluted:* ivory-white, odorless powder. *Undiluted:* white, crystalline rosettes.

Solubility—*Undiluted:* very slightly soluble in water; very soluble in acetone; freely soluble in chloroform; sparingly soluble in alcohol.

Uses—A so-called coronary vasodilator that is used in the prophylaxis of attacks of *angina pectoris*. It is the long-acting organonitrate of choice. Like the other organonitrates, its mechanism is not coronary vasodilation but rather arterial and arteriolar dilatation and venodilatation, which decrease cardiac work by decreasing arterial impedance and venous return. After sublingual administration, the onset of the effect is 2 to 3 min and the offset of effect is about 1 to 2 hr; after oral administration, the onset is about 30 min and the offset 4 to 6 hr. Therefore, nitroglycerin affords quicker relief, and isosorbide dinitrate is thus indicated only for the prophylaxis of attacks of angina in situations in which attacks can be anticipated. It is of no benefit in routine, long-term prophylaxis, owing to the development of tolerance, at least in part. Double-blind studies show chronic isosorbide dinitrate to be less effective than a placebo. The sustained-release forms have not been proven to be as effective as oral tablets for acute prophylaxis. Medical authorities recommend only the sublingual tablets.

The most frequent complaint by users of isosorbide dinitrate is headache. In some persons there is also a paradoxical increase in anginal pain. Mild gastrointestinal disturbances as well as vertigo and other signs of orthostatic hypotension may occur. It should be given cautiously in patients with glaucoma.

Bioavailability and efficacy by the oral route are erratic because of day-to-day changes in the hepatic drug-metabolizing system and differences among patients. Phenobarbital, and probably other inducers of the enzyme system, increase the metabolism and decrease efficacy.

Dose—*Sublingual* or *chewable tablets, adults*, **5** to **10 mg** as sublingual tablets 30 min in advance of an anticipated situation requiring prophylaxis; not recommended for relief of an acute anginal attack because nitroglycerin is more effective. The following doses are given in the USP. *Oral, adult, tablets*, **10 mg** 4 times a day, with dose adjustments as needed; or **40 mg** as an extended-release capsule or tablet every 6 to 12 hr, with dose adjustments as needed. *Sublingual*, or *chewable tablets, adult*, **5** to **10 mg** as a sublingual tablet every 2 or 3 hr, with dose adjustments as needed. The implication that the patient can be medicated continuously, if needed, is contrary to authoritative medical opinion that holds that long-acting organonitrates should be used only as prophylactics for predictable, moderately sustained attacks. Sustained use induces tolerance that jeopardizes all organonitrate therapy and necessitates a discontinuation in use for one or more weeks. Continuous prophylaxis should be managed with β-blockers or calcium entry blockers, relief of acute attacks and prophylaxis of brief attacks with nitroglycerin.

Dosage Forms—Tablets: 5, 10, and 20 mg; Chewable Tablets: 5 and 10 mg; Extended-Release Tablets: 40 mg.

Nitroglycerin

1,2,3-Propanetriol, trinitrate; Glyceryl Trinitrate; Glonoin; Trinitrin; (*Various Mfrs*)

$$\begin{array}{c} CH_2ONO_2 \\ | \\ H-C-ONO_2 \\ | \\ CH_2ONO_2 \end{array}$$

Nitroglycerin [55-63-0] $C_3H_5N_3O_9$ (227.09).

Preparation—By nitrating glycerin with a mixture of nitric and sulfuric acids called "nitration acid." This acid usually consists of 3 parts of concentrated nitric acid and 5 parts of sulfuric acid, the latter acid acting as a dehydrating agent thus making the nitration more complete.

Description—Practically colorless, odorless liquid with a sweet taste.

Packaging—Nitroglycerin is sufficiently volatile to require packaging of tablets in glass containers with tightly fitting metal screw caps, and holding no more than 100 tablets in each container; only original unopened containers may be dispensed. Patients should keep the tablets in the original container, close it tightly after each use, and avoid exposure to heat.

Uses—Like amyl nitrite, nitroglycerin is a general relaxant of smooth muscle. Its actions are directly on the smooth muscle and are independent of the type of innervation; the actions cannot be prevented by any known agent. In the doses used for prophylaxis or relief of acute attacks of stable *angina pectoris*, it dilates the capacitance veins, which decreases venous return, and the conducting arteries, which decreases arterial impedance. The former effect tends to decrease cardiac output and the latter to increase it, the net effect being a decrease in the short term but often an increase when plasma levels are sustained. Both effects decrease heart size, the major determinant of myocardial oxygen demand, and hence provide relief from anginal pain. The decrease in cardiac output lowers the blood pressure, which elicits reflex arteriolar constriction (which opposes the direct arteriolar dilating actions of the drug) and tachycardia. Normal coronary vessels may dilate but not the diseased ones. Nitroglycerin is erratic in variant (vasospastic) angina. The effect to decrease venous return and cardiac afterload ultimately decreases pulmonary arterial pressure and also left atrial pressure; these effects decrease pulmonary edema in left heart failure, and the drug is therefore used to relieve *paroxysmal nocturnal dyspnea*. It may also be used in *acute congestive heart failure* and after *myocardial infarction* to relieve pulmonary congestion; in the recumbent position the effect to decrease venous return is less marked and the effect to decrease cardiac afterload greater, so that cardiac output is maintained. Nitroglycerin is also used to relieve *biliary* and *ureteral spasm*.

After oral administration, nitroglycerin is rapidly metabolized in the intestinal wall and liver, so that systemic bioavailability is quite low. Consequently, oral doses are quite high and plasma levels are erratic. Bioavailability is much greater by the buccal and sublingual routes. Medical authorities do not recommend sustained-release forms of nitroglycerin, since oral bioavailability is so poor and tolerance is favored. By the sublingual route, the vasodilator effects of the drug appear in 2 to 3 min and last about 20 min, but exercise tolerance may be increased for as long as an hour in some patients. Buccal tablets, if retained in the mouth, release nitroglycerin for 3 to 5 hr. Sustained-release oral capsules and tablets maintain plasma levels for 8 to 12 hr. A nitroglycerin ointment can provide therapeutic blood levels for 2 to 12 hr per application but is not recommended for routine use. Transdermal preparations may sustain plasma levels for 24 hr or longer.

The volume of distribution is about 200 L! The distribution half-life is 1 to 4 min and the elimination half-life about 2 hr.

Cerebral vasodilation may cause transient headaches. Paradoxical angina occurs when the dose is too large and blood pressure falls too low to sustain coronary flow. Dizziness, nausea, and other symptoms of hypotension also occur.

Dose—*Buccal*, *adults*, extended-release tablets, **1 mg** 3 times a day, with dosage adjustments, if needed, by changing dose or frequency. *Oral*, *adults*, **1.3** to **9 mg** as an extended-release capsule or tablet every 12 hr, with adjustments at 12-hr intervals, if necessary. *Sublingual*, *adults*, **150** to **600 µg** (0.15 to 0.6 mg) as a sublingual tablet, repeated in 5 min, if needed, up to 10 mg a day. *Topical*,

adults, to the skin, as **0.2%** ointment, usually 2.5 to 5 cm, but up to 12.5 cm, of **2%** ointment every 3 to 4 hr, as needed **or 1 transdermal system**, *initially* the smallest, every 24 hr, with dosage adjustments by applying larger systems or by combinations of systems. *Intravenous infusion*, adults, *initially* **5 µg/min** (0.005 mg/min), adjusted at 5-min intervals by equal increments until the response is satisfactory or the rate is 20 µg/min, after which increments become 10 µg/min, then eventually 20 µg/min, if necessary.

Dosage Forms—Extended-Release Capsules: 2.5, 6.5 and 9 mg; Injection: 5 mg/1 mL, 8, 25 and 50 mg/10 mL; Ointment: 2%; Buccal Tablets: 1 and 2 mg; Extended-Release Tablets: 1.3, 2.6, 6.5 and 9 mg; Sublingual Tablets: 150, 300, 400, and 600 µg (0.15, 0.3, 0.4, and 0.6 mg). Transdermal Systems: to deliver 2.5, 5, 7.5, 10 and 15 mg per 24 hr.

Propranolol Hydrochloride—page 906.

Other Coronary Drugs

Dipyridamole [2,6-Bis(diethanolamino)-4,8-dipiperidinopyrimido-(5,4-*d*)pyrimidine [58-32-2] $C_{24}H_{40}N_8O_4$ (504.62); Persantine (*Boehringer Ingelheim*)]—Prepared from 2,4,6,8-tetrachloropyrimidopyrimidine by interactions with sodium iodide, aniline, and diethanolamine (Brit. Pat. 807,826). Yellow, crystalline powder; very slightly soluble in water; freely soluble in alcohol. *Uses:* Dipyridamole inhibits metabolism of adenosine, thus increasing the concentration of that nucleoside in the region of arterioles, where adenosine has a dilator action. It also inhibits phosphodiesterase, which promotes vasodilatation. Although it can induce coronary dilation after intravenous administration in normal subjects, it does not do so after oral administration, which is the route for which the commercial product is prepared. It also fails to cause coronary dilation after parenteral administration to patients with coronary insufficiency, which is not surprising, since diseased vessels have a fixed resistance. In carefully conducted clinical studies the drug has been shown to be no better than a placebo. It has antiplatelet activity. It causes dizziness, syncope, GI disturbances, and rashes. *Dose:* Oral, *adults*, usually 50 mg 3 times a day but up to 400 mg a day may be given.

Pentaerythritol Tetranitrate, Diluted [2,2-Bis(hydroxymethyl)-1,3-propanediol tetranitrate [78-11-5] $C(CH_2ONO_2)_4$ (316.14); Peritrate (*Parke-Davis*)]—A dry mixture of pentaerythritol tetranitrate (prepared by nitration of pentaerythritol) with lactose or other suitable inert excipient to permit safe handling of the explosive undiluted substance. *Uses:* A "so-called" long-acting organonitrate, the long duration of which is mainly the result of prolonged release and absorption from oral dosage forms. It is used in the prophylaxis of attacks of *angina pectoris* but not in the management of the acute attack. It is no better than a placebo as a routine chronic prophylactic in angina pectoris; tolerance develops with chronic use. Transient headache and nausea may accompany its use. It should be given cautiously to patients with glaucoma. Medical authorities state that the sustained-release forms are poorly effective. It is not absorbed sublingually. Since absorption by the oral route is erratic, efficacy is unpredictable. *Dose:* Oral, *adults*, usually 10 to 20 mg 4 times a day, increased to as much as 160 mg a day, if necessary, administered in four subdivided doses as regular tablets, or 30 to 80 mg as sustained-release tablets or capsules twice daily. For comment concerning "around-the-clock" dosage schedules see the dose statement under *Isosorbide Dinitrate* (page 853). *Dosage Forms:* Extended-Release Capsules: 30, 45, 60, and 80 mg; Tablets: 10, 20, and 40 mg; Extended-Release Tablets: 80 mg.

Perhexiline Maleate [2-(2,2-Dicyclohexylethyl)piperidine maleate (1:1) [6724-53-4] $C_{19}H_{35}N.C_4H_4O_4$ (393.57); Pexid (*Merrell-Dow*)]—For synthesis see *CA 65:* 2229f, 1966. White, crystalline powder; slightly soluble in water. *Uses:* An inhibitor of ion fluxes in general. In smooth muscle, tone is decreased; in cardiac muscle, automaticity, membrane responsiveness, conduction velocity, and responses to neurotransmitters and calcium are inhibited. Both arterioles and capacitance vessels are dilated, so that cardiac impedance and venous return are diminished, effects that decrease cardiac work and oxygen demand and hence tend to relieve or prevent anginal pain. To whatever extent coronary dilatation improves flow to the ischemic myocardium, the beneficial effect will be enhanced. In patients with angina pectoris, perhexiline decreases exercise tachycardia, and improves myocardial lactate extraction and the ECG signs of ischemia; such patients experience fewer anginal attacks and take fewer nitroglycerin tablets. The drug also decreases premature systoles and has other antiarrhythmic properties. It decreases pulmonary airway resistance, but no clinical use has been made of this effect. It also has thiazide-like diuretic activity. Perhexiline causes a relatively high incidence of dizziness and a lesser incidence of minor gastrointestinal upsets and malaise. It appears to cause a rise in SGOT and LDH activities in about 1 patient in 5, but no adverse consequences have been related to these effects. A case of polyneuropathy has been reported. *Dose:* Oral, *adults*, 100 mg twice a day.

Vasopressor Drugs

A number of drugs of classes treated elsewhere in this text have vasoconstrictor or cardiostimulator activity and can be used to elevate the blood pressure under appropriate conditions. The most important of these are sympathomimetics, which are treated in Chapter 45. In conditions in which the plasma volume is diminished, as in hypovolemic shock, fluid replacement tends to restore the blood pressure, but plasma extenders (Chapter 42) are not truly vasopressor, since they do not cause vasoconstriction.

The usefulness of vasoconstrictor agents in the treatment of shock has been intensely debated. In nearly every kind of shock, the body responds by reflex vasoconstriction, and it has been argued that if the arterioles and capacitance veins can respond to reflex sympathetic stimulation, vasoconstrictors are redundant; if arteriolar function has deteriorated to where it cannot respond to sympathetic impulses, it also cannot respond to vasoconstrictor drugs. Furthermore, there is much evidence that vasoconstriction increases the damage already in progress as the result of inadequate circulation. Consequently, the attention in the 1960s shifted to α-adrenergic blocking drugs and vasodilators and more recently to cardiostimulants. Dopamine comes closest to fulfilling the requirements of an ideal vasopressor drug for supporting blood pressure in shock; in appropriate dosage it dilates blood vessels in the renal, splanchnic, cerebral, and coronary beds, beds which are of vital importance, constricts in the cutaneous and skeletal muscle vascular beds, where very little flow is needed in shock, and stimulates the heart.

Lypressin—page 958.

Cardiac Glycosides (Digitalis)

The cardiac glycosides comprise a group of chemically and pharmacologically related drugs frequently referred to as digitalis. However, not all are glycosides, nor are they all derived from species of digitalis. But the aglycones, which are the noncarbohydrate portions of glycoside molecules (see page 401), are all chemically similar, and the actions of the various digitaloid agents are nearly identical except for onset and duration.

The primary action of digitalis on the heart is a direct *cardiotonic action* on the myocardium to *increase the force of contraction*. The increased contractility results from inhibition of the membrane sodium-potassium activated ATPase, which inhibition increases the intracellular stores of calcium. In congestive heart failure, stroke volume is increased, which more effectively empties the ventricles and lowers diastolic ventricular pressures and ultimately pulmonary and central venous pressures. Congestion is thus diminished. Increased cardiac output improves renal blood flow and glomerular filtration and decreases juxtaglomerular renin secretion, so that the renal resorption of sodium and water and hence of edema is diminished. Diuresis is promoted. Hepatic blood flow is also increased, which increases the clearance of aldosterone and contributes to the reduction in edema.

Slowing of the cardiac rate occurs only when the rate was originally rapid as the result of compensatory sympathetic reflexes consequent to failure. When the failure is abolished, there is no longer any need for the compensatory tachycardia, and consequently the heart rate slows to normal. This slowing has mistakenly been attributed to a "vagal action" of digitalis. However, digitalis does sensitize the sinoatrial node, atrium, and atrioventricular node to vagal impulses, and, in high therapeutic and toxic doses, increases vagal traffic by actions in the CNS and on the baroreceptors. High doses also may slow the ventricle by a direct action on atrioventricular conduction.

The chief therapeutic use for digitalis is in the treatment of *low output congestive heart failure*. It is of value regardless of whether the failure is predominantly of the right or left side of the heart. Arrhythmias and valvular defects may modify the response to digitalis, but their presence neither indicates nor contraindicates the use of the drug. However, it is generally true that the most dramatic responses are seen in patients with *both atrial fibrillation and congestive heart failure*. Badly damaged hearts do not respond well. When the failure is due to an acute toxic or infectious process, like typhoid fever or diphtheritic myocarditis, rather than to a chronic degenerative process like arteriosclerosis or failure secondary to hypertensive heart disease, digitalis may give poor results and may even be contraindicated. High output failure in patients with myxedema, hyperthyroidism, and thiamine deficiency is likewise not much benefited. Also, heart failure secondary to cardiovascular syphilis yields poorly to digitalis therapy. Digitalis has been advocated for use in peripheral circulatory collapse, shock, etc., but it is now clear that it promotes splanchnic ischemia, which may complicate and exacerbate shock and favor small bowel ischemia.

The signs and symptoms of heart failure in persons with mild heart failure are abolished by digitalis, but bed rest, sedatives, and often diuretics and restriction of salt intake may be required to obtain best results. Exertional and paroxysmal nocturnal dyspnea disappear; cough, cyanosis, ascites, edema, and chronic passive congestion of the lungs and abdominal viscera are relieved; the enlarged diastolic size of the heart is decreased; engorged veins due to increased venous pressure are returned to normal; and the diastolic rest period in each cardiac cycle is prolonged.

The action of digitalis to impair atrioventricular conduction is employed in the management of *atrial flutter, atrial fibrillation*, and *paroxysmal atrial tachycardia*. In patients with atrial fibrillation, digitalis may occasionally revert the arrhythmia if congestive heart failure is present. Digitalis glycosides do not directly cure the arrhythmia but by improving the condition of the heart and lessening stretch the fibrillation may cease in some instances. The atrial fibrillation usually persists. The action actually sought is second-degree heart block, which will decrease the ventricular rate toward a more optimal value. The same action is sought in atrial flutter, namely a partial heart block, to decrease the number of atrial impulses that pass through to the ventricles. In an occasional case of atrial flutter, the proper use of fairly large doses of digitalis may abolish the arrhythmia. In paroxysmal atrial tachycardia (PAT) a properly selected dose can interrupt one leg of the reentrant pathway within the AV node, thus terminating the "circus movement" yet allowing orthograde conduction of normal impulses. Cardiac glycosides are commonly used prophylactically against recurrences of PAT.

The choice of glycoside offers considerable difficulty to many practitioners. When absorbed in adequate amounts, all the active digitalis principles produce identical effects on the myocardium, and their toxic effects are essentially the same, although there is some evidence that digitoxin gains better access to the CNS and causes more neurological side effects and CNS-initiated arrhythmias. They differ from each other largely in speed of onset of action and duration of cardiac effects and in the degree of absorption by the oral route. With some glycosides (eg, digoxin), bioavailability varies widely from product to product, which imposes strict requirements for clinical or plasma-level monitoring when unfamiliar products are employed.

Initial digitalization may be accomplished rapidly or slowly, depending on the urgency of the case. The vast majority of patients with congestive heart failure are not *in extremis* and can be digitalized without a loading dose, so that about 5 half-lives are required to achieve a maintenance steady state.

In acute heart failure or incapacitating atrial tachydys-rhythmia, loading is desirable. The process of loading is known as *rapid digitalization*. It is not unusual to digitalize a patient in 12 or 24 hours by giving half the calculated dose at once, and the remainder in two or three divided doses at intervals of 6 hours. This principle is applied to other cardiac glycosides; only the timing differs. No fixed formula or rule of thumb can be employed. Each case is individualized, and the physician must constantly watch his patient to observe the developing effects of the drug, and to prevent unpleasant or serious toxic effects from overdosage. Optimal effects can be obtained without toxic effects, and the optimal dose is not necessarily the largest tolerated dose. It can be found only by careful observation of the patient. Usually the patient should be seen immediately before an additional dose is given, when rapid digitalization is employed.

In rare cases it may be necessary to inject intravenously ouabain, strophanthin, deslanoside, or some other purified parenteral preparation in order to save life. Such patients are usually *in extremis* and may die before digitalis given by mouth can exert its effect (within 2 hours) or they are patients who are unable to tolerate oral digitalis or who have gastrointestinal disorders that preclude oral dosage. Small doses are employed as a rule and digitalization with an orally efficacious preparation is then completed by the oral route.

Cardiac glycosides have a low margin of safety. They may cause nausea, vomiting, diarrhea, abdominal pain, headache, drowsiness, fatigue, malaise, backache, trigeminal neuralgia, "white vision" and other visual disturbances, convulsions, mental disturbances, eosinophilia, rashes, gynecomastia and, rarely, thrombocytopenia. Cardiac arrhythmias of all types are relatively common as a sign of excessive plasma levels. Heart block and premature ventricular contractions (PVC) are the most frequent, ventricular tachycardia the most ominous. Toxicity is more likely in the presence of hypokalemia, a common result of concomitant diuretic therapy for the cardiac edema. Amphotericin B and mineralocorticoids also cause hypokalemia and may promote digitalis toxicity. Intravenous calcium salts can also precipitate intoxication. Toxicity can be antagonized by edetate disodium, potassium (especially if hypokalemia exists), lidocaine, phenytoin, and, to a lesser extent, propranolol, quinidine, or procainamide. Toxic doses also give rise to serious ventricular arrhythmias.

Powdered Digitalis

Foxglove; Digitalis folium; Digitalis Leaf; Fairy Cap; Lady's Glove, Fingers, Thimbles, or Bells; Digifortis (*Parke-Davis*); Digitora (*Upjohn*)

The dried leaf of *Digitalis purpurea* Linné (Fam. *Scrophulariaceae*), the potency of 100 mg of which is equivalent to 1 USP Digitalis Unit.

Note—When Digitalis is prescribed, Powdered Digitalis is to be dispensed.

Constituents—The constituents which are of the greatest importance as cardiovascular agents are *digitoxin* [$C_{41}H_{64}O_{13}$] and *gitoxin* [$C_{41}H_{64}O_{14}$].

Digitonin, or *digitin* [$C_{56}H_{92}O_{29}$], a saponin-like glycoside of digitalis, is practically devoid of digitalis action but is widely used as a reagent for the determination of cholesterol. It is a specific precipitant for steroids having a 3-hydroxyl group with the β configuration as long as they do not contain a methyl group with an epi configuration at C_{16}.

Other constituents of digitalis are *digitoflavin*, *digitophyllin*, fat, etc. *German digitalin* is a purified mixture of the glycosides of digitalis seed. It is soluble in water but is much less active than French digitaline or Nativelle.

Apart from these glycosides, a number of other glycosides have been found. Among these are *digiproside*, *glucodigiproside*, *gitosin*, *gitaloxigenin monodigitoxoside*, and *glucogitaloxin*.

Uses—See the general statement.

The pharmacokinetics of digitalis and its glycosides approximate those of *Digitoxin* (see following monograph).

Dose—*Oral*, *adults*, *initially* usually **1.5 g** in divided doses over a period of 1 or 2 days, but as much as 2 g in one day may be given for more rapid loading; elderly and debilitated patients and persons with electronic cardiac pacemakers should be given the loading dose cautiously; *maintenance*, usually **100 mg** once a day, but as much as 200 mg a day may be given. These doses apply only if the patient has received no digitalis for at least 2 weeks. Not recommended for children.

Dosage Forms—Capsules: 100 mg; Tablets: 100 mg.

Digitoxin

Card-20(22)-enolide, 3-[(*O*-2,6-dideoxy-β-D-*ribo*-hexopyranosyl-(1 → 4)-*O*-2,6-dideoxy-β-D-*ribo*-hexopyranosyl-(1 → 4)-2,6-dideoxy-β-D-*ribo*-hexopyranosyl)oxy]-14-hydroxy-, (3β,5β)-, (*Various Mfrs*)

$C_{41}H_{64}H_{13}$ [71-63-6] (764.95); a cardiotonic glycoside obtained from *Digitalis purpurea* Linné, *Digitalis lanata* Ehrh, and other suitable species of *Digitalis*.

The side chain of Digitoxin consists of 3 molecules of digitoxose in glycosidic linkage. Removal of the side chain by hydrolysis yields the aglycone, digitoxigenin ($C_{23}H_{34}O_4$).

Description—White or pale buff, odorless, microcrystalline powder.

Solubility—Practically insoluble in water; 1 g in about 150 mL alcohol or 40 mL chloroform; very slightly soluble in ether.

Uses—See the general statement. Digitoxin is almost completely absorbed after oral administration except if cholestyramine is also being used. Action is maximal in 4 to 12 hr. After full digitalization, the duration of action is about 14 days. In plasma, about 97% is protein-bound. The volume of distribution is about 0.6 mL/g. Plasma concentrations of 15 to 25 ng/mL are considered to be therapeutic and 35 to 40 ng/mL or more to be toxic, but plasma potassium and calcium levels and other factors cause considerable variation. Hepatic metabolism accounts for 52 to 70% of elimination. The β-half-life ranges from 2.4 to 9.6 (av 7.6) days. Phenytoin and phenobarbital can induce hepatic microsomal enzymes and shorten the half-life, hence interfering with the efficacy of the drug.

Dose—*Oral*, *intramuscular*, or *intravenous*, *adults*, for *digitalization*, initially **600 μg** (0.6 mg), followed by **200 to 400** μg every 3 to 6 hr as needed, up to a total of no more than 1.6 mg in 1 or 2 days; for *maintenance*, usually **100 to 200 μg**, and no more than 300 μg a day. In the following *pediatric* doses, only the *digitalizing* dose is stated; the *maintenance* dose is calculated as 10% of the total digitalizing dose a day: *Oral*, *intramuscular*, or *intravenous*, *neonates*, **22 μg/kg** of body weight (or 300 to 350 μg/m² of body surface) divided into 3 or more doses at 6-hr intervals; *infants 2 weeks to 1 year of age*, **45 μg/kg** (or 750 μg/m²) divided into 3 or more doses at 6-hr intervals; *infants 1 to 2 years of age*, **40 μg/kg** (or 750 μg/m²) divided into 3 or more doses at 6-hr intervals; *children 2 years or older*, **30 μg/kg** (or 750 μg/m²) divided into 3 or more doses at 6-hr intervals.

The old practice of giving a single fixed digitalizing dose of 1.2 mg of digitoxin is not recommended. Few patients require such rapid digitalization; although this is approximately the average dose required, it is inadequate for some cases and causes overdigitalization in other patients. Loading and maintenance doses require reduction by 25 to 50% in small or elderly patients or in patients with renal, electrolyte, or metabolic disorders. The above doses apply only if the patient has received no digitalis for 2 weeks.

Dosage Forms—Injection: 200 μg/mL; Tablets: 50, 100, 150, and 200 μg.

Caution—Handle digitoxin with exceptional care, since it is highly potent.

Digoxin

Card-20(22)-enolide, 3-[(O-2,6-dideoxy-β-D-*ribo*-hexopyranosyl-
(1 → 4)-O-2,6-dideoxy-β-D-*ribo*-hexopyranosyl-(1 → 4)-2,6-dideoxy-
β-D-*ribo*-hexopyranosyl)oxy]-12,14-dihydroxy-, (3β,5β,12β)-,
Lanoxin (*Burroughs Wellcome*)

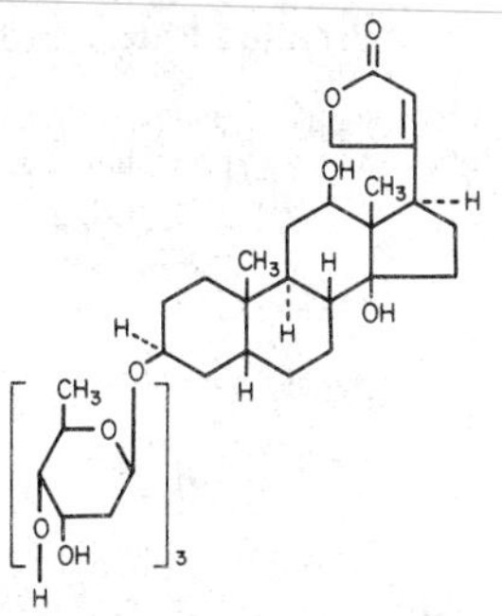

$C_{41}H_{64}O_{14}$ [20830-75-5] (780.95); a cardiotonic glycoside obtained
from the leaves of *Digitalis lanata* Ehrh. (Fam. *Scrophulariaceae*).

The side chain of digoxin consists of 3 molecules of digitoxose in
glycosidic linkage. Hydrolytic cleavage yields the aglycone, digoxigenin ($C_{23}H_{34}O_5$).

Description—Clear to white crystals or a white crystalline powder;
odorless; melts with decomposition above 235°.

Solubility—Practically insoluble in water and ether; slightly soluble
in diluted alcohol and chloroform.

Uses—See the general statement. Because digoxin is a purified
preparation, it is frequently used intravenously for very rapid digitalization. Intravenously its action becomes manifest in 15 to 30 min,
and the effect reaches its peak in 2 to 5 hr. Orally its action is manifest within 1 to 2 hr and reaches a peak in 6 to 8 hr. After full digitalization, the duration of action is about 6 days. In plasma 20 to 30%
is protein-bound. Digoxin has a high volume of distribution, with
a v_d^{ss} of about 5.1 mL/g in normal adults and neonates and even larger
in infants; in renal failure v_d^{ss} is approximately 3.3 mL/g. Extensive
intracellular binding accounts for the large volume of distribution.
The therapeutic concentration in plasma is 0.5 to 2.4 ng/mL, and
concentrations above 2.4 ng/mL are toxic, except that lower concentrations are toxic when hypokalemia, hypercalcemia, and certain other
conditions obtain. Therefore, blood-level assays have only a rough
significance; they are of especial utility in determining bioavailability.
Quinidine increases plasma concentrations. In adults, renal excretion
accounts for 60 to 90% of elimination; some digoxin is converted in
the liver to dihydrodigoxin. Infants appear to have a greater fraction
of extrarenal elimination. Biliary secretion and enterohepatic recirculation account for about 7 to 30% of the body burden. The
elimination half-life is 29 to 135 (usually 36 to 41) hr in normal adults;
in infants of 1 month to 2 years of age, it is sufficiently shorter to require a special dose regimen. In renal failure, the β-half-life may be
as long as 89 to 177 hr. Digoxin is often preferred to digitoxin because
of its shorter half-life; when loading is not used, the steady state is
reached earlier, and, when toxicity occurs, nontoxic levels are reached
earlier after discontinuation of the drug. However, it is easier to lose
control of digitalization if a dose is missed. Considerable attention
to appropriate spacing of maintenance doses is required for smooth
digitalization. By the oral route, about 50% to 85% of digoxin is absorbed from solid dosage forms, but it is 90 to 100% from hydroalcoholic solutions in capsules. Dietary fiber decreases bioavailability.
Increased gastrointestinal motility diminishes, and decreased motility
increases, absorption.

Dose—*Oral*, *adults* and *children over 10 yr of age*, for *rapid digitalization*, 1 to **1.5 mg** divided into 2 or more doses given at 6- to 8-hr
intervals, and, for *slow digitalization* and *maintenance*, 125 to 500
µg (0.125 to 0.5 mg) once a day; slow digitalization will require about
7 days to reach the steady state; *infants under 1 month of age*, for
digitalization, 40 to 60 µg/kg of body weight in 2 or more divided
doses every 6 to 8 hr; *infants, 1 month to 2 yr*, for *digitalization*, 60
to 80 µg/kg in 2 or more divided doses every 6 to 8 hr; *children 2 to
10 years of age*, for *digitalization*, 40 to 60 µg/kg in 2 or more divided
doses every 6 or 8 hr; for *maintenance*, all *infants* and *children under
10 yr*, ⅕ to ⅓ the total digitalizing dose a day. *Intramuscular* or
intravenous, *adults*, and *children over 10 yr of age*, for *digitalization*,
initially **600 µg** followed by **200 to 400 µg** every 3 to 6 hr as necessary,
and, for *maintenance*, 100 to 200 µg once a day; *infants under 2 weeks*

of age, for *digitalization*, 12 to 20 µg/kg of body weight followed by
6 to 10 µg/kg in 6 hr as necessary, to a total of 22 µg/kg; *infants 2
weeks to 1 yr of age*, for *digitalization*, 17.5 to 25 µg/kg followed by
4.5 to 12.5 µg/kg in 6 hr as necessary to a total of 45 µg/kg; *infants
1 to 2 yr* of age, for *digitalization*, a total of 40 µg/kg; *children 2 to
10 yr of age*, for *digitalization*, 12 to 20 µg/kg followed by 6 to 10
µg/kg every 6 hr as necessary to a total of 30 µg/kg; for *maintenance*,
all *infants and children under 10 yr*, ⅕ to ⅓ the total digitalizing dose
a day. None of the above doses are valid if the patient has received
a cardiac glycoside within the previous 2 weeks.

Dosage Forms—Capsules: 50, 100 and 200 µg; Elixir: 50 µg/mL;
Injection: 100 and 250 µg/1 mL, and 500 µg/2 mL; Tablets: 125, 250,
and 500 µg.

*Caution—Handle digoxin with exceptional care, since it is ex-
tremely poisonous.*

Other Cardiac Glycosides

Deslanoside—Desacetyllanatoside C; Cedilanid D (*Sandoz*) [17598-
65-1] $C_{47}H_{74}O_{19}$ (943.09). Deslanoside's side chain consists of 3 molecules
of digitoxose and 1 molecule of glucose in glycosidic linkage. Hydrolysis
yields the aglycone, digoxigenin ($C_{23}H_{34}O_5$)]. *Preparation:* By dea-
cetylating lanatoside C by treatment with alkali. *Description and Solubility:* Colorless or white crystals or a white, crystalline, odorless powder;
hygroscopic, absorbing about 7% of moisture when exposed to air; melts
indistinctly at about 220°. Very slightly soluble in water; 1 g in about 300
mL alcohol; very slightly soluble in chloroform. *Uses:* See the general
statement. By the intravenous route the onset of action is about 10 to 30
min, and the peak effect occurs in about 1 to 3 hr. The duration of action
is approximately 2 to 5 days. Elimination is primarily renal, and dosage
adjustments may be required in renal failure. The elimination half-life
is approximately 33 to 36 hr. Parenteral administration should be employed only in situations when rapid action is needed or when oral administration is not feasible. *Dose: Intramuscular, adults*, 1.6 mg at one
site or 800 µg (0.8 mg) at each of 2 sites, after which an orally administered
cardiac glycoside is substituted; *neonates*, 22 µg/kg of body weight (or 300
µg/m² of body surface) divided into 2 or 3 doses given at 3- or 4-hr intervals;
infants and *children 2 weeks to 3 years* of age, 25 µg/kg (or 750 µg/m²)
divided into 2 or 3 doses given at 3- to 4-hr intervals; *children 3 or more
years of age*, 22.5 µg/kg (or 750 µg/m²) divided into 2 or 3 doses given at
3- or 4-hr intervals. *Intravenous, adults*, initially 800 µg (0.8 mg), repeated in 4 hr, after which an orally administered cardiac glycoside is
substituted; *infants* and *children*, same as intramuscular dose. *Dosage
Forms:* Injection: 0.4 mg/2 mL.
*Caution—Handle deslanoside with exceptional care, since it is highly
potent.*

Gitalin [Gitaligin (*Schering*)]—A cardiotonic glycosidal mixture obtained from *Digitalis purpurea* Linné (Fam *Scrophulariaceae*); it contains 13–19% of gitoxin, 13–19% of gitaloxin, and 14–20% of digitoxin. A
cold-water extract of *Digitalis purpurea* is purified and evaporated to
dryness. The residue (gitalin) consists of the cardioactive glycosides gitaloxin (16-formylgitoxin), gitoxin, and digitoxin, with smaller amounts
of other glycosides and natural substances. A review of the preparation
and composition of gitalin is available in *Am J Pharm 136*: 71, 1964.
White or pale buff, amorphous powder; decomposes with liquefaction
between 120° and 150°. Slightly soluble in water; freely soluble in alcohol,
chloroform, and ether. *Uses:* See the general statement. It has an onset
of action of 2 to 4 hr and duration of 12 days. The drug is administered
only by the oral route; it is well absorbed. *Dose: Usual, initial, rapid
digitalization*, 2.5 mg followed by 0.75 mg every 6 hours until therapeutic
effect or toxicity develops with a total dose of about 6 mg being given in
24 hours; *slow digitalization*, 1.5 mg daily for 4 to 6 days; *maintenance*,
0.25 mg to 1.25 mg daily; *usual*, 0.5 mg daily. These doses apply only if
the patient has not had digitalis within 2 weeks. *Dosage Form:* Tablets:
0.5 mg.

Lanatoside C [3β-[(O-β-D-Glucopyranosyl-(1 → 4)-O-2,6-dideoxy-
β-D-*ribo*-hexopyranosyl-(1 → 4)-O-2,6-dideoxy-β-D-*ribo*-hexopyrano-
syl-(1 → 4)-2,6-dideoxy-β-D-*ribo*-hexopyranosyl)oxy]-12β,14-dihydrox-
y-5β-card-20(22)-enolide 3'''-acetate [17575-22-3] $C_{49}H_{76}O_{20}$ (985.13);
Digilanide C; Cedilanid (*Sandoz*)]—*Caution: Lanatoside C is extremely
poisonous.* A glycoside obtained from the leaves of *Digitalis lanata*
Ehrhart (Fam *Scrophulariaceae*). Its aglycone is identical with that of
digoxin. Colorless or white crystals or a white crystalline powder; odorless;
hygroscopic and will absorb 7% of water on exposure to air. Insoluble in
water; 1 g dissolves in about 45 mL alcohol, and about 2000 mL chloroform;
practically insoluble in ether. *Uses:* See the general statement. Protein
binding is 25% in plasma. The onset of action is 1 to 2 hr, the peak 4 to
6 hr and the duration 3 to 6 days. The half-life is 3 to 6 days. *Dose: Oral,
adults*, for *digitalization*, 3.5 mg the first day, 2.5 mg the second day, 2.0
mg the third day, and 1.5 mg a day thereafter until full digitalization is
obtained (the average total digitalizing dose is stated to be 10 mg); for
maintenance, 0.5 to 1.5 mg a day. These doses apply only if the patient
has not had digitalis for at least 2 weeks. *Dosage Form:* Tablets: 0.5
mg.

Ouabain—[G-Strophanthin; Ouabain octahydrate [11018-89-6] $C_{29}H_{44}O_{12} \cdot 8H_2O$ (728.78); *anhydrous* [630-60-4] (584.66).] *Caution—Ouabain is extremely poisonous.* A glycoside obtained from the seeds of *Strophanthus gratus* (Wall et Hook) Baillon and from the wood of *Acokanthera schimperi* (A DC) Schwf (Fam *Apocynaceae*). The side chain of ouabain consists of a molecule of rhamnose in glycosidic linkage. Hydrolytic cleavage yields the aglycone, ouabagenin ($C_{23}H_{34}O_8$). *Description:* White, odorless crystals, or a crystalline powder; stable in air, but is affected by light; its solutions are neutral to litmus paper; melts indistinctly and with decomposition at about 190°. *Solubility:* 1 g slowly in about 75 mL water, and in about 100 mL alcohol; slightly (and slowly) soluble in chloroform. *Uses:* See the general statement. Oral use is unsafe because of slow and irregular absorption from the gastrointestinal tract. Being water-soluble and rapidly acting, the chief use of ouabain is for parenteral administration when rapid digitalis-like effects are desired with *congestive heart failure, in extremis.* The actions and uses of cardiotonic glycosides and the choice of preparations are discussed under digitalis. After intravenous injection, the onset of action is 3 to 10 min, and the time of peak effect is 0.5 to 2 hr. Ouabain is almost entirely eliminated by renal excretion, with a β-half-life of about 21 hr in normal adults but longer in elderly persons and much longer in renal failure. *Dose: Intravenous, adults,* for *digitalization* only, initially 250 to 500 μg (0.25 to 0.5 mg) followed by 100 μg every hr, as needed, up to a total dose of 1 mg in 24 hr; *infants* and *children,* for *digitalization* only, initially 5 μg/kg of body weight (or 150 μg/m² of body surface) followed by 5 μg/kg in 2 or more divided doses administered at 30-min intervals until the end point is reached or the total dose is given. The above doses do not apply if the patient has received a cardiac glycoside within the previous 2 weeks. For treatment of supraventricular tachyarrhythmias the dose will usually be greater. In small or elderly patients or patients with metabolic, electrolyte or renal disturbances, the dose should be reduced by 25 to 50%. After initial digitalization by ouabain, digitalization is usually completed and maintained by the oral route. *Dosage Form:* Injection: 250 μg/mL.

Antidysrhythmic Drugs

Cardiac dysrhythmias may result from disturbances in pacemaker function of the sinoatrial node, from alterations in conduction path and velocity so that heart block or a self-perpetuating "circus" or reentrant rhythm occurs, or from activation of dormant pacemakers outside the sinus node. Dysrhythmias originating at the sinoatrial node may be tachycardia, bradycardia, and even cardiac arrest. Autonomic drugs are usually sufficient to manage such dysrhythmias. For example, sinus tachycardia may be slowed by β-adrenergic blocking drugs or by reflex action resulting from the pressor effects of certain vasoconstrictors, usually sympathomimetics that lack significant direct actions on the heart (see Chapter 45), or they may be slowed directly by cholinergic drugs or by anticholinesterases. $β_1$-Agonists are used to revive an arrested heart and to relieve certain types of heart block. Reentrant dysrhythmias include paroxysmal atrial tachycardia, atrial flutter, and atrial fibrillation. Circus rhythm may be terminated by drugs that increase atrial conduction velocity so that the circular-moving wave of excitation catches up with itself and thus dies in its own refractory zone, by *cardiac depressants* that increase the refractory period of the heart muscle and decrease membrane responsiveness (group 1: quinidine, procainamide, disopyramide) or change unidirectional conduction block in the reentrant path to bidirectional block, by drugs that improve myocardial cell responsiveness (group 2: lidocaine, phenytoin), such that unidirectional block is abolished, or drugs that shorten the relative refractory period, so that there is less time for a premature impulse to find a relatively refractory tissue and hence aberrant conduction path. Premature impulses from aberrant pacemakers, or ectopic foci, give rise to certain atrial tachycardias, some atrial flutters, some atrial fibrillations, nodal rhythms, ventricular tachycardias, ventricular extrasystoles, and ventricular fibrillation, and they also cause reentrant dysrhythmias by discharging at a time that finds the heart muscle relatively refractory. They may be suppressed by drugs (quinidine, procainamide, etc.) that decrease automaticity. Cardiac glycosides are also used to invoke heart block in unmanageable cases of atrial tachycardia, flutter, and

fibrillation, so that the ventricle is not overwhelmed with impulses of atrial origin.

Digitalis and Cardiac Glycosides—pages 856 to 858.

Disopyramide Phosphate

2-Pyridineacetamide, α-[2-[bis(1-methylethyl)amino]-ethyl]-α-phenyl-, phosphate (1:1);
Norpace (*Searle*)

$(CH_3)_2CH-NCH_2CH_2-\overset{\displaystyle|}{C}-CONH_2 \quad \cdot \; H_3PO_4$
$(CH_3)_2CH$

α-[2- (Diisopropylamino)ethyl] -α-phenyl-2- pyridineacetamide phosphate (1:1) [22059-60-5] $C_{21}H_{29}N_3O \cdot H_3PO_4$ (437.47).

Preparation—A patented process for synthesis of disopyramide converts 4-diisopropylamino-2-phenyl-2-(2-pyridyl)butyronitrile to the corresponding amide (disopyramide) by heating with concentrated H_2SO_4, followed by isolation and purification of the product (*CA 58:* 12522e, 1963).

Description—White, crystalline powder; pK_a 8.36.
Solubility—Freely soluble in water.

Uses—Disopyramide is an antidysrhythmic agent similar in properties to quinidine and procainamide, except that its antimuscarinic properties are more pronounced and are manifested at extracardiac as well as intracardiac sites. It decreases cardiac automaticity in non-nodal cells, increases the functional refractory period and shortens the relative refractory period in both atrial and ventricular cells, decreases the responsiveness of myocardial cells to electrical stimulation, decreases conduction velocity and increases the stimulus threshold. At the sinoatrial and atrioventricular nodes, its direct myocardial depressant actions are opposed by its antimuscarinic action (it has an antimuscarinic structure), so that at low to intermediate doses, especially, it may cause sinus tachycardia in some patients and decrease atrioventricular nodal capability to effect a second-degree block of high frequency atrial impulses passing through to the ventricle. For this reason, patients with supraventricular tachyarrhythmias are usually digitalized before disopyramide is administered. However, in the US, use in the treatment of supraventricular dysrhythmias is not approved. It is approved only as an oral preparation for suppression or prophylaxis of unifocal and multifocal *premature ventricular contractions, pulsus bigeminus* (coupled beats), and *ventricular tachycardia.* However, its efficacy against multifocal premature contractions and in the prevention of ventricular fibrillation as the end-sequel of ventricular dysrhythmias is in question. Given intravenously, it can sometimes arrest ventricular fibrillation, but an injection form is not marketed in the US.

Disopyramide has little of the serious immunologic toxicities of quinidine and procainamide and, in general, causes a lesser incidence of side effects. The most common are those reflecting its antimuscarinic properties, namely, dry mouth and skin. It can also cause blurred vision (from mydriasis and sometimes from cycloplegia), aggravation of narrow-angle glaucoma, constipation and urinary hesitancy. Nausea, vomiting, diarrhea, bloating, contractions of the pregnant uterus, urinary retention, dizziness, fatigue, headache, malaise, dermatoses, and nervousness also occur. Rarely, cholestasis and psychoses can occur. It has been implicated in one case of agranulocytosis. Like quinidine and procainamide, it can depress myocardial contractility and cause consequent hypotension, exacerbate heart failure, and cause heart block, usually in overdoses, and disopyramide must be used cautiously in patients with heart disease and conduction disturbances. The drug increases the dose requirement for warfarin.

Disopyramide is almost completely absorbed by the oral route. The onset of action is 30 to 180 min. Approximately 50% is excreted unchanged in the urine with a half-life of 5 to 7 hr in persons with normal renal function and adequate cardiac output; in renal failure, congestive heart failure and shock it may be as long as 34 hr, and dose adjustments are mandatory. About 10% is secreted into bile. A substantial fraction of a dose is eliminated by N-monodealkylation. Therapeutic plasma levels range from 2 to 4 μg/mL, and toxic levels are approximately 9 μg/mL.

Dose—*Oral, adults, initially,* **200 mg** (300 mg if loading is urgent), followed by **100** to **150 mg** every 6 hr. Pediatric dosage has not been established.

Dosage Forms—Capsules: 100 and 150 mg.

β-Adrenergic Blocking Drugs—page 876.

Calcium Entry Blockers—page 861.

Edrophonium Chloride—page 899.

Ephedrine Sulfate—page 883.

Epinephrine—page 883.

Hydroxyamphetamine Hydrobromide—page 885.

Isoproterenol—page 886.

Lidocaine Hydrochloride—page 1051.

Phenylephrine Hydrochloride—page 889.

Phenytoin—page 1081.

Procainamide Hydrochloride

Benzamide, 4-amino-*N*-[2-(diethylamino)ethyl]-, monohydrochloride;
Procan (*Parke-Davis*); Pronestyl Hydrochloride (*Squibb*)

$$NH_2\text{—}\langle\bigcirc\rangle\text{—}CONHCH_2CH_2N(C_2H_5)_2 \cdot HCl$$

p-Amino-*N*-[2-(diethylamino)ethyl]benzamide monohydrochloride [614-39-1] $C_{13}H_{21}N_3O.HCl$ (271.79).

Preparation—Among other ways, by condensing *p*-nitrobenzoyl chloride with β-diethylaminoethylamine and then reducing the nitro group to amino by any of the usual methods. The hydrochloride forms readily when a stream of hydrogen chloride is passed into a solution of the base in an appropriate organic solvent.

Description—White to tan, crystalline powder, odorless; pH (1 in 10 solution) between 5 and 6.5; melting range between 165° and 169°.

Solubility—Very soluble in water; soluble in alcohol; slightly soluble in chloroform; very slightly soluble in ether.

Uses—Procainamide is a group 1 antidysrhythmic drug with properties similar to those of *Quinidine*. Myocardial automaticity and excitability are depressed, conduction is slowed, and the effective refractory period, particularly that of the atrium, is increased. Procainamide is useful in suppressing *arrhythmias* of ventricular origin, including ventricular extrasystoles, and paroxysmal ventricular tachycardia. The drug is also effective against premature atrial contractions and atrial fibrillation but it is only moderately effective in arresting paroxysmal atrial tachycardia and atrial fibrillation. In cases of paroxysmal atrial tachycardia, other measures and agents of choice should be employed before procainamide is tried. Many cardiologists employ procainamide and quinidine interchangeably. However, either drug may be effective in an individual patient who has failed to respond to maximally tolerated doses of the other agent. Procainamide is effective immediately with intravenous injection whereas quinidine is not, so that procainamide is advantageous in arresting ventricular tachycardia. Procainamide is used in the management of *myotonia*.

Procainamide is usually well tolerated in the short term. Gastrointestinal distress manifested by nausea, vomiting, or anorexia may be noted when the drug is given orally, and hypotension, flushing, and giddiness almost always occur when the intravenous route is employed. Mental depression and hallucinatory psychoses have occurred. Hypersensitivity to the drug, with fever, urticaria, angioneurotic edema, rash, hepatomegaly, leukopenia, and fatal agranulocytosis occur; it is contraindicated in persons who have had these disorders. Cross-sensitivity to procaine and related drugs should be anticipated. In the long term, the most serious side-effect is a lupus-like syndrome. Ultimately, about 50% of chronic recipients must discontinue the drug because of adverse reactions. Procainamide depresses myocardial contractility and may cause hypotension; it should be used cautiously in patients with heart failure, valvular disease, or aortic stenosis. The drug has an antimuscarinic action on the atrioventricular node that may counteract its direct depressant action on that node. In patients with supraventricular tachydysrhythmias, the number of excessive impulses passing through the node may actually increase, especially at first. In addition, untoward responses may result from actions of the drug on an abnormal myocardium, such as ventricular asystole or fibrillation in patients with marked disturbances of atrioventricular conduction. Procainamide must be given cautiously if the patient is digitalized.

After oral administration, procainamide is almost completely absorbed, and peak plasma levels are reached in 1 to 2 hr. In plasma, about 15% is protein-bound. The volume of distribution is about 2 mL/g. Renal excretion, partly by tubular secretion, accounts for 50 to 60% of elimination. From 7 to 34% is metabolized as *N*-acetyl-procainamide, an active metabolite that can accumulate. There are slow and fast acetylators. The β-half-life of procainamide is 5 to 7 hr in patients with normal renal function but up to 25 hr in renal failure, shock, and congestive heart failure; doses must be adjusted in these conditions. Plasma concentrations of 4 to 10 $\mu g/mL$ correct 90% of responsive ventricular tachyarrhythmias without serious adverse effects.

Dose—*Oral, adults,* for *atrial dysrhythmias,* initially **1.25 g,** then **750 mg** 1 hr later, if necessary, followed by **500 mg** to **1 g** every 2 hr as needed or tolerated, except initially **1 g** every 6 hr with sustained-release tablets; for *maintenance,* **500 mg** to **1 g** every 4 to 6 hr; for *ventricular dysrhythmias,* initially **1 g,** followed by **250** to **500 mg** every 3 hr, except **12.5 mg/kg** every 6 hr, with adjustments; for *myotonia,* **250 mg** twice a day; *children,* **12.5 mg/kg** (or 375 mg per m² of body surface) 4 times a day. *Intramuscular, adults,* for *atrial* and *ventricular dysrhythmias,* **500 mg** to **1 g** every 6 hr. *Intravenous infusion, adults,* for *atrial dysrhythmias,* **500 mg** to **1 g,** infused at a rate of 25 to 50 mg/min; for *ventricular dysrhythmias,* **200 mg** to **1 g,** infused at a rate of 25 to 50 mg/min.

Dosage Forms—Capsules: 250, 375, and 500 mg; Injection: 1 g/2 mL and 1 g/10 mL; Tablets: 250, 375, and 500 mg; Sustained-Release Tablets: 250 and 500 mg.

Quinidine Gluconate

Cinchonan-9-ol, 6'-methoxy-, (9S)-, mono-D-gluconate (salt);
Quinidine Monogluconate (salt); Quinaglute (*Berlex*); Duraquin
(*Parke-Davis*)

Quinidine mono-D-gluconate [7054-25-3] $C_{20}H_{24}N_2O_2.C_6H_{12}O_7$ (520.58); the gluconate of an alkaloid that may be obtained from various species of *Cinchona* and their hybrids, or from *Remijia pedunculata* Flückiger (Fam *Rubiaceae*), or prepared from quinine. For the structure of quinidine, see page 417.

Description—White powder; odorless and has a very bitter taste.

Solubility—Freely soluble in water; only slightly soluble in alcohol.

Uses—An antiarrhythmic drug with the same actions, uses, and toxicity as *Quinidine Sulfate* (see below), but is preferred for *intramuscular* use, since it is nonirritating and stable in solution. The *intravenous* administration of quinidine is only occasionally warranted, but sometimes is a lifesaving measure in certain desperate conditions such as *ventricular tachycardia* with acute pulmonary edema or severe congestive failure. The cardiac effect may be observed in 15 to 20 min after intramuscular injection. Hypotension is frequent.

Dose—*Oral, adults,* as extended-release tablets, **324** to **660 mg,** every 6 to 12 hr; the higher doses should be used only after a trial with lower doses and clinical and laboratory reexamination and determination of plasma quinidine levels. *Intramuscular, adults,* initially **600 mg,** followed by **400 mg** at intervals as short as every 2 hr, if necessary, up to a maximum daily dose of 5 g. *Intravenous, adults,* **200** to **800 mg** in dilute solution (20 mg/mL in isotonic dextrose injection) given at a rate of no more than 1 mL/min (20 mg/min) with continuous monitoring of the electrocardiograph and blood pressure.

Dosage Forms—Injection: 800 mg/10 mL; Extended-Release Tablets: 324 and 330 mg.

Quinidine Polygalacturonate

A compound described as a polymer of quinidine and polygalacturonic acid and assigned the molecular formula $(C_{20}H_{24}N_2O_2.C_6H_{10}O_7.H_2O)_x$ [7681-28-9].

Preparation—From quinidine and polygalacturonic acid (from pectin); described in *Am J Pharm 130:* 190, 1958, also US Pat 2,878,252.

Description—Creamy white, amorphous powder; melts at about 180°, with decomposition.

Solubility—Sparingly soluble in water.

Uses—The actions, uses, and general toxicity of quinidine polygalacturonate are those of *Quinidine Sulfate*, except that it is not used in attempted conversion of ventricular dysrhythmias and it causes a lesser incidence and severity of gastrointestinal side effects and hence is gaining preference for oral use.

Dose—*Oral*, *adults*, *initially* **275** to **825 mg** for 4 or 5 doses at 3- to 4-hr intervals, after which upward adjustments in increments of 137.5 to 275 mg may be made on every third or fourth dose until the therapeutic end point is reached or toxicity supervenes, then **275 mg** 2 or 3 times a day for *maintenance*.

Dosage Form—Tablets: 275 mg, equivalent to 200 mg of quinidine sulfate.

Quinidine Sulfate

Cinchonan-9-ol, 6′-methoxy, (9S)-, sulfate (2:1) (salt), dihydrate; (*Various Mfrs*)

Quinidine sulfate (2:1) (salt) dihydrate [6591-63-5] $(C_{20}H_{24}N_2O_2)_2.H_2SO_4.2H_2O$ (782.95); *anhydrous* [50-54-4] (746.92); the sulfate of an alkaloid obtained from various species of *Cinchona* and their hybrids and from *Remijia pedunculata* Flückiger (Fam *Rubiaceae*), or prepared from quinine.

Quinidine is a stereoisomer of quinine (page 417) and occurs in cinchona bark in amounts ranging from 0.3 to over 1%, although in some barks it may be practically absent. Quinidine of commerce is usually accompanied by up to 20% of *hydroquinidine* (which is quinidine with an ethyl group replacing the vinyl) which, however, is therapeutically as potent as quinidine and no more toxic.

Preparation—Quinidine may be made by treating quinine with a metallic alkoxide (Doering WE, *et al: J Am Chem Soc 69:* 1700, 1947) or by oxidizing quinine to quininone and then reducing the latter with sodium isopropoxide (Woodward RB, *et al: J Am Chem Soc 67:* 1428, 1945). It may also be obtained directly from the mother liquors remaining after removal of quinine from extracts of *Cinchona*; separation from cinchonine and other alkaloids is effected by special processes.

Description—Fine, needle-like, white crystals, frequently cohering in masses; very bitter taste; darkens on exposure to light; solutions are neutral or alkaline to litmus; pK_{a1} 5.4; pK_{a2} 10.0.

Solubility—1 g in about 100 mL water, 10 mL alcohol, 15 mL chloroform; insoluble in ether.

Uses—Quinidine is a group 1 antidysrhythmic drug and hence decreases automaticity, membrane responsiveness, excitability, and conduction velocity. It prolongs the functional refractory period and shortens the relative refractory period and hence the vulnerable period for aberrant conduction. It is quite effective in suppressing chronic *atrial premature contractions*, and in converting and protecting against recurrences of *atrial fibrillation*. It is frequently given before attempted electroversion as a prophylactic against recurrence or new dysrhythmias. It is moderately effective against *paroxysmal atrial tachycardia*, *atrioventricular junctional premature systoles and tachycardia*, and *ventricular premature systoles*. It will sometimes convert atrial flutter and ventricular tachycardia.

Quinidine itself can cause dysrhythmias, in part because its effects to slow conduction favor reentrant impulses. Combined with digitalis, quinidine may induce bizarre abnormalities of rhythm. The effect on atrioventricular conduction is erratic, especially with low doses or early in the response to high doses. This is because not only does quinidine have an antimuscarinic action on the heart to relieve vagal influences on conduction but also it causes release of norepinephrine from adrenergic nerves. The result is an improvement in atrioventricular conduction and an increase in the ability of the ventricle to follow atrial beats, so that during supraventricular tachyarrhythmias there may be an increase in an already excessively high ventricular rate and a consequent further impairment of ventricular filling and cardiac output. As the plasma levels increase, the ventricular rate may fall again, as a result both of control of the atrial tachyarrhythmia and a quinidine-induced A-V block. Occasionally quinidine may cause ventricular tachycardia, fibrillation, or standstill.

Oral quinidine commonly causes nausea, diarrhea, abdominal discomfort and, less frequently, vomiting. It decreases myocardial contractility, hence cardiac output, and can cause hypotension, sometimes severe. It may also induce cinchonism (headache, vertigo, tinnitus, nausea, vomiting, diarrhea, palpitation, syncope, photophobia, diplopia, night blindness, disturbances of color vision, scotoma, mydriasis). It can also cause hypersensitivity, characterized by various rashes, thrombocytopenia and, rarely, angioedema and anaphylaxis. In the long term, about $1/3$ of all recipients discontinue the drug because of one or more of such side-effects, especially thrombocytopenia. One adverse effect is the result of its therapeutic action to terminate atrial flutter, namely, the dislodgement of mural thrombi with consequent embolism. Quinidine potentiates antihypertensive drugs, other antidysrhythmic drugs in both therapeutic and cardiovascular adverse effects, and the response to prothrombopenic anticoagulants. It also increases the effects of neuromuscular paralyzants; it has a neuromuscular depressant action of its own, which has found use in testing for myasthenia gravis and treating myotonia. Quinidine is contraindicated when there already is heart block, thrombocytopenia or other hypersensitivity, and should be used cautiously in heart failure and hypokalemia.

Quinidine is 90% absorbed by the oral route. In plasma 82% is protein-bound. The volume of distribution is 0.47 mL/g. Therapeutic plasma levels range from 3 to 6 µg/mL, and toxicity usually occurs by the time 8 µg/mL is reached. Elimination is 50 to 60% by hepatic biotransformation. The half-life is 3 to 17 hr, but usually it is 5 to 7 hr. An alkaline urine favors tubular resorption and hence prolongs the half-life and elevates plasma levels. Adjustments in dosage must be made when drugs (many antacids, carbonic anhydrase inhibitors) or diets that increase urine pH are used.

Dose—*Oral*, *adults*, initially **200** to **800 mg** every 2 or 3 hr up to 5 g on the first day, followed by **100** to **200 mg** 3 to 6 times a day; *infants* and *children*, **6 mg/kg** of body weight (or 180 mg/m² of body surface) 5 times a day. *Parenteral*, not recommended, although an injection is available.

Dosage Forms—Capsules: 200 and 300 mg; Injection: 200 mg/1 mL; Tablets: 100, 200, and 300 mg; Sustained-Release Tablets: 300 mg.

Verapamil—page 862.

Other Antidysrhythmic Drugs

Aprindine Hydrochloride [*N*-(2,3-Dihydro-1*H*-inden-2-yl)-*N*′,*N*′-diethyl-*N*-phenyl-1,3-propanediamine monohydrochloride [33237-74-0] $C_{22}H_{30}N_2.HCl$ (358.95) Fibocil (*Lilly*)]. *Uses:* An investigational drug expected to be released in the US. It has electrophysiological properties like those of lidocaine except that it slows conduction in the AV node and Bundle of His. The QRS complex may be widened. This property gives it a special usefulness in the treatment of the Wolf-Parkinson-White syndrome. It is also used to prevent or suppress premature ventricular impulses and ventricular tachydysrhythmias. Oral absorption is good, except that it may be erratic in persons with recent myocardial infarction. About 90% is bound in plasma. The drug is 100% metabolized in the liver. The half-life is about 28 hr. CNS side-effects mostly occur during intravenous loading. They include lightheadedness, vertigo, tremor and ataxia. The incidence is about 20%. Other common side-effects are anorexia, nausea, vomiting, and diarrhea. Reversible agranulocytosis and cholestatic jaundice occasionally occur. *Dose: Intravenous, adults*, for rapid control, 80 to 160 mg divided into 20-mg doses at 2-min intervals, after which oral dosage is begun; *oral, adults, initially*, 200 to 400 mg then, for *maintenance*, 100 to 200 mg once a day.

Bretylium Tosylate [2-Bromo-*N*-ethyl-*N*,*N*-dimethylbenzene-methanaminium 4-methylbenzenesulfonate [61-75-6] $C_{18}H_{24}BrNO_3S$ (414.39); Darenthin; Bretylol (*Arnar-Stone*)]—Prepared by interaction of *o*-bromobenzyl bromide and dimethylethylamine, the product being quaternized with *p*-toluenesulfonic acid. A white, crystalline powder; melts at about 98°; freely soluble in water and alcohol. *Uses:* Bretylium is presently indicated for the treatment of life-threatening ventricular dysrhythmias that are refractory to other antidysrhythmic drugs. It is particularly effective against ventricular tachycardia. It is also unique among antidysrhythmic drugs in the US in that it can sometimes revert a ventricular fibrillation without the use of concomitant electroversion. Bretylium is not recommended for suppression of asymptomatic premature ventricular contractions, and it has not been established that the drug has prophylactic value against ventricular dysrhythmias.

The mechanism of action of bretylium is incompletely known. It both depresses automaticity and increases the threshold to fibrillation-inducing electrical stimulation in both normal and infarcted myocardium. It also has antiadrenergic effects to impair release of and partially deplete norepinephrine in adrenergic nerve terminals and also to impair norepinephrine uptake, which should assist in suppression of automaticity, once the release phase is over. However, there is no temporal correlation between the onset and duration of the antiadrenergic action with those of the antidysrhythmic action. It also increases the functional refractory period and shortens the relative refractory period, effects which discourage reentry. Some side effects of bretylium can be severe, so that the drug is held in reserve for use after other treatment fails. However, in less than 10% of patients must the drug be discontinued because of intolerance.

Intravenous injection causes a high incidence of nausea and vomiting, which can be minimized by injection over a period of 10 to 30 min. Adrenergic neuron blockade by the drug causes orthostatic hypotension and severe hypotension even in the supine position in patients with inadequate heart function. During the onset of action, release of norepinephrine can cause hypertension, tachycardia, exacerbate ongoing dysrhythmias, and aggravate digitalis cardiotoxicity. Therefore, careful monitoring is required until sympathetic blockade ensues. In persons with severe pulmonary hypertension or aortic stenosis, adrenergic neuron blockade removes a compensatory response system necessary to adjust to the hypotension. Bretylium sometimes causes parotid enlargement and pain. Because of blockade of the neuronal catecholamine uptake system and chemical denervation supersensitivity, directly acting sympathomimetics should be administered cautiously. Bretylium is well absorbed from intramuscular sites. The plasma half-life averages about 10 hr but varies considerably. From excretion data, it can be surmised that it is completely eliminated by renal excretion. The dose should be adjusted in renal failure. *Dose: Intramuscular, adult*, initially 5 to 10 mg/kg, repeated in 1 or 2 hr, then 5 to 10 mg/kg every 6 to 8 hr for maintenance; *intravenous*, initially 5 mg/kg followed by additional doses of 10 mg/kg every 15 to 30 min up to a total of 30 mg/kg if necessary, then 5 to 10 mg/kg every 6 to 8 hr for maintenance. In ventricular fibrillation, the drug should be given by rapid intravenous injection. In all other uses, intravenous administration should be by a 10- to 30-min infusion at a rate of 1 to 2 mg/ min. *Dosage Form:* Injection: 500 mg/10 mL.

Encainide Hydrochloride [(±)-4-Methoxy-N-[2-[2-(1-methyl-2-piperidinyl)ethyl]phenyl]benzamide monohydrochloride [66794-74-9] $C_{22}H_{28}N_2O_2$.HCl (388.94) Enkade (*Mead Johnson*)]. *Uses:* An investigational drug expected to be released in the US. It is unique in that it slows conduction and prolongs the action potential in the Purkinje system and widens the QRS complex without affecting atrial, atrioventricular, or ventricular electrophysiological parameters. Its effect is greater in ischemic than in normal fibers. It is specifically indicated for the suppression of premature ventricular depolarizations and tachydysrhythmias. The main adverse effects are transient ataxia and diplopia at high plasma concentrations in patients with relatively resistant dysrhythmias. Although it is orally effective, it is rapidly metabolized during the first-pass to three metabolites, of which at least one, the O-desmethyl metabolite is active. The half-life of encainide is 0.3 to 3.3 hr and of the metabolite, 5 to 23 hr. *Dose: Oral, adult*, initially 25 mg every 4 to 6 hr, adjusted as needed to achieve control, then 25 to 100 mg every 6 to 8 hr for maintenance, up to a maximum of 300 mg/day.

Mexiletine [1-Methyl-2-(2,6-xylyloxy)ethylamine [31828-71-4] $C_{11}H_{17}NO$ (179.26); Mexitil (*Boehringer-Ingelheim*)] White crystals melting about 205°. *Uses:* An investigational drug expected to be released in the US. It resembles lidocaine in its electrophysiological effects in the heart and has the same uses and equal efficacy but is superior in that it may be used for chronic treatment. Its primary advantage is oral efficacy and relatively long half-life. Its useful actions are primarily limited to ventricular dysrhythmias. It has very little effect to decrease contractility but does cause some hypotension and bradycardia. Oral bioavailability is about 88%. Hepatic metabolism accounts for about 90% of elimination. The half-life is 10 to 12 hr. During intravenous loading, neurological adverse effects include lightheadedness, vertigo, tremor, nystagmus, and diplopia; cardiovascular effects include bradycardia and hypotension. Thrombocytopenia and antinuclear factor during long-term oral treatment have been reported. *Dose: Intravenous* or *oral*, for *loading*, 400 to 600 mg, then oral for *maintenance*, 200 to 400 mg every 8 hr.

Tocainide 2-Amino-N-(2,6-dimethylphenyl)propanamide [41708-72-9] $C_{11}H_{16}N_2O$ (192.26)]. *Uses:* An investigational drug expected to be released in the US. Tocainide is a homolog of the desethyl metabolite of lidocaine and hence lacks the first-pass vulnerability of lidocaine. It resembles lidocaine in its effects on transient sodium current but differs in that it only slightly shortens action potential duration. It decreases the excitability and automaticity of Purkinje fibers. Atrioventricular conduction is not affected. Effects are most notable in patients with conduction disturbances. The effect on myocardial contractility of non-failing hearts is negligible. Tocainide has a slight effect to increase vascular resistance. Like lidocaine, it is a local anesthetic. It is used to prevent and suppress premature ventricular depolarizations and ventricular tachydysrhythmias. Like lidocaine, tocainide has local anesthetic properties, to which are attributed to CNS adverse effects, such as lightheadedness, vertigo, tremor, twitching, paresthesia, sweating, hot flashes, mood alterations, blurred vision and diplopia. These effects occur only during intravenous loading. Gastrointestinal side effects with oral dosage include anorexia, nausea, vomiting, constipation and abdominal pain. These effects are diminished by giving the drug with food. Fever, rashes, and arthralgias occasionally occur. Rare occurrences of pulmonary edema, pneumonitis, hepatitis, bradycardia, and antinuclear antibody have been reported. About 90% is orally absorbed. The volume of distribution is 2.5 to 3.8 mL/g. Ten to 50% is protein-bound in plasma. The distribution half-life is 5 to 15 min and the elimination half-life is 11 to 17 hr. Sixty to 70% is metabolized in the liver. *Dose: Oral, adults, initially* 400 to 600 mg every 8 to 12 hr, subsequently adjusted to achieve the optimal response. *Intravenous*, 750 mg over 15 min, after which oral administration is begun.

Calcium Entry Blocking Drugs

Calcium entry blocking drugs are a heterogeneous group of agents whose main pharmacological effect is to prevent or slow the entry of calcium into cells via specialized calcium channels. Other names used for this class of drugs include calcium channel blockers, calcium antagonists, and slow channel blockers, since the entry of calcium into cells is slower than sodium entry after stimulation. Only three drugs in this group are now available in the US: verapamil, nifedipine, and diltiazem. However, this is an active area of drug development; several new agents are presently in various stages of investigation.

The entry of calcium into cells is of fundamental importance for the normal functioning of the cardiovascular system. In the SA node and AV node in the heart, the slow depolarization observed in these specialized tissue cells is a consequence of the slow inward movement of calcium ions. In atrial and ventricular muscle in the myocardium, the plateau phase of the action potential (phase 2) is the result of inward calcium movement which, in turn, couples the electrical excitation of these cells with muscle contraction. In vascular smooth muscle, calcium influx into cells is the excitation-contraction link that is necessary for smooth muscle contraction whenever smooth muscle is stimulated. Finally, inward calcium movements maintain the resting potential and may be responsible for action potentials in some smooth muscles. Although calcium entry into cells is also important for many tissue functions outside the cardiovascular system (eg, excitation-contraction coupling in skeletal muscle and nonvascular smooth muscle, excitation-release coupling at nerve endings, and excitation-secretion coupling in glands) calcium channels in the cardiovascular system appear to be the more sensitive to drugs. Thus, the clinical usefulness of these calcium entry blocking drugs is limited to their applications in the therapy of cardiovascular disease.

A useful working description of how these drugs act is possible, although their mechanism of action is not known in detail. Calcium enters cells through specialized pores in the membrane wall called calcium channels. There are two types of channels: one activated by membrane depolarization (voltage-operated) and a second activated by activation of a receptor (receptor-operated). Calcium entry blocking drugs decrease calcium entry in both the voltage-operated and receptor-operated channels, but the voltage-operated channel is the more sensitive to drug blockade. Exactly how the entry blockers "plug" the channels is the objective of much current research. Although all calcium entry blocking drugs have in common the ability to decrease calcium entry into cells, drug effects vary from site to site and from drug to drug. Whether this variation represents differences in calcium channels in the tissues or differences in the mechanisms of action of the drugs at various sites, or both, has not been clarified.

Calcium entry blocking drugs have been approved for the oral treatment of *variant (vasospastic)* and chronic *stable exertional angina pectoris*. They are useful in the therapy of these diseases for three reasons: They directly dilate coronary arteries and increase myocardial blood flow; they decrease myocardial oxygen demand by peripheral arteriolar dilatation, which decreases afterload; and they exert negative chronotopic and inotropic actions which also decreases oxygen demand. Verapamil has been approved for the intravenous therapy of *supraventricular tachyarrhythmias* because of its significant depressant effects on SA nodal automaticity and AV conduction. To the extent that calcium channel activity is important for spontaneous electrical discharges in diseased myocardium, calcium entry blocking drugs may also find use in the therapy of other arrhythmias. Some calcium entry blockers are effective in the therapy of *systemic hypertension* because they are potent arteriolar vasodilators, but as yet this is not an approved use in the US. They have been proposed for the treatment of *pulmonary hypertension*. Investigations of their use for the *preservation of the ischemic myocardium* are encouraging. Ischemic heart muscle is partially or completely depolarized, and excessive calcium enters through voltage-operated channels. The resulting high intracellular calcium concentrations activate ATPase and cause the depletion of ATP, cause mitochondrial damage, and activate various lytic enzymes that attack membrane and intracellular structures. Calcium entry blocking drugs retard the calcium entry and promote salvage of myocardium. Other unapproved and/or investigational uses of these agents include uses in patients with *active myocardial infarction, congestive heart failure* and *hypertrophic cardiomyopathy*. The choice of a drug for a particular purpose depends on the pharmacological properties of the drugs (see below), the presence of other drugs, and the cardiovascular status of the patient.

Untoward effects of the calcium entry blockers are consequences of calcium entry blockade and are primarily limited to the cardiovascular system. Drug-induced vasodilatation leads to hypotension and to dizziness, lightheadedness, flushing and headache. Decreased SA automaticity causes bradycardia, and decreased AV conduction sometimes can result in heart block. Decreased myocardial contractility can result in congestive heart failure, particularly, when these drugs are used with beta-adrenergic blocking drugs. Peripheral edema caused by these drugs may be due to a combination of heart failure and peripheral vasodilatation. Effects of the drug outside of the cardiovascular system are minimal. Constipation is sometimes reported and may be caused by excitation-contraction uncoupling in gastrointestinal smooth muscle. Excitation-secretion coupling in exocrine and endocrine glands is another important role of calcium, but the effects of calcium entry blocking drugs on glandular function have not proven to be clinically important, although nifedipine has been reported to decrease insulin secretion. In usual doses, calcium antagonists do not appear to affect norepinephrine release from sympathetic nerve endings although calcium is necessary for norepinephrine release. In sharp contrast to beta-adrenergic blockers, calcium entry blockers do not increase airway resistance.

Diltiazem Hydrochloride

Benzothiazepin-4(5*H*)-one, 3-(acetyloxy)-5-[2-(dimethylamino)ethyl]-2,3-dihydro-2-(4-methoxyphenyl)-, (+)-*cis*-, monohydrochloride; Cardizem (*Marion*)

[33286-22-5] $C_{22}H_{26}N_2O_4S \cdot HCl$ (450.98).
Preparation—*Chem Pharm Bull* 19, 595 (1971).

Description—White crystals melting about 188°.
Solubility—Freely soluble in water, alcohol or chloroform; slightly soluble in dehydrated alcohol.

Uses—See general statement. Diltiazem has less effect on peripheral resistance and myocardial contractility than do verapamil and nifedipine, but it is a more potent coronary vasodilator. Diltiazem slows conduction in the AV node but not as much as do verapamil. Heart rate is usually decreased by diltiazem because of its slight effects on SA node automaticity and because its modest peripheral vasodilatory effects do not evoke powerful reflex responses.

Diltiazem is 80% absorbed orally, but only 40 to 60% of an oral dose reaches the systemic circulation because of first-pass metabolism in

the liver. After administration, it is 70 to 80% bound to plasma protein. Displacement from protein binding sites by other drugs does not seem to be a clinical problem. Diltiazem is extensively metabolized by the liver to several metabolites, some of which have weak coronary vasodilator activity. Less than 4% of the drug appears unchanged in the urine. The plasma half-life is about 4 hours. The drug has been reported to have saturation kinetics after single doses greater than 60 mg.

Dose—*Oral, adults,* initially: **30 mg** 4 times a day to be increased to 240 mg day, as necessary.
Dosage Forms—Tablets: 30 and 60 mg.

Nifedipine

3,5-Pyridinecarboxylic acid, 1,4-dihydro-2,6-dimethyl-4-(2-nitrophenyl)-, dimethyl ester; Procardia (*Pfizer*)

[21829-25-4] $C_{17}H_{18}N_2O_6$ (346.34).
Preparation—See US Pat 3,485,847.

Description—Yellow crystals melting about 174°.
Solubility—Practically insoluble in water; slightly soluble in alcohol; very soluble in chloroform or acetone; solution are extremely light sensitive.

Uses—See general statement. Nifedipine is a potent peripheral vasodilator. This effect, coupled with its lack of significant effect to decrease SA node automaticity, causes reflex tachycardia. Sympathetic reflex activity also tends to negate the negative intropic effects of nifedipine.

About 90% of an oral dose of nifedipine is absorbed, but its bioavailability is 65 to 70%; there is significant hepatic first-pass metabolism. Greater than 90% of the drug is bound to plasma protein. Nifedipine is metabolized to inactive metabolites, probably by the liver. Most (80%) of the inactive metabolites are excreted in urine; 15% are excreted in the stool. The half-life of nifedipine is 4 to 6 hours.

Dose—*Oral, adults, initially,* **10 mg** 3 times a day, to be gradually increased to **20 to 30 mg** 3 or 4 times a day, if necessary. Doses exceeding 180 mg per day are not recommended.
Dosage Forms—Tablets: 10 mg.

Verapamil Hydrochloride

Benzeneacetonitrile, α-[3-[[2-(3,4-dimethoxyphenyl)ethyl]-methylamino]propyl]-3,4-dimethoxy-α-(1-methylethyl)-, hydrochloride; CALAN (*Searle*); Isoptin (*Knoll*)

Preparation—See *Arzneimittel-Forsch 12*: 563, 1962 and *Helv Chim Acta 58*: 2050, 1975.

Description—White to off-white crystals melting about 140°.
Solubility—1 g dissolves in about 15 mL of water; 25 mL of alcohol; 2 mL of chloroform. Soluble in most polar organic solvents. The pH of of a 7% (w/w) solution is about 4.2.

Uses—See general statement. Of the three available calcium entry blockers, verapamil has the greatest effects on the myocardium. Its effects on sinoatrial automaticity, AV conduction and myocardial contractility are greater than those of diltiazem. Verapamil dilates peripheral vascular smooth muscle more than diltiazem but not as much as does nifedipine. Effects on heart rate are variable and depend, in part, on the amount of reflex sympathetic activity evoked by peripheral dilatation. Verapamil is more than 90% absorbed, but only 20–35% of the dose reaches the system because of extensive hepatic first-pass metabolism. It is approximately 90% bound to plasma proteins.

Verapamil is rapidly metabolized by the liver to norverapamil and traces of several other metabolites. About 70% of a dose is excreted in urine as metabolites, and 16% of a dose appears in the feces within 5 days; less than 5% is excreted unchanged. The half-life of the drug is 2 to 5 hours in normal persons but may exceed 9 hr during chronic therapy. In patients with cirrhosis of the liver, the half-life may be increased to 14 to 16 hours. The half-life of verapamil in patients with liver disease may be three times normal, due, in part, to an increased volume of distribution in these persons. Saturation kinetics have been observed after repeated doses.

Dose: *Intravenous, adults, initially* **5 to 10 mg** (0.075 to 0.15 mg/kg) over a period of 2 min (3 min in the elderly), followed by **10 mg** (0.150 mg/kg) after 30 min, if necessary; *children, up to 1 yr of age, initially* **0.1 to 0.2 mg/kg** over 2 min (with EKG monitoring), repeated after 30 min, if necessary; *1 to 15 yr, initially* **0.1 to 0.3 mg/kg**, not to exceed 5 mg, repeated after 30 min, if necessary. *Oral, adults,* **80 mg** 3 or 4 times a day, gradually increased to as much as 480 mg/day, if necessary.

Dosage Forms—Injection: 5 mg/2 mL; tablets: 80 mg and 120 mg.

Drugs Affecting Blood Lipids

Drugs that affect blood lipids may be classified as cardiovascular drugs because of the probable relation of blood lipids to atherosclerosis. Atherosclerosis is regarded by many as a disorder in lipid metabolism or as a normal effect of a diet high in certain lipids. Since one of the major lipids in the atheroma is cholesterol, much attention has been centered upon cholesterol in the diet and blood. There is a correlation between blood cholesterol content and the incidence of coronary occlusion, although it is far from a perfect one. Experimentally, a diet high in cholesterol can promote or exacerbate atherosclerosis in certain species. Consequently, there has been interest in drugs that affect the absorption of cholesterol from the intestine. However, cholesterol is also synthesized from fatty acids in the body, and there has been great interest in the relative abilities of different fatty acids to elevate plasma cholesterol levels. Saturated fats induce higher blood cholesterol levels than do unsaturated fats, but it now appears that some of what was attributed to saturation is the result of cholesterol in fats derived from animals. Polyunsaturated fats have been thought to be not only the least offensive in elevating blood cholesterol but also to antagonize the cholesterologenic effects of saturated fatty acids. But the polyunsaturated fatty acids also undergo peroxidation and form epoxides, which have been suggested to be carcinogenic. The role of various fatty acids in atherogenesis now requires reevaluation. The blood β-lipoprotein and serum triglyceride levels also correlate somewhat with the incidence of coronary occlusion and with the type of fat in the diet. Since the first Framingham study, epidemiological studies and therapy have been preoccupied with the low-density (LDL) and the very-low-density (VLDL) lipoproteins and also with chylomicrons. It is now known, however, that a very important factor in atherogenesis is the plasma level of high-density lipoproteins (HDL), which serve as scavengers of cholesterol and not only protect the arteries from deposition of cholesterol but appear to be involved in the transport of cholesterol out of vessel walls. The blood lipids are only one of a number of factors that cause atherosclerosis and coronary occlusion. Thus it should not be expected that manipulation of the blood lipids will necessarily bring about improvement in the disease. In 1975, the results of a multicenter study on antilipidemic drugs was published. The essence of the report was that antihyperlipidemic drugs did not decrease the risk of coronary heart disease or lower mortality. However, many serious criticisms have been made of the study, one being that nearly half of the subjects in the study did not have a hyperlipidemia. A more recent study in Sweden has indicated a remarkable decrease in coronary reinfarction rate in patients treated with a combination of clofibrate and niacin. In the US, bile acid se-

questering resins have been shown to decrease the myocardial infarction rate. Furthermore, evidence continues to mount that low-fat diets in combination with antilipidemic drugs have a protective effect in coronary heart disease.

Aminosalicylic Acid—page 1213.

Cholestyramine Resin—page 813.

Clofibrate

Propanoic acid, 2-(4-chlorophenoxy)-2-methyl-, ethyl ester; Atromid S (*Ayerst*)

Ethyl 2-(*p*-chlorophenoxy)-2-methylpropionate [637-07-0] $C_{12}H_{15}ClO_3$ (242.70), calculated on the anhydrous basis.

Preparation—By condensing phenol with ethyl 2-chloro-2-methylpropionate in the presence of a suitable dehydrochlorinating agent and then chlorinating.

Description—Stable, colorless to pale-yellow liquid with a faint, characteristic odor and a characteristic taste; boiling point 158° to 160°.

Solubility—Insoluble in water; soluble in alcohol, and chloroform.

Uses—Clofibrate has a considerable effect in decreasing the VLDL levels in persons with hypertriglyceridemia. In the Coronary Drug Project, the average fall was 22%, but in combination with a fat-modified diet a lowering of 39% can be effected. The LDL (and cholesterol) levels usually decrease about 6%, but may actually be elevated in some cases. In persons with familial hypercholesterolemia it may lower the low-density lipoprotein levels by as much as 19% and in broad-beta disease by 23%. Clofibrate increases the HDL levels. Cholesterol is mobilized from xanthomata, but it has not yet been proven that it is also mobilized from atheromata. The mechanism of action appears to be that of suppressing release of free fatty acids from fat cells, thus decreasing precursor substrates for both triglyceride and cholesterol synthesis. It also decreases synthesis of glycerol and increases rate of conversion of VLDL to LDL. The principal uses are in the treatment of *hypertriglyceridemia* (or endogenous hyperlipidemia) and *broad-beta disease*. The drug does not affect the blood lipids in patients with untreated hypothyroidism.

Nausea, dyspepsia, and flatulence occur in about 10% of patients. Urticaria, pruritus, and stomatitis occasionally occur, and alopecia areata occurs rarely. Headache, vertigo, asthenia, myalgia, dermatitis, slight weight gain, breast tenderness in males, decrease in libido, elevation in SGOT and creatine phosphokinase levels in plasma, hypouricemia, and rare cardiomyopathy in the young also occur. In some women the drug causes the hair to be dry and brittle. In the Coronary Drug Project it was found that clofibrate increased the incidence of cholesterolic gallstones twofold, presumably as the result of transferring cholesterol from tissues to bile. It was also reported that there was a small increase in thromboembolic phenomena (clofibrate is antifibrinolytic), pulmonary embolism, intermittent claudication, and angina pectoris, but some of the conclusions have been cogently challenged. There is equivocal evidence that the drug may increase the incidence of bowel cancer. It has been reported to cause cardiac dysrhythmias. Clofibrate displaces weakly acidic drugs, such as thyroxine and warfarin, from plasma proteins; with warfarin the result is to increase the anticoagulant effect, and adjustments in dosage are required. It also decreases the efficacy of diuretics. Clofibrate is contraindicated in pregnant women and children unless there is a history of familial hyperlipidemia.

Clofibrate is hydrolyzed to clofibric acid during absorption and in its pass through the liver; it is the acid to which activity is attributed. The acid is strongly bound to plasma proteins. About 60% is metabolized, mostly to a glucuronide conjugate. The rest is mainly excreted into urine; there appears to be some renal tubular secretion, and clofibric acid can compete with other anions. Some is also secreted into bile and reabsorbed. The half-life is 10 to 20 (av 12) hr. Patients having better clinical responses have the slower rates of metabolism.

Warning—After reviewing results of recent studies which raised concerns about a possible carcinogenic effect and increased incidence of gastrointestinal disease associated with clofibrate use, the FDA in August 1979 required a boxed warning to be included in revised labeling for clofibrate, the warning to state, among other statements, the following: *Because of the hepatic tumorigenicity of clofibrate in rodents and the possible increased risk of malignancy associated with clofibrate in the human, as well as the increased risk of cholelithiasis, and because there is not, to date, substantial evidence of a beneficial effect on cardiovascular mortality from clofibrate, this drug should be utilized only for those patients described in the indications section* [of the labeling], *and should be discontinued if significant lipid response is not obtained.* (For the complete text of the warning see *FDA Drug Bulletin*, August 1979.)

Dose—*Oral, adults,* **500 mg** 3 times a day for persons weighing less than 120 lb, 4 times a day for those weighing 120 to 180 lb, and 5 times a day for those over 180 lb. It usually takes 1 to 3 months before an appreciable effect occurs; blood lipids return to pretreatment levels in 2 to 3 weeks after treatment is interrupted.

Dosage Form—Capsules: 500 mg.

Colestipol Hydrochloride

Tetraethylenepentamine polymer with 1-chloro-2,3-epoxypropane hydrochloride; Colestid (*Upjohn*)

Copolymer of diethylenetriamine and 1-chloro-2,3-epoxypropane, hydrochloride [37296-80-3].

Preparation—Colestipol hydrochloride is a high molecular weight, highly cross-linked, basic anion-exchange copolymer of diethylenetriamine and 1-chloro-2,3-epoxypropane, with approximately one of five amine nitrogens protonated (chloride form). Neither a structural formula nor a specific molecular weight has been assigned. US Pats. 3,692,895 and 3,803,237.

Description—Prepared in the form of light yellow beads; odorless; tasteless; hygroscopic.

Solubility—Insoluble in water, the beads swelling when placed in water or aqueous fluids.

Uses—Colestipol is an anion-exchange resin similar to *Cholestyramine Resin* (page 813) in its actions and uses, but there are differences in the anions for which it will exchange. Both resins bind and increase the fecal excretion of bile acids. The decrease in body content of bile acids is compensated by an increase in conversion of cholesterol to bile acids, thus decreasing the size of the cholesterol pool, but this is also partially compensated by an increased rate of synthesis. By sequestering bile acids in the intestines, the absorption of exogenous and biliary cholesterol is impaired, which also decreases the size of the cholesterol pool. The result is a lowering of LDL, which may decrease as much as 25% in *familial hypercholesterolemia*, the principal indication for colestipol. It also elevates HDL levels. It has not been established whether its use affects coronary heart disease, but there are reports that it decreases the mortality from coronary heart disease in men. It does not affect VLDL and plasma triglycerides. Colestipol can also be used in other disorders in which it is desirable to decrease the bile acid concentration in the intestines, such as in *bile-acid related diarrheas* resulting from ileal resection or disease, and in *biliary cirrhosis* or *obstructive jaundice*, in attempts to relieve pruritus that results from the accumulation of bile acids in the body.

The gritty nature and bulk of colestipol make it unpalatable. Despite its bulk it is constipating (about 10% of users), in part because of elimination of the intestinal mucosa-stimulating bile acids, fecal impaction can occur. Passing of stools may be more painful for patients with hemorrhoids, and it may increase stool strain, which is adverse in persons with heart disease and hypertension. It may exacerbate diverticulitis. The deficit in intraintestinal free bile acids leads to impairment of absorption of lipid-soluble, bile-requiring nutrients and drugs, such as vitamins A, D and K, fats, griseofulvin, etc., and even steatorrhea can result. Belching, bloating, diarrhea, nausea, vomiting and abdominal pain occur with an incidence of about 1–3%. Drugs with organic anion character may also be bound by the resin, but the selectivity appears to be capricious. It appears to interfere with the absorption of chlorothiazide, phenobarbital, tetracyclines, and penicillin G, but not with that of clofibrate, thyroxine, folic acid, aspirin, methyldopa, tolbutamide, warfarin or phenprocoumon (in contrast to cholestyramine). There are contradictions concerning interference with absorption of cardiac glycosides, namely that one investigation found colestipol decreased plasma levels of digitoxin in toxic patients (by capturing the glycoside during enterohepatic cycling) but another found no effect on bioavailability. It is presently advisable that other drugs be taken no later than 1 hour before or no sooner than 4 hr after ingestion of colestipol. Because the pool of chenodeoxycholic acid is diminished by colestipol, bile tends to become supersaturated with cholesterol, thus possibly increasing the risk of cholelithiasis (less than 0.5%). Safety in pregnancy or in children is unknown.

Dose—*Oral, adults,* 15 to **30 g** a day in 2 to 4 divided doses, each dose to be suspended in at least 90 mL of water or beverage and the glass rinsed with beverage to insure ingestion of entire dose. The resin should never be ingested dry.

Dosage Forms—Packets for Oral Suspension: 5 g; Bulk: 500 g.

Gemfibrozil

Pentanoic acid, 5-(2,5-dimethylphenoxy)-2,2-dimethyl-, Lopid (*Parke-Davis*)

[25812-30-0] $C_{15}H_{22}O_3$ (250.34).

Preparation—See US Pat 3,674,836.

Description—White crystals melting about 61°.

Uses—Gemfibrozil is structurally related to clofibric acid. It decreases the incorporatioin of long-chain fatty acids into triglycerides and thus decreases the hepatic synthesis of VLDL, and it also decreases the synthesis of VLDL carrier apolipoprotein. It thus decreases VLDL and, erratically, LDL. It also increases HDL and the HDL:cholesterol ratio, more than does clofibrate. At present, it is approved for use in type *IV hyperlipidemia* (hypertriglyceridemia) in which the patient is at risk of pancreatitis, although 90% of patients with types IIa and IIb hyperlipoproteinemia respond significantly.

The most frequent adverse effects are abdominal pain (6%), epigastric pain (5%), diarrhea (5%), nausea (4%), vomiting (1.6%) and flatulence (1%). Headache, malaise, fatigue, blurred vision, paresthesias, insomnia, dizziness, dry mouth, myalgia and arthralgia, mild hyperglycemia, rashes, dermatidides, urticaria, pruritis, leukopenia, anemia, and eosinophila also occur.

Gemfibrozil is well absorbed orally. It is mostly secreted into the urine, with a half-life of about 1.5 hr.

Dose—*Oral, adults,* **600 mg** twice a day, before breakfast and dinner.

Dosage Form—Capsules: 300 mg.

Neomycin—page 1181.

Niacin—pages 1015 and 1024.

Norethindrone Acetate—page 992.

Oxandrolone—page 999.

Probucol

Phenol, 4,4'-[(1-methylethylidene)bis(thio)]bis[2,6-bis(1,1-dimethylethyl)-, Biphenabid; Lorelco (*Merrell Dow*)

Acetone bis(3,5-di-*tert*-butyl-4-hydroxyphenyl)mercaptole [23288-49-5] $C_{31}H_{48}O_2S_2$ (516.84).

Preparation—By acid-catalyzed condensation of 4-mercapto-2,6-di-*tert*-butylphenol with acetone (*J Med Chem 13:* 722, 1970).

Description—White to yellow, crystalline powder; melts at about 125°.

Solubility—Practically insoluble in water; soluble in alcohol.

Uses—Probucol has a prominent effect to lower plasma LDL (and cholesterol) levels by decreasing cholesterol synthesis at an early stage.

In one clinical study, the plasma cholesterol content was decreased from 278 to 234 mg/dL, or 16%, after 3 months of treatment; however, after 9 months, the decrement was only 9%. It has a small and unpredictable effect on VLDL. Its effect on HDL is variable but slight. It is indicated for use in the treatment of *familial hypercholesterolemia* and *combined hyperlipoproteinemia* but not other hyperlipidemias. Although it has not been shown to reduce the atheromata or decrease coronary heart disease, it has been shown to effect the reduction or disappearance of xanthelasma and xanthomata.

Diarrhea occurs in about 10%, and transient flatulence, abdominal pain and nausea in less than 2% of patients. Hyperhidrosis, fetid sweat, and vomiting occur occasionally. Dizziness, chest pain, palpitations, and syncope are infrequent. Rare instances of angioneurotic edema have been reported. Other possibly drug-related but not established side effects include headache, insomnia, paresthesias, tinnitus, blurred vision, impotence, conjunctivitis, and various rashes. Probucol sensitizes the canine myocardium to catecholamine-induced dysrhythmias, but the effect has not been observed in other animals, so that the clinical significance is unknown. The safety of the drug in pregnancy, and in children, is not known.

About 8 to 10% of an oral dose is absorbed; absorption is increased by food. The drug accumulates in adipose tissue, and detectable amounts are found in blood for as long as 6 months after discontinuation of the drug.

Dose—*Oral, adults*, **500 mg** twice a day, with breakfast and evening meals.

Dosage Form—Film-coated Tablets: 250 mg.

Other Drugs Affecting Blood Lipids

Dextrothyroxine Sodium [*O*-(4-Hydroxy-3,5-diiodophenyl)-3-diiodo-, D-Tyrosine, monosodium salt hydrate; Choloxin (*Flint*) [7054-08-2] $C_{15}H_{10}I_4NNaO_4 \cdot x H_2O$; *anhydrous* [137-53-1] (798.86)]. *Preparation:* Using D-thyroxine, the process is analogous to that described for *Levothyroxine Sodium*, page 980. *Description and Solubility:* Light-yellow to buff-colored, odorless, tasteless powder; stable in dry air but may assume a slight pink color on exposure to light; pH (saturated solution) about 8.9. Soluble 1 g in about 700 mL water and about 300 mL alcohol; insoluble in chloroform, and ether. *Uses:* Thyroid hormones increase turnover of cholesterol, with catabolism increased more than biosynthesis. Furthermore they increase biliary secretion of neutral steroids and bile acids, which tends to lower plasma cholesterol levels. In addition to lowering the LDL levels, thyroid hormones lower those of the VLDL. The general metabolic actions of dextrothyroxine are proportionately less than with levothyroxine, so that it is possible to lower blood lipids with lesser increases in basal metabolic effect and other indices of thyrotoxicity. When used in combination with estrogenic substances, such as stilbestrol, the lipid-lowering effect is enhanced and the dose of dextrothyroxine may be reduced, but side effects of the estrogen may make use of the combination undesirable, especially in men. Untoward effects of dextrothyroxine include increased metabolic rate, tachycardia, and increased frequency of anginal attacks in persons with coronary insufficiency. Therefore the drug is not used in persons with coronary heart disease, the population that needs treatment most, and use is restricted mainly to young persons. It can elevate blood glucose levels in diabetics. It should be used cautiously in diabetics and persons with cardiac disease and in patients with hepatic or renal dysfunction. Dextrothyroxine suppresses TSH release and can thereby lower metabolic rate in hypothyroidism; therefore, thyroid hormones should be used first, instead of dextrothyroxine. Dextrothyroxine augments the action of anticoagulants, which requires that anticoagulant dosage be reduced appropriately. *Dose: Oral, adults*, initially 1 to 2 mg/day for 1 month, to be increased by increments of 1 to 2 mg at monthly intervals until either the desired effect is achieved or the daily dose is 8 mg. *Children*, initially 0.05 mg/kg/day, with increments of 0.05 mg/kg/day at monthly intervals, up to a maximum of 4 mg a day.

Sitosterols [Cytellin (*Lilly*)]—A mixture of β-sitosterol (stigmast-5-en-3β-ol) ($C_{29}H_{50}O$) (414.72) and related sterols of plant origin. It contains not less than 95% of total sterols and not less than 85% of unsaturated sterols, calculated as β-sitosterol. *Description* and *Solubility:* White, essentially odorless, tasteless powder. Freely soluble in chloroform and in carbon disulfide; practically insoluble in water; slightly soluble in alcohol. *Uses:* Because of their close structural relationship to cholesterol, the sitosterols have been studied as possible competitive inhibitors of cholesterol absorption; in patients with familial hypercholesterolemia they may lower the LDL by about 10%. They may cause diarrhea, bloating, and occasional nausea and vomiting. There is some evidence that the sitosterols may themselves be deposited in the vessels. *Dose:* 3 to 6 g, mixed in a beverage, 3 times a day before meals. *Dosage Forms:* Suspension: 3 g/15 mL.

Miscellaneous Cardiovascular Drugs

Alprostadil [(11α,13*E*,15*S*)-11,15-dihydroxy-9-oxoprost-13-en-1-oic acid [745-65-3] $C_{20}H_{34}O_5$ (354.49); Prostaglandin E₁; PGE₁; Prostin VR (*Upjohn*)]—Isolated from the seminal vesicle tissue of sheep. See *J Biol Chem 238:* 3555, 1963. For the synthesis refer to *J Org Chem 37:* 2921, 1974. White crystals melting about 115°; $[\alpha]_{578} - 61.6°$ (c = 0.56, THF). *Uses:* Endogenous prostaglandin E₁ helps maintain the patency of the ductus arteriosis of the fetus. After birth, prostaglandin production falls and the ductus closes. However, when there are congenital heart defects, such as the *tetralogy of Fallot, transposition of the great vessels, pulmonary atresia, pulmonary stenosis, coarctation of the aorta, tricuspid atresia*, or *imperfect aortic arch*, it is necessary that the ductus remain patent until corrective surgery can be accomplished. In such instances, infusion of alprostadil (PGE) helps maintain patency pending surgery. The following adverse effects may occur (incidence in parentheses): apnea (12%), bradypnea, tachypnea, respiratory depression, bronchial wheezing (all <1%); flushing (10%), bradycardia (7%), hypotension (4%), tachycardia (3%), cardiac arrest (1%), edema (1%), hyperemia, congestive heart failure, right ventricular spasm, second degree heart block, supraventricular tachycardia, ventricular fibrillation, shock (all <1%); fever (14%), convulsions (4%), opisthotomus, rigidity, hyperirritability, lethargy, hypothermia (all <1%); diarrhea (2%), regurgitation (<1%), hyperbilirubinemia (<1%); intravascular coagulopathy (1%); hemorrhage, anemia, thrombocytopenia, hematuria, anuria, hypokalemia, hyperkalemia, hypoglycemia, proliferation of cortex of long bones (all <1%) sepsis (2%), peritonitis (<1%). The drug must be used cautiously when any condition preexists that may add to or exaggerate any of the above effects. There should be monitoring of arterial pressure and pulmonary status especially when pulmonary flow is already compromised). *Dose: Intravenous infusion, neonates*, 500 μg/min.

CHAPTER 44

Respiratory Drugs

Ewart A Swinyard, PhD, DSc (Hon)

Professor Emeritus of Pharmacology
College of Pharmacy and School of Medicine, University of Utah
Salt Lake City, UT 84112

A number of pharmacologic agents have in common the property of acting on the respiratory system. Alcohol, anesthetic agents, barbiturates and other hypnotic drugs, morphine and other narcotic drugs, in addition to acetanilid and related antipyretic and analgesic drugs, exert undesirable side actions which depress the respiratory system. Although vomiting is a respiratory act, emetic drugs are discussed with the gastrointestinal drugs (see page 792) because they are used to evacuate the stomach in case of food and drug poisoning. Other agents, such as the nitrites, belladonna, stramonium, ephedrine, and epinephrine are powerful bronchodilators, but they also have other valuable therapeutic actions; consequently, these substances are described elsewhere. Included in this chapter are the respiratory stimulants, the expectorant and antitussive agents, bronchodilators, and the therapeutic gases.

Respiratory Stimulants

Respiration is controlled by a respiratory center in the medulla oblongata. This center is stimulated by the presence of carbon dioxide in the blood. An increase in the carbon dioxide content of blood, as in exercise, stimulates the respiratory center and increases the respiratory rate. Other drugs which act directly on the center to increase respiratory rate include atropine, caffeine, pentylenetetrazol, and picrotoxin. Respiration is partly controlled by both chemical and sensory stimuli from the carotid body and carotid sinus, and drugs such as nikethamide exert at least part of their respiratory effect through this mechanism. The rate of respiration is also modified by numerous forms of sensory stimuli reaching the brain from the skin, nose, mouth, throat, etc., and drugs such as ammonia act through this mechanism. Respiration may also be modified voluntarily through the higher brain centers, and drugs which restore the functional activity of depressed higher centers, such as pentylenetetrazol and picrotoxin, act to increase respiration.

The effectiveness of nonspecific analeptic drugs for the management of postanesthetic respiratory depression is controversial. Some clinicians believe that postanesthetic respiratory depression, irrespective of its cause, is best treated with manual or mechanical methods of respiratory assistance. Others believe respiration should be stimulated pharmacologically only if a specific antidote is available; for example, narcotic antagonists for respiratory depression induced by narcotics, anticholinesterases if due to a curariform muscle relaxant, etc. It is generally agreed that prolonged respiratory depression, such as that due to barbiturate poisoning, is best treated by methods which assure adequate ventilation and circulation and, when necessary, hemodialysis. Few clinicians find nonspecific analeptics useful in the above conditions.

Aromatic Ammonia Spirit—page 1310.

Ammonium Carbonate

Carbonic acid, monoammonium salt, mixt. with ammonium carbamate; Ammonia Crystal; Sal Volatile; Ammonium Sesquicarbonate

Monoammonium carbonate mixture with ammonium carbamate [8000-73-5]; consists of ammonium bicarbonate [NH_4HCO_3 = 79.06] and ammonium carbamate [NH_2COONH_4 = 78.07] in varying proportions. It yields 30–34% of NH_3.

Preparation—By subliming a mixture of ammonium sulfate and calcium carbonate.

Description—White powder or hard, white or translucent masses, having a strong odor of ammonia, without empyreuma, and with a sharp, ammoniacal taste; affected by light; on exposure to air, it loses ammonia and CO_2, becoming opaque, and is finally converted into friable, porous lumps or a white powder of ammonium bicarbonate; decomposed by hot water and by weak acids.

Solubility—1 g very slowly soluble in about 4 mL water and is partly (the carbamate portion) soluble in alcohol; decomposed by hot water; its solution has the odor of ammonia and is alkaline to litmus. For reactions occurring in water see under *Aromatic Ammonia Spirit* (page 1310).

Uses—A *pharmaceutical necessity* in the preparation of *Aromatic Ammonia Spirit* and as a source of ammonia in *smelling salts*. For the latter purpose, $\frac{1}{4}$ to 1 in. cubes are generally used. Both of these preparations are employed as *reflex respiratory stimulants* in hysterical syncope. Although ammonium carbonate has been used as an expectorant, ammonium chloride is preferred since it is less likely to cause gastric irritation.

Dose—Up to **300 mg** in dilute solutions.

Atropine Sulfate—page 913.

Caffeine—page 1133.

Caffeine and Sodium Benzoate—page 1135.

Camphor—page 780.

Carbon Dioxide

After-damp; Aer Fixus; Carbonic Acid Gas

Carbon dioxide [124-38-9] CO_2 (44.01).

Preparation—Various methods, eg, heating limestone, burning coke, and fermentation processes.

Description—Odorless, colorless gas; 1 L at 760 mm and 0° weighs 1.977 g. Its solutions are slightly acid to litmus and have a slightly acid taste.

Solubility—1 volume dissolves in about 1 volume water at 25°; it is more soluble at lower than at higher temperatures, also less soluble in alcohol and other solvents.

Uses—Carbon dioxide has few valid therapeutic uses. Its most valuable use is with oxygen in certain types of pump oxygenators to *avoid a reduction of carbon dioxide* tension of the blood. It is frequently used inappropriately when it is of little value and possibly even harmful. Carbon dioxide is often used to relieve persistent hiccups; it only occasionally produces transient relief. Its use has been suggested to *improve cerebral vascular disorders* (cerebral thrombosis), but it is of doubtful value and may be harmful because it increases intracranial pressure. Similarly, it has been used to induce deep breathing and coughing to avoid *postoperative* atelectasis, but is generally of little benefit. Carbon dioxide should not be used to resuscitate victims of carbon monoxide poisoning, drowning, electric shock, or asphyxiation; the carbon dioxide content of the blood is already high and further increases may only exacerbate the respiratory depression. It should not be used to treat overdosage with central nervous system depressants; the medullary chemoreceptors are depressed and will not respond.

Carbon dioxide is administered by inhalation, most conveniently through a tight-fitting mask. The gas is employed in conjunction with oxygen. Concentrations of 5 to 7.5% are employed; 5% is the usual concentration.

Dose—By *inhalation*, up to 7% in oxygen.

Doxapram Hydrochloride

2-Pyrrolidinone, 1-ethyl-4-[2-(4-morpholinyl)ethyl]-3,3-diphenyl-, monohydrochloride, monohydrate; Dopram (*Robins*)

1 - Ethyl - 4 - (2 - morpholinoethyl) -3,3- diphenyl -2- pyrrolidinone monohydrochloride monohydrate [7081-53-0] $C_{24}H_{30}N_2O_2 \cdot HCl \cdot H_2O$ (432.99); *anhydrous* [113-07-5] (414.97).

Preparation—1-Ethyl-3-pyrrolidinol is reacted with thionyl chloride to form the 3-chloro compound which is condensed with diphenylacetonitrile in toluene solution with the aid of sodamide. The resulting α-(1-ethyl-3-pyrrolidinyl)diphenylacetonitrile is hydrolyzed with 70% H_2SO_4 to the corresponding acid. On treatment with thionyl chloride, the acid is converted into the acid chloride which immediately isomerizes to 4-(2-chloroethyl)-3,3-diphenyl-1-ethyl-2-pyrrolidinone. Condensation of this with morpholine in a dehydrohalogenating environment yields doxapram (base) which, on reaction with HCl, gives the official salt.

Description—White to off-white, odorless, crystalline powder that is stable in light and air; melts at about 220°.

Solubility—1 g in 50 mL water; soluble in chloroform; sparingly soluble in alcohol; practically insoluble in ether.

Uses—For respiratory stimulation in *postanesthesia, chronic pulmonary disease associated with acute hypercapnia*, and as an adjunct to established supportive measures and resuscitative techniques in *drug-induced CNS depression*. The respiratory stimulation is thought to be mediated through the carotid chemoreceptors; as the dosage is increased, the respiratory centers in the medulla are stimulated with progressive stimulation in other areas of the brain and spinal cord. A pressor response, due to improved cardiac output, may also occur. An increased release of catecholamines has also been noted. The onset of respiratory stimulation after IV injection usually occurs in 20 to 40 seconds with peak effect in 1 to 2 minutes. The effect persists for 5 to 12 minutes. Doxapram is contraindicated in patients with epilepsy or other convulsive states, pulmonary disease such as pulmonary embolism, pulmonary incompetence due to muscle paresis, severe hypertension or cerebrovascular accidents, and coronary artery disease. It should also be administered cautiously to patients on sympathomimetic or monoamine oxidase inhibiting drugs (addictive pressor effects) and patients given anesthetic agents (holothane, cyclopropane, enflurane) known to sensitize the myocardium to catecholamines. Adverse reactions involve the autonomic system (headache, dizziness, apprehension, disorientation, etc), respiratory system (cough, dyspnea, tachypnea, laryngospasm, etc), cardiovascular system (phlebitis, variations in heart rate, arrhythmias, chest pain, etc.), gastrointestinal tract (nausea, vomiting, and diarrhea), genitourinary system (urinary retention and spontaneous voiding). Safe use during pregnancy has not been established. Doxapram is not recommended for use in children 12 years of age and younger.

Dose—Postanesthetic: *intravenous*, **0.5 to 1.0 mg/kg**, not to exceed **1.5 to 2.0 mg/kg** in multiple injections at 5 min. intervals. Drug-induced CNS depression: *intravenous*, **2.0 mg/kg** and repeated in 5 min; repeat same dose every 1 to 2 hours until patient awakens. Chronic obstructive pulmonary disease: *infusion*, 1 to 2 **mg/min** increased to a maximum of 3 mg/min.

Dosage Forms—Injection: 20 mg/mL in 20 mL vials.

Nikethamide—page 1136.

Pentylenetetrazol—page 1136.
Picrotoxin—page 1135.

Expectorant Drugs

Expectorants are drugs used to assist in the removal of secretion or exudate from the trachea, bronchi, or lungs, hence they are used in the treatment of cough. Such agents affect the respiratory tract in two ways: (1) by decreasing the viscosity of the bronchial secretions and facilitating their elimination so that local irritants are removed and ineffectual coughing is alleviated, and (2) by increasing the amounts of respiratory tract fluid a demulcent action is exerted on the dry mucosal lining, thus relieving the unproductive cough.

Many of the drugs that have expectorant activity are believed to act reflexly by irritating the gastric mucosa which, in turn, stimulates respiratory tract secretions. Included in this group are (1) the saline expectorants, ammonium salts, citrates, iodides, and antimony and potassium tartrate, (2) the ipecac expectorants, and (3) the creosotes and guaiacols. Although there is some experimental evidence that suggests that these substances do increase respiratory tract secretions, it is quite sparse and unconvincing. With few exceptions, most agents in this category do not exert specific local effects but usually possess other pharmacological actions, such as anesthetic, antiseptic, diuretic, or other activity. Moreover, clinical support for such use is based largely on tradition and subjective clinical impressions. Nevertheless, they continue to be used as adjuncts in numerous proprietary and prescription expectorant combinations. Consequently, many of these substances have become empiric remedies. It should be remembered, however, that water administered by a humidifier is probably the best agent available to facilitate the expectoration of secretions.

Acacia—page 1296.

Acetylcysteine

L-Cysteine, *N*-acetyl-, Mucomyst (*Mead-Johnson*)

N-Acetyl-L-cysteine [616-91-1] $C_5H_9NO_3S$ (163.19).
Preparation—By direct acetylation of L-cysteine.

Description—White, crystalline powder which has a very slight acetic odor and a characteristic sour taste; stable in ordinary light, nonhygroscopic (oxidizes in moist air), and stable at temperatures up to 120°; melts between 104° and 110°; pKa 3.24; pH (1 in 100) 2 to 2.75.

Solubility—1 g in 5 mL water; 4 mL alcohol; practically insoluble in chloroform and ether.

Uses—To reduce the viscosity of pulmonary secretions and facilitate their removal. Hence, it is used as adjuvant therapy in bronchopulmonary disorders when mucolysis is desirable. It is thought the sulfhydryl group in the molecule "opens" the disulfide bonds in mucus and lowers the viscosity. The mucolytic activity of acetylcysteine is related to pH; significant mucolysis occurs between pH 6 and 9. Clinical studies show that after a single oral dose of 100 mg, the drug is rapidly absorbed, reaches a peak concentration in 2 to 3 hours and is available in the lung in high concentrations in active form for at least 5 hours. Side effects are rare. However, bronchospasm, hemoptysis, and nausea and vomiting have been observed. Antimicrobial drugs, including all types of penicillin, should not be administered in acetylcysteine solution since it inactivates antibiotics.

Acetylcysteine has been used investigationally as an antidote to prevent or minimize hepatotoxicity in acute acetaminophen overdosage. It has also been used with some success as an ophthalmic solution for the treatment of keratoconjunctivitis sicca (dry eye) and as an enema for the management of bowel obstruction due to meconium ileus.

Dose—By *inhalation of nebulized solution*, **2 to 20 mL** of a **10%**

or 1 to **10 mL** of a **20%** solution every 2 to 6 hours; by *direct instilla-tion*, 1 to **2 mL** of a **10** or **20%** solution every 1 to 4 hours.
Dosage Forms—Solution: 10 and 20%.

Ammonium Carbonate—page 866.
Ammonium Chloride—page 934.
Antimony Potassium Tartrate—page 1238.
Creosote—RPS-15, page 1102.
Eucalyptol—page 1291.
Eucalyptus Oil—page 1286.
Glycerin—page 1308.
Glycyrrhiza—page 1286.

Guaifenesin

1,2-Propanediol, 3-(2-methoxyphenoxy)-, Glyceryl Guaiacolate
Breonesin (*Breon*); Various Mfrs

3-(*o*-Methoxyphenoxy)-1,2-propanediol   [93-14-1] $C_{10}H_{14}O_4$
(198.22).

Preparation—Guaiacol and 3-chloro-1,2-propanediol are condensed via dehydrochlorination by warming a mixture of the reactants with a base.

Description—White to slightly gray, crystalline powder having a bitter taste; may have a slight characteristic odor; stable in light and heat and is nonhygroscopic; melts within a range of 3° between 78° and 82°; pH (1 in 100 solution) between 5.0 and 7.0.
Solubility—1 g in 60–70 mL water; soluble in alcohol, chloroform, glycerin, and propylene glycol; insoluble in petroleum ether.

Uses—May be useful for the symptomatic relief of respiratory conditions characterized by dry, nonproductive cough and in the presence of mucous in the respiratory tract. Subjective clinical studies suggest that the expectorant action of guaifenesin ameliorates dry unproductive cough. In view of the lack of objective clinical studies, the clinical value of the drug must remain questionable. Experimentally, it increases respiratory tract secretions, but only when given in doses larger than those used clinically. Adverse effects are infrequent and usually consist of nausea and drowsiness. Guaifenesin may produce a false positive test for 5-hydroxyindoleacetic acid. It is an ingredient in a number of proprietary expectorant formulations.
Dose—*Usual, adult, oral,* **100** to **400 mg** every 4 to 6 hours. Maximum, **2.4 g**/day. *Usual, pediatric: children* 6 to 12 years of age, **50** to **100 mg** orally every 4 to 6 hours; do not exceed **600 mg/day**; *children* 2 to 6 years of age, **50 mg** every 4 hours; do not exceed **300 mg/day**.
Dosage Forms—Capsules: 200 mg; Syrup: 100 mg/5 mL; Tablets: 100 and 200 mg.

Hydriodic Acid Syrup—page 1320.

Ipecac

Ipecacuanha

The dried rhizome and roots of *Cephaëlis acuminata* Karsten, known in commerce as Cartagena, Nicaragua, or Panama Ipecac (Fam. *Rubiaceae*). Ipecac yields not less than 2% of the total ether-soluble alkaloids of ipecac, of which not less than 90% consists of emetine ($C_{29}H_{40}N_2O_4$) and cephaeline ($C_{28}H_{38}N_2O_4$), the content of the latter varying from an amount equal to, to not more than twice, the content of emetine.
Constituents—Ipecac contains *emetine (methylcephaëline)* [$C_{29}H_{40}N_2O_4$], *cephaëline,* [$C_{28}H_{38}N_2O_4$], *psychotrine* [$C_{28}H_{36}N_2O_4$], *O-methylpsychotrine* [$C_{29}H_{38}N_2O_4$], *emetamine* [$C_{29}H_{36}N_2O_4$], *ipecamine,* also *ipecacuanhic acid,* pectin, starch, resin, sugar, etc. All of the alkaloids are interrelated and may be synthesized from each other. Brazilian roots yield as much as 2.5% of total alkaloids and Cartagena root 2%.

Uses—Has *expectorant, emetic,* and *amebicidal properties.* The syrup is preferred for use as an expectorant and emetic; it is widely used as an emetic in accidental poisoning. Emetic doses of ipecac may be used in patients with *paroxysmal atrial tachycardia,* the vagal impulses arising from the excitation of the medullary vagal vomiting mechanism acting to bring about the cessation of the arrhythmia. Ipecac has amebicidal potency by virtue of its content of emetine, but is almost never used in the therapy of amebiasis.

Powdered Ipecac is ipecac reduced to a fine or a very fine powder and adjusted to a potency of 1.9–2.1% of the ether-soluble alkaloids of ipecac, by addition of exhausted marc of ipecac or of other suitable inert diluent or by addition of powdered ipecac of either a lower or a higher potency. *Description:* Pale brown, weak yellow, or light olive-gray powder.

Ipecac Syrup—yields, from each 100 mL, 123–157 mg of ether-soluble alkaloids of ipecac. *Preparation:* Exhaust powdered ipecac (70 g) by percolation, using a mixture of 3 volumes of alcohol and 1 volume of water as the menstruum, macerating for 72 hours, and percolating slowly. Reduce the entire percolate to a volume of 70 mL by evaporation at a temperature not exceeding 60° and preferably in vacuum, and add water (140 mL). Allow the mixture to stand overnight, filter, and wash the residue on the filter with water. Evaporate the filtrate and washings to 40 mL, and to this add hydrochloric acid (2.5 mL) and alcohol (20 mL), mix, and filter. Wash the filter with a mixture of 30 volumes of alcohol, 3.5 volumes of HCl and 66.5 volumes of water, using a volume sufficient to produce 70 mL of filtrate. Add glycerin (100 mL) and syrup (qs) to make the product measure 1000 mL, and mix. *Alcohol Content:* 1 to 2.5%. *Uses:* Emetic and *nauseant expectorant.* Ipecac syrup is probably the single most important item to have in the home for the treatment of poison ingestions. It is given orally to adults and children over 1 year of age in a dose of 1 tablespoonful (15 mL) followed by at least 1 glassful (8 oz) of liquid (water, juices, etc.); if the victim does not vomit within 15 to 20 min, the treatment should be repeated. The dosage should be recovered by gastric lavage if emesis does not occur after the second dose. The dose in children up to one year of age is 5 or 10 mL followed by the procedure described above. If activated charcoal is to be used, give the activated charcoal only after vomiting has been induced with ipecac syrup. Ipecac syrup is also useful for croupous *bronchitis* in children. *Dose: Emetic:* 10 to 30 mL; *usual,* 15 mL. Do not use in semiconscious, unconscious, or convulsing persons. Do not administer milk or carbonated beverages with this product. *Other Dose Information:* Expectorant, *oral, adults,* 0.5 to 2 mL every 6 hours.

Ipecac and Opium Powder—RPS 13, page 561.

Potassium Iodide

Potassium iodide [7681-11-0] KI (166.00).
Preparation—Potassium iodide may be prepared by reacting iodine with a hot solution of potassium hydroxide, the iodate simultaneously formed being subsequently reduced to iodide by heating the dry reaction mixture with carbon.

Description—Hexahedral crystals, either transparent and colorless or somewhat opaque and white, or a white, granular powder; slightly hygroscopic in moist air. The aqueous solution is neutral or slightly alkaline to litmus.
Solubility—1 g in 0.7 mL water, 22 mL alcohol, 2 mL glycerin, 75 mL acetone at 25°, and 0.5 mL boiling water. When dissolved in water heat is absorbed. 100 mL of a saturated aqueous solution at 25° contains 100 g of KI.

Uses—An *expectorant* and when the action of iodide is desired. It is used as an expectorant to liquefy thick and tenacious sputum in chronic bronchitis, bronchiectasis, bronchial asthma, and pulmonary emphysema. Also used as adjunctive treatment in cystic fibrosis, chronic senusitis, and after surgery to prevent atelectasis. Although a substantial number of patients respond well to potassium iodide, iodide-induced goiter and hypothyroidism have been observed. For this reason alternative drugs should be considered when an expectorant action is desired.

In regions where little iodine is obtained in the diet, iodides are completely effective in the *prevention of goiter.* Only minute doses are required and these small amounts can best be administered in the form of iodized salt (1 part of potassium iodide to 100,000 parts of salt). Saturated solution of potassium iodide may also be used with an antithyroid drug to prepare hyperthyroid patients for thyroidectomy and to treat thyrotoxic crisis or neonatal thyrotoxicosis. It is also used in place of Lugol's Solution for the treatment of *toxic goiter*, in the dose of 0.3 mL, 3 times daily. See *Strong Iodine Solution* (page 1161).

Potassium iodide solution (1 g/mL) is the drug of choice for cutaneous lymphatic sporotrichosis in patients who can tolerate the drug and do not have a history of iodism.

Mild untoward reactions occur frequently with iodide medication. The syndrome is known as iodism. The symptoms include salivation, lacrimation, coryza, soreness of the teeth and gums, swelling of the salivary glands and eruption of the skin. The symptoms disappear when the drug is discontinued. Serious reactions occur only very rarely. Concurrent use of potassium iodide with lithium and other antithyroid drugs may potentiate the hypothyroid and goitrogenic effects of these medications. Likewise, use with other potassium-containing medications and potassium-sparing diuretics may induce hyperkalemia and cardiac arrhythmias or cardiac arrest.

Dose—*Expectorant*, **300 mg** with a glassful of water every 4 to 6 hours; *antifungal*, **600 mg** 3 times a day, gradually increased to 12 g daily if tolerated. *Preoperative preparation for thyroidectomy*, 5 drops of a saturated solution 3 times daily for 10 days.

Potassium Iodide Solution [Saturated Potassium Iodide Solution] contains, in each 100 mL, 97–103 g of KI. *Preparation:* Dissolve potassium iodide (1000 g) in hot purified water (680 mL), cool to about 25°, and add sufficient purified water to make 1000 mL; filter, if necessary. *Note:* If the solution is not to be used within a short time, 500 mg of sodium thiosulfate should be added to each L. *Description:* Clear, colorless, and odorless solution having a characteristic, strongly salty taste; neutral or slightly alkaline to litmus paper; specific gravity about 1.700. *Uses:* Iodide supplement and expectorant; see *Potassium Iodide*. *Dose: Usual*, 0.3 mL, equivalent to 300 mg of potassium iodide.

Sodium Iodide

Sodium iodide [7681-82-5] NaI (149.89).

Preparation—From iodine and sodium hydroxide, or by metathesis between ferrosoferric iodide and sodium carbonate. See *Potassium Iodide.*

Description—Colorless, odorless crystals, or a white, crystalline powder. In moist air it cakes and then deliquesces, and frequently undergoes decomposition, developing a brown tint. Its solution in water is neutral or slightly alkaline to litmus and gradually becomes yellow because of the formation of free iodine. In contrast to potassium iodide, when sodium iodide is dissolved in water heat is liberated due to the formation of the dihydrate [NaI.2H$_2$O].

Solubility—1 g in 0.6 mL water, about 2 mL alcohol, and about 1 mL glycerin.

Uses—Can be used interchangeably with potassium iodide, as a therapeutic agent, except where sodium ion is contraindicated. See *Potassium Iodide.*

Dose—*Oral*, **300 mg** to **2 g** daily; *usual*, **300 mg** 2 to 4 times a day; *intravenous infusion*, **1** to **3 g** daily; *usual*, **1 g**.

Terpin Hydrate

Cyclohexanemethanol, 4-hydroxy-α,α-4-trimethyl-, monohydrate; Terpinum; Terpinol

p-Menthane-1,8-diol monohydrate [2451-01-6] C$_{10}$H$_{20}$O$_2$.H$_2$O (190.28); *anhydrous* [80-53-5] (172.27).

Preparation—By hydration of the pinenes in turpentine oil (or pine oil) in the presence of a strong acid.

Description—Colorless, lustrous crystals, or as a white powder; slight odor, and efflorescent in dry air; a hot 1:100 aqueous solution is neutral to litmus; when dried over H$_2$SO$_4$ in a vacuum, it melts at about 103°.

Solubility—1 g in about 200 mL water; 13 mL alcohol, 140 mL chloroform, and about 140 mL ether, at 25°; 1 g in about 35 mL boiling water and about 3 mL boiling alcohol.

Uses—In *bronchitis* as an *expectorant*. Terpin hydrate elixir contains too little of the compound to be effective alone and is employed mainly as a vehicle for cough mixtures such as *Terpin Hydrate and Codeine Elixir* and *Terpin Hydrate and Dextromethorphan Elixir*.

Dose—*Usual*, **125** to **300 mg** every 6 hours.

Terpin Hydrate Elixir: contains, in each 100 mL, 1.53–1.87 g of C$_{10}$H$_{20}$O$_2$.H$_2$O. *Preparation:* Dissolve terpin hydrate (17 g) in the alcohol (430 mL); add successively sweet orange peel tincture (20 mL), benzaldehyde (0.05 mL), glycerin (400 mL), syrup (100 mL), and purified water (qs) to make the product measure 1000 mL; mix well and filter, if necessary, until the product is clear. *Note*—The sweet orange peel tincture may be replaced by 1 mL orange oil dissolved in 15 mL alcohol. *Alcohol Content:* 39 to 44%. The high alcoholic content in this elixir is required for the solution of the terpin hydrate. *Incompatibilities:* Dilution of this elixir with water or liquids of low alcohol content causes precipitation of the terpin hydrate. *Dose: Usual, adult, oral*, the equivalent of 85 to 170 mg 3 or 4 times a day. *Usual, pediatric, oral*, children 1 to 4 years of age, 20 mg; children 5 to 9, 40 mg, and children 10 to 12, 85 mg. All children's doses may be repeated 3 or 4 times a day.

Terpin Hydrate and Codeine Elixir: contains, in each 100 mL, 1.53–1.87 g of C$_{10}$H$_{20}$O$_2$.H$_2$O (terpin hydrate), and 180–220 mg of C$_{18}$H$_{21}$NO$_3$.H$_2$O (codeine). *Preparation:* Dissolve codeine (2 g) in terpin hydrate elixir (qs) to make the product measure 1000 mL. *Alcohol Content:* 39 to 44%. *Uses:* This elixir is an *expectorant* and *sedative* used to allay excessive coughing. Its value resides primarily in its content of codeine. *Caution*—This elixir is sometimes used by addicts, by whom it is known as *GI Gin*, for its alcohol and codeine content. In some states pharmacists are required to register and limit its sale. Its repeated sale to an individual should be noted and stopped. *Dose: Usual*, 5 mL, equivalent to 10 mg of codeine and 85 mg of terpin hydrate.

Terpin Hydrate and Dextromethorphan Hydrobromide Elixir: contains, in each 100 mL, 1.53–1.87 g of C$_{10}$H$_{20}$O$_2$.H$_2$O (terpin hydrate), and 180–220 mg of C$_{18}$H$_{25}$NO.HBr.H$_2$O (dextromethorphan hydrobromide). *Preparation:* Dissolve dextromethorphan hydrobromide (2 g) in terpin hydrate elixir (qs) to make the product measure 1000 mL. *Uses:* The same indications as *Terpin Hydrate and Codeine Elixir*. It is used in the control of coughs associated with the common cold, laryngitis, tracheitis, and bronchitis. Dextromethorphan acts to elevate the threshold for coughing. Unlike codeine, it rarely produces drowsiness or gastrointestinal disturbances. *Dose: Usual*, 5 mL, equivalent to 10 mg dextromethorphan hydrobromide and 85 mg of terpin hydrate. *Other Dose Information:* The usual adult dose should not exceed 40 mL. Children, 4 to 12 years, 2.5 to 5 mL 4 times a day; total dose should not exceed 20 mL. Children, 2 to 4 years, 1 to 2.5 mL 1 to 4 times daily; total daily dose should not exceed 10 mL.

Tolu Balsam—page 1290.

Tolu Balsam Syrup—page 1291.

Tolu Balsam Tincture—page 1291.

Tyloxapol

Phenol, 4-(1,1,3,3-tetramethylbutyl)-, polymer with formaldehyde and oxirane; Various Mfrs

[*R* is CH$_2$CH$_2$O(CH$_2$CH$_2$O)$_m$CH$_2$CH$_2$OH; *m* is 6 to 8; *n* is not more than 5]

p-(1,1,3,3-Tetramethylbutyl)phenol polymer with ethylene oxide and formaldehyde [25301-02-4].

Preparation—*p*-(1,1,3,3-Tetramethylbutyl)phenol and formaldehyde are condensed by heating in the presence of an acidic catalyst and the polymeric phenol thus obtained is reacted with ethylene oxide at elevated temperature under pressure in the presence of NaOH. US Pat. 2,454,541.

Description—Amber, viscous liquid; may show a slight turbidity; slight aromatic odor; specific gravity about 1.072; stable at sterilization temperature; stable in the presence of acids, bases, and salts; oxidized by metals; pH (5% aqueous solution) between 4 and 7.

Solubility—Slowly but freely soluble in water; soluble in many organic solvents, including acetic acid, benzene, carbon tetrachloride, carbon disulfide, chloroform, and toluene.

Uses—A nonionic detergent that depresses both surface tension and interfacial tension. The hydrophobic alkyl groups impart oil solubility to the molecule and the large number of hydrophilic groups impart water solubility. Hence, it may be used as an emulsifying agent for both water-in-oil and oil-in-water systems. *Note—Precaution should be exercised to prevent contact of tyloxapol with metals.*

Tyloxapol is the active ingredient of certain preparations used to lower surface tension and help liquefy mucus. It has been reported to be useful for short-term management of many inflammatory and postoperative pulmonary conditions. Some reports indicate it has value when administered intermittently in long-term management of cystic fibrosis and other chronic pulmonary diseases. Some double-blind studies, however, indicate that agents of this type are no more effective than saline aerosols. Tyloxapol is also used in contact lens cleaner formulations.

Dose—*Mucolytic, usual, adult,* **0.125%** solution administered via aerosol nebulizer with pressurized oxygen or air into a tent or face mask, or by direct inhalation, as directed in package insert.

Other Expectorants

Calcium Iodide—[CaI$_2$.6H$_2$O; Calcidin (*Abbott*)]—Yellowish white, deliquescent powder, turning yellow in air due to liberation of iodine. Very soluble in water; soluble in alcohol. *Uses:* Adjunctive therapy in management of bronchial asthma, bronchitis, emphysema, and other respiratory disorders in which an expectorant action is desired. Adverse effects are similar to those of other iodides (see *Potassium Iodide*).

Creosote Carbonate—A mixture of carbonates of various constituents of wood-tar creosote. Clear, colorless or yellowish, viscid liquid; odorless or has a slight odor of creosote; tasteless. Insoluble in water; miscible with alcohol. *Uses:* Has been used as stimulant expectorant in doses of 1 g.

Guaiacol—Principally *o*-methoxyphenol when obtained from wood creosote; also synthesized. A white or slightly yellow crystalline mass or colorless to yellowish liquid; agreeable aromatic odor; the solid melts at about 28°; 1 g dissolves in about 65 mL water, 1 mL glycerin. *Uses:* Has been used as a stimulant expectorant in doses of 500 mg; also as a local anesthetic.

Antitussives

Antitussive agents are substances that specifically inhibit or suppress the act of coughing. Such inhibition may be induced in a variety of ways: (1) depression of the medullary center or associated higher centers, (2) increased threshold of the peripheral reflexogenous zones, (3) interruption of tussal impulses in the afferent limb of the cough reflex, (4) inhibition of conduction along the motor pathways, and (5) removal of irritants by facilitating bronchial drainage and mucociliary activity. The first four ways of inhibiting cough are believed to characterize the "antitussive" agents, whereas the latter one is more likely to be associated with some "expectorant" agents.

Antitussive agents may be classified in various ways. For example, *centrally acting antitussive* agents either depress the central nervous system and inhibit the "cough center" in the medulla or raise the threshold for central noxious stimuli and diminish the cough reflex, whereas *peripherally acting antitussive* agents act principally on the receptors within the respiratory tract. On the other hand, these substances may be classified as "narcotic antitussives" or "nonnarcotic antitussives." No such classification will be used in this section since most of the narcotic antitussives are discussed in Chapter 60, *Analgesics and Antipyretics.* Agents that have addiction potential will be identified, however, since the addiction liability of these substances is just as great whether administered for pain or for cough.

Apomorphine Hydrochloride—page 806.

Benzonatate

Benzoic acid, 4-(butylamino)-, 2,5,8,11,14,17,20,23,26-nonaoxaoctacosan-28-yl ester; Tessalon (*Ciba*)

CH$_3$(CH$_2$)$_2$CH$_2$NH—⟨benzene ring⟩—COOCH$_2$CH$_2$(OCH$_2$CH$_2$)$_n$OCH$_3$

Average: *n* = 8 [104-31-4] C$_{30}$H$_{43}$NO$_{11}$ (average: 603).

Benzonatate is a mixture of the *p*-butylaminobenzoate esters of the monomethyl ethers derived from a mixture of polyethylene glycols having the average composition of a nonaethylene glycol. The chemical name above is for the average compound.

Preparation—Ethyl *p*-(butylamino)benzoate is transesterified with a polyethylene glycol monomethyl ether fraction in a methanol solution of sodium methoxide. The crude ester is purified by extracting its benzene solution with sodium carbonate solution, the ester being retained in the benzene. US Pat 2,714,606.

Description—Pale yellow, clear, viscous liquid with a faint characteristic odor and a bitter taste followed by a sense of numbness.

Solubility—Freely soluble in chloroform, alcohol, and benzene; miscible with water in all proportions.

Uses—An *antitussive.* It acts peripherally by anesthetizing the stretch receptors in the respiratory passages, lungs, and pleura and thereby reducing the cough reflex at its source. It begins to act within 15 to 20 minutes and its effect lasts for 3 to 8 hours. Although its antitussive potency is essentially the same as for codeine when evaluated against experimentally induced cough in animals and man, it is somewhat less effective than codeine against cough associated with clinical illness.

Benzonatate is well tolerated in therapeutic doses. Untoward effects reported to date include headache, mild dizziness, pruritus and skin eruptions, nasal congestion, constipation, nausea, gastrointestinal upset, a sensation of burning of the eyes, and numbness or tightness in the chest. Hypersensitivity reactions have been reported. If the capsules are allowed to dissolve in the mouth, they exert a local anesthetic effect which is disagreeable to a few patients. Habituation, euphoria, respiratory depression, or constipation have not been reported.

Dose—**100** to **200 mg;** *usual,* **100 mg** 3 times a day. Capsules should not be chewed.

Dosage Forms—Capsules: 100 mg.

Codeine—page 1102.

Codeine Phosphate—page 1102.

Codeine Sulfate—page 1103.

Dextromethorphan Hydrobromide

Morphinan, 3-methoxy-17-methyl-, (9α,13α,14α)-, hydrobromide, monohydrate; Dormethan (*Dorsey*); Romilar (*Roche*); Various Mfrs.

[6700-34-1] C$_{18}$H$_{25}$NO.HBr.H$_2$O (370.33); *anhydrous* [125-69-9] (352.32).

Preparation—Dextromethorphan base (*d*-3-methoxy-*N*-methylmorphinan) is prepared from the corresponding *d*-3-hydroxy compound by methylation with phenyltrimethylammonium hydroxide. The procedure is analogous to that employed for the methylation of morphine to produce codeine. Treatment of the base with HBr yields the hydrobromide.

Description—Practically white crystals, or crystalline powder, having a faint odor; melts at about 126°, with decomposition, pH (1 in 100 solution) 5.2 to 6.5.

Solubility—1 g in about 65 mL water; freely soluble in alcohol and chloroform; insoluble in ether.

Uses—A synthetic morphine derivative employed exclusively as an *antitussive* agent. The drug acts centrally to elevate the threshold for coughing. Controlled studies in man indicate it has a cough suppression potency approximately one-half that of codeine. The oral administration of 30 mg to an adult provides effective antitussive activity over an 8- to 12-hour period. Unlike codeine, it is devoid of analgesic properties and produces little or no depression of the central nervous system. Addiction has not been observed after the administration of rather large doses for prolonged periods. The side effects include slight drowsiness and gastrointestinal upset; these are less severe and less frequent than with codeine. Accidental poisoning in children is characterized by stupor and ataxia with rapid recovery after emesis. Dextromethorphan hydrobromide should not be given to patients on monoamine oxidase inhibitors.

Dose—*Usual, Adult, oral,* **10** to **30 mg** every 4 to 8 hours; do not exceed **60** to **120 mg** in 24 hours. *Children (6 to 12),* **2.5** to **5 mg** every 4 hours or **7.5** to **15 mg** every 6 to 8 hours; do not exceed **40–60 mg** in

24 hours. *Children (2 to 6)*, **1.25** to **2.5 mg** every 4 hours or **3.75** to **7.5 mg** every 6 to 8 hours; do not exceed **30 mg** in 24 hours. *Adult, controlled release liquid*, **60 mg** twice daily; *children (6 to 12)*, **30 mg** twice daily; *children (2 to 6)*, **15 mg** twice daily.

Dosage Forms—Controlled release liquid: 30 mg/5 mL; Lozenges: 7.5 and 10 mg; Syrup: 2.5, 5, 10, and 15 mg/5 mL.

Diphenhydramine Hydrochloride—page 1128.
Ethylmorphine Hydrochloride—RPS-15, page 1040.
Hydrocodone Bitartrate—page 1104.

Levopropoxyphene Napsylate

Benzeneethanol, α-[2-(dimethylamino)-1-methylethyl]-α-phenyl-, propanoate (ester), [R-(R*,S*)]-, compd with 2-naphthalenesulfonic acid (1:1), monohydrate; Novrad (*Lilly*)

2-Naphthalenesulfonic acid compound with (−)-α-[2-(dimethyl-amino)-1-methylethyl]-α-phenylphenethyl propionate (1:1) monohydrate [55557-30-7] $C_{22}H_{29}NO_2 \cdot C_{10}H_8O_3S \cdot H_2O$ (565.72); *anhydrous* [5714-90-9] (547.71).

Preparation—The racemate of the α-diastereoisomer of the substituted butanol corresponding to propoxyphene is prepared as described on page 1115 and resolved with (+)-camphorsulfonic acid. The (−)-alcohol thus obtained is esterified with propionic anhydride to form (−)-propoxyphene base and combined with an equimolar quantity of 2-naphthalenesulfonic acid to form the salt.

Description—White powder; essentially odorless; bitter taste; melts within a range of 4° between 158° and 165° after drying.

Solubility—Very slightly soluble in water; 1 g in 17 mL alcohol, 2 mL chloroform.

Uses—An *antitussive* agent used in the symptomatic treatment of nonproductive cough. In contrast to *Propoxyphene* (1061), this isomer is devoid of analgesic activity. It is somewhat less potent than codeine in the treatment of cough; 50 to 100 mg appears to be as effective as 15 mg of codeine in experimental cough. If CNS stimulation or depression develop the dose should be reduced or the medication discontinued. Patients on this drug should be cautioned not to operate a motor vehicle or use hazardous machinery. Untoward effects are usually mild; nausea, epigastric burning, skin rash, urticaria, drowsiness, nervousness, and dizziness have been reported. Since the drug does not induce physical dependence, it is particularly valuable when long-term antitussive therapy is necessary.

Dose (base equivalent)—*Usual, adult, oral*, **100 mg** every 4 hours; maximum daily dose, **600 mg.** *Children, oral*, **0.5 mg/lb** every 4 hours; maximum daily dose, 25 to 75 lbs, **3 mg/lb.**

Dosage Forms (base equivalent)—Capsules: 100 mg.

Methadone Hydrochloride—page 1109.
Morphine Sulfate—page 1103.

Other Antitussive Agents

Chlophedianol Hydrochloride [2-Chloro-α-[2-(dimethylamino)-ethyl]benzhydrol hydrochloride; $C_{17}H_{20}ClNO \cdot HCl$; Ulo (*Riker*)]—White, crystalline powder; freely soluble in water. *Uses:* A nonnarcotic cough suppressant with some local anesthetic and anticholinergic properties. Side effects include excitation, hyperirritability, and nightmares. Tolerance or addiction have not been reported. Give with caution in patients on central nervous system depressants or stimulants. *Dose:* Usual, adult and children over 12 years of age, 25 mg (one teaspoonful of syrup) 4 times a day as required for cough; children 6 to 12 years of age 12.5 to 25 mg, and children 2 to 6 years of age 12.5 mg 3 or 4 times a day. *Dosage Form—* Syrup, 25 mg/5 mL.

Noscapine [*l*-Narcotine; $C_{22}H_{23}NO_7$; Nectadon (*MSD*)] Tusscapine (*Fisons*)—An alkaloid (see page 416 for formula) of opium, present in amounts ranging from 3 to 10%, from which source it is obtained. Both noscapine and noscapine hydrochloride occur as white to nearly white, crystalline powders; odorless, and of bitter taste. Noscapine is practically insoluble in water; its hydrochloride is freely soluble in water. *Uses:* Noscapine (and noscapine hydrochloride) is an antitussive that depresses the medullary centers and suppresses the cough reflex. It is used in the management of cough in bronchial asthma and pulmonary emphysema. The drug reduces the frequency and intensity of coughing paroxysms. Its antitussive potency and onset and duration of action have been reported to be approximately equal, milligram for milligram, to those of codeine; clinical evidence in support of this is lacking, and dosages have ranged from 5 to 90 mg 2 to 4 times a day. Therapeutically effective doses are essentially devoid of the unpleasant side effects of codeine and, except for occasional nausea and drowsiness, its side effects are negligible. Doses up to 90 mg have no effect on respiration in man. The drug has no morphine-like effects and has no effect on the morphine abstinence syndrome. Tolerance to the antitussive effect has not been observed. Noscapine is no longer controlled under the federal narcotic law. *Dose:* Oral, adult, 15 to 30 mg (of noscapine or noscapine hydrochloride) 3 or 4 times a day; children, 2 to 6 years of age, 7.5 to 15 mg, to a maximum of 4 times a day, do not exceed 120 mg in 24 hours; children (6 to 12), 15 mg 3 or 4 times a day, do not exceed 60 mg in 24 hours; children (2 to 6), 7.5 to 15 mg 3 or 4 times a day, do not exceed 4 doses a day.

Dosage Forms: Tablets, chewable, 15 mg; Syrup, 15 mg/5 mL.

Bronchodilators

Asthma is a disease characterized by increased responsiveness of the trachea and bronchi to various stimuli, manifested by widespread narrowing of the airways that changes in severity either spontaneously or as a result of therapy. The symptoms of asthma include recurrent, episodic bouts of coughing, shortness of breath, chest tightness, and wheezing. Its pathological features are contraction of airway smooth muscle, mucosal thickening from edema and cellular infiltration, and inspissation in the airway lumen of abnormally thick, viscid plugs of mucous. Drugs which reverse the contraction of smooth muscle, one of the common causes of airway obstruction, are referred to as bronchodilators.

A number of pharmacologically different groups of drugs possess bronchodilator properties. The bronchial muscles are controlled by the autonomic nervous system with parasympathetic fibers predominating in number and effect. Stimulation of parasympathetic nerves causes calcium-dependent contraction of the bronchi and enhances the release of chemical mediators that induce bronchospasm. Consequently, *anticholinergic* drugs (atropine) are useful for reducing bronchospasm. *Calcium antagonists*, such as verapamil and nifedipine, selectively inhibit calcium ion influx across the cell membrane and suppress calcium-dependent smooth muscle contraction.

Adrenergic drugs, such as *metaproterenol* and *albuterol*, exert a preferential effect on beta-2-adrenergic receptors and mediate relaxation of the smooth muscle of the respiratory tract. *Corticosteroids*, like beclomethasone dipropionate and prednisone, are not only effective anti-inflammatory agents, but also potentiate the bronchodilator effects of adrenergic drugs. The *xanthine drugs*, especially theophylline and related substances, are thought to be the most useful bronchodilators for moderate or severe reversible bronchospasm. Moreover, they also improve respiratory exchange by increasing diaphragmatic contractility. Theophylline competitively inhibits phosphodiesterase; this results in an increase in cyclic adenosine monophosphate (cAMP). This action increases the release of endogenous epinephrine. The methylxanthines are also thought to inhibit neural transmission at certain synapses, especially in the central nervous system, where adenosine, a structural analog, may be a neurotransmitter.

The effectiveness of the methyl xanthine preparations in the treatment of bronchial asthma depends on their conversion to theophylline, which is the active constituent. Consequently, the dosage of theophylline, its salts and dyphilline is usually expressed in terms of anhydrous theophylline base, despite the marked pharmacokinetic interpatient variability among these preparations. The approximate anhydrous theophylline content in the various theophylline derivatives is as follows:

84 to 86% of aminophylline anhydrous
74 to 82% of aminophylline hydrous
70% of dyphylline
62 to 66% of oxytriphylline
48 to 50% of theophylline calcium salicylate
91% of theophylline monohydrate
73 to 75% of theophylline olamine
55 to 65% of theophylline sodium acetate
45 to 47% of theophylline sodium glycinate

The anticholinergic drugs are discussed in Chapter 48, beta-2 and other adrenergic drugs in Chapter 47, cromolyn sodium in Chapter 61, and corticosteroids in Chapter 52. Theophylline and its various derivatives and combinations are presented in this section.

Albuterol—page 881.

Aminophylline

1*H*-Purine-2,6-dione, 3,7-dihydro-1,3-dimethyl-, compd with 1,2-ethanediamine (2:1)

Theophylline compound with ethylenediamine [317-34-0] $C_{16}H_{24}N_{10}O_4$ (420.43); *dihydrate* [49746-06-7] (456.46).

Preparation—By adding, with vigorous stirring, a weighed quantity of theophylline to a volume of solution containing the required equivalent quantity of the diamine in anhydrous alcohol. After a few hours, the precipitate of aminophylline is filtered off, washed with cold alcohol, and dried at a low temperature.

Description—White or slightly yellowish granules or powder, having a slight ammoniacal odor and a bitter taste; on exposure to air it gradually loses ethylenediamine and absorbs CO_2 with liberation of free theophylline; its solution is alkaline to litmus.

Solubility—1 g in about 5 mL water, but, owing to hydrolysis, separation of crystals of less aminated theophylline begins in a few minutes, these crystals dissolving on the addition of a small amount of ethylenediamine. When, however, 1 g is dissolved in 25 mL water, the solution remains clear; insoluble in alcohol and ether.

Incompatibilities—Aqueous solutions are alkaline and display the incompatibilities of the alkalies. *Acids* cause a precipitation of theophylline; even *carbon dioxide* of the air behaves thus.

Uses—Aminophylline is indicated for *bronchial asthma*, and for reversible bronchospasm associated with chronic bronchitis and emphysema. It is also useful as a diuretic agent. Absorption from the gastrointestinal tract after oral or rectal administration is incomplete, slow, and variable. Approximately 79% is converted to theophylline. Optimal serum therapeutic levels range from 10 µg/mL to 20 µg/mL. It is most effective when given intravenously; if given slowly in dilute solution, the drug is relatively nontoxic, although nausea, vomiting, and anorexia may appear in some patients. The simultaneous administration of aluminum hydroxide decreases the incidence of this side effect. See *Theophylline*.

Dose—*Usual, adult, bronchodilator, oral, loading:* Elixir, **7 mg/kg**; Tablets, **18.7 mg/kg** per day in 3 or 4 divided doses at 6 to 8 hour intervals; Enteric-Coated Tablets, see Tablets. *Intravenous, loading:* **6 mg/kg** over a period of 20 minutes. *Rectal, enema*, **300 mg** 3 times a day or **450 mg** twice a day; suppositories, **500 mg** 1 to 3 times a day. *Usual, adult, bronchodilator, oral, maintenance:* Elixir, **2.4 mg/kg** every 6 hours for 12 hours, then **2.4 mg/kg** every 12 hours; Tablets, increase 25% at 2 or 3 day intervals up to a maximum of **15.2 mg/kg** per day. *Intravenous, maintenance*, **600 µg/kg** per hour for 12 hours, then **300 µg/kg** per hour.

Pediatric, bronchodilator, rectal, enema, or *suppositories*, **3** to **5 mg/kg** every 6 to 8 hours, not to exceed **20 mg/kg/day**. *Pediatric, elixir, oral solution, tablets,* or *injection*, see package insert for information about the dose for a particular age group.

Dosage Forms—Enema: 60 mg/mL; Elixir, 83.3 mg/5 mL; Injection: 250 mg/10 mL, 500 mg/20 mL, and 500/2 mL (see below); Suppositories: 250 and 500 mg; Oral Solution: 105 mg/5 mL; Tablets: 100 and 200 mg; Extended-release tablets: 225 and 300 mg.

Aminophylline Injection [Theophylline Ethylenediamine Injection] is a sterile solution of aminophylline in water for injection, or is a sterile solution of theophylline in water for injection prepared with the aid of ethylenediamine. It contains, in each 100 mL, 2.5 g of $C_{16}H_{24}N_{10}O_4 \cdot 2H_2O$. Aminophylline Injection may contain an excess of ethylenediamine, but no other substance added for the purpose of pH adjustment; it contains 131 to 152 mg of $C_2H_8N_2$ per g of $C_{16}H_{24}N_{10}O_4 \cdot 2H_2O$. *Stabilization:* The aminophylline in this injection absorbs carbon dioxide from the air resulting in the liberation of free theophylline. The USP recognizes the difficulties experienced with the aminophylline injection and, for purposes of stabilization, permits the use of additional ethylenediamine. It appears to be advisable to prepare the solution directly from calculated quantities of theophylline and of ethylenediamine, thus entirely eliminating the possibility of previous absorption of CO_2. It has been found helpful to ampul the solution while hot, seal it at once, thus producing a slight vacuum in the ampul, and then sterilize the ampul immediately by autoclaving before seed crystals can start to form. Some operators prefer to repeat the sterilization operation, believing that this also helps to prevent subsequent precipitation.

Cromolyn Sodium—page 1131.

Dyphylline

1*H*-Purine-2,6-dione, 7-(2,3-dihydroxypropyl)-3,7-dihydro-1,3-dimethyl-, Neothylline (*Lemmon*); Lufyllin (*Carter-Wallace*)

7-(2,3-Dihydroxypropyl)theophylline $C_{10}H_{14}N_4O_4$ (254.25).

Preparation—By interaction of 1-chloro-2,3-dihydroxypropane with theophylline dissolved in a sodium hydroxide or potassium hydroxide solution. US Pat. 2,575,344 (see *CA 46:* 1722i, 1952).

Description—White, crystalline powder; bitter taste; melts at about 158°; pH (1 in 100 solution) 6.6 to 7.3.

Solubility—1 g in 3 mL water, 50 mL alcohol, 100 mL chloroform.

Uses—Indicated for relief of *bronchial asthma* and for reversible *bronchospasm* associated with *chronic bronchitis* and *emphysema*. It exhibits peripheral vasodilator and bronchodilator actions characteristic of theophylline. It also has some diuretic and myocardial stimulant effects, and is effective orally. Dyphylline is a derivative of theophylline and is not metabolized to theophylline *in vivo*. Following oral administration, dyphylline is 68 to 82% bioavailable. Peak plasma concentrations are reached in 1 hour; its half-life is 2 hours. The minimal therapeutic concentration is 12 µg/mL; 83% is excreted unchanged in the urine. Because of its somewhat shorter half-life, other theophylline derivatives are usually preferred for chronic bronchodilator therapy. Otherwise its pharmacological profile, effective and toxic serum levels, contraindications, precautions, adverse reactions, and drug interactions are similar to those for theophylline.

Dose—*Usual, adult, oral, acute attack*, **15 mg/kg** every 6 hours, up to 4 times a day. The dosage should be individualized by titration to the condition and response of the patient. *Intramuscular, adults*, **250 to 500 mg** injected slowly. *Children*, see package insert.

Dosage Forms—Elixir: 33.3 and 53.3 mg/5 mL; Injection: 250 mg/mL; Liquid: 100 mg/5 mL; Solution: 33.3 mg/5 mL; Tablets: 200 and 400 mg; Extended-Release Tablets: 400 mg.

Ephedrine—page 883.

Epinephrine—page 883.

Ethylnorepinephrine—page 891.

Isoetharine—page 885.

Isoproterenol—page 886.

Metaproterenol—page 887.

Oxtriphylline

Ethanaminium, 2-hydroxy-*N,N,N*-trimethyl-, salt with 3,7-dihydro-1,3-dimethyl-1*H*-purine-2,6-dione; Choline Theophyllinate; Choledyl (*Parke-Davis*)

Choline salt with theophylline (1:1) [4499-40-5] $C_{12}H_{21}N_5O_3$ (283.33).

Preparation—An aqueous solution of choline bicarbonate is reacted with theophylline in isopropanol. After concentration by vacuum distillation, the crude product is crystallized from isopropanol–methanol solution. US Pat 2,776,287 and 2,776,288.

Description—White, crystalline powder, having an amine-like odor; pH (1 in 100 solution) about 10.3.

Solubility—1 g in 1 mL of water; freely soluble in alcohol; very slightly soluble in chloroform.

Uses—Oxtriphylline, the choline salt of theophylline, is more soluble, more stable, better absorbed from the gastrointestinal tract, and produces less gastric irritation than aminophylline, but has pharmacological actions similar to other xanthine derivatives. (See *Theophylline*, this page). Hence, it is effective orally in the management of *acute bronchial asthma* and for *reversible bronchospasm*, associated with *chronic bronchitis* and *emphysema*. Development of tolerance is infrequent; therefore, it is useful for long-term therapy. Its usefulness in premenstrual tension or in dysmenorrhea has not been established. Untoward effects include gastric distress, and occasionally palpitation and central nervous system stimulation.

Dose—*Bronchodilator, usual, adult, oral,* **100 to 200 mg** every 6 hours; sustained-action, **400 to 600 mg** every 12 hours. *Pediatric,* children 2 to 12 years of age, **3.7 mg/kg** every 6 hours (dosage for children under 2 years of age has not been established).

Dosage Forms—Elixir: **100 mg/5 mL**; Pediatric Syrup: **100 mg/5 mL**; Tablets: 100 and 200 mg. Tablets, sustained-action: 400 and 600 mg.

Salbutamol (Albuterol)—page 886.
Terbutaline Sulfate—page 890.

Theophylline

1*H*-Purine-2,6-dione, 3,7-dihydro-1,3-dimethyl-, monohydrate or anhydrous; 1,3-Dimethylxanthine; Various Mfrs.

Theophylline monohydrate [5967-84-0] $C_7H_8N_4O_2.H_2O$ (198.18); *anhydrous* [58-55-9] (180.17); for the structural formula, see page 419.

Preparation—Present in tea but in too small an amount to make it an economical source. It has been made from caffeine, but is more successfully produced by total synthesis. See page 1134.

Description—White, odorless, crystalline powder having a bitter taste; stable in air; melts between 270° and 274°, and its saturated aqueous solution is neutral or slightly acid to litmus; weaker as a base than caffeine or theobromine and scarcely forms salts even with the strong acids, but is more "acidic" than those and readily dissolves in ammonia water.

Solubility—1 g in about 120 mL water and about 80 mL alcohol; more soluble in hot water; sparingly soluble in ether and chloroform; freely soluble in solutions of alkali hydroxides and ammonia.

Uses—Theophylline and its salts and derivatives are used as *bronchodilators* in the symptomatic treatment of *mild bronchial asthma* and *reversible bronchospasm* which may occur in association with *chronic bronchitis, emphysema,* and *other obstructive pulmonary diseases*. It relieves the primary manifestations of asthma, including shortness of breath, wheezing and dyspnea, and improves pulmonary function as measured by increased flow rates and vital capacity. The drug also suppresses exercise-induced asthma and, in doses that maintain therapeutic serum levels, prevents symptoms of chronic asthma. Theophylline is well absorbed after administration. Food has little effect on theophylline availability; absorption may be slower in the presence of food and more rapid in the presence of large volumes of fluid. Rectal suppositories are slowly and erratically absorbed regardless of the type of suppository base; retention enemas are absorbed more rapidly. The time required to reach peak plasma levels varies with the route and formulation used; following oral administration of liquids or uncoated tablets, peak plasma levels are reached in 2 hours. Average volume of distribution is 0.5 L/kg.

Theophylline plasma or serum levels of about 10 to 20 µg/mL are usually needed to produce optimum bronchodilator response. Some patients with mild pulmonary disease will experience relief of bronchospasm with theophylline plasma levels of 5 µg/mL. With plasma levels ranging from 8 to 20 µg/mL, a linear relationship exists between improvement in pulmonary function and the logarithm of theophylline plasma concentration. In premature infants, theophylline plasma levels of about 7 to 14 µg/mL may be sufficient to reverse apnea. Theophylline plasma levels of about 10 µg/mL produce a transient diuretic response. Theophylline is excreted by the kidneys. Less than 15% of the drug is excreted unchanged in the urine. Elimination kinetics vary greatly among individuals. The elimination half-life of theophylline averages about *7 to 9 hours in the adult nonsmoker* and *4 to 5 hours in the adult smoker* (one or two packs per day); 3 to 5 hours in children, and 20 to 30 hours in premature neonates. The premature neonate excretes about 50% unchanged theophylline and may accumulate the caffeine metabolite.

Theophylline, its salts, and dyphylline exert identical pharmacologic actions. Theophylline competitively inhibits phosphodiesterase, the enzyme that degrades cyclic 3′,5′-adenosine monophosphate (cyclic AMP). Increased levels of intracellular cyclic AMP may mediate most of the pharmacologic effects of the drug.

Theophylline has less stimulatory effect on the central nervous system and skeletal muscles than caffeine but has a greater effect on coronary dilatation, smooth muscle relaxation, diuresis, and cardiac stimulation than caffeine. In general, it has relatively more pharmacological activity in all categories than theobromine.

Theophylline produces central nervous system stimulation and gastrointestinal irritation following administration by any route. Theophylline and its salts and analogues are all somewhat irritating to gastric mucosa; the significance of reported differences among the individual agents is doubtful. The most common gastrointestinal side effects (both locally and centrally mediated) include nausea, vomiting, epigastric pain, abdominal cramps, anorexia, and rarely, diarrhea. Cardiovasular side effects of theophylline include palpitation, sinus tachycardia, and increased pulse rate. These side effects are usually mild and transient. Theophylline may also produce transiently increased urinary frequency, dehydration, twitching of fingers and hands, and elevated SGOT levels. Hypersensitivity reactions characterized by urticaria, generalized pruritus, and angioneurotic edema have been reported with aminophylline administration. Drug interactions are common in patients on theophylline. Agents which *decrease* the effects of theophylline include cigarette and marijuana smoking, phenobarbital, and charcoal-broiled foods. Agents which *increase* the effects of theophylline include cimetidine, erythromycin, influenza virus vaccine, troleandomycin, allopurinal, and thiabendazole. Theophylline *increases* the effects of sympathomimetic drugs, digitalis, and oral anticoagulants. Theophylline *decreases* the effects of phenytoin and lithium carbonate. Concomitant administration of theophylline with beta adrenergic blocking agents may result in antagonistic effects; theophylline with reserpine or halothane may induce tachycardia or cardiac arrhythmias, respectively.

Theophylline toxicity is most likely to occur when plasma levels exceed 20 µg/mL and becomes progressively more severe at higher serum concentrations. Tachycardia, in the absence of hypoxia, fever, or administration of sympathomimetic drugs, may be an indication of theophylline toxicity. Anorexia, nausea and occasional vomiting, diarrhea, insomnia, irritability, restlessness, and headache commonly occur. Fatalities in adults have occurred during or following IV administration of large doses of aminophylline in patients with renal, hepatic, or cardiovascular complications. In other patients, the rapidity of the injection, rather than the dose used, appears to be the more important factor precipitating acute hypotension, convulsions, coma, cardiac standstill, ventricular fibrillation, and death. There is no specific antidote for theophylline toxicity; therapy is usually supportive. Treatment includes stopping the drug, gastric lavage and/or emesis, and administration of antacids or demulcents and oxygen. Prompt restoration of fluid and electrolyte balance is essential. Other symptomatic procedures are instituted as necessary.

Dose—All dosages should be based on lean body weight since theophylline does not distribute into fatty tissue. Moreover, all dosage should be calculated on the basis of anhydrous theophylline content, regardless of the salt used. For the rapid control of acute symptoms in patients not on theophylline, an initial loading dose is required. *Adult (nonsmoker), oral loading,* **6 mg/kg** followed by 2 doses of **3 mg/kg** every six hours; *maintenance dose,* **3 mg/kg** every

8 hours. *Adult* (*smokers*), and *children* (*9 to 16 years*), *oral loading*, **6 mg/kg** followed by 3 doses of **3 mg/kg** every 4 hours; *maintenance dose*, 3 mg/kg every 6 hours. *Children* (*6 months to 9 years*), *oral loading*, **6 mg/kg** followed by 3 doses of **4 mg/kg** every 4 hours; *maintenance dose*, **4 mg/kg** every 6 hours. Consult package insert for detailed dosage regimen.

Dosage Forms—Capsules: 50, 100, 200, and 250 mg; Capsules extended-release: 50, 60, 65, 75, 100, 125, 130, 200, 250, 260, and 300 mg; Elixir: 80, 112.5, 150, and 225 mg/5 mL; Oral Liquid: 80 mg/15 mL; Oral Suspension: 100 mg/5 mL; Tablets: 100, 125, 200, 225, 250, and 300 mg; Tablets, extended-release: 100, 130, 200, 250, 260, 300, and 500 mg.

Theophylline, Ephedrine Hydrochloride, and Butabarbital

Tedral-25 (*Parke-Davis*)

Uses—Same as *Theophylline, Ephedrine Hydrochloride, and Phenobarbital*, including adverse effects, contraindications, and precautions. See below.

Dose—*Usual, adult, oral*, 1 **tablet** every 4 hours. *Usual, pediatric, oral,* children 6 to 12 years of age, ½ **tablet** every 6 hours; children under 6 years of age, dosage not established.

Dosage Forms—Tablets: 130 mg theophylline, 24 mg ephedrine hydrochloride, and 25 mg butabarbital.

Theophylline, Ephedrine Sulfate, and Hydroxyzine Hydrochloride

Marax (*Roerig*); Various Mfrs

Uses—Possibly effective in the management of *bronchospastic disorders*, such as *bronchial asthma*. It combines the bronchodilator effects of theophylline and ephedrine sulfate with the sedative and calming action of hydroxyzine hydrochloride. For adverse reactions, contraindications, precautions, and drug interactions, the monographs for each agent should be consulted (*Theophylline*, page 873, *Ephedrine Sulfate*, page 883; and *Hydroxyzine Hydrochloride*, page 1071).

Dose—*Usual, adult, oral,* 1 **tablet** 2 to 4 times daily. *Usual, pediatric, oral,* children over 5 years of age, **5 mL** of syrup 3 or 4 times daily; children 2 to 5 years of age, **2.5 to 5 mL** of syrup 3 or 4 times daily; not recommended for children under 2 years of age.

Dosage Forms—Syrup: 32.5 mg theophylline, 6.25 mg ephedrine sulfate, and 2.5 mg hydroxyzine hydrochloride per 5 mL. Tablets: 130 mg theophylline, 25 mg ephedrine sulfate, and 10 mg hydroxyzine hydrochloride.

Theophylline, Ephedrine Hydrochloride, and Phenobarbital

Tedral (*Parke-Davis*), Primatene "P" (*Whitehall*); Various Mfrs.

Uses—For the symptomatic relief of *bronchial asthma, asthmatic bronchitis*, and *bronchospastic disorders*. It is also used to abort or minimize *asthmatic attacks* and is of value in the management of seasonal or *perennial asthma*. The theophylline and ephedrine induce bronchodilation, whereas the phenobarbital is intended to counteract possible stimulation by ephedrine and as a mild, long-acting sedative for the apprehensive asthmatic patient. This combination should be used with caution in patients with cardiovascular disease, severe hypertension, prostatic hypertrophy, or glaucoma. Adverse reactions include epigastric distress, palpitation, tremulousness, insomnia, difficult micturition, and CNS stimulation. It should be remembered that phenobarbital may be habit-forming.

Dose—*Usual, adult, oral,* 1 or 2 **tablets** or 10 to 30 mL of the elixir or oral suspension every 4 hours or 1 extended-release tablet every 12 hours. *Usual, pediatric, oral,* **0.2 to 0.4 mL per kg** body weight or ½ to 1 **tablet** every 4 to 6 hours; children weighing less than 27 kg, dosage not established.

Dosage Forms—Elixir: 32.5 mg theophylline, 6 mg ephedrine hydrochloride, and 2 mg phenobarbital per 5 mL. Oral Suspension: 65 mg theophylline, 12 mg ephedrine hydrochloride, and 4 mg phenobarbital per 5 mL. Tablets: 130 mg theophylline, 24 mg ephedrine hydrochloride; and 8 mg phenobarbital. Extended-Release Tablets: the equivalent of 180 mg anhydrous theophylline, 48 mg ephedrine hydrochloride, and 25 mg phenobarbital.

Theophylline, Ephedrine Hydrochloride, Phenobarbital, and Guaifenesin

Tedral Expectorant (*Parke-Davis*); Bronkotabs (*Breon*)

Uses—Same as *Theophylline, Ephedrine Hydrochloride, and Phenobarbital* (see this page) with the addition of an expectorant. Guaifenesin increases the volume and decreases the viscosity of respiratory fluids, thus assisting the patient to cough up viscid mucus. Adverse reactions, contraindications, habituation liability, and precautions are similar to the combination without guaifenesin.

Dose—*Usual, adult, oral,* 1 or 2 **tablets** every 4 to 6 hours. *Pediatric,* over 6 years, **one-half** adult dose; children under 6, as directed by physician.

Dosage Forms—Tablets and Expectorant: 65, 100, or 130 mg theophylline, 24 mg ephedrine hydrochloride, 8 mg phenobarbital, and 100 mg guaifenesin per tablet or 5 mL of expectorant.

Theophylline and Guaifenesin

Quibron (*Mead Johnson*); Slo-Phyllin G.G. (*Rorer*), Theolair-Plus (*Riker*), Ashbron G (*Sandoz*); Various Mfrs

Uses—Same as *Theophylline* (see page 873), except it includes the expectorant action of guaifenesin. Guaifenesin increases the volume and decreases the viscosity of respiratory fluids. Thus, this combination induces bronchodilation and assists the patient in coughing up viscid mucus. Adverse reactions, contraindications, and precautions are the same as for theophylline.

Dose—*Usual, adult, oral,* 1 **capsule** every 6 to 8 hours for patients whose dosage has been adjusted upward to achieve therapeutic serum levels.

Dosage Forms—Capsules: 300 mg anhydrous theophylline and 180 mg of guaifenesin.

Theophylline Olamine

1*H*-Purine-2,6-dione, 3,7-dihydro-1,3-dimethyl-, compd with 2-aminoethanol (1:1); Theophylline Monoethanolamine (*Fleet*)

Theophylline compound with 2-aminoethanol (1:1) [573-41-1] $C_7H_8N_4O_2.C_2H_7NO$ (241.25).

Preparation—Analogous to the procedure for *Aminophylline*, except that 2-aminoethanol is used in place of ethylenediamine.

Description—White or practically white, crystalline powder with not more than a slight odor.
Solubility—1 g in 20 mL water.

Uses—The same actions, uses, and limitations as for *Aminophylline*.

Dose—*Adult, rectal,* **250** or **500 mg**; not to be repeated in less than 8 hours, and not more than 2 doses in 24 hours. Not recommended for children since dose has not been established.

Dosage Forms—Rectal Units delivering volumes equivalent to 250 and 500 mg.

Theophylline Sodium Glycinate

Glycine, mixt with 3,7-dihydro-1,3-dimethyl-1*H*-purine-2,6-dione, monosodium salt; Pemophyllin (*Merrell-Dow*)

Theophylline sodium mixture with glycine [8000-10-0]; an equilibrium mixture containing $C_7H_7N_4NaO_2$ (sodium theophylline) and $C_2H_5NO_2$ (aminoacetic acid) in approximately equimolecular proportions buffered with an additional mole of aminoacetic acid; yields 49–52% $C_7H_8N_4O_2.H_2O$ (theophylline).

Description—White, crystalline powder; has a slight ammoniacal odor, and a bitter taste; pH (saturated solution) between 8.5 to 9.5.
Solubility—1 g in 6 mL water; very slightly soluble in alcohol; practically insoluble in chloroform.

Uses—A solubilized, less irritating form of theophylline; it contains 49% theophylline. It is useful as a *smooth muscle relaxant* in the treatment of *bronchial asthma*. It should not be used in patients who might be harmed by myocardial stimulation. Adverse reactions include nausea, vomiting, burning epigastric pain, palpitation, dizziness, headache, nervousness, and similar minor complaints.

Dose—*Usual, adult, oral*, equivalent to **165** to **330 mg** of theophylline every 6 to 8 hours. *Usual, pediatric, oral*, expressed as equivalent of theophylline, children 6 to 12, **110 to 165 mg** every 6 to 8 hours; children 3 to 6, **55 to 82.5 mg** every 6 to 8 hours; children 1 to 3, **27.5 to 55 mg** every 6 to 8 hours; children under 1 year of age, dosage not established. See also package insert.

Dosage Forms—Elixir: 330 mg/15 mL; Tablets: 330 mg.

Other Theophylline Preparations

Theophylline, Ephedrine Sulfate, Phenobarbital and Guaifenesin [Bronkotabs, Bronkolixir (*Breon*)]—*Uses:* For prevention and relief of symptoms of asthma and bronchitis. For adverse reactions, precautions, contraindications, and habituation liability see respective drug monographs. *Dose: Usual, adult, oral*, 1 tablet or 10 mL of elixir every 3 or 4 hours; *pediatric, children over 6 years of age*, one-half adult dose. *Dosage Forms:* Elixir: 15 mg theophylline, 12 mg ephedrine sulfate, 4 mg phenobarbital, 50 mg guaifenesin in 5 mL; Tablets: 100 mg theophylline, 24 mg ephedrine sulfate, 8 mg phenobarbital, 100 mg guaifenesin (also available half-strength).

Theophylline Calcium Salicylate—A double salt or mixture of theophylline calcium and calcium salicylate, in equimolecular proportion, containing about 50% anhydrous theophylline. *Uses:* As for theophylline.

Theophylline Calcium Salicylate, Ephedrine Hydrochloride, Phenobarbital, and Guaifenesin [Verequad (*Knoll*)]—*Uses:* For bronchial asthma, chronic bronchitis, and pulmonary emphysema in which tenacious mucus and bronchospasm are troublesome symptoms. For adverse effects, contraindications, precautions, and habituation potential see respective drug monographs. *Dose: Usual, oral, adult* and *children over 12 years of age*, 1 tablet or 10 mL of suspension 3 or 4 times a day, repeated at bedtime if necessary; *children 6 to 12 years of age*, one-half tablet or 5 mL suspension 3 times a day. *Dosage Forms:* Tablets: equivalent of 65 mg anhydrous theophylline, 24 mg ephedrine hydrochloride, 8 mg phenobarbital, 100 mg guaifenesin; Suspension: 5 mL equivalent to one-half tablet.

Theophylline Calcium Salicylate, Ephedrine Hydrochloride, Phenobarbital, and Potassium Iodide [Quadrinal (*Knoll*)]—*Uses:* For bronchial asthma, chronic bronchitis, and pulmonary emphysema in which tenacious mucus and bronchospasm are dominant symptoms. For adverse effects, contraindications, precautions, and habituation potential see respective drug monographs. *Dose: Usual, oral, adult* and *children over 12 years of age*, 1 tablet or 10 mL of suspension 3 or 4 times a day; *children 6 to 12 years of age*, one-half tablet or 5 mL of suspension 3 times a day. *Dosage Forms:* Tablets: equivalent of 65 mg anhydrous theophylline, 24 mg ephedrine hydrochloride, 24 mg phenobarbital, 320 mg potassium iodide; Suspension: 5 mL equivalent to one-half tablet.

Theophylline Calcium Salicylate and Potassium Iodide [Theokin (*Knoll*)]—*Uses:* For symptomatic treatment of chronic obstructive pulmonary emphysema, bronchial asthma, and chronic bronchitis. Combines a well-tolerated bronchodilator with an effective expectorant that helps liquefy thick, tenacious mucus. For adverse reactions, precautions, and contraindications see *Theophylline*, and *Potassium Iodide*, in this chapter. *Dose: Usual, oral, adult*, 1 tablet or 15 mL of elixir 2 or 3 times a day at intervals no less than 6 hours; *pediatric, children over 12 years of age*, same as for adults; *children 6 to 12 years of* age, one-half tablet per 20 kg of body weight or 5 mL of elixir per 14 kg of body weight 2 or 3 times a day at intervals no less than 6 hours; *children under 6 years*, 2.5 mL of elixir per 7 kg of body weight, once or twice daily at intervals no less than 6 hours. *Dosage Forms:* Tablets: equivalent of 225 mg anhydrous theophylline, 450 mg potassium iodide; Elixir: 15 mL equivalent to one tablet.

Theophylline Sodium Acetate [A hydrated mixture of $C_7H_7N_4NaO_2$ (202.15) (sodium theophylline) and $C_2H_3NaO_2$ (82.03) (sodium acetate) in approximately equimolecular proportions; yields about 60% $C_7H_8N_4O_2$ (180.17) (anhydrous theophylline Theocin (*Winthrop*))]. *Preparation:* By heating an equimolecular mixture of theophylline and sodium hydroxide, in alcohol, to form theophylline sodium, then adding an equivalent amount of sodium acetate and evaporating to dryness. *Description and Solubility:* White, odorless, crystalline powder having a bitter, salty taste; gradually absorbs CO_2 from the air and liberates free theophylline; its solution is alkaline to phenophthalein TS. *Soluble* 1 g in about 25 mL water; insoluble in alcohol, ether, and chloroform. *Uses:* See *Theophylline*. *Dose: Usual*, **200** to **300 mg** 3 times a day. *Dosage Forms:* Tablets: 100 and 200 mg.

Therapeutic Gases

A number of pharmacologic agents are gaseous at normal temperatures and pressures, whereas others are liquids or even solids with such high vapor pressures that they yield vapors in sufficiently high concentration to exhibit pharmacological properties. Since these gases and vapors are absorbed by way of the respiratory tract, they could be included in this section. However, only those gases which have therapeutic application are presented here. Aside from the anesthetic gases and vapors, which are discussed elsewhere (see Chapter 55), the most important therapeutic gases are carbon dioxide, oxygen, and helium. Although helium is not a pharmacologically active agent, it does possess valuable therapeutic properties attributable to its unique physical properties; hence, it is included in this section.

Carbon Dioxide—page 866.

Helium

Helium [7440-59-7] He (4.003); contains not less than 99% by volume of He; the remainder consists mainly of nitrogen.

Preparation—See page 353.

Description—Colorless, odorless, tasteless, chemically inert gas; 1 L at 760 mm and 0° weighs 178–189 mg.

Solubility—Very slightly soluble in water.

Identification—A burning splinter of wood is extinguished when plunged into helium. It does not react with hydrogen.

Uses—A diluent for medicinal gases. Helium is inert with respect to body metabolism and has no physiologic function or pharmacologic toxicity. Its pharmacological actions are related exclusively to its physical properties; its density is about one-seventh that of oxygen. A mixture of 80 parts helium and 20 parts oxygen is only ⅓ as heavy as air. Such mixtures are used in the treatment of *respiratory obstruction* and are of great value in relieving *status asthmaticus* and the symptoms arising from inflammatory obstructions. When administered in *asphyxia*, the light mixture penetrates the air passages more readily than mixtures of nitrogen and oxygen. Helium may also be substituted for nitrogen in divers working at high ambient pressures; the helium eliminates the possibility of nitrogen narcosis on deep dives.

Dose—By *inhalation*, **60** to **80%**, with oxygen 20 to 40%.

Oxygen

Oxygen [7782-44-7], O_2 (32.00); contains not less than 99% by volume of O_2.

Preparation—See page 364.

Description—Colorless, odorless, tasteless gas; it supports combustion more energetically than air; 1 L at 760 mm and 0° weighs 1.429 g.

Solubility—1 volume in about 32 volumes water or in about 7 volumes alcohol at 20°C and 760 mm.

Identification—A glowing splinter of wood held in oxygen bursts into flame.

Uses—Oxygen is widely employed in the treatment and prevention of *hypoxia*. Hypoxia may result from an *inadequate oxygen content in inspired air* (high altitudes), *inadequate delivery of inspired air to the lungs* (asthma, obstruction of the airway, insufficiency of the respiratory muscles, or respiratory depression), *inadequate oxygenation of blood due to abnormal pulmonary gas exchange* (pulmonary fibrosis, pulmonary edema, pneumonia, tachypnea, etc), and *inadequate transport of oxygen by the circulation* (carbon monoxide poisoning, cardiac decompensation, shock, coronary occlusion, cerebrovascular accidents, etc.). In addition there are several miscellaneous uses, such as the treatment of abdominal distention, spontaneous pneumothorax and air embolism. Oxygen is also used by workers in pressurized spaces. Finally, in anesthesia, oxygen is a common diluent for gaseous and volatile anesthetic agents.

Dose—By *inhalation*, as required.

CHAPTER 45

Sympathomimetic Drugs

Stewart C Harvey, PhD

Professor of Pharmacology
School of Medicine, University of Utah
Salt Lake City, UT 84132

The next five chapters treat specifically of autonomic drugs, and several other chapters (eg, Chapters 41, 43, 59, and 62) include descriptions of or references to a number of autonomic drugs. Consequently, it will be helpful to review briefly the autonomic nervous system and the classification of drugs that act on or simulate components of that system.

Autonomic Nervous System and Autonomic Drugs

The *autonomic (involuntary) nervous system* is generally defined as that system of motor (efferent) nerves which contains cell bodies and corresponding synapses (ie, ganglia) outside of the cerebrospinal axis. The definition includes the sensory (efferent) nerves that subserve functions mediated by the autonomic motor nerves, although a given sensory nerve may also subserve somatic motor functions. This system modulates or controls the activities of smooth (involuntary) muscles of the body, including those that control the caliber of blood vessels, the heart muscle, and the digestive, salivary, sweat, and some endocrine glands. Unconsciously (without conscious control) it tends to maintain a constant state (homeostasis) of the vital functions of the body, constantly adjusting one or more factors to attempt to restore an equilibrium upset by external or internal influences; cerebral blood flow, body temperature, visual accommodation, blood sugar, and body fluid composition, for example, are kept remarkably constant by means of servoadjustments mediated through the autonomic nerves. However, it should be noted that the *somatic (voluntary) nervous system* also unconsciously subserves vital functions such as respiration, posture, swallowing, defecation, motor reflexes, body temperature, and many less vital but important unconscious modulations of skeletal muscle tone; however, the degree of conscious modulation of this control is much greater than in the autonomic nervous system. These involuntary somatic motor functions are coordinated with autonomic functions.

There are two main motor divisions to the autonomic nervous systems—the *sympathetic* (thoracolumbar) and the *parasympathetic* (craniosacral) divisions. Most organs or systems (effectors) receive innervation from both these divisions; generally, but not invariably, the two divisions are qualitatively opposed in their action on a given effector. An abridged list of responses is presented in Table I.

The opposition of the two divisions of the autonomic nervous system reflects the fact that the chemical substances (mediator, transmitter, or neurohumor) liberated by the postganglionic nerve terminals are not the same for the two divisions. Parasympathetic postganglionic nerves liberate acetylcholine, and hence are called *cholinergic* nerves. Most sympathetic postganglionic nerves liberate norepinephine; however, sympathetic postganglionic fibers to the sweat glands and a few fibers to the vascular beds of the mouth, face, and skeletal muscles liberate acetylcholine (ie, are cholinergic). The normal adrenal medulla, which is innervated by sympathetic preganglionics, liberates mostly epinephrine, originally known as adrenaline; since adrenaline was early thought to be the sympathetic transmitter, norepinephrine-releasing nerves are termed *adrenergic*.

At the ganglia, preganglionic nerves of either division liberate acetylcholine (ie, are cholinergic), but the character of the acetylcholine ganglionic receptors is different from those in the neuroeffectors, so that the two types of receptors are not blocked by the same drugs. Somatic motor nerves also liberate acetylcholine (ie, are cholinergic) and are similar to autonomic preganglionics in this regard.

Autonomic drugs are classified according to their relation to the chemical mediator that they either mimic or block. Thus, a drug is cholinergic if it either mimics or blocks stimulation by cholinergic nerves. The terms *cholinomimetic* and *adrenomimetic* have been advanced for the appropriate mimetic agents. There prevails, however, an older terminology based on the erroneous belief that all sympathetic postganglionic nerves yielded the same transmitter. Hence, adrenomimetics are usually called *sympathomimetics* (this chapter) and cholinomimetics are often called *parasympathomimetics* (Chapter 46); but it should be recalled that two types of cholinergic receptors exist, and the use of the term parasympathomimetic best fits those drugs that act upon the cholinergic neuroeffectors (ie, are muscarinic), not the ganglionic synapses. Agents that block the receptors are called *blocking agents*, according to the nature of the chemical transmitter with which they compete. Thus, there are *adrenergic blocking agents* (Chapter 47) and *antimuscarinic*

Table I—Response of Human Effector Organs to Autonomic Nerve Impulses

Effector system	Sympathetic nerve impulses	Parasympathetic nerve impulses
Systemic blood vessels	Constrict Dilate[a]	Innervate few systemic vessels, but dilate
Pulmonary blood vessels	Constrict	Dilate
Coronary blood vessels	Dilate	Dilate
Bronchioles	Dilate	Constrict
Stomach motility and tone	Decrease	Increase
Gastric secretion	Little effect	Increase
Intestinal motility and tone	Decrease	Increase
Urinary bladder sphincter	Constrict	Dilate
Heart	Increase rate and strength	Decrease rate and strength; block
Pupil of eye	Dilate	Constrict
Salivary glands	Stimulate to viscid saliva	Stimulate to watery saliva
Sweat glands	Stimulate[a]	Not innervated
Lacrimal glands	Not innervated	Stimulate

[a] *Cholinergic* sympathetic postganglionic nerves mediate response. Sympathetic cholinergic vasodilators are not prominent in man.

agents (Chapter 48), the latter term again restricted to those drugs that block acetylcholine at the neuroeffector receptors. Those agents that block acetylcholine at the ganglionic synapse are simply called *ganglionic blocking agents* (Chapter 43); their somatic motor counterparts (generally loosely included among the autonomic drugs) are called *neuromuscular blocking agents (curarimimetics)* (Chapter 49). The suffix *lytic* sometimes is used in lieu of the word *blocking*, thus a sympatholytic agent is an adrenergic blocking agent. No terminology has been developed for those agents that act at afferent (sensory or reflex) or central autonomic loci. Also, agents, such as the anticholinesterases, which enhance autonomic transmission by preserving the transmitter from enzymatic destruction, are endowed with no definitive designation; the *anticholinesterases* (Chapter 46) are awkwardly classified as cholinomimetics or parasympathomimetics.

An autonomic mediator not only is liberated at different sites and exerts different effects, but it may also act on different receptors. The actions of acetylcholine on the exocrine glands, smooth muscle and heart differ from those on autonomic ganglia and the voluntary neuromuscular junction. The former (and not the latter) effects are blocked by atropine, whereas the latter (and not the former) are blocked by tubocurarine. Since muscarine exerts the former actions (and not the latter), the corresponding receptors are called *muscarinic;* since nicotine exerts the latter reactions (and not the former), the corresponding receptors are called *nicotinic*. In the adrenergic system there are also two main types of receptors, α and β. There are two types of α-adrenoreceptors: α_1 and α_2. The α_1-adrenoreceptors subserve smooth muscular stimulant functions, adrenergic sweating, and adrenergic salivation. The α_2-adrenoreceptors serve to inhibit the presynaptic release of norepinephrine and other mediators and the postsynaptic activation of adenylate cyclase (and hence inhibit postsynaptic responses). The β-adrenoreceptors are subdivided into β_1- and β_2-adrenoreceptors, and perhaps more. They are characterized and defined by differences in responsiveness to sympathomimetics and blocking drugs. β_1-Adrenoreceptors effect cardiac stimulation and lipolysis; β_2-adrenoreceptors subserve adrenergic smooth muscle relaxation (eg, vasodilatation, bronchodilatation, and intestinal and uterine relaxation) and glycolysis. α-Adrenoreceptors are blocked by phenoxybenzamine. α_1-Adrenoreceptors are selectively blocked by prazosin and α_2-receptors by yohimbine and rauwolscine. β-Adrenoreceptors are blocked by propranolol. β_1-Adrenoreceptors are somewhat selectively blocked by metoprolol and β_2-receptors somewhat selectively by butoxamine. Dopamine excites a receptor that is blocked by haloperidol; this receptor does not appear to be activated by other adrenergic stimulants. There appear to be four types of dopamine receptors. There are also at least two receptors for histamine, H_1 and H_2.

Sympathomimetics

The abbreviated list of functions affected by sympathetic nerves, shown in Table I, indicates the potential complexity of the pharmacology of the sympathomimetics. It is, in fact, considerably more complex than might be surmised from the table, not only because of the several different receptors with different functions and structure-activity requirements but also because some sympathomimetics do not even act upon these receptors; some act indirectly by releasing norepinephrine from adrenergic nerve terminals. Furthermore, some sympathomimetics can pass through the blood-brain barrier into the central nervous system, where they may elicit a variety of effects, and others may not. Consequently, it is not possible to describe the actions, uses, adverse effects, etc of a prototype sympathomimetic that will apply to all sympathomimetics. The text, below, discusses prototypic actions

rather than prototypic drugs, in order to explain the varied behavior among the sympathomimetics. The dependent uses, adverse effects, and precautions are discussed in relation to the actions, in order that the pharmacodynamic bases of these be better comprehended.

Peripheral Actions and Uses—Not all sympathomimetics are capable of activating all adrenergic and dopaminergic receptors; even among those which are, there is marked variation in the relative intensities of activation of the several receptor types. Thus the natural mediator, dopamine, stimulates dopaminergic receptors strongly, β_1-adrenoreceptors moderately, α-adrenoreceptors weakly, and β_2-adrenoreceptors negligibly. The predominant sympathetic neurotransmitter, norepinephrine, stimulates α_1- and β_1-adrenoreceptors strongly, α_2-adrenoreceptors moderately, β_2-adrenoreceptors weakly and dopaminergic receptors negligibly. Epinephrine stimulates all of the α_1-, α_2-, β_1-, and β_2-adrenoreceptors strongly and dopaminergic receptors negligibly. Obviously, then, the pharmacodynamic profiles of these three natural sympathomimetics differ considerably from one-another. Only a few sympathomimetics act on only a single type of receptor.

α-Adrenoreceptor Agonists—α-Agonists cause arteriolar and venous constriction and hence have an action to increase blood pressure. This vasopressor action is used to *support blood pressure* in hypotensive states, such as in *orthostatic hypotension, carotid sinus syndrome, shock*, and during spinal *anesthesia*. In the treatment of hypovolemic *shock*, the constriction of the capacitance vessels (ie, large veins) increases the venous return to the heart and hence the cardiac output, but once the blood volume is repleted, they may not be necessary. In fact, the use of α-agonists in any kind of shock (except anaphylaxis) is controversial, because there is already ischemia of certain critical organs like the kidney and bowel, and vasoconstriction exacerbates the ischemia in these two organs and contributes to irreversible damage and life-threatening complications. Pancreatic ischemia results in the release of lysosomal enzymes that act upon a plasma substrate to generate a myocardial depressant peptide.

The systemic vasoconstrictor effects are also employed in the management of a variety of serious allergic conditions, such as *giant urticaria, serum sickness, drug reactions, angioneurotic edema*, and *anaphylaxis*. In these uses, epinephrine is the drug of choice. Also, the vasopressor effects of selective α-agonists (ie, devoid of significant β-activity) are sometimes used to elicit compensatory vagal reflexes, which slow the heart and block atrioventricular conduction and hence terminate *paroxysmal atrial* or *nodal tachycardia*.

The α-agonists are applied topically to induce local vasoconstriction in the nasopharyngeal, scleroconjunctival, and otic blood vessels in *vasomotor, rhinitis, acute rhinitis, acute coryza, nasopharyngitis, acute sinusitis, eustachian salpingitis, conjunctivitis, scleritis, hay fever, otitis media, barotitis media*, etc. This use to suppress hyperemia and the related edema is called *decongestion*. Conjunctival and scleral decongestion may relieve irritative *blepharospasm*. α-Agonists that are capable of penetrating the cornea may be used to relieve *uveal congestion*. By inhalation, α-agonists may be used for *bronchial congestion* in allergic, asthmatic, irritative or infectious conditions; relief of bronchiolar edema reduces peribronchiolar tissue turgor and thus enables a greater bronchodilatation. α-Agonists are also applied topically as *styptics* to arrest superficial hemorrhage. Lastly, they may be *combined with local anesthetics;* vasoconstriction keeps the local anesthetic at the injection site for a longer time.

Topically administered α-agonists are used to stimulate the radial smooth muscle of the iris and hence cause *mydriasis* for ophthalmologic examination or to break *posterior synechiae* in uveitis. Their effects on the ciliary body are slight, and they do not cause significant cycloplegia or increase intraocular pressure even in susceptible persons. However, they potentiate the cycloplegic actions of antimuscarinic drugs, with which they are sometimes combined, to enable a lower dose and thus shorten the duration of action of the antimuscarinic mydriatics. In *open-angle glaucoma*, intraocular vasoconstriction causes a decrease in the production of aqueous humor and hence in the intraocular pressure; they are sometimes used in combination with carbonic anhydrase inhibitors in this use.

In sufficient doses, α-agonists contract the trigone muscle and sphincter of the urinary bladder. They also decrease bowel tone. They are not employed for these actions because of the concomitant vasopressor actions; certain indirect or centrally acting sympathomimetics may be used.

The structural requirements for direct α-agonist-activity are a phenylethylamine skeleton to which at least two hydroxyl groups are attached; the optimal positions are ring 3- and sidechain L-2- (or L-β-), but ring 4- and L-β- and ring 3,4-dihydroxy compounds are active.

β_1-*Adrenoreceptor Agonists*—β_1-Agonists increase the heart rate, enhance atrioventricular conduction, and increase the strength of the heart beat (positive inotropic action). They also induce lipolysis and thus increase the concentration of plasma free fatty acids. These effects are achieved, in part, through the activation of the adenyl cyclase system and the intermediation of 3',5'-cyclic adenosine monophosphate (cyclic AMP). In the heart, especially, β_1-agonists also increase calcium ingress and storage, in part the result of mediation by cyclic AMP.

Use is made of the cardiostimulatory effects of β_1-agonists. They may be administered by intracardiac injection to restore the *heart beat* in *cardiac arrest* and *heart block with syncopal seizures* (as in Adams-Stokes syndrome) and by intravenous injection to sustain restored rhythm or to prevent a recurrence of arrests; however, β_1-agonists are not the treatment of choice, and physical and electrical measures take precedence. β_1-Agonists are also sometimes used for their positive inotropic actions in the treatment of *acute heart failure* and in *cardiogenic* or other types of *shock*, in which contractility is often diminished. However, they are somewhat controversial in the treatment of shock, not only because they favor arrhythmias, which are an especial threat in cardiogenic shock, but also because they promote a metabolic acidosis through the lipolytic actions.

β_2-*Adrenoreceptor Agonists*—β_2-Agonists relax smooth muscle and induce hepatic and muscle glycogenolysis, also by activating the adenyl cyclase system and increasing the intracellular levels of cyclic AMP. Thus they dilate the bronchioles, arterioles in vascular beds which are invested with β_2-receptors (such as in skeletal muscle, splanchnic and coronary but not renal or cutaneous beds), and veins, and they relax the uterus and intestines. The glycogenolytic effects in liver and muscle respectively result in hyperglycemia and hyperlactic acidemia. The hyperglycemic actions are sometimes used to treat *insulin overdosage*. At present, there are no "pure" β_2-agonists without some degree of β_1-agonist activity.

Some β_2-agonists are used as bronchodilators in the treatment of *bronchial asthma*, *emphysema*, *bronchitis*, and *bronchiectasis*, often in combination with theophylline. They increase ciliary activity and liquefy tenacious mucus and so have a mild expectorant action. These effects are usually beneficial, but they may cause mucus plugs. Tachyphylaxis to the bronchodilator effects sometimes occurs. In part, this may be due to acidosis, but with isoproterenol it is partly the result of the accumulation of an antagonistic metabolite.

Selective β_2-agonists, when administered by inhalation, may dilate bronchioles with a minimum of hypotensive side effects. However, some degree of cardiostimulation occurs with current drugs. Muscle tremor, by an action on the skeletal muscle fibers, also commonly occurs.

Certain β-agonists may be used as vasodilators in the treatment of peripheral vascular diseases. There are two preconditions for efficacy: (1) the disease process must predominantly have a vasospastic and not obliterative component, and (2) the vessels involved must have an effective population of β_2-receptors. Efficacy is thus essentially limited to selected cases of *intermittent claudication* and *thrombophlebitis*. Some of the presumed selective β_2-agonists for peripheral vascular disease relax vascular smooth muscle partly by a direct smooth muscle depressant mechanism. β_2-Agonists are sometimes promoted on the claim that they increase cerebral blood flow in arteriosclerosis or other cerebrovascular disorders. Although the cerebral vascular resistance may diminish slightly, the peripheral hypotensive effect usually diminishes perfusion pressure, which tends to decrease flow.

The vasodilator β_2-agonists are used in the treatment of *shock*. The splanchnic vasodilatation is beneficial, but there is reflex vasoconstriction in the renal vessels and marked vasodilatation in the muscle vessels, which are unwanted effects. Acidosis is also an adverse effect.

β_2-Agonists may be used to relax the uterus and delay delivery in *premature labor* and to treat *dysmenorrhea*.

The structural requirements for β_1- and β_2-agonist activities are not fully elucidated. An L-β-OH is essential to β_2- and important to β_1-activity. *N*-Alkyl substitution enhances both activities, isopropyl and terbutyl conferring optimal activity. A ring hydroxyl group at the 3- or 4-position is required; the 3-OH appears to be more favorable for β_2- and the 4-OH for β_1-activity, but there are important exceptions. Structural conformation is a key determinant. Since there are differences among β_2-agonists in selectivity for bronchioles and arterioles, there must be different structural requirements of the receptors involved.

Dopaminergic Agonists—Dopamine is the only marketed sympathomimetic with significant dopaminergic actions in the periphery; some sympathomimetics appear to act on dopamine receptors in the central nervous system. In the periphery, dopamine receptors are prominent in the splanchnic and renal vascular beds, where they mediate vasodilatation. Dilatation in these beds is important in the treatment of *shock* and *acute heart failure*, since these beds are often critically constricted in these conditions. Dopamine is used in the management of these disorders. It may also be used to induce diuresis, probably consequent to renal vasodilatation, at least in part.

Combined Agonist Activity—Most sympathomimetics act upon two or more receptor types, and the net effect is the algebraic sum of the α-, β_1-, and β_2-activities, and sometimes dopaminergic and serotoninergic activities as well. In describing the properties of a sympathomimetic, it is necessary to indicate the relative agonist activities in order to understand the overall effects.

Central Nervous System Actions and Uses—The actions of sympathomimetics in the central nervous system are exceedingly complex. Noradrenergic nerves are widely disseminated throughout the central nervous system, and dopaminergic nerves are crucial to some brain functions. Not only are there α-, β-, and dopamine receptors at the synapses, but the actions subserved may be either excitatory or inhibitory at a specific structure, which structure may, in turn, have facilitatory or inhibitory influences on other structures. Furthermore, some sympathomimetics appear to activate serotonin and possibly histamine receptors in the central nervous system. Also, some centrally acting sympathomimetics appear to act as agonists at some loci, antagonists at others, and transmitter-releasing agents at various loci. One drug may thus simultaneously display a number of activities.

The most prominent central nervous effects of centrally acting sympathomimetics are various manifestations of stimulation, which may give rise to nervousness, sleeplessness, hyperactivity, irritability, and increased respiration. In some users they may induce anxiety and in others a kind of euphoria that gives the user a feeling of accomplishment, expectation, and affectations for which some sympathomimetics may be widely abused. They allay the perception but not the reality of fatigue, and users often drive themselves to physical and emotional exhaustion (the "crash"). Large doses can cause hallucinations, and long, continued use may result in paranoia and other dangerous behavior, as well as exhaustion. Tolerance to the euphoric and certain other central actions occurs.

The effects to promote wakefulness are used in the treatment of *narcolepsy*. They are seldom any longer used to treat central nervous depression from overdoses of drugs, although the antagonism of respiratory depression is sometimes dramatic.

The centrally acting sympathomimetics may be beneficial in certain disorders of movement. In *parkinsonism* they often diminish rigidity, relieve oculogyric crises, and improve sleep. They may also provide relief in *spasmodic torticollis*. They also have a beneficial effect on mood in depressive states, but they have been superseded by other drugs. In the *abnormal behavioral syndrome* they have a paradoxical calming effect, but this use is controversial on social grounds.

A very widely used and greatly abused effect is that of the *suppression of appetite* (anorexiant, anorectic, or anorexigenic effect). The drugs may induce temporary weight loss in *exogenous obesity*. However, the weight loss is usually the least in those who need it most and seldom exceeds 10 lb, the effectiveness usually lasts but a few weeks (ie, tolerance develops), and there is danger of abuse; abuse potential varies among the sundry anorexiant drugs. At best, anorexiant drugs should be used only in a training program to condition the patient to new eating habits. Even so, the patient usually eventually resumes his hyperphagic behavior and may even show a rebound-like gain in weight.

Centrally acting sympathomimetics may exert autonomic actions by acting both in the periphery and upon the various autonomic nervous centers in the brain. Stimulants used for their pressor effects usually act in the periphery, but central sympathoadrenal stimulation may augment such effects and may be an important factor in the cardiovascular effects of intoxication. Some centrally acting sympathomimetics are used to *support blood pressure* in the *carotid sinus syndrome* or *orthostatic hypotension;* the oral efficacy and convenient duration of action offer advantages that partially offset disadvantages accruing to central stimulation. Their effects to suppress *urinary incontinence* and *enuresis* mostly derive from their central actions to increase the genitourinary autonomic nervous outflow. They may sometimes relieve the pain of *dysmenorrhea*, probably by central nervous and neuroendocrine mechanisms.

The structural prerequisites for central nervous activity are poorly defined, not only because of the complexities of the actions but also because penetrance through the blood brain barrier is also a key factor. Penetrance imposes the condition of lipid-solubility, which excludes polar molecules like those of the catecholamines. Except for ephedrine, the important centrally acting sympathomimetics are devoid of hydroxyl groups; consequently, they are essentially indirect sympathomimetics.

Indirect Sympathomimetics—Many sympathomimetics do not conform to the structural requirements for adrenergic agonist activity. The aliphatic and cycloaliphatic amine sympathomimetics, for example, deviate greatly from the prerequisite structure. These compounds derive their activity from an action to release norepinephrine from adrenergic nerve terminals, the final action, then, being mediated by norepinephrine. It might be expected that the pharmaco-

dynamics of the indirect sympathomimetics would be identical to those of exogenously administered norepinephrine, which, however, they are not. Firstly, the release from nerve endings may achieve high local concentrations of norepinephrine at the effector site that could not be safely achieved with injected norepinephrine. Thus therapeutic doses of ephedrine cause substantial bronchodilatation, while those of norepinephrine do not. Secondly, release is not everywhere equal. For example, ephedrine releases norepinephrine more effectively in the bronchioles and heart than elsewhere, hence considerable bronchodilatation and cardiostimulation can often be achieved with only mild to moderate vasoconstriction. Also, hydroxyamphetamine fails to release norepinephrine in the skin, although it does in the eye and the heart.

Disposition—Part of the norepinephrine or dopamine that is released from nerve terminals is returned to the interior of the nerve by a membrane transport system. This provides the principal means by which the action of adrenergic neurotransmitters is terminated. Neuronal uptake also assists in the termination of the action of small doses of exogenous norepinephrine. However, the predominant route of elimination in the periphery is O-methylation at the ring 3-OH group by the enzyme, catechol-O-methyltransferase (COMT). COMT is found throughout the peripheral tissues but is quite active in the liver. Other catecholamines, and, to a lesser extent, 3-OH monophenolic amines are also O-methylated. Ring hydroxyl groups are also conjugated in the liver. In the brain, both norepinephrine and dopamine are mostly eliminated by the mitochondrial enzyme, monoamine oxidase (MAO). In the periphery, MAO is not important to the elimination of catecholamines but is important to that of noncatecholic arylethylamines. The presence of sidechain substituents, as in ephedrine and amphetamine, renders the sympathomimetic amines resistant to oxidative deamination by MAO. Such drugs do, however, inhibit MAO.

By the oral route, a sympathomimetic must run the gamut of MAO, COMT and conjugases in the intestinal wall and liver. Sympathomimetics that are good substrates for these enzymes are ineffective or erratic orally. Most noncatecholamines are also oxidized by the cytochrome P450 system in the liver.

Adverse Effects, Precautions, and Contraindications—The multiple activities of sympathomimetics make for numerous side effects. Some of these, such as reflex homeostatic adjustments, which act to counter an effect or the elicitation of simultaneous physiologically antagonistic effects, are counterproductive but are not necessarily adverse. However, some reflex effects may be adverse, such as the prolonged reflex renal vasoconstriction that accrues to the use of isoproterenol infusion in shock. Some side effects, such as substernal pain, occur only in patients with a particular disease and indicate an adverse effect only in such patients.

The manufacturer's literature (package literature, *Physicians' Desk Reference*, etc) tends to list for each sympathomimetic drug all the collective side effects and contraindications of all sympathomimetics, without regard to the individual properties. In the discussion below, the adverse effects are enumerated according to the type of activity. For drugs with multiple activities, it will be necessary for the reader to synthesize the profile of adverse effects and contraindications from the component activities. However, certain precautions apply to all sympathomimetics, namely that elderly persons, infants and persons with thyrotoxicosis tend to be more sensitive to sympathomimetics, and that adverse effects of one kind or another are much more probable in persons with cardiovascular disease.

α_1-*Agonists*—One important adverse effect of *systemically* administered α_1-agonists is an excessive increase in blood pressure. In persons with weak or atheromatous blood vessels, a cerebrovascular accident (eg, stroke), coronary occlusion, aneurysm, or other serious event may occur. The heart works harder against the increased pressure, which may induce an attack of angina pectoris or precipitate or aggravate heart failure. *Hypertensive* or *elderly persons* may show an exaggerated pressor response. Vagal reflexes to the pressor response may cause bradycardia and various degrees of atrioventricular conduction block; the disturbed electrophysiology and myocardial stretch (the heart enlarges to work against the increased pressure) favor various serious cardiac arrhythmias in persons with certain types of heart damage. Therefore, except under the most careful medical supervision, α-agonists are contraindicated in persons with *hypertension*, *coronary heart disease*, *arteriosclerosis*, *atherosclerosis*, *diabetes* (because of vascular pathology), *cardiac arrhythmias*, or a history of *myocardial infarction*. They are also contraindicated in *venous thrombosis*, because venospasm may not only exacerbate the thrombosis but also may initiate thromboembolism.

The possible adverse effects of α_1-agonists in shock were mentioned under *Actions and Uses*. Prolonged infusion of some sympathomimetics can occasionally cause shock. Extravasation of α-agonists during intravenous administration may result in a slough; sometimes phentolamine is included in the solution to antagonize the perivascular vasoconstriction. Uterine and placental vasoconstriction in *pregnancy* may harm the fetus. α_1-Agonists interfere with *lactation*. Signs and symptoms of a strong vasoconstrictor effect are bradycardia with a strong pulse, occasional tingling in the extremities, headache and sometimes anxiety, which results from the enteroceptive detection of the altered cardiovascular status and other autonomic disturbances.

Other systemic side effects of α-agonists include mydriasis and photophobia (if the drug can penetrate into the eye), sweating, piloerection, and occasionally nausea and vomiting. Increased tension in the trigone muscle and urethral contraction may create a desire to urinate, but urination may be difficult; α-agonists should be used cautiously in elderly men, especially those with *prostatic hypertrophy*.

Adverse effects of α-agonists *applied topically* to the eye include photophobia (from mydriasis), browache, ocular pain, headache, aftercongestion, especially during chronic use, rebound miosis after the adrenergic effects wear off, floating opacities, and scleroconjunctival and especially corneal chemosis. Prolonged use, especially of epinephrine, may cause pigmentation in the cornea, conjunctiva and lids. Intense intraocular vasoconstriction can damage the retina; especial care must be exercised when there is no lens. Ophthalmologic sympathomimetics should be used cautiously when there is *retinal detachment* or before cataract surgery, because of possible rebound miosis. In *narrow-angle glaucoma*, mydriasis may close the angle sufficiently to increase the intraocular pressure. Adverse effects that may occur after topical application to the nasopharynx include aftercongestion and chemical rhinitis, with sneezing. Enough sympathomimetic may be absorbed after either conjunctival or nasopharyngeal application to cause serious hypertensive episodes in patients; *blood pressures of over 200 mm Hg are frequently observed in infants and small children*. Therefore, the precautions and contraindications that apply to systemic use also apply to topical use.

β_1-*Agonists*—The side effects of β-agonists with strong β_1-activity are tachycardia and palpitation. Substernal distress may occur if there is coronary heart disease, because tachycardia and a decrease in the efficiency of oxygen utilization increase the myocardial oxygen demand. There may also be premature atrial and ventricular contractions and tachyarrhythmias. The degree of vasodepression depends upon the degree of concomitant β_2-activity; with isoproterenol, there is usually diastolic hypotension and often systolic hypertension, with a net increase or decrease in blood pressure.

Because of the cardiostimulant effects, β_1-agonists are contraindicated in *coronary heart disease* and when there are *arrhythmias*. They are also contraindicated in *thyrotoxicosis*, because the heart is hyperreactive to adrenergic influences and may even already be in tachycardia. The potential detrimental consequences of the lipolytic effects have already

been mentioned. β_1-Agonists in high concentration can occasionally cause myocardial necrosis; this warrants caution after *coronary occlusion*. Myocardial necrosis may possibly occur after inhalation of β_1-agonists. An interesting adverse effect of β_1-agonist activity in chronic *obstructive pulmonary disease* is that of an increased perfusion of the nonfunctioning portions of the lungs (consequent to the increased cardiac output), which results in a decrease in mixed pulmonary venous oxygen saturation (pO_2).

β_2-*Agonists*—Because some β_2-agonists decrease the blood pressure, they cause reflex tachycardia and palpitation. Consequently, they must be used cautiously in the same cardiovascular diseases as must the β_1-agonists. When β_2-agonists are administered by inhalation, especially, pulmonary vasodilatation may cause shunting of blood and uneven circulation of the lung, which may have an effect to sometimes lower the mixed pulmonary venous pO_2 similar to that of β_1-agonists, above, despite the decrease in airway resistance. Also, pulmonary vasodilation favors peribronchiolar edema, which is counterproductive, and an α-agonist may be coadministered to antagonize the pulmonary vasodilation. Tolerance to the bronchodilator effects not only may occur, especially with high doses, but a rebound increase in airway resistance often occurs as the β_2-effects decline. Although β_2-agonists have a mild expectorant effect, they increase mucus secretion and may occasionally cause the development of mucus plugs.

When Freon-propelled inhalation aerosols of β-agonist bronchodilators were introduced, there was a sudden increase in the occurrence of both tolerance and sudden deaths. The development of metered sprays and a return to nebulization has reduced the incidence of such deaths. The deaths have been attributed to a combination of causes: a cardiotoxic effect of the propellant, an effect of the propellant (which may be regarded as a chlorocarbon) to sensitize the heart to the arrhythmiagenic effects of the component β_1-agonist activity of the bronchodilators (since the deaths mainly occurred with those agonists with combined β_1- and β_2-activity), and the ease of administration and hence ease of overdosing. Despite the improved safety of metered aerosols, it is important to stress the importance of waiting a few minutes between closely consecutive inhalations and of not exceeding the recommended frequency of dosing.

The hyperglycemic effects of β_2-agonists impose precautions when they are used in *diabetes*, and the increased metabolic rate requires caution in *thyrotoxicosis*. The detrimental effects of lactic acidosis in shock have been mentioned under *Actions and Uses*. Local and systemic acidosis from β_2-agonists decreases the bronchodilator response. β_2-Agonists may cause tremor, vertigo, and insomnia.

Both β_1- and β_2-agonists occasionally cause sweating, headache, and nausea and vomiting, probably indirectly the result of other effects. They may also cause anxiety, perhaps from central actions. The effects of β-agonists are unknown, and they should be avoided, if possible, in pregnancy.

Centrally Acting Sympathomimetics—Because these drugs may act both centrally and peripherally to stimulate the heart and to cause vasoconstriction, the same precautions that apply to systemic α- and β_1-agonists, both, should be observed. With central nervous therapeutic doses of the amphetamines, these cardiovascular side effects are often of a low order, but they may be a cause of death in intoxication. Centrally acting sympathomimetics must be used cautiously in the presence of *prostatic hypertrophy*. Other autonomic nervous system-mediated side effects include mydriasis, dry mouth, flushing, sweating, diarrhea, and impotence. Because of mydriasis, these drugs are contraindicated in *narrow-angle glaucoma*. Nausea, vomiting, and tremors are probably mostly of central nervous origin. With excessive doses, there may be hyperthermia, as the result of a combination of increased metabolic rate, increased physical activity, and vasoconstriction. They are contraindicated in *thyrotoxicosis*. Because of an increased sympathetic outflow to the liver hyperglycemia occasionally occurs; this and the increase in physical activity may change the insulin requirement in *diabetes*.

Relatively frequent central nervous side effects include restlessness, insomnia, agitation, and anorexia. REM sleep is disturbed. Dysphoria occurs in some persons. There is also sometimes headache, dizziness and dyskinesias. Respiratory stimulation may result in hyperventilation; this may precipitate absence seizures in persons with *petit mal*. There may be changes in libido as the result of changes in both endocrine and sympathetic nervous systems. When the centrally acting sympathomimetics are used chronically in children, endocrine disturbances may arrest growth; growth usually rebounds after discontinuation. The anxiety and psychotic states that occur after long, continued use and the potential for drug abuse have been mentioned. These drugs are especially contraindicated when there is a *history of drug abuse*, a state of *agitation* or in *pregnancy*. They are also contraindicated in *porphyria*.

All sympathomimetics can cause allergic reactions of various types, but they are more frequent with those that have polar moieties in the structure. Contact dermatitis especially, may occur from topical use. A history of *previous allergic reactions* to a particular or similar sympathomimetic contraindicates its use.

Drug Interactions—α-Agonists must not be given along with other *vasoconstrictor drugs*. Sympathomimetics with β_1-activity when used in the presence of *cardiac glycosides* may precipitate dangerous tachyarrhythmias. A hypertensive response to an α-agonist causes a vagal reflex which may combine with the action of a cardiac glycoside to increase heart block. Furthermore, cardiac glycosides themselves have vasoconstrictor actions, which not only may increase the hypertensive response to an α-agonist but the combined action may also result in bowel infarction, especially in the elderly. *Cyclopropane* and *chlorocarbon ether anesthetics* sensitize the heart to the arrhythmiagenic effects of β_1-agonists.

Since *reserpine* and *guanethidine*, respectively, deplete and prevent the release of norepinephrine from adrenergic nerve terminals, they tend to prevent the indirect sympathomimetics from acting. By a sort of chemical denervation supersensitivity, reserpine moderately and guanethidine and *methylphenidate* markedly increase the responses to direct sympathomimetics, especially norepinephrine and metaraminol. Dextroamphetamine and methamphetamine, and to a lesser extent other centrally acting sympathomimetics may hasten the offset of action of guanethidine.

Monoamine oxidase inhibitors (MAOI) increase the peripheral effects of noncatecholamine sympathomimetics which do not have substituents in the α-position; the effect is greater with primary than with secondary amines. MAOI also cause centrally acting sympathomimetics to evoke bizarre behavior. The use of MAOI should be discontinued two weeks in advance of the use of an interacting sympathomimetic. Like guanethidine and methylphenidate, *tricyclic antidepressants* (TCAD) block the neuronal reuptake system for catecholamines and metaraminol, and they may potentiate the peripheral actions of these drugs and the central actions of some centrally acting sympathomimetics. Although only certain sympathomimetics are affected by MAOI and TCAD, the manufacturer's and medical literature usually do not discriminate; in the absence of specific intelligence to the contrary, the reader should assume that the precautions apply to any sympathomimetic of interest.

Theophylline synergizes the β_1- and β_2- and centrally acting sympathomimetics, and should be used in combination with them only when there is a special rationale, as in asthma. Because certain *oxytocic* drugs (especially ergot alkaloids)

have vasoconstrictor actions, α-agonists and oxytocics should not be given together. β_2-Agonists relax the uterus and hence antagonize oxytocics. Some *ganglionic blocking drugs* increase the vasoconstrictor responses to α-agonists, and α-agonists and indirect sympathomimetics should be used cautiously during ganglionic blockade. *Mercurial diuretics* favor cardiac arrhythmias, so that β_1-agonist indirect and centrally acting sympathomimetics should not be given when such diuretics are in use. Systemic *carbonic anhydrase inhibitors* cause metabolic acidosis, which diminishes the responses to β_1- and β_2-agonists, especially. *Thyroxine, liothyronine*, etc. have the same effect as thyrotoxicosis to enhance the responses to the β_1- and β_2-agonists, especially, and to increase the basal metabolic effects of centrally acting sympathomimetics. *Central nervous stimulants* and centrally acting sympathomimetics should not be given at the same time; central stimulants may exacerbate anxiety, tremor, nausea and vomiting.

α-Adrenergic blocking agents, such as *phenoxybenzamine, prazosin*, and *phentolamine*, antagonize the α-agonists; if a sympathomimetics also has β_2-activity, the usual pressor response will be reversed to a depressor response. Large doses of *chlorpromazine* have the same effect. Chlorpromazine will also suppress some of the central nervous effects of sympathomimetics. *β-Adrenoreceptor blocking drugs*, such as propranolol, will suppress the actions of both β_1- and β_2-agonists. *Haloperidol* and related drugs will antagonize the vasodilator effects of dopamine and alter the central actions of some sympathomimetics.

Bromocriptine—page 929.

Albuterol Sulfate

1,3-Benzenedimethanol,
α^1-[[(dimethylethyl)amino]methyl]-4-hydroxy-, sulfate (2:1) (salt);
Proventil (*Schering-Plough*); Ventolin (*Glaxo*)

α^1-[(*tert*-Butylamino)methyl]-4-hydroxy-*m*-xylene-α,α'-diol,
sulfate (2:1) (salt) [51022-70-9] $(C_{13}H_{21}NO_3)_2 \cdot H_2SO_4$ (576.70).
Preparation—Refer to *J Med Chem 13:* 674, 1970.

Description—Off-white to white, crystalline powder; odorless; slightly bitter taste.
Solubility—One g dissolves in 4 mL of water; slightly soluble in alcohol, chloroform, and ether.

Uses—Albuterol has strong β_2- weak β_1- and no α-adrenergic agonist activity. It is used only as a *bronchodilator*. Many pulmonary specialists consider it to be the drug of choice in the treatment of *bronchospasm* in patients with reversible obstructive airway disease, such as bronchial asthma. Its side effects, contraindications and drug-interactions are those of β_2-agonists in general (see general statement); however, tremor is rare.

The half-life of albuterol is about 4 hr. By inhalation, the duration of action is 3 to 6 hr. The time of peak effect is 60 to 90 min. By the oral route, the duration of action is 4 to 8 hr.

Dose—*Oral, adults* and *children over 12 yr* or *60 lb*, **initially, 2** or **4 mg** 3 or 4 times a day, except only **2 mg** in elderly persons, to be cautiously increased to 8 mg/dose, if necessary, up to a total of 32 mg/day. *Oral inhalation, adults* and *children over 12 yr of age*, **90** or **180 µg** (**1** or **2 inhalations**) every 4 to 6 hr; dose for children under 12 yr has not been determined.
Dosage Forms—Metered Inhalation Aerosol: 17 g (90 µg per actuation); Tablets: 2 and 4 mg.

Dextroamphetamine Sulfate

Benzeneethanamine, α-methyl-, (*S*)-, sulfate (2:1); Dexamphetamine
Sulfate; *d*-1-Phenyl-2-aminopropane Sulfate;
Dexedrine Sulfate (*Smith Kline & French*)

(+)-α-Methylphenethylamine sulfate (2:1) [51-63-8]
$(C_9H_{13}N)_2.H_2SO_4$ (368.49).

Preparation—Analogous to *Dextroamphetamine Phosphate.*

Description—White, odorless, crystalline powder; pH (1 in 20 solution) between 5 and 6; specific rotation (4% aqueous solution of a dried sample) between +20° and +23.5°.

Solubility—1 g in about 10 mL water and about 800 mL alcohol; insoluble in ether.

Uses—Amphetamine is an *indirectly-acting sympathomimetic* with weak peripheral but strong central nervous system stimulant actions. As a central stimulant, the dextrorotatory isomer is approximately twice as potent as the racemic mixture (amphetamine) and 3 to 4 times as potent as the levorotatory isomer.

The approved uses are essentially limited to the treatment of *narcolepsy* and the *abnormal behavioral syndrome.* FDA approval of use as an anorexiant in the treatment of exogenous obesity will probably be rescinded shortly in favor of anorexiants with weaker euphoria and less rapidly developing tolerance.

Dextroamphetamine is addicting and is widely abused. It has been estimated that at the peak of the drug problem in the US nearly one-half of the dextroamphetamine manufactured in the US was being used illegally. During chronic abuse, tolerance to the euphoric effects may be as much as 25-fold, so that enormous quantities are used. With such high doses, repetitive, nonproductive activity and hallucinatory and paranoic psychoses are common.

The adverse effects of dextroamphetamine are those of the centrally acting sympathomimetics in general (see the general statement).

Dose—*Oral*, for *narcolepsy: adults*, 5 to 20 mg 1 to 3 times a day, *except* 5 to 30 mg once a day with *sustained-release* capsules; *children 6 to 12 yr* of age, 2.5 mg, twice a day (to be increased by increments of 5 mg at weekly intervals until the desired wakefulness is achieved), *except* 5 to 15 mg once a day with *sustained-release* capsules; *over 12 yr* of age, 5 mg once or twice a day (to be increased by increment of 10 mg at weekly intervals until the desired effect is achieved), *except* 10 or 25 mg once a day with *extended release* capsules. For *abnormal behavioral syndrome: children 3 to 6 yr* of age, 2.5 mg once a day (increased by increments of 2.5 mg at weekly intervals until the desired effect is achieved); *over 6 years* of age, 5 mg once or twice a day (increased by increments of 5 mg at weekly intervals until the desired effect is achieved), *except* 5 to 15 mg once a day with sustained-release capsules.

Sustained-release capsules are not to be used to initiate treatment and should not be substituted for conventional dose forms until the daily dose of the conventional form is equal to or exceeds the dosage provided by the sustained-release capsules.

Dosage Forms—Sustained-Release Capsules: 5, 10 and 15 mg; Elixir: 5 mg/5 mL; Tablets: 5 and 10 mg.

Dobutamine Hydrochloride

1,2-Benzenediol, 4-[2-[[3-(4-hydroxyphenyl)-1-methylpropyl]amino]-ethyl]-, hydrochloride, (±)-, Dobutrex (*Lilly*)

(±)-4-[2-[[3-(*p*-Hydroxyphenyl)-1-methylpropyl]amino]ethyl]-pyrocatechol hydrochloride [49745-95-1] $C_{18}H_{23}NO_3 \cdot HCl$ (337.85).

Preparation—For a summary of a patented process see *CA 80:* 14721z, 1974.

Description—White to off-white powder; melts at about 185°; pK_a (dobutamine) 9.4.

Solubility—Sparingly soluble in water, alcohol.

Uses—Dobutamine has strong β_1- and weak β_2- and α-adrenoreceptor agonist activity. Its positive inotropic actions and effects to enhance atrioventricular and intraventricular conduction are more prominent than its positive chronotropic effects, so that with appropriately low doses (ie, less than 20 μg/kg/min) it increases cardiac output considerably but affects heart rate only slightly. Heart rate is usually increased by only 5 to 15 beats/min, and an increase of more than 30/min occurs in only 10% of patients. Higher rates of infusion

can cause substantial tachycardia. The net effect of β_2- and α-adrenergic vascular actions is usually a slight decrease in peripheral resistance. However, the increase in cardiac output approximately compensates for decreased peripheral resistance, so that blood pressure is mildly affected, tending to increase slightly with low, and decrease slightly with high, doses. In clinical use, arterial pressure usually rises only 10 to 20 torr and rises by as much as 50 torr in only 7.5% of patients. Tachyphylaxis to the actions on cardiac output usually does not occur, but there is sometimes a slight diminution in response.

The principal clinical use is in the short-term treatment of *low output acute heart failure*, such as that after myocardial infarction or after cardiopulmonary bypass surgery. In heart failure the drug increases cardiac output, decreases pulmonary artery wedge pressure and increases urine output. It more consistently lowers pulmonary artery wedge pressure than does dopamine, but it less consistently causes diuresis.

Dobutamine is very rapidly biotransformed, mainly by catechol-*O*-methyltransferase, although some is also conjugated. The elimination half-life is only 2 min, so that the drug must be given by continuous intravenous infusion. After infusion is begun, the onset of action is 1 to 2 min; the effect requires 5 to 10 min to reach a steady state (plateau).

Dobutamine has been given safely in infusions lasting as long as 72 hr. Adverse effects other than usually mild hypertension and tachyardia (see above) occur in only 1 to 3% of patients. They include nausea, headache, palpitation, shortness of breath, anginal pain and nonspecific chest pain. Occasionally there is ectopic activity, mainly premature atrial and ventricular beats; other arrhythmias can occur. Because of facilitated AV conduction, the ventricular rate may be adversely increased in atrial fibrillation or flutter, and digitalis should be administered prior to dobutamine. The drug is contraindicated in idiopathic hypertropic subaortic stenosis. Thus far, few drug interactions are known. β-Adrenoreceptor-blocking drugs abolish the cardiac and vasodilator actions and unmask the vasoconstrictor effects. Sodium nitroprusside (and presumably any other vasodilator that substantially decreases cardiac afterload) enables a greater increase in cardiac output and decrease in pulmonary arterial wedge pressure. Neither reserpine nor tricyclic antidepressants affect the response to dobutamine. The safety of the drug in children is unknown.

Dose—*Intravenous, infusion, adult*, usually 2.5 to 10 μg/kg/min, but occasionally as much as 40 μg/kg/min is required.

Dosage Form—For Injection: 250 mg/20 mL.

Dopamine Hydrochloride

1,2-Benzenediol, 4-(2-aminoethyl-, hydrochloride;
Intropin (*Arnar-Stone*)

3,4-Dihydroxyphenethylamine Hydrochloride [62-31-7] $C_8H_{11}NO_2.HCl$ (189.64).

Preparation—Dopamine, which is 3-hydroxytyramine, may be prepared from tyramine by successive nitration to 3-nitrotyramine, reduction to 3-aminotyramine by catalytic hydrogenation, and diazotization to 3-hydroxytyramine.

Description—Dopamine hydrochloride occurs as a white, crystalline powder; decomposes at about 241°. To avoid oxidation of dopamine hydrochloride injection the air in containers is replaced with nitrogen. Yellow or brown discoloration of solutions indicates decomposition of the drug, and such solutions should not be used.

Solubility—Freely soluble in water; soluble in alcohol; practically insoluble in chloroform and ether.

Uses—Dopamine is a natural catecholamine formed by the decarboxylation of 3,4-dihydroxyphenylalanine (DOPA). It is a precursor to norepinephrine in noradrenergic nerves and is also a neurotransmitter in certain areas of the central nervous system, especially in the nigrostriatal tract, and in a few peripheral sympathetic nerves.

In the central nervous system and the splanchnic and renal vascular beds, it acts upon dopamine receptors that are distinct from α- and β-adrenoreceptors. At these dopamine receptors, haloperidol is an antagonist. In the above-named vascular beds it causes vasodilatation. The renal vasodilatation causes diuresis. Dopamine also has moderate β_1- and weak α-agonist activities, part of which is attributable to norepinephrine released by dopamine. During a low rate of intravenous infusion, only vasodilatation in the splanchnic and renal vascular beds usually predominates, and hypotension sometimes occurs. At an intermediate rate of infusion, the heart rate and force of contraction are increased, as is cardiac output, and blood pressure may increase accordingly. At high rates of infusion, α-adrenoreceptor-mediated vasoconstriction occurs, and the blood pressure may rise substantially; in contrast to other vasoconstrictor catecholamines, the skeletal muscle arterioles are well constricted. The α-adrenergic vasoconstriction in the splanchnic and renal vascular beds may overcome the dopaminergic vasodilatation in some recipients.

Dopamine is used in the treatment of *shock*, for which it has several advantages. Firstly, vasodilatation can often be effected in the two organs most likely to suffer ischemic damage in shock (kidney and small bowel); blood may be moved from the skeletal muscle to more vital organs, cardiac stimulation improves a usually deteriorated cardiac function, and diuresis also helps to preserve the renal tubules. Although dopamine is now the vasopressor agent of choice in shock, a substantial fraction of cases nevertheless fail to respond. Dopamine is also used to treat *acute heart failure;* the decreased vascular resistance decreases the cardiac afterload, the cardiostimulatory actions improve cardiac output, and the diuresis lessens edema.

The adverse effects, precautions, and drug interactions of dopamine are those expected from a β_1- and α-agonist (see the general statement). Hypotension, when it occurs, is not necessarily adverse, so long as the critical organs are adequately perfused. It can usually be counteracted by increasing the rate of infusion; if not, another pressor agent will be required. Haloperidol-like drugs suppress the vasodilator actions. Dopamine also causes nausea by a dopaminergic action at the chemoreceptor trigger zone.

The onset of action of dopamine following intravenous administration occurs within 5 min, and the duration of action is less than 10 min, but in patients receiving MAO inhibitors the duration of action may be prolonged to 1 hour.

Dose—*Intravenous infusion, initially* **0.5 to 5 µg per kg** of body weight per min, to be increased at 10- to 30-min intervals until the desired blood pressure is achieved; the effective rate usually does not exceed 15 µg per kg per min, but more than 50 µg/kg/min are occasionally required; if so, urine output should be monitored. The safety and efficacy of this drug in children has not been established.

Dosage Forms—For injection: 0.8, 1.6, 40, 80 and 160 mg/mL.

Ephedrine Sulfate

Benzenemethanol, α-[1-(methylamino)ethyl]-, [R-(R*,S*)]-, sulfate (2:1) (salt)

(−)-Ephedrine sulfate (2:1) (salt) [134-72-5] $(C_{10}H_{15}NO)_2.H_2SO_4$ (428.54).

Preparation—First obtained by Nagai in 1887 from a Chinese herb, *ma huang*, ephedrine is structurally related to epinephrine. Ephedrine may be obtained by alkalinizing powdered *ma huang* with milk of lime or sodium carbonate solution, and extracting the base with alcohol or benzene. It is now, however, almost exclusively produced by synthetic methods. The most economic process (Neuberg) for synthetic production commences with fermentation of a mixture of benzaldehyde and molasses to form the ketoalcohol, $C_6H_5CH(OH)COCH_3$, which is hydrogenated in a methylamine solution. The keto group is thereby reduced to —CHOH— which condenses with the methylamine.

Description—Fine, white, odorless crystals or a powder; affected by light, and its aqueous solution is practically neutral to litmus; rotation −30.5° to −32.5°.

Solubility—1 g in about 1.3 mL water and about 90 mL alcohol; insoluble in ether.

Incompatibilities—See *Ephedrine Hydrochloride.*

Uses—In ordinary doses ephedrine acts *indirectly* through release of norepinephrine from adrenergic nerves. In higher doses it has a direct sympathomimetic action. It penetrates membranes and into the brain, and hence has central nervous actions, which, however, are not as prominent as those of the amphetamines.

Although ephedrine mainly acts indirectly through the release of norepinephrine, its peripheral effects are as though it possessed weak α-agonist activity, except that it acts rather strongly on the trigone sphincter, and has moderate β_1- and β_2-agonist activity, except that the β_2-activity being limited to the bronchioles; its weak hyperglycemic effect results mainly from central nervous actions. Its uses have been all of those described in the general statement, except for those dependent on a vasodilator action. However, some actions and uses are more outstanding than others and deserve special mention. Its most important use has been that as a *bronchodilator*, for which its oral efficacy has special advantages; however, albuterol and other more selective, orally effective bronchodilators threaten to make ephedrine obsolete in this use. It will continue to be useful in the nonemergency, outpatient treatment of Adams-Stokes syndrome. It is occasionally used to treat *enuresis*. The weak vascular α-activity may actually have some advantages in the support of blood pressure during spinal anesthesia and in other non-shock hypotensions, since the weak vasoconstrictor effects may result in less ischemic damage than with stronger α-agonists; the moderate cardiac stimulation is beneficial. The weak vasoconstrictor effects also lend themselves to the ambulatory management of various *allergic conditions*, ephedrine being safer to use than stronger α-agonists; in allergic emergencies, it is inferior to epinephrine. As a topical decongestant it is not widely used, but it has the advantage of only slight after-congestion. It is no longer used as a mydriatic drug. Ephedrine has had an interesting use in the treatment of *myasthenia gravis*, in which disease it appears to improve muscular function by increasing the release of acetylcholine at the neuromuscular junction. The only central nervous use of importance is in the treatment of *narcolepsy*. However, ephedrine is used in various drug combinations with central depressants to counteract sedative effects. Also, sedatives may be included in ephedrine preparations to antagonize the central stimulant effects of ephedrine.

Ephedrine is resistant to monoamine oxidase (MAO) and is thus orally efficacious. By the oral route, its duration of action is 2 to 3 hours. The half-life is about 6 hours, but when the urine is alkaline it is longer, and, when acidic, it is shorter. Although it is not a substrate of MAO, it is said that MAO inhibitors may cause a hypertensive crisis in response to otherwise safe doses; therefore, caution is indicated. For other potential adverse effects and precautions, see the general statement.

As a rule, salts of ephedrine are employed instead of the free base.

Dose—*Oral, adults*, **25 to 50 mg** every 3 to 4 hours; *corrective for sedative effects* of antihistamines or anticonvulsants, **10 to 25 mg** every 3 to 4 hours, *except* **15 to 60 mg** every 8 to 12 hr with *extended-release* capsules; *children*, **500 µg/kg** (or **16.7 mg/m²** of body surface) every 4 to 6 hr, *except* **15 to 30 mg** every 8 to 12 hr with *extended-release* capsules. *Intravenous, adults*, **5 to 25 mg** *slowly*, repeated in 5 to 10 min, if necessary, up to a limit of 150 mg/day. *Intramuscular* or *subcutaneous, adults*, **25 to 50 mg**, repeated, if necessary, up to a limit of 150 mg/day; *children*, **500 µg/kg** (or **16.7 mg/m²**) every 4 to 6 hr. *Topical, intranasal, adults* and *children over 6 years* of age, **2 to 3 drops** of a 0.5 to 3% solution or a **small amount** of 0.6% jelly into each nostril 2 or 3 times a day.

Dosage Forms—Capsules: 25 and 50 mg; Injection: 25 and 50 mg/mL: Topical Jelly: 0.6%; Topical Solution: 0.5, 1 and 3%; Syrup: 11 and 20 mg/5 mL; Tablets: 7.5 mg (with 0.15 mg Atropine Sulfate).

Epinephrine

1,2-Benzenediol, 4-[1-hydroxy-2-(methylamino)ethyl]-, (R)-, Adrenaline; Suprarenalin; Nephridine; Adrenalin (*Parke-Davis*); (*Various Mfrs*)

(−)-3,4-Dihydroxy-α-[(methylamino)methyl]benzyl alcohol [51-43-4] $C_9H_{13}NO_3$ (183.21).

Preparation—Epinephrine may be synthesized by several processes. One of these starts with catechol (1,2-dihydroxybenzene), which is successively converted to (chloroacetyl)catechol with chloroacetyl chloride, then to (methylaminoacetyl)catechol with methylamine, and to racemic epinephrine by hydrogenation. The racemic form is resolved with D-tartaric acid.

Description—White to nearly white, microcrystalline, odorless powder, gradually darkening on exposure to light and air; combines with acids, forming salts that are readily soluble in water, and from these solutions the base may be precipitated by ammonia water or by alkali carbonates; solutions are alkaline to litmus; pK_a (apparent) 5.5.

Solubility—Very slightly soluble in water and in alcohol; insoluble in ether, chloroform, and fixed and volatile oils.

Incompatibilities—Solutions are usually prepared with the aid of HCl and an acid reaction is essential to the stability of such solutions not only because of possible precipitation but also because of the possibility of rapid oxidation to inert products. Oxidation is generally evidenced by development of a pink to brown color. Air, light, heat, and alkalies promote deterioration. Solutions buffered to a pH of 4.2 and containing a suitable antioxidant such as 0.1% sodium metabisulfite are stable for prolonged periods of time if protected from light, heat, and undue exposure to air. *Metals*, notably *copper*, *iron*, and *zinc*, destroy its activity.

Uses—Epinephrine is the predominant sympathomimetic in the adrenal medulla. It is liberated in conditions of stress and vigorous exertion. It possesses all of strong α_1-, α_2-, β_1-, and β_2-agonist activities (see the general statement). The β-adrenoreceptors respond to lower concentrations than the α-receptors, so that with low doses or low intravenous infusion rates it is possible to stimulate the heart and relax bronchioles and at the same time decrease the diastolic blood pressure; however, the vasoconstrictor effect is stronger than the vasodilator effect, so that at higher doses there is a net increase in vascular resistance, and extreme hypertensive crises can occur with overdoses. The uses are those of α- and β-agonists (see the general statement). Only the outstanding uses and failures require comment here.

Epinephrine is the drug of choice in the management of allergic emergencies, such as *anaphylaxis*, *angioneurotic edema*, *giant urticaria* and *serum sickness*. Despite new selective β_2-bronchodilators, epinephrine remains the drug of choice in the treatment of *status asthmaticus;* the vasoconstrictor activity assists the bronchodilator actions through a reduction in bronchiolar stiffness by decreasing edema and by diminishing bronchiolar secretions, and α_2-agonist activity suppresses vagal activity in the bronchioles. In chronic use as a bronchodilator, refractoriness often develops. Epinephrine has a poor record in the treatment of shock (very intense splanchnic and renal vasoconstriction and metabolic acidosis), and in general should not be used to support blood pressure. As a topical decongestant it causes too much aftercongestion to be a first-line drug. In *cardiac arrest*, epinephrine is an excellent resuscitant, but the concomitant vasoconstriction places an unwanted load on a compromised heart. It penetrates into the eye poorly from both blood stream and cornea, but high concentrations may be used to decrease the formation of the aqueous humor in *primary open-angle glaucoma;* it is used often in combination with a miotic and a carbonic anhydrase inhibitor. It is an excellent *styptic* because of both its local vasoconstrictor effects and the coagulant effects of its oxidation product, adrenochrome.

The adverse effects of epinephrine are those of a strong α-, β_1- and β_2-agonist (see general statement).

Orally administered epinephrine is destroyed by monoamine oxidase, catechol-O-methyltransferase, and is conjugated during its passage through the liver; consequently, oral dosage is ineffective. The plasma half-life of epinephrine is about 2.5 min. However, by the subcutaneous and intramuscular routes, local vasoconstriction retards absorption, so that the effects last much longer than the half-life would predict.

Note: Do not use any epinephrine dosage form if it is brown or pink in color or contains a precipitate; a hallucinatory reaction may occur.

Dose—*Intravenous, adult,* **100 μg** to **250 μg** of the diluted injection *slowly* for *vasopression*, repeated at 5- to 15-min intervals as needed, or **100 μg** to **1 mg** for *anaphylaxis* or *cardiac stimulation; children,* for *cardiac stimulation,* **5** to **10 μg per kg** of body weight (or **150** to **300 μg per m²** of body surface), and, for *anaphylaxis,* **300 μg** repeated at 15-min intervals for 3 or 4 doses, if necessary. *Intramuscular, adult, for anaphylaxis,* **200** to **500 μg** followed by 25 to 50 μg intravenously every 5 to 15 min, as needed, and, for *hypoglycemia* **300 μg** once; *children,* **300 μg**, repeated every 15 min for 3 or 4 doses, as needed, and for hypoglycemia, **10 μg per kg** (or 300 μg per m²) **200 μg** (0.2 mg) to **1 mg**, repeated as needed. *Intramuscular, in oil, adult,* **1** to **3 mg** in a 0.2% sterile oil suspension, repeated as needed; the duration of action may be 4 to 24 hours. *Subcutaneous, adult* and *children over 6 yrs of age,* for *bronchodilatation, initially* **200 μg** of the *injection,* repeated with doses up to **1 mg** at 20-min to 4-hour intervals, if necessary, *or initially* **500 μg** of the *Sterile Sus-*

pension, repeated with doses of up to 1.5 mg at 4-hour intervals or longer if necessary; the duration of action of the Injection is 15 to 30 min and the Sterile Suspension up to 10 hr; *children under 6 yr of age*, **10 to 25 μg per kg** (or **300 μg/m²**) of the injection, not to exceed 500 μg per dose, every 4 hr, if necessary or **25 μg per kg** (or **625 μg/m²**) of sterile suspension, repeated, if necessary, at intervals no less than 6 hr. *Intracardiac, adult,* as the diluted *Injection,* **100 μg** to **1 mg,** repeated every 5 min, if necessary; *children under 6 yr,* **5** to **10 μg per kg** (or **300 μg/m²**), repeated every 15 min for 2 doses then every 4 hr as needed. *Intraspinal, adults* and *children,* in combination with a local anesthetic, **200** to **400 μg,** to be added to the local anesthetic mixture. *Infiltration,* in combination with a local anesthetic, 1:100,000 to 1:20,000. *Oral Inhalation, adult* and *children over 6 yr* of age, as the *Inhalation Aerosol,* **200 μg** (1 metered spray), repeated in 2 or 3 minutes, if necessary, and not more frequently than every 4 hours thereafter, *or,* as the *Inhalation,* **1** to **2 sprays** of a 1% solution, repeated in 1 to 2 min, if necessary, then as required thereafter; inhalation doses for children over 6 must be individualized. *Topical, intranasal,* as a **0.1%** solution as needed; *topical, conjunctiva, adults* and *children,* for *glaucoma,* **1 drop** of a **0.5** to **2%** solution 1 to 2 times a day, and, for *mydriasis* and *ocular hemostasis,* **1 drop** of a **1%** solution for 1 to 3 doses, as needed.

All doses are as the equivalent of epinephrine; the actual ingredient may be the bitartrate, hydrochloride, sulfate or other salt. Epinephrine is rarely given intravenously in any form; the dose is usually less than 0.25 mg, given well diluted with isotonic solution and very slowly, so that the effects can be monitored. Topically, epinephrine can be used in ointment, suppository, jelly, or emulsion form, in addition to the solution. For topical application in operative procedures on the nose and throat, solutions of 0.002 to 0.05% freshly prepared from the 0.1% Injection may be used.

Dosage Forms—Inhalation: 1%; Inhalation Aerosol: 0.5% (200 and 270 μg per metered spray); Injection: 100 μg (0.1 mg)/mL, 1 mg/mL; Nasal Solution: 0.1%, nonsterile; Ophthalmic Solution: 0.1, 0.25, 0.5, 1, and 2%, nonsterile; Sterile Suspension (in oil): 5 mg/mL 0.2%.

Epinephrine Bitartrate

1,2-Benzenediol, 4-[1-hydroxy-2-(methylamino)ethyl]-, (R)-, [R-($R*,R$)]-2,3-dihydroxybutanedioate (1:1) (salt); Adrenaline Bitartrate BP; Epitrate (*Ayerst*); Lyophrin (*Alcon*); (*Various Mfrs*)

($-$)-3,4-Dihydroxy-α-[(methylamino)methyl]benzyl alcohol (+)-tartrate (1:1) salt [51-42-3] $C_9H_{13}NO_3 \cdot C_4H_6O_6$ (333.29).

For the structure of the base, see *Epinephrine*, above.

Preparation—By reacting epinephrine with an equimolar portion of tartaric acid and precipitating by the addition of alcohol.

Description—White, grayish white, or light brownish gray crystalline powder; odorless; slowly darkens on exposure to air and light; melting range 147° to 152°, with decomposition; pH (1% solution) 3.5.

Solubility—1 g in about 3 mL water and about 500 mL alcohol; practically insoluble in chloroform and in ether.

Uses—Epinephrine bitartrate is supplied only for use in *bronchial asthma, scleroconjunctival inflammation,* and *open-angle glaucoma.* For actions, uses, adverse effects, etc, see the general statement.

Dose—*Topical, adult,* to the *conjunctiva,* **1 drop** of the equivalent of a **0.25** to **2%** epinephrine (free base) solution once every 3 days to 2 times a day. *Oral inhalation, adult* and *children over 6 years of age,* **160 μg** as the base equivalent (1 metered spray), to be repeated in 1 min if necessary, and at intervals no shorter than 4 hr thereafter; the dose for children under 6 yr must be individualized.

Dosage Forms—Aerosol: Inhalation Aerosol: 300 μg (equivalent to 160 μg of base) per metered spray; Ophthalmic Solution: 0.25, 0.5, 1, 1.1 and 2%, epinephrine base equivalent; for Ophthalmic Solution: 55 mg base equivalent, to be constituted to 1.1%.

Epinephryl Borate Ophthalmic Solution

1,3,2-Benzodioxaborole-5-methanol, 2-hydroxy-α-[(methylamino)-methyl]-, (R)-, Epinal (*Alcon*)

($-$)-3,4-Dihydroxy-α-[(methylamino)methyl]benzyl alcohol, cyclic 3,4-ester with boric acid [5579-16-8] $C_9H_{12}BNO_4$ (209.01).

Preparation—Reported to be a 1:1 chelate formed in aqueous medium between boric acid and epinephrine (*J Pharm Sci 51:* 206, 1962). US Pat 3,149,035.

Uses—A preparation for ophthalmologic uses only. For actions, uses, adverse effects, etc. see the general statement.

Dose—*Topical,* to the *conjunctiva,* **0.1 mL** of the equivalent of a **0.5 to 1%** epinephrine solution twice a day.

Dosage Forms—Ophthalmic Solution: 0.25, 0.5, 1%, epinephrine base equivalent.

Fenfluramine Hydrochloride

Benzeneethaneamine, *N*-ethyl-α-methyl-3-(trifluoromethyl)-, hydrochloride; Pondimin (*Robins*)

N-Ethyl-α-methyl-*m*-(trifluoromethyl)phenethylamine hydrochloride [404-82-0] $C_{12}H_{16}F_3N.HCl$ (267.12).

Preparation—From α,α,α-trifluoro-*m*-tolualdehyde, which is condensed with nitroethane; the 1-nitroethylidene group reduced to the α-aminoethyl, then acetylated to the amide and reduced to fenfluramine. French Pat M1658.

Description—White, amorphous powder with a characteristic odor; melts between 165–170°.

Solubility—Sparingly soluble in water; pK_a is 9.92.

Uses—Fenfluramine is an anorexiant that differs from most other sympathomimetic anorexiants in not stimulating the central nervous system in the majority of users; instead, it usually exerts a mild sedative action. It appears to have a low drug-abuse potential. Doses of 80 to 400 mg can cause euphoria, derealization, and perceptual changes in persons with a history of drug abuse. It does not affect REM sleep during use, but insomnia may occur after withdrawal. Depression of mood has been noted in some patients after discontinuation of treatment with the drug. Unlike most sympathomimetic-related anorexiants, tolerance does not appear to develop, and after 6 to 8 weeks of treatment the body weight reaches a plateau that is relatively stable for at least another 16 weeks. Although weight loss is sometimes dramatic, with usual dosage and without strict dietary regulation, the loss averages only about 6 lb; the most obese patients tend to be those experiencing the smallest loss. When caloric intake is restricted by a deliberate program, fenfluramine enables the patient to endure the restrictions, and weight losses greater than those on an unrestricted diet can be achieved. On an unrestricted diet, the drug appears to be no more effective than dextroamphetamine in the early stages of management. Fenfluramine may differ from dextroamphetamine in its mechanism of action in that in addition to an effect in the hypothalamus to curb hunger it seems to promote uptake of glucose into muscle and so divert it from fat tissues. With therapeutic doses, fenfluramine appears to lack sympathomimetic cardiovascular actions; in fact, it appears to exert a masked inhibitory action on the sympathetic nervous system, since the drug increases the action of antihypertensive drugs.

In high doses, fenfluramine can cause an increase in blood pressure, tachycardia, and palpitations. Fenfluramine causes side effects in 2 to 20 times as many patients as does dextroamphetamine, the ratio depending on the particular effect. Drowsiness occurs in 67% of patients, gastrointestinal effects (nausea, diarrhea, constipation, abdominal discomfort, other) in about 37%, dry mouth in about 26%, insomnia in 22%, dizziness in 18%, headache in 15%, and skin rashes in about 3%. In children especially, urinary frequency and incontinence also occur. Fenfluramine should be used cautiously when methyldopa, oral hypoglycemics, or reserpine is also used.

Dose—*Oral, adults* and *children over 12 year of age, initially* **20 mg** 3 times a day, 30 min to 1 hr before each meal, with increments of 20 mg/day, if necessary, up to a maximum daily dose of 40 mg. If the drug initially is tolerated poorly, one dose a day may be temporarily dropped, and the dose gradually increased thereafter.

Dosage Forms—Tablets: 20 mg.

Hydroxyamphetamine Hydrobromide

Phenol, 4-(2-aminopropyl)-, hydrobromide; Paredrine (*SK&F*)

(±)-*p*-(2-Aminopropyl)phenol hydrobromide [306-21-8] $C_9H_{13}NO.HBr$ (232.12).

Preparation—Among other methods, by reducing *p*-methoxybenzyl methyl ketoxime followed by hydrolysis of the methoxy group with mineral acids. The free base may then be liberated with alkali, and, after extraction, may be converted into the salt by treatment with hydrobromic acid.

Description—White, crystalline powder; solutions are slightly acid to litmus, having a pH of about 5; melting range 189° to 192°.

Solubility—1 g in about 1 mL water and about 2.5 mL alcohol; slightly soluble in chloroform; insoluble in ether.

Uses—Hydroxyamphetamine is an indirect sympathomimetic, the actions of which are both α- and β₁-agonist in nature; it is essentially devoid of central nervous activity. It is used topically as a *mydriatic.* Mydrasis lasts several hours.

Although hydroxyamphetamine shares the general properties of other sympathomimetic amines, it also presents some interesting anomalies. The drug does not cause vasoconstriction when injected intradermally; consequently it does not prolong the duration of action of local anesthetics. In addition, its actions on the bronchi and gastrointestinal tract are of low intensity. For the adverse effects and precautions, see the general statement.

Dose—*Topical,* to the *conjunctiva,* 1 or **2 drops** of a **1%** solution, repeated as necessary.

Dosage Forms—Ophthalmic Solution: 0.5 and 1%.

Isoetharine Hydrochloride

1,2-Benzenediol, 4-[1-hydroxy-2-[(1-methylethyl)amino]butyl]-, hydrochloride; *N*-isopropylethylnorepinephrine hydrochloride; Bronkosol (*Breon*)

3,4-Dihydroxy-α-[1-(isopropylamino)propyl]benzyl alcohol hydrochloride $C_{13}H_{21}NO_3.HCl$ [2576-92-3] (275.77).

Preparation—Synthesis of isoetharine and other 1-(3,4-dihydroxyphenyl)-2-monoalkyl-1-butanols, starting with 3,4-dihydroxybutyrophenone, is described in German Pat 638,650 (*CA 31:* 32094, 1937). The base is converted to the hydrochloride or the mesylate (below).

Description—White to off-white, crystalline solid; odorless; melts between 196° and 208°, with decomposition.

Solubility—Soluble in water; sparingly soluble in alcohol; practically insoluble in ether.

Uses—Isoetharine possesses moderate α-, β₁- and β₂-agonist activities (see the general statement for actions, uses, adverse effects, precautions, and drug interactions). It is used only as a *bronchodilator,* mainly for *intermittent bronchospasm.* The duration of action is less than an hour. It is administered by inhalation; abroad it is also used orally in sustained release tablets formulated with a porous plastic base.

Dose—*Adult, inhalation,* by hand nebulizer, 3 to **7 inhalations** of a **1%** solution; by *oxygen aerosolization* (oxygen flow 4 to 6 L/min) or *intermittent positive pressure breathing* (1 ppb; inspiratory flow 15 L/min), **4 mL** of a **0.125%** solution, **2.5 mL** of a **0.2%** solution, **2 mL** of a **0.25%** solution, **0.5 to 1 mL** of a **0.5%** solution (dilute to 3 mL), and **0.25 to 5 mL** of a **1%** solution (dilute 1:3, ie, to 0.75 to 1.5 mL.

Dosage Forms—Solution for nebulization: 0.125, 0.2, 0.25 and 1%.

Isoetharine Mesylate

1,2-Benzenediol, 4-[1-hydroxy-2-[(1-methylethyl)amino]butyl]-, methanesulfonate (salt); *N*-isopropylethylnorepinephrine methanesulfonate; Bronkometer (*Breon*)

For the formula of isoetharine base, see under *Isoetharine Hydrochloride.*

3,4-Dihydroxy-α-[1-(isopropylamino)propyl]benzyl alcohol methanesulfonate [7279-75-6] $C_{13}H_{21}NO_3.CH_4O_3S$ (335.41).

Preparation—See *Isoetharine Hydrochloride.*

Description—White to off-white, crystalline solid; odorless; slightly bitter, salty taste; melts at about 165°.

Solubility—Freely soluble in water; soluble in alcohol; very slightly soluble in ether.

Uses—See *Isoetharine Hydrochloride,* above.

Dose—*Oral inhalation, adults,* **340 μg** (1 metered dose), to be repeated after 1 or 2 min, if necessary.

Dosage Form—Aerosol: 0.61% (340 μg/metered dose).

Isoproterenol Hydrochloride

1,2-Benzenediol, 4-[1-hydroxy-2-[(1-methylethyl)amino]ethyl]-, hydrochloride; Isopropylarterenol Hydrochloride; (*Various Mfrs*)

3,4-Dihydroxy-α-[(isopropylamino)methyl]benzyl alcohol hydrochloride [51-30-9] $C_{11}H_{17}NO_3.HCl$ (247.72).

Preparation—By the synthetic procedure given for *Epinephrine* (page 883), using isopropylamine in place of methylamine; the base is then converted to the hydrochloride without resolution.

Description—White to nearly white, odorless, crystalline powder, having a slightly bitter taste; gradually darkens on exposure to air and light; solutions become pink to brownish pink on standing exposed to air, and almost immediately so when rendered alkaline; pH (1% aqueous solution) about 5; melting range between 165° and 170°.

Solubility—1 g in 3 mL water and 50 mL alcohol; less soluble in dehydrated alcohol; insoluble in chloroform and ether.

Uses—Isoproterenol is a close congener of epinephrine; it has strong β_1- and β_2-agonist activities but lacks α-activity (see the general statement). Its primary use is in the treatment of *bronchial asthma*, for which it has supplanted epinephrine, but it in turn is being supplanted by metaproterenol and other selective β_2-agonists. It is mostly administered by oral inhalation for this purpose, the systemic and central nervous system side effects being much more prominent by other routes. The incidence of side effects by systemic routes is over 30% but by inhalation it is less than 10%. However, sudden death has occurred after inhalation, especially with aerosols. This has been attributed to the combination of a cardiotoxic action of the fluorocarbon propellant and the arrhythmiagenic action of isoproterenol, but it may also be, in part, the ease of overdosing. The incidence of sudden death has decreased dramatically after dosage metering was initiated. Chronic use of isoproterenol occasionally results in an increase in airway resistance. Isoproterenol is used to treat *ventricular bradycardia* and in the prophylaxis of *cardiac standstill*, but it will be displaced by more cardioselective sympathomimetics. In the treatment of *shock* it occasionally improves cardiovascular function, but it also sometimes worsens the condition. For the adverse effects and precautions of β-agonists, see the general statement.

Isoproterenol is erratically absorbed by the oral route. Absorption is somewhat less erratic by the sublingual and rectal routes. The duration of action by the sublingual and subcutaneous routes is 1 to 2 hours; by inhalation, it is 30 to 60 minutes.

Note—*Do not use any dosage form of isoproterenol hydrochloride if it is brown in color or contains a precipitate.*

Dose—*Oral inhalation, metered aerosol, adult* and *children,* **120 or 131 μg** as a metered spray, followed by a second dose in 1 to 5 min, if necessary, and repeated up to 4 to 6 times a day (i.e., no more than 6 inhalations in any one hour in a 24-hr period) for *asthma* or at intervals no shorter than 3 to 4 hr for *chronic obstructive pulmonary disease:* more than 3 applications per day require medical supervision. *Oral inhalation, hand nebulization, adult* and *children,* **5 to 15 sprays** of **0.5%** or **3 to 7 sprays** of **1%** solution, followed by a second dose in 5 to 10 min, if necessary, repeated up to 5 times a day; *compressed air* or *oxygen nebulization,* **2 mL** of a **0.125%** solution or **2.5 mL** of a **0.1%** solution delivered over a 15- to 20 min period up to 5 times a day. *Oral, extended release* tablets, *adult,* **15 to 30 mg** 2 to 6 times a day. *Sublingual, adult,* for *bronchodilatation,* **10 to 15 mg**

3 to 4 times a day; for *heart block, initially* **10 mg,** followed by **5 to 50 mg** as necessary; for *carotid sinus syndrome,* **10 to 30 mg** 4 to 6 times a day; *children,* for *bronchodilatation,* **5 to 10 mg** 3 times a day; for *heart block, initially* **5 mg,** subsequent doses determined by response. *Intracardiac, adults,* **20 μg,** repeated as needed. *Intravenous, adult,* **20 to 60 μg,** followed by **10 to 200 μg** as necessary. *Intravenous infusion, adult,* **0.5 to 5 μg** per min, the rate adjusted to maintain the desired blood pressure (solution usually contains 2 mg/500 mL, but 1 to 10 mg in 500 mL of 5% dextrose injection). *Intramuscular, adult, initially* **200 μg** (0.2 mg), followed by **20 μg** to **1 mg,** as necessary. *Subcutaneous, adult, initially* **200 μg,** followed by **150 to 200 μg,** as necessary. *Intracardiac, adult,* **20 μg,** to be repeated, if necessary. Unstated pediatric doses must be individualized.

Dosage Forms—Inhalation Aerosol: 0.25% w/w (120 or 131 μg per metered dose); Solution for Nebulization: 0.25, 0.5 and 1%; Injection: 200 μg/mL and 1 mg/5 mL; Sublingual Tablets: 10 and 15 mg; Extended Release Tablets: 15 and 30 mg.

Isoproterenol Hydrochloride and Phenylephrine Bitartrate—An aerosol device that delivers micronized particles of isoproterenol hydrochloride and phenylephrine bitartrate suspended in an inert mixture of sorbitan trioleate, cetylpyridinium chloride with fluorochlorohydrocarbons as propellants is marketed as Duo-Medihaler (*Riker*). Each valve actuation releases a uniform aerosolized dose of 0.16 mg of isoproterenol hydrochloride (equivalent to 0.137 mg of isoproterenol base) and 0.24 mg of phenylephrine bitartrate (equivalent to 0.126 mg of phenylephrine base). The action of isoproterenol is as a bronchodilator, and phenylephrine is included for its vasoconstrictor properties to reduce bronchiolar congestion. *Dose: Oral inhalation, adult,* 1 metered spray, to be followed by a second dose after 5 min, if necessary; for daily maintenance no more than 2 inhalations should be taken at any one time, or more than 6 inhalations in any one hour in a 24-hr period.

Isoproterenol Sulfate

1,2-Benzenediol, 4-[1-hydroxy-2-[(1-methylethyl)amino]ethyl]-, sulfate (2:1) (salt), dihydrate; Isopropylarterenol Sulfate; Norisodrine (*Abbott*); (*Various Mfrs*)

3,4-Dihydroxy-α-[(isopropylamino)methyl]benzyl alcohol sulfate (2:1) (salt) dihydrate [6700-39-6] $(C_{11}H_{17}NO_3)_2.H_2SO_4.2H_2O$ (556.62); anhydrous [299-95-6] (520.59).

For the structure of the base, see *Isoproterenol Hydrochloride.*

Preparation—An alcoholic solution of 2-chloro-3′,4′-dihydroxyacetophenone is condensed with isopropylamine. The 3′,4′-dihydroxy-2-(isopropylamino)acetophenone formed is isolated as the sulfate and its carbonyl group is reduced to carbinol by catalytic hydrogenation.

Description—White to nearly white, odorless, crystalline powder, having a slightly bitter taste; gradually darkens on exposure to air and light; solutions become pink to brownish pink on standing exposed to air, and almost immediately so when rendered alkaline; pH (1 in 100 solution) about 5; melting range 125° to 129°.

Solubility—1 g in 4 mL water; very slightly soluble in alcohol, benzene, and ether.

Uses—See *Isoproterenol Hydrochloride.* The sulfate is used only as a bronchodilator.

Dose—*Oral inhalation, aerosol powder, adults* and *children,* **1 or 2 metered inhalations** (45, 110 or 220 μg); a second dose may be given after 5 min, if necessary, and a third 10 min after the second; dosage should be limited to 3 doses per attack; the first trial should use the 10% concentration, the 25% concentration being held in reserve for use when the 10% concentration fails. *Aerosol solution, adults* and *children,* **1 metered spray** (80 μg); a second dose may be given after 2 to 5 min, if necessary, 4 to 6 times a day; no more than 6 doses should be given in any one hr during a 24-hr period.

Dosage Forms—Aerosol Powder: 10 and 25% (45 and 110 μg, respectively, per metered spray); Aerosol Solution: 2 mg/mL (80 μg per metered spray).

Lergotrile—page 932.

Norepinephrine Bitartrate

1,2-Benzenediol, 4-(2-amino-1-hydroxyethyl)-, (R)-[R-(R*,R*)]-2,3-dihydroxybutanedioate (1:1) (salt), monohydrate; Levarterenol Bitartrate; Noradrenaline Acid Tartrate; Levophed Bitartrate (*Winthrop*)

(−)-α-(Aminomethyl)-3,4-dihydroxybenzyl alcohol tartrate (1:1) (salt) monohydrate [69815-49-2] $C_8H_{11}NO_3.C_4H_6O_6.H_2O$ (337.28); *anhydrous* [51-40-1] (319.27).

Preparation—By the synthetic procedure given for *Epinephrine* (page 883), using ammonia in place of methylamine; the base is then converted to the bitartrate and resolved.

Description—White or faintly gray, crystalline powder; odorless; slowly darkens on exposure to air and light; solutions are acid to litmus, having a pH of about 3.5; melts, without previous drying, between 98° and 104° to form a turbid melt.

Solubility—1 g in about 2.5 mL water and about 300 mL alcohol; practically insoluble in chloroform and in ether.

Uses—Norepinephrine is the catecholamine released at almost all adrenergic nerve terminals in the periphery and in a large proportion of adrenergic nerve terminals in the central nervous system. It constitutes 10 to 18% of the catecholamine content of the adrenal medulla and as much as 97% of that of some pheochromocytomas.

Norepinephrine has strong α- and β_1- but weak β_2-agonist activity. It is used only for its α-activity, but β_1-activity contributes to its systemic usefulness and adverse effects (see the general statement for actions, uses, adverse effects and precautions of α- and β_1-agonists). Its principal use is to *support blood pressure* in various acute hypotensive states, especially in myocardial *shock*. In shock, despite adequate restoration of blood pressure, failure occurs in approximately 50% of cases. Prolonged infusions sometimes themselves cause shock. Even though norepinephrine possesses strong β_1-activity, an increase in heart rate often does not occur during intravenous infusion, because the vasoconstrictor actions marshal vagal reflexes that tend to slow the heart and nullify the direct effect to increase heart rate. However, the reflexes do not antagonize the effect on the strength of the heart beat, so that cardiac output is usually maintained, even though the rate is slowed. At the low blood pressures usually seen in shock, the baroreceptors are not operative, and an increase in heart rate is often seen after levarterenol. It is sometimes used in *cardiac arrest*. Like other β_1-agonists, norepinephrine is arrhythmiagenic. The β_2-activity is so weak that tolerated doses do not cause bronchodilatation or vasodilatation in muscle vascular beds; at the usual infusion rates, it also does not cause α-adrenergic bronchoconstriction.

Norepinephrine bitartrate is used as a vasoconstrictor in some local anesthetic solutions for dental use, usually in 0.0033% (1 in 30,000) concentration of norepinephrine.

Note—Do not use any dosage form of norepinephrine bitartrate if it is brown in color or contains a precipitate.

Dose—*Intravenous, adult*, by slow infusion, the equivalent of **1 to 10 μg/min** (of norepinephrine base), the rate being determined by the response. An initial rate of 8 to 12 μg/min is often used as a trial from which adjustments are made to achieve a systolic blood pressure of 80 to 120 torr; but many clinicians prefer to start with a low rate and increase the rate until response occurs, rather than risk a hypertensive crisis with the test rate. Especially if the patient has just had a pheochromocytoma removed, the rate may greatly exceed that given above. The average *maintenance* dose is **2 to 4 μg/min**, but the infusion rate will gradually need to be increased, which is in part a sign that volume replenishment is needed. Even after the initial rate-adjusting period, vigilant monitoring (at least every 15 minutes) is required. For *children*, *initially* **2 μg per min per m² of body surface**, the rate to be adjusted according to the response. The infusion is prepared by adding 8 mg of levarterenol bitartrate (equivalent to 4 mg of levarterenol) to 1 L of 5% dextrose or dextrose-sodium chloride injection. *If extravasation occurs, the exposed tissue should be infiltrated with 5 to 10 mg of phentolamine.*

Dosage Forms—Injection: 4 mg/4 mL. Procaine and Propoxycaine Hydrochlorides and Levarterenol Bitartrate Injection (2% procaine hydrochloride, 0.4% propoxycaine hydrochloride, 1 in 30,000 levarterenol): 1.8- and 2.2-mL cartridges; 30-mL vials. Procaine and Tetracaine Hydrochlorides and Levarterenol Bitartrate Injection (2% procaine hydrochloride, 0.15% tetracaine hydrochloride, 1 in 30,000 levarterenol): 2-mL cartridges.

Mephentermine Sulfate

Benzeneethanamine, N,α,α-trimethyl-, sulfate (2:1);
Wyamine Sulfate (*Wyeth*)

N,α,α-Trimethylphenethylamine sulfate (2:1) [1212-72-2] $(C_{11}H_{17}N)_2.H_2SO_4$ (424.60); *dihydrate* [6190-60-9] (460.63).

Preparation—Mephentermine may be prepared by a seven step synthesis starting with phenyl isopropyl ketone and conversion of the free base to the salt with sulfuric acid. US Pat 2,590,079.

Description—White, odorless crystals or a crystalline powder; solutions are acid to litmus, having a pH of about 6.

Solubility—1 g in 18 mL water, 220 mL alcohol, >1000 mL chloroform, >10,000 mL ether.

Uses—See *Mephentermine*. The sulfate is employed parenterally to *support blood pressure* during spinal anesthesia, or treatment with ganglionic blocking drugs, or in postural hypotension. It is not recommended for routine use in the management of shock, especially hypovolemic shock, although it can be given as an interim drug while preparations are being made for fluid replacement and other measures. Parenteral injections of the drug produce a very prompt and prolonged increase in blood pressure. Tachyphylaxis occurs, so that repeated injections lose their pressor effects. The central stimulant actions are weak relative to the cardiovascular action, and it is not possible to achieve a central effect without cardiovascular side effects; nevertheless, the drug has been used to elevate mood in geriatric patients and to antagonize the central depressant effects of certain antihistamines. See the general statement for the adverse effects, precautions, and drug interactions of indirect sympathomimetics and α- and β-agonists.

Mephentermine is absorbed orally and excreted in the urine. An alkaline urine favors retention of the drug and tends to elevate plasma levels. The duration of action is 1 to 2 hours.

Dose—*Intramuscular, adults*, in *spinal anesthesia*, **30 to 45 mg** 10 to 20 min prior to hypotensive procedure; *children*, **400 μg/kg**. *Intravenous, adults, initially* **30 to 45 mg**, then **30 mg** as needed; the dose should be half the above in cesarian section or hyperresponsive patients; *children*, **400 μg/kg**. Constant *intravenous infusion*, a 1% solution infused at a rate necessary to maintain blood pressure.

Dosage Forms—Injection (in closed injection system): 30 mg/mL; Injection: 30 mg/2 mL, and 150 mg and 300 mg/10 mL.

Metaproterenol Sulfate

1,3-Benzenediol, 5-[1-hydroxy-2-[(1-methylethyl)amino]ethyl]-, sulfate (2:1) salt; Orciprenaline Sulfate; Alupent (*Ciba-Geigy*); Metaprel (*Sandoz*)

3,5-Dihydroxy-α-[(isopropylamino)methyl]benzyl alcohol sulfate (2:1) [5874-97-5] $(C_{11}H_{17}NO_3)_2.H_2SO_4$ (520.59).

Preparation—One method involves condensing 2-chloro-3′,5′-dihydroxyacetophenone with isopropylamine, reducing the CO group to CHOH and reacting the resulting metaproterenol base with H_2SO_4. US Pat 3,341,594.

Description—White to off-white, odorless, bitter, crystalline powder; photosensitive and oxidizes in air; melts at about 202°.

Solubility—Freely soluble in water and in alcohol.

Uses—Metaproterenol possesses strong β_2-, weak β_1- and no α-agonist activity. The actions, uses, adverse effects, precautions, and drug interactions of β-agonists are discussed in the general statement. Because the cardiac stimulant effects are slight, metaproterenol is replacing isoproterenol and epinephrine in the management of *bronchial asthma*. Metaproterenol is not acted upon by catechol-O-methyltransferase, is only slightly degraded by monoamine oxidase, and is only slowly conjugated in the liver; consequently, it is orally effective. The duration of action after inhalation is about 4 hr and somewhat longer after oral administration. The duration of action but not the maximum effect may decrease with chronic use.

Dose—*Oral inhalation*, user *over 12 yr* of age only, *metered aerosol*, **2** or **3 inhalations** (1.3 or 1.95 mg) every 3 or 4 hr, up to a limit of 7.8 mg/day; hand *nebulization*, **5** to **15 inhalations** of a 5% solution every 3 or 4 hr for acute and 3 or 4 times a day for chronic bronchospasm; intermittant positive pressure breathing (ippb), **0.2** to **0.3 ml** of a **5%** solution, diluted to 2.5 mL, every 3 or 4 hr for acute and 3 or 4 times a day for chronic bronchospasm. *Oral*, user *over 9 yr* of age (or 27 kg of body weight), **20 mg** 3 or 4 times a day; *children 6 to 9 yr*, **10 mg** 3 or 4 times a day; *children under 6 yr*, **325 to 650 µg per kg** of body weight 4 times a day (syrup only).

Dosage Forms—Inhalation Aerosol (powder): 255 mg (650 µg per metered spray); Syrup: 10 mg/5 mL; Tablets: 10 and 20 mg.

Metaraminol Bitartrate

Benzenemethanol, α-(1-aminoethyl)-3-hydroxy-, [R-(R*,S*)]-, [R-(R*,R*)]-2,3-dihydroxybutanedioate (1:1) (salt); Aramine (*MSD*)

(−)-α-(1-Aminoethyl)-*m*-hydroxybenzyl alcohol tartrate (1:1) (salt) [33402-03-8] $C_9H_{13}NO_2 \cdot C_4H_6O_6$ (317.29).

Preparation—Among other methods, metaraminol may be synthesized by reactions utilizing *m*-hydroxybenzaldehyde and benzylamine as the principal reactants. The base obtained is converted to the bitartrate with an equimolar quantity of tartaric acid.

Description—White, practically odorless, crystalline powder; melts between 171° and 175°; pH (1 in 20 solution) between 3.2 and 3.5.

Solubility—Freely soluble in water; 1 g in about 100 mL alcohol; practically insoluble in chloroform and ether.

Uses—A directly acting *sympathomimetic* with strong α- and moderate β_1-agonist activity and virtually no β_2-agonist activity or actions on the central nervous system. See the general statement for actions, uses, adverse effects and precautions of α- and β_1-agonists. The drug is used mainly to support or elevate blood pressure during spinal or general anesthesia and in certain acute *hypotensive conditions*, such as anaphylactic shock (after initial management with epinephrine) or shock secondary to myocardial infarction, trauma, septicemia, gram-negative bacterial endotoxins, and adverse drug reactions. It is not recommended in hypovolemic shock. In the treatment of shock, metaraminol has largely been superseded by dopamine and dobutamine.

After prolonged infusion, a severe hypotensive episode often follows discontinuation, because the drug replaces norepinephrine in the adrenergic nerve terminals and becomes a false transmitter.

The duration of action is about 1.5 hr after intramuscular injection.

Dose (as metaraminol base)—*Intravenous*, *adult*, **0.5** to **5 mg** of metaraminol; *children*, **10 µg/kg** (or **300 µg/m²** of body surface). *Intravenous infusion*, *adults*, 15 to 100 mg/500 mL of 5% dextrose or dextrose-sodium chloride injection, infused at a rate adjusted to maintain systolic blood pressure at 80 to 100 torr; *children*, 400 µg/kg (or 12 mg/m²) in a parenteral solution such that there is 1 mg/25 mL, infused at the optimal rate. *Intramuscular adults*, **2** to **10 mg**; *children*, **100 µg/kg** (or **3 mg/m²**). *Subcutaneous* administration is not recommended because of the frequent occurrence of ischemic necrosis at the injection site; the dose is the same as for intramuscular injection.

Dosage Forms—Injection: 100 mg/10 mL (of metaraminol base).

Methoxamine Hydrochloride

Benzenemethanol, α-(1-aminoethyl)-2,5-dimethoxy-, hydrochloride; Vasoxyl Hydrochloride (*Burroughs Wellcome*)

(±)-α-(1-Aminoethyl)-2,5-dimethoxybenzyl alcohol hydrochloride [61-16-5] $C_{11}H_{17}NO_3 \cdot HCl$ (247.72).

Preparation—Among other ways, from 2′,5′-dimethoxypropiophenone through reaction with nitrous acid to form the 2-isonitroso derivative followed by catalytic hydrogenation which reduces both the carbonyl function to carbinol and the isonitroso function to amino. The methoxamine, dissolved in a suitable organic solvent, is readily converted to the hydrochloride by a stream of hydrogen chloride.

Description—Colorless or white, plate-like crystals, or a white, crystalline powder; odorless or has only a slight odor; solutions are acid to litmus, having a pH of about 5; melts between 214° and 219°.

Solubility—1 g in about 2.5 mL water and 12 mL alcohol; almost insoluble in chloroform and in ether.

Uses—A directly acting *sympathomimetic* amine with a prompt and prolonged pressor action which results almost exclusively from α-agonist activity to increase peripheral resistance. Not only does it not stimulate the heart but it has moderate beta-adrenergic receptor blocking properties. It actually causes bradycardia, mostly as the result of a reflex activation of the vagus nerve secondary to the increased blood pressure. The drug is useful for the treatment of *hypotensive states* when it is desired to raise blood pressure without cardiac stimulation. However, methoxamine has very little effect on the capacitance veins, so that its usefulness is compromised, especially in the treatment of various kinds of shock. It is mainly used to support blood pressure during anesthesia, including anesthesia by heart-sensitizing anesthetics. The reflex bradycardia is employed to terminate *paroxysmal supraventricular tachycardia*. Methoxamine has no inhibitory effect on bronchial muscles, causes no central stimulation, and does not increase the irritability of the cyclopropane-sensitized heart. The duration of action is 60 to 90 min. For the adverse effects, precautions, and contraindications of α-agonists, see the general statement.

Dose—*Intramuscular*, *adult*, *pre-* and *post-operative*, **5** to **10 mg**; with *spinal anesthesia* or *to correct hypotension*, **10** to **15 mg**; *children*, **250 µg/kg**. *Intravenous*, adult, for *hypotensive emergencies*, **3** to **5 mg** *slowly*; for paroxysmal supraventricular tachycardia, 10 mg *slowly*; children, **80 µg/kg** given slowly in divided doses.

Dosage Forms—Injection: 20 mg/mL.

Methylphenidate Hydrochloride—page 1136.

Naphazoline Hydrochloride

1*H*-Imidazole, 4,5-dihydro-2-(1-naphthalenylmethyl)-, monohydrochloride; Privine Hydrochloride (*Ciba-Geigy*)

2-(1-Naphthylmethyl)-2-imidazoline monohydrochloride [550-99-2] $C_{14}H_{14}N_2 \cdot HCl$ (246.74).

Preparation—In almost quantitative yields by heating 1-naphthylacetonitrile with ethylenediamine monohydrochloride at 175° to 200° for 1 hour. The 1-naphthylacetonitrile is made from naphthalene by chloromethylation with formaldehyde and HCl followed by treatment of the resulting 1-naphthylmethyl chloride with potassium cyanide.

Description—White, crystalline, odorless, bitter powder; melting range 253° to 258°, with decomposition; pH (1 in 100 solution) between 5.0 and 6.6.

Solubility—Freely soluble in water and alcohol; very slightly soluble in chloroform; practically insoluble in ether.

Uses—Although its structure differs markedly from that of most sympathomimetic agents, naphazoline is a directly acting *sympathomimetic* with only α-agonist activity. It is employed topically for relief of *nasal congestion*. It also may be used to relieve nasal congestion consequent to treatment with reserpine, etc., since its actions are mainly direct. Care should be exercised in its prolonged use, because naphazoline, in common with most locally applied vasoconstrictors, may cause a rebound congestion that simulates the condition for which it was originally employed; it also induces chemical rhinitis. Mere discontinuation of ill-advised vasoconstrictor therapy has been noted to produce dramatic relief of chronic nasal congestion in some cases. Naphazoline is also used as an ophthalmic solution for relief of *ocular congestion* and *blepharospasm*.

The common adverse effects include hypertension, bradycardia, sweating, sedation and, in children, occasional coma. For other potential adverse effects and precautions, see the general statement on α-agonists.

Dose—*Topical, adults*, to the *nasal mucosa*, **2 drops of 0.05%** solution every 3 to 4 hr, if necessary, or as **0.05% nasal spray** no more frequently than every 3 hr; to the *conjunctiva*, 1 to **2 drops** of **0.012** to **0.1%** ophthalmic solution every 3 to 4 hr or longer, if possible. Use in children is not recommended.

Dosage Forms—Nasal Solution: 0.05%; Ophthalmic Solution: 0.012, 0.02 and 0.1%.

Oxymetazoline Hydrochloride

Phenol, 3-[(4,5-dihydro-1*H*-imidazol-2-yl)methyl]-6-(1,1-dimethylethyl)-2,4-dimethyl-, monohydrochloride; Afrin (*Schering-Plough*)

6-*tert*-Butyl-3-(2-imidazolin-2-ylmethyl)-2,4-dimethylphenol monohydrochloride [2315-02-8] $C_{16}H_{24}N_2O \cdot HCl$ (296.84).

Preparation—2,4-Dimethyl-6-*tert*-butylphenol is converted into the benzyl cyanide intermediate, which is reacted with ethylenediamine *p*-toluenesulfonate whereby, through addition and deammoniation, the imidazoline ring is formed. The resulting oxymetazoline is converted to the salt through interaction with an equimolar quantity of hydrogen chloride. US Pat 3,147,275.

Description—White to nearly white, fine, crystalline powder; odorless; stable in light and heat, nonhygroscopic; melts at about 300° with decomposition; pH (1 in 20 solution) between 4.0 and 6.5.

Solubility—1 g in 6.7 mL water, 3.6 mL alcohol, 860 mL chloroform; practically insoluble in ether.

Uses—A directly acting sympathomimetic with only α-agonist activity. It is used only topically as a *nasal decongestant*. After-congestion is less prominent than with naphazoline, to which it is chemically related. For the action, adverse effects, and precautions of α-agonists, see the general statement.

Dose—*Intranasal, adults* and *children over 6 yrs of age,* **2 to 3 drops** or **sprays** of **0.05%** solution into each nostril every 4 to 12 hours; *children 2 to 5 yr of age,* **2 to 3 drops** of **0.025%** solution every 12 hr.

Dosage Forms—Nasal Solution: 0.025 and 0.05%; Nasal Spray: 0.05%.

Pergolide—page 932.

Phenylephrine Hydrochloride

Benzenemethanol, 3-hydroxy-α-[(methylamino)methyl]-, hydrochloride; Neo Synephrine Hydrochloride (*Winthrop*); (*Various Mfrs*)

(−)-*m*-Hydroxy-α-[(methylamino)methyl]benzyl alcohol hydrochloride [61-76-7] $C_9H_{13}NO_2 \cdot HCl$ (203.67).

Preparation—*m*-Hydroxyphenacyl bromide is condensed with methylamine and the carbonyl group is then reduced to carbinol via catalytic hydrogenation. The phenylephrine so formed is dissolved in a suitable solvent and neutralized with HCl.

Description—White or nearly white crystals; odorless; bitter taste; melts between 140° and 145°.

Solubility—Freely soluble in water and alcohol.

Uses—A directly acting sympathomimetic with strong α-agonist and negligible β-agonist and central nervous activity. See the general statement for the actions, uses, adverse effects, precautions, and drug interactions of direct α-agonists. Phenylephrine is used in the treatment of *paroxysmal supraventricular tachycardia* and to support *blood pressure*. Phenylephrine can be used in the presence of heart-sensitizing anesthetics because of its lack of significant beta-adrenergic cardiac stimulant actions. It is also used as a nasal,

sleroconjunctival, and uveal *decongestant*, as a *mydriatic* and to decrease aqueous humor formation in *open-angle glaucoma*. It is included in some local anesthetic preparations and in combination with inhaled bronchodilators.

Phenylephrine is absorbed orally, and, since it is not attacked by monoamine oxidase, it is effective by mouth for orthostatic hypotension. By the intravenous route the duration of action is about 15 to 20 minutes and by the intramuscular route 30 to 120 min.

Dose—*Intramuscular* or *subcutaneous, adults*, for *mild to moderate hypotension, initially,* **2 to 5 mg,** repeated at intervals no less than 10 to 15 min, *or,* for *prevention of hypotension during spinal anesthesia,* **2 to 3 mg** 4 min before anesthetic; *children, to treat hypotension,* **100 μg/kg** (or **3 mg/m²** of body surface), repeated in 1 to 2 hr, as needed, *or, prior to spinal anesthesia,* 44 to 88 **μg/kg**. *Intravenous, adults,* for *mild to moderate hypotension,* **500 μg,** repeated at intervals no less than 10 to 15 min *or,* for *severe hypotension during spinal anesthesia, initially* **200 μg,** with subsequent increments no greater than 200 μg, up to a total of 500 μg/dose, **or** for *paroxysmal supraventricular tachycardia, initially* **up to 500/μg** given over 0.5 min, with subsequent increments of 100 to 200 μg, up to a total of 1 mg/dose. To *prolong spinal* and *local anesthesia,* 2 to 5 mg added to a *spinal anesthetic* solution *or* 1 **mg** (as **0.005%** solution) to a *regional anesthetic* solution. *Topical, intranasal, adults,* **2 or 3 drops** or **1 or 2 sprays** of **0.2 to 0.5%** solution, repeated in 3 to 5 min after blowing, or a **small amount** of **0.5%** jelly into each nostril every 3 to 4 hr; *children, all age groups,* **2 or 3 drops** of solutions as follows: *up to 2 yrs,* **0.125%** every 3 to 4 hr; *2 to 6 yr,* **0.125%** every 3 to 4 hr or **0.16%** every 4 hr; *6 to 12 yr,* **0.25%** every 3 to 4 hr; *children 6 to 12* may use **1 or 2 sprays** of **0.25%** solution, repeated in 3 to 5 min after blowing, every 3 to 4 hr. *Topical,* to the *eye,* **1 drop** of 2.5 to 10% solution into the conjunctival sac, repeated once in 5 min, if necessary, for *opthalmoscopy* or 2 to 3 times a day for *chronic mydriasis*, or, 1 **drop** of **0.08** to **0.15%** solution 2 or 3 times a day for *scleroconjunctival decongestion* and *blepharospasm; children,* as adults, except 10% solution is not to be used.

Dosage Forms—Injection: 10 mg/1 mL; Ophthalmic Solution: 0.08, 0.120, 0.2, 0.25, 1, 2.5, and 10%; Nasal Solution: 0.125, 0.160, 0.2, 0.25, 0.5, and 1%.

Phenylpropanolamine Hydrochloride

Benzenemethanol, α-(1-aminoethyl)-, hydrochloride, (*R**,*S**)-, (±)-, Propadrine Hydrochloride (*MSD*); (*Various Mfrs*)

(±)-Norephedrine hydrochloride [154-41-6] $C_9H_{13}NO \cdot HCl$ (187.67).

Preparation—By reacting benzaldehyde with nitroethane to form α-(1-nitroethyl)benzyl alcohol and then reducing this nitroalcohol to the corresponding amino compound which is then converted to the hydrochloride. US Pat. 2,151,517. For an improved industrial process, see US Pat. 3,028,429.

Description—White, crystalline powder having a slight aromatic odor; affected by light; melts between 191° and 196°; pH (3 in 100 solution) between 4.2 and 5.5; pK_{a1} (0.10) 9.04; pK_{a2} (0.005) 9.06.

Solubility—1 g in 1.1 mL water, 7.4 mL alcohol, 4100 mL chloroform; insoluble in ether.

Uses—An indirectly acting sympathomimetic with prominent peripheral adrenergic effects and weak central stimulant actions. The principal uses of phenylpropanolamine are as a *nasal decongestant* in hay fever. Promotional claims that systemic (oral) phenylpropanolamine has a selective vasoconstrictor action in the nasopharyngeal and otic regions have not been substantiated in man; a substantial decongestant action in the above areas is accompanied by a hypertensive response. It is also used to treat *urinary incontinence*.

Phenylpropanolamine has mild CNS actions and is used as an anorexiant in the treatment of *endogenous obesity*.

The actions, adverse effects, precautions, and drug interactions of indirect and centrally acting sympathomimetics may be found in the general statement. Adverse effects are most likely to occur when the dose exceeds 75 mg/day. Notable side effects include the CNS effects of nausea, dizziness, nervousness, insomnia, headache, and tinnitus, and peripheral effects of palpitations, hypertension, and hyperglycemia.

Dose—*Oral, adults, for decongestion,* **25 mg** every 4 hr *or* **50 mg**

every 8 hr *or* **75 mg** in extended release form every 12 hr, not to exceed 15 mg/day: for *appetite suppression*, **25 mg** 3 times a day **or 75 mg** in extended-release form once a day; for urinary incontinence, **50** to **75 mg** 3 times a day. *Oral, children, for decongestion only, 2 to 6 yrs* of age, **6.25 mg** every 4 hr or **12.5 mg** every 8 hr, not to exceed 37.5 mg/day; *6 to 12 yrs*, **12.5 mg** every 4 hr or **25 mg** every 8 hr, not to exceed 75 mg/day; *under 2 yrs*, dose must be individualized.

Dosage Forms—Capsules: 25, 37.5 and 50 mg; Timed-Release Capsules: 75 and 150 mg; Drops: 25 mg/5 drops; Elixir: 20 mg/5 mL, Syrup: 12.5 mg/5 mL; Tablets: 25, 37.5 and 50 mg; Timed-Release Tablets: 75 mg.

Propylhexedrine

Cyclohexaneethanamine, *N*,α-dimethyl-, (±)-, Benzedrex (*SK&F*)

(±)-*N*-α-Dimethylcyclohexaneethylamine [101-40-6] $C_{10}H_{21}N$ (155.28).

Preparation—As described in US Pat 2,454,746, a solution of cyclohexylacetone in formic acid is reacted with *N*-methylformamide by heating for 4 hours at 160° to 180°. The resulting formyl derivative of propylhexedrine is then hydrolyzed by refluxing with 50% H_2SO_4 and the hydrolysate is extracted with ether to remove acid-insoluble material. The aqueous solution is then rendered strongly alkaline with sodium hydroxide and the propylhexedrine is extracted with ether and purified by distillation under reduced pressure.

Description—Clear, colorless liquid, having a characteristic, aminelike odor; volatilizes slowly at room temperature; solutions are alkaline to litmus; absorbs carbon dioxide from the air; specific gravity 0.848 to 0.852; boils at about 205°.

Solubility—1 g in >500 mL water, 0.4 mL alcohol, 0.2 mL chloroform, 0.1 mL ether.

Uses—A volatile *indirect sympathomimetic* amine which, because of its lack of central excitatory effects and addiction liability, was introduced as a substitute for amphetamine for use in inhaler cartridges. One or two inhalations through each nostril produce *vasoconstriction* and a *decongestant* effect on nasal mucous membranes. Because of its wide margin of safety and relative freedom from toxic side effects, the use of propylhexedrine by inhalation is not contraindicated in patients in whom an ephedrine-like action would be undesirable. It is considered safe for self-medication by adults, but children should not have unsupervised access to an inhaler. Because the action is indirect, it will have limited efficacy in the treatment of nasal stuffiness consequent to treatment with reserpine, guanethidine, and other adrenergic neuron-blockers and catecholamine-depletors. Untoward effects of propylhexedrine include after-congestion, headache, and rarely, increase in blood pressure.

Dose—1 or **2 inhalations** (approximately 250 or 500 μg), through each nostril, as required.

Dosage Forms—Inhalant: 50 and 250 mg.

Pseudoephedrine Hydrochloride

Benzenemethanol, α-[1-(methylamino)ethyl]-, [*S*-(*R**,*R**)]-, hydrochloride; *d*-Isoephedrine Hydrochloride; Ro-Fedrin (*Robinson*); Sudafed (*Burroughs Wellcome*); (*Various Mfrs*)

(+)-Pseudoephedrine hydrochloride [345-78-8] $C_{10}H_{15}NO.HCl$ (201.70).

Preparation—(−)-Ephedrine hydrochloride is acetylated to produce (+)-*N*-acetylpseudoephedrine hydrochloride which is then deacetylated to yield the official article. Ephedrine and pseudoephedrine are diastereoisomers, the former having the *erythro* and the latter the *threo* configuration.

Description—Fine, white to off-white crystals or powder having a faint, characteristic odor; melts between 182° and 186°; pH (1 in 20 solution) between 4.6 and 6.0.

Solubility—1 g in 0.5 mL water, 3.6 mL alcohol, 91 mL chloroform, 7000 mL ether.

Uses—Differs from ephedrine (page 883) in that it is relatively weaker in its pressor, cardiac, mydriatic, and central-stimulant actions. Its nasopharyngeal vasoconstrictor and bronchodilator actions are about the same. It is used as a *nasopharyngeal* and *otic decongestant*. Promotional statements imply that systemic pseudoephedrine can selectively constrict blood vessels in the head region without generalized vasoconstriction, but most medical authorities disagree; if the dose is insufficient to raise the blood pressure, it is also insufficient to act as a decongestant. Pseudoephedrine has an anomalous action to dilate renal blood vessels and increase urine output. It can also dilate vertebral arterioles, which is possibly a reflex to systemic vasopression. The adverse effects, precautions, and drug interactions are those of indirect and weak centrally acting sympathomimetics (see the general statement).

Dose—*Oral*, user *over 12 yr of age*, **60 mg** every 6 hr, not to exceed 240 mg/day, *or*, with *extended-release* forms, **120 mg** every 12 hr. *Children*, **4 mg/kg** (or **125 mg/m²** of body surface) per day in 4 divided doses, *or by age group: up to 2 yr*, dose to be individualized; *2 to 6 yr*, **15 mg** every 6 hr, not to exceed 60 mg/day; *6 to 12 yr*, **30 mg** every 6 hr, not to exceed 120 mg/day, *or*, in *extended-release* form, **60 mg** every 8 to 12 hr.

Dosage Forms—Syrup: 30 mg/5 mL; Tablets: 30 and 60 mg; Extended-Release Tablets: 120 mg.

Terbutaline Sulfate

1,3-Benzenediol, 5-[2-[(1,1-dimethylethyl)amino]-1-hydroxyethyl]-, sulfate (2:1) (salt); Brethine (*Ciba-Geigy*); Bricanyl (*Astra*)

α-[(*tert*-Butylamino)methyl]-3,5-dihydroxybenzyl alcohol sulfate (2:1) (salt) [23031-32-5] $(C_{12}H_{19}NO_3)_2.H_2SO_4$ (548.65).

Preparation—One method involves reduction of 2-(*tert*-butylamino)-3',5'-dihydroxyacetophenone (I) to the carbinol by catalytic hydrogenation, followed by neutralization of the base with H_2SO_4 (Brit Pat 1,199,630). Substance I may be prepared by various routes starting with 3,5-dihydroxybenzoic acid.

Description—White to gray-white, crystalline powder; odorless or has a faint odor of acetic acid; slightly bitter; unstable in light; melts at about 247°; pK_{a1} 8.8; pK_{a2} 10.1; pK_{a3} 11.2.

Solubility—1 g in 1.5 mL water, 250 mL alcohol.

Uses—Terbutaline possesses strong β$_2$- and weak β$_1$- and α-agonist activities. Terbutaline is used only as a *bronchodilator*. Of the β-agonists, terbutaline causes the greatest degree of tremor. By the subcutaneous route the onset of action is about 5 min, peak effect being reached in 30 to 60 min. The actions, uses, adverse effects, precautions, etc. of the β-agonists are discussed in the general statement.

Dose—*Oral, adult*, **2.5** to **5 mg** 3 times a day at approximately 6-hour intervals during the waking hours; *children, 12 to 15 yr of age*, **2.5 mg** 3 times a day; not advised for younger children. *Subcutaneous, adult*, **250 μg** to be repeated after 15 to 30 min, if necessary, and not to exceed 500 μg in any 4-hour period; not determined for children.

Dosage Forms—Injection: 1 mg/mL; Tablets: 2.5 and 5 mg.

Tetrahydrozoline Hydrochloride

1*H*-Imidazole, 4,5-dihydro-2-(1,2,3,4-tetrahydro-1-naphthalenyl)-, monohydrochloride; Tyzine (*Pfizer*); Visine (*Leeming*)

2-(1,2,3,4-Tetrahydro-1-naphthyl)-2-imidazoline monohydrochloride [522-48-5] $C_{13}H_{16}N_2.HCl$ (236.74).

Preparation—Ethyl phenylacetate and methyl acrylate undergo a Michael condensation and cyclization using sodium ethoxide as catalyst, followed by acidification to form 4-keto-1,2,3,4-tetrahydro-1-naphthoic acid. The keto group is reduced by catalytic hydrogenation to methylene, and the resulting 1,2,3,4-tetrahydro-1-

naphthoic acid is condensed with ethylenediamine in the presence of HCl.

Description—White crystals; odorless; melts with decomposition at about 256°.

Solubility—1 g in 3.5 mL water, 7.5 mL alcohol; very slightly soluble in chloroform, ether.

Uses—Tetrahydrozoline is chemically related to naphazoline but differs in its actions in that in addition to topical vasoconstrictor action it has a prominent vasodilator component in its systemic effects in man. It is used only as a *nasal* and *ophthalmologic decongestant*. The local and systemic adverse effects and precautions are those of topical α-agonists. In addition, profuse sweating, sedation, severe respiratory depression, coma and shock in young children after overdosage have been reported. Overdoses in adults cause hypotension and bradycardia.

Dose—*Topical, intranasal, user over 6 yr* of age, **2** to **4 drops** or **1 spray** of **0.05** or **0.1**% solution into each nostril twice a day, in the morning and in the evening; *children 2 to 6 yr* **2** to **3 drops** of **0.05**% solution at intervals no shorter than 3 hr. *To the eye,* 1 to **2 drops** of **0.05**% solution into the conjunctival sac 2 or 3 times a day.

Dosage Forms—Nasal Solution: 0.05 and 0.1%; Ophthalmic Solution: 0.05%.

Xylometazoline Hydrochloride

1*H*-Imidazole, 2-[[4-(1,1-dimethylethyl)-2,6-dimethylphenyl]methyl]-4,5-dihydro-, monohydrochloride; Otrivin Hydrochloride (*Ciba-Geigy*)

2-(4-*tert*-Butyl-2,6-dimethylbenzyl)-2-imidazoline monohydrochloride [1218-35-5] $C_{16}H_{24}N_2 \cdot HCl$ (280.84).

Preparation—Utilizing (4-*tert*-butyl-2,6-dimethylphenyl)acetonitrile as the participating nitrile, by the method described for *Naphazoline Hydrochloride*, page 888.

Description—White, odorless crystalline powder, melts above 300° with decomposition; pH (1 in 20 solution) between 5.0 and 6.6.

Solubility—1 g in about 30 mL water; freely soluble in alcohol; sparingly soluble in chloroform; practically insoluble in benzene and ether.

Uses—A direct sympathomimetic chemically related to *Naphazoline Hydrochloride* and *Tetrahydrozoline Hydrochloride*. It is used as a local vasoconstrictor for nasal decongestion. Its effects are prompt in onset and last for several hours but do not seem to be followed by as much reactive hyperemia (rebound congestion) as with naphazoline. Side effects are infrequent but are those of topical α-agonists (see the general statement for actions, uses, adverse effects, precautions, and drug interactions); in addition, overdoses may cause severe central nervous depression and even coma in children.

Dose—*Intranasal, adults* and *children over 12 yr* of age, **2** or **3 drops** or **1** or **2 sprays** of a **0.1**% solution into each nostril every 4 to 10 hr, as needed; *children, up to 6 mo,* **1 drop** of a **0.05**% solution every 6 hr, as needed; *6 to 12 yr,* **2** or **3 drops** of a **0.05**% solution every 4 to 10 hr, as needed.

Dosage Forms—Solution: 0.05 and 0.1%; Nasal Spray: 0.1%.

Other Sympathomimetic Drugs

Amphetamine Sulfate [(±)-α-Methylphenethylamine sulfate (2:1) [60-13-9] ($C_9H_{13}N)_2 \cdot H_2SO_4$ (368.49); Racemic Amphetamine Sulfate; Benzedrine Sulfate (*SK&F*)]—For the structural formula of the (+)-form of amphetamine see page 891. A white, odorless, slightly bitter, crystalline powder; 1 g dissolves in about 9 mL water and 500 mL alcohol. *Uses* and *Dose:* Amphetamine has actions and uses identical to those of *Dextroamphetamine* (see page 881). Although the potency is less than that of dextroamphetamine, the doses are the same. *Dosage Forms:* Sustained-Release Capsules: 15 mg; Tablets: 5 and 10 mg.

Benzphetamine Hydrochloride [(+)-*N*-Benzyl-*N*,α-dimethylphenethylamine hydrochloride [5411-22-3] $C_{17}H_{21}N \cdot HCl$ (275.82); Didrex (*Upjohn*)]—Prepared by benzylating (+)-desoxyephedrine with benzyl chloride in the presence of sodium carbonate, the resulting benzphetamine being separated by distillation and then converted to the hydrochloride. A white to off-white, crystalline powder; polymorphic, one form melting at about 130°, the other at 150° and higher, with decomposition. One g dissolves in about 1.5 mL water, 1.5 mL alcohol, 1.5 mL chloroform; slightly soluble in ether. *Uses:* An indirectly acting *sympathomimetic* and central nervous system stimulant. Its only approved use is as an *ano-*

rexiant, in which role it is about as efficacious as dextroamphetamine. Benzphetamine has euphoric action. For the limitations of anorexiant therapy and the adverse effects, precautions, and drug interactions of centrally acting sympathomimetics, see the general statement. *Dose: Oral,* user *over 12 yr* of age only, initially 25 mg once a day, to be increased, if necessary, to 25 to 50 mg, 1 to 3 times a day. *Dosage Forms:* Tablets: 25 and 50 mg.

Chlorphentermine Hydrochloride [*p*-Chloro-α,α-dimethylphenethylamine hydrochloride [151-06-4] $C_{10}H_{14}ClN \cdot HCl$ (220.14); Pre-Sate (*Warner-Chilcott*)]—Synthesized by grignardization of *p*-chlorobenzyl chloride with acetone, the resulting 1-(*p*-chlorophenyl)-2-methyl-2-propanol reacted with sodium cyanide in an acid medium to form the corresponding 2-formamido compound, which is hydrolyzed to chlorphentermine and then converted to the hydrochloride. A white to off-white powder; odorless and with a bitter taste; melts at about 235°. Freely soluble in water and alcohol; sparingly soluble in chloroform; practically insoluble in ether. *Uses:* An *anorexigenic sympathomimetic* with weak central stimulant activity. Its cardiovascular effects are also weak, so that the drug has been recommended especially for use in the treatment of obesity complicated by cardiovascular disorders. As an anorexigenic it appears to be as good as but not superior to other prominent anorexigenic drugs. Insomnia, nervousness, dizziness, and palpitation occasionally occur. Drug dependence can occur. For other possible adverse effects, precautions, and drug interactions, see the general statement on centrally acting sympathomimetics. *Dose: Oral,* user *over 12 yr* of age only, 65 mg of the base once a day, usually after breakfast. *Dosage Form:* Tablets: 65 mg chlorphentermine base.

Clortermine Hydrochloride [*o*-Chloro-α,α-dimethylphenethylamine hydrochloride [10389-72-7] $C_{10}H_{14}ClN \cdot HCl$ (220.14); Voramil (*USV*)]—An isomer of *Chlorphentermine* that differs in the position of the chlorine substituent in the base. *Uses:* An *anorectic drug* similar to chlorphentermine. Although it is a sympathomimetic, the cardiovascular actions are usually minimal in therapeutic doses. The actions, adverse effects, precautions, and drug interactions are those of centrally acting sympathomimetics (see the general statement). *Dose: Oral, adult* and *children over 12 yr* of age, 50 mg a day; not advised for use in children under 12. *Dosage Form:* Tablets: 50 mg.

Dextroamphetamine Saccharate—Dextroamphetamine is solubilized in an aqueous solution of saccharic (D-glucaric) acid. *Uses:* See *Dextroamphetamine Sulfate,* page 881. *Dose:* Not sold as a single-entity product.

Diethylpropion Hydrochloride 2-(Diethylamino)-1-phenyl-[1-propanone hydrochloride [134-80-5] $C_{13}H_{19}NO \cdot HCl$ (241.76). Tenuate (*Merrell*); Tepanil (*Riker*)]. White or creamy white, small crystals or crystalline powder; has a characteristic, mildly aromatic odor, and is stable in dry air; melts at about 175° with decomposition. Soluble 1 g in 0.5 mL water, 3 mL alcohol, 3 mL chloroform; practically insoluble in ether. *Uses:* The central nervous system stimulatory actions of diethylpropion occur at considerably lower doses than do the cardiovascular actions. Thus it is used only for its central effects. Its anorexiant effects are relatively more prominent than with dextroamphetamine, so that it is used only in the treatment of *obesity.* The adverse effects and precautions are those of centrally acting sympathomimetics in general (see the general statement). *Dose: Oral, adults* and *children over 12* years of age, 25 mg 3 times a day, 1 hour before each meal, or 75 mg in *sustained-release* form in the morning; 25 mg may be taken mid-evening if insomnia is not a problem. *Dosage Forms:* Extended-release Tablets: 75 mg; Tablets: 25 mg.

Dipivefrine Hydrochloride [2,2-Dimethylpropanoic acid (±)-4-[1-hydroxy-2-(methylamino)ethyl]-1,2-phenylene ester [5236-63-6] $C_{19}H_{29}NO_5$ (351.44)]. Prepared by selectively acylating the phenolic hydroxyl groups of epinephrine with pivaloyl chloride. *Uses:* The lipid solubility of dipivefrine gives the drug 17 times the penetrance of epinephrine. Once in the eye, it is converted to epinephrine. It is used in the treatment of *open-angle glaucoma.* After topical application, intraocular tension drops in about ½ hr and the effect is maximum at about 1 hr. The incidence of intolerance to the drug is $1/30$ that to epinephrine. See the general statement for the potential adverse effects of α, β-agonists. *Dose: Topical,* into the *conjunctival sac,* 1 drop of a 0.1% solution every 12 hr. *Dosage Form:* Ophthalmic Solution: 0.1%.

Ethylnorepinephrine Hydrochloride [4-(2-Amino-1-hydroxybutyl)-1,2-benzenediol hydrochloride $C_{10}H_{15}NO_3 \cdot HCl$ (233.70); ethylnoradrenaline hydrochloride, Bronkephrine (*Breon*)]—A crystalline substance, soluble in water. *Uses:* Possesses moderate α-, β₁-, and β₂-agonist activities. Its only use is as a *bronchodilator,* having about one-tenth the potency of isoproterenol. The α- and β-activities often roughly balance each other with respect to blood pressure but the distribution of blood flow is altered unfavorably. For actions, uses, adverse effects, precautions, and drug interactions, see the general statement. *Dose: Subcutaneous* or *intramuscular, adults,* 0.6 to 2 mg; *children,* 0.2 to 1 mg. In an emergency, by slow *intravenous injection,* 1 to 5 mg. *Dosage Form:* Injection: 2 mg/1 mL.

Isometheptene Mucate [*N*,6-Dimethyl-5-hepten-2-amine galactarate (2:1) (salt) ($C_9H_{19}N)_2 \cdot C_6H_{10}O_8$ (492.64)]—Bitter tasting white crystals melting about 150°; freely soluble in water; soluble about 1 g in 20 mL of alcohol; almost insoluble in ether or chloroform. *Uses:* Isometheptene is an indirectly-acting sympathomimetic (see general statement) which is claimed to constrict dilated cerebral and carotid vessels. It is marketed only in combination with dichloralphenezone and acetaminophen for the treatment of *migraine* or *tension headache*. *Dose: Oral, initially*, 65 or 130 mg, to be repeated every 4 hr, up to a maximal of 520 mg a day, if necessary, for tension headache and every hour, up to 320 mg per 12 hr, if necessary, for migraine headache.

Isoxsuprine Hydrochloride [*p*-Hydroxy-α-[1-[(1-methyl-2-phenoxyethyl)amino]ethyl]benzyl alcohol hydrochloride [579-56-6] $C_{18}H_{23}NO_3.HCl$ (337.85) Vasodilan (*Mead-Johnson*).] White, crystalline powder which is odorless and has a bitter taste; melts, with decomposition, at about 200°; pH (1 in 100 solution) between 4.5 and 6.0. Soluble 1 g in 500 mL water, 100 mL alcohol, >10,000 mL chloroform, >10,000 mL ether. *Uses:* Isoxsuprine is a β-agonist with a slight selectivity for the β_2-adrenoreceptors. However, a considerable portion of the vasodilator actions are attributable to a nonselective depression of vascular smooth muscle. It is considered to be "possibly effective" in Raynaud's disease, thromboangiitis obliterans, obliterative arteriosclerosis, and cerebrovascular insufficiency. See the general statement for the actions adverse effects and precautions of β-agonists. *Dose: Oral, adult*, **10** to **20** mg, 3 or 4 times a day. *Intramuscular, adult*, **5** to **10** mg 2 to 3 times a day.

Levonordefrin [(−)-α-(1-Aminoethyl)-3,4-dihydroxybenzyl alcohol [18829-78-2] and [829-74-3] $C_9H_{13}NO_3$ (183.21). *dl*-Nordefrin may be resolved by dissolving it in an alcoholic solution of *d*-tartaric acid and separating the enantiomorphs as the *d*-tartrates by fractional crystallization from which the levo isomer is obtained by treatment with alkali. White to buff-colored, odorless, crystalline solid; melts at about 210°. Practically insoluble in water; slightly soluble in acetone, chloroform, alcohol, and ether; freely soluble in aqueous solutions of mineral acids. *Uses:* A directly acting sympathomimetic α-agonist vasoconstrictor with negligible central effects as ordinarily used. Since dextronordefrin, which makes up ½ of the base of nordefrin, is negligibly active as a vasoconstrictor, levonordefrin is twice as potent as the racemic nordefrin base. On the other hand, dextronordefrin has weak central stimulant actions, and removal of the dextro isomer to yield levonordefrin greatly lessens central stimulant activity. However, as a *vasoconstrictor in local anesthetic solutions*, the central actions are of no significance, so that levonordefrin has no advantage over nordefrin hydrochloride. There is no reason why levonordefrin cannot be employed for its systemic vasopressor actions, although it is not marketed in a suitable form. See the general statement for actions, uses, adverse effects, etc. of α-agonists. *Dose:* In local anesthetic solutions, especially for dental use, in 0.005% concentration. *Dosage Forms—Injection:* 2% Mepivacaine, and 1:20,000 Levonordefrin, in 1-mL cartridges.

Mazindol [5-(*p*-Chlorophenyl-2,5-dihydro-3*H*-imidazo[2,1-*a*]isoindol-5-ol [22232-71-9] $C_{19}H_{13}ClN_2O$ (284.74); Sanorex (*Sandoz*)]—Prepared by catalyzed condensation/addition of *o*-(*p*-chlorobenzoyl)-benzoic acid and ethylenediamine; a white to off-white, crystalline powder; odorless or with a faint odor; insoluble in water and slightly soluble in alcohol. *Uses:* An *anorexiant* sympathomimetic with relatively weak cardiovascular actions and a variable effect on the central nervous system, causing signs of mild stimulation in some patients and mild depression in others. It causes little or no euphoria. In the treatment of obesity with mazindol about two-thirds of patients on a diet of 600 cal/day can adhere to the diet for over 12 weeks, which appears to be a better response than with any other anorexiant. Tolerance to mazindol is of a low order, and the abuse potential appears to be less than with most centrally acting sympathomimetics. The side effects, precautions, and drug interactions are those of other centrally acting sympathomimetics (see general statement) but some effects, such as drowsiness (20% of patients), weakness (14%), and moderate hypotension, differ. Reduction in blood pressure may be secondary to weight loss. Insulin requirements may change, mostly as a result of changed diet. Nausea occurs in about 10% of users. *Dose: Oral, adults* and *children over 12 yr;* 2 mg once a day 1 hr before lunch, or 1 mg 3 times a day, 1 hr before each meal. *Dosage Forms:* Tablets: 1 and 2 mg.

Methamphetamine Hydrochloride [(+)-*N*,α-Dimethylphenethylamine hydrochloride [51-57-0] $C_{10}H_{15}N.HCl$ (185.70); deoxyephedrine hydrochloride; methylamphetamine hydrochloride; (*Various Mfrs.*)]—Methamphetamine is prepared by catalytic hydrogenation of ephedrine and subsequently is converted to the hydrochloride. Occurs as white crystals or a white, crystalline powder; odorless; melts between 171° and 175°. One g dissolves in 2 mL of water, 3 mL alcohol, 5 mL chloroform; very slightly soluble in absolute ether. *Uses:* Actions are very similar to those of amphetamine, but at low doses the cardiovascular effects are less pronounced. It is mainly employed for its *central nervous system stimulant* actions in depressing appetite in the therapy of *obesity* and *abnormal behavioral states* in children. Tolerance to the normalizing effect in hyperkinetic children does not occur. Because it may elevate mood, it was once used as an antidepressant. At tolerated doses, the cardiovascular effects consist mainly of cardiac stimulation, which elevates blood pressure. Vasoconstriction makes a minor contribution to the pressor effect. The cardiovascular actions are elicited principally by the levo component in a racemic mixture; they are the result of an indirect, norepinephrine-releasing action. The side effects, contraindications, and drug interactions are those of centrally acting sympathomimetics. Methamphetamine is widely abused for its central stimulant actions. It is the drug usually called "speed" in drug abuse circles, although other centrally acting sympathomimetics are often given the same name. *Dose: Oral, adults* and *children over 12 yr* of age, for *endogenous obesity initially* 2.5 mg 3 times a day, 30 to 60 min before meals; the dose is increased as needed, but it seldom is necessary to exceed 5 mg. The drug is not recommended for use as an anorectic in children under 12 years of age. For *abnormal behavioral syndrome*, *children 6 yr and older*, 2.5 or 5 mg once or twice a day, with 5 mg/day-adjustments at weekly intervals, if needed *or*, in extended-release form, 5 to 15 mg once a day. *Dosage Forms:* Tablets, 5 and 10 mg; Extended-Release Tablets: 5, 10, and 15 mg.

Nylidrin Hydrochloride [*p*-Hydroxy-α-[1-[(1-methyl-3-phenylpropyl)amino]ethyl]benzyl alcohol hydrochloride [900-01-6; 849-55-8] $C_{19}H_{25}NO_2.HCl$ (335.87); Arlidin (*USV*)]—Nylidrin is prepared by reacting *p*-hydroxynorephedrine and benzylacetone in alcohol and catalytically hydrogenating the product. The hydrochloride occurs as a white, crystalline powder; odorless; practically tasteless. One g dissolves in about 65 mL water, and 40 mL alcohol; very slightly soluble in chloroform and ether. *Uses:* Nylidrin possesses β_2-agonist activity that is more selective for the skeletal muscle vasculature than the bronchioles. Some of the action appears to be a nonspecific smooth muscle relaxation. There is little effect on the cutaneous vasculature. It has mild β_1-agonist activity. See the general statement for the actions, uses, adverse effects, and precautions of β_2- and β_1-agonists. In normotensives, the drug has little effect on blood pressure, but it is hypotensive in hypertensive patients and hypertensive in hypotensive patients. It is used in the treatment of vascular disorders of the skeletal muscle vessels, such as *intermittent claudication*, *thrombophlebitis* and, to a lesser extent, *diabetic vascular disease*. However, it is effective only to the extent that there may be a vasospastic component in these disorders, which are otherwise mainly occlusive. It has been advocated for use in thromboangiitis obliterans, endarteritis obliterans, Raynaud's disease, and ischemic ulcers; inasmuch as the drug fails to increase significantly cutaneous blood flow, such use cannot be expected to be of benefit. *Dose: Oral*, 3 to 12 mg 3 or 4 times a day. *Dosage Forms:* Tablets: 6 and 12 mg.

Phendimetrazine Tartrate [(+)-3,4-Dimethyl-2-phenylmorpholine tartrate (1:1) [50-58-2] $C_{12}H_{17}NO.C_4H_6O_6$ (341.35); (*Various Mfrs.*)]—Phendimetrazine base may be prepared by interaction of *l*-ephedrine and ethylene chlorohydrin. The tartrate occurs as a white, crystalline powder; odorless; bitter taste; melts at about 186°, with decomposition; pK_a 7.2. Soluble in water and alcohol. *Uses:* Closely related to phenmetrazine, both chemically and pharmacologically, phendimetrazine is an indirectly acting *sympathomimetic* with predominantly central nervous stimulant actions. It is used as an *appetite suppressant* and not as a general central stimulant or sympathomimetic. Except for glossitis and cystitis, the adverse effects are those of centrally acting sympathomimetics (see the general statement for actions, uses, adverse effects, etc.). *Dose: Oral, adults* and *children over 12 yr* of age, 17.5 to 70 mg 2 or 3 times daily, 1 hr before meals, or 105 mg in extended-release form once a day. *Dosage Forms:* Extended-Release Capsules: 105 mg; Capsules: 35 mg; Tablets: 35 mg.

Phenmetrazine Hydrochloride [3-Methyl-2-phenylmorpholine hydrochloride [1707-14-8] $C_{11}H_{15}NO.HCl$ (213.71); Psychamine A66; Preludin (*Boehringer Ingelheim*)]—Phenmetrazine may be prepared by an addition reaction of norephedrine and ethylene oxide, the resulting alcohol being cyclized with a suitable dehydrant. The hydrochloride occurs as a white to off-white, crystalline powder; melts between 172° and 182°; pK_a 7.6. One g dissolves in about 0.4 mL water, 2 mL alcohol, 2 mL chloroform. *Uses:* A *sympathomimetic* with central nervous and weak cardiovascular activity. See the general statement for the actions, uses, adverse effects, precautions, and drug interactions of centrally acting sympathomimetics. It is employed as an anorexigenic agent, for which use it is about equal to dextroamphetamine. The side effects of euphoria, insomnia, headache, dizziness, nausea, urinary frequency, nervousness and hyperexcitability are claimed to be less frequent. However, some clinical studies indicate that phenmetrazine may have greater relative central stimulatory activity than amphetamine. Tolerance and drug dependence can occur. Abuse liability is low at recommended doses. *Dose: Oral, adults* and *children over 12 yr* of age, 25 mg once a day to 3 times a day administered 1 hr before meals or 50 or 75 mg a day as a single extended-relrease tablet taken 1 hr before breakfast. Not recommended for use in children under 12 yr of age. *Dosage Forms:* Tablets: 25 mg; Extended-Release Tablets: 50 and 75 mg.

Phentermine [α,α-Dimethylphenethylamine [122-09-8] $C_{10}H_{15}N$ (149.23)]—Synthesized by grignardization of benzyl alcohol with acetone, reacting the resulting α,α-dimethylphenethyl alcohol with sodium cyanide in acid to form the corresponding 2-formamido compound, and hydrolyzing this to phentermine. A colorless, mobile, oily liquid with an odor characteristic of amines; slightly soluble in water and soluble in alcohol, chloroform, and ether. *Phentermine Resin*, a cationic exchange resin complex of phentermine, and *Phentermine Hydrochloride*, a crystalline salt that is very soluble in water, are the two derivatives used in available dosage forms; the former is marketed under the name *Ionamin* (Pennwalt) and the latter as *Adipex* (Lemmon), *Fastin* (Beecham), and *Phentercot* (Truxton). *Uses:* Phentermine is a centrally acting sympathomimetic with weak cardiovascular activity. It is used an an *anorexiant.* The central stimulant actions are less prominent than with the amphetamines. Consequently, use of the drug is accompanied by a low incidence of side effects; however, the anorectic effects are also weaker. Clinical trials do not show unequivocal efficacy. Long-term use, particularly of doses larger than are recommended for therapy, can cause drug dependence. The adverse effects, precautions, and drug interactions are those of the centrally acting sympathomimetics (see the general statement). *Dose: Oral, adults* and *children over 12 yr* of age, *extended-release* forms, 15 to 30 mg (as phentermine base), to be taken on rising, or 8 mg 3 times a day 30 min before meals or 15 to 30 mg as a single dose before breakfast with *conventional* forms. *Dosage Forms:* Phentermine Resin Capsules: 15 and 30 mg; Phentermine Hydrochloride Capsules: 15, 30, 37.5 mg; Phentermine Hydrochloride Extended-Release Capsules: 15 and 30 mg; Tablets: 8 and 37.5 mg.

Pseudophedrine Sulfate [S-$(R*,R*)$]-α-[1-(Methylaminoethyl]benzenemethanol sulfate (2:1) (salt) [9460-12-0] $(C_{10}H_{15}NO)_2 \cdot H_2SO_4$ (428.54)]—Refer to the monograph on ephedrine for the synthesis of the base. *Uses:* Same as those of *Pseudoephedrine Hydrochloride* (page 890). *Dose: Oral, adults* and *children over 12 yr* of age, 120 mg of a sustained-release form every 12 hr. *Dosage Form:* Tablets: 120 mg (60 mg immediately available, 60 mg delayed release).

Racenephrine—Epinephrine obtained by synthesis is first isolated in racemic form, and is then resolved into the official highly active levorotatory isomer and the relatively inactive dextrorotatory isomer (see page 883). The racemic form, less costly to produce because of elimination of the resolution step, is available commercially and in approximately double the concentration of *l*-epinephrine is used (as the hydrochloride) in certain bronchodilator formulations. *Uses:* As a *bronchodilator* (see the general statement). The potency of the racemic mixture is about half that of *l*-epinephrine. *Dose: Oral inhalation, adult* and *children over 4 yr* of age, 2 or 3 sprays of a 2.25% solution, repeated in 5 min, if necessary, then 4 to 6 times a day; *children under 4 yr*, the dose must be individualized. *Inhalation* by *nebulizer/respirator*, 5 mL of a 0.1% solution for 15 min every 3 to 4 hr. *Dosage Form:* Inhalation containing 2.25% racemic epinephrine.

Racephedrine Hydrochloride [(±)-α-[1-(Methylamino)ethyl]benzyl alcohol hydrochloride [134-71-4] $C_{10}H_{15}NO \cdot HCl$ (201.70); *dl*-ephedrine hydrochloride; component of Amodrine (*Searle*)]—One of several methods for synthesizing this racemic form of ephedrine reacts 2-bromopropiophenone with methylamine and reduces the resulting 2-(methylamino)-propiophenone by catalytic hydrogenation. Occurs as fine, white crystals or powder; odorless; affected by light. One g dissolves in about 4 mL of water and about 25 mL of alcohol; insoluble in ether. *Uses:* Similar to those of *Ephedrine* (page 883). It is marketed only for its bronchodilator activity in mixtures containing other active ingredients. *Dose: Oral, adult, usual,* 25 mg.

CHAPTER 46

Cholinomimetic (Parasympathomimetic) Drugs

Stewart C Harvey, PhD

Professor of Pharmacology
School of Medicine, University of Utah
Salt Lake City, UT 84132

The terms *cholinomimetic* (*cholinergic*) and *parasympathomimetic* are not equivalent, but they are popularly treated as synonyms. It will be recalled (see General Statement on *Autonomic Nervous System and Autonomic Drugs*, page 876) that acetylcholine is liberated not only at parasympathetic *post*ganglionic nerve endings but also at all autonomic *pre*ganglionic nerve endings, at somatic motor nerve endings, and probably at certain central synapses. Thus, a cholinomimetic can be a ganglionic or neuromuscular stimulant (ie, can be *nicotinic*—see *Nicotine*, page 896), possibly even a centrally acting drug, with or without also being a parasympathomimetic. A parasympathomimetic drug is literally an agent whose cholinomimetic action is limited to the parasympathetic neuroeffectors (ie, it is *muscarinic*—see *Muscarine*, page 896). Most muscarinic substances also possess varying degrees of action on autonomic ganglia and neuromuscular junctions (ie, nicotinic actions). Even methacholine, which is generally held to be strictly muscarinic, exerts nicotinic actions on the neuromuscular junction in myasthenia gravis or on the adrenal medulla in pheochromocytoma. There are muscarinic receptors in autonomic ganglia. Their normal function is elusive and complex. There are sympathetic cholinergic neuroeffectors that are indistinguishable in receptor type from those of the parasympathetic system, so that every parasympathomimetic also is a mimetic of sympathetic cholinergic activity.

Acetylcholine is hydrolyzed to choline and acetic acid by the enzyme *acetylcholinesterase* at or near the site of liberation of the neurohumor. Similar specific and nonspecific esterases are also present in plasma, erythrocytes, and other tissues. Drugs that inhibit these enzymes prolong the life of acetylcholine at the cholinergic neuroeffectors and synapses and thereby facilitate the normal transmission of cholinergic nervous impulses. Although this action of anticholinesterases is one of support rather than mimicry of acetylcholine, the anticholinesterases are generally loosely classified as cholinomimetics. They are therefore included in this chapter also. The section on *Anticholinesterases* can be found on page 896.

Cholinomimetics

All therapeutic cholinomimetic drugs are used for their muscarinic actions. Muscarinic drugs dilate nearly all blood vessels, except that they constrict certain veins. In high doses they may decrease heart rate and atrioventricular conduction velocity and cause varying degrees of heart block; they may also decrease the strength of atrial, but not ventricular, contractions. However, in therapeutic doses, usually only vasodilatation occurs, and the heart rate and contractility may actually increase because of sympathetically mediated reflexes to the hypotension caused by vasodilatation. The muscarinic drugs stimulate gastrointestinal smooth muscle and increase peristalsis, thus decreasing bowel transit time and promoting defecation; in high doses, bowel and sphincter spasms can occur. The lower esophageal sphincter is also stimulated. There are also muscarinic actions to contract the smooth muscle of the detrusor muscle of the urinary bladder but relax that of the trigone sphincter, thus causing urination. The bronchial smooth muscle is contracted, and bronchospasm may result. Stimulation of the sphincter of the iris causes miosis (pupiloconstriction); stimulation of the ciliary body causes ciliary spasm and a decrease in intraocular tension in glaucoma. Miosis and ciliary spasm do not usually occur after systemic administration, since the muscarinic drugs penetrate poorly into the eye from the blood stream; topical or intraocular administration is employed to achieve therapeutic miosis. Most exocrine glands are stimulated; thus excessive salivation, rhinorrhea, bronchorrhea (and mucous plugs), increased gastric and pancreatic secretions, and copious sweating may be elicited.

All muscarinic drugs have some degree of nicotinic activity, although some may be considered devoid of such activity for practical purposes. Even with those that have relatively strong nicotinic activity, such as acetylcholine (the natural nicotinic neurotransmitter), nicotinic effects, such as neuromuscular stimulation and paralysis and sympathoadrenal discharge, are usually manifested only in highly toxic doses; however, in therapeutic doses, carbachol appears to exert some nicotinic actions at mural ganglia in the gut and perhaps at sacral parasympathetic ganglia.

Uses—The miotic and ciliary spastic effects are used in the topical treatment of *open-angle, acute congestive* and *narrow-angle glaucoma*, prior to or *during intraocular surgery*, such as cataract surgery (after the lens is delivered), iridectomy, penetrating keratoplasty, and other anterior segment surgery; they are also used in alternation with mydriatic drugs to *break adhesions between the iris and the lens*. They are occasionally used in the treatment of *accommodative strabismus*. Muscarinic drugs may be used to *antagonize mydriatics*.

In gastroenterology, certain muscarinic drugs are used in the treatment of *atonic constipation, congenital megacolon* (Hirschsprung's disease), postoperative and postpartum *adynamic intestinal ileus, postvagotomy gastric atony*, and *gastroesophageal reflux* (in which there is some residual function in the lower esophageal sphincter). They are also occasionally used to stimulate pancreatic secretion in tests of pancreatic function. In genitourinary practice, muscarinic drugs may be used to treat *functional urinary retention*. Their principal cardiovascular use is for the arrest of *paroxysmal atrial tachycardia*, although they have largely been replaced by superior drugs; even though therapeutic doses do not usually depress the normal functions of the heart, they often do induce a conduction block in the aberrant conduction pathway within the atrioventricular node that permits this reentrant arrhythmia to occur. *Vasospastic peripheral vascular disorders*, such as accompany Raynaud's disease and cold exposure or frostbite, have been successfully treated with these agents, but superior drugs are available. This is also true of their use to increase cutaneous blood flow in *scleroderma*. Muscarinic drugs are not useful in the management of occlusive vascular diseases.

Adverse Effects—The adverse effects of muscarinic drugs are simply extensions of their pharmacodynamic actions. Thus excessive salivary, nasopharyngeal, and bronchial secretions and bronchospasm are not only uncomfortable but may be life-threatening by way of impeding the movement of air to and from the lungs. Excessive sweating may cause discomfort, affect the clothing, and interfere with body temperature control. In low doses, vasodilatation may be mainly confined to the skin, causing flushing and prickly or burning sensations. Moderate to high doses may cause moderate to severe hypotension, leading to syncope and even shock. Excessive doses may cause severe bradycardia, even cardiac arrest, and atrioventricular conduction disturbances, especially heart block. Furthermore, reflex sympathoadrenal discharge coupled with direct muscarinic effects on conduction sets the stage for serious cardiac arrhythmias. Gastrointestinal adverse effects include epigastric distress, belching, diarrhea, involuntary defecation, nausea and vomiting (partly as the result of hypotension) and colic. There may also be a feeling of tightness in the urinary bladder, urinary frequency, and enuresis.

Topical muscarinic drugs applied to the conjunctiva or intraocularly may interfere with near vision (accommodative myopia) and cause blurred vision, ocular pain, browache, headache, ciliary and conjunctival congestion, twitching of the eyelids, and decreased vision in poor light. After conjunctival application, there may be enough local absorption into the blood stream and also nasolacrimal drainage to result in systemic side effects.

Precautions and Contraindications—Muscarinic drugs should be used cautiously in patients with hypertension, especially those under treatment with antihypertensive drugs, and when there is arteriosclerosis (since reflex adjustments to the hypotensive effects may be impaired). Systemic muscarinic drugs are contraindicated in the presence of atrioventricular conduction defects, coronary insufficiency, pheochromocytoma (catecholamine release and hypertensive crisis may be initiated), hyperthyroidism (atrial fibrillation may result), asthma, and peptic ulcer. Even in ophthalmologic use, care must be exercised in these conditions. After instillation of solutions into the conjunctival sac, the nasolacrimal duct should be occluded by digital pressure, to minimize drainage and oral absorption.

Atropine should be at hand, in case serious side effects occur. The muscarinic (parasympathomimetic) actions can be blocked by atropine and its congeners, which serve as antidotes to overdosage, and the ganglionic and neuromuscular (nicotinic) stimulant actions can be antagonized, respectively, by ganglionic blocking and neuromuscular blocking agents.

Acetylcholine Chloride

Ethanaminium, 2-(acetyloxy)-*N*,*N*,*N*-trimethyl-, chloride; Miochol (*Cooper Vision*)

$$CH_3CO(CH_2)_2N^+(CH_3)_3 \quad Cl^-$$

Choline chloride acetate [60-31-1] $C_7H_{16}ClNO_2$ (181.66).

Preparation—Trimethylamine is reacted with 2-chloroethyl acetate as described in *Bull Soc Chim France 15(4):* 544, 1914.

Description—Hygroscopic, crystalline powder.
Solubility—Very soluble in cold water and alcohol; decomposed by hot water or alkalies; practically insoluble in ether.

Uses—Principally a topical ophthalmological drug to *induce miosis* during certain intraocular surgical procedures, such as cataract surgery (*after* the lens is delivered), iridectomy, penetrating keratoplasty, and other anterior segment surgery. It is given as an irrigant into the anterior chamber. When applied to the intact cornea, acetylcholine penetrates too poorly to be a clinically useful miotic.

Because of the rapidity by which acetylcholine is destroyed by acetylcholinesterase, it has no systemic uses; even huge doses rarely cause death. When death occurs it is usually a hypoxic death from mucous plugs in the bronchial tree or a cardiac death from fibrillation caused by the combination of cholinergic and reflex sympathoadrenal stimulation.

Dose—*Topical*, into the anterior chamber of the eye, as a 1% solution.

Dosage Forms—for Ophthalmic Solution: 20 mg/2 mL in a 2-chamber vial.

Bethanechol Chloride

1-Propanaminium, 2-[(aminocarbonyl)oxy]-*N*,*N*,*N*-trimethyl-, chloride; Duvoid (*Norwich Eaton*); Urecholine Chloride (*MSD*)

$$\left[\begin{array}{c} CH_3CHCH_2N^+(CH_3)_3 \\ | \\ OCONH_2 \end{array} \right] \; Cl^-$$

(2-Hydroxypropyl)trimethylammonium chloride carbamate [590-63-6] $C_7H_{17}ClN_2O_2$ (196.68).

Preparation—By treating propylene chlorohydrin with phosgene, reacting the condensation product (2-chloro-1-methylethyl chloroformate) with ammonia in ether solution, and heating the resulting urethan with trimethylamine.

Description—Colorless or white crystals or a white crystalline powder, usually having a slight, amine-like odor. It is slightly hygroscopic. Its 1% solution has a pH between 5.5 and 6.5. Exhibits polymorphism; one form melts at about 211° and the other at about 219°.
Solubility—1 g in 1 mL water and 10 mL alcohol; less soluble in dehydrated alcohol; insoluble in chloroform and ether.

Uses—Bethanechol chloride has somewhat stronger muscarinic activity for the gastrointestinal and urinary tracts than for the cardiovascular system and hence is employed systemically only for the gastroenterological and genitourinary uses indicated in the general statement (page 894). It is the muscarinic drug of choice in the treatment of gastroesophageal reflux. It is also used in ophthalmology. See the general statement for ophthalmologic uses, adverse effects, precautions, and contraindications (this page). Bethanechol chloride is not hydrolyzed by the enzyme cholinesterase, and it has a relatively prolonged duration of action.

Bethanechol chloride is supplied for subcutaneous and for oral administration. It should be taken on an empty stomach. It should not be administered by the intravenous or intramuscular route. Even with subcutaneous administration, adverse systemic effects may occur.

Dose—*Oral, adult, initially* **5** to **10 mg** followed by hourly increments of 5 mg until a satisfactory response is achieved, then, for *maintenance*, **5** to **50 mg** 2 to 4 times a day. The *oral pediatric dose* is **200 µg** (0.2 mg) **per kg** of body weight (6.7 mg per m² of body surface) 3 times a day. *Subcutaneous, adult, initially* **2.5 mg**, repeated at 15- to 30-min intervals as necessary, up to **10 mg**, to obtain a satisfactory response, then **2.5** to **10 mg** 3 or 4 times a day. *Subcutaneous, pediatric*, **150** to **200 µg** (0.15 to 0.2 mg) **per kg** of body weight (or 5 to 6.7 mg per m² of body surface 3 times a day). *Topical*, into the conjunctival sac, as a 1% solution.

Dosage Forms—Injection: 5 mg/mL; Tablets: 5, 10, 25 and 50 mg.

Pilocarpine Hydrochloride

2(3*H*)-Furanone,3-ethyldihydro-4-[(1-methyl-1*H*-imidazol-5-yl)-methyl]-, monohydrochloride, (3*S-cis*)-, (*Various Mfrs*)

Pilocarpine monohydrochloride [54-71-7] $C_{11}H_{16}N_2O_2 \cdot HCl$ (244.72).

Preparation—It is prepared as described under *Pilocarpine Nitrate*, except that HCl is used in place of the HNO₃.

Description—Colorless, translucent, odorless, faintly bitter crystals; hygroscopic and affected by light; solutions acid to litmus; melts within a range of 3° between 199° and 204°; pK_{a1} 6.8, pK_{a2} 1.3.

Solubility—1 g in 0.3 mL water, 3 mL alcohol, 360 mL chloroform; insoluble in ether.

Incompatibilities—See *Alkaloids* (page 411). Since the free alkaloid is quite soluble in water, *alkalies* do not readily cause a precipitation when added to solutions of its salts. It reduces *silver nitrate*.

Uses—Pilocarpine is a tertiary amine and hence penetrates membranes better than quaternary ammonium drugs. Therefore it is used for topical administration in ophthalmology (see page 894). Systemically, it is not selective enough to lend itself to gastroenterological, genitourinary, or cardiovascular purposes. It was once used to cause salivary secretion or intense sweating, and it was also occasionally employed to overcome some of the antimuscarinic side effects of other drugs, especially those used in the treatment of parkinsonism. Because of lesser hygroscopicity, pilocarpine nitrate is more convenient to handle than the hydrochloride.

Pilocarpine is better tolerated than any other miotic. It is infrequently irritating or allergenic, and systemic responses to topical application are rare, but absorption from solutions of high concentration may result in systemic side effects. Lens opacities may follow prolonged use.

Dose—*Topical*, **1 drop** of **0.25 to 10%** solution into the conjunctival sac 1 to 6 times a day, as directed by a physician.

Dosage Forms—Ophthalmic Solution: 0.25, 0.5, 1, 1.5, 2, 3, 4, 5, 6, 8, and 10%.

Pilocarpine Nitrate

2(3*H*)-Furanone, 3-ethyldihydro-4-[(1-methyl-1*H*-imidazol-5-yl)-methyl]-, (3*S-cis*)-, mononitrate; P.V. Carpine (*Allergan*)

Pilocarpine mononitrate [148-72-1] $C_{11}H_{16}N_2O_2 \cdot HNO_3$ (271.27).

Preparation—The total alkaloids are extracted from the dried crushed leaves of *Pilocarpus microphyllus*, or other suitable *Pilocarpus* species, with alcohol containing a small amount of hydrochloric acid. The solvent is distilled off, the aqueous residue neutralized with ammonia, and allowed to stand until the resins are all deposited. It is then filtered, and the filtrate evaporated to a small bulk. Ammonia is added in excess and the free alkaloids extracted with chloroform. After removing the solvent by distillation, the residue is dissolved in a small quantity of dilute nitric acid and allowed to crystallize.

Description—Shining, white crystals; stable in air but is affected by light; solutions are acid to litmus; melts within a range of 3° between 171° and 176°.

Solubility—1 g in 4 mL water and 75 mL alcohol; insoluble in chloroform and ether.

Incompatibilities—See *Pilocarpine Hydrochloride*.

Uses—See *Pilocarpine Hydrochloride*.

Dose—*Topical, adult*, **1 drop** of a **0.5 to 6%** solution into the conjunctival sac 1 to 4 times a day. The 1 and 2% solutions are usually used.

Dosage Forms—Ophthalmic Solution: 0.5, 1, 2, 3, 4, and 6%.

Pilocarpine Ocular Controlled Release System—A system designed for continuous release of pilocarpine from a unit placed in the cul-de-sac of the eye. Each elliptically shaped unit contains a core reservoir of pilocarpine and alginic acid surrounded by a hydrophobic ethylene/vinyl acetate copolymer membrane that controls diffusion of pilocarpine into the eye at a constant rate (after an initial rapid release to achieve equilibrium concentration) for a week; the alginic acid remains in the core. Two rated-release systems are available (*Ocusert Pilo-20* and *Ocusert Pilo-40*, Ciba-Geigy), one containing 5 mg of pilocarpine and releasing 20 micrograms per hour for a week, and the other containing 11 mg of pilocarpine and releasing 40 micrograms per hour for a week. The faster rate of release of the latter system is achieved by adding di(2-ethylhexyl) phthalate to the membrane formulation, which increases the rate of diffusion of pilocarpine across the membrane. More pilocarpine is included in the core reservoir than diffuses into the eye, the excess serving as a diffusional energy source to release the drug at a constant rate.

Use: The system is indicated for control of elevated intraocular pressure in pilocarpine-responsive patients with narrow-angle glaucoma. Usually therapy is started with the 20 µg/hr system; if greater reduction of intraocular pressure is required than can be obtained with this system, the 40 µg/hr system may be prescribed by the ophthalmologist. Units should be changed every 7 days. Since pilocarpine-induced myopia may occur during the first several hours of therapy, the unit should be inserted at bedtime, to allow stabilization of the myopia before arising. Some patients may notice signs of conjunctival irritation, including mild erythema with or without a slight increase in mucous secretion when first using the units; these symptoms tend to lessen or disappear after the first week of therapy. In rare instances a sudden increase in pilocarpine effects has been reported during system use. Since the unit may slip out of the eye onto the cheek during initial use, the patient should be instructed to check for presence of the unit before retiring and on arising. The systems are available in packages containing 8 individual sterile units.

Other Cholinomimetics

Carbachol [Choline chloride carbamate [51-83-2]; carbamoylcholine chloride; [$NH_2COOCH_2CH_2N^+(CH_3)_3$]Cl⁻ (182.65); Miostat (*Alcon*)]—Prepared by reaction of ethylene chlorohydrin with phosgene, the resulting chloroethyl chloroformate treated with ammonia to produce chloroethyl urethan, which yields carbachol when reacted with aqueous trimethylamine. Occurs as white or faintly yellow crystals or crystalline powder; odorless or with a slight amine-like odor; hygroscopic; melts between 200° and 204°; pK_a 4.8. One g dissolves in about 1 mL water and 50 mL alcohol; practically insoluble in chloroform and ether. *Uses:* Carbachol has a moderate degree of selectivity for the gastrointestinal and urinary tracts, hence it was formerly widely used in gastroenterology and genitourinary practice. Today it is used in ophthalmology, mainly for the treatment of narrow angle glaucoma and to induce miosis prior to ocular surgery. It is not hydrolyzed by cholinesterase and hence has a longer duration of action than methacholine and acetylcholine. See the general statement (page 894) for actions, adverse effects, and contraindications. *Dose: Topical, adult*, 1 to 2 drops of 0.75 to 3% solution instilled into the conjunctival sac, 2 or 3 times a day; the nasolacrimal ducts should be occluded during application. *Intraocular, adult*, as an irrigant into the anterior chamber, 0.5 mL of 0.01% solution. *Dosage Forms:* Ophthalmic Solution: 0.75, 1.5, 2.25, and 3%; Intraocular Solution: 0.01%.

Muscarine—This alkaloid contains the quaternary ammonium ion, trimethyl(tetrahydro-4-hydroxy-5-methylfurfuryl)ammonium ion [300-54-9]. It exists as salts, e.g., muscarine chloride, [$C_9H_{20}N^+O$]Cl⁻. *Uses:* Muscarine was studied long before acetylcholine and other parasympathomimetics were discovered. Like acetylcholine it acts on smooth muscle, heart and exocrine glands, but it does not ordinarily stimulate postganglionic neurons of the neuromuscular junction. Hence on systemic administration it somewhat more faithfully simulates parasympathetic stimulation than does the real parasympathetic neurohumor, acetylcholine. Because of this and because of its temporal priority, muscarine has been a time-honored prototype of parasympathomimetics, and the neuroeffector actions of the parasympathomimetics are designated as *muscarinic* actions. These actions are readily blocked by atropine. Muscarine has no clinical uses, but it has clinical significance in that, in the form of a quaternary salt, it is the toxic agent in the red variety of the deadly mushroom *Amanita muscaris*.

Nicotine [1-Methyl-2-(3-pyridyl)pyrrolidine, $C_{11}H_{14}N_2$ [54-11-5]]—From *Nicotiana tabacum*. A poisonous, oily liquid. It has an unpleasant tobacco-like odor, a burning taste, and a strongly alkaline reaction.

Nicotine is the prototype of cholinomimetics of the so-called nicotinic type. The action of nicotine in the body is characterized by a primary transient stimulation followed by a persistent depression of all sympathetic and parasympathetic ganglia. The actions are explained by a common mechanism, namely, that of depolarization of the postsynaptic membrane. During the onset of depolarization, nerve action potentials are generated. Once the postsynaptic membrane becomes fully depolarized, further action potentials cannot be initiated, since they require a polarized postsynaptic membrane at their outset. Thus a block of synaptic transmission results from the persisting depolarization induced by nicotine. Even after the membrane is restored, the block may persist. The synaptic stimulatory and depressant effects of nicotine cannot be overcome by atropine.

Nicotine likewise stimulates then paralyzes skeletal muscles and thus induces a curariform action, which is the major reason for the toxic effect of the alkaloid on respiration. However, nicotine is more active on ganglia than on skeletal muscles, whereas the reverse is true of curare. In addition to the above well-established actions, nicotine also first stimulates then paralyzes the central nervous system. There is also evidence that the alkaloid possesses activity as a vasoconstrictor and that it increases intestinal motility.

Anticholinesterases

The term cholinesterase is a generic term that includes all enzymes capable of hydrolyzing acetylcholine. There are two main categories of cholinesterase. The term *acetylcholinesterase* is applied to any or all of a family of isoenzymes that very selectively hydrolyze acetylcholine and hence is called true, or specific, cholinesterase; it is not truly specific, since other choline esters may be hydrolyzed with low velocities. Acetylcholinesterase is concentrated in the region of the motor end plate, at autonomic ganglia, in cholinergic neurons in and outside the central nervous system, and in erythrocytes. The term *butyrocholinesterase* (also called cholinesterase, pseudocholinesterase, or nonspecific cholinesterase) is applied to a number of enzymes that may hydrolyze acetylcholine but for which butyrylcholine, not acetylcholine, is the optimal substrate. Butyrocholinesterase is present in glial and satellite cells in the central nervous system and autonomic ganglia, in smooth muscle, exocrine glands, and various organs, such as the liver, and plasma; its concentration in cholinergic neurons is usually insignificant.

Inhibition of acetylcholinesterase and butyrocholinesterase has various consequences according to where the enzymes are inhibited. Neither the butyrocholinesterase in plasma nor the acetylcholinesterase in erythrocytes has known functions, and their inhibition has no known physiological consequences, but inhibition may moderately increase the plasma half-life and concentration of acetylcholine and certain other hydrolyzable choline esters. The only important effects accrue to inhibition at sites of cholinergic neuroeffector transmission. The preservation of acetylcholine at such sites prolongs and intensifies the cholinergic activity there. Thus, at the neuromuscular junction, anticholinesterases facilitate neuromuscular transmission, with an early increase in muscle strength (by recruiting subliminal junctions) and a late decrease in muscle strength, even paralysis, if many motor end plates remain depolarized by persisting levels of acetylcholine. Excessive muscular fasciculations and fibrillations also occur, which also decrease muscle strength, by causing asynchrony among motor units and fibers. At the autonomic ganglia, the predominant effect is to facilitate transmission, and the final resultant effect depends on the effector organ system innervated by the excited postganglionic nerves. In the case of the atria and the atrioventricular node the activity in both adrenergic and cholinergic postganglionic nerves will be increased, so that the effects mediated by the parasympathetic nerves will be antagonized by those of the sympathetic nerves. However, in the parasympathetic innervation, acetylcholine is preserved by the anticholinesterase at two sites, the ganglia and the innervated heart cells, which amplifies the action, whereas in the sympathetic innervation transmission is facilitated only at the ganglia. Therefore, where there is dual and antagonistic innervation, as in the atria, atrioventricular node, pupil, stomach and intestines, urinary tract, etc, the parasympathetic effects predominate. Thus bradycardia, partial heart block, miosis, increased gastric secretion and motility, and tendency to urination all result from significant anticholinesterase activity. The blood pressure may be elevated, because there is little cholinergic innervation of the vascular tree, and the facilitation in the sympathetic pathway is not antagonized at the vascular smooth muscle. Ciliary spasm may be intense, because there is a negligible antagonistic sympathetic innervation of the ciliary body. Facilitation in both sympathetic and parasympathetic pathways adds to increase salivation and sweating (which, though sympathetic, is mostly cholinergic). Anticholinesterase action within the central nervous system may cause a bizarre mixture of stimulation and depression.

There are two main categories of cholinesterase inhibitors: those that are amine or quaternary ammonium compounds, which interact with the anionic sites of the cholinesterase as well as with the esteratic site, and those that are usually organophosphates (but may contain other nucleophilic moieties), which esterify the serine hydroxyl group at the esteratic site. The amine or ammonium anticholinesterases react reversibly with the enzymes, consistent with ionic bonding, even though some, like physostigmine or neostigmine, may have carbamate moieties that reversibly acylate

the esteratic serine hydroxyl; their durations of action are a few minutes to a few hours and are determined by elimination pharmacokinetics. The organophosphate-type anticholinesterases form a firmer bond, some so firm as to be essentially irreversible. With these, the duration of action is determined by the kinetics of dissociation at the esteratic site, or, with essentially irreversibly acting ones (like isoflurophate), the time for resynthesis of cholinesterase (weeks to months).

The organophosphate-type anticholinesterases have a moderate selectivity for butyrocholinesterase and hence cannot enhance neuromuscular transmission without excessive effects on glands and smooth muscle. They are un-ionized and hence also readily penetrate the blood-brain barrier and cause central nervous effects. They can also be absorbed from the skin. The amine and ammonium agents are more selective for acetylcholinesterase, and the quaternary ammonium anticholinesterases, especially, may often enhance neuromuscular function with only minimal to moderate autonomic side effects. The amine agents, like physostigmine, however, can pass the blood-brain barrier and elicit central effects. Consequently, physostigmine is not employed systemically but rather only topically to the eye. The quaternary ammonium compounds have a nicotinic agonist activity, which at ganglia and the neuromuscular junction adds to the indirect anticholinesterase effect; consequently, because of this dual effect they are the agents chosen to enhance neuromuscular function. Because of their confinement to the periphery, the quaternary agents are also chosen for any peripheral action.

Uses—The quaternary ammonium anticholinesterases are used systemically to abolish muscular paralysis from competitive *neuromuscular blocking drugs*, to improve muscle function in *myasthenia gravis*, to treat *intestinal distention*, such as congenital *megacolon*, postoperative and postpartum *adynamic intestinal ileus*, *postvagotomy gastric atony*, and *functional urinary retention*. They have also received desultory trials in the management of *gastroesophageal reflux*, to increase lower esophageal pressure. They have an erratic usefulness in the treatment of *delayed menstruation*. Edrophonium is used as an antiarrhythmic drug to interrupt the reentrant conduction pathway in *paroxysmal atrial tachycardia*. Edrophonium or neostigmine is also used in the differential *diagnosis of myasthenic crisis*, in which case it will improve muscle function, and *cholinergic crises*, in which case it will worsen function, and to diagnose *myotonia congenita*. Neostigmine at one time was used in the diagnosis of early pregnancy; three successive daily doses will initiate menstruation in 72 hr unless the patient is pregnant. Anticholinesterases, especially physostigmine, are used to treat atropine or tricyclic antidepressant poisoning.

The anticholinesterases are applied topically to the eye in the treatment of primary *wide-angle glaucoma*, *accommodative convergent strabismus*, *accommodative esotropia*, and for the *emergency treatment of acute congestive glaucoma*. They may also be used to *treat marginal corneal ulcers*. In *myasthenia gravis* topical application may be used to improve the function of the extraocular muscles and eyelids. The reversibly acting anticholinesterases may be alternated with mydriatics to *break adhesions between lens and iris*.

Adverse Effects and Intoxication—Conjunctivally applied anticholinesterases locally may cause stinging, lacrimation, ocular pain and browache (from ciliary spasm), blurring of vision, blepharospasm, conjunctival and intraocular hyperemia, transient early rise in intraocular pressure, iridocyclitis, pigment cysts of the iris, anterior and posterior synechiae, and, rarely, retinal detachment. Atropine can antagonize these effects. Allergies may also occur. In addition, organophosphate may cause fibrinous iritis, cataracts, especially in elderly patients (in 50% of cases chronically treated), and uveitis.

Adverse systemic effects, from systemic administration or systemic absorption after topical application, include excessive salivation, sweating, tracheobronchial secretion, lacrimation, bronchoconstriction, marked miosis, blurring of vision, nausea and vomiting, diarrhea, abdominal cramps and colic, involuntary defecation, pallor, hypertension or hypotension, bradycardia, and urinary frequency, urgency and enuresis. These effects can be antagonized with sufficiently large doses of atropine. Laryngospasm, tremors, muscle fasciculations and twitching, weakness (even respiratory paralysis), potentiation of succinylcholine, and dizziness are nicotinic effects that cannot be antagonized with atropine. These effects usually occur only after quite large overdoses. Pralidoxime will antagonize these actions if given early enough. Acute intoxication caused by large doses of physostigmine or organophosphates also induces central nervous effects, such as confusion, ataxia, loss of reflexes, slurred speech, Cheyne-Stokes respiration, convulsions, coma, and respiratory and circulatory paralysis. Huge doses of atropine and pralidoxime, if used early, can suppress these effects. General supportive measures are also necessary in the management of both peripheral and central toxicity.

Precautions and Contraindications—When systemic anticholinesterases are used, the margin between the first appearance of side effects and serious toxic effects is small. The first signs may be quite subtle. Furthermore, there is a wide variation among patients and in the same patient from time to time so that each patient must be approached cautiously. Therefore, careful medical supervision is mandatory. Anticholinesterases should be used cautiously or withheld in patients with bronchial asthma, mechanical intestinal or urinary obstruction, peptic ulcer, vagotonia, bradycardia, hypotension, recent myocardial infarction, epilepsy, parkinsonism or a known hypersensitivity to depolarizing neuromuscular blocking drugs and when cholinomimetics are to be used. Quinidine and quinine antagonize the neuromuscular effects of the anticholinesterases. They should not be given topically to the eye when there is a history of retinal detachment, uveitis or angle-closure glaucoma. Their potential systemic effects command the same precautions as for systemic anticholinesterases. Systemic anticholinesterases will antagonize ganglionic blocking drugs. The safety in mother and fetus of the amine and quaternary ammonium agents during pregnancy has not been established; systemic organophosphates are absolutely contraindicated.

Ambenonium Chloride

Benzenemethanaminium, N,N'-[(1,2-dioxo-1,2-ethanediyl)bis(imino-2,1-ethanediyl)]bis[2-chloro-N,N-diethyl-, dichloride; Mysuran; Mytelase (*Winthrop*)

[Oxalylbis(iminoethylene)]bis[(o-chlorobenzyl)diethylammonium] dichloride [115-79-7] $C_{28}H_{42}Cl_4N_4O_2$ (608.48); *tetrahydrate* [52022-31-8] (680.54).

Preparation—N,N-Diethylethylenediamine is reacted with ethyl oxalate to give N,N'-bis[2-(diethylamino)ethyl]oxamide which is doubly quaternized with 2-chlorobenzyl chloride. US Pat 3,096,373.

Description—White, odorless powder melting at about 200°.
Solubility—1 g in 5 mL water, 20 mL alcohol, >1000 mL chloroform and >1000 mL ether.

Uses—A quaternary ammonium *anticholinesterase* drug (see general statement) with actions similar to those of *Neostigmine* (see

page 899); ambenonium chloride is 2 to 4 times more potent and its duration of action after oral administration (4 hr) may be slightly longer. It is also claimed to have a lower incidence of side effects than neostigmine, particularly of the gastrointestinal tract. It is used in the treatment of *myasthenia gravis*. For side effects and precautions, see the general statement, above.

Dose—*Oral, adult, initially* **5 mg,** gradually increased as required up to **25 mg 3** or **4** times a day. Occasionally as much as 75 mg per dose may be required. Doses over 200 mg per day require careful medical supervision.

Dosage Forms—Tablets: 10 mg.

Demecarium Bromide

Benzenaminium, 3,3′-[1,10-decanediylbis(methylimino)carbonyloxy] bis[N,N,N-trimethyl-, dibromide; Tosmilen; Humorsol (*MSD*)]

(*m*-Hydroxyphenyl)trimethylammonium bromide decamethylenebis[methylcarbamate](2:1) [56-94-0] $C_{32}H_{52}Br_2N_4O_4$ (716.60).

Preparation—N,N'-Dimethyl-1,10-decamethylenediamine is added to molten 3-(dimethylamino)phenyl carbonate to produce 1,10-decamethylenebis[3-(dimethylamino)phenyl N-methylcarbamate]. This ester, a viscous oil, is dissolved in ethanol and doubly quaternized with an acetone solution of methyl bromide. US Pat 2,789,981.

Description—White, or slightly yellow, slightly hygroscopic, crystalline powder; melts at about 165°, with decomposition; pH (1 in 100 solution) between 5.0 and 7.0.
Solubility—Freely soluble in water and in alcohol; sparingly soluble in acetone; soluble in ether.

Uses—A quaternary ammonium *anticholinesterase* drug that has high topical penetrability into the eye. It is used topically for its ophthalmological actions (see the general statement). These actions may last 3 to 5 days.

Dose—*Topical, adult* and *pediatric*, to the conjunctiva, **1 drop** of **0.125** to **0.25**% solution twice a week to 1 or 2 times a day. For details of frequency and duration of application in the various uses of demecarium bromide see USP XX or the package literature.

Dosage Forms—Ophthalmic Solution: 0.125 and 0.25%.

Echothiophate Iodide

Ethanaminium, 2-[(diethoxyphosphinyl)thio]-N,N,N-trimethyl-, iodide; Phospholine Iodide (*Ayerst*)

(2-Mercaptoethyl)trimethylammonium iodide S-ester with O,O-diethyl phosphorothioate [513-10-0] [6736-03-04] $C_9H_{23}INO_3PS$ (383.22).

Preparation—β-(Dimethylamino)ethanol is reacted with sodium and the resulting sodium alkoxide is condensed with O,O-diethyl phosphorochloridothioate [ClP(S)(OC$_2$H$_5$)$_2$] to yield S-[2-(dimethylamino)ethyl] O,O-diethyl phosphorothioate. This ester is quaternized with methyl iodide. US Pat 2,911,430.

Description—White, crystalline, hygroscopic solid having a slight mercaptan-like odor. Its solutions have a pH of about 4.
Solubility—1 g in 1 mL water, 3 mL methanol, 25 mL dehydrated alcohol; practically insoluble in other organic solvents.

Uses—An *anticholinesterase* drug that is both a quaternary ammonium and organophosphate compound. It has a long duration of action. Applied topically to the eye it causes intense miosis and contraction of the ciliary body; the effects begin in 10 to 45 min and last 3 to 7 days. It is used for the treatment of *primary open-angle glaucoma* and *accommodative esotropia*. It should be used only when short-acting miotics have failed. For the adverse effects and precautions, see the general statement (this page). Echothiophate does not penetrate into the central nervous system.

Dose—*Topical, adult*, for *glaucoma*, **1 drop** of **0.03** to **0.25**% solution to the conjunctiva twice a day, in the morning and at bedtime;

for *accommodative esotropia*, **1 drop** of **0.06** to **0.125**% solution once a day or every other day for 3 weeks. Pediatric dosage has not been established.

Solutions are not marketed and must be prepared from the available powder by dissolution in isotonic sodium chloride solution containing 0.5% chlorobutanol; solutions are stable for over a year at 4° and for over a month at room temperature.

Dosage Forms—for Ophthalmic Solution: 1.5, 3, 6.25, and 12.5 mg.

Edrophonium Chloride

Benzenaminium, *N*-ethyl-3-hydroxy-*N*,*N*-dimethyl-, chloride; Tensilon (*Hoffmann-LaRoche*)

Ethyl(*m*-hydroxyphenyl)dimethylammonium chloride [116-38-1] [312-48-1] $C_{10}H_{16}ClNO$ (201.70).

Preparation—*m*-Dimethylaminophenol is dissolved in a suitable organic solvent and quaternized with ethyl iodide. The dimethyl-ethyl(3-hydroxyphenyl)ammonium iodide precipitates and is converted to the chloride in various ways, one of which involves treatment with moist silver oxide to form the quaternary base followed by neutralization with hydrochloric acid.

Description—White, odorless crystalline powder. Its 1 in 10 solution is practically colorless, pH (1 in 10 solution) between 4.0 and 5.0; melts between 165° and 170°, with decomposition.

Solubility—1 g in 0.5 mL water, 5 mL alcohol; insoluble in chloroform and ether.

Uses—Edrophonium chloride inhibits cholinesterase primarily at the neuromuscular junction and very little at other sites. It also has some direct nicotinic stimulant actions at the neuromuscular junction but not at the autonomic ganglia. The duration of action of a single small dose is only about 5 min, but large doses may act for 1 to 2 hr. It is used to *abolish neuromuscular paralysis due to d-tubocurarine* or similarly acting motor end-plate stabilizing drugs. It is also used as a *diagnostic agent for myasthenia gravis* or to differentiate a myasthenic crisis from a cholinergic crisis. Edrophonium chloride may be used occasionally to treat *myasthenic crises*. It also has an important use to arrest *paroxysmal atrial tachycardia*.

Transient blurring of vision, lacrimation, perspiration, and dizziness may accompany its use. It causes muscle fasciculations in the normal human. When it is used to differentiate myasthenic from cholinergic crisis, facilities for endotracheal intubation and artificial respiration must be available.

Dose—*Intravenous, adult*, as a *diagnostic agent, initially* **2 mg** injected within 15 to 30 sec, followed by **8 mg** if no response occurs within 45 sec; for *children, initially* **1 mg** if body weight is less than 34 kg, or **2 mg** if over 34 kg and, if no response occurs in 45 sec, up to a total of 5 mg if body weight is less than 34 kg and 10 mg if over 34 kg. The *infant* dose is **500 µg** (0.5 mg). For *myasthenic crisis*, by *intravenous drip*. To *antagonize curare-like* neuromuscular blocking drugs, initially **10 mg** repeated in 5 to 10 min as necessary; no more than a total of 40 mg should be given. *Intramuscular, adult, diagnostic*, **10 mg**; for *children*, **2 mg** if body weight is less than 34 kg and **5 mg** if over 34 kg.

Dosage Forms—Injection: 10 mg/mL, 100 mg/10 mL.

Hexafluorenium Bromide—page 923.

Isoflurophate

Phosphorofluoridic acid, bis(1-methylethyl) ester; DFP; Floropryl (*MSD*)

Diisopropyl phosphorofluoridate [55-91-4] $C_6H_{14}FO_3P$ (184.15).

Preparation—Isopropyl alcohol is reacted with PCl_3 to form diisopropyl phosphite. Oxidation with chlorine gives diisopropyl phosphorochloridate, which metathesizes with NaF to yield the phosphorofluoridate.

Description—Clear, colorless or faintly yellow liquid. It boils at 183°, and has a specific gravity of about 1.05. Its vapor is extremely irritating to the eye and mucous membranes. In the presence of moisture, it decomposes with formation of hydrogen fluoride.

Solubility—Sparingly soluble in water; soluble in alcohol.

Uses—An *organophosphate anticholinesterase;* consequently, it has a long duration of action. It is used topically in the treatment of *primary open-angle glaucoma*, but only when short-acting miotics have failed. It is also used in the treatment of *aphakic glaucoma* and *accommodative esotropia*. Within a day the intraocular tension drops, and it may remain depressed for as long as a week. Miosis lasts 2 to 4 weeks. For the adverse effects and contraindications, see the general statement, page 898.

Caution—When handling isoflurophate in open containers, protect the eyes, nose, and mouth with a suitable mask, and avoid contact with the skin.

Dose—*Topical, adult*, for *glaucoma*, a strip of **0.025**% ointment approximately **0.5 cm** long every third day to 3 times a day (pediatric schedule undetermined); diagnosis of *accommodative strabismus*, once a day at bedtime for 2 weeks; *uncomplicated esotropia*, once a day at bedtime, gradually decreasing to once a week for 2 months.

Dosage Forms—Ophthalmic Ointment: 0.025%.

Neostigmine Bromide

Benzenaminium, 3-[[(dimethylamino)carbonyl]oxy]-*N*,*N*,*N*-trimethyl-, bromide; Prostigmin Bromide (*Hoffmann-LaRoche*)

(*m*-Hydroxyphenyl)trimethylammonium bromide dimethylcarbamate [114-80-7] [59-99-4] $C_{12}H_{19}BrN_2O_2$ (303.20).

Preparation—It may be prepared by reacting dimethylcarbamoylchloride [$(CH_3)_2NCOCl$] with potassium *m*-(dimethylamino)phenolate, then quaternizing with methyl bromide.

Description—White, crystalline powder. It is odorless, and has a bitter taste. Its solutions are neutral to litmus. It melts between 171° and 176°, with decomposition.

Solubility—1 g in about 0.5 mL of water; soluble in alcohol; practically insoluble in ether.

Uses—Neostigmine is a quaternary ammonium anticholinesterase (see *Anticholinesterases*, page 896). It acts at the esteratic site of the enzyme to form the inactive dimethylcarbamoyl enzyme. Its effects are more prominent on certain structures than on others, being particularly effective on the bowel, urinary bladder, and skeletal muscle; the pupil, the heart, blood pressure, and secretions are affected to a much lesser extent in doses that are ordinarily effective on the structures listed above. The duration of action by the oral route is 3 to 6 hr and by the intramuscular route 2 to 4 hr.

Neostigmine is employed for the genitourinary, gastrointestinal, and neuromuscular uses indicated in the general statement. However, it is little used today to antagonize curare-like drugs or in the diagnosis of myasthenia gravis, because its duration of action is too long.

The adverse effects of neostigmine are those of quaternary ammonium anticholinesterases (see the general statement, page 898).

Neostigmine is poorly absorbed orally. Sometimes as little as 1% is absorbed. Changes in bowel condition can alter absorption considerably, which may make management difficult. Neostigmine is administered parenterally as the methylsulfate and orally as the bromide salt.

Dose—*Oral*, for *myasthenia gravis, initially* **15 mg** 3 times a day, gradually increased to **45 mg** every 2 to 4 hours if necessary (as much as 375 mg a day may be given); for *children, initially* **7.5** to **15 mg** 3 or 4 times a day or **330 µg** (0.33 mg) **per kg** of body weight 3 to 6 times a day, gradually increasing to as much as the adult dose.

Dosage Forms—Tablets: 15 mg.

Neostigmine Methylsulfate

Benzenaminium, 3-[[(dimethylamino)carbonyl]oxy]-*N*,*N*,*N*-trimethyl-, methyl sulfate; Prostigmin Methylsulfate (*Roche*)

(*m*-Hydroxyphenyl)trimethylammonium methyl sulfate dimethylcarbamate [51-60-5] [59-99-4] $C_{13}H_{22}N_2O_6S$ (334.39).

Preparation—It is made by the method outlined under *Neostigmine Bromide*, using dimethyl sulfate in place of methyl bromide.

Description—White, crystalline powder. It is odorless, and has a bitter taste. Its solutions are neutral to litmus. It melts between 144° and 149°.

Solubility—Very soluble in water; soluble in alcohol.

Uses—See *Neostigmine Bromide*.

Dose—*Intramuscular, adults, diagnostic,* **0.022 mg/kg** of body weight (along with atropine 0.011 mg/kg) on the first test and **0.03 mg/kg** (with 0.016 mg/kg atropine) on the second, if the first is equivocal; to control *exacerbations of myasthenia,* **1 to 2 mg** (with 0.2 to 0.6 mg atropine) every 3 to 6 hours; in *bladder atony* or *intestinal paresis,* **0.25 to 0.50 mg** every 4 to 6 hours; in *bladder* or *gastrointestinal atony,* **0.5 to 1 mg** as needed; *children, diagnostic,* **0.04 mg/kg** (with 0.01 mg/kg atropine). *Intravenous, adults, diagnostic,* **0.5 mg** (with 0.5 mg atropine); to control *exacerbations of myasthenia,* **1 to 2 mg** every 1 to 3 hours; to *treat overdosage of curare* or *ganglionic blocking drugs,* **0.5 to 2 mg;** *children, diagnostic,* **0.02 mg/kg** (with 0.01 mg/kg atropine). *Subcutaneous, adults,* in *bladder* or *gastrointestinal atony or spasm,* same as intramuscular; *infants,* to treat *myasthenia gravis,* **0.1 to 0.2 mg** 1 to 4 times a day (along with 0.01 mg/kg atropine).

Dosage Forms—Injection: 250 and 500 μg/mL, 5 and 10 mg/10 mL.

Physostigmine Salicylate

Pyrrolo[2,3-*b*]indol-5-ol, 1,2,3,3a,8,8a-hexahydro-1,3a,8-trimethyl-, methylcarbamate (ester); (3a*S-cis*)-, mono(2-hydroxybenzoate); Eserine Salicylate; Isopto-Eserine (*Alcon*)

Physostigmine monosalicylate [57-64-7] $C_{15}H_{21}N_3O_2.C_7H_6O_3$ (413.47).

Preparation—By extracting powdered *Physostigma* seeds with hot alcohol. After distilling off the alcohol, the residue is mixed with sodium carbonate and extracted with ether, from which solution the physostigmine is removed with dilute sulfuric acid. The free alkaloid may be obtained by alkalinizing the acid solution. The salicylate may be made by adding 2 parts of physostigmine to a solution of 1 part of salicylic acid in 35 parts of boiling distilled water, and allowing the salt to crystallize on cooling.

Description—White or faintly yellow odorless powder or shining crystals. It acquires a red tint when exposed to light and air; melts at about 184°.

Solubility—1 g in 75 mL water, 16 mL alcohol, 6 mL chloroform, and about 250 mL ether.

Incompatibilities—Aqueous solutions tend to develop a red color on standing; a pink solution does not necessarily indicate complete ineffectiveness but as the color deepens to red, the product rapidly loses its value. Boric acid retards the change but alkalies hasten decomposition. Alkali-free glass should be used. It is precipitated by the usual alkaloidal precipitants.

Uses—Physostigmine is the oldest of the anticholinesterases. It combines with the enzyme at the esteratic site to yield the inactive methylcarbamoyl enzyme. It shares with neostigmine marked stimulatory actions on the bowel, but causes more secretion of glands, more effect on blood pressure, more constriction of the pupil, and less action on skeletal muscle. Since it is a tertiary amine, it penetrates into the nervous system and can exert central action when given in overdoses. It also penetrates readily into the eye. Its main use in medicine is locally in the eye, for the purposes indicated in the general statement (page 897).

Because physostigmine can also enter the CNS, it is used as an antidote to CNS intoxication by drugs with antimuscarinic activity (antimuscarinic drugs, tricyclic antidepressants, H_1-antihistamines). Recent trials suggest that it may come to have a limited usefulness in the treatment of Alzheimer's disease.

For adverse effects and precautions, see the general statement, page 898.

The duration of the ocular effects after topical application is 6 to 12 hr; the duration of systemic effects is less than 2 hr.

Physostigmine is generally used as the salicylate or sulfate salt; the salicylate has the advantage of being less deliquescent than the sulfate. Addition of a small amount of boric acid to a solution of the salt is said to inhibit formation of the red decomposition product produced by alkalies and that frequently occurs in solutions of physostigmine salts dispensed on prescription. A solution that has developed a red color should not be used.

Dose—*Topical, adult,* for *open-angle glaucoma* or to *antagonize antimuscarinic mydriatics,* **1 drop** of **0.25 to 0.5%** solution instilled into the conjunctival sac 2 to 4 times a day; for *acute-angle closure glaucoma,* **1 drop** of **0.25%** solution every 5 min for 30 min, then at 30-min intervals until the angle opens. Pediatric doses have not been established. *Oral, adult,* **1 to 2 mg** three times a day. *Parenteral, adult,* **0.5 to 2 mg,** intramuscularly or intravenously, to be repeated in doses of 1 to 4 mg in life-threatening situations; *pediatric,* **0.5 mg** intravenously, very slowly over at least one min, to be repeated at 5- to 10-min intervals, if necessary, up to a total of 2 mg. Children should not receive the drug unless the situation is urgent.

Dosage Forms—Injection: 2 mg/2 mL; Ophthalmic Solution: 0.25 and 0.5%; Tablets: 1 mg.

Physostigmine Sulfate

Pyrrolo[2,3-*b*]indol-5-ol, 1,2,3,3a,8,8a-hexahydro-1,3a,8-trimethyl-, methylcarbamate (ester), (3a*S-cis*)-, sulfate (2:1); Physostigmine Sulfate (2:1)

Physostigmine sulfate (2:1) [64-47-1] $(C_{15}H_{21}N_3O_2)_2.H_2SO_4$ (648.77).

For structure of the amine base, see *Physostigmine Salicylate.*

Description—White, odorless, microcrystalline powder; melts at about 143°. Is deliquescent in moist air and acquires a red tint when long exposed to heat, light, air, or contact with traces of metals.

Solubility—1 g in 4 mL water, 0.4 mL alcohol, and about 1200 mL ether.

Uses—See *Physostigmine Salicylate.*

Dose—*Topical, adult,* to the conjunctiva, **1 cm** of **0.25%** ointment one or more times a day. Pediatric dosage has not been established.

Dosage Form—Ophthalmic Ointment: 0.25%.

Pyridostigmine Bromide

Pyridinium, 3-[[(dimethylamino)carbonyl]oxy]-1-methyl-, bromide; Mestinon (*Roche*)

3-Hydroxy-1-methylpyridinium bromide dimethylcarbamate [101-26-8] $C_9H_{13}BrN_2O_2$ (261.12).

For structure of physostigmine base, see *Physostigmine Salicylate.*

Preparation—3-Pyridinol is condensed with dimethylcarbamoyl chloride in the presence of a suitable basic catalyst such as dimethylaniline, magnesium oxide, etc. The resulting ester, 3-pyridyl dimethylcarbamate, is isolated, dissolved in a suitable organic solvent, and quaternized with methyl bromide.

Description—White or practically white, crystalline powder, having an agreeable, characteristic odor. It is hygroscopic. It melts between 154° and 157°.

Solubility—Freely soluble in water, alcohol, and chloroform; slightly soluble in solvent hexane; practically insoluble in ether.

Uses—A quaternary ammonium anticholinesterase drug that is approximately one-fourth as potent as neostigmine at the neuromuscular junction and about one-eighth as potent on the bowel, genitourinary tract, and exocrine glands. Its onset of action by the oral route is about 30 min, which is more than twice that of neostigmine and is a disadvantage, but its duration of action by the oral route is usually somewhat longer and absorption is less erratic than with neostigmine, which are advantages. Because of its relative affinity for the neuromuscular junction, its principal use is in the treatment of *myasthenia gravis,* in which use it causes fewer side effects than does neostigmine. It is also superior to neostigmine in that the patient may be carried through the night without the necessity of interrupting sleep to take medication. However, in some patients, it provides less control of muscular weakness than does neostigmine. Pyridostigmine is administered orally except when the patient is to undergo surgery or childbirth or is in myasthenic crisis. Neonates born of myasthenic mothers may also be given parenteral pyridostigmine to improve respiration, swallowing, and suckling. The drug is also used to antagonize competitive neuromuscular blocking drugs.

The adverse effects and precautions are listed in the general statement, page 898. Bromide sensitivity occasionally occurs.

Dose—*Oral, adult, initially* **60 mg** every 4 to 8 hr while the patient is awake; however, dosage usually has to be increased to **120 to 300 mg** every 4 hr. With sustained-release tablets, the dose is **180 to 540 mg** once or twice a day. In severe cases the dose often exceeds 1.5 g/day, and as much as 6 g/day has been recorded. The *oral pediatric* dose is **1.2 mg per kg** of body weight or **33 mg per m^2** of body surface, every 4 hr. *Parenteral, adult, intramuscularly* or by slow *intravenous* injection, 1/30 of the oral dose, except to antagonize competitive neuromuscular blocking drugs 10 to 20 mg is usually used; *pediatric, intrasmuscular,* **0.05 to 0.15 mg/kg.**

Dosage Forms—Injection: 5 mg/2 mL; Syrup: 60 mg/5 mL; Tablets: 60 mg; Sustained-Release Tablets: 180 mg.

Other Anticholinesterases

Guanidine Hydrochloride [Aminomethanamidine hydrochloride; carbamidine hydrochloride; iminourea hydrochloride; $(NH_2)_2C$=NH.HCl (95.54)Prioderm (*Purdue Frederick*)]—Guanidine may be variously prepared, as by interactions of ammonia, carbon dioxide, and sulfur dioxide, or from urea. The hydrochloride occurs as a crystalline powder; freely soluble in water and in alcohol. *Uses:* Although guanidine does not possess anticholinesterase activity, it does facilitate neuromuscular function in some disorders in a way reminiscent of the anticholinesterases, hence its inclusion here. It increases the sensitivity of skeletal muscle to acetylcholine. It is used in the treatment of myasthenic syndromes for which neostigmine is not of value; these are the *muscular weakness* in "*oat-cell*" carcinoma of the lung and the *Eaton-Lambert syndrome* of sarcoidosis. Excessive doses may cause hypertension and convulsions as well as hypotension, shock, and a curare-like muscle paralysis with respiratory depression. Chronic overdoses can cause dystrophic changes in muscle. *Dose: Oral*, 10 to 15 mg/kg/day in 3 to 4 divided doses.

Malathion [*S*-(1,2-Dicarbethoxyethyl) *O,O*-dimethyldithiophosphate [121-75-5]; $C_{10}H_{19}O_6PS_2$ (330.36)]—A deep brown to yellow liquid; characteristic odor; slightly soluble in water; miscible with many organic solvents. *Uses:* An organophosphate anticholinesterase used as a pediculicide and miticide for use on humans; it is a common garden insecticide. It has a low toxicity to humans because it is rapidly metabolized in the mammalian body. *Dose: Topical,* as a 0..5% lotion.

Cholinesterase Reactivators

Several substances are capable of displacing dialkylphosphate groups (from organophosphate anticholinesterases) and methyl- or dimethylcarbamoyl groups (from physostigmine or neostigmine) from the esteratic sites of cholinesterases poisoned by the anticholinesterases. At present, all such substances of value contain oxime groups, which engage in a nucleophilic attack on the attached phosphate or carbamoyl group and rupture the bond between the inhibiting group and the esteratic site. This action is especially important in the treatment of intoxication by organophosphate anticholinesterases, since the organophosphates have such a long duration of action. The reactivation of carbamoylated enzyme is less prominent. Unfortunately, within a period of minutes to hours after poisoning with an organophosphate, there is a change in the phosphorylated enzyme ("aging," dealkylation of the alkyl phosphate moiety), so that the alkylphosphate–enzyme bond becomes too stable to be displaced by reactivators. The efficacy of any one reactivator varies according to which anticholinesterase is involved because of differences in electrophilicity of the phosphorus in the various phosphate radicals; one anticholinesterase, octamethylphosphoramide, is refractory to displacement by cholinesterase reactivators. Atropine also must be used concomitantly with reactivators for optimal therapy. The reactivators may be used prophylactically.

Pralidoxime Chloride

Pyridinium, 2-[(hydroxyimino)methyl]-1-methyl-, chloride; 2-PAM Chloride; Protopam Chloride (*Ayerst*)

2-Formyl-1-methylpyridinium chloride oxime [51-15-0] $C_7H_9ClN_2O$ (172.61).

Preparation—Picolinal is converted to its oxime which is then quaternized with dimethyl sulfate. Metathesis of the resulting pralidoxime methosulfate with HCl yields the official chloride. US Pat 3,123,613.

Description—White to pale-yellow, crystalline powder; odorless; stable in air. Melts between 215° and 225°, with decomposition.

Solubility—Freely soluble in water.

Uses—A cholinesterase reactivator. The quaternary portion of the molecule attaches to the anionic site of the cholinesterase molecule and brings the oxime into close proximity to the poisoned esteratic site. The drug is used in the treatment of poisoning by organophosphate anticholinesterases; it has questionable value in poisoning by neostigmine or physostigmine. The therapeutic effect (remission) usually occurs within an hour. Pralidoxime is also given prophylactically to handlers of organophosphates, but the status of this use is in dispute. Pralidoxime does not antagonize all anticholinesterase compounds; the manufacturer's package literature should be consulted to ascertain whether the drug will be effective. After a period of time, organophosphate-inhibited cholinesterase undergoes a change that makes reactivation difficult; with isoflurophate this time is only about an hour.

The plasma half-life of pralidoxime is about 2.5 hours.

When pralidoxime is injected more rapidly than at the recommended rate, dizziness, nausea, headache, mild weakness, blurred vision, diplopia, or tachycardia may result.

Dose—*Intravenous, adult,* for accidental intoxication, 1 to **2 g** injected in a period of 15 to 30 min, to be repeated after an hour if muscle weakness persists. For a cholinergic crisis due to echothiophate it is often the practice to start with 50 mg and increase the dose every 5 min until a remission occurs. For cholinergic crisis due to neostigmine, ambenonium, or pyridostigmine, an initial dose of 1 to 2 g may be followed by 250 mg every 5 min until remission occurs. The *pediatric* dose is **20 to 40 mg per kg** of body weight, given in 5 min. *Intravenous infusion,* 1 to **2 g** in **100 mL** of sodium chloride injection over a period of 15 to 30 min; repeat in 1 to 2 hr if necessary. The pediatric dose is **20 to 40 mg per kg** of body weight in **100 mL.** *Oral,* 1 to **3 g,** repeated in 3 hr if necessary. If signs and symptoms of cholinesterase poisoning already exist, more than two doses will probably be of little extra value. If the drug is given prophylactically after exposure, before signs of poisoning ensue, up to 5 oral doses of 1 to 3 g each may be given, to protect against slowly absorbing anticholinesterase.

Dosage Forms—Sterile: 1 g; Tablets: 500 mg.

CHAPTER 47

Adrenergic and Adrenergic Neuron Blocking Drugs

Stewart C Harvey, PhD

Professor of Pharmacology
School of Medicine, University of Utah
Salt Lake City, UT 84132

The term *blockade* is rather loosely used to indicate interference with a response system such that the final effect is prevented. A *blocking drug* is the agent to that interference. *Adrenergic* blockade indicates that the particular response system affected is that which normally involves the catecholamine neurohumoral transmitters, epinephrine (*adren*aline) and norepinephrine (*noradren*aline, levarterenol). The term adrenergic refers to any of the cellular apparatus concerned with the elaboration, storage, release, transmission, reception or action of these catecholamines or to their mimetics. Thus the locus of action of a so-called adrenergic blocking agent might be any of these adrenergic sites. Until the discovery of the catecholamine-depleting effects of reserpine, the only adrenergic blocking agents were those that blocked at the adrenergic neuroeffector receptor as competitive antagonists to the catecholamines or their mimetics. Today, several drugs that block the adrenergic response system by inhibiting the synthesis, storage or release of catecholamines are used clinically. Such drugs prevent the response to stimulation of the sympathetic adrenergic nerves by preventing delivery of catecholamines to the neuroeffector receptor; they do not prevent the actions of catecholamines or sympathomimetics on the neuroeffector receptor as do the "classical" adrenergic blocking agents. Although no universal terminology has been adopted to distinguish those drugs that block the catecholamines and sympathomimetics from those that prevent the delivery of catecholamines to the receptor, the term *adrenergic blocking agent* is usually applied to the former class, in accordance with previous custom, and the term *adrenergic neuron blocking agent*, or antiadrenergic drug, applied to the latter class. The adrenergic blocking agents were once sometimes called *sympatholytics*, because they abolish ("lyse") the response to stimulation of the sympathetic nerves, or *adrenolytics*, because the classical adrenergic blocking drugs abolished certain responses to epinephrine (*adren*aline). Adrenergic neuron blocking agents are sympatholytic but not adrenolytic.

Adrenergic Blocking Agents

The classification of adrenoreceptors into α- and β-subtypes implies that there are possible two types of blocking drugs, α- and β-antagonists. In fact, inasmuch as there are subcategories, α_1-, α_2-, β_1-, and β_2-adrenoreceptors, there are four types of selective and three types of nonselective adrenergic antagonists. The classical adrenergic blocking drugs, ergotamine phenoxybenzamine, and phenotolamine block both α_1- and α_2-adrenoreceptors. Propranolol, nadolol, timolol, pindolol, and others block both β_1- and β_2-adrenoreceptors. Labetolol blocks both α- and β-receptors.

α-Adrenoreceptor Antagonists

Nonselective α-Antagonists—Only two nonselective α-adrenoreceptor antagonists, namely phenoxybenzamine and phentolamine, are presently marketed in the US. Other drugs, sometimes classified as α-blockers (eg, tolazoline, chlorpromazine) have other more prominent actions, for which they are used.

Blockade of α_1-adrenoreceptors causes readily apparent effects, whereas blockade of α_2-receptors causes subtle effects. Antagonism of α_1-adrenergic impulses to the arterioles decreases vascular resistance, thus tending to lower blood pressure, cause a pink warm skin, nasal and scleroconjunctival congestion and ptosis. α_1-Antagonism at the venules (capacitance vessels) not only increases venous capacitance, which necessitates fluid loading, but also causes postural and exercise hypotension. Other obvious effects of α_1-block are mild to moderate miosis and interference with ejaculation.

α-Antagonism causes tachycardia, palpitations and increased secretion of renin. These are β_1-adrenoreceptor responses not suppressable by α-blockade. They were formerly attributable solely to baroreflexes to the hypotension resulting from α_1-blockade. It is now known that there is also an abnormally large amount of norepinephrine released from adrenergic nerve endings (transmitter "overflow") as the result of concurrent block of α_2-adrenoreceptors, which receptors subserve both a negative feedback function to decrease the release of transmitter and a postsynaptic inhibitory function (by inhibiting adenylate cyclase) to decrease responsiveness to the transmitter. Consequently, tachycardia, palpitations and elevation of plasma renin levels may occur even when blood pressure falls very little. These reflex/overflow effects are counterproductive in the major uses of nonselective α-blocking drugs.

Nonselective α-adrenoreceptor antagonists are used in the treatment of peripheral vascular disorders in which there is an adrenergically-mediated vasospastic component, such as in *Raynaud's disease, acrocyanosis, frost bite, acute arterial occlusion, phlebitis, phlebothrombosis, diabetic gangrene, causalgia, shock* (to increase blood flow to intestines and kidney), and in *pheochromocytoma*. In shock, it is necessary first to expand the extracellular fluid volume in anticipation of increased venous capacitance. In pheochromocytoma, the drugs may be used well in advance of surgery, to accustom the patient to a lower blood pressure, and immediately before surgery, to prevent the occurrence of hypertensive crises caused by manipulation of the tumor, and for the long-term treatment of inoperable, metastatic pheochromocytoma.

Adverse effects of nonselective α-antagonists are postural hypotension, tachycardia, palpitations, fluid retention (from excess renin secretion), nasal and ocular congestion, and aggravation of the signs and symptoms of respiratory infections.

α-Antagonists are contraindicated in severe cerebral or coronary atherosclerosis and in renal insufficiency.

Selective α-Antagonists—Highly selective antagonists for both α_1- and α_2-adrenoreceptors are known. At present, only α_1-antagonists have known clinical uses. Only *prazosin* is available currently in the US, but the release of others is imminent. Theoretically, α_1-blockers should be useful for the same disorders as are the nonselective α-blockers, but prazosin is approved only for the treatment of *hypertension*. However, it enjoys a considerable use in refractory heart failure, to decrease the cardiac afterload.

α_1-Antagonists are advantageous in that they do not block α_2-receptors and hence do not cause overflow of transmitter and thus excessive tachycardia, stroke volume, and plasma renin levels; in some patients such side effects are almost nil. The most adverse side effect of α_1-blockade is sometimes severe postural hypotension and syncope, especially very early during treatment.

Selective α_2-antagonists include yohimbine and rauwolscine (α-yohimbine), but there are presently no therapeutic applications of α_2-blockade.

β-Adrenoreceptor Antagonists

Nonselective β-Antagonists—Drugs such as propranolol, nadolol, pindolol, and timolol suppress both β_1- and β_2-adrenoreceptor-mediated responses almost equally.

Blockade of myocardial β_1-receptors causes sinoatrial bradycardia, suppression of some ectopic pacemakers, decreased force of myocardial contraction, slowing of atrioventricular conduction, and increased atrioventricular refractoriness. The effect to slow the heart rate increases the duration of diastole (that segment of the heart cycle during which most left coronary blood flow occurs) and thus increases coronary blood flow to the subendocardial region. Therefore, β-blockers are of prophylactic value in the treatment of *stable angina pectoris*. Variant (vasospastic) angina may sometimes be exacerbated. Only propranolol and nadolol are approved currently in the USA as antianginal drugs, but all full β-antagonists are equally effective. It is widely held that the mechanism is that of decreasing myocardial oxygen demand, but the effect on oxygen utilization is mostly nullified by the exercise-induced increase in heart size, which increases oxygen need. The effect to decrease sinoatrial rate is also used to *suppress tachycardia in thyrotoxicosis and pheochromocytoma*. β-Antagonists are used in combination with vasodilators, to prevent reflex tachycardia and renin release. The effect to decrease myocardial contractility is employed in *hypertrophic subaortic stenosis*, in which a reduction in the rate of development of systolic tension decreases angina, palpitations and anxiety. The effect to decrease atrioventricular nodal conduction is employed in the chronic management of *paroxysmal supraventricular* tachycardia, in which β-antagonists may block one segment of the reentrant pathway within the AV node, and in *atrial flutter* and *atrial fibrillation*, in which a drug-induced second degree AV block diminishes the number of excessive impulses from reaching the ventricles, thus increasing filling time and improving stroke output.

β-Antagonists are used in the treatment of *essential hypertension*. Originally, the antihypertensive action was attributed to the decrease in cardiac output. This seems to be the mechanism of the early response, but it fails to explain the long-term effects. In the early stages of response, vascular resistance actually increases, reflexly. In a later stage, in which the greatest reduction in blood pressure occurs, the vascular resistance falls below premedication values and cardiac output returns partially toward premedication levels.

β-Blockers suppress that fraction of renin release that is sustained by sympathetic activity, but this effect occurs earlier than the major fall in vascular resistance. Only in high-renin hypertensive subjects do changes in plasma renin activity correlate with changes in blood pressure. The CNS must be ruled out as a locus of antihypertensive action, since not all effective β-blockers enter the CNS. β-Antagonists block presynaptic β-receptors and thus decrease transmitter release. At sympathetic terminals this would decrease norepinephrine release, but it occurs earlier than the antihypertensive action. This effect may contribute to postural hypotension.

β-Antagonists decrease morbidity and *increase survival after myocardial infarction*. Immediately after occlusion, their effects to suppress reflex tachycardia and increase in myocardial tension decreases oxygen need. This, along with a decrease in calcium entry into the myocytes (via β-receptor-operated channels), decreases myocardial necrosis. Certain fatal tachydysrhythmias are also prevented. Continuing β-blockade decreases the incidence of sudden death from dysrhythmias and reinfarction for as long as two years after an infarction.

The rate of formation of intraocular fluid is decreased by β-antagonists; this is useful in the treatment of open-angle *glaucoma*. Because timolol lacks local anesthetic activity and has a low irritancy it is applied topically in this disorder.

β-Antagonists have a varied usefulness in the prophylaxis of *migraine headache*, diminishing pain in many instances but increasing it in others. The locus of action is apparently peripheral rather than central. β-blockers also decrease spasm and pain in *spastic colon*, but clinical use of this effect remains investigational.

In the treatment of certain kinds of anxiety, such as stage fright and examination apprehension, β-antagonists are frequently effective. The efficacy is attributable to the prevention of the peripheral manifestations of sympathoadrenal discharge (eg, of tachycardia, palpitations, muscle tremor, etc) rather than to a central action. Their value in the treatment of pathological anxiety disorders is controversial. They appear to have little effect on the underlying disorder but only to decrease certain physical manifestations.

Not all β-antagonists penetrate into the CNS, and once there, they do not all behave similarly. Propranolol, but not metroprolol or timolol, block certain serotonin receptors. Central actions probably explain the increase in slow wave sleep, antiepileptic effects, suppression of tardive dyskinesias, the abolition of phantom limb, and possible improvement in schizophrenia after certain β-blockers. Both central and peripheral actions are probably involved in amelioration of the opiate, ethanol and amphetamine withdrawal syndromes, lessening of tremor, and of muscle spasms in tetanus.

Adverse effects accrue to both β_1- and β_2-antagonism. β_1-blockade in the sinoatrial node and myocardium prevents sympathetically-mediated increases in cardiac output during exercise, thus forcing cardiac output to adjust purely by a Starling mechanism. Consequently, pulmonary congestion occurs during vigorous exercise, even in athletes, and congestion limits performance. The antagonism of sympathetic nervous support to the heart may also convert a masked, compensated congestive heart failure to a frank congestive failure. However, if a tachydysrhythmia is present and the drug improves ventricular rate, congestion may actually diminish. At the AV node, β-antagonism may deepen a preexisting partial heart block and occasionally even cause ventricular asystole.

β-Antagonism in the bronchioles causes an increase in airway resistance. This can be expressed as a serious bronchospasm in bronchial asthma, bronchitis, emphysema, and chronic obstructive pulmonary disease. Laryngospasm may also occur. β_2-blockade in the liver may cause hypoglycemia in some persons. In insulin overdosage, β_2-blockade prevents the mobilization of glucose from the liver to offset hypoglycemia; furthermore, the prevention of reflex tachycardia deprives the patient of an early warning signal of impending insulin shock. β-Blockers may cause postural hypotension, with vertigo, weakness and syncope; this is more likely to occur in elderly persons or those with cerebrovascular disease or disorders of the inner ear. Prolonged use decreases renal perfusion.

Other adverse effects of β-blockade include impotence, increased very low density and decreased high density lipoproteins, occasional nausea and vomiting, mild diarrhea or constipation, and rare allergic responses, such as rashes, fever, and purpura. Centrally-acting β-blockers may cause drowsiness, decreased alertness, lassitude, vertigo, paresthesias, visual disturbances, insomnia, depression, mental confusion in the elderly, nightmares and hallucinations. Tolerance to these effects is frequent.

Abrupt withdrawal of β-blockers may precipitate rebound angina pectoris and/or hypertension. β-Blockers and clonidine should never be discontinued simultaneously.

Nonselective β-antagonists should be avoided, if possible, in the presence of bronchial asthma, bronchitis, emphysema, chronic obstructive pulmonary disease, sinus bradycardia, partial heart block, Raynaud's disease, diabetes, compensated and frank congestive heart failure, and variant (vasospastic) angina pectoris.

β-Antagonists interact with other drugs. They usually increase the fall in blood pressure caused by other antihypertensive drugs. They increase heart block caused by digitalis and may increase the dose requirement for the inotropic actions; exacerbate the myocardial depressant effects of halogenated general anesthetics and tricyclic antidepressants; augment the hypertensive actions of epinephrine and other α,β-adrenergic agonists; may cause monoamine oxidase inhibitors to become hypertensive; prolong the action of nondepolarizing neuromuscular paralysants; increase the hypoglycemic effects of insulin and oral hypoglycemic drugs; partially antagonize indirectly the bronchodilator effects of theophyllin and directly antagonize bronchodilator β_2-agonists. The effects of β-blockade are exaggerated in the presence of adrenergic neuronal blockade by reserpine, guanethidine, etc.

Selective β-Antagonists—At present there are available in the US two selective β_1-antagonists, atenolol and metoprolol. Others are acebutolol, practolol, and tolamolol. Advantages to selective β_1-blockade are lesser effects on bronchiolar airway resistance and a diminished effect to increase insulin-induced hypoglycemia. Although affinity for β_1-adrenoreceptors is many times that for β_2-receptors, care should be exercised when there is pulmonary disease or diabetes; these drugs block the reflex tachycardia that is premonitory to insulin shock.

Selective β_1-antagonists can be used for all the purposes listed under the nonselective blockers, although they have not been approved universally for these uses.

Partial Agonist β-Antagonists—Some β-antagonists also cause some stimulation of β-adrenoreceptors (ie, have *intrinsic sympathomimetic activity*. Of the β-antagonists presently available in the US, only pindolol has partial agonist properties. Most authorities hold that partial agonist activity offers no advantage over full antagonist activity. However, some advocates contend that partial agonism acts as a buffer to lessen the seriousness of the various adverse effects attributable to β-blockade. Statistically valid clinical comparisons have yet to be made.

Atenolol

Benzeneacetamide, 4-[2-hydroxy-3-[(1-methylethyl)amino]propoxy]-, Tenormin (*Stuart*)

2-[p-[2-Hydroxy-3-(isopropylamino)propoxy]phenyl]acetamide [29122-68-7] $C_{14}H_{22}N_2O_3$ (266.34).

Preparation—From p-hydroxyphenylacetamide, ethylene chlorohydrin and isopropylamine (US Pat 3,836,671).

Description—White crystals melting about 147°.

Uses—Atenolol is a selective β_1-antagonist (page 903) with very weak β_2-antagonist activity. It has less effect on airway resistance than metoprolol. It also has very little effect to decrease plasma renin activity.

Although it has all of the potential uses of β-antagonists, in the USA it has only been approved for the treatment of hypertension. Abroad, it is widely used as an antianginal drug. Investigational data suggest an efficacy in the management of acute anxiety attacks.

Atenolol can cause all the adverse effects common to β-antagonists (page 903), but it has almost no effect on airway resistance in persons with normal lungs and has sufficiently mild effects in persons with chronic obstructive pulmonary disease that the drug can be used cautiously in such patients. It can cause bronchoconstriction and thus is contraindicated in persons with bronchial asthma. Although atenolol poorly penetrates into the CNS, effects do occur in this system. Fatigue and depression are the most common noncardiovascular side effects. Allergic effects are infrequent; they include rash, fever, respiratory distress, and sore throat. Agranulocytosis and both thrombocytopenic and nonthrombocytopenic purpura occasionally occur.

The oral bioavailability is 50 to 60%. Plasma protein binding is 6 to 16%. The volume of distribution is 0.7 to 1.1 L/kg. Atenolol is eliminated mostly unchanged in the urine. The normal total body clearance is about 100 mg/min/1.73m² and the half-life is 6 to 7 hr. Dose adjustments are required when the glomerular filtration rate falls below 35 mL/min/1.73 m².

Dose—*Oral, adults, initially* **50 mg** once a day, to be increased after 2 weeks to 100 mg once a day, if necessary. Higher doses produce no further therapeutic effect. If creatine clearance is 15 to 35 mL/min/1.73 m² (half-life 16 to 27 hr), the maximum dose is **50 mg/day**; if it is less than 15 mL/min/1.73 m² (half-life 27 hr), it is **50 mg** every second day.

Dosage Forms—Tablets: 50 and 100 mg.

Labetalol Hydrochloride

Benzamide, 2-hydroxy-5-[1-hydroxy-2-[(1-methyl-3-phenylpropyl)-amino]ethyl]-, monohydrochloride; Trandate (*Glaxo*)

5-[1-Hydroxy-2-[(1-methyl-3-phenylpropyl)amino]ethyl]salicylamide monohydrochloride [32780-64-6] $C_{19}H_{24}N_2O_3$.HCl (364.87).

Preparation—Refer to US Pat 4,012,444.

Description and Solubility—White crystals soluble in water and ethanol; insoluble in ether and chloroform.

Uses—Labetalol combines both nonselective β- and α-antagonist activity, in a ratio of 3:1 by the oral and 7:1 by the intravenous routes. In addition, it has weak intrinsic β_2-adrenergic agonist activity, to which some investigators attribute its antihypertensive effects. The drug variably decreases heart rate and cardiac output but in conventional doses has very little effect on contractility. Plasma renin activity is usually decreased. Systemic vascular resistance is decreased and venous capacitance increased. The collective effect of these actions is a reduction in blood pressure, often without much change in heart rate.

Labetalol is used in the treatment of *essential* and *renal hypertension*, *toxemia of pregnancy* and other *hypertensive emergencies*, and *pheochromocytoma*. In essential hypertension it is often effective when other drugs have failed. It is also effective in *angina pectoris*.

The incidence of adverse effects is 6 to 25%. Effects of α-blockade include postural hypotension with accompanying dizziness, scleroconjunctival and injection and irritation, nasal stuffiness, and tingling of the scalp. Some tolerance to the α-blocking activity gradually occurs. Effects of β-blockade include bronchospasm (which is partly ameliorated by β_2-agonism) and occasional Raynaud's phenomenon, claudication and heart failure. Other effects include flushing yet cold extremities, palpitations, diarrhea, rare reversible alopecia, impotence, decreased libido, tremors, headache, lassitude, fatigue, rare myopathy, depression, and abnormal dreaming. After intravenous injection there is an occasional paradoxical pressor response. Allergic and immunologic effects include rashes, pruritis, increased antinuclear antibodies, and rare lupus-like syndrome.

The oral bioavailability of labetalol is about 25%, because of first-pass metabolism. Food, cimetidine, and liver disease increase bioavailability. In the liver, the drug is mostly conjugated to glucuronides, but the effect of oral administration selectively to decrease β-blocking activity implies an active metabolite. The elimination half-life is about 6 to 8 hr.

Dose—*Oral, adults, initially* **100 mg** twice a day, to be adjusted to a *maintenance* dose of **200 to 800 mg**/day in *mild to moderate hypertension* and **600 mg to 1.2 g**/day in *moderately severe* hypertension. *Intravenous, adults, initially* **20 mg** slowly over a 2-min period, then **40 to 80 mg** at 10-min intervals, if necessary.

Dosage Forms—Injection: 100 mg/20 mL; Tablets: 100, 200, 300 and 400 mg.

Metoprolol Tartrate

2-Propanol, 1-[4-(2-methoxyethyl)phenoxy]-3-[(1-methylethyl)amino]-, (±)-, [R-(R*,R*)]-2,3-dihydroxybutanedioate (2:1) (salt); Lopressor (*Ciba-Geigy*)

(±)-1-(Isopropylamino)-3-[p-(2-methoxyethyl)phenoxy]-2-propanol L-(+)-tartrate (2:1) (salt) [56392-17-7] $(C_{15}H_{25}NO_3)_2 \cdot C_4H_6O_6$ (684.83).

Preparation—From 4-(2-methoxyethyl)phenol, 3-chloro-1,2-propanediol and isopropylamine (Swedish Pat 368,004).

Description—White, odorless powder with a bitter taste melting about 120°.

Solubility—Very soluble in water; soluble in alcohol and chloroform; insoluble in acetone or ether.

Uses—Metoprolol is a selective β_1-antagonist with slight β_2-antagonist activity (see general statement). Its β_2-blocking activity is sufficient that in therapeutic doses it can suppress adrenergically-induced hyperglycemia and also frequently cause bronchospasm in asthmatic subjects. It only slightly increases airway resistance in normal persons and moderately in persons with obstructive airway disease.

The potential uses, adverse effects, contraindications and drug interactions are those of β-antagonists in general (page 903). However, it is presently approved only for the treatment of *hypertension*. Although it penetrates the CNS, its effects there are less intense than with propranolol. Nevertheless, about 10% of recipients will experience lassitude and dizziness. It may occasionally cause pruritis.

The oral bioavailability of metoprolol is about 40%. The volume of distribution is 3.5 to 5 L/kg. Only 12% is protein-bound in plasma. It is hydroxylated in the liver. There are slow and fast acetylator subjects; the eliminatioin half-life is about 1.7 to 4.2 hr in fast and 5 to 10 hr in slow hydroxylators.

Dose—*Oral, adults, initially* **100 mg**/day once or in 2 divided doses, with weekly adjustments in dosage up to a total of **450 mg**/day, if necessary. At the higher doses, β_2-antagonism may be significant.

Dosage Forms—Tablets: 50 and 100 mg.

Nadolol

2,3-Naphthalenediol, 5-[3-[(1,1-dimethylethyl)amino]-2-hydroxypropoxy]-1,2,3,4-tetrahydro-, *cis*-, Corgard (*Squibb*)

1-(*tert*-Butylamino)-3-[(5,6,7,8-tetrahydro-*cis*-6,7-dihydroxy-1-naphthyl)oxy]-2-propanol [42200-33-9] $C_{17}H_{27}NO_4$ (309.40).

Preparation—See US Pat 3,935,267.

Description—White crystalline powder melting about 125–135°. The pKa is 9.68.

Solubility—Freely soluble in alcohol; slightly soluble in chloroform; insoluble in acetone and hydrocarbon solvents.

Uses—Nadolol is a nonselective β-antagonist with all the actions, uses, adverse effects, contraindications and drug interactions characteristic of drugs in this class (see the general statement). However, nadolol differs from other β-blockers in that it increases, rather than decreases, renal blood flow by a direct vasodilator action. It is erratic in its effect to decrease plasma renin activity. It lacks CNS actions because it fails to penetrate into the CNS.

The oral bioavailability of nadolol is about 34%. Twenty to 30% is bound to plasma proteins. The volume of distribution is about 2 L/kg. Nadolol is eliminated unchanged in the urine and as conjugates in the bile, which are partially deconjugated in the small intestine and reabsorbed. The normal half-life is 10 to 24 hr but longer in renal failure.

Dose—*Oral, adults, for angina pectoris, initially* **40 mg** once a day, with increments of 40 to 80 mg/day at 3- to 7-day intervals, if necessary, up to a total dose of **240 mg**/day; for *hypertension, initially* **80 mg** once a day, with increments of **80 mg**/day at weekly intervals, if necessary, up to a total of **320 mg**/day. The plateau principle holds that dose adjustments at intervals of less than 5 days may result in excessive maintenance dosage. In renal failure, dosage must be adjusted.

Dosage Forms—Tablets: 40, 80, 120, and 160 mg.

Phenoxybenzamine Hydrochloride

Benzenemethanamine, N-(2-chloroethyl)-N-(1-methyl-2-phenoxyethyl)-, hydrochloride; Dibenzyline Hydrochloride (*SKF*)

N-(2-Chloroethyl)-N-(1-methyl-2-phenoxyethyl)benzylamine hydrochloride [63-92-3] $C_{18}H_{22}ClNO \cdot HCl$ (340.29).

Preparation—One method starts with phenol undergoing addition to propylene oxide to give 1-phenoxy-2-propanol, which is reacted with thionyl chloride to yield 1-phenoxy-2-chloropropane. Refluxing the latter with excess ethanolamine gives N-(phenoxyisopropyl)-ethanol and additional refluxing of this with benzyl chloride in the presence of $NaHCO_3$ yields 2-[N-benzyl-N-(1-methyl-2-phenoxyethyl)amino]ethanol. Treatment with thionyl chloride and HCl in $CHCl_3$ completes the synthesis. US Pat 2,599,000.

Description—White, crystalline, odorless powder; melts between 136° and 141°.

Solubility—1 g in 25 mL water, 6 mL alcohol, 3 mL chloroform, >1000 mL ether.

Uses—Phenoxybenzamine is a nonselective α-antagonist. It irreversibly alkylates sulfhydryl groups at the α_1-receptor site. Recovery from blockade can result only from synthesis of new receptors. The duration of action may be as long as 4 to 5 days. The effects and uses are those of α-blocking drugs in general, except that phenoxybenzamine has too unpredictable an efficacy in essential hypertension to be competitive with newer drugs. The long duration of action makes the drug especially useful in the management of inoperable pheochromocytoma.

In addition to the side effects of α-blockade, phenoxybenzamine causes drowsiness and has a local irritancy; by the oral route it may cause nausea, vomiting, and diarrhea. Contraindications are those of α-antagonists in general (page 903).

Dose—*Orally, initially* **10 mg**/day, taken with milk, for 4 days; thereafter, the dose is increased in increments of 10 mg until optimal dosage is achieved, which is usually 20 to 60 mg/day. To minimize gastrointestinal irritation, the daily dose should be divided into 10- and 20-mg fractions.

Dosage Form—Capsules: 10 mg.

Phentolamine Hydrochloride

Phenol, 3-[[(4,5-dihydro-1*H*-imidazol-2-yl)methyl](4-methylphenyl)-amino]-, monohydrochloride; Regitine Hydrochloride (*Ciba-Geigy*)

m-[*N*-(2-Imidazolin-2-ylmethyl)-*p*-toluidino]phenol monohydrochloride [73-05-2] $C_{17}H_{19}N_3O \cdot HCl$ (317.82).

Preparation—*m*-(*p*-Toluidino)phenol is refluxed with 2-chloromethylimidazoline hydrochloride.

Description—White or slightly grayish, crystalline, odorless powder. Its solutions are acid to litmus, having a pH of about 5, and foam on shaking. Melts at about 240°.

Solubility—1 g in 50 mL water, 100 mL alcohol; very slightly soluble in chloroform and in ether.

Uses—The same as those given for *Phentolamine Mesylate*; however, its use is limited mostly to oral medication prior to surgery to control and prevent paroxysmal hypertensive attacks in patients with pheochromocytoma.

Dose—*Oral, adult*, **50 mg** 4 to 6 times a day; *children*, **25 mg** 4 to 6 times a day. The dose may be doubled, if necessary.

Dosage Form: Tablets: 50 mg.

Phentolamine Mesylate

Phenol, 3-[[(4,5-dihydro-1*H*-imidazol-2-yl)methyl](4-methylphenyl)-amino]-, monomethanesulfonate (salt);
Regitine Mesylate (*Ciba-Geigy*)

Phentolamine mesylate [65-28-1] $C_{17}H_{19}N_3O \cdot CH_4O_3S$ (377.46). For the structure and chemical name of phentolamine, see *Phentolamine Hydrochloride*.

Preparation—By treating phentolamine base with an equimolar portion of methanesulfonic acid.

Description—White or off-white, odorless, crystalline powder. Its solutions are acid to litmus, having a pH of about 5, and slowly deteriorate. Melts at about 178°.

Solubility—1 g in 1 mL water, 4 mL alcohol, 700 mL chloroform.

Uses—Phentolamine is a nonselective α-adrenoreceptor antagonist. The blockade is reversible. In addition to α-blocking activity, it has mild to moderate sympathomimetic-like mydriatic and cardiostimulant (rate, force of contraction and dysrhythmias) activity, weak muscarinic activity in the gastrointestinal tract, and weak to mild histaminergic activity in the stomach (acid secretion) and arterioles (flushing and slight fall in blood pressure). These effects limit the dose that can be used so that α-blockade is usually incomplete. The effects of the α-blocking component of activity are those stated on page 902 and the uses those on page 903. Additional uses include the treatment or prevention of dermal necrosis and sloughing resulting from *extravasation of norepinephrine*, the treatment of *primary pulmonary hypertension*, and the management of *hypertensive crises* caused by drug interactions with *monoamine oxidase inhibitors* or the abrupt withdrawal of *clonidine*. It is used as a diagnostic agent for pheochromocytoma: a fall in diastolic blood pressure in excess of 25 torr is considered to be positive, although both false negative and positive responses occur. Analysis of urinary metanephrines is the preferred diagnostic method. In shock, it is sometimes combined with norepinephrine to block the α-vasoconstrictor effects and permit the uncomplicated β_1-effects to prevail.

The adverse effects are those of α-blockade (page 902), in addition to which there is weakness. The contraindications are those on page 904, with the addition that digitalis should be avoided in phentolamine-treated patients because of the danger of serious cardiac dysrhythmias.

Dose—*Intramuscular* or *intravenous, adults*, **5 mg;** as a hypertensive prophylactic in pheochromocytoma, it is to be given 1 to 2 hours prior to surgery. In *children*, **100 µg per kg** of body weight (or 3 mg per m² of body surface). *Regional infiltration*, after extravasation of levarterenol, **5 to 10 mg** in 10 mL of isotonic sodium chloride solution, injected into the area of extravasation, within 12 hours after occurrence. *With levarterenol*, to prevent dermal necrosis and sloughing, **10 mg/L** of levarterenol solution.

Dosage Form: for Injection: 5 mg/1 mL.

Prazosin—page 844.

Propranolol Hydrochloride

2-Propanol, 1-[(1-methylethyl)amino]-3-(1-naphthalenyloxy)-, hydrochloride; Inderal (*Ayerst*)

1-(Isopropylamino)-3-(1-naphthyloxy)-2-propanol hydrochloride [318-98-9] $C_{16}H_{21}NO_2 \cdot HCl$ (295.81).

Preparation—α-Naphthol is reacted with epichlorohydrin in aqueous alkali to form 2,3-epoxypropyl α-naphthyl ether and the epoxy ring ruptured by reaction with isopropylamine. The base is converted to hydrochloride with HCl.

Description—White or almost white powder that is odorless and has a bitter taste. It is stable to heat, unstable in light, and nonhygroscopic. It melts at about 161°. pK_a 9.45.

Solubility—1 g in 20 mL water and 20 mL alcohol; slightly soluble in chloroform; practically insoluble in ether.

Uses—Propranolol is a nonselective β-antagonist, with all the actions, uses, adverse effects and contraindications characteristic of this class of drugs (see general statement), except that it is not used to treat glaucoma. Only the (−)isomer has significant β-blocking activity. It is frequently stated that the drug has quinidine-like properties to decrease myocardial sodium entry, but it appears that such actions do not occur in therapeutic concentrations and that the antidysrhythmic actions are those of β_1-blockade alone.

Propranolol penetrates into the CNS and causes the central effects described on page 903. Propranolol has been reported to be of value in more than 20 noncardiovascular disorders, many of which are in the CNS. It also enters adrenergic neurons, from which it can be released by nerve impulses.

Propranolol can cause an erythematous rash with fever and sore throat.

By the oral route 30 to 60% reaches the systemic circulation, mainly because it is actively metabolized as it passes through the liver from the gut. Food increases the bioavailability. There are about 20 metabolites, at least one of which is also active. All of the propranolol is biotransformed in the liver. The volume of distribution is about 4 L/kg. Propranolol is 93% protein-bound. The minimal effective plasma concentration is in the range of 0.04 to 0.085 µg/mL. Plasma renin activity is suppressed at 0.10 to 0.20 µg/mL. The plasma half-life of a single dose of propranolol is about 2 to 3.5 hours, but it is about 3 to 5 hours with repeated dosage and also longer in congestive heart failure.

The oral route of administration of the drug is preferred.

Dose—*Intravenous*, for *arrhythmias, adult*, **1 to 3 mg** at a rate not to exceed 1 mg/min. The dose may be repeated in a few minutes if necessary. *Oral*, in *conventional form, adult*, for *arrhythmias*, **10 to 30 mg** 3 or 4 times a day, before meals and at bedtime; for *pheochromocytoma, preoperatively*, **20 mg** 3 times a day for 3 days prior to surgery; or, for the *management* of *inoperable tumor*, **10 mg** 3 times a day for 3 days before surgery but not to be given before an α-blocker has first been administered; for *essential hypertension*, *initially* **40 mg** twice a day, increased by 20-mg increments up to **160 mg**, 4 times a day (several days to several weeks of medication may be required before a substantial effect occurs); *for angina pectoris*, *initially* **10 to 20 mg**, 3 or 4 times a day to be increased to as much as **80 mg**, if necessary, 3 or 4 times a day; for *hypertrophic subaortic stenosis*, **20 to 40 mg**, 3 or 4 times a day; for *thyrotoxicosis*, **10 to 20 mg**, 3 or 4 times a day with adjustments as necessary; for *migraine*, **20 mg**, 4 times a day, with upward adjustments, up to a dose of 240 mg/day. *Oral, children*, **500 µg** to **1 mg/kg** of body weight/day in 3 or 4 divided doses. In *sustained-release form*, the total daily dose can be taken once a day.

Dosage Forms—Sustained-Release Capsules: 80, 120 and 160 mg. Injection: 1 mg/mL. Tablets: 10, 40 and 80 mg.

Timolol Maleate

2-Propanol, 1-[(1,1-dimethylethyl)amino]-3-[[4-(4-morpholinyl-1,2,5-thiadiazol-3-yl]oxy]-(S)-, (Z)-2-butenedioate (1:1) (salt); Blocadren, Timolate, Timoptic, Timoptol (*MSD*)

(−)-1-(*tert*-Butylamino)-3-[(4-morpholino-1,2,5-thiadiazol-3-yl)-oxy]-2-propanol maleate (1:1) (salt) [26921-17-5] $C_{13}H_{24}N_4O_4.S.-C_4H_4O_4$ (432.49).

Preparation—J Med Chem *15:*651 (1972).

Description—White crystals melting about 202°. The pH of a 5% aqueous solution is about 4.

Solubility—Freely soluble in water: soluble in alcohol; sparingly soluble in chloroform; practically insoluble in ether.

Uses—Timolol is a nonselective β-adrenoreceptor antagonist with all the potential uses, adverse effects, contraindications and drug interactions characteristic of this class of drugs (see the general statement), except that its CNS actions are very weak. Approved uses in the US include the treatment of hypertension, the prevention of reinfarction and/or sudden death *after myocardial infarction*, and the treatment of open-angle glaucoma. Timolol was the drug used in the Norwegian studies that convincingly demonstrated the value of β-blockers administered following myocardial infarction. Timolol differs from other β-blockers in that a fall in vascular resistance occurs with the first dose.

By the oral route the bioavailability of timolol is 60 to 75%. About 10% is bound to plasma proteins. β-Blocking concentrations are 5 to 10 ng/mL. Lipid solubility is low, so that concentrations in the CNS are low. Because of its high potency, topical efficacy in the eye is good. However, sufficient drug may be absorbed into the blood stream occasionally to cause adverse systemic effects, especially in infants. About 80% is eliminated by hepatic metabolism and 20% by renal excretion. The elimination half-life is about 3 to 4 hr.

Dose—*Oral*, *adults*, *initially* **10 mg** twice a day, to be maintained at that dose for prophylaxis after myocardial infarction but increased at one-week intervals, if necessary, up to a dose of 30 mg twice a day for hypertension. *Topical, to the eye, initially* **1 drop** of a **0.25%** solution twice a day, to be increased to 0.50%, if necessary; downward adjustment is made by dropping 1 dose/day.

Dosage Forms—Ophthalmic Solution: 0.25 and 0.50%; Tablets: 50 and 100 mg.

Trimazosin—page 845.

Other Adrenergic Blocking Drugs

Pindolol [1-(1H-Indol-4-yloxy)-3-[(1-methylethyl)amino]- 2-propanol [13523-86-9] $C_{14}H_{20}N_2O$ (248.32). Viskin (*Sandoz*)]—Preparation; Swiss Pat 472,404. An off-white almost odorless crystalline powder melting about 172°. It is practically insoluble in water; slightly soluble in anhydrous alcohol and chloroform. *Uses:* A nonselective β-antagonist with partial agonist activity (see general statement). The intrinsic sympathomimetic activity in man appears to be somewhat less than 0.5. When resting sympathoadrenal activity is low, the intrinsic activity is evident in that heart rate and force of contraction do not decrease to the extent expected from β-blockade or may actually slightly increase. When the sympathoadrenal activity is high, heart rate and force decline, as expected from β-blockade. With low doses, in hypertension, angina pectoris and ventricular tachydysrhythmias, its efficacy appears to be comparable to that of propranolol, but it is probably less effective against supraventricular tachydysrhythmias. With high doses, there may be a decrease in antihypertensive efficacy. The oral bioavailability of pindolol is about 90%. In plasma, about 57% is protein-bound. The volume of distribution is about 2.9 L/kg. The effective plasma concentration is 50 to 100 ng/mL. About 60% is eliminated by hepatic metabolism and 40% by renal excretion. The elimination half-life is 3 to 4 hr. *Dose: Oral*, *adults*, *initially* 10 mg twice a day, to be adjusted at 14- to 21-day intervals up to a maximum daily dose of 30 mg; above 30 mg/day, no further reductions in blood pressure are usually achieved and adverse effects are more prominent. *Dosage Forms:* Tablets: 5 and 10 mg.

Adrenergic Neuron Blocking Agents

(Antiadrenergic Drugs)

The biosynthesis of the adrenergic neurohumor, norepinephrine, takes place in the postganglionic sympathetic adrenergic neuron. The substrate is 3,4-dihydroxyphenylalanine (DOPA), which is formed in the adrenergic neuron by the hydroxylation of tyrosine. DOPA is acted upon by the enzyme dopa decarboxylase. The product of the decarboxylation is the catecholamine dopamine (3,4-dihydroxy-β-phenylethylamine). Within the adrenergic neuron in the region of the nerve endings are granular organelles that contain the enzyme dopamine β-oxidase, which introduces the side chain hydroxyl group into dopamine to make norepinephrine. The norepinephrine is stored in the same granular organelles. Nerve impulses cause the ingress of calcium, which releases norepinephrine from the storage granules. It can also be released by indirectly acting sympathomimetics (see Chapter 45) and drugs such as reserpine and guanethidine. After the norepinephrine is initially released from the granules by reserpine or guanethidine, newly formed or transported norepinephrine cannot be reincorporated into the depleted granules; furthermore, residual norepinephrine in the granules, of which there is considerable after guanethidine, cannot be released. The total effect is that norepinephrine is unavailable for delivery to the effector in response to nerve stimulation.

Drugs such as metyrosine, which suppress the biosynthesis of norepinephrine, also cause adrenergic neuronal block.

Guanadrel Sulfate

Guanidine, (1,4-dioxaspiro[4.5]dec-2-ylmethyl)-, sulfate (2:1); Hylorel (*Upjohn*)

[22195] $(C_{10}H_{19}N_3O_2)_2.H_2SO_4$ (524.63).
Preparation—US Pat 3,547,951.

Description—White solid melting about 213°.

Uses—Guanadrel is an adrenergic neuron-blocking drug with a mechanism of action and hemodynamic properties like those of guanethidine (below), to which it is chemically related. It has a shorter duration of action and consequently causes less severe morning postural hypotension, but postural hypotension during the rest of the day is comparable to that from guanethidine. Guanadrel causes somewhat less diarrhea and interferes less with ejaculation. Unlike guanethidine, guanadrel is used in the treatment of *mild* and *moderate essential hypertension*.

Guanadrel is well absorbed orally, the bioavailability of compressed tablets being about 85%. Peak effects are reached in 30 to 120 min after oral administration, although peak plasma concentrations are not achieved until 90 to 120 min. Less than 20% of plasma guanadrel is protein-bound. The drug does not penetrate into the brain or eye. The duration of action is 4 to 14 hr. Tricyclic antidepressants, amphetamines and other drugs that engage the amine uptake pump into the adrenergic neuron prevent recycling of guanadrel and hence shorten the duration of action or completely "deblock" the adrenergic neuron. Elimination is about 50% by hepatic metabolism and 50% by renal excretion. The distribution and elimination half-lives are 1 to 4 hr and 5 to 45 hr, respectively.

Dose—*Oral, adults, initially*, **5 mg** upon arising and again in the afternoon, to be gradually adjusted, if necessary, to a usual *maintenance* dose of 25 to 75 mg/day; some patients may require only one dose a day.

Dosage Forms—Scored tablets: 5 and 25 mg.

Guanethidine Sulfate

Guanidine, [2-(hexahydro-1(2H)-azocinyl)ethyl]-, sulfate (2:1); Ismelin Sulfate (*Ciba-Geigy*)

[60-02-6] $(C_{10}H_{22}N_4)_2 \cdot H_2SO_4$ (494.69).

Preparation—Cycloheptanone oxime undergoes Beckmann rearrangement to form hexahydro-2(1H)-azocinone [$\overline{CH_2(CH_2)_5CONH}$] which is then reduced to heptamethyleneimine [$\overline{CH_2(CH_2)_6NH}$]. This is condensed with chloracetonitrile and the resulting nitrile is hydrogenated to 1-(2-aminoethyl)heptamethyleneimine. Condensation with 2-methyl-2-thiopseudourea [$NH=C(SCH_3)NH_2$] sulfate eliminates CH_3SH to produce crude guanethidine sulfate.

Description—White, crystalline powder, having a strong, characteristic odor.

Solubility—Sparingly soluble in water; slightly soluble in alcohol; practically insoluble in chloroform.

Uses—An antiadrenergic neuron blocking agent that partially depletes the adrenergic nerve of its norepinephrine and prevents release of that which remains. The result is vasodilatation and a decrease in plasma renin activity, both of which act to lower blood pressure. The onset of action is slow, requiring several hours to 2 or 3 days for its full effect, and its duration of action may be 4 or more days. Guanethidine lowers the blood pressure more effectively than any other *antihypertensive* drug used in outpatient therapy, except, perhaps, the ganglionic blocking drugs. In fact, there is danger that the blood pressure will fall to dangerously low levels in some patients. Therefore, it is usually employed in submaximal doses and is combined with thiazides or hydralazine in order to permit some adrenergic function to remain. Guanethidine is usually not used to treat mild to moderate but only moderately severe to severe hypertension. Tolerance is rare and of low degree.

The most common untoward effects of guanethidine are those that obligatorily accrue to the effects of sympathetic blockade. They include orthostatic hypotension with its attendant vertigo, weakness, lassitude, nausea, and occasional syncope, bradycardia, nasal stuffiness, dry mouth, diarrhea, urinary incontinence, nocturia, failure of normal ejaculation. Fatigue and dyspnea from exertion also occur occasionally. Heart failure may also occur. Like reserpine, the drug may cause edema and azotemia as a result of a deficient renal blood flow consequent to decreased blood pressure and cardiac output. Adrenergic neuron blockage tends to exacerbate hypoglycemia in certain patients. Other effects include fatigue, ptosis, blurred vision, parotid tenderness, angina, muscle tremor, myalgia, alopecia, and mental depression.

Guanethidine potentiates the pressor effects of norepinephrine and certain other directly acting alpha sympathomimetics by inhibiting uptake into the adrenergic nerve terminals. It may also cause release of catecholamines from pheochrome tumors and hence precipitate hypertensive crises. It interferes with the pressor actions of indirectly acting sympathomimetics by inhibiting both uptake of the drugs into the adrenergic neuron and release of norepinephrine, but it potentiates whatever lesser amounts of levarterenol are released. Amphetamine-type central nervous stimulants, tricyclic antidepressants (except doxepin), antihistamines, levodopa, and chlorpromazine antagonize guanethidine. Tricyclic antidepressants and quinidine may cause cardiac arrest when given with guanethidine. The drug potentiates the hypoglycemic effects of oral hypoglycemics and insulin.

Guanethidine is contraindicated in pheochromocytoma, in patients hypersensitive to the drug, and when monoamine oxidase inhibitors are in use. It should be used cautiously in renal disease, cerebral vascular disease, coronary insufficiency, recent myocardial infarction, congestive heart failure, peptic ulcer, edematous states, diabetes, and anesthesia.

Only 3 to 30% of guanethidine is absorbed when administered orally. It is partly metabolized to two metabolites and partly excreted unchanged, (25 to 50%), mostly within a few hours; however, effective traces remain for up to 14 days. The onset of action is a few hours to a few days; the offset of action is several days.

Dose—*Oral, adult, ambulatory patients, initially* 10 or **12.5 mg** once a day, with 10- to 12.5-mg increments at 5- to 7-day intervals, if necessary to effect a fall in blood pressure, but not to exceed 200 mg/day; **25 to 50 mg**/day is the usual *maintenance* dose. In combination with other antihypertensives the usual dose will be lower. "Minidoses" of 5 mg are sometimes used in the treatment of moderate essential hypertension. *Hospitalized patients, initially* **25 to 50 mg**, with daily or bidaily increments of 25 to 50 mg if necessary. An initial large dose of 100 mg can be given without a hypertensive phase of action. Minidoses of 5 to 10 mg are now popular, especially in combination with other drugs. *Children*, **200 μg/kg** of body weight (or 6 mg per m² of body surface), with increments of 200 μg/kg at 7- to 10-day intervals, if necessary.

Dosage Forms—Tablets: 10 and 25 mg.

Reserpine

Yohimban-16-carboxylic acid, 11,17-dimethoxy-18-[(3,4,5-trimethoxybenzoyl)oxy]-, methyl ester, (3β,16β,17α,18β,20α)-, (*Various Mfrs*)

Methyl 18β-hydroxy-11,17α-dimethoxy-3β,20α-yohimban-16β-carboxylate 3,4,5-trimethoxybenzoate (ester) [50-55-5] $C_{33}H_{40}N_2O_9$ (608.69).

Reserpine, one of more than 20 alkaloids in *Rauwolfia serpentina*, was first isolated in pure crystalline form by Müller *et al.* (*Experientia* 8: 338, 1952). Subsequently it was found also in other species of *Rauwolfia*. A procedure for its separation is described in US Pat 2,833,771 (1958). Although it has been synthesized (Woodward *et al, J Am Chem Soc* 78: 2023, 1956) its production thus is not economically feasible.

Description—White or pale buff to slightly yellowish, odorless, crystalline powder. It darkens slowly on exposure to light, but more rapidly when in solution. It melts between 255° and 265° with decomposition.

Solubility—Insoluble in water; very slightly soluble in ether; 1 g in about 1800 mL alcohol and about 6 mL chloroform; slightly soluble in benzene; freely soluble in acetic acid.

Uses—Reserpine, the first rauwolfia alkaloid to be officially recognized, was first used for the symptomatic management of patients with anxiety or tension psychoneuroses or chronic psychoses involving anxiety, psychomotor hyperactivity, or compulsive aggressive behavior. Higher doses of the drug are required in the management of grossly disturbed psychoses than in anxiety-tension states. However, in both types of patients the drug must be administered for 1 or 2 weeks before the optimal level of dosage can be determined. The tranquilizing effect of the drug makes the patient more cooperative, less destructive, and more amenable to psychotherapy. Unless the dosage is carefully adjusted, the drug may induce a paradoxical form of anxiety and adverse reactive depression. In chronic psychoses, the drug does not appear to alter the basic psychopathological state. Because of the seriousness of side effects, reserpine is no longer used much as a tranquilizer.

Reserpine still has a firmly established position in modern antihypertensive therapy. Because the doses used are generally considerably smaller than those for its tranquilizing effects, the drug may be used for its hypotensive effects with more safety than as a psychopharmacologic drug. It exerts its antihypertensive effects through a partial depletion of the norepinephrine in the sympathetic postganglionic nerves. The effect is greater at the vascular smooth muscle than at the heart. Plasma renin activity is diminished. The drug is chiefly used in combination with thiazide diuretics for the management of mild, labile hypertension and in conjunction with potent hypotensive agents for the management of *essential hypertension* and *hypertensive emergencies.* The use of safe doses of oral reserpine alone is considered to be of little value for severe hypertension, but it is useful to augment or to prolong the action of potent hypotensive agents, to reduce dosage and side effects. The value of reserpine for routine use as a prophylactic against progressive vascular changes in patients with early hypertension is unwarranted. Intravenous reserpine is quite useful in the management of severe hypertension and hypertensive crises. The antihypertensive action of reserpine derives from adrenergic neuronal blockade consequent to depletion of the catecholamine-containing granules of the postganglionic sympathetic neuron. The mechanism of the central effects is similar. It depletes both brain serotonin and catecholamines. Reserpine is also used to treat *Raynaud's phenomenon.*

Reserpine is poorly and erratically absorbed from the gastrointestinal tract, which causes a considerable difference in efficacy of oral and intravenous doses. It characteristically has a long latency of onset and a prolonged duration of action. For example, with daily oral administration the effects of the drug usually are not fully manifest for several days to 2 weeks and may persist for as long as 4 weeks after oral medication is discontinued. Tolerance to the drug does not develop with continued administration.

Nasal congestion, scleroconjunctival congestion, drowsiness, bradycardia, lacrimation, excessive salivation, nausea, vomiting, anorexia, weight gain, and diarrhea are the most frequently noted side effects of reserpine. Dry mouth, headache, dizziness, dysuria, myalgia, and dull sensorium also occur. Suicidal depression is the most serious untoward effect. The drug may reactivate old peptic ulcers because it increases hydrochloric acid secretion by the stomach. Consequently, it should be used cautiously in patients with a history of peptic ulcer. Other serious reactions are orthostatic hypotension, fatigue, weakness, insomnia, nightmares, excitement, paradoxical anxiety, irrational behavior, parkinsonian rigidity (extrapyramidal syndrome), glaucoma, angina pectoris, dyspnea, deafness, uveitis, pruritus, rash, purpura, decreased libido, retrograde ejaculation, impotence, deafness, and optic atrophy.

Reserpine is contraindicated in pregnancy and in nursing mothers because it is transmitted to the offspring. It is also contraindicated in ulcerative colitis because of the increase in bowel motility, in biliary lithiasis, persons with suicidal tendencies or other mental depression, and persons receiving electroconvulsive treatment. It should be used cautiously in combination with quinidine, because of the danger of heart block, cardiac arrest, or arrhythmias. It may sensitize anesthetics and interfere with cardiovascular adjustments during surgery. It may decrease the response to indirect sympathomimetics.

Dose—*Oral, adults,* for *hypertension, initially* **0.1** to **0.25 mg**/day; when higher doses are used, the patient must be continuously monitored for mood depression; for *anxiety-tension, initially* **0.1** to **0.5 mg**/day for control, then adjusted to minimum effective dose; for *psychotic disorders, initially* **0.1** to **1 mg**/day, with subsequent adjustments to maintain control; *children,* for *hypertension,* **5 to 20 µg/kg** (or 150 to 600 µg/m^2 of body surface) a day, once or in 2 divided doses. *Intramuscular, adults,* for *hypertensive crises,* initially **0.5** to **1 mg**; if there is no response within 3 hr, follow with **2 mg**, then 3 hr later with **4 mg**, if necessary; if 4 mg fails to lower blood pressure substantially, another antihypertensive drug should be used; once the antihypertensive effect is achieved, the dose may be repeated 4 to 8 times a day until the crisis is over; *children,* weighing *less than 25 kg,* **20 µg/kg,** repeated every 4 to 6 hr, if necessary; *children* weighing *over 25 kg,* **0.5** to **1 mg** every 4 to 6 hr. *Intraarterial, adults,* for *Raynaud's phenomenon,* **0.5** to **1 mg.**

Dosage Forms—Extended-Release Capsules: 0.5 mg. Elixir: 0.2 mg/4 mL; Injection: 5 mg/2 mL, and 25 mg/10 mL; Tablets: 0.1, 0.25, 0.5, and 1 mg.

Other Adrenergic Neuron Blocking Agents

Alseroxylon [A fat soluble alkaloidal fraction isolated from R serpentina. A reddish-brown powder with a characteristic odor. Rautensin (*Dorsey*); Rauwiloid (*Riker*). *Uses:* The actions, potential uses and adverse effects are those of reserpine (page 908). However, alseroxylon is used only in the treatment of essential hypertension. *Dose: Oral, adults,* 2 to 4 mg/day.

Deserpidine [11-Desmethoxyreserpine [131-01-1]; $C_{32}H_{38}N_2O_8$ (578.64); Harmonyl (*Abbott*)]—An alkaloid from *Rauwolfia canescens* that differs structurally from reserpine in the absence of its 11-methoxy group. Occurs as a white to light yellow, crystalline powder; pK$_a$ 5.67; insoluble in water; slightly soluble in alcohol. *Uses:* An adrenergic neuron blocking drug; like reserpine it is used mainly for the treatment of mild to moderately severe essential hypertension in conjunction with thiazide diuretics. The effect of the drug is generally not evident for 10 to 14 days. It is occasionally used as a tranquilizer in the treatment of mild anxiety states. As with other rauwolfia alkaloids, higher doses are required for management of psychoses, which often cause serious side effects, so that this use is no longer common. Side effects and contraindications are the same as for reserpine. *Dose: Usual, oral,* for hypertension, 0.25 mg 1 or 2 times a day; for psychosis, 0.1 to 1 mg/day.

Ergoloid Mesylates [A mixture of equal amounts of the methanesulfonate (mesylate) salts of dihydroergocornine, dihydroergocristine, and dihydroergocryptine; Deapril ST (*Mead Johnson*); Hydergine (*Sandoz*)]—*Uses:* Lowers the blood pressure and obtunds pressor reflexes in part by a central depressant action at the vasomotor center and in part by an α-adrenergic blockage in the periphery, which causes vasodilatation. It also produces bradycardia by the combination of a stimulant action on the cardiodecelerator center and a depression of cardioaccelerator reflexes. Because the mixture of hydrogenated ergot alkaloids weakly dilates cerebral blood vessels, it was introduced for use in cerebral arteriosclerosis and dizziness, paresthesias, mood changes, nocturnal cramps, and senile dementia ("idiopathic cerebral dysfunction") in the aged (implied to be only secondary to arteriosclerosis). But arteriosclerotic vessels are incapable of much dilatation, and autopsies have failed to correlate such signs and symptoms with arteriosclerosis. Furthermore, no valid scientific studies are available to support the claim of efficacy. The drug may cause sublingual irritation, nasal stuffiness, nausea, vomiting, anorexia, other gastrointestinal upset, drowsiness, skin rash, headache, faintness, sore tongue (with sublingual form, and sinus bradycardia. Orthostatic hypotension sometimes occurs. *Dose: Oral* or *sublingual,* 1 mg 3 times a day.

Metyrosine [(−)-α-Methyl-L-tyrosine [672-87-7]; $C_{10}H_{13}NO_3$ (195.22); Demser (*MSD*)]—The synthesis is described in J Org Chem *32:* 4074 (1967). It is a white crystalline solid melting about 310° and is soluble about 1 g in 1750 mL of water. *Uses:* Metyrosine blocks tyrosine hydroxylase and thus suppresses the synthesis of catecholamines. This causes depletion of catecholamines in adrenergic neurons in both the sympathetic and central nervous systems and in the pheochrome cells in the adrenal medulla and accessory tissue. The drug is used to treat *pheochromocytoma.* It is too inconsistent in hypertension to be competitive with other drugs. Sedation is the most common side effect, but some tolerance occurs during the first week of treatment. Extrapyramidal dyskinesias occur in about 10% of recipients. Other adverse CNS effects include anxiety, confusion, depression, disorientation and hallucinations. Insomnia and hyperactivity may occur after withdrawal. Gastrointestinal side effects include diarrhea (about 10%), nausea, vomiting, and abdominal pain. Nasal stuffiness and impaired ejaculation result from sympathetic adrenergic neuron blockade. Other adverse effects are dry mouth, headache, gynecomastia, galactorrhea, peripheral edema, urticaria, pharyngeal edema, eosinophilia, and elevated SGOT. Crystalluria and nephrolithiasis and consequent hematuria and transient dysuria may occur. A daily urine output of over 2 L should be maintained. Metyrosine potentiates the extrapyramidal effects of phenothiazines and butyrophenones. The drug is mostly excreted unchanged in the urine. *Dose: Oral, adults* and *children over 12 yr, initially,* 250 mg, 4 times a day with daily increments of 250 to 500 mg up to a total daily dose of 4 g, if necessary. *Dosage Form: Capsules:* 250 mg.

Rauwolfia Serpentina The dried root of *Rauwolfia serpentina* (Linné) Betham ex Kurz (Fam *Apocynaceae*), sometimes with fragments of rhizome and aerial stem bases attached. It contains not less than 0.15% of reserpine–rescinnamine group alkaloids, calculated as reserpine. Powdered Rauwolfia Serpentina is rauwolfia serpentina reduced to a fine or very fine powder, and adjusted if necessary to conform to the official requirements for reserpine–rescinnamine group alkaloids by admixture with lactose or starch or with a powdered rauwolfia serpentina containing a higher or lower content of these alkaloids. It contains 0.15–0.20% of reserpine–rescinnamine group alkaloids, calculated as reserpine. *Uses:* Produces the sum of the actions of the total alkaloids contained in the whole root. The component alkaloids exhibit the sedative–antihypertensive–bradycrotic action characteristic of reserpine, the latter of which accounts for approximately 50% of the total activity. The actions, uses, and limitations are the same as those for *Reserpine,* page 908. *Dose: Oral, adult, initially* 100 to 200 mg twice a day for 1 to 3 weeks and thereafter for *maintenance,* 50 to 300 mg daily in divided doses. *Dosage Forms:* Powdered (see below); Tablets: 50 and 100 mg.

Rescinnamine [Methyl 18β-hydroxy-11,17α-dimethoxy-3β,20α-yohimban-16β-carboxylate 3,4,5-trimethoxycinnamate (ester) [24815-24-5]; $C_{35}H_{42}N_2O_9$ (643.72); Moderil (*Pfizer*)]—For the structural formula see page 421. Rescinnamine may be obtained by extraction from *Rauwolfia vomitoria* and other species of *Rauwolfia,* and it may also be synthesized from its more plentiful relative, reserpine, which differs only in being the 3,4,5-trimethoxybenzoic acid ester of methyl reserpate while rescinnamine is the 3,4,5-trimethoxycinnamic acid ester of methyl reserpate. Rescinnamine occurs as a white, or pale buff to cream-colored, crystalline powder, melting between 220° and 232°; practically insoluble in water, slightly soluble in alcohol, and soluble in chloroform. *Uses:* The same uses and order of effectiveness as reserpine. Thus, it is useful for the management of mild, labile hypertension and as a tranquilizing agent in agitated patients with simple neuroses and frank psychoses. Except that sedation and bradycardia occur less frequently and in milder form with rescinnamine, the incidence of other side effects such as weakness and fatigue, nasal congestion, dizziness, confusion, increased appetite, and weight gain is about the same as with reserpine. Both drugs are subject to the same precautions and contraindications. See *Reserpine. Dose:* 0.25 to 2 mg daily; *usual, initial,* 0.5 mg 1 or 2 times a day for up to 2 weeks; *maintenance,* 0.25 mg daily. The daily dose is increased or decreased by increments of 0.25 mg to achieve the desired therapeutic response. *Dosage Forms:* Tablets: 0.25 and 0.5 mg.

CHAPTER 48

Antimuscarinic and Antispasmodic Drugs

Stewart C Harvey, PhD

Professor of Pharmacology
School of Medicine, University of Utah
Salt Lake City, UT 84132

Antimuscarinic Drugs

Cholinergic transmission occurs not only at the neuroeffectors innervated by the parasympathetic and certain sympathetic postganglionic nerves but also at all autonomic ganglia, the somatic neuromuscular junction, and certain central synapses (see introductory statement, Chapter 45). *Antimuscarinic* drugs are competitive antagonists that act only on the cholinergic receptors at smooth muscle and secretory cells and certain central synapses. The term *cholinergic blocking drug* is loosely used by some as synonymous with antimuscarinic drug but it denotes any drug that can antagonize cholinergic stimuli at any cholinergic site, nicotinic or muscarinic. Other improper synonyms for the term antimuscarinic are *anticholinergic, cholinolytic, parasympatholytic*, and *parasympathetic blocking drugs.* Since "cholinergic," ganglionic, and neuromuscular blocking drugs have in common the antagonism of acetylcholine, it is to be expected that certain of these drugs may block at more than one kind of cholinergic receptor and that structural requirements for one type of blocking activity have some relationship to those for activity at other cholinergic sites.

Actions and Selectivity—The effects of antimuscarinic drugs on the whole are readily predicted by considering the consequences of interruption of parasympathetic (and sympathetic cholinergic) nerve stimulation. Thus, the effects are decreased gastrointestinal motility, decreased gastric secretion, dry mouth, drying of the mucous membranes in general, mydriasis, loss of accommodation (and a *pari passu* tendency to increased intraocular pressure), urinary retention, decreased sweating and compensatory cutaneous flush, bronchial and biliary dilation, tachycardia (although effective block of the cardiac inhibitory nerves is difficult to achieve), etc. Some antimuscarinics have important actions in the central nervous system (*vide infra*).

There are considerable differences among the antimuscarinic drugs in the extent to which the various effects are elicited, and it now appears that there are two or more types of muscarinic receptors, each with different structural requirements for blockade. Therefore, the selectivities (ie, profiles of activity and spectrum of efficacy) may differ considerably from drug to drug. For example, scopolamine has excellent mydriatic and cycloplegic activity yet cannot block cardiac vagal activity in nontoxic doses, whereas its derivative, methscopolamine, is the most efficacious drug for the antagonism of vagally mediated cardiac effects. Many structural features contribute to the different pharmacologic and therapeutic profiles of the antimuscarinic drugs, but the one of greatest importance is the amine function, the quaternary ammonium compounds differing in certain important respects from the secondary and tertiary amines.

Differences Between Tertiary and Quaternary Antimuscarinics—Tertiary (and secondary) amine antimuscarinic drugs can penetrate cell membranes in the nonionized form and hence can pass the blood-brain barrier. In the brain, they can exert both therapeutic and toxic actions. The quaternary ammonium antimuscarinic drugs do not easily pass the blood-brain barrier and hence usually lack prominent central nervous actions. Similarly, the quaternary ammonium compounds poorly penetrate into the eye from the bloodstream or cornea and are less likely than the tertiary amine antimuscarinic drugs to cause mydriasis and cycloplegia. Most topical mydriatic antimuscarinic agents are tertiary amines. Furthermore, the quaternary compounds are usually erratically and incompletely absorbed from the gut, in contrast to the tertiary amines.

The quaternary compounds have the greater affinity for nicotinic receptors, so that some degree of ganglionic blockade may result from therapeutic doses of some, but not all, quaternary ammonium antimuscarinic drugs. Some of the quaternary ammonium members also have a potential for neuromuscular paralysis, especially in drug interactions or in persons with myasthenia gravis.

The quaternary ammonium group seems to confer various degrees of selectivity for gastric secretory and perhaps for other gastrointestinal functions. The extent to which ganglionic blockade may be involved is not known.

The quaternary ammonium antimuscarinic drugs are mostly excreted into the urine unchanged, whereas the secondary and tertiary members are usually considerably biotransformed in the liver.

Uses—In ophthalmology, antimuscarinic drugs are used to *dilate the pupil* (cause *mydriasis*, in order to facilitate visualization) and to *paralyze accommodation* (cause *cycloplegia*, for refractive examination); some of these drugs (eg, eucatropine, homatropine) cannot effect a complete cycloplegia, so that they are not all equivalent. Generally, short-acting topical antimuscarinic drugs (cyclopentolate, tropicamide, eucatropine, homatropine) are preferred for examination, so that interference with vision or intraocular tension will last for the shortest possible time. They may be used in alternation with miotics to *break adhesions between the iris and lens*, to treat *acute iritis, uveitis, iridiocyclitis*, and *keratitis.*

Antimuscarinic drugs, especially atropine, are used almost routinely for *anesthetic premedication*, to *inhibit excessive salivary and bronchial* secretions and to *prevent bronchospasm* and *laryngospasm.* The antisecretory effects are also sought in the treatment of *sialorrhea, acute coryza, hay fever,* and *rhinitis;* proprietary "cold medicines" often contain various belladonna alkaloids for this purpose, but the doses are mostly subliminal. The effects to antagonize parasympathetically mediated bronchospasm and bronchorrhea are also employed in the treatment of *bronchial asthma;* given systemically, they are not as effective as certain sympathomimetic aerosols, but some antimuscarinic drugs given as aerosols are as effective.

In cardiology and anesthesiology, antimuscarinic agents are used to prevent or *suppress vagally mediated bradyarrhythmias* (such as occur after coronary occlusion), *heart block,* or *cardiac syncope* due to hyperactive carotid sinuses; in these, medical convention clings to atropine, which is less efficacious than methscopolamine (*not* scopolamine!)

In genitourinary practice, antimuscarinic drugs are used to relieve *urinary frequency and urgency,* to control *enuresis* in children, and to relieve *ureteral colic* (often in combination with opiates).

In gastroenterology, antimuscarinic drugs are widely used for their gastrointestinal effects, although parasympathetic effects in the bowel are difficult to suppress completely. In the *irritable colon syndrome* ("spastic colon") they provide some relief initially, but some refractoriness usually develops later. *Functional gastrointestinal disorders (functional diarrhea, spastic constipation, cardiospasm, pylorospasm, neurogenic colon,* general hypermotility) may respond as may mild to moderate irritative or infectious disorders, such as *mild diarrhea;* however, severe infectious dysenteries, regional enteritis and ulcerative colitis do not. *Acute enterocolitis, mucous colitis* and the *splenic flexure syndrome* may respond erratically. *Diverticulitis* sometimes may be considerably improved. Antimuscarinic drugs may be used in combination with meperidine in the relief of *biliary dyskinesia.* In these uses, belladonna alkaloids are commonly employed; although they are less expensive than nonsolanaceous antimuscarinic drugs, they also cause more intense side effects than many synthetic, especially quaternary ammonium, drugs. For gastrointestinal use, several antimuscarinic drugs are marketed in combination with barbiturates or other hypnotic-sedative drugs. This practice deserves to be condemned.

Antimuscarinic drugs are used in the adjunctive *treatment of peptic ulcer.* Since they *retard gastric emptying,* the flood of acid to a duodenal ulcer is lessened, but a gastric ulcer will continue to be exposed to acid and hence not be benefited. However, any delay in gastric emptying will *help retain antacids* in the stomach, which should be beneficial if the appropriate regimen of antacids is used. Many gastroenterologists will use antimuscarinic drugs only at bedtime, partly because nocturnal secretion presents the harder treatment problem and partly because side effects during rest and sleep are usually of less consequence to the patient than during the wake hours. It is generally not appreciated that there are antimuscarinic drugs of sufficient selectivity that side effects are often mild and tolerable even during wake time.

Even more controversy and confusion exists concerning the use of antimuscarinic drugs to *suppress gastric secretion.* There is a prevailing nihilistic medical mythopoeia that these drugs cannot suppress secretion in tolerated doses and that no drug is more selective or superior to atropine. This erroneous dogma mainly stems from early findings with methantheline and propantheline, which were promoted with great fanfare. Not only were their antisecretory effects in man found to be slight and inconsistent after oral administration but also patient acceptance was no better than with atropine. Since that time, authoritative gastroenterological opinion has asserted against a special status of nonsolanaceous antimuscarinic drugs in the treatment of ulcer. A careful reading of the original statements of opinion shows that there was no intent to deny that there were quantitative differences in selectivity for the gastrointestinal tract among antimuscarinic drugs but rather an intent to warn that suppression of gastric secretion cannot be achieved without side effects. Indeed, the same authorities have published data which show respectable differences in the incidence and intensity of side effects of even some older drugs and hence in their probable therapeutic indices. Furthermore, atropine is the worst of prototypes, since acid secretion is not affected in the therapeutic dose range and has never been used in high enough doses in comparative studies on side effects and patient acceptance. A more recent double-blind study which shows that oral anisotropine methylbromide can suppress gastric acid

secretion by 50 to 60% with an incidence of dry mouth of 10 to 50% and blurred vision 20 to 40% (accompanied by only slight decreases in visual acuity) and without cycloplegia or tachycardia clearly shows that a considerable gastrointestinal selectivity can be achieved. The advent of cimetidine has not made this matter moot, since cimetidine not only does not decrease nocturnal gastric secretion to a greater extent than the best of the antimuscarinic drugs but it does not promote ulcer healing more than the best of antacid regimens. Consequently, there is still a place for antimuscarinic drugs, especially in combination with antacids or, perhaps, cimetidine.

The secondary and tertiary amine antimuscarinic drugs may be used for their central nervous actions. In the treatment of *parkinsonism,* they play a secondary role but are quite important in combinations with first-choice drugs (see page 927). They may be of some occasional benefit in other *spastic and rigid conditions of cerebral origin.* They are also used to antidote muscarinic central nervous (and peripheral) toxicity in *anticholinesterase intoxication.* Scopolamine is used for its sedative and amnesic effects, but these effects are not typical of antimuscarinic drugs.

Other uses of antimuscarinic drugs include the treatment of *dysmenorrhea* (questionable efficacy), *hyperhidrosis,* and treatment of poisoning by *Amanita muscaria.*

Adverse Effects—With nearly all antimuscarinic drugs, *dry mouth* is the first and dry skin is the second most common side effect. *Thirst* and *difficulty in swallowing* occur when the mouth and esophagus become sufficiently dry; chronic dry mouth also fosters dental *caries.* Suppression of sweating causes reflexive *flushing* and *heat intolerance* and can result in heat exhaustion or heat stroke in a hot environment; it also contributes to the hyperthermia seen in intoxication. *Mydriasis* frequently occurs, especially with secondary and tertiary compounds; *photophobia* and *blurring* of *vision* are consequences of mydriasis. With the secondary and tertiary amines, *cycloplegia* (which exacerbates blurred vision) occurs approximately concomitantly with mydriasis, but usually higher doses are required with many quaternary ammonium antimuscarinic drugs. In susceptible persons, especially the elderly, cycloplegia may contribute to an *elevation of intraocular pressure.* *Difficulty in urination* and *urinary retention* may occur. Tachycardia is a common side effect. *Constipation,* even *bowel stasis,* may occur. Antimuscarinic drugs relax the lower esophageal sphincter and thus promote gastroesophageal reflux, heartburn, and reflux esophagitis.

In the larger therapeutic doses, the secondary and tertiary amine antimuscarinic drugs may cause *dizziness, restlessness, tremors, fatigue,* and *locomotor difficulties.* Serious systemic intoxication can occur even from topical ophthalmologic application, especially in children, since both local absorption and nasolacrimal drainage into the gut can deliver considerable amounts to the circulation. In serious intoxication, *hyperpyrexia, flushing, nausea, vomiting, drowsiness, disorientation, stupor, hallucinations, leukocytosis,* nonallergic *rashes, circulatory* or *respiratory collapse,* even *death,* in addition to all aforenamed effects, may occur. Children, especially infants and children with mongolism, spastic paralysis, or brain damage, are more sensitive than adults to the toxic effects. Blondes and people with light irides are also reputed to be more sensitive.

When barbiturates are included in an antimuscarinic product, adverse effects of the barbiturates must be anticipated and the possibility that chronic use will lead to dependence must be considered.

The quaternary ammonium drugs mostly have a low central nervous component of toxicity but instead may cause *orthostatic hypotension* (from ganglionic blockade) and *neuromuscular paralysis.*

Hypersensitivity with a variety of manifestations, usually *rash*, may follow use of any antimuscarinic drug, but it is more common with the solanaceous alkaloids.

Drug Interactions—Other drugs, such as phenothiazines, tricyclic antidepressants, certain antihistamines, meperidine, etc., which have weak antimuscarinic activity, may considerably intensify the effects of antimuscarinic drugs. Drugs with neuromuscular paralysant activity (neuromuscular blocking drugs, aminoglycosides, polymyxin, other) and ganglionic blocking drugs will summate with quaternary ammonium antimuscarinic drugs. Aluminum- and magnesium trisilicate-containing antacids have been shown to decrease the absorption of some antimuscarinic drugs and may possibly do so with all of them.

Precautions—If there is mydriasis and photophobia, *dark glasses* should be worn. The patient should also be warned that *driving* or *other vision-dependent capabilities* may be impaired. Appropriate dosage precautions must be taken with *infants, children, persons with mongolism, brain damage, spasticity,* or *light irides*. Elevated intraocular pressure, urinary difficulty and retention, and constipation are more probable in *elderly persons*. Men with *prostatic hypertrophy* should especially be monitored for urinary function. Antimuscarinics should be used cautiously in *toxic megacolon*. Because of the tachycardic effects of the drugs, care must be exercised when *tachycardia*, other *tachyarrhythmias, coronary heart disease, congestive heart disease,* or *hyperthyroidism* preexist. Persons with *hypertension* may experience both exaggerated orthostatic hypotension and tachycardia. Similarly, *autonomic neuropathy* requires caution. Persons with a history of *allergies* or *bronchial asthma* will show a higher than normal incidence of hypersensitivity reactions. Quaternary ammonium antimuscarinic drugs, especially, may cause neuromuscular paralysis (with fatal respiratory arrest) in persons with *myasthenia gravis*. Although these drugs are sometimes used in the treatment of *adhesions between lens and iris*, damage can occur, and expert precautions must be taken. Precautions are appropriate in *ulcerative colitis*. In *hiatus hernia* or *gastroesophageal reflux*, reflux and esophagitis are exacerbated by antimuscarinic drugs, because the lower esophageal sphincter is stimulated by cholinergic nerves. In a *hot environment*, the user is more susceptible to disruption of heat regulation. *Hepatic disease* for some and *renal disease* for other antimuscarinic drugs may decrease the rate of elimination. Cognizance should be taken of possible *drug interactions*. Lastly, until proven otherwise, it must be assumed that all antimuscarinic drugs can pass the placental barrier; the threat to the fetus *in utero* is unknown, but an infant born with an effective amount of drug aboard may have gastrointestinal difficulties and problems in early nutrition. When solutions of antimuscarinic drugs are applied topically to the eye, pressure should be applied just below the internal canthus of the eye to prevent nasolacrimal drainage.

Contraindications—An antimuscarinic drug is generally contraindicated in *narrow-angle glaucoma, pyloric* or *intestinal* obstruction, *intestinal atony* of the elderly, *paralytic ileus, achalasia of the esophagus*, frank *bladder neck obstruction*, or where there is *hypersensitivity* to the drug or a closely related one. There are specific exceptions according to the route employed and the degree of selectivity (profile of activity) of the drug used.

Anisotropine Methylbromide

8-Azoniabicyclo[3.2.1]octane, 8,8-dimethyl-3-[(1-oxo-2-propylpentyl)-oxy]-, bromide, *endo*-, Valpin (*Endo*)

8-Methyltropinium bromide 2-propylpentanoate [80-50-2] $C_{17}H_{32}BrNO_2$ (362.35).

Preparation—Tropine is esterified with 2-propylvaleryl chloride, and the ester is then quaternized with methyl bromide.

Description—White powder or plates; odorless; extremely bitter; melts at about 329°.

Solubility—Soluble in water, chloroform; slightly soluble in alcohol; insoluble in ether.

Uses—Anisotropine methylbromide is a quaternary ammonium antimuscarinic drug with high selectivity for the gastrointestinal tract. It can reduce gastric acid content by more than 50%, with only a 10% incidence of dry mouth or dry skin and no cycloplegia or tachycardia. It is used to treat various *spastic* or *hypermotile conditions of the gastrointestinal tract* (see page 911) and in adjunctive treatment of *peptic ulcer*. Although the incidence of side effects is low, the precautions and contraindications should be considered to be those of antimuscarinic drugs in general (see page 912).

Dose—*Oral, adult, usual,* **50 mg** 3 times a day.

Dosage Forms—Tablets: 50 mg.

Atropine Sulfate

Benzeneacetic acid, α-(hydroxymethyl)-, 8-methyl-8-azabicyclo[3.2.1]-oct-3-yl ester, *endo*-(±)-, sulfate (2:1) (salt), monohydrate

1αH,5αH-Tropan-3α-ol (±)-tropate (ester) sulfate (2:1) (salt) monohydrate [5908-99-6] $(C_{17}H_{23}NO_3)_2 \cdot H_2SO_4 \cdot H_2O$ (694.82); anhydrous [55-48-1] (676.82).

Caution—Atropine Sulfate is very poisonous.

Preparation—Atropine is dissolved in warm acetone, sufficient dilute sulfuric acid is added to form the 2:1 sulfate, and the atropine sulfate is crystallized from the solution.

Description—Colorless crystals or a white, crystalline powder; odorless; effloresces in dry air; slowly affected by light; when previously dried at 120° for 4 hours it melts not lower than 187°.

Solubility—1 g in 0.4 mL water, 5 mL alcohol, about 2.5 mL glycerin.

Uses—Atropine is a tertiary amine antimuscarinic drug with all of the actions, most uses, and adverse effects described in the general statement at the beginning of this chapter. By historical precedence, it has become the prototype and most widely used of antimuscarinic drugs, although in most respects it no longer deserves the special status it continues to enjoy.

Because atropine is obtained from species of *belladonna*, the word atropine has often been used as synonymous with belladonna. Actually, several genera of *Solanaceae* produce atropine and related alkaloids, so that atropine and other related natural or semisynthetic congeners are sometimes called *solanaceous* alkaloids.

Atropine is rapidly and completely absorbed from the gut, and it is rapidly distributed throughout the body. Following topical application it readily penetrates into the eye. It is metabolized, mainly in the liver, The plasma half-life is less than 4 hr. The half-life in the eye is long, and effects may last for 7 to 12 days after topical application to the eye. Intraocular inflammation, however, greatly shortens the life-life in the eye.

Dose—*Oral, antispasmodic,* **0.3** to **1.2 mg** every 4 to 6 hours, except **0.01 mg/kg** in *children* under 12 years of age; *antiparkinsonism, initially* **0.3 mg**/day with daily increments of 0.3 mg until the optimum dosage is achieved, which *usually* ranges from **0.1** to **0.25 mg** 4 times a day. *Parenteral, preanesthetic medicament to suppress secretions,* **0.2** to **0.6 mg**, except **0.01** to **0.015 mg/kg** up to a maximum of **0.4 mg** in *children* under 12 years of age; *preanesthetic, to block* *the cardiac vagus*, **1.5** to **2 mg**; *antispasmodic* (*usually subcutaneous*), **0.5 mg** every 4 to 6 hours, except **0.01 mg/kg** in children under 12 years of age. *Intravenous*, for treatment of intoxication by *Amanita muscaria* or *cholinomimetics*, **0.6** to **1 mg**; to treat *anticholinesterase poisoning*, initially **1** to **2 mg**, repeated at intervals of 3 to 8 min until signs and symptoms are controlled, which may require as much as 20 mg. *Topical*, to the eye, *adult*, **1** or **2 drops** of 1% solution or **0.3** to **0.5 cm** of 1% ointment into the conjunctival sac once for *refraction* and 3 times a day for *uveitis*. In *children*, **1 drop** of solution or **0.3 cm** of ointment of a strength depending on the age and color of the irides; solutions for refractive examination are **0.125%** for ages under 1 yr, **0.25%** for ages 1 to 5 yr and children over 5 yr who have blue irides, and **0.5** to 1% for children over 5 yr who have dark irides; for *uveitis*, **0.125** to 1%; ointments are **0.5%** for ages under 2 yr who have blue irides and 1% for all other children; for *uveitis*, **0.5** to 1%. Ointments are preferred for children because systemic intoxication is less likely than with solutions.

Dosage Forms—Injection: 0.8 mg/0.5 mL; 0.3, 0.4, 0.5, and 1.2 mg/1 mL; 0.25, 0.5 and 2.5 mg/5 mL; 4 and 10 mg/10 mL; 8 mg/20 mL; 15 mg/30 mL. Ophthalmic Ointment: 0.5 and 1%. Ophthalmic Solution: 0.5, 1, 2, and 3%. Tablets: 0.4 and 0.6 mg.

Atropine Sulfate and Diphenoxylate Hydrochloride Tablets—page 813.

Belladonna

Deadly Nightshade Leaf; Belladonna Herb; Black Cherry Leaf; Dwale; Dwayberry Leaf

The dried leaf and flowering or fruiting top of *Atropa belladonna* Linné or of its variety *acuminata* Royle ex Lindley (Fam. *Solanaceae*); it yields not less than 0.35% of the alkaloids of belladonna leaf. USP.

Uses—The actions of belladonna are those of its principal alkaloids, hyoscyamine and atropine (see the general statement and pages 917 and 918). Belladonna is used to decrease gastrointestinal activity in functional bowel disorders, to delay gastric emptying, and supposedly to decrease gastric secretion, which it cannot do in tolerated doses. It is also used in the treatment of nocturnal enuresis and dysmenorrhea. In all of these uses it is among the least selective of antimuscarinic drugs, and its wide use derives from historical precedence and habit rather than from therapeutic superiority.

Belladonna is included in a number of fixed-dose combinations, the value of the components of which mostly have not been proven and, in some, may actually entail hazard. Nonprescription combinations containing belladonna usually have a content too small for substantial activity.

The belladonna alkaloid content of the extract and tincture are much different, and doses are expressed in mg and mL rather than as the alkaloid equivalents. One mg of extract contains 1.25 µg of alkaloids. One mL of tincture contains 0.3 mg (300 µg) of alkaloids.

Dose—Of *extract*, *oral*, *adult*, **15 mg** 3 or 4 times a day ½ to 1 hr before meals and at bedtime, with dosage adjustment as needed. Fifteen mg is equivalent to 0.2 mg of atropine. Of *tincture*, *oral*, *adult*, **0.6** to **1 mL** 3 or 4 times a day, ½ to 1 hr before meals and at bedtime, with dosage adjustment as needed; *children*, **0.03 mL/kg** of body weight (0.8 mL/m² of body surface) 3 times a day.

Dosage Forms—Extract, Tablets: 15 mg; Tincture: 30 mg of belladonna alkaloids/100 mL.

Benztropine Mesylate—page 928.

Biperiden—page 928.

Chlorphenoxamine Hydrochloride—page 931.

Clidinium Bromide

1-Azoniabicyclo[2.2.2]octane, 3-[(hydroxydiphenylacetyl)oxy]-1-methyl-, bromide; Quarzan; ingredient of Librax (*Roche*)

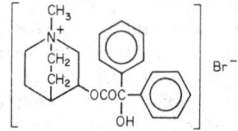

3-Hydroxy-1-methylquinuclidinium bromide benzilate [3485-62-9] C₂₂H₂₆BrNO₃ (432.36).

Preparation—3-Quinuclidinol is esterified to the benzilate either by transesterification with methyl benzilate or by reaction with benzilic acid methyl bromide, and the resulting 3-quinuclidinyl benzilate is quaternized with methyl bromide. US Pat. 2,648,667.

Description—White to nearly white, almost odorless, crystalline powder; melts to about 242°.

Solubility—Soluble in water and in alcohol; slightly soluble in ether and in benzene.

Uses—Clidinium bromide is a quaternary ammonium antimuscarinic drug with moderate selectivity for the *gastrointestinal tract*. Thus its uses are mainly in the treatment of *spastic* or *hypermotile conditions* of the gastrointestinal tract (see page 912) and in adjunctive treatment of *peptic ulcer*. In a combination with chlordiazepoxide it has been reported to reduce gastric secretion by 42 to 99% with only moderate side effects. Dry mouth is the principal side effect; mydriasis, and cycloplegia are less frequent. The precautions and contraindications are those of antimuscarinic drugs in general (see page 911).

Dose—*Oral*, *adult*, **2.5** to **5 mg** 3 or 4 times a day, before meals and at bedtime. Aged or debilitated persons and children should take only **7.5 mg**/day. More than **20 mg**/day is rarely required for maximum efficacy.

Dosage Forms—Capsules: 2.5 and 5 mg.

Chlorphenoxamine Hydrochloride—page 931.

Cyclopentolate Hydrochloride

Benzeneacetic acid, α-(1-hydroxycyclopentyl)-, 2-(dimethylamino)ethyl ester, hydrochloride; Cyclogyl (*Alcon*)

2-(Dimethylamino)ethyl 1-hydroxy-α-phenylcyclopentaneacetate hydrochloride [5870-29-1] C₁₇H₂₅NO₃.HCl (327.85).

Preparation—The acid moiety of the ester, 1-hydroxy-α-phenylcyclopentaneacetic acid (I), may be prepared by adding sodium phenylacetate to an ethereal solution of isopropyl magnesium bromide; treatment of the resulting sodium phenylacetate magnesium bromide with an ethereal solution of cyclopentanone produces a Grignard addition product that on hydrolysis yields I. The ester is produced by metathesis between the sodium salt of I and 2-dimethylaminoethyl chloride in isopropyl alcohol. After crystallization from acetone, the ester is converted to the hydrochloride with HCl.

Description—White, crystalline powder, which on standing develops a characteristic odor; melts between 137° and 141°; pH (1 in 100 solution) between 4.5 and 5.5.

Solubility—Very soluble in water; freely soluble in alcohol; insoluble in ether.

Uses—An *antimuscarinic* drug used primarily for its *ophthalmologic* actions (see page 911). After application to the cornea, cyclopegia is complete in 25 to 75 min; recovery is complete in 6 to 24 hr. The side effects and central nervous toxicity are those of antimuscarinic drugs (page 911) but the duration of the effects is very short.

Dose—*Topical*, *into the conjunctival sac*, *adult* for *mydriatic ophthalmoscopy* or *cycloplegic refraction*, **1 drop** of a 1 or 2% solution, repeated once in 5 min; 2% solution is recommended when the irides are dark; for *uveitis*, **1 drop** of a 0.5 or 1% solution 3 or 4 times a day. In *neonates* and *premature* and *small infants*, for *mydriatic ophthalmoscopy* or *cycloplegic refraction*, **1 drop** of a 0.5% solution once only. *Older infants* and *children*, for *mydriatic ophthalmoscopy*, **1 drop** of 0.5 or 1% solution once only; for *cycloplegic refraction*, **1 drop** of a 1 or 2% solution, repeated in 5 min; for *uveitis*, **1 drop** of a 0.5 or 1% solution 3 or 4 times a day. When phenylephrine is combined with cyclopentolate, a 0.2% concentration of the latter suffices for mydriatic ophthalmoscopy in all patients.

Dosage Forms—Ophthalmic Solution: 0.5, 1, and 2%.

Cycrimine Hydrochloride—RPS-16, page 870.

Dicyclomine Hydrochloride

[Bicyclohexyl]-1-carboxylic acid, 2-(diethylamino)ethyl ester, hydrochloride; Bentyl Hydrochloride (*Merrell-National*)

2-(Diethylamino)ethyl [bicyclohexyl]-1-carboxylate hydrochloride [67-92-5] $C_{19}H_{35}NO_2 \cdot HCl$ (345.95).

Preparation—Cyclohexanol is converted with hydrogen chloride to cyclohexyl chloride, which is grignardized with ethyl formate to dicyclohexyl carbinol (α-cyclohexylcyclohexanemethanol). The carbinol is oxidized with sodium dichromate to its ketone, which is chlorinated with sulfuryl chloride to 1-chlorocyclohexyl cyclohexyl ketone. This ketone, on reaction with the sodium derivative of 2-(diethylamino)ethanol, forms an intermediate that rearranges to dicyclomine base, which after purification is converted to the hydrochloride. US Pat 2,474,796.

Description—White, crystalline powder; practically odorless; very bitter; stable in air; melts between 169° and 174°; pH (1 in 100 solution) between 5.0 and 5.5.

Solubility—1 g in 13 mL water, 5 mL alcohol, 2 mL chloroform, 770 mL ether.

Uses—Dicyclomine possesses both antimuscarinic and nonspecific antispasmodic activities. It is used primarily for its effects on the gastrointestinal tract; in the treatment of *irritable colon, spastic constipation, mucous colitis, spastic colitis, pylorospasm,* and *biliary dyskinesia.* In the treatment of peptic ulcer it is used to *delay gastric emptying;* it does not suppress gastric secretion.

Side effects, precautions, and contraindications are those of antimuscarinic drugs in general (page 911), except that it does not appear to raise intraocular pressure in narrow-angle glaucoma; nevertheless, it is advisable to monitor the pressure in such patients.

Dose—*Oral, adult,* **10** to **20 mg** 3 or 4 times a day; *children,* usually as the syrup, **10 mg** 3 or 4 times a day; *infants,* **5 mg** 3 or 4 times a day. *Intramuscular, adult,* **20 mg** every 4 to 6 hr.

Dosage Forms—Capsules: 10 mg; Injection: 20 mg/2 mL and 100 mg/10 mL; Syrup: 10 mg/5 mL; Tablets: 20 mg.

Glycopyrrolate

Pyrrolidinium, 3-[(cyclopentylhydroxyphenylacetyl)oxy]-1,1-dimethyl-, bromide; Robinul (*Robins*)

3-Hydroxy-1,1-dimethylpyrrolidinium bromide α-cyclopentylmandelate [596-51-0] $C_{19}H_{28}BrNO_3$ (398.34).

Preparation—α-Phenylcyclopentaneglycolic acid is esterified by refluxing with methanol in the presence of hydrochloric acid and the resulting ester is transesterified with 1-methyl-3-pyrrolidinol using sodium as a catalyst. The transester is then reacted with methyl bromide to give glycopyrrolate.

Description—White, crystalline powder that is odorless and has a bitter taste; stable in light and heat and nonhygroscopic; melts within a range of 2° between 193° and 198°.

Solubility—1 g in 4.2 mL water, 30 mL alcohol, 260 mL chloroform; insoluble in ether.

Uses—A quaternary ammonium *antimuscarinic* drug that has a moderate degree of selectivity for the gastrointestinal tract. The drug not only prolongs gastric emptying time, which favors retention of antacids, but decreases gastric acid production in many patients in doses which cause minimal side effects. It is one of the four most selective drugs for suppressing gastric secretion. Consequently, glycopyrrolate is used especially in the treatment of *peptic ulcer.* It is also used for *preanesthetic medication, spastic colon, spastic duodenum, colitis, biliary spasm,* and other gastrointestinal disorders associated with spasm. It has been shown to be superior to atropine in the antagonism of the muscarinic side effects of neostigmine.

Although the incidence of side effects from glycopyrrolate is low

with recommended oral doses, they do occur; dry mouth and skin is the usual complaint. Ocular effects are uncommon and mild. The side effects, precautions, and contraindications should be considered to be those of antimuscarinic drugs in general (see page 911).

Dose—*Oral, adult, initially,* **1** to **2 mg** 3 to 4 times a day; once symptoms are controlled the dose is usually adjusted downward; *maintenance* usually **1 mg** 2 times a day. In acute severe conditions the total daily dose may exceed 8 mg. *Intramuscular, adult,* for *peptic ulcer,* **0.1** to **0.2 mg** 3 or 4 times a day; for *preanesthetic medication,* **0.044 mg/kg;** *children* under 12 years of age, for *preanesthetic medication,* **0.0044** to **0.0088 mg/kg.** *Intravenous, adult,* for *intraoperative medication,* **0.1 mg,** repeated at 2- to 3-min intervals, if necessary, and as a *corrective* to anticholinesterases, **0.2 mg/1 mg** of neostigmine or pyridostigmine equivalent; *children* under 12 years of age, for *intraoperative medication,* **0.0044 mg/kg** and for *corrective* for anticholesterases, adult dose.

Dosage Forms—Injection: 0.2 mg/1 mL, 0.4 mg/2 mL, 1 mg/5 mL, and 4 mg/20 mL; Tablets: 1 and 2 mg.

Homatropine Hydrobromide

Benzeneacetic acid, α-hydroxy-, 8-methyl-8-azabicyclo[3.2.1]oct-3-yl ester hydrobromide, *endo*-($\pm$)-,

$1\alpha H,5\alpha H$-Tropan-3α-ol mandelate (ester) hydrobromide [51-56-9] $C_{16}H_{21}NO_3 \cdot HBr$ (356.26); the hydrobromide of tropine mandelate. For the structural formula, see page 418.

Preparation—By heating *tropine* with *mandelic acid* in the presence of hydrochloric acid; ammonia is added, and the homatropine that is liberated is extracted with chloroform; the solution is evaporated, hydrobromic acid added, and the homatropine hydrobromide is crystallized.

Description—White crystals, or a white crystalline powder; affected by light; melts between 214° and 217° with slight decomposition; its aqueous solution is practically neutral or only faintly acid to litmus.

Solubility—1 g in 6 mL water, 40 mL alcohol, and about 420 mL chloroform; insoluble in ether.

Uses—Homatropine is used only for its effects in the eye (see page 911). It is sometimes preferred to atropine, because its effects are shorter in duration (0.5 to 2 days) and there is no protracted cycloplegia. It is often combined with sympathomimetics in ophthalmologic practice. Its systemic toxicity is considerably less than that of atropine, but rare systemic intoxication can occur from conjunctival instillation, especially in children.

Dose—*Topical,* to the conjunctiva, *adult,* for *cycloplegic refraction,* **1 drop** of a **2** or **5**% solution, repeated in 5 to 10 min, if necessary; for *uveitis,* **1 drop** of a **2** or **5**% solution 2 or 3 times a day; *children* use **1** or **2**% solution in lieu of adult concentrations.

Dosage Forms—Ophthalmic Solution: 1, 2, and 5%.

Hyoscyamine Hydrobromide

Benzeneacetic acid, α-(hydroxymethyl)-, 8-methyl-8-azabicyclo[3.2.1]-oct-3-yl ester, hydrobromide, [3(S)-*endo*]-

$1\alpha H,5\alpha H$-Tropan-3α-ol (−)-tropate (ester) hydrobromide [306-03-6] $C_{17}H_{23}NO_3 \cdot HBr$ (370.29); for the structure of hyoscyamine, see page 418.

Caution—Hyoscyamine Hydrobromide is extremely poisonous.

Preparation—By passing hydrogen bromide into a concentrated solution of hyoscyamine in ethanol and then diluting with ether.

Description—White, odorless, crystals or as a crystalline powder; does not melt below 149°; affected by light; pH (1 in 20 solution) about 5.4.

Solubility—Freely soluble in water, alcohol, and chloroform; very slightly soluble in ether.

Uses—Hyoscyamine is the levorotatory isomer of the racemic mixture known as atropine, and therefore ½ of atropine is hyoscyamine. Since the dextrorotatory isomer is nearly inactive, the potency of hyoscyamine is approximately twice that of atropine. The actions, uses, and toxicity are the same as those of antimuscarinic drugs in general (see page 911), except that hyoscyamine has not been used for ophthalmologic purposes and is of little use to suppress gastric secretion. In fact, its use mainly has been confined to that of an *antispasmodic* although it is sometimes used in rhinitis, cystitis and parkinsonism.

Hyoscyamine is marketed as the hydrobromide and sulfate salts. The hydrobromide is not marketed as a single-entity preparation but rather in a number of combinations, most of which have dubious rationales and efficacies.

Dose—*Oral* or *parenteral*, *adult*, **0.25** to **1 mg** in various combinations.

Hyoscyamine Sulfate

Benzeneacetic acid, α-(hydroxymethyl)-, 8-methyl-8-azabicyclo[3.2.1]-oct-3-yl ester, [3(*S*)-*endo*]-, sulfate (2:1), dihydrate

1αH,5αH-Tropan-3α-ol (−)-tropate (ester) sulfate (2:1) (salt) dihydrate [6835-16-1] ($C_{17}H_{23}NO_3$)$_2$.H_2SO_4.$2H_2O$ (712.85); *anhydrous* [620-61-1] (676.82); the sulfate of an alkaloid usually obtained from species of *Hyoscyamus* Linné or other genera of Fam *Solanaceae*. For the structural formula of hyoscyamine, see page 418.

Caution—Hyoscyamine Sulfate is extremely poisonous.

Description—White, odorless crystals or a crystalline powder; deliquescent; affected by light; when previously dried at 105° for 4 hours, does not melt below 200°; pH (1 in 100 solution) about 5.3.

Solubility—1 g in 0.5 mL water, 5 mL alcohol; practically insoluble in ether.

Uses—See *Hyoscyamine Hydrobromide* (above).

Dose—*Oral* or *sublingual*, *adult*, **0.125** to **0.25 mg** 2 to 4 times a day or **0.375 mg** in sustained-release form every 12 hr. *Intramuscular*, *intravenous*, or *subcutaneous*, *adult*, **0.25** to **0.5 mg** 3 or 4 times daily as needed. When parenteral medication is employed, oral medication should be substituted as soon as symptoms are controlled.

Dosage Forms—Timed-release Capsules: 0.375 mg; Elixir: 0.125 mg/5 mL; Injection: 0.5 mg/1 mL and 5 mg/10 mL; Solution: 0.125 mg/mL. Tablets: 0.125 and 0.25 mg.

Ipratropium Bromide

8-Azaniabicyclo[3.2.1]octane, 3-(3-hydroxy-1-oxo-2-phenylpropoxy)-8-methyl-8-(1-methylethyl)-, bromide monhydrate (*endo,syn*)-, (±)-, Atrovent (*Boehringer-Ingelheim*)

(8*r*)-3α-Hydroxy-8-isopropyl-1αH,5αH-tropanium bromide (±)-tropate monohydrate [66985-17-9]; anhydrous [22254-24-6] $C_{20}H_{30}BrNO_3$.H_2O (430.38)].

Preparation—Atropine is quaternized with isopropyl bromide.

Description—White, crystalline substance with a bitter taste.

Solubility—Freely soluble in water and alcohol; insoluble in chloroform and ether.

Uses—Ipratropium is a quaternary ammonium antimuscarinic drug (page 911). It is used for the treatment of *bronchial asthma* and *chronic obstructive pulmonary disease*, for which it is given as an inhalant aerosol. It appears to be approximately equivalent to β_2-agonists in its efficacy against these disorders, but the duration of action is longer. It seems to act mainly on the larger airways.

By inhalation, the incidence and severity of side effects is low, the most common effects being dry mouth, irritation in the throat, and unpleasant taste. Other effects are quite rare and include blurring of vision, drowsiness, dizziness, mild *brady*cardia (!) and airway obstruction caused by sputum made viscous by diminished tracheobronchial secretions.

By inhalation, ipratropium causes bronchodilatation in doses 1:1000 those of oral or intravenous doses, which avoids systemic side-effects. Bronchodilatation occurs within a few minutes, peaks at 1 to 2 hr and lasts 4 to 8 hr. About half the dose is eliminated in the feces. The half-life is 3 to 4 hr.

Dose—*Inhalation*, *adult*, **10 to 80 μg** 4 times day.

Isopropamide Iodide

Benzenepropanaminium, γ-(aminocarbonyl)-*N*-methyl-*N*,*N*-bis(1-methylethyl)-γ-phenyl-, iodide; Darbid (*Smith Kline Labs*)

(3-Carbamoyl-3,3-diphenylpropyl)diisopropylmethylammonium iodide [71-81-8] $C_{23}H_{33}IN_2O$ (480.43).

Preparation—4-(Diisopropylamino)-2,2-diphenylbutyronitrile is hydrated to the butyramide by heating with sulfuric acid. The amide is then quaternized with methyl iodide to form isopropamide iodide. The starting nitrile may be produced by condensing (3-chloro-2,2-dimethylpropyl)diethylamine with diphenylacetonitrile. US Pat 2,823,233.

Description—White to pale yellow, crystalline powder; practically odorless and has a bitter taste; melts at about 183°.

Solubility—1 g in 50 mL water, 10 mL alcohol, 5 mL chloroform; very slightly soluble in ether.

Uses—A quaternary ammonium *antimuscarinic* drug with very little ganglionic blocking action at regular doses. It is advocated for use in the adjunctive therapy of *peptic ulcer* and other conditions of *gastrointestinal hyperactivity*, but it has no special selectivity for the gastrointestinal system. However, its long duration of action (12 hours) makes it especially useful for managing the troublesome nocturnal secretion of the peptic ulcer patient. Even if it fails to reduce gastric secretion significantly, its effects to increase gastric retention assist antacid treatment.

The peripheral side effects, precautions, and contraindications of isopropamide are those of antimuscarinic drugs in general (page 911), except that the central effects are negligible. Hypersensitivity from the iodide may possibly occur; the iodide may also interfere with PBI and radioiodide uptake tests for thyroid function, and the drug should be discontinued one week prior to such tests.

Dose (isopropamide equivalent)—*Oral*, *adult and children over 12 years of age*, *initially*, **5 mg** 2 times a day, unless symptoms are severe, in which case **10 mg** is given; dosage is adjusted according to the response and the supervention of untoward effects.

Dosage Form—Tablets: 5 mg (isopropamide equivalent).

Mepenzolate Bromide

Piperidinium, 3-[(hydroxydiphenylacetyl)oxy]-1,1-dimethyl-, bromide; Cantil (*Merrell-National*)

3-Hydroxy-1,1-dimethylpiperidinium bromide benzilate [76-90-4] $C_{21}H_{26}BrNO_3$ (420.35).

Preparation—3-Pyridinol is quaternized with methyl bromide and the resulting 3-hydroxy-1-methylpyridinium bromide is catalytically reduced to 1-methyl-3-piperidinol. Transesterification of methyl benzilate with this alcohol in the presence of sodium methoxide produces 1-methyl-3-piperidyl benzilate which, on quaternization with methyl bromide, yields mepenzolate bromide. US Pat 2,918,408.

Description—White or light cream-colored powder; melts with decomposition at about 230°.

Solubility—1 g in 110 mL water, 120 mL ethanol, 630 mL chloroform; practically insoluble in ether.

Uses—Mepenzolate bromide has the same qualitative actions as other quaternary ammonium antimuscarinic drugs (see page 911), with some moderate selectivity for the gastrointestinal tract. It reduces motility in the colon, small intestine, and stomach, the effect on the colon supposedly being greatest. Given parenterally or in large oral doses, it can reduce gastric acid secretion of hydrochloric acid, but the effect does not occur during ordinary clinical use, promotion to the contrary. The drug also relaxes the sphincter of Oddi. Mepenzolate bromide is used in the treatment of *spastic colon*, *irritable bowel*, *regional ileitis*, *infectious diarrhea*, *ulcerative colitis*, *gaseous distention of the colon*, and *duodenal ulcer*.

Mepenzolate elicits all the side effects of antimuscarinic drugs (see page 912), but except for mild transient dry mouth and blurred vision, such side effects are uncommon. The central nervous effects of the drug are not observed except with extremely large doses. The precautions to be used are the same as those with antimuscarinic drugs in general.

Dose—*Oral, adult,* **25** to **50 mg** 4 times a day, preferably with meals and at bedtime.

Dosage Forms—Tablets: 25 mg.

Methscopolamine Bromide

3-Oxa-9-azoniatricyclo[3.2.1.0²,⁴]nonane, 7-(3-hydroxy-1-oxo-2-phenyl-propoxy)-9,9-dimethyl-, bromide; Scopolamine Methylbromide; Pamine Bromide (*Upjohn*)

$6\beta,7\beta$-Epoxy-3α-hydroxy-8-methyl-1αH,5αH-tropanium bromide (−)-tropate $C_{18}H_{24}BrNO_4$ (398.30). For the structural formula, see page 418.

Preparation—Benzene solutions of scopolamine and methyl bromide are mixed and allowed to stand. Quaternization occurs and the crystalline compound precipitates.

Description—White crystals, or as a white, odorless, crystalline powder; melts at about 225°, with decomposition.

Solubility—Freely soluble in water; slightly soluble in alcohol; insoluble in acetone and chloroform.

Uses—A quaternary ammonium derivative of scopolamine. It has greater selectivity than scopolamine or atropine in blocking vagal impulses to the gastrointestinal tract and the heart; it is used in the treatment of *vagally mediated bradyarrhythmias*, but there is danger of overshooting into tachydysrhythmias. It is also used especially in the treatment of *peptic ulcer* (since it decreases gastric emptying), *bowel hypermotility,* and *functional diarrhea.* In some persons it decreases the output of gastric acid secretion. It has been used against *hyperhidrosis* and *sialorrhea.* The side effects, precautions, and contraindications are those of antimuscarinic drugs in general (page 912), except that methscopolamine lacks the prominent central nervous toxicity of atropine and scopolamine. Systemic bioavailability is only 10 to 25%.

Doses—*Oral, adult,* **2.5** to **5 mg** 4 times a day, except **0.2 mg/kg/day** in 4 divided doses in *children.*

Dosage Forms—Tablets: 2.5 mg.

Orphenadrine Citrate—see page 932.

Oxyphencyclimine Hydrochloride

Benzeneacetic acid, α-cyclohexyl-α-hydroxy-, Daricon (*Pfizer*)

(1,4,5,6-Tetrahydro-1-methyl-2-pyrimidinyl)methyl α-phenylcyclohexaneglycolate monohydrochloride [125-52-0] $C_{20}H_{28}N_2O_3$·HCl (380.91).

Preparation—Glycolonitrile is heated with ethanol and hydrogen chloride in chloroform to form ethyl glycolimidate hydrochloride, which is condensed with *N*-methyltrimethylenediamine in ethanol to give 1,4,5,6-tetrahydro-1-methyl-2-pyrimidinemethanol. Reaction with thionyl chloride converts the methanol group to chloromethyl and the chloromethyl compound is refluxed with α-phenylcyclohexaneglycolic acid in isopropanol to yield oxyphencyclimine hydrochloride.

Description—White, odorless crystalline powder having a characteristic bitter taste; melts between 227° and 237° with decomposition.

Solubility—1 g in 100 mL water, 75 mL alcohol, 500 mL chloroform, >1000 mL ether.

Uses—Oxyphencyclimine is a tertiary amine antimuscarinic drug with actions and uses similar to those of quaternary ammonium drugs (see page 911 *et seq*). Its actions on the gastrointestinal and genitourinary systems are prominent. In large doses it can decrease secretion of gastric acid, but with the usual daytime dose its gastric ef-

fects are usually limited to decreased motility. After oral administration its effects are manifested in 1 to 2 hours and the peak effect is reached in 6 to 8 hours; the actions last longer than 12 hours. Its principal use is in the adjunctive treatment of *peptic ulcer.* Many gastroenterologists consider oxyphencyclimine to be among the best antimuscarinic drugs available for treatment of peptic ulcer.

Oxyphencyclimine can elicit all the side effects caused by tertiary amine antimuscarinic drugs (page 911), but the incidence and severity are much less in equieffective gastric antisecretory doses. Allergic responses, however, may be somewhat more frequent and occasionally more severe. The precautions and contraindications are those of antimuscarinic drugs in general.

Dose—*Adult, initially,* **5** or **10 mg** 2 or 3 times a day. The dose may be increased by daily increments of 10 mg up to **50 mg/day,** if necessary and if no serious effects supervene.

Dosage Form—Tablets: 10 mg.

Procyclidine Hydrochloride—page 932.

Scopolamine Hydrobromide

Benzeneacetic acid, α-(hydroxymethyl)-, 9-methyl-3-oxa-9-azatricyclo[3.3.1.0²,⁴]non-7-yl ester, hydrobromide, trihydrate, [7(*S*)-(1α,2β,4β,5α,7β)]-,

$6\beta,7\beta$-Epoxy-1αH,5αH-tropan-3α-ol (−)-tropate (ester) hydrobromide trihydrate [6533-68-2] $C_{17}H_{21}NO_4$·HBr·3H₂O (438.31); *anhydrous* [114-49-8] (384.27). For the structural formula of scopolamine see page 418.

Preparation—Scopolamine, an alkaloid occurring in several solanaceous plants, may be obtained from such plants by alkaloid extraction procedures followed by fractionation of the extract to remove other alkaloids, notably hyoscyamine.

Description—Colorless or white crystals or white, granular powder; odorless; slightly efflorescent in dry air; the anhydrous salt melts between 195° and 199°; pH (1 in 10 solution) between 4.0 and 5.5.

Solubility—1 g in 1.5 mL water, 20 mL alcohol; slightly soluble in chloroform; insoluble in ether.

Uses—Scopolamine differs from other antimuscarinic drugs in that in therapeutic doses it is a sedative and tranquilizing depressant to the central nervous system. In its peripheral actions, scopolamine differs from atropine in that it is a stronger blocking agent for the iris, ciliary body, and salivary, bronchial and sweat glands but is weaker in its action on the heart (in which it is incapable of exerting actions in tolerated doses), the intestinal tract, and bronchial musculature.

In addition to the usual uses for antimuscarinic drugs, scopolamine was formerly employed for its central depressant actions as a *sedative-hypnotic* drug. Frequently it is given as a *preanesthetic medicament* for both its sedative-tranquilizing and antisecretory actions. It is effective as a prophylactic against *motion sickness,* for which slow-release transdermal dosage forms have been devised. It is also sometimes used in other types of *vertigo.* It is occasionally used to suppress *delirium.* It is used as an *amnesic* agent in *obstetrics* (combined with morphine it was formerly used to produce "twilight sleep"). It is now rarely employed in *paralysis agitans, postencephalitic parkinsonism,* or *spastic states.* Although it is not selective for the gastrointestinal system, it continues to be promoted for management of pylorospasm, cardiospasm, "irritable" colon, mild diarrhea, and diverticulitis. As a *mydriatic* and *cycloplegic,* it has a somewhat shorter duration (3 to 7 days), and intraocular pressure is affected less markedly than with atropine.

Except for drowsiness, the side effects of scopolamine are those of tertiary amine antimuscarinic drugs (see page 911). Occasionally, with therapeutic doses a patient may experience excitement, restlessness, hallucinations, or delirium or disorientation, confusion, memory loss, stupor, and, rarely, coma. Infants and young children are quite susceptible to the CNS toxicity. Rarely there may be hypersensitivity, characterized by edema of the uvula, glottis, and lips. The toxic effects of overdoses, precautions, and contraindications are like those of tertiary amine antimuscarinic drugs.

Dose—Oral, adult, for *motion sickness,* **0.2** to **0.8 mg** 1 hr before departure, then 3 or 4 times a day; for *parkinsonism,* **0.3** to **1 mg** 3 or 4 times a day; for *vertigo* and *gastrointestinal hypermotility,* **0.4** to **0.8 mg** 3 or 4 times a day, with adjustments as necessary. *Intramuscular, intravenous* or *subcutaneous, adult,* antiemetic or amnesic, **0.3** to **0.65 mg**; *preanesthetic* (usually i.m.), **0.2** to **0.6 mg**;

sedative, **0.6 mg** 3 or 4 times a day; *children*, **0.006 mg/kg** of body weight up to a total of 0.3 mg. *Topical*, transdermal to the postauricular skin, *adults*, **1.5 mg** (from which 0.5 mg is delivered within 3 days). *Topical*, to the conjunctiva, *adult*, for *cycloplegic refraction*, 1 to **2 drops** of a **0.25** or **0.3%** solution of **0.3** to **0.5 cm** of a **0.2%** ointment 1 hr before refraction; for *uveitis*, apply same up to 3 times a day; *children*, for *cycloplegic refraction*, **1 drop** of a **0.25%** solution or **0.3 cm** of a **0.2%** ointment twice a day for 2 days before refraction; for *uveitis* **1 drop** of a **0.25%** solution of **0.3** to **0.5 cm** of a **0.2%** ointment 1 to 3 times day. *Topical*, to the *conjunctiva*, *adults* and *children*, **1 drop** of **0.25%** solution or **1 cm** of **0.2%** ointment 1 to 3 times a day for *uveitis* or **1 drop** of **0.25%** solution 45 min before refractive examination in children.

Dosage Forms—Injection: 0.2 mg/0.5 mL and 0.3, 0.4 and 1 mg/1 mL. Ophthalmic Ointment: 0.2%; Ophthalmic Solution: 0.25, and 0.3%; Tablets: 0.4 and 0.6 mg.

Trihexyphenidyl Hydrochloride—page 931.

Tropicamide

Benzeneacetamide, *N*-ethyl-α-(hydroxymethyl)-*N*-(4-pyridinylmethyl)-, Mydriacyl (*Alcon*)

N-Ethyl-2-phenyl-*N*-(4-pyridylmethyl)hydracrylamide [1508-75-4] $C_{17}H_{20}N_2O_2$ (284.36).

Preparation—Tropic acid is esterified with acetyl chloride and the resulting tropic acid acetate is converted to the corresponding acid chloride by reaction with thionyl chloride. Condensation of the acid chloride with 4-[(ethylamino)methyl]pyridine in the presence of an appropriate dehydrochlorinating agent yields the tropicamide acetate ester which saponifies readily to tropicamide. US Pat 2,726,245.

Description—White or practically white, crystalline powder; odorless, or has not more than a slight odor; melts between 96° and 100°.

Solubility—1 g in 500 mL water, 3 mL chloroform; freely soluble in alcohol, and solutions of strong acids.

Uses—An *antimuscarinic* drug that is used to induce *mydriasis* and *cycloplegia* in ophthalmologic practice. Applied topically to the eye it has short duration of action. The time to a maximal effect is usually 20 to 25 min. The duration of maximal effect is only about 15 to 20 min, but full recovery requires 5 to 6 hours. However, photophobia and other subjective indices of an effect may disappear as early as 2 hours after application. The drug thus has an obvious advantage over belladonna alkaloids in its shorter duration of action and over homatropine in its ability to induce cycloplegia. It is disadvantageous in that the ophthalmologist must time his examination to coincide with the time of maximal effect and that he has a brief time for examination or else that it is necessary to repeat administration at 30-min intervals in order to obviate the timing problem.

Although tropicamide does not increase intraocular pressure in normal persons, it may do so in patients with glaucoma or those who have certain structural deformities of the anterior chamber of the eye. It should thus be used cautiously in such patients. If an antimuscarinic must be employed in such patients, tropicamide is indicated because of its brief duration of action.

Side effects can occur from passage of solutions through the nasolacrimal duct and subsequent absorption. Dry mouth and tachycardia have occurred. Although intoxication in children has not been reported, it must be kept in mind. Tropicamide usually stings transiently when applied.

Dose—*Topical*, to the conjunctiva, *adult*, for *cycloplegic refraction*, **1** or **2 drops** of a **0.1%** solution, repeated in 5 min; for *ophthalmoscopy*, **1** or **2 drops** of a **0.5%** solution 15 to 20 min prior to examination. *Children*, **1 drop** of a **0.5** or **1%** solution repeated in 5 min.

Dosage Forms—Ophthalmic Solution: 0.5 and 1%.

Other Antimuscarinic Drugs

Levorotatory Alkaloids of Belladonna—A synthetic mixture of the pure salts of the levorotatory alkaloids found in belladonna. The ratio of the salts is such that a single dose contains the approximate amount of each of the following: scopolamine hydrobromide, 0.006 mg; atropine sulfate, 0.02 mg; hyoscyamine sulfate, 0.1 mg. *Uses:* Since the an-

timuscarinic activity of belladonna is only in the levorotatory isomers, the actions, uses and adverse effects of the levorotatory alkaloids are the same as those of *Belladonna*, page 914. Only the dose and dosage forms are different. *Dose: Oral, adult,* 0.25 to 0.5 mg 3 times day; *children over 6 years of age,* 0.125 to 0.25 mg 3 times a day. *Subcutaneous, adult,* 0.25 to 0.5 mg, once or twice a day.

Hexocyclium Methylsulfate [4-(β-Cyclohexyl-β-hydroxyphenethyl-1,1-dimethylpiperazinium methyl sulfate [115-63-9] $C_{21}H_{36}N_2O_5S$; Tral (*Abbott*)]—Synthesized from *N*-phenacyl-*N'*-methylpiperazine, cyclohexyl bromide and dimethyl sulfate. US Pat. 2,907,765. A white, crystalline powder, melting between 200° and 210°. One gram dissolves in about 2 mL water; slightly soluble in chloroform; insoluble in ether.

Uses: A quaternary ammonium antimuscarinic drug with a slight selectivity for gastric secretory cells; as with other drugs of this class suppression of gastric acid secretion in human subjects is readily demonstrable with parenteral administration or supraclinical doses but weak and unpredictable under outpatient conditions. It is promoted for adjunctive therapy in *peptic ulcer*, for which its true value still needs to be determined. Oral absorption of the drug is still erratic. Its side effects, precautions, and contraindications are those of antimuscarinic drugs in general (see page 911). Allergic reactions tend to be more frequent and severe, and idiosyncrasies are more common than with atropine. In elderly persons, it causes a relatively high incidence of confusion and/or excitement. In overdoses it also has a neuromuscular paralyzing effect; curare-like neuromuscular blocking drugs should be used cautiously in the presence of hexocyclium methylsulfate. *Dose: Adult,* 25 mg 4 times a day, before each meal and at bedtime. With sustained-release form, 50 mg twice a day, before breakfast and before the evening meal; to suppress nocturnal secretion, 75 mg may be taken at bedtime (in place of the second 50-mg dose). *Dosage Forms:* Tablets: 25 mg; Sustained Release Tablets: 50 and 75 mg.

Homatropine Methylbromide [3α-Hydroxy-8-methyl-1αH,5αH-tropanium bromide mandelate [80-49-9] $C_{17}H_{24}BrNO_3$ (370.29); Homapin (*Mission Pharmacal*); Novatrin (*Ayerst*)]—Prepared by quaternizing homatropine base with methyl bromide. A white, odorless powder which darkens slowly on exposure to light; melts about 190°; pH of a 1 in 100 solution between 4.5 and 6.5. Very soluble in water; freely soluble in alcohol; almost insoluble in ether and acetone; freely soluble in acetone containing 20% water. *Uses:* A quaternary ammonium antimuscarinic agent with typical actions and adverse effects. It is used only for the management of gastrointestinal hypermotility and spasm, for which it is more selective than atropine. It is not marketed as a single-entity product but only in combination with *three* barbiturates! *Dose:* The oral adult dose is commonly stated to be 2.5 to 5 mg 4 times a day, but the inclusion of phenobarbital, secobarbital, and butbarbital in the only product should prohibit round-the-clock medication and suggest 2.5 mg at bedtime only.

Methantheline Bromide [Diethyl (2-hydroxyethyl)methylammonium bromide xanthene-9-carboxylate [53-46-3] $C_{21}H_{26}BrNO_3$; Banthine Bromide (*Searle*)]—Synthesized from xanthene-9-carboxylic acid, diethylaminoethyl chloride, and methyl bromide. A white powder having a bitter taste; practically odorless; melts between 171° and 177°. Very soluble in water, alcohol, chloroform; practically insoluble in ether.

Uses: Methantheline bromide is the original quaternary ammonium antimuscarinic drug. Although it has some selectivity for the gastrointestinal tract, significant suppression of gastric secretion is rarely achieved with oral administration and is of brief duration when it occurs. It compares poorly with several more recent antimuscarinic drugs. It is promoted for adjunctive treatment of *duodenal ulcer* and it may relieve both the pain and the symptoms that accompany this condition. The mechanism whereby it relieves the pain of duodenal ulcer is probably mostly the reduction in gastrointestinal motility. Objective roentgenological improvement attributable to the drug remains to be shown, after all these years. Patients with gastric ulcer are not appreciably benefited. Instances of duodenal ulcer recurrence as well as development of gastric ulcer have been reported in individuals receiving prophylactic doses of the drug for healed duodenal ulcer. A large percentage of patients discontinue use of the drug because they refuse to tolerate the side effects. Of the numerous drugs used in the treatment of peptic ulcer, methantheline bromide appears to cause the highest incidence of intolerance (more than atropine!), and it is difficult to understand its continuing popularity in the face of overwhelming evidence of its inferiority compared to several more recently introduced antimuscarinic drugs. This is especially puzzling since it was the disappointing experience with methantheline that led so many medical authorities to assume an unjustified cynical attitude about the value of any antimuscarinic drug as a gastric antisecretory agent.

Side effects, precautions, and contraindications are those of quaternary ammonium antimuscarinic drugs in general (see page 911), although side effects may be mild and may become minimal with continuing use. Central nervous effects, as restlessness, euphoria, fatigue and rarely psychotic episodes can occur. *Dose: Oral, adult, initially,* 50 to 100 mg 4 times a day. The *maintenance dose* in peptic ulcer is usually 25 to 50 mg 4 times a day; the dose before bedtime can be larger than the maximal tolerated daytime dose. In *children, newborn,* 12.5 mg initially 2 times a day then 3 times a day; ages 1 to 12 mo, 12.5 mg gradually increasing to 25 mg 4 times a day; ages above 1 yr, 12.5 to 50 mg 4 times a day. *Dosage Form:* Tablets: 50 mg.

Methixene Hydrochloride [1-Methyl-3-(thioxanthen-9-ylmethyl)-piperidine hydrochloride $C_{20}H_{23}NS.HCl$; Trest (*Dorsey*)]—Synthesized from 3-pyridinemethanol, methyl iodide, thionyl chloride, and thioxanthene. US Pat 2,905,590. A white, crystalline powder; bitter taste; practically odorless; melts between 213° and 217°. Soluble in water, alcohol, chloroform; insoluble in ether. *Uses:* A tertiary amine antimuscarinic drug with some selectivity for the gastrointestinal tract which, however, is more the result of direct inhibition of smooth muscle than of selective muscarinic blockade. It is used in the management of conditions in which there is hypermotility, as in *pylorospasm*, *biliary dyskinesia*, *spastic colon*, *duodenitis*, and *gastritis*, and in other disorders in which it is desirable to diminish even normal motility, as in *duodenal ulcer*. It does not diminish gastric secretion. Although it is recommended for use in gastric ulcer, a decrease in motility can result in retention of acid and hence sometimes exacerbate the erosive process. Incidence of side effects is low with usual doses. The usual side effects are limited to dry mouth, blurred vision, and urinary retention. It potentially has all the side effects of antimuscarinic drugs (page 911), and the precautions and contraindications are the same. Although glaucoma is stated as a contraindication, low doses of methixene have been used in some glaucomatous patients without affecting intraocular tension. *Dose:* 1 to 2 mg 3 times a day. Dosage has not been established in children. *Dosage Form:* Tablets: 1 mg.

Oxybutynin Chloride [4-(Diethylamino)-2-butynyl α-phenylcyclo-hexaneglycolate hydrochloride [1508-65-2] $C_{22}H_{31}NO_3.HCl$; Ditropan (*Marion*)]—Oxybutynin base is synthesized by interaction of methyl phenylcyclohexaneglycolate and 4-diethylamino-2-butynyl acetate in *n*-heptane solution in the presence of sodium methylate, and converted to the hydrochloride by extraction with dilute hydrochloric acid. British Pat 940,540. A white to off-white, crystalline powder; melts at about 130°; pK_a 6.96. Freely soluble in water and in alcohol. *Uses:* An antispasmodic with weak antimuscarinic activity. In patients with uninhibited neurogenic and reflex neurogenic bladder cystometric studies have demonstrated that it increases vesical capacity, diminishes frequency of uninhibited contractions of the detrusor muscle, and delays initial desire to void. It is used for relief of symptoms associated with voiding (such as urgency, urge incontinence, frequency, nocturia, and incontinence) in patients confirmed by cystometry and other diagnostic procedures to have neurogenic bladder. The adverse effects, contraindications, warnings, and precautions are those of antimuscarinic drugs (see the general statement, page 911), except that it also causes drowsiness. Safety of use in women who are or who may become pregnant has not been established. Safety and efficacy in children under 5 years of age have not been established. *Dose: Oral, adult*, 5 mg 2 or 3 times daily, not exceeding 5 mg 4 times daily. *Children* over 5 years of age, 5 mg twice daily, not exceeding 5 mg 3 times daily. *Dosage Form:* Tablets: 5 mg.

Oxyphenonium Bromide [Diethyl(2-hydroxyethyl)methylammonium α-phenylcyclohexaneglycolate bromide [50-10-2] $C_{21}H_{34}BrNO_3$; Antrenyl Bromide (*Ciba*)]—A white, crystalline powder; melts at about 195°. Freely soluble in water and in alcohol; insoluble in ether. *Uses:* A quaternary ammonium antimuscarinic agent with a moderate selectivity for the gastrointestinal tract. It decreases gastric motility and in large doses transiently decreases gastric secretion; the effects on secretion are not elicited under ordinary conditions of use. It also reduces intestinal motility. Used in the treatment of *peptic ulcer*, in *intestinal hypermotility*, and *spastic colon*. The side effects, precautions, and contraindications are those of antimuscarinic drugs in general (page 911). *Dose: Oral, adult, initially*, 10 mg 4 times a day, subsequently adjusted according to the patient's initial response. Not for use in *children*. *Dosage Form:* Tablets: 5 mg.

Propantheline Bromide [(2-Hydroxyethyl)diisopropylmethylammonium bromide xanthene-9-carboxylate [50-34-0] $C_{23}H_{30}BrNO_3$; Pro-Banthine (*Searle*)]—Prepared by metathesis of sodium xanthene-9-carboxylate with β-diisopropylaminoethyl chloride and quaternization of the resulting ester with methyl bromide. White or nearly white crystals; melts between 156° and 162° with decomposition. Very soluble in water, alcohol, chloroform; practically insoluble in ether. *Uses:* A quaternary ammonium antimuscarinic agent (see general statement for actions and uses). It is closely related to methantheline, which it greatly resembles. Beneficial effects in *peptic ulcer* mostly derive from decreased gastric motility, although some suppression of gastric secretion may occur after parenteral administration. Propantheline bromide is metabolized in the liver; the half-life is about 9 hr. The incidence of side effects is about one-half that of methantheline, but is nevertheless considerably higher than that of several newer anticholinergic drugs. For potential side effects, precautions and contraindications see page 912. *Dose: Oral, adult*, 7.5 mg 3 times a day to 15 mg before each meal and 30 mg at bedtime. *Dosage Forms:* Tablets: 7.5 and 15 mg.

Thiphenamil Hydrochloride [2-Diethylaminoethyl diphenylthioacetate hydrochloride [548-68-5] $C_{20}H_{25}NOS.HCl$ (363.97); Trocinate (*Poythress*)]—White powder; bitter taste with a potent local anesthetic effect; melts at 129°; 1 g dissolves in 25 mL water; soluble in alcohol. *Uses:* A tertiary amine with weak *antimuscarinic* properties and very little selectivity; limited to the gastrointestinal uses of drugs of this class (page 912). It is used to decrease bowel hypermotility and spasm, as in the irritable colon syndrome, spastic colitis, mucous colitis, acute enterocolitis, and functional hypermotility of the gastrointestinal tract. The side effects, precautions, and contraindications are those of antimuscarinic drugs in general (page 911). *Dose: Oral, adult*, initially 400 mg, repeated in 4 hours if necessary and continued on a regimen determined by the conditions and the response, usually 4 times a day.

Tridihexethyl Chloride [(3-Cyclohexyl-3-hydroxy-3-phenylpropyl)-triethylammonium chloride [4310-35-4] $C_{21}H_{36}ClNO$ (353.98) Pathilon (*Lederle*). White, odorless, crystalline powder; melting range 196° to 202°. Soluble 1 g in 3 mL alcohol, 2 mL chloroform; practically insoluble in ether. *Uses:* A quaternary ammonium antimuscarinic agent (see page 911). By the oral route, effects on gastric acid secretion are only slight and transient, but by the parenteral route greater effects can be achieved; nevertheless, the antisecretory effect is not sufficient to be of much clinical significance. Delayed gastric emptying does sustain the action of antacids. Tridihexethyl chloride is used for the treatment of *irritable colon*, *spastic colon*, *mucous colitis*, *acute enterocolitis*, *splenic flexure syndrome*, and *neurogenic colon*. Side effects are low in incidence but are typical of antimuscarinic drugs. The precautions and contraindications are those of antimuscarinic drugs in general (page 911). *Dose: Oral, adult, initially*, 25 mg 3 times a day before meals and 50 mg before bedtime; the dose is subsequently adjusted according to the therapeutic response and occurrence of side effects, and may range from 30 to 225 mg/day.

Antispasmodic Drugs

Spasm may result from a local disorder, in which cellular injury initiates the contractile process, local hormones or other excitatory or irritant substances are released, or local reflexes are activated, or it may be the result of hyperactivity in efferent excitatory autonomic nerves or of electrolyte disturbances that favor increased neuronal and muscular activity. Therefore, according to the locus, cause, and mediators of a spastic condition, one or more of a number of classes of selective drugs may be employed, eg, neuromuscular blocking or centrally acting muscle relaxants for various spastic conditions of skeletal muscle, local anesthetics for some localized neurally mediated spasm, α-adrenoreceptor blocking drugs or β₂-adrenoreceptor agonists for vasospasm, β₂-agonists for bronchial and uterine spasms, antimuscarinic drugs for ciliary spasm or spastic bowel, calcium for hypocalcemic tetany, etc. Thus the term antispasmodic might apply to many different types of drug. The term should be reserved, however, for those drugs that relax smooth muscle nonselectively, that is, irrespective of the type of innervation and neurotransmitter and rather generally potentially affecting all smooth muscle, and only such drugs are included below. Calcium channel blocking drugs are discussed elsewhere. The selective antagonists are treated in the appropriate chapters. Long before the selective competitive antagonistic actions of antimuscarinic drugs were known, some antimuscarinic preparations and drugs were known to relieve certain spastic conditions of the bowel. Therefore, the term antispasmodic came to connote antimuscarinic drugs that have important gastrointestinal uses, and it has become common to include antispasmodics in chapters on antimuscarinic drugs. For want of a better alternative for this small group of agents, that tradition is maintained here.

Aminophylline—page 872.

Calcium Channel Blockers—page 861.

Ethaverine Hydrochloride—page 852.

Papaverine Hydrochloride—page 852.

Other Antispasmodic Drugs

Flavoxate Hydrochloride [2-Piperidinomethyl 3-methyl-4-oxo-2-phenyl-4*H*-1-benzopyran-8-carboxylate hydrochloride [3717-88-2] $C_{24}H_{25}NO_4$.HCl; Urispas (*SK&F*)]—For synthesis of this ester of 3-methylflavone-8-carboxylic acid see *J Med Pharm Chem 2:* 263, 1960; US Pat 2,291,070. Off-white, crystalline powder; melts at about 230° with decomposition. One gram dissolves in 6 mL water, 500 mL alcohol. *Uses:* A nonspecific smooth muscle relaxant with weak antimuscarinic properties; appears to have a selectivity for the urinary tract. It is promoted for the symptomatic relief but not the definitive treatment of dysuria, urinary urgency, nocturia, suprapubic pain, and urinary incontinence such as accompany urethrocystitis/urethrotrigonitis, urethritis, cystitis, and prostatitis. Untoward effects include nausea and vomiting, dry mouth, blurred vision, increased intraocular tension, dysuria, tachycardia, palpitation, hyperpyrexia, headache, drowsiness, mental confusion (particularly in elderly patients), eosinophilia, leukopenia, urticaria, and dermatoses. The precautions and contraindications are those of antimuscarinic drugs (page 912). Considering that the side effects and toxicity are all antimuscarinic in character, it is interesting that the actions on the urinary smooth muscle are not held to be antimuscarinic. *Dose: Oral, adult* or *children over 12 years old*, 100 to 200 mg 3 or 4 times a day; not recommended for children under 12 years of age. *Dosage Form:* Tablets: 100 mg.

CHAPTER 49

Skeletal Muscle Relaxants

Stewart C Harvey, PhD
Professor of Pharmacology
School of Medicine
University of Utah
Salt Lake City, UT 84132

Skeletal muscle may be relaxed by blocking the effect of somatic motor nerve impulses or by depressing the appropriate neurons within the central nervous system so that somatic motor nerve impulses fail to be generated. Interruption of certain afferent reflex pathways, as by local anesthesia, may also effect relaxation of circumscribed muscle groups; local anesthetic block of efferent somatic motor outflow is also sometimes employed to relieve localized skeletal muscle spasm. In this chapter only those drugs that act at the myoneural junction, the *neuromuscular blocking drugs*, and those drugs that act upon central neurons, the *centrally acting muscle relaxants*, will be treated.

Neuromuscular Blocking Drugs

Neuromuscular blocking drugs prevent somatic motor nerve impulses from initiating contractile responses in the effector skeletal (striated) muscles and hence cause a paralysis of the muscles. There are two categories of such drugs: the *competitive* (or *stabilizing*) paralysants and the *depolarizing* paralysants, to be discussed separately.

Uses—Competitive and depolarizing neuromuscular blocking drugs have the same major uses, in general. The pharmacokinetics and pattern of side effects, rather than their mechanism, determine the uses of any given agent. The principal use is to provide *adequate skeletal muscular relaxation* during surgery and during *orthopedic manipulations.* The short-acting drugs are used to relax the laryngeal muscles during *endotracheal intubation* and *bronchoscopy.* Neuromuscular paralysants may be employed to *decrease the severity* of muscle contraction during *electroconvulsive* or *pentylenetetrazol* treatment. Competitive neuromuscular paralysants have been used in the management of *tetanus* and in *various spastic disorders*, but the results have usually been disappointing. Competitive blocking drugs may be used in the *diagnosis of myasthenia gravis;* the myasthenic patient is extremely sensitive to the paralysant actions.

Competitive Neuromuscular Blocking Drugs

When impulses in the somatic motor nerves arrive in the nerve terminals in the motor endplate region, they evoke the release of acetylcholine, which diffuses to the postsynaptic motor endplate membrane. There acetylcholine combines with nicotinic cholinergic receptors to activate them, which leads to the opening of transmembrane ion channels, ion flow, and consequent membrane depolarization. Endplate membrane depolarization is followed by depolarization of the muscle membrane and subsequent contraction. Any interruption of the above sequence of events leads to muscular paralysis.

The competitive neuromuscular blocking drugs combine with the nicotinic receptors and occupy them without activating them. Acetylcholine cannot activate the already occupied receptors, so that motor nerve impulses cannot elicit contractions, and paralysis ensues.

Pharmacologic Antagonism—The interaction of blocking drug and receptor is reversible and dynamic. Drug molecules combine, dissociate, recombine, etc, thus leaving receptor molecules transiently unoccupied. The probability that an acetylcholine molecule will find an unoccupied receptor is directly proportional to the concentration. If the concentration is sufficiently elevated, dissociated blocking drug molecules will find the receptors occupied with acetylcholine and will be prevented from recombining with the receptors to maintain blockade. Thus a blockade can be competitively overcome. In practice, the acetylcholine concentration is raised by inhibiting acetylcholinesterase in the endplate region. Neostigmine and edrophonium are the most commonly employed anticholinesterases for antagonizing competitive neuromuscular paralysants. The anticholinesterases are discussed in Chapter 46 (page 894).

Side Effects and Precautions—The competitive neuromuscular blocking drugs are quite selective for the nonrespiratory muscles, so that it is possible to achieve surgical relaxation of the abdominal, limb, neck, or laryngeal muscles without significant loss of respiratory function. However, respiration may often be depressed to the point of danger, even apnea, so that *these drugs should be used only when facilities for prolonged respiratory assistance are at hand and the trachea is intubated,* in case respiratory assistance is needed.

The two other principal side effects are the release of histamine from mast cells and ganglionic blockade. The extent to which histamine release occurs varies among the several drugs; it is greatest with tubocurarine. The histamine released may cause vasodilatation and consequent hypotension and reflex tachycardia, bronchospasm, urticaria, rash, and rarely even angioneurotic edema. *Histamine-releasing neuromuscular blocking drugs should be avoided in persons with a history of bronchial asthma, angioneurotic edema, or anaphylaxis.*

Ganglionic blockade may occur, because the postsynaptic ganglionic cholinergic receptors are nicotinic. However, these receptors have somewhat different structural requirements from those at the neuromuscular junction, so that ganglionic blockade is only slight to moderate with the usual clinical doses of neuromuscular blocking drugs. The types of effects of ganglionic blockade depend upon which ganglia are blocked. Blockade of sympathetic ganglia contributes to hypotension and of vagal ganglia to tachycardia. Ganglionic blockade is salutary when adverse reflexes to surgical manipulation are attenuated.

All of the marketed neuromuscular blocking drugs are quaternary ammonium compounds; hence they do not penetrate the blood-brain barrier and thus lack central nervous actions.

Drug Interactions, Etc—Any drug with an effect to depress the excitability of the postsynaptic membrane at the motor endplate will increase the blocking effect of competitive neuromuscular blocking drugs. The anesthetic ethers, halothane, trimethaphan, and propranolol are among such drugs.

A number of antibiotics can cause neuromuscular paralysis in high doses and in therapeutic doses may increase neuromuscular blockade by the competitive blocking drugs. Some of these (gentamicin, kanamycin, neomycin, streptomycin, tobramycin, paromomycin, viomycin) apparently also act competitively on the nicotinic receptor and hence may be antagonized by anticholinesterases. Others (polymyxins, colistin, colistimethate, tetracyclines, lincomycin, clindamycin) have a more obscure action and are not antagonized by anticholinesterases, although anticholinesterases will antagonize the neuromuscular blocking drug and relieve the exaggerated paralysis; calcium partially antagonizes these drugs. Local anesthetics, quinine, quinidine, ganglionic blocking drugs and magnesium ion also potentiate the neuromuscular blocking actions of the competitive blocking drugs.

Hypothermia also increases the response to competitive neuromuscular blocking drugs.

Depolarizing Neuromuscular Blocking Drugs

The depolarizing neuromuscular blocking drugs are nicotinic agonists, which, like acetylcholine, interact with the postsynaptic nicotinic receptors to effect a depolarization of the membrane at the motor endplate. Unlike acetylcholine their sojourn at the endplate is long, so that the postsynaptic membrane may remain depolarized. Since the muscle membrane and consequent contraction can only be excited by a fresh depolarization, the muscle remains paralyzed; that is to say, the trigger for the conducted muscle impulse is the transient fall in endplate membrane potential and not the persisting depolarization.

Eventually, the motor endplate membrane repolarizes despite the continuing presence of the drug, owing to a shift in receptor conformation. Nevertheless, despite the fact that the membrane is poised for a new depolarization, motor nerve impulses and acetylcholine fail to elicit a response, because the nicotinic receptor is not in its perturbable conformation. During this phase, the neuromuscular blockade takes on some characteristics of competitive blockade and may even be partially antagonized by anticholinesterases. This second phase is erratic in onset among the various muscles, and blockade may be of a mixed type, thus complicating the treatment of overdoses. Furthermore, not all drug recipients respond alike. Electrolyte status, muscle condition, disease, genetic factors, the presence of other drugs and temperature all affect the time of onset and extent of phase two block. Moreover, not all depolarizing drugs are identical in the pattern of blockade. Clinically, phase two is usually significant only when the drug dose is repeated and blood-levels sustained beyond the normal single dose limit.

Side Effects and Precautions—During the onset of the drug-induced depolarization, as the membrane potential falls to the critical firing potential, there may arise conducted impulses that will cause random contraction (fibrillation) of the muscle fibers. In addition, the depolarizing neuromuscular blocking drugs stimulate both the intrafusal fibers and the muscle spindle afferent nerve endings, which results in facilitatory nerve traffic entering the spinal cord. Thus there is a more organized contraction pattern, namely discharge of whole motor units, or *fasciculations* and even *twitching*. The result is muscle soreness. Fasciculations and twitching can

exacerbate spasm and also cause damage in the presence of broken bones; consequently, the depolarizing drugs should be avoided in these conditions.

The muscles of respiration (intercostal and diaphragmatic) are more resistant to the paralyzing effects than are other skeletal muscles, and it is usually possible to achieve surgical relaxation of abdominal, limb, neck, or laryngeal muscles without significant loss of respiratory function. Nevertheless, respiration may often be depressed, sometimes to the point of apnea. This is especially likely after prolonged use, which favors considerable loss of potassium from the motor endplate region. Consequently, *the depolarizing neuromuscular blocking drugs should only be used with tracheal intubation and when facilities for prolonged assisted respiration are at hand.* Care should be used when respiration is already depressed and also when the lithotomy or Trendelenburg positions are employed, especially in young children and the aged.

During the depolarizing phase of neuromuscular block, potassium is rapidly lost from the muscles, which may cause hyperkalemia. If a sufficient amount of the mobilized potassium is excreted, there may be a later hypokalemia. Various cardiac arrhythmias, even cardiac arrest, may result, especially if the patient is digitalized.

The effects of depolarizing blocking drugs on autonomic ganglia and histamine stores are variable.

Drug Interactions, Etc.—Muscle paralysis with depolarizing neuromuscular blocking drugs is increased by hypothermia, hypokalemia, hypermagnesemia, polymyxin B, colistin, colistimethate, aminoglycoside antibiotics, (streptomycin, kanamycin, gentamicin, tobramycin, and neomycin).

Dantrolene Sodium

2,4-Imidazolidinedione, 1-[[[5-(4-nitrophenyl)-2-furanyl]methylene]-amino]-, sodium salt, hydrate (2:7); Dantrium (*Norwich-Eaton*).

1-[[5-(*p*-Nitrophenyl)furfurylidene]amino]hydantoin sodium salt hydrate [24868-20-0] $C_{14}H_9N_4NaO_5 \cdot 3\frac{1}{2}H_2O$ (399.29).

Preparation—See *J Med Chem 10*, 807(1967) and US Pat 3,415,821 for patent information.

Description—Orange powder; *free acid*, melts about 280°; pK_a about 7.5.

Solubility—Slightly soluble in water; more soluble in alkali.

Uses—Dantrolene differs from the classical neuromuscular blocking drugs in that its action is distal to the nicotinic receptors and neuromuscular junction. Instead, it suppresses excitation-contraction coupling by interfering with release of calcium from the sarcoplasmic reticulum. The muscle fibers still respond to nerve impulses, but the contractile response is lessened but not abolished. Therefore, muscle weakness, rather than paralysis, is the result. Fast muscle fibers (white) are affected more than slow muscle fibers (red). Because the contractility of the intrafusal fibers in the muscle spindles is also decreased, spinal cord-mediated stretch reflexes are attenuated, which provides the primary explanation of its ability to relieve certain types of spasm. Dantrolene is used to treat *spasticity resulting from upper motor neuron* lesions, such as those in *spinal cord injury*, *stroke*, *multiple sclerosis*, and *cerebral palsy* but not spasticity resulting from musculoskeletal injury, lumbago, or rheumatoid disorders. It is possible that a direct effect on the motor neuron may be involved in this limited spectrum of activity, since the drug does exert some CNS-depressant actions. In fact, the drug is used to treat the *neuroleptic malignant syndrome*. Its effect on intracellular calcium also lends itself to the treatment of *malignant hyperthemia*.

Interference with muscle function may cause weakness and fatigue, poor posture with consequent backache and myalgia, a feeling of suffocation, difficulties in swallowing, and diplopia and other visual disturbances. Effects on the CNS include drowsiness, dizziness, malaise, headache, nervousness, confusion, depression, and rarely convulsions. Other adverse effects include constipation, diarrhea, abdominal cramps, gastric irritation, gastrointestinal bleeding, increased urinary frequency, lacrimation, sweating, disorders of taste, urticaria, acneiform rash, eczematoid dermatitis, hepatitis, chills, and fever. Dantrolene is contraindicated in liver and pulmonary disease, in situations where alertness is essential, and when gross postural abnormalities result from its use. Dantrolene may color the urine orange to red.

Orally, dantrolene is absorbed poorly but more or less consistently, so that blood levels are proportional to the dose. It is metabolized in the liver to several products. It is stated that the plasma half-life is 5 hr by the intravenous route but 9 hr by the oral route. The former is probably an approximation of the *distribution* (α) half-life and the latter of the elimination (β) half-life.

Dose—*Oral, adult,* for *chronic spasticity,* initially **25 mg** once a day, to be increased at intervals of 4 to 7 days to as much as **100 mg** 2 to 4 times a day, if necessary; for *preoperative prophylaxis* of malignant hyperthermia, 4 to 8 **mg/kg/day** in 3 or 4 divided doses 1 or 2 days before surgery, so the last dose is taken 3 to 4 hr prior to surgery. *Children,* for *spasticity, initially,* **0.5 mg** twice a day, then gradually increasing the dose by increments of **0.5 mg/kg/day** up to **3 mg/kg** 2 to 4 times a day, not to exceed a total of 100 mg/day. *Intravenous, adult* and *children,* for *malignant hyperthermia, initially* **1 mg/kg** rapidly repeated, if necessary, up to total of **10 mg/kg**. Once the hyperthermia is controlled, 4 to 8 **mg/kg** is given orally for 1 to 3 days.

Dosage Forms—Capsules: 25, 50, and 100 mg. Powder for Injection: 22.4 mg, to make 70 mL solution of 0.32 mg/mL.

Gallamine Triethiodide

Ethanaminium, 2,2',2''-[1,2,3-benzenetriyltris(oxy)]tris[*N,N,N*-triethyl-, triiodide; 1,2,3-Tris(β-diethylaminoethoxy)benzene Triethiodide; Flaxedil (*Lederle*)

[*v*-Phenenyltris(oxyethylene)]tris[triethylammonium] triiodide [65-29-2] $C_{30}H_{60}I_3N_3O_3$ (891.54).

Preparation—Pyrogallol is condensed with 2-chlorotriethylamine and the resulting triamine is quaternized with ethyl iodide in boiling acetone.

Description—White, odorless, amorphous powder. It is hygroscopic.

Solubility—Very soluble in water; sparingly soluble in alcohol; very slightly soluble in chloroform.

Note—Gallamine triethiodide is pharmaceutically incompatible with meperidine hydrochloride (solutions must not be mixed).

Uses—Gallamine is a competitive neuromuscular blocking drug; see the general statement (page 921) for actions, uses, side effects, and drug interactions. In general, it has very little action on autonomic ganglia, but it usually blocks the cardiac vagus and hence causes tachycardia and occasionally hypertension. It releases histamine only in high doses. Hypersensitivity reactions occasionally occur, and serve anaphylaxis has been reported; the drug should be used cautiously in patients with a history of allergy, asthma, or atopy. It should be used cautiously if tachycardia preexists. Gallamine is eliminated mainly by renal excretion, and its action may be prolonged if there is renal dysfunction.

Dose—*Intravenous* or *intramuscular, initially,* **1 mg/kg** of body weight for *limb muscle paralysis* or **1.5 mg/kg** for *abdominal surgery,* not to exceed 100 mg, then **500 μg** to **1 mg** at 30- to 60-min intervals if necessary. The dose should be diminished if various ether anesthetics or halothane is used.

Dosage Forms—Injection: 200 mg/10 mL.

Hexafluorenium Bromide

1,6-Hexanediaminium, *N,N'*-di-9*H*-fluoren-9-yl-*N,N,N',N'*-tetramethyl-, dibromide; Mylaxen (*Mallinckrodt*)

Hexamethylenebis[fluoren-9-yldimethylammonium] dibromide [317-52-2] $C_{36}H_{42}Br_2N_2$ (662.55).

Preparation—*N,N,N',N'*-Tetramethyl-1,6-hexanediamine is dissolved in a suitable nonsolvolytic solvent and double quaternized with 9-bromofluorene. *J Am Chem Soc 76:* 1862, 1954.

Description—White, crystalline powder; melts between 188° and 189°.

Solubility—Sparingly soluble in water; soluble in alcohol; insoluble in ether and chloroform.

Uses—Hexafluorenium is a pharmacological enigma. It possesses weak neuromuscular blocking activity of the stabilizing type, but the actions are too weak to cause useful muscle relaxation except under deep ether anesthesia. Consistent with its stabilizing action, it potentiates neuromuscular blockade by tubocurarine and antagonizes that by decamethonium, but its effects on blockade by gallamine are erratic. Paradoxically, it markedly potentiates and prolongs the neuromuscular actions of succinylcholine. Hexafluorenium is a strong inhibitor of plasma (pseudo)cholinesterase, and, since destruction by plasma cholinesterase is usually the principal means whereby succinylcholine is degraded, the prolongation of action might be explained by the anticholinesterase action. However, the marked potentiation cannot be so explained, and various experimental observations indicate an unknown interaction at the neuromuscular junction. The drug is claimed to lessen the extent of fasciculation and later muscle soreness, which is not consistent with a simple anticholinesterase action. Clinically, hexafluorenium is used only to potentiate and prolong the effects of succinylcholine, so that it may be used in prolonged surgical procedures. The duration of action of a single dose is usually 20 to 30 min.

Adverse effects include prolonged paralysis, apnea and bronchospasm. Cardiovascular effects include hypertension or hypotension, bradycardia, rare cardiac arrest, tachycardia and tachydysrhythmias, hypersensitivity, salivation, increased intraocular pressure, and hyperthermia. In combination with succinylcholine, the adverse effects are those of large doses of succinylcholine and include effects, such as bronchospasm and varying degrees of atrioventricular block, that are rarely seen with succinylcholine alone. The bronchospasm may be due to histamine release. The combination is relatively contraindicated in bronchial asthma. It is claimed that prolonged apnea is less frequent in persons with atypical plasma cholinesterase which is not consistent with cholinesterase inhibition as the sole mechanism of the effect of hexafluorenium. Nevertheless, deep and prolonged muscle paralysis and apnea can occur. The drug should be used with caution in patients with any type of neuromyopathy and with cardiovascular, renal, hepatic, pulmonary, or metabolic disorder. The effect on the fetus is unknown.

Dose—Hexafluorenium bromide is given initially in a dose ratio of 2 mg for every mg of succinylcholine. *Intravenous, initially,* **300** to **400 μg/kg**; for prolonged procedures it may be necessary to administer an additional **100** to **200 μg/kg** at intervals of 30 min for the first repeated dose and 80 to 100 min thereafter. An interval of 3 min should separate administration of hexafluorenium and succinylcholine. For the dose of succinylcholine see *Succinylcholine Chloride.*

Dosage Form—Injection: 200 mg/10 mL.

Metocurine Iodide

Tubocuraranium, 6,6',7',12'-tetramethoxy-2,2,2',2'-tetramethyl-, diiodide; Dimethyl Tubocurarine Iodide; Metubine Iodide (*Lilly*)

(+)-*O*,*O*'-Dimethylchondrocurarine diiodide [7601-55-0] $C_{40}H_{48}I_2N_2O_6$ (906.64).

Preparation—By methylation of the naturally occurring *d*-tubocurarine, with methyl iodide or dimethyl sulfate, and conversion to the diiodide.

Description—White or yellow, crystalline powder.
Solubility—1 g in 400 mL water; very slightly soluble in alcohol; practically insoluble in chloroform and ether.

Uses—Metocurine iodide is a competitive neuromuscular blocking drug; see the general statement (page 921) for actions, uses, side effects, and drug interactions. In man, metocurine iodide is approximately three times more potent than *d*-tubocurarine chloride.

Dose—*Intravenous*, *initially*, **1.5 to 10 mg** given over a 30 to 60-sec period. The initial dose depends on the anesthetic employed: with ether, 1.5 to 3 mg; with cyclopropane, 2 to 4 mg; with nitrous oxide-thiopental, 3 to 10 mg. For limb muscle paralysis, dosage is in the lower range; for abdominal and respiratory muscle paralysis, it is at the upper end; for *endotracheal intubation*, **200 to 400 µg/kg.** Maintenance, **500 µg to 1 mg** every 25 to 90 min. For electroshock therapy, **1.75 to 5.5 mg.**

Dosage Forms—Injection: 40 mg/20 mL.

Pancuronium Bromide

Piperidinium, 1,1'-[(2β,3α,5α,16β,17β)-3,17-bis(acetyloxy)androstane-2,16-diyl]bis[1-methyl]-, dibromide; Pavulon (*Organon*)

1,1'-(3α,17β-Dihydroxy-5α-androstan-2β,16β-ylene)bis[1-methyl piperidinium]dibromide diacetate [15500-66-0] $C_{35}H_{60}Br_2N_2O_4$ (732.68).

Preparation—Described in US Pat 3,553,212.

Description—White, crystalline powder; hygroscopic; melts at about 215°.
Solubility—Freely soluble in water; soluble in alcohol and chloroform.

Uses—Pancuronium bromide is a competitive neuromuscular blocking drug; see the general statement (page 921) for actions, uses, side effects, and drug interactions. Its mechanism of action is usually assumed to be identical to that of tubocurarine, but the dose-response curve is steeper, which suggests a difference. It differs from tubocurarine in its side effects in that it does not block the autonomic ganglia and rarely releases histamine, so that it causes neither hypotension nor bronchospasm. In fact, it may cause a slight tachycardia and hypertension. Also, a slight transient rash may occasionally occur. Salivary secretion during light anesthesia is common. Drug interactions are the same as with tubocurarine, except that prior treatment with succinylcholine augments the paralysis and increases the duration; also, narcotic analgesics do not seem to affect actions of pancuronium. It may be used more safely in patients with cardiovascular disease or bronchial asthma than any other neuromuscular blocking drug. Indeed, it has actually been used in the *management of status asthmaticus*, to relax the muscles, thereby facilitating artificial respiration and decreasing oxygen demand.

After intravenous injection, the effects of pancuronium become maximal in less than 4.5 min in adults and 90 sec in children. The duration of action of usual doses is generally 30 to 60 min, but it depends on various factors, such as the anesthetic, or prior succinylcholine. The plasma half-life is probably slightly less than 2 hours. Pancuronium is excreted mostly unchanged into the urine, but up to one-third of a dose is deacetylated; thus it is advisable to use the drug cautiously in the presence of either renal or liver disease.

Dose—*Intravenous*, *adult*, *for surgical relaxation*, **20 to 100 µg/kg,** followed by supplemental doses of **10 µg/kg**; for *intubation*, **60 to 100 µg/kg.**

Dosage Form—Injection: 10 mg/10 mL, 4 mg/2 mL, 20 mg/5 mL.

Succinylcholine Chloride

Ethanaminium, 2,2'-[(1,4-dioxo-1,4-butanediyl)bis(oxy)]bis[*N*,*N*,*N*-trimethyl-, dichloride; Suxamethonium Chloride; Anectine (*Burroughs-Wellcome*); Quelicin (*Abbott*); Sucostrin (*Squibb*); Sux-Cert (*Travenol*)

Choline chloride succinate (2:1) *anhydrous* [71-27-2] $C_{14}H_{30}Cl_2N_2O_4$ (361.31); *dihydrate* [6101-15-1] (397.34); usually occurs as the dihydrate.

Preparation—It may be prepared by condensing succinyl chloride with β-dimethylaminoethanol and quaternizing the resulting ester with methyl chloride.

Description—White, odorless, crystalline powder. Its solutions are acid to litmus, having a pH of about 4. The dihydrate melts at about 160°; the anhydrous at about 190°, and is hygroscopic.
Solubility—1 g in about 1 mL water and about 350 mL alcohol; slightly soluble in chloroform; practically insoluble in ether.

Uses—Succinylcholine chloride is a depolarizing neuromuscular blocking agent; see the general statement (page 921) for actions, uses, side effects, and drug interactions. It usually has a very transient duration of action because of rapid hydrolysis of the drug by serum (pseudo)cholinesterases. The effects of a single injection usually last only a few minutes; consequently, it is of especial use for muscle relaxation during brief manipulations. Prolonged muscular relaxation is achieved by continuous intravenous infusion, and the intensity of muscle paralysis is readily controlled by adjustment of the infusion rate. Alternatively, prolonged muscular relaxation may be achieved with periodic injections when the drug is given in combination with hexafluorenium bromide (page 923). Although a stabilizing phase of action can occur, its occurrence is erratic and usually results only from prolonged use.

Succinylcholine chloride does not cause liberation of histamine but hypersensitivity reactions sometimes occur. As the drug depolarizes the motor end-plate, conducted impulses and contractions of motor units (fasciculations) may occur. Muscle aching resulting from its transient stimulatory action is minimized by slow administration. Hyperkalemia, due to potassium loss from muscle, and myoglobinemia sometimes result from these stimulatory actions. Excessive salivation may occur; this is preventable by premedication with atropine or scopolamine. It may induce a bradycardia that can be suppressed by atropine or methscopolamine but not by scopolamine. It may cause cardiac arrhythmias in patients with myocardial damage. Among neuromuscular blocking drugs, it is unique in its effect to increase intraocular pressure; it is contraindicated in persons with glaucoma or retinal detachment, and in persons with known hypersensitivity. Rarely, it may cause a severe (malignant) hyperthermia when an anesthetic such as halothane or cyclopropane is used. No specific pharmacological antagonist of the skeletal muscle effects is available but dantrolene can suppress malignant hyperthermia. Calcium channel blocking drugs also promise to be useful in this regard. Its actions may be prolonged in individuals with reduced plasma cholinesterase activity, such as results from a genetic defect or from liver disease or cachexia.

Dose—*Intravenous*, *adult*, *initially*, a test dose of **10 mg** to establish the sensitivity of the patient and the recovery time, then **10 to 80 mg**; intravenous infusion, **0.5 to 10 mg per min** (usually 2 to 3 mg per min). An alternative intravenous dose is **0.5 to 1 mg/kg.** After hexafluorenium bromide (above), the intravenous dose of succinylcholine is 0.2 mg/kg. *Intramuscular*, *infants*, *children*, and *adults*, up to **2.5 mg/kg,** not to exceed a total of **150 mg.**

Dosage Forms—Injection: 100 mg/5 mL, 200 and 500 mg and 1 g/10 mL, and 100 mg/20 mL; Sterile: 500 mg and 1 g.

Tubocurarine Chloride

Tubocuraranium, 7',12'-dihydroxy-6,6'-dimethoxy-2,2',2'-trimethyl-, chloride, hydrochloride, pentahydrate; (+)-Tubocurarine Dichloride; *d*-Tubocurarine Chloride

(+)-Tubocurarine chloride hydrochloride pentahydrate [6989-98-6] $C_{37}H_{41}ClN_2O_6 \cdot HCl \cdot 5H_2O$ (771.73); *anhydrous* [57-94-3] (681.65).

Preparation—Isolated from the stems and bark of the freshly gathered plant *Chondodendron tomentosum* which is extracted with small portions of water. Refer to RPS-16 for details.

Description—White or yellowish white to grayish white, odorless, crystalline powder; melts at about 270°, with decomposition.

Solubility—1 g in 20 mL water, 45 mL alcohol; insoluble in chloroform and ether.

Uses—Tubocurarine chloride is a competitive neuromuscular blocking agent; see the general statement (page 921) for the actions, uses, side effects and drug interactions.

Tubocurarine is not absorbed from the gut. After intravenous administration it rapidly disappears from the plasma, with a distribution half-life of about 12 min; however, its terminal plasma half-life is 1 to 3 hours. The duration of action of the first dose is 10 to 30 min, but a residual effect lasting several hours has been shown. Subsequent doses may have a longer action. It is both excreted into urine (43%) and degraded in the liver and kidneys, and either renal failure or hepatic failure can prolong the half-life.

Dose—*Intramuscular* or *intravenous*, for *paralysis of limb muscles*, *initially*, **6 to 10 mg** in 30 to 90 sec, followed in 5 min by **3 to 4.5 mg** more if necessary, and for profound *abdominal relaxation* and *apnea*, 15 to 27 mg; maintenance doses are usually about one-quarter to one-third of the initial doses, given at 45- to 60-min intervals. In the presence of ether, the dose should be one-third to one-half the standard dose. In *shock therapy*, 0.165 mg/kg of body weight may be given. In the diagnosis of *myasthenia gravis*, 0.007 to 0.022 mg/kg is given. In *children*, the dose for surgical relaxation is **0.1 to 0.25 mg/kg,** the larger dose producing apnea. Tubocurarine is occasionally given intramuscularly.

Dosage Forms—Injection: 30 mg/10 mL and 60 mg/20 mL.

Other Neuromuscular Blocking Drugs

Curare—A name applied to extracts principally of the bark and of other parts of plants of certain species of *Chondodendron* or *Strychnos*, especially *Chondodendron tomentosum* and *Strychnos toxiferin*, prepared by South American Indians of the Upper Amazon and Orinoco basins for use as arrow poisons. The extracts contain neuromuscular paralysant alkaloids and numerous other contaminants. The chondodendron alkaloids contain tertiary and quaternary benzylisoquinoline derivatives such as *d*-tubocurarine (see *Tubocurarine Chloride*), *curine*, and related compounds. The strychnos alkaloids contain β-carboline alkaloids such as the toxiferins and calabash *curarines*. None of the crude preparations is currently used in therapeutics. Only purified preparations or alkaloids from *Chondodendron tomentosum* are commercially available.

Atracurium Besylate—[2-(2-Carboxyethyl)-1,2,3,4-tetrahydro-6,7-dimethoxy-2-methyl-1-veratrylisoquinolinium benzenesulfonate, pentamethylene ester [64228-81-5] $C_{65}H_{82}N_2O_{18}S_2$ (1243.49) Tracrium (*Burroughs-Welcome*).]—For the preparation see US Pat 4,179,507. An off-white powder melting about 87°. *Uses:* Atracurium is a nondepolarizing neuromuscular blocking agent. Its duration of action is only 20 to 35 min (33 to 50% of that of tubocurarine), thus lending itself to short surgical procedures. Like tubocurarine, its potency is enhanced by diethyl ether, enflurane and isoflurane, and, to a lesser extent, by halothane. Prior treatment with succinylcholine shortens the onset of action and probably increases the degree of paralysis. Anticholinesterases antagonize the actions of atracurium. Aminoglycosides, polymyxins, magnesium, lithium, quinidine, and procainamide potentiate the drug. Atracurium is much less of a histamine releaser than is tubocurarine. The half-life is 20 min. *Dose: Adults*, intravenous, 0.4 to 0.5 mg/kg as a bolus, except 0.25 to 0.35 mg/kg after enflurane or isoflurane, and 0.3 to 0.4 mg/kg after succinylcholine or in patients with myocardial dysfunction.

Centrally Acting Muscle Relaxants

The cell bodies of the somatic motor nerves lie within the spinal cord and, hence, within the central nervous system. The activity of motor neurons is not only affected by facilitatory and inhibitory modulation through feedback from contralateral and ipsilateral stretch and other receptors but also from centers in the brain. Spasticity can arise from musculoskeletal injury, which may cause aberrant afferent impulse traffic into the spinal cord, from injury to or disease of the motor nerves or related interneurons within the cord or sensory neurons in the sensory ganglia, and from disorders in the brain which alter the flow of suprasegmental impulses to the motor neurons. Involuntary movement, such as is seen in palsies, chorea, or parkinsonism, is mostly the result of impairment of feedback control within the brain.

When the disorder is musculoskeletal or is within the spinal cord, the selectivity of drugs is relatively low, because the collective neurons involved in the reflex arcs are not sufficiently qualitatively different from the motor and sensory neurons in chemical sensitivity to permit a selective depression of the hyperactive influences on the motor neuron. However, some selectivity is achieved when interneurons are involved, simply because a small effect on each converging interneuron may summate to cause a moderate decrease in interneuron input to the motor neuron. Because the interneurons are involved in the fine tuning of neuronal activity, their influences are critically balanced and hence more susceptible to pharmacological action than the motor neuron itself. Consequently, most central relaxants are *interneuron depressants*, which, however, will manifest variable depressant actions throughout the central nervous system. Interestingly, many antianxiety and some sedative drugs possess muscle relaxant activity, probably because of the high sensitivity of the critically balanced interneurons to perturbation.

In tolerated doses, the centrally acting muscle relaxants are erratic, owing to their limited selectivity. Orally, they are usually ineffective (the tolerated doses being much too low); intravenously they have some established value in treating acute muscle spasms resulting from trauma or inflammation. Motor dysfunctions which accrue to spinal cord or brain disorders are little affected.

The central relaxant effects and uses of certain benzodiazepines, like diazepam, differ from those of interneuron depressants.

Baclofen

4-Amino-3-(4-chlorophenyl)butanoic acid; Lioresal (*Ciba-Geigy*)

β-(Aminomethyl)-*p*-chlorohydrocinnamic acid [1134-47-0] $C_{10}H_{12}ClNO_2$ (213.67).

Preparation—Synthesis of baclofen by hydrogenation of β-cyano-*p*-chlorohydrocinnamic acid, in acidified ethanol in the presence of platinic oxide catalyst, is described in Swiss Pat 449,046 (*CA 69:* 106273f, 1968).

Description—Crystalline powder; melts at about 207° (190°?).

Solubility—Slightly soluble in water; poorly soluble in organic solvents.

Uses—The muscle relaxant actions of baclofen are believed to result from an action within the spinal cord, where both monosynaptic and polysynaptic reflexes are inhibited by the drug. It is an analogue of gamma-aminobutyric acid, an inhibitory neurotransmitter, but it is not certain whether the actions of baclofen are attributable to a mimetic action. Its sedative and ataxic actions are consistent with such an action in the brain.

Baclofen is used in the relief of painful spasticity in *multiple sclerosis*, for which it is more effective than diazepam. Some residual ambulatory function must be present; the drug will not make nonambulatory patients ambulatory. Although spasticity may be lessened, the gait and posture of some patients may be worsened, because of the unmasking of incoordination. Baclofen may also afford some relief in patients with *spinal cord disease* and *traumatic transverse myelopathies*. It is not indicated in musculoskeletal spastic disorders. Its efficacy in stroke, cerebral palsy, parkinsonism and Huntington's chorea has not been fully investigated.

Sedation is the most frequent adverse effect, although it is less frequent and severe than with diazepam. Its use in combination with other CNS depressants or ethanol should be avoided, if possible. Weakness may occur, but it is less handicapping than with dantrolene. Other common side effects include dizziness, insomnia, pruritus, and rashes. The drug is contraindicated when a hypersensitivity exists. Less frequent side effects include hypotension and mental confusion. Abrupt withdrawal of baclofen has been reported to result in anxiety, tachycardia, and even visual hallucinations; therefore, dosage must be discontinued gradually. In patients with epilepsy, baclofen may increase the frequency of seizures. Overdoses may cause seizures, coma, loss of brain stem reflexes, and respiratory depression. It is teratogenic, and this risk must be considered in pregnancy. It also has been found to cause ovarian cysts and enlarged or hemorrhagic adrenal glands in experimental animals.

Baclofen is rapidly absorbed orally; absorption time is approximately 2 hr. More than 80% of the drug is excreted in the urine. The elimination half-life is 3 to 4 hr.

Dose—*Oral, adult, initially,* **5 mg** 3 times a day, with **5 mg**-increments per dose at 4-day intervals until relief is achieved or **20 mg** (4 times a day) is reached, whichever occurs first. Neither the dose nor the efficacy in children has been established. The drug should be withdrawn slowly.

Dosage Form—Scored Tablets: 10 and 20 mg.

Carisoprodol

Rela (*Schering*); Soma (*Wallace*)

$$(CH_3)_2CHNHCOOCH_2\underset{\underset{CH_2CH_2CH_3}{|}}{\overset{\overset{CH_3}{|}}{C}}CH_2\,OOCNH_2$$

N-Isopropyl-2-methyl-2-propyl-1,3-propanediol dicarbamate [78-44-4] $C_{12}H_{24}N_2O_4$ (260.33).

Preparation—Synthesis of carisoprodol, which is an isopropyl meprobamate, is described in US Pat 2,937,119.

Description—White, crystalline powder; melts at about 93°.
Solubility—1 g in about 3300 mL water; soluble in many common organic solvents.

Uses—Carisoprodol is a sedative drug with muscle relaxant properties that result from reticulospinal depression. It is used to treat muscle spasm of local origin, such as results from strains, sprains, and lumbago. Part of its action may result from analgesia, sedation, and alleviation of anxiety. Onset of relief takes about 30 min; duration of action is 4 to 6 hr.

Adverse effects of the first dose of carisoprodol may include sedation, diplopia, extreme weakness, ataxia, transient quadriplegia, tachycardia, postural hypotension, syncope, mydriasis, temporary loss of vision, dizziness, confusion, irritability, agitation, depression, disorientation, and dysarthria. Usually these subside within a few hours, but they may continue in milder form throughout treatment. Nausea and vomiting, hiccough, and epigastric distress may also occur. Sedation may occur throughout treatment. The patient should be advised not to operate a motor vehicle or machinery or attempt activities requiring alertness, judgment, or complex mentation. Addiction may occur; withdrawal signs and symptoms are abdominal cramps, chills, nausea, headache, and insomnia. Pregnant or lactating mothers should not use the drug. Hypersensitivity occasionally occurs, in part attributable to tartrazine in some products; manifestations may be smarting of the eyes, asthmatic episodes, pruritus, rash,

fixed drug eruption, eosinophilia, fever, angioneurotic edema, hypotension, or anaphylaxis.

Dose—*Oral, adult,* **350 mg** 4 times a day. The drug is not recommended for children.

Dosage Form—Tablets: 350 mg.

Chlorzoxazone

2(3*H*)-Benzoxazolone-, 5-chloro-, Paraflex (*McNeil*)

5-Chloro-2-benzoxazolol [95-25-0] $C_7H_4ClNO_2$ (169.58)

Preparation—From 2-amino-5-chlorobenzoxazole (US Pat 2,895,877).

Description—White, crystalline powder; melts about 192°.
Solubility—Sparingly soluble in water; freely soluble in aqueous solutions of alkali hydroxides or ammonia.

Uses—Chlorzoxazone inhibits polysynaptic reflexes within the spinal cord and subcortical regions of the brain. It is used to decrease muscle tone and tension and thus to relieve spasm and pain associated with musculoskeletal disorders such as fibrositis, bursitis, spondylitis, sprains and muscle injury. It is of little use in spasticity resulting from lesions involving motor neurons. It also exerts sedative actions, which aid in providing relief.

Adverse effects are infrequent and are generally mild. Central nervous effects include drowsiness, vertigo, lightheadedness, headache, malaise, and occasional stimulation. Manifestations of hypersensitivity are rash, petechiae, ecchymosis, and, rarely, angioneurotic edema or anaphylaxis. Liver damage possibly occurs, so that it is wise to avoid the drug if there is a history of liver disease. Nausea and vomiting are relatively frequent, and diarrhea and gastrointestinal bleeding can also occur, so that the drug is contraindicated in peptic ulcer. Ethanol or other CNS depressants should not be taken concomitantly.

Absorption time is about 3 to 4 hr. The elimination half-life is about 60 min. More than 90% of the drug is converted to the glucuronide in the liver.

Dose—*Oral, adult,* **250 mg** 3 or 4 times a day, except *initially* **500 mg** when pain is severe. It may be increased to **750 mg** 3 or 4 times a day, if necessary. *Children,* **125** to **500 mg** 3 or 4 times a day.

Dosage Forms—Tablets: 250 mg.

Cyclobenzaprine Hydrochloride

1-Propanamine, 3-(5*H*-dibenzo[*a,d*]cyclohepten-5-ylidene)-*N,N*-dimethyl-, hydrochloride; Flexeril (*MSD*)

N,N-Dimethyl-5*H*-dibenzo[*a,d*]cycloheptene-$\Delta^{5,\gamma}$-propylamine hydrochloride [6302-23-9] $C_{20}H_{21}N\cdot HCl$ (311.84).

Preparation—Cyclobenzaprine may be synthesized by Grignard addition of α-dimethylaminopropylmagnesium chloride to 10,11-dihydro-5*H*-dibenzo[*a,d*]cycloheptene-5-one, followed by elimination of water from the resulting tertiary carbinol (Villani *et al, J Med Pharm Chem 5:* 373, 1962; see also Winthrop *et al, J Org Chem 27:* 230, 1962).

Description—White, crystalline powder; melts at about 217°; pK$_a$ 8.47 (cyclobenzaprine).
Solubility—Freely soluble in water and alcohol.

Uses—Cyclobenzaprine depresses suprasegmental (upper) motor neurons in the brainstem and, to some degree, spinal motor neurons to decrease reflex skeletal muscle activity and tonus. It inhibits both the alpha and gamma motor systems. It is used to diminish spasm and pain associated with *musculoskeletal disorders* and to increase the range of movement. The drug also has weak antimuscarinic activity.

Frequent side effects include sedation (40%), dry mouth (28%), and dizziness (11%). Weakness, fatigue, insomnia, unpleasant taste and other paresthesias, blurred vision, tachycardia, nausea, and dyspepsia are less frequent. Rarely, there may be headache, nervousness, confusion, disorientation, tremors, ataxia, depression or euphoria, hallucinations, dyspnea, sweating, constipation, urinary difficulty and retention, dysarthria, and various allergic reactions (e.g. rash, urticaria, and facial edema). The drug should be used very carefully in the presence of monoamine oxidase inhibitors, CNS depressants (including ethanol), and when antimuscarinic drugs are also being given. It is contraindicated in narrow-angle glaucoma, when there is prostatic hypertrophy, after myocardial infarction, or during congestive heart failure, heart block, conduction disturbances, tachydysrhythmias, and thyrotoxicosis.

Cyclobenzaprine is erratically absorbed. The onset of action is about 1 hr. It is highly bound to plasma albumin. It is biotransformed and conjugated to glucuronides in the liver. The elimination half-life is 1 to 3 days. Very little is excreted unchanged.

Dose—*Oral, adult,* usually **10 mg** 3 times a day, but ranges from **20 to 60 mg** a day. The duration of treatment should not exceed 2 to 3 weeks.

Dosage Forms—Tablets: 10 mg.

Diazepam—page 1062.

Meprobamate—page 1072.

Methocarbamol

1,2-Propanediol, 3-(2-methoxyphenoxy)-, 1-carbamate; Neuraxin; Robaxin (*Robins*)

3-(*o*-Methoxyphenoxy)-1,2-propanediol 1-carbamate [532-03-6] $C_{11}H_{15}NO_5$ (241.24).

Preparation—3-(*o*-Methoxyphenoxy)-1,2-propanediol participates in a transesterification reaction with ethyl carbonate in the presence of an alkaline catalyst to eliminate ethanol and produce the cyclic carbonate of the starting diol. Subsequent treatment with ammonia ruptures the cyclic carbonate ring and forms the primary carbamate of the starting compound. US Pat 2,770,649.

Description—Fine, white powder; odorless or has a slight characteristic odor; melts between 93° and 97°.

Solubility—1 g in 40 mL water; freely soluble in alcohol; sparingly soluble in chloroform.

Uses—A *centrally acting muscle relaxant.* After parenteral administration, its action is prompt and intense enough to *facilitate orthopedic procedures.* Methocarbamol is used in the *treatment of muscle spasm* resulting from injury, musculoskeletal disorders, tetanus and other disorders. It has been used with limited success in the treatment of *paralysis agitans, cerebral palsy, multiple sclerosis,* and *cerebrovascular accidents* (with spastic manifestations). Like other centrally acting skeletal muscle relaxants, it has limited effectiveness, especially by the oral route. Side effects by the oral route include drowsiness, vertigo, headache, fever, rash, itching, urticaria, gastrointestinal upsets and rarely syncope. After parenteral administration there may also be flushing, headache, muscular incoordination, nystagmus, diplopia, hypotension, bradycardia and metallic taste. These effects are minimized if the injection is given slowly at a rate of less than 300 mg/min and no more than 200 mg/injection. Extravasated injections are locally irritating and may cause sloughing or thrombophlebitis. The vehicle for commercial solutions, 50% polyethylene glycol 300, causes uremia in persons with renal dysfunction, and parenteral administration is contraindicated in the presence of renal disease. It should be avoided in pregnancy and in nursing mothers.

Dose—*Oral, initially,* **1.5 to 2 g** 4 times a day for the first 2 or 3 days, then 2.25 to 4.5 g/day in 2 to 4 divided doses. For children, the daily oral dose should not exceed 15 mg/kg. *Intramuscular,* **1 g** every 8 hours. *Intravenous,* **1 to 3 g**/day given at a rate not exceeding 3 mL (0.3 g)/min. It should not be given for more than three consecutive days.

Dosage Forms—Injection: 1 g/10 mL; Tablets: 500 and 750 mg.

Other Centrally Acting Muscle Relaxants

Chlorphenesin Carbamate [3-(*p*-Chlorophenoxy)-1,2-propanediol 1-carbamate [886-74-8] $C_{10}H_{12}ClNO_4$; Maolate (*Upjohn*)]—Chlorophenol and glycidol (2,3-epoxy-1-propanol) form 3-(*p*-chlorophenoxy)-1,2-propanediol, which is esterified with carbamoyl chloride at the 1-hydroxy position. US Pats 3,161,567 and 3,214,336. A white, crystalline powder, melting between 89° and 91°. Very slightly soluble in water; freely soluble in alcohol; sparingly soluble in chloroform. *Uses:* A centrally active skeletal muscle relaxant similar in its actions to *Methocarbamol*. It is used to diminish *skeletal muscle spasms* resulting from trauma, inflammation, vertebral disk syndrome, osteoarthritis, and rheumatoid arthritis. (In the British Commonwealth, *chlorphenesin* is used topically to treat athlete's foot.) Side effects of chlorphenesin carbamate include drowsiness, dizziness, epigastric distress, nausea, skin rash, headache, insomnia, nervousness, and agitation. Rarely, leukopenia, thrombocytopenia, pancytopenia or agranulocytosis may occur. Anaphylaxis and drug fever also have been reported. The various hypersensitivity effects may be caused, in part, by tartrazine in the commercial product. Chlorphenesin carbamate probably has an addiction liability, as do other carbamates. Persons taking the drug should not drive, operate machinery, or undertake activities that require alertness, judgment, or mentation. *Dose:* Oral, 400 to 800 mg 2 to 4 times a day.

Metaxalone [5-[(3,5-Xylyloxy)methyl]-2-oxazolidinone [1665-48-1] $C_{12}H_{15}NO_3$; Skelaxin (*Robins*)]—Preparation described in *J Am Chem Soc 82:* 1166, 1960; US Pat 3,062,827. White, crystalline powder; melts at about 123°. Very slightly soluble in water; soluble in alcohol; freely soluble in chloroform. *Uses:* Reputed to have muscle relaxant properties with a central nervous focus of action. Marketed for relief of acute muscle spasm resulting from various injuries or strains, but its efficacy is in serious question, and there seems to be no reason to use the drug in lieu of drugs that are obviously more effective. Furthermore, the toxicity of metaxalone is greater than that of more efficacious drugs; toxic effects include anorexia, nausea, vomiting, vertigo, drowsiness, nervousness, mental confusion, dry mouth, urinary retention, pruritus, dermatitis, rarely leukopenia, anemia and jaundice, and possible pyuria, albuminuria, and nephrolithiasis. It may exacerbate grand mal epilepsy. It should not be used when there is anemia, liver or renal disease or in persons with a history of such disease. *Dose:* Oral, adult, 2.4 to 3.2 g daily in 3 or 4 divided doses for no more than 10 consecutive days. Safety and effectiveness in children 12 years and below have not been established. *Dosage Form:* Tablets: 400 mg.

Antiparkinson Drugs

Some kinds of spasticity and involuntary movement arise from disorders within discrete nervous structures which contain neurons predominately of only one or two transmitter types. These disorders may be controlled more selectively by drugs directed at the particular neurotransmitters. Parkinsonism (paralysis agitans) is an example of a disorder that lends itself to such specific treatment; the antiparkinson drugs are not interneuron depressants.

The disorder in parkinsonism lies mostly within the substantia nigra and corpus striatum. The cells in the substantia nigra, which connect to the corpus striatum, are dopaminergic; in parkinsonism, the substantia nigra is deficient in dopamine. A number of striatal interneurons are cholinergic. Therefore, intervention with either dopaminergic or antimuscarinic drugs is capable of enhancing nigrostriatal activity and improving the condition. Dopaminergic intervention is the more effective, especially against the spasticity. L-Dopa, amantadine, and the amphetamines exert dopaminergic influences. Used alone, the antimuscarinic drugs are second- or third-order drugs, showing efficacy in fewer than 25% of patients, but they are often used effectively in combination with L-dopa or amantadine.

The antimuscarinic drugs can suppress the extrapyramidal effects of the antipsychotic drugs (phenothiazines, reserpine, etc.), but since they mask the tardive dyskinesias, they should not be used chronically with such drugs.

Amantadine Hydrochloride

Tricyclo[3.3.1.1^{3,7}]decan-1-amine, hydrochloride; Symmetrel (*Endo*)

1-Adamantanamine hydrochloride [665-66-7] $C_{10}H_{17}N.HCl$ (187.71).

Preparation—Adamantane is brominated to the 1-bromo compound, which is then reacted with acetonitrile in the presence of sulfuric acid to produce N-(1-adamantanyl)acetamide. Alkaline hydrolysis liberates amantadine, which is reacted with hydrogen chloride in a suitable solvent to yield the official salt.

Description—White or nearly white, odorless, crystalline powder; bitter taste; stable in light, heat, and air; does not melt up to 300°, but sublimes slowly; pK_a (30°) 10.36; pH (1 in 5 solution) between 3.0 and 5.5.

Solubility—1 g in 2.5 mL water, 5.1 mL alcohol, 18 mL chloroform, 70 mL polyethylene glycol 400.

Uses—Amantadine possesses both antiparkinsonism and antiviral activity, having been introduced as an antiviral agent. Today, its principal use is to treat *parkinsonism* and drug-induced extrapyramidal syndromes. Its use in the *prophylaxis* of A_2 *influenza virus infection* (*Asian flu*) is less well established.

In the brain, amantadine appears to increase the dopamine released from dopaminergic neurons, thus facilitating the function of the remaining nigrostriatal neuronal pathways in patients with parkinsonism. Amantadine is inferior to levodopa but somewhat superior to the antimuscarinic drugs. Patients are sometimes dramatically improved, but the usual response is moderate to mediocre. Even when the response is excellent, usually after six to eight weeks of continuous treatment the efficacy gradually wanes, and control may be lost between the second and eighteenth months. Such tolerance is minimal if the drug is used for periods of only two to three weeks, separated by intervals of several weeks. Consequently, many physicians administer the drug only for short periods, when the patient requires additional treatment. In combination with levodopa, better control is maintained than with either agent alone.

Amantadine prevents the uncoating of certain viruses in the cell. Once the virus has gained entry into the cell, the drug does not prevent viral replication and interference with cell function. Indeed, there is evidence that amantadine actually facilitates viral replication. It is thus evident that the drug can only be of value when given prior to exposure to a virus. Although in tissue cultures amantadine is effective against several types of virus, clinically the drug appears to be useful only as a prophylactic against A_2 influenza virus. It protects approximately 50% of users. Failure, in part, is due to resistant strains. In some recipients, infection is not prevented, but symptoms are less severe. It is not effective against the B_2 virus, but, fortunately, B_2 is an infrequent cause of influenza. Since amantadine is inferior to influenza vaccine as a prophylactic and is ineffective if taken after exposure to the virus, the use of the drug is limited mostly to persons who refuse vaccination or to situations in which the supply of vaccine is limited or there is too little time to complete a course of vaccination.

Amantadine may cause hyperexcitability, tremors, anxiety, ataxia, slurring of speech, insomnia, drowsiness, lethargy, psychic depression, vertigo and postural hypotension. Less frequently, it may induce dry mouth, constipation, abdominal pain, nausea, vomiting, headache, dizziness, dyspnea, fatigue, and urinary retention. Dermatitis, pruritus, and livedo reticularis occasionally occur. Edema, which may precipitate cardiac congestion, is not infrequent. Confusion and visual hallucinations are seen, especially if the recommended dose is exceeded. Alkaline phosphatase in the blood may be elevated. Amantadine exaggerates the peripheral effects of the antimuscarinic drugs used during treatment. The drug is contraindicated in epileptics. There are indications that the drug may increase the incidence of measles. Medicated persons should avoid driving or other tasks in which safety depends upon alertness.

Oral amantadine is rapidly and completely absorbed. Over 90% is excreted in the urine unchanged. The elimination half-life is 10 to 37 hr; the half-life is pH dependent, being increased at higher urine pH. It is also increased in renal impairment. It crosses the placental barrier and is also excreted into milk.

Dose—*Oral*, **100 mg** twice a day. For *children* 9 to 12 years of age, **100 mg** twice a day; for *children* 1 to 9 years of age, **4** to **9 mg/kg;** for children 9 to 12 years of age, **100 mg** twice a day. The average duration of antiviral medication is 2 weeks, although it has been used for as long as 3 months. For parkinsonism, 1 dose is taken in the morning, and the 2nd mid-day.

Dosage Forms—Capsules: 100 mg; Syrup: 50 mg/5 mL.

Amphetamine Salts—page 891.
Atropine—page 913.

Benztropine Mesylate

8-Azabicyclo[3.2.1]octane, 3-(diphenylmethoxy)-, *endo*-, methanesulfonate; Benztropine Methanesulfonate USP XVI; Cogentin Mesylate (*MSD*)

3α-(Diphenylmethoxy)-1αH,5αH-tropane methanesulfonate [132-17-2] $C_{21}H_{25}NO.CH_4O_3S$ (403.54).

Preparation—Bromodiphenylmethane, formed by bromination of diphenylmethane, is condensed with tropine, using the sodium alkoxide derivative of tropine. After purification, the benztropine base thus obtained is dissolved in a suitable organic solvent and precipitated by reaction with methanesulfonic acid.

Description—White, colorless, slightly hygroscopic, crystalline powder. Melting range 141° to 145°.

Solubility—Very soluble in water; freely soluble in alcohol; very slightly soluble in ether.

Uses—The structure of benztropine resembles both atropine and antihistaminics of the diphenhydramine type. It is thus an *antimuscarinic* drug of potency one-quarter that of atropine sulfate and an antihistaminic of potency equal to that of pyrilamine maleate. It also possesses local anesthetic properties. However, only its central actions to suppress tremor and rigidity are employed therapeutically. These actions are similar to those of atropine; but unlike atropine, it possesses sedative and other effects similar to those of diphenhydramine. Since some patients, particularly the elderly, are often excited by other antiparkinson drugs, the sedative property is of special value. Benztropine mesylate is used mainly in the treatment of *paralysis agitans* (parkinsonism; see general statement, above) to control tremor and rigidity and also to relieve sialorrhea, oculogyric crises, mask-like facies and pain secondary to muscle spasm. It is also used to treat extrapyramidal dyskinesia resulting from the use of tranquilizers, such as reserpine or chlorpromazine. It may be used alone or in combination with other drugs.

Side effects of benztropine include dry mouth, mydriasis, blurred vision, nausea, and nervousness, and less frequently they may include vomiting, mental confusion, ataxia, sedation or excitement, hallucinations, paralysis of some muscle groups, dysphagia, hyperpyrexia, rash, and difficulty in urination. As with any antimuscarinic drug, benztropine must be used cautiously in the presence of bladder neck obstruction or glaucoma.

Dose—*Oral*, *adult*, *initially* **0.5 mg** at bedtime for a week; at weekly intervals the dose may be increased by 0.5 mg until the maximal effect is reached (usually 1 to **2 mg** 2 times a day) or side effects can not be tolerated (usually less than 8 mg/day). *Intravenous*, for drug-induced extrapyramidal dyskinesia, 1 to **4 mg** once or twice a day. *Intramuscular*, *adult*, for drug-induced extrapyramidal dyskinesia, *initially*, **2 mg** followed by *oral maintenance* of 1 to **2 mg** 1 or 2 times a day.

Dosage Forms—Injection: 2 mg/2 mL; Tablets: 500 µg and 1 and 2 mg.

Biperiden

1-Piperidinepropanol, α-bicyclo[2.2.1]hept-5-en-2-yl-α-phenyl-, Akineton (*Knoll*)

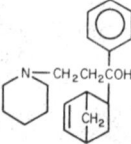

α-5-Norbornen-2-yl-α-phenyl-1-piperidinepropanol [514-65-8] $C_{21}H_{29}NO$ (311.47).

Preparation—Acetophenone undergoes Mannich condensation with formaldehyde and piperidine hydrochloride and the resulting 3-piperidinopropiophenone is grignardized in benzene with 5-chloro-2-norbornene to yield the tertiary carbinol, biperiden, which is extracted with methanol. US Pat 2,789,110.

Description—White, practically odorless, crystalline powder that is stable in light and nonhygroscopic. It melts between 112° and 116°.

Solubility—Practically insoluble in water; sparingly soluble in alcohol; freely soluble in chloroform.

Uses—Biperidin exerts *antimuscarinic* and *antiparkinson* actions similar to those of trihexyphenidyl, of which biperiden is a congener. In the treatment of *paralysis agitans* (parkinsonism) it reduces tremor, akinesia, muscle rigidity, drooling, and sweating. It also may decrease the incidence and severity of oculogyric crises. Biperiden sometimes appears to be of value in lessening spasticity in certain disorders of the pyramidal tract. In drug-induced extrapyramidal dyskinesia, biperiden may be given orally (as the hydrochloride) for mild symptoms or parenterally (as the lactate) for severe symptoms.

Untoward effects caused by biperiden result from the antimuscarinic properties and include dry mouth, blurring of vision, urinary retention, and heat stroke in hot weather. These effects are usually of low intensity and do not often result in intolerance. Less frequently, there occur drowsiness, dizziness, headache, dysuria, gastric irritation, and rash, and rarely confusion, disorientation, hallucinations, or psychotic episodes. The patient should be carefully monitored if glaucoma or urinary bladder neck obstruction exist.

Biperiden is not used as the free base but rather in salt form. The hydrochloride is used in oral medicaments and the lactate for parenteral administration (rarely necessary). Once a sufficient measure of control is obtained by parenteral administration, a switch to oral administration should be attempted.

Dose—See *Biperiden Lactate Injection* and *Biperiden Hydrochloride.*

Biperiden Hydrochloride

1-Piperidinepropanol, α-bicyclo[2.2.1]hept-5-en-2-yl-α-phenyl-, hydrochloride; Akineton Hydrochloride (*Knoll*)

α-5-Norbornen-2-yl-α-phenyl-1-piperidinepropanol hydrochloride [1235-82-1] $C_{21}H_{29}NO.HCl$ (347.93). For the structure of the base, see *Biperiden.*

Preparation—A methanolic solution of *Biperiden* is treated with a stream of hydrogen chloride.

Description—White, crystalline powder that is practically odorless and has a slightly bitter taste. It is stable in light, nonhygroscopic, and stable at ambient temperatures. It melts at about 275° with decomposition. It is optically inactive.

Solubility—Slightly soluble in water, alcohol, ether, and chloroform.

Uses—See *Biperiden.*

Dose—For *parkinsonism*, **2 mg** 3 or 4 times a day, except that *elderly patients* should begin with **1 mg** twice a day and gradually increase the dose; the above doses may be doubled, if necessary. For *drug-induced extrapyramidal dyskinesia*, **2 mg** 1 to 3 times a day.

Dosage Form—Tablets: 2 mg.

Biperiden Lactate Injection

1-Piperidinepropanol, α-bicyclo[2.2.1]hept-5-en-2-yl-α-phenyl-, compd. with 2-hydroxypropanoic acid (1:1); Akineton Lactate (*Knoll*)

α-5-Norbornen-2-yl-α-phenyl-1-piperidinepropanol lactate (salt) [7085-45-2] $C_{21}H_{29}NO.C_3H_6O_3$ (401.54). For the structure of the base, see *Biperiden.*

Preparation—*Biperiden* is reacted with aqueous lactic acid.

Uses—See *Biperiden.*

Dose—*Intramuscular*, **2 mg**. The dose may be repeated every ½-hour until symptoms are controlled, except that no more than four doses should be given in a 24-hour period. *Intravenous*, **5 mg**, injected *slowly*, no more than two doses should be given per day.

Dosage Form—Injection: 5 mg/1 mL.

Bromocriptine Mesylate

Ergotaman-3′,6′,18-trione methanesulfonate; Parlodel (*Sandoz*)

2-Bromoergocryptine monomethanesulfonate (salt) [22260-51-1] $C_{32}H_{40}BrN_5O_5.CH_3SO_3H$ (750.70).

Preparation—From N-bromosuccinimide and α-ergocryptine (US Pat 3,752,814).

Description—Yellowish-white, crystalline powder; melts about 194° with decomposition.

Solubility—Soluble in water; poorly soluble in most organic solvents.

Uses—Bromocriptine is the 2-bromo derivative of α-ergocryptine. Like all of the ergot alkaloids, it has dopamine-like agonist activity. In the treatment of *parkinsonism* it is used to supplement levodopa, when refractoriness to that agent develops. Bromocriptine also decreases the secretion of prolactin, presumably by its dopaminergic actions in the median eminence; some authorities consider dopamine to be the prolactin release-inhibiting hormone. Bromocriptine is used to treat *galactorrhea* and associated *amenorrhea* and *female infertility*. It decreases growth hormone secretion in *acromegaly* and is used to treat that disorder, mostly as an adjunct to radiotherapy or surgery; used alone, only a low percentage of remissions occur. Bromocriptine has also been used in the management of senile depression and related disorders.

The incidence of adverse effects seems to differ according to the particular clinical disorder, even when the same dosage regimen is used. When bromocriptine is used to treat galactorrhea/amenorrhea/female infertility, nearly 70% of recipients have adverse effects, whereas only about 23% have adverse effects when the drug is used to suppress physiological lactation. Adverse effect-related discontinuation of treatment occurs in 3 to 7% of cases. In parkinsonism, the incidence is complicated by the concomitant administration of levodopa. Nausea is the most frequent side effect (51%) in galactorrhea but occurs in only 7% in the postpartum patient. The incidences of other side effects are: headache, 10 to 18%; dizziness, 8 to 16%; postural hypotension, up to 28%; vomiting, 3 to 5%; fatigue, 1 to 7%; diarrhea, 0.4 to 3%; nasal congestion, up to 5%. Other less frequent side effects (mostly in parkinsonism) are occasional syncope, urinary frequency and incontinence, dyskinesias, visual disturbances, paresthesias, anxiety, nightmares, anorexia, depression, convulsions, cutaneous vasoconstriction, mottling of the skin and Raynaud's phenomenon, muscle cramps, ataxia, erythromyalgia, and rashes. There may be elevations in BUN, alkaline phosphatase, urate, CPK, SGOT, SGPT, and GPT, which are usually transient. Bromocriptine is teratogenic and may also induce spontaneous abortions. The drug is contraindicated in angina pectoris, peripheral vascular disease, pregnancy and if sensitivity to ergot alkaloids exists. Since it has been reported to cause delusions and hallucinations in postschizophrenics, it should also be withheld in patients with a history of psychoses.

The effects of bromocriptine last for 6 to 8 hr.

Dose—*Oral, adult*, for *galactorrhea* or *postpartum use*, **2.5 mg** a day with meals, to be gradually increased over a period of a week to as much as **2.5 mg** 2 or 3 times a day. In the postpartum patient, treatment is for 2 weeks; in galactorrhea/amenorrhea, treatment is for 6 months. In female infertility, barrier contraceptives should be used until a normal cycle has occurred (to protect a possible unknown pregnancy); if menstruation does not occur within 3 days of the expected date, the drug should be discontinued and a pregnancy test given. For *parkinsonism*, *initially* **2.5 mg** twice a day with meals, to be increased by increments of **2.5 mg**/day at bi- to quadra-weekly intervals, not to exceed a total of 100 mg a day.

Carbidopa

Benzenepropanoic acid, α-hydrazino-3,4-dihydroxy-α-methyl-, monohydrate, (*S*)-, Lodosyn (*MSD*); ing of Sinemet (*MSD*)

(−)-L-α-Hydrazino-3,4-dihydroxy-α-methylhydrocinnamic acid monohydrate [38821-49-7] $C_{10}H_{14}N_2O_4 \cdot H_2O$ (244.25); *anhydrous* [28860-95-9] (226.23).

Preparation—Condensation of 1-(4'-hydroxy-3'-methoxy-phenyl)-2-propanone with aqueous hydrazine and potassium cyanide forms the corresponding hydrazinenitrile, which is hydrolyzed first with HCl to convert the nitrile to amide and then refluxed with HBr to convert the amide to carboxyl and the methoxy group to OH, yielding the DL-form of carbidopa (Sletzinger *et al., J Med Chem 6:* 101, 1963). To obtain the L-form, one method involves acylation of the aforementioned hydrazinenitrile and treatment with 1-men-thoxyacetyl chloride, producing crystals which on hydrolysis yield the levorotatory compound (Karady *et al., J Org Chem 36:* 1946, 1949, 1971).

Description—White to creamy white, odorless or practically odorless, powder.
Solubility—Slightly soluble in water; practically insoluble in alcohol, chloroform, ether; freely soluble in $3N$ hydrochloric acid.

Uses—Carbidopa is an inhibitor of L-aromatic amino acid decarboxylase, often called dopa-decarboxylase. It has no direct therapeutic actions of its own but rather is used only to *protect levodopa* and L-*5-hydroxytryptophan*, both of which are decarboxylated by aromatic amino acid decarboxylase. Levodopa is 95% decarboxylated in the periphery.

Carbidopa does not enter the central nervous system in concentrations sufficient to inhibit aromatic amino acid decarboxylase there, so that its action is limited to the periphery, which is precisely what is desired. It is essential that levodopa and 5-hydroxytryptophan be decarboxylated in the brain to their respective biogenic amine products, dopamine and serotonin (5-hydroxytryptamine), which are the active agents. But in the periphery it is not desirable that these amino acids be decarboxylated, since decarboxylation not only lowers the concentration of aromatic amino acid available to the brain but also raises the concentrations of the amine products in the periphery, which give rise to some of the untoward effects of the aromatic amino acids. When carbidopa is given concomitantly with levodopa, only about 25% as much levodopa need be given, the onset of response is more rapid, pyridoxine no longer suppresses the efficacy, dietary control no longer is necessary, and certain side effects, such as nausea, vomiting, and natriuresis are diminished. The combination permits smoother control of parkinsonism than with levodopa alone.

The side effects that result from the levodopa-derived amines in the brain (psychic disturbances, dyskinesias) or the static hypotension, cardiac arrhythmias are not affected. Indeed, they may occur sooner and be more serious, if the dose of levodopa is not sufficiently reduced.

In the approved doses, carbidopa does not appear to cause adverse effects, even though the production in the periphery of dopamine and serotonin, which have natural physiological roles in the periphery, may be diminished. Therefore, side effects, precautions, and contraindications of a combination of levodopa and carbidopa are those of levodopa (see this page).

In the US, carbidopa is approved for use only in combination with levodopa. When carbidopa is added to levodopa, levodopa should first be discontinued for 8 hr, after which the combination should be given in a dose such that the levodopa component not exceed 25% of the previous daily dose. The dose may be adjusted gradually later, if necessary. The fixed-dose combination (1 carbidopa-10 levodopa) has the advantages of convenience and better patient compliance but the disadvantage that as the dose of the mixture is changed so is the degree of inhibition of the decarboxylase. Furthermore, the approved maximal daily dose of carbidopa is 200 mg, so that any daily dose of levodopa beyond 2 g/day must be made up by separate administration of levodopa, anyway.

Dose—As peripheral dopa decarboxylase is saturated by carbidopa at daily dosages of approximately 70 to 100 mg and since experience with daily dosages greater than 200 mg of carbidopa is limited, 200 mg has been established as the upper limit of carbidopa to be administered daily, in the form of *Carbidopa and Levodopa Tablets.* The *dose, oral,* of the tablets for *adults* (safety of use in patients under 18 years of age has not been established) is as follows: for persons not already taking levodopa, *initially* **10 mg** carbidopa/**100 mg** levodopa 3 times a day, adjusted upward daily or every other day until optimal dosage is reached; if nausea and vomiting (from the levodopa component) persists, tablets containing **25 mg** carbidopa/**100 mg** levodopa may be substituted, in order to increase the dosage of the carbidopa component. For persons already taking levodopa, after levodopa has been discontinued for 8 hours, a dose of Carbidopa and Levodopa Tablets that provides **25%** of the previous dose of levodopa, 3 times a day; an initial dose of **25 mg** carbidopa/**250 mg** levodopa 3 or 4 times a day is common. The dose of the combination tablets should not exceed that providing 200 mg/day of carbidopa; if more levodopa is needed than this limit permits, the excess levodopa should be administered separately. When supplemental doses of Carbidopa are needed, **25 mg** may be given *at the same time as Carbidopa/Levodopa Tablets.*

Dosage Forms—Carbidopa Tablets: 25 mg. Carbidopa and Levodopa Tablets: 10 mg carbidopa/100 mg levodopa, 25 mg carbidopa/100 mg levodopa, and 25 mg carbidopa/250 mg levodopa.

Dextroamphetamine Salts—page 891.

Diazepam—page 1062.

Diphenhydramine—page 1128.

Levodopa

L-Tyrosine, 3-hydroxy-; L-Dopa; Larodopa (*Roche*); Levopa (*SK&F*)

(−)-3-(3,4-Dihydroxyphenyl)-L-alanine [59-92-7] $C_9H_{11}NO_4$ (197.19).

Preparation—By indirect resolution of DL-3-(3,4-dihydroxyphenyl)alanine (DL-dopa). One method first converts this to DL-*N*-acetyl-3-methoxy-4-acetoxyphenylalanine and then resolves the latter with the aid of α-phenethylamine. Hydrolysis of the desired enantiomer with aqueous HBr yields levodopa. The starting DL-dopa may be synthesized commencing with vanillin and glycine.

Description—Fine, white to off-white, crystalline powder; oxidized by atmospheric oxygen in the presence of moisture and darkens.
Solubility—1 g in 10 mL $0.1N$ HCl, 250 mL water, about 555 mL alcohol, and 1000 mL chloroform.

Uses—Levodopa is the single most important drug in the treatment of incapacitating *paralysis agitans* (parkinsonism). The neurochemical basis was indicated in the introduction (page 921). It is also effective in nonincapacitating parkinsonism, but its cost and side effects are such that the use of levodopa is not warranted in many patients. Approximately 65 to 80% of patients are improved, some quite dramatically. The greatest effects are on rigidity and hypokinesia. Sialorrhea, dysphagia, seborrhea, postural instability, speech difficulties, and glabellar reflex are usually suppressed and may be abolished. Tremor and akinesia respond only erratically and require prolonged treatment, up to 6 months, before improvement ensues. All forms of parkinsonism respond; the idiopathic form responds best, but the postencephalitic form responds to lower doses; paradoxically, the postencephalitic patient may experience more severe adverse effects, including exacerbation of oculogyric crises, than patients with idiopathic or other forms of the disease. Consequently, postencephalitic patients require a conservative dose regimen that increases the dose quite slowly. Levodopa is also used to treat the parkinsonism-like neurological syndrome of *manganese intoxication*, in which there is also a deficiency of dopamine in the basal ganglia.

Levodopa is 40 to 70% absorbed orally. Less than 1% penetrates into the brain. There and throughout the body it is 99% decarboxylated to dopamine. Concurrent carbidopa (page 929) administration prevents peripheral decarboxylation and enhances availability to the brain. Peak concentrations of dopamine in the brain occur 1 to 2 hr after administration. The plasma half-life of levodopa alone is 0.5 to 1 hr; in combination with carbidopa it is 1.2 to 2.3 hr.

Nearly every patient experiences untoward effects, but only 5% find it desirable or necessary to discontinue medication. Nausea will occur in virtually all and anorexia, vomiting, flatulence, epigastric pain, and dry mouth in the majority of patients. Peptic ulceration and gastrointestinal bleeding sometimes occur. With a slow increase in dosage, the gastrointestinal side effects are less severe, and tolerance tends to develop. If nausea and vomiting are intolerable, they may be managed with non-phenothiazine, non-pyridoxine-containing antiemetics. The second most common type of side effect is the appearance of abnormal involuntary movements, which usually start with the face and tongue and gradually move downward to involve the arms, hands, and trunk. These dyskinesias are most severe 1 to 2 hr after administration. These effects are not seen immediately but progress slowly over a year's time. Eventually, nearly 75% of patients will show some such movements; however, most patients accept such movements as the price of increased mobility. The involuntary movements can be decreased by lowering the dose or the use of haloperidol or pyridoxine, but these recourses also abolish the therapeutic response to levodopa. Hypotension occurs in about 75% and orthostatic hypotension in about 30% of recipients of levodopa, but vertigo and syncope are uncommon. Cardiac arrhythmias occur occasionally. After 2 or 3 months, tolerance develops. Increased myocardial contractility, tachycardia, and atrial fibrillation may occur. Behavioral changes frequently accompany treatment with levodopa. Increased central nervous excitability, with nervousness, anxiety, insomnia, vivid dreams, tremor, and flushing occur. Paranoid ideation, delusions, hallucinations (often olfactory), delirium, and loss of judgment sometimes occur. Easy sexual arousal and loss of sexual inhibitions are common; in part this is the result of the emergence of normal desire long suppressed by physical incapacity. Serum glutamic oxaloacetate transaminase and glutamic pyruvate transaminase may be somewhat elevated early during therapy, but they usually subside later. Transient granulocytopenia may occur; agranulocytosis no longer seems to be an adverse effect since the dextro form was removed from the preparations. Dental caries is accelerated, and fillings often fall out, perhaps because the buffering effect of sialorrhea is diminished. Other miscellaneous side effects include increased pain when pain-producing pathology or headache exists, sweating, alopecia, cough, hoarseness, urinary frequency, incontinence or retention, nocturia, mydriasis, blurred vision, Horner's syndrome, fever, hot flashes, and loss or gain in weight. A mild natriuresis occurs, probably as the result of the action of dopamine formed in the kidney. Thrombocytopenia occurs rarely after long-term treatment.

Pyridoxine antagonizes levodopa, possibly by promoting premature decarboxylation (as a coenzyme to dopa decarboxylase), before the drug has penetrated into the brain. Some antagonism occurs with even as little as a Recommended Dietary Allowance, so that patients should not take multivitamin supplements containing pyridoxine. To what extent some of the central nervous side effects are attributable to pyridoxine deficiency is not known. Methyldopa and reserpine, which interfere with catecholamine synthesis and storage, exacerbate the parkinson syndrome and hence antagonize levodopa. Tricyclic antidepressants and monoamine oxidase inhibitors given concomitantly with levodopa evoke hypertensive crises and may precipitate many of the adverse central nervous side effects of levodopa, because they increase the local concentrations of dopamine formed from levodopa. Such drugs should be discontinued two weeks prior to taking levodopa. Antacids decrease gastric emptying time and thereby promote absorption, thus increasing efficacy in some patients. Levodopa is synergized by antimuscarinics.

Levodopa is contraindicated when there is evidence of uncompensated endocrine, renal, hepatic, pulmonary, or cardiovascular disease, narrow-angle glaucoma, blood dyscrasia, or hypersensitivity to the drug. It should be used cautiously in diabetes, hyperthyroidism, wide-angle glaucoma, epilepsy, hypotension, or when antihypertensives are being used. The drug should be discontinued 24 hours prior to anesthesia. Levodopa is a precursor of melanin and may activate latent malignant melanoma; it should be withheld from persons with a history of malignant melanoma or suspicious skin lesions.

Dose—*Initially*, **100 mg** to **1 g**/day in divided doses (usually **250 mg** 4 times a day) with meals. The dose is gradually increased in increments of **100** to **750 mg**/day at 3- to 7-day intervals until intolerable side effects occur, usually abnormal movements; the *maintenance* dose is usually **2.5** to **6 g**/day and should not exceed 8 g. After a prolonged period of stabilized response, the dose can sometimes be moderately decreased without loss of control.

Dosage Forms: Capsules: 100, 125, 250, and 500 mg; Tablets: 100, 250, and 500 mg.

Trihexyphenidyl Hydrochloride

1-Piperidinepropanol, α-cyclohexyl-α-phenyl-, hydrochloride; Artane (*Lederle*); Pipanol (*Winthrop*); Tremin (*Schering*)

α-Cyclohexyl-α-phenyl-1-piperidinepropanol hydrochloride [52-49-3] $C_{20}H_{31}NO.HCl$ (337.93).

Preparation—From a Mannich reaction of acetophenone, piperidine and formaldehyde. The piperidinopropiophenone formed is treated as for *procyclidine*.

Description—White or slightly off-white, crystalline powder, having no more than a very faint odor; melts between 247° and 253°, with slight decomposition.

Solubility—Slightly soluble in water; soluble in alcohol and chloroform.

Use—Trihexyphenidyl has weak *antimuscarinic* and *antispasmodic* activity. In the treatment of parkinsonism it is preferred to levodopa in patients with mild to moderate nonincapacitating symtoms, and most neurologists prefer to begin treatment of all cases with trihexyphenidyl. It is effective in all forms of the disease, although not uniformly. It is most effective against rigidity, but it is also useful in the relief of akinesia, tremor, sialorrhea, and oculogyria. Tolerance may develop, but not necessarily so. Trihexyphenidyl is also useful in the treatment of *drug-induced extrapyramidal symptoms*.

The adverse effects of trihexyphenidyl mostly derive from its antimuscarinic actions, but they are much less troublesome than with atropine. The most frequent are dry mouth, blurred vision, tachycardia, constipation, dry skin, nervousness, headache, sedation, and muscle weakness. Some of these effects subside after continued administration. Sometimes insomnia may occur. Urinary retention is infrequent, but it does occur. Occasionally, vomiting, severe tinnitus, vertigo, suppurative parotitis, or rash occur and may require discontinuation of medication. With large doses, inability to concentrate, impaired memory, disorientation, and confusion may occur, and if the dose is not reduced, they are followed by agitation, excitement, delirium, visual hallucinations, and psychoses. Elderly patients or persons with arteriosclerosis are especially susceptible to the adverse central effects. Trihexyphenidyl should be used cautiously in persons with cardiovascular or liver pathology, glaucoma, bladder neck obstruction, prostatitis, hyperthyroidism, or arteriosclerosis, and in elderly patients. There appear to be no likely important drug interactions. Trihexyphenidyl may be combined with other antiparkinson drugs.

Dose—*Oral, adult, initially* **1 mg** on the first day, after which the dose may be increased in increments of 2 mg/day at intervals of 3 to 5 days until symptoms are adequately controlled without the supervention of serious adverse effects; the *maintenance* dose is usually **6 to 10 mg**/day in 3 to 4 divided doses, but the dose may be even larger if necessary and required, up to a limit of 20 mg. Before timed-release forms are used, the dose with the normal tablet should be established. Timed-release forms are erratic.

Dosage Forms—Elixir: 2 mg/5 mL; Tablets: 2 and 5 mg; Sustained-release Capsules: 5 mg.

Phenelzine Sulfate—page 1096.

Other Antiparkinson Drugs

Chlorphenoxamine Hydrochloride—2-[(p-Chloro-α-methyl-α-phenylbenzyl)oxy]-N,N-dimethylethylamine hydrochloride [562-09-4] $C_{18}H_{22}ClNO.HCl$ (340.29) Phenoxene (*Dow*)]—Prepared from a methyl grignard reagent and p-chlorobenzoquinone; the resulting alcohol etherified with 2-(dimethylamino)ethyl chloride and converted to the hydrochloride (US Pat 2,785,202). A white crystalline powder melting about 133°. Very soluble in water or alcohol. *Uses:* Chlorphenoxamine is an antimuscarinic drug used for its central effects as an adjunct to other drugs to reduce muscle rigidity and akinesia in certain patients with *Parkinson's disease*. Speech, gait, and posture are frequently markedly improved, but it has little effect on tremor. Tolerance gradually develops. Chlorphenoxamine causes sedation (owing to diphenhydramine-like properties), vertigo, dry mouth, nausea, indigestion, or anorexia in one-fifth of cases. Other side effects include vomiting, burning sensation in the mouth, numbness and swelling of the extremities, epigastric pressure, nervousness, excessive sweating, blurred vision, confusion, apathy, asthenia, swelling of the feet, and urinary retention. It should not be used in patients with glaucoma, urinary retention, prostatic hypertrophy or other bladder neck obstruction, gastrointestinal obstruction, organic cardiospasm, or stenosing peptic ulcer. Because of the sedative effects, patients should be warned to drive carefully and should be warned about work hazards. Chlorphenoxamine increases the central depressant effects of barbiturates and probably all other sedative-hypnotic drugs, so that care must be taken to avoid adverse drug interactions. *Dose: Oral, adult, initially* 50 to 100 mg 3 to 4 times a day, followed by downward (by discontinuing one dose) or upward adjustments to as much as 100 mg 4 times a day.

Cycrimine Hydrochloride—α-Cyclopentyl-α-phenyl-1-piperidinepropanol hydrochloride [126-02-3] $C_{19}H_{29}NO.HCl$ (323.91) Pagitane (*Lilly*)—Prepared from piperidine, acetophenone, paraformaldehyde and hydrochloric acid in a typical Mannich reaction. The piperidinopropiophenone formed is treated with a cyclopentyl grignard reagent to produce the base with subsequent conversion to the hydrochloride. White, odorless solid; melts about 241° with decomposition. Soluble 1 g in about 175 mL of water or 50 mL of alcohol; a 1 in 200 aqueous solution has a pH between 5.2 and 5.8. *Uses:* Cycrimine is an antimuscarinic drug closely related to *Trihexyphenidyl* (page 931). It is one-half as potent as atropine as an antispasmodic and mydriatic and one-tenth as potent against the cardiac vagus and sialorrhea. It also has local anesthetic activity. It is slightly less potent than atropine in its central actions. It is used in the treatment of all forms of *paralysis agitans* (parkinsonism). Side effects of cycrimine include dry mouth, soreness of the mouth and tongue, blurred vision, epigastric distress, anorexia and nausea, weakness, and occasionally vertigo, restlessness, confusion or disorientation. Caution should be observed in elderly patients with arteriosclerosis, glaucoma, or any tendency toward urinary retention. *Dose: Oral, initially* 1.25 mg for idiopathic and arteriosclerotic and 5 mg for postencephalitic parkinsonism, to be given 2 to 3 times a day; at weekly intervals, the daily dose may be increased by 1.25 mg until symptoms are controlled or serious side effects supervene; the *maintenance* dose usually ranges from 3.75 to 15 mg/day, but it may be as high as 40 mg.

Ethopropazine Hydrochloride [10-[2-(Diethylamino)propyl]phenothiazine monohydrochloride [1094-08-2] $C_{19}H_{24}N_2S.HCl$; Parsidol (*Warner-Chilcott*)]—2-(Diethylamino)propyl bromide is converted to a Grignard complex and reacted with phenothiazine to give ethopropazine base. US Pat 2,607,773. A white or off-white, crystalline powder; melts at about 210°, with decomposition. Slightly soluble in water; soluble in alcohol and chloroform. *Uses:* A phenothiazine with both antimuscarinic and antihistaminic properties; used in the management of *paralysis agitans*, especially for control of rigidity. It may, however, also diminish spasm, tremor, and sialorrhea and prevent oculogyric crises. Except for its effects on oculogyric crises, authorities consider ethopropazine to be inferior to other antimuscarinic drugs used to treat parkinsonism; and it causes as many or more side effects, including exacerbation of parkinsonism. Side effects include sedation, vertigo, lassitude, inability to concentrate, confusion, dry mouth, blurred vision, and epigastric distress. Less frequent effects are paresthesias, heavy feeling in the limbs, ataxia, muscular cramps, rash, hypotention (in large doses) and, rarely, agranulocytosis; symptoms of parkinsonism are sometimes worsened. It should be used cautiously in patients who drive, operate machinery, or who have glaucoma, urinary tract obstruction, or gastrointestinal obstruction. It can enhance the central depression caused by sedative-hypnotic drugs or antihistamines, and such untoward drug interactions should be avoided. *Dose: Oral, initially* 50 mg once or twice a day; increase gradually if necessary. Patients with mild to moderate symptoms are frequently controlled with 100 to 400 mg daily. Severe cases may require doses gradually increased to 500 or 600 mg or more daily.

Lergotrile Mesylate—[2-Chloro-6-methyl-8β-acetonitrile monomethanesulfonate [51473-23-5] $C_7H_{18}ClN_3.CH_4S$ (395.90); (*Lilly*)].—A synthetic nonpeptide ergot derivative. *Uses:* Lergotrile has actions and uses like those of bromocriptine (page 929), except its usefulness in acromegaly remains to be demonstrated. Adverse effects include postural hypotension, various changes in CNS functions, including alterations in

behaviour and mood, and depression of liver function accompanied by changes in the index serum enzymes. It is probable that other side effects characteristic of bromocriptine will be reported. *Dose: Oral, adult*, 11 to 52 mg a day has been reported.

Orphenadrine Citrate—N,N-Dimethyl-2-[(o-methyl-α-phenylbenzyl)oxy]ethylamine citrate (1:1) [4682-36-4] $C_{18}H_{23}NO.C_6H_8O_7$ (461.51). Norflex (*Riker*)—Prepared from 2-methylbenzhydrol and 2-(dimethylamino)ethanol and the base converted to the salt with citric acid (US Pat 2,991,225). White, crystalline powder melting about 136°. Solubility about 1 g in 70 mL water or 400 mL alcohol. *Uses:* Orphenadrine, a methyl analogue of the antihistamine diphenhydramine, has weak antihistaminic and mild anticholinergic activities. Early pharmacologic reports noted that the drug reduces voluntary muscle spasm by a central effect, and possible utility in Parkinson's disease was suggested. Indications for the citrate are given as an adjunct for relief of discomfort associated with acute painful musculoskeletal conditions, by a mode of action not clearly identified but that may be related to the analgesic properties of the compound. Orphenadrine sometimes induces mild excitement and also a mild euphoria in fatigued or depressed patients. Peripheral atropine-like actions are weak, but blurred vision, dry skin, and dry mouth may occur. Other side effects include nausea, vertigo, rash, headache, dizziness, drowsiness, constipation, increased intraocular pressure, weakness, mental confusion, and occasional hallucinations. Orphenadrine is contraindicated in patients with acute-angle closure glaucoma or myasthenia gravis. It should be used cautiously in patients with gastrointestinal obstruction, urinary retention, urinary tract obstruction, or tachycardia; propoxyphene appears to interact to increase mental confusion, anxiety, and tremors. The manufacturer's recommendation of a longer interval between doses is based on the retarding effect of the plasticized matrix in which the citrate is compounded in the tablet dosage form. The citrate may be given parenterally. *Dose: Oral, adult*, initially 50 mg 3 times a day; may be increased to 100 mg 4 times a day.

Pergolide Mesylate [8-(Methylthio)methyl]-6-propylergoline [66104-23-2] $C_{19}H_{26}N_2S.CH_4O_3$ (410.59); (*Lilly*)].—A synthetic ergot derivative. *Uses:* Pergolide has actions and uses like those of bromocriptine (page 929). Side effects include nausea and vomiting, postural hypotension, premature ventricular contractions, confusion and hallucinations, dyskinesias, and elevated SGOT. It is likely that other side effects like those of bromocriptine will eventually be reported. The duration of action exceeds 24 hr. *Dose:* The optimal doses have yet to be established. *Oral, adult*, for *parkinsonism*, 0.1 to 10 mg a day, and, for *galactorrhea/amenorrhea/female infertility*, 0.15 to 0.25 mg a day have been reported.

Procyclidine Hydrochloride—[α-Cyclohexyl-α-phenyl-1-pyrrolidinepropanol hydrochloride [1508-76-5] $C_{19}H_{29}NO.HCl$ (323.91) Kemadrin (*Burroughs-Wellcome*).]—Prepared from the cyclohexyl grignard reagent and 3-(1-pyrrolidinyl)propiophenone; the resulting base then converted to the hydrochloride. White, crystalline powder melting about 226°. Solubility about 1 g in 33 mL of water; more soluble in alcohol. *Uses:* Procyclidine is an antimuscarinic drug used mostly as a substitute for trihexyphenidyl in the treatment of parkinsonism when the latter drug fails to control symptoms, but some physicians prefer to start with procyclidine. Sometimes procyclidine is used in combination with other drugs. The side effects, precautions, and contraindications of procyclidine are those of trihexyphenidyl. *Dose: Oral*, adult, initially 2 to 2.5 mg 2 or 3 times a day, after meals. The dose may be gradually increased by increments of 2.5 mg/day until symptoms are satisfactorily controlled or intolerable side effects supervene; the usual *maintenance* dose is 10 to 20 mg/day, but as much as 60 mg may be required.

CHAPTER 50

Diuretic Drugs

Ewart A Swinyard, PhD DSc (Hon)

Professor Emeritus of Pharmacology
College of Pharmacy and School of Medicine
University of Utah
Salt Lake City, UT 84112

Diuretics are drugs used to increase the volume of urine excreted by the kidneys. They are employed principally for the relief of edema and ascites. These conditions occur in diseases of the heart, kidneys, and liver. Diuretics are most effective in the treatment of cardiac edema, particularly that associated with congestive heart failure. They are also used in the ascites of cirrhosis, the nephrotic syndrome, diabetes insipidus, hypertension, edema of pregnancy, and to reduce cerebrospinal and intraocular fluid pressure. Some diuretics have highly *specialized* uses in glaucoma, hyperpotassemia, bromide intoxication, anginal syndrome, epilepsy, migraine, hypertension, and in premenstrual depression, conditions in which edema is not present or at least not definitely established.

The formation of urine from the blood, in simplest terms, consists of glomerular filtration and selective tubular reabsorption and secretion. As the glomerular filtrate passes through the tubules, substances essential to the blood and tissues—water, glucose, salts, and amino acids—are reabsorbed. Other substances in the glomerular filtrate, such as urea, are not as readily absorbed by the tubules. Thus, it is thought that in the renal tubule there is a specific mechanism for the transport of each ionic species, the capacities of which are quite different. For example, the capacity of the renal tubule to reabsorb sulfate ion is limited. The tubular capacity for the reabsorption of phosphate is such that sufficient is reabsorbed to maintain the normal extracellular level and any excess is excreted. On the other hand, much larger amounts of bicarbonate ion and chloride ion can be reabsorbed.

Under normal circumstances the glomerular filtration rate is about 100 mL/min. About 99 mL of the fluid is returned to the blood and only 1 mL is excreted as urine. It follows, therefore, that drugs may increase the rate of urine formation in two ways: (1) by increasing glomerular filtration and (2) by depressing tubular reabsorption. Increasing glomerular filtration is *not* an efficient mechanism and usually causes only a moderate increase in urine formation. If, for example, the percent of fluid reabsorbed by the renal tubules is assumed to remain constant, glomerular filtration rate would have to be increased twofold in order to double the urinary output. On the other hand, a 1% decrease in the tubular reabsorption of water, induced either by the administration of excessive quantities of electrolytes or nonelectrolytes (osmotic diuretics) or by agents which alter selective reabsorption of substances in the renal tubules, would double the urinary output.

Most diuretics block sodium and/or chloride reabsorption in the renal tubules. This results in natriuresis and diuresis. However, the mechanism(s) by which diuretics block the reabsorption and the site of action varies; they may act at either the proximal tubule, loop of Henle, distal tubule, collecting tubule or combinations of these sites. The *osmotic diuretics* are thought to produce diuresis by multiple mechanisms. Mannitol, the most widely used osmotic diuretic, is filtered at the glomerulus and is not reabsorbed by the renal tubules. Because of its osmotic action in the proximal tubules, mannitol prevents the reabsorption of water and impairs sodium reabsorption by lowering the concentration of sodium in the tubular fluid. In the loop of Henle, mannitol reduces medullary hypertonicity by increasing medullary blood flow. In the collecting duct, it reduces sodium and water reabsorption because of papillary washout, high flow rate, or some other factor. The *carbonic anhydrase inhibitors* (eg acetazolimide) act on the proximal convolution and possibly the collecting tubule, via the intermediate step of adenyl cyclase inhibition, to decrease bicarbonate reabsorption and passive forces favoring chloride reabsorption. The excess chloride (with accompanying sodium) is subsequently reabsorbed in the loop of Henle. Thus, sodium bicarbonate is excreted and the total diuretic effect is minimal. Although potassium excretion is increased during initial therapy with carbonic anhydrase inhibitors, clinically significant hypokalemia is seldom a problem. After several days of continuous administration, a mild hyperchloremic acidosis develops, which decreases the diuretic effect.

Thiazide diuretics act mainly to block sodium and chloride reabsorption at the *first (thick) portion* of the *distal tubules*. They also have a *mild anti-carbonic anhydrase* effect. The resulting natriuresis is accompanied by increased excretion of potassium, bicarbonate, chloride, and water. Unlike carbonic anhydrase inhibitors, thiazide diuretics are effective even though systemic acidosis or alkalosis may be present. The *antihypertensive* action of the *thiazides* is attributable to two factors: (1) *depletion of sodium* and subsequent reduction in *plasma volume* and (2) a *decrease in peripheral resistance*. The latter is thought to be due either to the loss of sodium from the arteriolar wall or a direct action on the vascular bed. In addition, there is some *inhibition* of the *pressor activity of norepinephrine*. In contrast, the antihypertensive effect of *chlorthalidone* is thought to be due to a *decreased cardiac output*.

The *potassium-sparing diuretics* (*spironolactone, triamterene*, and *amiloride*) interfere with sodium absorption in the late distal tubules and cortical collecting ducts, thereby promoting sodium excretion while conserving potassium. Spironolactone is a competitive inhibitor of aldosterone, whereas triamterene and amiloride interfere directly with electrolyte transport. These agents are not potent diuretics when used alone but, when combined with a thiazide (eg Aldactizide), they reduce potassium loss, increase sodium excretion, and minimize alkalosis. In addition, the onset of diuresis with combination therapy is much more rapid than with spironolactone alone (4 to 7 days). The *loop diuretics*, such as *furosemide, ethacrynic acid*, and *bumetanide*, act mainly on the medullary and cortical portions of the *thick ascending loop of Henle*. This action reduces the osmotic gradient in the renal medulla and impairs both the concentrating and diluting capacities of the kidney. Since furosemide also induces significant kaluresis, supplemental administration of potassium is often necessary. Ethacrynic acid induces a greater excretion of chloride than sodium; however, it can produce systemic alkalosis. Ethacrynic acid continues to be effective in the presence of alkalosis. It is also useful in cases of edema refractory to other drugs.

Contraindications and adverse effects resulting from diuretic therapy are usually due to electrolyte imbalance induced by these agents. All commonly employed diuretics can produce acute and chronic sodium depletion, hypokalemia, hyperglycemia, hyperuricemia, as well as alterations in chloride, magnesium, and calcium balance. Osmotic diuretics must be used with caution because they can produce a marked increase in extracellular fluid volume and may induce pulmonary edema. Hypersensitivity to diuretic agents is frequently encountered. Also, blood dyscrasias, pancreatitis (thiazides), decreased glucose tolerance (thiazides and ethacrynic acid), and ototoxicity (intravenous ethacrynic acid) are occasionally encountered during diuretic therapy.

Concurrent administration of diuretic agents and other drugs results in some of the most frequently encountered drug *interactions.* A common example is the prescribing of a *cardiac glycoside* and a *diuretic;* the diuretic-induced hypokalemia potentiates the cardiotoxicity of the glycoside. The adverse interaction can be minimized by either increasing potassium intake (potassium supplements, diet, or potassium-sparing diuretic) or by administering the diuretic intermittently (allows homeostatic mechanisms to correct imbalance). Other examples of adverse interactions include loss of blood sugar control in diabetic patients given thiazides, furosemide, or ethacrynic acid; more intensive skeletal muscle blockade in patients on certain muscle relaxants and hypokalemic-inducing diuretics; orthostatic hypotension induced by concurrent administration of methyldopa, guanethidine, or a ganglionic blocking agent and a diuretic; increased incidence of ototoxicity when patients on aminoglycoside antibiotics (gentamicin, kanamycin, neomycin, and streptomycin) are given diuretics reported to cause ototoxicity (ethacrynic acid and furosemide); increased incidence of nephrotoxicity when patients on cephaloridine are given diuretics which have nephrotoxic effects (ethacrynic acid and furosemide); hyperkalemia when potassium salts are administered with triamterene; disruption of uricosuric therapy by administration of a diuretic which increases plasma uric acid levels (thiazides); and an increased anticoagulant effect induced by displacement of warfarin from protein binding sites (thiazides). Thoughtful management of these interactions will not only result in improved patient response, but will also spare the patient unnecessary inconvenience and expense.

Agents employed clinically as diuretics may be divided into two groups: (1) osmotic diuretics and (2) renal tubular inhibiting diuretics. In this presentation a third category, miscellaneous renal agents, is provided for probenecid, an agent which is not a diuretic but inhibits renal tubule reabsorption of uric acid and blocks the renal excretion of a number of substances.

Osmotic Diuretics

The capacity of the renal tubule to reabsorb various electrolytes and nonelectrolytes is limited and, as previously mentioned, varies for each ionic species. If large amounts of these substances are administered to an individual, their concentration in the body fluids and, subsequently, in the glomerular filtrate exceeds the reabsorption capacity of the tubule, and the excess appears in the urine accompanied by an increased volume of water. Traditionally, substances which increase urine formation in this manner are called osmotic diuretics. It is now known, however, that osmotic diuretics, such as mannitol, exert several important mechanisms of action. For example, it has been shown to increase renal plasma flow and glomerular hydrostatic pressure secondary to vasodilatation of the afferent arteriole. Thus, it appears

that osmotic agents have multiple sites of action; nevertheless their major component probably is a decrease in medullary solute content resulting in less water reabsorption from the thin descending limb of Henle and collecting duct and less sodium chloride reabsorption in the ascending limb of Henle.

The major toxic effect of osmotic diuretics is related to the amount of solute administered and its effect on the volume and distribution of body fluids. For example, following the administration of mannitol it is distributed throughout the extracellular fluid; consequently, the administration of hypertonic solutions sufficient to make a significant contribution to extracellular osmolarity will be accompanied by a significant expansion of extracellular fluid volume, largely at the expense of intracellular fluid volume. In edematous states accompanied by diminished cardiac reserve, the use of mannitol introduces a risk which far outweighs any advantages. Also, a variety of signs and symptoms suggestive of hypersensitivity reactions have accompanied the use of some osmotic diuretics.

This group of diuretics includes osmotic electrolytes (potassium and sodium salts), osmotic nonelectrolytes (urea, glucose, sucrose, and mannitol), and acid-forming salts (ammonium and calcium salts). The acid-forming salts have only limited use as primary diuretics; their chief value is for the potentiation of mercurial diuretics.

Acacia—page 1296.

Ammonium Chloride

Muriate of Ammonia; Sal Ammoniac

Ammonium chloride [12125-02-9] NH_4Cl (53.49).

Preparation—By the following processes: 1. The ammoniacal liquid obtained from gas works during the destructive distillation of coal is neutralized with HCl and the crude product is subsequently purified. 2. The vapors of ammonia from synthetic processes are absorbed in HCl. 3. As a by-product in the Solvay process for sodium bicarbonate.

Description—Colorless crystals, or a white, fine or coarse crystalline powder; has a cool, saline taste, and is somewhat hygroscopic; when dissolved in water the temperature of the solution is lowered; a pH (1 in 20 solution) between 4.6 and 6.0.

Solubility—1 g in 3 mL water, 100 mL alcohol, 8 mL glycerin.

Uses—A *diuretic, systemic acidifier,* and *expectorant.* Ammonium chloride is a combination of a labile cation and a fixed anion. When the ammonium ion is converted to urea, the liberated hydrogen ion reacts with bicarbonate and other body buffers. The end result is that chloride ion displaces bicarbonate ion; the latter is converted to CO_2. Thus, the chloride load to the kidneys is increased and an appreciable amount escapes reabsorption along with an equivalent amount of cation (predominantly sodium) and an isoosmotic quantity of water. This is the basic mechanism by which ammonium chloride brings about a net loss of extracellular fluid and promotes the mobilization of edema fluid.

Ammonium chloride is sometimes employed alone for its diuretic action but usually it is given in conjunction with mercurial diuretics, the action of which it potentiates.

The fact that ammonium chloride causes systemic acidosis makes the salt of some value in the treatment of alkalosis. It also renders the urine acid and is prescribed for this purpose in conjunction with methenamine. In the rare instances when it is desired to produce an acidosis, ammonium chloride may be used. An example is in the treatment of lead poisoning where an acidosis is desired to hasten the excretion of lead.

Dose—*Oral,* 4 to 12 g daily; *usual, oral,* 1 to 2 g 4 times a day; *intravenous,* 100 to 1000 mL of 2% solution; *usual, intravenous,* 500 mL of a 2% solution is infused over a 3-hour period.

Other Dose Information—The oral dose may vary from 8 to 12 g daily in divided doses. The drug is usually taken with or after meals to avoid gastric irritation.

Dosage Forms—Injection: 160 mg/30 mL, 600 mg/100 mL, 10.7 g/500 mL, 21.4 g/1000 mL; Tablets: 500 mg and 1 g.

Glucose, Liquid—page 1313.

Mannitol

Mannite; Manna Sugar; Osmitrol (*Travenol*);
Resectisol (*Amer. McGaw*)

$$HOCH_2-\overset{\displaystyle H}{\underset{\displaystyle OH}{C}}-\overset{\displaystyle H}{\underset{\displaystyle OH}{C}}-\overset{\displaystyle OH}{\underset{\displaystyle H}{C}}-\overset{\displaystyle OH}{\underset{\displaystyle H}{C}}-CH_2OH$$

D-Mannitol [69-65-8] $C_6H_{14}O_6$ (182.17).

Preparation—May be extracted from manna and other natural sources with hot alcohol or other selective solvents. Commercially it is produced by catalytic or electrolytic reduction of certain monosaccharides such as mannose and glucose. Manufacture is somewhat complicated by the need for separation of stereoisomers.

Description—White, crystalline powder or free-flowing granules, odorless and having a sweetish taste; density about 1.52 at 20°; melts between 165° and 168°; pK_a (19°) 3.4.

Solubility—1 g in about 5.5 mL water; slightly soluble in pyridine; very slightly soluble in alcohol; soluble in alkaline solutions; practically insoluble in ether.

Uses—A *diuretic* and a *diagnostic agent for kidney function*. The intravenous administration of hypertonic solutions of mannitol is used to promote an *osmotic diuresis*. It is a useful adjunct in the treatment of acute renal failure before irreversible renal failure becomes established. It is also used to reduce intracranial pressure and to treat cerebral edema by reducing brain mass; to reduce intraocular pressure when elevated pressure is not amenable to other therapy, and to promote urinary excretion of toxic substances. Mannitol is superior to dextrose in that it is only slightly metabolized in the body and is only slightly reabsorbed by the renal tubule. Mannitol, although it requires a larger volume, produces fewer side effects than urea and is equally effective. Isolated cases of adverse reactions, such as pulmonary congestion, fluid and electrolyte imbalances, acidosis, electrolyte loss, dryness of the mouth, thirst osmotic nephrosis, marked diuresis, urinary retention, edema, headache, blurred vision, convulsions, nausea, vomiting, rhinitis, diarrhea, arm pain, thrombophlebitis, chills, dizziness, urticaria, dehydration, hypotension, hypertension, and anginal-like chest pains, have been reported during or following mannitol infusion. Its safe use during pregnancy and in children under 12 years of age has not been established.

Since only a negligible amount of mannitol which appears in the glomerular filtrate is reabsorbed by the renal tubule, mannitol has been employed for the measurement of *glomerular filtration rate*.

Dose—*Usual, intravenous infusion*, **50 to 200 g** daily.

Other Dose Information—The usual *diuretic* dose is 50 to 100 g, administered as a 5 to 20% solution.

Dosage Forms—Injection: 5 and 10% (in 500 and 1000 mL), 15% (in 150 and 500 mL), 20% (in 250 and 500 mL), 25% (in 50 mL); Mannitol and Sodium Chloride Injection (see below): *of each ingredient*—5 and 0.3% (in 500 and 1000 mL), 10 and 0.3% (in 500 and 1000 mL), 15 and 0.45% (in 150 and 500 mL), 20 and 0.45% (in 250 and 500 mL).

Mannitol and Sodium Chloride Injection [(*Various Mfrs*)]—A sterile solution of mannitol and sodium chloride in water for injection. It contains no bacteriostatic agents. *Description:* pH between 4.5 and 7. *Uses* and *Dose: See Mannitol.*

Potassium Acetate—page 837.

Potassium Chloride—page 834.

Potassium Citrate—RPS-16, page 777.

Sodium Bicarbonate—page 796.

Sodium Biphosphate—RPS-16, page 875.

Sodium Chloride—page 835.

Sodium Sulfate—page 804.

Sucrose—page 1290.

Urea

Carbonyldiamide; Ureaphil (*Abbott*); Urevert (*Travenol*)

$$CO(NH_2)_2$$

Carbamide [57-13-6] CH_4N_2O (60.06).

Preparation—Urea, a product of the metabolism of proteins, is excreted in human urine in average amounts of 30 g/day. In 1828 Wöhler obtained it on evaporating a solution containing potassium cyanate and ammonium sulfate, the ammonium cyanate first produced isomerizing to urea—reputedly the first synthesis of an organic compound from inorganic material.

A large-scale process for preparing urea is by heating calcium cyanamide with water under pressure:

$$CaNCN + 3H_2O \rightarrow CO(NH_2)_2 + Ca(OH)_2$$

Description—Colorless to white, prismatic crystals or a white, crystalline powder; almost odorless and has a cooling, saline taste; may gradually develop a slight odor of ammonia, especially in the presence of moisture; melts between 132° and 135°; aqueous solutions are neutral to litmus, but on standing or heating, decompose into NH_3 and CO_2; pK_a (21°) 0.1.

Solubility—1 g in 1.5 mL water, 10 mL alcohol; practically insoluble in chloroform or ether.

Uses—Urea is used *intravenously* as an *osmotic diuretic* for the reduction of intracranial pressure (in the control of cerebral edema) and of intraocular pressure. It is also used topically to hydrate and remove excess keratin from dry skin (see page 773). Adverse reactions include headache, nausea, vomiting, syncope, disorientation, transient confusion, and electrolyte depletion (hyponatremia and hypokalemia). Extravasation at the site of injection can cause local reactions. The infusion should never be mixed with blood in a transfusion set. Urea is contraindicated in patients with severely impaired liver and kidney function and in patients with active intracranial bleeding.

Dose—*Usual, intravenous infusion*, **100 mg** to **1 g/kg** daily, as a 30% solution in dextrose injection at a rate not exceeding 4 mL/min. *Children*, *over 2 years of age*, **0.5** to **1.5 g/kg** body weight; under 2 years of age, **0.1 g/kg** body weight may be adequate.

Dosage Forms—Sterile: 40 and 90 g.

Renal Tubular Inhibiting Diuretics

The most powerful and consistently effective diuretics are those which depress tubular mechanisms responsible for the active reabsorptive transport of certain ions. Drugs which induce diuresis in this way may be divided into five groups: carbonic anhydrase inhibitors, benzothiadiazine and related derivatives, potassium-sparing diuretics, loop diuretics, and other renal tubular inhibiting diuretics. The mechanisms, uses, and limitations of these several groups of diuretics will be discussed in the introductory statement to the respective section.

Carbonic Anhydrase Inhibitors

Carbonic anhydrase is an ubiquitous enzyme responsible for the catalytic reversible hydration of carbon dioxide and dehydration of carbonic acid, a process critical to the transport of carbon dioxide in the erythrocyte and its exchange in the parenchyma of the lungs. This enzyme is also found in the renal cortex, gastric mucosa, pancreas, eye, and central nervous system. The renal tubular cells also contain substantial amounts of carbonic anhydrase, and the CO_2 produced metabolically in the cells of the renal tubule is immediately converted to carbonic acid by the enzyme. Urine is acidified by secretion of hydrogen ions derived from carbonic acid formed in the proximal tubular cells in exchange for sodium ions in the lumen of the tubule. When carbonic anhydrase is inhibited, via adenyl cyclase stimulation, the amount of hydrogen ions available for exchange with sodium is decreased; the excess sodium ions retained in the tubule combine with bicarbonate and are excreted by the kidney with an increased volume of water and a loss of potassium. The diuretic effect is self-limiting when it is administered for longer than 48 hours, since the subsequent metabolic acidosis prevents further diuretic action by the carbonic anhydrase inhibitor.

Although carbonic anhydrase inhibitors were originally developed as diuretics, their *major usefulness is in glaucoma*.

Inhibition of carbonic anhydrase in the ciliary body of the eye markedly reduces secretion of aqueous humor; oral or parenteral administration of carbonic anhydrase inhibitors decreases intraocular pressure in most patients with this ocular defect. These agents have also been used in some cases of absence and generalized tonic-clonic epilepsy refractory to anticonvulsants.

Adverse reactions to carbonic anhydrase inhibitors are seldom serious and are rapidly reversible, since the drug is excreted rapidly. The most frequent adverse effects include: paresthesia, particularly tingling in the extremities; loss of appetite; polyuria; some drowsiness and confusion. During long-term therapy, an acidotic state may supervene; this can be corrected by administration of bicarbonate. Transient myopia has been reported. Other occasional reactions include urticaria, melena, flaccid paralysis, and convulsions. Drowsiness may impair ability to drive or perform other tasks requiring alertness; patients should be advised of this. Like other sulfonamide derivatives, the sulfonamide-type carbonic anhydrase agents may produce fever, rash, crystalluria, renal calculus, bone-marrow depression, thrombocytopenic purpura, hemolytic anemia, leukopenia, pancytopenia, and agranulocytosis. At the first signs of such reactions the drug should be discontinued and appropriate therapy instituted.

The safe use of these agents during pregnancy has not been established. These agents are contraindicated in patients with idiopathic renal hyperchloremic acidosis, renal failure, a known depletion of sodium and/or potassium, Addison's disease, and patients known to be sensitive to this class of drugs. Moreover, long-term therapy is contraindicated in patients with chronic noncongestive angle closure glaucoma.

Acetazolamide

Acetamide, N-[5-(aminosulfonyl)-1,3,4-thiadiazol-2-yl]-, Diamox (*Lederle*)

N-(5-Sulfamoyl-1,3,4-thiadiazol-2-yl)acetamide   [59-66-5] $C_4H_6N_4O_3S_2$ (222.24).

Preparation—Hydrazine hydrate is reacted with a double equimolar quantity of ammonium thiocyanate to produce 1,2-bis(thiocarbamoyl)hydrazine which yields, through loss of ammonia and rearrangement, 5-amino-2-mercapto-1,3,4-thiadiazole. This is acetylated and then oxidized to the 2-sulfonyl chloride with chlorine. The final step is amidation with ammonia.

Description—White to faintly yellowish white, crystalline, odorless powder.

Solubility—Very slightly soluble in water; sparingly soluble in hot water (90° to 100°); slightly soluble in alcohol.

Uses—Acetazolamide is a carbonic anhydrase inhibitor effective for adjunctive treatment of *edema due to congestive heart failure*, *drug-induced edema*, *absence* and other *centrencephalic epilepsies*, chronic simple (open-angle) *glaucoma*, secondary glaucoma, and *preoperatively in acute angle-closure glaucoma* where it is desired to lower intraocular pressure prior to surgery. When used orally in tablet form to lower intraocular pressure, it has a rapid onset of action (1 to 1½ hrs), reaches peak effect in 2 to 4 hrs, and the effect persists for 8 to 12 hrs. When sustained release capsules are employed, onset of action is approximately 2 hrs, peak effect varies from 8 to 12 hrs, and the effects persist for 18 to 24 hrs.

Acetazolamide is particularly useful where careful following of blood electrolytes is not possible, as in outpatients. It has low toxicity. For additional information on adverse effects and precautions see introductory statement, this page.

Dose—*Usual, adult, oral, diuretic* or *urinary alkalizer*, **500 mg** once a day in the morning for 1 or 2 days, alternating with 1 day of rest. *Usual pediatric*, dosage not established.

Other Dose Information—In *glaucoma*, 250 mg every 4 hours. In epilepsy, **375 to 1 g** in divided doses; when used in combination with other anticonvulsants, **250 mg** once daily.

Dosage Forms—Tablets: 125 and 250 mg. Substained release capsules: 500 mg.

Sterile Acetazolamide Sodium

Acetamide, N-[5-(aminosulfonyl)-1,3,4-thiadiazol-2-yl]-, monosodium salt; Diamox Sodium (*Lederle*)

N-(5-Sulfamoyl-1,3,4-thiadiazol-2-yl)acetamide monosodium salt [1424-27-7] $C_4H_5N_4NaO_3S_2$ (244.22); prepared from acetazolamide with the aid of NaOH. It is suitable for parenteral use.

For the structure of the base, see *Acetazolamide*.

Preparation—Acetazolamide is dissolved in aqueous NaOH solution containing an equimolar quantity of NaOH whereupon the acidic H of the —SO_2NH_2 group is replaced by Na. The solid sodium compound may then be produced by various drying or crystallization techniques.

Description—White solid, having the characteristic appearance of freeze-dried products; pH (freshly prepared solution, 1 in 10) between 9 and 10.

Uses—See *Acetazolamide*.

Dose—*Intravenous* or *intramuscular*, the equivalent of **250 mg** to **1 g** of acetazolamide daily; *usual*, **250 mg** 2 to 4 times a day.

Dosage Form—Sterile: 500 mg.

Dichlorphenamide

1,3-Benzenedisulfonamide, 4,5-dichloro-, Daranide (*MSD*); Oratrol (*Alcon*)

4,5-Dichloro-m-benzenedisulfonamide [120-97-8] $C_6H_6Cl_2N_2O_4S_2$ (305.15).

Preparation—*o*-Chlorophenol is reacted with chlorosulfonic acid to produce 5-chloro-4-hydroxy-1,3-benzenedisulfonyl chloride which is treated with PCl_5 to replace the 4-hydroxy with chlorine. Ammonolysis of the sulfonyl chloride yields the disulfonamide.

Description—White or nearly white, crystalline powder having not more than a slight characteristic odor; melts between 236.5° and 240°.

Solubility—Very slightly soluble in water; freely soluble in 1 N NaOH; soluble in alcohol; slightly soluble in ether.

Uses—A carbonic anhydrase inhibitor used in the treatment of *primary glaucoma*, the acute phase of *secondary glaucoma*, and in the preoperative control of intraocular tension. The drug lowers intraocular pressure by reducing the rate of secretion of aqueous humor. Although it has diuretic properties, it is not advocated for this purpose. Side effects and precautions are the same as other carbonic anhydrase inhibitors (see page 921).

Dose—*Initial, adult, oral, antiglaucoma*, **100 to 200 mg** followed by **100 mg** every 12 hours until desired response obtained. *Maintenance*, **25 to 50 mg** 1 to 3 times daily. *Urinary alkalizer or diuretic*, *oral*, **100 to 200 mg** once a day in the morning for 1 to 2 days, alternating with 1 day of rest.

Dosage Form—Tablets: 50 mg.

Methazolamide

Acetamide, N-[5-(aminosulfonyl)-3-methyl-1,3,4-thiadiazol-2(3H)-ylidene]-, Neptazane (*Lederle*)

N-(4-Methyl-2-sulfamoyl-Δ^2-1,3,4-thiadiazolin-5-ylidene)acetamide [554-57-4] $C_5H_8N_4O_3S_2$ (236.26).

Preparation—2-Acetamido-5-mercapto-1,3,4-thiadiazole, prepared as described under *Acetazolamide*, is treated with *p*-chlorobenzyl chloride to produce the *p*-chlorobenzylmercapto derivative which, on treatment with methyl bromide in the presence of sodium methylate, undergoes methylation and rearrangement to yield the acetylimino thiadiazoline derivative. This is oxidized with chlorine water to the 2-sulfonyl chloride which yields methazolamide on amidation with ammonia.

Description—White or faintly yellow, crystalline powder having a slight odor; melts at about 213°.

Solubility—Very slightly soluble in water and in alcohol; soluble in dimethylformamide; slightly soluble in acetone.

Uses—A *carbonic anhydrase inhibitor* chemically related to acetazolamide and used as *adjunctive treatment* of chronic simple glaucoma, secondary glaucoma, and preoperatively in acute angle-closure glaucoma where delay of surgery is desired to lower intraocular pressure. It is of doubtful value in glaucoma due to severe peripheral anterior synechiae or hemorrhage. It is sometimes used as a *urinary alkalizer*. Significant reduction in intraocular pressure occurs in 6 to 8 hours and persists for 8 to 10 hours. It is indicated in patients who do not respond to acetazolamide or in those who are intolerant to it. The contraindications, precautions, and adverse reactions are similar to those observed with acetazolamide and other carbonic anhydrase inhibitors (see page 921).

Dose—*Usual, adult, oral, glaucoma*, **50** to **100 mg** 2 or 3 times a day. *Urinary alkalizer*, **50** to **100 mg** once a day in the morning for 1 or 2 days, alternating with 1 day of rest.

Dosage Form—Tablets: 50 mg.

Organomercurial Diuretics

The introduction of more potent, less toxic, and orally effective diuretic agents has markedly reduced clinical use of mercurial diuretics. Indeed, the oral organomercurial diuretics are no longer marketed and the parenterally administered agents have largely been replaced by the more convenient loop diuretics (furosemide and ethacrynic acid).

The primary action of mercurial diuretics is to depress tubular reabsorption of sodium and fixed anion (primarily) chloride; water excretion occurs secondarily to this decreased electrolyte reabsorption. They have a dual action on potassium; urinary potassium secretion is increased or decreased, depending upon whether initial secretory rate is low or high. In the treatment of edema, mercurial diuretics usually slightly increase potassium secretion. The diuretic action is potentiated by ammonium chloride, theophylline preparations, and bed rest.

These agents are indicated for the treatment of *edema secondary* to *congestive heart failure*, the *nephrotic syndrome*, the *nephrotic stage* of *glomerulonephritis*, and *hepatic cirrhosis* or *portal obstruction*.

Mercurial diuretics are contraindicated in patients with acute and subacute nephritis, ulcerative colitis, dehydration, or a history of hypersensitivity to the mercurial ion. Patients should be cautioned to maintain sufficient sodium intake to avoid salt deficiency. Excessive dehydration may occur in the elderly patient. Serum electrolytes should be monitored periodically in order to avoid hyponatremia, hypokalemia, and hypochloremia.

Adverse effects include on rare instances idiosyncratic reactions characterized by flushing of the face, fever, chills, gastrointestinal disturbances, cutaneous eruptions, pruritus, and urticaria; mercurials should be discontinued in these patients. Other untoward effects observed with excessive use include weakness, somnolence, muscle pains, and, following excessive use, shock secondary to depletion of extracellular electrolytes.

The most predictable response occurs after the intravenous administration of the mercurials, *but this route is seldom used because severe reactions and sudden death may occur*. Intramuscular and subcutaneous administration are also effective and much safer.

Mersalyl With Theophylline

Uses—By parenteral administration for the treatment of edema secondary to congestive heart failure, the nephrotic syndrome, the nephrotic state of glomerulonephritis, and hepatic cirrhosis or portal obstruction. Mersalyl with theophylline is contraindicated in severe liver disease. Intravenous injection of this drug combination has caused rare, immediate cardiac reactions with sudden death, as well as tissue slough and phlebothrombosis from perivascular injection. Safety for use during pregnancy, in the nursing mother, or in women of childbearing age has not been established. See this page for drug interactions and adverse effects.

Dose—*To test susceptibility*, **0.5 mL** or less. *Usual intramuscular*, **1** or **2 mL** daily or every other day until "dry weight" has been attained. *Children*, to test susceptibility, **0.25 mL**. *Usual*, **0.5** to **1.0 mL**.

Dosage Form—2 mL ampuls, and 10 and 30 mL vials (contain 100 mg of mersalyl and 50 mg of theophylline per mL).

Benzothiadiazine and Related Diuretics

The benzothiadiazine diuretics resulted from efforts to develop more potent carbonic anhydrase inhibitors. Some very potent disulfonamides (see *Dichlorphenamide*, page 936) were synthesized, but were no more useful as diuretics than other members of the group, until a compound with ring closure of one of the sulfonamide groups was accomplished. This resulted in the introduction of the prototype thiazide, chlorothiazide, in 1958, a widely used, reliable, well-tolerated orally effective diuretic. The thiazide diuretics increase urinary excretion of sodium and water by inhibiting sodium reabsorption in the cortical (thick) portion of the ascending limb of Henle's loop and in the early distal tubules. They also increase excretion of chloride, potassium, and, to a lesser extent, bicarbonate ions. The latter effect is due to their slight carbonic anhydrase inhibitory action. Because of their site of action, they interfere with the dilution of urine but not the concentrating of urine.

The thiazide drugs are among the most widely used prescription drugs. They are usually the first drug to be employed in the treatment of *hypertension*. Since the thiazides induce only a limited (10%) reduction in blood pressure they are useful either in mild cases of hypertension or as adjunctive therapy to other drugs. The thiazide diuretics are *effective* as adjunctive therapy in *edema* associated with *congestive heart failure*, *hepatic cirrhosis*, and *corticosteroid* and *estrogen therapy*, as well as edema due to *various forms* of *renal dysfunction* (*nephrotic syndrome, acute glomerulonephritis*, and *chronic renal failure*). Thiazide diuretics have also been used on an *investigational basis* (alone or in combination with amiloride and/or allopurinol) to prevent the formation and recurrence of calcium stones in *hypercalciuric* and *normal calciuric patients*. Hydrochlorthiazide (50 mg, 1 or 2 times daily), trichloromethiazide (4 mg/day), and chlorthalidone (50 mg/day) have been used in these investigational studies.

Thiazide diuretics are contraindicated in anuria, patients hypersensitive to these and other sulfonamide drugs, and in otherwise healthy pregnant women with or without mild edema. Thiazides are excreted into breast milk; use by nursing mothers is not recommended. These drugs should be used with caution in patients with renal disease, since they may precipitate azotemia. They should also be used with caution in patients with impaired liver function, diabetes, gout, or a history of lupus erythematosus.

Adverse effects have been observed as follows: *gastrointestinal* (anorexia, gastric irritation, nausea, vomiting, cramping, diarrhea, constipation, jaundice, pancreatitis, sialadenitis), *central nervous system* (dizziness, vertigo, paresthesias, headache, xanthopsia), *hematologic* (leukopenia, agranulocytosis, thrombocytopenia, aplastic anemia), *cardiovascular* (orthostatic hypotension), *hypersensitivity* (purpura, photosensitivity, rash, urticaria, necrotizing angiitis, fever, respiratory distress, anaphylactic reactions), and *other* (hyperglycemia, glycosuria, hyperuricemia, muscle spasm, weakness, restlessness, and transient blurred vision). Periodic serum electrolyte determinations should be done on *all* patients in order to detect electrolyte imbalance such as hyponatremia, hypochloremic alkalosis, and hypokalemia.

Thiazides are involved in several clinically important drug interactions. They interact with adrenal corticosteroids to enhance hypokalemia, with vitamin D and calcium to induce hypercalcemia, with diazoxide to cause hyperglycemia, and with indomethacin to decrease the natriuretic and/or antihypertensive effect. Moreover, the thiazides *increase* lithium levels and the neuromuscular blocking effect of tubocurarine, but decrease the anticoagulant effect of the oral anticoagulants.

Three agents included in this section, chlorthalidone, metolazone, and quinethazone, are nonthiazide sulfonamide derivatives. Their mechanisms of action and therapeutic indications are similar to the benzothiadiazines. Demonstrable differences between these agents and the thiazide diuretics are largely dosage and duration of action. Hence their inclusion herein.

Bendroflumethiazide

2*H*-1,2,4-Benzothiadiazine-7-sulfonamide, 3,4-dihydro-3-, (phenylmethyl)-6-(trifluoromethyl)-, 1,1-dioxide; Naturetin (*Squibb*)

3-Benzyl-3,4-dihydro-6-(trifluoromethyl)-2*H*-1,2,4-benzothiadiazine-7-sulfonamide 1,1-dioxide [73-48-3] $C_{15}H_{14}F_3N_3O_4S_2$ (421.41).

Preparation—One method consists of cyclization of 4-amino-6-trifluoromethyl-*m*-benzenedisulfonamide through condensation with phenylacetaldehyde (*J Am Chem Soc 81:* 4807, 1959).

Description—White to cream-colored, finely divided, crystalline powder which is odorless or has a slight, characteristic floral odor; melts at about 220°.
Solubility—1 g in 23 mL alcohol, 200 mL ether; practically insoluble in water.

Uses—A potent, orally effective thiazide *diuretic* and *antihypertensive* agent. It is indicated as adjunctive therapy in *edema, congestive heart failure, nephrosis* and *nephritis, cirrhosis* and *ascites,* and other *edematous states.* It is also of value in *hypertension,* alone or when combined with other antihypertensive drugs, eg rauwolfia serpentina (Rauzide-*Squibb*) or nadolol (Corzide-*Squibb*). Diuresis occurs within 2 hours and lasts 6 to 12 hours. After 10 mg orally, peak plasma levels (86 ng/mL) are reached in 2 hours; the mean half-life is 3 hours and the apparent volume of distribution averages 1.48 L/kg. The major part of the drug is eliminated by nonrenal mechanisms; the nonrenal clearance is approximately 269 mL/min and renal clearance 105 mL/min. Urinary recovery of the thiazide averages 30%. Side effects and contraindications are similar to those reviewed above and on page 937.
Dose—*Usual, adult, oral, diuretic, initial,* **5** to **20 mg** daily; maintenance, **2.5** to **5 mg** daily. *Antihypertensive, initial,* **5** to **20 mg** daily; maintenance, **2.5** to **15 mg** daily. *Children, oral, initially,* up to **0.4 mg/kg** of body weight daily in 2 divided doses; *maintenance,* **0.05** to **0.1 mg/kg** daily in a single dose.
Dosage Forms—Tablets: 2.5, 5, and 10 mg.

Benzthiazide

2*H*-1,2,4-Benzothiadiazine-7-sulfonamide, 6-chloro-3-[[(phenylmethyl)thio]methyl]-, 1,1-dioxide; Aquatag, Proaqua (*Reid-Provident*); Exna (*Robins*)

3-[(Benzylthio)methyl]-6-chloro-2*H*-1,2,4-benzothiadiazine-7-sulfonamide 1,1-dioxide [91-33-8] $C_{15}H_{14}ClN_3O_4S_3$ (431.93).

Preparation—4-Amino-6-chloro-*m*-benzenedisulfonamide is reacted with chloroacetic anhydride to give 2,3′-dichloro-4′,6′-disulfamoylacetanilide which is then condensed and cyclized with benzyl mercaptan in the presence of sodium hydroxide. US Pat 3,111,517.

Description—Fine, white, crystalline powder having both a characteristic odor and taste; stable in both light and air; melts at about 240°.
Solubility—1 g in 41,000 mL water, 480 mL alcohol, 24,000 mL chloroform, 2900 mL ether.

Uses—A *diuretic* and *antihypertensive* agent with pharmacological characteristics and uses similar to the thiazides. Diuresis occurs within 2 hours, reaches peak activity in 4 to 6 hours, and lasts 12 to 18 hours. It is about 10 times as potent on a milligram basis as chlorothiazide. For a discussion of the action, precautions, side effects, and possible drug interactions see pages 933, 934, and 937.
Dose—*Usual, adult, oral, diuretic, initial,* **50** to **200 mg** daily; *maintenance,* **50** to **150 mg** daily; *usual, antihypertensive, initial,* **25** to **50 mg** twice daily; *maintenance,* adjust to the response of the patient with a maximal dose of **50 mg** 3 times a day. *Children, oral, initially,* 1 to **4 mg/kg** body weight daily divided into 3 doses. *Maintenance,* reduce as needed.
Dosage Forms—Tablets: 25 and 50 mg.

Chlorothiazide

2*H*-1,2,4-Benzothiadiazine-7-sulfonamide, 6-chloro-, 1,1-dioxide; Diuril (*MSD*)

6-Chloro-2*H*-1,2,4-benzothiadiazine-7-sulfonamide 1,1-dioxide [58-94-6] $C_7H_6ClN_3O_4S_2$ (295.72).

Preparation—3-Chloroaniline is acylated with chlorosulfonic acid to produce the 4,6-disulfonyl chloride which is amidated with ammonia to give the 4,6-disulfonamide. Heating the latter with formic acid results in cyclization through double condensation.

Description—White or practically white, odorless, crystalline powder which melts at about 340°, with decomposition.
Solubility—Very slightly soluble in water; freely soluble in dimethylformamide and dimethyl sulfoxide; slightly soluble in methanol and pyridine; practically insoluble in ether, benzene, and chloroform.

Uses—The prototype benzothiadiazine diuretic having the therapeutic indications, warnings, precautions, drug interactions, and adverse reactions described on pages 933–937. Diuretic effects are apparent within 2 hours after oral administration, reach peak activity in 4 hours, and persist for about 6 to 12 hours; after intravenous administration, effects are apparent in 15 min, reach a peak in 30 min, and persist for about 2 hours. Refractoriness to the drug is relatively uncommon even after prolonged periods of continuous administration. For information on drug interactions of benzothiazides, see page 937.
Dose—*Adult, oral, antihypertensive,* **250** to **500 mg**; *usual, antihypertensive,* **250 mg** 3 times a day; *diuretic,* **500 mg** to **1 g**; *usual, diuretic,* **500 mg** 1 or 2 times a day. *Children, oral,* **22 mg/kg** body weight daily in 2 divided doses; *infants,* under 6 months of age, up to **33 mg/kg** daily in 2 divided doses.
Other Dose Information—Dosage must be highly individualized according to the response of the individual patient and the severity of the condition under treatment.
Dosage Forms—Oral Suspension: 250 mg/5 mL; Tablets: 250 and 500 mg; Chlorothiazide Sodium for Injection: 500 mg.

Chlorthalidone

Benzenesulfonamide, 2-chloro-5-(2,3-dihydro-1-hydroxy-3-oxo-1*H*-isoindol-1-yl)-, Hygroton (*USV*)

2-Chloro-5-(1-hydroxy-3-oxo-1-isoindolinyl)benzenesulfonamide [77-36-1] $C_{14}H_{11}ClN_2O_4S$ (338.76).

Preparation—3-Amino-4-chlorobenzophenone-2-carboxylic acid is diazotized and the resulting diazonium chloride is reacted in the cold with sulfur dioxide in the presence of cupric chloride to form 4-chloro-2′-carboxybenzophenone-3-sulfonyl chloride (I). Heating I with thionyl chloride yields 3-chloro-3-(3′-chlorosulfonyl-4′-chlorophenyl)phthalide which is reacted with ammonia. Removal of the solvent and treatment of the residue with HCl yields chlorthalidone. US Pat 3,055,904.

Description—White to yellowish white, crystalline powder; melts with decomposition above 215°.

Solubility—Practically insoluble in water, chloroform, ether; slightly soluble in alcohol; soluble in methanol.

Uses—An orally effective nonthiazide *diuretic* useful in the treatment of edema associated with *congestive heart failure, renal disease, hepatic cirrhosis, obesity,* and the *premenstrual syndrome.* The diuretic effects start within 2 hours after administration, reach a peak in 6 hours, and persist for 48 to 72 hours. Therefore, the drug usually is given only every other day. Biochemical studies suggest that the prolonged duration of action is due to slow gastrointestinal absorption and enterohepatic recirculation. The drug is excreted unchanged by the kidney. Chlorthalidone also exerts an antihypertensive effect and may be administered with other agents, such as reserpine, ganglionic blocking agents, hydralazine, and guanethidine. Since chlorthalidone contains a sulfonamide group, its pharmacological actions and many of its untoward effects are similar to those of the other orally administered diuretics. See page 933. Chlorthalidone is contraindicated in patients with severe renal or hepatic disease. Patients on this drug should be watched closely for symptoms of renal damage or of electrolyte disturbance.

Dose—*Adult, oral, diuretic,* **50 to 100 mg** daily or **100 mg** on alternate days or 3 times weekly. Some patients may require 150 to 200 mg at these intervals.

Other Dose Information—Initial antihypertensive, 25 mg/day increased to 50 mg/day if necessary. Maximum, 100 mg/day. *Maintenance,* adjusted individually.

Dosage Form—Tablets: 25, 50 and 100 mg.

Cyclothiazide

2*H*-1,2,4-Benzothiadiazine-7-sulfonamide, 3-bicyclo[2.2.1]hept-5-en-2-yl-6-chloro-3,4-dihydro-, 1,1-dioxide; Anhydron (*Lilly*); Fluidil (*Adria*)

6-Chloro-3,4-dihydro-3-(5-norbornen-2-yl)-2*H*-1,2,4-benzothiadiazine-7-sulfonamide 1,1-dioxide [2259-96-3] $C_{14}H_{16}ClN_3O_4S_2$ (389.87).

Preparation—The process is analogous to that for *Chlorothiazide,* except that 5-norbornene-2-carboxaldehyde is employed in the cyclization step instead of formic acid. US Pat 3,275,625.

Description—White to nearly white, practically odorless powder; melts within a range of 4° between 217° and 225°.

Solubility—1 g in 70 mL alcohol, 30 mL methanol; practically insoluble in water, chloroform, and ether.

Uses—Cyclothiazide is an orally effective *diuretic* and *antihypertensive* agent. Diuresis occurs within 6 hours, reaches a peak in 7 to 12 hours, and lasts 18 to 24 hours. Its site and mechanism of action, pattern of electrolyte excretion, untoward effects, and clinical applications are similar to those of other thiazides. See page 933. Like other agents of this type, it may be used as an adjunct to other antihypertensive agents, such as reserpine and the ganglionic blocking agents.

Dose—*Usual, adult, oral, diuretic, initial,* **1** to **2 mg** daily; *maintenance,* **1** to **2 mg** every other day or 2 or 3 times a week; *usual, antihypertensive,* **2 mg** 1 to 3 times a day. *Children, initially,* **0.02** to **0.04 mg/kg** body weight daily; *maintenance,* dose reduced as needed.

Dosage Form—Tablets: 2 mg.

Hydrochlorothiazide

2*H*-1,2,4-Benzothiadiazine-7-sulfonamide, 6-chloro-3,4-dihydro-, 1,1-dioxide; Esidrix (*Ciba*); HydroDiuril (*MSD*); Oretic (*Abbott*); *Various Mfrs*

[58-93-5] $C_7H_8ClN_3O_4S_2$ (297.73).

Preparation—The process is identical with that for *Chlorothiazide* except that formaldehyde is employed in the final cyclization step instead of formic acid.

Description—White, or practically white, odorless, crystalline powder; melts with decomposition at about 268°. pK_{a1} 7.9; pK_{a2} 8.6.

Solubility—Slightly soluble in water; freely soluble in sodium hydroxide solution, dimethylformamide; sparingly soluble in methanol; insoluble in ether, chloroform.

Uses—Effective *diuresis,* comparable to that produced by 500 mg of chlorothiazide twice daily, is induced with 50 mg of hydrochlorothiazide twice daily; diuresis occurs within 2 hours, reaches a peak in 4 hours, and lasts 6 to 12 hours. Otherwise the pharmacological actions, clinical uses, drug interactions, and untoward effects are the same as for chlorothiazide. See pages 938, 939, 944, 945. Hydrochlorothiazide is also used in combination with potassium-conserving agents such as triamterene (Diazide, *SKF*) or amiloride (Moduretic, *MSD*).

Dose—*Adult, oral, antihypertensive,* initially **50** or **100 mg** a day as a single or divided dose; increased or decreased according to response, some patients requiring up to 200 mg a day in divided doses. *Adult, diuretic,* **25 to 100 mg** once or twice a day, or on alternate days. *Children, oral,* **2 mg/kg** of body weight daily, divided into 2 doses; *infants,* under 6 months of age, up to **3 mg/kg** daily in 2 doses.

Dosage Forms—Tablets: 25, 50, and 100 mg.

Hydroflumethiazide

2*H*-1,2,4-Benzothiadiazine-7-sulfonamide, 3,4-dihydro, 6-(trifluoromethyl)-, 1,1-dioxide; Diucardin (*Ayerst*); Saluron (*Bristol*)

[135-09-1] $C_8H_8F_3N_3O_4S_2$ (331.28).

Preparation—4-Amino-6-(trifluoromethyl)-*m*-benzenedisulfonamide is heated with formaldehyde in a sulfuric acid environment thus effecting concomitant condensation and cyclization to hydroflumethiazide. US Pat 3,254,076.

Description—White to cream-colored, finely divided, crystalline powder; odorless; melts between 270° and 275°; pH (1 in 100 dispersion in water) between 4.5 to 7.5.

Solubility—1 g in >5000 mL water, 39 mL alcohol, >5000 mL chloroform, 2500 mL ether.

Uses—A potent orally administered thiazide *diuretic* useful in the management of edema associated with *cardiac failure, hepatic cirrhosis, premenstrual tension,* and *steroid administration.* It is also recommended for the treatment of mild to moderate *hypertension* either alone or in combination with other antihypertensive agents. Diuresis occurs within 1 to 2 hours, reaches a peak in 2 to 4 hours, and lasts 6 to 12 hours. Since hydroflumethiazide potentiates the actions of other antihypertensive agents, the dose of other agents may need to be reduced when this drug is added to the regimen. Except for the fact that a smaller dosage is required for hydroflumethiazide, there is no convincing evidence of significant differences in therapeutic, metabolic, or toxic or sensitization in edematous or hypertensive patients over that of the parent compound, flumethiazide, or the prototype chlorothiazide. See pages 933 and 937.

Dose—*Adult, oral,* **25 to 200 mg;** *usual,* **50 to 100 mg/day.** *Children, initially,* **1 mg/kg** body weight daily; *maintenance,* adjusted as needed.

Other Dose Information—Refractory cases may require as much as 200 mg/day in divided doses. Dosage should be adjusted to provide the minimum effective dose for the individual patient.

Dosage Form—Tablets: 50 mg.

Methyclothiazide

2*H*-1,2,4-Benzothiadiazine-7-sulfonamide, 6-chloro-3-(chloromethyl)-
3,4-dihydro-2-methyl-, 1,1-dioxide; Enduron (*Abbott*);
Aquatensen (*Carter-Wallace*)

[135-07-9] $C_9H_{11}Cl_2N_3O_4S_2$ (360.23).

Preparation—By a process analogous to that for *Chlorothiazide*, 4-amino-6-chloro-N^3-methyl-*m*-benzenedisulfonamide is cyclized through condensation with monochloroacetaldehyde or an acetal thereof. US Pat 3,163,644.

Description—White or practically white, crystalline powder; odorless or has a slight odor and is tasteless; chars slightly below 220° and decomposes at 220°; pK$_a$ (extrapolated from water-acetone) 9.4.

Solubility—1 g in >10,000 mL water, 92.5 mL alcohol, >10,000 mL chloroform, 2700 mL ether; freely soluble in acetone.

Uses—An orally effective *diuretic* and *antihypertensive* agent of the thiazide group. Diuresis occurs within 2 hours, reaches a peak within 6 hours, and lasts 24 hours. Except for its enhanced potency and longer duration of action, its pharmacological actions, therapeutic uses, side effects, and contraindications are similar to chlorothiazide and related agents. See page 937. Diuresis comparable to that produced by 500 mg of chlorothiazide twice a day is induced with 2.5 mg once a day. See page 938.

Dose—*Usual, adult, oral*, **2.5 to 10 mg** once daily, 10 mg being the maximum single effective dose. *Usual maintenance and antihypertensive*, 2.5 to 5 mg once daily. *Children*, **0.05 to 0.2 mg/kg** body weight daily.

Dosage Forms—Tablets: 2.5 and 5 mg.

Metolazone

6-Quinazolinesulfonamide, 7-chloro-1,2,3,4-tetrahydro-2-methyl-3-(2-methylphenyl)-4-oxo; Zaroxolyn (*Pennwalt*)

[17560-51-9] $C_{16}H_{16}ClN_3O_3S$ (365.83).

Preparation—5-Chloro-*o*-toluidine is converted through a series of reactions into *N*-(*o*-tolyl)-2-amino-4-chloro-5-sulfamoylbenzamide, which undergoes ring closure through reaction with acetaldehyde. US Pat 3,360,518.

Description—Colorless, odorless, tasteless, crystalline powder; light-sensitive; pK$_a$ 9.72.

Solubility—Sparingly soluble in water and in alcohol.

Uses—A nonthiazide *diuretic* and *antihypertensive* drug. It acts primarily to inhibit sodium reabsorption at the cortical diluting site and in the proximal convoluted tubule. Sodium and chloride ions are excreted in approximately equal amounts; increased potassium excretion may also occur. Diuresis usually begins within 1 hour, reaches a peak in 2 hours, and persists for 12 to 24 hours. This long duration of action is attributed to protein binding and enterohepatic recycling. Metolazone is indicated for *hypertension*, *edema* accompanying *congestive heart failure*, *renal diseases* including the *nephrotic syndrome*, and other *conditions of diminished renal function*.

Clinical pharmacokinetic studies in normal patients and in patients with cardiac or renal failure reveal interesting differences. Approximately 65% of an administered oral dose (2.5 mg) is absorbed in normal control subjects. About 95% of the plasma metolazone is bound to plasma proteins in normal controls; about 90% is bound in patients with severe renal failure. Clearance of the drug is approximately equal to creatinine clearance and ranges from 110 mL/min in normal controls to 20 mL/min in patients with severe renal failure. About 10% of the administered dose is excreted in the bile in normal subjects. It is contraindicated in anuria, hepatic coma, known allergy or hypersensitivity, pregnancy, and nursing mothers. Adverse reactions are similar to those reported for thiazide agents.

Dose—*Usual, adult, oral, edema of cardiac failure*, **5 to 10 mg** once daily; *edema of renal disease*, **5 to 20 mg** once daily; *mild essential hypertension*, **2.5 to 5 mg** once daily.

Dosage Forms—Tablets: 2.5, 5, and 10 mg.

Polythiazide

2*H*-1,2,4-Benzothiadiazine-7-sulfonamide, 6-chloro-3,4-dihydro-2-methyl-3-[[(2,2,2-trifluoroethyl)thio]methyl]-, 1,1-dioxide;
Renese (*Pfizer*)

[346-18-9] $C_{11}H_{13}ClF_3N_3O_4S_3$ (439.87).

Preparation—6-Amino-4-chloro-N^1-methyl-*m*-benzenedisulfonamide is condensed with the dimethyl acetal of 2,2,2-trifluoroethylmercaptoacetaldehyde. The crude polythiazide, which precipitates when the reaction mixture is added to cold water, is recrystallized from 2-propanol. US Pat 3,009,911.

Description—White, crystalline powder with a characteristic odor; melts between 207° and 217°, with decomposition.

Solubility—1 g in >1000 mL water, 150 mL alcohol, 175 mL chloroform, >1000 mL ether; soluble in acetone.

Uses—An orally effective long-acting *diuretic* and *antihypertensive agent* of the thiazide class. Diuresis occurs within 2 hours, reaches a peak in 6 hours, and lasts 36 hours. Studies in 18 normal subjects receiving single 1-mg oral doses of polythiazide indicate a maximum plasma level of 3.22 ng/mL were reached 5 hours after drug administration. The mean plasma half-lives for absorption and elimination were 1.2 and 25.7 hr, respectively. The latter is consistent with the extended duration of action of polythiazide. Approximately 25% of the drug was excreted unchanged in the urine. Its clinical effectiveness, untoward reactions, and contraindications are similar to those of other benzothiadiazine diuretics. When compared on a milligram basis, 2 mg has approximately the same diuretic activity as 500 mg of chlorothiazide. See pages 938 and 944.

Dose—*Usual, adult, oral*, **1 to 4 mg** daily; *maintenance*, **0.5 to 8 mg** daily adjusted to optimal response. *Children, oral, initially*, **0.02 to 0.08 mg/kg** of body weight daily; *maintenance*, adjusted to need.

Other Dose Information—Antihypertensive, 2 to 4 mg daily, adjusted to achieve desired results.

Dosage Form—Tablets: 1, 2, and 4 mg.

Quinethazone

6-Quinazolinesulfonamide, 7-chloro-2-ethyl-1,2,3,4-tetrahydro-4-oxo-, Hydromox (*Lederle*)

[73-49-4] $C_{10}H_{12}ClN_3O_3S$ (289.74).

Preparation—4′-Chloro-*o*-acetotoluidide is subjected to chlorosulfonation and subsequent amination to form 2-amino-4-chloro-5-sulfamoylbenzamide. Refluxing with an acidulated alcoholic solution of the diethylacetal of propionaldehyde effects the required condensation cyclization to yield quinethazone. US Pat. 2,976,289.

Description—White to yellowish white, odorless, crystalline powder that has a bitter taste; discolors in the presence of strong light and alkaline materials; melts between 250° and 252°.

Solubility—1 g in 500 mL alcohol; freely soluble in solutions of alkali hydroxides and carbonates; very slightly soluble in water.

Uses—A quinazoline derivative with *diuretic* and *antihypertensive* action similar to the thiazides. It differs chemically from the benzothiazide type only in the replacement of a sulfur atom by a carbon. Diuresis occurs within 2 hours, reaches a peak in 6 hours, and lasts from 18 to 24 hours. Available clinical evidence indicates that its site, mechanism of action, electrolyte excretion pattern, therapeutic actions, and untoward effects are similar to those of chlorothiazide and related agents. See pages 933 and 937.

Dose—*Adult*, *oral*, **50 to 200 mg** daily; *usual*, **50 to 100 mg** once a day.
Dosage Form—Tablets: 50 mg.

Trichlormethiazide

2*H*-1,2,4-Benzothiadiazine-7-sulfonamide, 6-chloro-3-(dichloromethyl)-3,4-dihydro-, 1,1-dioxide; Metahydrin (*Merrell-Dow*); Naqua (*Schering-Plough*)

[133-67-5] $C_8H_8Cl_3N_3O_4S_2$ (380.65).

Preparation—By reacting 4-amino-6-chloro-*m*-benzenedisulfonamide with dichloroacetaldehyde, or an acetal thereof, in a suitable condensation environment. US Pats 3,163,645 and 3,264,292.

Description—White, crystalline powder that is odorless or has a slight characteristic odor; light-sensitive, but stable in air and heat; melts at about 274° with decomposition.
Solubility—1 g in 1100 mL water, 48 mL alcohol, 5000 mL chloroform, 1400 mL ether.

Uses—An orally effective and long-acting *diuretic* and *antihypertensive* of the thiazide class. Diuresis occurs within 2 hours, reaches a peak in 6 hours, and lasts 24 hours. As an antihypertensive, trichlormethiazide is also used in combination with reserpine (Metatensin, *Merrell-Dow;* Diutensin—R, *Carter-Wallace*). Pharmacological actions, therapeutic uses, untoward effects, and contraindications of trichlormethiazide are similar to those of the parent substance, chlorothiazide. See pages 937 and 938. On a milligram basis, it is approximately 250 times more active than chlorothiazide.
Dose—*Usual*, *adult*, *oral*, **2 to 4 mg** twice daily, then 1 to 2 mg once daily. *Children*, **0.07mg/kg** of body weight daily in single or divided doses.
Dosage Form—Tablets: 2 and 4 mg.

Potassium-Sparing Diuretics

The potassium-sparing diuretics include *spironolactone, triamterene* and *amiloride*. The effects of these agents on urinary electrolyte composition are similar in that they cause a mild natriuresis and decrease potassium and hydrogen-ion excretion. Despite this similarity, these agents actually compose two groups with respect to mechanism of action.

Spironolactone, the prototype agent of the so-called "aldosterone antagonists," is a specific competitive inhibitor of aldosterone at the receptor site level; hence, it is *effective only* when aldosterone is present. The other two potassium-sparing diuretics, triamterene and amiloride, exert their effect independent of the presence or absence of aldosterone. Triamterene, on the peritubular side, inhibits the potential in the collecting duct and not on the distal tubule. Amiloride, on the other hand, inhibits the potential in both the collecting duct and the distal tubule. In addition, amiloride also decreases sodium transport in the proximal tubule. The potassium-sparing action common to all three of these agents is due to alteration of passive forces controlling movement of these ions.

The potassium-sparing agents are used in the management of *edema* associated with *congestive heart failure, hepatic cirrhosis with ascites, the nephrotic syndrome* and *idiopathic edema*. In addition, they are used in combination with other drugs in the management of hypertension. Spironolactone is also used in *primary hyperaldosteronism.*

Potassium-sparing diuretics are contraindicated in patients with anuria, acute renal insufficiency, impaired renal function or hyperkalemia. Adverse reactions include diarrhea, nausea, vomiting, weakness, headache, erythematous rash, and urticaria. Gynecomastia and carcinoma of the breast have been

reported after spironolactone; however, no causal relationship between the latter and the drug has been established.

Amiloride Hydrochloride

Pyrazinecarboxamide, 3,5-diamino-*N*-(aminoiminomethyl)-6-chloro-, monohydrochloride; Midamor (*MSD*)

N-Amidino-3,5-diamino-6-chloropyrazinecarboxamide hydrochloride [2016-88-8] $C_6H_8ClN_7O.HCl$ (266.09).

Preparation—Pyrazine-2,3-dicarboxamide is converted to 3-amino-2-carboxamide through a Hoffman degradation using one equivalent of NaOBr; the carboxamide forming the ethyl ester by ethanolysis followed by reaction with sulfuryl chloride. This latter treatment forms the 5,6-dichloro derivative. As the 5-chloro is activated by the *p*-carboxyl it is readily converted to the amine with ammonia. Finally the ester group is condensed with guanidine to yield the product. See Belg Pat 639,386 [CA 62:14698f,1965].

Description—Odorless pale yellowish-green powder melting about 240°.
Solubility—Soluble 1 g in 200 mL of water; 350 mL of alcohol; practically insoluble in chloroform or ether.

Uses—Amiloride is a potassium-conserving drug with natriuretic, diuretic, and antihypertensive activity. It is approved only for concurrent use with other thiazide diuretics or other saliuretic-diuretic agents in the management of congestive heart failure or hypertension. It is used to restore normal serum potassium levels in patients who develop hypokalemia and in patients who would be exposed to a particular risk if hypokalemia were to develop. Its effect on electrolyte excretion reaches a peak between 6 and 10 hours and lasts about 24 hours. Peak plasma levels are reached in 3 to 4 hours and plasma half-life varies from 6 to 9 hours. The drug is not metabolized by the liver and is excreted unchanged in the urine. Amiloride is contraindicated in patients with hyperkalemia or those taking potassium supplements or other potassium-sparing drugs. It should be used with extreme care in patients with diabetes or impaired renal function.

Adverse effects include headache, nausea, anorexia, diarrhea, and vomiting (3 to 8%). Other adverse effects such as dizziness, encephalopathy, abdominal pain, constipation, weakness, muscle cramps, decreased libido, cough, and impotence occur less frequently. Serum potassium levels should be monitored.
Dose—*Single drug therapy:* **5 to 10 mg** daily; if persistent hypokalemia is documented with **10 mg/kg,** the dose can be increased to **15** and then **20 mg** daily.
Dosage Form—Tablets: 5 mg.
Dose—*Multiple drug therapy:* Amiloride and Hydrochlorthiazide (*Moduretic*, MSD), **1 tablet** daily. The dosage may be increased to **2 tablets** a day if necessary.
Dosage Form—Tablets: Amiloride hydrochloride, 5 mg, and hydrochlorthiazide, 50 mg.

Spironolactone

Pregn-4-ene-21-carboxylic acid, 7-(acetylthio)-17-hydroxy-3-oxo, γ-lactone (7α,17α)-, Aldactone (*Searle*)

17-Hydroxy-7α-mercapto-3-oxo-17α-pregn-4-ene-21-carboxylic acid γ-lactone acetate [52-01-7] $C_{24}H_{32}O_4S$ (416.57).

Preparation—By treating dehydroepiandrosterone (prepared from cholesterol or sitosterol) with acetylene to form the 17α-ethynyl-17β-hydroxy derivative which is carbonated to the 17α-propiolic acid. Reduction of the unsaturated acid in alkaline solution yields the saturated acid which cyclizes to the lactone on acidification. Bromination to the 5,6-dibromo compound, followed by oxidation of the 3-hydroxyl group to the ketone, then dehydrobromination to the 7α-hydroxyl derivative, produces spironolactone when esterified with thiolacetic acid.

Description—Light cream-colored to light tan, crystalline powder; faint to mild mercaptan-like odor; stable in air; melts between 198° and 207°, with decomposition.

Solubility—Practically insoluble in water; freely soluble in chloroform; soluble in alcohol; slightly soluble in fixed oils.

Uses—Spironolactone is a steroid that acts as a competitive antagonist of the potent endogenous mineral-corticosteroid, aldosterone. Spironolactone has a slower onset of action than triamterene or amiloride but its natriuretic effect is slightly greater during long-term therapy. Spironolactone is indicated in the treatment of *essential hypertension, edema* associated with *congestive heart failure, hepatic cirrhosis* with ascites, the *nephrotic syndrome, idiopathic edema*, and in the diagnosis of primary aldosteronism. Spironolactone, by blocking the sodium-retaining effects of aldosterone on the distal convoluted tubule, corrects one of the most important mechanisms responsible for the production of edema. Its onset of diuretic action is gradual and it requires 4 or 5 days to achieve full diuretic effect. It is a relatively weak diuretic and is usually employed as an adjunct to other diuretics, such as the thiazides. When used in this combined manner, it enhances the excretion of sodium and decreases the excretion of potassium. Further increase in diuresis may be obtained by the use of a glucocorticoid with spironolactone in combination with another diuretic. Spironolactone is rapidly metabolized after oral administration. The metabolites are excreted largely in the urine, but also in bile. The primary metabolite, canrenone, reaches peak plasma levels 2 to 4 hours after oral administration of spironolactone. The half-life of canrenone, following multiple doses of spironolactone, is 13 to 24 hours. Both spironolactone and canrenone are more than 90% bound to plasma proteins. Spironolactone is contraindicated in acute renal insufficiency, anuria, and hyperkalemia. It is also contraindicated in patients on digoxin; concurrent use elevates digoxin plasma levels and may induce digoxin toxicity. Similarly, concurrent use with lithium increases the risk of lithium toxicity. Side effects include hyponatremia, hyperkalemia, and drowsiness. Other adverse effects include headache, diarrhea, skin rashes and urticaria, mental confusion, drug fever, ataxia, gynecomastia, decreased libido in the male, and mild androgenic effects, such as hirsutism, irregular menses, and deepening of the voice.

Dose—*Usual, adult, oral,* **25 mg** 4 times a day; range, **25 to 200 mg** a day. *Children,* **3.3 mg/kg** body weight daily in divided doses.

Other Dose Information—If satisfactory diuretic effect is not achieved in 5 days, a thiazide diuretic should be added to the regimen.

Dosage Form—Tablets: 25 mg.

Triamterene

2,4,7-Pteridinetriamine, 6-phenyl-, Dyrenium (*SKF*)

2,4,7-Triamino-6-phenylpteridine [396-01-0] $C_{12}H_{11}N_7$ (253.27).

Preparation—5-Nitroso-2,4,6-triaminopyrimidine is refluxed with phenylacetonitrile in the presence of sodium methoxide. US Pat 3,081,230.

Description—Yellow, odorless, crystalline powder; stable to temperature and light.

Solubility—Practically insoluble in water, chloroform, ether; very slightly soluble in alcohol.

Uses—Triamterene inhibits reabsorption of sodium ions in exchange for potassium and hydrogen ions at that segment of the distal tubule under the control of adrenal mineralocorticoids. The effect is unrelated to the level of aldosterone secretion. After oral administration, 30 to 70% is absorbed. Diuresis appears 2 to 4 hours after ingestion; however, maximum therapeutic effect may not be seen for several days. It is metabolized primarily in the liver and about 3 to 5% is excreted unchanged in the urine. The half-life is 2 to 4 hours. Triamterene is also used in combination with hydrochlorothiazide (Diazide, *SKF*) in the treatment of edema associated with *congestive heart failure, cirrhosis,* and the *nephrotic syndrome*. It is also indicated in steroid-induced edema, idiopathic edema, edema due to secondary hyperaldosteronism, and in edematous patients unresponsive to other therapy. Triamterene directly inhibits the reab-

sorption of sodium and chloride independent of aldosterone. Although it promotes the excretion of sodium and chloride, it is believed to conserve potassium by reducing the transport of this ion from the tubular cell to the tubular lumen. Hence, it should not be used with potassium supplements and should be used with caution in patients with preexisting elevated serum potassium. It is also contraindicated in patients with severe kidney and liver disease. Side effects are usually mild and consist of nausea, vomiting, gastrointestinal disturbances, weakness, headache, dry mouth, and rash. Interstitial nephritis has also been reported.

Dose—*Adult, oral,* **100 mg** every other day to **300 mg** daily; *usual,* **100 mg** once a day.

Other Dose Information—The usual dose should be taken after meals. For *maintenance,* 100 mg daily or every other day. The total dose should not exceed 300 mg daily.

Dosage Forms—Capsules: 50 and 100 mg.

Loop Diuretics

The loop diuretics, ethacrynic acid (Edecrin), furosemide (Lasix), and bumetanide (Bumex), are the most potent currently available diuretic agents. Although differences do exist between these agents, they are similar in that their most important action is in the medullary and cortical (thick) ascending limb of Henle. Loop diuretics inhibit active chloride transport over the entire length of the ascending thick limb of Henle. The loop diuretics have a much greater diuretic effect than the thiazides. Unlike the mercurials, they are effective even in the presence of electrolyte and acid-base disturbances. These potent agents are usually reserved for patients with impaired renal function, acute pulmonary edema, or hypertensive crises.

Despite their similar actions, there are some essential differences between the loop diuretics. Furosemide is usually preferred to ethacrynic acid for a number of reasons; (1) it has a broader dose-response curve; (2) it is less ototoxic; (3) it causes fewer gastrointestinal side effects, (4) it is more convenient for intravenous use, and (5) it may be less likely to cause alkalosis.

Considerable controversy persists relative to their antihypertensive effectiveness as compared to the thiazides. There is little controversy relative to the superiority of the loop diuretics, in hypertension associated with renal insufficiency. Moreover, the loop diuretics *increase* renal blood flow, whereas the thiazides tend to *decrease* renal blood flow and further compromise renal function.

Adverse effects are similar for both thiazides and loop diuretics and the management of these effects are the same. However, because of the much greater potency of the loop diuretics as compared to thiazides, more strict monitoring is warranted to avoid severe electrolyte imbalances.

Ethacrynate Sodium for Injection

Acetic acid, [2,3-dichloro-4-(2-methylene-1-oxobutyl)phenoxy]-, sodium salt; Lyovac Sodium Edecrin (*MSD*)

Sodium [2,3-dichloro-4-(2-methylenebutyryl)phenoxy]acetate [6500-81-8] $C_{13}H_{11}Cl_2NaO_4$ (325.12); a sterile, cryodesiccated powder prepared by the neutralization of ethacrynic acid with NaOH.

Uses—See *Ethacrynic Acid.*

Dose—*Intravenous,* the equivalent of **50 to 100 mg** of ethacrynic acid; *usual,* the equivalent of **50 mg** of ethacrynic acid.

Dosage Form—Vials containing the equivalent of 50 mg of ethacrynic acid.

Ethacrynic Acid

Acetic acid, [2,3-dichloro-4-(2-methylene-1-oxobutyl)phenoxy]-, Edecrin (*MSD*)

[2,3-Dichloro-4-(2-methylenebutyryl)phenoxy]acetic acid [58-54-8] $C_{13}H_{12}Cl_2O_4$ (303.14).

Caution—Use care in handling Ethacrynic Acid, since it irritates the skin, eyes, and mucous membranes.

Preparation—2,3-Dichlorophenoxyacetic acid is subjected to a Friedel-Crafts reaction with butyryl chloride to form the 4-butyryl derivative. This undergoes a Mannich reaction with formaldehyde and dimethylamine, the product decomposing thermally to introduce the methylene group.

Description—White or practically white, crystalline powder that is odorless or practically odorless and has a bitter taste; relatively stable in light and at room temperature, and nonhygroscopic; melts between 121° and 125°.

Solubility—1 g in 1.6 mL alcohol, 3.5 mL ether, 6 mL chloroform; very slightly soluble in water.

Uses—A *diuretic agent* chemically unrelated to other oral or parenteral diuretics. Maximum water and sodium diuresis is similar to that with furosemide, but greatly exceeds that with thiazides or organomercurial diuretics. Ethacrynic acid is especially useful in patients who require an agent with greater diuretic potential than those commonly employed. It is used in the treatment of *fluid retentive states* caused by *congestive heart failure, cirrhosis of the liver*, and *renal disease*, including the nephrotic syndrome. It is also recommended for the short-term management of ascites due to malignancy, idiopathic edema, and lymphedema. In addition, it is useful for the short-term management of hospitalized pediatric patients with congenital heart disease or the nephrotic syndrome. It exerts its action on the cortical ascending (thick) loop of Henle and on the proximal and distal tubule, where it affects both the concentrating and diluting mechanisms of the kidney. Ethacrynic acid causes the excretion of virtually an isoosmotic urine by preventing sodium reabsorption from the loop of Henle; chloride excretion is even greater than sodium. After oral administration, diuresis begins within ½ hour, reaches a peak in 2 hours and persists for 6 to 8 hours. After intravenous administration, diuresis begins immediately and reaches a maximum within 30 minutes. Approximately 95% of ethacrynic acid is bound to plasma proteins. Plasma half-life is about 1 hour. Ethacrynic acid can be used with additive effect with diuretics having different sites of action. Adverse reactions include: *gastrointestinal* (anorexia, abdominal discomfort, dysphagia, nausea, vomiting, and diarrhea, gastrointestinal bleeding and pancreatitis have also occurred); *renal* (hyperuricemia, acute gout, and acute hypoglycemia with convulsions in uremic patients); *carbohydrate metabolism* (hyperglycemia in a few patients); *hemopoietic* (agranulocytosis or severe neutropenia, thrombocytopenia has been observed only rarely); *hepatic* (jaundice and abnormal liver function); *miscellaneous* (vertigo, deafness, and tinnitus with a sense of fullness in the ears; infrequently, skin rash, headache, fever, chills, hematuria, blurred vision, fatigue, apprehension and confusion). Patients on ethacrynic acid should have determinations of blood urea nitrogen, serum carbon dioxide and electrolytes, and white blood cell counts made frequently.

Dose—*Adult, oral*, **50** to **400 mg** daily; *usual*, **50 mg** 2 times a day or 2 times every other day. *Children, initial dose*, **25 mg**; increase by **25 mg** until desired effect obtained. Dose for infants has not been established.

Other Dose Information—Dosage must be carefully regulated to prevent excessive fluid and electrolyte loss.

Dosage Forms—Tablets: 25 and 50 mg.

Furosemide

Benzoic acid, 5-(aminosulfonyl)-4-chloro-2-[(2-furanylmethyl)amino]-, Lasix (*Hoechst-Roussel*)

4-Chloro-*N*-furfuryl-5-sulfamoylanthranilic acid [54-31-9] $C_{12}H_{11}ClN_2O_5S$ (330.74).

Preparation—2,4-Dichlorobenzoic acid is heated with chlorosulfonic acid and the resulting 5-chlorosulfonyl derivative is reacted with concentrated ammonia to convert it to the 5-sulfamoyl analogue (I). Refluxing I with furfurylamine in large excess or in the presence of sodium bicarbonate yields crude furosemide which is recrystallized from aqueous ethanol. US Pat 3,058,882.

Description—Fine, white to slightly yellow, crystalline powder that is odorless and practically tasteless; unstable in light but stable in air; melts between 203° and 205° with decomposition; pK_a 3.9.

Solubility—Practically insoluble in water; freely soluble in acetone, and solutions of alkali hydroxides; sparingly soluble in alcohol; slightly soluble in ether; very slightly soluble in chloroform.

Uses—A *diuretic* chemically related to the sulfonamide diuretics. It is characterized by high efficacy, rapid onset of action, comparatively short duration of action, and a tenfold ratio between minimum and maximum diuretic dose. Moreover, it is slightly more potent than the organomercurial agents, orally effective, and its diuretic action is independent of alterations in body acid-base balance. It acts not only on the proximal and distal tubules but also on the ascending limb of the loop of Henle.

Furosemide is indicated for the treatment of *edema* associated with *congestive heart failure, cirrhosis of the liver*, and *renal disease*, including the *nephrotic syndrome*. It is particularly indicated when a greater diuretic potential is needed than that produced by commonly employed diuretic agents. It is also useful in the management of selected patients with *hypertension*. Furosemide is given by both oral and parenteral routes of administration; parenteral administration should be reserved for those cases where oral therapy is not practical. Administered orally, the diuretic effect begins within 1 hour, reaches a peak in 1 or 2 hours, and persists for 6 to 8 hours. Administered intravenously, the diuretic effect begins within 5 min, reaches a peak in 30 min, and persists for 2 hours.

Clinical pharmacokinetic studies carried out after a single intravenous dose of 0.5, 1.0, or 1.5 mg/kg indicate that peak diuresis occurs between 20 and 60 min after injection. Apparent volume of distribution of the drug averages 11.4% of the body weight and is independent of the dose. Mean plasma half-life in these studies was 29.5 min with a clearance rate of 162 mL/min. Renal excretion was found to be the main route of elimination and averaged 92% of the administered dose with a mean renal clearance of 149 mL/min. Since this exceeds the glomerular filtration rate, it is thought that tubular secretion of furosemide occurs, despite the fact that 95% of the drug is bound to plasma protein.

Furosemide is known to be involved in a number of drug interactions. It increases the toxicity of lithium, digitalis, and theophylline. It decreases the arterial responsiveness of norepinephrine and antagonizes the skeletal muscle relaxant effects of tubocurarine and may potentiate the action of succinylcholine. Concomitant administration of indomethacin may reduce the natriuretic and antihypertensive effects of furosemide. This effect may also occur with other nonsteroidal anti-inflammatory drugs such as ibuprofen and naproxen. Metolazone acts synergistically with furosemide to stimulate profound diuresis in furosemide-resistant patients.

Furosemide is contraindicated in anuria, hepatic coma, and in patients known to be sensitive to the drug. Adverse effects which may result from therapy with furosemide include reduction of renal, cerebral, and cardiac blood flow, potassium loss with resultant cardiac and neuromuscular abnormalities, elevation of blood uric acid and blood sugar levels, allergic reactions, rare cases of exfoliative dermatitis, pruritus, and blood dyscrasias (thrombocytopenia and leukopenia). Paresthesia, blurring of vision, postural hypotension, nausea, vomiting, or diarrhea may occur. In addition, cases of reversible deafness and tinnitus have been reported. Diuresis induced by furosemide has also been accompanied by weakness, fatigue, lightheadedness or dizziness, muscle cramps, thirst, and urinary frequency. Excessive furosemide therapy can lead to profound diuresis with water and electrolyte depletion. Patients on this drug should be tested at frequent intervals for blood urea nitrogen, sodium, potassium, chloride, and carbon dioxide concentrations. The drug should not be used in cirrhotic patients, unless they do not respond to other therapy. Furosemide is contraindicated in women with child-bearing potential.

Dose—*Adult, oral*, **20** to **80 mg** daily; *usual*, **40** to **80 mg** once a day; *intramuscular or intravenous*, **20** to **40 mg**, after not less than 2 hours increased by 20 mg to desired effect. *Usual, pediatric*, **2 mg/kg** body weight as a single dose. If response is not adequate, increase by **1** or **2 mg/kg** after 6 to 8 hours; do not exceed **6 mg/kg**.

Dosage Forms—Injection and Oral Solution: 10 mg/mL; Tablets: 20, 40, and 80 mg.

Other Renal Tubular Inhibiting Diuretics

All of the xanthines (caffeine, theophylline, and theobromine) appear to induce diuresis by a direct action on the renal tubule. The increased urinary output involves an increase in the rate of sodium and chloride excretion, with no significant effect on urinary acidification. Although diuretic action is only slightly altered by changes in acid-base balance, it is potentiated by the coadministration of carbonic anhydrase inhibitors. In clinical practice, the xanthines are considered obsolete as diuretics and seldom used for three reasons: (1) they lack the efficacy of the newer agents, (2) their continued use leads to decreased effectiveness, and (3) they cause some gastric irritation. Therefore, caffeine, a powerful CNS stimulant is presented in Chapter 62 (*see* page 1133) and theophylline, a useful bronchodilator, is discussed in Chapter 44. Only theobromine will be presented in this section.

Aminophylline—page 872.

Caffeine—page 1133.

Theobromine

1*H*-Purine-2,6-dione, 3,7-dihydro-3,7-dimethyl-,

3,7-Dimethylxanthine [83-67-0] $C_7H_8N_4O_2$ (180.17); an alkaloid prepared from the dried ripe seed of *Theobroma cacao* Linné (Fam *Sterculiaceae*), or made synthetically.

For the structural formula, see page 419.

Description—White, crystalline powder with a bitter taste; sublimes at about 260°.
Solubility—1 g in 1800 mL water, 2400 mL alcohol, 6000 mL chloroform; soluble in solutions of fixed alkali hydroxides; insoluble in ether.

Uses—Theobromine has been employed as a *diuretic*, since its action on the kidney is more lasting than other xanthines. It acts by inhibiting reabsorption of sodium and chloride in the renal tubules. It is practically devoid of toxicity and thus can be employed on occasions when the more toxic diuretics are contraindicated, as, for example, when renal function is poor. The wide choice of more effective diuretics has markedly limited the use of theobromine even for this purpose.

Theobromine salts have been used to dilate the coronary arteries on the premise that they increase coronary blood flow. However, they also stimulate the heart and increase the oxygen needs of cardiac muscle. Unfortunately, the latter action severely compromises the effect on coronary arteries. For this reason, the use of theobromine and other xanthines in coronary artery disease is now obsolete. Xanthine preparations are apt to cause gastric irritation and are best given during meals. The salts are less irritating than the alkaloidal bases.

Dose—*Usual*, **500 mg**.

Theophylline—page 873.

Theophylline Sodium Acetate—page 875.

Miscellaneous Renal Agents

Indapamide

Benzamide, 3-(aminosulfonyl)-4-chloro-*N*-(2,3-dihydro-2-methyl-1*H*-indol-1-yl)-, Lozol (*USV*)

4-Chloro-*N*-(2-methyl-1-indolinyl)-3-sulfamoylbenzamide [26807-65-8] $C_{16}H_{16}ClN_3O_3S$ (365.83).
Preparation—*p*-Chlorotoluene is sulfonated and converted to the sulfonamide yielding 3-chloro-4-sulfamoylbenzoic acid. This acid

is reacted with thionyl chloride to form the carbonyl chloride and treated with 2-methylindole (skatole) to give the product. See US Pat 3,565,911.

Description—White crystals melting about 161°.

Uses—Indapamide is the first of a new class of diuretic/antihypertensives, the indolines. Its diuretic effect is similar to that induced by hydrochlorothiazide. Its antihypertensive effect results from decreased peripheral resistance, perhaps due to an alteration of transmembrane calcium events. Indapamide is used for the treatment of *hypertension*, alone or in combination with other antihypertensive drugs. It is also used in the management of *salt* and *fluid retention* associated with congestive heart failure.

Indapamide is preferentially and reversibly taken up by erythrocytes in peripheral blood. The whole blood/plasma ratio is about 6:1 at the time of peak concentration and decreases to 3.5:1 at 8 hours. From 71 to 79% of indapamide is bound to plasma proteins. Indapamide is extensively metabolized; only 7% of the unchanged drug is excreted by the kidneys. The half life in whole blood is 24 hours. Few drug interactions have been reported; indapamide reduces the renal clearance of lithium and tends to decrease arterial responsiveness to norepinephrine.

Adverse effects are usually mild and transient. Those most commonly observed include headache, dizziness, fatigue, muscle cramps, or numbness of the extremities. Orthostatic hypotension, premature ventricular contractions, impotence, reduced libido, and hypokalemia have been reported. Patients should advise their physician if muscle weakness, cramps, nausea, vomiting, or dizziness occur. The safe use in the pregnant or nursing mother has not been established.

Dose—*Usual, hypertension* and *edema of congestive heart failure*, **2.5 mg** as a single daily dose taken in the morning; if the response is not satisfactory after 1 (edema) to 4 (hypertension) weeks, the dose is increased to **5 mg** once daily. The dose of other agents should be reduced by 50% when used in combination with indapamide.

Dosage Form—Tablets: 2.5 mg.

Probenecid

Benzoic acid, 4[(dipropylamino)sulfonyl]-, Benemid (*MSD*)

[57-66-9] $C_{13}H_{19}NO_4S$ (285.36).
Preparation—Oxidation of the methyl group of *p*-toluenesulfonyl chloride produces *p*-carboxybenzenesulfonic acid. This acid is then converted into the corresponding sulfonyl chloride by treatment with chlorosulfonic acid, which is condensed with di-*n*-propylamine.

Description—White or nearly white, fine, crystalline powder; practically odorless; melts between 198° and 200°.
Solubility—Soluble in alcohol, chloroform, and acetone; practically insoluble in water.

Uses—An agent which selectively blocks both inward and outward renal transport of weak acids. With respect to the inward renal transport, it is an effective *uricosuric* agent for the treatment of gout and gouty arthritis. It inhibits tubular reabsorption of urate, thus increasing urinary excretion of uric acid and decreasing serum uric acid levels. With regard to outward renal transport (tubular secretion), it is effective as an adjuvant therapy with penicillin G, O, or V, or with ampicillin, methicillin, oxacillin, cloxacillin, or nafcillin, for elevation and prolongation of penicillin plasma levels by whatever route the antibiotic is given. Probenecid inhibits the renal excretion and may increase the plasma levels of methotrexate, sulfonamides, sulfonylureas, naproxen, indomethacin, rifampin, aminosalicylic acid, dapsone, clofibrate, and pantothenic acid. Patients concurrently taking any of these agents should be monitored closely and the dosage regimen appropriately adjusted.

Probenecid is rapidly and completely absorbed after oral administration. Plasma levels of 100 to 200 μg/mL are necessary for an adequate uricosuric effect, whereas plasma levels of only 40 to 60 μg/mL produce maximal inhibition of penicillin excretion. Plasma levels of 25 μg/mL are reached 30 min after a single 1-gram oral dose;

plasma levels reach a peak in 2 to 4 hours and remain above 30 μg/mL for 8 hours. Following a single 2-gram oral dose, peak plasma levels of 150 to 200 μg/mL are reached in 4 hours and levels of 50 μg/mL are sustained for 8 hours; the plasma half-life ranges from 4 to 17 hours. At a plasma concentration of 14 μg/mL, about 17% of the drug is bound to plasma protein.

Probenecid is contraindicated in hypersensitive individuals, children under 2 years of age, and persons with known blood dyscrasias or uric acid stones. Therapy with probenecid should not be started until an acute gouty attack has subsided. Exacerbation of gout following probenecid therapy may occur; in such cases, colchicine or other appropriate therapy is advisable. The drug should not be given with methotrexate, since plasma levels of the latter agent have been reported to be increased. Use of salicylates is also contraindicated because these substances antagonize the uricosuric action of probenecid. Patients who require a mild analgesic should be advised to use acetaminophen rather than salicylates. Probenecid is devoid of analgesic activity.

Probenecid is well tolerated, but an occasional patient may experience headache, anorexia, nausea, vomiting, urinary frequency, hypersensitivity reactions, sore gums, flushing, dizziness, and anemia. In gouty patients, exacerbation of gout and uric acid stones with or without hematuria, renal colic and costovertebral pain have been observed. Nephrotic syndrome, hepatic necrosis, and aplastic anemia occur rarely. Hemolytic anemia, which in some cases could be related to genetic deficiencies of red blood cell glucose 6-phosphate dehydrogenase, has been reported.

Dose—*Adult*, *oral*, **500 mg** to **2 g** daily; *usual*, **250 mg** twice a day for 1 week, then **500 mg** twice a day thereafter.

Dosage Form—Tablets: 500 mg.

Sulfinpyrazone—page 1115.

CHAPTER 51

Uterine and Antimigraine Drugs

Stewart C Harvey, PhD

Professor of Pharmacology
School of Medicine, University of Utah
Salt Lake City, UT 84132

Drugs that stimulate the smooth muscle of the uterus are known as *oxytocics*. Only two chemical types of oxytocics are clinically used: (1) the oxytocic fraction (oxytocin) of the posterior pituitary extract and (2) certain ergot alkaloids. However, a number of other agents possess mild to intense oxytocic actions. Some of these, eg, hydrastis and quinine, have been used formerly but are now archaic. The lay public, and sometimes also the physician, employ cathartics and abdominal congestants such as castor oil reflexly to induce uterine movement, but it is doubtful whether such agents are effective until the uterus is prepared to present the fetus normally. Certain prostaglandins have been used successfully as oxytocics and abortifacients.

The response of the uterus to oxytocics depends on estrogenic and progestational hormonal influences, the estrogenic influences being the more conducive to responsiveness near term. Progesterone hyperpolarizes the uterine smooth muscle and thus diminishes its responsiveness and coordination. Consequently, and fortunately, during the first two terms of pregnancy, oxytocics are generally incapable of inducing labor. Late in the third term, as the progesterone levels decline, uterine responsiveness rises sharply in advance of pelvic relaxation, cervical dilatation, and the coordination of uterine contractions necessary to proper delivery of the fetus. Consequently, the premature induction of labor by oxytocics can result in harm to both mother and infant and may result in stillbirth if premature separation of the placenta, placental vasoconstriction, or umbilical strangulation occur consequent to the actions of the oxytocic. Therefore, only under rare circumstances should oxytocics be used to induce labor; indeed, they are generally withheld *during* labor until the cervix is dilated and presentation of the fetus has occurred (ie, until the third stage of labor). The oxytocic is then given to hasten the delivery of the placenta and to diminish uterine bleeding, which diminution is the result of contractile compression of the blood sinuses and of vasoconstriction. Oxytocics may also be employed during the puerperium to aid in the involution of the uterus to normal. Oxytocin promotes and facilitates the normal phasic contractions which are characteristic of normal delivery. The ergot alkaloids induce prolonged contractions or contracture, which may be detrimental to safe delivery, and hence they are employed mainly in the third stage of labor to diminish bleeding. Prostaglandins, notably PGE_2 and PGF_2, promote normal type phasic contractions. However, the effects of the prostaglandins are not so dependent on the estrogen-progesterone balance as those of oxytocin, so that prostaglandins can induce labor considerably in advance of term and hence can be used to induce abortion.

Nonoxytocic ergot alkaloids are listed in this section because of their relationship to the oxytocic prototypes.

The so-called uterine sedatives comprise an ill-defined class of drugs that diminish or supposedly diminish uterine activity. They are employed to interrupt premature labor, to diminish pain in dysmenorrhea, and to diminish premenstrual discomfort. Some of these agents, such as central nervous sys-

tem sedatives, have a central locus, and it is questionable whether uterine activity is affected at all. Uterine activity and premature labor may be decreased after opiates have been administered. Ammonium chloride and other diuretics may give relief in dysmenorrhea, not by their effects on uterine activity, but by the relief of pelvic congestion and edema. Both estrogens and progestational hormones (see Chapter 52) have been employed in the treatment of dysmenorrhea. Though the estrogens may suppress uterine motility under certain circumstances, the prophylactic action in this instance is through the prevention of ovulation. Progestational hormones alone may decrease uterine motility in appropriate circumstances, but the mechanism of their action in dysmenorrhea is undetermined, except that it is not a proliferative effect. Usually, however, the progestins are used in combination with estrogens, to normalize a menstrual cycle and hence diminish dysmenorrhea. The balance between estrogens and progestational hormones may be more important to uterine activity than either type of hormone alone. Nonsteroidal anti-inflammatory drugs (which inhibit the synthesis of prostaglandins; see page 947) play a major role in the management of dysmenorrhea. β_2-Agonists, especially ritodrine, are also widely used. The hormone relaxin is claimed to decrease uterine motility. Miscellaneous "uterine sedatives," may be no more than placebos.

Most of the oxytocic ergot alkaloids also cause cerebral vasoconstriction. Since the painful phase of a migraine attack is the result of cerebral vasodilatation, a vasoconstrictor will often provide relief; this is the basis of the use of vasoconstrictor ergot alkaloids in the treatment of migraine headache. However, the migraine headache is preceded by vasoconstriction, which appears to set the stage for the later vasodilatation. This prodromal vasoconstriction is thought to be the result of excessive release, probably from platelets, of serotonin in the region of the vessels, and serotonin antagonists are effective in preventing not only the aura (vasoconstrictor phase) but also the subsequent headache.

Carboprost Tromethamine

Prosta-5,13-dien-1-oic acid, 9,11,15-trihydroxy-15-methyl-, (5Z,9α,11α,13E,15S)-, compound with 2-amino-2-(hydroxymethyl)-1,3-propanediol (1:1); Prostin/15M (*Upjohn*)

(15S)-15-Methylprostaglandin $F_{2\alpha}$ tromethamine [58551-69-2] $C_{21}H_{36}O_5 \cdot C_4H_{11}NO_3$ (489.65)

Preparation—By a series of complex alterations on a prostaglandin precursor. See US Pat 3,728,382.

Uses—Carboprost is a modified prostaglandin (see *Dinoprostone*, below) which occurs during normal term labor. It is used to *induce abortion* in weeks 12 to 20 of gestation. Successful induction is achieved in about 96% of trials, 78% being complete. It may be used during the second trimester to complete failed spontaneous or drug-induced abortions or to initiate delivery after premature rupture of the membranes. Advantages of carboprost over dinoprost are a longer duration of action and the consequent intramuscular, rather than intra- or extrta-amniotic, route of administration.

Vomiting and diarrhea occur in about 60% of cases and fever (to be differentiated from that of endometritis) in about 10%. Flushing and hot flashes, chills and/or shivering, hiccough, uterine pain, muscular pain, backache, eye pain, breast tenderness, pain at the injection site, paresthesias, and alteration of taste, tinnitus, vertigo, faintness, syncape, drowsiness, dry mouth and throat, thirst, respiratory distress and hyperventilation, coughing, weakness, hematemesis, chest pain or tightness, wheezing, sweating, blepharospasm, thyroid storm, tachycardia, palpitations, hypertension, and uterine rupture also may sometimes occur. Incomplete abortion is also adverse and requires D and C or suction. Carboprost is contraindicated in patients with a history of asthma, cardiovascular or renal disease, hypertension, diabetes, liver disease, jaundice, epilepsy, anemia, or uterine surgery.

Dose—*Intramuscular* (deep), initially, **250 μg** (0.25 mg) to be repeated at 1½ to 3½-hr intervals, or **100 μg** (0.1 mg) initially, followed by **250 μg** (0.25 mg) at 1½-hr intervals. Maintenance doses may be increased to 500 μg (0.5 mg), after several unsuccessful smaller doses. The total cumulative dose should not exceed 12 mg; the average dose is 2.6 mg. Continuous administration should not be longer than 2 days; the mean time to abortion is 16 hr.

Dosage Forms—250 μg of carboprost/1 mL.

Cyproheptadine—page 1132.

Dihydroergotamine Mesylate

Ergotaman-3′,6′,18-trione, 9,10-dihydro-12′-hydroxy-2′-methyl-5′-(phenylmethyl)-, (5′α)-monomethanesulfonate (salt); D.H.E. 45 (*Sandoz*)

Dihydroergotamine monomethanesulfonate [6190-39-2] $C_{33}H_{37}N_5O_5 \cdot CH_4O_3S$ (679.79).

For the structural formula of dihydroergotamine, see page 420.

Preparation—Dihydroergotamine, prepared by catalytic hydrogenation of ergotamine, is reacted with an equimolar portion of methanesulfonic acid in a suitable solvent.

Description—White, yellowish, or faintly red powder; pH (1 in 1000 solution) between 4.4 and 5.4.

Solubility—1 g in 125 mL water, 90 mL alcohol, 175 mL chloroform, 2600 mL ether.

Uses—A smooth muscle stimulant with somewhat weaker actions than those of ergotamine (see *Ergotamine Tartrate*, below). Its actions are erratic, and it is the least effective of the vasoactive drugs used in the treatment of *migraine headache*. However, when it does abolish headache, it usually does so without producing nausea and vomiting. Its greatest disadvantage is that it must be given parenterally. Dihydroergotamine has oxytocic activity and it has been used in the third stage of labor, but it is inferior to other ergot alkaloids used for this purpose. It depresses the vasomotor center more than does ergotamine and constricts the arterioles less, and its net effect is one of moderate hypotension. However, it is not useful as an antihypertensive because of its other side effects. Although dihydroergotamine is an α-adrenergic blocking agent, blockade is not achieved in therapeutic doses. It is an antagonist of serotonin (5-hydroxytryptamine), but it is doubtful that this activity contributes to the therapeutic effect against migraine, in the doses used.

The onset of action of dihydroergotamine mesylate is 15 to 30 min; the duration of action is 3 to 4 hr.

Adverse effects of dihydroergotamine include occasional nausea and vomiting, precordial "pressure" and pain (from coronary vasoconstriction), tachycardia or bradycardia, hypotension, muscle pain in the limbs, weakness in the legs, numbness and tingling in the digits, localized edema, and itching. Gangrene, especially of the extremities, can occur with chronic use or after a large overdose. Dihydroergotamine is contraindicated when there is peripheral vascular disease, coronary insufficiency, hypertension, renal impairment, hepatic dysfunction, sepsis, pregnancy, or hypersensitivity.

Dose—*Intramuscular*, *adult*, **1 mg** at the first sign of impending headache, then **1 mg** at the end of the first hour and *again* at the end of the second hour, making a total of 3 mg. Once the accumulative minimal effective dose is determined, it may be given as a single dose at the onset of an attack, *Intravenous*, *adult*, up to **2 mg.** No more than a total of 6 mg by any route should be given per week.

Dosage Form: Injection: 1 mg/mL.

Dinoprostone

Prosta-5,13-dien-1-oic acid, 11,15-dihydroxy-9-oxo-, (5Z,11α,13E,15S)-, Prostaglandin E₂; PGE₂; Prostin E₂ (*Upjohn*)

Prostaglandin E₂ [363-24-6] $C_{20}H_{32}O_5$ (352.47).

Preparation—The limited availability of the prostaglandins (see page 425) from natural sources has spurred efforts to synthesize them, and total synthesis of prostaglandins F₂ (dinoprost) and E₂ (dinoprostone) has been achieved. The complex syntheses are described in articles in *J Am Chem Soc 91:* 5675, 1969; *92:* 397, 1586, 1970; *94:* 2123, 4342, 1972.

Description—Colorless crystals or white to off-white crystalline solid; melts between 66° and 68°.

Solubility—1 g in about 1000 mL water; soluble in alcohol.

Uses—Dinoprostone is one of a family of over 30 natural, partially cyclic alkenoic acids, called *prostaglandins*, derived from arachidonic acid (see page 426). They are involved in the regulation of endocrine, reproductive, secretory, digestive, nervous, cardiovascular, respiratory, renal, and hemostatic systems. Certain prostaglandins are involved in the cyclical changes in uterine tone and activity and the changes consequent to pregnancy. Furthermore, prostaglandins in semen (whence the name prostaglandin) stimulate the myometrium and fallopian tubes in a way that facilitates the transport of sperm to the ovum. Not all prostaglandins have the same actions, some being vasodilator and others vasoconstrictor, etc. Some prostaglandins, eg, prostaglandins E₂ (PGE₂, dinoprostone) and F₂α (PGF₂α, dinoprost), are oxytocic and also induce cervical softening. Unlike oxytocin, they are oxytocic even in the second trimester of pregnancy and hence can be used as an early abortifacient. Dinoprostone is used to *terminate pregnancy* from the 12th week through the second trimester (80 to 90% effective), to *evacuate the uterus* in intrauterine fetal death or missed abortion up to 28 weeks after conception, and to *manage benign hydatidiform mole*. It is also used to induce labor in mid-trimester and later.

Endovaginal dinoprostone may be sufficiently absorbed into the bloodstream to cause systemic side effects; some of the effects attributed to the drug may possibly be the result of hormonal changes and of release of substances from the feto-placental unit or hydatidiform mole consequent to sloughing and movement or to movement itself. Adverse effects include the following, in decreasing order of frequency: nausea and vomiting (67%), transient fever (50%), diarrhea (40%), headache (10%), chills and shivering (10%), hypotension (10%), backache, arthralgia, flushing, vertigo, vaginal pain, chest pain, dyspnea, endometritis, faintness, syncope, vulvovaginitis, asthenia, muscle cramps and myalgia, tightness in the chest, breast tenderness, blurred vision, cough, rash, stiff neck, dehydration, tremor, paresthesias, impaired hearing, urinary retention, pharyngitis, laryngitis, sweating, wheezing, tachycardia, skin discoloration, vaginismus, tension, and convulsions (rare). Also, dinoprostone is not fetotoxic, and near the end of the second trimester a live fetus may be presented. Caution should be exercised when there is asthma or chronic obstructive pulmonary disease, hypotension, hypertension, other cardiovascular disease, renal or hepatic disease, anemia, jaundice, diabetes, a past history of epilepsy, endocervical disease, vaginitis or cervicitis. It is contraindicated in acute pelvic inflammatory disease and when there is hypersensitivity to the drug.

Dose—*Intrauterine*, high in the uterus, 20 mg, to be repeated at 3- to 4-hour intervals until delivery of the fetus.

Dosage Form—Suppository: 20 mg.

Ergoloid Mesylates—page 909.

Ergonovine Maleate

Ergoline-8-carboxamide, 9,10-didehydro-*N*-(2-hydroxy-1-methylethyl)-6-methyl-, [8β(S)]-, (Z)-2-butenedioate (1:1) (salt); Ergometrine Maleate; Ergotrate Maleate (*Lilly*)

9,10-Didehydro-N-[(S)-2-hydroxy-1-methylethyl]-6-methyl-ergoline-8β-carboxamine maleate (1:1) (salt) [129-51-1] $C_{19}H_{23}N_3O_2.C_4H_4O_4$ (441.48).

For the structural formula of ergonovine, see page 420.

Preparation—Ergonovine maleate may be prepared from the natural alkaloid ergonovine by dissolving the latter in a suitable solvent and reacting it with an equimolar portion of maleic acid.

Ergonovine alkaloid is also prepared synthetically from isolysergic acid obtained by alkaline hydrolysis of ergot alkaloids. One of the methods of synthesis involves the following steps: (1) conversion of the acid to its methyl ester by reaction with diazomethane; (2) hydrazinolysis of the ester to lysergic acid hydrazide; (3) condensation of the hydrazide with nitrous acid to form the azide; (4) metathesis of the azide with D-2-amino-1-propanol to form the amide; and (5) isomerization of the amide to the normal form by treatment with acetic or phosphoric acid.

Description—White to grayish white or faintly yellow, odorless, microcrystalline powder. It is affected by light.

Solubility—1 g in about 36 mL water and about 120 mL alcohol; insoluble in ether and chloroform.

Uses—Ergonovine is the most valued of the ergot alkaloids for obstetrical use. It is a powerful *uterine stimulant* and is active after both oral or parenteral administration. It is less toxic than the other natural alkaloids of ergot and is much less prone to cause gangrene (see *Ergot*, page 419). Ergonovine maleate is given after the delivery of the placenta for the purpose of inducing prolonged, nonphasic contractions of the uterus in order to *reduce postpartum bleeding*. It may also be administered during the puerperium to *promote involution of the uterus*. Ergonovine constricts the cerebral vessels and hence is used in the treatment of migraine headache, but it is inferior for this purpose and is not recommended.

Ergonovine may cause nausea and vomiting, especially when given intravenously. Like other oxytocics, it occasionally evokes severe hypertensive episodes, especially in hypertensive or toxemic patients or when regional anesthetics containing vasoconstrictors have been used. Such hypertensive episodes can be suppressed by chlorpromazine. Hypersensitivity, including anaphylactic shock, has been reported.

Ergonovine is contraindicated before the fetus has been presented, in persons with known allergy to ergot alkaloids, in uterine sepsis, toxemia of pregnancy, peripheral vascular disease, coronary insufficiency, kidney, or liver disease. It should be used cautiously if there is cardiac disease or hypertension. The actions are antagonized by hypocalcemia, and calcium gluconate can be used judiciously to improve the response.

Dose—*Oxytocic: intramuscular*, 200 μg, to be repeated in 2 to 4 hr, if necessary; *intravenous*, 200 μg, only in emergency when there is uncontrolled severe bleeding; *oral*, 200 to 400 μg 2 to 4 times a day, usually for 2 days postpartum but longer if necessary. *Migraine: oral, sublingual*, or *intramuscular, adult*, 200 to 400 μg at onset of headache; may be repeated at 2-hr intervals up to a total of 1.6 mg per day.

Dosage Forms—Injection: 200 μg/1 mL; Tablets: 200 μg.

Ergotamine Tartrate

Ergotaman-3′,6′,18-trione, 12′-hydroxy-2′-methyl-5′-(phenylmethyl)-, (5′α)-[R-(R^*,R^*)]-2,3-dihydroxybutanedioate (2:1) (salt); Ergomar (*Fisons*); Ergostat (*Parke-Davis*); Gynergen (*Sandoz*)

Ergotamine tartrate (2:1) (salt) [379-79-3] $(C_{33}H_{35}N_5O_5)_2.C_4H_6O_6$ (1313.43).

For the structural formula of ergotamine, see page 420.

Description—Colorless crystals or a white to yellowish white, crystalline powder, usually containing solvent of crystallization. These crystals lose the solvent of crystallization in a high vacuum. It melts at about 180° with decomposition.

Solubility—1 g in about 500 mL water and about 500 mL alcohol; slightly more soluble in the presence of a slight excess of tartaric acid.

Uses—Possesses the characteristic actions of ergot alkaloids (see *Ergot Alkaloids*, page 420). It is the drug of choice in the treatment of *migraine, cluster*, and other *vascular headaches*, and it affords relief in about 90% of cases. It contracts the painfully dilated cerebral vessels in these disorders. The drug is most effective if given early in the course of the attack. It is best administered by subcutaneous or intramuscular injection. Ergotamine also exerts oxytocic actions,

but it is no longer used as an oxytocic. There is no acceptable evidence that ergotamine is of benefit in menopausal disorders. Use of ergotamine to treat cardiovascular disorders could be dangerous.

Thirteen of 17 ergotamine-containing products are combinations. Caffeine (100 mg) is a time-honored adjuvant; it not only also constricts the affected cerebral vessels but is somewhat analgesic as well.

Some products contain belladonna alkaloids in marginally effective amounts, with the unsupported rationale that the alkaloids correct some hypothetical autonomic imbalance. Were there such an "imbalance", it would be uncorrectable with the drugs; indeed, the effects of ergotamine promote an imbalance reflexly. Products containing phenobarbital are also promoted with faulty rationale; if an anti-anxiety drug is justified, a benzodiazepine should be used. Cyclizine iş included in some combinations to suppress nausea and vomiting caused both by ergotamine and the migraine attack.

The duration of action averages 5 hr by the oral, and 15 min to 2 hr by the intramuscular and subcutaneous routes.

Adverse effect of ergotamine are most common after large doses or accumulation of small doses. They include nausea, vomiting, epigastric distress, diarrhea, muscle weakness, precordial distress and pain (indicative of coronary spasm), coldness of the skin (from vasoconstriction), bradycardia or tachycardia, paresthesias in the extremities, myalgia (especially in the thigh and neck muscles), localized edema (mostly in the face and extremities), itching and dermatitis. Occasionally hypertensive episodes occur. With continued administration, severe vasoconstriction, endarteritis, and gangrene may result. With combinations, the potential adverse effects of the other components must also be kept in mind. Ergotamine is contraindicated in pregnancy, peripheral vascular disease, coronary insufficiency or angina pectoris, thrombophlebitis, peptic ulcer, kidney disease, liver disease, sepsis, malnutrition, and when there is a history of hypersensitivity to ergot alkaloids.

Dose—*Oral, adult*, 1 to 2 mg; this dose may be repeated in 30 min and again in 1 hr. In subsequent attacks up to 3 or 4 mg may be taken, but no more than 6 mg should be taken in any one day. No more than 10 mg should be taken per week. *Sublingual or buccal, adult*, 2 mg; this dose may be repeated every 30 min up to a total of 6 mg in one day. No more than 10 mg should be taken per week. *Inhalation, adult*, 360 μg; this dose may be repeated at intervals no shorter than 30 min up to a total of 2.16 mg (6 inhalations) per day. A weekly limit is not stated, but it should probably not exceed 5 mg. *Rectal, adult*, 2 mg of ergotamine tartrate with 100 mg of caffeine; this dose may be repeated once only in 1 hour if necessary. No more than 5 suppositories (10 mg of ergotamine) should be taken/week.

Dosage Forms—Inhalation: 9 mg/mL; Suppositories: 2 mg (with 100 mg of caffeine); Tablets: 1 mg; Sublingual Tablets: 2 mg.

Methylergonovine Maleate

Ergoline-8-carboxamide, 9,10-didehydro-N-[1-(hydroxymethyl)propyl]-6-methyl-, [8β(S)]-, (Z)-2-butenedioate (1:1) (salt); Methergine (*Sandoz*)

9,10 - Didehydro - N-[(S)-1-(hydroxymethyl)propyl]-6-methyl-ergoline-8β-carboxamide maleate (1:1) (salt) [7054-07-1] [57432-61-8] $C_{20}H_{25}N_3O_2.C_4H_4O_4$ (455.51).

For the structural formula of methylergonovine, see page 420.

Preparation—Methylergonovine is synthesized by the method described above for ergonovine except that in step (4), D-2-amino-1-butanol is employed. The base, dissolved in a suitable solvent, yields the maleate by reaction with an equimolar quantity of maleic acid.

Description—White to pinkish tan, microcrystalline powder, which is odorless and possesses a bitter taste. It must be protected from light and heat. pH (1 in 5000 solution) between 4.4 and 5.2.

Solubility—1 g in 100 mL water, 175 mL alcohol, 1900 mL chloroform, 8400 mL ether.

Uses—Similar in its actions to ergonovine, and it shares the same uses as an *oxytocic* drug (see *Ergonovine Maleate* page 947). It may induce uterine contractions upon either oral or parenteral administration. The intensity and duration of its oxytocic action is greater than that of ergonovine but less than that of ergotamine. Despite a lesser incidence of side effects compared to other drugs used to treat migraine, authorities do not recommend this use because the efficacy is less.

The side effects of methylergonovine are the same as those of *Ergonovine* (page 947), but they are of a lesser intensity. The precautions and contraindications are also the same. Some obstetricians use methylergonovine even in the presence of toxemia of pregnancy, but this practice must be considered dangerous.

Dose—*Oxytocic: Oral, adult*, **200 μg** 3 to 4 times a day, usually for 2 days postpartum and no longer than 1 week. *Intramuscular*, **200 μg**, to be repeated in 2 to 4 hours if necessary. *Intravenous*, **200 μg** in a single dose in the emergency control of uterine bleeding.

Dosage Forms—Injection: 200 μg/mL; Tablets: 200 μg.

Methysergide Maleate

Ergoline-8-carboxamide, 9,10-didehydro-*N*-[1-(hydroxymethyl)propyl]-1,6-dimethyl-, (8β)-, (*Z*)-2-butenedioate (1:1) (salt); Sansert (*Sandoz*)

9,10-Didehydro-*N*-[1-(hydroxymethyl)propyl]-1,6-dimethylergoline-8β-carboxamide maleate (1:1) (salt) [129-49-7] $C_{21}H_{27}N_3$-$O_2.C_4H_4O_4$ (469.54).

For the structural formula of methysergide, see page 420.

Preparation—Methylergonovine (base) is methylated at the indole nitrogen with methyl iodide and the resulting methysergide (base) is dissolved in a suitable solvent and reacted with an equimolar portion of maleic acid. For the preparation of methylergonovine (base), see above. US Pat 3,113,133.

Description—White to yellowish white or reddish white crystalline powder; melting point is uncharacteristic showing decomposition above approximately 165°; odorless or has not more than a slight odor.

Solubility—1 g in 200 mL water, 165 mL alcohol, 3400 mL chloroform; practically insoluble in ether.

Uses—Methysergide is the *N*-methyl derivative of methylergonovine. However, its oxytocic activity is much weaker, and it is not employed as an oxytocic. Its principal therapeutic use is in the *treatment and prophylaxis of migraine headache*, for which the drug is quite effective, but it is of very little use during an acute attack. Since methysergide has only weak vasoconstrictor activity, cerebral vasoconstriction has been discounted as the mechanism of action against migraine; thus its action would differ from that of ergotamine (see *Ergotamine Tartrate*, page 948). However, direct proof in man that cerebral vasoconstriction does not occur has not been offered; the fact that methysergide induces anginal pain and intermittent claudication in some persons strongly suggests a significant degree of vasoconstrictor activity. It has been suggested that it may induce vasoconstriction indirectly through central vasomotor stimulation or through sensitization to other endogenous vasoconstrictors, but this hypothesis is unsatisfactory on both pharmacological and physiological grounds. Methysergide is a potent serotonin antagonist, and it has been suggested that its usefulness against migraine is based on this action; various facts contradict this suggestion. Methysergide has been used in suppressing gastrointestinal hypermotility and spasm and cardiovascular disorders that occur in patients with *carcinoid tumor*. These tumors release large amounts of serotonin into the bloodstream, and the antiserotonin actions of the drug are responsible for the beneficial effects. It has also been reported to be of some benefit in attenuating the *dumping syndrome*. The drug is not effective in tension and other types of headache.

Side effects of methysergide occur in more than a third of patients, but they are usually mild and of brief duration. They are severe enough in 20% of users to require discontinuation of the drug. The most common adverse effects are nausea, abdominal cramps, leg cramps, vertigo, restlessness, insomnia, drowsiness, confusion, epigastric pain (with increased secretion of gastric acid), and feelings of depersonalization. Less frequent effects include vomiting, diarrhea, constipation, muscle weakness, myalgia, arthralgia, paresthesias in the extremities, ataxia, facial flush, skin rash, telangiectasis, edema and weight gain, weakness, tachycardia, postural hypotension, coronary and peripheral arterial insufficiency, alopecia, and induction of premature labor. Neutropenia and eosinophilia are rare. Prolonged therapy has been known to cause retroperitoneal fibrosis. Patients should be instructed in the signs and symptoms of the syndrome, and a urogram should be taken at 6-month intervals during chronic use. It also causes pleuropulmonary, myocardial, and aortic fibrosis, the last-named to the point of obstruction. Methysergide suppresses sleep-related prolactin secretion and increases growth hormone secretion during sleep, effects that may be adverse or beneficial, de-

pending on circumstances. Many of the side effects diminish after continued administration of the drug. Methysergide is contraindicated during pregnancy, in patients with peripheral vascular disease, valvular heart disease, coronary artery disease, thrombophlebitis, severe hypertension, renal, hepatic, or pulmonary disorders, rheumatoid arthritis or other collagen diseases or any condition which may cause fibrosis. Methysergide should be taken with meals.

Dose—*Oral, adult*, 2 mg 2 to 4 times a day, preferably with meals. It should not be used continuously for a period longer than 6 months without a 1- to 2-month drug-free interval. When discontinuing use, the dose must be reduced gradually to avoid rebound headache.

Dosage Form—Tablets: 2 mg.

Oxytocin

Alpha-Hypophamine; Pitocin (*Parke-Davis*); Syntocinon (*Sandoz*); Uteracon (*Hoechst-Roussel*)

$$H-Cys-Tyr-Ile-Glu(NH_2)-Asp(NH_2)-Cys-Pro-Leu-Gly-NH_2$$

[50-56-6] $C_{43}H_{66}N_{12}O_{12}S_2$ (1007.19).

Preparation—It is obtained from the posterior lobe of the pituitary of healthy hogs or cattle. The material obtained from either source has the same aminoacid composition. Synthesis was achieved by du Vigneaud and is beyond the scope of this text (see *J Am Chem Soc* 76:3107 (1954)). Commercial preparation is described in US Pat 3,076,797.

Description—White powder; $[\alpha]_D^{22} - 26.2°$ (c = 0.53).

Solubility—Soluble in water, 1-butanol and 2-butanol.

Uses—See *Posterior Pituitary*, page 957. Natural, endogenous oxytocin is involved in normal parturition. The hormone stimulates guanyl cyclase in myometrial tissue, which promotes inward movement of sodium ion and the consequent increase in both the frequency and strength of contractions. The contractions that are induced are normal phasic contractions. It does not appear to initiate activity not already latent. Hence the drug is not very active until close to term, and it is less likely than ergonovine to cause harm to the fetus and mother. Nevertheless, unless the cervix is dilated, oxytocin can cause injury. Oxytocin is used antepartum when an early vaginal delivery is desired. It is the drug of choice for the *maintenance of labor* once the pregnancy is at term. It is used more frequently when there is prolonged *uterine inertia* than when labor is only somewhat sluggish. It may be used to *assist an ongoing abortion*. It cannot induce an abortion except in high doses (20 to 30 units) and usually not until after the 20th week of pregnancy. It may be used to *control postpartum hemorrhage* and *promote uterine involution*, but the appropriate ergot alkaloids are preferred. Oxytocin induces contraction of the myoepithelial cells around the breast alveoli, thus squeezing milk into the larger ducts and increasing flow through the nipple, and it is occasionally used in the treatment of breast engorgement or to increase milk flow to the infant.

Oxytocin has a weak antidiuretic hormone-like activity, and during prolonged infusion it can cause water intoxication with convulsions and coma, especially in patients with toxemia of pregnancy. Saline, rather than dextrose, for infusion lessens this danger. The drug also occasionally induces a hypertensive episode, which may cause subarachnoid hemorrhage or fetal death. Pelvic hematomas and allergic reactions may occur in the mother and cardiac arrhythmias and jaundice in the fetus. The drug is contraindicated in toxemia abruptio placentae, undilated cervix, over-distended uterus, abnormal presentation, and renal or cardiovascular disease.

Dose—*Intramuscular*, to control postpartum bleeding, **10 Units** after the delivery of the placenta. *Intravenous infusion*, for *induction and/or maintenance of labor*, *initially* 1 to **2 mUnits/min** then gradually increasing the rate by increments of 1 to 2 mUnits/min at 15- to 30-min intervals until a near-normal contraction pattern has been achieved or a rate of 20 mUnits/min has been established; to *control postpartum uterine bleeding*, **10 to 40 Units** in 1000 mL of isotonic sodium chloride solution with or without 5% dextrose infused at a *rate necessary to cause uterine contraction;* to *manage incomplete or impending abortion*, **20** to **40 mUnits/min.** *Intranasal*, to *stimulate milk flow*, **one spray into one or both nostrils** of a solution containing 40 Units/mL, to be administered 2 to 3 min prior to nursing or breast pumping.

Dosage Forms—Injection 10 Units/mL; Nasal spray: 40 Units/mL.

Other Uterine and Antimigraine Drugs

Dinoprost Tromethamine [$(5Z,9\alpha,11\alpha,13E,15S)$-9,11,15-Trihydroxyprosta-5,13-dien-1-oic acid comp. with 2-amino-2-(hydroxymethyl)-1,3-propanediol (1:1) [38562-01-5] $C_{20}H_{34}O_5.C_4H_{11}NO_3$ (475.62); Prostaglandin $F_{2\alpha}$ Tromethamine; Prostin F_2 Alpha Injectable (*Upjohn*)]—Dinoprost is a synthetic derivative of *dinoprostone* (see page 974) in which the O atom in 9-position of the latter is reduced to OH. Tromethamine (2-amino-2-hydroxymethyl-1,3-propanediol) converts dinoprost, which is slightly soluble in water, to a salt that is readily soluble and suitable for injection. It occurs as a white to off-white, crystalline powder; odorless and bitter tasting; stable in light, air, and heat; melts at about 100°. *Uses:* Dinoprost is a natural oxytocic prostaglandin that is active even during the second trimester of pregnancy and hence can be used as an early abortifacient (see *Dinoprostone*). Since the compound also has hypertensive actions, it is not given systemically but rather by intra-amniotic administration. Successful abortion occurs in about 86% of cases and incomplete abortion in about 12%. Untoward effects are those of dinoprostone, except hypertension rather than hypotension may occur. In addition, cough, burning sensations in eye and breast, dysuria, hematuria, hiccough, and polydipsia have been reported. Cervical perforation, rupture and retention of the placenta, and hemorrhage can occur. Dinoprost is contraindicated in acute pelvic inflammation. It should be used cautiously in patients with a history of hypertension, asthma, glaucoma, epilepsy, or cardiovascular disease. *Dose: Intra-amniotic*, 40 mg, by slow injection after previous removal of an appropriate volume of amniotic fluid; 10 to 40 mg may be repeated in 24 hr, if necessary. *Extra-amniotic*, initially 0.5 mg followed by 0.75 mg every 2 hr until abortion; or initially 0.25 mg followed by 0.75 mg in 5 min, 1 mg in 30 min, and 1 mg every 6 hr; or 1 mg/hr by continuous infusion; or 5 mg bolus every 2 to 3 hr to a total of 15 mg. *Dosage Form:* Injection: 5 mg/mL (dinoprost equivalent).

Ergot Alkaloids—Over 20 ergot alkaloids have been isolated, and a number of semisynthetic compounds have been made. The sources and a brief chemistry of the ergot alkaloids are discussed in Chapter 25. *Actions and Uses:* The pharmacology of the ergot alkaloids is quite complex. Although there are similarities among them, each possesses distinct properties. Natural alkaloids of the peptide type (ergotamine, ergosine, ergocornine, ergocryptine, ergocristine; see index) are potent vasoconstrictors and oxytocics of unknown mechanism and also weak α-adrenoreceptor blocking agents. They also possess weak dopaminergic activity, except bromocriptine, which has strong dopaminergic activity. 9,10-Hydrogenation considerably diminishes the vasoconstrictor activity, especially in the ergotoxine group (ergocornine, ergocryptine, and ergocristine) and moderately diminishes the oxytocic activity, but the α-blocking activity is increased; vasodepression, mostly due to a central action, obscures the residual vasoconstrictor action. Both the parent and dihydro alkaloids possess serotonin antagonist activity, but there is also some partial serotonin agonist activity with some. They also increase phosphodiesterase activity, and some ergot derivatives appear to block cyclic AMP, which gives some members the appearance of having β-adrenoreceptor blocking activity. The so-called amine alkaloids (which are actually alkanolamides), such as ergonovine and methylergonovine (see index), possess only slight vasoconstrictor activity but retain oxytocic activity, for which they are mainly used; they are nearly devoid of adrenergic or serotonin-blocking, serotonin-agonist, or dopaminergic activity, except that methysergide is an effective serotonin antagonist. The ergoline derivatives (LSD, lergotrile, lisuride, others) lack significant peripheral actions but have interesting central actions. LSD is a partial serotonin agonist, acting like serotonin at some loci and as antagonist at others, and it possesses dopaminergic activity as well; the hallucinogenic properties have been attributed to its serotoninergic activity. Other ergolines and some clavines have weak serotoninergic activity and lack hallucinogenic activity but have strong dopaminergic activity in some central loci and dopamine antagonist activity in others. Thus both the ergolines (especially lergotrile) and bromocriptine may cause remissions in parkinsonism, as the result of dopaminergic activity in the corpus striatum, but increase plasma levels of prolactin, growth hormone, and follicle-stimulating hormone, as the result of blocking dopamine receptors in the anterior pituitary gland (where dopamine inhibits release) and perhaps in the anterior hypothalamus (where dopamine promotes the release of the hormone-release factors). The emetic actions of the ergot alkaloids are probably attributable to dopaminergic activity at the chemoreceptor trigger zone on the floor of the fourth ventricle, and the hypotensive activity of the dihydrogenated ergot alkaloids possibly is attributable to dopaminergic and/or α-adrenergic activity in the vasomotor center. The effects of bromocriptine and lergotrile to diminish some senile dementia may also result from a dopaminergic action.

CHAPTER 52

Hormones

Stewart C Harvey, PhD
Professor of Pharmacology

C Dean Withrow, PhD
Associate Professor of Pharmacology

School of Medicine, University of Utah
Salt Lake City, UT 84132

Hormones are substances secreted by the endocrine, or ductless, glands which serve to integrate metabolic processes. The regulatory function of the hormones differs from other regulatory mechanisms (such as the nervous system and other glandular secretions) in that the hormones are transported to the affected tissues by the blood. Some of the hormones affect nearly all the tissues of the body; the action of others is restricted to but a few tissues or organs.

Chemically, the hormones represent a very diverse group of compounds. Some, like epinephrine and thyroxine, are relatively simple amino acid derivatives. Several groups of hormones, such as those produced by the adrenal cortex and the gonads, are steroids, while the pituitary, parathyroid, and pancreatic hormones are polypeptides or proteins; the molecular weights of the latter range from about 1000 to 30,000 or more. The gastrointestinal, thymic, renal, adrenal medullary, and cerebral (other than hypothalamic) hormones are not discussed in this chapter.

In most instances, the existence of a trophic hormone was usually first recognized when degeneration or destruction of a gland by disease or accident in humans or its experimental removal from animals was found to result in unfavorable physiological consequences. (The hypothalamic releasing and inhibitory hormones were anticipated on theoretical grounds and discovered as the result of theory-directed research.) Attempts were then made to reverse such untoward effects by implanting tissues from healthy animals (frequently at other sites) or by supplying extracts prepared from them. Once the type of physiological activity attributable to any one gland has been recognized and a biologically effective extract has been produced, the way is opened for the development of an assay method by means of which the hormone content of various preparations can be compared. The ultimate goal with each extract is to obtain a demonstrably pure active substance, to establish its chemical structure, and to develop either a method of synthesis or a convenient method of preparation from natural sources so as to make it available for therapeutic or experimental use. Frequently, the successful conclusion of attempts to isolate, purify, and identify a hormone has also permitted the development of chemical methods for its determination—for example, in body fluids. However, for some of the hormones, available chemical methods for identification and quantitative determination are still inferior to biological methods as regards specificity and sensitivity.

Standardization—Many of the hormones, or substances which possess nearly identical biological properties, have been prepared in chemically pure (usually crystalline) form, either from natural sources, or by synthesis. For such materials, the standard practice is prescription in terms of weight. With others, especially some of the polypeptide or protein hormones, potency is expressed in terms of biological activity. In such instances, a unit of biological activity is established as the amount necessary to produce a predetermined response in a test animal, or by comparison with an arbitrarily accepted standard preparation. For some preparations, eg, insulin and the posterior lobe hormones, the custom of designating dosage in terms of biological "units" has persisted even after the substance has become available in chemically pure form. The use of units is especially important when hormones of different sources differ in chemical composition and activity. In any event, no hormone preparation should be used therapeutically unless it is a pure substance or its activity can be assayed biologically.

Administration—A few of the hormones can be administered *orally* with full effect, as, for example, thyroid and certain steroid hormones. There is usually some loss due to destruction of the hormone in the digestive tract, its elimination from the circulation, or inactivation while it is in transit through the liver immediately after absorption. Some hormones must be administered by injection, either *hypodermically* or *intramuscularly*, because they are inactivated in the digestive tract. The intramuscular injection is usually chosen, and it gives rapid absorption if the hormone is in aqueous solution, or slower absorption if the hormone is in oil. This use of oil is not ideal, for oil is not readily removed from the site of injection, and oils are difficult to free from allergens. Suspensions of crystals of differing size also have variable repository actions. Another technique is the *implantation* of compressed pellets of those hormones which are only slightly soluble in tissue fluid; these pellets are placed in the subcutaneous tissues and are absorbed during a period of a few months. This technique has the disadvantage of requiring a careful surgical procedure, and, even with good technique, certain pellets may be extruded due to infection, or they may be of no value because of fibrous tissue barriers which develop about the pellets in some cases. Hormones entrained in degradable polymers, or even in silicones, can be used for slow-release forms. Still another form is the buccal tablet of very highly compressed steroid hormone which is held in the sublingual or buccal area for up to 45 min, and during this time there is absorption through the buccal mucous membrane, providing direct access of the steroid to the systemic circulation. This avoids the disadvantage of the oral route, by which steroids must pass through the liver where they are largely inactivated. Some of the synthetic or semisynthetic hormones are so structured as to greatly diminish enzymatic destruction in the liver and hence are effective orally. Notable among these are the oral contraceptives.

As with many other agents, the use of any of these drugs in food-producing animals by any method or route legally should be in accordance with the restrictions of the Bureau of Veterinary Medicine, Food and Drug Administration, wherein a specific "withdrawal time" lapse is required between the last drug dose and slaughter (or milk or egg production, as the case may be) to avoid drug residues in the human food supply.

The Pituitary Hormones

The pituitary body (hypophysis) comprises anterior, intermediate, and posterior portions or lobes, which have distinguishing structures and functions. Active principles have been discovered in extracts prepared in various ways from all three portions of the pituitary, and these will be listed and discussed separately.

The Anterior Pituitary

The pituitary body is known as the "master gland" because it has so many important actions in the body and it regulates the function of several of the other glands. Without the anterior portion of the pituitary gland, the sex functions and growth cease, and the functions of the adrenal cortex, the thyroid, and the parathyroids decrease markedly. The anterior lobe of the pituitary has at least *six* separate hormones. Some of the anterior pituitary hormones are also produced outside of the adenohypophysis and extrapituitary production plays a role in physiological functions of certain pituitary hormones. For example, a growth hormone-lactogenic hormone and ACTH elaborated by the placenta undoubtedly are important during pregnancy.

1. **Growth Hormone** (*GH, Somatropin, Somatotropin, STH*)—This hormone causes an increase in weight and length of the body. The increase in length is especially prominent, due to the bone growth, but its effect is manifested in nearly all the tissues of the body. Human growth hormone also possesses most of the activities of lactogenic hormone. For maximum action of growth hormone, all the essential and quasiessential amino acids must be present in abundance. Some, perhaps all, of the effects of GH are mediated by several *somatomedins*.

The growth hormone from human pituitaries has been isolated as a crystalline, apparently homogeneous protein containing 191 amino acid residues and of a molecular weight of 22,000 daltons. It is also found in a much larger molecule which is probably an association of the primary molecule with another protein. There are at least four isohormones of the primary molecule. Its biological properties can be assayed by observing the growth of hypophysectomized young rats in response to injections of the hormone, or by measuring the extent of bone growth (tibia) adjacent to the epiphyseal line. The daily injection of as little as 0.010 mg of purified growth hormone will cause a measurable increase in the weight of young hypophysectomized rats. In humans, the protein anabolic action of growth hormone is most readily measured by its nitrogen-retaining effect. Other assay methods involve the effect on the plasma sulfation factor, plasma phosphate, insulin tolerance, and especially radioimmunoassay.

In addition to effects upon protein metabolism, growth hormone affects the metabolism of carbohydrates and fats. These effects include (a) maintenance of a normal amount of muscle glycogen in hypophysectomized animals, (b) decreased responsiveness to insulin, and (c) increased concentration of nonesterified fatty acids in plasma. Human growth hormone also exerts prominent effects on the kidney and electrolyte metabolism. Human growth hormone has lactogenic activity, and for a long time it was thought that, in the human, growth hormone (STH) and prolactin (PrL) were the same substance. However in 1970 the two hormones were shown to be distinct and to be under separate regulation. Stimulation of lactation is an undesirable side effect of STH. Growth hormone produced in human placenta has an even greater lactogenic activity; 11 of the first 17 amino acids are the same and in identical sequence as those in lactogenic hormone, and the remaining 6 are similar.

Unlike corticotropin, insulin, and some of the other protein hormones, a considerable species difference has been observed in response to growth hormone administration. Thus, growth hormone active in fishes can be isolated from fish pituitaries, but this substance is inactive in mammals. Bovine growth hormone is active in fishes, rats, dogs (and presumably in cattle) but is inactive in monkeys and men, whereas growth hormone prepared from simian or human pituitaries is active in both primate species, as well as in nearly all lower orders of animals in which it has been tested. These differences appear to be reflections of significant differences in the chemical composition of the hormones from various sources. For example, the molecular weight of primate growth hormone is much smaller than that of the bovine variety (29,000 vs 46,000).

These facts explain why attempts to demonstrate beneficial effects when growth hormone preparations from domestic animals are used clinically have been disappointing. Human growth hormone from human pituitaries has been used successfully in stimulating growth (height and weight increase) in hypopituitary dwarfs for long periods. It has also been used

to treat other forms of retarded growth. An interesting diagnostic application of human growth hormone is based upon its ability to increase the concentration of free fatty acids in the blood. Patients suffering from acromegaly (a disease caused by excessive secretion of growth hormone) are sometimes treated by radiation therapy. In order to assess the effects of the treatment, growth hormone is administered and its effects upon plasma free fatty acid is determined. The administration of growth hormone to an untreated acromegalic causes no change in plasma free fatty acid, since the concentration of growth hormone in the circulation is already very high. If the treatment is successful, production of endogenous growth hormone diminishes or ceases; subsequent injection of growth hormone will cause an increase in free fatty acids in the plasma. The effect to increase blood glucose concentration has been used in the treatment of hypoglycemia (especially that which is lysine-sensitive) in children. The nitrogen-sparing anabolic effect has been employed to suppress catabolism from burns and other severe trauma.

2. **The Gonadotropic Hormones**—Three separate gonadotropins are secreted by the anterior pituitary. These three hormones, acting both in concert and sequentially, control the sexual (estrous) cycle in lower animals and the menstrual cycle in primates.

   a. Follicle-stimulating Hormone (*FSH*)—This substance promotes maturation of the primordial follicle and in combination with small amounts of LH (see below) stimulates secretion of estrogen by the developing follicle. Human FSH is a glycoprotein with a molecular weight of 17,000. The carbohydrate content is 8 to 9%. During the first 7 days of the estrous cycle, estrogens suppress the release of FSH, as a result of negative feedback actions on both the anterior pituitary and hypothalamus. In days 9 to 18, estrogens have a positive feedback effect to increase FSH secretion; progesterone blocks the positive but not the negative feedback effect.

   b. Luteinizing Hormone (*LH*)—The secretion of LH increases near the middle of the cycle. As noted above, small amounts of LH, acting with FSH, stimulate the secretion of estrogen by the ovarian follicle. As the amount of LH increases, ovulation occurs, and the corpus luteum begins to form.

   LH also acts upon the male gonads, specifically upon the interstitial cells of the testis, to produce testosterone. Because of this property, LS is also sometimes referred to as interstitial cell-stimulating hormone (ICSH).

   As with FSH, estrogens have a suppressant effect on LH secretion early and an augmenting effect later in the estrous cycle, but the time course of sensitivity is somewhat different from that with FSH. Progesterone similarly blocks the positive feedback effect. Androgens also suppress the secretion of LH.

   Human LH is a glycoprotein with a molecular weight of 35,000. The carbohydrate content is 3.5%.

   c. Prolactin (*PrL*; lactogenic hormone, mammotropin)—Prolactin is produced by the adenohypophysis. A related hormone, placental lactogen (PL; chorionic somatomammotropin) is produced by the placenta. Because the earliest known effects in mammals were the stimulation of breast growth and development and of milk secretion, there has been a preoccupation with these actions, but it is now recognized that PrL is a hormone with many different actions, perhaps more so than growth hormone, of which primitive prolactin appears to be the phylogenetic precursor.

   By itself, PrL does not cause breast development, but in concert with estrogens, progesterone, and permissive actions of hydrocortisone and insulin it is mammotropic. In the human, it also stimulates milk secretion by the mammary glands, but only after suitable priming by estrogens and progesterone. Other effects in humans include lipolysis, luteotropism and luteolysis, promotion of growth and secretion, increase in testicular steroidogenesis and development of the male accessory sex organs, and involvement in the regulation of gonadotropin release. Probably other, presently unidentified effects also occur, since in other mammals nitrogen anabolic, glycolytic, renotropic, erythropoietic, and somatotropic effects occur, along with effects to promote hair follicle and sebaceous gland development, vaginal mucification and behavioral changes. Many other effects are seen in non-mammalian vertebrates.

   Prolactin is a protein of MW 20,000, which is derived from a prohormone of MW 50,000. In the last 50 *N*-terminal aminoacids of prolactin there is 24% identity with growth hormone in the aminoacids and sequence. Human placental lactogen has an identity of 76%, which accounts for the greater growth hormone-like properties of the placental lactogen. Both prolactin and growth hormone have "big" and "little" circulating forms, the release of which appears to be under separate controls.

   Other Gonadotropic Preparations—In addition to the anterior pituitary glands, three other sources of gonadotropic activity are known. Two are produced by the chorionic cells of the placentae of women and mares, respectively. The third is a gonadotropin (human menopausal gonadotropin or HMG) present in the serum of postmenopausal women and is a mixture of FSH:LH in approximately a 1:1 ratio. Human chorionic gonadotropin (HCG) is secreted into the maternal blood and is excreted in the urine, where it may be detected within 48 hr after the ovum is implanted. The biological properties of HCG approximate most closely those of LH and PrL in combination, although it differs substantially from either in chemical properties. Thus, like PrL, HCG maintains the secretion of the corpus luteum, enabling pregnancy to continue. Like LH, it will act upon gonadal interstitial cells. Unlike FSH, it will not act upon the ovary of the hypophysectomized rat, although it will exert a marked synergism with FSH in this respect.

Human chorionic gonadotropin is a glycoprotein of molecular weight 35,000; the carbohydrate content is about 28%. The molecule has α and β subunits, the β-subunit conferring the special activity. There is about an 80% homology in structure and amino acid sequence to HLH-β. HCG-α is nearly identical to FSH-α, except for the terminal three aminoacids.

The international unit of HCG is defined as the activity of 0.1 mg of the international standard. Purified HCG contains approximately 12,000 IU/mg.

Uses of Gonadotropic Hormones—Although many attempts have been made to demonstrate in humans an effect of pituitary gonadotropins from domestic animals, the evidence obtained so far has been equivocal or frankly negative. This may be due to a species specificity of the kind already noted in connection with growth hormone preparations. Preparations of FSH from human pituitaries or menotropins from the serum of postmenopausal women, administered in conjunction with LH or HCG, have been found to induce ovulation in women suffering from diminished gonadotropin secretion. However, evidence of superovulation (production of more than one ovum) is sometimes obtained following administration of FSH or menotropins of human origin. Human chorionic gonadotropin is also used for stimulation of androgen secretion by testicular interstitial cells, and for expediting the descent of the testes in boys and young men with cryptorchidism. It has also been found to be effective in prolonging luteal function and in inducing ovulatory cycles in anovulatory women with metropathia hemorrhagica. However, human chorionic gonadotropin appears to induce ovulation only when a mature ovarian follicle is present. Unfortunately, a mature follicle is not common in anovulatory women. Prolactin has no clinical use. HCG is not effective in the treatment of obesity.

3. Thyrotropic Hormone (*Thyrotropin, TSH*)—This substance sustains the activity of the thyroid gland, promoting increased uptake of inorganic iodine and release of organically bound iodine. In the absence of TSH, the thyroid gland atrophies, producing only small amounts of thyroid hormone. An excess of TSH causes hypertrophy and hyperplasia of the thyroid, and a clinical picture resembling Graves' disease.

The most potent TSH preparations which have been obtained thus far are still impure. TSH obtained from beef pituitaries is a glycoprotein of molecular weight of about 28,000. The sugars are mannose, fucose, galactose and N-acetylglucosamine. Human TSH contains sialic acid. There are two subunits. The β subunit contains the specific activity; it has 113 amino acid residues, without carbohydrate moieties. The α subunit has 96 residues and the carbohydrate moieties. The α unit is functionally interchangeable with the α unit of LH or HCG, and the α units are nearly identical.

TSH assays depend upon the measurement of TSH-induced changes in the weight, acinar cell height, or iodine content of thyroids of chicks or guinea pigs. Methods based upon the discharge of thyroid iodine, which increases when TSH is administered, are to be preferred. The use of radioactive iodine as a tracer in the latter procedure represents an elegant refinement of this technique.

In Graves' disease an abnormal thyrotropic substance is present in the blood. Because of its long duration of action it is called long-acting thyroid stimulator (LATS). It is a 7S globulin of the immunoglobulin G (IgG) class. It may be an autoantibody to TSH which is capable of mimicking its antigen. It differs from TSH in that it crosses the placental barrier, and its production is not suppressed by thyroid hormone; the nonsuppressibility is the basis of a diagnostic test for borderline hyperthyroidism.

4. Adrenal Corticotropic Hormone (*Corticotropin, ACTH*)—ACTH is produced not only by the adenohypophysis but also by the placenta. This hormone maintains and controls the function of the adrenal cortex, and thus indirectly affects carbohydrate, protein, and mineral metabolism (see *Adrenal Hormones*, page 958). Adrenocorticotropin is a polypeptide containing 39 amino acid residues with a molecular weight of about 4500.

The hormones from pituitaries of various species of animals differ with respect to the sequence of amino acids 25–32, but these differences do not affect their biological actions. When corticotropin is treated briefly with pepsin, 11 amino acid residues at the C-terminal end are removed. The product (β-corticotropin) retains full biological activity. In contrast, even slight alteration of the N-terminal end of the molecule results in substantial inactivation.

A synthetic polypeptide containing the first 23 amino acid residues of naturally occurring corticotropin has essentially all of the biological and clinical properties of corticotropin. Several peptides have been synthesized which are more potent than natural ACTH.

Physiological Effects—Since the known physiological actions of corticotropin are mediated through the adrenal cortex, its effects are similar to those of the adrenal cortical hormones, especially the glucocorticoids (see *Adrenal Hormones*, page 958). ACTH also slightly enhances the adrenal cortical output of aldosterone and hence has a minor action on

mineral metabolism. However, aldosterone secretion is mostly under the control of the renin-angiotensin system.

The first 13 amino acids of ACTH are identical in sequence to those of α-MSH (melanocyte-stimulating hormone); consequently, ACTH causes some hyperpigmentation of the skin. ACTH also causes ketosis, fat mobilization (adipokinesis), hypoglycemia, and insulin resistance in high doses; these effects are not necessarily mediated through adrenal corticoids. There is evidence that both ACTH and α-melanotropin are contained in cerebral neurons and function as neurotransmitters and/or neuromodulators.

5. Other Pituitary Principles—From time to time the existence of anterior pituitary hormones other than those listed above has been postulated. Generally, the effects attributed to them have been shown to be referable to one or more of the known pituitary hormones. Thus, for example, the diabetogenic effect of anterior pituitary extracts has been shown to be due to the action of somatotropin under conditions of limited insulin supply. Several of the anterior lobe hormones possess adipokinetic properties as well as melanocyte-stimulating and adrenocorticotrophic activity. In addition, a unique peptide with adipokinetic activity has been isolated from pituitary residues remaining after corticotropin extraction. This substance is a peptide of molecular weight about 5000. Although it is very active in laboratory animals, as little as 1 mg causing persistent lipemia in rabbits, it has no demonstrable effect in human beings.

Hypothalamic Regulation of Anterior Pituitary Secretion: Releasing and Inhibiting Factors (*Hypothalamic Hormones*)—The secretion of an anterior pituitary hormone is not constant but rather undergoes intrinsic cyclical variations and is additionally affected by noncyclical factors, such as stress and input from sensory nerves. In some animals there are also extrinsic cyclical factors which are related to diurnal, seasonal, or other environmental cycles, but in man it is not clear to what extent cyclical hormone secretion is determined by such external cycles. The intrinsic cycles are mostly determined by what are called *negative feedback loops*, that is to say that a hormone eventually suppresses its own release indirectly by suppressing the secretion of a hormone from the tuberoinfundibular neuron system of the median eminence of the hypothalamus, which hormone stimulates the release of the anterior pituitary hormone. Such a hypothalamic hormone is called a *hypothalamic releasing factor* if its structure is unknown and as a *hormone* if its structure is known. For each anterior pituitary hormone there is one such factor (except that LH and FSH share the same factor); the designation RF (releasing factor) or RH (releasing hormone) is applied to each factor, CRF designating that for corticotropin, TRH for thyrotropin, LH-RH/FSH-RH for luteinizing and follicle-stimulating hormones, GH-RF for growth hormone, MRF for melanocyte-stimulating hormone, and PRF for prolactin. For growth hormone, prolactin and melanocyte-stimulating hormones there are also respective release inhibitory factors (GH-RIF, PIF, and MIF, respectively). These factors are secreted into the bloodstream of the pituitary portal system, by which route they reach the anterior hypophysis. To be effective, releasing factors must be released in pulses. GH-RIF, LHRH, and TRH are widely distributed in the brain and probably are also neurotransmitters; CRF is also produced in the periphery and is released during stress; GH-RIF (*somatostatin*) is also produced in the pancreas. There is also a pro GH-RIF which is a stronger inhibitor of insulin release but weaker inhibitor of glucagon release than is GH-RIH.

The negative feedback loop that goes from the anterior hypophysis to the hypothalamus is called the *short negative feedback loop*. There is also a *long negative feedback loop* that involves the appropriate target-gland hormone (cortisol for corticotropin, thyroid hormone for thyrotropin, estrogen for follicle-stimulating hormone, etc). The target hormone not only feeds back negatively on the hypothalamus but also directly on the anterior hypophysis, which appears to be the main locus of feedback for some target-cell hormones. Negative feedback to the hypothalamus apparently elicits both a decrease in secretion of a releasing factor and an increase in the secretion of the inhibitory factor. In the case of LH there is a *long positive feedback* loop in which secretion of estrogens favors secretion of LRF. The noncyclical perturbations in anterior pituitary hormone output are also effected through the hypothalamic releasing and inhibiting factors. PIF is thought to be two factors, namely, dopamine and gamma-aminobutyric acid (GABA).

The hypothalamic releasing factors are relatively small polypeptides with molecular weights ranging up to 8000 daltons. In man, the prolactin-releasing factor may be both norepinephrine and vasoactive intestinal polypeptide (VIP). The simplest releasing factor is TRF, the structure of which is *pyro*Glu-His-Pro-NH$_2$. *Pyro* means the glutamic acid is internally cyclized; this unit is common to several of the releasing factors.

The natural and synthetic hypothalamic releasing factors lend themselves to diagnostic as well as therapeutic uses. For example, if a hypothyroid patient responds to TRF with an increase in TSH, then the hypothyroidism may be a lesion in the hypothalamus or pituitary portal system rather than in the anterior hypophysis; this appears to be the situation in cretinism, and treatment with TRF rather than TSH or thyroid hormone may be indicated, because some releasing factors appear to have beneficial actions beyond that of releasing its pituitary hormone. If there is a limited pituitary response to TRF, even in large doses, then the pituitary reserve of TSH is limited. In thyrotoxicosis, TRF fails to affect plasma TSH or thyroid hormone concentrations, so that TRF may distinguish between thyrotoxicosis and apparent hyperthyroid states. LH-RH/FSH-RH can distinguish between hypothalamic and pituitary defects in hypogonadotropic hypogonadism in men but is not reliable in women. However, it does reveal the existence of primary gonadal failure and hypernormal negative feedback systems in amenorrheic women. LRF/FRF can be used to treat infertility if the defect is in the hypothalamus; even when the defect appears to be at the anterior pituitary level, after a course of treatment anovulatory women frequently go on to secrete normal amounts of LH. GH-RIF (*somatostatin*) may be used to treat acromegaly, gigantism, and diabetes mellitus associated with excess GH secretion. Structural analogues of the releasing factors are being studied for possible antagonists; an antagonist of LRF would have a considerable potential as a contraceptive.

The releasing and inhibiting factors are not only under the control of the various peripheral hormones but the brain as well, and the secretion of some has been demonstrated to be affected by neuropharmacologic drugs. Thus drugs such as reserpine and methyldopa that decrease the release of dopamine and/or norepinephrine increase the output of lactogenic and growth hormones. *Bromocriptine, lergotrile,* and *pergolide,* potent dopaminergic agonists, suppress the output of these two hormones and consequently have been tried, successfully, in the treatment of galactorrhea, prolactin-secreting tumors with hypogonadism in men, hyperprolactinemia-associated infertility in women, and acromegaly.

Chorionic Gonadotropin

Human Chorionic Gonadotropin; HCG (*Various Mfrs*)

A gonad-stimulating polypeptide hormone obtained from the urine of pregnant women. Its potency is not less than 1500 USP Chorionic Gonadotropin Units in each mg.

Description—White or practically white, amorphous powder.
Solubility—Freely soluble in water.

Uses—See *Uses of Gonadotropic Hormones* (page 953). Although chorionic gonadotropin alone rarely induces ovulation in anovulatory women, in sequence with *Menotropins* (page 955), which favors the maturation of ovarian follicles, or after clomiphene, ovulation may be effected in women with low gonadotropin secretion. There have been claims that chorionic gonadotropin may be effective in the treatment of infertility in women who have a luteal hypofunction and hence do not produce enough progesterone to develop a normal secretory endometrium, but acceptable evidence of a sufficient luteinizing effect is lacking. Likewise, there is a paucity of evidence of a usefulness of chorionic gonadotropin in the treatment of male sterility. The hormone stimulates testosterone secretion in the male, and some authorities consider chorionic gonadotropin to be superior to either oral or parenteral androgens for replacement therapy in androgenic insufficiency, but the necessity for the injection of chorionic gonadotropin is disadvantageous and such therapy is expensive. To achieve full spermatogenesis in *hypogonadotropic eunuchoidism*, the hormone is used in combination with menotropins. However, the spermatic tubules may be damaged by prolonged treatment. In *cryptorchidism*, chorionic gonadotropin usually promotes descent of the testicles if there is no anatomical obstruction. HCG is used as a *diagnostic* tool to assess the cause of delayed puberty in males, to test the responsiveness of the testes to gonadotropins, and to identify the source of androgens in hirsute females, for which HCG is unreliable.

Chorionic gonadotropin has been proposed as an aid to weight reduction, but evidence of efficacy and safety in this use is lacking.

Chorionic gonadotropin may cause virilization in prepuberal males, and such an effect is an indication to stop treatment. Ovarian hyperstimulation with abdominal discomfort occurs in about 7% of women given combined chorionic gonadotropin and menotropins. Some evidence exists that it may favor thromboembolism and rupture of ovarian cysts. In men, there may be edema from increased secretion of testosterone. It may also cause gynecomastia, headache, restlessness, depression, and pain at the injection site.

Dose—*Intramuscular*, for *cryptorchidism in boys*, one of **4000 USP Units** 3 times a week for 3 weeks, **5000 USP Units** every other day for 4 injections, 15 injections of **500 to 1000 USP Units** over a period of 6 weeks, or **500 USP Units** 3 times a week for 4 to 6 weeks; for *hypogonadism in men*, **500 to 1000 USP Units** for 3 weeks, then twice a week for 3 weeks *or* **4000 USP Units** 3 times a week for 6 to 9 months then **2000 USP Units** 3 times a week for 3 months; to *induce ovulation*, in combination with menotropins, **5000 to 10,000 USP Units** once following the last dose of menotropins; to *induce spermatogenesis* (in combination with menotropins), **5000 USP Units**

3 times a week for 4 to 6 mo; for *anovulation*, **8000 to 15,000 USP Units.**

Dosage Forms—For Injection: 2000, 2500, 5000, 10,000, and 20,000 Units.

Corticotropin Injection

ACTH Injection; Adrenocorticotropin Injection; (*Various Mfrs*)

A sterile solution, in a suitable diluent, or a sterile dry mixture (*Corticotropin for Injection*), containing the polypeptide hormone derived from the anterior lobe of the pituitary of mammals used for food by man, which increases rate of secretion of adrenal corticosteroids. Both forms may contain a suitable antimicrobial agent.

Preparation—Most commercial preparations of *corticotropin* are obtained from either hog or sheep pituitary glands, although beef and whale glands have also been used. Isolation of the hormonal principle(s) from swine and sheep pituitaries was reported in 1943 by Sayers *et al* (*J Biol Chem 149:* 425, 1943) and Li *et al* (*J Biol Chem 149:* 413, 1943). A process of purification of the hormonal substance is described in US Pat 3,124,509. For other information see *Adrenal Corticotropic Hormone*, page 953.

Two types of preparations are available: short- and long-acting. The short-acting preparations consist of a lyophilized powder or a stable aqueous solution containing 1% phenol. The powder is dissolved in physiological saline or other suitable medium before injection. Short-acting preparations are administered either intramuscularly or by intravenous infusion.

Long-acting preparations (repository corticotropin, corticotropin gel) contain *corticotropin* incorporated in a gelatin menstruum designed to delay the rate of absorption and increase the period of effectiveness. Combination of corticotropin with zinc hydroxide suspension also delays the rate of absorption. These are injected intramuscularly.

Corticotropin is standardized by the Sayers assay. The clinical effectiveness, however, varies with the mode of administration. The difference is particularly evident in comparisons of short-acting preparations injected intramuscularly with long-acting preparations similarly administered. For this reason, gel preparations are labeled in terms of "clinical units" to conform more nearly to their expected physiological potency. Fourteen USP Units in gelatin medium possess the approximate clinical efficacy of 40 USP Units of aqueous corticotropin solution by intermittent intramuscular injection.

Description—Colorless or light straw-colored liquid, or a white or practically white, soluble, amorphous solid having the characteristic appearance of substances prepared by freeze-drying. pH (of the liquid form or after reconstitution from the solid state) between 3 and 7.

Uses—Corticotropin is the hypophyseal hormone, ACTH, that stimulates the adrenal gland to produce hydrocortisone, desoxycorticosterone, and androgens. It is used as a *diagnostic* drug to assess the functional capacity of the adrenal gland. A rise in plasma cortisol or urinary 17-hydroxycorticosterone indicates a functional gland. This is at present the most important clinical use of this agent. However, cosyntropin is preferred because it is less allergenic. ACTH has been promoted as a therapeutic agent in a wide variety of glucocorticoid-responsive disorders (see page 961). In general, with the exception of primary adrenal insufficiency, ACTH is effective in all of the conditions for which glucocorticoids are found useful. Unlike the latter, however, corticotropin is ineffective when applied locally. There is no evidence that ACTH can achieve any therapeutic effect that cannot be achieved by appropriate doses of a glucocorticoid and its cost and allergenicity are definite disadvantages.

An interesting use of corticotropin in which the peptide hormone may be superior to glucocorticoids is in the management of severe myasthenia gravis. The hormone is given for 10 to 20 days, during which time muscle strength actually deteriorates to the extent that assisted respiration may be required. After treatment stops, the muscle strength returns to normal in 2 to 7 days and then increases above the pretreatment level for several months. Glucocorticoids cause less deterioration during administration but also bring about less improvement afterward. The margin between optimum clinical effectiveness and undesirable side effects is frequently narrow. The continued administration of large amounts of corticotropin may result in one or more of the manifestations of Cushing's syndrome, may exacerbate the symptoms of latent or frank diabetes, and, because of its anti-inflammatory action, may mask symptoms of infection.

The need for adequate medical supervision during its use, therefore, cannot be over-emphasized. Various side effects mediated by the glucocorticoids released from the adrenal gland are listed on page 960. They occur frequently when the dosage exceeds 40 Units a day.

Abrupt cessation of corticotropin injections may be followed by withdrawal effects which take the form of symptoms of adrenal insufficiency. These result from pituitary inhibition which occurs during treatment with corticotropin and may be minimized or eliminated by gradually reducing the amount injected. Corticotropin causes some side effects not caused by glucocorticoids, namely, hypersensitivity, salt and water retention, and androgenic effects (acne, hirsutism, and amenorrhea) in women. ACTH is contraindicated if there is osteoporosis, systemic mycosis, corneal herpes, or scleroderma.

Dose—*Replacement* or *therapeutic, adult, intramuscular* or *subcutaneous*, **20 USP Units**, 4 times a day, except 80 to 120 Units/day for 2 to 3 weeks for acute exacerbation of multiple sclerosis; *repository injection* (deep into the gluteus only), **40 to 80 Units** every 24 to 72 hr; *children, parenteral*, **0.4 Unit per kg** of body weight (or **12.5 Units per m²** of body surface), 4 times a day. *Diagnostic, adult, intravenous*, **10 to 25 Units** in several successive doses or *intramuscular* or *intravenous*, **80 Units** as a single dose, with plasma sampling 60 to 90 min after the last dose, or *intravenous* as an 8-hr infusion on each of two successive days, with 24-hr urine sampling; for infusion the dose is dissolved in 500 to 1000 mL of 5% dextrose solution.

Dosage Forms—Injection: 40 Units/1 and 2 mL, 200 and 400 Units/5 mL; for Injection: 25 and 40 Units; Repository Injection: 40 and 80 Units/1 mL, 200 and 400 Units/5 mL; Sterile Zinc Hydroxide Suspension: 200 Units/5 mL.

Cosyntropin

Cortrosyn (*Organon*)

Ser-Tyr-Ser-Met-Glu-His-Phe-Arg-Trp-Gly-Lys-Pro-Val-Gly-Lys-Lys-Arg-Arg-Pro-Val-Lys-Val-Tyr-Pro
1   2   3   4   5   6   7   8   9   10 11 12 13 14 15 16 17 18 19 20 21 22 23 24

α^{1-24}-Corticotropin [16960-16-0] $C_{136}H_{210}N_{40}O_{31}S$ (2933.46).

Preparation—This synthetic polypeptide is identical with the moiety of corticotropin containing the first 24 of its 36 amino acids. For detailed information concerning the synthesis see *Helv Chim Acta 44:* 1136, 1961; *46:* 1550, 1963.

Description—A white to off-white lyophilized mixture with 40 parts of mannitol; soluble in water.

Uses—The full adrenocorticotropic activity of corticotropin resides in the first 23 amino acids, whereas the allergenicity resides in the segment 22 to the C-terminal end. Thus cosyntropin has full corticotropic activity but negligible antigenicity. Consequently it is preferred for *diagnostic tests of adrenocortical sufficiency*. Repository preparations are unavailable, so that it is usually not used therapeutically.

Dose—*Intramuscular* or *intravenous*, **250 µg**, except **125 µg** in children 1 to 5 years of age and **100 µg** when less than 1 year of age. If the increase in plasma cortisol is at least 7 µg/100 mL and the absolute level is at least 18 µg/100 mL 30 to 60 min after injection, no further tests are made, the patient having normal adrenocortical function. If the response is subnormal, 250 µg is given as a 4- to 8-hr infusion (or corticotropin by the schedule under *Corticotropin Injection*) to distinguish between hypopituitarism, in which an adequate plasma cortisol or urinary 17-hydroxysterol response occurs, and Addison's disease, in which little response occurs.

Dosage Form—For Injection: 0.25 mg in 1-mL vial.

Menotropins

Pergonal (*Serono*)

Menotropins [9002-68-0]; an extract of postmenopausal urine containing the follicle-stimulating hormone (FSH) and luteinizing hormone (LH) in a 1:1 ratio.

Uses—Menotropins has the gonadotropic activities of FSH and LH (see page 952). It is used to *induce ovulation* in women with infertility consequent to insufficient endogenous production of gonadotropins. Clinical experience is that about 75% of anovulatory women ovulate after treatment and 25% become pregnant after 2 courses of treatment. Multiple gestation occurs in about 20% of completed pregnancies. The hyperstimulation syndrome occurs in 1 to 2% of cases. If urinary estrogen excretion is used to guide treatment with large doses and the need for concomitant chorionic gonadotropin, the ovulatory rate can be increased to 98% and the percentage of live births is improved, but multiple gestation is increased and hyperstimulation is more common. Menotropins is sometimes used to treat hypogonadotropic male infertility.

Side effects include ovarian enlargement, flatulence, abdominal discomfort, oliguria, weight gain, ascites, pleural effusion, hypotension, and hypercoagulability; these are all evidence of hyperstimulation. Occasionally, ovarian rupture and intraperitoneal hemorrhage occur, and surgery is required.

Dose—*Intramuscular*, in *females, initially* **75 IU** of each component/day for 9 to 12 days, followed by **5000 to 10,000 IU** of chorionic gonadotropin 1 day after the course of menotropins is stopped. If ovulation but not pregnancy occurs, the same course is repeated twice more. If there is no pregnancy, the dose is increased to **150 IU** for 9 to 12 days, and two such courses may be repeated, if necessary. Some clinicians stop the administration of menotropins when estrogen secretion reaches 50 to 100 µg/day and give 10,000 IU of chorionic gonadotropin 1 day later; others wait until the estrogen secretion is 100 to 150 µg/day. If the estrogen excretion is higher than 150 µg/day, chorionic gonadotropin is withheld, to minimize hyperstimulation. In *males*, **75 IU** of each component 3 times a week for 4 months; pretreatment and concomitant treatment with HCG is essential.

Dosage Form—For Injection: 75 IU of each component.

Somatropin

Somatotropin; GH; STH; Asellacrin (*Calbiochem-Behring*)

H—Phe-Pro-Thr-Ile-Pro-Leu-Ser-Arg-Leu-Phe-Asp-Asn-Ala-Met-Leu-Arg-Ala-His-Arg-
   1   5   10   15
Leu-His-Gln-Leu-Ala-Phe-Asp-Thr-Tyr-Gln-Glu-Phe-Glu-Glu-Ala-Tyr-Ile-Pro-Lys-Glu-
20   25   30   35
Gln-Lys-Tyr-Ser-Phe-Leu-Gln-Asn-Pro-Gln-Thr-Ser-Leu-Cys-Phe-Ser-Glu-Ser-Ile-Pro-
40   45   50   55
Thr-Pro-Ser-Asn-Arg-Glu-Glu-Thr-Gln-Gln-Lys-Ser-Asn-Leu-Gln-Leu-Leu-Arg-Ile-Ser-
60   65   70   75
Leu-Leu-Leu-Ile-Gln-Ser-Trp-Leu-Glu-Pro-Val-Gln-Phe-Leu-Arg-Ser-Val-Phe-Ala-Asn-
80   85   90   95
Ser-Leu-Val-Tyr-Gly-Ala-Ser-Asn-Ser-Asp-Val-Tyr-Asp-Leu-Leu-Lys-Asp-Leu-Glu-Glu-
100   105   110   115
Gly-Ile-Gln-Thr-Leu-Met-Gly-Arg-Leu-Glu-Asp-Gly-Ser-Pro-Arg-Thr-Gly-Gln-Ile-Phe-
120   125   130   135
Lys-Gln-Thr-Tyr-Ser-Lys-Phe-Asp-Thr-Asn-Ser-His-Asn-Asp-Asp-Ala-Leu-Leu-Lys-Asn-
140   145   150   155
Tyr-Gly-Leu-Leu-Tyr-Cys-Phe-Arg-Lys-Asp-Met-Asp-Lys-Val-Glu-Thr-Phe-Leu-Arg-Ile-
160   165   170   175
Val-Gln-Cys-Arg-Ser-Val-Glu-Gly-Ser-Cys-Gly-Phe—OH
180   185   190

[12629-01-5] $C_{990}H_{1529}N_{263}O_{299}S_7$ (18224.52)

Uses—For description, actions, and uses of somatotropin see *Growth Hormone* (page 952). Intramuscular administration of the hormone is preferred to subcutaneous injection because the hormone causes lipodystrophy or lipoatrophy at the cutaneous injection site. Pain and swelling usually occur on injection, so that sites should be rotated. Hypercalciuria occurs frequently but usually regresses in 2 to 3 months. Hyperglycemia and frank diabetes mellitus may occur. Myalgia and early morning headaches are relatively frequent. Antibodies to the hormone may be found in 30 to 40% of recipients in the first 3 to 6 months of treatment and may interfere with efficacy in about 5% of cases; subcutaneous administration favors the immune response. Occasionally, somatotropin causes hypothyroidism and supersaturation of cholesterol in bile. If the epiphyses are closed, the hormone should not be used because continued stimulation of growth of the phalanges and jawbone, but not other bones, can cause abnormal body proportions.

Dose—*Intramuscular, initially* **2 IU** 3 times a week at intervals no less than 48 hr; if the growth rate does not exceed 2.5 cm in the first 6 months, the dose should be doubled during the next 6 months, after which time it should either be continued or discontinued, according to the response.

Dosage Forms—For Injection: 4 IU.

Other Anterior Pituitary Hormones or Agents

Bromocriptine Mesylate [2-Bromoergocriptine monomethanesulfonate, $C_{32}H_{40}BrN_5O_5 \cdot CH_4O_3S$ (750.70); Parlodel (*Sandoz*)]—Bromocriptine may be prepared by heating a mixture of *N*-bromophthalimide (or *N*-bromosuccinimide) and α-ergocriptine in dioxane (*CA 72:* 43969b, 1970). A yellowish-white crystalline powder. *Uses:* Bromocriptine is a dopaminergic agonist with prolonged action. In the CNS not only does it stimulate postsynaptic dopamine receptors (as a partial agonist) but it also appears to block both the presynaptic dopamine reuptake system and the negative feedback presynaptic receptors that terminate dopamine release; therefore, it enhances the synaptic concentrations of dopamine in addition to its direct actions. Consequently, it increases the antiparkinson effects of levodopa (page 930) and has antiparkinson activity of its own. It also increases the turnover of brain serotonin and normalizes levodopa-depressed serotonin levels, thus decreasing some of the side effects of levodopa. It is used in combination with levodopa in parkinsonism to decrease the frequency of on-off effects and alone in levodopa-refractory cases. Its status is yet to be determined.

In the hypothalamus, dopamine is thought to be one of two prolactin-release inhibiting factors. As would be expected of a dopaminergic agonist, bromocriptine suppresses the anterior pituitary release of prolactin and decreases the blood levels; consequently it is used in the treatment of postpartum and drug-induced *galactorrhea* in females and *hyperprolactinemia* in males. It is also used to treat *amenorrhea* and *infertility* in hyperprolactinemic women; menstruation and fertility are sometimes promoted even in women with normal prolactin levels. It has not yet been established that bromocriptine is useful in treating breast tumors. It has been used successfully in the treatment of prolactin-secreting adenomas, such that surgery may be sometimes avoided. It also causes some regression of extrasellar pituitary tumors.

Although bromocriptine increases growth hormone levels in normal persons, it sometimes decreases them in persons with *acromegaly*. In about 25% of recipients there is a marked decrease in GH levels.

Bromocriptine is readily absorbed by oral administration, but first-pass metabolism destroys about 90% of the dose, most of that being excreted into bile. The half-life is about 3 hr. The duration of action of bromocriptine is 6 to 8 hr.

Adverse effects frequently include postural hypotension (occasionally with syncope), nausea, and constipation. When high doses are used, as in the treatment of parkinsonism, hallucinations, delusions, and changes in personality sometimes occur; 2 to 3 weeks are required for recovery after discontinuation of the drug. Peptic ulcer occurs in about 6% of recipients with acromegaly. Erythema, edema, ankle tenderness, and cold-induced digital vasospasm sometimes occur. Bromocriptine is teratogenic in humans. Phenothiazines antagonize bromocriptine.

Dose (bromocriptine equivalent): *Oral*, for *amenorrhea/galactorrhea*, *initially* 2.5 mg/day for one week followed by increments to achieve a dose of 2.5 mg 2 or 3 times a day, for up to 6 months; to *prevent physiological lactation*, 2.5 mg 2 to 3 times daily, with meals, for 14 to 21 days; to *relieve symptoms of premenstrual tension*, 2.5 to 7.5 mg/day in 1 to 3 divided doses; for *acromegaly*, 15 to 20 mg/day in 3 or 4 divided doses, but occasionally up to 60 mg/day; for *parkinsonism*, *initially* 2.5 mg twice a day with meals, to be increased, as necessary, at 2-week intervals by 2.5 mg/day up to 100 mg/day. *Dosage Form:* Tablets: 2.5 mg of bromocriptine.

Gonadorelin Hydrochloride—[The hydrochloride represents either the mono-, di- or a mixture of the mono- and dihydrochlorides, [51952-41-1] $C_{55}H_{75}N_{17}O_{13}.xHCl$; Factrel (*Ayerst*)] Gonadorelin is obtained by synthesis or from the hypothalamus. It is a faint yellow powder; 1 g is soluble in 25 mL of water, 50 mL of methanol, or 25 mL of 1% acetic acid. *Uses:* Gonadorelin is identical to natural LH-RH. It is used as a diagnostic agent to determine whether hypogonadism is the result of a defect in anterior pituitary release of LH or in hypothalamic release of LH-RH. If gonadorelin evokes a rise in LH levels, the disturbance is in the hypothalamus; if it does not, the disturbance is in the hypothalamus. Gonadorelin is used as an investigational drug to treat infertility, prostatic carcinoma, induction of puberty in hypogonadal males, metastatic breast cancer in premenopausal women, cryptorchidism, and endometriosis, and as a male contraceptive agent. Local swelling, itching or pain, and occasional rash at the injection site may occur after subcutaneous injection. Headache, nausea, lightheadedness, abdominal discomfort, and rare flushing may occur. *Dose: Intravenous* or *subcutaneous*, *adult*, 100 mg, usually per day for several days.

Lergotrile Mesylate [2-Chloro-6-methylergoline-8β-acetonitrile monomethanesulfonate [51473-23-5] $C_{17}H_{18}ClN_3.CH_4O_3S$ (395.90); (*Lilly*)]—A synthetic nonpeptide ergot derivative with actions very much like those of *Bromocriptine Mesylate* (above). Lergotrile has the higher affinity for dopamine receptors. *Dose: Oral*, for *galactorrhea*, *amenorrhea*, and *acromegaly*, initially 0.5 mg a day, increased as necessary to a maintenance dose of 2 mg 3 times a day; for *parkinsonism*, 11.2 to 52 mg/day.

Pergolide Mesylate [8-[(Methylthio)methyl]-6-propylergoline [66104-22-1] $C_{19}H_{26}N_2S.CH_4O_3S$ (410.59); (*Lilly*)]—Off-white crystals melting about 225°. For the preparation refer to US Pat 4,166,182. *Uses:* Pergolide has all of the actions and uses of Bromocriptine (above). Its advantage is a longer duration of action, namely, over 24 hr. *Dose: Oral*, *adults*, initially 50 μg, on the first day to be adjusted subsequently according to plasma prolactin levels.

Protirelin [5-Oxo-L-prolyl-L-histidyl-L-prolinamide [24305-27-9] $C_{16}H_{22}N_6O_4$ (362.39); Thypinone (*Abbott*) Relefact-TRH (*Hoechst-*

Roussel)]—Protirelin is the thyrotropin-releasing hormone or factor (TRH or TRF) elaborated in the hypothalamus, synthesis of which by several methods has been described (*J Med Chem 13*: 843, 1970; *14*: 481, 1971). *Uses:* Although protirelin mainly causes the release of thyrotropin (TSH) from the adenohypophysis, it also causes some release of prolactin (PrL) and growth hormone (GH). It activates the adenylate cyclase systems in the target pituitary cells, and cyclic AMP then causes hormonal release. Protirelin is used in the diagnosis of thyroid disorders, as discussed under *Hypothalamic Regulation of Anterior Pituitary Secretion* (page 953). In addition to the uses described there, TRH has other diagnostic uses. In thyrotoxicosis treated with antithyroid drugs, the TSH-response to TRH returns as thyroid function returns toward normal, so that the response is an indicator of the adequacy of treatment. When there is a deficiency of GH, the response is delayed, which is of diagnostic use. In GH-deficient children, the response of PrL to TRH is used as an indicator of whether the deficiency of GH is hypothalamic or pituitary in origin; if the PrL fails to rise, the deficiency is in the pituitary gland. The PrL response is sometimes used to evaluate hyperprolactinemic disorders. The response of GH and cortisol in anorexia nervosa (in which the TSH response is usually excessive) aids in assessing the hormonal factors in the disorder. TRH increases GH in acromegalic but not in normal persons, and it has been used in the diagnosis and monitoring of acromegaly. There are a considerable number of negative responses in some tests. For example, about 33% of responses are negative in goiter with a single nodule and 50% when multinodular.

Attempts have been made to use TRH as a therapeutic agent in primary hypothyroidism, but tolerance to the TSH—but not the PrL—response usually develops within a few weeks. Tolerance does not seem to develop in normal persons. *Dose: Intravenous*, 200 to 500 μg, with blood samples being removed at 30, 60, 90 and 120 min. Children 6 to 16 years of age, 7 μg/kg, up to 500 μg.

Thyrotropin [[9002-71-5] TSH; Thytropar (*Armour*)]—The thyrotropic hormone secreted by the basophilic cells of the bovine anterior pituitary. Prepared from extracts of the anterior lobe of the pituitary gland of domesticated animals by adjusting the pH to the isoelectric point and then either precipitating the hormone with a suitable buffer salt or extracting it with appropriate solvents. For a detailed discussion, see the monograph on *Thyrotropin*, Thomas, Springfield, IL, 1963. *Uses:* Exogenous thyrotropin increases the uptake of iodide into and the release of thyroid hormone from a functional thyroid gland. If the gland is incapable of proper function (primary thyroid failure), thyrotropin will not induce as much of an effect on iodine metabolism. Thus the hormone was once used diagnostically to *distinguish hypothyroidism secondary to anterior pituitary failure* to produce endogenous thyrotropin *from primary thyroid failure*, but it is little used for this purpose today. It was also used to *monitor thyroid function* in patients receiving thyroid treatment, to assess the degree of negative feedback on the pituitary, but assessment can be made by simply discontinuing treatment. Thyrotropin may also be given to enhance uptake of radioiodine in patients with neoplastic thyroid disorders, to distinguish normal thyroid tissue from neoplastic tissue. Thyrotropin is not used for replacement therapy in anterior pituitary failure. Untoward effects include nausea, vomiting, headache and urticaria. Occasionally more serious reactions, such as hypotension, tachyarrhythmias, thyroid enlargement, and, rarely, anaphylaxis occur. Thyrotropin is contraindicated in patients with coronary insufficiency and Addison's disease and should be used cautiously when there is angina pectoris or when glucocorticoids are being given. *Dose: Intramuscular* or *subcutaneous*, 10 IU. For diagnostic purposes, this dose may be repeated in 24 hours. For treatment prior to radioiodine treatment, the dose is given daily for 3 to 7 days. *Dosage Form:* For Injection: 10 IU/3 mL.

The Intermediate Lobe

The intermediate lobe of the pituitary produces a substance, *intermedin*, or *melanocyte-stimulating hormone* (MSH), which disperses the pigment granules in the melanophores and other chromatophores in some amphibians and fishes. The biological assay of MSH depends upon its capacity for darkening the skin of frogs either *in vivo* or *in vitro*.

Extracts of mammalian pituitaries contain two substances with MSH activity: α- and β-MSH. These are polypeptides containing 13 and 18 amino acids, respectively; the amino acid sequences in both are known. Although MSH has no known physiological role in mammals, alkali-treated MSH (which has a more prolonged action than the native material) will cause some darkening of the skin in man. Purified ACTH possesses intrinsic MSH activity, probably due to similarity of structure between ACTH and α-MSH. It has been suggested that the hyperpigmentation of Addison's disease is due to excessive ACTH secretion.

The hypothalamus produces both an MSH-releasing factor (MRF) and inhibitory factor (MIF).

The Posterior Pituitary (Neurohypophysis)

The posterior pituitary contains two peptide hormones, *oxytocin* and *vasopressin*. Neither is made in the posterior pituitary, but rather they are synthesized in neurons in the hypothalamus. Oxytocin is synthesized in the paraventricular nucleus and vasopressin the supraoptic nucleus. The axons of the hormone-secreting nerve cells pass from the hypothalamus to the internal infundibular zone of the posterior pituitary (hence the name neurohypophysis). The hormones flow down the axons as granules or vesicles composed of a hormone and a carrier protein called *neurophysin*. Their release at the nerve terminals is presumably effected by nerve impulses. Thus the control of release is actually in the appropriate hypothalamic nuclei.

Human and most mammalian vasopressin is Cys-Tyr-Phe-Gln-Asn-Cys-Pro-Arg-GlyNH$_2$, called *arginine vasopressin* or simply *vasopressin*. That from the pig contains lysine in place of arginine and hence is called *lysine vasopressin*, or *lypressin*. The two do not have identical activities. Vasopressin is usually called *antidiuretic hormone* (ADH) by physiologists and biochemists, because it decreases urine flow by increasing the resorption of water from the distal convoluted tubules and collecting ducts of the kidney. Not only does it promote water retention but under certain circumstances it increases the excretion of sodium and chloride. The effect is a decrease in the osmolarity of the extracellular fluid. When ADH secretion is suppressed (as from various physiological stimuli or ethanol) a watery diuresis ensues. When there is a defect in the hypothalamicopituitary secretion of ADH, *diabetes insipidus* results. Vasopressin is mainly used for its antidiuretic effects in this disease rather than for its vasoconstrictor actions, from which the name vasopressin comes. However, not only does vasopressin stimulate vascular smooth muscle, but also it increases bowel motility and it has been used to treat bowel stasis and to expel gas postsurgically; cholinergic drugs are considered to be superior. The vasoconstrictor and bowel spastic actions have special usefulness in arresting hemorrhage from peptic ulcers. The smooth muscle stimulant effects occur with higher doses than are necessary to affect renal function. Vasopressin also causes the release of ACTH much like the hypothalamic releasing hormone, CRF. Consequently, vasopressin is sometimes used diagnostically to assess the pituitary reserve of ACTH. Vasopressin also has weak oxytocic activity. Vasopressin has a brief half-life (less than 20 min). Lypressin has much weaker smooth-muscle stimulant activity than vasopressin, the ratio of antidiuretic to pressor activity being about 1000:1.

Oxytocin stimulates the contraction of smooth muscle in the uterus and alveoli of the lactating breast. At coitus, uterine stimulation by oxytocin causes peristaltic activity that assists the migration of spermatozoa. During parturition, the hormone enhances the uterine contractions. The uses of oxytocin in labor and breast engorgement are described in Chapter 51.

Neither vasopressin nor oxytocin survives the acid and enzymes of the gastrointestinal tract, so they must be given parenterally or intranasally.

Each of the octapeptides has been synthesized. Oxytocin has the structure:

Oxytocin

The structure of vasopressin from human, monkey, dog, cat, ox, camel, rabbit, and rat pituitaries is identical with that of oxytocin, except that the isoleucine and leucine residues are replaced by residues of phenylalanine and arginine, respectively. Vasopressin prepared from pig pituitaries (lypressin) contains lysine instead of arginine.

The synthesis of oxytocin by du Vigneaud and his students in 1953 represented the first synthesis of a peptide hormone. The synthetic product is qualitatively and quantitatively identical in biological properties with the purified natural hormone. Purified oxytocin contains 500 to 600 USP Units/mg.

The successful synthesis of the naturally occurring posterior lobe hormones has provided the impetus for the synthesis of a number of analogues of both oxytocin and vasopressin. Thus, substances in which one or more of the amino acids of the native hormones have been replaced by others, or containing fewer or additional amino acid residues, have been prepared and their pharmacological properties explored. One of these was the compound vasotocin, containing the pentapeptide ring of oxytocin and the tripeptide side chain of vasopressin. This substance possesses the biological properties of both neurohypophyseal hormones, although in lesser degree. Subsequently, it was shown that vasotocin is in fact the naturally occurring neurohypophyseal hormone of birds and amphibians.

It has become rather common practice to name those synthetic analogues of oxytocin and the two vasopressins in which one or more of the amino acids of the native hormones have been replaced by others by the simple expedient of assigning consecutive numbers to the amino acid residues in the native hormone and using these numbers to denote the alterations represented in the synthetic. Exemplifying with oxytocin, for which the numbering scheme is

```
        1           2          3
   cysteine—tyrosine—isoleucine
      | 6         5          4
   cysteine—asparagine—glutamine
        7           8          9
   proline—leucine—glycinamide,
```

a synthetic in which the leucine moiety is replaced by arginine is named simply 8-arginineoxytocin. Altered vasopressins are handled similarly; thus the name 2-(phenylalanine)-8-lysinevasopressin signifies a vasopressin which differs from native 8-lysinevasopressin in that the No. 2 amino acid residue (tyrosine) of the natural hormone has been replaced by phenylalanine.

Lypressin

Vasopressin, 8-L-lysine-, Diapid (*Sandoz*)

Cys-Tyr-Phe-Gln-Asn-Cys-Pro-Lys-Gly—NH₂
1   2   3   4   5   6   7   8   9

[50-57-7] $C_{46}H_{65}N_{13}O_{12}S_2$ (1056.22).

Preparation—Isolated from hog pituitaries and prepared synthetically (*J Biol Chem 222*: 951, 1956; *J Am Chem Soc 82*: 3195, 1960). One commercial synthetic method concludes by reacting the protected tripeptide, *N*-tosyl-*S*-benzyl-L-cysteinyl-L-tyrosyl-L-phenylalanylhydrazide, with the protected hexapeptide, L-glutaminyl-L-asparaginyl-*S*-benzyl-L-cysteinyl-L-prolyl- *N*-tosyl-L-lysyl-glycinamide, and then splits off the protecting groups with metallic sodium.

One mg of lypressin is stated to be equivalent to 270 USP Posterior Pituitary Units (1 Unit is equivalent to 3.7 µg).

Uses—Lypressin has strong antidiuretic but weak pressor activity. It is used only in the treatment of mild to moderate *diabetes insipidus* resulting from neurohypophyseal insufficiency. When the condition is severe, it does not give sufficient control because of its brief duration of action; even in moderate diabetes insipidus, control is only periodic, in accordance with the dosage regimen. In the severe condition, vasopressin tannate is used, although lypressin may be used as an adjunct between injections of the tannate. Diabetes insipidus from renal disorders is not affected. After nasal application of lypressin, antidiuresis peaks within ½ to 2 hr and lasts 3 to 8 hr.

When lypressin is used as recommended, untoward effects are infrequent and mild; they include nasal irritation and congestion, rhinorrhea, nasal pruritus, nasal ulceration, conjunctivitis, and headache. Overdosage may cause heartburn from postnasal drip, abdominal cramps, bowel hypermotility, and fluid retention. Inhalation of the spray can result in asthma-like tightness in the chest, dyspnea, and coughing. Thus far, allergic responses have not been reported. Because the marketed substance is synthetic and thus free of traces of foreign proteins, it may possibly lack allergenicity, even though its composition differs slightly from the human vasopressin.

Dose—*Intranasal*, 1 or 2 sprays (about 7 to 14 µg) to one or both nostrils whenever urinary frequency or substantial thirst indicates a need. The average interval is 6 hours. Increases in dosage should be achieved by more frequent administration rather than by increased number of sprays per application.

Dosage Form—Nasal Spray: 185 µg/mL in 8 mL.

Vasopressin Injection

Beta-Hypophamine; Pitressin (*Parke-Davis*)

H-Cys-Tyr-Phe-Glu(NH₂)-Asp(NH₂)-Cys-Pro-Arg*-Gly-NH₂
1   2   3   4   5   6   7   8   9

(*In pig vasopressin, Arg is Lys)

8-L-Lysine (or arginine) vasopressin: Lysine form-[50-57-7] $C_{46}H_{65}N_{13}O_{12}S_2$ (1056.22); Arginine form-[113-79-1] $C_{46}H_{65}N_{15}O_{12}S_2$ (1084.23).

A sterile solution in water for injection of the water-soluble, pressor hormone prepared by synthesis or obtained from the posterior lobe of the pituitary of healthy domestic animals used for food by man. Each mL possesses pressor activity equivalent to 20 USP Posterior Pituitary Units and not more than one unit of oxytocic activity.

Description—Clear, colorless or practically colorless liquid with a faint, characteristic odor.

Uses—The actions of vasopressin are discussed on page 957. The injection is employed for its *antidiuretic* effect and to dispel gas shadows in bowel roentgenography and pyelography. It should not be used as a pressor agent.

Untoward effects related to overdosage include water intoxication (with headache, nausea and vomiting, confusion, lethargy, coma, and convulsions), especially when patients drink excessive amounts of water or are given intravenous fluids, and stimulation of vascular, uterine, and intestinal smooth muscle, which may result in pallor, hypertension, coronary constriction (with anginal chest pain, electrocardiographic changes, and occasional myocardial infarction), uterine cramps, menorrhagia, and nausea, vomiting, diarrhea, and abdominal cramps. Hypersensitivity occasionally occurs; manifestations include urticaria, neurodermatitis, flushing, fever, wheezing, dyspnea, and rare anaphylactic shock. Large doses are oxytocic and also cause milk ejection. Alcohol, heparin, demeclocycline, lithium, and large doses of epinephrine antagonize vasopressin; glucocorticoids, urea, and oral hypoglycemic drugs potentiate it.

The plasma half-life is 10 to 20 min. However, the effect of an intramuscular injection lasts from 2 to 8 hr. From 10 to 15% is excreted unchanged.

Dose—*Intramuscular*, for *diabetes insipidus*, 5 to 10 USP Units (0.25 to 0.5 mL) 2 to 8 times a day; for *children*, 2.5 to 10 Units 3 or 4 times a day. May also be given *intranasally* on cotton pledgets, with a dropper, or as a spray, at intervals determined by return of polyuria or thirst. For *hypotonic bowel*, 5 Units, at 3- to 4-hr intervals, as needed.

Dosage Form—20 Units/0.5 and 1 mL.

Other Posterior Pituitary Preparations

Desmopressin Acetate [1-(3-Mercaptopropionic acid)-8-D-arginine vasopressin monoacetate (salt), trihydrate [62357-86-2] $C_{48}H_{68}N_{14}$-$O_{14}S_2.3H_2O$ (1183.22)]—A synthetic analogue of 8-arginine vasopressin (*Helv Chim Acta 49:* 695, 1966) that has the antidiuretic activity of vasopressin but less activity on smooth muscle. It is used in the treatment of *central* ("neurogenic") *diabetes insipidus*. It is also used to test the ability of the kidney to concentrate urine. Since desmopressin can raise the plasma levels of factor VIII (antihemophilic factor), it is sometimes used to increase factor VIII levels prior to surgery. Headache, mild hypertension, nasal congestion, mild abdominal cramping, water intoxication, and vulval pain sometimes occur. Chlorpropamide and clofibrate potentiate, and glyburide inhibits, antidiuretic action. *Dose:* For *diabetes insipidus, adult*, 10 to 40 µg a day in 1 to 3 divided doses; *children*, 5 to 30 µg a day. For *urine concentration test, intranasal*, 40 µg. *Dosage Form:* Sterile solution for intranasal use, 0.1 mg desmopressin acetate/mL, 2.5 mL/vial.

Posterior Pituitary [Pituitary; Hypophysis Sicca]—A powder prepared from the clean, dried, posterior lobe of the pituitary of domestic animals used for food by man. Each mg possesses oxytocic activity equivalent to not less than 1 USP Posterior Pituitary Unit. A yellowish or grayish, amorphous powder having a characteristic odor; partially soluble in water. *Uses:* To control postoperative ileus, in surgery as a hemostatic, for diabetes insipidus, and as an oxytocic. The preparation is very little used today. Adverse effects include pallor, hypertension, angina, uterine cramps, anxiety, tinnitus, coma, mydriasis, amaurosis, diarrhea, proteinuria, anaphylaxis, angioneurotic edema, and pruritis. *Dose: Intramuscular* or *subcutaneous*, 5 to 20 Units.

Vasopressin Tannate [β-Hypophamine Tannate; Pitressin Tannate (*Parke-Davis*)]—The water-insoluble tannate of the pressor principle of the posterior lobe of the pituitary of healthy domesticated animals used as food by man. A dark-brown, amorphous solid; insoluble in water and alcohol. *Uses:* For replacement therapy in *diabetes insipidus* but not for its action on the bowel (page 957). Vasopressin tannate has a longer duration of action than vasopressin, and it is more suitable for suspension in oil, so that depot preparations can be made conveniently from the tannate. Because of embolism, vasopressin tannate and its oil suspension should *never be given intravenously*. The untoward effects are the same as those of *Vasopressin Injection*, but the vascular effects are less frequent because of the slower rate of release into the blood stream. *Dose: Intramuscular*, 2.5 to 5 Units (except 1.5 to 2.5 Units in children) every 1 to 3 days. *Dosage Form:* Injection (in oil): 5 Units/1 mL.

The Adrenal Hormones

The adrenal hormones include both the adrenocorticoids from the adrenal cortex and epinephrine and norepinephrine from the adrenal medulla. The discussion below will deal only with the adrenocorticoids. Epinephrine and norepinephrine are treated in Chapter 45.

The cortex, or outer portion of the adrenal gland is one of the endocrine structures most vitally necessary for normal metabolic function. While it is possible for life to continue in the complete absence of adrenal cortical function, serious metabolic derangements ensue, and the capacity of the organism to respond to physiological or environmental stress is completely lost. The vital role of the adrenal cortex is due to its production of a group of hormones, all *steroid* in nature.

Physiology—Four general patterns of adrenal cortical hormone action have been described: (1) retention of sodium ions in extracellular fluid and potassium ions within cells, thus maintaining the normal distribution of water and chloride ion and resulting maintenance of blood volume and blood pressure; (2) maintenance of normal blood glucose levels and facilitation of liver glycogen deposition; and (3) enhanced mobilization of tissue protein and gluconeogenesis from protein; and (4) androgenic effects (see page 997) from androgenic steroids, mainly dehydroepiandrosterone, produced in the adrenal cortex. Steroids that affect the electrolyte metabolism as in (1) are called *mineralocorticoids;* those that affect carbohydrate and protein metabolism as in (2) and (3) and which favor lipolysis are called *glucocorticoids*. Glucocorticoids exert a regulatory influence upon lymphocytes, erythrocytes, and eosinophils of the blood, and upon the structure and function of lymphoid tissue. The relative or complete absence of adrenocortical function, known as *Addison's disease*, is accompanied by loss of sodium chloride and water, retention of potassium, lowering of blood glucose and liver glycogen levels, increased sensitivity to insulin, nitrogen retention, and lymphocytosis. The disturbances in electrolyte metabolism are the cause of morbidity and mortality in most cases of severe adrenal insufficiency. All of these disorders may be corrected by administration of adrenal cortical extract or the pure adrenal cortical steroids now available.

In its biosynthesis of the steroid hormones, the adrenal cortex uses cholesterol, which is present in large amounts in the gland; during periods of secretory activity it also consumes large quantities of ascorbic acid, which is likewise present in high concentration. Control of adrenal gland secretion appears to be of two kinds. The production of mineralocorticoids, chiefly aldosterone, appears to be controlled in part by sodium intake and consequent changes in intravascular fluid volume, in part by the anterior pituitary, and in part by the brain through its modulation of plasma renin activity. For normal development and normal capacity to meet the routine homeostatic requirements, adrenal cortical function must be stimulated by adrenocorticotropin (see *Pituitary Hormones*, page 952); adrenal cortical activity is enhanced through release of corticotropin from the anterior pituitary. In emergency states or during stress, adrenal cortical activity is increased, which prepares for a prolonged duration of the state of stress.

Structures—Over 50 steroids have been shown to be present in the adrenal cortex. Only seven of these, however, have been shown to exert a significant biological effect related to adrenal cortical function. However, the adrenal cortex also produces androgenic steroids. All of the adrenal cortical steroids, except the androgens, contain 21 carbon atoms, an α,β-unsaturated ketone in ring A, and an α-ketol chain ($—COCH_2OH$) attached to ring D. They differ in extent of oxygenation or hydroxylation at carbons 11, 17, or 19. Depending on whether the predominant biological effect is related to electrolyte and water metabolism, or to carbohydrate and protein metabolism, the cortical steroids are classified as either *mineralocorticoid* or *glucocorticoid*, respectively.

In general, clinical experience has indicated that the anti-inflammatory activity of adrenal cortical steroids in man correlates well with their glucocorticoid activity. The undesirable side effects of sodium retention and edema are associated with mineralocorticoid activity. Synthetic steroids possessing higher glucocorticoid and lower mineralocorticoid activity than cortisone or cortisol have been prepared and marketed. All adrenal corticoids require the 3-keto group and 4–5 unsaturation. Additional unsaturation in ring A enhances the anti-inflammatory and antirheumatic properties while at the same time reducing the sodium-retaining effect. Thus, prednisolone has 4 times the anti-inflammatory activity of cortisol and yet has only 0.8 of the mineralocorticoid activity.

The presence of oxygen at position 11 is necessary for significant glucocorticoid activity but not for mineralocorticoid activity; the 11β-hydroxy group is more potent than the 11-keto group; the 11-keto group is converted to the active β-hydroxy group in the body. The 17α-hydroxy group is also important to glucocorticoid activity. The 21-hydroxy group is essential to mineralocorticoid activity; it favors but is not required for glucocorticoid activity. Introduction of either methyl or hydroxyl groups at position 16 markedly reduces mineralocorticoid activity but only slightly decreases glucocorticoid and anti-inflammatory activity. Thus, paramethasone (16α-methyl), betamethasone (16β-methyl), dexamethasone (16α-methyl), and triamcinolone (16α-hydroxy) have no significant mineralocorticoid activity. 6α-Methylation has unpredictable effects. It enhances the mineralocorticoid activity of cortisol but virtually abolishes that of prednisolone. The 9α-fluoro group enhances both glucocorticoid and mineralocorticoid activities, but the effects of substituents at the 6 and 16 positions override this effect. Further examples will become apparent from the discussions provided in the following individual monographs.

Biological Activity—For biological testing of adrenal cortical hormones, a number of different types of assays have been used. All of the above compounds will prolong the lives of adrenalectomized animals, although their relative effectiveness varies widely, the mineralocorticoids being 10–30 times as potent as the glucocorticoids. Desoxycorticosterone and aldosterone are likewise considerably more effective in maintaining normal kidney function in adrenalectomized animals. One method of assaying effects on electrolyte metabolism involves the determination of the relative amounts of radioactive sodium (^{24}Na) and potassium (^{42}K) excreted during one hour after their injection. In adrenalectomized animals the ratio (^{24}Na:^{42}K) is high, but is restored to normal upon the injection of microgram amounts of mineralocorticoids. Glucocorticoid activity is most conveniently measured by determining the capacity to restore normal liver glycogen levels in adrenalectomized mice or rats. 17-Hydroxycorticosterone (hydrocortisone or cortisol) and 11-dehydro-17-hydroxycorticosterone (cortisone) are 2 to 5 times as active as corticosterone and 11-dehydrocorticosterone in this test; the 11-desoxycorticoids are essentially inactive. Topical glucocorticoids may also be assayed by their vasoconstrictor effect in the skin of the human.

The glucocorticoids appear to affect all cells, although not all in the same way. Interest primarily focuses on their anti-inflammatory and immunosuppressant effects. They prevent release of various lytic enzymes that not only extend tissue damage during inflammation but also that generate leukotactic substances. They decrease phagocytosis by macrophages and also the disruption of macrophages by ingested materials. Anti-inflammatory effects include the retardation of the migration of polymorphonuclear leukocytes, suppression of repair and granulation, reduction in the erythrocyte sedimentation rate, decreased fibrinogenesis, and diminished elaboration of C-reactive protein. Glucocorticoids do not affect antigen-antibody interaction or the release of the mediators of immediate hypersensitivity. The immunosuppressant effects may be partly the result of the suppression of phagocytosis and immunoinformation processing and partly of a decrease in the number of eosinophils and lymphocytes, suppression of delayed hypersensitivity reactions, decrease in tissue reaction to antigen-antibody interactions (but not in the interaction itself), and a reduction in plasma immunoglobulins.

In addition to the above-mentioned changes brought about by glucocorticoids are the so-called *permissive* effects. In these, the steroids do not themselves cause change but physiological amounts are required for certain organs or structures to respond to stimuli. For example, neither the kidney can respond to a water load nor the arterioles to epinephrine in the absence of adequate levels of glucocorticoids.

Once a steroid hormone has permeated a cell membrane, it combines with a cytosolic protein called a receptor, or aporeceptor. The steroid-protein complex then translocates to the cell nucleus, where it attaches to chromatin. The result is an enhancement or reduction of the transcription of both messenger RNA and ribosomal RNA, which, in turn, leads to an increased or decreased synthesis of certain proteins. The protein produced is probably determined by the aporeceptor, of which there is more than one kind within the cell. In renal tubular cells, mineralocorticoids appear mainly to induce the synthesis of a protein that decreases intracellular sodium content; it is not clear whether this protein acts directly to increase the activity of membrane $[Na^+\text{-}K^+]$-activated ATPase or indirectly to increase the mitochondrial production of ATP for the ATPase or whether it decreases sodium permease activity. Because of the manifold actions of the glucocorticoids, it is to be expected that many intracellular proteins would be induced, but this has been difficult to verify. Inhibitors of protein- and RNA-synthesis prevent the effects of glucocorticoids, and the cellular content of some enzymes is affected, but with a number of membrane-bound enzymes, only the activities, and not the content, are affected. The activities of some enzymes are increased and others decreased. These are enzymes that have phospholipid adjuvants. Since the glucocorticoids alter the phospholipid composition of a number of cell membranes, it is likely that the enzyme activities are altered through the phospholipid composition, possibly through the induction of phospholipid-synthesizing and/or lytic enzymes. Alterations in membrane composition may possibly explain the membrane-stabilizing effects. Some, but not all, lysosomal membranes are stabilized. Glucocorticoids also inhibit membrane lipid peroxidation, which possibly contributes to the salutary effects in brain edema; the effect appears to be one of decreasing the activity of membrane-bound, superoxide radical-generating mixed-function enzymes. Possibly related is an action to block phospholipase-A_2, which prevents the release of arachidonic acid from membrane phospholipids and its subsequent conversion to hydroxyeicosotetraenoic acid and ultimately prostaglandins, thromboxanes and leukotrienes. Alterations in the prostaglandin system change the cyclic nucleotide balance, often in favor of cyclic guanosyl phosphate. In the proliferative skin diseases, glucocorticoids decrease the markedly elevated arachidonic acid and cyclic AMP levels. Effects on the prostaglandin and cyclic nucleotide systems are undoubtedly involved in the anti-inflammatory response, as is also membrane stabilization. They also induce the production of an antileukokinetic (antichemotactic) peptide. This peptide may prevent the proper assembly of the microtubules, an effect that would also explain the antimitotic effect seen with lymphoblasts and certain other proliferating cells and hence explain certain immunosuppressant and antineoplastic activity and the effect to retard growth. The sundry anabolic (eg, gluconeogenic) and catabolic (eg, proteolytic) effects of the glucocorticoids are also probably indirect.

Side Effects—Certain side effects may appear during the first week of treatment with glucocorticoids; they include euphoria and a rare paradoxical suicidal depression, psychoses (especially with high doses), rare hypertension, anorexia, occasional hyperglycemia, rare colonic ulceration (even though the drugs are used to treat ulcerative colitis), increased susceptibility to infections (especially vaccinial, herpetic, varicellar, and other viral infections, fungal infections, tuberculosis), and acne. They also mask some of the signs of infections, thus causing a postponement of appropriate anti-infective treatment. Glucocorticoids appear to increase peptic ulceration, especially of the stomach. After 2 to 3 days of treatment, the pituitary release of ACTH is suppressed, and the adrenal secretion of cortisol is inadequate once glucocorticoid administration ceases; this condition is temporary after short-term treatment. In the case of a medical emergency, the depressed pituitary-adrenal response may make the patient unable to respond to stress. Consequently, patients on high-dose or long-term treatment should carry a card stating that he/she is under treatment with corticosteroids. Withdrawal of corticosteroids should be slow.

From the first week through the first year of therapy, additional side effects may appear, namely, fat redistribution to the nape of the neck ("buffalo hump") and lower abdomen, diabetes mellitus and hyperglycemia, "moon face" and other edematous states and renal potassium loss (from mineralocorticoid activity), alkalosis, additional infections (including tuberculosis), papilledema, glaucoma, posterior subcapsular cataracts, diplopia, 6th nerve palsies, osteoporosis, myopathy, ecchymoses and purpura, and cutaneous striae. Because of the long-loop negative feedback suppression of ACTH output, the normal adrenal production of corticosteroids from cholesterol is considerably decreased, and hypercholesterolemia results; some of the excess cholesterol is diverted to increase the production of adrenal and testicular androgens, so that masculinization of the female or virilization of the young male and premature cessation of growth may occur. After prolonged suppression of the anterior pituitary secretion of ACTH, there may be a permanent defect in pituitary-adrenal function. Continuous or repetitive use of glucocorticoids may cause painless joint destruction, especially if the drug is given intra-articularly.

After more than a year of glucocorticoid therapy, additional untoward effects include bone fractures and vertebral collapse (from marked osteoporosis), hyperlipidemia, possible premature atherosclerosis, and excessive dependence on the physician. Patients also become physically and psychically dependent upon glucocorticoids and engage in drug-seeking behavior characteristic of addicts.

Adverse effects of glucocorticoids applied to the skin include stinging or burning sensations, itching, irritation, dryness, scaliness, vasoconstriction, folliculitis, acne, bacterial or yeast infections, hypopigmentation, atrophy, and striae. Systemic effects can also occur, especially if occlusive dressings are used. Topical ophthalmologic glucocorticoids not only may cause serious exacerbations of viral, fungal, and bacterial infections of the eye but also glaucoma; examinations for intraocular tension and corneal integrity should be made every 4 to 6 weeks. From all of the above, it can be seen that glucocorticoids are dangerous drugs.

Because the mineralocorticoids are mainly used in physiological doses for replacement therapy, untoward effects are usually infrequent and mild. Sodium and water retention (with "moon face"), potassium loss, alkalosis, and hypertension can occur with excessive doses.

Drug Interactions—Glucocorticoids decrease the hypoglycemic activity of insulin and oral hypoglycemics, so that a change in dose of the antidiabetic drugs may be necessitated. In high doses, glucocorticoids also decrease the response to somatotropin. The usual doses of mineralocorticoids and large doses of some glucocorticoids cause hypokalemia and may exaggerate the hypokalemic effects of thiazide and high-ceiling diuretics. In combination with amphotericin B they also may cause hypokalemia. Glucocorticoids appear to enhance the ulcerogenic effects of nonsteroidal anti-inflammatory drugs. They decrease the plasma levels of salicylates, and salicylism may occur on discontinuing steroids. Glucocorticoids may increase or decrease the effects of prothrombopenic anticoagulants. Estrogens, phenobarbital, phenytoin, and rifampin increase the metabolic clearance of adrenal steroids and hence necessitate dose adjustments.

Other Precautions and Contraindications—Both glucocorticoids and mineralocorticoids must be used cautiously in congestive heart failure, hypertension, liver failure, renal failure, or nephrolithiasis. When glucocorticoids are used in persons with emotional instability or psychotic tendencies, hyperlipidemia, diabetes mellitus, hypothyroidism, myasthenia gravis, osteoporosis, peptic ulcer, ulcerative colitis, chronic infections (especially tuberculosis or a positive test), or a history of herpetic infections, periodic checks should be made. Topical application to the eye is absolutely contraindicated in the presence of ophthalmologic infections.

Absorption and Elimination—All corticosteroids are rapidly and completely absorbed from the gastrointestinal tract. Some, however, particularly the natural ones, are so rapidly destroyed as they pass through the liver that they are poorly effective by the oral route, hence must be given parenterally for systemic effects. Esterification with large hydrophobic organic acids decreases solubility and therefore slows systemic absorption from sites of injection. Esterification with water-soluble acids, such as phosphoric or succinic, increases the rate of absorption from injection sites and may even permit intravenous administration. All of the glucocorticoids are absorbed from the skin, but some slowly enough that metabolic destruction can limit systemic accumulation. Many glucocorticoids are also metabolized in the skin. Fluorination at the 9-position and various substituents at the 17-position make glucocorticoids resistant to local destruction and hence make these derivatives more likely to cause systemic effects. For this reason, topical use is usually avoided in children. In the liver, the carbonyl groups at positions 3, 11, 17, and 20 are reduced to hydroxyl, and the resulting compounds may be conjugated with sulfate or glucuronic acid. Double bonds in the A ring are also reduced. Less than 1% of unchanged steroid is excreted.

In the plasma, corticosteroids are bound to both corticosteroid binding globulin (CBG, transcortin, α_1-globulin) and albumin, which serve as transport vehicles. The extent of binding varies among the steroids. Various drugs and diseases can affect the concentration of transport proteins and their capacities.

Corticoids cross the placental barrier and may cause congenital malformations. They also appear in breast milk and may suppress growth of the infant.

Therapeutic Uses—The adrenal corticosteroids are used for replacement therapy in *adrenal insufficiency* (eg, *Addison's disease* and *congenital adrenal hyperplasia*). In this use, toxic effects are infrequent, since the aim is to approximate the equivalent of physiological body concentrations. Both mineralocorticoids and glucocorticoids may be required; sometimes adrenocortical extracts, which contain both, are used. Glucocorticoids are additionally used to treat rheumatic, inflammatory, allergic, neoplastic, and other disorders; the effects are only palliative and do not eradicate the underlying disorders. It is necessary to use supraphysiological doses, so that some untoward effects are unavoidable.

The anti-inflammatory actions of the glucocorticoids are employed in the treatment of *noninfectious acute ocular inflammation* (*allergic blepharitis, iritis, uveitis, choroiditis, conjunctivitis, sympathetic ophthalmia*) and certain infectious inflammations, especially in combination with antibiotics. Glucocorticoids are of value, in decreasing some *cerebral edemas*, eg, vasogenic, but are of dubious value in cerebral edema from other causes. In *infantile massive spasms* (minor motor epilepsy) glucocorticoids may be of benefit, but it is not clear how this derives from anti-inflammatory activity. In serious *acute allergic disorders*, glucocorticoids may be indicated; they should not be used chronically in allergic disorders, except in acute flare-ups. (However, they are approved for intranasal application for chronic noninfectious rhinitis.) Similarly, *acute bronchial asthma, status asthmaticus*, and some chronic *obstructive pulmonary disease*

may require glucocorticoids, but they should be avoided, if possible, in chronic asthma because of the implications for lifetime medication. These drugs suppress allergic and inflammatory manifestations of *trichinosis*.

Topical or systemic glucocorticoids often markedly improve certain skin diseases, such as *pruritus, psoriasis, dermatitis herpetiformis,* and *eczema; pemphigus, erythema multiforme, exfoliative dermatitis,* and *mycosis fungoides* usually require systemic treatment, which may be life-saving.

Probably the most widely known application of the anti-inflammatory actions of the glucocorticoids is in the treatment of the arthritides and rheumatic disorders. Immunosuppressant actions may also play a role in the treatment of such disorders. These disorders are *systemic lupus erythematosus, polyarteritis, temporal arteritis, Wegener's granulomatosis, polymyositis,* and *polymyalgia rheumatica.* Glucocorticoids may be indicated in severe cases of *rheumatoid arthritis* unresponsive to other treatment, *Still's disease, mixed connective tissue disease, drug-induced lupoid syndromes,* and *psoriatic arthropathy.* Rheumatic or arthritic conditions in which glucocorticoids may or may not provide temporary relief but are not justified chronically because of a high toxicity:benefit ratio are osteoarthritis, systemic ankylosing spondylitis, gout fibrositis, and Reiter's syndrome. Even though the *nephrotic syndrome* is not inflammatory, it may respond to treatment, perhaps as the result of immunosuppression. *Ulcerative colitis* sometimes may respond dramatically. The beneficial effects in *myasthenia gravis* are probably immunosuppressant. Chronic multiple sclerosis does not respond but acute relapses may.

Glucocorticoids may be palliative in *acute leukemia* and also in *chronic lymphocytic leukemia,* and they are components of certain curative antineoplastic combinations. They suppress the associated autoimmune hemolytic anemia and the nonhemolytic anemia, granulocytopenia, and thrombocytopenia that result from encroachment on the bone marrow, and also the cachexia and fever. The effects are only temporary, and the patient eventually becomes refractory to steroid therapy. *Hodgkin's disease, lymphosarcoma,* and *multiple myeloma* may also be temporarily suppressed, though most frequently only the pain is diminished. The mechanism of the palliative effects on these neoplasms is unknown.

In the treatment of *endotoxin shock,* massive doses of glucocorticoids suppress the vasculotoxic effects of the toxin. In all kinds of *shock,* massive doses decrease peripheral resistance, stimulate the heart, and decrease the amount of circulating myocardial depressant factor. To be optimally effective they must be given as a bolus.

Modalities and Regimens of Corticosteroid Therapy—*Replacement Therapy*—Treatment of primary and secondary adrenal insufficiency requires replacement of both glucocorticoids and mineralocorticoids in sufficient doses to relieve the signs and symptoms of insufficiency. However, when the patient experiences an additional stress, supplements of glucocorticoids may be required. The dose and dose-interval vary from patient to patient, but the doses are small and complications are infrequent and minimal; the most difficult challenge is in the adjustment of dosage in response to changes in stress.

Chronic Low-Dose Systemic Therapy of Disease—In mild inflammatory or collagen disorders, low doses of glucocorticoids are often sufficient to be palliative, and low-dose regimens are preferable, since adverse effects usually are of low intensity, provided that the therapeutic end point is only an amelioration and not elimination of the morbidity. Although low-dose therapy may cause some suppression of pituitary-adrenal function, the suppression is readily reversible, and some reserve in the system is extant. However, abrupt withdrawal of the drug not only may be followed by a return to the previous condition but an acute exacerbation of the disease. Pituitary-adrenal suppression and consequent acute flare-up after withdrawal may be lessened by avoiding round-the-clock administration and, instead, giving the drug between 8 and 9 am, in order that plasma levels and hence pituitary-adrenal suppression be at a minimum during the early morning sleeping hours, when pituitary adrenal function is at its diurnal peak.

Chronic High-Dose Systemic Therapy—In serious chronic inflammatory or immunologic disorders or in glucocorticoid-responsive neoplasia, large doses of glucocorticoids may be given for long periods of time. Consequently, side effects are frequent, and pituitary-adrenal suppression may be severe. The suppression may continue for weeks to months after cessation of treatment, so that withdrawal must be slowly tapered off to allow the pituitary-adrenal system to recover. Abrupt withdrawal will result in adrenal insufficiency, which may be life-threatening, as well as an acute recrudescence of the original disorder. Pituitary-adrenal suppression and systemic side effects may be less severe if the dose is given in the morning, so that nocturnal pituitary-adrenal activity is less inhibited. Another device to minimize such adverse systemic effects is that of *alternate day therapy*, in which twice the usual daily dose is given but only every other day, which permits the hypothalamico-pituitary segment of the pituitary-adrenal negative feedback system and various undiseased target organs time to recover partly toward normal between doses.

Intensive Short-Term Systemic Therapy—Massive doses of glucocorticoids may be required in certain acute conditions, such as bacteremic shock, status asthmaticus, etc. The short duration of such treatment, sometimes no longer than 48 hr, is not enough to give rise to pituitary-adrenal suppression, serious immunosuppression, or opportunistic infections, although in septic shock, suprainfections may occur. Psychosis, gastrointestinal bleeding, and hyperosmolar diabetic coma can occur in such short-term use.

Local Treatment—TOPICAL APPLICATION. Topical efficacy depends on the inherent glucocorticoid activity (or potency) of the steroid, the concentration in the preparation, permeability coefficient, the vehicle and excipients, and local metabolic processes. Except for serious conditions, low-potency glucocorticoids are preferred by many authorities, because adverse effects on the skin appear to be less severe than with high-potency agents, even if the latter are used at appropriately lower concentrations. Only hydrocortisone and its acetate are available for nonprescription topical use. Drugs with a high lipid-water distribution coefficient penetrate well from absorbable or nonoleaginous vehicles and tend to remain longer in the skin than water-soluble agents, exerting a more extended local action but lesser systemic side effects, especially if the drug is rapidly metabolized systemically. However, it is desirable that the agents be metabolized in the skin, so that less is delivered to the systemic circulation. Steroids that have the 17-OH group substituted and/or which are fluorinated are poorly metabolized locally and hence may have a significant potential for systemic effects; for this reason, especial caution is urged when such compounds are used in children. Occlusive dressings may be used, especially for low-potency, poorly penetrant steroids. The stratum corneum under the dressing becomes macerated and more permeable. However, such dressings increase absorption into the blood stream and hence favor systemic effects. LOCAL INJECTION. In order to achieve high, rapidly acting local concentrations of a glucocorticoid, it is sometimes injected as a very soluble derivative which rapidly generates the parent steroid. However, such soluble forms also rapidly leave the region of injection. For this reason, insoluble derivatives may be included or injected alone, so that a sustained action in parallel with slow dissolution may be effected.

Beclomethasone Dipropionate

Pregna-1,4-diene-3,20-dione, 9-chloro-11-hydroxy-16-methyl-17,21-bis(1-oxopropoxy)-, (11β,16β)-, Vanceril (*Schering-Plough*)

9-Chloro-11β,17,21-trihydroxy-16β-methylpregna-1,4-diene-3,20-dione 17,21-dipropionate [5534-09-8] $C_{26}H_{37}ClO_7$ (521.05).

Preparation—Synthesis of beclomethasone, a 9-chloro-16β-methyl derivative of prednisolone, and esters of beclomethasone, from steroid intermediates is described in British Pats 901,093 and 912,378 (*CA 58*: 3488e, 1963; *59*: 14082b, 1963).

Description—White to cream-white powder; odorless.
Solubility—Very slightly soluble in water; very soluble in chloroform; freely soluble in alcohol and acetone.

Uses—Beclomethasone dipropionate has 500 times the topical anti-inflammatory activity of dexamethasone but is less active as a systemic glucocorticoid and is almost inactive by the oral route. The low systemic activity is the result of rapid de-esterification and further metabolism in the liver. Also, it has a high lipid- but low water-solubility, so that it not only is well absorbed topically but also tends to remain at the site of application. Thus it may be administered by oral inhalation with usually negligible systemic side effects. It is indicated only in the treatment of *bronchial asthma* in which bronchodilators and cromolyn sodium are ineffective. As long as 2 to 4 weeks may be required for the onset of a beneficial effect. It is also employed in the treatment of *noninfectious rhinitis*.

The most common side effects of inhaled beclomethasone are dry mouth, hoarseness, sore throat, and pharyngeal or tracheal candidiasis. Usually, the effects on pituitary-adrenal function are negligible, but suppression of plasma cortisol levels occurs in a few percent of adult patients who receive 1600 µg/day and in all who receive 4000 µg/day. In children, doses of 400 to 800 µg/day have effects on adrenal function comparable to alternate-day therapy with prednisone. Patients who switch from continuous oral glucocorticoids to beclomethasone aerosols often show signs and symptoms of systemic glucocorticoid deficiency, and deaths from adrenal insufficiency have been reported. Adverse effects of intranasal beclomethasone include epistaxis, nasal irritation, sneezing and nasopharyngeal candidiasis. Hypersensitivity or other adverse effects to the propellants (CHF_3 and CH_2F_2) and oleic acid (a dispersing agent) may occur; hypersensitivity absolutely contraindicates use of the aerosol. The effects of beclomethasone on the fetus *in utero* and the extent of secretion into milk are not yet known.

Dose—*Oral inhalation*, adults and children over 12 yrs of age, initially, **84 µg** (2 metered inhalations) 3 or 4 times a day, to be adjusted later to the minimal number of daily inhalations that will control symptoms; in severe asthma, the initial dose is 100 µg 6 to 8 times a day and subsequently adjusted as needed, usually to a lower dose but occasionally to doses as high as 1000 µg per day or more; *children 6 to 12 yrs* of age, 42 to 84 µg (1 to 2 metered sprays) 3 or 4 times a day, not to exceed 500 µg per day. *Nasal insufflation*, adults and children over 12 yrs of age, initially 42 µg (1 metered insufflation) in each nostril 2 to 4 times a day; maintenance, 3 times a day. The mouth and throat should be rinsed after each oral or intranasal insufflation.

Dosage Form—Aerosol: 16.8 g/canister; each metered spray releases approximately 42 µg.

Betamethasone

Pregna-1,4-diene-3,20-dione, 9-fluoro-11,17,21-trihydroxy-16-methyl-, (11β,16β)-, Celestone (*Schering-Plough*)

9-Fluoro-11β,17,21-trihydroxy-16β -methylpregna-1,4-diene-3,20-dione [378-44-9] $C_{22}H_{29}FO_5$ (392.47).

Preparation—Betamethasone is prepared from 16-dehydropregnenolone (see *Progesterone*, page 993) by treatment with methyl magnesium iodide to insert the 16β-methyl group, catalytic reduction of the remaining double bond, enol acylation at position 20, and reaction with peracetic acid followed by hydrolysis to the 16β-methyl-17α-hydroxy compound. Bromination and acetoxylation gives the 3β-hydroxy-21-acetoxy derivative which is oxidized to the 3-oxo compound with chromic acid. Dibromination at positions 1 and 4 followed by dehydrobromination with dimethylformamide to the 1,4-diene, then incubation with *Pestalotia foedans* (or a similar organism) results in the 11α-hydroxy derivative. Esterification at the 11-position with ethyl chloroformate, elimination of the ester function with acetic acid to form the 1,4,9(11)-triene, treatment with *N*-bromoacetamide and perchloric acid gives the 9α-bromo-11β-hydroxy compound. Abstraction of HBr with potassium acetate affords the 9β,11β-epoxy derivative which by treatment with HF in a halogenated hydrocarbon yields the 9α-fluoro-11β-hydroxy analogue, betamethasone.

Description—White to practically white, odorless, crystalline powder; melts at about 240° with some decomposition.
Solubility—1 g in 5300 mL water, 65 mL alcohol, 325 mL chloroform; very slightly soluble in ether.

Uses—An extremely potent glucocorticoid with actions, uses, and side effects typical of this class of steroids (see introduction to this section). Its activity is 20 to 30 times that of cortisol. However, it only rarely induces sodium and water retention and potassium loss such as accompany treatment with cortisone and many other adrenal corticoids; on occasion, betamethasone may even increase sodium excretion and induce diuresis. In the usual doses, the incidence of characteristic adrenal corticoid untoward effects such as anorexia, protracted weight loss, vertigo, headache, and muscle weakness is quite low. The serum half-life of betamethasone is about 3 hr.
Dose—*Oral, adult, initially,* **0.6 to 7.2 mg** (usually **2.4 to 4.8 mg**) daily in single or divided doses; *maintenance,* **0.6 to 1.2 mg** daily or on alternate days; *pediatric, replacement,* **17.5 μg per kg** of body weight or **500 μg per m²** of body surface a day in 3 divided doses, and, for *disease,* **62.5 to 250 μg/kg** or **1.88 to 7.5 mg/m²** in 3 or 4 divided doses. *Topical,* as **0.2%** cream applied to skin 2 or 3 times a day in adults and once a day in children.
Dosage Forms—Cream: 0.2%; Syrup: 0.6 mg/5 mL; Tablets: 0.6 mg.

Betamethasone Acetate

Pregna-1,4-diene-3,20-dione, 9-fluoro-11,17-dihydroxy-16-methyl-21-(acetyloxy)-, (11β,16β)-, Betamethasone 21-Acetate

9-Fluoro-11β,17,21-trihydroxy-16β-methylpregna-1,4-diene-3,-20-dione 21-acetate [987-24-6] $C_{24}H_{31}FO_6$ (434.50).
For the structure of the base, see *Betamethasone.*
Preparation—*Betamethasone* 962 is acetylated with acetic anhydride in the presence of pyridine. US Pat 3,164,618.

Description—White to creamy white, odorless powder; sinters and resolidifies at about 165° and remelts with decomposition between 200° and 220°.
Solubility—1 g in 2000 mL water, 9 mL alcohol, 16 mL chloroform.

Uses—The actions are the same as those of the parent compound, *Betamethasone.* However, at present, the acetate is marketed only in combination with the sodium phosphate. The acetate is less soluble than the sodium phosphate, so that the acetate provides a sustained action after intramuscular or intra-articular injection.
Dose—See *Sterile Betamethasone Sodium Phosphate and Betamethasone Acetate Suspension.*

Betamethasone Sodium Phosphate

Pregna-1,4-diene-3,20-dione, 9-fluoro-11,17-dihydroxy-16-methyl-21-(phosphonooxy)-, disodium salt, (11β,16β)-, Betamethasone 21-(Disodium Phosphate)

9-Fluoro-11β,17,21-trihydroxy-16β-methylpregna-1,4-diene-3,-20-dione 21-(disodium phosphate) [151-73-5] $C_{22}H_{28}FNa_2O_8P$ (516.41).
For the structure of the base, see *Betamethasone.*

Preparation—Starting with *Betamethasone,* by the method described for *Dexamethasone Sodium Phosphate.* US Pat 3,164,618.

Description—White to practically white, odorless powder; hygroscopic.
Solubility—1 g in 2 mL water, 470 mL alcohol, >10,000 mL chloroform, >10,000 mL ether.

Uses—The actions are those of *Betamethasone,* to which the more soluble disodium phosphate is converted in the body. Following injection, the plasma or synovial fluid levels rise at a rapid rate to high levels, which effects a prompt response. Parenteral betamethasone sodium phosphate is employed when oral glucocorticoids cannot be used or when it is desirable to inject the drug directly into the affected structure.
Dose—The following doses are stated in terms of the *betamethasone equivalents,* but the content of ampules and vials is stated for betamethasone sodium phosphate itself. *To convert,* 4 mg of the sodium phosphate derivative is equivalent to 3 mg of betamethasone. *Intramuscular* or *intravenous, adult, initially* up to **9 mg**/day, to be adjusted downward as the disease responds; *intra-articular, intralesional,* or into *soft tissue,* up to **9 mg**/day as needed. *Children, intramuscular,* for *replacement,* **17.5 μg/kg** or **500 μg/m²** of body weight every third day *or* **5.8 to 8.75 μg/kg** or **166 to 250 μg** once a day; for *disease,* **20.8 to 125 μg/kg** or **625 μg** to **3.75 mg/m²** once or twice a day.
Dosage Forms—Injection: 4 mg/1 mL and 20 mg/5 mL, respectively equivalent to 3 mg/1 mL and 15 mg/5 mL of betamethasone. See also *Sterile Betamethasone Sodium Phosphate and Betamethasone Acetate Suspension.*

Sterile Betamethasone Sodium Phosphate and Betamethasone Acetate Suspension

Celestone Soluspan (*Schering*)

A sterile preparation of betamethasone sodium phosphate in solution and betamethasone acetate in suspension in water for injection.
Uses—See *Betamethasone Acetate* and *Betamethasone Sodium Phosphate.* The combination is intended for use in glucocorticoid-responsive disease (see page 961) in patients in whom oral medication cannot be achieved, in acute self-limiting disease in which a single dose is sufficient, and to initiate treatment in severe diseases where a prompt response is desired prior to switching to a drug with a slower onset and longer duration of action. Although the injection may be given intra-articularly, it must be remembered that repeated intra-articular glucocorticoids sometimes permit painless destruction of the joint. The suspension contains benzalkonium chloride, which may sensitize some recipients.
Dose—Doses are stated in terms of total glucocorticoid content. *Adult, intra-articular,* **1.5 to 12 mg** and *intrabursal,* **6 mg,** repeated as needed; *intradermal* or *intralesional,* **1.2 mg/cm²** of affected skin, up to a total of 6 mg, to be repeated once a week, if necessary; *intramuscular,* **500 μg** to **9 mg**/day. Pediatric doses not determined. Although the manufacturer's recommendations for parenteral therapy are for divided doses at 12-hr intervals, it is advisable to give all or nearly all of the daily dose between 8 and 9 am to minimize interference with the nocturnal activity of the pituitary-adrenal system.
Dosage Form—Sterile Suspension: Betamethasone phosphate equivalent to 15 mg of betamethasone and 15 mg of betamethasone acetate/5 mL.

Betamethasone Valerate

Pregna-1,4-diene-3,20-dione, 9-fluoro-11,21-dihydroxy-16-methyl-17-[(1-oxopentyl)oxy]-, (11β,16β)-, Betamethasone 17-Valerate; Valisone (*Schering-Plough*)

9-Fluoro-11β,17,21-trihydroxy-16β-methylpregna-1,4-diene-3,-20-dione 17-valerate [2152-44-5] $C_{27}H_{37}FO_6$ (476.58).
For the structure of the base, see *Betamethasone.*
Preparation—A solution of *Bethamethasone* in an organic solvent is treated with a lower alkyl orthovalerate such as trimethyl orthovalerate [$C_4H_9C(OCH_3)_3$] to produce betamethasone-17,21-ylene alkyl orthovalerate. This is then hydrolyzed with dilute acid and the resulting crude betamethasone 17-valerate is extracted and crystallized from a suitable organic solvent. US Pat 3,312,590.

Description—White to practically white, odorless, crystalline powder; melts at about 190°, with decomposition.

Solubility—1 g in 10,000 mL water, 16 mL alcohol, <10 mL chloroform, 400 mL ether.

Uses—The actions are the same as those of the parent compound, *Betamethasone*. However, the physicochemical properties of the compound favor penetration into the skin. It is thus employed for treatment of inflammatory and allergic dermatoses and dermatitides (see the general statement in this section).

Unless extensive areas of the skin are dressed with betamethasone valerate cream under occlusion, systemic effects are unlikely to occur. However, prolonged topical use may cause cutaneous and subcutaneous atrophy and consequent striae. Irritation, folliculitis, and sensitization are rare.

Dose—*Topical, adult*, as a cream, lotion, or ointment containing the equivalent of **0.01** or **0.1**% of betamethasone to the affected area 1 to 3 times a day or as an aerosol containing the equivalent of **0.15**% betamethasone 3 to 4 times a day. *Children*, as a **0.01**% cream 1 or 2 times a day or as a **1**% cream, lotion, or ointment, or **0.15**% aerosol once a day.

Dosage Forms (as the equivalent of betamethasone)—Aerosol: 0.15%; Cream: 0.01 and 0.1%; Lotion: 0.1%; Ointment: 0.1%.

Cortisone Acetate

Pregn-4-ene-3,11,20-trione, 21-(acetyloxy)-17-hydroxy-, Kendall's Compound E Acetate; Wintersteiner's Compound F Acetate; Reichstein's Substance Fa Acetate; Cortone Acetate (*MSD*)

17,21-Dihydroxypregn-4-ene-3,11,20-trione 21-acetate [50-04-4] $C_{23}H_{30}O_6$ (402.49).

Preparation—By a variety of methods using easily obtainable starting materials such as ergosterol, diosgenin or hecogenin from plant materials and cholesterol or desoxycholic acid from animal sources. The cortisone is esterified with acetic anhydride to give the acetate.

Description—White or practically white, odorless, crystalline powder; stable in air; melts at about 240° with some decomposition.

Solubility—Insoluble in water; 1 g in about 350 mL alcohol, 4 mL chloroform, 30 mL dioxane, and 75 mL acetone.

Uses—Cortisone is a natural glucocorticoid with a slight degree of mineralocorticoid activity; it has 0.8 the glucocorticoid activity of cortisol. Cortisone acetate is used specifically, in combination with desoxycorticosterone acetate, in *adrenal cortical insufficiency*. It may also be used for the numerous purposes described in the introduction to this section, where its untoward effects are also described. Although cortisone acetate is applied locally in some conditions, it requires conversion to cortisol to be substantially effective, and there is little to justify topical use. The plasma half-life of cortisone is about 30 min, which is shorter than the half-time for absorption of the acetate and conversion to cortisone. The plasma half-time for hydrocortisone, the active form of cortisone, is 1½ to 2 hr.

Dose—*Oral, adult*, for *replacement therapy*, **20** to **70 mg** daily, ⅔ taken in the morning and ⅓ in the afternoon, and, for *anti-inflammatory effects*, **25** to **50 mg** daily in mild chronic disorders and **75** to **300 mg** in acute and severe chronic disorders. *Children, replacement*, **700 µg/kg** of body weight (or **20 mg per m²** of body surface) a day every third day *or* **233** to **350 µg/kg** or **6.66** to **10 mg/m²** of body surface once a day; for *anti-inflammatory effects*, **2.5** to **10 mg/kg** of body weight (or **75** to **300 mg/m²** of body surface) a day. *Intramuscular, adult*, **20** to **30 mg** a day for serious chronic disorders; absorption is too slow and erratic by this route to lend itself to treatment of acute disorders. Once a satisfactory initial response has been obtained, the dose is gradually lowered to the satisfactory maintenance minimum. *Topical*, to the *conjunctiva, adult* and *children*, as a **1.5**% ointment, 3 or 4 times a day.

Dosage Forms—Ophthalmic Ointment: 1.5%; Sterile Suspension: 250 mg/10 mL and 500 mg/10 mL; Tablets: 5, 10, and 25 mg.

Desoxycorticosterone Acetate

Pregn-4-ene-3,20-dione, 21-(acetyloxy)-, Desoxycortone Acetate; Deoxycortone Acetate; Doca Acetate (*Organon*); Percorten (*Ciba*)

11-Deoxycorticosterone acetate [56-47-3] $C_{23}H_{32}O_4$ (372.50).

Preparation—Desoxycorticosterone, synthesized from the soya bean phytosterol stigmasterol, is condensed with acetyl chloride in pyridine solution. Dilution of the reaction product with water precipitates the ester.

Description—White, or creamy white, crystalline powder; odorless and stable in air; melts between 155° and 161°.

Solubility—Practically insoluble in water; sparingly soluble in alcohol, acetone, and dioxane; slightly soluble in vegetable oils.

Uses—A natural mineralocorticoid (see page 958 for actions, uses, and side effects). Physiologically it is of much less importance than aldosterone, but the cost of the latter is too prohibitive for clinical use. Treatment of *Addison's disease* has been greatly advanced by the use of desoxycorticosterone. Although the defects in carbohydrate and protein metabolism are not corrected by this particular compound, life can be maintained by its intelligent administration.

The serum half-life of desoxycorticosterone is about 70 min. Since Addison's disease is a permanent disorder, treatment is for life, and a long duration of action is therefore desirable. Desoxycorticosterone sometimes is administered in the form of subcutaneous pellets. With pellet implantation the hormone is slowly absorbed, and a single implantation of an adequate number of pellets may be effective for as long as 6 months or more. Signs of underdosage are corrected with intramuscular administration, and signs of overdosage by salt restriction. Addisonian patients usually take cortisone acetate or hydrocortisone along with desoxycorticosterone.

Patients receiving desoxycorticosterone should be careful to maintain an adequate intake of salt and carbohydrate and, during periods of acute adrenal insufficiency, carbohydrate must be specially administered. In crisis, extracts containing glucocorticoids should be administered.

Dose—*Intramuscular, adults*, for *Addison's disease*, initially **2** to **10 mg**/day, then **1** to **5 mg**/day for maintenance; for salt-losing *adrenogenital syndrome*, up to **6 mg** a day for 3 or 4 days, after which dosage is adjusted according to clinical response; *children*, **1** to **5 mg**/day or **1.5** to **2 mg/m²**/day, with frequent monitoring. *Subcutaneous implantation, adults* 1 pellet (**125 mg**) for each 0.5 mg of the injection required for daily maintenance, repeated at 8- to 12-month intervals.

Dosage Forms—Injection: 50 mg/10 mL; Pellets: 125 mg. The injection contains parabens, which can cause sensitization.

Desoxycorticosterone Pivalate

Pregn-4-ene-3,20-dione, 21-(2,2-dimethyl-1-oxopropoxy)-, Percorten Pivalate (*Ciba*)

11-Deoxycorticosterone pivalate [808-48-0] $C_{26}H_{38}O_4$ (414.59).

For the structure of the base, see *Desoxycorticosterone Acetate*.

Preparation—As described for the acetate except that trimethylacetyl chloride is employed.

Description—White, or creamy white, crystalline powder; odorless and stable in air; melts between 200° and 206°.

Solubility—Practically insoluble in water; soluble 1 g in 450 mL alcohol, 3 mL of chloroform, 160 mL of methanol. Soluble in ether and fixed oils.

Uses—The actions are the same as those of *Desoxycorticosterone Acetate*, except that intramuscular microcrystalline suspensions of the trimethylacetate (pivalate) have a very long duration of action. Consequently, it is used only for the treatment of chronic primary and secondary adrenal cortical insufficiency, usually only after a maintenance dose of desoxycorticosterone acetate is first established.

Dose—*Intramuscular, adults* and *children* **25 mg** for each mg of the oil solution of desoxycorticosterone acetate required for maintenance in the trial regimen (usually 25 to 100 mg), administered every 4 weeks.

Dosage Form—Sterile Suspension: 100 mg/4 mL.

Dexamethasone

Pregna-1,4-diene-3,20-dione, 9-fluoro-11,17,21-trihydroxy-16-methyl-, (11β,16α)-, (*Various Mfrs*)

9-Fluoro-11β,17,21-trihydroxy-16α-methylpregna-1,4-diene-3,-20-dione [50-02-2] $C_{22}H_{29}FO_5$ (392.47).

Preparation—In a manner quite similar to that for *Betamethasone*, the difference being that the 16-methyl group is inserted in the α-configuration.

Description—White to practically white, odorless, crystalline powder; stable in air; melts at about 250° with some decomposition.

Solubility—Soluble 1 g in 42 mL of alcohol, 165 mL of chloroform; sparingly soluble in acetone, dioxane, and methanol; very slightly soluble in ether; practically insoluble in water.

Uses—Dexamethasone possesses glucocorticoid activity, for which it is used clinically (see introduction to this section). It is especially used as an anti-inflammatory and antiallergic drug. Topically it is employed in the treatment of glucocorticoid-responsive dermatoses. Its systemic glucocorticoid potency is about 25 times that of cortisone. It is capable of inducing all the usual side effects of adrenal corticoids, except that the mineralocorticoid-like side effects are less pronounced than with cortisone acetate.

Its effect to suppress pituitary-adrenocortical function is used for differential diagnostic purposes in Cushing's syndrome. In the *rapid overnight test*, 1 mg of dexamethasone given at 11 or 12 pm will have a marked suppressant effect on plasma cortisol levels at 8 am in persons who do not have Cushing's syndrome but little effect on those who do. In the *low-dose 2-day test*, 0.5 mg every 6 hr for 2 days will fail to suppress 24-hr urinary output of 17-hydroxysteroids in patients with bilateral adrenal hyperplasia and autonomous adenomas but not in others. In the *high-dose 2-day test*, 2 mg every 6 hr for 2 days will suppress urinary 17-hydroxysteroids in adrenal hyperplasia (except multinodular hyperplasia) and most ACTH-responsive adrenal adenomas. Some multinodular hyperplasias and ACTH-responsive adrenal adenomas will not show suppression until the dose of dexamethasone is increased to 4 to 8 mg every 6 hr. When adrenal hyperplasia is secondary to an ACTH-producing tumor, no suppression will occur in any of these tests.

The plasma half-life of dexamethasone is 3 to 4 hr.

Dose—*Oral, adult, initially* **500 µg** to **9 mg** a day in single or divided doses, and usually less for *maintenance;* for *diagnostic doses,* see *Uses,* above; *children,* for *replacement,* **23** to **330 µg per kg** of body weight (or **670 µg** to **10 mg per m^2** of body surface) a day, and, for *disease,* **83** to **333 µg/kg** (or **2.5** to **10 mg/m^2**) a day in 3 or 4 divided doses. *Topical,* to the *skin,* as **0.01%** aerosol 2 to 4 times a day, **0.04%** cream or **0.1%** gel 3 or 4 times a day, except only 1 or 2 times a day with any preparation in children. *Topical,* to the *conjunctiva,* **1 drop** of **0.1%** suspension 3 or 4 times a day.

Dosage Forms—Aerosol: 0.01%; Cream: 0.04%; Elixir: 0.5 mg/5 mL; Gel: 0.1%; Ophthalmic Suspension: 0.1%; Tablets: 0.25, 0.5, 0.75, 1.5, 4 and 6 mg.

Dexamethasone Sodium Phosphate

Pregn-4-ene-3,20-dione, 9-fluoro-11,17-dihydroxy-16-methyl-21-(phosphonooxy)-, disodium salt, (11β,16α)-, Dexamethasone 21-(Disodium Phosphate); Decadron Phosphate (*MSD*); Dalalone (*O'Neal, Jones & Feldman*)

9-Fluoro-11β,17,21-trihydroxy-16α-methylpregna-1,4-diene-3,20-dione 21-(dihydrogen phosphate) disodium salt [2392-39-4] $C_{22}H_{28}FNa_2O_8P$ (516.41).

For the structure of the base, see *Dexamethasone.*

Preparation—Dexamethasone is esterified with methanesulfonyl chloride at the 21-position, and the ester is refluxed with sodium iodide in ethanol to form the 21-iodo derivative. This is treated with

silver dihydrogen phosphate and the resulting 21-(dihydrogen phosphate) is neutralized with sodium hydroxide.

Description—A white, or slightly yellow, crystalline powder; odorless or has a slight odor of alcohol; very hygroscopic; pH (1 in 100 solution) between 7.5 and 10.5.

Solubility—1 g dissolves in about 2 mL of water; slightly soluble in ether and chloroform.

Uses—The same actions as *Dexamethasone.* It is one of the most soluble adrenocortical compounds. Thus it lends itself well to intravenous administration, local injection, inhalation, and to solutions and water-based ointments for topical application, especially for ophthalmologic use. The inhalation aerosol is used in the management of bronchial asthma. Although it may be given intra-articularly, it is usually not recommended by this route because of the danger of painless joint destruction. The adverse effects and contraindications are those of other glucocorticoids (see the introduction in this section).

Dose—All doses below are stated in terms of dexamethasone equivalents. *Intravenous* or *intramuscular, adult,* **420 µg** to **7.5 mg** per day, the dosage being decreased when a response occurs; *intra-articular, intralesional,* or *soft-tissue injection,* **170 µg** to **5 mg**. *Oral inhalation,* **3 metered sprays (252 µg)** in *adults and* **2 metered sprays (168 µg)** in *children,* 3 or 4 times a day. *Intranasal, adult,* **2 metered sprays (168 µg)** into each nostril 2 or 3 times a day up to 1.2 mg/day; *children* over 6 years of age, **1** or **2 metered sprays** into each nostril twice a day. *Topical,* to the *skin,* as **0.1%** cream, 3 or 4 times a day for *adults* or once a day for *children;* to the *conjunctiva* as **0.05%** ointment 3 or 4 times a day or 1 drop of **0.05%** solution 4 to 6 times a day.

Dosage Forms—(as dexamethasone equivalents) Inhalation Aerosol: 84 µg/metered spray; Nasal Aerosol: 84 µg/metered spray; Cream: 0.1%; Injection: 3.3, 8.33 and 20 mg/mL; Ophthalmic Ointment: 0.05%; Ophthalmic Solution: 0.1%.

Fludrocortisone Acetate

Pregn-4-ene-3,20-dione, 21-(acetyloxy)-9-fluoro-11,17-dihydroxy-, (11β)-, Florinef Acetate (*Squibb*)

9-Fluoro-11β,17,21-trihydroxypregn-4-ene-3,20-dione 21-acetate [514-36-3] $C_{23}H_{31}FO_6$ (422.49).

Preparation—One method starts with *Cortisol Acetate* which is first dehydrated to the 4,9-diene. The 9α-fluoro and 11β-hydroxy groups are inserted by a method similar to that used for *Betamethasone.*

Description—Fine, white to pale-yellow powder that is odorless or practically odorless; hygroscopic; melts at about 225° with some decomposition.

Solubility—Insoluble in water; soluble 1 g in 50 mL of alcohol, 50 mL of chloroform, or 250 mL of ether.

Uses—A potent mineralocorticoid with considerable glucocorticoid activity. Its uses and side effects are those of mineralocorticoids (see page 958), except that when used for replacement therapy in adrenal insufficiency it may not always be necessary to use a glucocorticoid concurrently, although usually cortisol or cortisone are also administered. With the doses used for replacement therapy, glucocorticoid side effects of fludrocortisone acetate alone are mild and infrequent. The plasma half-life is about ½ hour.

Dose—*Oral, adult,* for *chronic adrenal insufficiency,* **0.05** to **0.2 mg** once a day to 3 times a week; for *congenital adrenogenital syndromes,* **0.1** to **0.2 mg/day**. In both of the above, a glucocorticoid is usually concomitantly administered.

Dosage Form—Tablets: 0.1 mg.

Flumethasone Pivalate

Pregna-1,4-diene-3,20-dione, 21-(2,2-dimethyl-1-oxopropoxy)-6,9-difluoro-11,17-dihydroxy-16-methyl-, (6α,11β,16α)-, Locorten (*Ciba-Geigy*); Locacorten (*Ciba-Geigy*)

6α,9-Difluoro-11β,17,21-trihydroxy-16α-methylpregna-1,4-diene-3,20-dione 21-pivalate [2002-29-1] $C_{27}H_{36}F_2O_6$ (494.57).

Preparation—The method described for *Betamethasone* (page 902) may be modified appropriately to cause the 16-methyl group to enter in α-configuration and to include one of several known methods for introducing the 6α-fluorine. The resulting flumethasone may be converted to the 21-pivalate by treatment with trimethylacetic anhydride in the presence of pyridine.

Description—White to off-white, crystalline powder.
Solubility—Practically insoluble in water; soluble 1 g in 90 mL of alcohol, 350 mL of chloroform, or 2800 mL of ether.

Uses—A glucocorticoid with about 800 times the potency of cortisone acetate. It is used only topically, for the treatment of glucocorticoid-responsive *dermatological disorders* (see the introduction in this section). When applied under occlusive dressings, it is especially used in the treatment of *nummular dermatitis*, *psoriasis* and *chronic neurodermatitis*. Since it contains fluorine substituents, metabolism in the skin is slow; nevertheless, systemic elimination is fast enough that systemic side effects are weak.

Dose—*Topical*, as **0.03%** cream applied as a film 3 or 4 times a day or under an occlusive dressing in *adults*, but only once a day in *children*.

Dosage Form—Cream: 0.03%.

Fluocinolone Acetonide

Pregna-1,4-diene-3,20-dione, 6,9-difluoro-11,21-dihydroxy-16,17-[(1-methylethylidene)bis(oxy)]-, (6α,11β,16α)-, Fluonid (*Herbert*); Synalar (*Syntex*)

6α,9-Difluoro-11β,16α,17,21-tetrahydroxypregna-1,4-diene-3,20-dione, cyclic 16,17-acetal with acetone [67-73-2] $C_{24}H_{30}F_2O_6$ (452.49).

Preparation—From the 21-acetate of 16α,17α-epoxy-3β,21-dihydroxypregn-5-en-20-one (available by synthesis from naturally occurring sapogenins such as diosgenin). Treatment of this pregnene with HF and N-bromoacetamide, followed by chromic acid oxidation and then treatment with HBr in acetic acid gives the Δ4-16β-bromo-6α-fluoro derivative. This latter compound on refluxing with potassium acetate in acetic acid and then saponifying with sodium carbonate yields the 6α-fluoro-16α,17α-dihydroxy compound which when incubated with minced, defatted bovine adrenals adds an 11β-hydroxyl group. From the 16,21-diacetate, with dimethylformamide and methanesulfonyl chloride, the 4,9-diene is synthesized, which is converted to the 9β,11β-epoxide and then to the 9α-fluoro-11β-hydroxy compound in a manner similar to that for *Betamethasone* (page 962). Oxidation of this product with selenium dioxide yields the 1,4-diene (fluocinolone) which on reaction with acetone and perchloric acid yields the acetonide.

Description—White, crystalline powder that is odorless; stable in light; melts at about 270°, with decomposition.
Solubility—1 g in >1000 mL water, 45 mL alcohol, 25 mL chloroform, 350 mL ether.

Uses—A glucocorticoid with potent anti-inflammatory and metabolic actions and negligible mineralocorticoid actions (see page 958). It is employed topically in the treatment of various *dermatoses*. In resistant nummular dermatitis, psoriasis, or chronic neurodermatitis it is usually used under occlusive dressings. Even in instances in which nearly the whole body has been covered by a cream containing

the corticoid, evidences of systemic side effects are rare. However, folliculitis or striae is a frequent complication, especially if occlusive dressings are used. Topical fluocinolone is contraindicated in the presence of tuberculosis, fungal infections, and most viral lesions of the skin (vaccinia, varicella, herpes simplex, etc.). Neomycin is often included in topical preparations of fluocinolone acetonide to suppress infections secondary to the inflammatory process or which result from the use of the glucocorticoid.

Dose—Topical, to the *skin*, *adult*, as **0.01** to **0.2%** cream, **0.025%** ointment, or **0.01%** solution, applied 2 to 4 times a day or under an occlusive dressing; *children*, as **0.01%** cream or solution once or twice a day or as **0.025** to **0.2%** cream or **0.025%** ointment once a day.

Dosage Forms—Cream: 0.01, 0.025, and 0.2%; Ointment: 0.025%; Topical Solution: 0.01%.

Fluocinonide

Pregna-1,4-diene-3,20-dione, 21-(acetyloxy)-6,9-difluoro-11-hydroxy-16,17-[(1-methylethylidene)bis(oxy)]-, (6α,11β,16α)-, Fluocinolide; Lidex, Topsyn (*Syntex*)

6α,9-Difluoro-11β,16α,17,21-tetrahydroxypregna-1,4-diene-3,20-dione, cyclic 16,17-acetal with acetone, 21-acetate [356-12-7] $C_{26}H_{32}F_2O_7$ (494.53).

Preparation—*Fluocinolone Acetonide* (this page) is esterified with acetic anhydride in the presence of pyridine. US Pats 3,126,375 and 3,592,930.

Description—White to creamy white, odorless, crystalline powder; stable in light, air, and at room temperature; melts, within a range of 3°, at about 300°, with decomposition.
Solubility—Insoluble in water; soluble 1 g in 70 mL of alcohol, 10 mL of acetone, or 10 mL of chloroform.

Uses—A glucocorticoid used only topically for its anti-inflammatory effects in glucocorticoid-responsive *dermatoses* (see introduction in this section). Systemic side effects are infrequent, but the local side effects are those of other glucocorticoids.

Dose—*Topical*, as 0.05% cream, gel, or ointment, applied 3 or 4 times a day for *adults* or once a day for *children*.

Dosage Forms—Cream: 0.05%; Gel: 0.05%; Ointment: 0.05%.

Fluorometholone

Pregna-1,4-diene-3,20-dione, 9-fluoro-11,17-dihydroxy-6-methyl-, (6α,11β)-, Oxylone (*Upjohn*)

9-Fluoro-11β,17-dihydroxy-6α-methylpregna-1,4-diene-3,20-dione [426-13-1] $C_{22}H_{29}FO_4$ (376.47).

Preparation—6α-Methyl-9α-fluoroprednisolone is esterified with p-toluenesulfonyl chloride to give the 21-p-toluenesulfonate. This is treated with sodium iodide in acetone solution to form the corresponding 21-iodo compound which is then reduced with sodium bisulfite to fluorometholone. US Pats 2,852,511 and 2,867,637.

Description—White to yellowish-white, odorless, crystalline powder; melts at about 280°, with decomposition.
Solubility—1 g in >10,000 mL water, 200 mL alcohol, 2200 mL chloroform, >10,000 mL ether.

Uses—A glucocorticoid with typical actions and side effects (see introduction in this section). By the oral route it is equipotent to cortisol, but by topical administration it is 40 times as potent. Consequently, it is used for topical treatment of glucocorticoid-responsive *dermatoses* and *ocular inflammations*. Under occlusive dressings it is particularly used to treat resistant nummular dermatitis, psoriasis, and chronic neurodermatitis.

Dose—*Topical*, to the *skin*, as **0.025%** cream, 1 to 3 times a day for *adults* and once a day for *children;* to the *conjunctiva*, *adults* and *children*, **1 drop** of **0.1%** ophthalmic suspension 2 to 4 times a day.

Dosage Forms—Cream: 0.025%; Ophthalmic Suspension: 0.1%.

Flurandrenolide

Pregn-4-ene-3,20-dione, 6-fluoro-11,21-dihydroxy-16,17-[(1-methylethylidene)bis(oxy)]-, (6α,11β,16α-)-, Flurandrenolone Acetonide; Cordran (*Lilly*)

6α-Fluoro-11β,16α,17,21-tetrahydroxypregn-4-ene-3,20-dione, cyclic 16,17-acetal with acetone [1524-88-5] $C_{24}H_{33}FO_6$ (436.52).

Preparation—Flurandrenolone (6α-fluoro-16α-hydroxycortisol) is condensed with acetone by treating its solution in acetone with 70% perchloric acid. US Pat 3,126,375.

Description—White to off-white, fluffy, odorless, crystalline powder.

Solubility—1 g in 72 mL alcohol, 10 mL chloroform; practically insoluble in water, ether.

Uses—A glucocorticoid that has high potency topically but low potency systemically because of rapid destruction in the liver. Consequently, its use is limited to management of *glucocorticoid-responsive dermatologic disorders*. Under occlusive dressings it is used especially to treat nummular dermatitis, psoriasis, and chronic neurodermatitis. Local side effects are uncommon but are typical of drugs of this class (see the introduction in this section). Neomycin is included in some topical preparations of flurandrenolide to suppress infections secondary to the inflammatory process or to the use of the glucocorticoid.

Dose—*Topical*, to the *skin*, *adult*, as **0.025** or **0.05%** cream or ointment or **0.05%** lotion 2 or 3 times a day or as a tape (plaster) containing **4 μg/cm²** 1 or 2 times a day. *Children*, as **0.025%** cream or ointment 1 or 2 times a day or as **0.05%** cream, lotion, or ointment, or as tape containing **4 μg/cm²** once a day.

Dosage Forms—Cream: 0.025 and 0.05%; Lotion: 0.05%; Ointment: 0.025 and 0.05%; Tape: 4 μg/cm².

Hydrocortisone

Pregn-4-ene-3,20-dione, 11,17,21-trihydroxy-, (11β)-, Compound F; Reichstein's "Substance M"; Cortef (*Upjohn*); Cortril (*Pfizer*); Hydrocortone (*MSD*); *Various Mfrs*

Cortisol [50-23-7] $C_{21}H_{30}O_5$ (362.46).

Preparation—The most attractive commercial synthesis involves the oxidation of 17α,21-dihydroxypregn-4-ene-3,20-dione, which is readily obtainable from diosgenin. Microbiological hydroxylation at the 11β-position is affected on the diacetate of the above compound employing organisms of the *Rhizopus*, *Aspergillus* or *Streptomyces* species. Saponification then yields hydrocortisone.

Description—White to practically white, odorless, crystalline powder; melts at about 215°, with decomposition.

Solubility—1 g in 40 mL alcohol; very slightly soluble in water and ether; slightly soluble in chloroform.

Uses—The principal natural glucocorticoid in man and thus the prototype of all glucocorticoids (for actions, uses, and side effects of

glucocorticoids, see the general statement in this section). Systemic side effects can result from topical application. Allergic bronchospasm after hydrocortisone in asthmatics has been reported. The plasma half-life is 1½ to 3 hr.

Some topical preparations include neomycin and/or other antibiotics to suppress emergence of infections.

Dose—*Adult*, *oral*, for *replacement*, 25 to 50 mg/day, ⅔ of which is to be taken in the morning and ⅓ in the afternoon; for *anti-inflammatory* use, **20 to 240 mg** a day in 3 or 4 divided doses. *Topical*, to the *skin*, as **0.125 to 2.5%** cream, **0.25 to 1%** gel, or **0.25 to 2.5%** lotion 3 or 4 times a day; to the *scalp*, as **0.5%** aerosol spray once a day initially and later decreased to 1 to 3 times a week; to the *eye*, as **0.2%** ophthalmic solution, as **1%** ophthalmic suspension containing antibiotics, or **0.5 to 1.5%** ointment containing antibiotics every hour during the day and every 2 hours at night; in the *ear* as **1%** otic ointment, solution, or suspension containing antibiotics; *rectal*, as **10-mg** suppository once a day; *enema*, **100 mg** once a day; *intravaginal*, **10 mg;** *intrasynovial* or *intralesional*, **10 to 50 mg;** to *oral mucosa*, as a **0.5%** paste 2 or 3 times a day after meals and at bedtime. *Children*, *oral*, for *replacement*, **0.56 mg per kg** of body weight (or **16 mg per m²** of body surface); for *anti-inflammatory* use, **2 to 8 mg** per kg of body weight (or **60 to 240 mg per m²** of body surface); *topical*, to the *skin*, as **0.125 to 1%** cream or lotion or **0.25 to 1%** gel or ointment 1 or 2 times a day or **2.5%** cream or ointment once a day; to the *scalp*, adult dose.

Dosage Forms—Cream: 0.5, 1, and 2.5%; Dental paste: 0.5%; Enema: 100 mg/60 mL; Gel: 0.25 and 1%; Lotion: 0.25, 0.5, and 1%; Ointment: 0.5, 1, and 2.5%; Ophthalmic Solution: 0.2%; Sterile Suspension: 50 mg/mL; Tablets: 5, 10, and 20 mg; Topical Aerosol: 0.5%.

Hydrocortisone Acetate

Pregn-4-ene-3,20-dione, 21-(acetyloxy)-11,17-dihydroxy-, (11β)-; Hydrocortisone 21-Acetate; Cortef Acetate (*Upjohn*); Cortril Acetate (*Pfizer*); Hydrocortone Acetate (*MSD*)

Cortisol 21-acetate [50-03-3] $C_{23}H_{32}O_6$ (404.50).

Preparation—Hydrocortisone is esterified with acetic anhydride to give the 21-acetate.

Description—White to practically white, odorless, crystalline powder; melts at about 220°, with decomposition.

Solubility—Insoluble in water; 1 g in 230 mL alcohol, 200 mL chloroform.

Uses—Has the actions of *Hydrocortisone*, to which it is converted in the body. However, it is not used for systemic therapy. It is used topically in the treatment of glucocorticoid-sensitive dermatoses, anorectal inflammations, inflammatory conditions of the eye, and intra-articularly in the treatment of arthritides. Systemic effects can result from local application.

The inclusion of neomycin or antifungal drugs in lotions and creams containing hydrocortisone acetate is for the purpose of protecting against bacterial or fungal infections that might be favored by the suppression of the inflammatory response and of clearing up infections secondary to the inflammatory condition.

Dose—*Intra-articular*, *intralesional*, or *soft-tissue injection*, *adult*, **5 to 75 mg** repeated at 1- to 3-week intervals, if necessary. *Topical, to the skin*, *adult*, as **0.5 to 1%** cream or **0.5 to 5%** lotion 3 or 4 times a day or 1 to 2.5% ointment 1 to 4 times a day; *children*, as **0.5 to 1%** cream or lotion or **1%** ointment 1 or 2 times a day or as a **2.5 to 5%** lotion or **2.5%** ointment once a day. *Topical*, to the *eye*, *adults* and *children*, a thin strip of **0.5 to 1.5%** ointment or **1 or 2 drops** of a **0.2%** solution or **2.5%** suspension every hour during the day and every 2 hours at night for the solution and 3 or 4 times a day for the other forms; *rectal*, *adult* as **1.0%** aerosol foam 1 to 3 times a day for 3 weeks, after which dosage is diminished every other day, or as suppository **15 to 25 mg** twice a day for 2 weeks, except 3 times a day or **30 to 50 mg** twice a day in severe proctitis.

Dosage Forms—Aerosol Foam: 1%; Cream: 0.5% or 0.5% of hydrocortisone equivalent, except 1% in certain combinations; Lotion: 0.5% of hydrocortisone equivalent; Ointment: 1 and 2.5%; Ophthalmic Ointment: 0.5 and 1.5%; Ophthalmic Suspension: 2.5%; Sterile Suspension: 25 and 50 mg/mL; Suppositories: 15 and 25 mg, except 10 mg in some combinations.

Hydrocortisone Cypionate

Pregn-4-ene-3,20-dione, 21-(3-cyclopentyl-1-oxopropoxy)-11,17-dihydroxy-, (11β)-, Cortisol Cypionate; Cortef Fluid (*Upjohn*)

Cortisol 21-cyclopentanepropionate [508-99-6] $C_{29}H_{42}O_6$ (486.65).

Preparation—*Hydrocortisone* is esterified by treatment with cyclopentanepropionyl chloride in the presence of pyridine.

Description—White to practically white, crystalline powder; odorless or has a slight odor.

Solubility—Insoluble in water; slightly soluble in ether; soluble in alcohol; very soluble in chloroform.

Uses—Actions and systemic uses are those of *Hydrocortisone*, to which it is converted in the body. Because of its low solubility, its absorption from the gastrointestinal tract is slower than that of hydrocortisone; also, its taste is more pleasant than that of hydrocortisone, so that it is used for oral therapy.

Dose—*Oral, adult*, the equivalent of **20** to **240 mg** of hydrocortisone daily, as a single dose or in divided doses; *children*, for *replacement*, the equivalent of **0.56 mg per kg** of body weight (or **16 mg per m²** of body surface) of hydrocortisone a day, or, for *anti-inflammatory* use, the equivalent of **2** to **8 mg per kg** of body weight (or **60** to **240 mg per m²** of body surface) a day.

Dosage Form—Oral Suspension: the equivalent of 10 mg of hydrocortisone/5 mL.

Hydrocortisone Sodium Phosphate

Pregn-4-ene-3,20-dione, 11,17-dihydroxy-21-(phosphonooxy)-, disodium salt, (11β)-, Cortisol Sodium Phosphate; Hydrocortone Phosphate (*MSD*); Corphos (*Cooper*)

Cortisol 21-(disodium phosphate) [6000-74-4] $C_{21}H_{29}Na_2O_8P$ (486.41).

For the structure of the base, see *Hydrocortisone*.

Preparation—From hydrocortisone by a method similar to that used for *Dexamethasone Sodium Phosphate*. US Pat 2,870,177.

Description—White to light-yellow, odorless or practically odorless, bitter-tasting powder; relatively stable in light and heat and very hygroscopic; pH (1% solution) 7.5 to 8.5.

Solubility—1 g in about 1.5 mL water; slightly soluble in alcohol; practically insoluble in chloroform, dioxane, and ether.

Uses—Has the same actions and uses as *Hydrocortisone*, to which it is converted in the body. However, the phosphate is quite soluble and hence has special usefulness as a parenteral form of cortisol in emergency situations in which a rapid response is essential or when oral medication cannot be tolerated.

Dose—The doses below are stated in terms of the hydrocortisone equivalents. *Intramuscular, intravenous*, or *subcutaneous, adult*, 15 to 240 mg a day until the condition responds, after which the dosage is gradually decreased; in *acute adrenal insufficiency*, **100 mg** is given *intravenously* followed by **100 mg** every 8 hr until the patient is out of danger. *Children, intramuscular*, for *replacement*, **560 µg/kg** or **16 mg/m²** of body surface a day in 3 divided doses every third day *or* **186** to **280 µg/kg** or **5.33** to **8 mg/m²** once a day; for *disease*, **660 µg** to **4 mg/kg** or **20** to **120 mg/m²** every 12 to 24 hr; *intravenous*, for *acute adrenal insufficiency, infants*, **1** to **2 mg/kg** followed by **25** to **150 g/kg/day** and *older children*, **1** to **2 mg/kg** followed by **150** to **250 µg/kg/day** in divided doses.

Dosage Form—Injection: the equivalent of 50 mg of hydrocortisone/mL.

Hydrocortisone Sodium Succinate

Pregn-4-ene-3,20-dione, 21-(3-carboxy-1-oxopropoxy)-11,17-dihydroxy-, monosodium salt, (11β)-, A-hydroCort (*Abbott*); Solu-Cortef (*Upjohn*)

Cortisol 21-(sodium succinate) [125-04-2] $C_{25}H_{33}NaO_8$ (484.52).

Preparation—Hydroxycortisone 21-(hydrogen succinate) is first prepared by reacting hydrocortisone with succinic anhydride dissolved in pyridine. When the reaction is complete, the mixture is added to cold, dilute HCl whereupon the acid ester precipitates. It is collected, washed with water, dried, and purified by recrystallizing from acetone. The sodium salt is then prepared by neutralizing the acid with dilute NaOH solution followed by drying the solution from the frozen state.

Description—White or nearly white, odorless, hygroscopic, amorphous solid.

Solubility—Very soluble in water and alcohol; insoluble in chloroform; very slightly soluble in acetone.

Uses—The actions and uses are the same as those of *Hydrocortisone*, into which it is converted in the body. However the sodium succinate derivative is highly soluble and hence is a desirable form for infusion concentrates and for intravenous or intramuscular administration when intense rapid action is desired. It is intended only for systemic short-term emergency therapy.

Dose—The same as that of *Hydrocortisone Sodium Phosphate*, above.

Dosage Forms—For Injection: the equivalent of 100, 250, and 500 mg and 1 g of hydrocortisone.

Methylprednisolone

Pregna-1,4-diene-3,20-dione, 11,17,21-trihydroxy-6-methyl-, (6α,11β)-, Medrol (*Upjohn*)

11β,17,21-Trihydroxy-6α-methylpregna-1,4-diene-3,20-dione [83-43-2] $C_{22}H_{30}O_5$ (374.48).

Preparation—*Progesterone* (page 993) is converted to the 6α-methyl derivative in the same manner as indicated in the synthesis of *Medroxyprogesterone Acetate* (page 992). Incubation of the 6α-methyl compound with an Ascomycete, such as *Pestalotia*, forms the 11α-hydroxy derivative which is oxidized to the 3,11-diketo compound with chromic acid. Further treatment with ethyl oxalate followed by bromination, rearrangement with sodium methoxide and debromination with zinc dust gives the methyl ester of the 4,17(20)-diene-21-carboxylate. With pyrrolidine, lithium aluminum hydride reduction and treatment with alkali, the 11β,21-dihydroxy-4,17(20)-diene is formed which is converted to the 21-acetate and then oxidatively hydroxylated to 6α-methylhydrocortisone acetate. Saponification, followed by dehydrogenation with *Septomyxa affinis* gives the 1,4,17(20)-triene, which is again converted to the 21-acetate, oxidatively hydroxylated to yield the 17α-hydroxy derivative and saponified to give methylprednisolone.

Description—White to practically white, odorless, crystalline powder; melts at about 240° with some decomposition.

Solubility—1 g in 10,000 mL water, 100 mL alcohol, 800 mL chloroform, 800 mL ether.

Uses—A glucocorticoid with actions, uses, and side effects typical of drugs of this class (see introduction in this section). It induces considerably less retention of sodium and water than the parent prednisolone. Because methylprednisolone possesses only weak mineralocorticoid activity, it is not employed in the management of acute adrenal insufficiency. The plasma half-life is 3 to 4 hours.

Dose—*Oral, adult*, 4 to 48 mg a day; *children*, for *replacement*, **117 µg** to **1.7 mg per kg** of body weight (or **3.3** to **50 mg per m²** of body surface) a day; for *disease*, **417 µg** to **1.67 mg/kg** (or **1.25** to **50 mg/m²** of body surface) a day in 3 divided doses.

Dosage Forms—Tablets: 2, 4, 8, 16, 24, and 32 mg.

Methylprednisolone Acetate

Pregna-1,4-diene-3,20-dione, 21-(acetyloxy)-11,17-dihydroxy-6-methyl-, (6α,11β)-, Methylprednisolone 21-Acetate; Depo-Medrol and Medrol Acetate; (*Upjohn*)

$11\beta,17,21$-Trihydroxy-6α-methylpregna-1,4-diene-3,20-dione 21-acetate [53-36-1] $C_{24}H_{32}O_6$ (416.51).

For the structure of the base, see *Methylprednisolone*.

Preparation—The 21-acetate compound obtained in the synthesis of *Methylprednisolone*, just prior to the final saponification.

Description—White or practically white, odorless, crystalline powder; melts at about 225° with some decomposition.

Solubility—1 g in 1500 mL water, 400 mL alcohol, 250 mL chloroform, 1500 mL ether.

Uses—Converted in the body to *Methylprednisolone*, over which it has no advantage in systemic therapy; thus the acetate is employed principally for local therapy. As a suspension it may be given intra-articularly or topically. Topical uses and adverse effects are discussed in the introduction in this section. Methylprednisolone acetate is combined with neomycin in some topical preparations.

Dose—*Intramuscular, adult, initially* 4 to 120 mg repeated at one-day to two-week intervals, if necessary; *children, for replacement,* 117 μg/kg (or 3.33 mg/m^2 of body surface) in 3 divided doses in one day, repeated every third day, *or* 39 to 58 μg/kg (or 1.11 to 1.66 mg/m^2) once a day; for *disease,* 139 to 835 μg/kg (or 4.16 to 25 mg/m^2 every 12 to 24 hr. *Intra-articular, intralesional* or into *soft tissue,* 4 to 80 mg. *Topical,* as 0.25% or 1% cream, applied 1 to 4 times a day on *adults* and 1 or 2 times a day on *children. Rectal, adult,* 40 mg as retention enema 3 to 7 times a week for 2 or more weeks; *children,* 500 μg to 1 mg/kg (or 15 to 30 mg/m^2) every 1 or 2 days for 2 or more weeks. *Topical,* to the *conjunctiva, as* 0.1% ophthalmic ointment 1 to 3 times a day.

Dosage Forms—Cream: 0.25 and 1%; for Enema: 40 mg; Ophthalmic Ointment: 0.1%; Sterile Suspension: 40 and 80 mg/1 mL, 100, 200 and 400 mg/5 mL, and 400 mg/10 mL.

Methylprednisolone Sodium Succinate

Pregna-1,4-diene-3,20-dione, 21-(3-carboxy-1-oxopropoxy)-11,17-dihydroxy-6-methyl-, monosodium salt, ($6\alpha,11\beta$)-, Methylprednisolone 21-(Sodium Succinate); Solu-Medrol (*Upjohn*); A-Methapred (*Abbott*)

$11\beta,17,21$-Trihydroxy-6α-methylpregna-1,4-diene-3,20-dione 21-(sodium succinate) [2375-03-3] $C_{26}H_{33}NaO_8$ (496.53).

For the structure of the base, see *Methylprednisolone*.

Preparation—*Methylprednisolone* is treated with succinic anhydride in pyridine and added to dilute HCl to precipitate the hemisuccinate which is neutralized with NaOH in aqueous acetone solution and the solvent removed by lyophilization.

Description—White, or nearly white, odorless, hygroscopic, amorphous solid.

Solubility—1 g in 1.5 mL water, 12 mL alcohol, >10,000 mL chloroform, >10,000 mL ether.

Uses—The actions are the same as those of *Methylprednisolone*, into which it is converted in the body; for actions, uses, and adverse effects of glucocorticoids see the introduction in this section. The solubility of methylprednisolone sodium succinate makes its use advantageous for parenteral and intra-articular administration when rapid and intense action is desired. It is used systemically only for short-term treatment.

Dose (as methylprednisolone equivalent)—*Intravenous* or *intramuscular, adult,* 10 to 40 mg as needed, except 5 mg per kg of body weight as a *bolus* every 4 hr in *shock. Intramuscular, children,* for *replacement* and *disease* therapy, see *Methylprednisolone Acetate. Intra-articular* or *intralesional,* 4 to 80 mg, as needed.

Dosage Forms—For Injection: 40, 125, 500 mg, and 1 g (as methylprednisolone).

Paramethasone Acetate

Pregna-1,4-diene-3,20-dione, 21-(acetyloxy)-6-fluoro-11,17-dihydroxy-16-methyl-, ($6\alpha,11\beta,16\alpha$)-, Haldrone (*Lilly*); Monocortone (*Syntex*)

6α-Fluoro-$11\beta,17,21$-trihydroxy-16α-methylpregna-1,4-diene-3,20-dione 21-acetate [1597-82-6] $C_{24}H_{31}FO_6$ (434.50).

Preparation—3-Hydroxy-16α-methylpregn-5-en-20-one acetate (16α-methylpregnenolone acetate) is subjected to a series of standard reactions to form 6α-fluoro-17,21-dihydroxy-16α-methylpregn-4-ene-3,20-dione, then hydroxylated at the 11β-position by incubation with bovine adrenal glands and converted to the 21-acetate. Dehydrogenation with selenium dioxide in the presence of pyridine completes the synthesis with creation of the 1,2-double bond.

Description—Fluffy, practically white, odorless, crystalline powder; exposure to light should be avoided. It melts at about 240° with decomposition.

Solubility—Very soluble in alcohol; soluble in acetone, chloroform, ether, and methanol; insoluble in water.

Uses—A glucocorticoid with actions, uses, and side effects typical of drugs of this class (see introduction in this section), except that it is almost devoid of mineralocorticoid side effects, although there may be occasional edema and rare hypertension. It is 10 times as potent as cortisone, but potency does not confer any particular advantages. Increased appetite and weight gain occur in only about $\frac{1}{3}$ of patients. The catabolic effects, such as protein depletion and osteoporosis, are only moderate with low to moderate doses of the drug.

Dose—*Oral, adult, initially* 2 to 8 mg a day in mild disorders, 8 to 12 mg a day in moderately severe disorders, and 20 to 40 mg a day in life-threatening illness, the dose being gradually reduced once the condition improves. *Children,* 58 to 800 μg per kg of body weight (or 1.67 to 25 mg per m^2 of body surface) a day.

Dosage Forms—Tablets: 1 and 2 mg.

Prednisolone

Pregna-1,4-diene-3,20-dione, 11,17,21-trihydroxy-, (11β)-, (*Various Mfrs*)

$11\beta,17,21$-Trihydroxypregna-1,4-diene-3,20-dione [50-24-8] $C_{21}H_{28}O_5$ (360.45); *sesquihydrate* [52438-85-4] (387.47); anhydrous or contains one and one-half molecules of water of hydration.

Preparation—From hydrocortisone by a microbiologic process utilizing *Corynebacterium simplex* which selectively dehydrogenates cortisol at the 1 and 2 positions.

Description—White to practically white, odorless, crystalline powder; melts at about 235°, with some decomposition.

Solubility—1 g in 30 mL alcohol, 180 mL chloroform; very slightly soluble in water.

Uses—A glucocorticoid with the actions, uses, and side effects typical of drugs of this class (see the introduction in this section). It is 4 times as potent as hydrocortisone but relatively somewhat weaker than hydrocortisone as a mineralocorticoid although sodium retention and potassium depletion can occur. The plasma half-life is about 3 hr. Except for its higher solubility, it may be considered equivalent to prednisone; it is the biologically active metabolite of prednisone.

Dose—*Oral, adult, initially* usually 5 to 60 mg but may be as high as 250 mg a day until a response occurs, when the dose is gradually diminished to the smallest effective maintenance dose; *children,* for *replacement,* 140 μg/kg (or 4 mg/m^2 of body surface) a day in 3 divided doses, or, for *disease,* 500 μg to 2 mg/kg (or 15 to 60 mg/m^2) a day in 3 divided doses. *Topical,* to the *skin,* as a 0.5% cream 3 or 4 times a day for adults and 1 or 2 times a day for children.

Dosage Forms—Cream: 0.5%; Tablets: 1 and 5 mg.

Prednisolone Acetate

Pregna-1,4-diene-3,20-dione, 21-(acetyloxy)-11,17-dihydroxy-, (11β)-, Prednisolone 21-Acetate; Meticortelone (*Schering*); Sterane (*Pfizer*); *Various Mfrs*

$11\beta,17,21$-Trihydroxypregna-1,4-diene-3,20-dione 21-acetate [52-21-1] $C_{23}H_{30}O_6$ (402.49).

Preparation—From *Prednisolone* by reaction with acetic anhydride.

Description—White to practically white, odorless, crystalline powder; melts at about 235° with some decomposition.

Solubility—1 g in 120 mL alcohol; practically insoluble in water; slightly soluble in chloroform and acetone.

Uses—The actions and uses are the same as those of *Prednisolone*, into which it is converted in the body. The acetate is relatively nonirritating to the tissues and hence is suitable for intramuscular or local injection; esterification also prolongs absorption. It may be used particularly in those situations in which oral prednisolone is not feasible, but there are no contraindications to substitution of the parenteral prednisolone acetate for oral prednisolone for any purpose.

Dose—*Intramuscular*, *adult*, *initially* **20** to **60 mg** a day in 4 divided doses until a satisfactory response occurs, then a gradual reduction to a minimal *maintenance* dose, which usually is in the range of 5 to **20 mg** a day; *children*, for *replacement*, **140 μg/kg** (or **4 mg/m²** of body surface) every third day, and, for *disease*, **166 μg** to **1 mg/kg** (or **5** to **30 mg/m²**) every 12 to 24 hr. *Intralesional*, or *soft-tissue injection*, 4 to **60 mg** every 1 to 4 weeks. *Topical*, to the *eyes*, as a **0.125** to 1% ophthalmic suspension or **0.5%** ointment; to the *skin*, as a **0.5%** ointment (containing 0.5% neomycin).

Dosage Forms—Ointment: 0.5% (with 0.5% neomycin); Ophthalmic Ointment: 0.25 and 0.5%; Ophthalmic Suspension: 0.125, 0.25, and 1%; Sterile Suspension: 25, 40, 50, 80, and 100 mg/mL.

Prednisolone Sodium Phosphate

Pregna-1,4-diene-3,20-dione, 11,17-dihydroxy-21-(phosphonooxy)-, disodium salt, (11β)-, Prednisolone 21-(Disodium Phosphate); Hydeltrasol (*MSD*)

11β,17,21-Trihydroxypregna-1,4-diene-3,20-dione 21-(disodium phosphate) [125-02-0] $C_{21}H_{27}Na_2O_8P$ (484.39).

Preparation—From *Prednisolone* by a method similar to that used for *Dexamethasone Sodium Phosphate*.

Description—White or slightly yellow, friable granules or powder; odorless or has a slight odor; slightly hygroscopic.

Solubility—1 g in 4 mL water and 13 mL methanol; slightly soluble in alcohol and chloroform; very slightly soluble in acetone and dioxane.

Uses—A soluble form of *Prednisolone*, into which it is converted in the body. It is employed parenterally in emergency situations in which an intense glucocorticoid action is required. Since absorption by the intramuscular route is quite rapid, the intravenous route is infrequently employed. The high solubility of the drug also lends itself well to intrasynovial injection in the treatment of arthritides and bursitides and to local injection for inflammatory cysts and soft-tissue inflammations. It is also employed in the local treatment of a number of inflammatory eye diseases and for inflammatory and pruritic dermatoses, bites, and burns.

Dose—Doses are stated in terms of the equivalents of *Prednisolone Phosphate*. *Intravenous* or *intramuscular*, *adult*, **40** to **60 mg** of the equivalent of prednisolone phosphate a day, except up to **2 g** a day intravenously in bacteremic shock. *Intramuscular*, *children*, for *replacement*, **140 μg/kg** (or **4 mg/m²** of body surface) in 1 day in 3 divided doses every third day, *or*, **46** to **70 μg/kg** (or **1.33** to **2 mg/m²**) per day; for *disease*, **166 μg** to **1 mg** (or **5** to **30 mg/m²**) every 12 to 24 hr. *Intra-articular*, *intralesional*, or *soft-tissue injection*, **2** to **30 mg** every 3 to 5 days to 2 to 3 weeks. *Topical*, to the *conjunctiva*, a thin strip of **0.25%** ointment of prednisolone phosphate equivalent 3 or 4 times a day or 1 drop of **0.113%** to **0.9%** ophthalmic solution, with or without antibacterial drugs, 4 to 6 times a day.

Dosage Forms (as equivalent of prednisolone phosphate)—Injection: 20 mg/mL; Ophthalmic Ointment: 0.25%; Ophthalmic Solution: 0.125, 0.5, and 1%; Ophthalmic/Otic Solution: 0.5%.

Prednisolone Tebutate

Pregna-1,4-diene-3,20-dione, 11,17-dihydroxy-21-[(3,3-dimethyl-1-oxobutyl)oxy]-, (11β)-, Prednisolone *tert*-butylacetate; Hydeltra T.B.A. (*MSD*) Prednalone T.B.A. (*O'Neal, Jones & Feldman*)

11β,17,21-Trihydroxypregna-1,4-diene-3,20-dione 21-(3,3-dimethylbutyrate) [7681-14-3] $C_{27}H_{38}O_6$ (458.59); *monohydrate* (476.61).

Preparation—From *Prednisolone* by esterification of the 21-hydroxyl group with 3,3-dimethylbutyryl chloride.

Description—White to slightly yellow powder; odorless or has not more than a moderate, characteristic odor; melts between 240° and 250°.

Solubility—Very slightly soluble in water; freely soluble in chloroform; soluble in acetone; sparingly soluble in alcohol.

Uses—Converted in the body to *Prednisolone*. At present, its use is confined to local injection into inflamed joints, tendons, and bursae or into soft-tissue lesions. Its low solubility results in a repository action, with an onset of action of 1 to 2 days and a duration of 2 to 3 weeks. Temporary local discomfort may follow injection.

Dose—*Intra-articular*, *intrasynovial*, *intralesional*, or *soft-tissue injection*, 4 to **40 mg** once every 2 or 3 weeks.

Dosage Form—Sterile Suspension: 20 mg/mL.

Prednisone

Pregna-1,4-diene-3,11,20-trione, 17,21-dihydroxy-, (*Various Mfrs*)

17,21-Dihydroxypregna-1,4-diene-3,11,20-trione [53-03-2] $C_{21}H_{26}O_5$ (358.43).

Preparation—As described for *Prednisolone* except that cortisone is used instead of hydrocortisone.

Description—White to practically white, odorless, crystalline powder; melts at about 230°, with some decomposition.

Solubility—1 g in 150 mL alcohol, 200 mL chloroform; very slightly soluble in water.

Uses—A dehydrogenated derivative of cortisone with actions, uses, and side effects typical of glucocorticoids (see introduction in this section). It has 3 to 5 times the glucocorticoid activity of hydrocortisone but somewhat less of mineralocorticoid activity, although sodium retention and potassium depletion may occur. It cannot be used alone for replacement therapy in adrenal insufficiency. Prednisone is the glucocorticoid predominantly used in *cancer chemotherapy*, always in combination with other drugs. It is also the glucocorticoid most used in the treatment of acute exacerbations of *multiple sclerosis*. In pediatrics it is widely used to treat *nephrosis*, *rheumatic carditis*, *leukemias*, *other tumors*, and *tuberculosis*.

The plasma half-life is 3 to 5 hr, but the effects last 12 to 36 hr.

Dose—*Oral*, *adult*, *initially* usually **5** to **60 mg** but may be as high as **250 mg** a day until a satisfactory response occurs, when the dose is gradually diminished to the smallest effective *maintenance* dose, usually **10** to **20 mg** a day; for acute exacerbations of *multiple sclerosis*, **200 mg/day** for 1 week, then **80 mg** every other day for 1 month. *Children*, **35** to **500 μg** per **kg** of body weight (or **1** to **15 mg per m²** of body surface), 4 times a day. However, dose regimens vary greatly with the use; for the details, see the USP DI, the AMA Drug Evaluations, the Physicians Desk Reference, or the package literature.

Dosage Forms—Syrup: 5 mg/5 mL; Tablets: 1, 2.5, 5, 10, 20, 25, and 50 mg.

Triamcinolone

Pregna-1,4-diene-3,20-dione, 9-fluoro-11,16,17,21-tetrahydroxy-, (11β,16α)-, Aristocort (*Lederle*); Kenacort (*Squibb*)

9-Fluoro-11β,16α,17,21-tetrahydroxypregna-1,4-diene-3,20-dione, [124-94-7] $C_{21}H_{27}FO_6$ (394.44).

Preparation—From hydrocortisone acetate via the 3,20-bisketal by treatment with thionyl chloride, refluxing with potassium hydroxide and acetylation to give 21-acetoxy-4,9,11(16)-pregnatriene-3,20-dione. Oxidation with osmium tetroxide to the 16α,17α-dihydroxy derivative and subsequent insertion of the 9α-fluoro and 11β-hydroxy groups as indicated for *Betamethasone* (page 962), gives a product lacking only a double bond at the 1-position. This latter step is accomplished by incubation with *Nocardia corallina*, followed by saponification of the acetate to yield triamcinolone. Alternatively, the compound can be made from *Fludrocortisone* by enzymatically inserting the 16α-hydroxyl group and dehydrogenating as above at the 1,2-position.

Description—Fine, white or practically white, crystalline powder having not more than a slight odor; its polymorphic forms and/or solvates melt between 248° and 250°, 260° 263°, 269° and 271°.

Solubility—1 g in about 5000 mL water, 70 mL propylene glycol, and less than 20 mL dimethyl sulfoxide; slightly soluble in alcohol and chloroform.

Uses—A glucocorticoid with actions, uses, and side effects typical of drugs of this class (see introduction in this section). As a glucocorticoid it is 7 to 13 times more potent than hydrocortisone. It has been claimed that therapeutic doses of triamcinolone are nearly devoid of mineralocorticoid and other side effects of hydrocortisone but the mineralocorticoid actions vary from patient to patient. It appears that the drug may induce naturesis, negative sodium balance with weight loss in most patients (along with headache, dizziness, and fatigue), and sodium retention with weight gain, moon face, etc. in others. Nearly every side effect seen with hydrocortisone has been observed with triamcinolone, but the relative frequencies are less; however, it does not increase appetite and thus differs from other glucocorticoids. By the oral route, more triamcinolone survives the first pass through the liver than does hydrocortisone, and blood levels are somewhat more predictable. The plasma half-life is about 5 hours.

Dose—*Oral, adult*, in *adrenal insufficiency*, 4 to 12 mg a day in single or divided doses (along with a mineralocorticoid); in *disease*, 4 to 48 mg a day. *Children*, in *adrenal insufficiency*, 117 μg per kg of body weight (or 3.3 mg per m² of body surface) a day; in *disease*, 416 μg to 1.7 mg per kg of body weight (or 12.5 to 50 mg per m² of body surface) a day.

Dosage Forms—Tablets: 1, 2, 4, 8, and 16 mg.

Triamcinolone Acetonide

Pregna-1,4-diene-3,20-dione, 9-fluoro-11,21-dihydroxy-16,17-[(1-methylethylidene)bis(oxy)]-, (11β,16α)-, Triamcinolone 16,17-Cyclic Acetal with Acetone; Aristocort Acetonide (*Lederle*); Aristoderm (*Lederle*); Kenalog (*Squibb*); (*Various Mfrs*)

9-Fluoro-11β,16α,17,21-tetrahydroxypregna-1,4-diene-3,20-dione cyclic 16,17-acetal with acetone [76-25-5] $C_{24}H_{31}FO_6$ (434.50).

Preparation—*Triamcinolone* is treated with acetone and perchloric acid followed by neutralization and vacuum concentration.

Description—White to cream-colored, crystalline powder having not more than a slight odor; melts between 290° and 294°.

Solubility—Practically insoluble in water; very soluble in dehydrated alcohol, chloroform, and methanol; sparingly soluble in acetone and ethyl acetate; slightly soluble in alcohol.

Uses—Triamcinolone acetonide is a high-potency glucocorticoid with the actions, uses, and side effects typical of that class of drugs (see introduction in this section). It has a higher lipid-water distribution coefficient than triamcinolone and is thus more suitable for topical use.

Dose—*Topical*, to the *skin, adult*, as 0.025, 0.1, or 0.5% cream or ointment, 0.1% aerosol foam or lotion, 0.1% gel, 0.025 or 0.1% lotion, or 0.015% aerosol solution, 2 to 4 times a day; *children*, as 0.025% cream, lotion, or ointment, or 0.015% aerosol solution 1 or 2 times a day, or 0.1 or 0.5% cream or ointment or 0.1% gel, lotion or aerosol lotion once a day. *Topical*, to the *oral mucous membranes*, as 0.1% paste 1 to 3 times a day (after meals or at bedtime). *Intramuscular*, 40 to 80 mg, repeated at 4-week intervals, in *adults* and 40 mg or 30

to 200 μg/kg (or 1 to 6.25 mg/m² of body surface), repeated at 7-day intervals, in *children*. *Intraarticular, intrabursal*, or into the *tendon sheath, adults* and *children*, 2.5 to 15 mg at weekly intervals or more frequently. *Intradermal* or *intralesional, adults*, up to 1 mg at intervals up to 1 week.

Dosage Forms—Cream: 0.025, 0.1, and 0.5%; Aerosol Foam: 0.1%; Gel: 0.1%; Aerosol Lotion: 0.1%; Lotion: 0.025 and 0.1%; Ointment: 0.025, 0.1, and 0.5%; Dental Paste: 0.1%; Aerosol Solution: 0.015%; Sterile Suspension: 10 and 40 mg/mL.

Triamcinolone Diacetate

Pregna-1,4-diene-3,20-dione, 16,21-bis(acetyloxy)-9-fluoro-11,17-dihydroxy-, (11β,16α)-, Triamcinolone 16,21-Diacetate; Aristocort Diacetate (*Lederle*); Kenacort (*Squibb*); Triamolone 40 (*O'Neal, Jones & Feldman*)

9-Fluoro-11β,16α,17,21-tetrahydroxypregna-1,4-diene-3,20-dione 16,21-diacetate [67-78-7] $C_{25}H_{31}FO_8$ (478.51).

For the structure of the base, see *Triamcinolone*.

Preparation—By direct acetylation of triamcinolone. Among other ways, it has also been prepared from 11β,16α,17,21-tetrahydroxypregn-4-en-3,20-dione (16α-hydroxycortisone) through the following sequence of reactions: (a) microbiological oxidation with *Nocardia corallina* or *Corynebacterium simplex* to the pregna-1,4-diene analogue, (b) acetylation yielding the 16α,21-diacetate, (c) selective dehydration involving the 11-hydroxy with thionyl chloride to form the 1,4,9(11)-pregnatriene compound, (d) addition of hypobromous acid to the 9,11-double bond followed by treatment with potassium acetate in ethanol to form the 9,11-epoxy compound, and (e) rupturing of the epoxy ring with hydrogen fluoride to introduce the 9α-fluorine.

Description—Fine, white or slightly off-white crystals that have not more than a slight odor and a slight, bitter taste. Prolonged heating above 100° will convert the hydrate to the anhydrous form.

Solubility—1 g in 13 mL alcohol, 80 mL chloroform; practically insoluble in water; slightly soluble in ether.

Uses—The actions and uses are identical with those of *Triamcinolone*. However, its slight solubility is such that on injection it has reasonably prompt onset of action yet a duration of action longer than that of more soluble preparations. It also has a more agreeable taste than triamcinolone and can thus be given in liquid oral preparations.

Dose (as triamcinolone equivalent)—*Oral, adult*, for *replacement*, 4 to 12 mg per day (along with a mineralocorticoid) and, for *anti-inflammatory* use, 8 to 48 mg a day. *Children*, for *replacement*, 117 μg per kg of body weight (or 3.3 mg per m² of body surface) a day (with a mineralocorticoid) and, for *anti-inflammatory* use, 416 μg to 1.7 mg per kg of body weight (or 12.5 to 50 mg per m² of body surface) a day. *Intra-articular, intrasynovial, intralesional* or into *soft tissue, adult*, 3 to 48 mg. *Intramuscular, adult* and *children* over 6 yrs of age, 40 mg once a week.

Dosage Forms—Sterile Suspension: 40 mg/1 mL and 125 and 200 mg/5 mL; Syrup: 2 and 5 mg/5 mL.

Triamcinolone Hexacetonide

Pregna-1,4-diene-3,20-dione, 21-(3,3-dimethyl-1-oxobutoxy)-9-fluoro-11-hydroxy-16,17-[(1-methylethylidene)bis(oxy)]-, (11β,16α)-, Aristospan (*Lederle*)

9-Fluoro-11β,16α,17,21-tetrahydroxypregna-1,4-diene-3,20-dione cyclic 16,17-acetal with acetone 21-(3,3-dimethylbutyrate) [5611-51-8] $C_{30}H_{41}FO_7$ (532.65). For the structure of the base, see *Triamcinolone*.

Preparation—*Triamcinolone Acetonide* is 21-esterified by reaction with 3,3-dimethylbutyryl chloride in the presence of pyridine.

Description—White to cream-colored, crystalline powder; odorless and tasteless to slightly bitter tasting; relatively stable to light, heat, and air; decomposes at about 295°; no polymorphs have been reported.

Solubility—1 g in 167 mL methanol and less than 20 mL chloroform; practically insoluble in water.

Uses—Gradually converted to *Triamcinolone* in the body and hence has the same potential actions, uses, and side effects. At present, it is used only for injection into inflamed joints and soft-tissue lesions. It is quite insoluble and hence has a repository action.

Dose—*Intra-articular* or *intrasynovial*, *adult*, **2** to **20 mg**, repeated at 3- or 4-week intervals, if necessary. *Intralesional* or *sublesional*, *adult*, up to **0.5 mg per in²** of diseased skin.

Dosage Forms—Sterile Suspension: 20 mg/1 mL and 25 and 100 mg/5 mL.

Other Adrenal Hormones

Amcinonide   [9-Fluoro-11β,16α,17,21-tetrahydroxypregna-1,4-diene-3,20-dione cyclic 16,17-acetal with cyclopentanone, 21-acetate [51022-69-6] $C_{28}H_{35}FO_7$ (502.58)]—A topical glucocorticoid that appears to have a slightly higher topical activity and bioavailability from topical formulations than triamcinolone acetonide and betamethasone valerate. *Dose: Topical*, to the *skin*, as 0.1% cream 2 or 3 times a day in adults and once a day in children.

Betamethasone Benzoate   [9-Fluoro-11β,17,21-trihydroxy-16β-methylpregna-1,4-diene-3,20-dione 17-benzoate [22298-29-9] $C_{29}H_{33}FO_6$ (496.57); Benisone (*Warner/Chilcott*); Flurobate (*Texas Pharmacal*); Uticort (*Parke-Davis*)]—A glucocorticoid with the actions of *Betamethasone* (page 962). It is used only topically for relief of inflammation in glucocorticoid-responsive dermatoses (see the general statement for topical uses and side effects). *Dose: Topical*, as 0.025% gel, cream, or lotion applied 2 to 4 times a day to adults but only once a day to children.

Betamethasone Dipropionate   [9-Fluoro-11β,17,21-trihydroxy-16β-methylpregna-1,4-diene-3,20-dione 17,21-dipropionate [5593-20-4] $C_{28}H_{37}FO_7$ (504.59); Diprosone (*Schering-Plough*)]—The actions of this glucocorticoid are those of Betamethasone (page 962), into which it is converted; its greater lipid-solubility makes it more suitable for topical therapy. It is used only to treat glucocorticoid-responsive dermatoses. For side effects of cutaneous use see the general statement in this section. *Dose: Topical*, to the *skin*, as 0.1% aerosol or 0.05% cream, lotion, or ointment (potency expressed as betamethasone) applied 3 times a day as the aerosol or 2 times a day as other dosage forms to adults but only once a day to children.

Clocortolone Pivalate   [9-Chloro-6α-fluoro-11β,21-dihydroxy-16α-methylpregna-1,4-diene-3,20-dione 21-pivalate [34097-16-0] $C_{27}H_{36}ClFO_5$ (495.03)]—Clocortolone pivalate is more than 10 times as potent as hydrocortisone when applied topically to the skin but has negligible systemic activity by this route. It has been used mainly in the treatment of eczema and atopic dermatitis but can probably be used to treat any glucocorticoid-responsive dermatosis or dermatitis. *Dose: Topical*, to the *skin*, *adults*, as 0.1% cream once or twice a day or by occlusive dressing.

Hydrocortisone Butyrate   [Cortisol 17-butyrate; Cortisol Butyrate [13609-67-1]; $C_{25}H_{36}O_6$ (432.56)]—As a topical anti-inflammatory drug, hydrocortisone 17-butyrate is about 10 times as potent as hydrocortisone valerate but it is considerably less potent in causing systemic effects, such as adrenal suppression. It also appears to cause less cutaneous atrophy than other steroids described above. *Dose: Topical*, to the *skin*, as 0.1% ointment.

Hydrocortisone Valerate   [11β,17,21-Trihydroxypregn-4-ene-3,20-dione 17-valerate [57524-89-7] $C_{26}H_{38}O_6$ (446.58); hydrocortisone 17-valerate; hydrocortisone valerate; Westcort (*Westwood*)]—Hydrocortisone valerate is used only for its topical anti-inflammatory properties. It is better absorbed than cortisol into the skin, from which site it is not transported as well into the blood. Consequently it has greater and longer-lasting local activity and lesser systemic activity and thus a greater therapeutic index than topical hydrocortisone. In the skin it is slowly converted to hydrocortisone; in the liver it is rapidly de-esterified and further metabolized. *Dose: Topical*, to the skin, as 0.2% cream 3 or 4 times a day to *adults* and once a day to *children*.

Desonide   [11β,16α,17,21-Tetrahydroxypregna-1,4-diene-3,20-dione, cyclic 16,17-acetal with acetone; 16-Hydroxyprednisolone 16,17-acetonide [638-94-8] $C_{24}H_{32}O_6$ (416.51); Tridesilon (*Miles*)]—A glucocorticoid of intermediate potency that is used only topically in the treatment of glucocorticoid-responsive skin diseases. It causes almost no systemic side effects; local side effects include burning sensations, itching, irritation, folliculitis, hypertrichosis, acneform eruptions, hypopigmentation, striae, cutaneous atrophy, miliaria, and skin infections. Maceration from occlusive film may occur. *Dose: Topical*, to *skin*, thin film of 0.05% cream or ointment 2 to 3 times a day to *adults* and once a day to *children*.

Desoximetasone   [9-Fluoro-11β,21-dihydroxy-16α-methylpregna-1,4-diene-3,20-dione [382-67-2] $C_{22}H_{29}FO_4$ (376.47); Topicort (*Hoechst-Roussel*)]—For syntheses see *CA 58*: 8388b, 1963; *Arzneimittel-Forschung 24*: 1, 1974. A white, crystalline powder; melts at about 217°. Insoluble in water; soluble in alcohol and chloroform; slightly soluble in water. A glucocorticoid of intermediate potency used only topically in the treatment of glucocorticoid-responsive dermatoses and dermatitides. As a 0.025% cream, it is approximately equieffective with 0.05% betamethasone dipropionate, 0.12% betamethasone valerate, and 0.1% triamcinolone. It

is fluorinated and lacks a 17-OH group, so that systemic effects such as adrenal suppression can occur, and it must be used cautiously in infants and children. For adverse effects see the general statement in this section. *Dose: Topical*, to the *skin*, as 0.05 or 0.25% cream twice a day in adults and once a day in children.

Dexamethasone Acetate   [Dexamethasone 21-acetate [1177-87-3] $C_{24}H_{31}FO_6$ (434.50); Decadron L.A. Suspension (*MSD*)]—The actions, uses, and side effects are those of dexamethasone (page 965). It is employed only as a repository form of dexamethasone, for systemic or intralesional use. *Dose* (dexamethasone equivalent): *Intramuscular*, *adults*, 8 to 16 mg every 1 to 3 weeks; *intralesional*, 0.8 to 1.6 mg/injection site; *intra-articular*, usually 4 to 16 mg every 1 to 3 weeks, if necessary.

Diflorasone Diacetate   [6α,9-Difluoro-11β,17,21-trihydroxy-16β-methylpregna-1,4-diene-3,20-dione   17,21-diacetate   [33564-31-7] $C_{26}H_{32}F_2O_7$ (494.53); Florone (*Upjohn*); Maxiflor (*Herbert*)]—A topical glucocorticoid of high potency. From clinical trials, it has been claimed both that the 0.05% cream or ointment is equivalent to 0.05% fluocinonide cream and more effective than 0.1% hydrocortisone cream or 0.1% betamethasone valerate ointment. Because it is fluorinated it can be expected to have more systemic activity than hydrocortisone and hence should be used cautiously in children. *Dose: Topical*, to the *skin*, as 0.05% cream or ointment 2 to 4 times a day to *adults* and once a day to *children*.

Flunisolide   [6α-Fluoro-11β,16α,17,21-tetrahydroxypregna-3,20-dione cyclic 16,17-acetal with acetone [3385-03-3] $C_{24}H_{31}FO_6$ (434.50); Syntaris (*Syntex*)]—For the synthesis refer to US Pat 3,124,571. *Uses:* A glucocorticoid used topically to treat *noninfectious rhinitis*. It has a half-life of 1 to 2 hr, which is about one-tenth that of beclomethasone, a steroid used for the same purpose. *Dose: Intranasal, adult*, initially 50 μg (2 metered sprays) into each nostril 2 times a day and, for *maintenance*, 25 μg (1 metered spray into each nostril once a day); *children 6 to 14 years* of age, initially 25 μg (one metered spray) into each nostril 3 times a day and, for *maintenance*, once a day. *Dosage Form:* Nasal spray: 25 μg/metered spray.

Fluprednisolone   [6α-Fluoro-11β,17,21-trihydroxypregna-1,4-diene-3,20-dione [53-34-9] $C_{21}H_{27}FO_5$ (378.44); Alphadrol (*Upjohn*)]—Synthesis of fluprednisolone is described in RPS-15, page 898. A white to off-white, odorless, crystalline powder; melts at about 210°. Practically insoluble in water; sparingly soluble in alcohol; slightly soluble in chloroform, ether. A glucocorticoid with typical actions, uses, and side effects (see introduction in this section). It is approximately 2.5 times as potent as prednisolone and 40 times as potent as cortisone. However, occasionally it does not appear to be able to control allergic or inflammatory conditions that can be controlled with other glucocorticoids. It also has erratic mineralocorticoid activity. *Dose: Oral, adult*, initially 2.5 to 30 mg a day followed by 1.5 to 12 mg a day for maintenance. *Children*, for *maintenance*, 70 μg/kg (or 2.5 mg per m² of body surface) per day in 3 divided doses; for *disease*, 250 μg to 1 mg/kg (or 7.5 to 30 mg/m²) a day in 3 or 4 divided doses. *Dosage Forms:* Tablets: 0.75 and 1.5 mg.

Halcinonide   [21-Chloro-9-fluoro-11β,16α,17-trihydroxypregn-4-ene-3,20-dione cyclic 16,17-acetal with acetone [3093-35-4] $C_{24}H_{32}ClFO_5$ (454.97); Halog (*Squibb*)]—For synthesis see *J Org Chem 27*: 690, 1962. A white, crystalline powder; melts at about 265°, with decomposition. Insoluble in water; slightly soluble in alcohol. A high-potency glucocorticoid used for topical treatment of glucocorticoid-responsive dermatoses and dermatitides. Its clinical status remains to be determined. The systemic side effects of topical application are usually of a low degree, but care must be exercised in children. The cutaneous side effects are somewhat more severe than with drugs of lower potency (see page 960 for adverse effects and contraindications). *Dose: Topical*, to the *skin*, as 0.025 or 1% cream or 1% ointment or solution 2 or 3 times a day in adults and once a day in children.

Medrysone   [11β-Hydroxy-6α-methylpregn-4-ene-3,20-dione [2668-66-8] $C_{22}H_{32}O_3$ (344.49); HMS Liquifilm (*Allergan*)]—A weak glucocorticoid effective in the treatment of allergic conjunctivitis and possibly in other mild superficial ocular inflammatory conditions. Untoward effects are stinging and burning sensations after instillation. *Dose: Topical*, to the eye, as 1% ophthalmic suspension. *Dosage Form:* Ophthalmic Suspension: 1%.

Methylprednisolone Sodium Phosphate   [11β,17,20-Trihydroxy-6α-methylpregna-1,4-diene-3,20-dione   21-(disodium   phosphate) [5015-36-1] $C_{22}H_{29}Na_2O_8P$ (498.42)]—The actions and uses of this water-soluble methylprednisolone derivative are essentially the same as those of methylprednisolone sodium succinate (page 969) except that the sodium phosphate is reported to yield about 20% higher plasma levels of methylprednisolone than the sodium succinate. *Dose:* See *Methylprednisolone Sodium Succinate*.

Prednisolone Acetate and Prednisolone Sodium Phosphate—When used in combination the soluble prednisolone sodium phosphate (see page 972) gives rise to rapidly achieved plasma or synovial fluid levels of prednisolone, whereas prednisolone acetate supposedly maintains the levels for a longer time because of its lower solubility. *Dose: Intramuscular, intra-articular,* or *intrasynovial*, in fixed ratio sterile suspension (1:4), 20 to 80 mg of prednisolone acetate and 5 to 20 mg of prednisolone sodium phosphate, repeated at 3 day- to 4-week intervals.

The Pancreatic Hormones

The larger portion of the pancreas consists of glandular tissue which secretes digestive enzymes, but there are also isolated groups of cells, called *Islets of Langerhans*, the beta cells of which produce an internal secretion known as *insulin* and the alpha cells a factor known as *glucagon*.

Insulin: *Chemistry*—Insulin is obtained by extraction of beef, sheep, swine, or whale pancreas; human insulin is now produced by chemical conversion from porcine insulin and by *E coli* into which the human genes for insulin have been inserted. Insulin was one of the first proteins obtained in crystalline form. Insulin (monomer) is a polypeptide of molecular weight 6000; it consists of two peptide chains containing 21 and 30 amino acids, respectively, the two chains being held together by disulfide (—S—S—) bonds of cystine. In aqueous solution, the insulin monomer polymerizes to form macromolecules of molecular weight 12,000 or 36,000, depending on pH and concentration. The isoelectric point of insulin is 5.3. Preparations of crystalline insulin contain about 0.5% zinc (USP limits: 0.27–1.08%), the function of which is unknown. The potency of crystalline insulin, calculated on the anhydrous basis, is not less than 26 USP Insulin Units in each mg.

The arrangement of the amino acids in each of the two chains of insulin has been determined for insulins from several species of animals, including man.* Although the species differences are relatively small, involving mainly substitutions among amino acids 8–10 of the shorter (A) chain, antibodies to insulin can be prepared in some animals.

Successful syntheses of both chains of bovine insulin has been achieved.

In patients with insuloma, an insulin of molecular weight 100,000 can be found in the plasma. It is probable that it represents a precursor to the regular insulin.

Physiology and Actions—Insulin is the hormone which facilitates the processes by which the various tissues in all parts of the body may use glucose, either as a fuel for the liberation of energy, or as a store, converted to the less soluble form known as glycogen or to the more permanent deposit in the form of a fat. When the supply of or response to insulin is inadequate, a disease known as *diabetes mellitus* occurs (see page 697). In this disorder, glucose accumulates rapidly in the body fluids, and as the blood glucose concentration increases beyond a certain point it is excreted by the kidneys. The amount of sugar in the urine is a rough index of the severity of the diabetes and may be used to approximate the amount of insulin necessary for treatment. Diabetic acidosis requires larger doses of insulin than does simple hyperglycemia. When there is diabetic coma, heroic doses are required. Although attention focuses on the intervention of insulin in glucose metabolism, it also has independent actions on lipid and protein metabolism.

Diabetes mellitus may also be produced by conditions other than a simple lack of insulin; but, even so, administration of adequate doses of insulin will save life and improve health as long as suitable insulin treatment is maintained. However, mild to moderate diabetes, as is much of maturity onset disease, can be managed with diet alone or in combination with oral hypoglycemics (page 976). Insulin is sometimes used to decrease protein catabolism after injury or myocardial infarction. The combination of insulin and glucose causes a fall in plasma potassium levels and is used for that effect.

When there is an excess of insulin, serious or dangerous symptoms from hypoglycemia may result, causing sweating,

hunger, incoherence, convulsions, coma, and death. Glucose administration relieves the symptoms of overdosage, and the diabetic patient often carries some source of glucose to alleviate hypoglycemia. Glucagon may be administered when hypoglycemia is severe.

Insulin interacts with receptors on the plasma membrane. Some receptors couple to the interior to release mediators of the actions of insulin. Others take the insulin into the cell, where it is released to interact with other receptors on various organellar membranes. Intracellularly, some proteins become phosphorylated and others dephosphorylated. The transport of mRNA out of the nucleus is decreased, and protein synthesis is altered.

Insulin is rapidly absorbed and exerts its maximum action within three hours. The plasma half-life is only 9 min. In severe diabetes, injections must be spaced throughout the day, usually being given before meals. During the night, when no insulin is available, the blood sugar rises and is usually at its highest point before the morning dose. This erratic behavior on the level of blood sugar can be controlled more adequately by the use of insoluble insulins, which are absorbed more slowly and thus can exert a continuous even action over a period as long as 24 hours (see below). Continuous infusion pumps for insulin are also available. Sustained blood levels have the disadvantage of suppressing glucagon-mediated homeostasis, thus favoring prolonged hypoglycemic episodes and encephalopathy.

Insulin is degraded locally, so that sometimes subcutaneous insulin has a low efficacy.

Preparations: *Crystalline Zinc Insulin*—By addition of appropriate amounts of zinc salts, insulin may be crystallized. This achieves a superior degree of purification, which is of advantage when treating diabetics who demonstrate an allergic sensitivity to Insulin Injection, the earlier and more commonly used, but less highly purified, type. The speed and duration of action of the zinc insulins depends on the crystal size. The microcrystalline form dissolves promptly and hence has an onset and duration of action (8 hr) nearly the same as that of zinc-free insulin (6 hr), and they may be used interchangeably. Either form meets USP standards. The Reference Standard of the USP consists of dried Zinc-Insulin Crystals, and is defined as containing 22 USP Units/mg. Zinc insulins of larger crystals size have slow-release properties that depend on crystal size. Thus Prompt Insulin Zinc Suspension, Insulin Zinc Suspension, and Extended Insulin Zinc Suspension, with durations of action of 14, 24, and 36 hours, respectively, represent increasing crystal sizes.

Insoluble Insulins—Insulin or zinc insulin may be combined with globin or protamine to yield complexes of larger molecular weight, and the complexes may be mixed in various proportions. The isoelectric point of globin zinc insulin, isophane insulin, or protamine zinc insulin is near pH 7.3. This means that at the pH of body fluids they are very insoluble. Crystalline zinc insulin has a higher solubility than the protein complexes but goes into solution at a very slow rate. Protamine zinc insulin is injected as a suspension. It goes into solution only slowly and this limits the rate of absorption. By the use of protamine zinc insulin the number of injections required to control the level of blood sugar can often be reduced to one daily. What is more important, wide fluctuations in the level of blood sugar are less likely to occur. In certain cases combinations of protamine zinc insulin and regular insulin may be employed.

Distinguishing Characteristics—FDA regulations require that the labels of various insulin preparations shall have distinctive colors.

The onsets and durations of action, purity and animal

---

* The determination of the structure of beef insulin by F Sanger in 1954 was the first example of the elucidation of the complete structure of a protein.

sources of the various commercial products vary, even among those of supposedly identical constitution. For details of the differences, see AMA Drug Evaluations, 5th edition, Chapter 47, Table 2, pp. 1030–1031.

Glucagon (*Hyperglycemic Factor*)—In addition to insulin, the pancreas also produces a substance which exerts an effect on blood sugar opposite to that of insulin. This *hyperglycemic factor*, or glucagon, is produced by the alpha cells of the Islets of Langerhans. It plays an important role in the physiological regulation of blood sugar, and defects in the control of glucagon secretion are a factor in certain types of diabetes mellitus. Contamination of an insulin preparation by glucagon is manifested by a transitory *increase* in blood glucose following insulin injection. Some insulins, for example the Danish *Novo* insulins, do not contain this hyperglycemic factor (HGF).

Somatostatin (*GH-RIF*)—Somatostatin (see page 953) is also produced in the pancreas, where it inhibits release of both insulin and glucagon; it is thought to be involved in the physiologic regulation of the secretion of these hormones. In diabetes mellitus, the persistence of glucagon output contributes to hyperglycemia and ketoacidosis; administration of somatostatin improves the metabolic condition by suppressing glucagon blood levels. Unfortunately, the half-life of somatostatin is very short, so that longer-lived congeners are being sought.

Glucagon

Glucagon (pig); (*Lilly*)

H - His - Ser - Glu(NH₂) - Gly - Thr - Phe - Thr - Ser - Asp - Tyr - Ser - Lys - Tyr - Leu - Asp - Ser -
1 2 3 4 5 6 7 8 9 10 11 12 13 14 15 16

Arg - Arg - Ala - Glu(NH₂) - Asp - Phe - Val - Glu(NH₂) - Trp - Leu - Met - Asp(NH₂) - Thr - OH
17 18 19 20 21 22 23 24 25 26 27 28 29

Glucagon [16941-32-5] $C_{153}H_{225}N_{43}O_{49}S$ (3482.78); a polypeptide occurring in the pancreas glands of domestic mammals used for food by man, which has the property of increasing the blood glucose concentration. It is employed as the hydrochloride.

Description—Fine, white or faintly colored, crystalline powder; practically odorless and tasteless.
Solubility—Soluble in dilute alkali and acid solutions; insoluble in most organic solvents.

Uses—Glucagon stimulates the hepatic adenylate cyclase system and hence promotes the breakdown of liver glycogen. The end result is the release of glucose and an elevation of blood glucose. Stimulation of adenylate cyclase in the heart causes positive inotropy and in intestinal muscle, relaxation. After parenteral injection the glucose response is quite prompt. The action lasts but 45 to 90 min. Glucagon is used primarily to *terminate hypoglycemic coma*, such as may occur from an overdose of insulin. It is dubious that it offers any compelling advantage over intravenous dextrose for this purpose, except when it is difficult to give an intravenous infusion. Its value in idiopathic hypoglycemia, islet cell carcinoma, and glycogen storage disease has not yet been fully determined. However, it can be used to diagnose glycogen storage disease. It must be used cautiously in islet cell carcinoma, because it stimulates the release of insulin and may cause hypoglycemia. Even in the diabetic patient it may cause rebound hypoglycemia, mostly, however, because of the persistence of insulin levels from the overdose for which glucagon was administered. It is used as an adjunct in hypotonic *radiography of the gastrointestinal tract*, to relax the smooth muscle. Side effects include nausea, vomiting, hypotension and rebound hypoglycemia, especially after intravenous administration.

Dose—*Parenteral, adult,* for *hypoglycemia,* **0.5 to 1 Unit** repeated as necessary; in hypoglycemia, if there is no response within 20 min. intravenous dextrose is mandatory; *children,* **0.025 Unit per kg** of body weight, repeated in 20 min, if necessary; for *diagnostic use,* **0.25 to 2 Units.**
Dosage Forms—For Injection: 1 and 10 Units (1 and 10 mg).

Insulin Injection

Regular Insulin; Crystalline Zinc Insulin; (*Various*)

A sterile, acidified or neutral solution of insulin. The solution has a potency of 40, 80, 100, or 500 USP Insulin Units in each mL.

Description—When containing in each mL not more than 100 USP Units, it is a colorless or almost colorless liquid; that containing 500 Units may be straw-colored; substantially free from turbidity and from insoluble matter; contains from 0.1 to 0.25% (*w/v*) of either phenol or cresol and 1.4 to 1.8% (*w/v*) of glycerin; pH, determined potentiometrically, between 2.5 and 3.5 for acidified injection, and 7.0 and 7.8 for neutral injection.

Uses—For the actions and uses, see the general statement. In diabetes mellitus, the dosage varies with the individual case. Insulin must be given by hypodermic injection, the hormone being destroyed in the gastrointestinal tract. Diabetic individuals are trained to inject themselves. For this purpose a special syringe measuring the dosage of insulin directly in units is employed.

Regular insulin is a *rapid acting* insulin. The time interval from a hypodermic injection of regular insulin until its action can be demonstrated is ½ to 1 hr. The duration of action is relatively short but longer than the plasma half-life, which is approximately 9 min. The duration of action is not linearly proportional to the size of the dose, but it is a simple function of the logarithm of the dose; if 1 unit will last 4 hr, 10 units will last 8 hr. Since the usual duration is from 5 to 8 hr after subcutaneous injection, the insulin injection usually is planned in 2 to 4 daily doses for proper control of severe diabetes. This is ordinarily timed a few minutes before the ingestion of food, in order to avoid an unpleasant reduction of the blood glucose level.

Dose—There is no standard dosage for insulin; each case must be studied individually. In practice, the amount of insulin given is based on the amount of glucose the patient utilizes from the diet, the response to treatment and whether insulin injection is used in combination with longer-acting insulins.

Subcutaneous, for a patient with newly diagnosed mild diabetes, *initially* **5 to 10 USP Units** 15 to 30 min before each meal. After the period of stabilization of dose, the dose is usually **10 to 20 Units** 3 or 4 times a day, but as much as **40 Units** is occasionally required. As an adjunct to intermediate-acting insulins, **5 to 10 Units** given in the same syringe, except with protamine zinc insulin. *Intravenous infusion, adult,* in coma or severe acidosis, **6 to 10 Units/hr.** Some physicians administer 1 g of dextrose for each unit of insulin used. The patient should never become hypoglycemic. The urine should be examined hourly for dextrose. If it becomes sugar-free, more dextrose must be given. More than 150 Units of insulin in 12 hours occasionally is needed. *Children,* **0.1 Unit/hr,** not to exceed the adult dose. *Intramuscular,* for diabetic ketoacidosis when facilities for intravenous infusion are inadequate, **5 to 10 Units/hr** following an *intravenous bolus* of **10 to 20 Units.**

Dosage of insulin should always be expressed in Units rather than in cubic centimeters or minims.

Dosage Forms—Injection, Beef *and* Pork: 400 and 1000 Units/10 mL; Pork: 400 and 1000 Units/10 mL, and 10,000 Units/20 mL; Human: 1000 Units/10 mL.

Isophane Insulin Suspension

Isophane Insulin; Isophane Insulin Injection; NPH Insulin (*Squibb*); NPH Iletin (*Lilly*)

A sterile suspension of zinc-insulin crystals and protamine sulfate in buffered water for injection, combined in a manner such that the solid phase of the suspension consists of crystals composed of insulin, protamine, and zinc. The protamine sulfate is prepared from the sperm or from the mature testes of fish belonging to the genus *Oncorhynchus* Suckley, or *Salmo* Linné (Fam *Salmonidae*).

Each mL is prepared from sufficient insulin to provide either 40, 80, or 100 USP Insulin Units of insulin activity.

Description—White suspension of rod-shaped crystals approximately 30 μm in length and free from large aggregates of crystals following moderate agitation; contains either (1) 1.4 to 1.8% (*w/v*) of glycerin, 0.15 to 0.17% (*w/v*) of metacresol, and 0.06 to 0.07% (*w/v*) of phenol, or (2) 1.4 to 1.8% (*w/v*) of glycerin, and 0.20 to 0.25% (*w/v*) of phenol; contains 0.15 to 0.25% (*w/v*) of dibasic sodium phosphate; contains also 0.01 to 0.04 mg of zinc and 0.3 to 0.6 mg of protamine for each 100 USP Insulin Units; when examined microscopically, the insoluble matter in the suspension is crystalline, and contains not more than traces of amorphous material; pH between 7.1 and 7.4, determined potentiometrically.

Uses—Isophane insulin is an insoluble, repository form of insulin (see introduction in this section). It is an *intermediate acting* insulin. The action begins in 1 to 2 hr, reaches a peak in 6 to 10 hr, and lasts 18 to 28 hr, except that human isophane insulin has a somewhat shorter duration of action. There may be occasional hypersensitivity to the protamine. *Isophane Insulin is never given intravenously.*

Dose—*Subcutaneous, initial,* usually **10 to 20 Units** ½ to 1 hr before breakfast; sometimes as much as **80 Units** daily may be required.

Note—*Isophane Insulin Suspension differs in its actions from that of other insulin injections in the USP in both time of onset and duration. To secure accuracy of dosage, the preparation must be brought into uniform suspension by careful shaking before use.*

Dosage Forms—Injection, Beef or Beef *and* Pork: 400 and 1000 Units/10 mL; Pork: 1000 Units/10 mL; Human: 1000 Units/10 mL.

Insulin Zinc Suspension

Lente Insulin (*Various Mfrs*)

A sterile suspension of insulin in buffered water for injection, modified by the addition of zinc chloride in a manner such that the solid phase of the suspension consists of a mixture of crystalline and amorphous insulin in a ratio of approximately 7 parts of crystals to 3 parts of amorphous material. Each mL is prepared from sufficient insulin to provide either 40, 80, or 100 USP Insulin Units of insulin activity.

Description—Almost colorless suspension of a mixture of characteristic crystals predominantly 10 to 40 μm in maximum dimension and many particles which have no uniform shape and do not exceed 2 μm in maximum dimensions; contains 0.15 to 0.17% (w/v) of sodium acetate, 0.65 to 0.75% (w/v) of sodium chloride, and 0.09 to 0.11% (w/v) of methylparaben; contains also, for each 100 USP Insulin Units, 0.12 to 0.25 mg of zinc of which 20 to 65% is in the supernatant liquid; pH between 7.2 and 7.5.

Uses—The "amorphous" zinc insulin component has a duration of action of about 6 to 8 hr and the crystalline zinc insulin component a duration of longer than 36 hr, owing to the slowness with which the larger crystals dissolve. An appropriate dose of the 3:7 mixture used in insulin zinc suspension has an onset of action of 1½ to 4 hr and an *intermediate* duration of action which is very close to that of isophane insulin suspension (18 to 28 hr), with which preparation it may be used interchangeably. The advantage of zinc insulin suspension is its freedom from foreign proteins, such as globin or protamine, to which certain patients are sensitive. For the actions and uses, see the introduction in this section.

Dose—*Subcutaneous,* usually **10 to 20** but sometimes as much as **80 USP Units** daily; the dose may be initially 10 Units daily with adjustments for newly developed moderate cases or 80% of an established dose of unmodified insulin (eg, *Insulin Injection*) or protamine zinc insulin for cases of longer standing. *Insulin Zinc Suspension must never be given intravenously!*

Dosage Forms—Injection, Beef, Beef *and* Pork: 400 and 1000 Units/10 mL; Pork: 1000 Units/10 mL; Human: 1000 Units/10 mL.

Extended Insulin Zinc Suspension

Ultra-Lente Iletin (*Lilly*); Ultralente Insulin/Ultratard (*Squibb-Novo*)

A sterile suspension of insulin in buffered water for injection, modified by the addition of zinc chloride in a manner such that the solid phase of the suspension is predominantly crystalline. In its preparation, sufficient insulin is used to provide either 40, 80, or 100 USP Insulin Units for each mL of the suspension.

Description—Almost colorless suspension of a mixture of characteristic crystals the maximum dimension of which is predominantly 10–40 μm; contains, for each 100 USP Units of insulin, 0.12–0.25 mg of zinc (of which 20–65% is in the supernatant liquid), and not more than 0.70 mg of nitrogen; contains also 0.15–0.17% (w/v) of sodium acetate, 0.65–0.75% (w/v) of sodium chloride, and 0.09–0.11% (w/v) of methylparaben; pH, between 7.2 and 7.5.

Uses—The actions and uses of the insulins are discussed in the introduction in this section. The crystals in extended insulin zinc

suspension are of sufficient size to have a slow rate of dissolution. It is a *long-acting* insulin with an onset of action of 4 to 6 hr, a peak at 10 to 14 hr, and duration usually in excess of 36 hr, which is slightly longer than that of *Protamine Zinc Insulin*. Since extended insulin zinc suspension is free of protamine and other foreign proteins, the incidence of allergic reactions is minimized. The dose needs to be individualized to the patient on the basis of a study of responses of blood and urine glucose to trial doses of the drug.

Dose—*Subcutaneous* (deep), usually **7 to 20** but sometimes as much as **80 USP Units** daily. *It must never be given intravenously!*

Dosage Forms—Injection, Beef: 1000 Units/10 mL; Beef *and* Pork: 400 and 1000 Units/10 mL.

Prompt Insulin Zinc Suspension

Semi-Lente Iletin (*Lilly*); Semitard (*Squibb-Novo*)

A sterile suspension of insulin in buffered water for injection, modified by the addition of zinc chloride in a manner such that the solid phase of the suspension is amorphous. In its preparation, sufficient insulin is used to provide either 40, 80, or 100 USP Insulin Units for each mL of the suspension.

Description—Almost colorless suspension of particles that have no uniform shape and the maximum dimension of which does not exceed 2 μm; contains, for each 100 USP Units of insulin, 0.12–0.25 mg of zinc (of which 20–65% is in the supernatant liquid), and not more than 0.70 mg of nitrogen; contains also 0.15–0.17% (w/v) of sodium acetate, 0.65–0.75% (w/v) of sodium chloride, and 0.09–0.11% (w/v) of methylparaben; pH between 7.2 and 7.5.

Uses—For the actions and uses of the insulins, see the introduction in this section. The zinc insulin in prompt insulin zinc suspension is a mixture of amorphous and extremely fine crystalline materials. Consequently, it is a *rapid-acting* insulin with an onset of ½ to 3 hr, a peak of 4 to 6 hr and a duration of 12 to 16 hr. Because prompt zinc insulin suspension is essentially free of foreign proteins, the incidence of allergic reactions is extremely low.

Dose—*Subcutaneous* (deep), usually **10 to 20** but sometimes as much as **80 USP Units** daily. *It should never be given intravenously!*

Dosage Forms—Injection, Beef or Pork: 1000 Units/10 mL; Beef *and* Pork: 400 and 1000 Units/10 mL.

Protamine Zinc Insulin Suspension

Protamine Zinc Insulin; Protamine Zinc Insulin Injection (*Squibb*); Protamine Zinc and Iletin (*Lilly*)

A sterile suspension of insulin in buffered water for injection, modified by the addition of zinc chloride and protamine sulfate. The protamine sulfate is prepared from the sperm or from the mature testes of fish belonging to the genus *Oncorhynchus* Suckley, or *Salmo* Linné (Fam *Salmonidae*). In the preparation, the amount of insulin used is sufficient to provide either 40, 80, or 100 USP Insulin Units for each mL of the suspension.

Description—White, or almost white, suspension, free from large particles following moderate agitation; must contain from 1.4 to 1.8% (w/v) of glycerin, and either from 0.18 to 0.22% (w/v) of cresol or from 0.22 to 0.28% (w/v) of phenol; contains from 0.15 to 0.25% (w/v) of Na_2HPO_4; must contain from 0.15 to 0.25 mg of zinc and from 1 to 1.5 mg of protamine for each 100 USP Insulin Units; pH, determined potentiometrically, between 7.1 and 7.4.

Uses—The actions and uses of the insulins are described in the introduction in this section. Protamine Zinc Insulin Suspension is a *long-acting* insulin with an onset of action of 4 to 6 hr, a peak at 10 to 12 hr, and a duration of about 36 hr. Consequently, it need not be given with any definite time relation to food intake, and it must not be depended upon when very prompt action is needed, as in diabetic acidosis and coma. Also, due to the prolonged action, the protamine zinc insulin need not be given more often than once daily, but this should be done at a fairly uniform, scheduled time. Since subliminal levels persist for three or four days, the dose should be adjusted at intervals of not less than 3 days.

Protamine zinc insulin and the more rapidly acting insulins have been mixed in various proportions and in different ways. Such variations produce mixtures that give intermediate patterns of speed and duration of physiological activity. This method, however, makes it possible through the long-acting insulin to take care of the sugar requirements during the night, while short-acting insulin causes full utilization of food taken during the day. It thus permits one to avoid large doses of the long-acting insulin such as might cause hypoglycemia in the early morning hours. However, the need to individualize the insulin schedule makes commercial fixed mixtures impractical and places the responsibility for the preparation in the hands of the physician. Except for the inconvenience of an extra injection, the short-acting insulin can just as well be administered by separate injection.

Protamine zinc insulin suspension is administered by injection usually into the loose subcutaneous tissue. *It is never administered intravenously.*

Dose—*Subcutaneous*, usually **7** to **20** but sometimes as much as **80 USP Units** daily.

Note—*Protamine Zinc Insulin Suspension differs in its action from that of other insulin injections in the USP in both time of onset and duration. To secure accuracy of dosage, the preparation must be brought into uniform suspension by careful shaking before use.*

Dosage Forms—Injection, Beef or Pork: 1000 Units/10 mL; Beef *and* Pork: 400 and 1000 Units/10 mL.

Secretin—page 1277.

Oral Hypoglycemic and Hyperglycemic Drugs

Compounds from several different chemical classes are capable of lowering blood sugar. The best known of these compounds are benzenesulfonylurea derivatives of the type $R_1C_6H_4SO_2NHCONHR_2$. Certain biguanides (formamidiniminoureas) also have such action, but are no longer used.

Oral hypoglycemics were received enthusiastically by the medical profession. However, the sulfonylureas especially have proved to be efficacious only in certain types of diabetes, primarily in noninsulin-dependent ("maturity onset") adult diabetes mellitus. Limitations to the usefulness of oral hypoglycemics are most certainly connected with the mechanism of their hypoglycemic action and with the nature of the metabolic deficiency in each of the various types of diabetes. The principal action of the sulfonylureas seems to be to increase secretion of insulin by sensitizing the pancreatic β-cell to circulating glucose, some β-cell function having to be present for sulfonylureas to lower blood sugar; in addition, hepatic glucogenesis is decreased, and also the number of insulin receptors per cell appears to be increased by certain agents. During chronic treatment tolerance may occur, so that neither insulin nor glucose blood levels may be much affected.

In 1970, the results of a collaborative study among a number of university medical centers were reported (University Group Diabetes Program, UGDP). The findings were that life expectancy with diet plus tolbutamide or phenformin was no greater than with diet alone, thus raising serious doubts about the advisability of using oral hypoglycemic agents at all. Furthermore, cardiovascular complications appeared to be higher when these drugs were used than in their absence, although the findings were by no means conclusive. Critics have pointed out serious defects in the design and execution of the study, and the American Diabetes Association no longer endorses the report. Consequently, the status of these drugs is uncertain. The usual advice is that the use of oral hypoglycemics should be limited to the management of noninsulin-dependent diabetes which does not respond to diet and in which the patient will not or can not tolerate insulin. Recent reports show glipizide to reverse thickening of the vascular basement membrane in diabetics.

A few drugs increase blood sugar and hence have received attention as possible agents for treating hypoglycemia. The monograph for glucagon is on page 974. Epinephrine and related catecholamines are not used for this purpose because of their strong cardiovascular effects and because they are poorly effective orally. Diazoxide, which has received considerable attention as an antihypertensive, also elevates blood sugar, especially in hypoglycemic patients, mostly infants and young children, who are responsive to leucine. The prognosis of leucine-sensitive hypoglycemic children is poor, so that diazoxide is used despite serious side effects.

Acetohexamide

Benzenesulfonamide, 4-acetyl-*N*-[[cyclohexylamino]carbonyl]-, Dymelor (*Lilly*)

1-[(*p*-Acetylphenyl)sulfonyl]-3-cyclohexylurea   [968-81-0] $C_{15}H_{20}N_2O_4S$ (324.39), calculated on the dried basis.

Preparation—*p*-Acetylbenzenesulfonamide is treated with anhydrous potassium carbonate and the resulting potassium salt of the sulfonamide is reacted with cyclohexyl isocyanate. After removal of acetone, the residue (potassium salt of acetohexamide) is dissolved in water and acidified with hydrochloric acid to precipitate acetohexamide. Purification is by recrystallization from aqueous ethanol. US Pat 3,320,312.

Description—White, practically odorless, crystalline powder; melts between 182.5° and 187°.

Solubility—1 g in 230 mL alcohol, 210 mL chloroform; practically insoluble in water and ether.

Uses—A sulfonylurea oral hypoglycemic drug with actions and uses similar to those of *Tolbutamide*. Thus it is used in the treatment of mild to moderately severe *diabetes mellitus* of the maturity-onset, nonketotic type in patients in whom diet alone cannot control glycosuria. It is ineffective in juvenile-onset, unstable, or brittle diabetes and is contraindicated in diabetes complicated by acidosis, ketosis, severe infections, coma, severe trauma, or major surgery.

The side effects of acetohexamide are similar to those of other sulfonylureas (see *Tolbutamide*, page 977). The incidence of adverse effects is low, and such effects are reversible. Contraindications and drug interactions are similar.

Acetoheximide is metabolized in the liver to a metabolite that has 2.5 times the activity of the parent compound. The metabolite is excreted in the urine; consequently, care must be exercised in renal failure. The plasma half-life of the parent drug is 6 to 8 hr, and the duration of action is 8 to 12 hr.

Dose—The dosage must be individualized; the *oral adult* dose ranges from **250 mg** to **1.5 g** daily; doses in excess of 1.5 g/day are not recommended. Doses below 1 g may be taken as a single dose in the morning, but larger doses should be divided into two separate doses.

Dosage Forms—Tablets: 250 and 500 mg.

Chlorpropamide

Benzenesulfonamide, 4-chloro-*N*-[(propylamino)carbonyl]-, Diabinese (*Pfizer*)

1-[(*p*-Chlorophenyl)sulfonyl]-3-propylurea   [94-20-2] $C_{10}H_{13}ClN_2O_3S$ (276.74).

Preparation—*p*-Chlorobenzenesulfonamide undergoes addition to propyl isocyanate by warming a solution of equimolar quantities of the two reactants.

Description—White, crystalline powder, having a slight odor; melts between 125° and 129°.

Solubility—Practically insoluble in water; soluble in alcohol; sparingly soluble in chloroform.

Uses—An oral hypoglycemic agent with actions and uses essentially the same as those of *Tolbutamide* (page 977). As with tolbutamide, its use is limited to patients with stable, mild to moderately severe diabetes mellitus who still have some residual pancreatic beta-cell function. If the patient requires more than 40 Units of insulin/day, he usually will not respond to chlorpropamide. Refractoriness sometimes develops. Elimination is mostly hepatic. The half-life (30 to 36 hr) and duration of action (*ca* 60 hr) are much longer than those of tolbutamide. The side effects are of the same type as with tolbutamide but have a somewhat higher incidence, namely, about 6%, half of which is cutaneous. Severe, refractory hypoglycemic coma occurs more often with chlorpropamide than with other oral hypoglycemic drugs. Chlorpropamide increases the endogenous release of vasopressin (ADH) and thus causes water retention with resultant hyponatremia and hypo-osmolality. Patients under treatment with chlorpropamide have a disulfiram-like intolerance to ethanol. Chlorpropamide is contraindicated in the presence of *renal* glycosuria because of the possibility of fatal hypoglycemia.

Dose—*Oral, adult, initially* **200** to **250 mg** in middle-aged patients and **100** to **125 mg** in elderly patients, given once a day, with breakfast. After 5 to 7 days, when the blood glucose response becomes constant, the dosage may be increased or decreased by 50 to 125 mg at weekly intervals. The *usual maintenance* dose is **100** to **500 mg** a day. Doses above 500 mg do not usually increase the response; the dose should not exceed 750 mg a day.

Dosage Forms—Tablets: 100 and 250 mg.

Diazoxide—page 847.

Tolazamide

Benzenesulfonamide, *N*-[[(hexahydro-1*H*-azepin-1-yl)amino]-carbonyl]-4-methyl-, Tolinase (*Upjohn*)

$$CH_3-\langle\bigcirc\rangle-SO_2NHCONH-N\langle\bigcirc\rangle$$

1-(Hexahydro-1*H*-azepin-1-yl)-3-(*p*-tolylsulfonyl) urea [1156-19-0] $C_{14}H_{21}N_3O_3S$ (311.40).

Preparation—Methyl *p*-tolylsulfonylcarbamate undergoes an ammonolysis type of reaction with 1-aminohexamethyleneimine. US Pat. 3,063,903.

Description—White to off-white, crystalline powder that is odorless or has a slight odor; melts between 161° and 169°, with decomposition; pK$_a$ (25°) 3.6; (37.5°) 5.68.

Solubility—Very slightly soluble in water; freely soluble in chloroform; soluble in acetone; slightly soluble in alcohol.

Uses—A sulfonylurea oral hypoglycemic drug with actions and uses similar to *Tolbutamide* (below). Thus it is used in the treatment of mild to moderately severe *diabetes mellitus* of the maturity-onset, nonketotic type in patients in whom glycosuria cannot be controlled by diet alone. It is ineffective in juvenile-onset, unstable or brittle diabetes and is contraindicated in diabetes complicated by acidosis, ketosis, severe infections, coma, severe trauma, or major surgery. After oral administration the plasma levels reach a peak in 4 to 8 hr. The plasma half-life is about 7 hr and the duration of action is 12 to 16 hr.

The total incidence of side effects is about 5%; about 2% of patients find it necessary to discontinue the drug. The side effects are the same types as those of *Tolbutamide*. Korsakoff-Wernicke encephalopathy has been reported; hypoglycemic episodes increase the need for thiamin.

Dose—*Oral, adult, initially* **100** to **200 mg** daily taken with breakfast; the dose is then adjusted every 4 to 6 days until a satisfactory response is achieved or toxicity requires discontinuation. Doses larger than 1 g/day will usually not increase the response. If the daily dose exceeds 500 mg, it should be given in 2 divided doses.

Dosage Forms—Tablets: 100, 250, and 500 mg.

Tolbutamide

Benzenesulfonamide, *N*-[(butylamino)carbonyl]-4-methyl-, Orinase (*Upjohn*)

$$CH_3-\langle\bigcirc\rangle-SO_2-NHCONH(CH_2)_3CH_3$$

1-Butyl-3-(*p*-tolylsulfonyl)urea [64-77-7] $C_{12}H_{18}N_2O_3S$ (270.35).

Preparation—Toluene is treated with chlorosulfonic acid and the resulting *p*-toluenesulfonyl chloride is converted into *p*-toluene-

sulfonamide by interaction with ammonia. Condensation of the sulfonamide with ethyl chloroformate in the presence of pyridine or another suitable basic catalyst produces ethyl *N*-*p*-toluenesulfonyl-carbamate. Aminolysis with butylamine in ethylene glycol monomethyl ether solutions yields tolbutamide.

Description—White, or practically white, crystalline powder; slightly bitter and practically odorless; melting range 126° to 132°.

Solubility—Practically insoluble in water, soluble in alcohol and chloroform.

Uses—A sulfonylurea that is orally active as a hypoglycemic drug. The drug releases somatostatin in the pancreatic islet beta cells which in turn cause the release of insulin. It also inhibits phosphodiesterase, which preserves cyclic AMP and thus favors glycogenolysis in a number of tissues. It is useful in the treatment of selected cases of *diabetes mellitus*, namely mild uncomplicated, stable diabetes of adult onset which cannot be controlled by diet alone. In order to respond patients must have some remaining functional islet beta cells which can be stimulated by the drug. If the patient requires more than 40 Units of insulin/day, he generally will not respond to tolbutamide. In diabetic patients the peak effect is reached in 5 to 8 hr. The duration of action is usually 8 to 12 hr (average plasma half-life 5.6 hr but longer in elderly patients; dose-dependent kinetics occur with high doses), so that two daily doses are required in most patients. The hypoglycemia induced by even high doses of tolbutamide is generally not as severe as can be induced by insulin, hence the incidence of acute hypoglycemic reactions is lower with tolbutamide; however, severe, refractory hypoglycemia sometimes does occur. Refractoriness to tolbutamide sometimes develops. See also page 976 for the findings of the UGDP.

Toxic effects of tolbutamide include diarrhea, nausea, vomiting, abdominal cramps, weakness, headache, tinnitus, paresthesias, allergic reactions (pruritus, erythema multiforme, maculopapular rash, all usually transient), photosensitivity and alcohol intolerance. Water retention and hyponatremia may result from enhancement of ADH (vasopressin) release. Cholestatic jaundice may occur (rarely), and the drug is contraindicated in the presence of liver damage. Rare leukopenia, thrombocytopenia, pancytopenia, and agranulocytosis occur. Furthermore, because the hypoglycemic action of tolbutamide is mild, the patient is more susceptible to loss of control of the blood sugar through dietary indulgence or infections. Hypoglycemic reactions are rare. Tolbutamide is contraindicated in nondiabetic patients with renal glycosuria and liver disease.

The sulfonylureas interact with a number of drugs. The following substances increase the hypoglycemic activity of sulfonylureas: dicumarol, phenylbutazone, oxyphenbutazone, several sulfonamides, chloramphenicol, large doses of salicylates, monoamine oxidase inhibitors, clofibrate, anabolic steroids, fenfluramine, guanethidine, β-adrenoreceptor blocking drugs and ethanol.

Dose—*Oral, adult, initially* **500 mg** twice a day. The dose is then gradually adjusted to the minimal *maintenance* dose that satisfactorily controls the hyperglycemia and glycosuria. Doses greater than 3 g are usually no more effective than smaller doses and greatly increase the likelihood of toxicity.

Dosage Form—Tablets: 250 and 500 mg.

Other Oral Hypoglycemic Drugs

Glipizide [1-Cyclohexyl-3-[[*p*-[2-(5-methylpyrazinecarboxamido)-ethyl]phenyl]sulfonyl]urea [29094-61-9] $C_{21}H_{27}N_5O_4S$ (445.54); Glibenese (*Pfizer*)]—A white odorless powder; practically insoluble in water and most organic solvents melting about 205°. For the synthesis refer to *Arzneimittel Forsch 21:* 200, 1971. *Uses:* A sulfonylurea oral hypoglycemic drug with actions and uses like those of tolbutamide (above). The incidence of adverse effects is about 12%. *Dose: Oral, Adult, initially* 2.5 to 5 mg/day, adjusted upward in increments of 2.5 mg/day, if necessary, to a maximum of 30 mg/day.

Glyburide [1-[[*p*-[2-(Chloro-*o*-anisamido)ethyl]phenyl]sulfonyl]-3-cyclohexylurea [10238-21-8] $C_{23}H_{28}ClN_3O_5S$ (494.00); Glibenclamide; Glybenclamide; Micronase (*Upjohn*); Diabeta (*Hoechst-Roussel*)]—For synthesis see *Arzneimittel-Forsch 16:* 1640, 1966; *CA 66:* 65289h, 1967. A white or nearly white, odorless or almost odorless, tasteless, crystalline powder; melts at about 173°. Sparingly soluble in water, ether; 1 g is soluble in 330 mL alcohol, 36 mL chloroform. *Uses:* A more potent sulfonylurea hypoglycemic drug than any on the market in the US. The side effects are of the same as those of *Tolbutamide* (above). It also appears to be superior in sustaining its effectiveness in long-term treatment. Transient leukopenia and hypoglycemia have been reported. The plasma half-life is 4.8 hr and the duration of action 5 to 16 hr. *Dose: Oral, adult, initially* 2.5 to 5 mg a day, adjusted upward in increments of 2.5 mg a day, if necessary, to a maximum of 20 mg a day.

The Parathyroid Hormone

Spontaneous atrophy, or injury (as at thyroidectomy), of the parathyroid glands is followed by a decrease in the concentration of serum calcium and an increase in serum phosphorus. These changes can be reversed by the parenteral administration of suitably prepared extracts of the parathyroids of domestic animals. The active principle of the parathyroid gland appears to be a protein of molecular weight 8500. Depending on the procedures used, active substances of lower molecular weight (3800 and 6900) can also be isolated from parathyroid tissue. These products possess $\frac{1}{4}$ to $\frac{1}{2}$ the specific calcium-mobilizing activity of the larger molecular-weight preparation, and probably represent partially degraded molecules.

Secretion of parathyroid hormone is stimulated by a fall in the free Ca^{2+} concentration of the plasma. The hormone then acts to restore Ca^{2+} concentration by: (1) increasing reabsorption of calcium and increasing the excretion of phosphate by the kidney, (2) increasing resorption of bone, with release of Ca^{2+}, and (3) increasing absorption of calcium and phosphate from the gastrointestinal tract. The gastrointestinal effects are mediated by $1\alpha,25$-dihydroxycholecalciferol, a metabolite of vitamin D_3; the parathyroid hormone is a trophin for renal synthesis of the metabolite. The metabolite also promotes the action of vitamin D_3 on bone. Vitamin D_2 (calciferol) and dihydrotachysterol can simulate the hypercalcemic effect of parathyroid hormone; these compounds, moreover, are active orally. Overdosage with any of these compounds can lead to dangerously high calcium concentrations in the blood, with attendant complications, such as calcification of kidneys and blood vessels. Their use, therefore, should have careful medical supervision and be controlled by frequent determinations of blood calcium.

The thyroid gland produces a hormone, *thyrocalcitonin* (see page 979), that reduces serum calcium concentration. A small amount of calcitonin is also produced in the parathyroid gland as well as the thymus, but the main source is the thyroid gland. The biological function of calcitonin seems to be to prevent excessive hypercalcemia from parathyroid hormone activity.

Calcitriol—page 1012.

Dihydrotachysterol

9,10-Secoergosta-5,7,22-trien-3-ol, (3β,5E,7E,10α,22E)-, Dihydrotachysterol; Hytakerol (*Winthrop*)

9,10-Secoergosta-5,7,22-trien-3β-ol [67-96-9] $C_{28}H_{46}O$ (398.67).

Preparation—Calciferol (activated ergosterol) is dissolved in a suitable organic solvent and subjected to catalytic hydrogenation until the proper amount of hydrogen has reacted.

Description—Colorless or white crystals, or a white, crystalline powder; odorless; melts between 123.5° and 129° for one form, or about 113° for the other form.

Solubility—Practically insoluble in water; soluble in alcohol; freely soluble in ether and chloroform; sparingly soluble in vegetable oils.

Uses—Chemically closely related to vitamin D_2 (calciferol) and is consequently frequently classified as a D vitamin. However, it possesses very weak antirachitic activity, being only about $\frac{1}{400}$ as potent as calciferol in this respect, mainly because its effects on calcium absorption from the intestine are quite weak. But it has potent calcemic activity (ie, raises plasma calcium concentration) and is similar to parathyroid hormone in this action. Consequently, it has long been used in lieu of parathyroid hormone in the treatment of *idiopathic* and *postoperative tetanies, hypocalcemia* and *hypoparathyroidism.* The drug should not be used in the presence of renal insufficiency or hyperphosphatemia. Extreme care must be used to prevent overdosage.

Adverse effects result mainly from hypercalcemia. They include anorexia, nausea, vomiting, diarrhea, languor, osteoporosis, weight loss, metastatic calcification, renal damage, anemia, band keratitis, and convulsions. In severe hypercalcemia there may be headache, vertigo, tinnitus, abdominal cramps, polyuria, thirst, ataxia, albuminuria, and xanthemia.

Dose—*Initially* **0.75** to **2.5 mg** a day for several days, after which adjustments are made according to plasma calcium concentrations; *maintenance, usual,* **0.25** to **1.75 mg**/day, but it may be as little as 0.25 mg/week.

Dosage Forms—Capsules: 0.125 mg; Solution (in oil): 0.25 mg/mL; Tablets: 0.125, 0.2, and 0.4 mg.

The Thyroid Hormones

The thyroid gland modulates the energy metabolism and certain nonenergetic metabolic functions of the body. In the absence of the thyroid gland the basal metabolic rate is less than 55% of normal, and growth and development are impaired. In the presence of a hyperactive gland the metabolic rate may be up to 160% of normal; the excitability of irritable tissues is increased, and tachycardia, nervousness, etc, result. Thyroid "hormone" is mainly used clinically to replenish the corporal hormone supply in conditions of thyroid insufficiency (hypothyroidism), such as may result from a natural thyroid or pituitary pathology or from thyroid surgery. The "hormone" is rarely administered to increase the metabolic rate and organic activity above normal, and such iatrogenic hyperthyroidism may indeed be dangerous.

The mediator by which the thyroid gland stimulates the tissues to a higher activity and rate of metabolism is called the *thyroid hormone,* but it is clear that not one but four active substances, all iodinated thyronines, are released by the gland. Thyroxine (L-3,5,3′,5′-tetraiodothyronine or T-4) is found in the greatest amount in blood (about 75% of the thyroid hormone content of the plasma), and the moderately less active

L-3,3′-*diiodothyronine* is present in the next greatest amount (25%). L-3,5,3′-*Triiodothyronine* (liothyronine or T-3), which is 3 to 10 times as active as thyroxine, and L-3,3′,5′-*triiodothyronine* comprise less than 3% of the plasma thyroid hormone content. But since the triiodothyronines disappear more rapidly from blood than thyroxine, they probably comprise a somewhat larger proportion of the glandular secretion; in the thyroid gland they account for about $\frac{1}{5}$ of the hormone content and as much as 40% of its hormone activity. Furthermore, in the tissues, some thyroxine is converted to liothyronine and perhaps as much as $\frac{1}{2}$ to $\frac{2}{3}$ of the body liothyronine is derived from thyroxine. Liothyronine is probably the principal hormone involved in the long negative feedback loop regulation of TSH (thyroid-stimulating hormone, or thyrotropin) release.

The thyroid gland concentrates iodide ion from the plasma and converts it to free iodine, which then reacts with tyrosine moieties within the substance of the gland eventually to produce the thyroid hormones. The glandular accumulation of iodine and the conversion to the intermediate, 3,5-diiodotyrosine, are under the control of the thyrotropic hormone (see page 952). Iodine deficiency results in a compensatory increase in the size of the thyroid gland in a usually fruitless homeostatic attempt to manufacture more hormone. Iodine administration corrects this type of goiter and permits the normal production of the thyroid hormones. The incorporation of sodium iodide into table salt helps protect against iodine-deficiency thyroid disorders.

In the colloid of the thyroid gland these thyronine derivatives are bound to a globulin, *thyroglobulin*, which was formerly thought to be the thyroid hormone. About 90% of the thyroid hormone content of the gland is in the thyroglobulin complex. The molecular weight of thyroglobulin is 650,000 daltons. Before thyroxine and liothyronine can be released into the bloodstream, the thyroglobulin must be assimilated by the thyroid follicular cells, within which the globulin is split by proteases to release the hormones. In the blood, the hormones are bound mainly to an albumin; the complex is dissociable, so that the hormones are free to pass into the body cells.

The thyroid hormones interact with nuclear receptors to increase RNA polymerase and also to increase the number of initiation sites for the polymerase. The result is an increase in transcription for a number of proteins, and the synthesis thereof is increased. Thyroid hormone also has a regulatory action on t-RNA. The synthesized proteins in turn regulate various enzymes and enzyme complexes, so that oxidative phosphorylation in the mitochondria may become partially uncoupled, membrane ATPase activity is increased, adenylate cyclase activity is enhanced, etc. There are also some direct actions on cellular functions, such as stimulation of amino acid transport systems, and inhibition of some zinc-dependent dehydrogenases, prostaglandin dehydrogenases, etc.

The uses and adverse effects of the thyroid hormones are indicated in the monograph on *Thyroid* (page 981). Thyroid hormones lower plasma lipid concentrations. However, because of their effect to increase the metabolic rate, they are not used clinically to lower blood lipids. The lipid-lowering action is also possessed by the dextro isomers of thyroid hormones, but the dextro forms have only a very weak effect on the metabolic rate. Consequently, dextrothyroxine is employed to lower blood lipids.

Calcitonin—Thyrocalcitonin is also a thyroid hormone, but its effects are to decrease plasma calcium concentration rather than to affect energy and lipid metabolism. It has an effect to decrease osteoclastic activity, thus inhibiting the movement of bone salts from bone to the blood. It decreases the renal tubular secretion of calcium and probably inhibits calcium pumping in many types of cells. It also increases renal excretion of phosphate. It has very little effect on the absorption of calcium from the intestine. It plays a role in the homeostasis of blood calcium. When plasma calcium levels are elevated, thyrocalcitonin is released in increased quantities. Thus it tends to oppose parathyroid hormone. The molecular weight of thyrocalcitonin is about 3600 daltons. It is a polypeptide of 32 amino acid units. In bovine calcitonin, 18 amino acid residues are different from those in human calcitonin, but the biological activity is about the same. Salmon calcitonin is biologically more potent than the hormone obtained from other non-human sources (see the next article).

Calcitonin

Calcitonin (Pork); Calcitonin (Salmon);
Calcimar (*USV*)

Cys-Ser-Asn-Leu-Ser-Thr-Cys-Val-Leu-Gly-Lys-Leu-Ser-Gln-Glu-Leu-His-
1   2   3   4   5   6   7   8   9   10 11 12 13 14 15 16 17

Lys-Leu-Gln-Thr-Tyr-Pro-Arg-Thr-Asn-Thr-Gly-Ser-Gly-Thr-Pro—NH2
18 19 20 21 22 23 24 25 26 27 28 29 30 31 32

[47931-85-1] $C_{145}H_{240}O_{48}S_2$ (3431.88).

A polypeptide hormone secreted by the parafollicular cells of the thyroid gland in mammals and by the ultimobranchial gland of birds and fish, isolated from various of these sources, all apparently containing the same 32 amino acid residues but differing in the linear sequence of the amino acids. It is stated that the calcitonin from salmon is biologically more potent than the hormone obtained from other sources.

A polypeptide containing the 32 amino acids in the same sequence as in calcitonin (salmon) has been synthesized and is commercially available in sterile, lyophilized form for uses described below. The source of the product is indicated in the labeling.

Description—White, fluffy powder; lyophilized.
Solubility—Very soluble in water; slightly soluble in alcohol; insoluble in chloroform, ether.

Uses—The actions of calcitonin are described in the preceding article. The hormone does not have much effect on normal plasma calcium, and patients with calcitonin-producing tumors of the thyroid medulla often do not manifest disturbances of calcium metabolism. It appears to act only in *hypercalcemia*, such as that caused by hyperparathyroidism, various carcinomas and multiple myeloma. It normalizes plasma calcium and causes a favorable change in bone structure in *Paget's disease*. Three to 12 months of treatment may be required to restore plasma electrolyte, alkaline phosphatase, and hydroxyproline to normal. Human calcitonin appears to be more effective than porcine or salmon calcitonin. Against osteoporosis the hormone has little effect, although there have been a few reports that bone pain was alleviated. Since few studies have been conducted with human calcitonin, no final judgment is yet possible. In combination with calcitriol, porcine calcitonin appears to be effective against senile and *postmenopausal osteoporosis*.

Side effects of calcitonin are mild nausea, vomiting, diarrhea, facial flushing, malaise, and rashes. Inflammation and pain at the injection site sometimes occur. Diuresis at the onset of treatment often occurs.

Isoproterenol and theophylline antagonize calcitonin.

Dose—*Intramuscular* or *subcutaneous*, *adult*, for *hypercalcemia*, initially **4 USP Units/kg** every 12 hr, to be increased as needed up to no more than **8 USP Units/kg** every 6 hr; for *Paget's disease*, initially **100 USP Units** once a day, then **50 to 1000 USP Units** every 1 or 2 days.

Dosage Form—Injection: 400 USP Units/2 mL. One USP Unit is equal to 1 MRC Unit.

Etidronate Disodium

Phosphonic acid, (1-hydroxyethylidene)bis-, disodium salt;
Didronel (*Procter & Gamble*)

Disodium (1-hydroxyethylidene)diphosphonate. $C_2H_6Na_2O_7P_2$ (249.99).

Preparation—Etidronic acid may be prepared in various ways, as by passing gaseous phosphorus trichloride into acetic acid at about 75°, by reaction of the same substances in a lower aliphatic tertiary amine such as tributylamine, or by reaction of an anhydrous mixture of phosphorous acid, acetic anhydride, and acetic acid.

Description—White powder.
Solubility—Very soluble in water.

Uses—The actions of etidronate disodium are unique, and there is no separate category in this volume into which the drug can logically be placed. Since it resembles calcitonin in its uses, it is placed here, but the drug is neither a hormone nor is its mechanism of action that of calcitonin. It is adsorbed onto hydroxyapatite (bone crystal), where it interferes with resorption of the crystals in osteoclasia and, in higher concentration, with new bone formation. In *Paget's disease* (osteitis deformans), for which it is mainly used, it slows the rate of turnover of bone, decreases excessive osteoclastic and osteoblastic cellular activities, and diminishes hydroxyproline levels in blood and urine and brings the elevated serum alkaline phosphate down toward normal. With appropriate (low) doses, bone pain is decreased, and mobility is increased. Where there is impairment of hearing or high-output heart failure, these also are improved. Deformity and fracturing are not prevented. Usually several months of treatment are required to effect a considerable improvement. Sometimes after a single course of treatment remission may be sustained for several years before another course becomes necessary. Etidronate is advantageous, relative to calcitonin, in not requiring parenteral administration, in freedom from antibody formation, and in cost.

In high doses (above 20 mg/kg and possible above 10 mg/kg) or after prolonged use, increased bone pain, decreased mineralization, and increased bone fractures may occur as the result of inhibition of osteoid formation. Etidronate is sometimes used deliberately to suppress heterotropic ossification after injury or bone surgery. Even with the usual dosage, there may be occasional nausea, vomiting, diarrhea and abdominal cramps, which can be lessened by dividing the dose into two or more doses. It should not be used if there is enterocolitis. The drug increases plasma levels of phosphate by an effect that increases renal resorption (probably indirectly through hormonal homeostasis), but no adverse effects have thus far been attributable to this effect. Etidronate does not appear to be teratogenic, but it increases the number of still-born fetuses in experimental animals, and it may also impair bone formation. Therefore, the drug should not be used during pregnancy, except in unusual circumstances.

Etidronate is absorbed by the oral route. Various constituents in food, especially calcium, impair absorption. The drug is eliminated entirely by renal excretion. Therefore, it should be used cautiously in renal failure. Urine hydroxyproline levels and serum alkaline phosphatase activity should be monitored periodically during treatment.

Dose—*Oral, adults, initially* **5 mg per kg** of body weight a day, usually as a single dose, to be taken two hours before eating. Treatment should not exceed 6 mo. When there is accelerated disease or high cardiac output, 10 to 20 mg/kg/day may be given, but for no longer than 3 mo.

Dosage Form—Tablets: 200 mg.

Levothyroxine Sodium

l-Tyrosine, *O*-(4-hydroxy-3,5-diiodophenyl)-3,5-diiodo-, monosodium salt, hydrate; Levothroid (*USV*); Synthroid (*Flint*)

Monosodium L-thyroxine hydrate [25416-65-3] $C_{15}H_{10}I_4N$-$NaO_4.xH_2O$; *anhydrous* [55-03-8] (798.86); the sodium salt of the levo isomer of thyroxine, an active physiological principle obtained from the thyroid gland of domesticated animals used for food by man, or prepared synthetically. It contains 61.6–65.5% of iodine, corresponding to 97–103% of levothyroxine sodium.

Preparation—L-Thyroxine is dissolved in dilute NaOH solution and the resulting sodium salt is precipitated by saturating the solution with NaCl.

Thyroxine may be prepared from thyroid glands and by synthesis. Preparation from the glands (fresh or desiccated) involves extraction with dilute sodium hydroxide followed by acidification with hydrochloric acid whereupon a very crude form of thyroxine is precipitated. Purification involves repeated solubilization by means of sodium hydroxide and reprecipitation with acid, these operations being conducted under increasingly refined conditions and with the aid of auxiliary operations designed to enhance the purity of the final precipitate of thyroxine.

I

II

III

The key compound in the synthesis of thyroxine is 3,5-diiodo-4-(*p*-methoxyphenoxy)nitrobenzene (I) which is readily formed by condensing *p*-methoxyphenol with 3,4,5-triiodonitrobenzene under the influence of anhydrous potassium carbonate. A series of subsequent operations involves (*a*) reduction of nitro to amino; (*b*) replacement of amino by cyano by treatment with cuprous cyanide and butyl nitrite; (*c*) hydration of cyano to carboxyl; and (*d*) reduction of carboxyl to formyl. The resulting aldehyde may be converted into thyroxine in various ways. One involves condensation with 2-phenyl-2-oxazolin-5-one to produce II which is then simultaneously hydrogenated, demethylated, and reductively cleaved by hydrogen iodide in the presence of phosphorus and acetic anhydride to give the DL-form of 3-[4-(4-hydroxyphenoxy)-3,5-diiodophenyl]alanine (III), which is resolved and the isolated L-enantiomorph is iodinated with ammoniacal potassium triiodide solution at the 3,5-positions on the phenoxy ring to give levothyroxine. Neutralization of this acid with NaOH yields the salt.

Description—Light yellow to buff-colored, odorless, tasteless, hygroscopic powder; stable in dry air but may assume a slight pink color upon exposure to light; pH (saturated solution) about 8.9.

Solubility—1 g in about 700 mL water and about 300 mL alcohol; insoluble in acetone, chloroform, and ether; soluble in solutions of alkali hydroxides.

Uses—Its actions, uses, side effects, and limitations are those of *Thyroid*. The sodium salt lends itself to intravenous administration in the treatment of myxedemic coma, although the more rapidly acting liothyronine is preferred. Approximately 50% of an oral dose is absorbed. The plasma half-life is about 9 to 10 days in hypothyroid, 6 to 7 days in euthyroid and 3 to 4 days in hyperthyroid persons, but the time for the intensity of its effect to fall to ½ of its initial value is 9 to 12 days, and some residual effects may be apparent for several weeks after the last dose. Although the L-form is twice as active as the racemic mixture, it offers no particular therapeutic advantage over the DL-form, and it has the disadvantage of being more expensive.

Dose—*Oral*, for *hypothyroidism* in *young* and *middle-aged adults, initially* **50** to **100 μg**/day, then adjusted by increments of 50 to 100 μg every 3 or 4 weeks until a satisfactory response occurs; in *severe* hypothyroidism the initial dose **12.5** to **25 μg**/day and increments are 25 μg until a total daily dose of **100 μg** is reached, after which the schedule for mild hypothyroidism is used. In *elderly adults, initially* **12.5** to **25 μg**/day for the first 6 weeks, after which the dose is doubled every 6 to 8 weeks until the desirable response is achieved. Adult *maintenance* doses range from **100** to **200 μg**/day or **2** to **3 μg/kg**/day up to 175 to 250 μg/day. *Children over 1 year* of age, **3** to **5 mg/kg**/day until the adult dose is reached, not to exceed 200 μg/day; *children under 1 year* of age, **25** to **50 μg**/day until 1 year of age; *premature infants*, **25 μg**/day for 4 to 6 weeks, then **50 μg**/day. *Intravenous*, for *myxedemic coma* in *adults*, **500 μg**; *maintenance is by oral administration*.

Dosage Forms—Injection: 100 μg/10 mL, 200 μg/6 and 10 mL, 500 μg/6 and 10 mL; Tablets: 25, 50, 100, 125, 150, 175, 200, 300, and 500 μg.

Liothyronine Sodium

L-Tyrosine, *O*-(4-hydroxy-3-iodophenyl)-3,5-diiodo-, monosodium salt; Cytomel (*SKF*)

Monosodium L-3-[4-(4-hydroxy-3-iodophenoxy)-3,5-diiodophenyl]alanine [55-06-1] $C_{15}H_{11}I_3NNaO_4$ (672.96).

Preparation—3,5-Diiodo-L-thyronine, the L-enantiomorph of compound (III) in the thyroxine synthesis described under *Levothyroxine Sodium*, is dissolved in methanol and iodinated only at the 3-position by treatment with ammonia and iodine at room temperature. The liothyronine (acid) is then liberated by acidifying the reaction mixture. It is purified and neutralized with NaOH to give the salt.

Description—Light-tan, odorless, crystalline powder.
Solubility—Very slightly soluble in water; slightly soluble in alcohol; practically insoluble in most other organic solvents.

Uses—It is 3 to 10 times more potent than *Levothyroxine Sodium.* The actions and uses are those of *Thyroid* and *Levothyroxine Sodium*, except that it is considered to be more suitable for treatment of a vague syndrome known as *metabolic insufficiency*, which perhaps is due to a deficiency in tissue utilization of thyroxine, and experimentally for treatment of *male infertility* and certain *menstrual disorders* associated with hypothyroidism. Liothyronine has also been used to *reduce goiter*, but it is less effective than Levothyroxine in suppressing TSH release. Because of the lesser pituitary suppression and the wide fluctuation in plasma levels, which negate monitoring, it is not the agent of choice for maintenance, especially after ablative radioiodine treatment. It is the treatment of choice to treat *myxedemic coma*, because of the rapid onset of action. It may be used to *suppress goiter* preparatory to surgery.

Liothyronine has a rapid onset of action. The peak effect occurs in 1 to 3 days, and the offset of action is about 3 days. The prompt onset and rapid offset are considered to be an advantage over thyroid or levothyroxine. The time for the intensity of its effect to fall to $\frac{1}{2}$ of its initial value is 4 to 10 days. Liothyronine is erratically absorbed from the gastrointestinal tract, and 30 to 40% may be recovered from the stools. Liothyronine is only loosely bound to plasma proteins and hence does not elevate the plasma protein-bound iodine (PBI) significantly. It crosses the blood-brain barrier and hence is not recommended for use in children.

Dose—(liothyronine equivalent)—*Oral*, for *mild hypothyroidism* in *young* and *middle-aged adults*, *initially* **25** μg/day for 1 to 3 weeks, after which the daily dose is increased by 12.5 to 25 μg at intervals of 1 to 3 weeks until the desired response is achieved (usually 25 to 50 μg); for *severe hypothyroidism*, *initially* **2.5** to **5** μg/day for 1 to 3 weeks, then increased by 5- to 10-μg increments to a *maintenance* dose of **50** μg/day; in *older adults* and in patients with cardiovascular disease, *initially* **5** μg/day for 3 to 6 weeks, after which the dose is doubled every 6 weeks until the desired response is obtained; in *simple nontoxic goiter*, *initially* **5** μg/day, then increased by 5 to 10 μg/day at 1- to 2-week intervals up to 25 μg/day, then by 12.5 to 25 μg/day every week to a *maintenance* dose of **50** to **100** μg/day. In *cretinism* in *children* of 7 kg or more of body weight, *initially* **5** μg a day for a week, then increased by 5 μg at weekly intervals until the daily dose is 15 to 20 μg; in cretins weighing less than 7 kg, **2.5** μg a day.

Dosage Forms—Tablets: 5, 25, and 50 μg.

Liotrix Tablets

Euthroid (*Warner-Chilcott*); Thyrolar (*Armour*)

A uniform mixture of synthetic levothyroxine sodium (T-4) and liothyronine sodium (T-3) in a 4:1 ratio by weight.

Uses—Since the endogenous thyroid hormone is actually not a single hormone but rather levothyroxine and liothyronine, some medical opinion holds that the 4:1 mixture in liotrix more closely approximates the normal physiological thyroid hormone in activity than either of the separate hormones. Furthermore, the effect on the protein-bound iodine more nearly correlates with the clinical response than that of either of the separate hormones, since the amount of iodine in equieffective doses of the two separate hormones differs by a factor of about 6 to 10.

Dose—*Oral*, *adult*, in *hypothyroidism without myxedema*, *initially* **50** or **60** μg of levothyroxine and **12.5** or **15** μg of liothyronine a day, with equal increments at monthly intervals until the desired effect is achieved; in *myxedema* or patients with *cardiovascular disease*, **12.5** μg of levothyroxine and **3.1** μg of liothyronine a day, with equal increments at 2- to 3-week intervals until the desired effect is achieved; for *maintenance* in both of the above, **50** to **120** μg of levothyroxine and **12.5** to **30** μg of liothyronine a day. In *elderly adults*, *initially* $\frac{1}{4}$ to $\frac{1}{2}$ the dose for young adults, doubled at 6- to 8-week intervals until a satisfactory response is obtained. In *children*, the same as in young adults, except the increments in dosage are made at intervals of 2 weeks.

Dosage Forms—(T-4:T-3)—12.5 μg:3.1 μg, 25 μg:6.25 μg, 30 μg:7.5 μg, 50 μg:12.5 μg, 60 μg:15 μg, 100 μg:25 μg, 120 μg:30 μg, 150 μg:37.5 μg, and 180 μg:45 μg.

Thyroglobulin

Proloid (*Warner-Chilcott*)

A substance obtained by the fractionation of thyroid glands from the hog, *Sus scrofa* Linné var. *domesticus* Gray (Fam. *Suidae*). It contains not less than 0.7% of organically bound iodine (I) [9010-34-8].

Preparation—Hog thyroid glands are grouped and extracted with dilute aqueous sodium chloride solution. Adjusting the pH to the isoelectric point with acetic acid and heating precipitates the crude product which is then defatted with an appropriate solvent, dried, milled, and blended.

Description—Cream- to tan-colored free-flowing powder that has a characteristic odor and taste; stable in air, heat, and light, although it may deteriorate on prolonged exposure to strong light.
Solubility—Insoluble in water, alcohol, and other common organic solvents.

Uses—A glycoprotein in the thyroid follicular lumen and epithelial cells that contains the iodinated thyroid hormones (see page 978). The actions and uses of thyroglobulin are the same as for *Thyroid*. However, it is less likely to cause hypersensitivity, although it is not completely free of contaminating proteins; to this extent it may have some advantage over thyroid, but it is difficult to see any advantage over levothyroxine sodium or liothyronine sodium. It is twice as expensive as *Thyroid*.

Dose—*Oral*, *adult*, in *hypothyroidism without myxedema*, *initially*, **32 mg**/day with equal increments at 1- or 2-week intervals until the desired effect is achieved; in *myxedema* or with *cardiovascular disease*, initially **16 to 32 mg**/day with equal increments at 2-week intervals until the desired effect is achieved; for *maintenance*, in both of the above, **32 to 200 mg**/day. For *children*, for cretinism use the adult dose for myxedema; otherwise use the appropriate adult dose.

Dosage Forms—Tablets: 32, 65, 100, 130 and 200 mg.

Thyroid

Desiccated Thyroid; Thyroid Extract; Thyroid Gland

The cleaned, dried, and powdered thyroid gland previously deprived of connective tissue and fat. It is obtained from domesticated animals that are used for food by man.

Thyroid contains 0.17–0.23% of iodine (I) in thyroid combination, and is free from iodine in inorganic or any form of combination other than that peculiar to the thyroid gland. A desiccated thyroid of a higher iodine content may be brought to this standard by admixture with a desiccated thyroid of a lower iodine content or with lactose, sodium chloride, starch, sucrose, or dextrose.

Description—Yellowish to buff-colored, amorphous powder, having a slight characteristic, meat-like odor and a saline taste.

Uses—The thyroid hormone is essential for normal metabolism and development. The congenital absence of thyroid hormone results in a condition known as *cretinism*. In childhood or adult life, absence of thyroid hormone causes *myxedema*. These conditions are characterized by an abnormally low basal metabolic rate. The primary therapeutic use of thyroid is in their treatment.

Thyroid preparations may be used to *suppress the secretion of thyrotropin* in simple *nonendemic goiter* (hence decreases thyroid size) and chronic lymphocytic thyroiditis (Hashimoto's disease). Thyroid hormones do not decrease hyperthyroid exophthalamus. The use of thyroid hormones in the *diagnosis* of hyperthyroidism is outlined under *Liothyronine Sodium*.

Thyroid is often given to individuals with *low metabolic rates* unassociated with myxedema. For example, patients with chronic constipation, menstrual disorders, sterility, arthritis, etc, associated with a low metabolic rate, are often benefited by thyroid hormone.

Employment of thyroid as an aid to reduce excessive weight is a frequent practice, often futile, and sometimes fraught with danger. In the absence of hypothyroidism, thyroid hormones do not improve skin conditions, mental depression, fatigue, lethargy, irritability, nervousness, menstrual irregularities, and other endocrine and reproductive disorders, and there is danger that untoward effects may be produced.

Untoward effects of overdoses of thyroid hormones include tachycardia, arrhythmias, angina pectoris, hypertension, insomnia, nervousness, hyperkinesis, tremors, diaphoresis, hot skin, gastrointestinal disturbances, and hypoadrenocorticism. Even with physiological doses, it may be advisable to administer glucocorticoids concurrently. Thyroid may cause allergic reactions.

Thyroid has a very slow onset of action. A given dose does not exert its maximum effect for several days and will continue to have some degree of action for 2 to 3 months. Therefore caution must be exercised in judging the dose of thyroid in that cumulative effects must be anticipated.

Dose—*Oral, adult*, for *hypothyroidism without myxedema*, ini-*tially* **60 mg**/day, with increments of 60 mg/day each month until the desired effect is achieved; for *myxedema* or with *cardiovascular disease*, *initially* **15 mg**/day for 2 weeks, 30 mg/day for 2 weeks, 60 mg/day for 2 weeks, then, if necessary, 120 mg/day for 2 months, then even 180 mg/day; *maintenance*, for both of the above, usually **60 to 180 mg**/day, but may range from 30 to 600 mg/day; in the *elderly*, *initially* **7.5 to 15 mg**/day, doubling every 6 to 8 weeks, if necessary; *children*, for *cretinism*, adult dose for myxedema; otherwise use the appropriate adult dose. Doses of *Thyroid Strong* should be ⅓ less, since the preparation is 50% stronger than Thyroid.

Dosage Forms—Tablets: 16, 32, 65, 98, 130, 195, 260, and 325 mg; Thyroid Strong Tablets: 32, 65, 130, and 195 mg.

Antithyroid Compounds

A number of linear and heterocyclic derivatives of thiourea inhibit the production of thyroid hormone by the thyroid gland. The mechanism of action is that of an interference with the incorporation of inorganic iodine into the organic form. The decline in thyroid hormone output and the resultant lowering of plasma levels of the thyroid hormones is sensed in the hypothalamus, which through the long loop feedback and intermediation of the thyrotropin-releasing factor stimulates the adenohypophysis to produce more thyrotropic hormone. Consequently, the thyroid gland is stimulated to enlarge, even though the enlarged gland cannot produce more thyroid hormone. Because of the thyroid enlargement consequent to the use of the thiourea class of antithyroid compounds, such compounds are called goitrogens. The goitrogens are employed in the control of hyperthyroidism. An enlarged thyroid gland is very vascular and friable, which makes surgery difficult. Therefore, iodine (or a thyroid hormone), which reduces the size of the gland, is added to the regimen preparatory to thyroid surgery.

Several other classes of compounds are also antithyroid agents. Compounds such as thiocyanates and perchlorates competitively inhibit the iodine uptake mechanism. Large doses of iodine inhibit the enzyme tyrosine iodinase and thus interfere with the production of thyroid hormone. Therefore, iodine also may be used in the treatment of hyperthyroidism. Curiously, this action of iodine is not goitrogenic; in fact, iodine opposes the goitrogenic effects of certain antithyroid drugs. Radioiodine (^{131}I) is antithyroid by virtue of tissue destruction caused by radiation. Thyroid hormones are antigoitrogenic by the long loop homeostatic feedback mechanism to reduce the hypothalamic release of thyrotropin-releasing factor.

Liothyronine Sodium—page 980.

Methimazole

2*H*-Imidazole-2-thione, 1,3-dihydro-1-methyl-, Tapazole (*Lilly*)

1-Methylimidazole-2-thiol [60-56-0] $C_4H_6N_2S$ (114.16).

Preparation—One method consists of cyclizing (methylamino)-acetaldehyde diethyl acetal with thiocyanic acid via de-ethanolation. Details are provided in *J Am Chem Soc 71:* 4000, 1949.

Description—White to pale buff, crystalline powder, having a faint characteristic odor; solutions are practically neutral to litmus; melting range 144° to 147°.

Solubility—1 g in 5 mL water, 5 mL alcohol, 4.5 mL chloroform, 125 mL ether.

Uses—An antithyroid drug that is employed for the preparation of the hyperthyroid patient for surgery and for the total treatment of *hyperthyroidism*. Methimazole is approximately 10 times as potent as *Propylthiouracil* and is more prompt in eliciting an antithyroid response. The drug also exhibits a more prolonged action than propylthiouracil; a single dose of 5 mg may inhibit the synthesis of thyroid hormone for 24 hr. The plasma half-life is 6 to 8.5 hr in hyperthyroid but 8 to 18 hr in hypothyroid patients; therefore, as the drug lowers the metabolic rate, its own metabolism is slowed, and accumulation will occur unless the dose is adjusted.

The toxic side effects are similar to those of *Propylthiouracil* (below). Approximately 6% of patients taking the drug experience some untoward effect. Thus, the incidence of untoward reactions is somewhat higher than with propylthiouracil, but considerably lower than with other antithyroid drugs. Cross-sensitization to other thiouracils can occur.

Dose—*Oral, adult, initially,* **15 mg**/day for *mild hyperthyroidism*, **30 to 40 mg** for *moderately severe hyperthyroidism*, and **60 mg** or more for *severe hyperthyroidism*, given in 3 divided doses; once the patient is euthyroid (may require up to 2 months!), the dose is diminished to **5 to 30 mg** a day for *maintenance*. In *children, initially,* **400 μg/kg**/day in 3 divided doses 8 hr apart and, for *maintenance,* **200 μg/kg**/day in 3 divided doses. For preparation *prior to thyroid surgery,* as above, except that when the patient becomes euthyroid **6 mg**/day of *iodine* for 10 days is added to the regimen. In *thyrotoxic crisis,* as above, except that iodine is added to the regimen a few hours after the initial dose of methimazole.

Dosage Form—Scored Tablets: 5 and 10 mg.

Potassium Iodide—page 868.

Propylthiouracil

4(1*H*)-Pyrimidinone, 2,3-dihydro-6-propyl-2-thioxo-, Propacil; (*Various Mfrs*)

6-Propyl-2-thiouracil [51-52-5] $C_7H_{10}N_2OS$ (170.23).

Preparation—By condensation of ethyl 3-oxocaproate with thiourea (*J Am Chem Soc 67:* 2197, 1945).

Description—White, powdery, crystalline substance; starch-like in appearance and to the touch; bitter taste; melting range 218° to 221°.

Solubility—Slightly soluble in water; sparingly soluble in alcohol; slightly soluble in chloroform and ether; soluble in ammonia and alkali hydroxides.

Uses—Interferes with the synthesis of thyroid hormone by the thyroid gland, an action which has been applied in the management of *hyperthyroidism*. Since the drug does not interfere with the release or utilization of stored thyroid hormone, the period which elapses between the beginning of medication and the manifestations of its antithyroid action is dependent upon the quantity of thyroid hormone stored in the gland. The marked hyperplasia of the thyroid gland which follows propylthiouracil administration is a result of a compensatory increase of thyrotropin release consequent to a reduction in the thyroid hormone titer of the blood. Propylthiouracil also blocks extrathyroidal conversion of thyroxine (T4) to liothyronine (T3), which in the periphery decreases the hypermetabolic condition and in the pituicytes interferes with short-loop negative feedback, thus favoring goitrogenesis.

Propylthiouracil is employed in the preparation of the hyperthyroid patient for surgery. When treatment with the drug has brought the basal metabolic rate to normal (euthyroidism) or nearly so, iodine is administered to reduce the marked vascularity and friability of the gland. Propylthiouracil is also used in the total (medical) treatment of hyperthyroidism. The duration of treatment usually ranges from 6 months to 3 years, after which time thyroid function may remain normal. However, at least half the patients so treated may be expected to have a recurrence 6 to 12 months after cessation of medication.

Propylthiouracil exerts toxic actions in a small but significant number of patients. The most serious of these toxic actions are granulocytopenia, leukopenia, drug fever, and dermatitis. Joint pains and urticaria may occur. Cross-sensitivity to other thiouracils may occur. A small percentage of patients experience nausea, abdominal discomfort, headache, drowsiness, vertigo, paresthesias and loss of taste sense. The overall incidence of untoward reactions to propylthiouracil is approximately 4%; the incidence of agranulocytosis approaches 0.5%. Therefore, the patient who receives chronic medication with this drug should be kept under close surveillance. The drug passes the placental barrier and may affect the fetus, so that during pregnancy the lowest possible dose should be used. It is also secreted into milk, and the drug should be withheld from nursing mothers.

Only about 75% of propylthiouracil is absorbed by the oral route. There is considerable confusion about the elimination half-life, probably because redistribution has been confused with elimination and because of analytical difficulties. The elimination half-life is probably about 3 to 5 hr in hyperthyroid, 6 to 8 hr in euthyroid, and 24 to 34 hr in hypothyroid persons, so that as the drug decreases the metabolic rate, the dose should be adjusted accordingly, to avoid accumulation.

Dose—*Oral, adult,* for *hyperthyroidism, initially* **300** to **1200 mg**/day in 3 or 4 divided doses at equal intervals, until the patient becomes euthyroid; *maintenance,* **50** to **800 mg**/day in 2 to 4 divided doses. *Neonates,* **10 mg/kg**/day in divided doses; *children 6 to 10 years* of age, **50** to **300 mg**/day in 2 or 3 divided doses; *children 10 years* of age *or older,* **150** to **600 mg**/day in 3 divided doses at 8-hr intervals. For *preparation* prior to *thyroid surgery,* as above, except that when the patient becomes euthyroid **6 mg**/day of *iodine* for 10 days is added to the regimen. In thyrotoxic crises, as above, except that iodine is added to the regimen a few hours after the initial dose of propylthiouracil.

Dosage Form—Tablets: 50 mg.

Sodium Iodide—page 869.
Sodium Iodide I 131—page 495.

The Sex Hormones

The sex hormones, like the hormones of the adrenal cortex, are steroids. They may be classified into the following groups, according to chemical structure and physiological activity:

1. Estrogenic hormones (female);
2. Progestational hormone (female);
3. Androgenic hormones (male).

Groups (1) and (2) are collectively known as the *ovarian hormones.* They include synthetic as well as natural products.

Structure—The natural estrogens are all steroids (see Chapter 25) containing 18 carbon atoms, oxygenated at carbons 3 and 17. Ring A of all the estrogens is aromatic; some estrogenic hormones found in the urine of *Equidae* possess further unsaturation in ring B.

Progesterone, the hormone of the corpus luteum, is a 21-carbon-atom steroid, possessing, like adrenal cortical steroids, an α,β-unsaturated ketone component in ring A. It differs from the latter in that its C_{17} does not carry hydroxyl.

The natural androgenic steroids are 19-carbon-atom compounds. They are characterized by a partly or completely saturated ring A, and by either a hydroxyl or a keto group at C_3 and C_{17}.

As with all other classes of steroids, stereoisomerism is of fundamental importance with the sex hormones; and the α- and β-configuration conventions are applied in drawing the structural formulas.

The Ovarian Hormones

The ovaries serve the dual purpose of secreting the female hormones and producing the ova which, after the menarche, are liberated normally at the rate of one every four weeks. The ovaries secrete two principal types of hormones which are intimately related to the entire process of sex development and function. The first category of these hormones is the group of steroids named *estrogens.* The second category of ovarian steroidal hormone is the *luteal* or *progestational hormone* named *progesterone.* The ovaries also secrete small amounts of androgens, adrenal steroids, and the nonsteroidal hormone relaxin (see below).

The ovarian production of hormones is regulated by the gonadotropic hormones of the anterior pituitary (see page 952). However, the control of pituitary gonadotropin production is, in turn, modulated by the estrogens and progesterone, which in low plasma concentrations appear to stimulate and at high concentrations inhibit the production of FSH, LH, and LtH. Thus a complex positive and negative feedback system subserves the cyclic phenomena of ovulation and menstruation. The exact details in this concert are not completely known for humans. It is known that in women ovulation can be prevented by estrogens as the result of suppression of FSH production. However, estrogen alone is not satisfactory for oral contraception, owing to what is termed "breakthrough" bleeding, except when dangerously high doses of estrogen are used. In impractically large doses, proges-

terone also inhibits ovulation, presumably because of suppression of the production of the hypothalamic luteinizing hormone releasing factor; furthermore, it can favor infertility by a second mechanism, namely, that of maintaining the endometrium in a hypoproliferative and hyposecretory state which is unfavorable to implantation of the fertilized ovum. It is now known that some progestins have an antifertility effect at doses well below those necessary to suppress endometrial proliferation and secretion. Interest in oral contraceptives originally started with progestins. However, intermenstrual bleeding occurs during continuous treatment with many progestogens, and it was found desirable to add estrogens, which, although they favor endometrial proliferation, have a hemostatic effect on uterine bleeding. Furthermore, the 19-norprogestogens were originally synthesized by a route that contaminated the intended product with an estrogen. It was gradually accepted that the estrogen not only helped normalize cyclic bleeding but also contributed to the contraceptive effect. In fact, some authorities argued that the estrogen was alone responsible for the antifertility effect and that the progestin was only promoting a normal mense. Now it is appreciated that progestins alone can be contraceptive in low doses which do not disturb the menses of many users. Progestins alone avoid the drawbacks of estrogens, namely nausea, vomiting, headache, a tendency to venous thrombosis, and other untoward effects, but they are less effective contraceptives than are the estrogens. The progestins have been combined with estrogens in oral contraceptives in a way such that anovulatory doses of estrogen are followed in sequence by a progestin, in order to simulate the sequence of hormone dominance during the estrous cycle and hence to allow a near-normal mense, but such sequential contraceptives are no longer available in the US.

In addition to the steroid hormones mentioned above, the ovary also produces one or more nonsteroid substances which are concerned in the reproductive physiology of various species of animals. A polypeptide compound present in aqueous extracts of the ovaries of pregnant sows and the blood of pregnant humans, to which the name *relaxin* has been given, causes relaxation of the symphysis pubis in estrogen-treated guinea pigs and mice. Other characteristic physiological properties of relaxin-containing extracts include effects upon uterine endometrium and myometrium and upon cervical musculature, although much of this activity is attributable to a contaminant, the *"uterine relaxing factor"* (Lututrin). Very active relaxin preparations which are substantially homogeneous electrophoretically have been isolated. Relaxin is a protein of molecular weight of about 6,000 which appears to be free of nonamino acid constituents. Relaxin preparations are standardized in terms of their ability to cause pelvic relaxation in estrogen-primed guinea pigs or mice. Another water-soluble ovarian preparation, lututrin, is assayed in terms of its ability to inhibit spontaneous contractions of the guinea pig uterus.

Much of the human physiology of relaxin and lututrin remains to be elucidated. There is considerable doubt that a deficiency of these hormones exists in the human and hence that there are rational indications for their use.

These preparations have been used in the treatment of dysmenorrhea, premature labor, cervical dystocia, and scleroderma, but evidence for their therapeutic effectiveness is still equivocal, and such preparations are no longer available.

Natural Estrogenic Hormones and Congeners

Natural estrogenic hormones are secreted by the ovarian follicles. They stimulate or regulate the growth and development of the uterus, the vaginal mucous membrane, and also other structures such as mammary glands, subcutaneous fat, axillary and pubic hair, and certain elements in the skin. These latter comprise the secondary sex characteristics. Therefore the estrogens are also called *female sex hormones.* Of the estrogens the most potent occurring naturally is *β-estradiol,* and its two principal metabolic products, *estrone* and *estriol,* which are also estrogenic. Several other products of metabolic change occur in smaller amounts, but these are not offered as single substances for therapy. Estrogens are secreted throughout the period of activity of the ovaries, but at varying rates at different times of the menstrual cycle.

The naturally occurring estrogens can be prepared synthetically, but at greater cost than by extraction from natural materials or by simple chemical processing of natural estrogens as they occur in urine. An interesting improvement of the natural estrogen has been the synthetic modification of β-estradiol, the most potent of natural estrogens, by the addition of a side chain, producing *ethinyl estradiol.* This has a very high activity when administered orally. The potencies of these estrogens were originally measured entirely in terms of biologically determined units, but in the cases of purified, crystalline products, weights may now be used. Biological units are still sometimes mentioned and are determined by the reaction of spayed rats to injections of the hormones, which induce rapid development of cornified cells in the vaginal mucosa, detectable by the vaginal smear technique.

Uses—Estrogens are used as *substitution therapy* when menopausal symptoms occur after cessation of ovarian function, following ovariectomy or X-ray or radium therapy, or in the natural menopause (also called the climacteric). The purpose of the treatment is to afford relief from any of a long list of complaints which are widely recognized as characteristic of the menopause. However, the use of estrogens for this purpose is the subject of debate. On the one hand, there is evidence that estrogens have clinically useful effects. There is general agreement that low-dose estrogen treatment will ameliorate the symptoms of vasomotor instability (hot flashes); prevent or reverse urogenital atrophy in menopausal women; and slow or prevent postmenopausal osteoporosis, especially when given with calcium supplements. The beneficial effects of estrogen therapy on irritability, depression, anxiety, memory and insomnia are more unpredictable. It is not clear whether or not estrogen administration can prevent arteriosclerotic cardiovascular disease. Several epidemiological and pathological studies suggest that coronary heart disease and arteriosclerosis are less severe in premenopausal women and estrogen-treated men than in women without ovarian function or normal men. However, other influences among the various treatment groups such as the presence or absence of hypertension have been invoked to explain these data. High-density lipoproteins are elevated by these drugs, but there is no evidence that changes in lipoprotein patterns decrease atherogenesis. On the other hand, any potential benefits of estrogen replacement therapy must be weighed against serious risk. There is a definite, at least six-fold, increase in the risk of endometrial cancer in estrogen users who have not had a hysterectomy. One collaborative study reported a small increase in gallbladder disease and in the incidence of breast tumors after estrogen treatment, but no increase in thromboembolic disease was observed. Estrogen may cause hypertension in some patients, but this appears to be reversible if drug therapy is stopped. A more complete description of estrogen side effects appears below and in the discussion of oral contraceptives (page 994). A reasonable position at present regarding estrogen therapy in postmenopausal women seems to be a cautious one. There is no compelling reason to withhold treatment from women suffering with debilitating vasomotor instability or in whom osteoporosis can be delayed. The use of estrogens to treat asymptomatic women is discouraged. Whether or not cyclic use of estrogens or use of different preparations will decrease side effects remains to be established. It is clear that even very low doses of estrogens are effective against menopausal symptoms and have low toxicity. However, such low doses do not provide optimal prophylaxis against osteoporosis. Careful monitoring for untoward effects is mandatory with estrogen use.

Estrogens are used in young women in whom there is *failure of steroidogenesis;* treatment brings about acceleration of delayed development of the uterus, the appearance of secondary sex characteristics, and subtle biochemical and behavioral changes. Applied locally, the estrogens are useful in the treatment of *atrophic* or *senile vaginitis, vulvovaginitis,* or *cervicitis* resulting from hypoestrogenesis but not from other causes.

A number of menstrual irregularities may be treated with estrogens. Some of these, such as *amenorrhea,* may be the result of steroid agenesis. Some have various causes, among them an asynchrony in the release of hypothalamic release factors and pituitary gonadotropin release. Estrogens used cyclically may regularize some of these conditions; *secondary amenorrhea* is such a condition. They are of value in decreasing electrolyte imbalance, headache, tension, breast engorgement, and nipple tenderness in *premenstrual tension,* but they are of dubious value in relieving neurological and mood changes in that disorder. In *dysmenorrhea* their efficacy is unproven, but if they are of value, it is in cyclic therapy. In *endometriosis,* estrogens are effective for only a short time, endometrial hyperplasia eventually resulting. In *dysfunctional uterine bleeding,* combined treatment with estrogens and progestogens is used, and normal withdrawal bleeding may follow the abrupt cessation of treatment.

Since estrogens suppress gonadotropin (FSH) release and also inhibit blastocyst implantation, they are used as *contraceptives* (see page 994). A contrasting use is to assist reproduction as an adjunct in the *prevention of habitual abortion.* They may be used in the *induction of parturition* and in the postpartum period to reduce *breast engorgement.*

Estrogens decrease plasma cholesterol and hence have been used as *hypocholesteremic* drugs, but side effects are usually unacceptable to the male recipient. Estrogens are also used to treat *acne vulgaris* and *hirsutism.* They are also used to inhibit the growth of *prostatic cancer* of men and *carcinoma of the breast* or carcinoma elsewhere in the reproductive tract of women who are more than 4 years beyond the menopause (see Chapter 63, page 1142).

There is a choice of compounds for estrogenic therapy. Estrone is commonly employed by intramuscular injection. Considerable activity is lost if the oral route is used. Ethinyl estradiol is the most active of all oral estrogens, and its oral activity is nearly equal to its parenteral activity. Per milligram, estradiol benzoate is more powerful in action than estrone. Its action is also more sustained. It is commonly given by intramuscular injection. Estriol is considerably less active than estrone when given hypodermically, and its activity following oral administration is probably too low to make it important. Conjugated estrogens (see page 986) retain much of their activity on oral administration and are used extensively by this route. Estrogens can also be given by inunction. In addition, various concentrates of estrogenic hormones are available.

Synthetic compounds, of which the best known is diethylstilbestrol, possess most of the actions of the natural estrogenic hormones and are often cheaper. Since they lose little activity after oral administration, they have replaced the natural estrogens in many fields of treatment.

Side Effects—Nausea and vomiting are frequent side effects of estrogens. These effects appear to be mainly of central nervous system origin and usually reflect only a small degree of local irritant action when administered orally. Anorexia also is frequent. Although estrogens may decrease salt and water accumulation in premenstrual tension, they may also cause such retention. This retention may be one factor in the breast tenderness caused by estrogens. They may also cause breast engorgement, in part by promoting the proliferation of the secretory acini and ducts. High doses of estrogens often cause dizziness. Headache is more frequent with high doses but does occur even with low doses. Malaise, irritability, and depression occasionally occur with small doses and frequently with large doses. Estrogens probably decrease folate absorption, an effect that could cause neurological impairment and megaloblastic anemia in elderly users; however, solid data are lacking. The effect on libido is erratic, being increased in some and decreased in others.

Estrogens effect changes in the concentration of some of the clotting factors in blood, and there is considerable evidence that they increase the incidence of thrombophlebitis and thromboembolism in both the superficial and deep veins. These disorders are additionally favored by venodilation caused by the drugs. Pulmonary embolism, cerebral embolism with stroke, and mesenteric vascular occlusion occur. Coronary thrombosis also seems to be increased among users of estrogens. The incidence of these pathologies is low but definite. Women over 35 years of age and having blood type O are most susceptible. Estrogens alter hepatic function, which may alter various tests of liver function as well as various synthetic and biotransformation processes. There may be a decrease in glucose tolerance, and diabetes mellitus may be exacerbated. Serum triglycerides rise, and dangerous hyperlipidemia may occur in persons who already have a type 4 hyperlipidemia.

The composition of the bile is altered, and there is an increased incidence of gallstones after long-term use. Although rare, porphyria may be provoked. Changes in the concentration of blood proteins may occur; thyroxine- and gluco-

corticoid-binding proteins are increased, which may alter endocrine relationships. Aldosterone secretion is increased, which not only accounts for sodium retention but also for an abnormal incidence of hypertension among users of estrogens.

Estrogens may induce changes in the skin, such as itching, increased pigmentation (in combination with progestins, causes chloasma), a tendency to candidiasis (also in the vagina), and spider angiomas. Although estrogens may improve acne, they only do so after a temporary worsening of the condition. Estrogens may cause a loss of scalp hair in some users and hypertrichosis in others.

It has long been held that estrogens increase the incidence of breast cancer in premenopausal women.

Estrogens increase the risk of cervical and uterine carcinoma, and periodic examinations are advisable. When diethylstilbestrol is taken during pregnancy, there is an increased likelihood of vaginal adenocarcinoma in the daughter after maturity. There is also an increased likelihood of functional abnormalities in the reproductive tracts in both female and male offspring.

It is thought that estrogens cause premature arrest of growth and epiphyseal closure in girls, but the subject requires greater study. Neuroophthalmic lesions during estrogen treatment have been described. Hypercalcemia may occur, especially in men taking large doses for prostatic carcinoma. Allergic reactions include rashes, erythema multiforme, erythema nodosum, and cholestatic jaundice. In women, chronic use may cause spotting or break-through vaginal bleeding; after discontinuation, withdrawal bleeding usually occurs.

Pharmacokinetics—Naturally occurring estrogens are not effective orally because they are destroyed almost totally in a single pass through the liver (first-pass effect). Oral effectiveness can be improved by administration of conjugated or esterified estrogens, by use of synthetic estrogens that are more slowly metabolized, or, in the case of estradiol, by preparation of the drug in a micronized form that is absorbed into the thoracic duct rather than into the portal circulation. Estrogens are rapidly absorbed from intramuscular sites, mucous membranes, skin and other sites of therapeutic application. The half-life of estradiol is 40–50 minutes, but other estrogens persist much longer.

Estrogens circulate in both free and conjugated forms. These are bound in varying amounts to albumin and to a specific sex hormone binding globulin (SSBG).

Estrogens are excreted primarily in the conjugated form in urine. Some free estrogen is secreted in bile from which some is excreted in feces and most return to the systemic circulation by the enterhepatic route. Estrogens are excreted in breast milk, so use in nursing mothers is not recommended.

Drug Interactions—Drugs that induce the hepatic microsomal mixed oxygenase system (eg, phenobarbital, phenytoin, rifampin, etc) will accelerate estrogen metabolism. Estrogens antagonize oral anticoagulants and also interfere with tests of coagulation. They also interfere with tests of thyroid function. By an unknown mechanism, estrogens increase the effects of tricyclic antidepressants.

Estradiol

Estra-1,3,5(10)-triene-3,17-diol, (17β)-, 17-Beta-estradiol; Dihydrotheelin; Estrace (*Mead Johnson*); Progynon (*Schering-Plough*)

[50-28-2] $C_{18}H_{24}O_2$ (272.39).

Preparation—Has been isolated from ovarian follicular fluid and from placental tissue, and is the most potent of the natural estrogens. It is usually prepared through reduction of the 17-keto group of *Estrone*.

It is curious that the urine of stallions and of the males of other *Equidae* contains 3 to 5 times as much estradiol as that of the female of the species.

Description—White or creamy white, small crystals or a crystalline powder; odorless and stable in air; hygroscopic; melts between 173° and 179°.

Solubility—1 g in 28 mL alcohol, 435 mL chloroform, 150 mL ether; practically insoluble in water.

Uses—See the general use statement under *Natural Estrogenic Hormones and Congeners* (page 984). Estradiol is mainly employed to supplement parenteral therapy with esters of estradiol. Parenteral estradiol may be used, but the hormone is rapidly destroyed, and the esters are superior. The plasma half-life is only about 1 hr. By the oral route, very little survives passage through the liver.

Dose—*Oral*, *adults*, for *replacement* therapy, **1** to **2 mg** a day for 21 days, to be repeated cyclically every 28 days; for *breast cancer*, **10 mg** 3 times a day for at least 3 months; *prostatic cancer*, **1** to **2 mg** 3 times a day.

Dosage Forms—Scored Tablets: 1 and 2 mg.

Estradiol Cypionate

Estra-1,3,5(10)-triene-3,17-diol, (17β)-, 17-cyclopentanepropanoate; Estradiol Cyclopentylpropionate NF XI; Depo-Testadiol (*Upjohn*)

Estradiol 17-cyclopentanepropionate [313-06-4] $C_{26}H_{36}O_3$ (396.57).

For the structure of the base, see *Estradiol*.

Preparation—Estradiol is esterified at both the 3- and 17-positions by treatment with cyclopentylpropionyl chloride in pyridine, the diester being recovered in the usual way by pouring the reaction mixture into an excess of cold, dilute hydrochloric acid. The solid 3,17-diester is collected and treated with potassium carbonate in aqueous methanol whereby saponification is effected only at the 3-position. Water is then added, and the crude 17-ester which precipitates is collected and crystallized from 80% methanol.

Description—White to practically white, odorless, crystalline powder; melting range 149° to 153°.

Solubility—1 g in >10,000 mL water, 40 mL alcohol, 7 mL chloroform, 2800 mL ether.

Uses—The same actions and uses as *Estradiol* and its other esters (see *Estradiol Benzoate*, *Valerate*). However, intramuscularly injected vegetable oil solutions of the cypionate have a more prolonged action than do those of the benzoate or valerate. The average duration of action is 3 to 8 weeks.

Dose—*Intramuscular*, *adults*, for female *hypogonadism*, **1.5** to **2 mg** once a month; *postmenopausal*, for vasomotor instability, **1** to **5 mg** every 2 to 4 weeks.

Dosage Forms—Injection (in oil): 10 and 50 mg/10 mL, 25 mg/5 mL.

Estradiol Valerate

Estra-1,3,5(10)-triene-3,17-diol, (17β)-, 17-pentanoate; Delestrogen (*Squibb*); (*Various Mfrs*)

Estradiol 17-valerate [979-32-8] $C_{23}H_{32}O_3$ (356.50).

For the structure of the base, see *Estradiol*.

Preparation—By the method described above for the cypionate, using valeryl chloride as the esterificant.

Description—White, crystalline powder; usually odorless but may have a faint, fatty odor; melts between 143° and 150°.

Solubility—Practically insoluble in water; sparingly soluble in sesame oil and peanut oil.

Uses—Its action, uses and contraindications are those of other estrogens (see page 984). It is very slowly absorbed from an oil suspension injected intramuscularly; the duration of action of suspensions in oil is about 3 weeks. In the management of primary or secondary amenorrhea and functional uterine bleeding, estradiol valerate may be administered along with the progestational agent employed.

Dose—*Intramuscular*, for *replacement*, **10** to **20 mg** every 4 weeks; for *postpartum breast engorgement* and to *suppress lactation*, **10**

to **25 mg,** at the end of the 1st stage of labor; for *prostatic carcinoma*, **30** to **40 mg** every 1 or 2 weeks.

Dosage Forms—Injection (in oil): 50, 100, and 200 mg/5 mL and 100, 200, and 400 mg/10 mL.

Conjugated Estrogens

Amnestrogen (*Squibb*); Menest (*Beecham*); Premarin (*Ayerst*)

A mixture containing the sodium salts of the sulfate esters of the estrogenic substances, principally estrone and equilin, that are of the type excreted by pregnant mares. Conjugated estrogens contains 50–65% of sodium estrone sulfate, and 20–35% of sodium equilin sulfate, calculated on the basis of the total estrogens content.

Preparation—The urine of pregnant mares is subjected to a solvent extraction process. US Pats 2,565,115 and 2,720,483.

Description—Buff-colored powder; odorless or with a slight, characteristic odor.

Solubility—Soluble in water.

Uses—See *Estrone*. Estrone sulfate, the principal constituent of conjugated estrogenic substances, retains a greater potency by the oral route than does estrone, so that it is superior for oral administration.

Conjugated estrogens has been advocated for rapid control of spontaneous "capillary bleeding" and to reduce "capillary bleeding" in surgery. However, in controlled studies no short-term hemostatic effect of the conjugated estrogens has been found, although such effects may result from chronic use.

Dose—*Oral*, in *menopause*, *postmenopause*, *primary ovarian failure*, or *postovariectomy*, **0.625** to **1.25 mg** a day for 21 days, to be repeated cyclically every 28 days; in *hypogonadism* (hypoestrogenesis) and *amenorrhea*, **2.5** to **7.5 mg** a day for 20 days followed by a rest for 10 days, to be repeated cyclically until menstruation occurs (a progestin may be added during days 16–20); for *dysfunctional uterine bleeding*, **2.5** to **5 mg** a day in divided doses for 1 week (along with a progestin); for *postcoital contraception*, **10 mg** 3 times a day for 5 days; for *prostatic carcinoma* **1.25** to **2.5 mg** 3 times a day; in *carcinoma* of the *breast*, **10 mg** 3 times a day for at least 3 months. *Intramuscular* or *intravenous*, in *dysfunctional uterine bleeding*, **25 mg,** repeated in 6 to 12 hours, if necessary. *Topical*, for *atrophic vaginitis* and *kraurosis vulvae*, **2** to **4 g** of a **0.0625**% cream a day.

Dosage Forms—Cream: 0.0625%; Injection: 25 mg/5 mL; Tablets: 0.3, 0.625, 1.25, and 2.5 mg.

Esterified Estrogens

A mixture of the sodium salts of the sulfate esters of the estrogenic substances, principally estrone, that are of the type excreted by pregnant mares. Esterified estrogens contains 75–85% of sodium estrone sulfate, and 6–15% of sodium equilin sulfate, calculated on the basis of the total esterified estrogens content.

Description—White or buff-colored, amorphous powder; odorless or has a slight characteristic odor.

Uses and **Dose**—See *Conjugated Estrogens*, oral administration only.

Dosage Forms—Tablets: 0.3, 0.625, 1.25, and 2.5 mg.

Estrone

Estra-1,3,5(10)-trien-17-one, 3-hydroxy-, Folliculin; Theelin (*Parke-Davis*)

[53-16-7] $C_{18}H_{22}O_2$ (270.37).

Preparation—The first sex hormone isolated in pure form (Doisy and Allen in 1929). It is present, along with traces of other estrogens, in the urine of pregnant mares to the extent of about 10 mg/liter and was formerly obtained exclusively from this source. It has also been prepared "synthetically" from stigmasterol, a phytosterol found in soya bean oil. Urinary estrone is regarded as resulting from the metabolic oxidation of the 17-hydroxy group of estradiol to a ketone group.

Estrone may be prepared from the Mexican yam (*Dioscorea*) via 16-dehydropregnenolone acetate as outlined in the synthesis of *Progesterone* (page 993). The side chain at position-17 is degraded by first forming the 20-oxime and then effecting Beckmann rearrangement with *p*-acetamidobenzenesulfonyl chloride to the 17-acetamido derivative which on treatment with dilute sulfuric acid forms the enamine acetate and is hydrolyzed to the 17-keto compound, estrone.

Note—The estrogenic activity of 0.1 μg of crystalline estrone constitutes the International Unit of estrogenic activity.

Description—Small, white crystals, or a white to creamy white, crystalline powder; odorless and stable in air; melts at about 260°.

Solubility—1 g in 250 mL alcohol (15°), 110 mL chloroform (15°); practically insoluble in water; soluble in vegetable oils.

Uses—See the general statement (page 984).

Dose—*Intramuscular*, in *menopause, postmenopause*, or *postovariectomy, initially* **0.1** to **2 mg** a week in 2 to 3 divided doses to gain relief, followed by gradual downward adjustments in dosage to the lowest possible effective dose for *maintenance;* for *postcoital contraception*, **5 mg** 3 times a day for 5 days; for *carcinoma of the prostate*, **2** to **4 mg** 2 or 3 times a week.

Dosage Forms—Sterile Solution in oil: 20 mg/10 mL and 60 mg/30 mL; Aqueous Suspension: 20 and 50 mg/10 mL, 60 and 150/30 mL. In several products, estrone potassium sulfate is included for a prompt action (see this page).

Estropipate

Estra-1,3,5(10)-trien-17-one, 3-(sulfooxy)-, compd with piperazine; Piperazine Estrone Sulfate (1:1); Ogen (*Abbott*)

Estrone hydrogen sulfate compound with piperazine (1:1) [7280-37-7] $C_{18}H_{22}O_5S.C_4H_{10}N_2$ (436.56).

Preparation—Estrone is reacted with SO_3 in *N,N*-dimethylformamide and piperazine is then added in excess whereby the product precipitates. US Pat 3,525,738.

Description—White to yellowish white, fine, crystalline powder; odorless or may have a slight odor; melts at about 190° to a light-brown viscous liquid which solidifies, on further heating, and finally melts at about 245° with decomposition.

Solubility—1 g in >2000 mL water, alcohol, chloroform, ether.

Uses—See *Estrone*. The cream is used in the treatment of atrophic vaginitis and kraurosis vulvae.

Dose (as estrone sodium sulfate equivalent)—*Oral, adults*, for *menopause, postmenopause*, or *postovariectomy, initially* **100 μg** a day for 1 week, a week of rest, then **100 μg** a week for *maintenance*, to be increased up to 200 μg a week, if necessary. *Topical*, to the *vagina*, **2** to **4 g** of a **0.15%** cream daily for 3 of every 4 weeks.

Dosage Forms—Tablets: 0.625, 1.25, 2.5, and 5 mg (of estrone sodium sulfate equivalent); Vaginal Cream: 0.15%.

Ethinyl Estradiol

19-Norpregna-1,3,5(10)-trien-20-yne-3,17-diol, (17α)-, 17-Ethynylestradiol; (*Various Mfrs*)

[57-63-6] $C_{20}H_{24}O_2$ (296.41).

Preparation—By the Nef reaction, or a modification thereof, whereby estrone is caused to react with sodium acetylide in liquid ammonia. Hydrolysis of the sodoxy addition complex yields the desired carbinol. It may also be prepared by a typical Grignard reaction from estrone and ethynyl magnesium bromide.

Description—White to creamy white, odorless, crystalline powder; melting range 180° to 186°; also exists in a polymorphic modification melting between 142° and 146°.

Solubility—Insoluble in water; soluble in alcohol, chloroform, ether.

Uses—Actions, uses, and limitations are those of the other estrogens (see page 984). It has an anovulatory effect at relatively low doses; for oral contraceptive action it is combined with a progestin. The ethinyl radical delays the decomposition of the estradiol molecule that occurs during absorption by the oral route. It is one of the most potent oral estrogens known.

Dose—*Oral*, for *replacement, menopausal*, **20** to **50 μg** a day for 21 days, to be repeated cyclically every 28 days; *post-ovariectomy* or irradiative *destruction of* the *ovary, initially* **50 μg** 3 times a day with subsequent reduction to the lowest effective dose; for *female hypogonadism*, **50 μg** 1 to 3 times a day for 14 days each month with progestin during the last 2 weeks to be repeated cyclically; for *secondary amenorrhea*, as above, except cycling is stopped after 3 to 6 cycles to see if normal cycling will take over; for *postcoital contraception*, **2.5 mg** twice a day for 5 days; for inoperable *prostatic cancer*, **150 μg** to **2 mg** a day; for inoperable *breast cancer* in postmenopausal women, *initially* **1 mg** 3 times a day.

Dosage Forms—Tablets: 20, 50, and 500 μg.

Ethinyl Estradiol and Ethynodiol Diacetate Tablets—page 995.

Ethinyl Estradiol and Norethindrone Acetate Tablets—page 996.

Ethinyl Estradiol and Norgestrel Tablets—page 996.

Polyestradiol Phosphate

Estra-1,3,5(10)triene-3,17-diol, (17β)-, polymer with phosphoric acid; Estradurin (*Ayerst*)

Estradiol phosphate polymer [28014-46-2] approx $(C_{18}H_{22})_m(O_4P)_n$.

Preparation—Consists essentially of a condensation polymerization of estradiol dihydrogen phosphate. Estradiol is reacted with phosphorus oxychloride in dry pyridine at −10° and the polymer precipitates when the viscous reaction mixture is treated with crushed ice and dilute HCl. US Pat 2,928,849. *Endocrinol 54*: 471, 1954.

Description—White, crystalline powder; melts between 195° and 202°.

Solubility—Very slightly soluble in water (increased by niacinamide), alcohol, chloroform, acetone.

Uses—A repository form of *Estradiol* (page 985); it is gradually depolymerized in the body to release the estradiol. It is specifically intended for use in the treatment of *prostatic carcinoma;* it is not recommended for use in replacement therapy.

Dose—*Intramuscular, initially* **40 mg** every 2 to 4 weeks, with subsequent adjustments in dosage being made by varying the dose interval; **80 mg**/dose may be given, but the duration is affected more than are the plasma levels by alterations in the dose/injection.

Dosage Form—For Injection: 40 mg (with 25 mg niacinamide and other ingredients).

Other Natural Estrogenic Hormones and Congeners

Estrone Potassium Sulfate [ing of Theelin R-P (*Parke-Davis*)]—The actions of this water-soluble estrogen are those of estrone. *Uses:* The aqueous solution of this compound is claimed to have a more rapid effect than that obtained from suspensions of insoluble estrogens. However, except for repository preparations, the rate of onset of estrogenic effect is determined mostly by the rate at which cellular changes can take place. Furthermore, the need for estrogens is not time-critical, and a few hours difference in onset of action makes no difference in the final outcome of treatment. Estrone potassium sulfate is not marketed as a single entity but only in a mixture containing 2 mg of estrone and 1 mg of estrone potassium sulfate in each mL.

Quinestrol [3-(Cyclopentyloxy)-19-nor-17α-pregna-1,3,5(10)-trien-20-yn-17-ol [152-43-2] $C_{25}H_{32}O_2$ (364.53) Estrovis (*Parke-Davis*)]—A white powder practically insoluble in water or organic solvents. *Uses:* For estrogen replacement therapy in the menopause, primarily for relief of vasomotor symptoms. *Dose:* Oral, *initially*, 100 mg daily for 7 days, followed after a 1-week interval by 100 mg weekly; dosage may be increased to 200 mg weekly, if necessary. *Dosage Forms:* Tablets: 100 mg.

Synthetic Estrogens

The exciting discovery by Dodds and co-workers in 1938 that diethylstilbestrol and other relatively simple nonsteroidal organic compounds possess estrogenic activity gave considerable impetus to research in this field during the next decade. This research was designed to discover compounds that had more favorable therapeutic indices because of either greater potency or lesser toxicity. Hundreds of compounds were synthesized and tested and numerous methods for the synthesis of these compounds starting with readily available materials have been devised.

Attempts to explain why such nonsteroidal compounds are estrogenically potent have been intriguing. Dodds pointed out that when the formulas are written appropriately there is a spatial resemblance between them and the true hormone estradiol. Others have focused attention on the closeness of the dimensions of the synthetics (especially length, width, and distance between OH groups) with those of estradiol. The synthetic estrogens combine with the same cytoplasmic receptors as natural estrogens and presumably also with the same nuclear receptor. The configuration of methallenestril does not conform to the hypothetical dimensions prerequisite to estrogenic activity.

Synthetic estrogens are less expensive than natural ones, and they also have a greater bioavailability. Regarding the latter it must be recalled that the oral doses of natural estrogens, with the possible exception of ethinyl estradiol (a derivative of a natural estrogen), may have to be five or more times that of the parenteral doses to secure similar results. This is the result of first-pass metabolism, excretion into bile, and destruction in the intestines. One disadvantage of some synthetic estrogenic compounds is that nausea follows use of even the minimum effective dose in some women, but probably not over 20% of those who use the materials carefully. In such women the synthetic materials must be replaced by natural products. One other slight difference which is possibly debatable is the general impression that the natural estrogens give the patient a greater feeling of well-being than do the synthetics.

Chlorotrianisene

Benzene, 1,1',1"-(1-chloro-1-ethenyl-2-ylidene)tris [4-methoxy]-, Tri-*p*-anisylchloroethylene; Tace (*Merrell-Dow*)

Chlorotris(*p*-methoxyphenyl)ethylene, [569-57-3] $C_{23}H_{21}ClO_3$ (380.87).

Preparation—An alcoholic solution of anisaldehyde is refluxed with potassium cyanide to yield anisoin which may be converted to deoxyanisoin (I) by reduction with zinc and hydrochloric acid. Performing a Grignard reaction on I with *p*-methoxyphenylmagnesium bromide yields 1,1,2-tri-*p*-anisylethanol (II). Dehydration of II by treatment with phosphoric acid produces 1,1,2-tri-*p*-anisylethene which is chlorinated directly in carbon tetrachloride solution. The resulting crude chlorotrianisene is purified by recrystallization from an acetone-alcohol mixture.

Description—Small white crystals, or as a crystalline powder; odorless and stable in air; exhibits polymorphism, one form melting at about 116° and the other at about 118°.

white powder practically insoluble in water or organic solvents. *Uses:* For estrogen replacement therapy in the menopause, primarily for relief of vasomotor symptoms. *Dose:* Oral, *initially*, 100 mg daily for 7 days, followed after a 1-week interval by 100 mg weekly; dosage may be increased to 200 mg weekly, if necessary. *Dosage Forms:* Tablets: 100 mg.

Solubility—1 g in about 4200 mL water, 360 mL ethanol, 28 mL ether, 1.5 mL chloroform.

Uses—An estrogen with most of the actions, uses and limitations of the other estrogens. See page 984. However, it is unique in that its potency is greater by the oral than by any other route, because drug is converted in the liver to a more active form. Also, it apparently induces less anterior pituitary and adrenal hyperplasia than other estrogens. In fact, it appears to be *anti*-estrogenic at the hypothalamic locus that regulates adenohypophyseal gonadotropin release. Furthermore, it causes a lesser incidence of withdrawal bleeding. It is stored in the fat, from which it is slowly released to give a sustained action. The consequent long duration of action makes this drug unsuitable for the treatment of menstrual disorders or other conditions in which cyclic therapy is desired.

Dose—*Oral, adults*, for *postmenopause, postovariectomy*, or *prostatic carcinoma*, **12 to 25 mg** a day; in female *hypogonadism* (hypoestrogenesis), **12 to 25 mg** a day for 21 days (with a progestogen on days 17 to 21), the cycle to be repeated after the 5th day of induced menstruation; for *senile vaginitis* or *kraurosis vulvae*, **12 to 25 mg** a day cyclically for 1 or 2 cycles; to *prevent postpartum breast engorgement*, **12 mg** 4 times a day for 7 days or **50 mg** every 6 hr for 6 doses or **72 mg** twice a day for 2 days, the first dose to be given within 8 hr of delivery for an immediate postpartum effect; for *prostatic carcinoma*, **12 to 25 mg** a day.

Dosage Forms—Capsules: 12, 25, and 72 mg.

Dienestrol

Phenol, 4,4'-(1,2-diethylidene-1,2-ethanediyl)bis-, Dienoestrol; DV (*Merrell-Dow*)

4,4'-(Diethylideneethylene)diphenol [84-17-3] $C_{18}H_{18}O_2$ (266.34).

Preparation—Among other methods, from diethylstilbestrol diacetate. Saturation of the olefinic bond with bromine yields the dibromo derivative which is then dehydrobrominated by refluxing with pyridine to yield dienestrol diacetate. Saponification then yields dienestrol.

Description—Colorless or white, or practically white, odorless needlelike crystals, or a white, crystalline powder; melts within a range of 3° between 227° and 234°.

Solubility—Practically insoluble in water; soluble in alcohol, ether; slightly soluble in chloroform.

Uses—Dienestrol, a potent estrogen, is now used only topically, for the treatment of *atrophic vaginitis* and *kraurosis vulvae*. It should not be used in patients with known or suspected cancer of the breast, known or suspected estrogen-dependent neoplasia, undiagnosed abnormal genital bleeding, active thrombophlebitis or thromboembolic disorders or a past history of such conditions, hypersensitivity to the ingredients of the cream or suppositories of dienestrol, or during pregnancy.

Dose—*Intravaginal*, as **0.01**% cream or **700 μg** to **1.4 mg** as suppository 1 or 2 times a day for 7 to 14 days, the frequency afterward gradually reduced to 1 to 3 times a week.

Dosage Forms—Cream: 0.01%; Suppositories: 0.7 mg.

Diethylstilbestrol

Phenol, 4,4'-(1,2-diethyl-1,2-ethenediyl)bis-, (*E*)-, DES; Diethylstilbestrol (*Lilly*); Stilboestrol

α,α'-Diethyl-(E)-4,4'-stilbenediol [56-53-1] $C_{18}H_{20}O_2$ (268.35).

Preparation—A synthetic estrogen first synthesized by Dodds *et al* in 1938. As to be expected, the compound exists in 2 geometric isomeric forms. The *cis*-isomer, which has less than one-tenth the activity of the *trans* and does not form readily, is unstable and tends to revert to the *trans*-isomer; hence the official product is *trans*-diethylstilbestrol.

Several methods of synthesis have been devised. That of Kharasch and Kleiman (*Medicinal Chemistry*, vol II, Wiley, New York, 1956) uses anethole hydrobromide as the starting material and is most convenient.

Description—White, odorless, crystalline powder; melts within a range of 4° between 169° and 175°.

Solubility—Practically insoluble in water; soluble in alcohol, ether, chloroform, fatty oils, and dilute alkali hydroxides.

Uses—For the same conditions for which natural estrogens are employed; see page 984 for uses, contraindications, and side effects. Diethylstilbestrol is advantageous because it is well absorbed orally. Because the rate of inactivation is slow, diethylstilbestrol can be administered orally in single daily doses even with large doses.

Diethylstilbestrol in large doses is used as an emergency postcoital contraceptive; it is not to be used routinely but only after rape or in other emergencies, because the total amount given is equivalent to a several-months' estrogen requirement. Success is 100% if the drug is used within 72 hr of insemination.

Nausea and vomiting appear to be caused, in part, by local actions of the drug. Enteric coatings on tablets slow the rate of release and lessen the incidence and intensity of such local effects. It is advised to start with the smaller doses for patients who tend to develop disagreeable symptoms such as nausea. Diethylstilbestrol is contraindicated in pregnancy because of the danger of inducing a latent vaginal carcinoma in female offspring and structural abnormalities in the genitourinary tract in male offspring.

Dose—*Oral*, in *female hypogonadism* (hypoestrogenesis) or *senile vaginitis* and *pruritus vulvae*, **1 mg** a day until a response occurs (may be combined with intravaginal administration); *postmenopausal* or *postovariectomy*, **0.2 to 0.5 mg** a day; for *prostatic carcinoma*, *initially* **1 to 3 mg** a day; for *breast carcinoma* in postmenopausal women, *initially* **15 mg** a day, then gradually adjusted upward to the limit of tolerance; for *postcoital emergency contraception*, **25 mg** twice a day for 5 days, starting within 72 hr of insemination. *Intravaginal*, as **0.1-mg** or **0.5-mg** suppository 1 to 2 times a day, up to **5 mg** a week (may be combined with oral administration).

Dosage Forms—Injection: 1 and 5 mg/mL, 50 and 250 mg/10 mL, 30, 60, 150, and 750 mg, and 1.5 g/30 mL; Tablets: 0.1, 0.25, 0.5, 1, and 5 mg; Extended-Release Tablets: 0.1, 0.25, 0.5, 1, and 5 mg; Vaginal Suppositories: 0.1 and 0.5 mg.

Diethylstilbestrol Diphosphate

Phenol, 4,4'-(1,2-diethyl-1,2-ethenediyl)bis-, bis(dihydrogen phosphate), (E)-, Stilphostrol (*Dome*)

α',α'-Diethyl-(E)-4,4'-stilbenediol bis(dihydrogen phosphate) [13425-53-1] $C_{18}H_{22}O_8P_2$ (428.31).

Preparation—*Diethylstilbestrol* is reacted with phosphorus oxychloride in the presence of pyridine.

Description—White, crystalline powder; decomposes between 204° and 206°; stable solutions at pH 10.

Solubility—Sparingly soluble in water (the disodium salt is soluble in water).

Uses—Indicated only for the treatment of *prostatic carcinoma*, in which it is claimed that it is more efficacious than other estrogens, and it has proven effective after tolerance to other estrogens has occurred. Whether it has a unique cytotoxic action on the cancer cells is not clear. It has been hypothesized that the drug enters the cell as the diphosphate and is hydrolyzed therein by the acid phosphatase that is in such high concentrations in prostatic carcinomatous cells, thereby precipitating diethylstilbestrol intracellularly. Present indications are that untoward effects are less frequent and less severe than with any other estrogen. Even with very large doses gynecomastia has been infrequent. Nausea, vomiting, dizziness, pain in the perineum, and transient pain at the sites of metastases are the most common side effects.

Dose—*Oral, initially* **50 mg** 3 times a day, gradually increased to as much as **200 mg** 3 times a day; *intravenous infusion, initially* **500 mg** in 300 mL of isotonic parenteral fluid over a 20- to 30-min period on the 1st day and **1 g** over a period of an hour on the next 5 days, then **250 to 500 mg** once or twice a week for maintenance.

Dosage Forms—Injection: 250 mg/5 mL (as the disodium salt); Tablets: 50 mg.

Mestranol

19-Norpregna-1,3,5(10)-trien-20-yn-17-ol, 3-methoxy-, (17α)-,

[72-33-3] $C_{21}H_{26}O_2$ (310.44).

Preparation—Estrone is converted to its 3-methoxy analogue by reaction with methyl sulfate. The ethynyl group may then be introduced at position 17 either through reaction with sodium acetylide in liquid ammonia followed by hydrolysis of the sodoxy compound, or through grignardization with ethynyl bromide. US Pat 2,666,769.

Description—White to creamy white, odorless, crystalline powder; melts within a range of 4° between 146° and 154°.

Solubility—Freely soluble in chloroform; sparingly soluble in ether; slightly soluble in alcohol; insoluble in water.

Uses—A contaminant in early preparations of norethynodrel. Such impure preparations were superior to pure norethynodrel for oral contraception. Therefore, mestranol was incorporated with norethynodrel in the historically famous oral contraceptive, *Norethynodrel with Mestranol* (page 996), and it is now combined with several progestins in oral contraceptives. When suppression of pituitary release of gonadotropins occurs with these preparations, it is likely that inhibition is more attributable to the mestranol than to the progestin. However, oral contraceptive preparations containing mestranol do not suppress ovulation in a large fraction of users, and the oral contraceptive effect cannot thus be correctly attributed to an anovulatory effect of the estrogen. Mestranol is an effective estrogen for the usual uses of estrogens, but it is not marketed as a single entity.

Dose and **Dosage Forms**—see *Hormonal Contraceptives* (page 994).

Ethynodiol Diacetate and Mestranol Tablets—page 996.

Norethindrone and Mestranol Tablets—page 996.

Norethynodrel and Mestranol Tablets—page 996.

Antiestrogens

In a broad sense, antiestrogens are substances which suppress the effects of estrogens, regardless of mechanism. Androgens and progestins would thus qualify as incomplete antiestrogens, since they are antagonists to estrogens in some of their effects. With the advent of competitive antagonists of estrogens, the term antiestrogen has become restricted in use to apply only to such drugs. A number of estrogens have been found which reduce the intensity of response to other estrogens, behaving as partial agonists, as it were. Some, such as tamoxifen, are complete antagonists; tamoxifen has been effective in the treatment of breast cancer in premenopausal women. Some substances appear to exert antiestrogenic effects only on some but not all target organs; for example, chlorotrianisene is estrogenic in the periphery but antiestrogenic in the hypothalamus, so that it interrupts the normal negative feedback system that modulates anterior pituitary gonadotropin release. A closely related compound, clomiphene, has even a stronger antiestrogenic action in the hypothalamus but is sufficiently weak in the periphery so as not to interfere with the peripheral effects of endogenously released estrogens. By blocking the effects of endogenous estrogen to suppress adenohypophyseal release of gonadotropins, antiestrogens allow the anterior pituitary to produce more gonadotropins than normally. The ovaries are thus stimulated to a greater extent and follicular development and maturation are enhanced. In cases of infertility resulting from failure to ovulate this effect may result in ovulation and the development of fertility.

Clomiphene Citrate

Ethanamine, 2-[4-(2-chloro-1,2-diphenylethenyl)phenoxy]-*N,N*-diethyl-, 2-hydroxy-1,2,3-propanetricarboxylate (1:1); Clomid (*Merrell-Dow*)

2-[*p*-(2-Chloro-1,2-diphenylvinyl)phenoxy]triethylamine citrate (1:1) [50-41-9] $C_{26}H_{28}ClNO.C_8H_8O_7$ (598.09).

Preparation—4-Hydroxybenzophenone is condensed with 2-(diethylamino)ethyl chloride in toluene in the presence of alkali. The 4-[2-(diethylamino)ethoxy]benzophenone thus formed is grignardized with benzyl chloride and the tertiary carbinol thus produced is dehydrated to give 2-[*p*-(1,2-diphenylvinyl)phenoxy]triethylamine. This compound is chlorinated to yield clomiphene and then reacted with an equimolar quantity of citric acid. Clomiphene citrate is a mixture of (*E*)- and (*Z*)-geometric isomers containing 30.0–50.0% of the latter isomer.

Description—White to pale yellow powder, essentially odorless; not appreciably hygroscopic; melts with decomposition between 117° and 119°.

Solubility—Sparingly soluble in alcohol; slightly soluble in water and chloroform; insoluble in ether.

Uses—An antiestrogenic drug that blocks the negative feedback action of endogenous estrogens on the hypothalamus by blocking cytosolic estrogen receptors and diminishing their number. The result is an increase in the secretion of LH-RH/FSH-RH and hence in gonadotropins. However, its effect is uneven, since it seems to be most effective in the late follicular and not in the luteal phase of the estrous cycle. The elevated LH levels bring about ovulation; sometimes more than one ovum is released, which may result in multiple pregnancies. Clomiphene is used to *induce ovulation* (increase fertility) in anovulatory and oligoovulatory women who have adequate endogenous estrogens and in whom the hypothalamic-anterior pitu-

itary has a latent capacity to function. In properly selected patients, 70 to 75% may be induced to ovulate, and successful pregnancy is achieved in 25 to 30%. The probability of multiple pregnancy is increased to 8 times normal. This is about the same order of success as with human chorionic gonadotropin (HCG); HCG plus clomiphene does not increase efficacy. Clomiphene is also under investigation as an agent to increase sperm production in oligospermic males.

In addition to multiple pregnancy, the major side effect is cystic enlargement of the ovaries. Increased cyclic ovarian pain, breast enlargement, and hot flashes which resemble those of the menopause also occur. Nausea is frequent. Blurred vision and scintillating scotoma may occur, and they require discontinuation of the treatment. Sulfobromophthalein retention may be increased. Desmosterol levels are elevated by high doses. All side effects are reversible, except pregnancy itself.

Dose—*Oral, initially* **50 mg** a day for 5 days, starting on the 5th day of the menstrual cycle or at any time in the amenorrheic patient. If ovulation occurs, the same dosage is continued cyclically until conception is achieved or 6 to 8 cycles have passed. If ovulation does not occur, the cycle is repeated with 100 mg a day; if necessary, up to 200 mg may be given, providing that appropriate monitoring is done. For *oligospermia*, **25 mg** a day for 25 days followed by a 5-day wait, to be repeated cyclically for 6 to 12 months or until conception is achieved.

Dosage Form—Tablets: 50 mg.

Tamoxifen Citrate

Ethanamine, 2-[4-(1,2-diphenyl-1-butenyl)phenoxy]-*N,N*-dimethyl-, (*Z*)-, Nolvadex (*Stuart*)

(*Z*)-2-[*p*-(1,2-Diphenyl-1-butenyl)phenoxy]-*N,N*-dimethylethylamine citrate (1:1) [54965-24-1] $C_{26}H_{29}NO.C_6H_8O_7$ (563.65).

Preparation—4-β-Dimethylaminoethoxy-α-ethyldesoxybenzoin by reaction with phenylmagnesium bromide or phenyl lithium is converted to 1-(4-β-dimethylaminoethoxyphenyl)-1,2-diphenylbutanol, which on dehydration yields a mixture of tamoxifen and its *cis*-isomer that may be separated with petroleum ether; tamoxifen is converted to the 1:1 citrate for dispensing use. See *Nature 212:* 733, 1966; *CA 67:* 90515g, 1967.

Description—White, crystalline powder; melts at about 140°.

Uses—Tamoxifen is a nonsteroidal antiestrogen used for palliative therapy of breast cancer in postmenopausal women. The drug competes with estrogens for cytosol estrogen receptors and thus blocks estrogen effects in the target tissue. Tumors with negative receptor assays do not respond to tamoxifen. The drug is also used to treat female infertility, the mechanism being that described for clomiphene (see above). Adverse effects frequently reported are hot flashes, nausea, and vomiting. The drug can also cause vaginal bleeding and discharge, skin rashes, transient leukopenia, and thrombocytopenia. Increased bone and tumor pain may occur. Infrequent side effects are anorexia and hypercalcemia. A few patients have developed retinal abnormalities.

Dose—*Oral, adult* for *breast cancer*, **10** or **20 mg,** twice daily; for *stimulating ovulation*, **5** to **40 mg** twice a day for 4 days.

Dosage Form—Tablets: 10 mg.

Progestational Substances (Progestins, Progestogens)

The second type of hormone produced in the ovaries is *progesterone*, which is excreted in the form of pregnanediol glucuronide. Although it originates in cells which also may produce estrogen and although it has a molecular structure very similar to that of the estrogens, progesterone has a unique physiological action. Under its influence the numerous minute glands which line the uterine cavity are transformed into secreting glands. This alteration is a part of the change which is essential to provide for the implantation of a fertilized ovum and for the continuing development of the placenta. This endometrial alteration requires the cooperation of an

estrogen; in the absence of an estrogen, a progestin that is devoid of estrogenic activity will exert an atrophic effect on the endometrium. Progestins also cause a change in the cervical secretions to suppress "ferning," a dendritic crystallization of cervical mucopolysaccharides. When the cervical mucus is not dendritic, it forms a tight net of fibers, through which it is believed sperm cannot pass. The antifertility effect of some progestins may possibly be due in part to the suppression of ferning. Progestins in high doses suppress the pituitary release of luteinizing hormone and the hypothalmic release of the LH-releasing factor (LRF), thus preventing ovulation. Progestins also decrease uterine motility, which may contribute to a contraceptive effect. Progestins also antagonize the endometrial actions of estrogens, especially the natural estrogens. Progestins have the ability to stimulate development of the glandular portions of the mammae. They also exert some effects upon the capacity of tissues to retain water in the intercellular spaces. They also have a thermogenic action.

Progestins may be used cyclically in the treatment of *infertility* in which the uterus is not receptive to implantation; the progestin sustains the secretory endometrium during the third and fourth weeks of the menstrual cycle. They are used cyclically with estrogens in the treatment of *secondary amenorrhea* and *dysfunctional uterine bleeding*. They may also be used to lessen *premenstrual tension*, although they cause salt and water retention, which is a factor in this disorder. The effect to suppress the release of LH and LRF is used to prevent ovulation, not only with some oral *contraceptives* but also in the treatment of *primary dysmenorrhea* and *endometriosis*. In *sexual infantilism* in the female, progestins may be combined with estrogens to bring about genital development and maturation. Progestins may decrease breast size in *mastodynia*. In *preeclampsia* and *toxemia* of pregnancy due to hormonal imbalance, progestins plus estrogens may improve the condition, even though both types of hormone can cause salt and water retention and estrogens can cause hypertension. Progestins may be used in huge doses as adjunctive treatment in *endometrial carcinoma*. Progestins have been used in the past to prevent habitual abortion or to treat threatened abortion. An intriguing use of progestins is to stimulate respiration in the *Pickwickian syndrome*.

The use of these agents during the first four months of pregnancy is not recommended because there is no evidence that the treatment is effective and there is evidence that the fetus may be harmed. In fact, the Food and Drug Administration now requires that women taking progestins must be informed that the use of these drugs during the first four months of pregnancy may increase the risk of heart defects and deformed arms and legs in their children.

Untoward effects of progestins include nausea, vomiting, diarrhea, edema and weight gain, headache, fatigue, hirsutism, urticaria, ulcerative stomatitis, pruritus vulvae, and a tendency to galactorrhea and vaginal candidal infections. Some are locally irritating. Some progestins have mild androgenic activity that may result in masculinization, especially in the female fetus. Others have a weak estrogenic component of activity. Some have both estrogenic and androgenic actions. Progestins increase the cutaneous pigmenting effect of estrogens, thus favoring cloasma (melasma) when used in combination. It is probable that progestins increase the intensity of adverse effects of estrogens, especially headache and hypertension. There may be breakthrough bleeding when continuous high doses are used which suppress menstruation, yet there may also be decreased menstrual flow in many patients.

Most oral contraceptives contain both an estrogen and a progestogen. Certain progestins may be used alone. The oral contraceptives are discussed on page 994.

Ethynodiol Diacetate

19-Norpregn-4-en-20-yne-3,17-diol, diacetate, (3β,17α)-,

19-Nor-17α-pregn-4-en-20-yne-3β,17-diol diacetate [297-76-7] $C_{24}H_{32}O_4$ (384.51).

Preparation—From *Norethindrone* by reducing the keto group to the carbinol state and then esterifying the 3- and 17-hydroxyls with acetyl chloride in the presence of pyridine.

Description—White, odorless, crystalline powder; stable in air; melts between 126° and 132°.

Solubility—Insoluble in water; very soluble in chloroform; freely soluble in ether; soluble in alcohol; sparingly soluble in fixed oils.

Uses—A *progestin* with actions and uses similar to *Norethindrone*, to which it is closely related chemically. However, because of the hydroxyl rather than keto character of the 3-position of the A ring, ethynodiol has stronger estrogenic activity and is essentially devoid of androgenic activity. It is useful in the treatment of all conditions in which progestins are indicated (see page 990). Ethynodiol diacetate is promoted as an *oral contraceptive*, for which purpose it is combined with an estrogen (marketed with mestranol or ethinyl estradiol); however, because of its inherent estrogenic activity, ethynodiol diacetate could probably be used alone. It suppresses the midcycle elevation of luteotropin that is the immediate stimulus to ovulation.

Dose and **Dosage Forms**—See *Ethynodiol Diacetate and Ethinyl Estradiol Tablets*, page 995.

Hydroxyprogesterone Caproate

Pregn-4-ene-3,20-dione, 17-[(1-oxohexyl)oxy]-, Delalutin (*Squibb*)

17-Hydroxypregn-4-ene-3,20-dione hexanoate [630-56-8] $C_{27}H_{40}O_4$ (428.61).

Preparation—Hydroxyprogesterone is esterified by heating with caproic anhydride in the presence of *p*-toluenesulfonic acid under an atmosphere of nitrogen. US Pat 2,753,360.

Description—White or creamy white, crystalline powder which is odorless or has a slight odor; melts between 120° and 124°.

Solubility—Insoluble in water; 1 g in about 20 mL ether and 800 mL benzene.

Uses—Possesses the actions and uses of the progestins (see page 933), except that it does not prevent ovulation. It is several times more potent than progesterone, and its duration of action is longer, but its onset of action is also slower. A single injection of a solution of hydroxyprogesterone caproate in oil will exert progestational effects for 1 to 2 weeks. It is not converted to progesterone or hydroxyprogesterone in the body. When used to regulate an irregular estrous cycle, it is usually combined with an estrogen.

In addition to a potential to cause the usual side effects of progestins, hydroxyprogesterone caproate occasionally causes hypersensitivity, coughing, or dyspnea. In rare instances it may cause virilization of the female fetus.

Dose—*Intramuscular*, cyclically, for *amenorrhea*, **375 mg** every 4 weeks for 4 cycles and, to *induce a secretory endometrium* and desquamation, **375 mg** every 4 weeks; to *test for endogenous estrogen production*, **250** mg; for *uterine carcinoma*, **1 g** once a day to once a week. AMA Drug Evaluations states the dose for menstrual disorders to be only 125 to 250 mg per cycle.

Dosage Forms—Injection: 125 and 250 mg/mL.

Levonorgestrel

18,19-Dinorpregn-4-en-20-yn-3-one, 13-ethyl-17-hydroxy-, (17α)-(−)-, Nordette, (*Wyeth*)

[797-63-7] $C_{21}H_{28}O_2$ (312.45). This compound is the (−)-isomer of norgestrel, but the D-configurational isomer. A former designation as the d-enantiomer is incorrect.

Preparation—Refer to *Experientia 19:* 394, 1963 for the (±)-form and US Pat 3,413,314 for both enantiomers.

Description—White crystals melting about 240°.

Solubility—Practically insoluble in water; soluble in chloroform; slightly soluble in ether or dioxane; sparingly soluble in ether.

Uses—This drug is the (−)-isomer of norgestrel (page 993). Levonorgestrel is the active form of norgestrel, hence levonorgestrel is twice as potent on a weight basis as is norgestrel. Otherwise, the pharmacological properties of norgestrel and levonorgestrel are the same. Levonorgestrel is used in combinations with ethinyl estradiol as an oral contraceptive.

Dosage Form—Tablets: Levonorgestrel/ethinyl estradiol, 0.15 mg/30 μg, in either 21- or 28-day packs.

Medroxyprogesterone Acetate

Pregn-4-ene-3,20-dione, 17-(acetyloxy)-6-methyl-, (6α)-, Provera, Depo-Provera (*Upjohn*); Curretab (*Reid-Provident*)

17-Hydroxy-6α-methylpregn-4-ene-3,20-dione acetate [71-58-9] $C_{24}H_{34}O_4$ (386.53).

Preparation—From 17α-hydroxyprogesterone by first forming the 3,21-bisethylene acetal with ethylene glycol, then treating with peracetic acid to give a mixture of the 5α,6α- and 5β,6β-epoxides. With methyl magnesium iodide the α-epoxide isomer yields the 5α-hydroxy-6β-methyl derivative which dehydrates and epimerizes with hydrogen chloride in chloroform to the Δ⁴-6α-methyl compound, medroxyprogesterone. Acylation with acetic anhydride and p-toluenesulfonic acid in acetic acid gives medroxyprogesterone acetate.

Description—White to off-white, odorless, crystalline powder; melts between 200° and 210°; stable in air.

Solubility—Insoluble in water; freely soluble in chloroform; soluble in acetone and dioxane; sparingly soluble in alcohol and methanol; slightly soluble in ether.

Uses—Actions, uses, and side effects are those of progestins in general (see page 990). Its oral efficacy is an advantage over progesterone. There is no clinical evidence to date confirming the supposed efficacy in threatened or habitual abortion. Furthermore, the drug is teratogenic during the first four months of pregnancy and hence should not be used for threatened abortion. In the British Commonwealth, medroxyprogesterone is used as an oral or injectable contraceptive. Aqueous suspensions administered intramuscularly have a duration of action of 2 to 4 weeks.

Dose—*Oral*, for *secondary amenorrhea* and *functional uterine bleeding*, **5** to **10 mg** a day for 5 to 10 days, starting on the assumed 16th to 21st day of the cycle, to be continued for 2 cycles in the case of bleeding; for *dysmenorrhea, premenstrual tension*, and *luteal infertility*, **2.5** to **10 mg** for 10 to 20 days, starting on the 6th to 16th day of each cycle; as an *adjunct to cyclical therapy with estrogen*, **10** to **20 mg** a day for the last 7 to 10 days of each cycle. *Intramuscular*, in *endometrial carcinoma, initially* **400 mg** to **1 g** a week, adjusted eventually to 400 mg a week, as an adjunct to other treatment.

Dosage Forms—Sterile Suspension: 100 and 400 mg/mL; Tablets: 2.5 and 10 mg.

Norethindrone

19-Norpregn-4-en-20-yn-3-one, 17-hydroxy-, (17α)-, Norethisterone; Micronor (*Ortho*); Nor-Q.D. (*Syntex*); Norlutin (*Parke-Davis*)

[68-22-4] $C_{20}H_{26}O_2$ (298.42).

Preparation—The methyl ether of estrone is reacted with lithium metal in liquid ammonia to reduce ring A to the 4-ene state and the reduced compound is oxidized with chromic acid in aqueous acetic acid to form estr-4-ene-3,17-dione (I). In order to prevent the 3-keto group from participating in the ensuing ethynylation reaction, I is reacted with ethyl orthoformate in the presence of pyridine hydrochloride to form the 3-ethoxy-3,5-diene compound (II). Acetylene is passed into a solution of II in toluene, previously admixed with a solution of sodium in *tert*-amyl alcohol, to form the 17-ethynyl-17-hydroxy compound. Hydrolysis at the 3-ethoxy linkage by heating with dilute HCl is accompanied by rearrangement of the 3-hydroxy-3,5-diene compound to the 3-oxo-4-ene state. US Pat 2,744,122.

Description—White to creamy white, odorless, crystalline powder; melts between 202° and 208°; stable in air.

Solubility—Practically insoluble in water; sparingly soluble in alcohol; soluble in chloroform and dioxane; slightly soluble in ether.

Uses—For the actions and uses, see page 990. In addition to its progestational actions, norethindrone has weak estrogenic actions, owing to biotransformation to an estrogenic metabolite. Among the progestational drugs, norethindrone ranks high in ability to postpone menstruation, and it is used for this purpose for both medical and social reasons. In high doses it prevents ovulation by suppressing pituitary gonadotropin output. In lower doses it suppresses the endometrium and decreases the fluidity of the cervical mucus. Consequently, the steroid is an important *oral contraceptive.* As an oral contraceptive, it is used alone or combined with an estrogen, especially *Mestranol* and *Ethinyl Estradiol;* when used alone, the pregnancy rate is about 3 times that when used in combination with an estrogen. In some women with type V hyperlipoproteinemia, norethindrone markedly decreases the concentrations of VLDL and chylomicrons; however, it also lowers HDL and hence is used only when the condition is refractory to other drugs. Norethindrone has weak androgenic properties and may cause deepening of the voice, hirsutism and acne, and it may cause masculinization of the fetus.

Dose—For *amenorrhea, dysfunctional uterine bleeding, premenstrual tension,* or *dysmenorrhea, cyclically,* **5** to **20 mg** a day for 21 days, starting on the 5th and ending on the 25th day of the menstrual cycle; for *endometriosis, initially* **10 mg** a day for 2 weeks, after which the dose is increased in increments of **5 mg** every 2 weeks until a *maintenance* dose of **30 mg** a day is reached; for *contraception,* **0.35 mg** (350 μg) a day continuously, starting on the first day of menstruation; for *hyperlipoproteinemia,* **5 mg** a day for the first 21 days of each menstrual cycle.

Dosage Form—Tablets: 0.375 mg; Scored Tablets: 5 mg.

Norethindrone Acetate

19-Norpregn-4-en-20-yn-3-one, 17-(acetyloxy)-, (17α)-, Norlutate (*Parke-Davis*)

17-Hydroxy-19-nor-17α-pregn-4-en-20-yn-3-one acetate [51-98-9] $C_{22}H_{28}O_3$ (340.46).

For the structure of the base, see *Norethindrone.*

Preparation—*Norethindrone* is acetylated by treatment with acetic anhydride in the presence of pyridine.

Description—White to creamy white, odorless, crystalline powder.

Solubility—1 g in >10,000 mL water, 10 mL alcohol, <1 mL chloroform, 18 mL ether, 2 mL dioxane.

Uses—The actions, uses, and side effects are identical to those of *Norethindrone.* However, it is 2 to 3 times as potent as the parent steroid. Although norethindrone acetate may be employed alone as a progestin, it is most commonly used in combination with an estrogen (ethinyl estradiol) for oral contraception or cyclic therapy.

Dose—For *amenorrhea, dysfunctional uterine bleeding, premenstrual tension* or *dysmenorrhea, cyclically,* **2.5** to **10 mg** a day for 21 days, starting on the 5th and ending on the 25th day of the menstrual cycle; for *endometriosis, initially,* **5 mg** a day for 2 weeks, with increments of 2.5 mg a day every 2 weeks until a *maintenance* dose of **15 mg** a day is reached.

Dosage Form—Scored Tablets: 5 mg.

Norethynodrel

19-Norpregn-5(10)-en-20-yn-3-one, 17-hydroxy-, (17α)-, ing of Enovid (*Searle*)

[68-23-5] $C_{20}H_{26}O_2$ (298.42).

Preparation—Dehydroepiandrosterone acetate is simultaneously saponified and oxidized by a series of reactions to 19-hydroxyandrost-6(6)-ene-3,17-dione. The hydroxymethyl group at the 10-position is then oxidized to carboxyl. The resulting acid is decarboxylated with simultaneous shifting of the double bond to give estr-5(10)-ene-3,17-dione. Selective addition of acetylene at the expense of the 17-one group yields norethynodrel. US Pat 2,725,389.

Description—White or nearly white, odorless, crystalline powder; stable in air; melts within a range of 3°, between 174° and 184°.

Solubility—Freely soluble in chloroform; sparingly soluble in alcohol and ether; very slightly soluble in water and solvent hexane.

Uses—A *progestin* which is isomeric with *Norethindrone*. However, the shift of the double bond in the A ring abolishes the weak androgenic properties found in norethindrone. In fact, norethynodrel exerts weak estrogenic actions, because it is biotransformed to an estrogenic metabolite. Nevertheless, for progestational therapy or for oral contraception it is usual to supplement norethynodrel with an estrogen, both to prevent withdrawal bleeding and to favor an anovulatory effect. The prevention of ovulation is the result of suppression of pituitary gonadotropin release. However, contraception results from other mechanisms. The drug is the primary ingredient of the oral contraceptive *Norethynodrel and Mestranol* (page 996). It is not advocated for infertility and maintenance of pregnancy, since it appears not to promote an endometrium which is favorable to nidation and support of the fetus. Furthermore, it causes some masculinization of the fetus, even though it otherwise lacks androgenic properties. This androgenic activity is somewhat antagonized by the estrogenic actions of mestranol and other estrogens. Norethynodrel is not used separately from its estrogenic adjuvant even in general progestational therapy.

Dose and **Dosage Forms**—see *Hormonal Contraceptives*, page 994.

Norgestrel

18,19-Dinorpregn-4-en-20-yn-3-one, 13-ethyl-17-hydroxy-, (17α)-(±)-, Ovrette, ing of Ovral (*Wyeth*)

[6533-00-2] $C_{21}H_{28}O_2$ (312.45).

Preparation—Described by the manufacturer as a total, stereoselective chemical synthesis. 6-Methoxy-α-tetralone is reacted with vinylmagnesium bromide and the resulting 1,2,3,4-tetrahydro-6-methoxy-1-vinyl-1-naphthol is condensed with 2-ethyl-1,3-cyclopentanedione to obtain initially a tricyclic intermediate (secosteroid) containing all of the gonane skeleton carbon atoms. Cyclization of the secosteroid via dehydration yields a 13-ethylgona-1,3,5(10),-8,14-pentaene structure which is then successively reduced and ethynylated.

Description—White or nearly white, practically odorless, crystalline powder; melts within a range of 4° between 205° and 212°.

Solubility—Insoluble in water; sparingly soluble in alcohol; freely soluble in chloroform.

Uses—Although a progestin with potentially all the actions, uses, and side effects of drugs of this class (see page 990), it is marketed only as an *oral contraceptive*, both as a single entity product and in combination with ethinyl estradiol. Its action is to make the endometrium unreceptive to implantation. It is free from estrogenic ac-

tivity. Although it has been demonstrated to have an androgenic effect in animals, such effects have not been reported in the human with the doses used.

Dose—*Oral*, as a single agent, **75 μg** a day, continuously, starting on the 1st day of menstruation.

Dosage Forms—Tablets: 75 μg.

Progesterone

Pregn-4-ene-3,20-dione; (*Various Mfrs*)

Progesterone [57-83-0] $C_{21}H_{30}O_2$ (314.47).

Preparation—From animal ovaries, synthesized from stigmasterol, or better from diosgenin (extracted from *Dioscorea mexicana*, a Mexican yam). The latter synthesis involves acetolysis, chromic acid oxidation, cleavage of the ketoester diacetate with boiling acetic acid to 16-dehydropregnenolone acetate, which on catalytic reduction yields pregnenolone acetate. Saponification of the acetate ester to the 3β-alcohol followed by Oppenauer oxidation affords progesterone. Progesterone in pure form was first isolated, from corpus luteum, in 1934 by Butenandt.

Description—White or creamy white, crystalline powder; odorless and stable in air; melts between 126° and 131°; a polymorphic modification melts at about 121°.

Solubility—Practically insoluble in water; soluble in alcohol, acetone, and dioxane; sparingly soluble in vegetable oils.

Uses—The natural endogenous progestin; its actions, uses, and side effects are described on page 990. However, its plasma half-life is only about 5 min, so that it is extremely difficult to achieve effective blood levels with any convenient dosage schedules. Authorities doubt its usefulness in the treatment of habitual or threatened abortion. It is not effective orally and is of limited and erratic efficacy buccally; consequently it is given intramuscularly as a suspension or solution in oil.

An intrauterine contraceptive device [*Progestasert* (*Alza*)] contains 38 mg of progesterone in silicone oil. The hormone is said to enhance the contraceptive effectiveness of the device by a local effect on the endometrium. Progesterone is released at an average rate of 65 μg daily for one year, at which time the device is replaced. It is not known whether or not progesterone will have adverse local or systemic effects when administered in this manner.

Dose—*Intramuscular*, for *primary* and *secondary amenorrhea*, **5 to 10 mg** a day for 6 to 8 days; in combination with an estrogen for *functional uterine bleeding* and *menorrhagia*, **5 to 10 mg** a day for the last 6 days of the cycle, or in *oil*, **2 to 10 mg** a day for 5 days or until hemostasis occurs or **50 mg** followed by **10 to 20 mg** a day for 4 days. *Intrauterine contraceptive system*, **38 mg** in silicone oil, once a year.

Dosage Forms—Injection (aqueous): 250, 500 and 1000 mg/10 mL; Injection (in oil): 250, 500 and 1000 mg/10 mL; Intrauterine Contraceptive System: 38 mg in silicone oil.

Other Progestins

Megestrol Acetate [17-Hydroxy-6-methylpregna-4,6-diene-3,20-dione acetate [595-33-5] $C_{24}H_{32}O_4$ (384.51); Megace (*Mead-Johnson*) Ovaban (*Veterinary*) (*Schering-Plough*)]—For synthesis see *RPS-15*, page 925. White or almost white, crystalline powder; odorless and tasteless; melts between 213° and 219° within a 3° range. Insoluble in water; sparingly soluble in alcohol; slightly soluble in ether; very soluble in chloroform. *Uses:* See the general statement in this section for actions, uses, and side effects. It is very potent in inhibiting ovulation, and is employed outside the US as an oral contraceptive. For such use it is supplemented by an estrogen, generally ethinyl estradiol. In the US it is used for palliative treatment of inoperable advanced carcinoma of the breast or endometrium, as an adjunct to other therapy. Megestrol has no estrogenic or androgenic properties of its own. Side effects include nausea and vomiting, headache, tiredness, breast discomfort, and weight gain. *Dose:* For *endometrial carcinoma*, 40 to 320 mg a day in divided doses; for *breast cancer*, 160 mg a day, divided into 4 doses. An adequate trial of the potential efficacy is at least 2 months. *Dosage Forms:* Tablets: 20 and 40 mg.

Hormonal Contraceptives

Mechanisms—The various mechanisms whereby hormonal contraceptives can prevent conception are complex. Knowledge in this field is still incomplete, but some mechanisms are relatively well understood. The mechanisms involved vary with the particular agent(s) in a preparation, the dose(s), and whether a cyclic or continuous schedule is used. It is probable that several mechanisms operate simultaneously with some preparations.

Suppression of Gonadotropic Output—During the menstrual cycle, there are two periods of elevated FSH secretion, a sharp peak just preceding ovulation and a long wave beginning just before menstruation. In sufficient doses, *estrogens* can suppress both phases by feedback actions on both the hypothalamus and the anterior hypophysis; FSH-LH output is desynchronized at the early peak, ovulation may be prevented, and the estrogen-progestin priming of the uterus is defective. Estrogens also suppress the hypophyseal output of LH. *Progestins* can also suppress the LH peak (by an action at the hypothalamus, only), but their action is weak, owing to their antiestrogenic effects, which oppose the suppressant actions of endogenous and exogenous estrogen. Very high doses of progestins are necessary to suppress LH output, unless the progestin is combined with an estrogen. A progestin alone desynchronizes the FSH and LH output, thus sometimes preventing ovulation; long-term use of a combination of progestin and estrogen depresses the output of both gonadotropins and more consistently prevents ovulation.

Ovarian Effects—Estrogens and progestins decrease the ovarian response to their respective gonadotropins, a short loop target hormone negative feedback, so to speak. The result may be a failure to ovulate, or, if ovulation does occur, a smaller, hyposecreting corpus luteum, the latter especially when a progestin is in the contraceptive preparation. This latter effect has been demonstrated with chlormadinone and megestrol.

Tubal Effects—In some species progestins and in others estrogens accelerate the ciliary and peristaltic egg transport in the fallopian tubes and increase secretions. Consequently, the ovum arrives in the uterus before the endometrium is prepared for nidation. The tubal effects of these hormones in man are unknown, but it is thought that the contraceptive effects of large postcoital doses of estrogens (see *Diethylstilbestrol*, page 988) may involve a tubal action.

Effects on Endometrium—Long-acting injectable progestins (see *Medroxyprogesterone*, page 992) in appropriate doses cause endometrial atrophy. Oral preparations vary according to the drug and the dose, some permitting a normal endometrium and others causing regression. In combination with estrogens, progestins effect a decrease in tortuosity and secretion of the endometrial glands and sometimes a regression to a stage of secretory exhaustion, with thinning of the endometrium after several cycles of use. With some combinations, the effect may be mainly an asynchrony in the development of the stroma and glands.

Effects on Cervix—Estrogens favor ferning (the parallel alignment of pinnate-structured mucoid cervical secretions), which creates open channels through which spermatozoa may pass. Progestins inhibit ferning and favor an impenetrable mucoid network. In the combination contraceptives, the progestins predominate.

Effects on Capacitance—Capacitance is the ability of the sperm to penetrate into the ovum. Progestins are thought to decrease capacitance, by an unknown mechanism, probably involving prostaglandins. It is speculated that the low-dose, continuously-administered progestin contraceptives are effective by the anticapacitant action.

Types of Preparations—The first oral contraceptives to be marketed were *progestin-estrogen combinations*, and the majority of currently marketed products are of this type. In these preparations, the progestin and estrogen are present in fixed amounts, so that blood levels rise and fall together, in contrast to the levels in the normal menstrual cycle, in which one estrogen peak appears 11 days in advance of the combined estrogen-progesterone peak. With the combined preparations, an artificial menstrual cycle is induced by using the contraceptive for only 20 to 21 days out of every 28; if they were to be used continuously, instead, no regular mense would occur, but breakthrough bleeding would eventually occur. The artificial mense caused by the cyclic use of combination contraceptives is usually not normal but oligemic. During the 7 to 8 days in which no hormones are taken, some products provide placebo or iron tablets in lieu of the combination; in these products, the pills are packaged to be taken serially by number to save the user the nuisance of keeping track of her pill consumption and of coordinating her consumption with her menstrual cycle. Over the years since combinations appeared on the market, the estrogen content has been considerably decreased in several products, because of the possible adverse effects of the estrogen component.

To provide a more normal mense and also possibly to decrease the incidence of adverse effects, *sequential* products were introduced. The estrogen was given alone during the first 14 to 16 days then combined with a progestin in the same pill for the next 5 to 7 days, thus covering 20 to 23 days of the cycle. These preparations have been removed from the market in the US because they were not acceptably effective as contraceptives and because their use was associated with elevated risk of adenocarcinoma and thromboembolic disease. Continued stimulation by estrogens unopposed by progestins during half of the cycle probably accounted for the increased risks associated with these drugs.

Continuous progestin-only oral products do not contain any estrogen and furthermore contain the progestin in amounts smaller (the so-called "mini-pill") than those used in combination or sequential products. The dose is small enough not to prevent ovulation and menstruation in most users, yet to act sufficiently on the uterus, cervix, or capacitance to prevent conception. However, the efficacy is less than with combination or sequential products. *Continuous-progestin injectable* products, repository forms of progestins, are also available, but they are not approved for contraceptive purposes.

Postcoital oral contraceptives (so-called "morning-after pills") have long been used in emergencies, such as rape, and they are now somewhat more widely used, as in student health services, to prevent pregnancy in girls or women who are caught without contraceptive preparation; these preparations, however, are not for routine use, inasmuch as the doses of estrogens employed are very high. They are effective if taken within 72 hours after coitus. *Postconception* "pills," still in the experimental stage, contain various antiluteal substances, so that the embryo is unable to remain implanted in the endometrium; there is great interest in prostaglandin congeners which may have antiluteal effects but minor gastrointestinal and other activity. Antagonist analogues of the gonadotropins and gonadotropin-releasing hormones provide the impetus for a way to prevent ovulation without the side effects of the steroid hormones. Oral contraception in the male has been approached experimentally by the use of drugs that inhibit sperm production, maturation, or transport. No safe drugs have yet been found. An interesting nonpharmacological development is immunization against the sperm or certain of its enzymes; in the female there seem to be few complications to such immunization, but there are in the male.

Efficacy and Failures—The efficacy of an oral contraceptive depends on the type and the dose of hormonal ingredients. The combined type which contains relatively high doses of estrogens is nearly 100% effective when taken correctly; failures can probably be attributed to the negligence of the user. There appears to be a finite, though small, probability of ovulation and hence of later conception if a single pill is missed, because of the rebound oversecretion of the gonadotropins. If one pill is skipped, the user should take it immediately upon discovery of the skip and take the rest on their schedule; if two or more are missed, she should additionally use other methods of contraception until her next cycle. Lowering the estrogen content in combination preparations decreases the side effects but increases the risk of pregnancy. The long-acting combinations have a relatively high failure rate. The continuous low-dose oral progestin products have a failure rate several times that of combination products.

The oral contraceptives provide excellent contraception when used by emotionally stable, intelligent, educated women, but are not as satisfactory among uneducated or emotionally labile women. This is because the demanding uninterrupted use requires understanding of the importance of the schedule as well as the consequences of pregnancy, and consistent determination. In underdeveloped countries, intrauterine devices are much more serviceable.

Adverse Effects—The medical and lay literature, alike, have been filled with accounts of adverse effects of the oral contraceptives, and many previous or potential users have been frightened away from these drugs. The adverse effects vary in incidence and severity according to the type of preparation. Most side effects are from the estrogens (see page 985) in combination contraceptives, but progestins also cause adverse effects. The estrogen-progestin ratio is important to the type and incidence of side effects.

Some side effects are of little consequence to the health of the user and present difficulties only as the user or physician reacts to them. Oligomenorrhea occurs in 20 to 80% of users of combination and some continuous progestin contraceptives, and amenorrhea occurs in some. The greatest offenders are the 19-nortestosterone derivatives. Some users consider oligomenorrhea a boon, yet others are emotionally disturbed by this innocuous effect. Spotting and breakthrough bleeding is more annoying, since its irregularity and unpredictability are inconvenient; sometimes such bleeding is more voluminous than in regular menstruation. Side effects such as tiredness, weakness, malaise, changes in libido, dizziness, nonspecific headaches, and psychiatric symptoms are often the result of suggestion and conditioning and occur frequently when placebos are used, so that it is difficult to state to what degree such effects are attributable to the oral contraceptives. An increase in the incidence of migraine headaches, however, is indisputable; the estrogen component appears to be responsible. Weight gain occurs with some but not all preparations; salt and water retention is mostly caused by estrogen components, whereas anabolic effects are caused by higher doses of the 19-nortestosterone-derived progestins (not the 17α-hydroxyprogesterones). Chloasma occurs in about 4% of users of combination contraceptives during the 1st year and 37% by the 5th year; it is attributable to the combined action of the two active components. Milk flow in lactating women may be decreased by an average of 50% when combination preparations are used. Changes in the color and secretions of the cervix may be misinterpreted as infection or carcinoma by the uninformed physician. Bacteriuria and urinary tract infections are more common in users than in nonusers. Estrogen-containing contraceptives also cause an uncommon choreiform movement.

Serious side effects of oral contraceptives are multiple. A reversible hypertension is observed in approximately 15% of users of estrogen-containing contraceptives; this is more than the incidence when estrogens are used alone for noncontraceptive purposes and suggests modulation by progestins. The prevalence of hypertension increases with duration of use and is greater in older women. Incidence of thromboembolic disorders, including stroke and myocardial infarction, is higher in women using oral contraceptives; the relative risk may be several times greater in users as compared to control populations. Further, the risk increases sharply in women over 35 years of age. Contraceptive use has also been associated with increased evidence of benign liver tumors. The relative risk of liver tumors appears to rise with duration of use of the drugs. In one study, mestranol-containing preparations were almost exclusively implicated, thus indicating that the type of synthetic estrogen might be important. Risk of gallbladder disease is increased two-fold in contraceptive users. Fetal abnormalities may result if the mother continues to take the pill after becoming pregnant. Neuroocular lesions have been associated with use of oral contraceptives. Some other possible complications of contraceptive use include breast cancer (pill use actually protects against the development of benign breast lesions), and cancer of the uterus, cervix and vagina. Any of the other side effects of estrogens or progestins given above may also be caused by these drugs. Patients taking oral contraceptives must be informed of their effectiveness and risks.

Perspectives—Oral contraceptives are potent drugs that are remarkably effective in prevention of pregnancy. They are not benign drugs and have many recognized and potential side effects. However, pregnancy itself is not without hazard, and it can be argued that risks of death and serious illness are less with oral contraceptives than with pregnancy in most women. Risks of serious complications with oral contraceptive use increase as the dose, duration of therapy and age of the patient increase, and as other risk factors, such as smoking, increase. Therefore, a prudent attitude toward oral contraceptives as a birth-control method would be as follows: There are relatively few contraindications to their use in young, healthy, sexually active women who seek careful control of family size and spacing. The risks associated with the low-dose combinations are less than with high-dose preparations. Once reproduction is completed or as a female approaches middle age, it probably would be wise to seek other methods of contraception.

Conjugated Estrogens—page 986.

Diethylstilbestrol—page 988.

Estrone—page 986.

Ethinyl Estradiol—page 987.

Ethynodiol Diacetate and Ethinyl Estradiol Tablets

Demulen (*Searle*)

Uses—For *combination oral contraception* (see page 994). For the actions of the separate components, see *Ethynodiol Diacetate* (page 991) and *Ethinyl Estradiol* (page 987). The adverse effects are mainly those of the ethinyl estradiol (see page 987); see also this page for adverse effects of combinations).

Dose—1 mg of ethynodiol diacetate and either 35 or 50 µg of ethinyl estradiol a day for 21 days, starting on the 5th day after the beginning of menstruation. One commercial product provides 7 placebo pills for the other 7 days of the cycle, in order to avoid interruption of the daily routine of pilltaking.

Dosage Form—Tablets: Ethynodiol Diacetate/Ethinyl Estradiol, 1 mg/35 or 50 µg.

Ethynodiol Diacetate and Mestranol Tablets

Ovulen (*Searle*)

Uses—For *combination oral contraception* (see page 994). For the actions of the separate components, see *Ethynodiol Diacetate* (page 991) and *Mestranol* (page 989). The mixture may also be used in various conditions in which progestogens are indicated, particularly in those situations in which anovulation is desired (see *Progestational Substances*, page 990). In large doses it may also be used to arrest dysfunctional uterine bleeding. Adverse effects in decreasing order of incidence are nausea, spotting, breakthrough bleeding, headache, dizziness, depression, edema, amenorrhea, breast tenderness, vomiting, and several miscellaneous effects of uncommon occurrence. Like all such mixtures, there is a possibility that the mixture favors rare venous thrombosis.

Dose—1 mg of *ethynodiol* acetate and 100 μg of *mestranol* daily for 20 or 21 days, starting on the 5th day after menstruation begins. One commercial product provides 7 placebo pills, in order to avoid interruption of the daily routine of pilltaking.

Dosage Form—Tablets: Ethynodiol Diacetate/Mestranol, 1 mg/100 μg.

Norethindrone—page 992.

Norethindrone and Ethinyl Estradiol Tablets

Ortho-Novum (*Ortho*)

Uses—For combination oral contraception (see page 994). For the action of the separate components, see *Norethindrone* (page 992) and *Ethinyl Estradiol* (page 987).

Dose—Combinations (norethindrone:ethinyl estradiol): **1 mg:50 μg** or **1 mg:35 μg** or **0.5 mg:35 μg** or **0.4 mg:35 μg** a day for 21 days, starting on the 5th day after beginning of menstruation. Several preparations are available in a 28-day pack in which 7 inert tablets are supplied for the other 7 days of the cycle so that the daily routine of pill taking is not altered. An exception for these routines is found in Ortho-Novum 10/11 (Ortho) in which **0.5 mg** norethindone and **35 μg** of ethinyl estradiol daily are taken for the first 10 days of the dose period and **1 mg** of norethindrone and **35 μg** of ethinyl estradiol daily are taken for the final 11 days of the dose period.

Dosage Forms—Tablets: Norethindrone/Ethinyl Estradiol, 1 mg/50 μg, 1 mg/35 μg, 0.5 mg/35 μg, 0.4 mg/35 μg.

Norethindrone and Mestranol Tablets

(*Various Mfrs*)

Uses—For *combination oral contraception* (see page 994). For the actions and uses of the separate components, see *Norethindrone* (page 992) and *Mestranol* (page 989). In the higher dose forms, at least, suppression of gonadotropin release by both components probably occurs, but in the products with low doses of norethindrone, the mestranol is the primary anovulatory agent. In addition to its role in the anovulatory effect, mestranol antagonizes some of the androgenic actions of norethindrone. The combination has been used in nearly all conditions in which progestins are indicated (see page 990), particularly in those situations where anovulation is desirable. It has also been used to regularize uterine bleeding.

These tablets were formerly used in a *sequential oral contraceptive* regimen in which the estrogen was given first and the progestogen was given after a proliferative endometrium was established.

For the side effects, see pages 985, 990, and 995.

Dose—*Combinations* (*norethindrone:mestranol*): *Oral*, for *contraception*, **2 mg:100 μg** a day for 20 or 21 days; **1 mg:80 μg** a day for 21 days, sometimes followed by a placebo tablet on days 22 through 28; **1 mg:50 μg** a day for either 20 or 21 days, with a placebo for 7 days in some 21-day products; all medication, above, is to start on the 5th day of the menstrual cycle. For *therapy*, **10 mg:60 μg** a day for 20 days.

Dosage Forms—Tablets: Norethindrone/Mestranol, 1/20, 1/50, 1/80, 2/100, and 10/60 mg/μg.

Norethindrone Acetate and Ethinyl Estradiol Tablets

Norlestrin (*Parke-Davis*); Zorane (*Lederle*)

Uses—For *combination oral contraception* (see page 994). Some products are quite low in estrogen content. For the actions of the separate components, see *Norethindrone Acetate* (page 992) and *Ethinyl Estradiol* (page 987). The antifertility effect appears to be due more to the progestogen than the estrogen. Adverse effects are essentially the same as those of the separate components (pages 987 and 992) and of combination preparations in general (page 994).

Dose—The following combinations of *norethindrone acetate: ethinyl estradiol* are used: **2.5 mg:50 μg, 1.5 mg:30 μg, 1 mg:50 μg,** and **1 mg:20 μg**. All are taken for 21 days, starting with the 5th day of menstruation, except for the 2.5 mg:50 μg combination which can be taken for only 21 days, if desired. Each of these combinations is available in a product which provides 7 iron tablets, to be taken on days 27 through 4, during which no hormones are given.

Dosage Forms—Tablets containing the combinations listed under *Dose*.

Norethynodrel and Mestranol Tablets

Enovid (*Searle*); Enovid E (*Searle*)

Uses—This combination became famous the world over as an oral contraceptive and has been dubbed "The Pill." See page 989. For the effects of the separate components, see *Norethynodrel* (page 993) and *Mestranol* (page 989). The contraceptive action is not entirely the result of prevention of ovulation; the endometrium is rendered inhospitable to the fertilized ovum, so that nidation cannot take place. In addition to oral contraceptive use, preparations containing 5 mg or more of norethynodrel may be used in the treatment of *dysmenorrhea* and *menorrhagia* and to produce cyclic withdrawal bleeding.

The side effects are those of the separate components as well as of combination contraceptives (page 995). The most frequent effects are bleeding irregularities, nausea, and vomiting in about $\frac{1}{4}$ of all users, breast fullness, chloasma, headache, weakness, dizziness, and diarrhea. The effects diminish with continual use. Sometimes fluid retention and acne occur. Cholestatic jaundice occurs rarely.

Dose—For *contraception*, norethynodrel (**2.5 or 5 mg**) plus *mestranol* (**100 or 75 μg,** respectively) daily for 20 or 21 days, starting on the 5th day after menstruation begins. For *cyclic therapy* in dysmenorrhea, functional uterine bleeding (once it is controlled), premenstrual tension, amenorrhea (once a menses has been accomplished), or idiopathic infertility, one 5:75 or 9.85:150 tablet daily for 20 days of each cycle, beginning on the 5th day after menstruation begins; for emergency control of *dysfunctional uterine bleeding*, one 9.85:150-mg tablet 2 or 3 times a day until bleeding is arrested, then once daily through the 24th day after menstruation began; for *endometriosis*, one 5:75 or 9.85:150 tablet daily for 2 weeks, beginning on the 5th day after menstruation begins, increasing in dosage every 2 weeks until 20 mg of norethynodrel a day is being given, to be continued for 6 to 9 months; to *delay menstruation*, one to two 9.85:150 tablets daily, beginning at least 1 week in advance of the expected menstruation; to *advance menstruation*, one 5:75 or 9.85:150 tablet for 10 days, beginning on the 5th day after the start of menstruation.

Dosage Forms—Tablets: Norethynodrel:Mestranol, 2.5:100, 5:75, and 9.85:150 mg:μg.

Norgestrel—page 993.

Norgestrel and Ethinyl Estradiol Tablets

Ovral (*Wyeth*)

Uses—For *combination oral contraception* (see page 994). For the actions of the separate components see *Norgestrel* (page 993) and *Ethinyl Estradiol* (page 987). The adverse effects are those of the estrogens (page 984), progestins (page 990), and combinations (page 995).

Dose—*Oral, adult,* for *contraception,* **500 μg** of *norgestrel* plus **50 μg** of *ethinyl estradiol* or **300 μg** of *norgestrel* plus **30 μg** of *ethinyl estradiol* a day for 21 days, starting on the 5th day of the menstrual cycle; for *postcoital contraception,* **1 mg** of *norgestrel* plus **100 μg** of *ethinyl estradiol* twice at 12-hr intervals.

Dosage Forms—Tablets: Norgestrel:Mestranol, 500:50 and 300:30 μg:μg.

Progesterone—page 993.

The Testicular Hormone

The testis has a dual function, to produce the germ cell (the *sperm*) and to supply the male hormone (*testosterone*). Two clearly defined groups of cells are found in the testes; the one group in the tubules produces the sperm, while the other, clustered in between the tubules, consists of interstitial cells (Leydig cells). The spermatogenic tissue produces an exocrine secretion and probably also androgens needed for spermatogenesis.

The interstitial cells are the seat of production of a steroid hormone, testosterone, which stimulates and maintains the secondary sex organs; these are the penis, prostate gland, seminal vesicles, vas deferens, and scrotum. It also exerts sustaining effects on the spermatogenic cells, and it stimulates the development of bone, muscle, skin, and hair growth, and emotional responses to produce the characteristic adult masculine traits. This group of combined actions of this hormone is termed *androgenic actions*. Testosterone also antagonizes a number of the effects of estrogens, and is sometimes employed clinically for this purpose. This is especially important in the suppression of metastatic carcinoma of the breast. Since it promotes development of the clitoris, which is an anatomic homologue of the penis, androgens may increase the libido of women.

The naturally occurring androgens (androsterone, testosterone) are derivatives of androstane. Testosterone and its esters (testosterone propionate) and derivatives (methyltestosterone) are the most commonly used androgenic steroids. In addition to their androgenic properties, however, these compounds exert widespread anabolic effects and promote the retention of calcium. In attempts to dissociate the virilizing and anabolic properties (for use in women) a number of compounds with high anabolic : androgenic ratios have been prepared. However, it has not yet been possible to abolish completely the androgenic effects.

Uses—For *substitutional therapy* in men who have climacteric symptoms, or in men or youths with *hypogonadism* (eunuchism, Klinefelter's syndrome). They have been employed to facilitate development of adult masculine characteristics when the adolescent process has been delayed. In *cryptorchidism* they may be used adjunctively with gonadotropins. They are also very useful in therapy of patients with *hypopituitarism* and with *Addison's disease*. They are of value in the treatment of *frigidity* and occasionally in *impotence*. Use of androgens for relief of impotence not associated with evidence of testicular underactivity (psychic causes) is known to be futile in most cases. Low doses of androgens have been used in pituitary dwarfism to *accelerate growth*, but care must be exercised not to arrest growth by epiphyseal closure. They are also sometimes used to *promote hematopoiesis*. The use of anabolic steroids to improve athletic performance has not only been condemned by the American College of Sports Medicine but is also of questionable efficacy in males; female performance may be improved, but at the expense of virilization.

With estrogens, androgen therapy may be efficacious in the treatment of the *menopause*. The anabolic effects are possibly of some benefit in the postclimacteric person, and they may retard *osteoporosis*, although many authorities do not believe that any lasting benefit is achieved. In functional *dysmenorrhea* androgens may give relief through an antiestrogenic action, although they also are often combined with estrogens to treat this disorder. They may be used to treat *endometriosis*. They may also be used in the treatment of *postpartum breast engorgement* and for *suppression of lactation*.

Testosterone and related compounds find widespread application in the palliative treatment of *cancer of the breast* in women. Its use in men with prostatic cancer, however, is contraindicated.

Side Effects—Androgens cause hirsutism, deepening or hoarseness of the voice, precocious puberty and epiphyseal closure in immature males, increased libido (in both male and female!), priapism, oligospermia (from negative feedback on LH and FSH production), enlargement of the clitoris in the female, flushing, decreased ejaculatory volume, gynecomastia, hypersensitivity, acne, weight gain, edema, and hypercalcemia. Biliary stasis and jaundice occur. There have been a few cases reported of hepatoma following long-term therapy. The 17α-methylated androgens are more prone to disturb liver function than are the nonsubstituted drugs. Hypercalcemia requires discontinuation of therapy, and edema requires diuretic therapy. Except in the treatment of breast cancer, a reduction in dosage is indicated upon virilization in women.

Administration of androgens to patients on anticoagulant therapy may increase the effect of anticoagulants and thus may require an adjustment of the dose of the latter. Likewise, dosage of insulin or of oral hypoglycemic agents may require adjustment when anabolic androgens are administered to diabetic patients.

Danazol

Pregna-2,4-dien-20-yno[2,3-d]isoxazol-17-ol, (17α)-, Chronogyn; Danocrine (*Winthrop*)

[17230-88-5] $C_{22}H_{27}NO_2$ (337.46).

Preparation—Danazol is a derivative of ethisterone (17α-ethynyltestosterone) in which an isoxazole ring is fused to the 2,3-position of the steroid nucleus. Methods for preparing such steroidal heterocycles have been described by Manson *et al*, *J Med Chem 6*: 1, 1963, also in US Pat 3,135,743.

Description—Pale yellow, crystalline powder; melts at about 225°.

Solubility—Practically insoluble in water; sparingly soluble in alcohol.

Uses—Danazol is a synthetic androgen with weak androgenic activity and no progestational or estrogenic effects. It suppresses the release of LH and FSH. It is used in the treatment of *endometriosis* in patients who do not respond to or cannot tolerate other drug therapy and in the management of *fibrocystic breast disease*. It may prevent attacks of *hereditary angioedema*. Androgenic side effects include acne, edema, mild hirsutism, decrease in breast size, oiliness of the skin and hair, weight gain, and clitoral hypertrophy. Hypoestrogenic manifestations include vasomotor instability, vaginitis with itching, burning and vaginal bleeding, and emotional lability. In doses over 400 mg/day, danazole may cause hepatic injury, including carcinoma. Danazol has been reported to lower serum levothyroxine levels.

Dose—*Oral, adult*, for *endometriosis*, **400 mg** twice a day for at least 3 to 6 months; for *fibrocystic breast* disease **50 to 200 mg** twice a day; for *angioedoma*, *initially* **200 mg** 2 or 3 times a day then, once the effect has been achieved, then decrements of no more than 50%, according to the frequency of attacks.

Dosage Form—Capsules: 50, 100, and 200 mg.

Dromostanolone Propionate

Androstan-3-one, 2-methyl-17-(1-oxopropoxy)-, (2α,5α,17β)-,
Drolban (*Lilly*)

17β-Hydroxy-2α-methyl-5α-androstan-3-one propionate [521-12-0] $C_{23}H_{36}O_3$ (360.54).

Preparation—Testosterone is reacted with ethyl formate and alkali metal hydride to form 2-(hydroxymethylene)testosterone (I) (*J Am Chem Soc 76:* 552, 1954). Refluxing a benzene suspension of I, methyl iodide, and sodium hydride under nitrogen produces 2-formyl-2-methyltestosterone which is then decarbonylated by passage through a column of alkalinized alumina to yield 2α-methyltestosterone (II). Esterification of II with propionic anhydride in pyridine solution forms II propionate which yields dromostanolone propionate on hydrogenation in the presence of palladium on barium sulfate or various other catalysts. US Pat 3,118,915.

Description—White to creamy white, crystalline powder; odorless or has a faint odor; melts, with a range of 4°, between 127° and 133°.

Solubility—1 g in 30 mL alcohol, 2 mL chloroform, 20 mL ether; practically insoluble in water.

Uses—An *androgen* similar in its actions to *Testosterone Propionate* (page 1001), but it appears to be somewhat less virilizing. Its use has been restricted to the treatment of *metastatic carcinoma of the breast*. With respect to efficacy in the regression of the carcinoma, it is about equivalent to testosterone propionate, but its lesser virilizing activity makes dromostanolone advantageous. The drug may improve anemia and the patient's sense of well-being, but these effects are unrelated to regression of the disease.

The untoward effects of dromostanolone are mainly those which result from virilization and include facial hair growth, deepening of the voice, acne, and enlargement of the clitoris, which occasionally may give rise to an increase in libido. The virilizing effects develop slowly and may not reach their peak for several months. Fluid retention with edema may occur. Effects on serum calcium are not untoward but rather reflect the success of the drug on osteolytic metastases; if regression occurs, serum calcium falls. Jaundice has not been reported, but the potential exists. Dromostanolone should be used with caution in the presence of liver disease, heart failure, kidney disease, and pregnancy.

Dose—*Intramuscular*, **100 mg** 3 times a week for 8 to 12 weeks or for the duration of a remission caused by the drug.

Dosage Forms—Injection: 500 mg/10 mL.

Fluoxymesterone

Androst-4-en-3-one, 9-fluoro-11,17-dihydroxy-17-methyl-, (11β,17β)-,
Halotestin (*Upjohn*); Ora-Testryl (*Squibb*)

9-Fluoro-11β,17β-dihydroxy-17-methylandrost-4-en-3-one [76-43-7] $C_{20}H_{29}FO_3$ (336.45).

Preparation—From 17-methyltestosterone first by introduction of a hydroxyl group at position 11 through oxidation with a microorganism (such as *Pestalotia* or *Aspergillus*), followed by dehydration, epoxidation and treatment with HF, as for *Betamethasone* (page 902).

Description—White or practically white, odorless, crystalline powder; melts at about 240°, with some decomposition.

Solubility—Practically insoluble in water; sparingly soluble in alcohol; slightly soluble in chloroform.

Uses—The same actions, uses, and limitations as androgens (page 997). It is approximately five times more potent than testosterone, and is orally effective. Nevertheless, it is less effective than testosterone in hypogonadism and is seldom used to initiate treatment but

rather for maintenance. In addition to the side effects of testosterone, fluoxymesterone may cause occasional cholestatic jaundice, gynecomastia, oligospermia after prolonged use, and hypersensitivity. Fluoxymesterone is sometimes combined with an estrogen for treatment of postmenopausal osteoporosis.

Dose—*Oral, adult, replacement therapy*, **1** to **5 mg** twice a day; for *delayed puberty*, initially **2 mg**/day followed by gradual increments, if necessary; for *anabolic effect* and treatment of *osteoporosis*, **2** to **5 mg** twice a day; for metastatic *breast cancer* in women, **5** to **10 mg** 3 times a day; in *hypoplastic* or *aplastic anemia*, **10** to **40 mg** a day; for *postpartum breast engorgement*, **2.5** to **5 mg** twice a day for 4 or 5 days postpartum.

Dosage Forms—Tablets: 2, 5 and 10 mg.

Methandrostenolone

Androsta-1,4-diene-3-one, 17-hydroxy-17-methyl-, (17β)-,
Methandienone; Dianabol (*Ciba*)

[72-63-9] $C_{20}H_{28}O_2$ (300.44).

Preparation—*Methyltestosterone* is dehydrogenated, either by microbial methods or by reaction with selenium dioxide, to create the Δ^1 double bond. US Pat 2,900,398.

Description—White to off-white crystals or crystalline powder; odorless; melts at about 165°.

Solubility—Insoluble in water; soluble in alcohol, chloroform, glacial acetic acid; slightly soluble in ether.

Uses—An androgenic steroid with relatively strong anabolic and weak androgenic activity. Consequently, it is employed mainly to *promote nitrogen anabolism* and weight gain in cachexia and debilitating diseases and after serious infections, burns, trauma, or surgery. It may relieve pain in certain types of *osteoporosis*, and it favors the retention of calcium, which assists in arresting the disease. It also helps to relieve pain and to promote a sense of well-being in the arthritides. Side effects include virilization and acne, especially in women and children, sodium retention and edema, and cholestatic jaundice. Methandrostenolone potentiates prothrombopenic anticoagulants and hence may favor hemorrhagic diatheses in persons taking such drugs.

Dose—*Oral, initially*, **5 mg** daily and, for *maintenance*, **2.5** to **5 mg** daily, except **10** to **20 mg**/day in *severe debilitation* and up to **50 µg/kg** a day in older children and adults with *pituitary dwarfism*. Continuous therapy should consist in repeated courses of no longer than 6 weeks, separated by intervals of 2 to 4 weeks.

Dosage Forms—Scored Tablets: 2.5 and 5 mg.

Methyltestosterone

Androst-4-en-3-one, 17-hydroxy-17-methyl-, (17β)-,
Metandren (*Ciba-Geigy*); Oreton Methyl (*Schering-Plough*)

[58-18-4] $C_{20}H_{30}O_2$ (302.46).

Preparation—Readily from dehydroepiandrosterone (prepared from cholesterol) by subjecting it to a Grignard reaction with CH_3MgI followed by an Oppenauer oxidation. The first reaction creates the tertiary carbinol structure at C_{17}, while the second oxidizes the secondary carbinol group at position 3 to carbonyl and causes a rearrangement of the double bond from the 5,6- to the 4,5- position.

Description—White or creamy white crystals or a crystalline powder; odorless, stable in air, but slightly hygroscopic; affected by light; melts between 162° and 167°.

Solubility—Practically insoluble in water; soluble in alcohol, methanol, ether, and other organic solvents; sparingly soluble in vegetable oils.

Uses—The actions, uses, and limitations are the same as those of androgens in general (page 997). Methyltestosterone is effective orally. It is also combined with various estrogens for treatment of menorrhagia, menopausal symptoms, dysmenorrhea, osteoporosis, malnutrition, and to suppress postpartum lactation. In addition to the side effects caused by testosterone, methyltestosterone may cause oligospermia, hypersensitivity with dermatologic manifestations, and a rare type of cholestatic jaundice. It is often stated that virilization in women does not occur unless the dose exceeds 300 mg/month, but virilization can occur with doses considerably less than this.

By the buccal route, potency is twice that by the oral route.

Dose—*Oral, adolescent* and *adult* for *replacement therapy*, **5 mg** 1 to 4 times a day; for *anabolic* effects, **10 to 20 mg** a day; for *inoperable breast cancer* in women, **25 mg** 4 times a day for the duration of improvement or for no longer than 3 months if there is no remission. *Buccal*, one-half the oral dose.

Dosage Forms—Capsules: 10 mg; Tablets: 10 mg; Tablets (buccal): 5 and 10 mg.

Nandrolone Decanoate

Estr-4-en-3-one, 17-[(1-oxodecyl)oxy]-, (17β)-,
Deca-Durabolin (*Organon*)

17β-Hydroxyestr-4-en-3-one decanoate [360-70-3] $C_{28}H_{44}O_3$ (428.65).

Preparation—A dry benzene solution of 17β-hydroxy-estr-4-en-3-one (19-nortestosterone) and pyridine is mixed with a dry benzene solution of decanoyl chloride and the esterification is allowed to proceed overnight in an atmosphere of nitrogen. After washing successively with acid, alkali, and water, the solvent is evaporated and the crude ester is recrystallized from petroleum ether or some other suitable solvent. US Pat 2,998,423.

Description—Fine, white to creamy white, crystalline powder; odorless or may have a slight odor; melts between 33° and 37°.

Solubility—Soluble in chloroform, alcohol, acetone, and vegetable oils; practically insoluble in water.

Uses—The actions and uses are the same as those of *Nandrolone Phenpropionate*. Oil solutions of the decanoate have a duration of action 3 to 4 times longer than that of the phenpropionate.

Dose—*Intramuscular, adult, anabolic* or for *osteoporosis*, **50 to 100 mg** every 3 to 4 weeks; *metastatic breast carcinoma* or *refractory anemias*, **100 to 200 mg** a week. *Children 2 to 13 years of age, anabolic*, **25 to 50 mg** every 3 to 4 weeks; other pediatric doses not determined.

Dosage Forms—Injection: 50 mg/1 mL, 100 mg/2 mL, 200 mg/1 mL, 200 mg/2 mL.

Nandrolone Phenpropionate

Estr-4-en-3-one, 17-(1-oxo-3-phenylpropoxy)-, (17β)-,
Durabolin (*Organon*)

17β-Hydroxyestr-4-en-3-one hydrocinnamate [62-90-8] $C_{27}H_{34}O_3$ (406.56).

For the structure of the steroid moiety, see *Nandrolone Decanoate*.

Preparation—19-Nortestosterone is esterified with hydrocinnamoyl chloride by the method described for *Nandrolone Decanoate*.

Description—Fine, white to creamy white, crystalline powder having a slight characteristic odor; melts between 95° and 99°.

Solubility—Practically insoluble in water; soluble in alcohol (1 g in 2 mL), chloroform, dioxane, and vegetable oils.

Uses—A synthetic androgen with actions intermediate to those of *Testosterone* and *Norethandrolone*. Although nandrolone phenpropionate is less androgenic than testosterone in doses which exert anabolic actions, virilization may occur after high doses or during chronic administration. Indeed, the androgenic virilizing actions are sought in the treatment with this agent of *inoperable breast cancer* in women. Nandrolone phenpropionate is mainly used in the treatment of *chronic wasting diseases, conditions in which negative nitrogen balance exists* and *osteoporosis*. Low doses may *accelerate growth of children* with retarded growth without excessively accelerating bone age; higher doses accelerate bone maturation more than body growth. The phenylpropionate ester moiety confers a long duration of action to suspensions in oil injected intramuscularly. The potential side effects are those of testosterone. Nandrolone phenpropionate does not appear to cause cholestatic jaundice, probably because it lacks an alkyl group on carbon 17.

Dose—*Intramuscular, adults, anabolic* or for *osteoporosis*, **25 to 50 mg** each week; *inoperable breast cancer* and *refractory anemias*, **50 to 100 mg** a week. For *children* 2 to 13 years of age, **12.5 to 25 mg** every 2 to 4 weeks; for *infants*, **1 mg/kg** of body weight every 2 to 4 weeks.

Dosage Forms—Injection: 25 mg/1 mL, 50 mg/2 mL, 125 mg/5 mL.

Oxandrolone

2-Oxaandrostan-3-one, 17-hydroxy-17-methyl-, (5α,17β)-,
Anavar (*Searle*)

17β-Hydroxy-17-methyl-2-oxa-5α-androstan-3-one [53-39-4] $C_{19}H_{30}O_3$ (306.44).

Preparation—Methyldihydrotesterone is converted into the corresponding 1,2-dehydro compound by bromination followed by dehydrobromination. Ring A is then ruptured through ozonization and subsequent hydrolysis to yield the aldehyde-acid (I). Reduction of the formyl group in I yields the expected hydroxy acid implied in the partial structure (II) which is lactonized to oxandrolone.

(I) (II)

Description—White, odorless, crystalline powder; stable in air but darkens when exposed to light; melts at about 225°.

Solubility—1 g in 5200 mL water, 57 mL alcohol, <5 mL chloroform, 860 mL ether, 69 mL acetone.

Uses—Although not strictly speaking a steroid, its configuration is that of a 17-methyl androgenic steroid. Its anabolic actions are strong relative to its androgenic actions. Consequently, it is used in the treatment of *chronic wasting diseases*, conditions in which *negative nitrogen balance* exists and *osteoporosis*, especially that caused by glucocorticoids. It lowers VLDL and is an investigational drug for hypertriglyceridemia in men. The drug may cause virilization in children or women, especially if the recommended doses are exceeded. The potential toxicity is that of the androgens but the incidence and severity are less than with testosterone. Oxandrolone may adversely affect liver function tests, and the possibility of cholestatic jaundice must be kept in mind. Leukopenia has also been reported. It is contraindicated in prostatic cancer, breast cancer in some women, pregnancy, nephrosis, and premature and newborn infants.

Dose—*Oral, adults, initially* **2.5 to 5 mg** 2 to 4 times a day, then **2.5 to 5 mg** a day for *maintenance*, not to be taken for more than 3 months in any one course; for *children*, **250 μg/kg** a day, repeated as indicated.

Dosage Form—Tablets: 2.5 mg.

Oxymetholone

Androstan-3-one, 17-hydroxy-2-(hydroxymethylene)-17-methyl-, (5α,17β)-, Anadrol (*Syntex*)

[434-07-1] $C_{21}H_{32}O_3$ (332.48).

Preparation—17β-Hydroxy-17-methylandrostan-3-one (17-methyldihydrotestosterone) is reacted with ethyl formate and sodium hydroxide by stirring the mixture under nitrogen for several hours thus forming the 2-(sodoxymethylene) derivative. Treatment of the washed sodium compound with cold dilute hydrochloric acid liberates the oxymetholone which may be purified by recrystallization from ethyl acetate. *J Am Chem Soc 81:* 427, 1959.

Description—White to creamy white crystals or crystalline powder; odorless and stable in air; tautomeric in nature and can exist as either tautomer or as a mixture of both, the exact composition depending on solvent and rate of crystallization; melts between 172° and 180°.

Solubility—1 g in >10,000 mL water, 40 mL alcohol, 5 mL chloroform, 82 mL ether, 14 mL dioxane.

Uses—An androgenic steroid with relatively greater anabolic activity than androgenic activity. Consequently, it is mainly employed to *promote nitrogen anabolism* and weight gain in cachexia and debilitating diseases and after serious infections, burns, trauma or surgery. It may relieve pain in certain types of *osteoporosis*, and it promotes calcium retention, so that the condition of the bone may improve. It may be used for its erythropoietic effects in the treatment of *hypoplastic* and *aplastic* anemias. Side effects include nausea, vomiting, anorexia, burning of the tongue, increased or decreased libido, acne, suppression of gonadotropin secretion, virilization (especially in women and children), gynecomastia in males, oligospermia, sodium retention and edema, abnormal liver function tests, cholestatic jaundice, decrease in several clotting factors, and hemorrhagic diathesis in the presence of anticoagulants.

Dose—*Oral, adults*, 1 to **5 mg/kg** of body weight a day, preferably for 3 weeks and never longer than 13 weeks/course, with rests of 2 to 4 weeks between courses; in *prepuberal children*, **2.5 to 5 mg** a day, for not more than 30 days/course.

Dosage Forms—Tablets: 50 mg.

Stanozolol

2′H-Androst-2-eno[3,2-c]pyrazol-17-ol, 17-methyl-, (5α,17β)-, Winstrol (*Winthrop*)

17-Methyl-2′H-5α-androst-2-eno[3,2-c]pyrazol-17β-ol [10418-03-8] $C_{21}H_{32}N_2O$ (328.50).

Preparation—17-Methyl-5α-androstan-17β-ol-3-one is converted into its 2-formyl derivative which is then condensed with hydrazine hydrate. US Pat 3,030,358.

Description—Nearly colorless, odorless, crystalline powder; exists in two forms: *needles*, melting at about 155°, and *prisms*, melting at about 235°.

Solubility—1 g in >1000 mL water, 41 mL alcohol, 74 mL chloroform, 370 mL ether.

Uses—An *androgenic steroid* with relatively strong anabolic and weak androgenic activity. Consequently, it is employed mainly to *promote nitrogen anabolism* and weight gain in cachexia and debilitating diseases and after serious infections, burns, trauma, or surgery. Although it may relieve pain in certain types of *osteoporosis*, it apparently does not affect bone density. It may have an erythropoietic effect in *hypoplastic* and *aplastic anemias*.

Side effects include increased or decreased libido, virilization (especially in women and children), sodium retention and edema, hypercalcemia, insomnia, restlessness, chills, hemorrhage in patients on anticoagulants, acne, and hepatic dysfunction. Potentially any of the side effects of *Testosterone* may occur.

Dose—*Oral, adults*, **2 mg** 3 times a day, except twice a day in women who are easily virilized by the usual dose. *Children under 6 years* of age, **1 mg** twice a day; *children 6 to 12 years* of age, up to 2 mg 3 times a day.

Dosage Form—Scored Tablets: 2 mg.

Testolactone

D-Homo-17a-oxaandrosta-1,4-diene-3,17-dione; Teslac (*Squibb*)

13-Hydroxy-3-oxo-13,17-secoandrosta-1,4-dien-17-oic acid δ-lactone [968-93-4] $C_{19}H_{24}O_3$ (300.40).

Preparation—By microbial transformation of progesterone, testosterone, and various other steroidal substances. US Pat 2,744,120; *J Org Chem 30:* 760, 1965.

Description—White to off-white, practically odorless, crystalline powder; stable in light, air, and normal temperatures; melts at about 218°.

Solubility—Slightly soluble in water and benzyl alcohol; soluble in alcohol and chloroform; insoluble in ether and solvent hexane.

Uses—Although structurally related to the androgens, it is essentially devoid of androgenic activity in therapeutic doses. It is used in the adjunctive and palliative treatment of inoperable *breast cancer* in women. When the tumor cells possess estrogen receptors and lesions are non-osseus, about 50% of cases will show some improvement. Remissions occur in approximately 15% of cases.

Except possibly for hypercalcemia, the side effects are not those of the androgens. There may be mild pain, irritation, and inflammation at the site of injection. Other reported side effects are nausea, vomiting, aches, myalgia, arthralgia, edema of the extremities, paresthesias, maculopapular rash, hypertension; these all subside without discontinuation of the drug, and it is not always clear to what extent the drug or the disease is responsible.

Dose—*Intramuscular*, **100 mg** 3 times a week; *oral*, usually **250 mg** 4 times a day.

Dosage Forms—Sterile Suspension: 500 mg/5 mL; Tablets: 50 and 250 mg.

Testosterone

Androst-4-en-3-one, 17-hydroxy, (17β)-, (*Various Mfrs*)

17β-Hydroxyandrost-4-en-3-one [58-22-0] $C_{19}H_{28}O_2$ (288.43).

Preparation—First isolated in crystalline form by Laquer in 1935 who obtained it from animal testes. Although small amounts of testosterone may be extracted from testicular material, the synthetic commercial supply is derived from cholesterol. The key intermediate in the synthesis is dehydroepiandrosterone which can be treated further, by either chemical or microbiological processes, to yield testosterone. US Pat 2,236,574.

Description—White or slightly creamy white crystals or crystalline powder; odorless; stable in air; melting range 153° to 157°.

Solubility—Practically insoluble in water; 1 g in about 6 mL of dehydrated alcohol, 1 mL chloroform, 100 mL ether; soluble in vegetable oils.

Uses—See the general statement, page 997. Testosterone is not effective orally because it is destroyed in the liver on absorption. Its plasma half-life is 10 to 20 min.

Dose—*Intramuscular*, in various *male hypogonadal states* and *postpubertal cryptorchidism*, **10** to **25 mg** 2 or 3 times a week; to *prevent postpartum breast engorgement*, **25 mg** once or twice a day for 3 or 4 days; in *metastatic breast cancer*, **100 mg** 3 times a week for low-grade and up to **1 g** a week in high-grade malignancy. *Subcutaneous implantation*, for *male hypogonadism*, **150** to **450 mg** (2 to 6 pellets) every 4 to 6 months.

Dosage Forms—Pellets: 75 mg; Sterile Suspension: 250, 500, 1000, and 3000 mg/10 mL; 750 and 1500 mg/30 mL.

Testosterone Cypionate

Androst-4-en-3-one, 17-(3-cyclopentyl-1-oxopropoxy)-, (17β)-,
Testosterone Cyclopentylpropionate USP XVI;
(*Various Mfrs*)

Testosterone cyclopentanepropionate [58-20-8] $C_{27}H_{40}O_3$ (412.61).

For the structure of the base, see *Testosterone*.

Preparation—Testosterone is esterified by interaction with 3-cyclopentylpropionyl chloride [$C_5H_{11}CH_2CH_2COCl$] in the presence of pyridine.

Description—White or creamy white, crystalline powder which is odorless or has a slight odor and is stable in air; melts between 98° and 104°.

Solubility—Insoluble in water; freely soluble in alcohol, chloroform, dioxane, and ether; soluble in vegetable oils.

Uses—The actions, uses, and limitations are the same as for androgens in general (see the general statement, page 997) but the cypionate has a much longer duration of action than testosterone when administered intramuscularly in oil. It is not used in women.

Dose—*Intramuscular*, in oil, in various *male hypogonadal states* and *impotence*, **200** to **400 mg** every 3 to 6 weeks initially and 4 to 6 weeks for maintenance once a response occurs; for *oligospermia*, **100** to **200 mg** every 3 to 6 weeks or 200 mg each week for 6 to 10 weeks, after which a rebound surge in sperm production may occur.

Dosage Forms—Injection: 50, 100, and 200 mg/1 mL, 500 mg and 1 and 2 g/10 mL.

Testosterone Enanthate

Androst-4-en-3-one, 17-[(1-oxoheptyl)oxy]-, (17β)-,
Delatestryl (*Squibb*)

Testosterone heptanoate [315-37-7] $C_{26}H_{40}O_3$ (400.60).

For the structure of the base, see *Testosterone*.

Preparation—A solution of enanthic acid in benzene is refluxed for about one hour after which it is allowed to cool, testosterone is added, and the mixture is refluxed for about 21 hours. The resulting light brown solution is cooled, extracted with a sodium hydroxide solution to remove surplus enanthic acid, washed with water, and dried over magnesium sulfate. After removal of solvent, the crude ester is purified by molecular distillation.

Description—White or creamy white, crystalline powder; odorless or has a faint odor characteristic of enanthic acid; melts between 34° and 39°, the initial temperature of the bath not exceeding 20°.

Solubility—Insoluble in water; 1 g in about 0.3 mL ether; soluble in vegetable oils.

Uses—The actions, uses, and limitations are the same as those of *Testosterone Cypionate*, except that the enanthate is also used for the treatment of osteoporosis. The effects of a single intramuscular injection may last 3 to 4 weeks.

Dose—*Intramuscular*, for replacement in *male hypogonadal states* and for *impotence*, **100** to **400 mg** every 4 to 6 weeks; for *oligospermia*, **100** to **200 mg** every 4 to 6 weeks or **200 mg** each week for 6 to 12 weeks, after which a rebound surge in sperm production may occur; *osteoporosis*, **200** to **400 mg** once every 4 weeks.

Dosage Forms—Injection: 200 mg/1 mL, 1 g/5 mL, 1 and 2 g/10 mL.

Testosterone Propionate

Androst-4-en-3-one, 17-(1-oxopropoxy)-, (17β)-,
Oreton Propionate (*Schering-Plough*)

17β-Hydroxyandrost-4-en-3-one propionate [57-85-2] $C_{22}H_{32}O_3$ (344.49).

For the structure of the base, see *Testosterone*.

Preparation—Readily from testosterone by refluxing with propionic anhydride.

Description—White or creamy white crystals or crystalline powder; odorless and stable in air; melts between 118° and 123°.

Solubility—Insoluble in water; freely soluble in alcohol, dioxane, ether, and other organic solvents; soluble in vegetable oils.

Uses—See the general statement. Intramuscular injection of the propionate provides a somewhat more intense action than with testosterone, but the duration of action is somewhat shorter, even though the half-life is about 4 hr. The parenteral route is not suited to long-term treatment. The other esters of testosterone and synthetic congeners have considerably diminished the importance of the propionate.

Dose—*Intramuscular*, for various *male hypogonadal states* and *postpubertal cryptorchidism*, **10** to **25 mg** 2 or 3 times a week; for *anabolic effects*, **5** to **10 mg** a day; for *metastatic breast cancer* in women, **100 mg** 3 times a week.

Dosage Forms—Injection (in oil): 25 and 50 mg/1 mL, 250, 500 and 1000 mg/10 mL, and 750, 1500, and 3000 mg/30 mL.

Other Androgenic Hormones

Calusterone   [17β-Hydroxy-7β,17-dimethylandrost-4-en-3-one [17021-26-0] $C_{21}H_{32}O_2$ (316.48); Methosarb (*Upjohn*)]—Reported to be synthesized by reduction of 6-dehydro-7,17α-dimethyltestosterone. White to off-white, odorless, tasteless, crystalline powder; stable in light and air; melts between 128° and 134°. Insoluble in water; freely soluble in alcohol. *Uses:* Has very weak androgenic actions yet is relatively effective in the palliation of *metastatic breast carcinoma* in which the tumor cells possess estrogen receptors. It is not used for androgenic therapy. Signs of virilization, such as deepening of the voice, acne, and facial hair growth occur in 20 to 25% of users. Edema, clitoral enlargement, and other androgenic effects occur occasionally but are mild. Hypercalcemia has been reported. Although some liver function tests may be altered, cholestatic jaundice is rare. Nausea and vomiting occur in 5 to 10% of patients. *Dose: Oral*, 150 to 300 mg a day in 3 or 4 divided doses. *Dosage Form:* Tablets: 50 mg.

Ethylestrenol [17α-Ethylestr-4-en-17-ol [965-90-2] $C_{20}H_{32}O$ (288.46); Maxibolin (*Organon*)]—A solution of 3-ethoxy-17α-ethylestradiol in ether is reacted in the cold with dry ethylamine to which lithium has been added. Following solvent extraction, the crude dry product is distributed between petroleum ether and 70% methanol. The petroleum ether layer is separated and evaporated to yield the ethylestrenol. US Pat 3,112,328. White to creamy white, crystalline powder that is odorless and tasteless; unstable in heat and light; melts between 83° and 95°. Freely soluble in alcohol; soluble in chloroform; practically insoluble in water. *Uses:* An anabolic steroid related to the androgens. It promotes tissue building, a renewal of vigor, a feeling of well-being, and bone matrix reconstruction. Consequently, there is an increase in appetite and body weight. It is used in treating the wasting diseases to facilitate convalescence from prolonged illness, and to arrest osteoporosis. It is also used to antagonize certain catabolic effects of corticosteroid therapy. Ethylestrenol potentially has all the side effects of *Testosterone* (page 1000), except that they are generally of lower incidence and weaker. Its most serious side effect is cholestatic jaundice, in common with other anabolic steroids. Although its androgenic actions are weak, the drug may induce withdrawal bleeding and amenorrhea in women, and it is contraindicated in prostatic carcinoma. *Dose: Oral, adult*, 4 mg once a day for up to 6 weeks; after a 4-week pause, an additional course may be administered if indicated. For *children*, 1 to 3 mg a day.

Methandriol [17α-Methylandrost-5-ene-3β,17β-diol [521-10-8] $C_{20}H_{32}O_2$ (304.47) Cytobolin (*McNeal, Jones & Feldman*)]—A white crystalline powder melting about 205°. It is practically insoluble in water; soluble in alcohol or ether. For the synthesis refer to *Helv Chim Acta* 18: 1487, 1935. *Uses:* An anabolic steroid "possibly effective" for the adjunctive treatment of senile and postmenopausal osteoporosis. *Dose: Intramuscular, adults*, 10 to 40 mg/day of the aqueous suspension or 50 to 100 mg once or twice a week of the suspension in oil; *children*, 5 to 10 mg/day of the aqueous suspension.

CHAPTER 53

Vitamins and Other Nutrients

Ernestine Vanderveen, PhD

National Institute of Alcohol Abuse and Alcoholism
ADAMHA
Rockville, MD 20875

John E Vanderveen, PhD

Division of Nutrition, Food and Drug Administration
Washington, DC 20204

Man consumes food to provide him with energy for growth, maintenance of normal body functions, and work. Energy is made available through conversion of carbohydrate, fat, and protein, which yield 4, 9, and 4 kilocalories per gram of the nutrient, respectively, when completely metabolized. The proportion of each of these nutrient sources in the human diet varies with environment, food availability, culture, and personal food behavior of the individual. In the United States the percent of total calories provided by carbohydrate, fat, and protein in most diets is approximately 50, 40, and 10 percent, respectively. Metabolism, growth, and tissue repair require adequate ingestion of protein, minerals, vitamins, water, and oxygen. The latter two are not generally classed as nutrients in the usual sense but are substances that must be supplied on a continuing basis and in sufficient amount to sustain life. Mineral elements present in organic compounds serve structural and catalytic roles in the metabolic process. Minerals are present as free ions in body fluids, where they act osmotically as electrolytes. The solid structure of the body, which is primarily bone tissue, contains mineral compounds. Vitamins are a heterogeneous group of organic compounds that participate in metabolic processes in minute amounts compared to other nutrients. The combination of complex processes through which living animal organisms obtain and utilize these materials is nutrition. The various disciplines of study aimed at elucidating those processes are collectively termed nutritional science. Understanding of the significance of nutrients in human physiology has evolved largely from research studies on lower forms of life, mainly bacteria and animals, such as the chicken, rat, guinea pig, mouse, dog, and monkey. These studies have been substantiated and enlarged by clinical observations on human populations in healthy states and various conditions of disease, in malnutrition, and by some experimental studies conducted with human subjects.

Misinformation About Food—A vast amount of confusion and nonscientific information surrounds the relationship of foods, as specially formulated food products, to health and prevention or cure of various disease conditions. Many persons do not accept the concept that consumption of appropriate amounts of food selected from a variety of plant and animal sources will, over a period of time, furnish adequate to abundant amounts of all known essential nutrients. Food behaviors of increasing numbers of people are influenced by misrepresentations and false claims made for "health" foods, fad diets, and miracle cures by individuals and groups who profit from sale of such foods or ideas. Often these purveyors are convincing in their approach, claiming to have experienced a "cure" or presenting evidence of their product's success in curing people of a variety of real or imagined illnesses. When the unwary consumer uncritically accepts the advice of the purveyors of falsely labeled products in place of needed medical treatment serious consequences can result. Risks incurred through following bizarre diet schemes for weight loss can be equally serious. Deaths have occurred from causes directly or indirectly associated with fad diets and other forms of self diagnosis and treatment.

The Food and Drug Administration (FDA) has the responsibility and authority to control interstate traffic of products which are falsely promoted through nutritional quackery practices. This includes authority to regulate nutritional supplements made from ingredients involved in interstate commerce. If labels include false or misleading statements, including claims of potency or activity that are incorrect, the FDA can initiate legal action to correct them. Through nationwide monitoring of labeling as well as of composition of the enormous number and variety of packaged foods in the market, some degree of compliance with regulations that pertain to fairness and honesty is accomplished. Pharmacists and others who are informed in the sciences that make up nutritional science should report instances of false and misleading claims in labeling to FDA.

Particularly in the field of nutrition, where misinformation may endanger the health of individuals, the consumer must be provided opportunity to learn to make sound decisions regarding his health and nutritional status. Effective nutrition education programs are perceived to be essential if consumers are to make decisions in their own best interest when faced with the complexities of the modern market place.

Pharmacists, because of their day-to-day contact with the public most directly concerned, have a responsibility to be well-informed to allay the fears that are created by pseudo-scientific writings of sensationalists, and to protect the health as well as the pocketbook of patrons.

Nutrient Requirements and Dietary Standards—The determination of quantitative human requirements for nutrients could be made if it were possible to correlate known nutrient intake with specific biological responses in precisely controlled studies. Although it is not possible, there are three kinds of studies which do yield information that can be used to closely estimate requirements. They are:

1. Balance studies, which employ a method of comparing nutrient intake and output and therefore measure body gain or loss of a stable component.
2. Biochemical measurements of a nutrient, nutrient metabolites, or related functional and structural components in a body fluid, compartment, tissue, or excreta.
3. Clinical evaluation and performance tests on subjects maintained on carefully controlled nutrient intakes to determine dietary levels that will prevent deterioration of physiological and cognitive functions.

Ideally, data from all three enable the investigator to determine the smallest amount of a nutrient that will prevent deficiency symptoms or support a well-defined physiological or biochemical response, eg, the maintenance of serum feritin levels in women of child bearing ages. An *average* requirement, however, is most often derived from such data to denote the amount of a nutrient that will support health in most persons of a given population group. It implies that the *true* requirement for *individuals* may be either above or below the average for the group. Obviously neither the perfect tool for determining human requirements nor the perfect criterion of physiological and cognitive responses have yet been devised or ascertained.

To utilize the knowledge about nutrient requirements in a practical way, ie, to develop dietary standards as goals for food selection, it is necessary to add amounts above estimated requirements as "safety factors" to cover both variation among individuals and the lack of precision inherent in the estimated requirement. The resulting values are called *allowances*, and the dietary standards used in the US are the Recommended Dietary Allowances (RDA) developed by the Food and Nutrition Board of the National Academy of Sciences-National Research Council (Table I). The Food and Nutrition Board also published Estimated Safe and Adequate Daily Dietary Intakes for 12 nutrients for which less information existed than was necessary to establish allowances (Table II).

In 1940 the FDA independently established a set of dietary standards called Minimum Daily Requirements, which were used in labeling to help consumers relate the nutrient content claimed for certain foods to their own nutrient needs. These have recently been replaced by the FDA with a new set of dietary standards, the US Recommended Daily Allowances (US RDA) (Table III), which include values for more nutrients and which were adapted and condensed from the Food and Nutrition Board's RDA, the latest revised edition published in 1979. Federal regulations require that manufacturers who make nutritional claims on the label of foods, including dietary supplements, must include a statement of the percentages of the US RDA's of the vitamins, minerals and protein supplied by an amount of the food usually consumed or recommended for consumption in 1 day.

Dietary standards are necessary and useful tools and are a means through which the findings in nutritional science can be applied for the improvement and maintenance of human health. They are assessed periodically and revised as new data become available.

Therapeutic Nutrition—Any interference with the body's ability to utilize the nutrients present in available food or, for that matter, its inability to obtain enough nutrients from the available food, calls for the intervention by professionals who are able to diagnose and treat the condition. The treatment, or therapy, may involve a range of actions from simple adjustment of nutrient intake to the intravenous feeding of special nutrient formulas. Diet therapy is practiced when a change in nutrition status of a patient can be effected gradually. This would be in cases where it is important to maintain optimal nutritional status during prolonged periods of physical stress, to bring about changes in body weight, and to adjust food intake (both qualitatively and quantitatively) when the body is functioning abnormally or when surgery or trauma have depleted the body's reserves. Specific kinds of diet therapy are also needed for long periods, if not for life, to compensate for inborn errors of metabolism.

Radical means of therapy in both the management and treatment of certain conditions is often necessary. For example, in correcting a nutritional deficiency such as pernicious anemia and preventing its recurrence in a susceptible individual, large doses of the missing nutrient are administered parenterally. Feeding by nasogastric tube or by gastrostomy or jejunostomy, is instituted when it is not possible for a patient to take food by mouth. Patients with extensive burns present nutritional problems much more far-reaching than those who have undergone major surgery or sustained severe hemorrhage. The first need for those individuals is for fluid and electrolyte replacement followed as quickly as possible by a diet or intravenous solution markedly increased in protein, calories, and vitamins. The focus in all these cases is on

restoration of nutrient supply commensurate with the specific need as soon as possible.

An understanding of the necessity for nutrient therapy is aided by recognizing the following factors which can affect nutrient needs:

1. Interference with food consumption (eg, impaired appetite, gastrointestinal disease, traumatic neurological disorders interfering with self-feeding, neuropsychiatric disorders, disease of soft or hard oral tissue, alcoholism, pregnancy anorexia and vomiting, food allergy, disease requiring a restricted diet).

2. Interference with absorption (eg, absence of normal digestive secretions, intestinal hypermotility, reduction of effective absorbing surface, impairment of intrinsic mechanism of absorption, drugs preventing absorption).

3. Interference with utilization or storage (eg, impaired liver function, hypothyroidism, neoplasm of gastrointestinal tract, drug therapy or radiation).

4. Increased destruction of tissues and/or function (eg, achlorhydria in the gastrointestinal tract, heavy metals and other metabolic antagonists).

5. Increased excretion or loss of nutrients (eg, lactation, burns, glycosuria and albuminuria, acute or chronic blood loss).

6. Increased nutrient requirements (eg, increased physical activity, periods of rapid growth, pregnancy and lactation, fever, hyperthyroidism, drug therapy).

Vitamins

Vitamins are organic compounds required for normal growth and maintenance of life by animals, including man. As a rule, animals are unable to synthesize these compounds by anabolic processes that are independent of environment other than air. These compounds are effective in small amounts, do not furnish energy, and are not utilized as building units for the structure of the organism, but are essential for transformation of energy and for regulation of the metabolism of structural units. They or their precursors are found in plants and, so far as is known, have specific metabolic functions to perform in plant cells. Plant tissues are sources for the animal kingdom of these protective nutritional factors. In addition to carbohydrates, fats, proteins, mineral salts, and water, it is essential that the food of man and animals contain small amounts of these organic substances called vitamins. If any one of at least 13 of these compounds is lacking in the diet, this breakdown results in a reduced rate or complete lack of growth in children and in symptoms of malnutrition that are known as deficiency diseases.

Vitamins are unlike each other in chemical composition and function. They are alike only in that they cannot be synthesized at all or at least not at an adequate rate in the tissues of animals or humans. The functions they serve fall into two categories, the maintenance of normal structure and of normal metabolic functions. For example, vitamin A is essential for the maintenance of normal epithelial tissue; vitamin D functions in the absorption of normal bone salts for the formation and growth of bone tissue. Certain vitamins of the water-soluble group, among them thiamin, riboflavin, pantothenic acid, and niacin, are known to be essential constituents of the respiratory enzymes that are required in the utilization of energy from oxidative catabolism of sugars and fats.

It is convenient in a discussion of this subject to divide these nutritional substances into two groups, the *fat-soluble* and the *water-soluble factors*. Vitamins A, D, E, and K fall into the fat-soluble group, since they can be extracted with fat solvents and are found in the fat fractions of animal tissues. The water-soluble vitamins include ascorbic acid and the B group of vitamins, which consists of some 10 or more well-defined compounds. Additional vitamin nomenclature can be found in Table IV. The characterization of vitamins as essential metabolic factors with discrete chemical structures required their isolation in pure form from natural sources and subsequent laboratory synthesis. Commercial chemical or microbiological syntheses, some from relatively simple com-

Table I—Food and Nutrition Board, National Academy of Sciences-National Research Council Recommended Daily Dietary Allowances, a Revised 1979*

Designed for the maintenance of good nutrition of practically all healthy people in the USA

	Age (yr)	Weight (kg)	Weight (lb)	Height (cm)	Height (in.)	Protein (g)	Vitamin A (µg RE)[b]	Vitamin D (µg)[c]	Vitamin E (mg α-TE)[d]	Ascorbic acid (mg)	Folacin (µg)[e]	Niacin (mg NE)[f]	Riboflavin (mg)	Thiamin (mg)	Vitamin B6 (mg)	Vitamin B12 (µg)[g]	Calcium (mg)	Phosphorus (mg)	Iodine (µg)	Iron (mg)	Magnesium (mg)	Zinc (mg)
Infants	0.0–0.5	6	13	60	24	kg × 2.2	420[d]	10	3	35	30	6	0.4	0.3	0.3	0.5[g]	360	240	40	10	50	3
	0.5–1.0	9	20	71	28	kg × 2.0	400	10	4	35	45	8	0.6	0.5	0.6	1.5	540	360	50	15	70	5
Children	1–3	13	29	90	35	23	400	10	5	45	100	9	0.8	0.7	0.9	2.0	800	800	70	15	150	10
	4–6	20	44	112	44	30	500	10	6	45	200	11	1.0	0.9	1.3	2.5	800	800	90	10	200	10
	7–10	28	62	132	52	34	700	10	7	45	300	16	1.4	1.2	1.6	3.0	800	800	120	10	250	10
Males	11–14	45	99	157	62	45	1,000	10	8	50	400	18	1.6	1.4	1.8	3.0	1,200	1,200	150	18	350	15
	15–18	66	145	176	69	56	1,000	10	10	60	400	18	1.7	1.4	2.0	3.0	1,200	1,200	150	18	400	15
	19–22	70	154	177	70	56	1,000	7.5	10	60	400	19	1.7	1.5	2.2	3.0	800	800	150	10	350	15
	23–50	70	154	178	70	56	1,000	5	10	60	400	18	1.6	1.4	2.2	3.0	800	800	150	10	350	15
	51+	70	154	178	70	56	1,000	5	10	60	400	16	1.4	1.2	2.2	3.0	800	800	150	10	350	15
Females	11–14	46	101	157	62	46	800	10	8	50	400	15	1.3	1.1	1.8	3.0	1,200	1,200	150	18	300	15
	15–18	55	120	163	64	46	800	10	8	60	400	14	1.3	1.1	2.0	3.0	1,200	1,200	150	18	300	15
	19–22	55	120	163	64	44	800	7.5	8	60	400	14	1.3	1.1	2.0	3.0	800	800	150	18	300	15
	23–50	55	120	163	64	44	800	5	8	60	400	13	1.2	1.0	2.0	3.0	800	800	150	18	300	15
	51+	55	120	163	64	44	800	5	8	60	400	13	1.2	1.0	2.0	3.0	800	800	150	10	300	15
Pregnant						+30	+200	+5	+2	+20	400	+2	+0.3	+0.4	+0.6	+1.0	+400	+400	+25	[h]	+150	+5
Lactating						+20	+400	+5	+3	+40	400	+5	+0.5	+0.5	+0.5	+1.0	+400	+400	+50	[h]	+150	+10

a The allowances are intended to provide for individual variations among most normal persons as they live in the US under usual environmental stresses. Diets should be based on a variety of common foods in order to provide other nutrients for which human requirements have been less well defined.

b Retinol equivalents. 1 Retinol equivalent = 1 µg retinol or 6 ng carotene.

c As cholecalciferol. 10 µg cholecalciferol = 400 IU vitamin D.

d Alpha tocopherol equivalents. 1 mg d-alpha tocopherol = 1 α-TE.

e Folacin allowances refer to dietary sources as determined by *Lactobacillus casei* assay after treatment with enzymes ("conjugases") to make polyglutamyl forms of the vitamin available to the test organism.

f 1 NE (niacin equivalent) is equal to 1 mg of niacin or 60 mg of dietary tryptophan.

g The RDA for vitamin B12 in infants is based on average concentration of the vitamin in human milk. Allowances after weaning are based on energy intake (as recommended by the American Academy of Pediatrics) and consideration of other factors such as intestinal absorption.

h Increased requirement during pregnancy cannot be met by the iron content of habitual American diets nor by existing iron stores of many women; therefore use of 30 to 60 mg of supplemental iron is recommended. Iron needs during lactation are not substantially different from those of nonpregnant women, but continued supplementation of the mother for 2 to 3 months after parturition is advisable in order to replenish stores depleted by pregnancy.

* Reproduced from *Recommended Dietary Allowances*, 9th Edition (1980), with permission of the National Academy of Sciences, Washington, DC

Table II—Estimated Safe and Adequate Daily Dietary Intakes of Additional Selected Vitamins and Minerals a*

	Age (yr)	Vitamins			Trace Elements[b]						Electrolytes		
		Vitamin K (µg)	Biotin (µg)	Pantothenic Acid (mg)	Copper (mg)	Manganese (mg)	Fluoride (mg)	Chromium (mg)	Selenium (mg)	Molybdenum (mg)	Sodium (mg)	Potassium (mg)	Chloride (mg)
Infants	0–0.5	12	35	2	0.5–0.7	0.5–0.7	0.1–0.5	0.01–0.04	0.01–0.04	0.03–0.06	115–350	350–925	275–700
	0.5–1	10–20	50	3	0.7–1.0	0.7–1.0	0.2–1.0	0.02–0.06	0.02–0.06	0.04–0.08	250–750	425–1275	400–1200
Children	1–3	15–30	65	3	1.0–1.5	1.0–1.5	0.5–1.5	0.02–0.08	0.02–0.08	0.05–0.1	325–975	550–1650	500–1500
and	4–6	20–40	85	3–4	1.5–2.0	1.5–2.0	1.0–2.5	0.03–0.12	0.03–0.12	0.06–0.15	450–1350	775–2325	700–2100
Adolescents	7–10	30–60	120	4–5	2.0–2.5	2.0–3.0	1.5–2.5	0.05–0.2	0.05–0.2	0.1–0.3	600–1800	1000–3000	925–2775
	11+	50–100	100–200	4–7	2.0–3.0	2.5–5.0	1.5–2.5	0.05–0.2	0.05–0.2	0.15–0.5	900–2700	1525–4574	1400–4200
Adults		70–140	100–200	4–7	2.0–3.0	2.5–5.0	1.5–4.0	0.05–0.2	0.05–0.2	0.15–0.5	1100–3300	1875–5625	1700–5100

a Because there is less information on which to base allowances, these figures are not given in Table I and are provided here in the form of ranges of recommended intakes.

b Since toxic levels for many trace elements may be only several times usual intakes, the upper levels for trace elements given in this table should not be habitually exceeded.

* Reproduced from *Recommended Dietary Allowances*, 9th Edition (1980), with permission of the National Academy of Sciences, Washington, DC.

Table III—US Recommended Daily Allowance (US RDA) for Labeling Purposes

	Unit	Infants	Children under 4 years of age	Adults and children 4 or more years of age	Pregnant or lactating women
Vitamin A	IU	1500	2500	5000	8000
Vitamin D	IU	400	400	400	400
Vitamin E	IU	5	10	30	30
Vitamin C	mg	35	40	60	60
Folacin	mg	0.1	0.2	0.4	0.8
Thiamin	mg	0.5	0.7	1.5	1.7
Riboflavin	mg	0.6	0.8	1.7	2.0
Niacin	mg	8	9	20	20
Vitamin B_6	mg	0.4	0.7	2	2.5
Vitamin B_{12}	μg	2	3	6	8
Biotin	mg	0.05	0.15	0.30	0.30
Pantothenic Acid	mg	3	5	10	10
Calcium	g	0.6	0.8	1.0	1.3
Phosphorus	g	0.5	0.8	1.0	1.3
Iodine	μg	45	70	150	150
Iron	mg	15	10	18	18
Magnesium	mg	70	200	400	450
Manganese[a]	mg	0.5	1.0	4.0	4.0
Copper	mg	0.6	1.0	2.0	2.0
Zinc	mg	5	8	15	15
Protein	g	...	20 (28)[b]	45 (65)[b]	...

[a] Proposed US RDA.
[b] Values in parentheses are US RDA's when Protein Efficiency Ratio (PER) of the protein is less than that of casein; the other values are used when PER is equal to or greater than that of casein. No claim may be made for a protein with a PER equal to or less than 20% that of casein.

pounds, are the source of most of the vitamins now used in pharmaceutical preparations, dietary supplements, and fortified foods.

Standardization—Vitamin activity or potency is measured by three principal types of methods:

1. *Biological*, in which rats, mice, guinea pigs, and chickens serve as the assay animals, have been exclusively used, and for some of the vitamins are the most reliable means of assay.
2. *Microbiological*, which employ bacteria that require certain of the water-soluble vitamins, are rapid, specific, and precise. Such methods are used for manufacturing and laboratory control of the production of some vitamins.
3. *Chemical*, utilizing a characteristic color or a sensitive reaction specific for the compounds, are available for most vitamins in uncomplicated mixtures.

The status of vitamin methods of assay is now such that manufacturers of vitamin preparations find it possible to state with precision the potency of their products, and tables of vitamin content of foods are, for most vitamins, quite complete. Methods of assay are described briefly in the individual vitamin sections.

In the interest of improvement and uniformity of expressing the results of such assays, the World Health Organization of the United Nations has sponsored the preparation and distribution of Standards. As a rule, an International Standard is no longer provided once the substance responsible for its characteristic activity has been isolated, identified, and made readily available. The USP has set up comparable Reference Standards in this country, and the biological potency of vitamins A and D is expressed in USP Units that are equal to International Units. However, availability of the vitamins in pure form encourages transition from use of units to use of weight in expressing amounts present in vitamin products.

The Fat-Soluble Vitamins

Vitamin A and Carotene

Vitamin A was the first fat-soluble vitamin discovered. Animal nutritionists observed growth failures in calves born of cows main-

tained on wheat or oats alone, whereas whole cornplant supported growth and development of the animals. The vitamin was found to be related to chlorophyll and carotenoid-containing plants. Later study revealed that the vitamin is essential for the maintenance of normal tissue structure and for other important physiologic functions such as vision and reproduction.

Chemistry and Assay—Vitamin A is represented primarily by the cyclic polyene alcohol vitamin A_1 (retinol) with an empirical formula of $C_{20}H_{30}O$ and whose four conjugated double bonds in the side chain are in the *trans* arrangement.

Vitamin A (Retinol) (Vitamin A₁)

Another representative of vitamin A occurring in nature is vitamin A_2, which has an additional double bond in the ring at the 3–4 position. It has only about $\frac{1}{4}$ to $\frac{1}{2}$ the biological activity of vitamin A_1 for the rat and has no commercial significance. A third such representative is neovitamin A-a in which the terminal double bond in the side chain of vitamin A_1 is *cis*. It has low biological activity.

Vitamin A_1 is a pale yellow crystalline compound, is soluble in fat solvents, and has an ultraviolet absorption maximum at 328 nm wavelength. The vitamin is not readily destroyed by heat but is easily oxidized and is less stable in acid than in alkaline solution. The esters of vitamin A_1 with the fatty acids, acetic and palmitic, are commercially important since they are considerably more stable than the alcohol.

The source of most of the vitamin A in animals, birds, and fish is the carotenoid pigments, the yellow-colored compounds in all chlorophyll-containing plants. At least 10 different carotenoids exhibit provitamin A activity, but only alpha- and beta-carotene and cryptoxanthin (found in yellow corn) are important in animal nutrition, beta-carotene being the most important.

β-Carotene

Table IV—Vitamin Nomenclature

Vitamin	Synonym or descriptive terms
A group	Antixerophthalmic vitamin
A₁	Retinol
A₂	Dehydroretinol
A acid	Retinoic acid (Tretinoin)
Provitamin A Carotenoids	Carotene (alpha & beta), cryptoxanthin (hydroxy beta-carotene)
B group	Formerly vitamin B complex
Thiamin	Vitamin B₁, aneurin, antiberiberi vitamin
Riboflavin	Vitamin B₂, lactoflavin
Niacin	Nicotinic acid and nicotinamide, pellagra-preventive factor
Pantothenic acid	Formerly vitamin B₃
B₆	Pyridoxine, pyridoxal, pyridoxamine
Biotin	Coenzyme R
Folacin	Folic acid (pteroylmonoglutamic acid, PGA) and folic acid polyglutamates, tetrahydrofolic acid, formyl tetrahydrofolic acid (formerly citrovorum factor, folinic acid)
B₁₂	Antipernicious anemia vitamin, cyanocobalamin, hydroxocobalamin (formerly vitamin B₁₂ᵦ), nitritocobalamin (formerly vitamin B₁₂ᵧ)
C	L-Ascorbic acid, antiscorbutic vitamin
D group	Antirachitic vitamin
D₂	Ergocalciferol (formerly calciferol), activated ergosterol
D₃	Cholecalciferol, activated 7-dehydrocholesterol
E group alpha- beta- gamma- delta-	tocopherols & tocotrienols — Possess vitamin E activity in varying degrees. Occur as fatty acid esters
K group	Antihemorrhagic vitamin
K₁	Phylloquinone } naturally occurring
K₂	Farnoquinone
K₃	Menadione, menaquinone
K₄₋₇	Biologically active } synthetic analogues of menadione

Theoretically one molecule of beta-carotene should yield two molecules of vitamin A₁; however, the availability of carotene in foods as sources of vitamin A for humans is low and extremely variable. Often, factors of ½, ⅓, ¼, or less are arbitrarily used to compensate for this. The utilization efficiency of carotene is generally considered to be ⅙ for humans; in other terms, 1 μg of beta-carotene would have the same biological activity as 0.167 μg of retinol. This conservatively takes into account the decremental effects on carotene utilization of absorption, transport and tissue conversion to the active vitamin. The conversion of the provitamin to vitamin A occurs primarily in the walls of the small intestine and perhaps to a lesser degree in the liver. Like vitamin A₁, the carotenes are soluble in fat solvents, in crystalline form appear deep orange or copper-colored, and have characteristic absorption spectra.

Total synthesis of vitamin A₁ and beta-carotene is achieved commercially, vitamin A usually being prepared as the acetate. Concentration of vitamin A from animal fats and fish liver oil is still important. The principal steps in the process are molecular distillation, saponification, and crystallization of the distillate and conversion to the desired ester.

The USP Unit for vitamin A is identical to the International Unit. The USP Reference Standard for vitamin A is a solution of crystalline vitamin A acetate in cottonseed oil such that there is contained 1 USP Unit (0.344 μg)/0.1 mg of solution. Although there is no USP Unit for carotene, there is an International Unit (IU); the relation between carotene and vitamin A is 6 to 3.44 by weight of the respective pure compounds.

Vitamin A can be assayed by direct measurement of its ultraviolet absorption, by photometric evaluation of the color reaction with antimony trichloride in chloroform (the Carr-Price reaction), or by a biologic method based on the resumption of growth of rats when the vitamin activity is added to a vitamin A-deficient diet. The chemical or physicochemical determination of beta-carotene depends on measurement of the yellow color of its solutions in organic solvents. Chromatographic separation of associated carotenoids is usually necessary before an accurate analysis of the biologically active compounds can be made.

Metabolic Functions—Of the known functions of vitamin A in the body, its role in the visual process is established best. The retina of man contains two distinct photo-receptor systems. The rods, which are the structural components of one system, are especially sensitive to light of low intensity. A specific vitamin A aldehyde is essential for the formation of rhodopsin (the high-molecular-weight glycoprotein part of the visual pigment within the rods) and the normal functioning of the retina. By virtue of this relation to the visual process, vitamin A alcohol has been named retinol and the aldehyde form named retinal. A vitamin A-deficient person has an impaired dark adaptation ("night-blindness").

Vitamin A also participates in the maintenance of the integrity of the epithelial membranes such that normal structures may be substituted by stratified keratinizing epithelium in the eyes and paraocular glands, respiratory, alimentary and genitourinary tracts under the stresses of a deficiency. The basal cells do not lose their function under such conditions, however, and are able to be restored to normal when sufficient vitamin A is absorbed. Abnormalities of nerve and connective tissue and of bones are further consequences of a dietary deficiency of the vitamin. In severe deficiency the affected epithelial and connective tissue may become the site of infections due to the cells' reduced resistance to bacterial invasion. This gave rise to the notion that administration of vitamin A was useful in the treatment of skin infections. However, expert medical opinion holds this application to be an abuse and that the vitamin has no anti-infective value in the absence of a specific deficiency. Nevertheless, both topical and oral vitamin A, and especially vitamin A acid, are prescribed by some physicians to treat acne vulgaris; however, further well controlled clinical trials are required to establish the efficacy of this practice.

The common severe deficiency symptoms are increased susceptibility to microbial infections, xerophthalmia and other eye disorders, loss of appetite and weight, and sterility, conditions which require a long time for their development. Although the recommended dietary allowance is no more than 6000 IU/day, in a deficiency much greater amounts are indicated. For example, the usual therapeutic oral dose range is from 10,000 to 20,000 IU daily for 7 to 10 days for infants and growing children and 25,000 to 100,000 IU daily for older children and adults.

If large doses of vitamin A are ingested for long periods of time, manifestations of toxicity develop. In the absence of a deficiency, chronic administration of vitamin A of 50,000 to 75,000 IU daily induces pathologic changes in bone and periosteal tissues, skin and mucous membranes, liver, and changes in behavior. Doses as low as 18,500 IU of a water-dispersed vitamin A preparation daily for 1 to 3 months are reported to be toxic for infants 3 to 6 months of age. Vitamin A toxicity has occurred in infants who were given liver daily for a period of three months.

Dietary Requirement and Food Sources—According to the National Research Council's "Recommended Dietary Allowances," the requirement for vitamin A appears to be proportional to body weight. The recommended allowances for the maintenance of good nutrition of healthy adults in the US is 1,000 Retinolequivalents (RE) for males and 800 RE for females per day (1,000 RE is equivalent to 5000 IU), although the adult requirement for maintenance of normalcy in important vitamin A functions is about ½ this value. Somewhat more vitamin A than the allowance should be provided during the latter two-thirds of pregnancy and even more during lactation. These increments would assure the nutritional well-being of the rapidly growing fetus and nursing infant, who are dependent on the mother's vitamin A intake.

About ½ of the vitamin A activity in the average American diet comes from beta carotene and related compounds. The other half is provided by the vitamin itself present in foods of animal origin. Not all of the carotene present in the food eaten is converted into vitamin A. Some passes through the digestive tract and is excreted as such. Of that absorbed, only the amounts necessary to meet requirements are converted to vitamin A. The rest is stored in the body or excreted. Intake of large amounts of carotene frequently causes a yellow or orange color to the skin which is considered to be harmless. The richest sources of carotene are yellow and green (leafy) vegetables and yellow fruits. Preformed vitamin A₁ is supplied primarily from the fat of dairy products and egg-yolk, but other important sources in some diets are liver, kidney, and fish. Federal regulations provide for the optional addition of 15,000 IU of vitamin A/lb of margarine. Almost all margarine is so fortified. There are also provisions for marketing vitamins A & D fortified nonfat dry milk containing 500 IU vitamin A and 100 IU vitamin D/reconstituted 8 fl oz.

Vitamin D

Vitamin D is the antirachitic vitamin effective in promoting calcification of the bony structures of man and animals. It is sometimes popularly known as the "sunshine" vitamin because it is formed by the action of the sun's ultraviolet rays on precursor sterols in the skin. Exposure to sunlight, therefore, has a powerful antirachitic effect. The term rachitic denotes the condition of a person or animal affected with the deficiency disease rickets.

Chemistry and Assay—The two immediate biological precursors (provitamins) to the vitamins D are the steroid alcohols ergosterol (ergosta-5,7,22E-trien-3β-ol) and 7-dehydrocholesterol (cholesta-5,7-dien-3β-ol). Under the influence of ultraviolet light, each undergoes scission of the 9(10) bond of the steroid nucleus with the simultaneous creation of a 10(19) double bond yielding, respectively, vitamin D_2 (ergocalciferol) and vitamin D_3 (cholecalciferol).

Vitamin D_2 (Ergocalciferol)
Vitamin D_3 (Cholecalciferol): same except C_{17} side chain is

Pure vitamins D_2 and D_3 are white, odorless crystals that are soluble in fat solvents such as ether, alcohol or chloroform, but insoluble in water. The compounds have characteristic absorption spectra, which property is useful in their identification. Both forms of the vitamin are stable to oxidation by air and to moderate heat in neutral and alkaline solutions. Upon alkaline saponification of fats, the vitamin appears in the nonsaponifiable fraction. It withstands autoclaving temperatures of 120° in the absence of air, but at this temperature is subject to oxidation, and it is completely destroyed by heating at 170°. Vitamin D is stable over long periods of storage in oil solution but is quite unstable in the presence of mineral salts, such as tricalcium phosphate, when compounded in tablet form. It may be stabilized by dispersion in gelatin or a similar protective coating.

The international standard for vitamin D is a crystalline preparation of pure vitamin D_3 assigned a potency of 40 million units/g. The USP adopted an equivalent standard of vitamin D_3 with the same assigned potency, distributed in the form of a cottonseed oil solution. The USP unit for vitamin D, therefore, is equivalent to the International Unit (IU).

The provitamins D are found in both plant and animal tissue; 7-dehydrocholesterol is principally found in animal skin and ergosterol in relatively large amounts in yeasts, although it was first isolated from ergot. The vitamin D which is absorbed through the intestinal wall from dietary sources or which is formed in the skin from 7-dehydrocholesterol enters the circulatory system, and excesses are stored. Like vitamin A, vitamin D is stored in animal body fats, principally in the liver. The liver oils, particularly of fish, are the most potent natural sources of the vitamin. The vitamin D of commerce is now principally synthesized from readily available structurally related compounds, such as cholesterol, which are often obtained as packinghouse by-products.

There are two methods for quantitative physicochemical assay of vitamin D; however, the biological assay based on the curative effects of the vitamin on experimental rickets in young rats is the method of choice for accurately measuring the total biological activity of the vitamin in complex materials of low potency. Minimal amounts of the vitamin are needed by the rat; therefore, the rachitic condition is produced by using an abnormal high-calcium, low-phosphorus diet. For relatively concentrated solutions of vitamin D in alcohol (but not in oil), ultraviolet spectrophotometric determination is made at the wavelength of maximum absorption. Antimony trichloride reacts with various vitamins D in a Carr-Price reaction yielding a yellow color whose intensity is proportional to the vitamin D present. The reaction is satisfactory only for concentrated preparations; cholesterol and vitamin A interfere only when present in amounts in excess of certain limits.

Metabolic Functions—The major part of the vitamin circulating in the blood is neither vitamin D_2 nor vitamin D_3 but the metabolite, 25-hydroxycholecalciferol (25-HCC) to which the ingested vitamin is converted in the liver by side-chain hydroxylation at carbon 25. 25-HCC appears to facilitate phosphate resorption in the renal tubule. A much more potent metabolite, 1,25-dihydroxycholecalciferol (1,25-DHCC), is synthesized in the kidney and finds its way to intestinal mucosal cells, bone and skeletal muscle where it is stored for regulating calcium absorption and mobilization. Vitamin D, therefore, is a precursor of a true hormone, 1,25-DHCC, which is secreted by an organ and performs a vital function. It is likely that some forms of vitamin D-resistant rickets can be explained by possible genetic inability of the body to produce adequate amounts of either 25-HCC or 1,25-DHCC. Conversely, some children may have an enhanced capacity to convert vitamin D to the more active metabolites and, thereby, manifest a hyperreactivity to amounts of the ingested vitamin very slightly in excess of recommended dietary allowances.

Vitamin D, through the action of these active metabolites, aids in the absorption of calcium from the intestinal tract and the resorption of phosphate in the renal tubule. Vitamin D is necessary for normal growth in children, probably having a direct effect on the osteoblast cells which influence calcification of cartilage in the growing areas of bone.

A deficiency of vitamin D leads to inadequate absorption of calcium from the intestinal tract and retention of phosphorus in the kidney and thence to faulty mineralization of bone structures. The inability of the soft bones to withstand the stress of weight results in skeletal malformations. Early rickets is difficult to diagnose, but fully developed cases in infants and children present characteristic signs. These include delayed closure of the fontanelles and softening of the skull, soft fragile bones with bowing of the legs and spinal curvature, enlargement of wrist, knee, and ankle joints, poorly developed muscles, restlessness, and nervous irritability. A form of "adult rickets" called osteomalacia similarly may occur. It, too represents a failure of the process of calcification caused by simple vitamin D lack and calcium inadequacy.

With adequate calcium-phosphorus intake, adult osteomalacia and uncomplicated rickets can be cured by the ordinary daily intake of 400 IU of vitamin D. Larger doses (about 1600 IU or more daily) are more rapidly effective, the first evidence of improvement—a rise in serum phosphorus—occurring in about 10 days.

Vitamin D has a serious toxic potential. There is a wide range of susceptibility to the toxic effects of vitamin D. Amounts of the order of 1000 to 3000 IU/kg of body weight per day, which are only about 80 to 100 times the recommended dietary intake, may lead to hypercalcemia and attendant complications, such as metastatic calcification and renal calculi in adults and as little as 2000 IU can inhibit linear growth of normal children. In advanced stages, demineralization of bones occurs, and multiple fractures may result from very slight trauma.

Dietary Requirement and Food Sources—The requirement for vitamin D can be met entirely by skin irradiation, so that the need for ingested vitamin D is influenced by the amount of exposure to ultraviolet light. There are few reliable data concerning minimum vitamin D requirements, except for infants. Long experience has shown that 400 IU/day is sufficient to meet the requirements of practically all healthy individuals, assuming no exposure to ultraviolet light. In normal full-term infants, intakes of as little as 100 IU/day have prevented rickets. There is no evidence that diets need supply more than 400 IU/day for normal growth of infants and children.

Vitamin D is the one vitamin of which conventional foods supply very little. Egg yolks, which are the best food source, vary in content from winter to summer depending most upon the content of the vitamin in the hen's diet. Dairy products contain some vitamin D, but again the potency varies with the season. Varieties of fish, whose muscle tissues contain substantial quantities of oil and fat, may supply an appreciable part of the dietary requirement. The livers of a number of fish, or the oils extracted from the livers, are extremely rich in vitamin D. Addition of vitamin D to appropriate foods has been an important factor in the prevention of any significant incidence of rickets in this country. Vitamin D-fortified whole milk, nonfat dry milk and evaporated milk containing 400 IU/qt (or reconstituted quart in the case of nonfat dry milk and evaporated milk) are particularly effective because of their use in infant feeding during the stage of growth most susceptible to rachitic changes. Fortification is accomplished by addition of vitamin D concentrates, mainly in the form of vitamin D_3. Fortification of other foods, such as processed cereals and margarine, is practiced to a limited degree.

Vitamin E

Vitamin E designates the group of compounds (tocol and tocotrienol derivatives) which exhibit qualitatively the biological activity of alpha tocopherol. Studies which led to its discovery as an essential factor in animal metabolism showed that it was, among other things, necessary for reproduction in rats. It is erroneously termed the antisterility vitamin, since it is not known to specifically function in this capacity in humans.

Chemistry and Assay—As with several of the other vitamins, there are a series of closely related compounds, tocopherols, known to occur in nature. Biological activity associated with the vitamin nature of the group is exhibited by four major compounds: alpha-, beta-, gamma- and delta-tocopherol, each of which can exist in various stereoisomeric forms. These are all methyl-substituted tocols; alpha tocopherol, the most important member of the series because of its activity and occurrence, is 5,7,8-trimethyltocol, ie, 2,5,7,8-tetramethyl-2-(4,8,12-trimethyltridecyl)-6-chromanol.

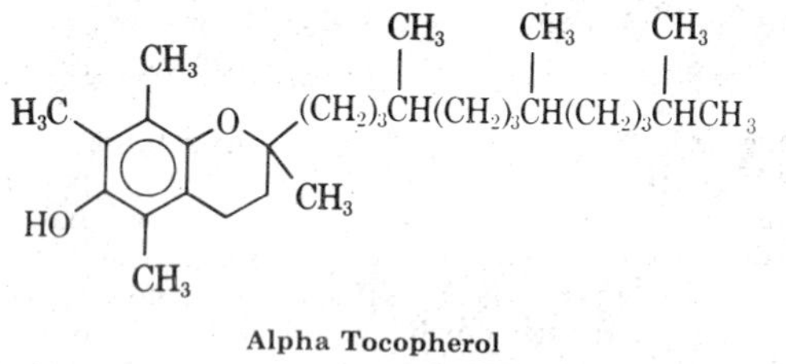

Alpha Tocopherol

The tocopherols are oily liquids at room temperature. High temperatures and acids do not affect the stability of vitamin E, but oxidation does take place readily in the presence of iron salts or in rancid fats. The tocopherols themselves act as antioxidants, the delta tocopherol having the greatest antioxidant power. Decomposition also occurs in ultraviolet light. Tocopherols are isolated on a commercial scale from vegetable oils, usually by molecular distillation, extraction with organic solvents, or absorption chromatography. Alpha tocopherol is usually the most important homologue isolated from these sources; it also can be prepared synthetically and made available as the acetate and acid succinate esters.

The international standard for vitamin E used as a reference in all assays for this vitamin is a solution of dl-alpha tocopheryl acetate in coconut oil. Each 0.1 g of this solution contains 1 mg of the acetate. Results of an assay are expressed in terms of mg of the vitamin. The following relationship exists between International Units (or the equivalent USP Units) of the vitamin and the respective weights of the common forms:

1 USP or IU = 1 mg dl-alpha tocopheryl acetate = 0.91 mg dl-alpha tocopherol = 0.735 mg d-alpha tocopheryl acetate (the ester of the natural form) = 0.671 mg d-alpha tocopherol (the natural form)

The International Unit represents biological activity as determined by the rat antisterility test.

The usual methods for quantitative assay of vitamin E depend either directly or indirectly upon the ease with which free alpha tocopherol is oxidized. The esters, which are almost exclusively used in pharmaceuticals, must first be hydrolyzed. The free alcohol then, because of its instability, must be handled with care in all other analytical operations. The physicochemical methods generally applied employ either of two oxidation-reduction reactions: (1) the formation of a red orthoquinone by treatment of the tocopherol with concentrated nitric acid and (2) the reduction of ferric chloride in the presence of α,α'-dipyridyl which forms a red-colored complex with ferrous ions. Both methods are relatively nonspecific and are suitable only when combined with adequate separation procedures.

The classical biological method is the rat assay in which female rats are depleted of vitamin E and mated with normal males. The dose of the material to be tested and of the standard is administered over a period of several days after conception. On the 20th day of pregnancy the female rats are killed and the numbers of living and dead fetuses, and resorption sites are recorded. Another more simple

bioassay is based on the dialuric acid hemolysis test in which the red blood cell fragility is measured as a criterion of vitamin E status in the rat.

Metabolic Functions, Dietary Requirement, and Food Sources—The exact biochemical mechanism whereby vitamin E functions in the body is still unknown; however, its most critical function occurs in the membranous parts of cells. Here it interdigitates with phospholipids, cholesterol, and triglycerides, the three main structural elements of membranes. Since vitamin E is an antioxidant, a favored reaction at this site is with very reactive and usually destructive compounds called free radicals. These are products of oxidative deterioration of such substances as polyunsaturated fat. Vitamin E converts the free radical into a less reactive and nonharmful form. In its role as a protector against oxidation, vitamin E shows nutritional interactions with a wide variety of nutrients: vitamin A, the trace element selenium, the sulfur amino acids methionine and cysteine/cystine, polyunsaturated fatty acids, and, to a lesser extent, vitamin C. Interestingly enough, the order of antioxidant power among the tocopherols, as measured by their effect on the rate of peroxide formation in fats, is the reverse of the order of biological potencies. Other physiological functions probably include participation in nucleic acid metabolism, and it also appears that the tocopherols may be a component of the cytochrome reductase segment of the terminal respiratory chain in intermediary metabolism. In general, it appears that vitamin E plays an important role in insuring the stability and integrity of cellular membranes; thus far in man, the only such demonstrated effect is on the red blood cell. The effect is also modified by the level of polyunsaturated fatty acids in the diet.

The therapeutic effectiveness of vitamin E in the prevention of abortion, in certain menstrual disorders, in the improvement of lactation, in muscular dystrophy, or in cardiovascular diseases has not been substantiated, and the promotion of vitamin E for such purposes is fraudulent. One usage that is established and sound is in hemolytic anemia in premature infants. Vitamin E also generally is considered to provide protection against pulmonary oxygen poisoning. Essentially all other examples of clinical indications of need for vitamin E at nutritional levels are related to malnourishment or malabsorption problems. The latter are found in humans with cystic fibrosis, liver cirrhosis, postgastrectomy, obstructive jaundice, pancreatic insufficiency, and sprue.

A clearly defined uncomplicated vitamin E deficiency disease has not been recognized as a public health problem. A deficiency state with respect to vitamin E has been demonstrated in human subjects, especially in premature and new-born infants and in infants with steatorrhea. The evidence rests mainly on determinations of *in vitro* hemolysis and blood tocopherol level. Vitamin E requirement apparently is not related to body weight directly or to caloric intake, but seems to be related to body weight in kilograms to the three-quarter power, sometimes designated as physiologic or metabolic size. According to the National Research Council's Recommended Dietary Allowances, the daily vitamin E activity allowances are as follows: infants, 3 to 5 IU; children, 5 to 7 IU; adults, 8 to 11 IU.

Vitamin E is ubiquitous in its distribution and is found particularly in vegetable fats and oils, dairy products and meat, eggs, cereals, nuts, and leafy green and yellow vegetables. *Vitamin E is so widely distributed in nature that it is difficult to prepare a diet deficient in it and hard to see how a vitamin E deficiency in diets for humans might occur.* In direct contrast to the more rapid turnover of some of the water-soluble vitamins, vitamin E is stored in fatty tissue and is removed from it only when the fat is mobilized. This means that many months of deprivation would have to pass in order to deplete the body stores.

Vitamin K

Vitamin K refers to a group of substances, widespread in nature, having similar biologic activity; one form was isolated first from alfalfa and the other from putrefied fish meal. The primary activity which makes the vitamin essential in human metabolism is its involvement in the blood-clotting system through synthesis of prothrombin and other clotting factors.

Chemistry and Assay—The parent structure of the K family of vitamins is 2-methyl-1,4-naphthoquinone or menadione. This fat-soluble compound and several water-soluble derivatives such as the sodium bisulfite and diphosphoric acid ester are the common commercial forms used in medical practice. Vitamin K_1 (isolated from alfalfa) is 2-methyl-3-phytyl-1,4-naphthoquinone.

Vitamin K₁—phylloquinone; phytonadione

Vitamin K_2 exists as a chemical series which, instead of the phytyl side-chain in the 3-position, have side-chains of varying number of unhydrogenated isoprene units depending on the bacterial source. The vitamin K_2 having a 35-carbon side-chain and originally isolated from the putrefied fish meal is 2-methyl-3-*all-trans*-farnesylgeran-ylgeranyl-1,4-naphthoquinone.

The naturally occurring substances in pure form are light-yellow solids or oils, insoluble in water, but soluble in fat solvents. Transparent colloidal solutions of vitamin K_1 can be prepared by means of nonionic surfactants. Although menadione, too, is fat-soluble, it is easily soluble in boiling water and it is also slightly volatile at room temperature. Vitamins K_1 and K_2 as well as menadione are redox substances stable in the quinone form. In this respect there is a structural analogy between the vitamins K and E and a recently isolated series of naturally occurring quinones called *ubiquinones*. The latter do not possess any vitamin activity. Vitamins K have characteristic absorption spectra in the ultraviolet and are sensitive to alkali, light, and ionizing radiation.

activity is sulfaquinoxaline, a sulfonamide drug used in veterinary medicine for treatment of various infectious intestinal diseases. It increases the animal's requirement for vitamin K in some undetermined manner probably by eliminating vitamin K-synthesizing enteric bacteria, upon which the animal depends, in part, for a source of the vitamin. Extended treatment with antibacterial drugs that alter the enteric flora also increases the dietary vitamin K requirement in man.

Optimal absorption of the vitamins K requires the presence of bile or bile salts in the intestine. Menadione, however, is easily absorbed in the absence of bile. The average diet apparently contains adequate amounts of vitamin K, since few if any malnourished humans have presented findings of dietary lack of vitamin K uncomplicated by intestinal disease, which prevents absorption. Because of the lack of reliable information concerning human intakes of vitamin K and because of other factors shown to be operative in experimental animals, but not yet evaluated in man, an absolute daily allowance for this vitamin has not been established. The daily requirement is probably below the equivalent of 2 mg of menadione administered intravenously.

The premature infant appears to be particularly sensitive to a lack of the vitamin, and also to an excess, particularly in the case of menadione. Because of this potential toxicity, the inclusion of menadione in over-the-counter dietary supplements for the gravid female is prohibited. Vitamin K_1 does not exhibit this toxicity and is the preferred form. For newborn infants and especially those born prematurely (and anoxic), a single dose of 1 mg of vitamin K_1, im-

Vitamin K₂₍₃₅₎ (farnoquinone)

There is neither an international nor USP standard (or Unit) for vitamin K. There is, however, a USP Reference Standard of menadione. The activity of test materials is generally measured in terms of biological equivalency to milligrams or micrograms of menadione in a chick feeding test.

After extraction and separation from interfering substances, the vitamins K can be determined by their ultraviolet spectra or by color reactions. They react with sodium ethylate to give a blue color, which changes to brown. A more sensitive reaction occurs with sodium diethyldithiocarbamate to give a transient blue color. A method for assay of menadione in injections is the photometric assay of Menotti, in which 2,4-dinitrophenylhydrazine in ethanol is heated with menadione in the presence of HCl. The vitamin is thus converted to the hydrazone, which when treated with ammonia yields a blue-green color.

The chick is particularly suited for the biological assay of vitamin K because of the ease in producing a dietary vitamin deficiency and the high requirement, and the criterion of activity (blood "prothrombin time") is readily measurable.

Metabolic Functions, Dietary Requirement, and Food Sources—Vitamin K is necessary for the formation of prothrombinogen and other blood clotting factors in the liver. During clotting, circulating prothrombin is required for the production of thrombin; in turn, the thrombin converts fibrinogen to fibrin, the network of which constitutes the clot. It is obvious from this description that interference with formation of prothrombin will reduce the clotting tendency of the blood. In a deficiency of the vitamin, a condition of hypoprothrombinemia occurs, and blood-clotting time may be greatly, or even indefinitely, prolonged. Internal or external hemorrhages may ensue either spontaneously or following injury or surgery.

A group of substances termed vitamin K antagonists are characterized by their property to decrease plasma prothrombin levels and their usefulness in medicine as anticoagulants (see page 766). Representative of this group is dicumarol, originally isolated from spoiled sweet clover hay, in which it is formed by bacterial action on coumarin. An important use of vitamin K is in the treatment of hypoprothrombinemia consequent to prothrombopenic anticoagulant therapy. Vitamin K_1 is the preferred form. Large doses of salicylates also antagonize vitamin K.

A few chemically related derivatives of dicumarol are commercially used as rodenticides. Another compound with similar antagonist

mediately after birth, is often a routine measure to prevent hemorrhagic disease. Vitamin K_1 may be administered to the mother 12 to 24 hours prior to the expected delivery, or at the first sign of labor, especially if the mother has been receiving prothrombopenic anticoagulants. Requirements normally decrease after the neonatal period, however it is important to ensure that adequate amounts of vitamin K are present in infant formulas, since these are likely to be the sole nutriment during this period. Milk substitute formulas containing less than 25 μg/L should have vitamin K_1 added to attain a level of at least 100 μg/L.

Although extensive measurements of dietary intakes and food content of the vitamins K have not been made, primarily because suitable analytical methods have not been developed, enough information is known to say that the vitamin is widely distributed in a variety of foods. The green, leafy vegetables, tomatoes, cauliflower, egg yolk, soybean oil, and liver of all kinds are good sources. Since it is insoluble in water, there is no loss in ordinary cooking. The human also utilizes vitamin K synthesized by certain enteric bacteria and probably obtains a large part of his need from this source.

Fat-Soluble Vitamin Preparations

Cholecalciferol

9,10-Secocholesta-5,7,10(19)-trien-3-ol, (3β)-, Vitamin D₃; Activated 7-Dehydrocholesterol

9,10-Secocholesta-5,7,10(19)-trien-3β-ol [67-97-0] $C_{27}H_{44}O$ (384.64); an antirachitic vitamin obtained from natural sources or prepared synthetically. See page 1007.

Description—White, odorless crystals; affected by air and light; melts between 84° and 88°.
Solubility—Insoluble in water; soluble in alcohol, chloroform, and fatty oils.

Uses—The only valid therapeutic uses of cholecalciferol are in the treatment of vitamin D *deficiency* or in the *prophylaxis* of deficiency in persons with a known deficiency, a high requirement, or an absorption defect. However, the substance may be employed to treat *hypocalcemic tetany* and *hypoparathyroidism*. Cholecalciferol should not be employed in the presence of renal insufficiency or hyperphosphatemia.

Dose—The same as for *Ergocalciferol*.

Cod Liver Oil

Oleum Morrhuae; Oleum Jecoris Aselli; Oleum Gadi

The partially destearinated fixed oil obtained from fresh livers of *Gadus morrhua* Linné and other species of the Family *Gadidae*; contains in each g, not less than 255 µg (850 USP Units) of vitamin A and not less than 2.125 µg (85 USP Units) of vitamin D.

Cod liver oil may be flavored by the addition of not more than 1% of a suitable flavoring substance or a mixture of such substances.

Preparation—The highest grade of medicinal cod liver oil is manufactured from fresh cod livers of healthy fish, removed from the fish within a few hours after they are caught. The oil is separated from the livers by heating with low-pressure steam. When livers of high quality are used and the manufacturing procedure is carried out under carefully controlled sanitary conditions the resulting crude oil is of a light yellow color, and of good flavor and odor. Such an oil requires no purification or chemical refining.

Due, however, to long-established trade demands, it is necessary to remove the cod liver stearin so that the oil will remain clear at temperatures above freezing. To accomplish this, the oil is chilled to precipitate the stearin, which is removed by pressure filtration. To preserve the natural vitamin content of cod liver oil, it should be stored out of contact with air and light, preferably in a cool place.

Constituents—Consists chiefly of unsaturated glycerides but contains *palmitin* and *stearin*, as well as traces of *chlorine, bromine, phosphorus,* and *sulfur*. American cod liver oils may contain as much as 3 ppm of arsenic, but there is little evidence as to how completely it may be assimilated. American cod liver oils are rich in *iodine*—one sample was found to contain nearly 15,000 parts of iodine/billion parts of oil.

The vitamins of cod liver oil occur in the unsaponifiable fraction. Since some persons object to taking oils, tablets and capsules containing the unsaponifiable fraction of cod liver oil are manufactured. In general the procedure consists of saponifying the cod liver oil, separating the unsaponifiable portion, and extracting it with suitable solvents. The extract is diluted with corn oil and filled into capsules or mixed with solid materials and manufactured into tablets. The vitamin potency of these preparations can be adjusted to the patient's requirements but obviously they do not supply the constituents present in the saponifiable portion of the cod liver oil from which they were prepared.

Description—Thin, oily liquid, with a characteristic, slightly fishy, but not rancid, odor and a fishy taste; specific gravity 0.918 to 0.927.

Solubility—Slightly soluble in alcohol; freely soluble in ether, chloroform, carbon disulfide, and ethyl acetate.

Uses—A source of vitamins A and D. The vitamins are present in such proportion that an oral dose of 5 mL provides the daily requirements for children or adults of both of these dietary essentials. However, it may not provide 100% of a US RDA. Cod liver oil has been employed in the prophylaxis of rickets in infants.

Dose—5 mL, to contain no less than **1170 µg** (3900 USP units) of vitamin A and **9.7 µg** (386 USP units) of vitamin D.

Note—Cod Liver Oil containing more than the minimum requirements for both vitamin A and vitamin D may be administered in proportionally smaller doses.

Dihydrotachysterol—page 978.

Ergocalciferol

9,10-Secoergosta-5,7,10(19), 22-tetraen-3-ol, (3β,5Z,7E,22E)-, Calciferol; Vitamin D₂; *Various Mfrs*

See page 1007 for the structure.

9,10-Secoergosta-5,7,10(19),22-tetraen-3β-ol [50-14-6] $C_{28}H_{44}O$ (396.65). Ergocalciferol is obtained by exposing ergosterol to ultraviolet light for the proper length of time. Insufficient irradiation results in the production of products with little or no antirachitic activity and prolonged exposure causes the production of toxic products. See page 1007.

Note—In stating the potency and dosage of vitamin D (cholecalciferol, ergocalciferol) dosage forms it is customary to use either the

International Unit (IU) or the equivalent USP Unit. One USP Unit (or International Unit) of vitamin D (cholecalciferol or ergocalciferol) is defined as the specific biologic activity of 0.025 µg of the crystalline international standard or pure vitamin D₃.

Description—White, odorless crystals; affected by light and air; melting range 115° to 118°.

Solubility—Insoluble in water; soluble in alcohol, chloroform, ether, and fatty oils.

Uses—Like other forms of vitamin D, it exhibits both antirachitic and calcemic effects. It has a relatively high potency and is thus especially useful for the treatment of severe or refractory *rickets*. It may also be used in the management of *hypocalcemia* and *hypoparathyroidism*. Care must be exercised to prevent overdosage. It should not be employed when renal insufficiency or hyperphosphatemia prevails. The serious toxic effects that may be caused by vitamin D are summarized in the general article on *Vitamin D* (see page 950, under *Metabolic Functions*).

Dose—*Prophylactic, to prevent rickets*, **10 µg** (400 USP Units)/day (see Tables I and III, this chapter); in the *treatment of vitamin D-resistant rickets* (*refractory rickets*), **300 µg** to **12.5 mg** (12,000 to 500,000 Units) daily; in *hypoparathyroidism*, **1.25** to **5 mg** (50,000 to 200,000 Units) daily, plus 4 g of calcium lactate administered 6 times a day. *Caution: dosage must be individualized under close medical supervision; the range between therapeutic and toxic doses is narrow.*

Dosage Forms—Capsules: 1.25 mg (50,000 USP Units); Solution; Tablets: 1.25 mg (50,000 USP Units).

Menadiol Sodium Diphosphate

1,4-Naphthalenediol, 2-methyl-, bis(dihydrogen phosphate), tetrasodium salt, hexahydrate; Vitamin K₄; Kappadione (*Lilly*); Synkavite (*Hoffmann-LaRoche*)

2-Methyl-1,4-naphthalenediol bis(dihydrogen phosphate) tetrasodium salt, hexahydrate [6700-42-1] $C_{11}H_8Na_4O_8P_2.6H_2O$ (530.18); *anhydrous* [131-13-5] (422.09).

Preparation—Reduction of menadione to the diol compound by treatment with zinc in the presence of acid followed by double esterification with HI, metathesis of the resulting 1,4-diiodo compound with AgH_2PO_4, and neutralization of the bis(dihydrogen phosphate) ester thus formed with NaOH.

Description—White to pink powder, having a characteristic odor; hygroscopic; solutions are neutral or slightly alkaline to litmus, pH about 8.

Solubility—Very soluble in water; insoluble in alcohol.

Uses—See *Menadione* and *Phytonadione*. Menadiol sodium diphosphate in the body is converted to menadione, and consequently it has the same uses and limitations, except that it is water-soluble and does not require the presence of bile salts for its absorption; therefore, it is especially useful in the presence of bile obstruction.

Dose—*Adult, oral, subcutaneous, intramuscular,* or *intravenous, usual,* for *hypoprothrombinemia*, **5** to **15 mg** daily; *intramuscular,* to *antagonize prothrombopenic anticoagulants,* up to **75 mg**, to be repeated as needed; to *antagonize the prothrombopenic actions of salicylates,* **10** to **25 mg** daily, in 3 divided doses.

Dosage Forms—Injection: 5 to 10 mg/mL, 75 mg/2 mL; Tablets: 5 mg.

Menadione

1,4-Naphthalenedione, 2-methyl-, Vitamin K₃

2-Methyl-1,4-naphthoquinone [58-27-5] $C_{11}H_8O_2$ (172.18).

Caution—*Menadione powder is irritating to the respiratory tract and to the skin, and a solution of it in alcohol is a vesicant.*

Preparation—By the action of chromic acid on 2-methylnaphthalene in the presence of H_2SO_4.

Description—Bright yellow, crystalline powder which is nearly odorless; affected by sunlight; melts between 105° and 107°.

Solubility—Practically insoluble in water; 1 g in 60 mL alcohol and 10 mL benzene; sparingly soluble in chloroform; soluble in vegetable oils.

Incompatibilities—Incompatible with alkalies. Reducing agents convert it to a hydroquinone. It is affected by light.

Uses—See *Phytonadione*. In some of its actions menadione appears to be more potent than phytonadione. However, menadione is inferior to natural vitamin K_1 in the antagonism of anticoagulants of the dicumarol type. Because of the insolubility of menadione, with oral doses bile salts should be coadministered when bile obstruction exists.

Dose—*Oral* and *intramuscular*, **2** to **10 mg** daily.

Dosage Forms—Injection (in oil): 2 and 10 mg/mL; Tablets: 2, 5, and 10 mg.

Menadione Sodium Bisulfite

2-Naphthalenesulfonic acid, 1,2,3,4-tetrahydro-2-methyl-1,4-dioxo-, sodium salt, trihydrate; Menadione Bisulfite

Sodium 1,2,3,4-tetrahydro-2-methyl-1,4-dioxo-2-naphthalenesulfonate trihydrate [6147-37-1] $C_{11}H_9NaO_5S.3H_2O$ (330.28); *anhydrous* [130-37-0] (276.24).

Preparation—By reacting menadione with sodium bisulfite. The reaction may be visualized as consisting of the typical addition of $NaHSO_3$ to a ketone forming the $R(OH)(SO_3Na)$ compound which then rearranges at the expense of one degree of unsaturation of the quinonoid nucleus. The compound readily regenerates menadione on treatment with mild alkali and thus behaves as a typical ketone-$NaHSO_3$ addition compound.

Description—White, crystalline, odorless, hygroscopic powder.

Solubility—1 g in 3 mL water, >1000 mL alcohol, >1000 mL chloroform, >2000 mL ether.

Uses—An addition product of menadione and sodium bisulfite, and it is converted in the body to menadione. Consequently, its actions and uses are those of menadione (see *Menadione* and *Phytonadione*).

Dose—*Usual, intravenous, intramuscular, subcutaneous*, **2** to **10 mg** daily. To antagonize prothrombopenic anticoagulants, 50 to 100 mg by slow intravenous injection has been given.

Dosage Forms—Injection: 5 and 10 mg/mL, 72 mg/10 mL.

Oleovitamin A and D

Concentrated Vitamins A and D Solution

A solution of vitamin A and vitamin D in fish liver oil or in an edible vegetable oil. The vitamin D is from natural sources or is present as ergocalciferol or cholecalciferol obtained by the activation of either ergosterol or 7-dehydrocholesterol; contains not less than 90% of the labeled amounts of vitamins A and D.

Description—Yellow to red oily liquid; clear liquid at temperatures above 65° and may crystallize on cooling; may be nearly odorless or may have a fish-like odor; does not have a rancid odor or taste; unstable in air and light.

Solubility—Insoluble in water and glycerin; very soluble in ether and chloroform; soluble in dehydrated alcohol and vegetable oils.

Uses—Since the vitamins A and D content of oleovitamin A and D may be varied, the uses also vary according to the composition. Thus it may be used to supply primarily either vitamin A or vitamin D. However, it is generally used as a source of both vitamins for use when the vitamin requirement is high or when there is a diminished absorption from the gastrointestinal tract.

Dose—To be determined by the physician according to the needs of the patient.

Dosage Forms—Capsules.

Phytonadione

1,4-Naphthalenedione, 2-methyl-3-(3,7,11,15-tetramethyl-2-hexadecenyl)-[R-[R*,R*-(E)]]-, 2-Methyl-3-phytyl-1,4-naphthoquinone; Vitamin K_1; Mephyton (*MSD*)

Phylloquinone [84-80-0] $C_{31}H_{46}O_2$ (450.70). Phytonadione is a mixture of *cis*- and *trans*-isomers; it contains not more than 20.0% of the *cis*-isomer. See page 1008.

Description—Clear, yellow to amber, very viscous, odorless or nearly odorless liquid; specific gravity about 0.967; stable in air but decomposes on exposure to sunlight; solution (1 in 20) in alcohol is neutral to litmus; refractive index 1.523 to 1.526 at 25°.

Solubility—Insoluble in water; soluble in dehydrated alcohol, benzene, chloroform, ether, and vegetable oils.

Uses—The natural product, vitamin K_1. For the metabolic functions of vitamin K, see page 1008.

Vitamin K_1 has a more prompt and prolonged action than menadione and other synthetic analogues of vitamin K, and it is the more reliable in restoring prothrombin to the blood in conditions of *hypoprothrombinemia. Hypoprothrombinemia in the newborn* may be prevented or treated by the administration of phytonadione to the mother shortly before parturition or by giving the infant a single dose shortly after birth. In *hypoprothrombinemia consequent to prothrombopenic anticoagulant therapy*, an adequate intravenous injection will usually stop hemorrhage within 3 to 4 hours and restore the plasma prothrombin level to normal in 12 to 24 hours. In hypoprothrombinemia resulting from liver disease it may have limited value, especially if the disease is hepatocellular; in *biliary obstruction or fistula*, in which only the absorption of vitamin K is impaired, hypoprothrombinemia responds promptly to parenteral phytonadione. In other enteric diseases in which absorption is defective—as in *sprue, regional enteritis, enterocolitis, ulcerative colitis, dysentery*, and in *extensive bowel resection*—phytonadione will correct hypoprothrombinemia if given parenterally.

It must be emphasized that phytonadione cannot be used to check bleeding irrespective of its origin. It is of no benefit in diseases of the blood-forming organs, thrombocytopenic purpura, hemophilia, etc.

Excessive doses of phytonadione may occasionally cause hyperprothrombinemia and a tendency toward thrombosis.

Dose—*Oral*, for *hypoprothrombinemia*, 2.5 to 10 mg or up to 25 mg (rarely 50 mg), repeated in 12 to 48 hr if necessary; *subcutaneous* or *intramuscular* (*intravenous* if unavoidable, at rate of 1 mg/min), **2.5** to **10 mg** or up to **25 mg** (rarely **50 mg**), repeated in 6 to 8 hr if necessary. For prophylaxis of hemorrhagic disease of the newborn, a single *intramuscular* dose of **0.5** to **1 mg**; less desirably, **1** to **5 mg** to mother 12 to 24 hr before delivery. For treatment of hemorrhagic disease of the newborn, **1 mg** subcutaneously or intramuscularly (higher doses if mother has been receiving oral anticoagulants).

Dosage Forms—Injection: 1 mg/0.5 mL, 10 mg/mL, 25 mg/2.5 mL, 50 mg/5 mL; Tablets: 5 mg.

Tretinoin—page 785.

Vitamin A

Contains a suitable form of retinol ($C_{20}H_{30}O$; vitamin A alcohol). It may consist of retinol or esters of retinol formed from edible fatty acids, principally acetic and palmitic acids. It may be diluted with edible oils, or it may be incorporated in solid, edible carriers or excipients, and it may contain suitable antimicrobial agents, dispersants, and antioxidants. See page 1005.

Note—In stating the potency and dosage of vitamin A dosage forms it is customary to use either the International Unit (IU) or the equivalent USP Unit. One USP Unit (or International Unit) of vitamin A is defined as the specific biologic activity of 0.3 μg of the all-*trans* isomer of retinol.

Description—Yellow to red, oily liquid that may solidify upon refrigeration; in solid form, it has the appearance of any diluent that has been added; may be nearly odorless or may have a fish odor, but has no rancid odor or taste; unstable to air and light.

Solubility—In liquid form, insoluble in water and glycerin; soluble in absolute alcohol and vegetable oils; very soluble in ether and chloroform. In solid form, may be dispersible in water.

Uses—The only valid therapeutic uses are in the treatment of vitamin A *deficiency* or in the *prophylaxis* of deficiency in persons with a known dietary deficiency, a high requirement, or an absorption defect. Large doses of vitamin A produce toxicity (see *Metabolic Functions* of *Vitamin A*, page 1005), symptoms of which may not be evident for 6 months or longer. Daily doses larger than 25,000 USP Units should not be prescribed unless severe deficiency exists.

Dose—*Prophylactic*, **1.2** to **2.4 mg** (4000 to 8000 USP Units) daily; see Tables I and III in this chapter for dosage variation with different age groups. *Therapeutic, oral, in severe deficiency*, adults and *children over 8 yr of age*, **30 mg** (100,000 Units) daily for 3 days, then **15 mg** (50,000 units) daily for 2 weeks, followed by **3** to **6 mg** (10,000 to 20,000 Units) daily for 2 months; *intramuscular, in severe deficiency, adults and children over 8 yr of age*, **15** to **30 mg** (50,000 to 100,000 Units) daily for 3 days, followed by **15 mg** (50,000 Units) daily for 2 weeks; *1 to 8 yr*, **1.5** to **4.5 mg** (5000 to 15,000 Units) daily for 10 days; *infants*, **1.5** to **3 mg** (5000 to 10,000 Units) daily for 10 days.

Dosage Forms—Capsules: 1.5, 3, 7.5 and 15 mg (5000, 10,000, 25,000 and 50,000 USP Units); Drops: 15 mg (50,000 USP Units)/mL; Tablets: 15 mg (50,000 USP Units); Injection: 15 mg (50,000 USP Units)/mL.

Vitamin E

A form of alpha tocopherol [$C_{29}H_{50}O_2$ = 430.71]. See page 1008. It includes the following: *d*- or *dl*-alpha tocopherol ($C_{29}H_{50}O_2$); *d*- or *dl*-alpha tocopheryl acetate [$C_{31}H_{52}O_3$ = 472.75]; *d*- or *dl*-alpha tocopheryl acid succinate [$C_{33}H_{54}O_5$ = 530.79].

The generic title *Vitamin E Preparation* is officially recognized for any single form of Vitamin E with one or more inert substances. The product may be in liquid or solid form, and it must contain not less than 95.0% and not more than 120.0% of the labeled amount of Vitamin E. For a Preparation labeled to contain a *dl*-form of Vitamin E allowance is made for it to contain a small amount of a *d*-form occurring as a minor constituent of an added substance.

Alpha tocopherol (also written α-tocopherol) is a trivial generic name (which embraces all stereoisomeric forms of 2,5,7,8-tetra-methyl-2-(4,8,12-trimethyltridecyl)-6-chromanol. The term *d*-alpha tocopherol is employed in the pharmaceutical field to designate that form of the compound which (a) occurs naturally and (b) is dextro-rotatory. The term *dl*-alpha tocopherol designates the mixture of stereoisomers prepared synthetically, commonly from racemic iso-phytol.

The phenolic hydroxyl is readily susceptible to acylation and the resulting esters, eg, the acetate and acid succinate, are much more resistant to oxidation and discoloration on exposure to air and light than the phenolic form.

Description—Little or no odor or taste. *The alpha tocopherols and alpha tocopheryl acetates:* clear, yellow, viscous oils. *d-Alpha tocopheryl acetate:* may solidify in the cold. *Alpha tocopheryl acid succinate:* white powder; the *d*-isomer melts at about 75°, and the *dl*-form melts at about 70°. *The esters:* stable to air and to light but are unstable to alkali; *the acid succinate:* also unstable when held molten.

Solubility—*Alpha tocopheryl acid succinate:* insoluble in water; slightly soluble in alkaline solutions; soluble in alcohol, ether, acetone, and vegetable oils; very soluble in chloroform. *Other forms of vitamin E:* insoluble in water; soluble in alcohol; miscible with ether, acetone, vegetable oils and chloroform.

Uses—The only valid therapeutic use is as a supplement to the diet of the newborn infant, especially if premature, or in the treatment of the infant with steatorrhea, in which the gastrointestinal absorption of vitamin E is impaired. No need for administration to children or adults has been demonstrated. For additional information see the general article on *Vitamin E* in this chapter.

Dose—*Usual, prophylactic*, from **5** to **30** USP Units of vitamin E. 30 IU corresponds to the US RDA (see Tables I and II in this chapter); only persons on diets high in polyunsaturated fatty acids or who have previously been on such diets for a long period of time actually require this daily intake. *Therapeutic*, to be determined by the physician according to the needs of the patient.

Dosage Forms—Capsules: 30, 37.5, 50, 75, 100, 200, 400, 500, 600, and 1000 IU.

Other Fat-Soluble Vitamins

Calcitriol [9,10-Seco(5Z,7E)-5,7,10(19)-cholestatriene-1α,3β,25-triol; 1,25-dihydroxycholecalciferol; 1,25-hydroxyvitamin D$_3$; 1,25-DHCC; $C_{27}H_{44}O_3$ (416.65); *Rocaltrol* (*Roche*)]—The biologically active form of vitamin D$_3$ (see page 1007) resulting from sequential hydroxylation of the vitamin at C-25 in the liver and at C-1 in the kidney; produced also synthetically. A colorless, crystalline compound. *Uses:* The form of vitamin

D$_3$ that stimulates intestinal calcium transport. Based on the observation that in acutely uremic rats calcitriol stimulates intestinal calcium absorption it has been suggested that a vitamin-D resistant state exists in uremic patients because of failure of the kidney to convert precursors to calcitriol, hence the indication for use of the latter compound in the management of hypocalciuria in patients undergoing chronic renal dialysis. Efficacy of calcitriol in reversing not only the calcium metabolic disorder but also of reducing elevated parathyroid hormone levels in some patients has been demonstrated. *Dose:* Optimal daily dose, administered *orally*, must be determined for each patient. The recommended initial dose is 0.25 μg/day; most patients undergoing hemodialysis respond to doses between 0.5 and 1 μg/day but dosages up to 2 μg/day have been reported. *Dosage Form:* Soft gelatin capsules containing 0.25 μg.

Vitamin A Acetate [Retinol Acetate; $C_{22}H_{32}O_2$]—Light-yellow to red oil with a slight fishy odor; light and oxygen cause deterioration; tasteless. Soluble in lipid solvents; insoluble in water. *Uses:* A form of vitamin A; 0.344 μg is equivalent to 1 USP unit or to 0.6 μg of beta-carotene. *Dose:* See *Vitamin A* (page 1005).

Vitamin A Palmitate [Retinol Palmitate; $C_{36}H_{60}O_2$]—Light-yellow to red oil; odorless in the pure state but otherwise has a slight fishy odor; unstable in light and air. Soluble in oils and lipid solvents; insoluble in water. *Uses:* A form of vitamin A. *Dose:* See *Vitamin A* (page 1005); by weight, the palmitate is approximately half as potent as vitamin A.

The Water-Soluble Vitamins

Except for ascorbic acid, all the vitamins in this water-soluble category belong to the B-group of vitamins. Some still retain their original individual designations, such as B$_1$, B$_6$, and B$_{12}$, whereas comparable names for other vitamins have become obsolete.

In 1930, when it was clear that vitamin B was of multiple nature, the term vitamin B complex was coined to refer to the group of water-soluble animal growth factors found in relatively high concentrations in such products as liver, yeast, and rice bran. This was a convenient term to use in the early scientific literature, but it was not intended to be a specific name for pharmaceutical preparations that contain varying proportions of the B vitamins. The term was intended to apply to a group of vitamins whose identity was being sought, rather than to a group of compounds whose identity had been established. Since the nature of the "complex" has been characterized, the term vitamin B complex is no longer appropriate.

Ascorbic Acid (Vitamin C)

Vitamin C, or ascorbic acid, is necessary for the prevention and cure of the deficiency disease scurvy (antiscorbutic vitamin).

Scurvy has been recognized since the Middle Ages and was found widespread in northern Europe and among the crews of sailing ships. During the 18th century it was learned that when fresh fruit was made available aboard sailing vessels, scurvy was avoided. In 1907 Holst and Frolich observed a scurvy-like syndrome in guinea pigs that was similar to human scurvy and cured it by feeding citrus juices. This gave an experimental means for the rapid development of our knowledge of vitamin C, to which many workers have contributed.

Chemistry and Assay—Ascorbic acid is a white, crystalline compound structurally related to the monosaccharides. It exists in nature in both a reduced and the oxidized form, dehydroascorbic acid. These substances are in a state of reversible equilibrium in biological systems, and both have the same biological activity.

L-Ascorbic Acid　　　　　**Dehydroascorbic Acid**

* marks the most active hydrogen, which is replaced by Na in sodium ascorbate.

Ascorbic acid is stable in the dry state but is easily oxidized in aqueous solution in the presence of air. Oxidation is accelerated by heat, light, alkalies, oxidative enzymes, and traces of copper and iron. Because of its relative instability, ascorbic acid is readily lost during cooking if simple precautions to avoid aeration are not taken. Also, because of its high aqueous solubility, the vitamin is lost to a considerable extent when large amounts of cooking water are discarded. Progressive loss of vitamin C in fresh fruits and vegetables occurs during storage.

Solutions of ascorbic acid are strongly reducing, and the vitamin is easily oxidized. In animal tissues the greater part of the vitamin is in the reduced form, but, as scurvy develops, the ratio of oxidized to reduced form rises. This property of reversible oxidation–reduction is the most likely basis for the role of the vitamin in biochemical reactions.

The article of commerce is produced exclusively by synthesis. Sorbitol, a hexose occurring in several fruits but commercially obtained by hydrogenating dextrose, is the raw material for production of ascorbic acid. Amounts of ascorbic acid are expressed in terms of weight, as milligrams. The USP provides a Reference Standard of L-ascorbic acid for assay purposes. The practical methods of ascorbic acid assay are based on its powerful reducing properties which enable determination by oxidimetric titration. The three most-used reagents for this titration are chloramine-T, 2,6-dichlorophenolindophenol, and iodine. Another practical assay is based on the conversion of ascorbic acid to oxalic acid 2-nitrophenylhydrazide by treatment with diazotized 2-nitroaniline. This yields a colored compound which is measured photometrically. Still another is the photometric assay of total ascorbic acid (ascorbic acid plus dehydroascorbic acid) by conversion of the vitamin to its 2,4-dinitrophenylhydrazone.

Metabolic Function, Dietary Requirement, and Food Sources—Vitamin C is known to be essential for the formation of intercellular collagen. In scorbutic tissues the amorphous ground substance, and the fibroblasts in the area between the cells appear normal but without the matrix of collagen fibers. These bundles of collagenous material appear within a few hours after the administration of ascorbic acid. This points to the relationship of the vitamin in maintenance of tooth structures, matrix of bone, and the walls of capillaries. In scurvy, these are the tissues found to be faulty.

The picture of clinical scurvy in humans is one that can be related to the general breakdown of intercellular collagen substance. Bleeding is common, particularly at sites of pressure. The occurrence of petechiae, pinpoint hemorrhages that occur in the skin under reduced pressure, has been used as a diagnosis of scurvy. This is an indication of weakness or fragility of the walls of capillaries. Bones become brittle and cease to grow, and normal structures are replaced by connective tissue that contains calcified cartilage. Anemia is a common occurrence in scurvy, caused by an impairment of hematopoiesis. Tooth enamel, cementum, and particularly dentin, change in structure, and the gums about the teeth become spongy and bleed easily. Keratoconjunctivitis sicca, xerostomia, salivary gland enlargement, xerosis, hyperpigmentation, ichthyosis, neuropathies, and mental depression may occur, even when the full-blown picture of scurvy is absent.

Vitamin C is essential for the healing of bone fractures. Such fractures heal slowly in a patient deficient in vitamin C. Wound healing is also impaired.

There is evidence to indicate that the vitamin functions in the metabolism of tyrosine. There is an abnormal excretion of homogentisic, p-hydroxyphenylpyruvic, and p-hydroxyphenyllactic acids in scorbutic guinea pigs following administration of tyrosine, which, of course, is corrected with ascorbic acid. The excretion of "tyrosyl" derivatives in humans on a vitamin C-low diet given 20 g of tyrosine daily is also affected by ascorbic acid administration. In some newborn, the occurrence of tyrosinemia possibly accruing to high protein intakes suggests that this relationship be taken into consideration in evaluating the ascorbic acid requirement for the infant.

An intake of 10 to 20 mg/day of ascorbic acid is sufficient to protect an adult from classical scurvy and 45 mg/day will maintain an adequate body pool of 1500 mg. Except for pregnant and lactating women, 60 mg is the recommended dietary allowance (Table I) for both men and women over the age of 11 years. For infants, 35 mg of ascorbic acid provides about the same amount as supplied daily by 850 mL of milk from mothers living in the US. The vitamin C requirements are increased following trauma, during infections, and during periods of vigorous physical activity; in such circumstances the requirement may be 100 to 200 mg daily.

The regular ingestion of from 1 to 4 g of ascorbic acid/day has been suggested as a means of shortening the illness period and alleviating the symptoms of the "common cold." A few clinical studies offer some support for this hypothesis, but definitive long-term studies with

large populations which might confirm the practice as a reliable public health measure have not been done. Although vitamin C in large amounts may have some pharmacologic effects, these are not related to the normal functioning of the vitamin at nutritional levels.

The prolonged ingestion of supplements of ascorbic acid in excess of about 3 g/day is not without potential danger. Gastrointestinal disturbances (nausea followed by diarrhea), kidney or bladder stone formation (resulting from an increased excretion of oxalate, urate, and calcium), prenatal conditioning of the fetus to deficiency symptoms, interference with simple tests for glycosuria, and interference with the anticoagulant effect of heparin are clinical problems which may occur.

For therapeutic purposes in treatment of adult scurvy, 1000 mg of ascorbic acid daily in divided doses for 1 week is recommended, then 500 mg until all signs disappear. It is also used in the treatment of idiopathic methemoglobinemia to reduce the ferric iron in heme to the ferrous state.

Ascorbic acid facilitates the absorption of iron by keeping the iron in the reduced form. A few microcytic anemias respond to ascorbic acid treatment, which may be in part due to improved absorption of iron.

Vitamin C is found in all living plant cells, is synthesized during the germination of seeds, and is relatively concentrated in the rapidly growing parts of the plant. It is present in all animal tissues as well, but only guinea pigs, primates, and a few exotic animal species, and man are unable to meet body needs by synthesis, and must rely upon a dietary source.

Although vitamin C appears to be present in all living tissues, our best sources of supply are fresh fruits such as citrus fruits, strawberries, melons, and green vegetables such as lettuce and cabbage. Potatoes do not contain large amounts of ascorbic acid, but, since relatively large quantities are consumed they are a reliable source. It is a common practice, and a sound one, to rely to a large extent on citrus fruits and juices as important vitamin C carriers, particularly in infant feeding. An ounce of orange or lemon juice/day is sufficient to prevent scurvy in humans on an otherwise vitamin C-low diet.

It is fairly common practice to add ascorbic acid to foods for technical purposes; eg, as an antioxidant to protect natural flavors and colors.

The B Vitamins

The "water-soluble B" of McCollum, or the "antiberiberi vitamine" of Funk, has now been differentiated into at least eleven separate and distinct chemical entities. It has been established that eight of these are required in human nutrition. They are *thiamin, riboflavin, niacin, folacin, pyridoxine, biotin, pantothenic acid, and vitamin B_{12}*. Para-aminobenzoic acid, choline, and inositol have an essential part in cellular metabolism in plants and animals, but this alone does not constitute presumptive evidence of their importance in human nutrition. When the dietary intake of methionine is adequate, choline can be synthesized endogenously; therefore, the human requirement is relative to the methionine intake, similar to the relationship between niacin and tryptophan. It can be stated categorically that the human does not require either an exogenous or endogenous source of para-aminobenzoic acid. Although inositol deficiency has not been demonstrated in humans, it may be an important nutrient in infant nutrition. Mammalian milk contains inositol and, since milk is the sole item of the diet of infants during this critical growth period, it may not be inappropriate to include it in non-milk-based formulas, a practice which has existed for over 20 years.

There is no one natural source of the B vitamins as a group that is necessarily superior to another source. No natural source contains all the water-soluble factors in the proportions that are needed in human nutrition, and the therapeutic value of any vitamin-containing material depends on the needs of the individual to whom it is being administered. Nevertheless, multiple deficiencies of B-vitamins often coexist. Furthermore, the repair of one B-vitamin deficiency may increase the need for another; thus, the administration of thiamin in clinical or subclinical beriberi increases the need for riboflavin. Consequently, there is some justification for multivitamin therapy with those five B vitamins for which *clinical* deficiencies occur (thiamin, niacin, riboflavin, folacin, and vitamin B_{12}). Human deficiencies in biotin and pantothenic acid have only been produced experimentally, and pyridoxine deficiency has occurred in infants fed an unfortified formula.

Biotin

cis-Hexahydro-2-oxothieno[3,4-*d*]imidazole-4-valeric acid

Before this nutritional factor was identified as a discrete chemical substance, it was variously called vitamin H, anti-egg-white injury factor, coenzyme R, Bios II, and others. Its discovery was an outgrowth of studies on the "toxicity" of large amounts of unheated egg white as the sole source of protein for rats.

Chemistry and Assay—Biotin is a colorless, crystalline monocarboxylic acid, only slightly soluble in water and alcohol (its salts are quite soluble). Water solutions are stable at 100°, and the dry substance is both thermostable and photostable. Biotin is unstable, however, in strong acids and alkaline solutions and in oxidizing agents. The vitamin is optically active and the natural isomer, which alone possesses biological activity, is the D-form (rings are *cis*-fused and the isomer is designated (+)-biotin).

Biotin

Although biotin with the above structure is the compound present in food sources, the sulfur atom can be replaced with an oxygen atom without reduction of its metabolic activity. Biotin occurs in animal and plant tissues primarily in combined forms which are liberated by enzymatic hydrolysis during digestion. One of the simplest such complexes is biocytin, ϵ-*N*-biotinyl-L-lysine. The amount of the vitamin in a product is expressed solely in terms of the weight of the chemically pure substance, the free monocarboxylic acid.

Only microbiological methods are feasible for the quantitative assay of biotin because of their sensitivity to the low concentrations usually encountered. After simple aqueous or acid extraction combined with heating, a microbiological assay using growth of the test organisms *Allescheria boydii* or *Lactobacillus arabinosus* as the criterion is carried out.

Metabolic Functions, Dietary Requirement, and Food Sources—Attempts to induce biotin deficiency in man by inclusion of large amounts (200 g) of dried unheated egg white for several days in the diet have resulted in the appearance of vague symptoms such as change in skin color and dermatoses, slight change in lingual papillae of the tongue, muscle pains, loss of appetite, sleeplessness, and extreme lassitude. Raw egg white contains a protein, avidin, which combines with biotin and prevents absorption of the vitamin from the intestine. Rapid relief from such symptoms was observed with administration of biotin. This condition is difficult to produce in human subjects and, since a frank and specific deficiency disease is not discernible, there is uncertainty as to the exact nature of the deficiency syndrome as well as the need for a dietary source of biotin in human nutrition. Intestinal synthesis is undoubtedly the important factor in the supply of biotin to the body.

Biotin functions in carbon dioxide fixation reactions in intermediary metabolism, transferring the carboxyl group to acceptor molecules. It similarly acts also in decarboxylation reactions. For its part in these vital enzymatic steps, in catalyzing deamination of amino acids, and in oleic acid synthesis, biotin is essential in human metabolism and presumed to be a dietary essential in the absence of adequate microbial synthesis in the intestine.

Diets providing a daily intake of 150 to 300 μg of biotin are considered adequate. And these amounts are readily met and exceeded when milk, meat, and eggs are frequent items of the diet.

Choline

The propriety of classifying choline as a vitamin and a member of the B group is questionable because it is synthesized in the human body, and there is no evidence that a lack of choline has a disturbing effect on human metabolism. Nevertheless, choline plays an important role both as a structural component of tissues and in biological methylation reactions. Dietary deficiency of it leads to gross pathology in several species of animals.

Chemistry—Choline is (β-hydroxyethyl)trimethylammonium hydroxide. Since it is completely dissociated, it is comparable to alkali hydroxides as a base. Consequently, it does not exist as a base at body pH but rather as a salt, the anion is that present in its immediate biological environment. The β-(hydroxyethyl)trimethylammonium cation is the biologically important moiety. The cation

is incorporated into phospholipids, such as lecithin and sphingomyelin, and acetylcholine, a substance released at cholinergic nerve junctions during transmission of nerve impulses. Acid hydrolysis of phospholipids yields the free choline salt which is very soluble in water, and to a lesser extent in ethanol.

Choline

Metabolic Functions, Dietary Requirement, and Food Sources—Besides its vital function as a precursor of acetylcholine, which is important in the sequence of nerve-muscle stimulations, choline is an important contributor of methyl groups needed for the *in vivo* synthesis of metabolites and perhaps some hormones. The biogenesis of choline appears to be universal in nature, and is the result of the three-step transfer of methyl groups to an acceptor, which may be either free aminoethanol or phosphatidyl aminoethanol. Such transfers require methionine as a methyl donor (actually, *S*-adenosylmethionine). Choline is indirectly a source of methyl groups; it is first oxidized to betaine, which then may transfer a methyl group to homocysteine to form methionine. By thus regenerating methionine lost in transmethylation reactions, exogenous choline can spare the amino acid for use in protein synthesis. Methionine is an essential amino acid.

Choline has the property of preventing the deposition of excess fat, or of causing the removal of excess fat from the liver of experimental animals fed high-fat diets and, because of this, is often classified as a "lipotropic agent." The lipotropic action probably relates to the incorporation of choline into phosphatidyl choline (lecithin), which, in turn, is incorporated into phospholipids and lipoproteins. The lipotropic action is independent of the function of choline as a reservoir of methyl groups.

There is presumptive evidence from nutritional and metabolic studies and teleological considerations that choline is important, if not essential, for the infant. It is appropriate to ensure, therefore, that choline is present in infant formulas at least to the level found in human milk. This is about 90 mg/L. Most infant formulas contain about 1½ times this amount. It is equally appropriate to include choline in chemically defined diets to be used as the sole source of nutrients for critically ill patients. An average mixed diet consumed by man in the US has been estimated to contain 500 to 900 mg choline/day, an amount known to be adequate when compared with animal requirements. Foods that supply large amounts of choline are liver, kidney, brain, muscle meats, fish, nuts, beans, peas, and eggs. Moderate amounts exist in cereals, milk, and a number of vegetables.

Folacin (Folic Acid)

The vitamin derives its name from the Latin work *folium*, leaf. It was first isolated from spinach leaves where it is now known to occur in relatively minute amounts, compared to other food sources. Several apparently unrelated factors had been isolated in various laboratories before realization that they had in common the same parent compound, pteroyl-L-glutamic acid: Factor U (a chick growth factor), vitamin M (a factor for monkeys), vitamin B_c (a chick anti-anemia factor), liver and yeast *L casei* factors (bacterial growth factors), and others. In 1972 the International Union of Nutritional Sciences Committee on Nomenclature decided that the term folacin should be used as the generic descriptor for folic acid pteroylmono-L-glutamic acid. However, the USP continues to call pteroylglutamic acid by the descriptor, folic acid, and common practice usually does the same.

Chemistry and Assay—Pteroylglutamic acid crystallizes from cold water, in which it is only slightly soluble, as yellow spear-shaped platelets. It is readily destroyed by boiling in acid solution and its solutions will deteriorate in sunlight. It is insoluble in alcohol and the usual organic solvents but readily dissolves in dilute solutions of alkali hydroxides and carbonates. The characteristic ultraviolet absorption spectrum of pteroylglutamic acid in dilute NaOH is used to aid in identification and measurement of the compound.

A series of compounds with several molecules of glutamic acid attached to the first glutamic acid radical in peptide linkage have been synthesized. Compounds with one, two, three and seven glutamic acid groups have been isolated. The latter three are known as conjugates. Some animals and man can utilize them as a source of pteroylglutamic acid, presumably because appropriate digestive enzymes can hydrolyze them. Microorganisms can use them to only a variable and limited extent, unless they are first hydrolyzed to the free form with liver, kidney, or pancreatic enzymes, called conjugases.

The functional form of this vitamin group is basically the 5,6,7,8-tetrahydrofolic acid in which a formyl group (—CHO), when present, is attached at either or both the N^5 or N^{10} positions. The hydrogenated N^5-formyl compound, formerly called *folinic acid*, or leucovorin, is available, as is the monosodium salt of folic acid, as a discrete pharmaceutical preparation. It is properly termed 5-formyltetrahydrofolic acid. These compounds similarly serve as standards during assay of the vitamin. A USP Reference Standard Folic Acid is available. Separately, the three moieties which make up the folic acid molecule (pteroic acid, *p*-aminobenzoic acid, and glutamic acid) have no vitamin activity.

The quantitative assay of folacin in natural products is mainly by biological or microbiological methods. In the chick assay, the birds are placed on a folic acid-free diet until they became anemic, after which folic acid supplements and the test material are administered. The degree of recovery is related to the quantity of reference folic acid fed. The two organisms most used in the microbiological method are *Lactobacillus casei* and *Streptococcus faecalis*. The method is based on the fact that pteroylglutamic acid is a required growth factor for each; however, the assay is complicated when biological material is analyzed, because naturally occurring folic acid derivatives do not all have the same biological activity for the two organisms.

Folic acid can be determined by either of two physicochemical methods, provided the compound is present in relatively pure form. One method is the spectrophotometric measurement of the extinction maxima of the ultraviolet absorption curve; the other is the photometric measurement after oxidative fission of folic acid to 4-aminobenzoylglutamic acid followed by diazotization and coupling to give an azo dye.

Metabolic Functions—Folic acid is one of the important hematopoietic agents necessary for proper regeneration of the blood-forming elements and their functioning. Although the mechanism whereby folic acid performs this vital role is not understood, much is known about the involvement of folic acid as a coenzyme in intermediary metabolic reactions in which one-carbon units are transferred. These reactions are important in interconversions of various amino acids and in purine and pyrimidine synthesis. This role is in contrast to that of choline in furnishing and transferring so-called labile methyl groups in transmethylation reactions. The biosynthesis of purines and pyrimidines is ultimately linked with that of nucleotides and ribo- and deoxyribo-nucleic acids, functional elements of all cells.

The concept of antivitamins or vitamin antagonists is exemplified in a particular aspect of folic acid metabolism. By virtue of its structural similarity, sulfanilamide competes with *p*-aminobenzoic acid in the biological synthesis of folic acid. The organism is thus deprived of needed folic acid. Sulfonamides act, therefore, as growth inhibitors of certain pathogenic organisms, a competitive antagonism which is responsible for the antibacterial action of sulfa drugs. Since mammals use preformed folic acid, sulfonamides do not disrupt the host metabolism.

Numerous analogues of pteroylglutamic acid have been prepared which exhibit potent anti-folic acid activity. Several compounds, notably aminopterin (4-aminopteroylglutamic acid) and methotrexate (4-amino-N^{10}-methylpteroylglutamic acid), compete with folic acid in nucleic acid synthesis and have been used in the treatment of leukemia and other cancers.

Dietary Requirement and Food Sources—Folacin deficiency results in megaloblastic anemia, glossitis, diarrhea, and weight loss. A deficiency is best diagnosed by the demonstration of low levels of the vitamin in serum or blood by microbiological assay or by the hematological response to a physiological dose of folic acid, 50 to 200

μg intramuscularly/day for 10 days. The condition of megaloblastic anemia arising as a result of dietary deficiency of folacin occurs most frequently after the age of 65 years, in persons suffering from malabsorption syndromes, in women during the last trimester of pregnancy, and in infants receiving unfortified proprietary formulas or goat's milk. In the treatment of megaloblastic or macrocytic anemia in the elderly, folic acid should be administered as the sole therapeusis *only* when the possibility of pernicious anemia and other primary diseases of the small bowel has been absolutely excluded, a restriction necessitated because of the vitamin's ability to mask other diagnostic signs of these conditions.

The minimum amount of folic acid required by the normal adult is about 0.05 mg/day, though pregnancy and other stressful situations, including various disease states and the consumption of alcohol, increase the requirement. Since the vitamin exists in nature predominantly in the combined form which has limited availability, the daily dietary allowances recommended by the Food and Nutrition Board, National Research Council takes this into account. Their recommendations are 0.4 mg for adolescents and adults, 0.8 mg during pregnancy, 0.6 mg during lactation, and from 0.05 to 0.3 mg for infants and children.

A balanced American diet for adults contains approximately 0.2 to 0.6 mg of total folic acid activity, and the intestinal microflora also provide some absorbable amounts of the vitamin. The best food sources of folic acid are liver, kidney, dry beans, asparagus, mushrooms, broccoli, and collards. Other good sources include spinach, peanuts, lima beans, cabbage, sweet corn, chard, turnip greens, lettuce, milk, and whole wheat products.

Inositol

Inositol is hexahydroxycyclohexane (1,2,3,5/4,6-cyclohexanol; *i*-inositol; *myo*-inositol; *meso*-inositol). Actually, there are nine stereoisomeric cyclohexanols, which are all now commonly referred to as inositols. Several occur in nature; the isomer described above is by far the most prevalent and is the only one that is biologically active.

Inositol

Inositol occurs normally in nearly all plant and animal cells, either free or combined, suggesting that it is an essential cell constituent. In animal tissues it occurs as a constituent of phospholipids. In plants it is usually found as *phytic acid*, the hexaphosphate ester of inositol. There has as yet been no demonstration of need for inositol in human nutrition. In fact, large amounts of phytic acid in the diet interfere with the absorption of minerals, especially calcium, zinc and iron.

Although inositol possesses weak lipotropic activity, it is not as effective as methionine or choline. There is no valid therapeutic use of the compound. It may, however, be important to ensure its presence, at levels customarily found in human milk, in foods which are fed to infants and critically ill patients as the sole item of the diet.

Niacin (Nicotinic Acid and Nicotinamide)

Nicotinic acid (niacin) and nicotinamide (niacinamide) have identical properties as vitamins. Both compounds had been known for sometime before their biological significance was realized. In 1867 nicotinic acid was synthesized by the oxidation of nicotine with nitric acid. But it was not until 1937 that it was isolated from biological sources and found to be effective in the cure of black tongue in dogs and, later, pellagra in humans. The vitamin has none of the pharmacological properties of nicotine, however. In the 1940s the term "niacin" was adopted as a synonym for food labeling purposes to avoid association with the nicotine of tobacco. The term "niacin" is used generically to include both nicotinic acid and nicotinamide.

Chemistry and Assay—Nicotinic acid is pyridine-3-carboxylic acid. The structures of nicotinic acid and nicotinamide are shown below.

Niacin, the most stable of the vitamins, is not destroyed by heating in acid or alkaline solution. It withstands mild oxidation, and retains its biological activity during the processing of food and the preparation and storage of pharmaceuticals. It is readily soluble in water and alcohol but insoluble in ether and chloroform. Niacinamide, on the other hand, may be extracted from water solution with ether. The amide is readily hydrolyzed to the free acid by heating in acid or alkaline solution.

The usual commercial synthesis of nicotinic acid used in foods and drugs is by the oxidation of quinoline with potassium permanganate or manganese dioxide, and monodecarboxylation of the purified quinolinic acid with controlled heating. Nicotinamide is usually prepared by esterifying nicotinic acid with methanol followed by ammonolysis.

The activity of both forms of the vitamin is expressed in milligrams of the chemically pure substance. Because they have identical biological activity and their molecular weights are nearly identical, they are equivalent on a weight basis. Reference Standard Niacin and also Niacinamide Reference Standard are available from the USP.

Niacin may be determined in food, drugs, and biological materials by microbiological assay or by chemical methods. No animal biological method exists. The chemical determination involves reaction of the pyridine ring with cyanogen bromide and coupling of the fission product with an aromatic amine. The yellow polymethine dye which is formed is measured in a photometer at 436 nm. In natural products niacin occurs mainly in combined form as a coenzyme and must be liberated by acid hydrolysis before assay.

The microbiological assays employs *Lactobacillus arabinosus* as the test organism. A quantitative discrimination between nicotinic acid and nicotinamide in a sample is possible by assaying with both this organism, which utilizes both forms, and *Leuconostoc mesenteroides*, which can utilize only nicotinic acid.

Metabolic Functions—In the body niacin is converted to niacinamide, which is an essential constituent of coenzymes I and II that occur in a wide variety of enzyme systems involved in the anaerobic oxidation of carbohydrates. The coenzyme serves as a hydrogen acceptor in the oxidation of the substrate. These enzymes are present in all living cells and take part in many reactions of biological oxidation.

Nicotinamide-adenine dinucleotide (NAD) is the inner salt of the 5′-ester of 3-carbamoyl-1-β-D-ribofuranosylpyridinium hydroxide with adenosine 5′-pyrophosphate, and has the structure shown below. Nicotinamide-adenine dinucleotide phosphate (NADP) differs only in that the adenosine moiety is esterified at its 2′-position with phosphoric acid.

NAD

These coenzymes are synthesized in the body and take part in the metabolism of all living cells. Since they are of such widespread and vital importance, it is not difficult to see why serious disturbance of metabolic processes occurs when the supply of niacin to the cell is interrupted.

The observations of numerous nutritionists that the daily requirement for niacin is influenced by the amount and kind of dietary protein led to the discovery that the amino acid tryptophan functions as a potential precursor of niacin. The efficiency of the conversion

indicates that 60 mg of dietary tryptophan is equivalent to 1 mg of niacin. This relationship has given rise to the use of the term "niacin equivalent," which is defined for the purpose of estimating the adequacy of diets in this vitamin as 1 mg of niacin or 60 mg of dietary tryptophan.

Niacin is readily absorbed from the intestinal tract, and large doses may be given orally or parenterally, with equal effect.

The principal excretory product of niacin in the urine is *N*-methylnicotinamide, a fluorescent compound formed in the liver. On a normal diet approximately one-fourth of the niacinamide ingested is excreted as *N*-methylnicotinamide. With increased levels of niacin intake the percent of ingested niacin excreted as the fluorescent substance is decreased.

Dietary Requirement and Food Sources—Pellagra, which means rough skin, is the primary deficiency disease due to lack of sufficient niacin in the diet, and it appears only after months of dietary deprivation. The condition involves the gastrointestinal tract, the skin, and the nervous system. Loss of weight, anorexia, weakness, insomnia, headache, and diarrhea are common and appear without obvious cause. Other early symptoms may include abdominal pain, nervousness, and mental confusion.

Typical manifestations of pellagra in a well-advanced stage are diarrhea, dermatitis, and dementia. Gastrointestinal difficulties vary in severity, and absence of gastric secretion is a common finding. In the more advanced state, diarrhea is severe. Dermatitis has a characteristic appearance and occurs at those sites subject to exposure or irritation. The skin lesions are usually bilaterally symmetrical and appear first as erythematous patches, changing to brown pigmented areas, followed by desquamation and thickening. Glossitis is common; it is characterized by swelling and redness at the margins and tip of the tongue. Because of inflammation and superficial desquamation, the tongue, gums, and lips appear scarlet and smooth. Mental symptoms vary in occurrence and intensity; they include irritability, mental depression, and emotional instability. A confused mental state with hallucinations, mania, and delirium is seen in advanced stages of the disease. Pellagra is a complex deficiency, and symptoms of riboflavin, thiamin and folacin deficiency frequently complicate the clinical picture.

Treatment of the disease requires immediate change to a nutritionally adequate diet and the administration of niacin or niacinamide. Where neurological symptoms are present, use of thiamin and riboflavin may be necessary as well. Recovery from the acute condition is dramatic in most instances, and occurs within 24 to 48 hours. Small doses given frequently during the day have been found to be more effective than a single large daily dose. Niacinamide is preferable to niacin because it does not produce vasodilation in the skin with sensations of itching, burning, or tingling. With severe nausea and diarrhea, intravenous injection of niacinamide is of additional advantage.

In considering dietary requirement and the foods which contribute to it, one must consider the content of preformed niacin and the niacin available by conversion from tryptophan, an essential amino acid present in all good-quality proteins. The minimum requirement to prevent pellagra is the equivalent of about 4.4 mg of niacin per 1000 kcal/day. The recommended dietary allowance of the Food and Nutrition Board is 6.6 mg per 1000 kcal and not less than 13 mg at caloric intakes of less than 2000 kcal. Most diets consumed in the US supply from 500 to 1000 mg or more of tryptophan daily and 8 to 17 mg of preformed niacin, equivalent to 16 to 33 mg of niacin.

Poultry, meats, and fish constitute the most important single food group source of niacin. Organ meats are somewhat superior to muscle tissue. Potatoes, legumes, and some green leafy vegetables contain moderate amounts of preformed niacin, as do whole grains. An important public health nutrition practice, begun in the 1940s, is the nutrient enrichment of cereal products: wheat flour, farina, corn products, rice, macaroni and noodle products, and bread. Niacin, thiamin, riboflavin, and iron are mandatory ingredients in products which are labeled "enriched." The level of enrichment for niacin is such that a significant proportion of the daily requirement is obtainable from a generous serving of these foods.

Pantothenic Acid

Knowledge of the identity and importance of pantothenic acid grew principally from experimental studies on microorganisms and chicks. Because of its wide distribution in nature it was named "pantothenic" from the Greek word *pantothen*, from all sides. The terms vitamin

B$_3$ and chick antidermatitis factor were once applied to variously purified concentrates of the factor, but they are now obsolete. No known therapeutic value exists for pantothenic acid, except perhaps in the treatment of frank or suspected cases of combined nutritional deficiencies.

Chemistry and Assay—Pantothenic acid is optically active. Maximum vitamin activity resides only in the D-form, and it is readily available as either the sodium or calcium salts which are crystalline substances. Another commercially available form used in liquid preparations is D-pantothenyl alcohol (panthenol). Chemically, pantothenic acid is a composite structure of β-alanine and 2,4-dihydroxy-3,3-dimethylbutyric acid γ-lactone, connected in peptide linkage.

$$HOCH_2-\underset{\underset{CH_3}{|}}{\overset{\overset{CH_3}{|}}{C}}-\underset{\underset{H}{|}}{\overset{\overset{OH}{|}}{C}}-\overset{\overset{O}{\parallel}}{C}-NHCH_2CH_2COOH$$

D-Pantothenic Acid

The free acid is fairly stable in neutral solution but sensitive to acids, bases, and heat. The salts are somewhat more stable, but even these are destroyed by autoclaving.

Pantothenic acid, its salts and alcohol, can be assayed by both chemical and microbiological methods. A chick growth method has been used but it is time-consuming and has been replaced since suitable methods are available for releasing the bound vitamin (a protein enzyme) from its firm combination in plant and animal tissue. The first step in chemical assay is acid or alkaline hydrolysis. This cleaves the molecule at the peptide linkage into an alanine part and a pantoic acid part. These fission products can then be determined photometrically by suitable color reactions. *Saccharomyces carlsbergensis* and *Lactobacillus plantarum* are used for the microbiological assay of pantothenic acid and its salts. There is available a USP Reference Standard Calcium Pantothenate.

Metabolic Functions, Dietary Requirement, and Food Sources—Pantothenic acid is of the highest biological importance because of its incorporation into coenzyme A (CoA), which is involved in many vital enzymatic reactions transferring a two-carbon compound (the acetyl group) in intermediary metabolism. It is involved in the release of energy from carbohydrate, in the degradation and metabolism of fatty acids, and in the synthesis of such compounds as sterols and steroid hormones, porphyrins, and acetylcholine. CoA is composed of one mole each of adenine, ribose, and β-mercaptoethylamine and three moles of phosphate for each mole of pantothenate.

Many microorganisms depend on the same metabolic pathways for their growth and reproduction as do animal species and humans and in this respect require pantothenic acid. Some have the ability to synthesize pantothenic acid at a life-sustaining rate from proper precursors. Synthesis by the bacterial flora of the intestine in man appears to be an important source of the vitamin and is the probable explanation, in part, that pantothenic acid deficiency in man is seldom encountered. A deficiency syndrome has been experimentally induced in human volunteers by the oral administration of a pantothenic acid antagonist, ω-methylpantothenic acid, imposed on a pantothenic acid-deficient diet. It has been impossible so far to induce an isolated deficiency of the vitamin in less than at least 9 months on anything resembling a natural diet alone because of the occurrence of significant amounts of pantothenic acid in such a wide variety of foods.

The symptoms which appear to be specific for a lack of available pantothenic acid from the studies using the antivitamin are neuromuscular disorders (paresthesias of the hands and feet and cramping of the legs and impairment of motor coordination), loss of normal eosinopenic response to adrenal corticotrophic hormone (ACTH), heightened sensitivity to a test dose of insulin, and, in concert with pyridoxine, a loss of antibody production. Fatigue, malaise, headache, sleep disturbances, nausea, abdominal cramps, epigastric distress, occasional vomiting and an increase in flatus were subjective observations of the pantothenic acid-deficient human volunteers.

Usual diets of adult Americans furnish about 10 to 15 mg of pantothenic acid daily, with a probable range of 6 to 20 mg. A daily intake of 5 to 10 mg is probably adequate for children and adults, and there is no evidence for or against a greater requirement during pregnancy or lactation. Human milk contains about 2 mg/L; cow's milk, about 3.5 mg/L. Liver and other organ meats and eggs are particularly good sources. Broccoli, cauliflower, white and sweet potatoes, tomatoes, and molasses are quite high in pantothenic acid. Muscle tissue of beef, pork, lamb, and chicken are also good sources.

Pyridoxine (Vitamin B$_6$)

Vitamin B-6 does not denote a single substance but is rather a collective term for a group of naturally occurring pyridines that are metabolically and functionally interrelated; namely, pyridoxine, pyridoxal, and pyridoxamine. They are interconvertible *in vivo* in their phosphorylated form. There is no information on the relative biologic activity of the three compounds in humans, and since pyridoxine is the most stable, it probably contributes the most vitamin activity to the diet.

Chemistry and Assay—Pyridoxine as the free base has a bitter taste and is readily soluble in water, alcohol, and acetone. It crystallizes as the hydrochloride and is prepared in this form for commercial use. Pyridoxine is one of the more stable vitamins and in the alcohol form withstands heating in acid or alkaline solution. Pyridoxal and pyridoxamine are less stable, however, and are known to undergo destruction in the more severe heat treatments sometimes used in food processing. Under most conditions of processing and storage of foods and pharmaceutical preparations the vitamin is well retained.

The structures of the three active forms of the vitamin and the phosphorylated form of one of them, pyridoxal phosphate, are shown below.

Pyridoxine   Pyridoxal

Pyridoxamine

Pyridoxal Phosphate

The biological activity of the vitamin is expressed in milligrams of the chemically pure substance, usually pyridoxine hydrochloride, for which a USP Reference Standard is available. Chicks and rats have been used for the biologic assay of vitamin B$_6$ by placing the animals on a deficient basal diet which, when supplemented with known amounts of the test vitamin, supports a degree of growth related to the amount present. Physicochemical methods can be used only to a limited extent for assaying vitamin B$_6$ quantitatively in natural products, because they are nonspecific for the three forms. Microbiological assays, however, will discriminate between the individual vitamin B$_6$ components and thus yield a more accurate estimate of total biologic activity. A very useful technique employed in this type of assay is the preliminary separation of the different vitamin forms by a column chromatographic procedure using an ion exchanger. The column eluates are then analyzed by procedures suited to the vitamin form present in the eluates. The organisms most commonly used are *Saccharomyces carlsbergensis*, *Lactobacillus casei*, and *Streptococcus faecalis*.

Metabolic Functions, Dietary Requirement, and Food Source—Vitamin B$_6$ in the form of pyridoxal phosphate or pyridoxamine phosphate functions in carbohydrate, fat, and protein metabolism; its major functions are most closely related to protein and amino acid metabolism. The vitamin is a part of the molecular configuration of many enzymes (a coenzyme), notably glycogen phosphorylase, various transaminases, decarboxylases and deaminases. The latter three are essential for the anabolism and catabolism of proteins.

The biological activity of vitamin B$_6$ seems to be a function of the molecule as a whole, since small changes in structure render it inactive. Deoxypyridoxine, a derivative of the vitamin in which one of the methanol groups is reduced to a methyl group, has potent antivitamin activity, but it is of limited experimental use in man because of its toxicity. The antivitamin isonicotinic acid hydrazide (isoniazid) has been widely used in the treatment of tuberculosis. It is chemically related to pyridoxine and acts also as an antagonist, thus requiring the physician to be alert to the pyridoxine nutriture of his patients so treated. A similar antagonism is possible during treatment of hypertension with the drug hydralazine.

No classic syndrome of pyridoxine deficiency exists, probably because it is widely distributed in nature and unique or unusual dietary habits have not so far produced an uncomplicated deficiency. That it is essential for the growth of animals and human infants is well established. Other manifestations of deficiency in humans are probably an acrodynia-like syndrome characterized by edema and loss of hair, nerve degeneration resulting in behavioral changes and, in infants, convulsive seizures. The latter symptom was shown to result when infants were fed a proprietary milk-based formula, unsupplemented with pyridoxine, in which the natural vitamin content was destroyed inadvertently during sterilization. Clearly, in this instance, marked changes in electroencephalogram patterns of the infants were produced; and they returned to normal minutes after pyridoxine administration.

In infants, although daily requirements of the vitamin are met by consumption of adequate quantities of normal breast milk, the protein-vitamin B_6 relationship is critical. General experience with proprietary formulas suggests that metabolic requirements are satisfied if the vitamin is present in amounts of 0.015 mg/g of protein, or 0.04 mg/100 kcal. The recommended dietary allowances of the Food and Nutrition Board for adolescents and adults, including conditions of pregnancy and lactation, range from 2.3 to 2.6 mg daily.

The best food sources of vitamin B_6 are muscle meats, liver, green vegetables and whole-grain cereals. The bran from the cereal grains has especially large amounts. Nuts, corn, eggs, and milk are also good sources.

Riboflavin

Riboflavin was formerly known as vitamin B_2 or G and lactoflavin. It owes its discovery as one of the components of the B vitamin group to its characteristic fluorescence and pigmenting quality in such common foods as milk and egg yolk. Isolation and characterization of the yellow protein enzyme originally from yeast led to studies on the essential nature of the flavin pigment part of the enzyme in human metabolism, growth, and health.

Chemistry and Assay—Riboflavin is a yellow to orange-yellow, crystalline powder having a slight odor. When dry, it is not appreciably affected by diffused light, but in solution, especially in the presence of alkalies, it deteriorates quite rapidly, the deterioration being accelerated by light.

In alkaline solution it is readily soluble, but quite unstable to heat and to light, forming lumiflavin, a fluorescent degradation product that is without biological activity. Riboflavin is more stable to heat in acid solution, particularly from pH 1 to 6.5, but upon irradiation forms lumichrome, also biologically inactive. Riboflavin is readily adsorbed from acid or neutral solution on such agents as frankonite, fuller's earth, and certain zeolites, and eluted with acetone or pyridine solutions. Adsorbates have been used in pharmaceutical preparations, but from some of these the vitamin has been found to be unavailable to the human because of difficulty of elution in the intestinal tract.

Solutions of riboflavin have a characteristic yellow-green fluorescence that has a maximum absorption at 565 nm in the acid pH range. This property is made use of in the chemical determination of riboflavin. It is rapidly reduced by hydrosulfite, or by hydrogen in the presence of zinc in acid solution, to the leuco form which is colorless and nonfluorescent. The leucoriboflavin is easily reoxidized by shaking in air. This oxidation–reduction property (see below) is the probable basis for the biological importance of riboflavin in the respiratory enzyme systems.

One g dissolves in from 3000 to about 20,000 mL of water, the variations in the solubility being due to differences in the internal crystalline structure of the riboflavin; it is more soluble in isotonic sodium chloride or alkaline solution than in water, and less soluble in alcohol. It is insoluble in most lipid solvents. Derivatives such as the phosphate or acetate have been prepared for use in pharmaceutical preparations when higher concentrations are desired.

Riboflavin   **Leucoriboflavin**

The activity of riboflavin is expressed in milligrams of the chemically pure substance, and a USP Reference Standard Riboflavin is available for assay purposes. In early work, the riboflavin content of substances was measured by a rat growth bioassay method, but this has been replaced by both physicochemical and microbiological methods.

Chemical determinations are based on colorimetric and fluorometric procedures. Straightforward measurement of the intrinsic yellow color of riboflavin is often sufficient for assaying pharmaceutical preparations. The fluorometric method is more sensitive and free of interferences and is therefore more suited to the assay of the vitamin in foods. It depends upon the extraction of the vitamin with dilute acid, filtration, treatment of the filtrate with permanganate and hydrogen peroxide to destroy interfering pigments, and measurement of the fluorescence.

Lactobacillus casei is used as the test organism for microbiological assay of riboflavin. It is determined by measurement of the growth stimulation of the organism or by alkaline titration of the acid produced during incubation.

Metabolic Functions—Riboflavin plays its physiological role as the prosthetic group of a number of enzyme systems that are involved in the oxidation of carbohydrates and amino acids. It functions in combination with a specific protein either as a mononucleotide containing phosphoric acid (FMN), or as a dinucleotide combined through phosphoric acid with adenine (FAD).

Flavin-adenine dinucleotide (FAD)

The specificity of each of the enzymes is determined by the protein in the complex. By a process of oxidation–reduction, riboflavin in the system either gains or loses hydrogen. The substrate, either carbohydrate or amino acid, may be oxidized by a removal of hydrogen. The first hydrogen acceptor in the chain of events is NAD or NADP, the di- or tri-nucleotide containing nicotinic acid and adenine. The oxidized riboflavin system then serves as hydrogen acceptor for the coenzyme system and in turn is oxidized by the cytochrome system. The hydrogen is finally passed on to the oxygen to complete the oxidative cycle. A number of flavoprotein enzymes have been identified, each of which is specific for a given substrate.

There is evidence now that some of the flavin enzymes contain metallic constituents. These metalloflavoproteins may contain iron, copper, or molybdenum. Succinic dehydrogenase, for example, contains iron, and xanthine oxidase contains molybdenum, as well as iron.

Riboflavin is absorbed after phosphorylation from the intestinal tract, and excreted in the urine. A human adult on an ordinary diet excretes from 0.5 to 1.5 mg in 24 hours, depending on the content of the diet. Of a 10-mg dose taken by mouth, 50 to 70% is excreted within 24 hours. In riboflavin deficiency there is little or none found in the urine. Measure of excretion has been used as a diagnostic sign of deficiency. Riboflavin, like thiamin, is stored to a limited extent, and constant dietary supply is needed to maintain normal body levels. Liver, kidney, and heart tissues contain relatively large amounts of riboflavin because of their high enzyme content.

Dietary Requirement and Food Sources—Symptoms of human ariboflavinosis include cheilosis (reddening of the lips and the appearance of fissures at the corners of the mouth), characteristic changes in color of the mucous membranes, inflammation of the tongue, and denuding of the lips. Lesions of a seborrheic nature have also been observed as a result of riboflavin deficiency. Ocular manifestations that appear in man and animals are characterized chiefly by corneal vascularization, in which the cornea is extensively invaded by small capillaries. This is usually accompanied by sensations of itching, burning, and roughness of the eyelid, lacrimation, photophobia, and visual fatigue. Some of these conditions may, of course, arise from other causes and are not necessarily indicative of riboflavin deficiency.

Riboflavin deficiency in humans has not been found to be widespread in any part of the world, but is undoubtedly a complicating factor in other deficiency diseases such as pellagra. For therapeutic purposes, doses of 1 to 10 mg daily have been given. Rapid disappearance of symptoms of ariboflavinosis occurs with 10-mg doses, and there is some question of the need for administering amounts larger than this.

Studies dealing with the quantitative riboflavin requirement of the human indicate that it is related to body size, metabolic rate, and rate of growth. And the parameter used to express these most closely is metabolic body size, represented as kg of body weight taken to the $\frac{3}{4}$ power. The recommended daily dietary allowance of the Food and Nutrition Board for riboflavin is 0.4 to 0.6 mg for infants, 0.8 to 1.2 mg for children up to 10 years, 1.0 to 1.7 mg for adolescents and adults and slightly higher for women during pregnancy and lactation. In general, the minimum requirement for riboflavin is about 0.3 mg for adults and 0.8 mg for infants on a 1000 kcal intake basis. From a physiological point of view, an intake of more than 0.5 to 0.6 mg/1000 kcal may be of little extra value in normal adult persons.

Riboflavin is widely distributed in nature, in both plants and animals, as an essential constituent of all living cells, and is therefore found widely distributed in small amounts in foods. It is quite stable during the processing of food, except where there is excessive exposure to light. Because of its water solubility, there is moderate loss of riboflavin in cooking when the cooking water is discarded. This loss, however, is generally smaller than that of thiamin, niacin, or ascorbic acid.

Foods that make important contributions of riboflavin to the diet are liver and other organ tissues, milk, and eggs. Vegetables and fruits furnish a small but constant supply.

Many species of microorganisms are capable of synthesizing riboflavin, and because of the extensive bacterial growth in the human intestinal tract, this may form an important and constant source of supply of riboflavin and may account for the limited occurrence of deficiency in humans.

When it was recognized that cereal products would be a good vehicle to use to improve the content of riboflavin in many diets, its mandatory addition as an enriching ingredient was adopted. In concert with thiamin, niacin and iron, riboflavin is present in nutritionally significant amounts in enriched wheat flour, farina, corn products, bread, macaroni, and noodle products. Because of certain cooking habits and the apparent unacceptability of the unnatural yellow color, the enrichment of rice with riboflavin has been resisted.

Thiamine

Concentrates of thiamine, often termed vitamin B_1, were given the latter name by early workers in this country who recognized that at least two accessory dietary factors were needed for normal growth of laboratory rats, one in butter fat and the other in "milk sugar." The names they suggested for these factors were fat-soluble vitamin A and

water-soluble vitamin B. It was shown subsequently by a number of investigators that the latter consisted of a group of substances rather than a single compound, but vitamin B_1 was finally the first pure compound of the group to be laboriously isolated from rice polishings. In the pioneer studies on this substance it was found that a thiamine concentrate prevented polyneuritis in chickens, which later was found to be caused by the absence of thiamine in their diet. Deriving from this observation, an early name for the factor is aneurin (from antineuritic), which has persisted in some countries.

Chemistry and Assay—Thiamine is a generic term applied to all substances possessing vitamin B_1 activity, regardless of the anion attached to the molecule. The cationic portion of the molecule, which is the part that may properly be called "thiamine," is made up of a substituted pyrimidine ring connected by a methylene bridge to the nitrogen of a substituted thiazole ring. A general structural formula is where A is any appropriate anion but usually chloride. In addition, ammonium salts may be formed with the amine substituent on the pyrimidine ring. The common nomenclature is confusing, but, in general, the term mono, as in thiamine mononitrate or thiamine monophosphate, designates the thiazolium type salt. Thiamine chloride hydrochloride is the ammonium salt formed by reacting thiamine chloride with hydrochloric acid (see page 1025).

Thiamine compounds are usually readily soluble in water and in alcohol but insoluble in fat solvents. They are stable in acid solution, and may be heated without decomposition, but unstable in neutral or alkaline solution. At neutral or alkaline pH splitting occurs at the methylene bridge upon heating in the presence of moisture. Splitting of the molecule takes place quantitatively in the presence of bisulfite ions, a reaction that is made use of in preparing dietary constituents free of thiamine for bioassay purposes.

Thiamine is oxidized in alkaline solution to thiochrome, a biologically inactive, highly fluorescent substance. This reaction is the basis for the chemical method of estimating thiamine. The pure vitamin is not readily oxidized in air.

An alternate commercial form of vitamin B_1 widely used because of its greater stability than the hydrochloride is the mononitrate.

The activity of the vitamin is expressed in milligrams of the chemically pure substance and a USP Reference Standard Thiamine Hydrochloride is available.

The determination of thiamine in food, biological materials, and pharmaceutical products is almost exclusively done by the thiochrome fluorometric method. On oxidation with ferricyanide in alkaline solution, thiamine is transformed into thiochrome which has a strong blue fluorescence. It is a very sensitive method and correlates well with bioassay results. The sequence in the determination involves extraction of the vitamin, enzyme hydrolysis, adsorption, elution and oxidation to thiochrome which is extracted with isobutanol and determined fluorometrically.

Before the development of suitable physicochemical methods, thiamine was determined in a typical rat-growth assay which is based on the growth response of young thiamine-depleted rats to supplemental doses of a reference standard and to the test material either fed in or separate from the diet or injected parenterally.

Metabolic Functions—In a phosphorylated form, thiamine (thiamine pyrophosphate; cocarboxylase) serves as the prosthetic group of enzyme systems that are concerned with the decarboxylation of α-ketoacids. For example, pyruvic acid is formed which is decarboxylated to form a two-carbon residue. This process of decarboxylation is catalyzed by the pyruvic acid decarboxylase enzyme system which consists of a specific protein, manganese ions, and diphosphothiamin. An α-hydroxyethyl group (the "acetaldehyde" residue of the decarboxylated pyruvic acid) attaches to the 2-carbon of the thiazole ring. The hydroxyethyl group (active "acetate," active "acetaldehyde," or two-carbon fragment) attaches to one of the sulfur atoms of lipoamide, from which it is removed by coenzyme A. Pyrophosphorylated thiamine is effective in the decarboxylation of other α-ketoacids as well. Some decarboxylation processes are reversible, so that synthesis (condensation) may be achieved; thus thiamine is also important to the biosynthesis of keto-acids. It is involved in transketolase reactions.

Thiamine is readily absorbed in aqueous solution from both the small and large intestine, and is then carried to the liver by the portal circulation. In the liver, as well as in all living cells, it normally combines with phosphate to form cocarboxylase. It may be stored in the liver in this form or it may combine further with manganese and specific proteins to become active enzymes known as carboxylases.

Thiamine is excreted in the urine in amounts that reflect the amount taken in and the amounts stored in the tissues. Measurement of the urinary excretion of thiamine after giving a small dose of thiamine is useful in determining whether body stores are adequate or deficient.

Dietary Requirement and Food Sources—Polyneuritis (dysfunctioning of the nervous system) or beriberi is the frank disease associated with thiamine deficiency in man. Peripheral neuritis is a pathological condition of the nerves of the extremities; usually both legs are affected and sometimes the arms as well. The symptoms include loss of sensation, muscle weakness, and paralysis. In beriberi this condition is also associated with edema and abnormal electrocardiogram patterns.

Severe cases of beriberi are commonly found in the Orient among people whose diets consist principally of milled or polished rice, from which the vitamin, contained in the bran and germ of the cereal, is largely removed during the milling process. American dietaries generally furnish sufficient thiamine to meet requirements, and with the use of a varied diet, including whole grain cereals or enriched bread or flour, adequacy of thiamine in most instances is beyond question. Symptoms of thiamine deficiency have been observed among chronic alcoholics, who use alcohol in place of food as a source of energy. Deficiency also occurs in cases of chronic diarrhea, in which absorption is interfered with over a period of time and during pregnancy complicated with anorexia and nausea.

In the diagnosis of thiamine deficiency, symptoms to be noted in particular are anorexia, fatigue, loss of weight, sensation of burning in the soles of the feet, tenderness in calf muscles, muscle cramps, and general muscular weakness. Such signs are not in themselves specific, however, without supplementary laboratory findings that indicate a reduced thiamine content of blood and urine.

For treatment of beriberi or thiamine deficiency in humans, the first requisite is a nutritionally complete, well-balanced diet. Good diet is essential, because beriberi in most instances results from a complex or multiple deficiency, and administration of thiamine alone may precipitate a condition resulting from a lack of other water-soluble factors. Doses of 10 to 100 mg of thiamine have been used in severe cases to bring about a cure, but evidence of superiority of the larger doses is lacking. As size of the dose is increased, the proportion of thiamine retained rapidly decreases, the excess being excreted rapidly in the urine. Frequent small doses are to be preferred to a single large daily dose. Only in the most severe cases, or in patients with impaired intestinal absorption, does parenteral administration appear advantageous. Pharmaceutical preparations of many types and potencies are available commercially.

It is generally assumed that thiamine need is related to calorie need, particularly to those calories derived from carbohydrate. The Food and Nutrition Board considers that 0.5 mg/1000 kcal will maintain satisfactory thiamine nutriture under normal conditions in the US. As the caloric allowance varies with age, so does the recommended daily dietary allowance for thiamine; for infants, 0.3 to 0.5 mg; for children up to 12 years, 0.7 to 1.4 mg; for adolescents and adults, 1.0 to 1.5 mg, the highest allowance being for boys and men 15 to 22 years. The literature on thiamine needs in maternal and child nutrition suggests an increased need for thiamine during pregnancy, and an additional 0.3 mg/day is recommended, in accordance with the increased calorie recommendation.

Thiamine is found widely distributed in foods. Thiamine is found in all plants, and is synthesized by some microorganisms, particularly yeasts. No one food can be considered of particular importance above all others, although the cereal grains, milk, legumes, nuts, eggs, and pork probably furnish the larger proportion of thiamine in diets used in this country. Sophistication and processing of foods generally tend to reduce the thiamine supply. For example, in the preparation of wheat flour, separation of the bran coat and germ removes $3/4$ or more of the thiamine present in the whole wheat. This is true for other cereal grains as well. Much of the white flour, corn grits, and rice used in this country is enriched to approximately the whole grain level. Because of the lability of thiamine to heat, cooking and baking processes reduce the raw food content of the vitamin.

The loss of thiamine in home cooking is not considered excessive, except with foods cooked in large amounts of water that is then discarded. Because of its solubility, the thiamine content of the cooking water is always appreciable.

Vitamin B$_{12}$

Vitamin B$_{12}$, the most recently discovered of the B group, was isolated from liver fractions in crystalline form in 1948 and was soon after shown to be specific for the treatment of Addisonian pernicious anemia. It has been established that extracts of liver, employed for more than 30 years in the control of pernicious anemia, contain vitamin B$_{12}$ as their active principle. Liver continues to be an important dietary source of the vitamin, but liver injection is no longer used in the treatment of pernicious anemia, because of the ready availability of crystalline forms of the vitamin.

Chemistry and Assay—Vitamin B$_{12}$ is a complex water-soluble compound which crystallizes as small red needles that have a specific rotation in dilute aqueous solution of $-59°$. Characteristic absorption spectrum maxima occur at 278, 361, and 550 nm. The crystalline substance blackens without melting at 300°. The compound is a cobalt coordination complex, in which the cobalt is trivalent and has a coordination number of six. The complex is neutral. Vitamin B$_{12}$ is composed of two heterocyclic systems, a benzimidazole and a modified porphyrin nucleus, with the following structure:

Cyanocobalamin

Actually, the cyanide group coordinated to the cobalt is not a part of the true vitamin but rather is an artifact caused by isolation of the vitamin on charcoal; in the liver the ligand is 5′-deoxyadenosyl anion. Nevertheless, by strict organic chemical definition, by virtue of the fact that the cyanide was the first form of the vitamin to be isolated, cyanocobalamin *is* vitamin B$_{12}$. When the ligand is hydroxide instead of cyanide, the compound is *vitamin B$_{12a}$* (hydroxocobalamin); when it is water, the substance is *vitamin B$_{12b}$;* (aquocobalamin); when it is nitro, the compound is *vitamin B$_{12c}$; the 5′-deoxyadenosyl form is coenzyme B$_{12}$;* if the ligand is methyl, the compound is *methyl B$_{12}$*. Sulfito- and thiocyanatocobalamins also are known. In practice, all of these compounds are vitamin B$_{12}$. A similar situation obtains with respect to the name *cobalamin*, which strictly is synonymous with cyanocobalamin but in loose practice applies to any active compound containing the α-(5,6-dimethylbenzimidazoyl)corrin nucleus. *Cobamides* is a generic term which has been used for these compounds.

Vitamin B$_{12}$ (cyanocobalamin) in an atmosphere of hydrogen with a platinum catalyst is reduced to a red crystalline compound with slightly changed ultraviolet absorption maxima, and a reduced stability to heat. Vitamin B$_{12a}$ results from such reduction. Vitamin B$_{12b}$, another reduced form, occurs in natural sources.

Commercially vitamin B$_{12}$ is obtained from the fermentation of *Streptomyces griseus.* The vitamin is precipitated from aqueous solutions saturated with ammonium sulfate by *n*-butanol. Purification is achieved by chromatography, using bentonite or aluminum silicate as the adsorbent. Sharply defined red bands are formed during the development of the chromatograms indicating the location of the vitamin. The red band is separated mechanically and eluted with water. The concentrated water solution on addition of acetone gives the crystalline vitamin which can be further purified by recrystallization from aqueous acetone.

The USP provides a Reference Standard Cyanocobalamin for use in assay of the vitamin. The most important physicochemical method for determining vitamin B$_{12}$ involves measurement of light absorbance at certain specific wavelengths characteristic for cyanocobalamin. This method is only applicable to relatively concentrated solutions of the compound, such as in pharmaceutical preparations.

Vitamin B$_{12}$ is one of the most active biological factors known; its activity for bacteria is measured in terms of millimicrograms. Because of this sensitivity of some bacteria to such low levels of the vitamin and the fact that foods contain exceptionally low concentrations of the vitamin, microbiological methods are widely used. The following three organisms, which require vitamin B_{12} for growth, are used: *Lactobacillus leichmannii*, *Ochramonas malhamensis*, and *Euglenia gracilis*.

Metabolic Functions, Dietary Requirement, and Food Sources—The vitamin is essential for the normal functioning of all cells, but particularly for cells of the bone marrow, the nervous system, and the gastrointestinal tract. It appears to facilitate reduction reactions and participate in the transfer of methyl groups. Evidence exists that vitamin B_{12} is involved in protein, carbohydrate, and fat metabolism, but its chief importance in mammalian tissues seems to be, together with folic acid, in the anabolism of deoxyribonucleic acid in all cells. Coenzyme forms of vitamin B_{12}, in which the vitamin is linked to adenine and a sugar, which catalyze specific reactions in intermediary metabolism have been isolated from bacterial cultures and probably have similar vitamin roles in mammalian cells.

The biochemical fault in pernicious anemia, a condition caused by a prolonged deficiency of vitamin B_{12}, is a failure of elaboration of the intrinsic factor, normally present in the secretions of the stomach mucosa. This intrinsic factor, which is essential for the absorption of the vitamin through the intestinal wall, is known to form a complex with vitamin B_{12}. Intrinsic factor, now available in a purified form, is reported to be a mixture of mucoproteins.

Vitamin B_{12} is a requisite for normal blood formation, and certain macrocytic anemias respond to its administration. In pernicious anemia, unless accompanied by intrinsic factor, the vitamin is not orally absorbed in effective amounts and must be administered parenterally in microgram quantities. Preparations containing vitamin B_{12} and intrinsic factor concentrate are now available for oral use, and have been shown for short-term use at least to be equivalent in value to the injections. Clinical studies indicate that if milligram amounts of the vitamin are administered orally, in the absence of intrinsic factor, enough of the vitamin passes through the intestinal wall to be effective in maintaining the pernicious anemia patient. However, the injectable form of vitamin B_{12} continues to be the drug of choice because of the desirability of regular attention of a physician to the condition of the patient.

The evidence indicating that vitamin B_{12} is the antipernicious anemia factor, and fully as effective in the treatment of macrocytic anemias as liver extract, appears to be complete. In treating pernicious anemia, vitamin B_{12} administered intramuscularly produces a maximal reticulocyte response in 4 to 9 days, and a restoration of red and white cell count in 4 to 6 weeks. The change in bone marrow, from a megaloblastic to a normoblastic state, is dramatic, and occurs within a few hours after the injection of as little as 1 µg of the vitamin. Vitamin B_{12} is considered to be the extrinsic factor of Castle, the absorption of which from the intestinal tract is facilitated by the intrinsic factor present in normal gastric juice. The biochemical defect in pernicious anemia then, is a failure of elaboration of the intrinsic factor. Because of this relationship, vitamin B_{12} given orally is much less effective in the pernicious anemia patient, and entirely ineffective if there is complete absence of intrinsic factor.

The vitamin is effective in preventing the occurrence of neurological changes common to pernicious anemia. Acute symptoms of combined system disease have been found to disappear rather promptly after B_{12} administration, but recovery appears to depend more on the chronicity of the disease than on the extent of neurological involvement, and conditions of long standing are less apt to show recovery.

A simple nutritional concept of pernicious anemia which seems valid is that of essentially an uncomplicated deficiency of vitamin B_{12} conditioned by the lack of intrinsic factor and, hence, the inability to absorb the vitamin from ingested food. This validation rests on several types of evidence, of which particularly convincing is the comparison of the clinical development of vitamin B_{12} deficiency in vegans, in patients following total gastrectomy (resulting in removal of intrinsic factor and interference with absorption of the vitamin) and the relapse following withholding of therapy from previously adequately treated patients with pernicious anemia. Simple experimental dietary deficiency of vitamin B_{12} has not yet been produced in the adult human under conditions of careful continuous observation. It seems probable that the requirements of parenterally administered (or absorbed) vitamin B_{12} by the patient with pernicious anemia or gastrectomy is similar to the requirements of the normal subject.

The recommended daily dietary allowance of the Food and Nutrition Board for vitamin B_{12} ranges from 0.5 to 3 µg; the lower value is for infants, and the higher value is for women during pregnancy.

Vitamin B_{12} occurs in meat and dairy products but is not present to any measurable extent in plants or cereal grains. It is probable that indigenous bacteria in plant foods synthesize sufficient vitamin B_{12} to meet the requirement of those individuals whose dietary habits preclude the use of animal food sources.

Water-Soluble Vitamin Preparations

Aminobenzoic Acid—page 787.

Ascorbic Acid

Vitamin C; Cecon (*Abbott*); Cevalin (*Lilly*);
Ce-Vi-Sol (*Mead-Johnson*)

L-Ascorbic acid [50-81-7] $C_6H_8O_6$ (176.13). See page 1012.

Preparation—The article in commerce is produced exclusively by synthesis. Sorbitol, a hexose sugar, occurring in several fruits but commercially obtained by hydrogenating dextrose in the presence of a Cu–Cr catalyst, is the raw material for the production of ascorbic acid. The D-sorbitol in aqueous solution is converted by the action of the organism *Acetobacter suboxydans* to L-sorbose, which is a ketose. The L-sorbose is then condensed with acetone by means of sulfuric acid to form diacetone sorbose. The object of the acetonation is to protect the hydroxyl group from oxidation in the subsequent steps. The diacetone sorbose, after suitable purification, is oxidized by potassium permanganate and then hydrolyzed forming 2 keto-L-gulonic acid. This acid is esterified with methanol and an intermediate sodio compound is formed with sodium methoxide. Hydrolysis with aqueous HCl removes the methyl group and sodium and lactonizes it yielding ascorbic acid. The process is illustrated on this page.

D-Glucose → (H₂) → D-Sorbitol → (*A. Suboxydans*) → L-Sorbose → ((CH₃)₂CO) → Diacetone L-Sorbose → (KMnO₄) → → (H₂O) → 2-Keto-L-gulonic Acid → (CH₃OH + HCl, then CH₃ONa) → [sodio intermediate] → (HCl) → L-Ascorbic Acid

Description—White or slightly yellow crystals or powder; odorless and on exposure to light gradually darkens; in the dry state, reasonably stable in air, but in solution rapidly deteriorates in the presence of air; melts at about 190°; specific rotation (1 in 10 aqueous solution) between +20.5° and +21.5°; aqueous solution has the acidic properties of a monobasic acid and it forms salts with metallic ions.

Solubility—1 g in about 3 mL water and 40 mL alcohol; insoluble in chloroform, ether, and benzene.

Incompatibilities—Stable in the dry state but in solution oxidizes rapidly in the presence of air. The reaction is accelerated by *alkalies* and certain *metals*, especially *copper;* it is retarded by acids. Aqueous solutions are strongly acidic, having a pH of 2 to 3.

Uses—In addition to the uses described on page 1012 vitamin C is sometimes given with iron salts in the treatment of iron-deficiency anemia; it functions to keep the iron in the ferrous state and hence to improve absorption. Apart from coadministration of vitamin C and iron preparations, a few cases of hypochromic anemia improve upon increasing the intake of vitamin. For additional information see the general article on *Ascorbic Acid* in this chapter.

No more than the recommended daily allowance should be given to the pregnant woman; the metabolism of the fetus adapts to high levels of the vitamin, and scurvy may develop after birth when the intake drops to normal levels.

Dose—*Daily, oral or parenteral,* **40 mg** to **1 g**; *usual, requirement,* **60 mg** once a day; *therapeutic,* **100** to **250 mg** 1 or 2 times a day.

Dosage Forms—Injection: 100 and 500 mg/mL, 100, 200, and 500 mg/2 mL, 500 mg and 1 g/5 mL, 1 g/10 mL; Tablets: 25, 50, 100, 250, and 500 mg.

Sodium Ascorbate

L-Ascorbic acid, monosodium salt; Cevalin (*Lilly*)

Monosodium L-ascorbate [134-03-2] $C_6H_7NaO_6$ (198.11).

Description—White or very faintly yellow crystals, or crystalline powder; odorless or practically odorless; relatively stable in air; on exposure to light it gradually darkens; pH (1 in 10 solution) between 7.5 and 8.

Solubility—1 g in 1.3 mL of water; very slightly soluble in alcohol; insoluble in chloroform and ether.

Uses—A pharmaceutical necessity for *Decavitamin Capsules* and *Decavitamin Tablets.* It is also used as an antioxidant in fruit and vegetable canning, and in the processing of meat.

Dose—See *Ascorbic Acid.*

Ascorbyl Palmitate—page 1278.

Calcium Pantothenate

β-Alanine, *N*-(2,4-dihydroxy-3,3-dimethyl-1-oxobutyl)-, calcium salt (2:1), (*R*-); Dextro Calcium Pantothenate; Pantholin (*Lilly*)

Calcium D-pantothenate (1:2) [137-08-6] $C_{18}H_{32}CaN_2O_{10}$ (476.54); the calcium salt of the dextrorotatory isomer of pantothenic acid.

Preparation—Several syntheses are available. In one, isobutyraldehyde is converted to the lactone of 2,4-dihydroxy-3,3-dimethylbutyric acid, the D-enantiomer of which obtained by resolution is combined with β-alanine to form D-pantothenic acid and then converted to the calcium salt.

Description—Slightly hygroscopic, white powder; odorless, has a bitter taste, and is stable in air; unstable to heat both in the dry state and in acid or alkaline solution; most stable at pH 5.5 to 6.5 and its solutions may be autoclaved at this pH for a short time without appreciable loss; solutions are neutral or slightly alkaline to litmus, having a pH of 7 to 9; specific rotation (calculated on the dried basis and in a 5% solution) +25° to +27.5°.

Solubility—1 g in about 3 mL water; soluble in glycerin; practically insoluble in alcohol, chloroform and ether.

Uses—See the article on *Pantothenic Acid*, in this chapter. Since a deficiency of pantothenic acid, alone, is virtually unknown, the primary indication for use is a general nutritional deficiency. Clinical cases have been too few to supply creditable data on dosage; consequently, the dose that follows is more customary than meaningful.

Dose—**10** to **100 mg** daily; *usual,* **10 mg** once a day.

Dosage Forms—Tablets: 10 and 30 mg.

Racemic Calcium Pantothenate

β-Alanine, *N*-(2,4-dihydroxy-3,3-dimethyl-1-oxobutyl)-, calcium salt (2:1), (±)-,

Calcium DL-pantothenate (1:2) [6281-63-1] $C_{18}H_{32}CaN_2O_{10}$ (476.54); a mixture of the calcium salts of the dextrorotatory and levorotatory isomers of pantothenic acid. It contains not less than 42.5% of dextrorotatory calcium pantothenate, calculated on the dried basis.

Preparation—As for *Calcium Pantothenate* except that the resolution is omitted.

Description—White, slightly hygroscopic powder; odorless, has a bitter taste, and is stable in air; solutions are neutral or alkaline to litmus, having a pH of 7 to 9; optically inactive.

Solubility—Freely soluble in water; soluble in glycerin; practically insoluble in alcohol, chloroform, and ether.

Uses—See *Calcium Pantothenate.* Since biological activity resides only in the dextro isomer, the racemic compound is only ½ as potent as calcium pantothenate.

Dose—**20** to **100 mg** daily; *usual,* **20 mg** (equivalent to approximately 10 mg of dextrorotatory calcium pantothenate) once a day.

Cyanocobalamin

α-5,6-Dimethylbenzimidazolylcobamide Cyanide; Vitamin B_{12}

Vitamin B_{12} [68-19-9] $C_{63}H_{88}CoN_{14}O_{14}P$ (1355.38). See page 1020.

Preparation—Vitamin B_{12} can be isolated from aqueous liver extracts and from *Streptomyces griseus* fermentation. Commercially, it is obtained from the latter source (see page 963).

Description—Dark red, hygroscopic crystals or amorphous or crystalline powder; when the anhydrous compound is exposed to air it may absorb about 12% of water.

Solubility—1 g in 80 mL of water; soluble in alcohol; insoluble in acetone, chloroform, and ether.

Uses—Cyanocobalamin and other forms of vitamin B_{12} are used to treat various megaloblastic anemias, especially *pernicious anemia* and other anemias in which the secretion of the intrinsic factor is impaired, as in *gastric cancer, gastric atrophy, total* or even *subtotal gastrectomy.* It may also be used to treat the megaloblastic anemias of *tropical sprue, idiopathic steatorrhea, gluten-induced enteropathy, regional ileitis, ileal resection, malignancies, granulomas, strictures, or other structural disorders of the ileum* in which vitamin B_{12} absorption is impaired; in most of these folacin deficiency is even more severe, and combined therapy is indicated. Vitamin B_{12} deficiencies untreated for periods of more than three months may result in permanent degenerative spinal cord lesions. The megaloblastic anemia associated with *fish tapeworm infestation* also responds to vitamin B_{12}. The megaloblastic anemias of pregnancy, infancy, alcoholism, and poverty are usually due to folacin deficiency and only infrequently respond to vitamin B_{12}. The vitamin is *not useful* in the treatment of infectious hepatitis, multiple sclerosis, trigeminal neuralgia, anorexia, miscellaneous neuropathies, thyrotoxicosis, retarded growth, aging, and various psychiatric disorders, and claims to the contrary and promotion therefore represent an abuse. This preparation should not be administered intravenously and is contraindicated in patients who are sensitive to cobalt or vitamin B_{12}. Patients with Leber's disease have been found to suffer severe and rapid opticatrophy when treated with vitamin B_{12}.

In addition to intrinsic factor, gastrointestinal absorption requires an alkaline pH. In the presence of pancreatic disease it may be necessary to administer oral vitamin B_{12} with bicarbonate or give the vitamin parenterally.

For additional information about cyanocobalamin see the general article on *Vitamin B_{12}* in this chapter.

Dose—*Intramuscular*, **30 μg** to 1 **mg**/dose; *maintenance*, **100 μg** once a month; *therapeutic*, **100 μg** once or twice a week.

The dose varies with the severity of the *anemia*, its response to therapy and with other signs and symptoms of the disease. For the patient with uncomplicated pernicious anemia in relapse, the initial intramuscular dose is 30 μg injected daily or every other day for 5 to 10 doses; then 15 to 30 μg injected once or twice weekly until the blood picture is normal. Maintenance dosage of 40 to 60 μg every 2 weeks or 80 to 100 μg every month usually suffices. Critically ill patients and those with intercurrent infection or with neurological complications require vigorous parenteral treatment, and larger doses for both initial and maintenance therapy must be employed. However, there is no acceptable evidence that doses in excess of 30 μg/day are necessary.

Dosage Forms—Injection: 100 μg and 1 mg/mL; 5 mg/5 mL; 300, 500, and 600 μg, 1000 μg and 1 and 10 mg/10 mL; 3 and 30 mg/30 mL.

Hydroxocobalamin

Cobinamide, dihydroxide, dihydrogen phosphate (ester), mono(inner salt), 3'-ester with 5,6-dimethyl-1-α-D-ribofuranosyl-1H-benzimidazole; Vitamin B_{12a}

Cobinamide dihydroxide dihydrogen phosphate (ester), mono(inner salt), 3'-ester with 5,6-dimethyl-1-α-D-ribofuranosylbenzimidazole [13422-51-0] $C_{62}H_{89}CoN_{13}O_{15}P$ (1346.37); an analogue of *Cyanocobalamin* in which a hydroxyl radical has replaced the cyano radical.

Preparation—Cyanocobalamin in solution is hydrogenated at room temperature with the aid of Raney nickel. The solution is then exposed to air and diluted with acetone. Oxidation takes place and, upon standing, the hydroxocobalamin crystallizes.

Description—Dark red crystals or red crystalline powder; odorless or has not more than a slight acetone odor; anhydrous form is very hygroscopic; pH (2 in 100 solution) between 8 and 10.

Solubility—1 g in 50 mL water, 100 mL alcohol, 10,000 mL chloroform, 10,000 mL ether. It is preferable to make aqueous solutions in acetate buffer at a pH between 3.5 and 4.5 in which 1 g dissolves in about 100 mL water.

Use and Dose—See *Cyanocobalamin*. When injected intramuscularly, hydroxocobalamin produces higher and more prolonged levels of vitamin B_{12} than the same doses of cyanocobalamin but this is not considered to be clinically important.

Dosage Forms—Injection: 1 mg/mL, 10 mg/10 mL.

Folic Acid

L-Glutamic acid, N-[4-[[(2-amino-1,4-dihydro-4-oxo-6-pteridinyl)-methyl]amino]benzoyl]-, PGA; Folacin; Pteroylglutamic Acid; Folvite (*Lederle*)

N-[p-[[(2-Amino-4-hydroxy-6-pteridinyl)methyl]amino]benzoyl]-L-glutamic acid [59-30-3] $C_{19}H_{19}N_7O_6$ (441.40). See page 1014.

Preparation—Commercial syntheses utilize different processes. In one of these 2,3-dibromopropionaldehyde, dissolved in a water-miscible organic solvent (alcohol, dioxane), is added to a solution of equal molecular quantities of 2,4,5-triamino-6-hydroxypyrimidine and p-aminobenzoylglutamic acid, maintaining a pH of about 4 by the controlled action of alkali as the reaction progresses. The scheme of the reaction is analogous to that described for *Methotrexate* (page 1152), the only difference being in the starting pyrimidine compound.

Description—Yellow or yellowish orange, odorless, crystalline powder.

Solubility—Very slightly soluble in water; insoluble in alcohol, chloroform, ether; readily dissolves in dilute solutions of alkali hydroxides and carbonates, and is soluble in hot diluted hydrochloric or sulfuric acid, forming very pale yellow solutions.

Uses—The only valid therapeutic use is in the treatment of a deficiency of the vitamin or prophylactically in instances in which the folacin requirement is increased, as in the third trimester of pregnancy. *Megaloblastic anemias* in which folic acid deficiency occurs may result from malabsorption syndromes, such as *sprue, idiopathic steatorrhea, celiac disease, intestinal reticulosis, regional jejunitis, jejunal diverticulosis, blind loop syndrome, and gastroenterostomy.* Megaloblastic anemia of infancy is generally the result of generalized malnutrition, as is nutritional megaloblastic anemia. In all of the

above-named megaloblastic anemias vitamin B_{12} deficiency often coexists, and folic acid, alone, may be inadequate. Pernicious anemia should be ruled out, lest the folic acid mask the disease (see below). In the megaloblastic anemias of deficiency, a low serum folic acid level will obtain. However, in megaloblastic anemias consequent to treatment with pyrimethamine, phenytoin, and related substances, or methotrexate, the serum folic acid levels may be normal; the signs of deficiency result from the antimetabolite effects of the drugs, and they may be overcome competitively by increasing the intake of folic acid. Folic acid is not effective in the treatment of aplastic anemia, leukemia, anemias of infection and nephritis, and general reduction in bone marrow activity of unknown origin.

The vitamin is readily absorbed from the gastrointestinal tract and from parenteral sites of administration. The portion of administered folic acid which is excreted in the urine varies directly with the dose; only a small fraction appears in the urine following the oral ingestion of 0.1 mg, but up to 90% may be excreted by the kidney when a single dose of 15 mg is ingested. The fate of the unrecovered folic acid is unknown. The indications for parenteral folic acid are rare. A solution of folic acid in water for injection, prepared with the aid of sodium hydroxide or sodium carbonate, is the preferred form for injection.

Folic acid is capable of bringing about an incomplete and temporary hematopoietic response in pernicious anemia, which may cause the physician to overlook the basic disorder. But folic acid does not affect the progressive neurological lesions of the disease, which may appear explosively and in an irreversible stage. Doses of folic acid which will correct a folacin deficiency but which will not generally cause a remission in pernicious anemia are on the order of 0.1 to 0.4 mg.

For additional information concerning folic acid see the general article on *Folacin (Folic Acid)* in this chapter.

Dose—*Usual, maintenance, oral intramuscular, intravenous, subcutaneous (deep)* **0.1** to **0.25 mg** (100 to 250 μg) once a day; *therapeutic, oral* or *parenteral,* **0.25 mg** (250 μg) to **1 mg** once a day.

Dosage Forms—Injection: 15 mg/mL, 150 mg/10 mL; Tablets: 100 and 400 μg and 1 mg.

Leucovorin Calcium

L-Glutamic acid, N-[[(2-amino-5-formyl-1,4,5,6,7,8-hexahydro-4-oxo-6-pteridinyl)methyl]amino]benzoyl]-, calcium salt (1:1), pentahydrate; Calcium Folinate SF (*Lederle*)

Calcium N-[p-[[(2-amino-5-formyl-5,6,7,8-tetrahydro-4-hydroxy-6-pteridinyl)methyl]amino]benzoyl]-L-glutamate (1:1) pentahydrate [6035-45-6] $C_{20}H_{21}CaN_7O_7.5H_2O$ (601.58); *anhydrous* [1492-18-8] (511.51).

Preparation—Folic acid is simultaneously hydrogenated and formylated in 90 to 100% formic acid under the influence of platinum oxide catalyst at low temperature and atmospheric pressure to yield leucovorin. Conversion to the calcium salt may be accomplished by dissolving the leucovorin in NaOH solution, treating with $CaCl_2$, and precipitating with ethanol.

Description—Yellowish white or yellow, odorless powder.
Solubility—Very soluble in water; practically insoluble in alcohol.

Uses—Leucovorin is folinic acid (see *Folic Acid*, page 1014). The calcium salt is a convenient pharmaceutical form that is preferred for intramuscular injection. Consequently, its uses and limitations in the *treatment of the megaloblastic anemias* are the same as for folic acid. However, it is superior to folic acid in *counteracting the excessive effects of the folic acid antagonists* (methotrexate, etc; see page 1152), since the antagonists competitively antagonize the conversion of folic acid to leucovorin and not the leucovorin itself.

Dose—*Intramuscular*, in *folate-deficiency anemia*, the equivalent of **1 mg** of leucovorin once daily; *folic acid antagonist antidote*, administer an amount of leucovorin equal to weight of antagonist given, as soon as possible.

Dosage Forms—Injection: 3 mg/mL.

Niacin

3-Pyridinecarboxylic acid; Nicotinic Acid

Nicotinic acid [59-67-6] $C_6H_5NO_2$ (123.11). See page 1015.

Preparation—Niacin may be variously prepared, as by oxidation of nicotine with nitric acid or potassium permanganate, by oxidation of quinoline, or synthesis from pyridine.

Description—White crystals or crystalline powder; odorless or has a slight odor; melts at about 235°.

Solubility—1 g in about 60 mL water; freely soluble in boiling water, boiling alcohol, and also solutions of alkali hydroxides and carbonates; practically insoluble in ether.

Uses—Chiefly in the treatment of pellagra, a disease common among the poor in subtropical countries due to diet deficiency. It has also been found useful in conjunction with vitamin B_1 and riboflavin in the treatment of nutritional deficiency in chronic alcoholism.

In doses of 20 mg or more in humans, niacin elicits a vasodilator effect that occurs a few minutes after oral ingestion, or immediately after intravenous injection, and lasts for a few minutes to an hour. Symptoms of flushing, itching, burning, or tingling occur, along with an increased skin temperature and increased motility and gastric secretion. Nicotinyl alcohol also shares this vasodilator property, and at one time both nicotinic acid and the alcohol were popularly used in the treatment of peripheral vascular disease and senility (as a cerebral vasodilator). These uses of nicotinic acid are obsolete and now are but an annoying side effect of large doses. The vasodilator effect of oral niacin is less if the niacin is given with a meal.

Larger doses of niacin lower blood cholesterol, phospholipids, triglycerides, and free fatty acids, and the drug is used in the treatment of hypercholesterolemia. Nicotinamide does not possess the hypolipemic or the vasodilator property.

Large doses of nicotinic acid, comparable to those used to lower blood lipids, cause abnormalities in liver function, including jaundice.

Niacin is well absorbed orally, and the oral and parenteral doses are the same. With large doses, a considerable amount is excreted into the urine, so that it is advisable to give several small doses during the day rather than one large one.

For additional information see the general article on *Niacin* in this chapter.

Dose—*Oral*, **20 mg** daily. For *treatment of deficiency*, *orally or parenterally*, **50 mg** 3 to 10 times daily; for *hypercholesterolemia*, **1.5 to 6 g** *orally* daily, in 3 to 10 divided doses.

Dosage Forms—Injection: 50 and 100 mg/mL; Tablets: 25, 50, 100, and 500 mg.

Niacinamide

3-Pyridinecarboxamide; Nicotinamide; Nicotinic Acid Amide

Nicotinamide [98-92-0] $C_6H_6N_2O$ (122.13). See page 1015.

Preparation—From niacin by various methods, as by reaction with thionyl chloride followed by treatment with ammonia, or by interaction of ammonia gas with molten niacin.

Description—White, crystalline powder; odorless or nearly so, and has a bitter taste; solutions are neutral to litmus paper; melts between 128° and 131°C.

Solubility—1 g in 1.5 mL water, 5.5 mL alcohol, and 10 mL glycerin.

Uses—See page 1016 and *Niacin*. Niacinamide lacks the vasodilator, gastrointestinal, hepatic, and hypolipemic actions of niacin. Consequently, it is preferred to niacin in the treatment of deficiency.

Dose—*Usual*, *oral* or *parenteral*, *prophylactic*, **10 to 20 mg** once a day; *therapeutic*, *parenteral*, **25 to 50 mg** 2 to 10 times a day, *oral*, **50 mg** 3 to 10 times a day.

Dosage Forms—Injection: 100 mg/2 mL, 500 mg/5 mL, 1 g/10 mL, 3 and 6 g/30 mL; Tablets: 25, 50, and 100 mg.

Pyridoxine Hydrochloride

3,4-Pyridinedimethanol, 5-hydroxy-6-methyl-, hydrochloride; Vitamin B_6 Hydrochloride; Hexa-betalin (*Lilly*)

Pyridoxol hydrochloride [58-56-0] $C_8H_{11}NO_3$·HCl (205.64).

Preparation—Several processes are available. One may be viewed as a cyclizing dehydration of ethyl glycinate (I), ethyl pyruvate (II), and 1,4-diethoxy-2-butanone (III) followed by saponification and decarboxylation at position 2 and cleavage of the three ethoxy groups with HI or another suitable reagent. Reaction of the base with HCl yields the hydrochloride. US Pats 2,904,551, 3,024,244, and 3,024,245.

Description—Colorless or white crystals or a white, crystalline powder; stable in air and slowly affected by sunlight; solutions are acid to litmus, having a pH of about 3; melting range 202° to 206° with some decomposition.

Solubility—1 g in 5 mL water and 115 mL alcohol; insoluble in chloroform and ether.

Uses—Pyridoxine deficiency in adults is extremely difficult to induce, and therapeutic need for pyridoxine, alone, in the adult is of rare occurrence. However, it is justified to give pyridoxine along with other B-vitamins when there is evidence of a *multiple B-vitamin deficiency*. Pyridoxine may be used prophylactically to prevent, or to treat, peripheral neuritis in *patients treated with isoniazid*. It has been claimed that pyridoxine controls the *nausea and vomiting of pregnancy* or of *radiation sickness*, but unequivocal proof has never been presented. In infants with *convulsive seizures due to pyridoxine dependency*, administration of the vitamin promptly corrects the condition (see the general article on *Pyridoxine* in this chapter). Pyridoxine has been claimed to be medically effective in treating the carpal-tunnel syndrome, however, more data is required to substantiate this claim. Extremely high doses (600 to 3000 mg per day) have been administered to schizophrenics, autistic children and children shown hyperkinesis. However, clear evidence of benefit has not been established. Caution needs to be exercised with these levels of administration because of recent reports of severe sensory-nervous-system dysfunction after daily consumption of 2 to 5 g of pyridoxine. Pyridoxine may be effective in correcting hypochromic or megaloblastic anemia in patients with adequate levels of iron who have not responded to other hematopoietic agents. As pyridoxine antagonizes levodopa, patients with Parkinson's disease treated with the latter drug should not take multivitamin supplements containing pyridoxine (see the article on *Levodopa*, in Chapter 49).

Dose—*Usual*, *oral*, *intramuscular*, or *intravenous*, *prophylactic*, **2 mg** once a day (for variations with age see Tables I and III, this chapter); for *deficiencies* in *adults* and *children*, **10 to 50 mg** daily. For *adults* and *children* with *refractory hypochromic* or *megaloblastic anemias* or *peripheral neuritis due to isoniazid or other drugs*, **100 to 200 mg** daily. For *convulsive seizures in children due to pyridoxine dependency*, **100 mg** daily.

Dosage Forms—Injection: 50 and 100 mg/mL, 500 mg and 1 g/10 mL, 3 g/30 mL; Tablets: 10, 25, 50, and 100 mg.

Riboflavin

Lactoflavin; Vitamin B_2

Riboflavine [83-88-5] $C_{17}H_{20}N_4O_6$ (376.37). See page 1018.

Preparation—Mostly by synthesis. In one method, 1-(6-amino-3,4-xylidino)-1-deoxy-D-ribitol (I) is condensed with alloxan (II) in acetic acid with boric acid as a catalyst. Among other ways, I may be prepared by condensing D-ribitol with 4,5-dimethylphenylenediamine. US Pat 2,807,611.

Description—Yellow to orange-yellow, crystalline powder having a slight odor; melts at about 280°; saturated solution is neutral to litmus; when dry not appreciably affected by diffused light, but when in solution, light induces quite rapid deterioration especially in the presence of alkalies.

Solubility—Very slightly soluble in water, alcohol, and isotonic sodium chloride solution; very soluble in dilute solutions of alkalies; insoluble in ether and chloroform.

Uses—To treat ariboflavinosis (riboflavin deficiency) and also to supplement other B vitamins in the treatment of pellagra and beriberi (see the general article on *Riboflavin* in this chapter).

Dose—*Usual*, *oral or parenteral*, *prophylactic*, **2 mg** once a day (for variation of dose with age see Tables I and II in this chapter); *therapeutic*, **5** to **10 mg** once a day.

Dosage Forms—Injection: 5 mg/mL, 350 mg/10 mL; Tablets: 1, 2, 5, 10, and 25 mg.

Thiamine Hydrochloride

Thiazolium, 3-[(4-amino-2-methyl-5-pyrimidinyl)methyl]-5-(2-hydroxyethyl)-4-methyl-, chloride, monohydrochloride; Vitamin B$_1$ Hydrochloride; Aneurine Hydrochloride; *Various Mfrs*

Thiamine monohydrochloride [67-03-8] C$_{12}$H$_{17}$ClN$_4$OS.HCl (337.27).

Preparation—This vitamin consists of two ring systems, a pyrimidine portion and a thiazole portion joined by a methylene bridge.

The *pyrimidine* may be prepared by several processes, one of which is as follows: Ethyl acrylate [CH$_2$=CHCOOC$_2$H$_5$] is heated with ethyl alcohol forming β-ethoxypropionic ester [C$_2$H$_5$O-CH$_2$CH$_2$COOC$_2$H$_5$] which is condensed in the presence of sodium metal with formic acid to form ethyl sodioformyl-β-ethoxypropionate [C$_2$H$_5$OCH$_2$CNa(CHO)COOC$_2$H$_5$]. This is then condensed with acetamidine yielding 2-methyl-5-ethoxymethyl-5-hydroxypyrimidine. This compound is treated with phosphorus oxychloride thereby replacing the OH on carbon 6 with Cl, and by reacting the resulting chloro derivative with ammonia, the Cl is replaced by NH$_2$. Finally, on treating the latter product with HBr, 2-methyl-5-bromomethyl-6-aminopyrimidine hydrobromide is produced.

The *thiazole* portion of the thiamine molecule may be built up in the following matter: Ethyl acetoacetate [CH$_3$COCH$_2$COOC$_2$H$_5$] is treated with ethylene oxide [C$_2$H$_4$O] and the resulting acetyl-butyryl lactone, when reacted with sulfuryl chloride, yields chloro-acetyl butyrolactone. This compound is decarboxylated when heated

Acetamidine   Enol form of Ethyl Sodioformyl-β-ethoxypropionate

2-Methyl-5-bromomethyl-6-aminopyrimidine Hydrobromide

Acetoacetic Ester

γ-Chloro-γ-acetyl Propanol   **4-Methyl-5-(β-hydroxyethyl)thiazole**

with HCl, splitting off CO$_2$ and forming chloroacetopropanol. The latter, when condensed with thioformamide yields the thiazole, 4-methyl-5-hydroxyethylthiazole.

The final step of this process is the combination of the pyrimidine and the thiazole to form a thiazolium halide. Since this is a simple addition of an alkyl halide (the bromo pyrimidine) to a tertiary amine (the thiazole) it is readily effected by bringing the two components together in a suitable solvent. The vitamin-bromohydrobromide so obtained is transformed into the corresponding chlorine compound, thiamine, with freshly precipitated silver chloride. The silver combines with the bromine to form the less soluble silver bromide and the chloride from the silver chloride replaces the bromine.

Description—Small white crystals or a crystalline powder usually having a slight, characteristic odor; when exposed to air, the anhydrous product rapidly absorbs about 4% of water; solutions are acid to litmus paper; pH (1 in 100 solution) between 2.7 and 3.4; melts, with some decomposition, at about 248°.

Solubility—1 g in about 1 mL water and about 170 mL alcohol; soluble in glycerin; insoluble in ether or benzene.

Incompatibilities—In the dry state, it is stable. Acidic solutions having a pH below 5.5, preferably from 5.0 to 3.5, are also relatively stable. *Alkalies* destroy it. It is precipitated from solution by several of the *alkaloidal reagents* such as *mercuric chloride*, *iodine*, *picric acid*, *tannin*, and *Mayer's reagent*. It is sensitive to both *oxidizing* and *reducing agents*.

Elixirs of thiamine hydrochloride are necessarily acid in reaction and are, therefore, incompatible with any acid-neutralizing substance. *Phenobarbital sodium* has been an occasional offender in this respect, the result frequently being such as to cause precipitation of the phenobarbital as well as a partial lowering of the acidity of the mixture with consequent deterioration of the vitamin. Phenobarbital, not the sodium derivative, may be dispensed in such an instance provided that sufficient alcohol is present to keep it in solution. If a part of the elixir is replaced with alcohol for this purpose, an amount of thiamine hydrochloride equivalent to that contained in the volume so replaced must be added to the product.

Uses—To treat *beriberi* and also *general B-vitamin deficiency*. The fact that thiamin cures the neuropathologies of beriberi has given rise to a widespread use of thiamine in nearly any type of neuropathology. Although such indiscriminatory use can do no organic harm to the patient, it constitutes an unnecessary expense; the promotion of the vitamin for such promiscuous use constitutes an abuse. For additional information see the general article on *Thiamine* in this chapter.

Dose—*Oral*, *prophylactic*, **5** to **10 mg** once daily (see also Tables I and III, this chapter); *therapeutic*, **10** to **35 mg** 3 times daily. *Intramuscular prophylactic*, **5** to **10 mg** once daily; *therapeutic*, **10** to **20 mg** 3 times daily. *Usual range of dose*, **5** to **200 mg** daily.

Dosage Forms—Injection: 100 mg/mL, 200 mg/2 mL, 500 mg and 1 g/10 mL, 2 g/20 mL, 2.5 g/5, 10, and 25 mL, 3 and 6 g/30 mL; Tablets: 5, 10, 25, 50, 100, and 250 mg.

Thiamine Mononitrate

Thiazolium, 3-[(4-amino-2-methyl-5-pyrimidinyl)methyl]-5-(2-hydroxyethyl)-4-methyl-, nitrate (salt); Thiamine Nitrate; Vitamin B$_1$ Mononitrate

Thiamine nitrate [532-43-4] C$_{12}$H$_{17}$N$_5$O$_4$S (327.36).

Preparation—In one method thiamine hydrochloride is reacted with sufficient NaOH to remove the HCl and replace the chloride ion by OH, and the resulting thiamine hydroxide is neutralized with nitric acid.

Description—White crystals or crystalline powder, usually having a slight, characteristic odor; pH (1 in 50 solution) between 6 and 7.5.

Solubility—1 g in about 44 mL water; slightly soluble in alcohol and chloroform.

Uses—More stable than the hydrochloride; solutions of the nitrate are practically neutral, while those of the hydrochloride are acid. Its vitaminergic actions and uses are identical to those of the hydrochloride. See *Thiamine Hydrochloride*.

Other Water-Soluble Vitamin Preparations

Choline Chloride [(2-Hydroxyethyl)trimethylammonium chloride; C$_5$H$_{14}$ClNO (139.62)]—*Preparation:* For the preparation of choline, see

Choline Dihydrogen Citrate. Description and Solubility: White, deliquescent crystals; a 10% aqueous solution has a pH of about 4.7. Very soluble in water or alcohol. *Uses:* For the metabolic effects of *Choline,* see page 1014. Choline chloride is used to reduce fatty infiltration of the liver and thus supposedly to prevent degeneration and cirrhosis. Such infiltration may occur after exposure to certain chemical intoxicants, such as carbon tetrachloride, chloroform, various other halogenated hydrocarbons (including several general anesthetics), divinyl ether, etc. Moderate to severe ethanol intoxication and habitual ingestion of ethanol also predispose to fatty infiltration of the liver. Patients who are acutely ill and cannot eat or persons on a high-fat diet frequently develop fatty livers, for which choline may be given. In none of these conditions has there been clearly demonstrable efficacy. Furthermore, a high-protein diet, especially one that includes eggs, meat, liver, and milk, not only provides some choline but also methionine, which promotes the endogenous synthesis of *Choline* (see page 1014). Once cirrhosis occurs, it is probably too late for any possible benefits. There is no evidence that choline is helpful in infectious hepatitis. For the above reasons, there is no longer any official preparation of choline. Since the anion is irrelevant to the metabolic effects, the chloride is neither superior nor inferior to other salts.

Choline Dihydrogen Citrate [(2-Hydroxyethyl)trimethylammonium Dihydrogen Citrate; $C_{11}H_{21}NO_8$ (295.29)]—*Preparation:* By treating aqueous trimethylamine with ethylene oxide. Conversion to the dihydrogen citrate is conveniently effected by dissolving the base in a suitable solvent such as ethanol and treating with an equimolar portion of citric acid. *Description and Solubility:* Colorless, translucent crystals, or a white, granular to fine, crystalline powder; odorless or may have a faint trimethylamine odor and has an acidic taste; hygroscopic when exposed to air; melts between 103° and 107.5°. 1 g dissolves in 1 mL water and 42 mL alcohol; very slightly soluble in ether, chloroform, and benzene. *Uses:* See *Choline Chloride,* above.

Sodium Folate [Monosodium Folate [6484-89-5] $C_{19}H_{18}N_7NaO_6$ (463.38); Folvite Sodium (*Lederle*)]—For the structure of the acid, see page 1014. *Preparation: Folic Acid* is reacted with $NaHCO_3$. *Description* and *Solubility:* Clear, mobile liquid having a yellow or orange-yellow color; pH between 8.5 and 11. *Uses:* Has the actions of *Folic Acid* (page 1023). However, the salt is preferred for parenteral use. *Dose: Parenteral,* 5 to 15 mg daily.

Multivitamin Preparations

In the preceding text and in various monographs, attention was called in several instances to the fact that it is desirable at times to administer more than one vitamin for what appear to be the symptoms of a single deficiency. The quotation "In the shadow of pellagra walks beriberi" has considerable substance in fact. Diets deficient in niacin are frequently also deficient in thiamin and certain other B vitamins of similar dietary source. The same relationship holds frequently for folacin and vitamin B_{12}. Malabsorption syndromes affect the assimilation of several vitamins. Furthermore, the repair of a deficiency of one vitamin may increase the requirement of another; for example, repletion of thiamin increases the need for riboflavin. Diseases in which there is increased metabolism, such as thyrotoxicosis, increase the need for more of the vitamins, as do periods of hard physical work, stress, pregnancy and lactation. Therefore, multivitamin therapy is often rational. However, most nondeprived persons, other than the aged and debilitated, consume a varied diet and routine multivitamin consumption is not indicated in the US. Advertising that suggests otherwise should be condemned.

A standard of identity for dietary supplements of vitamins has been published by the Federal Government. One of the primary motivations to standardize this kind of preparation was to protect consumers from an extant form of "economic adulteration." Such a situation exists when a product is sold as a dietary supplement which is inferior to that which should be expected for a product with this name. This is analogous to marketing a product for a particular therapeutic purpose, eg, the prevention of xerophthalmia, and having none or less than enough retinol present to do so, as judged by experienced clinical nutritionists. The composition of the preparation described below as Decavitamin complies with the requirements of the Federal standard for a dietary supplement for adults, except for the amount of folic acid (lower limit is 200 μg) and the absence of biotin (lower limit is 150 μg).

Official Multivitamin Preparations

Decavitamin Capsules

Various Mfrs

An official formulation is no longer provided; that of USP XVIII specified that each capsule contain

Retinol in the form of vitamin A	1.2 mg (4000 USP Units)
Vitamin D from natural sources or as ergocalciferol or cholecalciferol or the products obtained by the activation of either ergosterol or 7-dehydrocholesterol	10 μg (400 USP Units)
Ascorbic acid ($C_6H_8O_6$)	70 mg
Calcium pantothenate ($C_{18}H_{32}CaN_2O_{10}$) or its equivalent as racemic calcium pantothenate, D-panthenol or racemic panthenol	10 mg
Cyanocobalamin ($C_{63}H_{88}CoN_{14}O_{14}P$)	5 μg
Folic acid ($C_{19}H_{19}N_7O_6$)	100 μg
Niacinamide ($C_6H_6N_2O$)	20 mg
Pyridoxine hydrochloride ($C_8H_{11}NO_3$.HCl)	2 mg
Riboflavin ($C_{17}H_{20}N_4O_6$)	2 mg
Thiamine hydrochloride ($C_{12}H_{17}ClN_4OS$.HCl or its equivalent as thiamine mononitrate	2 mg
Alpha tocopherol, a suitable form, equivalent to 11 mg of (+)-α-tocopheryl acetate or 15 mg of (±)-α-tocopheryl acetate	

all amounts corresponding to not less than 100% of the molecular formula where stated.

Uses—*Multivitamin therapy* when a combined deficiency is suspected to exist.

Dose—*Usual,* 1 **capsule** daily.

Decavitamin Tablets

Various Mfrs

The content is identical to that of *Decavitamin Capsules.*
Uses—See *Decavitamin Capsules.*
Dose—*Usual,* 1 **tablet** daily.

Hexavitamin Capsules

Various Mfrs

Contain, in each capsule, not less than

Retinol in the form of vitamin A	1.5 mg (5000 USP Units)
Vitamin D as ergocalciferol or cholecalciferol obtained by the activation of ergosterol or 7-dehydrocholesterol or from natural sources	10 μg (400 USP Units)
Ascorbic acid	75 mg
Thiamine hydrochloride or an equivalent amount of thiamine mononitrate	2 mg
Riboflavin	3 mg
Niacinamide	20 mg

Uses—*Multivitamin therapy* when a combined deficiency of those vitamins contained in this preparation is suspected to exist.

Dose—As determined by the physician according to the needs of the patient.

Hexavitamin Tablets

Various Mfrs

The content is identical to that of *Hexavitamin Capsules.*
Uses—See *Hexavitamin Capsules.*
Dose—As determined by the physician according to the needs of the patient.

Amino Acids and Proteins

Nutritional Role—Protein hydrolysates, in which proteins have been reduced to short-chain peptides and amino acids, have long been used orally or in relatively dilute solutions intravenously as supplementary nutrients for patients unable to utilize intact protein adequately. More recently, patients in whom oral or tube feeding is contraindicated or inadequate, good nutrition may be achieved and maintained, for several months if necessary, by the procedure of intravenous feeding known as *total parenteral nutrition (TPN)*, sometimes called *intravenous* or *parenteral hyperalimentation*. Such feeding provides essential nutrients in a sufficiently concentrated form that does not exceed normal daily fluid requirements; this necessitates formulation of markedly hypertonic solutions (2000 mOsm/L and higher). Such solutions must be infused, at a constant rate throughout the entire day, into a large-diameter *central* vein where rapid dilution by high blood-flow minimizes vascular damage and the risk of phlebitis or thrombosis that is likely to occur on injection into a peripheral vein. The infusion route is generally through a surgically placed subclavian catheter into the superior vena cava, but in infants and small children it may be through a catheter in the jugular vein.

The most critical component in TPN is a nitrogen source available for repletion and/or maintenance of lean body mass and proteins essential for wound healing, tissue repair, and growth. Protein hydrolysate injections, sometimes supplemented with amino acids, are used as nitrogen sources, but in most hospitals solutions of mixed crystalline L-amino acids have replaced the former. Crystalline L-amino acids appear to be more efficiently utilized and better tolerated in the body than are the peptides of protein hydrolysates. Also, individual acids may be readily and reproducibly formulated to meet specific requirements of patients, such as those with renal failure and infants that are premature.

So that amino acids may be used for protein synthesis and to achieve positive nitrogen balance and weight gain in debilitated patients it is necessary to provide the equivalent of at least 150 nonprotein Calories per gram of nitrogen administered. Although fat is the richest calorie source, preparations suitable for parenteral nutrition have not been generally available,* and dextrose is commonly used for this purpose. Because of the large amounts of dextrose required to achieve caloric balance, and to avoid the fluid overload that would result from use of weaker solutions, markedly hypertonic concentrations of dextrose (25%—five times the isotonic concentration—or higher) must be supplied. As solutions so concentrated are prone to produce thrombosis when injected into a peripheral vein, they must be infused into a central vein, as described above.

In addition to dextrose and amino acids (or protein hydrolysate), TPN solutions may contain vitamins and electrolytes (often added to meet individual patient requirements). Various solutions for TPN use are commercially available, as are kits that include, for example, a 1-liter bottle containing 500 mL of 50% dextrose solution under vacuum, a 500-mL bottle of 8.5% solution of a crystalline amino acid mixture composed of 8 essential and 7 nonessential amino

acids in biologically utilizable proportion (FreAmine II,† McGaw), and a transfer set and additive cap for aseptic preparation of the final solution. Total parenteral nutrition solutions, which often require extemporaneous addition of compatible vitamins and/or electrolytes to solutions such as described above, should be prepared by a pharmacist experienced in parenterals production, using aseptic techniques performed under a laminar-flow, filtered-air hood (see Chapter 85, on *Intravenous Admixtures*).

Chemistry—The USP has provided monographs of standards and tests for each of the crystalline amino acids used in amino acid dosage forms. For comparative purposes the formulas and chemical names of the L-amino acids are given in Chapter 25, page 408, and other chemical data are provided in Table V of this chapter.

Each of the amino acids is readily synthesized, by a variety of methods, but always as a DL-mixture. While resolution to obtain the L-form can in some cases be conveniently accomplished, often it is easier and more economical to isolate individual acids from the mixed amino acids obtained by hydrolysis of selected proteins. Chromatographic fractionation of amino acids in such hydrolysates has generally replaced the tedious fractional precipitation and derivative distillation methods formerly employed.

The articles that follow describe certain amino acids which are used for certain nonnutritional purposes as well as components of nutritional formulations; also included are brief articles on Protein Hydrolysate Injection and on Oral Protein Hydrolysates.

Aminoacetic Acid

Glycocoll

NH_2CH_2COOH

Glycine [56-40-6] $C_2H_5NO_2$ (75.07).

Preparation—Aminoacetic acid is a constituent of many proteins. It may be synthesized by many processes; industrially it is prepared by interaction of ammonia with chloroacetic acid.

Description—White, odorless, crystalline powder, having a sweetish taste; solution is acid to litmus; pK_a 9.78.
Solubility—1 g in 4 mL water, 1254 mL alcohol; very slightly soluble in ether.

Uses—Aminoacetic acid has been occasionally used in the therapy of *myasthenia gravis* but most investigators doubt that the compound has any value in this disorder. Aminoacetic acid is used as an irrigating fluid in transurethral resection of the prostate. The acid is also used in various antacid preparations, sometimes as a complex salt. However, its limited buffering capacity does not warrant the expense of most of such preparations.

Dose—*Usual*, **30 g** daily, in divided doses; *application*, irrigating solution as a **1.5%** solution.

Dosage Forms—Irrigation: 1.5%/1500, 2000 and 3000 mL, 15% (concentrate)/1000 mL.

Arginine Hydrochloride

R-Gene (*Cutter*)

L-Arginine monohydrochloride [1119-34-2] $C_6H_{14}N_4O_2$.HCl (210.66). For the structural formula of arginine, see page 408.

---

* A 10% soybean emulsion (Intralipid), developed and used in Europe since 1961, that has an osmolarity of 280 mOsm/L (essentially isotonic with blood) and can be administered through peripheral veins, is now marketed in the US. The fat particles of this egg-yolk phospholipid emulsion are less than 0.5 μm in diameter, similar in size to naturally occurring chylomicrons. The emulsion is a useful source of calories and will also prevent and correct essential fatty acid deficiencies that may develop during long-term parenteral nutrition using nonlipid calorie sources. Its role in TPN is being evaluated.

† The composition of FreAmine II, in g/100 mL is: *Essential Amino Acids:* L-isoleucine 0.59; L-leucine 0.77; L-lysine acetate 0.87; L-methionine 0.45; L-phenylalanine 0.48; L-threonine 0.34; L-tryptophan 0.13; L-valine 0.56. *Nonessential Amino Acids:* L-alanine 0.60; L-arginine 0.31; L-histidine 0.24; L-proline 0.95; L-serine 0.50; aminoacetic acid 1.7; L-cysteine HCl <0.02. The calculated osmolarity of the solution is approximately 850 mOsm/L. Aminosyn (*Abbott*), a preparation of crystalline amino acids containing a somewhat different proportion of the same essential acids, and with the exception of L-tyrosine replacing L-cysteine the same nonessential amino acids, is supplied in concentrations of 5%, 7%, and 10% of the total acids, with calculated osmolarities of approximately 500, 700, and 1000 mOsm/L, respectively.

Table V — L-Amino Acids

Amino Acid[a]	Molecular Formula	Molecular Weight	Solubility in Water	pK Values
L-Alanine 56-41-7	$C_3H_7NO_2$	89.09	1 g in 6 mL	pK$_1$ 3.34 pK$_2$ 8.17
L-Arginine 74-79-3	$C_6H_{14}N_4O_2$	174.20	1 g in 5 mL	pK$_1$ 2.18 pK$_2$ 9.09 pK$_3$ 13.2
L-Aspartic Acid 56-84-8	$C_4H_7NO_4$	133.10	1 g in 200 mL	pK$_1{}'$ 1.88 pK$_2{}'$ 3.65 pK$_3{}'$ 9.60
L-Cysteine 52-90-4	$C_3H_7NO_2S$	121.16	Freely soluble	pK$_1$ 1.71 pK$_2$ 8.33 pK$_3$ 10.78
L-Cystine 56-89-3	$C_6H_{12}N_2O_4S_2$	240.30	1 g in 9000 mL	pK$_1$ 1 pK$_2$ 2.1 pK$_3$ 8.02 pK$_4$ 8.71
L-Glutamic Acid 56-86-0	$C_5H_9NO_4$	147.13	1 g in 115 mL	pK$_1{}'$ 2.19 pK$_2{}'$ 4.25 pK$_3{}'$ 9.67
L-Histidine 71-00-1	$C_6H_9N_3O_2$	155.16	1 g in 24 mL	pK$_1{}'$ 1.78 pK$_2{}'$ 5.97 pK$_3{}'$ 8.97
L-Hydroxyproline 51-35-4	$C_5H_9NO_3$	131.13	1 g in 3 mL (α-form)	pK$_1{}'$ 1.82 pK$_2{}'$ 9.65
L-Isoleucine* 73-32-5	$C_6H_{13}NO_2$	131.17	1 g in 25 mL	pK$_1$ 2.36 pK$_2$ 9.68
L-Leucine* 61-90-5	$C_6H_{13}NO_2$	131.17	1 g in 42 mL	K$_a$ 2.5×10^{-10} K$_b$ 2.3×10^{-2}
L-Lysine* 56-87-1	$C_6H_{14}N_2O_2$	146.19	Freely soluble	pK$_1$ 2.20 pK$_2$ 8.90 pK$_3$ 10.28
L-Methionine* 63-68-3	$C_5H_{11}NO_2S$	149.21	Soluble	pK$_1$ 2.12 pK$_2$ 9.28
L-Phenylalanine* 63-91-2	$C_9H_{11}NO_2$	165.19	1 g in 34 mL	pK$_1$ 2.16 pK$_2$ 9.18
L-Proline 147-85-3	$C_5H_9NO_2$	115.13	1 g in 0.7 mL	pK$_1$ 1.99 pK$_2$ 10.60
L-Serine 56-45-1	$C_3H_7NO_3$	105.09	1 g in 20 mL	pK$_1$ 2.19 pK$_2$ 9.21
L-Taurine 107-35-7	$C_2H_7NO_3S$	125.14	1g in 16 mL	pK$_1$ 1.50 pK$_2$ 8.74
L-Threonine* 72-19-5	$C_4H_9NO_3$	119.12	Freely soluble	pK$_1{}'$ 2.15 pK$_2{}'$ 9.12
L-Tryptophan* 73-22-3	$C_{11}H_{12}N_2O_2$	204.22	1 g in 88 mL	pK$_1$ 2.38 pK$_2$ 9.39
L-Tyrosine 60-18-4	$C_9H_{11}NO_3$	181.19	1 g in 2200 mL	pK$_1{}'$ 2.20 pK$_2{}'$ 9.11 pK$_3{}'$ 10.07
L-Valine* 72-18-4	$C_5H_{11}NO_2$	117.15	1 g in 12 mL	pK$_1$ 2.32 pK$_2$ 9.62

[a] The number below the name of each amino acid is its Chemical Abstracts Service (CAS) Registry Number. For structures and nomenclature see Chapter 25, page 408. Essential amino acids are identified by an asterisk.

Preparation—Arginine is present in the hydrolysis products of many proteins; for a method of separating it from gelatin hydrolysate see *J Biol Chem 132:* 325, 1940. It is converted to the hydrochloride by reaction with HCl.

Description—White crystals or crystalline powder; practically oderless.

Solubility—Soluble in water; slightly soluble in hot alcohol.

Uses—Arginine has been variously used in clinical practice. Intravenous administration in the symptomatic management of severe encephalopathies associated with ammoniacal azotemia, on the theory that arginine combines with ammonia to form asparagine, has not been of value in significantly reducing blood ammonia levels or in improving the clinical status of patients, and use of the amino acid for this purpose is no longer approved by the FDA. Oral administration to patients with cystic fibrosis to correct malabsorption and steatorrhea, and by inhalation as a mucolytic, have not been effective. Investigational use as a nutritional supplement in conditions in which its dibasic amino character or possible blood ammonia reducing power is useful has been reported.

Arginine stimulates pituitary release of growth hormone and prolactin, and pancreatic release of glucagon and insulin, and arginine hydrochloride is used diagnostically to evaluate pituitary growth hormone reserve and detect deficiency of the hormone in various conditions. It is administered by intravenous infusion and blood samples are taken at 30-min intervals after beginning infusion for 2.5 hr; the plasma growth hormone levels in these samples and in others taken 30 min before and at the start of infusion are determined and diagnostically evaluated.

Dose—*Intravenous infusion*, for *pituitary function test*, **30 g** of arginine hydrochloride, in 10% solution, infused at a constant rate over 30 min, preferably with the aid of an infusion pump; in *children* a dose of **500 mg/kg** of body weight is infused.

Dosage Form—Injection: 10% solution, 300 mL.

Glutamic Acid Hydrochloride—page 799.

Protein Hydrolysate Injection

A sterile solution of amino acids and short-chain peptides that represent the approximate nutritive equivalent of the casein, lactalbumin, plasma, fibrin, or other suitable protein from which it is derived by acid, enzymatic, or other method of hydrolysis. It may be modified by partial removal and restoration or addition of one or more amino acids. It may contain alcohol, dextrose, or other carbohydrate suitable for intravenous infusion. Not less than 50% of the total nitrogen present is in the form of α-amino nitrogen.

Description—Yellowish to reddish amber, transparent liquid.

Uses—Protein hydrolysates, as artificial hydrolytic digests of suitable proteins, supply, in the form of constituent amino acids and short-chain peptides, the approximate nutritive equivalent of the source protein. More than half of their total nitrogen is in the form of α-amino nitrogen. They are used for parenteral alimentation to maintain positive nitrogen balance in conditions in which there is interference with the ingestion, digestion, or absorption of food. Such conditions most frequently occur during severe illness, after surgical operations upon the gastrointestinal tract, or in cases of severe peptic ulcer. The protein hydrolysates are intended for repair and must be spared for such by adequate intake of other caloric foods; consequently, dextrose is frequently included in the preparations. Intravenous injection may induce nausea, vomiting, fever (especially after repeated administration), flushing and hypotension, abdominal pain, convulsions, phlebitis and thrombosis, and edema at the injection site. Protein hydrolysates may be given orally in conditions where absorption is adequate, but they are distasteful and frequently rejected by the patient. They are also used in nonallergenic diets for infants. Insufficient information exists to enable an exact statement of dose. 45 to 70 g of protein is sufficient to maintain positive nitrogen balance in the normal adult, but the needs may be greater in pathological conditions.

Dose—*Intravenous infusion, usual,* **2 to 3 L,** of **5%** solution daily.

Dosage Forms—5, 7, and 10% Protein Hydrolysate; 5% Protein Hydrolysate with 5% Dextrose; 5% Protein Hydrolysate with 5% Dextrose and 5% or 6.3% Alcohol; 5% Protein Hydrolysate with 12.5% Fructose; 5% Protein Hydrolysate with 12.5% Fructose and 2.4% Alcohol.

Sugars

Sugars are carbohydrates that are sweet to the taste and highly soluble in water. They may be either monosaccharides or disaccharides. The chemistry of the sugars is discussed in Chapter 25. In the section below are listed only those sugars that are used in medicine as aliments. Some of the sugars also have important uses as pharmaceutical necessities, in parenteral fluids, as diuretics, as osmotic "stuffing" for injection of other drugs, etc; consequently, the monographs of certain nutrient sugars may be found elsewhere in this volume.

Dextrose—page 1313.

Dextrose Injection—page 822.

Dextrose and Sodium Chloride Injection—page 822.

Fructose

D(−)-Fructose; Levulose

β-D-Fructopyranose

D-Fructose [57-48-7] $C_6H_{12}O_6$ (180.16); a sugar usually obtained by the inversion of aqueous solutions of sucrose and subsequent separation of fructose from glucose.

Preparation—Sucrose is inverted by treatment with dilute acid at moderate temperature, and the fructose is separated by precipitation of the lime-fructose complex. Fructose is released from the complex with carbon dioxide, which precipitates the calcium as carbonate. After filtering, the fructose solution is purified with activated carbon and ion-exchange resins and evaporated to dryness.

Description—Colorless crystals or as a white, crystalline or granular powder, which is odorless and has a sweet taste; specific rotation −89° to −91°.

Solubility—1 g in about 15 mL alcohol and about 14 mL methanol; freely soluble in water.

Uses—Fructose, a ketohexose, is used parenterally as a carbohydrate nutrient. It is converted to liver glycogen and metabolized more rapidly than dextrose, without requiring insulin, and thus may be utilized in diabetic patients. It is indicated in patients requiring fluid replacement and caloric feeding, but contraindicated in hypoglycemia, for which dextrose should be used. It is also contraindicated in patients with hereditary fructose intolerance.

Dose—*Intravenously* as required.

Dosage Forms—Injection: 100 g/1000 mL; Fructose and Sodium Chloride Injection: 100 g of fructose and 9 g of sodium chloride/1000 mL.

Lactose—page 1315.

Liquid Glucose—page 1313.

Sucrose—page 1290.

Syrup—page 1293.

Other Sugars

Invert Sugar [8013-17-0]—An equimolar mixture of glucose and fructose produced by hydrolysis of sucrose. Forms clear, colorless solutions having a pH of 3.5 to 6. *Uses:* Instead of dextrose, for parenteral administration of carbohydrate. While it has the same caloric value as dextrose (4 kcal/g), invert sugar is more rapidly utilized and may be administered intravenously twice as fast as dextrose. *Dose:* 1 L of a 5 or 10% solution in either water or isotonic sodium chloride solution.

Maltose [Malt Sugar; $C_{12}H_{22}O_{11}.H_2O$]—*Preparation:* By the action of diastase on starch. *Description* and *Solubility:* White crystalline powder; $[\alpha]D^{20}$ is +128.6°. Very soluble in water; slightly soluble in alcohol; insoluble in ether. *Uses:* Nutrient; sweetener; in culture media.

Fats and Oils

The role of fat in the nutritional physiology of man is both complex and contradictory. The unique and essential part it plays in metabolic processes and in the palatability of food points out its importance. Stored fat (adipose tissue) as well as dietary fat are concentrated sources of energy which the body can use efficiently for physical activity and in times of physical stress. Fat when oxidized to carbon dioxide and water yields nine kilocalories per gram whereas protein and carbohydrates both yield approximately four kilocalories per gram. Energy consumed in excess to metabolic needs is stored in the body as fat and represents the major body reserve of energy during periods of low calorie intake. Certain components of fat, called polyunsaturated fatty acids, are essential dietary components for tissue biosynthesis of prostaglandins, which perform vital hormone-like activities in the transmission of genetic information in all cells. Food fats are carriers, to varying degrees, of fat-soluble vitamins (A, D, E, and K). Also, a diet too restricted in fats lacks flavor and satiety value.

That fats are also involved or indicated in such significant pathologies as obesity and atherosclerosis or the syndrome called coronary heart disease (CHD) is well known. Epidemiologic, experimental, and clinical investigations have identified a number of "risk factors" associated with susceptibility to CHD that may be controlled. These include an elevation in plasma lipids, especially plasma cholesterol, high blood pressure (hypertension), heavy cigarette smoking, obesity, and physical inactivity. Persons falling into "risk categories" on the basis of their plasma lipid levels can be made aware of this during a physician's examination and appropriate professional dietary advice can then be followed. For such persons it is important, in addition to maintaining a desirable body weight, to decrease substantially the intake of saturated fat, and to lower cholesterol consumption. In practice, this entails substituting polyunsaturated vegetable oils for part of the saturated fat in the diet. Ordinary foods and some modified foods useful for this purpose are available on the market.

There are many abnormal conditions in which faulty digestion and absorption of fat occur and excessive amounts of fat are present in the feces. When these conditions exist, there is fecal fat loss, poor absorption of other nutrients, and diarrhea. As a result, there may be substantial weight loss and general malnutrition.

In recent years, it has been shown that the digestion and absorption of short- and medium-chain triglycerides (MCT's) are different from those of the long-chain triglycerides which are characteristic of most food fat. The hydrolysis and absorption of MCT's are faster than of long-chain triglycerides and it is possible for MCT's to be absorbed directly into the intestinal mucosa without first being hydrolyzed, making it possible to absorb MCT's in the absence of pancreatic juice and bile. Coconut oil contains more medium-chain fatty acids than other fats and oils and is used as a source for fractionation and preparation of MCT's. MCT's are commercially available as relatively pure 8-carbon or 10-carbon triglycerides and as a 4:1 mixture.

MCT's have been found to be useful in conjunction with the usual therapy in the treatment of such diseases as pancreatic insufficiency, cancer of the pancreas, cystic fibrosis of the pancreas, obstruction of the bile duct, certain abnormalities in the lymphatic system, regional enteritis, and in postoperative cases involving the removal of much of the stomach or small intestine. The most consistent beneficial effects reported from the use of MCT's are a decrease in the fecal loss of fat and less diarrhea.

Clinically, fats and oils have not been much used as parenteral aliments because their administration carries the danger of fat embolism and numerous other untoward effects; however, a soybean fat emulsion (*Intralipid*), developed and long used in Europe, which can be administered through peripheral veins as a source of calories, is now available in the US (see the first footnote in the preceding article on *Amino Acids and Proteins*).

Corn Oil—page 1295.

Olive Oil—page 1301.

Peanut Oil—page 1295.

Safflower Oil—RPS-16, page 803.

Fatty Acids

Arachidonic Acid [(*all-Z*)-5,8,11,14-Eicosatetraenoic Acid [506-32-1] $C_{20}H_{32}O_2$]—An *essential fatty acid*. Occurs in liver, brain, glandular organs, and depot fats of animals, small amounts in human depot fats. Melts at $-49.5°$. *Uses:* Has been recommended with other unsaturated fatty acids in infant eczema and dermatitis.

Linoleic Acid [(*Z,Z*)-9,12-Octadecadienoic acid [60-33-3]] and **Linolenic Acid** [(*Z,Z,Z*)-9,12-15-Octadecatrienoic acid [463-40-1] $CH_3(CH_2CH:CH)_3(CH_2)_7.COOH)$] are polyunsaturated fatty acids occurring as the glycerides in most vegetable oils. They are colorless or practically colorless liquids. Specific gravity of linolenic acid is about 0.91. Both acids are insoluble in water, but are soluble in organic solvents. *Uses:* Have been recommended in diets for infantile eczema and dermatitis.

Trace Elements

The trace elements are those inorganic nutrients that are required in small or "trace" amounts, a few micrograms to a few milligrams per day for man or per kilogram of diet for an experimental animal. The essentiality of several trace elements was established for animals and man during the 1930s. A resurgence of interest in this area has occurred in the past decade and a half due to technological advancements in analytical methodology and development of highly purified diets and "clean" environments for experimental animals.

Fourteen elements are now thought to be essential; however, evidence to support required functions in animals and man is still incomplete for nickel, silicon, tin and vanadium. It is expected that all fourteen of these, and possibly others, will be shown to be required by human beings. Some pertinent chemical and biological information on these elements is shown in Table VI. Some elements, notably manganese and chromium, can exist in several oxidation states; however, only one or two are compatible with a biological environment and function.

The amount of each element in a normal 70-kg adult man may vary considerably, depending on requirement and whether or not the element can be stored in certain tissues. Daily requirements ("allowances") have been established for

Table VI—Biological Data for the Essential Trace Elements

Element	Amount in 70-kg man, mg	Daily intake by man, range,[a] mg
Chromium	6.6	0.06–0.36
Cobalt	1.1	0.015–0.160
Copper	75–150	2.0[b]
Fluorine	2600	0.5–1.7[c]
Iodine	10–20	0.15[b]
Iron	4000–5000	18[b]
Manganese	12–20	1.25–6.5
Molybdenum	9.3	0.1–0.4
Nickel	10	0.30–0.60
Selenium	...	0.03–0.05
Silicon	18,000	...
Tin	17	1.5–3.5
Vanadium	10–25	1.0–4.0
Zinc	1400–2300	15[b]

[a] Values do not include amounts supplied by water.
[b] US RDA (See Table III, page 1005).
[c] Excludes high-fluoride areas.

Table VII—Distribution of Essential Trace Elements in Foods[a]

Element	Food source content	
	Average to high	Low
Chromium	Dried brewers' yeast, bran and germ of cereal grains, brown sugar, molasses, liver	Refined cereals, refined sugar
Cobalt	Leafy vegetables	Milk, refined cereals
Copper	Liver, kidney, fowl, fish, shellfish, nuts, dry legume seed, whole grain cereals	Milk, muscle meat, eggs, fruit, vegetables
Fluorine[b]	Seafish, red meat, eggs, tea	Milk
Iodine[b]	Seafish, shellfish, iodized salt	
Iron	Liver, kidney, shellfish, muscle meats, poultry, heart, egg yolk, dried legume seed, cane molasses, nuts	Milk, refined sugar
Manganese	Whole grain cereals, dried legume seed, tubers, fruits, non-leafy vegetables	Milk, poultry, fish
Molybdenum	Liver, kidney, dried legume seed, whole grain cereals, leafy vegetables	Fruits, root and stem vegetables, muscle meats, milk
Nickel	Whole grain cereals, vegetables	Muscle meats, fats, eggs, milk
Selenium[c]	Liver, kidney	
Silicon	Whole grain cereals, chicken skin, beer	Animal foods
Tin[d]	Cereals, muscle meats	Milk
Vanadium[b]	Liver, muscle meats, fish, bread, some cereal grains, nuts, a few root vegetables, oils from corn and soybeans	Milk, most vegetables
Zinc	Meat, egg yolk, whole grain cereals, oysters, fowl, milk	Fruits, fish vegetables

[a] Bioavailability is not taken into consideration; see text of individual elements.

[b] Most foods are highly variable.

[c] Selenium content is markedly affected by available selenium during growth of the plant or animal food. Cooking losses can occur.

[d] The tin content is markedly increased by exposure to tin-plated containers.

a few of the trace elements (Table III). Ranges of typical daily intakes of the other elements by healthy individuals provide a very rough guide to maximal needs. These values are based on limited data.

Information on trace-element distribution in foods is presented in Table VII. This is an attempt to indicate important sources of the elements or the level, particularly if low, in important foods. This table is of rather limited usefulness because it is based on so little information. At present, too little is known about the effect of agricultural practices and manufacturing processes on trace-element content.

Our understanding of trace-element function in man is less complete than that for vitamins. Study of a deficiency syndrome in animals often precedes recognition of deficiency or metabolic problems in man, particularly as related to a disease. For this reason, deficiency syndromes in animals are described for each element known to be essential.

Similarly, our knowledge of trace-element toxicity in man is limited and we must rely on animal data. Two problems must be considered. One is the effect of long-term supplementation with a "moderate" excess above requirement. For children and adults the Food and Drug Administration regulations on dietary supplements for each of four trace elements permit an excess of 50% above the US RDA (see Table III, page 1005). It is important to consider not only the amount of a single trace element, but also the balance among all required elements. This area requires periodic review as knowledge increases. The other toxicity problem relates to short-term intake of multiple recommended doses, either accidentally or purposefully. This must be regarded as undesirable, depending on the excess intake level. It is well

known to be very serious in the case of infants swallowing capsules containing ferrous sulfate.

Inorganic elements are very different from the various organic nutrients in that they cannot be destroyed or converted into another substance by the metabolic processes in the animal. In most cases the trace elements are bound to an organic ligand. This is the means for effecting elemental transport and function and minimizing toxicity. The binding may be very loose or very firm. Many of the elements are part of metalloenzymes. Nucleic acids also bind metal ions in a consistent pattern; however, the significance of this is not established. Other mechanisms of function are described for individual elements below.

Many pairs or larger groups of essential elements may have chemical properties that are closely similar. This can result in competition for binding sites that may alter transport, storage, excretion and function.

There are many elements in biological systems that have no known essential function but which have some chemical properties similar to those of required elements. These elements can become a health threat when they are present in sufficient quantity to replace a required element or to bind excessively to some organic ligand and cause a physiological aberration. Modern industrial technology has effected translocation of large quantities of many minerals from their native stores in the ground to the air, water and ultimately to the food supply. Three elements that have caused concern and some isolated severe problems for man are mercury, cadmium and lead. The nutritional status of an exposed person can modify the severity of adverse response to a toxic level of an element. A deficiency of certain nutrients can result in a more severe adverse effect while a moderate excess of other nutrients can afford some protection. The possibility must be kept in mind that elements now regarded only as toxic may have an essential function at a very low level of intake.

Chromium

Deficiency Syndrome and Function—The principal defect in chromium deficiency is an impairment of glucose utilization; however, disturbances in protein and lipid metabolism have also been observed. In the young animal, growth rate may be reduced. Corneal lesions have been observed in rats deficient in both chromium and protein; no lesions have been seen with either single deficiency.

Impaired glucose utilization occurs in many middle-aged and elderly human beings. In experimental studies, significant numbers of such persons have shown improvement in their glucose utilization after treatment with chromium. There have also been improvements in diabetic children and infants with kwashiorkor.

For biological activity, chromium must be trivalent. The most active form of chromium is that which is incorporated into a low-molecular-weight organic molecule that occurs in many foods. Its structure is not yet known. This compound has been designated GTF (glucose-tolerance-factor). From a variety of biochemical studies, it appears that the presence of insulin is required for all functions of chromium. GTF is the only one of many compounds tested that passed the rat placenta into the fetus.

Metabolism and Bioavailability—Chromium is transported by transferrin in the plasma and competes with iron for binding sites. The main excretory route is through the urine; however, some chromium is excreted in the bile and by the small intestine. The newborn animal has large stores of chromium that decline with age.

Toxicity—In animals, a wide margin of safety separates toxicity from the nutritional requirement of chromium (III).

Cobalt

Deficiency Syndrome, Function, and Metabolism—The only known essential function of cobalt is as a component of vitamin B_{12} (see page 1020).

Cobalt salts are poorly absorbed. Excretion is via the bile and through the intestinal wall. Cobalt is widely distributed in the body, with the highest concentrations in the liver, kidney and bone.

Toxicity—High levels of cobalt can produce a polycythemia in many species, an effect that is unrelated to vitamin B_{12}. Cobalt is usually considered relatively nontoxic; however, severe cardiac failure and some deaths in man resulted from consumption of large amounts of beer containing 1.2–1.5 ppm cobalt. The element was added to the beer to promote optimal foam stabilization.

Copper

Deficiency Syndrome and Function—The most common defect observed in copper-deficient animals is anemia. Other abnormalities include growth depression, skeletal defects, demyelination and degeneration of the nervous system, ataxia, defects in pigmentation and structure of hair or wool, reproductive failure and cardiovascular lesions, including dissecting aneurysms. Copper deficiency occurs very infrequently in human beings. A deficiency has been observed in some South American infants and a few in the United States receiving an artificial formula diet deficient in copper.

Several copper-containing metalloproteins have been isolated from animal tissues, including tyrosinase, ascorbic acid oxidase, laccase, cytochrome oxidase, uricase, monoamine oxidase, delta-aminolevulinic acid dehydrase and dopamine-β-hydroxylase. Copper functions in the absorption and utilization of iron, electron transport, connective tissue metabolism, phospholipid formation, purine metabolism and development of the nervous system. Ferroxidase I (ceruloplasmin), a copper-containing enzyme, effects the oxidation of Fe (II) to Fe (III), a required step for mobilization of stored iron. There is evidence that a copper-containing enzyme is responsible for the oxidative deamination of the epsilon amino group of lysine to produce desmosine and isodesmosine, the cross-links of elastin. In copper-deficient animals the arterial elastin is weaker and dissecting aneurysms may occur.

Metabolism and Bioavailability—Copper is absorbed from the small intestine. Most of the copper in the plasma is in ceruloplasmin; however, significant amounts are loosely bound to albumin, the fraction important in transport. The plasma copper level increases

in acute infections, pregnancy and in women taking birth-control pills. Small amounts of copper are excreted in the urine, but the major excretory pathway is via bile and feces.

Copper is present in high concentrations in the brain, liver, heart and kidney, with the highest levels occurring at birth. It is important that pregnant women receive adequate copper during pregnancy, so that the infant will have adequate stores of copper at birth.

A variety of salts of copper have been found to be available to experimental and domestic animals. These include the sulfate, nitrate, chloride, carbonate, oxide, hydroxide, iodide, glutamate, glycerophosphate, aspartate, citrate, nucleinate and pyrophosphate. Copper wire and copper sulfide were poorly utilized. The chemical form of copper in food is largely unknown. The absorption of copper can be decreased by large amounts of phytic acid, ascorbic acid, calcium, and zinc.

Toxicity—Wilson's disease, a genetic disease in man, leads to excess copper accumulation in the brain, liver and kidney, which leads to mental and neurological abnormalities. The disease is treated by administration of a chelating agent, penicillamine (β,β-dimethylcysteine), which removes excess copper from the tissues and results in its excretion.

Fluorine

Deficiency Syndrome and Function—The most important relationship of fluoride to health is that of preventing dental caries. Fluoride has been shown to enter the hydroxyapatite of teeth to form a more perfect crystal, which apparently resists acid attack more effectively. (See *Sodium Fluoride*, page 789). In areas where the fluoride content of the drinking water is unusually high, osteoporosis and calcification of the aorta of elderly persons are less than in control population groups not receiving high fluoride. In these areas the effective fluoride concentration is high enough to cause mottling of the tooth enamel in young children.

Metabolism and Bioavailability—The absorption of fluoride from the gastrointestinal tract is rapid and complete. Even the water-insoluble forms are absorbed fairly well. Fluoride can cross membranes easily, and it passes readily from the plasma into the tissues; however, the mammary gland and the placenta offer some resistance to transport. Excess fluoride is excreted in the urine.

Bones typically have high concentrations of fluoride, which gradually increase throughout life to about age 55 years. Of the soft tissues, the kidney is highest in fluoride. Calcium and aluminum can decrease the absorption of fluoride and sodium chloride can depress the skeletal uptake of fluoride.

Toxicity—Toxic doses of fluoride cause loss of appetite and body weight, muscular weakness, clonic convulsions, pulmonary congestion and respiratory and cardiac failure.

Chronic exposure to fluoride most often comes through consumption of drinking water, usually from deep wells drilled through or near fluoride-containing rocks. Levels of fluoride around 2 ppm or higher produce a permanent brownish mottling of tooth enamel when the exposure is during the time of tooth formation.

Iodine

Deficiency Syndrome, Function, and Metabolism—The iodine-deficiency disease is goiter (see *The Thyroid Hormones*, page 978). In iodine-deficient young, growth is depressed and sexual development is delayed, the skin and hair are typically rough and the hair becomes thin. Cretinism, feeble-mindedness and deaf-mutism occur in a severe deficiency. There is reproductive failure in the female and decreased fertility in the male.

Goiter has been observed in human beings in many areas of the world, with incidence in women and children usually higher than in the adult male. As a public-health measure, use of iodized salt has markedly reduced the incidence of goiter. Goitrogens can also cause goiter (see *Antithyroid Compounds*, page 982).

The only known function of iodine is for the production of the thyroid hormones, which regulate cellular oxidation.

The absorption of iodide can occur at all levels of the gastrointestinal tract. Iodinated amino acids can be absorbed as such, but less efficiently than iodide. Excretion of iodine is primarily via the urine, and the amount is a reasonably good indicator of thyroid status. Iodine in saliva is reabsorbed.

Iron

Deficiency Syndrome and Function—Hypochromic microcytic anemia is the characteristic result of iron deficiency. Depending on the severity, the anemia is accompanied by listlessness and tiredness, palpitation on exertion, sore tongue, angular stomatitis, dysphagia, and koilonychia.

Iron is an essential component of several important metalloproteins. These include hemoglobin, myoglobin, and many oxidation-reduction enzymes. In iron deficiency, there may be reduced concentrations of some of the iron-containing enzymes, such as cytochrome c in liver, kidney and skeletal muscle, and succinic dehydrogenase in the kidney and heart.

Metabolism—Iron is absorbed from the small intestine; however, the exact mechanism regulating the amount absorbed is still a matter of controversy. The proportion of dietary iron absorbed is greater in iron-deficient anemic individuals. Iron is transported via the blood, in which it is bound to transferrin, a β_1-globulin.

The iron from deteriorated red blood cells is reutilized. Under normal circumstances, the loss of iron from the body is very small, about 1 mg per day for men and an additional average daily loss of 0.5 mg/day by menstruating women. Iron is stored in the bone marrow, intestinal wall, liver and spleen, with the latter organs containing the largest amounts.

Bioavailability—The recognition of anemia as a major public-health problem for menstruating women and young children throughout the world has focused on the need for more extensive and better fortification of foods. This has stimulated a great deal of research on the availability of iron from foods and inorganic sources. Iron compounds that are readily utilized by experimental animals and man are ferric ammonium citrate, ferrous sulfate, ferrous gluconate, ferrous fumarate and ferrous ammonium sulfate. Average to poor sources of iron are reduced iron, ferric chloride and ferric pyrophosphate, whereas very poor sources are ferric oxide, ferrous carbonate, sodium iron pyrophosphate, and ferric orthophosphate. The availability of iron from foods can vary also.

Several dietary components can affect the availability of iron from many sources. Phytic acid can decrease iron absorption. The availability of iron is increased by a variety of reducing compounds such as ascorbic acid and molecules with sulfhydryl groups, as well as histidine and lysine. The smaller the particle size of reduced iron, the greater is the intestinal absorption and utilization. Heme iron is absorbed as such. Very high intakes of zinc, copper, manganese and cadmium can decrease the absorption of iron. Many additional studies are needed to evaluate adequately the availability of iron as influenced by composition of the diet and method of food preparation.

Toxicity—Since iron absorption is rather well-regulated, toxicity is not a common problem. Deaths have occurred, however, in children who swallowed capsules or tablets containing a readily available source of iron, such as ferrous sulfate. Acute effects include vomiting, hematemesis, hepatic damage, tachycardia, and peripheral vascular collapse.

Some individuals have a metabolic defect so that their iron absorption is not carefully controlled, and even a normal iron intake can lead to excess tissue accumulation. A disease known as hemochromatosis results. It usually can be controlled by phlebotomy at periodic intervals; however death can result if the disease is not treated.

Manganese

Deficiency Syndrome and Function—Manganese deficiency has been produced experimentally in many animals. Characteristics of the deficiency include growth depressions of the young animal, skeletal abnormalities (ranging from mild rarefaction to crippling deformities), mortality of the young, perosis (slipping of the Achilles tendon and accompanying joint deformity) in birds, depressed reproduction of both males and females, nutritional chondrodystrophy of the chick embryo, and ataxia in newborn mammals with head retraction, tremor, abnormal otoliths and semicircular canals in the ears. Newborn manganese-deficient guinea pigs have aplasia or marked hypoplasia of the pancreas. Manganese deficiency has never been recognized in man.

Manganese is required for the synthesis of mucopolysaccharides of cartilage and for the conversion of mevalonic acid to squalene. Glucose utilization is impaired in manganese deficiency. Pyruvate carboxylase is a manganese metalloenzyme.

Metabolism and Bioavailability—The homeostatic mechanism for regulating the concentration of manganese in the body is very precise. Manganese is absorbed from the small intestine and is then transported via the blood in the trivalent form bound to a β_1-globulin, transmanganin. Manganese is excreted in the bile and through the intestinal wall. The latter constitutes the principal mechanism for regulating the amounts of manganese in the tissues. With a high manganese intake, the element is also excreted in the pancreatic juice. The amount excreted in the urine is very small.

High levels of manganese occur in bone, liver, kidney, pancreas and the pituitary, whereas the concentration in the skeletal muscle is very low. The manganese in bone cannot be mobilized to meet a need. The stores of manganese, in the order of their importance, are found in the liver, skin and skeletal muscle. There is not a special store in the newborn.

In chick studies it was found that manganese was equally available from the oxide, carbonate, sulfate and chloride. High dietary intakes of calcium and phosphorus can decrease manganese absorption.

Toxicity—Miners exposed to manganese oxide dust for long periods of time develop psychiatric abnormalities that resemble schizophrenia. This is followed by crippling neurological disorders similar to those found in Parkinson's disease. Most young animals are unaffected by 1000 ppm manganese in the diet.

Molybdenum

Deficiency Syndrome, Function, and Metabolism—Adverse effects due to simple deficiency of molybdenum in man and in experimental animals have never been observed. Xanthine oxidase is an important molybdenum-containing enzyme. Due to a variety of indirect evidence and the importance of xanthine oxidase, molybdenum is considered to be an essential trace mineral for man, probably required in very small amounts.

Molybdenum supplied by water-soluble salts is readily absorbed. The element crosses the mammary gland easily. Excretion is into both urine and feces. The liver and kidney have the highest soft-tissue concentrations of molybdenum. Changes in level of dietary intake can be reflected in the concentrations in liver, kidney, skin, bones and hair. The newborn does not have special stores of the element. Sulfate can affect the absorption, tissue distribution and excretion of molybdenum. The content of molybdenum in erythrocytes decreases in many types of anemia.

Toxicity—The tolerance of animals to high intakes of molybdenum varies with species, age and the level of numerous other dietary components. The toxicity is decreased by copper, inorganic sulfate and the sulfur amino acids.

Nickel

Evidence that nickel is an essential element is based on abnormalities produced in chicks and rats fed diets containing 3–4 ppb nickel. Lipid metabolism was affected. Rats maintained through successive generations on the nickel-deficient diet had increased fetal mortality.

Absorption of nickel is small from ordinary diets. Excretion is primarily through the feces; however, significant amounts can be lost in sweat. Phytate can form a very stable complex with nickel so it is possible that phytate may decrease absorption of nickel. Further studies are required to establish clearly the essentiality of nickel and its significance to human health.

A low level of toxicity has been established for nickel in rats, mice, monkeys and chicks.

Selenium

Deficiency Syndrome and Function—Depending on species, age and specific diet composition, a deficiency of selenium can lead to one or more of the following abnormalities: growth depression, muscular dystrophy, degeneration of the myocardium, neurological lesions, liver necrosis, pancreatic fibrosis, exudative diathesis, ceroid-pigment deposition in adipose tissue, and death. Deficiency occurs in domestic animals with intakes below 0.02–0.05 ppm. Deficiency in man has only been demonstrated in China where extremely low intake causes a cardiomyopathy in children (Keshan disease). The NAS safe and adequate daily dietary intake of selenium are 10 to 80 µg for children and 50 to 200 µg for adults.

Most deficiency syndromes responsive to selenium also respond favorably to vitamin E. An exception is pancreatic fibrosis, which occurs only in selenium deficiency. Selenium is an essential component of the enzyme glutathione peroxidase. This provides a link between the antioxidant properties of vitamin E and the biological function of selenium in preventing most of the same selenium-deficiency problems. Animal studies have indicated that selenium may be useful as a chemoprevention agent but studies in man have not been accomplished. Experimentally, selenium has been shown to provide protection to pulmonary oxygen toxicity similar to that observed for vitamin E.

Metabolism—Selenium is absorbed from the duodenum. It can be metabolized to a variety of compounds and lost from the body via the bile, pancreatic and intestinal secretions, and ultimately through the feces, urine and expired air. Selenium can replace sulfur in the normal sulfur amino acids and selenite can also bind to sulfur amino acids. The highest tissue concentrations of selenium occur in the kidney, pancreas, pituitary and liver.

Toxicity—Acute selenium toxicity is characterized by abdominal pain, excess salivation, grating of the teeth, paralysis and blindness. Eventually disturbed respiration leads to death.

Selenium is one of the most toxic of the essential nutrients and the quantitative separation of required and chronic toxic levels is not very large. For domestic animals, the requirement is about 0.1–0.2 ppm, and 3 to 4 ppm in the diet are beginning levels for chronic toxicity. A reported carcinogenicity for selenium is an elusive association that has not been finally clarified.

Silicon

With highly purified diets it has been possible to produce a deficiency of silicon in chicks and rats. The deficiency affected growth rate, bones and integumental tissues. The primary biochemical lesion in the deficient animals was an effect on the cartilage matrix.

Silicon (as silicates) is easily absorbed from the intestinal tract and readily excreted in the urine, in part as SiO_2. Silicon is widely distributed in soil, plants, and animal tissues. It is relatively nontoxic; however, siliceous kidney stones have been reported in persons who chronically ingest magnesium trisilicate antacids.

Tin

Through rigid exclusion of environmental and dietary tin, it has been possible to produce growth retardation responsive to this element in rats. A maximal growth effect was obtained with 1 ppm tin in the diet, a level similar to that found in many foods.

Tin is poorly absorbed and most of that in the diet is excreted in the feces. Tin has a low order of toxicity.

Vanadium

Chicks and rats fed a diet containing less than 10 ppb vanadium had slow growth, defective bones and altered lipid metabolism. Vanadium is a rather toxic element. The addition of 25 to 50 ppm vanadium to the diet of rats causes diarrhea and mortality.

Zinc

Deficiency Syndrome and Function—Zinc is required for growth of every animal species studied; therefore, growth depression of young animals is invariably observed if the zinc deprivation is severe enough. Other characteristics of deficiency include skin lesions, alopecia, abnormal feathering in birds, deformed and poorly mineralized bones, hyperkeratinization of the esophagus, reduced numbers of circulating lymphocytes, impaired reproduction in males and females, fetal abnormalities and decreased learning ability. Persons with impaired taste acuity and discrimination and delayed healing of wounds and burns have responded favorably to therapeutic doses of zinc in some cases.

Nutritional dwarfism has been studied extensively in the Middle East. The syndrome includes delayed sexual development, reduced height and weight, hepatosplenomegaly, spoon nails, and usually anemia. Although the subjects were deficient to some degree in several nutrients, zinc was required for correcting the hypogonadism and growth depression. The syndrome occurs in both males and females. There is limited evidence that some young children in the United States do not receive adequate zinc.

Zinc is known to occur in many important metalloenzymes. These include carbonic anhydrase, carboxypeptidases A and B, alcohol dehydrogenase, glutamic dehydrogenase, D-glyceraldehyde-3-phosphate dehydrogenase, lactic dehydrogenase, malic dehydrogenase, alkaline phosphatase, aldolase and others. Impaired synthesis of nucleic acids and proteins has been observed in zinc deficiency. There is some evidence that zinc may be involved in the secretion of insulin and in the function of the hormone.

Metabolism and Bioavailability—Zinc can bind readily to sulfhydryl groups, amino groups and imidazole groups of proteins, amino acids and other organic molecules.

Zinc is absorbed primarily from the duodenum. It binds to all proteins of the plasma; however, it is most loosely bound to albumin and this may be important for transport to and from tissues. The concentration of zinc in plasma decreases rapidly when a low-zinc diet is fed, and it is reduced in pregnancy and in women taking birth control pills. The principal route of excretion is via the feces. Small amounts of zinc are excreted daily in the urine; these increase when there is tissue catabolism such as occurs in burns and in fasting. Significant losses of zinc can also occur in the sweat.

Zinc is present in all tissues, with very high concentrations in the prostate and choroid of the eye. Generally tissue concentrations are not greatly affected by zinc deficiency. The stores of zinc in the body are thought to be small.

Zinc is equally available to normal animals from a wide variety of inorganic salts as well as metallic zinc. Phytic acid can markedly decrease absorption of zinc, particularly in the presence of large amounts of calcium. Consumption of whole wheat bread, which contains phytic acid, has been shown to be primarily responsible for the zinc-deficiency dwarfism observed in the Middle East. The toxic effects of cadmium are probably partially related to interference with the normal physiological pathways and functions of zinc.

Toxicity—The taste threshold for a soluble salt of zinc in water is 15 ppm zinc, whereas 40 ppm have a very definite taste. A dose of 225 to 450 mg zinc has an emetic effect in an adult man. Acute toxicity of zinc is characterized by dehydration, electrolytic imbalance, stomach pain, lethargy, dizziness, muscular incoordination and renal failure.

Bibliography

Beaton GH, McHenry EW, eds: *Nutrition: A Comprehensive Treatise*, 3 vols, Academic, New York, 1964 (1st & 2nd vols), 1966 (3rd vol).

Beeson PB, McDermott W, Wyngaarden JB, eds: *Textbook of Medicine*, 15th ed, Saunders, Philadelphia, 1979.

Chaney MS, Ross ML: *Nutrition*, 8th ed, Houghton-Mifflin, Boston, 1971.

Davidson S, *et al*: *Human Nutrition and Dietetics*, 6th ed, Longman, London, 1975.

Fomon SJ: *Infant Nutrition*, 2nd ed, Saunders, Philadelphia, 1974.

Goodhard RS, Shils ME, eds: *Modern Nutrition in Health and Disease*, 6th ed, Lea & Febiger, Philadelphia, 1980.

Mitchell HS, *et al*: *Cooper's Nutrition in Health and Disease*, 15th ed., Lippincott, Philadelphia, 1968.

Pike RL, Brown ML: *Nutrition: An Integrated Approach*, Wiley, New York, 1975.

Robinson CH: *Normal and Therapeutic Nutrition*, 14th ed, Macmillan, New York, 1972.

Stanbury JB, *et al*: *The Metabolic Basis of Inherited Disease*, 5th ed, McGraw-Hill, New York, 1983.

Underwood EJ: *Trace Elements in Human and Animal Nutrition*, 4th ed, Academic, New York, 1977.

Recommended Dietary Allowances, NAS-NRC, Washington, DC, 1980.

Assay

Freed M, ed: *Methods of Vitamin Assay*, 3rd ed, Interscience, New York, 1966.

Joslyn MA, ed: *Methods in Food Analysis: Physical, Chemical and Instrumental Methods*, 2nd ed, Academic, New York, 1970.

Official Methods of Analysis, 13th ed, Assoc Off Anal Chem, Washington, DC, 1980.

The United States Pharmacopeia, XIth rev, Mack, Easton, PA, 1980.

Food Composition

Composition of Foods Raw-Processed-Prepared, USDA Handbook 8, Washington, DC, 1984; available from USGPO.

Nutritive Value of Foods, Handbook 456, USDA, Washington, DC, 1975; available from USGPO.

Pennington JAT, Church HN, Bower and Church: *Food Values of Portions Commonly Used*, 14th ed, Lippincott, Philadelphia, 1984.

CHAPTER 54

Enzymes

Michael R Franklin, PhD

Professor of Pharmacology
College of Pharmacy and School of Medicine
University of Utah
Salt Lake City, UT 84112

The functions of all living organisms depend on chemical reactions. For example, conversion of sugar to carbon dioxide and water with the release of energy proceeds through a series of chemical reactions each of which requires a biologic catalyst for the reaction to occur. Enzymes are proteins that serve as biologic catalysts. Without these enzymes conditions for reaction would be required which would be incompatible with the life of the cell. Thus, enzymes play a vital role in the function of the normal cell.

The importance of enzymes in normal body function is dramatically illustrated in conditions where one enzyme is nonfunctional as a result of a disease state or a congenital abnormality. Patients with these "inborn errors of metabolism" are strikingly abnormal. Phenylketonuric infants who are born without the enzyme phenylalanine hydroxylase (which is responsible for the conversion of phenylalanine to tyrosine) develop motor disturbances, light coloration of the skin, hair, and eyes, and in early childhood (if not in infancy) remain mentally retarded to the point of idiocy.

Since most chemical reactions in the body require the action of an enzyme, these biologic catalysts often serve as the focal point for regulation of body function. Increased enzyme activity accelerates the production of a given product that may be essential for a particular function. The synthesis of norepinephrine illustrates this principle well. Heart rate will increase when norepinephrine is released from the sympathetic nerves. Norepinephrine is synthesized through a series of enzymatic reactions of which the rate-limiting, and therefore the most important, regulating enzyme is tyrosine hydroxylase. Increased tyrosine hydroxylase activity brings about conversion of more tyrosine to dihydroxyphenylalanine (DOPA), which is converted by dopa decarboxylase to dopamine. Dopamine is converted to norepinephrine by the enzymatic activity of dopamine-β-hydroxylase. The formation of norepinephrine can be regulated by a number of factors, including a feedback mechanism. Increased levels of norepinephrine inhibit the enzyme tyrosine hydroxylase so that less norepinephrine is synthesized. Thus, levels of norepinephrine can control the amount of norepinephrine synthesized.

The actions of a considerable number of drugs representing a wide variety of pharmacologic agents depend on an enzyme-drug interaction. Notable examples demonstrating this diversity are given below. The hydrolysis of acetylcholine by cholinesterase is blocked in a competitive manner by physostigmine, and in a non-competitive manner by diisopropyl fluorophosphate, organophosphate insecticides, and several chemical warfare agents. The oxidation of norepinephrine and serotonin by monoamine oxidase is inhibited by the antidepressant, phenelzine. The oxidation of acetaldehyde to acetate by aldehyde dehydrogenase is inhibited by disulfiram. The oxidation of arachidonic acid to prostaglandins by cyclooxygenase is inhibited by and is the common mode of action of nonsteroidal antiinflammatory drugs such as aspirin and indomethacin. The hydrolysis of one of the cellular mediators

of hormonal action, cyclic 3',5'-adenosine monophosphate, by phosphodiesterase is inhibited by methylated xanthines, such as caffeine and theophylline. The 11β-hydroxylation reaction in the synthesis of cortisol, corticosterone, and aldosterone is inhibited by metyrapone. The thyroid peroxidase responsible for the synthesis of thyroxine is inhibited by propylthiouracil and methimazole. The conversion of xanthine to uric acid by xanthine oxidase is inhibited by allopurinol, which is used therefore in the treatment of gout. The bacterial synthesis of the essential vitamin folic acid is competitively inhibited by the sulfonamide antibiotics. The cancer chemotherapeutic agent fluorouracil is converted to a compound which inhibits the enzyme thymidylate synthetase which is needed for DNA synthesis.

These examples illustrate the importance of drug-enzyme interactions in the pharmacologic actions of therapeutic agents. The actions of drugs of the future also will undoubtedly depend on drug-enzyme interaction. Indeed, the pharmacologic action of many drugs currently being prescribed by the physician probably will eventually be found to involve such interplay. Since enzymes are so intricately involved in regulation of function, it is only logical to suppose that drugs may increase or decrease function by stimulating or depressing enzyme activity, respectively. A knowledge of enzymes and their properties, therefore, becomes increasingly important to the pharmacist in order to understand the action of drugs.

In addition to the action, the pharmacokinetics, drug interactions, and toxicities of many drugs are dependent upon enzyme activity. The enzymes responsible for these phenomena are those generally termed drug metabolizing enzymes and are predominately located in the liver. Contrary to most others, these enzymes typified by cytochrome P-450 and UDP-glucuronosyl transferase exhibit broad substrate specificity. The ability to metabolize a wide variety of drugs to more readily excretable products carries with it the potential for mutual competition when several drugs are administered simultaneously, thus altering the pharmacokinetics from that seen if a single drug is given. Toxicities arise from the two phase nature of drug metabolism; introduction of a reactive site suitable for conjugation and masking of that site with an endogenous polar molecule to form an excretable water-soluble conjugate. Failure to mask a reactive site allows it to interact with cell macromolecules (proteins, DNA, membranes) to produce cell damage, carcinogenesis, or cell death.

Properties—Four properties of enzymes make them exceptional catalysts.

1. Most enzymes will catalyze only a specific range of reactions and in many cases only one reaction will be catalyzed by a given enzyme. Some enzymes have a low degree of specificity; eg, pepsin hydrolyzes almost all soluble native proteins but the hydrolysis is limited to certain very specific peptide linkages. On the other hand, urease is a highly specific enzyme; its only known substrate is urea. Almost all enzymes show a high degree of spatial specificity. Arginase acts only on L-arginine; it does not attack

D-arginine. The specificity of enzymes is one of their most fundamental and important properties.

2. Enzymes are exceedingly efficient. Most enzymatic reactions, under optimal conditions, proceed 10^8 to 10^{11} times more rapidly than the corresponding nonenzymatic reactions.

3. Enzymes as a group are exceptionally versatile catalysts. For example, enzymes effectively catalyze hydrolytic reactions, dehydrations, acyl transfer reactions, oxidation–reduction reactions, polymerizations, aldol condensations, and free radical reactions.

4. Enzymes are subject to a variety of cellular controls. Their final concentration and rate of synthesis are under genetic control. In addition, enzymes are present in the cell in both inactive as well as active forms. The rate of conversion from inactive to active form is influenced by environmental changes; eg, phosphorylase *b* is converted to phosphorylase *a* very rapidly through a series of reactions which are triggered by release of catecholamines.

Nomenclature—Enzymes are usually named in terms of the reactions that are catalyzed. Usually the suffix "-ase" is added to the name of the substrate upon which the enzyme acts, ie, the enzyme which attacks urea is urease, and arginine is acted upon by arginase. Enzymes are also classified according to the reaction they catalyze, eg, reductases and dehydrogenases. Some older names, which are unrelated to the function of the enzyme, remain in usage, eg, rennin, trypsin, and pepsin.

The Commission on Enzymes of the International Union of Biochemistry has established a complete but rather complex system of classification and nomenclature. According to this classification enzymes are divided into six general groups:

1. *Oxidoreductases*—catalyzing oxidation–reduction reactions.
2. *Transferases*—catalyzing transfer of a chemical group from one molecule to another.
3. *Hydrolases*—catalyzing hydrolytic reactions.
4. *Lyases*—catalyzing the addition of groups to double bonds or *vice versa*.
5. *Isomerases*—catalyzing intramolecular rearrangements.
6. *Ligases* (also known as synthetases)—catalyzing the condensation of two molecules coupled with the cleavage of a pyrophosphate bond of ATP or similar triphosphate.

In this system every enzyme is coded in a four-number system according to the type of reaction catalyzed, type of isomerization, type of bond hydrolyzed, etc.

Many enzymes possess nonprotein chemical groups. Thus, an enzyme can often be dissociated into a protein component, *apoenzyme*, and a nonprotein component, *prosthetic group*. Prosthetic groups are also referred to as coenzymes or cofactors. Vitamins and certain metals are examples of these prosthetic groups.

Despite the ubiquity of enzymes in normal physiology, and as the basis of many drug effects and drug interactions, the use of enzymes as drugs is extremely limited. Being proteinaceous they can be inactivated by conditions and enzymes present in the GI lumen if given orally, and if given parenterally, can elicit immune responses. Most of the enzymes currently available on the market are hydrolases (Group 3 above). These enzyme preparations are of limited use in the following conditions: (1) debridement, ie, as aids in resolving and removing blood clots or fibrinous or purulent accumulations; (2) replacement therapy to correct certain gastrointestinal deficiencies; and (3) locally in certain inflammatory conditions after either topical application or hypodermic injection.

Asparaginase—page 1143.

Chymopapain

Chymodiactin (*Smith Labs*); Discase (*Baxter-Travenol*)

An enzyme of molecular weight approximately 27,000 isolated from papaya latex [9001-09-6].

An enzyme which rapidly hydrolyses proteoglycans, the major constituent of the nucleus pulposus. It does not affect collagen and does not dissolve ligaments.

Uses—For patients who have clear evidence of compression of the nerve root due to a herniated lumbar intervertebral disc. It is administered under general anesthesia by trained physicians by intradiscal injection. The enzyme is rapidly inactivated on leaving the disc. The major adverse effect is anaphylaxis (1% of patients), and chymopapain is contraindicated in patients sensitive to chymopapain, papaya, or in patients previously injected with any form of chymopapain.

Dose—2000 to 4000 units per disc in an injection of 1 to 2 mL. Maximum dose with multiple disc herniation is 10,000 units.

Dosage Forms—10,000 units per vial. Injection is 2000 units/mL.

Chymotrypsin

Avazyme (*Wallace*); Chymoral (*Armour*), Orenzyme (*Merrell-Dow*)

A proteolytic enzyme crystallized from an extract of the pancreas of the ox, *Bos taurus* Linné (Fam *Bovidae*). Potency: 1000 USP units/mg.

Description—White to yellowish white, odorless, crystalline or amorphous powder.

Solubility—An amount equivalent to 100,000 USP Chymotrypsin Units is soluble in 10 mL water or in 10 mL saline TS.

Uses—Promoted for use topically alone or in combination with trypsin for the debridement of necrotic wounds, ulcers, abscesses, empyemas, and fistulas. It has been used also for the liquefaction of blood and exudates that have not become organized by fibrous tissue. Chymotrypsin is inactivated rapidly when injected into closed cavities. The effectiveness of orally, buccally or intramuscularly administered chymotrypsin and other proteolytic enzymes for the treatment of inflammation and edema in traumatized tissue and other disease processes has not been adequately demonstrated clinically.

Chymotrypsin for Ophthalmic Solution is used as a proteolytic enzyme for zonule lysis (see *Alpha-Chymotrypsin*, under *Other Enzymes*).

Chymotrypsin causes local irritation and occasional ulceration. Its use has resulted in a variety of histamine-like allergic reactions including anaphylaxis which has been treated with antihistamine.

Dose—*Usual, intramuscular*, **2500** to **5000 USP units** 1 to 3 times a day. *Orally*, 50,000 to 100,000 units 4 times daily; *buccally*, 10,000 units 4 times daily.

Dosage Forms—Enteric coated tablets: 50,000 and 100,000 units chymotrypsin (Avazyme). Also in combination with trypsin (Chymoral, Orenzyme)

Hyaluronidase for Injection

Wydase (*Wyeth*)

A sterile, dry, soluble, enzyme product prepared from mammalian (bovine) testes and capable of hydrolyzing mucopolysaccharides of the type of hyaluronic acid; its potency is not less than the labeled potency in Hyaluronidase Units and it contains not more than 0.25 μg of tyrosine for each Hyaluronidase Unit. It may contain a suitable stabilizer.

Description—White, amorphous solid or a nearly colorless glass-like solid; it is destroyed by heat; its solutions are colorless and odorless.

Uses—Intercellular cement, which binds together the parenchymal cells of organs; appears to be a gel of highly polymerized polysaccharide, hyaluronic acid. The latter is present in all organs but is most abundant in tissues of mesenchymal origin (eg, connective tissue and blood vessels); the testis is the richest source of hyaluronidase in mammals. Hyaluronidase hydrolyzes hyaluronic acid by splitting the glucosaminidic bond between carbon-1 of the glucosamine moiety and carbon-4 of glucuronic acid. Hyaluronidase accelerates the subcutaneous spread of both particulate matter and solutions by depolymerizing the hyaluronic acid. This results in a larger area of distribution of drugs in the tissue spaces and facilitates their absorption.

The chief clinical use of hyaluronidase is to facilitate administration of fluids by hypodermoclysis. It has been used as an adjunct in subcutaneous urography for improving resorption of radiopaque agents to enhance absorption of drugs in tissue spaces, transudates, and various edemas. Its use with local anesthetics is not recommended. Hyaluronidase should not be used in infected areas because of the danger of spreading the infection.

Dose—*Usual*, *hypodermoclysis*, **150 units.**

Other Dose Information—A dose of 150 units is dissolved in 1 mL isotonic NaCl solution and either added to 1000 mL of hypodermoclysis fluid or injected at the proposed site of infusion. In order to avoid overhydration the rate of administration should not exceed that employed for intravenous infusion.

Dosage Forms—for Injection: 150 and 1500 units; Injection: 150 units/mL.

Malt Extract—page 1300.

Pancreatin

Viokase (*Viobin*); Pancreatin (*Lilly*)

A substance containing enzymes, principally amylase, protease, and lipase, obtained from the pancreas of the hog, *Sus scrofa* Linné var. *domesticus* Gray (Fam *Suidae*) or of the ox, *Bos taurus* Linné (Fam *Bovidae*). Pancreatin contains, in each mg, not less than 2 Units of lipase activity, not less than 25 Units of amylase activity, and not less than 25 Units of protease activity. Pancreatin of a higher digestive power may be labeled as a whole-number multiple of the three minimum activities or may be diluted by admixture with lactose, or with sucrose containing not more than 3.25% of starch, or with pancreatin of lower digestive power.

Description—Cream-colored, amorphous powder, having a faint, characteristic, but not offensive, odor. It hydrolyzes fats to glycerol and fatty acids, changes protein into proteoses and derived substances, and converts starch into dextrins and sugars. Its greatest activities are in neutral or faintly alkaline media; more than traces of mineral acids or large amounts of alkali hydroxides render it inert. An excess of alkali carbonate also inhibits its action.

Solubility—Slowly and incompletely soluble in water; insoluble in alcohol.

Incompatibilities—*Mineral acids* or excess *alkali hydroxides* or carbonates render it inert. It is precipitated by *strong alcoholic solutions* and by many *metallic salts.*

Uses—Indicated in the treatment of patients with cystic fibrosis (mucoviscidosis), chronic pancreatitis, partial or complete surgical pancreatectomy, and other conditions associated with exocrine pancreatic insufficiency. The administration of pancreatin decreases the nitrogen and fat content of the stool. The use of pancreatin except in pancreatic insufficiency is of no known value. The efficacy of pancreatin in the treatment of gaseous distention has not been demonstrated. When treating pancreatic insufficiency, a high-caloric diet which is high in protein and low in fat is recommended. A significant amount of the enzyme activity can be lost by peptic digestion during passage through the stomach. The efficacy of pancreatin is enhanced by simultaneous administration of cimetidine which increases intragastric pH. Dietary and enzyme regimens are best based on repeated clinical evaluation and, in hospitalized patients, periodic measurements of fecal fat and nitrogen loss. Since the underlying pancreatic deficiency is unchanged, replacement pancreatin therapy is permanent. At high doses, pancreatin can cause nausea, abdominal cramps, and diarrhea. The enzyme dust is irritating to the nasal membrane so inhalation should be avoided.

Dose—*Usual*, **325 mg** to **1 g,** taken before or with meal.

Dosage Forms—Capsules: 325 mg and 1 g; Granules: 12 and 20 gr; Tablets: 325 mg and 1 g.

Pancrelipase

Accelerase; Cotazym (*Organon*); Ilozyme (*Adria*); KuZyme (*Kremers-Urban*); Pancrease (*McNeil*)

A substance containing enzymes, principally lipase, with amylase and protease, obtained from the pancreas of the hog, *Sus scrofa* Linné var *domesticus* Gray (Fam *Suidae*). It contains, in each mg, not less than 24 Units of lipase activity, not less than 100 Units of amylase activity, and not less than 100 Units of protease activity.

Description—Cream-colored amorphous powder having a characteristic odor.

Solubility—Not completely insoluble in water forming a suspension.

Uses—Essentially the same actions as *Pancreatin*, of which it is a more concentrated form. However, the lipase activity is increased out of proportion to that of amylase and trypsin. It is employed as replacement therapy in *pancreatic insufficiency* to promote the absorption of fat and diminish steatorrhea. Adverse effects are similar to Pancreatin.

Dose—*Oral*, an amount of pancrelipase equivalent to **8000** to **24,000 units** of lipase activity prior to each meal or snack, or to be determined by the practitioner according to the needs of the patient.

Dosage Forms—Capsules: an amount of pancrelipase equivalent to 4000 to 8000 units of lipase activity (approximately 325 mg of pancrelipase); Packets: 16,000 and 40,000 units; Tablets: 9600 units (approximately 400 mg of pancrelipase).

Streptokinase

Streptase (*Hoechst-Roussel*); Kabikinase (*Pharmacia*)

An enzyme derived from beta-hemolytic streptococci.

Description—White powder; lyophilized.

Uses—Streptokinase activates plasminogen to plasmin, a proteolytic enzyme that degrades fibrin clots as well as fibrinogen and other plasma proteins. (Factors V and VII). [The route (method), duration, and dosage vary with each condition.] Streptokinase is indicated for the lysis of pulmonary emboli, deep vein thrombi, arterial thrombi and emboli, and acute coronary artery thrombosis (by intracoronary injection) associated with acute myocardial infarction. It is also indicated for clearance of occluded arteriovenous cannulae. Streptokinase may cause more rapid dissolution of the fresh thromboembolus than anticoagulant treatment, but the benefit of therapy must be weighed against the problem of increased hemorrhage associated with its use. If hemorrhage does occur with the drug, the antifibrinolysin, aminocaproic acid, can be given. Streptokinase is contraindicated in conditions where there is a predisposition to bleeding. Streptokinase also can cause fever and allergic reactions, including anaphylaxis.

Dose—Treatment should begin as soon as possible after the thrombus has formed. The usual loading dose is 250,000 IU intravenously over 30 minutes, followed by 100,000 IU per hour for 24 to 72 hours for pulmonary embolism, and 72 hours for deep-vein thrombosis. Heparin and oral anticoagulants are given after enzyme therapy has been completed. For recanalization in patients with acute coronary artery thrombosis, 20,000 IU of streptokinase is given by coronary catheter within 6 hours of the onset of symptoms, followed by 2000 to 4000 IU per minute until the vessel becomes patent, and continued at the rate of 2000 IU per minute for an additional 30 to 60 minutes.

Dosage Forms—Vials: 100,000, 250,000 and 750,000 IU, each vial also contains 25 mg cross-linked gelatin polypeptides and 25 mg sodium L-glutamate as stabilizers.

Sutilains

Travase (*Flint*)

A substance, containing proteolytic enzymes, derived from the bacterium *Bacillus subtilis*. Elaborated by fermentation with *B subtilis* and purified by filtration, salt and solvent precipitation, and lyophilization. Potency: not less than 2,500,000 Casein Units of proteolytic activity/g.

Description—Cream-colored odorless powder; *do not taste* (irritating to oral membranes); stable in light, hygroscopic, and decomposes in solvents.

Solubility—1 g dissolves in 100 mL water; insoluble in alcohol and other organic solvents.

Uses—Used as an adjunct to established methods of wound care for biochemical debridement of the following lesions: second and third degree burns, decubitus ulcers, incisional, traumatic, and pyrogenic wounds, and ulcers secondary to peripheral vascular disease. The enzyme digests necrotic soft tissues and a moist environment is essential to optimal enzyme activity. Detergents and antiseptics may render the substrate refractory, and heavy metal antibacterials may denature the enzyme. Sutilains is contraindicated for wounds communicating with body cavities or those containing exposed nerves or nervous tissue; for fungating neoplastic ulcers, and in wounds in women of childbearing potential. Sutilains should not be allowed to come in contact with the eyes. If this should inadvertently occur, the eyes should immediately be rinsed with copious amounts of water, preferably sterile water.

Dose—*Topical*, to the cleansed and moist wound, **2 to 4 times** daily.

Dosage Forms—Ointment: 82,000 Casein Units of proteolytic activity/g.

Urokinase

Abbokinase (*Abbott*); Breokinase (*Breon*)

Urokinase is an enzyme produced by the kidney and also found in urine; kidney tissue cultures and urine are sources of the enzyme. Two molecular forms (55,000 and 34,000 daltons), the smaller one derived by proteolysis of the larger one, are found in current therapeutic preparations [9039-53-6].

Description—White powder, lyophilized; soluble in water.

Uses—Urokinase is an activator of the endogenous fibrinolytic system which converts plasminogen to plasmin, which then degrades fibrin clots as well as fibrinogen and other plasma proteins. It is indicated for the lysis of acute massive pulmonary emboli and pulmonary emboli accompanied by unstable hemodynamics, and for clearance of IV catheters obstructed by clotted blood. Urokinase is markedly more expensive than is streptokinase. Since urokinase is derived from human cells, it is reportedly less antigenic than is streptokinase. This may be particularly important in the patient who requires a second course of treatment but who has developed antibodies to streptokinase.

Dose—The usual loading dose of 4400 IU per kilogram is given by intravenous infusion over 10 minutes, followed by a continuous infusion of 4400 IU per kg per hour for 12 hours. Heparin and oral anticoagulants are given after enzyme therapy has been completed.

Dosage Forms—Vials containing 250,000 IU urokinase activity, with 25 mg mannitol and 45 mg sodium chloride.

Other Enzymes

Alpha-Chymotrypsin [Alpha Chymar (*Barnes-Hind/Hydrocurve*), Zolyse (*Alcon*), Catarase (*Cooper Vision*)]—Chymotrypsin is obtained by a chymotrypsin-catalyzed cleavage of the dipeptide bonds of chymotrypsin [9004-07-3]. *Uses:* Chymotrypsin is the most stable member of the chymotrypsin family and has been used in cataract surgery. Following incision of the cornea, application of the enzyme for 2 to 4 minutes causes lysis of the zonules holding the lens, thus facilitating removal of the lens. Complications include temporary glaucoma, moderate uveitis, corneal edema, and striation. Delay of healing has been reported. *Dose:* Irrigation with 1–2 mL of a solution containing 75–150 units/mL.

Bromelains [Ananase (*Rorer*)]—A mixture of proteolytic enzymes derived from the stem of the pineapple plant, *Ananas comosus* (L.) Merr [9001-00-7]. *Uses:* Has been suggested for decreasing the inflammation and edema resulting from surgery and injury. The proposed rationale for its use is similar to papain and chymotrypsin. The oral effectiveness in reducing inflammation and edema is not yet established. *Dose:*

200,000 units daily. *Dosage form:* Enteric coated tablets; 50,000 or 100,000 units/tablet.

Collagenase [Biozyme C (*Armour*), Santyl (*Knoll*)]—A product of *Clostridium histolyticum*, which breaks down native collagen at physiological pH and temperature. It is a fermentation-produced enzyme complex. *Description* and *Solubility:* Amorphous and heat-labile. Soluble in water and alcohol. *Uses:* Collagen comprises about 75% of the dry weight of the skin and is the main constituent of necrotic debris and of the eschar which covers the surface of an ulcer; hence, collagenase is indicated for debridement of severely burned areas and dermal ulcers. Its effectiveness in the treatment of other necrotic skin lesions requires further investigation. The enzyme is compatible with antibiotics such as polymyxin B sulfate, neomycin or bacitracin. Collagenase is adversely affected by heavy metal antiseptics, detergents, and hexachlorophene so that these agents must be removed before using the enzyme. *Dose:* The ointment (250 units/g) is applied daily or every other day to the lesions and covered with sterile dressings.

Fibrinolysin and Desoxyribonuclease [Elase (*Parke-Davis*)]—This is a mixture of fibrinolysin of bovine plasma and desoxyribonuclease obtained from bovine pancreas. These two enzymes function together when used topically to lyse fibrin and liquefy pus, thus aiding in the removal of necrotic material both from the skin and certain body cavities. It is used as a debriding agent in surgical wounds, ulcerative lesions, and second and third degree burns and is used intravaginally in severe cervicitis and vaginitis. It is not suitable for parenteral use and is not to be used in thromboembolic diseases. The commercial product named above is supplied as a lyophilized powder (25 units of fibrinolysin and 15,000 units of deoxyribonuclease), from which a solution for topical use may be prepared, and in ointment form (30 units of fibrinolysin and 20,000 units of deoxyribonuclease).

Lactase [Lactaid (*Lact Aid*)]—A β-D-galactosidase derived from *Kluyveromyces lactis* yeast. Added to milk to convert the dissaccharide lactose into glucose and galactose for patients suffering from lactase insufficiency.

Papain [Papase (*Parke-Davis*)]—A proteolytic enzyme from the fruit of the tropical melon tree, *Carica papaya*. The enzyme exhibits broad spectrum specificity; peptides, amides, esters, and thioesters all being susceptible to papain-catalyzed hydrolysis. *Uses:* As an anti-inflammatory agent. It is considered possibly effective in relieving symptoms of episiotomy. *Dose:* Two chewable tablets (20,000 units/tablet) are taken buccally or orally, 4 times daily for 5 days.

Trypsin, Crystallized [Granulex (*Hickam*)]—A proteolytic enzyme crystallized from an extract of the pancreas gland of the ox, *Bos taurus Linné* (Fam *Bovidae*); its potency is not less than 25,000 Trypsin Units/mg. A white to yellowish white, odorless, crystalline or amorphous powder; an amount equivalent to 500,000 Trypsin Units is soluble in 10 mL of water or saline TS. *Uses:* Trypsin promotes proteolysis of a variety of protein substrates, including clotted blood, purulent exudates (pus), and necrotic tissue, but not living tissue. Especially in the presence of blood its duration of action is limited, because of the presence of inhibiting substances. Supplied in aerosol form (0.12 mg Trypsin per mL) together with balsam Peru and castor oil for debridement of eschar and other necrotic tissue.

Digestive Aids

Numerous preparations, both prescription and OTC, are available as aids for digestin, particulary for conditions where deficiencies of natural digestive enzymes exist. They contain some or all of the following categories of enzymes: amylolytic, proteolytic, cellulytic, and lipolytic. In addition, the preparations often include bile salts or bile extracts.

CHAPTER 55

General Anesthetics

Ewart A Swinyard, PhD, DSc(Hon)

Professor Emeritus of Pharmacology
College of Pharmacy and School of Medicine
University of Utah
Salt Lake City, UT 84112

Anesthetics are drugs which produce anesthesia, a condition of inability to appreciate sensation. Two types of anesthesia are usually recognized: local anesthesia and general anesthesia. In *local anesthesia*, the anesthesia is confined to a portion of the body and the patient is conscious (see Chapter 56). In *general anesthesia*, the anesthesia extends to the entire body and under which the patient is unconscious, in a state of muscular relaxation and insensibility to pain. This type of anesthesia is employed for most surgical operations and is the subject of this chapter.

The general anesthetic drugs may, for convenience in presentation, be divided into two groups: inhalation anesthetics and intravenous anesthetics. The first group includes the volatile liquids and gases; the second group, the rapidly-acting barbiturates and nonbarbiturates.

Halothane is the anesthetic agent preferred by many anesthesiologists to induce and maintain general anesthesia. Induction is fast and smooth. Halothane is a nonflammable, potent anesthetic. On the other hand, it is a relatively weak analgesic, exerts sympathomimetic action, produces hypotension and, on repeated administration, is toxic to the liver. It is expensive and requires a special vaporizer. Alternate preferred anesthetic agents include ether, enflurane, isoflurane, methoxyflurane, cyclopropane, nitrous oxide, and thiopental. The special features, advantages and disadvantages of these agents are briefly mentioned in the monographs which follow.

The safety, effectiveness, and general usefulness of general anesthesia have been greatly extended by the use of preanesthetic medications which are used to prepare the patient for anesthesia and by the development of dantrolene sodium (Dantrium: *Norwich–Eaton*) for the management of malignant hyperthermia. The barbiturates, benzodiazepines, and narcotics are given prior to anesthesia to produce serenity and amnesia for the events preceding the operation and to act as a base for the anesthetic to be given. The phenothiazine-type tranquilizers are used for their sedative actions, to increase effects of central nervous system depressants, and to reduce the incidence of postoperative nausea and vomiting. Atropine or scopolamine is used to lessen the secretion of saliva and to reduce undesirable reflex action through the vagus nerve. Scopolamine has the added effect of producing amnesia. Curare and related compounds are used to increase muscle relaxation. Malignant hyperthermia, an uncommon but devastating complication to inhalation anesthetics, usually appears during anesthesia but may occur several hours postoperatively. Clinical signs include tachycardia, cardiac arrhythmias, tachypnea, rapidly rising temperature, acidosis, and shock. Immediate intravenous treatment with dantrolene can be life-saving. These medications are mentioned elsewhere under the monograph for the particular agent (eg, see *Skeletal Muscle Relaxants*, page 921).

Drug Interactions and Anesthesia

The drugs a potential surgical patient may be taking for a chronic or acute illness and the several drugs usually employed before, during, and after surgery are not only a major factor in selecting both preanesthetic and anesthetic agents, but also present a unique problem in potential drug interaction. The family physician, anesthesiologist, and surgeon should thoughtfully consider this problem at least a week in advance of surgery and determine whether some drugs should be discontinued or the dose reduced. Although there are no rigid criteria for discontinuing drugs before surgery, the following possible drug interactions have been mentioned by *The Medical Letter* (*16:* 17–20, 1974) as worthy of consideration.

Anticoagulants may cause bleeding with spinal, epidural, dental, or other types of regional blocks or with tracheal intubations or other instrumentation, and may increase bleeding during and after surgery.

Antimicrobial Drugs—*Tetracyclines* predispose to renal insufficiency after methoxyflurane anesthesia. *Kanamycin, streptomycin, gentamicin, and neomycin* may cause neuromuscular block and apnea and therefore have an additive effect if *d*-tubocurarine or other nondepolarizing neuromuscular blocking agents are used.

Cardiovascular Drugs—Beta-adrenergic blockers such as *propranolol* may add to the myocardial depression of general anesthetics, induce bronchospasm, and prevent adequate circulatory response to blood loss. Despite these hazards, it may sometimes be preferable to continue the drug in patients with severe hypertension, severe angina, arrhythmias, or hyperthyroidism. *Digitalis and cardiac glycosides* should as a rule be continued, but the possibility of digitalis intoxication during general anesthesia should be kept in mind. *Quinidine, procainamide, and lidocaine* may aggravate myocardial depression, impair cardiac conduction, and cause peripheral vasodilatation. They may also potentiate neuromuscular blocking drugs. *Diuretics*, especially the thiazides, furosemide, and ethacrynic acid, can lead to hypovolemia, hypotension, alterations in sodium and potassium metabolism, and prolonged paralysis when used together with muscle relaxants. *Antihypertensive drugs* may cause additive hypotensive effects.

Corticosteroids should not be discontinued; sudden withdrawal may cause adrenal cortical insufficiency. In some cases, clinicians may increase the dosage of steroid for 24 to 48 hours before the operation.

Drugs Acting on the Nervous System—*Anticonvulsants* such as phenytoin and phenobarbital are inducers of hepatic microsomal enzymes and may enhance metabolism of inhalation anesthetics and diminish their effectiveness. Phenobarbital can also add to respiratory depression when sedatives are used in premedication. Tapering off anticonvulsants in too short a period before surgery, however, may result in convulsions, and sudden cessation may lead to status epilepticus. Respiratory depression may be more safely avoided by using lower doses of the sedative. *MAO inhibitors* (tranylcypromine, pargyline, and others) may cause hypertensive crises in conjunction with sympathomimetic amines. *Phenothiazines* in the large doses used for psychoses and the *tricyclic antidepressants* may add to the hypotensive effects of sedatives, narcotics, and general anesthetics. *Neostigmine* (for myasthenia gravis) is sometimes stopped before surgery to avoid respiratory failure due to cholinergic crisis postoperatively; if it is discontinued, however, other measures must be taken to prevent respiratory failure from myasthenic weakness. *Levodopa* can cause hypotension and occasionally arrhythmias. It need not be discontinued until a few hours before anesthesia, however, and can be restarted after surgery at the same dosage level.

Drugs for Glaucoma—Oral and topical drugs should generally be continued, particularly in narrow-angle glaucoma. When *echothiophate* has been used, the anesthesiologist must beware of inhibition of cholinesterase and prolonged paralysis which may occur after administration of succinylcholine.

Insulin dosage should be reduced at the time of surgery. Some anesthesiologists withhold insulin until the postoperative period, but hypoglycemia is rare in patients given insulin during surgery, as long as glucose is also administered. Patients who have been on oral hypoglycemics usually are not given insulin during surgery.

Oral Contraceptives should be stopped two to four weeks before surgery to minimize the risk of postoperative venous thrombosis.

The choice, dosage, and administration of anesthetic drugs require caution if the patient has been taking medication. A number of therapeutic, preanesthetic, and anesthetic drug interactions are possible. The importance of a drug in therapy must be weighed against the seriousness of the complications it may induce if it is continued during the administration of preanesthetic and anesthetic drugs.

Inhalation Anesthetics

Volatile liquids and gases are commonly used to induce anesthesia by progressively increasing the amount of volatile anesthetic in the inspired air and thus in the blood and brain. Three expressions are commonly used to characterize the movement of these substances from the inspired air to the blood and brain. (1) Vapor pressure (VP), in torr (1/760 of an atmosphere) at 20°, is used as a measure of volatility; (2) the blood gas partition coefficient at 37° (blood/gas) is used to show the rate at which the partial pressure of an inhalation anesthetic in the arterial blood approaches that in the alveoli (when solubility is low, equilibrium is approached rapidly); and (3) clinical potency is defined in terms of the minimal alveolar concentration (MAC) necessary to prevent movement in 50% of individuals subjected to a painful stimulus. Values for these expressions are shown in the respective monographs.

The administration of an anesthetic results in progressive depression of the central nervous system, which may be preceded by varying degrees of excitation. These drugs first depress the cerebral cortex and then the basal ganglia and cerebellum. This is followed first by sensory and then motor paralysis of the functions of the spinal cord from below, upward. If the administration of the anesthetic is continued, the medullary centers are involved, and death may result from paralysis of the respiratory and vasomotor centers.

Four more or less definite stages of anesthesia may be recognized. These stages vary considerably in character and duration, depending upon the nature of the anesthetic as well as the speed of induction and the manner in which it is administered. They are most clearly seen with ether. When induction is rapid, as with cyclopropane, the early stages are less clearly defined. When anesthesia is induced by intravenous administration, as with the thiobarbiturates, unconsciousness occurs so promptly that the preliminary stages of anesthesia are not observed. The four stages of anesthesia, as originally described by Dr A E Guedel, are presented below. These classical signs are reliable only for ether alone or in combination with nitrous oxide.

Stage I: Analgesia—This stage starts with the first inhalation of anesthetic gas and ends with the onset of unconsciousness. The patient is conscious and experiences sensations of warmth, remoteness, drifting, falling, and giddiness. There is a marked reduction in the perception of painful stimuli. This stage is often used in obstetrics and minor surgery.

Stage II: Delirium or Excitement—This stage begins with the loss of consciousness. The inhibitory control of the higher centers is removed, and the subconscious emotions take over. The responses in this stage vary with different individuals; some patients pass through this stage peacefully and quietly, others become very excited and may exhibit excessive and even violent, struggling movements. Blood pressure, heart rate, and respiratory rate are all increased. All reflexes are present. It is desirable to pass through this stage as quickly as possible.

Stage III: Surgical Anesthesia—This is the stage of unconsciousness and paralysis of reflexes. In this stage the patient reflects complete tranquillity. Respiration is full and regular; the pulse is slow, full, and strong; the face is calm and expressionless; the body's musculature becomes soft and pliable; and the pupils become constricted. This stage is divided into four planes on the basis of the disappearance of various reflexes and the degree of respiratory depression. All surgical procedures are carried out in this stage.

Stage IV: Medullary Paralysis—This stage begins with central respiratory paralysis and ends with cardiac failure and death unless restorative measures are instituted. This stage should be avoided, except under unusual circumstances controlled by a skilled anesthetist.

Recovery—If the anesthetic is removed and the respiration is reestablished and sustained before the heart stops, the symptoms may be reversed, and the body regains its normal physiological faculties. As recovery proceeds, the signs of the various stages occur in the reverse order, Stage I being the last stage to reappear.

The inhalation anesthetics are usually administered by one of two methods.

1. *Open Method*—The liquid anesthetic is dropped on a cotton or gauze mask held over the patient's nose or mouth. Air is the diluent and no anesthetic machine is required.

2. *Closed Method*—The gaseous or liquid anesthetic is contained in a special apparatus which, when attached to the patient's nose and mouth, constitutes a closed system. The patient is continually rebreathing the contents of the system. Provision is made for the removal of carbon dioxide with soda lime and the addition of oxygen as needed.

Sometimes, a semiclosed method, a modification of the second method, is used. This method employs a closed method type of apparatus, but a valve on the mask permits ready respiration outside the system, under which circumstances rebreathing is not excessive and no provision is made for removal of CO_2 or water.

Liquid Inhalation Anesthetics

The liquid inhalation anesthetics include chloroform, ether, ethyl chloride, halothane, methoxyflurane, fluroxene, enflurane, isoflurane and trichloroethylene. Chloroform, vinyl ether, and ethyl chloride have been supplanted by other agents because of their disadvantages, such as hepatotoxicity, adverse cardiovascular effects, and, except for chloroform, flammability. Except for ethyl chloride, which boils at 12°, the anesthetics in this group are liquids at room temperature and boil above 20°. All these agents are capable of producing surgical anesthesia when administered in appropriate concentrations and, unassisted by preanesthetic medication, can carry anesthesia to the stage of medullary paralysis. Hence, they are sometimes referred to as 100% anesthetic agents.

The inhalation anesthetics most used are halothane (Flu-

othane), methoxyflurane (Penthrane), enflurane (Ethrane), and isoflurane (Forane). Methoxyflurane is used infrequently because of its slow induction and renal toxicity. The use of halothane, for many years the most frequently employed halogenated inhalation anesthetic, has declined markedly because of reports of hepatitis, sometimes fatal, from its repeated use. Enflurane, introduced in 1973, has been the main substitute for halothane. Isoflurane is said to offer a number of advantages over other inhalation anesthetics; it is essentially free of any important toxicity (*Anesth Analg 60:* 666, 1981). Ether, at one time the standard of comparison for general anesthetics, is seldom used because it is inflammable and explosive. Chloroform, although still employed in the tropics, has been largely abandoned in this country as a general anesthetic; in this text it is classified as a pharmaceutical necessity. All of the fluorinated anesthetics, especially methoxyflurane, release inorganic fluoride during their metabolism; the fluoride concentrations can reach nephrotoxic levels after anesthesia with methoxyflurane. Serum inorganic fluoride levels from 50 to 80 μmol/liter may be associated with subclinical nephrotoxicity, and levels from 80 to 175 μmol/liter may be associated with clinical nephrotoxicity; patients with levels below 40 μmol/liter generally show no evidence of this toxic response. Animal studies suggest that trifluoroacetic acid is a major metabolite of halothane and fluroxene.

The ideal liquid anesthetic has yet to be discovered. An ideal anesthetic should have a high margin of safety, produce surgical anesthesia, have rapid and pleasant induction and recovery, be easily controlled and regulated, have no side effects or toxicity, not depress the cardiovascular and respiratory systems, be nonflammable and nonexplosive, provide good analgesia and muscle relaxation, and have low cost. Unfortunately, all available agents exhibit toxic properties that tend to limit their usefulness. Halothane and trichloroethylene sensitize the myocardium to sympathoadrenal discharges and to epinephrine. Consequently, serious and sometimes fatal cardiac arrhythmias may occur while patients are under the influence of these agents. Both enflurane and isoflurane are much less likely to sensitize the heart to epinephrine and sympathoadrenal discharges. Except for ether, which is not hepatotoxic, all halogenated liquid anesthetics are capable of producing liver damage.

Chronic, low-level exposure to the operating room atmosphere is an environmental hazard of increasing concern to operating-room personnel. Recent reports indicate a direct correlation between end-expired levels of anesthetic and operating-room concentrations of anesthetic times duration of exposure. The incidence of spontaneous abortion among operating-room personnel has been reported to vary from 19.5 to 37.9%, compared to 8.8 to 11.4% in a similar number of unexposed personnel. Other studies suggest that the liveborn offspring of both women directly exposed and wives of men chronically exposed to the operating-room environment have an increased incidence of congenital abnormalities. It is generally agreed that this health hazard should be carefully studied.

Chloroform—page 1312.

Enflurane

Ethane, 2-chloro-1-(difluoromethoxy)-1,1,2-trifluoro-, Ethrane (Ohio Medical)

$$H-\overset{\overset{\displaystyle F}{|}}{\underset{\underset{\displaystyle F}{|}}{C}}-O-\overset{\overset{\displaystyle F}{|}}{\underset{\underset{\displaystyle Cl}{|}}{C}}-\overset{\overset{\displaystyle F}{|}}{\underset{\underset{\displaystyle F}{|}}{C}}-H$$

2-Chloro-1,1,2-trifluoroethyl difluoromethyl ether [13838-16-9] $C_3H_2ClF_5O$ (184.49).

Preparation—May be synthesized by a series of reactions starting with trifluorochloroethylene. US Pats 3,469,011 and 3,527,813.

Description—Clear, colorless, volatile liquid; pleasant hydrocarbon-like odor; boils at 56.6°; nonflammable.

Solubility—Soluble in water to the extent of 0.275%, and water soluble in enflurane to the extent of 0.13%; miscible with organic solvents.

Uses—Enflurane (vp-180 torr, blood/gas-1.8, MAC-1.68%) is a pleasant-smelling, nonflammable halogenated ether *anesthetic* that provides rapid induction with little or no excitement. Pharyngeal and laryngeal reflexes are readily obtunded. Salivation and tracheo-bronchial secretions are mildly stimulated. It provides better analgesia and muscular relaxation than halothane, but high concentrations may cause cardiovascular depression and CNS stimulation, for which reason it is generally given with nitrous oxide. It does not appear to sensitize the heart to catecholamines. Enflurane is a respiratory depressant; spontaneous respiration may be adequate at light levels, but as the depth increases controlled ventilation may be nec-

essary. In common with other anesthetics of this chemical class, fluoride ions are liberated during its metabolism; the peak concentration is below that known to be associated with nephrotoxicity (>40 μM). Nevertheless, suspected nephrotoxicity has been reported. With deep anesthesia and hypocapnia, central nervous stimulation with increased electrical activity and seizure-like activity in the EEG have been reported. These effects can be terminated by reducing the anesthesia and the minute respiration or by substituting another anesthetic agent. This suggests that enflurane should not be used in patients with convulsive disorders. Recovery is rapid and uneventful; restlessness, delirium, nausea, and vomiting are seldom observed but shivering is quite common.

Dose—*Induction*, 2.0 to 4.5% in oxygen alone or with oxygen–nitrous oxide mixtures. Induction usually requires 7 to 10 minutes. Maintenance is usually accomplished with 0.5 to 3% concentrations.

Dosage Forms—Liquid: 125 and 250 mL.

Ether

Ethane, 1,1'-oxybis-, Diethyl Ether; Sulfuric Ether

$$C_2H_5OC_2H_5$$

Ethyl ether [60-29-7]; contains from 96.0–98.0% of $C_4H_{10}O$ (74.12), the remainder consisting of alcohol and water.

Caution—Ether is highly volatile and flammable. Its vapor, when mixed with air and ignited, may explode. Also, open or unopened containers stored for extended periods may develop peroxides which are explosive and shock sensitive.

History—Valerius Cordus in 1517 described ether or a very similar product under the name *Oleum Vitriolo Dulce*. Later it was called *Spiritus Vini Aethereius* and still later *Ether Sulphuricus*.

In 1842 Dr Crawford Long of Athens, GA, first used ether as a general anesthetic. In 1844 Dr Horace Wells, of Hartford, CT, used it independently for the same purpose. Drs C T Jackson and William Morton of Boston, MA, had also used it earlier. The first hospital operation under ether anesthesia was performed in Boston, in 1846, by Dr Warren.

Preparation—Ether may be made by reacting alcohol with sulfuric acid between the temperature of 130° and 137°, which is known as the etherifying temperature.

A large portion of the ether produced in the United States is made starting with ethylene. It is treated with sulfuric acid to form ethylsulfuric acid, which is decomposed by additional ethanol to ether, regenerating the sulfuric acid.

Description—Transparent, colorless, mobile liquid, having a characteristic odor, and a burning sweetish taste. It is highly volatile and flammable, and its vapor, when mixed with air and ignited, may explode violently. It is slowly oxidized by the action of air, moisture, and light, with the formation of peroxides. Specific gravity between 0.713 and 0.716 at 25°, corresponding to a $C_4H_{10}O$ content of 96 to 98%; the lower the specific gravity, the higher the absolute ether content; specific gravity of absolute ether 0.7097 at 25°. Boils at about 35°.

Solubility—Dissolves in about 12 times its volume of water at 25°C with slight contraction of volume; miscible with alcohol, benzene, chloroform, solvent hexane, and fixed and volatile oils.

Uses—Ether (vp-450 torr, blood/gas-12.1, MAC-1.92%) is a seldom used *anesthetic* with a pungent, irritating odor. It is flammable and explosive. Because of its high solubility in blood, induction is relatively slow and recovery is prolonged. It has a wide margin of safety, excellent analgesic properties, and produces profound skeletal muscle relaxation. The cardiovascular system is usually not adversely affected; it does not sensitize the heart to catecholamines, and ventricular arrhythmias are rare. Ether dilates the bronchi and stimulates bronchial secretion which may compromise airway patency. Excessive secretions can be controlled by premedication with an anticholinergic drug. Postoperative nausea and vomiting are common.

Caution—Ether to be used for anesthesia must be preserved in tight containers of not more than 3-kg capacity, and is not to be used for anesthesia if it has been removed from the original container longer than 24 hours.

Dose—By *inhalation* as required.

Ethyl Chloride

Ethane, chloro-, Chloroethane; Monochloroethane; Kelene

Chloroethane [75-00-3] C_2H_5Cl (64.51).

Caution—Ethyl Chloride is highly flammable. Do not use where it may be ignited.

Preparation—Ethyl chloride is generally prepared by distilling a mixture of alcohol, sodium chloride, and sulfuric acid.

Description—A gas at temperatures above 12°; below 12° or under sufficient pressure, it is a colorless, mobile, and very volatile liquid, boiling between 12° and 13° at ordinary pressure. Specific gravity about 0.921 at 0°. It has a characteristic ethereal odor and a burning taste. When it is liberated at ordinary room temperature from its sealed container it rapidly vaporizes and produces a lowering of the temperature. It burns with a smoky greenish flame and formation of hydrogen chloride.

Solubility—Slightly soluble in water; freely soluble in alcohol or ether.

Uses—Used as a *local anesthetic* by "freezing." It was formerly used topically as an alternate treatment of *creeping eruption* (*cutaneous larvae migrans*). Its great volatility requires special methods for dispensing; hermetically sealed tubes are used, so made that when the end is broken off, or the metallic orifice opened, and the tube held in the hand, the heat causes expansion and expels the liquid in a fine stream which is directed against the part to be anesthetized. When employed locally, ethyl chloride actually freezes the tissues, thawing is painful, healing is delayed, and tissues may be damaged.

Dose—*Topical*, as spray on intact skin.

Dosage Forms—Dispenseal bottle and Spray-Pak, 4 oz: metal tube, 100 g.

Fluroxene

Ethene, (2,2,2-trifluoroethoxy)-, Fluoromar (*Ohio Medical*)

$$CF_3CH_2-O-CH=CH_2$$

2,2,2-Trifluoroethyl vinyl ether [406-90-6] $C_4H_5F_3O$ (126.08). It contains a suitable stabilizer.

Caution—Fluroxene is highly volatile and flammable. Its vapor, when mixed with air and ignited, may explode.

Preparation—Under moderate pressure in the presence of a basic catalyst, 2,2,2,-trifluoroethanol undergoes addition to acetylene. US Pats. 2,830,007 and 2,870,218.

Description—Clear, colorless, volatile liquid having a mild ethereal odor. Boils at about 43°.

Solubility—1 mL in 222 mL water; miscible with alcohol, ether, acetone, and most halogenated solvents.

Uses—A fluorinated ether with a pungent odor used as a *general inhalation anesthetic*. It is flammable and explosive in concentrations above 4%. Muscular relaxation is difficult to obtain and concomitant use of relaxant drugs is usually necessary. When administered in combination with oxygen or nitrous oxide, induction is generally smooth and rapid; excessive salivation is not encountered. Recovery is rapid and postoperative nausea and vomiting may occur, but excitement or delirium is rare. Fluroxene is a good analgesic. It does not sensitize the myocardium to catecholamines, as often occurs with the halogenated hydrocarbons. It has been reported to cause hepatic and renal damage.

Dose—By *inhalation* as required.

Other Dose Information—For *induction*, 6 to 12% vaporized by a flow of oxygen or a nitrous oxide-oxygen mixture. For *surgical anesthesia*, concentrations of 3 to 8% are required.

Dosage Form—Liquid: 125 mL.

Halothane

Ethane, 2-bromo-2-chloro-1,1,1-trifluoro-, Fluothane (*Ayerst*)

$$\begin{array}{c} Br \quad F \\ | \quad | \\ H-C-C-F \\ | \quad | \\ Cl \quad F \end{array}$$

2-Bromo-2-chloro-1,1,1-trifluoroethane [151-67-7] $C_2HBrClF_3$ (197.38); contains 0.008–0.012% of thymol, by weight, as a stabilizer.

Preparation—Commercially available 2-chloro-1,1,1-trifluoroethane is subjected to direct bromination and halothane is isolated from the reaction product by fractional distillation.

Description—Colorless, mobile, nonflammable, heavy liquid, having a characteristic odor resembling that of chloroform. Its taste is sweet and produces a burning sensation; distils between 49° and 51°; specific gravity between 1.872 and 1.877 at 20°.

Solubility—Slightly soluble in water; miscible with alcohol, chloroform, ether, and fixed oils.

Uses—Halothane (vp-243 torr, blood/gas-2.3, MAC-0.77%) is a potent, relatively safe, frequently employed *general inhalation anesthetic*. Induction with halothane is smooth and relatively rapid with little or no excitement. It is not a potent analgesic. Therefore, it is frequently used in conjunction with nitrous oxide. Halothane alone does not produce good skeletal muscle relaxation. When muscle relaxation is required it must be used with succinylcholine, tubocurarine, or gallamine. Anesthesia is usually accompanied by hypotension; the degree of hypotension appears to be a function of the depth of anesthesia. Halothane sensitizes the myocardium to the action of epinephrine and norepinephrine; injection of these amines during halothane anesthesia may induce ventricular tachycardia or fibrillation. Although some hepatic damage has been reported after a single administration, more severe damage has been shown to occur after repeated use. Halothane should not be used in patients in whom previous exposure was accompanied by fever and/or jaundice. It is seldom used alone. It should be used with caution as an obstetrical anesthetic since it is not a potent analgesic and high concentrations relax the uterus and result in considerable uterine hemorrhage.

Dose—By *inhalation* as required.

Other Dose Information—For *induction*, 1 to 4% vaporized by a flow of oxygen or nitrous oxide-oxygen mixture. For *maintenance*, 0.5 to 1.5%.

Dosage Forms—Liquid: 125 and 250 mL.

Isoflurane

Ethane, 2-chloro-2-(difluoromethoxy)-1,1,1-trifluor-, Forane (*Ohio Medical*)

$$\begin{array}{c} F \\ | \\ HC-O-CHCF_3 \\ | \quad \quad | \\ F \quad \quad Cl \end{array}$$

1-Chloro-2,2,2-trifluoroethyl difluoromethyl ether [26675-46-7] $C_3H_2ClF_5O$ (184.49).

Preparation—Trifluoroethanol is methylated with dimethyl sulfate to form the methyl ether which is then chlorinated to the dichloromethyl ether, $CF_3CHClOCHCl_2$. This latter compound, on treatment with $HF/SbCl_5$ forms the product. See *J Med Chem 14*: 517 (1971).

Description—A low boiling liquid (48.5°) with a slight odor; nonflammable.

Solubility—Miscible with most organic solvents including fats and oils. Practically insoluble in water.

Uses—Isoflurane (vp-250 torr, blood/gas-1.38, MAC-1.3%), an isomer of enflurane, is a new nonflammable *inhalation anesthetic* for induction and maintenance of general anesthesia. Induction of and recovery from isoflurane anesthesia are rapid. However, its mild pungency limits the rate of induction; too rapid an increase in the inspired concentration can lead to breathholding, coughing, or laryngospasm. The levels of anesthesia can be rapidly and precisely altered to meet changing needs; respiration must be monitored closely and supported when necessary. Since isoflurane dilates constricted bronchial muscle, it is acceptable for use *in asthmatic patients*. Low doses of isoflurane decrease cardiac output to a lesser extent than enflurane and halothane. Both isoflurane and enflurane sensitize the heart to the arrhythmogenic effects of epinephrine, but are much less likely to do so than halothane. Isoflurane, if given in sufficiently high concentration, can induce sufficient muscle relaxation for any operation. Isoflurane is said to offer advantages over all previously available inhalation anesthetics, especially in its lack of any important toxicity (*Anesth Anal*, 60: 666, 1981). Less than 0.2% of administered isoflurane can be recovered as metabolites; this compares favorably with 2.4% for enflurane, 15 to 20% for halothane, and 50% for methoxyflurane. Because of this low rate of metabolism, isoflurane has little or no renal or hepatic toxicity. Isoflurane, like halothane and enflurane, can trigger malignant hyperthermia in susceptible patients.

Dose—*Induction:* Inspired concentrations of 1.5 to 3.0% usually produce surgical anesthesia in 7 to 10 minutes. *Maintenance:* Surgical levels of anesthesia can be sustained with 1.0 to 2.5% concentrations when nitrous oxide is used concomitantly.

Dosage Forms—Liquid: 100 mL.

Methoxyflurane

Ethane, 2,2-dichloro-1,1-difluoro-1-methoxy-, Penthrane (*Abbott*)

$$CHCl_2CF_2{-}O{-}CH_3$$

2,2-Dichloro-1,1-difluoroethyl methyl ether [76-38-0] $C_3H_4Cl_2F_2O$ (164.97). It may contain a suitable stabilizer.

Preparation—1,1-Dichloro-2,2-difluoroethane is reacted with methanol in the presence of strong alkali or a basic ion-exchange resin to produce a mixture consisting largely of methoxyflurane with small amounts of 2,2-dichloro-1-fluorovinyl methyl ether. US Pat. 3,264,356.

Description—Clear, mobile liquid having a characteristic fruity odor; boils at about 105°; specific gravity between 1.420 and 1.425.

Solubility—Very slightly soluble in water (at 37°); miscible with olive oil (in all proportions), chloroform, 95% ethyl alcohol, acetone, and benzene.

Uses—Methoxyflurane (vp-22.5 torr, blood/gas-13.0, MAC-0.16%) is the most potent of the liquid volatile anesthetic agents. A concentration of only 0.1–2.0% in the inspired mixture will maintain surgical anesthesia. Induction of anesthesia is relatively slow and recovery is prolonged. Relatively light anesthesia produces excellent muscle relaxation and analgesia. Because it depresses respiration, methoxyflurane is used mainly in short procedures, such as obstetrics, which require effective analgesia and muscle relaxation. Thus, it is valued mainly for its *analgesic potency* during the first stage of labor. Postoperative nausea and vomiting are infrequent. The anesthetic agent is contraindicated in patients with liver disease. It may cause renal failure or damage due to the release of the fluoride ions. Hence, it should not be used in patients receiving potentially nephrotoxic agents (eg, gentamicin, tetracyclines, etc), since concurrent use with these agents may induce irreversible renal failure.

Dose—By *inhalation* as required.

Other Dose Information—For *analgesia*, 0.5% in air. For *induction*, 1.5 to 3.0% vaporized by a 1:1 mixture of nitrous oxide and oxygen. For *maintenance*, 0.5% with appropriate supplementary drugs. Administered by the closed or semiclosed technique in a concentration of 1.5 to 3%.

Dosage Forms—Liquid: 15 and 125 mL.

Trichloroethylene

Ethene, trichloro-, Trilene (*Ayerst*); Trimar (*Ohio Medical*)

Trichloroethene [79-01-6] C_2HCl_3 (131.39). It contains 0.008–0.012%, by weight, of thymol. A dye certified for use in drugs by the FDA may be added to impart a blue color to trichloroethylene.

Preparation—Trichloroethylene may be prepared by abstraction of the elements of HCl from *sym*-tetrachloroethane by means of lime.

Description—Clear, colorless, or blue, mobile liquid with a characteristic, chloroform-like odor. It is not flammable, but is slowly decomposed by moisture, light accelerating the decomposition and is often stabilized with thymol. Specific gravity between 1.458 and 1.463 indicating a content of not less than 99.5% and not more than 100.0% of C_2HCl_3. Boils between 86° and 88°; solidifies at −83°.

Solubility—Practically insoluble in water; miscible with alcohol, chloroform, ether, and many other organic liquids; dissolves most fixed and volatile oils.

Uses—Has been sporadically employed as a *general inhalation anesthetic*. It is not a satisfactory anesthetic alone because of its slow induction and recovery rates. Moreover, it does not produce adequate muscle relaxation; hence, it is usually used to supplement nitrous oxide anesthesia. It appears to stimulate the pulmonary stretch receptors; this results in rapid, shallow, breathing. Moreover, it is slow in onset of analgesia and potentially cardiotoxic and hepatotoxic. It should not be used in a closed system with soda lime, because the heat generated by the combination of carbon dioxide with soda lime tends to decompose it to phosgene and hydrochloric acid. In the presence of alkali, it is broken down to dichloroacetylene, a compound that is both flammable and neurotoxic.

Dose—By *inhalation* as required.

Other Dose Information—Trigeminal neuralgia, a frangible glass ampul containing 1 mL is broken and the contents inhaled. A second inhalation may be necessary after a few minutes, if relief is not obtained, and further administrations are repeated 3 or 4 times daily for several weeks.

Dosage Form—Liquid: 300 mL.

Gaseous Inhalation Anesthetics

The gaseous anesthetic agents are in the vapor state at ordinary room temperature and, in general, have boiling points at less than 20°C. Consequently, they are confined under high pressure in cylinders and administered by the closed method with an anesthetic machine. These agents vary greatly in anesthetic potency, and their successful use often depends upon the proper premedication of the patient. For example, even under the most favorable circumstances, nitrous oxide–oxygen and ethylene–oxygen mixtures will carry patients only 15 and 25%, respectively, through the surgical stage of anesthesia. Thus, nitrous oxide and ethylene are referred to as 15 and 25% anesthetic agents, respectively. In marked contrast, cyclopropane, irrespective of previous preparation of the patient, will carry anesthesia through to medullary paralysis; hence, it is a 100% anesthetic agent. However, except for nitrous oxide, all of these gaseous anesthetics are flammable and/or explosive at concentrations necessary for anesthesia, particularly when given in oxygen-enriched mixtures. Although nitrous oxide is not flammable or explosive *per se*, it supports combustion as actively as does oxygen when it is present in proper concentrations with a flammable anesthetic. For this reason, these anesthetic agents are now essentially obsolete.

Cyclopropane

Trimethylene

Cyclopropane [75-19-4] C_3H_6 (42.08).

Caution—Cyclopropane is highly flammable. Do not use where it may be ignited. Use same precautions as those given under *Ethylene.*

Preparation—Among other methods, cyclopropane may be prepared by several patented processes which involve treating 1,3-dichloropropane with zinc in the presence of sodium iodide.

Description—Colorless gas resembling solvent hexane in odor; has a pungent taste. 1 L at 760 mm and 0° weighs about 1.88 g.

Solubility—1 volume dissolves in about 2.7 volumes of water at 15°; freely soluble in alcohol; soluble in fixed oils.

Uses—Cyclopropane (blood/gas-0.46, MAC-9.2%) is an anesthetic gas with a rapid onset of action. It may be used for either analgesia, induction, or maintenance of anesthesia. It produces skeletal muscle relaxation in full anesthetic doses. Cyclopropane must be administered in a closed system with oxygen by an experienced anesthetist. Disadvantages include difficulty in detection of the planes of anesthesia, occasional laryngospasm, and cardiac arrhythmias. Postanesthetic nausea, vomiting, and headache are frequent. Since it potentiates the effects of nondepolarizing neuromuscular blocking agents, these drugs should be used in reduced dosage with cyclopropane. *Cyclopropane/oxygen mixtures are explosive.* In view of these disadvantages, cyclopropane is rarely used.

Dose—By *inhalation* as required.

Nitrous Oxide

Dinitrogen Monoxide; Laughing Gas

Nitrogen oxide (N_2O) [10024-97-2]; contains not less than 99.0%, by volume, of N_2O (44.01). The remainder is chiefly nitrogen.

Preparation—Usually by heating ammonium nitrate to about 170° to produce nitrous oxide and water.

Nitrous oxide is furnished in compressed form in metallic cylinders.

Description—Colorless gas, without appreciable odor or taste. Specific gravity 1.53. 1 L, at a pressure of 760 mm at 0°, weighs about 1.97 g.

Solubility—1 volume dissolves in about 1.4 volumes of water at 20° under normal pressure; freely soluble in alcohol; soluble in ether and oils.

Uses—Nitrous oxide (blood/gas-0.47, MAC-101%) is the weakest but probably the safest inhalation *general anesthetic*. Therefore, its potency is increased by the use of halothane, methoxyflurane, enflurane, isoflurane, ether, or thiopental, and its muscle relaxant properties are enhanced by the concomitant use of a neuromuscular blocking drug. Thus, an anesthetic regimen is built around nitrous oxide, since it cannot by itself provide sufficient hypnosis and muscle relaxation. During its administration some patients become hysterical and because of this characteristic it is often called *laughing gas*. It causes only the lighter grades of anesthesia unless the patient has had considerable preanesthetic medication (morphine, scopolamine, barbiturate, etc) or unless supplemental anesthesia is used. Inasmuch as high concentrations of nitrous oxide are required, little room is left in the mixture for oxygen. This may result in serious anoxia and tissue damage, especially to the central nervous system. For this reason, considerable experience is required for the proper use of nitrous oxide as an anesthetic, and care must be exercised in the proper selection of patients. Due to the pleasant, rapid induction, nitrous oxide is often employed to initiate anesthesia, prior to the use of other anesthetic agents. It is also frequently used with halothane, methoxyflurane, enflurane, and isoflurane to assist in the maintenance of anesthesia. Nitrous oxide is also commonly used in dental surgery because of the rapid recovery which it allows. It is also employed in obstetrics to produce analgesia. One-time exposure of pregnant rats to nitrous oxide has demonstrated this anesthetic agent to be teratogenic. The FDA advises health professionals who are or may become pregnant that chronic occupational exposure to nitrous oxide may pose a risk to the fetus.

Dose—By *inhalation*, 60 to 80%, with oxygen 20 to 40%, as required.

Other Gaseous Inhalation Anesthetics

Ethylene [Ethene [74-85-1] CH_2=CH_2 (28.05); Olefiant Gas]—Prepared by catalytic dehydration of alcohol, or by cracking of petroleum, among 502 methods for making ethylene. A colorless, highly flammable gas, somewhat lighter than air; one volume dissolves in about 9 volumes of water at 25°, about 0.5 volume of alcohol at 25°, and about 0.05 volume of ether at 15.5°. *Uses:* A general inhalation anesthetic with rapid onset and recovery. It may be used for minor surgery and for analgesia in obstetrics. It is considerably weaker than cyclopropane but stronger than nitrous oxide. Unless sufficient preanesthetic medication is employed, ethylene will not produce adequate relaxation for the more painful surgical procedures. Inasmuch as high concentrations must be used (85 to 90%) the volume available for adequate amounts of oxygen is dangerously reduced. Disadvantages include unpleasant odor, inadequate muscle relaxation, hypoxia, and gas-oxygen mixtures are explosive. For these reasons it is now seldom used as a general anesthetic. *Dose:* By *inhalation* as required.

Intravenous Anesthetics

Intravenous anesthetics are receiving more attention than inhalation anesthetics for two reasons. Firstly, the development of new intravenous anesthetics appears to be more favorable both chemically and economically than does the development of inhalation anesthetics. Secondly, trace amounts of inhalation anesthetics polluting the operating-room environment have been implicated in a variety of ailments which affect operating room personnel. It is quite likely that this trend in developing new intravenous anesthetics will continue since present drugs have their shortcomings and the ideal intravenous anesthetic has yet to be developed.

Intravenous anesthetics differ from inhalation anesthetics in that, once injected, there is practically nothing that can be done to facilitate their removal or alter the course of effects. The time course of effects from induction and rapidly deepening anesthesia to gradual emergence depends almost entirely on progressive redistribution of these drugs within the body. Understanding the pharmacokinetics of the intravenous anesthetics is important to their sound, safe, and practical use. Pharmacokinetics allows predictions about drug concentrations in the body as related to dosage, time, and physiological and pathological alteration in biological functions. It may also provide preliminary indications of the likelihood and types of drug interactions that may be encountered. For these reasons appropriate kinetic data are included herein.

The rapidly acting barbiturates are most commonly injected intravenously to induce or sustain surgical anesthesia. Since they are poor analgesics, they are seldom used alone, but are usually supplemented with an inhalational anesthetic. Intravenous anesthetics are best suited for the induction of anesthesia and for short procedures, such as orthopedic manipulations and operations, genitourinary procedures, obstetric repair, and dilatation and curettage. A slow infusion of a dilute solution of an ultrashort-acting barbiturate can be employed to induce a sleep-like state in which the patient is amenable to psychotherapy and verbal suggestion.

The general principles which apply to the use of intravenous anesthetics are the same as those that govern the use of other general anesthetic agents.

Adverse reactions commonly encountered may include the following: *Induction complications:* Excitatory phenomena, that is tremors and involuntary muscle movements mostly involving the limbs; respiratory upset, that is cough, hiccup or laryngospasm; respiratory depression; cardiovascular changes. *Tissue irritation and damage* (drug and solvent): Pain on injection and venous complications. Effects of accidental arterial injection. *Recovery reactions:* Psychic phenomena—dreaming, hallucinations, dissociative phenomena, delirium, anxiety and agitation, emotional reactions, long-term effects of frequent repeated administrations; motor phenomena, for example, increased tone, tremors and convulsions; effects on pain; nausea and vomiting. *Hypersensitivity or idiosyncratic reactions:* True allergy–immune-based anaphylaxis; idiosyncratic–anaphylactoid. The most frequently encountered adverse reactions will be described in each monograph.

Droperidol—page 1087.

Etomidate

1*H*-Imidazole-5-carboxylic acid, 1-(1-phenylethyl)-, ethyl ester, (+)-, Amidate (*Abbott*)

(+)-Ethyl 1-(α-methylbenzyl)imidazole-5-carboxylate [33125-97-2] $C_{14}H_{16}N_2O_2$ (244.99).

Preparation—From α-methylbenzyl amine and ethyl chloroacetate in 8 steps.

Description—White or yellow crystals or amorphous; melting about 67°.

Uses—Etomidate is injected intravenously for *induction* of general anesthesia. It is also indicated for *supplementation* of less potent anesthetic agents, such as nitrous oxide in oxygen, during mainte-nance of anesthesia for short operative procedures (dilation and curettage or cervical conization). Intravenous etomidate produces a rapid induction of anesthesia with minimal cardiovascular and respiratory changes. It is a weak base (pK_a 4.24) with moderate lipophilic properties. Approximately 75% is bound to plasma protein. Pharmacokinetic studies in man (0.3 mg/kg) indicate that plasma concentrations fit a three-compartment model: distribution half-time, 2.81 min; intermediate $t_{1/2}$, 32.1 min; elimination $t_{1/2}$, 3.9 hr; total Vd, 4.6 L/kg; and total clearance, 954 mL/min. Adverse reactions include transient venous pain on injection and transient skeletal muscle movements, including myoclonus. Available data are not sufficient to justify its use in pregnancy, obstetrics, nursing mothers, or children under 10 years of age.

Dose—Intravenous: 0.2 to 0.6 mg/kg; *Usual:* 0.3 mg/kg intravenously over a period of 30 to 60 secs.

Dosage Form—Ampuls: 10 amd 20 mL, containing 2 mg/mL; Abbojet syringes, 20 mL.

Fentanyl Citrate—page 1108.

Fentanyl Citrate and Droperidol Injection

Innovar Injection (*Janssen*)

Uses—A fixed-dose combination of the narcotic analgesic fentanyl citrate (0.05 mg/mL), and the neuroleptic (tranquilizer) droperidol (2.5 mg/mL). The combined effect, sometimes referred to as *neuroleptanalgesia*, is characterized by general quiescence, reduced motor activity, and profound analgesia. Complete loss of consciousness usually does not occur. The combination is used to produce *tranquilization* and *analgesia* for *surgical* and *diagnostic procedures*. It may also be used as *anesthetic premedication*, for *induction of anesthesia*, and as an *adjunct* in the *maintenance of general* and *regional anesthesia*.

Fentanyl, a synthetic opiod analgesic, has a profile of action similar to morphine, except that it produces the same degree of analgesia with 1/50 the dose and is virtually devoid of emetic properties. The duration of analgesic action is about 30 minutes; after that time, patients given Innovar are without analgesia. Droperidol is a *neuroleptic* which produces general quiescence and decreased responsiveness to environmental stimuli. Its duration of action is 3 to 6 hours.

Since droperidol is a long-lasting drug with a relatively slow onset (10 to 15 min) and fentanyl citrate has a relatively rapid onset (1 to 2 min) with a short duration of action, the combination *should not* be used for maintenance therapy; fentanyl citrate alone should be used. Droperidol is 85 to 90% bound to plasma proteins and has a half-life of 2.2 hr. The half-life of fentanyl is said to be 1 to 4 hr, depending on the dose.

Common adverse reactions include respiratory depression, apnea, muscle rigidity and hypotension; if these remain untreated, respiratory arrest, circulatory depression, or cardiac arrest could occur. Extrapyramidal symptoms (dystonia, akathisia, and oculogyric crisis) have been observed. Restlessness, hyperactivity and anxiety may occur. Elevated blood pressure has also been reported. Other adverse reactions reported are dizziness, chills and/or shivering, twitching, blurred vision, laryngospasm, bronchospasm, bradycardia, tachycardia, nausea and emesis, diaphoresis, emergence delirium, and postoperative drowsiness and/or hallucinatory episodes.

Fentanyl citrate and droperidol injection is contraindicated in children under 2 years of age and in patients with bronchial asthma or myasthenia gravis. It should not be used in patients taking MAO inhibitors. The narcotic analgesic component, fentanyl citrate, can produce drug dependence of the morphine type and therefore has the potential for abuse. This fixed ratio combination can cause distressing and potentially lethal adverse effects (*Medical Letter, 22*, 74, 1981).

Dose—*Premedication, intramuscular,* 0.5 to 2 mL 45 to 60 min preoperatively; *induction, intravenous,* 1 mL/9 to 12 kg; *maintenance, intravenous,* combination not indicated; fentanyl alone in increments of 0.025 or 0.05 mg as indicated.

Dosage Forms—Injection (fentanyl as citrate 0.05 mg, droperidol 2.5 mg/mL): 2 and 5 mL.

Hexobarbital—page 1069.

Ketamine Hydrochloride

Cyclohexanone, 2-(2-chlorophenyl)-2-(methylamino)-, hydrochloride; Ketaject (*Bristol*); Ketalar (*Parke-Davis*)

(±)-2-(*o*-Chlorophenyl)-2-(methylamino)cyclohexanone hydrochloride [1867-66-9] Base [6740-88-1] $C_{13}H_{16}ClNO \cdot HCl$ (274.19).

Preparation—The product resulting from a Grignard reaction involving *o*-chlorobenzonitrile and bromocyclopentane is treated in the presence of strong alkali to form the epoxy compound (I). Reaction of this with methylamine yields the imine (II) which rearranges on heating in the presence of HCl. Belgian Pat 634,208

I   II

Description—White, crystalline powder with a characteristic odor. Its solutions are acid to litmus. Melts with decomposition between 258° and 261°. pH (1 in 10 solution) between 3.5 and 4.1.

Solubility—1 g dissolves in 5 mL water, 14 mL alcohol, 60 mL chloroform, and 60 mL absolute alcohol.

Uses—A rapidly acting nonbarbiturate *general anesthetic* that produces anesthesia characterized by profound analgesia, normal to hyperactive pharyngeal-laryngeal reflexes, normal or slightly enhanced skeletal muscle tone, cardiovascular stimulation, and an increase in cerebrospinal fluid pressure. Ketamine is the only intravenous anesthetic that routinely produces cardiovascular stimulation. Heart rate, arterial blood presure, and cardiac output are usually increased 2 to 4 min after intravenous injection and then slowly decline over the next 10 to 20 min. These pharmacologic effects result from excitation of the central sympathetic nervous system; increases in plasma epinephrine and norepinephrine levels are observed as early as 2 min after intravenous injection and return to control levels 15 min later. The clinical anesthetic state induced by ketamine is termed "dissociative anesthesia" since the patient may appear awake but is dissociated from the environment and does not respond to pain. Ketamine is used most frequently in children, particularly as an induction agent and as a noninhalation anesthetic for diagnostic and surgical procedures of short duration.

If skeletal muscle relaxation is necessary, a muscle relaxant must be used. It is also indicated for induction anesthesia prior to the administration of other anesthetic agents and for the supplementation of low-potency anesthetic agents such as nitrous oxide. Ketamine hydrochloride should be used by or under the direction of a physician familiar with the warnings and precautions to be observed when using this agent and experienced in administering general anesthetics, in the maintenance of a patent airway, and in the control of respiration.

After intravenous administration, the ketamine concentration has an initial slope (alpha phase) of 45 minutes with a half-life of 45 minutes. This phase corresponds clinically to the anesthetic effect of the drug. The anesthetic action is terminated by redistribution from the central nervous system and by hepatic biotransformation. The later half-life of ketamine (beta phase) is 2.5 hours. Intravenous doses (2 mg/kg) produce surgical anesthesia within 30 seconds and lasts about 10 minutes; intramuscular doses (9–13 mg/kg) produce surgical anesthesia in 3 to 4 minutes and lasts from 12 to 25 minutes.

It is contraindicated in patients with a significant elevation of blood pressure and those known to be hypersensitive to the drug. Prolonged recovery time may result if barbiturates and/or narcotics are used concurrently with the drug.

Adverse reactions include elevated blood pressure and pulse rate and occasionally hypotension, bradycardia, and arrhythmia; increased respiration or, if the drug is given too rapidly, severe respiratory depression, apnea, and laryngospasms; diplopia, nystagmus, and slight elevation in intraocular pressure; enhanced skeletal muscle tone manifest by tonic and clonic movements; anorexia, nausea, and vomiting; local pain at injection site, and transient erythema and/or morbilliform rash.

Special Note: Emergence reactions have occurred in approximately 12% of patients. The psychological manifestations vary in severity between pleasant dream-like states, vivid imagery, hallucinations, and emergence delirium. In some cases these states have been accompanied by confusion, excitement, and irrational behavior which a few patients recall as an unpleasant experience. The duration ordinarily lasts no more than a few hours; in a few cases, however, recurrences have taken place up to 24 hours postoperatively. No residual psychological effects are known to have resulted from use of ketamine. The incidence of these emergence phenomena is least in the young (15 years of age or less) and elderly (over 65 years of age) patient; also, they are less frequent when the drug is given intramuscularly. These reactions may be reduced if verbal, tactile, and visual stimulation of the patient is minimized during the recovery period. This does not preclude the monitoring of vital signs. In addition, the use of a small hypnotic dose of a short-acting or ultrashort-acting barbiturate or other agent such as diazepam may be required to terminate a severe emergence reaction. Certain drugs, such as droperidol or diazepam intramuscularly, have also been used in an attempt to reduce the incidence of emergence reactions. The incidence of emergence reactions is reduced as experience with the drug is gained. When ketamine is used on an outpatient basis, the patient should not be released until recovery from anesthesia is complete and then should be accompanied by a responsible adult.

Some reports indicate that ketamine hydrochloride may interact with thyroid medication to produce severe hypertension and tachycardia. It also potentiates the neuromuscular blocking effects of tubocurarine but not of succinylcholine. Large doses (over 2 mg/kg body wt) are likely to cause fetal depression. Although lower doses appear safe, it is not the preferred drug for obstetrical anesthesia.

Dose—*Induction, intravenous*, 1 to **4.5 mg/kg**. It usually requires 2 mg/kg to produce 5–10 min of anesthesia (*Note:* induction is so rapid in onset the drug should be administered only when the patient is in a supported position). *Intramuscular*, **6.5 to 13 mg/kg**. A dose of 10 mg/kg usually produces 12–25 min of surgical anesthesia. *Maintenance*, ½ of the full induction dose repeated as necessary for maintenance of desired level of anesthesia.

Dosage Forms—Injection: 10 mg/mL in 20- and 50-mL vials; 50 mg/mL in 10-mL vials; 100 mg/mL in 5-mL vials.

Magnesium Sulfate Injection—page 1078.

Methohexital Sodium

2,4,6(1*H*,3*H*,5*H*)-Pyrimidinetrione, 1-methyl-5-(1-methyl-2-pentynyl)-
5-(2-propenyl)-(±)-, monosodium salt; Brevital Sodium (*Lilly*)

Sodium 5-allyl-1-methyl-5-(1-methyl-2-pentynyl)barbiturate [309-36-4] $C_{14}H_{17}N_2NaO_3$ (284.29).

Preparation—1-Butynyl magnesium bromide is treated with acetaldehyde and the resulting alcohol is treated with PCl_5 to produce 2-chloro-3-pentyne. Condensation with ethyl cyanoacetate in the presence of sodium ethylate yields ethyl 1-methyl-2-pentynylcyanoacetate which, on similar further condensation with allyl bromide yields ethyl (1-methyl-2-pentynyl)allylcyanoacetate. Reaction with *N*-methylurea yields the iminobarbituric acid which on acid-catalyzed hydrolysis forms methohexital. Neutralization with NaOH produces the sodium salt.

The two diastereoisomers of the barbituric acid have been designated as α- and β-forms in the literature. The α-form is the one used medicinally (the β-form causes undesirable side effects) and is formed almost exclusively by the above process. The malonic ester synthesis described under *Barbital* is not used because it yields mainly the unwanted β-form.

Description—White to off-white hygroscopic powder; essentially odorless. Its solutions are alkaline to litmus.

Solubility—Soluble in water.

Uses—A rapidly acting intravenous barbiturate indicated for induction of anesthesia, supplementing other anesthetic agents, short surgical procedures and for inducing a hypnotic state. Although methohexital is less ionized than is thiopental (24% vs 39% at pH 7.4) its plasma protein binding is essentially the same (72 to 86%). It is thought the pattern of distribution of the two drugs immediately after injection and recovery following a single dose is due to the same mechanism, namely, redistribution of the drug from the brain into the muscle mass. Induction of anesthesia is about as rapid as with thiopental sodium, but recovery is more rapid. This is reflected in the short elimination half-life (70 to 125 min); this is a result of a high plasma clearance rate (657 to 999 mL plasma/min). However, complete psychomotor recovery seems to take the same length of time after the use of thiopental and methohexital in equianesthetic doses. Methohexital is particularly useful for brief procedures, such as *reduction of fractures, gynecologic examination, electroconvulsive therapy, genitourinary procedures*, and *oral surgery*. Adverse reactions include circulatory depression, thrombophlebitis, pain at injection site, respiratory depression, laryngospasm, bronchospasm, salivation, hiccups, muscle twitching, delerium, headache, nausea, and emesis. Acute allergic reactions, such as erythema, pruritus urticaria, rhinitis, dyspnea, hypotension, anxiety, abdominal pain, and peripheral vascular collapse, have also been reported. The drug is contraindicated when general anesthesia is not advisable, in patients with latent or manifest porphyria or in patients with a known hypersensitivity to barbiturates. Caution should be observed in debilitated patients or those with impaired respiratory, circulatory, renal, hepatic, or endocrine function. This drug should be administered only by persons trained in the use of intravenous anesthetics. Appropriate resuscitative equipment for prevention and treatment of anesthetic emergencies should be available. Solutions of methohexital sodium are incompatible with silicone and should not be allowed to come in contact with rubber stoppers or parts of disposable syringes that have come in contact with silicone.

Dose—*Usual, intravenous, induction*, 5 to **12 mL** of 1% solution, at the rate of **1 mL** every 5 sec; *maintenance*, **2 to 4 mL** every 4 to 7 min as required.

Dosage Forms—for Injection (with sodium carbonate buffer): 500 mg, 2.5 g, and 5 g of methohexital sodium with 30, 150, and 300 mg of sodium carbonate, respectively.

Paraldehyde—page 1073.

Pentobarbital Sodium—page 1068.

Secobarbital Sodium—page 1068.

Thiamylal Sodium for Injection

4,6-(1*H*,5*H*)-Pyrimidinedione, dihydro-5-(1-methylbutyl)-5-(2-propenyl)-2-thioxo-, monosodium salt; Surital Sodium (*Parke-Davis*)

Sodium 5-allyl-5-(1-methylbutyl)-2-thiobarbiturate [337-47-3] $C_{12}H_{17}N_2NaO_2S$ (276.33), with anhydrous sodium carbonate as a buffer.

Preparation—The thiobarbituric acid, thiamylal, may be prepared by the general process described under *Barbital*, page 1066, except using allyl bromide and 1-methylbutyl bromide as the alkylating agents instead of ethyl bromide, and condensing the resulting allyl 1-methylbutyl malonic ester with thiourea instead of urea. The free acid is neutralized with NaOH to form the sodium salt.

Description—Pale yellow, hygroscopic powder, having a disagreeable odor.

Uses—A rapidly-acting barbiturate indicated for *induction of anesthesia*, for *supplementing other anesthetic agents*, and for *intravenous anesthesia* for short surgical procedures, or as an agent for inducing a *hypnotic state*. Its anesthetic potency, profile of action and untoward effects are similar to those of thiopental.

Dose—*Usual, intravenous, induction*, 3 to **6 mL** of 2.5% solution at the rate of **1 mL** every 5 sec; *maintenance*, **0.5 to 1 mL** of 0.3% by continuous drip as required. The maximal total dose should not exceed 1 g or 40 mL of a 2.5% solution.

Dosage Forms—Injection: 1, 5, 10 g vials.

Thiopental Sodium

4,6-(1*H*,5*H*)-Pyrimidinedione, 5-ethyldihydro-5-(1-methylbutyl)-2-thioxo-, monosodium salt; Thiopentone Sodium; Pentothal Sodium (*Abbott*)

Sodium 5-ethyl-5-(1-methylbutyl)-2-thiobarbiturate [71-73-8] $C_{11}H_{17}N_2NaO_2S$ (264.32).

Preparation—In the same manner as *Thiamylal* (above), using 2-bromopentane as the alkyl halide and the ethyl 1-methylbutylmalonate is condensed with thiourea [$CS(NH_2)_2$].

Description—White to off-white, crystalline powder or a yellowish white to pale greenish yellow hygroscopic powder. It may have a disagreeable odor. Its aqueous solution is alkaline to litmus. Its solutions decompose on standing, and on boiling precipitation occurs. Carbon dioxide also causes precipitation in the solution.

Solubility—Soluble in water and alcohol; insoluble in absolute ether, benzene, and solvent hexane.

Incompatibilities—Thiopental precipitates in acid solutions.

Uses—The most commonly employed rapidly acting depressant of the central nervous system which induces *hypnosis* and *anesthesia*, but not analgesia. It produces anesthesia within 30 to 40 seconds after intravenous injection. Recovery after small doses is rapid with some somnolence and retrograde amnesia. Large or repeated doses of the drug result in prolonged anesthesia. It is indicated as the sole *anesthetic agent* for brief (15-min) procedures, for *induction* of *anesthesia* prior to administration of other anesthetic agents, to *supplement* regional or *low-potency anesthetic agents*, for the *control of convulsive states*, and for *narcoanalysis* and *narcosynthesis* in psychiatric disorders.

Thiopental is the barbiturate most highly bound to plasma protein. Approximately 72 to 86% of the plasma concentration is in bound form. Aspirin, phenylbutazone, and naproxen have been shown, in rats, to displace the anesthetic agent from plasma binding sites and cause reappearance of sleep. At a pH of 7.4, 61% of the drug is in nonionized form; since thiopental has a pK_a of 7.6 acidosis will favor penetration of the drug through the blood-brain barrier and alkalosis will have the opposite effect.

Thiopental confers a two- or three-compartment open-model system on the body, with an average half-life of 6.2 hours. A single intravenous injection of 3.5 to 4.0 mg/kg produces loss of consciousness within 10 seconds and a state of anesthesia followed by sleep which lasts about 3 to 5 minutes. The brain, because of its rich blood supply, will initially receive the major portion of the drug following injection. The blood level falls rapidly as a result of distribution of thiopental into muscle mass; in order to compensate, the drug is transferred rapidly out of the brain to maintain plasma equilibrium. This accounts for its short duration of action. Fat is the only compartment whose thiopental content continues to rise after 30 minutes postinjection. If repeated or large doses are administered the ultrashort action is lost, and awakening is prolonged. The drug effects are then terminated by sequestration in fat depots and by metabolism. Fat assumes the major role 0.5 and 2 hours following injection. Plasma concentrations will fall at a slow rate of 15% per hour due to metabolic degradation.

Untoward reactions include respiratory depression, myocardial depression, cardiac arrhythmias, prolonged somnolence and recovery, sneezing, coughing, bronchospasm, laryngospasm, and shivering. It must be administered by an anesthetist thoroughly trained in its use and well acquainted with its contraindications and dangers. Facilities for intratracheal oxygen administration should always be at hand when injecting thiopental sodium intravenously. It is contraindicated in patients with a complete absence of suitable veins or a history of barbiturate hypersensitivity, status asthmaticus, or porphyria.

Dose—*Usual, intravenous, induction*, 2 to 3 mL of a 2.5% solution at intervals of 30 to 60 sec; *maintenance*, 0.5 to 2 mL as required; *usual, rectal*, 30 to 50 mg/kg of body weight, in a 5 to 10% solution, or a 20% suspension in oil, to a total dose of 3 g. *Control of convulsive states*, 3 to 10 mL of 2.5% solution over 10-min period. For *narcoanalysis and narcosynthesis, adults*, 4 mL/min (100 mg/min) of a 2.5% solution; the injection may be preceded by the administration of an anticholinergic agent and a test dose of thiopental sodium.

Dosage Forms—for Injection: 500 mg; 1, 5, 6.25, 10, and 12.5 g.

Other Intravenous Anesthetics

Propanidid [Propyl {4-[(diethylcarbamoyl)methoxy]-3-methoxyphenyl}acetate [1421-14-3] $C_{18}H_{27}NO_5$ (377.40); Epontol(*Riker*)]—A colorless or pale greenish-yellow, viscous liquid with a slight odor; hygroscopic; boils at about 210°. Very slightly soluble in water; miscible with alcohol, chloroform, ether. *Uses:* A rapidly acting intravenous anesthetic that produces anesthesia within one arm-to-brain circulation time. It is very rapidly metabolised by plasma pseudocholinesterase and subsequently by hepatic microsomal cholinesterases. Thus, it is of particular value as a dental and outpatient anesthetic, since there is little residual depression. Adverse effects include myocardial depression, hypotension, and pain at the site of injection. It causes a slightly higher incidence of venous thrombosis at the injection site than barbiturates. It should be used with caution in poor risk patients, since the initial respiratory stimulation is followed by respiratory depression. Propanidid prolongs the action of suxamethonium, another agent that is hydrolyzed by pseudocholinesterase. *Dose: Usual, induction:* 5 to 10 mg/kg, intravenously. *Dosage Form:* Unavailable for general use in the US.

Unclassified Anesthetic

Phencyclidine Hydrochloride

Piperidine, 1-(1-phenylcyclohexyl)-, hydrochloride; Sernylan (*Parke-Davis*)

1-(1-Phenylcyclohexyl)piperidine hydrochloride [956-90-1] $C_{17}H_{25}N \cdot HCl$ (279.85).

Preparation—US Pat 3,097,136.

Description—White to creamy white, crystalline powder or granules that are odorless and have a slightly bitter taste; stable in light and air; melts between 222° and 228°.

Solubility—Freely soluble in water, alcohol, and chloroform; sparingly soluble in dilute HCl.

Uses—An *immobilizing agent* for subhuman primates only; effects are unlike those produced by the classical anesthetics. Although the animal is completely incapacitated, simple reflexes (patellar, palpebral, corneal, and pupillary) are not completely eliminated, the eyes remain open, muscle tone is increased in most cases, and respiration and blood pressure are not usually depressed except after deliberate overdosage. When phencyclidine hydrochloride is used prior to an anesthetic agent, such as ether or a barbiturate, a greatly reduced amount of the anesthetic will produce surgical anesthesia. Side effects observed include disorientation, euphoria, salivation, anxiety, restlessness, convulsions, muscular tremors, hyperpnea, respiratory arrest, cardiac arrest, and emesis. Decreased body temperature, shock, and death have also been observed in the *Macacus irus* monkey and *Anubis* baboon.

Phencyclidine, known among drug users as PCP, "hog" or "angel dust," is a drug seriously abused. It produces a feeling of numbness in the arms and legs, and hallucinations. Sprinkled on tobacco or marihuana cigarettes or taken in capsules, PCP can create a temporary psychosis very much like acute schizophrenia. It often leads to paranoia and has been linked with serious violence. (See also the article on *Phencyclidine* in Chapter 71.)

Dose—0.5 to 2 mg/kg; *usual, intramuscular*, 0.8 mg/kg.

CHAPTER 56

Local Anesthetics

Ewart A Swinyard, PhD, DSc (Hon)

Professor Emeritus of Pharmacology
College of Pharmacy and School of Medicine
University of Utah
Salt Lake City UT 84112

Although regional pain relief may be obtained by physical means (application of electric current to peripheral nerves, etc.), cooling an extremity, stimulation of α, β, and γ of the A fibers by needling (acupuncture), sonic waves, or application of pressure, it is most commonly obtained by the use of drugs that interrupt conduction of impulses when applied directly to peripheral nerves. Drugs that block nerve conduction are of two types: neurolytic agents that cause destruction of nervous tissue and provide long-lasting pain relief, and local anesthetic agents that induce a temporary conduction block and provide pain relief which lasts from a few minutes to a few hours. The neurolytic agents are occasionally used to relieve severe intractable pain, whereas the local anesthetics are frequently used to prevent pain in surgical procedures, dental manipulations, injury, and disease.

The synthetic local anesthetic agents may be divided into two groups: the slightly soluble compounds and the soluble compounds. The *slightly soluble* local anesthetics are used only for surface (topical) application, since their slow absorption renders them safe for use on ulcers, wounds, and mucous surfaces. The anesthesia which they induce is not as complete as that induced by soluble compounds, but the duration is longer. Many soluble anesthetics may also be used for topical anesthesia. On the other hand, only *soluble* local anesthetics of relatively low toxicity should be injected.

Local anesthesia induced by injectable agents is designated according to the technique or anatomic site of the injection. *Infiltration anesthesia* refers to injection directly into the area that is painful or to be subjected to surgical trauma. *Field block* is accomplished by setting up walls of anesthesia around an area rather than by direct infiltration. *Peripheral nerve block*, commonly called *regional anesthesia*, places the anesthetic agent in direct contact with the nerve. *Paravertebral nerve block* places the anesthetic agent in direct contact with the nerve at the site it leaves the intervertebral foramina. *Epidural block* and *caudal block* are similar; caudal block is an epidural block in the caudal region. *Subarachnoid block*, commonly called *spinal anesthesia*, but more correctly *spinal analgesia*, requires that the anesthetic be placed within the subarachnoid space so that the anesthetic agent mixes with spinal fluid. The use of a hyperbaric (heavy) solution or hypobaric (light) solution and proper positioning of the patient on the operating table permits anesthesia of various body areas.

Local anesthetics prevent both the generation and the conduction of the nerve impulse. When progressively increasing concentrations of a local anesthetic are applied to a nerve fiber, the threshold for excitation increases, the impulse conduction slows, the rate of rise of the action potential declines, the action potential amplitude decreases, and, finally, the ability to generate an action potential is abolished. All these effects result from the binding of the local anesthetic to sodium channels; this binding results in a blockade of the sodium current. If the sodium current is blocked over a critical portion of nerve, propagation of an impulse over the blocked area no longer is possible.

When infiltration, conduction, or regional techniques are employed, both nerve fibers and nerve endings are anesthetized. The ease in which a nerve fiber may be anesthetized is related to its type and size. Thus, myelinated nerves usually require a greater concentration of anesthetic solution and more time to be blocked than do nonmyelinated fibers, since the former are protected by an insulating barrier of myelin and can be reached only at the nodes of Ranvier, which interrupt the myelin sheath every 1 to 2 mm. Also, the size or nerve diameter is important because the larger the nerve fiber the greater will be the anesthetic concentration required to prevent nerve conduction. Accordingly, small nerve fibers concerned with vasoconstriction, temperature, and surface pain are most easily anesthetized, whereas large fibers associated with the sensation of touch, pressure, deep pain, and the sensations from joints and tendons are anesthetized with more difficulty. In spinal anesthesia, it is probable that both sensory and motor nerve fibers are anesthetized. In surface (topical) anesthesia, the sensory nerve endings are the chief nerve structures affected.

The duration of action of a local anesthetic is proportional to the time during which it is in actual contact with nervous tissues. Consequently, procedures that maintain localization of the drug at the nerve greatly prolong anesthesia. Cocaine itself constricts blood vessels, prevents its own absorption, and exhibits a duration of action longer than most local anesthetics. The addition of a vasoconstrictor drug, such as epinephrine, norepinephrine, nordefrin, levonordefrin, or phenylephrine, is almost always found in local anesthetic solutions. The presence of one of these drugs in the local anesthetic solution retards absorption of the local anesthetic solution, thereby reducing its systemic toxicity, increasing its duration of action, and increasing its efficiency by decreasing the volume of solution required. The pressor potency relative to epinephrine (shown in parentheses), maximal total dose, and usual concentration are as follows: epinephrine (1), 0.2 mg, 1:50,000 to 1:250,000; norepinephrine (0.6), 0.34 mg, 1:30,000; nordefrin (0.2), 1 mg, 1:10,000; levonordefrin (0.5), 1 mg, 1:20,000: and phenylephrine (0.2), 4 mg, 1:25,000. Except for solutions to be used for spinal anesthesia and for solutions to be injected in the fingers and toes, vasoconstrictor agents may be added to all local anesthetic solutions.

A number of precautions should be observed when injection anesthesia is contemplated. (1) Resuscitation equipment and appropriate drugs should be immediately available. (2) The safe use of these agents in pregnancy, with respect to adverse effects on fetal development, has not been established. (3) Local anesthetic procedures should be used with caution when there is inflammation and/or sepsis in the region of the proposed injection. (4) Local anesthetics containing epinephrine should be used with *extreme caution* in patients on MAO inhibitors, tricyclic antidepressants, phenothiazines, etc, as either severe hypertension or hypotension may occur. (5) Vasopressor agents used in caudal or other epidural blocks should be used with *extreme caution* in patients on oxytocic drugs, since the resulting interaction may produce severe persistent hypertension and/or rupture of cerebral blood vessels. (6) Serious dose-related cardiac arrhythmias may occur if local anesthetics containing a vasoconstrictor such as epinephrine are employed in patients during or following the administration of chloroform, halothane, cyclopropane, trichloroethylene or other inhalation anesthetics. Factors that must be given careful consideration prior to concurrent use of general and local anesthetics include effect of both agents on myocardium, the concentration and volume of the vasoconstrictor, and the elapsed time since injection.

Adverse reactions to local anesthetics may be divided into two groups: systemic and local adverse reactions. In general, these reactions are qualitatively similar for all local anesthetic agents. *Systemic adverse reactions* are usually associated with high blood levels of the drug and usually result from overdosage, rapid systemic absorption, or inadvertent intravenous injection. The reactions usually involve the central nervous and cardiovascular systems. The initial *central nervous system* reactions are excitatory and/or depressant, may be characterized by nervousness, dizziness, blurred vision and tremors, followed by drowsiness, convulsions, unconsciousness and possibly respiratory arrest. Other systemic effects may include nausea, vomiting, chills, pupil contraction, or tinnitus. The excitatory reactions may be very brief or absent, in which case the first manifestation of toxicity may be drowsiness, merging into unconsciousness and respiratory arrest. *Cardiovascular reactions* are depressant and may be characterized by hypotension, cardiovascular collapse, bradycardia, and possibly cardiac arrest. Treatment of a patient with toxic manifestations includes reassurance, maintaining a patent airway and supporting ventilation using oxygen and assisted or controlled respiration. Should circulatory depression occur, vasopressors such as ephedrine or metaraminol, and i.v. fluids may be used. Should a convulsion persist despite oxygen therapy, small increments of thiopental, pentobarbital, or diazepam may be given intravenously. *Allergic reactions* are characterized by cutaneous lesions, urticaria, edema, or anaphylactoid reactions. Untoward reactions from overdosage with epinephrine and other vasoconstrictor agents added to local anesthetics are relatively common. Anxiety, palpitation, dizziness, headaches, restlessness, tremors, tachycardia, anginal pain, and hypertension are frequently observed. These reactions may be differentiated from those caused by local anesthetics in that epinephrine does not produce convulsions and causes tachycardia rather than bradycardia. Reactions of this kind respond to sedatives, amyl nitrite, and oxygen.

Local adverse reactions to these anesthetic drugs, although infrequent, are either cytotoxic or allergic and are manifested by skin discoloration, pain, edema, slough, neuritis, or neurolysis. Eczematoid dermatitis, characterized by erythema and pruritus which proceeds to inflammation, swelling, vesiculation, and oozing, is the predominant local reaction. *Only the aminobenzoic acid* derivatives cause allergic sensitivity reactions; cross-sensitivity between members of this group is often reported. If a patient is allergic or does not tolerate a particular local anesthetic, it is advisable to use a drug from a different chemical family. Unfortunately, tests for sensitivity such as skin, conjunctival, and patch tests are not reliable for predicting the possibility of allergic reactions.

All local anesthetics are toxic, and the tolerance of patients varies. Safe dosage, therefore, is limited for each drug and must be individualized. Choice of drug, concentration, rate and site of injection, age, and emotional and physical status of the patient represent a few factors which must be considered. In general, the smallest amount of the least toxic drug that will serve the purpose should be used, if reactions are to be avoided. In some patients, premedication with either pentobarbital or diazepam may be advisable to minimize the incidence of toxic reactions. Many local anesthetics occasionally give rise to dermatitis. When this is severe, the use of the anesthetic should be discontinued.

The interested reader is referred to the following excellent reviews on the subject: *Symposium on Local Anesthetics, Br J Anesth, 47:* suppl 164, 1975; Tucker GT Mather LE Clinical pharmacokinetics of local anesthetics. *Clin Pharmacokinetics 4:* 241–278, 1979. Ruff RL. The kinetics of local anesthetic blockade of end-plate channels. *Biophys J 37:* 625–631, 1982, McLeskey CH. Rational use of local anesthetics. *NC Med J 43:* 496–500, 1982.

Injection Anesthetics

Injectable local anesthetic drugs can conveniently be divided into two groups: esters and nonesters. The esters include (1) benzoic acid esters (piperocaine, meprylcaine, isobucaine); (2) *para*-aminobenzoic acid esters (procaine, tetracaine, butethamine, propoxycaine, chloroprocaine); (3) *meta*-aminobenzoic acid esters (metabutethamine, primacaine); and (4) *para*-ethoxybenzoic acid ester (parethoxycaine). The nonesters are anilides (amides or nonesters) which include lidocaine, mepivacaine, pyrrocaine, and prilocaine. This classification is particularly important from the point of view of possible allergic reactions as well as biotransformation. Thus, local anesthetics with an *ester linkage* (aromatic acid + amino alcohol) such as procaine and those with an *amide linkage* (aromatic amine + amino acid) such as lidocaine, differ significantly in hypersensitivity, metabolism, and duration of action. Hypersensitivity seems to occur most prominently in response to local anesthetics of the *ester type* and frequently extends to chemically related compounds. Agents of the amide type are essentially free of this problem, and substitution of such a compound to avoid group specificity is usually possible. The *metabolic fate* of local anesthetics is of great practical importance because their toxicity depends largely on the balance between their rate of absorption and their rate of destruction. The *ester-type* local anesthetic appears to be hydrolyzed by both liver esterase and plasma esterase. Metabolic degradation by plasma esterase is particularly important in man; human plasma esterase can hydrolyze local anesthetics 4 to 20 times faster than can animal plasma esterases. Consequently, very little of the *ester-type* agent is available for hydrolysis by liver esterase. Spinal fluid contains little or no esterase; hence, anesthesia produced by intrathecal injection of a local anesthetic will persist until the local anesthetic agent is absorbed into the blood. On the other hand, *amide-type* local anesthetics are degraded by hepatic microsomes; the initial reactions involve *N*-dealkylation and subsequent hydrolysis. Consequently, the *amide-type* local anesthetics have a much longer duration of action than the ester-type.

Considerable pharmacokinetic data have been accumulated on the newer amide-type local anesthetics, particularly lidocaine, mepivacaine, bupivacaine and etidocaine. (The data will be presented in the respective monographs.) Comparatively little such information is available on the older ester-type agents; for the most part their rapid metabolism has compromised most attempts to measure their blood concentrations after less than heroic doses in man. Consequently, most studies with the latter agents deal with potency, toxicity, time for onset and duration of action. The descriptive phrase short-acting suggests a duration of 45 to 75 minutes, medium-acting, 90 to 150 minutes, and long-acting 180 minutes or longer.

With the exception of solutions for use in spinal anesthesia, local anesthetic solutions should be isotonic to avoid edema, local irritation, and inflammation at the site of injection. Solutions for spinal anesthesia may either be isobaric, hypobaric or hyperbaric depending on the desired level of anesthesia. The total maximal dosages employed with injection anesthetics vary markedly, depending on the technique used and the patients age, weight, and physical condition. In general, the physician should administer the least volume of the most dilute solution that is effective. For adverse effects and special warnings in the use of these agents refer to the introductory statement in this chapter.

Bupivacaine Hydrochloride

2-Piperidinecarboxamide, 1-butyl-*N*-(2,6-dimethylphenyl)-, hydrochloride; Marcaine Hydrochloride (*Breon*); Sensorcaine (*Astra*)

1-Butyl-2′,6′-pipecoloxylidide monohydrochloride [14252-80-3] $C_{18}H_{28}N_2O.HCl.H_2O$ (342.91).

Preparation—Similar to that of *Mepivacaine Hydrochloride*, except that butyl bromide instead of dimethyl sulfate is used for alkylation. US Pat 2,792,399.

Description—White, crystalline powder; odorless; melts with decomposition between 247° and 262°.

Solubility—1 g in 25 mL water, 8 mL alcohol; slightly soluble in chloroform.

Uses—An amide-type local anesthetic chemically related to lidocaine and a homologue of mepivacaine. All three of these anesthetics contain an amide linkage between the aromatic nucleus and the amino or piperidine group. They differ in this respect from the procaine-type local anesthetics which have an ester linkage.

Bupivacaine is used for *infiltration, field block; peripheral nerve block, paravertebral block, caudal,* or *epidural block.* The onset of action after local injection is rapid (5 min); onset may be delayed as long as 20 min when used for brachial plexus or peridural anesthesia. The duration of peripheral nerve blocks produced by bupivacaine may last up to 7 hr, compared to 3 or 4 hr when mepivacaine is used; the duration of peridural anesthesia is about 4 hr, compared to 1.5 to 2 hr with lidocaine. Epidural block with 0.75% solution induces complete motor block; hence, abdominal operations requiring complete muscle relaxation may be done. It has also been noted that a period of analgesia persists after the return of sensation; during this time the need for analgesics is reduced. Bupivacaine has a pKa of 8.05, $t_{1/2}$ of 2.7 hrs, V_d of 1.04, a partition coefficient of 130, and 84 to 95% of the drug is bound to plasma protein. Consequently, it has a low degree of placental transmission of parenteral local anesthetic and may cause the least fetal depression. After injection for caudal, epidural or peripheral nerve block in humans, peak blood levels of approximately 1.2 µg/mL are reached in 30 to 45 min, followed by a decline to insignificant levels within 3 to 6 hr. Bupivacaine, like other local anesthetics with an amide structure, is not detoxified by plasma esterases but is detoxified in the liver, via conjugation with glucuronic acid.

Contraindications, general warnings, precautions, and adverse reactions are similar to those of other amide-type local anesthetics (see Lidocaine, page 1051). It is not recommended for children under 12 years of age. The safe use in pregnancy, with respect to adverse effects on fetal development, has not been established.

Dose—*Infiltration anesthesia,* 1 to 30 mL of 0.25%; *epidural,* 10 to 20 mL of 0.25, 0.50, or 0.75%; (*Caution:* the unintentional intravenous injection of the 0.75% solution may cause cardiac arrest); *caudal,* 15 to 30 mL of 0.25 or 0.50%; *peripheral nerves,* 5 to 30 mL of 0.25 or 0.50%; *paravertebral block,* 20 to 50 mL of a 0.25% solution.

Dosage Forms—Ampuls or vials, 50-mL, 0.25%, with or without epinephrine 1:200,000; 30- or 50-mL, 0.5%, with or without epinephrine 1:200,000; and ampuls, 30-mL, 0.75% with or without epinephrine 1:200,000.

Chloroprocaine Hydrochloride

Benzoic acid, 4-amino-2-chloro-, 2-(diethylamino)ethyl ester, monohydrochloride; Nesacaine; Nesacaine-CE (*Pennwalt*)

2-(Diethylamino)ethyl 4-amino-2-chlorobenzoate monohydrochloride [3858-89-7] $C_{13}H_{19}ClN_2O_2.HCl$ (307.22).

Preparation—2-Chloro-4-nitrobenzoic acid is reacted with thionyl chloride and the resulting acid chloride is condensed with 2-(diethylamino)ethanol. Reduction of the nitro ester with iron and acidulated water yields chloroprocaine base which may be converted into the hydrochloride by dissolving in a suitable solvent and introducing hydrogen chloride.

Description—White, crystalline powder; odorless and stable in air; solutions are acid to litmus; exhibits local anesthetic properties when placed on the tongue; melts between 173° and 176°.

Solubility—1 g in about 20 mL water and about 100 mL alcohol; very slightly soluble in chloroform; practically insoluble in ether.

Uses—Chloroprocaine, a chlorinated analogue of procaine with similar pharmacologic properties, is used for *infiltration, field block, peripheral nerve block, paravertebral block,* and *epidural anesthesia.* It is not effective topically. Its onset of action is about 6 to 12 min and anesthesia lasts from 30 to 60 min; with the addition of epinephrine 1:200,000, duration is increased to 60 to 90 min. For adverse reactions see introduction.

Dose—*Maximum* **0.8 g** without epinephrine, **1.0 g** with epinephrine (1:200,000) as a **1** to **3**% solution. Repeated doses of up to 300 mg without epinephrine and 600 mg with epinephrine (1:200,000) may be given at 50 min intervals. *Usual, infiltration:* without epinephrine, up to **80 mL** of a **1**% solution; with epinephrine (1:200,000), up to **100 mL** of a **1**% solution. *Peripheral nerve block:* 1 or 2% with or without epinephrine. *Caudal:* 15 to 25 mL of a 2 or 3% (Nesacaine-CE) solution, repeated at 40- to 60-minute intervals as required. *Epidural:* 15 to 25 mL (2 to 2.5 mL per nerve segment to be blocked) of a 2 or 3% (Nesacaine-CE) solution; supplemental doses of 10 to 20 mL may be given at 40 to 50 min intervals; *peripheral nerve block,* **50 mL** of **1**% solution; *epidural,* **25 mL** of **3**% solution.

Dosage Forms—Injection: 1 and 2% in 30 mL (not for caudal or epidural anesthesia); 2 and 3% in 30 mL (for caudal and epidural).

Dibucaine

4-Quinolinecarboxamide, 2-butoxy-*N*-[2-(diethylamino)ethyl]-, Nupercainal (*Ciba-Geigy*)

2-Butoxy-*N*-[2-(diethylamino)ethyl]cinchoninamide [85-79-0] $C_{20}H_{29}N_3O_2$ (343.47).

Preparation—Dibucaine may be synthesized by the following sequence of reactions: (1) Acetylation of isatin (obtained by oxidation of indigo) to *N*-acetylisatin, (2) rearrangement to 2-hydroxycinchoninic acid by treatment with alkali, (3) formation of 2-chlorocinchoninoyl chloride by reaction with phosphorus pentachloride, (4) conversion to 2-chloro-*N*-[2-(diethylamino)ethyl]cinchoninamide with *asym*-diethylethylenediamine, (5) heating with sodium butoxide to produce dibucaine. US Pat 1,825,623.

Description—White to off-white powder; slightly characteristic odor; somewhat hygroscopic, and darkens on exposure to light; melts between 62° and 65°.

Solubility—Soluble in ether; slightly soluble in water.

Uses—See *Dibucaine Hydrochloride.*

Dose—*Topical,* as a **0.5**% cream or a **1**% ointment several times a day.

Dosage Forms—Cream: 0.5%; Ointment: 1%; Suppositories: 2.5%.

Dibucaine Hydrochloride

4-Quinolinecarboxamide, 2-butoxy-*N*-[2-(diethylamino)ethyl]-, monohydrochloride; Cinchocaine Hydrochloride; Nupercaine Hydrochloride (*Ciba-Geigy*)

For the formula of dibucaine base see the preceding article.

2-Butoxy-N-[2-(diethylamino)ethyl]cinchoninamide monohydrochloride [61-12-1] $C_{20}H_{29}N_3O_2 \cdot HCl$ (379.93).

Preparation—Dibucaine base is dissolved in an appropriate organic solvent or solvent mixture and precipitated with a stream of hydrogen chloride.

Description—Colorless or white to off-white crystals, or white to off-white crystalline powder; odorless, somewhat hygroscopic, and darkens on exposure to light; solutions have a pH of about 5.5; melts between 95° and 100°.

Solubility—1 g in about 2 mL water; freely soluble in alcohol, acetone, and chloroform.

Uses—Dibucaine hydrochloride, a quinoline derivative with a pK_a of 8.15, is the most potent and one of the most toxic of the long-acting local anesthetics. It is indicated for *surface* and *subarachnoid block* (spinal analgesia). Three solutions are available for spinal anesthesia: hyperbaric (heavy), hypobaric (light), and isobaric. Dibucaine is 15 to 20 times more potent and 15 times more toxic than procaine when injected. Onset of action is quite slow (15 min); duration of spinal anesthesia is 3 to 4 hr without epinephrine and 6 hr with epinephrine. For adverse reactions, see introduction.

Dose—*Injection, spinal, obstetrical* and *saddle block*, **2.5 to 5 mg** (1 to 2 mL hyperbaric solution); lower extremities, **4 mg** (6 mL of hypobaric solution); lower abdomen **7.5 to 10 mg** (11 to 15 mL of hypobaric solution); upper abdomen **10 to 12 mg** (15 to 18 mL of hypobaric solution). See manufacturer's literature for use of isobaric solution.

Dosage Forms—Aerosol: 0.25%; Ampuls: 1:200, 2 mL (isobaric); 1:1500, 20 mL (hypobaric); 5 mg dibucaine, 100 mg dextrose, 2 mL (hyperbaric).

Etidocaine Hydrochloride

Butanamide, N-(2,6-dimethylphenyl)-2-(ethylpropylamino)-, (±)-, monohydrochloride; Duranest Hydrochloride (*Astra*)

(±)-2-(Ethylpropylamino)-2′,6′-butyroxylidide monohydrochloride [3667-18-0 (free base)] $C_{17}H_{28}N_2O \cdot HCl$ (312.88).

Preparation—Etidocaine is synthesized by the interaction of 2,6-xylidine, 2-bromobutyric acid, and ethyl n-propylamine. German Pat. 2,162,744 (*CA 77:* 101244c, 1972).

Description—White, crystalline powder; pK_a 7.74 (etidocaine).

Solubility—Soluble in water; freely soluble in alcohol.

Uses—A local anesthetic of the amide-type chemically related to lidocaine. It is used for percutaneous *infiltration anesthesia* (in a concentration of 0.5%), *peripheral nerve blocks* (0.5 or 1.0%), *paravertebral nerve block* (0.5 to 1.5%), *caudal* or *epidural blocks*. Long-acting local anesthetics, such as etidocaine, have also been used instead of narcotics to relieve pain following abdominal operations or thoracotomy.

Etidocaine has a pK_a of 7.74, lipid solubility of 141 (in heptane/7.4 phosphate buffer system), $t_{1/2}$ of 2.7 hrs, Vd of 1.9 L/kg, and is 94% bound to plasma protein. In peripheral and epidural blocks, mean peak plasma levels of about 0.5–0.64 $\mu g/mL$ have been demonstrated following administration of 100 to 200 mg of the drug. Plasma half-life appears to be 1 to 2 hr after IV administration of 50 mg in normal adults. Etidocaine has a rapid onset (3 to 5 min) and a prolonged duration of action (5 to 10 hr). The duration of sensory analgesia is 1.5 to 2 times longer than that for lidocaine; duration in excess of 9 hr is not infrequent in peripheral nerve blocks. It also produces a significant degree of motor blockade and abdominal muscle relaxation when used for peridural analgesia.

Contraindications, warnings for use, precautions, and adverse reactions are similar to those for lidocaine (see this page). The safe use of etidocaine in pregnancy, with respect to adverse effects of fetal development, has not been established. The use of this agent in children under 14 years of age has not been investigated.

Dose—*Infiltration anesthesia*, 1 to **80 mL** of a **0.5%** solution with epinephrine 1:200,000; *peripheral nerve block*, **5 to 80 mL** of **0.5** or **1.0%** solution with epinephrine; *central neural block*,

10 to **30 mL** of **0.5 to 1.5%** solution with epinephrine; *caudal*, **10 to 30 mL** of **0.5 or 1.0%** solution with epinephrine.

Dosage Forms—0.5% with epinephrine 1:200,000, 50-mL multiple-dose vials; 0.5 or 1.0% with or without epinephrine 1:200,000, 30-mL single-dose vials; 1.0% with or without epinephrine 1:200,000, 30-mL ampul; 1.5% with epinephrine 1:200,000, 20-mL ampul.

Lidocaine

Acetamide, 2-(diethylamino)-N-(2,6-dimethylphenyl)-, Lida-Mantle (*Miles*); Xylocaine (*Astra*)

2-(Diethylamino)-2′,6′-acetoxylidide [137-58-6] $C_{14}H_{22}N_2O$ (234.34).

Preparation—By chloroacetylation of 2,6-xylidine and condensation of the resulting chloroacetoxylidide and diethylamine.

Description—White or slightly yellow, crystalline powder, with a characteristic odor; stable in air; melts between 66° and 69°; pK_a 7.86.

Solubility—Very soluble in alcohol and chloroform; freely soluble in benzene and ether; practically insoluble in water; dissolves in oils.

Uses—A *local anesthetic* used as an ointment topically on mucous membranes on minor burns, abrasions, and anorectal lesions; also used as an anesthetic lubricant for endotracheal intubation. See *Lidocaine Hydrochloride*.

Dose—*Topical*, as a **2.5 to 5%** ointment.

Dosage Forms—Ointment: 2.5 and 5.0%; Oral Spray: 10%; Cream: 2 and 3%; Suppositories: 100 mg.

Lidocaine Hydrochloride

Acetamide, 2-(diethylamino)-N-(2,6-dimethylphenyl)-, monohydrochloride, monohydrate; Dalcaine (*O'Neal, Jones & Feldman*); Dolicaine (*Reid-Provident*) Lignocaine Hydrochloride BP; Xylocaine Hydrochloride (*Astra*)

2-(Diethylamino)-2′,6′-acetoxylidide monohydrochloride [6108-05-0] $C_{14}H_{22}N_2O \cdot HCl \cdot H_2O$ (288.82); *anhydrous* [73-78-9] $C_{14}H_{22}N_2O \cdot HCl$ (270.80).

For the structure and preparation of the base, see *Lidocaine*.

Description—White, odorless, crystalline powder, having a slightly bitter taste; melts between 74° and 79°.

Solubility—Very soluble in water and alcohol; soluble in chloroform; insoluble in ether.

Uses—A widely employed amide-type *local anesthetic* and *antiarrhythmic* drug. As a local anesthetic, lidocaine hydrochloride is employed for *infiltration* and *field block anesthesia* in a concentration of 0.5%; for *peripheral nerve block* in a concentration of 0.5 and 1%; for *paravertebral nerve block* in a concentration of 0.5 to 1.5%; for *epidural or caudal anesthesia* in a concentration of 1.5% with 7.5% dextrose; and in *sub-arachnoid block* (*spinal analgesia*) in a concentration of 5% made hyperbaric with 7.5% dextrose. Lidocaine hydrochloride is also used topically on mucous membranes as a 1 to 4% aqueous solution, 2% jelly, 2.5% and 5% ointment, and 2.0% viscous. It is also used in the form of suppositories for temporary relief of pain associated with inoperative, irritated, or inflamed anorectal conditions. Some injections of lidocaine hydrochloride contain epinephrine to delay absorption, prolong its action, and reduce its toxic effects. Because it is also effective without a vasoconstrictor, it appears to be the anesthetic of choice for use in those individuals who are sensitive to epinephrine and its congeners. In addition, it is so dissimilar in chemical structure to procaine and related anesthetics that it is the agent of choice in individuals sensitive to procaine. The local anesthetic action of lidocaine is more rapid in onset, more intense, and of longer duration than that of procaine. It is also more potent than procaine. Lidocaine has a local vasodilating action but is usually used with epinephrine. When used alone, anesthesia after perineural injection lasts 60 to 75 min; with epinephrine, anesthesia lasts 2 hr or more. Lidocaine and procaine are approximately equally toxic when administered extravascularly in 0.5% solutions; when higher concentrations are used, lidocaine is $1\frac{1}{2}$ times as toxic as procaine. By the intravenous route, lidocaine is twice as toxic as procaine.

As an *antiarrhythmic agent* lidocaine hydrochloride is administered intravenously for the management of ventricular arrhythmias occurring during cardiac manipulation such as cardiac surgery, and life-threatening arrhythmias which are ventricular in origin, such as occur during acute myocardial infarction. For this purpose it is usually given in a dose of 50 to 100 mg intravenously at a rate of 25 to 50 mg/min. If the initial injection does not produce the desired clinical response, a second dose (⅓ to ½ the initial dose) may be given after 5 min. No more than 200 to 300 mg of lidocaine should be administered during a one-hour period. Smaller doses should be used in cardiac failure, a reduced cardiac output from any cause, and in patients over 60 years of age. Lidocaine exhibits a biphasic half-life. The distribution phase ($t_{1/2}$: 7 to 8 min) accounts for the short duration of action after intravenous administration (10 to 20 min). The terminal elimination half-life is 1 to 2 hours. Therapeutic antiarrhythmic plasma levels range from 1.5 to 5.5 μg/mL; subjective toxic effect levels range from 3 to 5 μg/mL; and objective adverse manifestations such as muscular irritability, convulsions, and coma appear at plasma lidocaine levels of 6 to 10 μg/mL. Thus, there is considerable overlap between therapeutic levels and subjective toxic effect levels. Moreover, toxicity may be significantly altered by the co-administration of other drugs. For example, co-administration with propranolol impairs the clearance of lidocaine and enhances toxicity; concomitant intravenous administration of phenytoin and lidocaine may induce excessive cardiac depression; and additive neurologic effects may be produced during concurrent administration of procainamide and lidocaine.

It should be emphasized that after administration as a local anesthetic agent, systemic absorption of lidocaine may result in blood concentrations in the usual therapeutic antiarrhythmic or even toxic ranges. Lidocaine plasma levels vary according to the site at which the local anesthetic is injected: subcutaneous, 1.2 μg/mL/100 mg; epidural, 1.1 μg/mL/100 mg; and subcutaneous (abdominal), 0.5 μg/mL/100 mg. Thus, the epidural injection of 25 mL of a 1.5% solution (375 mg) has the potential for producing a plasma level of 4.13 μg/mL of lidocaine, a value well within the range which induces subjective toxic effects (3 to 5 μg/mL) and approaching that which results in objective adverse manifestations (6 to 10 μg/mL). After absorption, lidocaine partitions extensively into body tissues. Studies in monkeys indicate lidocaine has a high affinity for spleen (tissue to plasma coefficient 3.5), lung (3.1), kidney (2.8), adipose tissue (2.0), brain (1.2), heart (0.96), and musculoskeletal tissues (0.6). Because of the avidity with which tissues take up lidocaine, only about 6% of a given dose is found in the blood at steady state. Lidocaine then redistributes to muscle and adipose tissue; these tissues then become the major storage reservoirs. For more detailed pharmacokinetic data on lidocaine, the interested reader is referred to the excellent review by Benowitz and Meister (*Clinical Pharmacokinetics 3:* 177, 1978).

Lidocaine is a weak base with a pK_a of 7.86, $t_{1/2}$ of 1.6 hrs, V_d of 1.3 L/kg, and 64% is bound to plasma protein. Maximal excretion in an acid urine is only 10%. The major portion of this agent is metabolized by the liver microsomal system. Two major metabolites have been identified: monoethylglycinexylidide and glycinexylidide. Animal experiments indicate both metabolites have antiarrhythmic and convulsant activities; the former has potency similar to lidocaine itself while the latter is only 10 to 26% as potent. Both metabolites, after further biotransformation in the liver, are excreted in the urine.

Some adverse central nervous system effects are frequently observed during lidocaine therapy. These commonly include drowsiness, dizziness, paresthesia, and euphoria. Typical symptoms with higher doses include confusion, agitation, dysarthria, vertigo, visual disturbances, tinnitus, and nausea. Sweating, muscle tremor, or fasciculations may also occur. Manifestations of severe toxicity include psychosis, seizures, respiratory depression, and coma. Seizures which persist after the administration of oxygen may be controlled by intravenous administration of small increments (50 to 100 mg) of thiopental, thiamylal, methohexital or 2.5 mg increments of diazepam. Caution must be exercised since overdosage may occur if sufficient time is not allowed for the anticonvulsant action of the individual doses to become apparent. Premedication with barbiturates has little or no value in averting central nervous system reactions. Diazepam has been recommended for prophylaxis of convulsions during local anesthetic therapy.

Dose—*Infiltration, peripheral nerve block,* or *epidural,* up to **60 mL** (100 mL with epinephrine), as a **0.5**% solution; up to **27 mg** (45 mL with epinephrine), as a **1**% solution; up to **20 mL** (33 mL with epinephrine), as a **2**% solution. *Usual, infiltration,* **50 mL** of a **0.5**%

solution. *Usual, peripheral nerve block,* **25 mL** of a **1.5**% solution. *Usual, epidural,* **15 to 25 mL** of a **1.5**% solution. *Topical,* up to **250 mg** as a **2 to 4**% solution or as a **2**% jelly, to mucous membranes.

Dosage Forms—*Injection: Single-dose vial,* 10 mL 2.0%; 20 mL 1.5%; 30 mL 1.0%; 50 mL 0.5%. *Single-dose vial with epinephrine* (1:200,000), 20 mL 2.0%; 30 mL 1.0 and 1.5%. *Multiple-dose vial,* 20 mL 1.0 and 2.0%; 50 mL 0.5, 1.0, and 2.0%. *Multiple-dose vial with epinephrine* (1:100,000), 20 mL 1.0 and 2.0%; 50 mL 1.0 and 2.0%. *Multiple-dose vial with epinephrine* (1:200,000), 50 mL 0.5%. *Ampules,* 2 mL 1.0 and 2.0%; 5 mL 1.0%; 30 mL 1.0%. *For cardiac arrhythmias, intravenous:* for direct IV injection, 5 mL (100 mg) prefilled syringe and ampule; for preparation of infusion solutions, 25 mL (1 g) single use vial (40 mg/mL); 50 mL (2 g) single use vial (40 mg/mL); 5 mL (1 g) additive syringe (200 mg/mL), 10 mL (2 g) additive syringe (200 mg/mL). *Spinal anesthesia:* 2 mL 1.5% with dextrose 7.5%; 2 mL 5% with glucose 7.5%. *Topical anesthesia: solution,* 5 mL ampule or prefilled disposable syringe 4%; 50 mL screw-cap bottle 4%; *oral spray,* 10%; *viscous solution,* 2%; *ointment,* 35 g tube 2.5 and 5%; *flavored ointment,* 3.5 g tubes 5%; *jelly,* 30 mL tubes 2%.

Mepivacaine Hydrochloride

2-Piperidinecarboxamide, *N*-(2,6-dimethylphenyl)-1-methyl-, monohydrochloride; Carbocaine (*Breon; Cook-Waite*)

1-Methyl-2′,6′-pipecoloxylidide monohydrochloride [1722-62-9] $C_{15}H_{22}N_2O.HCl$ (282.81).

Preparation—Picolinic acid (2-pyridinecarboxylic acid) is condensed with 2,6-xylidine to 2′,6′-picolinoxylidide which is reacted with dimethyl sulfate in xylene solution. Reduction of the pyridine ring followed by treatment with HCl yields the product.

Description—White, odorless, crystalline solid; melts with decomposition between 255° and 262°; pH (1 in 50 solution) about 4.5; pK_a 7.73 ± 0.08.

Solubility—Freely soluble in water and methanol; very slightly soluble in chloroform; practically insoluble in ether.

Uses—An amide anesthetic employed for *infiltration, field block, peripheral nerve block,* and *paravertebral nerve block anesthesia.* It is not effective topically, except in large doses; therefore it should not be used for this purpose. Mepivacaine has a pK_a of 7.69 $t_{1/2}$ of 1.9 hr, V_d of 1.2 L/kg, and a partition coefficient of 12.1. Approximately 65 to 77% of that in blood is bound to serum proteins. When used in obstetrics, maternal plasma concentrations vary from 2.9 to 6.9 μg/mL, whereas the umbilical vein concentration varies from 1.9 to 4.9 μg/mL; thus the fetus is exposed to only 60 to 70% of that in maternal plasma. Mepivacaine hydrochloride has an action similar to that of lidocaine hydrochloride; however, its duration of action is considerably longer than that of lidocaine. Anesthesia develops in 3 to 5 min and lasts 2 to 2½ hr. Mepivacaine may be used for many purposes without epinephrine. Thus, it is particularly indicated in circumstances in which epinephrine is contraindicated. Although systemic effects are similar to those produced by other local anesthetics, the drowsiness, lassitude, and amnesia observed after lidocaine do not occur with mepivacaine. For additional information see the introductory statement in this chapter.

Dose—*Injection, adults, maximum single dose,* **7 mg/kg** but not to exceed **550 mg;** total dose should not exceed **1 g** in any 24-hr period. *Children* tolerate the local anesthetic as well as adults; however, the dose should be carefully measured as a percentage of adult dose based on weight (5 to 6 mg/kg). *Usual dose, therapeutic block,* **1** to **5 mL** of **1** or **2**% solution; *infiltration,* up to **40 mL** of **1**% solution; *caudal* and *epidural,* 15 to **30 mL** of **1**%, **10** to **25 mL** of **1.5**%, or **10** to **20 mL** of **2**% solution; *paracervical block,* up to **40 mL** of **1**% solution; *nerve block,* **5** to **20 mL** of **1** or **2**% solution.

Dosage Forms—25 in 20 mL single-dose vials; 1 and 1.5% in 30 mL single-dose vials, and 1 and 2% in 50 mL multiple-dose vials.

Piperocaine Hydrochloride

[1-Piperidinepropanol, 2-methyl-, benzoate (ester), hydrochloride; Metycaine Hydrochloride (*Lilly*)

3-(2-Methylpiperidino)propyl benzoate (ester) hydrochloride [533-28-8] $C_{16}H_{23}NO_2 \cdot HCl$ (297.83).

Preparation—By interaction of 2-methylpiperidine and γ-chloropropyl benzoate.   US Pat 1,784,903.

Description—Small, white crystals or a white, crystalline powder; odorless; melts at about 174°.

Solubility—1 g in 1.5 mL water, 4.5 mL alcohol; freely soluble in chloroform; practically insoluble in ether.

Uses—An ester-type local anesthetic with intermediate duration of action. It has a more rapid onset and a longer duration of action than does procaine. Peak plasma levels following caudal administration are reached in 20 to 30 min and begin to decline within the next 10 min. It is used for *infiltration, field block, peripheral nerve block, paravertebral nerve block,* and for *caudal analgesia.* Injection should not be made into or through infected or inflamed tissues. It is also useful as a *topical anesthetic* in urology, rhinolaryngology, ophthalmology, and proctology. Piperocaine shares the toxic potentials of other local anesthetics, and the usual precautions for local anesthetics should be observed. See the introductory statement in this chapter.

Dose—*Usual, infiltration,* 0.5 to 1%; *regional,* and *large nerve block,* 0.5 to 2%; *instillation.* For detailed information, especially concerning use in caudal analgesia, see the manufacturer's literature.

Dosage Forms—Injection ampules 2% in 30-mL; Powder for solution: 4-oz bottles.

Prilocaine Hydrochloride

Propanamide, N-(2-methylphenyl)-2-(propylamino)-, monohydrochloride; Citanest Hydrochloride (*Astra*)

2-(Propylamino)-*o*-propionotoluidide   monohydrochloride [1786-81-8] $C_{13}H_{20}N_2O \cdot HCl$ (256.77).

Preparation—*o*-Toluidine is condensed with 2-bromopropionyl bromide and the resulting 2-bromo-*o*-propionotoluidide is condensed with propylamine to yield prilocaine (base). An acetone solution of the base treated with hydrogen chloride yields the official salt. Brit Pat 839,943.

Description—White, odorless, crystalline powder having an initially acid and then bitter taste, stable in light and air; melts between 166° and 169°; pK_a 7.89.

Solubility—1 g in 3.5 mL water, 4.2 mL alcohol, 175 mL chloroform; practically insoluble in ether.

Uses—An amide-type local anesthetic chemically related to lidocaine and mepivacaine. It has a pK_a of 7.89. It is used for *infiltration, nerve block, epidural,* and *caudal anesthesia.* It is not used topically or for spinal anesthesia. Onset of action after infiltration averages 1 or 2 min; duration of action is 60 min or longer. For major nerve blocks (epidural), the onset of analgesia is approximately 2 min longer than that for lidocaine; whereas the duration of action is 30–60 min longer than that for lidocaine. Approximately 55% of prilocaine hydrochloride is bound to plasma protein. After 600 mg of prilocaine hydrochloride peak plasma levels are reached in 20 min, at which time plasma levels average 4 μg/mL; the same dose with epinephrine also peaks at 20 min, but the plasma level is only 2μg/mL. Consequently, prilocaine is generally used without epinephrine. Hence, this local anesthetic is particularly useful for patients who cannot tolerate vasopressor agents, eg, patients with hypertension, diabetes, thyrotoxicosis, or other cardiovascular disorders. Prilocaine hydrochloride, like other amide-type local anesthetics, is not metabolized by plasma esterases; it is metabolized by both the liver and the kidney and excreted by the kidney. One of its metabolites is *o*-toluidine, a substance known to induce methemoglobinemia. Methemoglobin levels up to 15% and cyanosis have been reported following doses of 600 mg or more. Other clinical symptoms of methemoglobinemia, such as tachycardia, fatigue, headache, lightheadedness, and dizziness may occur at higher doses. Except for methemoglobinemia, side effects are similar to those observed with other local anesthetics. When

methemoglobinemia occurs, it can be reversed by intravenous injection of methylene blue, 1 to 2 mg/kg of a 1% solution administered over a 5-minute period. As with other local anesthetics, prilocaine hydrochloride is contraindicated in the presence of shock, severe cardiovascular disease, or heart block. For other adverse effects, see the introductory statement in this chapter.

Dose—*Usual, therapeutic nerve block,* for pain, **3** to **5 mL** of a 1 or **2%** solution; *infiltration,* **20** to **30 mL** of a 1 or 2% solution; *regional anesthesia, peridural,* and *caudal,* **15** to **20 mL** of a **3%** solution or **20** to **30 mL** of a 1 or 2% solution; *infiltration* and *nerve block in dentistry,* **0.5** to **5 mL** of a **4%** solution.

Dosage Forms—Injection: 1 and 2%/30 mL, 3%/20 mL, 4%/1.8 mL, 4% with epinephrine 1:200,000/1.8 mL.

Procaine Hydrochloride

Benzoic acid, 4-amino-, 2-(dimethylamino)ethyl ester, monohydrochloride; Novocain (*Winthrop*); Neocaine (*Fougera*)
(*Various Mfrs*)

2-(Diethylamino)ethyl *p*-aminobenzoate monohydrochloride [51-05-8] $C_{13}H_{20}N_2O_2 \cdot HCl$ (272.77).

Preparation—2-(Diethylamino)ethanol is made by reacting ethylene chlorohydrin or bromohydrin with diethylamine. The diethylaminoethanol is then heated with *p*-nitrobenzoyl chloride, forming diethylaminoethyl *p*-nitrobenzoate. The NO_2 group is reduced with iron or tin and HCl.

Description—Small, white, odorless crystals or a white crystalline powder; melts between 153° and 158°; pK_a 8.7.

Solubility—1 g in 1 mL water or 15 mL alcohol; slightly soluble in chloroform; practically insoluble in ether.

Uses—Procaine hydrochloride, an ester of *para*-aminobenzoic acid, was the preferred local anesthetic for many years, but it has now given up this position to lidocaine and other agents. It is used for *infiltration, field block, peripheral nerve block, paravertebral nerve block, epidural (caudal) block,* and *subarachnoid block (spinal analgesia) anesthesia.* It is ineffective when applied topically. Procaine hydrochloride has a slower onset of action than lidocaine or prilocaine; its duration of action is about one hr.

Procaine hydrochloride produces vasodilation and therefore vasoconstrictor drugs such as epinephrine, phenylephrine, levarterenol, or levonordefrin, may be required to retard absorption, prolong duration of action, and maintain homeostasis. Following absorption, procaine is rapidly hydrolyzed by esterases in both the plasma and liver (see introductory statement in this chapter). Since spinal fluid contains little or no esterase, procaine given by this route of administration remains active until it is absorbed into the general circulation. The products of metabolic degradation include *para*-aminobenzoic acid and diethylaminoethanol. The former inhibits the action of sulfonamides. Therefore, procaine and other ester-type local anesthetics should not be used in any condition in which therapy with sulfonamide is being employed. Procaine and its congeners also interfere with the laboratory determination of sulfonamide concentration in biological fluids. Local anesthetics other than derivatives of *para*-aminobenzoic acid should be used in all circumstances where sulfonamide therapy has been instituted. For adverse effects, see the introductory statement in this chapter.

Dose—*Infiltration:* maximum of **350** to **600 mg** as a **0.25** or **0.5%** solution. *Peripheral nerve block:* up to **200 mL** of a **0.5%** solution, **100 mL** of a **1.0%** solution, or **50 mL** of a **2%** solution. The initial dose should not exceed 1000 mg. *Subarachnoid block:* **0.5** to **2.0 mL** of a **10%** solution.

Dosage Forms—1% in 2 and 6 mL ampules, 1 and 2% in 30 mL vials, 10% in 2 mL ampules.

Tetracaine

Benzoic acid, 4-(butylamino)-, 2-(dimethylamino)ethyl ester; Pontocaine (*Breon*)

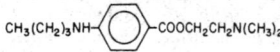

2-(Dimethylamino)ethyl   *p*-(butylamino)benzoate   [94-24-6] $C_{15}H_{24}N_2O_2$ (264.37).

Preparation—Ethyl p-aminobenzoate is butylated by refluxing with n-butyl bromide and ethanol in the presence of sodium carbonate. The resulting ethyl p-butylaminobenzoate is transesterified by heating with 2-(dimethylamino)ethanol in the presence of sodium ethoxide such that the liberated ethanol is continuously distilled from the reaction mixture.

Description—White, or light yellow, waxy solid; melting range 41° to 46°.

Solubility—1 g in 1000 mL water, 5 mL alcohol, 2 mL chloroform, 2 mL ether.

Uses—See *Tetracaine Hydrochloride.*

Dose—*Topical,* as a **0.5%** ointment, apply ¼ to 1 inch to lower conjunctival fornix. Prolonged use is not recommended.

Dosage Forms—Ointment: 0.5%; Ophthalmic Ointment: 0.5%.

Tetracaine Hydrochloride

Benzoic acid, 4-(butylamino)-, 2-(dimethylamino)ethyl ester, monohydrochloride; Amethocaine Hydrochloride; Pontacaine Hydrochloride (*Breon*); Anestaron (*Webcon*)

2-(Dimethylamino)ethyl p-(butylamino) benzoate monohydrochloride [136-47-0] $C_{15}H_{24}N_2O_2 \cdot HCl$ (300.83).

For the structure of the base see the preceding article.

Preparation—By dissolving tetracaine (base) in a solvent such as benzene and passing hydrogen chloride into the solution whereupon the salt precipitates. For the preparation of the base, see *Tetracaine.*

Description—Fine, white, crystalline, odorless powder with a slightly bitter taste followed by a sense of numbness; solutions are neutral to litmus. Melts at about 148°; 2 polymorphic modifications melt at about 134° and 139°, respectively. Mixtures of these may melt between 134° and 147°.

Solubility—Very soluble in water; soluble in alcohol; insoluble in ether and benzene.

Uses—An ester-type local anesthetic used topically on the eye and by *infiltration* for *subarachnoid block (spinal analgesia).* When used in the eye, it does not dilate the pupil, paralyze accommodation, or increase intraocular pressure. It is particularly suitable for *spinal anesthesia,* especially for surgical procedures requiring 2 to 3 hr. Tetracaine hydrochloride has a pK_a of 8.39. Although it is an ester-type local anesthetic, it is only slowly hydrolyzed by plasma and liver esterases. It has a delayed onset of action, often as long as 15 min, but a long duration of action; spinal anesthesia may last as long as 3 hr. It is also used in combination with procaine and levonordefrin to provide a rapid onset and prolonged duration of action in dental infiltration and nerve block anesthesia. Since the *para*-aminobenzoic acid metabolite of tetracaine may antagonize the activity of aminosalicylic acid and sulfonamides, it should not be used in patients receiving these drugs. For information on cautions, contraindications, and adverse effects, see the introductory statement in this chapter.

Dose—*Subarachnoid block (spinal analgesia):* **0.2** to a **1.0%** solution; *Niphanoid* (instantly soluble), perineum **5 mg,** perineum and lower extremeties **10 mg,** and up to costal margin **15 mg.** *Ophthalmic solution,* instil **1** or **2** drops.

Dosage Forms—*Injection:* 0.2 and 1.0% in 2 mL ampules, 0.3% in 5 mL ampuls, and *Niphanoid* (instantly soluble) 20 mg ampules. *Ophthalmic Solution:* 0.5% in 1, 2, and 15 mL. *Cream:* 1%.

Other Injection Anesthetics

Meprylcaine [2-Methyl-2-(propylamino)-1-propanol, benzoate ester, hydrochloride [956-03-6] $C_{14}H_{21}NO_2 \cdot HCl$ (271.79)].—*Description and Solubility:* White, odorless, crystalline solid; pH (1 in 50 solution) about 5.7. Soluble 1 g in 6 mL water, 5 mL alcohol, 3 mL chloroform, 12 mL ether; slightly soluble in acetone. *Uses:* A local anesthetic, used primarily in dentistry, with potency substantially greater than that of procaine. The drug is rapidly destroyed and hence the anesthesia induced is of relatively short duration. Acute toxicity is similar to that of procaine. See the introductory statement in this chapter. *Dose: Infiltration* and *nerve block,* 1 to 2 ml of a 2% solution with 1:50,000 epinephrine. *Dosage Forms:* Meprylcaine Hydrochloride and Epinephrine Injection: 2% meprylcaine hydrochloride and 1:50,000 epinephrine in 2, 2.5, and 20 mL containers.

Propoxycaine Hydrochloride [2-(Diethylamino)ethyl 4-amino-2-propoxybenzoate monohydrochloride [550-83-4] $C_{16}H_{26}N_2O_3 \cdot HCl$ (330.85)]—*Description and Solubility:* White, odorless, crystals which discolor on exposure to light and air; pH (2% w/v), about 5.4; pK_a 8.6.

Uses: An ester-type local anesthetic with an intermediate duration of action. When used as a *nerve block,* a 0.5% solution induces anesthesia which persists for about 2 hr. Hence, its duration of action is longer than that of procaine. Like other ester-type agents it is hydrolyzed primarily by plasma pseudocholinesterases and excreted by the kidneys. It is used for *infiltration anesthesia* and for *peripheral* and *sympathetic nerve block anesthesia.* Except for dental use, it is not usually administered with a vasoconstrictor agent. Propoxycaine hydrochloride should not be used for caudal, epidural, or spinal anesthesia. Since it shares the toxic potentials of other local anesthetics, it should be used with similar precautions. See the introductory statement in this chapter. *Dose: Usual,* 2 to 5 mL of a 0.5% solution; total dose should not exceed 20 mL. *Dosage Forms:* Injection: 150 mg/30 mL; Propoxycaine and Procaine Hydrochlorides and Norepinephrine Bitartrate Injection: 0.4%–2% and 1:20,000/2 mL.

Pyrrocaine Hydrochloride [1-Pyrrolidineacetamide, N-(2,6-dimethylphenyl)-, monohydrochloride; Endocaine Hydrochloride [2210-64-2] $C_{14}H_{20}N_2O \cdot HCl$ (268.79).]—*Description and Solubility:* White, odorless, crystals; soluble 1 g in 1.5 mL water, 12 mL alcohol, 8 mL chloroform; practically insoluble in ether. *Uses:* A 2% solution with epinephrine is used in dentistry for *infiltration* and *block anesthesia.* Clinical trials indicate that the intensity of anesthesia is similar to that obtained with the same formulation of lidocaine. Indeed, the two anesthetics appear to be approximately of the same potency and duration of action and to produce similar effects on blood pressure and heart rate. Since pyrrocaine differs in chemical structure from procaine and related compounds, it may be useful in those rare instances where the dentist or patient may be sensitive to the procaine type of local anesthetic. See introduction. *Dose: Usual, infiltration,* 1 mL of a 2% solution; *nerve block,* 1.5 to 2 mL of a 2% solution. *Other Dose Information—Usual,* 1 mL of a 2% Pyrrocaine Hydrochloride with Epinephrine (1:150,000 or 1:250,000) to be used for infiltration anesthesia and 1.5 to 2 mL to be used for nerve-block anesthesia. *Dosage Forms:* Pyrrocaine Hydrochloride and Epinephrine Injection: 2% and 1:100,000, 1:150,000 or 1:250,000/1.8 mL.

Topical Anesthetics

The salts and base forms of the esters and amides included in this section are used to produce topical (surface) anesthesia. The salts do not penetrate intact skin, but both forms penetrate abraded or raw granulated skin surfaces. The base forms relieve pruritus, burning, and surface pain on intact skin, but penetrate only to a limited degree. Wounds, ulcers, and burns are preferably treated with preparations that are relatively insoluble in tissue fluids. Mucous membranes of the nose, mouth, pharynx, larynx, trachea, bronchi, and urethra are readily anesthetized by both salt and base forms. Consequently, these agents are used prior to inserting intratracheal catheters, pharyngeal and nasal airways, nasogastric and endoscopic tubes, urinary catheters, laryngoscopes, proctoscopes, sigmoidoscopes, and vaginal specula. Many of these agents are also used in the eye for such procedures as tonometry, gonioscopy, and for removal of foreign bodies from the cornea, or for short operative procedures on the cornea or conjunctiva. For precautions, warnings, and adverse effects see the introductory statement in this chapter.

Benzocaine

Benzoic acid, 4-amino-, ethyl ester; Benzocaine; Anesthesin; Ethyl Aminobenzoate Solarcaine (*Plough*) and *Various Mfrs*

$$NH_2 - \langle \bigcirc \rangle - COOC_2H_5$$

Ethyl p-aminobenzoate [94-09-7] $C_9H_{11}NO_2$ (165.19).

Preparation—p-Nitrobenzoic acid, obtained by nitration of toluene and oxidation of the resulting p-nitrotoluene, is converted into the ethyl ester by heating with alcohol and sulfuric acid. The resulting ethyl p-nitrobenzoate is reduced with tin and hydrochloric acid.

Description—Small, white, odorless crystals or as a white crystalline powder; melts within a 2°-range between 88° and 92°.

Solubility—1 g in about 2500 mL water, 5 mL alcohol, 2 mL chloroform, 4 mL ether, 30 to 50 mL expressed almond oil or olive oil; also soluble in dilute mineral acids.

Uses—An insoluble *local anesthetic*. It is usually employed as an ointment to relieve pain associated with *ulcers*, *wounds*, and mucous surfaces. It is also used as a lubricant and anesthetic on intratracheal catheters, pharyngeal and nasal airways, nasogastric and endoscopic tubes, etc. Benzocaine is included in proprietary creams, lozenges, ointments, powders, sprays, and suppositories to relieve pain of denuded skin surfaces and inflamed mucous membranes, particularly those in the anorectal area. It acts only as long as it is in contact with the skin or mucosal surface. For adverse reactions, see the introductory statement in this chapter.

Dose—*Topical*, as a 1 to **20%** aerosol, cream, or ointment to the skin.

Dosage Forms—Aerosol: 9.4, 10, 13.6, and 20%; Cream: 1 and 5%; Lotion: 0.5%; Liquid or Gel: 2 and 6.3%; Ointment: 1, 2, 5, 10, and 20%; Spray: 20%.

Cocaine

8-Azabicyclo[3.2.1]octane-2-carboxylic acid, 3-(benzoyloxy)-8-methyl-, methyl ester, [1*R*-(*exo,exo*)]-,

Methyl 3β-hydroxy-1αH,5αH-tropane-2β-carboxylate benzoate (ester) [50-36-2] $C_{17}H_{21}NO_4$ (303.36); an alkaloid obtained from the leaves of *Erythroxylon coca* Lamarck and other species of *Erythroxylon* Linné (Fam. *Erythroxylaceae*), or by synthesis from ecgonine or its derivatives.

History—Isolated by Gaedken in 1844 from Brazilian coca leaves, which for many years was the only source of cocaine. At present the alkaloid is obtained principally from Java coca leaves. Brazilian coca leaves contain from 0.5 to 1% of methylbenzoylecgonine or cocaine, whereas the Java leaves contain very little cocaine as such. However, there are present in the latter such derivatives as benzoylecgonine, cinnamoylecgonine, methylecgonine, etc., to the extent of 1.5 to 2%, all of which are converted to cocaine in the manufacturing process. For the structural relationships among the ecgonine derivatives, see page 418.

Preparation—By moistening ground coca leaves with sodium carbonate solution, percolating with benzene or other solvents such as petroleum benzin, shaking the liquid with diluted sulfuric acid, and adding to the separated acid solution an excess of sodium carbonate. The precipitated alkaloids are removed with ether, and, after drying with sodium carbonate, the solution is filtered and the ether distilled off. The residue is dissolved in methyl alcohol and the solution heated with sulfuric acid or with alcoholic hydrogen chloride. This treatment splits off any acids from ecgonine and esterifies the carboxyl group. After dilution with water, the organic acids which have been liberated are removed with chloroform. The aqueous solution is then concentrated, neutralized, and cooled with ice, whereupon methylecgonine sulfate crystallizes. This is now benzoylated by heating with benzoyl chloride or benzoic anhydride at about 150°C. On adding water and sodium hydroxide, methylbenzoylecgonine or cocaine is precipitated. The cocaine is extracted with ether and the solution concentrated to crystallization. For the purification of cocaine, recrystallization from a mixture of acetone and benzene is generally preferred.

Total synthesis of cocaine was achieved by Willstätter *et al*, *Ann 434*: 111, 1923.

Description—Colorless to white crystals, or a white, crystalline powder that is odorless; melts between 96° and 98° and its solution in diluted HCl is levorotatory; saturated solution is alkaline to litmus.

Solubility—1 g in about 600 mL water, 7 mL alcohol, 1 mL chloroform, 3.5 mL ether, about 12 mL olive oil, and from 80 to 100 mL liquid petrolatum; very soluble in warm alcohol.

Uses—The first local anesthetic to be discovered. While it is considered too toxic for any anesthetic procedure requiring injection, it is still employed topically in a 1 or 2% solution for anesthesia of the ear, nose, throat, rectum, and vagina. Concentrations as high as 20% have been used to anesthetize the nose and throat. Toxic symptoms occur frequently because cocaine is absorbed readily and dosage is often not carefully monitored. Central nervous system effects include

euphoria and cortical stimulation manifested by excitement and restlessness. Stimulation of the lower motor centers causes hypertension, tachycardia, and tachypnea. Repeated use results in psychic dependence and tolerance, the euphoric effects of which are almost indistinguishable from those induced by amphetamines. Indeed, knowledgeable human subjects cannot distinguish between the subjective effects induced by the intravenous injection of 8 to 10 mg of cocaine and those induced by 10 mg of dextroamphetamine. Cocaine is listed under *Schedule II* of the *Controlled Substances Act*. For adverse reactions see the introductory statement in this chapter.

Dose—*Topical*, to mucous membranes, as a 1% solution.

Dosage Forms—Powder: in 7.5 and 30 g; Soluble Tablets: 135 mg.

Cocaine Hydrochloride

8-Azabicyclo[3.2.1]octane-2-carboxylic acid, 3-(benzoyloxy)-8-methyl-, methyl ester, hydrochloride, [1*R*-(*exo,exo*)]-, Neurocaine Hydrochloride

Methyl 3β-hydroxy-1αH,5αH-tropan-2β-carboxylate, benzoate (ester) hydrochloride [53-21-4] $C_{17}H_{21}NO_4 \cdot HCl$ (339.82).

Preparation—By adding cocaine to an alcoholic solution of hydrochloric acid and crystallizing.

Description—Colorless crystals or a white crystalline powder.

Solubility—1 g in 0.5 mL water, 3.5 mL alcohol, and 15 mL chloroform; soluble in glycerin and insoluble in ether.

Uses—In solution as a *local anesthetic* when applied to the mucous membrane or injected hypodermically; it is also a cerebral stimulant. For adverse effects, see the introductory statement in this chapter.

Dose—*Topical*, as a 1 to 4% solution, to mucous membranes.

Dosage Forms—Topical Solution: 2 to 10%; 40 or 100 mg per mL in 4 mL unit dose capsules.

Cyclomethycaine Sulfate

Benzoic acid, 4-(cyclohexyloxy)-, 3-(2-methyl-1-piperidinyl)propyl ester sulfate (1:1); Surfacaine (*Lilly*)

3-(2-Methylpiperidino)propyl *p*-(cyclohexyloxy)benzoate sulfate (1:1) [50978-10-4] $C_{22}H_{33}NO_3 \cdot H_2SO_4$ (457.58).

Preparation—One method esterifies *p*-chlorobenzoyl chloride with 2-methyl-1-piperidinepropanol, then introduces the cyclohexyloxy group through reaction with sodium cyclohexyl oxide, and treats the resulting cyclomethylcaine (base) with H_2SO_4.

Description—White, odorless, crystalline powder; melts between 162° and 165.5°.

Solubility—1 g in 50 mL water, 50 mL alcohol, 250 mL chloroform; very slightly soluble in dilute acids.

Uses—A topical anesthetic and lubricant used on nontraumatized, accessible mucous membranes prior to clinical examination and instrumentation. It is particularly useful for pain originating in mucous membranes of the rectum, vagina, urethra, and urinary bladder, and in various proctologic, gynecologic, and urologic manipulations. It is relatively ineffective in anesthetizing the mucous membranes of the mouth, nose, trachea, bronchi, eye, and ear. As with all topical anesthetic agents, cyclomethycaine sulfate carries a slight but predictable sensitizing potential when utilized on patients with allergies or in conditions of prolonged use. For adverse reactions, see the introductory statement in this chapter.

Dose—*Topical*, **0.25 to 1.0%** in suitable form.

Dosage Forms—Cream: 0.5%; Jelly: 0.75%; Ointment: 1%.

Dibucaine—page 1050.

Dibucaine Hydrochloride—page 1050.

Dimethisoquin Hydrochloride

Ethanamine, 2-[(3-butyl-1-isoquinolinyl)oxy]-*N*,*N*-dimethyl-, monohydrochloride; Quotane (*Menley & James*)

3-Butyl-1-[2-(dimethylamino)ethoxy]isoquinoline monohydrochloride [2773-92-4] $C_{17}H_{24}N_2O.HCl$ (308.85).

Preparation—A solution of α-n-butylphenethylamine in an organic solvent is reacted with phosgene to form α-butylphenethyl isocyanate which, on heating with anhydrous aluminum chloride, cyclizes through rearrangement to produce 3-n-butyl-3,4-dihydro-1(2H)-isoquinolone. Catalytic dehydrogenation at the 3,4-positions, followed by reaction of phosphorus oxychloride on the lactim form of the dehydrogenated compound, yields 3-n-butyl-1-chloroisoquinoline. Condensation with β-dimethylaminoethanol is then effected by treating a solution of the two compounds in an inert organic solvent with metallic sodium. The crude dimethisoquin base thus formed is purified by distillation under reduced pressure, and converted to the hydrochloride with HCl.

Description—White to off-white, odorless, crystalline powder; melting range 144° to 148°; pH (1 in 100 solution) between 3.5 and 5.5.

Solubility—1 g in about 8 mL water, 2 mL chloroform, and 3 mL alcohol; very slightly soluble in ether.

Uses—A quinoline-type surface anesthetic which is used topically in a 0.5% ointment for the relief of itching, irritation, burning or pain in dermatoses, including nonspecific pruritus, and mild sunburn. Onset of action is rapid (few minutes) and duration of action persists for 2 to 4 hr. It is less toxic than dibucaine, but somewhat more toxic than procaine. For adverse effects, see the introductory statement in this chapter.

Dose—*Topical*, to the skin, as a **0.5**% ointment 2 to 4 times a day.

Dosage Forms—Ointment: 0.5%.

Diperodon

1,2-Propanediol, 3-(1-piperidinyl)-, bis(phenylcarbamate) (ester), monohydrate; Diothane (*Merrell-Dow*)

3-Piperidino-1,2-propanediol dicarbanilate (ester) monohydrate [51552-99-9] $C_{22}H_{27}N_3O_4.H_2O$ (415.49); *anhydrous* [101-08-6] (397.47).

Preparation—Piperidine is condensed with 3-chloro-1,2-propanediol with the aid of alkali and the resulting 3-piperidino-1,2-propanediol undergoes addition to phenyl isocyanate to yield diperodon. US Pat 2,004,132.

Description—White to cream-colored powder having a characteristic odor.

Solubility—Insoluble in water.

Uses and **Doses**—See *Diperodon Hydrochloride*.

Dosage Forms—Ointment: 1%.

Diperodon Hydrochloride

1,2-Propanediol, 3-(1-piperidinyl)-, bis(phenylcarbamate) (ester), monohydrochloride; Diothane Hydrochloride (*Merrell-Dow*); Proctodon (*Rowell*)

3-Piperidino-1,2-propanediol dicarbanilate (ester) monohydrochloride [537-12-2] $C_{22}H_{27}N_3O_4.HCl$ (433.93).

Preparation—*Diperodon* is reacted with HCl.

Description—White crystals.

Solubility—Soluble in alcohol; slightly soluble in water.

Uses—A *local anesthetic*, particularly useful on damaged skin or mucous membranes, primarily the anus. Potency when used for surface anesthesia is similar to cocaine. Toxicity after intravenous injection is three times that of procaine. Therefore, its use has been restricted to surface anesthesia. Adverse reactions include burning or stinging of skin or mucous membrane and allergic manifestations.

Dose—*Local*, 1% solution.

Dosage Forms—Cream: 1%.

Dyclonine Hydrochloride

1-Propanone, 1-(4-butoxyphenyl)-3-(1-piperidinyl)-, Dyclone (*Merrell-Dow*)

4′-Butoxy-3-piperidinopropiophenone hydrochloride [536-43-6] $C_{18}H_{27}NO_2.HCl$ (325.88).

Preparation—p-Hydroxyacetophenone is reacted with butyl bromide in a basic environment to produce the butoxy compound, which is reacted with piperidine hydrochloride and formaldehyde in an organic solvent under acidic conditions. US Pat 2,771,391 and 2,868,689.

Description—White crystals or white, crystalline powder, which may have a slight odor; melts between 173° and 178°; pH (1 in 100 solution) between 4.0 and 7.0.

Solubility—Soluble in water, acetone, alcohol, and chloroform.

Uses—Dyclonine hydrochloride is used to anesthetize accessible mucous membranes (eg, the mouth, pharynx, larynx, trachea, esophagus, and urethra) prior to various endoscopic procedures. The 0.5% solution may also be used to block the gag reflex and to relieve pain associated with oral or anogenital lesions. It is contraindicated in cystoscopic procedures following intravenous pyelography; the drug precipitates iodine and interferes with visualization. When instilled into the conjunctival sac, it induces anesthesia without miosis or mydriasis. Dyclonine hydrochloride also has antimicrobial properties. The clinical significance of this property has not been determined. For adverse effects, see the introductory statement in this chapter.

Dose—*Topical*, as a **0.5** to **1**% solution, to the mucous membranes.

Dosage Forms—Solution: 0.5 and 1%.

Ethyl Chloride—page 1041.

Hexylcaine Hydrochloride

2-Propanol, 1-(cyclohexylamino)-, benzoate (ester), hydrochloride; Cyclaine (*MSD*)

1-(Cyclohexylamino)-2-propanol benzoate (ester) hydrochloride [532-76-3] $C_{16}H_{23}NO_2.HCl$ (297.82).

Preparation—A solution of 1-(cyclohexylamino)-2-propanol (I) in a solvent composed of benzene and tetrachloroethane is treated with benzoyl chloride. Esterification and salt formation occur simultaneously. I may be prepared by causing cyclohexylamine to undergo either addition to propylene oxide or condensation with α-propylene chlorohydrin.

Description—White powder, possessing a bitter taste and not more than a slight aromatic odor; melting range 182° to 184°; pH (1 in 20 solution) between 4.0 and 6.0.

Solubility—1 g in about 17 mL water; freely soluble in alcohol and chloroform; practically insoluble in ether.

Uses—A benzoic acid ester used for *surface anesthesia* of intact mucous membranes in endoscopy, intubations, and manipulations in the respiratory, upper gastrointestinal, and urinary tracts. Anesthesia is induced within 5 min and persists for about 30 min. Hexylcaine is not used by injection because of its great local and systemic toxicity when administered by this route. Hexylcaine is about $\frac{1}{4}$ as toxic as topically applied cocaine. Tissue irritation, burning, swelling, and tissue necrosis have been reported. For additional information on adverse reactions and precautions, see introductory statement in this chapter. Hexylcaine hydrochloride shares the toxic potentialities of other local anesthetic agents and should be employed with the same care and in accordance with established techniques of administration.

Dose—*Topical*, **5**%, according to site and condition.

Dosage Form—Solution: 5%.

Lidocaine—page 1051.
Lidocaine Hydrochloride—page 1051.

Phenacaine Hydrochloride

Ethanimidamide, N,N'-bis(4-ethoxyphenyl)-, monohydrochloride, monohydrate; Holocaine Hydrochloride

N,N'-Bis(p-ethoxyphenyl)acetamidine monohydrochloride monohydrate [6153-19-1] $C_{18}H_{22}N_2O_2.HCl.H_2O$ (352.86); *anhydrous* [620-99-5] $C_{18}H_{22}N_2O_2.HCl$ (334.84).

Preparation—Among other methods, by condensing phenetidine with acetophenetidine, using phosphorus oxychloride as the condensing agent.

Description—Small, white, odorless crystals or crystalline powder; faintly bitter taste; melts not below 190°.

Solubility—1 g in 50 mL water; freely soluble in alcohol or chloroform; insoluble in ether.

Uses—One of the oldest of the synthetic *local anesthetics*. It is used in a 1% solution mainly for producing local *anesthesia of the eye*. It is slightly irritating. Therefore, anesthesia is preceded by some smarting and discomfort. For adverse effects, see the introductory statement in this chapter.

Dose—To the conjunctiva as a 1% solution or as a 1 to 2% ointment.

Dosage Forms—Ophthalmic Ointment: 1 and 2%; Solution: 1%.

Piperocaine Hydrochloride—page 1052.

Pramoxine Hydrochloride

Morpholine, 4-[3-(4-butoxyphenoxy)propyl]-, hydrochloride; Tronothane; Tronolane (*Abbott*)

4-[3-(p-Butoxyphenoxy)propyl]morpholine hydrochloride [637-58-1] $C_{17}H_{27}NO_3.HCl$ (329.87).

Preparation—An aqueous mixture of 4-(3-chloropropyl)morpholine and p-butoxyphenol is refluxed until condensation is complete. The reaction mixture is cooled and the pramoxine (base) is extracted with benzene. After evaporation of the benzene, the purified base is converted to the hydrochloride with HCl.

Description—White to nearly white, crystalline powder, having a numbing taste; may have a slight aromatic odor; pH (1 in 100 solution) about 4.5; melting range 170° to 174°.

Solubility—1 g in about 35 mL chloroform; freely soluble in alcohol and water; very slightly soluble in ether.

Uses—A surface anesthetic which has low indices of sensitization and toxicity, and is unrelated structurally to either ester- or amide-type agents. Consequently, it may be useful in patients sensitive to these classes of drugs. Local anesthesia develops in 3 to 5 min; its potency is comparable to that of benzocaine. It is applied locally in a 1% concentration for the relief from discomfort and pain in hemorrhoids and rectal surgery, episiotomies, anogenital pruritus, itching dermatoses, and minor burns. It is too irritating to be used in the eye. For adverse effects, see introduction.

Dose—*Topical*, as a 1% cream or jelly every 3 to 4 hours.

Dosage Forms—Cream: 1%; Jelly: 1%. (Tronothane); Cream and Suppositories (Tronolane).

Proparacaine Hydrochloride

Benzoic acid, 3-amino-4-propoxy-, 2-(diethylamino)ethyl ester monohydrochloride; Alcaine (*Alcon*); Ophthaine (*Squibb*); Ophthetic (*Allergan*)

2-(Diethylamino)ethyl 3-amino-4-propoxybenzoate monohydrochloride [5875-06-9] $C_{16}H_{26}N_2O_3.HCl$ (330.85).

Preparation—p-Hydroxybenzoic acid is reacted with n-propyl chloride in alkaline solution and the resulting p-propoxybenzoic acid is nitrated to the 3-nitro compound. Treatment with thionyl chloride yields the acid chloride, which is coupled with 2-(diethylamino)ethanol. The resulting nitro ester is reduced to proparacaine base, which reacts with an equimolar quantity of HCl to form the hydrochloride.

Description—White to off-white, or faintly buff-colored, odorless, crystalline powder; on heating or exposure to air the compound tends to discolor; solutions exposed to air slowly discolor and finally become dark, with some loss of potency; crystals melt within a 2° range between 178° and 185°.

Solubility—1 g in about 30 mL water and 30 mL warm alcohol or methanol; insoluble in ether and benzene.

Uses—An effective surface anesthetic with a potency about equal to that of tetracaine. It is a useful anesthetic in ophthalmology and induces little or no initial irritation. Its onset of action is rapid; surface anesthesia of sufficient intensity to permit tonometry can generally be obtained within about 20 sec after the instillation of 1 or 2 drops of a 0.5% solution. The duration of such anesthesia is about 15 min. Proparacaine hydrochloride is useful for most ocular procedures that require topical anesthesia such as tonometry, removal of foreign bodies and sutures, gonioscopy, conjunctival scraping for diagnosis, and short operative procedures involving the cornea and conjunctiva. Deep anesthesia suitable for cataract extraction can be achieved by the instillation of 1 drop of a 0.5% solution every 5 to 10 min for 5 to 7 doses. Although proparacaine is too toxic for use as an injection anesthetic, its ophthalmic use has been relatively free from side effects of untoward reactions. For adverse effects, see the introductory statement in this chapter.

Dose—*Topically, removal of sutures:* 1 or 2 **drops** instilled 2 or 3 minutes before removal of sutures; *removal of foreign objects:* instill 1 or 2 **drops** prior to operating; *tonometry:* 1 or 2 **drops** immediately before measurement.

Dosage Forms—Ophthalmic Solution: 0.5%.

Tetracaine—page 1053.

Tetracaine Hydrochloride—page 1054.

Other Topical Anesthetics

Benoxinate Hydrochloride [4-Amino-3-butoxybenzoic acid, 2-(diethylamino)ethyl ester, monohydrochloride; Fluress (*Barnes-Hind*) [5987-82-6] $C_{17}H_{28}N_2O_3.HCl$ (344.88)].—*Description and Solubility:* White, odorless, crystals, or crystalline powder with a salty taste; melts at about 155°. Very soluble in water and chloroform; soluble in alcohol; insoluble in ether. *Uses:* A benzoic acid ester related to procaine, it is an effective *surface anesthetic* useful in ophthalmology. It also has bacteriostatic properties. Benoxinate hydrochloride is used in a 0.4% solution for tonometry, gonioscopy, and for short operative procedures involving the cornea and conjunctiva or in combination with the disclosing agent, Fluorescein Sodium (0.25%), for removal of foreign bodies in the cornea. A single instillation produces significant anesthesia within 60 sec and 2 drops in each eye at 90-sec intervals for 3 instillations induces sufficient anesthesia for removal of foreign objects from the cornea; full anesthesia persists for 20 to 30 min, and the sensitivity of the cornea returns to normal in 1 hr. Although signs of hypersensitivity have followed prolonged use in the eye, it should be used with the usual precautions for surface anesthesia, and should be used sparingly in patients with allergies, cardiac disease, hyperthyroidism, or open lesions. *Dose: Topical,* in the eye, 0.05 to 0.2 mL of 0.4% solution. *Dosage Forms:* Ophthalmic Solution: 0.4%; Ophthalmic Solution 0.4% with Fluorescein Sodium 0.25%.

Benzyl Alcohol [100-51-6] C_7H_8O (108.14).]—*Preparation:* Occurs in nature as the esters of benzoic and cinnamic acids in storax, Peruvian balsam, and tolu balsam. The commercial product is prepared by synthesis, as by hydrolysis of benzyl chloride, or from benzaldehyde. *Description and Solubility:* Colorless liquid with a sharp, burning taste and a faint aromatic odor; specific gravity between 1.042 and 1.047 at 25°; distils between 202.5° and 206.5°, and has a refractive index of 1.539 to 1.541; boils without decomposition at about 206°; slowly oxidizes in the air; aqueous solutions are neutral to litmus. *Soluble:* 1 g in about 30 mL water, or 1.5 mL diluted alcohol; miscible with alcohol, ether, and chloroform. *Uses:* Used in a 4% solution for *topical block anesthesia*. However, other agents such as lidocaine, hexylcaine, and tetracaine are more effective.

Butacaine Sulfate [3-(Dibutylamino)-1-propanol, 4-aminobenzoate (ester), sulfate (salt) (2:1); Butyn Sulfate (*Abbott*) [149-15-5] $(C_{18}H_{30}N_2O_2)_2.H_2SO_4$ (710.97)]— *Description and Solubility:* White to practically white, practically odorless, crystalline powder that is affected by light; solutions are very weakly acidic; melts at about 100°. *Soluble:* 1 g in 1.5 mL water, 2 mL alcohol, 2.5 mL chloroform, 2000 mL ether.

Uses: For *local anesthesia*, particularly of the eye. It is a more active local anesthetic than either cocaine or procaine. Its action is more prolonged and more rapid than that of cocaine. Locally, it is more toxic than procaine, but less toxic than cocaine. Parenterally, it is more toxic than cocaine. It acts through intact mucous membranes. *Dose:* Several instillations of a 2% solution about 3 min apart permit most surgical procedures. *Dosage Forms:* Solution: 2%; Ophthalmic Solution: 2%; Powder: 5 and 30 g.

Butamben [4-Amino-benzoic acid, butyl ester; Butesin (*Abbott*) [94-25-7] $C_{11}H_{15}NO_2$ (193.24).]—*Description and Solubility:* White, odorless, and tasteless crystalline powder; when boiled with water it slowly hydrolyzes to *para*-aminobenzoic acid and butyl alcohol: alkali hydroxides accelerate the hydrolysis. *Soluble:* 1 g in about 7000 mL water; soluble in dilute acids, alcohol, chloroform, or ether and in fixed oils. *Uses:* A *local anesthetic* of low solubility used on the skin to relieve pruritus and burning. See Butamben Picrate.

Chlorobutanol—page 1278.

Butamben Picrate [Butesin Picrate (*Abbott*)]—A compound of one molecule of trinitrophenol and two molecules of butyl *p*-aminobenzoate. *Uses:* For temporary relief of pain due to minor burns. The drug should be discontinued if a rash develops following its use. *Dose:* As a 1% ointment.

Clove Oil [Oleum Caryophylli BP; Oil of Cloves]—The volatile oil distilled with steam from the dried flower buds of *Eugenia caryophyllus* (Sprengel) Bullock et Harrison (formerly *E caryophyllata* Thunberg) (Fam *Myrtaceae*); contains not less than 85.0% by volume of total phenolic substances, chiefly eugenol ($C_{10}H_{12}O_2$). *Constituents:* The chief constituent is the phenol *eugenol* (this page) which occurs in amounts up to 85%. The odor of the oil is modified by the presence of less than 1% of *methyl pentyl ketone*. Other constituents include about 3% of *acetyleugenol*, a mixture of the sesquiterpenes α- and β-*caryophyllene*, and small amounts of *furfural, furfuryl alcohol, methyl heptyl ketone*, the methyl esters of *salicylic* and *benzoic acids*, the benzyl ester of *phenylacetic acid, vanillin*, and *caryophyllin* [$C_{30}H_{48}O_3$]. The percentage of eugenol present is regarded as an index to the oil's quality. *Description:* Colorless or pale yellow liquid, becoming darker and thicker by aging or exposure to air, and having the characteristic odor and taste of clove; specific gravity 1.038 to 1.060 at 25°; refractive index 1.527 to 1.535 at 20°; soluble in 2 volumes of 70% alcohol. *Uses:* A *germicide* but too irritant for most purposes. It is applied topically to alleviate toothache (see *Toothache Drops*, page 1507). It acts as an *obtundent*, relieving pain caused by exposed dentine. *Dose:* Topical, to dental cavities, as required.

Eugenol 2-Methoxy-4-(2-propenyl)phenol; Synthetic Clove Oil [97-53-0] $C_{10}H_{12}O_2$ (164.20); obtained from clove oil and from the other sources.]—*Preparation:* Found in the volatile oils from clove, pimenta, bay leaves, Ceylon cinnamon, camphor, sassafras, canella, and other oils. It is principally obtained, however, from clove oil. The oil is treated with an excess of NaOH solution which dissolves the eugenol and the mixture is then shaken with ether to remove the other constituents: The aqueous solution of sodium eugenol is acidified, and the separated eugenol is purified by distillation. *Description and Solubilities:* Colorless or pale yellow liquid, having a strongly aromatic odor of clove and a pungent, spicy taste; exposure to air causes it to become darker and thicker; specific gravity 1.064 to 1.070; refractive index 1.540 to 1.542 at 20°; distils between 250° and 255°. Slightly soluble in water; miscible with alcohol, chloroform, ether, and fixed oils; soluble in twice its volume of 70% alcohol. *Uses:* A *dental obtundent* and *topical anesthetic* used extensively to replace clove oil, principally by dentists, who also employ it for its disinfectant action in filing root canals. Eugenol is no longer administered internally. It is the basic material in one of the processes for the production of vanillin.

CHAPTER 57

Sedatives and Hypnotics

Ewart A Swinyard, PhD, DSc (Hon)
Professor Emeritus of Pharmacology
College of Pharmacy and School of Medicine
University of Utah
Salt Lake City, UT 84112

The term *sedative* refers to a quieting effect accompanied by relaxation and rest, but not necessarily sleep. Sedative drugs are used to allay excitement and reduce motor activity without inducing sleep. The term *hypnotic* refers to the production of sleep. Hence, hypnotic drugs are used to induce sleep when sleeplessness is not due to a definite stimulus, such as pain, dyspnea, or itching which prevents sleep or awakens the patient. Both sedative and hypnotic actions may reside in the same drug; a small dose of a drug may act as a sedative, whereas a large dose of the same drug may act as a hypnotic.

Agents used as sedatives and hypnotics include a large number of compounds of diverse chemical structure and pharmacological properties which have in common the ability to induce a nonselective, reversible depression of the central nervous system. Thus, inorganic salts (bromide), chloral derivatives (chloral hydrate), acetylenic alcohols (ethchlorvynol), cyclic ethers (paraldehyde), carbamic acid esters of alcohols (ethinamate), carbamic acid esters of glycols (meprobamate), diureides (barbiturates), piperidinedione derivatives (glutethimide), disubstituted quinazolones (methaqualone), benzodiazepines (chlordiazepoxide), and some miscellaneous aromatic tertiary alkylamines, such as antihistaminics (diphenhydramine), precursors of serotonin (L-tryptophan and 5-hydroxytryptophan), and parasympatholytics (scopolamine) all exhibit pronounced sedative and hypnotic effects. Some of these agents, such as diphenhydramine and scopolamine, exhibit primary pharmacological actions which dictate they should be classified in other sections of this text. On the other hand, agents such as flurazepam, nitrazepam, pentobarbital, meprobamate and related agents exhibit primary pharmacological actions which characterize them as sedative and hypnotic agents. Ideed, the benzodiazepines are the only class of hypnotic drugs proven effective for promoting sleep beyond 14 days of consecutive use. For convenience, the sedatives and hypnotics presented herein will be divided into three groups: benzodiazepines; barbiturates; and miscellaneous sedative and hypnotic agents.

Agents included in this chapter are used as *sedatives*, *hypnotics*, *anticonvulsants*, *preanesthetic medication*, and *diagnostic* and *therapeutic aids* in psychiatry. As *sedatives*, they are used in the management of neuroses and to allay the anxiety and apprehension which accompany various disease states, such as hypertension, cardiac failure, and coronary artery disease. Anxiety is perceived as a pervasive feeling of apprehension about some unspecified future threat to self esteem. This threat is assumed to arise within the person, perhaps based on a memory of a past threat triggered by some unrecognized present situation. The memory may signal the emotions and the somatic responses of the past fearful state. The somatic manifestations of anxiety include fatigue, dizziness, palpitations, indigestion, bowel disturbances, headaches, muscle aches, insomnia, excessive perspiration, tremulousness of the hands or voice, and other signs of nervous tension. Anxiety may be a primary symptom associated with emotional disorders or a secondary symptom of physical illness. In either case, it can be extremely disabling and worthy of careful diagnosis and treatment.

As *hypnotics*, they are used to induce sleep. The choice of hypnotic agent depends to a large extent on the characteristics of the insomnia. Some patients have difficulty only in falling asleep and, once asleep, need no drug assistance; a rapidly acting hypnotic drug with a short duration of action will suffice for these patients. Other patients fall asleep readily, but experience one or more periods of wakefulness during the night; a hypnotic drug with a long duration of action is usually indicated in such cases. Still other patients have trouble falling and in staying asleep; a rapidly acting hypnotic drug which exerts an effect throughout part or most of the night is required for such patients. In all cases, however, consideration should be given to what the patient does on the day following a night of drug-induced sleep. Persons who must be alert the following day will usually object to drugs which leave residual sedation, whereas hospitalized patients, or individuals with no place to go and nothing to do may actually benefit from such after effects.

It should be remembered that not all patients with insomnia require hypnotic drug therapy. Moreover, there are many instances where nonhypnotic drugs are superior to hypnotic drugs. For example, methylphenidate may improve sleep in some hyperkinetic patients, phenytoin in patients with insomnia due to paroxysmal nightmares, analgesics when sleep is impaired by pain, antithyroid drugs or beta-blockers when sleep is difficult due to hyperthyroidism, bethanechol or similar drugs in nocturnal gastroesophageal reflux, cimetidine in peptic ulcers, and others. Nonspecific hypnotic therapy should be employed only in those cases where specific causes of the insomnia *cannot* be identified and eliminated.

A number of these agents have *anticonvulsant* properties. Several benzodiazepines have excellent anticonvulsant actions and some are used in epilepsy. Clonazepam is used alone or as an adjunct in the management of absence (petit mal), petit mal variant, and, especially, akinetic and myoclonic seizures. Diazepam is used as adjunctive therapy in status epilepticus and severe recurrent seizures. All barbiturates exhibit anticonvulsant activity, but only phenobarbital, mephobarbital, and metharbital are sufficiently selective to be clinically useful *antiepileptics*. Phenobarbital is useful in the management of generalized tonic-clonic seizures and as adjunctive therapy in complex partial (temporal lobe) seizures.

Sedative and hypnotic agents are frequently used as *preanesthetic medication* and as *adjunctive therapy* in psychiatry. Benzodiazepines and barbiturates are commonly used to allay anxiety and apprehension prior to surgery. In psychiatry, barbiturates with a short half-life have been used in *narcoanalysis* and *narcotherapy*.

A number of the sedative-hypnotic drugs cross the placental barrier. Consequently, their chronic use during pregnancy may cause withdrawal effects in the newborn infant. Moreover, many of these substances are excreted in breast milk. Their chronic use during breast feeding may cause sedation in the nursing infant. Drowsiness is a side effect common to all sedative-hypnotic agents. Patients taking such substances should be cautioned about operating hazardous machinery or operating a motor vehicle while taking such medication. Concurrent use of sedative-hypnotic drugs with alcohol, other central nervous system depressants, MAO inhibitors or tricyclic antidepressants should be avoided. More detailed information with respect to adverse effects and drug interactions is provided in the introductory statement to each section and in the individual monographs.

Prolonged overdosage with most of these drugs can result in habituation and dependence liability. However, the "dependence risk" varies markedly among the various agents. For example, the dependence risk with benzodiazepines is very low and is estimated at one case per 5 million patient-months "at risk" for all recorded cases and probably one case per 50 million months in therapeutic use. Accordingly, flurazepam, chlordiazepoxide, diazepam and other benzodiazepines are listed in *Schedule IV* under the *Controlled Substances Act*. On the other hand, the dependence risk with methaqualone, amobarbital, pentobarbital and related substances is very high, with severe abuse potential. Consequently, these agents are listed in *Schedule II* under the *Controlled Substances Act*. It should be emphasized that with usual hypnotic doses and close medical supervision, the problem of dependence with these agents can be minimized. Nevertheless, they should be used with extreme caution, if at all, in patients with a history of previous drug dependence.

Benzodiazepines

This group includes the most frequently prescribed sedative-hypnotic agents. In 1980 the benzodiazepines accounted for 3.7% of all new prescriptions as compared with 0.8% for the barbiturates. Although physicians are only grudgingly giving up the barbiturates, it is now generally agreed that the benzodiazepines represent a significant advance in the management of the clinical conditions in which these agents are indicated.

The benzodiazepines are not general depressants of the central nervous system of the order of barbiturates, ethanol, various other sedative-hypnotic agents and general anesthetics. There are marked differences among the various agents in selectivity, pharmacological profile, and clinical usefulness. Moreover, they do not induce a true "anesthetic effect," since awareness is still present and muscular relaxation is not obtained even after large doses. Retrograde amnesia may occur and this creates the illusion that anesthesia has occurred. True surgical anesthesia can only be obtained when benzodiazepines are combined with other drugs which depress the central nervous system.

Gamma-aminobutyric acid (GABA) is a major inhibitory neurotransmitter in the mammalian central nervous system. It is generally believed that the benzodiazepines exert at least some of their actions via the inhibitory neurotransmitter GABA. The benzodiazepines potentiate GABA-mediated inhibitory neurotransmission and antagonize seizures caused by GABA depletion. *In vitro* binding studies support a GABA-benzodiazepine interaction. GABA stimulates [^{3}H]diazepam binding to synaptosomal membranes. The neurophysiological and biochemical evidence indicates that a GABA-benzodiazepine-chloride ionophore comprises a supramolecular structure. Therefore, an interaction between a benzodiazepine and its receptors stimulates GABA receptors and activates chloride channels. The cellular mechanisms of the benzodiazepines have been reviewed by Study and Barker (*JAMA*, *247*, 2147–2151, 1982).

The benzodiazepines are used in the symptomatic relief of anxiety and tension states resulting from a stressful environment or emotional factors. They are also useful in psychoneurotic states characterized by tension, anxiety, apprehension, fatigue, depression symptoms or agitation. Certain benzodiazepines (chlordiazepoxide and diazepam) are also useful in acute alcohol withdrawal to provide symptomatic relief from acute agitation, tremors, and impending delirium tremens and hallucinosis. Clonazepam is useful alone or as an adjunct in the management of several types of epileptic seizures. Diazepam is useful as an adjunct therapy to endoscopic procedures, to the management of acute skeletal muscle spasm, and, by parenteral injection, to status epilepticus, to control convulsions resulting from overdosage with local anesthetics, and other severe recurrent convulsive seizures. The benzodiazepines are also useful adjunct therapy in the management of apprehension and anxiety which precedes or accompanies surgical procedures and disease states.

Benzodiazepines markedly influence CNS activity of humans in both the waking and sleeping state. In the waking human EEG, alpha activity is decreased, fast activity (primarily beta) is increased and the energy content of the EEG is decreased. With respect to sleep, the benzodiazepines decrease sleep latency and decrease the number of awakenings and the time spent in stage 0 (wakefulness). They also increase the awakening threshold. The time spent in stage 1 (descending drowsiness) is decreased by flurazepam, lorazepam, and nitrazepam, but increased by chlordiazepoxide, diazepam, and oxazepam. The time spent in stage 2 (major fraction of non-REM sleep) is increased by all benzodiazepines. The time spent in stages 3 and 4 (slow wave sleep) is usually decreased; however, a few agents may increase these stages. The benzodiazepines increase the latency to REM sleep, decrease REM sleep time and increase the number of REM cycles. Total sleep time is increased by the benzodiazepines. The greatest increase is observed in subjects with the shortest base-line sleep time. In such individuals, total sleep time may increase three-fold.

After oral administration, the benzodiazepines are absorbed in from 1 to 6 hours, depending on the formulation given. Binding to serum albumin varies widely; after oral administration of flurazepam only a few percent is bound, whereas after nitrazepam 87% is in bound form. The extent to which benzodiazepines interact with other protein-bound drugs is not known; the absence of reports of such adverse interactions suggest that such competition is not of clinical significance. Biotransformation takes place in the liver by the microsomal drug metabolizing system. Clorazepate, chlordiazepoxide, diazepam, halazepam, flurazepam, and prazepam are transformed to active metabolites, primarily to N-desmethylated products with a longer half-life than the parent drug. This metabolite may be particularly significant in the elderly, newborn, or those with severe liver disease. Only lorazepam, oxazepam, temazepam, and triazolam do not form long-acting active metabolites; thus, their action is not significantly prolonged in the elderly and liver-diseased patient. Benzodiazepines cross the placental barrier and are excreted in human milk.

Patients on these drugs should be warned about potential effects induced by the concomitant use of alcohol or other CNS depressants such as other anti-anxiety and hypnotic drugs, tricyclic antidepressants, opiate analgesics, antipsychotics, antihistamines, including nonprescription sleep aids and cold remedies. They should also be warned not to operate a motor vehicle or hazardous machinery while on these drugs.

Side effects most commonly reported after benzodiazepines include drowsiness, fatigue, and ataxia; venous thrombosis and phlebitis at the site of the injection. Other less frequent side effects include blurred vision, diplopia, nystagmus; urticaria and skin rash; hiccups, changes in salivation, neutropenia and jaundice. Paradoxical reactions such as acute hyperexcited states, anxiety, hallucinations, increased muscle spasticity, insomnia, rage, sleep disturbances have also been reported; should these occur the drug should be discontinued. Since significant amounts of benzodiazepines are found in maternal and cord blood, these agents are not recommended for obstetrical use. The safe use of benzodiazepines in children under 12 years of age has not been established.

Although *physical* and *psychological* dependence have been reported, the incidence is relatively rare if the recommended dosage is followed. Nevertheless, individuals known to be addictive-prone, or those whom history suggests modify drug dosage on their own initiative, should not be given the drug. Withdrawal symptoms resemble those resulting from barbiturate withdrawal. The benzodiazepines are listed in *Schedule IV* under the *Controlled Substances Act*.

Chlordiazepoxide

3*H*-1,4-Benzodiazepin-2-amine, 7-chloro-*N*-methyl-5-phenyl-, 4-oxide; Libritabs (*Roche*)

7-Chloro-2-(methylamino)-5-phenyl-3*H*-1,4-benzodiazepine 4-oxide [58-25-3] $C_{16}H_{14}ClN_3O$ (299.76).

Preparation—For the preparation of chlordiazepoxide, see *Chlordiazepoxide Hydrochloride*.

Description—Yellow, practically odorless, crystalline powder; sensitive to sunlight; melts between 240° and 244°.

Solubility—1 g in >10,000 mL water, 50 mL alcohol, 6250 mL chloroform, 130 mL ether.

Uses—See *Chlordiazepoxide Hydrochloride*.
Dose—See *Chlordiazepoxide Hydrochloride*.
Dosage Forms—Tablets: 5, 10, and 25 mg.

Chlordiazepoxide Hydrochloride

3*H*-1,4-Benzodiazepin-2-amine, 7-chloro-*N*-methyl-5-phenyl-, 4-oxide, monohydrochloride; Librium (*Roche*); A-Poxide (*Abbott*); SK-Lygen (*SKF*); Murcil (*Reid-Provident*)

7-Chloro-2-(methylamino)-5-phenyl-3*H*-1,4-benzodiazepine 4-oxide monohydrochloride [438-41-5] $C_{16}H_{14}ClN_3O \cdot HCl$ (336.22).

For the structure of the base, see above.

Preparation—By condensation cyclization of 2-amino-5-chlorobenzophenone oxime with chloroacetyl chloride to form 6-chloro-2-chloromethyl-4-phenylquinazoline 3-oxide, which is subsequently reacted with methylamine in methanol solution. US Pat 2,893,992.

Description—White or nearly white, odorless, crystalline powder; sensitive to sunlight; melts between 212° and 218°, with decomposition.

Solubility—1 g in 10 mL water, 40 mL alcohol.

Uses—Indicated for the relief of anxiety and tension, withdrawal symptoms of acute alcoholism, preoperative apprehension and anxiety, and adjunct therapy in various disease states in which anxiety and tension are prominent features. Many clinicians consider chlordiazepoxide the drug of choice for these conditions, because of its long history of use. It has a pK_a of 4.6 and a half-life of 8 to 20 hr. During chronic administration, accumulation occurs, not only of the parent substance but also of three active metabolites (desmethylchlordiazepoxide, demoxepam, and desoxydemoxepam). Demoxepam has a half-life of 37 (range 28 to 63) hr and desoxydemoxepam of 44 (range 39 to 61) hr. These metabolites probably contribute to the overall activity of chlordiazepoxide, since they are pharmacologically active in animals. Steady-state plasma levels of chlordiazepoxide, desmethylchlordiazepoxide, and demoxepam average 0.75, 0.54, and 0.36 μmg/mL, respectively. Chlordiazepoxide is excreted in the urine; 1 to 2% is excreted unchanged and 3 to 6% as a conjugate.

As with other benzodiazepines, chlordiazepoxide hydrochloride requires the same warnings and precautions regarding its use in patients with known hypersensitivity, elderly and excessively depressed individuals, pregnant and lactating mothers, patients with known renal and hepatic impairment, patients on other CNS depressant drugs, and in patients with either a history of drug addiction or of indiscriminate alteration of drug dosage (page 1060). Adverse reactions include drowsiness, ataxia, confusion, skin eruptions, edema, menstrual irregularities, nausea and constipation, extrapyramidal symptoms and decreased libido in some patients; blood dyscrasias (agranulocytosis), jaundice, and hepatic dysfunction have occasionally been reported. Paradoxical reactions of rage, excitement, stimulation, hostility, and depersonalization have sometimes followed administration to severely disturbed patients. Skin rashes, nausea, headache, and decreased tolerance to alcohol have also been reported. The chronic administration of large doses of chlordiazepoxide hydrochloride may result in the development of tolerance and physical dependence.

Dose—*Oral*, 10 to 300 mg daily; *usual, oral*, 5 to 25 mg 3 or 4 times a day; *intramuscular* or *intravenous*, 25 to 300 mg in 6 hours; *usual, intramuscular* or *intravenous*, 50 to 100 mg, repeated in 2 to 6 hours if necessary. Elderly or debilitated patients should be restricted to 10 to 20 mg daily. Children 6 yr or older are usually given 5 to 10 mg 2 to 4 times daily.

Dosage Forms—Capsules: 5, 10, and 25 mg; Sterile: 100 mg.

Chlormezanone—page 1074.
Clobazam—page 1083.
Clonazepam—page 1077.

Clorazepate Dipotassium

1*H*-1,4-Benzodiazepine-3-carboxylic acid, 7-chloro-2,3-dihydro-2-oxo-5-phenyl-, potassium salt compd. with potassium hydroxide (1:1); Tranxene (*Abbott*)

[57109-90-7; 15585-90-7] $C_{16}H_{11}ClK_2N_2O_4$; $C_{16}H_{10}ClKN_2O_3 \cdot KOH$ (408.92).

Preparation—2-Amino-5-chlorobenzonitrile is grignardized with phenylmagnesium bromide and the resulting ketimine is condensed via deammoniation with diethyl aminomalonate. The diester is then saponified with KOH in aqueous methanol and the resulting dipotassium dicarboxylate cyclizes via isomerization. US Pat 3,516,988.

Description—Fine, light-yellow, practically odorless, crystalline powder; slightly burning taste; sensitive to light, moisture, and excessive heat; aqueous solutions are unstable (clear, light-yellow, and alkaline to litmus).

Solubility—Very soluble in water; very slightly soluble in alcohol; insoluble in chloroform, ether, benzene, and acetone.

Uses—For the symptomatic relief of anxiety associated with neurosis, psychoneuroses with symptoms of anxiety, and as an adjunct in disease states in which anxiety is a prominent feature. This substance is hydrolyzed in the stomach to desmethyldiazepam, a metabolic precursor of oxazepam and also a metabolite of both chlordiazepoxide and diazepam. The metabolite is rapidly absorbed (1 to 2 hours); the volume of distribution is 0.93 to 1.47 L/kg and the half-life ranges from 50 to 100 hours. Desmethyldiazepam accumulates for about 7 days, and then reaches a steady state. Consequently, the drug can be given once a day as well as in divided doses. Clorazepate potassium requires the same warnings and precautions regarding use with other drugs, use in hypersensitive individuals, use during pregnancy and in young children, use in elderly and excessively depressed patients, use in patients with impaired renal or hepatic function, and use in patients with a history of drug addiction as with other benzodiazepines (see page 1060). Drowsiness is the most common adverse effect. Less common untoward reactions include dizziness, various gastrointestinal complaints, nervousness, blurred vision, dry mouth, headache, and mental confusion. Other adverse reactions include insomnia, transient skin rashes, fatigue, ataxia, genitourinary complaints, irritability, diplopia, depression, and slurred speech. Hypotension, decreased hematocrit, and abnormal liver and kidney function have also been reported.

Dose—*Adult*, *oral*, **15** to **60 mg** daily; *usual*, **30 mg** daily in divided doses or 22.5 mg as a single-dose tablet every 24 hr. Elderly or debilitated patients, 7.5 to 15 mg daily. See also package insert.

Dosage Forms—Capsules: 3.75, 7.5, and 15 mg; Tablets, single dose: 3.75, 7.5, 15, and 22.5 mg. Half-Strength Tablets, 22.5 mg.

Diazepam

2*H*-1,4-Benzodiazepin-2-one, 7-chloro-1,3-dihydro-1-methyl-5-phenyl-, Valium (*Roche*)

[439-14-5] $C_{16}H_{13}ClN_2O$ (284.74).

Preparation—2-(Methylamino)-5-chlorobenzophenone in ethereal solution is reacted with bromoacetyl bromide to form 2-(2-bromo-*N*-methylacetamido)-5-chlorobenzophenone. The latter is then reacted with ammonia in methanol solution whereby the bromine is replaced by amino followed by cyclization through a dehydration involving the hydrogens of the amino group and the oxygen of the starting phenone. The crude diazepam may be purified by recrystallization from ether. US Pat 3,136,815.

Description—Off-white to yellow, practically odorless, crystalline powder which is stable in the air; melts between 131° and 135°.

Solubility—1 g in 333 mL water, 16 mL alcohol, 2 mL chloroform, and 39 mL ether.

Uses—A benzodiazepine indicated for the symptomatic relief of tension and anxiety, acute alcohol withdrawal, adjunct therapy in skeletal muscle spasms, and is preferred by many clinicians for the management of status epilepticus. Diazepam is well absorbed after single oral doses (pK_a 3.3), leading to rapid onset of clinical effects. Initially these effects may be transient, due to extensive distribution to body tissues. After distribution is complete, elimination is slow, with a half-life of 20 to 50 hr. Effective plasma levels vary from 0.2 to 0.5 μmg/mL. With chronic administration, diazepam and its major active metabolite, desmethyldiazepam, accumulate and reach a steady state in about 7 days. Consequently it may take this long to achieve maximal sedative and antianxiety effects, at which time the patient can usually be maintained by giving the drug once or twice daily. More details of its clinical uses as well as warnings, precautions, contraindications, addiction liability, and a detailed enumeration of its adverse reactions and side effects are given on page 1060. Patients on the drug should be cautioned not to drive an automobile or to operate dangerous machinery until a few days after the drug has been stopped.

Dose—*Adult*, *oral*, **2** to **10 mg** 2 to 4 times a day; *intramuscular* or *intravenous*, **2** to **15 mg**, repeated in 3 to 4 hours, if necessary, but no more than **30 mg** should be given in an 8-hour period. *Pediatric*, *oral*, over 6 months of age, 1 to **2.5 mg** 3 or 4 times a day.

Dosage Forms—Injection: 10 mg/2 mL; Tablets: 2, 5, and 10 mg.

Droperidol—page 1087.

Fentanyl Citrate—page 1108.

Flurazepam Hydrochloride

2*H*-1,4-Benzodiazepin-2-one, 7-chloro-1-[2-(diethylamino)ethyl]-5-(2-fluorophenyl)-1,3-dihydro-, dihydrochloride; Dalmane (*Roche*)

[1172-18-5] $C_{21}H_{23}ClFN_3O.2HCl$ (460.81).

Preparation—Aqueous CrO_3 is added dropwise to an acetic acid solution of 2-aminomethyl-5-chloro-1-[2-(diethylamino)ethyl]-3-(*o*-fluorophenyl)indole dihydrochloride and the mixture is stirred overnight.

Description—Off-white to yellow, crystalline powder; slight odor to odorless; melts with decomposition at about 212°; moderately hygroscopic.

Solubility—1 g in 2 mL water; freely soluble in alcohol; slightly soluble in chloroform.

Uses—A benzodiazepine widely used in all types of insomnia such as difficulty in falling asleep, frequent nocturnal awakenings, and/or early morning awakening. It is also used in acute and chronic medical situations in which restful sleep is desirable. Flurazepam is rapidly absorbed from the GI tract and rapidly metabolized by the liver. Following a single oral dose, peak plasma concentrations ranging from 0.5 to 4.0 ng/mL are reached in 30 to 60 min. The major metabolite, N^1-desalkylflurazepam, reaches steady-state levels after 7 to 10 days of treatment of 5- to 6-fold higher than the 24-hour levels observed on day 1. The parent compound disappears rapidly from the blood; *N*-desalkylflurazepam remains active and has a half-life that ranges from 47 to 100 hours. The major urinary metabolite is conjugated N^1-hydroxyethylflurazepam and accounts for 22 to 55% of the dose. Flurazepam is excreted primarily in the urine. Less than 1% is excreted in the urine as N^1-desalkylflurazepam. The onset of sleep ranges from 15 to 45 minutes. Maximum effectiveness may not be achieved for three or four nights. Thus, the metabolite is responsible for the clinical effect as well as the residual effects which persist after the drug is discontinued. Flurazepam hydrochloride requires the same warnings and precautions regarding use with other drug therapy, use in hypersensitive individuals, use during pregnancy, use in children under 12 years of age, use in elderly and excessively depressed patients, use in patients with impaired renal or hepatic function and use in patients with a history of drug addiction as with other benzodiazepines (see page 1060). Adverse reactions include dizziness, drowsiness, light-headedness, ataxia and falling (especially in elderly or debilitated persons), and severe sedation. The last is usually due to drug intolerance or overdosage. Other reported side effects include headache, heartburn, upset stomach, nausea, vomiting, diarrhea, constipation, gastrointestinal pain, nervousness, talkativeness, apprehension, irritability, weakness, palpitation, chest pains, body and joint pain, and genitourinary complaints. Less frequently sweating, flushes, blurred vision, difficulty in focusing, burning eyes, faintness, hypotension, shortness of breath, pruritus, skin rash, dry mouth, bitter taste, excessive salivation, anorexia, euphoria, depression, slurred speech, confusion, restlessness, hallucinations, and paradoxidal reactions (excitement, stimulation, and hyperactivity) have been observed.

Dose—*Usual*, *adult*, **15** to **30 mg** before retiring. Elderly and/or debilitated patients, initial **15 mg** until individual response is determined. The drug is not recommended for use in children under 15 yr of age.

Dosage Forms—Capsules: 15 and 30 mg.

Halazepam

2*H*-1,4-Benzodiazepin-2-one, 7-chloro-1,3-dihydro-5-phenyl-1-(2,2,2-trifluoroethyl)-, Paxipam (*Schering-Plough*)

[23092-17-3] $C_{17}H_{12}ClF_3N_2O$ (352.74).

Preparation—The synthesis is similar to that for diazepam, this page. See *J Med Chem*: **66**, 1354, 1973.

Description—A white crystalline solid melting about 165°. Physical properties are similar to diazepam.

Uses—Halazepam is indicated primarily for *anxiety* disorders or for the short-term relief of *symptoms of anxiety* not controlled by other more specific medication. Halazepam is rapidly and well absorbed after oral administration and excreted primarily in the urine. At least 90% of the absorbed drug is bound to plasma proteins.

Maximum plasma concentration is achieved within 1 to 3 hours after oral administration; half-life following a 40 mg oral dose is approximately 14 hours. The major active metabolite of halazepam is N-desmethyldiazepam; maximum plasma concentrations of this metabolite occur in 3 to 6 hours and has a half-life of elimination of approximately 50 to 100 hours. Less than 1% of the parent substance is excreted in the urine as unchanged drug. Common adverse effects include drowsiness, headache, apathy, psychomotor retardation, disorientation, confusion, euphoria, dysarthria, depression, and syncope. Ataxia, fatigue, and paraxodical agitation or rage have also been reported. No adverse drug interactions peculiar to halazepam have been reported. However, additive sedation with alcohol and other central nervous system depressant drugs would be anticipated, as well as those common to benzodiazepines (see page 1060). Halazepam should be used with caution in patients required to perform hazardous tasks and those with a history of drug abuse.

Dose—*Usual, adult, oral,* **20** to **40 mg** 3 or 4 times a day. *Elderly or sensitive patients*, **20 mg** once or twice a day. Information is inadequate to establish a dose for patients under 18 years of age.

Dosage Form—Tablets: 20 and 40 mg.

Lorazepam

2H-1,4-Benzodiazepin-2-one, 7-chloro-5-(2-chlorophenyl)-1,3-dihydro-3-hydroxy-, Ativan (*Wyeth*)

[846-49-1] $C_{15}H_{10}Cl_2N_2O_2$ (321.16).

Preparation—Syntheses of a number of substituted 1,4-benzodiazepin-2-ones, including lorazepam, have been described by Bell *et al.* (*J Med Chem 11:* 457, 1968; see also *J Org Chem 27:* 1691, 1962). Lorazepam differs from oxazepam in having a 5-*o*-chlorophenyl substituent in place of the 5-phenyl of oxazepam.

Description—White to off-white powder; no characteristic odor; melts at about 173°, with decomposition.

Solubility—Practically insoluble in water; slightly soluble in alcohol, chloroform.

Uses—A benzodiazepine used orally for *insomnia* due to anxiety and transient situational stress. It is used parenterally for *preanesthetic medication*, producing sedation and decreased ability to recall events related to the surgery. Lorazepam is rapidly absorbed after oral administration; peak plasma levels after a 2-mg dose are about 20 ng/mL and maximal clinical effects occur within 2 hours after administration. Its mean plasma half-life is about 12 hours, whereas that of its conjugated metabolite, lorazepam glucuronide, is about 18 hours. Approximately 85% is bound to plasma proteins. There is no evidence of accumulation of lorazepam on administration for up to 6 months. Preliminary clinical evaluation indicates that 2 to 4 mg of lorazepam is as effective an hypnotic as 30 mg of flurazepam. Adverse reactions, if they occur, usually appear at the beginning of therapy and disappear on continued medication or on decreasing the dose. Sedation is the most frequent adverse reaction (15.9%), followed by dizziness (6.9%), weakness (4.2%) and unsteadiness (3.4%). Less frequent adverse effects are disorientation, depression, nausea, headache, sleep disturbance, agitation, dermatological symptoms, eye function disturbance, gastrointestinal symptoms, and autonomic manifestations. Incidence of sedation and unsteadiness usually increases with age. Lorazepam requires the same warnings and precautions regarding use with other drugs, use in hypersensitive individuals, use during pregnancy and in young children, use in elderly and excessively depressed patients, use in patients with impaired renal or hepatic function, and use in patients with a history of drug addiction as with other benzodiazepines (see page 1060).

Dose—*Adult, oral,* 1 to **10 mg** daily, according to patient response; *usual*, **2** to **6 mg** in divided doses. In *anxiety*, **2** to **3 mg**, 2 or 3 times daily; in *insomnia*, **2** to **4 mg** at bedtime. A divided daily dose of **1** to **2 mg** initially is advised for elderly or debilitated patients. Dosage in children up to 12 yr not established.

Dosage Forms—Tablets: 0.5, 1, and 2 mg; Injection: 2 and 4 mg/mL vials.

Oxazepam

2H-1,4-Benzodiazepin-2-one, 7-chloro-1,3-dihydro-3-hydroxy-5-phenyl-, Serax (*Wyeth*)

[604-75-1] $C_{15}H_{11}ClN_2O_2$ (286.72).

Preparation—2-Amino-5-chlorobenzophenone is acylated with chloroacetyl chloride and the product is refluxed with sodium iodide to form the iodoacetamido compound (I). Reaction of I with hydroxylamine effects dehydration and dehydrohalogenation to form the benzodiazepine derivative (II). Treatment of II with acetic anhydride causes rearrangement to oxazepam which is simultaneously esterified to acetate. Saponification liberates oxazepam.

Description—Creamy white to pale-yellow powder that is practically odorless and has a bitter taste; stable in light and nonhygroscopic; melting point is indefinite; pH (1 in 50 suspension) between 4.8 and 7.0.

Solubility—1 g in >10,000 mL water, 220 mL alcohol, 270 mL chloroform, 2200 mL ether.

Uses—A congener of chlordiazepoxide and diazepam; it is a mild sedative useful in the management and control of anxiety, tension, agitation, irritability, and related symptoms, particularly in elderly patients. Also, it is useful for the control of acute tremulousness, inebriation, or anxiety associated with alcohol withdrawal. Unlike diazepam, oxazepam is slowly absorbed after oral administration (1 to 4 hours) and has a simple, one-step elimination pathway without active intermediate metabolites. Its half-life is short (5–15 hr), there is little accumulation, and full therapeutic effect can be expected with the first few doses. However, several daily doses may be necessary to reach a clinical steady state. Excessive and prolonged use may result in the development of physical dependence on the drug. Withdrawal symptoms following abrupt discontinuance of oxazepam are similar to those seen with barbiturates. As with other sedative agents, patients on this drug should be cautioned against driving automobiles or operating dangerous machinery. Other warnings, contraindications, and precautions are similar to those for other benzodiazepines (see page 1060). Untoward effects include transient mild drowsiness, dizziness, vertigo, headache, and rarely syncope. Mild paradoxical reactions such as excitement and excessive stimulation have also been recorded. Other side effects which have been observed include skin rashes, nausea, lethargy, edema, slurred speech, tremor, and altered libido. More severe reactions include leukopenia and jaundice. Fortunately, the latter reactions are only occasionally observed. Patients on the drug should be observed carefully for the appearance of other untoward effects characteristic of benzodiazepine drugs.

Dose—**10** to **30 mg**; *usual, adult, oral,* **10** to **15 mg** 3 or 4 times daily; severe anxiety and alcoholic patients with marked withdrawal effects, **15** to **30 mg** 3 or 4 times a day.

Dosage Forms—Capsules: 10, 15, and 30 mg; Tablets: 15 mg.

Prazepam

2H-1,4-Benzodiazepin-2-one, 7-chloro-1-(cyclopropylmethyl)-1,3-dihydro-5-phenyl-, Verstran (*Warner-Chilcott*); Centrax (*Parke-Davis*)

[2955-38-6] $C_{19}H_{17}ClN_2O$ (324.81).

Preparation—In one process 2-amino-5-chlorobenzophenone is acylated with cyclopropanecarboxylic acid chloride using triethylamine as acid-binder, reduced with lithium aluminum hydride to give 2-cyclopropylmethylamino-5-chlorobenzhydrol, and then oxidized with MnO$_2$ to the corresponding benzophenone. This is acylated with phthalimidoacetyl chloride and cyclized with hydrazine hydrate to produce prazepam. US Pats 3,192,199 and 3,192,200.

Description—Colorless, crystalline powder; melts at about 145°.
Solubility—Practically insoluble in water; soluble in alcohol, chloroform.

Uses—Prazepam is indicated for the management of *anxiety disorders* or for the short-term relief of the *symptoms of anxiety*. Prazepam is slowly absorbed after oral administration. Like diazepam and clorazepate, prazepam is converted primarily to desmethyldiazepam, which appears to be the principal active metabolite. This conversion occurs slowly in the liver and peak levels of this metabolite are observed approximately 6 hours after oral administration. A mean half-life of desmethyldiazepam, measured in subjects given 10 mg 3 times a day for one week, was 60 hours before and 70 hours after multiple dosing. It is excreted largely as metabolites. Prazepam is contraindicated in patients with known sensitivity to the drug and those with acute narrow-angle glaucoma. The warnings, precautions, drug interactions, and addiction liability for benzodiazepines are stated on page 1060.

Adverse reactions most frequently encountered with prazepam are fatigue, dizziness, weakness, drowsiness, lightheadedness, and ataxia. Of lesser frequency are headache, confusion, tremor, vivid dreams, slurred speech, palpitations, stimulation, dry mouth, diaphoresis, and various gastrointestinal complaints; also pruritus, skin rashes, swelling of feet, joint pains, genitourinary complaints, blurred vision, and syncope. The safety and effectiveness of the drug in patients under the age of 18 have not been established.

Dose—*Adult, usual, oral,* **30 mg** daily in divided doses, adjusted gradually within the range of **20** to **60 mg** daily, depending on patient response. Alternatively may be given as a single dose at bedtime, starting at **20 mg,** with a usual range of **20** to **40 mg**. A divided daily dose of **10** to **15 mg** initially is advised for elderly or debilitated patients.

Dosage Form—Capsules: 5 and 10 mg; Tablets: 10 mg.

Temazepam

2H-1,4-Benzodiazepin-2-one, 7-chloro-1,3-dihydro-3-hydroxy-1-methyl-5-phenyl-, Restoril (*Sandoz*); (*Wyeth*)

[846-50-4] $C_{16}H_{13}ClN_2O_2$ (300.74).
Preparation—The synthesis is similar to oxazepam using 2-(methylamino)-5-chlorobenzhydrol as the starting material. See *J Org Chem:* 27, 1691, 1962.

Description—White crystals melting about 120°.

Uses—Temazepam is a hypnotic drug indicated for the relief of *insomnia* associated with difficulty in falling asleep, frequent nocturnal awakenings, and/or early morning awakenings. Oral bioavailability is relatively slow (mean times to peak concentration, 2 to 3 hours); 96% is bound to plasma proteins. Volume distribution ranges from 1.4 to 1.5 L/kg and clearance from 1.10 to 1.36 mL/kg/min. The elimination half-life varies from 3 to 38 hours (mean, 14.7 hours). Temazepam is conjugated with glucuronic acid and excreted in the urine. Since metabolic enzyme induction does not appear to occur after 5 to 7 days of administration, tolerance to repeated use is not troublesome. Adverse effects are usually mild and diminish with continued administration. Those observed most frequently include morning drowsiness, dizziness, lethargy, confusion, and gastrointestinal disturbances (anorexia, diarrhea). Other less frequent adverse effects include vertigo, dryness of the mouth, paresthesias, tachycardia, panic reactions, nystagmus, paradoxical excitement, and hallucinations. Precautions for the use of temazepam and possible drug interactions are the same as those for other benzodiazepines (see page 1060). Dysmorphogenic changes in rib formation have been observed in two animal species given 50 to 100 times the human therapeutic dose. Use of temazepam during pregnancy should be avoided if possible.

Dose—*Usual, adult, hypnotic,* **30 mg** at bedtime. *Elderly* or *sensitive patients,* **15 mg**. Dosage in patients under 18 years of age has not been established.

Dosage Form—Capsule, 15 and 30 mg.

Triazolam

4H-1,2,4-Triazolo[4,3-a][1,4]benzodiazepine, 8-chloro-6-(2-chlorophenyl)-1-methyl-, Halcion (*Upjohn*)

8-Chloro-6-(*o*-chlorophenyl)-1-methyl-4H-*s*-triazolo[4,3-a]-[1,4]benzodiazepine. [28911-01-5] $C_{17}H_{12}Cl_2N_4$ (343.21).
Preparation—See Ger Pat 2,533,924.

Description—Tan crystals from isopropyl alcohol melting about 235°.
Solubility—Very slightly soluble in water; slightly soluble in alcohol.

Uses—Triazolam is useful in the short-term management of insomnia characterized by difficulty in falling asleep, frequent nocturnal awakenings, and/or early morning awakenings. Triazolam is rapidly absorbed after oral administration; approximately 90% is bound to plasma proteins. Time to peak concentration is 1.25 hours. Volume distribution ranges from 0.8 to 1.3 L/kg. The elimination half-life is 2.6 (1.7 to 5.2) hours. The metabolites of triazolam have little if any hypnotic activity. Common adverse effects include drowsiness, dizziness, and headache. Hallucinations and marked confusion have also been reported. No adverse drug interactions peculiar to triazolam have been reported; however, prescribers should be alert to the usual drug interactions common to benzodiazepines (see page 1060). The safe use of triazolam during pregnancy or lactation has not been established.

Dose—*Usual, adult, oral,* **0.25** to **0.5 mg** at bedtime; elderly or sensitive patients, **0.25 mg**. The dose for children under 18 years of age has not been established.

Dosage Form—Tablets, 0.25 and 0.5 mg.

Other Benzodiazepines

Bromazepam [7-Bromo-1,3-dihydro-5-(2-pyridinyl)-2H-1,4-benzodiazepin-2-one [1812-30-2] $C_{14}H_{10}BrN_3O$ (316.16); Lectopam (*Roche*)]—Colorless crystals, melting at about 238° with decomposition. *Uses:* A benzodiazepine under clinical investigation for use as a hypnotic and sedative. The pharmacokinetics of bromazepam, like those of diazepam and nitrazepam and perhaps other congeners, are complicated by its enterohepatic circulation. Elimination half-life appears to be about 8 to 19 hours. Contraindications, precautions, and side effects appear to be similar to those for other benzodiazepines. *Dose: Usual, adult, oral, sedative,* 6 to 12 mg 3 or 4 times a day; *hypnotic,* 24 mg at bedtime.

Flunitrazepam [5-(*o*-Fluorophenyl)-1,3-dihydro-1-methyl-7-nitro-2H-1,4-benzodiazepin-2-one [1622-62-4] $C_{16}H_{12}FN_3O_3$ (313.30); Rohypnol (*Roche*)]—Pale yellow, crystalline solid; melts at about 167°; sparingly soluble in water; readily soluble in alcohol. *Uses:* A benzodiazepine under clinical investigation for use as a hypnotic and preanesthetic medication. Elimination half-life has been reported to be 8 to 10 hours. The 7-amino derivative is the principal unconjugated metabolite. In the absence of contrary data, the contraindications, precautions, and side effects must be considered similar to other benzodiazepines. *Dose: Usual, adult, oral, hypnotic,* 1 to 2 mg.

Nitrazepam [1,3-Dihydro-7-nitro-5-phenyl-2H-1,4-benzodiazepin-2-one [146-22-5] $C_{15}H_{11}N_3O_3$ (281.26); Mogadon (*Hoffman-LaRoche*)]—Yellow, crystalline powder; odorless; tasteless; melts at about 227°; practically insoluble in water; 1 g dissolves in 120 mL alcohol, 45 mL chloroform, 990 mL ether. *Uses:* A benzodiazepine widely used in Europe and Canada as a sedative/hypnotic and in the management of myoclonic seizures. Nitrazepam is 80% bioavailable after oral administration. Peak concentrations are reached in 0.5 to 5.0 hours. It is widely distributed in the body; 10 to 15% is found in cerebrospinal fluid and 85 to 90% is bound to plasma proteins. It also crosses the placenta and is found in breast milk. It is extensively metabolized to inactive substances that are excreted in the urine. The elimination half-life is approximately 30 hours. Precautions, contraindications, and side effects are similar to those for other benzodiazepines. *Dose: Usual, oral, adult,* 2.5 to 10 mg.

Oxazolam [10-Chloro-2,3,7,11b-tetrahydro-2-methyl-11b-phenyloxazolo[3,2-d][1,4]benzodiazepin-6(5H)-one $C_{18}H_{17}ClN_2O_2$ (328.80); Serenal]—White or off-white, crystalline powder; almost odorless; tasteless; practically insoluble in water; slightly soluble in alcohol; soluble in chloroform. *Uses:* A benzodiazepine under clinical evaluation as a hypnotic agent. Elimination half-life is approximately 4.5 hours. Contraindications, precautions, and side effects resemble those of other benzodiazepines. *Dose, adult, oral, hypnotic,* for preoperative use 1 to 2 mg/kg has been administered.

Quazepam [7-Chloro-5-(2-fluorophenyl)-1,3-dihydro-1-(2,2,2-tri-fluoroethyl)-2*H*-benzodiazepine-2-thione [36735-22-5] $C_{17}H_{11}ClF_4N_2S$ (386.79); (*Schering-Plough*)]—*Uses:* Under investigation for use as a sedative/hypnotic for presurgical procedures and for short- to intermediate-term management of insomnia. Quazepam and its active metabolite, 2-oxoquazepam, have half-lives of approximately 40 hours. A second metabolite, *N*-desalkylflurazepam, has a half-life of 47 to 100 hours. The long half-lives of quazepam and its metabolites may be responsible for the drowsiness and hangover effects which persist for two or three days following discontinuation of the drug. Adverse effects, drug interactions, and precaution are probably similar to those for other benzodiazepines (see page 1060). *Dose: Usual, adult, oral,* 7.5 to 30 mg.

Barbiturates

The introduction of barbital in 1903 and phenobarbital in 1912 initiated the barbiturate era. For a period of over half a century they reigned as the preeminent sedative-hypnotic agents. Although several so-called nonbarbiturates attempted to displace the barbiturates from time to time, it was not until chlordiazepoxide was marketed in 1961 that their position was seriously challenged. During the ensuing 15 years the benzodiazepines have displaced the barbiturates as the sedative-hypnotics of choice. Indeed, a careful comparison of the barbiturates and the benzodiazepines reveals the following cogent reasons for this obsolescence: (1) dependence liability, (2) potential for suicide, (3) quality of sleep, (4) antianxiety selectivity, (5) propensity for drug interactions, (6) safety, and (7) side effects. Nevertheless, they continue to be prescribed by a significant number of physicians.

The development of clinical pharmacokinetic data on hypnotic drugs revealed that the traditional classification of barbiturates into long-, intermediate-, and short-acting compounds bears little relation to the rate of elimination of these agents in man. Moreover, these data indicate that onset (rate of absorption) and duration of action (rate of elimination) are essential factors to be considered in their use. In general, barbiturate salts are rapidly absorbed, in contrast to the free acids. Liver disease tends to decrease the elimination rate of these substances, whereas renal insufficiency may give rise to accumulation of polar metabolites. For these reasons and for ready reference, the elimination half-lives, apparent volumes of distribution, and clearance values of barbiturates are summarized in each monograph.

Although traditionally used as nonspecific central nervous system depressants for daytime sedation and short-term treatment of insomnia, the barbiturates have generally been replaced by the benzodiazepines. However, they are still given for preoperative medication to allay anxiety and facilitate induction of anesthesia. The anticonvulsant barbiturates, such as phenobarbital, mephobarbital, and metharbital, are used orally for the long-term management of generalized tonic-clonic and cortical focal seizures and intravenously for the management of acute convulsive episodes, such as status epilepticus, eclampsia, meningitis, tetanus, and toxic reactions to strychnine or local anesthetics. The barbiturates are also administered rectally in infants and children when oral or parenteral therapy may be undesirable.

Elixirs of certain barbiturates are still used as somnifacients and sedatives for children, despite the availability of more effective agents. They are also used in the relief of colic, excitation, and restlessness due to illness. Sedative doses may be administered as frequently as 3 to 4 times a day in cases of pylorospasm, whooping cough, nausea and vomiting of functional origin, etc.

Barbiturates are contraindicated in patients with a history of porphyria. They should be used with caution in patients with impaired hepatic or renal function, and in debilitated patients with depressed respiration. They are also contraindicated in persons with known previous addiction to the sedative/hypnotic drugs. Moreover, they should not be used in women of childbearing age, since their safe use in pregnancy has not been established. Patients on barbiturates should avoid alcoholic beverages and refrain from driving an automobile or operating hazardous machinery while receiving such drugs.

Drug interactions are relatively common in patients taking barbiturates along with other drugs. For this reason patients on these drugs should be monitored closely. The most common problems relate to the ability of barbiturates (especially phenobarbital) to induce the hepatic microsomal enzyme system and increase the rate of metabolism of coumarin anticoagulants, tricyclic antidepressants, oral contraceptives, corticosteroids, digitoxin, phenytoin, phenothiazines, doxycycline, and perhaps other agents. Accordingly, the effectiveness of these agents may be decreased when given to a patient already on a barbiturate and, contrariwise, patients on both a barbiturate and one of these agents may experience adverse effects if the barbiturate is discontinued during chronic therapy, *ie* a patient on coumarin may hemorrhage if the barbiturate is stopped and anticoagulant dosage is not readjusted. Barbiturates (especially phenobarbital) may competitively inhibit the metabolism of some drugs, such as phenytoin. Barbiturates have been shown to decrease the gastrointestinal absorption of dicumarol and griseofulvin. Some barbiturates potentiate the adverse effects of tricyclic antidepressants by competing for the same hydroxylating enzymes. Monoamine oxidase inhibitors, valproic acid, chloramphenicol, and acute alcoholic intoxication inhibit the metabolism of barbiturates. Chronic alcoholic intoxication, on the other hand, increases the metabolism of barbiturates. Concomitant use of ether or curare-like drugs may produce additive respiratory depression. It has also been suggested that sulfisoxazole competes with thiopental for plasma-protein binding sites and decreases the amount of the latter necessary for anesthesia. Finally, additive depressant effects may occur with concomitant use of barbiturates and other CNS depressant drugs.

Adverse reactions to barbiturates include the following: *CNS effects,* somnolence, agitation, confusion, hyperkinesia, ataxia, nightmares, lethargy, paradoxical excitement, nervousness, hallucinations, insomnia, anxiety, and dizziness; *respiratory effects,* apnea, hypoventilation, respiratory depression, bronchospasm, and circulatory collapse; *cardiovascular,* bradycardia, hypotension, and syncope; *hypersensitivity,* skin rashes, angioneurotic edema, fever, serum sickness, morbiliform rash, urticaria, exfoliative dermatitis, and Steven-Johnson syndrome; *other adverse effects,* headache, blood dyscrasias, myalgia, neuralgia, and arthritic pain. For these and other reasons mentioned in this section, their indiscriminate use should be avoided.

Accidental and suicidal deaths from acute barbiturate poisoning are encountered frequently. Treatment varies with the degree of intoxication. In general, emergency measures in *acute* poisoning are directed toward maintenance of respiration and cardiac function, followed by gastric decontamination. The latter is accomplished by gastric lavage, administration of activated charcoal (20 to 25 g in a child, 50 g in an adult) by gastric lavage tube, and a saline cathartic to clear the gut. In severe intoxication, measures to enhance elimination of absorbed barbiturate may be necessary, such as diuresis, urine alkalinization, dialysis, and hemoperfusion. The prognosis in barbiturate poisoning, with adequate medical care, is very good; mortality is less than 1%.

Chronic barbiturate poisoning involves a large number of individuals in this country. Some authorities consider the problem of chronic barbiturate poisoning as serious as morphine addiction. Consequently, three barbiturates (*amobarbital, pentobarbital,* and *secobarbital*) either alone or in combination have been placed under *Schedule II* of the

Controlled Substances Act. Serious withdrawal symptoms, including convulsions and psychoses, may occur when barbiturate is withheld from patients addicted to it. In some chronically intoxicated individuals, even though they have no previous history of epilepsy, major convulsive seizures follow sudden withdrawal of barbiturate. It is advisable to reduce the dose of barbiturate gradually in both epileptic and non-epileptic patients when cessation of chronic barbiturate medication is contemplated. It should also be emphasized that barbiturate therapy is contraindicated in patients with a history of drug addiction.

Amobarbital

2,4,6(1*H*,3*H*,5*H*)-Pyrimidinetrione, 5-ethyl-5-(3-methylbutyl)-, Amylobarbitone; Amytal (*Lilly*)

5-Ethyl-5-isopentylbarbituric acid [57-43-2] $C_{11}H_{18}N_2O_3$ (226.27).

Preparation—By the general method described under *Barbital*, using ethyl bromide and isopentyl as alkylating agents at the 5-position.

Description—White, crystalline, odorless, bitter powder; pH (saturated solution) about 5.6; melts within a 3° range between 156° and 161°.

Solubility—1 g in about 1300 mL water, 5 mL alcohol, about 17 mL chloroform, and 6 mL ether; soluble in solutions of fixed alkali hydroxides and carbonates.

Uses—A *sedative* and *hypnotic*. It may be used in any condition that requires sedation ranging from relief of anxiety and tension to hypnotic doses for preanesthetic medication. See the preceding general statement on *Barbiturates*. Amobarbital is a *Schedule II* drug under the *Controlled Substances Act.*

Dose—*Adult, usual:* Oral, *sedative*, **30 to 50 mg** 2 or 3 times daily, or **60 mg** as the extended-release tablet in the morning and on retiring; *hypnotic*; **100 to 200 mg**. *Pediatric, usual:* Oral, *sedative*, **2 mg/kg** or **60 mg/m²** body surface 3 times a day; *hypnotic*, dosage not established.

Dosage Forms—Elixir: 44 mg/5 mL; Tablets: 15, 30, 50, and 100 mg.

Ambobarbital Sodium

2,4,6(1*H*,3*H*,5*H*)-Pyrimidinetrione, 5-ethyl-5-(3-methylbutyl)-, monosodium salt; Amylobarbitone Sodium; Amytal Sodium (*Lilly*)

Sodium 5-ethyl-5-isopentylbarbiturate [64-43-7] $C_{11}H_{17}N_2NaO_3$ (248.26).

Preparation—By reacting amobarbital with a solution containing a chemically equivalent quantity of sodium hydroxide or sodium carbonate, evaporating to dryness, and crystallizing the residue from a solution in a suitable solvent such as alcohol.

Description—White, friable, hygroscopic, odorless, granular powder with a bitter taste; pH (1 in 20 solution) between 9.6 and 10.4.

Solubility—Very soluble in water; soluble in alcohol; practically insoluble in ether and chloroform.

Uses—A *hypnotic* and *sedative*. Amobarbital sodium is indicated for sedation and relief of anxiety, preanesthetic medication, and the control of acute convulsive disorders. The half-life is approximately 20 hours. See the general statement on *Barbiturates*. Amobarbital sodium is a *Schedule II* drug under the *Controlled Substances Act.*

Dose—*Adult, usual:* Oral, *sedative*, during *labor*, **200 to 400 mg** every 1 to 3 hours up to a total of 1 gram, *preoperative*, **200 mg** 1 or

2 hours before surgery; *hypnotic*, **65 to 200 mg** on retiring. *Intramuscular* or *intravenous*, *sedative*, **30 to 50 mg** 2 or 3 times a day; *intravenous*, *anticonvulsant* or *hypnotic*, **65 to 500 mg**; *intramuscular*, *hypnotic*, **65 to 200 mg**. *Pediatric, usual:* Oral, *sedative*, **2 mg/kg** or **60 mg/m²** body surface 3 times a day; *hypnotic*, dosage not established; *intramuscular* or *intravenous*, *anticonvulsant*, **3 to 5 mg/kg** or **125 mg/m²** body surface per dose; *intramuscular, hypnotic*, **3 to 5 mg/kg** or **125 mg/m²** body surface; dosage as *sedative* to be individualized by physician.

Dosage Forms—Capsules: 65 and 200 mg; Sterile Powder: 15 and 30 g vials.

Barbital

2,4,6(1*H*,3*H*,5*H*)-Pyrimidinetrione, 5,5-diethyl-, Barbitone; Diethylmalonylurea; Veronal (*Winthrop*)

5,5-Diethylbarbituric acid [57-44-3] $C_8H_{12}N_2O_3$ (184.19).

Preparation—A method for preparing barbital starts with monochloroacetic acid, which is treated with sodium cyanide to form cyanoacetic acid; the latter is reacted with hydrochloric acid in the presence of alcohol, yielding the diethyl ester of malonic acid. This ester, in absolute alcohol solution, is treated with the theoretical quantity of metallic sodium to replace one hydrogen of the CH_2 group, then a slight excess of the theoretical amount of an ethylating agent, such as ethyl bromide, is added. The second hydrogen is similarly replaced. The diethyl ester of diethylmalonic acid thus obtained is heated in an alcoholic solution, in the presence of sodium, with urea. Sodium barbital is formed, from which barbital is liberated with HCl.

The alkylation of the CH_2 group of the malonic ester, whether the alkyls are both the same as in barbital or different as in pentothal, may be done in two stages, introducing one alkyl group at a time.

Description—Colorless or white crystals or a white crystalline powder; odorless, has a slightly bitter taste, and is stable in the air; melts between 188° and 192°; aqueous solution is acid to litmus.

Solubility—1 g in 130 mL water, about 15 mL alcohol, 75 mL chloroform, 35 mL ether.

Uses—Barbital, the oldest of the barbiturates, is included here for historical reasons. It is seldom used in modern therapeutics. See the comprehensive general statement on *Barbiturates* in this section.

Dose—*Usual, adult, oral*, **300 mg**.

Dosage Forms—Elixir: 175 mg/5 mL; Tablets: 300 mg.

Butabarbital Sodium

2,4,6(1*H*,3*H*,5*H*)-Pyrimidinetrione, 5-ethyl-5-(1-methylpropyl)-, monosodium salt; Butisol Sodium (*Carter-Wallace*); Various Mfrs

Sodium 5-*sec*-butyl-5-ethylbarbiturate [143-81-7] $C_{10}H_{15}N_2NaO_3$ (234.23).

Preparation—By treating an alcoholic solution of butabarbital with an equimolar quantity of NaOH and removing the solvent by evaporation.

Description—White, butter powder; pH (1 in 10 solution) between 9.5 and 10.2.

Solubility—1 g in 2 mL water, 7 mL alcohol, 7000 mL chloroform, >10,000 mL ether.

Uses—A *sedative* and *hypnotic*. See the general statement on *Barbiturates* in this section. Butabarbital sodium is a *Schedule III* drug under the *Controlled Substances Act.*

Dose—*Adult, usual:* Oral, *sedative, daytime*, **15 to 30 mg** 3 or 4 times daily; *preoperative*, **50 to 100 mg**; *hypnotic*, **50 to 100 mg** on retiring. *Pediatric, usual:* Oral, *sedative*, **2 mg/kg** or **60 mg/m²**

body surface 3 times a day; *hypnotic*, dosage must be individualized by physician.

Dosage Forms—Capsules: 15 and 30 mg; Elixir: 30 mg/5 mL; Tablets: 15, 30, 50, and 100 mg.

Hexobarbital Sodium—RPS-15, page 983.

Mephobarbital

2,4,6(1*H*,3*H*,5*H*)-Pyrimidinetrione, 5-ethyl-1-methyl-5-phenyl-, Prominal; Phemitone; Mebaral (*Breon*)

5-Ethyl-1-methyl-5-phenylbarbituric acid [115-38-8] $C_{13}H_{14}N_2O_3$ (246.27).

Preparation—The diethyl ester of ethylphenylmalonic acid is prepared by the general method described under *Barbital*, and is then condensed with *N*-methylurea in the presence of sodium ethylate. The resulting sodium mephobarbital is treated with HCl, whereupon mephobarbital crystallizes.

The *N*-methylurea is prepared as follows. Methylamine is gassed into a mixture of sulfuric acid and absolute alcohol until the mixture is alkaline. Potassium cyanate is then added and the mixture is refluxed overnight whereupon the monomethyl ammonium cyanate produced initially by metathesis rearranges (Wöhler) to *N*-methylurea.

Description—White crystalline powder; odorless; bitter taste; saturated solution is acid to litmus; melts between 176° and 181°; pK$_a$ 8.8.

Solubility—1 g in >1000 mL water, >1000 mL alcohol, 50 mL chloroform, >1000 mL ether; soluble in solutions of fixed alkali hydroxides or carbonates.

Uses—A barbiturate with strong *sedative* and *anticonvulsant* actions but a relatively mild *hypnotic* action. Hence it is used for relief of anxiety, tension, and apprehension, and as an antiepileptic in the management of generalized tonic-clonic (grand mal) and absence (petit mal) seizures. See also the comprehensive general statement on *Barbiturates* in this section.

Dose—*Adult, usual, oral, anticonvulsant,* **400 to 600 mg** daily; *sedative,* **32 to 100 mg** 3 or 4 times a day; *delirium tremens,* **200 mg** 3 times a day. *Pediatric, usual, oral, anticonvulsant,* up to 5 years of age, **16 to 32 mg** 3 or 4 times a day; over 5 years, **32 to 64 mg** 3 or 4 times a day.

Dosage Forms—Tablets: 32, 50, 100, and 200 mg.

Metharbital—page 1078.

Methohexital Sodium for Injection—page 1046.

Pentobarbital

2,4,6(1*H*,3*H*,5*H*)-Pyrimidinetrione, 5-ethyl-5-(1-methylbutyl)-, Dorsital (*Dorsey*); Nembutal (*Abbott*)

5-Ethyl-5-(1-methylbutyl)barbituric acid [76-74-4] $C_{11}H_{18}N_2O_3$ (226.27).

Preparation—By the general method described under *Barbital* (page 1011) using ethyl bromide and 1-methylbutyl bromide as alkylating agents.

Description—White to practically white, fine powder; practically odorless; melts between 127° and 133°.

Solubility—1 g in >2000 mL water, 4.5 mL alcohol, 4 mL chloroform, 10 mL ether.

Uses—See *Pentobarbital Sodium.* Pentobarbital is a *Schedule II* drug under the *Controlled Substances Act.*

Dose—*Adult, usual: Oral, sedative,* equivalent of **20 mg** of pentobarbital sodium 3 or 4 times a day; *hypnotic,* equivalent of **100 mg**

of pentobarbital sodium on retiring, or **90 to 180 mg** as extended-release tablet 30 minutes before retiring. *Pediatric, usual: Oral, sedative,* equivalent of **2 mg/kg** or **60 mg/m²** of body surface of pentobarbital sodium 3 times a day; *hypnotic,* as individualized by physician.

Dosage Forms—Elixir: 18.2 mg/5 mL (equivalent to 20 mg/5 mL of pentobarbital sodium).

Pentobarbital Sodium

2,4,6(1*H*,3*H*,5*H*)-Pyrimidinetrione, 5-ethyl-5-(1-methylbutyl)-, monosodium salt; Pentobarbitone Sodium; Soluble Pentobarbital; Nembutal Sodium (*Abbott*); Palapent (*Bristol-Myers*)

Sodium 5-ethyl-5-(1-methylbutyl)barbiturate [57-33-0] $C_{11}H_{17}N_2NaO_3$ (248.26).

Preparation—By the process given for *Barbital*, using 2-bromopentane instead of ethyl bromide to react with one of the hydrogens in the CH_2 of the malonyl group. It is then converted into the soluble sodium salt by the addition of the required amount of NaOH.

Description—White, odorless, crystalline granules or a white powder with a slightly bitter taste; pH (1 in 10 solution) between 10.0 and 10.5 when for parenteral use; otherwise between 9.7 and 10.2; solutions decompose on standing, heat accelerating the decomposition; pK$_{a1}$ 8.17; pK$_{a2}$ 12.67.

Solubility—Very soluble in water; freely soluble in alcohol; practically insoluble in ether.

Uses—Widely used as a *sedative* or *hypnotic* and as preanesthetic medication. It is also indicated, in anesthetic doses administered intravenously, for control of certain convulsive syndromes. See also the general statement on *Barbiturates* in this section. Pentobarbital sodium is a *Schedule II* drug under the *Controlled Substances Act.*

Dose—*Adult, usual: Oral, sedative,* **30 mg** 2 to 4 times daily or **100 mg** as extended-release tablet once, in morning; *hypnotic,* **100 mg** at bedtime. *Intramuscular, preoperative sedative* or *hypnotic,* **150 to 200 mg**. *Intravenous, hypnotic* or *anticonvulsant,* **100 mg** given as initial dose, with additional small doses at 1-minute intervals, if necessary, up to a total of **500 mg.** *Rectal, sedative,* **30 mg** 2 to 4 times daily; *hypnotic,* **120** or **200 mg** on retiring. *Pediatric, usual: Oral, sedative,* **2 mg/kg** or **60 mg/m²** body surface 3 times daily; *preoperative sedative,* individualized by physician for children up to 10 years of age, **100 mg** for children 10 years of age and over; *hypnotic,* individualized by physician. *Intramuscular* or *intravenous, anticonvulsant,* **3 to 5 mg/kg** or **125 mg/m²** body surface per dose; *sedative* or *hypnotic,* individualized by physician. *Rectal, sedative,* same as oral dose; *hypnotic,* children up to 2 months of age, dosage not established, 2 months to 1 year (4.5 to 9 kg) **30 mg,** 1 to 4 years (9 to 18 kg) **30** or **60 mg,** 5 to 12 years (18 to 36 kg) **60 mg,** 12 to 14 years (36 to 50 kg) **60** or **120 mg.**

Dosage Forms—Capsules: 30, 50, and 100 mg; Injection: 50 mg/mL, in 1-, 2-, 20-, and 50-mL containers; 125 mg/mL in 10-mL vials; 300 mg/mL in 10-mL vials; Suppositories: 15, 30, 60, 120, 200 mg.

Phenobarbital

2,4,6(1*H*,3*H*,5*H*)-Pyrimidinetrione, 5-ethyl-5-phenyl-, Phenylethylmalonylurea; Phenobarbitone; Gardinal; Luminal; Various Mfrs

5-Ethyl-5-phenylbarbituric acid [50-06-6] $C_{12}H_{12}N_2O_3$ (232.24).

Preparation—Benzyl chloride is converted into phenylacetic ester (ethyl phenylacetate) by treating with sodium cyanide and then hydrolyzing with acid in the presence of alcohol. The ester is condensed in the presence of alcohol and metallic sodium with ethyl oxalate, forming diethyl sodium phenyloxaloacetate. HCl is added to liberate diethyl phenyloxaloacetate which, on being distilled at about 180°, splits off carbon monoxide, and forms phenylmalonic ester [$C_6H_5CH(COOC_2H_5)_2$]. The hydrogen of the CH in the phenylmalonic ester is then ethylated and the resulting ethylphenylmalonic ester condensed with urea as described under *Barbital*.

Description—White, odorless, glistening, small crystals, or a white crystalline powder, which may exhibit polymorphism; stable in air; pH (saturated solution) about 5; melts between 174° and 178°; pK_a 7.6.

Solubility—1 g in about 1000 mL water, 10 mL alcohol, about 40 mL chloroform, and 15 mL ether.

Uses—This classical barbiturate is a *sedative, hypnotic,* and *antiepileptic* drug. In appropriate doses it is used in neuroses and related tension states when mild, prolonged sedation is indicated, as in hypertension, coronary artery disease, functional gastrointestinal disorders, and preoperative apprehension. In addition, it has specific usefulness in the symptomatic therapy of *epilepsy*. It is especially useful in patients with generalized tonic-clonic seizures (grand mal) and complex partial (psychomotor) seizures. Effective doses usually produce a degree of drowsiness or sluggishness. Approximately 80% of an oral dose is absorbed and peak plasma levels are reached in 16 to 18 hours. Apparent volume of distribution is 0.7 to 1 L/kg. Therapeutic plasma levels range from 10 to 30 μg/mL. About 45 to 50% of the drug is bound to plasma protein. Apparent plasma half-life varies from 50 to 120 hours in adults and 40 to 70 hours in children. Approximately 65% of the drug is metabolized (largely to the inactive *p*-hydroxyphenyl derivative) and 35% is excreted by the kidney unchanged. Plasma clearance is slow and approximates 0.004 L/kg/hr. With the exception of metharbital and mephobarbital, phenobarbital is the only barbiturate effective in epilepsy. See the comprehensive general statement on *Barbiturates* in this section.

Dose—*Adult, usual: Oral, sedative,* **30** to **120 mg** in 2 or 3 divided doses; *hypnotic,* **100** to **320 mg;** *anticonvulsant,* **50** to **100 mg** 2 or 3 times a day. *Usual range of dose,* **30** to **600 mg** daily. *Pediatric, usual: Oral, sedative,* **2 mg/kg** or **60 mg/m²** body surface 3 times a day; *hypnotic,* individualized by physician; *anticonvulsant* or *antidyskinetic,* **3** to **5 mg/kg** or **125 mg/m²** body surface daily until a blood level of 10 to 15 μg/mL is attained.

Dosage Forms—Elixir (see below); Capsules: 15 mg; Capsules, extended release: 60 mg; Oral Solution: 7.5 and 100 mg/5 mL; Tablets: 8, 15, 30, 60, and 100 mg.

Phenobarbital Elixir contains 7.5 or 20 mg phenobarbital/5 mL. The USP XVIII formula for the latter was: Dissolve phenobarbital (4 g) in alcohol (150 mL), and add orange oil (0.75 mL), glycerin (450 mL), syrup (150 mL), and amaranth solution (10 mL), then add sufficient purified water to make 1000 mL. Mix, and filter, if necessary. *Alcohol content:* 12 to 15%. (Amaranth is no longer permitted to be used as a coloring agent.)

Phenobarbital Sodium

2,4,6(1*H*,3*H*,5*H*)-Pyrimidinetrione, 5-ethyl-5-phenyl-, monosodium salt; Sodium Phenobarbital; Soluble Phenobarbital; Phenobarbitone Sodium; Luminal Sodium (*Winthrop*)

Sodium 5-ethyl-5-phenylbarbiturate [57-30-7] $C_{12}H_{11}N_2NaO_3$ (254.22).

Preparation—By dissolving phenobarbital in an alcohol solution of an equivalent quantity of NaOH and evaporating at low temperature.

Description—Flaky crystals, or white, crystalline granules, or white powder; odorless; bitter taste; hygroscopic. Solutions are alkaline to phenolphthalein, and decompose on standing. pH (1 in 10 solution) between 9.2 and 10.2.

Solubility—Very soluble in water; soluble in alcohol; practically insoluble in ether, chloroform.

Uses—Phenobarbital sodium, because it is soluble in water, may be administered parenterally. It is given by slow intravenous injection for control of acute convulsive syndromes. For additional information see *Phenobarbital*, also the general statement on *Barbiturates* in this section.

Dose—*Adult, usual: Oral,* as for phenobarbital. *Intramuscular* or *intravenous, sedative,* **100** to **130 mg;** *anticonvulsant,* **200** to **300 mg** repeated in 6 hours if necessary; *preoperative medication,* **130** to **200 mg** every 6 hours; *postoperative sedation,* **32** to **100 mg.** *Pediatric, usual, intramuscular,* **60 mg/m²** 3 times daily; *anticonvulsant,* **125 mg/m²/dose;** *preoperative medication,* **16** to **100 mg;** *postoperative sedation,* **8** to **30 mg.**

Note: Doses should be reduced significantly in elderly or debilitated patients. No barbiturate should be given parenterally without full knowledge of its particular characteristics, dosage, and recommended rate of administration.

Dosage Forms—Injection: 30, 60, 65, and 130 mg/mL. Sterile powder, 120 mg ampuls.

Secobarbital

2,4,6(1*H*,3*H*,5*H*)-Pyrimidinetrione, 5-(1-methylbutyl)-5-(2-propenyl)-, Seconal (*Lilly*)

5-Allyl-5-(1-methylbutyl)barbituric acid [76-73-3] $C_{12}H_{18}N_2O_3$ (238.29).

Preparation—By the general method described under *Barbital* (page 1066) using allyl bromide and 1-methylbutyl bromide as alkylating agents at the 5-position.

Description—White, amorphous, or crystalline, odorless powder, having a slightly bitter taste; pH (saturated solution) about 5.6; melting range 96° to 100°.

Solubility—Very slightly soluble in water; freely soluble in alcohol, ether, and in solutions of alkali hydroxides; soluble in chloroform.

Uses—A *sedative* and *hypnotic*. See also *Secobarbital Sodium* and the general statement on Barbiturates in this section. Secobarbital is a *Schedule II* drug under the *Controlled Substances Act*.

Dose—See *Secobarbital Sodium*.

Dosage Forms—Elixir: 22 mg/5 mL; Capsules, 50 and 100 mg.

Secobarbital Sodium

2,4,6(1*H*,3*H*,5*H*)-Pyrimidinetrione, 5-(1-methylbutyl)-5-(2-propenyl)-, monosodium salt; Quinalbarbitone Sodium; Seconal Sodium (*Lilly*)

Sodium 5-allyl-5-(1-methylbutyl)barbiturate [309-43-3] $C_{12}H_{17}N_2NaO_3$ (260.27).

Preparation—By treatment with a chemically equivalent portion of NaOH as described under *Phenobarbital Sodium*.

Description—White, odorless, hygroscopic powder, having a bitter taste; pH (1 in 20 solution) between 9.7 and 10.5; solutions decompose on standing, heat accelerating the decomposition.

Solubility—Very soluble in water; soluble in alcohol; practically insoluble in ether.

Uses—A widely used *sedative* and *hypnotic*. The drug is also used, in anesthetic doses intravenously, for control of certain acute convulsive conditions, such as those associated with tetanus, status epilepticus, and toxic reactions to strychnine and local anesthetics. See the general statement on *Barbiturates* in this section. Secobarbital sodium is a *Schedule II* drug under the *Controlled Substances Act*.

Dose—*Adult, usual: Oral, sedative,* **30** to **50 mg;** *hypnotic,* **100 mg** at bedtime; *preoperative sedation,* **200** to **300 mg** 1 to 2 hours before surgery. *Intramuscular, hypnotic,* **100** to **200 mg;** *rectal, hypnotic,* **120** to **200 mg.** *Pediatric, usual, oral, sedation,* **6 mg/kg** daily in 3 divided doses; *intramuscular,* **3** to **5 mg/kg** maximum, **100 mg**); *rectal,* **6 mg/kg** daily in 3 divided doses.

Note: Doses should be reduced significantly in elderly or debilitated patients. No barbiturate should be given parenterally without full knowledge of its particular characteristics, dosage, and recommended rate of administration.

Dosage Forms—Capsules: 50 and 100 mg; Injection: 50 mg/mL; Sterile: 100 and 250 mg; Suppositories: 30, 60, 120, and 200 mg; Tablets: 60 mg, 100 mg (enteric-coated).

Talbutal

2,4,6(1*H*,3*H*,5*H*)-Pyrimidinetrione, 5-(1-methylpropyl)-5-(2-propenyl)-, Lotusate (*Winthrop*)

5-Allyl-5-*sec*-butylbarbituric acid [115-44-6] $C_{11}H_{16}N_2O_3$ (224.26).

Preparation—By the general method described under *Barbital*, using allyl bromide and *sec*-butyl bromide as alkylating agents.

Description—White, crystalline powder, which may have a slight odor of caramel; melts at about 108°, or may occur in a polymorphic form that melts at about 111°.

Solubility—1 g in 500 mL water, 1 mL alcohol, 2 mL chloroform, 40 mL ether.

Uses—A *hypnotic* which, in appropriate dose, induces sleep in 15 to 30 minutes that lasts 6 to 8 hours. See the general statement on *Barbiturates* in this section.

Dose—*Adult, usual, oral, hypnotic*, **120 mg** 15 to 30 minutes before retiring; *sedative*, **30** to **60 mg** 2 or 3 times a day. *Pediatric*, dosage not established.

Dosage Form—Tablets: 120 mg.

Thiamylal Sodium—page 1046.

Thiopental Sodium—page 1047.

Other Barbiturates

Aprobarbital [5-Allyl-5-isopropylbarbituric acid [77-02-1] $C_{10}H_{14}N_2O_3$ (210.23); Alurate (*Hoffman-LaRoche*)]—A white, crystalline powder; odorless; slightly bitter taste; melts at about 141°. Slightly soluble in cold water; soluble in alcohol, chloroform, ether. *Uses:* A *sedative* and *hypnotic*. See the general statement on *Barbiturates* in this section. *Dose: Usual, oral, sedative*, 20 to 40 mg 3 times daily; *hypnotic*, 40 to 160 mg on retiring. *Dosage Form:* Elixir: 40 mg/5 mL.

Hexobarbital [5-(1-Cyclohexen-1-yl)-1,5-dimethylbarbituric acid [56-29-1] $C_{12}H_{16}N_2O_3$ (236.27). Hexobarbitone; Sombulex (*Riker*)]. *Preparation*—By the general method described under *Barbital*, using methyl bromide and 1-cyclohexen-1-yl bromide as the alkylating agents and *N*-methylurea for the final condensation. The *N*-methylurea may be prepared as described under *Mephobarbital. Description and Solubility:* Colorless, odorless crystals or tasteless, white, crystalline powder; melts between 144° and 147°. Soluble in 3000 parts water, and about 45 parts alcohol; soluble in ether, chloroform, and solutions of alkali hydroxides. *Uses:* A *hypnotic* which in appropriate doses produces a satisfactory plasma-level profile of the intermittent type desirable in treating insomnia. See the comprehensive general statement on *Barbiturates* in this section. *Dose: Adult, oral, hypnotic*, 250 to 500 mg at bedtime; *sedative* in *obstetrics*, 250 to 500 mg every 2 or 3 hours as necessary. Pediatric dosage has not been established.

Secobarbital Sodium and Amobarbital Sodium Capsules (Tuinal, *Lilly*)—A mixture of equal parts of these barbiturates. *Uses:* A rapidly effective hypnotic for use when prompt and moderately sustained effect is required; not suitable for continuous daytime sedation. Adverse reactions, contraindications, and addiction liability are the same as for other barbiturates. See the general statement on *Barbiturates* in this section. This is a *Schedule II* drug under the *Controlled Substances Act. Dose:* 50 to 200 mg of the mixed barbiturates at bedtime or 1 hour preoperatively. *Dosage Forms:* Capsules containing 50, 100, and 200 mg of the mixed barbiturates.

Miscellaneous Sedatives and Hypnotics

In addition to the benzodiazepines and barbiturates discussed in the previous two sections, there are a number of other agents which possess useful sedative and hypnotic properties. These are derived from several heterogeneous structures, including alcohols (ethchlorvynol), carbamates (ethinamate, mebutamate, meprobamate), chloral hydrate

and related drugs (chloral betaine, triclofos), cyclic ether (paraldehyde), piperidinediones (glutethimide, methyprylon), and quinazolinone (methaqualone). In addition to sedative-hypnotic properties, several of these substances possess anticonvulsant, antispasmodic, local anesthetic, and weak antihistaminic properties. In general, the effective hypnotic dose of these substances is larger than that for either the benzodiazepines or barbiturates. Nevertheless, they do not differ qualitatively from the barbiturates in their desirable and undesirable effects. Hence, patients should be cautioned about concomitant use of alcohol or other CNS depressants and warned about operating a motor vehicle or hazardous machinery while on such drugs. It should be remembered that safe and effective use of many of these agents during pregnancy and in pediatric patients has not been established. Also, many of these agents will produce physical dependence and habituation when taken chronically in excessive doses. For this reason methaqualone is listed in *Schedule II* and glutethimide in *Schedule III* under the *Controlled Substances Act*. Other substances in this section have lower abuse potential and are listed in *Schedule IV*. Nevertheless, they should all be used with caution in patients with a previous history of drug dependence.

Disulfiram (Antabuse), an antioxidant agent devoid of sedative and hypnotic properties, is included in this section because of its use as an adjunct in the management of alcoholism.

Chloral Hydrate

1,1-Ethanediol, 2,2,2-trichloro-, Chloral; Noctec (*Squibb*)

$$CCl_3CH(OH)_2$$

Chloral hydrate [302-17-0] $C_2H_3Cl_3O_2$ (165.40).

Preparation—By hydration of trichloroacetaldehyde (chloral) obtained by action of chlorine on alcohol.

Description—Colorless, transparent, or white crystals; aromatic, penetrating, and slightly acrid odor; slightly bitter, caustic taste. Melts at about 55°; slowly volatilizes in air.

Solubility—1 g in 0.25 mL water, 1.3 mL alcohol, 2 mL chloroform, 1.5 mL ether; very soluble in olive oil.

Uses—A widely used hypnotic that is more effective for inducing sleep than prolonging it. Somnifacient doses promptly produce drowsiness and sedation, followed by quiet, sound sleep within an hour. Its effect on REM sleep is not well defined, but low doses of 500 to 1000 mg do not appear to decrease REM sleep, while high doses may do so. It is indicated for nocturnal and preoperative sedation. It is also used in combination with barbiturates in the first stage of labor. Chloral hydrate has also been used in the treatment of eclampsia and tetanus. In postoperative care it has been a valuable adjunct to opiates and analgesics. It has little or no analgesic action, and should not be used alone in the presence of pain.

Following oral administration, chloral hydrate is rapidly converted to trichloroethanol (TCE), which is largely responsible for its hypnotic action. Other metabolites are trichloroacetic acid (TCA) and trichloroethanolglucuronide (TCEG). Peak plasma levels of TCE and TCEG are reached in 20 to 60 minutes; plasma half-lives are 8.0 (7.0 to 9.5) hours and 6.7 (6.0 to 8.0) hours for TCE and TCEG, respectively. The half-life for TCA is 4 days. These data suggest that chloral hydrate has desirable properties, since the half-life of its active metabolite is short. The formation of TCA is a matter of concern, since its effect on the patient is unknown. Chloral hydrate must be used with caution in patients receiving oral anticoagulants because TCA displaces warfarin from plasma protein binding sites; it is likely that dicumarol is affected similarly. Also, concomitant administration of alcohol and chloral hydrate should be avoided; significant potentiation may occur. Gastric irritation occurs in some patients. Paradoxical excitement is observed rarely. The continued use of large doses causes peripheral vasodilation, hypotension, ventilatory depression, arrhythmias, and myocardial depression. Over-dosage may result in coma. Patients with serious heart, kidney, or liver disease should not be given chloral hydrate. If gastritis is present, the drug may be administered by rectum in olive oil as a retention enema. The acute toxic oral dose for adults is approximately 10 g; death has been reported after as little as 4 g and individuals have survived after ingesting 30 g.

For oral use, chloral hydrate is sometimes given in a flavored syrup. As alkali causes decomposition of chloral hydrate, it is important that the vehicle not be alkaline.

Dose—*Adult*, *oral*, *usual*, *sedative*, **250 mg** 3 times a day; *hypnotic*, **500 mg** to **1 g**, on retiring. *Usual range of dose*, **250 mg** to **2 g** daily. *Pediatric*, *usual*, *oral*, *hypnotic*, **50 mg/kg** or at the rate of **1.5 g/m²** body surface, up to **1 gram** per single dose, at bedtime; *sedative*, **8 mg/kg** or **250 mg/m²**, up to **500 mg** per dose, 3 times a day.

Dosage Forms—Capsules: 250 and 500 mg, and 1 g; Elixir: 500 mg/5 mL; Suppositories: 325, 500, and 650 mg. Syrup: 250 and 500 mg/5 mL.

Disulfiram

Thioperoxydicarbonic diamide, tetraethyl-, Tetraethylthiuram Disulfide; Antabuse (*Ayerst*)

$$(C_2H_5)_2NC-S-S-CN(C_2H_5)_2$$

Bis(diethylthiocarbamoyl) disulfide [97-77-8] $C_{10}H_{20}N_2S_4$ (296.52).

Preparation—A cold solution of diethylamine and carbon disulfide in alcohol is treated with an alcoholic solution of iodine. Ice water may be added to hasten separation of the disulfiram. *Ind Eng Chem* 20: 1173, 1928. US Pat 1,796,977.

Description—White to off-white, odorless, crystalline powder; melts between 69° and 72°.

Solubility—1 g in >5000 mL water, 30 mL alcohol, 15 mL ether; soluble in chloroform.

Uses—An adjunct in the treatment of selected chronic alcoholic patients who *want* to remain in a state of enforced sobriety. It is not a cure for alcoholism, when used alone without supportive therapy. It blocks the oxidation of alcohol at the acetaldehyde stage, which then accumulates in the body and produces unpleasant symptoms characterized by flushing, palpitation, dyspnea and hyperventilation, increased pulse rate, nausea and vomiting, cyanosis and decreased blood pressure, and occasionally profound collapse. These symptoms are usually followed by drowsiness and sleep, after which the patient fully recovers. The duration of the reaction varies from 30 to 60 min to several hours in the more severe cases, or as long as there is alcohol in the blood.

The drug should not be used without the patient's full knowledge and consent. Extreme caution is necessary during its use because severe and alarming reactions (and some deaths) have been reported in patients on disulfiram. These include cardiovascular complications involving unusual fall in blood pressure, cardiac arrhythmia, and electrocardiographic evidence of myocardial ischemia and even myocardial infarction. Some patients complain of mild drowsiness, fatigability, impotence, headache or peripheral neuritis, and occasionally skin rashes.

Patients on disulfiram should avoid contact with alcohol in a partially disguised form such as cough syrup or other medicinals containing it and alcoholic lotions applied to the skin. In addition to alcohol-induced reactions, physicians should be alert to drug-induced psychotic episodes that may occur during therapy. Disulfiram should not be used in patients recently treated with paraldehyde, and paraldehyde should not be given to patients receiving disulfiram. Disulfiram appears to decrease the rate at which certain drugs are metabolized and so may increase the blood levels and, thus, the clinical toxicity of drugs given concomitantly. Disulfiram should be given with caution in patients receiving phenytoin, oral anticoagulant drugs, metronidazole and isoniazid. Because of the possibility of an accidental disulfiram-alcohol reaction, it should be used with extreme caution in patients with diabetes mellitus, hypothyroidism, epilepsy, cerebral damage, chronic and acute nephritis, and hepatic cirrhosis or insufficiency. Patients should be informed of the reactions and cautions stated above.

Dose—*Usual*, *oral*, *initial*, up to **500 mg** daily for the first 2 or 3 weeks; *usual*, *maintenance*, **250 mg** daily.

Dosage Forms—Tablets: 250 and 500 mg.

Ethchlorvynol

1-Penten-4-yn-3-ol, 1-chloro-3-ethyl-, Placidyl (*Abbott*)

$$HC\equiv C-\underset{\underset{CH_2CH_3}{|}}{\overset{\overset{OH}{|}}{C}}-CH=CHCl$$

[113-18-8] C_7H_9ClO (144.60).

Preparation—By reacting ethyl chlorovinyl ketone (I) with lithium acetylide under Grignard reaction conditions. The alkoxide addition complex reacts readily with dilute acid to form crude ethchlorvynol which is extracted with a suitable, water-immiscible organic solvent such as ether and is subsequently purified by distillation. I may be prepared in good yield by addition of propionyl chloride to acetylene at a temperature of about 40° in the presence of zinc chloride.

Description—Colorless to yellow liquid possessing a characteristic pungent odor; darkens on exposure to light and air; specific gravity 1.068 to 1.071; refractive index 1.476 to 1.480.

Solubility—Immiscible with water; miscible with most organic solvents.

Uses—A mild hypnotic that induces sleep within 15 minutes to 1 hour and has duration of action of approximately 5 hours. Elimination half-life varies from 10 to 25 hours. Its effect is less profound and not as predictable as that obtained with benzodiazepines. It is indicated as short-term hypnotic therapy in insomnia. It is thought to have little effect on REM sleep; hence, REM rebound is not a problem. Ethchlorvynol has been reported to increase the metabolism of coumarin anticoagulants by enzyme induction; patients on oral anticoagulants should be monitored closely when ethchlorvynol is started or stopped. It is contraindicated in patients with porphyria and those with known hypersensitivity to the drug. Patients should be cautioned about concomitant use of alcohol, barbiturates, other CNS depressants, or MAO inhibitors, since such combinations may produce exaggerated depressant effects. Also, they should be warned against operating a motor vehicle or hazardous machinery while on the drug. The excessive chronic use of large doses of ethchlorvynol has been reported to cause psychic and physical dependence, tolerance, and withdrawal symptoms, including severe convulsions, when the drug is discontinued. It should not be used in patients with a history of drug abuse, and the drug should be gradually withdrawn from patients taking excessive quantities. The drug is metabolized primarily by the liver. Side effects, such as nausea, mental confusion, headache, and dermatitis, have been observed in some patients. In addition, hypotension, blurring of vision, dizziness, facial numbness, and allergic reactions have been reported. There have been rare reports of cholestatic jaundice and a few instances of thrombocytopenia. The safe and effective use of this agent during pregnancy and in pediatric-age patients has not been established.

Dose—*Hypnotic*, *adult*, **500 mg** at bedtime; **750 mg** may be used in patients whose sleep response to 500 mg is inadequate. Maximum, **1000 mg**. An additional 100 to 200 mg may be given to reinstitute sleep in patients who awaken after the usual 500 to 750 mg.

Dosage Forms—Capsules: 100, 200, 500 and 750 mg.

Ethinamate

Cyclohexanol, 1-ethynyl-, carbamate; Valmid (*Lilly*)

[126-52-3] $C_9H_{13}NO_2$ (167.21).

Preparation—By condensing 1-ethynylcyclohexanol with carbamoyl chloride in the presence of pyridine or another basic catalyst. The crude ester is obtained by treating the reaction mixture with dilute hydrochloric acid. It may be purified by crystallization from an ethanol-water mixture. The 1-ethynylcyclohexanol may be synthesized by a typical Grignard reaction using cyclohexanone and ethynylmagnesium bromide.

Description—White, essentially odorless powder; melting range 94° to 98°; pH (saturated solution) about 6.5.

Solubility—1 g in 400 mL water, 2.9 mL alcohol; freely soluble in chloroform and ether.

Uses—A mild hypnotic useful for the induction of sleep in simple insomnia. It is contraindicated in patients hypersensitive to the drug.

Ethinimate is rapidly absorbed after oral administration, inactivated by the liver, and excreted in the urine. Following a single dose of 1 g, peak plasma levels are reached in 36 minutes and decline to negligible values within 8 hours. Approximately 36% of the dose appears in the urine within 24 hours. Onset of action is 20 to 30 minutes. Therefore, it is more effective in inducing sleep than in maintaining sleep. Adverse effects are relatively infrequent. Rare cases of thrombocytopenic purpura and drug idiosyncrasy with fever have been reported. Paradoxical excitement in children, mild gastrointestinal disorders, and skin rashes have also been observed. Although no maternal or fetal adverse effects have been reported, sufficient laboratory work has not been done in this area to warrant its use in pregnant and lactating women. Ethinamate should not be taken concurrently with alcohol or other CNS depressants and patients on this drug should be warned against operating a motor vehicle or operating hazardous machinery for at least 4 or 5 hours after taking the drug. Ethinamate has not been studied in children; hence, it is not recommended for pediatric use. Habituation and physical dependence may result from excessive use of the drug. The abstinence syndrome is similar to that of the barbiturates. It should be used with caution in patients with a history of drug abuse.

Dose—*Adult, oral, usual,* **500 mg** to **1 g** 20 min before bedtime. Dosage in children not established.

Dosage Forms—Capsules: 500 mg.

Glutethimide

2,6-Piperidinedione, 3-ethyl-3-phenyl-, Doriden (*USV*)

2-Ethyl-2-phenylglutarimide [77-21-4] $C_{13}H_{15}NO_2$ (217.27).

Preparation—Benzyl cyanide in toluene solution is treated with ethyl chloride in the presence of sodamide to yield α-ethylbenzyl cyanide. This is then caused to undergo addition (Michael condensation) to methyl acrylate under the catalytic influence of piperidine or another suitable basic catalyst, thus forming methyl 4-cyano-4-phenylhexanoate (I). After purifying by low-pressure distillation, I is cyclized in acid medium. The cyclization may be represented as involving hydration of the cyanide group to amide and saponification of the ester, followed by dehydration between the amide and carboxyl groups.

Description—White, crystalline powder; saturated solution is slightly acid; melting range 86° to 89°.

Solubility—Freely soluble in ethyl acetate, acetone, ether, and chloroform; soluble in alcohol and methanol; practically insoluble in water.

Uses—A hypnotic useful for inducing sleep in all types of insomnia, and in medical conditions requiring sleep. It induces sleep without depressing respiration. The onset of action begins about one-half hour after the administration of a hypnotic dose and generally lasts from 4 to 8 hours. Oral absorption is variable with peak plasma level times between 1 and 6 hr. Elimination half-life varies from 5 to 22 hr, with an average value of 11.6 hr. Glutethimide is contraindicated in hypersensitive patients and patients should be warned about the concomitant use of alcohol and other CNS depressant drugs. Patients should also be cautioned about engaging in activities which require alertness until 4 or 5 hours have elapsed following ingestion of the drug. Glutethimide induces liver microsomal enzymes; therefore, glutethimide therapy in patients on coumarin anticoagulants may require adjustment of the coumarin dose during and upon cessation of glutethimide therapy. Adverse reactions include a generalized skin rash (in this case the drug should be withdrawn); occasionally, a purpuric or urticarial rash; exfoliative dermatitis has been rarely observed; nausea, hangover, paradoxical excitation, and blurred vision have occurred. Porphyria, blood dyscrasias (thrombocytopenic purpura, aplastic anemia, or leukopenia) have also been reported. Habituation and physical dependence may result from the prolonged administration of excessive doses. Glutethimide is a *Schedule III* drug under the *Controlled Substances Act*. The drug should be used with caution in patients with a history of drug abuse.

Dose—*Usual, hypnotic,* **250** to **500 mg** at bedtime. Elderly and debilitated patients, a maximum of **500 mg.** Not recommended in children under 12.

Dosage Forms—Capsules: 500 mg. Tablets: 125, 250, and 500 mg.

Hydroxyzine Hydrochloride

Ethanol, 2-[2-[4-[(4-chlorophenyl)phenylmethyl]-1-piperazinyl]ethoxy]-, dihydrochloride; Atarax (*Roerig*); Orgatrax (*Organon*); Durax (*Dermik*); Various Mfrs

2-[2-[4-(*p*-Chloro-α-phenylbenzyl)-1-piperazinyl]ethoxy]ethanol dihydrochloride [2192-20-3] $C_{21}H_{27}ClN_2O_2$·2HCl (447.83).

Preparation—By condensing *p*-chlorobenzhydryl chloride (I) with *N*-[2-(2-hydroxyethoxy)ethyl]piperazine (II). Conversion to the hydrochloride may be effected by dissolving the base in a double molar quantity of hydrochloric acid and evaporating the solution to dryness.

I may be synthesized by treating benzaldehyde with *p*-chlorophenylmagnesium bromide and reacting the resulting *p*-chlorobenzhydrol with a suitable halogenating agent. II may be synthesized by interaction of piperazine and ethylene oxide.

Description—White, odorless powder; melts with decomposition at about 200°.

Solubility—1 g in 1 mL water, 4.5 mL alcohol, 13 mL chloroform, >1000 mL ether.

Uses—For the management of neuroses and emotional disturbances characterized by anxiety, tension, agitation, apprehension or confusion. This includes its use in anxiety and apprehension associated with organic diseases, alcoholism, allergic conditions, pre- and postoperative conditions, and cardiac conditions. Hydroxyzine hydrochloride is contraindicated in early pregnancy and in patients who have shown a previous hypersensitivity to it. Like other minor tranquilizers it should be used with caution and proper dose adjustment in patients on other CNS depressant drugs. Therefore, when used as preanesthetic medication with other agents, such as meperidine and a barbiturate, the dosage should be adjusted on an individual basis. Atropine and other belladonna alkaloids are not affected by the drug. Since the drug may cause drowsiness, the patient should be warned not to drive a car or operate hazardous machinery while on the drug. Adverse reactions are relatively mild and include drowsiness and dryness of the mouth. Involuntary motor activity, including rare instances of tremor and convulsions have been reported. Clinical studies substantiate the absence of toxic effects on the liver or blood. *The potentiating effect of hydroxyzine hydrochloride must be taken into consideration when the drug is used in conjunction with central nervous system depressants such as narcotics and barbiturates.*

Dose—*Adult, oral, range,* **25** to **100 mg;** *usual,* **25 mg** 3 or 4 times daily, not to exceed 400 mg in a day. *Intramuscular, usual,* **25** to **100 mg** every 4 to 6 hours. *Pediatric, oral, usual,* under 6 years of age, **50 mg** daily in divided doses; over 6 years, **50** to **100 mg** daily in divided doses.

Dosage Forms—Injection: 25 and 50 mg/mL; 100 mg/2 mL; 250 and 500 mg/10 mL; Syrup: 10 mg/5 mL; Tablets: 10, 25, 50, and 100 mg.

Hydroxyzine Pamoate

Ethanol, 2-[2-[4-[(4-chlorophenyl)phenylmethyl]-1-piperazinyl]ethoxy]-, compd. with 4,4'-methylenebis[3-hydroxy-2-naphthalenecarboxylic acid] (1:1); Vistaril (*Pfizer*)

2-[2-[4-(*p*-Chloro-α-phenylbenzyl)-1-piperazinyl]ethoxy]ethanol 4,4'-methylenebis[3-hydroxy-2-naphthoate] (1:1) [10246-75-0] $C_{21}H_{27}ClN_2O_2$·$C_{23}H_{16}O_6$ (763.29).

Preparation—Hydroxyzine, prepared as described under *Hy-*

droxyzine Hydrochloride, is reacted with an equimolar portion of 4,4′-methylenebis[3-hydroxy-2-naphthoic acid].

Description—Light-yellow, practically odorless, powder.
Solubility—1 g in >1000 mL water, 700 mL alcohol, >1000 mL chloroform, >1000 mL ether, 10 mL dimethylformamide.

Uses and **Dose**—See *Hydroxyzine Hydrochloride.*
Dosage Forms—Capsules: 25, 50, and 100 mg; Oral Suspension: 25 mg/5 mL.

Magnesium Sulfate Injection—page 1078.

Meprobamate

1,3-Propanediol, 2-methyl-2-propyl-, dicarbamate; (*Various Mfrs.*)

$$NH_2COOCH_2 \overset{\overset{\displaystyle CH_3}{|}}{\underset{\underset{\displaystyle CH_2CH_2CH_3}{|}}{C}} CH_2 OOCNH_2$$

[57-53-4] $C_9H_{18}N_2O_4$ (218.25).
Preparation—2-Methyl-2-*n*-propyl-1,3-propanediol, in toluene solution, is condensed at about 0° with phosgene in the presence of dimethylaniline to yield the chloroformate diester, which is then subjected to ammonolysis to form the dicarbamate ester. The crude product is purified by crystallization from diluted alcohol.

Description—White powder, which has a characteristic odor and a bitter taste; melts within a range of 2° between 103° and 107°.
Solubility—Slightly soluble in water; freely soluble in alcohol and acetone; sparingly soluble in ether.

Uses—A propanediol derivative chemically related to mephenesin indicated for the management of *anxiety disorders* or for the short-term relief of the *symptoms of anxiety.* Anxiety or tension associated with the stress of everyday life usually do not require treatment with an anxiolytic. It is contraindicated in patients with acute intermittent porphyria and in patients allergic to meprobamate or related agents, such as carisoprodol, mebutamate, or carbromal. Physical and psychological dependence are known to occur after chronic use of high doses of meprobamate. Sudden withdrawal of the drug after prolonged, excessive use should be avoided in order to minimize withdrawal effects. Withdrawal symptoms usually appear 12 to 48 hours after discontinuation of meprobamate and usually cease within the next 12 to 48 hours. The drug should not be prescribed for patients with a history of drug abuse or those known to increase the dose of drugs on their own initiative. Patients should be warned not to attempt potentially hazardous tasks or take other CNS depressant drugs while on meprobamate. The drug should be used with caution in elderly or debilitated patients, epileptic patients, in patients with compromised hepatic or renal function, and in patients with suicidal tendencies. Meprobamate is capable of producing a variety of side effects and untoward reactions. Briefly, these include *CNS effects:* drowsiness, ataxia, dizziness, slurred speech, headache, vertigo, weakness, paresthesias, impaired visual accommodation, euphoria, over-stimulation and paradoxical excitement; *gastrointestinal:* nausea, vomiting, and diarrhea; *cardiovascular:* palpitation, arrhythmias, syncope, and hypotensive crises; a variety of *allergic or idiosyncratic* reactions including various skin, blood, and hypersensitivity reactions (also, Stevens-Johnson syndrome and bullous dermatitis) have been observed: *hematologic:* agranulocytosis, aplastic anemia, and rare cases of thrombocytopenic purpura have been reported. Exacerbation of porphyric symptoms has also been observed. Plasma half-life ranges from 6 to 17 hours (average 10 hours). Therapeutic blood levels range from 0.5 to 2.0 mg%; levels of 3 to 10 mg% usually correlate with mild to moderate symptoms of overdosage, ie, stupor or slight coma; and levels of 10 to 20 mg% with deeper coma requiring intensive therapy, with some fatalities occurring. At levels above 20 mg% more fatalities than survivors can be expected. It is evident, therefore, that the drug should be employed with the same discretion as other therapeutic agents and with due cognizance of the possibility of untoward effects.
Dose—*Adult, oral,* 1 to **2.4 g** daily; *usual, oral,* **400 mg** 3 or 4 times a day; *usual, intramuscular,* **400 mg** 3 or 4 times a day. *Pediatric, under 6 years* of age, use not recommended; *6 to 12 years,* **100 to 200 mg** 2 or 3 times a day.
Dosage Forms—Capsules: 200 and 400 mg; Capsules: (sustained release) 400 mg; Tablets: 200, 400, and 600 mg.

Methapyrilene Hydrochloride—RPS-16, page 1070.

Methaqualone

4(3*H*)-Quinazolinone, 2-methyl-3-(2-methylphenyl)-,

2-Methyl-3-*o*-tolyl-4(3*H*)-quinazolinone [72-44-6] $C_{16}H_{14}N_2O$ (250.30).

Preparation—*N*-Acetylanthranilic acid is cyclized through condensation with *o*-toluidine in the presence of phosphoryl chloride, and the mixture is then rendered alkaline to precipitate the crude product.

Description—White, crystalline powder with little or no odor and a bitter taste; stable in light and air; aqueous solution is alkaline to litmus; melts between 114° and 117°; pK_a (0.1, 22°) 2.54.
Solubility—1 g in 3300 mL water, 8 mL alcohol, 2.2 mL chloroform, 27 mL ether.

Uses—A substituted quinazolone indicated for use as a hypnotic, to induce sleep and as a daytime sedative. It has a rapid distribution half-life (1.8 to 2.1 hr) and a slow elimination half-life (10 to 42 hr). It induces sleep within 10 to 30 min which lasts 6 to 8 hr. Therapeutic doses are almost completely metabolized in the liver by hydroxylation. Very little unchanged drug is found in the urine. The drug should be taken only at bedtime and immediately before the patient retires. Also, patients on the drug should be warned against driving a car or operating hazardous machinery. The drug should be used with caution in patients with depression or suicidal tendencies and those with liver dysfunction. Also, patients on oral anticoagulants should be monitored closely if methaqualone is started or stopped. Side effects encountered are usually mild and transient and include headache, drowsiness, hangover, nausea, fatigue, epigastric discomfort, dizziness, dry mouth, emesis, restlessness, tachycardia, anorexia, diarrhea, urticaria, diaphoresis, bromhidrosis, exanthema, and paresthesia. Rare cases of aplastic anemia, possibly related to methaqualone, have been reported. The drug is contraindicated in women who are or may become pregnant; its safe use in children has not been established. Psychological dependence has occurred with methaqualone; physical dependence, at first believed to be of infrequent occurrence, has now reached alarming proportions, and some authorities on drug abuse believe that the potential for methaqualone addiction and abuse are as serious as those of barbiturates and heroin. Methaqualone should not be used for periods longer than three months. Furthermore, it should not be prescribed for addiction-prone patients or those whose history suggests they may increase the dosage on their own initiative. Methaqualone is a *Schedule II* drug under the *Controlled Substances Act.*
Dose—*Adult, oral, hypnotic,* **150** to **300 mg** at bedtime; *sedative,* **75 mg** 3 or 4 times daily. Pediatric dosage not established.
Dosage Forms—Tablets: 150 and 300 mg.

Methaqualone Hydrochloride

4(3*H*)-Quinazolinone, 2-methyl-3-(2-methylphenyl)-, monohydrochloride

2-Methyl-3-*o*-tolyl-4(3*H*)-quinazolinone monohydrochloride [340-56-7] $C_{16}H_{14}N_2O \cdot HCl$ (286.76).
Preparation—*Methaqualone* is combined with an equimolar quantity of HCl.

Description—White, odorless, crystalline powder; melts with decomposition at about 250°.
Solubility—1 g in 64 mL water; sparingly soluble in alcohol; soluble in chloroform and acetone; very slightly soluble in benzene and ether.

Uses—See *Methaqualone.*
Dose—*Hypnotic,* **200** to **400 mg** at bedtime; *sedative,* **100 mg** after each meal and at bedtime.
Dosage Forms—Capsules: 200 and 400 mg.

Methyprylon

2,4-Piperidinedione, 3,3-diethyl-5-methyl-,
Noludar (*Hoffmann-LaRoche*)

[125-64-4] $C_{10}H_{17}NO_2$ (183.25).

Preparation—3,3-Diethyl-2,4(1H,3H)-pyridinedione is hydroxymethylated at the 5-position by treatment with formaldehyde in the presence of an alkaline catalyst. The resulting methylol derivative is catalytically hydrogenated, whereupon the ring is saturated and the hydroxymethyl group is deoxygenated.

Description—White, or nearly white, crystalline powder that has a slight characteristic odor; melting range 74° to 77.5°.

Solubility—1 g in 11 mL water, 2 mL alcohol, 2 mL chloroform, 2 mL ether.

Uses—A hypnotic useful in the management of insomnia of varied etiology. It usually induces sleep within 45 min; it provides sleep for 5 to 8 hours. Mean plasma levels in patients following a single 650-mg dose peak 1 or 2 hours post-administration at approximately 7.8 to 10 μg/mL; the levels decline to 3.3 to 7.8 μg/mL after 4 hours. Side effects are usually infrequent and mild. There have been rare cases of morning drowsiness, dizziness, mild to moderate gastric upset (diarrhea, esophagitis, nausea, and vomiting), headache, paradoxical excitement, and skin rash. A few isolated cases of neutropenia and thrombocytopenia have been reported. Patients should be warned against the concomitant use of methyprylon and alcohol or other CNS depressants. Habituation and physical dependence have been reported to occur when excessive doses are taken over an extended period of time. Methyprylon is a *Schedule III* drug under the *Controlled Substances Act*. Its safe use during pregnancy and in children under 3 years of age has not been established.

Dose—*Adult, oral, hypnotic*, **200** to **400 mg** before retiring, individualized for maximum beneficial effect. *Children*, the effective dose varies greatly and should be individualized; initially **50 mg** may be given, increased up to **200 mg**, if required, at bedtime. Should not be given to children under 12 years of age.

Dosage Forms—Capsules: 300 mg; Tablets: 50 and 200 mg.

Paraldehyde

1,3,5-Trioxane, 2,4,6-trimethyl-, Paracetaldehyde
Paral (*O'Neal, Jones & Feldman*)

2,4,6-Trimethyl-*s*-trioxane [123-63-7] $C_6H_{12}O_3$ (132.16); a trimer of acetaldehyde.

Caution—Paraldehyde is subject to oxidation to form acetic acid. It may contain a suitable stabilizer.

Preparation—By treating acetaldehyde with small quantities of sulfur dioxide, hydrochloric acid, carbonyl chloride, or zinc chloride; almost complete conversion occurs, and by freezing the liquid and then distilling the crystallized material, if necessary, pure paraldehyde is produced.

Description—Colorless, transparent liquid with a disagreeable taste and a strong, characteristic, but not unpleasant or pungent odor; specific gravity about 0.99; congeals not below 11° and distils between 120° and 126°; in contact with air it slowly oxidizes to acetic acid.

Solubility—1 mL in about 10 mL water and about 17 mL boiling water; miscible with alcohol, chloroform, ether, and volatile oils.

Incompatibilities—*Acids* convert paraldehyde into acetaldehyde, which is prone to oxidation.

Uses—Paraldehyde is one of the oldest *sedatives* and *hypnotics*. It is rapidly absorbed after oral administration and produces sleep within 10 to 15 min. after a 4 to 8 mL dose. It is detoxified by the liver (70 to 80%) and 11 to 28% is excreted by the lungs. A negligible amount is excreted in the urine. Its chief disadvantage is that, being in part excreted through the lungs, it imparts an odor to the exhaled air. Also paraldehyde has an unpleasant taste and may irritate the throat and gastric mucosa unless dispensed in suitable vehicles. It is poorly soluble in water; hence, it is usually prescribed in combination with alcoholic liquors, elixirs, etc. The drug can also be taken in milk, fruit juices, iced tea, or with cracked ice. Finally, it can be administered as a rectal retention enema in olive oil. Paraldehyde

is effective in status epilepticus, but should be reserved for patients who do not respond to phenobarbital. It is occasionally employed as an *obstetrical analgetic*, in which case large doses are administered, usually by rectum. The drug is also frequently used in *delirium tremens*, and in patients undergoing *withdrawal therapy for alcoholism*.

Dose—*Adult, oral: hypnotic*, **4** to **8 mL** in milk or iced fruit juice; *delerium tremens*, **10** to **35 mL**. *Rectal*, **10** to **20 mL** with 1 or 2 parts olive oil. *Intramuscular, hypnotic*, **10 mL** (maximum **5 mL** per injection site) at a rate of 1 mL/minute; *sedation*, **2** to **5 mL** diluted with at least 100 mL of 0.9% sodium chloride. *Children, sedative*, **0.15 mL/kg** IM; *hypnotic*, **0.3 mL/kg**, IM.

Dosage Forms—Sterile: 2, 5, and 10 mL.

Promethazine Hydrochloride—page 1129.

Propranolol Hydrochloride—page 906.

Pyrilamine Maleate—page 1129.

Salicylamide—RPS-16, page 1064.

Scopolamine Hydrobromide—page 917.

Triclofos Sodium

Ethanol, 2,2,2-trichloro-, dihydrogen phosphate monosodium salt;
Triclos (*Merrell-Dow*)

[7246-20-0] $C_2H_3Cl_3NaO_4P$ (251.37).

Preparation—Chloral is reduced with sodium borohydride and the resulting trichloroethanol is esterified with polyphosphoric acid to give the dihydrogen phosphate. The ester is then reacted with an equimolar quantity of NaOH. US Pat 3,236,920.

Description—White or almost white, odorless powder with a saline taste; stable in light, hygroscopic in air, and unstable in heat above room temperature.

Solubility—1 g in 2 mL water and 250 mL alcohol; almost insoluble in ether.

Uses—A hypnotic agent suggested for insomnia characterized by difficulty in falling asleep, nocturnal awakening, and early morning awakening. The drug is rapidly dephosphorylated, principally in the gut, to trichloroethanol; the same pharmacologically active metabolite as obtained from chloral hydrate. Triclofos sodium produces a peak trichloroethanol level in 1 hour; it has a half-life of approximately 8 hours. It is contraindicated in patients with marked renal or hepatic impairment. Triclofos sodium may be habit forming and is subject to the same warnings, precautions, and drug interactions as chloral hydrate. Safe use during pregnancy has not been established. Except for a single dose to induce sleep during electroencephalography, the drug cannot be recommended in children under 12 years of age.

Dose—*Usual, hypnotic*, **1.5 g** 15 to 30 min before bedtime. *Sleep induction in electroencephalography (children under 12)*, **0.22 mL/kg**. Otherwise, triclofos is not recommended for use in children.

Dosage Forms—Tablets; 750 mg; Liquid: 100 mg/mL.

Other Nonbarbiturate Sedatives and Hypnotics

Acecarbromal [*N*-Acetyl-*N*-bromodiethylacetylurea; acetylcarbromal [77-66-7] (279.13); Sedamyl (*Riker*)]—Crystals, slightly bitter taste, melting at 109°; slightly soluble in water; freely soluble in alcohol. *Uses*: A sedative in hysteria and nervous irritability. *Dose*: *Usual*, 250 to 500 mg.

Buclizine Hydrochloride [1-(*p-tert*-Butylbenzyl)-4-(*p*-chloro-α-phenylbenzyl)piperazine dihydrochloride $C_{28}H_{33}ClN_2$.2HCl (505.96); Bucladin-S (*Stuart*)]—A white to slightly yellow, microcrystalline powder; odorless and tasteless; insoluble in water; slightly soluble in alcohol; soluble in chloroform. *Uses*: An agent similar in chemical structure and pharmacologic action to some antihistamines; it is used in the management of nausea, vomiting, and dizziness associated with motion sickness as well as labyrinthitis and Ménière's syndrome. Adverse effects include drowsiness, dryness of the mouth, headache, and jitteriness. Patients should be warned against engaging in activities that require mental alertness, as driving a car or operating heavy machinery or appliances. *Dose*: *Usual, oral*, 50 mg 1 to 3 times daily. The safe and effective dosage in children has not been established. *Dosage Forms*: Tablets: 25 and 50 mg.

Carbromal [Bromo-2-ethylbutyrylurea [77-65-6] (237.11)]—White, crystalline powder; odorless; melts at about 118°; 1 g dissolves in about 3000 mL water, 18 mL alcohol, 3 mL chloroform, 14 mL ether. *Uses:* A weak hypnotic that is now infrequently used. It is readily metabolized to urea in the body and is practically nontoxic, but it should be used with the same care as other bromine-containing compounds. *Dose: Usual, oral,* 500 mg. Available in combination with pentobarbital sodium as *Carbrital.*

Chlormezanone [2-(4-Chlorophenyl)tetrahydro-3-methyl-4H-1,3-thiazin-4-one 1,1-dioxide [80-77-3] $C_{11}H_{12}ClNO_3S$ (273.73); Trancopal (*Breon*)]—White, crystalline powder; melts at about 117°; soluble less than 0.25% in water and less than 1.0% in alcohol. *Uses:* A metathiazanone derivative indicated for management of mild anxiety and tension states. Clinical effects are usually seen within 15 to 30 minutes and may last up to 6 hours or longer. Adverse reactions include drug rash, dizziness, flushing, nausea, drowsiness, depression, edema, inability to void, and weakness. Jaundice has also been reported. *Dose: Usual, oral, adult,* 200 mg 3 or 4 times a day. *Children,* 5 to 12 years of age, 50 to 100 mg 3 or 4 times a day. *Dosage Forms:* Tablets: 100 and 200 mg.

Propiomazine Hydrochloride [1-[10-[2-(Diethylamino)propyl]phenothiazin-2-yl]-1-propanone monohydrochloride [1240-15-9] $C_{20}H_{24}N_2OS.HCl$ (376.94); Largon (*Wyeth*)]—Yellow powder; practically odorless; melts at about 203°; 1 g dissolves in less than 1 mL water, 6 mL alcohol, 2 mL chloroform. *Uses:* A sedative indicated for relief of restlessness and apprehension before and during surgery; also used as an adjunct to analgesics for apprehension and restlessness during labor. Adverse effects include dryness of mouth, moderate elevation in blood pressure, and rarely hypotension; tachycardia has been reported. Dose of barbiturates given concomitantly should be reduced 50%, and meperidine and morphine 25% to 50% because propiomazine enhances the effect of CNS depressants. *Dose: Adult,* intramuscular or intravenous, 10 to 40 mg; *usual,* 20 mg. *Dosage Form:* Injection: 20 mg/mL.

Tybamate [N-Butyl-2-methyl-2-propyl-1,3-propanediol dicarbamate [4268-36-4] $C_{13}H_{26}N_2O_4$ (274.36)] Tybatran (*Robins*)—White, crystalline powder, melting at about 50°, or a clear, viscous liquid that may congeal on standing; mild odor; bitter taste; very slightly soluble in water; very soluble in alcohol. *Uses:* A congener of meprobamate indicated for relief of anxiety and tension in psychoneurotic disorders. Except for a shorter half-life (tybamate, 8 hours; meprobamate, 10 hours), the pharmacological properties, contraindications, and untoward effects of tybamate are similar to those for *Meprobamate.* Dose: 250 or 500 mg 3 or 4 times daily; daily doses larger than 3000 mg are not recommended. *Children* (6 to 12), 20 to 35 mg/kg/day in 3 or 4 divided doses. Not recommended for children under 6 years. Dosage Forms: 250 and 350 mg capsules.

CHAPTER 58

Antiepileptics

Ewart A Swinyard, PhD, DSc (Hon)
Professor Emeritus of Pharmacology
College of Pharmacy and School of Medicine
University of Utah
Salt Lake City, UT 84112

Epilepsy may be defined as a paroxysmal, self-sustaining, and self-limiting cerebral dysrhythmia characterized by an abnormal and excessive EEG discharge and by a disturbance of consciousness; it may or may not be associated with body movements or hyperactivity of the autonomic nervous system. The epileptic attack is initiated by an abnormal focus of electrical discharge, originating either in the grey matter or other part of the brain. The discharge spreads to other parts of the central nervous system and results in convulsions and other manifestations of the disorder.

There are many conditions which result in seizures. These include the entire range of neurological diseases from infection to neoplasm to head injuries. Contrary to popular opinion, hereditary factors are involved in only a few subtypes of seizures. The antiepileptic drugs described in this chapter are also used in patients with febrile seizures or with seizures as a result of an acute illness such as meningitis, even though the term epilepsy is not applied to such patients unless they later develop chronic seizures. Seizures may also result from an acute toxic or metabolic disorder; in such cases appropriate therapy is directed to the specific abnormality, such as hypocalcemia. In most cases of epilepsy, the choice of medication is dictated by the seizure classification.

Based on a modification of the International Classification (*Epilepsia 11:* 102, 1970), epileptic seizures may be divided into two groups:

I. *Partial Seizures* (Focal Seizures).
  A. Partial seizures with elementary symptomatology (cortical focal). Generally without impairment of consciousness. Includes seizures confined to a single limb or muscle group (Jacksonian motor epilepsy), those with sensory or somatosensory symptoms (Jacksonian sensory epilepsy), and those with other limited symptoms depending upon the particular cortical area involved.
  B. Partial seizures with complex symptomatology (temporal lobe; psychomotor seizures). Generally with impairment of consciousness. Attacks of confused behavior with a wide variety of clinical manifestations, associated with bizarre generalized EEG activity during the seizure and temporal lobe abnormalities during the interseizure period.
  C. Partial seizures secondarily generalized.
II. *Generalized Seizures* (bilaterally, symmetrical seizures). Includes *absences* (petit mal), characterized by brief, abrupt loss of consciousness associated with synchronous, 3-per-second spike-and-wave pattern in the EEG, usually with symmetrical clonic motor activity (eyelid blinking or jerking of entire body). *Bilateral massive epileptic myoclonus*, isolated clonic jerks with brief burst of multiple spikes in EEG; *infantile spasms*, motor spasms with bizarre diffuse changes in the interseizure EEG, ie, hypsarrhythmia, and progressive mental retardation; *clonic seizures*, rhythmic clonic contraction of all muscles, loss of consciousness, and autonomic manifestations; *tonic seizures*, opisthotonus, loss of consciousness, and autonomic manifestations; *tonic-clonic seizures* (grand mal), characterized by a sequence of maximal tonic spasms of all body musculature followed by synchronous clonic jerking and profound depression of all central functions; *atonic seizures*, loss of postural tone with sagging of the head or falling; *akinetic seizures*, impaired consciousness and complete muscle relaxation, secondary to excessive inhibitory discharge.

The only effective way of controlling seizures is by the use of antiepileptic drugs. The many medical therapies of an-

tiquity have been replaced by a rational therapeutic approach which had its origin in the beginning of the nineteenth century. It has progressed from the use of bromides in 1857 and phenobarbital in 1912 to the modern era marked by introduction of diphenylhydantoin (phenytoin) in 1938. The clinical efficacy of the latter established the fact that chemicals effective in epilepsy need not be hypnotics and stimulated the laboratory search for other effective anticonvulsant agents. As a result, a number of anticonvulsant barbiturates, benzodiazepines, deoxybarbiturates, dipropylacetic acid derivatives, hydantoins, oxazolidinediones, and succinimides have been introduced in the last 45 years. As a result of these advances in drug therapy, it is generally stated that 50% of all victims of epileptic disorders can be satisfactorily controlled with available drugs and that the incidence of seizures can be reduced in another 25% of epileptic persons.

Knowledge of the underlying causes of various types of seizure disorders is still incomplete. Nevertheless, most experimental models of epilepsy are designed to simulate either in isolated animal brain tissues (*in vitro*) or in the intact laboratory animal (*in vivo*) various chemical, electrical, or overt manifestations of the disorder. *In vitro* procedures used to detect anticonvulsant drug activity include axons, intact single cells, groups of cells including pre- and post-synaptic events, and selected brain segments such as amygdaloid slices and isolated brain synaptosomes (the latter are especially useful for drug-receptor binding studies). *In vivo* studies employed to detect anticonvulsant activity include intracerebral injections and implants of substances in selected areas of the brain, kindling (repeated stimulation of the brain) procedures, sensory stimulation (light and sound), chemical stimulation (pentylenetetrazol, bicuculline, picrotoxin, strychnine, etc), and electrical stimulation (both threshold and maximal) in various species of laboratory animals. In the final analysis, all of these procedures (either *in vitro* or *in vivo*) measure the ability of the chemical substance to alter either seizure threshold or seizure spread.

Because of the variety of clinical types of epilepsy and their differences in response to drugs, a battery of tests is usually employed for the laboratory study of candidate anticonvulsant drugs in animals. In general, these tests measure the ability of drugs to elevate the threshold for minimal seizures or to modify the pattern of maximal convulsions induced in laboratory animals by electrical or chemical stimulation of the brain, to inhibit binding of a [^{3}H] ligand either to selected brain receptor sites, such as γ-aminobutyric acid (GABA) or benzodiazepine, or to a receptor site responsible for the activation of sodium channel ion flux. These tests not only reveal the spectrum of activity of candidate drugs with a view to detection of clinically useful properties, but also provide information as to the mechanism of action of drugs employed in the therapy of seizures. Suggested mechanisms of antiepileptic drug activity include inhibition of Na^+ and Ca^{2+} influx (phenytoin and carbamazepine); enhancement of Ca^{2+} binding to membrane phospholipids (phenytoin); potentiation of γ-aminobutyric acid inhibitory (GABA-ergic) activity and increase Cl^- conductance (phenobarbital and other barbiturates); inhibition of succinic semialdehyde dehydrogenase, aldehyde reductase, and/or γ-aminobutyric acid transaminase (valproate, ethosuximide); and selective interaction with benzodiazepine receptors, potentiation of GABA-ergic inhibitory neurotransmission, and increased chloride conductance (diazepam, clonazepam and other benzodiazepines). For a more detailed treatise on the mechanisms of action the reader should consult "Antiepileptic Drugs: Mechanisms of Action" edited by G H Glaser, J K Penry, and D M Woodbury (Raven Press, NY, 1980).

No one anticonvulsant drug is equally effective in all types of epilepsy. Hence, antiepileptic therapy must be individualized and drug therapy selected on the basis of seizure type. In generalized tonic-clonic seizures (grand mal), simple and complex partial (focal, psychomotor), the drugs of choice, listed in order of preference, are phenytoin or carbamazepine; in generalized absence seizures (petit mal), ethosuximide with valproate and clonazepam alternates. It should be noted that the same drugs are useful in both generalized tonic-clonic seizures and in complex partial seizures (temporal lobe; psychomotor). Status epilepticus, a succession of tonic-clonic seizures without intervening return of consciousness, requires prompt intravenous medication. The objective of treatment is suppression of the seizures, but all of the drugs used to treat this medical emergency can be lethal if they are given too rapidly or in overdosage. Intravenous diazepam (Valium) is preferred by many clinicians; since it is short-acting, maintenance medication must be started promptly. Some clinicians prefer intravenous phenytoin, especially in patients already on this drug. Phenobarbital is an effective alternative for the management of this disorder. If these drugs do not suppress the continuous seizure activity, general anesthesia may be used as an emergency treatment. For a thorough discussion of drug treatment of the epilepsies see "Antiepileptic Drugs" edited by D M Woodbury, J K Penry, and C E Pippinger (Raven Press, 1982).

Once the drug for a particular patient has been selected, administration should be started at a minimum dose and gradually increased until either seizures are controlled or toxic actions to the drug develop. If the latter occurs without seizure control, the dosage of the drug is reduced to a nontoxic level and a second drug is given following the same principle of increasing dosage. This system of pyramiding drug administration allows for the establishment of a reservoir of two or more anticonvulsant drugs, the combined action of which is more effective than any one drug by itself. When new drugs are introduced, previous medication should not be discontinued until an optimum dose level has been established for the new medicament; the drug to be discontinued should then be withdrawn gradually in order to minimize the possibility of inducing status epilepticus.

The monitoring of plasma levels of these drugs is now considered part of the routine management of patients with epilepsy. These drugs exert their action after forming reversible bonds with brain-tissue molecules ("receptors"). Consequently, their intensity of action tends to be proportional to the drug concentration in the biophase in the vicinity of the receptors. Antiepileptic drug molecules in cerebral extracellular water are in dynamic equilibrium with drug molecules in plasma water. Therefore, the antiepileptic drug concentration in plasma water is a measure of the drug concentration in brain and, hence, provides a measure of antiepileptic effect. The clinician needs to know the latter in order to manage his epileptic patients.

When should plasma antiepileptic drug levels be measured? Ideally, plasma levels should be measured in the steady state at fixed times in relation to the drug dosage interval. For most drugs which are eliminated according to processes which follow mono-exponential kinetics, virtually steady state plasma levels are achieved after approximately five drug elimination half-lives. In the case of antiepileptics, their elimination half-lives are so long in relation to dosage regimens that the change in plasma level over a dosage interval is likely to be within the experimental error in an individual drug concentration measurement. Therefore, unless the dosage is changed or other drug therapy added, the time of measurement of antiepileptic drug levels does not present too much of a problem.

The pertinent pharmacokinetic parameters of clinically useful antiepileptic drugs are summarized in each monograph. For more detailed information the reader is referred to "Antiepileptic Drugs: Quantitative Analysis and Interpretation" edited by C E Pippinger, J K Penry, and Knott (Raven Press, New York, 1978).

From a clinical standpoint antiepileptic drug levels should be monitored (1) at the outset of therapy, to see if a satisfactory plasma level has been obtained and (2) during the course of therapy. The latter is especially important if the seizures are not controlled, intercurrent illness develops, antiepileptic drug dosage is changed, dosage of any other drug is changed or symptoms occur which appear to be due to the drug. It is also important to monitor the epileptic patient during pregnancy, since antiepileptic drug levels tend to fall during pregnancy and to rise again during puerperium. Such monitoring increases the chances of controlling epilepsy in patients and decreases the risk of their being overdosed in the process.

Antiepileptic drugs may add to or potentiate the action of other central nervous system depressants, including other anticonvulsants and alcohol. A number of drugs, when concurrently administered with various antiepileptic agents, have been reported to alter the patient's response either to the antiepileptics or to the other drugs (see Chapter 102, on *Drug Interactions*, for additional information concerning specific interactions). Whether or not the effects are clinically significant cannot be categorically stated; they must be evaluated by careful observation of the individual patients, with monitoring of blood plasma levels of the concurrently administered drugs after which dosage adjustments of the interacting drugs may be necessary. For these reasons patients on antiepileptic medication should not take other drugs, either OTC or prescription, without the knowledge and approval of the physician responsible for their seizure therapy.

As tricyclic antidepressants may precipitate seizures, patients being treated with anticonvulsants should be observed closely for decreased seizure control if tricyclic antidepressant therapy is commenced; if necessary, dosage of the anticonvulsant should be adjusted.

The effects of anticonvulsant drugs in human pregnancy and nursing infants are unknown. Recent reports suggest an association between the use of anticonvulsant drugs by women with epilepsy and an increased incidence of birth defects in children born to these women. One such report indicates the use of antiepileptic drugs during pregnancy increases the incidence of birth defects from about 30/1000 to 90/1000. Data are more extensive with respect to phenytoin, phenobarbital, and trimethadione. More recent observations indicate that valproate may be associated with spinal defects in the fetus. Although systematic or anecdotal reports suggest a possible similar association with the use of all known anticonvulsant drugs, therapeutic abortion should be considered when trimethadione has been used during pregnancy. The great majority of mothers on anticonvulsant medication, however, deliver normal infants. It is also important to note that anticonvulsant drugs should not be discontinued in patients in whom the drug is administered to prevent generalized tonic-clonic seizures because of the strong possibility of precipitating status epilepticus with an attendant hypoxia and threat to life. In individual cases where the severity and frequency of the seizure disorder are such that the removal of medication does not pose a serious threat to the patient, discontinuation of the drug may be considered prior to and during pregnancy, although it cannot be said with any confidence that even minor seizures do not pose some hazard to the developing embryo or fetus. The prescribing physician will wish to weigh the risk/benefit of these considerations in treating or counseling epileptic women of child-bearing age.

Antiepileptic agents have several uses in the nonepileptic patient. They have been used to soften the seizures in patients undergoing electroshock therapy, to control convulsions occurring in dementia paralytica and tetanus, and to lessen muscular rigidity in certain cases of cerebral palsy. Phenytoin administered intravenously has been reported to be effective in suppressing recurrent cardiac arrhythmias. In addition, phenytoin, trimethadione, and phenacemide have been employed for the treatment of disturbed nonepileptic psychotic patients, particularly in catatonic excitement states, and in the management of children with behavioral disorders. The latter use is especially intriguing and warrants careful clinical study.

Acetazolamide—page 936.

Amphetamine Sulfate—page 891.

Carbamazepine

5*H*-Dibenz[*b,f*]azepine-5-carboxamide; Tegretol (*Ciba-Geigy*)

[298-46-4] $C_{15}H_{12}N_2O$ (236.27).

Preparation—5*H*-Dibenz[*b,f*]azepine, which may be prepared by thermal deammoniation of 2-(*o*-aminostyryl)aniline hydrochloride, is condensed with carbamoyl chloride by refluxing in an inert solvent in the presence of sodamide. US Pat 2,948,718.

Description—White to off-white powder; melts within a range of 3° between 187° and 193°.

Solubility—Practically insoluble in water; soluble in alcohol and acetone.

Uses—Carbamazepine is considered the drug of choice for complex partial seizures (temporal lobe, psychomotor). It is preferred by many physicians for *generalized tonic-clonic seizures* (grand mal) and simple partial (focal, Jacksonian) seizures, particularly in patients who have not responded to other less toxic anticonvulsants. It is also sometimes effective in patients with mixed seizure patterns which include the above, or other partial or generalized seizures. Carbamazepine is also useful in treatment of pain associated with true trigeminal neuralgia. Beneficial results have also been reported in glossopharyngeal neuralgia. Carbamazepine has a neutral pK$_a$; from 60 to 73% of the drug is bound to plasma protein, volume distribution is usually between 0.8 to 1.4 L/kg; and half-life varies from 10 to 25 hours in adults and 8.5 to 19 hours in children. Therapeutic plasma levels range from 4 to 10 μg/mL. Carbamazepine should not be used in combination with other drugs; for example, troleandomycin, erythromycin, cimetidine, isoniazid and propoxyphene inhibits the metabolism of carbamazepine and elevates the plasma concentrations of this agent. On the other hand, carbamazepine decreases the plasma levels of clonazepam, diazepam, ethosuximide, phenytoin, phenobarbital, primidone, and valproic acid.

To minimize adverse effects, initial dosage and daily increments should be limited to 200 mg. Adverse effects are encountered in approximately 50% of patients with serum carbamazepine levels from 8.5 to 10 μg/mL, but few occur with concentrations below 5 μg/mL. Diplopia, dizziness, drowsiness, and ataxia occur above 6 μg/mL; nystagmus may occur at serum levels below the therapeutic range. Other reactions include anorexia and nausea, rash (including the Stevens-Johnson syndrome), and edema. More serious adverse effects include aplastic anemia, agranulocytosis, thrombocytopenia, and transient leukopenia have been observed. Therefore, all patients should be subjected to a complete blood test before being placed on the drug; additional blood tests should be done at weekly intervals during the first month of therapy, every 2 weeks during the second and third month, and at monthly intervals as long as the patient is on the drug. Patients should be made aware of the early toxic signs and symptoms of hematological problems such as fever, sore throat, ulcers in the mouth, easy bruising, and petechial or purpuric hemorrhage. If any blood abnormality is observed, the drug should either not be used or stopped if the patient is already on the drug. If adverse effects are of such severity that the drug must be withdrawn, the physician must be aware that abrupt discontinuation of any anticonvulsant drug in a responsive patient may lead to increased seizure incidence or even status epilepticus.

The safe use of carbamazepine in pregnancy, lactation, and in women of child-bearing age has not been established. See introduction to this chapter.

Dose—*Range*, 200 to 1200 mg. *Usual, oral, anticonvulsant, adults and children over 12 years*—200 mg twice daily; increase gradually by 200 mg/day in divided doses until desired response is obtained. Do not exceed 1200 mg daily in patients over 15 years or 1000 mg daily in children 12 to 15 years. *Maintenance*—usually 800 to 1200 mg daily. *Usual, oral, analgesic*, 100 mg twice the first day, increased by 100 mg twice a day until desired response obtained; *maintenance, oral*, 100 to 400 mg twice a day as needed. *Usual, pediatric*, dose has not been established. *Maximum daily oral dose*, children 12 to 15 years, 1000 mg.

Dosage Form—Tablets: 200 mg; Tablets (Chewable) 100 mg.

Chlorpromazine Hydrochloride—page 1087.

Clonazepam

2*H*-1,4-Benzodiazepin-2-one, 5-(2-chlorophenyl)-1,3-dihydro-7-nitro-, Clonopin (*Hoffmann-LaRoche*)

[1622-61-3] $C_{15}H_{10}ClN_3O_3$ (315.72).

Preparation—*o*-Chlorobenzoyl chloride is reacted with *p*-nitroaniline to form 2-amino-5-nitro-2'-chlorobenzophenone, and this is condensed with bromacetyl bromide to form 2-bromoacetamido-5-nitro-2'-chlorobenzophenone, then treated with ammonia to form the corresponding acetamido compound. The acetamido compound is converted to its hydrochloride with anhydrous HCl in methanol, dissolved in boiling methanol and cyclized to clonazepam using pyridine as the catalyst.

Description—Light yellow, crystalline powder; faint odor; melts at about 238°; pK$_a$ 1.5 (deprotonation of nitrogen in 4 position), 10.5 (deprotonation of nitrogen in 1 position).

Solubility—Practically insoluble in water; slightly soluble in alcohol; sparingly soluble in chloroform; very slightly soluble in ether.

Uses—Clonazepam is one of the drugs of choice for the management of myoclonic epilepsy. It is also useful alone or as an adjunct in the management of several types of generalized seizures such as absence (petit mal) attacks not responsive to either valproate or ethosuximide, the Lennox-Gestaut syndrome (petit mal variant) and akinetic seizures. Clonazepam has a pK$_a$ of 10.5; 82% of the drug is bound to plasma protein; volume distribution is 2.5 L/kg; and half-life varies from 19 to 46 hours in adults and 13 to 33 hours in children. Therapeutic plasma levels range from 20 to 80 ng/mL. Like diazepam (Valium), which it resembles, tolerance develops in approximately 30% of patients as shown by a loss of anticonvulsant activity; adjustment of dosage may reestablish efficacy. Consequently, the drug should be withdrawn gradually during simultaneous substitution of another anticonvulsant. When used in patients with mixed seizure types, clonazepam may increase the incidence or precipitate the onset of generalized tonic-clonic seizures (grand mal). This may require the use of either increased dosage or addition of other antiepileptic medication. Clonazepam, like other benzodiazepines, is characterized in laboratory animals by its remarkable ability to antagonize pentylenetetrazol-induced seizures; it also has a taming effect in aggressive primates and induces muscle weakness and hypnosis.

The depressant effects of clonazepam may be potentiated by alcohol, narcotics, barbiturates, nonbarbiturate hypnotics, antianxiety agents, the phenothiazines, thioxanthene and butyrophenone classes of antipsychotic agents, monoamine oxidase inhibitors and the tricyclic antidepressants, and by other anticonvulsant drugs. Phenobarbital or phenytoin may decrease steady state plasma levels of clonazepam by enzyme induction. The concomitant use of clonazepam and valproate may produce absence status.

The most frequently occurring side effects are referable to central nervous system depression; drowsiness occurs in approximately 50% of patients and ataxia in approximately 30%. Other adverse reactions, listed by systems are: *Neurologic:* abnormal eye movements, aphonia, choreiform movements, coma, diplopia, dysarthria, dysdiadochokinesis, "glassy-eyed" appearance, headache, hemiparesis, hypotonia, nystagmus, respiratory depression, slurred speech, tremor, vertigo. *Psychiatric:* confusion, depression, forgetfulness, hallucinations, hysteria, increased libido, insomnia, psychosis and suicidal tendencies. *Respiratory:* chest congestion, rhinorrhea, shortness of breath, hypersecretion in upper respiratory passages. *Cardiovascular:* palpitations. *Dermatologic:* hair loss, hirsutism, skin rash, ankle and facial edema. *Gastrointestinal:* anorexia, coated tongue, constipation, diarrhea, dry mouth, encopresis, gastritis, hepatomegaly, increased appetite, nausea, sore gums. *Genitourinary:* dysuria, enuresis, nocturia, urinary retention. *Musculoskeletal:* muscle weakness, pains. *Miscellaneous:* dehydration, general deterioration, fever, lymphadenopathy, weight loss or gain. *Hematopoietic:* anemia, leukopenia, thrombocytopenia, eosinophilia.

The safe use of clonazepam in pregnancy, lactation, and in women of child-bearing age has not been established. See introduction to this chapter.

Dose—*Adults*, **1.5 mg** in 3 divided doses; dosage may be increased **0.5 to 1.0 mg** every 3 days until seizures are controlled or side effects preclude further increase. Maximum daily dose is **20 mg**. *Infants and children under 10 years*, **0.01 to 0.03 mg/kg/day**, but not to exceed **0.05 mg/kg/day** given in 3 divided doses. Dosage may be increased by **0.25 to 0.5 mg** every third day until a maintenance dose of **0.1 to 0.2 mg/kg** has been reached.

Dosage Form—Tablets: 0.5, 1.0, and 2.0 mg.

Clorazepate Dipotassium—page 1061.

Dextroamphetamine Sulfate—page 881.

Diazepam—page 1062.

Dimenhydrinate—page 808.

Diphenhydramine Hydrochloride—page 808.

Ephedrine Sulfate—page 883.

Divalproex Sodium

Pentanoic acid, 2-propyl-, sodium salt (2:1); Depakote (*Abbott*)

$$CH_3CH_2CH_2-CH-CH_2CH_2CH_3$$

Sodium hydrogen bis(2-propylvalerate) [76584-70-8] $C_{16}H_{31}NaO_4$ (310.41).

Preparation—Neutralization of a solution of valproic acid (page 1082) with ½ equivalent of sodium hydroxide and the solvent removed yields the product.

Uses—Divalproex is an antiepileptic agent that dissociates in the gastrointestinal tract into two mols of valproate. Hence, it has the same indications, adverse reactions, and contraindications as valproate. It differs from valproate, however, in that divalproex sodium is available in tablet form. See Valproate Sodium page 1082.

Dose—15 to 60 mg/kg/day. *Usual*, 15 mg/kg/day, increasing at weekly intervals by 5 to 10 mg/kg/day until seizures are controlled. A twice-a-day dosage is suggested wherever feasible.

Dosage Form—Tablets: 250 and 500 mg.

Ethosuximide

2,5-Pyrrolidinedione, 3-ethyl-3-methyl-, Zarontin (*Parke-Davis*)

2-Ethyl-2-methylsuccinimide [77-67-8] $C_7H_{11}NO_2$ (141.17).

Preparation—Methyl ethyl ketone is condensed with ethyl cyanoacetate to yield ethyl 2-cyano-3-methyl-2-pentenoate which, in ethanolic solution, adds hydrogen cyanide to form ethyl 2,3-dicyano-3-methylpentanoate. Proton-catalyzed saponification of the latter ester is accompanied by decarboxylation to produce 2-methyl-2-ethylsuccinonitrile. This, on heating with aqueous ammonia, forms the corresponding diamide which, through loss of ammonia, cyclizes to ethosuximide. US Pat 2,993,835.

Description—White to off-white-crystalline powder or waxy solid that has a characteristic odor; stable in light, air, and heat at 37°; melts between 47° and 52°.

Solubility—Very soluble in alcohol and ether; freely soluble in water and chloroform; very slightly soluble in solvent hexane.

Uses—Ethosuximide is the drug of choice for control of absence seizures (petit mal). It suppresses the paroxysmal three-cycle-per-second spike and wave activity associated with lapses of consciousness characteristic of this disorder. The frequency of attacks is reduced, apparently by depression of the motor cortex and elevation of the neuronal threshold to convulsive stimuli. Ethosuximide should not be used alone in mixed seizure types since it may increase the incidence of generalized tonic-clonic seizures in such patients. Ethosuximide is completely absorbed after oral administration. It has a pK_a of 9.5; the drug is not bound to plasma protein; volume distribution is 0.7 L/kg; and half-life is about 60 hours in adults and 30 hours in children. The drug is extensively metabolized to inactive substances. Therapeutic plasma levels range from 40 to 100 $\mu g/mL$. Maximal serum concentrations are usually achieved within five days after beginning oral therapy. Adverse effects involve the gastrointestinal, hemopoietic, nervous, and integumentary systems. Gastrointestinal symptoms occur frequently and include anorexia, nausea, vomiting, cramps, epigastric distress and abdominal pain; blood disturbances such as leukopenia, agranulocytosis, pancytopenia, aplastic anemia, eosinophilia have occurred; neurologic and sensory reactions observed include drowsiness, headache, dizziness, euphoria, hyperactivity, and ataxia; skin manifestations include urticaria, Stevens-Johnson syndrome, lupus erythematosus, and pruritic erythematous rashes; other reactions reported include myopia, vaginal bleeding, gum hypertrophy, and hirsutism. Periodic blood and urine tests should be made on patients on the drug. Ethosuximide should be administered with extreme caution in patients with known liver or renal disease. The safe use of ethosuximide in pregnancy, lactation, and in women of child-bearing age has not been established. See introduction to this chapter.

Dose—*Adults and children over 6 years of age*, **250 mg** orally twice daily, increased **250 mg** every 4 to 7 days until seizures are controlled or untoward effects develop. Children under 6 years, **250 mg** once a day. *Usual range of dose*, **500 mg** to **1.5 g** daily.

Dosage Forms—Capsules: 250 mg; Syrup: 250 mg/5 mL.

Magnesium Sulfate—page 803.

Magnesium Sulfate Injection

Sulfuric acid magnesium salt (1:1), heptahydrate;
Magnesium Sulfate Ampuls

A sterile solution of magnesium sulfate in water for injection. Magnesium sulfate (1:1) heptahydrate [10034-99-8] $MgSO_4.7H_2O$ (246.47); *anhydrous* [7487-88-9] (120.36).

Preparation—The magnesium sulfate is dissolved in water for injection, and the solution, suitably filtered until free from suspended matter, is placed in cleansed and sterile ampuls. These are sealed and suitably sterilized.

Since the water of hydration content of magnesium sulfate may vary sufficiently to be troublesome in making solutions of required concentration, some operators have found it advisable to prepare solutions slightly stronger than required and to have these assayed promptly, thereafter making up to final volume of the exact strength desired according to the assay results. The stock solution, in the meantime, is kept under refrigeration to protect it.

Uses—Magnesium sulfate is used to prevent or control convulsions in patients with pre-eclampsia and eclampsia. It acts at the myoneural junction to prevent the presynaptic release of acetylcholine and to decrease the motor endplate potential. Uterine contractions are inhibited and uterine blood flow enhanced. Since its action on the cardiovascular system is unpredictable, it is usually used concomitantly with an antihypertensive drug. Principal adverse reactions are related to the high plasma levels of magnesium and include flushing, sweating, hypotension, circulatory collapse, and cardiac and central nervous system depression. Respiratory depression is the most life-threatening effect. The magnesium ion rapidly crosses the placenta but rarely causes symptoms of toxicity in the neonate. Toxicity in the mother is indicated by loss of the pateller reflex; this occurs with magnesium plasma concentrations of 7 to 10 mEq/L. Plasma concentrations greater than 10 mEq/L affect the respiratory muscles. A salt of calcium, such as the gluconate, should be readily available for use as an antidote. The intravenous administration of 5 to 10 mEq of calcium (10 to 20 mL of 10% calcium gluconate) is usually adequate to reverse heart block or respiratory depression. In extreme cases peritoneal dialysis or hemodialysis may be necessary. Magnesium sulfate should not be administered parenterally to patients with heart block or myocardial damage. It should be used with extreme caution in patients with impaired renal function.

Magnesium sulfate injection is also used as an electrolyte replenisher for the treatment of magnesium deficiency.

Dose—*Anticonvulsant, adult: intravenous infusion,* **2** to **4 g** (**4** to **8 mL** of a 50% solution) over a 5-minute period; constant infusion, **1** to **2 g/hr** (**8 mL** of a 50% solution) in 230 mL of 5% dextrose injection. If the urine output falls below 30 mL/hour, the rate of administration should be reduced. Intramuscular administration should not be used because absorption is too variable.

Dosage Forms—Injection: 10% (*w/v*), 12.5% (*w/v*), and 50% (*w/v*) in containers of various sizes.

Mephenytoin

2,4-Imidazolidinedione, 5-ethyl-3-methyl-5-phenyl-, Mesantoin (*Sandoz*)

5-Ethyl-3-methyl-5-phenylhydantoin [50-12-4] $C_{12}H_{14}N_2O_2$ (218.25).

Preparation—5-Ethyl-5-phenylhydantoin, which may be prepared by condensing ethyl α-ethylmandelate with urea in the presence of sodium alcoholate, is monomethylated through reaction with dimethyl sulfate.

Description—White, crystalline powder; melts between 136° and 139°; pH (dissolve 500 mg in 10 mL alcohol, add 10 mL water, mix, and determine pH without delay) between 7.5 and 8.5.

Solubility—1 g in 1400 mL water, 15 mL alcohol, 3 mL chloroform, 90 mL ether.

Uses—An anticonvulsant with a spectrum of clinical activity similar to phenytoin. It may be useful in generalized tonic-clonic seizures (grand mal), complex partial seizures (temporal; psychomotor) and focal seizures (Jacksonian), and grand mal-type status epilepsy, particularly in those patients who have become refractory to or do not respond to less toxic anticonvulsants. Mephenytoin is demethylated to nirvanol, an anticonvulsant employed clinically in 1920 but abandoned because of a high incidence of serious toxicity. Approximately 8% of the total plasma level (mephenytoin and nirvanol) is mephenytoin, but this can vary widely. Approximately 40% of mephenytoin and 30% of nirvanol is bound to plasma protein and half-life varies from 18 to 34 hours. Therapeutic plasma levels range from 5 to 16 μg/mL for mephenytoin and 25 to 40 μg/mL for nirvanol. Drug interactons which may occur are similar to those for phenytoin sodium (see page 1081).

The major side effects are blood dyscrasias such as leukopenia, neutropenia, agranulocytosis, thrombocytopenia, and pancytopenia. Eosinophilia, monocytosis, and leukocytosis have been reported. Various kinds of anemia, including aplastic anemia, have occurred, but are uncommon. Severe skin manifestations, including maculopapular, morbilliform, scarlatiniform, urticarial, purpuric, and nonspecific skin rashes have been observed. Exfoliative dermatitis, Stevens-Johnson syndrome, toxic epidermal necrolysis and fatal dermatitides have been described as rare occurrences. Central effects

such as ataxia, diplopia, nystagmus, dysarthria, fatigue, irritability, choreiform movements, depression, and tremor have also occurred. Hepatitis, jaundice, and nephrosis have been reported, but not convincingly related to the drug. Polyarthropathy, pulmonary fibrosis, lupus erythematosus syndrome, and lymphadenopathy are extremely rare.

The safe use of mephenytoin in pregnancy, lactation, and in women of child-bearing age has not been established. See introduction to this chapter.

Dose—*Oral,* 50 to 100 mg daily and increasing the dose by 50 to 100 mg daily at weekly intervals in accordance with patients need; maximum daily dose 800 mg. Children usually require 100 to 450 mg orally in 3 divided doses daily, according to the nature of the seizure and the age and weight of the patient.

Dosage Form—Tablets: 100 mg.

Mephobarbital—page 1067.

Meprobamate—page 1072.

Metharbital

2,4,6(1*H*,3*H*,5*H*)-Pyrimidinetrione, 5,5-diethyl-1-methyl-, Gemonil (*Abbott*)

5,5-Diethyl-1-methylbarbituric acid [50-11-3] $C_9H_{14}N_2O_3$ (198.22).

Preparation—By the method described for *Mephobarbital* except that the diethyl ester of diethylmalonic acid is used instead of the diethyl ester of ethylphenylmalonic acid.

Description—White to nearly white, crystalline powder, possessing a faint aromatic odor; saturated solution has a pH of about 6.0; melting range 151° to 155°; pK$_a$ 8.45.

Solubility—1 g in 830 mL water, 23 mL alcohol, 40 mL ether.

Uses—Metharbital, an *N*-methylated derivative of barbital, is an alternative drug for generalized tonic-clonic seizures (grand mal), absence seizures (petit mal), myoclonic, and mixed types of seizures. It is rapidly demethylated to barbital by the liver, but its anticonvulsant activity appears to be independent of this degradation product. Unfavorable side effects, although relatively infrequent, include gastric distress, drowsiness, increased irritability, skin rash, and dizziness. These effects can usually be controlled by adjusting the dosage.

The safe use of metharbital in pregnancy, lactation, and in women of child-bearing age has not been established. See introduction to this chapter.

Dose—100 to 800 mg/day; *usual, initial,* 100 mg, up to 3 times a day. The usual pediatric dose is 50 mg 1 to 3 times daily depending on the age and weight of the patient.

Dosage Form—Tablets: 100 mg.

Methsuximide

2,5-Pyrrolidinedione, 1,3-dimethyl-3-phenyl, Celontin (*Parke-Davis*)

N,2-Dimethyl-2-phenylsuccinimide [77-41-8] $C_{12}H_{13}NO_2$ (203.24).

Preparation—2-Methyl-2-phenylsuccinic acid is dissolved in excess 40% methylamine. The water and excess amine are distilled off and the residue of the di(methylamine) salt of the acid is pyrolyzed at about 250° until no more distillate is formed. The residue of crude methsuximide may be purified by vacuum distillation. US Pat. 2,643,257.

Description—White to grayish white, crystalline powder; odorless or has not more than a slight odor; melts between 50° and 56°.

Solubility—1 g in 350 mL water, 3 mL alcohol, <1 mL chloroform, 2 mL ether.

Uses—An antiepileptic agent indicated for the control of absence seizures (petit mal) that are refractory to other drugs. When used in mixed types of epilepsy, methsuximide may increase the incidence of tonic-clonic seizures in some patients. Methsuximide, like ethosuximide, is not bound to plasma protein; volume distribution in dogs ranges from 13.5 to 22.5 L/kg; plasma half-life varies from 1.2 to 1.6 hours for methsuximide and from 28 to 36 hours for the *N*-desmethylmethsuximide metabolite. In view of its longer half-life, the desmethyl metabolite probably exerts the major antiepileptic effect. Adverse effects are similar to those of ethosuximide. Gastrointestinal disturbances, such as nausea, vomiting, anorexia, diarrhea, weight-loss, epigastric and abdominal pain, and constipation occur frequently. Hemopoietic complications including eosinophilia, leukopenia, monocytosis, and pancytopenia have been reported. Neurologic and sensory reactions observed include drowsiness, ataxia, irritability, nervousness, headache, blurred vision, photophobia, hiccups, and insomnia. Dermatologic disturbances include urticaria, Stevens-Johnson syndrome, and pruritic erythematous rashes. Periorbital edema and hyperemia have also been reported. Except for the skin and periorbital hyperemia, most untoward effects disappear when the dose of the drug is reduced. Patients on methsuximide therapy should be examined periodically for evidence of blood dyscrasias and for liver and kidney function.

The safe use of methsuximide in pregnancy, lactation, and in women of child-bearing age has not been established. See introduction to this chapter.

Dose—*Usual, initial,* **300 mg** daily; *maintenance,* **300 mg** to **1.2 g** daily. Optimum dosage must be determined by trial; a suggested schedule is 300 mg daily for first week increased 300 mg daily at weekly intervals until a daily dosage of 1.2 g daily is reached.

Dosage Forms—Capsules: 150 and 300 mg.

Oxazepam—page 1063.

Paraldehyde—page 1073.

Paramethadione

2,4-Oxazolidinedione, 5-ethyl-3,5-dimethyl-, Paradione (*Abbott*)

[115-67-3] $C_7H_{11}NO_3$ (157.17).

Preparation—Ethyl α-hydroxy-α-methylbutyrate and urea are refluxed for 24 hours in the presence of sodium methoxide, resulting in condensation cyclization with formation of the sodium derivative of 5-ethyl-5-methyl-2,4-oxazolidinedione. After distilling off the alcohol, dimethyl sulfate is slowly added to effect *N*-methylation.

Description—Clear, colorless liquid; may have an aromatic odor; pH (1 in 40 solution) about 6; refractive index 1.449 to 1.501.

Solubility—Sparingly soluble in water; freely soluble in alcohol, benzene, chloroform, and ether.

Uses—Paramethadione is used for control of absence seizures (petit mal) in patients refractory to other drugs. Its pharmacological properties, therapeutic uses, dosage, and toxicity are similar to those of trimethadione. However, the incidence of serious adverse effects may be less for paramethadione. More importantly, individuals who cannot tolerate one of the oxazolidinediones may tolerate the other. See *Trimethadione*, page 1082.

Dose—**300 mg** to **2.4 g** daily; *usual,* **300 mg** 3 or 4 times a day. It is generally advisable to start therapy at a dosage of **900 mg** daily and increase this by **300 mg** a day at weekly intervals until therapeutic effects are seen or until toxic. The initial dose for children under age 2 is 300 mg in 24 hr; 2 to 6 yr, 600 mg in 24 hr; over 6 yr, 900 mg in 24 hr.

Dosage Forms—Capsules: 150 and 300 mg; Solution: 300 mg/mL, 50 mL.

Phenacemide

Benzeneacetamide, *N*-(aminocarbonyl)-, Phenurone (*Abbott*)

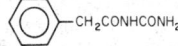

(Phenylacetyl)urea [63-98-9] $C_9H_{10}N_2O_2$ (178.19).

Preparation—Urea is reacted with phenylacetyl chloride. *J Am Chem Soc 70:* 4189, 1948.

Description—White to practically white, fine, crystalline powder; odorless, or practically so; melts at about 213°.

Solubility—1 g in >2000 mL of water, alcohol, chloroform, ether; 500 mL warm alcohol, 300 mL methanol.

Uses—Indicated in severe forms of epilepsy, particularly mixed forms of complex partial seizures (psychomotor), refractory to other drugs. Phenacemide can produce serious side effects as well as direct organ toxicity. Its use, therefore, entails the assumption of certain risks which must be evaluated against the potential benefit to the patient. This drug should be used *only* in those cases which do not respond to other anticonvulsant medication. Extreme caution must be exercised in treating patients who have previously shown personality disorders, liver dysfunction, or a history of allergy. Concurrent use with ethotoin is not recommended since paranoid symptoms have been reported in patients on this combination. The untoward effects which may occur include the following: gastrointestinal disturbances, anorexia and weight loss, headache, drowsiness, dizziness, insomnia, paresthesias, psychic changes, hepatitis, blood dyscrasias, skin rash, and nephritis. The safe use of phenacemide in pregnancy, lactation, or in women of child-bearing age has not been established. See introduction to this chapter. Liver function tests should be performed before and during therapy.

Dose—*Oral,* **0.5 g** 3 times a day with meals. After the first week, if seizures are not controlled and the drug is well tolerated, an additional 0.5 g may be taken on arising. In the third week, if necessary, the dosage may be further increased by 0.5 g at bedtime. The usual total adult dose ranges from 2 to 3 g daily, although some patients may require about $\frac{1}{2}$ the adult dose and others have required as much as 5 g daily. The usual initial dose for children 5 to 10 years of age is 250 mg 3 times daily the first week, additional 250 mg on arising the second week; a final 250 mg at bedtime may be added the third week.

Dosage Form—Tablets: 500 mg.

Phenobarbital Sodium—page 1067.

Phensuximide

2,5-Pyrrolidinedione, 1-methyl-3-phenyl-, Milontin (*Parke-Davis*)

N-Methyl-2-phenylsuccinimide [86-34-0] $C_{11}H_{11}NO_2$ (189.21).

Preparation—By the method described above for *Methsuximide* using phenylsuccinic acid as the starting compound, or by other methods. US Pat. 2,643,258.

Description—White to off-white, crystalline powder; odorless or has not more than a slight odor; melts between 68° and 74°.

Solubility—1 g in 210 mL water, 11 mL alcohol, <1 mL chloroform, 19 mL ether.

Uses—Phensuximide, the first succinimide introduced for the therapy of absence seizures (petit mal), is now relegated to secondary status. It is used for the control of severe epilepsy, particularly mixed forms of complex partial (psychomotor) seizures, refractory to other drugs. Its lesser effect is thought to be due to the fact that its desmethyl metabolite does not accumulate in the body. Phensuximide, although relatively free from serious toxic effects, may produce such side reactions as nausea, vomiting, anorexia, muscular weakness, drowsiness, ataxia, lethargy, and occasional skin disorders such as pruritus, skin eruptions, erythema multiforme, and erythematous rashes. Increased urinary frequency, renal damage, hematuria, granulocytopenia, transient leukopenia, and pancytopenia have been reported. Therefore, periodic urinalysis and blood studies are advisable in patients taking the drug for prolonged periods.

The safe use of phensuximide in pregnancy, lactation, and in women of child-bearing age has not been established. See introduction to this chapter.

Dose—*Usual,* **500 mg** to **1 g** 2 or 3 times a day, irrespective of age. As with other anticonvulsant medication, the dose should be adjusted to the individual patient.

Dosage Forms—Capsules: 250 and 500 mg; Oral Suspension: 62.5 mg/mL.

Phenytoin

2,4-Imidazolidinedione, 5,5-diphenyl-, Diphenylhydantoin; Dilantin (*Parke-Davis*)

5,5-Diphenylhydantoin [57-41-0] $C_{15}H_{12}N_2O_2$ (252.27).

Preparation—Phenytoin sodium, prepared as described in the preceding monograph, yields phenytoin on acidification of its aqueous solution.

Description—White powder; odorless; melts at about 295°.
Solubility—Practically insoluble in water; slightly soluble in cold alcohol, in chloroform, and in ether.

Uses—See *Phenytoin Sodium.*
Dose—*Range, oral,* **200** to **600 mg** daily; *usual,* **100 mg** 2 to 4 times a day.
Dosage Forms—Capsules: 100 mg; Oral Suspension: 6, 20, and 25 mg/mL; Tablets: 50 mg.

Phenytoin Sodium

2,4-Imidazolidinedione, 5,5-diphenyl-, monosodium salt; Diphenylhydantoin Sodium Salt; Diphenylhydantoin Sodium; Soluble Phenytoin; Alepsin; Epanutin; Eptoin; Dilantin Sodium (*Parke-Davis*)

5,5-Diphenylhydantoin sodium salt [630-93-3] $C_{15}H_{11}N_2NaO_2$ (274.25).

Preparation—By treating benzaldehyde with a solution of sodium cyanide, 2 moles of benzaldehyde are condensed (benzoin condensation) into one mole of benzoin, which is oxidized to benzil with nitric acid or cupric sulfate. The benzil is then heated with urea in the presence of sodium ethoxide or isopropoxide, forming phenytoin sodium.

Description—White, odorless powder; somewhat hygroscopic and on exposure to air gradually absorbs carbon dioxide with the liberation of diphenylhydantoin.
Solubility—Freely soluble in water, the solution usually being somewhat turbid due to partial hydrolysis and absorption of carbon dioxide; soluble in alcohol; practically insoluble in ether and chloroform.

Uses—Phenytoin is one of the drugs of choice for the management of generalized tonic-clonic (grand mal) seizures, complex partial (temporal lobe; psychomotor) seizures, and simple partial (focal, Jacksonian) seizures. Parenteral phenytoin is used for the control of status epilepticus of the generalized tonic-clonic (grand mal) type and in the management of seizures occurring during neurosurgery. Investigational uses of phenytoin include digitalis-induced cardiac arrhythmias, behavioral disorders, and, in large doses, the management of trigeminal neuralgia. It is much less effective in the latter than carbamazepine (see page 1077). Phenytoin has a pK_a of 8.31 to 8.33; 87 to 93% of the drug is bound to plasma protein; volume distribution ranges from 0.5 to 0.8 L/kg; and half-life is about 22 hours in adults and 18 to 22 hours in children. Therapeutic plasma levels range from 10 to 20 $\mu g/mL$ in adults and 5 to 20 $\mu g/mL$ in children. Toxic levels range from 30 to 50 $\mu g/mL$ and lethal levels approximate 100 $\mu g/mL$.

Phenytoin acts on the motor cortex where it stabilizes the neuronal membrane and inhibits the spread of the seizure discharge. Present evidence suggests that phenytoin enhances calcium binding to phospholipids in neuronal membranes; this results in a more stable membrane configuration. This event contributes to the regulation of calcium flux by reducing extracellular calcium concentration. Moreover, phenytoin inhibits voltage-sensitive sodium channels; this action also contributes to decreasing neuronal membrane excitability.

These observations are in harmony with the fact that the most easily demonstrated properties of phenytoin are its ability to limit the development of maximal seizure activity and to reduce the spread of the seizure process from the active focus. Both features are undoubtedly related to its clinical usefulness.

There are two distinct forms of Phenytoin Sodium Capsules: the rapid-release type (Prompt Phenytoin Sodium Capsules) and the slow-dissolution type (Extended Phenytoin Sodium Capsules). The former have a dissolution rate of not less than 85% in 30 minutes and are used for 3 or 4 times a day dosing, whereas the latter have a slow dissolution rate of 15 to 35% in 30 minutes, 45 to 65% in one hour, and not less than 85% in 2 hours and may be used for once-a-day dosing. Studies comparing doses of 100 mg three times daily of Prompt Phenytoin Sodium Capsules with a single, daily dose of 300 mg of Extended Phenytoin Sodium Capsules (Dilantin Kapseals, *Parke-Davis*) indicate that absorption, peak plasma levels, biologic half-life, difference between peak and minimum values, and urinary recovery are equivalent. Because of the differences in dissolution rates among various brands, *physicians should be cautioned to keep patients on one manufacturer's product.* For additional information, the reader is referred to the interesting articles by Shah and co-workers (*J Pharm Sci: 72,* 303–310, 1983).

Phenytoin metabolism may be significantly altered by concomitant use of other drugs. *Barbiturates* may enhance metabolism of phenytoin; however, the effect is variable and unpredictable. *Coumarin anticoagulants,* disulfiram, phenylbutazone, isoniazid, chloramphenicol, cimetidine, and sulfonamides may inhibit metabolism of phenytoin, thereby increasing serum levels of the drug. This may lead to an increased incidence of nystagmus, ataxia, or other toxic effects. *Tricyclic antidepressants* in high doses may precipitate seizures, and the dosage of phenytoin may have to be adjusted accordingly. Phenytoin may decrease the effects of dicumarol, disopyramide, and quinidine; in addition, it may inhibit the effect of prednisolone, dexamethasone, and corticosteroids. It has also been known to suppress protein-bound iodine, but no clinical cases of hypothyroidism have been reported. Phenytoin is a relatively safe anticonvulsant, although many adverse effects have been observed. Nystagmus may appear with serum concentrations of 8 to 20 $\mu g/mL$ and is nearly always present at higher levels. At concentrations greater than 30 $\mu g/mL$, ataxia and dysarthria commonly occur. Gingival hyperplasia and hirsutism are often intolerable, particularly in the young. A morbilliform rash may occur, usually in the first 10 days of treatment, and rarely progresses to exfoliative dermatitis or the Stevens-Johnson syndrome; the drug should be stopped if a rash appears. There are also reports of peripheral neuropathy, a lupus erythematosus syndrome, hepatitis, lymphadenopathy, megaloblastic anemia, and rickets and osteomalacia due to interference with vitamin D metabolism. Serum folic acid and vitamin K levels may also be depressed, and bleeding disorders have been reported in infants born to mothers taking the drug. Overdosage causes an acute cerebellar syndrome, delirium and, rarely, coma.

Phenytoin is contraindicated in patients with a history of sensitivity to hydantoins. Abrupt withdrawal of this medication may precipitate status epilepticus; when the dosage needs to be reduced or substitution of another antiepileptic appears desirable, such alteration in therapy should be done gradually. Recent reports suggest an association between the use of anticonvulsant drugs by women with epilepsy and an increased incidence of birth defects in children born to these women. The prescribing physician should weigh the benefit/risk potential of antiepileptic agents when treating or counseling epileptic women of child-bearing age. See introduction to this chapter.

Dose—*Range, oral,* **200** to **600 mg** daily; *usual, oral,* **100 mg** up to 4 times a day; *usual, intravenous,* **150** to **250 mg,** followed, if necessary, by **100** to **150 mg** 30 min later (intravenous administration should not exceed 50 mg/min); *usual, intramuscular,* **100** to **200 mg** every 6 to 8 hours for a total of 3 or 4 injections. *Usual pediatric dose, anticonvulsant,* **1.5** to **4 mg/kg** body weight or 125 mg/square meter of body surface, two times a day, not to exceed 300 mg daily; administered orally, intravenously, or less preferably intramuscularly. See package insert for detailed information concerning dosage for all patients. *Note*—If seizure control in *adults* is established with 100-mg capsules administered 3 times a day, once-a-day dosage with 300-mg Phenytoin Sodium Capsules SD (Dilantin Kapseals, *Parke-Davis*) may be considered as an alternative, but patients should be cautioned not to miss a dose inadvertently or to use another manufacturer's product (see under *Uses*).

Dosage Forms—Tablets (chewable): 50 mg; Oral Suspension: 30 mL (125 mg/5 mL); Capsules, Prompt: 30 and 100 mg; Capsules, Extended (one a day dosing): 30 and 100 mg; Injection: 50 mg/mL in 2- and 5-mL ampuls.

Primidone

4,6-(1*H*,5*H*)-Pyrimidinedione, 5-ethyldihydro-5-phenyl-, Primaclone; Mysoline (*Ayerst*)

[125-33-7] $C_{12}H_{14}N_2O_2$ (218.25).

Preparation—A solution of ethylphenylmalonamide (I) in a large molar excess of formamide (II) is refluxed for 2 hours. The cyclization may be looked upon as being brought about by a Cannizzaro type of disproportionation of II followed by a deammoniation and a dehydration between I and the highly reactive methanolamine resulting from the disproportionation.

Description—White, odorless, crystalline powder, which has a slightly bitter taste; melting range 279° to 284°.

Solubility—1 g in 2000 mL water, 200 mL alcohol; very slightly soluble in most organic solvents.

Uses—Primidone, either alone or in combination with other antiepileptics, is used as alternate therapy in the control of generalized tonic-clonic seizures (grand mal), complex partial seizures (temporal lobe; psychomotor) and focal epileptic seizures. Primidone is metabolized to phenylethylmalonamide (PEMA) and phenobarbital. Phenobarbital formation ranges from 15 to 25%. The plasma half-life of PEMA is 24–48 hours, whereas that of phenobarbital is 48 to 120 hours. Both substances tend to accumulate during chronic medication. PEMA is an active antiepileptic but is less potent and less toxic than phenobarbital. From 0 to 30% of primidone is bound to plasma protein; volume distribution averages 0.6 L/kg; and plasma half-life varies from 6 to 8 hours. Therapeutic plasma concentrations range from 6 to 12 µg/mL for primidone and from 15 to 45 µg/mL for phenobarbital. Few interactions with other drugs have been reported, but those for phenobarbital also apply to primidone. The ratio of phenobarbital to unmetabolized primidone in serum is significantly higher in epileptic patients treated with a combination of primidone and phenytoin than in patients on primidone alone. Primidone decreases the prothrombin response to dicumarol and warfarin. Also, concurrent treatment with valproate increases the plasma level of phenobarbital in patients on primidone. The most frequent side effects include ataxia and vertigo; these tend to disappear with continued or reduced therapy. Occasionally, nausea, anorexia, vomiting, fatigue, irritability, emotional disturbances, diplopia, nystagmus, drowsiness, and morbilliform rashes occur. Megaloblastic anemia may occur as a rare idiosyncrasy; this anemia responds to folic acid, 15 mg daily, without discontinuing the medication.

Dose—125 mg to 2 g daily; *usual*, 250 mg daily, at bedtime, the first week. The dose is increased in increments of 250 mg at weekly intervals to tolerance or therapeutic effectiveness; a total daily dose of 2 g should not be exceeded. For children under 8 years of age, ½ the adult dosage is given on a similar schedule.

Dosage Forms—Oral Suspension: 250 mg/5 mL; Tablets: 50 and 250 mg.

Quinacrine Hydrochloride—page 1220.

Sodium Bromide—RPS-16, page 1019.

Trimethadione

2,4-Oxazolidinedione, 3,5,5-trimethyl-, Tridione (*Abbott*)

[127-48-0] $C_6H_9NO_3$ (143.14).

Preparation—By a series of reactions beginning with acetone and involving the following steps: conversion with HCN to acetone cyanhydrin, hydrolysis and esterification with alcohol to ethyl dimethylglycolate, condensation with urea to 5,5-dimethyloxazolidine-2,4-dione, and methylation with dimethyl sulfate to trimethadione.

Description—White, crystalline granules having a slight, camphor-like odor; melting range 45° to 47°.

Solubility—Soluble in water; freely soluble in alcohol, ether, and chloroform.

Uses—Trimethadione, an alternative drug for absence seizures (petit mal), is not widely used because of its toxicity and the fact that reliable tests for plasma concentrations are not generally available.

A frequent troublesome effect is hemeralopia, a peculiar glare effect or photophobia; hemeralopia is managed by having the patient wear tinted glasses. Trimethadione is demethylated to an active more potent metabolite, dimethadione. Dimethadione is not further metabolized, but is excreted unchanged in the urine. Dimethadione has a pKa of 6.15; neither dimethadione nor trimethadione is bound to plasma protein and the half-life is 240 hours for dimethadione and 16 to 20 hours for trimethadione. Therapeutic plasma levels are >700 µg/mL for dimethadione and 20 µg/mL for trimethadione.

Clinically significant drug interactions with trimethadione have not been reported. Nevertheless, concurrent administration of drugs that produce similar adverse effects should be avoided.

Serious untoward effects may be associated with therapeutic doses of trimethadione. Gastrointestinal effects reported include hiccups, nausea, vomiting, abdominal pain, and gastric distress. Anorexia and weight loss have been reported. Central nervous system disturbances such as photophobia, diplopia, hemeralopia, vertigo, irritability, insomnia, drowsiness, paresthesia, headache, fatigue and malaise, and personality changes have been observed. Drowsiness appears to subside as therapy is continued. Skin rashes, bleeding gums, epistaxis, retinal and petechial hemorrhages, vaginal bleeding and blood dyscrasias including leukopenia, neutropenia, thrombocytopenia, pancytopenia, agranulocytosis and hypoplastic anemia, and fatal aplastic anemia have been reported. A lupus erythematosus-like syndrome has also been reported. In addition a syndrome simulating malignant lymphoma has been noted. Lymphadenopathy with hepatosplenomegaly associated with pruritus in hypersensitive individuals has also been observed. If lupus-like manifestations or lymph node enlargement should appear, therapy should be discontinued and the patient observed for a reversal of these symptoms before therapy is instituted for lupus erythematosus or lymphoma. Other reactions observed include changes in blood pressure, albuminuria, nephrosis, hepatitis, and precipitation of grand mal seizures. Since certain anticonvulsant drugs, including trimethadione and paramethadione, have been reported to be associated with an increased incidence of congenital malformations, the use of these drugs in pregnant women or in women of child-bearing age requires careful evaluation of the risks and benefits. See introduction to this chapter.

Dose—*Range*, 900 mg to 2.4 g daily; *usual*, 300 to 600 mg 3 or 4 times a day.

Other Dose Information—The adult dose for the treatment of epilepsy is 900 mg to 2.4 g daily, in divided amounts. Therapy is usually started at 900 mg daily and increased by 300 mg daily at weekly intervals until the desired therapeutic results are achieved or toxic symptoms appear. Fr infants and children the dose ranges from 300 to 900 mg daily, in 3 or 4 equally divided doses.

Dosage Forms—Capsules: 300 mg; Oral Solution: 40 mg/mL; Tablets (chewable): 150 mg.

Valproate Sodium

Pentanoic acid, 2-propyl-, sodium salt; Depakene (*Abbott*)

$$CH_3CH_2CH_2CHCOONa$$
$$CH_3CH_2CH_2$$

Sodium 2-propylpentanoate; sodium 2-propylvalerate [1069-66-5] $C_8H_{15}NaO_2$ (166.20).

Preparation—Valproic acid may be synthesized from 4-heptanol by successive conversions to 4-bromoheptane with HBr, to 4-cyanoheptane with HCN, and to 2-propylpentanoic (valproic) acid by alkaline hydrolysis of the 4-cyanoheptane.

Description—White, crystalline powder; odorless; saline taste.
Solubility—Soluble in water and in alcohol.

Uses—Valproic acid, an 8-carbon branched-chain fatty (carboxylic) acid, is unique in that its structure is unrelated to any other antiepileptic drug marketed in the United States. Clinical results indicate valproate sodium has a wide spectrum of antiepileptic activity. It is one of the drugs of choice in the management of pure absence seizures accompanied by a 3-per-second spike-and-wave in the electroencephalogram. Similarly, atypical absence seizures and myoclonic epilepsies respond well and, since there has never been an entirely satisfactory drug for these types of childhood epilepsy, this is an important advance. It is also effective in tonic-clonic seizures, but whether it is as effective as carbamazepine or phenytoin remains to be determined. Valproic acid has a pKa of 4.5; 90–95% of the drug is bound to plasma protein; volume distribution ranges from 0.1 to 0.5 L/kg, mean 0.2 L/kg; and half-life varies from 6 to 17 hours in adults and 4 to 14 hours in children. Therapeutic plasma levels range from 50 to 100 μg/mL; levels above 100 μg/mL are potentially toxic. More than ten metabolites have been identified in human blood and urine. Only 0.5 to 20% is excreted unchanged in the urine. Of the several metabolites, only 2-propyl-2-pentenoic acid (2-en-VPA) has been shown to accumulate in the brain. The 2-en-VPA metabolite is about 1.3 times more potent than the parent drug and may contribute significantly to the anticonvulsant effect of chronically administered valproate.

The precise mechanism of its anticonvulsant action is still unknown. It has been postulated that valproate administration inhibits GABA-transaminase, and thus, increases the concentration of cerebral GABA. However, other saturated straight-chain fatty acids (propionic, butyric, and pentanoic acids) which lack anticonvulsant properties are more potent inhibitors of GABA-transaminase than is valproic acid. It has also been reported that there is a strong correlation between the anticonvulsant potency of valproate and other branched-chain fatty acids and their ability to reduce the concentration of cerebral aspartate. The reports by M Goto *et al* (*J Pharm Dyn: 6*, 191–195, 1983) and A G Chapman *et al* (*Life Sciences: 32*, 2023–2031, 1983) provide interesting information on the relative importance of these changes and the anticonvulsant action of valproate.

Valproate sodium may decrease binding to serum proteins or block hepatic metabolism of phenobarbital. Administration of the drug to patients in a steady state while on phenobarbital (or primidone which is metabolized to phenobarbital) can increase the plasma levels of phenobarbital from 35 to 200%, causing excessive somnolence. Present evidence indicates this is due to an immediate decrease in the rate of elimination of phenobarbital. Valproate sodium interacts unpredictably with phenytoin; it has been associated not only with lowered serum phenytoin levels and increased seizure frequency, but also with increased free phenytoin levels and phenytoin toxicity. Conversely, phenobarbital, primidone, phenytoin, and other drugs may induce enzymes that metabolize valproate sodium and reduce its half-life.

Over 40 cases of fatal hepatic failure have been reported in patients on valproate therapy. Prodromal symptoms include weakness, anorexia, and vomiting followed in a few weeks by jaundice, ascites, then by hepatic encephalopathy and death. The mean duration of valproate therapy was two months. Consequently, tests of hepatic function should be performed prior to and every 2 months after initiation of valproate therapy.

The most commonly reported adverse effects are anorexia, nausea, and vomiting. These transitory gastrointestinal disturbances are dose related and occur in approximately 16% of patients treated with the drug. An unusual adverse effect is hair loss; fortunately this is reversible. Sedative effects have also been noted in patients receiving valproate alone, but are more intense in patients receiving other antiepileptic drugs, especially phenobarbital (see above). Other rarely observed untoward effects include skin rashes, headache, enuresis, insomnia, anxiety, fatigue, and paresthesias. Teratogenic effects have been reported in animals. Moreover, the use of valproate by women with epilepsy during the first trimester (3 months) of pregnancy has been reported by the Center for Disease Control, USPHS, to be associated with increased risk (1.2%) of spina bifida in their infants (*MMWR, 31*, Oct 28, 1982). Although the majority of women with epilepsy taking this drug will give birth to non-affected babies, it is recommended that they consider pre-natal testing for neural tube defects.

Dose (valproic acid equivalent)—*Adult* and *pediatric*, *initial*, **15 mg per kg** per day; increase at 1-week intervals by **5 to 10 mg per kg** per day; maximum daily dose, **30 mg per kg** (some patients may require up to **60 mg/kg** per day). If daily dose exceeds 250 mg it should be given in divided doses.

Dosage Forms—Capsules, 250 mg/kg. Syrup, 250 mg in 5 mL.

Other Antiepileptics

Clobazam [7-Chloro-1-methyl-5-phenyl-1*H*-benzodiazepine-2,4(3*H*,5*H*)-dione [22316-47-8] $C_{16}H_{13}ClN_2O_2$ (300.74); Urbanyl, Frisium (*Hoechst-Roussel*)]—White crystals melting about 180°; practically insoluble in water; sparingly soluble in alcohol; freely soluble in acetone or chloroform. See South African Pat 6,800,803 [*CA 70;* 10659f, 1969] for synthesis.] *Uses:* An investigational 1,5-benzodiazepine with anticonvulsant and acute-anxiety properties. Clobazam is effective against a wide variety of epileptic seizures; however, efficacy decreases in a few days to a few weeks in approximately one-third of patients. Clobazam is 85% bound to serum proteins; peak serum concentrations occur 1 to 4 hours after oral administration. It is metabolized to one active (*N*-desmethylclobazam) and several inactive metabolites. The mean half-life of the parent substance is 18 hours, whereas the half-life of the metabolites range up to 77 hours. The most frequent (10 to 40%) side effects include drowsiness, hangover effects, dizziness, and lightheadedness. Less frequent (5 to 10%) adverse reactions include weight gain, orthostatic hypotension, syncope, headache, dry mouth, and incoordination. *Dose:* Usual, adult, oral, 20 to 30 mg daily.

Ethotoin BP [3-Ethyl-5-phenylhydantoin $C_{11}H_{12}N_2O_2$ (204.22); Peganone (*Abbott*)]—A white, crystalline powder, melting at about 94°; sparingly soluble in water, freely soluble in alcohol. *Uses:* Management of grand mal and psychomotor seizures. With plasma levels below 8 μg/mL, the half-life ranges from 3 to 9 hours. Therapeutic plasma levels range from 15 to 50 μg/mL. Contraindicated in patients with hepatic and hematologic disorders. Should be used with extreme caution in combination with phenacemide, as paranoid symptoms have been reported with such use. Untoward effects include nausea, vomiting, fatigue, dizziness, headache, diplopia, nystagmus, skin rash, numbness, fever, diarrhea, and chest pain. Ataxia and gum hyperplasia have occurred rarely; lymphadenopathy has been reported in some patients. See general statement on use of antiepileptics during pregnancy. *Dose:* Initial, oral, adult, 1 g daily taken in 4 to 6 divided doses, after food; the usual adult maintenance dose is 2 to 3 g daily. Pediatric, initial, not over 750 mg daily, according to age and weight of patient; usual maintenance, from 500 mg to 1 g daily although occasionally 2 or (rarely) 3 g daily may be necessary. *Dosage Form:* Tablets, 250 and 500 mg.

Sulthiame [*p*-Tetrahydro-2*H*-1,2-thiazin-2-yl)benzenesulfonamide, *S,S*-dioxide [61-56-3] $C_{10}H_{14}N_2O_4S_2$ (290.37); Conadil; Trolone (*Riker*)]—A white, crystalline powder, melting at about 180°; very slightly soluble in water, slightly soluble in alcohol. *Uses:* This carbonic anhydrase inhibitor is used in Europe as an antiepileptic agent, usually in combination with other drugs; it has been shown to increase blood levels of concomitantly administered phenytoin. Daily doses of 600 mg to 1 g, in divided portions, have been given; doses greater than 600 mg appear to be accompanied by increased adverse effects. The drug is not produced in the US.

L-5-Hydroxytryptophan [$C_{11}H_{12}N_2O_3$]—A natural amino acid derived from tryptophan. Crystals; sparingly soluble in water. *Uses:* It is decarboxylated by L-aromatic amino acid decarboxylase to yield serotonin, a neurohumoral transmitter released by neurons in the brain, spinal cord, and sympathetic ganglia. In some psychiatric and neurological disorders, such as *depression* and *postanoxic intension myoclonus*, there seems to be a deficiency of neuronal serotonin, and 5-hydroxytryptophan appears to be of some benefit. It will probably prove to be useful in the treatment of mania, since the precursor tryptophan is somewhat effective. It seems to be most effective in cases in which the serotonin metabolite, 5-hydroxyindoleacetic acid, in the cerebrospinal fluid is low. Adjunct use of carbidopa (page 929) improves the responses by suppressing degradation in the periphery; the monoamine oxidase inhibitors suppress oxidation of serotonin, thus better sustaining brain levels. *Dose:* The optimal dose has not been established. *Oral*, in combination with carbidopa, initially 100 mg per day, followed by increments of 100 mg every 2 or 3 days.

CHAPTER 59

Psychopharmacologic Agents

Ewart A Swinyard, PhD, DSc (Hon)

Professor Emeritus of Pharmacology
College of Pharmacy and School of Medicine, University of Utah
Salt Lake City, UT 84112

Drugs that alter the mind and behavior have attracted the attention of man since the beginning of recorded history. Without the benefits of science and medicine, mankind has sought emotional comfort or novelty through the use of drugs for a venerable period of time. To cite two examples, alcohol and opium have been used for this purpose since antiquity. However, it was the inadvertent discovery of the unusual psychotomimetic properties of lysergic acid diethylamide in 1947 and the subsequent demonstration that these effects were similar to those induced by mescaline which marked the beginning of psychopharmacology. Additional interest in this new science was created with the introduction of chlorpromazine for the empiric treatment of mental disorders; the successful clinical use of this agent not only led to the realization that behavior can be objectively studied in laboratory animals, but also resulted in the discovery of a host of new drugs which stimulate, sedate, or otherwise change behavior. Indeed, over 1500 compounds classified as *psychoactive* or *psychotropic* drugs have been described, and approximately 20% of all prescriptions written in the United States are for medications intended to alter mental processes and alter behavior. Moreover, a large number of drugs prescribed for other purposes also modify thought, mood, and emotion. However, the primary characteristic of psychopharmacologic drugs, in contrast to the many other drugs that act on the central nervous system, is that they alter the mental state and behavior in a predictable way.

While pharmacotherapy does not cure mental disorders in the same sense that antibiotics cure infectious diseases, the available drugs do control most symptomatic manifestations and behavioral deviances, facilitate the patient's tendency toward remission, and improve his or her capacity for social, occupational, and familial adjustment. For example, the treatment of schizophrenic symptoms such as anxiety, delusions, hallucinations, paranoid states, catatonia, social withdrawal, and autonomic nervous system dysfunctions has been markedly changed by pharmacotherapy. The widespread use of these relatively safe compounds has greatly reduced the number of chronic patients residing in public mental hospitals, shortened the duration of hospitalization for acute episodes, and shifted the focus of treatment of mental disorders from institutional care to community based ambulatory treatment programs. Moreover, the advent of effective pharmacotherapy has also influenced research methodology and theory. Indeed, the important information gathered on the mechanism of action of psychoactive drugs has generated new hypotheses about the pathogenesis of these disorders.

Four theoretical models have been developed based on biogenic amine, endocrine, electrolyte, and genetic concepts. Most attention has been directed toward the biogenic amine model which is based on the relation between mood and the endogenous level of biogenic amines. Both catecholamines (epinephrine, norepinephrine, and dopamine) and indolamines (serotonin and histamine) have been implicated as having a possible role in the genesis of depression for at least four reasons: (1) Drugs used in the management of depression increase the level of amines in the brain. (2) Drugs which increase the level of brain amines induce alertness and overactivity in experimental animals. (3) Drugs (such as reserpine) known to deplete the brain amines produce sedation and inactivity in experimental animals. (4) Drugs that deplete brain amines cause depression in man. Thus, in its simplest terms the "catecholamine hypothesis" of affective disorders states that depression is associated with altered availability of one or another of the above amines at important receptor sites in the brain and, conversely, mania may be associated with an excess concentration of amines. It should be emphasized that biochemical changes in affective disorders are very complex and that other modalities such as acetylcholine, electrolyte disturbances, neuroendocrine changes, and other factors not yet investigated may play an important role. Nevertheless, this hypothesis is summarized here because of its possible value in understanding how certain agents in this chapter induce their salutary effects.

Drugs used in the treatment of behavioral disorders and those which are known to mimic certain of these disorders in man have been classified in various ways. For the purpose of this presentation, the psychopharmacologic drugs (psychoactive drugs) are divided into antipsychotic agents, antianxiety agents, antidepressant agents, and psychogenic agents.

Antipsychotic Agents

The several classes of drugs described in this section are used in the symptomatic treatment of psychoses, such as schizophrenia, organic psychoses, and the manic phase of manic-depressive illness. Drugs in this group act primarily on the lower brain areas to produce emotional calmness and relaxation without significant sedation, hypnosis, motor impairment, or euphoria. Structurally the antipsychotic drugs can be divided into six groups: (1) *phenothiazines* (chlorpromazine, etc.), (2) *thioxanthenes* (chlorprothixene and thiothixene), (3) *butyrophenones* (haloperidol), (4) *dihydroindolone* derivatives (molindone), (5) *dibenzoxazepines* (loxapine), and (6) *rauwolfia and its alkaloids*. Rauwolfia and its alkaloids are used primarily for their hypotensive action and are described in Chapter 47.

The numerous *phenothiazines* and related congeners have qualitatively similar effects, but their potency and side effects are markedly influenced by their chemical structure. For example, congeners with an aliphatic side chain, such as chlorpromazine, are relatively low in potency and high in sedative effects. Conversely, congeners with a piperazine constituent are more potent and have less sedative effects but more prominent extrapyramidal toxicity.

The mechanism of action of the antipsychotic agents is obviously complex, and many details remain to be established. Nevertheless, all antipsychotic agents currently employed clinically block postsynaptic dopaminergic receptors and act as competitive antagonists of dopamine centrally and peripherally. The desired antipsychotic and antiemetic effects and the undesired extrapyramidal effects are related, at least in part, to dopaminergic blockade. Extrapyramidal toxicity is also inversely related to the central anticholinergic properties of these agents. The various peripheral effects are also attributable to their anticholinergic properties, and peripheral alpha-adrenergic blockade, together with their central effects, and to the cardiovascular effects of some of these agents.

Experimentally, the *phenothiazines* suppress or abolish conditioned reflexes in trained rats, prevent morphine-induced mania in cats, and reduce the toxicity of amphetamine in aggregated mice. Many of these compounds also suppress vomiting from apomorphine, irradiation, and motion sickness, but, in laboratory animals, do not affect the emesis from morphine, veratrum alkaloids, digitalis, and copper sulfate. In addition, they decrease spontaneous motor activity, lower electroshock seizure threshold, and cause skeletal muscle relaxation. The phenothiazines also exhibit weak adrenolytic, hypotensive, antispasmodic, hypothermic, and antihistaminic effects and potentiate the action of many pharmacological agents.

Antipsychotic drugs are usually highly lipid-soluble and protein-bound (92–99%). They tend to have large volumes of distribution (usually more than 7 L/kg); bioavailability after oral administration is variable and quite low (25–35%). Plasma half-life tends to be short, ranging from 10 to 20 hours, but the duration of the antipsychotic action is much longer. Metabolites may be found in the urine weeks after the last dose of drug. This suggests that large amounts of the drug are sequestered in the tissues.

A *thioxanthene* is a phenothiazine in which the nitrogen at the 10-position is replaced by a carbon atom with a double bond to the side chain. The thioxanthene *chlorprothixene* has high sedative and adrenergic-blocking properties and a low to moderate tendency to induce extrapyramidal reactions. In contrast, *thiothixene* has low sedative and adrenergic-blocking properties and a high tendency to induce extrapyramidal reactions. Moreover, the former has a milligram for milligram potency somewhat less than most phenothiazines, whereas the latter has a potency essentially the same as the most potent phenothiazines.

The *butyrophenone haloperidol* is less sedative than the phenothiazines, but extrapyramidal symptoms occur even more frequently with this agent. It is also one of the most potent antipsychotic agents.

The *phenothiazines* are indicated for the management of *psychotic disorders*, control of *nausea and vomiting*, control of *manic depression*, relief of *intractable hiccups*, relief of *restlessness and apprehension* prior to surgery, *acute intermittent porphyria*, and as an adjunct in the treatment of *tetanus*. The thioxanthenes (chlorprothixene and thiothixene) are used for the management of the symptoms of *psychotic disorders*. The *butyrophenone* (haloperidol) is also employed for the management of symptoms of *psychoses*, including *schizophrenia*, the manic type of *manic depressive* illness, or *psychotic reactions* associated with organic brain syndrome or mental retardation. The dibenzoxazepine (loxapine succinate) is indicated for the management of *schizophrenia*.

Contraindications—Many of the contraindications to the use of these drugs are similar. For example, they are contraindicated in comatose patients who have received large amounts of CNS depressant drugs (alcohol, barbiturates, narcotics, etc), in patients with Parkinson's disease, and in patients with a known history of hypersensitivity to these agents. It is not known whether there is cross-sensitivity between the phenothiazines and the thioxanthenes, but this possibility should be kept in mind.

Warnings—The safe use of these agents during pregnancy has not been established with respect to possible adverse effects on fetal development. The safe use of butyrophenones and thioxanthenes in children has not been established. It is recommended that these agents not be used in children under 12 years of age. Geriatric or debilitated patients usually require a lower initial dose of these agents; the dose is then increased as needed and tolerated. Both phenothiazines and thioxanthenes have an anticholinergic effect; hence, should be used with extreme caution in patients with a history of glaucoma or prostatic hypertrophy. All agents in these groups tend to impair mental and physical ability required to operate a motor vehicle or complex hazardous machinery. Patients should be warned accordingly.

Precautions—Phenothiazines and thioxanthenes may significantly affect the actions of other drugs (see Chapter 102, on *Drug Interactions*, for additional information concerning specific interactions). They may increase, prolong, or intensify the action of CNS depressants (anesthetics, alcohol, barbiturates, narcotics, etc); therefore, appropriate adjustments in dosage of narcotics and barbiturates should be made when such agents are to be administered concomitantly. These agents also lower convulsive threshold; hence, they should be used with extreme caution in patients with a history of epilepsy. They should also be used cautiously in patients receiving atropine and related drugs, because of the possible additive anticholinergic effect. Since these agents have antiemetic properties, they may mask signs of drug overdosage and obscure symptoms of brain tumor or intestinal obstruction. These agents should also be used with extreme caution in patients with cardiovascular disease, chronic respiratory disorders, impaired liver function, or with a history of gastric ulcer; the aggravation of a preexisting ulcer has been reported.

Adverse Reactions—Although not all the adverse reactions listed herein have occurred following administration of either phenothiazines or thioxanthenes, the chemical and pharmacological similarities of the two groups suggest that *all* of the known side effects and toxicities associated with such therapy should be kept in mind. *CNS effects: drowsiness,* particularly during the first or second week of therapy; *extrapyramidal reactions* may be fairly common, usually three types (1) parkinsonian-like syndrome, (2) dystonia and dyskinesia, including torticollis, tics, and other involuntary muscle movements, and (3) akathisia, shown by restlessness and an urge to move about; *hyperreflexia*, reported in the newborn when phenothiazines are used during pregnancy; *grand mal seizures, catatonic-like states, psychotic symptoms,* and *cerebral edema* have also been reported. *Cardiovascular effects:* postural hypotension, tachycardia, bradycardia, faintness, dizziness, and cardiac arrest. *Hematological effects:* agranulocytosis, eosinophilia, leukopenia, hemolytic anemia, thrombocytopenic purpura and pancytopenia have been reported. *Liver:* jaundice has been observed but is usually reversible. *Allergic reactions:* urticaria or dermatitis in about 5% of patients. Three types have been identified, (1) hypersensitivity reactions, (2) contact dermatitis, and (3) photosensitivity resembling sunburn. *Endocrine effects:* these agents block ovulation, suppress the menstrual cycle, cause infertility and pseudopregnancy, lactation and breast engorgement in females. These agents reduce urinary levels of gonadotropins, estrogens, and progestins. In males, gynecomastia or change in libido have been observed. Cholesterol levels are also significantly increased. *Other reported reactions:* these include dry mouth, nasal congestion, constipation, myosis, mydriasis, urinary retention, increased appetite, weight gain, peripheral edema, fever, and suppression of cough reflex. The last may enhance the potential of aspiration and/or asphyxia. *Long-term effects:* prolonged therapy with high doses may cause pigmentation of exposed skin areas, ocular changes consisting of lenticular and corneal opacities, epithelial keratopathies, and pigmentary retinopathy; vision may be impaired.

Acetophenazine Maleate

Ethanone, 1-[10-[3-[4-(2-hydroxyethyl)-1-piperazinyl]propyl]-10H-
phenothiazin-2-yl]-, (Z)-2 butenedioate (1:2) (salt);
Tindal (*Schering-Plough*)

[5714-00-1] $C_{23}H_{29}N_3O_2S.2C_4H_4O_4$ (643.71).

Preparation—Piperazineethanol is condensed with 10-(3-chloropropyl)phenothiazin-2-yl methyl ketone (I) in the presence of a dehydrochlorinating agent such as sodamide. The resulting acetophenazine (base) is reacted with a double equimolar portion of maleic acid. I is prepared from phenothiazine through: (a) acetylation with acetic anhydride and aluminum chloride to the 2,10-diacetyl compound, (b) deacetylation at the 10-position with alkali, and (c) condensation of 2-acetylphenothiazine with 1-bromo-3-chloropropane. US Pat 2,985,654.

Description—A fine, yellow, powder that is odorless and has a bitter taste. It is sensitive to light and reasonably stable in dry air. It melts at about 165°, with decomposition.

Solubility—1 g in 10 mL water, 260 mL alcohol, 2850 mL chloroform, 6000 mL ether, 370 mL acetone, 11 mL propylene glycol.

Uses—A piperazine-substituted phenothiazine for the management of the manifestations of *psychotic disorders*. Contraindications, warnings, precautions, and adverse effects are similar to those for other phenothiazines, except extrapyramidal symptoms occur more frequently after administration of piperazine-substituted phenothiazines. See page 1085.

Dose—*Usual, adult, oral,* **20 mg** 3 times a day; range of total daily dose, **40 to 80 mg**. For hospitalized patients the optimum daily dosage ranges from **80 to 120 mg,** in divided doses, but patients with severe schizophrenia have received 400 to 600 mg daily. Not recommended for pediatric age group since safety and effectiveness in children have not been established.

Dosage Form—Tablets: 20 mg.

Carphenazine Maleate

1-Propanone, 1-[10-[3-[4-(2-hydroxyethyl)-1-piperazinyl]propyl]-
10H-phenothiazin-2-yl]-, (Z)-2-butenedioate (1:2);
Proketazine Maleate (*Wyeth*)

[2975-34-0] $C_{24}H_{31}N_3O_2S.2C_4H_4O_4$ (657.73).

Preparation—Phenothiazine is propionylated at the 2 and 10 positions through a Friedel-Crafts reaction with propionyl chloride and then depropionylated at the 10-position by alkaline hydrolysis. The resulting phenothiazin-2-yl-1-propanone is then condensed with trimethylene chlorobromide with the aid of sodium hydride to produce the 10-(3-chloropropyl) derivative, and the latter is further condensed with 1-piperazineethanol in a refluxing solvent to yield carphenazine. Treatment of an ethanolic solution of the base with maleic acid yields the maleate. US Pat 2,985,654.

Description—Yellow, fine powder; odorless or with a slight odor; melts within a range of 3° between 176° and 185°, with decomposition; pH (1 in 100 suspension) between 2.5 and 3.5.

Solubility—1 g in 600 mL water, 400 mL alcohol >10,000 mL chloroform, >10,000 mL ether.

Uses—A piperazine-substituted phenothiazine-antipsychotic drug structurally related to acetophenazine, fluphenazine, and perphenazine. It is used in the management of the manifestations of *psychotic disorders*. Untoward effects reported resemble those encountered with other phenothiazines. See page 1085 for a detailed review of the warnings, contraindications, precautions, and adverse effects characteristic of the phenothiazine agents.

Dose—*Usual*, **12.5 to 50 mg** 3 times a day; increased by 12.5 to 50 mg daily at intervals of from 4 days to 1 week. The maximal daily dose recommended is 400 mg. Dosage not established for children under 12 years of age.

Dosage Forms—Tablets: 25 mg.

Chlorpromazine

10H-Phenothiazine-10-propanamine, 2-chloro-N,N-dimethyl-,
Thorazine (*Smith Kline & French*)

2-Chloro-10-[3-(dimethylamino)propyl]phenothiazine [50-53-3] $C_{17}H_{19}ClN_2S$ (318.86).

Preparation—The base is prepared from 2-chlorophenothiazine and (3-chloropropyl)dimethylamine in the presence of sodamide, then filtering and distilling off the toluene.

Description—White, crystalline solid having an amine-like odor; darkens on prolonged exposure to light; melts at about 60°.

Solubility—1 g in 3 mL alcohol, 2 mL chloroform, 3 mL ether; practically insoluble in water.

Uses—See *Chlorpromazine Hydrochloride.*

Dose—*Antiemetic, rectal,* **50 to 100 mg** every 6 to 8 hours. *Dose range,* **50 to 400 mg** daily. *Pediatric, antiemetic,* children 6 months of age and older, **1 mg per kg** of body weight or ½ of a 25 mg suppository 3 or 4 times a day as necessary. Use in children under 6 months of age not recommended.

Dosage Forms—Suppositories: 25 and 100 mg.

Chlorpromazine Hydrochloride

10H-Phenothiazine-10-propanamine, 2-chloro-N,N-dimethyl-, monohydrochloride; Thorazine Hydrochloride (*Smith Kline & French*);
Promapar (*Parke-Davis*)

2-Chloro-10-[3-(dimethylamino)propyl]phenothiazine monohydrochloride [69-09-0] $C_{17}H_{19}ClN_2S.HCl$ (355.32).
See *chlorpromazine* for the structure of the base.

Description—White or slightly creamy white, odorless, crystalline powder; darkens on prolonged exposure to light; melts between 195° and 198°.

Solubility—1 g in 1 mL water, 1.5 mL alcohol, 1.5 mL chloroform; insoluble in ether and benzene.

Uses—The first *tranquilizer* of the phenothiazine group of compounds. It is *effective* in the management of manifestations of *psychotic disorders, nausea and vomiting,* manifestations of *manic depressive illness* (manic phase), *intractable hiccups, apprehension and anxiety* prior to surgery, *acute intermittent porphyria,* and as an adjunct in the treatment of *tetanus.* It is *probably effective* for control of symptoms in mild *alcohol withdrawal,* and for the control of *moderate to severe agitation,* hyperactivity, or aggressiveness in *disturbed children.* The volume of distribution of chlorpromazine has been reported to be 21.8 L/kg after intramuscular administration and 80.6 L/kg after a single oral dose. This 4-fold difference reflects the low bioavailability *via* the oral route (32%). At least 100 metabolites of chlorpromazine appear in man. Two of these, 11-hydroxy- and 7-hydroxychlorpromazine, are active in man. Effective plasma levels in acute schizophrenia have been reported to vary from 30 ng/mL to 300 ng/mL; plasma levels ranging from 750 to 1000 ng/mL are usually accompanied by neurotoxicity, manifest by tremors and convulsions. Because of great interindividual differences, plasma levels for this agent are largely of research interest. A detailed listing of contraindications, warnings, precautions, and adverse effects of this agent is given on page 1085.

Dosage is extremely variable and requires strict individualization. Administration is oral, intramuscular, or intravenous. Parenteral administration should be reserved for bedfast or hospitalized patients. If used in ambulatory patients, the patient must remain in a supine position for at least 1 hour after the injection. Alarming reactions with failure to respond to pressor agents have been reported from even small intravenous doses. Epinephrine should never be used in treating these cases since the adrenolytic action of the chlorpromazine may cause epinephrine reversal. Phenylephrine or levarterenol may be used to control the hypotension.

Dose—*Antiemetic: adults*, *oral*, **10 to 25 mg** every 4 to 6 hours; *intramuscular*, **25 to 50 mg** every 3 or 4 hours until vomiting ceases. *Children*, *oral*, **0.5 mg/kg** every 4 to 6 hours; *intramuscular*, **0.5 mg/kg** every 6 to 8 hours as required. *Tranquilizer: Adults, oral, usual*, **10 to 50 mg** 2 or 3 times/day to a total dose of **1 g** daily when indicated; *intramuscular*, **25 to 50 mg**, repeated in 1 hour if necessary to a total dose of **1 g** when indicated. *Children, oral*, **0.5 mg/kg** every 4 to 6 hours; *intramuscular*, **0.5 mg/kg** every 6 to 8 hours as required. Consult package literature for more specific information.

Dosage Forms—Injection: 25 mg/mL in 1, 2, and 10 mL; Capsules (timed release): 30, 75, 150, 200, and 300 mg; Syrup: 2 mg/mL; Concentrate: 30 and 100 mg/mL; Tablets: 10, 25, 50, 100, and 200 mg.

Chlorprothixene

1-Propanamine, 3-(2-chloro-9*H*-thioxanthen-9-ylidene)-
N,N-dimethyl-, (*Z*)-, Taractan (*Roche*)

(*Z*) - 2 - Chloro - *N,N* - dimethylthioxanthene - $\Delta^{9,\gamma}$ - propylamine [113-59-7] $C_{18}H_{18}ClNS$ (315.86).

Preparation—One method cyclizes 5-chloro-2-(phenylthio)benzoic acid with the aid of polyphosphoric acid to 2-chlorothioxanthen-9-one, followed by reaction with [3-(dimethylamino)propylidene]triphenylphosphorane to introduce the 9-substituent. US Pat 3,115,502 describes a process for converting the *cis* form of the compound to the therapeutically active *trans* form by heating in the presence of a strongly basic agent.

Description—Yellow, crystalline powder; slight amine-like odor and unstable when exposed to light and air; melts between 96.5° and 101.5°.

Solubility—1 g in 1700 mL water, 29 mL alcohol, 2 mL chloroform, 14 mL ether, 18 mL acetone.

Uses—A thioxanthene derivative chemically and pharmacologically related to chlorpromazine. In place of the nitrogen in the phenothiazine ring, chlorprothixene has a carbon atom with a double bond to the dimethylaminopropyl side chain. This structural difference is not associated with any striking pharmacological difference. It induces less sedation, adrenergic blockade and extrapyramidal reactions than does chlorpromazine. Chlorprothixene is indicated for the management of the manifestations of *psychotic disorders*. Thus, it has been used in the treatment of acute and chronic schizophrenia and in psychotic and other conditions in which anxiety, agitation, and tension predominate. Because of its structural similarity to the phenothiazines, all the known contraindications, warnings, precautions, and serious side effects associated with phenothiazine therapy should be borne in mind (see page 1085).

Dose—*Usual, adult, oral*, or *intramuscular*, **25 to 50 mg** 3 or 4 times a day; maximum, up to 600 mg daily. *Usual, pediatric, oral*, children 6 to 12 years of age, **10 to 25 mg** 3 or 4 times a day; children under 6 years of age, dosage not established. *Intramuscular*, not to be used in children under 12 years of age.

Dosage Forms—Injection: 25 mg/2 mL; Oral Suspension: 100 mg/5 mL; Tablets: 10, 25, 50, and 100 mg.

Droperidol

2*H*-Benzimidazol-2-one, 1-[1-[4-(4-fluorophenyl)-4-oxobutyl]-1,2,3,6-
tetrahydro-4-pyridinyl]-1,3-dihydro-,
Inapsine, ing of Innovar (*Janssen*)

1-[1-[3-(*p*-Fluorobenzoyl)propyl]-1,2,3,6-tetrahydro-4-pyridyl]-2-benzimidazolinone [548-73-2] $C_{22}H_{22}FN_3O_2$ (379.43).

Preparation—4-Chloro-4'-fluorobutyrophenone is prepared from γ-butyrolactone and reacted with 1-(1,2,3,6-tetrahydro-4-pyridyl)-

2-benzimidazolinone in the presence of a suitable condensing agent. US Pat. 3,161,645.

Description—White to light tan, amorphous or microcrystalline powder that is odorless and tasteless (*Note:* because this compound is extremely potent, no taste test is recommended); sensitive to light, air, and heat; hygroscopic; melts between 144° and 148° after drying in vacuum at 70° for 4 hours; pK_a 7.6.

Solubility—1 g in 10,000 mL water, 140 mL alcohol, 4 mL chloroform, 500 mL ether.

Uses—Droperidol, a butyrophenone derivative, is a *neuroleptic* used as an adjunct to anesthesia to produce sedation and reduce incidence of nausea and vomiting. It is more often used in combination with the analgesic fentanyl citrate (for uses, see *Fentanyl Citrate and Droperidol Injection*, page 1045).

Dose—*Premedication, intravenous* or *intramuscular*, **2.5 to 10 mg** 30 to 60 min before induction; *induction*, usually *intravenous*, **2.5 mg/20 to 25 lb**; *maintenance*, usually *intravenous*, **1.25 to 2.5 mg.**

Dosage Forms—Injection: droperidol lactate equivalent to 2.5 mg of droperidol/mL in 2- and 5-mL ampuls and 10-mL vials.

Fluphenazine Decanoate

Prolixin Decanoate (*Squibb*)

4-[3-[2-(Trifluoromethyl)phenothiazin-10-yl]propyl]-1-piperazineethanol decanoate (ester) [30909-31-4] $C_{32}H_{44}F_3N_3O_2S$ (591.77).

Preparation—Fluphenazine (see *Fluphenazine Hydrochloride*) is esterified with decanoyl chloride in the presence of pyridine. US Pats 3,194,733 and 3,394,131.

Description—Pale yellow to yellowish orange viscous liquid with a characteristic odor; light-sensitive.

Solubility—Insoluble in water; soluble in alcohol, acetone, benzene, and ether.

Uses—A trifluoromethyl phenothiazine derivative indicated for the management of *schizophrenia*. The basic effects of this drug are no different from *Fluphenazine Hydrochloride*, except for duration of action. The duration of action is essentially the same as *Fluphenazine Enanthate*.

Dose—*Intramuscular* or *subcutaneous*, **12.5 to 100 mg;** *usual*, **25 mg** every 2 weeks. Safety and efficacy of this drug in children have not been established.

Dosage Form—Injection: 25 mg/mL.

Fluphenazine Enanthate

Prolixin Enanthate (*Squibb*)

[2746-81-8] $C_{29}H_{38}F_3N_3O_2S$ (549.69).

Preparation—Fluphenazine is esterified through reaction with enanthoyl chloride in the presence of pyridine. For the preparation of fluphenazine, see *Fluphenazine Hydrochloride*. US Pat 3,058,979.

Description—Pale-yellow to yellow-orange, clear to slightly turbid, viscous liquid that has a characteristic odor; not recommended to be tasted; unstable in strong light, but stable in air at room temperature.

Solubility—1 g in <1 mL alcohol, <1 mL chloroform, 2 mL ether; insoluble in water.

Uses—Except for duration of action, it has actions, uses, contraindications, and untoward effects similar to those of fluphenazine hydrochloride. The esterification of fluphenazine with the enanthate moiety markedly prolongs the drug's duration of action without unduly attenuating its beneficial effects. The onset of action generally appears between 24 to 72 hours after injection, and the effects of the drug on psychotic symptoms become significant within 48 to 96 hours. Amelioration of symptoms continues for 1 to 3 weeks or longer, with an average duration of effect of about 2 weeks. It is especially useful when the patient or his family can not be relied upon to insure that an oral antischizophrenic drug will be given every day. See *Fluphenazine Hydrochloride*.

Dose—*Intramuscular* or *subcutaneous*, **12.5** to **100 mg** every 1 to 3 weeks; *usual*, **25 mg** every 2 weeks. Safety and efficacy of this drug in children have not been established.

Dosage Forms—Injection: 25 mg/mL.

Fluphenazine Hydrochloride

Permitil (*Schering-Plough*) Prolixin (*Squibb*)

4-[3-[2-(Trifluoromethyl)phenothiazin-10-yl]propyl]-1-piperazineethanol dihydrochloride [146-56-5] $C_{22}H_{26}F_3N_3OS.2HCl$ (510.44).

Preparation—Fluphenazine may be prepared by condensing 2-(trifluoromethyl)-10-(3-chloropropyl)phenothiazine with 1-piperazineethanol in toluene with the aid of sodamide. Reaction of the purified base with a double molar quantity of hydrogen chloride yields the official salt. The starting phenothiazine compound may be prepared by heating 3-(trifluoromethyl)diphenylamine with sulfur and condensing the resulting 2-(trifluoromethyl)phenothiazine with 1-bromo-3-chloropropane. US Pat 3,058,979.

Description—White or nearly white, odorless, crystalline powder; melts within a 5° range above 225°.

Solubility—1 g in 1.4 mL water, 6.7 mL alcohol; slightly soluble in chloroform; practically insoluble in ether.

Uses—A trifluoromethyl phenothiazine derivative intended for the management of manifestations of *psychotic disorders*. Although the pharmacologic effects of fluphenazine hydrochloride are, in general, similar to those of other phenothiazines, laboratory and clinical studies indicate that this drug exhibits several important differences. The drug is more potent, exhibits a more prolonged duration of action, is less likely to induce hypotension, is less sedative, and does not potentiate central nervous system depressants and anesthetics to the same degree as other phenothiazines. The intramuscular or subcutaneous administration of the enanthate salt has an average duration of 2 weeks. Therefore, it is useful in those patients who refuse to take the oral preparation. It appears to be particularly effective in modifying psychotic behavior patterns and ameliorating such symptoms as agitation, delusions, and hallucinations. Like other phenothiazines, fluphenazine hydrochloride should not be used in patients receiving large doses of hypnotics, and should be used with caution in patients with a history of convulsive disorders. Side effects induced by fluphenazine hydrochloride are similar to those encountered with other phenothiazines. Those most frequently encountered include reversible extrapyramidal symptoms (approximately 60% of patients) including parkinsonism, dystonia, dyskinesia, akathisia, oculogyric crises, opisthotonos, and hyperreflexia; liver damage manifest by jaundice or biliary stasis; blood dyscrasias, including leukopenia, agranulocytosis, thrombocytopenic purpura, eosinophilia, and pancytopenia; skin disorders such as itching, erythema, urticaria, and even exfoliative dermatitis; peripheral edema, endocrine disturbances, and autonomic reactions. Hypotension has rarely been a problem with fluphenazine hydrochloride. Patients given this drug should be under medical supervision and observed carefully for other untoward effects characteristic of phenothiazine agents (see page 1085).

Dose—*Usual, adult, oral, initial*, **0.5** to **10 mg** daily in divided doses; *maintenance*, **1** to **5 mg** as a single dose daily. *Intramuscular*, **1.25** to **10 mg** daily divided into 4 doses. Daily dosages exceeding 20 mg orally or 10 mg intramuscularly should be used with caution. Safety and efficacy of this drug in children have not been established.

Dosage Forms—Elixir: 1 mg/2 mL; Concentrate: 5 mg/mL; Injection: 25 mg/10 mL; Tablets: 250 μg, and 1, 2.5, 5, and 10 mg.

Haloperidol

1-Butanone, 4-[4-(4-chlorophenyl)-4-hydroxy-1-piperidinyl]-1-(4-fluorophenyl)-, Haldol (*McNeil*)

4-[4-(*p*-Chlorophenyl)-4-hydroxypiperidino]-4′-fluorobutyrophenone [52-86-8] $C_{21}H_{23}ClFNO_2$ (375.87).

Preparation—4-(*p*-Chlorophenyl)-4-piperidinol is condensed with 4-chloro-4′-fluorobutyrophenone in a toluene solution. The haloperidol thus formed is isolated and recrystallized from a solvent such as diisopropyl ether. The starting substituted piperidinol may be prepared from *p*-chloro-α-methylstyrene by the method described by Schmidle and Mansfield (*J Am Chem Soc 78*: 1702, 1956).

Description—White to faintly yellowish, odorless, amorphous or microcrystalline powder; light-sensitive and nonhygroscopic; saturated solution is neutral to litmus; melts between 147° and 152°; pK_a 8.2 to 8.3.

Solubility—1 g in >10,000 mL water, 60 mL alcohol, 15 mL chloroform, 200 mL ether.

Uses—A butyrophenone derivative that is an antipsychotic agent useful in the management of such symptoms as moderate to severe *agitation, anxiety* and *tension, assaultiveness, delusions, hallucinations, hostility*, and *hyperactivity*, when they are *manifestations of psychoses* including *schizophrenia*, the manic type of *manic depressive illness*, or *psychotic reactions* associated with organic brain syndromes or mental retardation. Haloperidol has been reported to be useful in *Gilles de la Tourette's disease* (motor tics, unusual barking, and hissing sounds). The bioavailability of this drug has been reported to be approximately 60% *via* the oral route. The half-life of elimination ranges from 10 to 19 hours after i.v. administration and 12 to 38 hours *via* the oral route. Therapeutic plasma levels range from 3 to 10 ng/mL, but some patients require significantly higher levels before adequate antipsychotic effects are observed. It has the same contraindications, warnings, and precautions as other drugs in this category (see page 1085). Like the phenothiazines, haloperidol frequently produces extrapyramidal reactions such as parkinsonism, dystonia, dyskinesia, oculogyric crises, and akathisia. Occasional adverse effects include blood dyscrasia, postural hypotension, and tachycardia. Rarely, cholestatic jaundice, photosensitivity reactions, and allergic skin reactions may occur. Care should be exercised when antihypertensive agents, general anesthetics, hypnotics, alcohol, analgesics, and other central nervous system depressants are used concomitantly with haloperidol, since it may potentiate their actions. See 1085 for a more detailed listing of potential adverse effects.

Dose—*Usual, adult, oral*, **0.5** to **5 mg** 2 to 3 times a day; maximum, **100 mg** daily. *Note: geriatric* or debilitated patients, *oral*, **0.5** to **2 mg** 2 or 3 times a day, increased gradually as needed and tolerated. *Intramuscular*, **2** to **5 mg** initially, repeat at hourly intervals if necessary, or at 4- to 8-hour intervals if symptoms are controlled; doses above 15 mg a day are seldom required. *Hyperkinesia* with mental retardation, *intramuscular*, **5 mg** 4 times a day initially, increased gradually to 60 mg a day if necessary. Not recommended for pediatric age group since safety and effectiveness in children have not been established.

Dosage Forms—Concentrate: 2 mg/mL; Solution: 2 mg/mL; Tablets: 0.5, 1, 2, 5, 10, and 20 mg; Injection: 5 mg/mL.

Lithium Carbonate

Carbonic acid, dilithium salt; Eskalith (*SKF*); Lithane (*Miles*); Lithonate (*Rowell*)

Dilithium carbonate [554-13-2] Li_2CO_3 (73.89).

Preparation—Lithium chloride is metathesized with sodium carbonate in aqueous solution.

Description—White, light, granular powder that melts at 618°.

Solubility—1 g in 78 mL cold water and 140 mL boiling water; very slightly soluble in alcohol; dissolved by dilute acids.

Uses—For the treatment of the manic phase of *manic-depressive psychoses*. Maintenance therapy prevents or diminishes the intensity of subsequent episodes in those manic-depressive patients with a history of mania. Other psychiatric conditions which may be benefited include recurrent severe depressions without manic episodes, schizo-affective psychosis, episodic alcoholism and periodic antisocial behavior, and periodic schizophrenic illness; its value in these conditions awaits further research. Lithium carbonate is water-soluble and is absorbed and excreted rather rapidly; consequently, it must be taken in divided doses over the day to maintain relatively constant plasma concentrations. Lithium carbonate has been used investigationally to improve the neutrophil count in patients with cancer-chemotherapy-induced neutropenia. Lithium alters sodium transport in nerve and muscle cells and effects a shift toward interneuronal metabolism of catecholamine. Lithium carbonate is completely absorbed 6 to 8 hours following oral administration. Its plasma half-life is about 24 hours. It is excreted by the kidneys; about 80% of filtered lithium is reabsorbed. The lithium ion is distributed in total body water, but is concentrated in various tissues to different degrees. After a steady state has been reached, about 40% is contained in cerebrospinal fluid and renal clearance is relatively constant. Serum levels should be maintained between 0.7 and 1.3 mEq/L. Adverse effects are noted at levels above 1.5 mEq/L and serious toxicity is common when concentrations exceed 2.0 mEq/L. Since toxicity develops at serum levels little higher than effective therapeutic levels frequent monitoring and dosage adjustments are mandatory for successful therapy.

Nausea, vomiting, and diarrhea are presumptive evidence of toxicity and indicate the dose should be reduced. The most common untoward effects are slight tremor and polyuria; these do not ordinarily require a reduction in dosages. Central nervous system effects, such as slurred speech, blurred vision, confusion, and lethargy, require immediate withdrawal of the drug and the administration of sodium chloride (at least 4 g extra/day) to facilitate the excretion of lithium. Adverse cardiovascular effects include arrhythmias and hypotension. Goiter, hypothyroidism, and diabetes insipidus have also been observed. Lithium carbonate should not be used in patients with cardiovascular or renal disease. Safe use of the drug during pregnancy has not been established; it can cause cardiac and other birth defects. The drug should not be used in children under 12 years of age.

Dose—*Usual, initial,* **600 mg** 3 times a day; *maintenance,* **300 mg** 3 times a day, to maintain a serum lithium level of 0.6 to 1.2 mEq/liter 8 to 12 hours following administration; *usual range of dose,* **900 mg** to **1.8 g** daily. Dosage for children under 12 years of age not established.

Warning, toxicity can occur at doses close to therapeutic levels.

Dosage Forms—Capsules: 300 mg; Syrup: 300 mg/5 mL. Tablets: 300 mg; Tablets (slow release): 300 and 450 mg.

Loxapine Succinate

Butanedioic acid, compd with 2-chloro-11-(4-methyl-1-piperazinyl)-dibenz[*b,f*][1,4]oxazepine (1:1); Daxolin (*Miles*)

2-Chloro-11-(4-methyl-1-piperazinyl)dibenz[*b,f*][1,4]oxazepine succinate (1:1) [27833-64-3], $C_{18}H_{18}ClN_3O.C_4H_6O_4$ (445.90).

Preparation—A method of synthesis of loxapine starting with xanthone oxime is described in US Pat 3,412,193. Other procedures are summarized in *CA 63:* 11592H, 1965.

Description—White to off-white, crystalline powder; pK_a 6.6 (loxapine base).

Solubility—Slightly soluble in water and in alcohol.

Uses—A dibenzoxazepine antipsychotic agent indicated for symptomatic control of schizophrenia; the mode of action has not been established. It is contraindicated in comatose or severe drug-induced depressed states, also in individuals with known hypersensitivity to the drug. Absorption following oral administration is virtually complete; after distribution to tissues it is metabolized and excreted in the urine and feces, mainly in the first 24 hours. In normal human volunteers, signs of sedation were seen within 20 to 30 minutes after administration, were most pronounced within 1.5 to 3 hours, and lasted through 12 hours.

Adverse reactions include drowsiness, dizziness, faintness, staggering gait, muscle twitching, weakness, confusional states, extrapyramidal symptoms, and persistent tardive dyskinesia as central nervous system effects; tachycardia; hypotension, hypertension, lightheadedness, and syncope as cardiovascular effects; dermatitis, edema, pruritus, seborrhea, and skin rashes as skin effects; dry mouth, nasal congestion, constipation, and blurred vision as anticholinergic effects; nausea, vomiting, weight gain or loss, dyspnea, ptosis, hyperpyrexia, flushed facies, headache, paresthesia, and polydipsia as other reactions.

It should be used with extreme caution in patients with a history of convulsive disorders since it lowers the convulsive threshold; seizures have been reported in epileptic patients receiving loxapine, even with maintenance of anticonvulsant therapy. As an antiemetic effect may occur in man, loxapine may mask signs of overdosage of toxic drugs and may obscure conditions such as intestinal obstruction and brain tumor. The drug should be used with caution in patients with cardiovascular disease. Increased pulse rates have been reported in most patients receiving antipsychotic doses; transient hypotension has been reported. In the presence of severe hypotension that requires vasopressor therapy, norepinephrine or angiotensin is preferred over epinephrine, which may be ineffective because of inhibition of its vasopressor effect by loxapine. Since the possibility of ocular toxicity from loxapine exists, careful observation for pigmentary retinopathy and lenticular pigmentation should be made. Because of possible anticholinergic action, loxapine should be used cautiously in patients with glaucoma or a tendency to urinary retention. Safe use during pregnancy or lactation has not been established; as studies have not been performed in children, use of the drug in children below the age of 16 is not recommended.

Dose—*Usual, adult, oral,* the equivalent of **10 mg** of loxapine 2 times a day; *maintenance, oral,* the equivalent of **15 to 25 mg** 2 to 4 times a day. Note: *Geriatric* or *debilitated patients,* the equivalent of **5 mg** of loxapine 2 times a day. *Maximum dose, adult, oral,* the equivalent of **250 mg** of loxapine daily. Not recommended for use in children below the age of 16.

Dosage Forms—Capsules: 5, 10, 25, and 50 mg of loxapine (as succinate); Oral Concentrate: 25 mg of loxapine (as hydrochloride)/mL; Injection: 50 mg/mL.

Mesoridazine Besylate

10*H*-Phenothiazine, 10-[2-(1-methyl-2-piperidinyl)ethyl]-2-(methylsulfinyl)-, monobenzenesulfonate; Serentil (*Sandoz*)

10-[2-(1-Methyl-2-piperidyl)ethyl]-2-(methylsulfinyl)phenothiazine monobenzenesulfonate [32672-69-8] $C_{21}H_{26}N_2OS_2.C_6H_6O_3S$ (544.74).

Preparation—Nitrophenide is converted by a series of reactions into 2-(methylthio)phenothiazine. Oxidation with H_2O_2 yields the corresponding sulfinyl compound which is reacted with 1-methyl-2-(2-chloroethyl)piperidine in the presence of a suitable condensing agent and the mesoridazine thus formed is converted, with benzenesulfonic acid, to the besylate salt. US Pat 3,084,161.

Description—White to pale yellow, crystalline powder with a faint odor; melts at about 178° with decomposition.

Solubility—1 g in 1 mL water, 11 mL alcohol, 3 mL chloroform, 6300 mL ether.

Uses—The salt of a metabolite of thioridazine, a phenothiazine derivative, indicated for the management of *schizophrenia, organic brain disorders,* symptoms of *alcohol withdrawal,* and *psychoneuroses.* It has pharmacologic properties similar to thioridazine, except that this agent has antiemetic activity and pigmentary retinopathy has not yet been associated with its use. Otherwise, it has warnings, precautions, contraindications, and adverse effects similar to those for other phenothiazines (see page 1085).

Dose—*Usual, adult, oral,* **50 to 400 mg** daily; *initial,* **50 mg** 3 times a day. *Intramuscular, usual,* **25 to 200 mg** daily; *initial,* **25 mg;** repeat in 30 to 60 min if necessary. Use in children under 12 years of age is not recommended because safe conditions for its use have not been established.

Dosage Forms—Concentrate: 25 mg/mL; Injection: 25 mg/mL; Tablets: 10, 25, 50, and 100 mg.

Perphenazine

1-Piperazineethanol, 4-[3-(2-chloro-10*H*-phenothiazin-10-yl)propyl]-,
Trilafon (*Schering*)

4-[3-(2-Chlorophenothiazin-10-yl)propyl]-1-piperazineethanol
[58-39-9] $C_{21}H_{26}ClN_3OS$ (403.97).

Preparation—A toluene solution of 2-chloro-10-(3-chloropropyl)phenothiazine and 1-piperazineethanol is refluxed with sodamide and the resulting perphenazine purified by high-vacuum distillation. US Pat 2,838,507.

Description—White to creamy-white powder which is almost odorless and has a bitter taste; melts between 94° and 100°.

Solubility—1 g in 7 mL alcohol, 13 mL acetone; practically insoluble in water; freely soluble in chloroform.

Uses—A phenothiazine compound, differing chemically from prochlorperazine only with respect to the substitution of a hydroxyethyl group for the methyl group of the latter drug. Perphenazine is indicated for the management of *psychotic disorders*, for the control of severe *nausea* and *vomiting*, and intractable hiccoughs in adults. Since it is a phenothiazine, it is subject to similar contraindications, warnings, and precautions as other members of this chemical class. Likewise, it should be considered capable of inducing similar adverse reactions. See page 1085 and *Chlorpromazine Hydrochloride*.

Dose—*Usual, oral,* nonhospitalized patients, **2 to 8 mg** 3 times a day; hospitalized patients, **8 to 16 mg** 2 to 4 times a day; *intramuscular,* **5 to 10 mg** initially, followed by **5 mg** in 6 hours. Severe *nausea* and *vomiting, adults, oral,* **8 to 16 mg** daily in divided doses or one Repetab twice a day. Not recommended for children under 12 years of age.

Dosage Forms—Injection: 5 mg/mL; Solution: 16 mg/5 mL; Tablets: 2, 4, 8, and 16 mg; Repetabs: 8 mg.

Piperacetazine

Ethanone, 1-[10-[3-[4-(2-hydroxyethyl)-1-piperidinyl]propyl]-10*H*-phenothiazin-2-yl]-, Quide (*Merrell Dow*)

10-[3-[4-(2-Hydroxyethyl)piperidino]propyl]phenothiazin-2-yl methyl ketone [3819-00-9] $C_{24}H_{30}N_2O_2S$ (410.57).

Description—Yellow, granular powder; melts between 102° and 106°.

Solubility—Practically insoluble in water; soluble in alcohol and dilute hydrochloric acid; freely soluble in chloroform.

Preparation—4-Piperidineethanol is condensed with 10-(3-chloropropyl)phenothiazin-2-yl methyl ketone (I) by refluxing in an inert solvent in the presence of sodamide. For the preparation of I see *Acetophenazine Maleate*.

Uses—Piperacetazine, a potent piperidine-substituted phenothiazine, is indicated for the management of the manifestations of *psychotic disorders*. It is also used for the management of manifestations of behavioral complications in patients with mental retardation. Side effects and contraindications are the same as those for other phenothiazines (see page 1085). Piperacetazine is contraindicated during pregnancy and lactation, in patients with preexisting thrombocytopenia, and other blood dyscrasias, bone-marrow depression, and liver impairment. It is not recommended in children under 12 years of age because conditions for its safe use have not been established.

Dose—*Initial,* **10 mg** 2 to 4 times daily; *maintenance,* up to **160 mg** daily in divided doses. If side effects appear, dosage should be reduced or discontinued. Use in children under 12 years of age is not recommended because safe conditions for its use have not been established.

Dosage Forms—Tablets: 10 and 25 mg.

Prochlorperazine—page 809.

Prochlorperazine Edisylate—page 809.

Prochlorperazine Maleate—page 809.

Promazine Hydrochloride

10*H*-Phenothiazine-10-propanamine, *N,N*-dimethyl-, monohydrochloride; Sparine (*Wyeth*)

10-[3-(Dimethylamino)propyl]phenothiazine monohydrochloride [53-60-1] $C_{17}H_{20}N_2S \cdot HCl$ (320.88).

Preparation—Phenothiazine is dissolved in an inert solvent and condensed with 3-chloro-*N,N*-dimethylpropylamine in the presence of sodium hydride to yield promazine. After purification, it is dissolved in an organic solvent and reacted with an equimolar quantity of HCl.

Description—White to slightly yellow, practically odorless, crystalline powder; oxidizes upon prolonged exposure to air, and acquires a blue or pink color; melts within a 3°-range between 172° and 182°; pH (1 in 20 solution) between 4.2 and 5.2.

Solubility—1 g in 3 mL water; freely soluble in chloroform.

Uses—An aliphatic phenothiazine used in the management of the manifestations of *psychotic disorders*. It is *probably effective* for the control of *nausea and vomiting*, for the relief of *apprehension prior to surgery*, and for *reducing agitation and tension associated with mild alcohol withdrawal* under supervision. Promazine hydrochloride has the same contraindications, warnings and precautions as other phenothiazines. Because of the close pharmacologic similarities among the various phenothiazines, each agent must be considered capable of inducing any untoward reaction common to this group of agents (see page 1085).

Promazine has the same therapeutic applications and limitations as chlorpromazine. Although some of the more serious toxic effects of chlorpromazine have not been encountered with promazine, it should be used with the same degree of caution. See *Chlorpromazine Hydrochloride*.

Dose—*Usual, adult, oral, intramuscular,* and *intravenous,* **10 to 200 mg,** every 4 to 6 hours. *Usual, pediatric, oral,* children 12 years of age and older, **10 to 25 mg** every 4 to 6 hours; under 12 years of age, dosage not established.

Other Dose Information—Total daily dose ranges from 25 to 300 mg to a maximum of 1 g daily.

Dosage Forms—Injection: 25 and 50 mg/mL, 50 and 100 mg/2 mL, 250 and 500 mg/10 mL; Solution: 30 and 100 mg/mL; Syrup: 10 mg/5 mL; Tablets: 10, 25, 50, and 100 mg.

Promethazine—page 1129.

Rauwolfia Serpentina—page 909.

Rescinnamine—page 909.

Reserpine—page 908.

Syrosingopine—RPS-16, p 849.

Thioridazine

10*H*-Phenothiazine, 10-[2-(1-methyl-2-piperidinyl)ethyl]-2-(methylthio)-, Mellaril (*Sandoz*)

[50-52-2] $C_{21}H_{26}N_2S_2$ (370.57).

Preparation—2-(Methylthio)phenothiazine, which may be prepared by reacting 2-chlorophenothiazine with (methylthio)sodium, is condensed with 2-(1-methyl-1-piperidyl)ethyl chloride with the aid of a dehydrochlorinating agent such as sodamide. US Pat. 3,239,514.

Description—Crystals that melt between 72° and 74°.

Uses and **Dose**—See *Thioridazine Hydrochloride*.

Thioridazine Hydrochloride

10*H*-Phenothiazine, 10-[2-(1-methyl-2-piperidinyl)ethyl]-2-(methyl-thio)-, monohydrochloride; Mellaril Hydrochloride (*Sandoz*)

[130-61-0] $C_{21}H_{26}N_2S_2 \cdot HCl$ (407.03).
For the structure and preparation of the base, see *Thioridazine*.

Description—White to slightly yellow, granular powder with a faint odor and a very bitter taste; stable in moderate heat, nonhygroscopic, and darkens on exposure to light; melts within a range of 3° between 157° and 163°; pH (1 in 100 solution) between 4.2 and 5.2.

Solubility—Freely soluble in water, chloroform, and methanol; slightly soluble in benzene; insoluble in ether.

Uses—A piperidyl-type phenothiazine tranquilizer with central sedative and behavioral effects similar to those of chlorpromazine. It has minimal antiemetic action and produces minimal extrapyramidal stimulation. Sedation and drowsiness are less intense with thioridazine than with chlorpromazine and related compounds. Thioridazine is *effective* in the management of manifestations of *psychotic disorders*. It is *probably effective* for relief of symptoms of *neurotic depressive reactions*, control of moderate to severe *agitation*, *hyperactivity*, or *aggressiveness in disturbed children*, and *possibly effective* in *alcohol withdrawal* syndrome, *intractable pain*, *psychoneuroses*, and *senility*. Half-life appears to be multiphasic with an early phase of 4 to 10 hours and a late phase of 26 to 36 hours; 96 to 99% is bound to plasma protein. The effective plasma level and the relation to clinical improvement remain to be established. The drug is sulfoxidized to mesoridazine and small amounts of sulforidazine; both are pharmacologically active. Contraindications, warnings and precautions are similar to those for other phenothiazines. Untoward effects, such as extrapyramidal reactions, sedation, and drowsiness are less intense and occur less frequently with thioridazine than with any other phenothiazine. Serious pigmentary retinopathy (decreased visual acuity, brownish color of vision, and impaired night vision), a complication attributed only to this drug, may occur with doses in excess of 800 mg a day. Other untoward effects are potentially the same as those for other agents in this chemical class. See page 1085.

Dose—*Adult*, *usual*, *initial*, **25 to 100 mg** 3 times a day; *maintenance*, **10 to 200 mg** 2 to 4 times a day. Total daily dose ranges from 200 to 800 mg, divided into two to four doses. *Usual*, *pediatric*, children 2 to 12 years of age, **0.5 to a maximum of 3.0 mg per kg** daily; dosage increased daily until optimum therapeutic effect obtained or the maximum dose reached; children under 2 years of age, not recommended.

Dosage Forms—Concentrate: 30 and 100 mg/mL; Suspension: 25 and 100 mg/5 mL; Tablets: 10, 15, 50, 100, 150, and 200 mg.

Thiothixene

9*H*-Thioxanthene-2-sulfonamide, *N*,*N*-dimethyl-9-[3-(4-methyl-1-piperazinyl)propylidene]-, (*Z*)-, Navane (*Pfizer*)

[5591-45-7 and 3313-26-6(*Z*)] $C_{23}H_{29}N_3O_2S_2$ (443.62).
Preparation—2-Chlorobenzoic acid is converted into its 5-dimethylsulfamoyl derivative by successive reaction with chlorosulfonic acid and dimethylamine. The chlorine is then replaced by phenylthio by treatment with benzenethiol in the presence of alkali and the resulting 2-phenylthio derivative is cyclized with polyphosphoric acid to form *N*,*N*-dimethyl-9-oxothioxanthene-2-sulfonamide. Reaction of this compound with [3-(4-methyl-1-piperidyl)propylidene]triphenylphosphorane replaces the oxo oxygen by the appropriately substituted propylidene group to yield thiothixene. US Pat 3,310,553.

Description—White to tan, crystalline powder that is practically odorless and has a very bitter taste; unstable in light; melts between 147° and 152°.

Solubility—Practically insoluble in water; very soluble in chloroform; slightly soluble in methanol and acetone.

Uses—A thioxanthene derivative used as an antipsychotic agent in the treatment of *psychotic disorders*. It is also helpful in the management of secondary symptoms of schizophrenia, such as, hallucinations, tension, and suspiciousness. Since thiothixene is closely related chemically to the phenothiazines, its contraindications, warnings, precautions, and adverse reactions are similar to the latter agents. See page 1085 for a detailed discussion of these factors.

Dose—*Usual*, *adult*, *oral*, **2 to 5 mg** 2 or 3 times a day; maximum 60 mg daily. Use in children under 12 years of age is not recommended because safe conditions for its use have not been established.

Dosage Forms—Capsules: 1, 2, 5, 10, and 20 mg.

Thiothixene Hydrochloride

9*H*-Thioxanthene-2-sulfonamide, *N*,*N*-dimethyl-9-[3-(4-methyl-1-piperazinyl)propylidene]-, dihydrochloride, dihydrate, (*Z*)-, Navane Hydrochloride (*Pfizer*)

[22189-31-7 and 49746-09-0(*Z*)] $C_{23}H_{29}N_3O_2S_2 \cdot 2HCl \cdot 2H_2O$ (552.57); *anhydrous* [49746-04-5] (516.54). For the structure of the base, see *Thiothixene*.

Preparation—*Thiothixene* is reacted with aqueous HCl and the hydrochloride is crystallized therefrom.

Description—White, or nearly white, crystalline powder, having a slight odor; affected by light.

Solubility—Soluble in water; slightly soluble in chloroform; practically insoluble in benzene, acetone, and ether.

Uses—See *Thiothixene*.

Dose—*Usual*, *adult*, *oral*, **2 to 5 mg** 2 or 3 times a day; *intramuscular*, **4 mg** 2 to 4 times a day; *daily range*, **16 to 30 mg**. Use in children under 12 years of age is not recommended because safe conditions for its use have not been established.

Dosage Forms—Injection: 2 mg/1 mL and 4 mg/2 mL; Oral Solution: 5 mg/mL.

Trifluoperazine Hydrochloride

10*H*-Phenothiazine, 10-[3-(4-methyl-1-piperazinyl)propyl]-2-(trifluoromethyl)-, dihydrochloride; Stelazine (*SKF*)

[440-17-5] $C_{21}H_{24}F_3N_3S \cdot 2HCl$ (480.42).
Preparation—By the process described for *Triflupromazine Hydrochloride* except that 1-(3-chloropropyl)-4-methylpiperazine is used as the condensing amine in place of (3-chloropropyl)dimethylamine. US Pat 2,921,069.

Description—White to pale-yellow, crystalline powder, practically odorless and has a bitter taste; melts at about 242° with decomposition.

Solubility—1 g in 3.5 mL water, 11 mL alcohol, 100 mL chloroform; insoluble in ether.

Uses—A piperazine phenothiazine *effective* in the management of the manifestations of *psychotic disorders*. It is possibly effective for the control of *excessive anxiety*, *tension*, and *agitation* seen in *neurosis* or associated with *somatic conditions*. The general profile of pharmacological action is similar to other phenothiazine derivatives. Bioavailability, time to peak effect, metabolism, and elimination half-life resemble those for chlorpromazine. Untoward effects such as hypotension, blurred vision, and other manifestations of autonomic blockade appear to be less troublesome than with other phenothiazines. Drowsiness is the most common minor untoward effect. Extrapyramidal symptoms occur much more frequently with trifluoperazine hydrochloride than with the dimethylaminopropyl-type phenothiazines. Other warnings, contraindications, precautions, and potential adverse effects have been reviewed in detail (see page 1085).

Dose—*Usual, oral, nonhospitalized patients*, 1 to 2 **mg** twice daily; *hospitalized patients*, 2 to 5 **mg** twice daily initially, gradually increasing to the optimum level of 15 to 20 **mg** daily, although a few patients may require 40 **mg** a day or more; *intramuscular*, 1 to 2 **mg** every 4 to 6 hours as required. (Doses stated in base equivalents.) *Usual, pediatric, oral, hospitalized children* 6 to 12 years of age, 1 **mg** once or twice a day, dosage gradually increased until symptoms controlled; maximum 15 mg daily.

Dosage Forms—Injection: 20 mg/10 mL; Concentrate: 10 mg/mL; Tablets: 1, 2, 5, and 10 mg. (Amounts stated in base equivalents.)

Trifluromazine

10*H*-Phenothiazine-10-propanamine, *N,N*-dimethyl-2-(trifluoromethyl)-, monohydrochloride; Vesprin (*Squibb*)

10-[3-(Dimethylamino)propyl]- 2-(trifluoromethyl)phenothiazine [146-54-3] $C_{18}H_{19}F_3N_2S$ (352.42).

Preparation—See *Trifluromazine Hydrochloride*.

Description—Viscous, light amber-colored, oily liquid, which crystallizes on prolonged standing into large irregular crystals.
Solubility—Practically insoluble in water.

Uses and **Dose**—See *Trifluromazine Hydrochloride*.
Dosage Forms—Oral Suspension: 50 mg/5 mL (hydrochloride equivalent).

Trifluromazine Hydrochloride

10*H*-Phenothiazine-10-propanamine, *N,N*-dimethyl-2-(trifluoromethyl)-, monohydrochloride; Vesprin Hydrochloride (*Squibb*)

10-[3-(Dimethylamino)propyl]-2-(trifluoromethyl)phenothiazine monohydrochloride [1098-60-8] $C_{18}H_{19}F_3N_2S.HCl$ (388.88). For the structure of the base see *Trifluromazine*.

Preparation—2-(Trifluoromethyl)phenothiazine is condensed with (3-chloropropyl)dimethylamine by refluxing in dry benzene in the presence of sodamide and the resulting base converted to the hydrochloride. The starting phenothiazine compound may be prepared by heating 3-(trifluoromethyl)diphenylamine with sulfur. US Pat 2,921,069.

Description—White to pale tan, crystalline powder with a slight, characteristic odor; melts between 170° and 178°.
Solubility—1 g in <1 mL water, <1 mL alcohol, 1.7 mL chloroform; insoluble in ether.

Uses—The 2-(trifluoromethyl) analogue of chlorpromazine hydrochloride. Indicated for the management of *psychotic disorders* (excluding psychotic depressive reactions) and for the control of *severe nausea* and *vomiting*. Except that it is somewhat more potent, trifluromazine has the same actions and limitations as chlorpromazine. See page 1085 for additional information on contraindications, warnings, precautions, and adverse reactions.
Dose—*Usual, oral*, 30 to 150 **mg** daily; *intramuscular*, 5 to 10 **mg,** repeated in 4 hours, if necessary; *intravenous*, 1 to 3 **mg,** repeated in 4 hours, if necessary. *Usual, pediatric, oral*, 2 **mg/kg** up to a maximum total daily dose of 150 mg in divided doses; *intramuscular*, 0.2 to 0.25 **mg/kg** up to a maximum total daily dose of 10 mg. Not to be administered to children under 2½ years of age.
Dosage Forms—Injection: 20 mg/mL, 100 mg/10 mL; Tablets: 10, 25, and 50 mg.

Other Agents for the Treatment of Psychoses

Bupropion hydrochloride [(±)-1-(3-chlorophenyl-2-(1,1-dimethylethyl)amino]-1-propanone hydrochloride [31677-93-7] $C_{13}H_{18}ClNO.HCl$ (276.21); Wellbutrin (*Burroughs-Wellcome*)]. *Description and solubility:* white crystals melting about 235°; 1 mg dissolves in 312 mL of water; 193 mL of alcohol. *Uses:* A second generation antidepressant under investigation for use in *depressed mood, cognitive impairments, insomnia, somatization, anxiety,* and *retardation.* Bupropion is structurally similar to amphetamine; but it does not effect the "classic" antidepressant pathways. Its mechanism of action is unknown; however, it does have weak dopaminergic effects. It is rapidly and extensively absorbed; peak plasma levels occur within 2 hours; it is 82 to 88% protein bound, highly

lipophilic, and widely distributed in the body. Bupropion is extensively metabolized (less than 1% excreted unchanged in 24 hours); some metabolites have minimal antidepressant activity; excretion is via the urine (87%) and feces (10%) with an elimination half-life of 10 to 21 hours. Side effects appear to be minimal. Daytime sedation, cardiotoxicity, anticholinergic, and antihistamine effects are not as common with bupropion as with conventional antidepressants. *Dose:* Usual, adult, oral, ranges from 150 to 750 mg/day; the maintenance dose is 150 to 450 mg/day. Onset of therapeutic effect is usually 5 to 21 days.

Ergoloids Mesylate [A mixture of equal amounts of the methanesulfonate (mesylate) salts of dihydroergocornine, dihydroergocristine, and dihydroergocryptine [8067-24-1; 11032-41-0]; Circanol (*Riker*); Deapril ST (*Mead Johnson*); Hydergine (*Sandoz*); Trigot (*Squibb*). *Uses:* For individuals over sixty who manifest signs and symptoms of an *idiopathic decline in mental capacity, ie, cognitive* and *interpersonal skills, mood, self-care,* and *motivation.* Pharmacokinetic studies in man indicate about 25% oral absorption; peak plasma levels of 0.5 ng Eq/mL/mg are achieved in 1.5 to 3 hours; elimination is apparently biphasic with half-lives of 4 and 13 hours. Ergoloids mesylate is contraindicated in indivuals who have previously shown hypersensitivity to the drug. The drug may cause sublingual irritation, nasal stuffiness, nausea, vomiting, and sinus bradycardia. orthostatic hypotension sometimes occurs. *Dose:* Sublingual or Oral, 1 mg 3 times a day. Alleviation of symptoms is gradual and may not be apparent for 3 or 4 weeks. *Dosage Forms:* Liquid: 1 mg/mL; Tablets: 1 mg; Tablets (sublingual): 0.5 and 1 mg.

Molindone Hydrochloride [3-Ethyl-6,7-dihydro-2-methyl-5-(morpholinomethyl)indol-4(5*H*)-one monohydrochloride [15622-65-8] $C_{16}H_{24}H_2O_2.HCl$ (312.84); Moban (*Endo*)]. *Description* and *Solubility:* White, crystalline powder. Freely soluble in water and alcohol. *Uses:* A dihydroindolone derivative indicated in the management of manifestations of acute or chronic schizophrenia. Reaches peak blood levels within 1.5 hours after oral administration; pharmacological action after a single oral dose persists for 24 to 36 hours. It has 36 recognized metabolites; only 2 to 3% is excreted unchanged in the urine and feces. Contraindicated in severe central nervous system depression and comatose states. Transient drowsiness is the most frequent adverse reaction; parkinsonian reactions, restlessness, insomnia, depression, blurred vision, dry mouth, nausea, and tachycardia occur less frequently. *Dose:* Mild symptomatology, 5 to 15 mg 3 or 4 times a day; moderate, 10 to 25 mg 3 or 4 times a day; severe, up to 225 mg may be required. *Dosage Forms:* Tablets: 5, 10, 25, 50, and 100 mg; Concentrate: 20 mg/mL.

Pimozide [1-[1-[4,4-bis(4-Fluorophenyl)butyl]-4-piperidinyl]-1,3-dihydro-2*H*-benzimidazol-2-one [2062-78-4] $C_{28}H_{29}F_2N_3O$ (461.55); Orap (*McNeil*)]. *Description and solubility:* Small crystals melting about 216°; almost insoluble in water; very slightly soluble in aqueous acid. It is a weak base, $pK_a = 7.32$. *Uses:* An investigational neuroleptic agent currently under clinical evaluation for use in acute and chronic *schizophrenia, Huntington's chorea, dyskinesias* resulting from excessive dopaminergic stimulation in the brain, *tardive and dyskinesias,* and *Tourette's syndrome.* Pimozide is a diphenylbutylpiperidine, an analog of butyrophenone and a derivative of the meperidine-like analgesics. Pimozide is a potent dopamine antagonist which selectively inhibits central dopaminergic receptors. It also alters dopamine release and increases turnover of brain dopamine, but not norepinephrine. Peak plasma concentrations are reached in 3 to 6 hours; plasma half-life is approximately 18 hours; it is excreted in the urine primarily as the butyric acid derivative. Although it produces extrapyramidal symptoms (incidence 10 to 15%) typical of other neuroleptic agents, it appears to have fewer sedative and automatic effects. *Dose:* Usual, adult, oral, is 16 mg/day. A dose of 1 mg is equivalent to 50 mg of chlorpromazine.

Antianxiety Agents

Antianxiety agents, or more precisely sedative-antianxiety drugs, have now surpassed antibiotics in sales and are the most widely prescribed of all drugs in the United States. Pharmacologically they are sedative-hypnotic in type. Anxiety is a universal human experience; it may permeate one's existence or be an intermittent transient phenomenon. The kinds of internal and external stimuli that can produce anxiety include most events in life. A wide range of sedative-antianxiety drugs is available. For example, certain antihistaminics (diphenhydramine), acetylenic carbinols (ethchlorvynol), monoureides (carbromal), barbiturates (phenobarbital), piperidinediones (methyprylon), propyl alcohol derivatives (meprobamate), benzodiazepines (chlordiazepoxide), etc., have in common the ability to induce various levels of sedation. All antianxiety agents produce mild sedation in doses unlikely to affect adversely the clarity of consciousness and the quality of psychomotor performance. Likewise, many of these drugs exhibit other pharmacological properties, such as hypnotic, muscle relaxant and anticonvulsant actions. For these reasons the antianxiety agents are discussed in Chapter 57 with the conventional sedative and hypnotic agents. They are mentioned here only to recognize their wide use in anxiety and neuroses.

Antidepressant Agents

Antidepressant agents are drugs which enhance alertness and may result in an increased output of behavior. When compared on the basis of their pharmacologic properties, these agents fall into two groups: *tricyclic antidepressants* (imipramine hydrochloride, imipramine pamoate, amitriptyline hydrochloride, amoxapine, desipramine hydrochloride, doxepin, protriptyline hydrochloride, trimipramine) and *monoamine oxidase inhibitors* (isocarboxazid, phenelzine sulfate, and tranylcypromine sulfate). The *tricyclic antidepressant* compounds are more effective and generally safer than the monoamine oxidase inhibitors in moderate and severe depression, especially the endogenous type. They also have antianxiety and sedative properties, which make them useful in the treatment of mild depression. In addition, some tricyclic antidepressants (imipramine and to a lesser extent amitriptyline and nortriptyline) are helpful in alleviating enuresis in children and adolescents. The monoamine oxidase inhibitors are used for symptomatic relief of severe reactive or endogenous depression in hospitalized or closely supervised patients who have not responded to other antidepressant therapy. They are more toxic and appear to be less effective than the tricyclic antidepressants. Therefore, the tricyclic compounds generally are the initial drugs of choice for patients who require antidepressant therapy.

Both tricyclic compounds and monoamine oxidase inhibitors potentiate central noradrenergic function, although they act through different mechanisms. Tricyclic compounds inhibit the re-uptake of norepinephrine and serotonin by neuron terminals. Monoamine oxidase inhibitors block intracellular metabolism of biogenic amines; this results in increased amine concentrations in the neuron terminals. The ability of both classes to facilitate adrenergic transmission and produce an antidepressant action is consistent with the hypothesis that depressive psychosis results from decreased activity of central noradrenergic pathways.

The antidepressant drugs induce a wide variety of *adverse effects*. The most common adverse effects induced by *tricyclic compounds* include dryness of the mouth, excessive perspiration, constipation, blurred vision, hypotension, drowsiness, and weight gain; occasionally, manic episodes, tremors, heart block, tachycardia and other arrhythmias, rashes, and facial sweating; rarely, cholestatic jaundice, bone marrow depression, epileptiform seizures, peripheral neuropathy and photosensitization. Urinary retention, especially in men, has also been reported. The untoward reactions produced by *monoamine oxidase* inhibitors include paradoxical hypertension. This hypertensive crisis is characterized by headache, palpitation, nausea and vomiting, and, occasionally, subarachnoid or intracranial hemorrhage. This reaction may be induced by the ingestion of certain kinds of sharp cheese, yeast extracts, broad beans, chicken livers, pickled herring, and chocolate. Other adverse reactions include hypotension, restlessness, insomnia, dry mouth, nausea, dizziness, constipation, and anorexia; occasionally, flushing, urinary retention, tremors, impotence, and paresthesias; rarely, skin rash, hepatitis, tinnitus, muscle spasms, and mania.

Special *precautions* should be taken when antidepressants are used with other medications. Patients should avoid all other medications including OTC preparations, unless specifically approved by their doctor. They should be advised to not use alcoholic beverages and to limit the amount of caffeine-containing beverages while on these medications.

The *tricyclic* compounds may decrease the effect of anticonvulsant medication, necessitating dosage adjustment; they potentiate the effects of antihistaminics, antimuscarinics, and other CNS depressants; they block the antihypertensive effects of clonidine and guanethidine; they alter blood glucose levels and decrease the effectiveness of hypoglycemic medication; their effectiveness is reduced by concurrent use of estrogens; their concurrent use with monoamine oxidase inhibitors should be avoided as a hyperpyretic crisis, severe convulsions, and death may occur, and a minimum of 14 days should elapse between the discontinuance of monoamine oxidase inhibitors and the initiation of tricyclic antidepressant therapy and vice versa; likewise, their concurrent use with sympathomimetics may result in severe hypertension or hyperpyrexia; and these agents may enhance the possibility of cardiac arrhythmias in patients on thyroid medication. The tricyclic compounds are contraindicated in patients with congestive heart failure, angina pectoris, and paroxysmal tachycardia; also, they should be used with caution in patients with urinary retention, glaucoma, diabetes, impaired liver function, asthma, and a history of convulsive seizures. *Monoamine oxidase inhibitors* potentiate a number of other drugs (barbiturates, insulin, procaine, adrenergic agents, methyldopa, thiazide diuretics, antiparkinson agents, phenothiazines, and morphine analgesics); thus, reduced dosage of each agent is necessary if the drugs are used concomitantly. The monoamine oxidase inhibitors should not be administered with or immediately following other MAO inhibitors or other antidepressants, such as dibenzazepines and phenothiazines. Such combinations can produce a hypertensive crisis, fever, marked sweating, excitation, delirium, tremor, twitching, convulsions, chorea, and circulatory collapse. At least 14 days should elapse between discontinuing an MAO inhibitor and the institution of another antidepressant or MAO inhibitor. A similar period of time should elapse before patients on MAO inhibitors undergo elective surgery. The MAO inhibitors should not be used in patients with cerebrovascular defects or in patients with cardiovascular disease, hypertension, or pheochromocytoma.

The safe use of tricyclic compounds or monoamine oxidase inhibitors during pregnancy or lactation has not been established. These agents should not be used in children under 12 years of age for the same reason. Also, geriatric, adolescent, and black patients on tricyclic compounds usually require reduced dosage; this is thought to be related to slower drug metabolism. Antidepressant drugs are toxic agents and should be employed only with a full knowledge of their precautions and potential adverse effects.

Amitriptyline Hydrochloride

1-Propanamine, 3-(10,11-dihydro-5*H*-dibenzo[*a,d*]cyclohepten-5-ylidene)-*N,N*-dimethyl-, hydrochloride; Elavil (*MSD*); Amitid (*Squibb*); Various Mfrs

10,11-Dihydro-*N,N*-dimethyl-5*H*-dibenzo[*a,d*]cycloheptene-$\Delta^{5,\gamma}$-propylamine hydrochloride [549-18-8] $C_{20}H_{23}N\cdot HCl$ (313.87).

Preparation—Phthalic anhydride is reacted with phenylacetic acid to form 3-benzylidenephthalide, which is hydrogenated to 2-phenethylbenzoic acid. Conversion to the acid chloride followed by intramolecular dehydrochlorination yields the ketone (5*H*-dibenzo[*a,d*]cyclohepten-5-one), which is grignardized with 3-(dimethylamino)propyl chloride. Dehydration of the resulting tertiary carbinol gives amitriptyline which is dissolved in a suitable solvent and converted to the hydrochloride by a stream of HCl. US Pat 3,205,264.

Description—White or practically white, odorless or practically odorless, crystalline powder or small crystals; melts between 195° and 199°; pH (1 in 100 solution) between 5.0 and 6.0.

Solubility—Freely soluble in water, alcohol, chloroform, and methanol; insoluble in ether.

Uses—A tricyclic antidepressant chemically and pharmacologically related to imipramine hydrochloride used for the relief of symptoms of *depression*. Endogenous depression is more amenable to therapy than other depressive states. It is useful in the management of depression accompanied by anxiety. It is also useful in temporarily alleviating enuresis in children and adolescents. It is rapidly absorbed after either oral or parenteral administration; (31 to 61% is bioavailable); peak plasma levels occur within 2–12 hours; 96% is bound to plasma proteins; pK_a is 9.4. The plasma half-life ranges from 31 to 46 hours; volume distribution is 5 to 10 L/kg; therapeutic plasma levels range from 80 to 200 ng/mL. It is metabolized via the same pathways as other tricyclic antidepressants. At least one active metabolite, nortriptyline, has been identified. Approximately 25 to 50% is excreted in the urine as inactive metabolites within 24 hours; small amounts are excreted in the feces *via* the bile. Although the incidence of adverse effects appears to be less with amitriptyline hydrochloride than with other effective antidepressants, drowsiness, xerostomia, tremor, fatigue, weakness, blurring of vision, constipation, urinary retention, edema, tachycardia, orthostatic hypotension, etc. have been observed. Most untoward effects can be controlled by a reduction in dosage. Patients taking large doses over an extended period of time should be watched closely for possible changes in liver and hematopoietic functions. See also page 1093.

Dose—*Usual, adult, oral, initial,* **75 mg** a day in divided doses, or **50 to 100 mg** once a day at bedtime; if necessary dose may be increased gradually to a total of **150 mg** a day; adolescent, elderly or black patients may require only **10 mg** 3 times a day and **20 mg** at bedtime; hospitalized patients may require 100 mg a day initially, increased gradually to 200 mg a day if necessary, and to as much as 300 mg a day in some patients. *Usual maintenance dose,* **50 to 100 mg** a day. *Usual, intramuscular,* **20 to 30 mg** 4 times a day initially. Not recommended for patients under 12 years of age.

Dosage Forms—Injection: 10 mg/mL; Tablets: 10, 25, 50, 75, 100, and 150 mg.

Deanol Acetamidobenzoate—page 1136.

Amoxapine

Dibenz[*b,f*][1,4]oxazepine, 2-chloro-11-(1-piperazinyl)-,
Asendin (*Lederle*)

[14028-44-5] $C_{17}H_{16}ClN_3O$ (313.79).
Preparation—See *Helv Chim Acta 50:* 245, 1967.

Description—White crystals melting about 175°.

Uses—An antidepressant with a mild sedative component. It is used for the relief of *depression* in patients with *neurotic and reactive depressive* disorders as well as *endogenous* and *psychotic depressions*. It is also used for *depression* accompanied by *anxiety* and *agitation*. The mechanism of its clinical action in man is not well understood. In animals, it reduces the uptake of norepinephrine and serotonin and blocks the response of dopamine receptors to dopamine. Amoxapine is rapidly absorbed and reaches peak plasma levels in about 90 minutes. Approximately 90% is bound to plasma proteins; half-life is about 8 hours and it is almost completely metabolized. The major metabolite is active and has a half-life of 30 hours. The metabolites are excreted in the urine as glucuronides. The most frequently encountered adverse effects are drowsiness (14%), dry mouth (14%), constipation (12%), and blurred vision (7%). Renal impairment may develop 3 to 5 days after substantial overdosage. Treatment is the same as that for non-drug renal impairment. Safety and effectiveness in children below the age of 16 have not been established.

Dose—*Adult, oral, initial,* **50 mg** 3 times daily, increased to **100 mg** 3 times a day on the 3rd day. When the effective dose has been established, the drug may be given in a single dose (not to exceed **300 mg**).

Dosage Form—Tablets: 25, 50, 100, and 150 mg.

Desipramine Hydrochloride

5*H*-Dibenz[*b,f*]azepine-5-propanamine, 10,11-dihydro-*N*-methyl-,
monohydrochloride; Norpramin (*Merrell-Dow*);
Pertofrane (*USV*)

10,11-Dihydro-5-[3-(methylamino)propyl]-5*H*-dibenz[*b,f*]azepine monohydrochloride [58-28-6] $C_{18}H_{22}N_2.HCl$ (302.85).

Preparation—Pyrolysis of the methanesulfonate of 4,4'-diaminobibenzyl results in cyclization with formation of 10,11-dihydro-5*H*-dibenz[*b,f*]azepine. This is condensed with *N*-(3-chloropropyl)-*N*-methylbenzylamine in the presence of alkali to form *N*-benzylated desipramine which, following debenzylation through reductive cleavage, is reacted with an equimolar quantity of HCl. Brit Pat 908,788; US Pat 3,454,698.

Description—White to off-white, crystalline powder that is odorless and has a bitter taste; unstable after long exposure to light, heat, and air; melts within a 5° range between 208° and 218°.

Solubility—1 g in 12 mL water, 14 mL alcohol, 3.5 mL chloroform, >10,000 mL ether.

Uses—A primary metabolite of imipramine used in the management of *depressive states.* It has pK_a's of 1.5 and 10.2. It is well absorbed after oral administration; 69 to 76% is bound to plasma protein. Approximately 60 to 70% is bioavailable. The plasma half-life ranges from 14 to 62 hours. Therapeutic plasma concentrations average 145 ng/mL. The plasma half-life ranges from 14 to 25 hours. Metabolism is *via* the same pathways as other tricyclic compounds. Desipramine is reported to be of benefit in endogenous *depressions* such as *manic depressive reactions,* and *reactive depressions.* Desipramine hydrochloride is contraindicated in patients on monoamine oxidase-inhibitor therapy. Since the drug possesses anticholinergic and epinephrine-potentiating properties, it should not be given to patients with glaucoma, urethral or ureteral spasm, or those who have had a myocardial infarction within 3 weeks. It is also contraindicated in patients with severe coronary heart diseases or with active epilepsy. See page 1093 for a more complete listing of precautions and adverse effects. Although not all those mentioned have been reported for desipramine hydrochloride, its pharmacological and chemical similarities suggest it should be suspect.

Dose—*Usual, adult, oral, initial,* **100 to 200 mg** a day in divided doses or as a single dose at bedtime; if necessary dose may be increased to a total of 300 mg a day; adolescent, elderly or black patients may require only **25 to 100 mg** daily in divided doses, to a maximum, if necessary, of 150 mg daily. Not recommended for patients under 12 years of age.

Dosage Forms—Capsules: 25 and 50 mg; Tablets: 25, 50, 75, 100, and 150 mg.

Doxepin Hydrochloride

1-Propanamine, 3-(dibenz[*b,e*]oxepin-11(6*H*)-ylidene)-*N,N*-dimethyl-,
hydrochloride; Adapin (*Pennwalt*); Sinequan (*Pfizer*)

N,N-Dimethyldibenz[*b,e*]oxepin-$\Delta^{11(6H),\gamma}$-propylamine hydrochloride [1229-29-4; 4698-39-9(*E*); 25127-31-5(*Z*)] $C_{19}H_{21}NO.HCl$ (315.84). Doxepin hydrochloride, an (*E*) and (*Z*) geometric isomer mixture, contains the equivalent of not less than 85.0% and not more than 92.0% of $C_{19}H_{21}NO$ (doxepin), calculated on the dried basis. It contains not less than 12.0% and not more than 16.0% of the (*Z*)-isomer, and not less than 72.0% and not more than 78.0% of the (*E*)-isomer.

Preparation—6,11-Dihydrodibenz[*b,e*]oxepin-11-one is prepared from phthalide and converted to 11-[3-(dimethylamino)propyl]-6*H*-dibenz[*b,e*]oxepin-11-ol through Grignard reaction with 3-

(dimethylamino)propyl chloride. Dehydration of the alcohol with mineral acid yields doxepin which is reacted with HCl.

Description—White, odorless, bitter, crystalline substance; decomposes slowly in light, nonhygroscopic up to 75% RH, and relatively stable in heat; melts between 185° and 191°.

Solubility—1 g in 1 mL water, 2 mL alcohol, and 10 mL chloroform.

Uses—A dibenzoxepin derivative that is a psychotherapeutic agent with antianxiety and antidepressant properties. It is recommended for the management of anxiety and/or depressive states associated with psychoneurosis, psychosis, alcoholism, and organic disease. Doxepin hydrochloride is apparently well absorbed from the gastrointestinal tract, but only 13 to 45% is bioavailable; volume distribution approximates 9–33 L/kg; therapeutic plasma levels range from 30 to 150 ng/mL. The plasma half-life is 8 to 24 hours. Metabolism appears to be *via* the same pathways as other tricyclic antidepressants; its *N*-demethylated metabolite is pharmacologically active. Adverse reactions, such as dry mouth, blurred vision, constipation, tachycardia, hypotension, and drowsiness, are usually mild and tend to subside as therapy is continued. Other side effects infrequently encountered include extrapyramidal symptoms, gastrointestinal disturbances, increased sweating, weakness, dizziness, fatigue, edema, paresthesia, flushing, chills, tinnitus, photophobia, decreased libido, rash, and pruritus. Doxepin hydrochloride is contraindicated in patients with glaucoma or a tendency to urinary retention. The drug should not be administered to patients either on MAO inhibitors or who have been on such agents within the prior 2 weeks. The drug may also potentiate the depressant effect of alcohol. The use of doxepin hydrochloride in the pregnant patient or in children under 12 years of age is not recommended, because safe conditions for its use have not been established.

Dose—*Usual, adult, oral,* **25 mg** 3 times a day; or up to **150 mg** once a day at bedtime; maximum, up to 300 mg daily. Dosage as low as **25** to **50 mg** daily suffices for some patients. Not recommended for patients under 12 years of age.

Dosage Forms—Capsules: 10, 25, 50, 75, 100, and 150 mg doxepin; Oral Concentrate: 10 mg doxepin/mL.

Imipramine Hydrochloride

5*H*-Dibenz[*b,f*]azepine-5-propanamine, 10,11-dihydro-*N,N*-dimethyl-, monohydrochloride; Presamine (*USV*); Tofranil (*Ciba-Geigy*); Imavate (*Robins*); Janimine (*Abbott*); SK-Pramine (*SKF*); *Other Mfrs*

5-[3-(Dimethylamino)propyl]-10,11-dihydro-5*H*-dibenz[*b,f*]azepine monohydrochloride [113-52-0] $C_{19}H_{24}N_2.HCl$ (316.87).

Preparation—2-(*o*-Aminophenethyl)aniline hydrochloride is heated to yield 10,11-dihydro-5*H*-dibenz[*b,f*]azepine which is condensed with 3-chloro-*N,N*-dimethylpropylamine by refluxing in benzene solution with the aid of sodamide. The basic constituents are then extracted with aqueous HCl and the extract is rendered alkaline and extracted with ether. After drying, the solvent is evaporated and the residue is vacuum-distilled to yield imipramine base. Treatment with alcoholic HCl produces the hydrochloride. US Pat. 2,554,736.

Description—White to off-white, odorless crystalline powder; melts between 170° and 174°.

Solubility—1 g in about 5 mL water, about 10 mL alcohol, and about 15 mL acetone; insoluble in ether and benzene.

Uses—A dibenzazepine-derivative tricyclic antidepressant effective in depressive syndromes, particularly those associated with *manic-depressive* and *involutional psychoses,* and to a lesser degree with *reactive depressions.* It may be useful as temporary adjunctive therapy in *reducing enuresis* (bed wetting) in children aged 6 years and older, after excluding possible organic causes. Imipramine has a pK$_a$ of 9.5. It is completely absorbed from the gastrointestinal tract. Peak plasma levels occur within 1 to 2 hours after oral administration and 30 minutes after intramuscular administration. Approximately 90% is bound to plasma proteins. Plasma half-life ranges from 8 to 16 hours. It is metabolized *via* the same pathways as other tricyclic compounds; desipramine, its *N*-monodemethylated metabolite, is pharmacologically active. About 40% is excreted in the urine as inactive metabolites within 24 hours and 70% within 72 hours; small

amounts are excreted in the feces *via* the bile. Side effects are common, especially in patients over 65. Most side effects occur in patients receiving more than 200 mg daily and include hypotension, seizures, tremors, diplopia, involuntary staring, visual hallucinations, and agitation. Because of possible congenital malformations associated with the use of this drug, imipramine hydrochloride should not be used during the first trimester of pregnancy. Imipramine should not be used in patients on monoamine oxidase inhibitors. For more detailed information on precautions and adverse effects, see page 1093.

Dose—*Usual, adult, oral, initial,* **75 mg** a day in divided doses, if necessary increased to a total of 150 mg a day (dosages over 200 mg a day are not recommended for outpatients); adolescent, elderly or black patients may require only **30** to **40 mg** a day initially and generally not over 100 mg a day; hospitalized patients may require 100 mg a day initially, increased gradually to 200 mg a day if necessary, and to as much as 250 to 300 mg a day if no response occurs after 2 weeks. *Usual maintenance* dose, for outpatients, **50** to **150 mg** a day. *Intramuscular, initial,* up to **100 mg** a day, in divided doses. Not recommended for children under 6 years of age. In *childhood enuresis,* an oral dose of **25 mg,** once a day one hour before bedtime, may be tried in children 6 years of age and older; after one week the dose may be increased, if necessary, to 50 mg nightly in children under 12 years and to 75 mg in children over 12 years.

Dosage Forms—Injection: 25 mg/2 mL; Tablets: 10, 25, and 50 mg.

Imipramine Pamoate

Tofranil-PM (*Ciba-Geigy*)

5-[3-(Dimethylamino)propyl]-10,11-dihydro-5*H*-dibenz[*b,f*]azepine compound (2:1) with 4,4-methylene-bis[3-hydroxy-2-naphthoic acid] [10075-24-8] $(C_{19}H_{24}N_2)_2.C_{23}H_{16}O_6$ (949.20).

Description—Yellow powder; tasteless; odorless.

Solubility—Insoluble in water; soluble in alcohol, ether, chloroform.

Uses—For relief of symptoms of depression. See *Imipramine Hydrochloride.*

Dose—*Usual, adult, oral,* the equivalent of **75 mg** of imipramine hydrochloride a day initially; optimum response is usually obtained with the equivalent of **150 mg** of imipramine hydrochloride daily, usually given at bedtime. Maximum dose, the equivalent of 200 mg of imipramine hydrochloride daily. Should not be used in children of any age because of the increased potential for acute overdosage due to the high potency of the capsule dosage forms.

Dosage Forms—Capsules: equivalent to 75, 100, 125, and 150 mg of imipramine hydrochloride.

Isocarboxazid

3-Isoxazolecarboxylic acid, 5-methyl-, 2-(phenylmethyl)hydrazide; Marplan (*Hoffmann-LaRoche*)

5-Methyl-3-isoxazolecarboxylic acid 2-benzylhydrazide [59-63-2] $C_{12}H_{13}N_3O_2$ (231.25).

Preparation—Acetonylacetone is reacted with nitric acid to form 5-methyl-3-isoxazolecarboxylic acid which is converted to its ethyl ester. The ester is reacted with hydrazine hydrate to form the acid hydrazide which is condensed with benzaldehyde to yield the 2-benzylidenehydrazide. This is reduced in anhydrous ether with lithium aluminum hydride to isocarboxazid. US Pat 2,908,688.

Description—White or nearly white, crystalline powder; slight, characteristic odor and stable in dry air; melts between 105° and 108°.

Solubility—1 g in 2000 mL water, 83 mL alcohol, 2 mL chloroform, 58 mL ether.

Uses—A monoamine oxidase inhibitor recommended only for *depressed* patients who are refractory to tricyclic antidepressants or electroconvulsive therapy and depressed patients in whom tricyclic antidepressants are contraindicated. As with other monoamine oxidase inhibitors, patients treated with isocarboxazid should be kept under close medical supervision. Untoward effects are those characteristic of monoamine oxidase inhibitors in general. See page 1093 for additional information on adverse reactions, and precautions and discussion on the use of isocarboxazid with other drugs. The drug should be discontinued at the first sign of jaundice or impaired liver function. It is contraindicated in patients with a history of liver disease or impaired liver function.

Dose—*Usual, initial,* **30 mg** daily as a single dose or in divided doses; *maintenance,* **10 to 20 mg** daily. If a favorable response is not obtained in 3 or 4 weeks, continued administration is unlikely to be beneficial. Use in patients under 16 years of age is not recommended since safety or efficacy in this group has not been established.

Dosage Form—Tablets: 10 mg.

Methylphenidate—page 1136.

Maprotiline Hydrochloride

9,10-Ethanoanthracene-9(10*H*)-propanamine, *N*-methyl-, Hydrochloride; Ludiomil (*Ciba-Geigy*)

$$CH_2CH_2CH_2NHCH_3$$

• HCl

[10262-69-8] $C_{20}H_{23}N.HCl$ (313.87).
Preparation—Refer to *Helv Chim Acta 52:* 1385, 1969.

Description—White crystals melting about 93°.

Uses—For the treatment of patients with *depressive neurosis (dysthymic disorder)* and *manic-depressive* illness, depressed type (major depressive disorder). It is also effective for the relief of *anxiety associated with depression.* Maprotiline hydrochloride belongs to a new chemical series, dibenzobicyclooctadienes. It has been postulated that it acts by potentiation of central adrenergic synapses by blocking reuptake of norepinephrine at nerve endings. This action is thought to account for its antidepressant action. The mean time to peak effect is 12 hours; half-life of elimination averages 51 hours; and steady state levels induced by 50 mg 3 times daily averages 238 ng/mL. Adverse reactions are similar to those observed with tricyclic antidepressants (see page 1093). Safety and effectiveness in children under the age of 18 have not been established.

Dose—*Adult, oral, mild to moderate depression,* **75 to 150 mg/day;** elderly, **25 mg/day;** maximum, **225 mg/day.** *Severe depression,* **100 to 150 mg/day;** maximum **300 mg/day.**

Dosage Forms—Tablets: 25, 50, and 75 mg.

Nortriptyline Hydrochloride

1-Propanamine, 3-(10,11-dihydro-5*H*-dibenzo[*a,d*]cyclohepten-5-yl-idene)-*N*-methyl-, hydrochloride; Aventyl Hydrochloride (*Lilly*); Pamelor (*Sandoz*)

• HCl

$$CHCH_2CH_2NHCH_3$$

10,11-Dihydro-*N*-methyl-5*H*-dibenzo[*a,d*]cycloheptene-$\Delta^{5,\gamma}$-propylamine hydrochloride [894-71-3] $C_{19}H_{21}N.HCl$ (299.84).

Preparation—10,11-Dihydro-5*H*-dibenzo[*a,d*]cyclohepten-5-one, which may be prepared as described under *Cyproheptadine Hydrochloride* (page 1132), is reacted with an alkali metal derivative of *N*-methyl-2-propynylamine and the product hydrolyzed to form the carbinol. The acetylenic bond in this is saturated by hydrogenation and the resulting carbinol is dehydrated to yield nortriptyline (base). Reaction of the base with hydrogen chloride produces the hydrochloride.

Description—White to off-white powder with a slight, characteristic odor; melts within a range of 3° between 215° and 220°.
Solubility—1 g in 90 mL water, 30 mL alcohol, 20 mL chloroform, 10 mL methanol.

Uses—A dibenzocycloheptene-derivative tricyclic antidepressant drug which is the active metabolite of amitriptyline. It is more likely to be effective in endogenous depressions than in other depressive states. It has a pK_a of 9.73. Peak plasma levels occur within 7 to 18.5 hours after oral administration; about 90% is bound to plasma protein. Therapeutic plasma levels range from 50 to 150 ng/mL. Plasma half-life ranges from 18 to 35 hours after oral administration. Approximately 30% is excreted in the urine in 24 hours, and small amounts are excreted in the feces *via* the bile. Pharmacological studies indicate it inhibits the activity of such diverse agents as histamine, 5-hydroxytryptamine, and acetylcholine. It also increases the pressor effect of norepinephrine but blocks the pressor response of phenethylamine. Studies suggest that nortriptyline hydrochloride interferes with the transport, release, and storage of catecholamines. Pharmacologic studies further show that nortriptyline hydrochloride has a combination of stimulant and depressant properties. In some clinical studies, the drug appeared to cause excitement or increased agitation in some patients and to have sedative effects in others. Similar effects have been observed with other drugs of this general type. Untoward side effects include dryness of the mouth, drowsiness, and a confusional state. Tremulousness and orthostatic hypotension have also been reported. Since drugs of this type can produce a sinus tachycardia and a first-degree heart block, they should be used with great caution in patients with vascular disease. Nortriptyline hydrochloride should not be used in combination with a monoamine oxidase inhibitor. The potentiation of adverse effects can be serious, even fatal. It is advisable to discontinue the monoamine oxidase inhibitor for at least 10 to 21 days before starting treatment with nortriptyline. Nortriptyline should be used with caution in patients with glaucoma or urinary retention. Epileptiform seizures may be associated with nortriptyline. Therefore, patients on this drug should be supervised closely during the initial phase of treatment. See page 1093 for additional information on the adverse reactions and precautions for tricyclic antidepressants.

Dose—*Usual, adult, oral,* **25 mg** 3 or 4 times a day (doses above 100 mg a day are not recommended); adolescent, elderly or black patients, **30 to 50 mg** a day, in divided doses. Not recommended for children since safety and effectiveness in pediatric age group have not been determined.

Dosage Forms—Capsules: 10 and 25 mg (base equivalent); Solution: 10 mg (base equivalent)/5 mL.

Pargyline Hydrochloride—page 850.
Pemoline—page 1137.

Phenelzine Sulfate

Hydrazine, (2-phenylethyl)-, sulfate (1:1); Nardil (*Warner-Chilcott*)

$$CH_2CH_2NHNH_2$$

• H_2SO_4

Phenethylhydrazine sulfate (1:1) [156-51-4] $C_8H_{12}N_2.H_2SO_4$ (234.27).
Preparation—Phenethyl alcohol is reacted with thionyl chloride to give phenethyl chloride which is then added to hydrazine hydrate to yield phenethylhydrazine hydrochloride. Reaction with sodium hydroxide liberates the base which is then reacted with sulfuric acid to form the sulfate. US Pat 3,314,855.

Description—White to yellowish white powder with a characteristic odor; subject to oxidation and must be protected from heat and light; melts between 164° and 168°; pH (1 in 100 solution) between 1.4 and 1.9.
Solubility—1 g in about 7 mL water; practically insoluble in alcohol, chloroform, and ether.

Uses—A monoamine oxidase inhibitor effective in depressed patients clinically characterized as "atypical," "nonendogenous," or "neurotic." Such patients often have mixed anxiety and depression and phobic or hypochondriacal features. Its use in endogenous depression is less convincing. It should rarely be the first drug used; it should be used in patients who fail to respond to the more commonly used antidepressant drugs. Maximal effects appear only after 1 to 2 weeks of therapy. Phenelzine sulfate is contraindicated in elderly, debilitated patients, or in patients with a cerebrovascular defect, cardiovascular disease, hypertension, history of headache, pheochromocytoma, or a history of liver disease. Phenelzine sulfate is a potent MAO inhibitor. Since this enzyme is widely distributed throughout the body, diverse adverse effects can be expected. These are summarized in the introductory statement to this section (see page 1093). Physicians should know and be alert for the more serious toxic effects which can be induced by these agents.

Dose—*Usual, adult, oral,* initially **15 mg** 3 times a day, increased with patient tolerance to **60 mg** a day and if necessary to **90 mg** a day; maintenance, **15 mg** a day or every second day. Not recommended for patients under 16 years of age since safety and effectiveness in this age group have not been established.

Dosage Form—Tablets: 15 mg (base equivalent).

Protriptyline Hydrochloride

5H-Dibenzo[a,d]cycloheptene-5-propanamine, N-methyl-, hydrochloride; Vivactil (MSD)

N-Methyl-5H-dibenzo[a,d]cycloheptene-5-propylamine hydrochloride [1225-55-4] $C_{19}H_{21}N.HCl$ (299.84).

Preparation—5H-Dibenzo[a,d]cyclohepten-5-one, prepared as described under *Cyproheptadine Hydrochloride* (page 1132), is reduced to the corresponding carbinol which is then converted to the 5-chloromethyl compound (I). Reaction with the Grignard reagent of (3-chloropropyl)dimethylamine converts I into the 5-(3-dimethylamino)propyl compound which, on monodemethylation with cyanogen bromide and hydrolysis, yields protriptyline. Reaction with HCl gives the hydrochloride.

Description—White to yellowish powder that is odorless or has not more than a slight odor and has a bitter taste; reasonably stable in light, stable in air, and stable in heat under the usual prevailing temperature conditions; melts at about 168°; pH (1 in 100 solution) between 5.0 and 6.5.

Solubility—1 g in 2 mL water, 4 mL alcohol, 2.3 mL chloroform, 2 mL methanol; practically insoluble in ether.

Uses—A tricyclic (dibenzocycloheptene) antidepressant drug useful in the management of mental *depression* in patients under close medical supervision. It also increases psychomotor activity; this property enhances its use in withdrawn and anergic patients. It is completely absorbed from the gastrointestinal tract. Peak plasma levels occur within 24 to 30 hours. About 92% is bound to plasma proteins. Therapeutic plasma levels range from 70 to 170 ng/mL. Metabolism and excretion are by the same pathways as other tricyclic antidepressants. The drug is eliminated slowly; 50% is excreted in the urine as metabolites within 16 days. Very little is excreted in the feces. Protriptyline also possesses anticholinergic properties and, hence, should not be used in patients with pyloric obstruction, glaucoma, or urinary retention. Tachycardia and postural hypotension occur more frequently with protriptyline hydrochloride than with other antidepressant drugs; hence, patients with cardiovascular disorders and elderly patients should be observed closely for these untoward effects. This agent is also contraindicated in patients taking any of the MAO inhibitor antidepressants, such as nialamide, isocarboxazid, tranylcypromine, or phenelzine. Antidepressants of this type reverse the effects of antihypertensive drugs such as guanethidine and should not be used concurrently with them. Adverse reactions attributable to antidepressant drugs are numerous and varied. The similar pharmacological properties of these agents suggest that each of these reactions should be considered when therapy with these agents is contemplated. See page 1093 for additional information on precautions and adverse reactions for this group of agents.

Dose—*Usual, adult, oral,* **15 to 40 mg** a day divided into 3 or 4 doses, increased to **60 mg** a day if necessary; adolescent, elderly or black patients, **5 mg** 3 times a day, increased gradually if necessary but in elderly patients the cardiovascular response should be closely monitored if the daily dose exceeds 20 mg. Not recommended for use in children because safety and effectiveness in this age group have not been established.

Dosage Forms—Tablets: 5 and 10 mg.

Tranylcypromine Sulfate

Cyclopropanamine, 2-phenyl-, *trans*-(±)-, sulfate (2:1); Parnate (SKF)

(±)-*trans*-2-Phenylcyclopropylamine sulfate (2:1) [13492-01-8] $(C_9H_{11}N)_2.H_2SO_4$ (364.46).

Preparation—Styrene is reacted with ethyl diazoacetate to form ethyl 2-phenylcyclopropanecarboxylate. Saponification of this ester

with sodium hydroxide and subsequent acidification yields a mixture of the *cis* and *trans* forms of the corresponding acid and the *trans* form is isolated by fractional crystallization from water. The *trans* acid is then subjected to the Curtius reaction whereby carboxyl is transformed successively through the acyl chloride, acyl azide, and isocyanate states to yield finally tranylcypromine. Reaction of the base with a ½ equimolar quantity of H_2SO_4 gives the sulfate. US Pat. 2,997,422.

Description—White, crystalline powder that is either odorless or has a faint, cinnamaldehyde-like odor and a slightly acid taste; stable in light, heat, and air; melts with decomposition at 218°.

Solubility—1 g in 25 mL water; very slightly soluble in alcohol and ether; practically insoluble in chloroform.

Uses—A nonhydrazine monoamine oxidase inhibitor used in the treatment of depression. It is probably effective for the symptomatic relief of severe reactive or endogenous depression in hospitalized or closely supervised patients who have not responded to other antidepressant therapy. Tranylcypromine sulfate is contraindicated in any patient over 60 years of age or in patients with confirmed or suspected cerebrovascular defects, cardiovascular disorders or pheochromocytoma; it should not be used concomitantly with other MAO inhibitors or sympathomimetic agents. In addition, patients on this drug should not eat cheese or other foods with a high tyramine content. Adverse effects most commonly observed include postural hypotension, dizziness, restlessness, insomnia, weakness, drowsiness, anxiety, agitation, manic symptoms, nausea, vomiting, diarrhea, abdominal pain, constipation, anorexia, dryness of the mouth, blurred vision, chills, tachycardia, edema, palpitation, impotence, and headaches not associated with a rise in blood pressure. A number of deaths have resulted in patients on tranylcypromine; death is usually attributed to intracranial hemorrhage. Severe reactions may appear without warning and develop rapidly. This drug, like other antidepressant agents, should only be used under close medical supervision. See page 1093 for additional information on precautions, warnings, and adverse reactions induced by this class of drugs.

Dose—*Usual, initial,* **10 mg** in the morning and afternoon daily for 2 weeks; if no response appears, increase dosage to **20 mg** in the morning and **10 mg** in the afternoon daily for another week; *maintenance,* **10 to 20 mg**/day.

Dosage Form—Tablets: 10 mg (base equivalent).

Trazodone Hydrochloride

1,2,4-Triazolo[4,3-a]pyridin-3(2H)-one, 2-[3-[4-(3-chlorophenyl)-1-piperazinyl]propyl]-, monohydrochloride; Desyrel (Mead-Johnson)

[25332-39-2] $C_{19}H_{22}ClN_5O.HCl$ (408.33).

Preparation—See US Patent 3,381,009.

Description—White crystals melting about 90°; pK_a in 50% ethanol, 6.14.

Solubility—Sparingly soluble in water or alcohol; soluble in chloroform.

Uses—Trazodone, a triazolopyridine derivative, is used for the treatment of *depression*. The mechanism responsible for its antidepressant action in man is not fully understood. In animals, trazodone selectively inhibits serotonin uptake by brain synaptosomes and potentiates the behavioral changes induced by 5-hydroxytryptophan. The drug is well absorbed after oral administration without selective localization in any tissue. Peak plasma levels occur in 1 hour when taken on an empty stomach and 2 hours when taken with meals. Elimination is biphasic; initial phase, half-life, 3 to 6 hours is followed by a slower phase, half-life, 5 to 9 hours. Clearance from the body is variable in some patients; the drug may accumulate in plasma. Trazodone may be arrhythmogenic in some patients. Consequently, it is not recommended for use during the initial recovery phase of myocardial infarction. The most frequently encountered adverse effects include blurred vision, dry mouth, dizziness/light-headedness, drowsiness, nausea/vomiting, fatigue, and headache. Safety and effectiveness in children below the age of 18 have not been established.

Dose—*Adults, oral, initial,* **150 mg/day,** increased by **50 mg/day**

every 3 or 5 days. Maximum dose: outpatients, **400 mg/day**; inpatients, **600 mg/day** in divided doses.

Dosage Form—Tablets: 50 and 100 mg.

Trimipramine Maleate

5*H*-Dibenz[*b,f*]azepine-5-propanamine, 10,11-dihydro-*N,N,β*-trimethyl-, (*Z*)-2-butenedioate (1:1); Surmontil (*Ives*)

Preparation—See *Compt Rend 252:* 2117, 1961.

Description—White crystals with bitter taste and slight numbing characteristic; melting about 143°.

Solubility—Slightly soluble in water and alcohol; freely soluble in chloroform.

Uses—Trimipramine is used to relieve the symptoms of *depression. Endogenous depression* is more likely to be alleviated than other depressive states. Clinical studies suggest that trimipramine is about equally as effective as amitriptyline in mild depression and less effective than amitriptyline in severely depressed patients. In view of the pharmacological similarities among tricyclic antidepressants, adverse effects may be similar to those listed on page 1093. The drug is not recommended for use in children, since the safety and effectiveness have not been established.

Dose—*Adult, outpatient, oral:* initially, **75 mg/day** in divided doses, increased to **150 mg/day**. Dosages over 200 mg are not recommended. *Adult, hospitalized patients, oral:* initially, **100 mg/day** in divided doses; this may be increased to **200 mg/day**. Maximum **250 to 300 mg/day**.

Dosage Forms—Capsules: 25 and 50 mg.

Psychogenic Agents

Psychogenic agents are drugs that consistently induce temporary abnormalities of the mental state of human subjects or the behavior of animals. This definition serves to separate the psychogenic agents from the many drugs which may produce similar effects when taken in excessive amounts or when given to susceptible individuals. Psychogenic drugs produce major disturbances of sensory perception and alter the ability of the subject to organize perceptions and thoughts for the purpose of adaptive behavior. In so doing they produce subjective effects such as hallucinations and alterations in gross behavior which bear some similarity to certain features of the major psychoses. For example, marihuana usually only produces mood changes, but in high doses it produces psychological syndromes that can be characterized as psychoses. Intensive investigation is directed toward elucidating those features which are common to both "clinical" and "experimental" psychoses. There are no recognized therapeutic applications for these agents. Consequently, they are listed in Schedule I of the Controlled Substances Act and are not available for prescription use. Nevertheless, they can be obtained for clinical and experimental research purposes. These agents are subjected to intensive abuse, a practice which can only be condemned. For a detailed discussion of the abuse potential of these agents see Chapter 71.

Cannabis [Marihuana]—The dried flowering tops of the pistillate plants of *Cannabis sativa* (Fam. *Moraceae*). *Uses:* No rational or indispensable therapeutic use in modern medicine. Formerly used in migraine, insomnia, neuralgia, and other syndromes. Currently, the active principles of the drug are under investigation for use as antiepileptic, anticancer, and immunosuppressive agents. The use of cannabis as an intoxicant and euphoric agent has increased sharply in recent years. It is frequently smoked in the form of cigarettes. It produces aggressive tendencies in some individuals and stimulates the senses so that external stimuli are magnified and distorted. Cannabis causes habituation but, unlike morphine, not true addiction. (See also pages 1347–1349).

Lysergic Acid Diethylamide [*d-N,N-*Diethyllysergamide; LSD-25; LSD $C_{20}H_{25}N_3O$]—Closely related structurally (page 420) to ergonovine, one of the principal alkaloids of ergot, but it is distinctly different in its physiological actions. It is an extremely potent agent; as little as 1 μg per kg of body weight will induce a hallucinogenic effect. Persons who have taken the drug experience a mental intoxication which has many of the features common with the perceptual disturbances of some cases of schizophrenia. Persons under the influence of lysergic acid diethylamide experience ataxia, tremors, auditory and visual hallucinations, depersonalization and disturbances in space, olfactory, and taste perception, but retain the knowledge that these unusual effects are induced by the drug. Contact with reality is not lost, except after massive doses. Repeated administration of the drug produces serious mental disturbances in some individuals.

The first effects from an oral dose of lysergic acid diethylamide appear within $\frac{1}{2}$ hour, reach a peak intensity in $1\frac{1}{2}$ hours, and disappear within 8 hours. Recovery is usually complete, except for some residual depression which may persist for as long as 24 hours after taking the drug. Tolerance to the drug develops within 3 to 7 days after repeated administration. When tolerance has developed a 4-fold dosage increase fails to evoke the hallucinatory syndrome.

Lysergic acid diethylamide should be considered, at least for the present, a tool for the study of "experimental psychoses." The indiscriminate use of the agent cannot be too severely condemned. (See also pages 1297–1299).

Mescaline [3,4,5-Trimethoxyphenethylamine $C_{11}H_{17}NO_3$]—Knowledge of mescaline psychosis dates back to antiquity, since, as the principal alkaloid of peyote, the dried flowering tops of the cactus *Lophophora Williamsii* Coulter, it has been used by various American Indian tribes for religious purposes. Interest in mescaline stems from its use as an experimental tool for the investigation of schizophrenia and other psychotic states, and for the study of visual hallucinations. It has also been used as an adjunct to psychotherapy in depth interviews.

Current interest in mescaline centers on the fact that when given orally or intravenously to normal subjects in doses of 5.0 to 7.0 mg/kg it causes unusual psychic effects and visual hallucinations. Diffuse anxiety is one of the early symptoms. Other symptoms include sympathomimetic autonomic effects, hyperreflexia of the limbs, static tremors, and vivid hallucinations which are usually visual and consist of brightly colored lights, geometric designs, animals, and, occasionally, human images; color and space perception is often impaired but, otherwise, the sensorium is normal and insight is retained. An extreme anxiety state may develop in some schizophrenic patients given mescaline, and the hallucinations in others may be sexual in character. The effects induced by a single full dose of mescaline appear within one hour and persist for about 12 hours. In some respects, the psychic changes are similar to those caused by lysergic acid diethylamide. Mescaline-induced psychoses are of academic interest only and the drug has no therapeutic application. (See also page 1297).

CHAPTER 60

Analgesics and Antipyretics

Ewart A Swinyard, PhD, DSc (Hon)

Professor Emeritus of Pharmacology
College of Pharmacy and School of Medicine, University of Utah
Salt Lake City, UT 84112

Analgesics are agents which relieve pain by acting centrally to elevate pain threshold without disturbing consciousness or altering other sensory modalities. Antipyretics are drugs which reduce elevated body temperature. Certain analgesics, aminopyrine and phenylbutazone, also possess antirheumatic and antiinflammatory properties; such substances, as well as gold compounds, are used in the treatment of arthritis. Drugs which exhibit one or more of these actions are considered in this chapter.

Despite the fact that pain is a universal experience of all mankind and everybody knows what is meant by it, attempts to define this term have not proved entirely satisfactory. Pain has been defined in psychologic language as a particular type of sensory experience perceived by nerve tissue distinct from sensations such as touch, pressure, heat, and cold. Since there are several types of pain (bright, dull, aching, pricking, cutting, burning, etc.) and it may arise from different causes (injury, body derangements, or disease), it is apparent that this definition is incomplete. Furthermore, it is now generally agreed that pain involves a large psychic component. Thus, it must be concluded that pain cannot be defined, except as one defines it introspectively for himself.

All persons in good health have the ability to perceive pain. The point at which pain is perceived is referred to as the "pain threshold." If this threshold is raised, more stimuli are required before pain is experienced. On the other hand, if this threshold is lowered, less stimuli induce the pain experience. Unfortunately, many factors such as sex, circulatory change, skin temperature, sweating, carbon dioxide tension, anxiety, fear, emotion, etc., alter the pain threshold. Consequently, pain threshold is not constant from individual to individual, or from one time to another in the same individual. Thus, data obtained from laboratory and clinical studies on the effect of drugs on pain threshold are difficult to interpret.

A possible mechanism by which analgesic drugs obtund pain (raise the pain threshold) has been formulated within recent years. The discovery of opiate receptors in selected portions of the central nervous system (Pert CB, Snyder SH, *Science 179:* 1011–1014, 1973) and the subsequent identification of an endogenous substance (*enkephalin*, one of a group of substances known as *endorphins*) from brain with properties similar to morphine (Hughes J, *Brain Res 88:* 295–308, 1975) not only make this possible but could lead to a host of treatments that will ease pain and suffering. Opiate receptors were located in the *medial thalamus* which processes deep, chronic, burning pain that is most susceptible to relief by narcotic analgesics, in the brain stem's *vagus nuclei* where coughing is triggered, and in *layers I and II* of the spinal cord at the point in the cord where the afferent nerves which carry pain perception first synapse. Interestingly, the greatest concentration of opiate receptors was found in the *amygdala*, that part of the limbic system which plays a major role in regulating emotions. Since these receptors bind morphine and related narcotic analgesic drugs as well as the narcotic antagonist naloxone, these observations markedly enlarge our understanding of the pharmacological profile of action of these drugs. Based on the assumption that there is no reason why the body should have evolved receptors for narcotic drugs unless it produces some narcotic-like substance of its own, pharmacologists John Hughes and Hans W. Kosterlitz at the University of Aberdeen in Scotland reported the isolation (from pig brain) and identification of such material (*Nature 258:* 577, 1975). It turned out to be two substances, both pentapeptides, which they called *enkephalins*. The two brain peptides differed only in the N-terminal amino acid, in one peptide being methionine and in the other leucine. The methionine-enkephalin is tyrosine-glycine-glycine-phenylalanine-methionine, while leucine-enkephalin is tyrosine-glycine-glycine-phenylalanine-leucine. *Endorphins* (a generic name contracted from endogenous and morphine, and used for all native brain peptides with opiate-like activity) probably regulate pain intensity by modulating the so-called pain threshold, the point at which one begins to perceive a stimulus as painful. Naloxone, on the other hand, tends to increase one's sensitivity to pain. These observations have not only markedly increased understanding of the mechanism by which narcotic analgesics obtund pain, but have also provided an explanation for the antitussive and euphoric action of these drugs as well as an insight into how tolerance and addiction develops. More importantly, perhaps, this kind of research has resulted in the development of a number of opiate and opiod analgesics with diverse pharmacological actions.

The available opiate and opiod analgesics are derivatives of five chemical groups (phenanthrenes, phenylheptylamines, phenylpiperidines, morphinans, and benzomorphans). Pharmacologically, these opiates and nonopiates differ significantly in activity. Some are strong agonists (morphine); others are moderate to mild agonists (codeine). In contrast, some opiate derivatives exhibit mixed agonist-antagonist activity (nalbuphine), whereas others are opiate antagonists (naloxone). The following table provides a classification of selected opiate and nonopiate analgesics and antagonists based on their agonist, agonist-antagonist, or antagonist properties.

Many drugs used to relieve pain are not analgesics. The general anesthetics obtund pain by producing a hiatus in consciousness, the local anesthetics prevent pain by blocking peripheral nerve fibers, the antispasmodics relieve certain kinds of pain by relaxing smooth muscle, and the adrenal corticoids relieve pain associated with rheumatoid arthritis by an anti-inflammatory action. These drugs are considered elsewhere.

Most of the drugs described in this section come under the control of the *Comprehensive Drug Abuse Prevention and Control Act of 1970.* This law, commonly referred to as the *"Controlled Substances Act,"* is designed to regulate the distribution of all drugs with abuse potential as designated by the *Drug Enforcement Administration*, Department of Justice (Chapter 107).

Morphine is the prototype of the opiate and opiod analgesics, all of which have similar actions on the central nervous system. Moreover, they have overlapping clinical usefulness.

Table I—Chemical and Pharmacological Classification of Selected Opiate and Nonopiate Analgesics and Antagonists

Chemical Group	Strong Agonists	Mild to Moderate Agonists	Mixed Agonist-Antagonist	Antagonists
Phenan-threne	Morphine	Codeine	Nalbuphine (Nubain)	Nalorphine[a] (Nalline)
	Hydromor-phone (Dilauded)	Oxycodone (Perco-dan)		
	Oxymor-phone (Numor-phan)	Hydrocodon (Hycodan)		Naloxone (Narcan)
Phenyl-heptyl-amines	Methadone (Dolo-phine)	Propoxy-phene (Darvon)		
Phenyl-piperi-dines	Meperidine (Demeral)			
	Fentanyl (Subli-maze)			
Morphinans	Levorphanol (Levo-Dromoran)		Butorphanol (Stadol)	Levallor-phan[a] (Lorfan)
Benzo-morphans			Pentazocine (Talwin)	

[a] Not a pure antagonist.

They are indicated in the management of *acute pain, chronic pain, severe pain of acute myocardial infarction, obstetric analgesia, preanesthetic medication, pulmonary edema, cough* (see Chapter 44), *gastrointestinal* and *urinary tract disorders* (see Chapter 41).

Agents used principally for symptomatic relief of pain may for convenience in presentation be divided into three groups: (1) opiate analgesics; (2) nonopiate analgesics; (3) analgesics and antipyretics; and (4) nonsteroidal antiinflammatory drugs. The drugs considered in this section are classified according to this scheme.

Opiate Analgesics

The opium group of narcotic drugs are among the most powerfully acting and clinically useful drugs producing depression of the central nervous system. Drugs of this group are used principally as analgesics, but possess numerous other useful properties. Morphine, for example, is used to induce sleep in the presence of pain, check diarrhea, suppress cough, ease dyspnea, and facilitate anesthesia.

Unfortunately, morphine also depresses respiration; it increases the activity and tone of the smooth muscles of the gastrointestinal, biliary, and urinary tracts causing constipation, gallbladder spasm, and urinary retention; it causes nausea and vomiting in some individuals; and it may induce cutaneous pruritus. In addition to these actions, morphine and related compounds have other qualities which tend to limit their usefulness. If these agents are given over a long period of time, tolerance to the analgesic effect develops so that the dose must be increased periodically to obtain equivalent pain relief. Tolerance and physical dependence develop, which combined with euphoria result in excessive use and addiction of those patients who have susceptible personalities. For these reasons, it is generally agreed that morphine and its derivatives should be taken only as directed by the physician (never in greater dose, more often, or longer than prescribed) and never used for pain when some other analgesic will suffice. Since drowsiness and decreased alertness are not uncommon, the patient taking any of these drugs should determine if the drug has such an effect before driving or performing any duty requiring mental alertness.

The opiate analgesics are generally *contraindicated* in patients with myxedema, Addison's disease, and hepatic cirrhosis. Such patients are highly sensitive to these agents. Consequently, respiratory depression, stupor, and even coma may result from relatively small doses of these agents. Since opiates decrease ventilation, which causes hypercapnia and progresses to cerebrovascular dilatation and increased intracranial pressure, they should be used with caution in head injuries, cerebral edema, and delirium tremens. These agents should also be used with caution in patients with cardiac arrhythmias, chronic ulcerative colitis, and impaired kidney function. Moreover, narcotic analgesics cross the placental barrier; hence, newborn infants whose mothers have been administered such analgesics during labor should be closely observed for signs of respiratory depression and treated for narcotic overdosage if necessary. Individual allergic sensitivity to a particular agent or group of agents also represents a significant reason for avoiding such agents.

The analgesic and depressant effects of these agents provide the basis for a number of *interactions* with other drugs. Alcohol, antihistamines, muscle relaxants, antipsychotics, tricyclic antidepressants, or sedative-hypnotics may interact with opiates to intensify their overlapping actions, such as respiratory depression and anticholinergic effects. Particular caution is necessary if monoamine oxidase inhibitors are administered concurrently with narcotic analgesics because of intensification of action (use of meperidine in patients treated with MAO inhibitors has produced severe and occasionally fatal reactions). Doses of the opiate analgesics should be adjusted to avoid these enhanced reactions. The combined use of propoxyphene and orphenadrine has been reported to cause mental confusion, anxiety, and tremors. Although clinical impressions regarding the seriousness of this problem differ widely, the problem can be avoided by using alternative analgesic and anticholinergic drugs. Further, anticholinergics, such as atropine, can partially reverse the biliary spasms induced by opiates, but are additive to the gastrointestinal and urinary tract effects of opiates. Consequently, severe constipation and urinary retention can occur during intensive anticholinergic-analgesic therapy.

The preparations of opium and its alkaloids are numerous and for convenience are divided into three groups: opium preparations, opium alkaloids, and semisynthetic opium alkaloids.

Opium and its preparations exhibit analgesic and narcotic effects which are directly proportional to their morphine content. Traditionally, opium is more frequently employed in the form of tinctures for diarrhea and dysenteries.

Opium

Gum Opium; Crude Opium; Raw Opium; Thebaicum; Meconium

The air-dried milky exudate obtained by incising unripe capsules of *Papaver somniferum* Linné or its variety *album* De Candolle (Fam *Papaveraceae*). It yields not less than 9.5% of anhydrous morphine.

History—Opium as a medicinal drug has been known and cultivated for many centuries, but it was not until the investigations of Sertürner, published in 1817, that it was known that the drug contained certain definite principles now called *alkaloids*.

Dioscorides, in the second century, was the first writer to discuss opium and its uses at length. He gave the recipe for a preparation called *diacodion*, which is the prototype of the formerly official syrup of poppies. Paracelsus used opium extensively in the fifteenth century and referred to it as the "stone of immortality." Van Helmont, early in the seventeenth century, used opium so freely that he was referred to as Doctor Opiatus. Sydenham, a little later in the same century, praised opium as the most valuable gift of God to man.

The principal opium exporting countries have been: Turkey, Iran

Table II—Alkaloidal Content of Opiums[a]

Exporting Country	% Morphine	% Narcotine	% Codeine	% Papaverine	% Thebaine
Turkey	11–12	3–4	0.8–1.4	1–1.5	1.0–1.5
Yugoslavia	13–15	3	1.1–1.5	1–1.5	0.8–1.2
Iran	9.5–10.5	5–6	2.5–4	2–2.5	3–4
India	10–11	...	2.5–3.5	0.8	0.5–1

[a] *Note*—For medicinal preparations only Turkish or Yugoslav opium is used.

(Persia), Yugoslavia, and India. The Turkish and Yugoslav products are nearly alike in their physical properties: color, odor, and consistency. Persian and Indian opiums, while closely resembling each other, differ from the former in physical properties—they are darker, have a somewhat different odor and consistency. There is also a marked difference between the two groups in the amounts of the principal opium alkaloids as shown in Table II.

Constituents—Opium owes its activity to the narcotic alkaloids in it. Twenty-five alkaloids have been found in various kinds of opium, and several more have been announced but their existence has not been confirmed. Three acids occur combined with the alkaloids in opium—*viz*, meconic, lactic, and sulfuric acids. Also present are *meconin* [$C_{10}H_{10}O_4$], pectin, glucose, mucilage, caoutchouc, wax, and odorous, fatty, and coloring matters. The known alkaloids are tabulated and classified on pages 412 to 413.

Description—More or less rounded, oval, brick-shaped, or elongated, somewhat flattened masses, usually about 8 to 15 cm in diameter and weighing about 300 g to 2 kg each; externally, it is pale olive-brown or olive-gray having a coarse surface and covered with a thin coating consisting of fragments of poppy leaves and, at times, with fruits of a species of *Rumex* adhering from the packing; it is more or less plastic when fresh, becoming hard or tough on keeping; internally, it is reddish brown and coarsely granular. It has a very characteristic odor, and a very bitter taste.

Uses—Owes its chief pharmacological effects to its content of morphine, other alkaloids not being present in sufficient amount to modify significantly the morphine type of action. Thus, opium has many of the same uses as morphine, but the latter drug is nearly always preferred, inasmuch as it can be given in a variety of ways. The average adult dose of opium is 60 mg, taken orally. This is the equivalent of 6 mg of morphine. Like morphine, opium has *analgetic* and *narcotic* effects. It acts as an *antiperistaltic* agent by causing spasm of the bowel musculature and preventing propulsive movements. Traditionally, opium is used for *diarrheas* and *dysenteries* rather than morphine. Opium produces *sedation* and *sleep*. It also controls *cough* and *dyspnea*. Opium thus has a variety of therapeutic uses in medicine and surgery.

Caution—Opium, and all opium derivatives and related synthetic compounds, are listed in *Schedule II* of the *Controlled Substances Act* (Chapter 107). It should not be dispensed except upon the presentation of a physician's prescription. See *Morphine*.

Powdered Opium is opium dried at a temperature not exceeding 70° and reduced to a very fine powder; yields 10.0–10.5% of anhydrous morphine. It may contain any of the diluents, with the exception of starch, permitted for powdered extracts under *Extracts* (page 1516). *Description:* Light brown to moderate yellowish brown, consisting chiefly of yellowish brown to yellow, more or less irregular and granular fragments of latex, varying from 15 to 150 μm in diameter; a few fragments of strongly lignified, thick-walled, 4- to 5-sided or narrowly elongated, epidermal cells of the poppy capsule; very few fragments of tissues of poppy leaves, poppy capsules, and occasionally *Rumex* fruits. In addition there will be the microscopic characteristics of the diluent if any has been used in the preparation of the powder. *Uses:* A pharmaceutical necessity for *Paregoric*. See *Opium* and *Morphine*.

Paregoric [Camphorated Opium Tincture USP XVI; Paregoric Elixir; Tinctura Opii Benzoica; Tinctura Thebaica Benzoica] yields, from each 100 mL, 35–45 mg of anhydrous morphine. *Preparation:* Macerate powdered opium (4.3 g), anise oil (3.8 mL), benzoic acid (3.8 g), and camphor (3.8 g) for 5 days, with occasional agitation, in a mixture of diluted alcohol (900 mL) and glycerin (38 mL). Then filter, and pass enough diluted alcohol through the filter to obtain 950 mL of total filtrate. Assay a portion of this filtrate as directed in the USP, and dilute the remainder with a sufficient quantity of diluted alcohol containing, in each 100 mL, 0.4 mL of anise oil, 400 mg of benzoic acid, 400 mg of camphor, and 4 mL of glycerin, to produce a solution containing, in each 100 mL, 40 mg of

anhydrous morphine. *History:* This preparation was originated by Professor LeMort of the University of Leyden about 1715. It was official in the 1721 edition of the London Pharmacopaeia as *Elixir Asthmaticum*, which was changed to *Elixir Paregoricum*, meaning soothing elixir, in 1746. It has also been known as *Tinctura Camphorae Composita* and *Tinctura Opii Benzoica*, and the formula has changed in minor details many times since its introduction into medicine. *Alcohol Content:* 44 to 46%. *Uses:* An *antidiarrheal agent* and mild *anodyne* in cough, nausea, and abdominal pains. It should never be used to quiet restless infants, as a habit may be induced. It contains 0.4% of opium. Paregoric is listed in *Schedule III* of the *Controlled Substances Act;* hence, it can only be obtained on a prescription order (either oral or written) of a licensed practitioner. *Dose: Usual, adult, oral,* 5 to 10 mL 1 to 4 times a day; *children,* 0.25 to 0.5 mL/kg 1 to 4 times daily.

Opium Alkaloids

The pharmaceutically important opium alkaloids are commonly subdivided into two chemical groups: (1) the isoquinoline derivatives which are, as a general rule, antispasmodic drugs, such as papaverine and narcotine (see page 412) and (2) the phenanthrene derivatives described in this section, such as morphine and codeine, which are analgesic and narcotic.* The Narcotic Act of 1956 required that all heroin in the hands of pharmacists, physicians, veterinarians, hospitals, etc, be surrendered to the federal government. Presently, heroin is under *Schedule I* of the *Controlled Substances Act.*

Morphine

History—Morphine was the first alkaloid discovered. In the 17th and 18th centuries many attempts were made to separate from opium the principle to which its activity was due. Preparations claimed to represent these active principles, but which were really extracts, were employed in medicine under the name of *Magisterium Opii*. Bucholz was the first to endeavor to obtain a crystalline product from opium. About 1800 a number of learned apothecaries of the time were devoting their attention to the separation of the suspected active principle. One of these apothecaries, Derosne, succeeded in isolating narcotine in 1803, and the following year Seguin read a paper to the Institute of France describing the isolation of a substance which is now recognized as morphine. He did not publish his paper however, until 1814 and in 1806, Friedrich William Adam Sertürner, an apothecary of Einbeck, Germany, announced the separation of a basic crystalline substance which existed in opium in combination with a special acid. He later published, in 1817, the results of further investigation in which he named the substance *morphium* and described it as a *vegetable alkali*. Liebig, in 1831, assigned to it the formula $C_{34}H_{36}N_2O_6$, which was later modified by Laurent to the present formula, $C_{17}H_{19}NO_3$ (285.34).

It was only after almost 100 years of intensive research by many able chemists that the correct structural formula (page 416), which adequately explains the chemical transformations of morphine, could be proposed. Final confirmation of this structure came with the successful total synthesis of morphine in 1952.

Preparation—Several processes are in use. In all or nearly all of them the morphine and most of the other opium alkaloids are extracted from the opium with water alone or with slightly acid water. In one of the processes, the extract after concentration is neutralized, a solution of calcium chloride is added, and the mixture is filtered and further concentrated. Crude morphine hydrochloride crystallizes and is purified by precipitation with ammonia and recrystallized as the sulfate or hydrochloride. In another process the concentrated water extract is mixed with alcohol and made strongly alkaline with ammonia. The morphine, being but slightly soluble in dilute alcohol, separates out while the greater part of the other alkaloids remain in solution. The crude morphine so obtained is purified by repeated crystallization as the sulfate or hydrochloride and reprecipitation if necessary in the presence of alcohol.

Description—Colorless or white, shining, rhombic prisms, fine needles, or a crystalline powder, permanent in the air; saturated aqueous solution is alkaline to litmus; melts with decomposition at about 250°.

---

* For a more detailed classification of the opium alkaloids, see page 412.

Solubility—1 g in about 5000 mL water, 210 mL alcohol (more soluble in methanol), 1220 mL chloroform, about 6500 mL ether, 100 mL lime water; insoluble in benzene; readily soluble in solutions of fixed alkali and alkaline earth hydroxides from which it is reprecipitated by ammonium chloride or sulfate.

Uses—Morphine is used as an *analgesic, adjunct to anesthesia, antitussive,* and *nonspecific antidiarrheal* agent. It is a strong analgesic, alters the psychological response to pain, and suppresses anxiety and apprehension. Consequently, it is used in small to moderate doses to relieve constant dull pain, and in moderate to large doses to alleviate intermittent, sharp pain of traumatic or visceral origin. Although effects may begin earlier, maximal analgesic effect occurs about 20 minutes after intravenous injection, 50 to 90 minutes after subcutaneous injection, and 30 to 60 minutes after intramuscular injection. Analgesia persists for approximately four hours but, in some patients, it may be as short as two and one-half hours or as long as seven hours. Although morphine has played a dominant and controversial role in *preanesthetic* medication, it is generally agreed it is of particular value when pain is present preoperatively, in selected types of cardiac surgery and in poor-risk patients in general. Morphine is an effective antitussive agent, but because of its erratic absorption after oral administration and its dependence liability, it should be used as an *antitussive* agent only when cough is associated with severe pain and cannot be controlled by antitussives having less potential for abuse. Morphine and other opiates such as paregoric are the most effective and prompt-acting *nonspecific antidiarrheal* agents. They act by enhancing tone in long segments of the longitudinal muscle and inhibiting propulsive contraction of both circular and longitudinal muscle. They are used to treat acute, self-limited diarrhea.

When administered orally, morphine is rapidly but incompletely absorbed and equally rapidly metabolized to morphine glucuronide; thus, the plasma levels after this route are usually only $\frac{1}{5}$ to $\frac{1}{3}$ those obtained after parenteral injection. The half-life of morphine in plasma or serum during the first 6 hours is between 2 and 3 hours; the serum half-life between 6 and 48 hours after intravenous administration ranges from 10 to 44 hours. Approximately 35% of the drug is bound, primarily to the albumin fraction. After parenteral administration 70 to 80% is excreted during the first 48 hours with 60% as conjugated morphine. Following oral administration, only about 60% of a given dose is excreted; this probably reflects the incomplete absorption from the gastrointestinal tract.

For a review of untoward effects, contraindications, interactions with other drugs, and precautions in the use of morphine see introductory statement, opiate analgesics, page 1100.

Overt symptoms of *morphine overdosage* include coma, pinpoint pupils, and depressed respiration. Shock, decreased body temperature, and pulmonary edema may occur. Treatment includes the establishment of a patent airway and ventilation of the patient. If significant respiratory depression occurs, a suitable narcotic antagonist, such as naloxone, should be administered. Other supportive measures should be applied as indicated.

Morphine is a *Schedule II* drug under the *Controlled Substances Act.*

Dose—See *Morphine Sulfate* below.

Morphine Sulfate

Morphinan-3,6-diol, 7,8-didehydro-4,5-epoxy-17-methyl-, (5α,6α)-, sulfate (2:1) (salt), pentahydrate

7,8-Didehydro-4,5α-epoxy-17-methylmorphinan-3,6α-diol sulfate (2:1) (salt) pentahydrate [6211-15-0] $(C_{17}H_{19}NO_3)_2.H_2SO_4.5H_2O$ (758.83); *anhydrous* [64-31-3] (668.76).

For the structural formula of morphine, see page 416.

Description—White, feathery, silky crystals, as cubical masses of crystals, or as a white crystalline powder; odorless and when exposed to air gradually loses water of hydration; darkens on prolonged exposure to light.

Solubility—1 g in 16 mL water, 570 mL alcohol, 1 mL water at 80°, and about 240 mL alcohol at 60°; insoluble in chloroform and ether.

Uses—See *Morphine* and *Morphine Sulfate Injection.*

Dose—*Usual, adult, oral,* 10 to 30 mg every 4 hours or as directed by physician.

Dosage Forms—Soluble Tablets: 10, 15, and 30 mg; Oral Solution: 10 and 20 mg/5 mL.

Morphine Sulfate Injection

A sterile solution of morphine sulfate in water for injection. It may contain suitable antimicrobial agents.

Preparation—Solutions of morphine sulfate at a pH above 7 decompose quickly even at room temperature. At a pH of less than 5.5 no change is reported in a 1% solution heated for 1 hour. The pH should be between 2.5 and 6.0. Sterilization should be conducted with a minimum of heat.

Uses—Morphine injection is indicated for the relief of severe pain. It is effective in the control of postoperative pain as well as for relieving preoperative apprehension. Its most important actions are on the brain, especially its higher functions. An initial transitory stimulation is followed by depression of the brain, its higher functions, and medullary centers. The reflexes and spinal functions are usually stimulated. Morphine injection affects psychic functions in such a way that the patient is more tolerant to discomfort and pain. In addition it appears to interfere with pain conduction. Morphine injection depresses the respiratory center, stimulates the vomiting center, depresses the cough reflex, constricts the pupils, increases the tone of the gastrointestinal and genitourinary tracts, and produces mild vasodilation. Morphine injection is contraindicated in bronchial asthma, respiratory depression, or idiosyncrasy to the drug. Overdoses may cause respiratory depression, coma, and death. The drug should be used with caution in the extremes of age (infants and aged) as well as in the debilitated patient, or in patients with increased intracranial pressure, toxic psychoses, myxedema, or prostatic hypertrophy. Untoward reactions may include allergic reactions, nausea, vomiting, constipation, urinary retention, depression, delirium and convulsions. Morphine Sulfate Injection is a *Schedule II* drug under the *Controlled Substances Act.*

Dose—*Usual, Adult, subcutaneous* or *intramuscular,* **5 to 20 mg/70 kg;** *Children,* **0.1** to **0.2 mg/kg**/dose. *Intravenous,* **4 to 10 mg** administered very slowly. Morphine should not be administered intravenously unless a narcotic antagonist is immediately available.

Dosage Forms—2, 4, 8, 10, and 15 mg/mL.

Codeine

Morphinan-6-ol, 7,8-didehydro-4,5-epoxy-3-methoxy-17-methyl-, monohydrate, (5α,6α)-, Methylmorphine

7,8-Didehydro-4,5α-epoxy-3-methoxy-17-methylmorphinan-6α-ol monohydrate [6059-47-8] $C_{18}H_{21}NO_3.H_2O$ (317.38); *anhydrous* [76-57-3] (299.37); an alkaloid obtained from opium or prepared from morphine by methylation.

For the structural formula, see page 416.

History—Isolated from opium by the French chemist Robiquet in 1832, and the name given it by the discoverer is derived from the Greek word meaning poppy capsules.

Preparation—While some codeine is obtained from opium directly the quantity is not sufficient to meet the extensive use of this alkaloid as a very valuable medicinal agent. Much more codeine is used than morphine. This need is met by making it by partial synthesis from morphine. The process involves methylating the phenolic OH of the latter. The methylating agent generally used is phenyltrimethylammonium hydroxide. Dry morphine is dissolved in a solution of potassium hydroxide in absolute alcohol, the required quantity of the methylating agent added, and the solution heated at about 130°. After cooling, water is added, the solution is acidified with sulfuric acid, the dimethylaniline formed is separated, and the alcohol is removed by distillation. Treatment with caustic soda solution precipitates the codeine, while any unreacted morphine is held in solution by the sodium hydroxide. The crude codeine is purified by crystallization as the sulfate.

Description—Colorless or white crystals, or a white, crystalline powder; effloresces slowly in dry air and is affected by light; when rendered anhydrous by drying at 80° it melts within a 2°-range between 154° and 158°; pH (saturated aqueous solution) about 9.8.

Solubility—1 g in 120 mL water, 2 mL alcohol, about 0.5 mL chloroform, 50 mL ether, and about 20 mL benzene. When heated in an amount of water insufficient for complete solution, codeine melts to oily drops which crystallize on cooling.

Incompatibilities—Precipitated from its aqueous solution by most *alkaloidal precipitants* but not by sodium, potassium, or ammonium carbonate or sodium bicarbonate. Aqueous solutions are sufficiently alkaline to precipitate other less soluble alkaloids from solutions of their salts. Ammonia may be liberated from *ammonium salts*. See also page 414.

Uses—May be viewed as a weakened morphine, which fails to produce proportionately greater narcotic effects as the dose is increased. Indeed, large amounts of codeine may cause excitement. Average doses are *sedative, analgetic,* and *antitussive.* When administered by the oral route 30 to 60 mg of codeine is approximately equivalent in analgesic effectiveness to 650 mg of aspirin; subcutaneously, 60 mg of codeine is somewhat less effective than 10 mg of morphine. Codeine is useful for inducing sleep in the presence of mild pain. Codeine is absorbed rapidly following oral administration. Peak plasma levels occur in about 1 hour and plasma half-life is about 3.5 hours. The bioavailability of codeine is greater than that of morphine after oral administration; its oral/parenteral analgesic potency ratio is 1:1.5. Like morphine, codeine also produces cortical and respiratory depression, but serious degrees of either are practically unknown. Codeine is less apt than morphine to cause nausea, vomiting, constipation, and miosis. Both tolerance and *addiction* to codeine occur, however, and the same precautions should be observed in its use as for morphine. *Naloxone* is a specific antagonist in cases of acute codeine intoxication.

Codeine, like morphine, is employed as an *analgetic, sedative, hypnotic, antiperistaltic,* and *antitussive* agent. It is commonly given in combination with aspirin or acetaminophen. It is a *Schedule II* drug under the *Controlled Substances Act.*

Dose—*Analgesic,* 15 to 60 mg; *usual, adult, oral, analgesic* **30 mg** every 4 hours; *usual, antitussive,* 5 to **10 mg** every 4 hours. *Usual, pediatric, oral,* **500 µg** (0.5 mg) **per kg** body wt or **16.7 mg per square meter** body surface every 4 hours.

Other Dose Information—The dose varies from 15 to 60 mg, and the drug may be taken orally or injected parenterally as a solution of one of its water-soluble salts, such as the phosphate or sulfate.

Codeine Phosphate

Morphinan-6-ol, 7,8-didehydro-4,5-epoxy-3-methoxy-17-methyl-, (5α,6α)-, phosphate (1:1) (salt), hemihydrate

7,8-Didehydro-4,5α-epoxy-3-methoxy-17-methylmorphinan-6α-ol phosphate (1:1) (salt) hemihydrate [41444-62-6] $C_{18}H_{21}NO_3 \cdot H_3PO_4 \cdot \frac{1}{2}H_2O$ (406.37); *anhydrous* [52-28-8] (397.36).

Preparation—By dissolving codeine in an equimolecular quantity of aqueous phosphoric acid, adding alcohol, and allowing the salt to crystallize from solution.

Description—Fine, white, needle-shaped crystals or a white, crystalline powder; odorless; readily loses water of hydration on exposure to air and is affected by light; solutions are acid to litmus and levorotatory.

Solubility—1 g in 2.5 mL water, 325 mL alcohol, 0.5 mL water at 80°, and 125 mL boiling alcohol.

Uses—See *Codeine, Morphine,* and *general statement* in this section. Being more soluble than codeine sulfate, the phosphate is preferred to the sulfate.

Dose—15 to 300 mg daily; *usual, adult, analgesic, oral* or *parenteral,* **30 mg** 4 to 6 times a day; *usual, antitussive, oral,* **10 mg** 6 to 8 times a day as necessary. *Usual, pediatric, oral,* **500 µg** (0.5 mg) **per kg** or **16.7 mg per square meter** body surface every 4 hours.

Dosage Forms—Injection: 15, 30, and 60 mg/mL, 600 mg and 1.2 g/20 mL; Tablets: 15, 30, and 60 mg.

Codeine Phosphate, Aspirin, Phenacetin, and Caffeine

APC with Codeine; Empirin Compound with Codeine
(Burroughs-Wellcome)

Uses—This popular combination has no advantage over codeine with aspirin; thus, the latter is preferred. Codeine phosphate, aspirin, phenacetin, and caffeine are used for the relief of pain of all degrees of severity, up to that which requires morphine.

Dose—*Usual,* 8 to **60 mg** codeine phosphate, **600 mg** aspirin, **300 mg** phenacetin, and **200 mg** caffeine. Additional dose information: *usual, adult, oral,* 1 or 2 tablets or capsules every 4 hours, as needed. Dosage for children has not been established.

Dosage Forms—Tablets: 8, 15, 30, or 60 mg codeine phosphate, 230 mg aspirin, 150 mg phenacetin, 32 mg caffeine; Capsules: 15, 30, or 60 mg codeine phosphate, 230 mg of aspirin, 160 mg phenacetin, 32 mg caffeine.

Codeine Sulfate

Morphinan-6-ol, 7,8-didehydro-4,5-epoxy-3-methoxy-17-methyl-, (5α,6α)-, sulfate (2:1) (salt), trihydrate

7,8-Didehydro-4,5α-epoxy-3-methoxy-17-methylmorphinan-6α-ol sulfate (2:1) (salt) trihydrate [6854-40-6] $(C_{18}H_{21}NO_3)_2 \cdot H_2SO_4 \cdot 3H_2O$ (750.86); *anhydrous* [1420-53-7] (698.81).

Preparation—By crystallization from a solution of codeine in diluted H_2SO_4.

Description—White crystals, usually needle-like, or a white, crystalline powder; effloresces in dry air and is affected by light; aqueous solution is practically neutral or only slightly acid to litmus.

Solubility—1 g in 30 mL water, 1300 mL alcohol, and in about 6.5 mL water at 80°; insoluble in chloroform and ether.

Incompatibilities—See *Alkaloids* (page 414). Codeine Sulfate reacts with *phenobarbital sodium* to produce the free alkaloid and phenobarbital, both of which may precipitate unless the vehicle contains a moderate proportion of alcohol.

Uses—See *Codeine, Morphine,* and *general statement* in this section.

Dose—*Analgesic,* 15 to 60 mg; *usual, adult, oral, analgesic,* **30 mg** every 4 hours; *usual, antitussive,* 5 to **10 mg** every 4 hours. *Usual, pediatric, oral,* **500 µg** (0.5 mg) **per kg** or **16.7 mg per square meter** body surface every 4 hours.

Dosage Forms—Tablets: 15, 30, and 60 mg.

Other Opium Alkaloids

Diacetylmorphine [Heroin; [561-27-3] $C_{21}H_{23}NO_5$ (369.40)]—An alkaloid prepared from morphine by acetylation. When alkaloidal morphine is heated with acetyl chloride, the synthetic alkaloid, diacetylmorphine, is produced. White crystalline powder without odor; saturated alcoholic solution is alkaline to moistened litmus paper. 1 g dissolves in about 1700 mL water, 31 mL alcohol, 1.4 mL chloroform, or 100 mL ether at 25°. *Uses:* Formerly used as a sedative in cough mixtures and to relieve moderate pain. Heroin is listed in *Schedule I* of the *Controlled Substances Act,* hence it cannot be prescribed. *Dose:* Was 3 mg. For the structure, see page 416.

Diacetylmorphine Hydrochloride [Heroin Hydrochloride; Diamorphine Hydrochloride BP; [1502-95-0] $C_{21}H_{23}NO_5 \cdot HCl \cdot H_2O$ (405.88)]— White, odorless, bitter, crystalline powder; melts between 229° and 233°. Soluble in 1.6 parts water or chloroform; soluble in alcohol; insoluble in ether. The manufacture or importation of this narcotic is prohibited by federal law. It was official and was used like morphine sulfate in doses of 3 to 5 mg.

Morphine Hydrochloride, BP, PhI $[C_{17}H_{19}NO_3 \cdot HCl \cdot 3H_2O]$— Odorless, white, crystalline powder or white, needle-like crystals having a bitter taste; when exposed to air it gradually loses a portion of its 3 molecules of water; darkens on prolonged exposure to light. 1 g is soluble in 18 mL water to give a solution having a pH of about 5. It is soluble in alcohol and glycerin but insoluble in chloroform and ether. It has the same actions, uses, and dose as *Morphine Sulfate* (page 1102).

Morphine Tartrate $[(C_{17}H_{19}NO_3)_2 \cdot C_4H_6O_6 \cdot 3H_2O]$—White, crystalline powder. Soluble in 11 parts of water; slightly soluble in alcohol; insoluble in chloroform, ether, and carbon disulfide. *Uses* and *Dose:* See *Morphine Sulfate* (page 1102).

Morphine and Atropine Sulfates Tablets—*Uses:* See *Morphine* (page 1101) and *Atropine* (page 913). This combination of alkaloids invites the same objection that all drug mixtures do; namely, that of fixed dosages. Nevertheless, atropine and morphine are commonly used together, especially for *preanesthetic medication,* and for relief of *visceral pain,* where atropine relaxes smooth muscles and hence counteracts the spasmodic effect of morphine. Thus, for example, morphine and atropine together give smoother relief of pain in *gallbladder colic* or *ureteral colic* than does morphine alone. The combination is also used to relieve the pain of acute coronary thrombosis. *Dose:* 5 to 20 mg morphine sulfate; 0.3 to 1.2 mg (atropine sulfate). *Dosage Forms:* 8, 10, 15, and 30 mg morphine sulfate and 0.4 mg atropine sulfate.

Semisynthetic Opiate Analgesics

In the effort to obtain an agent with the advantages of morphine or codeine without their disadvantages, chemists have modified the structure of these natural alkaloids of opium. Some of these modifications, eg, hydrocodone, hydromorphone, ethylmorphine, nalorphine, etc, result from making minor chemical alterations in the natural alkaloids, the characteristic nucleus (see page 416) remaining intact. Others, eg, dextromethorphan, levorphanol, levallorphan, etc, are truly synthetic compounds constructed around the nonopiate morphinan nucleus (see page 390) which is readily synthesizable from coal-tar derivatives. For pharmacologic convenience, all of these agents are classified here as semisynthetic opium alkaloids. In general, the pharmacological properties exhibited by these agents differ quantitatively from those of the parent substance, but qualitatively they are similar. The several semisynthetic agents that are clinically employed are described below.

Dextromethorphan Hydrobromide—page 870.

Hydrocodone Bitartrate

Morphinan-6-one, 4,5-epoxy-3-methoxy-17-methyl-, (5α)-, [R-(R,*R*)]-2,3-dihydroxybutanedioate (1:1), hydrate (2:5); Dihydrocodeinone Bitartrate USP XVI; (*Various Mfrs*)

4,5α-Epoxy-3-methoxy-17-methylmorphinan-6-one tartrate (1:1) hydrate (2:5) [34195-34-1] [6190-38-1] $C_{18}H_{21}NO_3.C_4H_6O_6.2\frac{1}{2}H_2O$ (494.50); *anhydrous* [143-71-5] (449.46).

For the structure of hydrocodone, see page 416.

Preparation—This synthetic alkaloid, 7,8-dihydrocodeinone, is prepared either by catalytic rearrangement of codeine or by controlled hydrolysis and oxidation of dihydrothebaine.

Description—Fine white crystals or a fine white crystalline powder; affected by light; pH (1 in 50 solution) between 3.2 and 3.8.
Solubility—1 g in 16 mL water; slightly soluble in alcohol; insoluble in ether and chloroform.

Uses—For the relief of moderate to severe pain and for the symptomatic relief of cough. It is a narcotic which is somewhat more addictive than codeine, and is listed as a *Schedule III* drug under the *Controlled Substances Act*.
Dose—5 to **50 mg** daily; *usual, adult, oral,* **5 to 10 mg** 3 to 4 times a day. *Usual, pediatric,* adequate dosing information is not available.
Dosage Form—Tablets: 5 mg.

Hydromorphone

Morphinan-6-one, 4,5-epoxy-3-hydroxy-17-methyl-, (5α)-, Dilaudid (*Knoll*)

4,5α-Epoxy-3-hydroxy-17-methylmorphinan-6-one [466-99-9] $C_{17}H_{19}NO_3$ (285.34).
For the structure, see page 416.

Description—Fine, white or practically white, odorless, crystalline powder; affected by light; melts at about 265°.
Solubility—Slightly soluble in water; freely soluble in alcohol; very soluble in chloroform.

Uses and **Dose**—See *Hydromorphone Hydrochloride* and *Hydromorphone Sulfate Injection*.

Hydromorphone Hydrochloride

Morphinan-6-one-, 4,5-epoxy-3-hydroxy-17-methyl-, (5α)-, hydrochloride, Dihydromorphinone Hydrochloride; Dilaudid Hydrochloride (*Knoll*)

4,5α-Epoxy-3-hydroxy-17-methylmorphinan-6-one hydrochloride [71-68-1] $C_{17}H_{19}NO_3.HCl$ (321.80).
Hydromorphone hydrochloride is 7,8-dihydromorphinone hydrochloride; for the structure, see page 416.
Preparation—By electrolytic reduction of morphine or by oxidation of dihydromorphine and then reacting with HCl. US Pat 2,649,454.

Description—Fine, white, odorless, crystalline powder, affected by light; aqueous solution is practically neutral or only slightly acid to litmus.
Solubility—1 g in about 3 mL water; sparingly soluble in alcohol; practically insoluble in ether.
Incompatibilities—Reactions characteristic of alkaloids are generally applicable to this substance.

Uses—A semisynthetic *analgetic,* chemically and pharmacologically similar to morphine, indicated for the relief of moderate to severe pain of myocardial infarction, cancer, trauma (soft tissue and bone), biliary and renal colic, burns, and postoperative pain. (See intro-

ductory statement, this section, page 1100). It is one-fifth as potent orally as intramuscularly; the peak effect occurs later and the duration of analgesia is longer after oral administration. After *parenteral* administration, analgesic action is apparent within 15 minutes and lasts for more than 5 hours. After *oral* administration, onset of analgesia is about 30 minutes. Slower absorption and hence longer relief from pain can be obtained from use of hydromorphone hydrochloride in suppository form. Hydromorphone hydrochloride causes less tendency to sleep than morphine when given in equivalent analgetic doses, and thus relief from pain can be obtained without sleep or stupefaction. It is contraindicated in bronchial asthma, respiratory depression, or idiosyncrasy to the drug. It is claimed that hydromorphone hydrochloride causes less constipation and vomiting than morphine; also, it produces less euphoria. However, *tolerance* and *addiction* do occur with hydromorphone hydrochloride, and the drug must be used with the same precautions as for morphine. It can be given by mouth, by rectum in suppository form, or injected subcutaneously or intravenously (in emergency).

Caution—This drug, being a morphine derivative, is classified as a *Schedule II* drug under the *Controlled Substances Act.* Naloxone (page 1106) is a specific antagonist in cases of acute hydromorphone intoxication.

Dose—*Oral* and *subcutaneous,* **1** to **4 mg;** *usual,* **2 mg** every 4 hours as necessary. The dose for children has not been established.
Dosage Forms—Injection: 1, 2, and 4 mg/mL; Tablets: 1, 2, 3, and 4 mg; Suppositories: 3 mg; Syrup: 1 mg/5 mL.

Levorphanol Tartrate

Morphinan-3-ol, 17-methyl-, [R-(R*,R*)]-2,3-dihydroxybutanedioate (1:1) (salt), dihydrate; Levo-Dromoran (*Roche*)

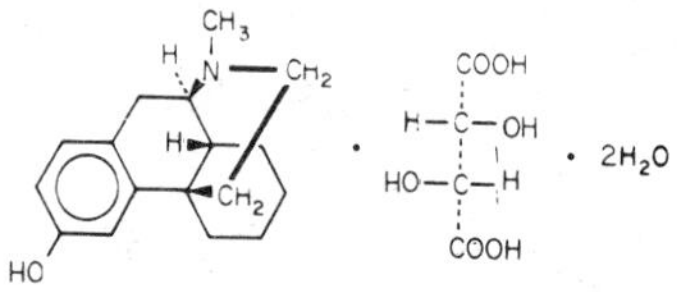

17-Methylmorphinan-3-ol tartrate (1:1) (salt) dihydrate [5985-38-6] $C_{17}H_{23}NO.C_4H_6O_6.2H_2O$ (443.49); *anhydrous* [125-72-4] (407.46).

Preparation—5,6,7,8-Tetrahydro-2-methylisoquinolinium bromide (I) is metathesized with *p*-methoxybenzyl magnesium bromide (II), and the product rearranges at the expense of the 1,2-double bond to form 1-(*p*-methoxybenzyl)-2-methyl-1,2,5,6,7,8-hexahydroisoquinoline (III). III may be redrawn as shown below to display the ensuing reactions more clearly. A solution of the hydrochloride of III is then hydrogenated at the 3,4-positions with the aid of platinized charcoal, and subsequent treatment with ammonia liberates the *dl*-1,2,3,4,5,6,7,8-octahydro compound (IV) which may be resolved into its *d*- and *l*-enantiomorphs by the usual procedures. The final step in the preparation of the base involves heating the *l*-enantiomorph with phosphoric acid at 150° whereby cyclization between the isoquinoline residue and the benzene ring occurs at the expense of the remaining double bond of the isoquinoline. During the treatment with phosphoric acid, the methoxy group is simultaneously converted to hydroxy, thus producing levorphanol (V).

The tartrate may be produced by dissolving the base in aqueous tartaric acid solution and crystallizing.

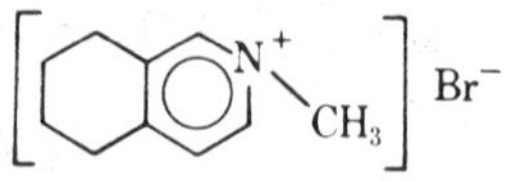

I

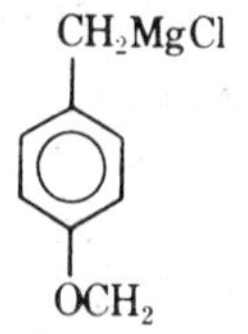

II

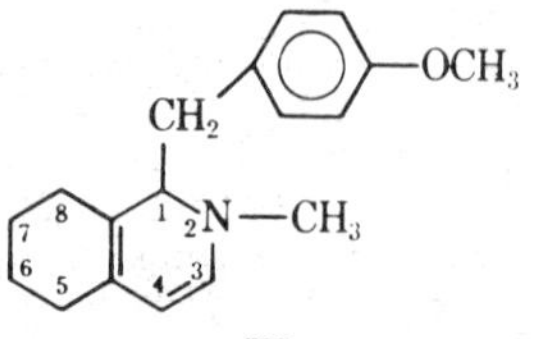

III

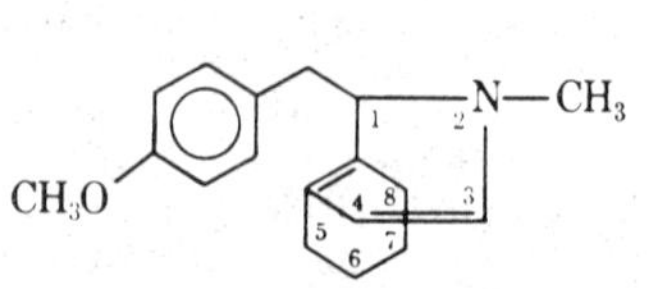

III (Redrawn)

IV   V

Description—Practically white, odorless, crystalline powder; melting range 114° to 117°.

Solubility—1 g in 50 mL water, 120 mL alcohol; insoluble in chloroform and ether.

Uses—A potent synthetic analgesic related chemically and pharmacologically to morphine (see *morphine*, page 1101 and introductory statement, this section, page 1100). It produces analgesia at least equal to that of morphine and greater than that of meperidine with much smaller doses than either. It also is longer-acting than either of the above; from 6 to 8 hours of pain relief can be achieved after either oral or parenteral administration. Its margin of safety is essentially the same as morphine, but it is less likely to produce nausea, vomiting, and constipation. Levorphanol tartrate is indicated whenever a narcotic analgesic is required; it is effective for both moderate and severe pain. The drug is contraindicated in acute alcoholism, bronchial asthma, increased intracranial pressure, respiratory depression, and anoxia. Other precautions and adverse reactions are similar to those induced by other narcotic analgesics. Levorphanol tartrate is a narcotic with addiction liability similar to that of morphine; therefore, the same precautions should be observed when prescribing this drug as for morphine. The drug is listed in *Schedule II* of the *Controlled Substances Act*.

Dose—*Oral* and *subcutaneous*, 1 to **3 mg**; *usual*, **2 mg.**

Dosage Forms—Injection: 2 mg/mL, 20 mg/10 mL; Tablets: 2 mg.

Oxymorphone Hydrochloride

Morphinan-6-one, 4,5-epoxy-3,14-dihydroxy-17-methyl-, (5α)-, hydrochloride; Numorphan (*Endo*)

4,5α-Epoxy-3,14-dihydroxy-17-methylmorphinan-6-one hydrochloride [357-07-3] $C_{17}H_{19}NO_4$·HCl (337.80).

For the structure, see page 416.

Preparation—Thebaine is dissolved in aqueous formic acid and treated with 30% hydrogen peroxide, after which neutralization with aqueous ammonia yields 14-hydroxycodeinone. This is then dissolved in acetic acid and hydrogenated with the aid of palladium-charcoal catalyst to form 14-hydroxy-7,8-dihydrocodeinone (oxycodone). In the form of its hydrochloride, this compound is demethylated by heating with pyridine hydrochloride to yield crude oxymorphone hydrochloride, which is then purified. US Pat 2,806,033.

Description—White, acicular crystals or as a white or slightly off-white powder; odorless; darkens on prolonged exposure to light; aqueous solutions are acid to litmus, having a pH of about 5.

Solubility—1 g in 4 mL water, 100 mL alcohol, >1000 mL chloroform, >1000 mL ether.

Uses—A semisynthetic narcotic analgesic agent with actions, uses, and side effects similar to those of hydromorphone and morphine, except it possesses no significant antitussive activity. After parenteral administration, 1 mg of oxymorphone hydrochloride is approximately equivalent in analgesic activity to 10 mg of morphine. Onset of action is rapid; initial effects are usually seen within 5 to 10 min, duration of action is approximately 3 to 6 hours. It satisfactorily controls postoperative pain, the more severe pain of advanced neoplastic diseases, and other types of pain that can ordinarily be controlled by morphine. Except that it is somewhat less constipating, the overall incidence and severity of side effects are similar to those of morphine. Its addiction liability is about the same as morphine. Oxymorphone hydrochloride is a *Schedule II* narcotic drug and subject to the regulations of the *Controlled Substances Act*.

Dose—*Usual, adult, oral; subcutaneous* and *intramuscular*, **1.0** to **1.5 mg** every 4 to 6 hours as needed; *intravenous*, **0.5 mg** *initially*, repeated in 4 to 6 hours if necessary. Dosage in children has not been established.

Dosage Forms—Injection: 1 and 1.5 mg/mL; Suppositories: 5 mg.

Other Semisynthetic Opiate Analgesics

Oxycodone Hydrochloride PhI [4,5α-Epoxy-14-hydroxy-3-methoxy-17-methylmorphinan-6-one Hydrochloride [124-90-3] $C_{18}H_{21}NO_4$·HCl (351.83); Dihydrohydroxycodeinone Hydrochloride; Eukodal]—For the structure, see page 416. Odorless, white, crystalline powder having a saline, bitter taste; melts between 274° and 278°. 1 g is soluble in 10 mL water and 60 mL ethyl alcohol. *Uses:* For the relief of moderate to severe pain. Like codeine and methadone, it retains one-half of its analgesic activity after oral administration. Listed in *Schedule II* under the *Controlled Substances Act*.

Dose—*Usual, adult, oral,* **5 mg** every 6 hours as needed for pain.

Dosage Forms—Solution: 5 mg/mL; Tablets: 5 mg (scored).

Opiate Antagonists

Although *N*-allylnorcodeine was observed in 1915 to prevent or abolish morphine- and heroin-induced respiratory depression, more than 25 years elapsed before it was demonstrated that *N*-allylnormorphine (nalorphine) had even more pronounced morphine-antagonizing properties. Even then the clinical significance of this antagonizing effect was not explored until 1951. Two years later it was shown that nalorphine would precipitate acute abstinence syndromes in postaddicts who had been given morphine, methadone, or heroin for brief periods. It was also shown that nonaddicted subjects given large doses of nalorphine exhibited dysphoria and anxiety rather than euphoria. Subsequently, it was noted that, although nalorphine antagonized the analgesic effects of morphine, it was a potent analgesic when given to patients with postoperative pain.

Except for meperidine, the substitution of an allyl group for the *N*-methyl group in most of the narcotics—eg, morphine, levorphanol, methadone, oxymorphone, and phenazocine—results in drugs with varying levels of narcotic antagonistic effect. It should be emphasized that this is not restricted to allyl substitution, since the substitution of other groups (methallyl, propyl, isobutyl, propargyl, or cyclopropargyl-methyl) for the *N*-methyl group of narcotic analgesics also produces substances that are antagonists.

The term *antagonist*, as used in this section, includes nalorphine hydrochloride and levallorphan hydrochloride, which are *antagonists* with partial *agonistic* activity, as well as naloxone which is a pure *antagonist* with virtually no agonistic actions. These competitive narcotic antagonists are effective in the management of *severe respiratory depression* induced by narcotic drugs, *asphyxia neonatorum* caused by administration of these drugs to the expectant mother, and for the *diagnosis of* possible *narcotic addiction*.

Levallorphan Tartrate

Morphinan-3-ol, 17-(2-propenyl)-, [*R*-(*R**,*R**)]-2,3-dihydroxybutanedioate (1:1) (salt); Lorfan Tartrate (*Roche*)

17-Allylmorphinan-3-ol tartrate (1:1) (salt) [71-82-9] $C_{19}H_{25}$NO·$C_4H_6O_6$ (433.50).

Preparation—The overall process involves demethylation of levorphanol (base) followed by allylation and conversion to the tartrate. The levorphanol (synthesized as described under *Levorphanol Tartrate*, page 1104) is reacted with cyanogen bromide (von Braun cleavage) whereby the *N*-methyl is converted to *N*-cyano. On alkaline hydrolysis, this cyano compound behaves as a typical cyanamide giving rise to the corresponding *sec*-amino compound (demethylated levorphanol). This may then be allylated in various ways, such as treating it with an equimolar quantity of allyl bromide in the presence of a suitable basic catalyst. The resulting levallorphan is reacted with an equimolar portion of tartaric acid and the bitartrate thus formed is purified by recrystallization.

Description—White or practically white, odorless, crystalline powder; melts between 174° and 177°.
Solubility—1 g in about 20 mL water and about 60 mL alcohol; practically insoluble in ether; insoluble in chloroform.

Uses—A potent narcotic antagonist indicated for use in the treatment of significant narcotic-induced respiratory depression. The actions of levallorphan are similar to those of nalorphine. It is used in obstetrics for the prevention and treatment of respiratory depression in the mother, fetus, and newborn infant caused by the administration of narcotics. It is also used to counteract respiratory depression when narcotics are employed preoperatively or postoperatively in the relief of pain, and to combat narcotic overdosage. If used in the absence of a narcotic-induced respiratory depression, levallorphan tartrate may *cause respiratory depression.* It is ineffective against the respiratory depression caused by barbiturates, anesthetics, other nonnarcotic agents, or diseased conditions. Levallorphan tartrate is contraindicated in mild respiratory depression and in narcotic addicts, since it may induce withdrawal symptoms. Adverse reactions include dysphoria, miosis, lethargy, dizziness, drowsiness, gastric upset and sweating. Pallor, nausea and a sense of heaviness in the limbs may occur. In high dosage, levallorphan tartrate may cause psychotomimetic manifestations, such as weird dreams, visual hallucinations, disorientation, and feelings of unreality.
Dose—*Intravenous,* **0.5 mg** (500 µg) to **2 mg,** repeated if necessary; *usual,* **1 mg,** followed by one or two **0.5 mg** doses at 10 and 15 minute intervals. *Neonatal respiratory depression,* secondary to narcotic administration to the mother, **0.05 to 0.1 mg** (approximately $\frac{1}{10}$ adult dose) into the umbilical cord vein immediately after delivery.
Dosage Forms—Injection: 1 mg/1 and 10 mL.

Nalorphine Hydrochloride

Morphinan-3,6-diol, 17-(2-propenyl)-7,8-didehydro-4,5-epoxy-, (5α,6α)-, hydrochloride; N-Allylmorphine Hydrochloride; Nalline Hydrochloride (*MSD*)

17-Allyl-7,8-didehydro-4,5α-epoxymorphinan-3,6α-diol hydrochloride [57-29-4] $C_{19}H_{21}NO_3$.HCl (347.84).
It is the N-allyl analogue of morphine. For the structure, see page 416.
Preparation—Commercially by allylation of normorphine (demethylmorphine).

Description—White or practically white, odorless, crystalline powder, slowly darkening on exposure to air and light; solutions are acid to litmus, having a pH of about 5; melting range 260° to 263°.
Solubility—1 g in about 8 mL water and about 35 mL alcohol; insoluble in chloroform and ether; soluble in diluted alkali hydroxide solution.

Uses—The prototype narcotic antagonist. Its pharmacological effects depend upon whether morphine or some related narcotic has previously been administered. In the nonmedicated individual, its effects resemble those of morphine and it is nearly as effective as morphine in relieving postoperative pain in human patients. Withdrawal following its chronic administration does not induce symptoms of abstinence.

The most useful property of nalorphine is its ability to antagonize many of the actions of morphine and related analgetics (meperidine, methadone, etc.). It is a *specific antidote in acute narcotic intoxication.* However, *naloxone* is preferred for this purpose. It is not effective against the respiratory depression produced by ether, cyclopropane, or barbiturate. Its use does not minimize the necessity for supportive therapy. When nalorphine (10 mg) is administered intravenously to narcotic-treated parturients a few minutes prior to delivery, neonatal respiratory depression is reduced. Alternatively, 0.2 mg may be injected into the umbilical vein after delivery.

Nalorphine also has diagnostic and experimental applications in the active narcotic addict. *Subcutaneous injection of 3 mg of nalorphine is usually sufficient to produce unequivocal evidence of physical dependence in the active addict not presenting symptoms of withdrawal at the time of examination.* If the signs of abstinence do not appear, additional increments of 5 and finally 8 mg may be injected at subsequent 20-min intervals. If withdrawal symptoms are severe, intravenous administration of a short-acting barbiturate may afford relief.

Nalorphine is listed in *Schedule III* of the *Controlled Substances Act.*
Dose—*Intravenous,* **2 to 10 mg**/dose; *usual,* **5 mg,** repeated 2 times at 3-min intervals if necessary.
Other Dose Information—The usual adult dose of 5 to 10 mg intravenously is repeated at intervals of 10 to 15 min until pulmonary ventilation is adequately increased. Excessive nalorphine may cause increased respiratory depression and total dosage should not exceed 40 mg.
Dosage Forms—Injection: 0.2 mg (200 µg) and 5 mg/mL, 10 mg/2 mL, 50 mg/10 mL.

Naloxone Hydrochloride

Morphinan-6-one, 4,5-epoxy-3,14-dihydroxy-17-(2-propenyl)-, (5α)-, hydrochloride, Narcan (*Endo*)

17-Allyl-4,5α-epoxy-3,14-dihydroxymorphinan-6-one hydrochloride [357-08-4] $C_{19}H_{21}NO_4$.HCl (363.84); *dihydrate* [51481-60-8] (399.87).
For the structure, see page 416.
Preparation—*Oxymorphone* (page 1105) is demethylated and the resulting 4,5α-epoxy-3,14-dihydroxymorphinan-6-one is N-allylated by reaction in ethanol with allyl bromide in the presence of $NaHCO_3$. The resulting naloxone is reacted with ethanolic HCl. US Pat 3,254,088.

Description—White to slightly off-white powder; aqueous solutions are acidic.
Solubility—Soluble in water; slightly soluble in alcohol; practically insoluble in chloroform and ether.
Incompatibilities—*Physical:* Long-chain or high-molecular-weight anions (forms relatively insoluble salts) and with alkaline solutions (base precipitates if concentration is high enough); however, injection is compatible with bulk IV solutions that are slightly alkaline. *Chemical:* Oxygen, oxidizing agents, bisulfites, and metabisulfites.

Uses—A synthetic congener of oxymorphone used as a narcotic antagonist essentially devoid of narcotic agonist properties. Hence, it does not possess morphine-like properties, such as respiratory depression, psychotomimetic effects, and pupillary constriction, characteristic of other narcotic antagonists. Naloxone hydrochloride is the drug of choice for management of respiratory depression induced by natural and synthetic narcotic analgesics, including depression induced by the partial agonist pentazocine. It is also indicated for diagnosis of acute narcotic overdosage. Naloxone hydrochloride is not effective against nonnarcotic respiratory depression. Naloxone rapidly disappears from serum in man. Following an intravenous dose naloxone is rapidly distributed in the body. The onset of activity is generally apparent within 2 minutes; the onset of action is only slightly less rapid when administered by the subcutaneous or intramuscular routes. The mean half-life in adults ranges from 30 to 81 minutes (mean 64 ± 12 minutes); the mean half-life in neonates is 3.1 ± 0.5 hours. It is metabolized in the liver, primarily by glucuronide conjugation, and excreted in the urine. This short duration of action necessitates multiple dosing and severely limits the value of naloxone. Hence, considerable research effort has been directed toward the development of antagonists with a much longer duration of action (*see Naltrexone* and *Nalbuphine,* following). Safe and effective use in children under 12 years of age and in pregnant women has not been established. Adverse effects are said to be rare and usually consist of nausea and vomiting. Naloxone is *unscheduled* under the *Controlled Substances Act.*
Dose—*Usual, parenteral,* **0.4 mg** (1 mL); if the desired level of response is not attained immediately, the same dose may be repeated at 2- or 3-min intervals. Lack of response after 2 or 3 injections suggests conditions may be due to other disease processes or nonnarcotic drugs. For postoperative respiratory depression caused by narcotic overdosage, *adults,* **0.1 to 0.2 mg** *intravenously* at 2- or 3-minute intervals until the desired effect is achieved. This dose may be repeated at one- or two-hour intervals as necessary. *Pediatric, intravenous,* **0.01 mg per kg** of body wt initially, repeated at 2- or 3-minute intervals as necessary. To reverse narcotic-induced respiratory depression in *newborn infants,* same as *pediatric, intravenous,* above.
Dosage Forms—Injection: 10-mL vials and 1-mL ampuls (0.4 mg/mL). Neonatal Injection: 0.02 mg/mL.

Other Opiate Antagonists

Cyclazocine [3-(Cyclopropylmethyl)-1,2,3,4,5,6-hexahydro-6,11-dimethyl-2,6-methano-3-benzocin-8-ol [3572-80-3] $C_{18}H_{25}NO$ (271.39); WIN 20,740]—An analogue of pentazocine, differing from the latter in having a cyclopropylmethyl substituent in place of 3-methyl-2-butenyl in the 3-position of the benzazocine nucleus common to both compounds. For synthesis of cyclazocine see *CA 58:* 2439c, 1963. Occurs as crystals melting at about 202°. *Uses:* A benzomorphan derivative 40 times more potent than morphine as an *analgesic.* It is also a potent morphine *antagonist.* The addiction potential of cyclazocine appears to be less than that of morphine, since in double-blind studies with former and current narcotic addicts the drug was identified less often than morphine as an opiate. Moreover, morphine produced twice the subjective feelings of elation. Cyclazocine is not yet available for general use.

Nalorphine Hydrobromide BP [$C_{19}H_{21}NO_3 \cdot HBr$]—White, crystalline powder; odorless; soluble in 24 parts of water and in 35 parts of alcohol. Its actions, uses, and dose are the same as for *Nalorphine Hydrochloride* (page 1106).

Naltrexone Hydrochloride [17-(Cyclopropylmethyl)-4,5α-epoxy-3,14-dihydroxymorphinan-6-one hydrochloride $C_{20}H_{23}NO_4 \cdot HCl$ (377.87) (*Endo*)]—Naltrexone, an analogue of nalbuphine (above), is an opiate *antagonist* suggested for use following methadone withdrawal to prevent relapse to heroin use. It is 17 times more potent than nalorphine as an antagonist in man. It is virtually devoid of agonistic activity, including ability to induce nalorphine-like dysphoric effects. Peak plasma levels one hour after a 100-mg oral dose are reported to be 43.6 ng/mL. Naltrexone has an apparent half-life of 96 hours. An oral 100-mg daily dose provides 2- to 3-day protection against a 25-mg intravenous heroin challenge. Thus its duration of action is longer than that of naloxone, but shorter than that of cyclazocine (above). Moreover, it is comparatively free of adverse effects, pharmacologic and metabolic tolerance, and abuse liabilities. It is currently under investigation for use in rehabilitation of well-motivated narcotic addicts.

Nonopiate Analgesics

The many undesirable side-actions of morphine and the dependence on the Mediterranean and Near East countries for opium stimulated the search for synthetic drugs as analgesic as morphine, but with fewer side-actions and less addiction liability. The ideal analgesic drug, as yet undiscovered but theoretically possible, conceivably could make morphine and other opium derivatives obsolete as analgesics.

It is generally agreed that an ideal analgesic drug should (1) not become ineffective through the development of tolerance, (2) not be habit-forming or addicting, (3) have a high ratio between the toxic dose and the effective analgesic dose, (4) be effective against all types of pain, (5) possess a short latent period and a long duration of action, (6) not alter sensory modalities, (7) not depress respiration or the cardiovascular system, (8) not affect the gastrointestinal tract, (9) be effective both orally and parenterally, and (10) be relatively inexpensive.

Since all the potent synthetic analgesics developed for clinical use are addicting, mimic some of the pharmacological properties of morphine, and are antagonized to some extent by nalorphine, it should be obvious that the ideal analgesic agent has yet to be developed. Nevertheless, currently available synthetic agents have valuable analgesic and pharmacological properties which are described in this section.

Alphaprodine Hydrochloride

4-Piperidinol, 1,3-dimethyl-4-phenyl-, *cis*-(±)-, propanoate (ester), hydrochloride, Nisentil Hydrochloride (*Roche*)

(±)-1,3-Dimethyl-4-phenyl-4-piperidinol propionate (ester) hydrochloride [14405-05-1; 49638-24-6] $C_{16}H_{23}NO_2 \cdot HCl$ (297.82).

Having two different centers of asymmetry the chemical exists in two diastereoisomeric forms which have come to be referred to commercially as the α and β forms. As the title indicates, it is the α form

which is official and the melting range provided identifies it as such.

Preparation—Under the influence of sodium ethoxide, the ethyl methyl ester of 2′-methyl-3,3′-(methylimino)dipropionic acid (I) undergoes intramolecular Claisen condensation to yield 1,3-dimethyl-4-piperidone (II). Reduction with lithium phenyl followed by hydrolysis yields the corresponding phenylated piperidinol which is esterified using propionic acid anhydride.

Description—White, crystalline powder; has a slight odor; melts between 218° and 220°.

Solubility—1 g in 2 mL water, 7 mL alcohol, 3 mL chloroform, 4700 mL ether.

Uses—A synthetic narcotic analgesic chemically similar to meperidine. Its analgesic potency is intermediate to that of morphine and meperidine, but its action is more prompt and of shorter duration. Following intravenous administration, analgesia appears within 1 or 2 minutes, with peak activity of 5 to 7 minutes and duration of $\frac{1}{2}$ to 1 hour. The volume of distribution is about 1.9 L/kg and elimination half-life 131 minutes. Subcutaneous administration provides analgesia within 5 to 10 minutes, with duration of action of approximately 2 hours. It is suited primarily for temporary analgesia in obstetrics, for urological examinations, for preoperative use in surgery and for minor surgical procedures, especially in orthopedics, ophthalmology, rhinology and laryngology, renal or biliary colic, and cardiovascular pain. The depressant effects of alphaprodine hydrochloride are potentiated by barbiturates, general anesthetic agents, and some phenothiazines. Thus, the dose should be reduced when used concomitantly with such agents. As with other narcotic analgesics, it should be used with caution in patients with increased intracranial pressure, hepatic insufficiency, severe CNS depression, myxedema, acute alcoholism, convulsive disorders, and in patients on MAO inhibitors. It should not be used in chronic pain, because its short duration of action requires frequent administration and enhances the possibility of addiction. Adverse effects include occasional respiratory depression, dizziness, drowsiness, sweating and urticaria; rarely, nausea, vomiting, restlessness, and confusion may occur. Alphaprodine hydrochloride is listed in *Schedule II* of the *Controlled Substances Act.* Tolerance and addiction may develop.

Dose—*Usual, adult, intravenous*, **400 to 600 µg** (0.4 to 0.6 mg) **per kg** of body weight; the initial intravenous dose should not exceed 30 mg; *subcutaneous*, **400 µg** (0.4 mg) to **1.2 mg per kg** of body weight; the initial subcutaneous dose should not exceed 60 mg. Maximal dose is 240 mg in 24 hours. *Usual, pediatric,* not established.

Dosage Forms—Injection: 40 and 60 mg/mL, 600 mg/10 mL.

Butorphanol Tartrate

Morphinan-3,14-diol, 17-(cyclobutylmethyl)-, (−)-, [R(R*,R*)]-2,3-dihydroxybutanedioate (1:1) salt; Stadol (*Bristol*)

(−)-17-(Cyclobutylmethyl)morphinan-3,14-diol tartrate (1:1) salt [54965-23-0] $C_{21}H_{29}NO_2 \cdot C_4H_6O_6$ (477.55).

Preparation—Total synthesis of *N*-substituted 3,14-dihydroxymorphinans, including butorphanol, from 7-methoxy-1-tetralone, has been reported by Monković *et al* (*J Am Chem Soc 95:* 7910, 1973).

Description—White, crystalline powder.
Solubility—Soluble in water.

Uses—A synthetic opioid *parenteral analgesic* with properties similar to those of pentazocine, but without demonstrated advantages over other narcotic analgesics. It is indicated for moderate to severe postsurgical pain. After intramuscular injection, analgesia begins within 10 minutes, reaches peak activity in 30 to 60 minutes, and persists for 3 to 4 hours. After intravenous administration, peak activity is reached within a few minutes. A 2-mg intramuscular dose of butorphanol tartrate is equivalent in analgesic effect to 10 mg of morphine. Adverse effects observed are similar to those observed after morphine, including dizziness, lightheadedness, and nausea. Transient but disturbing psychotomimetic reactions have been reported after doses of 2 to 4 mg. Two mg of butorphanol tartrate depresses the respiration to the same extent as 10 mg of morphine; slow, shallow respiration has been reported in patients taking recommended doses of the drug. The respiratory depression and other effects of butorphanol tartrate can be reversed by naloxone. Like pentazocine, the drug increases arterial resistance and the work of the heart; consequently, it is contraindicated in patients with acute myocardial infarction. Butorphanol tartrate is known to cause euphoria, and tolerance to the analgesic effect has been reported in animals. It is an *unscheduled drug* under the *Controlled Substances Act.*

Dose—*Usual, adult, intramuscular,* **2 mg** every 3 to 4 hours; *usual, dose range,* **1** to **4 mg.** *Usual intravenous,* **1 mg** every 3 or 4 hours; *usual dose range,* **0.5** to **2 mg** every 3 or 4 hours.

Dosage Forms—Injection: 1 or 2 mg/mL.

Fentanyl Citrate

Propanamide, N-phenyl-N-[1-(2-phenylethyl)-4-piperidinyl]-, 2-hydroxy-1,2,3-propanetricarboxylate (1:1); Sublimaze, ing of Innovar (*McNeil*)

N-(1-Phenethyl-4-piperidyl)propionanilide citrate (1:1) [990-73-8] $C_{22}H_{28}N_2O.C_6H_8O_7$ (528.60).

Preparation—One method consists of condensing propionyl chloride with N-(4-piperidyl)aniline, then condensing the resulting N-(4-piperidyl)propionanilide with phenethyl chloride, aiding each condensation by the presence of a suitable dehydrochlorinating agent. Reaction of the base with an equimolar portion of citric acid yields the (1:1) citrate. US Pat 3,164,600.

Description—White, crystalline powder or glistening crystals that are odorless and tasteless (*Note:* because this compound is extremely potent, no taste test is recommended); stable in air; melts between 147° and 152°; pK_a 8.3.

Solubility—1 g in about 40 mL water, 140 mL alcohol, and 350 mL chloroform.

Uses—A potent narcotic analgesic with rapid onset and short duration of action. It has a profile of pharmacologic action similar to morphine, except that it does not cause emesis or release histamine. Equianalgesia can be obtained with a dose $\frac{1}{150}$ that of morphine. After intravenous injection, peak analgesia appears within 3 to 5 min and lasts 30 to 60 min. Fentanyl produces signs and symptoms typical of narcotic analgesics, such as miosis, euphoria, and respiratory depression. Fentanyl is used primarily as an analgesic for the control of pain associated with all types of surgery. It can also be used as a supplement to all agents commonly employed for general and regional anesthesia. It is also an ingredient in *Fentanyl Citrate and Droperidol Injection*, page 1045. Fentanyl is contraindicated in children 2 years of age and younger, in asthmatic patients, and in patients with a history of myasthenia gravis. Other depressant drugs, such as barbiturates, major tranquilizers, tricyclic antidepressants, monoamine oxidase inhibitors, narcotics, and general anesthetics have an additive or potentiating effect on fentanyl citrate. Its safe use in pregnancy has not been established. Fentanyl crosses the placental barrier; use during labor may lead to respiratory depression in the newborn infant. Fentanyl citrate should be used with caution in patients with liver and kidney disease. Adverse reactions include respiratory depression, apnea, muscular rigidity, and hypotension. Less frequently, nausea and vomiting may occur. Infrequently, dizziness, visual disturbance, itching, euphoria, and spasms of the sphincter of Oddi have been observed. Fentanyl citrate is listed in *Schedule II* of the *Controlled Substances Act.*

Dose—*Usual, intramuscular,* as part of preoperative medication, **0.05** to **0.1 mg** 30 to 60 min prior to operation. For prompt analgesia

during induction, 0.05 to 0.1 mg intravenously, repeated at 2- to 3-min intervals until desired effect is achieved; dosage reduced to 0.025 to 0.05 mg in poor-risk and in very young and very old patients. For maintenance of analgesia during anesthesia, 0.025 to 0.05 mg intravenously. For control of postoperative pain, restlessness, and tachypnea, 0.05 to 0.1 mg intramuscularly; repeated in 1 to 2 hours as needed.

Dosage Forms—Injection: 0.05 mg/mL, in 2- and 5-mL ampuls (base equivalent).

Meperidine Hydrochloride

4-Piperidinecarboxylic acid, 1-methyl-4-phenyl-, ethyl ester, hydrochloride; Pethidine Hydrochloride; Dolantin, Dolantol, Eudolat, Isonipecaine; Demerol Hydrochloride (*Winthrop*)

Ethyl 1-methyl-4-phenylisonipecotate hydrochloride [50-13-5] $C_{15}H_{21}NO_2.HCl$ (283.80).

Preparation—One of several methods utilizes benzyl chloride, diethanolamine, and benzyl cyanide in the following principal steps:

Removal of the N-benzyl group is accomplished by catalytic hydrogenation in acetic acid solution using a palladium catalyst. The addition of formaldehyde to the reduction mixture followed by further catalytic hydrogenation leads to meperidine. The free base is converted to the hydrochloride by neutralization with HCl.

Description—Fine, white, crystalline, odorless powder; stable in air at ordinary temperatures; 1 in 20 solution is acid to litmus (pH about 5); melting range 186° to 189°; pK_a 7.7 to 8.15.

Solubility—Very soluble in water; soluble in alcohol; sparingly soluble in ether.

Uses—A synthetic narcotic analgesic with multiple actions qualitatively similar to those of morphine; the most prominent of these actions are on the CNS and on organs composed of smooth muscle. It acts principally to induce analgesia and sedation. Meperidine hydrochloride is indicated for preoperative use, relief of moderate to severe pain, support anesthesia, and for obstetrical analgesia. Meperidine crosses the placental barrier; use during labor may lead to respiratory depression in the newborn infant. Available evidence suggests it produces less smooth muscle spasm, constipation, and depression of cough reflex than equianalgesic doses of morphine. Meperidine hydrochloride in a 60- to 80-mg parenteral dose is essentially equal in analgesic effectiveness to 10 mg of morphine; the onset of action is slightly more rapid and the duration of action somewhat shorter than morphine. Meperidine hydrochloride is significantly less effective by the oral than by the parenteral route. Following intravenous administration of meperidine in healthy adults, the volume distribution at steady state was 269 L; plasma clearance was 1.06 L/min, and elimination half-life was 3.6 hours. There is evidence that the disposition of meperidine varies between day and night, with elimination half-life shorter and plasma clearance greater at night. Meperidine is contraindicated in patients on MAO inhibitors or who have received such agents within 14 days; meperidine has inconsistently precipitated severe and occasionally fatal reactions in patients who have received such medication within 14 days. Meperidine should be used with caution and in reduced dosage in patients on other narcotic analgesics, general anesthetics, phenothiazines, sedatives, tricyclic antidepressants, and other CNS depressants. Major adverse reactions include respiratory depression, circulatory depression, respiratory arrest, shock, and cardiac arrest. The most frequent untoward effects include dizziness, sedation, nausea, vomiting, and sweating. Other adverse reactions include euphoria, weakness, headache, agitation, tremor, transient hallucinations and disorientation. Other effects involving the gastrointestinal tract, cardiovascular system, and genitourinary tract are similar to morphine. Analgesia is possible with doses which do not cause stupefaction, a decided advantage over morphine. Pain is usually relieved within 20 minutes to 1 hour, analgesia lasting from 2 to 5 hours.

Naloxone is a specific antagonist in cases of acute meperidine intoxication.

Caution—Meperidine is a narcotic listed in *Schedule II* of the *Controlled Substances Act.*

Dose—*Oral* and *parenteral, adults, usual,* **50** to **150 mg** every three or four hours as necessary; *usual range of dose,* **50 mg** to **1.2 g** a day. *Children, oral,* **1.1** to **1.76 mg per kg** body wt, not to exceed adult dose, 6 to 8 times a day as necessary.

Dosage Forms—Injection: 25, 50, 75, and 100 mg/mL; multiple dose vials: 50 mg/mL in 30 mL vials, 100 mg/mL in 20 mL vials. Syrup: 50 mg/5 mL; Tablets: 50 and 100 mg.

Methadone Hydrochloride

3-Heptanone, 6-(dimethylamino)-4,4-diphenyl-, hydrochloride; Amidone Hydrochloride; Dolophine Hydrochloride (*Lilly*)

6-(Dimethylamino)-4,4-diphenyl-3-heptanone hydrochloride [1095-90-5] $C_{21}H_{27}NO.HCl$ (345.91).

Preparation—Diphenylacetonitrile is condensed with 2-chloro-1-dimethylaminopropane in the presence of sodamide, yielding 4-(dimethylamino)-2,2-diphenylvaleronitrile and an unwanted isomeric nitrile in approximately equal amounts. The isomers are separated and the former is subjected to Grignard addition with ethyl magnesium bromide. Subsequent hydrolysis in the presence of hydrochloric acid yields methadone hydrochloride.

Description—Colorless crystals or a white, crystalline, odorless powder; pH (1 in 100 solution) between 4.5 and 6.5; optically inactive (the official salt is a racemic mixture of which only the levo form has analgetic activity).

Solubility—1 g in 13 mL water, 8 mL alcohol, 3 mL chloroform; practically insoluble in ether and glycerin.

Uses—A synthetic *narcotic analgesic* with multiple actions quantitatively similar to morphine, the most prominent of which involve the CNS and organs composed of smooth muscle. The principal actions of therapeutic value are those of *analgesia, sedation,* and *detoxification* or *temporary maintenance* in narcotic addiction. Methadone also has significant *antitussive* properties. It is rapidly but probably incompletely absorbed after oral administration, since only 52% of a given dose appears in the urine. Mean plasma levels

of 182 and 420 ng/mL have been reported in patients maintained on a daily oral dose of 40 and 80 mg, respectively, 71 to 87% of which is in bound form. The half-life is approximately 25 hours, with a range of 13 to 47 hours. A parenteral dose of 8 to 10 mg is approximately equivalent in analgesic effectiveness to 10 mg of morphine; onset and duration of action of the two drugs are similar. Methadone is approximately ½ as potent orally as parenterally. It is indicated for the relief of moderate to severe pain, for detoxification treatment of narcotic addiction, and for temporary maintenance treatment of narcotic addiction. If methadone is administered for heroin treatment for more than three weeks, the procedure passes from treatment of the acute withdrawal syndrome (detoxification) to maintenance therapy; the latter use can be undertaken *only* in approved programs, unless the addict is hospitalized for conditions other than addiction. The methadone abstinence syndrome is qualitatively similar to that of morphine; however, the onset is slower, the course is more prolonged, and the symptoms less severe. Methadone can produce drug dependence of the morphine type; therefore, it should be prescribed and administered with the same degree of caution as morphine. Methadone is contraindicated in patients known to be sensitive to it. Methadone should be used with caution and in reduced dosage in patients on other narcotic analgesics, general anesthetics, phenothiazine and other tranquilizers, sedative-hypnotics, tricyclic antidepressants, monoamine oxidase inhibitors and CNS depressants; respiratory depression, hypotension, profound sedation or coma may result. Patients on a methadone maintenance program should not be given pentazocine or rifampin; these drugs may induce withdrawal symptoms. The safe use of methadone in pregnancy has not been established. It is not recommended for obstetrical analgesia, because its long duration may induce respiratory depression in the newborn. Adverse reactions are similar to those for other narcotic analgesics (see especially *Meperidine*).

Methadone is widely employed in the withdrawal management of patients addicted to morphine, heroin, and related narcotic drugs.

Naloxone is an effective antagonist in cases of acute methadone intoxication. Methadone is listed as a *Schedule II* drug.

Dose—*Analgesic: oral, intramuscular* or *subcutaneous, adults,* **2.5** to **10 mg** 6 to 8 times a day as necessary; *usual range of dose,* **15** to **80 mg** a day. *Children,* **0.175 mg/kg** 4 times a day as necessary. *Narcotic withdrawal management: adults, oral* for *detoxification,* 15 to 40 mg once a day, the dosage being decreased according to patient response; for *maintenance,* **40** to **120 mg** once daily.

Dosage Forms—Injection: 10 mg/mL and 200 mg/20 mL; Syrup: 10 mg/30 mL. Tablets: 5 and 10 mg; Dispersible Tablets: 40 mg; Oral Solution: 1 mg/mL.

Nalbuphine Hydrochloride

Morphinan-3,6,14-triol, 17-(cyclobutylmethyl)-4,5-epoxy-, hydrochloride, (5α,6α)-, Nubain (*Endo*)

[23277-43-2] $C_{21}H_{27}NO_4.HCl$ (393.91)
Preparation—Refer to US Pat 3,393,197.

Description—(Base)white crystals melting about 230°.

Uses—For the relief of moderate to severe pain. It may also be used for preoperative analgesia, as a supplement to surgical anesthesia, and for obstetrical analgesia during labor. Nalbuphine is related chemically to oxymorphone and the opiod antagonist, naloxone. It possesses both agonist and antagonist properties. Thus, it resembles pentazocine pharmacologically. The analgesic potency of parenteral nalbuphine on a milligram basis is approximately the same as that of morphine and about 3 to 4 times greater than that for pentazocine; its antagonistic potency is about ten times greater than that of pentazocine. The onset of action occurs within 2 to 3 minutes after intravenous administration and within 15 minutes after intramuscular or subcutaneous administration; the duration of effect is 3 to 6 hours. Adverse reactions induced by nalbuphine are the same as those for morphine and other potent analgesics (see page 1100). Those most frequently observed include sedation (56%) sweaty/

clammy (9%), nausea and vomiting (6%), dizziness and vertigo (5%), dry mouth (4%), and headache (3%). Respiratory depression may occur with usual doses of nalbuphine, but is not dose related. Naloxone reverses the respiratory depressant effect. The abrupt withdrawal of nalbuphine following prolonged administration causes opiate-like abstinence symptoms which are milder than those of morphine but more intense than those of pentazocine. Although nalbuphine possesses narcotic antagonist activity, there is evidence that in *nondependent* patients it will not antagonize a narcotic analgesic administered just before, concurrently with, or just after an injection of the drug. Therefore, patients receiving narcotic analgesics, general anesthetics, phenothiazines, other sedatives, hypnotics, or CNS depressants concomitantly with nalbuphine may exhibit additive effects. Thus, the dose of one or both agents should be reduced. Clinical experience to support use in children under 18 years of age is not presently available.

Dose—*Usual, adult, parenteral* (all routes), **10 mg/70 kg**, repeated every 3 to 6 hours as necessary. Dosage should be adjusted according to the severity of the pain, physical status of the patient, and other medications the patient may be receiving.

Dosage Forms—Injection: 10 mg/mL.

Pentazocine

2,6-Methano-3-benzazocin-8-ol, 1,2,3,4,5,6-hexahydro-6,11-dimethyl-3-(3-methyl-2-butenyl)-, $(2\alpha,6\alpha,11R*)$-, Talwin (*Winthrop*)

$(2R*,6R*,11R*)$-1,2,3,4,5,6-Hexahydro-6,11-dimethyl-3-(3-methyl-2-butenyl)-2,6-methano-3-benzazocin-8-ol [359-83-1] $C_{19}H_{27}NO$ (285.43).

Preparation—1,2,3,4,5,6-Hexahydro-6,11-dimethyl-2,6-methano-3-benzazocin-8-ol (I) is condensed with 1-bromo-3-methyl-2-butene by refluxing in N,N-dimethylformamide in the presence of sodium bicarbonate. The reaction mixture is filtered and the crude pentazocine is isolated by means of a suitable solvent extraction process and finally crystallized from aqueous methanol. US Pat 3,250,678.

Compound I may be prepared by the following sequence of reactions: 3,4-dimethylpyridine methiodide is converted to 1,3,4-trimethyl-2-(p-methoxybenzyl)-1,2-dihydropyridine with p-methoxybenzylmagnesium chloride, reduced to 1,3,4-trimethyl-2-(p-methoxybenzyl)-1,2,5,6-tetrahydropyridine with sodium borohydride, cyclized (with H_3PO_4 or HBr) to 1,2,3,4,5,6-hexahydro-3,6,11-trimethyl-2,6-methano-3-benzazocin-8-ol, esterified with acetic anhydride and reacted with cyanogen bromide to form 3-cyano-1,2,3,4,5,6-hexahydro-6,11-dimethyl-2,6-methano-3-benzazocin-8-ol acetate, and hydrolyzed with dilute HCl to compound I.

Description—White to very pale tan, crystalline powder that is odorless and has a slightly bitter taste; stable in light, heat (ambient room temperature), and air; melts between 147° and 158°; pK$_a$ about 8.95.

Solubility—1 g in >1000 mL water, 11 mL alcohol, 2 mL chloroform, 42 mL ether.

Uses—A synthetic *analgesic* agent. When administered orally in a 50-mg dose it appears to be equivalent in analgesic effectiveness to 60 mg of codeine. Significant analgesia occurs within 15 to 30 min after oral administration, 15 to 20 min after intramuscular injection, and 2 to 3 min after intravenous administration. Duration of action is usually 3 hours or longer. Half-life after intramuscular administration is 2.1 hours. Onset, duration of action, and degree of pain relief are related both to dose and the severity of pretreatment pain. Pentazocine weakly (about $\frac{1}{50}$ that of nalorphine) antagonizes the analgesic effect of morphine, meperidine, and phenazocine. It also produces incomplete reversal of the cardiovascular, respiratory, and behavioral depression induced by morphine and meperidine. It also has some sedative properties. Pentazocine is indicated for the control of moderate to severe pain. It is contraindicated in patients hypersensitive to it. Pentazocine should be used with caution in patients with head injuries and increased intracranial pressure; except during labor, its use during pregnancy has not been established; because of limited experience in children under 12 years of age, its use in this age group is not recommended; patients on the drug should be warned not to drive an automobile, operate machinery, or expose themselves

to hazards; and while some patients on therapeutic doses exhibit acute CNS manifestations (hallucinations, disorientation, and confusion), such instances are rare and usually clear spontaneously.

Adverse effects reported include: gastrointestinal (nausea, vomiting, diarrhea, infrequent constipation, and abdominal distress); CNS (dizziness, light-headedness, sedation, euphoria, headache, disturbed dreams, insomnia, syncope, visual blurring, and hallucinations); autonomic (sweating, flushing, and chills); allergic (rash, urticaria, and edema of the face); cardiovascular effects (hypotension and tachycardia); rarely, respiratory depression and urinary retention.

Pentazocine has been reported to cause psychological and physical dependence after both oral and parenteral use. This is more common in patients with a history of drug abuse. It is listed under *Schedule IV* of the *Controlled Substances Act*.

Dose—*Parenteral*, **20 to 60 mg** (as the lactate); *usual*, **30 mg** every 3 to 4 hours. Maximum daily dose, **360 mg.**

Dosage Forms—Lactate Injection: 30 mg (of base)/mL; Tablets: 50 mg.

Pentazocine Hydrochloride

2,6-Methano-3-benzazocin-8-ol, 1,2,3,4,5,6-hexahydro-6,11-dimethyl-3-(3-methyl-2-butenyl)-, hydrochloride, $(2\alpha,6\alpha\text{-}11R*)$-, Talwin Hydrochloride (*Winthrop*)

$(2R*,6R*,11R*)$-1,2,3,4,5,6-Hexahydro-6,11-dimethyl-3-(3-methyl-2-butenyl)-2,6-methano-3-benzazocin-8-ol hydrochloride [64024-15-3] $C_{19}H_{27}NO\cdot HCl$ (321.89).

For the structure of the base, see *Pentazocine*.

Preparation—*Pentazocine* is reacted with HCl.

Description—White, crystalline powder; it exhibits polymorphism, one form melting at about 254° and the other at about 218°.

Solubility—1 g in 30 mL water, 7 mL alcohol, >10,000 mL chloroform, 3 mL ether.

Uses—See *Pentazocine*.

Dose (base equivalent)—*Usual*, **50 mg** every 3 to 4 hours; may be increased to **100 mg** when needed. Total daily dose should not exceed **600 mg.**

Dosage Forms—Tablets: 50 mg. Pentazocine Hydrochloride and Aspirin (Tablets), equivalent to 12.5 and 325 mg, respectively.

Analgesics and Antipyretics

The analgesic and antipyretic drugs include a small, heterogeneous group of compounds which, unlike those presented in the two preceding sections, are without significant addiction liability, and therefore are not subject to regulation under the *Controlled Substances Act*. Most of these agents affect both pain and fever. Consequently, they are widely used for minor aches and pains, headaches, and the general feeling of malaise that accompanies febrile illnesses, and to alleviate symptoms of rheumatic fever, arthritis, gout, and other musculoskeletal disturbances. Several agents (allopurinol, colchicine, probenecid, etc) are included for their pain-relieving properties in various conditions (gout, arthritis, etc), but since they are of no value in other types of pain, they cannot be classed as true analgesic drugs.

The salicylate group of analgesics and antipyretics are by far the most commonly employed. Indeed, these are consumed at a rate in excess of 10,000 tons annually. In general, salicylates are *contraindicated* in hypersensitive individuals and in those with gastrointestinal disturbances, particularly hemorrhaging ulcers. They should also be used with caution in patients on anticoagulant therapy and avoided in patients on uricosurics. The *salicylates interact* with a wide variety of agents, some of which are clinically important while others are largely of theoretical interest. Nevertheless, the well-informed pharmacist will acquaint himself with the potential interactions between salicylate drugs and antidiabetic agents (increased hypoglycemia), oral anticoagulants (displacement of anticoagulants from protein binding sites, increased anticoagulant effect), uricosuric agents (relative effect of large and small doses of salicylates), antiarthritic drugs (may lower plasma concentrations of these agents), and the effect of salicylates on alcohol (the latter enhances gastrointestinal bleeding), tetracycline (may complex with buffering agent in some aspirin products) and other drugs (see Chapter 102).

Acetaminophen

Acetamide, *N*-(4-hydroxyphenyl)-, *N*-Acetyl-*p*-aminophenol; *p*-Acetamidophenol; Tylenol (*McNeil*); (*Various Mfrs*)

HO—⟨○⟩—NHCOCH₃

4'-Hydroxyacetanilide [103-90-2] $C_8H_9NO_2$ (151.16).

Preparation—*p*-Nitrophenol is reduced and the resulting *p*-aminophenol is acetylated by heating with a mixture of acetic anhydride and glacial acetic acid. The crude product may be purified by recrystallization from an ethanol–water mixture or from other suitable solvents.

Description—White, odorless, crystalline powder, possessing a slightly bitter taste; melts between 168° and 172°; pH (saturated solution) between 5.3 and 6.5; pK_a 9.51.

Solubility—1 g in 70 mL water, 20 mL boiling water, 10 mL alcohol, 50 mL chloroform, 40 mL glycerin; slightly soluble in ether.

Uses—A metabolite of phenacetin and acetanilid used as an analgesic and antipyretic. It is effective in a wide variety of arthritic and rheumatic conditions involving musculoskeletal pain as well as the pain of headache, dysmenorrhea, myalgias, and neuralgias. Acetaminophen is particularly useful as an analgesic-antipyretic in patients sensitive to aspirin and who experience other untoward reactions to aspirin. It rarely induces untoward effects and is usually well tolerated by aspirin-sensitive patients. Rarely, a sensitivity reaction may occur; in this case the drug should be stopped. Acetaminophen lacks the anti-inflammatory action of aspirin; hence, it is of only limited usefulness in inflammatory rheumatic disorders. It does not produce the methemoglobinemia, agranulocytosis, and anemia which sometimes result from long-continued use of acetanilid and phenacetin. Unlike aspirin, acetaminophen does not antagonize the effects of uricosuric agents. Although large doses have been reported to potentiate anticoagulants, small doses have no effect on prothrombin time.

Absorption of acetaminophen after oral administration is rapid and peak plasma levels are reached in 70 to 160 minutes. The therapeutic half-life is approximately 3 hours. Approximately 2% is excreted unchanged in the urine; the glucuronide and sulfate conjugates are nontoxic and account for about 95% of the drug. A much smaller amount, estimated to be 3%, is oxidized via the hepatic cytochrome P-450 system to a chemically reactive intermediate which combines with liver glutathione to form a nontoxic substance. However, after massive single doses of acetaminophen the supply of liver glutathione is exhausted and the excess reactive arylating intermediate covalently binds to vital hepatocellular macromolecules, leading to necrosis. Hepatic necrosis and death have been observed following overdosage; hepatic damage is likely if an adult takes more than 10 grams in a single dose or if a 2-year-old child takes more than 3 grams. Both *in vivo* and *in vitro* studies have shown that agents which stimulate metabolism, such as phenobarbital and phenytoin, potentiate acetaminophen-induced hepatotoxicity. The best indicator of potential liver injury is the half-life of acetaminophen elimination. A half-life greater than 4 hours is uniformly associated with liver injury. Also, plasma levels greater than 300 µg/mL at 4 hours post-ingestion are consistent with liver injury, whereas levels less than 120 µg/mL at 4 hours post-ingestion are usually not. Treatment of overdosage is largely supportive; no specific therapy is available.

The label on acetaminophen dosage forms carries the following (or equivalent) statement: *Warning—Do not give to children under 6 years of age or use more than 10 days unless directed by a physician. Keep this medication out of reach of children.*

Dose—*Usual, adult, oral*, **300 mg** to **1 g** 3 or 4 times a day. *Usual, pediatric, oral*, **175 mg per square meter** of body surface 4 times a day; or **60 mg** 3 or 4 times a day for children under 1 year of age, **60** to **120 mg** 3 or 4 times a day for children 1 to 2 years of age, **120 mg** 3 or 4 times a day for children 3 to 5 years of age, **150** to **325 mg** 3 or 4 times a day for children 6 to 12 years of age.

Dosage Forms—Capsules: 325 and 500 mg; Drops: 100 mg/mL and 120 mg/2.5 mL; Elixir: 120, 160, and 325 mg/5 mL; Liquid: 165 mg/5 mL; Suppositories: 120, 125, 325, and 650 mg; Syrup: 120 mg/5 mL; Tablets: 300, 325, 500, and 650 mg; Chewable Tablets: 80 mg; Wafers: 120 mg. *Acetaminophen and Codeine Phosphate*—Capsules: 325 mg acetaminophen with 15, 30, or 60 mg codeine phosphate; Oral Suspension: 125 mg acetaminophen with 12 mg codeine phosphate/5 mL; Tablets: 325 mg acetaminophen with 8, 15, 30, or 60 mg codeine phosphate.

Allopurinol

4*H*-Pyrazolo[3,4-*d*]pyrimidin-4-one, 1,5-dihydro-, Zyloprim (*Burroughs-Wellcome*)

[315-30-0] $C_5H_4N_4O$ (136.11).

Preparation—(Ethoxymethylene)malononitrile is reacted with hydrazine hydrate via deethanolation and addition thus cyclizing to form 3-aminopyrazole-4-carbonitrile. Controlled hydration of the nitrile forms the corresponding carboxamide which, on condensation with formamide, yields allopurinol. US Pat 2,868,803.

Description—Fluffy white to off-white powder which has only a slight odor and is tasteless; stable in light and air; melts above 300° with decomposition.

Solubility—Very slightly soluble in water and alcohol; soluble in solutions of fixed alkali hydroxides; practically insoluble in chloroform and ether.

Uses—A structural analogue of hypoxanthine used in the *treatment of gout*, primary or secondary *uric acid nephropathy*, *uric acid stone formation*, and to prevent urate deposition, renal calculi, or uric acid nephropathy in patients with leukemias, lymphomas, and malignancies who are receiving cancer chemotherapy with its resultant effect of increasing serum uric acid levels. It is not an analgesic *per se*; relief from pain is secondary to the reduction in blood uric acid levels. Allopurinol is not uricosuric; it inhibits the production of uric acid by blocking the biochemical reactions immediately preceding uric acid formation. Thus, it inhibits xanthine oxidase, the enzyme responsible for the conversion of hypoxanthine to xanthine and of xanthine to uric acid. In addition, allopurinol inhibits *de novo* purine synthesis by a feedback mechanism, which provides another benefit to the patient. Allopurinol is metabolized by xanthine oxidase to oxypurinol, which also inhibits xanthine oxidase. Oxypurinol has a much longer half-clearance time from plasma than allopurinol (18 to 30 hours and less than 2 hours, respectively). This accounts for its long duration of action and permits use of a single daily dose. Allopurinol is contraindicated in children (except those with hyperuricemia secondary to malignancy), and in nursing mothers; also contraindicated in patients who develop a severe reaction to the drug. A few cases of reversible hepatotoxicity have been observed; hence, periodic liver function studies should be done during the early stages of therapy. Allopurinol should not be given concomitantly with iron salts, since laboratory studies suggest increased hepatic iron concentration may occur. Moreover, allopurinol increases the effect of the oral anticoagulants and enhances the toxicity of azathioprine, cyclophosphamide, and mercaptopurine by decreasing the rate at which these agents are metabolized. It is particularly useful in patients who are resistant to or cannot tolerate uricosuric drugs and in patients with renal function so reduced as to not respond to conventional drugs. Allopurinol precipitates acute gouty arthritis in early therapy more frequently than uricosuric drugs. This can be minimized by giving maintenance doses of colchicine and by starting therapy on a small dose and increasing the dose gradually. Untoward effects include a rash, usually maculopapular; less frequently exfoliative, urticarial, or purpuric; the rash may be accompanied by fever, leukopenia, arthralgias, or other symptoms of hypersensitivity. Diarrhea is frequently observed. Isolated cases of peripheral neuritis, depression of the bone marrow, cataracts, and reversible hepatic damage have been reported.

Dose—**100** to **800 mg** daily; *usual, adult, oral, antigout*, **100** to **200 mg** 2 or 3 times a day; *oral, anti-urolithic*, **200 mg** 1 to 4 times a day. *Pediatric*, for use in *secondary hyperuricemia* associated with malignancies, children under 5 years of age, *oral*, **50 mg** 3 times a day; children 6 to 10 years of age, *oral*, **100 mg** 3 times a day.

Dosage Forms—Tablets: 100 and 300 mg.

Aspirin

Benzoic acid, 2-(acetyloxy)-,

Acetylsalicylic acid [50-78-2] $C_9H_8O_4$ (180.16).

Preparation—Salicylic acid is acetylated directly with acetic anhydride and the crude material is purified by recrystallization from benzene or various other nonaqueous solvents. A granulated form of aspirin, either white or colored, is also available commercially for compression into tablets.

Description—White crystals, commonly tabular or needle-like, or a white, crystalline powder; odorless or has a faint odor and is stable in dry air, but in moist air it gradually hydrolyzes into salicylic and acetic acids, the odor of the latter becoming noticeable; melts at about 135°, but the exact melting temperature varies with the conditions of the test; an alcoholic solution is not colored violet by ferric chloride (distinction from salicylic acid).

Solubility—1 g in about 300 mL water, 5 mL alcohol, 17 mL chloroform, and from 10 to 15 mL ether; less soluble in absolute ether; dissolves with decomposition in aqueous solutions of alkali hydroxides and carbonates.

Incompatibilities—Can form a damp to pasty mass when triturated with *acetanilid, acetophenetidin, antipyrine, aminopyrine, methenamine, phenol,* or *salol.* Powders containing aspirin with an alkali salt such as *sodium bicarbonate* may become gummy on contact with atmospheric moisture due to a partial solution and subsequent hydrolysis of the aspirin. Hydrolysis likewise occurs in admixture with salts containing water of crystallization. Solutions of alkali acetates and citrates, as well as alkalies themselves, dissolve aspirin, but the resulting solutions hydrolyze rapidly to form salts of acetic and salicylic acids. Sugar and glycerin have been shown to hinder the decomposition. Aspirin very slowly liberates hydriodic acid from *potassium* or *sodium iodide.* Subsequent oxidation by the air produces free iodine.

Uses—Aspirin, as well as the salts of salicylic acid (for example, sodium salicylate), is employed as an *antipyretic* and *analgetic* in a variety of conditions. It is indicated for the relief of pain from simple headache, discomfort and fever associated with the common cold, and minor muscular aches and pains. When drug therapy is indicated for the reduction of a fever, aspirin is one of the most effective and safest drugs. Epidemiological evidence has suggested the possibility of an association between the use of aspirin in the treatment of fever in children with varicella (chickenpox) or influenza virus infections and the subsequent development of Reye's syndrome. The current opinion of the Committee on Infectious Diseases of the Academy of Pediatrics is that "aspirin should not be prescribed under usual circumstances for children with varicella or those suspected of having influenza" (*Pediatrics 69:* 810–812, 1982). If control of fever is necessary alternative measures should be employed. Because aspirin inhibits platelet function, it has been used prophylactically to reduce the incidence of *myocardial infarction* and *transcient ischemic attacks.* In *gout* and in *acute rheumatic fever,* the salicylates, including aspirin, have a fairly specific action. In gout, large doses must be given fairly often, and the results obtained are somewhat less dramatic than with phenylbutazone or allopurinol. In acute rheumatic fever, full doses are given every hour until salicylism occurs (ringing in ears, dizziness), and then every 4 hours for days or weeks. In neither of the above-mentioned conditions are the salicylates a cure, and other forms of treatment are simultaneously employed. Following oral administration of aspirin, peak plasma levels are reached within 1 to 2 hours, and fairly constant levels are maintained for 4 to 6 hours. Plasma half-life following oral administration of one gram of aspirin ranges from 4.7 to 9 hours, with an average of 6 hours. With toxic doses (10 to 20 grams) the half-life may be increased to 22 hours. A direct correlation between plasma levels and clinical effectiveness has not been established, but analgesia is usually achieved at plasma levels of 15 to 30 mg/100 mL, anti-inflammatory activity at 20 to 30 mg/100 mL, and some symptoms of salicylism at 35 mg/100 mL. Aspirin is bound poorly to plasma protein; nevertheless, with therapeutic doses, from 50 to 80% is bound to plasma proteins.

Adverse effects from usual doses of aspirin are infrequent; most common are gastrointestinal disturbances (dyspepsia, nausea, vomiting, and occult bleeding). Prolonged administration of large doses (3.6 g daily) results in occult bleeding and may result in anemia. Massive gastrointestinal hemorrhage occurs rarely and, although its relationship to peptic ulcer is uncertain, a nonsalicylate analgesic may be preferred in high-risk patients.

As evidenced by substantial fecal blood loss, alcohol increases the gastric bleeding caused by aspirin in many patients. Concomitant use of aspirin and corticosteroids or pyrazolone derivatives (phenylbutazone, oxyphenbutazone) may increase the risk of gastrointestinal ulceration. Use of aspirin with fenoprofen, ibuprofen, indomethacin, or naproxen may cause lowering of plasma concentrations and thus reduce the effectiveness of the latter drugs. Aspirin displaces highly bound coumarin-type anticoagulants from protein-binding sites and thus increases the concentrations and effects of the anticoagulants. The hypoglycemic action of oral sulfonylureas may be increased by concurrent administration of aspirin. The uricosuric activity of probenecid and sulfinpyrazone are inhibited when either drug is administered simultaneously with aspirin. Buffered aspirin formulations that contain calcium, magnesium, or aluminum may form complexes with tetracycline from which absorption of the antibiotic is impaired.

Salicylates account for approximately 25% of all accidental poisonings, and may result from promiscuous use of large doses of these agents by the laity. To avoid accidental poisoning of children, aspirin and other salicylate drugs should be kept out of reach of children; also, caution in use of these drugs in children with fever and dehydration is necessary because they are particularly prone to intoxication from relatively small doses of the drugs. In addition, some few people manifest idiosyncrasy in the form of an allergic sensitivity to salicylates, especially aspirin, and may suffer from serious if not fatal asthma after ingestion of a single 300-mg dose. Consequently, aspirin should be used with great care in patients with asthma, nasal polyps, or allergens.

Aspirin crosses the placental barrier, and is excreted into breast milk. As use of aspirin prior to delivery may have inhibited platelet aggregation and diminished factor XII plasma levels in newborn infants, it has been suggested that no salicylate be ingested during the last month of pregnancy. Chronic high-dose aspirin therapy has been reported to increase the length of gestation and to prolong labor.

Dose—*Usual, adult, oral,* **300 to 650 mg** every 3 or 4 hours; or **650 mg to 1.3 g** as the extended-release tablet every 8 hours. *Rectal,* **200 mg to 1.3 g** 3 or 4 times a day. *Usual, pediatric, oral or rectal,* 1.5 g/m² of body surface a day in divided doses; or, children up to 2 yr of age, dosage to be individualized by physician; 2 to 4 yr of age, **160 mg** every 4 hr; 4 or 6 yr of age, **240 mg** every 4 hr; 6 to 9 yr of age, **320 mg** every 4 hours; 9 to 11 yr of age, **400 mg** every 4 hr; 11 to 12 yr of age, **480 mg** every 4 hr; 12 yr and over, **325 to 650 mg** every 4 hr. *Note:* No more than 5 doses should be given in a 24-hr period.

Dosage Forms—Capsules: 325 mg; Elixir: 325 mg/5 mL; Suppositories: 60, 120, 125, 150, 200, 300, 325, 600, and 650 mg, 1.2 and 1.3 g; Tablets: 65, 130, 300, 325, 500, and 650 mg; Tablets, Extended-Release: 650 mg; Tablets, Enteric-Coated: 325 and 650 mg; Tablets, Chewable: 81 mg. *Aspirin, Phenacetin, and Caffeine (APC)*—Tablets: 230 mg aspirin, 160 mg phenacetin, and 32 mg caffeine. *APC and Codeine Phosphate*—Capsules and Tablets: 8, 15, 30 or 60 mg codeine phosphate, 230 mg aspirin, 160 mg phenacetin, 16 or 32 mg caffeine. *APC and Codeine Sulfate*—Capsules and Tablets: 15 or 30 mg codeine sulfate, 230 mg aspirin, 160 mg phenacetin, and 32 mg caffeine. *Aspirin and Codeine Phosphate*—Tablets: 325 mg aspirin and 30 mg codeine phosphate.

Carbamazepine—page 1077.

Colchicine

Acetamide, *N*-(5,6,7,9-tetrahydro-1,2,3,10-tetramethoxy-9-oxobenzo[*a*]heptalen-7-yl)-, (*S*)-,

Colchicine [64-86-8] $C_{22}H_{25}NO_6$ (399.44); an alkaloid obtained from various species of *Colchicum.*

Caution—Colchicine is extremely poisonous.

Preparation—By extracting the corm or seed with alcohol. After distilling off the alcohol, the syrupy residue is diluted with water to precipitate fats and resins and filtered. The filtrate is digested with some lead carbonate, refiltered, evaporated to a small volume and the colchicine extracted with chloroform.

Description—Pale yellow to pale greenish yellow, amorphous scales, or powder or crystalline powder; odorless or nearly so, and darkens on exposure to light; melts at about 145°; pK$_a$ 12.35.

Solubility—1 g in 25 mL water and about 220 mL ether; freely soluble in alcohol and chloroform.

Uses—The agent of choice in the symptomatic treatment of *acute attacks* of *gouty arthritis*. When properly used, it will usually terminate an attack in 24 to 48 hours. It is also used in combination with either phenylbutazone, oxyphenbutazone, or allopurinol in the management of acute gout. The precise mechanism of action is unknown. Colchicine is thought to decrease leukocyte motility, phagocytosis, and lactic acid production, thereby decreasing the deposition of urate crystals and the inflammatory response. The drug is well absorbed after oral administration; 31% is bound to plasma protein. It is eliminated by both urinary and fecal routes. Its mechanism of action is unknown, and it appears to differ from the salicylates and cinchophen in its metabolic effects in gout. It is practically useless in chronic gout but its routine administration does lessen the frequency and severity of acute attacks. The alkaloid is very toxic, and it should be discontinued at the first evidence of toxicity, namely, diarrhea, nausea, vomiting, and abdominal pain. Patients taking colchicine for long periods are under some risk of occurrence of agranulocytosis, aplastic anemia, myopathy, and alopecia, hence should have periodic examinations for possible blood dyscrasias or other adverse effects. Caution should be exercised in prescribing colchicine for aged and debilitated patients, and for those with cardiac, renal, hepatic, gastrointestinal, or hematologic disease.

Dose—*Usual, adult, prophylactic, mild gout*, **0.5 to 0.65 mg** once a day for 1 to 4 days each week; *moderate to severe gout*, **0.3 to 0.65 mg** 1 to 3 times a day. For patients with gout scheduled for surgery, *oral*, **0.5 to 0.65 mg** 3 times a day for 3 days before and 3 days after surgery. *Therapeutic, oral*, **0.5 to 1.3 mg** initially, followed by **1 to 1.3 mg** every 2 hours until pain is relieved or until nausea, vomiting, or diarrhea occurs. Total accumulative dose ranges from 4 to 8 mg. Pediatric dosage has not been established. *Intravenous*, for acute attacks of gout, initially **2 mg**, followed by **0.5 mg** every 6 hours until a satisfactory response is achieved. The total intravenous dose for one course of treatment generally should not exceed 4 mg; subcutaneous extravasation may be painful.

Dosage Forms—Tablets: 0.432, 0.5, 0.6, and 0.65 mg; Injection: 1 mg/2 mL.

Magnesium Salicylate

Magnesium, bis(2-hydroxybenzoato-O^1,O^2)-, Magan (*Adria*); Mobidin (*Ascher*)

Magnesium salicylate [18917-95-8] $C_{14}H_{10}MgO_6$.4H$_2$O (370.60); *anhydrous* [34200-52-7] (298.53).

Preparation—Salicylic acid is reacted with a sufficient quantity of magnesium oxide in a hot mixture of isopropanol and water, and the hydrated salt crystallizes out on cooling.

Description—White to slightly pink, free-flowing crystalline powder; odorless or has a faint characteristic odor; aqueous solution is acid to litmus.

Solubility—1 g in 13 mL water; soluble in alcohol.

Uses—Although it has analgesic, antipyretic, and anti-inflammatory effects similar to those of aspirin and other salicylates, magnesium salicylate is indicated only for symptomatic relief of signs and symptoms of *rheumatoid arthritis, osteoarthritis, bursitis*, and other *musculoskeletal* disorders. Salicylates inhibit the synthesis of prostaglandins; the importance of this mechanism in analgesia and anti-inflammatory effect has not been fully elucidated. Following ingestion of 524 mg of magnesium salicylate, a peak concentration of 3.6 mg salicylic acid/dL is reached in 1½ hours with a half-life of 2 hours. Except for the danger of hypermagnesemia in advanced chronic renal disease and the fact that safe use of this agent in children under 12 years of age has not been established, the contraindications, warnings, precautions, drug interactions, and treatment of overdosage are the same as for *Aspirin* (page 1112) and *Sodium Salicylate* (page 1115).

Dose—*Usual, adult, oral*, **600 mg**, 3 or 4 times daily. May be increased to **3.6 to 4.8 g**/day in divided doses at intervals of 3 to 6 hours. In rheumatic fever, as much as **9.6 g**/day may be required.

Dosage Form—Tablets: 480, 545, and 650 mg (salicylic acid equivalent 75%).

Methysergide Maleate

Ergoline-8-carboxamide, 9,10-didehydro-N-[1-hydroxymethyl)-propyl]-1,6-dimethyl-, (8β)-, (Z)-2-butenedioate (1:1) (salt); Sansert (*Sandoz*)

9,10-Didehydro-N-[1-(hydroxymethyl)propyl]-1,6-dimethyl-ergoline-8β-carboxamide maleate [129-49-7] $C_{21}H_{27}N_3O_2$.$C_4H_4O_4$ (469.54).

Preparation—See US Pat 3,218,324.

Description—Off-white to pinkish white crystals melting with decomposition above 165°.

Solubility—1 g in about 500 mL of water, 125 mL of methanol, 165 mL of ethanol, 10,000 of chloroform. A 0.2% aqueous solution has a pH of about 4.

Uses—For the *prevention* or *reduction of intensity* and *frequency* of vascular headaches in patients suffering from one or more severe vascular headaches per week. It is also indicated in patients suffering from vascular headaches that are either uncontrollable or so severe that preventive therapy is indicated regardless of the frequency of the attack. It may prove beneficial in the prophylaxis of migraine. *Warning: Retroperitoneal fibrosis, pleuropulmonary fibrosis, and fibrotic thickening of cardiac valves may occur in patients receiving long-term methysergide maleate therapy. Therefore, this preparation should be reserved for prophylaxis in patients whose vascular headaches are frequent and/or severe and uncontrollable and who are under close medical supervision.* Other adverse effects include *vasoconstrictor effects* (angina-like pain, vascular insufficiency), *central nervous system effects* (insomnia, nervousness, euphoria, dizziness, ataxia, hallucinations, drowsiness, mental depression, etc), *gastrointestinal reactions* (nausea, vomiting, diarrhea, abdominal pain), and *miscellaneous reactions* (dermatitis, alopecia, edema, weight gain, arthralgia, and myalgia). *Methysergide should not be used for more than six months without imposing a three or four week drug-free period* (the dosage should be reduced gradually two or three weeks before discontinuation of the drug).

Dose—*Usual, adult, oral*, **4 to 8 mg** daily in divided doses taken with food. No pediatric dose has been established.

Dosage Form—Tablets: 2 mg.

Methotrimeprazine

10H-Phenothiazine-10-propanamine, 2-methoxy-N,N,β-trimethyl-, (−)-, Levoprome (*Lederle*)

(−)-10-[3-(Dimethylamino)-2-methylpropyl]-2-methoxyphenothiazine [60-99-1] $C_{19}H_{24}N_2OS$ (328.47).

Preparation—By (1) condensation of *o*-chlorobenzoic acid with *m*-anisidine via dehydrochlorination with potassium carbonate and a copper catalyst to form 2-(*m*-anisidino)benzoic acid; (2) decarboxylation of the acid via pyrolysis to form 3-methoxydiphenylamine; (3) cyclization of the amine by heating with sulfur to form 2-methoxyphenothiazine; and (4) condensation of the 2-methoxyphenothiazine with 2-methyl-3-(dimethylamino)propyl chloride via dehydrochlorination with sodamide.

Description—Fine, white, practically odorless, crystalline powder; unstable in light and nonhygroscopic; melts at about 126°.

Solubility—Practically insoluble in water; sparingly soluble in methanol; freely soluble in chloroform and ether; sparingly soluble in alcohol at 25° but freely soluble in boiling alcohol.

Uses—A *nonaddicting analgesic drug* with some sedative, tranquilizer, antihistaminic, anticholinergic, and antiadrenergic effects. It is available only in a form for intramuscular administration. It is indicated for the relief of pain of moderate to marked degree of severity in nonambulatory patients. It is also indicated for obstetrical analgesia and sedation where respiratory depression is to be avoided. It can also be used as preanesthetic medication for producing sedation, and for relieving anxiety and apprehension. It is as effective as morphine or meperidine in severe pain; 20 mg of methotrimeprazine is approximately as effective as 10 mg of morphine or 75 mg of meperidine. Maximum analgesic effect usually occurs within 20 to 40 minutes after intramuscular injection and lasts for about four hours. Unlike potent analgesics it does not induce psychic or physical dependence; it does not suppress the symptoms of morphine withdrawal. Methotrimeprazine does not depress respiration; thus, it may be particularly useful for obstetrical analgesia and in patients with pulmonary insufficiency.

Methotrimeprazine is contraindicated for use with an unusually large number of agents: anesthetics, aspirin, central nervous system depressants, reserpine or tricyclic antidepressants (may potentiate the effects of either these medications or methotrimeprazine; dosage adjustments may be necessary); anticholinergics (may produce paralytic ileus); antihypertensives or monoamine oxidase (MAO) inhibitors (concurrent use is not recommended); atropine, scopolamine, or succinylcholine (may produce tachycardia and hypotension, and aggravate other CNS effects such as stimulation, delirium, and extrapyramidal symptoms); epinephrine (may produce paradoxical hypotension). The potential usefulness of methotrimeprazine must be weighed against its major adverse reactions, *orthostatic hypotension and sedation;* the former may last from 12 to 16 hours after drug administration. Other untoward effects include dizziness, disorientation, amnesia, slurred speech, blurred vision, light-headedness, nausea, vomiting, dry mouth, nasal congestion, pain at site of injection, difficulty in urination, chills, and uterine inertia. Leukopenia, agranulocytosis, jaundice, and extrapyramidal symptoms have also been reported. Since this is a phenothiazine, the physician should be alert for other untoward effects characteristic of these agents.

Dose—*Intramuscular,* **5 to 40 mg;** *usual,* **10 mg** initially followed by **10 to 20 mg** every 4 to 6 hours. *Ambulation should be avoided or carefully supervised for at least 6 hours following the initial dose.*

Other Dose Information—For preanesthetic medication, intramuscular, 10 to 20 mg.

Dosage Form—Injection: 20 mg/mL (as the hydrochloride).

Phenacetin

Acetamide, *N*-(4-ethoxyphenyl)-, Acetphenetidin; *p*-Ethoxyacetanilid

$$C_2H_5O-\langle\bigcirc\rangle-NHCOCH_3$$

p-Acetophenetidide [62-44-2] $C_{10}H_{13}NO_2$ (179.22).

Preparation—*p*-Nitrophenol, dissolved in sodium hydroxide solution, is condensed with ethyl bromide or another suitable ethylating agent and the *p*-nitrophenetole so obtained is reduced with sodium sulfide or other suitable reductant. The resulting *p*-phenetidine is acetylated by refluxing with acetic anhydride.

Description—White, glistening crystals, usually in scales, or as a fine, white, crystalline powder; odorless, has a slightly bitter taste, and is stable in air; saturated solution is neutral to litmus; melting range 134° to 136°.

Solubility—1 g in about 1300 mL water, 15 mL alcohol, 15 mL chloroform, and about 130 mL ether.

Incompatibilities—Forms eutectics with *aspirin, aminopyrine, chloral hydrate,* etc. It is decomposed by *alkalies* or *strong acids. Oxidizing agents* usually produce a red color.

Uses—An *analgetic* and *antipyretic* having approximately the same effectiveness as aspirin, however, it has little anti-inflammatory activity and lacks the uricosuric effect of aspirin. It is mainly used for mild to moderate pain associated with the musculoskeletal system. Acetaminophen is the principle active metabolite of phenacetin. Although phenacetin is an effective analgesic-antipyretic, it has greater potential for toxicity (methemoglobinemia and hemolytic anemia) than acetaminophen. Kidney disease, often irreversible, has been noted with doses of phenacetin of 1 g or more per day taken for one to three years and with total ingestion of 2 kg or more. For this reason all preparations containing phenacetin must carry the following statement. *Warning—This medication may damage the kidneys when used in large amounts or for a long period of time. Do not take more than the recommended dosage, nor take regularly for longer than 10 days without consulting your physician.*

Dose—**300 mg** to **2 g** daily; *usual, adult, oral,* **300 to 600 mg** every 3 or 4 hours as needed. If this does not relieve the pain, the drug should be discontinued.

Dosage Form—Phenacetin is available only as a component of combination products. The dose is 300 mg repeated up to 6 to 8 times daily.

Probenecid—see page 944.

Propoxyphene Hydrochloride

Benzeneethanol, α-[2-(dimethylamino)-1-methylethyl]-α-phenyl-, propanoate (ester), [*S*-(*R**,*S**)]-, hydrochloride, Darvon (*Lilly*); (*Various Mfrs*)

(2*S*,3*R*)-(+)-4-(Dimethylamino)-3-methyl-1,2-diphenyl-2-butanol propionate (ester) hydrochloride [1639-60-7] $C_{22}H_{29}NO_2 \cdot HCl$ (375.94).

Preparation—The Mannich base formed by condensing propiophenone and dimethylamine with formaldehyde is grignardized with benzyl magnesium chloride to produce a mixture of the racemates of the two diastereoisomers (designated commercially as α and β) of the alcohol. The desired α-*dl* form is isolated by fractional crystallization and resolved by means of *d*-camphorsulfonic acid. The desired α-*d* enantiomorph is propionylated with propionic acid in the presence of trimethylamine to form propoxyphene which adds an equivalent of HCl in forming the hydrochloride.

Description—White, crystalline powder which is odorless, and has a bitter taste: melts within a 3°-range between 163.5° and 168.5°.

Solubility—Freely soluble in water; soluble in alcohol, chloroform, and acetone; practically insoluble in benzene and ether.

Uses—A mild analgesic structurally related to the narcotic analgesic methadone. Although its pharmacologic properties resemble those of the narcotics as a group, it does not compare with them in analgesic potency. Well-controlled studies indicate that the milligram potency of propoxyphene is about ½ to ⅔ that of codeine. It appears that the effectiveness of propoxyphene in a dose of 32 mg is questionable and in a dose of 65 mg it is not more, and usually less, effective than the same dose of codeine or 650 mg of aspirin. It has no anti-inflammatory or antipyretic action and little antitussive activity, despite the fact its levo isomer is used for this purpose. It is indicated for the control of *mild to moderate pain.* Propoxyphene is completely absorbed after oral administration; however, first-pass elimination of 30 to 70% markedly reduces its bioavailability. The apparent volume of distribution is 700 to 1800 L; oral clearance is 1.3 to 3.6 L/minute, and half-life 14.6 hours. Propoxyphene is contraindicated in patients hypersensitive to it and to aspirin, phenacetin, or caffeine. The drug should not be used during pregnancy, unless in the physician's judgment the potential benefits exceed the potential hazards. The most frequent adverse effects are dizziness, sedation, nausea, and vomiting. Other adverse reactions include constipation, abdominal pain, skin rashes, light-headedness, headache, weakness, euphoria, dysphoria, and minor visual disturbances. The chronic ingestion of 800 mg/day has caused toxic psychoses and convulsions. Confusion, anxiety and tremors have also been reported in patients receiving propoxyphene concomitant with orphenadrine. The depressant effects of propoxyphene may be additive with those of other depressant drugs, such as alcohol, tranquilizers, and sedative-hypnotics. Since both psychic and physical dependence have been induced with this agent, it should be prescribed with the same degree of caution as codeine.

Dose—**32 to 520 mg** daily; *usual,* **65 mg** 6 times a day as necessary. Drowsiness or dizziness may occur which may impair ability to drive or perform other tasks requiring alertness. Propoxyphene is not recommended for children.

Dosage Forms—Capsules: 32 and 65 mg. *Propoxyphene Hydrochloride and Acetaminophen*—Tablets: 65 mg and 650 mg, respectively. *Propoxyphene Hydrochloride and APC*—Capsules: 32 or 65 mg of propoxyphene hydrochloride, with 227 mg of aspirin, 162 mg of phenacetin, and 324 mg of caffeine. *Propoxyphene Hydrochloride and Aspirin*—Capsules, Tablets: 65 mg and 325 mg, respectively.

Propoxyphene Napsylate

Benzeneethanol, α-[2-(dimethylamino)-1-methylethyl]-α-phenyl-, propanoate (ester), [S-(R*,S*)]-, compound with 2-naphthalenesulfonic acid (1:1) monohydrate; Darvon-N
(*Lilly*)

(αS,1R)-α-[2-(Dimethylamino)-1-methylethyl]-α-phenylphenethyl propionate compound with 2-naphthalenesulfonic acid (1:1) monohydrate [26570-10-5] $C_{22}H_{29}NO_2.C_{10}H_8O_3S.H_2O$ (565.72); anhydrous [17140-78-2] (547.71).

For the structure of the base, see *Propoxyphene Hydrochloride*.

Preparation—*Propoxyphene* is reacted with an equimolar quantity of aqueous 2-naphthalenesulfonic acid and the salt is crystallized therefrom.

Description—White, bitter, crystalline powder with essentially no odor; melts in a 4° range between 158° and 165°.

Solubility—1 g in 10,000 mL water, 15 mL alcohol, 10 mL chloroform; soluble in ether.

Uses—Actions and uses are the same as *Propoxyphene Hydrochloride*, except that, because of its larger molecular weight, a dose of 100 mg is required instead of the 65 mg dose of the hydrochloride. This compound permits more stable liquid and tablet dosage forms because of its very slight solubility in water.

Dose—*Usual*, **100 mg** every 4 hours as needed for pain. The maximum recommended dose is 600 mg per day.

Dosage Forms—Oral Suspension: 50 mg/5 mL; Tablets: 100 mg. *Propoxyphene Napsylate and Acetaminophen*—Tablets: 50 mg and 100 mg, 325 mg and 650 mg, respectively. *Propoxyphene Napsylate and Aspirin*—Tablets: 100 mg and 325 mg, respectively; Capsules: 65 mg and 325 mg, respectively.

Salsalate

Benzoic acid, 2-hydroxy-, 2-carboxyphenyl ester; Disalacid (*Riker*); Arcylate (*Hauck*); Saloxium (*Whitehall*)

Preparation—By condensation of 2 moles of salicylic acid in the presence of thionyl chloride. See Ger Pat 214,044.

Description—A crystalline solid melting about 148°.
Solubility—Only slightly soluble in water but hydrolyzes slowly into 2 molecules of salicylic acid. Soluble in alcohol or ether; sparingly soluble in benzene; insoluble in dilute acids.

Uses—For the relief of the signs and symptoms of rheumatoid arthritis, osteoarthritis, and related rheumatic disorders. Salsalate, salicylsalicylic acid, is a dimer of salicylic acid. It is insoluble in gastric juice, but soluble in the small intestine where it is partially hydrolyzed to two molecules of salicylic acid. On a molar basis, the amount of salicylic acid available from salsalate is about 15% less than that from aspirin. Biotransformation of salsalate is saturated at anti-inflammatory doses; hence, the half-life of salicylic acid is increased from 3.5 to more than 16 hours. Thus, twice a day dosing with salsalate will maintain blood levels within the desired therapeutic range (10–30 mg/100 mL) throughout 12-hour intervals. Therapeutic blood levels continue for up to 16 hours after the last dose. The mechanism of anti-inflammatory action of salsalate and other anti-inflammatory drugs remains unclear. In contrast to aspirin, salsalate does not cause gastrointestinal blood loss and can be given to aspirin-sensitive patients. Otherwise, precautions and adverse effects resemble those of the salicylates (see page 1110).

Dose—*Usual, adult, oral,* **325** to **1000** mg 2 or 3 times daily. If necessary, adjust frequency of dosage based on response.

Dosage Forms—Capsules: 500 mg; Tablets: 325, 500, and 750 mg.

Sodium Salicylate

Benzoic acid, 2-hydroxy-, monosodium salt

Monosodium salicylate [54-21-7] $C_7H_5NaO_3$ (160.10).

Preparation—Salicylic acid is mixed with sufficient distilled water to form a paste, then sufficient pure sodium carbonate is added in small portions to neutralize all but a small fraction of the salicylic acid. The resulting solution is filtered through a filter free from iron, as even slight contact with iron will discolor the product. The filtered solution is evaporated at a low temperature to dryness, preferably in a vacuum.

Description—Amorphous or microcrystalline powder or scales; colorless or has not more than a faint, pink tinge; odorless, or has a faint, characteristic odor, and a sweet, saline taste; affected by light; aqueous solution is neutral or acid to litmus.

Solubility—1 g in 1 mL water, 10 mL alcohol, and about 4 mL glycerin; very soluble in boiling water and boiling alcohol.

Incompatibilities—Solutions of salicylates slowly darken in color due to an *oxidation reaction* influenced by the presence of *alkalies* or *iron* and leading to a quinoid structure. The reaction is retarded by the presence of more easily oxidized substances such as sodium bisulfite, sodium hypophosphite, or sodium thiosulfate.

Uses—The analgetic, antipyretic actions and limitations of the salicylates are presented in detail under *Aspirin* (page 1112). Like the latter compound, sodium salicylate is employed for the *relief of pain* and the *reduction of fever*. It is also serviceable in the symptomatic therapy of *gout* and in acute *rheumatic fever*. It is about ⅓ less potent, on a weight basis, than aspirin, and therefore the equivalent analgetic dose is somewhat higher. The sodium salt tends to cause gastric irritation due to the liberation of free salicylic acid by the acid gastric juice. For this reason, an equivalent amount of sodium bicarbonate is usually employed along with sodium salicylate. The drug does not affect platelet function but, like aspirin, it does increase prothrombin time. It should not be used by patients on a low-sodium diet.

Dose—**300 mg** to **4 g** daily; *usual, adult, oral,* **300** to **650 mg** every 4 hours as needed.

Dosage Forms—Tablets: 325 and 650 mg; Tablets, Enteric-Coated: 324, 325, 650 mg; Injection: 1 g and 1.5 g/10 mL.

Sodium Thiosulfate—see RPS-16, page 1176.

Sulfinpyrazone

3,5-Pyrazolidinedione, 1,2-diphenyl-4-[2-(phenylsulfinyl)ethyl]-, Anturane (*Ciba-Geigy*)

[57-96-5] $C_{23}H_{20}N_2O_3S$ (404.48).

Preparation—[2-(Phenylsulfinyl)ethyl]malonic acid diethyl ester is condensed with hydrazobenzene with the aid of a solution of sodium ethoxide in absolute ethanol. The reaction is completed by adding xylene and heating at about 130° whereby the residual ethanol and that liberated during the condensation is removed. The sulfinpyrazone is isolated by a solvent extraction process and recrystallized from ethanol. US Pat 2,700,671.

Description—White to off-white powder; melts between 130.5° and 134.5°.
Solubility—Practically insoluble in water and solvent hexane; soluble in alcohol and acetone; sparingly soluble in dilute alkali.

Uses—A pyrazolone derivative chemically related to phenylbutazone used as a potent uricosuric agent in the prevention, rather than the treatment, of acute gouty arthritis. In chronic gout, sulfinpyrazone suppresses formation of new tophi and may reduce the size of old tophaceous deposits and alleviate joint pain and stiffness. It is less effective than allopurinol in reducing serum uric acid. Moreover, the drug is of no value in treating acute gouty arthritis. Consequently, most patients require concomitant use of colchicine or of other drugs for adequate symptomatic relief, since sulfinpyrazone has only weak, if any, analgesic or anti-inflammatory action. Salicylates, even in small doses, antagonize the uricosuric action of sulfinpyrazone. Therefore, patients should be advised not to take aspirin or other salicylates except on authorization of their physician. Also, patients on the drug should be advised to maintain a high fluid intake. The drug is contraindicated in patients with active peptic ulcer, renal impairment or a history of renal calculi, especially uric acid stones, because of the possibility of aggravating these conditions. Sulfinpyrazone should be used with caution in patients on sulfa drugs, sulfonylurea hypoglycemic agents, and insulin since it may potentiate these agents. Side effects include upper gastrointestinal disturbances, rash (reported in about 3% of patients), and, rarely, anemia, leukopenia, agranulocytosis, and thrombocytopenia.

Dose—200 to 800 mg daily; *usual, initial,* **100 to 200 mg** 1 or 2 times a day; *maintenance,* **100 to 400 mg** 2 times a day, with meals or milk.

Dosage Forms—Capsules: 200 mg; Tablets: 100 mg.

Other Nonaddicting Analgesics and Antipyretics

Antipyrine [2,3-Dimethyl-1-phenyl-3-pyrazolin-5-one [60-80-0] $C_{11}H_{12}N_2O$ (188.23); Phenazone]—Variously prepared, in one method by condensing ethyl acetoacetate and phenylhydrazine to 1-phenyl-3-methylpyrazolone, followed by methylation of the product. Colorless crystals or white, crystalline powder; odorless; slightly bitter taste; melts at about 111°. One g dissolves in less than 1 mL of water, 1.3 mL alcohol, 1 mL chloroform, 43 mL ether. *Uses:* An early and long popular oral analgesic and antipyretic, now largely replaced by safer and more effective agents. A solution of antipyrine (5.4%) and benzocaine (1.4%) in anhydrous glycerin (*Auralgan,* Ayerst) is used as a topical decongestant and analgesic for relief of pain and reduction of inflammation in the congestive and serous stages of acute otitis media. It is instilled into the ear canal every 1 or 2 hours as needed (or 3 or 4 times a day). The solution is also used to facilitate removal of excessive or impacted cerumen.

Ethoheptazine Citrate [Ethyl hexahydro-1-methyl-4-phenyl-1*H*-azepine-4-carboxylate citrate (1:1) [6700-56-7] $C_{16}H_{23}NO_2 \cdot C_6H_8O_7$ (453.49); Zactane Citrate (*Wyeth*)]—Synthesis of the compound is described in US Pat 2,666,050. A white to nearly white powder; practically odorless; melts within a 3°-range between 135° and 145°. One g dissolves in about 30 mL water, 140 mL alcohol; insoluble in chloroform, ether. *Uses:* A nonnarcotic analgesic of moderate potency considered *possibly effective* for relief of mild to moderate pain. It is ineffective in relieving severe pain and less effective than aspirin for postpartum pain. Ethoheptazine is apparently devoid of antipyretic, anti-inflammatory, and addicting properties. Incidence of side effects after usual doses is relatively low. Nausea, vomiting, epigastric distress, dizziness, and pruritus have been observed. Its metabolic fate and routes of excretion are uncertain. *Dose:* 75 to 150 mg; *usual,* 75 mg 3 or 4 times a day. *Dosage Form:* Tablets: 75 mg.

Nonsteroidal Anti-inflammatory Drugs

The number of nonsteroidal anti-inflammatory drugs (NSAIDs) has increased to the point where they warrant separate classification. In addition to aspirin, the NSAIDs available in this country include meclofenamate sodium, oxyphenbutazone, phenylbutazone, indomethacin, piroxicam, sulindac, and tolmetin for the treatment of arthritis; mefenamic acid and zomepirac for analgesia; and ibuprofen, fenoprofen, and naproxen for both analgesia and arthritis. Ibuprofen, mefenamic acid and naproxen are also used for the management of dysmenorrhea.

The clinical usefulness of NSAIDs is restricted by a number of adverse effects. Phenbutazone has been implicated in hepatic necrosis and granulomatous hepatitis; and sulindac, indomethacin, ibuprofen, and naproxen with hepatitis and cholestatic hepatitis. Transient increases in serum aminotransferases, especially alanine aminotransferase, have been reported. All of these drugs, including aspirin, inhibit synthesis of prostaglandins which help regulate glomerular filtration and renal sodium and water excretion. Thus, the NSAIDs can cause fluid retention, decrease sodium excretion, followed by hyperkalemia, oliguria, and anuria. Moreover, all of these drugs can cause peptic ulceration. Blood dyscrasias associated with NSAIDs are rare, but death has been attributed to the use of these drugs. All of these drugs can

interfere with platelet function and may cause bleeding in patients taking anticoagulants. In addition, agranulocytosis or aplastic anemia have been reported in patients on indomethacin, ibuprofen, fenoprofen, naproxen, tolmetin, and piroxicam. Oxyphenbutazone and phenylbutazone have caused agranulocytosis and aplastic anemia, especially in the elderly, and may cause leukemia. Other adverse effects attributed to these drugs include dermatitis, headaches, tinnitus, and allergic reactions. Available data are not sufficient to recommend any one of these agents as safer than the others. Patients taking these drugs should have periodic white cell counts and determinations of serum creatinine levels and hepatic enzyme activities.

Amodiaquine—see page 1217.

Aspirin—see page 1112.

Diflunisal

[1,1′-Biphenyl]-3-carboxylic acid, 2′,4′-difluoro-4-hydroxy-, Dolobid (*MSD*)

[22494-42-4] $C_{13}H_8F_2O_3$ (250.20).

Preparation—Refer to US Pat 3,714,226.

Description—White crystals melting about 210°.

Solubility—Sparingly soluble in water; soluble in most organic solvents or dilute aqueous base.

Uses—Diflunisal is a prostaglandin inhibitor and nonsteroidal analgesic, antiinflammatory, and antipyretic drug used in the management of *mild* to *moderate* pain and osteoarthritis. Double blind studies indicate that a 500 mg dose of flunisal is more effective in the control of post-operative episiotomy pain than 600 mg of aspirin, in post-operative oral surgery 500 to 1000 mg of flunisal was more potent than 600 mg of acetaminophen alone and comparable to 600 mg of acetaminophen with 60 mg of codeine, and more effective than 100 mg of propoxyphene napsylate. Moreover, flunisal had a longer duration of action. Following oral administration, peak plasma levels occur within 2 to 3 hours. Approximately 99% is bound to plasma proteins. Plasma half-life is 8 to 12 hours. About 90% of the drug is excreted in the urine as two soluble glucuronide conjugates. Although diflunisal is a derivative of salicylic acid it is not metabolized to salicylic acid. The drug is contraindicated in patients in whom acute asthmatic attacks, urticaria, or rhinitis are precipitated by aspirin. Diflunisal prolongs the clotting time in patients on anticoagulant therapy, significantly increases plasma levels of hydrochlorathiazide and acetaminophen, decreases the hyperuricemic effect of furosemide, and significantly decreases the urinary excretion of naproxen and its glucuronide metabolite. The most prominent side effects include nausea, dyspepsia, gastrointestinal pain, and diarrhea; dizziness, headache, and rash have also been reported in 3 to 9% of patients. Flunisal appears to cause less gastrointestinal bleeding than aspirin.

Dose—*Usual, adult, oral, mild to moderate pain, initial,* **1000 mg** followed by **500 mg** every 12 hours. *Osteoarthritis,* **500 to 1000 mg** daily in two divided doses; *maintenance,* maximum of **1500 mg**/day. Take with water, milk, or meals.

Dosage Form—Tablets (film coated): 250 and 500 mg.

Dihydroergotamine Mesylate—see page 947.

Ergotamine Tartrate—see page 948.

Fenoprofen Calcium

Benzeneacetic acid, α-methyl-3-phenoxy-, calcium salt (2:1), (±)-, dihydrate; Nalfon (*Lilly*)

(±)-Calcium *m*-phenoxyhydratrope dihydrate [53746-45-5] $C_{30}H_{26}CaO_6.2H_2O$ (558.64); *anhydrous* [34597-40-5] (522.61).

Preparation—Synthesis of fenoprofen and other aryl- and alkyl-substituted phenoxyacetic acids, some of which exhibit anti-inflammatory properties, is described in US Pat 3,600,437 (see *CA 75:* 49707m, 1971).

Description—White, crystalline powder; pK_a 4.5 (fenoprofen).
Solubility—Slightly soluble in water; sparingly soluble in alcohol.

Uses—A nonsteroidal compound that has *anti-inflammatory*, (antiarthritic), and *analgesic* properties. Its mechanism of action is unknown, except that it has been shown to inhibit prostaglandin synthetase. Although it is known to reduce joint swelling, relieve pain, and decrease the duration of morning stiffness, there is no evidence that fenoprofen alters the progressive course of the underlying disease.

Fenoprofen calcium is rapidly absorbed after oral administration. Peak plasma levels (of about 50 μmg/mL) are reached within 2 hours after oral administration of a 600-mg dose. The plasma half-life is approximately 3 hours. It is highly bound (99%) to albumin. About 90% of a single oral dose is eliminated within 24 hours as fenoprofen glucuronide and 4'-hydroxyfenoprofen glucuronide, the major urinary metabolites of the agent.

Fenoprofen calcium is indicated for relief of the symptoms of *rheumatoid arthritis* and *osteoarthritis*. It is also indicated for acute flares and exacerbations and in the long-term management of these diseases. The safety and effectiveness of this agent has not been established for patients bedridden or confined to a wheelchair, permitting little or no self-care (Functional Class IV rheumatoid arthritis). Fenoprofen is contraindicated in patients sensitive to aspirin and other nonsteroidal anti-inflammatory drugs. The safety of this drug in pregnancy and lactation has not been established. Likewise, the safety and effectiveness in children are unknown. Fenoprofen calcium interacts with a number of drugs. Patients receiving hydantoins, sulfonamides or sulfonylureas should be observed for signs of toxicity to these drugs. Fenoprofen prolongs prothrombin time in patients receiving coumarin-type anticoagulants. Peripheral edema, platelet aggregation and prolonged bleeding time have been observed. Adverse reactions most commonly encountered include dyspepsia, constipation, nausea, vomiting, abdominal pain, anorexia, occult blood in the stool, diarrhea, flatulence and dry mouth. Other adverse effects related to the skin are pruritus, rash, increased sweating and urticaria; those related to the nervous system include somnolence, dizziness, tremor, confusion and insomnia; those related to the cardiovascular system, palpitations, tachycardia and occasionally anemia.

Dose (fenoprofen equivalent)—*Usual, adult, oral, rheumatoid arthritis,* **600 mg** 4 times a day; *osteoarthritis,* **300** to **600 mg** 4 times a day; the dosage to be adjusted in accordance with the patient's age, condition, and changes in disease activity. *Maximum daily dosage,* not to exceed 3200 mg. For best results, the drug should be administered 30 minutes before or at least 2 hours after meals.
Dosage Forms (fenoprofen equivalent)—Capsules: 300 mg; Tablets: 600 mg.

Hydroxychloroquine Sulfate—see page 1220.

Ibuprofen

Benzeneacetic acid, α-methyl-4-(2-methylpropyl)-,
Motrin (*Upjohn*); Rufen (*Boots*); Nuprin (*Bristol-Myers*); Advil (*American Home Prod*)

(±)-*p*-Isobutylhydratropic acid; (±)-2-(*p*-isobutylphenyl)propionic acid [15687-27-1] $C_{13}H_{18}O_2$ (206.28).
Preparation—A process for synthesis of ibuprofen from isobutylbenzene is described in US Pat 3,385,886.

Description—White to off-white, crystalline powder; slight characteristic odor and taste; melts at about 75°; apparent pK_a 5.2.
Solubility—Very slightly soluble in water; very soluble in alcohol and other organic solvents.

Uses—A nonsteroidal *anti-inflammatory agent* that possesses *analgesic* and *antipyretic* activities. In mild to moderate pain, such as dysmenorrhea, 200 mg of ibuprofen appears to be as effective as 650 mg of aspirin. Like other nonsteroidal anti-inflammatory agents its mechanism of action is not known. However, its therapeutic action is not due to pituitary-adrenal stimulation. Evidence that it does have a salutary effect is shown by a reduction of joint swelling, decrease in pain, decrease in duration of morning stiffness and by improved functional capacity as indicated by an increase in grip strength, a delay in the time to onset of fatigue, and a decrease in the time to walk 50 feet.

The drug is rapidly absorbed after oral administration and peak plasma serum levels are generally attained within one to two hours after oral administration. With single doses from 200 mg to 800 mg, a dose-response relationship exists between the amount of drug administered and the integrated area under the serum drug concentration vs time curve. It is rapidly metabolized and eliminated in the urine; excretion is virtually complete 24 hours after the last dose of drug. The serum half-life is 1.8 to 2.0 hours.

Ibuprofen is indicated for relief of symptoms of *rheumatoid arthritis* and *osteoarthritis*. It is also indicated in the treatment of *acute* flares and in the *long-term management* of these diseases. The safety and effectiveness of this agent has not been established for patients bedridden or confined to a wheelchair, permitting little or no self care (Functional Class IV rheumatoid arthritis). Ibuprofen is contraindicated in individuals sensitive to the drug or in individuals with the syndrome of nasal polyps, angioedema, and bronchospastic reactivity to aspirin or other nonsteroidal anti-inflammatory agents. Peptic ulceration and gastrointestinal bleeding have been reported. Consequently, ibuprofen should be given under close supervision to patients with a history of upper gastrointestinal tract disease. Blurred and/or diminished vision, scotomata, and other changes in color vision have been noted; the drug should be discontinued and the patient given an ophthalmologic examination. Patients should be cautioned to report to their physicians signs or symptoms of gastrointestinal ulceration or bleeding, blurred vision or other eye symptoms, skin rash, weight gain, or edema.

Ibuprofen, like aspirin and other NSAID'S can inhibit platelet function and prolong bleeding time, but the effects are reversible and not as long lasting as those of aspirin. Nevertheless, ibuprofen should be administered with caution to patients on anticoagulants. Ibuprofen is not recommended for use during pregnancy or in nursing mothers.

Adverse reactions with an incidence greater than 1% may be categorized as follows: *gastrointestinal*, (4 to 16%), nausea, epigastric pain, heartburn, diarrhea, abdominal distress, nausea and vomiting, indigestion, constipation and abdominal cramps or pain; *central nervous system*, dizziness (3 to 9%), headache, nervousness and tinnitus; *dermatologic*, rash (3 to 9%) and pruritus; *metabolic*, decreased appetite, edema, and fluid retention.

Adverse effects with an incidence of less than 1% may be categorized as follows: *gastrointestinal*, gastric or duodenal ulcer with bleeding and/or perforation; *dermatologic*, vesiculobullous eruptions, urticaria, erythema multiforme; *central nervous system*, depression, insomnia; *special senses*, amblyopia (blurred and/or diminished vision, scotomata and/or other changes in vision); *hematologic*, leukopenia and decreases in hemoglobin and hematocrit; *cardiovascular*, congestive heart failure in patients with marginal cardiac function, and elevated blood pressure. Other reactions have been reported but under circumstances where a causal relationship could not be established.

Dose—*Usual, adult, oral, analgesia* (dysmenorrhea), **200** to **400 mg** every 4 to 6 hours as needed; *rheumatoid arthritis*, and *osteoarthritis*, including flareups of chronic disease, **300** or **400 mg** 3 or 4 times a day, adjusted to meet the need of the patient. *Maximum total daily dosage*, 2400 mg.
Dosage Forms—Tablets: 200, 300, 400, and 600 mg.

Indomethacin

1*H*-Indole-3-acetic acid, 1-(4-chlorobenzoyl)-5-methoxy-2-methyl-,
Indocin (*MSD*)

1-(*p*-Chlorobenzoyl)-5-methoxy-2-methylindole-3-acetic acid
[53-86-1] $C_{19}H_{16}ClNO_4$ (357.79).

Preparation—*p*-Anisidine is diazotized and the diazonium compound reduced with sodium sulfite. The resulting *p*-methoxyphenylhydrazine undergoes the Fisher indole synthesis with methyl levulinate. The steps involved include formation of the hydrazone (I), rearrangement of I to the enamine compound II, and cyclization of II through loss of ammonia to form III. III is then hydrolyzed to the acid which is re-esterified via the anhydride to give the *tert*-butyl ester. Acylation with *p*-chlorobenzoyl chloride followed by debutylation yields indomethacin. US Pat 3,161,654.

Description—Pale-yellow to yellow-tan, crystalline powder that is odorless, or has a slight odor, and has a slightly bitter taste; light-sensitive, stable in air, and stable in heat under the usual prevailing temperature conditions; one polymorphic form melts at about 155°, the other at about 162°.

Solubility—1 g in 50 mL alcohol, 30 mL chloroform, 40 mL ether; practically insoluble in water.

Uses—A nonsteroid drug with anti-inflammatory, antipyretic, and analgesic properties. *It is not a simple analgesic and because of its potential serious untoward effects should not be used for trivia.* Indomethacin is indicated for the treatment of *rheumatoid arthritis, ankylosing (rheumatoid) spondylitis, osteoarthritis,* and *gouty arthritis.* The drug is rapidly absorbed after oral administration; peak plasma levels are reached in 2 hours: 97% of the drug is protein-bound. It has a half-life of 2.6 to 11.2 hours; 10 to 20% of the drug is excreted unchanged in the urine. Since it is a potent drug and has a potential to cause adverse effects, it should be carefully considered for active disease unresponsive to adequate trial with salicylates and other established measures, such as appropriate rest. The drug is contraindicated in children, pregnant women and nursing mothers, patients with gastrointestinal problems, and in patients allergic to aspirin. The incidence of untoward effects has been reported to vary from a few percent to 75% of patients. Most frequent untoward actions include *gastrointestinal reactions* (single or multiple ulcerations, hemorrhage, gastrointestinal bleeding, increased pain in ulcerative colitis, gastritis, nausea, vomiting, epigastric distress); *eye reactions* (corneal deposits and retinal disturbances, and blurring of vision); *hepatic reactions* (toxic hepatitis, jaundice, some fatalities have been reported), *hematologic reactions* (aplastic anemia, hemolytic anemia, depression of the bone marrow, agranulocytosis, leukopenia, and thrombocytopenia purpura), *hypersensitivity reactions* (acute respiratory including asthma and dyspnea, angiitis, pruritus, urticaria, skin rashes, etc); *ear reactions* (deafness rarely, tinnitus); *central nervous system reactions* (psychic disturbances, depersonalization, depression, mental confusion, coma, convulsions, peripheral neuropathy, drowsiness, light-headedness, dizziness, and

headache); *cardiovascular-renal reactions* (edema, hypertension, hematuria); *dermatologic reactions* (loss of hair, erythema nodosum); and *miscellaneous reactions* (vaginal bleeding, hyperglycemia, glycosuria, ulcerative stomatitis, and epistaxis). Both the incidence and severity of side effects appear to be dose related.

The high potential for dose-related adverse reactions (see above) makes it imperative that the smallest effective dosage be determined for each patient. Gastrointestinal reactions may be reduced by giving the drug with food, immediately after meals, or with antacids. The occurrence of ocular and/or hematologic disturbances in some patients on prolonged therapy with indomethacin indicates the need for periodic ophthalmologic examination and appropriate blood tests. As probenecid appears to enhance the effect of indomethacin, adjustment of the dose of the latter may be necessary when the two drugs are prescribed concurrently. Whether or not indomethacin has any effect on anticoagulants is uncertain, but concurrent administration may be hazardous because of increased risk of gastrointestinal bleeding.

Indomethacin may aggravate psychiatric disturbances, epilepsy, and parkinsonism; it should be used with considerable caution in patients with these conditions. Patients should be warned that ability to drive or perform other activities requiring alertness may be adversely affected. The drug should be discontinued if any of the untoward effects listed above occurs, pending consultation with the physician.

Dose—*Usual, adult, in gout, oral,* 100 mg initially, then **50 mg** 3 times a day until pain is relieved, then dosage is rapidly reduced until discontinued. *Antipyretic, oral,* **25** to **50 mg** 3 times a day. *Antirheumatic, oral,* **50 mg** 2 or 3 times a day; if well tolerated increase by 25 mg weekly until satisfactory response is obtained or until a total daily dose of 150 to 200 mg is reached.

Other Dose Information—The dose is gradually increased until optimum control is achieved. A dose of 200 mg a day should not be exceeded because of the high incidence of adverse effects. It should not be administered to children under 14 years of age.

Dosage Forms—Capsules: 25 and 50 mg.

Meclofenamate Sodium

Benzoic acid, 2-[(2,6-dichloro-3-methylphenyl)amino]-, monosodium
salt, monohydrate; Meclomen (*Parke-Davis*)

Monosodium *N*-(2,6-dichloro-*m*-tolyl)anthranilate monohydrate
[6385-02-0] $C_{14}H_{10}Cl_2NNaO_2 \cdot H_2O$ (336.15).

Preparation—By the Ullman condensation of *o*-iodobenzoic acid and 2,6-dichloro-*m*-toluidine in the presence of copper-bronze, *J Med Chem* **11:** 1009, 1968.

Description—White crystals melting about 290°.

Solubility—A saturated solution in water (1 g in 65 mL) is slightly turbid and has a pH of about 7.5.

Uses—Meclofenamate sodium is used for the treatment of *acute* and *chronic rheumatoid arthritis* and *osteoarthritis.* Following oral administration, peak plasma levels are reached in one-half to one hour. Plasma half-life after 4 days chronic dosing is 3.3 hours. The drug does not accumulate in the body; it is metabolized to an active hydroxymethyl derivative (25%) and an inactive carboxy derivative (6%); both metabolites are excreted as glucuronides. Approximately two-thirds of the dose is excreted in the urine and one-third is excreted in the feces. It is not recommended as the initial drug because of gastrointestinal side effects which are sometimes severe (see page 1117). It is not recommended for use in children. Patient selection should be based on a careful assessment of the benefit/risk ratio.

Dose—*Usual, oral,* **200 to 400 mg**/day in 3 or 4 equal doses. After satisfactory response has been obtained, adjust dosage as required. May be taken with meals or milk. Terminate therapy if any severe adverse reactions occur.

Dosage Form—Capsules: 50 and 100 mg.

Mefenamic Acid

Benzoic acid, 2-[(2,3-dimethylphenyl)amino]-,
Ponstel (*Parke-Davis*)

N-(2,3-Xylyl)anthranilic acid [61-68-7] $C_{15}H_{15}NO_2$ (241.29).

Preparation—*o*-Chlorobenzoic acid is condensed with 2,3-xylidine with the aid of potassium carbonate and the resulting potassium salt is treated with mineral acid to liberate the desired acid. US Pat 3,138,636.

Description—White to off-white, crystalline powder that is odorless and has very little initial taste, but it has a bitter aftertaste; darkens on prolonged exposure to light, is nonhygroscopic, and is stable at 25°, 37°, and 45°; decarboxylates at temperatures above its melting point (at 300°, 100% is decarboxylated in 3 min); melts between 227° and 232°.

Solubility—1 g in 220 mL alcohol; insoluble in water; sparingly soluble in chloroform and ether.

Uses—An analgesic drug indicated for the relief of mild to moderate pain when *therapy will not exceed 1 week* and for the treatment of *primary dysmenorrhea.* Mefenamic acid is also indicated for the relief of pain resulting from dental extractions. It is contraindicated in patients with ulceration of the upper or lower intestinal tract, children under 14 years of age, women during pregnancy, and patients known to be hypersensitive to the drug. Untoward effects include diarrhea which may be severe and indicates the drug should be stopped, autoimmune hemolytic anemia, thrombocytopenic purpura, leukopenia, pancytopenia, agranulocytosis, and bone-marrow hypoplasia. Minor reactions include drowsiness, gastrointestinal discomfort, dizziness, headache, vomiting, urticaria, rash, eosinophilia, blurred vision, insomnia, and perspiration. Rarely, palpitations, facial edema, dyspnea, eye pain, ear pain, dysuria, hematuria, reversible loss of color vision, and increased insulin need in diabetic patients. Mild renal and hepatic toxicity have also been reported (see page 1117). Since this drug is useful in mild to moderate pain, physicians would be well advised to consider its use only in cases which either can not tolerate or do not respond to less toxic agents.

Dose—*Usual, adults* and *children over 14 years of age, oral,* **500 mg,** followed by **250 mg** every 6 hours, as needed. Take with food. *Caution:* Do not use for more than 7 days.

Dosage Form—Capsules: 250 mg.

Naproxen

2-Naphthaleneacetic acid, 6-methoxy-α-methyl-, (+)-,
Naprosyn (*Syntex*)

(+)-6-Methoxy-α-methyl-2-naphthaleneacetic acid [22204-53-1] $C_{14}H_{14}O_3$ (230.26).

Preparation—6-Methoxynaphthalene is acetylated in the 2-position and the acetyl group is then converted to —CH(CH₃)COOH by a sequence of reactions—Willgerodt-Kindler, esterification, alkylation, and hydrolysis—yielding DL-naproxen (*CA 71:* 91162j, 1969). Resolution of the racemate may be effected through precipitation of the more potent D-enantiomer as the cinchonidine salt (*J Med Chem 13:* 203, 1970).

Description—White to off-white, crystalline powder; bitter taste; melts at about 155°; apparent pK_a 4.15.

Solubility—Practically insoluble in water at pH 2; freely soluble in water at pH 8 or above; sparingly soluble in alcohol.

Uses—Naproxen is a nonsteroidal compound that has anti-inflammatory, analgesic, and antipyretic activities. As with the structurally related compounds fenoprofen and ibuprofen, the mode of action is unknown, except that inhibition of prostaglandin synthesis may have an action role. While various manifestations of anti-inflammatory and analgesic actions are evident in patients with rheumatoid arthritis under treatment with naproxen or its congeners, there is no evidence that the progressive source of the underlying disease is altered.

Naproxen appears to be completely absorbed from the gastrointestinal tract after oral administration. Peak plasma levels (about 55 µg/mL) are reached in 2 to 4 hours after a 500-mg dose, and steady-state levels are attained after 4 or 5 doses at 12-hour intervals.

More than 99% is bound to serum albumin. The mean plasma half-life is about 13 hours. Approximately 95% of a dose is excreted in the urine, principally as conjugates of naproxen and its inactive metabolite 6-demethylnaproxen.

It is indicated for relief of symptoms of rheumatoid arthritis, both of acute flares and long-term management of the disease. Safety and effectiveness in patients who are incapacitated, largely or wholly bedridden or confined to a wheelchair, with little capacity for self care (Functional Class IV rheumatoid arthritis) have not been established. Symptomatic improvement, where use of the drug is indicated, usually begins within 2 weeks but a longer trial period may be necessary. Naproxen is comparable to aspirin in controlling disease symptoms, but with lesser frequency and severity of nervous system and milder gastrointestinal adverse effects. The adverse effects, precautions, contraindications, and drug interactions are essentially the same as for fenoprofen calcium (page 1117).

Dose—*Adult, rheumatoid arthritis, osteoarthritis, ankylosing spondylitis: initially,* **250 to 375 mg** twice daily (morning and evening), increased or decreased according to response of patient. Daily dosage in excess of 1000 mg is not recommended. *Acute gout,* **750 mg** followed by **250 mg** every 8 hours until relieved.

Dosage Form—Tablets: 250, 375, and 500 mg.

Naproxen Sodium

2-Naphthaleneacetic acid, 6-methoxy-α-methyl-, sodium salt
Anaprox (*Syntex*)

[26159-34-2] $C_{14}H_{13}NaO_3$ (252.24).

Uses—See Naproxen.

Dose—*Adult, rheumatoid arthritis, osteoarthritis, ankylosing spondylitis: initially,* **275 mg** twice daily (morning and evening). Adjust dose according to clinical response. Daily doses in excess of 1000 mg have not been studied. *Acute gout: initially,* **825 mg** followed by 275 mg every 8 hours until the attack has subsided.

Dosage Forms—Tablets: 275 mg.

Oxyphenbutazone

3,5-Pyrazolidinedione, 4-butyl-1-(4-hydroxyphenyl)-2-phenyl-,
monohydrate; Oxalid (*USV*); Tandearil (*Ciba-Geigy*)

4-Butyl-1-(*p*-hydroxyphenyl)-2-phenyl-3,5-pyrazolidinedione monohydrate [7081-38-1] $C_{19}H_{20}N_2O_3.H_2O$ (342.39); *anhydrous* [129-20-4] (324.38).

Preparation—Diethyl butylmalonate is condensed with *p*-benzyloxyhydrazobenzene, with the aid of a solution of sodium ethoxide in anhydrous ethanol, to form 1-(*p*-benzyloxy)-2-phenyl-4-butyl-3,5-pyrazolidinedione (I). Completion of the reaction is effected by adding xylene and heating the mixture to about 140° for several hours, thus removing the alcohol released by the cyclizing condensation. Debenzylation of I is effected by Raney nickel hydrogenation at ambient temperature and pressure. Recrystallization of the initial product is from ether/petroleum ether. US Pat 2,745,783.

Description—White to yellowish white, odorless, crystalline powder; melts over a wide range between about 85° and 100°.

Solubility—1 g in >10,000 mL water, 1.5 mL alcohol, 4 mL chloroform, 15 mL ether.

Uses—A derivative of phenylbutazone which exhibits the same analgesic, antipyretic, anti-inflammatory and mild uricosuric properties as the parent drug. Like phenylbutazone, it should not be considered a simple analgesic and should not be administered casually. Oxyphenbutazone is rapidly and completely absorbed after oral administration. Protein binding *is high;* time to peak serum concentration is 6 hours and peak serum concentration after 300 mg is 35 µg/mL; elimination half-life is 72 hours; and excretion is primarily by the kidneys. Except that oxyphenbutazone causes less gastrointestinal distress, its effectiveness, indications, contraindications, and adverse reactions are the same as those for *Phenylbutazone,* (page 1120).

Dose—*Usual, adult, oral, antirheumatic,* **100** or **200 mg** three times a day. *Maintenance,* **100 mg** one to four times a day; *antigout, initially,* **400 mg** as a single dose; then **100 mg** every 4 hours or until desired response is obtained.

Other Dose Information—It should always be taken immediately after meals or with a full glass of milk, to minimize gastric irritation. Oxyphenbutazone should not be used in children under 14 years of age.

Dosage Form—Tablets: 100 mg.

Penicillamine—see page 1225.

Phenylbutazone

3,5-Pyrazolidinedione, 4-butyl-1,2-diphenyl-, Azolid (*USV*); Butazolidin (*Ciba-Geigy*)

4-Butyl-1,2-diphenyl-3,5-pyrazolidinedione [50-33-9] $C_{19}H_{20}N_2O_2$ (308.38).

Preparation—Butylmalonyl chloride is condensed with hydrazobenzene in ether solution at 0° with the aid of pyridine. After extracting the pyridine with aqueous HCl, the phenylbutazone is extracted with aqueous Na_2CO_3 and then precipitated by addition of HCl. US Pat 2,562,830.

Description—White to off-white, odorless, crystalline powder; melts between 104° and 107°.

Solubility—1 g in about 20 mL alcohol; very slightly soluble in water; freely soluble in acetone and ether.

Uses—A synthetic pyrazoline derivative chemically related to aminopyrine which has anti-inflammatory, antipyretic, analgesic, and mild uricosuric properties. It is indicated for the symptomatic relief of *gout, rheumatoid arthritis, rheumatoid spondylitis, osteoarthritis, psoriatic arthritis, acute superficial thrombophlebitis,* and *painful shoulder.* The disease process of these conditions is unaltered by the drug.

Therapy should not be started until the patient has been subjected to a complete physical and laboratory examination, including hemogram and urinalysis. It should not be given to patients in whom it is contraindicated or those not available for frequent observation. Patients should be warned not to exceed the recommended dosage and to immediately report any fever, sore throat or lesions in the mouth (symptoms of blood dyscrasia); dyspepsia, epigastric pain, symptoms of anemia, unusual bleeding, bruising, black or tarry stools (symptoms of intestinal lesions); and significant weight gain or anemia. The goal of therapy should be *short-term* relief of *severe* symptoms to a level tolerable with the *smallest* possible drug dosage. If a favorable response is not observed within one week, the drug should be discontinued. The drug is contraindicated in patients with gastrointestinal problems, a history of drug allergy, and in children under 14 years of age. Phenylbutazone is also contraindicated in patients on other concurrent therapy, such as potent chemotherapeutic drugs and anticoagulant medication.

Phenylbutazone is rapidly absorbed after oral administration and very highly bound to plasma protein. Time to peak serum concentration approximates 2.5 hours; however, usual time for onset of antigout activity varies from 1 to 4 days and that for antirheumatic activity 3 to 7 days. Therapeutic serum concentrations average about 43 mg/mL; elimination half-life is about 84 hours. The drug (1%) and its major metabolite (oxyphenbutazone, 2%) are excreted by the kidneys.

Phenylbutazone produces untoward effects in about 40% of patients; approximately 15% have to discontinue the drug because of toxic effect. Consequently, phenylbutazone should be employed only in those patients who fail to respond adequately to less hazardous substances. The most frequently encountered untoward effects are water retention, nausea, rash, epigastric pain, vertigo, and stomatitis. Other less frequent but more severe effects include hepatitis, hypertension, transient psychosis, moderate leukopenia, agranulocytosis, and thrombocytopenia. Central nervous system stimulation, visual symptoms, anemia, lethargy, constipation, diarrhea, gastrointestinal

hemorrhage, fever, and cardiac arrhythmias have also been observed.

Numerous drug interactions have been reported. In general, phenylbutazone should not be administered to patients taking anticoagulants, anti-inflammatory agents, bone marrow depressants, digitoxin, hypoglycemics, methotrexate, phenytoin, or sulfonamides.

Since phenylbutazone is a potent drug and misuse can lead to serious results, physicians are well advised to familiarize themselves with its gastrointestinal, acid-base balance, hepatic, dermatologic, allergic, renal, cardiovascular, ocular, metabolic, and endocrine effects before prescribing this drug. The drug should be used with caution in pregnant women, nursing mothers, elderly patients, and patients known to have other illnesses.

This drug should be taken with milk or with meals to minimize gastric irritation.

Dose—100 to 600 mg daily; *usual, Antirheumatic, initial,* **100 mg** 3 to 6 times a day; *maintenance,* **100 mg** 1 to 4 times a day. *Antigout,* **400 mg** as a single dose, then **100 mg** every 4 hours for approximately four days or until desired response is obtained, with duration not exceeding one week.

Dosage Form—Tablets: 100 mg; Capsules: 100 mg.

Piroxicam

2*H*-1,2-Benzothiazine-3-carboxamide, 4-hydroxy-2-methyl-*N*-pyridinyl-, 1,1-dioxide; Feldene (*Pfizer*)

[36322-90-4] $C_{15}H_{13}N_3O_4S$ (331.35).

Preparation—See *J Med Chem 15;* 848, 1972.

Description—White crystals melting about 200°.

Solubility—Very slightly soluble in water. A saturated solution in dioxane:water (2:1) has a pK_a of about 6.3.

Uses—For acute or long-term use in the relief of signs and symptoms of *osteoarthritis* and *rheumatoid arthritis.* In patients with osteoarthritis, piroxicam 20 mg/day was as effective against pain and improving joint movement as aspirin 3.9 g/day or indomethacin 75 mg/day. Like other nonsteroidal anti-inflammatory drugs, piroxicam inhibits prostaglandin synthesis and inhibits chemotaxis and release of liposomal enzymes. Piroxicam is rapidly absorbed after oral administration; peak plasma levels occur within 3 to 5 hours. Chronic administration with 20 mg/day produces steady state plasma levels of 3 to 5 mcg/mL in 7 to 12 days. Volume distribution approximates 0.12 to 0.14 L/kg; mean half-life is about 50 hours (range, 30 to 86 hours). It is metabolized primarily by hydroxylation and excreted in the urine. For adverse effects and precautions, see page 1116. Safety and efficacy in children has not been established.

Dose—*Usual, adult, oral,* **20 mg/day.** Because of its long half-life, the effect of therapy should not be assessed for two weeks.

Dosage Form—Capsules: 10 and 20 mg/kg.

Sulindac

1*H*-Indene-3-acetic acid, 5-fluoro-2-methyl-1-[[4-(methylsulfinyl)-phenyl] methylene]-, (*Z*)-, Clinoril (*MSD*)

(*Z*)-5-Fluoro-2-methyl-1-[*p*-(methylsulfinyl)benzylidene]indene-3-acetic acid [38194-50-2] $C_{20}H_{17}FO_3S$ (356.41).

Preparation—Synthesis of sulindac is described in US Pat 3,647,858 and 3,654,349.

Description—Yellow crystals, melting at about 183°, with decomposition; pK_a 4.5.

Solubility—Practically insoluble in water; sparingly soluble in alcohol.

Uses—An indene-type anti-inflammatory agent indicated for acute and long-term relief of signs and symptoms of *osteoarthritis, rheumatoid arthritis, ankylosing spondylitis, acute painful shoulder,* and *acute gouty arthritis.* It also possesses analgesic and antipyretic properties. Its precise mechanism of action is unknown; however, it is thought the sulfide metabolite may inhibit prostaglandin synthesis. Sulindac is approximately 90% absorbed after oral administration. Peak plasma levels are achieved in about 2 hours in the fasting patient and 3 to 4 hours when administered with food. The mean half-life of sulindac is 7.8 hours; the mean half-life of the sulfide metabolite is 16.4 hours. Sulindac is contraindicated in Functional Class IV arthritis (incapacitated, largely or wholly bedridden, or confined to a wheelchair; little or no self-care), patients in whom acute asthmatic attacks, urticaria, or rhinitis are precipitated by aspirin or other nonsteroidal anti-inflammatory agents, and in patients sensitive to the drug.

Adverse reactions include gastrointestinal pain (in 10% of patients); dyspepsia, nausea with or without vomiting, diarrhea, constipation, rash, dizziness, headache (in 3 to 9% of patients); flatulence, anorexia, gastrointestinal cramps, pruritus, nervousness, tinnitus, edema (in 1 to 3% of patients); gastritis or gastroenteritis, peptic ulcer, gastrointestinal bleeding, liver function abnormalities associated with jaundice, stomatitis, sore or dry mucous membranes, vertigo, hypersensitivity (including fever which may be accompanied by chills, skin rash, leukopenia or eosinophilia) (in less than 1% of patients). In the November 1979 issue of its *Drug Bulletin,* the FDA announced that it had received reports of the following reactions to sulindac: congestive heart failure, Stevens-Johnson syndrome, toxic epidermal necrolysis, bone-marrow depression, thrombocytopenia, leukopenia, gastrointestinal perforation, nephropathy, and pancreatitis; also adverse ocular effects including diplopia, cloudy vision, eyeball swelling, noninflammatory ulceration of the cornea, retinal hemorrhage, blurred vision, and spots before the eyes. Also, see page 1116.

Although sulindac has less effect on platelet function and bleeding time than aspirin, it should be used with caution in patients who may be adversely affected by this action. It should also be used with caution in patients with impaired liver and kidney function. Its safe use during pregnancy and in nursing mothers has not been established.

Dose—*Usual, adult, oral,* **150 mg** twice a day with food. *Usual, maximum dose,* **400 mg** per day. *Pediatric* indications and dosage have not been established.

Dosage Forms: Tablets: 150 and 200 mg.

Tolmetin Sodium

1*H*-Pyrrole-2-acetic acid, 1-methyl-5-(4-methylbenzoyl)-, sodium salt, dihydrate; Tolectin (*McNeil*)

Sodium 1-methyl-5-*p*-toluoylpyrrole-2-acetate dihydrate [64490-92-2] $C_{15}H_{14}NNaO_3 \cdot 2H_2O$ (315.31).

Preparation—Tolmetin, as the acetonitrile, is obtained by a Friedel-Crafts reaction between 1-methylpyrrole-2-acetonitrile and *p*-methylbenzoyl chloride; after separation from the 4-aroyl isomer simultaneously produced, by fractional crystallization and/or adsorption chromatography, the tolmetin acetonitrile is converted to tolmetin by saponification and subsequently to its sodium salt (*J Med Chem* 14: 646, 1971).

Description—Light yellow, crystalline powder; pK_a 3.5 (tolmetin).
Solubility—Freely soluble in water; slightly soluble in alcohol.

Uses—Tolmetin is a nonsteroidal compound that has anti-inflammatory, analgesic, and antipyretic activities. Its mode of action is unknown; inhibition of prostaglandin synthesis may be responsible for its anti-inflammatory action. In patients with rheumatoid arthritis various manifestations of its anti-inflammatory and analgesic actions are observed, but there is no evidence of alteration of the progressive course of the underlying disease.

The drug is rapidly and almost completely absorbed with peak plasma levels being reached within 30–60 minutes after an oral therapeutic dose (40 μg/mL after a 400-mg dose). It is approximately 99% bound to plasma proteins; the mean plasma half-life is about 1 hour. Essentially all of a dose is excreted in urine within 24 hours either as an inactive oxidative metabolite or as conjugates of tolmetin.

Tolmetin sodium is indicated for the relief of signs and symptoms of rheumatoid arthritis, both of acute flares and long-term management of the disease. Safety and effectiveness in patients who are incapacitated, largely or wholly bedridden or confined to a wheelchair, with little capacity for self care (Functional Class IV rheumatoid arthritis) have not been established. The drug is comparable to aspirin and to indomethacin in controlling disease activity but the frequency of the milder gastrointestinal adverse effects is reported to be less than in aspirin-treated patients and the incidence of central nervous system adverse effects less than in indomethacin-treated patients. Concomitant administration of tolmetin and aspirin is not recommended since there does not appear to be any greater benefit from the combination over that achieved with aspirin alone and the potential for adverse reactions is increased. Tolmetin is contraindicated in patients demonstrated to be hypersensitive to the drug, and also in those in whom aspirin and other nonsteroidal anti-inflammatory drugs induce symptoms of asthma, rhinitis, or urticaria. In patients with active rheumatoid arthritis who also have an active peptic ulcer, treatment with nonulcerogenic drugs should be attempted; if tolmetin must be given, the patient should be closely observed for signs of ulcer perforation or severe gastrointestinal bleeding. As tolmetin is eliminated primarily by the kidneys, patients with impaired renal function should be closely monitored and dosage reduced or discontinued if necessary. As tolmetin prolongs bleeding time, patients who may be adversely affected thereby should be carefully observed when treated with the drug. Patients with compromised cardiac function should be treated with caution because the drug causes some retention of water and sodium, with resultant mild peripheral edema.

The most frequent adverse reactions are gastrointestinal and include, in descending order of frequency, epigastric or abdominal pain or discomfort (in about 1 of 6 patients), nausea, vomiting, indigestion, heartburn, constipation, and dyspepsia. The most common nervous system reactions are headache (1 of 15 patients), followed by dizziness and lightheadedness, tension and nervousness, and drowsiness. Tinnitus occurs in 1 of 40 patients. Mild edema is observed in about 1 in 50 patients. Rash, including maculopapular eruptions or urticaria, develops in 1 of 30 patients; pruritus in about 1 in 50 patients. Small and transient decreases in hemoglobin and hematocrit not associated with gastrointestinal bleeding occur infrequently; also a few cases of granulocytopenia. Also, see page 1116.

Studies in children have been inadequate to evaluate the safety and effectiveness of the drug in this age group. Use of tolmetin in pregnancy is not recommended, and since it is not known if it is secreted in human milk use by nursing mothers is also not recommended.

Dose (tolmetin equivalent)—*Adult, initial,* **400 mg** 3 times a day, subsequently adjusted to patient's response. Symptom control is usually achieved with a daily dosage of **600 to 1800 mg,** given in 3 or 4 divided doses. Daily dosage exceeding **2000 mg** has not been studied and therefore is not recommended. Therapeutic response can be expected in a few days to a week, with progressive improvement in succeeding weeks of therapy. If gastrointestinal symptoms occur, the drug should be given with meals, milk, or antacids other than sodium bicarbonate.

Dosage Form—Tablets (tolmetin equivalent): 200 mg. *Note:* each tablet contains 18 mg (0.784 mEq) of sodium.

Other Nonsteroidal Anti-Inflammatory Drugs

Dimethyl Sulfoxide [Methyl sulfoxide [67-68-5] CH_3SOCH_3 (78.13); DMSO]—Prepared by air-oxidation of dimethyl sulfide in the presence of nitrogen oxides. A practically colorless and odorless liquid, very hygroscopic, boiling at 189°, and with a density of 1.100. It is soluble in water, alcohol, ether, and chloroform. *Uses:* An aprotic solvent with remarkable properties to enhance penetrance of many locally applied drugs. During the course of its agricultural use as a solvent it was discovered to relieve arthritic pain, and it soon became rather widely and promiscuously used in the topical treatment of various collagen diseases. The discovery of DMSO-induced lens opacities in animals resulted in termination of these uses. At present it is approved only for the treatment of *interstitial cystitis.* Locally applied DMSO, in concentrations above 50%, breaks down collagen, and has anti-inflammatory and local anesthetic effects, all of which probably contribute to relief of pain and improvement in bladder function and mucosal cytology. DMSO is converted to dimethyl sulfide, which imparts to the skin and breath a foul odor described as "garlic-like," but more offensive. No other side effects of intravesical instillation of 50% solutions have been reported but transient disturbances of color vision, photophobia, headache, nausea, diarrhea, urethral burning sensation on urination, and allergies have occurred from topical application to the skin. *Dose: Intravesical*, as a 50% solution.

Gold Compounds

Most authorities prefer the gold compounds over the adrenal steroids or nonsteroidal anti-inflammatory drugs for the adjunctive treatment of selected cases of active rheumatoid arthritis. Gold compounds suppress or prevent, but do not cure arthritis and synovitis. Although their exact mechanism is not known, localized high concentrations of gold are found in Kupffer cells and synoviocyte liposomes; this suggests that gold therapy may inhibit liposomal enzyme activity in macrophages and decrease macrophage phagocytic activity. Accumulation occurs with repeated administration and levels persist for many years in subsynovial tissues and in macrophages of many tissues. Macrophages are thought to be involved in the antigen process and in the interaction of helper T-lymphocytes with antibody forming B-lymphocytes. Whether or not this action is responsible for the effectiveness of gold compounds in arthritis is unknown.

Before gold therapy is initiated, the patient's hemoglobin, erythrocyte, leucocyte, differential, and platelet counts should be determined and a urinalysis should be done to serve as a basic reference. Urine should be analyzed for protein and sediment changes prior to each injection and complete blood counts should be done prior to every second injection throughout the course of treatment.

Adverse reactions to gold therapy may occur at any time during treatment or many months after therapy has been discontinued. Common adverse reactions include *cutaneous* (dermatitis, pruritic eruptions, erythema, vesicular and exfoliative dermatitis, alopecia, loss of nails); *mucous membranes* (stomatitis, buccal ulcers, glossitis or gingivitis); *pulmonary* (interstitial pneumonitis, fibrosis, fever, rash, cough, shortness of breath, etc); *renal* (nephrotic syndrome, glomerulitis with hematuria, and rarely renal failure); *hematologic* (granulocytopenia, thrombocytopenia, leukopenia, eosinophilia, hemorrhagic diathesis, hypoplastic and aplastic anemia); and *miscellaneous reactions* (flushing, dizziness, sweating, nausea, vomiting, and malaise).

If toxicity develops, gold therapy should be discontinued immediately. Treatment includes topical or systemic corticosteroids as appropriate and the chelating agent dimercaprol (BAL) to increase the excretion of gold.

Auranofin

Gold, (2,3,4,6-tetra-*O*-acetyl-1-thio-β-D-glucopyranato-*S*)-(triethylphosphine)-, Ridaura (*SKF*)

(1-Thio-β-D-glucopyranosato)(triethylphosphine)gold [34031-32-8] $C_{20}H_{34}AuO_9PS$ (678.48).

Preparation—By condensation of the tetraacetate ester of aurothioglucose with triethylphosphine to form the coordination complex; see US Pat 3,635,945.

Description—Colorless crystals melting about 110°.

Uses—Auranofin, an investigational compound in which gold is complexed with triethylphosphine, is used in the treatment of rheumatoid arthritis. The value of gold salts in rheumatoid arthritis is well established; however, most available gold preparations must be administered intramuscularly. Although auranofin is administered orally, it appears to retain the efficacy of the parenteral gold substances without causing major side effects. Auranofin is well absorbed following oral administration. Following 3 mg of auranofin twice daily (1.7 mg elemental gold/day) mean blood levels reached at 12 days were 0.7 µg/mL and half-life was 2 to 3 weeks (range, 10 to 173 days). The mechanism by which auranofin exerts its therapeutic effect in rheumatoid arthritis is unknown. However, pharmacologic actions of auranofin include inhibition of antibody (lgb) production, inhibition of liposomal enzyme release from phagocytizing leukocytes, and inhibition of mediator release in immediate hypersensitivity reactions. In contrast to parenteral gold preparations, auranofin is not a potent inhibitor of sulfhydryl group reactivity. Adverse effects noted in the limited clinical studies conducted in the United States include diarrhea (34%) and microscopic hematuria; skin reactions (pruritus, rash) were mild and occurred in about 30% of patients; and mucosal ulcerations in approximately 10%; proteinuria was observed in 4% and was serious enough in 0.7% of patients to discontinue therapy. Liver function test abnormalities occurred in 0.4% of patients. The contraindications for auranofin are the same as those for parenteral gold compounds.

Dose—*Usual, adult, oral*, **3 mg** twice a day.

Dosage Form—Capsules: 3 mg (Investigational drug).

Aurothioglucose

Gold, (1-thio-D-glucopyranosato)-, Gold Thioglucose; Solganal (*Schering-Plough*)

(1-Thio-D-glucopyranosato)gold [12192-57-3] $C_6H_{11}AuO_5S$ (392.18). It is stabilized by addition of not more than 5% of sodium acetate.

Preparation—By refluxing an aqueous solution of thioglucose with gold tribromide in the presence of sulfur dioxide. The compound is thus precipitated, and is purified by dissolving in water after which it is reprecipitated by the addition of alcohol.

Description—Yellow powder, odorless or nearly so, and stable in air; pH (1 in 100 solution) about 6.3; aqueous solutions are unstable on long standing.

Solubility—Freely soluble in water; practically insoluble in acetone, alcohol, chloroform, and ether.

Uses—An *antirheumatic* used for treatment of active and progressing *rheumatoid arthritis* and nondisseminated *lupus erythematosus*. The adrenal steroids once largely displaced gold compounds from the therapeutic armamentarium, but recognition of the dangers of steroid therapy and the potential curative properties of gold has restored the use of gold. No other antirheumatic drug is capable of arresting the progression of the disease, as gold can do in some cases. The best therapy is based on the daily excretion rate of gold in the individual patient. The aim is to build up slowly the body burden of gold to the point of obvious improvement of the condition or of minimal toxicity, then maintain with doses that just balance the amount of gold excreted. In the absence of determinations of urinary gold to guide maintenance therapy, it is best to increase the weekly dosage in small steps so that more than 12 weeks are required to reach a maximum dose. Maintenance is then achieved by lengthening the interval between doses to 3 or 4 weeks.

Pruritus is generally the first sign of toxicity. Other toxic manifestations are listed in the introduction to this section (see this page). Although side effects can occur after the first dose, severe side effects do not usually occur until at least 300 to 500 mg has been administered; sometimes they do not occur until several months after treatment has been discontinued. Glucocorticoids increase toxicity yet protect against serious consequences such as nephrosis. Dimercaprol and penicillamine increase excretion of gold.

Dose—*Intramuscular, adult*, **10 mg** in the 1st week, **25 mg** in the 2nd and 3rd weeks, and **50 mg** a week thereafter until a total of **800 mg** to **1 g** has been given; if there has been no response, the drug is discontinued; if there has been improvement and no toxicity has occurred, **25** to **50 mg** every other week is given for 4 doses, every 3 weeks for 4 doses, then every 3 to 4 weeks thereafter. *Children*, 6 to 12 yr of age, **2.5 mg** the first week, **6.25 mg** the second and third weeks, and

12.5 mg a week until **200 to 250 mg** has been given, after which **6.25 to 12.5 mg** every 3 to 4 weeks is used for maintenance. A relapse during the lengthening intervals requires a shortening of the intervals. Toxicity requires discontinuation.

Dosage Form—Suspension: 50 mg/mL.

Gold Sodium Thiomalate

Butanedioic acid, mercapto-, monogold(1+) sodium salt; mercaptosuccinic acid, monogold(1+) sodium salt; Myochrysine (*MSD*)

$$Au-S-\overset{\displaystyle CH_2COO^-}{\underset{\displaystyle CHCOO^-}{|}} \cdot xNa^+ \cdot (2-x)H^+$$

A mixture of mono- and di-sodium salts of gold thiomalic acid, $C_4H_4AuNaO_4S$ (368.09) and $C_4H_3AuNa_2O_4S$ (390.07).

Preparation—Sodium thiomalate is reacted with gold chloride. US Pat 1,994,213.

Description—White to yellowish white, odorless, fine powder; affected by light; pH (1 in 10 solution) between 5.8 and 6.5.

Solubility—Very soluble in water; insoluble in alcohol, ether.

Uses—An *antirheumatic* with the same uses and toxicity as *Aurothioglucose*, except for reported nitritoid reactions with gold sodium thiomalate. It is given intramuscularly only.

Dose—Many authorities consider the dose to be that of *Aurothioglucose*. However, the manufacturer's recommended and hence USP adult dose is: *intramuscular, initially* **10 mg** in the first and **25 mg** in the second week, then **50 mg** once a week for 20 weeks and, for *maintenance*, **50 mg** every 2 weeks for 4 doses, **50 mg** every 3 weeks for 4 doses, then **50 mg** a month, if tolerated. *Children*, up to 12 yr of age, **1 mg per kg** of body weight, not to exceed **25 mg** per dose, once a week for 6 months, then once a month.

Dosage Forms—Injection: 10, 25, 50, and 100 mg/mL.

CHAPTER 61

Histamine and Antihistamines

Ewart A Swinyard, PhD, DSc (Hon)

Professor Emeritus of Pharmacology
College of Pharmacy and School of Medicine
University of Utah
Salt Lake City, UT 84112

Despite the fact that histamine is of relatively little therapeutic importance few agents have commanded more attention from biochemists, pharmacologists, and physiologists. This ubiquitous substance is a natural constituent of many tissues in man. It is found in at least three types of storage sites. One fraction is held in the granules of mast cells and basophils, the equivalent cells in peripheral blood. Histamine in these granules is bound with heparin and cannot exert an effect or be metabolized. The mast cells are degranulated and the histamine released by the antigen-antibody complex formed as the first step in an immediate allergic reaction and by histamine-liberating chemicals. A second fraction of histamine is held in the mucosal layer of the gastrointestinal tract, where it is not contained in mast cells and not depleted by histamine liberation. The third fraction is held in the hypothalamus and area postrema; the histamine in this site is released by reserpine. These observations suggest that the endogenous release of this substance may be the causative agent in a number of physiologic and pathologic reactions, such as allergy and anaphylactic shock.

The demonstration that histamine was the factor responsible for allergic and anaphylactic phenomena stimulated the search for histamine antagonists. In 1937, Bovet and Staub demonstrated that certain phenolic ethers were able to block many of the pharmacological actions of histamine. This observation provided the stimulus that resulted in the discovery and development of many useful antihistaminic agents.

Subsequently it was established that typical antihistamine drugs (such as pyrilamine maleate) in low concentrations suppress histamine contractions of smooth muscle in various organs, such as the gut and bronchi. The pharmacological receptors involved in these mepyramine-sensitive histamine responses have been defined as H_1-receptors. Based on a single analogy with catecholamine β-receptors and their antagonists and on the structure of histamine, Black and coworkers in 1964 (Black, *et al Nature 236:* 385, 1972) initiated a systematic search for antagonists that would block the histamine-induced gastric acid secretion, increases in heart rate, and inhibition of uterine contractions. This investigation resulted in the identification of burimamide (N-methyl-N'-(4-(4(5)-imidazolyl)butyl)thiourea), an H_2 receptor antagonist, and led to the development of a new class of drugs, the histamine H_2-receptor antagonists. Burimamide and metiamide block the effects of histamine not inhibited by older H_1-receptor antagonists, such as those to be discussed in this chapter. The newer H_2-antagonist drugs, such as cimetidine and ranitidine, inhibit gastric secretion stimulated not only by histamine, but also by insulin, pentagastrin, food, or physiological vagal reflex. These agents are discussed on pages 797, 798.

Another amine, 5-hydroxytryptamine, is also widely distributed in animals and is present in some plants. This substance, discovered independently by three groups of workers, is also known as *enteramine*, and *serotonin*. It is found in largest amounts in brain, blood, spleen, stomach, intestine,

lungs, and skin. It has been suggested that 5-hydroxytryptamine may be involved in the regulation of vascular tone, motor and secretory activity of the gastrointestinal tract, and kidney function. It has been postulated also that 5-hydroxytryptamine serves as a neurotransmitter in the brain and that it may be involved in mental function. These observations and the demonstration that tumors of the argentaffin cells of the intestinal mucosa (argentaffinomas or carcinoids) secrete large amounts of 5-hydroxytryptamine have stimulated the search for 5-hydroxytryptamine antagonists. A number of substances, including ergot alkaloids and derivatives, indole derivatives, adrenergic blocking agents, anticholinergic drugs, morphine-like analgesics, and some phenothiazines have been shown to possess this property. In addition, at least two agents that exhibit both antihistaminic and anti-5-hydroxytryptamine properties are available to clinicians and more selective 5-hydroxytryptamine antagonists are under clinical investigation. Therefore, 5-hydroxytryptamine antagonists also will be included in this chapter.

Betazole Hydrochloride

1H-Pyrazole-3-ethanamine, dihydrochloride; Histalog (*Lilly*)

3-(2-Aminoethyl)pyrazole dihydrochloride [138-92-1] $C_5H_9N_3$.2HCl (184.07).

Preparation—Betazole may be synthesized by catalytic reduction of 3-pyrazoleacetaldehyde hydrazone, which is obtained by treating 4H-pyran-4-one with hydrazine. The betazole base is dissolved in alcohol and converted to the dihydrochloride with anhydrous HCl, which is precipitated with ether.

Description—White, crystalline, nearly odorless powder; solutions are acid to litmus; pH (1 in 20 solution) about 1.5; softens at a temperature not lower than 215°, and finally melts at a temperature not higher than 240°.

Solubility—Soluble in water; practically insoluble in chloroform.

Uses—An isomer of histamine (a pyrazole rather than an imidazole derivative) which induces maximal stimulation of gastric secretion without the high incidence of side effects that occurs with histamine. A subcutaneous injection of 50 mg of betazole hydrochloride is equivalent to 0.3 mg of histamine. It is *effective* in the clinical testing of gastric secretion. The maximum response to betazole begins about 45 minutes after administration and lasts approximately 2½ hr. The secretory volume and acidity are usually increased 100 to 200% in the normal patient. A specimen obtained during a 15-min period of maximal response usually contains 3 to 13 milliequivalents (average 8.5) of free acid. High values are found in duodenal ulcer and pyloric obstruction; low values in gastric ulcer, carcinoma of the stomach, and chronic gastritis, and in chronic diseases and debilitated states. Absence of free hydrochloric acid is always found in pernicious anemia. The most commonly observed side effect is flushing of the face accompanied by a sense of warmth. Headache and urticaria may also occur. Weakness and syncope have been reported. Although H_1-antihistamines have been reported of value in the management of betazole hydrochloride-induced urticaria, they have no effect on the stimulation of gastric secretion produced by betazole hydrochloride. The drug should be used with caution in patients with bronchial asthma.

Dose—*Subcutaneous* or *intramuscular*, **40 to 60 mg;** *usual*, either **0.5 mg/kg** or a single total dose of **50 mg.** In either case the dose is equivalent to about ½ the standard dose of histamine.

Dosage Forms—Injection: 50 mg/mL.

Histamine Phosphate

1*H*-Imidazole-4-ethanamine, phosphate (1:2); Histamine Phosphate

4-(2-Aminoethyl)imidazole phosphate (1:2) [51-74-1] $C_5H_9N_3.2H_3PO_4$ (307.14).

Preparation—Histamine occurs in very small amounts in ergot. It is among the products of bacterial decomposition of histidine, and this constitutes one of the methods for its production. It is also produced synthetically from imidazolylpropionic acid by several methods.

Description—Colorless, odorless, long prismatic crystals; stable in air but is affected by light; its aqueous solution is acid to litmus; when dried at 105° for 2 hours, it melts at about 140°.

Solubility—1 g in about 4 mL water.

Pharmacology—Although many tissues contain a lethal amount of histamine in a bound or inactive form, no effect is produced until it is released in free form into body fluids as a result of certain stimuli. Since histamine is destroyed in the intestinal tract by the enzyme histaminase, it is ineffective when taken orally. After injection, histamine constricts certain smooth muscles such as the bronchi, uterus, and intestines and dilates the capillary bed. Characteristically, increased capillary permeability accompanies the dilation, and there is a seepage of fluid, plasma proteins, and even some cellular elements of the blood into extracellular spaces. Dilation of the capillaries and arterioles produces flushing of the face, fall in blood pressure, and increase in skin temperature.

Histamine stimulates all types of glandular secretions—gastric, duodenal, salivary, and lacrimal. An important effect in man is stimulation of the gastric glands, which increases the hydrochloric acid of the stomach. This effect is the basis of a diagnostic test to differentiate between nonspecific hypochlorhydria and that caused by pernicious anemia (see page 1273).

One highly characteristic effect of histamine is the "triple response" induced by the intracutaneous injection of small amounts of this agent. It consists of (1) local reddening at the site of the injection, (2) a wheal or patch of localized edema which obscures the original red spot, and (3) the scarlet flare that surrounds the wheal. The initial red spot is mostly due to local capillary dilatation, and the wheal develops from arteriolar dilation and increased capillary permeability. The flare is a local phenomenon produced by an axon reflex involving peripheral sensory nerves. Since the flare does not appear in the presence of atrophy or degeneration of the nerve, this reaction has been used as a diagnostic test to distinguish between real and pseudoanesthesia.

When injected intravenously, histamine provokes an increased output of epinephrine from the adrenal medulla as indicated by a secondary rise in blood pressure. Clinical use is made of this action on the adrenals by employing histamine as a test agent in the diagnosis of pheochromocytoma.

Uses—Histamine is used as a *diagnostic* agent for testing the *functional capacity of the gastric glands.* If no acid is secreted following the injection of 0.25 to 0.5 mg (usually as a 1:1000 solution), a true gastric achylia exists. Histamine is also employed in the *diagnosis of pheochromocytoma.* In patients with adrenal medullary tumors, intravenous administration of the compound is followed by a dramatic rise in blood pressure due to the release of excessive quantities of epinephrine and norepinephrine from the neoplasm. Histamine has a few other minor diagnostic applications. Since the "flare" that results from intracutaneous injection of this agent is mediated by an axon reflex, this approach has been used as a test for the integrity of sensory nerves; the wheal that results has been used as a test for circulatory competency.

Adverse reactions are observed even after small doses such as em-

ployed in gastric analysis (0.01 mg/kg subcutaneously). These include flushing, dizziness, headache, bronchial constriction, dyspnea, visual disturbances, faintness, syncope, urticaria, asthma, marked hypertension or hypotension, palpitation, tachycardia, nervousness, abdominal cramps, diarrhea, vomiting, metallic taste, allergic manifestations, or collapse with convulsions. The hypotension is usually postural and requires no treatment other than the recumbent position. If treatment is required, epinephrine (0.3 mg SC) is an effective physiologic antagonist.

Dose—*Diagnostic, gastric test, subcutaneous,* **27.5 μg** (equivalent to 10 μg of histamine)**/kg.** *Usual range of dose,* **10 to 40 μg/kg.** *Pheochromocytoma test, intravenous,* **10 μg** and monitor blood pressure and pulse every 30 sec; if no response within 5 min, repeat with **50 μg** and monitor blood pressure and pulse as above for 15 min.

Dosage Forms—Injection: 0.275, 0.55, 1, and 2.75 mg/mL.

Antihistamines

Following the suggestion by Dale and Laidlaw in 1911 that the symptoms of histamine shock resembled those in anaphylaxis, many experimenters added findings tending to substantiate the concept that release of histamine from tissues is responsible for the anaphylactic reaction. It is true that some manifestations of anaphylaxis cannot be explained by histamine effect, but it was argued that histamine is at least the major mechanism. The histamine concept was gradually adopted to explain the allergic reaction in man after Lewis, in 1924, claimed that histamine effects in man were identical with those of allergy. Many attempts were then made in animals and man to raise the tolerance to histamine by injections of the latter. The preponderance of evidence indicates that tolerance to histamine only infrequently can be acquired in that manner. Evidence that obtaining such tolerance in man can be obtained by administration of conjugated histamine (histamine-azoprotein or *Hapamine*) has not been established.

Although many substances had been previously demonstrated to antagonize responses to histamine and certain manifestations of antigen–antibody reactions, it was not until 1942 that sufficiently specific and nontoxic agents became available for this action to be of clinical importance. As a result of intensive research in this field, an excessive number of effective agents are now on the market. All conventional antihistamines antagonize histamine to approximately the same extent, regardless of their chemical class (ethanolamine, ethylenediamine, alkylamine, phenothiazine). The clinical and pharmacological differences, therefore, are related chiefly to variations in adverse effects and to nonhistamine antagonizing actions, such as their atropine-like effects, central nervous system effects (depression, stimulation, antiemetic, anti-tremor and motion sickness) and local anesthetic properties. A knowledge of these factors is essential for proper drug selection.

All presently available antihistamines (H_1-receptor antagonists) act by competitively antagonizing the effects of histamine at receptor sites; they do not block the release of histamine and, hence, offer only palliative relief of allergic symptoms. After oral administration, effects are apparent within 15 to 30 min, are maximal within 1 hr and persist for 4 to 6 hr. The liver is the principal site of metabolism; the agents are excreted in urine as unidentified metabolites.

Clinically, indications for use of the various antihistaminic drugs vary considerably. The majority of these agents are *effective* in *perennial* and *seasonal allergic rhinitis, vasomotor rhinitis, allergic conjunctivitis, urticaria and angioedema, allergic reactions to blood and plasma, dermographism,* and as adjuncts to conventional therapy in *anaphylactic reactions.* A few antihistamine drugs are probably effective in mild, local *allergic reactions to insect bites, physical allergy,* and minor *drug* and *serum* reactions characterized by *pruritus*. Selected antihistamines (eg, diphenhydramine hydrochloride) reduce rigidity and tremors in *paralysis agitans* (Parkinson's disease) and in *drug-induced extrapyramidal symptoms*. Some antihistamine agents (eg, buclizine, cyclizine, dimenhydrinate, diphenhydramine, meclizine, and others) are also effective in the *active and prophylactic* management of *motion sickness*. The more sedative agents (eg, diphenhydramine, doxylamine, promethazine, and others) are sometimes used as substitutes for barbiturates in *insomnia* and *insomnia* predominant in certain medical disorders. Certain antihistaminic drugs, such as chlorpheniramine, doxylamine succinate, and pyrilamine maleate, are used in proprietary medication advertised as daytime sedatives and sleep aids. Methapyrilene, formerly used in virtually all nonprescription sleep aids in the United States, was removed from these products in 1979 because of its possible carcinogenic properties.

The phenothiazine antihistaminic drugs possess other useful clinical properties not shared by conventional antihistaminic drugs. For example promethazine hydrochloride is useful for *preoperative, postoperative,* and *obstetric sedation,* prevention and control of *nausea* and *vomiting* associated with certain types of anesthesia and surgery, and as *adjunctive therapy* to meperidine or other analgesics for the *control of postoperative pain*.

The usefulness of antihistaminic drugs in various other clinical conditions, such as bronchial asthma, atopic dermatitis, neurodermatitis, allergic eczema, various contact and chemotoxic dermatitides, generalized pruritus, and use in cardiac arrhythmias, spasmolysis in gastrointestinal allergies, prophylaxis of drug reactions, etc, must await further clinical investigation before a final assessment can be made.

It is generally agreed that *most* antihistamine drugs are *ineffective* in migraine and histamine headache, prevention or reduction of the sequelae of pain, edema, and hemorrhage in oral surgery, potentiation of narcotic analgesic drugs, as antiemetic agents in postoperative patients, as antitussive agents, or for treatment of nocturnal leg cramps, leg cramps of pregnancy, and functional dysmenorrhea.

The most common side effect of antihistamines is sedation, evidenced principally by drowsiness, and diminished alertness and ability to concentrate. Less common effects—unless large doses are used—include dryness of the mouth, blurred vision, vertigo, and gastrointestinal distress (see also above). The sedative effect may be so intense as to impair driving ability and performance of duties requiring mental alertness. Other side reactions elicited by these drugs include nausea, headache, and restiveness. Dermatologic complications and skin eruptions have followed local application or oral administration of antihistamines. In a few individuals, certain antihistamines produce signs of central excitation such as insomnia and nervousness. Since the depressant effects of alcoholic beverages and other drugs that depress the central nervous system (tranquilizers, hypnotics, sedatives, antianxiety agents, depressants, analgesics, etc) are increased by antihistamines, the physician may proscribe concurrent use or modify the conditions of such use. Patients being treated with monoamine oxidase inhibitors, or who have been treated with such drugs within the preceding two weeks, should not be given antihistamines.

Because of their drying effect on mucous membranes, antihistamines may exacerbate wheezing and therefore should not be used during an asthmatic attack. Because of the anticholinergic action of antihistamines, their use in the following diseases may be contraindicated or subject to great caution: narrow-angle glaucoma, prostatic hypertrophy, stenosing peptic ulcer, pyloroduodenal obstruction, bladder-neck obstruction, increased intraocular pressure, history of bronchial asthma, hyperthyroidism, cardiovascular disease, hypertension. Antihistamines should not be given to pre-

mature or newborn infants, and may be proscribed by the physician for patients breast-feeding infants.

These brief observations call attention to the enormous number of clinical conditions for which antihistaminic drugs have been suggested. They also point up the fact that these drugs vary from *effective* to *ineffective* in these conditions. When one considers the multiplicity of available antihistaminic drugs, their numerous untoward reactions, and their propensity to induce sedation of variable intensity, one can appreciate the complex therapeutic problem that confronts the thoughtful physician in the selection of an antihistaminic drug for a particular patient with a histamine-related clinical condition.

Brompheniramine Maleate

2-Pyridinepropanamine, γ-(4-bromophenyl)-*N,N*-dimethyl-, (*Z*)-butenedioate (1:1); Dimetane (*Robins*)

2-[*p*-Bromo-α-[2-(dimethylamino)ethyl]benzyl]pyridine maleate (1:1) [980-71-2] $C_{16}H_{19}BrN_2.C_4H_4O_4$ (435.32).

Preparation—α-(*p*-Bromophenyl)-2-pyridineacetonitrile is converted to its sodium derivative with sodium amide and condensed with 2-chloro-*N,N*-dimethylethylamine. The resulting nitrile is converted to its corresponding acid, which is decarboxylated by treatment with H_2SO_4. Brompheniramine base, obtained on alkalinization, is solvent-extracted and reacted with maleic acid.

Description—White, odorless, crystalline powder; melts between 130° and 135°; pH (1 in 100 solution) between 4.0 and 5.0.

Solubility—1 g in 5 mL water, 15 mL alcohol, 15 mL chloroform; slightly soluble in ether and benzene.

Uses—The bromine analogue of chlorpheniramine; an antihistaminic agent with anticholinergic (drying) and sedative side effects. It is *probably effective* for temporary relief of hay fever and upper respiratory allergy symptoms, such as itchy, watery eyes, sneezing, itching nose or throat and for amelioration and prevention of allergic reactions to blood or plasma in patients with a known history of such reactions. See also article on *Antihistamines*.

Dose—*Usual, adult, oral,* 4 to **8 mg** 3 or 4 times a day; extended-release tablets, 8 or **12 mg** every 12 hr. Do not exceed 24 mg in 24 hrs. *Parenteral, intramuscular, intravenous,* or *subcutaneous,* **10 mg** 2 times a day; maximum, 40 mg. *Pediatric, children* under 5 yr, *oral,* **125 µg per kg** of body wt or **3.75 mg per m²** of body surface every 6 hr; *children* over 6 yr, *oral,* **2 to 4 mg** 3 or 4 times a day or **8 to 12 mg** as extended-release tablet every 12 hr; *parenteral, children* 11 yr and under, **125 µg per kg** of body wt or **3.75 mg per m²** of body surface every 6 hr; contraindicated for premature and full-term neonates.

Dosage Forms—Elixir: 2 mg/5 mL; Injection: 10 mg/mL; Tablets: 4 mg; Extended-release Tablets: 8 and 12 mg.

Carbinoxamine Maleate

Ethanamine, 2-[(4-chlorophenyl)-2-pyridinylmethoxy]-*N,N*-dimethyl-, (*Z*)-2-butenedioate (1:1); Clistin (*McNeil*)

2-[*p*-Chloro-α-[2-(dimethylamino)ethoxy]benzyl]pyridine maleate (1:1) [3505-38-2] $C_{16}H_{19}ClN_2O.C_4H_4O_4$ (406.87).

Preparation—Picolinaldehyde and *p*-chlorophenylmagnesium bromide undergo a Grignard reaction to produce *p*-chloro-α-(2-pyridyl)benzyl alcohol. This is converted into its sodium alkoxide derivative with sodamide. β-Dimethylaminoethyl chloride is added to form carbinoxamine; the base is converted into the maleate by reaction with maleic acid.

Description—White, odorless, crystalline powder; melting range 116° to 121°; pH (1 in 100 solution) 4.6 to 5.1; pK_a 8.7.

Solubility—1 g in <1 mL water, 1.5 mL alcohol, 1.5 mL chloroform, 8300 mL ether.

Uses—An antihistaminic agent with weak atropine-like anticholinergic activity and a low incidence of side effects. It is *probably effective* in allergic rhinitis, vasomotor rhinitis, allergic conjunctivitis, mild uncomplicated allergic skin manifestation of urticaria and angioedema. Adverse reactions are relatively mild and rarely occur; dizziness, drowsiness, nausea, and dryness of the mouth have been observed. Other precautions and contraindications are the same as those for other antihistaminic drugs (see page 1125).

Dose—*Usual, adult, oral,* 4 to **8 mg** 3 or 4 times a day. *Pediatric, children,* 1 to 3 yrs, **2 mg** 3 or 4 times daily; 3 to 6 yrs, **2** to **4 mg** 3 or 4 times daily; over 6 yrs, 4 to **6 mg** 3 or 4 times daily; contraindicated for premature and full-term neonates.

Dosage Forms—Tablets: 4 mg.

Chlorpheniramine Maleate

2-Pyridinepropanamine, γ-(4-chlorophenyl)-*N*,*N*-dimethyl-, (*Z*)-2-butenedioate (1:1); (*Various Mfrs*) Chlor-Trimeton (*Schering-Plough*)

2-[*p*-Chloro-α-[2-(dimethylamino)ethyl]benzyl]pyridine maleate (1:1) [113-92-8] $C_{16}H_{19}ClN_2.C_4H_4O_4$ (390.87).

Preparation—Chlorpheniramine may be prepared by condensing 2-[*p*-chloro-α-(2-chloroethyl)benzyl]pyridine with dimethylamine in the presence of sodamide. Treatment of the base with an equimolar portion of maleic acid results in the formation of the maleate.

Description—White, odorless, crystalline powder; its solutions are acid to litmus having a pH between 4 and 5; melts between 130° and 135°.

Solubility—1 g in 4 mL water, 10 mL alcohol, 10 mL chloroform; slightly soluble in ether and benzene.

Uses—An *antihistaminic* agent which is *probably effective* in allergic and vasomotor rhinitis, allergic conjunctivitis, mild urticaria and angioedema, allergic reactions to blood and plasma in sensitive patients, dermographism, and as adjunct therapy in anaphylactic shock. Chlorpheniramine maleate is widely used as an ingredient in proprietary antitussive formulations. It has a low incidence of side effects, which are similar to those induced by other antihistamines. See article on *Antihistamines.*

Dose—*Usual, adult, oral,* **4 mg** 4 to 6 times a day; extended-release capsules or tablets, 8 to **12 mg** every 8 to 12 hr; *parenteral,* 5 to **20 mg** as a single dose, with a maximum of 40 mg in 24 hr. *Pediatric, children* 11 yr and under, *oral,* **2 mg** 3 to 6 times a day; do not exceed **12 mg** in 24 hours. Extended-release forms not recommended for children under 12 years.

Dosage Forms—Injection: 10, 20, and 100 mg/mL; Tablets: 4 mg; Extended-release Capsules: 8 mg; Extended-release Tablets: 8 and 12 mg; Syrup: 2 mg/5 mL.

Clemastine Fumarate

Pyrrolidine, 2-[2-[1-(4-chlorophenyl)-1-phenylethoxy]ethyl]-1-methyl-, [*R*-(*R**,*R**)]-, (*E*)-2-butenedioate (1:1); Tavist, Tavegyl (*Dorsey*)

(+)-(2*R*)-2-[2-[(*R*)-*p*-Chloro-α-methyl-α-phenylbenzyl)oxy]-ethyl]-1-methylpyrrolidine fumarate (1:1) [14976-57-9] $C_{21}H_{26}ClNO.C_4H_4O_4$ (459.97).

Preparation—Various benzhydryl ethers that have histamine-inhibiting action, of which clemastine is one, may be prepared by heating a mixture of the appropriate benzhydryl bromide and *N*-methyl-2-piperidylethanol in the presence of sodium carbonate. Details of the process, as well as of an alternate synthesis, are described in British Pat 942,152 (see *CA 60*: 9250g, 1964).

Description—White to faintly yellow, crystalline powder; practically odorless; melts at 176° to 181°, with decomposition.

Solubility—Very slightly soluble in water, chloroform, ether; slightly soluble in alcohol.

Uses—A long-acting *antihistamine* with anticholinergic (drying) and sedative side effects. Indicated for relief of symptoms associated with seasonal allergic rhinitis and mild uncomplicated allergic skin manifestations of urticaria and angioedema. Side effects and contraindications are similar to those of other agents in this group (see page 1125).

Dose—*Usual, adult, oral,* 1 *to* **2 mg** (clemastine base) daily; may be repeated as required but not to exceed **6 mg** daily. *Children under 12 years,* safety and efficacy have not been established.

Dosage Form—Tablets: 1.34 and 2.68 mg of clemastine fumarate (equivalent to 1 and 2 mg of clemastine base).

Cyclizine—page 807.

Dexchlorpheniramine Maleate

2-Pyridinepropanamine, γ-(4-chlorophenyl)-*N*,*N*-dimethyl-, (*S*)-, (*Z*)-2-butenedioate (1:1); Polaramine (*Schering*)

(+)-2-[*p*-Chloro-α-[2-(dimethylamino)ethyl]benzyl]pyridine maleate (1:1) [2438-32-6] $C_{16}H_{19}ClN_2.C_4H_4O_4$ (390.87).

Preparation—Racemic chlorpheniramine (see *Chlorpheniramine Maleate*) is resolved with the aid of *d*-phenylsuccinic acid. The *d*-enantiomorph of the base is then liberated from its *d*-phenylsuccinate by treatment with sodium hydroxide and reacted with an equimolar portion of maleic acid.

Description—White, odorless, crystalline powder; melts between 110° and 115°; pH (1 in 100 solution) between 4.0 and 5.0.

Solubility—1 g in 1.1 mL water, 2 mL alcohol, 1.7 mL chloroform, 2500 mL ether.

Uses—The dextro isomer of chlorpheniramine; it is an antihistaminic agent which has about twice the potency of chlorpheniramine and a wide margin of safety. Its uses and limitations are similar to those for chlorpheniramine maleate (see this page). See also the article on *Antihistamines.*

Dose—*Usual, adult, oral,* **2 mg** every 4 to 6 hours, or 4 to **6 mg** as extended-release tablets every 8 to 12 hr. *Pediatric, infants, oral,* **500 µg** (0.5 mg) every 4 to 6 hours; *children* 6 to 12 years, **1 mg** every 4 to 6 hours, or a **4 mg** extended-release tablet once daily at bedtime; *children* 2 to 5 years, **500 µg** (0.5 mg) every 4 to 6 hours. Do not use extended-release form; contraindicated for premature and full-term neonates.

Dosage Forms—Syrup: 2 mg/5 mL; Tablets: 2 mg; Extended-release Tablets: 4 and 6 mg.

Dimenhydrinate—page 808.

Dimethindene Maleate

1*H*-Indene-2-ethanamine, *N*,*N*-dimethyl-3-[1-(2-pyridinyl)ethyl]-, (*Z*)-2-butenedioate (1:1); Forhistal (*Ciba-Geigy*); Triten (*Marion*)

2-[1-[2-[2-(Dimethylamino)ethyl]inden-3-yl]ethyl]pyridine maleate (1:1) [3614-69-5] $C_{20}H_{24}N_2.C_4H_4O_4$ (408.50).

Preparation—1-(2-Pyridyl)ethyllithium, obtained by interaction of phenyllithium and 2-ethylpyridine, undergoes addition to 2-[2-(dimethylamino)ethyl]indan-1-one. Acid-catalyzed hydrolysis yields the tertiary carbinol, which dehydrates on warming to form dimethindene (base). Reaction with maleic acid yields the maleate.

Description—White to off-white, crystalline powder with a characteristic odor; stable in dry air, but sensitive to light; melts with decomposition at about 161°.

Solubility—1 g in about 200 mL water; freely soluble in methanol; soluble in chloroform; practically insoluble in ether.

Uses—An indene compound that is a potent antihistaminic agent used in perennial and seasonal allergic rhinitis; vasomotor rhinitis;

allergic conjunctivitis; mild, uncomplicated allergic skin manifestations of urticaria and angioedema; amelioration of allergic reactions to blood or plasma; dermographism; anaphylactic reactions as adjunctive therapy to epinephrine and other standard measures after the acute manifestations have been controlled. Since it is chemically different than other antihistamines, it may be useful in patients not responding to other agents. See page 1125.

Dose—*Usual, adult* and *children* over 6 yr of age, *oral*, Extended-release tablet, **2.5 mg** 1 or 2 times a day.

Dosage Forms—Extended-release tablets: 2.5 mg.

Diphenhydramine Hydrochloride

Ethanamine, 2-(diphenylmethoxy)-*N,N*-dimethyl-, hydrochloride;
β-Dimethylaminoethyl Benzhydryl Ether Hydrochloride;
Benadryl Hydrochloride (*Parke-Davis*); Bendylate (*Reid-Provident*)

2-(Diphenylmethoxy)-*N,N*-dimethylethylamine hydrochloride [147-24-0] $C_{17}H_{21}NO.HCl$ (291.82).

Preparation—By heating diphenylbromomethane, β-dimethylaminoethanol, and sodium carbonate in toluene. After distilling off the toluene, the purified diphenhydramine is converted to the hydrochloride with hydrogen chloride.

Description—White, odorless, crystalline powder; slowly darkens on exposure to light; its solutions are practically neutral to litmus; melting range 167° to 172°.

Solubility—1 g in 1 mL water, 2 mL alcohol, 2 mL chloroform, 50 mL acetone; very slightly soluble in benzene and ether.

Uses—A potent antihistaminic agent that possesses anticholinergic (drying), antitussive, antiemetic and sedative effects. Diphenhydramine is *effective* for use in perennial and seasonal allergic rhinitis; vasomotor rhinitis; allergic conjunctivitis due to inhalant allergens and foods; mild, uncomplicated allergic skin manifestations of urticaria and angioedema; amelioration and prevention of allergic reactions to blood or plasma in patients with a known history of such reactions; dermographism; therapy for anaphylactic reactions adjunctive to epinephrine and other standard measures after the acute manifestations have been controlled; parkinsonism (including drug-induced) in the elderly unable to tolerate more potent agents; mild cases of parkinsonism (including drug-induced) in other age groups; other cases of parkinsonism (including drug-induced) in combination with centrally acting anticholinergic agents; and active and prophylactic treatment of motion sickness. It also has significant antitussive activity; the syrup is used as a cough suppressant for the control of cough due to colds or allergy.

Diphenhydramine hydrochloride is *probably effective* for use in mild, local allergic reactions to insect bites; physical allergy; minor drug and serum reactions characterized by pruritus; and intractable insomnia and insomnia dominant in certain medical disorders. Other suggested uses require further investigation.

Numerous side effects are observed by patients on this drug, such as drowsiness, confusion, restlessness, nausea, vomiting, diarrhea, blurring of vision, diplopia, difficulty in urination, constipation, nasal stuffiness, vertigo, palpitation, headache, insomnia, urticaria, drug rash, photosensitivity, hemolytic anemia, hypotension, epigastric distress, anaphylactic shock, tightness of the chest and wheezing, thickening of bronchial secretions, dryness of the mouth, nose, and throat, and tingling, heaviness, and weakness of the hands.

Dimenhydrinate (Dramamine) contains approximately 50% diphenhydramine. The former agent is capable of masking symptoms of ototoxicity; therefore, dimenhydrinate and diphenhydramine should be used with caution in patients receiving aminoglycoside antibiotics (streptomycin, neomycin, or kanamycin) or other ototoxic drugs.

Since diphenhydramine has an atropine-like action, it should be used with caution in patients with asthma. Likewise, patients should be cautioned about taking this drug with other depressant substances, because of the additive effect. Persons should also be advised not to operate a motor vehicle, fly an airplane, or operate hazardous machinery while on this drug. The incidence of side effects is about 30 to 60%.

Dose—*Usual, adult, oral*, **25** to **50 mg** 3 or 4 times a day, with maximum of 400 mg daily; *intravenous* or deep *intramuscular*, **10** to **50 mg**/dose, with maximum of 400 mg daily; *topical*, to skin, **2%** cream 3 or 4 times a day. *Pediatric, children, oral, intravenous* or deep *intramuscular*, **1.25 mg/kg** of body wt or **37.5 mg per m²** of body surface 4 times a day not to exceed 300 mg daily; *topical*, to skin, same as adult; contraindicated for neonates.

Dosage Forms—Capsules: 25 and 50 mg; Elixir: 12.5 mg/5 mL; Injection: 10 and 50 mg/mL; Syrup: 12.5 mg/5 mL; Tablets: 50 mg.

Diphenylpyraline Hydrochloride

Piperidine, 4-(diphenylmethoxy)-1-methyl-, hydrochloride;
Diafen (*Riker*)

4-(Diphenylmethoxy)-1-methylpiperidine hydrochloride [132-18-3] $C_{19}H_{23}NO.HCl$ (317.86).

Preparation—Diphenylpyraline is formed when a xylene solution of 1-methyl-4-piperidinol and benzhydryl bromide is refluxed. Reaction with HCl in a suitable solvent yields the hydrochloride. US Pat 2,479,843.

Description—White, crystalline powder; melts at about 206°.
Solubility—Soluble in water, alcohol, and isopropyl alcohol; insoluble in ether and benzene.

Uses—An antihistaminic agent with anticholinergic (drying) and sedative effects. It is *effective* for use in perennial and seasonal allergic rhinitis, vasomotor rhinitis, allergic conjunctivitis due to inhalant allergens and foods, mild uncomplicated allergic skin manifestations of urticaria and angioedema: angioedema, dermographism, and amelioration of reactions to blood or plasma. Untoward effects, contraindications, and precautions are similar to other antihistamines. See article on *Antihistamines*.

Dose—*Usual, adult, oral*, **5 mg** extended-release capsule every 12 hours. *Children* (6 to 12), **5 mg** daily. Not recommended for children under 6.

Dosage Forms—Tablets: 2 mg; Extended-release Capsules: 5 mg.

Doxylamine Succinate

Ethanamine, *N,N*-dimethyl-2-[1-phenyl-1-(2-pyridinyl)ethoxy]-,
butanedioate (1:1); Decapryn Succinate (*Merrell-National*);
Unisom (*Pfizer*)

2-[α-[2-(Dimethylamino)ethoxy]-α-methylbenzyl]pyridine succinate (1:1) [562-10-7] $C_{17}H_{22}N_2O.C_4H_6O_4$ (388.46).

Preparation—Methylphenyl-2-pyridylcarbinol is converted into its sodium alcoholate and refluxed in toluene with 2-(dimethylamino)ethyl chloride. The doxylamine thus formed is reacted with an equimolar quantity of succinic acid in warm acetone.

Description—White or creamy white powder, having a characteristic odor; melts within a range of 3° between 103° and 108°.
Solubility—Very soluble in water and alcohol; freely soluble in chloroform; very slightly soluble in ether and benzene.

Uses—An antihistaminic agent *probably effective* for the symptomatic treatment of seasonal and perennial allergic rhinitis, vasomotor rhinitis, allergic conjunctivitis due to inhalant allergens and foods, mild, uncomplicated allergic skin manifestations of urticaria and angioedema, and the amelioration and prevention of allergic reactions to blood or plasma in patients with a known history of such reactions. The drug is *ineffective* for the prevention and symptomatic relief of measles. Untoward effects and contraindications are similar to those for other members of this group of drugs. See article on *Antihistamines*.

Dose—*Usual, adult, oral,* **12.5 to 25 mg** every 4 to 6 hr as needed. *Pediatric, children* 12 yr and over, *oral,* **12.5 to 25 mg** every 4 to 6 hr as needed; *children* 6 to 12 years, **6.25 to 12.5 mg** every 4 to 6 hr, not to exceed **75 mg** daily; contraindicated for premature and full-term neonates.

Dosage Forms—Syrup: 6.25 mg/5 mL; Tablets: 12.5 and 25 mg.

Hydroxyzine Hydrochloride—page 1071.

Methdilazine

10*H*-Phenothiazine, 10-[(1-methyl-3-pyrrolidinyl)methyl]-, Tacaryl (*Westwood*)

10-[(1-Methyl-3-pyrrolidinyl)methyl]phenothiazine [1982-37-2] C₁₈H₂₀N₂S (296.43).

Preparation—Methdilazine may be prepared by condensation of phenothiazine with 1-methyl-3-pyrrolidinylmethyl chloride. US Pat 2,945,855.

Description—Light-tan, crystalline powder; characteristic odor; melts within a range of 2° between 83° and 88°; pKₐ 7.45.

Solubility—1 g in >10,000 mL water, 2 mL alcohol, 1 mL chloroform, 8 mL ether.

Uses—See *Methdilazine Hydrochloride.*

Dose—*Usual, adult, oral,* **7.2 mg** (equivalent to 8 mg of methdilazine hydrochloride) 2 to 4 times a day. *Pediatric, children* over 3 yr, **3.6 mg** 2 to 4 times a day.

Dosage Form—Tablets (chewable): 3.6 mg.

Methdilazine Hydrochloride

10*H*-Phenothiazine, 10-[(1-methyl-3-pyrrolidinyl)methyl]-, monohydrochloride; Tacaryl Hydrochloride (*Westwood*)

10-[(1-Methyl-3-pyrrolidinyl)methyl]phenothiazine monohydrochloride [1229-35-2] C₁₈H₂₀N₂S.HCl (322.89). For the structure of the base, see *Methdilazine.*

Preparation—Methdilazine is reacted with an equimolar quantity of hydrogen chloride in a nonaqueous solvent.

Description—Light-tan, crystalline powder which has a slight characteristic odor and a bitter anesthetic taste; melts between 184° and 190°; pH (1 in 100 solution) between 4.8 and 6.0.

Solubility—1 g in 2 mL water, 2 mL alcohol, 6 mL chloroform, >10,000 mL ether.

Uses—A phenothiazine antihistaminic *effective* for the symptomatic relief of urticaria. It has also been used for the therapy of migraine headache. It is contraindicated in asthma, narrow-angle glaucoma, prostatic hypertrophy, peptic ulcer, pyloroduodenal obstruction, and newborn infants; also in acutely ill or dehydrated children, because of the greater susceptibility of dystonias with phenothiazines. It should not be given concomitantly with other phenothiazines, antihistamines, or MAO inhibitors. Adverse effects include drowsiness, dizziness, gastrointestinal disturbances, dryness of the mucous membranes, headache and skin rash. Extrapyramidal symptoms have also been reported. Other untoward reactions may include those for phenothiazines in general (see page 1125).

Dose—*Usual, adult, oral,* **8 mg** 2 to 4 times a day. *Children* over 3 yr, **4 mg** 2 to 4 times a day.

Dosage Forms—Syrup: 4 mg/5 mL; Tablets: 8 mg.

Promethazine Hydrochloride

10*H*-Phenothiazine-10-ethanamine, *N,N,α*-trimethyl-, monohydrochloride; Phenergan (*Wyeth*); Remsed (*Endo*); (*Various Mfrs*)

10-[2-(Dimethylamino)propyl]phenothiazine monohydrochloride [58-33-3] C₁₇H₂₀N₂S.HCl (320.88).

Preparation—Promethazine may be prepared by reacting phenothiazine with 1-chloro-2-(dimethylamino)propane hydrochloride in the presence of sodamide and sodium hydroxide in xylene. The base is extracted, purified, and converted to the hydrochloride.

Description—White to faint yellow, practically odorless, crystalline powder; it is slowly oxidized, particularly when moistened, on prolonged exposure to air, becoming blue in color; pH (1 in 20 solution) between 4.0 and 5.0; melts within a 3° range between 215° and 225°.

Solubility—Very soluble in water, hot dehydrated alcohol, and chloroform; practically insoluble in ether, acetone, and ethyl acetate.

Uses—A phenothiazine antihistaminic of marked potency and prolonged duration of action. It is *effective* for use in perennial and seasonal allergic rhinitis; vasomotor rhinitis; allergic conjunctivitis due to inhalant allergens and foods; mild, uncomplicated allergic skin manifestations of urticaria and angioedema; amelioration and prevention of allergic reactions to blood or plasma in patients with a known history of such reactions; dermographism; therapy for anaphylactic reactions adjunctive to epinephrine and other standard measures after the acute manifestations have been controlled; preoperative, postoperative or obstetric sedation; prevention and control of nausea and vomiting associated with certain types of anesthesia and surgery; therapy adjunctive to meperidine or other analgesics for control of postoperative pain; sedation in both children and adults as well as relief of apprehension and production of light sleep from which the patient can be easily aroused; active and prophylactic treatment of motion sickness; antiemetic action in postoperative patients.

Untoward reactions include dryness of the mouth, blurring of vision and, rarely, dizziness. Rare cases of leukopenia and one case of agranulocytosis have been reported. Minor increases in blood pressure and occasional mild hypotension have been documented. The appearance of photosensitivity may contraindicate further treatment. Excessive doses in adults have resulted in deep coma, sedation and, rarely, convulsions; in children, hyperexcitability and nightmares. See page 1125.

Dose—*Antihistaminic: adults, oral, parenteral, or rectal,* **12.5 to 25 mg** 4 to 6 times a day, not to exceed 150 mg daily. *Pediatric, oral, parenteral, or rectal,* **6.25 to 12.5 mg** 3 times a day or **25 mg** once a day at bedtime; contraindicated in premature and full-term neonates. *Sedative: adults, oral, parenteral, or rectal,* **25 to 50 mg** at bedtime. *Pediatric, oral, parenteral, rectal,* **12.5 to 25 mg** at bedtime. *Antiemetic: adults, parenteral, rectal,* **12.5 to 25 mg** 4 to 6 times a day as needed. *Pediatric, oral, parenteral, rectal,* **250 to 500 μg per kg** or **7.5 to 15 mg per m²** body surface 4 to 6 times a day as needed. *Preoperative: adults, oral,* **50 mg** given the night before surgery. *Pediatric,* **12.5 to 25 mg** the night before surgery. *Postoperative sedation and adjunctive use with analgesics: adults,* **25 to 50 mg;** *children,* **12.5 to 25 mg.**

Dosage Forms—Injection: 25 and 50 mg/mL; Suppositories: 12.5, 25, and 50 mg; Syrup: 6.25 and 25 mg/5 mL; Tablets: 12.5, 25, and 50 mg.

Pyrilamine Maleate

1,2-Ethanediamine, *N*-[(4-methoxyphenyl)methyl]-*N',N'*-dimethyl-*N*-2-pyridinyl-, (*Z*)-2-butenedioate (1:1); Antallergan Maleate; Anthisan Maleate; Pyranisamine Maleate; (*Various Mfrs*)

2-[[2-(Dimethylamino)ethyl](*p*-methoxybenzyl)amino]pyridine maleate (1:1) [59-33-6] C₁₇H₂₃N₃O.C₄H₄O₄ (401.46).

Preparation—Pyrilamine may be prepared by condensing 2-[[2-(dimethylamino)ethyl]amino]pyridine with *p*-methoxybenzyl chloride in the presence of sodamide. Treatment of the base with maleic acid yields the maleate.

Description—White, crystalline powder, usually having a faint odor; its solutions are acid to litmus, melts between 99° and 103°.

Solubility—1 g in 0.5 mL water, 3 mL alcohol, 2 mL chloroform; slightly soluble in ether and benzene.

Uses—An antihistaminic agent with a low incidence of sedative effects. The effectiveness and clinical applications are essentially the same as those for diphenhydramine, except it is not recommended for use in the management of parkinsonism or drug-induced extrapyramidal symptoms. Pyrilamine maleate is also employed in a number of proprietary antitussive formulations. See *Diphenhydramine*, page 1128, and article on *Antihistamines.*

Dose—*Adults, oral,* **25** to **50 mg** 3 or 4 times daily. *Pediatric,* (6 yrs and older), **12.5** to **25 mg** 3 to 4 times daily.

Dosage Forms—Tablets: 25 mg.

Trimeprazine Tartrate

10*H*-Phenothiazine-10-propanamine, *N,N,β*-trimethyl-, [*R*(*R*,R**)]-, 2,3-dihydroxybutanedioate (2:1); Temaril (*Smith Kline*)

10-[3-(Dimethylamino)-2-methylpropyl]phenothiazine tartrate (2:1) [41375-66-0; 4330-99-8] ($C_{18}H_{22}N_2S$)$_2$.$C_4H_6O_6$ (746.98).

Preparation—A xylene solution of phenothiazine is refluxed with sodamide and then with (3-chloro-2-methylpropyl)dimethylamine. The trimeprazine thus formed is extracted with aqueous acid, liberated with alkali, and extracted with ether. After removal of the ether, the base is distilled under reduced pressure and reacted with tartaric acid. US Pat 2,837,518.

Description—White to off-white, odorless, crystalline powder which darkens on exposure to light; melts between 160° and 164°.

Solubility—1 g in 2 mL water, 20 mL alcohol, 5 mL chloroform, 1800 mL ether.

Uses—A phenothiazine compound more active than promethazine and less active than chlorpromazine in histamine-induced bronchospasm in guinea pigs. Its tranquilizing properties are of a low order and its chief use is as an antipruritic drug. It is considered *effective* for use in the treatment of pruritic symptoms due to urticaria; and *possibly effective* for prolonged relief of pruritic symptoms in a variety of allergic and nonallergic conditions, including neurodermatitis, allergic dermatitis, contact dermatitis, pityriasis rosea, eczematous dermatitis, poison ivy dermatitis, drug rash, pruritus ani and vulvae. Side effects may mimic both phenothiazines and antihistamines; drowsiness, dryness of mucous membranes, and gastrointestinal disturbances are commonly observed. Patients on therapy lasting over one month should be monitored for possible agranulocytosis, hypotension, or parkinson-like symptoms. MAO inhibitors and thiazide diuretics intensify these symptoms. For a more detailed description of untoward reactions see *Chlorpromazine Hydrochloride* (see 1085, 1086).

Dose (base)—*Usual, adult, oral,* **2.5 mg** 4 times a day or **5 mg** as extended-release capsules every 12 hrs. *Pediatric, oral,* 6 mo to 3 yr, **1.25 mg** 1 to 4 times a day; 4 to 6 yr, **2.5 mg** 1 to 4 times a day; 7 yr and over **2.5 mg** 1 to 4 times a day or the equivalent of **5 mg** as an extended-release capsule once daily.

Dosage Forms (base)—Capsules (extended-release): 5 mg; Syrup: 2.5 mg/5 mL; Tablets: 2.5 mg.

Tripelennamine Citrate

1,2-Ethanediamine, *N,N*-dimethyl-*N'*-(phenylmethyl)-*N'*-2-pyridinyl-, 2-hydroxy-1,2,3-propanetricarboxylate (1:1); Pyribenzamine Citrate (*Ciba-Geigy*)

2-[Benzyl[2-(dimethylamino)ethyl]amino]pyridine citrate (1:1) [6138-56-3] $C_{16}H_{21}N_3.C_6H_8O_7$ (447.49).

Preparation—Tripelennamine is reacted with an equimolar portion of citric acid in a suitable solvent that may then be removed by evaporation. For the preparation of the base, see *Tripelennamine Hydrochloride.*

Description—White, crystalline powder; solutions are acid to litmus; melts at about 107°.

Solubility—1 g in about 1 mL water; freely soluble in alcohol; very slightly soluble in ether; practically insoluble in chloroform and benzene.

Uses—An antihistamine agent said to be more palatable by the oral route of administration than the hydrochloride. Otherwise, its actions and uses are the same. See *Tripelennamine Hydrochloride.*

Dose (tripelennamine hydrochloride equivalent)—*Usual, adult, oral,* **25** to **50 mg** every 4 to 6 hr, up to 600 mg daily. *Pediatric, oral,* equivalent of **1.25 mg per kg** body wt. or **37.5 mg per m²** of body surface every 6 hr, not to exceed 300 mg daily.

Dosage Form (tripelennamine hydrochloride equivalent)—Elixir: 25 mg/5 mL.

Tripelennamine Hydrochloride

1,2-Ethanediamine, *N,N*-dimethyl-*N'*-(phenylmethyl)-*N'*-2-pyridinyl-, monohydrochloride; Pyribenzamine (*Ciba*)

2-[Benzyl[2-(dimethylamino)ethyl]amino]pyridine monohydrochloride [154-69-8] $C_{16}H_{21}N_3.HCl$ (291.82). For the structure of the base, see *Tripelennamine Citrate.*

Preparation—Tripelennamine may be prepared as follows: *o*-aminopyridine, prepared by the action of sodamide on pyridine, is reacted with *β*-dimethylaminoethyl chloride in the presence of sodamide, and the resulting 2-[2-(dimethylamino)ethylamino]pyridine is condensed with benzyl bromide in the presence of sodamide. The hydrochloride is formed from the base by treatment with hydrogen chloride in an organic solvent.

Description—White, crystalline powder which slowly darkens on exposure to light; its solutions are practically neutral to litmus; melting range 188° to 192°.

Solubility—1 g in 1 mL water, 6 mL alcohol, 6 mL chloroform, and about 350 mL acetone; insoluble in benzene, ether, and ethyl acetate.

Uses—An antihistaminic agent *effective* in perennial and seasonal allergic rhinitis, vasomotor rhinitis, allergic conjunctivitis due to inhalant allergens and foods, mild uncomplicated allergic skin manifestations of urticaria and angioedema, amelioration and prevention of allergic reactions to blood or blood plasma in patients with known history of such reactions, dermographism, anaphylactic actions adjunctive to epinephrine and other standard measures after the acute manifestations have been controlled.

Tripelennamine hydrochloride has a low incidence (20 to 35%) of side reactions; gastrointestinal irritation is common, but not severe; sedation is moderate, and central nervous system stimulation occurs occasionally. See general statement (pages 1125–6).

Dose—*Usual, adult, oral,* **25** to **50 mg** every 4 to 6 hr or **100 mg** as extended-release tablet every 8 to 12 hr; range **25** to **600 mg** daily. *Pediatric, oral, children,* **1.25 mg per kg** body wt or **37.5 mg per m²** of body surface every 6 hr, not to exceed 300 mg daily, or **50 mg** as extended-release tablet every 8 to 12 hr. The 100 mg extended-release tablet should not be used in children.

Dosage Forms—Tablets: 25 and 50 mg. Extended-release Tablets: 50 and 100 mg.

Triprolidine Hydrochloride

Pyridine, 2-[1-(4-methylphenyl)-3-(1-pyrrolidinyl)-1-propenyl]-, monohydrochloride, monohydrate, (*E*)-, Actidil (*Burroughs-Wellcome*)

(*E*)-2-[3-(1-Pyrrolidinyl)-1-*p*-tolylpropenyl]pyridine monohydrochloride monohydrate [6138-79-0] $C_{19}H_{22}N_2.HCl.H_2O$ (332.87); *anhydrous* [550-70-9] (314.86).

Preparation—4'-Methylacetophenone is reacted with formaldehyde and pyrrolidine to form 3-(1-pyrrolidinyl)-4'-methylpropiophenone. Reaction with 2-pyridylsodium and subsequent hydrolysis produces the tertiary carbinol, *α*-[2-(1-pyrrolidinyl)-ethyl]-*α*-*p*-tolyl-2-pyridinemethanol, which is dehydrated with sulfuric acid to introduce the propenyl double bond. Alkalinization liberates triprolidine, which is purified and reacted with an equimolar portion of HCl. US Pats 2,712,020 and 2,712,023.

Description—White, crystalline powder having no more than a slight, but unpleasant, odor and a bitter taste. Its solutions are alkaline to litmus, and it melts at about 115°. It is light-sensitive, nonhygroscopic, and stable to reasonable heat.

Solubility—1 g in 2.1 mL water, 1.8 mL alcohol, 1 mL chloroform, 2000 mL ether.

Uses—An unusually potent antihistaminic agent with a rapid onset and long duration of action. The maximum effect occurs in about 3½ hours; the duration of effect is about 12 hours. The actions, uses, and incidence of side effects are comparable to those of *Doxylamine Succinate* (page 1128).

Dose—*Usual, adult, oral,* **2.5 mg** 3 or 4 times daily. *Children* (6 to 12 years), **1.25 mg** 3 or 4 times daily; (4 to 6 years), **0.9 mg** (syrup only) 3 or 4 times daily; (2 to 4 years), **0.6 mg** (syrup) 3 or 4 times daily; (4 months to 2 years), **0.3 mg** (syrup) 3 or 4 times daily.

Dosage Forms—Syrup: 1.25 mg/5 mL; Tablets: 2.5 mg.

Other Antihistamines

Pheniramine Maleate [2-[α-[2-(Dimethylamino)ethyl]benzyl]pyridine maleate (1:1); $C_{16}H_{20}N_2 \cdot C_4H_4O_4$ (356.43) Trimeton (*Schering-Plough*)]. *Preparation:* The base may be prepared by condensing 1-phenyl-1-(2-pyridyl)-3-chloropropane with dimethylamine in the presence of sodamide. Treatment of the base with an equimolar portion of maleic acid results in the formation of the maleate. *Description and Solubility:* White, crystalline powder with a faint, amine-like odor; pH (1 in 100 solution) 4.5 to 5.5; melts between 104° and 108°. 1 g dissolves in 5 mL water; very soluble in alcohol; slightly soluble in benzene and ether. *Uses:* An antihistaminic with a profile of clinical use similar to chlorpheniramine maleate (see page 1127). It induces moderate sedation and side effects similar to other members of this group of drugs. See page 1125. *Dose: Usual,* 40 mg.

Inhibitors of Histamine Release

The antihistamines described in the previous section antagonize in varying degree most but not all pharmacological effects of histamine. These agents appear to accomplish this by occupying the "receptor sites" on the effector cell to the exclusion of the agonist, histamine, without initiating a response. Typically they are competitive antagonists. They do not prevent the release of histamine in response to injury, drugs, or antigens. However, a relatively new drug, cromolyn sodium, can prevent the release of histamine from mast cells which have been sensitized by specific antigens. This inhibitor of histamine release is described in this section.

Cromolyn Sodium

4*H*-1-Benzopyran-2-carboxylic acid, 5,5′-[(2-hydroxy-1,3-propanediyl)-bis[4-oxo-, disodium salt; DSCG; Sodium Chromoglicate; Intal (*Fisons*)

5,5′-[(2-Hydroxytrimethylene)dioxy]bis[4-oxo-4*H*-1-benzopyran-2-carboxylic acid] disodium salt [15826-37-6] $C_{23}H_{14}Na_2O_{11}$ (512.34).

Preparation—2,6-Dihydroxyacetophenone is reacted with epichlorohydrin in the presence of a basic catalyst to yield the diether, 2′,2‴-[(2-hydroxytrimethylene)dioxy]bis[6′-hydroxyacetophenone]. Reaction with diethyl oxalate effects dehydration and deethanolation of each hydroxyacetophenone portion thus introducing the fused oxopyrancarboxylate groups as ethyl esters. This diester is then saponified with NaOH. US Pat 3,419,578.

Description—White, odorless, crystalline powder; tasteless but with a slightly bitter aftertaste; hygroscopic; pK_a believed by analogy with similar monochromes to be about 1.5 to 2; melts at about 261°; does not exhibit polymorphism.

Solubility—1 g dissolves in 20 mL water; insoluble in alcohol and in chloroform.

Uses—A useful and unique adjunct in the management of severe perennial bronchial asthma in patients who have a significant bronchodilator-reversible component to their airway obstruction; however, it has no role in treating an acute attack of asthma, especially status asthmaticus, and the patient should be so instructed. Cromolyn has no intrinsic bronchodilator, antihistaminic, anticholinergic, antiserotonin, or corticosteroid-like properties.

Cromolyn sodium is effective only when administered with a special inhaler, according to accompanying instructions. To be effective it should be used every day as prescribed by the physician. Beneficial results may not be apparent for 2 to 4 weeks. During use, hoarseness or cough may develop; gargling and rinsing the mouth after each dose may help prevent hoarseness. If skin rash develops, or the breathing problem worsens, the physician should be consulted. Patients being treated also with adrenocorticoids (as cortisone or prednisone) should not discontinue such therapy unless directed to do so by the physician.

It is poorly absorbed following oral administration and is administered only by inhalation. After inhalation about 8% of the total dose is deposited in the lungs, absorbed, and rapidly excreted unchanged in urine and bile. The remainder of the dose is either exhaled or deposited in the oropharynx, swallowed and excreted via the alimentary tract. It should be used with caution in patients with impaired renal and hepatic function.

Cromolyn sodium appears to act primarily through a local effect on the lung mucosa, inhibiting the degranulation of sensitized mast cells occurring after exposure to specific antigens. It prevents the release of the mediators of Type I allergic reactions, including histamine and SRS-A (slow-reacting substance of anaphylaxis). See Chapter 72. Cromolyn sodium may also be used to reduce and/or eliminate the long-term dependence on corticosteroids; however, if adrenocorticoid insufficiency occurs following a stress situation, corticosteroid therapy may have to be reinstituted.

Its safety in pregnancy has not been established and its use in children under 5 years of age is not recommended.

Adverse reactions are uncommon. Maculopapular rash and urticaria clear promptly on discontinuation of therapy. Occasional patients may experience cough and/or bronchospasm following inhalation. Symptoms of asthma may recur if the drug is reduced below recommended dosage, or discontinued. There have been rare reports of eosinophilic pneumonia and therapy should be discontinued if this condition occurs. Proliferative arterial lesions have been reported in both treated and untreated animals.

Dose—*Usual, adult, inhalation,* **20 mg** 4 times a day, maximum, up to 160 mg daily. If the patient becomes symptom-free, the dose may be reduced by 20 mg/day over a period of 1 week. *Usual, pediatric, oral inhalation,* under 5 yr, not recommended; 5 yr and over, **20 mg** 4 times a day.

Dosage Form—Capsules (for inhalation), 20 mg; Solution (for neubilizer), 20 mg/2 mL.

5-Hydroxytryptamine (Serotonin) Antagonists

The pharmacologic actions of 5-hydroxytryptamine are varied and complex. Liberation of excessive amounts in man, as in argentaffin cell tumors, produces episodic flushing, tachycardia, and hypertension followed by cyanosis and diarrhea, asthma, and pulmonary stenosis. 5-Hydroxytryptamine antagonists have been employed in the management of this malignancy as well as certain skin diseases and psychoses. The most likely effective clinical application of these antagonists, however, is in the treatment of malignant carcinoid.

In addition to the agents described below, methysergide maleate exhibits 5-hydroxytryptamine antagonist properties. It also has other more prominent actions and uses; consequently, it is described in another chapter (see page 949).

Azatadine Maleate

5*H*-Benzo[5,6]cyclohepta[1,2-*b*]pyridine, 6,11-dihydro-11-(1-methyl-4-piperidinylidene)-, (*Z*)-2-butenedioate (1:2); Optimine (*Schering-Plough*)

6,11-Dihydro-11- (1-methyl-4-piperidylidene)- $5H$-benzo[5,6]-cyclohepta[1,2-b]pyridine maleate (1:2) [3978-86-7] $C_{20}H_{22}N_2.2C_4H_4O_4$ (522.55).

Preparation—Azatadine is a chemical relative of cyproheptadine, differing from the latter in that a pyridine ring replaces one of the benzene rings of cyproheptadine and in the saturation of the cycloheptane ring of the latter compound. It may be prepared by dehydrating the condensation product formed in the presence of sodium and liquid ammonia from 4-chloro-N-methylpiperidine and 5,6-dihydro-11H-benzo[5,6]cyclohepta[1,2-b]pyridine-11-one. Treatment of azatadine base with a bimolar quantity of maleic acid forms the maleate salt. US Pat 3,326,924.

Description—White to off-white powder; not hygroscopic.
Solubility—Very soluble in water; soluble in alcohol.

Uses—Azatadine, like its prototype cyproheptadine, is an antihistamine with antiserotonin, anticholinergic, and sedative effects. Stated indications for the drug are treatment of perennial and seasonal allergic rhinitis, and chronic urticaria. In general, the same contraindications, warnings, and precautions apply to this drug as to the antihistamines (page 1125). The most frequent adverse reactions are sedation, sleepiness, dizziness, disturbed coordination, epigastric distress, and thickening of bronchial secretions. Some of lesser occurrence are anaphylactic shock, hypotension, hemolytic anemia, fatigue, blurred vision, wheezing, and nasal stuffiness. Use in pregnancy is inadequate to determine possible harmful effects.

Dose—*Usual, adult, oral,* **1** or **2 mg** twice a day. Not intended for use in children under 12 yr of age.
Dosage Form—Tablets: 1 mg.

Cyproheptadine Hydrochloride

Piperidine, 4-(5H-dibenzo[a,d]cyclohepten-5-ylidene)-1-methyl-, hydrochloride, sesquihydrate; Periactin Hydrochloride (*MSD*)

4-(5H-Dibenzo[a,d]cyclohepten-5-ylidene)-1-methylpiperidine hydrochloride sesquihydrate [41354-29-4] $C_{21}H_{21}N.HCl1\frac{1}{2}H_2O$ (350.89); *anhydrous* [969-33-5] (323.86).

Preparation—Phthalic anhydride is reacted with phenylacetic acid to form 3-benzylidenephthalide which, on isomerization and hydrogenation, gives 2-phenethylbenzoic acid. This is converted to its acid chloride, which then undergoes condensation to close the 7-membered ring and give 10,11-dihydro-5H-dibenzo[a,d]cyclohepten-5-one. Bromination at the 10 position followed by dehydrobromination introduces the 10,11 double bond. Grignardization of this ketone with 4-chloro-1-methylpiperidine followed by dehydration of the resulting carbinol yields cyproheptadine (base) which, on reacting with an equimolar quantity of hydrogen chloride, forms the hydrochloride. US Pat 3,014,911.

Description—White to slightly yellow, crystalline powder that is odorless or practically odorless and has a slightly bitter taste; relatively stable in light, stable at room temperature, and nonhygroscopic; the ses-

quihydrate is stable in air; the anhydrous form melts at about 250° and the sesquihydrate melts at about 162°.

Solubility—1 g in 275 mL water, 35 mL alcohol, 26 mL chloroform; practically insoluble in ether.

Uses—An antihistamine with antiserotonin, anticholinergic, anti-aldosterone, and sedative effects. It is *effective* for the treatment of perennial and seasonal allergic rhinitis, vasomotor rhinitis, allergic conjunctivitis due to inhalant allergens and foods, mild uncomplicated allergic skin manifestations of urticaria and angioedema, amelioration and prevention of reactions to blood or plasma in patients with a known history of such reactions, cold urticaria, dermographism, and as therapy for anaphylactic reactions adjunctive to epinephrine and other standard measures after the acute manifestations have been controlled. It is *probably effective* in mild, local allergic reactions to insect bites, physical allergy, and minor drug and serum reactions characterized by pruritus. It is *possibly effective* in pruritus of allergic dermatoses including contact dermatitis and pruritus of chicken pox. It is also under investigation for use as prophylaxis therapy for patients subject to migraine and to stimulate the appetite in underweight patients and those with anorexia nervosa. In general the same contraindications, warnings, and precautions apply to this drug as do to the antihistamines (page 1125). Untoward effects that appear frequently include drowsiness, and somnolence. Dry mouth, dizziness, jitteriness, faintness, dryness of the mucous membranes, headache, nausea, and allergic skin manifestations have also been reported to occur in low incidence. Rarely, central nervous system stimulation may appear.

Dose—*Usual, adult, oral,* **4 mg** 3 or 4 times a day, with a maximum of **500 μg** (0.5 mg) **per kg** per day. *Pediatric, children* 2 to 6 yr, *oral,* **2 mg** 2 or 3 times a day, with a maximum of **12 mg** daily; 7 to 14 yr, *oral,* **4 mg** 2 or 3 times daily, with a maximum of **16 mg** daily; contraindicated for premature and full-term neonates.
Dosage Forms—Syrup: 2 mg/5 mL; Tablets: 4 mg.

Other Histamines, Antihistamines

Chlorcyclizine Hydrochloride 1-[(4-Chlorophenyl)phenylmethyl]-4-methylpiperazine, monohydrochloride [1620-21-9] $C_{18}H_{21}ClN_2.HCl$ (337.29). *Description:* White, odorless or almost odorless, crystalline powder; its solutions are acid to litmus; pH (1 in 100 solution) between 4.8 and 5.5; melts at about 225°. *Soluble:* 1 g in 2 mL water, 11 mL alcohol, 4 mL chloroform; practically insoluble in ether and benzene. *Uses:* A mildly sedative antihistaminic agent with slight anticholinergic, antispasmodic, and local anesthetic action. It has a long action and a low incidence of toxic side effects. An ingredient in proprietary cold and allergy preparations. See article on *Antihistamines. Dose:* 25 to 100 mg; *usual,* 50 mg up to 4 times a day. *Dosage Forms:* Tablets: 25 and 50 mg.

Dexbrompheniramine Maleate [(S)-γ-(4-Bromophenyl)-N,N-dimethyl-2-pyridinepropanamine, (Z)-2-butenedioate (1:1); (+)-2-[p-Bromo-α-[2-dimethylamino)ethyl]benzyl]pyridine maleate (1:1) [2391-03-9] $C_{16}H_{19}BrN_2.C_4H_4O_4$ (435.32).] *Description and Solubility:* White, odorless, crystalline powder; pH (1 in 100 solution) about 5; melts between 103° and 113°. *Soluble:* 1 g in 1.2 mL water, 2.5 mL alcohol, 2 mL chloroform, 3000 mL ether. *Uses:* The dextro isomer of brompheniramine maleate. The major portion of the antihistaminic activity is said to reside in the dextro isomer; the levo form is relatively inactive. It has actions, untoward effects, and therapeutic applications similar to brompheniramine maleate. See *Brompheniramine Maleate* (page 1126) and also the article on *Antihistamines. Dose: Usual, adult, oral,* 2 mg 3 or 4 times a day to 6 mg as extended-release tablet every 8 to 12 hr. *Pediatric,* dosage not established. *Dosage Forms:* Tablets: 2 mg; Extended-release Tablets: 6 mg.

CHAPTER 62

Central Nervous System Stimulants

Ewart A Swinyard, PhD, DSc (Hon)
Professor Emeritus of Pharmacology
College of Pharmacy and School of Medicine
University of Utah
Salt Lake City, UT 84112

Central nervous system stimulants are drugs which increase the activity of some portion of the brain or spinal cord. Drugs which act upon the cerebral cortex and subcortical structures including the thalamus (eg, methylphenidate etc.) increase motor activity and enhance mental alertness; those which act upon the sensory areas in the brain (eg, caffeine and its various combinations) increase alertness, brighten spirits, and combat mental fatigue; those which act directly or reflexly on the medulla (eg, nikethamide, pentylenetetrazol, and picrotoxin) stimulate the respiratory center; those which act on the spinal cord (eg, nux vomica and strychnine) facilitate and exaggerate spinal reflexes.

The excitability of the central nervous system reflects a balance between excitatory and inhibitory influences that is normally maintained within relatively narrow limits. Drugs can increase excitability either by blocking inhibition (strychnine, picrotoxin) or by enhancing excitation (caffeine, pentylenetetrazol, and probably most other analeptic agents). The central nervous system stimulants are sometimes dramatic in their pharmacological effects, but they are much less important therapeutically than the central nervous system depressants. Central nervous system stimulants are among the most commonly prescribed drugs for childhood disorders, such as hyperactivity, minimal brain dysfunction, and attention deficit disorders. At one time they were frequently employed for the emergency management of drug-induced central depression, post anesthesia respiratory depression or apnea, and chronic pulmonary disease associated with acute hypercapnia. In most instances, these conditions can best be managed with mechanical ventilatory support. At one time pentylenetetrazol was used to activate the EEG in order to facilitate the diagnosis of epilepsy and as a convulsant for the treatment of schizophrenia. Since the latter can be accomplished more effectively with electroshock, pentylenetetrazol is seldom used for this purpose. Pentylenetetrazol is also available in over 20 oral formulations for the management of a number of non-specific symptoms in the elderly. The validity of its use for this purpose has yet to be established.

A number of central nervous system stimulants have therapeutically useful actions on other parts of the body, and a number of drugs not included in this chapter stimulate the central nervous system when administered in toxic doses. For example, caffeine, a classical central nervous system stimulant, has clinically useful actions on the heart, blood vessels, and kidneys. On the other hand, atropine and ephedrine, drugs with primary actions on the peripheral autonomic nervous system, stimulate the central nervous system.

Only those drugs which have central stimulation as their predominant action are listed in this section. Those agents whose central stimulant properties are secondary (atropine, sympathomimetic amines, cocaine, nicotine, lobeline, carbon dioxide, cyanide, apomorphine, and emetine) and those whose central stimulant properties are induced only with toxic doses (phenol, salicylates, local anesthetics, ergot alkaloids, etc.) are listed in other chapters. For convenience, the drugs described are divided into four groups: xanthine derivatives, analeptics, psychostimulants, and miscellaneous central nervous system stimulants.

Xanthine Derivatives

Stimulation of the central nervous system can be produced in man and animals by a large number of natural and synthetic substances. None, however, occupy as prominent a place in the environment of man as do the xanthine derivatives. The most popular sources of these substances are the xanthine beverages, which include coffee, tea, cocoa, and cola-flavored drinks. Coffee and tea contain caffeine, whereas cocoa contains theobromine. The caffeine content of tea leaves (about 2.0%) is higher than that of coffee beans (0.7 to 2.0%) but the beverages as finally prepared contain about equal amounts of this stimulant. Caffeine is present in amounts of about 100–150 mg/180 mL of brewed coffee; 60–80 mg/180 mL of instant coffee; 40–100 mg/180 mL of tea; and 17–55 mg/180 mL of cola beverage. There is little doubt that the popularity of these beverages depends on their stimulant action, although most people are unaware of any stimulation.

Xanthine derivatives include caffeine, theobromine, theophylline and a number of related synthetic derivatives, all of which have similar pharmacological properties that differ markedly in the intensity of their actions in various structures. For example, the stimulant effects of caffeine on the central nervous system and on skeletal muscle are greater than those of the other xanthines; theophylline and theobromine surpass caffeine in their diuretic, cardiac, and smooth muscular actions, whereas theophylline surpasses theobromine in diuretic efficacy. Therefore, in the therapeutic application of these drugs for a specific effect, side actions can be minimized and the desired effect intensified by careful selection of the xanthine employed.

The principal therapeutic application of caffeine is as a central nervous system stimulant. Therefore, caffeine and its congeners which possess this effect will be discussed in this section. The principal therapeutic use of theophylline and related compounds is as a bronchodilator in the management of asthma. For this reason, oxtriphylline, theobromine, theophylline and their various derivatives and combinations are discussed in Chapter 44, *Respiratory Drugs*.

Aminophylline—page 872.

Caffeine

1*H*-Purine-2,6-dione, 3,7-dihydro-1,3,7-trimethyl-, Theine

1,3,7-Trimethylxanthine [58-08-2] $C_8H_{10}N_4O_2$ (194.19); *monohydrate* [5743-12-4] (212.21).

For the structural formula, see page 419.

Preparation—Caffeine may be prepared from tea or coffee by boiling with water in the presence of lime or magnesium oxide, which serves to precipitate the tannins and some of the coloring matter. After filtration, the crude caffeine that separates is recrystallized from hot water after treatment with decolorizing charcoal. A source of the commercial supply is tea dust or sweepings; increasing quantities of caffeine are now obtained as a by-product in the manufacture of "decaffeinized coffee." It is also produced by methylation of theobromine (partial synthesis) and by total synthesis from urea or dimethylurea by variations of Traube's classic process (*Ber 33:* 3052, 1900). The essential steps of a synthesis of theophylline and caffeine from urea are shown below:

Theophylline

Description—White powder or white, glistening needles, usually matted; odorless and has a bitter taste; solutions are neutral to litmus; the hydrate is efflorescent in air and loses all its moisture at 80°; when rendered anhydrous by drying, melts between 235° and 237.5°.

Solubility—1 g of hydrous caffeine dissolves in about 50 mL water, 6 mL water at 80°, 75 mL alcohol, about 25 mL alcohol at 60°, about 6 mL chloroform, and 600 mL ether. Being a weak base, caffeine does not form stable salts, and even its salts of strong acids, such as the hydrochloride or hydrobromide, are readily hydrolyzed by water. The solubility of caffeine in water is increased by the presence of organic acids or their alkali salts, eg, benzoates, salicylates, cinnamates, or citrates and this is the reason for the use of several such preparations.

Uses—Caffeine is used orally as a mild *central nervous system stimulant* to aid in staying awake and to restore mental alertness in fatigued patients. In combination with ergotamine tartrate it is used to abort *vascular headaches* such as migraine and cluster headaches (histamine cephalalgia). It is used alone or in combination with analgesics (acetaminophen, aspirin, phenacetin, etc) for the treatment of headache; since it has no analgesic activity the validity of this use must remain suspect. It is used in combination with antihistamines and other sedative agents to overcome the sedative properties of such drugs; however, effective dosage for this purpose has not been adequately established. It is used parenterally in the form of caffeine and sodium benzoate for the treatment of *respiratory depression* associated with overdosage of central nervous system depressant drugs (narcotic analgesics, alcohol, etc). Because of the questionable benefit of such use and its transient action, most authorities believe caffeine and other analeptics should not be used in these conditions and recommend other supportive therapy. Finally, caffeine is used orally either alone or in combination with other drugs (analgesics, diuretics, etc) to relieve tension and fluid retention associated with menstruation; in view of its minimal diuretic action, its usefulness in this condition is questionable.

Caffeine and citrated caffeine are well absorbed following oral administration. Absorption by the oral route is more rapid than that after intramuscular injection. Absorption from suppositories following rectal administration is slow and erratic. Following the oral administration of 100 mg of caffeine (as in coffee), peak plasma levels of about 1.5 to 1.8 µg/mL are reached after 50 to 75 minutes. Following oral administration of 250 mg to "caffeine-naive" subjects, peak plasma levels of 4.2 to 26 µg/mL are reached in a mean time of 60 minutes. Therapeutic plasma concentrations range from 6 to 13 µg/mL; concentrations >20 µg/mL commonly produce adverse reactions. The lethal concentration is >100 µg/mL. It is rapidly distributed throughout all body tissues, readily crossing the placenta and blood-brain barrier. Approximately 17% of the drug is bound to plasma proteins. Plasma half-life is 3 to 4 hours in adults. Plasma half-life in neonates born of women given caffeine prior to delivery has been estimated to be about 80 hours. The drug is rapidly metabolized by the liver to 1-methyluric acid, 1-methylxanthine, and 7-methylxanthine. About 10% is excreted unchanged by the kidneys.

Caffeine competitively inhibits phosphodiesterase, the enzyme that breaks down cyclic 3′,5′-adenosine monophosphate (cyclic-AMP). Increased levels of intracellular cyclic-AMP is thought to mediate most of the pharmacologic actions induced by caffeine.

In one double-blind clinical study, oral administration of 250 mg of caffeine to nine healthy young non-coffee drinkers who had no coffee, tea, or cola in the previous 3 weeks *increased plasma renin activity* 57%, plasma *norepinephrine* 75%, and plasma *epinephrine* by 207%; urinary *normetanephrine* and *metanephrine* were *increased* 52 and 100%, respectively; mean *blood pressure increased* 14/10 mm Hg within one hour; *heart rate* first *decreased* and then *increased;* and *respiratory rate increased* 20%. Whether habitual ingestion has similar effects remains to be determined.

Caffeine stimulates all levels of the central nervous system. In oral doses of 100 to 200 mg, it stimulates the cerebral cortex producing a more rapid and clear flow of thought, wakefulness or arousal in fatigued patients, and improved psychomotor coordination. Its cortical effects are milder and of shorter duration than those of the amphetamines. In slightly larger doses, caffeine stimulates medullary vagal, vasomotor and respiratory centers, inducing bradycardia, vasoconstriction, and an increased respiratory rate.

Caffeine exerts multiple effects on the heart. It has a positive inotropic effect on the myocardium and a positive chronotropic effect on the sinoatrial node, causing a transient increase in heart rate, force of contraction, cardiac output, and work of the heart. In doses in excess of 250 mg, the centrally mediated vagal effects of caffeine may be masked by increased sinus rates; tachycardia, extrasystoles, or other ventricular arrhythmias may result.

Caffeine constricts the cerebral blood vessels but directly dilates peripheral blood vessels; thus, it decreases peripheral vascular resistance. The effect of this decrease in vascular resistance on blood pressure is compensated for by increased cardiac output. Thus, the overall effect of caffeine on heart rate and blood pressure is dependent on whether the central nervous system or peripheral effects predominate. In most instances, therapeutic doses of caffeine increase blood pressure only slightly.

Other pharmacological effects of caffeine include the following: it stimulates voluntary skeletal muscle, increasing the force of muscle contraction and decreasing muscular fatigue; it stimulates parietal cells, increasing gastric acid secretion; it induces a mild diuresis by increasing renal blood flow and glomerular filtration rate and decreasing proximal tubular reabsorption of sodium and water; and stimulates glycogenolysis and lipolysis, but the increases in blood glucose and plasma lipids are usually not significant in normal patients. Repeated use of this substance may result in the development of tolerance to its diuretic, cardiovascular, and central nervous system effects.

Caffeine and other xanthines may enhance the cardiac inotropic effects of beta-adrenergic stimulating agents and decrease the effect of benzodiazepines. It has also been reported to increase its own metabolism and that of other drugs such as phenobarbital and aspirin. The clinical importance of these drug interactions remains to be determined. Caffeine also interferes with some laboratory tests. It produces false-positive elevations of serum urate; a slight increase in urine levels of vanillylmandelic acid, catecholamines, and 5-hydroxyindoleacetic acid. Since high urine levels of vanillylmandelic acid or catecholamines may result in a false-positive diagnosis of pheochromocytoma or neuroblastoma, caffeine intake should be avoided during these tests.

Acute toxicity involving caffeine has only rarely been reported. Overdosage is usually associated with gastrointestinal pain, mild delirium, insomnia, diuresis, dehydration, and fever. More serious symptoms include cardiac arrhythmias and convulsions. The acute lethal dose of caffeine in adults appears to be about 5 to 10 g either intravenously or orally. Death has occurred in a child following oral ingestion of 3 grams of caffeine.

Prolonged, high intake of caffeine may produce tolerance, habituation, and psychological dependence. Abrupt discontinuation of the stimulant may result in headache, irritation, nervousness, anxiety and dizziness.

The ingestion of large amounts of combinations containing aspirin, phenacetin, and caffeine has been associated with analgesic nephropathy, characterized by sterile pyuria, asymptomatic bacteriuria, pyelonephritis, papillary necrosis, interstitial fibrosis and nephritis. The role of caffeine in the etiology of this condition has not been conclusively established. For an indepth review of "The Health Consequences of Caffeine" the interested reader is referred to the interesting article by Curatolo and Robertson (*Ann. Int. Med. 98*, 641–653, 1983).

Dose—100 to **500 mg**; *usual*, **200 mg** as necessary.
Dosage Forms—Capsules, Extended Release: 200 and 250 mg; Tablets: 100, 150, 200, and 250 mg.

Citrated Caffeine

Caffeine citrate (1:1) [69-22-7]; a mixture of caffeine and citric acid containing 50% $C_8H_{10}N_4O_2$ (anhydrous caffeine) and 50% $C_6H_8O_7$ (anhydrous citric acid).
Preparation—The formula of USP IX was:

Caffeine	50 g
Citric Acid	50 g
Distilled Water, hot	100 mL

Dissolve the citric acid in the hot distilled water, add the caffeine, and evaporate the resulting solution to dryness on a water bath, constantly stirring towards the end of the operation. Reduce the product to a fine powder and transfer it to well-closed containers. It is, however, usually prepared by mixing equal proportions of finely powdered anhydrous caffeine and anhydrous citric acid.

Description—White, odorless powder having a slightly bitter, acid taste, and an acid reaction.
Solubility—1 g in about 4 mL warm water, the caffeine gradually precipitating on diluting the solution with an equal volume of water but redissolving on further dilution with sufficient water.
Incompatibilities—Neutralization of the citric acid by *alkalies* or *alkaline salts* will cause precipitation of caffeine if in sufficient concentration. The alkali salts of organic acids may release either caffeine or the free organic acid. In general, it displays the incompatibilities of the citric acid which it contains.

Uses—See *Caffeine*.
Dose—100 to **500 mg**; *usual*, **300 mg** as necessary.
Dosage Forms—Tablets: 65 mg.

Caffeine and Sodium Benzoate Injection

A sterile solution of caffeine and sodium benzoate in water for injection; contains an amount of anhydrous caffeine ($C_8H_{10}N_4O_2$) equivalent to 45–52%, and an amount of sodium benzoate ($C_7H_5NaO_2$) equivalent to 47.5–55.5%, of the labeled amounts of caffeine and sodium benzoate.

Description—pH between 6.5 and 8.5.

Use—See *Caffeine*, page 1133.
Dose—*Parenteral*, **200 mg** to **1 g**; *usual*, **500 mg**, repeated as necessary.
Dosage Form—Injection: 250 mg (Caffeine Anhydrous 125 mg and Sodium Benzoate 125 mg) per mL.

Dyphylline—page 872.
Oxtriphylline—page 872.
Theobromine—page 944.
Theobromine Calcium Salicylate—RPS-15, page 1070.
Theobromine Sodium Acetate—RPS-15, page 1070.
Theobromine Sodium Salicylate—RPS-15, page 1070.
Theophylline—page 873.
Theophylline Calcium Salicylate—page 875.
Theophylline, Ephedrine Hydrochloride, and Phenobarbital—page 874.
Theophylline Olamine—page 874.
Theophylline Sodium Acetate—page 875.
Theophylline Sodium Glycinate—page 874.

Analeptics

Analeptics are agents which stimulate various areas of the central nervous system. Excessive doses of these drugs may cause the stimulation to spread to the motor areas of the brain and precipitate convulsions. Analeptics were formerly employed to counteract severe intoxication by general depressants. However, no safe, selective respiratory stimulant is currently available. Moreover, depressant drug intoxications can be managed more effectively with more conservative measures that stress intensive supportive care. Hence, the airway is kept clear by suction or by endotracheal tube, the patient is turned regularly, and oxygen is administered as needed. Shock is overcome by the use of blood or plasma expanders and vasopressors. Where available, dialysis is used to remove the drug. Thus, only a few very specialized applications remain for these agents.

Doxapram Hydrochloride—page 867.

Picrotoxin

Cocculin

Picrotoxin [124-87-8] $C_{30}H_{34}O_{13}$ (602.59); an active principle obtained from the seed of *Anamirta cocculus* (Linné) Wight et Arnott (Fam. *Menispermaceae*).
Preparation—The ground berries (seeds) of *A. cocculus* are boiled with alcohol and filtered hot. The filtrate is concentrated and two volumes of hot water added. After cooling with ice it is filtered and the filtrate evaporated under reduced pressure. Picrotoxin crystallizes out during evaporation and is purified by solution in hot acetone and precipitation with water. The yield is about 1.4%.

Description—Flexible, shining, prismatic crystals or a microcrystalline powder; odorless; stable in air, but affected by light; solutions are neutral to litmus; melts between 198° and 200°.
Solubility—1 g in about 350 mL water, about 30 mL boiling water, and about 3 mL boiling alcohol; more readily soluble in diluted acids and alkalies; sparingly soluble in ether and chloroform.

Uses—A powerful *central nervous system stimulant* which affects all parts of the nervous system to some extent. Formerly employed as a respiratory stimulant in the *treatment of acute barbiturate intoxication*. Picrotoxin is not a selective respiratory stimulant and is not considered a useful therapeutic agent. The onset of action is 3 to 20 min and the duration of action is 45 to 60 min. The difference between a therapeutic and a toxic dose of picrotoxin is very small and convulsions are easily produced. Picrotoxin appears to block GABA (gamma aminobutyric acid) at postsynaptic sites. In mammalian systems the block is not good enough to establish it as a selective antagonist of GABA at a given site. Nevertheless, it is a valuable pharmacological tool for the study of drug mechanism.
Dose—*Usual, intravenous*, to be determined by the physician according to the needs of the patient.
Other Dose Information—Picrotoxin is injected intravenously in a continuous infusion at a rate of 1 to 2 mg/min, or intermittently (6 to 12 mg every 10 to 20 min) until corneal and swallowing reflexes appear; subsequently, the drug is injected intramuscularly in doses of 3 to 6 mg at intervals of 15 to 30 min, as needed.
Dosage Forms—Injection: 3 mg/mL.

Pipradrol Hydrochloride—RPS-15, page 1034.

Racephedrine Hydrochloride—page 893.

Other Stimulants Acting on the Medulla

Nikethamide [*N,N*-Diethylnicotinamide [59-26-7] $C_{10}H_{14}N_2O$ (178.23); Coramine (*Ciba*); Nikethyl (*Abbott*)]—*Preparation:* By treating the ethyl or methyl ester of nicotinic acid with diethylamine, or by reacting nicotinyl chloride with the amine. *Description* and *Solubility:* clear, colorless to pale yellowish, somewhat viscous liquid which crystallizes on standing in the cold and melts again as the temperature rises; a faint, aromatic odor, and a bitter taste; specific gravity 1.058 to 1.066; congealing range 22° to 24°. Miscible with water, alcohol, and ether. *Uses:* A weak analeptic used to overcome *central nervous system depression, respiratory depression*, and *circulatory failure*, particularly when due to central depressant drugs. It is indicated in the management of anesthetic overdosage, asphyxia in the newborn, narcotic, hypnotic, and carbon monoxide poisoning, cardiac decompensation and coronary occlusion, shock, central depression of acute alcoholism, and respiratory depression following electroshock therapy in psychotic patients. Nikethamide is well absorbed from all routes of administration. It is converted to nicotinamide and then excreted as *N*-methylnicotinamide. Pharmacokinetic data in humans are not available. The difference between the clinically effective dose and that producing side effects varies but is often small. With severe overdosage, as may occur with injection, generalized muscle spasms and convulsive seizures may occur. *Dose:* Usual, *intramuscular* and *intravenous*, 1 to 15 mL of the 25% parenteral solution, repeated as needed. For oral maintenance therapy, 3 to 5 mL every 4 to 6 hrs, when indicated. *Dosage Form:* Injection and Oral Solution: 25% (by wt) aqueous solution.

Pentylenetetrazol [6,7,8,9-Tetrahydro-5*H*-tetrazolo[1,5-*a*]azepine [54-95-5] $C_6H_{10}N_4$ (138.17); Leptazol; Pentetrazol; Pentamethylenetetrazol; Metrazol (*Knoll*)]—*Preparation:* From hydrazoic acid and cy-

clohexanone. *Description* and *Solubility:* White, odorless crystals with a slightly pungent bitter taste; a 1 in 10 solution is neutral to litmus; melting range 58° to 61°. Freely soluble in water and alcohol; soluble in ether and chloroform. *Uses:* A central nervous system stimulant *administered orally* to enhance the *mental* and *physical activity* of elderly patients. It is also available in combination with a vasodilator (niacin), antihistamines with prominent antiemetic/antivertigo activity (dimenhydrinate or pheniramine maleate), and, in some formulations, various vitamins; these products are intended for use in a wide variety of nonspecific symptoms of the elderly, such as *senile confusion, depression, functional memory defects*, and *general debilitation*. The validity of such combinations has yet to be established. The drug has been used in convulsant doses given by *parenteral administration* for the treatment of *schizophrenia*. Since this can be accomplished more effectively by electroshock, pentylenetetrazol is seldom used for this purpose. It has also been used to activate the EEG in the diagnosis of epilepsy. Pentylenetetrazol may interact with antihypertensive agents and other drugs frequently administered to aged patients, resulting in serious adverse effects. Pentylenetetrazol is readily absorbed after both oral and parenteral administration. It is rapidly metabolized by the liver and excreted by the kidneys. At recommended dosage, adverse effects occur infrequently, although insomnia, anorexia, nausea, vomiting, and headache have been reported. Overdosage produces toxic symptoms typical of those induced by CNS stimulants which act upon the higher motor centers and the spinal cord. Convulsions may result; these are spontaneous, last several minutes, and are followed by profound depression. Death characterized by anoxia, medullary depression, and respiratory paralysis, has been reported from the ingestion of 10 g. The drug should not be used during pregnancy or lactation. Safe use in children has not been established. *Dose—Usual, oral*, 100 to 200 mg 3 times daily. *Parenteral*, in depression from barbiturates, 500 mg IV within 3 to 5 seconds; subsequent IM injections of 100 or 200 mg may be given as needed. *Dosage Forms—Oral:* Elixir, 100 mg/5 mL; Liquid, 50 mg/5 mL; Tablets, 100 mg. Parenteral: 100 mg/mL.

Psychostimulants

A number of drugs that stimulate the central nervous system are promoted for treatment of hyperactive behavior in children (psychostimulants). A degree of hyperactivity which is not acceptable either at home or at school is often accompanied by difficulty in learning and sometimes by other neurological signs, such as "clumsiness." Although the usefulness of psychostimulant drugs in treatment of "hyperactivity" has been controversial, there is a patient group with severe, persistent hyperactivity and a short attention span that is likely to benefit from treatment with these agents. The psychostimulants most frequently used for this purpose include *deanol acetamidobenzoate, methylphenidate,* and *pemoline;* these agents will be presented in this section. Other drugs that also have psychostimulant actions, such as amphetamine and dextroamphetamine, have other more prominent pharmacological activities; consequently, these substances are presented in Chapter 45 (see page 881).

Amphetamine Phosphate—RPS-15, page 822.

Amphetamine Sulfate—page 891.

Deanol Acetamidobenzoate

Benzoic acid, 4-(acetylamino)-, compd. with 2-(dimethylamino)ethanol (1:1); Deaner (*Riker*)

(CH$_3$)$_2$NCH$_2$CH$_2$OH · HOOC———⟨○⟩——— NHCOCH$_3$

2-(Dimethylamino)ethanol *p*-acetamidobenzoate (salt) [3635-74-3] $C_{14}H_{11}NO.C_9H_9NO_2$ (268.31).

Preparation—Deanol, prepared by reacting equimolar quantities of dimethylamine and ethylene oxide, is dissolved in a suitable solvent and reacted with an equimolar quantity of *p*-acetamidobenzoic acid.

Description—White to off-white crystalline powder with little or no odor; melts between 159° and 163°.

Solubility—1 g in about 2 mL water and 25 mL alcohol; slightly soluble in ether and chloroform; insoluble in benzene.

Uses—A mild central nervous system stimulant that is *possibly*

effective in the management of *hyperactive children* with behavior problems and learning difficulties. It is also proposed for the symptomatic relief of underachievers, reading and speech difficulties, impaired motor coordination, hyperactive, impulsive behavior, often described as social, antisocial, impulsive or stimulus-governed. The mechanism(s) and site(s) of action in humans have not been determined. Studies with carbon-14 labeled deanol indicate that it crosses the blood-brain barrier and is probably converted intracellularly to acetylcholine. Information on the absorption, distribution, metabolism, and excretion in humans is not provided by the manufacturer. In one study, oral administration of 200 mg or 1 g significantly increased cerebral electrical activity, as measured by an electroencephalograph, within 60 to 70 minutes and persisted for 90 to 120 minutes. When administered to hyperactive children, it has a gradual onset of action; full therapeutic effects are not usually apparent until after 2 to 3 weeks of therapy. Relative contraindications include epilepsy with a tonic-clonic component. Side effects are relatively mild; overstimulation, headache, constipation, insomnia, muscle twitching and tenseness, and rarely postural hypotension have been reported. Prolonged administration to children causes temporary suppression of normal weight and/or height patterns in some patients. Unlike amphetamines, it does not depress appetite or cause jitteriness. Although no absolute contraindications are known, grand mal epilepsy and mixed epilepsy with a grand mal component are relative contraindications. The drug should be administered early in the day to avoid insomnia.

Dose (base equivalent)—*Oral, initial,* **500 mg** daily. If satisfactory improvement occurs, the patient may be maintained on **250 to 500 mg** daily.

Dosage Forms—Tablets: 25, 100 and 250 mg (of the base).

Dextroamphetamine Phosphate—RPS-16, p 820.

Dextroamphetamine Sulfate—page 881.

Methylphenidate Hydrochloride

2-Piperidineacetic acid, α-phenyl-, methyl ester, hydrochloride, (*R**,*R**)-(±)-, Ritalin (*Ciba*)

Methyl α-phenyl-2-piperidineacetate hydrochloride [298-59-9] $C_{14}H_{19}NO_2\cdot HCl$ (269.77).

Preparation—2-Chloropyridine is condensed with phenylacetonitrile and the resulting α-phenyl-2-pyridineacetonitrile is hydrated to its corresponding amide. The pyridine ring is then catalytically hydrogenated and the amide converted to its corresponding carboxylic acid. Esterification with methanol with the aid of HCl yields the final product.

Description—White, odorless, fine, crystalline powder melting about 75°; solutions are acid to litmus.

Solubility—Freely soluble in water and methanol; soluble in alcohol; slightly soluble in chloroform and acetone.

Uses—A mild central nervous system stimulant with a potency intermediate to caffeine and amphetamine. Methylphenidate hydrochloride is *effective* as adjunctive therapy to other remedial measures (psychological, educational, and social) in the management of *minimal brain dysfunction* (*hyperkinetic behavior disorders*) in *carefully selected children*. Drug treatment is not indicated for all children with this disorder; stimulants are not intended in the child who exhibits symptoms secondary to environmental factors or primary psychiatric disorders. Consequently, these should be ruled out and available psychological, educational, and social resources should be utilized before drug therapy is instituted. Methylphenidate hydrochloride is also *effective* in *narcolepsy* and *possibly effective* in *mild depression* as well as *apathetic* or *withdrawn senile behavior*.

Methylphenidate hydrochloride appears to be well absorbed from the gastrointestinal tract. Peak blood levels are reached in 1 to 3 hours. Its effects persists for 3 to 6 hours. The extent of its distribution in man is unknown. However, plasma half-life ranges from 2 to 7 hours. Following oral administration of 20 mg of C 14-labeled methylphenidate hydrochloride, approximately 50, 80, and 95% of the dose was recovered as metabolites in the urine within 6, 24, and 90 hours, respectively. The pharmacologic actions of the drug are qualitatively similar to those of the amphetamines. The mechanism of action has not been determined. It is thought to act on the cerebral cortex and subcortical structures, including the thalamus; stimulation by methylphenidate causes an increase in motor activity, mental alertness, diminished sense of fatigue, brighter spirits, and mild euphoria. It also produces an anorexigenic effect.

The drug is contraindicated in patients with anxiety, tension, and agitation or those known to be sensitive to the drug. The safe use in children under 6 years of age has not been established. It is also contraindicated in patients with a prior history of epilepsy or those with EEG abnormalities in absence of seizures. Methylphenidate hydrochloride may decrease the hypotensive effect of guanethidine. It should be used with caution in patients on pressor agents or MAO inhibitors. Human pharmacologic studies indicate the drug may inhibit metabolism of coumarin anticoagulants, anticonvulsants, and tricyclic antidepressants. Dosage of these agents may require downward adjustment when given concomitantly with methylphenidate.

Adverse reactions include nervousness, insomnia, hypersensitivity reactions (including various skin manifestations), anorexia, nausea, dizziness, palpitations, headache, dyskinesia, blood pressure and pulse changes, tachycardia, angina, cardiac arrhythmias, abdominal pain, and weight loss. Toxic psychoses, leukopenia, anemia, and a few cases of scalp hair loss have been reported. Tolerance, psychic dependence, and abnormal behavior have been reported in patients who have abused this drug. Consequently, it should be administered cautiously, if at all, in emotionally unstable patients, those with a history of drug dependency, and those known to alter drug dosage on their own initiative.

Dose—*Oral*, **10** to **60 mg** daily; *usual*, **10 mg** 2 or 3 times a day. Sustained-release tablets have an 8-hour duration of action; these may be used when the dose of SR tablets correspond to the 8 hour dose of methylphenidate hydrochloride.

Dosage Forms—Tablets: 5, 10, and 20 mg. Sustained-Release Tablets: 20 mg.

Pemoline

4(5*H*)-Oxazolone, 2-amino-5-phenyl-, Cylert (*Abbott*)

2-Imino-5-phenyl-4-oxazolidinone   [2152-34-3] $C_9H_8N_2O_2$ (176.17).

Preparation—Ethyl mandelate, $C_6H_5CH(OH)COOC_2H_5$, is reacted with guanidine, $HN{=}C(NH_2)_2$, in boiling alcohol solution. US Pat 2,892,753.

Description—White, crystalline powder; odorless and tasteless; melts at about 256°, with decomposition.

Solubility—Practically insoluble in water, chloroform, ether; slightly soluble in alcohol.

Uses—A central nervous system stimulant with minimal sympathomimetic effects. Although laboratory studies indicate that pemoline may act through dopaminergic mechanisms, the mechanism and site of action in man are not known. Indicated as adjunctive therapy in children with minimal *brain dysfunction* (*hyperkinetic behavior disorders*). Pemoline (50 to 200 mg in two divided doses daily) has been used investigationally for the treatment of narcolepsy and excessive daytime sleepiness. Peak serum levels of the drug are reached 2 to 4 hours after ingestion of a single oral dose; the serum half-life is approximately 12 hours, and a steady state level is reached in 2 to 3 days of multiple dosage. About 50% of the drug is bound to serum proteins. Approximately 75% of an oral dose is excreted in the urine within 24 hours, about 43% unchanged and 22% as pemoline conjugates.

Insomnia, usually transient, is the principal adverse effect. Anorexia with weight loss may occur during early weeks of therapy; weight gain usually resumes within 3 to 6 months. Stomachache, skin rashes, increased irritability, mild depression, nausea, dizziness, headache, drowsiness, and hallucinations have been reported. Reports of jaundice, dyskinetic movements, and convulsive seizures have not been established as having a causal relationship to pemoline therapy.

Pemoline is contraindicated in patients with hypersensitivity or idiosyncrasy to the drug. It is not recommended for children less than 6 years of age since safety and efficacy in this age group have not been established. Sufficient data on safety and efficacy of long-term use in children are not yet available. Safety for use during pregnancy and lactation has not been established.

Dose—*Oral*, *initial*, **37.5 mg** given as a single dose each morning; may be increased by **18.75 mg** daily at weekly intervals until desired clinical response is obtained. The effective dose for most patients is **56.25** to **75 mg** daily; the maximum recommended dose is **112.5 mg** daily. Significant benefit from the drug may not be evident until the third or fourth week of treatment.

Dosage Forms—Tablets: 18.75, 37.5, and 75 mg.

Miscellaneous Central Nervous System Stimulants

A number of drugs that stimulate the central nervous system may quite properly be classified as either sympathomimetic or anorexigenic agents. Cross references to these substances are listed below. Other drugs, such as flurothyl and strychnine, act primarily on the central nervous system and are described herein. There are no official preparations of strychnine. Although strychnine has no valid place in modern therapeutics, it is important, not only from a historical point of view but also as a physiological tool for the study of the mechanism of action of other drugs, as a pesticide for destroying agricultural rodents and predatory animals, and as a frequently encountered cause of poisoning in man.

Benzphetamine Hydrochloride—page 891.

Camphor—page 780.

Clortermine Hydrochloride—page 891.

Diethylpropion—page 891.

Fenfluramine—page 885.

Strychnine

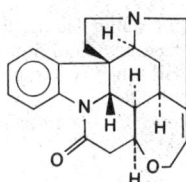

Strychnine [57-24-9] $C_{21}H_{22}N_2O_2$ (334.42); an alkaloid obtained chiefly from *Nux Vomica*, the dried ripe seed of *Strychnos Nux-vomica* Linné (Fam *Loganiaceae*), which contains 1–2% of the alkaloid.

Preparation—Comminuted nux vomica is moistened with sodium carbonate solution and extracted with hot mineral oil or toluene. The alkaloids are removed from these solvents with diluted H_2SO_4 and the acid solution is concentrated. The less soluble brucine bisulfate crystallizes from solution first. On neutralization and concentration of the mother liquor, strychnine sulfate crystallizes and is purified. The alkaloidal base is obtained by precipitation with ammonia.

Description—Colorless, transparent, prismatic crystals, or a white, crystalline powder; odorless, has a very bitter taste, and stable in the air; saturated solutions are alkaline to litmus.

Solubility—1 g in 6420 mL water, 136 mL alcohol, 5 mL chloroform, 180 mL benzene; very slightly soluble in ether.

Uses—Has no important therapeutic use, but has proved useful in the investigation of the mode of action of anticonvulsant drugs. Its most striking effects are on the central nervous system and consist of stimulation followed by depression of reflexes. After strychnine the motor effects of spinal reflexes are increased and the latent period is decreased. Reflexes become more generalized and, after large doses, small sensory disturbances send all the voluntary muscles in the body into violent and painful convulsions. Strychnine acts mainly on the spinal cord and convulsions occur after removal of the rest of the central nervous system. Strychnine does not excite by direct action, but acts as a competitive antagonist of the inhibitory transmitter (glycine) at postsynaptic inhibitory sites in the same manner as curare blocks acetylcholine at the neuromuscular junction. It has no effect on presynaptic inhibition. Strychnine has an excitatory action on the medulla, where it stimulates the vasomotor and vagal centers. It also enhances the sensations of touch, smell, hearing, and sight.

The alkaloid is used as a pesticide for destroying agricultural rodents and predatory animals and for trapping fur animals. Occasionally, domestic animals and man are poisoned by this agent.

The symptoms of strychnine poisoning are primarily those of stimulation of the central nervous system. The first symptom begins 10 to 30 min following ingestion, and is usually stiffness of the muscles of the neck and face. The patient next exhibits heightened reflex activity or excitability. This progresses to spontaneous muscle twitchings, and sensory stimuli may result in spinal convulsions. The characteristic picture is one of opisthotonos, trismus, and risus sardonicus. The convulsions may involve all voluntary muscles, including the diaphragm, thus interfering with the ability to breathe and resulting in cyanosis. Death is by respiratory failure.

Treatment of strychnine poisoning consists of prevention of asphyxia by maintaining a patent airway and adequate pulmonary ventilation, controlling the convulsions by the administration of a soluble barbiturate, ridding the body of the unabsorbed poison by gastric lavage with 1:10,000 potassium permanganate solution, and general supportive therapy. If the patient can be kept alive for 5 to 6 hours after ingestion of the drug, the prognosis is very good.

Caution—Strychnine is extremely poisonous.

Dose—*Usual*, 1.5 mg.

Other Central Nervous System Stimulants

Flurothyl [Bis(2,2,2-trifluoroethyl) ether [333-36-8] $C_4H_4F_6O$ (182.07) Indoklon (*Ohio Medical*)]. *Preparation:* 2,2,2-Trifluoroethyl *p*-toluenesulfonate is metathesized with sodium 2,2,2-trifluoroethoxide and the crude ether thus obtained is distilled and purified. US Pat 3,363,006. *Description and Solubility:* Clear, colorless, volatile liquid having a pleasant, mild, etheral odor; boils at about 64°; specific gravity between 1.415 and 1.419. Soluble 1 g in 500 mL water; miscible with alcohol, ether, propylene glycol, and halogenated solvents. *Uses:* Flurothyl, an agent known to produce clonic and tonic convulsions in laboratory animals, is used as an alternate for electroconvulsive therapy in the treatment of mental disorders. Clinical studies suggest the two procedures are similar in safety, efficacy and side effects. Flurothyl is effective after either inhalation or parenteral administration. Convulsions start within 15 to 20 sec after administration of the drug; the initial myoclonic jerks are followed by an intense tonic phase which lasts from 30 to 90 sec. Recovery is prompt and uneventful. Many patients are said to prefer the drug to electroshock. On the other hand, flurothyl convulsions are less predictable and less easily induced than are electroshock seizures. Memory impairment, skeletal fractures, and prolonged apnea are occasional complications of both electroconvulsive therapy and drug-induced convulsions. Arterial spasm and gangrene may follow perivenous administration. Furthermore, the possibility that repeated administration of the halogenated compound might induce liver damage should not be ignored. *Dose—Usual*, up to 1 mL by special inhalation. *Other Dose Information*—Intravenous, 6 to 8 mL of a 10% solution. *Dosage Forms*—Inhalation: 2 mL.

Mazindol—page 892.

Phendimetrazine Tartrate—page 892.

Phenmetrazine Hydrochloride—page 892.

Phentermine—page 892.

CHAPTER 63

Antineoplastic and Immunosuppressive Drugs

Stewart C Harvey, PhD

Professor of Pharmacology
College of Medicine, University of Utah
Salt Lake City, UT 84132

Antineoplastic Drugs

Prior to the 1940s the principal nonsurgical treatment of neoplasms was X-ray and radium therapy, although certain arsenicals and urethane were also in use. During the 1940s there were three main developments: radioisotopes, nitrogen mustards, and antifolic acid agents. The use of sex hormones for the treatment of certain types of neoplasms and of adrenal corticoids and ACTH for the treatment of leukemia also developed considerably during these years.

Much excitement was generated by these early developments in antineoplastic therapy, but it was later tempered by the realization that not only were the drugs not curative but also that, for the most part, life-expectancy was negligibly increased, the drugs being mainly palliative. Subsequently, there has been a great proliferation in both the number and classes of anticancer drugs and in the theory of cell kinetics and cell-population statistics, so that with the consequently improved armamentarium and regimens, long-term disease-free remissions are achievable with several neoplasms, and a few carcinomata can even be cured.

Tumor Growth and Kinetics

The principal difference between mature normal tissues and tumors is not in the rate of cell replication but in that in most normal tissues the rate of proliferation equals the rate of cell death, whereas in neoplasms proliferation exceeds the death rate. Proliferation in normal tissue responds to subtle signals that indicate when proliferation is needed for repair, regeneration, or growth and development. Neoplasms seem to lack such an autoregulation of proliferation, and the rate of cell-replication appears to depend on mostly an intrinsic rate modulated by the adequacy of the vascular supply.

Exponential Growth and Doubling Times—In the early stages, the growth of a tumor is approximately constant. The doubling time is the mean ("average") interval between successive mitoses. It is characteristic of the particular type of tumor cell. Doubling time varies markedly among various kinds of tumors. In Burkitt's tumor, it is approximately 24 hr; in acute leukemia, 2 weeks; in breast cancer, 3 months; and in multiple myeloma, 6 to 12 months. Contrary to common belief, these doubling times are within the range of those for normal tissues. For example, white cell precursors divide approximately every 12 hr and mucosal cells of the rectum every 24 hr.

A tumor cell becomes detectable when the number of cells reaches about 10^9 to 10^{10} cells. This requires 30 to 33 doubling times. The neoplasm becomes lethal when the population reaches about 5×10^{11} to 5×10^{12} cells, after 39 to 42 doubling times.

Phases of the Cell Cycle—Some drugs can exert a lethal action only when a cell is in a particular stage of activity and growth. Therefore, a resumé of cell kinetics will be useful. After mitosis and cell division, the new daughter cells are in a resting state, termed phase G_0 (G for gap). The length of time spent in G_0 depends on both the type of cell and the autoregulatory factors. In some tissues, such as bone marrow, gastrointestinal mucosae, and skin, G_0 is only moderately prolonged during maturation and aging, whereas with others, such as nerve and skeletal muscle cells, G_0 becomes essentially infinitely long well in advance of maturity. In solid tumors, G_0 is longer when the cell mass is large than when small, because the vascular supply cannot keep pace with the rate of growth. Ultimately the cell enters a post-resting phase, called G_1. In this phase, metabolism appears to be normal, but the cell is committed to divide. After a latency, the cell enters the S-phase, in which DNA synthesis is activated, in preparation for mitosis. The cell then enters another phase, G_2, the premitotic phase, in which DNA synthesis is essentially at rest but protein synthesis and other metabolic activities are increased and the cell volume grows. Finally, the cell undergoes mitosis (phase M) and cellular fission.

The cell cycle can be thought of as existing in two superstages: G_0 as one, and all of $G_1 + S + G_2 + M$ as the other, the latter comprising all phases committed to cellular division. The entity $(G_1 + S + G_2 + M)/(G_0 + G_1 + S + G_2 + M)$ is known as the *growth fraction*. In tumors, it usually lies between 0.2 to 0.7. The growth fraction tends to be greater in the more rapidly proliferating tissues and tumors, but not always.

Chemotherapeutic Intervention

Phase Specificity—Antineoplastic drugs are of two general categories: (1) Those that can act upon the cell throughout its cycle; such drugs are said to be *phase-nonspecific*. (2) Those that act preferentially during one or more of the non-resting phases; these drugs are said to be *phase-specific*. Even phase-nonspecific drugs have greater activity during the growth phases. The particular phase during which a drug acts depends on the lethal mechanism. Those that combine irreversibly with DNA can do so at any time and hence are phase-nonspecific; however, more DNA is exposed during the growth phases than during G_0, so that even these drugs have some phase selectivity. Drugs that interfere with DNA synthesis will be specific to the S-phase, those that block protein synthesis mainly to phases S and G_2, and those that inhibit microtubule assembly mainly to M.

Tumor Selectivity and Response—Especially for phase-specific drugs, the probability of a lethal action on a tumor cell (or normal cell) is directly proportional to the percent of time spent in the vulnerable phase. It follows that the percent of time spent in the vulnerable phase will be an important determinant of the susceptibility of tumors of different cell types. Even without reference to any particular growth phase, the generality that *those tumors with a large growth fraction are more susceptible to chemotherapy than* *those with a low fraction* is an important precept. Examples of tumors that respond well to chemotherapy are acute leukemia in children,* Burkitt's lymphoma,* choriocarcinoma,* chronic myelogenous leukemia, lymphocytic leukemia, Hodgkin's disease, Wilms' tumor, and breast cancer. Examples of neoplasms that respond poorly are malignant melanoma, carcinoma of the gastrointestinal tract, bronchogenic carcinoma, and tumors of the uterus and cervix.

Different cell types spend different proportions of time in one as opposed to another phase (i.e., more in G_2 than S, etc.). Therefore, the most effective drug would be expected to be of a type that is specific to the phase of longest duration. In part, this may account for the differences in efficacy among drugs of different mechanisms and phase specificity.

At present, there is great interest in and investigation of the possibility of *synchronizing* tumor cells so that all cells are in the same phase of the cycle. If the cells were synchronized and the host cells were not, then the tumor could be made more vulnerable to appropriate drugs given at the proper time and the therapeutic index could be increased. Synchronization is attempted by a holding "pulse" of a mitostatic or some other drug that holds the cells in a given phase until the out-of-phase cells also come into that phase. Discontinuation of the synchronizing drug simultaneously releases the cells to resume their cycle, all starting from the same phase.

Determinants of Sensitivity and Selectivity—In addition to the growth fraction or vulnerable phase time of a tumor, other factors also determine the selectivity of drugs for certain cell types. The demand for nutrients varies among tumor types but also differs between tumor cells and normal cells. For example, many tumors require more asparagine than normal cells, so that if the plasma asparagine is enzymatically destroyed (see *Asparaginase*, page 1143), the tumor cells are selectively "starved" to death. Some drugs are metabolized in the peripheral cells as well as in the liver, and the different cell types differ in their ability to metabolize these drugs. For example, with bleomycin there is evidence to suggest that the drug is metabolized less in susceptible tumor cells than in other cells, thus permitting higher local concentrations. Several drugs are converted to active metabolites by the target cells ("lethal synthesis"), and differences in the rates of conversion may contribute to selectivity. Also, differences in penetrance account for some differences among drugs; lipid-soluble antineoplastic drugs are more effective than water-soluble ones for neoplasms in the central nervous system. An unassessed factor in selectivity is that of effects on the immune system. There are not only tumor cell-attacking "killer" T-cells but also suppressor T-cells and blocking factors from B-cells which protect certain neoplastic cells from immune attack. According to which immune cells are the most suppressed, some antineoplastic drugs might antagonize the immune response to neoplastic cells and other drugs augment it.

Requirements for "Kill"—A remission can usually be achieved with a kill of 90 to 99% of the neoplastic cells. A kill of 99% would leave at least 10^7 to 10^8 surviving cells to carry on tumor growth, and the remission would last only 3 to 4 doubling times. With those neoplasms against which the immune system is ineffective, a 100% kill is necessary to effect a true cure, since it has been shown experimentally that a single implanted neoplastic cell can develop into a tumor. However, a true cure may not always be necessary. For example, with a tumor the doubling time of which is 12 months, a kill of 99.99% (which would leave perhaps 10^6 surviving cells) would require about 13 years for the tumor cell population to recover to the number extant at the time of treatment. A second course of an appropriate chemotherapy might add

another 13 years which, with middle-aged or elderly patients, might be beyond the normal life-expectancy. However, with a rapidly doubling tumor like Burkitt's tumor, the survival time in the untreated patient is measured in days, not years; even if all but a single cell were killed by an antineoplastic drug, survival would be prolonged less than two months; therefore, either a complete kill or sustained or frequently repeated courses are imperative. Fortunately, 50 to 60% of Burkitt's tumor cells are in the S-phase and are thus highly susceptible to drugs that are S-phase-specific.

Combination Chemotherapy—One way of increasing the percent of kill is to combine two or more antineoplastic drugs. There are three criteria to optimize such combinations: (1) Each component drug must have some efficacy by itself. (2) Each component drug should have a different mechanism of cytotoxic activity and, preferably, phase-specificity. (3) Each component drug should have a different spectrum of toxicity than the other components, in order to avoid overwhelming toxicity of a given type.

Log Cell-Kill Principle—Antineoplastic drugs may be characterized by their *log cell-kill index*, that is, by the negative log of the fraction of the tumor cell population that survives a single course of treatment. Thus a drug that kills 99.9% of the tumor cell population, ie, leaves 0.0001 (or $1/10^4$) of the population, is known as a 4-log drug; a second drug that kills 99.9% is known as a 3-log drug. The log cell-kill index is a tenuous number, but it serves a usefulness in predicting the effects of combinations that meet criteria 1 and 2. The predicted effect of a combination is obtained by adding the indices of the component drugs. Thus a 4-log drug plus a 3-log drug should provide a 7-log combination, that is, kill 99.99999% or leave $1/10^7$ of the population. A third drug that kills 99% (2-log drug) would further reduce the remaining population to $1/10^9$, which comes close to complete eradication of a tumor caught early.

Drug Resistance—Unfortunately, resistance develops to chemotherapeutic agents. It has not been unequivocally ascertained whether the resistant cell type is present as a minor type in the tumor cell population prior to treatment or whether treatment itself induces resistant cells through mutagenesis, or both. In any event, the usefulness of a given agent is often terminated by the transformation to a resistant tumor. Four mechanisms of resistance have been identified: (1) Loss of the endocellular transport system for the drug, as appears to happen with methotrexate. (2) Disappearance of the enzyme necessary for "lethal synthesis." (3) An increase in the production of the enzyme inhibited by the drug, as sometimes happens with methotrexate. (4) The development of an active transport system that removes the drug from the cell. Other mechanisms are easy to conceive and undoubtedly will be discovered.

Toxicity—Neoplastic cells have composition and activities very much like those of the host cells. This has made it thus far impossible to design antineoplastic drugs that will not also attack normal cells. Every antineoplastic drug has a therapeutic index less than 1.0. The principles that apply to antitumor efficacy also apply to the toxicity. Thus the tissues most affected are those with high growth fractions, and the integrity of the highly proliferative tissues can be considerably disturbed. Consequently, the bone marrow, lymphoblasts, mucous membranes, skin, and gonads are affected to a greater extent than are other cells. Since the myelogenous leukocyte turnover is faster and the growth fraction is greater than those of erythrocytes, *bone-marrow depression* usually causes a more severe neutropenia and thrombocytopenia than anemia. Bone-marrow depression is a major adverse effect of 31 of 36 current antineoplastic drugs. Suppression of proliferation of mucosal cells causes *mucositis*, characterized by aphthous and gastrointestinal ulceration. Fifteen of the current 36 drugs prominently cause mucositis. Arrest of the prolifera-

---

* These neoplasms are now considered to be curable.

tion of the cutaneous epithelial cells may cause *alopecia* (18 of 36 drugs), scaliness of the skin, and sometimes even desquamation. Some drugs that lack significant dermatologic actions may nevertheless recall cutaneous toxicities induced by previous drugs or radiation. Aspermia may result from actions on the seminiferous tubules and amenorrhea from actions on the ovaries (where the growth fraction but not the turnover rate is high). The immune cells have a rapid turnover and are highly susceptible to certain cytotoxic agents. *Immunosuppression* makes the patient more vulnerable to *infection;* it is noteworthy that 50% of cancer patients die of intercurrent infections rather than from the terminal phases of the neoplastic disease. Immunosuppression probably enhances the growth of certain neoplasms. Since they interfere in genetic mechanisms, certain antineoplastic drugs are mutagenic and carcinogenic, and the patient is subjected to the risk of future neoplasia. The incidence of acute leukemia is considerably higher in persons who have been treated with antineoplastic drugs than in the general population. Theoretical considerations predict that all neoplastic drugs are teratogenic, and teratogenic activity has been shown with some.

There are also other toxicities related to antineoplastic actions. For example, massive cell destruction results in the release of large quantities of purine bases from the nucleic acids of the dead cells, which purine bases are metabolized to uric acid. Hyperuricemia, renal damage consequent to hyperuricuria, and also some neurological damage may result. It is common to give allopurinol along with antineoplastic drugs. Massive destruction of certain leukemic cells may also cause an acute hypotensive crisis which is sometimes called "anaphylaxis", although it is not a true allergic response.

Some of the local adverse effects are also related to the antineoplastic mechanisms. Extravasation or accidental contamination of the skin or lungs may present very high concentrations to the cells in the local area, such that the cells will be killed by the cytotoxic actions, leading to vesication, ulceration, sloughing, bronchitis, etc. With the nitrogen mustards, the drugs need not interact with DNA to be caustic, since the nitrogen mustards readily alkylate critical chemical groups in the cell membranes and in the cytoplasm. Local toxicity in the gastrointestinal tract prevents certain antineoplastic drugs from being administered orally. Local gastrointestinal toxicity may cause nausea, vomiting, diarrhea, cramping, etc, but these are also acute side-effects of many antineoplastic drugs administered intravenously, and it is not clear whether they relate to the antineoplastic actions.

Precautions and Contraindications—With all drugs that cause bone-marrow depression, it is essential to monitor the blood cell count, which may serve both as a guide to adequate dosage and as a precaution against overdoses. The minimum advisable leukocyte and platelet count varies somewhat among the drugs but is usually 3000 to 4000 leukocytes and 20,000 to 100,000 platelets. When the count falls below these limits, the drug dosage should be reduced or the drug discontinued until there is recovery. It is usually inadvisable to begin treatment with a bone-marrow depressant drug within 4 weeks of the administration of another bone-marrow depressant drug or radiation therapy. When two bone-marrow depressant drugs are used in combination, it is necessary to reduce the dose and to monitor more frequently. Although other toxicities are usually not as life-threatening as bone-marrow depression, analogous precautions should be observed, although monitoring cannot be as quantitative as cell counts. However, aphthous ulcers can be visualized and monitored. With patients in poor condition, it is imperative to proceed cautiously and to monitor more closely than with patients in good condition. Not only may elderly patients be more susceptible to the adverse actions of antineoplastic drugs but toxicity will be more incapacitating and life-threatening, so

that therapy should be undertaken most cautiously. Antineoplastic drugs should not be used during pregnancy unless alternatives are exhausted.

Classes and Mechanisms of Drugs—Antineoplastic drugs may be grouped into seven categories. Some of the categories are based on chemical and mechanistic properties and others on the origins of natural products.

Alkylating Agents—There are three subgroups of the alkylating agents: nitrogen mustards, ethylenimines, and alkylsulfonates. The nitrogen mustards are all bis(β-chloroethyl)amines. The ethylenimines contain three ethylenimine groups per molecule, and the alkylsulfonates are bismethylsulfonates. Thus these compounds are all polyfunctional alkylating agents, a fact that relates importantly to the mechanism of action. The alkylating groups react with nucleophilic centers in many different kinds of molecules. However, their bi- or tri-functional character allows them to cross-link double-stranded DNA, thus preventing the strands from separating for replication.

Nitrosoureas—The nitrosoureas are usually classified as alkylating agents. Carmustine is bifunctional and may be able to cross-link double-stranded DNA. Lomustine and semustine each contain a single β-chloroethyl group, but can cross-link DNA by using the nitroso group as a second electrophilic group. Streptozocin lacks an alkylating moiety. Carbamoylation of nucleoside bases in nucleic acids has been suggested as a possible mechanism of action. However, the nitroso group is also a free radical and ion generator, which could confer radiomimetic properties.

Methylhydrazines—Procarbazine and dacarbazine are sometimes classified as alkylating agents, because an "alkylating" moiety supposedly is liberated within the target cell. However, like other hydrazines, they generate free hydroxyl radicals and ions and are thus also considered to be radiomimetic.

Antimetabolites—There are three subcategories of antimetabolites: purine analogues, pyrimidine analogues, and folinic acid analogues. The purine analogues are incorporated into DNA as the deoxyribotides and into RNA as the ribotides, where they interfere with coding and replication. They also act like the natural purine bases in inhibiting synthesis of purine bases by acting through the allosteric feedback systems (pseudo-feedback). The pyrimidine analogues inhibit enzymes in the biosynthetic pathways for pyrimidine ribotides and deoxyribotides; thymidylate synthetase, orotic acid decarboxylase, aspartate carbamoyltransferase, and dihydroorotase are inhibited. Methotrexate is the only folinic acid analogue in use; it binds very tightly to dihydrofolate reductase and thereby prevents the conversion of dihydrofolate (folinate) to tetrahydrofolate.

Antibiotics—This is a miscellaneous group of drugs with respect to mechanism of action. Mitomycin appears to be an alkylating agent, daunorubicin and dactinomycin bind to DNA and inhibit DNA synthesis, and mithramycin inhibits DNA-dependent RNA polymerase. Bleomycin both acts as an antimetabolite of thymidine and causes fragmentation of DNA.

Steroid Hormones—The steroid hormones are transported to the cell nucleus, where they attach to chromatin and usually stimulate transcription and hence protein synthesis. However, the glucocorticoids suppress mitosis in lymphocytes and fibroblasts and appear to inhibit transcription. This so-called lympholytic effect is employed in the chemotherapy of the lymphocytic leukemias and in immunosuppression. The estrogens, progestins, and androgens probably also inhibit transcription and prevent mitosis in those cell types which are derived from normal cells that are suppressed by these hormones in the natural hormonal physiology. Thus the normal prostate gland is suppressed by estrogens, apparently by a competitive antagonism of androgens, and estrogens are used to treat cancer of the prostate gland, etc. Similarly, androgens exert an antiestrogen effect on certain breast tumors; only tumors of a cell type that contains estrogen receptors are responsive. Antiestrogens are also used to suppress such tumors. Estrogens also suppress the growth of some breast tumors, but the mechanism of the effect is poorly understood. Progestins behave as antiestrogens in the endometrium and

hence may be employed in the chemotherapy of endometrial carcinoma. The hormones are described in Chapter 52. Drugs that induce local inflammation and fibrosis may suppress effusions secondary to various neoplasms. Thus, quinacrine may be given into the pleural and peritoneal cavities to control such effusions. Since the neoplastic process is unaffected, quinacrine is not truly antineoplastic.

Immunosuppressive Drugs

The immune system is quite complex. Several types of cells are involved. These are cells the ancestral line of which has derived from bone-marrow stem cells. Some of the descendants of the stem cells migrate to sites elsewhere in the body, where they become small lymphocytes. There are two general types of small lymphocytes involved in the immune responses: the B-cells and the T-cells. The B-lymphocytes get the designation B from the fact that in birds they derive from stem cell clones in the bursa of Fabricus; in man, the location of analogous clones may be in the intestinal mucosal Peyer's patches. The T-cells get their designation from the fact that they are derived from stem cells cloned in the thymus gland. Undifferentiated small lymphocytes take up residence in lymph tissue in the spleen, tonsils, intestines, and other sites. B- and T-cells respond to antigen by cellular transformation, proliferation, and differentiation. Proliferation increases the population of immunocompetent cells and differentiation creates cells with various roles to play in the immune response. Both B- and T-cells differentiate into what may be broadly termed effector cells and memory cells. The memory cells revert to an inactive state (G_0) but respond to later immune challenge by accelerated proliferation, differentiation, and activity. During their residence in the bursa equivalent, the future effector B-cells become programmed to respond to an antigen by transformation into plasma cells, which produce antibodies (immunoglobulins I_A, I_D, I_E, I_G and I_M), the role of which is to combine with circulating antigens. The immunity conferred by B-cells is known as *humoral immunity*. Hypersensitivity mediated through the humoral immune system is called immediate hypersensitivity, since the response is rapid. T-cells become programmed in the thymus to respond in various ways to antigen that has become fixed to cell surfaces or engulfed by macrophages. The cytotoxic T-cell (effector cell, "killer" cell), with the aid of complement, attacks and lyses those cells to which the offending antigen is attached. There are different cytoxic T-cells for different antigens. There are also helper T-cells, which promote B-cell activity, and suppressor T-cells, which restrain both the cytotoxic T-cells and the B-cells. Helper and suppressor B-cells also exist. T-Cell-mediated immunity is known as cell-mediated immunity. It is the immune response involved in graft-rejection, autoimmunity, and delayed hypersensitivity.

The priming of lymphocytes in response to antigen is known as the primary response. The final effector response is known as the secondary, or efferent, response.

There are other bone-marrow stem-cell derived cells, such as macrophages and K-cells, that participate in the immune response. In the primary response, the macrophages phagocytose antigens and alter them in ways that the antigen becomes capable of activating T- and B-cell precursors. Thus the macrophages are an integral part of the afferent limb of the primary response. They also appear to be involved in the efferent response; they fix and alter antigen prior to its recognition by the T-cells.

An immunosuppressive drug is one that can attenuate the expression of at least one type of immune response. The numerous cell types involved in the immune system afford an

equal number of places of immunosuppressive drugs to intervene, and it is conceivable that a T-cell responsive to one antigen may be affected more than another T-cell specific to another antigen or that suppressor T-cells might be affected more than cytoxic or helper T-cells. In general, information on drug selectivity is lacking. However, the increase in the incidence of lymphomas in persons with a past history of immunosuppression lends credence to the hypothesis of a selectivity for suppressor T-cells. The ability of indomethacin to delay graft rejection also suggests a selective action on suppressor cell function, since prostaglandins are suppressor mediators. In general, though, cells involved in the primary response seem to be more susceptible to immunosuppressive treatment than those in the secondary response. The overall effect of an immunosuppressive drug probably depends on its phase specificity and the differences and similarities of the cell cycle phasing among the various cell types.

The immunosuppressive drugs comprise a number of classes of drugs, not all of which are antineoplastic drugs. For example, the antimalarial drug pyrimethamine, and the antibacterial drug trimethopterin, have immunosuppressant properties and have been used clinically as immunosuppressants. Also penicillamine and gold salts are employed as immunosuppressants in the treatment of rheumatoid arthritis. Biological agents, such as lymphocyte immune globulin and antimacrophage serum are actively under investigation. Physical interventions, such as radiation, desensitization, and surgery are still used in the management of certain immune diseases, which testifies to the present limitations of the drugs.

The alkylating agents mainly affect the short-lived and not the long-lived small lymphocytes. They also suppress proliferation of macrophages but do not interfere with phagocytosis. Therefore, the primary immune response is mainly affected, although cyclophosphamide acts on both afferent and efferent limbs in certain immune disorders. The antipurines, 6-mercaptopurine and azathioprine, have a strong effect on cellular immunity and act mainly on the efferent limb (according to their program of use), although they also have suppressant effects on macrophage proliferation and display afferent activity in certain circumstances. The antipyrimidines mainly behave as efferent suppressants. Experimentally, methotrexate has mixed properties, but in man it behaves mostly as an efferent suppressant. Adrenalcorticoids both suppress macrophage activity and decrease the population of small lymphocytes. Clinically, they behave mostly as afferent suppressants, but they are adjuvant to efferent and mixed suppressants.

The adverse effects and precautions of the primary immunosuppressant drugs are those of the antineoplastic drugs.

A great deal of publicity has been given the use of immunosuppressive drugs to prevent rejection of organ and bone-marrow transplants. However, they have a greater potential usefulness in the management of the autoimmune diseases. Diseases in which they are of established benefit include systemic lupus erythematosus, rheumatoid arthritis, nonglomerular nephrosis, psoriasis, and chronic active hepatitis.

Diseases for which these drugs have not been unequivocally proven sufficiently efficacious for general use include ulcerative colitis, Crohn's disease, Behçet's disease, chronic glomerulonephritis (membranous), chronic thrombocytopenic purpura, and autoimmune hemolytic anemia.

Aminoglutethimide

2,6-Piperidinedione, 3-(4-aminophenyl)-3-ethyl-, Cytadren (*Ciba-Geigy*).

2-(*p*-Aminophenyl)-2-ethylglutaramide [125-84-8] $C_{13}H_{16}N_2O_2$ (232.28)

Preparation—By a procedure similar to glutethamide (page 1071) with nitration of the α-ethylbenzyl cyanide to the *p*-nitro derivative. This is then reduced to the amine after ring closures. US Pat 2,848,455.

Description—White crystals melting at 149–150°.

Solubility—Very slightly soluble in water but freely soluble in many organic solvents.

Uses—Aminoglutethimide inhibits the first step in adrenalcorticoid biosynthesis by inhibiting the conversion of cholesterol to Δ^5-pregrenolone. It also inhibits the aromatase that converts androstenedione to estrone and estradiol, thus eliminating the adrenal source, the only source of estrogens in postmenopausal and oophorectomized women. Consequently, treatment with aminoglutethimide is preferred to adrenalectomy in postmenopausal women with *estrogen receptor-positive breast carcinoma*. Hydrocortisone is concomitantly administered to suppress the counterproductive, counterregulatory increase in ACTH release that accrues to the drug-induced lowering of plasma hydrocortisone. The regime, however, causes more adverse effects than does tamoxifen and hence is a second-choice treatment. Aminoglutethimide is also useful in the management of certain cases of *Cushing's syndrome*.

Early adverse effects include lethargy (in 40% of recipients), ataxia (in 10%), nausea, vomiting, and anorexia, to all of which tolerance develops in 1 to 6 weeks, and morbilliform rash. Delayed adverse effects mostly relate to mineralocorticoid insufficiency and include orthostatic hypotension (in 10%; symptoms are dizziness and weakness) so that mineralocorticoids may require supplementation. Occasional adverse effects include pruritis, myalgia, headache, masculinization and hirsuitism in women, precocious sexual development in boys, hypothyroidism with goiters after long-term use, leucopenia, thrombocytopenia, granulocytopenia, and pancytopenia. Alkaline phosphatase and SGOT activities in serum frequently occur, and cholestatic jaundice occurs rarely. Aminoglutethimide induces the metabolism of dexamethasone, thus that particular glucocorticoid should not be used concomitantly.

Aminoglutethimide is well-absorbed orally. Initially, about 50% is excreted in the urine unchanged, but induction of liver metabolism diminishes the importance of renal elimination. The elimination half-life is initially about 13 hr but decreases to about 7 hr after 1 to 2 weeks.

Dose—*Oral*, *initial*, **20 mg** 2 to 4 times a day for 2 weeks; if serum hydrocortisone levels are inadequately suppressed, the dose may be increased by 250 mg/day at weekly to biweekly intervals up to a maximum of **2 g/day**.

Dosage Forms—tablets: 250 mg.

Asparaginase

L-Asparagine amidohydrolase; E.C. 3.5.1.1.; Elspar (*MSD*)

L-Asparaginase [9015-68-3], an enzyme of molecular weight 133,000 ± 5000, believed to consist of four equivalent subunits.

Preparation—L-Asparaginase, an enzyme that catalyzes hydrolysis of L-asparagine to L-aspartate and ammonia, occurs in many bacteria, fungi, yeasts, plants, and animal tissues. Isolated in pure form from several sources, it is usually obtained from *Escherichia coli*, which produces also an asparaginase devoid of antileukemic activity that is removed on purification of the enzyme. See Mashburn and Wriston, *Arch Biochem Biophys 105:* 450, 1964.

Description—White, crystalline powder.

Solubility—Freely soluble in water; practically insoluble in chloroform, methanol.

Uses—Protein synthesis in several normal as well as malignant cell types is partly dependent upon exogenous asparagine, and, in a few cells, such as lymphoblasts and certain other leukemic cells, is essentially totally dependent. The enzymatic destruction of asparagine by asparaginase injected into plasma deprives the dependent cells of the essential asparagine and thus not only arrests their growth but may even result in some cell death and tumor regression.

At present, asparaginase is used mainly in chemotherapy of *acute lymphocytic leukemia*, in sequential combinations with other drugs. When asparaginase is administered immediately after a course of vincristine and a glucocorticoid (usually prednisone or dexamethasone) for the induction of the first remission in children, the median duration of remission is more than doubled. Some, but not other, studies indicate a small increase in the incidence of complete remissions. The enzyme is also useful for induction of remission in children with relapse of acute lymphocytic leukemia. It is not recommended for maintenance.

Sixty to 90% of recipients of asparaginase will show laboratory evidence of an impairment of liver function; plasma fibrinogen and other clotting factors may be diminished, and most patients will have a considerable elevation of blood ammonia. Effects on the pancreas are also common; insulin production is diminished and there may be hyperglycemia, serum amylase activity may increase, and acute pancreatitis, sometimes hemorrhagic, may occur in as many as 5% of the recipients. There are also actions on the central nervous system, to cause impairment of the sensorium, mental depression and rare coma. Nausea, vomiting, chills and fever also occur frequently. Hypersensitivity reactions, ranging from mild rash to anaphylaxis and death, occur in 5 to 20% of recipients, so that sensitivity testing before administration is necessary and desensitization may be required before a second course is administered. *Erwina* (Porton) asparaginase is less sensitizing than that from *E coli*. Asparaginase also has immunosuppressant activity.

Asparaginase must be administered parenterally. Its half-life is about 16 hr.

Dose—*Intravenous*, **1000 IU per kg** of body weight per day for 10 days. *Intramuscular*, **6000 IU/m²** of body surface at 3-day intervals for a total of 9 doses.

Dosage Forms—For Injection: 10,000 units.

Azathioprine

1*H*-Purine, 6-[(1-methyl-4-nitro-1*H*-imidazol-5-yl)thio]-, Imuran (*Burroughs-Wellcome*)

6-[(1-Methyl-4-nitroimidazol-5-yl)thio]purine   [446-86-6] $C_9H_7N_7O_2S$ (277.26).

Preparation—*N,N'*-Dimethyloxaldiamide is reacted with phosphorus pentachloride to give 5-chloro-1-methylimidazole. This is nitrated and the resulting 5-chloro-1-methyl-4-nitroimidazole is condensed with purine-6-thiol (mercaptopurine) in an appropriate dehydrohalogenating environment. US Pat 3,056,785.

Description—Yellow, matted powder that is odorless and has a slightly bitter taste; light-sensitive, nonhygroscopic, and stable to reasonable temperatures; decomposes at about 245°.

Solubility—Insoluble in water; very slightly soluble in alcohol and chloroform; soluble in dilute solutions of alkali hydroxides (unstable); sparingly soluble in dilute mineral acids.

Uses—A derivative of *Mercaptopurine* into which it is largely converted in the body, but not all of its actions are those of mercaptopurine. It is used only as an *immunosuppressive* drug. It probably has been used more than any other immunosuppressive drug in *kidney transplantations*. At present, about one-half of kidney transplants survive for longer than 3 years when azathioprine is used, but other measures also contribute to this rate of success. It also is used in other organ transplantations, but since such operations are less frequent, reliable data are not yet available. Azathioprine also appears to bring about a satisfactory response in a high percentage of patients with *ulcerative colitis*, *regional enteritis*, or *refractory idiopathic thrombocytopenic purpura*. Azathioprine may reduce the adrenalcorticosteroid requirement in *rheumatoid arthritis*, but its potential toxicity is greater than that of gold or chloroquine, so that azathioprine is not recommended for early therapy. It is usually of little benefit in *systemic lupus erythematosus*.

Toxicity or intercurrent infection (see introduction) occurs in about one-third of patients under treatment with azathioprine. Bone-marrow depression is the most frequent, occurring in about 11% of patients; leukopenia (28 to over 50%, as much as 16% serious), thrombocytopenia, and to a lesser extent anemia or pancytopenia are manifested. Pancreatitis, alopecia, arthralgia, skin rashes, serum sickness, stomatitis, esophagitis, steatorrhea, retinopathy, peritoneal hemorrhage, and pulmonary edema may also occur in a small percent of cases. Occasionally, hepatic damage, with elevation of the plasma content of liver enzymes and jaundice, is seen, but damage seems to be slight and to disappear during the course of treatment. However, in the presence of liver dysfunction the drug should be withheld. Although the incidence is rare, an increase in reticulum cell sarcoma and lymphoma has been noted in transplant patients receiving azathioprine; it is not clear whether this is from immunosuppression or from the successfully sustained transplant. However, the drug is carcinogenic in experimental animals. Although azathioprine is rapidly degraded in the liver, the kidney importantly regulates the plasma concentration of the effective metabolites, so that toxicity is greatly increased in the presence of allopurinol or renal impairment, unless the dosage is properly adjusted. It should not be used during pregnancy, if possible.

Dose—*Oral or intravenous*, if treatment is begun at the time of transplantation, *initially*, 3 to **5 mg per kg body weight per day**, after which adjustments are made to attempt to maintain the homograft without toxicity; the *maintenance dose* may be as low as 1 **mg per kg** but usually is **2 to 3 mg per kg per day**. Treatment must be started within 24 hr of transplantation. When treatment is started 1 to 5 days before transplantation, 1 to **5 mg per kg per day**. In the presence of renal damage or allopurinol the dose should be reduced to $\frac{1}{4}$ to $\frac{1}{3}$ of the above. Reduce dose or stop treatment at the first sign of bone-marrow depression. For rheumatoid arthritis, initially **1.0 mg per kg** as a single or twice daily dose to be increased by **0.5 mg/kg/day** after 6 to 8 weeks and thereafter at 4-week intervals to a total of **2.5 mg/kg/day** or the supravention of severe toxicity.

Dosage Forms—For Injection (as sodium salt): 100 mg of azathioprine equivalent; Tablets: 50 mg.

Bleomycin Sulfate

Blenoxane (*Bristol*)

(Main component: Bleomycin A₂, in which **R** is (CH₃)₂S⁺CH₂CH₂CH₂—)

Bleomycin Sulfate (salt) [9041-93-4]

A mixture of the sulfates salts of a group of related basic glycopeptide antibiotics, notably bleomycin A_2 and bleomycin B_2, obtained from cultures of *Streptomyces verticillus;* bleomycin A_2 is the main component of the bleomycin used clinically.

Preparation—For the purification and separation of the bleomycins see Umezawa *et al*, *J Antibiot 19:* 200, 210, 1966, also Takita *et al*, *ibid. 21:* 79, 1968 and *22:* 237, 1969.

Description—Bleomycin sulfate occurs as a cream-colored, hygroscopic powder.

Solubility—Very soluble in water; sparingly soluble in alcohol.

Uses—Bleomycin causes fragmentation of DNA and also inhibits incorporation of thymidine into DNA. It stops the progression of cells through the G_2 and M phases of the cell cycle. In spite of these actions, it has only very little effect on bone marrow, a circumstance that gives bleomycin a special usefulness in drug combinations. Its selectivity appears to be related to distribution. With vinblastine and cisplatin it is a component of one of two first-choice combinations for the treatment of *testicular carcinoma*. It is the drug of second choice for the treatment of *squamous cell carcinoma of the cervix* and, in combination with cisplatin, also of *squamous cell carcinoma of the head and neck*. It has also been used successfully in the treatment of squamous cell carcinomas of the skin, penis, and vulva. In combination with doxorubicin and prednisone, it is the treatment of second choice for *Hodgkin's disease*. Non-Hodgkin's lymphomas have also been reported to respond to the drug. It has shown efficacy against reticulum cell sarcoma, lymphosarcoma, choriocarcinoma, and teratocarcinoma.

Bleomycin is very toxic, and about 10% of patients develop a pneumonitis which progresses to pulmonary fibrosis; 1% of bleomycin-treated patients die of pulmonary complications. The effect is most likely to occur in elderly patients or those who have received a total of 400 units. The drug must be used extremely cautiously in the presence of pulmonary disease. Acute hyperpyrexia and cardiorespiratory collapse also occur, especially in patients with lymphomas; for this reason, patients with lymphomas are given two test doses of 5 units or less and are observed for a day before treatment is begun. Bleomycin commonly causes nausea, vomiting, chills, and fever, and in half of the patients it causes erythema and hyperkeratosis, which sometimes progresses to vesication. Other occasional adverse effects are cutaneous desquamation, hyperesthesia, pruritus, tenderness, alopecia, and aphthous ulcers. Cutaneous toxicity is most likely to occur when the total cumulative dose exceeds 150 units.

Bleomycin is poorly absorbed orally and is also inactivated in the gut and liver. Consequently, it must be administered parenterally. Higher concentrations are reached in certain neoplasms (carcinomas more than sarcomas), lungs and skin than in other tissues, which accounts for the selectivity and the loci of toxicities. In the tissues, the drug appears to be deaminated and possibly also hydrolyzed by peptidases. The enzymatic destruction is less in those tissues in which the higher concentrations are reached. Sixty to 70% is excreted in the urine. In patients with normal renal function, the elimination half-life is about 2 hr; in renal failure the half-life may be as long as 21 hr. Care must be exercised in the presence of renal impairment.

Dose—*Intravenous*, *intramuscular*, or *subcutaneous initially*, **10 to 20 units per m²** of body weight (or 0.25 to 0.5 unit per kg) once or twice a week. In Hodgkin's disease, once a remission of 50% is achieved, the *maintenance* dose is **1 unit** per day or 5 units once a week. Pulmonary toxicity can be monitored by the occurrence of dyspnea and by X-ray; infiltrates in the roentgenogram mean dosage must be discontinued.

Dosage Form—Sterile: 15 units (1 unit is equivalent to the activity, microbiologically determined, of 1 mg of a bleomycin A_2 reference standard).

Bromocriptine—page 929.

Busulfan

1,4-Butanediol, dimethanesulfonate; Tetramethylene Dimethanesulfonate; Myleran (*Burroughs-Wellcome*)

CH₃SO₂O(CH₂)₄OSO₂CH₃

1,4-Butanediol dimethanesulfonate [55-98-1] $C_6H_{14}O_6S_2$ (246.29).

Caution—Busulfan is very poisonous. Great care should be taken to prevent inhaling particles of Busulfan and exposing the skin to it.

Preparation—By esterifying 1,4-butanediol with methanesulfonyl chloride in the presence of pyridine.

Description—White, crystalline powder; melting range 115° to 118°.

Solubility—Very slightly soluble in water; slightly soluble in alcohol; 1 g in about 45 mL acetone.

Uses—An alkylating radiomimetic which is efficacious in certain cases as a *neoplastic suppressant*. Its principal distinction is that in the usual doses it exerts very little action on rapidly proliferative tissues other than bone marrow. With low doses, granulocytopoiesis can be selectively suppressed without affecting erythropoiesis. Thus, it is employed for the palliative treatment of *chronic granulocytic* (myelogenous, myeloid, myelocytic) *leukemia*, for which it is the drug of choice. It is not to be used in terminal or acute phases of the disease. It is also quite effective in the treatment of *polycythemia vera* and *primary thrombocytosis*. Since it has little effect on lymphopoiesis, it is of no value in lymphocytic leukemia, Hodgkin's disease, or malignant lymphoma. It is useless against solid tumors.

The principal toxicity of busulfan is pancytopenia and long-lasting thrombocytopenia. *Lymphocytopenia* is uncommon. A complete differential blood count (including thrombocytes) once a week is mandatory. Nausea, vomiting, diarrhea, impotence, amenorrhea, sterility, and fetal malformation occasionally occur. Granulocyte destruction results in a high rate of excretion of urates, the precipitation of which may cause renal damage; cotreatment with *Allopurinol* (page 1111) may avoid such damage. Busulfan also sometimes causes cheilosis, glossitis, interstitial pulmonary fibrosis, anhidrosis, skin pigmentation (which may be the result of adrenalcortical hypofunction), alopecia, and gynecomastia.

Busulfan is not immunosuppressive.

The elimination half-life is 2 to 3 hr.

Dose—*Adult*, *oral*, for *chronic intermittent therapy*, **0.1 mg per kg body weight** (usually 4 to 8 mg) **per day** in two divided doses until leukocyte count drops to 10,000 to 20,000 cells/mm³; for *chronic continuous therapy*, initially as above but with dose reduction to maintain the leukocyte count at 10,000 to 20,000/mm³ (usually about 2 mg/day), keep leukocyte count in the normal range, the dose varying from **2 mg per week** to 2 to **4 mg per day**. The drug must be discontinued if there is a precipitous decrease in leukocyte count. The *pediatric dose initially* is 60 μg **per kg body weight** or **1.8 mg per m² of body surface per day;** *maintenance*, the dose necessary to maintain the leukocyte count at about 20,000/mm³.

Dosage Form—Tablets: 2 mg.

Calusterone—page 1001.

Carmustine

Urea, *N,N'*-bis(2-chloroethyl)-*N*-nitroso-, BiCNU (*Bristol*)

$$ClCH_2CH_2N-\overset{\overset{O}{\|}}{C}-NCH_2CH_2Cl$$
$$\underset{H}{\quad}\quad\underset{N=O}{\quad}$$

1,3-Bis(2-chloroethyl)-1-nitrosourea [154-93-8] $C_5H_9Cl_2N_3O_2$ (214.05).

Preparation—Carmustine, like other cytotoxic nitrosoureas, may be synthesized by nitrosation with sodium nitrite of the appropriate substituted urea—in this case 1,3-bis(2-chloroethyl)urea—in a cold, acid medium (eg, formic acid). Methods of synthesis of nitrosoureas have been published by Johnston *et al: J Med Chem 6:* 669, 1963.

Description—White or light yellow powder; melts, with decomposition, to an oily liquid at about 30°.

Solubility—Slightly soluble in water; freely soluble in alcohol; highly soluble in lipids. Decomposes rapidly in acid and in aqueous solutions above pH 7.

Uses—Although carmustine is an alkylating drug, it is also thought to carbamoylate amino and other groups and to effect condensations through the nitroso group. Synthesis of DNA and RNA is inhibited. The drug is used mainly in the treatment of *brain tumors* (for which it shares drug-of-choice status with its congener lomustine), *Hodgkin's disease* and other *lymphomas* and *multiple myeloma*. It has been reported to have a high efficacy against *Burkitt's tumor*. Although it has activity against various other carcinomas, including melanoma and renal cell carcinoma, it is not among the usual choices for such diseases. Carmustine is usually given in combination with radiotherapy in the treatment of brain tumors and with vincristine, procarbazine, and glucocorticoids (eg, prednisone) in the treatment of the various lymphomas and multiple myeloma.

Within 2 hr after administration and lasting for 4 to 6 hr, nausea and vomiting occur frequently. Rapid intravenous infusion causes

intense flushing and conjunctival suffusion with a similar time-course. There may be a burning sensation but rarely thrombosis at the site of injection. Delayed bone-marrow toxicity occurs; also thrombocytopenia that reaches a nadir in about 4 wk and a less severe leukopenia in about 6 wk, each lasting 2 to 7 wk; mild anemia may occur. With repeated doses, bone-marrow depression is cumulative. Leukocyte and platelet counts and signs of intercurrent infections should be carefully monitored throughout treatment. Severe dyspnea and a sometimes fatal interstitial pulmonary fibrosis occasionally occur. There may also be a mild, reversible hepatotoxicity in about 25% of recipients. Other adverse effects include slight nephrotoxicity (with a transient elevation of BUN) to severe nephrotoxicity and renal failure with large cumulative doses, vertigo, and ataxia.

By the oral route, carmustine is almost completely metabolized as it passes through the liver; consequently, it must be given intravenously. Even after intravenous administration, its plasma half-life is only 2 to 3 min. Because the drug is highly lipid-soluble, it readily passes the blood-brain barrier, and concentrations of metabolites in the cerebrospinal fluid range from 115 to 117% of those in plasma.

Dose—*Intravenous*, **200 mg per m²** of body surface in a single dose or divided into two doses on successive days once every 6 wk. Subsequent adjustments of dosage are determined according to the therapeutic and toxic response (see the manufacturer's literature or *Drug Facts* and *Comparisons*). A preexisting bone-marrow depression or concomitant use of other myelosuppressive drugs requires that lower doses be used.

Dosage Form—For Injection, 100 mg.

Other Dose Information—Into each vial is injected 3 mL of sterile, absolute ethanol and 27 mL of sterile water, to yield a solution containing 3.3 mg/mL. This solution is then added to an injection of isotonic sodium chloride or dextrose solution.

Chlorambucil

Benzenebutanoic acid, 4-[bis(2-chloroethyl)amino]-,
Leukeran (*Burroughs-Wellcome*)

$$(ClCH_2CH_2)_2N-\bigcirc-CH_2CH_2CH_2COOH$$

4-[*p*-[Bis(2-chloroethyl)amino]phenyl]butyric acid [305-03-3] $C_{14}H_{19}Cl_2NO_2$ (304.22).

Caution—*Chlorambucil is very poisonous. Great care should be taken to prevent inhaling particles of Chlorambucil and exposing the skin to it.*

Preparation—4-Phenylbutyric acid is nitrated and the resulting *p*-nitro acid is esterified with isopropyl alcohol. The nitro ester is then hydrogenated to the aminoester. Reaction with ethylene oxide converts the —NH_2 into —$N(CH_2CH_2OH)_2$ which is then converted into —$N(CH_2CH_2Cl)_2$ by treatment with $POCl_3$. Hydrolysis of the ester yields the acid, chlorambucil.

Description—Off-white, slightly granular powder.
Solubility—Very slightly soluble in water; soluble in dilute alkali; 1 g in 2 mL acetone.

Uses—Chlorambucil is an alkylating agent effective by the oral route. It is more completely and predictably absorbed than is triethylenemelamine. It is the agent of choice in the treatment of *chronic lymphocytic leukemia*. It is also effective in the treatment of Waldenstrom's *macroglobulinemia, multiple myeloma, lymphosarcoma, giant cell follicular lymphoma* and to a lesser degree in choriocarcinoma, Hodgkin's disease and ovarian and testicular tumors. As an immunosuppressant it has been reported to be of value in the treatment of *vasculitis* associated with rheumatoid arthritis, *autoimmune hemolytic anemias, scleroderma, systemic lupus erythematosus, systemic sclerosis*, and *Behçet's disease*.

Chlorambucil is the slowest-acting and least toxic of currently used nitrogen mustards. Its toxicity is mainly bone-marrow depression, although in therapeutic doses it is generally moderate and reversible. Most patients will have some neutropenia after the third week of treatment until about 10 days after discontinuation of treatment. Slowly progressing lymphopenia also occurs, but it repairs itself quickly after treatment. Thrombocytopenia and anemia also occur sometimes. When the total accumulated dose exceeds 6.5 mg/kg the incidence of severe bone-marrow damage becomes high, and even irreversible toxicity may occur. It is mandatory that hemoglobin, leukocyte, and platelet counts be monitored closely. Chlorambucil is contraindicated for four weeks after radiotherapy or other drugs that depress bone marrow. If possible, chlorambucil should be avoided during the first trimester of pregnancy.

The elimination half-life of chlorambucil is about 2.5 hr.

Dose—*Adult*, *oral*, *initially* **0.1 to 0.2 mg per kg body weight** (usually 4 to 10 mg) **per day** for 3 to 6 weeks, as necessary to effect remission. Lymphocytic leukemia usually requires only **0.1 mg/kg**, but Hodgkin's disease may require **0.2 mg/kg**. When there is already some evidence of bone-marrow depression or lymphocytic infiltration of bone marrow, the daily dose should not exceed **0.1 mg/kg**. *Maintenance* may not be necessary, but, if it is, the dose ranges from **0.03 to 0.1 mg/kg/day**. The drug should be taken one hour before breakfast or 2 hours before dinner. *Pediatric*, **0.1 to 0.2 mg/kg body weight** or **4.5 mg/m²** of body surface once a day.

Dosage Form—Tablets: 2 mg.

Chloroquine—page 1218.

Chloroquine Phosphate—page 1218.

Chromic Phosphate P32—page 489.

Cisplatin

Platinum, diamminedichloro-, (*SP*-4-2)-, Platinol (*Bristol*)

cis-Diamminedichloroplatinum [15663-27-1] $Cl_2H_6N_2Pt$ (300.06).

Preparation—A solution of potassium tetrachloroplatinate(II), which is prepared by reduction of the hexa chloroplatinate(II) salt with hydrazine, is neutralized with ammonium chloride and ammonium hydroxide. The *cis*-isomer precipitates (*Inorg Synth 7:* 239, 1963).

Description—White, lyophylized powder melting about 207°.

Solubility—1 g in about 1000 mL of water or normal saline; 1 g in about 42 mL of dimethylformamide.

Uses—Cisplatin cross-links DNA and hence acts like alkylating agents. It is used in various first choice combinations for the treatment of *metastatic carcinomas of the testes*, *cervix*, and *ovary*, *squamous cell carcinoma of the head and neck*, *non-small cell cancer of the lung*, and *advanced cancer of the bladder*. It is also used alone in the treatment of bladder cancer.

Acute toxicity includes severe nausea, vomiting, and anorexia, which occur in almost all recipients, and occasional anaphylactoid reactions. Delayed toxicity includes ototoxicity (tinnitus and/or hearing loss in about 30% of patients), which requires audiometric monitoring; serious nephrotoxicity, which requires monitoring of serum creatinine and urate and of BUN and avoidance of other nephrotoxic drugs; bone marrow depression (in 25 to 30% of recipients), which requires leukocyte and platelet counts; occasional peripheral neuropathies, loss of taste, and convulsions. Electrolyte deficits, perhaps from hemodilution by fluids, have been reported.

Cisplatin is not absorbed orally and must be given intravenously. About 90% is bound to plasma proteins. It does not cross the blood-brain barrier. Elimination is mainly renal. The distribution half-life is 25 to 49 min and the elimination half-life 58 to 73 hr. However, platinum can be identified in tissues for prolonged periods of time. It is incompatible with aluminum.

Dose—*Intravenous*, for *metastatic testicular tumors* (in combination with bleomycin and vinblastine), **20 mg/m²** for 5 days every 3 weeks for three courses; then, for *maintenance*, **0.2 mg/kg** every 4 weeks for 3 or 4 courses; for *metastatic ovarian tumor* (in combination with doxorubicin), **50 mg/m²** every 3 weeks or, *as a single agent*, **200 mg/m²** every 4 weeks; for *bladder cancer*, or, as a single agent, **50 to 70 mg/m²** every 3 or 4 weeks. All regimens are subject to modification according to hematologic, nephrologic, audiometric, and other indices of toxicity.

Cyclophosphamide

2*H*-1,3,2-Oxazaphosphorin-2-amine, *N*,*N*-bis(2-chloroethyl)tetrahydro-, 2-oxide, monohydrate; Cytoxan (*Mead-Johnson*); Tymtran (*Adria*)

[6055-19-2] $C_7H_{15}Cl_2N_2O_2P.H_2O$ (279.10); anhydrous [50-18-0] (261.09).

Caution: Great care should be taken to prevent inhaling particles of Cyclophosphamide and exposing the skin to it.

Preparation—3-Amino-1-propanol is condensed with *N*,*N*-bis(2-chloroethyl)phosphoramidic dichloride [(ClCH₂CH₂)₂-N—POCl₂] in dioxane solution under the catalytic influence of triethylamine. The condensation is double, involving both the hydroxyl and the amino groups, thus effecting the cyclization.

Description—White, crystalline powder; liquefies on loss of its water of crystallization.

Solubility—1 g in about 25 mL water; soluble in alcohol.

Uses—Cyclophosphamide is an alkylating agent. Unlike other β-chloroethylamino alkylators, it does not readily cyclize to the active ethyleneimonium form until activated by hepatic enzymes. Thus the substance is stable in the gastrointestinal tract, is well tolerated and effective by the oral and parenteral routes, and does not cause local vesication, necrosis, phlebitis, or even pain.

Alone or in combination, cyclophosphamide is the drug of choice for treatment of *Burkitt's tumor*. It is a component of various first-choice combinations for treatment of *multiple myeloma*, *squamous cell* and *large cell anaplastic carcinomas*, and *adenocarcinoma of the lung*, *small cell lung cancer*, *soft tissue sarcomas*, *neuroblastoma*, *pediatric solid tumors*, *Ewing's sarcoma*, *non-Hodgkin's lymphomas*, *breast tumor*, *oat-cell bronchogenic carcinoma*, *ovarian tumors*, and *testicular tumors*. In combination, it shares drug-of-choice status with various other drugs for chemotherapy of *acute* and *chronic lymphocytic leukemia*, *prostatic carcinomas*, *choriocarcinoma*, and miscellaneous carcinomas. It is a drug of third choice for treating *bladder tumors* and shares third-choice with other drugs for *endometrial tumors*.

Cyclophosphamide is an *immunosuppressive drug*. It has been shown to be of value in the treatment of *rheumatoid arthritis*, *Wegner's granulomatosis*, *idiopathic thrombocytopenic purpura* (alone or in combination), *erythroid aplasia*, *childhood nephrotic syndrome*, *pemphigus vulgaris*, and *dermatomyositis* (in combination). It appears to be erratic against *systemic lupus erythematosus*. It may possibly be efficacious in the management of *uveitis*. It improves the survival of *bone marrow* and probably of *heart transplants*.

Alpoecia occurs in about 50% of patients receiving maximal prolonged treatment. Leukopenia is the inevitable side effect and is used as an index of dosage. Other side effects include anorexia, nausea and vomiting (regardless of route of administration), mucosal ulcerations, dizziness, occasional thrombocytopenia, hypoprothrombinemia, nail ridging, cutaneous pigmentation, sterile hemorrhagic cystitis, water intoxication, aspermia in males (3 to 6 months or longer in onset), anovulation in 30 to 50% of females, and occasional hepatic dysfunction. Bladder telangiectasis and abnormal urinary cytology occur; in long-term use, bladder fibrosis and carcinoma occasionally occur. The blood count should be monitored closely during induction and at least weekly thereafter.

Cyclophosphamide is absorbed orally. It is distributed to the tissues with a volume of distribution greater than the total body water. The plasma half-life is 4 to 6 hr.

Dose—*Adult*, *oral*, 1 to **5 mg/kg/day**, depending on gastrointestinal tolerance to the drug. The oral route usually is not recommended for loading because of the limited amount usually tolerated. *Intravenous*, *initially* **10 to 20 mg/kg/day** until a total of 40 to 50 mg/kg has been given (2 to 6 days), except less if the blood count is already low; *maintenance* may be (1) *oral*, 1 to **5 mg/kg/day**, (2) *intravenous*, **10 to 15 mg/kg** every 7 to 10 days, or (3) *intravenous*, **3 to 5 mg/kg** twice a week. A leukocyte count of 3000 to 4000/mm³ is usually desired. *Pediatric*, *oral or intravenous*, *initially* **2 to 8 mg/kg/day** or **60 to 250 mg/m²/day**; *oral*, *maintenance*, **2 to 5 mg/kg** or **50 to 150 mg/m²** twice a week.

Cyclophosphamide may also be given intramuscularly, into body cavities, or by infiltration.

Dosage Forms—For Injection: 100, 200, and 500 mg; Tablets: 25 and 50 mg.

Cyclosporine

Sandimmune (*Sandoz*)

Cyclosporin A [59865-13-3] $C_{62}H_{111}N_{11}O_{12}$ (1202.63).

Preparation—A metabolite of *Cylindrocarpon lucidum* and *Trichoderma polysporum*. It is practically insoluble in water but is soluble in ethanol and fixed oils.

Uses—Cyclosporine suppresses helper T-lymphocyte activity without affecting suppressor T-lymphocytes or B-lymphocytes. Thus, it is a selective immunosuppressive drug without the cytotoxicity characteristic of most other immunosuppressive drugs. Since it works only on the primary (afferent) immune process, it must be administered before exposure to the specific antigen to be protected against. The drug appears to be more effective than conventional therapy in *renal transplantation*. It has also been used in *transplantation of liver, pancreas, heart, lung,* and *bone marrow*. It is usually employed in combination with glucocorticoids and other immunosuppressive drugs.

The most serious adverse effects are depressed renal function (which must be distinguished from graft rejection), benign breast tumors, and psychic depression. Other adverse effects include hirsuitism, tremors, neurasthenia, an increase in serum liver enzymes, and gingival hyperplasia. Convulsions in children also treated with methylprednisolone have been reported. Cyclosporine should not be given with aminoglycosides, amphotericin B, or ketoconazole.

Cyclosporine is readily absorbed from the gut. It is almost completely metabolized in the liver to a number of metabolites.

Dose—*Oral,* 15 to 20 mg/kg, when used in conjunction with other immunosuppressive drugs.

Dosage Forms—Oral Solution: 100 mg/50 mL and 50 mg/5 mL.

Cytarabine

2(1*H*)-Pyrimidinone, 4-amino-1-β-D-arabinofuranosyl-, Cytosine Arabinoside; Cytosar-U (*Upjohn*)

1-β-D-Arabinofuranosylcytosine [147-94-4] $C_9H_{13}N_3O_5$ (243.22).

Preparation—Cytidine is reacted with fuming HNO_3 and the resulting cytidine 2′,3′,5′-trinitrate is boiled in alcohol containing dilute alkali hydroxide to form the inverted 2′-hydroxy compound. Remaining nitrate groups are removed via saponification. *CA 75:* 130077q, 1971.

Description—White to off-white, odorless, crystalline powder; nonhygroscopic and stable at 40°; melts between 210° and 222°.

Solubility—1 g in 5 mL water, 500 mL alcohol, 1000 mL chloroform, 300 mL methanol.

Uses—A pyrimidine nucleoside antimetabolite that is cytotoxic to a number of cell types. It competes with deoxycytidine and also interferes with incorporation of uridine into deoxycytidine nucleotides. Cytarabine is S-phase specific. It is especially used in the treatment of *acute granulocytic, myelomonocytic,* or *monocytic leukemias,* particularly in adults; in combination with thioguanine, and daunorubicin, it is the drug of choice. It is also a component of a first-choice combination to treat the *acute phase of chronic myelocytic leukemia.* With other drugs it shares third-choice status for *non-Hodgkin's lymphomas* and *acute lymphocytic leukemia.* There does not appear to be cross-refractoriness to mercaptopurine, methotrexate, or prednisone. It is also effective in the treatment of *preleukemic syndromes.*

As an immunosuppressant, cytarabine suppresses primary (afferent) responses in doses that cause little or no other toxicity. It is under active clinical investigation.

Cytarabine is not sufficiently absorbed orally to be maximally effective by this route. Oral bioavailability is less than 0.2. However, it does penetrate into the cerebrospinal fluid and reaches a concentration up to 40% of that in plasma. In the body, 90% is destroyed by deamination; the plasma half-life is 1 to 3 hr. Since detoxification takes place throughout the body, the drug may be given in the presence of renal impairment, but the dose should be reduced in hepatic failure.

The primary adverse effects are leukopenia (66%), thrombocytopenia (62%), and, less frequently, anemia and megaloblastosis, which are actually closely related to the therapeutic response and hence are essentially unavoidable. Bone-marrow depression is more severe when the drug is given by continuous intravenous infusion than by single injection. Other side effects are nausea, vomiting, diarrhea, aphthous ulceration, abdominal pain, esophagitis, chest pain, thrombophlebitis at the site of injection, neuritis, arthralgias, flushing, rash, alopecia, and teratogenicity. Liver damage may occur. Cytarabine should be given cautiously and in reduced doses to patients with liver impairment or bone-marrow depression. It must not be given in combination with methotrexate. Leukocyte and platelet counts should be made daily during the initial course of treatment and at regular intervals during maintenance.

Dose—*Adult, rapid intravenous injection,* initially **100 mg/ m^2/day** for 7 to 10 days; if an antileukemic response (neutrophils less than 1000/mm^3) or hematologic toxicity (platelets less than 50,000/mm^3) has not occurred within 10 days, the dose is increased to **200 mg/ m^2/day** until a therapeutic response or hematologic toxicity occurs. *Constant intravenous infusion, initially* **200 mg/ m^2/day** for 5 days; courses are repeated at intervals of about 2 weeks. In *combination* with thioguanine, initially thioguanine 2.5 mg/kg orally twice a day and cytarabine **3 mg/kg** by intravenous drip twice a day for 7 to 10 days; courses are repeated after 20 days of rest. In combination with cyclophosphamide, vincristine, and prednisone, **100 mg/ m^2/day** in 3 divided doses for 5 days; courses are repeated every 2 weeks. *Subcutaneous, for maintenance,* **1 mg/kg/week** or semiweekly. *Intrathecally,* for acute central nervous system leukemia, **30 mg/ m^2** of body surface every 1 to 7 days; this application has not yet been approved by FDA. *Pediatric, initial, intravenous,* **2 mg/kg** or *intravenous infusion,* **0.5 to 1 mg/kg** once a day for 10 days; *maintenance, subcutaneous,* **1 mg/kg** twice a week. All doses are subject to modification if the platelet count falls below 50,000/mm^3 or the granulocyte count below 1000/mm^3.

Dosage Forms—Sterile: 100 and 500 mg.

Dacarbazine

1*H*-Imidazole-4-carboxamide, 5-(3,3-dimethyl-1-triazenyl)-, DIC; DTIC-Dome (*Miles*)

5-(3,3-Dimethyl-1-triazeno)imidazole-4-carboxamide [4342-03-4] $C_6H_{10}N_6O$ (182.18).

Preparation—5-Diazoimidazole-4-carboxamide, obtained by reaction between 5-aminoimidazole-4-carboxamide and sodium nitrite in acid solution, is reacted with an anhydrous solution of dimethylamine in methanol at 5° to produce dacarbazine (Shealy *et al., J Org Chem 27*: 2150, 1962).

Description—Colorless to ivory-colored microcrystalline powder, sensitive to light and heat; reported to melt at 205° and decompose explosively at 250° to 255°; pK$_a$ 4.42.

Solubility—Slightly soluble in water and in alcohol.

Uses—Dacarbazine has a cytotoxic action of unknown mechanism. It shares a first-choice status with semustine in the treatment of *metastatic malignant melanoma.* The success rate is only about 20%. It is also a component of a first-choice combination (dacarbazine-doxorubicin-vinblastine-cyclophosphamide) for soft tissue tumors. The combination of dacarbazine-doxorubicin-bleomycin-vinblastine-cyclophosphamide is the treatment of second choice for *Hodgkin's disease.* With several drugs it shares third-choice status for *neuroblastoma.*

The most serious adverse effect of dacarbazine is bone-marrow depression, which is occasionally fatal; the myelogenous leukocytes and platelets are the most affected, anemia being mild, when it occurs. Careful monitoring of leukocytes, platelets, and erythrocytes is required. If there is preexisting bone-marrow depression or if another bone-marrow suppressant drug is in use or has been used within 4 weeks, the dose of dacarbazine must be reduced. Anorexia, nausea, and vomiting lasting 1 to 12 hr occur in over 90% of recipients of the drug; tolerance occurs after the first few doses; phenobarbital or prochlorperazine often will arrest the vomiting. Diarrhea is also frequent; it may be partially prevented by restriction of food and fluids prior to the administration of drug. An influenza-like syndrome accompanied by fever up to 39°, myalgia, and malaise, sometimes occurs approximately 1 week after large doses and may continue for 1 to 3 weeks. Facial flushing, facial paresthesias, and alopecia have also been observed. Abnormalities in liver or renal function have been reported, and the drug should be used cautiously in patients with liver or renal damage. Extravasation of dacarbazine may cause pain and local necrosis.

Dacarbazine is eliminated with a half-life of 35 min. Approximately 50% of an intravenous dose is metabolized in the liver; by the oral route, very little remains unchanged, thus making the intravenous route necessary. The unmetabolized drug is excreted in the urine by tubular secretion. The volume of distribution is larger than total body water.

Dose—*Intravenous*, for *malignant melanoma*, **2 to 4.5 mg per kg** of body weight per day for 10 days; the higher doses do not appear to be more efficacious than the lower ones. The course is repeated at 4-week intervals. An alternative regimen is **150 mg/m²/day** for 5 days, repeated every 3 weeks. For *Hodgkin's disease*, **150 mg/m²/day** for 5 days, repeated every 4 weeks (in combination with other drugs); alternatively, **375 mg/m²/day**, every 15 days.

Dosage Forms—Sterile for Injection: 100 and 200 mg.

Other Dose Information—100 mg and 200 mg are reconstituted with 9.9 and 19.7 mL of sterile water, respectively. The duration of injection should be no less than 1 min.

Dactinomycin

Dactinomycin; Meractinomycin; Cosmegen (*MSD*)

Actinomycin D [50-76-0]; C$_{62}$H$_{86}$N$_{12}$O$_{16}$ (1255.43).

Caution—Handle Dactinomycin with exceptional care, to prevent inhaling particles of it and exposing the skin to it.

Preparation—Elaborated during the culture of *Streptomyces antibioticus*. After extracting from the fermentation broth, it is purified through chromatographic and crystallization processes. US Pat 2,378,876.

Description—Bright-red crystalline powder; light-sensitive and should be protected appropriately; it should also be protected from excessive heat and moisture; melts between 245° and 248° with decomposition. Contains in each mg an amount of antibiotic activity of not less than 900 μg of dactinomycin.

Solubility—1 g in about 8 mL alcohol, 25 mL water (at 10°), 1000 mL water (at 37°), and about 1666 mL ether.

Uses—An antineoplastic drug that inhibits DNA-dependent RNA polymerase. In combination with vincristine it provides the chemotherapy of choice for treatment of *Wilms' tumor*, and the combination dactinomycin-methotrexate is first choice for *choriocarcinoma*. In combination with other drugs it has second-choice status for chemotherapy of *testicular tumors* and *Ewing's sarcoma*. It has been reported to have limited value in the treatment of *osteogenic sarcoma*, *malignant melanoma*, *sarcoma botyroides*, *neuroblastoma*, *lymphomas*, and *breast* and *lung cancers*, but it does not even rank as drug-of-third choice in these disorders. Dactinomycin-vincristine in combination appears to suppress metastases in embryonal rhabdomyosarcoma and to prolong survival. Tumors that fail to respond to systemic treatment sometimes respond to local perfusion. Dactinomycin potentiates radiotherapy. Dactinomycin is a secondary (efferent) immunosuppressive.

Nausea and vomiting are usual and occur within the first few hours after administration of dactinomycin. Anorexia, abdominal pain, diarrhea, proctitis, and gastrointestinal ulceration follow. The pa-

tient may also experience malaise, fatigue, lethargy, myalgia, and fever. Cheilitis, ulcerative stomatitis, pharyngitis, esophagitis and proctitis are common. Because agranulocytosis, leukopenia, pancytopenia, thrombocytopenia, and anemia frequently occur, *the blood picture must be monitored daily.* Cutaneous eruptions, alopecia, hyperpigmentation, and erythema also occur. Anaphylaxis has been reported. Side effects appear to be reversible. The drug is locally toxic, and phlebitis and cellulitis may occur at the site of injection; extravasation may cause serious local tissue damage. Venous thrombosis may also result from local effects.

Dactinomycin is mostly eliminated by biliary and renal excretion; the half-life is about 36 hr. The drug does not pass the blood-brain barrier.

Dose—*Intravenous*, *adults*, **0.01 mg** (10 μg)/**kg** or **0.5 mg** (500 μg) once a day and *children*, **0.015 mg** (15 μg)/**kg**, divided into 4 doses, for no more than 5 days. An alternative schedule is 2.5 mg/m² of body surface in 3 or 4 divided doses over the course of a week. Single doses of 2 mg/week for 3 weeks also have been successfully employed. Courses can be repeated at intervals as short as 3 weeks if no sign of residual toxicity is present, but courses are usually repeated every 6 weeks to 3 months. The injection should be made into the tubing of a running intravenous infusion, so as to avoid extravasation. When dactinomycin is used in combination with radiation treatment or other antineoplastic drugs, the dose of it and usually of the other therapy needs to be reduced.

Dosage Form—For Injection: 0.5 mg (500 μg).

Diethylstilbestrol Diphosphate—page 988.

Daunorubicin Hydrochloride

5,12-Naphthacenedione, 8-acetyl-10-[(3-amino-2,3,6-trideoxy-α-L-*lyxo*-hexanopyranosyl)oxy]-7,8,9,10-tetrahydro-6,8,11-trihydroxy-10-methoxy-, (8S-*cis*)-, hydrochloride; Cerubidine (*Ives*).

[23541-50-6] C$_{27}$H$_{29}$NO$_{10}$.HCl (563.99).

Preparation—An antibiotic produced by *S peuceticus* or *S coeruleorubidus*.

Description—Red needles decomposing about 190°.

Solubility—Soluble in water, methanol and ethanol; insoluble in ether or chloroform. The pH of an aqueous solution containing 5 mg per mL is 4.5–6.5.

Uses—Daunorubicin intercalates into DNA, blocks DNA-directed RNA polymerase, and inhibits DNA synthesis. It can prevent cell division in doses that do not interfere with nucleic acid synthesis.

In combination with other drugs daunorubicin is included in the first choice chemotherapy of *acute myelocytic leukemia* in adults (for induction of remission), the *acute phase of chronic lymphocytic leukemia*, the second choice treatment of *acute lymphocytic leukemia*, and sometimes in the chemotherapy of neuroblastoma.

Acutely, daunorubicin causes nausea, vomiting, fever, and rare convulsions, cardiac dysrhythmias and S-T depression, and pulmonary edema, occasionally fatal. Phlebitis at the site of injection or a slough from extravasation may occur. It also colors the urine red. Delayed toxicity includes frequent bone marrow depression (with leukopenia and thrombocytopenia), which may be severe, stomatitis and aphthous ulceration, anorexia, hemorrhagic mucositis enterocolitis, abdominal pain, fever, rashes, usually reversible alopecia (in 80% of recipients), renal tubular damage, and hematuria. Cardiotoxicity may also be delayed. Rhythm disturbances are not related to cumulative dose, but a late congestive heart failure is frequent when the cumulative dose exceeds 550 mg/m². The onset of failure may occur as long as 1 to 6 months after discontinuation of treatment. Daunorubicin is teratogenic, mutagenic, and carcinogenic. Monitoring of blood cell counts, renal function, and ECG is required.

Oral absorption is poor, and daunorubicin must be given intravenously. The half-life of distribution is 45 min and of elimination, about 55 hr. It is mostly metabolized in the liver and also secreted into bile (ca. 40%). Dosage must be reduced in liver or renal insufficiencies.

Dose (base equivalent)—*Intravenous*, as a *single agent*, **30 to 60 mg/m²/day** for 3 days every 3 or 4 weeks; *in combination* (usually with cytarabine and other drugs), **45 mg/m²/day** for 3 days for the first course and 2 days for subsequent courses at 3- to 6-week intervals.

Dosage Forms (base equivalent)—For injection: 20 mg (as the base equivalent to 21.4 mg of the hydrochloride).

Doxorubicin Hydrochloride

5,12-Naphthacenedione, 10-[(3-amino-2,3,6-trideoxy-α-L-*lyxo*-hexopyranosyl)oxy]-7,8,9,10-tetrahydro-6,8,11-trihydroxy-8-(hydroxyacetyl) - 1-methoxy-, (8S-*cis*)-, hydrochloride; Hydroxydaunorubicin Hydrochloride; Adriamycin (*Astra*)

14-Hydroxydaunorubicin hydrochloride [25316-40-9] $C_{27}H_{29}NO_{11}$·HCl (579.99).

Preparation—Doxorubicin is an anthracycline antibiotic isolated from cultures of *Streptomyces peucetius* var *caesius* (US Pat 3,590,028). It differs from daunorubicin (see page 1148) only in having a hydroxyacetyl group in place of the acetyl group in daunorubicin, in position 8.

Description—Red-orange, crystalline powder; almost odorless; hygroscopic; melts at about 205°, with decomposition; pK_a 8.22.

Solubility—1 g dissolves in about 10 mL water and about 2000 mL alcohol.

Uses—Doxorubicin has proven to have the widest antineoplastic spectrum and usefulness of the antineoplastic drugs. It binds to DNA and inhibits nucleic acid synthesis, inhibits mitosis, and promotes chromosomal aberrations. Administered alone, it is the drug of first choice for the treatment of *thyroid adenoma* and *primary hepatocellular carcinoma*. It also shares with cisplatin a first-choice status for the treatment of *bladder tumors*. It is a component of several first-choice combinations for the treatment of *ovarian* and *breast tumors*, *non-Hodgkin's lymphomas*, *bronchogenic oat-cell carcinoma*, *gastric adenocarcinoma*, *retinoblastoma*, *neuroblastoma*, *mycosis fungoides*, and *pancreatic carcinoma*. It is the drug of second choice against *Wilms' tumor*, and shares second-choice status in combination with other drugs for treatment of *breast cancer*, *endometrial cancer*, *Hodgkin's disease*, *adrenal tumors*, *rhabdomyosarcoma*, and induction of remission in *acute lymphocytic leukemia*. It is a third-choice agent for the treatment of brain tumors, testicular cancer, islet cell carcinoma, squamous cell carcinoma of the head and neck, prostatic carcinoma, and multiple myeloma. It is also an immunosuppressant, but its status remains to be determined.

There is a high incidence of bone-marrow depression, which manifests itself mainly as a neutropenia that is most severe 10 to 14 days after treatment and lasts about 7 days; a white cell count as low as 1000/mm³ is to be expected. Monitoring of leukocytes and erythrocytes and signs of intercurrent infection is mandatory. Other frequent adverse effects are nausea and vomiting and reversible alopecia. Stomatitis and esophagitis may occur 5 to 10 days after treatment. Anorexia and diarrhea occur occasionally. Rarely, there may be hypersensitivity (fever, chills, urticaria), hyperpigmentation of the nails, lacrimation, conjunctivitis, and recurrence of skin reactions caused by prior radiotherapy. Hyperuricemia from rapid lysis of neoplastic cells may occur. An uncommon but serious toxicity is acute left-ventricular cardiomyopathy, which is refractory to digitalis. A persistent decrease in the voltage of the QRS complex is the most reliable prodromal sign. This cardiotoxicity is most likely to occur in patients in whom the cumulated dose is 550 mg/m². Prior radiotherapy to the chest, concomitant cyclophosphamide therapy, or hyperthermia may cause the cardiomyopathy to occur with a total dose as low as 400 mg/m². Doxorubicin is locally toxic and causes venous streaking, and extravasation results in pain, cellulitis and

sloughing. Its natural color may cause the urine to be red. Doxorubicin may potentiate hemorrhagic cystitis caused by cyclophosphamide, mucositis by radiotherapy, hepatotoxicity by 6-mercaptopurine, and add with the bone-marrow depressant actions of other antineoplastic drugs.

Doxorubicin is poorly absorbed and must be administered intravenously.

The major route of elimination is biliary secretion, which accounts for 40 to 50% of the elimination. Most of the remainder is metabolized in the liver, partly to an active metabolite (adriamycinol), but a few percent is excreted into the urine. In the presence of liver impairment, the dose should be reduced.

Dose—*Intravenous*, **60 to 75 mg per m²** of body surface at 21-day intervals or **30 mg per m²** on each of 3 successive days repeated at 28-day intervals. The lowest dose should be used in elderly patients, when there is prior bone marrow depression caused by prior chemotherapy or neoplastic marrow invasion, or when the drug is combined with other myelopoietic suppressant drugs. The dose should be reduced by 50% if the serum bilirubin lies between 1.2 and 3 mg/dL and by 75% if above 3 mg/dL. The total dose should not exceed 550 mg/m² in patients with normal heart function and 400 mg/m² in persons having received mediastinal irradiation.

Dosage Forms—For Injection: 10 and 50 mg.

Other Dose Information—The contents of the vial should be reconstituted to a final concentration of 2 mg/mL. The solution should then be injected into a freely running intravenous infusion of sodium chloride injection or 5% dextrose injection at a rate such that the dose not be administered in less than 5 min.

Dromostanolone Propionate—page 998.

Ethinyl Estradiol—page 987.

Fluorouracil

2,4(1*H*,3*H*)-Pyrimidinedione, 5-fluoro-, 5-FU; Adrucil (*Adria*); Efudex (*Hoffmann-LaRoche*); Fluoroplex (*Herbert*)

5-Fluorouracil [51-21-8] $C_4H_3FN_2O_2$ (130.08).

Caution—Great care should be taken to prevent inhaling particles of Fluorouracil and exposing the skin to it.

Preparation—Potassium fluoroacetate is reacted with methyl bromide to form methyl fluoroacetate which is then subjected to a Claisen condensation with methyl formate and sodium ethoxide to produce the potassium enolate of the methyl ester of α-fluoromalonaldehydic acid (I). Cyclization of I is effected through condensation under anhydrous conditions with *S*-benzylisothiourea. The resulting 2-(benzylthio) compound is readily hydrolyzed in the presence of acid to fluorouracil. US Pat 2,802,005.

Description—White to practically white, practically odorless, crystalline powder; stable when exposed to air; decomposes at about 282°.

Solubility—1 g in 80 mL water, 170 mL alcohol, and 55 mL methanol; practically insoluble in chloroform, ether, and benzene; solubility in aqueous solutions increases with increasing pH of the solution.

Uses—A congener of uracil that acts both as a surrogate and as an antimetabolite of that nucleotide. Its metabolite, 5-fluorouridine-5'-monophosphate (FUMP), blocks the synthesis of thymidylic acid and hence of deoxyribonucleic acid; as fluorouridine diphosphate it is also incorporated into ribonucleic acid. Uracil is preferentially utilized by neoplastic tissue; thus the antimetabolite has some degree of selectivity for the neoplasm. It is not curative, but it may bring about regression of a number of neoplasms. It is the antineoplastic of choice in the treatment of *carcinoma of the pancreas*. In combination with other drugs it provides chemotherapy of first choice in the treatment of *breast cancer*, *islet cell tumors*, *colorectal cancer* and *gastric carcinoma*. It is a component of second choice combinations for chemotherapy of *primary hepatocellular carcinoma*, and it shares second-choice rank with other drugs for treatment of *prostatic carcinoma* and *bladder tumors*. It shares third-choice status for the treatment of *endometrial carcinoma*, *squamous cell tumor of the cervix*, *head and neck*, and *ovarian tumors*. Fluorouracil may be useful in the treatment of *neoplasms of the gallbladder* and, to a lesser extent, those of the esophagus, larynx, thyroid, and pharynx. Remissions of as long as 4 years have been noted in a few instances, although the average is a few months.

Fluorouracil is also used topically in the treatment of precancerous dermatoses, especially *actinic keratosis*, for which it is the treatment of choice if the lesions are multiple. Even lesions that are not clinically discernible respond. For this reason, the drug is applied to the entire affected area. Healing continues for one to two months after treatment. The drug does not affect nonkeratotic lesions. Fluorouracil is a secondary (efferent) immunosuppressive agent and therefore has not been used in organ transplantation.

The drug is quite toxic, about two-thirds of patients showing signs of toxicity; the mortality rate is about 3% when treatment is initiated by daily doses. When the drug is administered by intravenous bolus, leukopenia is the principal adverse effect, usually occurring between the 7th and 14th days but readily recovering if the dose is promptly lowered. Thrombocytopenia is less frequent; the nadir occurs between the 7th and 17th days Aphthous ulceration may occur and is a sign that therapy should be temporarily discontinued. Other toxic effects include diarrhea, vomiting, nausea, gastrointestinal ulceration (the dose-limiting effect of constant infusion), alopecia, dermatitis, hyperpigmentation, pharyngitis, esophagitis, cerebellar ataxia (sometimes irreversible), and epistaxis. Lassitude and asthenia, lasting from 12 to 35 hr after an injection, may occur. When fluorouracil causes death, it is usually from septicemia, so that concomitant antibiotic therapy is advisable. Topically, fluorouracil may induce photosensitization and always erythema, scaling, fissuring, tenderness and usually erosion, ulceration, necrosis and reepithelialization as the result of the therapeutic action, although some persons appear to be resistant to this effect.

By the oral route, there is a first-pass elimination of the drug by the gut and liver, so that intravenous administration is required. At least 60% is metabolized to CO_2, but over 15% is excreted into the urine. The drug enters the cerebrospinal fluid and effusions. The plasma half-life is about 10 minutes, but the active metabolite, FUMP, may be detectable for days.

Dose—*Intravenous, initial* course, **12 mg/kg/day** (not to exceed 800 mg) for 4 days. If toxicity has not occurred, **6 mg/kg/day** on days 6, 8, 10 and 12; poor risk patients should receive **6 mg/kg/day** for 3 days and, if no toxicity, **3 mg/kg/day** on days 5, 7, and 9. For *maintenance*, if toxicity to the first course was minimal, either **repeat the course** every 30 days or give **10 to 15 mg/kg** (not to exceed 1 g) once a week, after recovery from the initial toxicity is complete. USPDI (1980) adopted an initial course of 7 to 12 mg/kg/day for 4 days, to be repeated every 3 to 4 days for 2 weeks, and, for maintenance, 7 to 12 mg/kg every 7 to 10 days; this regimen has not been widely accepted. When fluorouracil is used in combination with nitrosoureas, only 75% of the full dose should be used; the dose should also be reduced when it is used in other combinations. *Topical*, as a 1% cream or solution, applied once or twice a day to the entire affected area until necrosis, erosion, and ulceration occur.

Dosage Forms—Cream: 1 and 5%; Injection: 500 mg/10 mL; Topical Solution: 1 and 2%.

Fluoxymesterone—page 998.

Gold Au 198—page 491.

Hydroxyprogesterone Caproate—page 991.

Interferons—page 1231.

Lomustine

Urea, *N*-(2-chloroethyl)-*N'*-cyclohexyl-*N*-nitroso-, CCNU; CeeNU (*Bristol*)

1-(2-Chloroethyl)-3-cyclohexyl-1-nitrosourea   [13010-47-4] $C_9H_{16}ClN_3O_2$ (233.70).

Preparation—Lomustine, a cytotoxic nitrosourea, may be prepared by nitrosation of its substituted urea moiety (see preparation of *Carmustine*).

Description—Yellow powder.
Solubility—Practically insoluble in water; soluble in alcohol; highly soluble in lipids.

Uses—Lomustine is a chemical congener of *Carmustine* (page 1145) and has similar mechanisms of action and shares some of the same uses. Like carmustine, it reaches high concentrations in the cerebrospinal fluid and hence shares with carmustine a first-choice status for the treatment of *brain neoplasms*. It is the drug of second choice to treat *colorectal* and *renal* cancers and is a component of a second-choice combination for oat-cell lung cancer. It has third-choice status for treatment of both *Hodgkin's* and *non-Hodgkin's lymphomas, multiple myeloma,* and *non-small cell lung cancers.*

The adverse effects are similar to those of carmustine except that interstitial pulmonary fibrosis has not been reported. Nausea and vomiting occur later (3 to 6 hr) and last longer (24 hr). Thrombocytopenia and leukopenia reach nadirs in 4 and 6 weeks, respectively, and last 1 to 2 weeks. Stomatitis, alopecia, anemia, and mild, transient hepatotoxicity occasionally occur. Dysarthria, ataxia, lethargy, and disorientation have been reported. Monitoring of leukocyte counts is required. When other myelosuppressive drugs are in use or have been used within the prior 4 weeks, the dose of lomustine should be reduced.

Lomustine is well absorbed orally and survives the first pass through the liver to be effective by the oral route. It is distributed among the tissues with a volume of distribution greater than total body water. In the cerebrospinal fluid, the concentration of metabolites reaches 150% of that in plasma. Biotransformation occurs throughout the body; the half-life is less than 1 hr.

Dose—*Oral, adult* and *pediatric*, **130 mg per m²** of body surface every 6 weeks, except 100 mg per m² if bone-marrow function is depressed. Repeat courses should not be given until the platelet count has returned to 100,000/mm³ and the leukocyte count to 4,000/mm³, and they should never be given at intervals less than 6 weeks.

Dosage Forms—Capsules: 10, 40, and 100 mg.

Mechlorethamine Hydrochloride

Ethanamine, 2-chloro-*N*-(2-chloroethyl)-*N*-methyl-, hydrochloride; Nitrogen Mustard; HN2; Mustargen (*MSD*)

$$CH_3N(CH_2CH_2Cl)_2 \cdot HCl$$

2,2'-Dichloro-*N*-methyldiethylamine hydrochloride [55-86-7] $C_5H_{11}Cl_2N \cdot HCl$ (192.52).

Caution—Mechlorethamine Hydrochloride is a vesicant, and the powder or its solution is irritating to the respiratory tract.

History—The medical uses for nitrogen mustards were discovered as a result of chemical warfare research on vesicant agents during World War II. After noting that these agents brought about dissolution of lymphoid tissue, L Goodman, A Gilman, and T Dougherty were prompted to study the effect of nitrogen mustards on transplanted lymphosarcoma in mice. The first clinical trial with these agents was conducted in collaboration with GE Lindskog at Yale University in the fall of 1942.

Preparation—Among other ways, mechlorethamine (base) may be synthesized by reacting methylamine with a double equimolar portion of ethylene oxide to produce *N*-methyldiethanolamine, which is then reacted with thionyl chloride. After purification, the base may then be converted conveniently to the hydrochloride by dissolving it in a suitable organic solvent and passing HCl into the solution.

Description—White, crystalline, hygroscopic powder; melts between 108° and 111°; pH (1:500 aqueous solution) between 3.0 and 5.0.
Solubility—Very soluble in water; soluble in alcohol.

Uses—Mechlorethamine is the prototype of a series of alkylating agents called the nitrogen mustards. The β-chloroethyl groups lose chloride ions to generate carbonium and azaridium (ethylenimonium) ions, which are very reactive and alkylate many biologically important chemical groups. In DNA they alkylate guanine groups; if one "arm" alkylates one guanine moiety and the second arm another guanine on the opposing strand of double-stranded DNA, the DNA becomes irreversibly cross-linked. This inhibits mitosis and may also cause chromosomal breakage. Relatively undifferentiated germinal cells are nonproliferative and hypertrophied during exposure to the drug, but the more differentiated germinal cells disintegrate. Certain neoplastic growths, particularly of the lymph nodes and bone marrow, are somewhat more sensitive to the drug than are the normal more slowly proliferative tissues.

Although mechlorethamine was the drug that ushered in the era of cancer chemotherapy, it has only limited uses today. The combination known as MOPP (mechlorethamine, vincristine, procarbazine, prednisone) is the treatment of choice for *Hodgkin's disease*. It is also a component of a first-choice combination to treat *medulloblastoma*. Mechlorethamine's only other therapeutic status of note is as the drug of second choice in the topical treatment of *mycosis fungoides* and the systemic treatment of *neuroblastoma*. In *polycythemia vera*, remissions of several months to two years have been achieved. All of the above diseases eventually develop resistance to nitrogen mustards. Mechlorethamine is an immunosuppressive drug, but the requirement for intravenous administration and its high toxicity have discouraged its use. In the treatment of *"malignant" rheumatoid arthritis* it effects a good initial response in nearly all patients; maintenance is carried on with cyclophosphamide or other immunosuppressive drugs. It has also been reported to improve the condition of a high percentage of patients with *ulcerative colitis*.

Nausea and vomiting commonly occur within 30 to 180 min after administration, but sedative agents greatly diminish the incidence of such untoward actions originating centrally. Diarrhea also frequently occurs. Bone-marrow depression may result in leukopenia and thrombocytopenia and thus in bleeding tendencies; hyperheparinemia also may rarely lead to hemorrhagic complications. Serious and potentially lethal hematologic responses mainly occur when the total accumulated dose in a course of therapy exceeds 0.4 mg (400 μg)/kg. Skin eruptions are rarely noted, but herpes zoster (shingles) commonly occurs, especially in the treatment of malignant lymphoma. Sometimes temporary menstrual irregularities occur in females. In patients with large tumor masses which rapidly involute with treatment, there may be hyperuricemia, and adequate fluid intake is required to prevent crystalluria and kidney damage. Alopecia, metallic taste, headache, drowsiness, asthenia, tinnitus, and deafness sometimes occur. Mechlorethamine is teratogenic and carcinogenic and should not be used during the first trimester of pregnancy. Severe local reactions to mechlorethamine, as well as rapid chemical breakdown of the drug, require that therapy be limited to the intravenous route; even so, extravasation may cause tender local induration and sloughs, and irritation from within the lumen of the vessel may cause phlebothrombosis or thrombophlebitis, especially if the infusion rate is too rapid or the concentration of solution is too high.

Dose—*Intravenous, adult* and *pediatric*, **0.4 mg** (400 μg)/**kg** per course, as a single dose or divided into 2 doses given on 2 separate days or 4 doses on 4 successive days; after prior radiation or chemotherapy, the dose should be 0.2 mg (200 μg) to 0.3 mg (300 μg)/kg. The single dose is preferable, since it spares the patient the unnecessary repetition of bouts of nausea and vomiting. Patients with normal bone-marrow function can sometimes tolerate up to twice the usual dose, although serious bone-marrow depression will result at the higher doses. Courses may be repeated only when bone-marrow function has recovered, as indicated by the cellular composition of the peripheral blood; the required wait is usually not less than 6 weeks. The drug is best injected (as a 1 mg/mL solution) into intravenous tubing which is rapidly conducting some isotonic fluid; the injection should be made slowly but completed within a few minutes. *Intracavity*, **0.4 mg/kg** in an isotonic solution to which is added a 1 mg/mL solution of the drug; accumulated fluids are removed, and the solution instilled, after which the position of the patient is changed every minute for several minutes, to spread the solution around.

Dosage Form—For Injection: 10 mg.

Medroxyprogesterone Acetate—page 992.

Megestrol Acetate—page 993.

Melphalan

L-Phenylalanine, 4-[bis(2-chloroethyl)amino]-,
Alkeran (*Burroughs-Wellcome*)

L-3-[*p*-[(Bis(2-chloroethyl)amino]phenyl]alanine   [148-82-3] C$_{13}$H$_{18}$Cl$_2$N$_2$O$_2$ (305.20).

Caution—Do not inhale.

Preparation—L-3-Phenylalanine is nitrated and the *p*-nitro compound is reduced to L-3-(*p*-aminophenyl)alanine. This is reacted with ethylene oxide to form the corresponding bis(2-hydroxyethyl)-amino compound which is then treated with phosphoryl chloride to yield melphalan.

Description—Off-white to buff powder having a faint odor; sensitive to light, heat, and moisture; melts at about 180° with decomposition.

Solubility—Practically insoluble in water, chloroform, ether; slightly soluble in alcohol; soluble in dilute mineral acids.

Uses—Melphalan is an alkylating agent of the nitrogen-mustard type. In combination with prednisone either it or cyclophosphamide is the drug of choice for treatment of *multiple myeloma*. Seventy to 80% of patients show subjective improvement and 33 to 50% show objective improvement for periods from 6 months to 2 years, and life expectancy may be increased even when no objective signs of improvement obtain. It is a component of the combination of choice against *ovarian carcinoma*. It is occasionally used in the treatment of *tumors of the testis, osteogenic sarcoma*, and *chronic granulocytic leukemia*.

Melphalan is a primary (afferent) immunosuppressive drug.

Adverse effects include mild nausea and vomiting after large doses, bone-marrow depression with anemia, neutropenia, thrombocytopenia, and occasional azotemia. Aphthous ulceration, gastrointestinal hemorrhage, skin eruptions, and bronchopulmonary dyplasia also occur occasionally. Regular blood-cell counts are required. Melphalan should be given cautiously if the patient has been receiving radiation or other cancer chemotherapy. It is contraindicated in thrombocytopenia, anemia, leukopenia, and during the first trimester of pregnancy. In the presence of impaired renal function the drug should be used cautiously.

Melphalan is well absorbed by the oral route, being as efficacious as by the intravenous route. It is transformed into metabolites in probably all tissues. The elimination half-life is about 1 to 3 hr.

Dose—*Daily schedule, initially* **0.1** to **0.15 mg/kg/day** for one week followed by a rest until the leukocyte count begins to rise again (2 to 6 weeks); *maintenance*, **0.05 mg/kg/day**, to be subsequently adjusted to 1 to 3 mg per day, according to hematologic toxicity. *Intermittent schedule, initially* **0.25 mg** (250 μg)/**kg/day** for 4 days; every 6 weeks the course is repeated, except that the dose is adjusted according to the leukocyte and platelet count; it is desired to keep the leukocyte count slightly below 3500 cells/mm^3 and the platelet count below 100,000/mm^3. Various other regimens can be found in the package literature and *Drug Facts and Comparisons*.

Dosage Form—Tablets: 2 mg.

Mercaptopurine

6*H*-Purine-6-thione, 1,7-dihydro-, monohydrate; 6 MP;
Purinethol (*Burroughs-Wellcome*)

Purine-6-thiol monohydrate (tautomer) [6112-76-1] C$_5$H$_4$N$_4$S.H$_2$O (170.19); *anhydrous* [50-44-2] (152.17).

Preparation—Thiourea and ethyl cyanoacetate are reacted in the presence of sodium methylate to give 2-thiol-4-amino-6-hydroxy-pyrimidine (I) which is then converted to the 5-nitroso derivative (II) by treating with sodium nitrite and acetic acid. Reduction of II with sodium hydrosulfite yields the corresponding diamino compound (III) which is then desulfurized by hydrogenolysis in the presence of Raney nickel to yield 4,5-diamino-6-hydroxypyrimidine (IV). The imidazole ring closure is then effected by double condensation of IV with formic acid (V), and the resulting hypoxanthine is thiolated with P$_2$S$_5$.

Description—Yellow, crystalline powder which is odorless or practically odorless; melts with decomposition above 308°.

Solubility—Insoluble in water, acetone, and ether; soluble in hot alcohol and dilute aqueous alkali; slightly soluble in diluted H$_2$SO$_4$.

Uses—Mercaptopurine is an antimetabolite precursor that is converted to 6-thioinosinic acid, which acts as an antimetabolite to inhibit synthesis of adenine and guanine and also to prevent conversion of purine bases into nucleotides. It also mimics inosinic acid in exerting a negative feedback suppression of the synthesis of inosinic acid. Some mercaptopurine is also converted to thioguanine, which is incorporated into DNA and RNA to generate defective nucleic acids. Thus nucleic acid synthesis and functions are impaired several ways. Cell mitosis is inhibited.

Mercaptopurine in combination with methotrexate provides a combination of first choice in the *maintenance chemotherapy of acute lymphocytic leukemia*. It is one of several drugs of third-choice for the treatment of stable *chronic granulocytic leukemia;* the remission rate is about 80% if the disease is caught early, but cures are not achieved. Induction is sometimes accomplished with busulfan and maintenance with mercaptopurine. There is no cross-resistance between mercaptopurine and non-purine antineoplastic drugs.

Mercaptopurine is mostly a secondary (efferent) *immunosuppressive* drug that is capable of eliciting a high percentage of favorable responses in *ulcerative colitis* and *psoriatic arthritis*. It is also moderately effective in the treatment of *systemic lupus erythematosus, dermatomyositis*, and *polymyositis*. However, it will probably not become the drug of choice for any of these disorders. Immunosuppression predisposes to intercurrent infections.

Bone-marrow depression occurs during treatment. Leukopenia and thrombocytopenia (with hemorrhage) are common and may be severe, but anemia is rare. Frequent monitoring of the blood-cell population is mandatory. Nausea, vomiting, and anorexia may occur; they signal onset of gastrointestinal toxicity, which may take the form of mucositis and ulceration. Oral, pharyngeal, and esophageal mucositis may also occur, with thrush-like stomatitis or aphthous ulceration. Diarrhea and sprue-like symptoms occasionally occur. There may also be jaundice in 10 to 40% of patients with acute leukemia. In patients with high white-cell counts or massive disease, cellular destruction leads to hyperuricemia and sometimes to tubular clogging with urate crystals and consequent oliguria, thus necessitating use of allopurinol.

Only about 50% of mercaptopurine is orally absorbed. It is mainly inactivated by xanthine oxidase, an enzyme that is inhibited by allopurinol, so that a drug interaction may occur. The elimination half-life of mercaptopurine is slightly less than 1 hr in adults and about $\frac{1}{2}$ hour in children.

Dose—*Oral, adult* or *pediatric, initially*, **2.5 mg per kg** of body weight or **70 mg** per **m²** of body surface per day in single or divided doses, to be continued for 4 weeks. At this time the effect of treatment is evaluated and the maintenance dose determined accordingly; the usual *maintenance* dose is **1.5 to 2.5 mg/kg/day.** If serious toxic effects occur, the drug should be withheld until signs of toxicity disappear, after which the dose is continued at one-half the previous dose. In the treatment of ulcerative colitis, 1.5 mg/kg/day is often used. In the presence of allopurinol, the dose should be reduced to $\frac{1}{4}$ to $\frac{1}{3}$ of the usual dose.

Dosage Form—Tablets: 50 mg.

Methotrexate

L-Glutamic acid, *N*-[4-[[(2,4-diamino-6-pteridinyl)methyl]methylamino]benzoyl]-, Amethopterin; (*Lederle*)

4-Amino-10-methylfolic Acid; [59-05-2]; a mixture of 4-amino-10-methylfolic acid and closely related compounds and contains not less than 85.0% of $C_{20}H_{22}N_8O_5$ (454.44).

Caution—Methotrexate is extremely poisonous.

Preparation—2,3-Dibromopropionaldehyde (I) is condensed in an aqueous medium with 2,4,5,6-tetraminopyrimidine (II). The condensation is multiple, consisting of: (*a*) dehydrobromination, involving a hydrogen of the 5-amino group and the 2-bromine; (*b*) dehydration, involving two hydrogens of the 6-amino group and the oxygen in II; and (*c*) dehydrogenation, involving the remaining hydrogen of the 5-amino group and the 2-hydrogen of II. The dehydrogenation in step *c* is brought about by another molecule of II which, by effecting the dehydrogenation, is reduced to 2,3-dibromo-1-propanol. The overall effect of these condensations is the cyclization of I with II to produce 6-bromomethyl-2,4-diaminopteridine (III). Further condensation (dehydrobromination involving the bromine in III and the hydrogen of the methylamino group in *N*-[*p*-(methylamino)benzoyl]glutamic acid) yields crude methotrexate, which is purified.

Description—Orange-brown, crystalline powder.

Solubility—Practically insoluble in water, alcohol, chloroform, ether; freely soluble in dilute solutions of alkali hydroxides and carbonates; slightly soluble in dilute hydrochloric acid.

Uses—Methotrexate inhibits dihydrofolate reductase, and it thus prevents conversion of deoxyuridylate to thymidylate and blocks the synthesis of new DNA needed for cellular replication. It is the drug of choice for treatment of trophoblastic tumors, such as *choriocarcinoma, hydatidiform mole*, and *chorioadenoma destruens*, in which cases the rate of response is about 80% and survival is greatly prolonged. It is also the drug of choice for *CNS prophylaxis* in *acute lymphocytic leukemia*. In combination with other drugs it provides the therapy of choice for induction and maintenance in *acute lymphocytic leukemia*. It is also included in first-choice combinations for treatment of *cervical cancer, medulloblastoma, osteogenic sarcoma*, and *breast cancer*. It is included in second-choice combinations for the treatment of *non-Hodgkin's lymphomas, oat-cell* and *non-small cell lung cancers, soft tissue sarcomas*, and *embryonal rhabdomyosarcoma*. It is a component of a second-choice combination for *Burkitt's lymphoma*. It is a drug of third choice against *mycosis fungoides*.

Methotrexate may be given by intra-arterial infusion into the affected region in the treatment of a variety of carcinomata of the head, neck, pelvis, and limbs; the local concentrations achieved may be high enough to be effective and yet low enough in the rest of the body not to be toxic. Folinic acid (leucovorin) is also often given systemically to prevent generalized toxicity.

Methotrexate is a secondary (efferent) immunosuppressive drug. It is one of a few drugs used to treat *Reiter's syndrome*, although results range from poor to good. It is employed to treat *psoriasis* refractory to other drugs; with methotrexate about 50% of affected joints and 65% of skin lesions improve. Methotrexate has provided improvement in *dermatomyositis* and *polymyositis* (40 to 100% improvement), *Wegner's granulomatosis, pemphigus vulgaris, pityriasis rubra pilaris, bullous pemphigoid*, and *thrombocytopenic purpura*, but other drugs appear to be equal or superior.

The toxic effects of methotrexate are extensions of its antimetabolite effects; sometimes toxicity occurs first. They include bone-marrow hypoplasia with leukopenia, thrombocytopenia (with hemorrhage), and anemia. Depression of cellular proliferation along the gastrointestinal tract results in diarrhea, ulcerative stomatitis, hemorrhagic enteritis, and perforation. Alopecia may also occur. Dosage schedules in which methotrexate is chronically given daily may cause liver damage. The drug must not be used when there is preexisting liver damage or bone-marrow depression, or in the first trimester of pregnancy. Daily blood counts and triweekly creatinine determinations are mandatory. The toxicity and therapeutic effects may be antagonized by leucovorin (leucovorin "rescue"); if the leucovorin is given after an appropriate delay, it can prevent the toxic but not the therapeutic effect on certain tumors or the immune system.

In doses below 30 mg/m² of body surface, methotrexate is well absorbed by the oral route, but about $\frac{1}{3}$ of an oral dose is metabolized by intestinal bacteria, and antibiotics affect the amount absorbed. In doses above 80 mg/m², the amount absorbed is further reduced by 30 to 50%. Only about 50% of the drug is bound to plasma protein, but it does not gain much access to the cerebrospinal fluid because it is strongly ionized; consequently, it must be administered intrathecally for use in the CNS. In the usual doses, it appears to be actively transported into other tissues. Plasma clearance is triexponential, with a distribution half-life of about 45 min, a second phase of about 3.5 hr (possibly an enterohepatic component, since 10% of the drug is secreted into bile), and an elimination half-life of 6 to 69 hr. Renal tubular secretion accounts for about 80% of elimination, and probenecid, salicylate, etc, interfere with excretion. The dose must be adjusted in renal failure.

Dose—Methotrexate is administered by the oral, intravenous, and intramuscular routes. Not only are there substantially different regimens for different uses but also for the same use. The reader is referred to the package literature, *Drug Facts and Comparisons*, *USP Dispensing Information*, and *AMA Drug Evaluations*, ed 5.

Dosage Forms—Tablets: 2.5 mg; Methotrexate Sodium Injection: 2.5 mg/mL and 25 mg/mL (methotrexate equivalent) in 2-mL vials. Methotrexate Sodium Powder for Injection: 20, 50 and 100 mg.

Mitotane

Benzene, 1-chloro-2-[2,2-dichloro-1-(4-chlorophenyl)ethyl]-, *o,p'*-DDD; Lysodren (*Calbiochem*)

1,1-Dichloro-2-(*o*-chlorophenyl)-2-(*p*-chlorophenyl)ethane [53-19-0] $C_{14}H_{10}Cl_4$ (320.05).

Preparation—Chlorobenzene is condensed with 2,2-dichloro-1-(*o*-chlorophenyl)ethanol with the aid of H_2SO_4.

Description—White, tasteless, crystalline powder having a slight, aromatic odor; stable in light, air, and heat; melts between 75° and 81°.

Solubility—Practically insoluble in water; soluble in alcohol, ether, solvent hexane, and fixed oils and fats.

Uses—Since it is toxic to the adrenal cortex, it is used in the treatment of *inoperable adrenal cortical carcinoma*. Nearly 50% of patients will respond to treatment. Adverse effects include anorexia, nausea, vomiting (in 80%), diarrhea, lethargy, somnolence (25%), dizziness (15%), headache, confusion, asthenia, tremors, ataxia, speech difficulties, neuropathies, dermatitis (15%), hypersensitivity, flushing, hyperpyrexia, postural hypotension, alopecia, pigmentation, leukopenia, thrombocytopenia, hyperbilirubinemia, albuminuria, hemorrhagic cystitis, elevated serum transaminase, blurred vision, diplopia, lens opacities, and retinopathy. The drug should be used with caution in the presence of liver damage, bone-marrow depression, dermatitis, or neuropathy.

Dose—*Oral, adults,* 2 to **16 g** daily; *usual initial,* **9** to **10 g** a day in 3 or 4 divided doses, gradually increased until clinical improvement or serious adverse effects occur; *maintenance,* **0.5** to **20 g** (usually 2 to 10 g)/day for as long as 2 years. Discontinue after 3 months if no improvement has taken place.

Dosage Form—Tablets: 500 mg.

Penicillamine—page 1225.

Podophyllum—page 783.

Polyestradiol Phosphate—987.

Prednisolone Sodium Succinate—RPS-16, p 910.

Prednisone—page 970.

Procarbazine Hydrochloride

Benzamide, *N*-(1-methylethyl)-4-[(2-methylhydrazino)methyl]-, monohydrochloride; Matulane (*Roche*)

N-Isopropyl-α-(2-methylhydrazino)-*p*-toluamide monohydrochloride [366-70-1] $C_{12}H_{19}N_3O\cdot HCl$ (257.76).

Preparation—1,2-Bis(carbobenzoxy)-1-methylhydrazine is reacted with 4-(bromoethyl)benzoic acid methyl ester ultimately to yield 4-[[2-methyl-1,2-di(carbobenzoxy)hydrazino]methyl]benzoic acid. Thionyl chloride is used to obtain the acid chloride which is reacted with isopropylamine to give the *N*-isopropylamide compound. Treatment with 33% HBr in glacial acetic acid removes the protecting carbobenzoxy groups and the resulting procarbazine hydrobromide may be converted to the hydrochloride by the usual process. US Pat 3,520,926.

Description—White to pale yellow, crystalline powder having a slight odor and a bitter taste; solutions are acid to litmus; stable in light, slowly oxidized in air, and stable at room temperature (in the presence of oxygen, oxidation is accelerated by increased temperature); melts at about 223° with decomposition; pK_a at room temperature 6.8.

Solubility—1 g in 7 mL water, 100 mL alcohol; slightly soluble in chloroform; insoluble in ether.

Uses—Auto-oxidation of procarbazine generates hydrogen peroxide and hydroxyl radicals, the latter being thought to cause the observable degradation of DNA and chromosomal breaks; DNA synthesis, and hence protein synthesis, is impaired. The most important use of procarbazine is as a component of MOPP (mechlorethamine, vincristine, procarbazine, prednisone), the chemotherapy of choice for *Hodgkin's disease*. It is also a component of a first-choice combination of *non-Hodgkin's lymphomas* and of a second-choice combination for *medulloblastoma*. It is among third-choice agents to treat *primary brain neoplasms* and *oat-cell bronchogenic carcinoma*. Cross-resistance with other agents or radiation apparently does not occur.

Untoward reactions include frequent leukopenia, thrombocytopenia, anemia, less frequent nausea, vomiting, and, rarely, anorexia, dry mouth, stomatitis, dysphagia, diarrhea, constipation, myalgia and arthralgia, chills and fever, sweating, fatigue, asthenia, lethargy, and drowsiness. Ascites, edema, effusions, cough, intercurrent infections, epistaxis, hemorrhaging, melena, pruritus, allergic dermatitis, allergic pneumonitis, flushing, alopecia, pigmentation, herpes, jaundice, headache, vertigo, depression, paresthesias, neuropathies, insomnia, nightmares, ataxia, confusion, coma, tremors, and convulsions may occur. Rarely there may be hoarseness, hypotension, tachycardia, syncope, hemolysis, nystagmus, photophobia, photosensitivity, retinal hemorrhage, diplopia, papilledema, impaired hearing, and slurred speech. Procarbazine is mutagenic, and is teratogenic and carcinogenic in experimental animals. Thus, procarbazine must be regarded as a dangerous drug.

Central nervous system depressants should not be given at the same time except under supervision. Since procarbazine is a monoamine oxidase inhibitor, tricyclic antidepressants, various sympathomimetics, and tyramine-containing foods should be avoided. Since procarbazine has disulfiram-like activity, patients should be warned against ingestion of alcoholic beverages. Caution must be exercised in the presence of liver damage, respiratory disorders, renal impairment, or bone-marrow depression.

Procarbazine is almost completely absorbed by the oral route. It penetrates readily into the cerebrospinal fluid. It is rapidly metabolized and auto-oxidized, with an elimination half-life of only about 7 min. Almost none is excreted unchanged.

Dose—*Adult, oral, initially,* **2** to **4 mg/kg/day** of procarbazine equivalent, in divided doses if desired, for one week, then **4** to **6 mg/kg/day** until the leukocyte count falls below 4000/mm³ or the platelet count falls below 100,000/mm³ or a remission occurs. If hematological toxicity occurs, treatment is suspended until the blood picture is normal, then resumed at **1** to **2 mg/kg/day**. Once remission has occurred, the dose is maintained at **1** to **2 mg/kg/day**. The *pediatric* dose is **50 mg** once a day for one week, then **100 mg/m²/day** until the response reaches its maximum, and **50 mg** once a day thereafter.

Dosage Form—Capsules containing the equivalent of 50 mg of procarbazine.

Sodium Iodide I 131—page 495.

Sodium Phosphate P 32—page 496.

Tamoxifen—page 990.

Testolactone—page 1000.

Testosterone Propionate—page 1001.

Thioguanine

H-Purine-6-thione, 2-amino-1,7-dihydro-, Tabloid (*Burroughs-Wellcome*)

2-Aminopurine-6(1*H*)-thione [154-42-7] $C_5H_5N_5S$ (167.19); *hemihydrate* [50322-14-0] (176.20).

Preparation—By thionation of guanine with phosphorus pentasulfide. US Pat 2,884,667.

Description—Pale yellow, crystalline powder; odorless or practically odorless.

Solubility—Insoluble in water, alcohol, chloroform; freely soluble in dilute solutions of alkali hydroxides.

Uses—Thioguanine is an antimetabolite of guanine which is converted into 6-thioguanine-ribose-phosphate; this not only is incorporated into DNA and RNA but also interferes with guanine synthesis. It acts mainly in the S-phase of the cell cycle, but cell replication is ultimately prevented. Although its actions are very similar to those of mercaptopurine, some of which is converted to thioguanine, and cross-resistance occurs between the two drugs, the actions and uses are not identical. With other drugs, thioguanine is a component of combinations that are treatments of choice for *acute myelocytic leukemias* and the *acute* phase of *chronic granulocytic leukemia*. It is a second-choice drug for use against *acute lymphocytic leukemia*. It is sometimes used in the stable phase of *chronic myelocytic leu-*

kemia. It is also a potent *immunosuppressive drug*, but its status has yet to be settled. It has especially been used in the treatment of *nephrosis* and *collagen-vascular disorders*.

The adverse effects of thioguanine are virtually the same as those for mercaptopurine (see page 1151), except that the incidence of gastrointestinal toxicity is less and there is no adverse interaction with allopurinol.

Thioguanine is nearly completely metabolized in the body; the 6-thiol group is methylated and the 8-amino group removed to yield 6-methylmercaptopurine. Xanthine oxidase is not involved.

Dose—*Oral, adult* and *pediatric, initially* **2 mg/kg/day** (to the nearest 20 mg) or **100 mg/m²** of body surface/day for 4 weeks, after which the dose may be cautiously advanced to as much as **3 mg/ kg/day** if the response has been inadequate; if response is still inadequate, treatment is stopped and another drug tried. In combination with daunorubicin and vincristine for induction of remission of *acute myelocytic leukemia*, **100 mg/m²** of body surface twice a day for 7 days, to be repeated every 28 days.

Dosage Form—Tablets: 40 mg.

Vinblastine Sulfate

Vincaleukoblastine, sulfate (1:1) (salt); Velban (*Lilly*)

(*R* is CH₃)

[143-67-9] C₄₆H₅₈N₄O₉·H₂SO₄ (909.06).

Preparation—By extracting the leaves, bark, or stems of *Vinca rosea* with aqueous or aqueous–alcoholic sulfuric acid, isolating the alkaloid from the extract by the usual precipitation and solvent techniques, and purifying by chromatography on aluminum oxide. Conversion to the (1:1) sulfate may be effected by dissolving the alkaloid in an equimolar quantity of dilute H₂SO₄ and either evaporating to dryness or precipitating with a suitable organic solvent. US Pat 3,097,137.

Description—White to slightly yellow, amorphous or crystalline powder; odorless; hygroscopic.

Solubility—Freely soluble in water.

Uses—Vinblastine interferes with the assembly of the microtubules, supposedly by combining with tubulin; the result is mitotic arrest in metaphase. However, there is evidence that vinblastine exerts its antineoplastic effect by interfering with glutamate and aspartate metabolism. The antineoplastic spectrum and toxicity are much different than for vincristine, which also interacts with tubulin. Vinblastine is a component of a three-drug combination that is the treatment of choice for *testicular carcinoma*. It is a component of combinations that provide second-choice treatment for *Hodgkin's disease*, *choriocarcinoma*, *squamous cell carcinoma* of the head and neck, and *renal-cell carcinoma*. It is among the third-choice drugs for *neuroblastoma*, *breast tumors*, and neck, and *mycosis fungoides*. It has also been used to treat lymphosarcoma, lymphocytic lymphoma, Kaposi's sarcoma reticulum-cell sarcoma, and Letterer-Siwe's disease. There is no cross-resistance between vinblastine and other classes of antineoplastics.

Vinblastine is a secondary (efferent) immunosuppressive drug, but it has not been exploited for this purpose.

Nausea, vomiting, headache, and paresthesias occur within 4 to 6 hr and last from 2 to 10 hr. Diarrhea, constipation, adynamic ileus, anorexia, and stomatitis also may occur and are premonitory of neurotoxic effects, such as severe headache, malaise, mental depression, paresthesias, and loss of deep tendon reflexes. Neurotoxicity occurs in 5 to 20% of cases, depending on the dose. Central nervous system damage is occasionally permanent when excessive doses have been used. Blindness and death have been reported. Alopecia occurs in about 30 to 60% of users, but it is generally reversible. Mild bone-marrow depression with leukopenia occurs in a high percentage

of patients and may require discontinuation of the drug. The thrombocytes are less affected, unless other thrombocytogenic drugs are also being given or have recently been given. Anemia is rare. The blood cell count must be determined each week. The drug is locally toxic, and extravasation should be avoided. It may cause phlebitis at the site of injection. Inappropriate secretion of ADH may occur. It is teratogenic in animals, and it probably should not be used during the first trimester of pregnancy.

Dose—*Adult, intravenous, initially* **0.1 mg** (100 µg)/**kg**; 7 days later and each week thereafter the dose is increased by 0.05 mg (50 µg)/kg until the leukocyte count falls to 3000 cells/mm³, the tumor regresses, or a maximal dose of 0.5 mg (500 µg)/kg is reached (usually 0.15–0.2 mg/kg). Thereafter the dose is *maintained* at a level one increment smaller than the last dose, given at intervals of 1 to 2 weeks. Some authorities use a maintenance dose of 10 mg once or twice a month. *Pediatric, intravenous,* **0.1** to **0.2 mg** (100 to 200 µg)/**kg** or **3** to **6 mg/m²** once a week. For adult and pediatric doses based on body surface, see the USPDI.

Dosage Form—Sterile: 10 mg.

Vincristine Sulfate

Vincaleukoblastine, 22-oxo-, sulfate (1:1) (salt); Oncovin (*Lilly*)

Leurocristine sulfate (1:1) (salt) [2068-78-2] C₄₆H₅₆N₄O₁₀·H₂SO₄ (923.04).

The structure is the same as for *vinblastine sulfate*, except that *R* is CHO, an aldehyde.

Preparation—Using suitable modifications in the chromatographic part of the process, vincristine sulfate may be prepared as described above for *Vinblastine Sulfate*. US Pat 3,205,220.

Description—White to slightly yellow, amorphous or crystalline powder; odorless; hygroscopic.

Solubility—Freely soluble in water.

Uses—Vincristine combines with the protein tubulin and prevents assembly of microtubules, thus disrupting various cellular processes, including spindle-formation and mitosis. Synthesis of RNA and proteins is also suppressed. The alkaloid is the most widely used of the antineoplastic drugs. It is especially useful in the treatment of hematological malignancies. In combination with other drugs it is the preferred treatment for inducing *remission* in *acute lymphocytic leukemia*. It is a component of a combination of choice for *acute myelogenous leukemias*, alone or as a component of MOPP (mechlorethamine, vincristine, procarbazine, prednisone; the O is for Oncovin, the tradename of vincristine), the first-choice treatment for *Hodgkin's disease*, and it is also a component of the second-choice combination. It is included in several first-choice combinations for *non-Hodgkin's lymphomas*. It is also a component of first-choice combinations for *oat-cell bronchogenic carcinoma*, *Wilms' tumor chronic myelocytic leukemia* (acute phase) *medulloblastoma*, *oat-cell lung carcinoma*, *soft tissue sarcomas*, *Ewing's sarcoma*, and *embryonal rhabdomyosarcoma*. Vincristine-containing combinations are second-choice treatments for *breast carcinoma neuroblastoma* and *chronic lymphocytic leukemia*. Vincristine is also sometimes employed in the treatment of breast cancer, multiple myeloma, cervical cancer and primary brain tumors. Some authorities prefer to use vincristine only to induce remissions and not for maintenance, because chronic use favors neurotoxicity. Cross-resistance to other drugs does not occur, not even to vinblastine.

Vincristine differs from most other antineoplastics in that bone-marrow depression does not frequently occur; this is one reason why vincristine is used in combinations. However, leukopenia does occur, and white-cell counts should be made before each dose. Treatment is usually limited by the neurotoxic effects. Adverse effects usually begin with nausea, vomiting, constipation, abdominal cramps, and weight loss; these effects are readily reversible. The drug may also cause slowly reversible reactions, such as alopecia and peripheral neuropathy. Serious neuropathic effects may occur; they include loss of deep tendon reflexes, neuritic pain, numbness of extremities, headache, ataxia, and visual defects; paresis or paralysis and atrophy of certain extensor muscles may occur late; paralysis of cranial nerves 2, 3, 6, and 7 may occur. Neuropathies may persist for several months. Severe hypertension, agitation, or mental depression also may transiently occur. The drug is locally toxic, and extravasation should be avoided. It is best given into the tubing for a running intravenous solution.

Vincristine is rapidly cleared from the blood. It manifests 3-compartment kinetics, with half-lives of 0.08, 2.3 and 85 hr. Seventy percent is secreted into the bile. In obstructive jaundice the toxicity is greater, and the dose should be reduced. About 12% is excreted in urine. It does not penetrate into the brain, hence it cannot be used for CNS leukemias.

Dose—*Intravenous, for acute lymphatic leukemia in children under 12 years of age,* initially **1.5 mg/m²** (approximately 0.03 to 0.075 mg/kg for a 10-year-old and 0.05 to 0.15 mg/kg for a 1-year-old) as a single dose the first week, followed by weekly increments of 0.025 mg/kg up to a maximum dose of 2 mg/m² (0.15 mg/kg), thereafter, for *maintenance; in patients 12 to 20 years of age,* **1.5 to 4.5 mg/m²** once a week, along with prednisone (40 mg/m² orally once a day) until a remission occurs, with other drugs used for *maintenance; adults,* **1.4 mg/m²** (0.025 to 0.075 mg/kg) once a week with adjustments in dosage as necessitated by toxic effects and therapeutic response. When vincristine is used in combination with drugs other than prednisone, the recommended dose is 1 to 1.5 mg/m².

Dosage Forms—For Injection: 1 and 5 mg.

Other Antineoplastic and Immunosuppressive Drugs

Amsacrine [*N*-[4-(9-Acridinylamino)-3-methoxyphenyl]methanesulfonamide; [51264-14-3] $C_{21}H_{19}N_3O_3S$ (393.46)]—Prepared from 2′-methoxy-4′-nitrobutyranilide. The nitro group is reduced to the amine, converted to the methanesulfonamide, deacylated and the resulting free amino group reacted with 9-acridinyl chloride to yield the product. US Pat Appl 25,157; *CA* 95:97615b (1981). *Uses:* Amsacrine intercalates into DNA and inhibits DNA synthesis. Phases S and G_2 of the cell cycle are the most sensitive. It is currently the primary drug for the treatment of *acute myelocytic leukemia* of adults, which disease has become refractory to standard regimens; complete remissions are achieved in 10 to 20% of such patients. It is also effective in refractory *non-Hodgkin's lymphomas.* Immediate toxicity includes nausea, vomiting, local irritation at the injection site, acute cardiotoxicity, and occasional convulsions. Delayed toxicity includes leukopenia in almost all recipients, mucositis, and delayed cardiotoxicity. The drug is not absorbed effectively by the oral route. It is metabolized in the liver and secreted into the bile. The elimination half-life is 2 to 3 hr. *Dose: Intravenous,* for induction of remission in acute myelocytic leukemia, 75 mg/m² a day for a week, to be repeated every 4 weeks.

5-Azacytidine [4-Amino-1-ribofuranosyl-1,3,5-triazin-2(1*H*)-one; $C_8H_{12}N_4O_5$ (244.20)]—A ring analogue of cytidine, obtained by synthesis or produced microbiologically. *Uses:* 5-Azacytidine is an antimetabolite used investigationally to treat refractory *acute myelogenous leukemias* and the *acute phase of chronic myelogenous leukemias.* Acutely it causes nausea, vomiting, diarrhea, and fever. Delayed toxicity includes prolonged leukopenia, thrombocytopenia, and hepatotoxicity, not dose-related. The mortality rate has been reported to be about 6%. *Dose: Intravenous,* 50 to 400 mg/m²/day for 5 days, repeated at intervals of 2 to 3 weeks, the length of the interval being determined by the time required for the white blood cell count to pass its nadir, or 150 to 200 mg/m² twice weekly for 2 to 8 weeks, or 200 to 633 mg/m² per week. The least amount of nausea and vomiting occurs when the drug is given by continuous infusion over the entire 5-day period, but if each daily dose is infused over 18 hr, the acute toxicity is negligibly increased. If the daily dose is given in 15 to 30 min, the acute toxicity is greatly enhanced and will result in a substantial proportion of patients refusing treatment.

Etoposide [9-[(4,6-*O*-Ethylidene-β-D-glucopyranosyl)oxy]-5,8,-8a,9-tetrahydro-5-(4-hydroxy-3,5-dimethoxyphenyl)furo[3′,4′:6,7]-naphtho[2,3-*d*]-1,3-dioxol-6(5a*H*)-one; [33419-42-0] $C_{29}H_{32}O_{13}$ (588.56) Vepesid (*Bristol*)]—A semisynthetic derivative of podophyllotoxin. A white to yellow-brown powder melting about 221°. It is poorly soluble in water but soluble in organic solvents. *Uses:* Etoposide and teniposide arrest the cell cycle in late S and G_2 phases. Etoposide effects remissions in about 40% of patients with *oat-cell carcinoma* of the lung. It is currently the drug of third choice in *testicular cancer,* behind two standard combinations, and is active against *choriocarcinoma.* Both etoposide and teniposide are active against acute *lymphocytic leukemia, acute myelocytic leukemia, Hodgkin's disease,* and *non-Hodgkin's lymphomas.* Acute toxicity includes nausea, vomiting, chills and fever. Intravenous etoposide may cause hypotension, tachycardia, and palpitations. Late toxicity includes myelosuppression (mostly leukopenia, with a nadir between 8 and 14 days), alopecia, fever, and peripheral neuropathy. The oral bioavailability is about 50%. Approximately 94% is bound to plasma proteins, and cerebrospinal fluid levels are correspondingly low (less than 10% of those in plasma). Only about 30% is excreted unchanged. The distribution half-life is 3 hr and the elimination half-life 15 hr. *Dose: Oral,* 100 mg/m² a day for 5 days; *intravenously* (slowly), 50 to 75 mg/m² a day for 5 days.

Estramustine Phosphate Sodium [Estradiol 3-bis(2-chloroethyl)-carbamate 17-hydrogen phosphate; $C_{23}H_{30}Cl_2NNa_2O_6P$ (564.35) Emcyt (*Roche*)]—A compound of estradiol with a nitrogen mustard moiety. *Uses:* Estramustine is an alkylating agent that is among several drugs of second choice for treatment of *cancer of the prostate* gland. It causes nausea and vomiting, delayed bone-marrow depression, mild gynecomastia, perianal anesthesia, thrombophlebitis, occasional myocardial infarction, hypertension, hypoglycemia and hepatotoxicity. It is carcinogenic in animals. *Dose: Oral, 600 mg/m²/day* (10–16 mg/kg/day) in 3 divided doses; treatment has been continued for as long as 3 years. In combinations, the dose may be the same, but when combined with other bone-marrow depressant drugs it may have to be reduced.

Floxuridine [Uridine, 2′-deoxy-5-fluoro-, FUDR (*Roche*) [50-91-9] $C_9H_{11}FN_2O_5$ (246.19)]. *Description and Solubility:* White to off-white, odorless solid; melts between 149° and 153°. Soluble 1 g in 3 mL water, 12 mL alcohol, >10,000 mL chloroform, >10,000 mL ether. *Uses:* In the body it is converted into a false nucleotide which interferes with the synthesis of DNA. It is also converted to fluorouracil, so that it potentially has all the actions and uses of *Fluorouracil* (page 1149). However, at present its use is restricted to regional intra-arterial infusion of carcinomata which are judged incurable by surgery or other chemotherapy, mainly colorectal cancer and *adenocarcinoma metastatic to the liver.* In these uses, it does not appear to be superior to fluorouracil. The most frequent adverse effects are nausea, vomiting, diarrhea, enteritis, localized erythema along the course of infused artery, leukopenia, and elevation in serum transaminase, alkaline phosphatase, bilirubin, and lactic dehydrogenase. Other effects are abdominal cramps, anorexia, duodenal ulcer, duodenitis, gastroenteritis, pharyngitis, glossitis, gastritis, alopecia, dermititis, hyperpigmentation, edema, peeling of the skin, pruritus, various rashes and skin ulceration, abscesses, ataxia, blurred vision, convulsions, depression, hemiplegia, hiccoughs, lethargy, nystagmus, malaise, pain, vertigo, asthenia, dysuria, fever, hypoadrenalism, thrombocytopenia, prothrombinopenia, hypoproteinemia, and aberrations in the sedimentation rate and BSP test. Floxuridine is contraindicated in patients with cachexia, potentially serious infections, or bone-marrow depression. The drug is mainly metabolized in the body, but some is excreted unchanged in the urine. *Dose: Continuous arterial infusion,* 0.1 to 0.6 mg (100 to 600 µg)/kg/day. The higher end of the dose range (0.4 to 0.6 mg/kg/day) is reserved for hepatic artery infusion, since the liver metabolizes the drug and so decreases systemic toxicity.

Hexamethylmelamine [2,4,6-Tris(dimethylamino)-1,3,5-triazine; $C_9H_{18}N_6$ (210.28)]—*Uses:* An investigational alkylating agent related to triethylenemelamine, an early alkylating agent. Hexamethylmelamine is one of several secondary drugs for treatment of *ovarian tumors.* It has also proven useful in the treatment of both *Hodgkin's* and *non-Hodgkin's lymphomas, oat-cell bronchogenic carcinoma,* and *breast tumor.* Nausea and vomiting are the main acute adverse effects. Delayed toxicity includes bone-marrow depression, CNS depression, peripheral neuritis, ataxia, hallucinations, psychoses, pruritus, and dermatitis. *Dose: Oral, 100 mg* a day for 14 days, repeated at 4-week intervals.

Hydroxyurea [$H_2NCONHOH$ (76.06); Hydrea (*Squibb*)]—A white powder prepared by interaction of hydroxylamine hydrochloride and potassium cyanide; odorless and essentially tasteless; melts at about 135°; freely soluble in water. *Uses:* Inhibits synthesis of DNA but not of RNA. It is lethal to cells in the S-phase and also holds cells in the G_1-phase, in which they are more sensitive to irradiation. Hydroxyurea is not the drug of first choice for any neoplasia; it is the drug of second choice only for *chronic agranulocytic leukemia.* Even as a back-up drug for busulfan in chronic granulocytic leukemia, its value may be limited by cross-resistance to busulfan. It is sometimes combined with radiation to treat squamous cell carcinoma of the head and neck, or used alone to treat inoperable ovarian carcinoma, in which it has erratic palliative actions; superior chemotherapy is retiring it from such uses. As an *immunosuppressant,* it may be used in the treatment of *psoriasis.* It appears to improve the condition of the patient in a high percentage of cases, but the quality of the response may not be as good as with some other drugs. Thus it has an unsettled status. Its most serious side effect is bone-marrow depression, in which the neutrophils are most affected; the leukocyte count drops about 50% in 2 to 4 days but recovers within a week. Thrombocytopenia and anemia are uncommon. Megaloblastosis may occur. Aphthous ulceration, nausea, vomiting, diarrhea, headache, vertigo, disorientation, hallucinations, convulsions, minor rashes, and pruritus also may occur. Elevated BUN and hyperuricemia and urate nephrolithiasis have been reported. Hydroxyurea is mainly eliminated by renal excretion. The drug is contraindicated in renal failure and when there is prior bone-marrow depression. The blood-cell population, and kidney and liver functions must be monitored weekly. *Dose: Oral,* for *chronic granulocytic leukemia* or *continuous therapy of solid tumors,* 20 to 30 mg/kg/day and for *intermittent therapy* of solid tumors or *combined with radiation* therapy for carcinoma of the head and neck, 80 mg/kg every third day.

Ifosfamide [3-(2-Chloroethyl)-2-(2-chloroethylamino)perhydro-2*H*-1,3,2-oxazaphosphorine 2-oxide; $C_7H_{15}Cl_2N_2O_2P$ (261.09)]—*Uses:* An investigational alkylating agent isomeric with cyclophosphamide. It has been reported to be superior to cyclophosphamide for treatment of *oat-cell bronchogenic carcinoma.* It has also shown promise in the treatment of *Burkitt's tumor.* Nausea and vomiting occur acutely. Delayed toxicity includes bone-marrow depression, hemorrhagic cystitis, alopecia, and a usually temporary sterility. Ifosfamide is slowly converted to an active metabolite, the half-life being approximately 3 days. The active metabolites are rapidly bound to proteins. The volume of distribution is larger than that of total body water. *Dose: 1 g/m²* of body surface once a day for 5 days; courses are repeated at approximately 3-week intervals, depending on whether the blood cell count has passed its nadir. Ascorbic acid is coadministered, to diminish the cystitis.

Levamisole Hydrochloride [2,3,5,6-Tetrahydro-6-phenylimidazole[2,1-*b*]thiazole monohydrochloride [16595-80-5] $C_{11}H_{12}N_2S.HCl$ (240.75)]—*Preparation:* US Pat 3,274,209; 3,579,530. *Description and Solubility:* White to cream colored crystals; soluble 1 g in 2 mL water, 5 mL methanol; practically insoluble in ether. *Uses:* Levamisole is an investigational drug that both stimulates and inhibits immune responses to a variety of antigens, depending upon dose and timing of administration. Its effects are thought to be through muscarinic receptor-guanylate cyclase coupled modulation of hormonal influences on lymphocytes. Clinical interest focuses on the immune-stimulatory actions, especially in cancer. Favorable clinical results have been reported for its use against *bronchogenic carcinoma*, *Hodgkin's disease*, *breast cancer*, *Crohn's disease*, *rheumatoid arthritis*, *lupus erythematosis*, *recurrent herpes infections*, and *aphthous stomatitis*. Adverse effects are mild and not frequent. They include nausea, vomiting, headache, fever, vertigo (especially with alcohol), and rare reversible granulocytopenia. The drug is readily absorbed orally. It is nearly completely metabolized in the liver. The elimination half-life is about 4 hr. *Dose: Oral*, to be individualized; a common regimen is 150 mg/day for 4 days each week or every other week.

Lymphocyte Immune Globulin (Equine) [Antithymocyte Globulin]—A preparation of equine immunoglobulin containing antibodies to human lymphocytes and obtained from antilymphocyte serum. *Uses:* Antithymocyte globulin suppresses T-cell activity but does not affect B-lymphocytes. It is used mostly to prevent allograft rejection in *renal transplantation*. It has also been reported to be of value in the treatment in *T-cell leukemias*, *graft-vs-host disease*, and *aplastic anemia*. Adverse effects include chills, fever, urticaria, generalized rashes, pruritis, dyspnea, tachycardia, hypotension, and anaphylaxis. Infrequently, it causes nausea, vomiting, diarrhea, stomatitis, pain and thrombophlebitis at the injection site, arthralgia, chest pain, and back pain. A skin test for sensitivity to horse serum prior to use is advisable. *Dose:* To be individualized.

Mithramycin [Aureolic acid; $C_{52}H_{76}O_{24}$ (1085.16); Mithracin (*Pfizer*)]—An antibiotic elaborated during culture of certain strains of *Streptomyces;* a yellow, crystalline powder; odorless; hygroscopic; slightly soluble in water; very slightly soluble in alcohol. *Uses:* Mithramycin binds to guanine-rich DNA and thus inhibits DNA-dependent RNA polymerase. It acts mainly during the S-phase. It also blocks parathormone. It is a minor drug for treatment of *testicular carcinoma*. It is often used to treat *malignant hypercalcemia* (neoplasms that cause dissolution of bone salts) not responsive to conventional treatment. Mithramycin is quite toxic, and drug-induced mortality ranges from 0.09 to 0.7%, depending on dose. Death results from hemorrhagic diatheses resulting from prothrombinopenia, thrombocytopenia, increased clotting and bleeding times, and abnormal clot retraction. The hemorrhagic episode usually begins with nosebleed, but it may begin with hematemesis. The most common untoward effects are nausea, vomiting, diarrhea, anorexia, and stomatitis. Less frequently there occur fever, facial flushing, rash, phlebitis, malaise, headache, drowsiness, asthenia, lethargy, depression, hepatic dysfunction, renal insufficiency, hypocalciuria, hypopotassemia, hypophosphatemia, and leukopenia. The hemorrhagic syndrome occurs in about 5% of patients who receive no more than 30 μg/kg/day for no more than 10 doses, whereas it is about 12% for higher doses. *Dose: Intravenous infusion*, for *testicular tumors*, *0.025 to 0.03 mg* (25 to 30 μg)/*kg* in 1 L of 5% dextrose injection, infused over a 6-hr period, once a day for 8 to 10 days, unless toxicity supervenes; additional courses of treatment are given at monthly intervals until the tumor completely regresses or begins to regrow. For *hypercalcemia* and *hypercalciuria*, *0.025 mg* (25 μg)/*kg/day* for 3 or 4 days; additional courses or 2 to 4 doses/week may be given, if necessary.

Mitobronitol [1,6-dibromo-1,6-dideoxy-D-mannitol; $C_6H_{12}Br_2O_4$ (308.000)]—A white, crystalline powder; melts at about 178°; soluble in water. *Uses:* Dibromomannitol is an investigational drug that has already attained a drug-of-second-choice status for treatment of *chronic granulocytic leukemia*. Various gastrointestinal disturbances occur acutely. Delayed toxicity includes bone marrow depression, hyperpigmentation of the skin, and alopecia. *Dose: Oral, adult, initial, 5 mg/ kg/day* until a total cumulated dose of 10 to 15 g, then 5 to 10 mg/kg once a week for maintenance. An alternative schedule is 250 mg per day every 2 to 3 days, whenever the leukocyte count exceeds 20,000/mm³.

Mitomycin [Mitomycin C; $C_{15}H_{18}N_4O_5$ (334.34); Mitocin-C (*Bristol*); Mutamycin (*Bristol*)]—One of three closely related entities isolated from the antibiotic complex produced by *Streptomyces caespitosus*, an organism from Japanese soil. A blue-violet, crystalline powder; soluble in water. *Uses:* Mitomycin inhibits DNA synthesis by cross-linking double-stranded DNA through guanine and cytosine. The combination of fluorouracil-doxorubicin-mitomycin provides the first choice treatment of *gastric cancer*. Mitomycin is one of two drugs of second choice for treatment of tumors of the *bladder* (by instillation) and *pancreatic adenocarcinoma*. It has some efficacy against breast tumors, osteogenic sarcoma, squamous cell carcinoma of the head and neck, colorectal cancer, and non-small cell carcinoma of the lung. Acute adverse effects occur in

about 14% of patients; they include nausea, vomiting, anorexia, fever, and local irritation and cellulitis from extravasation at the site of injection. Delayed toxicity includes cumulative, frequently irreversible, bone-marrow depression (in 64% of recipients), stomatitis, alopecia, and renal impairment (in 20% of recipients). *Dose: Intravenous*, either *10 to 20 mg/m²* of body surface as a single dose or *2 mg/m²/day* for 5 days, an interval of 2 days, then again 2 mg/m²/day for 5 days. The course is repeated at 6- to 8-week intervals, recovery of the blood picture permitting; treatment should be resumed until the platelets recover to 75,000/mm³ and the leukocytes to 3000/mm³.

Pipobroman [1,4-Bis(3-bromopropionyl)piperazine; $C_{10}H_{16}Br_2N_2O_2$ (356.06); Vercyte (*Abbott*)]—Prepared by condensation of piperazine with 3-bromopropionyl chloride; a white or practically white, crystalline powder; melts at about 103°; 1 g dissolves in 230 mL water, 35 mL alcohol, 5 mL chloroform. *Uses:* An antineoplastic drug of the alkylating type. Its use is mainly limited to treatment of *polycythemia vera* and *chronic granulocytic leukemia*. Even in these disorders, however, it is generally not as effective as older modes of treatment. Consequently, it is held in reserve for use in patients who have become refractory to x-irradiation and busulfan in the case of leukemia, and phlebotomy and radiophosphate in the case of polycythemia vera. Adverse effects include severe anemia, in part of a hemolytic nature, and reticulocytosis. Leukopenia and thrombocytopenia are the result of the intended action of the drug, but the leukocyte count should be kept above 3000/mm³ and the platelet count above 100,000/mm³. Transient nausea, vomiting, abdominal cramps, and diarrhea sometimes occur. There is an occasional rash. The drug is contraindicated in patients whose bone-marrow function remains depressed from radiation or previous chemotherapy. It should not be used in pregnancy. *Dose: Oral*, for *polycythemia vera*, initially, *1 mg/kg/day* for at least 30 days, after which the dose may be increased to *1.5 to 3 mg/kg* if there was no previous response; once the hematocrit has been reduced by 50%, maintenance is begun at *0.1 to 0.2 mg* (100 to 200 μg)/*kg/day*. For *chronic myelocytic leukemia*, initially *1.5 to 2.5 mg/kg/day* until the optimal therapeutic response or serious untoward effects occur; *maintenance* doses range from *7 to 175 mg/day*. Maintenance is withheld until the leukocyte count rises again to 10,000 cells/mm³.

Semustine [1-(2-Chloroethyl)-3-(4-methylcyclohexyl)-1-nitrosourea; methyl lomustine; methyl-CCNU; $C_{10}H_{18}ClN_3O_2$ (247.71)]—*Uses:* Semustine is an investigational nitrosourea that has quickly become a drug of first choice for treatment of *gastric adenocarcinoma* (in combination with fluorouracil and doxorubicin) and one of two drugs of first choice against *malignant melanoma* and of second choice for *colorectal cancer* and *primary brain neoplasms*, an efficacy it shares with other lipid-soluble nitrosoureas, and for *Lewis lung carcinoma*. It has a lesser efficacy against osteogenic sarcoma and gall bladder cancer and non-islet cell pancreatomas. Nausea and vomiting occur acutely. With lipid emulsion forms, chest pain may occur. Delayed toxicity includes bone-marrow depression, with leukopenia and prolonged thrombocytopenia and alopecia. *Dose: Oral*, 175 to 200 mg/m² of body surface once every 6 weeks, except 100 mg/m² in combination with other bone-marrow depressant drugs; *intravenous*, in a lipid emulsion, for *brain tumors*, 130 to 150 mg/m² once every 6 weeks.

Streptozocin [Streptozotocin; $C_8H_{15}N_3O_7$ (265.22)]—A nitrosourea antibiotic isolated from *Streptomyces achromogenes* fermentation broth; also synthesized. Very soluble in water; soluble in alcohol. *Uses:* Streptozocin has become the drug of first choice (in combination with fluorouracil) for treatment of *malignant pancreatic insulinoma* and *malignant carcinoid tumor*. It is a component of a second-choice combination for *colon cancer*. It has also shown promise in the treatment of *Hodgkin's disease* and *non-islet cell pancreatic cancer*. Acute adverse effects include nausea and vomiting, local pain at the site of administration, and chills. Renal damage is the principal delayed toxicity but hepatotoxicity also occurs. Bone-marrow depression occurs in about 20% of recipients. The drug is mainly metabolized; its half-life is about 15 minutes. *Dose: Intravenous* or *intra-arterial, 1 g/m²* of body surface per week for 2 weeks; dosage is adjusted according to the therapeutic and toxic responses.

Teniposide [Of similar structure to etoposide, except the methyl substituent of the ethylidene group is replaced by 2-thienyl. [29767-20-2] $C_{32}H_{32}O_{13}S$ (656.66)]. *Uses:* Teniposide is similar to etoposide (page 1155) in mechanism of action, uses, toxicity, and pharmacokinetics, except that it is additionally used against *breast cancer* and *neuroblastoma* but is not used against testicular cancer, choriocarcinoma, and oat-cell carcinoma of the lung. *Dose:* The optimal dose has yet to be determined.

Triethylenethiophosphoramide [Tris(1-aziridinyl)phosphine sulfide; Thio-Tepa (*Lederle*) [52-24-4] $C_6H_{12}N_3PS$ (189.21). *Caution—Thiotepa is extremely poisonous.*] *Preparation*—Ethylenimine is condensed with thiophosphoryl chloride ($PSCl_3$) in the presence of triethylamine as the acid receptor. *Description and Solubility:* Fine, white, crystalline flakes having a faint odor; melts between 52° and 57°. Soluble 1 g in 13 mL water, 8.3 mL alcohol, 1.9 mL chloroform, 4.1 mL ether. *Uses:* Triethylenethiophosphoramide is an alkylating agent. However, it has a much lower chemical reactivity than the β-chloroethylamines and hence has a low degree of local irritancy and lacks the vesicant properties. For this reason it is presently used mainly for local application, where appropriate. Local instillation into the urinary bladder for *papillary carcinoma* is sometimes quite effective. It may also be instilled into other cavities to control serous infusions consequent to certain neoplasms. It may occasionally be infiltered directly into tumors, especially obstructive lesions. Given systemically, its bone-marrow toxicity is quite unpredictable, so that such use is dangerous; consequently, it is nearing obsolescence for systemic treatment. The neoplasms for which it is still a possible desperation choice are *ovary carcinomas* and *embryonal rhabdomyosarcoma*. Local adverse effects include local pain, weeping and occasional perforation through the lesion. The most serious systemic adverse effect is bone-marrow depression, characterized by neutropenia, thrombocytopenia, and usually low-grade anemia. It is mandatory to monitor the blood cell counts. The effects may not appear for 5 to 30 days, which complicates management. Anorexia, nausea and vomiting are not as common as with other alkylating agents. Headache, dizziness, fever, and tightness in the throat may occur. Hyperuricemia may result from massive cell destruction, and crystalluria and oliguria are possible. Hypersensitivity is uncommon, but hives, skin rash, and even anaphylaxis can occur. Depression of spermatogenesis and ovarian function have been reported. Systemic side effects from local instillation can occur. Thiotepa is excreted mostly unchanged, so that the dose should be reduced in renal failure. It is contraindicated if there is prior bone-marrow depression or pregnancy. *Dose: Parenteral*, 0.3 to 0.4 mg/kg at intervals of 1 to 4 weeks. *Intrapleural*, *intraperitoneal*, or *intrapericardial* or *intratumor*, 0.6 to 0.8 mg/kg once a week; if the leukocyte count is below 3000 cells/mm^3, treatment is discontinued until the count rises above that value (preferably until about 10,000 cells/mm^3). For *maintenance*, 0.07 to 0.8 mg/kg every 1 to 4 weeks. In malignant ascites the *intraperitoneal* dose is 10 to 15 mg once a week as long as leukocyte and platelet counts are sufficient. For instillation into the *bladder*, 60 mg in 30–60 mL distilled water once a week for 4 weeks; the solution should be retained in the bladder for 2 hr at each instillation. Solutions for topical application can be mixed with 2% procaine and/or 1:1000 epinephrine.

Uracil Mustard [5-[Bis(2-chloroethyl)amino]uracil; $C_8H_{11}Cl_2N_3O_2$ (252.10)]—Prepared from 5-aminouracil, ethylene oxide, and thionyl chloride as reactants. An off-white, crystalline powder; odorless; melts at about 200°, with decomposition; 1 g dissolves in >1000 mL water, 150 mL alcohol. *Uses:* An alkylating agent of the nitrogen mustard type. It is essentially an obsolete drug, having been displaced by the more efficacious and less toxic chlorambucil. However, uracil mustard may still have a special use in the treatment of *primary thrombocytosis*. Other neoplasms for which the drug is occasionally used are Hodgkin's disease, non-Hodgkin's lymphomas, chronic lymphocytic leukemia, chronic myelogenous leukemia, and polycythemia vera. The most common untoward effects are nausea, vomiting, and diarrhea. Pruritus, dermatitis, and partial alopecia do occur, but less frequently than with cyclophosphamide. Nervousness, irritability, depression, amenorrhea, and oligospermia occur infrequently. Bone-marrow depression with leukopenia, thrombocytopenia, and even anemia may occur, and the blood picture must be monitored twice a week during the first month of treatment. The bone-marrow damage may become irreversible when the cumulative dose approaches 1 mg per kg. Rapid involution of tumors may cause hyperuricemia and consequent nephropathy and renal failure, so that plasma uric acid levels should be determined regularly and the patients should drink much water. *Dose: Schedule A: Initially 1 to 2 mg/day* until a therapeutic response or hematopoietic toxicity occurs. The drug is then withdrawn until adverse effects subside or the clinical condition deteriorates. The *maintenance* dose is *1 mg/day* for 3 weeks out of each 4-week period. *Schedule B: Initially 3 to 5 mg/day* for 1 week, the total dosage not to exceed 0.5 mg/kg of body weight. The *maintenance* dose is 1 mg/day for 3 weeks out of each 4-week period. Critical bone marrow toxicity is indicated by a leukocyte count below 1500 cells/mm^3, platelet count below 50,000/mm^3, or a hemoglobin concentration less than 70% of pretreatment values.

Vindesine Sulfate [3-Aminocarbonyl)-O^4-deacetyl-3-methoxycarbonyl)vincaleukoblastine sulfate (1:1) (salt) Eldisine (*Lilly*); [59917-39-4] $C_{43}H_{55}N_5O_7 \cdot H_2SO_4$ (852.01)]—A semisynthetic derivative of the *Vinca* alkaloids. The pH of the reconstituted solution for injection is 4.2–4.5; above pH 6 the free base precipitates. *Uses:* Vindesine is an investigational drug that combines the therapeutic and toxic properties of vincristine and vinblastine. Its therapeutic status is quite promising. It is active against vinca-resistant *acute lymphocytic leukemia*, the *blast crisis* of *chronic myelocytic leukemia, malignant glioma, melanoma, Hodgkin's* and *non-Hodgkin's lymphomas*, and *colorectal, breast*, and *esophageal carcinomas*. In combination with cisplatin it is especially effective against *bronchogenic carcinoma*. Toxicity includes occasional nausea and vomiting, common but moderate myelosuppression (especially leukopenia), alopecia, constipation, ileus, muscle aches, paresthesias, weakness, occasional chills and fever, phlebitis, and rare confusion and lassitude. Vindesine is poorly absorbed orally. It manifests 3-compartment pharmacokinetics, with half-lives of 2 min, 1 hr, and 24 hr. *Dose: Intravenous*, rapid injection or continuous infusion, either 3 to 4 mg/m^2 a week for induction and every 2 weeks for maintenance or 1.2 to 2 mg/m^2 on days 1, 3, and 5 every 3 weeks.

CHAPTER 64

Antimicrobial Drugs

Stewart C Harvey, PhD

Professor of Pharmacology
School of Medicine, University of Utah
Salt Lake City, UT 84132

The antimicrobial drugs occupy a unique niche in the history of medicine. The germ theory of disease was the vehicle of a dramatic revolution in medicine, and aseptic procedures and antiseptic drugs were its agents. During the entire preceding history of medicine, fewer than a handful of drugs had a known locus of action, and even fewer had been submitted to systematic laboratory investigation. The first systemic antimicrobial drugs revolutionized the treatment of certain protozoal infections, especially syphilis, but the second major revolution in medicine in which the antimicrobial drugs played a major role awaited the appearance of sulfanilamide and penicillin; the exponential development in the antibiotic and systemic antibacterial field is the inevitable result of the momentum created by those two agents.

The term *microbe* is sometimes applied only to the unicellular microphytes. However, in its broader sense it includes not only the multicellular microphytes but the microzoa as well. Therefore, this chapter includes the antifungal and antiprotozoal agents as well as the antibacterial agents.

The uses of the drugs in this chapter are extracted from a world literature, and, since this book is not specifically addressed to any particular national readership, uses may be listed that are not approved by the United States FDA. In the United States, the package literature should be used as the guide to approved uses. However, the approved indications are often vague, such as "infections caused by susceptible organisms." Although the monographs may give some indication as to the probable susceptibility of various infectious organisms, it is incumbent upon the user to apply standard sensitivity tests and clinical acumen, rather than the monographs, to define the suitability of an antimicrobial drug in a given clinical case.

Antiseptics, Disinfectants, and Spermaticides

The words *antiseptic*, *disinfectant*, and *germicide* all connote an agent which kills microbes upon contact, although certain denotations are more rigid and discriminatory. Drugs in this category are applied locally, although a few may be applied systemically as well. Thousands of chemical compounds have germicidal properties, and hundreds are now available. Unfortunately, many of these are poorly effective in the presence of serum or other organic media, or else they are excessively damaging to the tissues. Tissue damage, of course, is not of concern when such agents are employed for the disinfection of inanimate objects; on the other hand, corrosiveness, stain, and other effects then become important considerations. Some of the popular antiseptics listed below do not warrant their exalted status, and many excellent antiseptics are unexploited.

It is commonly believed that antiseptics are nonselective and that they have a continuous spectrum of activity. Although this is approximately true, certain significant absolute exceptions exist, and the relative susceptibilities of the numerous microorganisms must be considered in antiseptic use. For example, hexachlorophene is primarily effective against gram-positive organisms, cationic antiseptics are not effective against sporulating organisms, etc. Certain bacteria are even capable of growing in 70% ethanol. But bichloride of mercury and iodine have very broad and therapeutically complete spectra of efficacy.

Many antiseptics are also antifungal agents, and certain antiseptics will be treated in the section on antifungal drugs.

No really satisfactory classification of antiseptics exists. The most widely used scheme is the chemical classification. Nevertheless, the drugs listed below are not arranged according to chemical type. However, it will be noted that the major chemical categories represented are oxidizing agents (including the halogens and halogen-releasing compounds), phenols and related compounds, compounds of heavy metals (especially of mercury), surface-active agents (especially the cationic detergents), and a variety of dyes. Scattered representatives from the alcohols and glycols, aldehydes, and acids may also be noted. Locally effective antibiotics are discussed with the antibiotics.

It should be kept in mind that systemic antimicrobial drugs are often superior to topical ones. This is because topical agents usually do not penetrate into infected sites as well as systemic agents do. Nevertheless, topical drugs are often efficacious, simply by limiting surface infections so that tissue defenses can clean up below without continual reinfection from superficial foci. Furthermore, some superficial disorders do not seem to respond to safe systemic agents, or, if they do, there may be cogent reasons for withholding systemic drugs, for example, to avoid sensitizing the patient or creating resistant microorganisms. Therefore, there is still an important place for topical antiseptics. However, topical antiseptics can damage tissue defenses, so that sometimes they may exacerbate lesions. Such occasions are not always predictable, and they evidently depend in part on the condition of the patient and the activity of the immunological response to infection.

Many antiseptics have spermaticidal activity, although not all of these can be safely administered into the vagina. There are only two spermaticides that are not also used as antiseptics, too few a number to warrant a separate chapter or section. Consequently, spermaticides are included here.

Acetic Acid, Diluted—page 1309.

Acetic Acid Solutions

A sterile solution of glacial acetic acid in water for injection. It contains, in each 100 mL, 237.5–262.5 mg of $C_2H_4O_2$.

Description—pH between 2.9 and 3.3.

Uses—Microorganisms will not proliferate at low pH, and all acids are bacteriostatic at low concentrations and bactericidal at high concentrations. However, the small, lipid-soluble, weak acids penetrate intracellularly and will exert a greater antimicrobial effect at a given pH than will a mineral acid. Acetic acid is used to discourage bacterial infections in surgical wounds, to suppress growth by *Pseudomonas aeruginosa* in extensive burns of the skin, as a component of a number of dermatologic lotions. It is used to treat external otitis caused by *Pseudomonas*, *Candida* and *Aspergillus*, and vaginal infections caused by *Candida*, *Trichomonas*, or *Hemophilus vaginalis*. Acetic acid has a long history of lay use as a spermatocide. The 0.25% solution is used for bladder irrigation, especially during catheterization. Acetic acid is also used in mouthwashes/gargles, but the contact time is much too short for the acid to have an effect.

Acetic acid can cause irritation and inflammation, especially in the vagina.

Dose—Acetic acid is used *topically* as a 1% surgical dressing, 5% solution in burn therapy, 0.1% dermatologic lotion, 2 to 5% solution for otitis, and 0.25% for irrigation.

Acrisorcin—page 1226.

Alcohol—page 1159.

Rubbing Alcohol

Rubbing alcohol and all preparations coming under the classification of *Rubbing Alcohols* must be manufactured in accordance with the requirements of the US Treasury Department, Bureau of Alcohol, Tobacco, and Firearms, using *Formula 23-H* (8 parts by volume of acetone, 1.5 parts by volume of methyl isobutyl ketone, and 100 parts by volume of ethyl alcohol). It contains 68.5–71.5% by volume of absolute ethyl alcohol, the remainder consisting of water and the denaturants, with or without color additives, and perfume oils. Rubbing Alcohol contains in each 100 mL not less than 355 mg of sucrose octaäcetate or not less than 1.40 mg of denatonium benzoate. The preparation may be colored with one or more color additives, listed by the FDA for use in drugs. A suitable stabilizer may also be added. Rubbing Alcohol complies with the requirements of the Bureau of Alcohol, Tobacco, and Firearms, of the US Treasury Department.

Note—Rubbing Alcohol must be packaged, labeled, and sold in accordance with the regulations issued by the US Treasury Department, Bureau of Alcohol, Tobacco, and Firearms.

Description—Transparent, colorless or colored as desired, mobile, volatile liquid, with an extremely bitter taste, and in the absence of added odorous substances, a characteristic odor; flammable; specific gravity of *Formula 23-H* is between 0.8691 and 0.8771 at 15.56°.

Uses—Applied externally as a *cooling, soothing* application for bedridden patients and athletes. It is also widely used for cleansing the surgeon's hands and instruments and for disinfection of the skin prior to penetration of the skin by a hypodermic needle. As an *antiseptic* it is good against vegetative bacteria and fair against fungi and viruses. It is ineffective against spores. It is widely believed that 70% ethanol provides the greatest reduction in bacterial count; however, this is in error. Other concentrations may be more effective, but their rate of kill is slower. In order to reduce the skin bacterial count to 5% of normal, 70% ethanol must be left on the skin for at least 2 min. Ethanol is also a feeble *anesthetic* and a mild *counterirritant*. See *Alcohol* (page 1306). *It is not potable.*

Aluminum Acetate Solution—page 778.

Aluminum Subacetate Solution—page 778.

Bacitracin—page 1201.

Benzalkonium Chloride

Ammonium, alkyldimethyl(phenylmethyl)-, chloride;
Zephiran Chloride (*Winthrop*); Mercurochrome II

Alkylbenzyldimethylammonium chloride [8001-54-5]; a mixture of alkylbenzyldimethylammonium chlorides of the general formula $[C_6H_5CH_2N(CH_3)_2R]Cl$, in which R represents a mixture of alkyls, including all or some of the group beginning with n-C_8H_{17} and extending through higher homologs, with n-$C_{12}H_{25}$, n-$C_{14}H_{29}$ and n-$C_{16}H_{33}$ comprising the major portion. On the anhydrous basis, the content of n-$C_{12}H_{25}$ homolog is not less than 40%, and the content of the n-$C_{14}H_{29}$ homolog is not less than 20%, of the total alkylbenzyldimethylammonium chloride content. The amounts of the n-$C_{12}H_{25}$ and n-$C_{14}H_{29}$ homolog components comprise together not less than 70% of the total alkylbenzyldimethylammonium chloride content.

Preparation—By treating a solution of *N*-alkyl-*N*-methylbenzylamine in a suitable organic solvent with methyl chloride, the solvent being so chosen that the quaternary compound precipitates as it is formed.

Description—White or yellowish white, thick gel or gelatinous pieces; aromatic odor, and a very bitter taste; solutions are alkaline to litmus and foam strongly when shaken.

Solubility—Very soluble in water and alcohol; 1 g of the anhydrous form dissolves in about 6 mL benzene and in about 100 mL ether.

Incompatibilities—Like other cationic surface-active agents, benzalkonium chloride is incompatible with *soap* and other *anionic agents*. The large organic ions of the two agents, being oppositely charged, are attracted to each other and, in sufficient concentration, precipitate from solution. *Nitric acid* and *nitrates* cause precipitation.

Uses—Benzalkonium chloride is bacteriostatic in low and bactericidal in high concentrations. Gram-positive bacteria are more sensitive than gram-negative bacteria. Indeed, some gram-negative bacteria, especially *Pseudomonas cepacia*, have been known to grow in solutions of benzalkonium chloride and thus to cause epidemics of hospital infections. *Mycobacterium tuberculosis* is also relatively resistant. The antiseptic has a slow action. It requires 7 min for the bacterial count on the skin to be decreased by a mere 50%, while only 36 sec is required by 70% ethanol; to effect a 90% reduction, 25 min is required for benzalkonium chloride compared to 2 min for the ethanol. Some gram-negative bacteria require hours of exposure to be killed.

Benzalkonium chloride is used for application to skin and mucous membranes. It is widely used in over-the-counter ophthalmic solutions and as applications to contact lenses. It is also used for the sterilization of inanimate articles, such as surgical instruments. Solutions of benzalkonium chloride have low surface tension and possess detergent and emulsifying actions. It is also a mild astringent and is used as such. It has relatively low systemic toxicity, but poisoning from oral ingestion has been reported. After repetitive use it sometimes may cause dermatitides. Like other cationic surface-active agents, it has certain limitations. It cannot be relied upon to kill clostridial spores, it is ineffective against some viruses, it is inactivated by soap and other anionic surface-active agents, and when applied to the skin it has a tendency to form a film under which bacteria remain viable. Organic matter from tissue inactivates the drug, so that it has limited efficacy in the disinfection of wounds. Benzalkonium chloride is adsorbed by various organic substances, so that the concentration in a sterilizing solution may drop below the antibacterial level, and the sterilization of surgical gloves, sponges, etc. may be erratic. The drug can cause irritation and damage the epidermis, and it can also cause allergies. In view of the availability of more reliable and more rapidly acting antiseptics, there is little to commend continued use of benzalkonium chloride.

Dose—*Topical*, 0.02 to 0.5% solution; to the *conjunctiva*, 0.1 mL of 0.01% solution. For *preoperative disinfection* of unbroken skin or treatment of superficial injuries or fungous infections, 1:1000 to 1:750 tincture. For *preoperative disinfection* of mucous membranes and denuded skin, 1:10,000 to 1:2000; for instillation or irrigation of the *vagina*, 1:5000 to 1:2000; for irrigation of widely *denuded surfaces*, 1:10,000 to 1:5000; to the *eye*, 1:10,000 to 1:5000; for irrigation of the *urinary bladder* and *urethra*, 1:20,000; for retention lavage of the bladder, 1:40,000; for disinfection of *deep lacerations*, 1:1000; for irrigation of *deep wounds*, 1:3000; for treatment of infected denuded areas with wet dressings, 1:5000; as a detergent solubilizer of water-insoluble drugs, up to 0.5%; for sterile storage of *metallic instruments* and *rubber articles*, 1:1000 to 1:750. When the drug is used for sterile storage of metal instruments, sodium nitrite (0.5%) is added to the solution to prevent corrosion of metal.

Dosage Forms—Vaginal Gel: 0.05%; Solution: 0.1 (1 in 1000) and 0.133% (1 in 750); Tincture: 0.133%; Tincture Spray: 0.133%; Concentrates: 12.8, 17, 17.5, and 50% aqueous, and 17% tincture.

Benzoic Acid—page 1230.

Benzyl Alcohol—page 1057.

Boric Acid—page 1310.

Chlorhexidine Gluconate

D-Gluconic acid, compd with *N,N″*-bis(4-chlorophenyl)-3,12-diimino-2,4,11,13-tetraazatetradecanediimidamide (2:1); Hibiclens (*Stuart*)

1,1'-Hexamethylenebis[5-(p-chlorophenyl)biguanide] di-D-gluconate [18472-51-0] $C_{22}H_{30}Cl_2N_{10} \cdot 2C_6H_{12}O_7$ (897.77).

Preparation—Chlorhexidine base may be prepared by refluxing a mixture of hexamethylenebis[dicyandiamide], [NCNHC(:NH)-NH(CH$_2$)$_3$]$_2$, and p-chloroaniline hydrochloride in 2-ethoxyethanol at 130°–140° for two hours (Rose and Swain, *CA 50:* 1082h, 1956). The digluconate, diacetate, and dihydrochloride salts may be obtained by neutralizing the base with the respective acids.

Uses—Chlorhexidine is bactericidal to both gram-positive and gram-negative bacteria, although it is not as potent against the latter. It disrupts the plasma membrane of the bacterial cell, and cellular contents are lost.

In a 4% aqueous solution as a surgical scrub, it decreases the cutaneous bacterial population more than either hexachlorophene or povidone-iodine. It is slightly less effective than povidone-iodine if the skin is contaminated with certain gram-negative bacteria. A 1% aqueous solution has erratic antiseptic effects, but a 0.5% solution in 95% ethanol is more effective than a 4% aqueous solution. Chlorhexidine solutions leave a residue on the skin which gives a persistent antibacterial effect lasting 1 or 2 days. Its actions are not affected by blood, pus, or soaps.

Chlorhexidine is used for the preoperative preparation of both surgeon and patient, for the treatment of *superficial skin infections*, *burns*, *acne vulgaris*, and the *irrigation of wounds* and *surgical infections*. It can be used in the hospital nursery to bathe neonates for prophylaxis against staphylococcal and streptococcal infections. Abroad, it is used as a mouthwash for *oral hygiene* and *oropharyngeal infections*, especially *aphthous ulcers*. Chlorhexidine is absorbed onto tooth enamel, where it exerts a persisting action to *decrease the growth of dental plaque*.

Chlorhexidine is negligibly absorbed from the skin and mucous membranes; it has low systemic toxicity. Thus it would not be expected to cause systemic intoxication from topical application, and none has been noted thus far. A few cases of sensitization have been reported. Bacterial resistance to the drug has not been reported, but overgrowth (superinfection) by naturally resistant gram-negative bacteria may sometimes occur. Instances of hospital epidemics caused by *Pseudomonas maltophilia* actually growing in aqueous solutions of chlorhexidine have been reported. The substance is considerably adsorbed by new glass, and the concentration of weak solutions may thus be lowered; it is not adsorbed by polyethylene.

Dose—*Topical*, as a 4% cleanser or **0.5%** tincture.
Dosage Forms—Aqueous Emulsion: 4%; Tincture: 0.5%.

Ethylene Oxide

Oxirane

$$H_2C\!\!-\!\!CH_2$$
$$\diagdown\;\diagup$$
$$O$$

Ethylene oxide [75-21-8] C_2H_4O (44.05).
Preparation—Ethylene is catalytically oxidized with air at high temperature.

Description—Colorless, flammable gas; liquid below 12°.
Solubility—Soluble in water, alcohol, and ether.

Uses—An alkylating agent that has a very broad germicidal spectrum, including spores and viruses. Since it is reactive at room temperature, it may be used for the disinfection and sterilization of heat-labile objects, such as certain catheters and endoscopes in the hospital and various materials in the pharmaceutical and other industries. Because it is applied as a gas, it is advantageous for the sterilization of objects that would be harmed by immersion in aqueous or other media.

Because of the high chemical reactivity of ethylene oxide, it reacts with many pharmaceutical substances and with vitamins, amino acids, and other food constituents, so that its use needs to be carefully limited. It is no longer legal to treat fruit with this gas. Because it reacts with tissue constituents, it is toxic. Inhalation of the gas causes nausea, vomiting, and neurological disorders, and severe exposures can cause death. Consequently, sterilization must be done only in appropriate chambers or rooms. Chemical burns can result from the wearing of ethylene oxide-sterilized clothing, shoes, or gloves that have been inadequately aired after sterilization; thrombophlebitis or hemolysis can result from the use of catheters, and tracheitis from endotracheal tubes which have retained a residue of the gas. Polyvinyl

tubing, bags, and ware are especially dangerous because of the formation of chlorohydrin. Therefore, after exposure, such items should be aired for 5 days at room temperature or 8 hours at 120°C. The gas is also used as a fumigant.

The gas is highly explosive at concentrations above 3%, so that it needs to be mixed with CO_2 or fluorocarbons before use.

The gas kills vegetative bacteria very rapidly, but desiccated microorganisms and spores are killed only slowly, so that a 3-hour exposure at 30°C is advised. The optimal humidity for action is 30 to 40%.

Ethylene oxide is also discussed on pages 1256 and 1446.

Application—**120 mg/L** to pure ethylene oxide, depending upon the use, temperature, humidity, and gaseous diluents.

Glutaral

Pentanedial; Glutaraldehyde; Glutaric Dialdehyde;
Cidex (*Surgikos*)

OCH(CH$_2$)$_3$CHO

Pentanedial [111-30-8] $C_5H_8O_2$ (100.12).
Preparation—The 1:1 Diels-Alder adduct of acrolein and a vinyl alkyl ether is hydrolyzed, forming glutaral and an alkanol.

Description—Colorless liquid with a pungent odor; boils at about 188° with decomposition; stable in light; oxidizes in air; polymerizes on heating. *Glutaral Concentrate* is a 50% (w/w) solution in water.
Solubility—Soluble in water and in alcohol.

Uses—Glutaral is a *disinfectant* superior to formaldehyde. It is microbicidal against all microorganisms, including spores and viruses. Of low volatility, it does not release odorous and irritant vapor as does formaldehyde solution, and it is much more rapidly acting than the latter. It does not damage endoscopes. A 2% alkaline solution in 70% isopropanol kills dried spores in 10 hours, but an acid-stabilized solution kills them in 20 minutes. Solutions can be aerosolized to kill bacteria in the air and also on surfaces (tables, floors, walls, etc.). Glutaral is also employed as a tissue fixative for optical and electron microscopy; being bifunctional, glutaral cross-links proteins in tissue and thus limits movement during staining and handling.

Alkaline and neutral solutions of glutaral polymerize and have shelf lives of less than two weeks. Acid-stabilized solutions have a somewhat longer shelf life. When poloxamers or polyethylene glycols are used to stabilize solutions, the shelf life is increased to as long as several months, and antimicrobial activity is also enhanced.

Application—As a 2% solution, applied directly or aerosolized.

Halazone

Benzoic acid, 4-[(dichloroamino)sulfonyl]-,

HOOC—⟨benzene ring⟩—SO$_2$NCl$_2$

p-Dichlorosulfamoyl)benzoic acid [80-13-7] $C_7H_5Cl_2NO_4S$ (270.09).
Preparation—p-Toluenesulfonylchloride obtained by the reaction of toluene and chlorosulfonic acid is converted to the amide, which is treated with hypochlorite to form p-toluenesulfondichloramide. The methyl group is then oxidized with dichromate or permanganate to form halazone.

Description—White, crystalline powder having a chlorine-like odor; melts with decomposition at about 194° and is affected by light.
Solubility—1 g in >1000 mL water, 140 mL alcohol, >1000 mL chloroform, >2000 mL ether; soluble in solutions of alkali hydroxides or carbonates, forming the corresponding salts; soluble in glacial acetic acid.

Uses—For the extemporaneous *disinfection of drinking water*, as tablets. The chemical hydrolyzes to yield HClO and Cl$_2$. Organic matter in the water competes with microorganisms for the active molecules, so that dirty water requires more halazone than clear water.

Application—**2 to 10 ppm** (0.0002 to 0.001%), in drinking water. Tablets for Solution: 4 mg. One 4-mg tablet to 1 pint of water theoretically yields 8 ppm. For polluted water, use two or three tablets. A 30-min wait is required before the water may be considered potable. The HClO and Cl$_2$ can be removed with sodium thiosulfate to remove the odor and improve the taste.

Hexachlorophene

Phenol, 2,2'-methylenebis[3,4,6-trichloro-, G-11; AT-7;
(*Various Mfrs*)

2,2'-Methylenebis[3,4,6-trichlorophenol] [70-30-4] C$_{13}$H$_6$Cl$_6$O$_2$
(406.91).

Preparation—By the Baeyer condensation reaction involving two molecules of 2,4,5-trichlorophenol, and one molecule of formaldehyde. Sulfuric acid is employed as the dehydrant.

Description—White to light tan, crystalline powder; odorless or only slightly phenolic odor; melting range 161° to 167°.

Solubility—Insoluble in water; freely soluble in acetone, alcohol, and ether; soluble in chloroform and dilute solutions of fixed alkali hydroxides.

Uses—Hexachlorophene is an effective *bactericidal antiseptic* against gram-positive bacteria but it has low activity against gram-negative organisms; *in vitro* a 3% solution will kill *Staphylococcus aureus* in 15 to 30 sec, but as long as 24 hr may be required to kill some gram-negative organisms. On the skin the bacterial population will initially decrease by only 30 to 50% but within an hour the decrease will exceed 90%. When washes are repeated two or more times a day, the decrease will reach an asymptote of 95 to 99% in 3 or 4 days from a persisting residuum of hexachlorophene in the skin. This reservoir can be removed by ethanol, isopropyl alcohol, and soap and water washes or other detergents. The drug is effective whether applied as a tincture, detergent emulsion, or soap; the tincture is the most effective and a 0.23% tincture foam has been reported to be more effective than a 3% soap. In soaps, one hydroxyl group is neutralized, which moderately decreases activity.

Preparations containing hexachlorophene are widely used as antiseptic scrubs by physicians, dentists, food handlers, and others. The incidence and severity of *pyogenic skin infections* are reduced by routine use of a hexachlorophene preparation. Such preparations, however, are not available over-the-counter because of concern over potential toxicity. Hexachlorophene is only moderately effective for sterilization.

It has been common practice to bathe newborn infants regularly with 3% hexachlorophene solution to prevent staphylococcal epidemics in nurseries, a practice now in dispute. Neurological damage is acknowledged as a possible danger, but the practice does appear to suppress fatal epidemics. Chlorhexidine, triple-dye, and lactic acid offer alternative treatments.

In infants, hexachlorophene can cause myelinopathy and spongiform encephalomalacia following topical application. Neuropathy in adult burn patients has resulted from topical application. By the oral route hexachlorophene can cause nausea, vomiting, and abdominal cramps with associated water and electrolyte derangements. Topically the drug can cause sensitization. Hexachlorophene is teratogenic. Hospital epidemics have resulted from resistant gram-negative bacteria actually growing in nonalcoholic preparations of hexachlorophene. Superinfections caused by gram-negative bacteria or *Candida* sometimes result from repetitive applications.

Dose—*Topical*, to the *skin*, as a **0.25, 1,** or **3**% emulsion, **0.25**% solution, **0.23**% foam tincture, or **3**% sponge. Aqueous preparations containing less than 2% have low efficacy. Two or more applications a day are required. As a disinfectant of inanimate objects, 3%.

Dosage Forms—Cleansing Emulsion: 0.25, 1 and 3%; Foam: 0.23%; Sponge: 3%. Some products also contain parachlorometaxylenol to prevent contamination by gram-negative bacteria and to broaden the antibacterial spectrum.

Iodine

Iodine [7553-56-2] I (126.90).

Preparation—From the iodide in the ashes of seaweed by chlorination, from the iodate in chile saltpeter by reduction with sulfite ion, or from the iodide in oil well brines by oxidation with chlorine or nitrite ion.

Description—Heavy, grayish black plates or granules, having a metallic luster and a characteristic odor; specific gravity about 4.9; melts at about 114° but volatilizes even at room temperature.

Solubility—1 g in 3000 mL water, 13 mL alcohol, 80 mL glycerin; freely soluble in chloroform, carbon tetrachloride, ether, and glacial acetic acid; soluble in solutions of iodides.

Incompatibilities—Oxidizes *hypophosphites*, *sulfites*, the lower valence forms of some *metals*, and *other reducing agents*, the iodine being reduced to an iodide. *Thiosulfates* (hyposulfites) also react with free iodine. It reacts with *fixed oils* to form addition compounds, and with *volatile oils* to form various derivatives. The reaction with *turpentine oil* is violent. An explosive iodide of nitrogen may be formed with *ammonia water* or *ammoniated mercury*. *Alkali hydroxides* and *carbonates* react with iodine to form iodides and iodates. Many *alkaloids* are precipitated from aqueous solutions of their salts. In *alcoholic solution* iodine slowly forms hydrogen iodide if alkali iodide is absent.

Uses—Iodine is one of the three best all-around antiseptics. It is active against bacteria, fungi, yeasts, protozoa, and viruses. A solution of 1:20,000 kills most bacteria within 1 min. Wet bacterial spores require about 15 min, but dry spores may require hours, even with high concentrations. On the skin, a 1% tincture will kill 90% of the bacteria in 90 sec. Iodine complexes with amino groups in tissue compounds to form iodophores from which the iodine is slowly released to have a sustained action. It maintains its peak efficacy for nearly an hour and exerts some action for several hours.

Iodine may be used to "purify" drinking water. Five to 10 drops of 2% iodine tincture to a quart of water left for 1 hr is both amebacidal and bactericidal; there is controversy over its ability to kill *Giardia*. Some communities use iodine in lieu of chlorine for water purification because organic matter has little effect to antagonize iodine, as it does chlorine, and carcinogenic compounds are not generated.

Iodine has a high therapeutic index, especially with the 2% aqueous solution, which may be applied to open wounds with little or no stinging and interference with body defenses. Potassium ion and hypertonicity in the 5% solution cause local pain in wounds. Tinctures sting and may cause some tissue damage in open wounds. The 7% tincture occasionally causes chemical burns of the skin. There is little need to use a preparation stronger than 2% aqueous solution or 1% tincture.

Iodine Solution contains, in each 100 mL, 1.8–2.2 g of I, and 2.1–2.6 g of NaI. *Preparation:* Dissolve iodine (20 g) and sodium iodide (24 g) in purified water (50 mL), then add sufficient purified water to make the product measure 1000 mL. *Description:* Transparent liquid, having a reddish brown color and the odor of iodine. *Incompatibilities:* See *Iodine*. *Uses:* An effective nonirritating *germicide* and *fungicide* despite its relatively low content of free iodine. Indeed, it may be diluted severalfold and still remain one of the most effective antiseptics. Irritation or "iodine burns" are uncommon with this concentration. See also *Strong Iodine Solution*. *Dose: Topical*, to the *skin* in full strength or diluted to as low as 0.1% for application to wounds.

Strong Iodine Solution [Lugol's Solution; Aqueous Solution of Iodine; Solutio Iodi Aquosa; Compound Iodine Solution] contains, in each 100 mL, 4.5–5.5 g of iodine (I), and 9.5–10.5 g of potassium iodide (KI). *Preparation:* Dissolve iodine (50 g) and potassium iodide (100 g) in purified water (100 mL), then add sufficient purified water to make the product measure 1000 mL. The potassium iodide is added only to increase the solubility of the iodine. *Description:* Transparent liquid having a deep brown color, and the odor of iodine. *Incompatibilities:* See *Iodine*. *Uses:* Traditionally in the treatment of many conditions in which the action of the iodide ion is desired. For example, in the treatment of *thyrotoxicosis* strong iodine solution is employed in order to reduce the metabolic rate prior to operation on the thyroid. For such purposes, however, potassium iodide is equally effective. The presence of free iodine in strong iodine solution makes this preparation of great value as a *germicide* and *fungicide*. Thus, it retains most of the desirable properties of tincture of iodine without the attending irritation which results from the presence of alcohol in the latter preparation. Either strong iodine solution or iodine solution can be used for the treatment of those conditions described under the tincture. Aqueous solutions of iodine have the advantage of being less painful than alcoholic solutions when applied to cuts, and they can be made isotonic with the blood (a 2% solution of iodine with alkali iodide is isotonic), but they are subject to freezing and they do not dry rapidly. On the other hand, alcoholic solutions dry rapidly and do not freeze. The solution is also keratolytic, probably because of its content of potassium iodide. It is used to treat keratitides associated with excessive keratin. *Dose: Oral*, 0.1 to 3 mL daily, but usually not exceeding 0.3 mL; *topical*, strong solution may be applied directly to the *intact skin*, but *Iodine Solution* is usually preferred, except in keratitis.

Iodine Tincture [Mild Tincture of Iodine; Weak Solution of Iodine] contains, in each 100 mL, 1.8–2.2 g of iodine (I), and 2.1–2.6 g of sodium iodide (NaI). *Preparation:* Dissolve iodine (20 g) and sodium iodide (24 g) in alcohol (500 mL) and then add sufficient purified water to make the product measure 1000 mL. Sufficient sodium iodide is present to stabilize the tincture and make it miscible with water in all proportions. More than enough iodide is present to combine, theoretically, with all the iodine to form NaI$_3$, and thus the iodine does not react with the alcohol to form acetaldehyde and hydrogen iodide. If hydriodic acid was formed, the solution would be more painful when applied to wounds. Sodium iodide is used in this tincture, instead of the potassium salt, as it is less irritating than KI when applied to open wounds. *Description:* Transparent liquid having a reddish brown color and the odors of iodine and alcohol. *Alcohol Content:* 44 to 50%. *Incompatibilities:* See *Iodine. Uses:* One of the oldest and most effective of the *germicides* and *fungicides.* For disinfection of the skin, the alcoholic vehicle facilitates spreading and penetration. If the stronger tinctures are employed, vesication and desquamation may occur, if the excess iodine is not removed with alcohol. For application to wounds and abrasions, the more dilute tinctures or aqueous solutions of iodine and iodide should be employed. The dilute tincture is also the preparation of choice in the treatment of skin infections due to bacteria and fungi. Elemental iodine is effective for the *purification of drinking water* in emergencies; 5 to 10 drops of tincture to a quart of water is both *amebicidal* and *bactericidal,* if allowed to stand for 15 min; iodine solution in the same dilution is equally effective. Elemental iodine is also an alkaloidal precipitant and the tincture or solution may be employed as a chemical antidote in the treatment of *poisoning by alkaloids* in the dilution of 1 scant teaspoonful to a quart of water. It should be administered by stomach tube and removed by gastric lavage. *Dose: Topical,* to the *skin* 2 or 3 times a day.

Isopropyl Alcohol

2-Propanol

CH₃CH(OH)CH₃

Isopropyl alcohol [67-63-0] C_3H_8O (60.10).

Preparation—Most of the isopropyl alcohol prepared commercially is obtained by treating propylene with H_2SO_4 followed by hydrolysis. The olefin is obtained in the cracking of petroleum.

Some of the alcohol is also obtained by the reduction of acetone through high-pressure hydrogenation.

Description—Transparent, colorless, mobile, volatile liquid with a characteristic odor and slightly bitter taste; specific gravity 0.783 to 0.787; distilling range 81° to 83°; refractive index 1.376 to 1.378 at 20°.

Solubility—Miscible with water, alcohol, ether, and chloroform.

Uses—For the disinfection of hypodermic syringes and needles and, as the rubbing alcohol, it is used as a skin antiseptic. Isopropyl alcohol is superior to ethyl alcohol in regard to its *antiseptic* properties. All concentrations greater than 70% are effective skin disinfectants. The 91% concentration does not appear to affect the potency of subcutaneous insulin and hence may be used to prepare the skin for injection. It does promote bleeding at an injection site, which may make reading of allergic tests difficult. Isopropyl alcohol can not be relied on to destroy the spores of organisms such as *Clostridium tetani, Clostridium welchii,* or *Bacillus anthracis.* It has a greater effect than ethanol to dry and irritate the skin. It is not potable and should not be given by mouth. It is also used in hair and scalp preparations, hand and face lotions, aftershave lotions, liniments, various antiseptic and antifungal mixtures, cleansers, and in the *Isopropyl Rubbing Alcohol* described below. The isopropyl rubbing alcohol is recognized as a rubefacient, although it is more widely used as an antiseptic.

Dose—As an antiseptic it is applied to the skin in concentrations greater than 70% *v/v.* It should be left on the skin for at least 2 min.

Dosage Forms—Isopropyl Rubbing Alcohol: 70%; Isopropyl Alcohol: 91% and 100%.

Isopropyl Rubbing Alcohol contains 68–72% of isopropyl alcohol, by volume, the remainder consisting of water, with or without color additives certified by the FDA for use in drugs, suitable stabilizers, and perfume oils. *Description:* Transparent, mobile, volatile liquid with a slightly bitter taste and, in the absence of odorous constituents, a characteristic odor; specific gravity between 0.872 and 0.883. *It is not potable.*

Lactic Acid—page 1314.

Mafenide Acetate

Benzenesulfonamide, 4-(aminoethyl)-, monoacetate; Sulfamylon (*Winthrop*)

H₂NCH₂—⟨benzene ring⟩—SO₂NH₂ · C₂H₄O₂

α-Amino-*p*-toluenesulfonamide monoacetate [13009-99-9] $C_7H_{10}N_2O_2S.C_2H_4O_2$ (246.28).

Preparation—*p*-Cyanobenzenesulfonamide is dissolved in ethanolic HCl and hydrogenated using Pd-charcoal catalyst (*J Am Chem Soc 62:* 2099, 1940) yielding the hydrochloride; ammonia is added to an aqueous solution of the hydrochloride and the base thus liberated is collected and reacted with acetic acid.

Description—White, crystalline powder melting about 167°; pH (1 in 10 solution) between 6.4 and 6.8.

Solubility—Freely soluble in water.

Uses—Mafenide has an irregular antibacterial spectrum that includes both gram-positive and gram-negative microorganisms. Although it is generally more active against the gram-positive organisms, a higher percentage of strains of *Pseudomonas aeruginosa* respond than of staphylococci and streptococci. Since *Ps aeruginosa* is the most common pathogenic invader in burned surfaces, mafenide is especially useful in the management of the burned patient. Staphylococci and streptococci are also common invaders in burned tissue, but many of the strains do not respond to mafenide, so that combination treatment is generally necessary. Mafenide is also quite effective against anaerobes, such as the clostridia, and the German army first employed the drug to prevent gas gangrene.

Although mafenide is a sulfonamide, the para-substituent differs from the sulfa drugs, and its mechanism of action is much different. Thus there is no correlation between bacterial sensitivities to mafenide and those to sulfa drugs. Mafenide is only bacteriostatic, not bactericidal, so that at best it only holds the growth of the sensitive bacteria in check to allow the body defenses a chance to recover. The drug is more effective if it is applied early, before bacterial colonization has become extensive.

Mafenide is applied topically. It penetrates tissues well without loss of potency, so that it reaches most of the infected sites.

In common with the sulfa drugs, mafenide inhibits carbonic anhydrase. Consequently, the treated burn patient with a large burn surface (usually over 30%) may suffer from systemic hyperchloremic acidosis with an alkaline urine. Hyperventilation results. Since burn patients often get pneumonia or renal complications, the acidotic action can be serious. Recovery follows removal of the drug by bathing; mafenide should not be reapplied for several days. Other untoward effects include frequently pain at the site of application, which pain lasts for 20 to 30 min, and occasional allergic reactions, which usually appear as some form of dermatitis, but agranulocytosis has been reported. Also, certain fungi tend to grow beneath the cream.

Dose—*Topical,* as 8.5% cream, to be applied in a layer approximately 2 mm thick, once or twice daily. Recovery is facilitated if the old layer is washed away, to aid debridement and the removal of microorganisms, before each reapplication. Also, whenever the cream is prematurely wiped away, as by patient movement, it should be reapplied.

Dosage Form—Cream: The equivalent of 8.5% of free base.

Methenamine

1,3,5,7-Tetraazatricyclo[3.3.1.1³,⁷]decane; Aminoform; Cystamin; Cystogen; Hexamine; Uritone; *Various Mfrs*

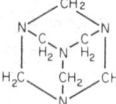

Hexamethylenetetramine [100-97-0] $C_6H_{12}N_4$ (140.19).

Although a cyclic tetramine, the therapeutic action of this compound depends exclusively on its ability to liberate formaldehyde under suitable environmental conditions.

Preparation—By adding a moderate excess of ammonia water to formaldehyde solution, and evaporating to dryness.

Description—Colorless, lustrous crystals or a white crystalline powder; practically odorless; aqueous solution is alkaline to litmus; sublimes at about 260°; when ignited it burns with a smokeless flame.

Solubility—1 g in 1.5 mL water, 12.5 mL alcohol, 10 mL chloroform, 320 mL ether.

Incompatibilities—Alkaline in reaction and forms salts with weak acids. *Strong acids* and concentrated solutions of organic acids decompose it with liberation of formaldehyde. With prolonged contact, weak acids also decompose it, as do acidic vehicles.

It liquefies, in some cases with decomposition, when rubbed with *aspirin, antipyrine, benzoic acid, lithium carbonate, menthol, phenol, potassium acetate, sodium benzoate, sodium salicylate* etc. *Ammonium salts* and *alkalies* darken it. In capsules, it may slowly combine with the gelatin, rendering it insoluble.

Uses—Methenamine is a *urinary tract anti-infective*, provided it is acting in an acid medium. It is rapidly excreted and thus reaches effective antiseptic concentrations in the urine. The drug depends for its action on the liberation of free formaldehyde. This occurs to the extent of 20% of theoretical at pH 5, 6% at pH 6 and almost not at all at pH 7.6. Consequently, precaution must be taken to maintain an acid urine (pH 6 or below) during medication with methenamine. This is usually accomplished by administration of sodium biphosphate, mandelic acid, hippuric acid, ascorbic acid, or cranberry juice. At a pH of 6, a daily dose of methenamine of 2 g will yield an average 24-hour urine concentration of about 18 to 60 $\mu g/mL$, which is about 40 times the minimum to inhibit the growth of most bacteria that cause urinary tract infections. However, it will not prevent growth of *Candida albicans*. It is improbable that products which provide only 40.8 to 81.6 mg/dose can provide a high enough concentration of formaldehyde, since the urine contains substances that bind some of the formaldehyde.

Methenamine is of particular value in the treatment of *E coli* infections of the urinary tract. It also is especially useful in patients with renal insufficiency. Because of its low systemic toxicity, failure to excrete the drug causes no harmful consequences, unless renal insufficiency is severe.

Approximately 10 to 30% is converted to formaldehyde in the acid stomach contents unless enteric capsules are employed. Even with enteric coatings, nausea, vomiting, diarrhea and other gastrointestinal distress often occur when the dose exceeds 500 mg 4 times a day. Formaldehyde liberated from the compound presumably is the cause of the distress. Other untoward effects are occasional pruritis and skin rashes and bladder irritation, painful and frequent urination, and hematuria in persons who have taken the drug longer than 3 to 4 weeks. Dyspnea, lipoid pneumonitis, and headache occur rarely. In persons with acidosis or renal failure, the acid salts usually given concomitantly may be detrimental. The drug should not be used if hepatic insufficiency exists.

Dose—*Oral, adults*, **500 mg** to **1.5 g**; *usual*, **1 g** 4 times a day. *Children*, 6 to 12 years of age, **500 mg** 4 times a day; under 6 years of age, **18.3 mg/kg** 4 times a day; oddly, the convenient elixir form is no longer available, so that the mandelate is the preferred pediatric preparation. If therapy has begun with a high dose of methenamine, it should be reduced for long-term treatment, once the urine is bacteriologically clear. When methenamine and sodium biphosphate tablets are administered the usual dose is 500 mg. Products which contain as little as 40.8 mg/tablet contain other antiseptics in addition to methenamine. The doses of methenamine as methenamine mandelate and methenamine hippurate are given in the separate monographs.

Dosage Forms—Tablets: 500 mg; Methenamine/Sodium Biphosphate: 325 mg/325 mg and 300 mg/500 mg.

Methenamine Mandelate

Benzeneacetic acid, α-hydroxy-, compd with 1,3,5,7-tetraazatricyclo[3.3.1.1.^{3,7}]decane (1:1); Mandelic Acid Hexamethylenetetramine Compound (1:1); Mandelamine (*Warner-Chilcott*)

Hexamethylenetetramine monomandelate [587-23-5] $C_6H_{12}N_4.C_8H_8O_3$ (292.34); contains not less than 95.5% of $C_6H_{12}N_4.C_8H_8O_3$ and not less than 50% of mandelic acid [$C_8H_8O_3$ = 152.15].

For the structure of the base, see *Methenamine*.

Preparation—By reacting equimolar quantities of methenamine and mandelic acid in water or alcohol and concentrating until crystallization occurs.

Description—White, crystalline powder, practically odorless and having a sour taste; melts at about 127°, with decomposition; solutions are acid to litmus (pH about 4).

Solubility—Very soluble in water; 1 g in about 10 mL alcohol, 20 mL chloroform, and 350 mL ether.

Uses—A *urinary tract anti-infective*. See *Methenamine*. Mandelic acid alone also possesses antiseptic activity at a pH below 5.5, which action synergizes the action of the formaldehyde released from methenamine. Furthermore, mandelic acid itself tends to decrease urine pH and aid the action of both components. In some preparations sodium biphosphate is added to further lower urine pH.

Because mandelic acid is excreted into urine, methenamine mandelate is contraindicated in renal insufficiency, though methenamine alone is not. Methenamine mandelate has been used experimentally with some success in the topical treatment of infections in burned skin.

Dose—*Oral, adults*, **1 g** 4 times a day; *children 6 to 12 yr of age*, **0.5 g** 4 times a day; *children under 6 yr of age*, **18.3 mg/kg** of body weight 4 times a day.

Dosage Forms—Granules (for reconstitution): 0.5 and 1 g; Oral Suspension: 250 and 500 mg/5 mL; Tablets: 500 mg and 1 g; Enteric Coated Tablets: 250 and 500 mg and 1 g.

Methylene Blue—page 842.

Nitrofurazone

Hydrazinecarboxamide, 2-[(5-nitro-2-furanyl)methylene]-, Furacin (*Eaton*); Amifur (*SKF*)

$$NO_2 \underset{}{\overset{O}{\diagup\!\!\!\diagdown}} CH=NNHCONH_2$$

5-Nitro-2-furaldehyde semicarbazone [59-87-0] $C_6H_6N_4O_4$ (198.14).

Preparation—By condensing 5-nitro-2-furaldehyde with semicarbazide hydrochloride in the presence of sodium acetate.

Description—Odorless, lemon-yellow, crystalline powder; nearly tasteless, but develops a bitter aftertaste; darkens slowly on exposure to light; melts at about 236° with decomposition; pH (saturated solution) between 5 and 7.5.

Solubility—1 g in 4200 mL water, 590 mL alcohol, 350 mL propylene glycol, and polyethylene glycol mixtures up to about 1%; practically insoluble in chloroform and ether.

Uses—A local antibacterial agent with a broad spectrum of activity. Most bacteria of surface infections of the skin or mucosal surfaces are sensitive to the drug. It is applied topically in the treatment of mixed, superficial infections of the skin. It finds use, especially, in the treatment of second and third degree burns and in skin grafting in which there are complications from bacterial infections that are refractory to the usual drugs of choice but in which bacterial sensitivity to nitrofurazone is demonstrable. It has not yet been shown to be useful in the treatment of minor burns, wounds, or cutaneous ulcers which are infected. Nitrofurazone retains its antibacterial activity in blood, serum, and pus; phagocytosis is not inhibited and nitrofurazone does not interfere with healing. However, it is a slowly acting drug, and at least 24 hours are required for it to take effect properly. Therefore, no treatment should be less than 2 or 3 days in duration.

Approximately 0.5 to 2% of patients become sensitized to the drug, sometimes within 5 days of initiation of treatment. The systemic toxicity is low.

Dose—*Topical*, **0.2%**. The dosage interval and duration of treatment vary with the particular use and dosage form. Five days is the usual duration, except for severe burns. Except in burn therapy, a duration of less than 1 week is usually desirable, to avoid sensitization.

Dosage Forms—Cream: 0.2%; Soluble Dressing: 0.2%.

Caution (for all Nitrofurazone dosage forms)—Avoid exposure at all times to direct sunlight, excessive heat, or alkaline materials.

Nonoxynol 9

α-(*p*-Nonylphenyl)-ω-hydroxytetra(oxyethylene); Igepal CO-630 (*GAF*); Conceptrol (*Ortho*)

$$C_9H_{19}\!-\!\langle\bigcirc\rangle\!-\!(OCH_2CH_2)_n OH$$

(*n* = approx 9)

[26027-38-3] $C_{15}H_{24}O(C_2H_4O)_n$.

Preparation—Reaction between nonylphenol and ethylene oxide.

Description—Almost colorless liquid.

Solubility—Soluble in water, alcohol, polar or chlorinated organic solvents, xylene or corn oil; insoluble in aliphatic hydrocarbons (kerosene).

Uses—Nonoxynol is the most widely used spermaticide in the US. It is 100% effective *in vitro*, but the failure rate in practice probably lies between 2 and 4%, depending on the dosage form, concentration, user care in application and compliance. It appears to be effective in the treatment of cold sores and canker. It also is an ingredient in some products for feminine hygiene.

Dose—*Topical*, high in the vaginal vault, as a **2 to 5%** cream, **8** or **12.5%** foam, **1 to 5%** gel, or **100 mg** as a suppository.

Dosage Forms—Cream: 2, 4, and 5%; foam: 8 and 12.5%; suppositories: 2.27%, 5.56% and 100 mg.

Octoxynol 9

Poly(oxy-1,2-ethanediyl, α-[4-(1,1,3,3-tetramethylbutyl)phenyl]-ω-hydroxy-, Octylphenoxy Polyethoxyethanol NF XII

Polyethylene glycol mono[*p*-(1,1,3,3-tetramethylbutyl)phenyl]-ether [9002-93-1]; an anhydrous liquid mixture of mono-*p*-(1,1,3,3-tetramethylbutyl)phenyl ethers of polyethylene glycols in which *n* varies from 5 to 15, and which has an average molecular weight of 647, corresponding to the formula $C_{34}H_{62}O_{11}$.

Preparation—By reacting *p*-(1,1,3,3-tetramethylbutyl)phenol with ethylene oxide at elevated temperature under pressure in the presence of NaOH.

Description—Clear, pale yellow, viscous liquid, having a faint odor and a bitter taste; specific gravity between 1.059 and 1.068; pH (1 in 100 aqueous solution) between 6 and 8.

Solubility—Miscible with water, alcohol, and acetone; soluble in benzene and in toluene; insoluble in solvent hexane.

Uses—Octoxynol is a nonirritating spermaticide that is widely used in vaginal creams and jellies. It is highly spermaticidal in vitro, but the exact failure rate in practice remains to be determined accurately. It is probably about 2.5% with the cream and 4% with the jelly, rates that reflect differences in dispersion, concentration, and user practice in application.

Octoxynol is a nonionic detergent, emulsifier, and dispersing agent that is a pharmaceutical necessity for *Nitrofurazone Solution*.

Dose—*Topical*, high in the vaginal vault, as **3%** cream or **1%** gel.

Dosage Forms—Concentrate: 50%; cream: 3%; gel: 1%.

Phenazopyridine Hydrochloride

2,6-Pyridinediamine, 3-(phenylazo)-, monohydrochloride; Pyridium (*Parke-Davis*)

2,6-Diamino-3-(phenylazo)pyridine monohydrochloride [136-40-3] $C_{11}H_{11}N_5$.HCl (249.70).

Preparation—Aniline is diazotized with sodium nitrite and excess HCl, and the resulting benzenediazonium chloride is coupled with 2,6-diaminopyridine.

Description—Light or dark red to dark violet, crystalline powder; odorless or has a slight odor; melts at about 235° with decomposition.

Solubility—1 g in <10 mL water, 59 mL alcohol, 331 mL chloroform, >5000 mL ether, 100 mL glycerin.

Uses—An antiseptic drug used in the management of *genitourinary tract infections*. When taken systemically it is quickly excreted into the urine, so that a high local concentration is reached. Thus the drug may be administered either orally or instilled locally. However, a considerable proportion of the drug is metabolically converted to an inactive form, so that large oral doses are required to exert a therapeutic effect. Although the drug may often bring about rapid relief of discomfort, such as pain, burning, urgency, and frequency, in the urinary tract infections, the relief of discomfort is mostly attributable to a local anesthetic action rather than to an antibacterial action. When instilled locally in cystitis, the anesthetic effect may allow other therapeutic measures to be executed with a minimum of pain. Phenazopyridine may occasionally cause gastrointestinal irritation. Jaundice, hemolytic anemia, and methemoglobinemia have been reported. After oral administration the color of the urine may be orange red to dark red, if the urine is acidic. Large doses and prolonged treatment can give rise to renal stones of phenazopyridine. The drug is contraindicated in renal insufficiency, severe hepatitis,

and pyelonephritis of pregnancy, and it should be used cautiously in the presence of gastrointestinal disturbances. Phenazopyridine is often combined with sulfonamides or methenamine salts.

Dose—*Oral, adults*, **50 to 200 mg** 3 or 4 times a day; *usual*, **200 mg** 3 times a day. *Children*, **4 mg/kg** 3 times a day after meals.

Dosage Form—Tablets: 100 and 200 mg.

Phenol—page 1315.

Phenylethyl Alcohol—page 1289.

Pine Tar—page 782.

Polymyxin B Sulfate—page 1202.

Povidone-Iodine

2-Pyrrolidinone, 1-ethenyl-, homopolymer, compd with iodine; Betadine (*Purdue-Frederick*); PVP-Iodine (*GAF*)

1-Vinyl-2-pyrrolidinone polymer compd with iodine [25655-41-8]; contains 9–12% of available iodine.

Preparation—Povidone having an average molecular weight of 40,000 is heated with elemental iodine in the presence of a little water whereby a small amount of the iodine enters into loose organic union with the polymer to form a compound which contains approximately 10% of available iodine.

Description—Yellowish-brown, amorphous powder, having a slight, characteristic odor; aqueous solution is acid to litmus.

Solubility—Soluble in water and alcohol; practically insoluble in chloroform, carbon tetrachloride, ether, solvent hexane, and acetone.

Uses—Povidone-iodine kills both gram-positive and gram-negative bacteria, fungi, viruses, protozoa, and yeasts. The povidone component serves the functions of iodide in iodine solution and tincture, namely, to increase the solubility of iodine and to provide a slow-release form of iodine. The affinity of povidone for iodine is greater than that of iodide, so that the concentration of free iodine is less than 1 part per million. Consequently the immediate bactericidal action of povidone-iodine is only moderate compared to that of iodine solutions. A 10% povidone-iodine solution (1% of available iodine) kills only about 85% of cutaneous bacteria, much less than with iodine solutions or tinctures of comparable iodine content. In fact, the FDA category for povidone-iodine is III. Although it takes 6 to 8 hr for the skin bacterial population to return to normal, which is longer than with iodine solutions, the effective duration of action for surgical purposes is only about an hour, which is about the duration of effective antisepsis with iodine solution or tincture. It is claimed that povidone-iodine stings less than iodine preparations. This is not true; it is iodine tincture that stings, and tinctures of povidone-iodine also sting. Iodine solutions are more effective in wound irrigation. Povidone-iodine stains the skin and clothing less than iodine solutions and is also less irritant under occlusive dressings, which simply reflect that there is less free iodine. Povidone-iodine is sufficiently absorbed from the skin to cause hypothyroidism in infants. It is mutagenic in the Ames test. Therefore, there is no clear advantage of povidone-iodine over iodine solutions or tinctures.

Povidone-iodine antiseptic preparations are clinically indicated for prevention and treatment of surface infections as well as to degerm the skin prior to injection and hyperalimentation procedures; for seborrhea; for disinfection of wounds, burns, lacerations, and abrasions; for preoperative and postoperative scrubbing and washing of hospital operating-room personnel; for preoperative skin preparation of patients.

Dose—*Topical*, **0.5 to 10%** (0.05 to 1% available iodine equivalent). To the skin, 7.5 to 10%, in various liquid forms, as ointment, or as aerosol; to the mouth and pharynx, 0.5 to 1% solution; to the vaginal mucosa as 0.5 to 1% solution or gel; for baths, from 30 to 50 ppm. Available iodine equivalents can be calculated by dividing the povidone-iodine concentration by 10; actual free-iodine concentrations are less than available iodine concentrations.

Dosage Forms—Aerosol: 5%; Solution: 5, 7.5, 10, and 30% (some are diluted before use). Also available as Foam, Gauze, Mouthwash-Gargle (0.5%), Ointment (10%), Shampoo (7.5%), Surgical Scrub/Skin Cleanser (7.5%), Scrub Applicator (2%), Scrub Solution

(2%), Swab (10%), Vaginal Douche (10%), Vaginal Gel (10%), Perineal Wash (10%), Whirlpool Concentrate, for bathing patients (10%).

Salicylic Acid—page 785.

Selenium Sulfide

Selenium Disulfide; Selsun (*Abbott*); Exsel (*Herbert*)

Selenium sulfide (SeS$_2$) [7488-56-4] SeS$_2$ (143.08); contains 52.0 to 55.5% of selenium.

Preparation—Among other ways, by adding an aqueous solution of selenious acid to an aqueous solution containing a stoichiometric excess of hydrogen sulfide.

Description—Reddish brown to bright-orange powder, having not more than a faint odor.

Solubility—Practically insoluble in water and organic solvents.

Uses—An *antibacterial, antifungal,* and *mildly keratolytic* agent used in the local treatment of nonexudative *seborrheas* of the scalp, eyelids, external ear, and glabrous skin. It is effective in the treatment of *pityriasis versicolor*. It is also useful in the management of *acne vulgaris* and *juvenilis* and *atopic eczema*, but it has not been approved for these uses. Some authorities attribute its efficacy to irritant rather than to antibacterial properties; others attribute the effect to cytostatic actions. It induces inflammation of the mucous membranes and exposed tissues, so that care should be exercised in the application of the compound. It also causes "rebound" oiliness of the scalp. It should not be allowed to get into the eyes. Occasionally it causes loss of hair. Although selenium sulfide has considerably lower toxicity than selenites and some other selenium compounds and is available over-the-counter, care should nevertheless be taken to keep preparations away from the mouth.

Dose—*Topical*, to the scalp, **5** or **10 mL** of 1 to **2.5%** lotion and massage, after 2 or 3 min rinse thoroughly and repeat application and rinsing. The 1% cream or lotion is applied in sufficient amount to lather, afterward rinsed, and the treatment repeated.

Dosage Forms—Lotion Shampoo: 1 and 2.5%.

Silver Nitrate

Nitric acid silver(1+) salt; Argenti Nitras

Silver(1+) nitrate [7761-88-8] AgNO$_3$ (169.87).

Preparation—By the action of nitric acid on metallic silver.

Description—Colorless or white crystals; on exposure to light in the presence of organic matter it becomes gray or grayish black; pH of solutions about 5.5.

Solubility—1 g in 0.4 mL water, 30 mL alcohol, about 250 mL acetone, slightly more than 0.1 mL boiling water, and about 6.5 mL of boiling alcohol. It is slightly soluble in ether.

Incompatibilities—Easily reduced to metallic silver by most *reducing agents*, including *ferrous salts, arsenites, hypophosphites, tartrates, sugars, tannins, volatile oils,* and other *organic substances*. In neutral or alkaline solutions, precipitated by *chlorides, bromides, iodides, borax, hydroxides, carbonates, phosphates, sulfates, arsenites,* and *arsenates*. *Potassium permanganate, tannic acid,* and *soluble citrates and sulfates* may cause a precipitate if sufficiently concentrated. In acid solution, only the *chloride, bromide,* and *iodide* are insoluble. *Ammonia water* dissolves many of the insoluble silver salts through formation of the silver diammine complex, Ag(NH$_3$)$_2$$^+$.

Uses—Silver nitrate is an *antiseptic, disinfectant, astringent,* and *caustic*. Silver ion readily combines with proteins, which changes their physical properties. The astringent, caustic, and possibly the germicidal properties are attributable to this action. As an antiseptic, silver ion has a very broad spectrum, which includes staphylococci, streptococci, pseudomonas, and other species that commonly invade burn wounds. Consequently silver nitrate has been used quite successfully in the management of the severely burned patient. However, because silver ion combines with chloride ion in the serum and wound exudates, hypochloremia and other electrolyte disturbances occur, which require constant attention and correction. In the treatment of burns silver nitrate has been replaced by silver sulfadiazine. The compound has also been used in the treatment of traumatic wounds, but present evidence indicates that silver nitrate may actually increase the infection rate. Because of the activity of silver ion against gonococci, the nitrate is still used to prevent gonococcal eye infections in the newborn and was once used by urethral or intravaginal instillation as a venereal prophylactic.

Silver nitrate stains clothing, linens, etc. and may cause argyria, a permanent silver pigmentation of the tissues.

Silver nitrate is a pharmaceutical necessity for the preparation of other therapeutic silver salts, such as *silver sulfadiazine, silver allantoinate,* and *silver protein*. The uses of silver nitrate as a caustic are described under *Toughened Silver Nitrate*, page 784.

Dose—*Topical*, as a **0.5%** solution to *burned areas* of the *skin;* **0.1 mL** of a 1% solution to the *conjunctiva*. A 1:10,000 solution is mildly antiseptic and astringent. It is employed for irrigation of the bladder and urethra. Solutions as strong as 10% are used for local treatment of infected ulcers of the mouth.

Dosage Forms—Applicators: 10%; Solution: 1 and 10%; Ophthalmic solution: 1%.

Silver Sulfadiazine

Benzenesulfonamide, 4-amino-*N*-2-pyrimidinyl-, monosilver (1+) salt; Silvadene (*Marion*)

N^1-2-Pyrimidinylsulfanilamide monosilver(1+) salt [22199-08-2] C$_{10}$H$_9$AgN$_4$O$_2$S (357.13).

Description—A white powder.

Solubility—Practically insoluble in water.

Uses—Silver sulfadiazine combines in one compound the *antibacterial* properties of silver ion and sulfadiazine; it is especially effective against *Pseudomonas aeruginosa*. It is indicated for topical use as an adjunct for prevention and treatment of wound sepsis in patients with second- and third-degree burns. The solubility product of silver sulfadiazine is lower than that of silver chloride, thus insoluble silver chloride is not formed when the drug comes in contact with body fluids and, also, the electrolyte disorders that result from use of silver nitrate in the topical treatment of burns are avoided. Silver sulfadiazine can penetrate the eschar. Although some sulfadiazine is absorbed, it is rarely sufficient to cause crystalluria. However, bacterial resistance to sulfonamides can occur. The drug does not cause pain at the site of application.

Dose—*Topical*, to the affected skin, as 1% cream, applied once or twice daily with sterile, gloved hand.

Dosage Form—Cream, water-miscible: 1%.

Zinc Sulfate

Sulfuric acid, zinc salt (1:1), heptahydrate; White Vitriol; Zinc Vitriol

Zinc sulfate (1:1) heptahydrate [7446-20-0] ZnSO$_4$.7H$_2$O (287.54); *anhydrous* [7733-02-0] (161.44); contains 55.6–61% of ZnSO$_4$, corresponding to 99–108.7% of the hydrated salt.

Preparation—By reacting metallic zinc or zinc oxide with diluted sulfuric acid. It is also prepared by roasting zinc sulfide in a limited supply of oxygen and extracting the sulfate with water.

Description—Colorless, transparent prisms, or small needles, or a granular, crystalline powder; odorless and has an astringent metallic taste; efflorescent in dry air; solutions are acid to litmus.

Solubility—1 g in 0.6 mL water and about 2.5 mL glycerin; insoluble in alcohol.

Incompatibilities—See *Zinc Chloride* (page 779). Combinations of zinc sulfate and *sodium borate* with or without *boric acid* to be used as collyria are frequently troublesome due to precipitation of zinc borate. A quantity of glycerin, equal in weight to the borate, suffices to maintain a clear solution. There is also a tendency for solutions of zinc sulfate to form a slight cloudiness due to the separation of a basic salt formed through partial hydrolysis.

Insoluble sulfates are formed with *lead, barium, strontium,* and *calcium salts. Silver* and *mercury* form slightly soluble salts. Zinc sulfate has a dehydrating action on *methylcellulose* suspensions which leads to precipitation of the latter. *Acacia, proteins,* and *tannins* may also be precipitated.

Uses—An *astringent, emetic,* and weak *antiseptic*. Its antiseptic and astringent properties make it a valuable agent for use as an eyewash (aqueous solution) for the treatment of *conjunctivitis* caused by Morax-Axenfeld bacillus. Antibiotics have largely replaced it in general ophthalmic antiseptics. It may also be applied to the skin as a solution or as *White Lotion* (see page 779) for the treatment of *acne, dandruff, ivy poisoning, lupus erythematosus,* and *impetigo*.

It is the principal ingredient in some deodorant anhidrotics. It is included in some *vulvovaginal deodorants*. Large (but subemetic) doses of zinc accelerate the healing of chronic lesions or wounds, especially in patients with low serum-zinc concentrations. Topical zinc preparations also seem to accelerate the heating of chronic ulcers of the skin. Other disorders reported to respond to oral zinc sulfate are *rheumatoid arthritis* and *acrodermatitis enteropathica*.

Dose—*Topical, ophthalmic*, **0.1 mL** of **0.21** or **0.25%** aqueous solution to the *conjunctiva* 3 or 4 times a day; *dermatologic*, as an *astringent*, **0.5%**, or *antiseptic*, **1%**. As a *deodorant*, **7.5%**. *Oral, adult*, **220 mg** 1 to 3 times a day; *infants*, **50 mg** twice a day. Some physicians have given 660 mg a day, in divided doses, to adults for as long as 4 months. Zinc sulfate is a prompt emetic in doses of 0.6 to 2 g. As a trace element nutrient, see page 1034.

Dosage Forms—Ophthalmic Solution: 0.21 and 0.25%.

Other Antiseptics

Aminacrine Hydrochloride [9-Aminoacridine hydrochloride monohydrate [134-50-9] $C_{13}H_{10}N_2.HCl.H_2O$ (248.72) Monacrin (*Winthrop*)]—Synthesized from *N*-phenylanthranilic acid; a pale yellow, crystalline powder; highly fluorescent. One g is soluble in 300 mL water, 150 mL alcohol; soluble in glycerin. *Uses:* A *broad-spectrum antimicrobial* effective against many gram-positive and gram-negative bacteria, trichomonads, and various fungi, especially *Monilia*. It retains activity in the presence of body fluids, pus, and secretions. Its principal use is in the treatment of infections of the vagina and exocervix, such as moniliasis, trichomonal vaginitis, and infections caused by *Hemophilus vaginalis*, or as a prophylactic agent in various gynecological procedures. *Dose: Intravaginal*, as a 0.2% cream, or 12 mg in a suppository or tampon.

Benzethonium Chloride [*N,N*-Dimethyl-*N*-[2-[2-[4(1,1,3,3-tetramethylbutyl)phenoxy]ethoxy]ethyl]ammonium chloride [121-54-0] $C_{27}H_{42}ClNO_2$ (448.09)]—Prepared from *p*-diisobutylphenol with dichlorodiethyl ether, dimethylamine, and benzyl chloride. *Description and solubility:* Colorless crystals melting about 160°; soluble about 1 g in about 1 mL of water; 1 mL of alcohol; 1 mL of chloroform; 6000 mL of ether. *Uses:* A quaternary ammonium detergent antiseptic and spermaticide once widely used. It has the same limitations and erratic behavior that characterize benzalkonium chloride (page 1159). Its present uses are as a vaginal douche and as a preservative in ophthalmic preparations. *Dose:* To the vagina, as a 3.17% solution of the monohydrate. As a preservative, 0.01%.

Butylparaben [Butyl *p*-hydroxybenzoate [94-26-8] $C_{11}H_{14}O_3$ (194.23)]—Prepared by esterification of *p*-hydroxybenzoic acid with butanol; small, colorless crystals or white powder; melts at about 69°. Very slightly soluble in water; freely soluble in alcohol, ether, chloroform. *Uses:* An antiseptic and preservative, with actions and uses similar to those of methylparaben, with which it is sometimes used in combination. Butylparaben appears to be the best antifungal agent among the parabens. It is used in antiseptic creams and ointments, and in many pharmaceutical products as a preservative. It may occasionally cause hypersensitivity, usually manifested as dermatitis.

p-tert-Butylphenol [4-(1,1-Dimethylethyl)phenol; $C_{10}H_{14}O$ (150.21); ing of Vestal LpH (*Vestal*)]—Prepared by heating phenol with isobutanol; crystalline powder; melts at about 98°. Practically insoluble in cold water; soluble in alcohol, ether, and in sodium hydroxide solution. *Uses:* This phenol has broad-spectrum antibacterial activity against vegetative organisms. It is used as a hospital disinfectant, in about 3% concentration, in mixtures containing other agents.

Cetalkonium Chloride [Benzylhexadecyldimethylammonium chloride [122-18-9] $C_{25}H_{46}ClN$ (396.12)]—Prepared by action of benzyl chloride on (*N,N*-dimethyl)hexadecylamine; colorless crystals; melts at about 59°. Sparingly soluble in cold water; soluble in alcohol, glycerin, ether, chloroform. *Uses:* A *quaternary ammonium disinfectant* with actions similar to those of *Benzalkonium Chloride*. It is used primarily for intended antisepsis of the oral-pharyngeal mucosa and as a preservative. *Dose:* Topical, 0.033% solution; lozenges or troches containing 2.4 or 4 mg.

Cetyldimethylethylammonium Bromide [$C_{20}H_{44}BrN$; ing of Cetacaine, Cetylcide (*Cetylite*)]—White, crystalline powder; soluble in water, alcohol; slightly soluble in chloroform, ether. *Uses:* A *quaternary ammonium disinfectant* with properties similar to those of other agents of that group. Its actions are antagonized by soaps and tissue components. It can cause dermatitides after repeated contact. It is used for sterilization of surgical and dental instruments and in oral topical anesthetics. *Dose:* Topical, as an ingredient in topical anesthetics, 0.005%; for instrument sterilization, 6.5%, with other disinfectants.

Cetylpyridinium Chloride [1-Hexadecylpyridinium chloride monohydrate [6004-24-6] $C_{21}H_{38}ClN.H_2O$ (358.01); Anhydrous [123-03-5] (339.99) Ceepryn, Cepacol (*Merrell-Dow*)]. *Preparation:* From cetyl chloride and pyridine. *Description and solubility:* White powder melting about 72°; soluble 1 g in about 4.5 mL of water, 2.5 mL alcohol, 4.5 mL chloroform. *Uses:* A local anti-infective with surface-active and antiseptic properties against sensitive nonsporulating bacteria. Its antimicrobial spectrum and limitations are those of Benzalkonium Chloride (page 1159). It is used in lozenges, troches and mouthwashes. *Dose:* Topical,

to the mouth and throat, as a 0.5 or 0.05% solution or 0.5, 2.5, or 5 mg in lozenges or troches.

Chlorothymol [4-Chloro-5-methyl-2-(1-methylethyl)phenol; 1-methyl-3-hydroxy-4-isopropyl-6-chlorobenzene [89-68-9] $C_{10}H_{13}ClO$ (184.66)]—Prepared by action of sulfhydryl chloride on thymol in carbon tetrachloride. White crystals or crystalline, granular powder with characteristic odor and an aromatic and very pungent taste; melts at about 62°. One g dissolves in 0.5 mL alcohol, 2 mL chloroform, 1.5 mL ether, practically insoluble in water. *Uses:* An *antiseptic* with greater antibacterial activity than thymol. It is occasionally used in over-the-counter oral antiseptics, mouthwashes, hemorrhoid agents, and preparations for treatment of athlete's foot. It is included in some packaged wash cloths or papers, such as Zephiran Towelettes. Its antibacterial activity is considerably reduced in the presence of organic matter.

Cloflucarban [4,4'-Dichloro-3-(trifluoromethyl)carbanilide [369-77-7] $C_{14}H_9Cl_2F_3N_2O$ (349.15); trifluoromethyldichlorocarbanilide; Irgasan CF3 (*Ciba-Geigy*)]—A white, crystalline powder; melts at about 215°. Insoluble in water; soluble in organic solvents. *Uses:* An *antiseptic* and *disinfectant* agent with greater activity against gram-positive than against gram-negative organisms. It is incorporated into antiseptic soaps, cleaning preparations, and disinfectants. Like other carbanilides, it probably has a potential for sensitization and photosensitization. In a soap formulation it is used in 0.5% concentration, together with 1% of triclocarban.

Clorophene [4-Chloro-α-phenyl-*o*-cresol; *o*-benzyl-*p*-chlorophenol [120-32-1] $C_{13}H_{11}ClO$ (218.69); ing of Vestal LpH (*Vestal*); ing of Lysol (*Lehn & Fink*)]—Prepared by chlorination of *o*-benzylphenol. White or off-white crystals; slight phenolic odor; melts at about 49°. Practically insoluble in water; soluble in solutions of alkali hydroxides. *Uses:* This phenol has broad-spectrum *antibacterial* activity against most vegetative organisms. It is used in combination with other disinfectants in hospital and household disinfectant preparations, in 6.4% concentration in over-the-counter products for the treatment of dandruff, seborrhea, and diaper rash.

Cloroxine [5,7-Dichloro-8-quinolinol [773-76-2] $C_9H_5Cl_2NO$ (214.05)]. *Description and solubility:* Yellowish crystals melting about 180°; slightly soluble in most organic solvents; soluble in fixed acids or bases (amphoteric) forming yellow solutions. *Uses:* A mild antibacterial and antifungal drug that is used for dandruff and seborrheic dermatitis. It is irritating to the eyes. About 0.5% of users will have a form of contact dermatitis. *Dose:* Topical, to the scalp as a 2% shampoo.

Cresol [[1319-77-3] $CH_3C_6H_4OH$ (108.14); Cresylol; Tricresol]—A mixture of isomeric cresols obtained from coal tar or from petroleum; contains not more than 5% of phenol. Colorless, or yellowish to brownish yellow, or a pinkish, highly refractive liquid, becoming darker with age and on exposure to light; phenol-like, sometimes empyreumatic odor; specific gravity 1.030 to 1.038; not less than 90% distils between 195° and 205°; saturated solutions are neutral or slightly acid to litmus. 1 mL dissolves in about 50 mL water, usually forming a cloudy solution; miscible with alcohol, ether, and glycerin; dissolved by solutions of fixed alkali hydroxides. *Uses:* A *disinfectant* and *antiseptic* substance. It resembles phenol in its medicinal properties. Compared to modern antiseptics, its potency is low and its continued use rests mainly on force of habit and low cost. Owing to its greater insolubility in water, it is nearly always employed in combination with alkalies associated with fats or oils, or soaps which render it very soluble but less effective. Saponated cresol solution was an official preparation for several decades. Cresol is a good disinfectant against vegetative bacteria and fungi, but it is poor against viruses and ineffective against spores. Its only medicinal use is in burn and sunburn creams and lotions, in combination with camphor. It is used as a disinfectant on dishes, utensils, and other inanimate objects. It is still used as a disinfectant of floors in hospitals. It is no longer much used as a preservative for injection or other pharmaceutical materials. It is a component of mercocresols. *Application:* 1 to 5% solution on dishes, utensils, and other inanimate objects.

Ethoxazene Hydrochloride [4-[(*p*-Ethoxyphenyl)azo]-*m*-phenylenediamine monohydrochloride [2313-87-3] $C_{14}H_{16}N_4O.HCl$ (292.77); Serenium (*Squibb*)]—A reddish powder; insoluble in water. *Uses:* Ethoxazene hydrochloride has actions, uses, and side effects almost identical to those of *Phenazopyridine Hydrochloride* (page 1164). *Dose:* Oral, *adults* and *children 8 yr of age or older*, 100 mg 3 times a day, before meals; *children under 8 yr of age*, 100 mg twice a day, before meals.

Ethylparaben [Ethyl-*p*-hydroxybenzoate [120-47-8] $C_9H_{10}O_3$ (166.18)]—Prepared by esterification of *p*-hydroxybenzoic acid with ethanol; small, colorless crystals or white powder; melts at about 116°. Slightly soluble in water and in glycerin; freely soluble in alcohol, ether. *Uses:* An antiseptic and preservative, with actions and uses similar to those of methylparaben, with which it is sometimes used in combination. It is used in antiseptic creams, ointments and cosmetics. Like other parabens it may occasionally cause hypersensitivity, usually manifested as dermatitis.

Formaldehyde Solution [Formol; Formalin]—Contains not less than 37%, by weight, of formaldehyde [50-00-0] HCHO (30.03), with methanol added to prevent polymerization. Formaldehyde is prepared by catalytic vapor phase oxidation of methanol, the gas being dissolved in water to produce the required concentration of the solution. Formaldehyde solution is a clear, colorless or nearly colorless liquid having a pungent, irritating odor; on long standing, especially in the cold, it sometimes becomes cloudy due to separation of paraformaldehyde (trioxymethylene). *Uses:* A *disinfectant* and *deodorant.* The solution was once extensively used for disinfecting rooms, which have been subjected to infection, by spraying it on sheets hung in the room, or by releasing formaldehyde vapor into the room from a generator. Formaldehyde is an effective disinfectant against vegetative bacteria, fungi, spores, and viruses only if an adequate time of exposure is provided: in 8% concentration 18 hr are required to kill spores; in 0.5% concentration 2 to 4 days are required for spores and 6 to 12 hr for bacteria. A solution of 20% formaldehyde and 50% ethanol is superior to formaldehyde alone for disinfecting sputa; the ethanol both enhances antimicrobial activity and retards polymerization. It is also used to preserve zoological specimens and cadavers. Formaldehyde can cause dermatitis, allergic reactions and possibly cancer. *Application:* For disinfection of inanimate objects, 10 to 37%.

Gentian Violet [C.O. Basic Violet 3; [4-[bis[*p*-(dimethylamino)phenyl]methylene]-2,5-cyclohexadien-1-ylidene]dimethylammonium chloride [548-62-9] $C_{25}H_{30}ClN_3$ (407.99); methylrosaniline chloride USP XVI; methyl violet; crystal violet]—Hexamethylpararosaniline chloride, usually admixed with pentamethylpararosaniline chloride and tetramethylpararosaniline chloride; generally prepared by oxidizing a mixture of aniline and *p*-toluidine. Pure hexamethylpararosaniline may be obtained by action of carbonyl chloride (phosgene) on *N,N*-dimethylaniline. A dark green powder or greenish glistening pieces having a metallic luster and not more than a faint odor. Sparingly soluble in water; 1 g in about 10 mL alcohol, 15 mL glycerin; soluble in chloroform; insoluble in ether.

Uses: A dye *bactericidal* to gram-positive organisms in very high dilutions. It also acts against the causative organism of Vincent's angina and against many strains of *Monilia, Torula, Epidermophyton,* and *Trichophyton.* Among many conditions once treated with the dye are listed *Vincent's angina, cystitis* and *urethritis, suppurating joint infections, eczematoid dermatitis, furunculosis, recurrent dermatomycosis, monilial paronychia, chronic ulcers, bed sores, impetigo, pruritus ani, leukorrhea* and *vaginitis,* etc. The drug has been largely outmoded by the antibiotics and systemic antibacterial drugs, not so much because of its inefficacy but because of its cosmetic effects and staining of clothing. Gentian violet has also been used in the treatment of *burns,* forming a pliable eschar and helping to control infection from gram-positive organisms; it is little used at present for this purpose. It is mainly used to treat vaginal infections caused by *Candida. Dose: Topical,* 0.25 to 1% solution twice a day. For instillation in closed cavities a 0.01% solution should be used. A vaginal tampon containing 5 mg is inserted and retained for 3 or 4 hours, once or twice daily, for 12 days. A 2-mg vaginal tablet is used nightly, or morning and night. For treatment of burns a 1% solution is sprayed over the burned tissue at 2-hour intervals.

Hexylresorcinol [4-Hexylresorcinol [136-77-6] $C_{12}H_{18}O_2$ (194.27); AT37]—*Caution—Hexylresorcinol is irritating to the oral mucosa and respiratory tract and to the skin, and its solution in alcohol has vesicant properties. Preparation:* Resorcinol is heated with caproic acid [$CH_3(CH_2)_4COOH$] in the presence of zinc chloride as a condensing agent. The resulting caproylresorcinol is then heated with amalgamated zinc and hydrochloric acid (Clemensen's reduction) whereby the CO of the caproyl group is reduced to CH_2 yielding hexylresorcinol. *Description:* White, or yellowish white, needle-shaped crystals; has a faint odor and a sharp, astringent taste, and produces a sensation of numbness when placed on the tongue; acquires a brownish pink tint on exposure to light and air; melts between 62° and 67°. *Solubility:* 1 g in about 2000 mL water; freely soluble in alcohol, methanol, glycerin, ether, chloroform, benzene, and vegetable oils. *Uses:* Hexylresorcinal has a high phenol coefficient and was once widely employed as an antiseptic. As a skin wound cleanser, it was placed in category I by the FDA Advisory Panel on Antimicrobial Drugs. In addition to bactericidal activity, it has fungicidal activity. It is presently marketed only as a minor antiseptic for cuts, abrasions, minor burns, mouthwash and for sore throat. In part, relief is attributable to local anesthetic activity. It can cause irritation. *Dose: Topical,* to the skin or mouth as a 0.1% glycerine-aqueous solution or as 2.4 or 4 mg lozenge.

Hydrogen Peroxide Solution [Hydrogen peroxide [7722-84-1] H_2O_2 (34.01); hydrogen dioxide]—Hydrogen peroxide may be prepared by many methods, one of the important ones involving electrolysis of sulfuric acid in a solution containing sulfate, whereby persulfate is formed, which is hydrolyzed to hydrogen peroxide. Solutions containing up to about 90% H_2O_2 may be obtained by distillation, higher concentrations by fractional crystallization. The official hydrogen peroxide solution contains 2.5 to 3.5 g of H_2O_2 in each 100 mL. *Description:* Clear, colorless liquid, odorless or having an odor resembling that of ozone. Usually deteriorates on standing or on protracted agitation; decomposes rapidly when in contact with many oxidizing or reducing substances. When rapidly heated, it may decompose suddenly. *Uses:* A much overrated *germicide* active by virtue of release of nascent oxygen; it is short-acting because the release occurs rapidly. It is a relatively feeble germicide with poor penetrability. Its chief value is in cleansing of wounds where the effervescence caused by release of oxygen provides for mechanical removal of tissue debris from inaccessible regions. It is somewhat effective as a mouthwash in the treatment of *Vincent's stomatitis;* continued use for this purpose may lead to the condition known as "hairy tongue." The solution may be employed in the treatment of *Trichomonas vaginalis vaginitis* and of *balanitis,* but it is much inferior to metronidazole. It is also popularly used as a hair bleach. *Dose: Topical,* for cleansing wounds, 1.5 to 3% solution; as mouthwash, 3% solution; for intravaginal use, 2% solution.

Lime, Chlorinated [Bleaching powder; "chloride of lime"]—Prepared by passing chlorine over calcium hydroxide; a complex compound of indefinite composition that rapidly decomposes on exposure to air. It contains not less than 30% *w/w* of available chlorine. Partially soluble in water and in alcohol. *Uses:* A *disinfectant, deodorant,* and *bleach,* variously used for these purposes: to disinfect feces, urine, and sanitary utensils; for purification of drinking water (1 oz to 2000 gal); for disinfection of swimming pool water (0.25 to 1 ppm of free chlorine); for removal of dyes from the skin. It is used as a household bleach.

Merbromin [2′,7′-Dibromo-4′-(hydroxymercuri)fluorescein disodium salt [129-16-8] $C_{20}H_8Br_2HgNa_2O_6$ (750.67); Mercurochrome]—Iridescent, green scales or granules; freely soluble in water, forming a red solution with a yellow-green fluorescence. *Uses:* Formerly a popular and highly regarded antiseptic. On the skin or in wounds it cannot be relied on to reduce the bacterial population by more than half. It has the lowest therapeutic index of the organomercurials. It is inactivated by serous fluids and tissue constituents. It never deserved a place in first aid kits and in the medicine cabinet.

Mercuric Oxide, Yellow [[21908-53-2] HgO (216.59); Yellow Precipitate]—For preparation see RPS-15, page 1103. A yellow to orange-yellow, heavy, impalpable powder; becomes discolored and decomposes on exposure to air. Practically insoluble in water; insoluble in alcohol. *Uses:* In the form of a 1% ointment used for *inflammation of the eyes, pruritus ani,* and *epidermophytosis;* now largely replaced by other and safer agents.

Mercury, Ammoniated [[10124-48-8] $HgNH_2Cl$ (252.07); White Precipitate]—Prepared by adding an aqueous solution of mercury bichloride to a large excess of an aqueous solution of ammonia. White, pulverulent pieces, or a white, amorphous powder; stable in air but darkens on exposure to light. Insoluble in water and alcohol. *Uses:* Applied as an ointment, ammoniated mercury was once used in the treatment of cutaneous infections, *impetigo, ringworm, pruritus ani, pinworm,* and *crab louse infestation.* Its present use is mainly in the treatment of psoriasis. The drug sensitizes the skin, and patients need to be watched for drug-induced lesions. It is capable of causing chronic mercury intoxication with prolonged use. Preparations containing iodine enhance absorption of the mercurial, so that they should not be applied shortly before or concomitantly with ammoniated mercury. Since superior or less toxic drugs are available to treat conditions for which ammoniated mercury is most efficacious, there is no need to use this drug at present. *Dose: Topical,* as a 5% ointment 2 or 3 times a day.

Methenamine Hippurate [Hexamethylenetetramine monohippurate [5714-73-8] $C_6H_{12}N_4.C_9H_9NO_3$ (319.36); Hiprex (*Merrell-National*); Urex (*Riker*)]—Prepared by the interaction of methenamine and hippuric acid in methanol solution. US Pat 3,004,026. Fine, white, crystalline powder; practically odorless; melts at about 115°. Freely soluble in water, alcohol, chloroform. *Uses:* A *urinary tract antiseptic* which depends on release of formaldehyde from methenamine for its antibacterial action, the hippuric acid component lowering urine pH and thus facilitating conversion of methenamine to formaldehyde. Hippuric acid is secreted by the renal tubular anion transport system, so that urine concentrations are initially higher than those of mandelic acid from methenamine mandelate. Wide fluctuations in urine levels of hippuric acid are detrimental to the therapeutic action of the methenamine unless the pH of urine stays below 6. Nausea, dysuria, and rash occasionally occur. *Dose:* 1 g 2 times a day. The dose for children of ages 6 to 12 is 500 mg to 1 g 2 times a day.

Methylbenzethonium Chloride [Benzyldimethyl[2-[2-[[4-(1,1,3,3-tetramethylbutyl)tolyl]oxy]ethoxy]ethyl]ammonium chloride monohydrate [1320-44-1] $C_{28}H_{44}ClNO_2.H_2O$ (480.13); *anhydrous* [25155-18-4] (462.11). Diaparene Chloride (*Breon*)]. *Preparation:* By the method described for *Benzethonium Chloride* except that cresol is employed instead of phenol. Inasmuch as the starting cresol contains both the *o*- and *m*-isomers, the corresponding isomers of the quaternary are both present in the final product. *Description:* White, hygroscopic crystals, mild odor, very bitter taste; solutions are neutral or slightly alkaline to litmus; melts between 159° and 163°. *Solubility:* 1 g in 0.8 mL water, 0.9 mL alcohol, >10,000 mL chloroform, 0.7 mL ether. *Uses:* A quaternary ammonium antiseptic with actions and limitations like those of *Benzalkonium Chloride.* It is ineffective against sporulating organisms. At present, its primary use is in the treatment of *ammonia dermatitis* (diaper rash), by application both to the skin and to diapers, undergarments, and bed linens. Like other quaternary detergent antiseptics, it is inactivated by soap and inhibited by organic matter. Quaternary ammonium antiseptics can cause sensitization, usually manifested as rashes. *Dose: Topical,* as a 0.1 or 0.2% cream or 0.067, 0.1, or 0.13% ointment and as a powder, in combination with various other ingredients.

Methylparaben [Methyl *p*-hydroxybenzoate [99-76-3] $C_8H_8O_3$ (152.15); Methyl Parasept; Nipagin M; Solbrol]—Prepared by esterification of *p*-hydroxybenzoic acid with methanol. Colorless crystals or white, crystalline powder; faint, characteristic odor; melts at about 126°. One g dissolves in 400 mL water, 3 mL alcohol, 10 mL ether, soluble in glycerin, oils, fats. *Uses:* An antiseptic and preservative used in various pharmaceutical preparations in concentrations of 0.05 to 0.25%; also used in cosmetic preparations containing vegetable and animal fats and oils that are susceptible to decomposition. Where a strong antiseptic effect is desired, 3 to 5 times the usual concentration may be used. Combinations of two or more esters of *p*-hydroxybenzoic acid have a "synergistic" antiseptic action; thus a preparation containing 0.15% of the propyl ester (propylparaben) and 0.05% of the benzyl ester is said to have a stronger antiseptic action than 0.2% of either ester alone. All parabens are capable of sensitizing the skin and inducing cutaneous allergic responses, although the incidence of such reactions is low. Allergy from oral ingestion or parenteral administration has not been reported. Topical antibiotic or corticosteroid preparations may contain 0.3% of parabens. A combination of 0.18% methylparaben and 0.02% propylparaben is approved for use as a preservative for certain parenteral solutions. Methylparaben is used in combination with propylparaben as a preservative in artificial tears.

Oxychlorosene [[8031-14-9] $C_{20}H_{35}ClO_4S$ (407.02); Clorpactin XCB (*Guardian*)]—Described as a buffered hypochlorous acid derivative of a mixture of long-chain alkylbenzenesulfonates; an antiseptic and surfactant. *Uses:* A topical antiseptic by virtue of its hypochlorite component. Effective against most bacteria and their spores, viruses, yeasts, and fungi. A 0.4% solution in sodium chloride injection is used as a local irrigant during surgery of neoplasms. Solutions of *oxychlorosene sodium* are used topically for treating localized infections and for removing necrotic debris. For bladder irrigation 0.1 to 0.2% solutions are used.

Oxyquinoline [8-Hydroxyquinoline [148-24-3] C_9H_7NO (145.14)]—White crystals or crystalline powder; melts at about 76°. Almost insoluble in water, ether; freely soluble in alcohol, chloroform. *Uses:* A *bacteriostatic* and *fungistatic* compound. It is included in preparations for the treatment of acne and cold sores (1.82%) and canker and in vaginal douches (0.1%). *Oxyquinoline sulfate*, which is freely soluble in water and in about 100 parts of glycerin, is used in the treatment of athlete's foot; it is used in concentrations of 0.06 to 0.25%. It is also used in burn and sunburn medicaments.

Parachlorometaxylenol [4-Chloro-3,5-xylenol [88-04-0], Chloroxylenol; C_8H_9ClO (156.61)]—Prepared by treating 3,5-dimethylphenol with chlorine. White crystals or crystalline powder that discolors readily; melts at about 115°. One g dissolves in 3000 mL water, 1 mL alcohol; soluble in ether, fixed oils. *Uses:* A disinfectant active against streptococci but less active against staphylococci and almost inactive against certain gram-negative organisms; inactive against spores; activity reduced in contact with blood or serum. Used for topical antisepsis in the treatment of minor burns, acne, seborrhea, and in the treatment of athlete's foot. It is used as a counterirritant in some topical analgesic preparations. The substance is allergenic. *Dose: Topical*, as 0.3 to 1% ointment, cream, or lotion or 2% shampoo.

Parachlorophenol [*p*-Chlorophenol [106-48-9] C_6H_5ClO (128.56)]—Prepared by chlorination of melted phenol with sulfuryl chloride. White or pink crystals with a characteristic phenolic odor; melts at about 42°. Very soluble in alcohol, glycerin, chloroform, ether, fixed and volatile oils; sparingly soluble in water. *Uses:* A *local antibacterial* agent similar in properties and uses to phenol; the introduction of chlorine in the molecule of phenol increases germicidal activity but the toxicity and caustic action are also increased. It is used principally in dental practice for root canal therapy, in 1 to 5% concentration in various solutions or as *camphorated parachlorophenol*, which is prepared by triturating 35% of parachlorophenol with 65% camphor until they liquefy.

p-tert-Pentylphenol [[80-46-6] $C_{11}H_{16}O$ (164.24)]—A crystalline powder, melting at about 95°. Practically insoluble in water; soluble in alcohol, ether, chloroform. *Uses:* This phenol has broad-spectrum *antibacterial* activity against vegetative organisms. It is marketed in a lubricant jelly for lubricating endoscopes and for application to the skin and mucous membranes; the jelly contains 0.02% of the phenol and also other antiseptic drugs.

Phenylmercuric Acetate [(Acetato)phenylmercury [62-38-4] $C_8H_8HgO_2$ (336.74).] *Preparation:* Readily formed by heating benzene with mercuric acetate. *Description and Solubility:* White to creamy white, crystalline powder or as small white prisms or leaflets; odorless; melts between 149° and 153°; soluble 1 g in 180 mL water, 225 mL alcohol, 6.8 mL chloroform, 200 mL ether. *Uses:* Actions are similar to those of *Phenylmercuric Nitrate*. It is used in contraceptives and vaginal douches, eyewashes and ophthalmological preparations. It serves as a preservative in various drug preparations. *Dose:* For *application* to the *skin*, as a 0.2% solution in 50% alcohol; as a *preservative*, in concentrations of 0.002 to 0.125%; in *vaginal suppositories* and *jellies*, 0.02%.

Phenylmercuric Nitrate [Nitratophenylmercury [55-68-5]; a mixture of phenylmercuric nitrate [$C_6H_5HgNO_3$ (339.70)] and phenylmercuric hydroxide [C_6H_5HgOH (249.70)] containing 87–87.9% of $C_6H_5Hg^+$ (phenylmercuric ion), and 62.75–63.5% of Hg (mercury). This chemical is a basic salt. The normal nitrate [$C_6H_5HgNO_3$] has also been prepared, but it is unstable, decomposing into the basic compound on contact with water.] *Preparation: Phenylmercuric Acetate* is refluxed in benzene with ammonium nitrate and the normal phenylmercuric nitrate thus formed is subjected to hydrolysis to form the basic salt. *Description and solubility:* White, crystalline powder; affected by light; saturated aqueous solution is acid to litmus; melts between 175° and 185°; soluble 1 g in 600 mL water; slightly soluble in alcohol or glycerin; more soluble in the presence of either nitric acid or alkali hydroxides. *Uses:* A *local antibacterial* agent for external use in solution or ointment as an antiseptic for prophylactic and therapeutic disinfection of the *skin, superficial abrasions, lacerations, wounds,* and *infections.* It is also used in vaginal

preparations to reduce odor and to maintain bacterial, trichomonal, and fungal growth at a minimum. It is used in several preparations for treatment of hemorrhoids. Phenylmercuric nitrate is used as a preservative in solutions employed to clean or wet contact lenses. Like all mercurials, it is inferior to iodine, iodophors, and chlorhexidine against staphylococci of the skin. It can cause skin rashes. Prolonged topical application can result in mercury intoxication. *Dose:* For *topical application* to the *skin* or *mucosae*, as a 0.1 to 0.033% tincture; as a *preservative in pharmaceuticals*, 0.0025%.

Poloxamer-Iodine—A compound of a type of poly(oxypropylene)-poly(oxyethylene) copolymer (a poloxamer) with iodine; contains approximately 10% of available iodine. *Uses:* An iodophor very similar to *Povidone-Iodine* in its *antiseptic* properties and uses. When the two compounds are compared in equal concentrations, poloxamer-iodine yields about twice as high a free-iodine concentration, but the clinical efficacies appear to be the same. *Dose: Topical*, to the skin, the equivalent of 0.75 to 1% iodine (7.5 to 10% of the complex). *Dosage Forms:* Concentrated Liquid: 5%; Surgical Scrub Liquid: 0.75%; Solution: 1%; Swabs: 1%; Whirlpool Additive: 1%. The concentrations indicated are of titratable iodine; for equivalent concentrations of the complex, multiply by 10.

Potassium Permanganate [Permanganic acid ($HMnO_4$), potassium salt [7722-64-7] $KMnO_4$ (158.03)]—May be prepared by oxidizing manganese dioxide with potassium chlorate in potassium hydroxide solution, then completing the oxidation with chlorine or air and carbon dioxide. Dark purple crystals or small crystals of dark bronze-like color; 1 g dissolves in 15 mL water. A powerful oxidizing agent that may produce an explosion when triturated with organic matter or other readily oxidizable substances. *Uses:* A strong *oxidizing agent*, exerting antibacterial and antifungal actions against organisms susceptible to nascent oxygen. When 0.01% solutions are used the action is slow and may require an hour to be effective; solutions of 0.02% concentration are irritating to tissues. Thus the agent has a low therapeutic index and is best forgotten. It is occasionally used in the treatment of *urethritis.* Irrigation of the bladder with a solution is sometimes effective in the treatment of persistent urinary infections. It is sometimes employed for the vesicular lesions of epidermophytosis, in the vesicular stage of eczema dermatitis, and in the treatment of ivy poisoning; manganous and manganic ions resulting from reduction of permanganate exert astringent actions in these uses. Potassium permanganate is capable of oxidizing certain drugs and venoms. In the treatment of poisoning following oral ingestion of barbiturates, chloral hydrate, and many alkaloids, gastric lavage with a solution of potassium permanganate helps to destroy the poison and thus prevent absorption. Permanganate solution should not be left in the stomach. Application of permanganate crystals to snake bites to promote oxidation of the venom probably does not destroy the venom sufficiently to affect its actions. *Dose: Topical*, 0.004 to 1% solution 2 or 3 times a day or in a wet dressing. For urethritis, 0.025%; for bladder irrigation, 0.02%; for ivy poisoning or eczema, 0.01%; for epidermophytosis, 1%; for gastric lavage, 0.02%. *Dosage Form:* Tablets for Solution: 300 mg.

Propylene Oxide [Methyloxirane [75-56-9] C_3H_6O (58.08)]—Prepared by action of aqueous potassium hydroxide solution on propylene chlorohydrin. A colorless, ethereal liquid, extremely flammable; boils at about 34°. Miscible with water (to the extent of about 40% by weight), with alcohol and with ether. *Uses:* Propylene oxide is *microbicidal* to all microorganisms, including viruses and spores. Because it is a liquid, it is easier to handle than ethylene oxide, but because its boiling point is quite low it can also be used in the vapor phase like ethylene oxide. Its high solubility in water permits its use in solutions. It has the same toxic potential as ethylene oxide, and careful rinsing and/or desorption after its use are necessary. *Application:* As 5% solution with 70% isopropanol or other antiseptics with which it does not react.

Propylparaben [Propyl *p*-hydroxybenzoate [94-13-3] $C_{10}H_{12}O_3$ (180.20)]—Prepared by esterification of *p*-hydroxybenzoic acid with propanol. Colorless crystals or white powder; melts at about 96°. One g dissolves in 2500 mL water, 1.5 mL alcohol, 3 mL ether. *Uses:* An *antifungal* preservative, often used with *Methylparaben.*

Pyrithione Zinc [Bis[1-hydroxy-2(1*H*)-pyridinethionato]zinc [13463-41-7] $C_{10}H_8N_2O_2S_2Zn$ (317.68); Danex (*Herbert*); Head & Shoulders (*Procter & Gamble*); Zincon (*Lederle*)]—Pyrithione may be prepared by oxidizing 2-bromopyridine to its *N*-oxide with perbenzoic or peracetic acid, followed by treatment with sodium sulfide or sodium hydrosulfide; the water-soluble sodium salt thus obtained is converted to the relatively insoluble zinc salt by reaction with zinc ion. An off-white powder with a slight odor. Practically insoluble in water; very slightly soluble in alcohol. *Uses:* Possesses *antibacterial* and *antifungal* activity. Used in the treatment of *seborrhea sicca;* a mild cytostatic action is believed to be responsible for the antiseborrheic action. It is reported to be strongly bound to both hair and skin and that the binding is correlated with clinical effectiveness. Zinc pyrithione is the active ingredient of many antidandruff shampoo formulations, in which is used in 1 to 2% concentration, along with anionic surfactants.

Silver Protein, Mild [9008-39-3] Mild Silver Protein; Mild Protargin; Argyrol (*Smith, Miller & Patch*)]—Prepared by interaction of silver oxide with a protein in the presence of alkali; contains 19–23% silver, largely nonionized. Dark brown or almost black, shining scales or granules; odorless, frequently hygroscopic, and affected by light. Freely soluble in water, forming a dark-colored solution; practically insoluble in alcohol, chloroform, ether. *Uses:* Formerly widely used in the treatment of conjunctivitis, cystitis, nose and throat infections, and in prophylaxis of gonorrhea. It is now considered archaic. Both local and generalized argyria can follow indiscriminate or long-continued application to mucous membranes. *Dose: Topical,* in 5 to 25% solution to the skin or mucous membranes up to several times a day as required.

Sodium Benzoate [[532-32-1] $C_7H_5NaO_2$ (144.11)]—White, granular or crystalline powder; 1 g dissolves in 2 mL water, 75 mL alcohol. *Uses:* Extensively as a *food* and *pharmaceutical preservative,* the only one permitted to be used for many classes of food products. To be effective the pH of the preparation in which it is used must not be above 4. It is not bactericidal, only bacteriostatic. It also has fungistatic activity. Sodium benzoate is sometimes used as a test for liver function by measuring the amount of hippuric acid, its metabolite, excreted in urine.

Sodium Hypochlorite Solution—An aqueous solution containing 4.0 to 6.0% w/w of sodium hypochlorite [7681-52-9] NaClO (74.44). Prepared by electrolysis of a solution of sodium chloride in a cell permitting reaction of chlorine with sodium hydroxide; an equivalent quantity of sodium chloride is simultaneously produced. A clear, pale greenish yellow liquid having a slight odor of chlorine; affected by light. *Uses:* A powerful *disinfectant* and *deodorant,* also a *bleaching agent.* Not only is it effective against vegetative bacteria, but also against viruses and to some degree against spores and fungi. It is used for disinfecting utensils and apparatus. The 5% solution is not usually used on or in the human, although it is sometimes used in root canal therapy and is considered by some authorities to be much better than parachlorophenol for this purpose. For therapeutic uses it is employed in the form of *Diluted Sodium Hypochlorite Solution,* described in the following article.

Sodium Hypochlorite Solution, Diluted—An aqueous solution of chlorine compounds of sodium containing, in each 100 mL, the equivalent of 450 to 500 mg of NaClO. The solution may be prepared by diluting *Sodium Hypochlorite Solution* with nine volumes of purified water and adding sufficient 5% sodium bicarbonate solution until no red color is produced with powdered phenolphthalein. The resulting solution is assayed and diluted with sufficient purified water to make the final solution contain, in each 100 mL, 450 to 500 mg of NaClO. *Uses:* Employed in full strength, as a freshly prepared solution. It is used in the treatment of suppurating wounds, often by continuous irrigation (Carrel technique). Not only does the solution exert a *germicidal action* but it also dissolves *necrotic tissue.* Disadvantages are that sodium hypochlorite solutions dissolve blood clots, delay clotting, and are irritating to the skin. For prophylaxis of *epidermophytosis,* diluted sodium hypochlorite solution is sometimes employed as a foot bath. The solution is also a *deodorant.* *Dose: Topical,* as solution containing 0.15 to 0.5% of NaClO. The full-strength solution contains 0.5% NaClO; to prepare the 0.15% solution it should be diluted 1 to 3.

Succinic Dialdehyde [Butanedial; $C_4H_6O_2$ (86.09)]—By any method of synthesis a polymer is formed that must be distilled *in vacuo* to obtain the monomer. A solid, melting at 65° and boiling at 169°. *Uses:* Succinic dialdehyde is microbicidal to all microorganisms, including spores and viruses. Its properties and uses are closely similar to those of *glutaral* (glutaraldehyde), page 1160. *Application:* As a 10% solution containing 2,5-dimethyloxytetrahydrofuran as a stabilizing agent.

Thimerosal [Ethyl (sodium-*o*-mercaptobenzoato)mercury [54-64-8] ($C_9H_9HgNaO_2S$ (404.81); Merthiolate (*Lilly*)]—*Preparation:* An ethanolic solution of thiosalicylic acid is treated with ethylmercuric chloride (or hydroxide) in the presence of NaOH. *Description and solubility:* Light cream-colored, crystalline powder with a slight characteristic odor; pH (1% solution) about 6.7; affected by light; soluble 1 g in 1 mL water, 12 mL alcohol; almost insoluble in ether. *Uses:* A relatively nontoxic *antibacterial* agent with both weak bacteriostatic and mild fungistatic properties. Spore-forming bacteria are particularly resistant. On the skin, thimerosal tincture is less effective than is the solvent alone. However, it is somewhat more effective than the aqueous solution. It is used to *disinfect skin surfaces.* It is also applied to wound and abrasions, and also the eye, nose, throat, and urethra. Thimerosal is quite inferior to iodine, iodophors, and chlorhexidine. Because of this, it is surprising that thimerosal is still included in first-aid kits and used by physicians. Thimerosal can be used in a concentration of 1:10,000 in whole blood, plasma, or serum as a preservative; no untoward effects caused by such mercurial-containing blood products have been reported. Mercury poisoning has occurred from prolonged application to oral-pharyngeal or rectal mucosae. *Dose: Topical,* 0.1% to the *skin* as a solution, tincture, cream, aerosol or glycerite.

Thymol [*p*-Cymen-3-ol [89-83-8] $C_{10}H_{14}O$ (150.22)]—Obtained from volatile oil of *Thymus vulgaris* Linné (Fam *Labiatae*) by fractional distillation, also from other botanical sources. May be synthesized from *p*-cymene, also by interaction of *m*-cresol and isopropyl chloride. Colorless crystals or white, crystalline powder; aromatic, thyme-like odor; pungent taste; melts at about 50°. When triturated with camphor, menthol, chloral hydrate, and some other substances, the mixture liquefies. One g dissolves in about 1000 mL water, 1 mL alcohol, 1 mL chloroform, 1.5 mL ether, 2 mL olive oil. *Uses:* An *antifungal* and *antibacterial* agent. Its phenol coefficient is about 50. It is incorporated in some lotions and creams for treatment of acne; also in ointments for treatment of hemorrhoids. Thymol is included in mouthwashes for its antiseptic action, but such preparations have been shown to have little germicidal efficacy. It is included as a counterirritant in topical analgesic mixtures. *Dose: Topical,* 0.5% to the skin and 1% to the vagina.

Triclocarban [3,4,4'-Trichlorocarbanilide [101-20-1] $C_{13}H_9Cl_3N_2O$ (315.59)]—Prepared from 3,4-dichloroaniline and 4-chlorophenyl isocyanate. Fine, white to off-white powder; slight characteristic odor; melts at about 256°. Practically insoluble in water. *Uses:* An *antifungal* and *antibacterial* agent incorporated in some antiseptic and deodorant soaps and other cleansing preparations, and into some preparations for treatment of acne. It is capable of causing photoallergic reactions. Used in 0.5 to 1.5% concentration in marketed products.

Triclosan [2,4,4'-Trichloro-2'-hydroxydiphenyl ether [3380-34-5] $C_{12}H_7Cl_3O_2$ (289.54); Irgasan DP 300 (*Ciba-Geigy*)]—White to off-white, crystalline powder or soft agglomerates, melting at about 56°. Practically insoluble in water; soluble in dilute sodium hydroxide solution. *Uses:* Has broad-spectrum *antibacterial* activity against vegetative organisms. It is used in soaps for disinfection of the skin, in surgical scrubs, and in deodorants, in concentrations of 0.1 to 2%.

Systemic Antibacterial Drugs

During the early part of this century, giant strides were made in the systemic treatment of certain microzoal infections. Nevertheless, these advances did not greatly affect directly the overall practice of medicine. The advent of sulfanilamide in 1935 marked the beginning of a major revolution in the practice of medicine. The subsequent profusion of antibacterial agents overwhelmed the physician with golden tools. Several leading causes of death were deposed to a minor status and some to a mere nuisance. The consequent lengthening of the life span turned medicine toward the degenerative diseases and the problems of aging. The social, economic, and political consequences of these effects will reverberate for generations. Meanwhile, certain of the arts of "non-drug" management of infection have nearly been forgotten, and carelessness has been fostered by the glitter and security of the "wonder drugs." The realization that certain microorganisms are successfully resisting the "wonder drugs" not only impels a ceaseless search for new systemic antibacterial agents but also forces a sober return to certain ancillary arts of the medical and surgical management of infectious disease.

Although certain of the drugs listed in this section are used only for their local actions, their obvious relationship to parent systemic agents warrants their inclusion.

In the dose statements under the various drugs, the permissible range of doses is usually indicated. The reader can assume the low dose is for use in mild infections or in patients with abnormally low rates of elimination and that the high dose is for use in serious or very serious infections or in patients with abnormally high rates of elimination. With many drugs, oral medication should never be used in serious infections, either because of intolerance to appropriately high doses or to erratic or limited absorption; thus parenteral administration may be obligatory. Serious untoward effects are much more likely to occur with parenteral, especially intravenous, administration, so that for most drugs intravenous use should be replaced by oral or intramuscular use at the earliest possible time that the patient's condition permits.

Treatment should always extend at least 2 or 3 days after signs of infection have cleared, and in some types of infections for weeks or months. There are rare exceptions, such as the single-dose treatment of acute gonorrhea. These details are not given in the monographs, but they are usually found in the package inserts or other descriptive literature.

Sulfonamides

History—The compound *p*-aminobenzenesulfonamide, now known as *sulfanilamide*, was first synthesized in 1908, but it was many years before its therapeutic value was discovered. In 1932, a German firm prepared a red dye, 4-(4′-sulfamylphenylazo)-*m*-phenylenediamine or, *p*′-sulfamylchrysoidine, and in 1935 Domagk reported remarkable curative effects of this compound and named it *Prontosil*. In the same year, a group of French investigators found that the antibacterial property of the drug resided in the *p*-aminobenzenesulfonamide portion of the molecule. In 1937 Ewins and Phillips of England synthesized sulfapyridine, which was the first sulfonamide used with great success in combating pneumonia. Then followed sulfathiazole, sulfadiazine, and a large number of other sulfonamides. Over 3300 sulfonamides have since been prepared, but only a few have been accepted for medicinal use.

All the official, and generally all the therapeutically useful, antimicrobial sulfonamides are characterized by the following structure:

Preparation—*p*-Acetamidobenzenesulfonyl chloride, made by treating acetanilide with chlorosulfonic acid, is the basic intermediate of all the sulfonamides. This is treated with the desired amine in the presence of a weak base such as pyridine, and the resulting acetyl compound is deacetylated via proton- or hydroxyl-catalyzed hydrolysis. The reactions taking place in the synthesis of sulfadiazine are illustrated in the following:

Antimicrobial Properties—The sulfonamides originally possessed a wide antimicrobial spectrum which included all gram-positive cocci, except enterococcus, all gram-positive bacilli, nearly all *Enterobacteriaceae* and gram-negative cocci, *H influenzae*, *B pertussis*, *Pasteurella*, some *Pseudomonas*, *Chlamydia* (psittacosis, *Trachoma*, *Lymphogranuloma venereum*), *Actinomycetes*, *Nocardia*, and some *Toxoplasma* and malaria. However, resistance to the drugs has greatly limited the spectrum. The extent of acquired resistance to sulfonamides varies among communities, so that sensitivity testing is essential to the optimal use of these drugs. In most circumstances, these agents exert only a bacteriostatic action, and ultimate elimination of the invading microorganisms is dependent upon the cellular and humoral defense mechanisms of the host, which are neither enhanced nor inhibited by the sulfonamides. However, bactericidal concentrations of these agents are sometimes attained in the urinary and intestinal tracts, where the concentration of drug may be quite high.

The mechanism of the antimicrobial action of the sulfonamides has been analyzed extensively. The sulfonamides compete with *p*-aminobenzoic acid and prevent its normal cellular utilization, particularly its incorporation into folic acid

(pteroylglutamic acid, PGA). Thus, sulfonamide-sensitive organisms are primarily those which synthesize their own folic acid. Organisms able to utilize preformed folic or tetrahydrofolic acid or the tetrahydrofolate-dependent pyrimidines and thymidine are not generally affected by these agents. This mechanism is of importance as an example of the general concepts of *biological antagonism* and *antimetabolites*. The efficacy of sulfonamides is generally enhanced when the drugs are used in combination with the folic acid antagonist trimethoprim.

Microorganisms initially sensitive to the sulfonamides may become resistant to these drugs. The clinical importance of such acquired bacterial resistance is attested by the fact that the majority of the strains of *Neisseria gonorrhoeae* now isolated from patients with gonococcal urethritis are resistant to these agents, whereas the sulfonamides were once the agents of choice against such organisms. *Enterobacteriaceae* have especially become resistant. Numerous other examples could be cited, including the occurrence of epidemics among military populations caused by sulfonamide-resistant microorganisms after mass oral prophylactic use of these drugs. While such epidemics have fortunately not yet been of importance in civilian medicine, they do emphasize the necessity for proper precautions to minimize the development of acquired bacterial resistance. The sulfonamides should be employed only when specific indications exist for such medication. Further, when these agents are employed, they should be administered in adequate dosage as early as possible in the course of the infection.

Certain combinations of the sulfonamides with various antibiotics minimize the development of bacterial resistance and achieve chemotherapeutic results not attainable with either agent alone. However, not all combinations of chemotherapeutic agents have a rational basis. The microbe must be sensitive to both drugs used in combination; however, regardless of original sensitivity, neither the tetracyclines nor chloramphenicol delay the emergence of resistance. Occasionally antibacterial drugs in combination are antagonistic. Specific examples of valid combinations of the sulfonamides with other chemotherapeutic agents are indicated below.

Absorption, Distribution, and Fate—Sulfonamides in which the para-amino group is free are readily absorbed into the blood stream, mostly via the small intestine. Although only a small amount may remain unabsorbed, the local concentration in the bowel may be high enough to exert a prominent antibacterial action on some of the bowel flora. Sulfonamides with ionizable *N*-acyl groups (eg, phthalyl or succinyl) are poorly absorbed and hence exert a more pronounced effect on the bowel flora. Absorption from the skin and vagina is erratic. Once into the bloodstream, sulfonamides bind to serum albumin to varying degrees, ranging from less than 10 to over 90%, depending on the particular drug. Protein-binding limits penetrance into the tissues and glomerular filtration and hence is a determinant of the distribution and rate of excretion. Concentrations in tissue fluids usually range from about 50 to 80% of those in the plasma. Highly polar sulfonamides do not penetrate tissues well, but they are excreted rapidly. Thus sulfisoxazole is mainly extracellular in distribution and thus is of limited usefulness in systemic infections; because it is rapidly filtered in the renal glomerulus and is poorly resorbed by the renal tubules (being lipid-insoluble), high concentrations are reached in the urine, and it is of especial use in the treatment of urinary tract infections. Nevertheless, when the urinary tract infection is extraluminal, more penetrant sulfonamides, such as sulfadiazine, may be more effective. Sulfonamides are acetylated in the liver to an extent of 30 to 85% depending on the sulfonamide and the patient. The fraction of the acetylate conjugate in the urine varies accordingly. Crystallization of sulfonamide, conjugate, or both may occur in the urine, depending on the solubility properties of each form of the drug at the pH of the urine and on the volume of urine. In general, both parent and acetylated sulfonamides are more soluble in alkaline than acid urine.

Toxicity—Untoward effects during therapy with sulfonamides represent the major limitation to their clinical use. The most frequently observed side effects are crystalluria and related renal damage, hematuria being noted in approximately 2% of patients receiving sulfadiazine or other pyrimidine congeners. Gastrointestinal side effects include nausea, vomiting, abdominal pain, diarrhea, anorexia, stomatitis, and rare pancreatitis. Of the neurological effects, headache, vertigo, and insomnia are the most frequent, but tinnitus, psychic depression, ataxia, hallucinations, peripheral and optic neuritis, acute myopia, and convulsions occasionally occur. This incidence is less when adjuvant alkali and fluid therapy is instituted or when sulfonamide mixtures or the newer, more soluble, congeners are employed. Hypersensitivity reactions, such as drug fever, dermatitis, hepatitis, polyarteritis nodosa, lupoid syndrome, pulmonary eosinophilia, rare myocarditis, etc., occur in about 2% of patients receiving most present-day sulfonamides. The incidence of hypersensitivity reactions is higher in patients receiving sulfapyridine. Agranulocytosis, aplastic anemia, leukopenia, and thrombocytopenia have been noted during sulfonamide therapy, but the incidence is low when sulfadiazine and the other newer congeners are employed. Hemolytic anemia may occur; persons whose erythrocytes are deficient in glucose 6-phosphate dehydrogenase (G6-PD) are especially susceptible. Sulfonamide-induced hepatocellular jaundice is now rare. Long-acting sulfonamides, especially, may cause exudative erythema multiforme (Stevens-Johnson syndrome), a very serious reaction; conjunctival and corneal scarring may occur as a part of the syndrome. Central nervous system effects are infrequently observed during current sulfonamide therapy, and cyanosis, acid-base disturbances, and other miscellaneous toxic effects formerly common during therapy with sulfanilamide, sulfathiazole, or sulfapyridine are only rarely observed during administration of sulfadiazine.

Sulfonamides displace bilirubin from plasma proteins and hence can cause kernicterus in the newborn. It is not recommended that sulfonamides be administered to infants younger than two months. Consequently, sulfonamides should be avoided in pregnant women near term and in newborn or premature infants. Some sulfonamides have been shown to be teratogenic in rats. If at all possible, then, sulfonamides should be avoided in pregnancy.

Because the sulfonamides may cause serious untoward effects, they should be administered only when bacteriological diagnosis indicates that these agents can be expected to be superior to drugs of other classes. Constant medical surveillance, preferably daily, is necessary, and periodic blood counts and urinalysis are mandatory.

Uses—In spite of the dominance of antibiotics, sulfonamides still retain a place in the chemotherapy of infectious diseases. In only a few infections, a sulfonamide remains the agent of choice; in others, particularly in serious infections, a sulfonamide is occasionally employed in combination with an appropriate antibiotic. In addition, sulfonamides have certain important prophylactic uses. Major advantages of sulfonamides are their low cost and ease of administration; major disadvantages are their untoward effects and limited efficacy.

Sulfonamides are the drugs of choice only for the treatment of *nocardiosis*. The combination, trimethoprim-sulfamethoxazole is the treatment of choice for infections caused by *Shigella*, *H ducreyi* (chancroid), *Ps pseudomallei* (melioidosis), and *Pneumocystis carinii*. Sulfonamides are drugs of second choice for infections caused by *Chlamydia trachomatis;* if the chlamydial infection is superficial, as in trachoma or inclusion conjunctivitis, both oral and topical administration are employed. Sulfonamides share second-choice status with other drugs in the treatment of infections caused by *H influenzae* (if not life-threatening), and *lymphogranuloma venereum*, and *meningococcal meningitis*, for which trisulfapyrimidines is indicated. Trimethoprim-sulfamethoxazole is an alternative treatment for infections caused by *Enterobacter*, *E coli*, *Pr mirabilis*, indole positive *Proteus*, *Providencia*, *Salmonella*, *Klebsiella*, *Serratia*, *Acinetobacter*, *Brucella*, *H influenzae*, *Vibrio cholerae* (cholera), and *Nocardia*. Sulfonamides are sometimes combined with penicillin in the treatment of otitis, and with streptomycin in meningitis caused by *H influenzae*, and may be combined with pyrimethamine in toxoplasmosis. Strains of *meningococcus* are more sensitive to sulfonamides, but the occurrence of resistant strains has made penicillin G the drug of first choice. They are of use in some urinary tract infections caused by *E coli*, *Salmonella*, *Shigella*, *Staphylococcus*, *Klebsiella-Enterobacter*, *Pr mirabilis* and *Pr vulgaris*. Sulfonamides may be combined with penicillin in certain *selected* cases of *subacute bacterial endocarditis* not responsive to antibiotics alone. In regions in which there is a problem of resistance of malarial parasites to the usual antimalarials, sulfonamides may be given in combination with trimethoprim and other antimalarials. Prolonged treatment with sulfapyridine but not other sulfonamides is often useful in the treatment of *dermatitis herpetiformis;* the mechanism is unknown. Similarly, the beneficial effect of sulfasalazine in *ulcerative colitis* is poorly understood.

Important prophylactic uses of sulfonamides include their employment to reduce the *meningococcal* carrier rate and thus decrease the spread of meningococcal infections in congested populations, and for mass chemoprophylaxis during outbreaks of *bacillary dysentery*. They offer an alternative to penicillin in the prevention of recrudescences of rheumatic fever.

The insoluble sulfonamides intended for intestinal chemotherapy are employed for *preoperative* preparation of the bowel prior to surgery. Indications for bowel sterilization are now considered to be few, and there are superior antibiotics when such sterilization is elected. Certain of these unabsorbed sulfonamides have been employed alone or combined with systemic sulfonamide therapy in acute and chronic *bacillary dysentery*, in *ulcerative colitis*, and *regional enteritis*. These sulfonamides may also be employed as adjuvant agents in the therapy of *intestinal amebiasis*.

Types and Choice of Preparations—The antimicrobial spectrum of all sulfonamides is essentially the same. However, on the basis of solubility and degree of absorption from the gastrointestinal tract, the sulfonamides can be divided into two broad classes, namely, those employed for systemic chemotherapy and those intended only for intestinal chemotherapy. Sulfonamides employed for their systemic actions include sulfacytine, sulfadiazine, sulfamerazine, sulfamethazine, sulfamethizole, sulfamethoxazole, sulfisoxazole, sulfisomidine, sulfapyridine and the sulfonamide mixtures (see below). These agents are readily absorbed from the gastrointestinal tract and adequate blood concentrations are easily maintained. All of these agents yield sufficiently high concentrations in urine to be useful against some urinary tract infections, but the more rapidly excreted ones yield higher concentrations and are generally preferred, except where tissue penetrance is also important.

Differences exist among these sulfonamides regarding distribution among the tissues and especially penetration into the cerebrospinal fluid. Differences in distribution have not been well formulated into guidelines for clinical choice. This is partly because such differences are partly illusory; that is, differences resulting from protein-binding are irrelevant to defining the penetrance of the free, or active, form of the drug, and not enough is yet known about the complete distribution of the free form of most of the sulfonamides.

Plasma half-lives have some bearing on choice, other than the simple matter of the convenience to the patient of the dose-interval. The relevance of rapid excretion has been noted. Very-long-acting sulfonamides bind strongly to proteins, which favors allergic responses.

Systemic sulfonamides and their conjugates differ in solubility in urine, and sulfonamide mixtures and particularly certain congeners cause a lower incidence of crystalluria and related renal toxicity than do the other sulfonamides.

Oral administration of the sulfonamides is preferred. However, when medication cannot be taken by mouth, the soluble sodium salts may be given parenterally.

Because topical chemotherapy is rarely effective, except in the most superficial infections, and may be dangerous because of sensitization and the development of acquired bacterial resistance, topical administration of the sulfonamides, with the possible exception of sulfacetamide sodium, is not recommended and is strongly discouraged, except in trachoma and inclusion conjunctivitis, in which both topical and systemic treatment are used.

An important consideration in the choice of sulfonamide should be cost to the patient.

Sulfonamide Mixtures—Sulfonamide mixtures are designed to minimize the incidence of crystalluria and related renal injury associated with systemic use of sulfonamides. Since the solubility of a particular sulfonamide is not influenced by the presence of others in the same solution, a higher total concentration of sulfonamide can be attained in the urine without precipitation after administration of a mixture than is possible if a single sulfonamide is given. Employment of mixtures reduces the dose of sodium bicarbonate necessary to maintain the sulfonamides in solution in the urine and may obviate such need completely. Mixtures of equal weights of two or three sulfonamides are commonly employed. Those most frequently used include sulfadiazine, sulfamerazine, sulfamethazine, or sulfacetamide. Sulfonamide mixtures are available only for oral administration, but mixtures of parenteral preparations have been prepared extemporaneously and employed to advantage.

The antimicrobial potencies of the components of a mixture are additive, and the spectrum and the therapeutic uses of sulfonamide mixtures are the same as those of the individual components. The incidence of renal toxicity is reduced, even without concomitant administration of alkalinizing salts. It can be reduced further if adjuvant urine alkalinization is employed. The incidence of hypersensitivity reactions is not enhanced and may be reduced. Precautions for use of sulfonamide mixtures are the same as those for use of the individual congeners. Adequate 24-hour urine volume should be assured by fluid therapy if necessary. The dosage for the sulfonamide mixtures is essentially the same as that for the components.

Incompatibilities—The sodium derivatives are soluble in water, invariably imparting to the solution a marked alkalinity. Hence such solutions are incompatible with all acidic substances and with precipitable amines.

Local anesthetics related to para-aminobenzoic acid antagonize the action of the sulfonamides. *Ethyl aminobenzoate*, *procaine*, *isocaine*, *butacaine*, and *tetracaine*, are so related.

Sulfacetamide Sodium

Acetamide, *N*-[(4-aminophenyl)sulfonyl]-, monosodium salt, monohydrate; Soluble Sulfacetamide; *Various Mfrs*

N-Sulfanilylacetamide monosodium salt monohydrate [6209-17-2] $C_8H_9N_2NaO_3S.H_2O$ (254.24); *anhydrous* [127-56-0] (236.22).

Preparation—By reacting sulfanilamide with acetic anhydride, followed by controlled alkaline hydrolysis to remove the N^1-acetyl group and subsequent acidification to a pH of about 4 to form sulfacetamide which is dissolved in the required quantity of NaOH solution and the solution is evaporated to dryness or precipitated with alcohol.

Description—White, crystalline, odorless powder with a bitter taste; pH (1 in 20 solution) between 8 and 9.5.
Solubility—1 g in 2.5 mL water; sparingly soluble in alcohol; practically insoluble in benzene, chloroform, and ether.
Incompatibilities—See above.

Uses—Its *antibacterial* spectrum is similar to that of the other sulfonamides, but it is less potent, owing to poor penetration into both tissues and bacteria. Employed in high concentration by local application, it is of benefit in various *ophthalmologic infections*, especially those caused by pyogenic cocci, gonococcus, *E coli*, and Koch-Weeks' bacillus. *Trachoma* may also sometimes respond well. Since the drug is nonirritating even in high concentration, it can be employed in sufficient concentration to achieve penetration of the ocular tissues. Although the high local concentrations thus attained obviate certain of the undesirable aspects of local chemotherapy, the usual limitations and dangers of such therapy are not completely eliminated. It is used also in the topical treatment of *acne vulgaris*, *seborrheic dermatitis*, and various bacterial infections of the skin caused by susceptible organisms. Sulfacetamide is a component of mixtures for the treatment of vaginal infections caused by *Candida*, *Trichomonas*, and *Gardnerella*, but there is no clinical evidence that proves its efficacy for this purpose. In many infections, systemic chemotherapy may also be necessary. Sulfacetamide sodium is contraindicated if sensitivity to any sulfonamide exists. It is capable of causing sensitivity.

Dose—*Topical*, as **10%** ointment to the *conjunctiva* and lash margins 5 times a day or **1 drop** of a 10 to 30% solution every 1 to 3 hours during the day and less frequently at night; to the *skin*, as **10%** lotion.
Dosage Forms—Lotion: 10%; Ophthalmic Ointment: 10%; Ophthalmic Solution: 10, 15, and 30%.

Sulfacytine

Benzenesulfonamide, 4-amino-*N*-(1-ethyl-1,2-dihydro-2-oxo-4-pyrimidinyl)-, Renoquid (*Parke-Davis*)

1-Ethyl-*N*-sulfanilylcytosine [17784-12-2] $C_{12}H_{14}N_4O_3S$ (294.34).

Preparation—Sulfacytine, one of a group of *N*-sulfanilyl-1-alkylcytosines synthesized by Doub *et al* (*J Med Chem 13*: 242, 1970), may be prepared by interaction of *N*-acetylsulfanilyl chloride and 1-ethylcytosine, the resulting *N*-(*N*-acetylsulfanilyl)-1-ethylcytosine being subsequently hydrolyzed to *N*-sulfanilyl-1-ethylcytosine (sulfacytine). US Pat 3,375,247.

Description—White to cream-colored, crystalline powder; melts at about 169°; pK_a 6.9.
Solubility—Slightly soluble in water.

Uses—Sulfacytine is rapidly excreted unchanged into the urine and reaches high concentrations in the urine; with recommended doses, the average maintenance urine concentration has been reported to be approximately 420 µg/mL, or more than 10 times the minimal inhibitory concentration for sensitive strains of *E coli*, *Enterobacter*, and *Proteus*. It is indicated for the treatment of uncomplicated, acute urinary tract infections caused by susceptible strains of bacteria (see page 1171). Because sulfacytine is more lipid-soluble than sulfisoxazole, it should have a more favorable tissue penetrance and hence will probably prove to be of greater efficacy than sulfisoxazole in treating complicated and chronic urinary tract and prostatic infections.

Following oral administration, sulfacytine is rapidly absorbed, and peak plasma levels occur in 2 to 3 hr. It is about 85% protein-bound in plasma. About 88% is excreted into the urine; very little is acetylated. The elimination half-life is 4 to 4.5 hr; it is prolonged in renal failure, and care must be exercised.

The potential adverse effects are those of the sulfonamides in general, (see page 1170); headache, gastrointestinal disturbances and rashes are the most frequent. It may exacerbate ongoing bronchial asthma and allergies. The effects on the fetus and children under 14 years of age are unknown.

Dose—Oral, *children* over 14 years of age and *adults*, *initially* **500 mg** then **250 mg** 4 times a day for *maintenance*, for 10 days. The dose range will undoubtedly be expanded as more experience with the drug is gained. Up to 2 g a day have been administered safely.

Sulfadiazine

Benzenesulfonamide, 4-amino-N-2-pyrimidinyl-,
Microsulfon (*CMC*); *Various Mfrs*

N^1-2-Pyrimidinylsulfanilamide [68-35-9] $C_{10}H_{10}N_4O_2S$ (250.27).

Preparation—By combining *p*-acetamidobenzenesulfonyl chloride (see page 1170) with 2-aminopyrimidine (2-amino-1,3-diazine) in the presence of a mild alkaline agent, then splitting off the acetyl group by hydrolyzing with acid or alkali.

Description—White or slightly yellow powder; odorless or nearly so; stable in air, but slowly darkens on exposure to light; melts between 251° and 254°.

Solubility—1 g in about 13,000 mL water; sparingly soluble in alcohol and acetone; 1 g in about 620 mL human serum at 37°; freely soluble in dilute mineral acids, solutions of potassium and sodium hydroxides, and ammonia TS.

Incompatibilities—See page 1172.

Uses—The therapeutic uses of sulfadiazine have been described on page 1171. Minimal therapeutic blood levels of the drug are in the range of 100 to 150 μg/mL. Sulfadiazine serves as the prototype for comparison of other sulfonamides and their mixtures.

Sulfadiazine is bound to plasma proteins to the extent of 40 to 50%, and concentrations of the drug in the cerebrospinal fluid vary from 50 to 60% of those in the plasma; this is a good tissue concentration, as antibacterial agents go. A dose of about 60 mg/kg will provide a therapeutic concentration in cerebrospinal fluid. Higher concentrations are attained when the meninges are inflamed, and intrathecal administration of the drug is usually not necessary. Thus sulfadiazine is the sulfonamide of choice for CNS infections susceptible to sulfonamides and for which superior agents are not available; nocardiosis is an example, as is antibiotic-resistant meningococcal meningitis. Sulfadiazine readily enters cells, and the volume of distribution is slightly greater than total body water. The tissue-penetrating properties of sulfadiazine have proven to be of importance in combatting urinary tract infections, so that in some such infections it may be superior to the more soluble sulfonamides.

Sulfadiazine is acetylated in the liver to the extent of 30 to 50%; both the free and acetylated forms are excreted in the urine. The elimination half-life is about 12 to 17 hr but varies considerably.

Untoward effects occur in approximately 6 to 8% of patients receiving sulfadiazine therapy. Crystalluria and related renal damage can be minimized by administration of adjuvant alkalinizing salts and by maintenance of an adequate 24-hr urine volume. Urinary volume in the adult should be maintained at more than 1500 mL/24 hr. If adjuvant alkali therapy is employed, an initial dose of 4 g of sodium bicarbonate and subsequent doses of 2 g at intervals of 4 hr are necessary to achieve adequate alkalinization of the urine. To minimize crystalluria, sulfadiazine is also commonly combined with other sulfonamides (see *Trisulfapyrimidines*, page 1176). Hypersensitivity reactions are observed in 1 to 2% of patients, but agranulocytosis and other serious blood dyscrasias have been reported only rarely.

Dose—Oral, *adult*, *initially*, **2** to **4 g** and, for *maintenance*, **500 mg** to **1 g** every 6 hr; *infants* older than 2 months and *children*, initially **75 mg per kg** of body weight (or **4 g per m²** of body surface) per day, divided into 4 or 6 even doses, up to a maximum of 6 g per day. For the *prophylaxis* of rheumatic fever, **0.5 g** for persons weighing less than 30 kg, and **1 g** for persons weighing more than 30 kg, once a day. In severe infections, the initial oral dose for adults of 100 mg/kg

is followed by 1 to 1.5 g every 4 hr day and night until the temperature has been normal for 5 to 7 days. In severe infections in children, the initial dose is 100 to 150 mg/kg. Subsequent doses of ¼ the initial dose are administered every 6 hr. In moderate or mild infections in both adults and children, an initial dose of 50 mg/kg and maintenance dose ⅓ of the initial dose at intervals of 4 to 6 hr are adequate.

Dosage Forms—Tablets: 500 mg.

Sulfamerazine

Benzenesulfonamide, 4-amino-N-(4-methyl-2-pyrimidinyl)-,
Sulfamethyldiazine

N^1-(4-Methyl-2-pyrimidinyl)sulfanilamide   [127-79-7]
$C_{11}H_{12}N_4O_2S$ (264.30).

Preparation—By the method described for *Sulfadiazine*, using 4-methyl-2-aminopyrimidine instead of 2-aminopyrimidine.

Description—White or faintly yellowish white crystals or powder; slightly bitter taste and odorless or nearly so; stable in air, but slowly darkens on exposure to light; melts between 234° and 239°.

Solubility—1 g in about 6250 mL water, readily soluble in dilute mineral acids and solutions of potassium, ammonium, and sodium hydroxides; slightly soluble in alcohol; very slightly soluble in ether and chloroform.

Incompatibilities—See page 1172.

Uses—Closely resembles sulfadiazine in its *antibacterial* properties, toxicity, and therapeutic uses. It has a minimal effective concentration of 3 to 20 μg/mL. It is widely employed in sulfonamide mixtures in those infections in which the systemic antimicrobial actions of the sulfonamides are indicated (see introduction to this section, and also *Sulfadiazine*).

Sulfamerazine is more completely absorbed from the gut and more slowly excreted by the kidneys than is sulfadiazine. Hence doses of sulfamerazine required to maintain effective blood levels are smaller and are administered at slightly greater intervals than are those of sulfadiazine. About 75% of sulfamerazine is bound to plasma proteins, which is a greater extent than with sulfadiazine, and its concentration in the cerebrospinal fluid is only about 25% of that in plasma. Consequently, it is necessary to maintain a higher blood level with sulfamerazine in order to achieve efficacy equal to that of sulfadiazine. The elimination half-life is about 24 hr. Approximately 35 to 60% of the drug in the urine is in the inactive acetylated form. Both the free and acetylated forms are less soluble than those of sulfadiazine, so that crystalluria may occur, even despite a lower rate of excretion than with sulfadiazine. Consequently it is presently only used in combination with other sulfonamides (see *Trisulfapyrimidines* in this section).

Dose—There is no single entity dosage form of sulfamerazine, and it is used only in the *Trisulfapyrimidines* preparations.

Sulfamethazine

Benzenesulfonamide, 4-amino-N-(4,6-dimethyl-2-pyrimidinyl)-,
Sulphadimidine

N^1-(4,6-Dimethyl-2-pyrimidinyl)sulfanilamide   [57-68-1]
$C_{12}H_{14}N_4O_2S$ (278.33).

Preparation—By the general method for N^1-substituted sulfanilamides described on page 1170 using 2-amino-4,6-dimethylpyrimidine for the condensation with the sulfonyl chloride.

Description—White or yellowish white, almost odorless powder which may darken on exposure to light; slightly bitter taste; melts between 197° and 200°.

Solubility—Very slightly soluble in water and ether; slightly soluble in alcohol; soluble in acetone.

Uses—Closely resembles *Sulfamerazine* in its antimicrobial properties, toxicity, and therapeutic uses. It has a minimal effective concentration of 10 to 100 μg/mL. It is employed as a component of sulfonamide mixtures in those infections in which the systemic antimicrobial actions of sulfonamides are indicated (see introduction to this section, and also *Sulfamerazine*).

Sulfamethazine, like sulfamerazine, is usually considered to be more slowly excreted by the kidney than is sulfadiazine, yet its half-life is reported to be only 7 hr. A longer half-life is consistent with the fact that doses of sulfamethazine required to maintain effective blood levels are smaller and are administered at slightly longer intervals than are those of sulfadiazine. The drug is 70 to 90% acetylated in the liver. About 80% is bound to plasma proteins.

Sulfamethazine is a component of *Trisulfapyrimidines*, described in this section.

Dose—There is no single entity dosage form of sulfamethazine and it is used only in the *Trisulfapyrimidines* preparations.

Sulfamethizole

Benzenesulfonamide, 4-amino-*N*-(5-methyl-1,3,4-thiadiazol-2-yl)-, Thiosulfil (*Ayerst*)

N[1]-(5-Methyl-1,3,4-thiadiazol-2-yl)sulfanilamide [144-82-1] $C_9H_{10}N_4O_2S_2$ (270.32).

Preparation—By the general method for *N*[1]-substituted sulfanilamides described on page 1170 using 5-methyl-2-amino-1,3,4-thiadiazole for the condensation with the sulfonyl chloride.

Description—White crystals or powder; slightly bitter taste and almost odorless; it has no odor of hydrogen sulfide; melting range 208° to 212°; pK_a 5.45.

Solubility—1 g in 2000 mL water, 38 mL alcohol, 1900 mL chloroform, 1900 mL ether; freely soluble in solutions of ammonium, potassium, and sodium hydroxides; soluble in dilute mineral acids.

Uses—The bacterial actions and toxicity of sulfamethizole are those of other sulfonamides (see introduction to this section). The degree of protein binding in plasma is very low, so that the drug is rapidly filtered in the glomerulus and excreted; the rate of excretion is only 10 to 20% slower than that of creatinine. About 95% is excreted unmetabolized. The half-life is about 4 hr. The rapid rate of excretion (and consequent high concentrations in urine) and high solubility (hence low incidence of crystalluria) make the drug useful in the treatment of urinary tract infections caused by sulfonamide-susceptible organisms. It is excreted too rapidly to be of use in systemic infections. There is very little cross-sensitization between sulfamethizole and other sulfonamides, so that it often may be used when sensitivity exists to other sulfonamides. The drug has been reported to inhibit the metabolism of phenytoin, warfarin, and tolbutamide.

Dose—*Oral, adult, usual,* **0.5** to **1 g** 3 or 4 times daily. *Children and infants* (over 2 months of age), **30** to **45 mg/kg/24 hr**, divided into 4 doses.

Dosage Forms—Tablets: 250, 500 mg and 1 g.

Sulfamethoxazole

Benzenesulfonamide, 4-amino-*N*-(5-methyl-3-isoxazolyl)-, Gantanol (*Hoffmann-LaRoche*)

N[1]-(5-Methyl-3-isoxazolyl)sulfanilamide [723-46-6] $C_{10}H_{11}N_3O_3S$ (253.28).

Preparation—By the general method for *N*[1]-substituted sulfanilamides (page 1170) using 3-amino-5-methylisoxazole as the coupling amine. The latter may be prepared by heating ethyl 5-methylisoxazole-3-carbamate with aqueous sodium hydroxide. US Pat 2,888,455.

Description—White to off-white, crystalline powder; practically odorless and stable in air; melts between 168° and 172°.

Solubility—1 g in 3400 mL water, 50 mL alcohol, 1000 mL chloroform, 1000 mL ether.

Uses—Chemically closely related to *Sulfisoxazole;* has high aqueous solubility and low tissue penetrance, with the volume of distribution being considerably less than the extracellular space. Sulfamethoxazole is bound to plasma proteins to the extent of about 68%. Thus it is best suited to treatment of *urinary tract infections* caused by susceptible organisms. It is not rational to use sulfamethoxazole for systemic infections when there are other sulfonamides with more favorable distribution, although it has been used successfully against gonorrhea, meningitis, and serious respiratory-tract infections, and prophylactically against susceptible meningococci. Despite its unfavorable pattern of distribution, it is the sulfonamide most used around the world in combination with trimethoprim or pyrimethamine for treatment of various systemic infections. The combination with trimethoprim is discussed in the following article, on *Sulfamethoxazole and Trimethoprim.* (The main use, however, is for the treatment of urinary tract infections.) With pyrimethamine it is used in the treatment of chloroquine-resistant falciparum malaria. Sulfamethoxazole is slowly and incompletely absorbed and is excreted more slowly than is sulfisoxazole, so that its duration of action is longer. Conjugation in the liver to the *N*-acetyl metabolite accounts for about 70% of elimination. The plasma half-life of sulfamethoxazole is 9 to 12 hr. The minimal effective concentration is 0.2 to 50 μg/mL. The toxicity is typical of sulfonamides, including crystalluria (see page 1171).

Dose—*Oral, adult, initially* **2 g,** followed by **1 g** 2 or 3 times a day. *Infants* over 1 month of age and *children, initially* **50** to **60 mg/kg** of body weight, followed by **25** to **30 mg/kg** every 12 hr.

Dosage Forms—Oral Suspension: 500 mg/5 mL; Tablets: 500 mg.

Sulfamethoxazole and Trimethoprim

Bactrim (*Roche*); Septra (*Burroughs Wellcome*)

Uses—Sulfamethoxazole and trimethoprim inhibit sequential steps in the formation of tetrahydrofolic acid, the sulfonamide that of formation of dihydrofolic acid, and trimethoprim that of conversion of dihydrofolate to tetrahydrofolic acid and thence to folinic acid. Thus the inhibition is magnified by the independent actions at two consecutive metabolic steps, and bacteriostasis may be altered to that of bactericide. The minimal inhibitory concentration of the sulfamethoxazole is decreased to $\frac{1}{2}$ to $\frac{1}{15}$ that of sulfamethoxazole alone, depending on the microorganism. Moreover, even if resistance develops to the action at one step, inhibition at the other step helps to maintain the antibacterial action; incidence of resistance is low but has been increasing with widespread use of the drug. The double blockade also widens the antibacterial spectrum from that of either agent alone. Thus some strains of sulfonamide-insensitive *Pseudomonas aeruginosa* may become sensitive to the combination. All strains of *Streptococcus pneumoniae, Neisseria meningitidis,* and *Corynebacterium diphtheriae* are sensitive to the combination. Also, 50 to 95% of strains of *Staphylococcus aureus* and *epidermidis; Streptococcus pyogenes, fecalis,* and *viridans; Hemophilus ducreyi; Proteus mirabilis, vulgaris, morganii,* and *rettgeri; Pseudomonas cepaciae* and *pseudomallei; Salmonella; Shigella; Enterobacter; Serratia,* and *Alcaligenes* are inhibited. Other bacteria that show a considerable incidence of sensitivity are *Brucella abortus, Pasteurella haemolytica,* various *Klebsiella, Nocardia asteroides, Pneumocystis carinii,* and some species of *Yersinia.* The frequent sensitivity of methicillin-resistant *Staph aureus* is noteworthy.

The predominant use of sulfamethoxazole-trimethoprim is in the treatment of *urinary tract infections,* especially recurrent, chronic, or complicated infections not considered controllable by single drugs. With these limitations of use, the rate of development of resistant strains in a community can be retarded. Urinary tract infections caused by *E coli, Klebsiella-Enterobacter,* and *Proteus* species are the ones mostly treated. Treatment of *pneumonitis* caused by *Pneumocystis carinii* is approved. However, tissue distribution of sulfamethoxazole is poor, and the pharmacokinetics of the mixture is not optimal for treatment of systemic infections; use of *Sulfadiazine and Trimethoprim* (page 1174) is more appropriate. Nevertheless, the combination has been successfully used to treat cholera, brucellosis, typhoid fever and the carrier state, gonorrhea, streptococcal pharyngitis, and various pulmonary infections (including abscesses) caused by *Streptococcus pneumoniae* and *Hemophilus influenzae.*

Trimethoprim is absorbed in about 2 hr and sulfamethoxazole in about 4 hr. During maintenance at steady state, 400 mg of sulfamethoxazole and 80 mg of trimethoprim (5:1 ratio) yield plasma levels

(C_{min}^{ss}) of about 20 and 1 μg/mL of unbound drug, respectively. Trimethoprim enters the cerebrospinal fluid and tissues more readily than does sulfamethoxazole, so that the ratio is less than 20:1 at these sites. In the presence of the sulfonamide, trimethoprim is poorly bound by plasma proteins, so that it filters rapidly into the urine, and less than 40% is metabolized. Consequently the urine concentration may be 100 times that in plasma, whereas the sulfamethoxazole concentration may be only 3 times higher, thus departing from the supposedly optimal 20:1 ratio. The half-life of trimethoprim is about 9 hr. Impairment of renal function increases the half-life of each drug, the greater effect being on that of sulfamethoxazole.

The adverse effects of recommended doses are those of short-acting sulfonamides (page 1170), except that crystalluria is rare. Nausea, vomiting, glossitis, and stomatitis also occur and are probably attributable to trimethoprim. In persons with subclinical folate deficiency, trimethoprim may precipitate megaloblastic anemia and leukopenia and exaggerate the probability of thrombocytopenia. Headache, peripheral neuritis, depression, convulsions, ataxia, hallucinations, fatigue, and muscle weakness may occur. The combination is immunosuppressant in humans, and teratogenic or fetucidal in animals. The combination increases the effects of the coumarin anticoagulants, sulfonylurea oral hypoglycemics, phenytoin, and methotrexate. Diuretics increase the risk of thrombocytopenia, especially in elderly patients with heart failure. Alkalinization of the urine decreases elimination of trimethoprim.

Dose—*Oral, adults and children over 40 kg* (over 32 kg for *Pneumocystis carinii*), **800 mg** of sulfamethoxazole and **160 mg** of trimethoprim every 12 hr for 10 to 14 days. *Children under 40 kg*, for *urinary tract infections*, **20 mg** of sulfamethoxazole and **4 mg** of trimethoprim **per kg** of body weight every 12 hr; *children under 32 kg* for pneumonitis caused by *Pneumocystis carinii*, **25 mg** of sulfamethoxazole and **5 mg** of trimethoprim **per kg** of body weight every 6 hr.

Dosage Forms—Oral Suspension: 200 mg sulfamethoxazole and 40 mg trimethoprim in 5 mL; Tablets: 400 mg sulfamethoxazole and 80 mg of trimethoprim, and 800 mg sulfamethoxazole and 160 mg trimethoprim.

Sulfasalazine

Benzoic acid, 2-hydroxy-5-[[4-[(2-pyridinylamino)sulfonyl]phenyl]-azo]-, Salicylazosulfapyridine; Azulfidine (*Pharmacia*)

5-[[p-(2-Pyridylsulfamoyl)phenyl]azo]salicylic acid [599-79-1] $C_{18}H_{14}N_4O_5S$ (398.39).

Preparation—N^1-2-Pyridylsulfanilamide is diazotized and coupled with salicylic acid.

Description—Light brownish yellow to bright yellow, practically tasteless, odorless, fine powder; melts at about 255° with decomposition.

Solubility—1 g in >10,000 mL water, 2900 mL alcohol, >10,000 mL chloroform, >10,000 mL ether.

Uses—Poorly absorbed from the small intestine, so that the drug passes into the colon where bacterial enzymes release both 5-aminosalicylic acid and sulfapyridine from the sulfasalazine. It has a suppressive effect on *ulcerative colitis*, which effect was once attributed to the local antibacterial effect of sulfapyridine in decreasing anaerobic bacteria. The drug inhibits prostaglandin synthesis, which is the most probable mechanism of the local anti-inflammatory effect. The contribution of locally released 5-aminosalicylic acid is conjectural.

Since some sulfapyridine is absorbed from the colon, sulfasalazine has the toxic potential of *Sulfapyridine* (see under *Other Sulfonamides*). Adverse effects mostly occur when plasma levels exceed 50 μg/mL of sulfapyridine. Heinz-body and acute hemolytic anemias occur, so that the hematological status of the patient must be regularly monitored. Folic acid absorption is also impaired by the drug. Toxic epidermal necrolysis has been reported. If the initial dose does not exceed 2 g/day, the toxic potential is said to be minimized without seriously compromising therapeutic action. Sulfasalazine imparts a yellow color to alkaline urine. Iron compounds decrease absorption of sulfasalazine, the therapeutic significance of which is unknown.

Relapses occur in about 33% of cases, so that continuous prophylactic use is often advocated. However, after a year of continuous successful suppression, the relapse rate is about the same as when no prophylaxis is used.

Dose—*Oral, adults, initially* 1 to **2 g** a day, then **500 mg** every 6 hr for maintenance. The adult dose should never exceed 8 g a day. *Children, initially* 40 to 60 **mg/kg** of body weight a day, in 3 to 6 divided doses and **30 mg/kg** a day in 4 divided doses for maintenance; occasionally initial doses of up to 150 mg/kg/day are required to achieve control.

Dosage Form—Oral Suspension: 250 mg/5 mL; Enteric-Coated Tablets: 500 mg; Tablets: 500 mg.

Sulfisoxazole

Benzenesulfonamide, 4-amino-*N*-(3,4-dimethyl-5-isoxazolyl)-, Gantrisin (*Roche*); SK-Soxazole (*SKF*); Sulfizin (*Reid-Provident*)

N^1-(3,4-Dimethyl-5-isoxazolyl)sulfanilamide [127-69-5] $C_{11}H_{13}N_3O_3S$ (267.30).

Preparation—By the general method for N^1-substituted sulfanilamides described on page 1170 using 3,4-dimethyl-5-aminoisoxazole for the condensation with the sulfonyl chloride.

Description—White to slightly yellowish, odorless, crystalline powder; melts between 194° and 199°.

Solubility—1 g in about 6700 mL water; soluble in diluted hydrochloric acid.

Uses—The *antibacterial* properties and therapeutic uses of sulfisoxazole resemble those of sulfadiazine. The minimum inhibitory concentrations for bacteria to be treated in urinary tract infections are 1 to 20 μg/mL. However, sulfisoxazole does not penetrate cells and pass barriers as well as most sulfonamides; the volume of distribution is only 0.16 mL/g. Consequently, it is not always effective against systemic infections which are sensitive to other sulfonamides. Urinary tract infections caused by sulfonamide-susceptible bacteria respond favorably, and the drug finds favor in the treatment of many such infections. However, in genitourinary tract infections in which penetration into the involved tissues is required, sulfisoxazole may not be as effective as sulfadiazine. It is secreted into prostatic fluid, but it is not known whether it is secreted into other genitourinary fluids. The extent of protein binding in plasma is 86%. About 47% of sulfisoxazole is acetylated in the liver. Both it and the conjugate are rapidly excreted by the kidney and reach high concentrations in the urine. The half-life is about 6 hr. Since both the free and acetylated forms of sulfisoxazole are highly soluble, even in acidic urine, adjuvant alkali therapy is not necessary and fluids need not be forced. The incidence of renal toxicity is lower than that caused by sulfadiazine or sulfonamide mixtures. With this exception, untoward effects during sulfisoxazole therapy are similar to those caused by other sulfonamides (see page 1171). Topical use may compromise subsequent use of sulfonamides by causing occasional sensitization or bacterial resistance.

Dose—*Oral, adult, initially* 2 to **4 g,** followed by **750 mg** to **1.5 g** every 4 hr or 1 to **2 g** every 6 hr. *Infants* over 1 month of age and *children, initially* 75 **mg/kg** of body weight (or 2 g/m² of body surface), followed by **25 mg/kg** (or 667 mg/m²) every 4 hr or **37.5 mg/kg** (or 1 g/m²) every 6 hr, not to exceed 6 g a day.

Dosage Forms—Tablets: 500 mg. Vaginal Cream: 10%.

Sulfisoxazole Acetyl

Acetamide, *N*-[(4-aminophenyl)sulfonyl-*N*-(3,4-dimethyl-5-isoxazolyl)-, Acetyl Gantrisin; Lipo Gantrisin (*Hoffmann-LaRoche*)

N-(3,4-Dimethyl-5-isoxazolyl)-*N*-sulfanilylacetamide [80-74-0] $C_{13}H_{15}N_3O_4S$ (309.34).

Preparation—Sulfisoxazole is selectively acetylated at the *N*-position by converting it into its sodium salt which may then be metathesized with an equimolar quantity of acetyl chloride.

Description—White or slightly yellow, crystalline powder; melting range 192° to 195°.

Solubility—Practically insoluble in water; 1 g in 176 mL alcohol, 35 mL chloroform, 1064 mL ether.

Uses—Converted to sulfisoxazole in the gastrointestinal tract. Thus its actions and toxicity are identical to those of *Sulfisoxazole* (see preceding article). Sulfisoxazole acetyl is tasteless, hence is more suitable for liquid oral preparations. The half-life is about 10 hr. When it is incorporated into a vegetable oil suspension, oral absorption is slowed, and the duration of action is prolonged.

Dose (base equivalent)—With the Oral Suspension and the Syrup, the dose is the same as that of Sulfisoxazole. With the Delayed Absorption Oral Suspension, the *adult* dose is **4** to **5 g** every 12 hr, and the *pediatric* dose is **60** to **75 mg/kg** of body weight every 12 hr, not to exceed 6 g a day.

Dosage Forms (base equivalent)—Oral Suspension: 500 mg/5 mL; Extended-Release Oral Suspension: 1 g/5 mL; Syrup: 500 mg/5 mL.

Sulfisoxazole Diolamine

Benzenesulfonamide, 4-amino-*N*-(3,4-dimethyl-5-isoxazolyl)-, compd with 2,2′-iminobis[ethanol] (1:1)

N^1-(3,4-Dimethyl-5-isoxazolyl)sulfanilamide compound with 2,2′-iminodiethanol (1:1) [4299-60-9] $C_{11}H_{13}N_3O_3S.C_4H_{11}NO_2$ (372.44).

Preparation—Sulfisoxazole is dissolved in an aqueous solution containing an equimolar portion of diethanolamine [HN(CH₂CH₂OH)₂] and the solution is evaporated to dryness.

Description—White to off-white, fine, crystalline powder; odorless; melts between 119° and 124°.

Solubility—1 g in 2 mL water, 16 mL alcohol, 1000 mL chloroform, >10,000 mL ether.

Uses—Its actions and uses are the same as those of *Sulfisoxazole*, except that the diolamine salt is more soluble and hence is suitable for injection and for ophthalmic application. The ophthalmic preparations are employed in the treatment of corneal ulcers, conjunctivitis, and other superficial ocular infections caused by sensitive organisms and as an adjunct in the treatment of trachoma.

Dose (base equivalent)—The *initial* dose, **50 mg/kg** (or 1.125 g/m² of body surface), is the same for all parenteral routes. *Maintenance* doses are as follows: *intramuscular*, **33 mg/kg** (or 750 mg/m²) every 8 hr *or* **50 mg/kg** (or 1.125 g/m²) every 12 hr; *intravenous*, **25 mg/kg** (or 562.5 mg/m²) every 6 hr; *subcutaneous*, **33 mg/kg** (or 750 mg/m²) every 8 hr. The injection must be diluted 1 + 6 to make a 5% solution for subcutaneous or intravenous administration. Intravenous administration should be by slow infusion. *Topical*, to the conjunctiva and lid margin, **0.5** to **1 in** of 4% ointment or **1 drop** of 4% solution every 8 hr or more frequently with solution.

Dosage Forms (sulfisoxazole equivalent)—Injection: 400 mg/mL in 5 mL; Ophthalmic Ointment: 4%; Ophthalmic Solution: 40 mg/mL.

Trisulfapyrimidines

Various Mfrs

Each dose unit contains 162 or 167 mg of each of sulfadiazine, sulfamerazine, and sulfamethazine. The suspension may contain either sodium citrate or sodium lactate, and a suitable antimicrobial agent.

Uses—The *antibacterial* spectrum and therapeutic uses of sulfonamide mixtures are the same as the sum of the individual components. An advantage of such mixtures is the lesser incidence of crystalluria and renal injury associated with use of sulfonamides (see page 1171).

Dose—*Oral*, *adult*, *initially* **2** to **4 g** of sulfonamides, followed by **2** to **4 g** a day in 3 to 6 divided doses. *Infants* over 2 months of age and *children*, initially **75 mg/kg** of body weight (or 2 g/m² of body surface), followed by **150 mg/kg** (or 4 g/m²) a day in 4 to 6 divided doses, not to exceed 6 g a day.

Dosage Forms—Oral Suspension: 167 mg of each component; Tablets: 162 or 167 mg of each component.

Other Sulfonamides

Sulfabenzamide [*N*-Sulfanilylbenzamide [127-71-9] $C_{13}H_{12}N_2O_2S$ (276.31); ing of Sultrin (*Ortho*); Trysul (*Savage*)]—A crystalline powder; melts at about 182°; nearly insoluble in water. *Uses:* A sulfonamide employed topically, in combination with other sulfonamides, for treatment of *Gardnerella* (*Hemophilus*) *vaginalis* vaginitis. It can cause sensitization, and development of drug resistance that may compromise future systemic therapy with other sulfonamides. Available dosage forms include a "triple-sulfa" cream containing as one of the ingredients 3.7% of sulfabenzamide and a vaginal tablet containing 184 mg of sulfabenzamide and other sulfonamides.

Sulfacetamide [N^1-Sulfanilylacetamide [144-80-9] $C_8H_{10}N_2O_3S$ (214.24); ing of Sultrin (*Ortho*) and Trysul (*Savage*)]—Prepared by reacting sulfanilamide with acetic anhydride, followed by controlled alkaline hydrolysis to remove the N^1-acetyl group and subsequent acidification to a pH of about 4. White, crystalline powder; melts at about 183°. pK_a 1.78. 1 g dissolves in about 140 mL water; soluble in alcohol; insoluble in ether. *Uses:* Employed topically in combination with sulfabenzamide and sulfathiazole for the treatment of vaginitis caused by *Gardnerella* (*Hemophilus*) *vaginalis*. *Dose:* Topical as vaginal cream containing 2.86% sulfacetamide (with other sulfonamides) twice a day for 4 to 6 days or as a vaginal tablet containing 144 mg of sulfacetamide (with other sulfonamides) twice a day for 10 days.

Sulfadoxine [N^1-(5,6-Dimethoxy-4-pyrimidinyl)sulfanilamide [2447-57-6] $C_{12}H_{14}N_4O_4S$ (310.34); Fanasil; Fanzil]—A white, crystalline powder; melts at about 192°. *Uses:* Sulfadoxine has antimicrobial activity similar to that of *Sulfadiazine*. Its principal use, however, is in the prophylaxis or suppression of malaria caused by chloroquine-resistant *P falciparum*. It is used only in combination with pyrimethamine, in a fixed-dose formulation. *Dose: Oral*, for *acute attack*, *adults*, 2 to 3 tablets, alone or in sequence with primaquine or quinine. *Children* 9 through 14 yr, 2 tablets; 4 through 8 yr, 1 tablet; under 4 yr, ½ tablet. For *prophylaxis*, *adults*, 1 tablet a week or 2 tablets every other week. *Children*, 9 through 14 yr, ¾ tablet for each tablet used by adult; 4 through 8 yr, ½ tablet for each tablet used by adult; under 4 yr, ¼ tablet for each used by adult. Each tablet contains 500 mg of sulfadoxine and 25 mg of pyrimethamine.

Sulfanilamide [*p*-Aminobenzenesulfonamide [63-74-1] $C_6H_8N_2O_2S$ (172.21)]—Prepared by action of ammonia on acetylsulfanilyl chloride, followed by hydrolysis of the resulting N^4-acetylsulfanilamide. White crystals, granules, or powder; melts at about 165°. 1 g dissolves in about 125 mL water, 37 mL alcohol; soluble in glycerin; insoluble in chloroform, ether; soluble in solutions of hydrochloric acid and alkali hydroxides. *Uses:* One of the first sulfonamides, introduced into US medicine in 1936, now largely replaced by more effective and less toxic congeners. It is now only of historic interest and cannot be recommended for systemic therapeutic use. It is still marketed in combination with aminacrine hydrochloride and allantoin for the treatment of vaginitis caused by *Garderella* (*Hemophilus*) *vaginalis*, *Trichomonas*, and *Candida*. *Dose: Topical*, into the vagina, as 15% cream or 1-g suppository.

Sulfapyridine [N^1-2-Pyridylsulfanilamide [144-83-2] $C_{11}H_{11}N_3O_2S$ (249.29)]—Prepared by the general method for N^1-substituted sulfanilamides, using 2-aminopyridine as the coupling amine. White or faintly yellowish crystals, granules, or powder; melts at about 191°. 1 g dissolves in 3500 mL water, 440 mL alcohol; freely soluble in dilute mineral acids and aqueous solutions of alkali hydroxides. *Uses:* Largely replaced by equally effective and less toxic congeners. It induces a high incidence of leukopenia, agranulocytosis, drug fever, and dermatoses. It is now mainly of historical interest and cannot be recommended for therapeutic use, except in *dermatitis herpetiformis*, for which use this drug has maintained a special status. *Dose: Oral*, *adult*, 500 mg 4 times a day until improvement occurs, to be then diminished by 500 mg/day every 3 days until symptom-free maintenance obtains. Recrudescences may require higher doses. *Dosage Form:* Tablets: 500 mg.

Sulfathiazole [N^1-Thiazolylsulfanilamide [74-14-0] $C_9H_9N_3O_2S_2$ (255.32); ing of Sultrin (*Ortho*) and Trysul (*Savage*)]—White or faintly yellow crystals, granules, or powder; melts at about 202°. 1 g dissolves in about 1700 mL water, 200 mL alcohol. *Uses:* Largely now only of historical interest and not recommended for therapeutic use. Its continued use in topical preparations can only be condemned, especially since sulfathiazole is one of two sulfonamides most likely to cause hypersensitivity. It is an ingredient in a combination with sulfabenzamide and sulfacetamide for the topical treatment of vaginitis caused by *Gardnerella* (*Hemophilus*) *vaginalis*.

Antibiotics

Antibiotic substances are chemical compounds produced as a result of the metabolic activities of living cells and which inhibit, in very low concentrations, the growth of micro-organisms. While antibiotics have been isolated from tissues of higher plants and animals, the term generally has come to refer to inhibitory substances of microbial origin. The antagonistic effect of one microorganism upon the development of others has been recognized since the early days of bacteriology, and the formation of inhibitory substances is but one expression of microbial antagonism.

From the standpoint of chemotherapy and pharmacology, two milestones mark the historical development of the field of antibiotics: (1) discovery by Chain, Florey, and associates at Oxford University of the unusually favorable therapeutic and pharmacological properties of extracts of cultures of the mold *Penicillium notatum*, found to produce *penicillin* by Fleming in 1929; and (2) Dubos' discovery in 1939 of *tyrothricin* and its *in vivo* efficacy against certain virulent bacterial infections. As a result of these studies, and particularly because of the demands due to World War II, a remarkable impetus was imparted to the search for new antibiotics. During the decade 1940–1950 a large number were described, and in the following nine years still more were reported and research in this field continues unabated. More than 4000 are known today.

The increased use of antibiotics in man and animals and the extension of uses to areas other than the treatment and prophylaxis of disease have created serious problems. More and more strains of organisms have become resistant to the available antibiotics, and this is particularly true of the penicillins, the most widely used. The staphylococci have created the greatest problem, and in "closed populations," such as hospitals, frequently more than 90% of the strains isolated are resistant to penicillin G. In most communities, the incidence of resistance is about 70%. Therefore, hospital controls are required to discourage the unnecessary use of antibiotics, so that the incidence of resistant strains in the hospitals can return toward that in the surrounding communities. The incidence in the community could also be lowered by a more selective, less frequent, use.

The wide use of antibiotics in animal nutrition and disease has resulted in the sensitization of a relatively large number of the susceptible people, many of whom have serious reactions upon contact with these drugs. Such agricultural use also contributes to the pool of antibiotic-resistant bacteria in a community.

In this chapter penicillin is considered in considerable detail since it is the historical prototype. It was the first antibiotic to be produced commercially and still assumes a position of major importance in this field.

Detection and Isolation of Antibiotic-Producing Organisms

The detection of productive organisms is based on the ability of cultures of the candidate organism to inhibit certain concomitantly cultured test bacteria under controlled conditions *in vitro*. A number of different test organisms are used, because no one organism is representative of the antibiotic susceptibilities or organisms in general. Thus, the use of a certain strain of *S aureus* as the test organism will detect all antibiotics inhibitory to that organism, but the antibiotic may or may not also be effective against *E coli*, for example, or even against various other strains of *S aureus*. To insure securing a valid antibacterial spectrum, a number of species and types of strains must be used in the testing.

Antibiotic-producing organisms can be obtained by: (1) testing pure cultures of organisms available in culture collections or isolated from natural sources, and (2) "screening," or selection through suitable techniques from the vast heterogeneous mixed population of the soil or other natural habitations of microorganisms. In the first case the practice consists simply of adding to broth or agar cultures, seeded with the test organism, suitable quantities or culture filtrates of the cultures being examined, incubating, and inspecting for inhibition of the test organism. The screening method involves plating out in serial dilution an aqueous extract of soil or other natural substrate using a medium, usually agar, previously seeded with the test organism. During incubation the various organisms of the soil population develop, and those forming antibiotic substances are distinguished by a clear zone or halo around the colony, indicative of inhibition of the test organism which, in the region beyond the clear zone, grows abundantly in the form of a marked turbidity throughout the agar. Many modifications of this principle are employed. Thus, use of different media, pH, temperature, and substrates will expose for screening different types of soil organisms. These conditions must be compatible with the growth of the particular test organism employed. Theoretically, the best chance for detecting the largest possible number of antagonists lies in the preincubation for a few days of the agar cultures containing the soil dilutions, but without the test bacteria. This is followed by a secondary incubation after the test organism is applied to the plate by streaking or spraying. In this manner slow-growing soil organisms are given the opportunity to develop and manifest antibiotic-producing ability.

Once detected, the antagonist is isolated in pure culture and identified, and the optimal conditions for production of the antibiotic substance produced by it are investigated. The composition of the medium is important. Different organic and inorganic nitrogenous substances are tested, with and without various carbohydrates, minerals, heavy metals, etc. Once a favorable medium is established, other known strains of the antagonist, obtained either from stock culture collections or isolated from nature, are compared for the character and amount of the antibiotic produced, and the highest yielding strain selected for further work. The antibacterial spectrum is obtained, ie, the relative effectiveness of the antibiotic in inhibiting the growth of a large variety of gram-positive and gram-negative bacteria, rickettsiae, viruses, and fungi, especially those which are pathogenic. This indicates those infections in which it may be useful chemotherapeutically. Several concentrates or isolates of the antibiotic, not necessarily pure, are then examined for toxicity in mice. Only low toxicity preparations and, in particular, those in which toxicity is inversely proportional to the antibacterial potency are of interest. Toxicity and pharmacological data are obtained in animals and, if favorable, in clinical trials on human beings. If the clinical trials show the antibiotic to be a promising therapeutic agent, attention is turned to large-scale manufacture. Chemical studies of the structure of the pure compound will indicate the feasibility of chemical synthesis. Generally, antibiotics are complex, rather large-molecular-weight substances whose synthesis may be extremely difficult, or at least uneconomical, compared to microbiologic production. This is the case now with most of the successful antibiotics, such as penicillin, streptomycin, chlortetracycline, etc.

The gradual increase in numbers of strains of microorganisms resistant to antibiotics, especially the staphylococci, and the numbers of individuals developing sensitivity to them make it extremely desirable that screening programs for the isolation and development of new agents be continued.

Production of Antibiotics

The development and operation of the large-scale commercial production of antibiotic substances may be exemplified by a description of the manufacture of penicillin. In general, the approach and methods employed are typical. Two types of processes for the microbiological production of antibiotics are known: (1) *the surface process*, in which the antibiotic-producing organism grows in the form of a pad on the surface of a liquid medium in trays or bottles, or on the surface of a finely divided moist solid substrate such as wood shavings, wheat bran, etc; (2) *the submerged process*, in which the organism develops in a liquid medium, maintained continuously under mechanical agitation and aeration, so that the organism develops uniformly and homogeneously in the form of a suspension of single cells, or small aggregates or colonies, throughout all portions of the culture liquid. The penicillin is excreted into the culture fluid. The molds used industrially today are derived from *Penicillium chrysogenum*.

The Submerged Process—This process, in which growth is greatly accelerated and the handling of large quantities greatly facilitated, is considerably more efficient than surface processes, and hence is the only feasible method for large-scale commercial production. Stationary, closed, iron, or stainless steel cylindrical-shaped tanks, known as fermenters, of 5000 to 30,000 gal capacity, are used in penicillin manufacture. Most of these are equipped with vertical single-shaft propeller or turbine-type agitators and with a mechanical means of comminuting and distributing sterile air, introduced for maximum dispersal effect in the region of the agitator. Some use sterile air only for agitation. The tanks have a detachable manhole on the top, sight glasses, and outlets to valve-closed sampling lines and accessory feed chambers, enabling inoculation by hand if necessary, particularly in small seed tanks, and the addition whenever necessary of other (sterile) materials, such as antifoam agents, during the fermentation. All outlets from the tank are exposed continuously to flowing steam to minimize chances of contamination. The culture medium is sterilized by high-pressure steam and cooled by brine. Temperature control during growth of the mold is maintained automatically at 23–25°. The compressed air, which is introduced into the fermenters, is sterilized by filtration through steam-sterilized cartridges of suitable size and filled, for example, with glass wool.

Inoculum for large tanks is obtained by building up the amount of growth successively through a series of seed tanks, from tank to tank, and transferring under air pressure through sterile pipe lines. Generally this massive inoculum amounts to 5 to 10% of the main batch and, consequently, seed tanks are about $\frac{1}{10}$ the volume of the next larger tank. The first and smallest seed tank is inoculated with a laboratory-prepared culture, consisting either of spores or of a small flask of submerged growth obtained on a laboratory, rotary, or reciprocal-type shaking machine.

The stock or master culture of the penicillin-producing mold is dry and cold-preserved in the form of spores. Continuous vegetative transfer of the mold on artificial media leads to loss of penicillin-producing power (physiological degeneration). Hence, the number of intermediate transfers between master culture and the final batch is kept at a minimum.

A Typical Production Medium

Corn-steep liquor (solids)	2 to 5%
Crude lactose	2 to 3%
Calcium carbonate	0.5 to 1%

The culture medium used for commercial production of penicillin generally contains natural nitrogenous material, nitrate, α-aminoadipic acid, cottonseed meal or corn-steep liquor, which is a by-product of the corn-milling industry, lactose, side-chain precursor, surface-active agent, and mineral salts (including sulfate). The penicillin potency is followed by assay every 3 to 6 hours and, at the time when the potency stops rising, the batch is harvested. Maximum activity generally is reached in 50 to 90 hours. Due to the instability of penicillin at ordinary temperatures, the batch is cooled to 5° and the mycelium filtered off by pressure filtration.

The penicillin is extracted and concentrated by two general processes: (1) charcoal adsorption, and (2) solvent extraction.

In the *charcoal adsorption process*, activated charcoal absorbs the penicillin and, after filtration, the penicillin is eluted with a solvent such as an 80% solution of acetone in water. The eluate is concentrated by evaporation, cooled to 0°, and acidified with mineral acid to pH 2. Penicillin, a rather strong acid, is extractable at this pH into organic solvents; amyl acetate is generally used. The low temperature minimizes losses due to the extremely instability of penicillin at pH 2.

In the *solvent extraction process* the penicillin is extracted from the filtrate by a water-immiscible solvent after the solution has been adjusted to pH 2 to liberate the acid form of penicillin, which is soluble in organic solvents while the sodium salt is insoluble. A number of successive extractions, at carefully adjusted pH values, reduces the volume and separates the large majority of impurities. From the immiscible solvents the penicillin is reextracted with a dilute solution of sodium bicarbonate, thus forming *penicillin sodium*, which is soluble in water but not in the immiscible solvent. This aqueous solution ("rich water") is rendered sterile and pyrogen-free by passage through suitable filters, and a sample taken for the determination of the potency. The liquid is frozen to prevent any decomposition while the analysis is being made. After the analysis is completed, the frozen liquid is melted and again filtered through suitable filters to further insure freedom from bacterial and pyrogenic contaminations. The penicillin is extracted by an appropriate solvent and crystallized.

Improvements in Production—The greatest advancements in the production of penicillin have been (1) the use of the submerged or tank method of production, (2) the use of corn-steep liquor, and (3) progressive improvement in the penicillin-producing capacity of the mold.

The earliest widely used strain in tank production was *Penicillium notatum*, No 832, which yielded 50 to 60 units per mL. Later, a strain of *Penicillium chrysogenum*, No 1951B25, with maximum yields of 250 units per mL, was discovered. Spores of this organism, exposed to X-ray irradiation and tested from single spore isolates, led to selection of a mutant strain X1612 producing approximately 500 units per mL. Strain X1612 was subjected to ultraviolet irradiation and strain Q176, yielding penicillin potencies of more than double that of X1612, was obtained. This strain has been widely used in commercial production, but industry has even improved on it. Some variant strains produce several thousand units per mL. The improvement in strains suitable for the surface production of penicillin followed a similar path although these were obtained by testing single spore isolates from parent cultures. A strain excellent in submerged culture is not necessarily good for surface culture, and *vice versa*. Surface culture methods are no longer used for commercial production of any of the presently useful antibiotics.

A large number of different fungi are now known to produce penicillin. Over 20 different species of *Aspergillus* and *Penicillia* produce penicillin, as do the dermatophyte *Trichophyton mentagrophytes* and a thermophilic fungus, *Malbranchea pulchella*.

Antibiotic Control

Federal control of antibiotics dates back to an amendment of the 1938 Food, Drug and Cosmetic Act (Section 507) under which the Food and Drug Administration was required to pretest all forms of penicillin and its preparations before releasing them for sale. This certification covered potency, demonstration of nontoxicity, and moisture content (the presence of excess moisture makes penicillin less stable). When intended for parenteral use, it was also tested for freedom from pyrogens, for sterility, and for the clarity and pH of its solutions.

This amendment included the provision that when it was found by the Federal Security Administrator (now Secretary of the Department of Health, Education, and Welfare) that the pretesting of penicillin or its preparations was no longer necessary to insure safety and efficacy of such drugs, they could be exempted from the pretesting requirement.

Under this provision of the Act the Federal Security Agency, FDA Division, finding that certain new, highly purified forms of penicillin no longer required pretesting, issued a notice in the Federal Register of April 13, 1949, exempting Crystalline Penicillin G Potassium and Crystalline Penicillin G Sodium from this provision.

In March, 1947, the Congress of the US placed streptomycin under the certification system and in July of 1949 included chlortetracycline, chloramphenicol, and bacitracin. Since these amendments include all derivatives as well, both dihydrostreptomycin and tetracycline, as well as pyrrolidinomethyl tetracycline and demeclocycline, were certifiable drugs.

In May, 1963, the Drug Amendments passed by Congress in 1962 became effective and superseded all previous rulings. These now provide that *all* antibiotics used in humans are subject to certification. Furthermore, those certifiable prior to passage of these latest amendments, ie, chlortetracycline, bacitracin, streptomycin, penicillin, and chloramphenicol, must also be certified for veterinary use.

Classes and Agents

Antibiotics are classified by various schemes, the two most important being according to mechanism of action and according to chemical relationship. The antibiotic monographs that follow will be arranged according to chemical relationship.

Aminoglycosides

The aminoglycosides each contain one or more aminosugars, such as glucosamine or neosamine, linked by glycoside linkages to a basic (amino or guanidino) 6-membered carbon ring, eg, streptidine or streptamine.

Antibacterial Spectrum—Aminoglycosides may be classified as broad-spectrum antibiotics. In general, they have greater activity against gram-negative than gram-positive bacteria. Although there are similarities among them with respect to the antibacterial spectrum there are also marked differences, and it is not possible to make a general statement that will apply to all members sufficiently accurately that serious errors and misconceptions will not be encouraged. For example, gentamicin will inhibit over 90% of strains of *Pseudomonas aeruginosa* but kanamycin will inhibit almost none; similarly, *Actinobacillus mallei* is among the bacteria most predictably sensitive to streptomycin and least to gentamicin. It is easier to state what organisms are not affected: anaerobes (*Bacteroides, Clostridium, Entameba histolytica, Trichomonas vaginalis*), *Rickettsia*, fungi, *Trypanosoma*, and viruses. The important antibacterial activities will be described for each agent in its monograph.

Mechanism—The aminoglycosides combine with bacterial (not mammalian) ribosomes to arrest protein synthesis. The initiation complex can be formed but cannot pass into subsequent stages of protein synthesis. The binding is quite firm, so that inhibition is severe enough that a bactericidal effect can result. The drugs also appear to interfere with the binding of aminoacetyl-t-RNA, which prevents chain elongation. They further appear to cause misreading of some RNA codons, such that inappropriate proteins can be formed when protein synthesis is not completely prevented.

Resistance—Resistance to aminoglycosides develops very rapidly with some bacteria, sometimes as a single-step high resistance. With meningococcus, *Hemophilus*, and some other bacteria, even dependence on the drug can occur. Although resistance to one aminoglycoside often confers resistance to others, there are important exceptions that may determine the choice of aminoglycoside for the treatment of certain infections. Both acquired and natural resistance is often the result of bacterial elaboration and aminoglycoside-destructive enzymes; nine such enzymes have been identified. Because of the rapid acquisition of resistance, it is common to employ aminoglycosides only in combination with other antibacterial drugs when the organism is one that rapidly develops high resistance.

Uses—Some uses of aminoglycosides are common to all members of the group, but there are also considerable differences; consequently the uses will be described for each drug.

Toxicity—Most of the toxic actions are common among all aminoglycosides, although there are important quantitative differences in incidence and severity. Hypersensitivity, mostly manifested as rashes but sometimes as drug fever and blood dyscrasias, occurs in 5–10% of recipients. Eosinophilia is relatively common. A history of sensitization contraindicates use. Cross-sensitization occurs. Vestibular and auditory function may be impaired; in the early stages it may be reversible, but often it becomes irreversible if medication is not stopped. Headaches, dizziness, and nausea and vomiting during movement are early signs of impairment of vestibular function. Loss of auditory perception of high-frequency sound signals onset of auditory toxicity. Aminoglycosides vary with respect to whether auditory or vestibular function is most affected. High-ceiling diuretics increase risk of ototoxicity. Nephrotoxicity, manifested by albuminuria, hematuria, cylindruria, azotemia, tubular necrosis and renal failure, is common to all aminoglycosides, although there are marked differences in incidence and severity. Aminoglycosides should not be used in combination with other nephrotoxic substances. Neuromuscular blockade also occurs with high doses, as the result of both postjunctional and prejunctional inhibitory actions, probably as the result of interference with movement of calcium into nerve terminals and motor endplate. Low plasma-calcium predisposes to the blockade. Aminoglycosides will greatly increase neuromuscular paralysis induced by curarizing drugs and ether anesthetics. Superinfections ("overgrowth"), most often candidal, may occur during prolonged use, as the result of interference with microbial ecology.

Pharmacokinetics—At the pH of the lower small bowel, aminoglycosides are polycationic and hence are poorly absorbed from the gut. For the same reason, they are mostly confined to the extracellular space and penetrate cells poorly. The distribution coefficients (Δ') range from 0.19 to 0.28 mL/g. Aminoglycosides penetrate the blood-brain barrier only slightly, unless the meninges are inflamed. Binding to plasma protein is low and ranges from 0 to 34%. The drugs are mostly excreted into urine, the amount ranging from 60 to 100%. The average clinically significant half-lives are about 2 to 2.5 hr, but there is a much slower phase of elimination that relates to the gradual release of tissue-bound drug; there is greater variation among individuals than there is among the drugs. Renal failure greatly prolongs the half-life. Half-lives in the inner ear are 4 to 5 times those in plasma; the half-lives in the renal cortex range from 25 to 700 hr. These facts help explain the predisposition to vestibular, auditory, and renal toxicities.

Amikacin Sulfate

D-Streptamine, O-3-amino-3-deoxy-α-D-glucopyranosyl-(1→6)-
O-[6-amino-6-deoxy-α-D-glucopyranosyl-(1→4)]-N^1-(4-amino-
2-hydroxy-1-oxobutyl)-2-deoxy-, (S)-sulfate (1:2) salt
Amikin (*Bristol*)

[39831-55-5] $C_{22}H_{43}N_5O_{23}\cdot2H_2SO_4$ (781.78).

Preparation—Amikacin, the 1-L-(−)-4-amino-2-hydroxybutyryl derivative of kanamycin, is obtained by acylation of the C-1 amino group of the 2-deoxystreptamine moiety of kanamycin with L-(−)-4-amino-2-hydroxybutyric acid. German Pat 2,234,315, corresponding to US Pat 3,781,268 (*CA 78:* 136615x, 1973).

Description—Amikacin base occurs as a white to off-white flocculent powder, which is converted to the sulfate salt in preparing injection dosage forms.

Solubility—Amikacin base is freely soluble in water; insoluble in alcohol.

Uses—The N-(4-amino-2-hydroxy-1-oxobutyl) group protects the aminoglycoside from all but one of the nine aminoglycoside-inactivating enzymes and acetyltransferase. In one study, more than 80% of strains of bacteria resistant to one or more aminoglycosides were sensitive *in vitro* to amikacin. The greatest differences are shown with *Ps aeruginosa* and to a lesser extent with various *Enterobacteriaceae*. Most streptococci and a number of strains of otherwise sensitive gram-negative organisms are naturally resistant to the drug by virtue of mechanisms other than drug-destructive enzymes.

The most important bacterial species that are usually sensitive are *E coli*, *Ps aeruginosa*, *Proteus spp* (regardless of indole character), *Klebsiella pneumoniae*, *Serratia marcescens*, *Providencia stuartii*, *Citrobacter freundii*, and *Acinetobacter* species. Various staphylococci are also susceptible, irrespective of penicillinase production. The minimum effective concentration is 2 to 4 μg/mL for 90% of "sensitive" bacteria.

It is important that amikacin be held in reserve to treat only serious infections caused by the above-named gram-negative bacteria that are resistant not only to other aminoglycosides but other classes of antibacterial drugs. In this way, the development of resistant strains of bacteria can be retarded and the special usefulness of the drug not jeopardized. Septicemia, and serious infections of burns, urinary tract, respiratory tract, and various soft tissues, meningitis, peritonitis, osteomyelitis, omphalitis in neonates, and serious surgical infections are indications for use, provided the criteria of bacterial sensitivity to amikacin and insensitivity to both less toxic drugs and other aminoglycosides are met.

The toxicity is that of the aminoglycosides in general (this page). Tremors, paresthesias, arthralgia, and hypotension also occur. Plasma levels should be monitored where possible, and auditory tests and examination of the urine are mandatory. It is desirable to keep the plasma levels below 35 μg/mL. The effect on the fetus is unknown, and use in pregnancy should be avoided, if possible.

The absorption, distribution, and elimination is that of aminoglycosides in general (see general statement). Intramuscular injection of 7.5 mg/kg will yield a peak plasma concentration of 8 to 25 μg/mL in about 1 hr, and intravenous infusion of 500 mg in 30 min yields a mean level of 38 μg/mL. Amikacin is totally eliminated unchanged in the urine. The half-life is 2 to 2.5 hr in adults with normal renal function but up to 30 hr in renal failure. In neonates it is 4 to 8 hr. Because of the short half-life, it has been suggested that the usually suggested dose interval of 8 to 12 hr may be too long, but the effect on bacterial protein synthesis outlasts the time above the minimum inhibitory concentration.

Dose—*Intramuscular or intravenous, adults, children*, and *older infants*, **5 mg/kg** every 8 hr or **7.5 mg/kg** every 12 hr for 7 to 10 days, not to exceed 1.5 g a day, except in *urinary tract infections*, in which case the dose is 250 mg every 12 hr; in *neonates*, *initially* **10 mg per kg** followed with **7.5 mg/kg** every 12 hr, not to exceed 15 mg per kg

per day. In renal failure, the dose is based on creatinine clearance, assuming 100% renal elimination (or see package literature). For intravenous administration, 5% dextrose or physiological saline is used. The duration of infusion should be 30 to 60 min, except 1 to 2 hr in infants.

Dosage Forms—Injection: 100 mg/2 mL, 500 mg/2 mL, and 1 g/4 mL.

Gentamicin Sulfate

Gentamicin, sulfate; *Various Mfrs*

Gentamycins sulfate [1405-41-0]; the sulfate salt of the antibiotic substances produced by the growth of *Micromonospora purpurea*. Potency: not less than 590 μg of gentamicin/mg, on the anhydrous basis.

Gentamicin is a mixture of gentamicin C_1, gentamicin C_2, and gentamicin C_{1A}. Gentamicin C_{1A} is O-3-deoxy-4-C-methyl-3-(methylamino)-β-L-arabinopyranosyl-(1→6)-O-[2,6-diamino-2,3,4,6-tetradeoxy-α-D-*erythro*-hexopyranosyl-(1→4)-2-deoxy-D-streptamine.

Preparation—Gentamicin is recovered from a fermentation broth produced when submerged cultures of two subspecies of *Micromonospora purpurea* are grown in a yeast extract-cerelose medium. US Pat 3,136,704.

Description—White to buff powder that is odorless; stable in light, air, and heat; melts with decomposition between 200° and 250°.

Solubility—Soluble in water; insoluble in alcohol, acetone, and benzene.

Uses—Gentamicin is currently the most important aminoglycoside for use in the treatment of infections caused by gram-negative bacteria. It has broad-spectrum antibacterial activity. In concentrations of 1 μg/mL it will inhibit many strains of *Staph aureus;* in 1.5 μg/mL most indole-negative and some indole-positive *Proteus*, nonpigmented *Serratia*, and *Mycobacterium tuberculosis;* in 5 μg/mL, all penicillin-resistant and some methicillin-resistant *Staph aureus*, group A streptococci, *Strep pneumoniae*, *Past multocida*, *H influenzae*, *Acinetobacter*, and *Bacteroides;* in 10 μg/mL, about 90% of *Ps aeruginosa*. *Enterobacter-Klebsiella* and *E coli* are also usually highly sensitive. *Citrobacter*, *Pr inconstans*, *Salmonella*, *Shigella*, *Listeria*, *Brucella* and some *Streptococcus* have variable sensitivities. *Neisseria*, *Clostridia*, *Corynebacterium*, and *Ps pseudomallei* are relatively resistant. For more infections, plasma levels of 4 to 6 μg/mL should be achieved. It is frequently used, somewhat promiscuously, in the treatment of urinary tract infections.

The action of gentamicin against *Pseudomonas* is of especial interest, since species of that genus resistant to other antibiotics have become an important cause of surgical infections they almost always invade burned skin. They also cause some serious urinary tract infections. However, because of systemic toxicity, present systemic use is mainly limited to life-threatening infections caused by *Pseudomonas*, *Klebsiella-Enterobacter-Serratia*, *Citrobacter*, and *Proteus*. Since gentamicin has a narrower range of safety than kanamycin, if the organisms are sensitive to the latter it is preferred. In these infections gentamicin may be combined with an appropriate cephalosporin or penicillin; carbenicillin in high doses can *inhibit* the action of gentamicin. The promiscuous use of gentamicin in the treatment of urinary tract infections amenable to other agents must be condemned.

Gentamicin is used topically in the treatment of *impetigo*, infected *bed sores*, *burns*, and nasal *staphylococcal carrier state*, *pyodermata*, and in infections of the external eye and adnexa. Its use in minor infections is an abuse. This also applies to its use in preoperative bowel sterilization in most instances. The toxicity and precautions of gentamicin are those of the aminoglycosides in general (see introduction in this section). The peak serum concentration should be kept below 12 μg/mL. Cutaneous sensitizing potential is low, but allergic skin reactions and photosensitivity have been reported. Systemic toxicity includes auditory and vestibular impairment (2.3%), nephrotoxicity (2%; if the kidneys are previously normal, nephrotoxicity occurs only with high dose), and neuromuscular blockade, which may interact with neuromuscular blocking drugs.

The absorption, distribution, and elimination of gentamicin are those of aminoglycosides in general (see introduction).

Dose (base equivalent)—*Intramuscular* or *intravenous, adults,* **1 to 1.7 mg/kg** of body weight every 8 hr or **0.75 to 1.25 mg/kg** every 6 hr for 7 to 10 days; for *urinary tract infections,* body weight less than 60 kg, **3 mg/kg** once a day or **1.5 mg/kg** every 12 hr. *Infants and children,* **2.5 mg/kg** of body weight every 8 hr; *neonates* less than 7 days old, **2.5 mg/kg** of body weight every 12 hr. In renal failure, dosage is adjusted according to the creatinine clearance, based on the assumption of 100% excretion. Intravenous infusion should be made over a 1- to 2-hr period. *Intrathecal, adults,* **4 to 8 mg** once a day; *infants* and *children over 3 mo* of age, **1 to 2 mg** once a day. *Topical,* to eye, **0.05 to 1 mL** of solution every 4 hr or a small amount of ointment every 8 to 12 hr; *topical,* to skin, as **0.1%** cream or ointment 3 to 4 times a day. Except for enterococcal infections, the urine should be alkalinized in urinary tract infections.

Dosage Forms—Cream: 1 mg/g; Injection: 1, 10 and 40 mg/mL; Ointment: 1 mg/g; Ophthalmic Ointment: 3 mg/g; Ophthalmic Solution: 3 mg/mL.

Kanamycin Sulfate

D-Streptamine, *O*-3-amino-3-deoxy-α-D-glucopyranosyl-(1→6)-*O*-[6-amino-6-deoxy-α-D-glucopyranosyl-(1→4)]-2-deoxy-, sulfate (1:1); Kantrex (*Bristol*)

Kanamycin sulfate [133-92-6; 25389-94-0] $C_{18}H_{36}N_4O_{11} \cdot H_2SO_4$ (583.58); contains kanamycin sulfate equivalent to not less than 75% of kanamycin (484.50) (the antibiotic activity of 750 μg of kanamycin in each mg) and not more than 5% of kanamycin B sulfate, on the anhydrous basis.

Kanamycin A (kanamycin) is *O*-3-amino-3-deoxy-α-D-glycopyranosyl-(1→6)-*O*-[6- amino-6-deoxy-α-D-glucopyranosyl-(1→4)]-2-deoxy-D-streptamine. Kanamycin B differs only in that the (1→4) carbohydrate residue is 2,6-diamino-2,6-dideoxy-α-D-glucopyranosyl.

Kanamycin is produced solely by fermentation using *Streptomyces kanamyceticus.*

Description—White, odorless, crystalline powder.
Solubility—Freely soluble in water; insoluble in alcohol, acetone, ethyl acetate, and benzene.

Uses—Active against gram-negative organisms such as *Klebsiella, Enterobacter, Acinetobacter, Brucella, Neisseria, Hemophilus, Shigella, Salmonella, E coli, Serratia marcescens,* and many strains of *Proteus.* Unfortunately, *Pseudomonas aeruginosa* and *Bacteroides* are resistant. It is also effective against some *Mycoplasma* and gram-positive bacteria, especially *Staph pyogenes* and *Staph epidermidis,* most of which strains are inhibited by 1 μg/mL and many others by 2 to 2.5 μg/mL; others, such as streptococci and pneumococci, are not inhibited at levels usually attained in body fluids. However, in combination with penicillin it is effective against *Strep fecalis.* It is also effective against mycobacteria in a concentration of 2.5 to 10 μg/mL. Most sensitive organisms can develop resistance to kanamycin. Furthermore, there is almost complete cross-resistance with neomycin and paromomycin.

Kanamycin is used only when there is resistance to safer drugs. It is used in the treatment of *gram-negative septicemias,* particularly in *shock,* serious *urinary tract infections,* gram-negative *bacterial*

endocarditis, peritonitis, *Klebsiella pneumoniae,* and *neonatal meningitis.* It is often used in combination with other drugs for use against serious staphylococcal infections and tuberculosis. Kanamycin is used orally for bowel sterilization in hepatic coma and prior to bowel surgery.

The toxicity is that of aminoglycosides in general (see introduction in this section). About 30% of patients will manifest a hearing deficit and 7% disturbed vestibular function. Ototoxicity is highly probable if the total (cumulative) dose exceeds 10 g. With oral administration, vomiting, diarrhea, steatorrhea, and other malabsorption syndromes can occur. Pain occurs at the injection site. Because of its toxicity, kanamycin is not widely used, and its status is that of a second-order "back-up" drug.

The absorption, distribution, and elimination of kanamycin are those of aminoglycosides in general (see introduction). Intramuscular injection of 1 g yields a plasma concentration of 20 to 35 μg/mL in about 1 hr. Although the half-life is about 2.5 hr in adults, it is 18 hr in premature infants less than 2 days old, and 6 hr in infants 5 to 22 days old. The half-life is prolonged in renal failure, and doses must be adjusted according to creatinine clearance assuming 100% renal elimination.

Dose (base equivalent)—*Oral, adult* for therapy in *intestinal infections,* **1 g** 3 times a day for 5 to 7 days; for *preoperative preparation,* **1 g** every hr for 4 doses, then **1 g** every 6 hr for 36 to 72 hr; in *hepatic coma,* **2 to 3 g** every 6 hr; *infants* and *children, oral,* any use **8.3 mg/kg** every 4 hr or **12.5 mg/kg** of body weight every 6 hr for 5 to 7 d. *Intramuscular, adults* and *children,* **3.75 mg/kg** every 6 hr, **5 mg/kg** every 8 hr, or **7.5 mg/kg** every 12 hr. *Intravenous, adults* and *children,* **3.75 mg/kg** every 6 hr, **5 mg/kg** every 8 hr, or **7.5 mg/kg** every 12 hr for 7 to 10 days. *Intraperitoneal, adults,* **0.5 g;** the dose is to be diluted with sterile water to a volume of 20 mL. By any parenteral route, the dose should not exceed 1.5 g/day for up to 5 days. *Inhalation, adults,* **250 mg** every 6 to 12 hr.

Dosage Forms—Capsules: 500 mg; Injection: 75 and 500 mg/2 mL, 1 g/3 mL.

Neomycin Sulfate

Mycifradin Sulfate (*Upjohn*); *Various Mfrs*

Neomycin sulfate [1405-10-3]; the sulfate of an antibacterial substance produced by the growth of *Streptomyces fradiae* Waksman (Fam. *Streptomycetaceae*). Potency: equivalent to not less than 600 μg of neomycin/mg, calculated on the dried basis.

Neomycin consists almost entirely of a pair of $C_{23}H_{46}N_6O_{13}$ epimers designated as neomycin B and neomycin C, and the ratio of B to C has been observed to vary widely among different production lots. The total structure and the common names of the component parts of neomycin C are shown below.

Neomycin B

Systematically, it is *O*-2,6-diamino-2,6-dideoxy-α-D-glucopyranosyl-(1→3)-*O*-β-D-ribofuranosyl-(1→5)-*O*-[2,6-diamino-2,6-dideoxy-α-D-glucopyranosyl- (1→4)]-2-deoxy-D-streptamine. Neomycin B is identical except that the α-D-glucopyranosyl residue in the neobiosamine moiety is β-L-idopyranosyl.

Description—White to slightly yellow powder or cryodesiccated solid; odorless or practically odorless, and hygroscopic; pH (aqueous solution, 33 mg/mL) between 5 and 7.5.
Solubility—1 g in about 1 mL water; very slightly soluble in alcohol; insoluble in acetone, chloroform, and ether.

Uses—Gram-negative bacteria that are sensitive to neomycin are: *E coli, Klebsiella-Enterobacter, Proteus, Pasteurella, Hemophilus, Salmonella, Shigella, N meningitidis, V cholerae,* and *Bordetella pertussis; Ps aeruginosa* is usually not sensitive. Sensitive gram-positive organisms are: *B anthracis, C diphtheriae, Listeria, Borellia, Leptospira, M tuberculosis, Staph aureus,* and *Strep fecalis;* group A *Strep pyogenes* and *Strep viridans* are resistant. Concentrations of 5 to 10 µg/mL are usually adequate to inhibit susceptible organisms. The antibiotic is used in a wide variety of local infections, including *infected dermatoses, burns, wounds, ulcers, impetigo, furunculosis, otitis externa, conjunctivitis,* and *sty;* also for irrigation of the bladder and urethra during catheterization, as prophylaxis. It is often combined with other antibiotics, especially polymyxin B sulfate, bacitracin zinc, and gramicidin. It is also incorporated into topical steroid preparations, to control secondary infections in inflammatory disorders; however, evidence indicates that neomycin in such preparations often fails to control the infections. Orally, the drug is used to produce intestinal antisepsis prior to large bowel surgery, for the treatment of gastroenteritis caused by toxigenic *E coli,* and to suppress ammonia-producing bowel flora in the management of hepatic coma. Oral neomycin interferes with the absorption of cholesterol, and hence it is used in the treatment of *hypercholesterolemia.* Because of rapid overgrowth of nonsusceptible bacteria, including staphylococci, oral neomycin therapy should not be continued for longer than 72 hr; this is not possible for antihyperlipidemic therapy, so a less than maximal dose is used in order to cause less disruption of the enteric floral ecology. Because neomycin has high toxicity, it is used systematically only in very desperate situations in which the usual antibiotics are ineffective. These are usually septicemias or serious urinary tract or respiratory infections caused by gram-negative bacilli. In some countries neomycin is used as an aerosol in the treatment of respiratory infections.

Although orally administered neomycin rarely causes systemic toxic effects, it frequently produces loose stools, nausea, vomiting, and malabsorption syndromes. Applied topically, the drug is well tolerated, relatively nonirritating, and has a low index of sensitivity. However, contact dermatitis occasionally occurs. Injected parenterally, neomycin causes serious nephrotoxic, ototoxic, and neurotoxic effects. The renal injury is usually reversible and is manifested by albumin and granular casts in the urine and an elevation of nonprotein nitrogen in the blood; ototoxicity is mainly auditory and may be additive to that produced by streptomycin. Because of the potential toxicity, parenteral injection and prolonged oral administration of neomycin are assiduously avoided, if possible.

About 97% of orally administered neomycin is eliminated unchanged in the feces; an oral dose of 3 g produces a peak serum level of only 1 to 4 µg/mL. An intramuscular dose of 1 g produces a peak serum level of 20 µg/mL. Unlike other aminoglycosides, only 50% of neomycin is excreted unchanged. The half-life is 2 hr.

Dose (base equivalents)—*Oral,* for *preoperative bowel sterilization, adults,* **0.7 g** or for *infants, children* and *adults,* **10.3 mg/kg** of body wt, every 4 hr for 4 doses, then every 4 hr for the remainder of 24 to 72 hr; for *E coli enterocolitis,* for *infants, children,* and *adults,* **8.75 mg/kg,** every 6 hr for 2 to 3 days; for *hepatic coma, adults,* **0.7** to **2.1 g** and for *infants* and *children,* **10** to **30 mg/kg** or 0.428 to 1.28 g/m² of body surface every 6 hr for 5 to 6 days; for *hyperlipidemia; adults,* **350 mg** 4 times a day; *neonates* and *premature infants* should receive **2.5** to **12.5 mg/kg** 4 times a day for any oral use. *Intramuscular,* for *urinary tract infections, adults,* **1.3** to **2.6 mg/kg** every 6 hr. *Topical,* to the skin, as **0.35%** cream or ointment 1 to 3 times a day; to the conjunctiva, as **0.35%** ophthalmic ointment 1 to 3 times a day.

To calculate doses in terms of neomycin sulfate, multiply by 1.43 (500 mg of neomycin sulfate is equivalent to 350 mg of neomycin base).

Dosage Forms (as base equivalents)—Cream: 3.5 mg/g; Ointment: 3.5 mg/g; Ophthalmic Ointment: 3.5 mg/g; Oral Solution: 87.5 mg/5 mL; Sterile Powder, to be reconstituted to 2 mL: 350 mg; Tablets: 350 mg.

Streptomycin Sulfate

D-Streptamine, *O*-2-deoxy-2-(methylamino)-α-L-glucopyranosyl-(1→2)-*O*-5-deoxy-3-*C*-formyl-α-L-lyxofuranosyl-(1→4)-*N,N'*-bis(aminoiminomethyl)-, sulfate (2:3) (salt); Streptomycin Sulfate (2:3)

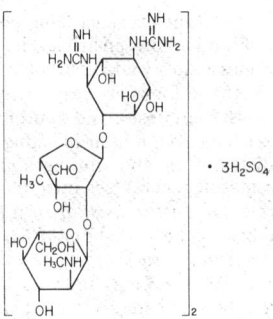

Streptomycin sulfate (2:3) (salt) [3810-74-0] $(C_{21}H_{39}N_7O_{12})_2$·$3H_2SO_4$ (1457.38). Potency: equivalent to 650 to 850 µg of streptomycin $(C_{21}H_{39}N_7O_{12})$/mg.

Streptomycin is an organic base, consisting of *N*-methyl-*l*-glucosamine and streptidine linked through the carbohydrate streptose. The overall structure is portrayed above.

Preparation—Isolated from soil by Waksman and his colleagues of Rutgers University in 1943.

Streptomycin is produced in organic or synthetic media, in surface or submerged cultures of an actinomycete, *Streptomyces griseus,* a mold-like organism with filaments (mycelium) of bacterial thickness.

Commercially, streptomycin is manufactured like penicillin, microbiologically in tank fermenters with aeration and agitation.

Description—White or practically white powder; odorless or has not more than a faint odor; hygroscopic, but stable toward air and light; pH (1 in 5 solution) between 4.5 and 7.0.

Solubility—Freely soluble in water; very slightly soluble in alcohol; practically insoluble in chloroform.

Uses—In low concentrations streptomycin is bacteriostatic and in high concentrations bactericidal to a large number of gram-negative and gram-positive bacteria. *Brucella, Erysipelothrix, H ducreyi, L monocytogenes, Actinobacillus mallei, Nocardia, Yersinia pestis, Francisella tularensis,* many strains of *M tuberculosis* and of *Shigella* are sensitive to concentrations that are usually achievable in man. Strains of *E coli, H influenzae, N pertussis, N gonorrhea, Salmonella, Staph aureus* and *epidermidis, Strep fecalis, pneumoniae, pyogenes* (Group A) and *viridans,* and *V cholerae* are variably sensitive and insensitive.

The only infections in which streptomycin alone is the drug of choice are *tularemia* and *bubonic plague.* In combination with a tetracycline it is first choice in the treatment of *brucellosis,* infections caused by *Actinobacillus mallei* and with ampicillin or penicillin G infections caused by *enterococci* (especially endocarditis). It is an alternate choice drug in the treatment of chancroid, *rat-bite fevers* (*Spirillum* and *Streptobacillus,* and *tuberculosis;* in tuberculosis, however, it is never used alone, because of the rapidity of development of resistance. Occasionally, streptomycin is used in combination with other drugs in desperate situations, such as meningitides, in which the sensitivity is marginal.

The toxicity is that of aminoglycosides in general (see introduction in this section). In addition, malaise and myalgia may occur. Vestibular disturbances are more frequent than loss of hearing.

The absorption, distribution, and elimination of streptomycin are those of aminoglycosides in general. An intramuscular dose of 1 g causes a peak plasma concentration of 25 to 30 µg/mL in the adult.

Dose (base equivalent)—*Intramuscular, adults,* for *tuberculosis,* in combination with one or more of the drugs isoniazid, ethambutol, rifampin, or aminosalicylic acid, **1 g** a day, to be reduced to **1 g** 2 to 3 times a week, until toxicity or resistance supervenes; for *tularemia,* **1** to **2 g/day** in 2 or 4 divided doses until the patient has been afebrile for 5 to 7 days (total of about 7 to 10 days); for *plague,* **2** to **4 g/day** in 2 to 4 divided doses until the patient has been afebrile for at least 3 days; for susceptible bacterial *endocarditis* (in combination with penicillin), **1 g** twice a day for the first week, then **0.5 g** twice a day for the second week, except 0.5 g twice a day for 2 wk in patients over 60 yr of age; for *enterococcal endocarditis* (in combination with penicillin), **1 g** twice a day for 2 weeks and **0.5 g** twice a day for 4 weeks; for various *fulminating infections,* **2** to **4 g/day** in divided doses for variable periods; for less severe infections, **1** to **2 g** a day in two divided doses. *Intramuscular, children,* for *tuberculosis,* in combination with other antitubercular drugs, **20 mg/kg** once a day, not to exceed

1 g/day; for *other infections*, in combination with other antibacterial drugs, **5 to 10 mg/kg** every 6 hr or **10 to 20 mg/kg** every 12 hr.

Dosage Forms (base equivalent)—Injection: 1 g/2.5 mL and 5 g/10 and 12.5 mL; sterile powder: 1 and 5 g. 1.25 g of streptomycin sulfate is equivalent to 1 g of streptomycin.

Paromomycin—page 1221.

Tobramycin

D-Streptamine, O-3-amino-3-deoxy-α-D-glucopyranosyl-(1→6)-
O-[2,6-diamino-2,3,6-trideoxy-α-D-*ribo*-hexopyranosyl-
(1→4)]-2-deoxy-, Nebcin (sulfate) (*Lilly*)

O-3-Amino-3-deoxy-α-D-glucopyranosyl-(1→4)-O-[2,6-diamino-2,3,6-trideoxy-α-D-*ribo*-hexopyranosyl-(1→6)]-2-deoxy-L-strepta-mine [32986-56-4] $C_{18}H_{37}N_5O_9$ (467.52). Potency: Not less than 900 μg of $C_{18}H_{37}N_5O_9$ per mg, calculated on the anhydrous basis.

Preparation—An antibiotic entity separated from an antibiotic complex produced by *Streptomyces tenebrarius*. In its injection dosage form tobramycin is present as a sulfate.

Description—White or off-white, hygroscopic powder.
Solubility—Freely soluble in water; very slightly soluble in alcohol; practically insoluble in chloroform, ether.

Uses—Tobramycin is bactericidal to most strains of *Klebsiella-Enterobacter-Serratia* organisms in concentrations of 0.75 μg/mL or less, *Staph aureus* in 1 μg/mL, and most other gram-negative organisms in 2 μg/mL, except 50% *Proteus* spp and *E coli* in 3 μg/mL and *Pseudomonas* in 5 to 10 μg/mL. Thus it is generally less active than gentamicin, but it is approximately 4 times as active against *Pseudomonas*. Carbenicillin and certain other penicillins synergize its actions against *Pseudomonas*. Strains with low-level resistance to gentamicin are sensitive to tobramycin, but strains with high-level resistance are not. Because of its efficacy against *Pseudomonas* infections, tobramycin should be used only in the treatment of such infections when they are caused by organisms insensitive not only to gentamicin but other less toxic antimicrobial drugs as well. In this way, the development of resistant strains is discouraged, and the future value of the drug is not likely to be jeopardized. Despite this precept, the drug is promoted for the treatment of serious infections caused by generally sensitive strains of *Pseudomonas*, *E coli*, *Proteus* spp (irrespective of indole character), *Providencia*, *Klebsiella-Enterobacter-Serratia*, *Citrobacter*, and *Staph aureus*. Although a few staphylococci are susceptible, it is not used for staphylococcal infections, except in combination with penicillin G against identified susceptible strains of *Strep fecalis*.

The toxic effects of tobramycin are those of aminoglycosides in general (see introduction in this section). Both auditory and vestibular functions may be affected. Plasma concentrations should be monitored and concentrations above 12 μg/mL avoided. Urine should be regularly examined.

The absorption, distribution, and elimination is that of aminoglycosides in general (see introduction). Intramuscular injection of 1 mg/kg will yield a peak plasma concentration of about 4 μg/mL. Elimination is impaired in renal failure.

Dose (base equivalent)—*Intramuscular* or *intravenous infusion*, adults, **0.75 to 1.25 mg/kg** every 6 hr *or* 1 to **1.7 mg/kg** every 8 hr for 7 to 10 days or longer, except up to 8 mg/kg per day, divided in 3 or 4 equal doses, in life-threatening infections; *neonates up to 1 wk of age* and *premature infants*, up to **2 mg/kg** of body weight every 12 hr; *older infants* and *children*, **1.5 to 1.9 mg/kg** every 6 hr *or* 2 to **2.5 mg/kg** every 8 hr. In renal failure the dose must be adjusted according to the creatinine clearance, based on 100% excretion.

Dosage Forms (base equivalent; the injection is prepared with the aid of sulfuric acid to solubilize the tobramycin and it exists, therefore, as the sulfate salt)—Injection: 20, 40 and 80 mg/2 mL and 60 mg/1.5 mL. Sterile Powder: 1.2 g.

Other Aminoglycosides

Netilmicin Sulfate [[56391-57-2] $(C_{21}H_{41}N_5O_7)_2.5H_2O$ (1441.54) Netromycin (*Schering-Plough*)]. A synthetic derivative of sisomicin; see *Chem Commun* 206, 1976. *Uses:* Netilmicin has an antibacterial spectrum of activity much like that of gentamicin and tobramycin. However, it is not degraded by certain bacterial enzymes that degrade gentamicin and tobramycin, so that it may be effective at times when there is resistance to gentamicin and tobramycin, especially by *Enterobacteriaceae*. At present, its clinical status remains to be determined. It does not appear to offer advantages over amikacin. Its toxicity, contraindications, and pharmacokinetics are like those of aminoglycosides in general (page 1179); dose adjustments must be made in renal failure. *Dose: Intramuscular* or *intravenous infusion*, *adults*, for serious *systemic infections*, 1.3 to 2.2 mg/kg every 8 hr or 2 to 3.25 mg/kg every 12 hr; for serious *urinary tract infections*, 1.5 to 2 mg/kg every 12 hr. *Infants older than 6 weeks* and *children* up through 12 yr, 1.8 to 2.7 mg/kg every 8 hr *or* 2.7 to 4 mg every 12 hr. *Neonates less than 6 wk* of age, 2 to 3.25 mg/kg every 12 hr.

Sisomicin Sulfate [[32385-11-8] $C_{19}H_{37}N_5O_7$ (447.53)]—An antibiotic closely related to gentamicin C_{1A}; produced by *Micromonospora inyoensis*. See *J Antibiot 23:* 551, 555, 1970. *Uses:* Similar to gentamycin in antibacterial spectrum and pattern of drug resistance. Occasionally it is effective when bacteria are resistant to all other aminoglycosides. However, it is not considered to offer any advantages over tobramycin. Its toxicity, contraindications, and pharmacokinetics are those of aminoglycosides in general (page 1179). Sisomicin is approved for use in the US but is not yet marketed here. *Dose: Intramuscular* or *intravenous infusion*, *adults*, 1 mg/kg every 8 hr. In renal failure, the dose is adjusted according to the creatinine clearance; plasma concentrations should be no higher than 10 μg/mL at the peak and no less than 2 μg/mL at the trough.

Cephalosporins

The cephalosporins are a group of antibiotics closely related to the penicillins. The cephalosporanic acid moiety characteristic of cephalosporins is an analogue of the penicillanic acid moiety characteristic of penicillins; cephalosporanic acid contains a dihydrometathiazine ring, while penicillanic acid contains a tetrahydrothiazole (thiazolidine) ring. Both have a β-lactam ring. 7-Aminocephalosporanic acid derivatives are much more acid-stable than the corresponding 6-amino-penicillanic acid compounds. Moxalactam has a dihydro-metaoxazine ring in lieu of the thiazine ring.

Antibacterial Actions—The cephalosporins have a mechanism of action very similar to that of the penicillins, namely, they inhibit the cross-linking of the peptidoglycan units in the bacterial cell wall by occupying the D-alanyl-D-alanine substrate site of the transpeptidase. There is some evidence, however, that the site of action is not identical to that of penicillins. Because of the similar mechanisms, it is to be expected that the antibacterial spectra would be very similar, as they are. Cephalosporins are presently classified as first-, second- and third-generation cephalosporins. The first-generation drugs have the highest activity against gram-positive and the lowest against gram-negative bacteria. Thus, they are active against most staphylococci (even penicillinase-producers, but not methicillin-resistant staphylococci). They are also active against most streptococci, including *S pyogenes*, *viridans*, and *pneumoniae*. They are not active against *S faecalis*. Other susceptible gram-positive bacteria are *Cl perfringens*, *Listeria*, and *Corynebacterium*. First-generation cephalosporins also are moderately active against certain gram-negative bacteria, such as *Neisseria gonorrheae* and *meningitidis*, many *E coli*, some *H influenzae*, and non-hospital acquired *Klebsiella* and *Pr mirabilis* and some *Salmonella* and *Shigella*. First-generation cephalosporins include cefadroxil, cefazolin, cephalexin, cephaloglycin, cephaloridine, cephalothin, cephalexin, cephapirin, and cephradine.

The second-generation cephalosporins are more active against gram-negative and less active against gram-positive bacteria than are first-generation members, except that cefoxitin has very high activity against gonococci. Notable of the increased activity against gram-negative organisms is greater efficacy against most *H influenzae*, the efficacy of cefoxitin against *B fragilis* and indole-positive *Proteus* and the activity of cephamandole against *Enterobacter* and indole-positive *Proteus*. Like the first-generation, members of this group are inactive against *Ps aeruginosa*. Cefaclor, cefamandole, cefoxitin, and cefuroxime belong in this group.

The third-generation cephalosporins are considerably less active than first-generation drugs against gram-positive but have a much expanded spectrum of activity against gram-negative organisms. They are quite active against gram-negative anaerobes, and, except for cefsulodin, are frequently active against *Enterobacteriaceae* (*E coli*, *Enterobacter*, *Klebsiella pneumoniae*). Of special interest is the activity against *Ps aeruginosa*, although only cefoperazone has high activity. These drugs are inactive against *Acinetobacter*. Drugs in this group include cefoperazone, cefmenoxime, cefotaxime, cefsulodin, ceftazidime, ceftizoxime, ceftriaxone, and moxalactam.

Resistance—As with the penicillins one common mechanism of resistance is that of elaboration of a β-lactamase. Although some cephalosporins are inactivated by penicillinase-types of β-lactamase, some are not but are affected by cephalosporinase types. Therefore, there may be cross-resistance between penicillins and cephalosporins, but not necessarily so. In addition to β-lactamase-related resistance, other types of resistance, analogous to methicillin resistance, occur.

Indications—No cephalosporin is the *a priori* drug of choice for any infection, even when used in combination with another agent, but a cephalosporin may sometimes be used when hypersensitivity or resistance to penicillin obtains in an infection in which a penicillin would have been otherwise the drug of choice. No cephalosporin is even the unequivocal drug of second choice. Therefore, the following indications are ones in which a cephalosporin is only one of two or more second-choice drugs which equally could be selected (but only on the basis of *in vitro* tests); in some indications, another drug should be combined with a cephalosporin: infections caused by *Staph aureus* (both penicillinase-producing and methicillin-resistant), *Staph epidermidis*, *Strep viridans*, *bovis*, *pneumoniae*, *Cl tetani*, *Kl pneumoniae*, and *Pr mirabilis*. Second-generation cephalosporins provide alternate drugs for the treatment of infections caused by *H influenzae* and *N gonorrhoeae*. Occasionally, third-generation cephalosporins may be used in infections caused by *E coli*, *Salmonella*, *Shigella*, *Pseudomonas*, *Serratia*, *Enterobacter*, indole-positive *Proteus*, and *Bacteroides fragilis*. Some third-generation cephalosporins penerate into the cerebrospinal fluid well enough to be useful in certain infections of the central nervous system.

Adverse Effects—Hypersensitivity occurs in about 5 to 10% of recipients of cephalosporins; manifestations are eosinophilia, drug fever, maculopapular rash, urticaria, serum sickness, angioneurotic edema, anaphylaxis, positive Coombs test associated with rare hemolytic anemia, and infrequent transient hepatic abnormalities (increased SGOT, SGPT, and total bilirubin), thrombocytopenia, neutropenia, and interstitial nephritis. There is an appreciable incidence of cross-sensitization with penicillin; when previously manifested penicillin sensitivity has not been serious, a cephalosporin, especially cefazolin, may be administered cautiously after sensitivity testing, but *only if necessary;* skin tests often give false negatives. If the previous reaction to penicillin was severe, such as with anaphylaxis or angioneurotic edema, or if the patient reacts to penicillin minor determinants, a cephalosporin is contraindicated.

Other adverse effects of cephalosporins include pain, induration, sterile abscess and sloughing at the site of intramuscular injection, thrombophlebitis after intravenous administration, nausea, vomiting, glossitis, diarrhea, loose stools, abdominal pain and heartburn, especially with oral admin-

istration, sodium load and water retention with sodium salts, antibiotic-associated colitis (especially with poorly absorbed members) and a false-positive urine test for glucose (Benedict, Fehling and Clinitest, but not Tes-Tape). Present cephalosporins are not significantly nephrotoxic alone but may considerably increase the nephrotoxicity of an aminoglycoside. Cephalosporins should not be used in combination with other antibiotics that cause nephrotoxicity or ototoxicity. High-ceiling diuretics (eg, furosemide and ethacrynic acid) also enhance nephrotoxicity and make certain cephalosporins ototoxic. The acquisition costs of some cephalosporins is very high, up to $1600 for a 10-day course; however, costs to the patient are not necessarily proportional and substitution for some costly penicillins sometimes is economical. Superinfections by gram-negative bacteria and *Candida* may occur.

Pharmacokinetics—Cephalosporins vary considerably in their peroral bioavailability (15 to 86%), protein binding (14 to 96%), and half-lives (45 to 150 min). Elimination is mainly by glomerular filtration and tubular secretion (except for cefoperazone) and some biliary secretion (and reabsorption), except that most of cephaloglycin and some of cefotaxime, cephalothin, cephapirin, and cephacetrile are deacetylated and subsequently further transformed; consequently, renal failure may greatly increase the half-lives of most cephalosporins. Cephalosporins vary in their penetrance into tissues. Only cephalothin and third-generation cephalosporins achieve therapeutic concentrations in cerebrospinal fluid, and then only in inflammation of the meninges. Cephalosporins cross the placental barrier and reach plasma concentration in the fetus in about 10% of maternal concentrations; effects on the fetus are unknown, but it is advisable to avoid treatment of pregnant women with cephalosporins if possible.

Cefaclor

5-Thia-1-azabicyclo[4.2.0]oct-2-ene-2-carboxylic acid, 7-[(aminophenylacetyl)amino]-3-chloro-8-oxo-, [6*R*-[6α,7β(*R**)]]-, monohydrate; Ceclor (*Lilly*)

[[70356-03-05] $C_{15}H_{14}ClN_3O_4S.H_2O$ (385.82)] Cefaclor is a semisynthetic cephalosporin related to cephalexin.

Preparation—See *J Med Chem* 18: 403, 1975.

Description—White crystalline solid. Aqueous solutions are most stable at pH of about 3.5, which is the pH of a 2% solution.

Solubility—Soluble in water (1 in 100); practically insoluble in most organic solvents.

Uses—Cefaclor is a second-generation cephalosporin with typical antibacterial activities and adverse effects (see the general statement). It is the only *orally* efficaceous member of its group. It is approved for use in the treatment of *upper respiratory tract infections, pharyngitis* and *tonsillitis* caused by *Str pyogenes; lower respiratory tract infections* caused by *Str pneumoniae, pyogenes,* and *H influenzae; otitis media* caused by *Str pneumoniae, Str pyogenes,* staphylococci, and *H influenzae; cutaneous infections* caused by *Staph Aureus* and *Str pyrogenes;* and *urinary tract infections* caused by *E coli, Pr mirabilis, Klebsiella* spp and coagulase-negative staphylococci. A 250-mg dose causes a peak plasma concentration of about 7 μg/mL. In plasma, 40% is bound to protein. The volume of distribution is 0.21 mL/g. About 60 to 80% is excreted unchanged into the urine. The half-life is 0.6 to 0.9 hr, except longer in renal failure.

Dose—*Oral, adults,* **250** to **500 mg** every 8 hr; *infants 1 month* and *older* and *children,* **6.7** to **13.4 mg/kg** every 8 hr.

Dosage Forms—Capsules: 250 and 500 mg; for *oral* suspension: 125 and 250 mg/5 mL (reconstituted).

Cefadroxil

5-Thia-1-azabicyclo[4.2.0]oct-2-ene-2-carboxylic acid, 7-[[amino(4-hydroxyphenyl)acetyl]amino]-3-methyl-8-oxo-, monohydrate, [6R-[6α,7β(R*)]]-, Duricef (*Mead Johnson*); Ultracef (*Bristol*)

[66592-87-8] $C_{16}H_{17}N_3O_5S.H_2O$ (381.40)
Preparation—See US Pat 3,864,340.

Description—White crystals melting about 197°.
Solubility—Soluble in water; the pH of a 5% aqueous solution is about 5.

Uses—Cefadroxil is a first-generation cephalosporin with typical actions, uses, adverse-effects, etc. (see the general statement). It is approved for use in *pharyngitis* and *tonsillitis* caused by *Str pyrogenes* (group A, beta-hemolytic), *cutaneous infections* caused by staphylococci and streptococci, and *urinary tract infections* caused by *E coli*, *Pr mirabilis*, and *Klebsiella* spp. It is absorbed by the oral route. In plasma, 20% is bound to proteins. The volume of distribution is 0.26 mL/gm. About 90% is eliminated unchanged in the urine. The half-life is about 1.5 hr.

Dose—*Oral, adults, urinary tract infections*, **0.5 to 1 g** every 12 hr *or* **1 g** once a day; for *pharyngitis* and *tonsilitis*, **0.5 g** every 12 hr for 12 days. *Children*, **15 mg/1 kg** every 12 hr.

Dosage Forms—Capsules: 500 mg; for Oral Suspension: 125, 250, and 500 mg/5 mL (reconstituted); Tablets: 1 g.

Cefamandole Nafate

5-Thia-1-azabicyclo[4.2.0]oct-2-ene-2-carboxylic acid, 7-[[(formyloxy)phenylacetyl]amino]-3-[[(1-methyl-1H-tetrazol-5-yl)thio]methyl]-8-oxo-, monosodium salt, [6R-[6α,7β(R*)]-, Mandol (*Lilly*)

[42540-40-9] $C_{19}H_{17}N_6NaO_6S_2$ (512.49).
Uses—Cefamandole is a second-generation cephalosporin. It is active against 80 to 90% of indole-positive strains of *Proteus* and is also active against *H influenzae*, *E coli*, *Klebsiella*, *Enterobacter*, *Serratia*, and *Providencia*. However, it is not as effective as amikacin, gentamicin, or tobramycin. Cefamandole is effective against enteric anerobes such as *B. fragilis* and clostridia, but it is not as effective as cefoxitin. There is no cross-resistance to ampicillin or methicillin. In general, indications for use are those of the cephalosporins as a group (see introduction in this section).

The adverse effects of cefamandole are those of other cephalosporins (see introduction) but it has low nephrotoxicity and causes less pain on intramuscular, and less phlebothrombosis on intravenous, injection than with most other cephalosporins. The sodium content of cefamandole and of the sodium carbonate added to it, amounting to a total of approximately 77 mg of sodium per gram of cefamandole activity, should be taken into account when the drug is used in persons with low sodium tolerance.

Cefamandole is not absorbed when administered orally. It is 67 to 80% bound to plasma proteins and has a volume of distribution of 0.16 mL/g. An intramuscular dose of 500 mg yields a peak plasma concentration of 12 to 15 µg/mL in 0.5 to 1 hr. About 85% is secreted into the urine; the half-life is 0.75 to 1 hr.

Dose (cefamandole equivalent)—*Intramuscular* or *intravenous*, *adults*, for *various infections*, **0.5 to 2 g** every 4 to 6 hr; for *pneumonia* and *skin infections*, **0.5 g** every 6 hr; for urinary tract infections, **0.5 to 1 g** every 8 hr; for surgical *prophylaxis*, **1 to 2 g** 0.5 to 1 hr before and every 6 hr after surgery; *infants 1 month* of age or *older* and *children*, for *all infections*, **8.3 to 16.7 mg/kg** every 4 hr *or* **12.5 to 25 mg/kg** every 6 hr *or* **16.7 to 33.3 mg/kg** every 8 hr; for surgical *prophylaxis*, **12.5 to 25 mg/kg** 0.5 to 1 hr before and every 6 hr after surgery.

Dosage Forms—Injection: 0.5 and 1 mg/10 mL and 2 g/20 mL. There are 3.3 mEq of sodium per g.

Cefazolin Sodium

5-Thia-1-azabicyclo[4.2.0]oct-2-ene-2-carboxylic acid, 3-[[(5-methyl-1,3,4-thiadiazol-2-yl)thio]methyl]-8-oxo-7-[[(1H-tetrazol-1-yl)acetyl]-amino]-, monosodium salt (6R-*trans*)-, Ancef (*SKF*); Kefzol (*Lilly*)

[27164-46-1] $C_{14}H_{13}N_8NaO_4S_3$ (476.48). Potency: Not less than 850 µg and not more than 1050 µg of cefazolin ($C_{14}H_{14}N_8O_4S_3$) per mg, calculated on the anhydrous basis.

Preparation—The sodium salt of 7-aminocephalosporanic acid is acylated with 1H-tetrazole-1-acetyl chloride and the acetoxy group is then displaced by reaction with 5-methyl-1,3,4-thiadiazole-2-thiol; the resulting cefazolin is converted to the sodium salt.

Description—White to off-white, crystalline powder.
Solubility—Freely soluble in water, in saline TS, and in dextrose solutions; very slightly soluble in alcohol; practically insoluble in chloroform and in ether.

Uses—The actions and uses of cefazolin are those of first-generation cephalosporins (see introductory statement in this section). It is less active than cephalothin against gram-positive, but more active against gram-negative, bacteria. Organisms resistant to both penicillin G and methicillin are sensitive to cefazolin. Cefazolin resistance also can occur.

The drug can be used to treat *infections of the respiratory tract*, *skin*, *soft tissues*, *bones*, *joints*, and *urinary tract*, and *endocarditis* and *septicemia* caused by susceptible organisms. Among urinary tract infections, cystitis responds much better than pyelonephritis. Cefazolin is the preferred cephalosporin for surgical prophylaxis, because of its (relatively) long half-life.

The adverse effects of cefazolin are those of cephalosporins in general (see introduction). It causes less pain at the site of injection and less phlebitis than cephalothin, but it appears to cause more oral, genital, and vaginal candidiasis, and anal pruritus. It causes a transient increase in blood urea nitrogen yet seems to have negligible nephrotoxicity.

Cefazolin is not absorbed orally. It is bound to the extent of 70 to 85% by plasma proteins and has a low volume of distribution of only 0.10 to 0.14 mL/g. An intramuscular dose of 500 mg will yield a peak plasma concentration of 37 µg/mL at 1 hr; intravenously 500 mg will yield a concentration of >94 µg/mL. From 95% is excreted into urine. The half-life is 1.5 to 2 hr in normal persons.

Dose (cefazolin equivalent)—*Intramuscular* or *intravenous*, *adults*, for *most infections*, **0.25 to 1 g** every 6 to 8 hr; for *pneumococcal pneumonia*, **0.5 g** every 12 hr; for *urinary tract infections*, **1 g** every 12 hr; for surgical *prophylaxis*, **1 g** 0.5 to 1 hr before, **0.5 to 1 g** during and every 6 hr after surgery; *infants over 1 month* of age and *children*, all infections, **6.25 to 25 mg/kg** every 6 hr *or* **8.3 to 33.3 mg/kg** every 8 hr.

Dosage Forms (cefazolin equivalent)—Sterile Powder: 250 and 500 mg, and 1, 5, and 10 g.

Cefoperazone Sodium

5-Thia-1-azabicyclo[4.2.0]oct-2-ene-2-carboxylic acid, 7-[[[[(4-ethyl-2,3-dioxo-1-piperazinyl)carbonyl]amino](4-hydroxyphenyl)acetyl]amino]-3-[[(1-methyl-1H-tetrazol-5-yl)thio]methyl]-8-oxo-, monosodium salt, [6R-[6α,7β(R*)]]-,

[62893-20-3] $C_{25}H_{26}N_9NaO_8S_2$ (667.65).
Preparation—See Belg Pat 837,682; *CA 87*: 6002v, 1977.

Description—White powder.

Uses—Cefoperazone is a third-generation cephalosporin with antibacterial activities typical of that class. It is the most active member against *Ps aeruginosa* but is not active against β-lactamase-producing *B fragilis*. It is less active than cefotaxime or moxalactam against most gram-negative enteric bacteria but is more active against *Ps aeruginosa*. It is unique among cephalosporins in that dosage adjustments are not required in renal failure.

Cefoperazone is approved for use in *urinary tract infections* caused by *Enterobacter*, *Ps aeruginosa*, and anaerobic cocci and bacilli; *respiratory tract infections* caused by *Enterobacter*, *E coli*, *H influenzae*, *K pneumoniae*, pneumococci, *Proteus*, *Ps aeruginosa*, *Staph aureus*, and *Strep pyogenes; cutaneous infections* by *Ps aeruginosa*, *Staph aureus*, and *Strep pyogenes; gynecological infections* by *Bacterioides*, *Clostridia*, anaerobic cocci, *E coli*, gonococcus, *Staph aureus* and *epidermidis*, and *Strep agalactiae; bone* and *joint infections* by *Enterobacter*, *E coli*, *Klebsiella*, *Proteus*, *Pseudomonas*, and *Staph aureus;* and *septicemina* from anaerobic gram-positive cocci, *Clostridium*, *E coli*, *H influenzae*, *Klebsiella*, pneumonococcus, *Ps aeruginosa*), *Staph aureus*, and *Strep agalactiae* and *pyogenes*. In serious infections by gram-negative bacilli, it is customary to combine cefoperazone with an aminoglycoside.

The adverse effects are those of cephalosporins in general (page 1184), but the incidence is low. There is a tendency towards hypoprothrombinemia. It causes a disulfiram-like reaction to ethanol. A 10-day treatment with cefoperazone costs over $1400.

Cefoperazone is poorly absorbed orally. An intravenous dose yields a peak plasma concentration of 250 to 357 μg/mL depending on the rate of delivery, an intramuscular dose 80 to 120 μg/mL. In plasma, 82 to 93% is protein-bound. The volume of distribution 0.13 to 0.20 mL/g in adults but 0.5 mL/g in neonates. Biliary secretion eliminates 70% and urinary excretion 30% of the drug. Dose adjustments are needed in hepatic but not in renal failure.

Dose (Cefoperazone equivalent)—*Intramuscular* or *intravenous infusion*, *adults*, for *mild infections*, 1 to **2 g** every 12 hr and, for *severe infections*, **1.5** to **3 g** every 6 hr, **2** to **4 g** every 8 hr or **3** to **6 g** every 12 hr. Pediatric dosage has not been determined.

Dosage Form (cefoperazone equivalent)—Powder for injection: 1 and 2 g. Each g contains 1.5 mEq of sodium.

Cefotaxime Sodium

5-Thia-1-azabicyclo[4.2.0]oct-2-ene-2-carboxylic acid, 3-[(acetyloxy)methyl]-7-[[(2-amino-4-thiazolyl)(methoxyimino)acetyl]amino]-8-oxo-, monosodium salt, [6R-[6α,7β(Z)]]-, Claforan (*Hoechst-Roussel*)

[64485-93-4] $C_{16}H_{16}N_5NaO_7S_2$ (477.44).
Preparation—See US Pat 4,098,888.

Description—White to off-white solid melting about 163°.
Solubility—Freely soluble in water; practically insoluble in most organic solvents. The pH of a 10% solution is about 5.5.

Uses—Cefotaxime is a third-generation cephalosporin with an antibacterial spectrum characteristic of its class (see general statement). Against gram-negative bacilli it is equal or superior to the aminoglycosides, except against *Ps aeruginosa*, *Acinetobactor*, and some *Enterobacter*. It is more active against multiple-drug-resistant gram-negative bacilli than are moxalactam and cefoperazone. It is more resistant to β-lactamases than are earlier generation drugs. Against *Staph aureus*, it is less active than other cephalosporins. It has more indications than any other cephalosporin presently available. It is approved for use against *genitourinary infections* caused by gonococcus, *Enterococcus*, *Atrobacter*, *Enterobacter*, *E coli*, *Klebsiella*, indole-positive *Proteus*, *Serrata* and *Staphylococcus; lower respiratory tract infections* from *Strep pneumoniae* and *pyogenes*, *H influenzae*, *E coli*, *Klebsiella*, *Serratia Enterobacter*, and *Staph aureus; gynecological infections* caused by *E coli*, *Enterococcus*, *Klebsiella*, *Pr mirabilis*, *Bacterioides*, *Clostridium*, anaerobic cocci, and *Staph epidermidis; cutaneous infections* caused by *Staph aureus* and *epidermidis*, *Strep pyogenes*, *Enterococcus*, *Enterobacter*, *E coli*, *Klebsiella*, *Serratia*, *Pr mirabilis*, indole-positive *Proteus*, *Pseudomonas*, *Bacterioides*, and anaerobic streptococci; *intra-abdominal infections* from *Bacterioides*, *E coli*, *Klebsiella*, and anaerobic streptococci; *bone* and *joint* infections from *Staph aureus;* *CNS infections* caused by meningococcus, *H influenzae*, *K pneumoniae*, *Strep pneumoniae*, and *E coli;* and *septicemia* caused by *E coli*, *Klebsiella*, and *Serratia*. It is used for surgical prophylaxis.

When appropriate, it may be combined with an aminoglycoside. Cefotaxime has no unique toxicity (see page 1184). It is very expensive, with a daily acquisition cost of over $150.

Cefotaxime is poorly absorbed by the oral route. A plasma level of 80 to 90 μg/mL results from 2 g intravenously. In plasma, 40 to 50% is protein-bound. The volume of distribution is 0.25 to 0.39 mL/g. Cefotaxime penetrates into the cerebrospinal fluid. About 90% is eliminated in the urine and 8% in the feces. The half-life is 1 to 1.2 hr.

Dose—*Intramuscular*, *adults*, for *gonorrhea*, **1 g** as a single dose. *Intramuscular* or *intravenous* for *various infections*, **1** to **2 g** every 4 to 8 hr, except **1 g** every 12 hr for *pneumonococcal pneumonia; surgical prophylaxis* in *cesarian section*, **1 g** intravenously when the umbilical cord is clamped then **1 g** intramuscularly or intravenously at 6 and 12 hr; *other surgical prophylaxis*, **1 g** 0.5 to 1 hr before, once during, and every 6 to 8 hr after surgery; *infants* and *children up to 50 kg*, **8.3** to **30 mg/kg** every 4 hr or **12.5** to **45 mg/kg** every 6 hr. *Intravenous*, *neonates up to 4 wk*, **50 mg/kg** every 8 hr.

Dosage Forms (Cefotaxime equivalent)—Powder for injection: 0.5, 1, and 2 g. Each g contains 2.2 mEq of sodium.

Cefoxitin Sodium

5-Thia-1-azabicyclo[4.2.0]oct-2-ene-2-carboxylic acid, 3-[[(aminocarbonyl)oxy]methyl]-7-methoxy-8-oxo-7-[(2-thienylacetyl)-amino]- (6R-*cis*)-, monosodium salt; Mefoxin (*MSD*)

[33564-30-6] $C_{16}H_{16}N_3NaO_7S$ (449.44).
Preparation—See *J Amer Chem Soc 94:* 1410, 1972.

Description—White crystals with a very characteristic odor; slightly hygroscopic; pK$_a$ 2.2 (acid).
Solubility—Very soluble in water; soluble in methanol; slightly soluble in acetone; sparingly soluble in ethanol or ether.

Uses—Cefoxitin is a second-generation cephalosporin with antibacterial activity typical of that class (see general statement). It is approved for use against the following infections, by organism and location: *Bacterioides* (skin, respiratory tract, endometrium, pelvis, peritonitis, septicemia), *Clostridia* (endometrium, pelvis, skin), *E coli* (urinary tract, peritonitis, endometrium and pelvis, skin, lower respiratory tract, septicemia), *H influenzae* (lower respiratory tract), *Klebsiella* (lower repiratory tract, urinary tract, peritonitis, skin, septicemia), *N gonorrhea* (endometrium, pelvis, urinary tract), *Peptococcus* and *Peptostreptococcus* (endometrium, pelvis, skin), indole-positive *Proteus* spp (urinary tract), *Pr mirabilis* (urinary tract, skin), *Staph aureus* (skin, lower respiratory tract, bones and joints, septicemia), *Staph epidermidis* (skin), *Strep pneumoniae* (lower respiratory tract, septicemia), group B streptococci (endometrium, pelvis), streptococci, other than enterococci, (skin), and for surgical prophylaxis. Its toxicity is that of other cephalosporins (page 1184), but pain at the injection site is less than with first-generation cephalosporins.

Cefoxitin is poorly absorbed orally. In plasma, 70 to 80% is protein-bound. The volume of distribution is 0.16 mL/g. Intramuscularly, 500 mg yields a plasma level of about 11 μg/mL in 0.5 hr. More than 85% is eliminated in the urine with a half-life of 0.75 to 1 hr.

Dose—(Cefoxitin equivalent) *Intramuscular*, *adults*, for *gonorrhea*, **2 g** (0.5 hr after 1 g probenecid) once only; *various infections*, intramuscular or intravenous, *adults*, **1** to **2 g** every 4 to 8 hr; *surgical prophylaxis* with *cesarean section*, **2 g** intravenously at the time the umbilical cord is clamped, **2 g** *intravenously* or *intramuscularly* twice at 4-hr intervals then every 7 hr for 1 day; with *transurethral prostatectomy*, **1 g** *intravenously* just before surgery, then every 8 hr for 5 days; *other* surgical prophylaxis, **2 g** intramuscularly or intravenously, 0.5 to 1 hr before and every 6 hr thereafter. *Intramuscular* or *intravenous*, *infants 3 mo* or *older* and *children*, **13.3** to **26.7** mg/kg every 4 hr or **20** to **40 mg/kg** every 6 hr; for *surgical prophylaxis*, **30** to **40 mg/kg** 0.5 to 1 hr before and every 6 hr after surgery.

Dosage Forms (Cefoxitin equivalent)—Powder for injection: 1 and 2 g. Each g contains 2.3 mEq of sodium.

Cefuroxime Sodium

(6R,7R)-7-[2-(2-Furyl)glyoxylamido]-3-(hydroxymethyl)-8-oxo-5-thia-1-azabicyclo[4.2.0]oct-2-ene-2-carboxylic acid (Z)-mono(O-methyloxime) carbamate (ester).

[56238-63-2] $C_{16}H_{15}N_4NaO_8S$ (446.39).
Preparation—See US Pat 3,974,153.

Description—Off-white to white powder; unbuffered aqueous solutions are stable for about 12 hours at room temperature; about 15% decomposition occurs after 24 hours. Suspensions for IM use and solutions for IV infusion are usually stable for 48 hrs if stored between 2° and 10°. May become yellowish on standing.

Solubility—1 g in 5 mL of water; slightly soluble in alcohol. A 10% aqueous solution has a pH of about 7.

Uses—Cefuroxime is a second-generation cephalosporin with antibacterial activity typical of that class (see general statement). Its activity against *H influenzae* and ability to penetrate into the cerebrospinal fluid make it particularly useful for treating meningitis caused by that organism; it is also approved to treat *meningitis* caused by *Strep pneumoniae*, *N meningitidis*, and *Staph aureus*. It has excellent activity against all gonococci, hence is used to treat *gonorrhea*. It may be used to treat lower *respiratory tract infections* caused by *H influenzae*, *Klebsiella* spp, *E coli*, *Strep pneumoniae* and *pyogenes*, and *Staph aureus*. It is approved for use against *urinary tract infections* caused by *E coli* and *Klebsiella*, a more limited approval than for other second-generation drugs. It may be used against *cutaneous infections* caused by *Enterobacter* spp, *E coli*, *Klebsiella* spp, *Staph aureus* and *Strep pyogenes*. *Septicemias* that may be treated with cefuroxime are those caused by *E coli*, *H influenzae*, *Klebsiella*, and *Staph aureus*. It is approved for surgical prophylaxis. The adverse effects are those of cephalosporins in general (page 1184). Pain at the injection site is usually slight. However, suprainfections caused by *Pseudomonas* and *Candida* may occur more frequently than with first- and other second-generation cephalosporins.

Cefuroxime is poorly absorbed by the oral route. A 0.5 g-dose will yield a plasma level of over 8 µg/mL. In plasma, 33% is protein-bound. The volume of distribution is 0.19 mL/g. It penetrates into cerebrospinal fluid. More than 85% is eliminated by the oral route; the half-life is 1 to 1.5 hr but may be as much as 24 hr in renal failure.

Dose (cefuroxime equivalent)—*Intramuscular* or *intravenous*, *adults*, for *cutaneous*, *disseminated gonococcal*, and *urinary tract infections* and *pneumonia*, **0.75 to 1.5 g** every 8 hr; for uncomplicated *gonorrhea*, **1.5 g** (intramuscularly) as a single dose; for *serious infections* or those from *less sensitive organisms*, **1.5 g** every 6 hr; for *meningitis*, **3 g** every 8 hr; for *surgical prophylaxis*, **1.5 g** intravenously 0.5 to 1 hr before and **1.5 g** intramuscularly or intravenously every 8 hr, if a prolonged procedure (for open heart surgery, begin when anesthesia is induced and continue every 12 hr for a total of 6 g). *Infants 3 months* and *older* and *children*, **50 to 100 mg/kg/day** in 3 or 4 divided doses, except in *meningitis*, **200 to 240 mg/kg/day** until the condition improved.

Dosage Forms (Cefuroxime equivalent)—Powder for injection: 0.75 and 1.5 g. Each g contains 2.4 mEq of sodium.

Cephalothin Sodium

5-Thia-1-azabicyclo[4.2.0]oct-2-ene-2-carboxylic acid, 3-[(acetyloxy)-methyl]-8-oxo-7-[(2-thienylacetyl)amino]-, monosodium salt, (6R-trans)-, Keflin (*Lilly*)

[58-71-9] $C_{16}H_{15}N_2NaO_6S_2$ (418.41). Potency: equivalent to not less than 850 µg of cephalothin ($C_{16}H_{16}N_2O_6S_2$)/mg, calculated on the anhydrous basis.

Preparation—7-Aminocephalosporanic acid is *N*-acetylated through condensation with 2-thiopheneacetyl chloride in a dehydrochlorinating environment. The starting acid may be prepared

from the natural antibiotic, cephalosporin C, by either proton-catalyzed or enzymatic hydrolysis. The cephalothin thus prepared may be converted into its sodium salt by interaction with sodium acetate in a suitable organic solvent.

Description—White to off-white, practically odorless, crystalline powder that is moderately hygroscopic; decomposes on heating.

Solubility—Freely soluble in water, saline TS, and dextrose solution; slightly soluble in alcohol; insoluble in most organic solvents.

Uses—The actions, uses, and toxicity of cephalothin are primarily those of first-generation cephalosporins (see introductory statement in this section). Cephalothin is not affected by penicillinase and hence is active against many penicillinase-producing strains against which penicillin G is ineffective, so that cephalothin can be used when penicillin fails. The drug should be reserved for treatment only of serious infections resistant to penicillin or in patients allergic to penicillin. *Bacteremias*, *infections of the respiratory tract*, *urinary tract infections*, *soft-tissue infections*, *infections of the bones and joints*, and *cardiovascular infections* caused by susceptible organisms may be treated with the drug. It has also been reported to be effective in the treatment of peritonitis and staphylococcal and pneumococcal meningitides; it yields the highest concentrations in the cerebrospinal fluid of any first-generation cephalosporin.

Cephalothin sodium may cause occasional urticaria, rash, eosinophilia, or fever; leukopenia or neutropenia are rare. Superinfections (overgrowth) may occur, especially with *Pseudomonas*. The drug is irritant and may cause pain, induration, sterile abscesses, or thrombophlebitis. Acute tubular necrosis is rare, but granular casts in the urine are common after large doses. The sodium can cause adverse effects in persons with congestive heart failure or renal failure. High plasma levels interfere with the determination of creatinine.

Cephalothin is destroyed in the gastrointestinal tract and must be given parenterally. It is bound by plasma proteins to the extent of 70%. The volume of distribution is 0.26 mL/g. An intravenous dose of 1 g will effect a concentration in normal cerebrospinal fluid of 0.4 to 1.4 µg/mL and up to 5.6 µg/mL when the meninges are inflamed. Plasma half-life is 0.75 to 1 hr; it may be as long as 3 to 8 hr in severe renal failure.

Dose (cephalothin equivalent)—*Intramuscular* or *intravenous*, *adults*, *cellulitis-furunculosis* or *pneumonia*, **500 mg** every 6 hr; *other infections*, 1 to 2 g every 6 hr; *surgical* prophylaxis, 1 to 2 g. 0.5 to 1 hr before, during, and every 6 hr after surgery. *Children*, **13.3 to 26.6 mg/kg** every 4 hr *or* 20 to 40 mg/kg every 6 hr; *surgical prophylaxis*, 20 to 30 mg/kg 0.5 to 1 hr before, during, and every 6 hr after surgery. See package literature for other doses and for dose adjustments in renal failure.

Dosage Forms—Powder for Injection: 1, 2, 4, and 20 g.

Cephapirin Sodium

5-Thia-1-azabicyclo[4.2.0]oct-2-ene-2-carboxylic acid, 3-[(acetyloxy)-methyl]-8-oxo-7-[[(4-pyridinylthio)acetyl]amino]-, monosodium salt, (6R-trans)-, Cefadyl (*Bristol*)

[24356-60-3] $C_{17}H_{16}N_3NaO_6S_2$ (445.44). Potency: the equivalent of 855-1000 µg of cephapirin/mg.

Preparation—7-Aminocephalosporanic acid, prepared from cephalosporin C by hydrolysis, is acylated with (4-pyridylthio)acetyl chloride in a dehydrochlorinating environment, and the resulting cephapirin is converted to its sodium salt by interaction with sodium 2-ethylhexanoate in an organic solvent.

Description—White to off-white, crystalline powder; decomposes on heating; pK_{a1} 2.15; pK_{a2} 5.44.

Solubility—1 g in about 1.7 mL water; very soluble in dilute hydrochloric acid; insoluble in chloroform, ether.

Uses—Cephapirin is a first-generation cephalosporin with properties and uses almost identical to those of cephalothin sodium. However, it is more soluble and consequently causes less pain at the site of injection and has a lower incidence of thrombophlebitis. Also, it is less expensive, so that in many hospital formularies it has replaced cephalothin.

Dose (cephapirin equivalent)—*Intramuscular* or *intravenous*, *adults*, **500 mg** to **1 g** every 4 to 6 hr, except **7.5 to 15 mg/kg** of body weight in renal failure; for *surgical prophylaxis*, **1** to **2 g** 0.5 to 1 hr before, during, and every 6 hr after surgery. *Infants* over 3 months old and *children*, **10** to **20 mg/kg** of body weight every 6 hr.

Dosage Forms (cephapirin equivalent)—Sterile: 1, 2, 4, and 20 g.

Cephradine

5-Thia-1-azabicyclo[4.2.0]oct-2-ene-2-carboxylic acid, 7-[(amino-1,4-cyclohexadien-1-ylacetyl)amino]-3-methyl-8-oxo-, [6R-[6α,7β(R*)]]-, Anspor (*SKF*); Velosef (*Squibb*)

(6R,7R) - 7-[(R)-2-Amino-2-(1,4-cyclohexadien-1-yl)acetamido]-3-methyl-8-oxo-5-thia-1-azabicyclo[4.2.0]oct-2-ene-2-carboxylic acid [38821-53-3] $C_{16}H_{19}N_3O_4S$ (349.40). Potency: 900 to 1050 µg of $C_{16}H_{19}N_3O_4S$/mg (anhydrous basis).

Preparation—Preparation of cephradine starting with 7-amino-desacetoxycephalosporanic acid is described in *J Med Chem* 14: 117, 1971.

Description—White, crystalline powder; polymorphic; pK_{a1} about 2.6, pK_{a2} about 7.3.

Solubility—Sparingly soluble in water; very slightly soluble in alcohol; practically insoluble in chloroform and ether.

Uses—Cephradine is a first-generation cephalosporin (see introductory statement in this section) but differs in that it has activity against enterococci. It is indicated for the treatment of *upper and lower respiratory tract* and *urinary tract infections, prostatitis, pharyngitis, otitis media,* staphylococcal and streptococcal *endocarditis, osteomyelitis,* and *infections of the skin* and *soft tissues* caused by susceptible organisms.

The adverse effects of cephradine are those indicated in the introduction; in general, they are mild.

Cephradine is almost completely absorbed from the gut. As an oral suspension, 500 mg yields a peak plasma concentration of about 20 µg/mL in 30 min, but from capsules the peak is 6 to 24 µg/mL at about 1 hr. Food delays the peak time to about 2 hr and diminishes the concentration by about 50%. Interestingly, with intramuscular injection, the absorption time is as long and the peak concentration even lower than with oral cephradine administered with food. The drug is bound approximately 14% by plasma proteins. The volume of distribution is 0.25 mL/g. Elimination is almost entirely by renal excretion, the half-life being 0.7 to 1.5 hr in normal subjects.

Dose—*Oral, adults,* either **250** to **500 mg** every 6 hr or **500 mg** to **1 g** every 12 hr, up to 4 g a day; *children,* **6.25** to **12.5 mg/kg** of body weight every 6 hr, except twice that amount if necessary, not to exceed 4 g a day; the dose for children over 9 months of age may be doubled if the interval is also doubled to 12 hr. *Intramuscular* or *intravenous, adults,* **500 mg** to **1 g** every 6 hr; *infants 1 yr* and *older* and *children,* **6.25** to **25 mg/kg** of body weight every 6 hr, not to exceed 8 g a day; however, in severely ill infants and children, up to **75 mg/kg** every 6 hr may be given. In renal failure, all doses require appropriate adjustment (see the package literature).

Dosage Forms—Capsules: 250 and 500 mg; for Injection: 250 and 500 mg and 1, 2, and 4 g; for Oral Suspension: 125 and 250 mg/5 mL (reconstituted).

Moxalactam Disodium

5-Oxa-1-azabicyclo[4.2.0]oct-2-ene-2-carboxylic acid, 7-[[carboxy(4-hydroxyphenyl)acetyl]amino]-7-methoxy-3-[[(1-methyl-1H-tetrazol-5-yl)thio]methyl]-8-oxo-, disodium salt; Moxam (*Lilly*)

[64953-12-4] $C_{20}H_{18}N_6Na_2O_9S$ (564.44).
Preparation—See *J Med Chem* 22: 757, 1979.

Description—White to off-white powder with faint characteristic odor.

Solubility—Very soluble in water.

Uses—Moxalactam is a third-generation cephalosporin with antibacterial activities typical of this class (see general statement). It has limited activity against group-B streptococci and is inactive against *Listeria.* It is highly active against β-lactamase-producing gonococcus and *H influenzae.* It has moderate activity against *Ps aeruginosa.* It is approved for use against *lower respiratory tract infections* caused by *Staph aureus, Strep pneumoniaea, H influenzae, Pr mirabilis, Enterobacter, E coli,* and *Klebsiella; urinary tract infections* by *Enterobacter, E coli,* and *Klebsiella,* and *Proteus; cutaneous infections* by *Staph aureus, Strep pyogenes, E coli, Serratia,* and mixed infections by aerobes and anaerobes involving *Bacterioides, Clostridium, Enterobacter, Klebsiella, Peptococcus,* and *Streptopeptococcus;* simple or mixed *intra-abdominal infections* caused by *Bacterioides, Clostridium, Enterobacter, E coli, Eubacterium, Fusobacterium, Klebsiella, Peptococcus, Pr mirabilis, Ps aeruginosa,* and *Strep agalactiae; bone* and *joint infections* caused by *Ps aeruginosa, Serratia,* and *Staph aureus; CNS infections* by *E coli, H influenzae,* and *Klebsiella;* and *septicemia* from *B fragilis, E coli, Klebsiella, Pseudomonas, Serratia, Staph aureus,* and pneumococcus. In serious gram-negative infections it is usually combined with an aminoglycoside.

Adverse effects are those of cephalosporins in general (page 1184) but also include prolonged prothrombin time and a dilsulfiram-like effect to cause ethanol intolerance. The daily acquisition cost is over $150.

Moxalactam is poorly absorbed orally. An intravenous dose of 1 g yields peak plasma levels of 60 to 85 µg/mL and an intramuscular dose yields 28 to 52 µg/mL. In plasma 40 to 50% is protein-bound. The volume of distribution is 0.26 to 0.40 mL/g. Even in the absence of inflammation, moxalactam penetrates into the cerebrospinal fluid sufficiently to reach concentrations active against some organisms. About 90% is eliminated in the urine with a half-life of 2 to 2.5 hr, except longer in renal failure. The active R epimer has a somewhat shorter half-life.

Dose (Moxalactam equivalent)—*Intramuscular* or *intravenous, adults, mild* to *moderate* infections, **0.5** to **2 g** every 12 hr; *cutaneous infections,* **0.5 g** every 8 hr; *urinary tract infections,* **0.25** to **0.5 g** every 8 to 12 hr; *severe infections* and infections by bacteria of low to moderate susceptibility, up to **4 g** every 8 hr; *neonates, infants,* and *children,* **50 mg/kg** every 12 hr for infants up to 1 wk of age, every 8 hr to 4 wk, every 6 hr for older infants, and every 6 to 8 hr for children; for *severe infections,* **up to 200 mg/kg** (not to exceed the adult dose).

Dosage Forms (Moxalactam equivalent)—Powder for injection: 1 g/10 mL and 2 g/20 mL (reconstituted). Each g contains 3.8 mEq of sodium.

Other Cephalosporins

Cefsulodin Sodium [[6R-[6α,7β(R*)]]-4-(Aminocarbonyl)-1-[[2-carboxy-8-oxo-7-[(phenylsulfoacetyl)amino]-5-thia-1-azabicyclo[4.2.0]oct-2-en-3-yl]methylpyridinium hydroxide, inner salt, monosodium salt. [52152-93-9] $C_{22}H_{19}N_4NaO_8S_2$ (554.52); Cefomonil (*Takeda-Abbot*)]—For preparation see *J Med Chem* 17: 1312, 1974. Colorless needles melting about 175° with decomposition. *Uses:* Cefsulodin does not fit into any of the subclasses of cephalosporins. It has fair activity against *Staph aureus* and poor activity against all other important pathogenic bacteria except *Ps aeruginosa,* against which it has good activity. It is indicated for use in staphylococcal and pseudomonal infections. Its development is in phase III. It is not orally effective. After an intramuscular dose of 1 g, the peak plasma level is about 19 µg/mL. In plasma, 30% is protein-bound. The volume of distribution is 0.33 mL/g. About 65 to 70% is eliminated by renal excretion, with a half-life of 1.3 to 2.7 hr, except up to 13 hr in renal failure.

Ceftazidime Sodium [1-[[6R,7R]-7-[2-(2-Amino-4-thiazolyl)glyoxylamido]-2-carboxy-8-oxo-5-thia-1-azabicyclo[4.2.0]oct-2-en-3-yl]methyl]pyridinium hydroxide, inner salt, 7^2-(Z)-[O-(1-carboxy-1-methylethyl)oxime] $C_{22}H_{21}N_6NaO_7S_2$ (568.56)]—For the preparation see Ger Pat 2,921,316. *Uses:* Ceftazidime is a third-generation cephalosporin with antibacterial activities and adverse effects characteristic of its class (see general statement). Its development is in phase III. Its antibacterial spectrum is very similar to that of cefoperazone (page 1185), except that it is more active against *Bacterioides* and especially against *Ps aeruginosa,* the best of any cephalosporin. Its approved indications will be those of cefoperazone, and it will likely be the cephalosporin of choice for infections caused by *Ps aeruginosa.* It is not orally effective. In plasma, 17 to 20% is protein-bound. The volume of distribution is 0.23 mL/g. About 75 to 85% is eliminated by renal excretion, with a half-life of 1.8 hr, except longer in renal failure.

Ceftizoxime Sodium [Sodium (6*R*,7*R*)-7-[2-(2-imino-4-thiazolin-4-yl)glyoxylamido]-8-oxo-5-thia-1-azabicyclo[4.2.0]oct-2-ene-2-carboxylate 7²-(*Z*)-(*O*-methyloxime). [68401-82-1] $C_{13}H_{12}N_5NaO_5S_2$ (405.38)]—For the preparation see US Pat 4,166,115. *Uses:* Ceftizoxime is a third-generation cephalosporin with antibacterial activity typical of this class (see general statement). It is about as active as cefotaxime or moxalactam and more active than cefoperazone against gram-negative enteric bacilli but is less active than cefoperazone against *Ps aeruginosa*. It has spotty activity against anaerobes; it has activity against several strains of *B fragilis*. It is not active against *Enterococcus*. Ceftizoxime has been used effectively in lower respiratory tract, genitourinary, and soft-tissue infections, osteomyelitis, gonorrhea, intra-abdominal infections, and some cases of meningitis. It is infrequently effective in infections caused by *Ps aeruginosa*. In serious infections by gram-negative bacilli, ceftizoxime is usually combined with an aminoglycoside. Its adverse effects are those of cephalosporins in general (page 1184). Over 40% of recipients experience transient dizziness and headache. The drug is not effective orally. In plasma, only 30% is protein-bound. The volume of distribution is 0.26 mL/g. Intramuscular and intravenous doses of 1 g yield respective plasma levels of 36 and 61 µg/mL 30 min after administration. About 90% of elimination is renal, with a half-life of 1.3 to 1.6 hr. *Dose: Intramuscular or intravenous, adults*, 500 mg every 12 hr for simple urinary tract infections, 1 g every 8 hr or 2 g every 12 hr in severe infections, and 3 to 4 g intravenously every 8 hr in life-threatening infections. Pediatric dosage has not been established.

Ceftriaxone Sodium [(6*R*,7*R*)-7-[2-(2-Amino-4-thiazolyl)glyoxylamido]-8-oxo-3-[[(1,2,5,6-tetrahydro-2-methyl-5,6-dioxo-*as*-triazin-3-yl)thio]methyl]-5-thia-1-azabicyclo[4.2.0]oct-2-ene-2-carboxylic acid, 7²-(*Z*)-(*O*-methyloxime), disodium salt. [74578-69-1] $C_{18}H_{16}N_8Na_2O_7S_3$ (598.53); Rocephin (*Hoffmann-LaRoche*).] *Description and solubility:* For the preparation see *J Antibiot 33:* 793, 1980. White crystals melting about 155° (3½ H₂O); very soluble in water. *Uses:* Ceftriaxone is a third-generation cephalosporin with antibacterial activities and adverse effects characteristic of its class (see general statement). Its development is in phase III. The approved uses will probably be similar to those of cefotaxime (page 1186). It is not orally effective. Pharmacokinetics are distinctly two-compartmental, the redistribution time being about 2 hr. An intravenous dose of 500 mg yields a peak plasma level of about 50 µg/mL before and about 30 immediately after redistribution. In plasma, 83 to 96% is protein-bound. The volume of distribution is 0.13 mL/g. Elimination is 60 to 80% renal. The half-life is about 8 to 12 hr, which is unique among cephaloporins and which will probably result in a prominent clinical status for this drug. In anephric patients, the half-life is 20 to 34 hr.

Cephalexin [(6*R*,7*R*)-7-[(*R*)-2-Amino-2-phenylacetamido]-3-methyl-8-oxo-5-thia-1-azabicyclo[4.2.0]-oct-2-ene-2-carboxylic acid monohydrate [23325-78-2] $C_{16}H_{17}N_3O_4S.H_2O$ (365.40); Keflex (*Lilly*).] *Preparation: J Med Chem 12:* 310, 1969. *Description and solubility:* White crystals; pK$_a$ 5.2, 7.3; soluble 1 g in 100 mL of water; soluble in dilute aqueous alkaline solutions; the pH of a 0.5% solution is about 4.5; very slightly sol to practically insoluble in organic solvents. *Uses:* Cephalexin is a first-generation cephalosporin with antimicrobial activity and adverse effects characteristic of that class. It is approved for use against respiratory infections caused by pneumococcus and group A beta-hemolytic streptococci; otitis media by *H influenzae, N catarrhalis*, pneumococcus, staphylococci, and streptococci; bone and joint infections caused by *Pr mirabilis* and *staphylococci;* skin and soft tissue infections caused by staphylococci and streptococci; and urinary tract infections by *E coli, Klebsiella*, and *Pr mirabilis*. It is effective orally. Elimination is by renal excretion with a half-life of 0.6 to 0.9 hr, except 5 to 30 hr in renal failure. *Dose: Oral, adults*, 250 to 500 mg every 6 hr, except 500 mg every 12 hr for skin and soft-tissue infections; *children*, for otitis media, 18.8 to 25 mg/kg every 6 hr; for skin and soft-tissue infections, 12.5 to 50 mg/kg; and for other infections, 6.25 to 25 mg/kg every 6 hr.

Miscellaneous—*Cefonicide* is a second-generation cephalosporin with a somewhat broader spectrum than cephalothin (page 1187). It will be promoted because of its favorable half-life of about 4.9 hr, so that it may be given once a day. *Ceforanide* is a second-generation cephalosporin with a spectrum of antibacterial activity much like that of cefamandole (page 1185). It differs in having a longer and more favorable elimination half-life, namely 3.0 hr, except about 25 hr in renal failure. *Cefmanoxime* is a third generation cephalosporin (see page 1183) with high activity against *Ps aeruginosa*. Like all third-generation cephalosporins, it is not effective orally. About 75 to 80% is eliminated by renal excretion, with a half-life of 1 hr. There are other cephalosporins in various phases of development.

Macrolides

The macrolides are hydroxylated macrocyclic lactones containing 12 to 20 carbon atoms in the primary ring. There are 37 known members of this class but only one, namely, erythromycin (and its derivatives), is of clinical importance. Other macrolides that have been marketed for use are mitasamycin, oleandomycin, spiramycin, and troleandomycin.

Macrolides bind to the 50s subunit of the bacterial ribo-some. The main effect seems to be inhibition of the translocation step in protein synthesis, so that the synthesis itself is inhibited. The complex has a low-enough affinity constant that some protein synthesis can take place, so that these drugs are mainly bacteriostatic in therapeutic concentrations. Macrolides bind equally to ribosomes from gram-positive and gram-negative bacteria; the much greater effect on gram-positive organisms is the result of greater permeation of the cell membrane. Macrolides do not bind to mammalian ribosomes. The activities and uses of erythromycin-type macrolides are discussed mainly under the prototype, erythromycin.

Erythromycin

Ilotycin (*Lilly*); E-Mycin (*Upjohn*); *Others*

(3*R**,4*S**,5*S**,6*R**,7*R**,9*R**,11*R**,12*R**,13*S**,14*R**)-4-[(2,6-Dideoxy - 3-*C*-methyl-3-*O*-methyl-α-L-*ribo*-hexopyranosyl)oxy]-14-ethyl - 7,12,13 - trihydroxy-3,5,7,9,11,13-hexamethyl-6-[[3,4,6-trideoxy-3 -(dimethylamino)-β-D-*xylo*-hexopyranosyl]oxy]oxacyclotetradecane-2,10-dione [114-07-8] $C_{37}H_{67}NO_{13}$ (733.94). Potency: not less than 850 µg of $C_{37}H_{67}NO_{13}$/mg, calculated on the anhydrous basis.

Preparation—Elaborated during the growth of a strain of *Streptomyces erythreus*. US Pat 2,823,203.

Description—White or slightly yellow crystals or powder; odorless or practically odorless; slightly hygroscopic; pK$_a$ 8.7.

Solubility—1 g dissolves in about 1000 mL of water; soluble in alcohol, chloroform, ether.

Uses—Erythromycin has a spectrum of activity that resembles the activity of penicillin. It is most effective against gram-positive cocci, such as enterococci, group A hemolytic streptococci, pneumococci, and *Staph aureus*. *Neisseria meningitidis* and *gonorrhoeae, Listeria, Corynebacterium diphtheria* and *acnes*, and some strains of *H influenzae* are also sensitive. Mycoplasma and the agent of Legionnaires' disease are inhibited by low concentrations of the drug. Enterococci are resistant. The drug is equally sensitive against both penicillin-sensitive and penicillin-resistant strains of staphylococci; it is also active against bacteria that have developed resistance to streptomycin. It has been shown to have *in vivo* activity against amebae, treponemes, and pinworms. The activity demonstrated by erythromycin against certain of the large viruses and rickettsia places this drug in the so-called "broad-spectrum" group, since it attacks three types of microorganisms (bacteria, rickettsia, and viruses) although showing low activity against some of the important disease-producing organisms of the gram-negative group. There is no cross-resistance between erythromycin and other antibiotics except to other macrolides. However, bacteria that are multiple-resistant to erythromycin and one or more other antibiotics are of frequent occurrence.

Erythromycin is the drug of choice in the treatment of infections caused by *Campylobacter, Chlamydia* (pneumonia only), *Corynebacterium diphtheriae, Bordetella pertussis, Legionella pneumophila* and *micdadei, Mycoplasma pneumoniae*, and *Ureoplasma ureolyticum*. It has been successfully employed in systemic infections caused by susceptible organisms, infections which include *pneumonia, empyema, gonorrhea, anthrax, oropharyngeal Bacterioides infection, meningitis, bacteremia, osteomyelitis*, and *wound infections* and in the prophylaxis of rheumatic fever. However, its use is secondary to penicillin for these purposes. Erythromycin serves mainly as a back-up drug when penicillin resistance or allergy occurs. The antibiotic is not particularly effective against *Strep fecalis* infections and is not uniformly curative in subacute bacterial endocarditis, but it may be useful in the treatment of urinary tract infections caused by *Strep fecalis* and gram-negative bacilli. Miscellaneous infections responding to erythromycin therapy include *otitis media* and *bronchitis* caused by pneumococci or *H influenzae, pertussis, pneumonia, clostridial infections, nongonorrheal urethritis, erythrasma, syphilis, Vincent's stomatitis, granuloma inguinale, psittacosis,* the *diphtheria* carrier state, and enterococcal *enteritis.* Local infections susceptible to erythromycin include *impetigo, wound* and *burn infections, infected eczema, acne vulgaris,* and *sycosis vulgaris.* Because of the possibility of producing resistant strains of staphylococci, indiscriminate use of erythromycin should be avoided. A large number of staphylococci have acquired resistance to the drug since it was introduced. Use of erythromycin in the treatment of intestinal *amebiasis* has been superseded by metronidazole.

Untoward reactions attributable to erythromycin therapy are uncommon and usually are of little consequence. Nausea, vomiting, and, occasionally, diarrhea and stomatitis may occur, particularly with large doses. Serious systemic toxicity has not been observed and there are no absolute contraindications to use of erythromycin except hypersensitivity; skin eruptions, fever and eosinophilia occasionally occur. Superinfections, especially of *Candida,* may occur. Because hepatic dysfunction, with or without jaundice, occurs in some patients receiving oral erythromycin products (especially the estolate), the FDA requires all manufacturers of such products to include in package literature a statement that caution should be exercised in administering the antibiotic to patients with impaired hepatic function.

Erythromycin is variably absorbed after oral administration. In part this variability is the result of various types of enteric coatings and in part of biological variation. Absorption appears to be of zero reaction order, especially with higher doses. Food interferes with absorption. The antibiotic is destroyed by gastric acid. Peak plasma levels are attained in 1 to 4 hr, following which the concentration declines sharply by the 4th to 6th hr. It is 73% bound to plasma proteins. The volume of distribution is 0.53 mL/g. The plasma half-life is 1.2 to 1.6 hr, except that it may be up to 5 to 6 hr in renal insufficiency. A single oral dose of 200 to 300 mg usually provides a plasma concentration of 0.6 to 0.8 μg/mL. The antibiotic does not readily diffuse into cerebrospinal fluid, but attains antibacterial concentrations in peritoneal and pleural fluids. Only 2% of oral and 20% of parenteral erythromycin is excreted in active form by the kidney. Alkalinization favors resorption and thus lowers urine concentration (pK_a = 8.6), but it also increases potency disproportionately, so that the urine should be alkalinized for treatment of urinary tract infections. Alkalinization also broadens the spectrum, so that urinary tract infections caused by gram-negative bacilli respond. The antibiotic is concentrated in the liver and excreted in active form in the bile; the feces of patients given large oral doses of erythromycin contain about 0.5 mg/g. Erythromycin increases the plasma levels of theophylline, so that the dose of theophylline may have to be decreased.

Dose—*Oral, adults,* **250 mg** every 6 hr, **333 mg** every 8 hr, or or **500 mg** every 12 hr (for *bacterial infections* only). The usual adult oral dose is 250 mg every 6 hr, but the dose may be doubled for more severe infections and infections caused by *Legionella.* In *gonorrhea,* the dose is **500 mg** every 6 hr for 6 or 7 days and in *syphilis* **1 g** every 6 hr for 10 to 15 days, except 30 days in late syphilis. In *intestinal amebiasis* (obsolete), **250 mg** every 6 hr or **333 mg** every 8 hr for 10 to 14 days. *Oral, children,* **7.5** to **25 mg/kg** of body weight every 6 hr or **15** to **50 mg/kg** every 12 hr for bacterial infections; the 6-hr schedule is mandatory for intestinal amebiasis. The dose can be doubled, if necessary. For prophylaxis against streptococci in rheumatic fever and chorea, **250 mg** every 12 hr. *Topical,* to the *skin,* as 1% ointment 3 or 4 times a day or **1.5** or **2%** solution twice a day and to the *conjunctiva* as a thin strip (about 1 cm) of **0.5%** ointment one or more times a day.

Dosage Forms—Capsules Enteric-Coated: 250 mg; Ointment: 10 mg/g; Ophthalmic Ointment: 5 mg/g; Tablets: 250 and 500 mg; Tablets, Enteric-Coated: 250, 333, and 500 mg.

Erythromycin Ethylsuccinate

Erythromycin 2'-(ethyl butanedioate); E.E.S. (*Abbott*); Pediamycin (*Ross*); *Other Mfrs*

Erythromycin 2'-(ethyl succinate) [41342-53-4] $C_{43}H_{75}NO_{16}$ (862.06). Potency: the equivalent of not less than 765 μg of erythromycin ($C_{37}H_{67}NO_{13}$)/mg, calculated on the anhydrous basis.

For the structure of *Erythromycin,* see page 1189.

Preparation—Erythromycin is esterified at the 2'-position by reacting it with ethyl 3-chloroformylpropionate [ClCO-CH$_2$CH$_2$CO$_2$Et] in dry acetone in the presence of sodium bicarbonate.

Description—White or slightly yellow, crystalline powder; odorless or practically so; practically tasteless; pK_a 7.1.

Solubility—Very slightly soluble in water; freely soluble in alcohol, chloroform, and polyethylene glycol 400.

Uses—Erythromycin ethylsuccinate is relatively tasteless and hence is also used in flavored oral "suspensions" for pediatric use. Except as noted above, its actions and uses are essentially those of *Erythromycin,* into which it is converted in the body.

Dose (base equivalent)—*Oral, adults,* for disseminated *gonorrhea,* **800 mg** every 6 hr for 7 days; for *Legionella,* **400 mg** to **1 g** every 6 hr; for *syphilis,* **800 mg** every 6 hr for 15 days in early and 30 days in late syphilis; for *other bacterial infections,* **400 mg** every 6 hr or **800 mg** every 12 hr; for *intestinal amebiasis,* **400 mg** every 6 hr for 7 days; for prophylaxis against streptococci in rheumatic fever and chorea, **400 mg** every 12 hr. *Children, see* under *Erythromycin.*

Dosage Forms (base equivalent)—Oral Suspension: 200 and 400 mg/5 mL; Powder for Oral Suspension: 100 mg/2.5 mL and 200 and 400 mg/5 mL; Tablets: 400 mg; Tablets, Chewable: 200 mg.

Erythromycin Gluceptate

Erythromycin monoglucoheptonate (salt); Ilotycin Glucoheptonate (*Dista*)

Erythromycin glucoheptonate (1:1) (salt) [304-63-2] $C_{37}H_{67}NO_{13}.C_7H_{14}O_8$ (960.12). Potency: the equivalent of not less than 600 μg of erythromycin ($C_{37}H_{67}NO_{13}$)/mg, calculated on the anhydrous basis.

Preparation—By dissolving erythromycin in an aqueous solution containing the proper amount of glucoheptonic acid and removing the solvent under reduced pressure.

Description—White powder which is odorless or practically odorless and slightly hygroscopic; its 1 in 20 solution is neutral or slightly acid.

Solubility—Freely soluble in water, alcohol; slightly soluble in chloroform; practically insoluble in ether.

Uses—See *Erythromycin.* This salt is particularly suited for intravenous administration. There may be reversible hearing loss when the intravenous dose exceeds 4 g a day.

Dose (base equivalent)—*Intravenous, adults,* **250** to **500 mg** or **3.75** to **5 mg/kg** of body weight every 6 hr, but may be as much as 4 g or more a day, if necessary; *children,* **3.75** to **5 mg/kg** every 6 hr. Intravenous doses should be administered slowly over a period of 20 to 60 min. As soon as the patient's condition indicates an effect on the infection, the erythromycin should be changed to an oral form.

Dosage Forms (base equivalent)—Sterile: 250 and 500 mg, and 1 g.

Erythromycin Lactobionate

Erythrocin Lactobionate (*Abbott*)

Erythromycin mono(4-*O*-β-D-galactopyranosyl-D-gluconate) (salt) [3847-29-8] $C_{37}H_{67}NO_{13}.C_{12}H_{22}O_{12}$ (1092.23); contains not less then 90% of labeled amount of $C_{37}H_{67}NO_{13}$ (erythromycin).

Preparation—Using lactobionic acid, erythromycin lactobionate (1:1) (salt) is prepared as described above for the glucoheptonate.

Description—White or slightly yellow crystals or powder, having a faint odor; its 1 in 20 solution has a pH between 6.5 and 7.5.

Solubility—Freely soluble in water, alcohol; slightly soluble in chloroform; practically insoluble in ether.

Uses—The water solubility of this erythromycin salt allows it to be given parenterally, either intravenously or intramuscularly. It has the same uses and actions as erythromycin base (see *Erythromycin*). Intravenous doses in excess of 4 g a day may cause reversible hearing loss. The parenteral route should be employed only if the patient cannot tolerate the base by the oral route. Once some control of the infection is obtained the preparation should be changed to an oral one if the patient is then able to tolerate it.

Dose (base equivalent)—*Intravenous, see Erythromycin Gluceptate.*

Dosage Forms (base equivalent)—for Injection: 500 mg and 1 g.

Erythromycin Stearate

Erythromycin octadecanoate (salt); Erythrocin Stearate (*Abbott*); *Various Mfrs*

Erythromycin stearate (salt) [643-22-1] $C_{37}H_{67}NO_{13}.C_{18}H_{36}O_2$ (1018.42); the stearic acid salt of erythromycin, with an excess of stearic acid. Potency: equivalent to not less than 550 μg of erythromycin ($C_{37}H_{67}NO_{13}$)/mg, calculated on the anhydrous basis.

Preparation—By reacting erythromycin with the proper quantity of stearic acid in acetone solution and then diluting the solution with water to precipitate the salt.

Description—White or slightly yellow crystals or powder; practically odorless and has a slightly bitter taste; pH (1% aqueous suspension) between 6.0 and 11.0.

Solubility—Practically insoluble in water; soluble in alcohol, chloroform, and ether.

Uses—Its actions and uses are identical to those of *Erythromycin*. It is insoluble in water and hence is supposedly destroyed to a lesser extent in the stomach. It is hydrolyzed in the small intestine and in the tissues to yield erythromycin. It is claimed to give the same blood levels as oral erythromycin, but there is considerable variation, which is partly biological and partly pharmaceutical in cause.

Dose (base equivalent)—*Oral*, same as that of *Erythromycin*.

Dosage Forms (base equivalent)—Tablets, Film-Coated: 250 and 500 mg.

Other Macrolides

Erythromycin Estolate [Erythromycin 2′-propionate dodecyl sulfate (salt) [3521-62-8] $C_{40}H_{71}NO_{14}.C_{12}H_{26}O_4S$ (1056.39) Ilosone (*Dista*).]—Potency: equivalent to not less than 600 μg of erythromycin ($C_{37}H_{67}NO_{13}$)/mg, calculated on the anhydrous basis. For the structure of the base see *Erythromycin*. *Preparation:* Erythromycin is reacted with propionic acid anhydride in acetone solution to form the 2′-propionate ester which is then converted to its hydrochloride. The ester salt is then metathesized with sodium dodecyl sulfate. *Description and solubility:* White, crystalline powder; odorless or practically odorless; practically tasteless. Practically insoluble in water; 1 g in 20 mL alcohol, 10 mL chloroform. *Uses:* The actions and uses are those of *Erythromycin*. The estolate is very insoluble in water, and it is more acid-stable and less affected by presence of food in the stomach than are other erythromycin preparations. About 20% of erythromycin estolate is absorbed as the base, and 80% as the ester; the latter undergoes continuing hydrolysis to maintain approximately this ratio. Further hydrolysis at the bacterial cell level contributes to the activity of the drug.

Hepatic dysfunction, with or without jaundice, has occurred in association with erythromycin estolate administration, chiefly in adults. The drug is contraindicated in patients with hepatic dysfunction or preexisting liver disease. *Dose: Oral*, see under *Erythromycin*.

Troleandomycin [Oleandomycin triacetate (ester) [2751-09-9] $C_{41}H_{67}NO_{15}$ (813.98); Triacetyloleandomycin; TAO (*Roerig*)]—Prepared by acetylating oleandomycin with acetic anhydride in the presence of pyridine. White, crystalline powder; 1 g dissolves in about 10 mL alcohol; slightly soluble in water, ether. *Uses:* Converted in the body to oleandomycin, which has the actions of *Erythromycin*, but is only ¼ as potent. It is indicated only for treatment of infections of the upper respiratory tract caused by group A β-hemolytic streptococci and pneumococcal pneumonia and to eradicate streptococci from the nasopharynx. Cross-resistance occurs to erythromycin, but some erythromycin-resistant bacteria respond to oleandomycin. The adverse effects are those of erythromycin. Anaphylaxis has been reported. It elevates serum concentrations of theophylline. It also interacts with ergotamine to cause vasospastic ischemia. In hepatic failure the dose interval must be increased. *Dose: Oral, adults*, 250 to 500 mg every 6 hr; *children*, 125 to 250 mg *or* 6.6 to 11 mg/kg every 6 hr.

Penicillins

History—During an inspection of some culture plates in the laboratory of St Mary's Hospital London, in 1928, Professor Alexander Fleming observed the lysis of staphylococcus organisms by a contaminating mold. Upon subculturing the mold he found in the broth a powerful, but nontoxic, antibacterial substance. He gave it the name "penicillin" from the organism *Penicillium notatum* which caused the generation of the antibiotic.

Chemistry—The name "penicillin" now designates a number of antibiotic substances produced by the growth of various *Penicillium* species or by other means. The better

Table I—Some Natural Penicillins

Natural penicillin	Radical (R)
Penicillin G	benzyl
Penicillin F	2-pentenyl
Penicillin dihydro-F	*n*-amyl
Penicillin K	*n*-heptyl
Penicillin O	(allylthio)methyl
Penicillin V	phenoxymethyl
Penicillin X	*p*-hydroxybenzyl
Penicillin N	D-4-amino-4-carboxybutyl
Penicillin S	γ-chlorocrotylmercaptomethyl
Penicillin BT	butylmercaptomethyl

known natural penicillins are listed in Table I. Penicillins F, G, and X were formerly referred to as I, II, and III, respectively.

The parent compound is (2*S*-*cis*)-4-thia-1-azabicyclo[3.2.0]heptane-2-carboxylic acid (I). The 3,3-dimethyl-7-oxo derivative of I is commonly known by the trivial name penicillanic acid (II), and the penicillins are α-carboxamido derivatives of it (III):

Penicillins are variously named in the literature as derivatives of I, II, and III above. Nomenclature by I is purely systematic, whereas that by II and III is trivial. As derivatives of II, it is merely necessary to identify the specific 6α-carboxyamido group; as derivatives of III, only the R of the 6α-carboxamido group is identified.

The introduction of various acids, amines, or amides into the medium in which the mold is developing leads to the production of biosynthetic penicillins which differ only in R. Dozens of biosynthetic *penicillins* have been prepared in this manner in an attempt to obtain compounds superior to penicillin G with respect to various physical, microbiological, or pharmacological properties. In 1958 methods were devised for preparing the penicillin nucleus, thus making it possible to biosynthesize penicillins that could not be formed in a more normal medium. The resulting compounds were often more acid-stable, more penicillinase-resistant, or had a wider antibacterial spectrum.

Much of the penicillin of commerce is pure crystalline G. It occurs in fermentation liquors together with variable amounts of K and F penicillins and smaller amounts of others, and is separated from the other penicillins during purification. Commercial practice suppresses to a certain extent the natural tendency of the mold to form penicillins other than the desired G by the incorporation of a precursor of G, namely phenylacetic acid, phenylacetamide, phenylethylamine, or other substance containing the phenylacetyl radical, which is built directly into the penicillin G molecule. Penicillin G has the additional advantage of being much easier to crystallize than K or F.

As seen in the figure of structures, penicillins are acids. The potassium salt predominates in use, with the sodium salt next. These salts are very soluble in water. The acid moiety can be used to combine penicillins with various bases, such as procaine or benzathine, to create insoluble salts, for repository use, or for the purpose of decreasing solubility so as to make the compound more resistant to gastric acid.

Penicillin in solution is very unstable at pH 5 or less and at 8 or above. Solutions of penicillin begin to deteriorate upon standing a few days, even in the cold. Certain penicillins are more resistant to acid hydrolysis and thus lend themselves better to oral administration.

Spectrum—Penicillins are bacteriostatic at low and bactericidal at high concentrations. According to their antibacterial spectrum (and roughly to their dates of introduction), penicillins have been classified as first-, second-, third-, and fourth-generation penicillins. All the early penicillins are of the *first-generation* and have a *narrow spectrum* of activity limited mostly to gram-positive bacteria and gram-negative cocci and a few miscellaneous bacteria. The first-generation includes penicillin G, penicillin V, methicillin, nafcillin, oxacillin, cloxacillin, and dicloxacillin. They are especially active against many gram-positive bacteria, particularly *Strep pyogenes, anaerobic streptococci*, most *pneumococci, Cl tetani, Cl perfringens (Welchii), Coryn diphtheriae, B anthracis* and *Listeria monocytogenes.* Staphylococci, especially *Staph aureus*, are mostly resistant, although they were originally mostly sensitive. *Strep viridans* is variably sensitive to penicillins. *Strep fecalis (enterococcus)* is usually resistant. Strains in which resistance is attributable to bacterial elaboration of penicillinase are usually sensitive to penicillinase-refractory penicillins such as methicillin. A second kind of resistance, not dependent on a penicillinase, is called methicillin-resistance. The gram-negative cocci, *N meningitidis* and *N gonorrhea*, are sensitive to penicillins, although resistant gonococci are on the increase. The activity of first-generation (narrow spectrum) penicillins against the gram-negative bacilli is usually too low to be of clinical significance, but over 80% of strains of *E coli*, most *Pr mirabilis*, and some *Salmonella* and *Shigella* are sufficiently sensitive to respond in the urinary tract, where penicillin concentration is high. Since the concentration is also high in bile, first-generation penicillins may be used to treat biliary tract infections caused by some gram-negative enterobacteria as well as by enterococci. These drugs are also active against *Treponema pallidum, Leptospira, Streptobacillus moniliformis, Spirillum minus*, and *Actinomycetes.*

The *second-generation* penicillins have a greater efficacy than first-generation penicillins against enterococcus, meningococcus, and several aerobic gram-negative bacilli, such as community-acquired *E coli, H influenzae, Pr mirabilis, Salmonella* (including *S typhi*), and *Shigella.* Members of this group have somewhat less activity against most gram-positive bacteria. All of the present second-generation penicillins are *aminopenicillins* (2-phenyl-2-aminoacetyl, other), and this term is often applied to this group. Members include amoxicillin, ampicillin, cyclicillin, epicillin, and several propenicillins (eg, bacampicillin) that yield active aminopenicillins in the body.

Third-generation penicillins manifest a further extension of the spectrum to include some strains of *P aeruginosa* and increased activity against *Enterobacter.* Activity against these bacilli is not high enough to be used against systemic infections but is sufficient for the treatment of uncomplicated urinary tract infections. They are even less active than second-generation drugs against most gram-positive bacteria. Third-generation penicillins include carbenicillin, ticarcillin, and the propenicillin, indanylcarbenicillin.

Fourth-generation penicillins, also called *antipseudomonal penicillins*, have sufficiently increased activity against *Ps aeruginosa* that they may be used against systemic infections, although only in combination with an aminoglycoside. They are also active against *Acinetobacter* and some strains of

Klebsiella and *Serratia.* Activity against gram-positive bacteria is further diminished. Members of this group include azlocillin, mezlocillin, and piperacillin. Sometimes mezlocillin and piperacillin are called *extended-spectrum* penicillins because of their heightened activity against enterococcus and the anaerobic bacillus, *B fragilis.* Both third- and fourth-generation (antipseudomonal) penicillins have antiplatelet actions that may favor bleeding episodes.

Sometime penicillins are classified in other ways. It is common to call the penicillinase-resistant penicillins, "antistaphyococcal," the second through fourth generations together "broad-spectrum," and the third and fourth generation together "antipseudomonal" penicillins.

Resistance—The penicillin resistance of many gram-positive and gram-negative bacteria is due to their elaboration of penicillin-destroying enzymes called *penicillinases*, members of a group called beta-lactamases. Penicillinases are produced by large numbers of bacteria and actinomycetes and convert penicillin into inactive *penicilloic acid* by liberation of a second carboxyl group. Resistance of bacteria to penicillin cannot be explained entirely on penicillinase production because many resistant organisms produce little or no penicillinase. With some bacteria, eg, *Staph aureus*, resistance develops very fast clinically, but some microorganisms, eg, *T pallidum*, never become resistant. More resistant bacteria dwell in hospital personnel than in the community at large, because such personnel are close to patients under treatment. Acquired resistance is the result of the selection of natural penicillin-resistant strains that are ordinarily held in check by the sensitive parent strain. Resistant genes may be acquired by mutation, transduction by viruses, transformation, and conjugative transfer of resistant-gene-containing plasmids.

Mechanism—Penicillin is known to interfere with the synthesis of peptidoglycans, which are part of the cell-wall material. Consequently, the growing protoplast cannot form a protective cell wall. Several wall enzymes are reversibly inhibited, the most important being a D,D-carboxypeptidase which also functions as a transpeptidase. Conditions favoring rapid growth of bacteria are best for the inhibitory action of penicillin. Under favorable conditions, penicillin exerts a direct bactericidal action, and successful penicillin therapy may be relatively independent of immunity mechanisms of the host.

Potency—The potency of penicillin is expressed in units per mg. *One International Unit is equivalent to the activity of 0.6 μg of pure crystalline sodium penicillin G* to which, by international conference, a potency of 1667 *units/mg* has been assigned. See Table II. Because of the large doses now used, it is common to speak in terms of megaunits, ie, 1 megaunit equals 10^6 Units.

Table II—Potencies of Some Penicillin Products

Drug	MW	Units/mg
Penicillin G Benzathine	981.2	1211
Penicillin G Potassium	372.5	1595
Penicillin G Procaine	588.7	1009
Penicillin G Sodium Reference Standard	356.4	1667
Penicillin V Reference Standard	350.4	1695

Assay—See *Biological Testing* (page 557).

Uses—First-generation penicillins are especially effective in the treatment of infections caused by gram-positive bacteria, particularly staphylococcal, streptococcal, pneumococcal, and clostridial infections. Penicillin G is the drug of choice in the treatment of gram-negative *gonococcal, fusobacterial*, and *meningococcal infections.* It is the drug choice in the treatment of pneumonia and other respiratory tract infections caused by *Strep pneumoniae*, groups A, B, C and G streptococci, *Staph aureus* (sensitive strains) and *B anthracis*. Penicillin G is also the drug of choice in the treatment of infections by *Cl perfringens* and *tetani*, *Spirillum* and *Streptobacillus* (rat-bite fevers), *Pasteurella* (multocide), *Leptotrichia*, oropharyngeal *Bacterioides*, *Actinomyces*, and *Listeria monocytogenes*. It is presently the chief therapeutic agent in the treatment of both *gonorrhea* and *syphilis*, although gonococci resistant to penicillin have become a serious problem. Penicillin is often lifesaving in the treatment of *subacute bacterial endocarditis* when the causative organism is penicillin-sensitive. It is especially valuable when the organism is *Strep viridans*, but it has been used successfully when the endocarditis is caused by *E coli*. As much as 10 to 100 million units of penicillin may be injected daily in this disease. Massive doses of broad-spectrum penicillins are also often used successfully to treat septicemias caused by *E coli* and some other gram-negative bacteria, especially if the focus is thought to be in the biliary tract. Aminopenicillins are the drugs of choice in infections caused by *Pr mirabilis*, *Shigella*, *Salmonella* (other than *typhi*), and nonlife-threatening infections caused by *H influenzae*. Carbenicillin and ticarcillin are drugs of choice in *urinary tract infections* caused by *Ps aeruginosa*. Penicillin G is an alternate drug in the treatment of *diphtheria*. The drug is used in the *prophylaxis* of rheumatic fever and of *pneumonia* in patients with croup.

Penicillin is sometimes employed in *combination* with other agents. The results of such therapy are often, but not invariably, superior to those obtainable with penicillin alone. When it is administered with the tetracyclines, chloramphenicol, or the sulfonamides, antagonism may be noted if the microorganism is highly susceptible to penicillin when it is administered alone. Nevertheless, it is often used in combination with chloramphenicol in the treatment of bacterial meningitis caused by *H influenzae*.

The number of bacteria and the quantity of pus appear to have only a minor influence upon the antibacterial action of penicillin, except when the organism produces penicillinase.

Adverse Effects—Penicillin is practically nontoxic. However, hypersensitivity reactions occur in several percent of patients, depending on the type of preparation employed and the route of administration. The most common manifestation of this allergic response is a skin rash. Nondermatologic manifestations of allergy include serum sickness, angioedema, nephropathy, rare hemolytic anemia, Arthus reaction, rare pericarditis, enteropathy, hepatotoxicity and anaphylaxis. It is estimated that several hundred persons die each year in the US from penicillin-induced anaphylaxis. Neutropenia, which occasionally results from high-dose therapy, does not appear to involve an immune process.

Side effects of oral administration of penicillins are nausea, vomiting, epigastric distress, diarrhea, and black "hairy" tongue.

Like other antibiotics, penicillin can markedly alter the normal bacterial flora of man. As a result, superimposed infection by a penicillin-resistant microorganism may develop during the course of treatment, and appropriate chemotherapy should be instituted as soon as possible. Overgrowth even occurs in the bowel, because penicillin is secreted into the bile, which keeps the intestinal levels high. Coagulation disorders may also occur as the result of the suppression of enteric bacteria which synthesize vitamin K.

Very high concentrations of penicillin are neurotoxic, and nerve damage has resulted from intramuscular administration. Crystalline penicillin has an irritating effect when applied directly to the central nervous system. Symptoms following intrathecal administration include listlessness, headache, nausea, vomiting, respiratory difficulty, cyanosis, fall in blood pressure, thready pulse, muscular twitching and convulsions. These are reduced or eliminated by lowering dosage.

With sodium and potassium salts, the effect of the cation load must be considered. Lastly, untoward effects sometimes result from the rapid bactericidal effects, because of the release of endotoxins and other bacterial cell components.

Absorption, Distribution, and Excretion—Penicillin G in the form of its sodium or potassium salt is rapidly absorbed from subcutaneous and intramuscular sites. The intramuscular route is preferred. Penicillin G is given intravenously by continuous infusion only when it is imperative to maintain very high blood concentrations such as in the treatment of subacute *bacterial endocarditis*. The rate of absorption from intramuscular sites of injection may be markedly slowed by the use of repository (depot) preparations consisting of relatively insoluble salts of penicillin in a suitable vehicle. For example, therapeutic blood levels (for some purposes) persist 12 to 24 hours after a single 300,000-unit dose of *Procaine Penicillin in Aqueous Suspension*, 24 to 48 hours after *Procaine Penicillin in Oil*, and 1 week or more after 1.2 million units of *Benzathine Penicillin G*. However, the slower the absorption, the lower the peak plasma level, and some uses are precluded.

The absorption of penicillin G from the gastrointestinal tract is incomplete and irregular, but some acid-stable penicillins are well absorbed. To obtain the same blood concentrations as by the intramuscular route, 3 to 5 times the parenteral dose of penicillin G must be employed. Penicillin G should be ingested when the stomach is empty because an empty stomach empties rapidly and because penicillin binds to food substances. Although hydrochloric acid in the gastric juice destroys penicillin G, buffer agents have not proved to be necessary for successful oral medication, since the dose can be raised to compensate. Oral penicillin G therapy should never be relied upon alone in severe infections.

Penicillins distributed are in the extracellular water, but they penetrate cells poorly. Tissue concentrations are about $1/4$ the plasma concentration *at equilibrium*. Plasma levels fall so fast that there is not enough time for the build-up of high concentrations in many tissues. Most penicillins not readily penetrate the subarachnoid space from the blood stream, although meningeal inflammation increases penetrance; hence, in *meningitis* it may be advisable to use both the intrathecal and intramuscular routes. For intrathecal administration a soluble salt is used. In neurosyphilis the concentration in the cerebrospinal fluid afforded by conventional doses is sometimes inadequate. Local instillation may also be necessary in various body cavities and in abscesses, etc. as a supplement to systemic administration.

Penicillins mostly are secreted into the urine, partly by glomerular filtration but mostly by tubular secretion (80%). Substances which interfere with renal tubular excretion of penicillin (see *Probenecid*, page 944) serve to enhance and prolong the effective blood levels of the antibiotic. Probenecid can completely block the renal tubular secretion of penicillin into the tubular urine; this markedly slows the excretion of the antibiotic. Phenylbutazone also interferes with excretion to a degree comparable to probenecid; sulfinpyrazone, aspirin, indomethacin and some sulfonamides also moderately interfere with the excretion of penicillin. The normal plasma half-time of penicillin G is about 45 min, but in persons over 60 years old it is up to twice as long. In oliguria, it may be 7 to 10 hours.

Amoxicillin

4-Thia-1-azabicyclo[3.2.0]heptane-2-carboxylic acid, 6-[[amino(4-hydroxyphenyl)acetyl]amino]-3,3-dimethyl-7-oxo-, [2S-[2α,5α,6β(S*)]]-, D(−)-α-Amino-*p*-hydroxybenzylpenicillin; Amoxil; Larotid (*Beecham*)

[61336-70-7] $C_{16}H_{19}N_3O_5S\cdot 3H_2O$ (419.45); *anhydrous* [26787-78-0] (365.30).

Preparation—By acylation of 6-aminopenicillanic acid with D-(−)-2-(*p*-hydroxyphenyl)glycine.

Description—Fine, white to off-white, crystalline powder; bitter taste; high humidity and temperature over 37° adversely affect stability.

Solubility—1 g in 370 mL water, 2000 mL alcohol.

Uses—Amoxicillin, chemically *p*-hydroxyampicillin, has an antibacterial spectrum identical to that of *Ampicillin*, except that it is less active against *Shigella*. Like ampicillin, it is destroyed by penicillinase and hence cannot be used to treat infections caused by resistant strains of bacteria of the penicillinase-producing type. However, it is more acid-stable than ampicillin and hence is better suited for oral use. The indications for use and status are those of ampicillin, except that ampicillin is preferred in infections caused by *Shigella* and also it cannot be given parenterally for severe infections. The toxicity is that of ampicillin, but there is less diarrhea.

By the oral route, nearly 100% is absorbed. An oral dose of 250 mg will provide a peak plasma concentration of about 4 μg/mL. In plasma, amoxicillin is 17% protein-bound. The volume of distribution is 0.4 mL/g. From 50 to 72% is eliminated by renal tubular secretion. The half-life is about 1 hr when renal function is normal and 7 to 10 hr in renal failure.

Dose (anhydride equivalent)—*Oral, adults,* and *children weighing 20 kg* or more, **250** to **500 mg** every 8 hr, but as much as **4.5 g** a day may be given, if necessary; for *gonorrhea* **3 g** is given as a single dose along with 1 g of probenecid. *Infants weighing less than 6 kg,* **25** to **50 mg** every 8 hr; *infants weighing 6 to 8 kg,* **50** to **100 mg** every 8 hr; *infants weighing 8 to 20 kg,* **6.7** to **13.3 mg/kg** of body weight every 8 hr.

Dosage Forms (anhydride equivalent)—Capsules: 250 and 500 mg; for Oral Suspension: 50 mg/mL, and 125 and 250 mg/5 mL; Chewable Tablets: 125 and 150 mg.

Ampicillin

4-Thia-1-azabicyclo[3.2.0]heptane-2-carboxylic acid, 6-[(aminophenylacetyl)amino]-3,3-dimethyl-7-oxo-, [2S-[2α,5α,6β(S*)]]-, *Various Mfrs*

[69-53-4] $C_{16}H_{19}N_3O_4S$ (349.40); *trihydrate* [7177-48-2] (403.45). Potency: 900 to 1050 μg of $C_{16}H_{19}N_3O_4S$/mg, calculated on the anhydrous basis.

Preparation—6-Aminopenicillanic acid is acylated with D-(−)-glycine. US Pat 2,985,648.

Description—White, practically odorless, crystalline powder; occurs as the trihydrate, which is stable at room temperature.

Solubility—1 g in about 90 mL water, 250 mL absolute alcohol; practically insoluble in ether, and chloroform.

Uses—Ampicillin was the first *second-generation* penicillin (see the general statement). It is useful in the treatment of infections due to sensitive strains of *Shigella, Salmonella, E coli, H influenzae, Aerobacter,* enterococci, *N gonorrheae, N meningitidis,* and *Pr mirabilis.* These bacteria readily acquire resistance by elaboration of penicillinase, so ampicillin is often given in combination with cloxacillin. Its *in vitro* spectrum against gram-positive cocci is similar to but generally somewhat less effective than that of penicillin G except that it is somewhat more effective against *Strep faecalis* (enterococcus). It is ½ as effective against *Staph aureus* and ¹⁄₂₀ against *Strep pyogenes.* It is poorly effective against penicillinase-producing organisms. Ampicillin is useful in the treatment of *genitourinary tract infections* caused by *E coli, Pr mirabilis, N gonorrheae,* nonhemolytic streptococci, and penicillin G-resistant enterococci. It is often combined with cloxacillin for this purpose. It is especially indicated in respiratory tract infections caused by *H influenzae* and *D pneumoniae* together. Since ampicillin is excreted in the bile, it is valuable in treating *biliary tract infections* due to *E coli* or penicillin-resistant salmonellae, shigella, or enterococci. Intestinal salmonellosis responds erratically. Ampicillin often effects a satisfactory response in *meningitis* in children in which the bacterium is meningococcus, pneumococcus, or *H influenzae.* In mixed infections containing ampicillin-sensitive cocci and bacilli, ampicillin may be preferred to a combination of penicillin G and an aminoglycoside.

Ampicillin causes allergic reactions typical of other penicillins. It is 5 times as allergenic as phenoxymethyl penicillin. The incidence of rashes is about 7%, but most of these are not allergenic; they are especially prevalent in patients with infectious mononucleosis. Patients allergic to penicillin G are often also allergic to ampicillin. The drug may also cause nausea and vomiting, diarrhea, glossitis, and stomatitis.

Ampicillin is acid-resistant and is about 40% absorbed by the oral route. Bioavailability is dose-dependent. It is bound to plasma proteins to the extent of 8 to 20%. The volume of distribution is 0.17 to 0.31 mL/g. About 45% is excreted unchanged in the urine. Its half-life in plasma is about 0.5 to 1 hr, but it may be as long as 20 hr in renal failure.

Ampicillin may be used in the anhydrous form or as the trihydrate but commercial ampicillin is usually the trihydrate.

Dose (anhydrous equivalent)—*Oral, adults,* and *children weighing 20 kg or more,* **12.5** to **25 mg/kg** of body weight (or **250** to **500 mg**) every 6 hr; as much as 4 g per day may be given, if necessary. For *gonorrhea,* a single dose of **3.5 g,** with 1 g of probenecid. *Infants and children weighing up to 20 kg,* **12.5** to **25 mg/kg** every 6 hr *or* **16.7** to **33.3 mg/kg** every 8 hr.

Dosage Forms (anhydrous equivalent)—Capsules: 250 and 500 mg; for Oral Suspension: 100 mg/mL and 125, 250, and 500 mg/5 mL on reconstitution.

Ampicillin Sodium

4-Thia-1-azabicyclo[3.2.0]heptane-2-carboxylic acid, 6-[(aminophenylacetyl)amino]-3,3-dimethyl-7-oxo-, monosodium salt, [2S-[2α,5α,6β(S*)]]-, *Various Mfrs*

[69-52-3] $C_{16}H_{18}N_3NaO_4S$ (371.39). Potency: not less than 845 μg of ampicillin/mg, on the anhydrous basis.

Preparation—*Ampicillin* is dissolved in a suitable organic solvent and precipitated as the sodium salt by the addition of sodium acetate.

Description—White to off-white, crystalline powder; hygroscopic; pK_{a1} 2.66; pK_{a2} 7.24.

Solubility—Very soluble in water and isotonic NaCl and dextrose solutions.

Uses—Has the actions and uses of *Ampicillin,* and is the form in which ampicillin is employed for intramuscular and intravenous administration.

Dose (anhydrous ampicillin equivalent)—*Intramuscular or intravenous, adults* and *children weighing 20 kg or more,* **250** to **500 mg** every 6 hr; for bacterial *meningitis* or *septicemia,* **1** to **2 g** every 3 or 4 hr *or* **18.8** to **25 mg/kg** every 3 hr *or* **25** to **33 mg/kg** every 4 hr; for *gonorrhea* **500 mg** repeated in 8 to 12 hr; daily limit is 300 mg/kg (or 16 g) a day. *Infants* and *children weighing less than 20 kg,* usually **6.25** to **25 mg/kg** of body weight every 6 hr, *or* **8.3** to **33.3 mg/kg** every 8 hr; for *meningitis* or *septicemia,* **adult dose.**

Dosage Forms (anhydrous ampicillin equivalent)—Sterile: 125, 250, and 500 mg, and 1, 2, and 10 g. Each g contains 3 mEq of sodium.

Carbenicillin Disodium

4-Thia-1-azabicyclo[3.2.0]heptane-2-carboxylic acid, 6-[(carboxyphenylacetyl)amino]-3,3-dimethyl-7-oxo-, disodium salt, [2S-(2α,5α,6β)]-, (α-Carboxybenzyl)penicillin Disodium; Geopen (*Pfizer*); Pyopen (*Beecham*)

[4800-94-6] $C_{17}H_{16}N_2Na_2O_6S$ (422.36). Potency: the equivalent of not less than 770 μg of carbenicillin/mg, calculated on the anhydrous basis.

Preparation—One method consists of hydrolyzing esters of the type

(R = alkyl, aryl, or benzyl) with the aid of a suitable esterase such as α-chymotrypsin or pancreatin, and extracting the acid and reacting it with aqueous NaHCO₃. *CA 72:* 41674a, 1970. The starting esters may be prepared by acylating 6-aminopenicillanic acid with monoesters of phenylmalonic acid. US Pats 3,282,926 and 3,492,291.

Description—White to off-white, crystalline powder with a bitter taste; hygroscopic; odorless, pH (1% solution, w/v) between 6.5 and 8.0. pK_{a1} 2.76; pK_{a2} 3.5.

Solubility—1 g in 1.2 mL water, 25 mL alcohol; practically insoluble in chloroform and ether.

Uses—Carbenicillin is a third-generation penicillin (see page 1192). Penicillin G-resistant species and strains are also resistant to carbenicillin. Since both penicillin G and ampicillin are more potent and effective against the gram-positive bacteria, carbenicillin is not for use in the treatment of infections caused by them. Against the gram-negative bacteria, the spectrum of activity of carbenicillin differs not only from penicillin G but also from ampicillin in being moderately effective in high doses against most strains of *Ps aeruginosa;* however, these bacteria rapidly acquire resistance to the drug. Nevertheless, the use of carbenicillin in the treatment of pseudomonas infections is what primarily distinguishes this drug among the penicillins. Carbenicillin shares with ticarcillin drug of choice status in treating urinary tract infections caused by this bacterium. It is never used alone, but rather in combination with an aminoglycoside, against systemic pseudomonal infections. Although it is approved for use against severe systemic infections, septicemia, intraabdominal, pelvic, and soft-tissue infections caused by *H influenzae, Strep pneumoniae,* and other susceptible organisms and urinary tract infections caused by *N gonorrhoeae, Enterobacter,* and *Strep faecalis,* better, or less expensive drugs, are recommended.

Adverse effects are those of penicillins in general (page 1193). The rare penicillin-type coagulopathy has been reported. Reversible elevated serum SGOT levels occasionally occur. Carbenicillin has a heparin-like action. Cation toxicity can occur. Intramuscular injections cause pain; intravenous injections occasionally cause thrombophlebitis. Suprainfections caused by *Klebsiella* may occur. Carbenicillin can cause hypokalemic alkalosis. In persons with a low sodium tolerance, the sodium content must be taken into account. Carbenicillin is expensive.

Carbenicillin is unstable in acid and hence is not suited for oral administration; about 50% of an oral dose is absorbed. An indanyl ester (see following article) is more stable and is used for oral therapy. The volume of distribution is 0.18 mL/g. About 85% is secreted into the urine, but it is also partly destroyed in the liver and also excreted into the bile. The normal half-life of carbenicillin is about 1 hr, but in severe renal insufficiency it may be as long as 13 to 15 hr. If liver failure simultaneously exists, the half-life may be as long as 23 hr.

Dose (carbenicillin equivalent)—*Intramuscular* or *intravenous, adults,* for *urinary tract infections,* up to **50 mg/kg** or 1 to **2 g** every 6 hr; for *respiratory tract* and *soft-tissue infections, septicemia,* and *meningitis,* **50** to **83.3 mg/kg** every 4 hr; for *gonorrhea,* **4 g** divided between two intramuscular sites and with 1 g of probenecid. The maximum daily dose recommended is 42 g. If the creatinine clearance is less than 5 mL/min, the dose should be 2 g intravenously every 8 to 12 hr; if both renal and hepatic failure exist, it is 2 g intravenously every 24 hr. *Older infants* and *children,* for *urinary tract infections,* **12.5** to **50 mg/kg** of body wt every 6 hr (or **8** to **33 mg/kg** every 4 hr); for *respiratory tract* and *soft-tissue infections, septicemia,* and *meningitis,* use the adult dose. Some infants and children may require as much as 600 mg/kg per day (in divided doses), and as much as 800 mg/kg per day has been given. *Neonates over 2 kg of body weight,* for *respiratory tract* and *soft-tissue infections, septicemia,* and *meningitis,* initially **100 mg/kg** of body weight, followed by **75 mg/kg** every 6 hr during the first 3 days of life and **100 mg/kg** every 6 hr thereafter; *neonates up to 2 kg,* same as larger neonates except every 8 hr during the first 3 days.

Dosage Forms (carbenicillin equivalent)—Powder for Injection: 1, 2, 5, 10, 20, and 30 g. Each g contains 4.7 to 5.3 mEq of sodium.

Carbenicillin Indanyl Sodium

4-Thia-1-azabicyclo[3.2.0]heptane-2-carboxylic acid, 6-[[3-[(2,3-dihydro-1*H*-inden-5-yl)oxy]-1,3-dioxo-1-phenylpropyl]amino]-3,3-dimethyl-7-oxo-, monosodium salt, [2*S*-(2α,5α,6β)]-, Geocillin (*Pfizer*)

[26605-69-6] $C_{26}H_{25}N_2NaO_6S$ (516.54). Potency: 659 to 769 µg of carbenicillin/mg, calculated on anhydrous basis, at time of certification, and not less than 630 µg at any time during expiration period.

Preparation—6-Aminopenicillanic acid is coupled with 5-indanyl α-chloroformylphenylacetate (prepared from phenylmalonic acid), producing carbenicillin indanyl, which is neutralized with NaOH.

Description—White, or nearly white, powder; hygroscopic; bitter tasting.

Solubility—Soluble in water; insoluble in chloroform, ether.

Uses—Converted to carbenicillin in the body, so that its actions and adverse effects are those of *Carbenicillin.* However, the indanyl derivative is stable in gastric juice and can be administered orally. Its uses are limited to treatment of uncomplicated *urinary tract infections* caused by carbenicillin-sensitive organisms. Oral doses of 500 mg and 1 g give rise to peak plasma concentrations of about 2 and 6 µg/mL, respectively, of carbenicillin. The amount of unchanged carbenicillin secreted into urine is 35 to 40%, which is inconsistent with the belief that all of the indanyl derivative is converted to carbenicillin during its rapid absorption.

Dose (carbenicillin equivalent)—*Oral, adults,* **382** to **764 mg** every 6 hr. Pediatric dosage has not been established.

Dosage Form (carbenicillin equivalent)—Tablets: 382 mg.

Cloxacillin Sodium

4-Thia-1-azabicyclo[3.2.0]heptane-2-carboxylic acid, 6-[[[3-(2-chlorophenyl)-5-methyl-4-isoxazolyl]carbonyl]amino]-3,3-dimethyl-7-oxo-, monosodium salt, monohydrate, [2*S*-(2α,5α,6β)]-, Cloxacillin Sodium Monohydrate; Tegopen (*Bristol*); Cloxapen (*Beecham*)

[7081-44-9] $C_{19}H_{17}ClN_3NaO_5S \cdot H_2O$ (475.88); *anhydrous* [642-78-4] (457.86). Potency: the equivalent of not less than 825 µg of cloxacillin/mg.

Preparation—6-Aminopenicillanic acid is acylated with 3-(*o*-chlorophenyl)-5-methyl-4-isoxazolecarboxylic acid and the resulting cloxacillin is purified by recrystallization and converted to the sodium salt.

Description—White, odorless, crystalline powder having a bitter taste; stable in light and only slightly hygroscopic; decomposes between 170° and 173°; pH (1 in 100 solution) between 4.5 and 7.5.

Solubility—Freely soluble in water; soluble in alcohol; slightly soluble in chloroform.

Uses—A penicillinase-resistant first-generation penicillin (see general statement). The drug shares a first-choice status with other penicillinase-resistant penicillins in the treatment of staphylococcal infections caused by penicillin G-resistant strains. However, it is less active than penicillin G against non-penicillinase-producing bacteria, especially streptococci. It is not effective against gram-negative organisms. Consequently, its use should be limited to treating infections caused by penicillinase-producing susceptible microorganisms which are resistant to penicillin G. However, it can be used in combination with ampicillin in the treatment of urinary tract infections caused by gram-negative bacilli. By thus limiting its use, the development of resistance to cloxacillin ("methicillin resistance") is discouraged.

The adverse effects caused by cloxacillin are virtually identical to those caused by other penicillins (see page 1193). Rash and urticaria are the principal allergic manifestations. Not all patients allergic to penicillin G are sensitive to cloxacillin, but cross-sensitization is usual. Cloxacillin may also cause occasional nausea, vomiting, abdominal discomfort, epigastric fullness or diarrhea. Superinfections occasionally occur. In persons with a low sodium tolerance, the sodium content must be taken into account.

Cloxacillin is relatively stable in gastric acid. Its absorption by the oral route is about 37 to 80%, which is better than that of nafcillin, but it is nevertheless erratic; the recommended dose is high enough to compensate for irregularity in the affected blood levels. Food in the stomach interferes with absorption. About 90% is bound to plasma proteins. The volume of distribution is 0.15 mL/g. Only 30% is excreted unchanged in the urine. The half-life is about 0.5 hr in persons with normal renal function.

Dose (cloxacillin equivalent)—*Oral, adults* and *children weighing 20 kg or more*, **250** to **500 mg** every 6 hr; *infants* and *children weighing less than 20 kg*, **12.5** to **25 mg/kg** of body weight every 6 hr. Adults may be given up to 6 g a day, if necessary.

Dosage Forms (cloxacillin equivalent)—Capsules: 250 and 500 mg; for Oral Solution: 125 mg/5 mL (reconstituted).

Dicloxacillin Sodium

4-Thia-1-azabicyclo[3.2.0]heptane-2-carboxylic acid, 6-[[[3-(2,6-dichlorophenyl)-5-methyl-4-isoxazolyl]carbonyl]amino]-3,3-dimethyl-7-oxo-, monosodium salt, monohydrate, [2S-(2α,5α,6β)]-, Dicloxin (*Bristol*); Pathocil (*Wyeth*); Veracillin (*Ayerst*)

[13412-64-1] $C_{19}H_{16}Cl_2N_3NaO_5S \cdot H_2O$ (510.32); *anhydrous* [343-55-5] (492.31). Potency: the equivalent of not less than 850 µg of dicloxacillin/mg.

Preparation—6-Aminopenicillanic acid is acylated with 3-(2,6-dichlorophenyl)-5-methyl-4-isoxazolecarboxylic acid and the resulting dicloxacillin (acid) is purified by recrystallization and converted to the sodium salt.

Description—White to off-white, crystalline powder with a faint, characteristic odor; melts between 222° and 225° with decomposition; pK_a 2.67.

Solubility—Freely soluble in water; soluble in alcohol.

Uses—A penicillinase-resistant first-generation penicillin (see general statement). As with all penicillinase-resistant penicillins, it is not as effective as penicillin except against those organisms whose resistance depends on penicillinase production. Therefore, its use should be limited to the treatment of susceptible penicillinase-producing strains, mostly of *Staph pyogenes* var *aureus* resistant to penicillin G, for which it shares first-choice status with the other penicillinase-resistant penicillins.

The toxicity of dicloxacillin is the same as that of penicillins in general (see page 1193). Many patients allergic to penicillin G are not allergic to dicloxacillin, but others are, so that appropriate precautions must be taken. Nausea and diarrhea sometimes occur, but they usually do not necessitate discontinuation of the drug. Elevated serum SGOT is seen in some patients, as with other penicillins, but the significance is not clear; rare hepatotoxicity has been observed. In persons with a low sodium tolerance, the sodium content must be taken into account.

Among the currently available penicillinase-resistant penicillins, dicloxacillin is the best absorbed by the oral route; the amount absorbed is 74 to 80%. Dicloxacillin is bound to plasma proteins to the extent of 90 to 97%, the highest among the penicillins. The volume of distribution is only 0.1 mL/g. About 60% of dicloxacillin is excreted into the urine. Its half-life in plasma is 0.5 to 1.5 hr in normal patients but is longer in renal insufficiency.

Dose (dicloxacillin equivalent)—*Oral, adults* and *children weighing 40 kg or more*, usually **125** to **500 mg** every 6 hr, but may be taken up to **6 g** a day, if necessary; *infants* and *children under 40 kg*, **3.125** to **6.25 mg/kg** of body weight every 6 hr. Dosage for neonates has not been established.

Dosage Forms (dicloxacillin equivalent)—Capsules: 125, 250, and 500 mg; for Oral Suspension: 62.5 mg/5 mL (reconstituted).

Mezlocillin Sodium

4-Thia-1-azabicyclo[3.2.0]heptane-2-carboxylic acid, 3,3-dimethyl-6-[[[[[3-(methylsulfonyl)-2-oxo-1-imidazolidinyl]carbonyl]amino]phenyl-acetyl]amino]-7-oxo-, [2S[2α,5α,6β(S*)]]-, monosodium salt; Mezlin (*Miles*)

[51841-65-3] $C_{21}H_{24}NaN_5O_8S_2$ (561.56).
Preparation—See Ger Pat 2,318,955.
Description—Yellowish-white powder.
Solubility—Very soluble in water; soluble in DMF or methanol; very slightly soluble in alcohol or acetone.

Uses—Mezlocillin is a fourth-generation penicillin (see general statement). It has greater activity than either ampicillin or carbenicillin against *Acinetobacter*, *B fragilis*, *Citrobacter*, *Enterobacter*, *E coli*, *Klebsiella*, *Ps aeruginosa*, and *Serratia*. Its activity against entercocci is comparable to that of ampicillin. Against *Ps aeruginosa* its activity is equal to that of ticarcillin but less than that of piperacillin; it is recommended for use against systemic pseudomonal infections only in combination with an aminoglycoside. Although mezlocillin is approved for use against a variety of infections caused by the above bacteria at different sites, the drug has not been proven to have a clear-cut advantage over any other appropriate drug; even against *Ps aeruginosa*, its activity is less than that of piperacillin and about that of ticarcillin. For this and the reason that resistance of *Pseudomonas* and some other *Enterobacteriaceae* develops rapidly, mezlocillin should probably be held in reserve for infections sensitive to this drug but insensitive to the longer-established antibiotics, except when certain other antibiotics may excessively increase body sodium content in persons with sodium intolerance.

Mezlocillin causes no adverse effects unique to penicillins. The overall incidence is about 10%, local reactions accounting for about 3% and skin reactions about 2%. Pseudomembranous colitis, interstitial nephritis, hepatitis, and bleeding diathesis have not been reported, although thrombocytopenia has.

The oral bioavailability of mezlocillin is low and erratic. In plasma, 16 to 42% is protein-bound. The volume of distribution is about 0.1 mL/g. The drug penetrates into cerebrospinal fluid, especially in meningitis. Urinary excretion eliminates 55 to 65% of the drug and biliary excretion 5 to 25%. The remainder is metabolized; this fraction of elimination is dose-dependent. The half-life is 0.8 to 1.5 hr, except longer in either renal or hepatic insuficiency.

Dose (Mezlocillin equivalent)—*Intramuscular*, or *intravenous*, *adults*, *uncomplicated gonorrheal urethritis*, **1** or **2 g** as a single dose 0.5 hr after 1 g of probenecid; *uncomplicated urinary tract infections*, **25** to **31.3 mg/kg** or **1.5** to **2 g** every 6 hr; *other infections*, **33.3** to **58.3 mg/kg** every 4 hr, **50** to **87.5 mg/kg** every 6 hr, or **3** to **4 g** every 4 to 6 hr; *infants over 1 mo of age* and *children up to 12 yr*, **50 mg/kg** every 4 hr; *younger infants*, **75 mg/kg** every 6 to 8 hr for infants up to 8 days of age and every 12 hr for infants younger than 8 days. *Intravenous*, *adults*, for *complicated urinary tract infections*, **37.5** to **50 mg/kg** or **3 g** every 6 hr. Dosage adjustments are required in renal failure.

Dosage Forms (mezlocillin equivalent)—Powder for injection: 1, 2, 3 and 4 g. Each g contains 1.85 mEq of sodium.

Nafcillin Sodium

4-Thia-1-azabicyclo[3.2.0]heptane-2-carboxylic acid, 6-[[(2-ethoxy-1-naphthalenyl)carbonyl]amino]-3,3-dimethyl-7-oxo-, monosodium salt, monohydrate, [2S-(2α,5α,6β)]-, Unipen (*Wyeth*); Nafcil (*Bristol*)

[7177-50-6] $C_{21}H_{21}N_2NaO_5S.H_2O$ (454.47); *anhydrous* [985-16-0] (436.46). Potency: equivalent to not less than 820 μg of nafcillin/mg.

Preparation—6-Aminopenicillanic acid is acylated by treatment with 2-ethoxy-1-naphthoyl chloride in an anhydrous organic solvent containing triethylamine. An aqueous extract of this product is admixed with a water-immiscible solvent and nafcillin is precipitated by the addition of sulfuric acid. Nafcillin sodium is precipitated by mixing ethanolic solutions of the acid and sodium ethylhexanoate. US Pat 3,157,639.

Description—White to yellowish white powder having not more than a slight characteristic odor.

Solubility—Freely soluble in water and chloroform; soluble in alcohol.

Uses—Nafcillin is a penicillinase-resistant first-generation penicillin, the use of which is restricted to the treatment of infections caused by penicillinase-producing cocci (mostly staphylococci), although it is sometimes used in children against streptococcal infections. These restrictions are intended to minimize the development of "methicillin" resistance.

Nafcillin is partly destroyed by gastric acid, and about 36% is absorbed from the gut, somewhat erratically. For serious infections, initial therapy should be by parenteral administration. About 90% is bound to protein in plasma. The volume of distribution is 0.10 to 0.29 mL/g. Only about 27% is eliminated unchanged in the urine. The half-life is 0.5 to 1 hr.

Untoward reactions are similar to those shown by other penicillins. It causes occasional nausea and diarrhea. It is irritating and may cause pain and an increase in serum transaminase activity after intramuscular injection. Thrombophlebitis can occur with intravenous injection. Cross-sensitivity between nafcillin and other penicillins may occur, but penicillin-sensitive patients often can tolerate nafcillin. The sodium content must be considered when the drug is used in persons with a low sodium tolerance.

Dose (nafcillin equivalent)—*Oral, adults,* **250 mg** to **1 g** every 4 to 6 hr; *older infants* and *children,* **6.25** to **12.5 mg/kg** every 6 hr, except **250 mg** every 8 hr in *streptococcal pharyngitis; neonates,* **10 mg/kg** every 6 to 8 hr. *Intramuscular, adults,* usually **500 mg** every 4 to 6 hr, but as much as 12 g/day may be given; *older infants* and *children,* usually **25 mg/kg** every 12 hr; *neonates,* usually **10** to **20 mg/kg** every 12 hr. *Intravenous, adults,* usually **500 mg** to **1.5 g** every 4 to 6 hr, but as much as 20 g/day may be given; *neonates, older infants* and *children,* usually **10** to **20 mg/kg** every 4 hr *or* **20** to **40 mg/kg** every 8 hr, but up to 200 mg/kg/day may be given.

Dosage Forms (nafcillin equivalent)—Capsules: 250 mg; for Oral Solution: 250 mg/5 mL; for Injection: 500 mg and 1, 1.5, 2, 4, and 10 g; Tablets: 500 mg. Each g contains 2.9 mEq of sodium.

Oxacillin Sodium

4-Thia-1-azabicyclo[3.2.0]heptane-2-carboxylic acid, 3,3-dimethyl-6-[[(5-methyl-3-phenyl-4-isoxazolyl)carbonyl]amino]-7-oxo-, monosodium salt, monohydrate, [2S-(2α,5α,6β)]-, Bactocill (*Beecham*); Prostaphlin (*Bristol*)

[7240-38-2] $C_{19}H_{18}N_3NaO_5S.H_2O$ (441.43); *anhydrous* [1173-88-2] (423.42). Potency: equivalent to 815 to 950 μg of oxacillin $(C_{19}H_{19}N_3O_5S)$/mg.

Preparation—Fermentation-produced 6-aminopenicillanic acid is condensed with 5-methyl-3-phenyl-4-isoxazolyl chloride in a suitable organic solvent and the resulting oxacillin is precipitated as the sodium salt by the addition of sodium acetate.

Description—Fine, white, crystalline powder, odorless or having a slight odor.

Solubility—Freely soluble in water; slightly soluble in absolute alcohol, chloroform; insoluble in ether.

Uses—Oxacillin is a penicillinase-resistant first-generation penicillin (page 1192). Its actions and uses are nearly identical to those of *Nafcillin Sodium.* Its absorption is equal to that of nafcillin but less than that of *Dicloxacillin.* It is less potent than penicillin G

against *Strep pyogenes* and nonresistant *Staph aureus.* Like methicillin, dicloxacillin, and nafcillin, it should be restricted to treatment of penicillin G-resistant *staphylococci* infections, to minimize the development of resistant strains. Because of the variation in absorption after oral administration, oral oxacillin sodium is not the antistaphylococcal penicillin of choice for most serious infections such as bacteremia and osteomyelitis, but the drug may be given parenterally. It may be given orally after the infection is under control.

About 30% of oxacillin is absorbed orally. The presence of food in the stomach interferes with absorption. About 93% of oxacillin in plasma is bound to protein. The volume of distribution is 0.19 mL/g. About 30 to 50% of oxacillin is excreted in the urine, the remainder into the bile and destroyed in the body. Its half-life is 0.5 hr, except in oliguria it is only 2 hr.

Allergenic effects are similar to those of other penicillins, although cross-reactions do not always occur. Oxacillin may also cause nausea, vomiting, diarrhea, fever, eosinophilia, hairy tongue, and, rarely, moniliasis. Because an increased plasma concentration of SGOT occasionally occurs it is suggested that special attention be paid to the use of oxacillin in newborn infants and in patients with hepatic dysfunction. The sodium content of the drug must be considered when the drug is to be used in persons with a low sodium tolerance.

Dose (oxacillin equivalent)—*Oral, adults* and *children weighing more than 40 kg,* usually **500 mg** to **1 g** every 4 to 6 hr, but up to 6 g/day may be given; *infants* and *children less than 40 kg,* **12.5** to **25 mg/kg** of body weight every 6 hr. *Intramuscular or intravenous, adults* and *children weighing over 40 kg,* usually **1** to **2 g** every 4 hr, but up to 20 g/day may be given; *infants* and *children weighing less than 40 kg,* **12.5** to **25 mg/kg** of body weight every 6 hr *or* **16.7 mg/kg** every 4 hr; *neonates* **25 mg/kg** every 6 hr if *over 2 kg* and 15 to 30 days of age, every 8 hr if under 2 kg and 15 to 30 days of age, and every 12 hr if under 2 kg and 1 to 14 days of age.

Dosage Forms (oxacillin equivalent)—Capsules: 250 and 500 mg; for Injection: 250 and 500 mg, and 1, 2, 4, and 10 g; for Oral Solution: 250 mg/5 mL. Each g contains 2.8 mEq of sodium.

Penicillin G Benzathine

4-Thia-1-azabicyclo[3.2.0]heptane-2-carboxylic acid, 3,3-dimethyl-7-oxo-6-[(phenylacetyl)amino]-, [2S-(2α,5α,6β)]-, compd with N,N'-bis-(phenylmethyl)-1,2-ethanediamine (2:1), tetrahydrate; Bicillin (*Wyeth*)

[41372-02-5] $C_{16}H_{20}N_2.2C_{16}H_{18}N_2O_4S.4H_2O$ (981.19); *anhydrous* [1538-09-6] (909.13). Potency: 1090 to 1272 Penicillin Units/mg. One mg of Penicillin G Benzathine represents 1211 Penicillin G Units.

Preparation—Precipitates on mixing aqueous solutions containing N,N-dibenzylethylenediamine diacetate and sodium penicillin G in the required molar proportion.

Description—White, odorless, crystalline powder; saturated solution is slightly acid or is neutral to litmus, having a pH of 5 to 7.5.

Solubility—1 g in about 5000 mL water and about 65 mL alcohol.

Uses—Has low water-solubility, hence on intramuscular injection it is released slowly and yields prolonged blood levels of penicillin, generally for 1 to 4 weeks. Its antibacterial activity is that of the penicillin G moiety (see page 1191), except that its long duration of action makes it especially suitable for prophylaxis of rheumatic fever. However, by the intramuscular route the blood levels are quite low and are not suitable for most of the uses of penicillin G. For example, 1.2 million units will yield an average plasma level of only 0.15 unit/mL on the first day, and by the 14th day it will have fallen to 0.03 unit/mL. Cerebrospinal fluid concentrations are negligible. With probenecid the levels will be somewhat higher. Consequently, it is indicated *only* for the *prophylaxis* and *treatment* of *infections* caused by highly susceptible *group A streptococcus, syphilis, yaws, bejel,* and *pinta.*

Dose (penicillin G equivalent)—*Intramuscular, adults,* **1,200,000 units** as a single dose for upper *respiratory tract infections;* **2,400,000 units** for *primary, secondary* and *latent syphilis,* as a single dose, or **2,400,000** to **3,000,000 units** once a week for 2 to 3 weeks for *late* *syphilis*, but as much as 2,400,000 units a day can be given, if necessary; for *continuous prophylaxis* against streptococcal infections, **1,200,000 units** once a mo or **600,000 units** every 2 wks. *Children weighing more than 27.3 kg (60 lb)*, for upper *respiratory tract infections*, **900,000 units** as a single dose; *infants* and *children weighing less than 27.3 kg*, for upper *respiratory tract infections*, **300,000** to **600,000 units** as a single dose; *infants* and *children up to 2 yr of age*, for *congenital syphilis*, **50,000 units/kg** of body weight as a single dose; *children 2 to 12 yr of age* with *congenital syphilis*, the adult dose diminished according to relative body weight. *Oral, adults* and *children over 12 yr of age*, usually **400,000** to **600,000 units** every 4 to 6 hr, but as much as 12,000,000 units a day may be given, if necessary; *infants* and *children up to 12 years of age*, **4167** to **15,000 units/kg** of body weight every 4 hr or 6250 to 22,500 units/kg every 6 hr or 8333 to 30,000 units/kg every 8 hr.

Dosage Forms (penicillin G equivalent)—Sterile Suspension: 600,000 units/1 mL, 900,000 units/1.5 mL, 1,200,000 units/2 mL, 2,400,000 units/4 mL, 3,000,000 units/10 mL; Tablets: 200,000 units.

Penicillin G Potassium

4-Thia-1-azabicyclo[3.2.0]heptane-2-carboxylic acid, 3,3-dimethyl-7-oxo-6-[(phenylacetyl)amino]-, monopotassium salt, [2S-(2α,5α,6β)]-, Benzylpenicillin Potassium

[113-98-4] $C_{16}H_{17}KN_2O_4S$ (372.48). Penicillin G Potassium has a potency of not less than 1440 and not more than 1680 Penicillin G Units per mg.

Description—Colorless or white crystals, or a white, crystalline powder; odorless or practically so, and moderately hygroscopic; decomposed by prolonged exposure to temperatures of about 100°, moisture accelerating decomposition; not appreciably affected by air or by light; solutions deteriorate at room temperature, but solutions stored below 15° remain stable for several days; rapidly inactivated by acids and alkalies, and also by oxidizing agents; pH (aqueous solution, 30 mg/mL) between 5 and 7.5.

Solubility—Very soluble in water, saline TS, and dextrose solutions; soluble in alcohol (but is inactivated by this solvent), glycerin, and many other alcohols.

Uses—See the uses of penicillins in the introductory statement in this section (page 1192). The potassium salt has no advantage over the sodium salt except when high doses are used in patients on sodium restriction. The potassium salt also avoids the hypokalemic alkalosis that sometimes occurs during treatment with high doses of penicillins. The possibility of potassium intoxication from massive doses in oliguric patients should be kept in mind. The bioavailability by the oral route is 20 to 33%. In plasma 50 to 65% is protein-bound. The volume of distribution is 0.47 mL/g. Renal elimination is 60 to 90% of the total, the remainder being mostly biliary. The half-life is 0.5 hr, except longer in renal failure or after probenecid.

Dose (penicillin G equivalent)—*Oral, adults* and *children 12 yr of age or older, for treatment of infections*, usually **200,000** to **500,000** units every 6 to 8 hr, but up to 12,000,000 units a day may be given, if necessary; *infants* and *children under 12 yr of age*, **4167** to **15,000 units/kg** of body weight every 4 hr, *or* 6250 to 22,500 **units/kg** every 6 hr, *or* 8333 to 30,000 **units/kg** every 8 hr; for *prophylaxis of rheumatic fever* and/or *chorea*, **200,000** to **250,000 units** twice a day. The drug should be taken with a full glass of water on an empty stomach. *Intramuscular* or *intravenous, adults*, usually **1,000,000** to **5,000,000 units** every 4 to 6 hr; *neonates* and *premature infants*, usually **30,000 units/kg** of body weight every 12 hr, except 500,000 to 1,000,000 units/day for neonates with *Listeria infections; older infants* and *children*, usually **4167** to **16,667 units/kg** of body weight every 4 hr, or **6250** to **25,000 units/kg** every 6 hr, except up to 400,000 units/kg/day for life-threatening infections. Intravenous infusion, adults, for actinomycosis, fusospirochetosis, rat-bite fever, erysipeloid endocarditis, gonorrheal endocarditis and arthritis, and *Pasteurella* bacteremia and meningitis, **10,000,000** to **20,000,000 units/day;** for clostridial infections, **20,000,000 units/day;** for *Listeria* endocarditis and meningitis, **15,000,000** to **20,000,000 units/day;** for meningococcal meningitis, **20,000,000** to **30,000,000 units/day** or **1,000,000** to **2,000,000 units** every 2 hr. Such high daily doses or rapid intravenous injection of doses of 5,000,000 units or higher may occasionally cause convulsive seizures. A few doses are smaller than the above. Consult the package literature or USP XX for details of dosage in various infections.

Dosage Forms (penicillin G equivalent)—for Injection: 200,000, 500,000, 1,000,000, 5,000,000, 10,000,000, and 20,000,000 units; for Oral Solution: 200,000, 250,000, and 400,000 units/5 mL (reconstituted); Tablets for Oral Solution: 100,000, 200,000, and 250,000 units; Tablets: 200,000, 250,000, 400,000, 500,000, and 800,000 units.

Penicillin G Procaine

4-Thia-1-azabicyclo[3.2.0]heptane-2-carboxylic acid, 3,3-dimethyl-7-oxo-6-[(phenylacetyl)amino]-, [2S-(2α,5α,6β)]-, compd with 2-(diethylamino)ethyl 4-aminobenzoate (1:1) monohydrate
Various Mfrs

[6130-64-9] $C_{16}H_{18}N_2O_4S.C_{13}H_{20}N_2O_2.H_2O$ (588.72); *anhydrous* [54-35-3] (570.70). Potency: 900 to 1050 Penicillin Units/mg. One mg represents 1009 Penicillin G units.

Preparation—An aqueous solution of sodium (or potassium) penicillin G undergoes metathesis with an equimolar quantity of procaine hydrochloride.

Description—White, fine crystals or a white, very fine, microcrystalline powder; odorless or practically so, and not appreciably affected by air or light; pH (saturated solution) between 5.0 and 7.5; rapidly inactivated by acids and by alkali hydroxides, also by oxidizing agents.

Solubility—1 g in 250 mL water, about 30 mL alcohol, and about 60 mL chloroform.

Uses—Upon intramuscular injection procaine penicillin G slowly releases the penicillin G and provides prolonged duration of effective blood levels. An intramuscular dose of 300,000 units yields a peak plasma concentration of 1.5 units/mL at 1 to 3 hr, and the level is about 0.2 unit/mL at 24 hr and 0.05 unit/mL at 48 hr. Because of the relatively low peak blood levels, the drug is indicated only for mild to moderately severe infections by very susceptible organisms. For its uses and toxicity see the introductory statement in this section (page 1192). Allergies can occur due to the procaine component but other toxic effects of procaine are very rare. Intravenous injection will cause embolism.

Dose (penicillin G equivalent)—*Intramuscular, adults* and *children over 12 yr of age*, usually **600,000** to **1,200,000** units once a day, but up to 4,800,000 units a day may be given; for *diphtheria*, **300,000** to **600,000** units/day (with antitoxin); in *gonorrhea*, **4,800,000 units** in a single dose divided between 2 sites plus 1 g of probenecid is usually given; for *syphilis*, **600,000 units**/day for 8 days when early, secondary or latent or 10 to 15 days when tertiary or neurosyphilis; *infants* and *children up to 32 kg of weight*, for *congenital syphilis*, **50,000 units/kg** of body weight a day for 10 days; for some infections the pediatric dose may be as much as 100,000 units/kg of body weight a day. Consult the package literature for dosage for specific infections. For most mild to moderately severe infections, 600,000 to 1,200,000 units a day suffices. Severe infections should be treated with parenteral penicillin G potassium.

Dosage Forms (penicillin G equivalent)—Sterile Suspension: 300,000, 500,000, and 600,000 units/mL.

Penicillin G Sodium

4-Thia-1-azabicyclo[3.2.0]heptane-2-carboxylic acid, 3,3-dimethyl-7-oxo-6-[(phenylacetyl)amino]-, monosodium salt, [2S-(2α,5α,6β)]-, Benzylpenicillin Sodium

[69-57-8] $C_{16}H_{17}N_2NaO_4S$ (356.37). Penicillin G Sodium has a potency of not less than 1500 and not more than 1750 Penicillin Units per mg.

The structure is analogous to that for *Penicillin G Potassium*.

Description—Colorless or white crystals, or as a white to slightly yellow, crystalline powder; odorless or practically so, and is moderately hygroscopic; relatively stable in air, but is inactivated by prolonged heating at about 100°, especially in the presence of moisture; solutions lose potency fairly rapidly at room temperature, but retain substantially full potency for several days at temperatures below 15°; solutions are rapidly inactivated by acids, alkali hydroxides, oxidizing agents, and penicillinase.

Solubility—1 g in 40 mL water.

Uses—See the uses of penicillins in the introductory statement in this section (page 1191). When massive doses of penicillin G sodium are used, a considerable sodium load is introduced, which expands the extracellular space and may cause edema in patients with heart failure. Massive doses can also cause hypokalemic alkalosis.

Dose (penicillin G equivalent)—*Intramuscular* and *intravenous*, identical to those of *Penicillin G Potassium* (1 mg represents 1667 units).

Dosage Forms (penicillin G equivalent)—for Injection: 5,000,000 units; Sterile: 1,000,000 units. Each 1,000,000 units contains 1.69 mEq of sodium.

Penicillin V Potassium

4-Thia-1-azabicyclo[3.2.0]heptane-2-carboxylic acid, 3,3-dimethyl-7-oxo-6-[(phenoxyacetyl)amino]-, monopotassium salt, [2S-(2α,5α,6β)]-, Penicillin Potassium Phenoxymethyl; *Various Mfrs*

[132-98-9] $C_{16}H_{17}KN_2O_5S$ (388.48). Penicillin V Potassium has a potency of not less than 1380 and not more than 1610 Penicillin V units per mg.

Description—White, odorless, crystalline powder; pH (aqueous solution, 30 mg/mL) between 4 and 7.5; pK_a 2.73.
Solubility—Very soluble in water; 1 g in about 150 mL alcohol.

Uses—The antibacterial spectrum of penicillin V is essentially that of penicillin G, but penicillin V is less potent and effective. Consequently, it shares the same uses (see page 1192), except that in severe acute infections parenteral penicillin G is mandatory. Penicillin V is inactivated less by gastric juice than is penicillin G. Thus it may be administered orally without the use of buffers. But it offers no therapeutic advantage over appropriate oral preparations of penicillin G and it is more expensive. Like penicillin G, it may cause allergic reactions, and it frequently shows cross-sensitivity to the other penicillins. However, allergic reactions are much less common with administration of oral penicillin than with intramuscular forms. Its other toxicities are also those of penicillin G. The bioavailability varies and is about 60% at best (from solutions). Bioavailability not only varies from preparation to preparation and product to product but also from patient to patient. Consequently, plasma levels are unpredictable. A dose of 1,000,000 units of the acid gives peak plasma levels of about 2 to 3 µg/mL, but the potassium salt will provide levels of 4.5 to 9 µg/mL. Food interferes with absorption. Penicillin V is 75 to 80% bound to plasma proteins. The volume of distribution is 0.73 mL/g, which is considerably larger than that of penicillin G. Only 20 to 40% is excreted unchanged in the urine. The half-life is 0.5 to 0.6 hr.

Dose (penicillin V equivalent)—*Oral, adults* and *children 12 yr of age or older*, usually **125 to 500 mg** (200,000 to 800,000 units) every 6 to 8 hr, except **125 to 250 units** every 12 hr for prophylaxis of rheumatic fever. Up to 7.2 g (11,520,000 units) a day may be given. *Children under 12 yr*, **15 to 50 mg** (25,000 to 90,000 units)/kg/day in 3 to 6 equally divided and equally spaced doses.

Dosage Forms (penicillin V equivalent)—for Oral Solution: 125 and 250 mg/5 mL (reconstituted); Tablets: 125, 250, and 500 mg.

Piperacillin Sodium

4-Thia-1-azabicyclo[3.2.0]heptane-2-carboxylic acid, 6-[[[[(4-ethyl-2,3-dioxo-1-piperazinyl)carbonyl]amino]phenylacetyl]amino]-3,3-dimethyl-7-oxo-, [2S-[2α,5α,6β(S*)]]-, monosodium salt; Pipracil (*Lederle*)

[59703-84-3] $C_{23}H_{26}N_5NaO_7S$ (539.54).
Preparation—See US Pat 4,087,424.

Description—White crystals melting about 185°.
Solubility—1 g in about 1.5 mL water or methanol; 5 mL of ethyl alcohol.

Uses—Piperacillin is a fourth-generation penicillin with antibacterial activities characteristic of its class (see general statement). It is the most active penicillin against *Ps aeruginosa*, with a potency nearly that of gentamicin. It is more potent against *Klebsiella* and several other enteric bacilli than is carbenicillin or ticarcillin. It has a low efficacy against penicillinase- and other β-lactamase-producing bacteria. Resistance can develop rapidly to piperacillin during use, so that it should be administered only in combination with an aminoglycoside when used against *Ps aeruginosa* and other hard-to-suppress bacilli. Present authoritative medical opinion holds that piperacillin should be reserved for use against various pseudomonal and severe enteric bacillary infections. Although piperacillin is approved for use in gonorrhea, penicillin G is a superior choice. Piperacillin causes no unique adverse effects. It is expensive.

The oral bioavailability of oral piperacillin is too low and erratic to be of use. In plasma, 16 to 22% is protein-bound. The volume of distribution is about 0.2 mL/g. Renal excretion accounts for 60 to 80% of elimination. The half-life is 0.6 to 1.2 hr, except longer in renal failure.

Dose (piperacillin equivalent)—*Intramuscular, adults,* for *gonorrhea*, **2 g** as a single dose (after 1 g of probenecid. *Intramuscular* or *intravenous, uncomplicated urinary tract infections*, **1.5 to 2 g** (or **25 to 31.3 mg/kg**) every 6 hr or 3 to 4 g every 4 to 6 hr. *Intravenous infusion adults,* for *gynecological, intra-abdominal, skin,* and *soft-tissue infections*, hospital-acquired *pneumonia*, and *septicemia*, **2 to 3 g** (or **33.3 to 50 mg/kg**) every 4 hr or 3 to 4 g (or 50 to 75, mg/kg) every 6 hr; for *complicated urinary tract infections*, **3 to 4 g** or **31.25 to 50 mg/kg**, every 6 to 8 hr or **41.7 to 66.7 mg/kg** every 8 hr. Dosage adjustments are required in renal failure.

Dosage Forms (piperacillin equivalent)—Powder for Injection: 2, 3, and 4 g. Each g contains 1.85 mEq of sodium.

Ticarcillin Disodium

4-Thia-1-azabicyclo[3.2.0]heptane-2-carboxylic acid, 6-[(carboxy-3-thienylacetyl)amino]-3,3-dimethyl-7-oxo-, disodium salt, [2S-[2α,5α,6β(S*)]]-, Ticar (*Beecham*)

[4697-14-7] $C_{15}H_{14}N_2Na_2O_6S_2$ (428.38). Potency: equivalent to not less than 800 µg of ticarcillin ($C_{15}H_{16}N_2O_6S_2$)/mg, calculated on the anhydrous basis.

Description—White to pale yellow powder; hygroscopic.
Solubility—Very soluble in water.

Uses—Ticarcillin is a third-generation penicillin almost identical to carbenicillin in its antibacterial spectrum and potency, except that it is twice as active against *Ps aeruginosa*. However, resistance to carbenicillin automatically confers resistance to ticarcillin and *vice versa*. Resistance develops rapidly. The drug is usually combined with gentamicin or tobramycin to enhance activity and delay resistance. With carbenicillin it shares drug of first-choice status for the treatment of urinary tract infections caused by *Ps aeruginosa*, and in combination with gentamicin or tobramycin first-choice status in the treatment of all other infections caused by the bacterium.

The adverse effects are those of penicillins in general (see introductory statement in this section), and cross-sensitivity to penicillin occurs. Sodium overload and hypokalemia can occur, especially with high doses. In renal failure, high doses may inhibit platelet aggregation, and hemorrhagic phenomena may result. Ticarcillin is expensive, but less so than carbenicillin.

Ticarcillin is not absorbed orally. An intravenous dose of 3 g provides a serum concentration of 260 µg/mL. In plasma, 55 to 65% is protein-bound. The volume of distribution is 0.22 mL/g. It is 60 to 70% eliminated by renal excretion. The half-life is 1.2 hr, except longer in renal failure.

Dose (ticarcillin equivalent)—*Intramuscular* or *intravenous, adults* and *children 40 kg in weight or more*, for *uncomplicated urinary tract infections*, **1 g** every 4 to 6 hr; *children up to 40 kg* in weight, for *uncomplicated urinary tract infections*, **12.5** to **25 mg/kg** every 6 hr *or* **16.7** to **33.3 mg/kg** every 8 hr; *neonates*, for *intra-abdominal, female pelvic* and *genital tract, respiratory* tract, *skin*, and *soft-tissue* infections and *septicemia, initially* **100 mg/kg** followed by **75 mg/kg** every 4 to 6 hr for neonates over 2 kg in weight and every 8 hr for those under 2 kg for the first two weeks of life then **100 mg/kg** every 4 hr thereafter. *Intravenous infusion, adults* and *children over 40 kg*, for *intra-abdominal, female pelvic* and *genital tract, respiratory tract, skin and soft-tissue* infections, and *septicemia*, **25** to **37.5 mg/kg** every 3 hr, **33.3** to **50 mg/kg** every 4 hr, or **50** to **75 mg/kg** every 6 hr; for complicated urinary tract infections, **25** to **33.3 mg/kg** every 4 hr or **37.5** to **50 mg/kg** every 6 hr; *infants* and *children up to 40 kg*, for *intra-abdominal, female pelvic* and *genital tract, respiratory tract, skin* and *soft-tissue* infections and *septicemia*, **33.3** to **50 mg/kg** every 4 hr or **50** to **75 mg/kg** every 6 hr; for *complicated urinary tract* infections, **25** to **33.3 mg/kg** every 4 hr or **37.5** to **50 mg/kg** every 6 hr.

Dosage Forms (ticarcillin equivalent)—Sterile: 1, 3, 6, and 20 g.

Other Penicillins

Azlocillin Sodium [Sodium (2*S*,5*R*,6*R*)-3,3-Dimethyl-7-oxo-6-[(*R*)-2-(2-oxo-1-imidazolidinecarboxamido)-2-phenylacetamido]-4-thia-1-azabicyclo[3.2.0]heptane-2-carboxylate [*CAS-37091-66-0.*] $C_{20}H_{22}N_5NaO_6S$ (483.48); Azlin (*Miles*).] *Preparation: Eur J Med Chim Ther 17:* 59, 1982. *Description and solubility:* White to off-white powder soluble in water, methanol or DMF; slightly soluble in alcohol. *Uses:* Azlocillin is a ureido penicillin that does not fit into the usual classes of penicillins. It is active against most gram-positive cocci (including *Str faecalis*) except for penicillinase producers and anaerobes such as *B fragilis, Clostridia, Peptococcus, Peptostretococcus,* and *Fusobacterium.* Among the gram-negative enterobacteria it is active against *E coli, Enterobacter, Citrobacter*, indole-positive and indole-negative *Proteus, Shigella* and some strains of *Acinetobacter, Klebsiella, Salmonella,* and *Serratia;* against these enterobacteria it is less active than mezlocillin or piperacillin. It is more active against *Ps aeruginosa* than is carbenicillin, mezlocillin, or ticarcillin but slightly less active than is piperacillin. It is active against *H influenzae* and *Neisseria.* It probably does not offer any advantages over other penicillins. It is approved for use against respiratory tract infections caused by *E coli, H influenzae, Pr mirabilis, Strep faecalis,* and *Ps aeruginosa* and skin and soft-tissue, bone and joint infections, and septicemia caused by *Ps aeruginosa.* Against systemic pseudomonal infections, it should always be combined with an aminoglycoside. Except for a low sodium content, azlocillin probably does not offer any advantages over other older appropriate penicillins. The adverse effects are those of penicillins (page 1193). However, it has been reported that 40% of patients with cystic fibrosis develop a serum sickness-like syndrome. It also has antiplatelet activity. The acquisition cost is currently about $120 a day. Oral bioavailability is low. In plasma, about 40% is protein-bound. The volume of distribution is 0.2 mL/g. About 65% is eliminated by renal excretion, with a half-life of about 1 hr, except longer in renal failure. *Dose* (azlocillin equivalent): *Intravenous, adults*, for *uncomplicated urinary tract infections*, 25 to 31.3 mg/kg or 2 g every 6 hr; for *complicated urinary tract infections*, 37.5 to 50 mg/kg or 3 g every 6 hr; for *systemic infections*, 33.3 to 50 mg/kg or 3 g every 4 hr *or* 50 to 75 mg/kg or 4 g every 6 hr. *Children*, for *acute plumonary* complications of cystic fibrosis, 75 mg/kg every 4 hr. Dosage adjustments are required in renal failure.

Bacampicillin Hydrochloride [(2*S*,5*R*,6*R*)-6-[(*R*)-(2-Amino-2-phenylacetamido)]-3,3-dimethyl-7-oxo-4-thia-1-azabicyclo[3.2.0]heptane-2-carboxylic acid ester with ethyl 1-hydroxyethyl carbonate, monohydrochloride [*CAS-37661-08-8*] $C_{21}H_{27}N_3O_7S.HCl$ (501.98); Spectrobid; Ambaxin (*Upjohn, UK*).]—*Preparation:* See US Pat 3,939,270. *Description and solubility:* White crystals melting about 175°. Soluble 1 g in about 15 mL of water, 7 mL of alcohol, or 10 mL of chloroform. *Uses:* Bacampacillin is converted in the body to ampicillin, so that its antibacterial efficacy, uses, and adverse effects are those of ampicillin (page 1192). By the oral route, it is almost 100% absorbed, so that an oral dose equal (mole for mole) to that of ampicillin or amoxicillin will yield a plasma concentration of ampicillin nearly 200% higher than will ampicillin itself and about 30% higher than that of amoxicillin. After 4 hr there are no significant differences in levels. The drug is administered in a "pulsed" (twice-a-day) dosing regiman (plasma levels return nearly to zero between doses). In such a regimen, bacampicillin has an efficacy equal to that of ampicillin or amoxicillin at 6- or 8-hr intervals; it has not been shown whether ampicillin or amoxicillin in pulsed regimens would not also be equally efficacious, especially if doses were used to achieve equivalent plasma levels. The greater bioavailability results in a lower incidence of diarrhea. Bacampicillin costs two to four times as much as a molar equivalent dose of ampicillin and more than twice as much as a bioequivalent dose; it is 2 to 3 times as expensive as a bioequivalent dose of amoxicillin. Medical authority does not hold bacampicillin to offer any advantages over amoxicillin. Other than the differences in absorption and systemic bioavailability, the pharmacokinetics should be that of ampicillin. However, there are reported differences that require confirmation. *Dose: Oral, adults*, for *lower respiratory tract infections*, 560 mg every 12 hr; for *skin, soft-tissue* and *upper respiratory tract infections*, 280 to 560 mg every 12 hr; for *uncomplicated gonorrhea*, 1.12 g (and 1 g of probenecid) as a single dose; *infants* and *children* weighing *up to 25 kg*, for *lower respiratory tract* infections, 17.5 mg/kg every 12 hr; for *skin, soft-tissue*, and *upper respiratory tract infections*, 8.8 to 17.5 mg/kg every 12 hr. Dosage adjustments are required in renal failure.

Clavulanic Acid [(*Z*)-(2*R*,5*R*)-3-(2-Hydroxyethylidene)-7-oxo-4-oxa-1-azabicyclo[3.2.0]heptane-2-carboxylic acid [58001-44-8] $C_8H_9NO_5$ (199.16).]—In combination with amoxicillin marketed as Augmentin (*Beecham*-UK). *Uses:* Although clavulanic acid is not a penicillin, it is placed here because of its close relationship to the penicillins. It is a β-lactam that inhibits β-lactamases. The plasmid-mediated β-lactamases (penicillinases) are inhibited more strongly than are the chromosomally mediated β-lactamases, so that penicillins are preserved better than cephalosporins. In combination with a penicillinase-susceptible penicillin, clavulanic acid considerably increases the effectiveness of such a penicillin against penicillinase-producing gram-positive and gram-negative bacteria, including *Enterobacteriaceae, Hemophilus*, and *Neisseria.* Enhanced efficacy against urinary tract infections has particularly been noted in clinical trials. The activity of antipseudomal penicillins against *Pseudomonas* is not affected. Side effects occur in 6 to 14% of recipients. They include nausea (6%), diarrhea (4%), vomiting (1.5%) and rashes (1.5%). *Dose:* A combination of 125 mg of clavulanic acid (as the potassium salt) with 250 mg of amoxicillin, three times a day; with severe infection the dose may be increased.

Cyclacillin [6-(1-Aminocyclohexanecarboxamido)-3,3-dimethyl-7-oxo-4-thia-1-azabicyclo[3.2.0]heptane-2-carboxylic acid [3485-14-1] $C_{15}H_{23}N_3O_4S$ (341.43); Cyclapen-W (*Wyeth*)]—White, crystalline powder; 1 g dissolves in about 35 mL of water (at 38°). A second-generation penicillin (*see* general statement) with less *in vitro* activity than other antibiotics of the ampicillin class but being efficacious for treatment of the following infections when caused by organisms demonstrated to be susceptible to the action of cyclacillin: Tonsillitis and pharyngitis caused by Group A beta-hemolytic streptococci; bronchitis and pneumonia caused by *S pneumoniae;* otitis media caused by *S pneumoniae* and *H influenzae;* acute exacerbation of chronic bronchitis caused by *H influenzae;* skin and soft-tissue infections caused by Group A beta-hemolytic streptococci and staphylococci, non-penicillinase producers; urinary tract infections caused by *E coli* and *P mirabilis.* Cyclacillin should not be used in any infections caused by *E coli* and *P mirabilis* other than those of the urinary tract. Possible adverse effects include allergic reactions typical of penicillins; diarrhea, nausea and vomiting, skin rash, and isolated instances of headache, dizziness, abdominal pain, vaginitis, and urticaria have been reported. *Dose: Oral, adults*, 250 to 500 mg every 6 hr, depending on the infection and its severity; *infants over 2 mo of age* and *children up to 20 kg*, for *otitis media*, 16.7 to 33.3 mg/kg every 8 hr; *respiratory tract infections, tonsillitis*, and *pharyngitis*, 125 mg every 8 hr; *children over 20 kg*, for *respiratory tract infections, tonsillitis* and *pharyngitis*, 250 mg every 8 hr; *infants* and *children, other infections* 12.5 to 25 mg/kg every 6 hr.

Hetacillin [6-(2,2-Dimethyl-5-oxo-4-phenyl-1-imidazolidinyl)-3,3-dimethyl-7-oxo-4-thia-1-azabicyclo[3.2.0]heptane-2-carboxylic acid [3511-16-8] $C_{19}H_{23}N_3O_4S$ (389.47); Versapen (*Bristol*)]—Prepared by acylation of 6-aminopenicillanic acid with D-(−)-phenylglycyl chloride and condensing the product with acetone. White, crystalline powder; practically insoluble in water. *Uses:* In the body hetacillin is rapidly converted to ampicillin, so that its actions, uses, and adverse effects are those of *Ampicillin.* In the acid form, hetacillin is administered only orally and its uses are thus limited to mild to moderate, uncomplicated infections. A dose of 500 mg will yield a peak plasma concentration of 3 to 4 μg/mL, which is only 10% higher than that achieved by an equal dose of ampicillin. *Dose* (ampicillin equivalent): *Oral, adults*, and *children weighing more than 40 kg*, usually 225 to 450 mg every 6 hr, but as much as 3.6 g a day may be given; *infants* and *children under 40 kg*, 5.6 to 11.3 mg/kg every 6 hr.

Hetacillin Potassium [Potassium salt of *Hetacillin* [5321-32-4] $C_{19}H_{22}KN_3O_4S$ (427.56); Versapen-K (*Bristol*)]—White to light-buff, crystalline powder; freely soluble in water. *Uses:* See *Hetacillin* (above). *Dose:* Identical to that of *Hetacillin.*

Methicillin Sodium [Monosodium 6-(2,6-dimethoxybenzamido)-3,3-dimethyl-7-oxo-4-thia-1-azabicyclo[3.2.0]heptane-2-carboxylate monohydrate [7246-14-2] $C_{17}H_{19}N_2NaO_6S.H_2O$ (420.41); *anhydrous* [132-92-3] (402.40), Potency: not less than 815 μg of methicillin ($C_{17}H_{20}N_2O_6S$)/mg Staphcillin (*Bristol*); Celbenin (*Beecham*).]—*Preparation:* Fermentation-produced 6-aminopenicillanic acid is condensed with 2,6-dimethoxybenzoyl chloride in a suitable organic solvent and the resulting methicillin is precipitated as the sodium salt by the addition of sodium acetate. *Description and solubility:* Fine, white, crystalline powder, odorless or having a slight odor. Freely soluble in water; slightly soluble in chloroform; insoluble in ether. *Uses:* Methicillin is a first-generation penicillinase-resistant penicillin. It is about 1/20 as potent as penicillin G against non-penicillinase-producing but 10 times as potent as penicillinase-producing gram-positive cocci. Its use is limited to treatment of infections caused by penicillinase-producing cocci. Methicillin is destroyed by gastric acid and must be given parenterally. About 40% is bound to plasma proteins. The volume of distribution is 0.31 mL/g. Approximately 67% is eliminated by renal tubular secretion; the half-life is about 1.1 hr. There is more pain after its intramuscular injection than after similar injections of other penicillins. Methicillin can cause the well-known allergic reactions typical of all penicillins. However, many patients allergic to penicillin G are not sensitive to methicillin, but the drug should be used cautiously if penicillin-sensitivity exists. Methicillin sodium occasionally causes depression of red bone marrow functions resulting in anemia, neutropenia, or granulocytopenia. These symptoms are reversible after prompt termination of therapy. Allergic hemolytic anemia also can occur. Allergic nephropathy has been reported. When used in persons with low sodium tolerance the sodium content must be taken into account. Because of the side-effects, need for frequent injections, and lower potency than nafcillin, methicillin is not the antistaphylococcal penicillin of choice. *Dose:* (methicillin equivalent)—*Intramuscular, adults, usually* 1 g every 4 to 6 hr; *infants* and *children,* 25 mg/kg every 6 hr. *Intravenous, adults, usually* 1 to 2 g every 4 hr, but in severe infections the dose can be increased to as much as 24 g/day; *infants* and *children,* 16.7 to 33.3 mg/kg every 4 hr *or* 25 to 50 mg/kg every 6 hr, but in severe infections the dose may be as high as 300 mg/kg/day.

Investigational and Foreign Penicillins—*Carindacillin* and *carfecillin* are esters that yield carbenicillin on hydrolysis in the body. Their properties and potential uses closely resemble those of carbenicillin indanyl sodium; however, they do not pass as much unchanged carbenicillin into urine. *Epicillin* closely resembles ampicillin in structure, antibacterial activity, adverse effects, absorption, distribution, and elimination and, consequently, in therapeutic efficacy and dose. Only in the treatment of *E coli* has a difference been reported, epicillin being superior. *Floxacillin* (Flucloxacillin) is very similar to dicloxacillin in properties and uses. *Amdinocillin* (Mecillinam) has activity against many β-lactamase-producing enterobacteria, such as *Klebsiella, Proteus,* and *E coli,* and its discovery represents a step forward in the development of improved broad-spectrum penicillins. It is poorly absorbed by the oral route but two esters, *bacmecillinam* and *Amdinocillin Pivoxil* (Pivmecillinam) are orally effective. They are especially useful in combination with amoxicillin, their primary beneficial actions appearing to be that of inhibiting β-lactamase and thus preserving amoxicillin. *Pirbenicillin* has a broad spectrum of antibacterial activity much like that of carbenicillin, but it is 3 to 4 times as potent against *Ps aeruginosa,* against which it is especially indicated. *Pivampicillin,* like bacampicillin, is an ester which is hydrolyzed to ampicillin during intestinal absorption. By the oral route it yields plasma concentrations of ampicillin 2 to 3 times those from unesterified ampicillin, which gives the ester a distinct advantage in efficacy by the oral route. *Sulbenicillin* has an antibacterial spectrum of activity and potency very close to those of carbenicillin. Like carbenicillin, it is not absorbed orally. Its chief distinction is that renal failure affects its half-life (1 hr) considerably less than that of carbenicillin. *Talampicillin* is also an ester that is hydrolyzed to ampicillin in the body.

Polypeptides

The polypeptides differ from each other in their mechanism of action and antibacterial spectrum, and grouping them together is only an organizational convenience. Only colistin and polymyxin B have close chemical and antibacterial relatedness.

Bacitracin

Ayfivin; Penitracin; Topitracin; Zutracin

Bacitracin [1405-87-4]; polypeptide produced by the growth of the *licheniformis* group of *Bacillus subtilis* (Fam *Bacillaceae*). It has a potency of not less than 40 USP Units* of bacitracin/mg. Sterile bacitracin has a potency of not less than 50 Units/mg.

Bacitracin is a mixture of at least nine polypeptides, principally bacitracin A, $C_{66}H_{103}N_{17}O_{16}S$ (1411). The structure of bacitracin A has been shown to be

---

* The USP Unit of Bacitracin is the bacitracin activity exhibited by the weight of USP Bacitracin Reference Standard indicated on the label of the Standard. The USP unit and that defined by the FDA are equivalent.

in which the detailed structure at the upper right represents a cyclic condensation moiety derived from cysteine and isoleucine.

Preparation—Several methods for isolation and purification of this antibiotic have been published. For details of certain of these multi-step procedures see US Pats 2,498,165, 2,828,246, and 2,915,432.

Description—White to pale buff powder, odorless, or has a slight odor; hygroscopic; solutions rapidly deteriorate at room temperature; precipitated from its solutions and is inactivated by salts of many of the heavy metals; solutions retain their potency for several weeks if kept in a refrigerator.

Solubility—Freely soluble in water; soluble in alcohol; insoluble in chloroform, and ether.

Uses—Bacitracin is effective mainly against gram-positive bacteria. It is largely limited in its use to infections which can be treated by topical application or local infiltration. The high incidence of nephrotoxicity (albuminuria, cylindruria, azotemia, accumulation of drug) which follows its parenteral administration precludes systemic use except in life-endangering staphylococcal infections in which other antibiotics have proved to be ineffective.

Bacitracin is employed in *surgical infections* caused by pathogens sensitive to the antibiotic; these infections include carbuncles, felons, superficial and deep abscesses, infected traumatic and operative wounds, infected ulcers, and chronic osteomyelitis.

Bacitracin is effective topically in the treatment of the following *cutaneous bacterial infections* where the pathogen is bacitracin-sensitive: Impetigo contagiosa, folliculitis, pyoderma, ecthyma, furunculosis, decubitus ulcer, infectious eczematoid dermatitis, scabies, and dermatophytosis. The drug is used in the treatment of *ophthalmological conditions* including styes, acute and chronic conjunctivitis, corneal ulcer, keratitis, and dacryocystitis. *Infections of the ear, mouth, and nasopharynx* such as Vincent's angina, pharyngitis, chronic suppurative otitis media, and mastoiditis have been successfully treated with bacitracin. The zinc salt is often preferred for topical therapy and is the form most often incorporated into combinations. It is usually combined with neomycin and polymyxin B sulfate.

Development of bacterial resistance is much less frequent and slower for bacitracin than for penicillin, and for most organisms is essentially nil. The drug is not inactivated by the metabolic products of mixed infections.

In addition to renal damage, toxic effects of parenteral bacitracin include pain, induration and petechiae at the site of injection, skin rash, malaise, anorexia, nausea, and vomiting. In a few instances tinnitus and a peculiar taste may be noted. Topical application is usually not irritating and rarely induces allergic reactions.

Bacitracin is not effective by the oral route. Systemically, the half-life of bacitracin is about 1.5 hr. Approximately 30% is excreted into the urine unchanged.

Dose—*Intramuscular, infants less than 2.5 kg in weight,* **900 units/kg** of body weight per day in 2 or 3 divided doses; *infants more than 2.5 kg, up to 1 yr of age,* **1000 units/kg** in 2 or 3 divided doses. *Topical,* to the *conjunctiva,* a thin strip (about 1 cm) of ointment containing 500 units/g every 3 hr or more frequently; to the skin, ointment containing 500 units/g 2 or 3 times a day. Procaine, 2%, in isotonic sodium chloride solution may be used as a diluent for solutions injected intramuscularly, using a quantity sufficient to provide a concentration of 10,000 units/mL. Procaine should not be used in bacitracin solutions injected into cerebral tissue or into spinal fluid.

Dosage Forms—Ointment: 500 units/g; There is no single entity ophthalmic dosage form for bacitracin; combinations contain 400 or 500 units/g; Sterile: 50,000 units.

Bacitracin Zinc

Bacitracins, zinc complex

Zinc bacitracin [1405-89-6]; the zinc salt of a kind of bacitracin or a mixture of two or more such salts. Potency: not less than 40 Units of bacitracin activity/mg.

Description—White to pale tan powder; odorless or has a slight odor; hygroscopic.
Solubility—Sparingly soluble in water.

Uses—Bacitracin zinc is incorporated into various ointments used for topical antibiotic therapy (see *Bacitracin*). It is more stable than bacitracin, and the zinc may enhance the activity of the antibiotic. The astringent properties of zinc may reduce inflammation. It is frequently combined with polymyxin B and/or neomycin.

Dose—*Topical*, as ointment containing 500 units/g 2 or 3 times a day.

Dosage Forms (bacitracin equivalent)—In combination with other antibacterial drugs and/or steroids, 89 units/g in an aerosol, 400 and 500 units/g in ointments, and 400 units/g in a powder.

Polymyxin B Sulfate

Polymyxin B, sulfate; Aerosporin (*Burroughs-Wellcome*);
Various Mfrs

Polymyxin B sulfate [1405-20-5]; the sulfate salt of a substance produced by the growth of *Bacillus polymyxa* (Prazmowski) Migula (Fam *Bacillaceae*). It has a potency of not less than 6000 Units of polymyxin B/mg, calculated on the anhydrous basis.

Preparation—The filtered broth from the fermentation step (see page 1178) is treated with a certified dye and the polymyxin B–dye salt complex thus precipitated is collected by filtration, washed with water, and treated with an alcoholic solution of a lower aliphatic amine sulfate. The polymyxin B sulfate thus formed is filtered off, purified, and lyophilized.

There are several polymyxins each of which is an *N*-monoacylated decapeptide with seven of the amino acid residues in cyclic union. Polymyxin B is a mixture of polymyxin B_1 ($C_{56}H_{98}N_{16}O_{13}$) and polymyxin B_2 ($C_{55}H_{96}N_{16}O_{13}$) the only difference being in the composition of the *N*-acyl group:

$$
\begin{array}{c}
\text{O} \\
\parallel \\
\text{Dbu-Thr-Dbu-C-R} \\
\end{array}
$$

Dbu·Dbu·Thr·Dbu·Dbu·DPhe·Leu

(Dbu = 2,4-diaminobutyric acid)
Polymyxin B_1 R = (+)-5-methylheptyl
Polymyxin B_2 R = 5-methylhexyl

The close relationship between these polymyxins and the colistins (see preceding article) is readily apparent.

Description—White to buff-colored powder; odorless or has a faint odor; solutions are slightly acid or are neutral to litmus, having a pH of 5.0 to 7.5; pK_a 8 to 9.

Solubility—Freely soluble in water; slightly soluble in alcohol.

Uses—Its *in vitro* and *in vivo* antimicrobial spectrum of activity is restricted to gram-negative bacteria, including *Aerobacter*, *Escherichia*, *Hemophilus*, *Klebsiella*, *Pasteurella*, *Pseudomonas*, *Salmonella*, *Shigella*, and most *Vibrio*; all strains of *Proteus* and most of *Serratio marcescens* are unaffected by the antibiotic. Some strains of *Neisseria* and *Brucella* are also resistant. All gram-positive bacteria are resistant. Bacteria initially sensitive to the antibiotic rarely acquire resistance to it.

Systemic polymyxin B is indicated only when other drugs cannot be employed. It is used to treat *meningitis* caused by *Ps aeruginosa* and *H influenzae*, *septicemia* caused by *Ps aeruginosa Enterobacter aerogenes*, and *K pneumoniae*, serious *urinary tract* infections caused by *Ps aeruginosa*, and other pseudomonal infections. In meningitis, it must be given intrathecally. In systemic therapy it is as effective and no more toxic as colistimethate, despite popular belief to the contrary. The drug is also used topically for the treatment or the prevention and treatment of *external ocular infections* caused by susceptible microorganisms, especially *Ps aeruginosa*. In topical therapy, it is often combined with neomycin, gramicidin, and bacitracin. It is also included in glucocorticoid ophthalmologic topical preparations.

Polymyxin is readily absorbed when injected subcutaneously or intramuscularly. Peak levels are attained within 30 min to 2 hours after injection; the plasma half-life is about 6 hours, but it varies considerably. When the half-life is appreciably longer, the usual doses are cumulative and may lead to toxicity. The drug does not gain access to the cerebrospinal fluid. Gastrointestinal absorption is slow and negligible. The antibiotic is excreted by the kidney; a total of 60% of the administered drug can be recovered from the urine. In renal failure the half-life is longer, and the dose needs to be diminished.

Polymyxin B sulfate, when given parenterally, can adversely affect the nervous system and the kidney, especially if the total daily dose

exceeds 3 mg (30,000 units)/kg. Neurological disturbances are usually subjective and include dizziness, mild weakness, and paresthesias of the mouth, face, and the extremities. Symptoms are rarely severe when recommended doses are employed; but larger amounts have caused incoordination, ataxia, dysarthria, and dyssynergia. Nephrotoxic effects, with damage to the kidney glomerular and tubular epithelium, are manifested by albumin, red blood cells, leukocytes, and, occasionally, granular casts in the urine; in severe cases, oliguria and elevated level of serum nonprotein nitrogen are noted. Toxic effects usually clear within 4 days after the last dose of the drug. Substances such as soap, which antagonize cationic surface-active agents, impair the action of the antibiotic.

Dose—*Intramuscular*, *adults* and *children*, **2.5** to **3 mg/kg** of body weight a day in 4 to 6 equally divided doses; *infants* can be given **4 mg/kg** a day without adverse effects, and *neonates* and *premature infants* have been given **4.5 mg/kg/day** in serious infections caused by *Ps aeruginosa*. The intramuscular route is not recommended because of pain at the site of injection. *Intravenous*, *adults* and *children*, **0.75** to **1.25 mg/kg** every 12 hr; infants with normal renal function may be given up to 4 mg/kg a day. It is imperative to adjust all systemic doses in renal insufficiency. *Topical*, to the *conjunctiva* as a thin strip (about 1 cm) of 0.05, or 0.1% ointment or 1 to 3 drops of 0.1 to 0.163% solution every hr. *Intrathecal*, the following doses are suggested: children under 2 yr of age, 2 mg daily for 3 or 4 days, then 2.5 mg every other day; children over 2 yr and adults, 5 mg daily for 3 or 4 days, then 5 mg every other day. The intrathecal solution should contain 3 to 5 mg in 1 mL of 0.9% sterile sodium chloride solution. (1 mg represents 10,000 units.)

Dosage Forms—Injection: 50 mg/20 mL; Ophthalmic Ointment: 0.5, and 1 mg/g; Ophthalmic Solution: 1 and 1.63 mg/mL; Ophthalmic Sterile: 50 mg, to be reconstituted to 20 to 50 mL. 1 mg equals 10,000 units.

Other Polypeptides

Capreomycin Sulfate—Capreomycin sulfate [1405-37-4], an antibiotic produced by *Streptomyces capreolus*, is a mixture of polypeptides, a structure for one of which has been proposed (*Nature 231*: 301, 1971). A white to slightly yellowish white, amorphous powder; essentially odorless; freely soluble in water. *Uses*: Possesses antibacterial activity, especially toward acid-fast bacilli, hence used in the treatment of *tuberculosis*. When it is used alone, resistance readily develops. It should be administered only in combination with other antitubercular drugs, such as isoniazid or ethambutol. Capreomycin is a fourth- or fifth-choice drug in tuberculotherapy. It should not be used unless bacteriological sensitivity tests demonstrate its potential usefulness and need. Although capreomycin is not chemically related to the aminoglycosides, cross-resistance to kanamycin occurs, and also to viomycin.

As with aminoglycosides, loss of hearing may develop with chronic use; the reported incidence is 11%. Hearing should be tested regularly. Also, as with kanamycin, renal toxicity may occur during treatment; such toxicity includes transient proteinuria, cylindruria, and azotemia. Severe renal failure attributable to the drug is rare. Other untoward effects include pain and sterile abscesses at the site of injection, tinnitus, hypokalemia, skin rashes, eosinophilia, leukocytosis, leukopenia, and partial neuromuscular blockade that can potentiate that of anesthetics and neuromuscular paralysants.

Capreomycin is not absorbed after oral administration, so that parenteral administration is required. The half-life is 3 to 6 hr, except longer in renal insufficiency. *Dose* (base equivalent): *Intramuscular*, 1 g/day (not to exceed 20 mg/kg/day) for 60 to 120 days, then 1 g 2 or 3 times a week for 18 to 24 months. It is always used in combination with other antitubercular drugs.

Colistimethate Sodium [Pentasodium colistinmethanesulfonate [21362-08-3; 8068-28-8] contains the pentasodium salt of the penta-(methanesulfonic acid) derivative of colistin A, $C_{58}H_{105}N_{16}Na_5O_{28}S_5$ (1749.81), as the major component, with a small proportion of the pentasodium salt of the same derivative of colistin B, $C_{57}H_{103}N_{16}Na_5O_{28}S_5$ (1735.78). Potency: the equivalent of not less than 390 μg of colistin base activity per mg Coly-Mycin M Injectable (*Warner-Chilcott*).]—*Preparation*: Purified colistin is treated with formaldehyde in aqueous solution, and the resulting colistin-formaldehyde complex (pentamethylolcolistin) is reacted with sodium bisulfite to generate the penta(methanesulfonate). *Description and solubility*: White to slightly yellow, odorless, fine powder. Freely soluble in water; insoluble in ether. *Dose*: Must generate colistin in the body to be effective. Since it is water-soluble, it is a suitable form of colistin for intramuscular injection. By the intravenous route, it has no advantage over polymyxin B sulfate. It has nearly the same antibacterial spectrum as polymyxin B against most gram-negative bacilli and it also elicits the same renal and neural toxic symptoms. The incidence of nephrotoxicity is about 20%. Like polymyxin B sulfate the drug is especially useful in the treatment of infections caused by *Pseudomonas* and *Serratia* spp. It may also be used to treat serious infections caused by *Ent aerogenes*, *Esch coli*, and *K pneumoniae*. It is used only when other drugs cannot be used. It is mainly eliminated by renal excretion. It has a plasma half-life of 1.6 to 2.7 hours, except that it may be 2 to 3 days in severe renal failure. Blood levels should be monitored in renal insufficiency. *Dose:* (colistin equivalent)—*Intramuscular, adults* and *children*, 1.25 mg/kg of body weight 2 to 4 times a day. In moderate renal insufficiency (creatinine clearance greater than 20 mL/min), 1.8 to 2.5 mg/kg every 12 hours; in severe renal failure (creatinine clearance 5 to 20 mL/min), 1.25 mg/kg every 12 hours; with negligible renal function (creatinine clearance less than 5 mL/min), 0.75 mg/kg every 12 to 18 hours.

Colistin Sulfate [Colistins sulfate [1264-72-8]; the sulfate salt of an antibacterial substance produced by the growth of *Bacillus polymyxa* var *colistinus*. It consists primarily of colistin A with small amounts of colistin B. Potency: not less than 500 µg of colistin/mg. The colistins are monoacylated decapeptides with seven of the amino acid residues in cyclic union. Colistin B [$C_{52}H_{98}N_{16}O_{13}$ = 1155.45] is a des-homolog of colistin A [$C_{53}H_{100}N_{16}O_{13}$ = 1169.47] Coly-Mycin S (*Warner-Chilcott*).] *Preparation:* Information concerning isolation of colistin from cultures of *Bacillus colistinus* (obtained from Japanese soil), synthesis of colistin A, structure of colistins, and probable identity of colistins and polymyxins E is available in reviews by Vogler and Studer (*Experientia 22:* 345, 1966) and in several articles in *Medicamenta 61* (509): 177–234, 1973. *Description and solubility:* White to slightly yellow, odorless, fine powder; solutions are more stable at an acid pH than at an alkaline pH; the dry powder is stable indefinitely. Freely soluble in water; insoluble in acetone or ether. *Uses:* The antibacterial spectrum of colistin is very similar to that of polymyxin B (page 1202), but colistin is usually less potent, except against *Klebsiella pneumoniae* and *Serratia marcescens*. Colistin is marketed only for oral administration in the treatment of intestinal infections. It is especially indicated in the treatment in children of acute enteritis caused by *Pseudomonas*, *Shigella*, and *E coli* refractory to other drugs. Resistance rarely occurs. It is also used topically in the treatment of some external ear infections. Colistin has the same toxicity as polymyxin B sulfate (below), but adverse effects by the oral route rarely occur, except in infants. Infants receiving colistin sulfate should be examined frequently for impairment of renal function. Colistin sulfate is not absorbed by the oral route except in infants, in whom significant blood levels can be obtained by this route of administration. The drug is excreted in the urine. The plasma half-life is about 1.6 to 2.7 hr but it may be 2 to 3 days in severe renal failure. *Dose:* (colistin equivalent)—*Oral*, 1.67 to 5 mg/kg 3 times a day; *topical*, to external ear, **0.2 mL** of a **0.3%** suspension, 3 times a day

Gramicidin—Gramicidin [1405-97-6] is an antibacterial substance produced by growth of *Bacillus brevis* Dubos (Fam *Bacillaceae*); it has a potency of not less than 900 µg of gramicidin/mg. It is a polypeptide antibiotic complex of four components—gramicidin A, B, C, and D— formerly believed to have cyclic structures but probably existing as chains of 15 amino acids in alternating D- and L-forms. A white, or nearly white, odorless, crystalline powder; insoluble in water, soluble in alcohol. *Uses:* Gramicidin is active against gram-positive organisms, except the gram-positive bacilli, and against certain gram-negative organisms, such as the *Neisseria*. It is bacteriostatic to some organisms, and bactericidal to others. It is effective only by topical application; not only is it ineffective systemically, but it is highly toxic. Serum and body fluids inhibit its activity. The antibiotic is useful in the local treatment of various infections of the eye. However, it is never used alone, but rather in combination with other substances, such as polymyxin B, neomycin, and nystatin. Ointments for ophthalmic use generally contain 0.0025%.

Tetracyclines

The tetracyclines are all very much alike with respect to their antimicrobial spectra and the untoward effects they elicit. They differ mainly in their absorption, duration of action, and suitability for parenteral administration.

Antimicrobial Actions—The tetracyclines are broad-spectrum antibiotics. They are mainly bacteriostatic. They bind to the bacterial 30s ribosomes and prevent t-RNA from combining with m-RNA. Thus protein synthesis is inhibited. The drugs have activities against both gram-positive and gram-negative bacteria, mycobacteria, *Mycoplasma*, treponemas, leptospira, rickettsia, actinomycetes, *Coxiella*, *Chlamydiae*, and plasmodia. Among the susceptible gram-positive bacteria are *Staph pyogenes*, *Staph epidermidis*, *Strep pyogenes*, *Strep viridans*, *Strep fecalis* (enterococcus), anaerobic streptococci, *D pneumoniae*, *E anthracis*, *Cl tetani*, *Cl perfringens*, and *Listeria monocytogenes*. Susceptible gram-negative bacteria include *Enterobacteriaceae* such as, *Esch coli*, *Salmonella*, *Shigella*, and *Klebsiella-Enterobacter Neisseria* (gonococci and meningococci), *H influenzae*, *B pertussis*, *Brucella*, *Pasteurella*, *Vibrio cholerae*, *Bacteroides* and *Pseudomonas*, *Serratia marcescens* and *Proteus* are

usually resistant. The acid-fast *Mycobacterium tuberculosis* is poorly susceptible. *Mycoplasma pneumoniae* and the T-strains are sensitive. The tetracyclines are second-choice drugs against Legionnaires' disease. They have variable efficacy in the treatment of infections caused by anaerobic bacteria (*Clostridium*, *Bacteroides*). The tetracyclines do not have a direct action against amebas, but they suppress amebic dysentery by altering the intestinal bacterial flora. Although resistance to the tetracyclines is not acquired as rapidly as to penicillin, it does, nevertheless, readily occur. Among the gram-positive bacteria, staphylococci become most easily resistant; in hospital populations the incidence of resistance among strains of *Staph aureus* may run from 30 to 50% but may increase to as high as 75% after several days of treatment. Various streptococci and pneumococci also become resistant. The incidence of resistance among various gram-negative bacteria is also very high, especially among the *Enterobacteriaceae*, which in the intestine can pass resistance-controlling genes from one species, even genus, to another (infectious drug resistance). Resistance to one tetracycline usually confers resistance to all others, except that some tetracycline-resistant strains of streptococci and *E coli* may retain sensitivity to minocycline. Cross-resistance between penicillin and tetracyclines or between other classes of antibiotics and tetracyclines is uncommon, except in infectious drug resistance, in which the acquired episome or plasmid contains more than one gene for resistance to other drugs.

Uses—A tetracycline alone is the *drug of choice* in the treatment of *cholera*, *relapsing fever* and infections caused by *rickettsia*, *Mycobacterium fortuitum* and *marinum*, and *Chlamydia psittaci* and *trachomatis* (except pneumonia and inclusion conjunctivitis). With other drugs it shares *first-choice* status for the treatment of *Mycoplasma pneumonia* (primary atypical pneumonia) and gonorrhea. A tetracycline is a component of (*first-choice combinations* for the treatment of *brucellosis* and *glanders*. It is a *second-choice* drug for the treatment of *actinomycosis*, *anthrax*, *chancroid*, *mellioidosis*, *plague*, *rat-bite fevers*, *syphilis*, *yaws*, and infections caused by *Cl tetani*, *Leptospira*, *Leptotrichia buccalis*, *Listeria*, and *Ureaplasma*. Tetracyclines may be used in the treatment of minor *staphylococcal infections*, but other drugs take precedence. However, in the treatment of acne, tetracyclines maintain a favored but challengeable status; if there is inflammation with pustules and cysts, an antibiotic may be indicated. In the treatment of *peritonitis*, tetracyclines may be of use, but the incidence of resistance is now quite high among the offending organisms, so that other drugs are usually preferred. When susceptible bacteria are causative, tetracyclines may be used to treat *biliary tract infections*. The tetracyclines are the drugs of choice in the antibacterial phase of treatment of *cholera*. In *urinary tract infections*, other drugs are usually preferred, unless sensitivity testing especially indicates tetracyclines. However, tetracyclines are usually the drugs of choice in *nongonococcal urethritis* and in *prostatitis* (often a mycoplasma). In urinary tract infections and urethritis, the urine should be acidified to favor antibacterial action. In the treatment of the meningococcal carrier state, minocycline, but not other tetracyclines, appears to be effective.

Chlortetracycline was once used as an antimalarial. There has been renewed interest in the usefulness of tetracycline in the treatment of falciparum malaria.

Adverse Effects—The tetracyclines cause a number of untoward effects. *Gastrointestinal toxicity* is common with oral use; it is probably the combined effect of local irritation and alteration of the intestinal flora. Manifestations are heartburn, epigastric distress, nausea, vomiting, diarrhea and rare esophageal ulceration in persons with esophageal obstruction or spastic disease. Claims that some tetracyclines cause less gastrointestinal distress have not yet been supported by objective clinical evidence, but it is probable that those that are used in the lower doses cause a lesser incidence of such effects. Some tetracyclines occasionally cause *antibiotic-associated* (peudomembranous) *colitis*.

The broad-spectrum antibacterial activity of the tetracyclines causes marked alterations in the floral ecology, so that microorganisms formerly held in check overgrow to cause *superinfections*. This occurs most frequently in the bowel but it may also occur readily in the mouth, lungs, and vagina and occasionally elsewhere. The most common superinfection is candidiasis, but overgrowth from staphylococci, enterococci, *Proteus*, *Pseudomonas*, or *Cl dificile* (cause of colitis) occurs. Staphylococcal enteric superinfections are frequently fatal. Staphylococcal enteritis is especially likely to happen to children. The usual effect of an overgrowth in the bowel is diarrhea. However, in debilitated patients or patients with very high numbers of monilia in the gut, the yeast can enter the blood stream and disseminate to various locations.

Various *hypersensitivity* reactions, especially urticaria, asthma, or facial edema, occur, but they are uncommon. *Phototoxicity* occurs, to a very high extent with demeclocycline but to a low extent with minocycline and other tetracyclines

Hepatotoxicity, which is sometimes fatal, occasionally results when the daily dose in adults exceeds 1 g/day, especially if the tetracycline is given intravenously; pregnancy and renal failure predispose to this toxicity. Tetracyclines may also increase the risk of hepatic damage by other hepatotoxic drugs.

Although tetracyclines probably do not affect normal kidney function, they *aggravate preexisting renal insufficiency*, which can lead to extreme azotemia, but without oliguria. Doxycycline appears to be free of this effect. Old preparations that have undergone decomposition on the shelf are serious offenders in causing nephrotoxicity. Tetracyclines also interact with diuretics to cause azotemia. They may promote nephrotoxicity caused by methoxyflurane. Minocycline can cause ototoxicity.

Tetracyclines *pigment developing teeth* and reversibly *impair bone growth* through complexation with the bone salts and fixation to matrix proteins. Whether tooth defects in fact result has not yet been unequivocally proven. The implication is that tetracyclines should be avoided in children under 6 years old, in whom the cosmetically important permanent teeth have not erupted. It should also be avoided in pregnancy.

A rare, reversible *cerebral toxicity* which causes a bulging fontanelle in infants and headache, irritability, vomiting, blurred vision, and papilledema in children and adults has been observed in tetracycline-treated patients. There are also rare ocular toxicities, such as transient myopia, diplopia, papilledema, and blurred vision.

Intravenous tetracyclines may cause *thrombophlebitis*, caused mainly by the acid required to effect solution. The soluble tetracyclines like rolitetracycline rarely cause this complication. Polyvinylpyrrolidone and phosphate in intravenous preparations lessen the irritant action. Because of the various dangers from intravenous tetracyclines (local, hepatic, and renal), administration by this route should be withheld unless the illness is so severe that the necessary dose cannot be tolerated by mouth, the patient is unable to take oral medication, or oral therapy is inadequate. Intramuscular injections cause local pain, unless a local anesthetic is included.

Absorption, Distribution, and Elimination—The extent of gastrointestinal absorption is 70 to 90%. Tetracyclines complex with bivalent and trivalent metal ions, so that their absorption is greatly impaired by calcium-, magnesium-, and

aluminum-containing antacids and by iron preparations. If possible, such drugs should be withheld during tetracycline therapy or at least not administered within 1 hour before or after the tetracycline. Food, especially milk products or other high calcium foods, also interferes with oral absorption of tetracyclines. Phosphate appears to improve absorption, in part by removing calcium.

Bioavailabilities (oral) of tetracyclines range from 30 to 95%. All tetracyclines are bound to plasma proteins, to an extent ranging from 35 to 91%. There is no correlation between protein binding and volume of distribution or half-life. Volumes of distribution range from 0.5 to 1.28 mL/g. Half-lives vary from 8 to 18 hr. Renal excretion is the principal mode of elimination, except that chlortetracycline is mostly excreted in the feces and doxycycline is more than 50% metabolized and/or excreted into the colon. The tetracyclines penetrate well into the tissues and body fluids, but penetration into the cerebrospinal fluid is low by the oral route, so that concentrations may be no more than $\frac{1}{50}$ to $\frac{1}{10}$ of those in the plasma; with intravenous administration, higher levels can be achieved. The tetracyclines are excreted into the bile and mostly resorbed in the intestine, but even intravenous doses are capable of altering the bowel flora.

Demeclocycline Hydrochloride

2-Naphthacenecarboxamide, 7-chloro-4-(dimethylamino)-
1,4,4a,5,5a,6,11,12a-octahydro-3,6,10,12,12a-pentahydroxy-1,11-dioxo-,
monohydrochloride, [4S-(4α,4aα,5aα,6β,12aα)]-, 7-Chloro-6-
demethyltetracycline Hydrochloride; Demethylchlortetracycline
Hydrochloride NF XII; DMCT; Ledermycin; Declomycin (*Lederle*)

Demeclocycline monohydrochloride [64-73-3] $C_{21}H_{21}ClN_2O_8 \cdot HCl$ (501.32). Potency: not less than 900 μg of $C_{21}H_{21}ClN_2O_8 \cdot HCl/mg$, calculated on the anhydrous basis.

Preparation—An appropriate mutant strain of *Streptomyces aureofaciens* is grown in an appropriate liquid nutrient medium under controlled conditions of temperature, pH, and aeration. The harvested broth is acidified and filtered, and the antibiotic is isolated from the filtrate, either by solvent extraction or by chemical precipitation, and converted into the hydrochloride.

Description—Yellow, crystalline powder; odorless and has a bitter taste; pH (1 in 100 solution) about 2.5.
Solubility—1 g in about 60 mL water and about 980 mL alcohol; sparingly soluble in solutions of alkali hydroxides and carbonates; practically insoluble in chloroform.

Uses—Has a spectrum of activity similar to other tetracyclines (see introductory statement in this section). Its potency *in vitro* against most of the organisms susceptible to the group is equal to that of tetracycline, except that it is twice as potent against *Strep viridans*, *Klebsiella*, *Serratia*, *Ps aeruginosa*, gonococcus, and *H influenzae*. It is better absorbed (66%) after oral administration than oxytetracycline but not as well as tetracycline. In plasma it is protein-bound 75 to 91%. Its volume of distribution is 1.8 mL/g. It readily penetrates into body cavities, fluids, and cells. Its half-life is about 10 to 17 hr, except up to 60 hr in renal failure. About 42% is eliminated in urine. Because of its slow rate of excretion, its efficacy against urinary tract infections is compromised. In general, demeclocycline has the same uses as other tetracyclines. However, it has unique usefulness in the treatment of inappropriate antidiuretic hormone secretion; the mechanism is not understood. The incidence and type of side effects encountered with this drug are similar to those of other tetracyclines, except that the incidence of gastrointestinal side effects may be lower than with tetracycline, possibly because of the smaller doses used. However, it causes antibiotic-associated colitis more than does tetracycline, and it can also impair renal function. Photodynamic and photosensitivity reactions appear more frequently with demeclocycline. Nonsystemic antacid preparations, milk, or food should not be taken with the drug, since these interfere with its gastrointestinal absorption.

Dose—*Oral, adults,* usually **150 mg** every 6 hr or **300 mg** every 12 hr, but as much as 2.4 g a day may be given, if necessary; for *gonorrhea*, initially **600 mg**, then 300 mg every 12 hr until a total dose of 3 g has been given; for *syphilis,* a total of 18 to 24 g in divided doses over 10 to 15 days in males and perhaps longer in females; for *acne,* initially **300 mg** twice a day until improvement, then a gradual reduction to **75** to **300 mg** a day; for inappropriate *ADH secretion,* **3.25** to **3.75 mg/kg** every 6 hr. *Children 8 yr and older,* **1.65** to **3.3 mg/kg** of body weight every 6 hr or **3.3** to **6.6 mg/kg** every 12 hr; not recommended for children under 8 yr because of tooth discoloration and effects on bone growth.

Dosage Forms—Capsules: 150 mg; Tablets: 150 and 300 mg.

Doxycycline

2-Naphthacenecarboxamide, 4-(dimethylamino)-1,4,4a,5,5a,6,11,12a-octahydro-3,5,10,12,12a-pentahydroxy-6-methyl-1,11-dioxo-, [4*S*-(4α,4aα,5α,5aα,6α,12aα)]-, monohydrate; Vibramycin (*Pfizer*)

[17086-28-1] $C_{22}H_{24}N_2O_8.H_2O$ (462.46); *anhydrous* [564-25-0] (444.44). Potency: 880 to 980 μg of $C_{22}H_{24}N_2O_8$/mg.

Preparation—6 - Deoxy - 6-demethyl-6-methylene-5-oxytetracycline (*see Methacycline*) is dissolved or suspended in an inert liquid such as methanol and hydrogenated under the influence of catalytic amounts of noble metals such as rhodium or palladium to give a mixture of the 6α- and 6β-methyl epimers. The desired epimer is then isolated by chromatographic processes. US Pat 3,200,149.

Description—Yellow, crystalline powder.
Solubility—Very slightly soluble in water; freely soluble in dilute acid and alkali hydroxide solutions; sparingly soluble in alcohol; practically insoluble in chloroform and ether.

Uses—Doxycycline has actions and uses generally the same as other tetracyclines (see the introductory statement in this section). Against gram-positive bacteria it is about twice as potent as tetracycline, except that it is up to 10 times as potent against *Strep viridans.* Furthermore, strains of *Strep fecalis* that are resistant to other tetracyclines may be sensitive to doxycycline. Against gram-negative bacteria doxycycline is as potent to twice as potent as tetracycline. Doxycycline is the drug of first choice for *prophylaxis* of "travelers' diarrhea," a disorder caused by several organisms. It is the best of the tetracyclines against anaerobes.

Doxycycline is more completely absorbed (90 to 100%) after oral administration than other tetracyclines, and its absorption does not appear to be inhibited by foods. Plasma-protein binding is about 93%. It has a volume of distribution of 0.75 mL/g. It readily penetrates cells, body fluids and cavities. Elimination is about 65% by hepatic metabolism and 35% by biliary/renal excretion. The rate of excretion is slow and the half-life is the longest of the tetracyclines, namely, 13 to 23 hr. The slow rate of excretion means that urine concentrations are lower than with other tetracyclines, which compromises its efficacy in urinary tract infections in which urine concentration is important. Nevertheless, doxycycline has been used successfully in the treatment of urinary tract infections, especially those, such as pyelonephritis or prostatitis, in which tissue concentration may be more important than urine concentration. Renal insufficiency has little influence on plasma levels or duration of action.

The toxicity of doxycycline is that of tetracyclines in general, but there is lesser incidence of gastrointestinal effects, including alteration in bowel flora populations, than with other tetracyclines. Photosensitization occurs much more frequently than with shorter-acting tetracyclines. Although doxycycline complexes calcium to a lesser extent than other tetracyclines, absorption is hindered by calcium-containing as well as by other nonsystemic acids and by iron preparations.

Dose (anhydrous equivalent)—*Oral, adults* and *children weighing over 45 kg,* to *treat infections, usually* **100 mg** every 12 hr on the first day followed by either **50** to **100 mg** every 12 hr or **100** to **200 mg** a day, but up to 300 mg a day may be given; for *gonorrhea, initially* **200 mg** followed by **100 mg** every 12 hr for 3 days in males and perhaps longer

in females, or 2 doses of **300 mg** one hour apart; for *syphilis,* **300 mg** a day in divided doses for at least 10 days; for *prophylaxis of traveller's diarrhea,* **100 mg** once a day for 3 weeks. *Children weighing 45 kg or less, initially* 2 doses of **2.2 mg/kg** of body weight at 12-hr intervals the first day followed by either **1.1** to **2.2 mg/kg** every 12 hr or 2.2 to 4.4 mg/kg once a day. Not recommended for children under 8 yr of age because of tooth discoloration and effects on bone growth.

Dosage Form (anhydrous equivalent)—for Oral Suspension: 25 mg/5 mL (reconstituted).

Doxycycline Hyclate

2-Naphthacenecarboxamide, 4-(dimethylamino)-1,4,4a,5,5a,6,11,12a-octahydro-3,5,10,12,12a-pentahydroxy-6-methyl-1,11-dioxo-, [4*S*-(4α,4aα,5α,5aα,6α,12aα)]-, monohydrochloride, compd with ethanol (2:1), monohydrate, Vibramycin Hyclate (*Pfizer*)

See *Doxycycline* for structure of the parent compound [24390-14-5] $(C_{22}H_{24}N_2O_8.HCl)_2.C_2H_6O.H_2O$ (1025.89). Potency: the equivalent of 800–920 μg of doxycycline/mg.

Preparation—Doxycycline hydrochloride is crystallized from a solution in ethanol containing hydrochloric acid.

Description—Yellow, crystalline powder.
Solubility—Soluble in water and solutions of alkali hydroxides and carbonates; slightly soluble in alcohol; practically insoluble in chloroform and ether.

Uses—see *Doxycycline.*
Dose (base equivalent)—*Oral,* the same as for *Doxycycline. Intravenous infusion, adults* and *children* weighing *over 45 kg, initially* **200 mg** once or **100 mg** twice on the first day followed by **100** to **200 mg** once a day or **50** to **100 mg** twice a day; *children up to 45 kg,* **4.4 mg/kg** once or **2.2 mg/kg** twice on the first day followed by **2.2** to **4.4 mg/kg** once a day or **1.1** to **2.2 mg/kg** twice a day. Not recommended for children under 8 yr of age because of effects on tooth coloration and bone growth.

Dosage Forms (base equivalent)—Capsules: 50 and 100 mg; for Injection: 100 and 200 mg; Film-Coated Tablets: 100 mg.

Meclocycline Sulfosalicylate

2-Naphthacenecarboxamide, 7-chloro-4-(dimethylamino)-1,4,4a,5,5a,6,11,12a-octahydro-3,5,10,12,12a-pentahydroxy-6-methylene-1,11-dioxo-, [4*S*-(4α,4aα,5α,5aα,12aα)]-, mono(2-hydroxy-5-sulfobenzoate) (salt); Meclan (*Ortho*)

[73816-42-9] $C_{22}H_{21}ClN_2O_8.C_7H_6O_6S$ (695.05).
Preparation—see *J Am Chem Soc 83:* 2773, 1961.
Uses—Meclocycline has the antibacterial activities of the tetracyclines in general (see general statement). It is used only topically, for the treatment of *acne vulgaris.* It is not absorbed from the skin into the blood. Contact dermatitis occurs very rarely. However, there is cross-sensitivity with other tetracyclines. It can also sensitize to formaldehyde. Phototoxicity has not yet occurred. It can stain the follicles temporarily and also clothing. Ultraviolet fluorescence of the skin occurs, as with other topical tetracyclines.

Dose—*Topically,* to the *skin,* as a 1% cream to the affected area twice a day.

Dosage Form—Cream: 1%.

Methacycline Hydrochloride

2-Naphthacenecarboxamide, 4-(dimethylamino)-1,4,4a,5,5a,6,11,12a-octahydro-3,5,10,12,12a-pentahydroxy-6-methylene-1,11-dioxo-, [4*S*-(4α,4aα,5α,5aα,12aα)]-, monohydrochloride; 6-Methylene-5-hydroxytetracycline; Rondomycin Hydrochloride (*Wallace*)

[3963-95-9] $C_{22}H_{22}N_2O_8$.HCl (478.89). Potency: equivalent to not less than 832 μg of methacycline/mg.

Preparation—5-Hydroxytetracycline is reacted with a halogenating agent such as N-chlorosuccinimide to form 11a-chloro-5-hydroxytetracycline-6,12-hemiketal (I). Dehydration of I with polyphosphoric acid yields 11a-chloro-6-methylene-5-hydroxytetracycline. Dechlorination at 11a may be accomplished by catalytic hydrogenation or by usual reduction processes. The methacycline (base) thus obtained is dissolved in methanol and treated with HCl to form the salt.

Description—Yellow to dark yellow, crystalline powder; pH (1% solution) between 2 and 3; odorless and has a bitter taste; unstable in light, nonhygroscopic, and stable at room temperature; decomposes without melting at about 225°.

Solubility—1 g in 100 mL water, 300 mL alcohol, >1000 mL chloroform, >1000 mL ether.

Uses—Methacycline has the actions and uses of tetracyclines in general (see introductory statement in this section). Organisms sensitive to methacycline will be sensitive to any other tetracycline and *vice versa*. Likewise, development of resistance is mutual among methacycline and all other tetracyclines. Furthermore, any patient hypersensitive to another tetracycline will be allergic to methacycline. Toxicity and side effects are those of other tetracyclines, but photosensitivity is more frequent than with tetracycline, chlortetracycline, or oxytetracycline. Thus the only advantage of methacycline is its longer duration of action. The half-life is approximately 14 to 17 hr, which is about that of demeclocycline but less than that of doxycycline. The long duration of action is in part due to greater binding by plasma and tissue proteins, which binding diminishes the effective plasma level of the drug and slows excretion in urine. It is 79 to 90% protein-bound in plasma. The volume of distribution is 0.97 mL/g. The low rate of excretion results in a low urine concentration, so that it is less effective in urinary-tract infections than the shorter-acting tetracyclines. Methacycline should not be used in patients with impaired renal function, but if its use cannot be avoided, the dose-interval must be increased to as long as 3 to 4 days in anuria. Non-systemic antacids and food interfere with absorption.

Dose—*Oral, adults, usually* either **150 mg** every 6 hr or **300 mg** every 8 hr but up to 2.4 g a day may be given; for *gonorrhea, initially* **900 mg** followed by **300 mg** every 6 hr for a total of 5.4 g, except that females may require a longer treatment; for *syphilis*, a total of 18 to **24 g** in equally divided doses over 10 to 15 days; for *Mycoplasma pneumonia*, **450 mg** every 12 hr for 6 days. *Children 8 or more yr of age*, either **1.65 to 3.3 mg/kg** of body weight every 6 hr or **3.3 to 6.6 mg/kg** every 12 hr. Not recommended for children under 8 yr of age because of effects on teeth and bone.

Dosage Forms—Capsules: 150 and 300 mg.

Minocycline Hydrochloride

2-Naphthacenecarboxamide, 4,7-bis(dimethylamino)-1,4,4a,5,5a,6,11,12a-octahydro-3,10,12,12a-tetrahydroxy-1,11-dioxo-, [4*S*-(4α,4aα,5aα,12aα)]-, monohydrochloride; 7-Dimethylamino-6-demethyl-6-deoxytetracycline; Minocin (*Lederle*)

[13614-98-7] $C_{23}H_{27}N_3O_7$.HCl (493.94). Potency: equivalent to not less than 785 μg of minocycline ($C_{23}H_{27}N_3O_7$)/mg.

Preparation—6-Demethyltetracycline, dissolved in tetrahydrofuran containing methanesulfonic acid, is reacted with dibenzyl azodicarboxylate to form 7-[1,2-bis(carbobenzoxy)hydrazino]-6-demethyltetracycline. Palladium-catalyzed hydrogenation in the presence of formaldehyde yields minocycline which reacts with an equimolar quantity of HCl to form the monohydrochloride. US Pats 3,148,212 and 3,226,436.

Description—Yellow, odorless, crystalline powder with a slightly bitter taste; slightly hygroscopic; stable in air when protected from light and moisture (strong light and/or moist air causes it to darken); potency in solution affected primarily due to epimerization; pH (1 in 100 solution) between 3.5 and 4.5; pK_{a1} 2.8; pK_{a2} 5.0; pK_{a3} 7.8; pK_{a4} 9.3.

Solubility—1 g in about 60 mL water and about 70 mL alcohol; soluble in solutions of alkali hydroxides and carbonates; practically insoluble in chloroform and ether.

Uses—Actions and uses are essentially the same as those of the tetracyclines in general (see introductory statement in this section). Against most gram-positive organisms it appears to be generally 2 to 4 times as potent as tetracycline, but it shares an equally low potency against *Strep fecalis*. Against *Strep viridans* it is about 8 times as potent. Against gram-negative bacteria it is generally 2 to 4 times as potent as tetracycline. It is especially effective against *Mycobacterium marinum*, and it is now the drug of choice for treating infections caused by that bacterium.

In addition to being used for treatment of all the infections for which other tetracyclines are used, minocycline appears to be unique in successfully eliminating sulfonamide-resistant meningococci from the nasopharynx. It also differs from other tetracyclines in that bacterial resistance to the drug is of a lower order and incidence; this is especially true of staphylococci, in which cross-resistance has been reported to be as low as 4%. Thus it may sometimes be used to treat staphylococcal infections that have become resistant to other tetracyclines. For this reason, some authorities contend that minocycline ought not to be used as the outset in staphylococcal infections but rather should be held in reserve until resistance to other tetracyclines occurs. As a prophylactic against rheumatic fever, chorea, and nasopharyngeal streptococcal infections, minocycline may become the tetracycline of choice. Although minocycline is slowly excreted and does not yield high urine concentrations, present evidence indicates that it is about as efficacious in the treatment of urinary tract infections as the rapidly excreted tetracyclines.

The incidence and severity of the usual side effects of tetracyclines, effects like phototoxicity and gastrointestinal upsets, are less than with other tetracyclines. Diarrhea, abdominal pain and flatus are experienced by only 2 to 5% of patients. However, nausea and vomiting are frequent, as the result of ototoxicity and CNS effects. There are also autonomic nervous disorders; dry mouth and cycloplegia occur in 2 to 10% of recipients, and caution is advised in persons with glaucoma or males with partial obstruction of the urinary tract. Headache occurs in 33% and myalgia in 12% of patients. Lethargy, fatigue, vertigo, confusion, and disorientation occur in about 25% of users. Insomnia occurs in 9%, hot flashes in 8%, and tinnitus in 4%. Impairment of hearing and vestibular function can result from use in patients with meningitis, the various manifestations of CNS toxicity and ototoxicity occurring in 50 to 90% of recipients of minocycline.

Minocycline is 90 to 100% absorbed by the oral route. Its absorption is diminished slightly by food and milk and markedly by non-systemic antacids and iron preparations. It is 70 to 75% protein-bound in plasma. The volume of distribution is 0.97 mL/g. The half-life is 11 to 17 hr. Only 10% is reported to be excreted unchanged, but the half-life has been reported to be greatly prolonged in renal failure.

Dose (minocycline equivalent)—*Oral, adults*, usually either **200 mg** initially followed by **100 mg** every 12 hr or **100 to 200 mg** initially followed by **50 mg** every 6 hr; as much as 350 mg can be given the first day and 200 mg a day on subsequent days; in the *meningococcal carrier* state, **100 mg** every 12 hr for 5 days; for infections by *M marinum*, **100 mg** every 12 hr for 6 to 8 wk. *Children 8 yr of age or older*, initially **4 mg/kg** of body weight followed by **2 mg/kg** every 12 hr. Not recommended in children under 8 yr because of effects on teeth and bone. *Intravenous*, same as usual oral dosage.

Dosage Forms (minocycline equivalent)—Capsules: 50 and 100 mg; Sterile: 100 mg to be reconstituted to 5 mL; Oral Suspension: 50 mg/5 mL; Tablets: 50 and 100 mg.

Oxytetracycline

2-Naphthacenecarboxamide, 4-(dimethylamino)-1,4,4a,5,5a,6,11,12a-octahydro-3,5,6,10,12,12a-hexahydroxy-6-methyl-1,11-dioxo-, [4*S*-(4α,4aα,5α,5aα,6β,12aα)]-, dihydrate; Oxytetracycline Dihydrate Terramycin (*Pfizer*); *Various Mfrs*

[6153-64-6] $C_{22}H_{24}N_2O_9$.2H$_2$O (496.47); *anhydrous* [79-57-2] (460.44). Potency: not less than 832 μg of $C_{22}H_{24}N_2O_9$/mg.

Preparation—By the growth of a selected strain of *Streptomyces rimosus* on a medium consisting of water, proteins, and nutrient salts.

Description—Pale yellow to tan, odorless, crystalline powder; stable in air, but exposure to strong sunlight causes it to darken; deteriorates in solutions of pH below 2, and is rapidly destroyed by alkali hydroxide solutions; saturated solution is nearly neutral to litmus, having a pH of about 6.5.

Solubility—1 g in 4150 mL water, 100 mL alcohol, >10,000 mL chloroform, 6250 mL ether; freely soluble in diluted hydrochloric acid or alkaline solutions.

Uses—The actions, toxicity, and uses of oxytetracycline are essentially those of tetracycline in general (see introductory statement in this section). The relative susceptibilities of various microorganisms to oxytetracycline are virtually the same as for chlortetracycline and tetracycline, with a few possible exceptions. Bacterial resistance to oxytetracycline automatically confers resistance to chlortetracycline or tetracycline. Oxytetracycline is also used in the treatment of intestinal amebiasis; it removes both cysts and motile forms from the intestine and compares favorably with halogenated quinolines. However, all these drugs have been superseded by metronidazole. Approximately 58% of an oral dose is absorbed in the fasting state. It is bound to plasma proteins only about 35%. The volume of distribution is 1.9 mL/g. About 70% is eliminated by renal excretion. The biologic half-life is 6 to 10 hr; it may be 3 to 4 days in anuria. The gastrointestinal side effects are greater than with other tetracyclines. Food, milk, nonsystemic antacids and iron preparations interfere with oral absorption.

Dose (anhydrous oxytetracycline)—*Oral, adults,* **250** to **500 mg** every 6 hr; *children, 8 years or older,* **6.25** to **12.5 mg/kg** every 6 hr. *Intramuscular, adults,* **100 mg** every 8 hr, **150 mg** every 12 hr, *or* **250 mg** once a day; up to 500 mg a day may be given, if necessary; *children 8 or more yr of age,* usually either **5** to **8.3 mg/kg** of body weight every 8 hr *or* **7.5** to **12.5 mg/kg** every 12 hr, except that no dose should exceed 250 mg. Not recommended for children under 8 yr because of effects on teeth and bone.

Dosage Forms (anhydrous oxytetracycline)—Injection: 50 and 125 mg/mL; Tablets: 250 mg.

Oxytetracycline Hydrochloride

2-Naphthacenecarboxamide, 4-(dimethylamino)-1,4,4a,5,5a,6,11,12a-octahydro-3,5,6,10,12,12a-hexahydroxy-6-methyl-1,11-dioxo-, [4S-(4α,4aα,5α,5aα,6β,12aα)]-, monohydrochloride; 5-Hydroxytetracycline Monohydrochloride; *Various Mfrs*

[2058-46-0] $C_{22}H_{24}N_2O_9 \cdot HCl$ (496.90). Potency: equivalent to not less than 835 μg of oxytetracycline ($C_{22}H_{24}N_2O_9$)/mg, calculated on the anhydrous basis.

For the structure of the base, see *Oxytetracycline.*

Description—Yellow, crystalline powder; odorless, has a bitter taste, and is hygroscopic; decomposes above 180°, and exposure to strong sunlight or to temperature above 90° in moist air causes darkening, but no appreciable loss in potency; potency is affected in solutions of pH below 2, and is rapidly destroyed by alkali hydroxide solutions; pH (1% solution) between 2 and 3.

Solubility—1 g in 2 mL water, but the solution becomes cloudy or turbid due to liberation of oxytetracycline base; 1 g in 35 mL alcohol, less soluble in dehydrated alcohol; insoluble in chloroform and ether.

Uses—See *Oxytetracycline.*

Dose (oxytetracycline equivalent)—*Oral,* identical to that of *Chlortetracycline Hydrochloride* (above). *Intravenous, adults,* usually **250** to **500 mg** every 12 hr, but up to 2 g a day may be given; *children, 8 yr of age or more,* usually **5** to **10 mg/kg** of body weight every 12 hr. Not recommended for children under 8 yr because of effects on teeth and bone. Plasma concentrations should not exceed 15 μg/mL, especially in pregnant women or postpartum women with pyelonephritis. *Topical,* in combination with polymyxin B and/or hydrocortisone, 3% ointment or 0.5% ophthalmic ointment.

Dosage Forms (oxytetracycline equivalent)—Capsules: 125 and 500 mg; for Injection: 250 and 500 mg.

Tetracycline

2-Naphthacenecarboxamide 4-(dimethylamino)-1,4,4a,5,5a,6,11,12a-octahydro-3,6,10,12,12a-pentahydroxy-6-methyl-1,11-dioxo-, [4S-(4α,4aα,5α,5aα,6β,12aα)]-, *Various Mfrs*

[60-54-8] $C_{22}H_{24}N_2O_8$ (444.44). Potency: equivalent to not less than 975 μg of tetracycline hydrochloride ($C_{22}H_{24}N_2O_8 \cdot HCl$)/mg, calculated on the anhydrous basis.

Preparation—By removal of chlorine from chlortetracycline by hydrogenation. Also obtained from a *Streptomyces* species cultured in an appropriate nutrient medium.

Description—Yellow, odorless, crystalline powder; stable in air, but exposure to strong sunlight causes it to darken; potency is affected in solutions of pH below 2, and is rapidly destroyed by alkali hydroxide solutions; more soluble than chlortetracycline and within the physiological and moderately alkaline range of pH is more stable; its solutions darken more rapidly than chlortetracycline but less than oxytetracycline; pH (aqueous suspension, 10 mg/mL) between 3.0 and 7.0.

Solubility—1 g in about 2500 mL water and about 50 mL alcohol; freely soluble in dilute HCl and alkali hydroxide solutions; practically insoluble in chloroform and ether.

Uses—The antibiotic spectrum, actions, toxicity, absorption, fate and excretion, doses, and uses are essentially the same as those of the tetracyclines in general (see introductory statement in this section). Tetracycline has been reported to be useful in the treatment of *toxoplasmosis;* it is not known whether this use can be extended to all tetracyclines. The gastrointestinal side effects from tetracycline are less than those from chlortetracycline and oxytetracycline but more than from demeclocycline. About 77% of an oral dose is absorbed. In the plasma 25 to 55% is bound to proteins. The volume of distribution is 1.5 mL/g. About 60% is eliminated by renal excretion. The plasma half-life is 6 to 11 hr in patients with normal renal function; in oliguria it may be as long as 2 to 4 days, and dosage must be adjusted accordingly.

Dose (tetracycline hydrochloride equivalent)—*Oral, adults, most infections,* **250** to **500 mg** every 6 hr or **500 mg** to **1 g** every 12 hr; for *acne, initially* **500 mg** to **2 g** a day in divided doses, then, after improvement, gradually reduced to **125 mg** to **1 g** a day; for *gonorrhea,* **500 mg** every 6 hr for 5 days; for *syphilis,* **500 mg** every 6 hr for 15 days for early and 30 days for late syphilis; *children 8 yr of age and older,* **6.25** to **12.5 mg/kg** every 6 hr or **12.5** to **25 mg/kg** every 12 hr. Not recommended for children under 8 yr because of effects on bone and teeth.

Dosage Form (tetracycline hydrochloride equivalent)—Oral Suspension: 125 mg/5 mL.

Tetracycline Hydrochloride

2-Naphthacenecarboxamide, 4-(dimethylamino)-1,4,4a,5,5a,6,11,12a-octahydro-3,6,10,12,12a-pentahydroxy-6-methyl-1,11-dioxo-, monohydrochloride, [4S-(4α,4aα,5aα,6β,12aα)]-, *Various Mfrs*

[64-75-5] $C_{22}H_{24}N_2O_8 \cdot HCl$ (480.90). Potency: not less than 900 μg of $C_{22}H_{24}N_2O_8 \cdot HCl$/mg.

For the structure of the base, see *Tetracycline.*

Description—Yellow, odorless, crystalline powder; moderately hygroscopic; stable in air, but exposure to strong sunlight in moist air causes it to darken; potency affected in solutions of pH below 2, and is rapidly destroyed by alkali hydroxide solutions; pH (1 in 100 solution) between 1.8 and 2.8.

Solubility—1 g in 10 mL water and about 100 mL alcohol, the aqueous solution becoming turbid after some time because of hydrolysis; soluble in solutions of alkali hydroxides and carbonates; practically insoluble in chloroform and ether.

Uses—As for *Tetracycline.* Since the hydrochloride is the more soluble form of tetracycline it is used for parenteral administration and in solution for topical use.

Dose—*Oral,* same as for *Tetracycline* (above). *Intramuscular,* same as for *Oxytetracycline* (above). *Intravenous,* same as for *Oxytetracycline Hydrochloride* (above). Not recommended for use in children under 8 yr of age because of effects on teeth and bones. *Topical,* to the *skin* as **3%** ointment once or twice a day or as **0.22%** solution 2 or more times a day; to the conjunctiva as a thin strip (about 1 cm) of **1%** ointment 6 or more times a day or 1 or 2 drops of **1%** suspension into conjunctival sac 2 to 4 times a day.

Dosage Forms—Capsules: 100, 250, and 500 mg; for Intramuscular Injection: 100 and 250 mg; for Intravenous Injection: 250 and

500 mg; Ophthalmic Ointment: 1%; Topical Ointment: 3%; for Topical Solution: 0.22% when reconstituted; Ophthalmic Suspension: 1%; Tablets: 250 and 500 mg.

Other Tetracyclines

Chlortetracycline Hydrochloride [[64-72-2] $C_{22}H_{23}ClN_2O_8$.HCl (515.35) Aureomycin Hydrochloride (*Lederle*).]—*Preparation: Streptomyces aureofaciens*, Duggar, is grown in an appropriate nutrient medium under controlled conditions of temperature, pH, and aeration. The chlortetracycline produced is recrystallized from various solvents at controlled acidity and is converted to the hydrochloride. *Description and solubility:* Yellow, odorless, bitter, crystalline powder, which is stable in air; slowly affected by light. Potency: not less than 900 μg of $C_{22}H_{23}ClN_2O_8$.HCl/mg. Soluble 1 g in 75 mL water and about 560 mL alcohol; soluble in solutions of alkali carbonates or hydroxides; practically insoluble in chloroform or ether. *Uses:* The antibacterial spectrum, uses, and adverse effects of chlortetracycline are those of tetracyclines (see the preceding introductory statement). At present it is used only for the treatment of ocular infections and of pyodermas, such as *folliculitis*, *carbuncles*, *bullous impetigo*, *ecthyma*, *cellulitis*, *erysipelas*, and *nonbullous impetigo* caused by staphylococci and beta-hemolytic streptococci. Hypersensitivity can occur. *Dose: Topical*, to the *skin* as **3%** ointment 1 to 3 times a day, or to the *conjunctiva* as a thin strip (about 1 cm) of **1%** ointment every 2 hr or more frequently if needed.

Doxycycline Calcium [A complex prepared from doxycycline (p 1205) and calcium chloride.] *Uses* and *Dose:* the same as for Doxycycline.

Oxytetracycline Calcium—A calcium chelate salt of oxytetracycline [15251-48-6] $C_{44}H_{48}CaN_4O_{18}$ (960.96), in which an atom of calcium binds two molecules of oxytetracycline.]—Prepared by interaction of aqueous solutions of oxytetracycline hydrochloride and calcium chloride. A yellow to light-brown, crystalline powder, insoluble in water. *Uses:* Has the actions of *Oxytetracycline*, its low solubility being utilized to prepare a syrup dosage form in which the suspended calcium salt lacks the disagreeable taste of the soluble oxytetracycline hydrochloride. The syrup contains the equivalent of 125 mg of oxytetracycline in 5 mL.

Tetracycline Phosphate Complex—A relatively insoluble complex prepared by interaction of solutions of tetracycline hydrochloride and sodium metaphosphate. A yellow, fine, crystalline powder, having a potency of not less than 750 μg/mg, as tetracycline hydrochloride, calculated on the anhydrous basis. *Uses:* Has the actions, uses, and toxicity of *Tetracycline*. It has been claimed that this complex, for oral administration, produces faster and higher blood levels than obtained with tetracycline or tetracycline hydrochloride. The difference, if any, is minor and does not change the dosage schedule of this agent from that of tetracycline. *Dose: Oral*, see *Tetracycline*.

Miscellaneous Antibiotics

Because of similarities among bacteria and fungi in biosynthetic mechanisms, antibiotics tend to fall into chemical groups. Furthermore, similarities among the target organisms in physiology and metabolism tend to select certain types of molecules as effective antibiotics. Nevertheless, there is species and strain individuality which lends itself to exploitation. Thus some of the miscellaneous antibiotics are the result of the biosynthetic uniqueness of the generating organism and others of the unique requirements for activity of some specific target organisms.

Some of the drugs in this section have distant relationships with antibiotics in distinct chemical classes; for example, lincomycin and clindamycin might be considered by some to be aminoglycosides. Interestingly, in their antibacterial actions they closely resemble the chemically unrelated macrolides. The similarities in spectrum, mechanism, and toxicity of some miscellaneous antibiotics to chemically unrelated drugs are the result of actions at different points in the same general biochemical or physiological function.

Amphotericin B—page 1226.

Candicidin—page 1226.

Chloramphenicol

Acetamide, 2,2-dichloro-*N*-[2-hydroxy-1-(hydroxymethyl)-2-(4-nitrophenyl)ethyl]-, [R-(R*,R*)]-, Chloromycetin (*Parke-Davis*); *Various Mfrs*

D-*threo*-(−)-2,2-Dichloro-*N*-[β-hydroxy-α-(hydroxymethyl)-*p*-nitrophenethyl]acetamide [56-75-7] $C_{11}H_{12}Cl_2N_2O_5$ (323.13). Potency: not less than 900 μg of $C_{11}H_{12}Cl_2N_2O_5$/mg.

Preparation—Chloramphenicol is believed to be the first naturally occurring compound known to contain a nitro group or to be a derivative of dichloroacetic acid. Its stereochemical configuration is analogous to that of (−)-norpseudoephedrine, and is the only one of the four related stereoisomers that has antibiotic activity.

Chloramphenicol can be obtained from the filtrate of a *Streptomyces venezuelae* culture by extraction with ethyl acetate. If the charcoal extract is rich in chloramphenicol, the latter can be crystallized from the ethyl acetate by diluting with many volumes of kerosene.

Several synthetic methods of preparation are known. One of the better known commences with *p*-nitroacetophenone and, after converting it into *p*-nitro-2-aminoacetophenone, proceeds through the following steps: (a) acetylation of the —NH$_2$ group, (b) reaction with HCHO to introduce the terminal —CH$_2$OH group, (c) reduction with aluminum isopropoxide to give a mixture of the racemates of the *threo* and *erythro* forms of *p*-NO$_2$PhCH(OH)CH(NH$_2$)CH$_2$OH, (d) isolation of the *threo* racemate and resolution of it using *d*-camphorsulfonic acid, and (e) condensing the (−) enantiomorph with methyl dichloroacetate.

Description—Fine, white to grayish white or yellowish white, needle-like crystals or elongated plates; odorless; intensely bitter taste; pH (saturated solution) between 4.5 and 7.5; reasonably stable in neutral or moderately acid solutions but rapidly destroyed in alkaline solutions; melts between 149° and 153°.

Solubility—1 g in about 400 mL water; freely soluble in alcohol; slightly soluble in ether and chloroform.

Uses—Has a wide spectrum of antibacterial activity. The drug is effective in the following: *rickettsial diseases* including epidemic, murine, and scrub typhus, Rocky Mountain spotted fever, rickettsial pox, and Q fever; *virus diseases* including the psittacosis-lymphogranuloma group; and many *bacterial infections* including those caused by *A aerogenes*, *E coli*, *K pneumoniae*, *H pertussis*, *E typhosa*, *Brucella*, *V cholerae*, staphylococci, streptococci, corynebacteria, mycoplasmas, actinomycetes, and *T pallidum*. Because of serious toxic reactions, the systemic use of the drug should be limited only to very serious infections that cannot be managed by other drugs. However, it is still used much too promiscuously. It is still the drug of choice for typhoid fever, and, in combination with ampicillin, for meningitis, fulminating respiratory infections, or life-threatening septicemias caused by *H influenzae*. It is the drug of second choice for brucellosis, shigellosis, paratyphoid fever, ornithosis, psittacosis, and (in combination) various pseudomonal infections. *It should never be used in trivial or mild infections.* Chloramphenicol is used topically for superficial conjunctival infections and blepharitis caused by *E coli*, *H influenzae*, *Moraxella lacunata*, *Staph aureus* and *Strep hemolyticus*.

Bone-marrow injury is the major toxic effect of chloramphenicol. Thrombocytopenia, granulocytopenia, and aplastic anemia are the most serious hematopoietic disturbances observed and have resulted in a number of fatalities. Aplastic anemia has occurred even after ophthalmic use. Any patient under treatment with chloramphenicol must be given a leukocyte and differential count every other day. Bone-marrow depression is more serious in pregnancy and in infants than in other persons. Optic atrophy and blindness occur in a small number of cases, mainly in children on prolonged therapy. Minor untoward effects such as transient mild euphoria, skin rash, and gastrointestinal disturbances (occasional nausea and vomiting, gaseous distention, loose stools, and pruritus ani) have been observed; the drug is contraindicated in patients with a history of previous sensitization. Occasional untoward effects include glossitis, stomatitis, and pharyngitis. The use of chloramphenicol, as with other antibiotics, may result in an overgrowth of microorganisms not susceptible to the drug. In neonates chloramphenicol may cause fatal cyanosis, vomiting, abdominal distention, and loose, green stools, owing to the inability of the infant to metabolize the drug in consequence of glucuronyl transferase deficiency. Chloramphenicol interacts adversely with other drugs that depress bone-marrow (antineoplastics, colchicine, gold salts, penicillamine, phenylbutazone). Oral anticoagulants, oral hypoglycemics, and phenytoin inhibit the metabolism of chloramphenicol and increase the risk of intoxication; appropriate dose adjustments should be made.

Chloramphenicol is rapidly absorbed from the gastrointestinal tract, with a bioavailability of about 90%. Significant serum levels are obtained in 30 min, peak blood concentrations of 10 to 15 $\mu g/mL$ (after 1-g dose) are reached in about 2 hr, and a therapeutic concentration is maintained for about 6 to 8 hr. 60% of chloramphenicol in blood is bound to serum albumin. The volume of distribution is about 0.7 mL/g. From 85 to 95% is biotransformed in the liver. The half-life is 1.5 to 5 hr, except over 24 hr in neonates 1 to 2 days old and 10 hr in infants 10 to 16 days old. Because of considerable variability, plasma levels must be monitored. Also, the clearance increases with continuous use, and dose adjustments are necessary. When there is impaired hepatic function, and sometimes of renal function as well, the dosage must be reduced, according to determined plasma concentrations. Chloramphenicol can cross the placental barrier and intoxicate the fetus, so that the drug should be avoided in pregnancy, if possible. The drug interferes with the elimination of phenytoin.

Dose—*Oral, adults, children,* and *infants over 2 weeks of age,* usually **12.5 mg/kg** of body weight every 6 hr or **25 mg/kg** every 12 hr; up to 100 mg/kg/day may be given to adults. *Infants up to 2 weeks of age* and infants with *immature hepatic metabolic function,* **6.25/kg** every 6 hr. The desired plasma concentration is in the range of 5 to 20 $\mu g/mL$. *Topical,* as **1%** dermatologic cream 3 or 4 times a day, as **0.5%** otic solution 3 times a day, or as **0.5%** ophthalmic solution or **1%** ophthalmic ointment every 2 to 3 hr for the first 3 days and every 3 to 4 hours thereafter, as required.

Dosage Forms—Capsules: 50, 100, and 250 mg; Cream: 0.5%; Ophthalmic Ointment: 1%; for Ophthalmic Solution: 25 mg; Ophthalmic Solution: 0.5%; Otic Solution: 0.5%.

Chloramphenicol Palmitate

Hexadecanoic acid, 2-[(2,2-dichloroacetyl)amino]-3-hydroxy-3-(4-nitrophenyl)propyl ester, [R-(R*,R*)]-, Chloromycetin Palmitate (*Parke-Davis*)

Chloramphenicol α-palmitate [530-43-8] $C_{27}H_{42}Cl_2N_2O_6$ (561.54). Potency: 550 to 595 μg of chloramphenicol ($C_{11}H_{12}Cl_2N_2O_5$)/mg.

Preparation—Chloramphenicol is esterified by treatment with palmitoyl chloride [$CH_3(CH_2)_{14}COCl$] in the presence of pyridine. The crude ester is obtained by pouring the reaction product into a large excess of dilute hydrochloric acid and filtering. It is then purified by recrystallization from an appropriate solvent.

Description—Fine, white, unctuous, crystalline powder, having a faint odor and a bland, mild taste; melts between 87° and 95°.

Solubility—Insoluble in water; very slightly soluble in solvent hexane; soluble in ether; sparingly soluble in alcohol; freely soluble in acetone and chloroform.

Uses—The drug is insoluble and hence lacks the bitter flavor of chloramphenicol. It is hydrolyzed in the upper intestinal tract to chloramphenicol. Therefore, its oral uses are those of the parent drug (see *Chloramphenicol*); however, it does not share the topical efficacy of the parent drug. Its toxicity is likewise that of chloramphenicol; it should not be used unless certain severe criteria of indication are met. Since the absorption of the chloramphenicol palmitate depends on the hydrolysis of the palmitate ester to chloramphenicol, the blood levels of chloramphenicol rise more slowly after an oral dose than with the parent chloramphenicol, and its duration of action is somewhat longer.

Dose—*Oral,* same as for *Chloramphenicol,* expressed as chloramphenicol equivalent.

Dosage Form (chloramphenicol equivalent)—Oral Suspension: 150 mg/5 mL.

Chloramphenicol Sodium Succinate

Butanedioic acid, mono[2-[(2,2-dichloroacetyl)amino]-3-hydroxy-3-(4-nitrophenyl)propyl]ester, [R-(R*,R*)]-, monosodium salt; Chloromycetin Succinate (*Parke-Davis*)

Chloramphenicol α-(sodium succinate) [982-57-0] $C_{15}H_{15}Cl_2N_2NaO_8$ (445.19). Potency: equivalent to 650 to 765 μg of $C_{11}H_{12}Cl_2N_2O_5$ (chloramphenicol)/mg.

Preparation—Chloramphenicol is reacted with an equimolar portion of succinic acid anhydride to yield chloramphenicol hydrogen succinate which, after purification by recrystallization, is neutralized with sodium hydroxide to give the ester-salt.

Description—Light yellow, crystalline powder.
Solubility—Freely soluble in water and alcohol.

Uses—Useful for parenteral administration by virtue of its high aqueous solubility. Its effectiveness *in vivo* depends on the liberation of the parent compound by hydrolysis, and, therefore, its uses are similar to those of chloramphenicol. Paradoxically, parenteral bioavailability, as chloramphenicol, is higher with the succinate than with chloramphenicol itself. Also, the volume of distribution (2.1 mL/g) is higher. Chloramphenicol sodium succinate may be preferred when oral therapy is not feasible, or when rapid attainment of a high blood level is desired. The toxicity of chloramphenicol sodium succinate is that of the parent drug; thus it should not be used unless certain severe criteria of indication are met.

Dose (chloramphenicol equivalent)—*Intravenous, adults,* **12.5 mg/kg** every 6 hr, but up to 100 mg/kg a day in life-threatening infections; *infants 2 wk* of age and older, **12.5 mg/kg** every 6 hr or **25 mg/kg** every 12 hr; *infants under 2 wk,* **6.25 mg/kg** every 6 hr; in severe infections, up to 100 mg/kg a day may be given.

Dosage Forms—Sterile: 1 g.

Clindamycin Hydrochloride

L-*threo*-α-D-*galacto*-Octopyranoside, methyl 7-chloro-6,7,8-trideoxy-6-[[(1-methyl-4-propyl-2-pyrrolidinyl)carbonyl]amino]-1-thio-, (2S-*trans*)-, monohydrochloride; Cleocin Hydrochloride (*Upjohn*)

(*) Indicates site of esterification to form the palmitate or phosphate derivatives.

[21462-39-5] $C_{18}H_{33}ClN_2O_5S \cdot HCl$ (461.44). Potency: equivalent to not less than 800 μg of clindamycin/mg.

Preparation—*Lincomycin* is treated with a solution of Rydon reagent prepared from triphenylphosphine, acetonitrile, and chlorine. The base is ultimately reacted with HCl. *CA 73:* 15185*v*, 1970.

Description—White or practically white, crystalline powder with a strong, characteristic taste; odorless or has a faint mercaptan-like odor; stable in air and light; pK_a 7.72.

Solubility—Freely soluble in water; soluble in alcohol.

Uses—Clindamycin has an antibacterial spectrum very much like that of *Lincomycin,* from which it is derived. However, among staphylococci and several streptococci it may be as much as 20 times more potent than lincomycin. It is also more potent against certain gram-negative organisms, but not against gram-negative cocci; with the recommended doses the plasma levels usually are not high enough to be effective against gram-negative bacteria. Clindamycin is especially useful in the treatment of several infections caused by anaerobes; it is the drug of choice for treatment of gastrointestinal infections caused by *B fragilis* and is one of several second choices for treatment of infections caused by oropharyngeal strains of *B fragilis,* *Fusobacterium,* anaerobic streptococci, and *Cl perfringens* (but not other clostridia). It is important as an alternate drug for treating infections caused by penicillin-resistant *Staph aureus.* It is also used for treatment of respiratory tract infections and pharyngitis or tonsillitis caused by *Strep pyogenes.* It is perhaps the best drug for the topical treatment of *acne vulgaris* (used as the phosphate).

Clindamycin may cause abdominal pain, nausea, vomiting, diarrhea, and loose stools, which may occasionally contain blood and mucus. Incidence of benign diarrhea is about 10 to 20%. Incidence of pseudomembranous colitis is estimated to be 1:10,000 (by clinical criteria) to 10% (by endoscopy). Allergic rashes and urticaria occur with an incidence of about 10%. Rarely, a Stevens-Johnson-like syndrome occurs. Anaphylaxis has also occurred. Transient neutropenia and eosinophilia occur, and thrombocytopenia and agranulocytosis have been reported.

By the oral route, bioavailability is about 90% with low doses (150 mg) but 23 to 38% with higher doses. The presence of food in the stomach and intestines does not appear to interfere with absorption. In plasma clindamycin is 60 to 95% protein-bound. Its volume of distribution is about 1 mL/g. Most of the clindamycin is eliminated in the liver, only about 10% being excreted in the urine. The half-life is 2.4 to 3 hr, except 3.5 to 5 hr in anuria and 7 to 14 hr in liver disease. Hepatic failure can be expected to reduce the dose requirement more than renal failure.

Dose (base equivalent)—*Oral, adults,* for *moderately severe* infections, **150 to 300 mg** every 6 hr; for *very severe* infections, **300 to 450 mg** every 6 hr; *infants 1 mo* of age and *older*, **2 to 6.3 mg/kg** every 6 hr or **2.7 to 8.3 mg/kg** every 8 hr. In children under 10 kg in weight the dose should be no less than a total of 37.5 mg. Use cautiously in infants less than 1 mo old. To avoid esophageal irritation, take each dose with a full glass of water. Treatment of infections caused by anaerobes should be initiated with parenteral clindamycin (clindamycin phosphate), then switched to oral medication when the condition shows improvement.

Dosage Forms (clindamycin equivalent)—Capsules: 75 and 150 mg.

Clindamycin Palmitate Hydrochloride

L-*threo*-α-D-*galacto*-Octopyranoside, methyl 7-chloro-6,7,8-trideoxy-6-[[(1-methyl-4-propyl-2-pyrrolidinyl)carbonyl]amino]-1-thio-2-hexadecanoate, (2S-*trans*)-, monohydrochloride;
Cleocin Pediatric (*Upjohn*)

[25507-04-4] $C_{34}H_{63}ClN_2O_6S \cdot HCl$ (699.86). Potency: equivalent to not less than 540 μg of clindamycin ($C_{18}H_{33}ClN_2O_5S$)/mg.

Preparation—The 3- and 4-OH groups of clindamycin are protected by condensation with cuminaldehyde and the 2-OH group is then condensed with palmitoyl chloride at the marked hydroxyl group (see structure for *clindamycin hydrochloride*). The protecting group is then removed through appropriate hydrolytic procedure and the clindamycin palmitate is finally reacted with an equimolar quantity of HCl.

Description—White to off-white, amorphous powder with a characteristic odor and taste; may form lumps and glass-like crystals when drying; stable in light, heat (up to 50°), and air.

Solubility—1 g in 5 mL water, 3 mL alcohol, 4 mL chloroform; freely soluble in ether.

Uses—Converted to clindamycin in the small intestine. It has the same actions and uses as *Clindamycin Hydrochloride*. The palmitate lacks the bitter taste of clindamycin and is thus suited to use in an oral solution for pediatric use. The absorption time, plasma levels, and plasma half-life are identical to those of clindamycin hydrochloride; the half-life in young children is about 2 hours.

Dose (clindamycin equivalent)—*Oral, children*, as for *Clindamycin Hydrochloride;* the palmitate is not usually used in adults.

Dosage Form (clindamycin equivalent)—for Oral Solution: 75 mg/5 mL.

Clindamycin Phosphate

L-*threo*-α-D-*galacto*-Octopyranoside, methyl-7-chloro-6,7,8-trideoxy-6-[[(1-methyl-4-propyl-2-pyrrolidinyl)carbonyl]amino]-1-thio-, (2S-*trans*)-, 2-(dihydrogen phosphate), Cleocin Phosphate (*Upjohn*)

[24729-96-2] $C_{18}H_{34}ClN_2O_8PS$ (504.96). Potency: equivalent to not less than 758 μg of clindamycin/mg.

Preparation—The 3- and 4-OH groups of clindamycin are protected by condensation with cuminaldehyde and the 2-OH* group (refer to the structure of the hydrochloride, p 1209) is then condensed with $POCl_3$. Appropriate hydrolytic procedures finally convert the —$OPOCl_2$ residue to —$OPO(OH)_2$ and remove the protecting group.

Description—White to off-white, hygroscopic, crystalline powder; odorless or nearly so; bitter taste; stable in light and air but unstable in temperature of 50° (degrades to free clindamycin); melts with decomposition at about 175°.

Solubility—1 g in 2.5 mL water, >1000 mL alcohol.

Uses—Rapidly hydrolyzed in the plasma to clindamycin. Thus it has the same actions and uses as *Clindamycin Hydrochloride*, except that the phosphate is given parenterally, which avoids the gastrointestinal side effects of the oral forms of clindamycin. However, the dangers of anaphylaxis are greater. Although the phosphate is promoted for treatment of infections of all grades of severity, it would seem advisable to withhold its use in mild infections, unless the oral forms cannot be tolerated. In infections caused by anaerobes, treatment with clindamycin should be initiated with this derivative given parenterally. Clindamycin phosphate is also applied topically in the treatment of acne vulgaris.

Dose (clindamycin equivalent)—*Intramuscular* or *intravenous, adults, usually* **300 to 600 mg** every 6 to 8 hr; up to 2.7 g/day may be given, if necessary; *children over 1 month old*, **3.75 to 10 mg/kg** (or

87.5 to 112.5 mg/m² of body surface) every 6 hr *or* **5 to 13.3 mg/kg** (or 116.7 to 150 mg/m²) every 8 hr; irrespective of body weight, for severe infections the minimum daily dose is 300 mg. *Topical*, to the *skin*, as 0.1% solution twice a day.

Dosage Forms (clindamycin equivalent)—Injection: 300 mg/2 mL and 600 mg/4 mL; Topical Solution: 1 mg/mL.

Cycloserine

3-Isoxazolidinone, 4-amino-, (R)-, Seromycin (*Lilly*); Oxamycin (*MSD*)

(+)-4-Amino-3-isoxazolidinone [68-41-7] $C_3H_6N_2O_2$ (102.09); a substance produced by the growth of *Streptomyces orchidaceus* or obtained by synthesis. Potency: not less than 900 μg of $C_3H_6N_2O_2$/mg.

Preparation—Cycloserine may be isolated from the fermentation of *Streptomyces orchidaceus* or made synthetically from DL-serine (see RPS-15, page 1146).

Description—White to pale yellow, crystalline powder; odorless or has a faint odor; hygroscopic and deteriorates upon absorbing water.
Solubility—Freely soluble in water.

Uses—Inhibits a wide variety of both gram-positive and gram-negative bacteria, and mycobacteria. However, *Pseudomonas*, *Proteus*, and gonococci are resistant. It has been used successfully against stubborn *urinary tract infections* caused by streptococci, staphylococci, *E coli* and *Enterobacter aerogenes*. However, interest mainly centers on its moderate usefulness in the therapy of *tuberculosis* resistant to other drugs; it is a "back-up" drug secondary to isoniazid, streptomycin, and aminosalicylic acid. It is always combined with other antituberculosis drugs. It should not be used unless other antitubercular drugs have become ineffective or are contraindicated. Resistance to cycloserine does develop.

Depending on the dose, toxic effects referable to the central nervous system occur within the first 2 weeks (usually) in a large percentage of patients. These are reversible on discontinuance of therapy. Such effects are headache, vertigo, paresis, dysarthria, lethargy, somnolence, depression, confusion, irritability, behavioral changes, psychotic episodes with suicidal tendencies, hyperreflexia, tremors, twitching, ankle clonus, and convulsions. Central nervous system toxicity can be controlled by the administration of pyridoxine, anticonvulsants, sedatives, and tranquilizing agents. Toxic effects are minimized if blood levels of the drug do not exceed 25 to 30 μg/mL. Skin rashes may occur.

Oral bioavailability is 70 to 90%. Cycloserine penetrates into all body fluids, cavities, and tubercles. The levels in cerebrospinal fluid are 50 to 80% of those in plasma, except 80 to 100 in meningitis. About 70% is eliminated in urine; the half-life is 10 hr but longer in renal failure.

Dose—*Oral, adults* and *children over 10 yr* of age, **250 mg** every 12 hr; in tuberculosis, after the first 2 weeks the dose-interval is cautiously shortened to as short as every 6 hr, according to plasma levels and adverse effects; *children 2 to 10 yr*, **125 mg** every 12 hr for urinary tract infections and **5 to 20 mg/kg** a day in divided doses for tuberculosis; *infants* and *children up to 2 yr*, **62.5 mg** every 12 hr, except **5 to 20 mg/kg** a day in tuberculosis.
Dosage Form—Capsules: 250 mg.

Rifampin

Rifamycin, 3-[[(4-methyl-1-piperazinyl)imino]methyl]-, Rifampicin; Rifadin (*Dow*); Rimactane (*Ciba-Geigy*)

[13292-46-1] $C_{43}H_{58}N_4O_{12}$ (822.95). Potency: not less than 900 μg of $C_{43}H_{58}N_4O_{12}$/mg.

Preparation—Rifamycin SV, which may be prepared by the method of Sensi, et al (US Pat 3,313,804), is converted to the 8-carboxaldehyde derivative, known also as 3-formylrifamycin SV, and this is condensed with 1-amino-4-methylpiperazine in a Schiff base reaction to yield rifampin.

Description—Red-brown, crystalline powder; odorless; unstable in light, heat, air, and moisture; melts between 183° and 188° with decomposition.

Solubility—1 g in about 762 mL water; freely soluble in chloroform; soluble in ethyl acetate and methanol.

Uses—A broad-spectrum antibiotic effective against most gram-positive bacteria, especially *Staph pyogenes*, *Strep pyogenes*, *Strep viridans*, and *D pneumoniae*, and variably active against gram-negative organisms, especially *H influenzae*, meningococci and gonococci. Both *Mycobacterium tuberculosis* and *Mycobacterium leprae* are very susceptible to the drug. Unfortunately, many bacteria very rapidly acquire resistance to rifampin; this, along with the superiority of other antibiotics against many of the above-cited bacteria and the desire to avoid inadvertent development of resistance of mycobacteria to the drug, is an important reason why rifampin enjoys a very limited range of use. Its clinical use is mainly in the treatment of tuberculosis. The rate of development of resistance of the mycobacterium is low. Nevertheless, rifampin is always used in combination with other antitubercular drugs; it may be added to isoniazid and ethambutol to make a first-choice combination for treatment of infections caused by *Mycobacterium tuberculosis*, to isoniazid for those caused by *atypical mycobacteria*, and to dapsone for *leprosy*. It also appears to be an excellent drug for *prophylaxis of meningococcal* disease and treatment of meningococcal carrier state.

Rifampin may cause heartburn, epigastric distress, gas, cramps, diarrhea, anorexia, and nausea and vomiting. Headache, drowsiness, and fatigue commonly occur, and inability to concentrate, confusion, muscular weakness, ataxia, pain in the extremities, visual disturbances, and generalized numbness are other CNS side effects. Immunologic disturbances may occur, such as occasional rheumatoid and lupoid syndromes, allergic rashes, eosinophilia, leukopenia, and hemolytic anemia. Thrombocytopenia is frequent and a monthly thrombocyte count is advisable. Avoidance of high doses also helps to obviate thrombocytopenia. Jaundice and other manifestations of hepatotoxicity have occurred during treatment. Where possible, it is wise to avoid using rifampin in combination with ethionamide, prothionamide, pyrazinamide, or *p*-aminosalicylates, which can also cause hepatic dysfunction. Rifampin induces the hepatic drug metabolizing enzyme system and accelerates the metabolism of digitoxin, methadone, phenytoin, oral contraceptives and estrogens, oral anticoagulants, barbiturates, tolbutamide, and itself. However, it is also a competitive inhibitor of cytochrome P450 and hence may inhibit the metabolism of some of these same and other drugs. Probenecid inhibits metabolism of rifampin by blocking uptake into hepatocytes. Rifampin is teratogenic in laboratory animals and should therefore be withheld in pregnancy.

Rifampin is 100% absorbed after oral administration, but food in the stomach delays absorption of the drug. Bentonite in granules of *p*-aminosalicylic acid also interferes with absorption, and the granules should not be given close to the time of rifampin administration. Rifampin is widely distributed in the body, even into cerebrospinal fluid. In plasma 98% is protein-bound. The volume of distribution is 0.9 mL/g. About 85% of the drug is eliminated by biotransformation in the liver. An active metabolite is secreted into bile, where it is therapeutically effective. Metabolism is dose-dependent with doses above 300 to 450 mg, so that with therapeutic doses the serum half-life is 1.5 to 5 hr. Even so, the drug is usually administered at 8- to 12-hr intervals, because absorption is slow enough to sustain effective levels for 8 to 10 hours. Nevertheless, patients who eliminate the drug rapidly probably should be considered for a different schedule. About $\frac{1}{3}$ of a dose is excreted in the feces via the bile. Although rifampin does not appear to accumulate in patients with hepatic insufficiency, the hepatic metabolism and the fact that the drug may be hepatotoxic suggest that rifampin should be used cautiously in hepatic dysfunction. The risk of hepatotoxicity is increased when rifampin is used with isoniazid. Rifampin colors the urine red, and the patient should be forewarned.

Dose—*Oral, adults*, **600 mg** once a day, taken with a glass of water at least 1 hr before a meal; against the meningococcal carrier state, only 4 days of use are required; *children over 5 yr of age*, **10 to 20 mg/kg** of body weight once a day. Some authorities recommend 2 or 3 divided doses. Schedules based on single daily or twice weekly doses are incompatible with the brief sojourn of this drug in the body. Furthermore, if the single doses are high, massive hemolysis is favored. The drug should always be used in combination with at least one other antitubercular drug.

Dosage Forms—Capsules: 150 and 300 mg; in combination with isoniazid, Capsules: 300 mg rifampin and 150 mg isoniazid; Tablets: 300 mg.

Spectinomycin Hydrochloride

4*H*-Pyrano[2,3-*b*][1,4]benzodioxin-4-one, decahydro-4a,7,9-trihydroxy-2-methyl-6,8-bis(methylamino)-, [2*R*-(2α,4aβ,5aβ,6β,7β,8β,9α,9aα,10aβ)]-, dihydrochloride, pentahydrate; Trobicin (*Upjohn*)

[22189-32-8]; $C_{14}H_{24}N_2O_7 \cdot 2HCl \cdot 5H_2O$ (495.35); *anhydrous* [21736-83-4] (405.27). Potency: equivalent to not less than 603 μg spectinomycin/mg.

Preparation—By growth of the soil microorganism *Streptomyces spectabilis*. Reaction with a double equimolar quantity of HCl yields the hydrochloride. *Antibiot Chemother 11:* 118 and 661, 1961. US Pat 3,234,092.

Description—White, odorless, crystalline powder with a slightly bitter taste; stable in light, nonhygroscopic, and stable in air at room temperature.

Solubility—1 g in about 7 mL water; practically insoluble in alcohol, chloroform, and ether.

Uses—Spectinomycin is a wide-spectrum antibiotic with moderate activity against both gram-positive and gram-negative bacteria. However, it is employed clinically for only one purpose, namely, to treat or prevent acute gonorrhea when the organism is resistant to penicillin, or when the patient is allergic to penicillin. Clinical studies have shown it to be no more efficacious than tetracycline and possibly no better against some strains of gonococcus than ampicillin or erythromycin. It is advantageous, however, in that a single dose usually suffices.

The drug is poorly absorbed orally and must be given intramuscularly; 2 g will provide a plasma concentration of about 100 μg/mL. The distribution coefficient is 0.12 mL/g. About 75% is excreted into urine unchanged. Plasma half-life is approximately 1 day.

Untoward effects caused by spectinomycin include frequent pain at the site of injection and infrequent headache, nausea, vomiting, insomnia, chills, fever, mild pruritus, and urticaria. Undoubtedly the toxicity would be much greater if the drug were administered repetitively rather than as a single dose. Spectinomycin does not eradicate *Treponema*, but it may delay or mask signs of early syphilis and thus engender a false sense of security.

Dose (base equivalent)—*Intramuscular, adults*, as a single injection, usually **2 g**, but **4 g** is used in regions in which partial resistance to the drug is known to occur; *children* weighing *less than 45 kg*, **40 mg/kg.**

Dosage Forms—for Injection: 2 and 4 g.

Vancomycin Hydrochloride

Vancomycin, hydrochloride; Vancocin (*Lilly*)

Vancomycin hydrochloride [1404-93-9] is a substance produced by growth of *Streptomyces orientalis* (Fam *Streptomycetaceae*). Potency: equivalent to not less than 900 μg of vancomycin per mg, calculated on the anhydrous basis.

The structure of vancomycin, a glycopeptide, has been intensively studied and continues to be investigated. A molecular weight of about 3300 has been proposed; analyses show that it contains about 7% nitrogen, 16% carbohydrate, and about 4.4% of chlorine; a branched-chain aminosugar, *vancosamine*, obtained by acid hydrolysis of vancomycin, has received structural study, as have also aromatic rings in the compound.

Preparation—Vancomycin is produced by the submerged fermentation process (page 1178). After purification the base is converted to the soluble hydrochloride with HCl.

Description—Tan to brown, free-flowing powder; odorless; bitter taste.

Solubility—Freely soluble in water; insoluble in ether, chloroform.

Uses—Vancomycin is highly active against gram-positive cocci, neisseria, and clostridia. It inhibits synthesis of peptidoglycan in cell-wall formation. It is the drug of choice in the treatment of antibiotic-associated colitis and other infections caused by *Cl dificile*. It has proved valuable in the treatment of severe staphylococcic infections. Development of resistance to vancomycin is virtually unknown, and there is no cross-resistance from other antibiotics. This is extremely important, since staphylococci are capable of resisting all the major systemic antibiotics, and a "back-up" drug is needed. Streptococcal, micrococcal, and pneumococcal infections have also been successfully treated with vancomycin. It should not be used alone in treating enterococcal endocarditis. Used systemically, the drug may cause deafness, skin rashes, and fever. Renal failure predisposes to these effects. Consequently the drug is held in reserve for serious infections unresponsive to other antibacterial agents.

Vancomycin is poorly absorbed from the gastrointestinal tract, so that it may be used orally against staphylococcal and enterococcal enteritis. However, severe enteritis often requires concomitant systemic therapy and hence parenteral administration. In plasma, 10% is protein-bound. The volume of distribution is 0.47 mL/g. The plasma half-life is 2 to 6 hr. Since the drug is 95% eliminated by excretion in urine, the half-life in anuric patients ranges from 3 to 10 days and doses must be appropriately adjusted. Vancomycin is irritating and may cause thrombophlebitis, or pain at the site of injection; also chills, fever, occasional urticaria and maculopapular rashes, nephrotoxicity and ototoxicity, and, rarely, neuropathy. The drug is contraindicated in patients taking, or who have recently taken, ototoxic or nephrotoxic drugs, except that it is used in combination with streptomycin for surgical prophylaxis against bacterial endocarditis in penicillin-sensitive patients. Elderly persons should have serial auditory tests and determinations of plasma levels of the drug.

Dose (vancomycin equivalent)—*Oral* and *intravenous, adults,* usually either **500 mg** every 6 hr *or* **1 g** every 12 hr; as much as 2 g may be given per day in very serious infections. *Neonates* and *premature infants* (intravenous only), **5 mg/kg** of body weight every 12 hr; *older infants* and *children,* **10 to 11 mg/kg** (or 300 mg per m^2 of body surface) every 6 hr. Intravenous doses should be dissolved in 100 to 250 mL of an isotonic solution and infused over a period of 20 to 30 min. It is desirable to maintain C_{min} above 15 μg/mL and C_{max} below 30 to 40 μg/mL, except lower in combination with an aminoglycoside.

Dosage Forms (vancomycin equivalent)—Sterile: 500 mg; for Oral Solution: 10 g.

Other Miscellaneous Antibiotics

Fosfomycin   [(−)-(1*R*,2*S*)-(1,2-Epoxypropyl)phosphoric   acid [23155-01-4] $C_3H_7O_4P$ (138.06)]—An antibiotic produced by *Streptomyces fradiae;* crystals that melt at about 94°; soluble in water. *Uses:* Has activity against both gram-positive and gram-negative bacteria. Among enteric organisms (*E coli, Klebsiella, Proteus, Pseudomonas, Serratia,* and *S fecalis*) over 80% of strains are sensitive, and most of the remainder are sensitive in combination with an aminoglycoside, amoxicillin, or carbenicillin. The drug has been used successfully in the treatment of urinary tract infections, infantile acute gastroenteritis, and pneumonia, bronchitis, and other respiratory infections caused by susceptible organisms. The drug is only about 37% absorbed by the oral route. It has a volume of distribution of about 0.39 mL/g. Renal excretion accounts for approximately 75% of elimination. The elimination half-life is about 2 hr. Side-effects include rashes, diarrhea, and induration at intramuscular sites of injection. *Dose: Intramuscular* or *intravenous* (as the sodium salt), *adults,* 500 mg every 6 hr; *children,* 37.5 mg/kg every 6 hr. *Oral* (as the calcium salt), tentatively the same as the parenteral dose.

Fusidate   Sodium   [Sodium   3α,11α,16β-trihydroxy-29-nor-8α,9β,13α,14β-dammara-17(20),24-dien-21-oate 16-acetate, [751-94-0] $C_{31}H_{47}NaO_6$ (538.67); Fucidin (*Squibb*)]—A steroid antibiotic obtained from the fermentation broth of *Fusidium coccineum.* White powder; concentrated neutral sterile solutions are stable for several weeks, but concentrations below 0.1 μg/mL are stable for only a few days: less stable in alkaline than in neutral or acid media. Freely soluble in water. *Uses:* Active primarily against gram-positive bacteria and gram-negative cocci but very low activity against gram-negative bacilli and fungi. Clostridia and corynebacteria are especially sensitive. It is highly effective against both penicillin-resistant and penicillin-sensitive strains of *Staphylococcus aureus* and is thus clinically useful in the treatment of infections caused by penicillin-resistant staphylococci. Although staphylococci and other

bacteria become resistant, *in vitro* resistance is uncommon in the clinic. No cross-resistance has been observed with any clinically used antibiotics. The drug is excreted into the bile and is also metabolized in the body; only 10% is excreted in the urine. The only side effects are due to local irritation and these seldom necessitate discontinuance of treatment. *Dose:* 500 mg 3 times daily. Sodium fusidate is available in Canada and abroad but not in the US.

Lincomycin   Hydrochloride   [Methyl   6,8-dideoxy-6-(1-methyl-*trans*-4-propyl-L-2-pyrrolidinecarboxamido)-1-thio-D-*erythro*-α-D-*galacto*-octopyranoside   monohydrochloride   monohydrate [7179-49-9] $C_{18}H_{34}N_2O_6S.HCl.H_2O$ (461.01) Lincocin (*Upjohn*); a substance produced by the growth of a member of the *lincolnensis* group of *Streptomyces lincolnensis* (Fam *Streptomycetaceae*) Potency: equivalent to not less than 790 μg of lincomycin/mg.]—*Description and solubility:* White or practically white, crystalline powder; odorless or has a faint odor and a bitter taste; stable in light and air; pK_a 7.92. Freely soluble in water. *Uses:* The antibacterial activity of lincomycin resembles that of *Erythromycin.* It has a rather broad spectrum of activity against gram-positive organisms, especially staphylococci, pneumococci, pyogenic streptococci, clostridia, and corynebacteria. Unlike erythromycin, it has little efficacy against enterococci. Gram-negative cocci, such as gonococci and meningococci, are also very little affected by the drug, and gram-negative bacilli are unaffected. Lincomycin has been essentially displaced by clindamycin because of the greater potency of the latter and also because it has been thought that clindamycin was safer. Lincomycin is effective against actinomycosis. It is used to treat serious pneumococcal, staphylococcal and streptococcal infections of the respiratory and urinary tracts or of soft tissues when the infecting organism is susceptible and other antibiotics cannot be used, as in penicillin allergy or resistance. Since there is no cross-resistance between penicillin and lincomycin and infrequently between erythromycin and lincomycin, the drug is useful when resistance to other antibiotics emerges. Resistance to lincomycin does develop, although slowly. Resistance develops faster if the bacterium is already resistant to erythromycin. Lincomycin may cause nausea and vomiting, abdominal cramps, or diarrhea in some patients, and it may induce pseudomembranous colitis which lasts for 1 to 2 weeks after the drug is stopped. It now appears that the incidence is no higher and may be even less than with clindamycin, so that the status of lincomycin should be reevaluated. Less frequently there may be headache, tinnitus, dizziness, malaise and aching, pruritus, rash, proctitis, vaginitis, or moniliasis. Jaundice, leukopenia, or neutropenia rarely occur. Rapid intravenous infusion can cause syncope and even cardiopulmonary arrest. Phlebitis can also result from intravenous infusion. Lincomycin is about 30% absorbed from the gut; food in the stomach decreases absorption. The drug is eliminated about 30% by renal excretion and partly by hepatic metabolism. The plasma half-life is 4 to 7 hr, except that it may be as long as 10 to 13 hr in renal failure and 9 hr in hepatic insufficiency. *Dose:* (base equivalent), *oral, adults,* 500 mg every 8 hr for serious infections and 500 mg or more every 6 hr for more severe infections; *children over 1 month of age,* 30 mg/kg of body weight per day in 3 or 4 divided doses in serious infections and 60 mg/kg per day in more severe infections. *Intramuscular, adults,* 600 mg every 24 hr in serious infections and every 12 hr or more often in more severe infections; *children over 1 month of age,* 10 mg/kg of body weight every 24 hr in serious and every 12 hr in more severe infections. *Intravenous, adults,* 600 mg to 1 g every 8 to 12 hr in serious infections and up to 8 g a day in more severe or fulminating infections; *children over 1 month of age,* 10 to 20 mg/kg per day, depending on the infection, to be given in divided doses. Intravenous doses should be infused over a period of at least 1 hr. *Subconjunctival,* 75 mg.

Novobiocin   Sodium   [Novobiocin monosodium salt [1476-53-5] $C_{31}H_{35}N_2NaO_{11}$ (634.61); Albamycin (*Upjohn*)]—Contains the equivalent of not less than 80% of novobiocin. White or practically white, crystalline powder; odorless or practically odorless and hygroscopic; pH between 6.5 and 8.5. Very soluble in water; freely soluble in alcohol. *Uses:* Mainly active against gram-positive organisms, especially *Staphylococcus aureus.* It usually has little or no activity against gram-negative organisms, but certain strains of *Proteus vulgaris* and coliform bacteria are moderately susceptible to the drug. It is only moderately active against gram-negative cocci. Its use should be reserved for treatment of infections caused by staphylococci that have proved resistant to all other safe antibiotics or for other infections in the occasional patient that is allergic to all the common effective antibiotics. Since staphylococci readily become resistant to novobiocin, it is imperative that its use be limited by the above conditions, lest its usefulness as a drug-in-reserve be destroyed. Novobiocin has a relatively high index of sensitization with both dermatologic and hematologic manifestations. Leukopenia, anemia, pancytopenia, agranulocytosis, and thrombocytopenia have occurred. The drug may also induce nausea and vomiting, diarrhea, abdominal pain, intestinal hemorrhage, vertigo, drowsiness, arthritis, conjunctivitis, alopecia, pneumonitis, jaundice, hyperbilirubinemia, and myocarditis. The principal route of administration is oral, although intravenous or intramuscular injection may be used when oral therapy is not feasible. Intramuscular deposition is painful. *Dose* (equivalent of novobiocin): *Intravenous,* by infusion, or *intramuscular, adults,* 500 mg every 12 hr; *children,* 7.5 mg/kg every 12 hr for moderate acute infections and 15 mg/kg every 12 hr in very severe infections.

Viomycin   Sulfate   [Viomycin   sulfate   (salt)   [37883-00-4]

$C_{25}H_{43}N_{13}O_{10} \cdot xH_2SO_4$; Viocin Sulfate (*Pfizer*) the sulfate salt of an antibacterial substance produced by the growth of *Streptomyces puniceus*, *Streptomyces floridae*, or *Actinomyces vinaceus*, or by other means. It contains an amount of viomycin sulfate equivalent to not less than 700 μg of viomycin/mg, calculated on the anhydrous basis.]—*Description and solubility:* White to slightly yellow, crystalline powder; hygroscopic; odorless or practically so. Freely soluble in water; very slightly soluble in alcohol; insoluble in chloroform, or ether. *Uses:* Unlike other antibiotics, viomycin is relatively more active against mycobacteria than against any other genus of microorganisms. However, it is not as potent as streptomycin, and its toxicity is relatively greater. But, it is active against streptomycin- and isoniazid-resistant strains of tubercle bacilli, so that it finds uses as an *antituberculous agent* when the causative organisms become resistant to other antituberculous drugs. Because of its toxicity, viomycin should not be used for routine therapy of minimal or primary pulmonary tuberculosis, unless other therapy has failed. However, it may be used as an adjunct to the therapy of extrapulmonary tuberculosis, pneumonic tuberculosis or progressive exudative tuberculosis with hematogenous lesions. It may also be employed prophylactically with chest surgery in tuberculous patients. Other antituberculous agents should be combined with viomycin. Viomycin may cause renal damage, edema or fluid retention, allergic reactions, ototoxicity, with both vestibular dysfunction (eg vertigo) and partial loss of hearing, and electrocardiographic abnormalities. Toxic manifestations are fewer and less severe with intramuscular than with intravenous injection; thus the intramuscular route is mandatory. Viomycin is not absorbed by the oral route. About 80% is eliminated by renal excretion. The half-life is 2 hr in persons with normal renal function. *Dose: Intramuscular*, 1 g 2 times in one day twice a week. A course of therapy is 4 to 6 months. During the first month 2 g may be given daily, if necessary, only if laboratory facilities to monitor toxicity are available. The drug is not recommended for children.

Miscellaneous Systemic Antibacterial Drugs

Aminosalicylate Calcium

Benzoic acid, 4-amino-2-hydroxy-, calcium salt (2:1), trihydrate

Calcium 4-aminosalicylate (1:2) trihydrate [133-15-3 (*anhydrous*)] $C_{14}H_{12}CaN_2O_6 \cdot 3H_2O$ (398.38).

Preparation—From *p*-aminosalicylic acid and calcium carbonate.

Description—White crystals with a distinctive taste.

Solubility—1 g dissolves in 7 mL of water; aqueous solutions slowly darken, with decomposition.

Uses—See *Aminosalicylate Sodium* (below). The calcium salt avoids the problem of sodium overloading. However, it may contribute to hypercaliuria.

Dose (aminosalicylate equivalent)—See *Aminosalicylic Acid* (below).

Aminosalicylate Sodium

Benzoic acid, 4-amino-2-hydroxy-, monosodium salt, dihydrate;
Sodium 4-Aminosalicylate; Sodium Para-aminosalicylate;
Sod. PAS; *Various Mfrs*

Monosodium 4-aminosalicylate dihydrate [6018-19-5] $C_7H_6NNaO_3 \cdot 2H_2O$ (211.15); *anhydrous* [133-10-8] (175.12).

Caution—Prepare solutions of Aminosalicylate Sodium within 24 hours of administration. Under no circumstances use a solution if its color is darker than that of a freshly prepared solution.

Preparation—This salt is ordinarily prepared by neutralizing the free acid with sodium hydroxide or sodium carbonate, and precipitating the sodium salt by addition of ethanol.

Description—White to cream-colored, crystalline powder; practically odorless; taste sweet and saline; aqueous solutions decompose slowly and darken in color; pH (aqueous 1:50 solution) between 6.5 and 8.5.

Solubility—1 g in about 2 mL water; sparingly soluble in alcohol; very slightly soluble in ether and chloroform.

Uses—One of two salts of para-aminosalicylic acid (PAS) used in the treatment of *tuberculosis*. PAS is bacteriostatic, so that it only arrests but does not eradicate the tubercle bacillus. Used alone, it can sometimes successfully manage the disease, but resistance emerges and also toxicity limits the dose. Therefore, PAS is always used in combination with 1 or 2 other antitubercular drugs. In such combinations, the PAS supports the other drugs and delays emergence of resistance. It is not in any first-choice combination and is considered to be a third- or lower-choice component.

The incidence of adverse effects is about 20%. PAS frequently causes epigastric discomfort, anorexia, nausea, vomiting, diarrhea, and peptic ulceration. High-capacity antacids and aluminum hydroxide gel lessen the incidence of gastrointestinal symptoms, but aluminum hydroxide interferes with absorption. By converting PAS to aminosalicylate sodium, some buffering is achieved in the stomach, which lessens the incidence and intensity of gastrointestinal distress. It also prevents systemic acidosis caused by PAS. Occasionally, soft stools and diarrhea occur. PAS tends to crystallize in the urine when it is acidic; the resulting crystalluria can cause renal tubular damage. With aminosalicylate sodium, the urine may be neutral or slightly alkaline, depending on the diet. Crystalluria is thus less common; nevertheless, a good fluid intake and fruit juices or bicarbonate may still be indicated. When sodium intake should be restricted, the drug is contraindicated. About 4% of recipients manifest some form of hypersensitivity: eosinophilia, malaise, myalgia, sore throat, dermatoses, drug fever, leukopenia, agranulocytosis, thrombocytopenia, hemolytic anemia, jaundice, pancreatitis, myeloradiculoneuritis, vasculitis, Loeffler's pulmonic syndrome, encephalopathy, goiter, or hypokalemia may occur. Salicylism does not occur. PAS displaces oral anticoagulants from plasma proteins.

PAS is excreted in urine to an extent of about 50%; the remainder is acetylated PAS. The plasma half-life is 45 to 6 min, except up to 23 hr in renal failure; patients fall into one or the other groups of fast and slow acetylators.

Dose (aminosalicylate equivalent)—See *Aminosalicylic Acid* (below).

Dosage Forms—Tablets (regular, enteric-coated): 500 and 1 g; Powder for Oral Solution: 4.18 g. Each g contains 4.8 mEq of sodium.

Aminosalicylic Acid

Benzoic acid, 4-amino-2-hydroxy-, PAS

4-Aminosalicylic acid [65-49-6] $C_7H_7NO_3$ (153.14).

Caution—Under no circumstances use a solution if its color is darker than that of a freshly prepared solution.

Preparation—From *m*-aminophenol by a modification of the Kolbe-Schmitt reaction which involves heating the phenol under pressure with a source of carbon dioxide such as ammonium carbonate or potassium bicarbonate.

Description—White, or nearly white, bulky powder; darkens on exposure to light and air; odorless, or has a slight acetous odor; melts between 135° and 140° with decompositioin; pH (saturated aqueous solution) between 3 and 3.7.

Solubility—1 g in about 600 mL water and about 21 mL alcohol; slightly soluble in ether.

Uses—See *Aminosalicylate Sodium* for *antitubercular* actions, uses, adverse effects, and pharmacokinetics. It is also used to lower blod lipids; it can lower the low-density lipoproteins (and cholesterol) by 15 to 20%, and the very-low-density lipoproteins (and triglycerides) by 25%. It is used mainly in the treatment of *familial* hypercholesterolemia. The drug impairs absorption of cholesterol. The incidence of gastrointestinal disturbances and of crystalluria is greater than with the sodium salt. A preparation of aminosalicylic acid stated to have much of its irritant impurities removed by recrystallization with ascorbic acid (PAS-C, *Hellwig*) is reported to induce a lesser incidence of gastrointestinal side effects. Aminosalicylic acid can cause systemic acidosis in children. The urine should be alkalinized.

Dose—*Oral, adults*, for *tuberculosis*, **3 g** to **4 g** every 8 hr or **5 to 6 g** every 12 hr, but up to 20 g a day; for *antihyperlipidemia* therapy, **6 to 8 g** a day in 1 or 2 doses. In adults, 4 g may provide plasma levels of about 75 µg/mL in 1½ to 2 hr; *children*, for *tuberculosis*, **50 to 75 mg/kg** every 6 hr or **66.7 to 100 mg/kg** every 8 hr, not to exceed 12 g a day. Dosage adjustments may be required in renal failure.

Dosage Forms—Tablets (regular, buffered or enteric-coated): 500 mg.

Dapsone

Benzenamine 4,4′-sulfonylbis-, Avlosulfon (*Ayerst*)

$$H_2N\text{—}\bigcirc\text{—}\underset{O}{\overset{O}{\underset{\|}{\overset{\|}{S}}}}\text{—}\bigcirc\text{—}NH_2$$

4,4′-Sulfonyldianiline [80-08-0] $C_{12}H_{12}N_2O_2S$ (248.30).

Preparation—Benzene is condensed with sulfuric acid to yield phenyl sulfone $[(C_6H_5)_2SO_2]$ which is then nitrated by standard procedures to yield the 4,4′-dinitro derivative. Reduction with tin and HCl or with various other appropriate reductants yields dapsone.

Description—White or creamy white, crystalline powder; odorless and has a slightly bitter taste; melts between 175° and 181°.

Solubility—Very slightly soluble in water; freely soluble in alcohol; soluble in dilute mineral acids.

Uses—Dapsone has an antibacterial spectrum and mechanism of action similar to that of sulfanilamide (see *Sulfonamides*, page 1170), of which dapsone was originally studied as a congener. Limited success against tuberculosis has been achieved with dapsone, but it is far surpassed by other agents. However, dapsone is a useful drug in the chemotherapy of *leprosy*. Most of the sulfones used in the treatment of this disease owe both their activity and toxicity to dapsone released from the molecule. For this reason, dapsone is the preferred sulfone, since it is cheaper than and equally efficacious to the other sulfones. Dapsone is of some limited value in the treatment of *malaria*, especially that caused by *P falciparum;* it may be combined with other antimalarial drugs, especially pyrimethamine. It is also useful as a suppressant in the treatment of *dermatitis herpetiformis*.

Dapsone is absorbed by the oral route. Absorption is more efficient with low than with high doses; 50 mg per day will give a steady-state concentration of 5 to 7 µg/mL, and 100 mg only 7 to 9 µg/mL. It is eliminated in the liver by acetylation. There are slow and fast acetylators among patients. The half-life is 10 to 50 hr, and 4 to 20 days are required to reach plateau concentrations.

Dapsone may cause hemolytic anemia in glucose 6-phosphate dehydrogenase-deficient persons, methemoglobinemia, gastrointestinal upset, headache, nervousness, giddiness, tachycardia, motor neuropathy, blurred vision, paresthesias and pruritus, hematuria, liver damage, and jaundice or rash which may become exfoliative. The dermatitis frequently occurs during the 5th week of therapy. Hypermelanosis follows. Lepra reactions (erythema nodosum-like) may occur from a flooding of the body with endotoxins released from killed organisms. Careful initial grading of dose and rest periods avoids much of the toxicity.

Dose—*Oral, adults*, for *leprosy*, **50 to 100 mg** (or 0.9 to 1.4 mg/kg) once a day; for *dermatitis herpetiformis, initially* **50 mg** a day with gradual increments up to 300 mg a day, if necessary; *children*, for *leprosy* and *dermatitis herpetiformis*, **0.9 to 1.4 mg/kg** once a day.

Dosage Forms—Tablets: 25 and 100 mg.

Ethambutol Hydrochloride

1-Butanol, 2,2′-(1,2-ethanediyldiimino)bis-, [R-(R*,R*)]-, dihydrochloride; *Myambutol* (*Lederle*)

$$CH_3CH_2\text{—}\underset{H}{\overset{CH_2OH}{\underset{|}{\overset{|}{C}}}}\text{—}NHCH_2CH_2NH\text{—}\underset{CH_2OH}{\overset{H}{\underset{|}{\overset{|}{C}}}}\text{—}CH_2CH_3 \cdot 2HCl$$

(+)-2,2′-(Ethylenediimino)di-1-butanol dihydrochloride [1070-11-7] $C_{10}H_{24}N_2O_2 \cdot 2HCl$ (277.23).

Preparation—(±)-2-Aminobutanol is resolved via its tartrate and the (+)-enantiomorph is condensed with 1,2-dichloroethane in an appropriate dehydrochlorinating environment. The ethambutol thus formed is dissolved in a suitable solvent and reacted with HCl. US Pat 3,297,707.

Description—White, crystalline powder that is essentially odorless and has a bitter taste; stable in light and heat but is hygroscopic when exposed to high relative humidities; melts between 198° and 202°.

Solubility—Freely soluble in water; soluble in alcohol; slightly soluble in ether and chloroform.

Uses—A tuberculostatic drug that is effective against tubercle bacilli resistant to isoniazid or streptomycin. It acts only on proliferating cells, apparently by interfering with synthesis of RNA. When used alone in the treatment of tuberculosis, the drug may clear the sputum of mycobacteria within 3 months in the majority of patients, but bacterial resistance occurs in 35% of cases, and relapses frequently occur. In combination with isoniazid or other tuberculostatic drugs, relapses are uncommon. It should be used as a companion drug to isoniazid. Ethambutol may also be used in combination with one of the lesser tuberculostatic drugs, such as cycloserine, pyrazinamide, or ethionamide. The ethambutol-isoniazid rifampin combinations, with or without rifampin, are now the most frequently used.

Ethambutol occasionally causes optic neuritis, with blurred vision and diminished visual acuity to green light; the effect relates to the duration of use of the drug. Although these effects disappear on discontinuation, the drug should be discontinued at the first indication of a loss in visual acuity. Eye tests should be made before and at monthly intervals after the onset of therapy. Other untoward effects include dermatitis, pruritus, anorexia, nausea, vomiting, abdominal pain, pyrosis, fever, headache, vertigo, malaise, mental confusion, disorientation, hallucinations, paresthesias, elevated serum urate levels, and gout, and abnormal liver function. Multivitamins should be given concurrently with ethambutol. Leukopenia and anaphylaxis are rare occurrences.

The oral bioavailability is 75 to 80%. Ethambutol is well distributed to most tissues and fluids but poorly in cerebrospinal fluid. The volume of distribution is 1.6 mL/g. Over 80% is eliminated in the urine. The half-life is 3 to 4 hr but up to 8 hr in renal failure.

Dose—*Oral, adults* and *children over 13 yr* of age, in combination with other tuberculostatic drugs, for *initial treatment*, **15 mg/kg** of body weight once a day; for *retreatment* of relapsed cases, **25 mg/kg** once a day for 60 days, then reduced to **15 mg/kg** once a day.

Dosage Forms—Tablets: 100 mg, 400 mg (film-coated).

Isoniazid

4-Pyridinecarboxylic acid, hydrazide; Isonicotinylhydrazine; Niconyl (*Parke-Davis*); Nydrazid (*Squibb*); Hyzyd (*Mallinckrodt*)

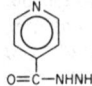

Isonicotinic acid hydrazide [54-85-3] $C_6H_7N_3O$ (137.14).

Preparation—By heating isonicotinic acid or its ethyl ester with anhydrous hydrazine. Isonicotinic acid may be synthesized by various oxidative processes starting with 4-methylpyridine.

Description—Colorless or white crystals, or a white, crystalline powder; odorless; slowly affected by exposure to air and light; solutions are practically neutral to litmus; melts between 170° and 173°.

Solubility—1 g in about 8 mL water and about 50 mL alcohol; slightly soluble in chloroform and ether.

Uses—Isoniazid is most potent and selective of the known *tuberculostatic antibacterial* agents, and it is regarded as the most effective agent in the therapy of tuberculosis. It has also been employed as a prophylactic for use in persons constantly exposed to tubercular patients. The fact that isoniazid gains access to all organs and to all body fluids, including cerebrospinal fluid, renders the drug of special value in treating tuberculous meningitis and other extrapulmonary forms of the disease. The drug is never used alone because of rapid emergence of resistance. Used in combination with other antitubercular drugs, it enhances the clinical response, permits lower doses of the other active agent(s) to be used, and retards emergence of resistant tubercle bacilli. It is the central drug around which various combinations are formulated. The first-choice combination contains isoniazid and ethambutol, with or without rifampin; streptomycin may be included to initiate treatment.

Untoward effects from isoniazid are relatively few except in persons who are slow acetylators, when the dose must be lowered. The effects may include restlessness, insomnia, muscle twitching, hyperreflexia, paresthesia, and even convulsions, toxic encephalopathy, optic neuritis and atrophy, and psychoses. These neurological disorders result from competition of isoniazid with pyridoxine; pyridoxine administration suppresses the neurological disorders without antagonizing the antitubercular action. Other signs of pyridoxine deficiency may occur. The drug may also cause nausea, vomiting, epigastric distress, agranulocytosis, hemolytic or aplastic anemia, thrombocytopenia, eosinophilia, fever, various rashes and dermatoses, and rheumatoid and lupoid syndromes. Hepatitis, with jaundice, occurs in about 2% of recipients over 50 years of age, but 10 to 20% will show elevations in SGOT and SGPT. The hepatic, hematologic, and dermatologic effects are probably all allergic.

Isoniazid is mostly acetylated by the liver; the rate varies considerably. In fast acetylators, the half-life is 1 to 1½ hours; in slow ones, it is 2 to 5 hours. Intramuscular injections cause local irritation.

Dose—*Oral* or *intramuscular*, *adults*, for *treatment*, **5 mg/kg** of body weight once a day up to 300 mg a day; for *prophylaxis* in persons with a positive tuberculin test, **300 mg** once a day. *Infants* and *children*, for treatment, **10 to 20 mg/kg** of body weight a day, up to 300 to 500 mg of total dose a day, except **30 mg/kg** a day in the first week of treatment of tubercular meningitis; for *prophylaxis*, **10 mg/kg** once a day, up to a maximum of 300 mg a day.

Dosage Forms—Injection: 100 mg/mL in 10-mL containers; Tablets: 100 and 300 mg. For Isoniazid and Rifampin Capsules, see *Rifampin*, page 1210.

Nitrofurantoin

2,4-Imidazolidinedione, 1-[[(5-nitro-2-furanyl)methylene]amino]-, Furadantin (*Norwich-Eaton*); *Other Mfrs*

1-[(5-Nitrofurfurylidene)amino]hydantoin [67-20-9] $C_8H_6N_4O_5$ (238.16).

Caution—Nitrofurantoin is discolored by alkali and by exposure to light, and is decomposed upon contact with metals other than stainless steel or aluminum.

Preparation—5-Nitro-2-furaldehyde (I) readily undergoes condensation with 1-aminohydantoin (II) to yield nitrofurantoin. I is synthesized by direct nitration of "2-furfural diacetate" [2-furanmethanediol diacetate (III), prepared by the addition reaction between 2-furaldehyde and acetic anhydride] followed by saponification to regenerate the formyl group which, had it not been so protected, would have been oxidized to carboxyl during the nitration. II may be synthesized by effecting the addition of cyanic acid to hydrazinoacetic acid (IV) to produce the 3-carbamoyl derivative (V) which cyclizes by dehydration to II.

Description—Lemon-yellow, odorless crystals or fine powder; bitter aftertaste.

Solubility—Very slightly soluble in water and alcohol.

Uses—Nitrofurantoin is effective against a majority of urinary tract pathogens, including certain strains of *E coli*, *Klebsiella*, *Proteus* sp, *Pseudomonas*, and *Aerobacter* sp. It is also effective against many staphylococci, clostridia, and *B subtilis*. It is indicated for the treatment of infections of the urinary tract: pyelonephritis, cystitis, and pyelitis. An acid urine favors activity. It is not the drug of first choice in the treatment of any acute infection and it is rarely used. In chronic bacteriuria, it is a second- or third-choice agent. However, as a prophylactic in the prevention of recurrences it is effective, being slightly superior to methenamine mandelate but inferior to sulfamethizole. Nitrofurantoin is not indicated for treatment of associated perinephric or renal cortical abscesses, prostatitis, or other genitourinary-tract infections, since in these the blood level is more important than urine concentration.

Microcrystalline nitrofurantoin is rapidly and completely absorbed; the macrocrystalline form is more slowly and less completely absorbed. About 67% of nitrofurantoin is metabolized in the body, and 33% is excreted into the urine unchanged. The half-life is only 0.3 to 1 hr; slow absorption helps to sustain urine levels. Dose adjustment must be made in renal failure.

Nausea, vomiting, and diarrhea occur in an appreciable number of patients. Reduction in dosage, or administration with food or milk, lessens the incidence; it is claimed that use of a "macrocrystalline" product diminishes the incidence and intensity of gastrointestinal upsets without affecting potency. Absorption is delayed, but bioavailability is not diminished. Gastrointestinal effects also occur in some patients receiving the drug intravenously. Hypersensitivity reactions with dermatologic manifestations also occur. Headache, vertigo, drowsiness, malaise, muscular aches, nystagmus, and polyneuropathy occasionally occur. Neuropathies appear to be more likely to occur if there is renal insufficiency; they appear to be caused by metabolites. Hemolytic anemia, megaloblastic anemia, granulocytopenia, leukopenia, eosinophilia, and maculopapular rashes occur occasionally. Nitrofurantoin also causes infrequent cholestatic jaundice and hepatocellular damage. Pneumonitis and pulmonary fibrosis can occur, especially in elderly patients. Occasionally there is transient alopecia. Superinfections may occur. A course of nitrofurantoin ordinarily should not exceed 2 weeks, and courses should be separated by rest periods. The drug is mutagenic in the Ames test. Nitrofurantoin interferes with the action of nalidixic acid.

Dose—*Oral*, *adults*, **50 to 100 mg** or **1.25 to 1.75 mg/kg** every 6 hr; *children over 1 month of age*, **1.25 to 1.75 mg/kg** of body weight every 6 hr for 10 to 14 days, to be decreased to half that dose for another 10 to 14 days, then decreased to one-fourth the initial dose for prolonged maintenance; for prevention of recurrences in persons with a normal pyelogram, a single dose of **200 mg** at nighttime appears sufficient. *Intravenous infusion*, patients *over 54.5 kg*, **180 mg** twice a day; *patients under 54.5 kg*, **3.3 mg/kg** every 12 hr.

Dosage Forms—*Capsules:* 50 and 100 mg; Capsules, macrocrystals: 25, 50, and 100 mg; Powder for Injection: 180 mg. Oral Suspension: 25 mg/5 mL; Tablets: 50 and 100 mg.

Trimethoprim

2,4-Pyrimidinediamine, 5-[(3,4,5-trimethoxyphenyl)methyl]-, Syraprim, Proloprim (*Burroughs-Wellcome*); Trimpex (*Hoffman-LaRoche*)

2,4-Diamino-5-(3,4,5-trimethoxybenzyl)pyrimidine [738-70-5] $C_{14}H_{18}N_4O_3$ (290.32).

Preparation—By interaction of α-(ethoxymethyl)-3,4,5-trimethoxycinnamonitrile and guanidine, the former prepared by condensing 3,4,5-trimethoxybenzaldehyde with β-ethoxypropionitrile. US Pat 3,049,544.

Description—White to cream-colored crystals or crystalline powder; odorless; bitter taste; melts at about 199°; pK_a about 6.6.

Solubility—Very slightly soluble in water; 1 g dissolves in about 285 mL absolute alcohol, 53 mL chloroform.

Uses—Trimethoprim is a congener of pyrimethamine and it similarly inhibits dihydrofolate reductase, although it is considerably less potent. It was introduced as an antimalarial drug (mostly against *P falciparum*) and is still used somewhat for that purpose, usually in combination with an appropriate sulfonamide. However, its most important use is as an antibacterial agent. Bacterial dihydrofolate reductases are generally more susceptible than are the plasmodial ones. Therefore, the drug is effective against all bacteria that must synthesize their own folinic acid (leucovorin). This gives it a wide spectrum of activity that includes *Strep pyogenes*, *viridans*, and *pneumoniae*, *Staph aureus* and *epidermidis*, *H influenzae*,

Klebsiella-Enterobacter-Serratia, E coli, various *Shigella* and *Salmonella, Bordetella pertussis, V cholerae* and others. It is not effective against *Ps aeruginosa* but is against *Ps cepaciae* and *pseudomallei.* Many of these same organisms must also synthesize their own folic acid. Sulfonamides block the incorporation of *p*-aminobenzoate into folate, thus inhibiting a crucial biosynthetic step just previous to that where trimethoprim acts. Therefore, the combination of trimethoprim and sulfonamides is supposedly more effective than either drug alone, although clinical confirmation of significant synergism is lacking. Nevertheless, it is widely used in combination with sulfamethoxazole. Trimethoprim alone is approved for the same uses as the above combination (see page 1174). It would seem prudent to use the combination for urinary tract infections, even though the cost is greater, but the pharmacokinetics are such that sulfamethoxazole in the present formulation adds little to trimethoprim alone for systemic infections. Mammalian dihydrofolate reductase is about 1:10,000 to 1:50,000 as sensitive to trimethoprim as the bacterial enzymes, so that there is little interference with folate metabolism in man. The toxicity is low. It includes occasional nausea and vomiting, diarrhea, malaise, immunosuppression and, rarely, rash, leukopenia and thrombocytopenia. By the oral route, it is well-absorbed and reaches a peak in 2 to 3 hr. A blood level of 1 to 2 μg/mL in an adult is provided by 160 mg. About 45% is protein-bound in plasma. The volume of distribution is about 1.4 mL/g. The concentration in cerebrospinal fluid reaches 30 to 50% of that in plasma. Trimethoprim is mainly excreted into the urine. The half-life is 9 to 12 hr in normal subjects, but may be increased 2- to 3-fold when the creatinine clearance falls below 10 mL/min.

Dose—*Oral, adults* and *children over 12 yr* of age, for *prophylaxis* of *urinary tract infections,* **100 mg** once a day; for *treatment* of *urinary tract infections,* **100 mg** every 12 hr or **200 mg** once a day for 10 days; tentative doses for: *chancroid,* 100 mg every 12 hr; *other infections,* 200 mg every 12 hr.

Dosage Forms—Oral Suspension: 40 mg/5 mL; Tablets: 100 mg.

Other Miscellaneous Systemic Antibacterial Drugs

Acetohydroxamic Acid [*N*-Hydroxyacetamide [546-88-3] $C_2H_5NO_2$ (75.07); AHA]—For the synthesis see *Synthesis,* 654, 1980. *Description and solubility:* White solid melting about 90°; pK$_a$ 8.7; soluble in water; pH of aqueous solution is about 9.4. *Uses:* AHA is not an antibacterial drug but rather an inhibitor of bacterial urease. Its inclusion here is for want of a better location. Urease-producing bacteria convert urea to NH$_3$ and H$_2$CO$_3$. The consequent alkalinization of the urine favors further bacterial growth and antagonizes most urinary tract antiinfectives (except aminoglycosides, which work best in alkaline media). The ammonia also favors the formation of struvite renal stones, which both interferes with effective antimicrobial treatment and causes renal pathologies. AHA decreases urine pH, helps dissolve and prevents struvite stones. The drug is used as an adjunct to antimicrobial therapy of urinary tract infections caused by urease-producing bacteria (mostly *Proteus*). Adverse effects occur in up to 30% of long-term recipients. Transient, mild headache is the most frequent. Depression, anxiety, nervousness, tremulousness and malaise occur with a frequency of 20%. Nausea, vomiting, and anorexia also occur in about 20% of cases. Laboratory evidence of hemolytic anemia occurs in about 15% of cases, although frank anemia is rare. Rashes occur after the ingestion of alcohol. Phlebitis may be exacerbated by the drug. AHA is teratogenic in rats. Consequently, AHA is a drug of last resort to be used when surgery is contraindicated and other measures have been ineffective. From 36 to 65% of AHA is excreted in urine. The half-life is 5 to 10 hr. *Dose: Oral, adults, initially,* 12 mg/kg a day in 3 or 4 divided doses; *then,* 250 mg 3 or 4 times a day, not to exceed a total daily dose of 10 to 15 mg/kg; *children,* 10 mg/kg a day in 3 or 4 divided doses. Dosage must be adjusted in renal failure.

Aztreonam [(*Z*)-2-[[[(2-Amino-4-thiazolyl)[[(2*S*,3*S*)-2-methyl-4-oxo-1-sulfo-3-azetidinyl]carbamoyl]methylene]amino]oxy]-2-methyl-propionic acid. [78110-38-0] $C_{13}H_{17}N_5O_8S_2$ (435.43)]—Synthesis: Neth Pat Appl 81 00571 (*CA 96:* 181062x, 1982). *Uses:* Aztreonam is the first monobactam (monocyclic β-lactam) to be used in humans. Monobactams are β-lactams without the adjacent 5- or 6-member ring characteristic of penicillins and cephalosporins. When there is an appropriately electronegative substituent on the lactam nitogen, the β-lactam ring is resistant to the β-lactamases. Aztreonam has high activity against gram-negative bacteria, and it has been used effectively in various systemic and urinary tract infections caused by such organisms. Its exact indications remain to be defined. Aztreonam is eliminated mainly by renal excretion, in part by tubular secretion. Probenecid has a moderate effect to slow excretion. The half-life is about 1.8 hr.

Cinoxacin [1-Ethyl-1,4-dihydro-4-oxo[1,3]dioxolo[4,5-*g*]cinnoline-3-carboxylic acid [28657-80-9] $C_{12}H_{10}N_2O_5$ (262.22); Cinobac (*Lilly*)]—For synthesis see US Pat 3,669,965. Buff crystals melting about 265°. Insoluble in water but soluble in most polar organic solvents. *Uses:* Cinoxacin is active against many gram-negative urinary tract pathogens, such

as *E coli, Klebsiella, Enterobacter, Proteus, Serratia,* and *Citrobacter.* It is not effective against *Ps aeruginosa* or gram-positive pathogens. Cross-resistance occurs between it and nalidixic acid but not to any antibiotic. It is used only for the treatment of urinary tract infections caused by susceptible organisms. It is almost completely absorbed by the oral route. Food in the stomach delays absorption. In plasma, 60 to 70% is protein-bound. Cinoxacin is almost completely eliminated by renal excretion. Probenecid impairs excretion. The half-life is 1.5 to 3.5 hr but longer in renal failure. Adverse effects are infrequent and usually mild. They include nausea, vomiting, dizziness, rashes, restlessness, insomnia, tinnitus, paresthesis, photophobia, anorexia, colic, diarrhea, and perineal burning. *Dose: Oral, children over 12 yr* of age and *adults,* 250 mg every 6 hr or 500 mg every 12 hr for 7 to 14 days.

Ethionamide [2-Ethylthioisonicotinamide [536-33-4] $C_8H_{10}N_2S$ (166.24); Trecator (*Ives*)]—Prepared from 2-ethylisonicotinamide by dehydration and subsequent reaction with hydrogen sulfide. A bright yellow powder with a mild sulfide-like odor; melts at about 160°. Slightly soluble in water, chloroform, ether; sparingly soluble in alcohol. *Uses:* Chemically related to *Isoniazid* and shares with it usefulness against tuberculosis. However, it is less potent and more toxic than isoniazid so that its general use should be avoided; rather, it should be used only when the usual combinations of streptomycin, aminosalicylic acid, and isoniazid are ineffective or cannot be tolerated. Ethionamide should be used only in combination with other primary antitubercular drugs and only after the microorganism has been shown *in vitro* to be susceptible to the drug. Resistance develops rapidly when ethionamide is used alone. Untoward effects include gastrointestinal distress (nausea, vomiting, anorexia), thrombocytopenia, stomatitis, occasional hepatotoxicity, gynecomastia, possible damage to the inner ear, drowsiness, depression, peripheral and optic neuritis, impotence, postural hypotension, pellagra-like syndrome, difficulty in the control of diabetes, acne, and allergic dermatitides. Pyridoxine can prevent most of the neurotoxicities. Ethionamide may increase the toxicity of drugs with which it is given in combination. *Dose: Oral, adults,* 250 mg every 8 to 12 hr; *children,* 4 to 5 mg/kg every 8 hr.

Nalidixic Acid [1-Ethyl-1,4-dihydro-7-methyl-4-oxo-1,8-naphthyridine-3-carboxylic acid [389-08-2] $C_{12}H_{12}N_2O_3$ (232.24); NegGram (*Winthrop*); Cybis (*Breon*)]—The principal steps in the synthesis of this compound are given in RPS-15, page 1152. A white to slightly yellow, crystalline powder; melts at about 228°; pK$_a$ 8.6. *Solubility:* 1 g dissolves in >1000 mL water, 910 mL alcohol, 29 mL chloroform, >1000 mL ether. *Uses:* An antibacterial agent effective against gram-negative organisms, especially Enterobacteriaceae like most *E coli,* several *Proteus, Klebsiella-Enterobacter, Aerobacter,* and paracolon group, a few *Pseudomonas,* some *Salmonella,* and a few *Shigella* sp. It is not effective against *Ps aeruginosa* or *Serratia marcescens.* By the oral route is difficult to achieve effective plasma levels. Furthermore, binding to plasma protein inhibits activity. The drug reaches effective concentrations in the urine, and it is used for treatment of acute urinary-tract infections. This is the only approved use in the US. The drug has a minor status today; authoritative tables and most reviews do not mention it. Bacterial resistance develops rapidly, and escape from control occurs in 6 to 25% of patients. About 96% of nalidixic acid is absorbed. It is conjugated in the liver, and only 10 to 15% is excreted unchanged into the urine. The half-life is about 8 hr. It can displace from plasma proteins oral anticoagulants and probably a number of other drugs with weak-acid, lipid-soluble properties.

The majority of patients tolerate nalidixic acid without untoward effects. Abdominal pain, nausea, vomiting, skin rashes, pruritus, and urticaria are the most frequent side effects. Occasionally fever, severe prolonged photosensitivity, or eosinophilia occur. Headache, vertigo, drowsiness, malaise, disturbances of vision, muscle weakness, or myalgia may occur infrequently. Cholestasis, thrombocytopenia, leukopenia, hemolytic anemia, and paresthesias and toxic psychosis occur rarely. Convulsions have occurred in patients with parkinsonism or cerebral vascular insufficiency and in children receiving excessive doses. Overdoses may cause metabolic acidosis. Nalidixic acid gives false positive tests for urine glucose by some tests. *Dose: Oral, adults* and *children over 12 yr of age,* 1 g every 6 hr for 1 to 2 weeks, which for prolonged treatment is reduced at the end of 2 weeks to 500 mg every 6 hr; *infants over 3 mo* of age and *children, initially* 13.8 mg/kg every 6 hr for 1 or 2 weeks then 8.3 mg/kg every 6 hr for maintenance.

Pyrazinamide [Pyrazinecarboxamide [98-96-4] $C_5H_5N_3O$ (123.11); Aldinamide (*MSD*)]—Prepared by thermal decarboxylation of 2,3-pyrazinedicarboxylic acid to form the monocarboxylic acid, which is esterified with methanol and then subjected to controlled ammonolysis. A white to practically white, crystalline powder; melts at about 190°. *Solubility:* 1 g is soluble in 67 mL water, 135 mL chloroform, 1000 mL ether; slightly soluble in alcohol. *Uses:* An antituberculosis drug more effective than aminosalicylic acid, cycloserine, or viomycin, but not streptomycin, isoniazid, ethambutol, or rifampin. It is generally administered with isoniazid, which it potentiates. However, it is quite toxic and should be held in reserve until other therapy fails. It may cause fever, anorexia, malaise, and hepatic damage, with or without jaundice, and death can occur. All patients intended to be treated with this drug should have prior liver-function tests, which tests must also be repeated periodically during therapy. All patients should be hospitalized during treatment. Pyrazinamide may cause retention of uric acid. *Dose: Oral, adult,* 5 to 8.75

mg/kg of body weight every 6 hr or 6.7 to 11.7 mg/kg every 8 hr; the total daily dose should not exceed 3 g. The dose for children has not been established.

Sulfoxone Sodium [Disodium [sulfonylbis(*p*-phenyleneimino)dimethanesulfinate [144-75-2] $C_{14}H_{14}N_2Na_2O_6S_3$ (448.43); Diasone Sodium (*Abbott*) a mixture of sulfoxone sodium and suitable buffers and inert ingredients; contains 73–81% of sulfoxone sodium.]—*Preparation:* *p*-Chloronitrobenzene is treated with sodium sulfide and the resulting 4-nitro-4'-aminodiphenylsulfide with HCl and tin to form 4,4'-diaminodiphenylsulfide. After acetylation with acetic anhydride, the resulting *N,N'*-diacetyl compound is oxidized to the sulfone with potassium dichromate and H_2SO_4. Deacetylation is accomplished by acid hydrolysis, and the resulting 4,4'-diaminodiphenyl sulfone is condensed with sodium formaldehyde sulfoxylate. *Description and solubility:* White to pale yellow powder with a characteristic odor; pK_{a1} 11.51; pK_{a2} 12.70. Soluble 1 g in 13.5 mL water, >1000 mL alcohol, >1000 mL chloroform, >2000 mL ether. *Uses:* See *Dapsone* (page 1214), into which sulfoxone is largely converted in the body. *Dose: Oral, adults, for leprosy,* 330 mg twice a week or 165 mg 4 times a week during the first 2 weeks, then 4 times a week or 165 mg a day in the third and fourth weeks, and 330 mg every day 6 days a week thereafter; for *dermatitis herpetiformis*, 330 to 660 mg a day. *Children*, one-half the adult dose.

Antimalarials

Until World War II, malaria has been the world's greatest scourge, its steady accumulated toll far exceeding that of the more explosive plague. Even today probably over 125 million people are afflicted, and about million die each year from malaria. Knowledge of mosquito control, insecticides, and antimalarials, however, have all but eradicated the disease in the more advanced countries, such as the US; similar strides have been made in certain relatively undeveloped countries, so that malaria now ranks second to tuberculosis in many of these countries.

The export of cinchona from Peru in 1643 allowed the European countries and their colonies some means of suppressing the disease, and the introduction of quinine in the 19th century improved therapy somewhat. However, great advances were not made until the introduction of pamaquine in 1926 and quinacrine (atabrine) in 1930, as the result of screening by I G Farben of over 12,000 candidates. These synthetics did not immediately displace quinine. Only when the supplies of quinine were cut off in World War II did it become imperative to supply synthetic antimalarials to our armed forces in the Pacific and Mediterranean. The US Office of Scientific Research and Development coordinated a study of about 7000 new, and an equal number of old, synthetic compounds. Not only were the older German compounds "rediscovered," but several new and superior agents (especially amodiaquine, chloroquine, pentaquine, and primaquine) resulted. The British counterpart of this program brought forth *chloroguanide*. The continued search in this field has yielded other antimalarials, but the pace has recently been slow. However, because of the emergence of resistant strains of plasmodia, the effectiveness of several of the "newer" agents is rapidly diminishing, so that not only are new drugs again being actively sought, but combinations of old drugs are on trial. In this connection, it is of interest that various sulfonamides (mostly sulfadoxine or sulfadiazine) and tetracycline are being used.

Malaria is caused by several species of the protozoan *Plasmodium*, of which *P vivax* and *P falciparum* are the most common. They all have complex life cycles involving both the anopheles mosquito and the erythrocyte of the human host. In vivax, a persisting tissue phase continues to infect the blood at intervals for many years. Thus, the ideal antimalarial not only should eradicate the microzoan from the blood, (ie, to "suppress" the clinical attack) but from the tissues as well, to effect a "radical cure." The several antimalarials differ in their point of interruption of the cycle of the parasite and in the type of malaria affected.

The 4-aminoquinolines (amodiaquine, choroquine, hydroxychloroquine) and quinacrine cause similar adverse effects. Gastrointestinal side effects such as nausea, vomiting, diarrhea, and sialorrhea are common; they can be diminished by administering the drugs with meals and milk. Oropharyngeal and dermatologic side-effects may occur, especially during protracted therapy. They include pigmentation of the skin, nailbeds and palate (especially quinacrine), bleaching of hair, pruritus, and lichenoid and pleomorphic skin eruptions. They may precipitate severe attacks of psoriasis in patients with that disease. The drugs should not be coadministered with phenylbutazone or gold salts, which have similar dermatotoxicities. There is cross-sensitization among all the 4-aminoquinolines. The drugs may cause neurological disturbances, such as fatigue, lassitude, neuromyopathy, polyneuritis, toxic psychosis, and ototoxicity with vertigo and/or decreased auditory sensitivity. The knee and ankle reflexes should be monitored periodically. Ocular disorders, such as corneal opacities, keratopathy and retinopathy (the drugs are concentrated in the retina) occur, especially during long-term treatment. Periodic ophthalmologic examinations are advised. The drugs are contraindicated if retinal or visual field disease is present. The 4-aminoquinolines are concentrated in the liver and may cause hepatotoxicity, and they may precipitate attacks of porphyria; they must be used cautiously in persons with liver disease or who are under medication with other potentially hepatotoxic drugs (carbarsone, gold salts, erythromycin estolate, indomethacin, phenylbutazone, certain anabolic steroids, etc). Hematologic disorders occasionally caused by the 4-aminoquinolines include leukopenia, pancytopenia and agranulocytosis; periodic white blood counts are necessary. The drugs may depress the electrocardiographic T-wave. They pass the placental barrier and can cause cochleovestibular paresis in the fetus; they should be withheld in pregnancy, if possible.

Amodiaquine Hydrochloride

Phenol, 4-[(7-chloro-4-quinolinyl)amino]-2-[(diethylamino)methyl]-, dihydrochloride, dihydrate; Camoquin Hydrochloride (*Parke-Davis*)

4-[(7-Chloro-4-quinolyl)amino]-α-(diethylamino)-*o*-cresol dihydrochloride dihydrate [6398-98-7] $C_{20}H_{22}ClN_3O.2HCl.2H_2O$ (464.82); *anhydrous* [69-44-3] (428.79).

Preparation—4,7-Dichloroquinoline is condensed with 2-(diethylamino)methyl-4-aminophenol. The base is isolated and converted into the dihydrochloride.

Description—Yellow, crystalline powder; odorless and has a bitter taste.

Solubility—Soluble in water; sparingly soluble in alcohol; very slightly soluble in chloroform, and ether.

Uses—Amodiaquine is very similar to chloroquine (see *Chloroquine Phosphate*) in its *antimalarial* actions. Thus, it is capable only of eradicating the parasite from the erythrocytes, so that malaria caused by *P falciparum* can be cured, but only the *suppression of acute attacks* in the other types of malaria can be effected. Unfortunately, resistance to amodiaquine occurs, and in some regions successful management of malaria caused by *P falciparum* is achieved in less than 25% of cases. When there fails to be an unfavorable clinical response, quinine, pyrimethamine, sulfonamides, or dapsone may be added, although authorities are as yet uncertain which of these or which combinations are best. Like quinacrine and chloroquine, amodiaquine is of value in the treatment of *lupus erythematosus*, *giardiasis*, and extraintestinal *amebiasis*.

The adverse effects of amodiaquine and precautions of use are described in the introduction to this section.

Dose (base equivalent)—*Oral, adults, prophylactic,* **400 mg** once a week; *therapeutic*, initially **600 mg** followed by **400 mg** 6, 24, and 48 hr later. *Children, 9 to 12 yr* of age *prophylactic*, **300 mg**; *5 to 8 yr*, 150 to 200 mg; *2 to 4 yr*, 50 to 100 mg; and *1 yr or less*, 50 mg once a week; *therapeutic*, initially **10 mg/kg** then **5 mg/kg** at 6, 24 and 48 hr. Suppressive therapy should begin 2 weeks in advance of entering a malarious region and continue for 8 weeks after departure.

Dosage Form (base equivalent)—Tablets: 200 mg.

Chloroquine Hydrochloride

1,4-Pentanediamine, N^4-(7-chloro-4-quinolinyl)-N^1,N^1-diethyl-, dihydrochloride; Aralen Hydrochloride (*Winthrop*)

7-Chloro-4-[[4-(diethylamino)-1-methylbutyl]amino]quinoline dihydrochloride [3545-67-3]; a sterile solution of chloroquine in water for injection prepared with the aid of hydrochloric acid. It contains, in each mL, 47.5–52.5 mg of $C_{18}H_{26}ClN_3 \cdot 2HCl$ (392.80).

Preparation—The base is prepared by heating a mixture of 4,7-dichloroquinoline and N,N-diethylpentyl amine.

Description—A colorless liquid; pH between 5.5 and 6.5.

Uses—Its actions and uses are those of *Chloroquine Phosphate*, except that the hydrochloride lends itself better to solutions for intramuscular injection. The intramuscular route may be indicated in patients who cannot tolerate oral chloroquine or in cerebral malaria, in which a very rapid response is desired. The toxicity is like that of the phosphate (see next article), even to the occurrence of gastrointestinal complaints; in addition, respiratory depression, hypotension, or shock may occur consequent to too rapid a rate of injection or after an overdose.

Dose—*Intramuscular, adults,* for *malaria*, **200 to 250 mg**, to be repeated in 6 hr, if necessary, but not to exceed 1 g in the first 24 hr; for *extraintestinal amebiasis*, **200 to 250 mg** once a day for 10 to 12 days. *Children*, for *malaria*, **6.25 mg/kg** of body weight and no more, to be repeated in 6 hr, if necessary, but not to exceed 12 mg/kg in any 24-hr period; for *extraintestinal amebiasis*, **7.5 mg/kg** a day for 10 to 12 days.

Dosage Form—Injection: 50 mg, equivalent to 40 mg of chloroquine.

Chloroquine Phosphate

1,4-Pentanediamine, N^4-(7-chloro-4-quinolinyl)-N^1,N^1-diethyl-, phosphate (1:2); Aralen Phosphate (*Winthrop*)

7-Chloro-4-[[4-(diethylamino)-1-methylbutyl]amino]quinoline phosphate (1:2) [50-63-5] $C_{18}H_{26}ClN_3 \cdot 2H_3PO_4$ (515.87).

For the structure of the base, see *Chloroquine Hydrochloride*.

Preparation—By addition of concentrated phosphoric acid to a hot ethanolic solution of chloroquine base.

Description—White, crystalline powder; odorless; bitter taste; slowly discolors on exposure to light; aqueous solution has a pH of about 4.5; melting ranges 193° to 195° (usual form) or 210° to 215° (other polymorphic form); pK_{a1} 7; pK_{a2} 9.2.

Solubility—Freely soluble in water; practically insoluble in alcohol, chloroform, and ether.

Uses—Chloroquine phosphate is used both for control of acute attacks of *vivax malaria* and for suppression against all plasmodia except chloroquine-resistant *P falciparum*. The drug is neither a prophylactic nor a radical curative agent in vivax malaria. In regions where *P falciparum* is generally sensitive to chloroquine, it is markedly effective in terminating acute attacks of *falciparum malaria* and usually bring about complete cure in this type of malaria. However, in some regions a high incidence of resistance exists, as high as 89% in Vietnam, so that other drugs, such as amodiaquine, pyrimethamine plus sulfadiazine, sulfadoxine, or quinine (with or without tetracycline) may have preference. Resistant strains of *P vivax* also occur.

Chloroquine was once the most generally useful of all antimalarial agents, but it now appears that emerging resistance is relegating the drug to secondary status.

Although not useful in intestinal amebiasis, chloroquine is an effective agent in the treatment of extraintestinal amebiasis, especially *amebic hepatitis*. It is not used alone but rather in combination with dihydroemetine or emetine. The combination is only the treatment of second choice, behind metronidazole-diiodohydroxyquin. Since chloroquine is well tolerated, it has been recommended that it be employed routinely even in cases of amebiasis without demonstrable hepatic involvement. Like quinacrine, it may also be of value in chronic discoid *lupus erythematosus* and *rheumatoid arthritis*. Chloroquine is quite effective in the treatment of *photoallergic* reactions.

The adverse effects of chloroquine are those of the 4-aminoquinolines (see introductory statement in this section). The incidence is low, except for the gastrointestinal side-effects of the oral forms.

Chloroquine is almost completely absorbed from the gastrointestinal tract and is usually administered orally. Chloroquine (as the hydrochloride) is given intramuscularly when necessary to resort to parenteral administration. Tissues bind chloroquine, although not quite to the same degree of quinacrine. It is degraded in tissues to unknown products. The drug is slowly excreted in the urine with an initial half-life of 1 wk, changing to 17 days after 4 wks, then ultimately becoming months.

Dose—*Oral, adults,* for *malaria*, as a *prophylactic*, **500 mg** once a week, and for *therapy*, initially **1 g** followed by **500 mg** in 6 to 8 hr, then **500 mg** once a day on the second and third days; for *extraintestinal amebiasis*, **250 mg** 4 times a day for 2 days followed by **250 mg** twice a day for at least 2 or 3 weeks; for *lupus erythematosus*, **250 mg** twice a day for 2 weeks then once a day thereafter; to suppress *photoeruptions*, **250 mg** twice a day for 2 wk then once a day. *Children*, for *malaria*, as a *prophylactic*, **8.3 mg/kg** of body weight, not to exceed 500 mg, once a week, and for *therapy*, initially **16.7 mg/kg**, not to exceed 1 g, then **8.3 mg/kg**, not to exceed 500 mg, 6, 24, and 48 hr later; for *extraintestinal amebiasis*, **10 mg/kg**; not to exceed 600 mg, every day for 3 wk. Suppressive treatment should begin 2 weeks in advance of entering into a malarious region and continue for 8 weeks after departure; rapid loading for suppression can be achieved by giving the two weekly doses in a single day, 6 hr apart.

Dosage Forms: Tablets: 250 and 500 mg, equivalent to 150 and 300 mg, respectively, of chloroquine base.

Dapsone—page 1214.

Primaquine Phosphate

1,4-Pentanediamine, N^4-(6-methoxy-8-quinolinyl)-, phosphate (1:2); (*Winthrop*)

8-[(4-Amino-1-methylbutyl)amino]-6-methoxyquinoline phosphate (1:2) [63-45-6] $C_{15}H_{21}N_3O \cdot 2H_3PO_4$ (455.34).

Preparation—2-Chloropentylamine is condensed with 8-amino-6-methoxyquinoline and the resulting primaquine base is reacted with a double molar quantity of phosphoric acid.

Description—Orange-red, crystalline powder; odorless and has a bitter taste; solutions are acid to litmus; melts at about 200°.

Solubility—1 g in about 15 mL water; insoluble in chloroform and ether.

Uses—An antimalarial which is very important for the *radical cure* (ie, prevention of relapse) *of relapsing vivax malaria;* it is not employed for suppressive therapy or for control of the acute clinical attacks of the disease. It is also used to treat *toxoplasmosis*, although it is not among the two top choices. Incidence of serious untoward effects is low. In Caucasians, therapeutic doses of primaquine are adequately tolerated. Mild to moderate abdominal cramps and occasional epigastric distress, dizziness, weakness occur in some individuals. Administration of the drug with milk, food, or antacids lessens these effects; however, aluminum-containing antacids interfere with absorption. Mild hemolytic anemia, cyanosis (methemoglobinemia), and leukocytosis may also be observed. At higher dose levels these symptoms are accentuated, and leukopenia may be noted. Toxicity is not increased by concurrent administration of quinine or chloroquine, which are often given concurrently. However, quinacrine greatly enhances the toxicity of primaquine and must not be given at the same time. Impairment of liver function has not been noted, even in patients with infectious hepatitis. Persons with tendencies toward granulocytopenia (eg, lupus erythematosus or rheumatoid diseases) should not take primaquine because the blood dyscrasia may be precipitated. Other hemolyzing drugs should not be administered concurrently. Untoward effects in non-Caucasians are similar, but the incidence and degree of anemia and intravascular hemolysis are greater. A daily dose of 15 mg of primaquine (base) can be safely administered for 14 days to both Caucasian and non-Caucasian adults without special medical supervision. Larger doses are too toxic for those non-Caucasians and other persons whose erythrocytes are deficient in glucose 6-phosphate dehydrogenase, but usually can be administered to Caucasian subjects, who should be carefully supervised. A sudden darkening of the urine, leukocytosis, or severe skin reaction are indicators of hemolysis, and the drug must be discontinued immediately. Bone-marrow depressant drugs (eg, antineoplastics, colchicine, gold salts, penicillamine, phenylbutazone, hydroxyphenylbutazone, quinacrine) given concurrently can cause excessive bone-marrow depression.

Dose—*Oral, adults,* **26.3 mg** once a day for 2 weeks, except **52.6 mg** against resistant organisms; to eliminate gametocytes of *Pl falciparum,* **78.9 mg** as a single dose; *infants* and *children,* **667 μg** (0.67 mg)/**kg** of body weight once a day for 2 weeks.

Dosage Form—Tablets: 26.3 mg, equivalent to 15 mg of primaquine base.

Pyrimethamine

2,4-Pyrimidinediamine, 5-(4-chlorophenyl)-6-ethyl-, Daraprim (*Burroughs-Wellcome*)

2,4-Diamino-5-(*p*-chlorophenyl)-6-ethylpyrimidine [58-14-0] $C_{12}H_{13}ClN_4$ (248.71).

Preparation—Ethyl propionate is condensed with *p*-chlorophenylacetonitrile in the presence of sodium methylate. The resulting α-propionyl-*p*-chlorophenylacetonitrile is reacted with isoamyl alcohol to form the hemiacetal which undergoes dehydration to α-(*p*-chlorophenyl)-β-ethyl-β-isoamyloxylacrylonitrile (I). I is reacted with guanidine whereupon cyclization occurs due to (*a*) the liberation of isoamyl alcohol by condensation involving the imino hydrogen of guanidine and the isoamyloxy group of I, and (*b*) an addition reaction involving an amino group of guanidine and the nitrile group of I.

Description—White, crystalline powder; odorless; melting range 238° to 242°.

Solubility—Practically insoluble in water; 1 g in about 200 mL alcohol, 125 mL chloroform.

Uses—Pyrimethamine is chemically related to chloroguanide and is similar to it in mechanism of action. It inhibits dihydrofolate reductase in plasmodia; thus the developing parasite cannot utilize nucleic acid precursors needed for growth. Its action in preventing the development of the erythrocytic phase of the parasite is slow, so that it is of little value in suppression of acute attacks, except as an adjunct to quinine; rather it is used mainly as a suppressive prophylactic for the prevention of clinical attacks by *P falciparum* in regions where the organism is resistant to chloroquine, in which use it is combined with sulfadoxine. It also renders the parasites incapable of sporulating in the mosquito, so that the life cycle of the parasite is broken. In some regions, treatment with pyrimethamine is successful in up to 90% of cases; addition of quinine increases the success rate to about 95%. Combination of pyrimethamine and trisulfapyrimidines is the treatment of choice for *toxoplasmosis.* Pyrimethamine is also of use as an *immunosuppressive.*

The toxicity of pyrimethamine is low. Anorexia and vomiting are common with large doses. Skin rashes are rare. In high doses pyrimethamine may cause megaloblastic anemia and, less commonly, leukopenia, thrombocytopenia, and pancytopenia as the result of antagonism of folic acid. Atrophic, pharyngitis, and esophagitis oc-

casionally results. CNS signs of folate deficiency may occur. Because of the intensive dose regimen for toxoplasmosis, semiweekly blood-cell and platelet counts should be made. The hematopoietic toxicity can be reversed by leucovorin. The antifolate actions are damaging to the fetus, so that the drug should be avoided in pregnancy, if possible, or be coadministered with leucovorin.

Dose—*Oral, adult, antimalarial,* for *prophylaxis* or *suppression,* in combination with sulfadoxine, **25 mg** once a week and for *treatment* of uncomplicated attacks, in combination with quinine and sulfadiazine, **25 mg** twice a day for 3 days; for *toxoplasmosis,* in combination with trisulfapyrimidines, *initially* **50 to 100 mg** once a day for 2 days then **25 mg** once a day for 4 to 6 weeks. *Infants* and *children, antimalarial,* for *prophylaxis* or *suppression,* in combination with sulfadoxine, **0.9 mg/kg** (not to exceed adult dose) once a week and for *treatment* of uncomplicated attack, in combination with quinine and sulfadiazine, **0.3 mg/kg** 3 times a day for 3 days; for *toxoplasmosis,* in combination with trisulfapyrimidines, *initially* **1 mg/kg** twice a day for 1 to 3 days then **0.5 mg/kg** twice a day for 4 to 6 weeks.

Dosage Form—Tablets: 25 mg.

Quinine Sulfate

Cinchonan-9-ol, 6'-methoxy-, (8α,9R)-, sulfate (2:1) (salt), dihydrate

Quinine sulfate (2:1) (salt) dihydrate [6119-70-6] $(C_{20}H_{24}N_2O_2)_2 \cdot H_2SO_4 \cdot 2H_2O$ (782.95); *anhydrous* [804-63-7] (746.92); the sulfate of an alkaloid obtained from the bark of *Cinchona officinalis* Linné (*C ledgeriana* Moens) (Fam *Rubiaceae*) or other species of *Cinchona.* Contains not more than 10.0% of dihydroquinine. For the structural formula of quinine see page 417.

Preparation—The crude sulfate, obtained when quinine is isolated from the bark of *Cinchona* sp, is recrystallized once or twice from hot water slightly acidified with sulfuric acid.

Description—White, fine, needle-like crystals, usually lusterless, making a light and readily compressible mass; odorless, and has a persistent, very bitter taste; when exposed to light, it acquires a brown tint.

Solubility—1 g in about 500 mL water, 120 mL alcohol, 35 mL water at 100°, and about 10 mL alcohol at 80°; slightly soluble in chloroform and ether.

Uses—As an antimalarial drug, quinine was largely replaced by less toxic and more effective drugs, except in areas where quinine was available locally and was less expensive than the newer agents. However, the occurrence of resistance to the newer and usually superior antimalarial drugs has left a place for the use of quinine. Quinine only affects the erythrocytic form of the plasmodia and hence is used only as a suppressive in the management of acute attacks of *vivax, malariae,* or *ovale* malaria. It may cure up to 50% of infections caused by *falciparum* plasmodia, but some strains are resistant. Quinine may be combined with pyrimethamine, but it appears to be antagonized by chloroquine. The quinine-pyrimethamine-sulfadiazine combination is presently the treatment of choice for infections caused by chloroquine-resistant *P falciparum;* an alternative is quinine with tetracycline. In severe infections, intravenous quinine dihydrochloride is the drug of choice.

Quinine has an effect to suppress neuromuscular transmission. In the symptomatic treatment of a rare myopathy known as *myotonia congenita,* or Thomsen's disease, quinine exerts a neuromuscular depressant action. Quinine is also used as a diagnostic test for myasthenia gravis, in which syndrome the symptoms are markedly aggravated by quinine but characteristically relieved by neostigmine. It occasionally benefits patients with spasmodic torticollis (torsion spasm) and also persons with nocturnal leg cramps. Quinine is an *oxytocic* and enjoys some lay popularity as an abortifacient, but is most unreliable in this regard. Quinine is a frequent constituent of bitter *tonics* and *stomachic* preparations. A syndrome of toxic effects known as "cinchonism," follows the repeated use of full therapeutic doses of quinine. Mild cinchonism is characterized by tinnitus, headache, nausea, and slight disturbance of vision. In severe cinchonism the skin is hot and flushed, rashes are frequent, and the central nervous system is involved; headache, fever, vomiting, apprehension, excitement, confusion, delirium, and syncope are common. The emesis is due to a central action of quinine as well as to the local irritant action of the drug on the intestinal mucosa. In a few cases, renal damage, photosensitivity, and hypoprothrombinemia may occur. Agranulocytosis has rarely been observed. Transient ventricular tachycardia is noted in rare instances after massive acute overdosage. Although quinine generally exerts vasodilator actions, retinal vasoconstriction, leading to loss of vision, has been described; these effects have mostly followed rapid intravenous injections or large overdoses.

Quinine is readily absorbed from the gastrointestinal tract. The drug is only moderately concentrated in tissues and undergoes degradation particularly in the liver. Quinine and its degradation products are rapidly excreted in the urine and for this reason the drug must be given every 6 hours in order to maintain relatively constant plasma levels.

The drug is given after meals to minimize gastric irritation. Intramuscular and subcutaneous injections of quinine are painful and are frequently followed by local tissue injury. The intravenous route is rarely used and only in emergencies.

Dose—*Oral, adults, antimalarial*, infections by chloroquine-resistant *Pl falciparum*, **650 mg**, every 8 hr for 10 to 14 days; for *other malarial infections*, **200 mg** to **1 g** every 8 hr for 6 to 12 days; for *myotonia*, **300** to **600 mg** every 8 or 12 hr; for *nocturnal leg cramps*, **200** to **300 mg** at bedtime and also after the evening meal, if necessary. *Children, antimalarial*, **8.3 mg/kg** every 8 hr or the following total daily doses given in 2 or 3 divided doses: *12 to 15 yr of age*, 1 to 2 g; *7 to 11 yr*, 500 mg to 1 g; *4 to 6 yr*, 300 to 500 mg; *1 to 3 yr*, 200 to 300 mg; *under 1 yr*, 100 to 200 mg.

Dosage Forms—Capsules: 130, 195, 200, 260, and 300 mg; Oral Suspension: 110 mg/5 mL; Tablets: 260, 300, and 325 mg.

Sulfadiazine—page 1173.

Sulfadoxine—page 1176.

Other Antimalarials

Chloroguanide Hydrochloride [1-(*p*-Chlorophenyl)-5-isopropyl-biguanide monohydrochloride [637-32-1] $C_{11}H_{16}ClN_5$.HCl (290.19); Proguanil Hydrochloride; Paludrine (*Ayerst*)]—May be prepared by reactions of isopropylamine, dicyanamide, and *p*-chloroaniline hydrochloride as the main reactants. White, crystalline powder, melts at about 243°. 1 g is soluble in 75 mL water, 30 mL alcohol; insoluble in chloroform, ether. *Uses:* Against *P falciparum* malarial parasites has an effect not only to suppress acute clinical attacks but also to destroy extraerythrocytic forms and hence to eradicate the infection. It also renders the gametocyte incapable of encysting itself in the mosquito vector. Against this plasmodium, chloroguanide is used as a causal prophylactic, a suppressive, and a radical curative drug. Against *P vivax* it acts only on the erythrocytic phase and hence is of value only as a suppressive drug in the control of acute attacks; against vivax it has no advantage over other suppressive antimalarials. Resistance to chloroguanide has occurred to such an extent that in some parts of the world the value of the drug has been seriously compromised, and it is very little used today. However, after a decade of disuse of chloroguanide, organisms should regain sensitivity to it. For additional information, including dosage, see RPS-15, page 1154. A new, related drug, *cycloguanil* has undergone successful field trials, but resistance occurs rapidly, so that its ultimate status is not clear.

Hydroxychloroquine Sulfate [2-[[4-[(7-Chloro-4-quinolyl)amino]pentyl]ethylamino]ethanol sulfate (1:1) [747-36-4] $C_{18}H_{26}ClN_3O.H_2SO_4$ (433.95); Plaquenil (*Winthrop*).]—*Preparation:* Hydroxychloroquine is prepared by condensing 4,7-dichloroquinoline with N^1-ethyl-N^1-(2-hydroxyethyl)-1,4-pentanediamine. After isolation and purification, the base may be dissolved in absolute ethanol or other organic solvent and precipitated as the sulfate by reaction with sulfuric acid. *Description and solubility:* White or nearly white, crystalline powder; odorless, and has a bitter taste; solutions are acid to litmus, having a pH of about 4.5; exists in two forms, the usual form melting at about 240° and the other form melting at about 198°. Freely soluble in water; practically insoluble in alcohol, chloroform, or ether. *Uses:* A drug similar in action and uses to *Chloroquine Phosphate* (see 1218). It mainly attacks the erythrocytic phase of the malaria parasite (ie, it is a suppressant), and therefore is not radically curative for *P vivax* infections. Like chloroquine, it is of use in the treatment of *lupus erythematosus* and *rheumatoid arthritis*, for which it is preferred. Toxicity is similar to that of chloroquine phosphate (see the introductory statement in this section). Early claims that hydroxychloroquine is less toxic have not been substantiated. Skin and retinopathy rashes occur with equal frequency with either drug. *Dose:* Oral, *adults*, for *antimalarial prophylaxis*, 400 mg once a week; for *antimalarial therapy*, *initially* 800 mg followed by 400 mg in 6 to 8 hr, then at 24 and

48 hr; *antirheumatic*, initially 400 to 800 mg once a day, then 200 to 400 mg once a day after a response has been achieved; for *lupus erythematosus*, 400 mg once or twice a day; for photosensitivity, 200 mg 2 or 3 times a day. *Children*, as an *antimalarial prophylactic*, 6.4 mg/kg (not to exceed 400 mg) once a week; for *antimalarial* therapy, *initially* 12.9 mg/kg (not to exceed 800 mg), then 6.4 mg/kg (not to exceed 400 mg) at 6, 24 and 48 hr.

Mefloquine   [(DL-*erythro*-α-2-Piperidyl-2,8-bis(trifluoromethyl)-4-quinolinemethanol [53230-10-7] $C_{17}H_{16}F_6N_2O$ (378.32)].   *Uses:* Mefloquine can eliminate fever and parasitemia and cause a radical cure in infections caused by *Pl falciparum* and can suppress infections caused by *Pl vivax*; with *Pl vivax*, infections usually recur at a later time. Its mechanism is unknown; it is not by intercalation into DNA. Mefloquine is well absorbed orally. In plasma, it is extensively bound to plasma proteins and is concentrated in the liver and lungs. It is eliminated mainly in the feces, mostly after biliary secretion. The half-life is about 17 days. *Dose: Oral, adults*, for suppressive cure of infections by *Pl falciparum*, 250 mg a week or 1 g every 4 weeks; for *suppression* of infections by *Pl vivax*, 250 mg a week.

Quinacrine Hydrochloride [6-Chloro-9-[[4-(diethylamino)-1-methylbutyl]amino]-2-methoxyacridine dihydrochloride dihydrate [6151-30-0] $C_{23}H_{30}ClN_3O.2HCl.2H_2O$ (508.91); *anhydrous* [69-05-6] (472.88); Atabrine Hydrochloride (*Winthrop*).]—*Preparation:* 2,4-Dichlorobenzoic acid is condensed in alkaline solution with *p*-anisidine, and the product, on treatment with phosphorus oxychloride, is cyclized to methoxydichloroacridine. This is heated with 2-amino-5-diethylaminopentane in phenol solution and the reaction mixture is added to acetone containing hydrochloric acid. Quinacrine is precipitated as the dihydrochloride while the phenol is held in solution by the acetone. *Description and solubility:* Bright yellow, odorless, bitter, crystalline powder; pH (1 in 100 solution) about 4.5; melts at about 250°, with decomposition. Soluble 1 g in about 35 mL water; soluble in alcohol; almost insoluble in chloroform. *Uses:* Inhibits the erythrocytic stage of development of the malarial parasite (suppressive action) and controls clinical attacks. It is neither a true causal prophylactic agent (an agent lethal to sporozoites or succeeding exoerythrocytic stages of development) nor a radical curative agent (an agent lethal to both erythrocytic and exoerythrocytic parasites). It does not prevent relapses in *vivax* malaria. However, suppressive doses of the drug at times *may* cure *falciparum malaria*. The drug is more effective and less toxic than quinine, but less effective and more toxic than chloroquine. It is the drug of choice for the treatment of *giardiasis*. Quinacrine is now virtually obsolete for the treatment of dwarf, beef, pork, and fish tapeworm infestations. A small percentage of patients treated with quinacrine exhibit untoward effects. These effects are essentially the same as those caused by the 4-aminoquinolines (see introductory statement in this section), of which quinacrine can be considered to be an analogue. The gastrointestinal irritancy is higher than with the 4-aminoquinolines, and it is common to give sodium bicarbonate concomitantly. Quinacrine is readily absorbed from the gastrointestinal tract and from intramuscular and intracavitary sites of injection. It is very slowly excreted in the urine and accumulates in tissue on chronic administration. Quinacrine is usually administered orally; each dose is given with water after a meal. If the oral route cannot be employed, intramuscular injection is preferred over the intravenous route of administration. *Dose: Oral, adults, antimalarial*, as a *suppressive*, 100 mg once a day for 1 to 3 months, and for *therapy*, initially 200 mg every 6 hr for 5 doses followed by 100 mg 3 times a day for 6 days; for *beef, fish, and pork tapeworms*, 200 mg every 10 min for 4 doses; for *dwarf tapeworm*, 300 mg every 20 min (on an empty stomach) for 3 doses on the first day followed by 100 mg 3 times a day for 3 days; for *giardiasis*, 100 mg after meals 3 times a day for 5 to 7 days. *Infants* and *children*, see package literature; *Drug Facts and Comparisons* or *The Medical Letter Handbook of Antimicrobial Therapy*.

Quinine Dihydrochloride [Acid quinine hydrochloride [60-93-5] $C_{20}H_{24}N_2O_2.2HCl$ (397.34)]—White powder; odorless; very bitter taste; solutions are strongly acid. 1 g dissolves in about 0.6 mL water. *Uses:* For the treatment of severe malarial attacks by chloroquine-resistant *P falciparum*. For actions, uses, and adverse effects of quinine, see *Quinine Sulfate*. Extravasation of the dihydrochloride can cause irritation. It was once common to combine the drug with urea to make a sclerosing mixture for closing inguinal rings, etc, a practice now considered obsolete but continued by some practitioners. *Dose: Intravenous, adults*, 600 mg, to be repeated in 6 to 8 hr; infants and children, 12.5 mg/kg of body weight, repeated in 6 to 8 hr provided oral therapy cannot be started, the maximal total dose not to exceed 1800 mg. For infusion, the dose is dissolved in sterile isotonic solution (300 mL for adults, less for children) and infused over a period of no less than an hour.

Amebicides

The incidence of amebiasis in the US has been estimated to be from 5 to 20%, depending on the locality. Most infections are essentially asymptomatic, but the number of severe infections is still large.

Amebic infections generally remain confined to the intestines, where they may give rise to dysentery; but in an appreciable fraction of cases the amebae may locate elsewhere, especially in the liver. The chemotherapy of amebiasis thus must provide drugs to treat both the intestinal and extraintestinal forms of the disease. In addition, the ideal amebicide also is capable of eliminating amebic cysts from the intestine. No safe drug exists that will eradicate all of motile forms, cysts, and extraintestinal amebas, but judicious combined therapy can eliminate the parasite from all sites.

Dehydroemetine Dihydrochloride

Emetan, 6',7',10,11-tetramethoxy-2,3-didehydro-, dihydrochloride

2,3-Dehydroemetine   dihydrochloride $C_{29}H_{38}N_2O_4 \cdot 2HCl$ (551.56).

The structure of dehydroemetine differs from that of emetine (see the next monograph) only in having two less hydrogen atoms, in the 2- and 3-positions, a double bond replacing the single bond in the emetine structure.

Preparation—Synthesis of dehydroemetine and its isomeric forms is described in publications of Brossi *et al*, *Helv Chim Acta 42:* 772, 1959; *ibid 45:* 2219, 1962; *Experientia 18:* 18, 211, 1962.

Description—White, crystalline powder; odorless; bitter taste.
Solubility—1 g in 30 mL water.

Uses—The actions and uses of dehydroemetine are those of emetine (see the following monograph). It is equally efficacious and less cardiotoxic than emetine and hence combinations containing dehydroemetine are preferred to those with emetine.

Dose—*Intramuscular* or *subcutaneous, adults* and *children*, 1 to **1.5 mg/kg** of body weight a day, not to exceed 90 mg a day, for no more than 5 days. Adults may be given the daily dose as a single or divided injection, but it should be divided into 2 doses in children.

Dosage Form—Injection: 60 mg/2 mL. In the US the drug is available only from the Parasitic Disease Drug Service, Centers for Disease Control, Atlanta, GA 30333.

Emetine Hydrochloride

Emetan, 6',7',10,11-tetramethoxy-, dihydrochloride

Emetine dihydrochloride [316-42-7] $C_{29}H_{40}N_2O_4 \cdot 2HCl$ (553.57); the hydrochloride of an alkaloid obtained from ipecac, or prepared by methylation of cephaeline, or prepared synthetically.

Description—White or very slightly yellowish, crystalline powder; odorless; affected by light.
Solubility—Freely soluble in water and in alcohol.

Uses—Emetine eradicates amebae from both intestinal and extraintestinal sites. At one time it was the principal drug in the antiamebic armamentarium. However, it has been replaced by less toxic and equally effective drugs, including its derivative dehydroemetine. In combinations (with paromomycin for severe intestinal amebiasis and chloroquine for amebic hepatitis), it ranks only as an alternative when other drugs fail. Emetine is concentrated in the liver, and for that reason it has been used especially for *amebic* hepatitis; it is also of considerable value in the treatment of amebic abscesses in other locations. Occasionally emetine may be life-saving. It rapidly relieves symptoms of intestinal amebiasis by destroying motile amebas, but the percentage of cures is below 15% since cysts are little affected: other agents are not only safer but superior. Emetine may be used initially to control quickly severe intestinal amebiasis; the drug is then followed by treatment with other agents. It has no place in the therapy of mild ambulatory or chronic cases.

The incidence of toxic effects from emetine is very high, both by local and systemic administration. Large doses produce acute lesions in the heart, liver, kidney, and intestines, and the dose is now restricted. Nevertheless, deaths still sometimes occur, often because of repeated courses of treatment at close intervals; the drug has a probable half-life on the order of weeks to months. The intravenous

route is contraindicated. Diarrhea, nausea, and vomiting are frequent, as are also skeletal muscle weakness, stiffness, and aching. Sensory disturbances also occur. By far the most important toxic effects are cardiovascular; they include hypotension, precordial pain, dyspnea, tachycardia, and long-persisting electrocardiographic changes; electrocardiographic and blood-pressure recordings at daily intervals are necessary. Emetine is contraindicated in patients with organic disease of the heart or kidney, unless there is no therapeutic alternative, in pregnancy, and when there has been a previous course of therapy within 6 weeks.

A course of emetine should not continue for more than 5 days. The patient should be kept in bed, and carefully watched for toxic effects.

Dose—*Subcutaneous* or *intramuscular, adults* and *children*, 1 **mg/kg** of body weight (up to maximum of 60 mg) a day, in one or two doses in adults and always in 2 divided doses in children.

Dosage Forms—Injection: 30 and 60 mg/mL.

Iodoquinol

8-Quinolinol, 5,7-diiodo-, Diiodohydroxyquinoline; Diodoquin; Diiodoquin, Floraquin (*Searle*); Yodoxin (*Glenwood*)

[83-73-8] $C_9H_5I_2NO$ (396.95).

Preparation—8-Quinolinol is iodinated by treatment with iodine monochloride or with a solution of iodine in potassium iodide.

Description—Light yellowish to tan, microcrystalline powder; wetted by water with difficulty, odorless or nearly so; stable in air; melts with decomposition.
Solubility—Practically insoluble in water; sparingly soluble in alcohol and ether.

Uses—Iodoquinol is the drug of choice for the treatment of asymptomatic infections caused by *Entameba histolytica*. In symptomatic intestinal disease, it is combined with metronidazole to treat mild to moderate infections and with metronidazole dehydroemetine, emetine, or paromomycin to treat severe *intestinal amebiasis*. It is ineffective in the treatment of extraintestinal amebiasis such as hepatic abscess. Bed rest is not required. It is the drug of choice in the treatment of infections caused by *Dientameba fragilis*. It is a second-choice drug in the treatment of balantidial dysentery. It also has been used in the local and systemic treatment of a *Trichomonas vaginalis vaginitis* and infections caused by *Trichomonas hominis* (intestinalis). It is used in the topical treatment of certain *fungal cutaneous infections* and in eczema in which fungal infection is a complication. Iodoquinol was once thought to have a low order of toxicity, but it now appears that a gastrointestinal-neurologic syndrome of obscure etiology, common in regions where iodoquinol is used, is caused by the drug and other halogenated hydroquinolines. For this reason, Japan withdrew such drugs from the market. Long-term, high-dosage (more than 1300 mg/day) should be avoided. Iodine toxicoderma, chills, fever, mild to severe dermatitis, irritation, abdominal discomfort, diarrhea, and headache occur. The drug may cause goiter. It can also interfere with certain thyroid tests, and protein-bound iodine may remain elevated for as long as 6 months after termination of a course of treatment. Systemic toxicity can result from topical, especially intravaginal, application. Because of gastrointestinal irritation, it should be taken after meals.

Dose—*Oral, adults*, **630** or **650 mg** 2 to 3 times a day for 20 days; *children*, **13.3 mg/kg** of body weight (or 333 mg/m^2 of body surface), not to exceed 195 mg/day, 3 times a day for 20 days.

Dosage Forms—Tablets: 210 and 650 mg; Powder: 25 g.

Metronidazole—page 1222.

Paromomycin Sulfate

D-Streptamine, *O*-2-amino-2-deoxy-
α-D-glucopyranosyl-(1→4)-*O*-[*O*-2,6-diamino-2,6-dideoxy-β-L-idopyr-
anosyl-1(1→3)-β-D-ribofuranosyl-(1→5)]-2-deoxy, sulfate (salt);
Humatin (*Parke-Davis*)

O-2,6-Diamino-2,6-dideoxy-β-L-idopyranosyl-(1→3)-O-β-D-ribo-
furanosyl-(1→5)-O-[2-amino-2-deoxy-α-D-glucopyranosyl-(1→4)]-
2-deoxystreptamine   sulfate   (salt)   [1263-89-4]
$C_{23}H_{45}N_5O_{14}.xH_2SO_4$; the sulfate of an antibiotic substance or substances produced by the growth of *Streptomyces rimosus* var *paro-
momycinus*, or a mixture of two or more such salts. Potency:
equivalent to not less than 675 μg of paromomycin ($C_{23}H_{45}N_5O_{14}$) per
mg, calculated on the anhydrous basis.

Preparation—Paromomycin [7542-37-2] is isolated from fermentation broths by ion-exchange adsorption.

Description—Off-white to light-yellow, amorphous powder that is
odorless or practically odorless; very hygroscopic.

Solubility—1 g in <1 mL water; >10,000 mL alcohol, chloroform,
ether.

Uses—Effective against most clinically significant gram-negative
bacteria, especially various species of *Shigella* and *Salmonella* and
strains of *E coli*. It is not effective against *Ps aeruginosa*. Among
the gram-positive organisms, only staphylococci are sufficiently
sensitive to be of clinical significance. It has been used to treat gastroenteritis or bacterial dysentery caused by these organisms, but
resistance develops rapidly and relapse rate is high, and other antibiotics are more successful. It has also been used to reduce the bacterial content of the intestine prior to surgery on the bowel or to rid
the bowel of nitrogen-forming bacteria in patients with hepatic coma.
Currently there is a great deal of interest in its use for bowel "sterilization" in patients with leukemia under treatment with antineo-

plastic drugs. Its principal and approved use (US) is in the treatment
of *amebiasis*. In the treatment of asymptomatic and mild to moderate intestinal disease, it is an alternative drug. It alters the ecology
of the intestinal flora in such a way that growth of intestinal amebas
is discouraged and it also helps to prevent secondary infections that
may follow or facilitate amebic invasion of the intestinal walls. It is
of no value in treating hepatic or other extraintestinal abscesses. It
is the drug of second choice for treatment of infestations of beef,
dwarf, fish, and pork *tapeworms*.

Paromomycin often causes gastrointestinal hypermotility, nausea,
diarrhea, and abdominal cramps, which generally appear on the second or third day of treatment and when the daily dose exceeds 2 g.
Occasionally the drug may cause headache, vertigo, vomiting, abdominal pain, or skin rash. Overgrowth of enteric staphylococci and
other pathogenic bacteria rarely occurs, but may if treatment is prolonged. Malabsorption syndromes have not been reported. There
is mutual cross-resistance to kanamycin and neomycin, and often to
streptomycin. Although paromomycin is poorly absorbed from the
gut, there is potential nephrotoxicity, especially in the presence of
renal disease.

Dose (base equivalent)—*Oral*, for *intestinal amebiasis*, *adults* and
children, **25 to 35 mg/kg** of body weight per day, in 3 divided doses,
for 5 to 10 days; for *dwarf tapeworm*, *adults* and *children*, **45 mg/kg**
once a day for 5 to 7 days; for *fish*, *beef*, and *pork tapeworms*, **1 g** every
15 min for 4 doses in *adults* and **11 mg/kg** every 4 hr for 4 doses in
children; for *hepatic coma*, *adults*, **4 g** a day in divided doses for 5
or 6 days.

Dosage Forms (base equivalent)—Capsules: 250 mg.

Other Amebicides

Diloxanide Furoate [2,2-Dichloro-4'-hydroxy-N-methylacetanilide,
2-furoate [3736-81-0] $C_{14}H_{11}Cl_2NO_4$ (328.19); Furamide (*Boots-
UK*).]—*Preparation:* See US Pat 2,912,438. *Uses:* Diloxanide has a
wide range of limited anti-infective activity against amebae, bacteria, fungi,
and helminths. Against *Entameba histolytica* it can arrest active intestinal infection but does so erratically. It is consistent only in suppressing
asymptomatic intestinal amebiasis and in eradicating cysts from the stools
of infected persons. It is alternative to iodoquinol in this use. Adverse
effects are mild or infrequent. Flatulence mainly occurs, but nausea,
vomiting, esophagitis, diarrhea, abdominal cramps, tingling sensations,
pruritis and urticaria sometimes occur. *Dose: Adults*, 500 mg 3 times
a day for 10 days; *children over 2 yr* of age, 20 mg/kg a day in 3 divided
doses for 10 days. Courses may be repeated if necessary. In the US, diloxanide furoate is available only from the Parasitic Disease Drug Service,
Centers for Disease Control, Atlanta, GA 30333.

Miscellaneous Antiprotozoal Drugs

Among the protozoal infections that are endemic to the US
are trichomoniasis, amebiasis, giardiasis, and malaria, in decreasing order of incidence. Other protozoal infections, uncommon in the US, nevertheless constitute serious public
health and agricultural problems within the possessions and
elsewhere. Until the advent of the antibiotics all the protozoal
infections were managed very similarly, with heavy metals
providing the backbone of therapy, except for malaria.
However, the heavy metals are no longer employed in the
treatment of syphilis and yaws and are not essential to the
management of amebiasis or trichomoniasis. The amebicides
and antimalarials are useful in the treatment of a number of
other protozoal infections. The antimalarials and amebicides
have been treated in separate sections above. The antisy-
philitics are largely included among the antibiotics. Consequently, the drugs listed below are a miscellaneous group of
compounds.

Amodiaquine Hydrochloride—page 1217.

Antimony Potassium Tartrate—page 1238.

Iodoquinol—page 1221.

Metronidazole

1*H*-Imidazole-1-ethanol, 2-methyl-5-nitro-, Flagyl (*Searle*)

2-Methyl-5-nitroimidazole-1-ethanol   [443-48-1] $C_6H_9N_3O_3$
(171.16).

Preparation—2-Methyl-5-nitroimidazole is condensed with
ethylene chlorohydrin by heating with a large excess of the chlorohydrin. After removing the surplus chlorohydrin, the residue is
extracted with water and the extract is alkalinized and extracted with
chloroform. Evaporation of the chloroform yields crude metronidazole which is recrystallized from ethyl acetate. US Pat
2,944,061.

Description—White to pale yellow, odorless, crystals or crystalline
powder; stable in air, but darkens on exposure to light; melts between 159°
and 163°.

Solubility—Sparingly soluble in water, alcohol, and chloroform; slight
soluble in ether.

Uses—Metronidazole is bactericidal to anaerobic and microaerophilic microorganisms, including *Bacteroides*, *Clostridium* species,
Endolimax nana, *Entameba histolytica*, *Fusobacterium vincentii*,
Gardnerella vaginalis, *Giardia lamblia*, *Peptococcus*, *Peptostreptococcus*, and *Trichomonas vaginalis*. These organisms reduce the
nitro group and generate metabolites that inhibit DNA synthesis.
Metronidazole has long been the drug of choice for the treatment of
trichomoniasis and more recently in combination with iodoquinol
for the treatment of symptomatic *amebiasis* (except in brain). Be-

cause it is well absorbed orally, concentrations in the lower bowel sometimes are not high enough to eradicate amebas, so that it is *combined with iodoquinol* to make a first-choice combination. It is also the drug of choice for the treatment of vaginitis caused by *Gardnerella vaginalis*. It is the alternative drug to treat *giardiasis* (although some authorities consider it the drug of first choice) and *guinea worm (Dracunculus)* infection. The drug is currently of interest for the *treatment* and *prophylaxis of infections caused by anerobic bacteria* (especially *B fragilis*). Metronidazole has also been reported to be of value in Crohn's disease. The drug sensitizes hypoxic tumor cells to radiation and has been employed as an adjunct to radiation therapy.

The most common untoward effects are nausea, diarrhea, anorexia, epigastric distress, and abdominal cramps. Unpleasant taste, vomiting, furry tongue and stomatitis are fairly frequent. Urticaria, pruritus, flushing, dysuria, cystitis, dry mouth, dry vulva and vagina, feeling of pelvic pressure, vaginal burning, rash, vertigo, headache, numbness, paresthesias, and insomnia occur occasionally. Incoordination and ataxia are rare. Sudden overgrowth of monilia sometimes occurs. The urine sometimes turns a dark color. During metronidazole treatment the patient should refrain from drinking alcoholic beverages, since metronidazole has a mild effect similar to *Disulfiram* (page 1070). Neutropenia occurs, so that a blood count should be made, especially before a second course of the drug. In patients with blood dyscrasias great care must be exercised. Metronidazole should not be used in patients with diseases of the central nervous system. The drug has been found to be carcinogenic in mice and rats, and mutagenic. Substances mutagenic in the Ames test have been found in the urine of recipients. Metronidazole has been used in pregnancy without consequence, but it is advisable to withhold it during pregnancy, if possible.

Metronidazole is usually about 80% absorbed by the oral route, but in some patients absorption is low. Both unchanged drug and metabolites are excreted into the urine. The half-life is about 6 to 12 hr. The drug inhibits the oxidation of warfarin.

Dose—*Oral, adults*, for *trichomoniasis*, **2 g** once only, **1 g** twice in a single day, or **250 mg** 3 times a day for 7 days; for *amebiasis*, **500 to 750 mg** 3 times a day for 5 to 10 days; for *giardiasis*, **2 g** once a day for 3 days *or* 250 to **500 mg** 3 times a day for 5 to 7 days; for *balantidiasis*, **750 mg** 3 times a day for 5 to 6 days; for *anaerobic infections*, **7.5 mg/kg** (up to a total dose of 1 g) every 6 hr for 7 or more days; for *dracunculiasis*, **250 mg** 3 times a day for 10 days. *Children*, for *trichomoniasis*, **5 mg/kg** for 7 days; for *amebiasis*, **11.6 to 16.7 mg/kg** 3 times a day for 10 days; for *giardiasis*, **5 mg/kg** 3 times a day for 5 to 7 days; for *dracunculiasis*, **8.3 mg/kg** (up to a total of 250 mg) 3 times a day for 10 days. *Intravenous, adults*, for *anaerobic infections*, initially **15 mg/kg** followed by **7.5 mg/kg** (up to a total of 1 g) every 6 hr for 7 or more days.

Dosage Forms—Injection (buffered with phosphate and citrate to pH of about 6): 500 mg/100 mL. Each 100 mL contains 1.4 mEq of sodium. Tablets: 250 and 500 mg.

Metronidazole Hydrochloride

1*H*-Imidazole-1-ethanol, 2-methyl-5-nitro-, hydrochloride; Flagyl IV
(Searle)

[69198-10-3] $C_6H_9N_3O_3 \cdot HCl$ (207.62).

Uses—See *Metronidazole* (above). The hydrochloride is used for the systemic treatment of infections by anaerobic bacteria.

Dose—*Intravenous*, see *Metronidazole*.

Dosage Forms—Powder for injection: 500 mg.

Stibogluconate Sodium

Gluconic acid, diester with antimonic acid ($H_8Sb_2O_9$), trisodium salt, nonahydrate

D-Gluconic acid, cyclic 3,4,5-Sb:3′,4′,5′-Sb′-ester with antimonic acid ($H_8Sb_2O_9$), trisodium salt, nonahydrate [16037-91-5] $C_{12}H_{17}Na_3O_{17}Sb_2 \cdot 9H_2O$ (907.86); *anhydrous* (745.73). *Note:* Although recorded in the literature, this composition is not in complete agreement with the manufacturer's analytical data.

Description—Odorless, colorless, amorphous powder.
Solubility—Very soluble in water; insoluble in alcohol and ether.

Uses—Stibogluconate is the drug of choice for the treatment of all forms of *leishmaniasis*. It is not known whether the active form is

the pentavalent or trivalent form. Some of the pentavalent antimony is reduced to trivalent antimony in the body.

Stibogluconate sodium is considerably less toxic than tartar emetic. Vomiting and coughing are thus uncommon. Late in a course of treatment, muscle and joint pains occasionally occur. Bradycardia and electrocardiographic changes are infrequent. Hypersensitivity reactions, such as various rashes, facial edema, hypotension (even rare anaphylaxis), hemolytic anemia, hepatitis, etc can occur after several doses, but such occurrences are not common. Headache, syncope, and abdominal pain also occasionally occur. Liver function may be depressed. Locally the drug is fairly well tolerated, but pain and other evidences of local toxicity can occur. Dimercaprol will diminish the toxic effects and arrest the development of allergy. Stibogluconate sodium is contraindicated with hepatitis, nephritis, or myocarditis are present.

Dose (antimony equivalent)—*Intramuscular* or *intravenous, adults*, **600 mg** a day for 6 to 10 days; *children*, **10 mg/kg** of body weight per day for 6 to 10 days. It may be necessary to repeat the course 2 or 3 times, with 10-day rest intervals in between courses. With debilitated persons, it may be advisable to give the drug every other day. In oriental sore, the lesion may be infiltrated around the edges with the equivalent of 200 mg of antimony. In the US this drug is available only from the Parasitic Disease Drug Service, Centers for Disease Control, Atlanta, GA 30333.

Sulfadoxine—page 1176.

Suramin Sodium

1,3,5-Naphthalenetrisulfonic acid, 8,8′-[carbonylbis[imino-3,1-phenylenecarbonylimino(4-methyl-3,1-phenylene)carbonylimino]]bis-, hexasodium salt; Germanin; Antrypol (*ICI-UK*)

Hexasodium 8,8′-[ureylenebis[*m*-phenylenecarbonylimino(4-methyl-*m*-phenylene)carbonylimino]]di-1,3,5-naphthalenetrisulfonate [129-46-4] $C_{51}H_{34}N_6Na_6O_{23}S_6$ (1429.15).

Preparation—8-Amino-1,3,5-naphthalenetrisulfonic acid is condensed with *m*-nitro-*p*-toluoyl chloride in the presence of sodium acetate. The resulting nitro compound is reduced, and the amino derivative is condensed with *m*-nitrobenzoyl chloride; the product is reduced to the corresponding amino compound which is then reacted with carbonyl chloride in the ratio of two moles of the former to one of the latter. The suramin acid thus obtained is neutralized with NaOH to produce the sodium salt.

Description—White or slightly pink powder, which is odorless and has a slightly bitter taste; very hygroscopic and affected by light; pH (1 in 100 solution) between 5.5 and 7.
Solubility—Soluble in water; slightly soluble in alcohol; insoluble in ether, chloroform.

Uses—One of the few nonmetallic compounds effective in the treatment and prophylaxis of *trypanosomiasis* caused by *T rhodesiense, T hippicum*, and *T gambiense*. If it is used early, it can be used alone, but if there is central nervous system involvement, arsenicals also must be used. *T cruzi* (agent of Chagas' disease) does not respond. Suramin is also an effective agent for the treatment of *onchocerciasis*. It has also been effectively employed in the treatment of *pemphigus*.

In some patients, suramin may cause nausea and vomiting, shock, and loss of consciousness immediately after injection. Later, sensory disturbances (photophobia, paresthesias, etc), papular eruptions, and palpebral edema may occur. Still later, albuminuria, hematuria, and casts may occur. Hemolytic anemia and agranulocytosis are rare but possible. It is irritating upon intramuscular injection.

Suramin is not absorbed from the gastrointestinal tract. After intravenous injection, the blood level falls in three phases: rapidly for a few hours, more slowly for several days, then very slowly, such that the blood concentration may persist for up to 3 months. Suramin binds to plasma protein. It does not penetrate the central nervous system. It is concentrated in the kidney.

Dose—*Intravenous, adults*, for *prophylaxis*, **1 g** by slow infusion every 3 months; for *active trypanosomiasis*, **1 g** on days 1, 3, 7, 14 and 21; *children;* **20 mg/kg** of body weight on days 1, 3, 7, 14, and 21. Initially, try 200 mg to test for sensitivity before giving the full dose. A second course of therapy should not be repeated until 3 months after the end of the 1st course. For *onchocerciasis, adults*, **1 g** weekly for 7 to 10 weeks.

Dosage Forms—for Injection: 1 g of sterile powder. Available in the US from the Parasitic Disease Drug Service, Centers for Disease Control, Atlanta, GA 30333.

Other Miscellaneous Antiprotozoal Drugs

Meglumine Antimoniate [1-Deoxy-1-methylamino-D-glucitol antimonate [133-51-7] $C_7H_{18}NO_8Sb$ (365.97).]—*Uses:* In the treatment of cutaneous and mucocutaneous leishmaniasis, meglumine antimoniate is considered by tropical disease authorities to be the drug of choice in lieu of sodium stibogluconate. Against visceral forms (kala azar) it is somewhat less effective. Oriental and Brazilian organisms are more sensitive than African and Mediterranean forms. The drug has a lesser toxicity than stibogluconate, but antimony poisoning can occur.

Melarsoprol [2-[*p*-[(4,6-Diamino-*s*-triazin-2-yl)amino]-phenyl]-1,3,2-dithiarsolane-4-methanol [494-79-1] $C_{12}H_{15}AsN_6OS_2$ (398.34).]—Slightly cream or grayish cream powder with a slight odor and a bitter taste; melts at about 217° with decomposition. Insoluble in water, alcohol, and ether. *Uses:* In the treatment of advanced African trypanosomiasis with CNS involvement. It has replaced other arsenicals for this purpose. *Dose: Intravenous, adults*, initially 2.6 to 3.6 mg/kg daily for 3 days followed after 1 wk by 3.6 mg/kg a day for 3 doses, to be repeated after 10 to 21 days; children, initially 0.36 mg/kg, to be gradually increased at 1- to 5-day intervals to 3.6 mg/kg, for a total of 9 to 10 doses and 18 to 25 mg/kg over 1 mo. In the US melarsoprol is available only from the Parasitic Disease Drug Service, Centers for Disease Control, Atlanta, GA 30333.

Nifurtimox [4-[(5-Nitrofurfurylidene)amino]-3-methylthiomorpholine-1,1-dioxide [23256-30-6] $C_{10}H_{13}N_3O_5S$ (287.29); Bayer 2502.]—Orange-red crystals, melting at about 181°; soluble in water. *Uses:* Nifurtimox is presently the only drug effective against infections caused by *Trypanosoma cruzi* (South American trypanosomiasis). It destroys only the extracellular organisms in blood. *Dose:* The dose schedule is complex; for information concerning it, and for the drug, contact the Parasitic Disease Drug Service, Centers for Disease Control, Atlanta, GA 30333.

Ornidazole [α-(Chloromethyl)-2-methyl-5-nitroimidazole-1-ethanol [16773-42-5] $C_7H_{10}ClN_3O_3$ (219.63).]—*Uses:* Ornidazole is the chloromethyl analogue of metronidazole (page 1222), which it closely resembles in spectrum of antimicrobial action, clinical efficacy, and pharmacokinetics, except that its half-life (14.5 hr) is longer. It is very similar to tinidazole in usefulness and single-dose schedules.

Pentamidine Isethionate [*p,p′*-(Pentamethylenedioxy)dibenzamidine bis(β-hydroxyethanesulfonate) [140-64-7] $C_{19}H_{24}N_4O_2.2C_2H_6O_4S$ (592.68)]—Crystals, hygroscopic, melting at about 180°. Soluble in water; slightly soluble in alcohol; insoluble in ether, chloroform. *Uses:* Pentamidine is the alternate drug to suramin for treatment of the hemolymphatic stage of African sleeping sickness (trypanosomiasis) caused by *T brucei gambiense* and *T brucei rhodesiense*. It is the alternate drug for the treatment of infections caused by *Pneumocystis carinii*. Frequent adverse effects include pain at the site of injection, hypotension, vomiting, blood dyscrasias, and renal damage. Occasional effects are diabetes, shock, and liver damage. Herxheimer reactions are rare. *Dose: Intra-*

muscular, adults and *children*, 4 mg/kg of body weight a day for 10 days for trypanosomiasis and 12 to 14 days for *Pneumocystis carinii*. In the US the drug is available only from the Parasitic Disease Drug Service, Centers for Disease Control, Atlanta, GA 30333.

Spiramycin [Leucomycin [8025-81-8]; An antibiotic of the erythromycin/carbomycin type produced by *Streptomyces ambofaciens* from the soil of northern France. It is composed of spiramycins I, $C_{45}H_{78}N_2O_{15}$ (63%); II, $C_{47}H_{80}N_2O_{16}$ (24%); and III, $C_{48}H_{82}N_2O_{16}$ (13%). See *J Org Chem 39*: 2474, 1974. *Description and solubility:* Yellowish-white powder with a bitter taste; 1 g is soluble in 50 mL of water; very soluble in chloroform or alcohol; soluble in dilute aqueous acid; insoluble in hydrocarbon solvents. *Uses:* A macrolide antibiotic with an antibacterial spectrum resembling that of erythromycin but having greater activity against certain protozoa. It is an alternative drug for the treatment of *toxoplasmosis*. It is often given in combination with pyrimethamine-sulfamethoxazole. *Dose: Oral, adults*, 2 to 4 g a day for 3 to 4 wk; *children*, 50 to 100 mg/kg a day for 3 to 4 wk.

Tinidazole [1-[2-(Ethylsulfonyl)ethyl]-2-methyl-5-nitroimidazole [19387-91-8] $C_8H_{13}N_3O_4S$ (247.26) Fasign; Simplotan (*Pfizer*).]—*Preparation:* For information concerning preparation of tinidazole see *CA 71:* 3384e, 1969; also US Pat 3,376,311. *Description:* Colorless crystals, melting at about 127°. *Dose:* Tinidazole is the ethylsulfonyl derivative of metronidazole and has the same antimicrobial spectrum and uses (see page 1222). It has about the same or slightly greater efficacy in the treatment of *amebiasis* and *trichomoniasis*. In *giardiasis*, tinidazole has been found to be effective against strains resistant to metronidazole. It has yet to be compared with metronidazole in the treatment or prophylaxis of infections caused by anaerobic bacteria. Tinidazole has two advantages over metronidazole which may cause replacement of the older by the newer drug, namely, a relatively high single-dose efficacy in some infections and a lower incidence and intensity of side effects. It has all the side-effects of metronidazole, but, in clinical use they are less frequent and less intense. Epigastric pain occurs in about 6% of recipients; nausea, dry mouth, and candidal overgrowth in the vagina in 4%; vomiting in 1%. Tinidazole is well absorbed by the oral route, but with the large single daily dose, sufficient unabsorbed drug remains in the intestines to exert an amebicidal action that may possibly be superior to that of metronidazole. In plasma, 20% is bound to protein. Elimination is essentially by renal excretion. The half-life averages about 12.5 hr in normal subjects but is probably much longer in renal failure. *Dose: Oral, adults*, for *trichomoniasis, male and female*, 2 g as a single dose and again after 3 to 5 days rest, if the first dose did not effect a cure; for *intestinal amebiasis*, 600 mg twice a day for 5 to 10 days *or* 2 g as a single dose a day for 2 to 6 days; for *extraintestinal amebiasis*, 800 mg 3 times a day for 5 days *or* 2 g as a single dose a day for 3 days; for *giardiasis*, 150 mg twice a day *or* 2 g as a single dose.

Tryparsamide [Monosodium *N*-(carbamoylmethyl)arsanilate [554-72-3] $C_8H_{10}AsN_2O_4Na$ (296.08)]—Prepared by the interaction of arsanilic acid and chloroacetamide. White, crystalline powder. 1 g is soluble in 2 mL water; slightly soluble in alcohol; insoluble in ether, chloroform. *Uses:* Tryparsamide with suramin is an alternative to melarsoprol in the treatment of late trypanosomal infections with CNS involvement caused by *T brucei gambiense* and *T brucei rhodesiense*. Adverse effects are frequent and include nausea and vomiting, occasional fever, hypersensitivity, exfoliative dermatitis, impaired vision, and optic atrophy. *Dose: Intravenous, adults*, 30 mg/kg of body weight every 5 days to a total of 12 injections; the course may be repeated after a rest period of 1 month. Tryparsamide is available in the US only from the Parasitic Disease Drug Service, Centers for Disease Control, Atlanta, GA 30333.

Antidotes to Heavy Metals

During the time when the use of arsenicals in war gases and in antiluetics was at its peak, no successful antidote to heavy metal poisoning existed, although the erratic sodium formaldehyde sulfoxylate antidote to mercury had been developed. Dimercaprol appeared at the end of the era of arsenical antiluesis, but the continued use of arsenic, antimony, and bismuth for other purposes has left a place for this agent. Because arsenic, antimony, and bismuth are still used, somewhat, in the treatment of protozoal infections, antidotes to the heavy metals are included here, rather than in a separate chapter. Edetate calcium disodium is discussed below because it is useful as an antidote to lead and several other heavy metals, even though such metals have no antimicrobial applications. Penicillamine was originally introduced as a chelating agent for heavy metals, but it has become important in the treatment of various autoimmune and other diseases.

Deferoxamine Mesylate—page 838.

Dimercaprol

1-Propanol, 2,3-dimercapto-, British Anti-Lewisite; BAL in Oil (*Hynson, Westcott & Dunning*)

$$CH_2CHCH_2OH$$
$$SH \quad SH$$

[59-52-9] $C_3H_8OS_2$ (124.22) and not more than 1.5% of 1,2,3-trimercaptopropane ($C_3H_8S_3$).

Preparation—A methanol solution of NaOH is saturated with hydrogen sulfide resulting in the formation of sodium hydrogen sulfide [NaSH]. 2,3-Dibromopropanol is added and the mixture heated at 40° under pressure. 2,3-Dibromopropanol is prepared by bromination of allyl alcohol.

Description—Colorless or almost colorless liquid; offensive, mercaptan-like odor; specific gravity 1.242 to 1.244; boiling range 66° to 68° (0.2 mm Hg).

Solubility—1 g in about 20 mL water; soluble in alcohol, benzyl benzoate, and vegetable oils.

Uses—In oil solution it is an *antidote* used in the treatment of *arsenic, gold, and mercury poisoning.* The drug also may be of value in the treatment of antimony, thallium, and bismuth poisoning. It is used in the treatment of acute *lead encephalopathy* only in conjunction with *Edetate Calcium Disodium.* The thiol groups of dimercaprol compete with the physiologically essential —SH groups found in the tissues, and thus remove the metal ions. The combination of heavy metal and dimercaprol is a stable compound which is excreted. Dimercaprol is particularly useful in hemorrhagic encephalitis resulting from arsenotherapy, in arsenical or gold dermatitis, and possibly in postarsenical jaundice.

Dimercaprol usually causes hypertension and tachycardia, which lasts for about 2 hours. It also often causes nausea, vomiting, headache, burning sensations in the mouth and throat, and a feeling of pressure in the throat, chest and hands. It may also cause conjunctivitis, lacrimation, salivation and rhinorrhea, sweating, and abdominal pain. Sterile abscesses often occur at the site of injection. In children, fever frequently occurs; it appears after the 3rd dose and remains throughout the course.

Dose—*Intramuscular, adults,* and *children,* for *mild arsenic* or *gold* intoxication, **2.5 mg/kg** every 8 hr for 2 days then once a day for 10 days; for *severe arsenic* or *gold intoxication,* **3 mg/kg** every 4 hr for 2 days, every 8 hr on the 3rd day, then every 12 hr for 10 days; for *mercury intoxication, initially* **5 mg/kg** followed by **2.5 mg/kg** once or twice daily for 10 days; for *acute lead encephalopathy, initially* **4 mg/kg** then 3 to 4 mg/kg every hr (in combination with calcium disodium edeate at separate sites twice a day) for 2 to 7 days.

Dosage Form—Injection (in oil): 300 mg/3 mL.

Edetate Calcium Disodium

Calciate(2-), [[N,N'-1,2-ethanediylbis[N-(carboxymethyl)glycinato]]-(4-)-$N,N',O,O',O^N O^{N'}$]-, disodium, hydrate (OC-6-21)-, Calcium Disodium Versenate (*Riker*); Versene CA (*Merrell-Dow*)

Disodium[(ethylenedinitrilo)tetraacetato]calciate(2-) hydrate; calcium disodium ethylenediaminetetraacetate hydrate [23411-34-9] $C_{10}H_{12}CaN_2Na_2O_8.xH_2O$; *anhydrous* [62-33-9] (374.27); a mixture of the dihydrate and trihydrate of calcium disodium ethylenediaminetetraacetate (predominantly the dihydrate).

Preparation—Among other ways, by boiling an aqueous solution of edetate disodium (page 838) with slightly more than an equimolar quantity of calcium carbonate until carbon dioxide is no longer evolved, filtering while hot, and crystallizing.

Description—White, crystalline granules or white, crystalline powder; odorless, slightly hygroscopic, and has a faint, saline taste; stable in air.
Solubility—Freely soluble in water.

Uses—Primarily in the diagnosis and treatment of *lead poisoning,* but may be used for removing certain other heavy metals from the body. As a diagnostic agent, it causes a surge of lead into the urine, the magnitude of which reveals the extent of the body burden of lead. Treatment is usually by intravenous infusion, but in lead encephalopathy the infusion fluid exacerbates the cerebral edema, so that the drug is given, instead, by the intramuscular route in a hyperosmotic concentration. Since this agent already contains calcium it is useless as an anticoagulant or for treatment of hypercalcemia.

During infusion there may be transitory hypotension, inversion of the T-wave of the ECG, and prolongation of prothrombin time. Fever sometimes occurs 4 to 8 hr after an infusion. It is accompanied by malaise, fatigue, thirst and chills. Myalgia, headache, vomiting, and increased urinary urgency often follow. Sneezing, nasal congestion,

lacrimation, glycosuria, anemia, and dermatitis also occasionally occur. Edetate sometimes causes a usually reversible hydropic degeneration of the renal tubular epithelium, especially in the lower nephron.

Edetate calcium disodium is entirely eliminated in the urine with a half-life of 1 hr, except longer in renal insufficiency.

Dose—*Intravenous infusion, adults,* **1 g** in 250 to 500 mL of isotonic solution over a period of 1 hr 2 times a day for 3 to 5 days; the total daily dose should not exceed 50 mg/kg when symptoms are only mild; for *children,* up to **35 mg/kg** of body weight (or 850 mg/m^2 of body surface) as 0.2 to 0.4% solution in an isotonic injection twice a day. *Intramuscular, adults,* **1 g** in 0.5% procaine hydrochloride solution twice a day; *children,* up to **35 mg/kg** (or 850 mg/m^2) in 0.5% procaine hydrochloride solution twice a day.

Dosage Form—Injection: 200 mg/mL.

Penicillamine

D-Valine, 3-mercapto-, β,β-Dimethylcysteine; Cuprimine (*MSD*); Depen (*Wallace*)

$$HS-\underset{\underset{CH_3}{|}}{\overset{\overset{CH_3}{|}}{C}}---\underset{\underset{NH_2}{|}}{\overset{\overset{H}{|}}{C}}--COOH$$

D-3-Mercaptovaline [52-67-5] $C_5H_{11}NO_2S$ (149.21).

Preparation—By acid hydrolysis of penicillin. It is precipitated from the hydrolysis mixture as the mercuric salt which is then collected, suspended in water, and treated with hydrogen sulfide to liberate the free acid. Purification involves only recrystallization from water. Penicillamine is also obtained by synthesis.

Description—Fine, white or practically white, crystalline powder, having a slight characteristic odor and a slightly bitter taste; relatively stable in both light and air; melts at about 200° with decomposition; pH (1 in 100 solution) between 4.5 and 5.5.
Solubility—Freely soluble in water; slightly soluble in alcohol; insoluble in chloroform and ether.

Uses—A chelating agent useful in the treatment of *Wilson's disease* and *biliary cirrhosis* (in which the serum and liver copper concentration, respectively, are excessively high), and *lead, gold,* or *mercury poisoning.* It is especially useful in the long-term treatment of lead poisoning because of its oral efficacy, which the edetates lack. Penicillamine is also useful in the treatment of *cystinuria* and *rheumatoid arthritis;* plasma cystine levels fall in the former during treatment but rise in the latter. The mechanism in rheumatoid arthritis is unknown.

Side effects most often appear shortly after therapy has begun. It may cause ecchymosis, dermatitis, eruptions of the mucous membranes, leukopenia, thrombocytopenia, agranulocytosis, fever, nephrosis, lymphadenopathy, and optic neuritis. Anorexia, nausea, epigastric pain, diarrhea, vomiting, stomatitis, peptic ulcer, and disorders of taste are also common effects. Cholestatic jaundice, toxic hepatitis and pancreatitis occur rarely. Blood counts must be made every 2 weeks during the first 6 months of therapy.

Dose—*Oral, adults,* as an *antidote* to heavy metals, **500 mg** 4 times day for 1 to 2 mo; *antirheumatic,* initially **125 mg** once or twice a day, followed by increments of **125 to 250 mg/day** at 1- to 3-month intervals up to a maximum of **1.5 g** a day; in *cystinuria,* **500 mg** 4 times a day; for *Wilson's disease* and *biliary cirrhosis,* **250 mg** 4 times a day. *Children,* as an antidote, **10 to 13.3 mg/kg** 3 times a day for 1 to 6 mo; in *cystinuria,* **7.5 mg/kg** of body weight 4 times a day; in *Wilson's disease* and *biliary cirrhosis,* **250 mg** a day in fruit juice for infants over 6 mo of age and young children and adult dose in older children.

Dosage Forms—Capsules: 125 and 250 mg; Tablets: 250 mg.

Sodium Formaldehyde Sulfoxylate—page 1279.

Antifungal Drugs

The fungi comprise five widely differing classes of primitive flora, including the bacteria; the variations in cell physiology and biochemistry are extreme among fungi. Thus, antifungal agents include a wide variety of chemical types of rather narrow antifungal spectrum. Broad-spectrum antifungal

agents in general are toxic and are irritants, as expected from their nonselectivity; however, many of these have limited absorption through the epidermis and so may be employed in dermatologic preparations. Not all antifungal agents are fungicidal; many are only fungistatic, and certain of them may owe their efficacy to a keratolytic action that causes a sloughing of the stratum corneum with its entrained fungi.

Acrisorcin

1,3-Benzenediol, 4-hexyl-, compd with 9-acridinamine (1:1); Akrinol (*Schering-Plough*)

4-Hexylresorcinol compound with 9-aminoacridine (1:1) [7527-91-5] $C_{12}H_{18}O_2.C_{13}H_{10}N_2$ (388.51).

Preparation—9-Aminoacridine is combined directly with an equimolar quantity of 4-hexylresorcinol in a solvent such as acetone.

Description—Yellow, odorless powder; melts with decomposition at about 190°.

Solubility—1 g in 1000 mL water, 18 mL alcohol, 320 mL chloroform, 55 mL acetone.

Uses—Possesses antifungal activity, especially against *Malassezia furfur*. Therefore, it is used in the treatment of *tinea* (pityriasis) *versicolor*, which is caused by *Pityrosporon orbiculare* (*Malassezia furfur*). Permanent cures are not always effected. Although acrisorcin has mild antibacterial activity, it is not used for such properties.

By topical application, the toxicity is low. It may produce hives, erythematous vesicles, and blisters. It sometimes causes burning sensations when placed on eczematous lesions. After acrisorcin, exposure to ultraviolet light may promote itching. It should not be used around the eyes.

Dose—*Topical*, apply to the affected area 2 times a day for at least 6 weeks after the lesions disappear. Vigorous prewashing is important to good results.

Dosage Form—Cream: 0.2%.

Aminacrine Hydrochloride—page 1166.

Amphotericin B

Fungizone (*Squibb*)

[1R-(1R*,3S*,5R*,6R*,9R*,11R*,15S*,16R*,17R*,18S*,19E,21E, 23E,25E,27E,29E,31E,33R*,35S,36S*,37S*)]-33-[(3-Amino-3,6-dideoxy-β-D-mannopyranosyl)oxy]-1,3,5,6,9,11,17,37-octahydroxy-15,16,18-trimethyl-13-oxo-14,39-dioxabicyclo[33.3.1]nonatriaconta-19,21,23,25,27,29,31-heptaene-36-carboxylic acid [1397-89-3] $C_{47}H_{73}NO_{17}$ (924.09); a substance produced by the growth of *Streptomyces nodosus*. Potency: not less than 750 µg of amphotericin B/mg.

Preparation—By the growth of selected strains of *Streptomyces nodosus* in an appropriate medium under controlled conditions of temperature, pH, and aeration. After extracting from the medium, the crude product is purified by treatment with various solvents at controlled acidity.

Description—Yellow to orange powder; odorless or practically so.
Solubility—Insoluble in water, anhydrous alcohol, ether.

Uses—Has the widest spectrum of antifungal activity of any systemic antifungal drug. By the intravenous route it is an extremely useful drug for therapy of *systemic fungous diseases*, especially coccidiomycosis, cryptococcosis, systemic moniliasis, histoplasmosis,

aspergillosis, rhodotorulosis, sporotrichosis, phycomycosis (mucormycosis) and North American blastomycosis. It is also used topically in the treatment of *superficial monilial infections*. It is not effective against viruses, protozoa, or bacteria. However, it is effective against some species of *Leishmania* (*L braziliensis* and *mexicana*), for which it is the drug of second choice. Acquired resistance to the drug has not been observed.

Amphotericin B is very poorly absorbed from the gastrointestinal tract. It is slowly excreted by the kidneys but neither renal failure nor hemodialysis has a consistent effect on plasma levels. The plasma half-life is 18 to 24 hours.

Amphotericin B may induce chills and fever, nausea and vomiting, diarrhea, abdominal "cramps," hemorrhagic gastroenteritis, dyspepsia, headache, vertigo, pain in the vein injected, thrombophlebitis, muscle and joint pains, anemia, purpura, hypertension, hypotension, cardiac arrest, ventricular fibrillation, skin rashes, hypokalemia, renal damage, blood dyscrasias, loss of hearing, and other untoward effects. When given intrathecally it may cause grand mal convulsions, radiculitis, arachnoiditis, paralysis of the extremities, urinary retention, and other difficulties. Because of the potential seriousness of its toxic effects, intravenous use of amphotericin B should be primarily for patients with progressive, potentially fatal infections, and the patient should always be hospitalized during a course of therapy and renal function should be monitored. Hypokalemia may favor digitalis toxicity and sensitize to neuromuscular blocking drugs.

Dose—*Intravenous infusion, adults, infants*, and *children*, initially **250 µg/kg** of body weight a day, increased by daily increments of **5 to 10 mg,** if tolerated, up to a maximum of **1.5 mg/kg** (or 45 mg/m² of body surface in infants and children); the dose is prepared as a solution of 100 µg/mL in 5% dextrose and infused over a period of 6 hr. *Intrathecal*, **25** to **100** µg every 48 to 72 hr, with gradual increments up to a single-dose maximum of **500 µg** and total accumulated dose of **15 mg.** *Topical*, as 3% cream, lotion, or ointment.

Dosage Form—for Injection: 50 mg; Cream: 3%; Lotion: 3%; Ointment: 3%.

Anthralin—page 780.

Butyl Paraben—page 1166.

Candicidin

Candeptin (*Schmid*); Vanobid (*Merrell-National*)

Candicidin [1403-17-4]; a substance produced by the growth of *Streptomyces griseus* Waksman and Henrici (Fam *Streptomycetaceae*); contains not less than 1000 µg/mg.

Candicidin is a polyene antibiotic reported to be a conjugated heptaene complex containing also residues of mycosamine and *p*-aminoacetophenone. It has been separated into three fractions designated A, B, and C. A is reported to be simply the sodium salt of B and both A and B are actively antifungal. Fraction C possesses little activity and is thought to be a degradation product. The antifungal activity of candicidin is highly pH-dependent, maximal at 7 to 8.

Description—Yellow to brown powder that has a fatty acid-type odor and a bitter taste; unstable in light in the UV range, unstable to moisture and sensitive to oxidation, and unstable to elevated temperatures; pH (1% aqueous suspension) between 8 and 10.

Solubility—1 g in 75 mL water, 260 mL alcohol, 10,000 mL chloroform, 33,000 mL ether.

Uses—An antibiotic with a rather broad spectrum of activity similar to that of amphotericin B. However, it is not active against filamentous fungi, including the ringworm varieties, and coccidioides. It is very active against *Candida* (*Monilia*) *albicans* and other *Candida* sp, hence the origin of its name. The drug is used topically for the treatment *candidal vulvovaginitis*.

Candicidin is not absorbed from the gastrointestinal tract. Candicidin occasionally causes a mild irritation of the vulva. Irritation of the skin has not been reported. The drug may rarely cause an allergic reaction.

Dose—*Intravaginal*, as a **0.06**% ointment or **3-mg** vaginal tablet inserted twice daily for 14 days.

Dosage Forms—Ointment: 0.06%; Vaginal Tablets: 3 mg.

Clioquinol

8-Quinolinol, 5-chloro-7-iodo-, Iodochlorhydroxyquin; Vioform (*Ciba-Geigy*); *Various Mfrs*

[130-26-7] C_9H_5ClINO (305.50).

Preparation—By chlorination of 8-quinolinol with sulfuryl chloride [SO_2Cl_2] followed by iodination of the 5-chloro-8-hydroxyquinoline with iodine.

In the chlorination step, a dichloroquinoline is also formed. The 5-chloro-8-hydroxyquinoline is separated from the by-product by extraction with hot water.

Description—Voluminous, spongy, yellowish white or brownish yellow powder having a slight, characteristic odor; melts with decomposition at about 180°; affected by light.
Solubility—1 g in >100,000 mL water, 3500 mL alcohol, 120 mL chloroform, 4500 mL ether.

Uses—Possesses antimicrobial and mildly irritant properties. It is used for topical *antifungal* actions on the skin and in the vagina. It is possibly effective in *mucocutaneous mycoses* such as tinea capitis, tinea cruris, tinea corporis, tinea pedis, intertrigo, and moniliasis. It has been claimed to be effective against *trichomonal infections*. In all of these uses the FDA has classified the drug as possibly effective. Some of the promoted cutaneous indications are disorders in which an infectious component is not prominent and is probably not primarily etiologic. In these, as with ichthammol, tars, etc, the mild irritant properties may be more important than the antimicrobial properties. Since most of the *dermatologic preparations* of clioquinol in the US also contain hydrocortisone, it is difficult to assess the true contribution of the clioquinol component. Examples of such disorders are atopic dermatitis, stasis dermatitis, contact dermatitis, nummular eczema, infantile eczema, lichen simplex, and neurodermatitis. Also possibly effective in cutaneous disorders of a more infectious nature, such as bacterial dermatoses, folliculitis, acne urticata, pyoderma, impetigo, impetiginized eczema, seborrhea, and anogenital pruritus.

On mucocutaneous surfaces the drug may cause local burning sensations and itching, which tend to disappear upon repetitive administration. The drug is sufficiently absorbed through the skin to interfere with thyroid tests based upon protein-bound iodine. Orally, the drug may cause diarrhea and anal pruritus. It may be sufficiently absorbed to cause rare irreversible myeloptic neuropathy and a gastrointestinal-neurological syndrome. It is contraindicated in liver disease and in persons with a history of iodine-sensitivity. Clioquinol may cause iodism by any route.

Dose—*Topical*, to the *skin*, as a **3%** cream, lotion or ointment 2 to 4 times a day.
Dosage Forms—Cream: 3%; Lotion: 3%; Ointment: 3%. The cream and ointment are available with or without and the lotion only with 0.5 or 1% hydrocortisone.

Clotrimazole

1*H*-Imidazole, 1-[(2-chlorophenyl)diphenylmethyl]-, Lotrimin (*Schering-Plough*); Mycelex (*Dome*)

1-(*o*-Chloro-α,α-diphenylbenzyl)imidazole   [23593-75-1] $C_{22}H_{17}ClN_2$ (344.84).

Preparation—For information concerning synthesis see *CA 71*: 91473m, 1969; 72: 66939f, 1970.

Description—White, to pale yellow, crystalline powder; melts at about 142°, with decomposition.
Solubility—Slightly soluble in water; soluble in alcohol, chloroform; slightly soluble in ether.

Uses—Clotrimazole is a broad-spectrum antifungal agent that inhibits growth of pathogenic dermatophytes, yeasts, and *Pityros-*

poron obiculare (*Malassezia furfur*). It exhibits fungicidal activity *in vitro* against isolates of *Trichophyton rubrum, T mentagrophytes, Epidermophyton floccosum, Microsporum canis*, and *Candida albicans*. It shares with miconazole first-choice status for topical treatment of *tinea pedis, tinea cruris*, and *tinea corporis* due to any of the aforementioned organisms, *candidiasis* due to *Candida albicans*, and *tinea versicolor* due to *Pityrosporon obiculare;* also for local treatment of *vulvovaginal candidiasis*. In Europe the drug is also used systemically; however, most clinical studies indicate that used orally the drug has limited efficacy yet considerable CNS toxicity.

Adverse effects from topical use include erythema; stinging, blistering, and peeling of the skin; pruritus; and urticaria. Swallowed (investigational) troches may evoke colic, epigastric pain, nausea, vomiting, and diarrhea.

Dose—*Topically*, to the skin, as 1% cream or solution twice daily, morning and evening. *Intravaginally*, **5 g** of 1% cream or one **100-mg** tablet daily, preferably at bedtime, for 7 to 14 consecutive days.
Dosage Forms—Cream: 1%; Vaginal Cream: 1%; Topical Solution: 1%; Vaginal Tablets: 100 mg.

Econazole Nitrate

1*H*-Imidazole, 1-[2-[(4-chlorophenyl)methoxy]-2-(2,4-dichlorophenyl)ethyl]-, (±)-, mononitrate, Ecostatin (*Squibb*)

(±)-1-[2,4-Dichloro-β-[(*p*-chlorobenzyl)oxy]phenethyl]imidazole mononitrate [68797-31-9] $C_{18}H_{15}Cl_3N_2O.HNO_3$ (440.70).
Preparation—See *J Med Chem 12*: 784, 1969.

Description—White crystals melting about 162°.
Solubility—Very slightly soluble in water or most organic solvents.

Uses—Econazole has antifungal activity against the dermatophytes (*Epidermophyton floccosum, Microsporon auduoni, canis* and *gypseum*, and *Trichophyton rubrum, mentagrophytes*, and *tonsurans*), *Pityrosporon obiculare* (*Malasserzia furfur*) and *Candida albicans*. It is employed in the treatment of *cutaneous Candidiasis*, and *tineas corporis, cruris, pedis*, and *versicolor* (*pityriasis versicolor*). It readily penetrates into the stratum corneum, where effective concentrations persist for up to several days. In about 3% of recipients, local erythemia, burning sensation, stinging and itching occur.

Dose—*Topical* to the *skin*, as a 1% cream twice a day, except only once a day for pityriasis versicolor. Treatment should be maintained for at least 2 wk for pityriasis versicolor, tinea corporis, tinea cruris and candidiasis, and 1 mo for tinea pedis.

Flucytosine

Cytosine, 5-fluoro-, Ancobon (*Hoffmann-LaRoche*)

[2022-85-7] $C_4H_4FN_3O$ (129.09).
Preparation—5-Fluorouracil (page 1149) is reacted with $POCl_3$ to form 2,4-dichloro-5-fluoropyrimidine which is reacted with NH_3 to produce 2-chloro-4-amino-5-fluoropyrimidine. Heating the latter in concentrated HCl yields flucytosine. US Pat 3,368,938.

Description—White to off-white, crystalline powder; odorless or has a slight odor; melts at about 295° with decomposition; stable in light, nonhygroscopic, and stable for at least 3 months at 45°.
Solubility—1 g in about 83 mL water and about 12 mL 0.1 *N* HCl; slightly soluble in alcohol; practically insoluble in chloroform and ether.

Uses—Flucytosine is converted in the fungus to 5-fluorouridylic acid, which is incorporated into RNA, where it interferes with normal protein synthesis. Certain fungal organisms are more sensitive to interference from the drug than are human cells, so that the drug is useful in the treatment of some fungal infections. Most clinical isolates of *Cryptococcus* and 40 to 92% of *Candida* are sensitive to the drug. *Torulopsis glabrata*, *Sporotrichum schenckii*, *Aspergillus*, *Chromomyces*, and *Phialophora* are also frequently sensitive. Flucytosine is the drug of choice to treat *chromomycosis* and of second choice to treat *systemic candidiasis*. It may be combined with amphotericin B for first-choice treatment of *cryptococcosis*, especially with meningitis. It may also be used effectively to treat candidiasis of the urinary tract. Since resistance to the drug can develop, not only should sensitivity tests precede therapy but they should be conducted also throughout the course of treatment. The culture medium is very important in the testing; incorrect media make resistance appear to be greater than it is.

Some patients may be given as much as 5 g a day without toxic effects, and the drug has also been given for as long as 820 days without untoward effects. Nevertheless, nausea, vomiting, diarrhea, and rash are rather commonly caused by the drug. There have been a few cases of intestinal perforation. Bone-marrow depression, manifested by anemia, leukopenia, and thrombocytopenia, occur in about 10% of patients; there have been a few fatalities. Flucytosine should not be used with antineoplastics or immunosuppressants. Sedation, confusion, hallucinations, headache, and vertigo occur infrequently. Mild azotemia and an increase in liver enzymes in the plasma are rather common effects, but hepatic necrosis seems to be a rare effect. Nausea can be lessened if the several capsules in a dose are taken separately at 10- to 15-min intervals. Nephrotoxicity from concurrently administered amphotericin B will increase the plasma levels and hence the toxicity of flucytosine.

About 90% of flucytosine is absorbed orally. It is distributed well among all the tissues, including the CNS. About 63 to 84% is excreted unchanged in the urine with a half-life 2.5 to 8 hr. The dose needs to be adjusted if renal function is abnormal. If there is any reason to suspect a decrease in renal sufficiency, function tests should be made at the outset.

Dose—*Oral, adults, infants,* and *children,* **12.5 to 37.5 mg/kg** (or 375 to 563 mg/m² of body surface for infants and children) every 6 hr. The duration of treatment varies from a few days to months. In very severe infections, 50 mg/kg/dose may be given.

Dosage Forms—Capsules: 250 and 500 mg.

Formaldehyde Solution—page 1166.

Gentian Violet—page 1167.

Griseofulvin

Spiro[benzofuran-2(3*H*),1′-[2]cyclohexene]-3,4′-dione, 7-chloro-2′,4,6-trimethoxy-6′-methyl-, (1′*S-trans*)-, Fulvicin (*Schering-Plough*); Grifulvin (*McNeil*); Grisactin (*Ayerst*)

7-Chloro-2′,4,6-trimethoxy-6′*β*-methylspiro[benzofuran-2(3*H*)-1′-[2]-cyclohexene]-3,4′-dione [126-07-8] C₁₇H₁₇ClO₆ (352.77); a substance produced by the growth of *Penicillium griseofulvum* or by other means. It has a potency equivalent to not less than 900 µg of C₁₇H₁₇ClO₆/mg.

Preparation—By the submerged process using selected strains of *Penicillium patulum.*

Description—White to creamy white, odorless powder, in which particles of the order of 4 µm in diameter predominate.

Solubility—Soluble in chloroform; sparingly soluble in alcohol; very slightly soluble in water.

Uses—An effective agent in the treatment of superficial fungus infections. It is fungistatic and not fungicidal. Administered systemically, the drug is highly effective in the management of *tinea capitis, tinea corporis, tinea unguium* (onychomycosis) and the chronic form of *tinea pedis* caused by the dermatophytes, *Microsporon, Trichophyton,* and *Epidermophyton.* It also may be dramatically effective against *favus.* Infections caused by *T rubrum* may respond, but relapses are frequent. Part of the reason for relapses is that some of the fungi, at least, grow in dead and dying squamous epithelial cells and their keratin residues. Since griseofulvin does not kill but only arrests reproduction of the organism, it is necessary to continue medication long enough for the entire epi-

dermis to be shed and replaced in order to remove reinfecting organisms. When there is hyperkeratosis, the time for desquamation may be long. Griseofulvin is deposited in the basal cells and is carried outwards into the epidermis as normal skin growth proceeds. This also makes for a long latency from the time medication is begun until evidence of improvement occurs. Because griseofulvin disrupts microtubules it has anti-inflammatory properties and has been used successfully in the management of cutaneous inflammatory conditions and several polyarthritic syndromes.

Serious untoward reactions are infrequent, but skin eruptions, leukopenia, granulocytopenia, and allergic reactions such as serum sickness or angioneurotic edema are among the serious side effects reported. It is recommended that the drug be reserved for use in infections not amenable to conventional topical measures and for those in which the causative organism has been shown to be susceptible to its effect. Griseofulvin may also cause nausea, vomiting, epigastric distress, and diarrhea; these may often be avoided by giving the drug with or shortly following a meal. Headache is also relatively frequent. Infrequently, phototoxicity, proteinuria, lassitude and fatigue occur, and rarely there is mental confusion, and motor incoordination. It is advisable to monitor kidney, blood, and liver functions. Ingestion of alcohol during treatment with griseofulvin causes tachycardia and flushing.

Only a few percent of an oral dose is absorbed, and there is a great deal of variation. Absorption is greater if the drug is administered with a high-fat meal. The smaller the crystal size, the more complete the absorption. The principal route of elimination may be transepidermal loss, although a considerable loss in feces probably also occurs. The amount of unchanged drug in the urine is relatively small. The half-life is 24 hr. Griseofulvin induces the hepatic microsomal system, and the metabolism of warfarin is increased, thus necessitating dosage adjustments. Phenobarbital decreases plasma levels of griseofulvin, but it is not clear whether the action is through hepatic enzyme induction or an influence on absorption via alterations in bile acid secretion.

Dose—*Oral, adult,* for *tinea capitis corporis* or *cruris, microcrystalline* form, **500 mg** a day in a single dose or divided doses, or *ultramicrocrystalline* form, **250 to 330 mg** a day in a single dose or divided doses; for *tinea pedia* or *unguium, microcrystalline* form, **1 g** a day in divided doses, or *ultramicrocrystalline* form, **500 to 660 mg** a day in divided doses. *Children , microcrystalline* form, **10 mg/kg** (or 300 mg/m² of body surface a day); *or, 14 to 23 kg* in weight, **125 to 250 mg** a day; *over 23 kg,* **250 to 500 mg** a day; *ultramicrocrystalline* form, **5.5 to 7.3 mg/kg** a day; or, *14 to 23 kg* in weight, **62.5 to 165 mg** a day; *over 23 kg,* **125 to 330 mg** a day.

Dosage Forms—*Microsize Griseofulvin* Capsules: 125 and 250 mg; Oral Suspension: 125 mg/5 mL; Tablets: 250 and 500 mg. *Ultramicrosize Griseofulvin* Tablets: 125, 165, 250 and 300 mg.

Haloprogin

Benzene, 1,2,4-trichloro-5-[(3-iodo-2-propynyl)oxy]-, ing of Halotex (*Westwood*)

3-Iodo-2-propynyl 2,4,5-trichlorophenyl ether [777-11-7] C₉H₄Cl₃IO (361.39).

Preparation—For synthesis of haloprogin see *CA 58:* 14635g, 1963.

Description—White or pale yellow, crystalline powder; melts at about 114°.

Solubility—Very slightly soluble in water; soluble in alcohol.

Uses—Haloprogin is fungicidal to various species of *Candida, Epidermophyton, Malassezia, Microsporon,* and *Trichophyton.* It is employed topically in the treatment of *tinea pedis* (athlete's foot), *tinea cruris, tinea corporis, tinea manuum,* and *tinea versicolor.* In the treatment of athlete's foot, the cure rate is about 80%. It has also been used to treat *cutaneous candidiasis,* for which it has about the same efficacy as nystatin.

Haloprogin has a low order of toxicity. Deliberate attempts to induce contact dermatitis and phototoxicity have been unsuccessful. However, irritation, burning sensation, pruritus, vesiculation, increased maceration, and so-called "sensitization" occasionally occur during treatment, especially if occlusive footwear is worn; the apparent sensitization is possibly a response to debris and endotoxins from killed fungi, such as often occurs with other effective antifungal drugs. These reactions give the appearance of the exacerbation of the infection, but mycological examinations show the fungal population to be decreasing. Haloprogin is poorly absorbed from the skin. That which is absorbed is converted to trichlorophenol. There have been no reports of systemic intoxication from topical application. One 4-year old child was treated with 12.1 kg of a 1% preparation over a period of 3 years without evidences of systemic effects.

Dose—*Topical*, to the *skin*, *adults*, *infants* and *children*, as a 1% cream or solution twice a day for 2 to 4 weeks.

Dosage Forms—Cream: 1%; Topical Solution: 1%.

Ichthammol—page 781.

Iodine—page 1161.

Ketoconazole

Piperazine, 1-acetyl-4-[4-[[2-(2,4-dichlorophenyl)-2-(1*H*-imidazol-1-ylmethyl)-1,3-dioxolan-4-yl]methoxy]phenyl]-, *cis*-, Nizarol (*Janssen*)

[65277-42-1] $C_{26}H_{28}Cl_2N_4O_4$ (531.44).

Preparation—See *J Med Chem 22:* 1003, 1979.

Description—White crystals melting about 146°.

Uses—Ketoconazole blocks the fungal synthesis of ergosterol, which is essential to the integrity of the cell membranes of nearly all the pathogenic fungi. Consequently, ketoconazole has a broad spectrum of antifungal activity, which includes *Blastomyces dermatitidis*, *Candida spp*, *Chromomyces*, *Coccidioides immitis*, dermatophytes, *Histoplasma capsulatum*, and *Paracoccidioides braseliensis*. *Aspergillus*, *Cryptococcus neoformans*, and *Sporothrix schenckii* are moderately affected but *Mucor* is not. Except against *Aspergillus*, *Mucor* and *Sporothix*, ketoconazole is an alternative drug for the systemic treatment of mucocutaneous or systemic infections caused by the above organisms and onychomycosis caused by dermatophytes, but it is considerably less effective than the present drugs of choice, and successful treatment sometimes requires months. It is most effective against candidiasis.

Nausea and vomiting are the most frequent (ca 3%) side effects; these can be avoided by taking the drug with food. Pruritis is the next most frequent (1.5%) and abdominal cramps third (1.2%). Other effects are pruritis, sleepiness, headache, diarrhea, photophobia, fever, thrombocytopenia, gynecomastia, impotence, and oligospermia (from low testosterone levels). Hepatitis is rare. Most adverse effects are transient and all are reversible, except that three cases of liver necrosis have been fatal. Monitoring of liver function is mandatory. In rats, ketoconazole is teratogenic; thus it should not be used during pregnancy.

Ketoconazole is well absorbed by the oral route. A dose of 2 g with a meal will cause a peak plasma level of about 3.5 μg/mL, but up to 50 μg/mL have been reported. In plasma, 99% is protein-bound. The principal route of elimination is biliary secretion, less than 4% being renal excretion. There are a number of metabolites. Enterohepatic circulation complicates the pharmacokinetics. During the first 10 hr (alpha-phase), the half-life is 1.4 to 3.3 hr; thereafter (beta-phase) it is 8 hr.

Dose—*Oral*, *adults* 200 to 400 mg once a day; *infants* and *children*, weighing *less than 20 kg*, 50 to 150 mg; *20 to 40 kg*, 100 to 200 mg; *more than 40 kg*, 200 to 300 mg. (Manufacturer's recommended dose is 3.3 to 6.6 mg/kg for children over 2 yr, undetermined for younger children.)

Mercuric Oxide, Yellow—page 1167.

Mercury, Ammoniated—page 1167.

Miconazole

1*H*-Imidazole, 1-[2-(2,4-dichlorophenyl)-2-[(2,4-dichlorophenyl)-methoxy]ethyl]-, Monistat (*Ortho*)

1-[2,4-Dichloro-β-[(2,4-dichlorobenzyl)oxy]phenethyl]imidazole [22916-47-8] $C_{18}H_{14}Cl_4N_2O$ (416.12).

Preparation—For synthesis of miconazole see *J Med Chem 12:* 784, 1969.

Uses—Miconazole is fungicidal to various species of *Aspergillus*, *Blastomyces*, *Candida*, *Cladosporium*, *Coccidioides*, *Epidermophyton*, *Histoplasma*, *Madurella*, *Pityrosporon* (*Malassezia*), *Microsporon*, *Paracoccidioides*, *Phialophora*, and *Trichophyton*. It also has activity against gram-positive bacteria. It inhibits ergosterol synthesis, which disrupts fungal cell membranes. Sulfonamides enhance the antifungal action in *Candida*. The drug readily penetrates into the stratum corneum and remains there in high concentration for as long as 4 days, which probably contributes to its efficacy against the dermatophytoses. In *tinea pedis* (athlete's foot) a mycological cure rate of 96% has been reported with topical miconazole nitrate, which considerably exceeds that of any other drug except clotrimazole. Comparable efficacy has been reported in use against *tinea versicolor*, ringworm, onychomycosis, and *cutaneous candidiasis*. Topically, for *vulvovaginal candidiasis*, the reported cure rate varies from 80 to 95%, considerably superior to that with nystatin (65%) and amphotericin B (75%). Often pruritus is relieved after a single application. It is also effective against some vaginal infections caused by *T glabratus*. The free base is useful in the topical treatment of various ophthalmic mycoses. Miconazole base has been used successfully in the systemic treatment of several deep or systemic mycoses, especially those of *candidiasis* and *cryptococcosis*. It is the drug of second choice for the treatment of *coccidiomycosis*. It is also useful against *paracoccidioidomycosis*. Systemic use against minor, self-limiting infections, should be avoided.

Burning, itching, and maceration sometimes occur after application of the nitrate to the skin, as happens frequently with effective antifungal drugs; the effect, at least in part, seems to result from irritating debris released from killed organisms. Intravaginally, burning, itching, pelvic discomfort, urticaria, and headache occur in 6 to 7% of users, especially during the first few days of treatment. Experimental and clinical studies suggest that the drug is safe for use in pregnancy, but systemic use during pregnancy should probably be avoided, if possible. Oral miconazole appears to be well tolerated, but nausea, vomiting, and diarrhea occur; no evidence of renal or hepatic toxicity has been observed. Intravenous administration may cause phlebitis, hypercholesterolemia and hypertriglyceridemia (caused by the vehicle), hyponatremia (from ADH secretion), nausea, vomiting, diarrhea, anorexia, and infrequent allergic and immune reactions, such as fever, chills, pruritis, rashes, thrombocytopenia, anaphylaxis, and anemia. Wheezing and tachypnea and sinoatrial and ventricular tachycardias occur, which can be avoided by slower rates of infusion. Intrathecally, it may cause some meningeal irritation, but the route appears to be safe.

From topical sites, only trace amounts of miconazole appear in the blood or urine. Slightly less than 50% of an oral dose is absorbed. In plasma, about 93% is bound to proteins. Less than 1% of an oral dose appears unchanged in urine. The drug manifests three-compartment pharmacokinetics. The terminal (elimination, β) half-life is about 1 day. Systemic miconazole inhibits the metabolism of warfarin.

Dose—*Intravenous infusion*, *adults*, for *candidiasis*, 200 to 600 mg every 8 hr for 1 to 20 wk; for *coccidiomycosis*, 600 mg to 1.2 g every 8 hr for 3 to 20 wks; for *cryptococcosis*, 400 to 800 mg every 8 hr for 3 to 12 or more wk; for *paracoccidioidomycosis*, 66.7 to 400 mg every 8 hr for 2 to 16 or more wk; for *petriellidosis*, 200 mg to 1 g 3 times a day for 5 to 20 wk. *Children 1 year* of age or over, 20 to 40 mg per kg of body weight a day, up to a maximum of 15 mg per kg per dose. *Oral*, *adults* (not yet approved) 500 mL to 1 g 3 times a day. *Intrathecal*, 20 mg every 3 to 7 days. *Bladder irrigation*, 200 mg, as a diluted injection.

Dosage Forms—Injection: 200 mg/10 mL, solubilized with a polyethylene glycol and lactic acid, in water for injection.

Miconazole Nitrate

Micatin (*Johnson & Johnson*); Monistat (*Ortho*)

The mononitrate salt of *Miconazole* [22832-87-7] $C_{18}H_{14}Cl_4N_2O\cdot HNO_3$ (479.15).

Description—White, crystalline powder; melts at 170°.
Solubility—Very slightly soluble in water.

Uses—The actions, uses, and side effects of miconazole nitrate are discussed under *Miconazole* (above).

Dose—*Topical*, to the *skin* as a **2%** cream or lotion twice a day, except only once a day for *tinea versicolor*, and to the *vagina* as a **2%** cream or **100 mg** as a suppository once a day at bedtime for 14 days.

Dosage Forms—Cream: 2%; Lotion: 2%; Vaginal Cream: 2%; Vaginal Suppository: 100 mg.

Tolnaftate

Carbamothioic acid, methyl(3-methylphenyl)-, *O*-2-naphthyl ester; Tinactin (*Schering-Plough*)

O-2-Naphthyl *m*,*N*-dimethylthiocarbanilate [2398-96-1] $C_{19}H_{17}NOS$ (307.41).

Preparation—*N*-Methyl-*m*-tolylamine is condensed with 2-naphthyl chlorothionoformate in the presence of sodium bicarbonate or other dehydrochlorinating agent. French Pat 1,337,797.

Description—White to creamy white, odorless, fine powder; melts between 110° and 113°.
Solubility—Practically insoluble in water; slightly soluble in alcohol; freely soluble in chloroform; sparingly soluble in ether.
Uses—For the treatment of superficial *mycoses of the skin* (*tinea pedis, tinea cruris, tinea corporis, tinea manuum*) caused by *Epidermophyton floccosum, Malassezia furfur*, and several species of *Microsporon* and *Trichophyton*. In the treatment of *tinea pedis* (athlete's foot), the mycological cure rate is about 80%. It is not effective alone against infections of the hair or nails. When *T rubrum* is the infecting agent, relapses are common. Tolnaftate is administered only topically and may be unable to reach infections in hyperkeratotic lesions or in the normally thick horny layers of the palms or soles, so that a keratolytic should be employed concurrently or systemic treatment with griseofulvin should be employed. No adverse effects caused by tolnaftate have been reported; other than occasional burning sensations and maceration at the site of the lesion, probably caused by endotoxins from killed fungi. Sensitization to other ingredients of the commercial product has been observed.

Dose—*Topical*, as a 1% aerosol, cream, gel, ointment, powder, or solution twice a day. Treatment usually lasts from 3 to 6 weeks.

Dosage Forms—Cream: 1%; Gel: 1%; Powder: 1%; Topical Solution: 1%; Topical Aerosol Powder: 1%; Topical Aerosol Solution: 1%.

Potassium Iodide—page 868.

Potassium Permanganate—page 1168.

Propylparaben—page 1168.

Resorcinol—RPS-16, page 1107.

Resorcinol Monoacetate—RPS-16, page 1107.

Salicylic Acid—page 785.

Sodium Benzoate—page 1169.

Sodium Hypochlorite Solution—page 1169.

Other Antifungal Drugs

Benzoic Acid [[65-85-0] $C_7H_6O_2$ (122.12).]—*Preparation:* Occurs naturally in benzoin and in various other balsamic substances, from which it may be obtained by sublimation, but in small amounts. It is synthesized from a variety of starting compounds, as toluene, phthalic anhydride, benzaldehyde, etc. *Description and solubility:* White needles or scale-like crystals; odorless or with a slight benzaldehyde-like odor; somewhat volatile at moderately warm temperatures; congeals between 121° and 123°. Soluble 1 g in 300 mL water, 3 mL alcohol, 5 mL chloroform, 3 mL ether. *Uses:* Benzoic acid is *fungistatic*. It is used in combination with salicylic acid, as in Benzoic and Salicylic Acids Ointment (below). It is used especially in the treatment of *athlete's foot* and to a lesser extent for

management of *ringworm*. As sodium benzoate it is extensively used as a preservative for various food products.

Benzoic and Salicylic Acid Ointment [Whitfield's Ointment. Benzoic acid and salicylic acid, present in a ratio of about 2 to 1, in a suitable ointment base.]—*Uses:* Combines the fungistatic activity of benzoic acid and the keratolytic activity of salicylic acid. It is used mainly in the treatment of *epidermophytosis interdigitalis* (athlete's foot), but it is also sometimes used in the treatment of ringworm of the scalp. Since the benzoic acid only keeps the fungus from growing and spreading, eradication of the organism is dependent on gradual desquamation of the stratum corneum in which the fungus is embedded and the keratin on which it subsists; the salicylic acid hastens the desquamation through its keratolytic action. Keratolysis also aids penetration by benzoic acid into hyperkeratotic sites. *Dose: Topical*, to the affected area twice a day as an ointment usually containing 6% benzoic acid and 3% salicylic acid.

Calcium Undecylenate [Ca($C_{11}H_{19}O_2$)$_2$; ing of Caldecort (*Pennwalt*); Caldesene (*Pharmacraft*).]—*Uses:* An antifungal agent with actions resembling *Zinc Undecylenate*. The undecylenate moiety has antifungal and weak antibacterial activity, and the calcium moiety has mild astringent activity. The drug is not promoted for use in the treatment of athlete's foot but rather for prophylaxis and treatment of diaper rash, intertrigo, prickly heat, and dyshidrosis and for its soothing action to relieve itching or burning skin sensations in minor cutaneous irritations. It is also combined with neomycin and hydrocortisone acetate for the purpose of suppressing fungal infections that complicate other dermatologic conditions. The principal side effect is a transient mild stinging at the site of application when the site is excoriated. *Dose: Topical*, as a 10% ointment or powder.

Ciclopirox Olamine [6-Cyclohexyl-1-hydroxy-4-methyl-2(1*H*)-pyridone compound with 2-aminoethanol (1:1) [41621-49-2] $C_{12}H_{17}NO_2\cdot C_2H_7NO$ (268.36); Loprox (*Hoechst-Russel*).]—Ciclopirox has a spectrum of antifungal activity similar to that of miconazole (page 1229). Against dermatophytosis its efficacy seems to be comparable to that of haloprogin (page 1228). It is effective against candidal infections. Adverse effect occur in about 0.4% of users; they include pruritis and maceration but not rashes as yet. *Dose: Topical*, as 1% solution twice a day.

Hydroxystilbamidine Isethionate [2-Hydroxy-4,4′-stilbenedicarboxamidine bis(2-hydroxyethanesulfonate) (salt) [533-22-2] $C_{16}H_{16}N_4O\cdot 2C_2H_6O_4S$ (532.58); (*Merrell-National*).]—*Preparation:* Dry hydrogen chloride is passed into a solution of 2-hydroxy-4,4′-vinylenedibenzonitrile and absolute ethanol in anhydrous ether whereby the nitrile groups are converted into iminoether hydrochlorides. Treatment with excess alcoholic ammonia removes the HCl and effects ammonolysis at the ethoxy linkage, thus yielding the diamidine. This is then reacted in alcohol solution with a double equimolar portion of isethionic acid to form the readily crystallizable diisethionate. *Description and solubility:* Fine, yellow, crystalline powder; odorless; stable in air but decomposes upon exposure to light; pH (1 in 100 solution) between 4.0 and 5.5; melts at about 280°. Soluble in water; slightly soluble in alcohol; and insoluble in ether. *Uses:* Hydroxystilbamidine is occasionally useful in treatment of North American *blastomycosis*, especially when there is a renal disorder or when the infection is limited to the skin. It can eradicate severe pulmonary and systemic forms of the disease, but the relapse rate is high. Prior to use of the diamidines, this disease was incurable. At present, hydroxystilbamidine ranks behind amphotericin B and ketoconazole because of their lesser toxicity and superiority. On injection, hydroxystilbamidine may cause hypotension, tachycardia, dyspnea, flushing, sialorrhea, sweating, formication, vertigo, headache, nausea, vomiting, syncope, facial and palpebral edema, urinary and fecal incontinence, liver damage, and neuropathies. Renal and hepatic functions should be monitored. These effects may be minimized by slow intravenous infusion. The drug is rarely given intramuscularly; there are pain and swelling at the site of injection. *Dose: Intravenous infusion, adults*, 225 every 24 hr; *infants* and *children*, 3 to 4.5 mg/kg of body weight every 24 hr. *Intramuscular, adults*, 225 every 24 hr. The infusion should take 2 to 3 hr, and the solution should contain the dose in 200 mL of isotonic dextrose or saline injection. For intramuscular injection, the dose is dissolved in 10 mL of isotonic saline solution. A course of treatment may sometimes be as long as 2 to 3 months.

Natamycin [Pimaricin, an antibiotic produced by *Streptomyces natalensis*, [$C_{33}H_{47}NO_{13}$] (665.75); Myprozine (*American Cyanamide*); Natacyn (*Alcon*).]—A polyene macrolide with antifungal activity like that of amphotericin B (page 1226). However, solutions of natamycin are more stable than those of amphotericin B. It is employed topically in the treatment of susceptible fungal keratitis, blepharitis, and conjunctivitis. It is the treatment of choice in keratitis caused by *Fusarium solani*. Natamycin has also been used to treat superficial fungal infections of the skin and vagina. *Dose: Topical*, to the *eye*, as 5% suspension, *initially* every 2 hr then every 3 or 4 hr after 3 or 4 days; to the *skin* as 2% cream, *vagina*, as 25-mg tablet, and to the respiratory tract as an aerosol for inhalation.

Nystatin [Nystatin [1400-61-9] is a substance produced by the growth of *Streptomyces noursei* Brown, *et al* (Fam *Streptomycetaceae*). It contains not less than 4400 Units of nystatin activity/mg. Nystatin is a mixture, the composition of which has not been completely elucidated. Nystatin A$_1$ [34786-70-4] $C_{47}H_{75}NO_{17}$ is closely related to *Amphotericin*

B. Each is a macrocyclic lactone containing a ketal ring, an *all-trans* polyene system, and a mycosamine (3-amino-3-deoxyrhamnose) moiety.] *Description and solubility:* Yellow to light tan powder, having an odor suggestive of cereals; hygroscopic; affected by long exposure to light, heat, and air. Very slightly soluble in water; slightly soluble in alcohol; insoluble in ether, chloroform. *Dose:* Nystatin is active *in vitro* against a number of yeasts and molds, but its clinical usefulness is limited to the treatment of *candidiasis.* The antibiotic is poorly absorbed from the gastrointestinal tract; consequently it is not effective against systemic infections but is effective against *intestinal candidiasis.* It may prevent emergence of candidal superinfections resulting from oral therapy with broad-spectrum antibiotics, although such superinfections are so infrequent that routine "prophylactic" use of nystatin is not worthwhile. It does *not* prevent diarrhea from oral broad-spectrum antibiotics. Nystatin has been employed with variable success in the treatment of oral "thrush" (moniliasis). It is used alone to treat vulvovaginal candidiasis. For use on the skin, it may be combined with neomycin, gramicidin and triamcinolone acetonide. It is not the drug of first or second choice in any use. Nystatin is relatively nontoxic, but nausea, vomiting, and diarrhea may occur with oral therapy. *Dose: Topical, to the skin, adults* and *children,* to the affected area 2 or 3 times a day as a cream, ointment, or powder containing 100,000 units/g with or without other agents; *intravaginal,* 100,000 units high into the vagina once or twice a day.

Sodium Propionate [Sodium propionate hydrate [6700-17-0] $C_3H_5NaO_2.xH_2O$; anhydrous [137-40-6] (96.06); Mycoban]—Prepared by neutralization of propionic acid. Colorless, deliquescent crystals or granular, crystalline powder. 1 g is soluble in 1 mL water, 24 mL alcohol. *Uses:* Propionic acid and its soluble salts are fungistatic and bacteriostatic against a number of gram-positive cocci. Clinically sodium propionate is used in the treatment of otomycosis. It is also used in the treatment of epidermophytosis but it is not as effective as most other agents used for this condition. It is not fungicidal, so that other hygiene measures must be emphasized. Sodium propionate is often compounded with antibiotics or antiseptics. Sodium and calcium propionate are used in preventing molding of bread. *Dose: Topical,* in dosage forms containing 0.5 to 10% of sodium propionate.

Tioconazole [1-[2,4-Dichloro-β-[(2-chloro-3-thenyl)-oxy]phenethyl]imidazole [65899-73-2] $C_{16}H_{13}Cl_3N_2OS$ (387.71).]—*Preparation:* See US Pat 4,062,966. *Uses:* Tioconazole is related to *Miconazole* (page 1229) and has a similar antifungal spectrum. It is effective topically in the treatment of *candidiasis* and various *dermatophytic infections* (especially the tineas). It appears to have an efficacy comparable to miconazole in the treatment of tinea infections.

Triacetin [Glyceryl triacetate [102-76-1] $C_9H_{14}O_6$ (218.21); Enzactin (*Ayerst*)]—Prepared by esterification of glycerin with acetic anhydride. Colorless liquid with a slight fatty odor; boils at about 260°; soluble in 14 parts of water; soluble in alcohol, chloroform, ether. *Uses:* Marketed as an antifungal drug for treatment of superficial fungous infections of the skin, especially for trichophyta, *Epidermophyton,* and *Microsporon.* Hydrolysis of the ester by mycoenzymes releases acetic acid, and any antimycotic action is attributable to the drop in pH. It is fungistatic only and does not obviate other hygiene measures. Although it is mildly effective *in vitro,* medical authorities are dubious of its clinical efficacy, which is insignificant compared to that of the newer antifungal drugs. *Dose:* Topical, to affected area twice daily as 15% aerosol, as 25% cream, or as 33% powder.

Undecylenic Acid [10-Undecenoic acid [112-38-9] $C_{11}H_{20}O_2$ (184.28)]—Obtained by pyrolysis of ricinoleic acid, the principal fatty acid of castor oil. A colorless to pale yellow liquid with a characteristic odor; practically insoluble in water; miscible with alcohol, chloroform, ether. *Uses:* An antifungal agent employed in treatment of *dermatophytosis* and *tinea capitis;* it is only fungistatic, not fungicidal. Astringents assist in reducing rawness and irritation; thus zinc, in the form of *Zinc Undecylenate,* is often incorporated into powders, ointments, or aerosols of undecylenic acid. *Compound Undecylenic Acid Ointment* contains the zinc salt, and is prepared by stirring into melted polyethylene glycol ointment (750 g) undecylenic acid (50 g) and zinc undecylenate (200 g). Responses of athlete's foot to the drug are sometimes dramatic, but at other times the infection persists despite treatment. Efficacy in the treatment of tinea capitis is generally poor, although sometimes the condition seems to respond readily. With prolonged treatment with undecylenic acid in powder form, the cure rate in *tinea pedia* (athlete's foot) is about 53%, substantially less than that with tolnaftate and halogrogin and only half that with miconazole. Undecylenic acid rarely causes irritation or sensitization. *Dose: Topical,* as Cream, Compound Undecylenic Acid Topical Aerosol Powder, Ointment, Powder, or Soap applied as needed until a therapeutic response obtains or until it is evident that the medicament is ineffective. Two weeks to several months may be required for eradication of the organism.

Zinc Undecylenate [Zinc 10-undecenoate [557-08-4] $C_{22}H_{38}O_4Zn$ (431.92); Zinc Undecenoate]—A fine, white powder; practically insoluble in water and alcohol. *Uses:* See *Undecylenic Acid,* above.

Antiviral Agents

Despite intensive efforts to discover drugs that may be of value in the systemic treatment of virus infections, such infections have been singularly resistant to chemotherapy, except for those caused by certain of the "large viruses," which yield a number of antibiotics and sulfonamides. The intracellular and intimate relation to nuclear metabolism of virus reproduction makes it difficult to destroy a virus without irreparable damage also to the host cell. Nevertheless, in recent years there has been considerable success in the development of drugs relatively selective for viruses and/or their intracellular repication. There is also a continuing strong interest in *interferon.* An interferon is a proteinaceous substance, produced in response to exposure to active or inactivated viruses, or even certain bacteria, which enables cells to become refractory to infection by other viruses which are not necessarily serologically related. Interferons also stimulate T-lymphocytes. Unfortunately, clinical successes with interferons have been confounded by their antigenicity. Purification by monoclonal antibodies and isolation of and transfer of the genes for human leukocyte interferon to bacteria not only resulted in the bacterial production of an interferon of low antigenicity but also of enough quantity for large-scale investigational use. There is also considerable interest in substances, such as *statolon,* which can stimulate the *in vivo* production of interferons.

Many antiseptics and astringents are virucidal and may be used for purposes of disinfection of virus-contaminated objects or substances. Also, β-propiolactone and certain other substances are specifically employed to destroy the virus of serum hepatitis that may contaminate human blood products.

Acyclovir

6*H*-Purin-6-one, 2-amino-1,9-dihydro-9-[(2-hydroxyethoxy)methyl]-, Zovirax (*Burroughs-Wellcome*)

9-[(2-Hydroxyethoxy)methyl]guanine [59277-89-3] $C_8H_{11}N_5O_3$ (225.21).

Preparation—See Ger Pat 2,539,963.

Uses—Acyclovir has activity against *Herpes simplex* viruses (HSV) 1 and 2, varicella-zoster, Epstein-Barr viruses, and cytomegalovirus. Inside an infected cell, acyclovir is changed into the triphosphate, which is then incorporated into DNA; this terminates elongation of the DNA and prevents viral replication. Acyclovir sodium is approved in the US for the systemic treatment of recurrent mucosal and cutaneous infections caused by HSV-1 and HSV-2 in immunocompromised adults and children and for severe initial herpes genitalis infections in immunocompetent patients. However, the drug has been employed effectively in the treatment of HSV encephalitis and neonatal infections and in the treatment of chicken pox and herpes-zoster infections. Resistant but less virulent strains of HSV have developed during treatment. Acyclovir is also approved for the topical treatment of nonfulminating HSV-1 and HSV-2 infection (except in the eye), but it is not very effective, especially against genital herpes in women. It does not eradicate latent herpes.

Acyclovir is usually well tolerated. The most frequent adverse effect of systemic treatment is irritation at the site of injection. The drug may crystallize in the urine, cause hematuria, and impair renal function if fluid intake is inadequate, glomerular filtration rate is low, the dosage-interval is too short, or the drug is given as a bolus.

Metabolic encephalopathy with hallucinations, confusion, tremors, and seizures, bone marrow depression and alterations in hepatic function have also resulted from parenteral therapy. The drug is mutagenic and should be avoided in pregnancy, if possible. Topically, adverse effects occur in about 30% of recipients and consist of local stinging, burning or pain (28%), itching (4%) and rash (0.3%).

Infusions of 5 mg/kg at 8-hr intervals at steady-state achieve peak plasma concentrations of 5.5 to 13.8 μg/mL and trough concentrations of 0.7 to 1.0 μg/mL. In plasma, only 9 to 33% is protein-bound. Renal excretion accounts for 62 to 91% of elimination. The half-life is about 2.5 hr but may be as long as 19.5 hr in renal failure.

Dose—*Topical*, to the affected skin or mucous membranes (not conunctival) every 3 hr except during sleep.

Dosage Forms—Ointment: 5% in a polyethylene glycol base.

Acyclovir Sodium

Uses—See *Acyclovir* (above). The sodium salt is used for intravenous administration.

Dose—*Intravenous infusion*, *adults*, and *children over 12* yr of age, **5 mg/kg** at constant rate over 1 hr repeated every 8 hr for 5 days in immunocompetent patients and 7 days for immunocompromised patients.

Dosage Form—Powder for injection: 500 mg/10 mL (reconstituted).

Amantadine Hydrochloride—page 927.

Cytarabine—page 1147.

Idoxuridine

Uridine, 2'-deoxy-5-iodo-, IDU; Dendrid (*Alcon*); Herplex (*Allergan*); Stoxil (*Smith Kline & French*)

2'-Deoxy-5-iodouridine [54-42-2] $C_9H_{11}IN_2O_5$ (354.10).

Preparation—By refluxing a solution of deoxyuridine in aqueous mineral acid in the presence of iodine. Brit Pat 1,024,156. For the preparation of deoxyuridine, see *J Chem Soc 1958:* 3035.

Description—White, practically odorless, crystalline powder; turns black between 168° and 171°; a 0.1% aqueous solution has a pH of about 6; a 0.1% solution in distilled water and preserved with 1:50,000 thimerosal is stable at room temperature for over a year.

Solubility—Slightly soluble in water and alcohol; practically insoluble in chloroform and ether.

Uses—An antimetabolite of thymidine. It may also be incoparated into desoxyribonucleic acid in lieu of thymidine, thus interfering with normal nuclear functions. It was first studied as an *antineoplastic drug*. However, its *antiviral* activity has received the greater clinical scrutiny. At present its use is limited to the topical therapy of *herpes simplex keratitis of the eye;* the dendritic type responds readily, but the stromal type does not respond unless adrenal steroids are given concurrently. Anterior uveitis and adenovirus conjunctivitis have been reported to respond to the drug. Herpetic lesions of the skin do not respond. The drug has been given intravenously in successful treatment of herpetic encephalitis.

Local treatment to the eye may occasionally cause reversible epithelial edema and corneal stippling, inflammation, stinging, itching, or photophobia. Allergic reactions are rare. It may interfere with the healing of deep lesions of the cornea. When applied to the cornea, idoxuridine does not produce systemic toxicity. When given systemically, idoxuridine may cause depression of bone marrow and alopecia, especially if a total of more than 20 g is given.

The ointment does not require as frequent administration as the solution and hence is especially advantageous for use at night.

Dose—*Topical*, to the conjunctiva, as a **0.5%** ointment every 4 hr during the day and just before bedtime, or **0.1 mL** of a **0.1%** solution every hr during the day and every 2 hr at night. This schedule is continued until the lesions no longer stain with fluorescein; thereafter, the intervals between applications may be doubled. The solution may

be applied at 4-hour intervals if at each application 1 drop is instilled every minute for 5 min.

Dosage Forms—Ophthalmic Ointment: 0.5%; Ophthalmic Solution: 0.1%.

Trifluridine

Thymidine, α,α,α-trifluoro-, Viroptic (*Burroughs-Wellcome*)

2'-Deoxy-5-(trifluoromethyl)uridine [70-00-8] $C_{10}H_{11}F_3N_2O_5$ (296.20).

Preparation—See *J Amer Chem Soc 84:* 3597, 1962.

Description—White crystals melting about 188°.

Uses—Trifluridine is an analog of thymidine which not only inhibits thymidylic phosphorylase and specific DNA polymerases which are involved in the incorporation of thymidine into DNA but is also itself incorporated into viral DNA, so that "nonsense" DNA is formed. It is active against *Herpes simplex* viruses (HSV) 1 and 2 and some adenoviruses. It also has antineoplastic activity. In the US, it is approved for use only in the topical treatment of *herpetic keratitis*.

Nearly 5% of recipients experience transient mild stinging or burning of the conjunctiva and sclera and 3% palpebral edema after instillation into the conjunctival sac. Less frequently there may be irritation, hyperemia, stromal edema, keratitis sicca, epithelial keratopathy, punctate keratopathy, and hypersensitivity. There is a rare cross-sensitivity to idoxuridine. Trifluridine is mutagenic, but its oncogenic potential is unknown.

Dose—*Topical*, to the *conjunctiva*, *adults* and *children*, **1 drop** of a **1%** solution every 2 hr during waketime; after re-epithelialization, the dose interval may be lengthened to 4 hr, application continuing for 7 days.

Dosage Form—Ophthalmic Solution: 1%.

Vidarabine

9*H*-Purin-6-amine, 9-β-D-arabinofuranosyl-, monohydrate; Adenine Arabinoside; Vira-A (*Parke-Davis*)

9-β-D-Arabinofuranosyladenine monohydrate [24356-66-9] $C_{10}H_{13}N_5O_4.H_2O$ (285.26); *anhydrous* [5536-17-4] (267.24). Potency: not less than 845 μg and not more than 985 μg of $C_{10}H_{13}N_5O_4$/mg.

Preparation—Production of vidarabine by culturing a strain of *Streptomyces antibioticus* is described in British Pat 1,159,290 (*CA 71:* 79757z, 1969). Several methods of synthesis have been published. In one of these 2,3,5-tri-*O*-benzyl-β-D-arabinofuranose, readily preparable from D-arabinose, is converted to 2,3,5-tri-*O*-benzyl-D-arabinofuranosyl chloride, which is condensed with *N*-benzoyladenine; subsequent removal of the protecting groups yields vidarabine. *J Org Chem 28:* 3004, 1963.

Description—White to off-white powder.

Solubility—Very slightly soluble in water.

Uses—Vidarabine is active against *Herpes simplex* viruses, types 1 and 2, varicella-zoster, Epstein-Barr vaccinia, B viruses, and cytomegalovirus. In cells, it and its hypoxanthine metabolite are phosphorylated; the several phosphorylated metabolites inhibit the viral DNA polymerase and viral-induced ribonucleotide reductase. It is indicated for topical treatment of superficial *herpetic keratitis* and *conjunctivitis*, especially if idoxuridine has proved to be ineffective or cannot be tolerated. Its efficacy is approximately equal to that of idoxuridine. It is not effective against other ocular viral or microbial infections. It is also indicated for the treatment of *herpes simplex encephalitis*, and it has been shown to decrease mortality in this disease. It is the least toxic antiviral drug for the purpose. It has also been used to treat cytomegalovirus infections, but efficacy appears to be low. If the drug is started within the first 3 days of herpes zoster, it is effective in reducing complications.

Topically to the eye, adverse effects include a blurring of vision (from chemosis, typical of ophthalmic ointments), and possible drug-related burning, irritation, pain, photophobia, punctal occlusion and sensitization. These effects are less severe than with idoxuridine. By the intravenous route, nausea and other gastrointestinal disturbances are common. Weakness, tremor, dizziness, ataxia and confusion have been reported but may have been disease-related; however, probably drug-related neurological deterioration, coma, and death have occurred in renal transplant patients. Decreases in hemoglobin and white cell and platelet counts have been observed, but severe bone-marrow depression or renal and hepatic toxicities have not occurred. The blood-cell counts should be monitored during treatment. Vidarabine is oncogenic and mutagenic in mice and rats.

In the body, vidarabine is deaminated to the hypoxanthine analog (Ara-HX). The half-life of vidarabine is about 1 hr and that of Ara-HX 3.3 hr. Ara-HX penetrates into cerebrospinal fluid and is the primary active agent in viral encephalitis. The CSF/plasma ratio is about 3.3. Ara-HX is primarily eliminated by renal excretion, and dose adjustments are required in renal failure. Topically, only small amounts are absorbed from the conjunctiva and too little through the normal cornea to be useful in treating herpetic uveitis, but penetrance through the infected cornea appears to be greater.

Dose (as monohydrate)—*Topical*, to the *conjunctiva* as a thin strip (about 1 cm) of **3%** ointment 5 times a day at 3-hour intervals until reepithelialization, then with decreased frequency for at least 7 more days. *Intravenous*, by infusion, **15 mg/kg** of body weight a day for 10 days; infusion should be made over a 12- to 24-hr period.

Dosage Forms (as monohydrate)—Ophthalmic Ointment: 3%; Sterile: 1 g/5 mL.

Other Antiviral Agents

Human Leukocyte A and Other Interferons *Uses:* Viruses and certain non-viral substances induce various cells to depress genes that code for a number of virus-suppressing proteins called interferons (IFNs). They are of three types: leukocyte (α-IFN), fibroblast (β-IFN), and immune (γ-IFN; produced by T-lymphocytes). The interferons promote the synthesis of proteins that not only interfere with virus replication but also which affect host cell functions. Ultimate cellular effects are inhibition of: cell division, tumor growth, antibody formation, erythroporesis, genesis of adipocytes and cytochrome-P450 activity; and enhancement of: macrophagocytosis, activity of certain "killer" and "memory" T-lymphocytes and other "killer" cells, formation of "memory" T-lymphocytes, expression of surface antigens, and the production of antibodies. Some of these effects appear to be mediated by prostaglandins. The multiplicity of effects imply a potential for a variety of uses, antiviral, antineoplastic, and immune-suppressant activities having received the most experimental and investigational attention. The cloning of the gene for the production of human leukocyte A interferon and its successful

incorporation into DNA of bacteria is providing a means for large scale production such that definitive adequate clinical trials will be enabled. Earlier work with mixtures of impure interferons has been inconclusive and adverse effects have been overwhelming in some instances. Human leukocyte A interferon has been shown to be effective in the treatment of varicella in immunocompromised children, the prevention of recurrences of cytomeglovirus and even possibly opportunistic bacterial infections in renal and other transplant recipients, and the treatment of hairy-cell leukemia, Kaposi's sarcoma, metastatic carcinoid tumors, and ovarian cancer. Human fibroblast interferon has been successfully used against viral encephalitis (intrathecal), herpes-zoster, genital herpes, and hepatitis B viremia, and encouraging results have been obtained in the therapy of a number of tumors. Recombinant DNA technology, DNA sequencing, and purification of interferons by monoclonal antibodies is enabling the determination of the aminoacid sequences of various interferons. This may enable large-scale chemical synthesis of interferons not successfully produced in bacteria. Interferons cause headache, myalgia and fever and elevate plasma amyloid A levels. It is not clear whether the deaths that occurred in some clinical trials were from interferons or impurities, but probably the latter.

Methisazone [1-Methylindole-2,3-dione 3-(thiosemicarbazone) [1910-68-5] $C_{10}H_{10}N_4OS$ (234.28) Marboran (*Burroughs-Wellcome*).]— *Preparation:* A mixture of 1-methylindole-2,3-dione and thiosemicarbazide in 50% aqueous ethanol is refluxed for several hours (*Brit J Pharmacol 15:* 101, 1960). *Description and solubility:* Fine, orange-yellow powder; melts at about 245°, with decomposition. Practically insoluble in water. *Uses:* An antiviral drug which has prophylactic value against smallpox and alastrim and may be of some benefit in eczema vaccinatum and vaccinia gangrenosa, especially in combination with gamma globulin. It appears to interfere with the synthesis of a protein required for assembly and morphogenesis of the virus. It does not affect replication of viral DNA or affect RNA. The drug may cause severe nausea and vomiting, and anorexia, in about half of the recipients. It occasionally causes diarrhea, transient fluid retention, and allergic reactions. Rarely, it causes hyperbilirubinemia. It also causes occasional reversible amnesia. Alcohol increases the adverse effects. *Dose: Oral*, 1.5 to 3 g twice a day for 4 days; as a prophylactic against smallpox, it must be given before the 8th or 9th day of the 12-day incubation period. Complications of vaccinia have been treated with an initial dose of 200 mg/kg, followed by 50 mg/kg every 6 hours for 8 doses. The drug is not marketed in the US but is available from the manufacturer for use in emergencies.

Miscellaneous Investigational Antiviral Agents—*Rimantidine*, a derivative of amantidine, is more active than is amantadine against influenza A virus and is widely used in the Soviet Union. Trials in the US indicate it to be the superior congener. *Ribavirin* (1-β-D-ribofuranosyl-1,2,4-triazole-3-carboxamide) has activity against a variety of RNA and DNA viruses. It has been used successfully against respiratory syncytial viral infections and infectious hepatitis. It may be of benefit in the treatment of *Herpes simplex*) infections. Against influenza A it is only of marginal benefit. *Isoprinosine* has prophylactic activity against rhinoviruses, *Herpes simplex* and influenza A. *6-Azauridine*, which suppresses several RNA and DNA viruses, has undergone encouraging trials in the treatment of measles and subacute sclerosing viral panencephalitis. *Acetylpyridine thiosemicarbazones* have a remarkable effect to eradicate the lesions caused by *Herpes simplex* viruses; however, they do not eradicate the viruses within the nerves and hence do not prevent recurrences. *Bromodeoxyuridine, fluoroidodoaracytosine*, and *phosphonoformic acid* are other investigational drugs that inhibit the replication of *Herpes simplex* and varicella-zoster viruses. *Rifamipin* blocks the assembly of viral envelopes and is currently under investigation as an antiviral drug. Applied topically in vaccinia, it can suppress the pox lesions. *Levamisole* continues to be investigated, but clinical trials are not encouraging.

CHAPTER 65

Parasiticides

Ewart A Swinyard, PhD, DSc (Hon)
Professor Emeritus of Pharmacology
College of Pharmacy and School of Medicine
University of Utah
Salt Lake City, UT 84112

Parasitic infections are now a world-wide problem. Consequently, the subject is an important part of pharmacology. In its broadest aspects, it includes the problem of eradication of all organisms that live within or upon man. However, discussion in this chapter will be limited to the anthelmintics and to those agents which are applied directly to the skin of the human host in the treatment of pediculosis and scabies. The antimalarials, amebicides, and fungicides are discussed in Chapter 64.

Anthelmintics

The term anthelmintic frequently is restricted to drugs acting locally to expel parasites from the gastrointestinal tract. However, there are several types of worms which penetrate other tissues; drugs which act on these parasitic infections are also known as anthelmintics. Furthermore, drugs that kill worms are commonly referred to as vermicides; those that affect the worm in such a manner that peristaltic activity or catharsis expels it from the intestinal tract are referred to as vermifuges. This arbitrary division serves no useful purpose since many anthelmintics manifest both actions, according to the dose employed. Therefore, the anthelmintics are more properly defined as drugs used to combat any type of helminthiasis.

The worm parasites of man belong to two phyla: *Nemathelminthes* (roundworms) and *Platyhelminthes* (flatworms). The roundworms include the hookworm, roundworm, whipworm, pinworm, *Strongyloides stercoralis*, *Trichinella spiralis*, and *Wuchereria bancrofti*. There are two common varieties of hookworm, *Necator americanus*, the American variety, and *Ancylostoma duodenale*, the European variety. They are cylindrical worms, 1 to 2 cm long, with two pairs of hooks near the mouth. They attach themselves to the mucosa of the duodenum and derive their nourishment by sucking blood from the surrounding blood vessels. The common roundworm, *Ascaris lumbricoides*, is the most prevalent of human helminths. It may be 5 to 15 in. long, ⅛ to ¼ in. in diameter, grayish to reddish in color, and inhabits the upper part of the small intestine; therefore it is occasionally vomited up. The whipworm, *Trichuris trichiura*, is about 2 in. long and resembles a whip; it inhabits the cecum principally, but is also found in the lower part of the ileum and the appendix. The pinworm or threadworm, *Enterobius vermicularis*, is 1/16 to ½ in. long and inhabits the small intestine, cecum, and colon. *Strongyloides stercoralis* is only about 1/12 in. long. It inhabits the duodenum chiefly, but may be found in the stomach, biliary passages, pancreatic ducts, and various parts of the intestinal tract. Infection with *Trichinella spiralis* causes trichinosis, a condition which results from eating incompletely cooked pork infested with the larvae of the worm. When such meat is eaten, the cysts dissolve, the parasites mature, and a new crop of larvae develop which penetrate the intestinal mucosa and eventually lodge in the muscles. The most important filarial worm is *Wuchereria bancrofti*, which is transmitted by the bite of the mosquito. Symptoms result from the blocking of the lymphatic ducts with the adult worms.

The flatworms are of two types, segmented (cestodes) and nonsegmented (trematodes). The cestodes include the tapeworms and the trematodes include the flukes. Four common varieties of parasitic tapeworms are found in man; *Taenia saginata* (beef tapeworm), *Taenia solium* (pork tapeworm), *Diphyllobothrium latum* (fish tapeworm), and *Hymenolepis nana* (dwarf tapeworm). Except for the dwarf tapeworm, they are from 6 to 30 ft in length and may contain 3000 to 4000 segments, each segment being capable of producing hundreds of eggs. The dwarf tapeworm is only ¼ to ½ in. in length, but consists of 150 to 200 segments. The larval stage of all tapeworms is spent in the muscles of the intermediate host, and human infection occurs through eating imperfectly cooked meat and fish. Three varieties of blood fluke inhabit the blood stream of man causing schistosomiasis: *Schistosoma haematobium*, *Schistosoma mansoni*, and *Schistosoma japonicum*. These parasites cause epigastric distress, abdominal pain, anorexia, diarrhea with blood and mucus in the stools, enlarged and tender liver, pyrexia, and ascites. The intermediate host is either a fresh water snail or a fresh water mollusk. Transmission is by way of contaminated water.

Parasitic worms are harmful to the human host for a number of reasons. They deprive the host of food, they injure organs or obstruct ducts, they may elaborate substances toxic to the host, and they may provide a portal of entry for other organisms. It is desirable, therefore, to eradicate the parasites as soon as they have been discovered. Nevertheless, the need for treatment must be carefully weighed against the toxicity of the drug; the mere presence of a parasite does not necessarily demand that it must be treated.

Proper choice of the anthelmintic is important, as most drugs are more effective against some species than others and virtually all antiparasitic drugs induce some adverse effects. The drug selected should offer the best combination of effectiveness and relative safety. An excellent review of the choice of drugs for parasitic infections was published in *The Medical Letter* (20: 17–24, 1978 and 24: 5–12, 1982).

Many of the newer drugs require little or no change in the patient's normal routine. When the patient has a tapeworm infestation, a thorough examination of the stools produced by the second purgation is necessary. Unless the head of the worm has been expelled and identified, the worm will regenerate. Usually three specimens of stools are examined one week after administration of the anthelmintic. If ova or parasites are still present, the treatment should be repeated.

All drugs which are poisonous to the worms are also poisonous to the patient. Therefore, the recommended methods of treatment for each drug should be followed carefully and the patient watched closely for the appearance of any untoward drug effects.

Bithionol

2,2'-Thiobis(4,6-dichlorophenol); Lorothidol (*Winthrop*), Bitin (*Tanaba, Japan*)

Bis(2-hydroxy-3,5-dichlorophenyl)sulfide [97-18-7] $C_{12}H_6Cl_4O_2S$ (356.07).

Preparation—By reaction of 2,4-dichlorophenol and sulfur chloride.

Description—White or off-white, crystalline powder; melts at 188°.
Solubility—Practically insoluble in water; freely soluble in alcohol and ether; soluble in solutions of alkali hydroxides.

Uses—An alternative drug for infections caused by *Fasciola hepatica* (sheep liver fluke) and by *Paragonimus westermani* (lung fluke). Untoward reactions are frequent and include photosensitivity skin reactions, vomiting, diarrhea, abdominal pain, and urticaria.

Dose—*Usual, adult, oral,* 30 to 50 mg per kg of body weight on alternate days for 10 to 15 doses. *Pediatric,* as for adults.

Dosage Form—Available from the Parasitic Disease Drug Service, Center for Disease Control, Atlanta, GA 30333.

Diethylcarbamazine Citrate

1-Piperazinecarboxamide, *N,N*-diethyl-4-methyl-, 2-hydroxy-1,2,3-propanetricarboxylate; 1-Diethylcarbamoyl-4-methylpiperazine Dihydrogen Citrate; Filarabits (*SK&F*)

N,N-Diethyl-4-methyl-1-piperazinecarboxamide citrate (1:1) [1642-54-2] $C_{10}H_{21}N_3O.C_6H_8O_7$ (391.42).

Preparation—By acylating piperazine with diethylcarbamoyl chloride, and then methylating at the N^4-position by treatment with formaldehyde and formic acid. Treatment of the purified base with an equimolar portion of citric acid yields the official citrate.

Description—White, crystalline powder; odorless, or has a slight odor; slightly hygroscopic; melts between 134° and 139°.
Solubility—Very soluble in water; sparingly soluble in alcohol; practically insoluble in acetone, chloroform, and ether.

Uses—The drug of choice for treating filariasis infections (*Wuchereria bancrofti, Brugia malayi, Acanthocheilonema perstans, Loa loa,* and *tropical eosinophilia*). It is also the drug of choice in *Onchocerca volvulus* infections, but more intensive therapy is required. In adequate dosage it rapidly clears the blood of the microfilariae and it appears to be curative. The drug should be administered with special caution in *Loa loa*, because it can provoke an encephalopathy. It is also the drug of choice in onchocerciasis; antihistamines or corticosteroids may be required to control the allergic reactions due to the disintegration of microfilariae. The adult forms of *Onchocerca* are *not* killed by diethylcarbamazine citrate; they must either be removed surgically or treated with suramin sodium. Untoward reactions are frequent but not serious; they include severe allergic or febrile reactions, due to the filarial infection, and gastrointestinal disturbances. Rarely, encephalopathy and loss of vision are encountered.

Dose—*Usual,* 2 mg/kg 3 times a day for 10–30 days. In *Wuchereria bancrofti* and *Acanthocheilonema perstans* (*Loa loa*) 50 mg, day 1; 50 mg, 3 times, day 2; 100 mg, 3 times on day 3; 2 mg/kg 3 times a day, day 4 through day 21. In *Onchocerca volvulus* infections 25 mg/day for 3 days, then 50 mg/day for 5 days, 100 mg/day for 3 days, and 150 mg/day for 12 days. *Pediatric,* except for *Onchocera volvulus*, the dose is the same as for adults; in *Onchocerca volvulus* infections, 0.5 mg/kg 3 times a day for 3 days (maximum 25 mg/day), 1 mg/kg 3 times a day for 3 or 4 days (maximum 50

mg/day), 1.5 mg/kg 3 times a day for 3 or 4 days (maximum 100 mg/day), and then 2 mg/kg 3 times a day for 2 or 3 weeks (maximum 150 mg/day). *Tropical eosinophilia* 2 mg/kg for 7 to 10 days.
Dosage Forms—Syrup: 120 mg/5 mL; Tablets: 50 mg.

Emetine Hydrochloride—page 1221.

Gentian Violet—page 1167.

Mebendazole

Carbamic acid, (5-benzoyl-1*H*-benzimidazol-2-yl)-, methyl ester; Vermox (*Janssen*)

Methyl 5-benzoyl-2-benzimidazolecarbamate [31431-39-7] $C_{16}H_{13}N_3O_3$ (295.30).

Preparation—Synthesis of mebendazole and related anthelmintic benzimidazolecarbamates is described in German Patent 2,029,637 (corresponding to US Patent 3,657,267). See *CA 74:* 100047s, 1971.

Description—White to slightly yellow powder; melts at about 290°.
Solubility—Practically insoluble in water, alcohol, ether, chloroform.

Uses—The anthelmintic of choice in hookworm (*Ancylostoma duodenale, Necator americanus*), pinworm (*Enterobius vermicularis*), roundworm (*Ascaris lumbricoides*), and whipworm (*Trichuris trichiura*) infestations. It is an alternative anthelmintic in guinea worm (*Dracunculus medinensis*), filariasis (*Onchocerca volvulus*), Gnathostomiasis, and under investigation for use in Trichinosis (*Tricohinella spiralis*) and *Capillaria philippinensis*. Mebendazole blocks the glucose uptake by susceptible helminths, thereby depleting glycogen stored within the parasite. The glycogen depletion results in a decreased formation of adenosine triphosphate (ATP); the latter is required for survival and reproduction of the helminth. Side effects are usually mild and transient; abdominal pain and diarrhea have occurred in cases of massive infection and expulsion of worms. Leucopenia is rare but has been reported. Mebendazole is contraindicated in pregnancy and in persons who have shown hypersensitivity to the drug.

Dose—*Usual, adults* and *children, oral,* for control of *pinworm infestation,* 100 mg administered once; for other infestations, 100 mg, morning and evening, for 3 consecutive days. If necessary, a second course of treatment may be given in 3 weeks. A single dose of 11 mg/kg (1 g maximum) may be used. In *Trichinosis,* 200 to 400 mg is given 3 times a day for 3 days and then 400 to 500 mg 3 times a day for 10 days. Tablets may be chewed, swallowed or crushed and mixed with food. The drug has not been adequately studied in children under 2 yr of age and benefit/risk should be considered before use in children of this age.

Dosage Form—Tablets: chewable, 100 mg.

Metronidazole—page 1222.

Metrifonate

Dimethyl (2,2,2-trichloro-1-hydroxyethyl) phosphate; Bilarcil (*Bayer*)

[52-68-6] $C_4H_8Cl_3O_4P$ (257.44).

Preparation—By the reaction between chloral and dimethyl phosphite. (*JACS 76:* 4186, 1964.)

Description—White crystal melting about 84°.
Solubility—1 g in 6.5 mL water, 33 mL chloroform, 5.9 mL ether, 6.6 mL benzene; solutions in fixed alkali decompose readily.

Uses—The drug of choice for *Schistosoma haematobium.* Adverse effects observed include nausea, vomiting, bronchospasm, weakness, diarrhea, and abdominal pain.

Dose—*Adults* and *children,* three doses of 10 mg/kg given every other week.

Dosage Form—Available from the Parasitic Disease Division, Center for Disease Control, Atlanta, GA 30333.

Niclosamide

Benzamide, 5-chloro-N-(2-chloro-4-nitrophenyl)-2-hydroxy-, Niclocide (*Miles*); Yomesan (*Bayer*)

2′,5-Dichloro-4′-nitrosalicylanilide [50-65-7] $C_{13}H_8Cl_2N_2O_4$ (327.12).

Preparation—PCl_3 is slowly introduced into a boiling xylene solution containing 5-chlorosalicylic acid and 2-chloro-4-nitroaniline in equimolar ratio and the heating continued for 3 hours. Crystals of niclosamide separate on cooling and are recrystallized from ethanol. US Pat 3,079,297.

Description—Pale yellow crystals; melting range 225° to 230°.
Solubility—Practically insoluble in water; sparingly soluble in alcohol, chloroform, ether.

Uses—The anthelmintic of first choice in the treatment of beef tapeworm (*Taenia saginata*), fish tapeworm (*Diphyllobothrium latum*), pork tapeworm (*Taenia solium*), and dwarf tapeworm (*Hymenolepis nana*) infections. Niclosamide inhibits phosphorylation in the mitochondria of cestodes. Both *in vitro* and *in vivo*, the scolex and proximal segments are killed on contact with the drug. The loosened scolex may be digested in the intestine; hence, it may be impossible to identify the scolex in the feces. Untoward effects occur only occasionally; nausea and abdominal pain have been reported most frequently. Other side effects include oral irritation, fever, rectal bleeding, weakness, bad taste, sweating, palpitations, and irritability.

Dose—*Usual, oral; adult*, a single dose of 4 tablets (**2 grams**) chewed thoroughly. *Pediatric*, 11 to 34 kg, a single dose of 2 tablets (**1 gram**); >34 kg, a single dose of 3 tablets (**1.5 grams**). For dwarf tapeworm infection, the drug should be taken for 6 to 7 days. The patient should omit breakfast but may eat 2 hours after the last dose. The tablets should be chewed thoroughly and then washed down with water.

Dosage Forms—Tablets: 500 mg.

Niridazole

2-Imidazolidinone, 1-(5-nitro-2-thiazolyl)-, Ambilhar (*Ciba-Geigy*)

1-(5-Nitro-2-thiazolyl)-2-imidazolidinone [61-57-4] $C_6H_6N_4O_3S$ (214.22).

Preparation—By condensation of 2-amino-5-nitrothiazole with β-chloroethylisocyanate in the presence of base to achieve cyclization of the intermediate compound (*Experientia 20*: 452, 1964).

Description—Yellow, crystalline powder; odorless; tasteless; melts at about 260°.
Solubility—Practically insoluble in water and most organic solvents.

Uses—The drug of choice for guineaworm (*Dracunculus medinensis*) infestation and an alternative antischistosomal drug for *Schistosoma japonicum*. Adverse effects include vomiting, cramps, dizziness, and headaches; occasionally diarrhea, slight electrocardiographic changes, rash, insomnia, paresthesia; rarely psychosis, hemolytic anemia, and convulsions. Niridazole is absolutely contraindicated in the presence of hepatocellular disease, portal hypertension, or a history of mental disorders or seizures.

Dose—*Usual, adults* and *children, oral*, **25 mg/kg** of body weight daily (with a maximum of **1.5 g** daily) in two divided doses for 5 to 7 days in schistosomiasis and for 7 to 10 days in dracunculiasis.

Dosage Form—Tablets: 500 mg, available from the Parasitic Disease Drug Service, Center for Disease Control, Atlanta, GA 30333.

Oxamniquine

6-Quinolinemethanol, 1,2,3,4-tetrahydro-2-[[(1-methylethyl)amino]-methyl]-7-nitro-, Vansil (*Pfizer*).

1,2,3,4-Tetrahydro-2-[(isopropylamino)methyl]-7-nitro-6-quinolinemethanol [21738-42-1] $C_{14}H_{21}N_3O_3$ (279.34).

Preparation—From 6-methoxymethylquinaldinic acid to form the acyl chloride, which with diethylamine yields the amide. Reduction of the amide with lithium aluminum hydride and Raney nickel produces the diethylaminomethyl derivative. Nitration of the latter compound in the 7-position followed by demethylation of the 6-position yields oxaminiquine (US Pat 3,821,228).

Description—A light orange crystalline powder melting about 151°.
Solubility—Soluble in 3300 in water; soluble in acetone, chloroform, and methanol.

Uses—The drug of choice for infection caused by *Schistosoma mansoni*. Especially effective in the immediate post infection stage. Oxamniquine significantly reduces the egg load of *S. mansoni*. There are no known contraindications. Adverse effects observed include occasional headache, fever, dizziness, somnolence, nausea, diarrhea, rash, insomnia, ECG changes. Convulsions have also been observed, but are rare.

Dose—*Schistosoma mansoni*, adults and children, 15 mg/kg once.

Dosage Forms—Capsules, 250 mg/kg.

Piperazine Citrate

Piperazine 2-hydroxy-1,2,3-propanetricarboxylate (salt) (3:2), hydrate; Antepar Citrate (*Burroughs-Wellcome*)

Piperazine citrate (salt) (3:2) hydrate [41372-10-5] $(C_4H_{10}N_2)_2 \cdot 2C_6H_8O_7 \cdot xH_2O$; *anhydrous* [144-29-6] (642.66).

Preparation—Piperazine and citric acid, in 3:2-molar proportion, are reacted in aqueous solution, from which piperazine citrate is crystallized.

Description—White, crystalline powder, having not more than a slight odor; a 1 in 10 solution is acid to litmus, having a pH of about 5.
Solubility—Soluble in water; insoluble in alcohol and ether.

Uses—An alternate *anthelmintic* used for the treatment of *roundworm* (*Ascaris lumbricoides*) and pinworm (*Enterobius vermicularis*) infections. Piperazine citrate, as well as other piperazine salts, form piperazine hexahydrate in solution. Consequently the citrate, phosphate, and the chelated form are thought to be equally effective. Piperazine hyperpolarizes the Ascaris muscle by blocking acetylcholine and alters membrane permeability to ions responsible for maintaining the resting potential. The paralyzed Ascaris is expelled via peristalsis. The mechanism of action against Enterobius is unknown. The drug is relatively nontoxic. Occasionally, dizziness, urticaria and gastrointestinal disturbances, are observed. Rare untoward effects include visual disturbances, ataxia and hypotonia. Piperazine citrate may increase seizure incidence in epileptic patients. Excessively prolonged or repeated treatment should be avoided. The drug is contraindicated in patients with impaired renal or hepatic function, convulsive disorders, or a history of hypersensitivity reactions from piperazine and its salts.

Dose (piperazine hexahydrate equivalent)—For *ascariasis: usual, adult, oral*, a single daily dose of **3.5 g** (75 mg/kg) for 2 days; *pediatric*, a single daily dose of **75 mg/kg** for 2 days, with a maximum daily dose of **3.5 g**. For *enterobiasis: adult* and *pediatric*, a single daily dose of **65 mg/kg** for 7 days, with a maximum daily dose of **2.5 g**. In severe infections (ascariasis or enterobiasis) the treatment course may be repeated after an interval of two weeks.

Dosage Forms—Syrup: 550 mg piperazine citrate/5 mL (equivalent to 500 mg piperazine hexahydrate); Tablets: 250 and 500 mg piperazine citrate (equivalent to 250 and 500 mg piperazine hexahydrate).

Praziquantel

4*H*-Pyrazino[2,1-*a*]isoquinolin-4-one, 2-(cyclohexylcarbonyl)-
1,2,3,6,7,11b-hexahydro-, Biltricide (*Miles*)

[55268] $C_{19}H_{24}N_2O_2$ (312.41).

Preparation—Aminomethyltetrahydroisoquinoline, cyclohexanecarbonyl chloride, acetonitrile, and aqueous hydrochloric acid are refluxed in the presence of pyridine to first form the cyclohexanecarbamoylmethyl derivative which cyclizes to form the product (Ger Pat 2,504,250).

Uses—The drug of choice for infections caused by *Schistosoma japonicum*, *S. mekongi*, and various kinds of flukes (Chinese liver, sheep liver, intestinal and lung). It is an alternative drug for the treatment of *Hymenolepis nana* (dwarf tapeworm), *Schistosoma haematobium*, and *S nansoni*. Praziquantil increases the permeability of the worm's cell membrane to calcium ions; this causes massive contraction and paralysis of its musculature and disintegration of its tegumental layer. Adverse effects include sedation, abdominal discomfort, fever, sweating, nausea, eosinophilia, headache, and dizziness. Available in US only on investigational basis.

Dose—*Usual, adult or children, S Haematobium* and *mansoni*, one dose of 40 mg/kg; *S japonicum*, 30 mg/kg twice in one day; *S mekongi*, 20 mg/kg three times in one day; flukes, 25 mg/kg three times a day for one day.

Pyrantel Pamoate

Pyrimidine, 1,4,5,6-tetrahydro-1-methyl-2-[2-(2-thienyl)ethenyl]-, (*E*), compd. with 4,4′-methylenebis[3-hydroxy-2-naphthalenecarboxylic acid] (1:1); Antiminth (*Roerig*); Combantrin (*Pfizer*)

(*E*) - 1,4,5,6-Tetrahydro-1-methyl-2-[2-(2-thienyl)vinyl]pyrimidine 4,4′-methylenebis[3-hydroxy-2-naphthoate] (1:1) [22204-24-6] $C_{11}H_{14}N_2S.C_{23}H_{16}O_6$ (594.68).

Preparation—Thiophene is converted to 2-thiophenecarboxaldehyde (I) via a Vilsmeier-Haack reaction. *N*-Methyl-1,3-propanediamine is condensed with acetonitrile to yield 1,4,5,6-tetrahydro-1,2-dimethylpyrimidine which is then coupled with I in the presence of methyl formate to yield pyrantel (base). The pyrantel is isolated as the tartrate and metathesized with a soluble alkali metal pamoate.

Description—Yellow to tan powder that is tasteless and free of characteristic odor; decomposes slowly in light; nonhygroscopic in air under ordinary conditions; relatively stable in heat; melts with decomposition between 247° and 261°.

Solubility—Insoluble in water; very slightly soluble in alcohol.

Uses—The anthelmintic of choice in the treatment of hookworm (*Necator americanus* and *Ancylostoma duodenale*), pinworm (*Enterobius vermicularis*), and roundworm (*Ascaris lumbricoides*) infestations. It is recommended also as an alternate drug in the treatment of *Trichostrongylus* sp. infections. Side effects occur only occasionally and are relatively mild; gastrointestinal disturbances, headache, dizziness, rash, and fever have been reported.

Dose—*Usual, oral, children* and *adults*, **11 mg** pyrantel base/**kg**, with a maximum of 1 g, as a single dose for infestations with *Ancylostoma duodenale*, *Ascaris lumbricoides*, *Nectar americanus*, and *Trichostrongylus* sp.; for *Enterobius vermicularis* infestation the same dose is employed, but repeated in two weeks. *Note:* Light hookworm infestations need not be treated in the absence of symptoms or anemia. Members of the family of patients with pinworm infestations should also be treated to prevent recurrence.

Dose Form—Oral Suspension containing 50 mg pyrantel base/mL.

Pyrvinium Pamoate

Quinolinium, 6-(dimethylamino)-2-[2-(2,5-dimethyl-1-phenyl-1*H*-pyrrol-3-yl)ethenyl]-1-methyl-, salt with 4,4′-methylenebis[3-hydroxy-2-naphthalenecarboxylic acid] (2:1); Povan (*Parke-Davis*)

6 - (Dimethylamino)-2-[2-(2,5-dimethyl-1-phenylpyrrol-3-yl)vinyl]-1-methylquinolinum 4,4′-methylenebis-[3-hydroxy-2-naphthoate] (2:1) [3546-41-6] $C_{75}H_{70}N_6O_6$ (1151.41).

Preparation—6-(Dimethylamino)-1-methylquinaldinium methyl sulfate (I) is condensed with 2,5-dimethyl-1-phenyl-3-pyrrolecarboxaldehyde (II) in methanol. The resulting pyrvinium methyl sulfate is then metathesized with disodium 4,4′-methylenebis[3-hydroxy-2-naphthoate]. I is readily prepared from 6-aminoquinaldine by methylation followed by quarternization with dimethyl sulfate. II may be prepared by condensing 2,5-dimethyl-1-phenylpyrrole with formamide and degrading the resulting 3-carboxamide to the aldehyde. US Pat 2,515,912.

Description—Bright orange or orange-red to almost black, crystalline powder.

Solubility—Practically insoluble in water and ether; slightly soluble in chloroform and methoxyethanol; very slightly soluble in alcohol.

Uses—An anthelmintic, recommended as an alternate drug in the treatment of pinworm (*Enterobius vermicularis*) infections. Pyrvinium pamoate is well tolerated and causes few untoward effects. Nausea, vomiting, diarrhea, and transient photosensitization have been reported. The drug resembles a cyanine dye and colors the stools bright red and will stain clothing if vomited.

Dose—*Usual*, for *pinworm* the equivalent of **5 mg** of pyrvinium base/**kg** (maximum 350 mg) in a single dose; repeat in 2 weeks. *Pediatric*, same as for adults.

Dosage Forms—Tablets: film seal, 50 mg.

Quinacrine Hydrochloride—page 1220.

Thiabendazole

1*H*-Benzimidazole, 2-(4-thiazolyl)-, Mint (*MSD*);
Thibenzole (*Merck*)

2-(4-Thiazolyl)benzimidazole [148-79-8] $C_{10}H_7N_3S$ (201.25).

Preparation—Ethyl pyruvate is brominated and the resulting 2-bromo ester is reacted with thioformamide whereby cyclization occurs with formation of ethyl 4-thiazolecarboxylate. This ester is saponified and condensed with *o*-phenylenediamine to introduce the benzimidazole moiety. US Pat 3,017,415.

Description—White to practically white, odorless or practically odorless, tasteless powder; stable in light and nonhygroscopic; melts between 296° and 303°.

Solubility—Practically insoluble in water; slightly soluble in acetone and alcohol; very slightly soluble in chloroform and ether.

Uses—The *anthelmintic* of choice in *Strongyloides stercoralis*, *Trichostrongylus sp*, cutaneous larva migrans (creeping eruption), *Angiostrongylus cantonensis*, and *visceral larva migrans*, trichinosis (*Trichinella spiralis*). In severe trichinosis, steroids should also be used to control the symptoms. It is also recommended as an alternate drug in the treatment of *hookworm* (*Necator americanus*), and *Capillaris philippensis* infections. In the latter, it appears to be effective during the intestinal phase but its effect on larvae which have migrated is questionable. No special diet or purgation is needed with thiabendazole. Side effects usually include nausea, vomiting, vertigo, headache, and weakness. Leukopenia, crystalluria, rash, disturbance of color vision, and hallucinations have also been reported. In rare instances, shock, tinnitus and Stevens-Johnson syndrome have been observed. Since from $\frac{1}{3}$ to $\frac{1}{2}$ of patients are usually incapacitated for several hours after receiving the drug, the drug should be given on days when the patient does not have to go to school or to work. Patients on the drug should be cautioned not to engage in activities requiring mental alertness.

Dose—*Usual, oral, adults* and *children,* **25 mg/kg** twice daily after meals; the daily dose should not exceed 3 g. For *Strongyloides stercoralis, Trichostrongylus* sp., and *Necator americanus* infections this dosage is given 2 days; for trichinosis and severe visceral larva migrans, the dosage is continued for 5 days. For cutaneous larva migrans (creeping eruption), thiabendazole is applied topically or administered orally in the above dosage for 2 to 5 days. For *Capillaris philippensis* **25 mg/kg** is given each day for 30 days.

Dosage Forms—Oral Suspension: 500 mg/5 mL; Chewable tablets, 500 mg.

Other Anthelmintics

Antimony Potassium Tartrate [Tartar Emetic Dipotassium bis[μ-tartrato(4-)]diantimonate(2-) trihydrate [28300-74-5] $C_8H_4K_2Sb_2O_{12}.3H_2O$ (667.85); *anhydrous* [11071-15-1] (613.81)]—*Preparation:* By dissolving a mixture of 10 parts of potassium bitartrate with 8 parts of antimony trioxide [Sb_2O_3] in 75 parts of boiling water, filtering the solution while hot and allowing it to crystallize. *Description:* Colorless, odorless, transparent crystals, or a white powder; the crystals effloresce upon exposure to air; solutions are acid to litmus. 1 g in 12 mL water and about 15 mL glycerin, and about 3 mL boiling water; insoluble in alcohol. *Incompatibilities—Mineral acids,* when added to aqueous solutions of antimony potassium tartrate, precipitate basic salts of antimony, with possibly some potassium bitartrate. *Alkali hydroxides* and *carbonates* of sufficient concentration precipitate antimony trioxide. Precipitation is retarded by citrates, tartrates, glycerin, and sugar. Many metallic salts form insoluble tartrates. Addition of *alcohol* to an aqueous solution may cause precipitation. An insoluble tannate is formed with *tannic acid.* *Uses:* Formerly used for infections caused by *Schistosoma japonicum.* It is also an *emetic,* chiefly by virtue of its irritant action on the gastrointestinal mucosa. Subemetic doses produce an *expectorant* action due to reflex stimulation of the salivary and bronchial glands. Toxic effects induced by antimony potassium tartrate frequently include painful local inflammation, coughing and vomiting when intravenous injection is rapid, muscle and joint stiffness, and bradycardia. Occasional adverse effects include colic, diarrhea, rash, pruritus, and myocardial damage. Rarely, liver damage, hemolytic anemia, renal damage, shock, and sudden death are encountered. *Dose: Usual, intravenous,* as a 0.5 to 1% solution, *initial,* 40 mg, repeated every 2 days, each dose increased by 20 mg until 140 mg is reached, then 140 mg every other day for a total course-of-treatment dose of 2 g.

Hycanthone Mesylate [9*H*-Thioxanthen-9-one, 1-[[2-(diethylamino)ethyl]amino]-4-(hydroxymethyl)-, monomethanesulfonate (salt); Etrenol Mesylate (*Winthrop*) [23255-93-8] $C_{20}H_{24}N_2O_2S.CH_4O_3S$ (452.58). *Preparation:* Hycanthone (base) may be prepared from lucanthone by microbiological transformation using any of various molds. Reaction with an equimolar quantity of methanesulfonic acid yields the mesylate. *Uses:* Formerly used against *Schistosoma haematobium* and *S mansoni;* it is *ineffective* in *S japonicum* infections. Adverse effects include anorexia, nausea and vomiting, abdominal colic, constipation, dizziness, myalgia, headache, and pain at the site of the injection. Transient changes in liver function and in the ECG have also been reported. *Dose: Usual, intramuscular, adults* and *children 2 years and older,* single dose of 3.5 mg/kg; total dose should not exceed 200 mg given in gluteus minimus. *Dosage Forms:* for Injection: Obtainable from the

Parasitic Disease Drug Service, Center for Disease Control, Atlanta, GA 30333.

Piperazine [Piperazine [110-85-0] $C_4H_{10}N_2$ (86.14).] *Preparation:* By catalytic deamination of diethylenetriamine and of ethylenediamine. US Pat 2,267,686. *Description:* White to slightly off-white lumps or flakes having an ammoniacal odor; melts between 109° and 113°; boils between 145° and 146°; in water it crystallizes with $6H_2O$ in colorless crystals called *piperazine hydrate,* melting at 44° and boiling between 125° and 130°. *Solubility:* Soluble in water and alcohol; insoluble in ether. *Incompatibilities:* With salts of heavy metals, alkaloidal salts, and with acetanilid, phenacetin, and nitrites. *Uses:* Piperazine and several of its salts—*piperazine adipate, piperazine calcium edetate, piperazine citrate, piperazine phosphate,* and *piperazine tartrate*—are used as anthelmintics. For further information see *Piperazine Citrate.*

Sodium Stibocaptate [2,3-Dimercaptosuccinic acid cyclic ester with antimonic acid, diester with 2,3-dimercaptosuccinic acid hexasodium salt; Astiban (*Hoffmann-La-Roche*) $C_{12}H_6Na_6O_{12}S_6Sb_2$ (787.74).] *Preparation:* By reaction of disodium 2,3-dimercaptosuccinate and Sb_2O_3 (*CA 65:* 17580e, 1966; see also *CA 53:* 16158a, 1959). *Description and Solubility:* White or slightly yellowish green powder; hygroscopic; unstable after being moistened. Soluble in water to form a clear, colorless, odorless solution that decomposes at room temperature with formation of an orange-reddish precipitate. *Uses:* Sodium Stibocaptate is sometimes used for the treatment of infections caused by *Schistosoma mansoni,* and *Schistosoma haematobium,* and *Schistosoma japonicum.* Adverse effects are similar to those of antimony potassium tartrate but except for rash and pruritus are less frequent and usually less severe. *Dose: Usual, adult,* 8 mg/kg *intramuscularly* (10% solution) given once or twice a week for a total of 5 doses. *Pediatric,* as for adults. *Dosage Form:* Powder, available from the Parasitic Disease Drug Service, Center for Disease Control, Atlanta, GA 30333.

Stibophen [Pentasodium bis[4,5-dihydroxy-*m*-benzenedisulfonato-(4)antimonate(5-) heptahydrate; Fuadin (*Winthrop*) [15489-16-4] $C_{12}H_4Na_5O_{16}S_4Sb.7H_2O$ (895.20); *anhydrous* [23940-36-5] (769.09).] *Preparation:* By reaction between antimony trioxide, sodium catechol-3,5-disulfonate, and NaOH. *Description and Solubility:* White, slightly yellow or pink, odorless, crystalline powder. It is affected by light and is oxidized upon prolonged exposure of its solution to air; therefore, unused portions of its solution should be discarded. Its aqueous solution is alkaline and stable when autoclaved; however, prolonged storage should be avoided since this may cause its dissociation and resultant increasing toxicity. Owing to its phenolic character and the presence of sulfonic acid groups it is discolored by ferric iron. 1 g in 1 mL water, >10,000 mL alcohol, >10,000 mL chloroform, 10,000 mL ether. *Uses:* Formerly used as an alternative *antischistosomal* drug for the treatment of *Schistosoma mansoni* infections. It is contraindicated in renal and cardiac disease, and in hepatic disease not caused by schistosomiasis. Treatment should be stopped if recurrent vomiting, albuminuria, intercurrent febrile infection, or blood dyscrasias occur. Heart damage has occurred occasionally with long use of the drug. Severe, sometimes fatal, hypersensitivity reactions have been reported. Sulfhemoglobinuria and encephalopathy are among other adverse effects of rare occurrence. *Dose: Adults,* 1.5 to 2 mL of a 6.3% solution on the first day, 3.5 mL the second day, 5 mL the third day, then 5 or 6 doses of 5 mL each on alternate days. The drug may also be given in daily doses of 4 to 5 mL 5 days a week for 4 weeks. *Children,* 0.5 mL on the first day. If no adverse reactions are noted, 0.5 mL/10 kg of body weight on the second day, and then 1 mL/10 kg every second or third day until a total of 1 mL/kg has been given. Courses should not be repeated in less than 6 to 12 weeks and not unless viable eggs of *Schistosoma* are found in the stool or demonstrated in rectal biopsy. *Dosage Form:* Injection: 6.3% solution in 5-mL containers.

Pediculicides and Scabicides

Pediculicides are compounds effective in the treatment of pediculosis. Pediculosis in man is caused by three species of sucking lice known as *Pediculus humanus* variety *capitis,* the head louse, *Pediculus humanus* variety *corporis,* the body louse, and *Phthirius pubis,* the crab louse. These parasitic, wingless insects thrive where personal hygiene is neglected. The eggs (nits) of the body louse are attached to the fibers of clothing while those of the other two species are attached to hairs by a chitin-like cement. Cutting the hair short or shaving the area is helpful in destroying the eggs. The period of development from egg to adult is about 2 to 4 weeks. To be effective completely, an antipedicular agent must kill both parasites and eggs. Should the latter fail to be destroyed,

repeated applications of the agent may be necessary to destroy the newly hatched lice.

Scabicides are compounds that are effective against *Sarcoptes scabiei,* the animal parasite that causes scabies in man. The parasite, a mite, thrives where personal hygiene is neglected. After copulation takes place on the surface of the skin, the female mite excavates a sinuous inward-sloping burrow in the corneous layer of the skin. The eggs are laid in the burrow and, after hatching, the larvae and nymphs may exit. In order to eradicate this infestation, an antiscabious agent must kill both parasites and eggs. If the eggs are not destroyed, repeated applications of the antiscabious agent may be necessary. The life cycle from egg to adult parasite is from 8 to 15 days. Sulfur ointment has been a time-honored scabicide, but has now been replaced by more effective agents.

Since many agents possess both antipedicular and anti-scabious properties, the pediculicides and scabicides are listed together.

Benzyl Benzoate

Benzoic acid, phenylmethyl ester; Benylate (*Breon*)

Benzyl benzoate [120-51-4] $C_{14}H_{12}O_2$ (212.25).

Preparation—Benzyl benzoate is one of the active constituents of Peruvian Balsam. It is also present in small quantities in other natural balsamic substances. The market supply of it, however, is produced synthetically by the esterification of benzoic acid with benzyl alcohol in a manner similar to the production of ethyl acetate.

Description—Clear, colorless, oily liquid having a slight, aromatic odor and a sharp, burning taste; specific gravity 1.116–1.120; congeals at a temperature not below 18.0°.

Solubility—Practically insoluble in water or glycerin; miscible with alcohol, ether, or chloroform.

Uses—Applied externally in concentration of 10 to 30% as a scabicide. It is employed as an alternative drug in the treatment of *scabies* and is also useful in the treatment of *pediculosis*. Severe skin irritation may occur in some patients. It is usually employed as *Benzyl Benzoate Lotion*.

Dose—*Topical*, as lotion over previously dampened skin of entire body, except face.

Benzyl Benzoate Lotion [Benzyl Benzoate Application] contains 26–30% (*w/w*) of $C_{14}H_{12}O_2$. *Preparation:* Mix triethanolamine (5 g) with oleic acid (20 g), add benzyl benzoate (250 mL), and mix. Transfer the mixture to a suitable container of about 2000-mL capacity, add purified water (250 mL), and shake the mixture thoroughly. Finally add the remaining purified water (500 mL), and again shake thoroughly.

Uses: This lotion is used for the treatment of *scabies*. It is applied with a brush after the entire body has been thoroughly scrubbed with soft soap and hot water. A second coat is applied when the first is dry and the lotion is left on the body for 24 hours. At the end of that time the body is again thoroughly bathed and dressed in clean clothes. Adults require from 120 to 180 mL; a child from 60 to 90 mL. Do not apply to the face.

Chlorophenothane

1,1,1-Trichloro-2,2-bis(*p*-chlorophenyl)ethane Dicophane; Gesarol; GNB; DDT; Neocid; SBLY

1,1'(2,2,2-Trichloroethylidene)bis[4-chlorobenzene; [50-29-3] $C_{14}H_9Cl_5$ (354.49).

Preparation—By condensing chloral and chlorobenzene in the presence of sulfuric acid. There are several grades of the product. Technical DDT is a mixture containing about 70% of *p,p'*-DDT and 30% *o,p'*-DDT. Purified DDT (aerosol DDT) is a purer grade containing a higher percentage of the *p,p'*-isomer. Medicinal DDT consists of this highly purified DDT, suitable for use in solution directly upon the skin.

Description—Colorless or white crystals, or a white to slightly off-white crystalline powder; odorless or has a slight aromatic odor and a bitter taste; stable in air; slowly discolored by light; congeals at a temperature not lower than 89°.

Solubility—Insoluble in water; 1 g in 40 to 60 mL alcohol, 2.5 mL acetone, 3.5 mL chloroform, 4 mL ether (the greater the purity, the lower is its solubility in alcohol).

Uses—Sometimes effective in *pediculosis*, although lindane is the treatment of choice. It is effective against *head lice*, *body lice*, and *crab lice*. A simple, effective, and safe preparation is a mixture of 10% DDT powder with talc or any other suitable diluent. For the treatment of head or pubic lice, the powder is rubbed into the hair and allowed to remain for several days. For the treatment of body lice, the underclothes are dusted with the preparation. All contaminated clothing should be thoroughly laundered or dry cleaned to prevent reinfestation. One application is usually sufficient to control pediculosis, but treatment may be repeated after a week, if necessary.

DDT is not an effective miticide, (lindane is the drug of choice) and should not be employed alone for the treatment of scabies. See also Chapter 65.

Toxicity—When applied locally as a powder, the compound is nonirritating and is not absorbed through intact skin. However, when it is dissolved in organic solvents, appreciable percutaneous absorption occurs. The compound is only slowly absorbed from the gastrointestinal tract; absorption is greatly facilitated in the presence of fats and oils. The fatal oral dose of DDT for man is not known; a dose of 20 g has produced severe poisoning, but not death. The signs and symptoms of DDT poisoning in humans are vague and ill-defined; vomiting, numbness, and partial paralysis of the extremities, mild convulsions, loss of proprioception and vibratory sensation of the extremities, and hyperactive knee jerk reflexes are commonly observed. Treatment consists in gastric lavage followed by a saline laxative. Symptomatic therapy includes the judicious use of phenobarbital or pentobarbital to calm the patient.

DDT formerly found broad application in the fields of agriculture and public health and as a household insecticide. See Chapter 66.

Dose—*Topical*, **5** or **10%** (in an inert base as a dusting powder) 1 or 2 times a week.

Crotamiton

2-Butenamide, *N*-ethyl-*N*-(2-methylphenyl)-, Eurax (*Westwood*)

N-Ethyl-*o*-crotonotoluidide [483-63-6] $C_{13}H_{17}NO$ (203.28).

Preparation—By condensation of a crotonyl halide, ester, salt or a derivative thereof with *N*-ethyl-*o*-toluidine.

Description—Colorless to slightly yellowish oil, with a faint amine-like odor.

Solubility—Practically insoluble in water; miscible with alcohol.

Uses—A scabicidal and antipruritic agent; highly effective in eradicating scabies infestations and useful for symptomatic treatment of pruritic skin. Allergic sensitivity or primary irritation reactions may occur in some patients. It should not be applied to acutely inflamed skin, raw, weeping surfaces, or in the eyes or mouth.

Dose—In *scabies*, thoroughly massage into the skin of the entire body, from the chin down, a **10%** cream or lotion; a second application 24 hr later is advised to assure complete eradication of mites. A cleansing bath should be taken 48 hr after the last application. In *pruritus* the cream is massaged gently into affected areas until absorbed; repeated as needed.

Dosage Form—Cream: 10%; Lotion 10%.

Lindane

Cyclohexane, 1,2,3,4,5,6-hexachloro-, (1α,2α,3β,4α,5α,6β)-, Gamma Benzene Hexachloride; Gammexane; BHC; 666; Kwell (*Reed & Carnrick*); Scabene (*Stiefel*)

γ-1,2,3,4,5,6-Hexachlorocyclohexane [58-89-9] $C_6H_6Cl_6$ (2⨯

Gamma benzene hexachloride, as this compound was for officially called, is one of the nine theoretical stereoisomeric of 1,2,3,4,5,6-hexachlorocyclohexane. It has been shown to ha conformation and, in terms of equatorial-axial notation, becomes 1*e*,2*e*,- 3*e*,4*a*,5*a*,6*a*-hexachlorocyclohexane.

Preparation—By the chlorination of benzene in the presence of light. The reaction product is a mixture of stereoisomers containing from 10 to 15% of the insecticidally active gamma isomer which may be separated by solvent extraction processes.

Description—White, crystalline powder having a slight musty odor.

Solubility—Practically insoluble in water; slightly soluble in ethylene glycol; 1 g in 20 mL dehydrated alcohol, 3.5 mL chloroform, 40 mL ether.

Uses—Widely used as an ectoparasiticide and ovicide. It is an alternative drug for the treatment of *Pediculosis capitis* (head lice), *Phthirus pubis* (crab lice), and *Sarcoptes scabiei* (scabies). As a *scabicide*, it is employed in a 1% concentration in a vanishing cream or lotion. The mixture is applied in a thin layer over the entire cutaneous surface from the neck down. One ounce is usually sufficient for an adult. Leave on for at least 12 hours; remove by thorough washing. One application is usually curative; retreatment is indicated only if living mites can be demonstrated.

Lindane is an alternative treatment for *Pediculosis pubis* and *capitis*. Sufficient lotion or cream (1%) is applied to cover the affected and adjacent hair areas; leave in place for 8 to 12 hours; follow by thoroughly washing treated area. Retreatment is seldom necessary unless living lice can be demonstrated 7 days after treatment.

Adverse effects include occasional eczematous skin rash and conjunctivitis; rarely, convulsions and aplastic anemia have been observed.

Dose—*Topical*, 1% in cream or lotion, or in an inert base as a dusting powder once or twice a week.

Dosage Forms—Cream: 1%; Lotion: 1%/60 and 500 mL; Shampoo: 1%.

Malathion

Diethyl mercaptosuccinate *S*-ester with *O,O*-dimethyl phosphorodithioate; Prioderm (*Purdue Frederick*)

$$(CH_3)_2 \overset{\overset{S}{\|}}{P}-S-\underset{\underset{CH_2COOC_2H_5}{|}}{CH}-COOC_2H_5$$

Diethyl 2-(dimethoxyphosphinothioylthio)succinate [121-75-5] $C_{10}H_{19}O_2PS_2$ (330.35).

Preparation—From *O,O*-dimethyl phosphonyl chloride and dimethyl mercaptosuccinate in the presence of sulfur; US Pat 2,578,652.

Description—Dark brownish-yellow liquid melting about 3° with a very characteristic odor.

Solubility—Slightly soluble in water but very soluble in most organic solvents. Hydrolyzes rapidly at a pH below 5 or above 7. Aqueous solutions and lotions are usually buffered to a pH of about 5.4.

Uses—Malathion is lousicidal and ovicidal *in vitro*. Louse eggs succumb to 3 seconds of exposure to 0.062% malathion in acetone and lice to about 0.003%. Consequently, it is used as a lotion for the treatment of head lice and their ova. Adverse effects are usually restricted to irritation of the scalp. However, it is a weak organophosphate and will induce symptoms of cholinesterase depletion after accidental ingestion.

Dose—Sprinkle malathion, in the form of a lotion, on the *dry* hair; rub gently until hair and scalp are thoroughly wet; allow to dry naturally (avoid heat); 8 to 12 hours after application, shampoo the hair thoroughly; use a fine-toothed comb to remove dead lice and eggs. If required, repeat with a second application in 7 to 12 days.

Dosage Form—Lotion, 0.5% malathion.

Precipitated Sulfur

Precipitated Sulphur; Lac Sulfuris; Milk of Sulfur

Sulfur [7704-34-9] S (32.06).

Preparation—To a slurry of 1 part of lime and 10 parts of water, 2 parts of sublimed sulfur are added, thoroughly mixed, and the mixture is boiled with frequent agitation until all of the sulfur is dissolved:

$$12S + 3Ca(OH)_2 \rightarrow 2CaS_5 + CaS_2O_3 + 3H_2O$$

After allowing it to cool, the clear liquid is decanted through a filter, and a slight excess of HCl, calculated from the quantity of lime used, is added to the filtrate. The acid decomposes the calcium pentasulfide and the thiosulfate with the precipitation of sulfur:

$$2CaS_5 + CaS_2O_3 + 6HCl \rightarrow 3CaCl_2 + 12S + 3H_2O$$

Description—Very fine, pale yellow, amorphous or microcrystalline powder; odorless and tasteless.

Solubility—Practically insoluble in water; very slightly soluble in alcohol; slightly soluble in olive oil. Distinguished from other forms of sulfur by more rapid solubility in carbon disulfide: on shaking 1 g of precipitated sulfur with 5 mL carbon disulfide it should dissolve quickly except for a small amount of insoluble matter usually present.

Incompatibilities—Sufficiently hydrophobic that it sometimes causes trouble in lotions where it tends to float on the surface. Among substances which have been shown to promote the wetting of sulfur and thus aid its dispersion are triethanolamine oleate and benzoin tincture. Trituration of the sulfur with a few drops of alcohol, glycerin, or a dilute solution of a wetting agent is also of some service.

Uses—Sulfur is an active parasiticide; a 10% sulfur paste or ointment is used as an alternative treatment for *Sarcoptes scabei* (mites). Sulfur is also actively *keratolytic* and, in the form of full-strength ointment or in combination with other keratolytic agents such as salicylic acid, it is used in the treatment of skin disorders such as *psoriasis, seborrhea, eczema-dermatitis*, and *lupus erythematosus*. The percentage of sulfur in an ointment should be reduced in the event that a patient's skin shows intolerance. Prolonged use of sulfur may result in a characteristic dermatitis venenata.

Dose—*Topical, as a* **10%** ointment every night for 3 nights.

Sulfur Ointment USP contains 10% of S.

Pyrethrins with Piperonyl Butoxide

Rid Shampoo (*Pfipharmeca*); Triple X Shampoo (*Youngs Drug*); and various others

Pyrethrins are the insecticidal extracts of the pyrethrum flower and are usually synthesized from pyrethrolone [(Z)-(+)-4-hydroxy-3-methyl-2-(2,4-pentadienyl)-2-cyclopentene-1-one, $C_{11}H_{14}O$] and chrysanthemic acid [2,2-dimethyl-3-(2-methyl-1-propenyl)cyclo-propanecarboxylic acid, $C_{10}H_{17}O_2$] to yield a mixture of pyrethrins I and II. Piperonyl butoxide, [5-[[2-(2-butoxyethoxy)ethoxy] methyl]-6-propyl-1,3-benzodioxazole, $C_{19}H_{30}O_5$] has a synergistic effect on pyrethrins and rotenone, another floral insecticide.

Use—This combination (pyrethrins 0.3%, piperonyl butoxide 3.0%) is the treatment of choice for *Pediculosis humanis*, *P capitis*, and *Phthirus pubis*. Contraindicated in individuals sensitive to the ingredients or ragweed. Harmful if swallowed or inhaled. May be irritating to the eyes and mucous membranes. Discontinue use and notify physician if irritation or skin rash occurs.

Dose—Apply topically only once; it may be necessary to apply a second time 5 to 7 days later to kill hatching progeny.

Dosage Form—Liquid: 60 and 120 mL; Shampoo: 60 and 120 mL; Gel: 30 g.

Other Pediculicides

Copper Oleate [Cuprex (*Beecham*)]—*Use:* An alternative treatment for *Pediculus humanus capitis*, and *Phthirus pubis*. Contraindicated in individuals sensitive to copper oleate and/or tetrahydronaphthalene. Discontinue and notify physician if irritation or skin rash occurs. *Dose:* Apply topically. *Dosage Form:* Liquid: 0.03% copper oleate and 30.97% tetrahydronaphthalene; 90 and 480 mL.

CHAPTER 66

Pesticides

Ara H Der Marderosian, PhD

Professor of Pharmacognosy
Philadelphia College of Pharmacy and Science
Philadelphia, PA 19104

Pesticides may be defined simply as chemical agents used to control pests. In its broadest sense it includes insecticides, rodenticides, fungicides and herbicides. These substances represent big business, with the US being the largest producer in the world (34% of the total). As of 1980, the US produced 660 million kg of synthetic organic pesticides with a value of $4.2 billion. Over 50 US companies manufacture pesticides, with 14 concerns accounting for some 85% of all pesticide sales. The majority of the 50 basic producers prepare one or more ready-to-use forms of their products, while another 3250 formulators throughout the US prepare 35,000 different items for retail sales. It has been estimated that this amounts to something like 2 kg (4.4 lb) per person in terms of the production of food, clothing, and durable goods for the 270 million persons living in this country.

Even though domestic use has grown significantly, other countries are also using pesticides at an increasingly faster rate as they develop their agricultural and industrial economies. In 1980 the US exported 335 million kg and at the same time increased imports of other pesticides at least sevenfold in the last decade.

In terms of market breakdown, the agricultural sector uses about 72% of the pesticides sold in the US, while the government and industry use some 21%. Home and garden use is at a level of only 7%. Some of the areas in which householders currently depend on pesticides are: weed control on lawns; mildew control in laundries; algae control in swimming pools; flea control on pets; outdoor powders and sprays to control garden insects and pests; indoor sprays for roaches and ants; aerosols for mosquitoes and flies; wood and soil treatments for termite control; various baits for control of mice, rats, and other rodents; treatment of wool for moth control; and various repellents against chiggers, biting flies, and mosquitoes. Pharmacies throughout the US stock a myriad of consumer pesticide products used for these purposes. This represents an important area in which pharmacists can exercise their knowledge and skills, particularly for proper use, handling, and disposal of pesticides.

As of 1980, the US Environmental Protection Agency (EPA) registered over 2600 pesticide active ingredients found in some 575 herbicides, 670 fungicides and nematicides, 610 insecticides, 630 disinfectants, and 125 rodenticides. Further, the EPA lists numerous solvents, surfactants, stabilizers, and similar substances. In 1981, at least 1100 pesticide active ingredients were still being produced. Some 200 of these are in the major active ingredient group. Various economic, political, and toxicological considerations which crop up routinely in the pesticide business preclude any more accurate figures within a given year.

For those who question the use of pesticides at all it is important to know something about what damage pests can do

Acknowledgment is made of helpful comments and suggestions by David Steiger, Pennsylvania State Department of Agriculture, Randy Hirschorn, and R Sutton of the City of Philadelphia, Department of Public Health, and Dudley Thompson, Information Services Section, Office of Pesticide Programs, US Environmental Protection Agency.

on a worldwide basis. First it should be understood that plants are the world's major source of food. These plants are susceptible to between 80,000 to 100,000 diseases caused by everything from viruses to bacteria, fungi, algae, and even other higher plants. Food plants have to compete with some 30,000 different species of weeds world-wide, of which at least 1800 species are capable of causing serious economic losses. Various higher organisms like nematodes and insects also devastate crops routinely around the world. It has been estimated that about one-third of the food crops of the world is destroyed by these various pests at various stages, viz, growth, harvest, and storage. The rates of destruction often are higher in less developed nations. The Food and Agriculture Organization (FAO) estimates that one-half of cotton production in developing countries would be lost to pests without the use of pesticides. Even in the US crop devastation due to pests is estimated to be about 30% ($20 billion annually) even though pesticides are used widely here. Several studies have shown that this country could not survive as a nation without pesticides. Without herbicides alone, at least 10 to 12% of the US population would be working on our farms instead of the current 3%.

Another important consideration of recent origin is the concept of minimum or reduced tillage. In this relatively new farming practice herbicides help promote savings of energy and soil conservation by drastically reducing plowing and cultivation. Now, farmers till only enough to plant new crops. Previous crop debris and weeds are left on the soil and insects and weeds are controlled chemically rather than mechanically through unnecessary plowing. This method of control requires some 80% less energy. There have been many who have argued for the return of what is called "organic" farming. Generally, organic farmers prefer to avoid the use of synthetic chemical products at all. They prefer naturally occurring chemicals such as rock phosphate and limestone and the manure of domestic animals. Also, leguminous plants are used as a nitrogen source as well as other plants which contain natural pesticidal compounds. While these are laudable practices, they generally result in higher prices because of the costs of these less available materials and the higher costs involved in the more labor intensive practices of organic farming. In addition, more land with lower yielding capability would have to be farmed to make up for the lower efficiency of organic farming. From a scientific point of view all natural materials are not necessarily organic and organic substances are not necessarily natural. All things on earth are made up of chemicals and plants do not really differentiate between what is made by man or nature. However, organic farming practices are sensible for the smaller farmer who wishes to avoid excess use of unnecessary chemicals and does not mind the use of extra labor practices to save money on materials.

Perhaps the major reason for use of pesticides has been the long world history of mass destruction of crops by disease and insects. One is constantly reminded that it would not take long to return to a primitive agriculture status by the numerous reports of crop devastation and disease which appear in various underdeveloped countries. Some of the recent examples of pest effects include the destruction of 3 million tons of wheat by stem rust in western Canada in 1954; the continuous problem of arthropod-borne encephalitides which caused an average of 205 human cases in the US annually between 1964 and 1973; and the reduction of the annual death rate of malaria through the use of pesticides (down from 6 million in 1939 to 2.5 million in 1965 to less than 1 million today). There are at least two dozen common diseases (encephalitis, typhus, anthrax, dysentery, etc) still of concern to man transmitted by a myriad of insects, ticks, or mites.

As with all substances used by modern man, pesticides offer a risk-benefit ratio which must be assessed for each application. A modern concerned society should always advocate very specific, carefully planned usage of pesticides, well integrated with other control practices. This approach has become quite popular today and is referred to as Integrated Pest Management (IPM). It consists of determining a workable combination of the best parts of all possible control procedures and applying them to a specific problem. The concept is to keep pests at a controllable level within the confines of sound ecological principles so that economic injury to plants or man is avoided. Overall, while mistakes have been made (eg, DDT) pesticides have contributed significantly to the increased productivity of the US farmer. In 1981, each American farmer produced enough food and fiber for 78 people as opposed to only 14 people in 1950. Currently at least one-third of today's crops are saved through the use of pesticide chemicals in agriculture. On the world scale it is widely known that current food supplies are inadequate. Estimates are given that at least 56% of the population of the world is undernourished with the situation in some countries being much worse. With world population continuing to explode (4.4 billion in 1980; expected 5.4 billion in 1990) there is little doubt that agriculture needs all the help it can get. Comparisons between foreign and US farmers is enlightening. The Asian farmer produces about 19,964 kg of food a year, the Russian farmer 14,973 kg, the European farmer 15,880 kg, while the American farmer produces 170,145 kg. This makes it easy to understand why the US can grow 48% of the world's corn and 63% of the world's soybeans with only 2% of the population involved in agriculture. Viewed from the point of view of health alone, millions of humans around the world are killed or made sick annually from a myriad of insect-borne diseases. The overall worldwide losses from insects, weeds, rats, and diseases is estimated to be in the vicinity of $90 billion annually. Without pesticides the world population could not exist.

Pesticides and Law

In the US, numerous federal laws protect the user of pesticides as well as the consumers. Many of these laws are quite old and many have been amended from time to time for obvious reasons. Since they are all complex and change with time a brief summary is presented here so that the pharmacist will be aware who is responsible for which laws and what the current status of pesticide registration is.

Federal Insecticide, Fungicide and Rodenticide Act (FIFRA)

1. Became law in 1947; superseded 1910 Federal Insecticide Act
2. Extended coverage to include herbicides and rodenticides
3. Required these products to be registered with USDA before marketing for interstate commerce
4. Basically required good and useful labeling to promote safe use (manufacturer's name and address; name, brand, and trademark of product; net contents; ingredient statement; an appropriate warning statement; etc.)

The Miller Amendment to the Food, Drug, and Cosmetic Act (1906, 1938) passed in 1954

1. Provided that any raw agricultural product would be condemned as adulterated if it contains any pesticide chemical whose safety has not been formally cleared or is present in amounts above the tolerance levels
2. Basically set allowable amounts of all pesticides in food products eg, 10.0 ppm carbaryl in lettuce

The Food Additives Amendment to the Food, Drug and Cosmetic Act (1906, 1938, 1954) passed and added in 1958

1. Extended to all types of food additives the same philosophy that had been applied to the pesticide residues on raw agricultural commodities by the 1954 Miller amendment
2. Included the Delaney clause, which states that any chemical found to cause cancer in humans or animals when administered in appropriate tests may not appear in foods consumed by humans.

Amendment to FIFRA (1947), 1959

1. Amended to include nematocides, plant regulators, defoliants, and desiccants as economic poisons (pesticides). (Poisons and repellants used against amphibians, reptiles, birds, fish, mammals, and invertebrates have since been included as economic poisons.)

Amendment to FIFRA (1947, 1959), 1964

1. Amended to require that all pesticide labels contain the federal registration number
2. Also required caution words, such as Warning, Danger, Caution, and Keep Out of Reach of Children, to be included on the front label of all poisonous pesticides
3. Manufacturers also had to remove safety claims from all labels.

In December 1970, the responsibility for the administration of FIFRA transferred from the Pesticide Regulation Division of USDA to the newly created Environmental Protection Agency (EPA). Also, the authority to establish pesticide tolerances was transferred from FDA to the EPA; however, the enforcement of tolerances remains the responsibility of the FDA, Federal Environmental Pesticide Control Act (FEPCA).

In 1972, FIFRA (1947, 1959, 1964) was revised to the current FEPCA, but still commonly referred to as FIFRA, amended 1972. Its major provisions are:

1. The use of any pesticide inconsistent with the label is prohibited.
2. Any deliberate violations of the FEPCA by growers, applicators, or dealers can result in heavy fines and/or imprisonment.
3. All pesticides are classified into (a) general use or (b) restricted categories.
4. Anyone applying the restricted-use category of pesticides must be certified by the state in which he or she resides. This provision includes both farmers and commercial applicators.
5. All pesticide manufacturing plants must be registered and inspected by the EPA.
6. States may register pesticides on a limited basis when intended for special local needs.
7. All pesticide products must be registered by EPA whether shipped in interstate or intrastate commerce.
8. In order for a product to be registered, the manufacturer is required to provide scientific evidence that the product, when used as directed will (a) effectively control those pests listed on the label, (b) not injure humans, crops, livestock, wildlife, or damage the total environment, and (c) will not result in illegal residues in food or feed.

The Environmental Protection Agency Responsibilities

1. Interpret its laws and implement its provisions.
2. Has established by regulation, ten categories of certification for commercial applicators. These include: (1) agricultural pest control (plant and animal); (2) forest pest control; (3) ornamental and turf pest control; (4) seed treatment; (5) aquatic pest control; (6) right-of-way pest control; (7) industrial, institutional, structural, and

health-related pest control; (8) public health pest control; (9) regulatory pest control; and (10) demonstration and research pest control.

3. Set general standards of knowledge for all categories of certified commercial applicators of pesticides. In each state, the certification is carried out by an appropriate regulatory agency, usually the State Department of Agriculture. Pesticide applicators are trained through the various Cooperative Extension Service of the State.

FIFRA was further amended in 1975, 1978, 1980, and 1981 to further clarify the intent of new laws. The most important provisions (summarized) are given below:

1. Generic standards are to be set for the active ingredients, rather than for each product. (This will help speed registration since there are only some 1000 active ingredients in over 35,000 formulations on the market.)
2. Reregistration of all older products is required in the light of new knowledge.
3. The EPA may grant a conditional registration for a pesticide where justified.
4. Efficacy data may be waived and a product granted registration where justified. Final proof will depend on product performance.
5. The use of data from one registrant may be used by another manufacturer or formulators, if paid for.
6. Trade secrets will be protected, however, EPA may reveal general data on pesticide effects, efficacy, and environmental chemistry. The categories of data kept confidential are such proprietary data as manufacturing and quality control processes; methods of testing, detecting, or measuring deliberately added inert components; and production, distribution, sale, and inventories of pesticides.
7. "State primacy" is advocated by EPA. This means that the states have the primary enforcement responsibility. The state must indicate that its regulatory methods (against suspected misuse of pesticides) will meet or exceed federal requirements. The state has 30 days to act before EPA will step in. State authority can be rescinded if it consistently fails to act.
8. States can register pesticides for Special Local Needs (SLN) wherever unusual situations require it.
9. The phrase, "to use any registered pesticide in a manner inconsistent with its labeling" is carefully defined in the new regulations.

Rebuttable Presumption Against Registration (RPAR)
(RPAR changed to Special Review (SR) as of July 1982)

This process was designed by EPA to ensure full gathering of scientific information on pesticide safety. It is a means of cataloging and updating all risks and benefits of pesticides through time. The definitions of the risk criteria, which when met or exceeded, can trigger RPAR or SR analysis may be found in the Federal Register (July 3, 1975); 40 CFR 162.11.

Pre-RPAR or SR

The initial study of risk involves an intensive review of the scientific studies which suggest that the RPAR or SR criteria have been exceeded by the chemical in question. All possible risk indicators are sought. The validation of risk indicator studies, the overall literature search, and the exposure analysis form the EPA's preliminary position on the potential risk of the pesticide. This document is referred to as Position Document one (PD 1). This is published in the Federal Register along with a formal notice of Presumption Against Registration.

Issuance of a RPAR

After PD 1 is published, the public response process begins. A period of 45 days is allowed for comments on the presumptions against registration presented in PD 1. Another 60 day extension may be granted if justified. Most risk rebuttals are conducted by the registrant of the pesticide, but anyone can participate, eg, USDA, states, growers, private parties, EPA, etc.

As a standard policy, the National Agricultural Pesticide Impact Assessment Program (NAPIAP) team determines benefits assessment and determination of exposure under various use conditions. The NAPIAP rebuttal, which involves every state, provides a means for people to be heard in this regulatory process. More details on the process are available through the EPA.

Tolerances, Acceptable Daily Intake (ADI) and No Observable Effect Level (NOEL)

The tolerance level of a pesticide is the maximum amount of the pesticide that can legally be present on a food or feed. This is expressed in parts per million (ppm) of the pesticide in the food by weight. These levels are set by EPA and enforced by FDA or USDA (meat, poultry, and eggs).

The tolerance in each foodstuff is set low enough so that daily consumption will not result in an exposure that exceeds the acceptable daily intake (ADI) for the pesticide. The ADI is that level of residue to which daily exposure over the course of an average human life span appears to be without appreciable risk, based on currently available facts. This is usually set arbitrarily one hundred times lower than the no observable effect level (NOEL).

For the most part, pesticide residues on crops at the time of harvest are usually less than the tolerances. Also, residues generally decrease during storage and transit and are reduced further by washing, peeling, and cooking procedures.

State Regulation

Since these vary considerably for each state there is little room to include them in this chapter. For the most part, these laws are similar to the federal regulations. Reference is made to local state agricultural agencies for specific information.

Pesticides & The Law

At the international level, the World Health Organization (WHO) and the Food and Agriculture Organization of the United Nations continue to press for wider use of certain pesticides to help raise the level of efficiency in agriculture. Recent WHO literature relates international concern on safe use of pesticides and pesticide residues in food.

Interest in pesticides extends beyond their use simply to increase crop yields, specifically in their use in the control of pests as vectors of disease. For example, it is well known that insects such as chiggers, itch mites, and ticks transport disease to man directly or via foodstuffs, and that mosquitoes, tsetse flies, rat fleas, and others are capable of directly injecting disease organisms into his blood stream. Pest control also enters into areas where livestock must be protected against predatory animals such as coyotes, wolves, and bobcats.

It should be stated at the outset that the various pesticides discussed in this chapter are subject to numerous constraints under new and continually changing rulings. For this reason it is suggested that reference be made directly to the EPA for definitive information on specific pesticides and their registered uses.

While it is difficult to classify all pesticides chemically or biologically it will be useful to list some of the major categories with a few examples in each class:

Insecticides
  Stomach poison or protective insecticides—Chlorinated hydrocarbons (methoxychlor, kelthane, chlordane); miscellaneous (carbaryl, guthion, trichlorfon).
  Contact insecticides—Botanicals (nicotine sulfate, pyrethrum, rotenone); organic phosphorus compounds (parathion, malathion); miscellaneous (carbaryl).
  Fumigants—Gaseous materials used in tightly closed spaces such as warehouses, ship holds, mills, grain elevators, boxcars, vaults,

and in the soil; these include hydrocyanic acid gas, methyl bromide, phosphine, and paradichlorobenzene.

Acaricides (Miticides)
Phosphate insecticides, tetradifon, chlorobenzilate.

Fungicides
Construed under FEPCA (1972) as those chemicals and formulations used to control fungi and bacteria on living and nonliving plants and plant parts, as well as on or in all materials and surfaces but *excluding* all uses on living humans or animals and all uses on or in processed foods, beverages or pharmaceuticals. A *localized fungicide* is dodine; examples of *complete fungicides* are benomyl and thiabendazole.

Nematicides
Construed under FEPCA (1972) as those chemicals and formulations used to control nematodes (roundworms) inhabiting soil and water that are associated with damage to plants or plant parts. *Postplanting nematicides* are fumazone, nemagon, VC-13; *systemic nematicides* are aldicarb, demeton.

Herbicides
Selective—Dalapon, siduron, 2,4-D.
Nonselective—Erbon, bromacil, ammonium sulfamate.
Contact—Cacodylic acid, paraquat, DNBP.
Translocated—2,4-DB; MCPA.

Plant Regulators
All preparations intended to alter the behavior or products of plants through physiological action, such as gibberellic acid, maleic hydrazide, succinic acid.

Defoliants and Desiccants
Preparations intended to cause leaves or foliage of plants to drop prematurely, and are usually used to aid harvesting of certain crops as cotton. Endothall, arsenic acid, sodium chlorate, and tributyl phosphorotrithioate are in this class.

Rodenticides
Strychnine, zinc phosphide, warfarin, bromodialone, chlorophacinone.

Sex Pheromones
Chemical substances produced and released by one sex of an insect (usually the female) that elicit a sexual response in an individual of the opposite sex. *cis*-7,8-Epoxy-2-methyloctadecane (Disparlure) is a gypsy moth lure.

Juvenile Hormones (Insect Growth Regulators)
A relatively new type of pest control agent that regulates insect growth. Isopropyl-11-methoxy-3,7,11-trimethyldodeca-2,4-dienoate (generic name, methoprene; brand name Altosid) is used to arrest mosquito development at the pupal stage.

Many of the chemical names given to pesticides are contractions of longer systematic nomenclature that usually serve as nonproprietary names. As with drugs, many proprietary names are featured.

According to the major purpose for which pesticides are used, they may be classified in the following way:

Acaricides—Control ticks or mites.
Algicides—Destroy algae and other aquatic vegetation.
Antiseptics—Protect objects from damage by microorganisms.
Arboricides—Defoliate and/or destroy trees or shrubby vegetation.
Bactericides—Control bacterial infection in plants.
Fungicides—Control fungal infection in plants.
Herbicides—Control weeds or undesirable species of plants.
Insecticides—Control harmful insects. Several specific terms named for the insect group have been coined; eg, aphicide—agents which control aphids.
Larvicides—Control larval stages of insects.
Limacides or **Molluscicides**—Control mollusks, including gastropods.
Nematicides—Control round worms (nematodes).
Predacides—Control predatory mammals or birds.
Zoocides—Control rodents (rodenticides).

General Suggestions to Pharmacists

The pharmacy is a logical source to obtain pesticide and pest-control information. However, if the pharmacist desires to handle pesticides and build a permanent patronage, he should acquaint himself with the common pest problems, with chemicals recommended, and how such materials should be used. In particular, the pharmacist should be acquainted with the classification of pesticides since he will be handling and selling the "general use" type and not the "restricted use" group.

The pharmacist should also keep abreast of new laws which will influence the ways in which chemicals may be used legally. Particular attention should be placed on becoming familiar with the FEPCA discussed above and the Pesticide Chemicals Amendment to the Food, Drug, and Cosmetic Act dealing with the safety determination needed on the residue of pesticides on raw agricultural commodities. This amendment is commonly known as the "Miller Bill" and was passed in 1954. The pharmacist should also study the Chemical Additives Amendment to that same Act passed in 1958 and fully effective in 1960. An annual updating of federal and state pesticide legislation may be obtained through the most recent edition of *Pesticide Handbook-Entoma* published by the Entomological Society of America. This publication also contains such information as how to use pesticides safely, antidotes and emergency treatments for poisons, poison control centers in the US, rates of application and table of measures, commercial analytical/toxicological and field testing laboratories, agricultural chemistry leaders and coordinators, EPA regional pesticide contacts, types of pesticides, structural pest control, pesticides and the environment, wildlife and pollenators, microbial control, product resistance to insects, insect growth regulators, animal and plant protection, regulation of pesticides at national and local levels, and numerous other data. Another excellent guide is *Farm Chemicals Handbook*, Meister Publ Co, 37841 Euclid Ave, Willoughby, OH 44094. For information on pesticide toxicity reference is made to the 3rd edition of the EPA publication; *Recognition and Management of Pesticide Poisoning*, Jan 1982 (EPA-540/9-80).

The entomologist and plant physiologist of the State Agricultural Experiment Station, and the county agent of the state's Cooperative Extension Service, should be consulted for identification of insects and up-to-date information about plant diseases. Publications on weed, insect, and plant disease control may be obtained from the state experiment station. Also, the Office of Information, US Department of Agriculture, Washington, DC, supplies on request a publications list from which may be selected for ordering those needed for a personal reference library. To learn about applicator certification, contact the local State Department of Agriculture.

Meetings of insecticide dealers, held annually in many states, also can be important sources of knowledge of new developments in the field of insecticides. Information about the scheduling of such meetings may be obtained from the local county agricultural agent. Each year the Cooperative Extension Service in each state publishes recommendations on pesticides.

Since there are many dependable sources of pesticides, the pharmacist will generally find it advantageous to stock packaged materials for his sales. To aid in contacting wholesalers, the guide known as ENTOMA, prepared and distributed by the Entomological Society of America, 4603 Calvert Rd, College Park, MD 20740, is invaluable.

Guidance on methods of rodent and predatory animal control may be obtained from the US Fish and Wildlife Service, Department of the Interior, Washington, DC.

Authority for promulgating regulations establishing tolerances for pesticide chemicals in or on raw agricultural commodities, or exempting any pesticide chemical from the necessity of such a tolerance, is vested in the Secretary of Health, and Human Services, through the Federal Food, Drug, and Cosmetic Act, as amended. It should be emphasized that both FEPCA and state laws require that pesticides be used according to label directions. Failure to do so can result in civil and criminal penalties.

Since garden insecticides are of fair importance in suburban areas, the pharmacist should be aware of the numerous inexpensive publications that are available from the Superintendent of Documents, US Government Printing Office, Washington, DC 20402. These include discussion of such topics as diseases and pests of garden and ornamental plants.

Finally, it has been noted that pharmacists are frequently consulted on venereal diseases, which have increased dramatically in recent years. Beyond the usual recommendation to consult a physician, the pharmacist may be of direct service in recommending agents for body lice infestation.

Control of Insects

Insects may be controlled through proper application of chemicals by means of suitable techniques.

Classification of Insect Control Chemicals

Insect control chemicals may be classified as insecticides, fumigants, repellants, and attractants.

Insecticides—Insecticides are often classified according to the type of action that results in destruction of the insect. Three broad categories, namely *stomach poisons, contact insecticides,* and *fumigants,* are generally recognized. Among older insecticides such classification was rather distinct. However, with the new synthetic organic compounds, a single material often produces insecticidal action in several ways. Certain materials are often selected and used, however, in such a manner as to accomplish control primarily by stomach, contact, or fumigating action.

Stomach Poisons—For control of insects by this method it is usually necessary to apply the insecticide to the food that they consume. Stomach poisons are widely used to control leaf-feeding insects or other pests of plants that will result in consumption of the surface-contaminated material. Stomach poisons are also used in specially prepared baits for controlling a variety of insects. With the rapid advances in employing systemic insecticides it is now feasible to destroy by stomach action certain insects which feed on plant juices or blood and tissues of animals, which in the past were considered vulnerable only to contact insecticides. Systemic insecticides are those chemicals which move in plants and animals from one location where applied to another location where the insect may be feeding. Some of the more widely used systemic insecticides include Systox (demeton; O,O-diethyl O (and S)-[2-(ethylthio)ethyl]phosphorothioates), Meta Systox R, and dimethoate (O,O-dimethyl S-methylcarbamoylmethyl-phosphorodithioate). Stomach poisons include a variety of *arsenicals, fluosilicates, rotenone,* various *chlorinated hydrocarbons,* and the *organic phosphates* and *carbamates.*

Contact Insecticides—Most of the insecticides in use today depend largely on contact action to destroy insects. *Pyrethrum, rotenone, oil emulsions, nicotine,* and *soaps* have been used for this purpose for many years. The *chlorinated hydrocarbon* insecticides (BHC, chlordane, dieldrin, and endrin, etc), the *organic phosphates* (parathion, TEPP, malathion, etc), and the *carbamates* (eg, carbaryl (Sevin)) have been employed extensively for many years but many of these will soon be unavailable for lack of reregistration or because of cancellation. Some now have restricted use for specific purposes as stated in the EPA suspended and cancelled pesticide list of May 1977. Contact insecticides are employed against chewing as well as sucking insects.

Often insecticides appear on the market with added compounds called synergists, which may enhance the effects of the insecticides considerably. Some, like piperonyl butoxide, help block metabolic degradation of the insecticide by the insect.

Fumigants—Fumigants are gases or vapors used for the control of insects, usually in enclosed spaces. The fumigants include *hydrocyanic acid, ethylene dichloride, carbon tetrachloride, methyl bromide, chloropicrin,* and many others. A number of the *chlorinated hydrocarbon* and *organic phosphorus* insecticides have sufficiently high vapor toxicity to cause marked fumigating action against insects particularly in enclosed spaces and in soils, but many of these, like lindane, have been cancelled for use in vaporizers.

Repellants—A variety of insect control chemicals possess repellant action. *Citronella* and *creosote* are examples of older materials. *Dimethyl phthalate, ethohexadiol,* and *diethyltoluamide* are examples of materials more recently developed. Such materials often cause insects to avoid contact with treated surfaces. Repellancy in a strict sense might vary greatly as to mode of action. Some insecticides such as pyrethrum have little or no repellent action except on contact. However, the action of *pyrethrum* is so rapid that the spraying of animals may cause flies and mosquitoes to leave after alighting and before biting.

Attractants—The use of attractants to lure insects to poisons or traps has been employed as a means of control for many years. The attractants employed are usually favorite foods for the particular insect involved, such as *molasses, sugar,* or *milk* for houseflies, sugar or *grease* for ants, *bran* for cutworms, *bananas* for cockroaches, decaying *meats* for blowflies, and protein hydrolysate materials for tropical fruit flies such as the Mediterranean fruit fly. In some cases specific chemicals prove highly attractive. Notable examples are *methyl eugenol* for attracting males of the oriental fruitfly, a serious pest of fruits in some tropical areas, and many synthetic substitutes like 10-dodecadienol, the codling moth sex attractant, and *cis*-7,8-epoxy-2-methyloctadecane (Disparlure), the gypsy moth sex attractant.

A new trap for Japanese beetles now on the market, combines a controlled release strip containing a furanone sex attractant and a eugenol odor attractant.

Qualifications of Suppliers of Insecticides

Mere stocking of insecticides is not enough to establish a professionally recognized and economically successful enterprise as a supplier of insecticides, for three basic services must be provided in addition to physical supplies. These services, principally of information, are:

1. Recognition of the type of insect causing the damage, either from examination of the insect or the injury it produces.
2. Recommendation of a remedy, based on knowledge of the action of various insecticides or other insect-control chemicals and of the life history, habits, and structure of the insect responsible.
3. Familiarity with methods of application of the remedy, for which the user is largely responsible but who may need instruction in such methods.

Pharmacists will find the following specific information useful in developing the aforementioned services.

1. An understanding of the relative importance of different insects and the relation of the cost of treatment to the increase in value resulting therefrom to the product injured is necessary. Not infrequently the cost will exceed the damage that might be done. If the value of the product is small, the insect may not cause appreciable loss even though it may be conspicuously evident. Again, the damage may have been done before its recognition and the delayed treatment will not affect the insect or aid in preventing the damage.
2. A knowledge of the life history, and of the habits of the common insects is desirable, as all insect control methods are based on a knowledge of these things.
3. The ability to recognize the common insects is a great aid as it is the first step in providing suitable control. The county agents, federal entomologists, and the members of the staff of the respective State Agricultural Experiment Stations are usually available to aid in the identification of insect pests.

4.   A knowledge of how insecticides kill, of the relation of types of mouth parts to the kind of insecticide to use, and when and how the material should be applied is useful.

5.   A knowledge of the usual insect problems of a community will enable the supplier to carry in stock the insecticides likely to be needed. This will eliminate surplus stocks and will provide the materials which so often fill emergency needs.

6.   A knowledge of the toxicity of an insecticide to warm-blooded animals, persistence of residues on plants or in animal tissues, hazard of the materials to bees, or fish and wildlife is important in order that advice can be given on precautions which should be taken in the use of certain chemicals. A wide variety of chemicals is in use today. They vary in their toxicity and hazards to different organisms. The degree of danger is not only governed by the inherent toxicity to higher animals and beneficial organisms in a lower category but also by the manner of use and extent of exposure. A highly toxic material properly applied in small amounts may be less hazardous than a material low in toxicity which is applied in larger amounts. The variety of insect control chemicals is clearly apparent by mentioning some of the materials in wide use today. They include: some arsenicals, nicotine compounds, a few chlorinated hydrocarbon insecticides (methoxychlor, lindane), and the insecticides grouped under the name *organic phosphates*, which at present includes *parathion*, *malathion*, *dipterex*, *diazinon*, *dursban*, *imidan*, and the newer carbamates, which include *Sevin* (*carbaryl*, 1-naphthyl-*N*-methylcarbamate) and others. Several pamphlets are available from EPA that deal with pesticide disposal, pesticide dust avoidance respirators, and diagnosis and treatment of poisoning by pesticides. These should be kept on hand for reference by pharmacists providing poison control information on pesticides.

7.   It is important to follow the recommendations for each locality. An insecticide effective in one region may not be in others.

8.   It is essential to understand the labels on trade-named preparations and to follow the directions very carefully.

9.   Knowledge of the essentials of a good insecticide, its effect on insects, and its availability and cost, is important.

10.   Those manufacturing and offering preparations such as insecticides, rodenticides, etc for sale on the open market, must familiarize themselves with the various regulations of the individual states where the products are being manufactured or are to be sold. If such products are shipped in interstate commerce, these preparations must also comply with the various federal regulations, especially the FEPCA of 1972 and subsequent EPA amendments.

11.   Many states require dealers in pesticides to be licensed. Some require the dealer to pass a written test to obtain the license. The test usually focuses on pesticide laws and regulations.

Mouth Parts and Relation to Insect Control—In general, pests have two kinds of mouth parts: chewing and sucking. An understanding of the mouth parts and how they relate to the use of different chemical insecticides will often aid in recommending a satisfactory insecticide treatment.

Chewing insects include the *grasshoppers*, *cockroaches*, *crickets*, *bird lice*, *beetles*, *slugs*, and *caterpillars*. Such insects have mandibles or jaws that enable them to cut off and take into their stomachs solid tissue. Consequently, an insecticide can be used that kills when taken into the stomach with food eaten by the insect. Most of the newer insecticides, however, are active both as contact and as stomach poisons.

Sucking insects include *plant bugs*, *leafhoppers*, *scale insects*, *aphids*, *fleas*, *mosquitoes*, *flies*, and *sucking lice* on animals. Such an insect punctures the plant or animal but does not take any of the surface tissue into its stomach; consequently, stomach poisons that have no contact action will be ineffective when applied to the surface. During recent years, however, a variety of compounds have been found that are absorbed through the roots, stems, or leaves and transported to various parts of the plant where the chemical is available to sucking insects or chewing insects that feed inside or on the plant or fruit. This class of compounds is referred to as systemics. Insecticides having systemic action offer great promise for controlling insects, and a number of such compounds are now being employed on both plants and animals.

Plants that have been attacked by chewing pests are frequently recognized by the appearance of the eaten areas. Some plant feeders eat the entire tissue, as do *potato beetles;* others eat holes in leaves, as do *flea beetles;* while some chewing insects skeletonize the leaves, as do *slugs* and the *Mexican bean beetle.*

Sucking insects injure plants in different ways and it is often difficult to determine the kind of insect responsible for the damage unless specimens are available. Sucking insects or mites may remove the sap and cause the plant to "stand still," wilt, or drop its foliage; or they may deform the plant, causing the leaves or shoots to curl and become deformed. Some sucking insects, such as the *potato leafhopper*, the *tarnished plant bug*, and *plant lice* (*aphids*) inject toxic secretions at the time of feeding, causing the death of plant cells while others—*plant lice*, *leafhoppers*, and *striped cucumber beetles*—may injure plants directly by feeding as well as through the transmission of plant diseases. Sucking insects may also affect animals by removing the blood, injecting toxic secretions, causing swelling and irritation, or carrying disease organisms.

Life History and Habits of Insects—In general, there are two types of metamorphosis or development among insects, known as incomplete and complete. Those with incomplete metamorphosis, such as aphids, grasshoppers, plant bugs, and scale insects, have only three stages in development: the *egg* or *embryo*, the *nymph* and the *adult* or *imago*. Insects with complete metamorphosis, such as beetles, butterflies, moths, flies, bees, ants, and wasps, have four stages in development. In this type, the larva hatching from the egg has no resemblance to the adult, there being also an intermediate resting stage known as the *pupa*, during which remarkable changes in structure take place.

The interrelation of insects, where they hibernate, when they are actively feeding, where they lay their eggs, natural enemies which feed on destructive pests, etc, all have an important bearing on controls. The ant is essential to the life of the corn root aphid and cultural practices which eliminate the ant will likewise eliminate the aphid; the fact that anopheles mosquitoes often rest in homes and other sheltered areas explains the great success of residual type sprays such as malathion and baytex for controlling malaria which such mosquitoes transmit; a knowledge of the preferred oviposition sites for grasshoppers permits surveys of egg abundance or abundance of newly hatched nymphs to forecast impending outbreaks of grasshoppers.

Methods of Insect Control

For convenience, insect controls can be grouped as follows:

Natural Controls—Those that are usually present and that normally tend to hold insects in check:

1.   *Natural Enemies*—Parasitic and predacious insects. Every insect is more or less hindered in its increase by other insects as well as by predacious birds, mammals, and other animal life. Although insect-eating birds and certain mammals are important, the insect parasites, predators, and insect diseases are usually the most important factors in natural insect control. In fact, it is probable that outbreaks of insects, such as the army worm, are often due not so much to favorable conditions for the pests as to unfavorable conditions for the insect parasites and predators which normally hold them in check. The use of a specific insecticide against a major pest on a crop might lead to a serious outbreak of a secondary pest because of the destruction of natural enemies which normally keep it in check, particularly if the pesticide chosen were largely ineffective against the secondary pest. Such an upset in the balance between destructive and useful insects is a problem of increasing concern in developing insect control chemicals.

2.   *Weather and Topographic Influences*—Summer and winter temperatures, rainfall, soil and atmospheric humidity, and all similar natural factors have their effect on insects and their hosts. No definite statement can be made concerning the effect of these factors on all insects. A severe winter may be harmful to some insects such as those which winter in an exposed condition; on the other hand, such conditions may have little effect on insects which are well protected. Similarly, a severe winter may weaken trees and make them more susceptible to insect attack, or it may kill the fruit buds and deprive fruit-infesting insects of their food. However, it should be remembered that insects have a high reproductive capacity and the seasonal conditions, especially spring and early summer conditions, may aid insects in becoming destructively abundant even though they pass the winter few in numbers. On the other hand, an insect overwintering in large numbers may not be important the following season

if the weather is not favorable for increase. In tropical, temperate, and frigid climates there are to be found insect pests peculiar to these areas due to their adaptation to prevailing weather and topographic influences. Topographic features, such as mountain ranges, act as rather effective barriers to insect migration. However, the great increase in the amount and speed of national and international travel and commerce during the last few decades has provided greater opportunities for hitch-hiking insect species to overcome such barriers.

Artificial Controls—Those that are scientific developments of man:

1. *Farm Practices*—Many of our most effective aids to insect control are those called farm practices. These include rotations, cultivation, time of planting, time of harvesting, sanitation, good seed, good fertility, good planting conditions, and drainage. In general, it may be said that the practices recognized as the best garden, agronomic, orchard, greenhouse, or other farm practices, are likewise the best for holding insects in check. Certain insect problems are intensified, however, because of changes in practices such as irrigation, prolonged fruiting periods, etc. It is generally recognized, for example, that supplemental irrigation, increased use of fertilizers and the planting of higher-yielding varieties of cotton have increased the boll weevil problem.

2. *Mechanical Devices*—Aside from devices for applying insecticides, there are mechanical devices of value in fighting insect pests. The house screens, fly swatters, insect-proof packages for cereals, and other contrivances may be included in this classification.

3. *Insecticides*—An insecticide may include any material used for the purpose of killing insects or of protecting crops, animals, or other property against insect attack. Insect repellants, fumigants, and attractants are considered insecticides in a broad sense. It is important to note that some insecticides may destroy only certain insect pests and are not effective against all insects.

4. *Parasiticides*—These substances kill animal parasites such as itch mites, ticks, etc.

5. *Sterilizing Agents*—The release of large numbers of insects treated by radioisotopes or chemicals to interfere with reproduction has produced high degrees of control of native populations with whom the sterilized individuals mate, particularly where the insect may mate only one time. Intensive research to extend this insect control concept is underway.

6. In the 1920's, entomologists experimenting with moths and butterflies found that there were natural chemicals internal to the insects which controlled their development. The release of these natural chemicals was controlled by the brain. These findings encouraged the development of so-called biological pesticides. Further work in the 1970's showed that synthetic analogs could react similarly. For example, methoprene can prevent adult moth emergence from pupae. It has been found to be useful in many areas eg, it can have an effective life of up to 4 years in controlling stored product pests like beetles in tobacco.

Application of Insecticides

How Insecticides Kill—An understanding of how insecticides affect insects will assist in explaining methods and timing of applications.

Stomach poisons kill by being taken into the stomach where they are acted upon by the digestive juices, absorbed through the stomach walls, and assimilated by the blood. Details of the mode of action that leads to the death of the insect are not too well known, even for our most common insecticides. However, much information is being obtained on the general nature of toxic action.

Contact insecticides kill by direct or indirect contact with the insect. Sometimes the insecticide may penetrate directly through the body integument; in other cases it causes oxidation and suffocates the insect, dissolves the insect covering, or may prevent settling of the young, as in scale insects, when lime-sulfur has been used. Some contact insecticides are effective only when applied in the presence of the insect, a fact that explains the necessity of the proper timing of applications as well as the importance of directing the spray or dust to the insect itself. Other contact insecticides of the residual type may persist on the treated surfaces where insects rest, such as barn walls, leaves of plants, etc, and kill pests that contact the insecticide deposit.

Fumigants can be applied only in enclosed spaces. Fumigants surround the insect and, being in a gaseous state, readily enter the breathing pores of the insect and kill much as do all volatile insecticides. The systemic insecticides like the

phosphates are taken up by the plants. These kill insects, which in turn can cause a residual phosphate problem.

Essentials of a Good Insecticide—There are certain important factors that have a definite bearing on the practicability of insecticides. These are:

1. Insecticidal or killing properties.
2. Effect on the plant or animal or environment being treated under varying conditions.
3. Physical properties, such as color, odor, staining properties, adhesiveness, spreading properties, stability under varying seasonal and storage conditions, reaction with other insecticides or with fungicides, consistency, and cost of preparing suitable formulations.
4. Availability.
5. Cost.
6. Safety in the hands of the user.
7. Safety and palatability of the food products exposed to the insecticide.
8. Ease of application.
9. Flammability or explosive character.

All of these factors must be kept in mind by those interested in insect control by the use of insecticides, whether researcher, manufacturer, dealer, or user.

Insecticide Formulations—Most of the contact and stomach insecticides cannot be used for insect control as manufactured. They must be compounded in forms that will permit the user to apply them directly or in a manner that requires simple mixing with water or some other diluent before application. Many insect repellants, however, are applied to the skin or clothing without being formulated. The fumigants are also used without special preparation before use.

Insecticides are generally employed in three ways—as dusts, sprays, or baits.

Dust Preparations—Prepared dusts ready for use may contain from 1 to 20% of the active insecticide in a carrier such as talc, bentonite, or pyrophyllite. When the insecticide compound is a crystalline material, it usually has to be ground to a fine state so that the finished product will readily flow from the dusting equipment and disperse readily. In dusts made from insecticide chemicals that are liquid, such as chlordane or parathion as examples, the concentration of the active material seldom can exceed 5% and still have good dusting qualities. Special conditioning agents may be necessary and special equipment might be required to make a satisfactory dust product. For this reason the ultimate user is seldom in position to make his own insecticidal dusts from the manufactured insecticide chemical. Dusts are used mainly for home purposes.

Insecticide dusts are used for controlling pests on agricultural crops, in homes, on man, or on animals.

In some instances where it is desired to limit the drift of dust particles and to prevent particles from adhering to vegetation, dry preparations are prepared so that the particles are about the size of sugar granules. Such preparations, called "granular insecticides," are used for treating soils for soil-inhabiting pests and for certain other pests such as the European corn-borer where the granules collect in whorls or leaf axilla and destroy the young larvae before they bore into the stalk. They are also employed to some extent for controlling mosquito larvae, sand-fly larvae, and other insects affecting man. In general, however, dusts and granular insecticides are not used as extensively as are sprays.

Spray Preparations—Insecticidal sprays are formulated in three ways—as solutions, emulsions, or suspensions.

In preparing *solutions* the material may be dissolved in a suitable solvent such as crude or refined kerosene. The solutions are then ready for use. Many insecticide preparations containing pyrethrum, Lethane, malathion, Thanite, chlordane, lindane, methoxychlor, etc for household use are distributed in solution form ready for application. Ultra-low volume (ULV) spraying by airplanes makes use of some of these.

When employed as *emulsions*, the chemical is dissolved in a solvent in combination with an emulsifying agent. It is usually highly concentrated. Such a concentrate is intended for dilution with water before use. Emulsion concentrates, for example, may contain 40 to 50% carbaryl, 45 to 50% xylene, and 10% of an oil-soluble emulsifying agent. Depending on the intended use this concentrate is added to water at rates varying from 1 part of concentrate to 4 or as much as 100 parts of water. Emulsion sprays are used widely in the agricultural field for controlling both plant and animal pests and for controlling household and industrial pests.

Suspensions are prepared in dry form similar to dusts but contain a wetting agent which makes it possible to prepare suspensions in water. These preparations in concentrate form are usually called wettable powders. The wettable powders may contain from 15 to 75% of the active ingredient depending on the insecticide formulated.

Wettable powder concentrates (25–85%) are added to water for application at concentrations ranging from about 0.1 to 2.5% of the active ingredient. Wettable powder sprays are used on crops, livestock, and as barn sprays. Such sprays are particularly useful for application to plants that might be sensitive to the oils employed for emulsions or solutions.

Bait Preparation—Many of the active ingredients have been formulated into insect baits. Baygon bait, and Magikil Jelly are two effective examples. In very restrictive areas, a new product, Amdro (amidinohydrazone) has been packaged as a bait inside a self-contained stick-on bait station. These can be effective in restaurant kitchen ceilings and similar areas.

Other Insecticide Preparations—Insecticides are employed in several other ways. Heat is used to produce vapors or smokes for dispensing lindane for insect control. This method is also employed for treating greenhouses with azobenzene and other insecticides for controlling insects and mites.

One of the most widely used methods of dispensing insecticides is the aerosol form. The *aerosol bomb* developed just prior to and during World War II and employed by the military services has gained general favor by civilians. Millions of the aerosol "bombs" are now sold annually for dispensing insecticides in homes and industrial establishments for controlling flies, mosquitoes, and other household pests. Pyrethrum, allethrin, organic thiocyanates, and methoxychlor in various formulations are used most frequently as the insecticides. The insecticides are dissolved in a liquefied gas, such as Freon 12, plus a suitable solvent under pressure in the container. Producers are now allowed to substitute a nonchlorofluorocarbon propellant. When applied, the Freon volatilizes instantly, leaving the insecticide and nonvolatile solvent suspended in the air as minute droplets that contact the insects present. Aerosols are also employed for applying insecticides in greenhouses. Methyl chloride may be substituted for the Freon for such uses. Vinyl chloride may not be used in pesticide aerosols as it was cancelled for this use in 1975. Since late 1979, chlorofluorocarbons have not been allowed for most aerosol propellant uses.

The liquefied gas propellant is also used to apply "wet aerosols" or so-called "self-propelled" sprays. The water droplets here are larger than those usually obtained with aerosol propellants. The amount of nonvolatile solvent is increased so that the droplets are larger and will readily wet the surface treated. Such wet aerosol sprays are used for applying insect repellants to the skin or clothing or for applying insecticides as residual sprays for controlling various household insects.

The development of systemic insecticides for controlling plant and animal pests has led to other special methods of use. For control of cattle grubs in cattle, boluses containing the insecticide are administered orally. In using plant systemics the treatment of soils prior to planting with a slurry of the insecticides or insecticide granules is one of the methods of use.

Insecticidal strips of polymer impregnated with DDVP (Vapona) emit vapors for long periods of time. In areas of little human or animal activity these can be effective.

Equipment for Applying Insecticides—Often failure to obtain satisfactory results with insecticide preparations is due to improper equipment for their application. A knowledge of the type of equipment to employ is therefore important to the supplier of insecticides. Equipment might vary from small hand sprayers or even paint brushes for use in homes to large power sprayers for treating livestock, field crops, fruit or large shade trees. Use of airplanes and helicopters for insecticide dispersal is steadily increasing. The manufacturers of equipment, also county agents, entomologists, and agricultural engineers with state and federal governments, as well as suppliers of insecticides, are in a position to give advice on insect control equipment to the potential user.

Control of Household Pests and Insects Attacking Man

The pharmacist is often asked to provide materials or to advise on the control of insects, ticks, and mites affecting man or those that are pests in homes or industrial establishments. Suggestions for the control of such arthropods are presented below.

General Considerations

The most important measure to follow in minimizing insect problems in the home or on the person is to practice *sanitation* and *good housekeeping*. Many of the pests in homes and industrial establishments, including mice, rats, cockroaches, ants, and silverfish, depend on exposed foods or scraps of food for their existence. Cleanliness will therefore go a long way toward reducing the insect problem within homes, restaurants, and other buildings. Pantry pests, such as grain moths, and weevils of various kinds develop in flour, corn meal, dog biscuits, and many other food products. An open container of oatmeal or dog biscuits hidden away in a pantry for several months can produce hundreds of moths or other pests that may continue to emerge over a period of weeks or months. Obviously, the simplest and best solution for such a problem is to destroy the source of the infestation rather than to use insecticides repeatedly.

A homeowner might be alarmed, and rightly so, when an infestation of fleas is detected in his home. In most modern dwellings the odds are great that the source of the fleas is the cat or dog which has not had proper care. The householder can minimize the danger of flying pests such as mosquitoes and flies getting into the premises by maintaining screen doors and windows in proper condition and by closing any openings into the home. Poorly cared-for garbage containers can be responsible for serious fly problems by attracting adult flies and by providing places for fly breeding. A few tin cans or tire casings that catch rainwater can provide the moisture essential for mosquito breeding on the premises.

Among the four general control measures for the prevention of insect and mite damage without chemicals are: physical control measures, mechanical methods, cultural control procedures, and biological methods. Physical control measures simply involve direct action by hand, such as removal of insect nests or egg masses. Mechanical control methods involve use of equipment specifically designed to control insects, as applying sticky bands around tree trunks to trap tent caterpillars, frequent hosing of foliage to prevent red spider mites and mealybugs from taking hold. Cultural control methods are based on knowledge of the life history and habit pattern of insects and controlling these in various ways, like cultivating the soil when many insects are in the pupal stage, or breeding insect-resistant plants, or interplanting. Interplanting marigolds, which discourage nematode growth, with tomatoes is an example. Use of the praying mantis, which devours insects, is an example of biological control.

It is recognized, however, that in spite of proper precautions, every home owner is likely to be faced with insect problems that must be solved by applying insect control chemicals. In some cases, however, the solution is not simple. It may require knowledge of the habits of the pest, a thorough survey of the problem, and know-how to control the pest involved. Often it is not practical for the owner to attempt to do the job himself. In such circumstances the services of a licensed pest control operator (listed in the yellow pages of telephone directories) should be sought. The National Pest Control Association is in a position to advise on qualified pest control firms in almost every city. County agents, entomologists in State Experiment Stations, and with the Federal Government are prepared to give advice and furnish publications which will be helpful in many cases.

For insect control in living quarters, in food-handling establishments, and on the person, the factor of safety in handling and applying toxic chemicals must be considered fully. Fortunately a number of efficient insecticides have low levels of hazard to man and animals, although no insecticide can be considered completely harmless. The petroleum oil solvent most commonly used as the carrier in household sprays is in itself sufficiently hazardous to cause toxic effects if the operator is careless in use and permits overexposure to it.

Foods and food utensils should not be left uncovered while insecticides are being used. All food preparation surfaces, utensils and food serving areas should be cleaned thoroughly before the next use to avoid contamination by pesticide residues. Care is needed in handling and applying pesticides to avoid excessive inhalation or skin contact. All poisons should be stored so that they are inaccessible to children and unauthorized people or where they cannot be mistaken for food. It must also be kept in mind that many preparations containing petroleum oil are flammable or the vapors are explosive.

While stressing necessary precautions, it must be kept in mind that the proper use of insecticides should not be discouraged. Many pests in and around homes are capable of transmitting diseases, and experience has shown that the disease hazard may be far greater than that of the chemicals needed to control the insects responsible for propagating an epidemic.

Ants—Several species of ants are pests in the home or around the premises. In the past, poison baits of various kinds containing *arsenicals*, *thallium*, or other poisons were used to destroy them. The use of thallium sulfate is no longer permitted as ant poison or for any other use around the home due to its excessive toxicity. Such methods are still effective under certain conditions but the use of newer sprays or dusts provides more effective and more rapid results.

Efforts should be made to locate the colony and destroy it if possible, although inside buildings the colony often cannot be found or may be inaccessible for treatment. The use of dusts and suitable sprays applied to the point of runoff on runways and other surfaces where ants have been seen, and along baseboards, borders of floors, window frames, doorsills, and similar places will usually give satisfactory control, although follow-up treatments may be necessary. In general, the procedure for poisoning ants is similar to that for controlling roaches.

For ant control on lawns or in gardens, the best procedure is to locate the ant colony and apply Baygon, Dursban, Ficam or one of the other pyrethrin derivatives. Baygon, a carbamate insecticide, and Dursban, an organic phosphate insecticide, have become popular for this use. These are currently formulated at higher concentrations for use by professional applicators only. The material may be applied with a sprinkling can, sprayer, or any other convenient method being sure to follow product labels, particularly those allowed for lawn use only. A concentration of 0.25% of these insecticides is suggested for treating individual mounds. The amount to apply varies with the size of the colony. A quart may be sufficient for small colonies and up to 3 gal may be necessary for large fire ant colonies a foot high and 2 to 3 feet in diameter at the base. The surface of the mound or soil should be disturbed by raking and the material poured on and around the nest.

Children and pets should not be permitted to play on the lawns until the area has been watered or rained on and allowed to dry. It is advised that the insecticide be washed off vegetation, into the ground, by sprinkling; this will not reduce the efficacy of the treatment.

Chlordane solution use has been suspended except for subsurface termite control and specific cases of fire ant and beetle control.

Chlorpyrifos (*Dursban*), and synergized pyrethrum sprays, may be employed for ant control in homes, but use of lindane in vaporizers has been cancelled.

Bedbugs—The bedbug is effectively controlled by spraying thoroughly the bed frame, springs, edges, and ticking of mattresses with 1 to 3% malathion by a professional applicator. Cracks and crevices, and surfaces behind objects near a wall should also be treated. Bedbugs stay well hidden in such places. Spraying the bed and other hiding places to the point of running off of the solution will provide long-lasting control. The treated mattress should be well aired before use.

Chiggers—Chiggers or red bugs cause severe annoyance to many people. These mites are most common in southern and midwestern areas. Some individuals are particularly susceptible to chigger bites, especially if they have not previously been exposed to them.

The insect repellants dimethyl phthalate, dimethyl carbate, diethyltoluamide, 2-ethyl-1,3-hexanediol, Indalone, and benzyl benzoate, when applied to clothing, are excellent in preventing attack by chiggers. The repellants may be applied by hand to socks, inside cuffs of trousers and sleeves, and the edges of any other openings in the clothing. Additional application of the repellant to the skin on the legs and forearms and base of neck will increase the probability of complete protection. Chiggers seldom attack the exposed portion of the body and are killed or repelled while crawling over treated clothing or exposed skin.

Clothing may be made repellant by light spraying, by drawing the mouth of the bottle along the parts of cloth to be treated (cuffs, fly, etc), or by complete impregnation of the cloth.

Although the repellants are highly effective in providing protection against chigger attack, persons often become exposed in areas where they do not expect chiggers to be present. After chiggers attack, there is no known treatment of the bites that will destroy the toxic substance which causes the irritation, although certain local anesthetics such as benzocaine will provide relief for several hours. A thorough soapy bath as soon as chigger irritation is noted, which may be within a few hours after exposure, will reveal those attached and thus allow for removal and subsequent reduction of irritation.

Cockroaches—The German, American, and brown-banded are the most common cockroach species found in homes and industrial establishments. Although the efficacy of different insecticides varies with the species, those in common use can be employed effectively in most instances. The German roach accounts for 98% of the problem in the US.

Most aerosol formulas contain pyrethrum, allethrin, or resmethrin. Although intended primarily for flying insects, the aerosols can be used fairly effectively for roach control if applied in considerable amounts directly into the hiding places or released in high concentration in closed rooms. A thorough spray or dust treatment is considered more effective and longer-lasting. Many purchasers of aerosols expect roach control in the home by a light treatment. Such treatment, although satisfactory for flies, mosquitoes, and similar pests, is inadequate for good roach control.

Boric acid and borax in finely powdered form, applied to hiding places and runways, are used for roach control, although they are less effective and slower to produce results than most other insecticides. The materials are also used in tablet form mixed with food baits which the roaches must eat. When well distributed in office buildings or rooms where there is little food for roaches, they often provide satisfactory control.

Baygon (o-isopropoxyphenyl methylcarbamate) and *Dursban* (*chlorpyrifos*) sprays and dusts are widely used insecticides for roach control. The sprays, either oil-base or prepared from an emulsifiable concentrate, should contain about 2% and dusts about 5% of the insecticide as described on the label. During the day, roaches usually remain well hidden in cracks, crevices, and behind objects. It is important to know where the roaches hide and where they run. The coarse, wet insecticide sprays are applied into these runways and hiding places. A few puffs of a mist spray will not provide satisfactory control. A paint brush may be used to apply the solution instead of a sprayer, if label directions allow it. A dust should be blown directly into hiding places and placed along runways. In those situations where Baygon is ineffective professional use of Dursban [O,O-diethyl-O-(3,5,6-tri-chloro-2-pyridyl)phosphorothionate] may be recommended. *Ficam* (2,2-dimethyl-1,3-benzodioxol-4-yl) or *bendiocarb* (generic name) is also useful and is popular as a highly effective broad-spectrum carbamate insecticide for control of at least six species of cockroach.

Pyrethrum sprays or dusts usually will provide satisfactory roach control. It is necessary, however, to treat with pyrethrum often to obtain and maintain control. The use of synergists with this insecticide has made it more effective.

When chlorinated hydrocarbon resistance is encountered in roaches, malathion as a 1 to 2% spray has proved to be an effective substitute. Diazinon [O,O-diethyl-O-(2-isopropyl-4-methyl-6-pyrimidinyl)phosphorothioate] has also proved useful where roach resistance has been a problem. The residual life of malathion is generally less than that obtained with methoxychlor prior to the appearance of insecticide-resistant strains.

Fleas—Fleas often are pests in homes and even in lawns in some areas. Infestations are usually associated with the presence of cats, dogs, rats, or other animals. To prevent recurrence of fleas, the source of the trouble should be treated. For dogs, powders containing 1% lindane, pyrethrum, or rotenone are used per label directions. For cats, only rotenone or pyrethrum insecticides are recommended, because these animals are very susceptible to toxic effects of chlorinated hydrocarbons. If the source of the fleas is rats, the host animals should be eliminated by following suitable rodent control measures. Actual flea control in homes is usually not difficult. Bedding where dogs sleep should be removed and the area thoroughly cleaned. Ordinary household sprays containing pyrethrum may also be used although several repeat treat-

ments may be required. Certain volatile organophosphate insecticides are the active ingredients of "flea collars" for dogs and cats. A new insect growth regulator, methoprene, is giving effective indoor flea control. This agent interferes with the life cycle of insects undergoing complete metamorphosis.

Finally, attention must be given to the pesticide label precautions. Some dogs and many cats are allergic to collars. Malathion as well as Sevin (carbaryl) are excellent materials for the control of fleas in the home or in infested yards.

Flies—For most homes or industrial establishments flies can be eliminated by using ordinary household sprays or aerosols. The most common ones consist of deodorized kerosene, about 0.1% pyrethrins or allethrin, and 0.75% of a synergist such as piperonyl butoxide or sulfoxide. Many variations in percentages of such insecticides are included in different formulations. Aerosol formulas often contain from 0.25 to 0.6% pyrethrins or allethrin, 0.8 to 1% of a synergist, and from 1 to 2% methoxychlor. The method of using the sprays or aerosols is generally known and usually well described on the labels.

If flies are a serious problem on the premises other methods of control must be followed. During recent years the use of poison baits has become more widespread. Dry sugar containing 1% Bayer L 13/59, malathion, or Diazinon sprinkled around the premises where flies congregate has given good control. The use of these materials in sweetened liquid bait (syrup in sugar) sprinkled in such places has also been used with good success.

Malathion and Diazinon sprays used as residual treatments outdoors around homes, in livestock buildings (including inside dairy barns), and similar places have recently come into use. When used according to label directions, these materials often provide good fly control up to several weeks after application.

Itch Mite—Many preparations have been employed for controlling the itch mite, or *scabies*. One of the most successful was the NBIN emulsion employed for head-louse control. It is important that all portions of the body be treated, and that a bath be delayed for about 12 hours after treatment. A second treatment may be needed after one week although one thorough treatment will usually eliminate the infestation.

Lice—Three kinds of lice attack man: the *body louse*, *head louse*, and *crab* (*pubic*) *louse*. In the US head louse and pubic louse infestations are more common than those of the body louse.

Body louse infestations can be controlled by regular changes of clothing and sterilization of all wearing apparel and bedding. When the use of insecticides is indicated, a thorough dusting of the clothing with 1% lindane dust is recommended, according to label directions. The Department of Defense and the World Health Organization are considering the adoption of a 1% malathion dust if final toxicological clearance is obtained. This substitute treatment if approved will provide a highly efficient material for louse control. Synergized pyrethrum dusts are also highly effective for body louse control. A formula known as MYL developed during World War II consisted of 0.2% pyrethrins, 2% n-butyl undecylenamide, 2% benzocaine (ovicide), 0.25% of an antioxidant in a pyrophyllite carrier. Recent investigations have shown that the synergists piperonyl butoxide or sulfoxide are equally as effective as the n-butyl undecylenamide. It has also been found that allethrin is about as effective as pyrethrins in such formulations.

Head louse infestations are readily controlled with benzyl benzoate followed by a thorough shampoo the next morning. Weekly treatments may be needed. Since eggs are not easily destroyed treatments should be repeated. One treatment applied to the hair on the head before bedtime will kill all motile stages of the lice, which may be brushed or washed out of the hair in the morning.

Crab louse infestations are effectively controlled with any of the preparations discussed under *head louse*. It is important that all hairy portions of the body be treated.

Mosquitoes—Mosquitoes which occasionally enter homes can be killed easily with the type of space sprays and aerosols discussed in connection with fly control. Mosquitoes often breed in areas several miles from the places where they are serious nuisances. Community mosquito control programs are the only real solution to this problem. The problem of achieving satisfactory mosquito control in a community is usually so complex and extensive that the help and advice of specialists are necessary.

Persons exposed to mosquitoes, biting gnats, and flies outdoors in connection with work or recreation can obtain relief by applying skin repellants. The most common individual repellants available on the market are diethyltoluamide, dimethyl phthalate, ethohexadiol (Rutgers 612), dimethyl carbate, and Indalone. Various combinations of these are also available. All of these materials used as directed on container labels will provide transient relief from insect attack.

In some circumstances treatment of the exposed skin alone is inadequate because the mosquitoes may also bite through clothing. The application of repellants to clothing by impregnation, by light spraying, or by hand will prevent attack. The same repellant materials intended for skin application may be used. Most of the repellants are plasticizers. They should not be applied to rayons and similar synthetic clothing.

Moths and Carpet Beetles—Every home owner is likely to encounter damage due to clothes moths or carpet beetles, often called "buffalo" moths. The damage caused by these insects to woolens and other items such as furs, materials made of animal hair, feathers, etc is very great.

For many years the fumigants naphthalene and paradichlorobenzene were the chief means of control. It takes a high concentration of vapor to kill clothes moths or carpet beetles, however. Many pounds of these fumigants are needed to eliminate infestations in closets that are not tight or where the doors are opened too often to permit sufficient concentration of vapor. In using these fumigants add crystals, flakes, or balls at the rate of 1 lb/100 feet^3 and make closets tight by sealing cracks and edges of doors. Since the gas is considerably heavier than air, the fumigant should be placed high in the closet. For protecting clothing, furs, etc in trunks and other storage spaces for long periods, about 1 lb for an average size trunk is sufficient.

In stuffed furniture it is often difficult to get the insecticide to the infestation. Fumigation in vaults by companies prepared to do such work may be necessary. The use of methoxychlor, and lindane sprays as contact insecticides and as residual sprays is a great aid in controlling moth infestations in homes. All of these materials will kill the different stages on contact. Methoxychlor is not highly effective as a residual deposit, however, for killing carpet beetles which crawl over treated surfaces. Lindane is superior for this purpose.

As a surface spray or dust to eliminate general infestations in a home, Ficam (bendiocarb), Dursban, diazinon or resmethrin are effective; the spray or dust being applied to the edges of rugs, floor area between rug and wall, and baseboards. In closets, the floors, corners, walls, etc should be treated; also behind pictures, radiators, and other hard-to-clean places. The entire rug may be sprayed with methoxychlor. Lindane is not recommended for general treatments in homes because of possible excessive vapors or skin contact that might be hazardous. Limited spot treatment is advocated for these materials. Other materials, such as fluoride solutions, are also satisfactory for treatment of rugs and similar items. Directions on the label should be followed at all times.

Moth infestations are destroyed and woolen items effectively protected against subsequent infestations by treating with paradichlorobenzene, naphthalene, or DDVP (dichlorvos).

Silverfish—For control of silverfish, use carefully applied residual insecticide sprays and dusts such as bendiocarb, chlorpyrifor, diazinon, propoxur, silica gel, and other similar products. Silverfish may be found in many places in the home—basement, attic, around books, and behind wall paper. They feed on the starchy material used as glues or for sizing paper.

Ticks—Ticks are serious pests in some areas. If the infested areas must be used, it is possible to kill the ticks by following the procedures suggested for area chigger control. Protection of individuals from tick attack, however, is fairly effective if clothing is thoroughly impregnated with certain repellants. Emulsions of dimethyl phthalate, and diethyltoluamide, may be used for such treatment.

Insecticides, Fumigants and Repellants

The number of insecticides and repellants currently in use has increased greatly during the past quarter-century. New synthetic compounds have come into use for many pests for which practical chemical control methods were unknown, and in some cases have largely replaced certain inorganic compounds and insecticides of plant origin. However, some of the more recently developed chemicals are being replaced by even newer materials because of development of resistance by various insects to insecticides. This is a problem of major significance in insect control. The housefly, for example, became resistant to DDT and to other chlorinated hydrocarbon insecticides within 5 to 10 years after they came into extensive use. Organic phosphorus insecticides were developed as substitutes but within a few years evidence of resistance to them became apparent. A wide variety of insects affecting man, livestock, fruits, vegetables, and cotton are resistant to one or more of the newer insecticides. Currently the resistant strains are still generally restricted to certain localities. However, authorities in insect control are generally agreed that such local resistance problems are likely to become more widespread with continued use of the materials.

The more widely employed insect control chemicals and their areas of use will be discussed briefly. The extensive literature on the many insecticides may be consulted for further details and the US Department of Agriculture, State Experiment Stations, the US Public Health Service, and manufacturers of specific insecticides are all prepared to provide more detailed information. The EPA should be consulted for the latest information about a particular pesticide since its status may change at any time. A chart for emergency treatment of acute pesticide poisoning is available from the US Navy Disease Vector Ecology and Control Center, Jacksonville, FL 32212.

Common Insecticides

Allethrin (*dl*-2-allyl-4-hydroxy-3-methyl-2-cyclopenten-1-one esterified with a mixture of *cis* and *trans dl*-chrysanthemum monocarboxylic acids)—This synthetic pyrethrin-like compound has been developed as the result of basic studies on the complex composition of the active principles in pyrethrum insecticides. It has many of the desirable features of pyrethrum—high insecticidal activity with low toxicity to warm-blooded animals. In general allethrin is effective against the same insects as pyrethrum. For some species such as the *housefly* and the *body louse* it is equally as effective, but against others it is less effective than pyrethrum. At present it can be produced commercially at a cost somewhat lower than the cost of the pyrethrins (principal active ingredients in pyrethrum). This advantage in practical use is offset, however, due to the fact that the insecticidal activity of allethrin is not increased to the same degree as the pyrethrins when combined with synergists available at present.

The development of allethrin is of great significance however. It is now used in household sprays and aerosols as a substitute for pyrethrins or to supplement the pyrethrins. The Department of Defense uses the insecticide in sprays and aerosols supplied to troops. Research has shown that allethrin is highly efficient for the control of lice affecting man. The availability of allethrin assures a supply of a pyrethrum-like insecticide in the event our source of supply of pyrethrum is cut off or greatly reduced as during World War II.

Arsenicals—The arsenicals, including *Paris green* (an acetoarsenite of copper), *lead arsenate*, *calcium arsenate*, *calcium arsenite*, and *sodium arsenite*, are among the older insecticides. Arsenicals are still employed to a limited extent as dusts and sprays for controlling a variety of *chewing insects*, for use as dips for *ticks* and other livestock pests, in poison baits for *fly* control or for controlling *cutworms*, and as larvicides for *Anopheles mosquitoes*. Due to the development and availability of many new insecticides equally as effective and often less hazardous to plants and animals the arsenicals have been largely replaced by other insecticides. Some use is seen in herbicides, wood preservatives and plant dessicants though not widespread. In the suspended and cancelled list of the EPA (May 1978) and Oct 1979, arsenic trioxide in excess of 1.5% and sodium arsenite in excess of 2.0% are listed as unacceptable for home use. The following statements must appear prominently on labels: "Do not use or store in or around the home" and "Do not allow domestic animals to graze treated area."

Fluorine Compounds—*Sodium fluoride*, one of several fluorine compounds, has served a useful purpose for controlling *roaches* and *silverfish* in homes and industrial establishments, but it is not much used today. In the suspended and cancelled list of the EPA (May 1978), sodium fluoride is cancelled for home use if the product contains more than 40% of this compound. Sodium fluoroacetate has been cancelled for use in mammalian predator control; the label should have instructions for predator use blocked out. The Oct 1979 suspended and cancelled list of EPA lists only fluoroacetamide which is allowed for use only inside of sewers against the Norway and roof rat by a certified applicator.

Lime-Sulfur—Originally used as a *sheep dip* for the control of *mites* and *ticks*, lime-sulfur in liquid and dry form is now better known as a dormant spray for the control of *scale insects* and as a summer spray for the control of certain *plant diseases*. For the methods of using the lime-sulfur liquid concentrate, follow recommendations on the container. Generally used to control Apple scab and powdery skin irritation mildews.

Nicotine—This, the volatile liquid alkaloid of tobacco (*Nicotiana tabacum*), is a powerful insecticide; however, it is highly toxic to the nervous system of man and other animals. Nicotine extracts are usually obtained from the stems and refuse parts of tobacco. It is available in two forms, namely, free nicotine and nicotine sulfate. The latter is available mainly as an aqueous solution, containing 40% of nicotine. For the common garden sprays to control *aphids* (*plant lice*) and similar insects, the nicotine sulfate is the form commonly used although dusts containing nicotine sulfate are also available. It kills a wide range of both chewing and sucking insects. Soap or saponin (obtainable from Merck & Co) should always be used with nicotine sulfate unless combined with an alkaline solution such as Bordeaux mixture or lime-sulfur. This is needed to release the nicotine, which is the active killing agent.

Nicotine is effective as a destructive agent for *plant lice* and also serves as an efficient stomach poison for some pests. It is water-soluble, but should be kept in tightly stoppered containers as it decomposes very quickly. Nicotine, as used, does not injure the most delicate foliage. It is generally considered to be most effective as a contact insecticide when used during the warm part of the day.

Free nicotine is used for fumigating greenhouses because the nicotine is immediately volatilized.

Nicotine has lost much of its popularity in recent years, due to the introduction of new, synthetic chemicals having improved effectiveness and equal or greater safety. It is no longer produced in the US.

Oil Sprays—Oils made from petroleum are among the insecticides that have been used for many years, chiefly as contact insecticides for *scale insects* and *mites* attacking plants. They are very important today. Oils will destroy other insects however, including *aphids*, *thrips*, *leafhoppers*, and *eggs of* certain *Lepidopterous species*.

There are two classes of oils used as insecticides: the *dormant oils* and *summer oils*. The dormant oils are applied to more hardy trees during the dormant period. The summer oils are used on fruit and vegetable crops during the growing season. The chief differences between the two types are the degree of refinement and their heaviness or viscosity, which determine in part the degree of phytotoxicity. The oils are applied as emulsions which permit dilution with water and more uniform distribution on the plants. The concentration of oil in the finished spray for citrus usually ranges from 1.66 to 2.0%. Small amounts of insecticides such as parathion added to the oil sprays increases their efficacy against various insects.

Pyrethrum—Pyrethrum flowers, the first widely used insecticide, possess unusually fast contact action against many insects causing paralysis in a few minutes. Their low mammalian toxicity and rapid toxic action against many pests are features that are not present in the newer materials.

The active substances, pyrethrins I and II, occur in the oleoresin secretion of certain floral parts (achenes) of the closed or partially open flowers. A maximum of about 1.4% of pyrethrins has been adopted by the foremost manufacturers of pyrethrum insecticides.

Formerly, pyrethrum insecticides were prepared as dusts by using the finely ground flowers or were prepared and used as liquids by extracting the active ingredients from the flowers with special fractions of light petroleum oil, preferably odorless kerosene. Today manufacturers extract and concentrate the active ingredients in products containing about 20% pyrethrins. This concentrate is used to prepare the various preparations employed by the public including dusts, petroleum oil solutions, emulsion concentrates, wettable powders, and aerosol formulations.

Pyrethrum is still used as an ingredient in most household sprays and aerosols chiefly for its *knockdown* effects against insects. It is also used in dusts and liquid preparations for controlling a variety of garden pests and *fleas*, *lice*, and *ticks* on pets.

The continued prominent place of pyrethrum as an insecticide has been maintained chiefly because of the development of chemicals which when combined with pyrethrum have the remarkable property of increasing the insecticidal activity of the insecticide even though the material added alone has little or no insecticidal properties. This cooperative potentiation is known as *synergism*.

These compounds include sesamin, piperonyl butoxide, sulfoxide, and others and are called "synergists." The development of these synergists has increased the range of activity of pyrethrins and at the same time permits reduction in the cost of formulas containing it.

"Synergized" pyrethrum combinations, although not so long-lasting as the chlorinated hydrocarbon insecticides, are used chiefly in household sprays and aerosols for *flies*, *mosquitoes*, and other *household pests*, in liquid and dust preparations for controlling *external parasites* on pets, as sprays for flies on dairy cattle, and as dusts and sprays for controlling certain *vegetable pests*. Synergized pyrethrum powders and liquids were employed extensively for a time in controlling *lice* attacking man during World War II. Some newer preparations include Pyrefume, Pyrellin, Pyrenone, Pyrexcel, and Pyrocide. Most of these contain pyrethrins in varying concentrations and other materials such as piperonyl butoxide, rotenone, or ryania. Many pyrethroid synthetics have been found effective and are now registered for use. These include newer allethrin derivatives, resmethrin products, and *S*-bioallethrin. A 2% aerosol formulation of resmethrin has been approved by the World Health Organization as a replacement for a pyrethrum-DDT formulation in aircraft disinfection.

Rotenone—This is a useful botanical insecticide and represents the chief chemical constituent of derris (*D elliptica* and *D chinensis*) and cubé roots (species of *Lonchocarpus*) and other sources. Rotenone ($C_{23}H_{22}O_6$) is commercially available as such or in the form of derris and cubé roots, sold with assayed rotenone content, usually 5%.

Rotenone is incorrectly classified as a nontoxic insecticide. It can cause skin irritation. Its use for louse control on humans is not recommended since irritation is often produced, especially in the groin region. On internal administration in moderately large doses, especially in the presence of fatty foods, it is very toxic to higher animals. In general, however, rotenone insecticides are considered low in hazard. The relatively small amounts applied and rapid loss of toxic action results in minor residues on food crops.

Its paralyzing action on insects is slower than that of pyrethrum but more certain, with usually no recoveries. As a dry, crystalline powder, rotenone is odorless and relatively stable. It is soluble in alcohol, oils, chloroform, and carbon tetrachloride (used in the extraction from the crude drug and its quantitative determination). It is slightly soluble in water, but aqueous sprays, particularly in the presence of alkaline soaps, quickly deteriorate and must be prepared fresh before use.

Rotenone dusts at concentrations ranging from 0.75 to 1.0% are still used to control pests such as the *Mexican bean beetle*, *cabbage worms*, *leaf hoppers*, and other insects attacking a variety of vegetables. It is especially useful for application to vegetables near the time for harvest when certain of the effective newer insecticides cannot be used because of potentially excessive residues.

Rotenone is also used for controlling insect parasites of animals. It is effective for controlling *cattle grubs*, and is employed also for *lice*, *fleas*, and *ticks* on pets and livestock.

Sulfur is widely used in insecticide preparations. It was formerly used for controlling such insects as *plant mites*, *fleahoppers* on cotton, *lice* on livestock, and *chiggers*. The new insecticides available today are far more efficient than sulfur for most insects. However, it is still one of the more effective insecticides for certain species of plant mites. Sulfur is also used in combination with many other insecticide dusts as a diluent. It serves a useful purpose in such combinations in controlling or preventing a buildup of mites and for the control of *plant diseases*. Sulfur is employed as a spray made from wettable sulfur or is used in wettable powder preparations containing other insecticides.

Thiocyanates—Several organic thiocyanates, on the market under trade names, have proved rather successful as substitutes for pyrethrum and other contact insecticides, when used in sprays. The common thiocyanates are lauryl thiocyanate (Lor), β-butoxy-β'-thiocyanodiethyl ether (Lethane 384), β-thiocyanoethyl esters of fatty acids (Lethane 60), and fenchyl and bornyl thiocyanoacetates.

Other materials—A number of other insecticides that have been used as pesticides, but for limited purposes, include: *Pentachlorophenol*

(C_6Cl_5OH), widely used as a wood preservative to control termites, other wood infesting insects, and wood rots; it is currently under investigation for dioxin contamination and the health ramifications of this contaminant. *Ryania*, a plant product containing alkaloids, is used to some extent for controlling corn borers and codling moths on apples; and *sabadilla*, another plant product, which is effective for controlling squash bugs, lygus bugs, and harlequin bugs.

Chlorinated Hydrocarbon Insecticides

The advances in insect control since about 1940 have been phenomenal because of the development and extensive use of a variety of chemical compounds broadly classified as synthetic chlorinated hydrocarbons. The use of this class of insecticides began with DDT, which was first employed in Switzerland, but within a decade a number of new similar insecticides of comparable, or in some instances greater, insecticidal activity came into use. These materials, although effective against similar pests in many instances, vary in their usefulness for controlling insects. Insect species vary in their susceptibility to the different compounds. In addition, a factor of great significance that limits the practical use of many insecticides is the hazard associated with their use. Some of the insecticides possess long residual action—which may be of great advantage in controlling certain pests—but which is an objectionable feature when applied to food plants consumed by man and animals. Some of the materials are stored in fat or are excreted in milk of animals when the residues are consumed on forage treated for insect control or when the insecticides are applied to the animals for controlling pests. Such residues of some insecticides may persist for months while others are eliminated within a few days or weeks.

Because of the residue problem, DDT use was cancelled, and aldrin and dieldrin have been cancelled for all uses except subsurface ground insertion for termite control, dipping of nonfood roots and tops, and mothproofing by manufacturing processes in a closed system.

Obviously it is not possible in this chapter to discuss in detail the many uses for the various chlorinated hydrocarbon insecticides. The formulation to use, amount to apply, method and time of application, precautions that must be observed in avoiding harmful residues on the harvested crop, and many other aspects must be considered. Only a brief discussion of the more important compounds in this class and their areas of use follows:

Aldrin [The *endo-exo* isomer of 1,2,3,4,10,10-hexachloro-1,4,4a,5,8,8a-hexahydro-1,4:5,8-dimethanonaphthalene]—This compound is chemically and physically somewhat similar to dieldrin. It is almost equally toxic to the same kinds of insects and the acute toxicity to animals of the same general order, but it is much less persistent. Therefore, it does not possess the long residual action. Aldrin changes into dieldrin after application to soil or plants. This permits its use for controlling certain *pests on agricultural crops* when timed so that the residues disappear before harvest, but this feature limits its use where a persistent poison is needed. As of August, 1974 the EPA suspended manufacture of all pesticides containing aldrin or its metabolite dieldrin as an "imminent hazard to the public." However, the EPA will continue the use of these compounds against termites, as a dip for roots and tops of nonfood plants, and against clothes moths under certain circumstances. This status still holds as of the May 1978 list of suspended and cancelled pesticides published by EPA and the subsequent revision on October 1979.

Benzene Hexachloride [BHC, Lindane, 666, Gammexane, Gexane]—The insecticidal properties of this compound were discovered in France and England. The product as manufactured consists of a mixture of isomers. The gamma isomer is most active against insects, but the product sold to formulators may contain from 12 to 99% of the gamma isomer. The almost pure gamma isomer, called *lindane*, is recognized as a different insecticide from BHC, although all grades of BHC depend on the gamma isomer for insecticidal activity. Lindane, because of its purity, is most desirable where the musty odor of the cruder products is objectionable. It is also regarded safer from the standpoint of chronic toxicity because some of the other isomers present in the cruder grades are regarded more toxic chronically and are more persistent as residues on foods. It is the official (USP) form.

Gamma BHC is active against a wider variety of *insects*, *ticks*, and *mites* and is generally effective at lower dosages than is DDT. In practical insect control, however, it may or may not be more useful. The chief advantage of DDT over BHC in this regard is its longer residual action. BHC has wide uses for controlling *pests on cotton* and other crops where the odor is not a factor. Many food products retain the musty odor when exposed to BHC; therefore, its use on food and field crops is restricted. Several states have banned the use of BHC products and its use may eventually be discontinued.

Lindane is used in household sprays and dusts on livestock and other animals and for controlling some *pests on fruits and vegetables*. When *lice* resistant to 10% DDT powder appeared in Korea the Department of Defense substituted a 1% lindane dust for controlling this insect attacking man.

The acute oral toxicity of lindane to animals is somewhat higher than DDT, but when absorbed through the skin it is more toxic than DDT. Lindane possesses high insecticidal activity in vapor form. This property has resulted in certain restricted use for the compound in devices that generate vapors with the aid of heat.

Chlordane [Velsicol 1068, CD-68, Octachlor, Octa-Klor; 1,2,4,5,6,7,8,8-octachloro-2,3,3a,4,7,7a-hexahydro-4,7-methanoindene]—This insecticide, developed in the US, is a viscous amber-colored liquid, nearly odorless. It is readily soluble in a wide variety of solvents.

As of Oct 1979, the EPA lists chlordane as suspended for all uses except subsurface ground insertion for termite control, dipping of roots or tops of nonfood plants, in Federal/State quarantine programs for the Japanese beetle and imported fire ant, control of blackvine weevil on Japanese yew in Michigan, control of Texas Harvester ant in Oklahoma, control of white-fringed beetle attacking food crops in eight southwestern states of the US, control of soil insects attacking Florida citrus root weevils, control of strawberry root pests by preplant treatments, and control of white grubs in Michigan. Other specific uses are still allowed but it is being phased out completely.

DDT [dichlorodiphenyltrichloroethane; 1,1,1-trichloro-2,2-bis(*p*-chlorophenyl)ethane]—This crystalline substance is practically odorless, with low vapor pressure and high toxic action to a wide range of insects. One of its chief uses was in the field of medical entomology, particularly for controlling *mosquito larvae* and *adults, flies, body lice, bedbugs*, and *fleas*. It was also used extensively for controlling pests of livestock, farm crops, forest and shade trees and stored products. Due to its persistence and ubiquitous nature, and its accumulation and storage in various members of the food chain, with possible deleterious results, its use in the US was cancelled in 1972. Emergency use is permitted only with EPA approval (see introduction). The Oct 1979 Suspended and Cancelled Pesticides list, published by EPA, classifies DDT as cancelled except for use by the US Public Health Service and other health service officials for control of vector diseases, for the US Department of Agriculture or the military for health quarantine, in drugs for controlling body lice (to be dispensed by a physician), and in the formulation of prescription drugs for controlling body lice.

Dieldrin [the *endo-exo* isomer of 1,2,3,4,10,10-hexachloro-6,7-epoxy-1,4,4a,5,6,7,8,8a-octahydro-1,4:5,8-endomethanonaphthalene]—A white, granular substance. One of the most potent chlorinated hydrocarbons; used until recently. It can control a wider range of pests than DDT. The main disadvantage of dieldrin is its rather high toxicity, both orally and dermally, as well as its high chronic toxicity in animals. It is similar to DDT in its accumulation in fatty tissues of animals and its excretion in milk. These disadvantages seriously limited its use and resulted in its minimal use today.

Dieldrin is employed in some parts of the world as a residual spray for Anopheles mosquito control where malaria is a serious problem. The May 1978 and Oct 1979 Suspended and Cancelled Pesticides list published by EPA currently classifies dieldrin as cancelled for all uses except for subsurface ground insertion for termite control, dipping of nonfood roots and tops, and mothproofing by manufacturing processes in a closed system. No longer made in the US.

Endrin [1,2,3,4,10,10-hexachloro-6,7-epoxy-1,4,4a,5,6,7,8,8a-octahydro-1,4:5,8-*endo-endo*-dimethanonaphthalene]—Endrin is a chlorinated hydrocarbon insecticide that is highly effective against many pests, but it has high toxicity for man and animals. It is used for controlling most *cotton insects*. The EPA has cancelled its use on tobacco and practically everything else except for specific cases (Oct 1979). It is on a special restricted use list in New Jersey.

Ethyl 4,4-Dichlorobenzilate [Chlorobenzilate]—This is an effective ascaricide-miticide, marketed as Ascaraben for the use on citrus only.

Heptachlor [1,4,5,6,7,8,8-heptachloro-3a,4,7,7a-tetrahydro-4,7-methanoindene]—A crystalline compound chemically related to chlordane, highly active against a wide range of insects. Heptochlor has been suspended by EPA for all uses except subsurface ground insertion for termite control, dipping of roots or tops of nonfood plants, control of narcissus bulb fly, for certain seed treatments, and ant control to achieve pineapple mealybug control in Hawaii.

Methoxychlor [1,1,1-trichloro-2,2-*bis*(*p*-methoxyphenyl)ethane]—This insecticide has chemical and physical properties similar to those of DDT. The chief advantage of methoxychlor over other chlorinated hydrocarbon insecticides is its low hazard to animals. It is satisfactory for controlling *flies* and other *household pests*, including *clothes moths*, and *flies* and *lice* on livestock, *Mexican bean beetles*, and a variety of other insects attacking fruit, vegetable, and forage crops. Methoxychlor is available in 25 to 50% concentration in various application forms.

Methoxychlor is one of the few chlorinated hydrocarbon insecticides that is not readily stored in animal fat or excreted in milk when consumed as residues on forage crops. For this reason it is used for controlling various insects on livestock feeds and forage. It was also used as a spray for controlling flies and lice on dairy cows but is no longer used thus because small amounts of the insecticide occur in milk.

Toxaphene—This substance is a reproducible mixture of 175 or more polychloro derivatives of camphene produced by chlorination of the latter to a content of 67–69% chlorine, representing the empirical formula $C_{10}H_{10}Cl_8$. It is a yellow, waxy solid, practically insoluble in water. This product has had most of its uses suspended by the EPA except for scabies control on cattle and sheep.

Miticides

A variety of synthetic organic insecticides are used for controlling mites on plants, in addition to older insecticides such as sulfur and the organic phosphates discussed in the next section. Among the compounds used are *Ovex* (*p*-chlorophenyl *p*-chlorobenzenesulfonate), *Dimite* (4,4′-dichloro-*alpha*-methylbenzhydrol), and *Kelthane* (1,1-bis(*p*-chlorophenyl)-2,2,2-trichloroethanol), used extensively on fruits and vegetables. These miticides may be used as dusts or sprays, and they are often combined with other insecticide applications or in insecticide-fungicide formulations.

Organic Phosphorus Compounds

A large variety of organic compounds of phosphorus possess high insecticidal activity. They are often referred to as organophosphorus compounds. Some of these compounds also have unusually high potency as miticides, and many are also extremely toxic to man and other warm-blooded animals because of their action as irreversible inhibitors of cholinesterase.

A number of human fatalities in the US and other parts of the world have occurred as a result of exposure to phosphate insecticides and many other persons have suffered ill effects. It is important, therefore, that the more toxic of these insecticides be handled with extreme caution and strictly in accordance with recommendations outlined by the manufacturer and federal and state agencies.

The reputation of the organic phosphorus insecticides is such that to the uninformed most compounds in this class are regarded as being dangerous to use. This is a misconception. The mammalian toxicity of some of the compounds is of a low order and they can be handled with no more danger than that associated with the use of a number of the synthetic chlorinated hydrocarbon insecticides which are employed without serious toxic reactions.

The organophosphorus compounds will control a wide range of pests and disease carriers. Certain of these compounds possess systemic action, a characteristic that offers great promise for controlling important insect pests of crops as well as livestock.

The organic phosphorus insecticides are used extensively, in many instances replacing in part, at least, some of the chlorinated hydrocarbons and older insecticides such as rotenone. This trend is due to several factors. Resistance to the chlorinated hydrocarbons by a number of pests has necessitated substitute materials possessing a different mode of insecticidal action. Several of the organic phosphorus compounds do not accumulate in meat and milk as readily as do certain chlorinated hydrocarbon insecticides when consumed as residues on forage crops.

The phosphorus insecticides have not been in use as long as the older materials and relatively few insects have become resistant to them. There is no assurance, however, that many pests will not in time become resistant to the phosphorus materials. A number of species of mites on plants became resistant within a few years, and, as already mentioned, the house fly has also developed resistance to certain organic phosphorus compounds. There is some evidence, however, that in some insect species, resistance to the phosphorus in-

secticides does not develop to the high level of the chlorinated hydrocarbons.

Organic phosphorus insecticides generally destroy a wide range of insect species. Consequently, their use often kills many parasites, predators, and pollinating insects as well as the destructive pests.

The more widely used organic phosphorus insecticides are briefly described, and some of their more important uses are given.

Ciodrin [3-hydroxycrotonic acid α-methylbenzyl ester dimethyl phosphate; Crotoxyphos]—An insecticide for control of animal parasites and for premises use.

Co-Ral [Bayer 21/199; *O*-3-chloro-4-methylumbeliferone *O,O*-diethylphosphorothioate; coumaphos]—An effective organophosphorus insecticide for systemic control of cattle grubs (*Hyoderma* spp). It is a slightly brownish crystalline material with a weak pleasant odor. Co-Ral is best known at present for its systemic action for cattle grub control when applied as a dermal spray, but it is also an excellent contact insecticide. It is employed for fly control in barns and for application to livestock for the control of the screw-worm, lice, horn flies, and ticks. Co-Ral is moderate in toxicity, being much less toxic than parathion but more toxic than malathion. When applied to livestock as a spray, it is employed in concentrations ranging from 0.25 to 0.5%.

Demeton—This is a mixture of *O,O*-diethyl *S* (and *O*)-[2-(ethylthio)-ethyl] phosphorothioates. A commercial product called Systox contains demeton. Demeton possesses systemic action. It is an amber-colored liquid with a somewhat unpleasant odor. Demeton is absorbed by plants when applied to foliage, to trunks of the plant, or to the seed. It is also taken up by the roots when mixed with soil. When absorbed by the plant, it becomes available to sucking insects such as plant lice, scale insects, leafhoppers, thrips, and the mites. It has also been shown experimentally to kill certain leaf-feeding lepidopterous larvae, larvae of fruit flies, and even boll weevils on cotton. It is employed in insect control on potatoes, apples, cotton, walnuts, and certain ornamental plants primarily as a foliage spray or dust. It possesses contact action, but its main action is systemic.

Demeton is regarded as one of the most desirable insecticides for controlling aphids on alfalfa because, through systemic action, the aphids are controlled without serious kill of the parasites and predators. This is an example of successful integration of an insecticide with biological control agents to obtain satisfactory control of insects. Demeton is in the same category as parathion and TEPP so far as mammalian toxicity is concerned. It must, therefore, be used with equal caution. The methyl analogue of demeton, called methyldemeton, has also come into use as a systemic. It has insecticidal action similar to demeton. For certain aphids it seems to provide longer lasting control.

Diazinon [*O,O*-diethyl *O*-(2-isopropyl-4-methyl-6-pyrimidinyl)-phosphorothioate; Spectracide]—This compound, an amber-colored liquid with a somewhat objectionable odor in its technical form, is an excellent insecticide. It is less toxic than parathion but more so than malathion to warm-blooded animals. Diazinon is highly toxic to flies as a contact and residual spray as well as a stomach poison and is in use for controlling these insects both as sprays and in poison baits. It is also effective against aphids, mites, leafhoppers, the codling moth, fruitflies, cabbage worms, mosquitoes, roaches, and other insects. Some resistant strains of houseflies have been reported.

Dibrom (1,2-dibromo-2,2-dichloroethyl dimethylphosphate; Naled)—A broad-spectrum insecticide for both plant protection and premises use.

Dipterex [*O,O*-dimethyl 2,2,2-trichloro-1-hydroxyethylphosphonate; *trichlorofon*]—White, crystalline solid; soluble in water. The material also known as Bayer L 13/59 is used in poison baits for controlling flies. The toxicity of Dipterex to warm-blooded animals is reported to be of a low order.

EPN [*O*-ethyl *O-p*-nitrophenyl phenylphosphonothioate; Velsicol]—EPN, an amber liquid, is effective against a wide range of pests, including aphids, mites, scale insects, the European corn borer, mosquito larvae, boll weevil, pink bollworm, codling moth, plum curculio, and others. It is slightly less toxic to warm-blooded animals than parathion but merits the same degree of extreme caution in its use.

Guthion [*O,O*-dimethyl *S*-(4-oxo-3*H*-1,2,3-benzotriazine-3-methyl) phosphorodithionate; *azinphosmethyl*]—This compound, also known as Bayer 17147, is a crystalline material relatively insoluble in water. It has a wide spectrum of activity as a contact insecticide for the control of insect pests. It is generally more persistent on plants than other commonly used organophosphorus insecticides. The material is employed as a dust or spray. Although the toxicity of Guthion is somewhat lower than that of parathion, it is in the class of highly toxic materials and must be handled with extreme caution. Guthion is finding wide use for controlling cotton insects, particularly the boll weevil, which has become resistant to chlorinated hydrocarbon insecticides. Guthion is also highly effective for the control of fruit pests such as the plum curculio, codling moth, stink bugs, aphids, and mites. This has proven useful in integrated fruit pest control.

Malathion—This phosphorus compound, *S*-(1,2-dicarbethoxyethyl)

O,O-dimethyldithiophosphate, as produced commercially, is a light amber liquid, having a sulfur-like odor. It is relatively low in toxicity to most warm-blooded animals and is active against a wide range of insects, although in general it is less effective than parathion or TEPP. The much lower toxicity to warm-blooded animals and rapid loss of residues on plants make it an acceptable insecticide for many uses.

Malathion is used extensively for controlling insects on vegetables, fruits, and cereal and forage crops as well as for controlling insects affecting man and animals. The residues disappear in a few days to two weeks, thus permitting application near the harvest period. The compound is available commercially as emulsifiable concentrates, wettable powders, dusts, and for ultra-low-volume spraying.

Parathion [*O,O*-diethyl *O-p*-nitrophenyl phosphorothioate]—This compound is a brownish liquid. It is highly active against most insects. Its use is restricted, however, by its high toxicity to man and animals. Parathion insecticides are available commercially as dusts and as emulsifiable and wettable powder concentrates for mixing sprays.

Parathion is especially useful for controlling aphids, spider mites, and scale insects but is also effective against many other insect pests, including leaf-feeding insects, certain soil pests, corn borers, and mosquitoes. The insecticidal action is primarily by contact, but it also has powerful stomach action. Its vapor pressure and toxicity in vapor form are sufficiently high to result in marked fumigating action against some insects although the compound is not classed as a fumigant. Parathion is not excreted in milk or stored in tissues of animals when consumed as residues on feed crops. It is, therefore, of considerable interest for use on feed crops for insect control.

The hazards of parathion are so great that it is often advocated that the compound be used only by or under the supervision of persons who fully understand the precautions that should be followed in handling and applying the insecticide. There is danger in handling and mixing the insecticide. It is readily absorbed through the skin. When sprays are used without protective equipment, toxic reactions may result; also there is danger in prolonged exposure to the usual dusts or sprays. The May 1978 and Oct 1979 Suspended and Cancelled Pesticides list of EPA adds restrictions on the use of parathion, and requires that registration be limited to preparations packed in one-gallon containers or larger and that manufacturers and formulators of registered parathion products be in compliance with the standardized safety label enclosed with PR 71-2.

Methyl Parathion—This is a compound closely related to parathion and has insecticidal and toxic properties somewhat similar to it. Methyl parathion is employed for controlling mites, aphids, thrips, and other insects, including such pests as the boll weevil. A new special encapsulated formulation has been well received.

Phorate [*O,O*-diethyl *S*-(ethylthio)methyl phosphorodithioate; Thimet]—Thimet is a liquid material with an objectionable odor. It is relatively insoluble in water. It is one of the more toxic of the organophosphorus insecticides and must be handled with extreme caution. Thimet is primarily systemic in action and is readily absorbed by the roots of plants when applied to the seeds or when added to the soil. Thimet has had limited use for controlling aphids, spider mites, thrips, leafhoppers, and certain other insects on cotton and sugar beets.

Phosdrin [1-methoxycarbonyl-1-propen-2-yl dimethyl phosphate; Mevinphos]—Contact and systemic insecticide-acaricide with broad range of use on vegetable, fruit, field, forage crops. Phosdrin is a liquid material, miscible with water and quite volatile. The toxicity of Phosdrin is high, and it must be employed with extreme caution such as that required for parathion.

The insecticide destroys insects both as a contact and stomach poison. The residue disappears rapidly from treated plants which makes it particularly desirable for controlling pests on crops near the harvest time. The insecticide is useful for controlling such pests as aphids, mites, flea beetles, cutworms, and army worms.

Phosphamidon [2-chloro-2-diethylcarbamoyl-1-methylvinyl dimethyl phosphate]—An organic phosphate, a water-miscible oil, used as a systemic insecticide in small grains, cotton, and other field crops.

Carbamate Insecticides

Carbamate insecticides, like the organic phosphorus insecticides, inhibit insect cholinesterases. Their mode of action is sufficiently different, however, for them to be considered a separate class of insecticides. The carbamates of interest as insecticides include:

Carbaryl [1-naphthyl *N*-methylcarbamate; Sevin]
Dimetan [5,5-dimethyl-3-oxo-1-cyclohexen-1-yl dimethylcarbamate]
Isolan [1-isopropyl-3-methyl-5-pyrazolyl dimethylcarbamate]
Pyrolan [3-methyl-1-phenyl-5-pyrazolyl dimethylcarbamate]

Carbaryl, occurring as crystals slightly soluble in water, is highly effective against a wide range of insects, including the codling moth, Mexican bean beetle, cabbage worms, gypsy moth, boll weevil, and pink bollworm. It is not highly effective against most insects of medical importance or against mites affecting plants. Although the carbamate insecticides are considered to be of moderate to low toxicity to higher animals, carbaryl is highly toxic to the honey bee. Has the greatest range of controlled pests of any insecticide; vegetables, fruits, field crops, ornamentals, and pets.

Newer Methods of Insect Control

Extensive research continues on new methods of insect control that reduce or avoid the dangers of toxic insecticide residues. Three experimental procedures that illustrate how such control may be achieved are described below.

1. The use of irradiation to destroy the breeding capacity of the insect. Certain insects breed only once, and when the female of such a species is mated with a sterile mate, that female will not produce fertile eggs. Advantage has been taken of this biological fact in controlling the screw worm—a serious pest of cattle in the Southern US. In this operation males are irradiated with controlled doses of radioactive cobalt and are then released in tremendous numbers in the areas to be protected. Preliminary results have been so promising that this procedure is being considered for use against other species of insects with the same biological characteristics.

2. Distribution of the spores of organisms which are pathogenic for certain insect species only. A strain of spores, *Bacillus thuringiensis*, *Berliner*, has been shown to have value in controlling a small number of insect species and is now commercially available as *Teknar*, *Bactimos*, and others. Another is *Bacillus popilliae* available in *Doom* and *Japidemic*.

3. The use of certain of the silica aerogels which act on soft-bodied insects by desiccation. Since the silica aerogels are exceedingly low in toxicity to humans, residues may be insignificant.

Pheromones are potentially important for monitoring insect populations. They are chemical substances produced and released by one sex of an insect (usually the female) that elicit a sexual response in an individual of the opposite sex. The specificity of pheromones makes them valuable for detecting and estimating insect populations before an infestation can enlarge or spread. There are at least 90 different pheromones currently available eg boll weevil (*granlure*), codling moth (*codlelure*), house fly (*muscalure*), Mediterranean fruit fly (*trimedlure*), etc.

Insect population suppression can also be achieved by using large numbers of attractant-bated traps (mass-trapping), by disruption of normal communication between sexes ("confusion technique"), and by using a mixture of pheromone and a chemical sterilant.

Fumigants

Fumigants have and still are being used extensively for controlling a wide range of insects. Homes, industrial establishments, ships, and other structures may be fumigated to control household or structural pests. Large amounts of fumigants are employed to control pests in grains and woolens, in soil, and in living plants or plant products such as nursery stock, fruits, and vegetables.

The most common fumigants and their uses are briefly discussed below.

Aluminum Phosphide—A pelletized source of phosphine plus fire retardant. Presently used widely in grain fumigation. Available as *Phostoxin*.

Carbon Disulfide [CS_2]—This is one of the older fumigants. It is a colorless to slightly yellow liquid with a disagreeable odor. The vapor is heavy (about 2.6 times that of air). The chief disadvantage of carbon disulfide is its extreme explosiveness. It is also toxic to animals and lengthy exposure must be avoided.

To reduce its flammability, carbon disulfide is used in combination with carbon tetrachloride, usually in the ratio of 1 part carbon disulfide to 4 parts carbon tetrachloride. Carbon disulfide is most often used for *treatment of grains in storage bins*. It has limited use in emulsion form for controlling *soil-infesting insects*.

Carbon Tetrachloride [CCl_4]—This is a liquid with a heavy vapor (5 times that of air). This fumigant alone does not have extensive use because it does not possess a high degree of fumigating action to most insects. It is, however, used in combination with other fumigants, because the vapor is nonflammable; its use with such fumigants as carbon disulfide and ethylene dichloride reduces the fire hazard. It is employed also in combination with methyl bromide or ethylene dibromide to aid in the distribution of the vapor. Combinations of carbon tetrachloride and other fumigants are employed most extensively in *grain fumigation. Caution: Carbon tetrachloride can be toxic on inhalation.* It is no longer allowed for home use.

Chloropicrin, Trichloronitromethane [CCl$_3$NO$_2$]—This is a colorless liquid which causes intense irritation of the eyes and throat and induces vomiting. Chloropicrin is used chiefly as a *soil fumigant.* It may be injected in the soil in combination with xylene, carbon tetrachloride, or ethylene dichloride to help distribute the gas. It is also used in combination with certain other fumigants for *treating stored products* by sprinkling or spraying the infested materials. Since the gas is only slowly volatilized thorough airing after use is required.

D-D Mixture—This is a mixture of 1,3-dichloropropene and 1,2-dichloropropene. It is a dark colored liquid having a sharp disagreeable odor. The material is flammable and is highly toxic to humans. The chief use of D-D Mixture is for *soil fumigation* to control *nematodes,* etc. It is toxic to most plants and is therefore applied to the soil several weeks before planting the crop.

Ethylene Dibromide [CH$_2$BrCH$_2$Br]—This is a colorless liquid, having a sharp chloroform-like odor. Its vapor is 6.5 times as heavy as air. There is no explosive hazard associated with its use, but it is highly toxic to humans. Prolonged breathing of the vapor even at low temperatures should be avoided and if the liquid is spilled on clothing the clothing should be removed immediately.

Ethylene dibromide is highly effective for controlling many pests. It is useful *for treating soils.* For such use it may be emulsified with water and applied to the soil surface, or mixed into soil in a xylene or light petroleum oil solution. Certain fruits and vegetables are treated with the fumigant to destroy insect infestations, although there is often only a narrow margin of safety between the dosage that does not adversely affect the commodity and that required to destroy the insects. The fumigant is also effective against most *grain insects.* It is usually applied by spraying, in combination with other fumigants, on top of the grain in tight bins.

As of 1983, the EPA banned certain uses of EDB and is moving to end others because of evidence that it can cause cancer, mutations, and reproductive disorders in laboratory animals at low tolerances.

Ethylene Dichloride [CH$_2$ClCH$_2$Cl]—This is a colorless liquid. The vapor is 3.5 times as heavy as air. Although not flammable under most conditions of use it is a fire hazard and is often used in combination with carbon tetrachloride. Like most fumigants it is toxic to humans. Ethylene dichloride is used against a wide variety of pests especially *grain insects.* Emulsions of the chemical are also employed to destroy *soil insects.*

Ethylene Oxide [CH$_2$CH$_2$O]—This is a gas at ordinary temperatures and is relatively light (1.5 times as heavy as air). Because the vapor readily forms an explosive mixture in air, it is usually combined with carbon dioxide to reduce the explosive hazard. An ethylene oxide-carbon dioxide mixture (ratio of 1 to 9) is available in metal cylinders. This gas is especially useful for fumigating insects in packaged cereals, bagged rice, tobacco, and clothing and furs in vaults. It leaves no odor or harmful residues in the products. It may injure foods like nuts, and dried fruits or fresh fruits. It is also used in vaults for fumigating valuable *packaged documents.*

Hydrocyanic Acid [HCN]—This is a colorless gas lighter than air, with an odor of almond. It is perhaps the best known of the fumigants. HCN is deadly to most living things. Therefore, its use as a fumigant is extremely hazardous. Nevertheless it is widely used and when employed with necessary precautions it is one of the most useful fumigants available. The gas is released from cylinders under pressure or by the addition of sodium or potassium cyanide to sulfuric acid and water. Calcium cyanide as dusts or granules is also used and generates the gas slowly in moist air.

For many years HCN was used under tents to control *scale* and other *citrus pests.* Its use for this purpose has been discontinued because the California red scale developed resistance to the gas. HCN is used in warehouses and other industrial establishments, shops, homes, etc to destroy *pests.* Certain foodstuffs and a wide range of non-foods may be treated in warehouses or special vaults for insect control.

Methyl Bromide [CH$_3$Br]—This is a colorless and usually odorless gas at ordinary temperatures approximately three times as heavy as air. The gas is nonflammable and is sometimes used as a fire extinguisher. The gas is highly toxic to humans; and the absence of odor and slow toxic action are characteristics which increase its hazard. Methyl bromide is among the most widely used fumigants. It destroys a wide range of *pests.* It is not highly toxic to most plants and leaves no objectionable odor in food. Since the chemical is a gas at ordinary temperatures it is applied from containers into which it has been compressed as a liquid. It readily vaporizes at temperatures ordinarily encountered in fumigating. Methyl bromide is usually formulated with a small amount of chloropicrin to recognize the presence of this colorless and odorless gas.

Some important uses of methyl bromide are for *fumigating warehouses, ships, railroad cars, residences, grains, living plants* shipped under quarantine regulations, *tobacco,* and many other products. The fumigant is also used to destroy *soil pests.* During World War II it was used successfully to *fumigate clothing of refugees and prisoners of war* to control *body lice.*

Naphthalene [C$_{10}$H$_8$]—This is a white crystalline material with vapor about 4.4 times as heavy as air, and a characteristic odor not unpleasant to most people. Naphthalene is perhaps the most commonly used fumigant for protecting clothing and furs from *moth* attack. It is used in flake form or as "moth balls."

Orthodichlorobenzene [C$_6$H$_4$Cl$_2$]—This is a colorless liquid with a strong characteristic odor. The vapor is about 5 times as heavy as air. Although it will burn, the chemical does not have a great explosive hazard. The chemical is toxic to animals and spillage on the skin or prolonged breathing of the vapors should be avoided. The fumigant is too toxic to plants to be used in soil where plants are to be grown. The chief use of orthodichlorobenzene is *to treat logs or timber* to destroy insect infestations. The chemical is also an effective *larvicide for flies.* It can be used successfully in emulsion form to destroy fly larvae in latrines or on carcasses of animals.

Paradichlorobenzene [C$_6$H$_4$Cl$_2$]—This is a white crystalline compound with a characteristic odor which at low temperature is not unpleasant. The vapor is about 5 times as heavy as air. It is not explosive under most conditions.

Paradichlorobenzene crystals are used extensively in homes to destroy *moths.* Woolen clothing treated with the crystals and stored away in reasonably tight boxes will be well protected from moth attack.

Paradichlorobenzene is also used to control such insects as the *peach tree borer.* It is placed in a shallow trench about 2 to 4″ from the base of the trunk and covered with soil.

Sulfur Dioxide [SO$_2$]—This is one of the oldest fumigants. The gas is formed by burning sulfur or it may be furnished in commercial cylinders. It has been replaced by other more desirable fumigants. The chief objections to its use are the tarnishing effects of the gas in moist air and its powerful bleaching action.

Sulfuryl Fluoride [SO$_2$F$_2$]—Vikane (*Dow*). An odorless, colorless gas used for the control of pests in dwellings, buildings, construction materials, furnishings, and vehicles.

Insect Repellants

Repellants are substances used to protect humans, animals, and plants from insects by making the hosts objectionable or unattractive by disguising the characteristic odor of the hosts.

During World War II troops on many fronts in tropical and semitropical regions employed repellants effectively in the preventive campaign to keep away mosquitoes and other annoying and disease-carrying insect pests. The problem here was to use compounds that not only had effective staying and nonirritating properties when applied to the skin of man and animals, but also were without pronounced and penetrating odors that would give the enemy information about patroling or combat activities and locations of hideouts, etc. During and since World War II more than 10,000 chemicals were tested for utility as insect repellants.

A repellant that was found quite effective by the Armed Services was official in USP XV under the title *Compound Dimethyl Phthalate Solution,* also known as *622 Mixture,* which consists of 60% (w/w) of *dimethyl phthalate,* 20% (w/w) of *ethohexadiol,* and 20% (w/w) of *butopyronoxyl.* It is relatively nonirritating to the skin but somewhat irritating to mucous membranes; care must be taken to avoid contact with the eyes. The three ingredients of this solution are sometimes used separately, in various application forms. Perhaps the best all-purpose repellant, developed since World War II, is *diethyltoluamide,* which in various tests has been shown to be the most effective agent against a wide variety of insects.

Repellants, single- or multi-ingredient, are generally compounded in solution, emulsion, cream, or semisolid stick application forms. Most will provide relief from attack from mosquitoes, biting flies, and gnats for periods of 30 minutes to 2 hours or longer.

The volatile oils of citronella, cedarwood, eucalyptus, pennyroyal, bergamot, cassia, clove, wintergreen, and lavender are to some degree repellent to mosquitoes and other annoying insects but are not nearly as effective as the aforementioned chemicals.

Individuals who are allergic or sensitive to repellants may show various skin reactions, such as burning, itching, and swelling. Most repellants cause smarting when applied to broken skin or mucous membranes, hence care should be exercised when applying them around the eyes or other sensitive areas.

A brief chemical and physical description of the principal repellants follows.

Butopyronoxyl [n-butyl-3,4-dihydro-2,2-dimethyl-4-oxo-1,2H-pyran-6-carboxylate; Indalone; $C_{12}H_{18}O_4$]—A yellow to pale reddish brown liquid of aromatic odor; reasonably stable in air but slowly affected by light; insoluble in water; miscible with alcohol.

n-Butyl phthalate [1,2-benzenedicarboxylic acid dibutyl ester; $C_{16}H_{22}O_4$]—An oily liquid used as an insect repellant for impregnation of clothing.

n-Butylacetanilide [BAA] $C_{12}H_{17}NO$—A clothing impregnant repellant for ticks and chiggers.

Di-n-butyl succinate $C_{12}H_{22}O_4$; *Tabatrex*—A liquid insect repellent against ants, cockroaches and flies used in buildings only.

Diethyltoluamide [N,N-diethyl-m-toluamide; N,N-diethyl-3-methylbenzamide; (*Delphene*); $C_{12}H_{27}NO$]—A colorless liquid with a faint, pleasant odor; practically insoluble in water, miscible with alcohol.

Dimethyl Phthalate [dimethyl 1,2-benzenedicarboxylate; phthalic acid dimethyl ester; $C_{10}H_{10}O_4$]—A colorless or practically colorless, oily liquid having a slight aromatic odor; insoluble in water, miscible with alcohol.

Ethohexadiol [2-ethyl-1,3-hexanediol; Rutgers 612; $C_8H_{18}O_2$]—A colorless, oily liquid, odorless or with a slight odor; 1 mL dissolves in about 50 mL water, miscible with alcohol.

2-Undecanone—MGK—A dog and cat repellant.

Control of Rodents

The following compounds are commonly employed to control rodents. They are dangerous and must be handled with caution.

Bromadiolone—Yellowish powder, rather insoluble and used in baits or tracking powder for rodent control.

Brodifacoum—Offwhite powder. An anticoagulant rodenticide. Available in pellets and bait blocks.

Chlorophacinone (*Rozol*)—White crystalline material made in grain bait, water bait, paraffin blocks and tracking powder.

Diphenadione [Diphacinone; 2-diphenylacetyl-1,3-indandione]—This is the most toxic of the anticoagulants in use at present. While other chemicals in this class are usually used, in bait, at a concentration of 0.025%, diphacinone is effective in 0.005% concentration.

Endrin—This chlorinated hydrocarbon insecticide (see page 1253) is used also as a ground spray to control orchard mice. A dosage rate of 2 lb/acre is applied, and about ½ of the ground surface is treated. This practice has been questioned because it risks injury in livestock and wildlife, but it has gained wide acceptance in apple-growing areas of Eastern US. Its status is being reviewed; use in New York and New Jersey is restricted. The EPA has cancelled its use on tobacco.

Phosphorus—White or yellow phosphorus is available in the form of prepared baits for rat or mouse control. It is often packaged in a low-concentration paste for use in treating bread or other palatable rat food. Phosphorus is a dangerous poison toxic to all animals that ingest it. Great care must be used in placing baits containing phosphorus. Not much in general use today.

Pindone [Pival; 2-pivaloyl-1,3-indandione]—This anticoagulant rodenticide resembles warfarin in its action and methods of use. It is available in concentrates, solutions, and prepared baits, which must be used as directed.

Red Squill (*Dethdiet*, *Rodine*)—Because of its relative safety for humans, pets, and domestic animals, properly standardized red squill powders and extracts were generally recommended poisons for rats. Red squill contains, scilliroside, a cardiac glycoside and strong emetic which causes humans and most species of domestic animals to void the poison promptly. Its specific toxicity is due to the inability of rats to vomit. This allows the absorption of the toxicant. Other animals do vomit, allowing them to survive accidental poisoning. Red squill has never been more than a mediocre rodenticide and is little used in the US today.

Strychnine—Strychnine is another powerful alkaloidal poison but seldom used in rat baits because it is so readily detected by them. It was once used to control *field* and *house mice*, *prairie dogs*, *pocket gophers*, *ground squirrels* (sometimes called gophers in sections of the West where

they are common), and similar animals and certain species of birds. The EPA has cancelled and suspended the use of strychnine for mammalian predator control.

Valone (*PMP*; 2-isovaleryl-1,3-indandione)—This anticoagulant is used to formulate rat and mouse poisons.

Viruses—Rat viruses are not registered for use in the US at present. Governmental agencies responsible for protecting human and animal health have recommended against the general sale of bacterial cultures for pest mammal control.

Warfarin [*WARF-42*, *Compound 42*; 3-(α-acetonylbenzyl)-4-hydroxycoumarin]—This chemical relative of dicumarol acts by causing a loss of clotting power of the blood, and the animals die of exhaustion from multiple hemorrhages. The product was the first successful anticoagulant rodenticide and was unique in that it had to be eaten repeatedly to cause death. For rats, the feeding time is usually from 3 to 10 days, and for mice a much longer period of daily feeding is needed. Fantastically low percentages of the poison in food are effective, and food baits now on the market contain 0.025 to 0.05% of the poison, and concentrates for making solutions of the sodium salt of warfarin containing 0.005% of warfarin equivalent are available. At these levels rats and mice do not detect the material in the baits and will continue to come back to eat or drink until too weak to do so.

Warfarin itself is a highly toxic poison, but the fact that it is needed at such low concentrations in baits and that these must be eaten repeatedly to cause symptoms makes it less likely to injure pets and children than certain other poisons. It has had a good record of safety and is considered one of the less dangerous rat and mouse control materials.

Several other coumarin derivatives are available; eg, 3-(1-furyl-3-acetylethyl)-4-hydroxycoumarin, known by the nonproprietary name coumafuryl and marketed under several tradenames (eg, Fumarin, Fumasol, Krumkil, Lurat, and Rat-A-Way). This was developed and produced by Amchem Products, Inc.

Zinc Phosphide [Zn_3P_2]—This is a phosphorus preparation which has found a definite place in a specialized rodent control problem in the United States. It is blended with a diluent to permit its easier use as a dusting powder over cut apples in the preparation of a highly effective orchard mouse bait. Just enough of the perishable bait is made to supply an afternoon's work, and it is placed by uncovering mouse tunnels and making a bait spot of two or three apple sections placed directly in the runway. This is repeated at several points in the trails around each orchard tree, and when properly done is quite effective. The same zinc phosphide blend can be used on other types of food bait for domestic rat or mouse control. It is dangerous to animals other than rats or mice, and should be handled carefully.

Control of Fungi and Bacteria

Fungicides are chemical compounds used to prevent or retard the deleterious action of a varied group of plants called fungi, which for the most part are microscopic, devoid of green coloring matter, and reproduce by spores.

Fungi are present throughout the world. They attack other living and dead plants, animals, human beings, and such diversified inanimate objects as foodstuffs, cloth, paper, lumber, paint, plastic coverings, and leather, to mention only a few of the substances affected.

Some fungicide materials are also toxic to bacteria but in general the term is limited to those materials used for pro-

tection against fungi. For many years fungicides have been used extensively in agriculture for the protection of crops.

The prevalence of fungi fluctuates with environmental conditions. Early historical and religious writings contain references to the blasting, blighting, rusting, or mildewing of the crops. From the dawn of civilization down to the present day there has been a constant battle between the agriculturist on one hand and the fungi on the other, with the environmental conditions swinging the balance to one side and then to the other. Prior to 1853 losses resulting from the attacks of fungi were accepted as inevitable since the true cause was not understood but in that year Anton de Bary established the parasitism of the fungi associated with the rust and smut diseases. This discovery, establishing the science of plant pathology, has been followed by an increasing number of investigations into the cause of plant diseases and by the development of a wide variety of materials used for the control of these diseases.

Fundamental Requirements of a Fungicide—To protect plants against the attack of fungi the compounds used must be toxic to the parasite yet relatively noninjurious to the host plant. These materials may be applied in either liquid or powder form. The process of applying substances in liquid form is termed spraying; that of applying them in powder form, dusting.

Irrespective of the method of application a fungicide, to be entirely satisfactory, must be

1. Capable of destroying, controlling or preventing the growth of the fungus.
2. Relatively noninjurious to the host plant.
3. Easy to apply.
4. Easy to prepare.
5. Reasonable in cost.

Types of Fungicidal Action—Fungicide materials are of varied composition and their exact mode of action against specific organisms is beyond the scope of this discussion. In general, however, all materials fall into two general categories; ie, (1) *protective* and (2) *eradicative*.

In the *protective type* the material does not necessarily kill the fungus spores but does prevent their germination. The various forms of elemental *sulfur* used as spray or dust are protective in their action against the spores of the apple scab fungus (*Venturia inaequalis*) and are widely used by commercial orchardists to prevent numerous infections from developing on the apple leaves and fruit. However, the same materials used against certain rust fungi are definitely eradicative in their action upon the rust spores. This diverse effect on different fungi is but one example of the complexity of the problem.

In the *eradicative type* the material kills the fungus and in this way stops the disease either before or soon after initial infection has occurred. The complex *calcium polysulfides* or newer agents like the Captan, Thiram, or Benlate preparations, for example, have a definite eradicative effect on the apple scab fungus. Unfortunately, most of the eradicative materials are rather caustic in their action and they can be used only under certain conditions since they are apt to produce injury often more serious in consequence than the disease they are being used to combat. However, whenever it is possible to use an eradicative type of fungicide without incurring serious injury to the plant, this procedure should be adopted as it is productive of the most satisfactory control results.

Commonly Used Fungicides

It is realized that the pharmacist is not expected to have the detailed knowledge of a technically trained plant pathologist regarding the use of fungicide materials. However, he is frequently asked for advice and he should familiarize himself with directions on pesticide labels and recognize the importance of having his patrons understand and follow the directions; also, he should utilize the services of state or county extension pathologists when label information is insufficient to deal with specific problems that might arise.

The following list of commonly used materials should enable him to answer intelligently the majority of questions with which he is confronted. Requests for information concerning large-scale usage of fungicides should be referred to the State Agricultural Experiment Station, to the US Department of Agriculture, or to the EPA.

Ammoniacal Copper Carbonate—A copper fungicide of especial value when a material is needed that does not discolor the foliage. It is water-soluble and is readily washed off by rain. Readily prepared in small quantities by dissolving 1 level teaspoonful of copper carbonate in 2 tablespoonfuls of ammonia water and adding 1 gal of water, as the label directs. Also available in commercial forms for uses on vegetable and field crops.

Arasan—see *Tetramethylthiuram Disulfide.*

Benomyl [Methyl 1-(butylcarbamoyl)-2-benzimidazolecarbamate]—A carbamate type of fungicide of broad spectrum with both protective and curative qualities. Shows local systemic activity within leaf system and from soil applications where root system stays within treated zone. Registered for use on roses, other ornamentals, turf, stone fruits, melons, beans, cucumbers, grapes, pome fruits, and peanuts. LD50, rat oral dose is over 10,000 mg/kg.

Bioquin I—see *Copper 8-Quinolinolate.*

Bismuth Subsalicylate—Used at the rate of 1½ lb/100 gal plus a spreader sticker, this material has given effective control of downy mildew (blue mold) of tobacco.

Bluestone—see *Bordeaux Mixture.*

Blue Vitriol—see *Bordeaux Mixture.*

Bordeaux Mixture—A complex chemical compound resulting from the mixing of a dilute solution of copper sulfate with a dilute suspension of lime in water. Once widely popular, Bordeaux mixture is used very little if at all in the US.

Botran—This trade name and others (DCNA, Allisan) refer to *2,6-dichloro-4-nitroaniline*, which was developed in England. This substituted amine is formulated as a yellow, wettable powder used for spraying (75%) and for dipping (50%); it is also used as dust. It is generally used as a soil and foliar fungicide to control *Sclerotinia* mold, *Monilinia* rot, *Rhizopus* rot, *Sclerotium* and *Botrytus* mold, including storage or transit on vegetables, fruits, and ornamentals. It is almost nontoxic to rats but phytotoxic to strawberries, wilted leaf lettuce, asters, petunias and some other greenhouse plants, and to some germinating seeds and annual seedlings. It is persistent on leaf surfaces for 1 to 2 weeks and involves low hazard generally.

Caution—Avoid inhalation of dust and spray mist; occasional cases of contact dermatitis have been reported.

Calcium Hypochlorite—The activity of this compound as a general disinfectant is based on its ability to release chlorine. Various forms of this are used to sanitize swimming pools.

Captan [*N*-trichloromethylthio-4-cyclohexene-1,2-dicarboximide]—An organic fungicide used at the rate of 1 to 2 lb/100 gal of water for control of diseases of fruits, vegetables, and ornamental plants. Excellent for summer spraying of apple trees. Used extensively on fruits and vegetables and on field and ornamental crops. Do not use with lime or other strong alkali.

Copper 8-Quinolinolate—An organic copper compound (sold under the tradename Bioquin I) is used for the control of alternaria blight, botrytis blight, powdery mildew on carnations, chrysanthemums and roses. Also has some industrial fungicide use. Generally recommended to be used at the rate of 1 lb/100 gal of water. *Zinc and magnesium compounds* of similar composition have also been tested as well as *8-hydroxyquinoline sulfate, 8-quinolinol benzoate*, and *8-quinolinol.*

Copper Sulfate—In addition to being the principal ingredient of Bordeaux mixture, copper sulfate is the essential component of many commercial copper fungicides.

Corrosive Sublimate—*Bichloride of mercury*, or corrosive sublimate, has long been used as a general disinfectant and fungicide until recent cancellation. Corrosive sublimate is a very poisonous compound and it must be used with proper precautions. Its only registered use is on non-grazed turf grasses and other specific applications allowed by EPA.

Cycloheximide [(3-[2-(3,5-dimethyl-2-oxocyclohexyl)-2-hydroxy-ethyl]glutarimide; Acti-Dione-PM (-RZ,-BR, and -S); Actispray]—This antibiotic-type compound is noncorrosive and is formulated as an oil solution, a wettable powder, and water-soluble tablets. It is generally used for white pine blister rust, some turf fungi, and powdery mildew on ornamentals. Its toxicity varies according to formulation. It is highly toxic to rats with some phytotoxicity, particularly in producing some injury to fruit when used with flowable parathion. Injury has also been reported to sour cherry when the fruit was ¼ in. or less in diameter. In addition, early sprays may cause injury to tender foliage. It has some phytotoxicity to numerous rose cultivars. There are no particular hazards except with concentrated formulations. *Caution*—It will irritate the skin on prolonged contact.

Dichlone [2,3-dichloro-1,4-naphthoquinone (*Quintar*)]—This organic spray preparation, sold under the trade name *Phygon XL*, has been found to be an effective substitute for both sulfur and copper in the control of the various fungus diseases of fruit trees and on vegetables. It is generally used at a dosage of ¾ to 1 lb/100 gal of spray. It has also been employed dry as a seed treatment at rates varying from 1 to 4 oz/100 lb of seed. *Caution*—One serious drawback to its use is that the chemical may cause skin irritations.

Difolatan [(*Chevron; Captafol*); *cis-N*-[(1,1,2,2-tetrachloroethyl)-thio]-4-cyclohexene-1,2-dicarboximide]—This sulfenimide is a solid of low toxicity which is insoluble in water. It is formulated as an 80% wettable powder and a 7.5% dust. It is generally used as a fungicidal protectant-eradicant particularly for the control of early and late blight on potatoes. Also extensively used on fruits, melons, tomatoes, onions. It is slightly toxic to rats, fish, and birds. Foliage of some roses may be injured with this fungicide. It is persistent on plant surfaces for 7 to 10 days. No hazard occurs in its use. It is not compatible with strongly alkaline materials. It should not be used in combination with or closely following oil sprays.

Diphenyl (biphenyl)—Used as a preservative for citrus in storage and transit.

Disodium Ethylenebisdithiocarbamate Hexahydrate—See *Nabam*.

Dithane D 14—See *Nabam*.

Dithane M 22—See *Maneb*.

Dithane M 45—A zinc ion and manganese ethylene bisdithiocarbamate compound. Broad-spectrum fungicide used on vegetables, fruits, turf, and ornamentals for leafspot, early and late blight, crown rot, damping off, anthracnose, and others. One of the most commonly used vegetable fungicides.

Dithane Z 78—See *Zineb*.

Dodine [(*Am Cyanamid*); *N*-dodecylguanidine acetate; Cyprex, Melprex; Doquadine]—This agent is a fairly stable fungicide formulated as a 65% wettable powder and a protectant and eradicant fungicide, particularly for apple and pecan scab, cherry leaf spot, sycamore anthracnose, and other tree diseases. It may cause foliage or fruit injury, particularly if applied at freezing or near-freezing temperatures. *Caution*—It may produce eye and skin irritation. If exposed, flush eyes for at least 15 min.

Dyrene [2,4-dichloro-6-(*o*-chloroanilino)-*s*-triazone; anilazine; Kemate (*Chemagro*)]—It is used as a foliar fungicide for the control of turf diseases, some vegetable diseases, berries, and gladiolus. It may be phytotoxic to some fruit and ornamentals and potentially hazardous to animals. It can cause skin irritation.

Ferbam—This iron organic compound, *ferric dimethyldithiocarbamate*, is used extensively as a substitute for sulfur and copper compounds in the control of fungus diseases of fruit trees. It is employed as a specific for the control of the apple cedar rust. In the Pacific Northwest it is used instead of sulfur for the control of pear scab since it does not russet the fruit. Likewise, it is used for the control of the fungi causing apple scab, apple blotch, and bitter rot since it reduces the risk of spray injury and at the same time gives satisfactory control of these fungi.

It is also used for the control of tomato anthracnose, and is especially effective for the control of anthracnose leaf blight, downy mildew, and fruit rot of cucumbers and melons. It causes less leaf injury than copper compounds on tomatoes, cucumbers, and melons.

Caution—Ferbam is a flammable material and must not be mixed near an open flame. In mixing sprays the operator should avoid inhaling ferbam. It is not safe to apply ferbam just before or just after applications of Bordeaux mixture.

Fermate—See *Ferbam*.

Ferric Dimethyldithiocarbamate—See *Ferbam*.

Folpet [(*Stauffer*); (*N*-trichloromethylthio)phthalimide; Phaltan; Rose and Garden Fungicide (*Ortho; Stauffer*)]—It is generally used as a protectant-eradicant fungicide for fruit, vegetables, ornamentals, and turf. It is especially good for black spot of rose. It is slightly more phytotoxic than captan. It is not recommended for apples before the 4th cover spray, it may burn grape leaves in hot, dry seasons, and it may also severely injure sweet cherry leaves and snapdragons. It has a low health hazard. Concentrated solutions may cause skin irritation. Its use is limited to the western states.

Formaldehyde [Formalin (*Celanese*); D&P77 (*Allied*); Karsan (*Du Pont*)]—It is generally used in seed and plant bed treatments for damping off, in mushroom houses, vegetables, ornamentals, and a soil treatment for onion smut. It also possesses germicidal properties. Concentrated solutions can be phytotoxic to plants both on contact and when injected into soil. It is not persistent in that it breaks down quickly in soil and water. It can be very irritating on prolonged breathing and on contact with the skin.

Glyodin [2-heptadecylglyoxalidine acetate]—An organic spray compound used by commercial growers to control cherry leaf spot.

Karathane [(*Rohm & Haas*); 2-(1-methylheptyl)-4,6-dinitrophenol crotonate and other nitrophenols or derivatives; Iscothan]—A dark-brown liquid available as a 25% wettable powder, a 48% liquid concentrate, and a dust. Its formulation is water-soluble and therefore is washed off by rain. Used as a fungicide on apples, apricots, grapes, peaches, pears, melons, and a few ornamentals. It also has miticidal properties. It is less effective than sulfur but safer on sulfur-sensitive plants.

Karbam Black—See *Ferbam*.

Karbam White—See *Ziram*.

Krenite—(*Sodium Dinitro-ortho-cresylate*.)—A plant growth regulator which stops treated plants from refoliating during the next growing season.

Lime-Sulfur Solution—A widely used spray material consisting of approximately 30% *calcium polysulfides* prepared by heating sulfur and lime together with appropriate quantities of water.

Lime-sulfur solution has proved especially effective for the control of the apple scab fungus, and has been used widely for the control of many other plant diseases. The water dilution for use during the growing season

varies from 1 gal of the concentrate for 50 gal of spray to 1 gal for 100 gal. Used at a concentration of 12 gal for 100 gal of spray during the winter months lime-sulfur has long been used on peach trees for the combined control of San Jose scale and the leaf curl fungus.

Since the calcium polysulfides are likely to produce spray injury, lime-sulfur is being replaced by less injurious forms of sulfur and various organic materials in large-scale commercial spraying operations.

Maneb [manganese ethylenebisdithiocarbamate; Manzate, Dithane M-22, Chem-Neb, MEB, etc]—The manganese salt of dithiocarbamic acid is used at the rate of 1–2 pounds per 100 gal of water for the control of potato, tomato, celery, carrot, and onion diseases. It has also been used to control grape black rot; and is used on many fruits and vegetables. Currently an important fungicide.

Mercaptobenzothiazole—Used on apples as a plant fungicide by pesticide formulators in their products.

Mercurous Chloride and **Mercuric Chloride Mixture**—A mixture of 65% mercurous chloride, 32% mercuric chloride, and 3% of an activator substance had been used as a turf fungicide in the prevention of snow mold. The EPA, however, had cancelled all uses of mercury salts except as a fungicide in the treatment of textiles and fabrics intended for continuous outdoor use; as a fungicide to control brown mold on freshly sawed lumber; as a fungicide to control Dutch elm disease; as an in-can preservative in water-based paints and coatings; as a seed disinfectant for treating such farm seeds as wheat, oats, barley, flax, sorghum, and cotton; as a fungicide to treat "summer turf" diseases; as a fungicide to control "winter turf" diseases. Also, subject to the following: (a) The use of these products shall be prohibited within 25 feet of any body of water where fish are taken for human consumption; (b) these products can be applied only by or under the direct supervision of golf-course superintendents; (c) the products will be classified as restricted-use pesticides when they are reregistered and classified in accordance with section 4(c) of FEPCA.

Nabam—Disodium ethylenebis[dithiocarbamate] used for industrial applications only; not for food crops.

Pentachloronitrobenzene [PCNB; Terraclor; Brassicol]—A nitrobenzene compound used as a soil fungicide effective against many soil pathogens which attack vegetables, turf, and ornamentals. Also used as foliar spray on young lettuce, cabbage, and cauliflower as well as on fruit trees.

Phygon XL—See *Dichlone*.

Polyramcombi—This is a mixture of 5.2 parts by weight (83.9%) of ammoniates of [ethylenebis(dithiocarbamato)] zinc with 1 part by weight (16.1%) ethylenebis[dithiocarbamic acid], bimolecular and trimolecular cyclic anhydrosulfides and disulfides. These dithiocarbamates are solids and are insoluble in most common solvents. They decompose under strongly basic or acidic conditions. It is available as an 80% wettable powder and several dusts. Moisture can cause deterioration. It is generally used as blight control on potatoes and tomatoes. It can control apple scab, cedar apple rust, sooty blotch, and fly speck and is also used on ornamentals. Also useful on certain other vegetables and some field crops. It has no known phytotoxicity and is persistent on plant surfaces for 10 to 14 days. This agent is compatible with chlorinated hydrocarbons, coppers, sulfurs, and phosphates except parathion oil sprays. Karathane or Diazinon should be added just before use. It is safer than lead arsenate on apples. It has low hazard potential.

Sodium *o*-Phenylphenate [*o*-phenylphenol; Dowicide-1]—Used on a variety of fruits and vegetables to increase storage life.

Sulfur—The element sulfur has long been one of the standard fungicide materials and is still widely used to control a wide variety of plant diseases. Sulfur is sold as a dry powder ground to varying degrees of fineness, as a paste, or fused with clay (bentonite) and subsequently ground. Many special brands are available and each manufacturer claims special virtues for his particular product. They all depend for their effectiveness on the inherent toxic property of sulfur in affecting the growth processes of various fungi. The directions on the packages will be a guide to their use. Sulfur is one of the cheapest fungicide materials and will probably continue to be used extensively as spray or dust for many years to come.

Combined with lime and water and heated for a considerable period sulfur forms complex *polysulfides*. This reaction product called *lime-sulfur* has been described in a preceding paragraph. If sulfur is added to slaking stone lime and the only heat supplied is that of the stone lime combining with water, another type of spray called *self-boiled lime-sulfur* results. Properly prepared self-boiled lime-sulfur has a very low calcium polysulfide content and produces very little injury. Self-boiled lime-sulfur can be used with safety on peaches during the growing season whereas lime-sulfur used at that time would cause excessive injury to the trees.

Tersan—[1,4-dichloro-2,5-dimethoxybenzene; chloroneb; Demosan]—Used in systemic seed treatment, in-furrow soil treatment, and turf diseases.

Tetramethylthiuram Disulfide [Thiram; bis(dimethylthiocarbamoyl) disulfide]—A pink powder available in wettable and nonwettable forms under trade-names of *Arasan* and *Tersan*. Used extensively as a seed treatment for the control of seed decay and damping off. Also has uses on several fruits, vegetables and ornamentals. Dosage for this purpose should be in accord with manufacturer's directions. Used also as a spray for the control of turf and lawn grass diseases, such as dollar spot and brown patch.

Yellow Cuprous Oxide—This material, containing 47% of metallic copper, is sold under the tradename of *Yellow Cuprocide* and may be used as a spray or dust. Used at the rate of 1½ lb/100 gal it is effective against celery blight, Alternaria blight of tomato, early and late blights of potato, anthracnose, downy mildew, and other leaf diseases of cucurbits and is recommended for a variety of vegetable crops wherever a copper spray is needed.

Zerlate—See *Ziram.*

Zinc Dimethyldithiocarbamate—See *Ziram.*

Zinc Ethylenebisdithiocarbamate—See *Zineb.*

Zinc Sulfate—Zinc sulfate and hydrated lime, 8 pounds of each to 100 gallons of water, are used to prepare a spray called *zinc-lime* which is the zinc equivalent of Bordeaux Mixture. Zinc-lime is used extensively for the control of the bacterial spot disease of peaches.

Zineb—This compound, *zinc ethylenebisdithiocarbamate*, has proved to be exceptionally effective in the control of potato and tomato late blight in Florida. It has not been much superior to copper compounds in the more northern tomato-growing sections. Zineb is less injurious to the tomato and potato plants than copper compounds, a factor of considerable importance in the South where numerous spray applications are required during the long growing season.

Zineb has also been used on cucumbers, muskmelons, and watermelons for downy mildew and anthracnose control, especially in Florida. The lack of injury on these plants is an especially valuable feature of this compound, since cucumbers and melons are extremely susceptible to copper injury. For the same reason this compound has proved of value for the control of cabbage and cauliflower diseases and also has many uses on fruits. It is sometimes used to control fire blight on apple and pear trees. It has also been applied as a dust containing 8 to 10% of the fungicide.

Ziram—Ziram, *zinc dimethyldithiocarbamate*, is a white powder and does not leave an objectionable residue. It has found extensive use in the control of vegetable diseases (celery leaf blight, downy mildew of cucurbits, bean anthracnose, cabbage downy mildew, and squash black rot). Ziram has also been used for peach brown rot control, but is apt to produce leaf injury and fruit russet when used on apples, sour cherries, pears and several other fruits. It is not an effective material for the control of potato or tomato late blight.

Relatively crude, denatured forms of streptomycin and oxytetracycline are being used to control many bacterial diseases of plants. Cycloheximide, under the name Acti-Dione, is used to control cherry leaf spot and dollar spot of turf.

Antibiotics

Streptomycin—This antibiotic is marketed as the sulfate or nitrate under the trade names Agrimycin 17, AG-Strep, and Phytomycin by Pfizer, Merck, and Olin Mathieson. It is formulated as a dry, wettable powder (sulfate) and liquid (nitrate). Its salts are very soluble in water. It has general use as an antibacterial against fire blight of apples and pears and similar infections on ornamentals including woody and herbaceous plants. It is persistent on plant surfaces for up to 4 months, but is considered of low general toxicity. It can produce allergenic reactions such as rashes, conjunctivitis, and bronchial asthma. This agent should not be applied following Bordeaux mixture and it is incompatible with lime sulfur, pyrethrane, and aldrin.

Other animal and plant diseases can be controlled with aureomycin, terramycin, and phytoactin.

Control of Weeds and Plants

Many herbicides are used for weed control, and others are being evaluated experimentally to determine their usefulness. Only those of current general interest and usefulness are described below.

Available information on the degree of toxicity of herbicides is listed in the descriptions of chemicals used for weed control. The symbol LD50 (lethal dose that kills 50% of the experimental animals) precedes each number that indicates relative oral toxicity. For example, the single acute oral dose for calcium cyanamide, LD50 = 1400 mg/kg, indicates a relatively low oral toxicity. The larger the LD50 number, the less poisonous the herbicide.

All LD values listed in this guide are based on a single dose of material orally administered to animals, followed by observation of the treated animals for a definite period of time. However, these findings do not indicate the possible hazards that may arise from skin contact or inhalation of the substance or substances indicated. Likewise, these data do not accurately predict the toxicity of a formulation which may differ according to the solvent or diluent employed.

Phenoxy Compounds

Several compounds in this group, including 2,4-dichlorophenoxyacetic acid (2,4-D), 2-methyl-4-chlorophenoxyacetic acid (MCPA), and 2,4,5-trichlorophenoxypropionic acid (Silvex) are used as postemergence selective herbicides to control broad-leaved weeds in corn, small grains, sorghum, rice, flax, lawns, and to control brush and weeds in pastures, along roadsides, rights-of-way, and drainage and irrigation ditches. Some of the phenoxy compounds also may be applied to the surface of the soil as a preemergence treatment to control grasses and broad-leaved weeds in corn and other crops. Silvex is also used on lawns. The use of 2,4,5-trichlorophenoxyacetic acid (2,4,5-T) has been cancelled.

Phenoxy compounds usually are formulated and marketed as two basic types. They are of low to intermediate oral toxicity (LD50 = 375 to 1200 mg/kg) for the various formulations. There are now certain restrictions on these.

1. Salts

The most widely used salts of 2,4-D, MCPA, and other phenoxy acids include such organic amine salts as diethanolamine, triethanolamine, alkanolamine, dimethylamine, triethylamine, isopropylamine, and others. These organic amine salt formulations are available chiefly as water-soluble liquids. The amine salt formulations are more phytotoxic per pound of acid equivalent than the other salt forms, and are more effective in controlling a wider range of weeds.

Some of the phenoxy compounds also are commercially available as sodium and ammonium salt formulations, chiefly as water-soluble powders, but also as water-soluble liquids. These salt formulations are satisfactory to use on easy-to-kill weeds, such as mustard, pigweed, and lambs-quarters, but they are less phytotoxic per pound of acid equivalent than the amine salts and are not as effective in controlling as wide a range of weeds.

The salt formulations of 2,4-D, MCPA, and other phenoxy compounds are practically nonvolatile, and are much safer to use near valuable susceptible plants than ester formulations if spray drift is avoided.

4-(2,4-Dichlorophenoxy)butyric acid [4-(2,4-DB)] and 4-(2-methyl-4-chlorophenoxy)butyric acid [4-(MCPB)] have shown promise for postemergence control of broad-leaved weeds in (a) cereals underseeded with certain forage legumes; (b) establishment of pure stands of forage legumes; (c) forest legume seed-production fields; (d) flax; (e) other weed-crop situations. Legumes that are relatively tolerant to 4-(2,4-DB) include white clover, alsike clover, red clover, alfalfa, and bird's-foot trefoil. Butoxone (*Amchem*) and Butyrac (*Chipman*) are marketed preparations.

2. Esters

(a) *Relatively high-volatility esters*—This type includes methyl, ethyl, isopropyl, butyl, amyl, and other esters known to possess relatively high vapor activity. These esters of 2,4-D, MCPA, and other phenoxy compounds are liquids which, when properly formulated, form emulsions when mixed with water. Because they are highly volatile, they should not be used under high temperature conditions for weed control in areas adjacent to susceptible plants, such as cotton, tomatoes, grapes, flowers, and ornamentals. These volatile esters are more phytotoxic per pound of acid equivalent, than the amine or other salts of 2,4-D and MCPA, to most crops, annual weeds, and hard-to-kill weeds and brush, especially in the more arid regions and under conditions adverse to rapid plant growth. They penetrate leaves rapidly and their effectiveness is not reduced by rain unless it occurs immediately after application. If a range of rates of application is suggested, the esters should be applied at the lower rates and the amine or other salts at the higher rates.

(b) *Relatively low-volatility esters*—This type includes the butoxyethanol, butoxyethoxypropanol, capryl, ethoxyethoxypropanol, isooctyl, propylene glycol butyl ether, and other esters known to be of low volatility. The low-volatility esters are less hazardous than highly volatile esters in areas adjacent to susceptible crops when temperatures are 95°F or less. When temperatures exceed 95°F, the vapors of both the high and low-volatility esters will cause injury. Even under such high temperatures the low-volatility esters are less hazardous to adjacent susceptible crops.

Phenols

The dinitroalkyl phenols and chloro-substituted phenols have been used widely as contact selective and nonselective postemergence herbicides. They have also been used for selective preemergence weed control in a number of large-seeded crops, including peanuts, soybeans, lima beans, snapbeans, and cotton. The substituted phenols consist mainly of two types.

1. Dinitro Compounds

These include the parent compounds 4,6-dinitro-*o-sec*-butylphenol (DNBP), 4,6-dinitro-*o-sec*-amylphenol (DNAP), and 3,5-dinitro-*o*-cresol (DNC). They are not soluble in water but are soluble in oil and may be applied in an oil carrier, or emulsified with water and applied as an emulsion. The parent compounds are used for preemergence and non-selective postemergence weed control. The salts of these compounds, including sodium, ammonium, various amines, and others, are water-soluble, and are used for selective preemergence and postemergence weed control in some crops. DNC has been cancelled for crop use.

The dinitro compounds are yellow dyes that impart a yellow coloration to clothes and skin. These compounds can be used for weed control without danger if precautions are taken to avoid inhaling the vapors or coming in contact with the spray drift or spray solution. When these materials are used as preemergence sprays, severe injury to the crop often results if extremely high temperatures occur in the 2-week period following treatment.

The dinitro compounds are highly toxic (LD50 = 26 to 45 mg/kg) for rats.

2. Chloro-Substituted Phenols

These include pentachlorophenol (PCP), which is soluble in oil but not in water, and its sodium salt (sodium pentachlorophenate), which is soluble in water. PCP is used as a fortifying agent in oil sprays for nonselective weed control. PCP in oil and sodium PCP in water have been used for selective preemergence weed control in several crops. PCP has recently been cancelled for crop use.

The pentachlorophenols are of relatively intermediate to high oral toxicity (LD50 = 50 to 500 mg/kg for the various formulations) when fed to rats.

Carbamates

The carbamates at present include isopropyl *N*-phenylcarbamate (IPC), isopropyl *N*-(3-chlorophenyl)carbamate (CIPC), and 2-chloroallyl diethylthiocarbamate (CDEC), *Eptam* or *S*-ethyl dipropylthiocarbamate (EPTC); *Tillam* or *S*-propyl butylethylthiocarbamate (PEPC), and *Vernam* or *S*-propyl dipropylthiocarbamate. They are relatively insoluble in water but are formulated with organic solvents as emulsifiable concentrates. The carbamates form emulsions with water and may be applied as either low- or high-gallonage sprays. They are effective as selective dormant postemergence sprays for the control of annual grasses, chickweed, and some other broad-leaved weeds in alfalfa and clovers. CIPC is less volatile than IPC and possesses greater residual weed control properties. Both are now being used effectively in some areas for preemergence weed control in cotton, snapbeans, lima beans, spinach, and certain other field and horticultural crops. The carbamates also are used as preplanting sprays for weed control in canning peas and sugar beets. Absolute soil incorporation of many of these is necessary to obtain satisfactory results.

The carbamates are of relatively low oral toxicity (LD50 = 3000 to 5000 mg/kg) for rats.

Ethyl di-n-propylthiocarbamate (*EPTC*) has been used successfully in preliminary trials as a preemergence herbicide to control annual grasses and many broad-leaved weeds in forage legume seedlings and in other field and horticultural crops. It remains active in the soil for short periods. EPTC is formulated as an emulsifiable concentrate, is stable, and apparently noncorrosive. It is marketed as Eptam (*Stauffer*).

S-Ethyl cyclohexylethylthiocarbamate (Ro-neet; Cycloate) is a thiocarbamate effective as a selective preemergence herbicide. Applied to a well-prepared seed bed, incorporated into soil to a depth of 2 to 3 inches, just before planting. It should be used on mineral soil only. The compound is volatile.

Urea and Uracil Herbicides

The substituted urea herbicides include 3-(*p*-chlorophenyl)-1,1-dimethylurea (monuron); 3-(3,4-dichlorophenyl)-1,1-dimethylurea (diuron); 3-(phenyl)-1,1-dimethylurea (fenuron), and 1-*n*-butyl-3-(3,4-dichlorophenyl)-1-methylurea (neburon). These compounds are only slightly soluble in water. They are formulated as wettable powders or as liquids and must be applied as suspensions in high volumes of water. They are the first group of organic chemicals to possess sufficient residual properties to be used as soil sterilants. At present they are being used for nonselective weed control on cultivated land and have registration for crop use. However, diuron and monuron also have shown considerable experimental promise and are being used as selective preemergence herbicides in cotton and certain other crops. Neburon has the least herbicidal activity and is least toxic of the substituted urea herbicides listed above to many crops, particularly perennial grasses.

The substituted urea herbicides are relatively low in oral toxicity (LD50 = 3400 to 7500 mg/kg) for rats.

3-tert-Butyl-5-chloro-6-methyluracil (Sinbar; Terbacil) is a urea derivative used as a selective preemergence herbicide. It is effective against most annual weeds, and is usually applied at a rate of 0.5 to 6 lb/acre. It should not be used on sandy or gravelly soils.

Trichloroacetic Acid (TCA)

Several salts of trichloroacetic acid (TCA) are used as weed killers, including the ammonium and sodium salts. Sodium TCA is used most widely. It has shown varying degrees of effectiveness in controlling quack grass, Bermuda grass, Johnson grass, and other annual and perennial grasses. Best results are obtained when it is applied in combination with tillage and cultural practices. Sodium TCA also is being used as a preemergence spray for the control of annual grasses and several broad-leaved weeds in flax, sugar beets, sugarcane, and certain other crops. The residual toxicity from high rates of TCA for the control of perennial grasses may disappear within a few weeks or may persist for a year or longer depending on the rate of application, soil type, temperature, and soil-moisture relations. Sodium TCA is highly soluble in water, somewhat caustic, and will corrode spray equipment. Recently TCA has been placed in crop use cancellation.

TCA has low oral toxicity (LD50 = 5000 mg/kg) for rats.

2,2-Dichloropropionic Acid (Dalapon)

This herbicide possesses properties somewhat similar to TCA. In contrast with TCA, when dalapon is applied to the foliage of grasses in the vegetative stages of growth, it is translocated from the leaves to the roots of most species. Dalapon has proved less erratic and more effective than TCA when applied as a foliage spray for the control of most of the annual grasses. It is much more effective on quack grass, Bermuda grass, Johnson grass, and other perennial grasses. The sodium salt of dalapon, which is highly soluble in water, is the most widely used formulation. Research indicates that it is most effective as a preemergence or postemergence spray for controlling perennial grasses when applied in combination with tillage and cultural practices. Dalapon apparently possesses less residual toxicity than TCA; but further research is needed to determine the rate of disappearance of the herbicide from the soil. Dalapon has shown promise in experiments for weed control in sugarcane, sugar beets, bird's-foot trefoil, alfalfa, and for spot treatment control of Johnson grass and other grasses in cotton. It has given effective control of cattails and phragmites on irrigation and drainage canals. Dalapon is now registered for a broad range of uses.

Dalapon is low in oral toxicity (LD50 = 6590 to 8120 mg/kg) for rats.

3-Amino-1,2,4-triazole (Amitrol)

This herbicide is available as a white, crystalline powder; soluble in water. It has shown promise for control of Canada thistle, leafy spurge, Russian knapweed, quack grass, Bermuda grass, sedges, horsetail rush, cattails, and tules, and several woody plants such as poison ivy, poison oak, white ash, and prickly ash. Amitrol is translocated throughout the plant and affects the growing points, producing chlorosis and inhibition. It is quickly inactivated in most soils and appears promising for control of certain perennial weeds in apple and pear orchards and in cornland.

Amitrol is low in acute oral toxicity (LD50 = 15,000 mg/kg) for mice. This chemical is the one responsible for the widely publicized seizure of cranberries in 1959. It is no longer used in cranberry culture. Amitrol has been recently cancelled for food crop use.

N-(1-Naphthyl)phthalamic Acid (NPA; Naptalam; Alanap)

This chemical is formulated for experimental herbicidal use as the sodium salt, imide, and acid. The sodium salt of NPA is available as a wettable powder and as a liquid concentrate. Presently, NPA is being used for preemergence control of grasses and broad-leaved weeds in cucumbers, squash, cantaloupes, and other crops in the cucurbit group. It also has shown some promise for weed control in irrigated cotton in the West. NPA has been recently cancelled for food crop use.

NPA has low oral toxicity (LD50 = 8200 mg/kg).

3,6-Endoxohexahydrophthalic Acid (Endothall)

The disodium salt of this acid is used for control of certain weeds in turf, alfalfa, sugar beets, and in certain other crops. It is being used as a preharvest aid, a general contact herbicide, and chemical defoliant. Also helpful for submerged aquatic weeds and on turf.

Endothal has high oral toxicity (LD50 = 35 to 120 mg/kg) for rats.

1,2-Dihydro-3,6-pyridazinedione (Maleic Hydrazide, MH)

This chemical is formulated as a water-soluble sodium or diethanolamine salt for use as a herbicide. It has shown promise for control of several annual and perennial grasses when applied in combination with tillage and cultural treatments. It has been used also as a grass inhibitor to reduce mowing on areas such as roadsides. The chemical, however, has performed erratically both as a herbicide and as a grass inhibitor. Additional research is needed to determine the place of this compound in the field of weed control. Limited use since EPA suspended it pending further tests.

MH has low oral toxicity (LD50 = 5800 mg/kg) for rats.

Ammonium Sulfamate (NH₄SO₃NH₂)

This water-soluble, white, crystalline powder is most widely used for control of woody plants in areas adjacent to cotton, grapes, tomatoes, and other plants that are susceptible to the phenoxy compounds. It will prevent stumps from sprouting when applied to the cut surface, and will kill large trees and sprouting stumps when the crystals or concentrated solutions are used in cups (ax chips) made around the base of a tree or stump. Tolerances have been announced for food crop use.

Ammonium sulfamate has relatively low oral toxicity (LD50 = 3900 mg/kg) for rats.

Herbicidal Oils

Herbicidal oils usually are obtained in the distillation of petroleum and coal tar. Aromatic constituents usually have the greatest influence on their herbicidal properties. Recent research, however, has shown that a number of constituents of oils affect both total herbicidal activity and selectivity. Several herbicidal oils are known under a variety of names such as aromatic solvent, solvent naphtha, and petroleum naphtha. These oils vary widely in their herbicidal toxicity and selectivity depending on their origin and composition. One specific example is a petroleum-naphtha with A. P. I. gravity 49 to 50, boiling range 300° to 400°F, unsaturated compounds 0.5 to 1.0%, aromatic content 22 to 24%, sulfur compounds 0.25 to 0.30%, and a maximum aniline point to 128°F, which is being used extensively as a directed postemergence spray for control of seedling annual grasses and broad-leaved weeds in cotton.

Stoddard solvent and light aromatic oils have been used extensively as selective herbicidal oils for weed control in crops of the carrot family. Nonselective herbicidal oils of high aromatic content are being used effectively to control Johnson grass on ditchbanks in the Southwest. Aromatic solvents also are being used to control aquatic weeds in irrigation canals and ditches in the Western States. Diesel oil, fuel oil, stove oils, and other oils are used as carriers for herbicides. Oil sprays usually are more effective than water sprays in wetting leaf surfaces and in penetrating waxy leaf surfaces. Oil-water emulsions fortified with dinitrophenols or chlorophenols are used rather extensively for control of annual weeds in orchards and alfalfa, as well as weeds on ditchbanks and other noncrop areas.

Herbicidal oils are relatively low in oral toxicity; for example, Stoddard solvent: LD50 = 2000 mg/kg for rats.

Chlorates

A number of chlorates, including sodium and calcium, are used to control deep-rooted perennial weeds. They also are used for temporary and semipermanent soil sterilization to prevent growth of all types of vegetation. Sodium chlorate is used most extensively. It is a white, crystalline, water-soluble powder. Sodium chlorate can be applied in dry form by hand or with various types of spreaders, or as a spray using high-volume spray equipment.

Sodium chlorate leaves the soil unproductive for 1 to 4 years, depending on the precipitation, prevailing temperatures, soil type, and other soil and climatic factors. For semipermanent sterilization, higher rates of application are required on the sandy soils of humid regions than on the heavy soils of lower rainfall areas. To kill all vegetation, higher initial rates of application are necessary on the heavy soils of arid regions than on soils of humid areas. The chlorates have use as cotton defoliants. Toxicity persists for longer periods in arid regions because there is less leaching and slower decomposition than in humid regions.

Sodium chlorate has low oral toxicity (LD50 = 700 mg/kg) for rats.

Caution. The manufacturer's directions for use of sodium chlorate should be followed carefully. This chemical, particularly in spray solutions, must be handled with extreme caution. Flammable articles, such as clothing, shoes, hay, wood, or weeds, that have dried after having been wet with a sodium chlorate solution become violently flammable and even explosive. They can be ignited easily by friction, sparks, or even by the heat from the sun. *Serious injury or property damage* may result from carelessness or failure to observe caution.

Boron Compounds

A number of boron compounds, including borax, sodium pentaborate, boron trioxide, anhydrous sodium diborate, and mixtures of these compounds with 2,4-D, sodium chlorate, and/or a substituted urea compound are used to control deep-rooted perennial weeds, and for temporary and semipermanent soil sterilization to prevent growth of all vegetation. The boron compounds also have use as cotton defoliants. Addition of 2,4-D, sodium chlorate, or a substituted urea herbicide to boron compounds will greatly influence the rate of application required for killing all vegetation. Careful attention should be given to label directions. Boron compounds normally are applied as dry granular formulations, but mixtures of boron

and 2,4-D, and boron and sodium chlorate also are formulated for spray application.

Glyphosphate—isopropylamine salt of *N*-(phosphonomethyl)glycine. A non-selective post-emergence herbicide. In wide use today since it is effective only when striking the green parts of growing plants. Used as a liquid spray.

Picloram—4-Amino-3,5,6-trichloropicolinic acid. A long term residual control agent for broad leaved plants available in liquid and granular form.

Arsenicals

Arsenical herbicides include sodium arsenite, arsenic trioxide, arsenic pentoxide, disodium methanearsonate (DSMA), monosodium acid methanearsonate (MSMA), and other compounds of arsenic. Sodium arsenite was used to a limited (restricted) extent as a soil sterilant, to kill trees and stumps, and to remove bark from trees. It also has been used to control vegetation beneath areas to be paved. Sodium arsenite leaves soil unproductive for 1 to 4 years, depending on the type of soil and climatic conditions. Areas frequented by livestock should not be treated with sodium arsenite because of the hazard of poisoning.

The methanearsonates are used as selective postemergence contact herbicides, and also on food crops within certain tolerances.

EPA restrictions as to use of, and requirements for labeling, arsenicals are given in the discussion of *Arsenicals* under *Common Insecticides.* Their current uses are not widespread.

N,N-Diallyl-2-chloroacetamide

N,N-Diallyl-2-chloroacetamide (CDAA; *Randox*) formulated as an emulsifiable concentrate, is used for preemergence control of weed grasses for soybeans, corn, and certain other crops; it is less effective on broad-leaved weeds than on grasses. The compound may cause serious irritation of the eyes, and goggles and gloves should be worn during its application.

Methyl Bromide

Methyl bromide applied at heavy rates as a volatile temporary soil sterilant will kill most weed seeds and plants. It has a boiling point of 38°F, and is sold in sealed cans as a liquid under pressure. When released at 68°F, it becomes a gas 3.2 times heavier than air. The gas must be released under an airtight cover for use as a soil sterilant. Confining the gas under an airtight cover for 24 hours is usually sufficient for weed control if soil in the treated area is moist and has been loosened to aid gas penetration. It is safe to plant crops 2 to 3 days after the airtight cover is removed. *Methyl bromide gas is poisonous to man and animals.* Effects of exposures within a 24-hour period are cumulative. Skin contact can produce severe burns. The gas is colorless with a slight, sweetish odor, and warning traces of other gases, such as chloropicrin, are sometimes added.

Methyl bromide is relatively toxic, having the power to be absorbed by the skin as well as by inhalation. Since ethylene dibromide (EDB) has come into question since carcinogenicity questions have arisen, methyl bromide use may be likewise questioned.

2,3-Dichloro-1,4-naphthoquinone (Dichlone)

Dichlone is available as a dry, wettable powder that wets and disperses readily in water. It is used for control of blue-green and green algae in lakes and ponds. It mixes well with oil, is chemically stable, and, as an algicide, remains active in water with a pH up to 9 or 10. It is currently being considered for restrictions.

Dichlone is relatively low in oral toxicity (LD50 = 1500 mg/kg) for rats.

Paraquat

1,1′-Dimethyl-4,4′-bipyridinium ion. A contact herbicide and desiccant with a broad scope of uses as an herbicide. Recently used (with much controversy) to control illegal growing of marihuana.

Rosin Amine D Acetate (RADA)

RADA is a water-soluble material that effectively controls fresh-water algae in irrigation canals. It also prevents algae from forming on surfaces of such structures as humidification systems and irrigation installations.

Triazines

2-Chloro-4,6-bis(ethylamino)-s-triazine (simazin) is a wettable powder with low solubility in water and in organic solvents. It is employed for preemergence weed control in corn, transplanted tomatoes, and fruit crops. As a soil sterilant, simazin has been effective when applied at heavy rates. Simazin is marketed as Simazine 80WP (*Geigy*) and other formulations. It is used to control both broadleaf weeds and grasses in ornamentals, fruits, and corn, and for noncrop uses. It is not recommended that crops be planted the same season as application was made as injury may result. Several plants are sensitive to this chemical. See label cautions. Other substituted triazines, including Ametryn, Cyanazine, and Propazine, are available.

Simazin has low oral toxicity (LD50 = 5000 mg/kg) for mice.

Benzoic Acids (Benzoics)

2,3,6-Trichlorobenzoic acid (2,3,6-TBA) and several other isomers of benzoic acid have shown promise as herbicides. The herbicide 2,3,6-TBA is translocated in plants and is effective against a number of weeds that other herbicides have failed to control. It has been used with some success as a preemergence spray for weed control in corn. It is effective as a postemergence spray for the control of wild garlic, annual weed brome grasses, quack grass, some species of brush, several perennial weeds, and certain other weeds that are serious pests in lawns and turf. It has residual herbicidal activity in the soil. 3-Amino-2,5-dichlorobenzoic acid, marketed as Amiben (*Amchem*), is used as a selective preemergence herbicide on vegetables, corn, and soybeans. A related compound in this class is Banval (3,6-dichloro-2-methoxybenzoic acid).

Plant Regulators

A plant growth regulator is a preparation which, in minute amounts, alters the behavior of ornamental or crop plants, or the products thereof, through physiological (hormone) action rather than physical action. It may act to accelerate or retard growth, to prolong or break a dormant condition, to promote rooting, or in other ways. A classification of plant growth regulators usually includes: auxins—2,4-D, MCPB, BNOA; Gibberillins; cytokinins—kinetin; ethylene generators—ethylene ethephon; inhibitors—benzoic acid, MH; retardants—A-Rest, Atrinal. Gibberellic acid is used extensively on seeds to aid in uniform germination and growth and on grapes to increase size. 2-Methyl-4-chlorophenoxyacetic acid (MCPA) and a number of related chemicals are used to thin blossoms, to stop the premature drop of fruits or vegetables before harvest, to increase the uniformity of ripening, and for a wide variety of other purposes. For example, when applied properly, 2,4-D will increase the red color in potatoes, and other chemicals will produce pineapples of more uniform shape than untreated ones. This field of chemical usage is expanding and appears to have a future limited only by the necessity to prove that the uses will be safe, from both the toxicological and nutritional viewpoints. Also, 2,4-D is used on tomatoes to cause all fruits to ripen at the same time for machine harvesting. According to the EPA Suspended and Cancelled Pesticides List of May 1978, products containing 2,4-D for use on grains must include the following label statement: "Do not forage or graze treated grain fields within 2 weeks after treatment with 2,4-D."

The identification of vegetable growth inhibitors may yield improved storage methods for crops. Growth inhibitors for onions and cabbage have been identified but further studies are necessary to determine their ultimate value. Other growth regulators of potential value include: *Ethrel* (2-chloroethylphosphonic acid), which functions by releasing ethylene in plant tissues; it can increase appearance of fruit on pineapple with rates of 1 to 4 lbs/acre. *Captan* (N-(trichloromethylthio)-4-cyclohexene-1,2-dicarboximide) is registered for use in increasing the fruit set of both oranges and tangelos

at the relatively high rate of 5 lbs/acre. *Ripenthol*, which contains *endothall* (7-oxabicyclo[2.2.1]heptane-2,3-dicarboxylic acid), can delay sucrose breakdown in mature sugarcane, giving planters a longer harvest period; this has increased yields of sugar in sugarcane up to 25%.

Desiccants and Defoliants

Desiccants and defoliants become increasingly important as mechanical harvesting gains popularity in farming. In the same way that removal of weeds by use of herbicides just before the combines are put into the fields to harvest wheat will prevent clogging of the machines with weed debris, the removal of cotton leaves by chemical treatment aids mechanical harvesting of cotton and other leafy crops. Arsenic acid, pentachlorophenol and more complex chemicals such as *S,S,S*-tributylphosphorotrithionate and *S,S,S*-tributylphosphorotrithioite, and others are being used for this purpose. Requests for information concerning developments in this field should be addressed to the United States Department of Agriculture, state Experiment Stations, or manufacturers of specific products. Questions on the legal status of pesticides should be sent to Director, Pesticides Regulation Division, Environmental Protection Agency (EPA), Washington, DC 20460.

Bibliography

Biological effects of pesticides in mammalian systems. *Ann NY Acad Sci 160* (art 1): 1–422, 1969.

Melnikov NN: *Chemistry of Pesticides*, Springer-Verlag, New York, 1971.

De Ong ER, *et al: Insect Disease and Weed Control*, Chem. Pub, New York, 1972.

Stevens-White R, ed: *Pesticides in the Environment*, vol 1, part 1, Dekker, New York, 1071; vol 1, part 2, 1971.

Djerassi C, *et al:* Insect control of the future: operational and policy aspects. *Science 186:* 596, 1974.

Klingman GC, Ashton FM, Noordhoff LJ: *Weed Science: Principles and Practices*, Wiley, New York, 1975.

Edwards CA: *Persistent Pesticides in the Environment*, Chem. Rubber Press, Cleveland, OH, 1970.

Brooks GT: *Chlorinated Insecticides*, vol I, *Technology and Application*, Chem. Rubber Press, Cleveland, OH, 1974; vol II, *Biological and Environmental Aspects*, 1975.

Street JC, ed: *Pesticide Selectivity*, Dekker, New York, 1975.

Deichmann WB, ed: *Pesticides Symposia* (Toxicology), Halos and Assoc., Miami, 1970.

Matsumura F, ed: *Environmental Toxicology of Pesticides*, Academic Press, New York, 1972.

Eto M: *Organophosphorus Pesticides: Organic and Biological Chemistry*, Chem. Rubber Press, Cleveland, OH, 1974.

Jacobson M: *Pesticides of the Future*, Dekker, New York, 1975.

Morgan DP: *Recognition and Management of Pesticide Poisonings*, EPA-540/9-80, Washington, DC, Jan 1982, 3rd Edition.

EPA Suspended and Cancelled Pesticides, EPA, Office of Public Awareness (A-107), Washington, DC, May 1978.

Farm Chemicals Handbook, Meister Publ Co, 37841 Euclid Ave., Willoughby, OH 44094, Published annually.

Pesticides, Theory and Application by George W Ware, WH Freeman and Co., San Francisco, 1983.

Wiswesser, WJ, ed: Pesticide Index, 5th Edition, Entomological Society of America, 4603 Calvert Rd, Box AJ, College Park, MD 20740, 1976.

CHAPTER 67

Diagnostic Drugs

Ewart A Swinyard, PhD, DSc (Hon)
Professor Emeritus of Pharmacology
College of Pharmacy and School of Medicine, University of Utah
Salt Lake City, UT 84112

Diagnostic methods have become increasingly complex and frequently involve the use of drugs. For many years inorganic substances were used for visualization of the gastrointestinal tract. More recently a variety of organic substances have been employed for visualization of the liver, gallbladder, urinary tract, bronchi, lungs, heart, blood vessels, and spinal canal. Drugs of varying chemical structure have been used for the study of blood flow, blood volume, and for the diagnosis of diseases such as pernicious anemia and myasthenia gravis. A number of radioactive substances have been introduced to measure *organic function*. These are discussed in Chapter 29.

Although some drugs employed as diagnostic agents are innocuous, others possess pharmacologic activity and/or undesirable side actions. Indeed, no diagnostic test or drug is completely devoid of risk. Sudden death from anaphylactic reaction has followed intravenous injection of such a relatively inert substance as dehydrocholic acid. Alarming pharmacological responses have been observed to follow use of more active agents, such as the more effective iodine-containing compounds. Iodism quite commonly follows use of diagnostic agents with a high iodine content. Therefore, it is generally agreed that the clinician should evaluate carefully the need of every test and should reserve diagnostic drugs for those situations where effective management of the patient depends on their use. In addition, appropriate facilities should be available for coping with situations that may arise as a result of the procedure, as well as for emergency treatment of severe reactions to the contrast agent itself. After intravascular administration of a radiopaque agent, competent personnel and emergency facilities should be available for at least 30 to 60 min, since severe delayed reactions have been known to occur.

Some of the more commonly employed diagnostic drugs are listed in this chapter. For convenience in presentation, they are divided according to use into four groups as follows: drugs used as X-ray contrast media, drugs used to test organ function, drugs used to determine blood volume and hemopoietic function, and drugs used for miscellaneous diagnostic tests.

Drugs Used as X-ray Contrast Media

Barium sulfate and compounds containing iodine are opaque to X-rays. By administering these preparations in various ways it is possible to visualize with the fluoroscope or to photograph by X-rays various structures such as the blood vessels, gastrointestinal tract, gallbladder and ducts, ureters and kidney pelvis, and uterus and fallopian tubes, etc.

Hence, drugs described in this section help to reveal anatomic evidence of disease.

Drugs Used for Outlining the Gastrointestinal Tract
Previous to the introduction in 1910 of barium sulfate as a contrast medium, insoluble bismuth salts were used in roentgen examination of the gastrointestinal tract. Bismuth subcarbonate was preferred over the subnitrate because of its lower toxicity. In modern medical practice, barium sulfate has replaced the bismuth salts, because it is completely innocuous even when taken in very large doses, and it is inexpensive. Since the soluble barium salts are highly toxic, it is recommended that when barium sulfate is prescribed the title should be written out in full.

Barium Sulfate

Sulfuric acid, barium salt (1:1); Synthetic or Artificial Barytes; Various Trade Names

Barium sulfate (1:1) [7727-43-7] $BaSO_4$ (233.39).
Caution—When Barium Sulfate is prescribed, the title always should be written out in full to avoid confusion with the poisonous barium sulfide or barium sulfite.
Preparation—Barium sulfate precipitates when an aqueous solution containing barium ion is mixed with a solution containing sulfate ion. It also can be obtained by suitable purification of native barium sulfate.

Description—Fine, white, odorless, tasteless, bulky powder, free from grittiness; its suspension in water is neutral to litmus paper.
Solubility—Practically insoluble in water, solutions of acids and of alkalies, and organic solvents.

Uses—Medicinally used in roentgenography (page 487) for the purpose of making the intestinal tract opaque to the X-ray so that it may be photographed. As the amount required is large, 60 to 250 g (2 to 8 oz), and as soluble salts of barium are extremely poisonous, it is highly important to be sure that the sulfate dispensed is of USP quality. When preparing barium sulfate mixtures for X-ray diagnosis, they should be strained through gauze or mixed well with food, otherwise lumps of the salt may give false indication of an ulcer niche. The following suggestions are offered if specific directions are not given by the attending physician:
For the Roentgen-Ray Examination of the Stomach—The evening before the examination, the patient receives 30 mL of castor oil or other suitable cathartic. In the morning an ordinary portion of wheat-meal porridge, with which 60 g of barium sulfate has been well mixed, together with a little sugar and cream, is administered by mouth. The patient is then directed to abstain from further food. The examination is made six hours later.
For the Roentgen-Ray Examination of the Colon—An enema containing barium sulfate and one or more suitable dispersing and/or suspending agents is warmed to body temperature and injected into the rectum from a height of from 3 to 6 ft (90 to 180 cm). The examination is made with a fluoroscope while the injection is passing into the rectum.
Suspensions of barium sulfate can be very constipating; impaction has occurred after such use.
Dose—*Usual, oral,* **60 to 450 g** in suitable suspension; *usual, rectal,* **150 to 750 g** in suitable suspension.
Dosage Forms—for Suspension: a dry mixture containing not less than 90.0% $BaSO_4$, with one or more suitable dispersing and/or suspending agents and that may contain suitable colors, flavors, fluidizing agents, and preservatives; in bulk or single-dose powder and disposable, prefilled cups or enema kits.

Drugs Used for Outlining the Gallbladder and Bile Ducts
(*Cholecystography and Cholangiography*)

Certain radiopaque substances are excreted in the bile and, hence, are used for visualization of the gallbladder (cholecystography) and bile ducts (cholangiography). They are generally organic iodine compounds that cast a shadow on the X-ray film. Hence, use of these agents is accompanied by some risk and a considerable number of untoward effects. These include mild transient symptoms such as restlessness, sensations of warmth, sneezing, perspiration, salivation, flushing, pressure in the upper abdomen, dizziness, nausea, vomiting, chills, fever, headache, pallor and tremors. Rarely, swollen eyelids, laryngospasm, respiratory difficulties, hypotension, cardiac reactions and cyanosis have been reported. Hypersensitivity reactions may occur. In rare instances, despite the most careful sensitivity testing, anaphylactoid reactions may also occur. In addition, renal function tests may be altered and renal failure may occur. Moreover, these drugs should be administered with extreme caution to patients known or suspected to have pheochromocytoma. These materials have been shown to promote the phenomenon of sickling in individuals who are homozygous for sickle-cell disease. Iodine-containing contrast agents may alter the results of thyroid function tests; such tests, if indicated, should be performed prior to the administration of the contrast agent. Safe use of iodinated drugs during pregnancy has not been established; therefore these agents should be used in pregnant patients only when, in the judgment of the physician, such use is deemed essential to the welfare of the patient (see Introduction, this chapter).

Ceruletide Diethylamine—page 1274.

Cholecystokinin—page 1274.

Iocetamic Acid

Propanoic acid, 3-[acetyl(3-amino-2,4,6-triiodophenyl)amino]-2-methyl-, Cholebrine (*Mallinckrodt*)

A mixture of two diastereoisomers (A and B). *N*-Acetyl-*N*-(3-amino-2,4,6-triiodophenyl)-2-methyl-β-alanine [16034-77-8] $C_{12}H_{13}I_3N_2O_3$ (613.96).

Preparation—*m*-Nitroaniline is heated with methacrylic acid and the resulting *N*-(3-nitrophenyl)-2-methyl-β-alanine is *N*-acetylated with a mixture of acetic anhydride and acetic acid. After reducing the NO_2 to NH_2 with the aid of Raney nickel, iodination is effected with $NaICl_2$.

Description—White to creamy white powder; odorless or has a faint acetic acid odor; unstable in light; melts between 190° and 222° (isomer A at about 232°, isomer B at about 201°); pK$_a$ (isomer A) 4.25; pK$_a$ (isomer B) 4.10.

Solubility—Insoluble in water; slightly soluble in alcohol, acetone, and chloroform; very slightly soluble in ether and benzene.

Uses—An oral *cholecystographic* agent indicated for the radiographic visualization of the gall bladder. It is rapidly absorbed following oral administration, conjugated with glucuronic acid in the liver, secreted into the bile as radiopaque glucuronide, and concentrated in the functioning gallbladder. Contraction of the gall bladder also may provide visualization of the biliary ducts. Contraindications, warnings, precautions, and adverse reactions are similar to other iodinated diagnostic agents (see this page).

Dose—*Usual, oral, adult,* **3 g** (4 tablets) or **4.5 g** (6 tablets) as a single dose. Cholecystography is done 10–15 hours.

Dosage Form—Tablets: 750 mg.

Iodipamide

Benzoic acid, 3,3'-[(1,6-dioxo-1,6-hexanediyl)diimino]bis[2,4,6-triiodo-, Cholografin (*Squibb*)

3,3'-(Adipoyldiimino)bis[2,4,6-triiodobenzoic acid] [606-17-7] $C_{20}H_{14}I_6N_2O_6$ (1139.77).

Preparation—From benzoic acid by: (*a*) nitration to 3-nitrobenzoic acid; (*b*) reduction by means of stannous chloride or other reducing agent to 3-aminobenzoic acid; (*c*) iodination with iodine monochloride in acetic acid to the 2,4,6-triiodo derivative; (*d*) acylation of the amino group with adipoyl chloride [ClCO(CH₂)₄COCl].

Description—White, nearly odorless, crystalline powder.
Solubility—Very slightly soluble in water, chloroform, and ether; slightly soluble in alcohol.

Uses—Radiopaque component of *Iodipamide Meglumine Injection.*

Iodipamide Meglumine Injection

Benzoic acid, 3,3'-[(1,6-dioxo-1,6-hexanediyl)diimino]bis[2,4,6-triiodo-, compd. with 1-deoxy-1-(methylamino)-D-glucitol (1:2); Cholografin Meglumine (*Squibb*)

1-Deoxy-1-(methylamino)-D-glucitol 3,3'-(adipoyldiimino)-bis-[2,4,6-triiodobenzoate] (2:1) (salt) [3521-84-4] $C_{20}H_{14}I_6N_2O_6$). $2C_7H_{17}NO_5$ (1530.20).

Preparation—Iodipamide is reacted with a double equimolar quantity of methylglucamine (meglumine), using sufficient water for injection to produce a solution of the required concentration.

Description—Clear, colorless to pale yellow, slightly viscous liquid.

Uses—For *intravenous cholangiography* and *cholecystography* as follows: visualization of the gallbladder and biliary ducts in the differential diagnosis of acute abdominal conditions, visualization of the biliary ducts especially in patients with symptoms after cholecystectomy, and visualization of the gallbladder in patients unable to take oral contrast media or to absorb media from the gastrointestinal tract. The contrast medium appears in the bile within 10 to 15 min after injection and the biliary ducts are visualized within 25 min; the gallbladder begins to fill within 1 hr, maximum filling occurring in 2 to 2.5 hr. Adverse reactions and contraindications are similar to those common to iodine-containing compounds.

Dose—*Usual, intravenous, adult,* **20 mL** of **52%** solution administered over a period of 10 min. *Infants* and *children*, **0.3 to 0.6 mL/kg** of body weight; total dosage should not exceed 20 mL.

Dosage Form—Injection: 52% solution.

Iodoxamate Meglumine

Benzoic acid, 3,3'-[(1,16-dioxo-4,7,10,13-tetraoxahexadecane-1,16-diyl)-diimino]bis]2,4,6-triiodo-, compound with 1-deoxy-1-(methylamino)-D-glucitol (1:2); Cholovue (*Squibb*)

[51764-33-1] $C_{26}H_{26}I_6N_2O_{10}.2C_7H_{17}NO_5$ (1678.36).

Uses—Intravenously as a radiopaque medium for *cholecystocholangiography* for rapid visualization of the gallbladder and biliary ducts. Iodoxamate, following intravenous injection or infusion, is carried to the liver and rapidly excreted in the feces. Less than 15% is excreted by the kidneys. It is contraindicated in patients with severe impairment of hepatic and renal function, as well as with a known sensitivity to iodine. Although animal studies performed with doses up to 12 times the human dose have revealed no evidence of teratogenic effects, the safe use in pregnant women has not been established. Therefore, this drug should not be used during pregnancy unless clearly needed. Likewise, safety and effectiveness in children remain undetermined. Contraindications and adverse effects are similar to other iodine-containing substances (see page 1265). The admixture of iodoxamate meglumine and an antihistamine may cause a precipitate to form in the syringe or infusion bottle. If antihistamines are administered concomitantly, they should *not* be mixed with the contrast medium but should be administered at another site.

Dose—Intravenous: **20 mL; Drip** Infusion, **100 mL** at a rate of **3 mL/min.** These doses should not be repeated until four days have elapsed.

Dosage Form—20 mL single-dose vials and 100 mL single-dose infusion bottles.

Iopanoic Acid

Benzenepropanoic acid, 3-amino-α-ethyl-2,4,6-triiodo-, Telepaque (*Winthrop*)

3-Amino-α-ethyl-2,4,6-triiodohydrocinnamic acid [96-83-3] $C_{11}H_{12}I_3NO_2$ (570.93).

Preparation—A mixture of *m*-nitrobenzaldehyde, butyric anhydride, and sodium butyrate is heated in xylene to effect a Perkin condensation yielding *m*-nitro-α-ethylcinnamic acid. The acid is reduced with hydrogen in the presence of Raney nickel. The resulting *m*-amino-α-ethylhydrocinnamic acid is iodinated with iodine monochloride in acetic acid solution.

Description—Cream-colored powder; tasteless or nearly so; faint characteristic odor; affected by light; melts with decomposition between 152° and 158°.

Solubility—Insoluble in water; soluble in alcohol, chloroform, and ether; soluble in solutions of alkali hydroxides and carbonates.

Uses—Orally as a *radiopaque medium* in *cholecystography*. Although not the method of choice, it may also be used for oral *cholangiography*. It is promptly absorbed from the gastrointestinal tract, concentrated in the gallbladder, and subsequently excreted, approximately two-thirds through the gastrointestinal tract and one-third through the kidneys. About 50% of an administered dose is excreted within 24 hr and the remainder in about 5 days. It is relatively free from undesirable reactions and has low toxicity. Occasionally, nausea and diarrhea and, rarely, dysuria have followed its administration. A mild stinging sensation during urination may occur. Hypersensitivity reactions involving the skin, mucous membranes, and a systemic serum sickness-type reaction have been reported. It is contraindicated in patients with acute nephritis and uremia, since it is eliminated by the kidneys. It should not be administered when disorders of the gastrointestinal tract exist which prevent absorption of the medium.

The usual regimen is to give the patient a fat-free evening meal following which the iopanoic acid is administered approximately 14 hr before the time scheduled for roentgenography. Immediately after the roentgen examination, the patient is given a high-fat meal and additional exposures are made in order to evaluate the contraction of the gallbladder and to visualize the patency of the extrahepatic ducts. When the latter structures are of particular interest, the dose of iopanoic acid may be increased to 5 or 6 g.

Dose—3 to 6 g; *usual*, **3 g.**

Dosage Form—Tablets: 500 mg.

Ipodate Calcium

Benzenepropanoic acid, 3-[[(dimethylamino)methylene]amino]-2,4,6-triiodo-, calcium salt; Oragrafin Calcium (*Squibb*)

Calcium 3-[[(dimethylamino)methylene]amino]-2,4,6-triiodohydrocinnamate [1151-11-7] $C_{24}H_{24}CaI_6N_4O_4$ (1233.98).

Preparation—By precipitation using aqueous solutions of sodium ipodate and calcium chloride. The crude precipitate is recrystallized from a suitable solvent, such as aqueous dimethylformamide. The preparation of *Ipodate Sodium* is described in the next monograph.

Description—White to off-white, fine crystalline powder that is odorless and has a chalky, very bitter taste. It should be stored at room temperature in a tightly closed container protected from light. It melts at 300° with decomposition.

Solubility—1 g in 1700 mL water, 2.6 mL chloroform; slightly soluble in alcohol.

Uses—A water-insoluble substance that contains 61.7% iodine and is used as a contrast medium for *cholecystography*. It may also be used for *cholangiography*, but is not the drug of choice. The agent is rapidly absorbed from the gastrointestinal tract and excreted in the bile in sufficient quantity to outline the biliary ducts within 30 min after administration; optimal opacification of the ducts occurs 1 to 3 hr after ingestion. Maximal visualization of the gallbladder occurs 10 hr after administration of the salt. Untoward effects reported include abdominal cramping, diarrhea, nausea, vomiting, dysuria, urticaria, headache, heartburn, and epigastric pain. Although rare, hypotension and circulatory collapse have been reported. The drug is contraindicated in patients with severe renal disease and in patients known to be allergic to iodine. It also interferes with thyroid function tests based on uptake of radioactive iodine by the gland.

Dose—*Usual*, **3** to **6 g** as a single dose given 10 to 12 hr before the examination.

Dosage Form—for Oral Suspension: 3 g.

Ipodate Sodium

Benzenepropanoic acid, 3-[[(dimethylamino)methylene]amino]-2,4,6-triiodo-, sodium salt; Oragrafin Sodium (*Squibb*)

Sodium 3-[[(dimethylamino)methylene]amino]-2,4,6-triiodohydrocinnamate [1221-56-3] $C_{12}H_{12}I_3N_2NaO_2$ (619.94).

Preparation—3-Amino-2,4,6-triiodohydrocinnamic acid is condensed with *N,N*-dimethylformamide with the aid of iodomethanesulfonyl chloride to produce 3-[[(dimethylamino)methylene]-amino]-2,4,6-triiodohydrocinnamic acid. Neutralization of the acid with sodium hydroxide yields the sodium salt (*Chem Ber 93:* 2347, 1960).

Description—White to off-white, crystalline powder that is odorless. It should be stored at room temperature in a tightly closed container protected from light. It melts between 303° and 304° with decomposition.

Solubility—1 g in 1 mL water, 2 mL alcohol; very slightly soluble in chloroform.

Uses—A radiopaque medium for the visualization of the gallbladder and biliary tract. Except that ipodate sodium is somewhat less rapidly absorbed from the gastrointestinal tract, is soluble in water, and contains slightly less iodine (61.4%), its actions, uses, onset and duration of effects, and contraindications are similar to those for *Ipodate Calcium*.

Dose—3 to 6 g; *usual*, **3 g** given 12 hr before examination.

Dosage Form—Capsules: 500 mg.

Drugs Used for Outlining Various Cavities

A number of radiopaque preparations are available which consist of iodine addition products of vegetable oils. These preparations are nonirritating and can be injected as contrast media into various cavities of the body such as the urinary and genital tracts, bronchi, fistulous tracts, and the spinal canal.

Thus, they are useful in the X-ray diagnosis of gynecologic conditions, bronchial and pulmonary lesions, and tumors of the spinal cord. They are removed slowly from closed cavities and may give rise to foreign-body reactions; some reports indicate blood iodine level may be elevated for 2 to 4 years after the use of one of these agents. Other untoward reactions are characteristic of iodine compounds (see page 1264).

Ethiodized Oil

Ethiodol (*Savage*)

An iodine addition product of the ethyl ester of the fatty acids of poppyseed oil, containing 35.2–38.9% of organically combined iodine. It is sterile.

Preparation—By saponifying poppy-seed oil and subjecting the resulting fatty acids to iodination and subsequent esterification with ethanol.

Description—Straw-colored to amber-colored, oily liquid; may have an alliaceous odor.

Solubility—Insoluble in water; soluble in acetone, chloroform, and ether.

Uses—A *contrast medium* used in *lymphography, hysterosalpingography, sialography*, and visualization of *sinus* and *fistulous tracts*. It is contraindicated in acute parotitis. It should not be used for bronchography or myelography, or in the presence of intrauterine bleeding, pelvic infection, or pregnancy. Likewise, it should not be used in patients known to be sensitive to iodine. Except for pulmonary embolism resulting from accidental intravasation of the medium, other side effects, such as transient fever, allergic dermatitis, lipogranuloma formation, and delayed wound healing, are rare and of little consequence.

Dose—*Usual, hysterosalpingography, by special injection*, **5 mL** followed by increments of **2 mL** until tubule patency is established or limit of tolerance is reached. *Lymphography, by special injection, lower extremity*, **6 to 8 mL** per extremity, at a rate of 0.1 to 0.2 mL per minute; *upper extremity*, **2 to 4 mL** per extremity, at a rate of 0.1 to 0.2 mL per minute. *Usual, pediatric, dose, lymphography*, **1 mL** to a maximum of **6 mL**. *Usual, sialography* and visualization of *sinus* and *fistulous tracts*, slowly in **1-mL** increments, depending on the size of the area being examined.

Dosage Form—10 mL.

Iodized Oil Injection

Iodised Oil Viscous Injection; Lipiodol (*Savage*)

An iodine addition product of vegetable oil or oils, containing 38–42% of organically combined iodine. It is sterile.

Preparation—The methods of preparing iodized oil involve addition of elemental iodine to the unsaturated fatty constituents of a vegetable oil, the resulting oil containing chemically saturated iodoglycerides. The oil most generally used is poppy-seed oil.

Description—Thick, viscous, oily liquid, having an alliaceous odor and an oleaginous taste. It is light to dark brown in color, and on exposure to air and light it becomes darker due to liberation of iodine. Specific gravity about 1.35.

Solubility—Insoluble in water; soluble in ether, chloroform, or petroleum benzin; 1 mL of iodized oil should yield a clear solution with 10 mL of solvent hexane.

Uses—The injection is assigned the category *diagnostic aid (radiopaque-hysterosalpingographic)*. Formerly used for visualization of various internal cavities, the stated indications are now restricted to hysterosalpingography, sialography, visualization of sinus and fistulous tracts, and, with great caution, bronchography. Many reports of adverse and toxic effects from use of iodized oils have been published, including deaths from use in bronchography (primarily due to anoxia associated with emphysema or bronchospasm) and in hysterosalpingography (primarily due to cerebral oil embolism). Use of this injection is contraindicated in the presence of active bleeding, in patients with disease in which there is inflammation (pelvic inflammatory disease, pulmonary tuberculosis), and in individuals with known or suspected iodine sensitivity.

Dose—*Usual*, 1 to **30 mL** by special injection, depending on procedure.

Dosage Forms—Injection: 1, 5, 10, and 20 mL.

Iophendylate

Benzenedecanoic acid, iodo-*i*-methyl-, ethyl ester; Pantopaque (*Lafayette*)

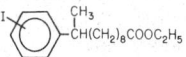

Iophendylate is a mixture of isomers of ethyl iodophenylundecanoate, consisting chiefly of ethyl 10-(iodophenyl)undecanoate [1320-11-2] $C_{19}H_{29}IO_2$ (416.34).

Preparation—This substance is reported to be manufactured as follows. Benzene is reacted with undecylenic acid forming a mixture of isomers of phenylundecyclic acid. The mixture is iodinated and finally esterified with ethyl alcohol. After decolorization, the desired fraction is separated by distillation.

Description—Colorless to pale yellow, viscous liquid; darkens on long exposure to air; odorless or possesses a faintly ethereal odor; specific gravity between 1.248 and 1.257.

Solubility—Very slightly soluble in water; freely soluble in alcohol, benzene, chloroform, and ether.

Uses—A *radiopaque medium* for *myelography*. It is commonly used for visualization of tumors or herniation of the intervertebral disc or other lesions compressing the spinal cord. It is absorbed at a rate of about 1 mL/year, varying with the condition of the tissues; persistent levels in the body interfere with tracer studies with radioactive iodine. The incidence of adverse reactions is low.

Dose—*Usual, myelography, intrathecal* or by special injection, **3 to 12 mL**.

Dosage Forms—Injection (sterile iophendylate): 3, 6, and 12 mL.

Other Drugs Used for Outlining Various Cavities

Propyliodone [Propyl 3,5-diiodo-4-oxo-1(4*H*)-pyridineacetate [587-61-1] $C_{10}H_{11}I_2NO_3$ (447.01) (Dionosil (*Glaxo*).] *Preparation:* 4(1*H*)-Pyridone, as the nitrate in aqueous solution, is iodinated with a mixture of sodium iodide and sodium iodate in the presence of sulfuric acid. The 3,5-diiodo-4(1*H*)-pyridone thus formed is isolated and condensed with chloroacetic acid to yield 3,5-diiodo-4-oxo-1(4*H*)-pyridineacetic acid, which is esterified with propyl alcohol. *Description and Solubility:* White, or almost white, crystalline powder; odorless or has a faint odor; melts between 187° and 190°. Practically insoluble in water; soluble in acetone, alcohol, and ether. *Uses:* A *radiopaque medium* for *bronchographic* use. Direct instillation into the bronchi results in well-defined bronchograms for at least 30 min. It is usually eliminated from the lungs in 7 to 10 days. Because of its toxicity, it should only be used if absolutely essential. Propyliodone is contraindicated in patients with pulmonary emphysema or bronchiectasis. *Dose: Usual, bronchography, intrathecal*, 0.75 to 1 mL of 60% oil suspension, to a maximum of 12 to 18 mL. *Dosage Form:* Sterile Oil Suspension: 20 mL of 60%.

Drugs Used for Intravenous Pyelography and Angiography

Satisfactory X-ray pictures of the urinary tract, blood vessels, or heart may be obtained by the intravenous injection of soluble iodine compounds of low toxicity which are rapidly excreted in the urine. The inorganic iodide, sodium iodide, is too toxic for intravenous injection; however, there are organic iodine compounds available for this use. All of these organic iodine compounds can interfere with thyroid function tests based on glandular uptake of radioactive iodine. Also, serious adverse effects are sometimes encountered.

The *most frequent* adverse reactions are nausea, vomiting, facial flush and a feeling of body warmth. These are usually of brief duration. *Allergic-type reactions* include: dermal manifestations of urticaria with or without pruritus, erythema and maculopapular rash; dry mouth; sweating; conjunctival symptoms; facial, peripheral and angioneurotic edema. Symptoms relating to the respiratory system include sneezing, nasal stuffiness, coughing, choking, dyspnea, chest tightness and wheezing, which may be initial manifestations of more severe and infrequent reactions including asthmatic attack, laryngospasm and bronchospasm with or without edema, pulmonary edema, apnea and cyanosis. Rarely, these allergic-type reactions can progress into anaphylaxis with loss of consciousness and coma and severe cardiovascular disturbances. *Cardiovascular reactions* include: generalized vasodilation, flushing and venospasm. Occasionally, thrombosis or, rarely, thrombophlebitis, as well as red blood cell clumping and agglutination, crenation and interference in clot formation. Severe cardiovascular responses include rare cases of hypotensive shock, coronary insufficiency, cardiac arrhythmia, fibrillation and arrest. *Neurological reactions* include: spasm, convulsions, aphasia, syncope, paresis, paralysis resulting from spinal cord injury and pathology associated with the syndrome of transverse myelitis, visual field losses that are usually transient but may be permanent, coma and death. *Other reactions* may consist of: headache, trembling, shaking, chills without fever and lightheadedness; temporary renal shutdown or other nephropathy. These agents should be used with extreme caution in patients with a positive history of bronchial asthma or allergy, a family history of allergy, or a previous reaction or hypersensitivity to a contrast agent, those with combined renal and hepatic disease, severe hypertension or congestive heart failure. Safe use of these agents during pregnancy has not been established. Also, it is not known whether they are excreted in human milk. Therefore, these agents should be used in pregnant patients only when, in the judgment of the physician, their use is deemed essential to the welfare of the patient. In general, nursing should not be continued following administration of any of these iodinated substances. In addition, emergency facilities and competent personnel should be available for at least 30 to 60 min after administration of the agents. See also the introduction to this chapter, page 1264.

Diatrizoate Meglumine

Benzoic acid, 3,5-bis(acetylamino)-2,4,6-triiodo-, compd. with 1-deoxy-1-(methylamino)-D-glucitol (1:1); Cardiografin, Cystografin (*Squibb*); Hypaque Meglumine, Hypaque-Cysto (*Winthrop*); Reno-M (*Squibb*)

1-Deoxy-1-(methylamino)-D-glucitol 3,5-diacetamido-2,4,6-triiodobenzoate (salt) [131-49-7] $C_7H_{17}NO_5.C_{11}H_9I_3N_2O_4$ (809.13).

Preparation—Diatrizoic acid is reacted with an equimolar quantity of methylglucamine (meglumine), usually in water for injection to produce a solution of the required concentration.

Uses—In different concentrations for many diagnostic tests. The 85% injection is used for adult *angiocardiography* and *thoracic aortography*. On injection into a vessel or into the heart, it is rapidly diffused in the vascular system and excreted by the kidneys. As the contrast medium enters the cardiac chambers, the vessels and aorta, lesions or malformations of the heart, and obstructions or anomalies are visualized. The drug should be used with great care in patients known to have multiple myeloma; anuria resulting in progressive uremia, renal failure, and eventually death has occurred. Also, it should be used with extreme caution in patients known to have pheochromocytoma, severe hepatic and renal disease, patients who are homozygous for sickle-cell disease, and patients known to be sensitive to iodine compounds. Safe use in pregnancy has not been established. A 85% solution is used for adult *angiocardiography* and *thoracic aortography;* a 76% solution is used in *excretion urography, aortography, pediatric angiocardiography* and *peripheral arteriography;* a 60% solution is used for *excretory urography, cerebral angiography, peripheral arteriography, venography, splenoportography, arthrography,* and *discography,* and a 30% solution for *retrograde cystourethrography* and *infusion urography,* and enhancement of *computed tomography* of the brain. Adverse reactions, precautions, and contraindications are similar to those for other iodinated diagnostic agents (see page 1265, this section).

Dose—As the dosage and concentration of injections of diatrizoate meglumine vary greatly with the many diagnostic uses and techniques

of administration of the agent, and often with the physical condition and preliminary preparation of the patient, the *latest* package insert should be consulted for adult and pediatric dosages and other information concerning uses of this diagnostic drug.

Dosage Forms—Injection: 30, 60, 70, 76, and 85%.

Diatrizoate Sodium

Benzoic acid, 3,5-bis(acetylamino)-2,4,6-triiodo-, monosodium salt; Hypaque Sodium (*Winthrop*)

Monosodium 3,5-diacetamido-2,4,6-triiodobenzoate [737-31-5] $C_{11}H_8I_3N_2NaO_4$ (635.90).

Preparation—Diatrizoic acid is reacted with an equimolar quantity of NaOH, usually in water for injection to produce a solution of the required concentration.

Uses—A radiopaque agent with uses, profile of toxicity, and precautions similar to those for *Diatrizoate Meglumine* and other iodinated diagnostic agents (see page 1265, this section). Diatrizoate sodium contains somewhat more iodine (59.87%) than the meglumine salt (47.01%); consequently, it is somewhat more toxic. Solutions of diatrizoate sodium are considerably less viscous than those prepared from diatrizoate meglumine. Also, diatrizoate sodium should not be used in coronary angiography because it is more likely to cause serious cardiac arrhythmias than is the meglumine salt. When administered orally or given as an enema, it is used as a radiopaque medium to outline the upper and lower gastrointestinal tract.

Dosage—As the dosage and concentration of injections, oral solutions, and enemas of diatrizoate sodium vary considerably with the diagnostic uses and techniques of administration of the agent, the *latest* package insert should be consulted for adult and pediatric dosages and other information concerning uses of this diagnostic drug.

Dosage Forms—Powder; Injections: 20, 25, and 50%; Solution: 41.7%.

Diatrizoate Meglumine and Diatrizoate Sodium Injection

Hypaque-M (*Winthrop*); Renografin (*Squibb*); Renovist (*Squibb*)

A sterile solution of diatrizoate meglumine and diatrizoate sodium in water for injection, or a sterile solution of diatrizoic acid in water for injection prepared with the aid of NaOH and meglumine. It may contain small amounts of suitable buffers and of edetate calcium disodium or edetate disodium as a stabilizer. When intended for intravascular use, it contains no antimicrobial agents.

Description—Clear, colorless to pale yellow, slightly viscous liquid; may crystallize at room temperature or below.

Uses—Designed to combine the lower toxicity of the meglumine salt with the lower viscosity and higher iodine content of the sodium salt. In appropriate concentrations it is used as a radiopaque medium for *angiocardiography, aortography, angiography, excretion urography, hysterosalpingography, peripheral arteriography* and *venography,* and other radiographic procedures. Contraindications, general warnings and adverse effects are similar to those for other iodinated diagnostic agents (see page 1265, this section).

A solution containing 66% of diatrizoate meglumine and 10% of diatrizoate sodium (Gastrografin, *Squibb*) is used as a contrast medium for radiographic examination of the gastrointestinal tract following oral or rectal administration. The preparation is particularly indicated where use of barium is not feasible or is potentially dangerous. It is contraindicated in patients sensitive to salts of diatrizoic acid and should be used with caution in patients sensitive to iodine. The safety of the oral solution in pregnancy has not been established. It is usually well tolerated; occasionally some diarrhea occurs.

Dose—As the dosage and concentration of diatrizoate meglumine and diatrizoate sodium injection vary greatly with the many diagnostic uses and techniques of administration of the injection, and often with the physical condition and preliminary preparation of the patient, the *latest* package insert should be consulted for adult and pediatric dosages and other information concerning uses of this diagnostic drug, as well as of the oral solution used for radiographic examination of the gastrointestinal tract.

Dosage Forms—Injection, containing the following percentages of diatrizoate meglumine and diatrizoate sodium, respectively: 50/25, 60/30, 52/8, 66/10, 34.3/35, 28.5/29.1; Oral Solution: 66/10.

Diatrizoate Meglumine and Iodipamide Meglumine Injection—A sterile, aqueous solution of diatrizoate meglumine equivalent to 40% diatrizoic acid and iodipamide meglumine equivalent to 20% iodipamide, containing approximately 38% of bound iodine (*Sinografin*, Squibb). *Uses*: A radiopaque medium indicated for *hysterosalpingography*. Following intrauterine administration immediate visualization of the uterus and tubes is achieved. Medium spilled into the peritoneal cavity is absorbed within 20 to 60 minutes. The preparation is contraindicated during pregnancy or in patients with acute pelvic inflammatory disease. The test should not be performed within 30 days following curettage or conization. Otherwise the precautions, adverse effects, and contraindications are similar to those for other iodinated diagnostic agents (see page 1265, this section). *Dose: Usual, uterus,* 3 to 4 mL; an additional 3 to 4 mL will outline the *fallopian tubes.* Total dose varies from 1.5 to 10 mL. *Dosage Form:* Single-dose vials: 10 mL.

Diatrizoic Acid

Benzoic acid, 3,5-bis(acetylamino)-2,4,6-triiodo-,

3,5-Diacetamido-2,4,6-triiodobenzoic acid [117-96-4] $C_{11}H_9I_3N_2O_4$ (613.92); *dihydrate* [50978-11-5] (649.95).

Preparation—From benzoic acid by: (*a*) nitration to the 3,5-dinitro acid; (*b*) reduction by means of stannous chloride or other reducing agent to the corresponding diamino acid; (*c*) iodination with iodine monochloride in acetic acid to the 2,4,6-triiodo derivative; (*d*) acetylation of the amino groups using acetic anhydride.

Description—White, odorless powder.
Solubility—Very slightly soluble in water and alcohol; soluble in dimethylformamide and alkali hydroxide solutions.

Uses—Radiopaque component of *Diatrizoate Meglumine Injection*, *Diatrizoate Meglumine and Diatrizoate Sodium Injection*, *Diatrizoate Sodium Injection*, *Diatrizoate Sodium Oral Solution.*

Iodamide Meglumine

Benzoic acid, 3-(acetylamino)-5-[(acetylamino)methyl]-2,4,6-triiodo-, compound with 1-deoxy-1-(methylamino)-D-glucitol(1:1); Renovue-65, Renovue-Dip (*Squibb*)

α,5-Diacetamido-2,4,6-triiodo-*m*-toluic acid, compound with 1-deoxy-1-(methylamino)-D-glucitol(1:1) [18656-21-8] $C_{12}H_{11}I_3N_2O_4$.$C_7H_{16}NO_5$ (823.16).

Preparation—For the synthesis of iodamic acid see *Helv Chim Acta 48:* 259, 1965; this material is converted to the salt in the same fashion as diatrizoate meglumine previously described.

Uses—A diagnostic agent for *excretion urography* administered either by intravenous infusion (Renovue-Dip) or intravenous injection (Renovue-65). Following either intravenous infusion or injection it is rapidly transported to the kidneys and excreted essentially unchanged, principally by glomerular filtration. However, at least one-third of the intravenous dose is secreted by the renal tubules. Thus, it permits visualization of the kidneys and urinary passages through normal physiologic mechanisms of excretion. There are no absolute contraindications to the use of this diagnostic agent. However, urography should be performed with extreme caution in patients with severe hepatic and renal disease, or anuria. Otherwise, the precautions, adverse effects, and contraindications are similar to those for other iodinated diagnostic agents (see page 1265, this section).

Dose—*Excretory urography:* by *drip IV infusion* − **4.5 mL/kg** (maximum **300 mL**), infused over 10 min period; by *intravenous injection* − **0.8 mL/kg** (maximum **50 mL**) injected within 1 to 2 minutes.

Dosage Forms—IV infusion, 300 mL bottles; IV injection, 50 mL vials.

Iothalamic Acid

Benzoic acid, 3-(acetylamino)-2,4,6-triiodo-5-[(methylamino)carbonyl]-,

5-Acetamido-2,4,6-triiodo-*N*-methylisophthalamic acid [2276-90-6] $C_{11}H_9I_3N_2O_4$ (613.92).

Preparation—By oxidizing *m*-xylene with potassium permanganate, condensing the resulting isophthalic acid with an equimolar quantity of methylamine, and iodinating with iodine monochloride in acetic acid.

Description—White, odorless powder.
Solubility—Slightly soluble in water and alcohol; soluble in solutions of alkali hydroxides.

Uses—Radiopaque component for *Iothalamate Meglumine Injection*, *Iothalamate Meglumine and Iothalamate Sodium Injection*, and *Iothalamate Sodium Injection.*

Iothalamate Meglumine Injection

Benzoic acid, 3-(acetylamino)-2,4,6-triiodo-5-[(methylamino)carbonyl]-, compd with 1-deoxy-1-(methylamino)-D-glucitol (1:1); Conray Cysto-Conray (*Mallinckrodt*)

1-Deoxy-1-(methylamino)-D-glucitol 5-acetamido-2,4,6-triiodo-*N*-methylisophthalamate (salt) [13087-53-1] $C_{11}H_9I_3N_2O_4$.$C_7H_{17}NO_5$ (809.13).

Preparation—Iothalamic acid is reacted with an equimolar quantity of methylglucamine (meglumine), using sufficient water for injection to produce a solution of the required concentration.

Uses—One of the least toxic radiopaque media used parenterally as a 17.2% sterile solution for retrograde *cystography*, and *cystourethrography;* a 30% sterile solution for *intravenous infusion urography* and for contrast enhancement of computed *tomographic brain images;* a 43% sterile solution for use in *venography, infusion urography, retrograde pyelography, cystography, cystourethrography;* a 60% sterile solution for use in *excretory urography, cerebral angiography, peripheral arteriography,* and *venography.* It is contraindicated in patients with a known sensitivity to salts of iothalamic acid and should not be used for urography in patients with anuria. Intravenous urography is hazardous to patients with multiple myeloma; anuria, progressive uremia, renal failure and death have occurred. No form of therapy, including dialysis, has been effective in reversing this effect. The diagnostic agent should also be used with extreme caution in patients with pheochromocytoma and individuals homozygous for sickle cell disease. Iodine-containing contrast agents may also alter the result of thyroid function tests. Adverse effects, precautions, and contraindications are similar to those for other iodinated diagnostic agents (see page 1265, this section). The safety of iothalamate meglumine in pregnancy has not been established.

Dose—As the dosage and concentration of iothalamate meglumine injection vary considerably with the diagnostic uses and techniques of administration of the injection, the *latest* package insert should be consulted for adult and pediatric dosages and other information concerning uses of this diagnostic drug.

Dosage Forms—Injection: 17.2, 30, 43, and 60%.

Iothalamate Meglumine and Iothalamate Sodium Injection

Vascoray (*Mallinckrodt*)

A sterile solution of iothalamic acid in water for injection, prepared with the aid of meglumine and NaOH. It may contain small amounts of suitable buffers and of edetate calcium disodium or edetate disodium as a stabilizer. When intended for intravascular use, it contains no antimicrobial agents.

Description—Clear, colorless to pale yellow, slightly viscous liquid.

Uses—In *intravascular angiocardiography*, *aortography*, selective *renal arteriography*, selective *coronary arteriography*, *renal arteriography*, *excretory urography*, and *computed tomography*. The warnings, contraindications, and adverse effects are the same as for other iodinated diagnostic agents (see page 1265, this section).

Dose—As the dosage of this injection varies with its diagnostic uses and techniques of administration, the *latest* package insert should be consulted for adult and pediatric dosages and other information concerning uses of the injection.

Dosage Form—Injection containing 52% iothalamate meglumine and 26% iothalamate sodium.

Iothalamate Sodium Injection

Benzoic acid, 3-(acetylamino)-2,4,6-triiodo-5-[(methylamino)carbonyl]-, monosodium salt; Conray 325, Conray 400, Angio-Conray (*Mallinckrodt*)

Monosodium 5-acetamido-2,4,6-triiodo-*N*-methylisophthalamate [1225-20-3] $C_{11}H_8I_3N_2NaO_4$ (635.90).

Preparation—Iothalamic acid is reacted with an equimolar quantity of NaOH, using sufficient water for injection to produce a solution of the required concentration.

Uses—For *intravascular angiocardiography*, *aortography*, *excretory urography*, and enhancement of *computerized tomography*. It is contraindicated in cerebral angiography, and in patients with sensitivity to iothalamic acid. Adverse effects and precautions are similar to those for other iodinated diagnostic agents (see page 1265, this section).

Dose—As the dosage and concentration of iothalamate sodium injection vary considerably with the diagnostic uses and techniques of administration of the injection, the *latest* package insert should be consulted for adult and pediatric dosages and other information concerning uses of this diagnostic drug.

Dosage Forms—Injection: 54.3, 66.8, and 80%.

Metrizamide

D-Glucose, 2-[[3-(acetylamino)-5-(acetylmethylamino)-2,4,6-triiodobenzoyl]amino]-2-deoxy-, Amipaque (*Winthrop*)

2-[3-Acetamido-2,4,6-triiodo-5-(*N*-methylacetamido)benzamido]-2-deoxy-D-glucopyranose [31112-62-6] $C_{18}H_{22}I_3N_3O_8$ (789.10).

Preparation—The acyl halide of metrizoic acid (see this page) and glucosamine are reacted under conditions whereby the amine portion of the glucosamine is preferentially acylated in lieu of the hydroxyl groups.

Solubility—Freely soluble in water; protect aqueous solutions from light.

Uses—Metrizamide is a radiopaque agent injected into the subarachnoid space for *lumbar*, *thoracic*, *cervical*, and *total columnar myelography* and *computerized tomography*. It is absorbed from cerebrospinal fluid into the blood stream. Approximately 60% of the administered dose is excreted unchanged through the kidneys within 48 hours. Following subarachnoid injection conventional radiography will continue to provide good diagnostic contrast for at least 30 minutes; after 1 hour the degree of diagnostic contrast is not adequate. Metrizamide should not be given to patients known to be hypersensitive to it. The concurrent administration of corticosteroids and metrizamide is contraindicated. Lumbar puncture should not be

performed in the presence of significant bacteremic infections. This agent should be used with caution in patients with a history of epilepsy, severe cardiovascular disease, chronic alcoholism, or multiple sclerosis. Adverse reactions are similar to those for other iodinated diagnostic agents (see page 1265).

Dose—As the dosage and concentration of Metrizamide injection varies with the diagnostic use and position of the patient, the *latest* package insert should be consulted for concentrations and dosage.

Dosage Forms—3.75 g/20 mL and 6.75 g/50 mL single dose vials.

Tyropanoate Sodium

Benzenepropanoic acid, α-ethyl-2,4,6-triiodo-3-[(1-oxobutyl)amino]-, monosodium salt; Bilopaque Sodium (*Winthrop*)

Sodium 3-butyramido-α-ethyl-2,4,6-triiodohydrocinnamate [7246-21-1] $C_{15}H_{17}I_3NNaO_3$ (663.01).

Preparation—Iopanoic acid is reacted with butyric anhydride in the presence of H_2SO_4 as a catalyst. The reaction product is converted to the sodium salt with NaOH, and purified by recrystallization from a solvent such as isopropanol.

Description—Off-white, odorless, hygroscopic powder with a bitter taste; decomposes on heating.

Solubility—Soluble in water and in alcohol; very slightly soluble in acetone and ether.

Uses—An oral radiopaque agent used in *cholecystography*. Optimal visualization occurs in 10 to 12 hr after oral administration. The drug is contraindicated in patients with advanced hepatorenal disease, severe impairment of renal function, or severe gastrointestinal disease which prevents absorption. Common side effects include nausea, vomiting, abdominal cramps, or discomfort. Other allergic responses characteristic of iodine-containing compounds have been observed (see page 1265, this section). Tyropanoate sodium is not recommended for use in children under 12 years of age. Although no teratogenic effects have been observed in animals, safe use of this agent in pregnant women has not been established.

Dose—*Usual, oral, adult* **3 g** administered with water in a single dose. For best results, drug administration is preceded by a diet containing some fat in order to empty the gallbladder. The meal immediately prior to drug administration should be fat free. If no visualization occurs, the dose is repeated the next day.

Dosage Form—Capsules: 750 mg.

Other Radiopaque Drugs

Metrizoic Acid [3-(Acetylamino)-5-(acetylmethylamino)-2,4,6-triiodo-benzoic acid] [1949-45-7]; $C_{12}H_{11}I_3N_2O_4$ (627.95) Isopaque (*Winthrop*). *Preparation:* Metrizoic acid differs from diatrizoic acid only in having a 5-(acetylmethylamino) group in place of the 5-(acetylamino) group of diatrizoic acid. Synthesis of various triiodinated derivatives of 3-alkylamino-5-aminobenzoic acid, of the type of metrizoic acid, is described by Pitre and Fumigalli, *Farmaco* (Pavia) *Ed Sci* 17: 340, 1962 (see *CA* 58: 8955h, 1963). *Description and Solubility:* White or off-white, crystalline powder; odorless; decomposes and becomes yellow on exposure to light. 1 g in 1200 mL water, 600 mL alcohol; insoluble in chloroform and ether; soluble in solutions of alkali hydroxides and carbonates. *Uses:* Metrizoic acid is a radiopaque agent similar to diatrizoic acid in structure and use. Like diatrizoic acid, it is used as the meglumine and sodium salts, usually with small amounts of calcium or calcium and magnesium metrizoates in the ratio present in human serum, a combination claimed to improve tolerance to the diagnostic agent. Two combination solutions used in the US are described in the following paragraphs. *Meglumine and Calcium Metrizoates Solution:* A sterile, aqueous solution of the meglumine and calcium salts of metrizoic acid. Each mL of the solution supplied as *Isopaque 280* (Winthrop) contains 140.1 mg meglumine, 0.35 mg calcium, and 461.8 mg metrizoic acid; the solution contains approximately 280 mg of organically bound iodine per mL. *Uses:* This solution is indicated for *excretory urography* and for *cerebral angiography* and *peripheral arteriography*. It is contraindicated for myelography and for examination of dorsal cysts or sinuses that might communicate with the subarachnoid space; injection into the subarachnoid space may produce convulsions and result in death. Other warnings and adverse effects are similar to those for other iodinated radiopaque materials (see page 1265, this section). *Dose:* The *latest* package insert should be consulted for dosage and other information. *Dosage Forms:* Vials containing 20, 30, and 50 mL. *Meglumine, Sodium, Calcium and Magnesium Metrizoates Solution:* A sterile, aqueous solution of the meglumine, sodium, calcium, and magnesium salts of metrizoic acid. Each mL of the solution supplied as *Isopaque 440* (Winthrop) contains 75.9 mg meglumine, 16.6 mg sodium, 0.78 mg calcium, 0.15 mg magnesium, and 730 mg metrizoic acid; the solution contains approximately 440 mg of organically bound iodine per mL, and the ratio of calcium to magnesium is similar to that found in normal human serum. *Uses:* This solution is indicated for *angiocardiography* in adults and children and *aortography* and *peripheral arteriography* in adults. Contraindications, precautions, and adverse reactions are similar to those described for *Meglumine and Calcium Metrizoates Solution* and for other iodinated diagnostic agents (see page 1265, this section). *Dose:* The *latest* package insert should be consulted for dosage and other information. *Dosage Form:* Vials containing 50 mL.

Drugs Used to Test Organ Function

The classic studies of Abed and Rowntree in 1909 demonstrated that parenterally administered phenoltetrachlorophthalein was excreted only in the bile, while phenolsulfonphthalein was excreted almost exclusively in the urine. These findings were promptly adopted by Rowntree and his associates as a means of testing liver and kidney function. The importance of these early observations is attested by the several drugs that are now commonly used to test organ function. Described in this section are those drugs used to test liver, kidney, and gastric function.

Sodium Iodide I 131 Capsules—page 495.
Sodium Iodide I 131 Solution—page 495.

Drugs Used to Test Liver Function

Unfortunately, available methods for estimating the extent of liver damage by various measurements of decreased liver function are still comparatively unsatisfactory. The liver itself has such a large reserve of functional capacity that most methods of determining decreased function do not reveal such a state until 70 to 90% of the liver cells have been damaged. Most liver function tests involve the intravenous injection of a standardized amount of substance, such as bilirubin, rose bengal, or sulfobromophthalein, agents which depend almost wholly on the liver for excretion. The rate of clearance of the substance from the plasma becomes a measure of the excretory capacity of the liver.

Indocyanine Green

1*H*-Benz[*e*]indolium, 2-[7-[1,3-dihydro-1,1-dimethyl-3-(4-sulfobutyl)-2*H*-benz[*e*]indol-2-ylidene]-1,3,5-heptatrienyl]-1,1-dimethyl-3-(4-sulfobutyl)-, hydroxide, inner salt, sodium salt;
Cardio-Green (*Hynson, Westcott & Dunning*)

2-[7-[1,1-Dimethyl-3-(4-sulfobutyl)benz[*e*]indol-2-ylidene]-1,3,5-heptatrienyl] -1,1-dimethyl-3-(4-sulfobutyl) -1*H*-benz[*e*]indolium hydroxide, inner salt, sodium salt [3599-32-4] $C_{43}H_{47}N_2NaO_6S_2$ (774.96).

Preparation—By reacting 1,1,2-trimethyl-3-(4-sulfobutyl)-1*H*-benz[*e*]indolium hydroxide inner salt (I) with a bis(Schiff base) derived from glutaconic aldehyde. The starting indolium compound I is prepared by heating 1,1,2-trimethyl-1*H*-benz[*e*]indole with 4-hydroxy-1-butanesulfonic acid δ-sultone. Details for preparing these tricarbocyanine dyes are provided in US Pats 2,251,286 and 2,895,955.

Description—Dark green, blue-green, olive brown, dark blue, or black powder; odorless or with a slight odor; solutions are deep emerald-green in color; pH (1 in 200 solution) about 6; unstable in solution.
Solubility—Soluble in water and methanol; practically insoluble in most other organic solvents.

Uses—To determine *cardiac output*, *hepatic function*, and *liver blood flow*, and for *ophthalmic angiography*. Following intravenous injection, the distribution volume is relatively constant among individuals and approximates that of plasma volume, because tissue binding is negligible and the fraction of unbound drug in blood is very small. Indeed, indocyanine green is so highly bound to plasma proteins, particularly alpha lipoproteins, that it does not distribute extravascularly and its clearance is not limited by binding. The intrinsic clearance of bound and unbound drug is high, hepatic extraction ratios in man vary from 50 to 80%. It is not metabolized, but is entirely eliminated by active uptake into hepatic parenchymal cells. It is then transported to bile and once excreted in the small intestine is not reabsorbed; consequently, it imparts a green color to the stool. These properties, together with low toxicity and easy measurement in plasma, have made it a commonly used indicator for the measurement of liver blood flow.

For hepatic function studies, the calculated amount of the diagnostic agent is injected into an arm vein. Twenty minutes after injection, 6 mL of venous blood is withdrawn from the opposite arm. After coagulation and centrifugation, the clear serum is read in a photometer at 800 to 810 nm. A dye retention of less than 4% is found in healthy subjects. Failure to remove the dye, as indicated by serum levels in excess of 4%, is indicative of impaired hepatic function. Indocyanine green contains a small amount of sodium iodide; thus, it should be used with caution in patients allergic to iodides and radioactive iodine uptake studies should not be performed for at least one week following its use. Since probenecid has been shown in dogs to affect hepatic uptake, this possibility should be kept in mind. The safe use of this drug in pregnancy has not been established.

Dose—*Usual, adult, intravenous, cardiac output determination, via cardiac catheter,* **5 mg** in **1 mL;** *children,* **2.5 mL** in **1 mL;** *infants,* **1.25 mg** in **1 mL**. *Hepatic function determination,* **0.5 mg/kg**. *Ophthalmic angiography,* **40 mg** in **2 mL**.

Dosage Forms—Sterile: 25 and 50 mg vials; 10 and 40 mg disposable units.

Sodium Benzoate—page 1169.

Sulfobromophthalein Sodium

Benzenesulfonic acid, 3,3′-(4,5,6,7-tetrabromo-3-oxo-1(3*H*)-isobenzofuranylidene)bis[6-hydroxy-, disodium salt; Bromsulphalein R Sodium; Bromtetragnost; B.S.P.;
Bromsulphalein (*Hynson, Westcott & Dunning*)

4,5,6,7-Tetrabromo-3′,3″-disulfophenolphthalein disodium salt [71-67-0] $C_{20}H_8Br_4Na_2O_{10}S_2$ (837.99).

Preparation—Tetrabromophthalic anhydride, made by brominating phthalic anhydride in alkaline solution and precipitating with acid, is condensed with phenol. The resulting phenoltetrabromophthalein is sulfonated with sulfuric acid, and the disulfonic acid so obtained converted into the sodium salt with sodium carbonate.

Description—White, crystalline powder; odorless, has a bitter taste, and is hygroscopic.
Solubility—Soluble in water; insoluble in alcohol and acetone.

Uses—One of the best agents for testing *liver function*. It is injected intravenously and 30 min later a sample of blood is drawn and the dye content of the alkalinized serum is compared with a series of standards. The normal liver excretes most of the dye within a period of 30 min. Sulfobromophthalein should be used with caution in patients where a previous paravascular infiltration has occurred, in known asthmatics, and in patients with a history of allergy or urticaria.
Dose—*Usual, intravenous,* **5 mg/kg** (500 mg maximum); *usual dose range,* **2** to **5 mg/kg** body weight.
Dosage Form—Injection: 50 mg/mL.

Other Drugs Used to Test Liver Function

Galactose [$C_6H_{12}O_6.H_2O$]—First prepared by Pasteur in 1856 from milk sugar. Occurs as a component of pectins, gums, and mucilages. Obtained by hydrolysis of milk sugar. Colorless or white crystals. Melts at 118° to 120°, 165° when anhydrous. Soluble in about 3.5 parts of water; soluble in pyridine; slightly soluble in alcohol. *Uses:* For diagnosing hepatic function. The patient takes 40 g galactose in 420 mL tea in the morning and fasts until urine has been passed every hour for 4 hours. The sugar in the urine is then quantitatively determined.

Phenoltetrachlorophthalein [$C_{20}H_{10}Cl_4O_4$]—Formed by the condensation of phenol and tetrachlorophthalic acid or its anhydride. *Uses:* For the determination of functional activity of the liver; excretion is determined by disappearance from the blood stream, excretion in the duodenum by means of a duodenal tube, or excretion in the stool. Sodium salt given intravenously; should not be given subcutaneously or intramuscularly. *Dose: Intravenous,* 5 mg/kg.

Drugs Used to Test Kidney Function

The rate of excretion of a number of drugs in the urine has been proposed as a means of measuring the functional capacity of the kidney. Glomerular filtration rate can be measured by the renal plasma clearance of inulin, thiosulfate, mannitol, or endogenous creatinine. The inulin clearance is thought to be most reliable since mannitol is subject to some tubular reabsorption, thiosulfate to some tubular excretion and reabsorption, and endogenous creatinine to some tubular excretion. Effective renal plasma flow and tubular functional capacity can be measured by the use of sodium aminohippurate and iodohippurate. Because of the greater accuracy and facility of chemical methods for the determination of the compound, sodium aminohippurate is considered the drug of choice. Although the excretion of phenolsulfonphthalein is accomplished by the same mechanisms as the excretion of sodium aminohippurate, its plasma clearance averages about two-thirds of the effective renal plasma flow, and its toxicity prevents its use for the determination of functioning tubular capacity.

Aminohippurate Sodium

Glycine, *N*-(4-aminobenzoyl)-, monosodium salt; (*MSD*)

Monosodium *p*-aminohippurate [94-16-6] $C_9H_9N_2NaO_3$ (216.17).

Preparation—By reacting *p*-aminohippuric acid with NaOH and adjusting the pH of the resulting solution to 7 to 7.2 with citric acid. In preparing the injection, the salt is not isolated from the solution.

Uses—A *diagnostic aid (kidney function).* See *Aminohippuric Acid.*

Dose—*Usual, intravenous,* **2 g.**

Dosage Forms—Injection: 2 g/10 mL, 10 g/50 mL.

Aminohippuric Acid

Glycine, *N*-(4-aminobenzoyl)-, PAH; PAHA; *N*-(*p*-Aminobenzoyl)glycine

p-Aminohippuric acid [61-78-9] $C_9H_{10}N_2O_3$ (194.19).

Preparation—By reacting *p*-nitrobenzoyl chloride with glycine and then reducing the *p*-nitro group with tin and HCl.

Description—White, crystalline powder; discolors in light; melts at about 195°, with decomposition.

Solubility—1 g in 45 mL water, 50 mL alcohol, and 5 mL diluted HCl; very slightly soluble in chloroform, and ether; freely soluble in solutions of alkali hydroxides or carbonates with some decomposition.

Uses—Aminohippuric acid (PAH) is secreted into the urine by the renal tubules. The capacity of the tubules to transport this acid (the transport maximum or *Tm*) is limited and measurement of this *Tm* is employed as a *diagnostic aid in evaluating kidney function.* The *Tm* of PAH and other compounds such as penicillin and probenecid is mutually lowered since all employ the same excretory mechanism, ie, all compete for an essential intermediary in the tubular transport system. *Probenecid* (page 944), for example, lessens renal tubular

transport of penicillin and thus maintains efficient blood levels of the antibiotic. Similarly, the excretion of other diagnostic agents, e.g., phenolsulfonphthalein, may be depressed by PAH.

Known quantities (sufficient to produce 2 mg/100 mL of blood plasma) of PAH are administered intravenously to the patient. The urine formed during a definite but short period is collected and the average amount of PAH eliminated is calculated in mg/min. This value divided by the PAH plasma content in mg/mL is equivalent to the *effective renal plasma flow* in mL/min. The normal rate for men is 697 ± 136 mL/min and for women 594 ± 102 mL.

To determine *tubular excretory mass,* a sterile solution of the sodium salt of PAH is injected intravenously in a volume sufficient to "saturate" the capacity of the tubular cells to excrete PAH (above 60 mg/100 mL of plasma), and the PAH content of the plasma is determined in mg/mL. The amount excreted in urine is determined in mg/min, this value including both glomerular filtration and tubular excretion. The glomerular filtration rate, using *Mannitol* (page 935), is determined in mg/min. From the glomerular filtration rate and the PAH content per mL of plasma is calculated the amount of PAH that was filtered through the glomeruli in one minute (mL/min × mg/mL). Then the total number of mg/min excreted in the urine minus the amount filtered through the glomeruli per minute equals the amount of PAH in mg/min excreted by the tubules (tubular excretory mass or *Tm*). The mean normal value for both men and women is 77.5 ± 13 mg/min.

Indigotindisulfonate Sodium

1*H*-Indole-5-sulfonic acid, 2-(1,3-dihydro-3-oxo-5-sulfo-2*H*-indol-2-ylidene)-2,3-dihydro-3-oxo-, disodium salt; Soluble Indigo Blue; Indigo Carmine

Disodium 3,3′-dioxo[$\Delta^{2,2'}$-biindoline]-5,5′-disulfonate [860-22-0] $C_{16}H_8N_2Na_2O_8S_2$ (466.35).

Preparation—Anthranilic acid is treated with chloroacetic acid to form phenylglycine-*o*-carboxylic acid. The latter is fused with KOH or NaOH and the resulting indoxylacetic acid loses carbon dioxide to form *indoxyl,* which is oxidized by air to *indigo blue.* Indigo carmine is prepared from indigo blue by sulfonating with H_2SO_4 and neutralizing the SO_3H groups with sodium carbonate.

Description—Dusky, purplish blue powder, or blue granules with a coppery luster; affected by light; solutions have a blue or bluish purple color.

Solubility—1 g in about 100 mL water; slightly soluble in alcohol; practically insoluble in most other organic solvents.

Uses—In a *kidney function test.* This dye usually appears in the urine in 10 min after intravenous injection and is entirely excreted within 3 hours. The rate of excretion of the dye in the urine after injection (usually intravenously) is determined colorimetrically by comparison of the color of the urine with color standards. Occasionally an allergic-type of idiosyncratic response has occurred. Patients with a history of allergy should be tested for sensitivity before the drug is given. Indigo carmine is also employed as a *reagent,* as a *stain* for microscopic specimens, and as a *dye.*

Dose—*Usual, intravenous,* **40 mg**; *usual, intramuscular,* **50 to 100 mg.**

Dosage Form—Injection: 40 mg/5 mL.

Inulin

(Arnar-Stone)

Inulin [9005-80-5] $C_6H_{11}O_5(C_6H_{10}O_5)_nOH$. A substance, occurring in some plants of the *Compositae* family, closely allied to starch except that it is a levulan rather than a dextran. It differs from starch in the following particulars: it is colored yellow by iodine, does not gelatinize with water, and is not found in plants in the form of granules having concentric layers. When hydrolyzed with acid, fructose is produced.

Preparation—Isolated from various *Compositae* members, eg, Inula, Taraxacum, Pyrethrum, Lappa, etc.

Uses—Inulin is filtered only by the glomeruli and is neither secreted nor reabsorbed by the tubules. Therefore, it is used as a *diagnostic agent for evaluation of glomerular filtration*. Usually, the patient is hydrated with 1000 mL of water followed by 200 mL every 30 min until the test is completed. Two hours following the first intake of water, a control blood sample is taken, the inulin is administered intravenously, and the exact time noted. One hour later the bladder is emptied, the urine discarded, the time noted, a blood sample taken, and the time once more noted. Urine and blood samples are then collected hourly for 2 hours. The samples are analyzed for inulin. Appropriate calculations are then made. Although considerable variation occurs, normal clearance values are 130 ± 20 mL/min in the male and 120 ± 15 mL/min in the female. Untoward reactions are infrequent and usually mild.

Dose—*Usual, intravenous*, **10 g** dissolved in 100 mL sodium chloride injection and injected at the rate of 10 mL/min.

Dosage Form—Injection: 5 g/50 mL.

Iodohippurate Sodium I 131—page 492.
Iodohippurate Sodium I 131 Injection—page 492.
Mannitol—page 935.

Phenolsulfonphthalein

Phenol, 4,4′-(3*H*-2,1-benzoxathiol-3-ylidene)bis-, (*S,S*-dioxide); Phenol Red; P.S.P.; Sulfonphthal

4,4′-(3*H*-2,1-Benzoxathiol-3-ylidene)diphenol *S,S*-dioxide [143-74-8] $C_{19}H_{14}O_5S$ (354.38).

Preparation—By fusing the anhydride of *o*-sulfobenzoic acid with phenol. The *o*-sulfobenzoic anhydride may be obtained by heating the acid with phosphorus pentoxide.

Description—Crystalline powder, varying in color from bright to dark red; stable in air.

Solubility—1 g in about 1300 mL water, and about 350 mL alcohol and about 500 mL acetone; almost insoluble in chloroform and ether; freely soluble in solutions of alkali hydroxides and their carbonates.

Uses—A *diagnostic aid* used for determining *kidney function*. When injected intramuscularly or intravenously, it begins to be excreted in patients with normal kidneys in from 5 to 10 min. In patients with deficient renal function, the first appearance of its secretion is delayed. In normal cases, after intramuscular injection, almost the total amount (from 60 to 80%) is excreted within 2 hours. Failure to excrete nearly the full amount within 2 hours indicates a deficient functional activity, and the degree of this functional deficiency may be estimated by the proportionate amount excreted within 2 hours. The average normal eliminations after intravenous administration are from 35 to 45% in 15 min, from 50 to 65% in 30 min, and from 65 to 80% in the first hour.

From 20 to 30 min before the test, the patient is given 300 to 400 mL of water to insure free urinary excretion; otherwise delayed appearance may be due to lack of excretion.

Under aseptic precautions a catheter is introduced and the bladder is completely emptied, or the patient is allowed to empty it voluntarily. The time is noted, and 1 mL of a solution of phenolsulfonphthalein containing 6 mg/mL is administered intramuscularly into the lumbar muscles, or intravenously, by means of a graduated syringe. Care must be taken that all of the solution is injected.

The urine is allowed to drain into a test tube containing a drop of 25% NaOH solution, and the time of appearance of the first faint pinkish tinge is noted.

In patients having no urinary obstruction, the catheter is withdrawn at the time of appearance of the drug in the urine. If injection is made *intramuscularly*, the patient is instructed to void into a receptacle

at the end of 1 hour and 10 min, and into a second receptacle at the end of the second hour. If injection is made *intravenously*, the patient is instructed to void into a receptacle at the end of 15 or 30 min or 1 hour.

The urine collected is made alkaline with a 25% solution of NaOH and then diluted to 1 L; a small filtered portion is taken to compare with the standard used for all estimations. Comparison is made in a colorimeter devised for this purpose.

Dose—*Usual, intramuscular* or *intravenous*, **6 mg.**

Dosage Form—Injection (see below): 6 mg/1 mL.

Phenolsulfonphthalein Injection—*Preparation*: It may be prepared by the USP XV procedure, using proportional quantities of phenolsulfonphthalein and sodium bicarbonate for other concentrations.

To phenolsulfonphthalein (6 g) contained in a beaker of about 500-mL capacity, add water for injection (100 mL), then dissolve sodium bicarbonate (1.43 g), added in small portions, by stirring. Add sodium chloride (9 g), and boil the mixture gently until the volume of the solution has been reduced to about 70 mL. Filter through a pledget of sterile cotton into a suitable flask, and wash the filter with water for injection. Dilute to about 950 mL with water for injection, and test the solution for sensitiveness (as directed in the USP). If necessary, adjust the solution so that it will conform to the test for sensitiveness by adding sufficient weak solution of sodium hydroxide. Then dilute with water for injection to 1000 mL, mix well, distribute into suitable containers, and sterilize. *Note*: The 1.43 g of sodium bicarbonate may be replaced by 17 mL of 1 *N* NaOH.

Drugs Used to Test Gastric Function

In some clinical situations it is important to know whether the stomach can secrete hydrochloric acid. Proof of the absence of hydrochloric acid in the stomach is essential to the diagnosis of pernicious anemia and, in some circumstances, offers presumptive evidence of gastric cancer. On the other hand, the presence of hydrochloric acid contributes to the diagnosis of peptic ulcer and peptic esophagitis, which conversely can be virtually excluded by the demonstration of true achlorhydria.

Because the volume of acid secreted by the normal stomach covers the entire range of volume encountered in disease and because there is no sharp line of demarcation in the secretory capacity of the stomach variously diseased, the quantity of acid secreted even in response to a controlled stimulus is seldom of any diagnostic importance. Therefore, it is usually important only to establish the presence or absence of free hydrochloric acid in the stomach. The gastric stimulants included in this section and those listed below are frequently of value for this purpose.

Alcohol—page 1159.
Betazole Hydrochloride—page 1124.
Caffeine—page 1133.
Caffeine and Sodium Benzoate—page 1135.
Histamine Phosphate—page 1125.

Pentagastrin

L-Phenylalaninamide, *N*-[(1,1-dimethylethoxy)carbonyl]-
β-alanyl-L-tryptophyl-L-methionyl-L-α-aspartyl-, Peptavlon (*Ayerst*)

$$N\text{-}(CH_3)_3COC\overset{O}{\overset{\|}{-}}\beta Ala\text{-}Trp\text{-}Met\text{-}Asp\text{-}Phe\text{-}NH_2$$

N-Carboxy-β-alanyl-L-tryptophyl-L-methionyl-L-aspartylphenyl-L-alaninamide *N-tert*-butyl ester [5534-95-2] $C_{37}H_{49}N_7O_9S$ (767.90).

Description—Fine colorless needles melting about 230° with decomposition.

Solubility—Soluble in dimethyl sulfoxide and dimethylformamide; slightly soluble in alcohol and dilute solutions of ammonia; practically insoluble in water, ether or benzene.

Uses—A diagnostic agent used to evaluate gastric acid secretory function. It is useful in testing for *anacidity* in patients with suspected pernicious anemia, atrophic gastritis, or gastric carcinoma; for *hypersecretion* in patients with possible duodenal ulcer or postoperative stomal ulcer, for the diagnosis of Zollinger-Ellison tumor; and for determining the adequacy of acid reducing operations for peptic ulcer. Acid secretion is increased within 10 min after a subcutaneous injection of pentagastrin and reaches a peak in most patients within 20 to 30 min. Excessive doses may inhibit gastric acid secretion. Pentagastrin is contraindicated in patients hypersensitive to the drug. Likewise, it should be used with caution in patients with pancreatic, hepatic, or biliary disease. Adverse reactions include abdominal pain, nausea, vomiting, flushing, tachycardia, dizziness, faintness, lightheadedness, drowsiness, blurred vision, and headache. The use of pentagastrin in pregnant women and children has not been studied.

Dose—*Usual, subcutaneous, adult:* **6 mcg/kg.**
Dosage Forms—0.25 mg (250 μg) per mL in 2 mL ampules.

Drugs Used to Determine Blood Volume

The estimation of blood volume is important in detecting impending shock and as a guide to the amount of plasma or other fluids to be used in order to avoid inadequate or excessive dosage. Certain radioisotopes (see Chapter 29), are used for the determination of blood volume, as is the dye Evans Blue, described hereunder.

Evans Blue

1,3-Naphthalenedisulfonic acid, 6,6'-[(3,3'-dimethyl[1,1'-biphenyl]-4,4'-diyl)-bis(azo)]bis[4-amino-5-hydroxy]-, tetrasodium salt

C.I. direct blue 53 tetrasodium salt [314-13-6] $C_{34}H_{24}N_6Na_4O_{14}S_4$ (960.79).

Preparation—By diazotizing *o*-tolidine and coupling the resulting diazo compound with 1-amino-8-naphthol-2,4-disulfonic acid.

Description—Green, bluish green, or brown powder; odorless; the dried product is hygroscopic; exhibits a maximum absorbance at about 610 nm.

Solubility—Very soluble in water; very slightly soluble in alcohol; practically insoluble in benzene, carbon tetrachloride, ether, and chloroform.

Uses—A *diagnostic agent* employed in *blood volume estimation.* A known quantity of the dye is quantitatively injected into the blood stream. It combines firmly with plasma protein and remains within the intravascular compartment. After allowing time for thorough mixing, withdrawal of a sample of blood and determination of the concentration of the dye in the sample enables the clinician to calculate the volume of blood in the patient. No adverse effects—either acute or chronic—have been reported. Massive doses stain the sclerae and skin; disappear over a period of several weeks.

Dose—*Usual, intravenous,* 2 to 4 mL of injection containing 4.52 mg dried Evans Blue/mL.
Dosage Forms—Injection: 22.6 mg/5 mL.

Miscellaneous Diagnostic Drugs

A number of drugs have useful diagnostic applications. Others, such as ceruletide diethylamine and cholecystokinin are useful as adjuncts in cholecystokinetic cholecystography. These diagnostic aids are described herein. Some agents, such as fluorescein sodium, guaiac, and congo red, are used either as reagent solutions or reagent strips primarily for diagnostic purposes, whereas other drugs exert major pharmacological actions which are described in other chapters of this text, but are also used more or less incidentally for certain specific diagnostic tests. Phentolamine, piperoxan, phenoxybenzamine, and tetraethylammonium chloride are used in the differential diagnosis of hypertension and pheochromocytoma. The vasoconstrictor ergot alkaloids are useful adjuncts in the determination of coronary function. Edrophonium chloride, quinine sulfate, and neostigmine are employed in the diagnosis of myasthenia gravis, and the latter drug is sometimes used in a pregnancy test. Sodium Phos-

phate P 32 is used for the diagnosis and localization of brain and intraocular tumors. Although most of these applications are mentioned in the monograph for each drug, they are mentioned here as a reminder of these uses.

Arginine—page 1027.
Dehydrocholate Sodium—page 799.

Ceruletide Diethylamine

Caerulin compound with *N*-ethylethaneamine; Tymtran (*Adria*)

5-Oxo-L-prolyl-L-glutaminyl-L-α-aspartyl-*O*-sulfo-L-tyrosyl-L-threonylglycyl-L-tryptophyl-L-methionyl-L-α-aspartyl-L-phenylalaninamide compound with *N*-ethylethaneamine [71247-25-1] $C_{58}H_{73}N_{13}O_{21}S_2 \cdot x C_4H_{11}N$ (1352.41 − free acid; the diethylamine salt is not a true stoichiometric compound and the composition varies to contain from 1 to 3 moles of the base).

Preparation—The free acid has been isolated from the skin of the Australian tree toad, *Hyla caerulea* as described in *Experientia 23:* 700, 1967. The salt is formed on treatment with diethylamine.

Uses—As an aid in oral *cholecystokinetic cholecystography* whenever contraction of the gallbladder would facilitate diagnostic visualization, particularly when the gallbladder is opacified or in any way obscured. This drug is qualitatively identical to cholecystokinin. It contracts the gallbladder, stimulates pancreatic exocrine and gastric secretion, delays gastric emptying, inhibits motility of the proximal duodenum, and stimulates motility of the distal duodenum, jejunum, ileum, and to a lesser extent, the colon. Gallbladder contraction is evident 10 minutes after IM injection and contraction exceeding 40% occurs within 15 to 20 minutes. Adverse reactions are usually mild and of brief duration. Abdominal pain or cramps and nausea occur in about 10% of patients. Other systemic effects include eructation, regurgitation, weakness, flushing, dizziness, hypotension, diarrhea, sweating, an urge to defecate and urinate, hiccoughs and gas. Safe use in pregnant women, lactating mothers, and children has not been established.

Dose—0.3 mcg/kg, IM.
Dosage Forms—*Injection:* 40 mcg (20 mcg/mL) in 2 mL amps.

Cholecystokinin

CCK (*Pharmacia*)

Pancreozymin [9011-97-6]. A polypeptide isolated from the mucosa of the intestine which induces contraction and emptying of the gall bladder. Porcine cholecystokinin contains 33 peptide residues; the *C*-terminal peptide is identical to cerulitide (*Eur J Biochem 6:* 156, 1968). Both the *C*-terminal dodecapeptide and the *N*-terminal hexapeptide have been synthesized; see *J Org Chem 37:* 2303, 1972.

Uses—As adjunctive therapy in *cholecystography,* preoperative and secondary *cholangiography,* and X-ray studies of the small bowel. Adverse effects are rare. If the drug is given too rapidly, flushing may occur. See Ceruletide Diethylamine, page 1274.

Dose—*Intravenous:* **1 to 75 IDU** (see package insert).
Dosage Form—Powder for injection: 75 Ivy Doz Units/vial.

Congo Red

1-Naphthalenesulfonic acid, 3,3'-[[1,1'-biphenyl]-4,4'-diylbis(azo)]bis[4-amino-, disodium salt; Direct Red

C. I. direct red 28 disodium salt [573-58-0] $C_{32}H_{22}N_6Na_2O_6S_2$ (696.67).

Preparation—Benzidine is doubly diazotized and coupled with

4-amino-1-naphthalenesulfonic acid. The resulting bisazo acid is then converted to the disodium salt.

Description—Dark red or reddish brown powder; odorless and decomposes on exposure to acid fumes; solutions have a pH of 8 to 9.5.

Solubility—1 g in about 30 mL water; slightly soluble in alcohol; practically insoluble in ether.

Uses—Has been used in a wide variety of diagnostic tests. However, it is recognized only for its use in the detection of *amyloidosis*. As much as 80% of an injected dose can be retained by the abnormal amyloid deposit. Thus, the dye will disappear more rapidly from the blood of affected patients than it does from the normal individual. In amyloid growths in the liver, no dye appears in the urine; in amyloid growths in the kidneys, substantial amounts appear in the urine. The drug should be injected slowly to prevent thrombosis. Except for rare idiosyncratic reactions which may cause death, the drug is relatively free from toxic effects.

Dose—*Intravenous*, **100 to 200 mg** as a 1% solution in water for injection.

Dosage Form—Injection: 1%.

Edrophonium Chloride—page 899.

Erythrosine Sodium

Spiro[isobenzofuran-1(3*H*),9′-[9*H*]xanthen]-3-one, 3′,6′-dihydroxy-2′,4′,5′,7′-tetraiodo-, disodium salt; Trace (*Lorvic*)

2′,4′,5′,7′-Tetraiodofluorescein disodium salt monohydrate [49746-10-3] (897.88); *anhydrous* [568-63-8 or 16423-68-0] $C_{20}H_6$-$I_4Na_2O_5$ (879.86); a dye consisting principally of erythrosine sodium, with smaller amounts of lower iodinated fluoresceins; contains not less than 87% of erythrosine sodium.

Preparation—Fluorescein is dissolved in NaOH solution and treated with iodine in KI solution.

Description—Odorless, red or brownish red powder, which dissolves in water to form a bluish red solution that shows no fluorescence in ordinary light.

Solubility—Soluble in water, glycerin, and propylene glycol; sparingly soluble in alcohol; insoluble in fats and oils.

Uses—Dental disclosing agent used to identify areas of plaque on the teeth. When the solution is applied topically to the teeth or the tablets chewed, areas of plaque to be removed are colored red. The identified plaque is removed and the test repeated as necessary.

Dose—For *external use*, apply **solution** *topically* to the teeth or chew **1 tablet** thoroughly. Following use, rinse the mouth with water. Do not swallow.

Dosage Forms—Solution: 2%; Tablets: 3.5 and 8.5 mg.

Fluorescein Sodium

Spiro[isobenzofuran-1(3*H*),9′-[9*H*]xanthene]-3-one, 3′,6′-dihydroxy-, disodium salt; Soluble Fluorescein; Resorcinolphthalein Sodium; Uranin; Uranine Yellow

Fluorescein disodium salt [518-47-8] $C_{20}H_{10}Na_2O_5$ (376.28).

Preparation—By heating resorcinol with phthalic anhydride at about 200°. After purifying, the phthalein is dissolved in the required amount of sodium hydroxide solution and evaporated to dryness.

Description—Orange-red, odorless powder; hygroscopic; aqueous solution is strongly fluorescent even in extreme dilution; the fluorescence disappears when the solution is made acid, and reappears when the solution is again made alkaline.

Solubility—Freely soluble in water; sparingly soluble in alcohol.

Uses—Either as an ophthalmic strip or as a 2% aqueous solution as an ophthalmic *diagnostic aid*. It is applied topically for the diagnosis of *corneal lesions*, pressure points on the surface of the cornea under contact lenses, and the detection of minute *foreign bodies* embedded in the cornea. While a weak solution of fluorescein will not stain the normal cornea, ulcers or parts deprived of epithelium and pressure points will become green and remain so for a time; foreign bodies will appear surrounded by a green ring; loss of substance in the conjunctiva is indicated by a yellow hue. Fluorescein also reveals defects or disease of the endothelium of the cornea, producing a deep coloration of the diseased area. It is also used to outline and demarcate *tumors*, particularly in the central nervous system. Fluorescein sodium is sometimes used intravenously as a diagnostic aid for various purposes, particularly to determine circulation time (see *Fluorescein Sodium Injection*, below).

In using sodium fluorescein in the eye, it is particularly important that the preparation be sterile and that no accidental contamination of the solution with *Pseudomonas aeruginosa* take place. A diseased or injured eye is readily infected with this organism that can cause blindness. Fluorescein sodium, being anionic, is not compatible with preservatives such as benzalkonium chloride or substances known to be effective against *Pseudomonas aeruginosa*, such as polymyxin B sulfate. The solution is best used as a unit-dose package or dispensed from a container which protects the contents from contamination. It is also available as paper strips impregnated with sodium fluorescein which are dried, heat-sterilized, and packaged in hermetically sealed unit-dose packets. One of these dipped into the lacrimal fluid of the eye to be examined releases enough of the highly soluble drug to permit examination of the eye for lesions or injury.

Dose—*Topical*, **0.1 to 0.3 mL** of a 2% solution, to the conjunctiva. *Ophthalmic strip*, moistened with sterile water and applied to conjunctiva.

Dosage Forms—Injection (see below); 5 and 10%; Ophthalmic Strips: 0.6, 1, and 9 mg.

Fluorescein Sodium Injection [Fluorescite (*Alcon*); Funduscein (*Smith, Miller and Patch*)]—*Uses*: A diagnostic aid in *ophthalmic angiography* which includes examination of the fundus, evaluation of the iris vasculature, distinction between viable and nonviable tissue, and observation of the aqueous flow. It is useful in the differential diagnosis of malignant and nonmalignant ocular tumors. Fluorescein sodium injection is also used to determine *circulation time* and *circulation adequacy*. To determine circulation time, 5 mL of the injection is administered rapidly via the antecubital vein; the lips of the patient are viewed under longwave ultraviolet light and the time from the injection to the time the lips acquire a greenish yellow hue noted. The circulation time in adults varies from 15 to 20 sec; the circulation time is prolonged in right heart failure and hypothyroidism; it is shortened in hyperthyroidism and anemia, but is essentially normal in bronchial asthma. Adverse reactions include cardiac arrest, basilar artery ischemia, severe shock, and thrombophlebitis at the site of injection. Transient nausea, vomiting, and allergic reactions have been reported in sensitive patients. A strong taste may develop following high dosage. Epinephrine 1:1000 and antihistamines should be available for use in event of an emergency. *Dose: Usual, adult, intravenous*, for *determination of circulation time*, 500 mg as a 10% solution injected rapidly in the antecubital vein (doses up to 1250 mg have been well tolerated); *usual, pediatric, intravenous*, 15.4 mg per kg of body weight, as a 5% solution.

Methacholine Chloride—RPS-16, page 837.

Gonadorelin Hydrochloride

Factrel (*Ayerst*)

5-oxoPro-His-Trp-Ser-Tyr-Gly-Leu-Arg-Pro-Gly-NH$_2$ · xC$_2$H$_4$O$_2$ · yH$_2$O
  1   2   3   4   5   6   7   8   9   10

Leutinizing hormone-releasing factor hydrochloride [51952-41-1] $C_{55}H_{75}N_{17}O.x$HCl (1182.33; free base − the *hydrochloride* may be either the mono- or dihydrochloride or a mixture thereof).

Preparation—Isolated from the hypothalamus of pigs or sheep. The industrial preparation is described in German Pat 2,213,737.

Description—The base is a white to very pale yellowish powder containing not less than 85% of active peptide and not more than 6% acetic acid.

Uses—Diagnostic agent used for evaluating *hypothalamic-pituitary gonadotropic* function. The test should be conducted in the absence of other drugs which directly effect pituitary secretion of the gonadotropins, including preparations that contain androgens, estrogens, progestins, or glucocorticoids. Adverse reactions include headache, nausea, lightheadedness, abdominal discomfort, and flushing. Localized swelling may occur at the site of injection. Safety for use during pregnancy has not been established.

Dose—*Subcutaneous or intravenous:* **100 mcg.** (See latest package insert).

Dosage Form—Powder for injection: 100 and 500 μg (as HCl) per vial (accompanied by 2 mL amp. of 2% benzyl alcohol and water for injection).

Metyrapone

1-Propanone, 2-methyl-1,2-di-3-pyridinyl-,
Metopirone (*Ciba-Geigy*)

2-Methyl-1,2-di-3-pyridyl-1-propanone [54-36-4] $C_{14}H_{14}N_2O$ (226.28).

Preparation—Methyl 3-pyridyl ketone is electrolytically reduced to the corresponding pinacol, 2,3-bis(3-pyridyl)-2,3-butanediol; heating with a strong inorganic acid results in dehydration of the pinacol with subsequent rearrangement to form metyrapone. US Pat 2,966,493.

Description—White to light amber, fine, crystalline powder, having a characteristic odor; darkens on exposure to light.

Solubility—Sparingly soluble in water; soluble in methanol and chloroform; forms water-soluble salts with acids.

Uses—A synthetic compound that has the unique ability to inhibit 11-beta-hydroxylation in the biosynthesis of cortisol, corticosterone, and aldosterone. Hence, it is used to test for *hypothalamic-pituitary* function. In the normal individual, metyrapone blocks the enzymatic step that leads to cortisol and corticosterone synthesis, produces an intense stimulation of ACTH secretion, and induces a marked increase in urinary excretion of 17-hydroxycorticosteroids. In patients with abnormal pituitary function, the ability to increase ACTH production is lacking and no significant increase in 17-hydroxycorticosteroids is seen. The drug is particularly valuable as a diagnostic aid in patients suspect of hypopituitarism and Cushing's syndrome. Metyrapone has a $T_{1/2}$ of about 20–26 min. The drug is rapidly metabolized in the liver and excreted by the kidneys. Untoward effects include anorexia, nausea, abdominal discomfort, diarrhea, dizziness, vertigo, headache, sedation, and allergic rash. The drug is contraindicated in patients with adrenal cortical hypofunction. Since several drugs modify the results obtained in the test, the test should be performed in patients receiving no other medication.

Dose—*Usual, adult, oral,* **750 mg** every 4 hours for 6 doses. *Pediatric dose*, **15 mg per kg** of body weight every 4 hours for 6 doses.

Dosage Form—Tablets: 250 mg.

Metyrapone Tartrate Injection

1-Propanone, 2-methyl-1,2-di-3-pyridinyl-, [R-(R*,R*)]-2,3-
dihydroxy-, butanedioate (1:2);
Metopirone Ditartrate (*Ciba-Geigy*)

2-Methyl-1,2-di-3-pyridyl-1-propanone tartrate (1:2) [908-35-0] $C_{14}H_{14}N_2O.2C_4H_6O_6$ (526.45).

Preparation—*Metyrapone* is combined with a double molar quantity of tartaric acid.

Uses—To test *pituitary* function. Except that an occasional thrombophlebitis is encountered when metyrapone tartrate is used intravenously as an injection, its contraindications, untoward effects, and limitations are the same as *Metyrapone.*

Dose—*Usual, adults* and *children,* **30 mg/kg** in 1000 mL of sodium chloride injection or dextrose injection (5%) infused over a 4-hour period beginning between 8 and 10 A.M. The 24-hour urine collection should begin at the start of the test.

Dosage Form—Injection (formulated with the base): 100 mg/mL in 10-mL ampuls.

Neostigmine Bromide—page 899.
Phenoxybenzamine—page 905.
Phentolamine Hydrochloride—page 906.
Phentolamine Mesylate—page 906.
Quinine Sulfate—page 1219.

Protirelin

L-Prolinamide, 5-oxo-L-propyl-L-histidyl-, TRH; Thypinone (*Abbott*);
Relefact (*Hoechst-Roussel*)

Thyrotropin releasing factor [24305-27-9] $C_{16}H_{22}N_6O_4$ (362.39).

Preparation—Protirelin obtained from most mammals appears to be identical and is apparently not species specific. A review of synthetic methods is found in *Methods in Enzymology 37:* 408, 1975.

Solubility—Highly purified material is partially soluble in chloroform and very soluble in methanol.

Uses—As an adjunct in the diagnostic assessment of *thyroid function* and *pituitary or hypothalamic dysfunction.* Protirelin is a synthetic tripeptide believed to be structurally identical to the naturally occurring thyrotropin-releasing hormone produced by the hypothalmus. Following IV administration, $T_{1/2}$ is approximately 5 min; TSH levels reach a peak in 20 to 30 min and declines slowly over a period of 3 hours to baseline levels. Adverse effects occur in about 50% of patients and include hypertension or hypotension with or without syncope and breast enlargment. Other reactions include nausea, urge to urinate, flushing, lightheadedness, bad taste, abdominal discomfort, headache, and dry mouth. It should only be used in pregnant women when clearly indicated.

Dose—*Intravenous, adult,* **500 mcg;** *children* (6 to 16 years), 7 **mcg/kg,** up to **500 mcg;** *infants and children* (up to 6 years), 7 mcg/kg.

Dosage Form—500 mcg per mL in 1 mL amps.

Saralasin Acetate

Sarenin (*Norwich-Eaton*)

Sar - Arg - Val - Tyr - Val - His - Pro - Ala   •   x CH₃COOH   •   xH₂O
 1   2   3   4   5   6   7   8

Angiotensin II, 1-(*N*-methylglycine)-5-L-valine-8-L-alanine-, acetate (salt) hydrate [39698-78-7] $C_{42}H_{65}N_{13}O_{10}.xC_2H_4O_2.xH_2O$ (912.06; free base).

Use—For the detection of *angiotensin II dependent hypertension.* It is intended to be used as one of several tests (plasma renin activity, intravenous pyelogram, renal arteriogram, and renal vein renin) to help detect a renal cause of hypertension. It has a dual action depending on the levels of circulating angiotensin II. In the presence of high levels of circulating angiotensin II, it competively inhibits the binding of angiotensin II to the receptor sites and lowers blood pressure. In the presence of low levels of circulating angiotensin II, the drug behaves as an agonist and raises the blood pressure. Like other tests of the renin-angiotensin system, the saralasin test has a demonstrated error rate (false-positive and false-negative). Therefore, the test accuracy is highly dependent upon fluid and electrolyte status, use of hypertensive drugs, and precise testing technics. Saralasin, an angiotensin II analog that binds to angiotensin II receptors, is metabolized in the body by aminopeptidases. It has a mean plasma $T_{1/2}$ of about 3 min. and a mean pharmacologic $T_{1/2}$ of about 8 min. The biological effects, once attained, last at least 30 min. The saralasin test should not be used in patients known to have pheochromocytoma. Adverse reactions include exaggerated depressor or pressor responses, headache, malaise, nausea, lightheadedness, and local discomfort at the injection site. Safe use during pregnancy has not been established.

Dose—*Intravenous constant rate infusion:* **18 mg (30 mL)** over a period of 20 to 30 min (see package insert).

Dosage Form—*Injection:* 18 mg per 30 mL amp.

Secretin

Secretin-Boots (*Warren-Teed*)

Secretin [1393-25-5] is a polypeptide hormone, secreted by the duodenal mucosa and to a lesser extent by the upper jejunal mucosa, which stimulates secretion of water and bicarbonate from the pancreas. As isolated from porcine mucosa and purified, the hormone consists of 27 amino acid units from 12 different amino acids, and has the molecular formula $C_{122}H_{220}N_{44}O_{41}$; it has been synthesized (Bodanszky *et al*, *J Am Chem Soc 89*: 685, 6753, 1967). The hormone supplied for diagnostic use is of porcine origin; it is a sterile, refined, freeze-dried powder, stable for 2 years when stored in its original, unopened vial at 2° to 7°, but unstable in solution.

Uses—Secretin is used in the diagnosis of *pancreatic disorders*. Intravenous injection of the hormone in persons with normal pancreatic secretion increases the bicarbonate content and volume of secretion from the pancreas. Reduced secretory volume and diminished bicarbonate concentration are signs of pancreatic insufficiency. Volume reductions are indicative of pancreatic duct obstruction as seen in neoplasms; bicarbonate concentration reductions indicate pancreatic inflammatory disease.

In performing the test a double-lumen tube is passed through the mouth after a 12- to 15-hour fast, under fluoroscopic guidance so that a proper placement of the proximal tube in the gastric antrum and of the distal tube beyond the papilla of Vater is accomplished. Constant suction is applied to both outlets of the tube throughout the test. After a control period of collection of fluid for 10 to 20 minutes, and skin testing of the patient for sensitivity to secretin to avoid an anaphylactic reaction, a standard dose of 1 clinical unit per kg of body weight of secretin is injected intravenously. A 60-minute collection period of aspirated secretions, fractioned into 4 periods, the first two at 10-minute intervals and the last two at 20-minute intervals, provides separate duodenal and stomach specimens that are analyzed for volume variations, bicarbonate concentrations, and other constituents.

Secretin is contraindicated in patients with a history of atopic asthma, allergy, and those showing a positive skin test. It should be used with great caution, if at all, in patients with acute pancreatitis.

Dose—See above.

Dosage Form—Vials containing approximately 100 units.

Sincalide

Caerulein, 1-de(5-oxo-L-proline)-2-de-L-glutamide-5-L-methionine;
Kinevac (*Squibb*)

SO₃H
|
Asp - Tyr - Met - Gly - Trp - Met - Asp - Phe — NH₂
 1   2   3   4   5   6   7   8

L-Aspartyl-L-tyrosyl-L-methionylglycyl-L-tryptophyl-L-methionyl-L-aspartylphenyl-L-alaninamide hydrogen sulfate (ester) [25126-32-3] $C_{49}H_{62}N_{10}O_{16}S_3$ (1143.27).

Sincalide is the synthetic C-terminal octapeptide of cholecystokinin.

Description—White, lyophilized powder.

Solubility—Very slightly soluble in water; practically insoluble in alcohol.

Uses—Sincalide, a synthetic fragment of cholecystokinin, is reported to be at least five times more active than the physiological hormone that stimulates contraction of the gallbladder and increases intestinal motility. Sincalide is used to obtain a *specimen of gallbladder bile*, in conjunction with secretin to *stimulate pancreatic secretion* for analysis, and for *postevacuation cholecystography* in cases where the physician wishes to avoid the usual fatty meal. Untoward reactions include mild, transient, abdominal discomfort and an urge to defecate, and occasional dizziness, flushing, and nausea. Safety of sincalide in pregnant women or for children has not been established.

Dose—*Usual, adult, intravenous,* for *contraction of gallbladder,* **0.02 µg per kg** of body weight injected over a period of 30 to 60 seconds; if satisfactory contraction does not occur in 15 minutes, a second dose, **0.04 µg per kg** may be administered. For the *secretin-sincalide* test, **0.25 unit per kg** of secretin infused over a period of 60 minutes, followed in 30 minutes with **0.02 µg per kg** of sincalide administered over a 30-minute period.

Dosage Form—Vials containing 5 µg.

Sodium Phosphate P 32—page 496.
Tetraethylammonium Bromide—RPS-15, page 782.

Thromboplastin

Thrombokinase

[9002-05-5] A powder or a liquid suspension that exhibits thrombokinase activity derived from the acetone-extracted brain and/or lung tissue of freshly killed rabbits. It may contain added sodium chloride and calcium chloride in suitable proportions. It is used in the form of a suspension for the determination of the prothrombin time and activity of the blood.

The thrombokinase activity is such that the addition of thromboplastin gives a clotting time of 11 to 16 sec with normal human plasma and the proper concentration of calcium ion.

Description—In the dry form, it is a buff-colored powder. In the liquid form, it is an opalescent or a turbid suspension from which some solid matter may be deposited on standing. It may have a characteristic odor of dried animal tissue. It may contain a suitable antibacterial agent.

Uses—A necessary reagent in the determination of prothrombin activity or prothrombin time of the plasma. It is active by virtue of its content of thrombokinase, a factor that is necessary, along with calcium ions, for the conversion of prothrombin to thrombin. It is used in the form of a suspension adjusted to a concentration such that in the standard prothrombin determination with normal human plasma and calcium concentration the clotting time lies between 11 and 16 sec. It has also been used in surgery as a hemostatic to arrest hemorrhage, but it is little used for this purpose.

Other Miscellaneous Diagnostic Drugs

Azuresin; [Azure A Carbacrylic Resin; A complex combination of 3-amino-7-(dimethylamino)phenothiazin-5-ium chloride [$C_{14}H_{14}ClN_3S$ (291.80)] known as azure A dye, and a carbacrylic cation-exchange resin. It contains, in each g, 50–70 mg of the dye. Diagnex Blue (Squibb). *Preparation:* The resin component is prepared by catalytic polymerization of a suitable carbacrylic monomer. The azure A dye component may be prepared by the method described for methylene blue on page 842 except that an equimolar mixture of *N,N*-dimethyl-*p*-phenylenediamine and *p*-phenylenediamine is employed instead of the former alone. *Description:* Moist, irregular, dark blue or purple-colored granules; it has a slightly pungent odor. *Uses:* An ion-exchange resin used as an indicator for detection of achlorhydria without the discomfort of intubation. A stimulant of gastric secretion (caffeine) is given one hour before administration of 2 g of the resin. If hydrochloric acid is secreted, the hydrogen ions displace the blue dye (azure A) from the resin. The dye is absorbed and excreted in the urine within 2 hours after administration of the resin. The urine specimen collected 2 hours after administration of the resin is tested for the concentration of dye as an indication of the presence or absence of free hydrochloric acid in the stomach; a color comparator is supplied with each test unit of the drug. Azuresin is of negligible toxicity and no cases of idiosyncrasy have been reported. Inaccurate results may result in patients with pyloric obstruction, severe hepatic or renal disease, impaired intestinal absorption, vomiting, marked dehydration, bladder obstruction, or subtotal gastrectomy. *Dose: Usual,* 2 g preceded by 500 mg of *Caffeine and Sodium Benzoate. Dosage Form:* for Injection: 500 mg.

CHAPTER 68

Pharmaceutical Necessities

Ewart A Swinyard, PhD, DSc (Hon)

Professor Emeritus of Pharmacology
College of Pharmacy and School of Medicine
University of Utah
Salt Lake City, UT 84112

Werner Lowenthal, PhD

Professor of Pharmacy and Pharmaceutics and Professor of Educational Planning and Development
School of Pharmacy
Virginia Commonwealth University
Richmond, VA 23298

This chapter describes substances that are of little or no therapeutic value, but which are useful in the manufacture and compounding of various pharmaceutical preparations. Hence, they are referred to as pharmaceutical necessities. The substances described include antioxidants and preservatives; coloring, flavoring, and diluting agents; emulsifying and suspending agents; ointment bases; pharmaceutical solvents; and miscellaneous agents. For a more detailed review of the uses of these agents, the interested reader is referred to the various chapters in Part 8 of this book.

Antioxidants and Preservatives

An antioxidant is a substance capable of inhibiting oxidation and that may be added for this purpose to pharmaceutical products subject to deterioration by oxidative processes as, for example, the development of rancidity in oils and fats or the inactivation of some medicinals in the environment of their dosage forms. A preservative is, in the common pharmaceutical sense, a substance that prevents or inhibits microbial growth and may be added to pharmaceutical preparations for this purpose to avoid consequent spoilage of the preparations by microorganisms. Both antioxidants and preservatives have many applications in making medicinal products.

Alcohol—page 1159.

Ascorbyl Palmitate

L-Ascorbic acid, 6-hexadecanoate; Ascorbic Acid Palmitate (ester)

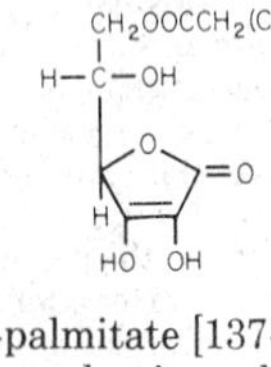

L-Ascorbic acid 6-palmitate [137-66-6] $C_{22}H_{38}O_7$ (414.54).

Preparation—By condensing palmitoyl chloride with ascorbic acid in the presence of a suitable dehydrochlorinating agent such as pyridine.

Description—White to yellowish white powder having a characteristic odor; melts between 107° and 117°.

Solubility—1 g in >1000 mL water, 125 mL alcohol, >1000 mL chloroform, >1000 mL ether.

Uses—An *antioxidant* used in foods and pharmaceuticals. It is also used to prevent rancidity, to prevent the browning of cut apples, in meat curing, and in the preservation of canned or frozen foods.

Benzoic Acid—page 1230.

Butylated Hydroxyanisole

Phenol, (1,1-dimethylethyl)-4-methoxy-, Tenox BHA (*Eastman*)

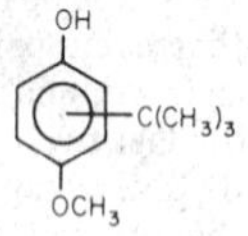

tert-Butyl-4-methoxyphenol [25013-16-5] $C_{11}H_{16}O_2$ (180.25).

Preparation—By an addition interaction of *p*-methoxyphenol and 2-methylpropene. US Pat 2,428,745.

Description—White or slightly yellow, waxy solid having a faint, characteristic odor.

Solubility—Insoluble in water; 1 g in 4 mL alcohol, 2 mL chloroform, 1.2 mL ether.

Uses—An *antioxidant* in cosmetics and pharmaceuticals containing fats and oils.

Butylated Hydroxytoluene

Phenol, 2,6-bis(1,1-dimethylethyl)-4-methyl-, Butylated Hydroxytoluene Crystalline (*Diamond-Shamrock*); Tenox BHT (*Eastman*)

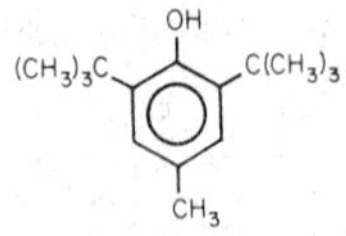

2,6-Di-*tert*-butyl-*p*-cresol [128-37-0] $C_{15}H_{24}O$ (220.35).

Preparation—By an addition interaction of *p*-cresol and 2-methylpropene. US Pat 2,428,745.

Description—White, tasteless crystals with a mild odor; stable in light and air; melts at 70°.

Solubility—Insoluble in water; 1 g in 4 mL alcohol, 1.1 mL chloroform, 1.1 mL ether.

Uses—An *antioxidant* employed to retard oxidative degradation of oils and fats in various cosmetics and pharmaceuticals.

Chlorobutanol

2-Propanol, 1,1,1-trichloro-2-methyl-, Chlorbutol; Chlorbutanol; Acetone chloroform; Chloretone (*Parke-Davis*)

$(CCl_3)C(CH_3)_2OH$

1,1,1-Trichloro-2-methyl-2-propanol [57-15-8] $C_4H_7Cl_3O$ (177.46); *hemihydrate* [6001-64-5] (186.46).

Preparation—Chloroform undergoes chemical addition to acetone under the catalytic influence of powdered potassium hydroxide.

Description—Colorless to white crystals, of a characteristic, somewhat camphoraceous odor and taste; anhydrous melts at about 95°; hydrous melts at about 76°; boils with some decomposition between 165° and 168°.

Solubility—1 g in 125 mL water, 1 mL alcohol, and about 10 mL glycerin; freely soluble in chloroform, ether, and volatile oils.

Incompatibilities—The anhydrous form must be used in order to prepare a clear solution in liquid petrolatum. It is decomposed by *alkalies; ephedrine* is sufficiently alkaline to cause its breakdown with the formation of ephedrine hydrochloride which will separate from a liquid petrolatum solution. It is only slightly soluble in water, hence alcohol must be used to dissolve the required amount in certain vehicles. A soft mass is produced by trituration with *antipyrine, menthol, phenol,* and other substances.

Uses—Topically as a solution in clove oil as a *dental analgesic.* It has *local anesthetic* potency to a mild degree and has been employed as an anesthetic dusting powder (1 to 5%) or ointment (10%). Chlorobutanol has antibacterial and germicidal properties. It is chiefly used as a *preservative* in solutions of epinephrine, posterior pituitary, etc. When administered orally, it has much the same therapeutic use as chloral hydrate. Hence, chlorobutanol has been employed as a sedative and hypnotic. It has been taken orally to allay vomiting due to gastritis.

Dose—*Topical,* as a **25%** solution in clove oil.

Other Dose Information—The dose by mouth is 300 mg to 1 g, given in tablets or capsules.

Ethylenediamine

1,2-Ethanediamine

$$H_2NCH_2CH_2NH_2$$

Ethylenediamine [107-15-3] $C_2H_8N_2$ (60.10).

Caution—*Use care in handling Ethylenediamine because of its caustic nature and the irritating properties of its vapor.*

Note—*Ethylenediamine is strongly alkaline and may readily absorb carbon dioxide from the air to form a nonvolatile carbonate. Protect Ethylenediamine against undue exposure to the atmosphere.*

Preparation—By reacting ethylene dichloride with ammonia, then adding NaOH and distilling.

Description—Clear, colorless, or only slightly yellow liquid, having an ammonia-like odor and strong alkaline reaction; miscible with water and alcohol; anhydrous boils between 116° and 117° and solidifies at about 8°; volatile with steam; a strong base and readily combines with acids to form salts with the evolution of much heat.

Uses—A *pharmaceutical necessity* for *Aminophylline Injection.* Ethylenediamine is irritating to skin and mucous membranes. It may also cause sensitization characterized by asthma and allergic dermatitis.

Ethylparaben—page 1166.

Ethyl Vanillin—page 1286.

Glycerin—page 1308.

Methylparaben—page 1167.

Monothioglycerol

1,2-Propanediol, 3-mercapto-,

$$HSCH_2CH(OH)CH_2OH$$

3-Mercapto-1,2-propanediol [96-27-5] $C_3H_8O_2S$ (108.15).

Preparation—An ethanolic solution of 3-chloro-1,2-propanediol is heated with potassium bisulfide.

Description—Colorless or pale yellow, viscous liquid having a slight sulfidic odor; hygroscopic; specific gravity between 1.241 and 1.250; pH (1 in 10 solution) between 3.5 and 7.

Solubility—Freely soluble in water; miscible with alcohol; insoluble in ether.

Uses—A pharmaceutic aid stated to be used as a preservative. It has been used in 1:5000 solution to stimulate healing of wounds, and as a 1:1000 jelly in atrophic rhinitis.

Phenol—page 1315.

Phenylethyl Alcohol—1289.

Phenylmercuric Nitrate—1168.

Potassium Sorbate

2,4-Hexadienoic acid, (*E,E*)-, potassium salt; 2,4-Hexadienoic acid, potassium salt; Potassium 2,4-Hexadienoate

Potassium (*E,E*)-sorbate; potassium sorbate [590-00-1] [24634-61-5] $C_6H_7KO_2$ (150.22).

Preparation—*Sorbic Acid* is reacted with an equimolar portion of KOH. The resulting potassium sorbate may be crystallized from aqueous ethanol. US Pat 3,173,948.

Description—White crystals or powder with a characteristic odor; melts at about 270° with decomposition.

Solubility—1 g in 4.5 mL water, 35 mL alcohol, >1000 mL chloroform, >1000 mL ether.

Uses—A water-soluble salt of sorbic acid used in pharmaceuticals to *inhibit the growth of molds and yeasts.* Its toxicity is low, but it may irritate the skin.

Propylparaben—page 1168.

Sassafras Oil—page 1292.

Sodium Benzoate—page 1169.

Sodium Bisulfite

Sulfurous acid, monosodium salt; Sodium Hydrogen Sulfite; Sodium Acid Sulfite; Leucogen

Monosodium sulfite [7631-90-5] $NaHSO_3$ and sodium metabisulfite ($Na_2S_2O_5$) in varying proportions; yields 58.5–67.4% of SO_2.

Description—White or yellowish white crystals or granular powder having the odor of sulfur dioxide; unstable in air.

Solubility—1 g in 4 mL water; slightly soluble in alcohol.

Uses—An *antioxidant* and *stabilizing agent.* Epinephrine hydrochloride solutions may be stabilized by the addition of small quantities of the salt. It is also used to help solubilize kidney stones. Sodium bisulfite is useful for removing permanganate stains and for solubilizing certain dyes and other chemicals (see *Menadione Sodium Bisulfite,* page 1011).

Sodium Formaldehyde Sulfoxylate

Methanesulfinic acid, hydroxy-, monosodium salt

Monosodium hydroxymethanesulfinate [149-44-0] CH_3NaO_3S (118.08); *dihydrate* [6035-47-8] (154.11).

Preparation—Zinc dust is reacted with sulfur dioxide in the presence of formaldehyde and water to form zinc formaldehyde sulfoxylate and zinc formaldehyde bisulfite

$$2Zn + 4SO_2 + 4CH_2O + 2H_2O \rightarrow Zn(HOCH_2SO_2)_2 + Zn(HOCH_2SO_3)_2$$

On addition of NaOH, the zinc salts are converted to sodium salts, and further reaction with zinc dust reduces the bisulfite component to sulfoxylate. US Pat 2,013,125.

Description—White crystals or as hard, white masses having the characteristic odor of garlic; pH (1 in 50 solution) between 9.5 and 10.5.

Solubility—1 g in 3.4 mL water, 510 mL alcohol, 175 mL chloroform, 180 mL ether.

Uses—A locally acting *antidote* that reduces mercuric chloride to insoluble mercurous chloride or to metallic mercury. Administered as a 5% solution (250 mL) with a stomach tube; after removal of the lavage a second 250-mL portion of solution is left in the stomach. It is not nearly as effective as *Dimercaprol* (page 1224) in systemic mercury poisoning, and the latter antidote should be used to counteract mercury that is absorbed.

Sodium Metabisulfite

Disulfurous acid, disodium salt

Disodium pyrosulfite [7681-57-4]$Na_2S_2O_5$ (190.10).

Preparation—Formed when sodium bisulfite undergoes thermal dehydration. It may also be prepared by passing sulfur dioxide over sodium carbonate.

Description—White crystals or white to yellowish crystalline powder having an odor of sulfur dioxide; on exposure to air and moisture, it is slowly oxidized to sulfate.

Solubility—1 g in 2 mL water; slightly soluble in alcohol; freely soluble in glycerin.

Uses—A *reducing agent*. It is used in easily oxidized pharmaceuticals, such as epinephrine hydrochloride and phenylephrine hydrochloride injections, to retard oxidation.

Sorbic Acid

2,4-Hexadienoic acid, (*E,E*)-, 2,4-Hexadienoic acid

(*E,E*)-Sorbic acid; Sorbic acid [22500-92-1] [110-44-1] $C_6H_8O_2$ (112.13).

Preparation—By various processes. Refer to US Pat 2,921,090.

Description—Free-flowing, white, crystalline powder, having a characteristic odor; melts between 132° and 135°.

Solubility—1 g in 1000 mL water, 10 mL alcohol, 15 mL chloroform, 30 mL ether, 19 mL propylene glycol.

Uses—A *mold and yeast inhibitor*. It is also used as a fungistatic agent for foods, especially cheeses.

Sulfur Dioxide

Sulfur dioxide [7446-09-5] SO_2 (64.06).

Preparation—By burning sulfur or sulfides and by reacting a bisulfite or a sulfite with a strong acid.

Description—Colorless, nonflammable gas, with a strong, suffocating, odor characteristic of burning sulfur; 1 L weighs 2.927 g at 760 mm and 0°; readily liquefies under pressure forming a colorless liquid with a density of approximately 1.5 g/mL and a boiling point of −10°.

Solubility—1 volume of water dissolves approximately 36 volumes of sulfur dioxide at 760 mm and 20°; 1 volume of alcohol dissolves approximately 114 volumes under the same conditions; soluble in ether and in chloroform.

Note—*Sulfur dioxide is used mostly in the form of a gas in pharmaceutical applications, and is described herein for such purposes. However, it is usually packaged under pressure, hence the USP specifications* (*Water, Nonvolatile residue, and Sulfuric acid*), *are designed for the testing of its liquid form.*

Uses—The gas in the presence of moisture forms sulfurous acid which is a *bleaching agent*, *fungicide*, and *bactericide*. For this reason fruits are often exposed to the gas before drying to prevent darkening and the growth of molds and bacteria. The gas is also an *antioxidant* and a pharmaceutical necessity for *Injections*. It may be intensely irritating to the eyes and respiratory tract.

Thimerosal—page 1169.

Other Antioxidants and Preservatives

Maleic Acid BP [*cis*-Butenedioic acid $C_4H_4O_4$ (116.07); Toxilic acid] —*Preparation:* Benzene vapor is oxidized by passage over heated vanadium pentoxide. Odorless, white, crystalline powder having a strongly acid taste; melts between 132° and 140°. Soluble in 1.5 parts water, 2 parts alcohol, and 12 parts ether. *Uses:* In the preparation of ergometrine maleate injection; as a rancidity retardant in fats and oils (1:10,000).

Propyl Gallate BP [Propyl 3,4,5-Trihydroxybenzoate]—White to creamy-white crystalline powder; odorless; slightly bitter taste. Soluble in 1000 parts water and 3 parts alcohol. *Uses:* A preservative.

Coloring, Flavoring, and Diluting Agents

The use of properly colored and flavored medicinal substances, although offering no particular therapeutic advantage, is of considerable importance psychologically. A water-clear medicine is not particularly acceptable to most patients, and, in general, is thought to be inert. Many very active medicinal substances are quite unpalatable, and the patient may fail to take the medicine simply because the taste or appearance is objectionable. Disagreeable medication can be made both pleasing to the taste and attractive by careful selection of the appropriate coloring, flavoring, and diluting agents. Therefore, judicious use of these substances is important in securing patient cooperation in taking or using the prescribed medication and continued compliance with the prescriber's intent.

Coloring Agents or Colorants

Coloring agents may be defined as compounds employed in pharmacy solely for the purpose of imparting color. They may be classified in various ways, eg, inorganic or organic. For the purpose of this discussion two subdivisions are used: (1) *Natural Coloring Principles* and (2) *Synthetic Coloring Principles*. The members of these groups are used as colors for pharmaceutical preparations, cosmetics, foods, and as bacteriological stains and diagnostic agents.

Natural Coloring Principles

Natural coloring principles are obtained from mineral, plant, and animal sources. They are used primarily for artistic purposes, as symbolic adornments of natives, as colors for foods, drugs, and cosmetics, and for other psychological effects.

Mineral colors are frequently termed *pigments* and are used to color lotions, cosmetics, and other preparations, usually for external application. Examples are *Red Ferric Oxide* (page 1320) and *Yellow Ferric Oxide* (page 1320), titanium dioxide (page 790) and carbon black.

The term pigment is also applied generically to plant colors by phytochemists. Many plants contain coloring principles that may be extracted and used as colorants, eg, chlorophyll. Anattenes are obtained from annatto seeds and give yellow to orange water-soluble dyes. Natural beta-carotene is a yellow color extracted from carrots and used to color margarine. Alizarin is a reddish-yellow dye obtained from the madder plant. The indigo plant is the source of a blue pigment called indigo. Flavones, such as riboflavin, rutin, hesperidin, and quercetin, are yellow pigments. Saffron is a glycoside that gives a yellow color to drugs and foods. Cudbear and red saunders are two other dyes obtained from plants. Most plant colors have now been characterized and synthesized, however, and those with the desirable qualities of stability, fastness, and pleasing hue are available commercially as synthetic products.

Animals have been a source of coloring principles from the earliest periods of recorded history. For example, *Tyrian purple*, once a sign of royalty, was prepared by air oxidation of a colorless secretion obtained from the glands of a snail (*Murex brandaris*). This dye is now known to be 6,6'-dibromoindigo, and has been synthesized, but cheaper dyes of the same color are available. Cochineal from the insect *Coccus cacti* contains the bright red coloring principle *carminic acid*, a derivative of anthraquinone. This dye is no longer used in foods and pharmaceuticals due to *Salmonella* contamination.

Synthetic Coloring Principles

Synthetic coloring principles date from 1856 when W H Perkin accidentally discovered *mauveine*, also known as a *Perkin's purple*, while engaged in unsuccessful attempts to synthesize quinine. He obtained the dye by oxidizing aniline containing *o*- and *p*-toluidines as impurities. Other discoveries of this kind followed soon after, and a major industry grew up in the field of coal-tar chemistry.

The earliest colors were prepared from aniline and for many years all coal-tar dyes were called aniline colors, irrespective of their origin. The coal-tar dyes include more than a dozen well-defined groups among which are *nitroso-dyes, nitro-dyes, azo-dyes, oxazines, thiazines, pyrazolones, xanthenes, indigoids, anthraquinones, acridines, rosanilines, phthaleins, quinolines*, and others. These in turn are classified, according to their method of use, as *acid dyes* and *basic dyes*, or *direct dyes* and *mordant dyes*.

Certain structural elements in organic molecules, called chromophore groups, give color to the molecules, eg, azo (—N==N—), nitroso (—N==O), nitro (—NO$_2$), azoxy (—N==N—O—), carbonyl (>C==O), and ethylene (>C==C<). Other such elements augment the chromophore groups, eg, methoxy, hydroxy, and amino groups.

Stability—Most dyes are relatively unstable chemicals due to their unsaturated structures. They are subject to fading due to light, metals, heat, microorganisms, oxidizing and reducing agents, and strong acids and bases. In tablets, fading may appear as spotting and specking.

Uses—Most synthetic coloring principles are used in coloring fabrics and for various artistic purposes. They also find application as indicators, as bacteriological stains, diagnostic aids, and as reagents in microscopy, etc.

Many coal-tar dyes were originally used in foodstuffs and beverages without careful selection or discrimination between those that were harmless and those that were toxic and without any supervision as to purity or freedom from poisonous constituents derived from their manufacture.

After the passage of the Food and Drugs Act in 1906, the US Department of Agriculture established regulations by which a few colors came to be known as *permitted colors*. Certain of these colors may be used in foods, drugs, and cosmetics, but only after certification by the Food and Drug Administration that they meet certain specifications. From this list of permitted colors may be produced, by skillful blending and mixing, other colors that may be used in foods, beverages, and pharmaceutical preparations. Blends of certified dyes must be recertified.

The word "permitted" is used in a restricted sense. It does not carry with it the right to use colors for purposes of deception, even though they be "permitted" colors; for all food laws have clauses prohibiting the coloring of foods and beverages in a manner so as to conceal inferiority or to give false appearance of value.

The certified colors are classified into three groups as follows: (1) FD&C dyes which may legally be used in foods, drugs, and cosmetics, (2) D&C dyes which may legally be used in drugs and cosmetics, and (3) External D&C dyes which may legally be used only in externally applied drugs and cosmetics. There are specific limits for the pure dye, sulfated ash, ether extractives, soluble and insoluble matter, uncombined intermediates, oxides, chlorides, and sulfates. As the use status of these colors is subject to change, the latest regulations of the FDA should be consulted to determine how they may be used—especially since several FD&C dyes formerly widely used have been found to be carcinogenic even when "pure" and therefore have been banned from use.

The Coal-Tar Color Regulations specify that the term "externally applied drugs and cosmetics" means drugs and cosmetics which are applied only to external parts of the body and not to the lips or any body surface covered by mucous membrane. No certified dye, regardless of its category, may legally be used in any article which is to be applied to the area of the eye.

Lakes are calcium or aluminum salts of certified dyes extended on a substrate of alumina. They are insoluble in water and organic solvents, hence are used to color powders, pharmaceuticals, foods, hard candies, and food packaging.

The application of dyes to pharmaceutical preparations is an art that can be acquired only after an understanding of the characteristics of dyes and a knowledge of the composition of the products to be colored have been obtained. Specific rules for the choice or application of dyes to pharmaceutical preparations are difficult to formulate. Each preparation may present unique problems.

Preparations which may be colored include most liquid pharmaceuticals, powders, ointments, and emulsions. Some general hints may be offered in connection with solutions and powders, but desired results can usually be obtained only by a series of trials. In general, an inexperienced operator tends to use a much higher concentration of the dye than is necessary, resulting in a dull color. The amount of dye present in any pharmaceutical preparation should be of a concentration high enough to give the desired color and low enough to prevent toxic reactions and permanent staining of fabrics and tissues.

Liquids (Solutions)—The dye concentration in liquid preparations and solutions should usually come within a range of 0.0005% (1 in 200,000) and 0.001% (1 in 100,000), depending upon the depth of color wanted and the thickness of column to be viewed in the container. With some dyes, concentrations as low as 0.0001% (1 in 1,000,000) may have a distinct tinting effect. Dyes are most conveniently used in the form of stock solutions.

Powders—White powders usually require the incorporation of 0.1% (1 in 1000) of a dye to impart a pastel color. The dyes may be incorporated into the powder by dry blending in a ball mill or, on a small scale, with a mortar and pestle. The dye is incorporated by trituration and geometric dilution. Powders may also be evenly colored by adding a solution of the dye in alcohol or some other volatile solvent having only a slight solvent action on the powder being colored. When this procedure is employed, the solution is added in portions, with thorough mixing after each addition, after which the solvent is allowed to evaporate from the mixture.

Many of the syrups and elixirs used as flavoring and diluting agents are colored. When such agents are used no further coloring matter is necessary. The use of colored flavoring agents is discussed in a subsequent section. However, when it is desired to add color to an otherwise colorless mixture, one of the agents described in the first section may be used.

Incompatibilities—FD&C dyes are mainly anionic (sodium salts), hence are incompatible with cationic substances. Since the concentrations of these substances are generally very low, no precipitate is evident. Polyvalent ions such as calcium, magnesium, and aluminum may also form insoluble compounds with dyes. A pH change may cause the color to change. Acids may release the insoluble acid form of the dye.

Caramel

Burnt Sugar Coloring

A concentrated solution of the product obtained by heating sugar or glucose until the sweet taste is destroyed and a uniform dark brown mass results, a small amount of alkali, alkaline carbonate, or a trace of mineral acid being added while heating.

Description—Thick, dark brown liquid with the characteristic odor of burnt sugar, and a pleasant, bitter taste; specific gravity not less than 1.30; 1 part dissolved in 1000 parts of water yields a clear solution having a distinct yellowish orange color which is not changed and no precipitate is formed after exposure to sunlight for 6 hours; when spread in a thin layer on a glass plate, it appears homogeneous, reddish brown, and transparent.

Solubility—Miscible with water in all proportions and with dilute alcohol up to 55% by volume; immiscible with ether, chloroform, acetone, benzene, solvent hexane, or turpentine oil.

Uses—To produce a brown color in elixirs, syrups, and other preparations.

Flavoring Agents

Flavor

The word flavor refers to a mixed sensation of taste, touch, smell, sight, and sound, all of which combine to produce an infinite number of gradations in the perception of a substance. The four primary tastes—*sweet*, *bitter*, *sour*, and *saline*—appear to be the result partly of physicochemical and partly of psychological action. Taste buds (see Fig 68-1), located mainly on the tongue, contain very sensitive nerve endings that react, in the presence of moisture, with the flavors in the mouth and as a result of physicochemical activity electrical impulses are produced and transmitted via the seventh, ninth, and tenth cranial nerves to the areas of the brain which are devoted to the perception of taste. Some of the taste buds are specialized in their function, giving rise to areas on the tongue which are sensitive to only one type of taste. The brain, however, usually perceives taste as a composite sensation, and accordingly the components of any flavor are not readily discernible. Children have more taste buds than adults, hence are more sensitive to tastes.

As mentioned above, taste is partly dependent on the ions which are produced in the mouth, but psychologists have demonstrated that sight (color) and sound also play a definite role when certain reflexes become conditioned through custom and association of sense perceptions. Thus in the classic experiments of Pavlov demonstrating "conditioned reflexes," the ringing of a bell or the showing of a circle of light caused the gastric juices of a dog to flow although no food was placed before it, and much of the enjoyment derived from the eating of celery is due to its crunchy crispness as the fibrovascular bundles are crushed. The effect of color is just as pronounced; oleomargarine is unpalatable to most people when it is uncolored, but once the dye has been incorporated gourmets frequently cannot distinguish it from butter. Color and taste must coincide, eg, cherry flavor is associated with a red color.

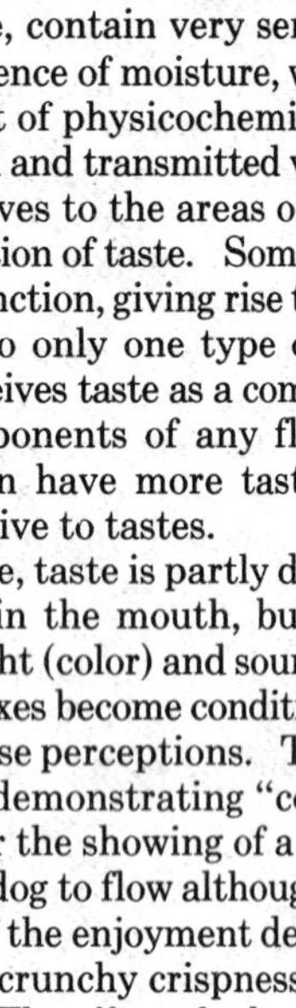

A person suffering from a head cold finds his food much less palatable than usual because his sense of smell is impaired, and if the nostrils are held closed raw onions taste sweet and it is much easier to ingest castor oil and other nauseating medicines. The volatility of a substance is an important factor that is influenced by the warmth and moisture of the mouth since the more volatile a compound the more pronounced is its odor. The sense of smell detects very minute amounts of material and is usually much more sensitive in detecting the presence of volatile chemicals, but the tongue is able to detect infinitesimal amounts of some vapors if it is protruded from the mouth so that solution of the gases in the saliva may take place. In this manner traces of sulfur dioxide can be detected in the air since it dissolves in the saliva and creates a sour taste.

Flavors described as hot are those that exert a mild counterirritant effect on the mucosa of the mouth, those that are astringent and pucker the mouth contain tannins and acids that produce this effect by reacting with the lining of the mouth, and wines possess a bouquet due to the odor of the volatile constituents. Indian turnip (Jack-in-the-pulpit) owes its flavor largely to the stinging sensation caused by the minute acicular crystals of calcium oxalate which penetrate the mucous membrane.

Other physiological and physical factors that also may affect taste are coarseness or grittiness due to small particles, eg, ion-exchange resin. Antidiarrheal preparations have a chalky taste. Menthol imparts a cool taste because it affects the coldness receptors. Mannitol gives a cool sensation when it dissolves because its negative of heat of solution will cause the temperature to drop. For this reason, mannitol is often used as the base for chewable tablets.

There is a definite threshold of taste for every substance, which varies somewhat with the individual and with the environment. The experienced chef tastes his delicacies at the temperature at which they will be served since heat and cold alter the flavor of many preparations. Thus, lemon loses its sour taste entirely at an elevated temperature and other flavors become almost nonvolatile, tasteless, and odorless when cooled sufficiently. In addition to the influence of temperature the sensitivity of each individual must be considered. For example, it has been determined by experiment that the

Fig 68-1.   Upper Surface of the tongue.   a: Taste receptors for all tastes; b: sweet, salty, and sour tastes; c: salty and sour; d: sour only; e: no taste sensation; f: sweet and sour; and g: bitter, sweet, and sour tastes (adapted from Crocker EC: *Flavor*, McGraw-Hill, New York, 22, 1945).

amount of sugar that can just be detected by the average individual is about 7 mg. However, this amount cannot be tasted by some and it is definitely sweet to others.

People are more sensitive to odor than to taste. There are about 10,000 to 30,000 identifiable scents, of which the average person can identify about 4000. Women are more sensitive to odors than men. Additional insights can be obtained by reading, *Biochemistry of Taste and Olfaction*[1] and *Handbook of Sensory Physiology*[2].

Preservation of Flavors—Most monographs of official products contain specific directions for storage. Proper methods of storage are essential to prevent deterioration which in many instances results in destruction of odor and taste. Under adverse conditions undesirable changes occur due to one or a combination of the following: enzymatic activity, oxidation, change in moisture content, absorption of odors, activity of microorganisms, and effects of heat and light. In certain products some of the changes wrought by these factors are desirable, as when esters are formed due to the activity of enzymes and when blending and mellowing results from the interchange of the radicals of esters (*transesterification*).

One method for protecting readily oxidizable substances, such as lemon oil, from deteriorating, and thus preserving their original delicate flavor, is to microencapsulate them by spray drying. The capsules containing the flavors are then enclosed in various packaged products (eg, powdered gelatins) or tablets which are deliciously flavored when the capsule is disintegrated by mixing and warming with water or saliva.

Correlation of Chemical Structure with Flavor and Odor—The compounds employed as flavors in vehicles vary considerably in their chemical structure, ranging from simple esters (methyl salicylate), alcohols (glycerin), and aldehydes (vanillin) to carbohydrates (honey) and the complex volatile oils (anise oil). Synthetic flavors of almost any desired type are now available. These frequently possess the delicate flavor and aroma of the natural products and also the desirable characteristics of stability, reproducibility, and comparatively low cost. Synthetic products such as cinnamaldehyde and benzaldehyde, first officially recognized when several of the essential oils became scarce during war years, have been widely used.

There is a close relationship between chemical structure and taste. Solubility, the degree of ionization, and the type of ions produced in the saliva definitely influence the sensation interpreted by the brain.

Sour taste is caused by hydrogen ions and it is proportional to the hydrogen-ion concentration and the lipid solubility of the compound. It is characteristic of acids, tannins, alum, phenols, and lactones. Saltiness is due to simultaneous presence of anions and cations, eg, KBr, NH_4Cl, and sodium salicylate. High-molecular-weight salts may have a bitter taste. Sweet taste is due to polyhydroxy compounds, polyhalogenated aliphatic compounds and α-amino acids. Amino and amide groups, especially if the positive effect is balanced by proximity of a negative group, may produce a sweet taste. Sweetness increases with the number of hydroxy groups, possibly due to increase in solubility. Imides such as saccharin and sulfamates such as cyclamates are intensely sweet. Cyclamates have been removed from the market because they reportedly cause bladder tumors in rats. Free bases such as alkaloids and amides such as amphetamines give bitter tastes. Polyhydroxy compounds with a molecular weight greater than 300, halogenated substances, and aliphatic thio compounds may also have bitter tastes. Unsaturation frequently bestows a sharp, biting odor and taste upon compounds.

No precise relationship between chemical structure and odor has been found. There are no primary odors, and odors blend into each other. Polymerization reduces or destroys odor; high valency gives odor and unsaturation enhances odor. A tertiary carbon atom will often give a camphoraceous odor; esters and lactones have a fruity odor, and ketones have a pleasant odor. Strong odors are often accompanied by volatility and chemical reactivity.

Selection of Flavors

The proper selection of flavors for disguising nauseating medicines aids in their ingestion. Occasionally, sensitive patients have become sufficiently nauseated to vomit at the thought of having to take disagreeable medication, and it is particularly difficult to persuade children to continue to use and retain distasteful preparations. There is a need to know the allergies and idiosyncrasies of the patient; thus, it is foolish to use a chocolate-flavored vehicle for the patient who dislikes the flavor or who is allergic to it, notwithstanding the fact that this flavor is generally acceptable.

Flavoring Methodology

Each flavoring problem is unique and requires an individual solution. The problem of flavoring is further complicated because flavor and taste depend on individual preferences. In solving flavoring problems the following techniques have been used:

1. *Blending*—Fruit flavors blend with sour taste; bitter tastes can be blended with salty, sweet and sour tastes; salt reduces sourness and increases sweetness; chemicals such as vanillin, monosodium glutamate, and benzaldehyde are used for blending.
2. *Overshadow*—Addition of a flavor whose intensity is longer and stronger than the obvious taste, eg, methyl salicylate, glycyrrhiza, and oleoresins.
3. *Physical*—Formation of insoluble compounds of the offending drug, eg, sulfonamides; emulsification of oils; effervescence, eg, magnesium citrate solution; high viscosity of fluids to limit contact of drug with the tongue, and mechanical procedure such as coating tablets, are physical methods to reduce flavoring problems.
4. *Chemical*—Adsorption of the drug on a substrate, or formation of a complex of the drug with ion-exchange resins or complexing agents.
5. *Physiological*—The taste buds may be anesthetized by menthol or mint flavors.

Flavors, as used by the pharmacist in compounding prescriptions, may be divided into four main categories according to the type of taste which is to be masked, as follows:

1. *Salty Taste*—Cinnamon syrup has been found to be the best vehicle for ammonium chloride; and other salty drugs such as sodium salicylate and ferric ammonium citrate. In a study of the comparative efficiency of flavoring agents for disguising salty taste, the following additional vehicles were arranged in descending order of usefulness: orange syrup, citric acid syrup, cherry syrup, cocoa syrup, wild cherry syrup, raspberry syrup, glycyrrhiza elixir, aromatic elixir, and glycyrrhiza syrup. The last-named is particularly useful as a vehicle for the salines by virtue of its colloidal properties and the sweetness of both glycyrrhizin and sucrose.
2. *Bitter Taste*—Cocoa syrup was found to be the best vehicle for disguising the bitter taste of quinine bisulfate; then followed, in descending order of usefulness, raspberry syrup, cocoa syrup, cherry syrup, cinnamon syrup, compound sarsaparilla syrup, citric acid syrup, licorice syrup, aromatic elixir, orange syrup, and wild cherry syrup.
3. *Acrid or Sour Taste*—Raspberry syrup and other fruit syrups are especially efficient in masking the taste of sour substances such as hydrochloric acid. Acacia syrup, and other mucilaginous vehicles are best for disguising the acrid taste of substances, such as capsicum, since they tend to form a colloidal protective coating over the taste buds of the tongue. Tragacanth, unlike acacia, may be used in an alcoholic vehicle.
4. *Oily Taste*—Castor oil may be made palatable by emulsifying with an equal volume of aromatic rhubarb syrup or with compound sarsaparilla syrup. Cod liver oil is effectively disguised by the addition of wintergreen oil or peppermint oil. Lemon, orange, and anise or combinations of these are also useful. It is better to mix most of the flavor with the oil before emulsifying it, and then the small remaining quantity can be added after the primary emulsion is formed.

Those flavors that are most pleasing to the majority of people are associated with some stimulant of a physical or physiological nature. This may be a central nervous stimulant such as caffeine, which is the reason so many enjoy tea and coffee as a beverage, or it may be a counterirritant such as one of the spices that produce a "biting" sensation, or an agent which "tickles" the throat such as soda water. Sherry owes its sharp flavor to its acetaldehyde content and some of the volatile oils contain terpenes that are stimulating to the mucous surfaces.

Selection of Vehicles

Too few pharmacists realize the unique opportunity they have in acquainting physicians with a knowledge of how to increase both the palatability and efficacy of their prescribed medicines through judicious selection of vehicles. Because of the training which a pharmacist receives, his knowledge of the characteristics of various pharmaceuticals and therapeutic agents and his technique and skill in preparing elegant preparations are well developed, so that he is admirably qualified to advise concerning the proper use of vehicles.

A large selection of flavors is available as well as a choice of colors, so that one may prescribe a basic drug for a prolonged period, but by changing the vehicle from time to time, the taste and appearance are so altered that the patient does not tire of the prescription or show other psychological reactions to it.

The statement of the late Dr Bernard Fantus that "the best solvent is the best vehicle" helps to explain the proper use of a flavoring vehicle. For example, a substance that is soluble in alcohol, eg, phenobarbital, will not readily leave an alcoholic vehicle to dissolve in the aqueous saliva.

Waters—These are the simplest of the vehicles and are available with several flavors. They contain no sucrose, a fact to be considered at times, since sucrose under certain circumstances may be undesirable. They are likewise nonalcoholic, another fact which frequently influences vehicle selection.

Elixirs—These have added sweetness that waters lack, and they usually contain alcohol, which imparts an added sharpness to the flavor of certain preparations, making the latter more pleasing to the taste. Elixirs are suitable for alcohol-soluble drugs.

Syrups—These vehicles, like elixirs, offer a wide selection of flavors and colors from which to choose. Their specific value, however, lies particularly in the fact that they are intensely sweet and contain little or no alcohol, a combination which makes them of singular value as masking agents for water-soluble drugs.

Vehicles consisting of a solution of pleasantly flavored volatile oils in syrup or glycerin (1:500) have been successfully employed in producing uniform and stable preparations. These vehicles are prepared by adding 2 mL of the volatile oil, diluted with 6 mL of alcohol, to 500 mL of glycerin or syrup, which has been gently warmed. The solution is added a little at a time with continuous shaking, and then sufficient glycerin or syrup is added to make 1000 mL; and mixed well.

Alcohol solutions of volatile oils are sometimes used as "stock solutions" for flavoring pharmaceuticals.

A listing of substances, most of them official, used as flavors, flavored vehicles, or as sweeteners, is given in Table I. Additional information on flavoring ingredients may be obtained in *Fenaroli's Handbook.*[3]

References

1. Cagan RH and Kare MR: *Biochemistry of Taste and Olfaction,* Academic Press, 1981.
2. Beidler LM ed: *Handbook of Sensory Physiology* Vol IV, Parts 1 and 2, Springer-Verlag 1971.
3. Furia TE, Bellanca N: *Fenaroli's Handbook of Flavor Ingredients* The Chemical Rubber Co, Cleveland, OH, 1971.

Table I—Flavoring Agents

Acacia syrup	Honey
Anethole	Iso-Alcoholic elixir
Anise oil	Lavender oil
Aromatic elixir	Lemon oil
Benzaldehyde	Lemon tincture
Benzaldehyde elixir, compound	Mannitol
	Methyl salicylate
Caraway	Nutmeg oil
Caraway oil	Orange, bitter, elixir
Cardamom oil	Orange, bitter, oil
Cardamom seed	Orange flower oil
Cardamom spirit, compound	Orange flower water
	Orange oil
Cardamom tincture, compound	Orange peel, bitter
	Orange peel, sweet, tincture
Cherry juice	Orange spirit, compound
Cherry syrup	Orange syrup
Cinnamon	Peppermint
Cinnamon oil	Peppermint oil
Cinnamon water	Peppermint spirit
Citric acid	Peppermint water
Citric acid syrup	Phenylethyl alcohol
Clove oil	Raspberry juice
Cocoa	Raspberry syrup
Cocoa syrup	Rosemary oil
Coriander oil	Rose oil
Dextrose	Rose water
Eriodictyon	Rose water, stronger
Eriodictyon fluidextract	Saccharin
Eriodictyon syrup, aromatic	Saccharin calcium
	Saccharin sodium
Ethyl acetate	Sarsaparilla syrup, compound
Ethyl vanillin	
Fennel oil	Sorbitol solution
Ginger	Spearmint
Ginger fluidextract	Spearmint oil
Ginger oleoresin	Sucrose
Glucose	Syrup
Glycerin	Thyme oil
Glycyrrhiza	Tolu balsam
Glycyrrhiza elixir	Tolu balsam syrup
Glycyrrhiza extract	Vanilla
Glycyrrhiza extract, pure	Vanilla tincture
Glycyrrhiza fluidextract	Vanillin
Glycyrrhiza syrup	Wild cherry syrup

Acacia Syrup—see page 1293.

Anethole

Benzene, 1-methoxy-4-(1-propenyl)-, (*E*)-, Anethol; Anise Camphor

(*E*)-*p*-Propenylanisole [4180-23-8] $C_{10}H_{12}O$ (148.20); obtained from anise oil and other sources, or prepared synthetically.

Preparation—Anethole is the principal constituent of anise and fennel oil and is usually obtained from these sources by fractionating and chilling the proper fraction whereby it crystallizes out.

Description—Colorless or faintly yellow liquid at or above 23°; aromatic odor of anise and a sweet taste; affected by light; specific gravity 0.983 to 0.988; distils completely between 231° and 237° and congeals at not less than 20°; its alcohol solution is neutral to litmus.

Solubility—Very slightly soluble in water; freely soluble in alcohol; miscible with chloroform or ether; yields a clear solution with 2 volumes of alcohol.

Uses—A *flavoring agent.* The uses of anethole are similar to those of anise oil. It is sometimes sold as *Synthetic* or *Artificial Anise Oil* for flavoring and is a licorice-like flavor used in *Diphenhydramine Hydrochloride Elixir.*

Anise Oil

Aniseed Oil; Star Anise Oil

The volatile oil distilled with steam from the dried, ripe fruit of *Pimpinella anisum* Linné (Fam *Umbelliferae*) or from the dried, ripe fruit of *Illicium verum* Hooker filius (Fam *Magnoliaceae*).

Note—If solid material has separated, carefully warm the oil until it is completely liquefied, and mix it before using.

Constituents—The official oil varies somewhat in composition, depending upon whether it was obtained from *Pimpinella anisum* or the star anise, *Illicium verum*. *Anethole* is the chief constituent of both oils, occurring to the extent of 80 to 90%. *Methyl chavicol*, an isomer of anethole, and *anisic ketone* [$C_{10}H_{12}O_2$] are also found in both oils, as are small amounts of many other constituents.

Description—Colorless or pale yellow, strongly refractive liquid, having the characteristic odor and taste of anise; specific gravity 0.978 to 0.988; congeals not below 15°.

Solubility—Soluble in 3 volumes 90% alcohol.

Uses—Extensively as a *flavoring agent*, particularly for licorice candies. It has been given as a *carminative* in a dose of about 0.1 mL.

Aromatic Elixir—page 1294.

Aromatic Elixir, Red—RPS-15, page 1240.

Benzaldehyde

Artificial Essential Almond Oil

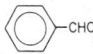

Benzaldehyde [100-52-7] C_7H_6O (106.12).

Preparation—By the interaction of benzal chloride with lime in the presence of water. Benzal chloride is obtained by treating boiling toluene with chlorine.

Description—Colorless, strongly refractive liquid, having an odor resembling that of bitter almond oil, and a burning aromatic taste; affected by light; specific gravity 1.041 to 1.046; boils at about 180°, solidifies at about −56.5°, and on exposure to air it gradually oxidizes to benzoic acid.

Solubility—Dissolves in about 350 volumes water; miscible with alcohol, ether, chloroform, fixed and volatile oils.

Uses—In place of bitter almond oil for *flavoring* purposes; it is much safer than the latter because it contains no hydrocyanic acid. It is also extensively used in *perfumery* and in the manufacture of dyestuffs and many other organic compounds, such as aniline, acetanilid, mandelic acid, etc.

Compound Benzaldehyde Elixir—*Preparation:* Dissolve benzaldehyde (0.5 mL) and vanillin (1 g) in alcohol (50 mL); add syrup (400 mL), orange flower water (150 mL), and sufficient purified water, in several portions, shaking the mixture thoroughly after each addition, to make the product measure 1000 mL; then filter, if necessary, until the product is clear. *Alcohol Content:* 3 to 5%. *Uses:* A useful vehicle for administering bromides and other salts, especially when a low alcoholic content is desired.

Camphor Water—RPS-13, page 436.

Caraway

Carum; Caraway Seed; Caraway Fruit; Kümmel

The dried ripe fruit of *Carum carvi* Linné (Fam *Umbelliferae*).

Constituents—About 5% of *volatile oil*, with a little *fixed oil* and other constituents.

Uses—A *flavor*. It has also been used empirically as a *carminative* and *stimulant*.

Caraway Oil [Oleum Cari]—A volatile oil distilled from the dried, ripe fruit of *Carum carvi* Linné (Fam *Umbelliferae*); yields not less than 50% (v/v) of $C_{10}H_{14}O$ (carvone). The chief odoriferous component of the oil is the ketone *d-carvone* [$C_{10}H_{14}O$], which is the optical isomer of the levorotatory variety occurring in spearmint oil. The remainder of the oil consists mainly of the terpene *d-limonene* [$C_{10}H_{16}$]. Colorless or pale yellow liquid, with the characteristic odor and taste of caraway; specific gravity 0.900 to 0.910. *Uses:* In making caraway water and as a flavor and *carminative* in other pharmaceutical preparations.

Cardamom Seed

Cardamom Fruit; Cardamom; Ceylon or Malabar Cardamom

The dried ripe seed of *Elettaria cardamomum* (Linné) Maton (Fam. *Zingiberaceae*).

Cardamom seed should be recently removed from the capsule.

Constituents—A *volatile oil*, the yield of which is 1.3% from Malabar Ceylon Seeds and 2.6% from Mysore-Ceylon Seeds. *Fixed oil* is present to the extent of 10%, also starch, mucilage, etc.

Uses—A *flavor*. For many years it was empirically employed as a *carminative*.

Cardamom Oil—The volatile oil distilled from the seed of *Elettaria cardamomum* (Linné) Maton (Fam *Zingiberaceae*). Varieties of the oil contain *d-α-terpineol* [$C_{10}H_{17}OH$] both free and as the acetate, 5 to 10% *cineol* [$C_{10}H_{18}O$], and *limonene* [$C_{10}H_{16}$]. The Ceylon Oil, however, contains the alcohol 4-*terpineol* (4-carbomenthenol) [$C_{10}H_{17}OH$], the terpenes *terpinene* and *sabinene*, and *acetic* and *formic acids*, probably combined as esters. Colorless or very pale yellow liquid possessing the aromatic, penetrating, and somewhat camphoraceous odor of cardamom, and a persistently pungent, strongly aromatic taste; affected by light. Specific gravity 0.917 to 0.947; miscible with alcohol; dissolves in 5 volumes 70% alcohol. *Uses:* A *flavor*.

Cardamom Tincture, Compound—page 1294.

Cherry Syrup—page 1292.

Cinnamon

Saigon Cinnamon; True Cinnamon; Saigon Cassia

The dried bark of *Cinnamomum loureirii* Nees (Fam. *Lauraceae*).

Cinnamon contains, in each 100 g, not less than 2.5 mL of volatile oil.

Uses—A *flavoring agent*. Formerly, it was used as a carminative.

Cinnamon Oil [Cassia Oil; Oil of Chinese Cinnamon]—The volatile oil distilled with steam from the leaves and twigs of *Cinnamomum cassia* (Nees) Nees ex Blume (Fam *Lauraceae*), rectified by distillation; contains not less than 80%, by volume, of the total aldehydes of cinnamon oil. Cinnamaldehyde is the chief constituent. Yellowish or brownish liquid, becoming darker and thicker on aging or exposure to the air, and having the characteristic odor and taste of cassia cinnamon; specific gravity 1.045 to 1.063. Soluble in an equal volume of alcohol, 2 volumes 70% alcohol, and an equal volume of glacial acetic acid. *Uses:* A *flavor*. It was formerly used in a dose of 0.1 mL for flatulent colic.

Cocoa

Cacao USP XVI; Prepared Cocoa; Powdered Cocoa; Cocoa Powder; Medium-Fat Cocoa

A powder prepared from the roasted, cured kernels of the ripe seed of *Theobroma cacao* Linné (Fam *Sterculiaceae*).

Cocoa yields 10–22% of nonvolatile, ether-soluble extractive.

Preparation—The cocoa bean is dark as the result of a fermentation and roasting process which it undergoes. *Plain chocolate* consists of shelled cocoa beans (*cocoa nibs*) ground to a smooth paste which forms a hard cake when it cools because of the high fat content (50 to 58%).

Cocoa is the food prepared by pulverizing the residue remaining after part of the fat has been removed by expression from plain chocolate. Cocoa may be flavored by the addition of ground spice, ground vanilla bean, vanillin, ethylvanillin, coumarin, salt, and other flavors as long as they do not imitate the flavor of chocolate, milk or butter. Three types of cocoa are recognized depending on fat content: *breakfast cocoa* or *high fat cocoa* (22% minimum), *cocoa* or *medium-fat cocoa* (10 to 22%), and *low-fat cocoa* (less than 10%).

Sweet chocolate is plain chocolate plus added sugar and flavor (usually vanilla).

Milk chocolate is a mixture of sweet chocolate and milk powder or other dairy product. Chocolate and the products described above contain the purines theobromine and caffeine, and considerable quantities of fat (cocoa butter or theobroma oil), as well as protein and starch. These factors are lowered in sweet chocolate because of the large amount of added sugar (more than 50% of the final product).

Description—Weak reddish to purplish brown to moderate brown powder having a chocolate-like odor and taste, free from sweetness.

Uses—A food and pharmaceutically as a flavor in tablets, syrups, pill and tablet coatings, troches, etc.

Cocoa Syrup—page 1285.

Coriander Oil

The volatile oil distilled with steam from the dried ripe fruit of *Coriandrum sativum* Linné (Fam *Umbelliferae*).
Constituents—The alcohol *d-linalool* (formerly termed "*coriandrol*") is the chief constituent of this oil, occurring in amounts varying from 60 to 80%. Other constituents include *l-borneol*, *geraniol*, *pinenes*, *terpinenes*, and *p-cymene*.

Description—Colorless or pale yellow liquid, having the characteristic odor and taste of coriander; specific gravity 0.863 to 0.875.
Solubility—Soluble in 3 volumes 70% alcohol.

Uses—A flavoring agent. It was formerly employed in a dose of 0.1 mL as a *carminative*.

Eriodictyon

Consumptives' Weed; Mountain Balm; Yerba Santa

The dried leaf of *Eriodictyon californicum* (Hooker et Arnott) Torrey (Fam *Hydrophyllaceae*).
Constituents—A bitter *resin*, *volatile oil*, *eriodictyonone* [$C_{16}H_{14}O_6$, also called *homoeriodictyol*], *fixed oil*, *tannin*, *gum*, etc.
Uses—A pharmaceutical necessity. It is used in the preparation of *Eriodictyon Fluidextract.*

Eriodictyon Fluidextract [Yerba Santa Fluidextract]—*Preparation:* Using Eriodictyon (in moderately coarse powder, 1000 g), prepare the fluidextract by Process A (page 1516), using a mixture of 4 volumes of alcohol and 1 volume of water as the menstruum. Macerate the drug during 48 hours, then percolate at a moderate rate, and reserve the first 800 mL of percolate. *Alcohol Content:* 57 to 62%. *Uses:* A peculiar, aromatic *flavor*, used in syrups and elixirs, especially for masking the taste of bitter drugs like quinine. Because of its resinous character it requires an alkali to render it soluble in aqueous mixtures.

Eriodictyon Syrup, Aromatic—page 1286.

Ethyl Acetate

Acetic acid, ethyl ester; Acetic Ether

$$CH_3COOC_2H_5$$

Ethyl acetate [141-78-6] $C_4H_8O_2$ (88.11).
Preparation—By slow distillation of a mixture of alcohol and acetic acid in the presence of sulfuric acid.

Description—Transparent, colorless liquid with a fragrant and refreshing, slightly acetous odor, and a peculiar acetous, burning taste; specific gravity 0.894 to 0.898; distils between 76° and 77.5°.
Solubility—1 mL in about 10 mL water; miscible with alcohol, acetone, ether, chloroform, fixed and volatile oils.

Uses—Chiefly as a *flavoring agent*. It is used industrially in artificial fruit essence, as a *solvent* for nitrocellulose varnishes and lacquers, and as a solvent in organic chemistry.

Eucalyptus Oil

The volatile oil distilled with steam from the fresh leaf of *Eucalyptus globulus* Labillardière or of some other species of *Eucalyptus* L'Heritier (Fam *Myrtaceae*). Eucalyptus oil contains not less than 70% of $C_{10}H_{18}O$ (eucalyptol).
Constituents—The most important constituent is *eucalyptol* (*cineol*). Other compounds include *d-α-pinene*, *globulol*, *pinocarveol*, *pinocarvone*, and several aldehydes.

Description—Colorless or pale yellow liquid, having a characteristic, aromatic, somewhat camphoraceous odor, and a pungent, spicy, cooling taste; specific gravity 0.905 to 0.925 at 25°.
Solubility—Soluble in 5 volumes 70% alcohol.

Uses—A *flavoring agent* and an *expectorant* in chronic bronchitis. It also has *bacteriostatic* properties. This oil may be toxic.

Ethyl Vanillin

Benzaldehyde, 3-ethoxy-4-hydroxy-, Bourbanal; Ethovan; Vanillal; Vanirome

3-Ethoxy-4-hydroxybenzaldehyde [121-32-4] $C_9H_{10}O_3$ (166.18).
Preparation—By reacting *o*-ethoxyphenol with formaldehyde and *p*-nitrosodimethylaniline in the presence of aluminum and water.

Description—Fine, white or slightly yellowish crystals; odor and taste similar to vanillin; affected by light; solutions are acid to litmus; melting range 76° to 78°.
Solubility—1 g in about 100 mL water at 50°; freely soluble in alcohol, chloroform, ether, and solutions of fixed alkali hydroxides.

Uses—A *flavor*, like vanillin, but stronger.

Fennel Oil

The volatile oil distilled with steam from the dried ripe fruit of *Foeniculum vulgare* Miller (Fam *Umbelliferae*).
Note—If solid material has separated, carefully warm the oil until it is completely liquefied, and mix it before using.
Constituents—Anethole [$C_{10}H_{12}O$] is the chief constituent, occurring to the extent of 50 to 60%. Some of the other constituents are *d*-pinene, phellandrene, dipentene, fenchone, methylchavicol, anisaldehyde, and anisic acid.

Description—Colorless or pale yellow liquid, having the characteristic odor and taste of fennel; specific gravity 0.953 to 0.973; congealing temperature is not below 3°.
Solubility—Soluble in 8 volumes 80% alcohol and in 1 volume 90% alcohol.

Uses—A flavoring agent. It was formerly employed in a dose of 0.1 mL as a *carminative*.

Glycyrrhiza

Licorice Root; Liquorice Root; Sweetwood; Italian Juice Root; Spanish Juice Root

The dried rhizome and roots of *Glycyrrhiza glabra* Linné, known in commerce as Spanish Licorice, or of *Glycyrrhiza glabra* Linné var *glandulifera* Waldstein et Kitaibel, known in commerce as Russian Licorice, or of other varieties of *Glycyrrhiza glabra* Linné, yielding a yellow and sweet wood (Fam *Leguminosae*).
Constituents—This well-known root contains 5 to 7% of the sweet principle *glycyrrhizin*, or *glycyrrhizic acid* which is 50 times as sweet as cane sugar. There is also present an oleoresinous substance to which its slightly acridity is due. If alcohol or an alkali is used as a menstruum for the root and the preparation not treated to deprive it of acridity, it will have a disagreeable after-taste. For this reason boiling water is used for its extraction in both the extract and the fluidextract.

Description—The USP/NF provides descriptions of *Unground Spanish and Russian Glycyrrhizas*, *Histology*, and *Powdered Glycyrrhiza*.

Uses—Valuable in pharmacy chiefly for its *sweet flavor*. It is one of the most efficient substances known for masking the taste of bitter substances, like quinine. Acids precipitate the glycyrrhizin and should not be added to mixtures in which glycyrrhiza is intended to mask disagreeable taste. Most of the imported licorice is used by tobacco manufacturers to flavor tobacco. It is also used in making candy.

Pure Glycyrrhiza Extract [Pure Licorice Root Extract]—*Preparation:* Moisten 1000 g of glycyrrhiza, in granular powder, with boiling water, transfer it to a percolator, and percolate with boiling water until the glycyrrhiza is exhausted. Add enough diluted ammonia solution to the percolate to impart a distinctly ammoniacal odor, then boil the liquid under normal atmospheric pressure until it is reduced to a volume of about 1500 mL. Filter the liquid, and immediately evaporate the filtrate until the residue has a pilular consistency. Pure extract of glycyrrhiza differs from the commercial extract in that it is almost completely soluble in aqueous mixtures. The large amount of filler used in the commercial extract to give it firmness renders it unfit to use as a substitute for the pure extract. *Description:* Black, pilular mass having a characteristic, sweet taste. *Uses:* A *flavoring agent.* One of the ingredients in *Aromatic Cascara Sagrada Fluidextract.*

Glycyrrhiza Fluidextract [Licorice Root Fluidextract; Liquid Extract of Liquorice]—*Preparation:* To 1000 g of coarsely ground glycyrrhiza add about 3000 mL of boiling water, mix, and allow to macerate in a suitable, covered percolator for 2 hours. Then allow the percolation to proceed at a rate of 1 to 3 mL/min, gradually adding boiling water until the glycyrrhiza is exhausted. Add enough diluted ammonia solution to the percolate to impart a distinctly ammoniacal odor, then boil the liquid actively under normal atmospheric pressure until it is reduced to a volume of about 1500 mL. Filter the liquid, evaporate the filtrate on a steam bath until the residue measures 750 mL, cool, and gradually add 250 mL alcohol and enough water to make the product measure 1000 mL, and mix. *Alcohol Content:* 20 to 24%, by volume. *Uses:* A pleasant *flavor* for use in syrups and elixirs to be employed as vehicles and correctives.

Glycyrrhiza Elixir—page 1286.

Glycyrrhiza Syrup—page 1286.

Honey—page 1320.

Hydriodic Acid Syrup—page 1320.

Iso-Alcoholic Elixir—page 1319.

Lavender Oil

Lavender Flowers Oil

The volatile oil distilled with steam from the fresh flowering tops of *Lavandula officinalis* Chaix ex Villars (*Lavandula vera* DeCandolle) (Fam *Labiatae*) or produced synthetically. It contains not less than 35% of esters calculated as $C_{12}H_{20}O_2$ (linalyl acetate).

Constituents—Lavender oil is a product of considerable importance in perfumery. *Linalyl acetate* is the chief constituent. *Cineol* appears to be a normal constituent of English oils. Other constituents include: *amyl alcohol, d-borneol* (small amount); *geraniol, lavandulol* ($C_{10}H_{18}O$); *linaloöl; nerol; acetic, butyric, valeric,* and *caproic acids* (as esters); traces of *d-pinene, limonene* (in English oils only), and the sesquiterpene *caryophyllene; ethyl n-amyl ketone;* an aldehyde (probably *valeric aldehyde); and coumarin.*

Description—Colorless or yellow liquid, having the characteristic odor and taste of lavender flowers; specific gravity 0.875 to 0.888.

Solubility—1 volume dissolves in 4 volumes 70% alcohol.

Uses—Primarily as a *perfume.* It was formerly used in doses of 0.1 mL as a *carminative.*

Lemon Oil

The volatile oil obtained by expression, without the aid of heat, from the fresh peel of the fruit of *Citrus limon* (Linné) Burmann filius (Fam *Rutaceae*), with or without the previous separation of the pulp and the peel. The total aldehyde content, calculated as citral ($C_{10}H_{16}O$), is 2.2–3.8% for California-type lemon oil, and 3.0–5.5% for Italian-type lemon oil.

Note—Do not use lemon oil that has a terebinthine odor.

Constituents—From the standpoint of odor and flavor, the most noteworthy constituent is the aldehyde *citral*, which is present to the extent of about 4%. About 90% of *d-limonene* is present; small amounts of *l-α-pinene, β-pinene, camphene, β-phellandrene,* and γ-terpinene also occur. About 2% of a solid, nonvolatile substance called *citroptene, limettin,* or *lemon-camphor,* which is dissolved out of the peel, is also present. In addition, there are traces of several other compounds: *α-terpineol;* the *acetates of linaloöl* and *geraniol; citronellal, octyl* and *nonyl aldehydes;* the sesquiterpenes *bisabolene* and *cadinene;* and the ketone *methylheptenone.*

When fresh, the oil has the fragrant odor of lemons. Because of the instability of the terpenes present, the oil readily undergoes deterioration by oxidation, acquiring a terebinthinate odor.

Description—Pale yellow to deep yellow or greenish yellow liquid, with the characteristic odor and taste of the outer part of fresh lemon peel; specific gravity 0.849 to 0.855.

Solubility—Soluble in 3 volumes alcohol; miscible in all proportions with dehydrated alcohol, carbon disulfide, or glacial acetic acid.

Uses—A *flavor* in pharmaceutical preparations and in certain candies and foods.

Methyl Salicylate

Benzoic acid, 2-hydroxy-, methyl ester; Gaultheria Oil; Wintergreen Oil; Betula Oil; Sweet Birch Oil; Teaberry Oil; Artificial Wintergreen Oil; Synthetic Wintergreen Oil

Methyl salicylate [119-36-8] $C_6H_4(OH)COOCH_3$ (152.15); produced synthetically or obtained by maceration and subsequent distillation with steam from the leaves of *Gaultheria procumbens* Linné (Fam *Ericaceae*) or from the bark of *Betula lenta* Linné (Fam *Betulaceae*).

Note—Methyl salicylate must be labeled to indicate whether it was made synthetically or distilled from either of the plants mentioned above.

Preparation—Found naturally in gaultheria and betula oils and in many other plants but the commercial product is usually synthetic, made by esterifying salicylic acid with methyl alcohol in the presence of sulfuric acid and distilling.

Description—Colorless, yellowish, or reddish liquid, having the characteristic odor and taste of wintergreen; specific gravity (synthetic), 1.180 to 1.185, (from gaultheria or betula), 1.176 to 1.182; boils between 219° and 224° with some decomposition.

Solubility—Slightly soluble in water; soluble in alcohol and glacial acetic acid.

Uses—A pharmaceutical necessity and *counterirritant* (local analgesic). As a pharmaceutical necessity, it is used to flavor the official *Aromatic Cascara Sagrada Fluidextract,* and it is equal in every respect to wintergreen oil or sweet birch oil. As a counterirritant, it is applied to the skin in the form of a liniment, ointment or cream; care should be exercised since salicylate is absorbed through the skin.

Caution—Because it smells like wintergreen candy, methyl salicylate is frequently ingested by children and has caused many fatalities. *Keep out of the reach of children.*

Dose—*Topical,* in lotions and solutions in **10** to **25%** concentration.

Nutmeg Oil

Myristica Oil NF XIII; East Indian Nutmeg Oil; West Indian Nutmeg Oil

The volatile oil distilled with steam from the dried kernels of the ripe seeds of *Myristica fragrans* Houttuyn (Fam *Myristicaceae*).

Constituents—Nutmeg oil contains about 80% of *d-pinene* and *d-camphene,* 8% of *dipentene,* about 6% of the alcohols *d-borneol, geraniol, d-linaloöl,* and *terpineol,* 4% of *myristicin,* 0.6% of *safrol,* 0.3% of *myristic acid* free and as esters, 0.2% of *eugenol* and *isoeugenol* and traces of the alcohol *terpineol-4,* a citral-like aldehyde, and several acids, all present as esters.

Description—Colorless or pale yellow liquid having the characteristic odor and taste of nutmeg; specific gravity (East Indian Oil) between 0.880 and 0.910, (West Indian Oil) between 0.854 and 0.880.

Solubility—Soluble in an equal amount of alcohol; 1 volume of East Indian Oil in 3 volumes of 90% alcohol; 1 volume of West Indian Oil in 4 volumes of 90% alcohol.

Uses—Primarily as a *flavoring agent.* It is used for this purpose in *Aromatic Ammonia Spirit* (page 1507). The oil is also employed as a *flavor* in foods, certain alcoholic beverages, dentifrices, and tobacco; to some extent, it is also used in perfumery. It was *formerly* used as a *carminative* and *local stimulant* to the gastrointestinal tract in a dose of 0.03 mL. In overdoses, it acts as a narcotic poison. *This oil is very difficult to keep and even if slightly terebinthinate is unfit for flavoring purposes.*

Orange Oil

Sweet Orange Oil

The volatile oil obtained by expression from the fresh peel of the ripe fruit of *Citrus sinensis* (Linné) Osbeck (Fam *Rutaceae*). The total aldehyde content, calculated as decanal ($C_{10}H_{20}O$), is 1.2 to 2.5%.

Note—Do not use Orange Oil that has a terebinthine odor.

Constituents—Consists of *d-limonene* to the extent of at least 90%; in the remaining 5 to 10% are the odorous constituents, among which, in samples of American origin, are *n-decylic aldehyde, citral, d-li-naloöl, n-nonyl alcohol*, and traces of *esters* of *formic, acetic, caprylic*, and *capric* acids.

In addition to most of these compounds, Italian-produced oil contains *d-terpineol, terpinolene, α-terpinene*, and *methyl anthranilate*.

Kept under the usual conditions orange oil is very prone to decompose, and rapidly acquires a terebinthine odor.

Description—Intensely yellow, orange, or deep orange liquid, which possesses the characteristic odor and taste of the outer part of fresh sweet orange peel; specific gravity 0.842 to 0.846.

Solubility—Miscible with dehydrated alcohol and with carbon disulfide; dissolves in an equal volume of glacial acetic acid.

Uses—A *flavoring agent* in elixirs and other preparations.

Orange Flower Oil

Neroli Oil

The volatile oil distilled from the fresh flowers of *Citrus aurantium* Linné (Fam *Rutaceae*).

Constituents—*β-Ocimene, l-α-pinene, l-camphene, dipentene, l-linaloöl, geraniol, farnesol, d-terpineol, phenylethyl alcohol, nerol, nerolidol, decylic aldehyde, jasmone, methyl anthranilate, indole, acetic esters of the alcohols* present, and traces of *esters of benzoic, phenylacetic,* and *palmitic acids.*

Description—Pale yellow, slightly fluorescent liquid, which becomes reddish brown on exposure to light and air; distinctive, fragrant odor, similar to that of orange blossoms, and an aromatic, at first sweet, then somewhat bitter, taste; may become turbid or solid at low temperatures; specific gravity 0.863 to 0.880; neutral to litmus paper; an alcoholic solution has a *violet fluorescence.*

Uses—A *flavor* and *perfume.* Several less valuable varieties of the oil are commercially known. These are designated as *Bigarade* (from the fresh flowers of bitter orange, the ordinary neroli oil), *Portugal* (from the fresh flowers of sweet orange), and *Petit-grain* (from the leaves and young shoots of the bitter orange). The finest variety is known as *Petale.*

Orange Flower Water—page 1292.

Sweet Orange Peel Tincture

Preparation—From sweet orange peel, which is the outer rind of the non-artificially colored, fresh, ripe fruit of *Citrus sinensis* (Linné) Osbeck (Fam *Rutaceae*), by Process M (page 1516). Macerate 500 g of the sweet orange peel (*Note—Exclude the inner, white portion of the rind*) in 900 mL of alcohol, and complete the preparation with alcohol to make the product measure 1000 mL. Use talc as the filtering medium.

The white portion of the rind must not be used, as the proportion of oil, which is only in the yellow rind, is reduced, and the bitter principle *hesperidin* is introduced.

Alcohol Content—62 to 72%.

Uses—A *flavor*, used in syrups, elixirs, and emulsions. This tincture was introduced to provide a delicate orange flavor direct from the fruit instead of depending upon orange oil which so frequently is terebinthinate and unfit for use. The tincture keeps well.

Compound Orange Spirit

Contains, in each 100 mL, 25–30 mL of the mixed oils.

Orange Oil	200 mL
Lemon Oil	50 mL
Coriander Oil	20 mL
Anise Oil	5 mL
Alcohol, a sufficient quantity,	
To make	1000 mL

Mix the oils with sufficient alcohol to make the product measure 1000 mL.

Alcohol Content—65 to 75%.

Uses—A *flavor* for elixirs. An alcoholic solution of this kind permits the uniform introduction of small proportions of oils and also preserves orange and lemon oils from rapid oxidation. These two oils should be bought in small quantities by the pharmacist, since the spirit is most satisfactorily made from oils taken from bottles not previously opened. This will insure that delicacy of flavor which should always be characteristic of elixirs.

Orange Syrup

Syrup of Orange Peel

Contains, in each 100 mL, 450–550 mg of citric acid ($C_6H_8O_7$).

Sweet Orange Peel Tincture	50 mL
Citric Acid (anhydrous)	5 g
Talc	15 g
Sucrose	820 g
Purified Water, a sufficient quantity,	
To make	1000 mL

Triturate the talc with the tincture and citric acid, and gradually add 400 mL of purified water. Then filter, returning the first portions of the filtrate until it becomes clear, and wash the mortar and filter with enough purified water to make the filtrate measure 450 mL. Dissolve the sucrose in this filtrate by agitation, without heating, and add enough purified water to make the product measure 1000 mL. Mix, and strain.

Note—Do not use Orange Syrup that has a terebinthine odor or taste or shows other indications of deterioration.

Alcohol Content—2 to 5%.

Uses—A pleasant, acidic vehicle.

Peppermint

American Mint; Lamb Mint; Brandy Mint

Consists of the dried leaf and flowering top of *Mentha piperita* Linné (Fam *Labiatae*).

Uses—The source of green color for *Peppermint Spirit* (page 814). The odor of fresh peppermint is due to the presence of about 2% of a volatile oil, much of which is lost on drying the leaves in air. Peppermint is widely cultivated both in the US and France. It was formerly used as a carminative.

Peppermint Oil—The volatile oil distilled with steam from the fresh overground parts of the flowering plant of *Mentha piperita* Linné (Fam *Labiatae*), rectified by distillation and neither partially nor wholly dementholized. It yields not less than 5% of esters, calculated as menthyl acetate [$C_{12}H_{22}O_2$], and not less than 50% of total menthol [$C_{10}H_{20}O$], free and as esters. *Constituents:* This is one of the most important of the group of volatile oils. The chief constituent is *Menthol* (page 781) which occurs in the levorotatory form; its ester, *menthyl acetate*, is present in a much smaller amount. Other compounds which are present include the ketone *menthone, piperitone, α-pinene, l-limonene, phellandrene, cadinene, menthyl isovalerate, isovaleric aldehyde, acetaldehyde, menthofuran, cineol,* an unidentified *lactone* [$C_{10}H_{16}O_2$], and probably *amyl acetate.* Colorless or pale yellow liquid, having a strong, penetrating odor of peppermint, and a pungent taste, followed by a sensation of cold when air is drawn into the mouth; specific gravity 0.896 to 0.908; 1 volume dissolves in 3 volumes 70% alcohol. *Uses:* A *flavoring agent, carminative, antiseptic,* and *local anesthetic.* It is also extensively used as a *flavor* in candy, chewing gum, etc.

Peppermint Spirit—page 814.

Peppermint Water—page 1292.

Phenylethyl Alcohol

Benzeneethanol; 2-Phenylethanol

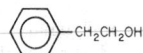

Phenethyl alcohol [60-12-8] $C_8H_{10}O$ (122.17); occurs in a number of essential oils such as those of rose, neroli, hyacinth, carnation, and others.

Description—Colorless liquid with a rose-like odor and a sharp, burning taste; solidifies at $-27°$; has a specific gravity between 1.017 and 1.020.

Solubility—1 g in 60 mL water; <1 mL alcohol, chloroform, ether; very soluble in fixed oils, glycerin, propylene glycol; slightly soluble in mineral oil.

Uses—Introduced for use as an antibacterial agent in ophthalmic solutions but it is of limited effectiveness.

It is used in *flavors*, as a *soap perfume*, and in the preparation of synthetic oils of rose and similar flower oils. It is also a valuable perfume fixative.

Pine Needle Oil

Dwarf Pine Oil

The volatile oil distilled with steam from the fresh leaf of *Pinus mugo* Turra and its variety *pumilio* (Haenke) Zenari (Fam *Pinaceae*); contains 3–10%, by weight, of esters calculated as $C_{12}H_{20}O_2$ (bornyl acetate).

Constituents—It contains the terpenes *l-α-pinene*, *β-pinene*, *l-phellandrene*, *l-limonene*, *dipentene*, and possibly *sylvestrene*, the ester *bornyl acetate*, and several unidentified terpene and sesquiterpene alcohols.

Description—Colorless to yellowish liquid, having a pleasant, aromatic odor and a bitter, pungent taste; specific gravity 0.853 to 0.871 at 25°.

Solubility—Dissolves in 4.5 to 10 volumes of 90% alcohol, often with turbidity.

Uses—Chiefly as a *perfume* and *flavoring agent*. It is also employed as an inhalant in bronchitis.

Raspberry Syrup—page 1294.

Rose Oil

Otto of Rose; Attar of Rose

The volatile oil distilled with steam from the fresh flowers of *Rosa gallica* Linné, *Rosa damascena* Miller, *Rosa alba* Linné, *Rosa centifolia* Linné, and varieties of these species (Fam *Rosaceae*).

Constituents—From the quantitative standpoint the chief components are the alcohols *geraniol* [$C_{10}H_{18}O$] and *l-citronellol* [$C_{10}H_{20}O$]. The sesquiterpene alcohols *farnesol* and *nerol* occur to the extent of 1% and 5 to 10%, respectively. Together, the four alcohols constitute 70 to 75% of the oil. *Phenylethyl alcohol*, which comprises 1% of the oil, is an important odoriferous constituent. Other compounds present are *linaloöl*, *eugenol*, *nonyl aldehyde*, traces of *citral*, and two solid hydrocarbons of the paraffin series.

Description—A colorless or yellow liquid, which has the characteristic odor and taste of rose; at 25°, a viscous liquid; on gradual cooling it changes to a translucent, crystalline mass, which may be easily liquefied by warming; specific gravity 0.848 to 0.863 at 30° compared with water at 15°; 1 mL mixes with 1 mL chloroform without turbidity; on the addition of 20 mL 90% alcohol to this solution, the resulting liquid is neutral or acid to moistened litmus paper and deposits a crystalline residue within 5 min on standing at 20°.

Uses—Principally as a *perfume*. It is officially recognized for its use as an ingredient in *Rose Water Ointment* and cosmetics.

Stronger Rose Water

Triple Rose Water

A saturated solution of the odoriferous principles of the flowers of *Rosa centifolia* Linné (Fam *Rosaceae*), prepared by distilling the fresh flowers with water and separating the excess volatile oil from the clear, water portion of the distillate.

Note—Stronger rose water, diluted with an equal volume of purified water, may be supplied when *Rose Water* is required.

Description—Nearly colorless and clear liquid which possesses the pleasant odor and taste of fresh rose blossoms; must be free from empyreuma, mustiness, and fungal growths.

Uses—An ingredient in *Rose Water Ointment*. It is sometimes prepared extemporaneously from concentrates or from rose oil, but such water is not official and rarely compares favorably with the fresh distillate from rose petals.

Saccharin

1,2-Benzisothiazol-3(2H)-one, 1,1-dioxide; Gluside; *o*-Benzosulfimide

1,2-Benzisothiazolin-3-one 1,1-dioxide [81-07-2] $C_7H_5NO_3S$ (183.18).

Preparation—Toluene is reacted with chlorosulfonic acid to form *o*-toluenesulfonyl chloride, which is converted to the sulfonamide with ammonia. The methyl group is then oxidized with dichromate yielding *o*-sulfamoylbenzoic acid which, when heated, forms the cyclic imide.

Description—White crystals or a white crystalline powder; odorless or has a faint aromatic odor; in dilute solution it is intensely sweet; solutions are acid to litmus; melting range 226° to 230°.

Solubility—1 g in 290 mL water, 31 mL alcohol, or 25 mL boiling water; slightly soluble in chloroform and in ether; readily dissolved by dilute solution of ammonia, by solutions of alkali hydroxides, and by solutions of alkali carbonates with the evolution of CO_2.

Uses—A sweetening agent in *Aromatic Cascara Sagrada Fluidextract* and highly alcoholic preparations. It is an intensely sweet substance. A 60-mg portion is equivalent in sweetening power to approximately 30 g of sucrose. It is used as a *sweetening agent* in vehicles, canned foods, beverages, and in diets for diabetics to replace the sucrose. The relative sweetening power of saccharin is increased by dilution.

Saccharin Calcium

1,2-Benzisothiazol-3(2H)-one, 1,1-dioxide, calcium salt, hydrate (2:7)
Calcium *o*-Benzosulfimide

1,2-Benzisothiazolin-3-one 1,1-dioxide calcium salt hydrate (2:7) [6381-91-5] $C_{14}H_8CaN_2O_6S_2.3\frac{1}{2}H_2O$ (467.48); *anhydrous* [6485-34-3] (404.43).

Preparation—Saccharin is reacted with a semimolar quantity of calcium hydroxide in aqueous medium and the resulting solution is concentrated to crystallization.

Description—White crystals or a white, crystalline powder; odorless or has a faint aromatic odor; and an intensely sweet taste even in dilute solutions; in dilute solution it is about 300 times as sweet as sucrose.

Solubility—1 g in 2.6 mL water, 4.7 mL alcohol.

Uses and **Dose**—See *Saccharin*.

Saccharin Sodium

1,2-Benzisothiazol-3(2H)-one, 1,1-dioxide, sodium salt, dihydrate; Soluble Saccharin; Soluble Gluside; Sodium *o*-Benzosulfimide

1,2-Benzisothiazolin-3-one 1,1-dioxide sodium salt dihydrate [6155-57-3] $C_7H_4NNaO_3S.2H_2O$ (241.19); *anhydrous* [128-44-9] (205.16).

Preparation—Saccharin is dissolved in an equimolar quantity of aqueous sodium hydroxide and the solution is concentrated to crystallization.

Description—White crystals or a white crystalline powder; odorless or has a faint aromatic odor and an intensely sweet taste even in dilute solutions; in dilute solution it is about 300 times as sweet as sucrose; when in powdered form it usually contains about 1/3 the theoretical amount of water of hydration due to efflorescence.

Solubility—1 g in 1.5 mL water, 50 mL alcohol.

Uses—Same as *Saccharin* but has the advantage of being more soluble in neutral aqueous solutions.

Application—**15 to 60 mg** as necessary.

Dosage Form—Tablets: 15, 30, and 60 mg.

Sarsaparilla Syrup, Compound—RPS-13, page 445.

Sherry Wine—RPS-15, page 1240.

Sorbitol

Sionin; Sorbit; D-Sorbitol; D-Glucitol Sorbo (*Atlas*)

$$HO-\overset{\overset{\displaystyle H}{|}}{\underset{\underset{\displaystyle H}{|}}{C}}-\overset{\overset{\displaystyle OH}{|}}{\underset{\underset{\displaystyle H}{|}}{C}}-\overset{\overset{\displaystyle H}{|}}{\underset{\underset{\displaystyle OH}{|}}{C}}-\overset{\overset{\displaystyle OH}{|}}{\underset{\underset{\displaystyle H}{|}}{C}}-\overset{\overset{\displaystyle OH}{|}}{\underset{\underset{\displaystyle H}{|}}{C}}-\overset{\overset{\displaystyle H}{|}}{\underset{\underset{\displaystyle H}{|}}{C}}-OH$$

D-Glucitol [50-70-4] $C_6H_{14}O_6$ (182.17); it may contain small amounts of other polyhydric alcohols.

Preparation—Commercially by reduction (hydrogenation) of certain sugars, such as glucose.

Description—White, hygroscopic powder, granules, or flakes, having a sweet taste; the usual form melts at about 96°.

Solubility—1 g in about 0.45 mL water; slightly soluble in alcohol, methanol, and acetic acid.

Uses—An *osmotic diuretic* given intravenously in 50% (*w/v*) solution to diminish edema, to lower cerebrospinal pressure, or to reduce intraocular pressure in glaucoma. It is also used as a laxative, sweetener, humectant, plasticizer, and, in 70% (*w/w*) solution, as a vehicle.

Dose—**50 to 100 mL** of a **50%** solution; as a *laxative*, *oral*, **30 to 50 g.**

Sorbitol Solution is a water solution containing, in each 100 g, 69–71 g of total solids consisting essentially of D-sorbitol and a small amount of mannitol and other isomeric polyhydric alcohols. The content of D-sorbitol [$C_6H_8(OH)_6$] in each 100 g is not less than 64 g. *Description:* Clear, colorless, syrupy liquid, having a sweet taste and no characteristic odor; neutral to litmus, and has a specific gravity of not less than 1.285 and a refractive index at 20° of 1.455 to 1.465. *Uses:* It is not to be injected. It has been used as a replacement for propylene glycol and glycerin.

Spearmint

Spearmint Leaves; Spearmint Herb; Mint

The dried leaf and flowering top of *Mentha spicata* Linné (*Mentha viridis* Linné) (Common Spearmint) or of *Mentha cardiaca* Gerard ex Baker (Scotch Spearmint) (Fam *Labiatae*).

Uses—A flavoring agent. Fresh spearmint is used in preparing mint sauce, and also the well-known mint julep. The volatile oil is the only constituent of importance in this plant; the yield is from 1/2 to 1%.

Spearmint Oil is the volatile oil distilled with steam from the fresh over-ground parts of the flowering plant of *Mentha spicata* or of *Mentha cardiaca;* contains not less than 55%, by volume, of $C_{10}H_{14}O$ (carvone = 150.22). The chief odoriferous constituent is the ketone *l-carvone*. American oil also contains *dihydrocarveol acetate* [$CH_3COOC_{10}H_{17}$], *l-limonene* [$C_{10}H_{16}$], a small amount of *phellandrene* [$C_{10}H_{16}$], and traces of *esters of valeric* and *caproic acids*. Colorless, yellow, or greenish yellow liquid, having the characteristic odor and taste of spearmint; soluble in 1 volume of 80% alcohol, but upon further dilution may become turbid; specific gravity 0.917 to 0.934. *Uses:* Primarily as a flavoring agent. It has also been used as a *carminative* in doses of 0.1 mL.

Sucrose

α-D-Glucopyranoside, β-D-fructofuranosyl-; Sugar; Cane Sugar; Beet Sugar

Sucrose [57-50-1] $C_{12}H_{22}O_{11}$ (342.30); a sugar obtained from *Saccharum officinarum* Linné (Fam *Gramineae*), *Beta vulgaris* Linné (Fam *Chenopodiaceae*), and other sources. It contains no added substances.

For the structural formula, see page 399.

Preparation—Commercially from the sugar cane, beet root, and sorghum. Originally sugar cane was the only source; but at present the root of *Beta vulgaris* is largely used in Europe, and to an increasing degree in this country, for making sucrose.

The sugar cane is crushed and the juice amounting to about 80% is expressed with roller mills. The juice after "defecation" with lime and removal of excess of lime by carbonic acid gas, is run into vacuum pans for concentration and the saccharine juice is evaporated in this until it begins to crystallize. After the crystallization is complete, the warm mixture of crystals and syrup is run into centrifuges, in which the crystals of raw sugar are drained and dried. The syrup resulting as a by-product from raw sugar is known as *molasses.* Raw beet sugar is made by a similar process, but is more troublesome to purify than that made from sugar cane.

The refined sugar from either raw cane or beet sugar is prepared by dissolving the raw sugar in water, clarifying, filtering, and finally decolorizing the solution by passing it through bone-black filters. The water-white solution is finally evaporated under reduced pressure to the crystallizing point and then forced to crystallize in small granules which are collected and drained in a centrifuge.

Description—Colorless or white crystals, crystalline masses or blocks, or a white, crystalline powder; odorless, has a sweet taste, is stable in air, and its solutions are neutral to litmus; melts with decomposition between 160° and 185°, and has a specific gravity of about 1.57; specific rotation at 20° is not less than +65.9°; unlike the other official sugars (dextrose, fructose, and lactose), sucrose does not reduce Fehling's solution even in hot solutions; also differs from these sugars in that it is darkened and charred by sulfuric acid in the cold; fermentable, and in dilute aqueous solutions it ferments into alcohol and eventually acetic acid.

Sucrose is hydrolyzed by dilute mineral acids, slowly in the cold, and rapidly on heating into one molecule each of dextrose and levulose. This process is technically known as "inversion" and the product is referred to as "invert sugar"; the term inversion being derived from the change, through the hydrolysis, in the optical rotation from dextro of the sucrose to levo of the hydrolyzed product. The enzyme *invertase* also hydrolyzes sucrose.

Solubility—1 g in 0.5 mL water, 170 mL alcohol, and in slightly more than 0.2 mL boiling water; insoluble in chloroform and ether.

Uses—Principally as a pharmaceutical necessity for making syrups and lozenges. It gives viscosity and consistency to fluids.

Intravenous administration of hypertonic solutions of sucrose has been employed chiefly to initiate *osmotic diuresis.* Such a procedure is not completely safe and renal tubular damage may result, particularly in patients with existing renal pathology. Safer and more effective diuretics are available.

Compressible Sugar

Sucrose that may contain some starch, malto-dextrin, or invert sugar; contains 95.0–98.0% sucrose.

Description—White, crystalline, odorless powder having a sweet taste; stable in air.

Solubility—The sucrose portion is very soluble in water.

Uses—A *pharmaceutic aid* as a *tableting excipient* and *sweetening agent.* See also *Sucrose.*

Confectioner's Sugar

Sucrose ground together with corn starch to a fine powder; contains 95.0–97.0% sucrose.

Description—Fine, white, odorless powder having a sweet taste; stable in air; specific rotation not less than +62.6°.

Solubility—The sucrose portion is soluble in cold water; Confectioner's Sugar is entirely soluble in boiling water.

Uses—A *pharmaceutic aid* as a *tableting excipient* and *sweetening agent.* See also *Sucrose.*

Syrup—page 1294.

Tolu Balsam

Tolu

A balsam obtained from *Myroxylon balsamum* (Linné) Harms (Fam *Leguminosae*).

Constituents—Up to 80% *resin*, about 7% *volatile oil*, 12 to 15% free *cinnamic acid*, 2 to 8% benzoic acid, and 0.05% *vanillin*. The volatile oil is composed chiefly of *benzyl benzoate* and *benzyl cinnamate*, *ethyl benzoate*, *ethyl cinnamate*, a terpene called *tolene* (possibly identical with *phellandrene*), and the sesquiterpene alcohol *farnesol* have also been reported to be present.

Description—Brown or yellowish brown, plastic solid; transparent in thin layers and brittle when old, dried, or exposed to cold temperatures; pleasant, aromatic odor resembling that of vanilla and a mild, aromatic taste.
Solubility—Nearly insoluble in water and in solvent hexane; soluble in alcohol, chloroform, and ether, sometimes with slight residue or turbidity.

Uses—In the form of a syrup, it is used as a *vehicle, flavoring agent*, and stimulating *expectorant*. It is also an ingredient of *Compound Benzoin Tincture* (page 776).

Tolu Balsam Syrup [Syrup of Tolu; Tolu Syrup]—*Preparation:* Add tolu balsam tincture (50 mL, all at once) to magnesium carbonate (10 g) and sucrose (60 g) in a mortar, and mix intimately. Gradually add purified water (430 mL) with trituration, and filter. Dissolve the remainder of sucrose (760 g) in the clear filtrate with gentle heating, strain the syrup while warm, and add purified water (qs) through the strainer to make the product measure 1000 mL. Mix thoroughly. *Note:* May be made also in the following manner: Place the remaining sucrose (760 g) in a suitable percolator, the neck of which is nearly filled with loosely packed cotton, moistened after packing with a few drops of water. Pour the filtrate, obtained as directed in the formula above, upon the sucrose, and regulate the outflow to a steady drip of percolate. When all of the liquid has run through, return portions of the percolate, if necessary, to dissolve all of the sucrose. Then pass enough purified water through the cotton to make the product measure 1000 mL. Mix thoroughly. *Alcohol Content:* 3 to 5%. *Uses:* Chiefly for its agreeable *flavor* in cough syrups. *Dose:* 10 mL.
Tolu Balsam Tincture [Tolu Tincture]—*Preparation:* With tolu balsam (200 g), prepare a tincture by Process M (page 1516), using alcohol as the menstruum. *Alcohol Content:* 77 to 83%. *Uses:* A balsamic preparation employed as an addition to expectorant mixtures. Also used in the preparation of *Tolu Balsam Syrup*. *Dose:* 2 mL.

Vanilla

Vanilla Bean

The cured, full-grown, unripe fruit of *Vanilla planifolia* Andrews, often known in commerce as Mexican or Bourbon Vanilla, or of *Vanilla tahitensis* J W Moore, known in commerce as Tahiti Vanilla (Fam *Orchidaceae*); yields not less than 12% of anhydrous extractive soluble in diluted alcohol.
Constituents—Contains a trace of a volatile oil, fixed oil, 4% resin, sugar, *vanillic acid*, and about 2.5% *vanillin* (this page). This highest grade of vanilla comes from Madagascar; considerable quantities of the drug are also produced in Mexico.
Uses—A flavor.
Note—Do not use Vanilla which has become brittle.

Vanilla Tincture [Extract of Vanilla]—*Preparation:* Add water (200 mL) to comminuted vanilla (cut into small pieces, 100 g) in a suitable covered container, and macerate during 12 hours, preferably in a warm place. Add alcohol (200 mL) to the mixture of vanilla and water, mix well, and macerate about 3 days. Transfer the mixture to a percolator containing sucrose (in coarse granules, 200 g), and drain; then pack the drug firmly, and percolate slowly, using diluted alcohol (qs) as the menstruum. If the percolator is packed with an evenly distributed mixture of the comminuted vanilla, sucrose, and clean, dry sand, the increased surface area permits more efficient percolation. This tincture is unusual in that it is the only official one in which sucrose is specified as an ingredient. *Alcohol Content:* 38 to 42%. *Uses:* A flavoring agent. See *Flavors*, page 1280.

Vanillin

Benzaldehyde, 4-hydroxy-3-methoxy-,

4-Hydroxy-3-methoxybenzaldehyde [121-33-5] $C_8H_8O_3$ (152.15).
Preparation—From vanilla, which contains 2 to 3%. It is also found in many other substances, including tissues of certain plants,

crude beet sugar, asparagus, and even asafetida. The vanillin of commerce is made synthetically, and, while chemically identical with the product obtained from the "vanilla bean," because vanilla contains other odorous products, "flavoring preparations" made from vanillin never equal in flavor the preparation in which vanilla alone is used. Vanillin is synthesized by oxidation processes from either coniferin or eugenol, by treating guaiacol with chloroform in the presence of an alkali, and by other methods.

Description—Fine, white to slightly yellow crystals, usually needle-like having an odor and taste suggestive of vanilla; affected by light; solutions are acid to litmus; melts between 81° and 83°.
Solubility—1 g in about 100 mL water and about 20 mL glycerin, and 20 mL water at 80°; freely soluble in alcohol, chloroform, ether, and solutions of the fixed alkali hydroxides.
Incompatibilities—Combines with *glycerin*, forming a compound which is almost insoluble in alcohol. It is decomposed by *alkalies* and is slowly oxidized by the *air*.

Uses—Only as a *flavor*. Solutions of it are sometimes sold as a synthetic substitute for vanilla for flavoring foods but it is inferior in flavor to the real vanilla extract.

Water—page 1292.

Water, Purified—page 1293.

Wild Cherry Syrup—page 1294.

Other Flavoring Agents

Anise NF IX [Anise Seed; European Aniseed; Sweet Cumin]—The dried ripe fruit of *Pimpinella anisum* Linné. It contains about 1.75% of volatile oil. *Uses:* A flavor and carminative.
Ceylon Cinnamon—The dried inner bark of the shoots of coppiced trees of *Cinnamomum zeylanicum* Nees (Fam *Lauraceae*); contains, in each 100 g, not less than 0.5 mL volatile oil. *Uses:* A *carminative* and *flavor*.
Clove—The dried flower-bud of *Eugenia caryophyllus* (Sprengel) Bullock et Harrison (Fam *Myrtaceae*). It contains, in each 100 g, not less than 16 mL of clove oil. *Uses:* An *aromatic* in doses of 0.25 g and as a condiment in foods.
Coriander—The dried ripe fruit of *Coriandrum sativum* Linné (Fam *Umbelliferae*); yields not less than 0.25 mL volatile coriander oil/100 g. *Uses:* Seldom used alone, but is sometimes combined with other agents, chiefly as a *flavor*. It is also used as a condiment and flavor in cooking.
Eucalyptol [Cineol; Cajeputol; $C_{10}H_{18}O$ (154.25)]— Obtained from eucalyptus oil and from other sources. Colorless liquid, having a characteristic, aromatic, distinctly camphoraceous odor, and a pungent, cooling, spicy taste. 1 volume is soluble in 5 volumes 60% alcohol; miscible with alcohol, chloroform, ether, glacial acetic acid, and fixed or volatile oils; insoluble in water. *Uses:* Primarily as a *flavoring agent*. Locally it is employed for its *antiseptic* effect in inflammations of the nose and throat and in certain skin diseases. It is sometimes used by inhalation in bronchitis.
Fennel [Fennel Seed]—The dried ripe fruit of cultivated varieties of *Foeniculum vulgare* Miller (Fam *Umbelliferae*); contains 4 to 6% of an oxygenated volatile oil and 10% of a fixed oil. *Uses:* A *flavor* and *carminative*.
Ginger NF [Zingiber]—The dried rhizome of *Zingiber officinale* Roscoe (Fam *Zingiberaceae*), known in commerce as Jamaica Ginger, African Ginger, and Cochin Ginger. The outer cortical layers are often either partially or completely removed. *Constituents:* A pungent substance, *gingerol;* volatile oil (Jamaica Ginger, about 1%; African Ginger, 2 to 3%), containing the terpenes *d-camphene* and *β-phellandrene* and the sesquiterpene *zingiberene; citral cineol*, and *borneol*. *Uses:* A *flavoring agent*. It was formerly employed in a dose of 600 mg as an intestinal stimulant and carminative in colic and in diarrhea.
Ginger Oleoresin—Yields 18–35 mL of volatile ginger oil/100 g of oleoresin. *Preparation:* Extract the oleoresin from ginger, in moderately coarse powder, by percolation, using either acetone, alcohol, or ether as the menstruum.
Glycyrrhiza Extract [Licorice Root Extract; Licorice]—An extract prepared from the rhizome and roots of species of *Glycyrrhiza* Tournefort ex Linné (Fam *Leguminosae*). *Description:* Brown powder or in flattened, cylindrical rolls or in masses; the rolls or masses have a glossy black color externally, and a brittle, sharp, smooth, conchoidal fracture; the extract has a characteristic and sweet taste which is not more than very slightly acrid. *Uses:* A *flavoring agent*.
Lavender [Lavandula]—The flowers of *Lavandula spica* (*Lavandula officinalis* or *Lavandula vera*); contains a volatile oil with the principal constituent *l*-linalyl acetate. *Uses:* A *perfume*.
Lemon Peel USP XV, BP [Fresh Lemon Peel]—The outer yellow rind of the fresh ripe fruit of *Citrus limon* (Linné) Burmann filius (Fam *Rutaceae*); contains a volatile oil and hesperidin. *Uses:* A *flavor*.

Lemon Tincture USP XVIII [Lemon Peel Tincture]—*Preparation:* From lemon peel, which is the outer yellow rind of the fresh, ripe fruit of *Citrus limon* (Linné) Burmann filius (Fam *Rutaceae*), by *Process M* (page 1516), 500 g of the peel being macerated in 900 mL alcohol and the preparation being completed with alcohol to make the product measure 1000 mL. Use talc as the filtering medium. The white portion of the rind must not be used, as the proportion of oil, which is found only in the yellow rind, is reduced and the bitter principle, hesperidin, introduced. *Alcohol Content:* 62 to 72%. *Uses:* A flavor, its fineness of flavor being assured as it comes from the fresh fruit, and being an alcoholic solution it is more stable than the oil.

Myrcia Oil [Bay Oil; Oil of Bay]—The volatile oil distilled from leaves of *Pimenta racemosa* (Miller) J W Moore (Fam *Myrtaceae);* contains the phenolic compounds eugenol and chavicol. *Uses:* In the preparation of bay rum as a *perfume.*

Orange Oil, Bitter—The volatile oil obtained by expression from the fresh peel of the fruit of *Citrus aurantium* Linné (Fam *Rutaceae);* contains primarily *d*-limonene. Pale yellow liquid with a characteristic; aromatic odor of the Seville orange; if it has a terebinthinate odor, it should not be dispensed; refractive index 1.4725 to 1.4755 at 20°. It differs little from *Orange Oil* (page 1288) except for the botanical source. Miscible with anhydrous alcohol and with about 4 volumes alcohol. *Uses:* A *flavor.*

Orange Peel, Bitter [Bitter Orange; Curacao Orange Peel; Bigarade Orange]—The dried rind of the unripe but fully grown fruit of *Citrus aurantium* Linné (Fam *Rutaceae). Constituents:* The inner part of the peel from the bitter orange contains a volatile oil and the glycoside *hesperidin* ($C_{28}H_{34}O_{15}$). This, upon hydrolysis in the presence of H_2SO_4, yields *hesperetin* ($C_{16}H_{14}O_6$), *rhamnose* ($C_6H_{12}O_5$), and D-glucose ($C_6H_{12}O_6$). *Uses:* A *flavoring agent.* It has been used as a bitter.

Orange Peel, Sweet USP XV—The fresh, outer rind of the non-artificially colored, ripe fruit of *Citrus sinensis* (Linné) Osbeck (Fam *Rutaceae);* the white, inner portion of the rind is to be excluded. Contains a volatile oil but no hesperidin, since the glycoside occurs in the white portion of the rind. *Uses:* A *flavor.*

Orris [Orris Root; Iris; Florentine Orris]—The peeled and dried rhizome of *Iris germanica* Linné, including its variety *florentina* Dykes (*Iris florentina* Linné), or of *Iris pallida* Lamarck (Fam *Iridaceae);* contains about 0.1 to 0.2% of a volatile oil (orris butter), myristic acid, and the ketone irone; irone provides the fragrant odor of orris. *Uses:* A *perfume.*

Pimenta Oil [Pimento Oil; Allspice Oil]—The volatile oil distilled from the fruit of *Pimenta officinalis* Lindley (Fam *Myrtaceae*). *Uses:* A *carminative* and *stimulant* and also as a *condiment* in foods.

Rosemary Oil—The volatile oil distilled with steam from the fresh flowering tops of *Rosmarinus officinalis* Linné (Fam *Labiatae);* yields not less than 1.5% of esters calculated as bornyl acetate ($C_{12}H_{20}O_2$), and not less than 8% of total borneol ($C_{10}H_{18}O$), free and as esters. *Constituents:* The amount of esters, calculated as bornyl acetate, and of total borneol, respectively, varies somewhat with the geographic source of rosemary oil. Cineol is present to the extent of about 19–25%, depending on the source. The terpenes *d*- and *l*-α-*pinene, dipentene*, and *camphene*, and the ketone *camphor* also occur in this oil. *Description:* Colorless or pale yellow liquid, having the characteristic odor of rosemary, and a warm, camphoraceous taste; specific gravity 0.894 to 0.912. Soluble in 1 volume of 90% alcohol, by volume, but upon further dilution may become turbid. *Uses:* A *flavor* and *perfume*, chiefly, in rubefacient liniments such as *Camphor and Soap Liniment.*

Sassafras—The dried bark of the root of *Sassafras albidum* (Nuttall) Nees (Fam *Lauraceae*). *Uses:* Principally because of its high content of volatile oil which serves to disguise the taste of disagreeable substances. An infusion (*sassafras tea*) was formerly extensively used as a home remedy, particularly in the southern states.

Sassafras Oil—The volatile oil distilled with steam from *Sassafras. Uses:* A *flavor* by confectioners, particularly in hard candies. Either the oil or safrol is used as a *preservative* in mucilage and library paste, being far superior to methyl salicylate for this purpose. Since the oil is *antiseptic*, it is sometimes employed in conjunction with other agents for local application in diseases of the nose and throat; safrol is also so used.

Wild Cherry [Wild Black Cherry Bark]—The carefully dried stem bark of *Prunus serotina* Ehrhart (Fam *Rosaceae*), free of borke and preferably having been collected in autumn. *Constituents:* A glucoside of *d*-mandelonitrile ($C_6H_5.CHOH.CN$) known as *prunasin* (page 403), the enzyme *emulsin*, tannin, a bitter principle, starch, resin, etc. In the BP and the English literature this drug has been termed "Virginian Prune"—a literal but incorrect translation of the older botanical name, *Prunus virginiana. Uses:* A *flavoring agent*, especially in cough preparations. It is an ingredient in *Wild Cherry Syrup.* As with bitter almond, contact with water, in the presence of emulsin, results in the production of benzaldehyde and HCN. All preparations of wild cherry should be made without heat in order to avoid destruction of the enzyme which is responsible for the production of the free active principles.

Diluting Agents

Diluting agents (vehicles or carriers) are indifferent substances which are used as solvents for active medicinals. They are of primary importance for diluting and flavoring drugs which are intended for oral administration, but a few such agents are specifically designed for diluting parenteral injections. The latter group is considered separately.

The expert selection of diluting agents has been an important factor in popularizing the "specialties" of manufacturing pharmacists. Since a large selection of diluting agents is available in a choice of colors and flavors, the prescriber has an opportunity to make his own prescriptions more acceptable to the patient. The best diluting agent is usually the best solvent for the drug. Water-soluble substances, for example, should be flavored and diluted with an aqueous agent and alcohol-soluble drugs with an alcoholic vehicle. Thus, the diluting agents presented herein are divided into three groups on the basis of their physical properties: aqueous, hydroalcoholic, and alcoholic.

Aqueous Diluting Agents

Aqueous diluting agents include aromatic waters, syrups, and mucilages. Aromatic waters are used as diluting agents for water-soluble substances and salts, but cannot mask the taste of very disagreeable drugs. Some of the more common flavored aqueous agents and the official forms of water are listed below.

Orange Flower Water

Stronger Orange Flower Water; Triple Orange Flower Water

A saturated solution of the odoriferous principles of the flowers of *Citrus aurantium* Linné (Fam. *Rutaceae*), prepared by distilling the fresh flowers with water and separating the excess volatile oil from the clear, water portion of the distillate.

Description—Should be nearly colorless, clear, or only faintly opalescent; the odor should be that of the orange blossoms; it must be free from empyreuma, mustiness, and fungoid growths.

Uses—A *vehicle flavor* and *perfume* in syrups, elixirs, and solutions.

Peppermint Water

A clear, saturated solution of peppermint oil in purified water, prepared by one of the processes described under *Aromatic Waters* (page 1495).

Uses—A *carminative* and *flavored vehicle.*
Dose—15 mL.

Tolu Balsam Syrup—page 1291.

Water

Water [7732-18-5] H_2O (18.02).

Drinking water, which is subject to federal Environmental Protection Agency regulations with respect to drinking water, and which is delivered by the municipal or other local public system or drawn from a private well or reservoir, is the starting material for all forms of water covered by Pharmacopeial monographs.

Drinking water may be used in the preparation of USP drug substances (eg, in the extraction of certain vegetable drugs and in the manufacture of a few preparations used externally) but not in the preparation of dosage forms, or in the preparation of reagents or test solutions. It is no longer the subject of a separate monograph (in the USP), inasmuch as the cited standards vary from one community to another and generally are beyond the control of private parties or corporations.

Purified Water

Water obtained by distillation, ion-exchange treatment, reverse osmosis, or any other suitable process; contains no added substance.

Caution—Do not use Purified Water in preparations intended for parenteral administration. For such purposes, use Water for Injection, Bacteriostatic Water for Injection, or Sterile Water for Injection, page 1295.

Preparation—From water complying with federal Environmental Protection Agency regulations with respect to drinking water. A former official process for water, when prepared by distillation, is given below. The pharmacist who is preparing sterile solutions, and must have freshly distilled water of exceptionally high grade, not only free from all bacterial or other microscopic growths but also free from the products of metabolic processes resulting from the growth of such organisms in the water, may advantageously follow this plan. The metabolic products are commonly spoken of as pyrogens and usually consist of complex organic compounds which cause febrile reactions if present in the solvent for parenteral medicinal substances.

Distillation Process

Water	1000 Vol
To make	750 Vol

Distil the water from a suitable apparatus provided with a block-tin or glass condenser. Collect the first 100 volumes and reject this portion. Then collect 750 volumes and keep the distilled water in glass-stoppered bottles, which have been rinsed with steam or very hot distilled water immediately before being filled. The first 100 volumes are discarded to eliminate foreign volatile substances found in ordinary water and only 750 volumes are collected, since the residue in the still contains concentrated dissolved solids.

Description—Colorless, clear liquid, without odor or taste.

Uses—A *pharmaceutic aid* (vehicle and solvent). Purified water must be used in the compounding of dosage forms for internal (oral) administration as well as sterile pharmaceuticals applied externally, such as collyria and dermatological preparations, but these must be sterilized before use.

Whenever water is called for in official tests and assays, purified water must be used.

Syrups Used as Diluting Agents

Syrups are useful as diluting agents for water-soluble drugs and act both as solvents and flavoring agents. The flavored syrups usually consist of simple syrup (85% sucrose in water) containing appropriate flavoring substances. *Glycyrrhiza Syrup* is an excellent vehicle for saline substances because of its colloidal properties, sweet flavor, and lingering taste of licorice. *Acacia Syrup* is valuable in disguising the taste of urea. Fruit syrups are especially effective for masking sour tastes. *Aromatic Eriodictyon Syrup* is the diluting agent of choice for masking the bitter taste of alkaloids. *Cocoa Syrup* and *Cherry Syrup* are good general flavoring agents.

Acacia Syrup

Acacia, granular or powdered	100 g
Sodium Benzoate	1 g
Vanilla Tincture	5 mL
Sucrose	800 g
Purified Water, a sufficient quantity,	
To make	1000 mL

Mix the acacia, sodium benzoate, and sucrose; then add 425 mL of purified water, and mix well. Heat the mixture on a steam bath until solution is completed. When cool, remove the scum, add the vanilla tincture and sufficient purified water to make the product measure 1000 mL, and strain if necessary.

Uses—A *flavored vehicle* and *demulcent.*

Cherry Syrup

Syrupus Cerasi

Cherry Juice	475 mL
Sucrose	800 g
Alcohol	20 mL
Purified Water, a sufficient quantity,	
To make	1000 mL

Dissolve the sucrose in cherry juice by heating on a steam bath, cool, and remove the foam and floating solids. Add the alcohol and sufficient purified water to make 1000 mL, and mix.

Alcohol Content—1 to 2%.

Uses—A pleasantly *flavored vehicle* which is particularly useful in masking the taste of saline and sour drugs.

Cocoa Syrup

Cacao Syrup; Chocolate-flavored Syrup; Chocolate Syrup

Cocoa	180	g
Sucrose	600	g
Liquid Glucose	180	g
Glycerin	50	mL
Sodium Chloride	2	g
Vanillin	0.2	g
Sodium Benzoate	1	g
Purified Water, a sufficient quantity,		
To make	1000	mL

Mix the sucrose and the cocoa, and to this mixture gradually add a solution of the liquid glucose, glycerin, sodium chloride, vanillin, and sodium benzoate in 325 mL of hot purified water. Bring the entire mixture to a boil, and maintain at boiling temperature for 3 min. Allow to cool to room temperature and add sufficient purified water to make the product measure 1000 mL.

Note—Cocoa containing not more than 12% nonvolatile, ether-soluble extractive ("fat") yields a syrup having a minimum tendency to separate. "Breakfast cocoa" contains over 22% "fat."

Uses—A pleasantly *flavored vehicle.* It should not be used for patients who are allergic to it.

Aromatic Eriodictyon Syrup

Aromatic Yerba Santa Syrup; Syrupus Corrigens

Eriodictyon Fluidextract	32	mL
Potassium Hydroxide Solution (1 in 20)	25	mL
Compound Cardamom Tincture	65	mL
Lemon Oil	0.5	mL
Clove Oil	1	mL
Alcohol	32	mL
Sucrose	800	g
Magnesium Carbonate	5	g
Purified Water, a sufficient quantity,		
To make	1000	mL

Dissolve the oils in the alcohol, add the fluidextract and the tincture, then the potassium hydroxide solution and 325 mL of purified water. Add the magnesium carbonate, shake the mixture, allow it to stand overnight, filter, and add sufficient purified water through the filter to make the liquid measure 500 mL. Pour this filtrate upon the sucrose contained in a bottle, and dissolve by placing the bottle in hot water, and agitating the contents frequently. Cool the solution, and add sufficient purified water to make the product measure 1000 mL.

Alcohol Content—6 to 8%.

Incompatibilities—Alkaline in reaction due to the potassium hydroxide used in its manufacture. *Acids* are neutralized with usually a concurrent precipitation of the resins of the syrup. The tannin which it contains introduces the incompatibilities of that substance.

Uses—A pleasantly *flavored vehicle*, especially adapted to the administration of bitter substances like quinine.

Syrup

Simple Syrup

Sucrose	850 g
Purified Water, a sufficient quantity,	
To make	1000 mL

May be prepared by using boiling water or, preferably, without heat, by the following process:

Place the sucrose in a suitable percolator the neck of which is nearly filled with loosely packed cotton moistened, after packing, with a few drops of water. Pour carefully about 450 mL of purified water upon the sucrose, and regulate the outflow to a steady drip of percolate. Return the percolate, if necessary, until all of the sucrose has dissolved. Then wash the inside of the percolator and the cotton with sufficient purified water to bring the volume of the percolate to 1000 mL, and mix.

Specific Gravity—Not less than 1.30.

Uses—A *sweet vehicle*, sweetening agent, and as the basis for many flavored and medicated syrups.

Other Syrups Used As Diluting Agents

Citric Acid Syrup USP XVIII [Syrup of Lemon]—*Preparation:* Dissolve citric acid (hydrous, 10 g) in purified water (10 mL), and mix the solution with syrup (950 mL). Add lemon tincture (10 mL), and enough syrup to make the product measure 1000 mL, and mix. *Note: Do not dispense Citric Acid Syrup if it has a terebinthine odor or taste or shows other indications of deterioration. Alcohol Content:* Less than 1%. *Incompatibilities:* Reactions characteristic of the acid which it contains; hence, it is not a suitable vehicle for alkaline ingredients such as phenobarbital sodium from which it precipitates phenobarbital. *Uses:* Solely as a *pleasant vehicle*, the formula making it possible to prepare extemporaneously and quickly a syrup having the flavor of lemon.

Glycyrrhiza Syrup USP XVIII [Licorice Syrup]—*Preparation:* Add fennel oil (0.05 mL), and anise oil (0.5 mL) to glycyrrhiza fluidextract (250 mL) and agitate until mixed. Then add syrup (qs) to make the product measure 1000 mL, and mix. *Alcohol Content:* 5 to 6%. *Incompatibilities:* The characteristic flavor is destroyed by acids due to a precipitation of the glycyrrhizin. *Uses:* A *flavored vehicle*, especially adapted to the administration of bitter or nauseous substances.

Hydriodic Acid Syrup—Contains, in each 100 mL 1.3 to 1.5 g HI (127.91). *Preparation:* Mix diluted hydriodic acid (140 mL) with purified water (550 mL), and dissolve dextrose (450 g) in this mixture by agitation. Add purified water (qs) to make the product measure 1000 mL, and filter. *Caution: Hydriodic Acid Syrup must not be dispensed if it contains free iodine, as evidenced by a red coloration. Description:* Transparent, colorless, or not more than pale straw-colored, syrupy liquid; odorless and has a sweet, acidulous taste; specific gravity about 1.18; hydriodic acid is easily decomposed in simple aqueous solution (unless protected by hypophosphorous acid) free iodine being liberated, and if taken internally, when in this condition, it is irritating to the alimentary tract. The dextrose used in this syrup should be of the highest grade obtainable. *Incompatibilities:* The reactions of the *acids* (page 1496) as well as those of the water-soluble iodide salts. Oxidizing agents liberate iodine; alkaloids may be precipitated. *Uses:* Traditionally as a *vehicle for expectorant* drugs. Its therapeutic properties are those of the iodides. *Dose:* Usual, 5 mL.

Raspberry Syrup USP XVIII—*Preparation:* Dissolve sucrose (800 g) in raspberry juice (475 mL) by heating on a steam bath, cool, and remove the foam and floating solids. Add alcohol (20 mL) and purified water (qs) to make 1000 mL, and mix. *Alcohol Content:* 1 to 2%. *Incompatibilities:* Raspberry juice is prepared to contain not less than 1.5% citric acid; the syrup, therefore, has reactions characteristic of this acid, notably its incompatibility with alkaline substances. *Uses:* A pleasantly *flavored vehicle* used to disguise the salty or sour taste of saline medicaments.

Wild Cherry Syrup USP XVIII—*Preparation:* Pack wild cherry (in coarse powder, 150 g), previously moistened with water (100 mL), in a cylindrical percolator, and add water (qs) to leave a layer of it above the powder. Macerate for 1 hour, then proceed with rapid percolation, using added water, until 400 mL of percolate is collected. Filter the percolate, if necessary, add sucrose (675 g) and dissolve it by agitation, then add glycerin (150 mL), alcohol (20 mL), and water (qs) to make the product measure 1000 mL. Strain if necessary. *Wild cherry syrup may be made also in the following manner:* The sucrose may be dissolved by placing it in a second percolator as directed for preparing *Syrup*, and allowing the percolate from the wild cherry to flow through it and into a graduated vessel containing the glycerin and alcohol until the total volume measures 1000 mL. *Note:* Heat is avoided, lest the enzyme emulsin be inactivated. If this should happen, the preparation would contain no free HCN, upon which its action as a sedative for coughs mainly depends. For a discussion of the chemistry involved, see *Wild Cherry* (page 1292). *Alcohol Content:* 1 to 2%. *Uses:* Chiefly as a *flavored vehicle* for cough syrups.

Mucilages Used as Diluting Agents

Mucilages are also suitable as diluting agents for water-soluble substances, and are especially useful in stabilizing suspensions and emulsions.

The following mucilage used for this purpose is described under *Emulsifying and Suspending Agents*, page 1296.

Acacia Mucilage—page 1296.

Hydroalcoholic Diluting Agents

Hydroalcoholic diluting agents are suitable for drugs soluble in either water or diluted alcohol. The most important agents in this group are the elixirs. These solutions contain approximately 25% alcohol. *Medicated* elixirs which have therapeutic activity in their own right are not included in this section. Listed below are the common, nonmedicated elixirs which are used purely as diluting agents or solvents for drugs.

Aromatic Elixir

Simple Elixir

Orange Oil	2.4 mL
Lemon Oil	0.6 mL
Coriander Oil	0.24 mL
Anise Oil	0.06 mL
Syrup	375 mL
Talc	30 g
Alcohol,	
Purified Water, each, a sufficient quantity,	
To make	1000 mL

Dissolve the oils in alcohol to make 250 mL. To this solution add the syrup in several portions, agitating vigorously after each addition, and afterwards add, in the same manner, the required quantity of purified water. Mix the talc with the liquid, and filter through a filter wetted with diluted alcohol, returning the filtrate until a clear liquid is obtained.

Alcohol Content—21 to 23%.

Uses—A pleasantly *flavored vehicle*, employed in the preparation of many other elixirs. The chief objection to its extensive use is the high alcohol content (about 22%) which at times may counteract the effect of other medicines.

Cardamom Spirit, Compound—RPS-15, page 1236.

Other Hydroalcoholic Diluting Agents

Glycyrrhiza Elixir [Elixir Adjuvans; Licorice Elixir]—*Preparation:* Mix glycyrrhiza fluidextract (125 mL) and aromatic elixir (875 mL) and filter. *Alcohol Content:* 21 to 23%. *Uses:* A *flavored vehicle.*

Flavored Alcoholic Solutions

Flavored alcoholic solutions, of high alcoholic concentration, are useful as flavors to be added in small quantities to syrups or elixirs. The alcohol content of these solutions is approximately 50%. There are two types of flavored alcoholic solutions: tinctures and spirits. Only nonmedicated tinctures and spirits are used as flavoring agents.

Compound Cardamom Tincture

Cardamom Seed, in moderately coarse powder	20 g
Cinnamon, in fine powder	25 g
Caraway, in moderately coarse powder	12 g
To make	1000 mL

Prepare a tincture by Process M (page 1516), macerating the mixed powders in 750 mL of a mixture of 50 mL of glycerin and 950 mL of diluted alcohol, and completing the preparation by using first the remainder of the mixture of alcohol and glycerin prepared as directed above, and then diluted alcohol.

Note—Compound cardamom tincture may be colored with one or more colors (page 1280).

Alcohol Content—43 to 47%.

Uses—A useful vehicle because of its pleasant *flavor* and color.

Lemon Tincture—page 1292.

Myrcia Spirit, Compound—RPS-13, page 452.

Orange Spirit, Compound—page 1288.

Orange Peel, Sweet, Tincture—page 1288.
Peppermint Spirit—page 814.

Diluting Agents for Injections

Injections are liquid preparations, usually solutions or suspensions of drugs, intended to be injected through the skin into the body. Diluting agents used for these preparations may be aqueous or nonaqueous and must meet the requirements for sterility and also of the pyrogen test. Aqueous diluting agents include such preparations as *Sterile Water for Injection* and various sterile, aqueous solutions of electrolytes and/or dextrose. Nonaqueous diluting agents are generally fatty oils of vegetable origin, fatty esters, and polyols such as propylene glycol and polyethylene glycol. These agents are used to dissolve or dilute oil-soluble substances and to suspend water-soluble substances when it is desired to decrease the rate of absorption and, hence, prolong the duration of action of the drug substances. Preparations of this type are given intramuscularly. See *Parenteral Preparations*, page 1522.

Corn Oil

Maize Oil

The refined fixed oil obtained from the embryo of *Zea mays* Linné (Fam *Gramineae*).

Preparation—Expressed from the Indian corn embryos or germs separated from the grain in starch manufacture.

Description—Clear, light yellow, oily liquid with a faint characteristic odor and taste; specific gravity 0.914 to 0.921.
Solubility—Slightly soluble in alcohol; miscible with ether, chloroform, benzene, and solvent hexane.

Uses—Main official use is as a *solvent* and *vehicle for injections.* It is used as an edible oil substitute for solid fats in the management of hypercholesterolemia. Other uses include making soaps and for burning. It is a semidrying oil and therefore unsuitable for lubricating or mixing paint.

Cottonseed Oil

Cotton Seed Oil; Cotton Oil

The refined fixed oil obtained from the seed of cultivated plants of various varieties of *Gossypium hirsutum* Linné or of other species of *Gossypium* (Fam *Malvaceae*).

Preparation—Cotton seeds contain about 15% oil. The testae of the seeds are first separated, and the kernels are subjected to high pressure in hydraulic presses. The crude oil thus has a bright red to blackish red color. It requires purification before it is suitable for medicinal or food purposes.

Description—Pale yellow, oily liquid with a bland taste; odorless or nearly so; particles of solid fat may separate below 10° and the oil solidifies at about 0° to −5°; specific gravity 0.915 to 0.921.
Solubility—Slightly soluble in alcohol; miscible with ether, chloroform, solvent hexane, and carbon disulfide.

Uses—Official as a *solvent* and *vehicle for injections.* It is sometimes taken orally as a mild cathartic in the dose of 30 mL or more. Taken internally, digestible oils retard gastric secretion and motility and increase the caloric intake. Cottonseed oil is also used in the manufacture of soaps, oleomargarine, lard substitutes, glycerin, lubricants, and cosmetics.

Ethyl Oleate

9-Octadecenoic acid, (*Z*)-, ethyl ester

$$HC-CH_2(CH_2)_6\ COOC_2H_5$$
$$\|$$
$$HC-CH_2(CH_2)_6\ CH_3$$

Ethyl oleate [111-62-6] $C_{20}H_{38}O_2$ (310.52).
Preparation—Among other ways, by reacting ethanol with oleoyl chloride in the presence of a suitable dehydrochlorinating agent.

Description—Mobile, practically colorless liquid, having an agreeable taste; specific gravity 0.866 to 0.874; acid value not greater than 0.5 and an iodine value of 75 to 85; sterilized by heating at 150° for 1 hour; properties similar to those of almond and arachis oils, but is less viscous and more rapidly absorbed by the tissues; boils between 205° and 208°.
Solubility—Does not dissolve in water; miscible with vegetable oils, mineral oil, alcohol, and most organic solvents.

Uses—A *vehicle* for certain intramuscular injectable preparations.

Peanut Oil

Arachis Oil; Groundnut Oil; Nut Oil; Earth-Nut Oil

The refined fixed oil obtained from the seed kernels of one or more of the cultivated varieties of *Arachis hypogaea* Linné (Fam *Leguminosae*).

Description—Colorless or pale yellow, oily liquid, with a characteristic nutty odor and a bland taste; specific gravity 0.912 to 0.920.
Solubility—Very slightly soluble in alcohol; miscible with ether, chloroform, and carbon disulfide.

Uses—A *solvent* in preparing oil solutions for injection (page 1522). It is also used for making liniments, ointments, plasters, and soaps, as a substitute for olive oil.

Sesame Oil

Teel Oil; Benne Oil; Gingili Oil

The refined fixed oil obtained from the seed of one or more cultivated varieties of *Sesamum indicum* Linné (Fam *Pedaliaceae*).

Description—Pale yellow, almost odorless, oily liquid with a bland taste; specific gravity 0.916 to 0.921.
Solubility—Slightly soluble in alcohol; miscible with ether, chloroform, solvent hexane, and carbon disulfide.

Uses—A *solvent* and *vehicle* in official injections. It is used much like olive oil both medicinally and for food. It does not readily turn rancid. Sesame oil is also used in the manufacture of cosmetics, iodized oil, liniments, ointments, and oleomargarine.

Water for Injection

Water purified by distillation or by reverse osmosis. It contains no added substance.
Caution—Water for Injection is intended for use as a solvent for the preparation of parenteral solutions. For parenteral solutions that are prepared under aseptic conditions and are not sterilized by appropriate filtration or in the final container, first render the Water for Injection sterile and thereafter protect it from microbial contamination.

Description—Clear, colorless, odorless liquid.

Uses—*Pharmaceutic aid* (vehicle and solvent).

Bacteriostatic Water for Injection

Sterile water for injection containing one or more suitable antimicrobial agents.
Note—Use Bacteriostatic Water for Injection with due regard for the compatibility of the antimicrobial agent or agents it contains with the particular medicinal substance that is to be dissolved or diluted.
Uses—*Sterile vehicle* for parenteral preparations.

Sterile Water for Injection

Water for Parenterals

Water for injection sterilized and suitably packaged. It contains no antimicrobial agent or other added substance.

Description—Clean, colorless, odorless, liquid.

Uses—For the preparation of *all aqueous parenteral solutions*, including those used in *animal assays*. See page 1521 for a detailed discussion.

Sterile Water for Irrigation

Water for injection that has been sterilized and suitably packaged. It contains no antimicrobial agent or other added substance.

Description—Clear, colorless, odorless liquid.

Uses—An *irrigating solution.*

Emulsifying and Suspending Agents

An emulsion is a two-phase system in which one liquid is dispersed in the form of small globules throughout another liquid that is immiscible with the first liquid. Emulsions are formed and stabilized with the help of emulsifying agents, which are surfactants and/or viscosity-producing agents. A suspension is defined as a preparation containing finely divided insoluble material suspended in a liquid medium. The presence of a suspending agent is required to overcome agglomeration of the dispersed particles and to increase the viscosity of the medium so that the particles settle more slowly. Emulsifying and suspending agents are used extensively in the formulation of elegant pharmaceutical preparations for oral, parenteral, and external use. For the theoretical and practical aspects of emulsions the interested reader is referred to pages 317 and 1507. More detailed information on the use of suspending agents is given on page 1422.

Acacia

Gum Arabic

The dried gummy exudate from the stems and branches of *Acacia senegal* (Linné) Willdenow or of other related African species of *Acacia* (Fam *Leguminosae*).

Constituents—Principally calcium, magnesium, and potassium salts of the polysaccharide *arabic acid*, which on acid hydrolysis yields L-arabinose, L-rhamnose, D-galactose, and an aldobionic acid containing D-glucuronic acid and D-galactose.

Description—*Acacia*—Spheroidal tears up to 32 mm in diameter or angular fragments of white to yellowish white color; translucent or somewhat opaque; very brittle; almost odorless; produces a mucilaginous sensation on the tongue. *Flake Acacia*—White to yellowish white, thin flakes. *Powdered Acacia*—White to yellowish white, angular microscopic fragments. *Granular Acacia*—White to pale yellowish white, fine granules. *Spray-dried Acacia*—White to off-white compacted microscopic fragments or whole spheres.

Solubility—Insoluble in alcohol, but almost completely soluble in twice its weight of water at room temperature; the resulting solution flows readily and is acid to litmus.

Incompatibilities—*Alcohol or alcoholic solutions* precipitate acacia as a stringy mass when the alcohol amounts to more than about 35% of the total volume. Solution is effected by dilution with water. The mucilage is destroyed through precipitation of the acacia by *heavy metals. Borax* also causes a precipitation which is prevented by glycerin. Acacia contains calcium and, therefore, possesses the incompatibilities of this ion.

Acacia contains a *peroxidase* which acts as an oxidizing agent and produces colored derivatives of *aminopyrine, antipyrine, cresol, guaiacol, phenol, tannin, thymol, vanillin,* and other substances. Among the alkaloids affected are *atropine, apomorphine, cocaine, homatropine, hyoscyamine, morphine, physostigmine,* and *scopolamine.* A partial destruction of the alkaloid occurs in the reaction. Heating the solution of acacia for a few minutes at 100° destroys the peroxidase and the color reactions are avoided.

Uses—Extensively as a *suspending agent* for insoluble substances in water (page 1511), in the preparation of emulsions (pages 317 and 1507), and for making pills and troches (page 1631).

It is used for its *demulcent* action in inflammations of the throat or stomach.

Acacia solutions should not be used as a substitute for serum protein in the treatment of *shock* and as a *diuretic* in hypoproteinemic edema, since acacia produces serious syndromes that may result in death.

Acacia Mucilage [Mucilage of Gum Arabic]—*Preparation:* Place acacia (in small fragments, 350 g) in a graduated bottle having a wide mouth and a capacity not greatly exceeding 1000 mL, wash the drug with cold purified water, allow it to drain, and add enough warm purified water, in which benzoic acid (2 g) has been dissolved, to make the product measure 1000 mL. After stoppering, lay the bottle on its side, rotate it occa-

sionally, and when the acacia has dissolved strain the mucilage. *May also be prepared as follows:* dissolve benzoic acid (2 g) in purified water (400 mL) with the aid of heat, and add the solution to powdered or granular acacia (350 g), in a mortar, triturating until the acacia is dissolved. Then add sufficient purified water to make the product measure 1000 mL, and strain if necessary. This second method is primarily for the extemporaneous preparation of Acacia Mucilage. *Uses:* A *demulcent* and a *suspending agent*. It has also been employed as an *excipient* in making pills and troches, and as an *emulsifying agent* for cod liver oil and other substances. *Caution—Acacia Mucilage must be free from mold or any other indication of decomposition.*

Agar

Agar-Agar; Vegetable Gelatin; Gelosa; Chinese or Japanese Gelatin

The dried, hydrophilic, colloidal substance extracted from *Gelidium cartilagineum* (Linné) Gaillon (Fam *Gelidiaceae*), *Gracilaria confervoides* (Linné) Greville (Fam *Sphaerococcaceae*), and related red algae (Class *Rhodophyceae*).

Constituents—Chiefly of the calcium salt of a galactan mono(acid sulfate).

Description—Usually in bundles of thin, membranous, agglutinated strips or in cut, flaked, or granulated forms; may be weak yellowish orange, yellowish gray to pale yellow, or colorless; tough when damp, brittle when dry; odorless or with a slight odor; produces a mucilaginous sensation on the tongue. Also supplied as a white to yellowish white or pale yellow powder.

Solubility—Insoluble in cold water; soluble in boiling water.

Incompatibilities—Like other gums, agar is dehydrated and precipitated from solution by *alcohol. Tannic acid* causes precipitation; *electrolytes* cause partial dehydration and decrease in viscosity of sols.

Uses—A relatively ineffective bulk-producing laxative used in a variety of proprietary cathartics. In mineral oil emulsions it acts as a stabilizer. The usual dose is 4 to 16 g once or twice a day.

It is also used in culture media for bacteriological work, as a stabilizer in emulsions, and in the manufacture of ice cream, confectionaries, etc.

Alginic Acid

Alginic acid [9005-32-7] (average equivalent weight 200); a hydrophilic colloidal carbohydrate extracted with dilute alkali from various species of brown seaweeds (*Phaeophyceae*).

Preparation—Precipitates when an aqueous solution of *Sodium Alginate* is treated with mineral acid.

Description—White to yellowish white, fibrous powder; odorless or practically odorless, and tasteless; pH (3 in 100 dispersion in water) between 1.5 and 3.5; pK$_a$ (0.1N NaCl, 20°) 3.42.

Solubility—Insoluble in water and organic solvents; soluble in alkaline solutions.

Uses—A *pharmaceutic aid* (tablet binder and emulsifying agent). It is used as a sizing agent in the paper and textile industries.

Sodium Alginate

Alginic acid, sodium salt; Algin; Manucol; Norgine; Kelgin (*Kelco*)

Sodium alginate [9005-38-3] (average equivalent weight 220); the purified carbohydrate product extracted from brown seaweeds by the use of dilute alkali. It consists chiefly of the sodium salt of alginic acid, a polyuronic acid composed of beta-D-mannuronic acid residues linked so that the carboxyl group of each unit is free while the aldehyde group is shielded by a glycosidic linkage.

Description—Nearly odorless and tasteless, coarse or fine powder, yellowish white in color.

Solubility—Dissolves in water, forming a viscous, colloidal solution; insoluble in alcohol and in hydroalcoholic solutions in which the alcohol content is greater than about 30% by weight; insoluble in chloroform, ether, and acids, when the pH of the solution becomes lower than about 3.

Uses—A *thickening* and *emulsifying agent.* This property makes it useful in a variety of areas. For example, it is used to impart smoothness and body to ice cream and to prevent formation of ice particles.

Bentonite

Wilhinite; Soap Clay; Mineral Soap

Bentonite [1302-78-9]; a native, colloidal, hydrated aluminum silicate.

Occurrence—Bentonite is found in the Midwest of the US and Canada. Originally called *Taylorite* after its discoverer in Wyoming, its name was changed to bentonite after its discovery in the Fort Benton formation of the Upper Cretaceous of Wyoming.

Description—Very fine, odorless powder with a slightly earthy taste, free from grit; the powder is nearly white, but may be a pale buff or cream-colored.

The US Geological Survey has defined bentonite as "a transported stratified clay formed by the alteration of volcanic ash shortly after deposition." Chemically, it is $Al_2O_3.4SiO_2.H_2O$ plus other minerals as impurities. It consists of colloidal crystalline plates, of less than microscopic dimensions in thickness, and of colloidal dimensions in breadth. This fact accounts for the extreme swelling that occurs when it is placed in water, since the water penetrates between an infinite number of plates. A good specimen swells 12 to 14 times its volume.

Solubility—Insoluble in water or acids, but it has the property of adsorbing large quantities of water, swelling to approximately twelve times its original volume, and forming highly viscous thixotropic suspensions or *gels.* This property makes it highly useful in pharmacy. Its gel-forming property is augmented by the addition of small amounts of alkaline substances, such as magnesium oxide. It does not swell in organic solvents.

Incompatibilities—*Acids* and *acid salts* decrease the water-absorbing power of bentonite and thus cause a breakdown of the magma. Suspensions are most stable at a pH above 7.

Uses—A *protective colloid* for the *stabilization of suspensions.* It also has been used as an emulsifier for oil, as a base for plasters, ointments, and similar preparations.

Bentonite Magma USP—*Preparation:* Sprinkle bentonite (50 g), in portions, on hot purified water (800 g), allowing each portion to become thoroughly wetted without stirring. Allow it to stand with occasional stirring for 24 hours. Stir until a uniform magma is obtained, add purified water to make 1000 g, and mix. The magma may be prepared also by mechanical means such as by use of a blender, as follows: Place purified water (about 500 g) in the blender, and while the machine is running, add bentonite (50 g). Add purified water to make up to about 1000 g or up to the operating capacity of the blender. Blend the mixture for 5 to 10 min, add purified water to make 1000 g, and mix. *Uses:* A *suspending agent* for insoluble medicaments.

Carbomer

Carboxypolymethylene

A synthetic high-molecular-weight cross-linked polymer of acrylic acid; contains 56 to 68% of carboxylic acid (—COOH) groups. The viscosity of a neutralized preparation (2.5 g/500 mL water) is 30,000 to 40,000 centipoises.

Description—White, fluffy powder with a slight characteristic odor; hygroscopic; pH (1 in 100 dispersion) about 3; specific gravity about 1.41.

Solubility (neutralized with alkali hydroxides or amines)—Dissolves in water, alcohol, and glycerin.

Uses—A *thickening, suspending, dispersing,* and *emulsifying agent* for pharmaceuticals, cosmetics, waxes, paints, and other industrial products.

Carboxymethylcellulose Sodium

Carbose D; Carboxymethocel S; C.M.C. Cellulose Gum (*Hercules*)

Cellulose, carboxymethyl ether, sodium salt [9004-32-4]; contains 6.5–9.5% of sodium (Na), calculated on the dried basis. It is available in several viscosity types: low, medium, high, and extra high.

Description—White to cream-colored powder or granules; the powder is hygroscopic; pH (1 in 100 aqueous solution) between 6.5 and 8.5.

Solubility—Easily dispersed in water to form colloidal solutions; insoluble in alcohol, ether, and most other organic solvents.

Uses—*Pharmaceutic aid* (suspending agent; tablet excipient; viscosity-increasing agent). In tablet form it is used as a hydrophilic colloid laxative.

Dose—*Usual, adult, laxative,* **1.5 g** 3 or 4 times a day.
Dosage Form: Tablets: 500 mg.

Carrageenan

Carrageenan [9000-07-1].

Preparation—Carrageenan is the hydrocolloid extracted with water or aqueous alkali from certain red seaweeds of the class *Rhodophyceae*, and separated from the solution by precipitation with alcohol (methanol, ethanol, or isopropanol), or by drum-roll drying, or by freezing.

Constituents—Carrageenan is a variable mixture of potassium, sodium, calcium, magnesium, and ammonium sulfate esters of galactose and 3,6-anhydrogalactose copolymers, the hexoses being alternately linked α-1,3 and β-1,4 in the polymer. The three main types of copolymers present are *kappa*-carrageenan, *iota*-carrageenan, and *lambda*-carrageenan, which differ in the composition and manner of linkage of monomeric units and the degree of sulfation (the ester sulfate content for carrageenans varies from 18% to 40%). *Kappa*-carrageenan and *iota*-carrageenan are the gelling fractions; *lambda*-carrageenan is the nongelling fraction. The gelling fractions may be separated from the nongelling fraction by addition of potassium chloride to an aqueous solution of carrageenan. Carrageenan separated by drum-roll drying may contain mono- and di-glycerides or up to 5% of polysorbate 80 used as roll-stripping agents.

Description—Yellow-brown to white, coarse to fine powder; odorless; tasteless, producing a mucilaginous sensation on the tongue.

Solubility—All carrageenans hydrate rapidly in cold water, but only *lambda*-carrageenan and sodium carrageenans dissolve completely. Gelling carrageenans require heating to about 80° for complete solution where potassium and calcium ions are present.

Uses—Carrageenan is used in the pharmaceutical and food industries as an emulsifying, suspending, and gelling agent.

Powdered Cellulose

Cellulose [9004-34-6] $(C_6H_{10}O_5)_n$; purified, mechanically disintegrated cellulose prepared by processing alpha cellulose obtained as a pulp from fibrous plant materials.

Description—White, odorless substance, consisting of fibrous particles, which may be compressed into self-binding tablets which disintegrate rapidly in water; exists in various grades, exhibiting degrees of fineness ranging from a free-flowing dense powder to a coarse, fluffy, nonflowing material; pH (supernatant liquid of a 10 g/90 mL aqueous suspension after 1 hour) between 5 and 7.5.

Solubility—Insoluble in water, dilute acids, and nearly all organic solvents; slightly soluble in NaOH solution (1 in 20).

Uses—*Pharmaceutic aid* (tablet diluent; adsorbent; suspending agent).

Cetyl Alcohol—page 1304.

Cholesterol

Cholest-5-en-3-ol, (3β)-, Cholesterin

Cholest-5-en-3β-ol [57-88-5] $C_{27}H_{46}O$ (386.66).
For the structural formula, see page 406.
A steroid alcohol widely distributed in the animal organism. In addition to cholesterol and its esters, several closely related steroid alcohols occur in the yolk of eggs, the brain, milk, fish oils, wool fat (10 to 20%), etc. These closely resemble it in properties. One of the methods of commercial production involves extraction of cholesterol from the unsaponifiable matter in the spinal cord of cattle, with petroleum benzin. Wool fat is also used as a source of cholesterol.

Description—White or faintly yellow, almost odorless pearly leaflets or granules; usually acquires a yellow to pale tan color on prolonged exposure to light or to elevated temperatures; melts between 147° and 150°.

Solubility—Insoluble in water; 1 g slowly dissolves in 100 mL alcohol, and about 50 mL dehydrated alcohol; soluble in acetone, hot alcohol, chloroform, dioxane, ether, ethyl acetate, solvent hexane, and vegetable oils.

Uses—To enhance incorporation and emulsification of medicinal products in oils or fats. It is a *pharmaceutical necessity* for *Hydrophilic Petrolatum*, in which it enhances water-absorbing capacity. See Chapter 21.

Dioctyl Sodium Sulfosuccinate (Docusate Sodium)—page 806.

Gelatin

White Gelatin

A product obtained by the partial hydrolysis of collagen derived from the skin, white connective tissues, and bones of animals. Gelatin derived from an acid-treated precursor is known as Type A and exhibits an isoelectric point between pH 7 and pH 9, while gelatin derived from an alkali-treated precursor is known as Type B and exhibits an isoelectric point between pH 4.7 and pH 5.2.

Gelatin for use in the manufacture of capsules in which to dispense medicines, or for the coating of tablets, may be colored with a certified color, may contain not more than 0.15% of sulfur dioxide, may contain a suitable concentration of sodium lauryl sulfate and suitable antimicrobial agents, and may have any suitable gel strength that is designated by Bloom Gelometer number.

Regarding the special gelatin for use in the preparation of emulsions, see *Emulsions* (page 1507).

Description—Sheets, flakes, or shreds, or a coarse to fine powder; faintly yellow or amber in color, the color varying in depth according to the particle size; slight, characteristic bouillon-like odor; stable in air when dry, but is subject to microbic decomposition when moist or in solution.

Solubility—Insoluble in cold water, but swells and softens when immersed in it, gradually absorbing from 5 to 10 times its own weight of water; soluble in hot water, acetic acid, and hot mixtures of glycerin and water; insoluble in alcohol, chloroform, ether, and fixed and volatile oils.

Uses—In pharmacy to coat pills and form capsules, and as a vehicle for suppositories. It is also recommended as an emulsifying agent. See under *Emulsions* in Chapters 21 and 84, also *Suppositories* (page 1580), and *Absorbable Gelatin Sponge* (page 832). It has also been used as an adjuvant protein food in malnutrition.

Glyceryl Monostearate—page 1304.

Hydroxyethyl Cellulose

Cellulose, 2-hydroxyethyl ether; Cellosize (*Union Carbide*); Natrosol (*Hercules*)

Cellulose hydroxyethyl ether [9004-62-0].
Preparation—Cellulose is treated with NaOH and then reacted with ethylene oxide.

Description—White, odorless, tasteless, free-flowing powder; softens between 135° and 140°; refractive index (2% solution) about 1.336; pH about 7; solutions are nonionic.
Solubility—Dissolves readily in cold or hot water to give clear, smooth, viscous solutions; partially soluble in acetic acid; insoluble in most organic solvents.

Uses—Resembles carboxymethylcellulose sodium in that it is a cellulose ether, but differs in being nonionic and, hence, its solutions are unaffected by cations. It is used pharmaceutically as a thickener, protective colloid, binder, stabilizer, and suspending agent in emulsions, jellies and ointments, lotions, ophthalmic solutions, suppositories, and tablets.

Hydroxypropyl Cellulose

Cellulose, 2-hydroxypropyl ether; Klucel (*Hercules*)

Cellulose hydroxypropyl ether [9004-64-2].
Preparation—After treating with NaOH, cellulose is reacted with propylene oxide at elevated temperature and pressure.

Description—Off-white, odorless, tasteless powder; softens at 130°; burns out completely between 450° and 500° in N_2 or O_2; refractive index

(2% solution) about 1.337; pH (aqueous solution) 5 to 8.5; solutions are nonionic.
Solubility—Soluble in water below 40° (insoluble above 45°); soluble in many polar organic solvents.

Uses—A broad combination of properties useful in a variety of industries. It is used pharmaceutically as a binder, granulation agent, and film-coater in the manufacture of tablets; an alcohol-soluble thickener and suspending agent for elixirs and lotions; and a stabilizer for emulsions.

Hydroxypropyl Methylcellulose

Cellulose, 2-hydroxypropyl methyl ether

Cellulose hydroxypropyl methyl ether [9004-65-3], available in grades containing 16.5–30.0% of methoxy and 4.0–32.0% of hydroxypropoxy groups, and thus in viscosity and thermal gelation temperatures of solutions of specified concentration.

Preparation—The appropriate grade of methylcellulose (see below) is treated with NaOH and reacted with propylene oxide at elevated temperature and pressure and for a reaction time sufficient to produce the desired degree of attachment of methyl and hydroxypropyl groups by ether linkages to the anhydroglucose rings of cellulose.

Description—White to slightly off-white, fibrous or granular, free-flowing powder.
Solubility—Swells in water and produces a clear to opalescent, viscous colloidal mixture; undergoes reversible transformation from sol to gel on heating and cooling, respectively. Insoluble in anhydrous alcohol, ether, chloroform.

Uses—A protective colloid that is useful as a dispersing and thickening agent, and in ophthalmic solutions to provide the demulcent action and viscous properties essential for contact lens use and in "artificial tear" formulations. See *Hydroxpropyl Methylcellulose Ophthalmic Solution* (page 776).

Lanolin, Anhydrous—page 1303.

Methylcellulose

Cellulose, methyl ether; Methocel (Dow); Cellothyl (*Warner-Chilcott*); Hydrolose (*Upjohn*); Syncelose (*Blue Line*)

Cellulose methyl ether [9004-67-5]; a methyl ether of cellulose containing 27.5–31.5% of methoxy groups.

Preparation—By the reaction of methyl chloride or of dimethyl sulfate on cellulose dissolved in sodium hydroxide. The cellulose methyl ether so formed is coagulated by adding methanol or other suitable agent and centrifuged. Since cellulose has 3 hydroxyl groups/glucose residue, several methylcelluloses can be made varying, among other properties, in solubility and viscosity. Types useful for pharmaceutical application contain from 1 to 2 methoxy radicals/glucose residue.

Description—White, fibrous powder or granules; aqueous suspensions are neutral to litmus; stable to alkalies and dilute acids.
Solubility—Insoluble in ether, alcohol, and chloroform; soluble in glacial acetic acid and in a mixture of equal parts of alcohol and chloroform; swells in water, producing a clear to opalescent, viscous colloidal solution; insoluble in hot water and saturated salt solutions; salts of minerals acids and particularly of polybasic acids, phenols, and tannins coagulate solutions of methylcellulose, but this can be prevented by the addition of alcohol or of glycol diacetate.

Uses—A synthetic substitute for natural gums that has both pharmaceutic and therapeutic applications. Pharmaceutically, it is used as a *dispersing, thickening, emulsifying, sizing,* and *coating agent*. It is an ingredient of many nose drops, eye preparations, burn medications, cosmetics, tooth pastes, liquid dentifrices, hair fixatives, creams, and lotions. It functions as a protective colloid for many types of dispersed substances and is an effective stabilizer for oil-in-water emulsions.

Therapeutically, it is used as a *bulk laxative* in the treatment of *chronic constipation*. Taken with 1 or 2 glassfuls of water, it forms a colloidal solution in the upper alimentary tract; this solution loses water in the colon, forming a gel that increases the bulk and softness of the stool. The gel is bland, demulcent, and nonirritating to the gastrointestinal tract. Once a normal stool develops, the dose should be reduced to a level adequate for maintenance of good function. Although methylcellulose takes up water from the gastrointestinal tract quite readily, tablets of methylcellulose have caused fecal impaction and intestinal obstruction when taken with a limited amount of water. Methylcellulose is also used as a topical ophthalmic protectant, in the form of 0.5 to 1% solution serving as artificial tears or a contact lens solution applied to the conjunctiva, 0.05 to 0.1 mL at a time, 3 or 4 times a day as needed.

Dose—*Usual*, as laxative, 1 to **1.5 g**, with water, 2 to 4 times daily.

Dosage Forms—Tablets: 500 mg; Ophthalmic Solution: 0.5 and 1%; Syrup: 5.91 g/30 mL.

Octoxynol 9

Poly(oxy-1,2-ethanediyl), α-[4-(1,1,3,3-tetramethylbutyl)phenyl]-ω-hydroxy-, Octylphenoxy Polyethoxyethanol NF XII

Polyethylene glycol mono[p-(1,1,3,3-tetramethylbutyl)phenyl]-ether [9002-93-1]; an anhydrous liquid mixture of mono-p-(1,1,3,3-tetramethylbutyl)phenyl ethers of polyethylene glycols in which n varies from 5 to 15, and which has an average molecular weight of 647, corresponding to the formula $C_{34}H_{62}O_{11}$.

Preparation—By reacting p-(1,1,3,3-tetramethylbutyl)phenol with ethylene oxide at elevated temperature under pressure in the presence of NaOH.

Description—Clear, pale yellow, viscous liquid, having a faint odor and a bitter taste; specific gravity between 1.059 and 1.068; pH (1 in 100 aqueous solution) between 6 and 8.

Solubility—Miscible with water, alcohol, and acetone; soluble in benzene and in toluene; insoluble in solvent hexane.

Uses—A nonionic detergent, emulsifier and dispersing agent. It is an ingredient in *Nitrofurazone Solution*. See *Polyethylene Glycol 400* (page 1305).

Oleyl Alcohol

9-Octadecen-1-ol, (Z)-, Aldol 85 (*Sherex*)

(Z)-9-Octadecen-1-ol [143-28-2] $C_{18}H_{36}O$ (268.48); a mixture of unsaturated and saturated high-molecular-weight fatty alcohols consisting chiefly of oleyl alcohol.

Preparation—One method reacts ethyl oleate with absolute ethanol and metallic sodium (*Org Syntheses Coll Vol III:* 673).

Description—Clear, colorless to light yellow, oily liquid; faint characteristic odor and bland taste; iodine value between 85 and 95; hydroxyl value between 205 and 215.

Solubility—Soluble in alcohol, ether, isopropyl alcohol, and light mineral oil; insoluble in water.

Uses—*Pharmaceutic aid* (emulsifying agent; emollient).

Polyvinyl Alcohol

Ethenol, homopolymer

Vinyl alcohol polymer [9002-89-5] $(C_2H_4O)_n$.

Preparation—Polyvinyl acetate is approximately 88% hydrolyzed in a methanol-methyl acetate solution using either mineral acid or alkali as a catalyst.

Description—White to cream-colored powder or granules; odorless.

Solubility—Freely soluble in water; solution effected more rapidly at somewhat elevated temperatures.

Uses—A *suspending agent* and *emulsifier*, either with or without the aid of a surfactant. It is commonly employed as a lubricant and protectant in various ophthalmic preparations, such as decongestants, artificial tears, and contact lens products (see page 1565).

Povidone

2-Pyrrolidinone, 1-ethenyl-, homopolymer; Polyvinylpyrrolidone; PVP

1-Vinyl-2-pyrrolidinone polymer [9003-39-8] $(C_6H_9NO)_n$; a synthetic polymer consisting of linear 1-vinyl-2-pyrrolidinone groups, the degree of polymerization of which results in polymers of various molecular weights. It is produced commercially as a series of products having mean molecular weights ranging from about 10,000 to about 700,000. The viscosity of solutions containing 10% or less of povidone is essentially the same as that of water; solutions more concentrated than 10% become more viscous, depending upon the concentration and the molecular weight of the polymer used. It contains 12–13% of nitrogen.

Preparation—1,4-Butanediol is thermally dehydrogenated with the aid of copper to γ-butyrolactone which is then reacted with ammonia to form 2-pyrrolidinone. Addition of the latter to acetylene yields vinylpyrrolidinone (monomer) which is thermally polymerized in the presence of hydrogen peroxide and ammonia.

Description—White to creamy white, odorless powder, hygroscopic; pH (1 in 20 solution) between 3 and 7.

Solubility—Soluble in water, alcohol, and chloroform; insoluble in ether.

Uses—A *dispersing* and *suspending* agent in pharmaceutical preparations.

Propylene Glycol Monostearate

Octadecanoic acid, monoester with 1,2-propanediol

1,2-Propanediol monostearate [1323-39-3]; a mixture of the propylene glycol mono- and diesters of stearic and palmitic acids. It contains not less than 90% of monoesters of saturated fatty acids, chiefly propylene glycol monostearate $(C_{21}H_{42}O_3)$ and propylene glycol monopalmitate $(C_{19}H_{38}O_3)$.

Preparation—By reacting propylene glycol with stearoyl chloride in a suitable dehydrochlorinating environment.

Description—White, wax-like solid or white, wax-like beads or flakes; slight, agreeable, fatty odor and taste; congeals not lower than 45°; acid value not more than 2; saponification value between 155 and 165; hydroxyl value between 150 and 170; iodine value not more than 3.

Solubility—Dissolves in organic solvents such as alcohol, mineral or fixed oils, benzene, ether, and acetone; insoluble in water but may be dispersed in hot water with the aid of a small amount of soap or other suitable surface-active agent.

Uses—A *surfactant*. It is particularly useful as a dispersing agent for perfume oils or oil-soluble vitamins in water, and in cosmetic preparations.

Silicon Dioxide, Colloidal—page 1317.

Sodium Lauryl Sulfate

Sulfuric acid monododecyl ester sodium salt; Irium; Duponol C (*Du Pont*); Gardinol WA (*Procter & Gamble*)

Sodium monododecyl sulfate [151-21-3]; a mixture of sodium alkyl sulfates consisting chiefly of sodium lauryl sulfate. The combined content of sodium chloride and sodium sulfate is not more than 8%.

Preparation—The fatty acids of coconut oil, consisting chiefly of lauric acid, are catalytically hydrogenated to form the corresponding alcohols. The latter are then esterified with sulfuric acid (sulfated) and the resulting mixture of alkyl bisulfates (alkylsulfuric acids) is converted into a mixture of sodium salts by reacting with alkali under controlled conditions of pH.

Description—Small, white or light yellow crystals having a slight, characteristic odor.

Solubility—1 g in 10 mL water, forming an opalescent solution.

Incompatibilities—Reacts with *cationic surface-active agents* with loss of activity, even in concentrations too low to cause precipitation. Unlike soaps, it is compatible with dilute acids, and calcium and magnesium ions.

Uses—An emulsifying, detergent, and wetting agent in ointments, tooth powders, and other pharmaceutical preparations, and in the metal, paper, and pigment industries. See Chapters 21 and 88.

Sorbitan Esters

Spans (*Atlas*)

Sorbitan esters (*monolaurate* [1338-39-2]; *monooleate* [1338-43-8]; *monopalmitate* [26266-57-9]; *monostearate* [1338-41-6]; *trioleate* [26266-58-0]; *tristearate* [26658-19-5]).

Preparation—Sorbitol is dehydrated to form a *hexitan* which is then esterified with the desired fatty acid. See *Polysorbates*, page 1306, which are polyethylene glycol ethers of sorbitan fatty acid esters.

Description—*Monolaurate:* Amber, oily liquid; may become hazy or form a precipitate; viscosity about 4250 cps; HLB no 8.6; acid no 7.0 max; saponification no 158 to 170; hydroxyl no 330 to 358. *Monooleate:* Amber liquid; viscosity about 1000 cps; HLB no 4.3; acid no 8.0 max; saponification no 145 to 160; hydroxyl no 193 to 210. *Monopalmitate:* Tan, granular waxy solid; HLB no 6.7; acid no 4 to 7.5; saponification no 140 to 150; hydroxyl no 275 to 305. *Monostearate:* Cream to tan beads; HLB no 4.7; acid no 5 to 10; saponification no 147 to 157; hydroxyl no 235 to 260. *Trioleate:* Amber, oily liquid; viscosity about 200 cps; HLB no 1.8; acid no 15 max; saponification no 170 to 190; hydroxyl no 55 to 70. *Tristearate:* Tan, waxy beads; HLB no 2.1; acid no 12 to 15; saponification no 176 to 188; hydroxyl no 66 to 80.

Solubility—*Monolaurate:* Soluble in methanol and alcohol; dispersible in distilled water and hard water (200 ppm); insoluble in hard water (20,000 ppm). *Monooleate:* Soluble in most mineral and vegetable oils; slightly soluble in ether; dispersible in water; insoluble in acetone. *Monopalmitate:* Dispersible (50°) in distilled water and hard water (200 ppm); soluble in ethyl acetate; insoluble in cold distilled water and hard water (20,000 ppm). *Monostearate:* Soluble (above melting point) in vegetable oils and mineral oil; insoluble in water, alcohol, and propylene glycol. *Trioleate:* Soluble in mineral oil, vegetable oils, alcohol, and methanol; insoluble in water. *Tristearate:* Soluble in isopropyl alcohol; insoluble in water.

Uses—Nonionic *surfactants* used as *emulsifying agents* in the preparation of water-in-oil emulsions.

Stearic Acid—page 1304.

Stearyl Alcohol

1-Octadecanol [112-92-5] $C_{18}H_{38}O$ (270.50); contains not less than 90% of stearyl alcohol, the remainder consisting chiefly of cetyl alcohol [$C_{16}H_{34}O$ = 242.44].

Preparation—Through the reducing action of lithium aluminum hydride on ethyl stearate.

Description—White, unctuous flakes or granules having a faint, characteristic odor and a bland taste; melts between 55° and 60°.

Solubility—Insoluble in water; soluble in alcohol, chloroform, ether, and vegetable oils.

Uses—A surface-active agent used to *stabilize emulsions* and increase their ability to retain large quantities of water. See *Hydrophilic Ointment* (page 1304). *Hydrophilic Petrolatum* (page 1303), and Chapters 21 and 88.

Sterculia Gum—page 805.

Tragacanth

Gum Tragacanth; Hog Gum; Goat's Thorn

The dried gummy exudation from *Astragalus gummifer* Labillardière, or other Asiatic species of *Astragalus* (Fam. *Leguminosae*).

Constituents—60 to 70% bassorin and 30 to 40% soluble gum (*tragacanthin*). The bassorin swells in the presence of water to form a gel and tragacanthin forms a colloidal solution. Bassorin, consisting of complex methoxylated acids, resembles pectin. Tragacanthin yields glucuronic acid and arabinose when hydrolyzed.

Description—Flattened, lamellated, frequently curved fragments or straight or spirally twisted linear pieces 0.5 to 2.5 mm in thickness; white to weak yellow in color; translucent; horny in texture; odorless; insipid, mucilaginous taste. Powdered tragacanth is white to yellowish white.

Introduced into water, tragacanth absorbs a certain proportion of that liquid, swells very much, and forms a soft adhesive paste, but does not dissolve. If agitated with an excess of water, this paste forms a uniform mixture; but in the course of one or two days the greater part separates, and is deposited, leaving a portion dissolved in the supernatant fluid. The finest mucilage is obtained from the whole gum or *flake* tragacanth. Several days should be allowed for obtaining a uniform mucilage of the maximum gel strength. Tragacanth is wholly insoluble in alcohol. A common adulterant is *Karaya Gum*, and the USP/NF has introduced tests to detect its presence.

Uses—A *suspending agent* in lotions, mixtures, and extemporaneous preparations and prescriptions. It is used with emulsifying agents largely to increase consistency and retard creaming. It is sometimes used as a *demulcent* in sore throat and the jelly-like product formed when the gum is allowed to swell in water serves as a basis for pharmaceutical jellies, eg, *Ephedrine Sulfate Jelly*. It is also used in various confectionery products. In the form of a glycerite, it has been used as a pill excipient.

Tragacanth Mucilage—*Preparation:* Mix glycerin (18 g) with purified water (75 mL) in a tared vessel, heat the mixture to boiling, discontinue the application of heat, add tragacanth (6 g) and benzoic acid (0.2 g), and macerate the mixture during 24 hours, stirring occasionally. Then add enough purified water to make the mixture weigh 100 g, stir actively until of uniform consistency, and strain forcibly through muslin. *Uses:* A suspending agent for insoluble substances in internal mixtures. It is also a *protective* agent.

Xanthan Gum

Keltrol (*Kelco*)

A high-molecular-weight polysaccharide gum produced by a pure-culture fermentation of a carbohydrate with *Xanthomonas campestris*, then purified by recovery with isopropyl alcohol, dried, and milled; contains D-glucose and D-mannose as the dominant hexose units, along with D-glucuronic acid, and is prepared as sodium, potassium, or calcium salt; yields 4.2–5% of carbon dioxide.

Preparation—See above and US Pats 3,433,708 and 3,557,016.

Description—White or cream-colored, tasteless powder with a slight organic odor; powder and solutions stable at 25° or less; does not exhibit polymorphism; aqueous solutions are neutral to litmus.

Solubility—1 g in about 3 mL alcohol; soluble in hot or cold water.

Uses—A hydrophilic colloid to thicken, suspend, emulsify, and stabilize water-based systems.

Other Emulsifying and Suspending Agents

Chondrus [Irish Moss; Carrageenan]—The dried sun-bleached plant of *Chondrus crispus* (Linné) Stackhouse (Fam *Gigartineaceae*). *Uses:* Principally as an emulsifying agent for liquid petrolatum and for cod liver oil. It is also a protective.

Malt—The partially germinated grain of one or more varieties of *Hordeum vulgare* Linné (Fam *Gramineae*) and contains amylolytic enzymes. Yellowish or amber-colored grains, having a characteristic odor and a sweet taste. The evaporated aqueous extract constitutes malt extract.

Malt Extract—The product obtained by extracting malt, the partially and artificially germinated grain of one or more varieties of *Hordeum vulgare* Linné (Fam *Gramineae*). *Uses:* An infrequently used emulsifying agent.

Ointment Bases

Ointments are semisolid preparations for external application to the body. They should be of such composition that they soften, but not necessarily melt, when applied to the skin. Therapeutically, ointments function as protectives and emollients for the skin, but are used primarily as vehicles or bases for the topical application of medicinal substances. Ointments may also be applied to the eye or eyelids.

Ideally, an ointment base should be compatible with the skin, stable, permanent, smooth and pliable, nonirritating, nonsensitizing, inert, and able readily to release its incorporated medication. Since there is no single ointment base which possesses all these characteristics, continued research

in this field has resulted in the development of numerous new bases. Indeed, ointment bases have become so numerous as to require classification. Although ointment bases may be grouped in several ways, it is generally agreed that they can be classified best according to composition. Hence, the following four classes are recognized herein: oleaginous ointment bases, emulsifiable ointment bases, emulsion ointment bases, and water-soluble ointment bases.

For completeness, substances are included that, although not used alone as ointment bases, contribute some pharmaceutical property to one or more of the various bases.

Oleaginous Ointment Bases and Components

The oleaginous ointment bases include fixed oils of vegetable origin, fats obtained from animals, and semisolid hydrocarbons obtained from petroleum. The vegetable oils are used chiefly in ointments to lower the melting point or to soften bases. These oils can be used as a base in themselves when a high percentage of powder is incorporated.

The vegetable oils and the animal fats have two marked disadvantages as ointment bases: (1) Their water-absorbing capacity is low and (2) they have a tendency to become rancid. Insofar as vegetable oils are concerned, the second disadvantage can be overcome by hydrogenation; a process which converts many fixed oils into white, semisolid fats, or into hard, almost brittle, waxes.

The hydrocarbon bases comprise a group of substances with a wide range of melting points so that any desired consistency and melting point may be prepared with representatives of this group. They are stable, bland, chemically inert, and will mix with virtually any chemical substance. Oleaginous bases are excellent emollients.

White Ointment

Ointment USP XI; Simple Ointment

White Wax .... 50 g
White Petrolatum .... 950 g
To make .... 1000 g

Melt the white wax in a suitable dish on a water bath, add the white petrolatum, warm until liquefied, then discontinue the heating, and stir the mixture until it begins to congeal. It is permissible to vary the proportion of wax to obtain a suitable consistency of the ointment under different climatic conditions.

Uses—An emollient and vehicle for other ointments.

Yellow Ointment

Yellow Wax .... 50 g
Petrolatum .... 950 g
To make .... 1000 g

Melt the yellow wax in a suitable dish on a steam bath, add the petrolatum, warm until liquefied, then discontinue the heating, and stir the mixture until it begins to congeal. It is permissible to vary the proportion of wax to obtain a suitable consistency of the ointment under different climatic conditions.

Uses—An emollient and vehicle for other ointments. Both white and yellow ointment are known as "simple ointment." White ointment should be used to prepare white ointments and yellow ointments should be used to prepare colored ointments when simple ointment is prescribed.

Cetyl Esters Wax

"Synthetic Spermaceti"

A mixture consisting primarily of esters of saturated fatty alcohols (C_{14} to C_{18}) and saturated fatty acids (C_{14} to C_{18}). It has a saponification value of 109–120 and an acid value of not more than 5.

Description—White to off-white, somewhat translucent flakes having a crystalline structure and pearly luster when caked; it has a faint odor and a bland, mild taste; free from rancidity; specific gravity between 0.820 and 0.840 at 50°; iodine value not more than 1; melts between 43° and 47°.
Solubility—Insoluble in water; practically insoluble in cold alcohol; soluble in boiling alcohol, ether, chloroform, and fixed and volatile oils; slightly soluble in cold solvent hexane.

Uses—A replacement for spermaceti used to give consistency and texture to ointments, as *Cold Cream* and *Rose Water Ointment.*

Oleic Acid

9-Octadecenoic acid, (Z)-, Oleinic Acid; Elaic Acid

$$HC-CH_2(CH_2)_6COOH$$
$$\| $$
$$HC-CH_2(CH_2)_6CH_3$$

Oleic acid [112-80-1] obtained from tallow and other fats, and consists chiefly of (Z)-9-octadecenoic acid (282.47). Oleic acid used in preparations for internal administration is derived from edible sources.

It usually contains variable amounts of the other fatty acids present in tallow such as linolenic and stearic acids.

Preparation—Obtained as a by-product in the manufacture of the solid stearic and palmitic acids used in the manufacture of candles, stearates, and other products. The crude oleic acid is known as "red oil," the stearic and palmitic acids being separated by cooling.

Description—Colorless to pale yellow, oily liquid with a lard-like odor and taste; specific gravity 0.889 to 0.895; congeals at a temperature not above 10°; pure oleic acid solidifies at 4°; at atmospheric pressure it decomposes when heated at 80° to 100°; on exposure to air it gradually absorbs oxygen, darkens, and develops a rancid odor.
Solubility—Practically insoluble in water; miscible with alcohol, chloroform, ether, benzene, and fixed and volatile oils.
Incompatibilities—Reacts with *alkalies* to form soaps. *Heavy metals* and *calcium salts* form insoluble oleates. *Iodine solutions* are decolorized by formation of the iodine addition compound of oleic acid. Oleic acid is oxidized to various derivatives by *nitric acid*, *potassium permanganate*, and other agents.

Uses—Oleic acid is classified as an emulsion adjunct, which reacts with alkalis to form soaps that function as emulsifying agents; it is used for this purpose in such preparations as *Benzyl Benzoate Lotion* and *Green Soap.* It is also used to prepare oleate salts of bases.

Olive Oil

Sweet Oil

The fixed oil obtained from the ripe fruit of *Olea europaea* Linné (Fam *Oleaceae*).

Preparation—By crushing recently collected ripe olives in a mill without breaking the putamen, then moderately pressing the pulpy mass. This produces the highest grade oil, known as *virgin oil*, "sublime oil," or "first expressed oil." The mass in the press is then mixed with water and again expressed with greater pressure, an oil of second quality resulting. Any oil remaining in the press cake is finally extracted with carbon disulfide, or the mass is thrown into large cisterns, mixed with water, and the oil allowed to separate. This is sometimes called "Pyrene oil," "bagasse oil," or "huile d'enfer." When bought in bulk or from unlabeled containers, cottonseed oil, colza oil, grapeseed oil, sesame oil, or other bland oils are not uncommonly found as adulterants. Large quanties of olive oil are imported from Italy and other countries bordering the Mediterranean, and it is produced to a limited extent in the Southern US, chiefly in California.

Description—Pale yellow or light greenish yellow, oily liquid, having a slight characteristic odor and taste, with a faintly acrid aftertaste; specific gravity 0.910 to 0.915.

Solubility—Slightly soluble in alcohol; miscible with carbon disulfide, chloroform, and ether.

Uses—In making cerates, ointments, liniments, and plasters. It is a bland oil, well suited for *emollient* purposes and for food. Olive oil is also used as an emollient laxative; sufficient must be given so that enough escapes digestion to soften the stool. The usual dose is 30 mL.

Paraffin

Paraffin Wax, Hard Paraffin

A purified mixture of solid hydrocarbons obtained from petroleum.

Description—Colorless or white, more or less translucent mass, with a crystalline structure; slightly greasy to the touch; odorless and tasteless; congeals between 47° and 65°.

Solubility—Freely soluble in chloroform, ether, volatile oils, and most warm fixed oils; slightly soluble in dehydrated alcohol; insoluble in water and alcohol.

Uses—Mainly to increase the consistency of some ointments.

Petrolatum

Yellow Soft Paraffin; Amber Petrolatum; Yellow Petrolatum; Petroleum Jelly; Paraffin Jelly

A purified mixture of semisolid hydrocarbons obtained from petroleum. It may contain a suitable stabilizer.

Preparation—The "residuums," as they are termed technically, which are obtained by the distillation of petroleum, are purified by melting, usually treating with sulfuric acid, and then percolating through recently burned bone black or adsorptive clays; this removes the odor and modifies the color. Selective solvents are also sometimes employed to extract impurities.

It has been found that the extent of purification required to produce *Petrolatum* and *Light Mineral Oil* of official quality removes antioxidants that are naturally present, and the purified product subsequently has a tendency to oxidize and develop an offensive odor. This is prevented by the addition of a minute quantity of α-tocopherol, or other suitable antioxidant, as is now permissible.

Description—Unctuous mass of yellowish to light amber color; not more than a slight fluorescence after being melted; transparent in thin layers; free or nearly free from odor and taste; specific gravity 0.815 to 0.880 at 60°; melts between 38° and 60°.

Solubility—Insoluble in water; almost insoluble in cold or hot alcohol and in cold dehydrated alcohol; freely soluble in benzene, carbon disulfide, chloroform, and turpentine oil; soluble in ether, solvent hexane, and in most fixed and volatile oils, the degree of solubility in these solvents varying with the composition of the petrolatum.

Uses—A base for ointments. It is highly occlusive and therefore a good emollient but it may not release some drugs readily.

White Petrolatum

White Petroleum Jelly; White Soft Paraffin

A purified mixture of semisolid hydrocarbons obtained from petroleum, and wholly or nearly decolorized. It may contain a suitable stabilizer.

Preparation—In the same manner as petrolatum, the purification treatment being continued until the product is practically free from yellow color.

Description—White or faintly yellowish, unctuous mass; transparent in thin layers, even after cooling to 0°; specific gravity 0.815 to 0.880 at 60°; melts between 38° and 60°.

Solubility—Similar to that described under *Petrolatum*.

Uses—Similar to yellow petrolatum but is often preferred because of its freedom from color. It is employed as a protective and as a base for ointments and cerates and to form the basis for burn dressings. See *Petrolatum Gauze* (page 774).

Spermaceti

A waxy substance obtained from the head of the sperm whale, *Physeter macrocephalus* Linné (Fam *Physeteridae*).

Constituents—A mixture of several constituents of which cetin, or cetyl palmitate [$C_{15}H_{31}COOC_{16}H_{33}$], predominates. When recrystallized from alcohol, *cetin* is obtained, while the mother liquor on evaporation deposits an oil, *cetin elain*, which when saponified yields *cetin elaic acid*, an acid resembling, but distinct from, oleic acid.

Preparation—By pumping the oleaginous material from the head of the sperm whale, separating the liquid portion known as sperm oil, and purifying the remaining crude solid, which is spermaceti.

Description—White, somewhat translucent, slightly unctuous masses with a crystalline fracture and pearly luster; faint odor and a bland, mild taste; free from rancidity; specific gravity about 0.94; melts between 44° and 52°.

Solubility—Insoluble in water; practically insoluble in cold alcohol; slightly soluble in cold solvent hexane; soluble in boiling alcohol, ether, chloroform, and fixed and volatile oils.

Uses—One of the solid fatty substances formerly employed to give consistency and texture to cerates and ointments, as in *Cold Cream* and *Rose Water Ointment*. In the interest of whale conservation, spermaceti has been replaced by *cetyl esters wax* (also known as *synthetic spermaceti*).

Dose—*For external use*, topically as required.

Starch Glycerite

Starch Glycerin

Starch	100 g
Benzoic Acid	2 g
Purified Water	200 mL
Glycerin	700 mL
To make about	1000 g

Rub the starch and the benzoic acid with the purified water in a porcelain dish until a smooth mixture is produced, then add the glycerin, and mix well. Heat the mixture on a sand bath to a temperature between 140° and 144°, with constant but gentle stirring until a translucent, jelly-like mass results, and then strain through muslin.

Starch Glycerite should be freshly prepared.

Uses—Although not an oleaginous base, this *emollient* preparation is sometimes used as a substitute for a fatty ointment. It has also been used as a *pill excipient*.

Dose—*For external use*, *topically* as required.

White Wax

Bleached Beeswax; White Beeswax; Bleached Wax

The product of bleaching and purifying yellow wax that is obtained from the honeycomb of the bee [*Apis mellifera* Linné (Fam *Apidae*)].

Preparation—The color of yellow wax is discharged by exposing it with an extended surface to the combined influence of air, light, and moisture. In one process a stream of melted wax is directed on a revolving cylinder kept constantly wet, upon which it congeals in thin layers. These layers are spread on linen cloths stretched on frames and exposed to the air and light, care being taken to wet and occasionally turn them. In a few days they are partially bleached; but to remove the color completely it is necessary to repeat the whole process one or more times. When sufficiently bleached, it is melted and cast into small circular cakes.

Description—Yellowish white, nearly tasteless, somewhat translucent solid with a faint, characteristic odor; free from rancidity; melting range 62° to 65°; specific gravity about 0.95.

Solubility—Insoluble in water; sparingly soluble in cold alcohol; boiling alcohol dissolves the cerotic acid and a portion of the myricin, which are constituents of white wax; completely soluble in chloroform, ether, and fixed and volatile oils; partly soluble in cold benzene and cold carbon disulfide; completely soluble in these liquids at about 30°.

Uses—A stiffening agent in many preparations such as cerates, pastes, and ointments.

Yellow Wax

Beeswax; Yellow Beeswax

The purified wax from the honeycomb of the bee, *Apis mellifera* Linné (Fam *Apidae*).

Constituents—A mixture of three substances: (1) *myricin*, insoluble in boiling alcohol and consisting chiefly of *myricyl palmitate* [$C_{30}H_{61}(C_{16}H_{31}O_2)$] and *myricyl alcohol* [$C_{30}H_{61}OH$]; (2) *cerin* or *cerotic acid* [$C_{26}H_{52}O_2$], formerly called *cerin* when obtained only in

an impure state, which is dissolved by boiling alcohol, but crystallizes out on cooling; (3) *cerolein*, which remains dissolved in the cold alcoholic liquid. This latter is probably a mixture of fatty acids.

Preparation—Yellow wax is a natural secretion of bees. It is obtained on the large scale by first abstracting the honey from the combs by shaving off the ends of the cells, draining, and then placing them in centrifuges. The honey is rapidly whirled out, water is added, and the wax is thoroughly and quickly cleaned; it is then melted and strained and run into molds to cool and harden.

Description—Yellow to grayish brown solid with an agreeable, honeylike odor, and a faint, characteristic taste; when cold it is somewhat brittle and when broken it presents a dull, granular, noncrystalline fracture; becomes pliable from the heat of the hand; specific gravity about 0.95; melts between 62° and 65°.

Solubility—Insoluble in water; sparingly soluble in cold alcohol; completely soluble in chloroform, ether, and fixed and volatile oils; partly soluble in cold benzene and carbon disulfide; completely soluble in these liquids at about 30°.

Uses—A stiffening agent in many pharmaceutical preparations and ingredient of many polishes.

Absorbent Ointment Bases

The term absorbent is used here to denote the water-absorbing or emulsifying properties of these bases and not to describe their action on the skin. These bases, sometimes called *emulsifiable ointment bases*, are generally anhydrous substances which have the property of absorbing (emulsifying) considerable quantities of water and still retaining their ointment-like consistency. Preparations of this type do not contain water as a component of their basic formula, but if water is incorporated, when and as desired, a water-in-oil emulsion results. The following official products fall into this category.

Anhydrous Lanolin

Wool Fat USP XVI; Refined Wool Fat

Lanolin that contains not more than 0.25% of water.

Constituents—Contains the sterols *cholesterol* [$C_{27}H_{45}OH$] and *oxycholesterol* as well as triterpene and aliphatic alcohols. About 7% of the alcohols are found in the free state, the remainder occurring as esters of the following fatty acids: *carnaubic*, *cerotic*, *lanoceric*, *lanopalmitic*, *myristic*, and *palmitic acids*. Some of these acids are found free. The emulsifying and emollient actions of lanolin are due to the alcohols that are found in the unsaponifiable fraction when lanolin is treated with alkali. Constituting approximately one-half of this fraction and known as *lanolin alcohols*, the latter is comprised of *cholesterol* (30%), *lanosterol* (25%), *cholestanol* (*dihydrocholesterol*) (3%), *agnosterol* (2%), and various other alcohols (40%).

Preparation—By purifying the fatty matter (*suint*) obtained from the wool of the sheep. This natural wool fat contains about 30% of free fatty acids and fatty acid esters of *cholesterol* and other higher alcohols. The cholesterol compounds are the important constituents and, to secure these in a purified form, many processes have been devised. In one of these the crude wool fat is treated with weak alkali, the saponified fats and emulsions centrifuged to secure the aqueous soap solution, from which, on standing, a layer of partially purified wool fat separates. This product is further purified by treating it with calcium chloride and then dehydrated by fusion with unslaked lime.

It is finally extracted with acetone and the solvent subsequently separated by distillation. Anhydrous lanolin differs from lanolin in that the former contains practically no water.

Description—Yellow, tenacious, unctuous mass having a slight, characteristic odor; melts between 36° and 42°.

Solubility—Insoluble in water, but mixes without separation with about twice its weight of water; sparingly soluble in cold alcohol; more soluble in hot alcohol; freely soluble in ether and chloroform.

Uses—An ingredient of ointments, especially when an aqueous liquid is to be incorporated. It gives a distinctive quality to the ointment, increasing absorption of active ingredients and maintaining a uniform consistency for the ointment under most climatic conditions. However, anhydrous lanolin has been omitted from many ointments on the recommendation of dermatologists who have found that many patients are allergic to this animal wax.

Hydrophilic Petrolatum

Cholesterol	30 g
Stearyl Alcohol	30 g
White Wax	80 g
White Petrolatum	860 g
To make	1000 g

Melt the stearyl alcohol, white wax, and white petrolatum together on a steam bath, then add the cholesterol, and stir until it completely dissolves. Remove from the bath, and stir until the mixture congeals.

Uses—A *protective* and *water-absorbable ointment base*. It will absorb a large amount of water of aqueous solutions of medicating substances, forming a water-in-oil type of emulsion. See *Ointments* (page 1573).

Other Absorption Ointment Bases

Hydroxystearin Sulfate [Sulfated Hydrogenated Castor Oil; SHCO]—A substance prepared by sulfating hydrogenated castor oil. Pale, yellow-brown, unctuous semisolid mass with a faint odor containing about 9% organically bound SO_3. Dispersible in water and glycerin; miscible with propylene glycol, petrolatums, and fixed oils. *Uses:* A surface-active agent used in preparing hydrophilic ointment bases and other emulsions.

Emulsion Ointment Bases and Components

Emulsion ointment bases are actually semisolid emulsions. These preparations can be divided into two groups on the basis of emulsion type: emulsion ointment base water-in-oil (w/o) type and emulsion ointment base oil-in-water (o/w) type. Bases of both types will permit the incorporation of some additional amounts of water without reducing the consistency

of the base below that of a soft cream. However, only oil-in-water emulsion ointment bases can be readily removed from the skin and clothing with water. Water-in oil emulsions are better emollients and protectants than are oil-in-water emulsions. Water-in-oil emulsions can be diluted with oils.

Cetyl Alcohol

Cetostearyl Alcohol; "Palmityl" Alcohol; Aldol 52 (*Sherex*)

$$CH_3(CH_2)_{14}CH_2OH$$

1-Hexadecanol [124-29-8] $C_{16}H_{34}O$ (242.44); a mixture of not less than 90% of cetyl alcohol, the remainder chiefly stearyl alcohol.

Preparation—By catalytic hydrogenation of palmitic acid, or saponification of spermaceti, which contains cetyl palmitate.

Description—Unctuous, white flakes, granules, cubes, or castings, having a faint characteristic odor and a bland, mild taste; melts between 45° and 50° and not less than 90% distils between 316° and 336°.

Solubility—Insoluble in water; soluble in alcohol, chloroform, ether, and vegetable oils.

Uses—Similar to *Stearyl Alcohol* (page 1300). Cetyl alcohol also imparts a smooth texture to the skin, and is widely used in cosmetic creams and lotions.

Cold Cream

Petrolatum Rose Water Ointment USP XVI

Cetyl Esters Wax	125 g
White Wax	120 g
Mineral Oil	560 g
Sodium Borate	5 g
Purified Water	190 mL
To make about	1000 g

Reduce the cetyl esters wax and the white wax to small pieces, melt them on a steam bath with the mineral oil, and continue heating until the temperature of the mixture reaches 70°. Dissolve the sodium borate in the purified water, warmed to 70°, and gradually add the warm solution to the melted mixture, stirring rapidly and continuously until it has congealed.

If the ointment has been chilled, warm it slightly before attempting to incorporate other ingredients (see USP for allowable variations).

Uses—Useful as an emollient, cleansing cream, and ointment base. It resembles *Rose Water Ointment*, differing only in that mineral oil is used in place of almond oil and omitting the fragrance. This change produces an ointment base which is not subject to rancidity like one containing a vegetable oil. This is a water-in-oil emulsion.

Glyceryl Monostearate

Octadecanoic acid, monoester with 1,2,3-propanetriol

Monostearin [31566-31-1]; a mixture chiefly of variable proportions of glyceryl monostearate $[C_3H_5(OH)_2C_{18}H_{35}O_2 = 358.56]$ and glyceryl monopalmitate $[C_3H_5(OH)_2C_{16}H_{31}O_2 = 330.51]$.

Preparation—Among other ways, by reacting glycerin with commercial stearoyl chloride.

Description—White, wax-like solid or occurs in the form of white, wax-like beads, or flakes; slight, agreeable, fatty odor and taste; does not melt below 55°; affected by light.

Solubility—Insoluble in water, but may be dispersed in hot water with the aid of a small amount of soap or other suitable surface-active agent; dissolves in hot organic solvents such as alcohol, mineral or fixed oils, benzene, ether, and acetone.

Uses—A thickening and emulsifying agent for ointments. See *Ointments* (page 1573).

Hydrophilic Ointment

Methylparaben	0.25 g
Propylparaben	0.15 g
Sodium Lauryl Sulfate	10 g
Propylene Glycol	120 g
Stearyl Alcohol	250 g
White Petrolatum	250 g
Purified Water	370 g
To make about	1000 g

Melt the stearyl alcohol and the white petrolatum on a steam bath, and warm to about 75°. Add the other ingredients, previously dissolved in the water and warmed to 75°, and stir the mixture until it congeals.

Uses—A *water-removable ointment base* for the so-called "washable" ointments. This is an oil-in-water emulsion.

Lanolin

Hydrous Wool Fat

The purified, fat-like substance from the wool of sheep, *Ovis aries* Linné (Fam *Bovidae*); contains 25 to 30% water.

Description—Yellowish white, ointment-like mass, having a slight, characteristic odor; when heated on a steam bath it separates into an upper oily and a lower water layer; when the water is evaporated a residue of *Lanolin* remains which is transparent when melted.

Solubility—Insoluble in water; soluble in chloroform and ether with separation of its water.

Uses—Largely as a vehicle for ointments, for which it is admirably adapted, on account of its compatibility with skin lipids. It emulsifies aqueous liquids. Lanolin is a water-in-oil emulsion.

Rose Water Ointment

Cold Cream; Galen's Cerate

Cetyl Esters Wax	125 g
White Wax	120 g
Almond Oil	560 g
Sodium Borate	5 g
Stronger Rose Water	25 mL
Purified Water	165 mL
Rose Oil	0.2 mL
To make about	1000 g

Reduce the cetyl esters wax and the white wax to small pieces, melt them on a steam bath, add the almond oil, and continue heating until the temperature of the mixture reaches 70°. Dissolve the sodium borate in the purified water and stronger rose water, warmed to 70°, and gradually add the warm solution to the melted mixture, stirring rapidly and continuously until it has cooled to about 45°. Then incorporate the rose oil.

Rose water ointment must be free from rancidity. If the ointment has been chilled, warm it slightly before attempting to incorporate other ingredients (see USP for allowable variations).

History—Originated by Galen, the famous Roman physician-pharmacist of the 1st century AD, was known for many centuries by the name of *Unguentum* or *Ceratum Refrigerans*. It has changed but little in proportions or method of preparation throughout many centuries.

Uses—An *emollient* and *ointment base*. It is a water-in-oil emulsion.

Stearic Acid

Octadecanoic acid; Cetylacetic Acid; Stearophanic Acid

Stearic acid [57-11-4]; a mixture of stearic acid $[C_{18}H_{36}O_2 = 284.48]$ and palmitic acid $[C_{16}H_{32}O_2 = 256.43]$, which together constitute not less than 90.0% of the total content. The content of each is not less than 40.0% of the total.

Purified Stearic Acid USP is a mixture of the same acids which together constitute not less than 96.0% of the total content, and the content of $C_{18}H_{36}O_2$ is not less than 90.0% of the total.

Preparation—From edible fats and oils (see exception below) by boiling them with soda lye, separating the glycerin and decomposing the resulting soap with sulfuric or hydrochloric acid. The stearic acid is subsequently separated from any oleic acid by cold expression. It is also prepared by the hydrogenation and subsequent saponification of *olein*. It may be purified by recrystallization from alcohol.

Description—Hard, white or faintly yellowish somewhat glossy and crystalline solid, or a white or yellowish white powder; an odor and taste suggestive of tallow. Stearic acid melts at about 55.5° and should not congeal at a temperature below 54°; the purified acid melts at 69° and 70° and congeals between 66° and 69°; stearic acid slowly volatilizes between 90° and 100°.

Solubility—Practically insoluble in water; 1 g in about 20 mL alcohol, 2 mL chloroform, 3 mL ether, 25 mL acetone, or 6 mL carbon tetrachloride; freely soluble in carbon disulfide; also soluble in amyl acetate, benzene, and toluene.

Incompatibilities—Insoluble stearates are formed with many *metals*. Ointment bases made with stearic acid may show evidence of drying out or lumpiness due to such a reaction when *zinc* or *calcium* salts are compounded therein.

Uses—In the preparation of sodium stearate which is the solidifying agent for the official glycerin suppositories, in enteric tablet coating, ointments, and for many other commercial products, such as toilet creams, vanishing creams, solidified alcohol, etc. (Stearic acid labeled solely for external use is exempt from the requirement that it be prepared from edible fats and oils.)

Other Emulsion Ointment Base Component

Wool Alcohols BP—Prepared by the saponification of the grease of the wool of sheep and separation of the fraction containing cholesterol and other alcohols. It contains not less than 30% cholesterol. *Description*

and *Solubility:* Golden-brown solid, somewhat brittle when cold but becoming plastic when warm, with a faint characteristic odor; has a smooth and shiny fracture; melting point not below 58°; acid value not more than 2; saponification value not more than 12; emulsions made with this material do not darken on the surface or acquire an objectionable odor in hot weather. Insoluble in water; moderately soluble in alcohol; completely soluble in 25 parts boiling anhydrous alcohol; freely soluble in ether, chloroform, and petroleum ether. *Uses:* An emulsifying agent for the preparation of water-in-oil emulsions; as a water absorbable substance in ointment bases; to improve the texture, stability, and emollient properties of o/w emulsions. It is known also as *Lanolin Alcohols*.

Water-Soluble Ointment Bases and Components

Included in this section are bases prepared from the higher ethylene glycol polymers (PEG). These polymers are marketed under the trademark of Carbowax. The polymers have a wide range in molecular weight. Those with molecular weights ranging from 200–700 are liquids; those above 1000 are wax-like solids. The polymers are water-soluble, non-volatile, and, unctuous agents. They do not hydrolyze or deteriorate and will not support mold growth. These properties account for their wide use in washable ointments. Mixtures of PEG are used to give bases of various consistency, such as very soft to hard bases for suppositories.

Glycol Ethers and Derivatives

This special class of ethers is of considerable importance in pharmaceutical technology. Both mono- and poly-functional compounds are represented in the group. The simplest member is ethylene oxide [CH_2CH_2O], the internal or cyclic ether of the simplest glycol, ethylene glycol [$HOCH_2CH_2OH$]. External mono- and di-ethers of ethylene glycol [$ROCH_2CH_2OH$ and $ROCH_2CH_2OR'$] are well known due largely to research done by the Carbide and Carbon Chemicals Co.

Preparation—In the presence of NaOH at temperatures of the order of 120° to 135° and under a total pressure of about 4 atmospheres, ethylene oxide reacts with ethylene glycol to form compounds having the general formula $HOCH_2(CH_2OCH_2)_nCH_2OH$, commonly referred to as condensation polymers and termed polyethylene (or polyoxyethylene) glycols. Other glycols besides ethylene glycol function in similar capacity, and the commercial generic term adopted for the entire group is polyalkylene (or polyoxyalkylene) glycols.

Nomenclature—It is to be noted that these condensation polymers are bifunctional; ie, they contain both ether and alcohol linkages. The compound wherein $n = 1$ is the commercially important diethylene glycol [$HOCH_2CH_2OCH_2CH_2OH$], and its internal ether is the familiar dioxane [$CH_2CH_2OCH_2CH_2O$]. The mono- and di-ethers derived from diethylene glycol have the formulas $ROCH_2CH_2O$-CH_2CH_2OH and $ROCH_2CH_2OCH_2CH_2OR'$. The former are commonly termed "*Carbitols*" and the latter "*Cellosolves*," registered trademarks belonging to the Carbide and Carbon Chemicals Co.

Polyethylene glycols are differentiated in commercial nomenclature by adding a number to the name which represents the average molecular weight. Thus, polyethylene glycol 400 has an average molecular weight of about 400 (measured values for commercial samples range between 380 and 420) corresponding to a value of n for this particular polymer of approximately 8. Polymers have been produced in which the value of n runs into the hundreds. Up to n = approximately 15, the compounds are liquids at room temperature, viscosity and boiling point increasing with increasing molecular weight. Higher polymers are waxy solids and are termed commercially *Carbowaxes* (another Carbide and Carbon Chemicals Co trademark).

It should be observed that the presence of the two terminal hydroxyl groups in the polyalkylene glycols makes possible the formation of both ether and ester derivatives, several of which are marketed products.

Uses—Because of their vapor pressure, solubility, solvent power, hygroscopicity, viscosity, and lubricating characteristics, the polyalkylene glycols or their derivatives function in many applications as effective replacements for glycerin and water-insoluble oils. They find considerable use as plasticizers, lubricants, conditioners, and finishing agents for processing textiles and rubber. They are also important as emulsifying agents and as dispersants for such diverse

substances as dyes, oils, resins, insecticides, and various types of pharmaceuticals. In addition, they are frequently employed as ingredients in ointment bases and in a variety of cosmetic preparations.

Polyethylene Glycols

Poly(oxy-1,2-ethanediyl), α-hydro-ω-hydroxy-,
Carbowaxes (*Carbide & Carbon*); Atpeg (*ICI Americas*)

$$H[OCH_2CH_2]_nOH$$

Polyethylene glycols [25322-68-3].

Preparation—Ethylene glycol is reacted with ethylene oxide in the presence of NaOH at temperatures in the range of 120° to 135° under pressure of about 4 atm.

Description—*Polyethylene glycols 200, 300, 400,* and *600* are clear, viscous liquids at room temperature. *Polyethylene glycols 900, 1000, 1450, 3350, 4500,* and *8000* are white, waxy solids. The glycols do not hydrolyze or deteriorate under typical conditions. As their molecular weight increases, their water solubility, vapor pressure, hygroscopicity, and solubility in organic solvents decrease; at the same time, freezing or melting range, specific gravity, flash point, and viscosity increase. If these compounds ignite, small fires should be extinguished with carbon dioxide or dry chemical extinguishers and large fires with "alcohol" type foam extinguishers.

Solubility—All members of this class dissolve in water to form clear solutions and are soluble in many organic solvents.

Uses—Polyethylene glycols possess a wide range of solubilities and compatibilities, which makes them useful in pharmaceutical and cosmetic preparations. Their blandness renders them highly acceptable for hair dressings, hand lotions, sun-tan creams, leg lotions, shaving creams, and skin creams (eg, a peroxide ointment which is stable may be prepared using polyethylene glycols, while oil-type bases inactivate the peroxide). Their use in washable ointments is discussed under *Ointments* (page 1573). They are also used in making suppositories, hormone creams, etc. See *Polyethylene Glycol Ointment* (below) and *Glycol Ethers* (this page). The liquid polyethylene glycol 400 and the solid polyethylene glycol 3350, used in the proportion specified (or a permissible variation thereof) in the official Polyethylene Glycol Ointment, provide a water-soluble ointment base used in the formulation of many dermatologic preparations. The solid, waxy, water-soluble glycols are often used to increase the viscosity of liquid polyethylene glycols and to stiffen ointment and suppository bases. In addition, they are used to compensate for the melting point lowering effect of other agents, ie, chloral hydrate, etc, on such bases.

Polyethylene Glycol Ointment USP—*Preparation:* Heat polyethylene glycol 3350 (400 g) and polyethylene glycol 400 (600 g) on a water bath to 65°. Allow to cool, and stir until congealed. If a firmer preparation is desired, replace up to 100 g of polyethylene glycol 400 with an equal amount of polyethylene glycol 3350. If 6 to 25% of an aqueous solution is to be incorporated in this ointment, replace 50 g of polyethylene glycol 3350 by 50 g of stearyl alcohol. *Uses:* A water-soluble ointment base.

Polyoxyl 40 Stearate

Poly(oxy-1,2-ethanediyl), α-hydro-ω-hydroxy-, octadecanoate;
Myrj (*ICI Americas*)

$$RCOO(C_2H_4O)_nH$$

(*RCOO* is the stearate moiety;
n is approximately **40**)

Polyethylene glycol monostearate [9004-99-3]; a mixture of monostearate and distearate esters of mixed polyoxyethylene diols and corresponding free glycols, the average polymer length being equivalent to about 40 oxyethylene units. *Polyoxyethylene 50 Stearate* is a similar mixture in which the average polymer length is equivalent to about 50 oxyethylene units.

Preparation—One method consists of heating the corresponding polyethylene glycol with an equimolar portion of stearic acid.

Description—White to light-tan waxy solid; odorless or has a faint fat-like odor; congeals between 37° and 47°.

Solubility—Soluble in water, alcohol, ether, and acetone; insoluble in mineral and vegetable oils.

Uses—Contains ester and alcohol functions that impart both lyophilic and hydrophilic characteristics to make polyoxyl 40 stearate useful as a surfactant and emulsifier. It is an ingredient of some water-soluble ointment and cream bases.

Polysorbates

Sorbitan esters, poly(oxy-1,2-ethanediyl) derivs., Monitans (*Ives-Cameron*); Sorlates (*Abbott*); Tweens (*ICI Americas*)

$$HO(C_2H_4O)_w \quad (OC_2H_4)_x OH$$

$$\begin{array}{c} H \\ | \\ C(OC_2H_4)_y OH \\ | \\ H_2C(OC_2H_4)_z R \end{array}$$

[Sum of *w*, *x*, *y*, and *z* is 20;
R is $(C_{11}H_{23})COO$]

Sorbitan esters, polyoxyethylene derivatives; fatty acid esters of sorbitol and its anhydrides copolymerized with a varying number of moles of ethylene oxide. The NF recognizes: *Polysorbate 20* (*structure given above*), a laurate ester; *Polysorbate 40*, a palmitate ester; *Polysorbate 60*, a mixture of stearate and palmitate esters; *Polysorbate 80*, an oleate ester.

Preparation—These important nonionic surfactants (page 267) are prepared starting with sorbitol by (1) elimination of water forming sorbitan (a cyclic sorbitol anhydride); (2) partial esterification of the sorbitan with a fatty acid such as oleic or stearic acid yielding a hexitan ester known commercially as a *Span;* and (3) chemical addition of ethylene oxide yielding a *Tween* (the polyoxyethylene derivative).

Description—*Polysorbate 80:* Lemon- to amber-colored, oily liquid having a faint, characteristic odor, and a warm, somewhat bitter taste; specific gravity between 1.07 and 1.09; pH (1:20 aqueous solution) between 6 and 8.

Solubility—*Polysorbate 80:* Very soluble in water, producing an odorless and nearly colorless solution; soluble in alcohol, cottonseed oil, corn oil, ethyl acetate, methanol, and toluene; insoluble in mineral oil.

Uses—Because of their hydrophilic and lyophilic characteristics, these nonionic surfactants are very useful as emulsifying agents forming o/w emulsions in pharmaceuticals, cosmetics, and other types of products. Polysorbate 80 is an ingredient in *Coal Tar Ointment* and *Solution.* See *Glycol Ethers* (page 1305).

Other Water-Soluble Ointment Base Component

Polyethylene Glycol 400 Monostearate USP XVI—It is an ether, alcohol, and an ester. Semitransparent, whitish, odorless, or nearly odorless mass; melting range 30° to 34°. Freely soluble in carbon tetrachloride, chloroform, ether, and petroleum benzin; slightly soluble in alcohol; insoluble in water. *Uses:* A nonionic surface-active agent in the preparation of creams, lotions, ointments, and similar pharmaceutical preparations, which are readily soluble in water.

Pharmaceutical Solvents

The remarkable growth of the solvent industry is attested by the more than 300 solvents now being produced on an industrial scale. Chemically, these include a great variety of organic compounds, ranging from hydrocarbons through alcohols, esters, ethers, and acids to nitroparaffins. Their main applications are in industry and the synthesis of organic chemicals. Comparatively few, however, are used as solvents in pharmacy, because of their toxicity, volatility, instability, and/or flammability. Those commonly used as pharmaceutical solvents are described in this section.

Acetone

2-Propanone; Dimethyl Ketone; β-Ketopropane

$$CH_3COCH_3$$

Acetone [67-64-1] C_3H_6O (58.08).

Caution—Acetone is very flammable. Do not use where it may be ignited.

Preparation—Formerly obtained exclusively from the destructive distillation of wood. The distillate, consisting principally of methanol, acetic acid, and acetone was neutralized with lime and the acetone was separated from the methyl alcohol by fractional distillation. Additional quantities of acetone were obtained by pyrolysis of the calcium acetate formed in the neutralization of the distillate.

Acetone is now largely obtained as a by-product of the butyl alcohol industry. This alcohol is formed in the fermentation of carbohydrates such as corn starch, molasses, etc, by the action of the bacterium *Clostridium acetobutylicum* (Weizmann fermentation) and acetone is always one of the products formed in the process. It is also obtained by the catalytic oxidation of isopropyl alcohol, which is prepared from propylene resulting from the "cracking" of crude petroleum.

Description—Transparent, colorless, mobile, volatile, flammable liquid with a characteristic odor; specific gravity not more than 0.789; distils between 55.5° and 57°; congeals at about −95°; aqueous solution is neutral to litmus.

Solubility—Miscible with water, alcohol, ether, chloroform, and with most volatile oils.

Uses—As an *antiseptic* in concentrations above 80%. In combination with alcohol it is used as an antiseptic *cleansing* solution. It is employed as a menstruum in the preparation of oleoresins in place of ether. It is used as a *solvent* for dissolving fatty bodies, resins, pyroxylin, mercurials, etc., and also in the manufacture of many organic compounds such as chloroform, chlorobutanol, and ascorbic acid.

Alcohol

Ethanol; Spiritus Vini Rectificatus; S. V. R.; Spirit of Wine; Methylcarbinol

Ethyl alcohol [64-17-5]; contains 92.3–93.8%, by weight (94.9–96.0%, by volume), at 15.56° (60°F) of C_2H_5OH (46.07).

Preparation—Alcohol has been made for centuries by fermentation of certain carbohydrates in the presence of *zymase*, an enzyme present in yeast cells. Utilizable carbohydrate-containing materials include molasses, sugar cane, fruit juices, corn, barley, wheat, potato, wood, and waste sulfite liquors. As yeast is capable of fermenting only D-glucose, D-fructose, D-mannose, and D-galactose it is essential that more complex carbohydrates, such as starch, be converted to one or more of these simple sugars before they can be fermented. This is variously accomplished, commonly by enzyme- or acid-catalyzed hydrolysis.

The net reaction that occurs when a hexose, glucose for example, is fermented to alcohol may be represented as

$$C_6H_{12}O_6 \rightarrow 2C_2H_5OH + 2CO_2$$

but the mechanism of the process is very complex. The fermented liquid, containing about 15% of alcohol, is distilled to obtain a distillate containing 94.9% of C_2H_5OH, by volume. To produce *absolute alcohol*, the 95% product is dehydrated by various processes.

Alcohol may be produced also by hydration of ethylene, abundant supplies of which are available from natural and coke oven gases, from waste gases of the petroleum industry, and other sources. In another synthesis acetylene is catalytically hydrated to acetaldehyde, which is then catalytically hydrogenated to ethyl alcohol.

Description—Transparent, colorless, mobile, volatile liquid with a slight, but characteristic odor and a burning taste; boils at 78° but volatilizes even at a low temperature, and is flammable; when pure, it is neutral towards all indicators; specific gravity at 15.56° (the US Government standard temperature for Alcohol) not above 0.816, indicating not less than 92.3% of C_2H_5OH by weight or 94.9% by volume.

Solubility—Miscible with water, acetone, chloroform, ether, and many other organic solvents.

Incompatibilities—Alcohol and preparations containing a high percentage of alcohol will precipitate many inorganic salts from an aqueous solution. *Acacia* is generally precipitated from a hydroalcoholic medium when the alcohol content is greater than about 35%.

Strong *oxidizing agents* such as *chlorine*, *nitric acid*, *permanganate*, or *chromate* in acid solution react, in some cases violently, with alcohol to produce oxidation products.

Alkalies cause a darkening in color due to the small amount of aldehyde usually present in alcohol.

Uses—In pharmacy principally for its solvent powers (page 216). It is also used as the starting point in the manufacture of many important compounds, like ether, chloroform, etc. Alcohol is also used as a fuel, chiefly in the denatured form.

Alcohol is a central nervous system depressant. Consequently, it has been occasionally administered intravenously for preoperative and postoperative sedation in patients in whom other measures are ineffective or contraindicated. The dose employed is 1 to 1.5 mL/kg. The intravenous use of alcohol is a specialized procedure and should be employed only by one experienced in the technique of such use.

Alcohol is widely used and abused by lay persons as a sedative. It has, however, no medically approved use for this purpose. Moreover, alcohol potentiates the central nervous system effects of numerous sedative and depressant drugs. Hence, it should not be used by patients taking certain prescription drugs or OTC medications (see page 1807).

Externally, alcohol has a number of medical uses. It is a solvent for the toxicodendrol causing *ivy poisoning*, and should be used to wash the skin thoroughly soon after contact. Alcohol (25%) is employed for bathing the skin for the purpose of *cooling* and *reducing fevers*. In high concentrations it is a *rubefacient* and an ingredient of many liniments. Alcohol (50%) is used to prevent sweating in *astringent* and *anhidrotic* lotions. It is also employed to cleanse and harden the skin and is helpful in preventing *bedsores* in bedridden patients. Alcohol in a concentration of 60 to 90% is germicidal. At optimum concentration (70% by weight) it is a good *antiseptic* for the skin (*local anti-infective*) and also for instruments. Alcohol is also used as a *solvent* to cleanse the skin splashed with phenol. High concentrations of alcohol are often injected into nerves and ganglia for the *relief of pain*, accomplishing this by causing nerve degeneration.

Denatured Alcohol

An act of Congress June 7, 1906, authorizes the withdrawal of alcohol from bond without the payment of internal revenue tax, for the purpose of denaturation and use in the arts and industries. Denatured alcohol is ethyl alcohol to which have been added such denaturing materials as to render the alcohol unfit for use as an intoxicating beverage. Denatured alcohol is divided into two classes, namely, *completely denatured alcohol* and *specially denatured alcohol*, prepared in accordance with approved formulas prescribed in Federal Industrial Alcohol Regulations 3.

Information regarding the use of alcohol and permit requirements may be obtained from the Regional Director, Bureau of Alcohol, Tobacco, and Firearms, in any of the following offices: Cincinnati, OH; Philadelphia, PA; Chicago, IL; New York, NY; Atlanta, GA; Dallas, TX; and San Francisco, CA. Federal regulation provides that completely and specially denatured alcohols may be purchased by properly qualified persons from duly established denaturing plants or bonded dealers. No permit is required for the purchase and use of completely denatured alcohol unless the purchaser intends to recover the alcohol.

Completely Denatured Alcohol—This term applies to ethyl alcohol to which have been added materials (methyl isobutyl ketone, pyronate, gasoline, acetaldol, kerosene, etc) of such nature that the products may be sold and used within certain limitations without permit and bond.

Specially Denatured Alcohol—This alcohol is intended for use in a greater number of specified arts and industries than completely denatured alcohol and the character of the denaturant or denaturants

used in such that specially denatured alcohol may be sold, possessed, and used only by those persons or firms that hold basic permits and are covered by bond.

Formulas for products using specially denatured alcohol must be approved prior to use by the Regional Director, Bureau of Alcohol, Tobacco, and Firearms in any of the regional offices listed above.

Uses—Approximately 50 specially denatured alcohol formulas containing combinations of more than ninety different denaturants are available to fill the needs of qualified users. Large amounts of specially denatured alcohols are used as raw materials in the production of acetaldehyde, synthetic rubber, vinegar, and ethyl chloride; as well as in the manufacture of proprietary solvents and cleaning solutions. Ether and chloroform can be made from suitably denatured alcohols and formulas for the manufacture of Iodine Tincture, Green Soap Tincture, and Rubbing Alcohol are set forth in the regulations.

Specially denatured alcohols are also used as solvents for surface coatings, plastics, inks, toilet preparations, and external pharmaceuticals. Large quantities are used in the processing of such food and drug products as pectin, vitamins, hormones, antibiotics, alkaloids and blood products. Other uses include supplemental motor fuel, rocket and jet fuel, antifreeze solutions, refrigerants, and cutting oils. Few products are manufactured today that do not require the use of alcohol at some stage of production. Specially denatured alcohol may not be used in the manufacture of foods or internal medicines where any of the alcohol remains in the finished product.

Diluted Alcohol

Diluted Ethanol

A mixture of alcohol and water containing 41.0–42.0%, by weight (48.4–49.5%, by volume), at 15.56°, of C_2H_5OH (46.07).

Preparation—

Alcohol	500 mL
Purified Water	500 mL

Measure the alcohol and the purified water separately at the same temperature, and mix. If the water and the alcohol and the resulting mixture are measured at 25°, the volume of the mixture will be about 970 mL.

When equal volumes of alcohol and water are mixed together, a rise in temperature and a contraction of about 3% in volume take place. In small operations the contraction is generally disregarded; in larger operations it is very important. If 50 gal of official alcohol are mixed with 50 gal of water, the product will not be 100 gal of diluted alcohol, but only 96¼ gal, a contraction of 3¾ gal. US *Proof Spirit* differs from diluted alcohol and is stronger; it contains 50%, by volume, of absolute alcohol at 15.56° (60°F). This corresponds to 42.5% by weight, and has a specific gravity of 0.9341 at the same temperature. If spirits have a specific gravity lower than that of "proof spirit" (0.9341), they are said to be "*above proof*," if greater, "*below proof*."

Diluted alcohol may also be prepared from the following:

Alcohol	408 g
Purified Water	500 g

Rules for Dilution—The following rules are applied when making an alcohol of any required lower percentage from an alcohol of any given higher percentage:

I. By Volume—Designate the volume percentage of the stronger alcohol by V, and that of the weaker alcohol by v.

Rule—Mix v volumes of the stronger alcohol with purified water to make V volumes of product. Allow the mixture to stand until full contraction has taken place, and until it has cooled, then make up the deficiency in the V volumes by adding more purified water.

Example—An alcohol of 30% by volume is to be made from an alcohol of 94.9% by volume.—Take 30 volumes of the 94.9% alcohol, and add enough purified water to produce 94.9 volumes at room temperature.

II. By Weight—Designate the weight-percentage of the stronger alcohol by W, and that of the weaker alcohol by w.

Rule—Mix w parts by weight of the stronger alcohol with purified water to make W parts by weight of product.

Example—An alcohol of 50% by weight is to be made from an alcohol of 92.3% by weight.—Take 50 parts by weight of the 92.3% alcohol, and add enough purified water to produce 92.3 parts by weight.

Description—As for *Alcohol*, except its specific gravity is between 0.935 and 0.937 at 15.56°, indicating that the strength of C_2H_5OH corresponds to that given in the official definition.

Uses—A menstruum in making tinctures, fluidextracts, extracts, etc. Its properties have been already fully described in connection with the various preparations. Its value consists not only in its *antiseptic* properties, but also in its possessing the *solvent* powers of both water and alcohol. See *Alcohol.*

Nonbeverage Alcohol

Nonbeverage alcohol is tax-paid alcohol or distilled spirits used in the manufacture, by approved formula, of such medicines, medicinal preparations, food products, flavors, or flavoring extracts as are unfit for beverage purposes. Internal Revenue Service Regulations provide that qualified holders of Special Tax Stamps who use tax paid alcohol or distilled spirits in the types of products listed above, may file a claim for *alcohol tax drawback* or refund of a considerable part of the tax paid.

Amylene Hydrate

2-Butanol, 2-methyl-, Tertiary Amyl Alcohol; Dimethylethylcarbinol

$$CH_3CH_2\underset{\underset{OH}{|}}{\overset{\overset{CH_3}{|}}{C}}CH_3$$

tert-Pentyl alcohol [75-85-4] $C_5H_{12}O$ (88.15).

Preparation—Amylene is mixed with 2 volumes of 60% H_2SO_4, both previously cooled to 0°, for about 1 hour; then neutralized with soda, distilled, and the first half of the distillate containing most of the amylene hydrate is treated with anhydrous potassium carbonate and redistilled.

Description—Clear, colorless liquid of camphoraceous odor; solution is neutral to litmus; specific gravity between 0.803 and 0.807; distils completely between 97° and 103°.

Solubility—1 g in about 8 mL water; miscible with alcohol, chloroform, ether, and glycerin.

Uses—Chiefly as a *pharmaceutic necessity for Tribromoethanol Solution* (RPS-15, page 985). It has been used as a *sedative-hypnotic* in doses of 1 to 4 g administered in glycerin.

Chloroform—page 1312.

Ether—page 1041.

Ethyl Acetate—page 1286.

Glycerin

1,2,3-Propanetriol; Glycerol

$$HOCH_2\underset{\underset{OH}{|}}{C}HCH_2OH$$

Glycerol [56-81-5] $C_3H_8O_3$ (92.09).

Chemically, glycerin is the simplest trihydric alcohol. It is worthy of special note because the two terminal alcohol groups are primary whereas the middle one is secondary. Glycerol thus becomes the first polyhydric alcohol which can yield both an aldose (*glyceraldehyde*) and a ketose (*dihydroxyacetone*).

Preparation—
1. By saponification of fats and oils in the manufacture of soap.
2. By hydrolysis of fats and oils through pressure and superheated steam.
3. By fermentation of beet sugar molasses in the presence of large amounts of sodium sulfite. Under these conditions a reaction, expressed as follows, takes place:

$$C_6H_{12}O_6 \rightarrow C_3H_5(OH)_3 + CH_3CHO + CO_2$$
Glucose　　　Glycerin　　　Acetaldehyde

4. Glycerin is now prepared in large quantities from propylene, a petroleum product. This hydrocarbon is chlorinated at about 400° to form allyl chloride, which is converted to allyl alcohol. Treatment of the unsaturated alcohol with hypochlorous acid [HOCl] yields the chlorohydrin derivative. Extraction of HCl with soda lime yields 2,3-epoxypropanol which undergoes hydration to glycerin.

Description—Clear, colorless, syrupy liquid with a sweet taste and not more than a slight, characteristic odor, which is neither harsh nor disagreeable; when exposed to moist air it absorbs water and also such gases as H_2S and SO_2; solutions are neutral; specific gravity not below 1.249 (not less than 95% $C_3H_5(OH)_3$); boils at about 290° under 1 atmos pressure, with decomposition but can be distilled intact in a vacuum.

Solubility—Miscible with water, alcohol, and methanol; 1 g in about 12 mL ethyl acetate and about 15 mL acetone; insoluble in chloroform, ether, and fixed and volatile oils.

Incompatibilities—An explosion may occur if glycerin is triturated with strong *oxidizing agents* such as *chromium trioxide*, *potassium chlorate*, and *potassium permanganate*. In dilute solutions the reactions proceed at a slower rate forming several oxidation products. Iron is an occasional contaminant of glycerin and may be the cause of a darkening in color in mixtures containing *phenols*, *salicylates*, *tannin*, etc.

With *boric acid* or *sodium borate*, glycerin forms a complex, generally spoken of as glyceroboric acid, which is a much stronger acid than boric acid.

Uses—One of the most valuable products known to pharmacy by virtue of its *solvent* property. Glycerin is useful as a *humectant* in keeping substances moist, owing to its hygroscopicity. Its agreeable taste and high viscosity adapt it for many purposes. Some modern ice collars and ice bags contain glycerin and water hermetically sealed within vulcanized rubber bags. The latter are sterilized by dipping in a germicidal solution and are stored in the refrigerator until needed. Glycerin also has some therapeutic uses. In pure anhydrous form, glycerin is used in the eye to reduce corneal edema and to facilitate ophthalmoscopic examination. It is used orally as an evacuant and, in 50 to 75% solution, as a systemic osmotic agent.

Isopropyl Alcohol—page 1162.

Methyl Alcohol

Methanol; Wood Alcohol

$$CH_3OH$$

Methanol [67-56-1] CH_4O (32.04).

Caution—Methyl alcohol is poisonous.

Preparation—By the catalytic reduction of carbon monoxide or carbon dioxide with hydrogen. A zinc oxide-chromium oxide catalyst is commonly used.

Description—Clear, colorless liquid having a characteristic odor; flammable; specific gravity not more than 0.790; distills within a range of 1°, between 63.5° and 65.7°.

Solubility—Miscible with water, alcohol, ether, benzene, and most other organic solvents.

Uses—*Pharmaceutic aid* (solvent). It is toxic. Ingestion may result in blindness; vapors also may cause toxic reactions.

Methyl Isobutyl Ketone

2-Pentanone, 4-methyl-

$$(CH_3)_2CHCH_2COCH_3$$

4-Methyl-2-pentanone [108-10-1]; contains not less than 99% of $C_6H_{12}O$ (100.16).

Description—Transparent, colorless, mobile, volatile liquid having a faint, ketonic and camphoraceous odor, distils between 114° and 117°.

Solubility—Slightly soluble in water; miscible with alcohol, ether, and benzene.

Uses—A *denaturant* for rubbing alcohol and also as a *solvent* for gums, resins, nitrocellulose, etc. It may be irritating to the eyes and mucous membranes, and, in high concentrations, narcotic.

Monoethanolamine

Ethanol, 2-amino-; Ethanolamine; Ethylolamine

$$HOCH_2CH_2NH_2$$

2-Aminoethanol [141-43-5] C_2H_7NO (61.08).

Preparation—This alkanolamine is conveniently prepared by treating ethylene oxide with ammonia.

Description—Clear, colorless, moderately viscous liquid having a distinctly ammoniacal odor; affected by light; specific gravity between 1.013 and 1.016; distillation range 167° to 173°.

Solubility—Miscible in all proportions with water, acetone, alcohol, glycerin, and chloroform; immiscible with ether, solvent hexane, and fixed oils; dissolves many essential oils.

Uses—A *solvent* for fats, oils, and many other substances, it is a pharmaceutical necessity for *Thimerosal Solution* (page 1169). It combines with fatty acids to form soaps which find application in various types of emulsions such as lotions, creams, etc.

Propylene Glycol

$$CH_3CH(OH)CH_2OH$$

1,2-Propanediol [57-55-6] $C_3H_8O_2$ (76.10).

Preparation—Propylene is converted successively to its chlorohydrin (with HOCl), epoxide (with Na_2CO_3), and glycol (with water in presence of protons).

Description—Clear, colorless, viscous, and practically odorless liquid having a slightly acrid taste; specific gravity 1.035 to 1.037; completely distils between 184° and 189°; absorbs moisture from moist air.

Solubility—Miscible with water, alcohol, acetone, and chloroform; soluble in ether; dissolves many volatile oils; immiscible with fixed oils.

Uses—A *solvent, preservative*, and *humectant*. See *Hydrophilic Ointment* (page 1304).

Trolamine

Ethanol, 2,2′,2″-nitrilotris-, Triethanolamine

2,2′,2″-Nitrilotriethanol [102-71-6] $N(C_2H_4OH)_3$ (149.19); a mixture of alkanolamines consisting largely of triethanolamine, containing some diethanolamine [$NH(C_2H_4OH)_2$ = 105.14] and monoethanolamine [$NH_2C_2H_4OH$ = 61.08].

Preparation—Along with some mono- and diethanolamine, by the action of ammonia on ethylene oxide.

Description—Colorless to pale yellow, viscous, hygroscopic liquid having a slight odor of ammonia; aqueous solution is very alkaline; melts at 20° to 21°; specific gravity between 1.120 and 1.128; a strong base and readily combines even with weak acids to form salts.

Solubility—Miscible with water or alcohol; soluble in chloroform; slightly soluble in ether or benzene.

Uses—In combination with a fatty acid, eg, oleic acid (see *Benzyl Benzoate Lotion*, page 1239), as an *emulsifier*. See *Monoethanolamine*.

Water—page 1292.

Other Pharmaceutical Solvents

Alcohol, Dehydrated, BP, PhI [Dehydrated Ethanol; Absolute Alcohol]—A transparent, colorless, mobile, volatile liquid having a characteristic odor and a burning taste; specific gravity not more than 0.798 at 15.56°; hygroscopic, flammable, and boils at about 78°C. Miscible with water, ether, and chloroform. *Uses:* A pharmaceutical solvent; also used by injection for relief of pain (see *Alcohol*, page 1159).

Coconut Oil [Coconut Oil; Copra Oil]—The fixed oil obtained by expression or extraction from the kernels of the seeds of *Cocos nucifera* Linné (Fam. *Palmae*). Pale yellow to colorless liquid between 28° to 30°, semisolid at 20°, and a hard, brittle crystalline solid below 15°; odorless and tasteless or has a faint odor and taste characteristic of coconut; it must not be used if it has become rancid; melting range 22° to 25°; specific gravity between 0.918 and 0.923. Readily soluble in alcohol, ether, chloroform, carbon disulfide, and petroleum benzin; insoluble in water.

Petroleum Benzin [Petroleum ether; Purified benzin]—Clear, colorless, volatile liquid having an ethereal or faint, petroleum-like odor, and a neutral reaction; specific gravity between 0.634 and 0.660. Practically insoluble in water; miscible with ether, chloroform, benzene, and fixed oils. *Caution:* Highly flammable, and its vapor, when mixed with air and ignited, may explode. *Uses:* A solvent for fats, resins, oils, and similar substances.

Miscellaneous Pharmaceutical Necessities

The agents listed in this section comprise a heterogeneous group of substances with both pharmaceutical and industrial applications. Pharmaceutically, some of these agents are used as diluents, enteric coatings, excipients, filtering agents, and as ingredients in products considered in other chapters. Industrially, some of these agents are used in various chemical processes, in the synthesis of other chemicals, and in the manufacture of fertilizers, explosives, etc.

Acetic Acid

Acetic acid; a solution containing 36–37%, by weight, of $C_2H_4O_2$ (60.05).

Preparation—By diluting with distilled water an acid of higher concentration, such as the 80% product, or more commonly glacial acetic acid, using 350 mL of the latter for the preparation of each 1000 mL of acetic acid.

Description—Clear, colorless liquid, having a strong characteristic odor and a sharply acid taste; specific gravity about 1.045; congeals at about −14°; acid to litmus.

Solubility—Miscible with water, alcohol, and glycerin.

Uses—In pharmacy as a *solvent* and *menstruum*, and for making diluted acetic acid. Acetic acid is also used as a starting point in the manufacture of many other organic compounds, eg, acetates, acetanilid, sulfonamides, etc. It is official primarily as a *pharmaceutic necessity* for the preparation of *Aluminum Subacetate Solution* (page 778).

Diluted Acetic Acid

Dilute Acetic Acid

A solution containing, in each 100 mL, 5.7–6.3 g of $C_2H_4O_2$.

Preparation—

Acetic Acid	158 mL
Purified Water, a sufficient quantity,	
To make	1000 mL

Mix the ingredients.

Note—This acid may also be prepared by diluting 58 mL of glacial acetic acid with sufficient purified water to make 1000 mL.

Description—Essentially the same properties, solubility, purity, and identification reactions as *Acetic Acid*, but its specific gravity is about 1.008 and it congeals at about −2°.

Uses—*Bactericidal* to many types of microorganisms and is occasionally used in 1% solution for surgical dressings of the skin. A 1% solution is actively *spermatocidal*. It is also used in vaginal douches for the management of *Trichomonas*, *Candida*, and *Hemophilus* infections.

Glacial Acetic Acid

Concentrated Acetic Acid; Crystallizable Acetic Acid; Ethanolic Acid; Vinegar Acid

$$CH_3COOH$$

Glacial acetic acid [64-19-7] $C_2H_4O_2$ (60.05).

Preparation—This acid is termed "glacial" because of its solid glassy appearance when congeals. In one process it is produced by distillation of weaker acids to which has been added a water-entraining substance such as ethylene dichloride. In this method, referred to as "azeotropic distillation," the ethylene dichloride distils out with the water before the acetic acid distils over, thereby effecting concentration of the latter.

In another process aqueous acetic acid is mixed with triethanolamine and heated. The acetic acid combines with the triethanolamine to form a triethanolamine acetate. The water is driven off first; then, at a higher temperature, the triethanolamine compound decomposes to yield glacial acetic acid.

A greater part of the glacial acetic acid now available is made synthetically from acetylene. When acetylene is passed into acetic acid containing a metallic catalyst such as mercuric oxide, ethylidene diacetate as produced which yields, upon heating, acetic anhydride and acetaldehyde. Hydration of the former and air oxidation of the latter yield glacial acetic acid.

Description—Clear, colorless, liquid with a pungent, characteristic odor; when well diluted with water, it has an acid taste; boils at about 118°; congeals at a temperature not lower than 15.6°, corresponding to a minimum of 99.4% of CH_3COOH; specific gravity about 1.05.
Solubility—Miscible with water, alcohol, acetone, ether, and glycerin; insoluble in carbon tetrachloride and in chloroform.

Uses—A *caustic* and *vesicant* when applied externally and is often sold under various disguises as a *corn solvent*. It is an excellent *solvent* for fixed and volatile oils as well as for many other organic compounds.

It is official primarily as a *pharmaceutic aid*, for use as an acidifying agent.

Almond Oil—RPS-16, page 720.

Aluminum

Aluminim Al (26.98); the free metal in the form of finely divided powder. It may contain oleic acid or stearic acid as a lubricant. It contains not less than 95% of Al, and not more than 5% of *Acid-insoluble substances*, including any added fatty acid.

Description—Very fine, free-flowing, silvery powder free from gritty or discolored particles.
Solubility—Insoluble in water and alcohol; soluble in hydrochloric and sulfuric acids and in solutions of fixed alkali hydroxides.

Uses—A *protective*. An ingredient in *Aluminum Paste* (RPS-14, page 772).

Aluminum Monostearate

Aluminum, dihydroxy(octadecanoato-*O*-)-

Dihydroxy(stearato)aluminum [7047-84-9]; a compound of aluminum with a mixture of solid organic acids obtained from fats, and consists chiefly of variable proportions of aluminum monostearate and aluminum monopalmitate. It contains the equivalent of 14.5–16.5% of Al_2O_3 (101.96).
Preparation—By interaction of a hydroalcoholic solution of potassium stearate with an aqueous solution of potassium alum, the precipitate being purified to remove free stearic acid and some aluminum distearate simultaneously produced.

Description—Fine, white to yellowish white, bulky powder, having a faint, characteristic odor.
Solubility—Insoluble in water, alcohol and ether.

Uses—A *pharmaceutic necessity* used in the preparation of *Sterile Procaine Penicillin G with Aluminum Stearate Suspension* (see page 1198).

Strong Ammonia Solution

Stronger Ammonia Water; Stronger Ammonium Hydroxide Solution; Spirit of Hartshorn

Ammonia [1336-21-6]; a solution of NH_3 (17.03), containing 27.0–31.0% (*w/w*) of NH_3. Upon exposure to air it loses ammonia rapidly.
Caution—Use care in handling Strong Ammonia Solution because of the caustic nature of the Solution and the irritating properties of its vapor. Cool the container well before opening, and cover the closure with a cloth or similar material while opening. Do not taste Strong Ammonia Solution, and avoid inhalation of its vapor.
Preparation—Ammonia is obtained commercially chiefly by synthesis from its constituent elements, nitrogen and hydrogen, combined under high pressure and at high temperature in the presence of a catalyst.

Description—Colorless, transparent liquid, having an exceedingly pungent, characteristic odor; miscible with alcohol; even when well diluted it is strongly alkaline to litmus; specific gravity about 0.90.

Uses—Only for chemical and pharmaceutical purposes. It is used primarily in making ammonia water by dilution and as a chemical reagent. It is too strong for internal administration. It is an ingredient in *Aromatic Ammonia Spirit* (page 1507).

Barium Hydroxide Lime

A mixture of barium hydroxide octahydrate and calcium hydroxide. It may contain also potassium hydroxide and may contain an indicator that is inert toward anesthetic gases such as ether, cyclopropane, and nitrous oxide, and that changes color when the barium hydroxide lime no longer can absorb carbon dioxide.
Caution—Since Barium Hydroxide Lime contains a soluble form of barium, it is toxic if swallowed.

Description—White or grayish white granules; may have a color if an indicator has been added.

Uses—A carbon dioxide adsorbent. See *Soda Lime* (page 1317).

Boric Acid

Boric acid (H_3BO_3); Boracic Acid; Orthoboric Acid

Boric acid [10043-35-3] H_3BO_3 (61.83).
Preparation—Lagoons of the volcanic districts of Tuscany formerly furnished the greater part of the boric acid and borax of commerce. Borax is now found native in California and some of the other western states; calcium and magnesium borates are found there also. Boric acid is produced from native borax, or from the other borates, by reacting with hydrochloric or sulfuric acid.

Description—Colorless scales of a somewhat pearly luster, or crystals, but more commonly a white powder slightly unctuous to the touch; odorless and stable in the air; volatilizes with steam.
Solubility—1 g in 18 mL water, 18 mL alcohol, 4 mL glycerin, 4 mL boiling water, and 6 mL boiling alcohol.

Uses—A buffer, and it is this use that is officially recognized. Boric acid is a very weak *germicide* (*local anti-infective*). Its nonirritating properties make solutions of boric acid suitable for application to such delicate structures as the cornea of the eye. Aqueous solutions are employed as an eye wash, mouth wash, and for irrigation of the bladder. A 2.2% solution is isotonic with lacrimal fluid. Solutions of boric acid, even if they are made isotonic, will hemolyze red blood cells. Boric acid is also employed as a dusting powder, when diluted with some inert material. It can be absorbed through irritated skin, eg, infants with diaper rash.

Although boric acid is not significantly absorbed from intact skin, it is absorbed from damaged skin and fatal poisoning, particularly in infants, has occurred with topical application to burns, denuded areas, granulation tissue and serous cavities. *Serious poisoning can result from oral ingestion* of as little as 5 g. Symptoms of boric acid poisoning are nausea, vomiting, abdominal pain, diarrhea, headache, and visual disturbance. Toxic alopecia has been reported from the chronic ingestion of a mouth wash containing boric acid. The kidney may be injured and death may result. Its use as a preservative in beverages and foods is prohibited by national and state legislation. *There is always present the danger of confusing boric acid with dextrose when compounding milk formulas for infants. Fatal accidents have occurred.* For this reason boric acid in bulk is colored, so that it cannot be confused with dextrose.

Boric acid is used to prevent discoloration of physostigmine solutions.
Dose—*Topically*, as required.

Calcium Hydroxide

Slaked Lime; Calcium Hydrate

Calcium hydroxide [1305-62-0] $Ca(OH)_2$ (74.09).
Preparation—By reacting freshly prepared calcium oxide with water.

Description—White powder, possessing an alkaline, slightly bitter taste absorbs carbon dioxide from the air forming calcium carbonate; solutions exhibit a strong alkaline reaction.

Solubility—1 g in 630 mL water and 1300 mL boiling water; soluble in glycerin and in syrup; insoluble in alcohol; the solubility in water is decreased by the presence of fixed alkali hydroxides.

Uses—In the preparation of *Calcium Hydroxide Solution*.

Calcium Hydroxide Topical Solution

Calcium Hydroxide Solution; Lime Water

A solution containing, in each 100 mL, not less than 140 mg of Ca(OH)₂ (74.09).

Note—The solubility of calcium hydroxide varies with the temperature at which the solution is stored, being about 170 mg/100 mL at 15°, and less at a higher temperature. The official concentration is based upon a temperature of 25°.

Preparation—

Calcium Hydroxide	**3 g**
Purified Water	**1000 mL**

Add the calcium hydroxide to 1000 mL of cool, purified water, and agitate the mixture vigorously and repeatedly during 1 hour. Allow the excess of calcium hydroxide to settle. Dispense only the clear, supernatant liquid.

The undissolved portion of the mixture is not suitable for preparing additional quantities of calcium hydroxide solution.

The object of keeping lime water over undissolved calcium hydroxide is to insure a saturated solution.

Description—Clear, colorless liquid with an alkaline taste, and a strong alkaline reaction; absorbs carbon dioxide from the air, a film of calcium carbonate forming on the surface of the liquid; when heated, it becomes turbid, owing to the separation of calcium hydroxide, which is less soluble in hot than in cold water.

Uses—This solution is too dilute to be effective as a gastric antacid. It is employed *topically* as a *protective* in various types of lotions. In some lotion formulations it is used with olive oil or oleic acid to form calcium oleate that functions as an emulsifying agent. The USP classes it as an *astringent*.

Dose—*Topically*, in astringent solutions and lotions as required (see *Calamine Lotion*, page 778).

Calcium Pantothenate, Racemic—page 1022.

Calcium Stearate

Octadecanoic acid, calcium salt

Calcium stearate [1592-23-0]; a compound of calcium with a mixture of solid organic acids obtained from fats and consists chiefly of variable proportions of stearic and palmitic acids [calcium stearate, $C_{36}H_{70}CaO_4 = 607.03$; calcium palmitate, $C_{32}H_{62}CaO_4 = 550.92$]; contains the equivalent of 9–10.5% of CaO (calcium oxide).

Preparation—By precipitation from interaction of solutions of calcium chloride and the sodium salts of the mixed fatty acids (stearic and palmitic).

Description—Fine, white to yellowish white, bulky powder having a slight, characteristic odor; unctuous and free from grittiness.

Solubility—Insoluble in water, alcohol, and ether.

Uses—A *lubricant* in the manufacture of compressed tablets. It is also used as a conditioning agent in food and pharmaceutical products. Its virtually nontoxic nature and unctuous properties makes it ideal for these purposes.

Calcium Sulfate

Sulfuric acid, calcium salt (1:1); Gypsum; Terra Alba

Calcium sulfate (1:1) [7778-18-9] CaSO₄ (136.14); *dihydrate* [10101-41-4] (172.17).

Preparation—From natural sources or by precipitation from interaction of solutions of calcium chloride and a soluble sulfate.

Description—Fine, white to slightly yellow-white, odorless powder.

Solubility—Dissolves in diluted HCl; slightly soluble in water.

Uses—A *diluent* in the manufacture of compressed tablets. It is sufficiently inert that few undesirable reactions occur in tablets made with this substance. It is also used for making plaster casts and supports.

Carnauba Wax

Obtained from the leaves of *Copernicia cerifera* Mart (Fam *Palmae*).

Preparation—Carnauba wax, which consists chiefly of *myricyl cerotate* with smaller quantities of *myricyl alcohol*, *ceryl alcohol*, and *cerotic acid*, is obtained by treating the leaf buds and leaves of *Copernicia cerifera*, the so-called *Brazilian Wax Palm*, with hot water.

Description—Light-brown to pale yellow, moderately coarse powder, possessing a characteristic bland odor, and free from rancidity; specific gravity about 0.99; melts between 81° and 86°.

Solubility—Insoluble in water; freely soluble in warm benzene; soluble in warm chloroform and toluene; slightly soluble in boiling alcohol.

Uses—A pharmaceutic aid used as a *polishing agent* in the manufacture of coated tablets.

Microcrystalline Cellulose

Cellulose [9004-34-6]; purified, partially depolymerized cellulose prepared by treating alpha cellulose, obtained as a pulp from fibrous plant material, with mineral acids.

Preparation—Cellulose is subjected to the hydrolytic action of 2.5 *N* HCl at the boiling temperature of about 105° for 15 min whereby amorphous cellulosic material is removed and aggregates of crystalline cellulose are formed. These are collected by filtration, washed with water and aqueous ammonia, and disintegrated into small fragments, often termed cellulose crystallites, by vigorous mechanical means such as a Waring blendor. US Pat 3,141,875.

Description—Fine, white, odorless, crystalline powder; consists of free-flowing, nonfibrous particles which may be compressed into self-binding tablets which disintegrate rapidly in water.

Solubility—Insoluble in water, dilute acids, and most organic solvents; slightly soluble in NaOH solution (1 in 20).

Uses—A tablet diluent and disintegrant. It can be compressed into self-binding tablets which disintegrate rapidly when placed in water.

Microcrystalline Cellulose and Sodium Carboxymethylcellulose—A colloid-forming, attrited mixture of microcrystalline cellulose and sodium carboxymethylcellulose. *Description* and *Solubility:* Tasteless, odorless, white to off-white, coarse to fine powder; pH (dispersion) between 6 and 8. Swells in water, producing, when dispersed, a white, opaque dispersion or gel; insoluble in organic solvents and dilute acids. *Uses:* Pharmaceutic aid (suspending agent). *Grades Available* (amounts of sodium carboxymethylcellulose producing viscosities in the concentrations designated); 8.5%, 120 cps in 2.1% solution; 11%, 120 cps in 1.2% solution; 11%, 65 cps in 1.2% solution.

Powdered Cellulose—page 1297.

Cellulose Acetate Phthalate

Cellulose, acetate, 1,2-benzenedicarboxylate

Cellulose acetate phthalate [9004-38-0]; a reaction product of the phthalic anhydride and a partial acetate ester of cellulose. When dried at 105° for 2 hours, it contains 19–23.5% of acetyl (C₂H₃O) groups and 30–36.0% of phthalyl (*o*-carboxybenzoyl, C₈H₅O₃) groups.

Preparation—Cellulose is esterified by treatment with acetic and phthalic acid anhydrides.

Description—Free-flowing, white powder; may have a slight odor of acetic acid.

Solubility—Insoluble in water and alcohol; soluble in acetone and dioxane.

Uses—An *enteric tablet coating material*. Coatings of this substance disintegrate due to the hydrolytic effect of the intestinal esterases, even when the intestinal contents are acid. *In vitro* studies indicate that cellulose acetate phthalate will withstand the action of artificial gastric juices for long periods of time, but will readily disintegrate in artificial intestinal juices.

Cherry Juice

The liquid expressed from the fresh ripe fruit of *Prunus cerasus* Linné (Fam *Rosaceae);* contains not less than 1% of malic acid [$C_4H_6O_5$ = 134.09].

Preparation—Coarsely crush washed, stemmed, unpitted, sour cherries in a grinder so as to break the pits but not mash the kernels. Dissolve 0.1% of benzoic acid in the mixture, and allow it to stand at room temperature (possibly for several days) until a small portion of the filtered juice remains clear when mixed with one-half of its volume of alcohol and the resulting solution does not become cloudy within 30 min.   Then press the juice from the mixture, and filter it.

Description—Clear liquid with an aromatic, characteristic odor, and a sour taste; affected by light; the color of the freshly prepared juice is red to reddish orange; pH between 3 and 4; specific gravity between 1.045 and 1.075.

Uses—To prepare *Cherry Syrup* (page 1293).

Carbon Tetrachloride

Methane, tetrachloro-, Tetrachloromethane

Carbon tetrachloride [56-23-5] CCl_4 (153.82).
Preparation—One method consists of catalytic chlorination of carbon disulfide.

Description—Clear, colorless liquid having a characteristic odor resembling that of chloroform; specific gravity between 1.588 and 1.590; boils at about 77°.
Solubility—Soluble in about 2000 volumes water; miscible with alcohol, acetone, ether, chloroform, and benzene.

Uses—Carbon tetrachloride is officially recognized as a *pharmaceutical necessity* (solvent).   Formerly used as a cheap *anthelmintic* for the treatment of *hookworm* infections but causes severe injury to the liver if absorbed.

Chloroform

Methane, trichloro-, Trichloromethane

Trichloromethane [67-66-3] $CHCl_3$ (119.38); contains 99–99.5% of $CHCl_3$, the remainder consisting of alcohol.
Caution—Care should be taken not to vaporize Chloroform in the presence of a flame, because of the production of harmful gases (hydrogen chloride and phosgene).
Preparation—Chloroform is made by the reduction of carbon tetrachloride with water and iron and by the controlled chlorination of methane.

Pure chloroform readily decomposes on keeping, particularly if exposed to moisture and sunlight, resulting in formation of phosgene (carbonyl chloride [$COCl_2$]) and other products.   The presence of a small amount of alcohol greatly retards or prevents this decomposition; hence the requirement that chloroform contain 0.5% to 1% of alcohol.   The alcohol combines with any phosgene forming ethyl carbonate which is nontoxic.

Description—Clear, colorless, mobile liquid of a characteristic, ethereal odor and a burning, sweet taste; not flammable but its heated vapors burn with a green flame; affected by light and moisture; specific gravity between 1.474 and 1.478, indicating 99–99.5% of $CHCl_3$; boils at about 61°; not affected by acids, but is decomposed by alkali hydroxide into alkali chloride and sodium formate.
Solubility—Soluble in 210 volumes of water; miscible with alcohol, ether, benzene, solvent hexane, acetone, and with fixed and volatile oils.

Uses—An obsolete *inhalation anesthetic.*   Although it possesses advantages of nonflammability and great potency, it is rarely used due to the serious toxic effects it produces on the heart and liver. Internally it has been used, in small doses, as a *carminative.*   Externally it is an *irritant* and when used in liniments it may produce blisters.

Chloroform is categorized as a pharmaceutic aid.   It is used as a *preservative* during the aqueous percolation of vegetable drugs to prevent bacterial decomposition in the process of manufacture.   In most instances it is evaporated before the product is finished.

Chloroform is an excellent solvent for alkaloids and many other organic chemicals, and is used in the manufacture of these products and in chemical analyses.

Citric Acid

1,2,3-Propanetricarboxylic acid, 2-hydroxy-

$$CH_2COOH$$
$$|$$
$$HOCCOOH$$
$$|$$
$$CH_2COOH$$

Citric acid [77-92-9] $C_6H_8O_7$ (192.12); *monohydrate* [5949-29-1] (210.14).

Preparation—Citric acid is found in many plants.   It was formerly solely obtained from the juice of limes and lemons and from pineapple wastes.   Since about 1925 the acid has been largely produced by fermentation of sucrose solution, including molasses, by fungi belonging to the *Aspergillus niger* group, theoretically according to the following reaction:

$$C_{12}H_{22}O_{11} + 3O_2 \rightarrow 2H_3C_6H_5O_7 + 3H_2O$$

| Sucrose | Oxygen | Citric Acid | Water |

but in practice there are deviations from this stoichiometric relationship.

Description—Colorless, translucent crystals, or a white, granular to fine crystalline powder; odorless and has a strongly acid taste; the hydrous form effloresces in moderately dry air, but is slightly deliquescent in moist air; loses its water of crystallization at about 50°; dilute aqueous solutions are subject to molding (fermentation), oxalic acid being one of the fermentation products.
Solubility—1 g in 0.5 mL water, 2 mL alcohol, and about 30 mL ether; freely soluble in methanol.

Uses—In the preparation of *Anticoagulant Citrate Dextrose Solution, Anticoagulant Citrate Phosphate Dextrose Solution, Citric Acid Syrup,* and *effervescent salts.*   It has also been used to dissolve urinary bladder calculi, and as a mild astringent.

Cocoa Butter

Cacao Butter; Theobroma Oil; Oil of Theobroma

The fat obtained from the roasted seed of *Theobroma cacao* Linné (Fam *Sterculiaceae*).
Preparation—By grinding the kernels of the "chocolate bean" and expressing the oil in powerful, horizontal hydraulic presses.   The yield is about 40%.   It has also been prepared by dissolving the oil from the unroasted beans by the use of a volatile solvent.
Constituents—Chemically it is a mixture of stearin, palmitin, olein, laurin, linolein, and traces of other glycerides.

Description—Yellowish, white solid with a faint, agreeable odor and a bland (if obtained by extraction) or chocolate-like (if obtained by pressing) taste; usually brittle below 25°; specific gravity between 0.858 and 0.864 at 100°/25°; refractive index between 1.454 and 1.458 at 40°.

Solubility—Slightly soluble in alcohol; soluble in boiling dehydrated alcohol; freely soluble in ether and chloroform.

Uses—By virtue of its low fusing point and its property of becoming solid at a temperature just below the melting point, theobroma oil is valuable in pharmacy for making suppositories.   See *Suppositories* (page 1580).   In addition to this use, cocoa butter is an excellent emollient application to the skin when inflamed; it also is used in various skin creams, especially the so-called "*skin foods.*"   It is also used in massage.

Titanium Dioxide—page 790.

Denatonium Benzoate

Benzenemethanaminium *N*-[2-[(2,6-dimethylphenyl)amino]-2-oxoethyl]-*N,N*-diethyl-, benzoate;

Benzyldiethyl [(2,6-xylylcarbamoyl)methyl]ammonium benzoate [3734-33-6] $C_{28}H_{34}N_2O_3$ (446.59).

Preparation—2-(Diethylamino)-2',6'-xylidide is quaternized by reaction with benzyl chloride. The quaternary chloride is then treated with methanolic potassium hydroxide to form the quaternary base which, after filtering off the KCl, is reacted with benzoic acid. The starting xylidide may be prepared by condensing 2,6-xylidine with chloroacetyl chloride and condensing the resulting chloroacetoxylidide with diethylamine. US Pat 3,080,327.

Description—White, odorless, crystalline powder; an intensely bitter taste; melts between 166° and 170°.

Solubility—1 g in 20 mL water, 2.4 mL alcohol, 2.9 mL chloroform, 5000 mL ether.

Uses—A *denaturant* for ethyl alcohol.

Dextrin

British Gum; Starch Gum; Leiocom

Dextrin [9004-53-9] $(C_6H_{10}O_5)_n$.

Preparation—By the incomplete hydrolysis of starch with dilute acid, or by heating dry starch.

Description—White or yellow, amorphous powder (*white:* practically odorless; *yellow:* characteristic odor); dextrorotatory; $[\alpha]_D^{20}$ generally above 200°; does not reduce Fehling's solution; gives a reddish color with iodine.

Solubility—Soluble in 3 parts boiling water, forming a gummy solution; less soluble in cold water.

Uses—An *excipient* and *emulsifier*.

Dextrose

Anhydrous Dextrose; Dextrose Monohydrate; Glucose; D(+)-Glucose; α-D(+)-Glucopyranose; Medicinal Glucose; Purified Glucose; Grape Sugar; Bread Sugar; Cerelose; Starch Sugar; Corn Sugar

D-Glucose monohydrate [5996-10-1] $C_6H_{12}O_6.H_2O$ (198.17); *anhydrous* [50-99-7] (180.16). A sugar usually obtained by the hydrolysis of starch. For the structure, see page 399.

Preparation—See *Liquid Glucose* (page 1313).

Description—Colorless crystals or a white, crystalline or granular powder; odorless, and has a sweet taste; specific rotation (anhydrous) +52.5° to +53°; anhydrous dextrose melts at 146°; dextrose slowly reduces alkaline cupric tartrate TS in the cold and rapidly on heating, producing a red precipitate of cuprous oxide (difference from *sucrose*).

Solubility—1 g in 1 mL water, 100 mL alcohol; more soluble in boiling water and boiling alcohol.

Uses—See *Dextrose Injection* (page 822). It is also used, instead of lactose, as a supplement to milk for infant feeding.

Dichlorodifluoromethane

Methane, dichlorodifluoro-,

CCl_2F_2

Dichlorodifluoromethane [75-71-8] CCl_2F_2 (120.91).

Preparation—Carbon tetrachloride is reacted with antimony trifluoride in the presence of antimony pentafluoride.

Description—Clear, colorless gas having a faint, ethereal odor; vapor pressure at 25° about 4883 mm of mercury.

Uses—A *propellant* (No 12, see page 1664) in aerosols.

Dichlorotetrafluoroethane

Ethane, 1,2-dichloro-1,1,2,2-tetrafluoro-,

$CClF_2CClF_2$

1,2-Dichlorotetrafluoroethane [76-14-2] $C_2Cl_2F_4$ (170.92).

Preparation—By reacting 1,1,2-trichloro-1,2,2-trifluoroethane with antimony trifluorodichloride [SbF_3Cl_2] whereupon one of the 1-chlorine atoms is replaced by fluorine. The starting trichlorofluoroethane may be prepared from hexachloroethane by treatment with SbF_3Cl_2 (Henne AL: *Org Reactions II:* 65, 1944).

Description—Clear, colorless gas having a faint, ethereal odor; vapor pressure at 25° about 1620 mm of mercury; usually contains 6–10% of its isomer, $CFCl_2$—CF_3.

Uses—A *propellant* (No 114 and 114a, see page 1662) in aerosols.

Edetic Acid

Glycine, N,N'-1,2-ethanediylbis[N-(carboxymethyl)-,

$(HOOCCH_2)_2NCH_2CH_2N(CH_2COOH)_2$

(Ethylenedinitrilo)tetraacetic acid [60-00-4] $C_{10}H_{16}N_2O_8$ (292.24).

Preparation—Ethylenediamine is condensed with sodium monochloroacetate with the aid of sodium carbonate. An aqueous solution of the reactants is heated to about 90° for 10 hours, then cooled and acidified with HCl whereupon the acid precipitates. US Pat 2,130,505.

Description—White, crystalline powder; melts with decomposition above 220°.

Solubility—Very slightly soluble in water; soluble in solutions of alkali hydroxides.

Uses—A *pharmaceutic aid* (metal complexing agent). The acid, rather than any salt, is the form most potent in removing calcium from solution. It may be added to shed blood to prevent clotting. It is also used in pharmaceutical analysis and the removal or inactivation of unwanted ions in solution. Salts of the acid are known as edetates. See *Edetate Calcium Disodium* (page 1225) and *Edetate Disodium* (page 1225).

Ethylcellulose

Cellulose ethyl ether [9004-57-3]; an ethyl ether of cellulose containing 44–51% of ethoxy groups. The *medium-type* viscosity grade contains less than 46.5% ethoxy groups; the *standard-type* viscosity grade contains 46.5% or more ethoxy groups.

Preparation—By the same general procedure described on page 1297 for *Methylcellulose* except that ethyl chloride or ethyl sulfate is employed as the alkylating agent. The 45 to 50% of ethoxy groups in the official ethylcellulose corresponds to from 2.25 to 2.61 ethoxy groups/$C_6H_{10}O_5$ unit, thus representing from 75 to 87% of the maximum theoretical ethoxylation, which is 3 ethoxy groups/$C_6H_{10}O_5$ unit.

Description—Free-flowing, white to light tan powder; forms films that have a refractive index of about 1.47; aqueous suspensions are neutral to litmus.

Solubility—The medium-type is freely soluble in tetrahydrofuran, methyl acetate, chloroform, and mixtures of aromatic hydrocarbons with alcohol; the standard-type is freely soluble in alcohol, methanol, toluene, chloroform, and ethyl acetate; both types are insoluble in water, glycerin, and propylene glycol.

Uses—A *pharmaceutic aid* as a tablet binder and for film-coating tablets and drug particles.

Gelatin—page 1297.

Liquid Glucose

Glucose; Starch Syrup; Corn Syrup

A product obtained by the incomplete hydrolysis of starch. It consists chiefly of dextrose [D(+) glucose, $C_6H_{12}O_6$ = 180.16] dextrins, maltose, and water.

Preparation—Commercially by the action of very weak H_2SO_4 or HCl on starch.

One of the processes for the manufacture of glucose is as follows: The starch, usually from corn, is mixed with 5 times its weight of water containing less than 1% of HCl, the mixture is heated to about 45°, and then transferred to a suitable reaction vessel into which steam is passed under pressure until the temperature reaches 120°. The temperature is maintained at this point for about an hour, or until tests show complete disappearance of starch. The mass is then heated to volatilize most of the hydrochloric acid, sodium carbonate or calcium carbonate is added to neutralize the remaining traces of acid, the liquid is filtered, then decolorized in charcoal or bone-black filters, as is done in sugar refining, and finally concentrated in vacuum to the desired consistency.

Liquid glucose, when made by the above process, contains about 30 to 40% of dextrose mixed with about an equal proportion of dextrin, together with small amounts of other carbohydrates, notably maltose. By varying the conditions of hydrolysis, the relative proportions of the sugars also vary.

If the crystallizable dextrose is desired, the conversion temperature is higher and the time of conversion longer. The term "glucose" as customarily used in the chemical or pharmaceutical literature usually refers to dextrose, the crystallizable product.

The name "grape sugar" is sometimes applied to the solid commercial form of dextrose because the principal sugar of the grape is dextrose, although the fruit has never been used as a source of the commercial supply.

Description—Colorless or yellowish, thick, syrupy liquid; odorless, or nearly so, and has a sweet taste; differs from sucrose in that it readily reduces hot alkaline cupric tartrate TS producing a red precipitate of cuprous oxide.

Solubility—Miscible with water; sparingly soluble in alcohol.

Uses—As an ingredient of *Cocoa Syrup* (page 1293), as a tablet binder and coating agent, and as a diluent in pilular extracts; it has replaced glycerin in many pharmaceutical preparations. It is sometimes given *per rectum* as a *food* in cases where feeding by stomach is impossible. It should not be used in the place of dextrose for intravenous injection.

Hydrochloric Acid

Chlorhydric Acid; Muriatic Acid; Spirit of Salt

Hydrochloric acid [7647-01-0] HCl (36.46); contains 36.5–38.0%, by weight, of HCl.

Preparation—By the interaction of NaCl and H_2SO_4 or by combining chlorine with hydrogen. It is obtained as a by-product in the manufacture of sodium carbonate from NaCl by the Leblanc process in which common salt is decomposed with H_2SO_4. HCl is also a by-product in the electrolytic production of NaOH from NaCl.

Description—Colorless, fuming liquid having a pungent odor; fumes and odor disappear when it is diluted with 2 volumes of water; strongly acid to litmus even when highly diluted; specific gravity about 1.18.

Solubility—Miscible with water or alcohol.

Uses—Officially classified as a pharmaceutic aid that is used as an acidifying agent. It is used in preparing *Diluted Hydrochloric Acid* (page 799).

Hypophosphorous Acid

Phosphinic acid

Hypophosphorous acid [6303-21-5] HPH_2O_2 (66.00); contains 30–32% by weight, of H_3PO_2.

Preparation—By reacting barium or calcium hypophosphite with sulfuric acid or by treating sodium hypophosphite with an ion-exchange resin.

Description—Colorless or slightly yellow, odorless liquid; solution is acid to litmus even when highly diluted; specific gravity about 1.13.

Solubility—Miscible with water or alcohol.

Incompatibilities—Oxidized on exposure to air and by nearly all *oxidizing agents. Mercury, silver,* and *bismuth salts* are reduced partially to the metallic state as evidenced by a darkening in color. *Ferric compounds* are changed to ferrous.

Uses—An *antioxidant* in pharmaceutical preparations.

Isopropyl Myristate

Tetradecanoic acid, 1-methylethyl ester

$$CH_3(CH_2)_{12}COOCH(CH_3)_2$$

Isopropyl myristate [110-27-0] $C_{17}H_{34}O_2$ (270.45).

Preparation—By reacting myristoyl chloride with 2-propanol with the aid of a suitable dehydrochlorinating agent.

Description—Liquid of low viscosity that is practically colorless and odorless; congeals at about 5° and decomposes at 208°; withstands oxidation and does not readily become rancid.

Solubility—Soluble in alcohol, acetone, chloroform, ethyl acetate, toluene, mineral oil, castor oil, and cottonseed oil; practically insoluble in water, glycerin, and propylene glycol; dissolves many waxes, cholesterol, and lanolin.

Uses—*Pharmaceutic aid* used in cosmetics and topical medicinal preparations as an emollient, lubricant, and to enhance absorption through the skin.

Kaolin—see page 811.

Lactic Acid

Propanoic acid, 2-hydroxy-, 2-Hydroxypropionic Acid; Propanoloic Acid; Milk Acid

$$CH_3CH(OH)COOH$$

Lactic acid [50-21-5] $C_3H_6O_3$ (90.08); a mixture of lactic acid and lactic acid lactate ($C_6H_{10}O_5$) equivalent to a total of 85–90%, by weight, of $C_3H_6O_3$.

Discovered by Scheele in 1780, it is the acid formed in the souring of milk, hence the name *lactic*, from the Latin name for milk. It results from the decomposition of the lactose (milk sugar) in milk.

Preparation—A solution of glucose or of starch previously hydrolyzed with diluted sulfuric acid is inoculated, after the addition of suitable nitrogen compounds and mineral salts, with *Bacillus lactis*. Calcium carbonate is added to neutralize the lactic acid as soon as it is formed, otherwise the fermentation stops when the amount of acid exceeds 0.5%. When fermentation is complete, as indicated by failure of the liquid to give a test for glucose, the solution is filtered, concentrated and allowed to stand. The calcium lactate that crystallizes is decomposed with dilute sulfuric acid and filtered with charcoal. The lactic acid in the filtrate is extracted with ethyl or isopropyl ether, the ether is distilled off and the aqueous solution of the acid concentrated under reduced pressure.

Description—Colorless or yellowish, nearly odorless, syrupy liquid; acid to litmus; absorbs water on exposure to moist air; when a dilute solution is concentrated to above 50%, lactic acid lactate begins to form; in the official acid the latter amounts to about 12 to 15%; specific gravity about 1.20; decomposes when distilled under normal pressure but may be distilled without decomposition under reduced pressure.

Solubility—Miscible with water, alcohol, and ether; insoluble in chloroform.

Uses—Lactic acid is used in the preparation of *Sodium Lactate Injection* (page 835). It is also used in babies' milk formulas, as an acidulant in food preparations, and in 1–2% concentration in some spermatocidal jellies. A 10% solution is used as a bactericidal agent on the skin of neonates. It is corrosive to tissues on prolonged contact. A 16.7% solution in flexible collodion is used to remove warts and small cutaneous tumors.

Lactose

D-Glucose, 4-*O*-β-D-galactopyranosyl-, Milk Sugar

Lactose [63-42-3] $C_{12}H_{22}O_{11}$ (342.30); *monohydrate* [10039-26-6] (360.31); a sugar obtained from milk.

For the structural formula, see page 399.

Preparation—From skim milk, to which is added diluted HCl to precipitate the casein. After removal of the casein by filtration, the reaction of the whey is adjusted to a pH of about 6.2 by addition of lime and the remaining albuminous matter is coagulated by heating; this is filtered out and the liquid set aside to crystallize. Animal charcoal is used to decolorize the solution in a manner similar to that used in purifying sucrose.

Another form of lactose, known as β-lactose, is also available on the market. It differs in that the D-glucose moiety is β instead of α. It is reported that this variety is sweeter and more soluble than ordinary lactose and for that reason is preferable in pharmaceutical manufacturing where lactose is used. Chemically, β-lactose does not appear to differ from ordinary α-lactose. It is manufactured in the same way as α-lactose up to the point of crystallization, then the solution is heated to a temperature above 93.5°, this being the temperature at which the *alpha* form is converted to the *beta* variety. The *beta* form occurs only as an anhydrous sugar whereas the *alpha* variety may be obtained either in the anhydrous form or as a monohydrate.

Description—White or creamy white, hard, crystalline masses or powder; odorless, and has a faintly sweet taste; stable in air, but readily absorbs odors; pH (1 in 10 solution) between 4.0 and 6.5; specific rotation between +54.8° and +55.5°.

Solubility—1 g in 5 mL water and 2.6 mL boiling water; very slightly soluble in alcohol; insoluble in chloroform or ether.

Uses—A *diluent* largely used in medicine and pharmacy. Lactose is generally an ingredient of the medium used in penicillin production. It is extensively used as an addition to milk for infant feeding.

Magnesium Chloride

Magnesium chloride hexahydrate [7791-18-6] $MgCl_2.6H_2O$ (203.30); *anhydrous* [7786-30-3] (95.21).

Preparation—By treating magnesite or other suitable magnesium minerals with HCl.

Description—Colorless, odorless, deliquescent flakes or crystals, which lose water when heated to 100° and lose hydrochloric acid when heated to 110°; pH (1 in 20 solution in carbon dioxide-free water) between 4.5 and 7.

Solubility—Very soluble in water; freely soluble in alcohol.

Uses—*Electrolyte replenisher; pharmaceutic necessity* for hemodialysis and peritoneal dialysis fluids.

Magnesium Stearate

Octadecanoic acid, magnesium salt

Magnesium stearate [557-04-0]. A compound of magnesium with a mixture of solid organic acids obtained from fats, and consists chiefly of variable proportions of magnesium stearate and magnesium palmitate. It contains the equivalent of 6.8–8.0% of MgO (40.30).

Description—Fine, white, bulky powder, having a faint, characteristic odor. Is unctuous, adheres readily to the skin, and is free from grittiness.

Solubility—Insoluble in water, alcohol, and ether.

Uses—A *pharmaceutical necessity* (*lubricant*) in the manufacture of compressed tablets.

Meglumine

D-Glucitol, 1-deoxy-1-(methylamino)-,

$$HOCH_2-\overset{\overset{\displaystyle H}{|}}{C}-\overset{\overset{\displaystyle H}{|}}{C}-\overset{\overset{\displaystyle OH}{|}}{C}-\overset{\overset{\displaystyle H}{|}}{C}-CH_2NHCH_3$$

1-Deoxy-1-(methylamino)-D-glucitol [6284-40-8] $C_7H_{17}NO_5$ (195.21).

Preparation—By treating glucose with hydrogen and methylamine under pressure and in the presence of Raney nickel.

Description—White to faintly yellowish white, odorless crystals or powder; melts between 128° to 132°.

Solubility—Freely soluble in water; sparingly soluble in alcohol.

Uses—In forming salts of certain pharmaceuticals, surface-active agents, and dyes. See *Diatrizoate Meglumine Injection* (page 1268), *Iodipamide Meglumine Injection* (page 1265), and *Iothalamate Meglumine Injection* (page 1269).

Light Mineral Oil

Light Liquid Petrolatum NF XII; Light Liquid Paraffin; Light White Mineral Oil

A mixture of liquid hydrocarbons obtained from petroleum. It may contain a suitable stabilizer.

Description—Colorless, transparent, oily liquid, free, or nearly free, from fluorescence; odorless and tasteless when cold, and develops not more than a faint odor of petroleum when heated; specific gravity between 0.818 and 0.880; kinematic viscosity not more than 33.5 centistokes at 40°.

Solubility—Insoluble in water and alcohol; miscible with most fixed oils, but not with castor oil; soluble in volatile oils.

Uses—Officially recognized as a *vehicle*. Once it was widely used as a vehicle for nose and throat medications; such uses are now considered dangerous because of the possibility of lipoid pneumonia. It

is sometimes used to cleanse dry and inflamed skin areas and to facilitate removal of dermatologic preparations from the skin. It should never be used for internal administration because of "leakage." See *Mineral Oil* (page 805).

Nitric Acid

Nitric acid [7697-37-2] HNO_3 (63.01); contains about 70%, by weight, of HNO_3.

Preparation—May be prepared by treatment of sodium nitrate (Chile saltpeter) with sulfuric acid, but usually produced by catalytic oxidation of ammonia.

Description—Highly corrosive fuming liquid having a characteristic, highly irritating odor; stains animal tissues yellow; boils at about 120°; specific gravity about 1.41.

Solubility—Miscible with water.

Uses—*Pharmaceutic aid* (acidifying agent).

Nitrogen

Nitrogen [7727-37-9] N_2 (28.01); contains not less than 99%, by volume, of N_2.

Preparation—By the fractional distillation of liquified air.

Uses—A diluent for medicinal gases. Pharmaceutically it is employed to replace air in the containers of substances which would be adversely affected by air oxidation. Examples include its use with fixed oils, certain vitamin preparations, and a variety of injectable products. It is also used as a propellant.

Persic Oil

Apricot Kernel Oil; Peach Kernel Oil

The oil expressed from the kernels of varieties of *Prunus armeniaca* Linné (Apricot Kernel Oil), or from the kernels of varieties of *Prunus persica* Sieb et Zucc (Peach Kernel Oil) (Fam *Rosaceae*).

Description—Clear, pale straw-colored or colorless, almost odorless, oily liquid with a bland taste; specific gravity between 0.910 and 0.923; not turbid at temperatures above 15°.

Solubility—Slightly soluble in alcohol; miscible with ether, chloroform, benzene, and solvent hexane.

Uses—A *vehicle*. It is also used in preparing cold creams.

Phenol

Carbolic Acid

C_6H_5OH

Phenol [108-95-2] C_6H_6O (94.11).

Preparation—For many years made only by distilling crude carbolic acid from coal tar and separating and purifying the distillate by repeated crystallizations, it is now prepared synthetically.

A more recent process utilizes chlorobenzene as the starting point in the manufacture of phenol. The chlorobenzene is produced in a vapor phase reaction, with benzene, HCl, and oxygen over a copper catalyst, followed by hydrolysis with steam to yield phenol and HCl (which is recovered).

Description—Colorless to light pink, interlaced, or separate, needleshaped crystals, or a white or light pink, crystalline mass; characteristic odor; when undiluted, it whitens and cauterizes the skin and mucous membranes; when gently heated, phenol melts, forming a highly refractive liquid; liquefied by the addition of 10% of water; vapor is flammable; gradually darkens on exposure to light and air; specific gravity 1.07; boils at 182°; congeals at a temperature not lower than 39°.

Solubility—1 g in 15 mL water; very soluble in alcohol, glycerin, chloroform, ether, and fixed and volatile oils; sparingly soluble in mineral oil.

Incompatibilities—Phenol produces a liquid or soft mass when triturated with *camphor*, *menthol*, *acetanilid*, *acetophenetidin*, *aminopyrine*, *antipyrine*, *ethyl aminobenzoate*, *methenamine*, *phenyl salicylate*, *resorcinol*, *terpin hydrate*, *thymol*, and several other substances including some *alkaloids*. It also softens *cocoa butter* in suppository mixtures.

Phenol is soluble in about 15 parts of water; stronger solutions may be obtained by using as much glycerin as phenol. Only the crystallized phenol is soluble in fixed oils and liquid petrolum, the liquefied phenol is not all soluble due to its content of water. *Albumin* and *gelatin* are precipitated by phenol. *Collodion* is coagulated by the precipitation of pyroxylin. Traces of *iron* in various chemicals such as *alum*, *borax*, etc, may produce a green color.

Uses—A *caustic*, *disinfectant*, *topical anesthetic*, and pharmaceutical necessity as a *preservative* for injections, etc. At one time widely used as a germicide and still the standard against which other antiseptics are compared, it has few legitimate uses in modern medicine. Nevertheless, it is still used in several proprietary antiseptic mouthwashes, hemorrhoidal preparations, and burn remedies. In full strength, a few drops of liquefied phenol may be used to cauterize small wounds, dogs bites, snake bites, etc. Phenol is commonly employed as an *antipruritic*, either in the form of phenolated calamine lotion (1%), phenol ointment (2%), or a simple aqueous solution (0.5 to 1%). Phenol has been used for sclerosing hemorrhoids, but more effective and safer drugs are available. A 5% solution in glycerin is used in simple earache. Crude carbolic acid is an effective, economical agent for disinfecting excrement. Phenol is of some therapeutic value as a *fungicide*, but more effective and less toxic agents are available. If accidentally spilled, phenol should be removed promptly from the skin by swabbing with alcohol.

Liquefied Phenol [Liquefied Carbolic Acid] is phenol maintained in a liquid condition by the presence of 10.0% of water. It contains not less than 89.0%, by weight, of C_6H_6O. *Note—When phenol is to be mixed with a fixed oil, mineral oil, or white petrolatum, use crystalline Phenol, not Liquefied Phenol. Preparation:* Melt phenol (a convenient quantity) by placing the unstoppered container in a steam bath and applying heat gradually. Transfer the liquid to a tared vessel, weigh, add 1 g of purified water for each 9 g of phenol, and mix thoroughly. *Description:* Colorless liquid, which may develop a red tint upon exposure to air and light; characteristic, somewhat aromatic odor; when undiluted it cauterizes and whitens the skin and mucous membranes; specific gravity about 1.065; when it is subjected to distillation, the boiling temperature does not rise above 182°, which is the boiling temperature of phenol; partially solidifies at about 15°. *Solubility:* Miscible with alcohol, ether, and glycerin; a mixture of liquefied phenol and an equal volume of glycerin is miscible with water. *Uses:* A formulation which facilitates the dispensing of concentrated phenol. Its therapeutic uses are described above under *Phenol.* It is a *pharmaceutic necessity for Phenolated Calamine Lotion* (page 778).

Phenyl Salicylate—RPS-15, page 1269.

Phosphoric Acid

Orthophosphoric Acid; Syrupy Phosphoric Acid;
Concentrated Phosphoric Acid

Phosphoric acid [7664-38-2] H_3PO_4 (98.00); contains 85–88%, by weight, of H_3PO_4.
Preparation—Phosphorus is converted to phosphorus pentoxide [P_2O_5] by exposing it to a current of warm air, then the P_2O_5 is treated with water to form phosphoric acid. The conversion of the phosphorus to the pentoxide takes place while the phosphorus, distilling from the phosphorus manufacturing operation, is in the vapor state.

Description—Colorless, odorless liquid of a syrupy consistency; specific gravity about 1.71.
Solubility—Miscible with water or alcohol, with the evolution of heat.

Uses—To make the diluted acid and as a weak acid in various pharmaceutical preparations. Industrially it is used in dental cements and in beverages as an acidulant.

Diluted Phosphoric Acid [Dilute Phosphoric Acid] contains, in each 100 mL, 9.5–10.5 g of H_3PO_4 (98.00). *Preparation:* Mix phosphoric acid (69 mL) and purified water (qs) to make 1000 mL. *Description:* Clear, colorless, odorless liquid; specific gravity about 1.057. Miscible with water and alcohol. *Uses:* A *pharmaceutical necessity.* It has also been employed in *lead poisoning* and in other conditions in which it is desired to administer large amounts of phosphate and at the same time produce a mild acidosis. It has been given in the dose of 60 mL daily (5 mL/hour) under carefully controlled conditions.

Potassium Metaphosphate

Metaphosphoric acid (HPO_3), potassium salt

Potassium metaphosphate [7790-53-6] KPO_3 (118.07); a straight-chain polyphosphate, having a high degree of polymerization; contains the equivalent of 59–61% of P_2O_5.

Preparation—By thermal dehydration of monopotassium phosphate (KH_2PO_4).

Description—White, odorless powder.
Solubility—Insoluble in water; soluble in dilute solutions of sodium salts.

Uses—*Pharmaceutic aid* (buffering agent).

Monobasic Potassium Phosphate

Phosphoric acid, monopotassium salt; Potassium Biphosphate; Potassium
Acid Phosphate; Potassium Dihydrogen Phosphate;
Sørensen's Potassium Phosphate

Monopotassium phosphate [7778-77-0] KH_2PO_4 (136.09).
Preparation—H_3PO_4 is reacted with an equimolar quantity of KOH and the solution is evaporated to crystallization.

Description—Colorless crystals or a white, granular or crystalline powder; odorless and stable in air; pH (1 in 100 solution) about 4.5.
Solubility— Freely soluble in water; practically insoluble in alcohol.

Uses—A component of various buffer solutions. Medicinally it has been used as a urinary acidifier.

Pumice

Pumex

A substance of volcanic origin, consisting chiefly of complex silicates of aluminum, potassium, and sodium.

Description—Very light, hard rough, porous, grayish masses or a gritty, grayish powder of several grades of fineness; odorless, tasteless, and stable in the air.
Three powders are available:
Pumice Flour or *Superfine Pumice*—Not less than 97% passes through a No 200 standard mesh sieve.
Fine Pumice—Not less than 95% passes through a No 150 standard mesh sieve, and not more than 75% passes through a No 200 standard mesh sieve.
Coarse Pumice—Not less than 95% passes through a No 60 standard mesh sieve, and not more than 5% passes through a No 200 standard mesh sieve.
Solubility—Insoluble in water and is not attacked by acids or alkali hydroxide solutions.

Uses—A *filtering* and *distributing medium* for pharmaceutical preparations. Because of its grittiness, powdered pumice is used in certain types of soaps and cleaning powders and also as a *dental abrasive*.

Pyroxylin

Cellulose, nitrate; Soluble Guncotton

Pyroxylin [9004-70-0]; a product obtained by the action of a mixture of nitric and sulfuric acids on cotton, and consists chiefly of cellulose tetranitrate [$(C_{12}H_{16}N_4O_{18})_n$].
Note—Pyroxylin available commercially is moistened with about 30% of alcohol or other suitable solvent. The alcohol or solvent must be allowed to evaporate from the Pyroxylin to yield the dried substance described in the Pharmacopeia.
Preparation—Shönbein, in 1846, found that nitric acid acts on cotton and produces a soluble compound. It was subsequently proved that this substance, pyroxylin, or guncotton, belongs to a series of closely related nitrates in which the nitric acid radical replaces the hydroxyl of the cellulose formula. This is usually indicated by taking the double empirical formula for cellulose $C_{12}H_{20}O_{10}$ and indicating replacement of four of the OH groups thus:

$$C_{12}H_{20}O_{10} + 4HNO_3 \rightarrow C_{12}H_{16}O_6(NO_3)_4 + 4H_2O$$

Cellulose   Cellulose
                   Tetranitrate

The pyroxylin used in preparing collodion is a varying mixture of the di-, tri-, tetra-, and pentanitrates, but is mainly tetranitrate. The hexanitrate is the true explosive guncotton, and is insoluble in ether, alcohol, acetone, or water.

Description—Light yellow, matted mass of filaments, resembling raw cotton in appearance, but harsh to the touch; *it is exceedingly flammable* burning, when unconfined, very rapidly and with a luminous flame; when kept in well-closed bottles and exposed to light, it is decomposed with the evolution of nitrous vapors, leaving a carbonaceous residue.

Solubility—Insoluble in water; dissolves slowly but completely in 25 parts of a mixture of 3 volumes of ether and 1 volume of alcohol; soluble in acetone and glacial acetic acid, and is precipitated from these solutions by water.

Uses—A *pharmaceutic necessity* for *Collodion* (RPS-16, page 717).

Rosin

Resina; Colophony; Georgia Pine Rosin; Yellow Pine Rosin

A solid resin obtained from *Pinus palustris* Miller, and from other species of *Pinus* Linné (Fam *Pinaceae*).

Constituents—American rosin contains *sylvic acid* [$C_{20}H_{30}O_2$], α-, β-, and γ-*abietic acids* [$C_{20}H_{30}O_2$], γ-*pinic acid* (from which α- and β-pinic acids are gradually formed), and *resene*. Some authorities also include *pimaric acid* [$C_{30}H_{20}O_2$] as a constituent. French rosin is called *galipot*.

Description—Sharply angular, translucent, amber-colored fragments, frequently covered with a yellow dust; fracture brittle at ordinary temperatures, shiny and shallow-conchoidal; odor and taste are slightly terebinthinate; easily fusible and burns with a dense, yellowish smoke, specific gravity between 1.07 and 1.09.

Solubility—Insoluble in water; soluble in alcohol, ether, benzene, glacial acetic acid, chloroform, carbon disulfide, dilute solutions of sodium hydroxide and potassium hydroxide, and some volatile and fixed oils.

Uses—A pharmaceutical necessity for *Zinc-Eugenol Cement* (page 1319). Formerly, and to some extent still, used as a component of plasters, cerates, and ointments, to which it adds adhesive qualities.

Purified Siliceous Earth

Purified Kieselguhr; Purified Infusorial Earth; Diatomaceous Earth; Diatomite

A form of silica [SiO_2] [7631-86-9] consisting of the frustules and fragments of diatoms, purified by boiling with acid, washing, and calcining.

Occurrence and Preparation—Large deposits of this substance are found in Virginia, Maryland, Nevada, Oregon, and California, usually in the form of masses of rocks, hundreds of feet in thickness. Under the microscope it is seen to consist largely of the minute siliceous frustules of diatoms. It must be carefully purified in a manner similar to that directed for *Talc* (page 1319), and thoroughly calcined. The latter treatment destroys the bacteria which are present in large quantities in the native earth.

Description—Very fine, white, light gray, or pale buff mixture of amorphous powder and lesser amounts of crystalline polymorphs, including quartz and cristobalite. Is gritty, readily absorbs moisture, and retains about four times its weight of water without becoming fluid.

Solubility—Insoluble in water, acids, or in dilute solutions of alkali hydroxides.

Uses—Introduced into the USP as a distributing and *filtering medium* for aromatic waters; also suitable for filtration of elixirs. Like talc, it does not absorb active constituents.

Colloidal Silicon Dioxide

Silica [7631-86-9] SiO_2 (60.08); a submicroscopic fumed silica prepared by the vapor-phase hydrolysis of a silicon compound.

Description—Light, white, nongritty powder of extremely fine particle size (about 15 nm).

Solubility—Insoluble in water and acids (except hydrofluoric); dissolved by hot solutions of alkali hydroxides.

Uses—A *tablet diluent* and as a *suspending* and *thickening agent* in pharmaceutical preparations.

Soda Lime

A mixture of calcium hydroxide and sodium or potassium hydroxide or both.

It may contain an indicator that is inert toward anesthetic gases such as ether, cyclopropane, and nitrous oxide, and that changes color when the soda lime no longer can absorb carbon dioxide.

Description—White or grayish white granules; if an indicator is added, the soda lime may have a color; absorbs carbon dioxide and water on exposure to air.

Uses—Neither a therapeutic nor a pharmaceutical agent. It is a *reagent for the absorption of carbon dioxide* in anesthesia machines, in oxygen therapy, and in metabolic tests. Because of the importance of the proper quality of soda lime for these purposes it has been made official and standardized.

Sodium Carbonate

Carbonic acid, disodium salt, monohydrate; Monohydrated Sodium Carbonate USP XVII

Disodium carbonate monohydrate [5968-11-6] $Na_2CO_3.H_2O$ (124.00); *anhydrous* [497-19-8] (105.99).

Preparation—The initial process for the manufacture of sodium carbonate was devised by Leblanc, a French apothecary, in 1784, and consists of two steps: first, the conversion of common salt [NaCl] into sodium sulfate by heating it with sulfuric acid, and second, the decomposition of the sulfate by calcium carbonate (limestone) and charcoal (coal) at a high temperature to yield sodium carbonate and calcium sulfide. The carbonate is then leached out with water.

Sodium carbonate is currently prepared by the electrolysis of sodium chloride, whereby sodium and chlorine are produced, the former reacting with water to produce sodium hydroxide and this solution treated with carbon dioxide to produce sodium carbonate. The process is most extensively used in localities where electric power is very cheap.

The monohydrated form is made by crystallizing a concentrated solution of sodium carbonate at a temperature above 35° (95°F), and stirring the liquid so as to produce small crystals. It contains about 15% of water of crystallization.

Soda ash is a term designating a commercial quality of anhydrous sodium carbonate. Its annual production is very large, and it has a wide variety of applications, among which are the manufacture of glass, soap, and sodium salts; it is also used for washing fabrics.

Washing soda, or *sal soda* is sodium carbonate with 10 molecules of water. It is in the form of colorless crystals which rapidly effloresce in the air.

Description—Colorless crystals or a white, crystalline powder; stable in air under ordinary conditions; when exposed to dry air above 50° the salt effloresces, and at 100° becomes anhydrous; decomposed by weak acids forming the salt of the acid and liberating carbon dioxide; aqueous solution is alkaline to indicators (pH about 11.5).

Solubility—1 g in 3 mL water and 1.8 mL boiling water; insoluble in alcohol.

Incompatibilities—*Acids*, *acid salts*, and *acidic preparations* cause its decomposition. Most *metals* are precipitated as carbonates, hydroxides, or basic salts. *Alkaloids* are precipitated from solutions of their salts.

Uses—Occasionally used topically for dermatitides as a lotion; it has been used as a mouthwash and a vaginal douche. It is used in the preparation of the sodium salts of many acids. The USP recognizes it as a pharmaceutic aid used as an alkalizing agent.

Sodium Hydroxide

Caustic Soda, Soda Lye

Sodium hydroxide [1310-73-2] NaOH (40.00); includes not more than 3% of Na_2CO_3 (105.99).

Caution—Exercise great care in handling Sodium Hydroxide, as it rapidly destroys tissues.

Preparation—By treating sodium carbonate with milk of lime, or by the electrolysis of a solution of sodium chloride as explained under *Potassium Hydroxide* (page 783). It is now largely produced by the latter process. See also *Sodium Carbonate*, above.

Description—White, or nearly white, fused masses, small pellets, flakes, sticks, and other forms; hard and brittle and shows a crystalline fracture; exposed to the air, it rapidly absorbs carbon dioxide and moisture; melts at about 318°; specific gravity 2.13; when it is dissolved in water or alcohol, or when its solution is treated with an acid, much heat is generated; aqueous solutions, even when highly diluted, are strongly alkaline.

Solubility—1 g in 1 mL water; freely soluble in alcohol or glycerin.

Incompatibilities—Exposed to air, it absorbs *carbon dioxide* and is converted to sodium carbonate. With *fats* and *fatty acids*, it forms soluble soaps; with *resins* it forms insoluble soaps. See *Potassium Hydroxide* (page 783).

Uses—Too alkaline to be of medicinal value but is occasionally used in veterinary practice as a caustic. It is extensively used in pharmaceutical processes as an alkalizing agent and is generally preferred to potassium hydroxide because it is less deliquescent, and less expensive; in addition, less of it is required since about 40 parts of it are equivalent to 56 parts of KOH. It is a pharmaceutical necessity in the preparation of *Glycerin Suppositories* (page 802).

Sodium Stearate

Octadecanoic acid, sodium salt

Sodium stearate [822-16-2] $C_{18}H_{35}NaO_2$ (306.47) consists chiefly of sodium stearate and sodium palmitate [$C_{16}H_{31}NaO_2$ = 278.41).

Preparation—Stearic acid is reacted with an equimolar portion of NaOH.

Description—Fine, white powder, soapy to the touch; usually has a slight, tallow-like odor; affected by light; solutions are alkaline to phenolphthalein TS.

Solubility—Slowly soluble in cold water and cold alcohol; readily soluble in hot water and hot alcohol.

Uses—The USP includes sodium stearate as a pharmaceutic aid used as an emulsifying and stiffening agent. It is an ingredient of glycerin suppositories. In dermatologic practice it has been used topically in sycosis and other skin diseases.

Starch

Corn Starch; Wheat Starch; Potato Starch

Starch [9005-25-8]; consists of the granules separated from the mature grain of corn [*Zea mays* Linné (Fam *Gramineae*)] or of wheat [*Triticum aestivum* Linné (Fam *Gramineae*)], or from tubers of the potato [*Solanum tuberosum* Linné (Fam *Solanaceae*)].

Preparation—In making starch from corn, the germ is separated mechanically and the cells softened to permit escape of the starch granules. This is generally done by permitting it to become sour and decomposed, stopping the fermentation before the starch is affected. On the small scale, starch may be made from wheat flour by making a stiff ball of dough and kneading it while a small stream of water trickles upon it. The starch is carried off with the water, while the *gluten* remains as a soft, elastic mass; the latter may be purified and used for various purposes to which gluten is applicable. The quality of commercial starch largely depends on the purity of the water used in its manufacture. Starch may be made from potatoes by first grating them, and then washing the soft mass upon a sieve, which separates the cellular substances and permits the starch granules to be carried through. The starch must then be thoroughly washed by decantation, and the quality of this starch also depends largely on the purity of the water that is used in washing it.

Description—Irregular, angular, white masses or fine powder; odorless; slight, characteristic taste. *Corn starch:* Polygonal, rounded or spheroidal granules up to about 35 μm in diameter which usually have a circular or several-rayed central cleft. *Wheat starch:* Simple lenticular granules 20 to 50 μm in diameter and spherical granules 5 to 10 μm in diameter; striations faintly marked and concentric. *Potato starch:* Simple granules, irregularly ovoid or spherical, 30 to 100 μm in diameter, and subspherical granules 10 to 35 μm in diameter; striations well marked and concentric.

Solubility—Insoluble in cold water and in alcohol; when it is boiled with about 20 times its weight of hot water for a few minutes and then cooled a translucent, whitish jelly results; its aqueous suspension is neutral to litmus.

Uses—Has absorbent and demulcent properties. It is used as a dusting powder and in various dermatologic preparations; also as a pharmaceutic aid (filler, binder, and disintegrant). *Note—Starches obtained from different botanical sources may not have identical properties with respect to their use for specific pharmaceutical purposes, eg, as a tablet-disintegrating agent. Therefore, types of starch should not be interchanged unless performance equivalency has been ascertained.*

Under the title *Pregelatinized Starch* the NF recognizes starch that has been chemically or mechanically processed to rupture all or part of the granules in the presence of water, and subsequently dried. Some types of such starch may be modified to render them compressible and flowable.

Storax

Liquid Storax; Styrax; Sweet Gum; Prepared Storax

A balsam obtained from the trunk of *Liquidambar orientalis* Miller, known in commerce as Levant Storax, or of *Liquidambar styraciflua* Linné, known in commerce as American Storax (Fam *Hamamelidaceae*).

Constituents—The following occur in both varieties of storax: *styracin* (*cinnamyl cinnamate*), *styrol* (*phenylethylene*, C_8H_8), *α- and β-storesin* (the cinnamic acid ester of an alcohol called *storesinol*), *phenylpropyl cinnamate*, free *cinnamic acid*, and *vanillin*. In addition to these, Levant storax contains *ethyl cinnamate*, *benzyl cinnamate*, free *storesinol*, *isocinnamic acid*, *ethylvanillin*, *styrogenin*, and *styrocamphene*. This variety of storax yields from 0.5 to 1% of *volatile oil;* from this have been isolated *styrocamphene*, *vanillin*, the cinnamic acid esters of *ethyl*, *phenylpropyl*, *benzyl*, and *cinnamyl alcohols*, *naphthalene*, and *styrol*.

American storax contains, in addition to the aforementioned substances common to both varieties, *styaresin* (the cinnamic acid ester of the alcohol *styresinol*, an isomer of storesinol) and *styresinolic acid*. It yields up to 7% of a dextrorotatory volatile oil, the composition of which has not been completely investigated; styrol and traces of vanillin have been isolated from it.

Description—Semiliquid, grayish to grayish brown, sticky, opaque mass, depositing on standing a heavy dark brown layer (Levant storax); or a semisolid, sometimes a solid mass, softened by gently warming (American storax); transparent in thin layers, has a characteristic odor and taste, and is more dense than water.

Solubility—Insoluble in water, but soluble, usually incompletely, in an equal weight of warm alcohol; soluble in acetone, carbon disulfide, and ether, some insoluble residue usually remaining.

Uses—An *expectorant* but is used chiefly as a local remedy, especially in combination with benzoin; eg, it is an ingredient of *Compound Benzoin Tincture* (page 776). It may be used, like benzoin, to protect fatty substances from rancidity.

Sucrose Octaacetate

α-D-Glucopyranoside, 1,3,4,6-tetra-*O*-acetyl-β-D-fructofuranosyl-, tetraacetate

Sucrose octaacetate [126-14-7] $C_{28}H_{38}O_{19}$ (678.60).

Preparation—Sucrose is subjected to exhaustive acetylation by reaction with acetic anhydride in the presence of a suitable condensing agent such as pyridine.

Description—White, practically odorless powder having an intensely bitter taste; hygroscopic; melts not lower than 78°.

Solubility—1 g in 1100 mL water, 11 mL alcohol, 0.3 mL acetone, 0.6 mL benzene; very soluble in methanol and chloroform; soluble in ether.

Uses—A *denaturant* for alcohol.

Sulfurated Potash

Thiosulfuric acid, dipotassium salt, mixt. with potassium sulfide $(K_2(S_x))$; Liver of Sulfur

Dipotassium thiosulfate mixture with potassium sulfide (K_2S_x) [39365-88-3]; a mixture composed chiefly of potassium polysulfides and potassium thiosulfate. It contains not less than 12.8% of S (sulfur) in combination as sulfide.

Preparation—By thoroughly mixing 1 part of sublimed sulfur with 2 parts of potassium carbonate and gradually heating the mixture in a covered iron crucible until the mass ceases to swell and is completely melted. It is then poured on a stone or glass slab and, when cold, broken into pieces and preserved in tightly-closed bottles. When the heat is properly regulated during its production, the reaction is approximately represented by the equation:

$$3K_2CO_3 + 8S \rightarrow 2K_2S_3 + K_2S_2O_3 + 3CO_2$$

As this product rapidly deteriorates on exposure to moisture, oxygen, and carbon dioxide, it is important that it be recently prepared to produce satisfactory preparations.

Description—Irregular pieces, liver-brown when freshly prepared, changing to a greenish yellow; decomposes upon exposure to air; has an odor of hydrogen sulfide and a bitter, acrid, and alkaline taste; even weak acids cause the liberation of H_2S from sulfurated potash; a 1 in 10 solution is light brown in color and is alkaline to litmus.

Solubility—1 g in about 2 mL water, usually leaving a slight residue; alcohol dissolves only the sulfides.

Uses—Extensively in dermatologic practice, especially in the official *White Lotion* or *Lotio Alba* (page 779). The equation for the reaction of the potassium trisulfide in preparing the lotion is:

$$ZnSO_4 + K_2S_3 \rightarrow \underline{ZnS} + 2\underline{S} + K_2SO_4$$

The mixture of insoluble zinc sulfide and sulfur gives the lotion its creamy white appearance.

Talc

Talcum; Purified Talc; French Chalk; Soapstone; Steatite

A native, hydrous magnesium silicate, sometimes containing a small proportion of aluminum silicate.

Occurrence and Preparation—Native talc, called *soapstone* or *French chalk*, is found in various parts of the world. An excellent quality is obtained from deposits in North Carolina. Deposits of a high grade of talc, conforming to the USP requirements, are also found in Manchuria. Native talc is usually accompanied by variable amounts of mineral substances. These are separated from it by mechanical means, such as flotation or elutriation. The talc is then finely powdered, treated with boiling dilute HCl, washed well, and dried.

Description—Very fine, white, or grayish white crystalline powder; unctuous to the touch, adhering readily to the skin, and free from grittiness.

Uses—The USP recognizes talc as a dusting powder and pharmaceutic aid; in both categories it has many specific uses. Its medicinal use as a dusting powder depends on its desiccant and lubricant effects. When perfumed, and sometimes medicated, it is used extensively for toilet purposes under the name *talcum powder;* for such use it should be in the form of an impalpable powder. When used as a filtration medium for clarifying liquids a coarser powder is preferred to minimize passage through the pores of the filter paper; for this purpose it may be used for all classes of preparations with no danger of adsorption or retention of active principles. It is used as a lubricant in the manufacture of tablets, and as a dusting powder when making handmade suppositories. Although it is used as a lubricant for putting on and removing rubber gloves it should not be used on surgical gloves because even small amounts deposited in organs or healing wounds may cause granuloma formation.

Tartaric Acid

Butanedioic acid, 2,3-dihydroxy-, Butanedioic acid,
2,3-dihydroxy-, [R-(R*,R*)]

```
        COOH
         |
    H — C — OH
         |
   HO — C — H
         |
        COOH
```

L-(+)-Tartaric acid [87-69-4] $C_4H_6O_6$ (150.09).

Preparation—From *argol*, the crude cream of tartar (potassium bitartrate) deposited on the sides of wine casks during the fermentation of grapes, by conversion to calcium tartrate which is hydrolyzed to tartaric acid and calcium sulfate.

Description—Large, colorless or translucent crystals, or a white granular to fine crystalline powder; odorless, has an acid taste, is stable in the air, and its solutions are acid to litmus; dextrorotatory.

Solubility—1 g in 0.8 mL water, 0.5 mL boiling water, 3 mL alcohol, 250 mL ether; freely soluble in methanol.

Uses—Chiefly as the acid ingredient of preparations in which it is neutralized by a bicarbonate, as in effervescent salts, and the free acid is completely absent or present only in small amounts in the finished product. It is also used as a buffering agent.

Trichloromonofluoromethane

Methane, trichlorofluoro-,

$CFCl_3$

Trichlorofluoromethane [75-69-4] CCl_3F (137.37).

Preparation—Carbon tetrachloride is reacted with antimony trifluoride in the presence of a small quantity of antimony pentachloride. The reaction produces a mixture of CCl_3F and CCl_2F_2 which is readily separable by fractional distillation.

Description—Clear, colorless gas having a faint, ethereal odor; vapor pressure at 25° is about 796 mm of Hg; boils at approximately 24°.

Solubility—Practically insoluble in water; soluble in alcohol, ether, and other organic solvents.

Uses—A *propellant* (No 11, see page 1662) in aerosols.

Zinc-Eugenol Cement

Zinc Compounds and Eugenol Cement NF XI

The Powder

Zinc Acetate	0.5 g
Zinc Stearate	1 g
Zinc Oxide	70 g
Rosin	28.5 g

Powder the rosin and incorporate it with about an equal weight of zinc oxide until thoroughly mixed. Sift the mixture on a sieve of not less than 100-mesh. Regrind the material which does not pass through the sieve with more of the zinc oxide and sift again; repeat the process until all of the material readily passes through the sieve. Thoroughly mix the zinc stearate and zinc acetate with a portion of the zinc oxide and pass through a 100-mesh sieve. Thoroughly mix the two mixtures with the remainder of the zinc oxide.

The Liquid

Eugenol	85 mL
Cottonseed Oil	15 mL

The Cement

To prepare the cement mix 10 parts of the powder with 1 part of the liquid to a thick paste immediately before use. *Note:* The amount of liquid may be varied to give any desired consistency.

Description—*Powder:* yellowish white to white in color; *Liquid:* thin and colorless to weak yellow, having a strong aromatic odor of clove and a pungent, spicy taste; affected by light; specific gravity between 1.043 and 1.048; refractive index between 1.528 and 1.531 at 20°.

Solubility—*Liquid:* miscible with alcohol, chloroform, and ether; only slightly soluble in water.

Uses—In general dental practice as a *dental protective*, ie, as a pulp capping or a *temporary filling.*

Iso-Alcoholic Elixir

Iso-Elixir

Low-Alcoholic Elixir
High-Alcoholic Elixir ....of each a calculated volume
Mix the ingredients.

Low-Alcoholic Elixir

Compound Orange Spirit	10 mL
Alcohol	100 mL
Glycerin	200 mL
Sucrose	320 g
Purified Water, a stufficient quantity,	
To make	1000 mL

Alcohol Content—8 to 10%.

High-Alcoholic Elixir

Compound Orange Spirit	4 mL
Saccharin	3 g
Glycerin	200 mL
Alcohol, a sufficient quantity,	
To make	1000 mL

Alcohol Content—73 to 78%.

Uses—Intended to serve as a general *vehicle* for various medicaments that require solvents of different alcohol strengths. When iso-alcoholic elixir is specified in a prescription, the proportion of its two ingredients to be used is that which will produce a solution of the required alcohol strength.

The alcohol strength of the iso-alcoholic elixir to be used with a single liquid galenical in a prescription is approximately the same as that of the galenical. When galenicals of different alcohol strengths are used in the same prescription, the iso-alcoholic elixir to be used is to be of such alcohol strength as to secure the best solution possible. This will generally be found to be the average of the alcohol strengths of the several ingredients.

For nonextractive substances, the lowest alcohol strength of iso-alcohol elixir that will yield a perfect solution should be chosen.

Other Miscellaneous Pharmaceutical Necessities

Bucrylate [Propenoic acid, 2-cyano-, 2-methylpropyl ester; Isobutyl 2-cyanoacrylate [1069-55-2] $C_8H_{11}NO_2$ (153.18); (*Ethicon*)]—*Preparation:* One method reacts isobutyl 2-chloroacrylate with sodium cyanide. *Uses:* Surgical aid (tissue adhesive).

Ceresin [Ozokerite; Earth Wax; Cerosin; Mineral Wax; Fossil Wax]—A hard, white odorless solid resembling spermaceti when purified, occurring naturally in deposits in the Carpathian Mountains, especially in Galicia. It is a mixture of natural complex paraffin hydrocarbons. Melts between 61° and 78°; specific gravity between 0.91 and 0.92; stable toward oxidizing agents. Soluble in 30% alcohol, benzene, chloroform, petroleum, benzin, and hot oils. *Uses:* Substitute for beeswax; in dentistry for impression waxes.

Ethylenediamine Hydrate BP, PhI [$H_2NCH_2CH_2NH_2.H_2O$]—Clear, colorless or slightly yellow liquid with an ammoniacal odor and characteristic alkaline taste; solidifies on cooling to a crystalline mass (mp 10°); boils between 118° and 119°; specific gravity about 0.96; hygroscopic and absorbs CO_2 from the air; aqueous solutions are alkaline to litmus. Miscible with water and alcohol; soluble in 130 parts chloroform; slightly soluble in benzene and ether. *Uses:* In the manufacture of aminophylline and in the preparation of aminophylline injections.

Ferric Oxide, Red—Contains not less than 90% Fe_2O_3. It is made by heating native ferric oxide or hydroxide at a temperature which will yield a product of the desired color. The color is governed by the temperature and time of heating, the presence and kind of other metals, and the particle size of the oxide. A dark colored oxide is favored by prolonged heating at high temperature and the presence of manganese. A light-colored oxide is favored by the presence of aluminum and by finer particle size. *Uses:* Imparting color to neocalamine and cosmetics.

Ferric Oxide, Yellow—Contains not less than 97.5% Fe_2O_3. It is prepared by heating ferrous hydroxide or ferrous carbonate in air at a low temperature. *Uses:* As for *Red Ferric Oxide* (above).

Honey NF XII [Mel; Clarified Honey; Strained Honey] is the saccharine secretion deposited in the honeycomb by the bee, *Apis mellifera* Linné (Fam *Apidae*). It must be free from foreign substances such as parts of insects, leaves, etc, but may contain pollen grains. *History:* Honey is one of the oldest of food and medicinal products. During the 16th and 17th centuries it was recommended as a cure for almost everything. *Constituents: Invert sugar* (62–83%), *sucrose* (0–8%), and *dextrin* (0.26–7%). *Description:* Thick, syrupy liquid of a light yellowish to reddish brown color; translucent when fresh, but frequently becomes opaque and granular through crystallization of dextrose; characteristic odor and a sweet faintly acrid taste. *Uses:* A sweetening agent and pharmaceutic necessity.

Hydriodic Acid, Diluted, contains, in each 100 mL 9.5–10.5 g of HI (127.91), and 600 mg to 1 g of HPH_2O_2 (66.00). The latter is added to prevent the formation of free iodine. *Caution: Diluted Hydriodic Acid must not be dispensed or used in the preparation of other products if it contains free iodine. Preparation:* On a large scale, by the interaction of iodine and hydrogen sulfide. *Description* and *Solubility:* Colorless or not more than pale yellow, odorless liquid; specific gravity, about 1.1. Miscible with water or alcohol. *Uses:* In *Hydriodic Acid Syrup* (page 1294). The latter has been used as an expectorant. It is also used in the manufacture of inorganic iodides and disinfectants. The 57% acid is also used for analytical purposes, such as methoxyl determinations.

Lime [Calx; Calcium Oxide; Quicklime; Burnt Lime; Calx Usta; CaO (56.08)]—*Preparation:* Lime (calcium oxide) is made by calcining *limestone* (a native calcium carbonate) in kilns with strong heat. *Description and Solubility:* Hard, white, or grayish white masses or granules, or a white or grayish white powder; odorless; solution is strongly alkaline. 1 g is soluble in about 840 mL water and 1740 mL boiling water; soluble in glycerin and syrup; insoluble in alcohol. *Uses:* In making mortar, whitewash, and various chemicals and products. It is an ingredient in *Sulfurated Lime Solution* (RPS-16, page 1187). In the USP, calcium hydroxide has replaced lime, as it is more stable and more readily available of a quality suitable for medicinal use than the lime usually obtainable. Unless protected from air, lime soon becomes unfit for use, due to the action of carbon dioxide and moisture in the air. See *Calcium Hydroxide* (page 1310).

Peach Oil—An oil resembling almond oil obtained from *Persica vulgaris* (Fam *Rosaceae*). See *Persic Oil* (page 1315).

Polacrilin Potassium [Methacrylic acid polymer with divinylbenzene, potassium salt [39394-76-5]; Amberlite IRP-88 (*Rohm & Haas*)]—*Preparation:* Methacrylic acid is polymerized with divinylbenzene and the resulting resin is neutralized with KOH. *Description* and *Solubility:* Dry, buff-colored, odorless, tasteless, free-flowing powder; stable in light, air, and heat. Insoluble in water. *Uses: Pharmaceutic aid* (tablet disintegrant).

Poloxalene [Glycols, polymers, polyethylene-polypropylene [9003-11-6]; Bloat Guard (*SK&F*)]—*Preparation:* Polypropylene glycol is reacted with ethylene oxide. *Uses: Pharmaceutic aid* (surfactant).

Raspberry Juice—The liquid expressed from the fresh ripe fruit of *Rubus idaeus* Linné or of *Rubus strigosus* Michaux (Fam *Rosaceae*); contains not less than 1.5% of acids calculated as citric acid. *Preparation:* Express the juice from the washed, well-drained, fresh ripe red raspberries. Dissolve 0.1% of benzoic acid in the expressed juice and allow it to stand at room temperature (possibly for several days) until a small portion of the filtered juice produces a clear solution when mixed with $\frac{1}{2}$ of its volume of alcohol, the solution remaining clear for not less than 30 min. Strain the juice from the mixture or filter it, if necessary. *Description:* Clear liquid with an aromatic, characteristic odor and a characteristic, sour taste; the freshly prepared juice is red to reddish orange; affected by light; specific gravity between 1.025 and 1.045; pH between 2.7 and 3.8; refractive index not less than 1.3445. *Uses:* In the preparation of *Raspberry Syrup* (page 1294), a *flavored vehicle.*

Sarsaparilla—The dried root of *Smilax aristolochiaefolia* Miller, known in commerce as Mexican Sarsaparilla; or of *Smilax regelii* Killip et Morton, known in commerce as Honduras Sarsaparilla; or of *Smilax febrifuga* Kunth, known in commerce as an Ecuadorian Sarsaparilla; or of undetermined species of *Smilax* Linné, variously known in commerce as Ecuadorian and Central American Sarsaparilla (Fam *Liliaceae*). *Constituents:* Contains glycosides of the saponin group, *sarsasaponin* (*parillin*) and *smilasaponin* (*smilacin*) which are related structurally to the digitalis glycosides, and possess the steroid nucleus. When hydrolyzed with dilute acids, they split into sugars and the corresponding sapogenin. Sarsasaponin yields *sarsasapogenin* (*parigenin*) plus one rhamnose and two glucose molecules, and smilacin yields *smilagenin* plus sugar molecules. There are also present starch, resin, coloring matter, and volatile oil. *History:* This drug was first used in Europe in the 16th century as a much-vaunted remedy for syphilis. The origin of the name is in doubt. *Uses:* This agent is without pharmacological actions, and is not employed in modern therapeutics, although the laity is inclined to attribute certain therapeutic virtues to its use.

Sodium Glutamate [Sodium Acid Glutamate [142-47-2] $HOOCCH(NH_2)CH_2CH_2COONa$]—White or nearly white, crystalline powder. Very soluble in water; sparingly soluble in alcohol. *Uses:* Imparts a meat flavor to foods.

Sodium Thioglycollate [Sodium Mercaptoacetate; $HSCH_2COONa$] —Hygroscopic crystals which discolor on exposure to air or iron. Freely soluble in water; slightly soluble in alcohol. *Uses:* Reducing agent in Fluid Thioglycollate Medium for sterility testing.

Suet, Prepared [Mutton Suet]—Internal fat of the abdomen of the sheep, *Ovis aries* (Fam *Bovidae*), purified by melting and straining. White solid fat with a slight, characteristic odor and taste when fresh; melts between 45° and 50° and congeals between 37° and 40°; must be preserved in a cool place in tight containers. *Uses:* In ointments and cerates.

CHAPTER 69

Adverse Effects of Drugs

Joseph A Linkewich, Pharm D

Director, Pharmacy Service
Jeanes Hospital
Philadelphia, PA 19111

We are the beneficiaries of a continuous expansion of medical capability. Contributing largely to this expanding capability, specifically in providing the means to alter the course of many diseases, has been the great improvement in the quality and quantity of drugs used in medical practice. This favorable development has not been entirely benign, for drugs produce adverse as well as beneficial effects. As we shall see, many have attempted to characterize the extent to which drugs induce disease. As an overview, Jick[1] has suggested that 30% of hospitalized medical patients experience at least one adverse drug reaction during their hospital stay. He also indicates that approximately 3% of hospital admissions to medical services are due to adverse drug reactions. Precise measurement of the extent to which drugs contribute to patient morbidity and mortality is very difficult. Few disagree, however, that drug toxicity is a significant health problem in terms of patient suffering and resultant economic consequences.

Indicative of the growing awareness of deleterious effects of drugs is the increased library shelf-space assigned to the now numerous texts and catalogs devoted to discussion and retrieval of adverse drug reaction information (see the *Bibliography* for a partial listing of these publications).

It has been stated that drug-induced adverse effects are the price to be paid for more effective medicinals. There can be no quarrel with this statement; however, it is the *high* price that is of concern. Empiricism in therapeutics and shoddy therapeutics should no longer be tolerated; the powerful drugs used today must be properly prescribed, dispensed and administered. On the bright side, studies with drugs at molecular, pharmacological, and clinical levels are continuing to yield data which facilitate proper drug use.

This chapter was prepared with the objective of providing students and practitioners a realization of the magnitude of the adverse-drug-reaction problem. It will not serve as the single reference source of documented adverse reactions; for information concerning specific drug-induced reactions the publications listed in the *Bibliography* should be consulted. In preparing the several sections of the discussion on *Drug-Induced Diseases by Systems* in this chapter, selected authoritative current reviews were used to provide illustrative information and a port of entry into this expanding literature.

Studies of Adverse Reactions

Studies or systems designed to determine the types of adverse reactions experienced by hospitalized or ambulatory patients, or the incidence of untoward reactions in the general "pill-consuming" population, have yielded conflicting information.

Most studies in which investigators actively followed or directly monitored patients' therapy have disclosed alarming rates of adverse events accompanying drug use, a finding in marked contrast to those from systems in which physicians voluntarily reported adverse reactions as they occur.

The earliest investigations are those of Schimmel[2] and of Cluff.[3] A 10% incidence of adverse drug reactions was found by Schimmel when his group actively monitored medical inpatients. Cluff and associates validated Schimmel's data, and in a series of reports called attention to the grave nature of the adverse-drug-reaction problem, as well as to the "tip-of-the-iceberg" character of existing systems designed for reporting of reactions.

Most early studies (conducted in the mid-60s through early-70s) were constructed as intense short-term monitoring programs. Typically, data on adverse reactions in a series of inpatients, or patients being admitted to a hospital, would be collected by physicians, trained epidemiologists, or other health workers. Association of an adverse clinical event with drug exposure usually rested with the investigator and/or other physicians in charge of the patient's care. After several months (in few cases, years) of data collection, analyses would be performed to delineate the most common side effects observed, severity of these effects, drugs implicated, contributing patient, drug, or environmental predispositions, etc. These early surveys served best to alert the health community to a problem which, up to today, is denied or minimized by some.[4] Experience with these short-term adverse reaction monitoring programs led to the development of more comprehensive surveillance projects, such as the Boston Collaborative Drug Surveillance Program (BCDSP). The development and methodology of this surveillance program has been described in detail,[5] and its major findings to date have been compiled and published.[6,7] Basically, this system records all drug exposures and all beneficial and adverse events in monitored inpatients. Thus, the BCDSP is directed toward the discovery of all clinical effects of drugs during use in normal medical practice (nonexperimental use) in various clinical situations. All surveillance tasks are performed by trained nurse or pharmacist monitors. Each monitor is assigned to a ward where data are abstracted from medical records and from interviews with patients and physicians. Data are collected on all consecutively admitted patients, and include the following information: age, sex, race, weight, consumption of tobacco and beverages (alcohol, coffee, tea), previous drug reactions, and results of routine blood and urine tests. A drug history for the period of one month prior to admission is compiled. Drug administration records include names of drugs, dates of initiation of therapy, dosages, dosage forms, routes of administration, indications for use, etc. When a drug is discontinued, reasons for termination, information on efficacy of the drug, and adverse reactions to it are obtained. If an adverse reaction is suspected, supplementary information is obtained by the monitor, and final judgment is made by the Program's staff concerning a possible causal relationship between use of the drug and an adverse event. The judgment is expressed in the terms "definite," "probable," "doubtful," or "don't know." On discharge, information concerning all instances of certain adverse events is obtained, whether or not these were attributable to a drug; discharge diagnoses are also recorded. These data are added to the computer master file, which is periodically surveyed to evaluate suspected and unsuspected drug effects. Special analyses of the data, designed to find answers to questions suggested by the routine surveys or by published reports of other investigators, are also undertaken.

Basic findings generated by this comprehensive program include information on drug utilization, such as magnitude of drug use, relative frequencies of various drug indications, most commonly prescribed drugs, and frequency of adverse reactions (at one analysis point 5.5% of 103,770 drug exposures were associated with adverse effects[5]). As drug efficacy information is also obtained from prescribers, this method permits clinical evaluation of new drugs. Individual drugs can be evaluated for incidence of known or suspected adverse effects. For example, one report of the BCDSP revealed that rashes were substantially more common in patients receiving ampicillin than in patients receiving penicillin G or drugs other than penicillin.

Adverse reactions previously believed to occur infrequently, and previously unsuspected adverse drug reactions, are detected by the monitoring system; for example, the detection of the relationship between intravenously administered ethacrynic acid and gastrointestinal bleeding in monitored hospitalized patients.[8] Of 105 patients receiving this treatment, 26% were observed by the attending physician to develop gastrointestinal bleeding, yet in no instance in the clinical environment was the bleeding attributed to administration of ethacrynic acid notwithstanding that the incidence of bleeding in other hospitalized (or control) patients was 4.5%. This illustrates what can be revealed by the routine computerized analysis of data obtained by careful monitoring of patients' drug regimens.

A startling report from the BCDSP described fatal drug reactions occurring in participating hospitals.[9] In this series of over 26,000 consecutively monitored patients, deaths due to drugs occurred in 24 cases (nearly 1 per 1000), most of the fatalities being attributed to commonly used drugs. Hyperkalemia from potassium supplements, and pulmonary edema from parenteral fluid therapy were prominent causes of deaths judged to be preventable. Antineoplastic drugs, digoxin, and heparin were associated with multiple deaths. Other investigators using varying methods have reported roughly comparable drug-associated mortality statistics.[10] Most have concluded that drug-associated deaths are relatively uncommon and usually occur in patients who are seriously or terminally ill and are being treated with toxic compounds.

The BCDSP has published more than 110 reports as of January, 1978. As of October, 1977, about 35,000 consecutively admitted patients have been monitored and disease, drug use, and adverse event data recorded in the master file. Surveillance was conducted in 22 institutions, most of which were in the U.S., but some hospitals in Ontario, New Zealand, and Israel were included. A wide variety of subject matter has been treated in the reports published thus far, including information concerning adverse reactions to propranolol, spironolactone, tricyclic antidepressants, quinidine, procainamide, furosemide, and flurazepam. The clinical significance of the interaction between chloral hydrate and warfarin, the potentiation of ampicillin rash by allopurinol or hyperuricemia, and increase in BUN due to concurrent administration of tetracycline and diuretics have also been reported. Environmental or patient-characteristic factors which influence the efficacy or toxicity of drugs have been the subject of several reports. Examples include: the effects of age and sex on the toxicity of heparin; the relationship between ABO bloodtype and thromboembolic phenomena associated with oral contraceptive intake; the effects of serum-albumin levels on the side effects of prednisone and phenytoin; the relationship between dose and acute reactions to prednisone; the effect of cigarette smoking on the efficacy of pro-

poxyphene, on the sedative effects of diazepam and chlordiazepoxide, and on the clinical toxicity of theophylline; and the relationship of age with toxicity from flurazepam. In addition, the BCDSP has accumulated information on the incidence and categories of hospitalized patients at risk of developing drug-induced convulsions, deafness, anaphylaxis, extrapyramidal reactions, and renal dysfunction. References 6 and 7 should be consulted for a more thorough review of the outputs from the BCDSP.

The BCDSP is a unique monitoring system, since all drug exposures in the wards monitored are tabulated, and an intensive effort is made to quantitate accurately the number of adverse events occurring in patients exposed. No other approach has been able to present clinical adverse-drug-reaction-data which provide both numerator (number of adverse events) and denominator (number of patients exposed) information. This kind of patient-at-risk information is vital if prescribers are to balance "benefits versus risks" in their goal to achieve rational prescribing. The expertly designed BCDSP will continue to offer health professionals much useful therapeutic information in future years from continued analysis of this large data base.

Data have been developed in recent years by both the BCDSP[11] and others on hospital admissions attributed to adverse drug reactions which occur in ambulatory patients. One[12] prospective epidemiologic study of over 6000 patients consecutively admitted to a medical service indicated that 2.9% of these admissions were due to drug reactions. Remarkably, eight drugs accounted for 35% of these admissions. These eight pharmaceuticals were aspirin, digoxin, warfarin, hydrochlorothiazide, prednisone, vincristine, norethindrone, and furosemide. In 18% of the cases, OTC drugs were implicated. Drug hypersensitivity (allergic) mechanisms were judged to be responsible for the reactions only 18% of the time.

Strikingly similar results were reported from the BCDSP's series of over 7000 monitored medical admissions. Drug reactions were the cause for admission in 3.7% of these patients. This total excluded patients admitted for complications due to drug abuse (an additional 0.5%) and patients admitted with accidental or intentional overdoses (an additional 0.7% of admissions). In this series, five drugs were implicated in 37% of the drug-induced admissions; these included digoxin, aspirin, prednisone, warfarin, and guanethidine. It is not comforting to note that "old," "familiar" pharmaceuticals seem to be the primary culprits insofar as outpatient reaction rates are concerned.

Some Specific Problems

An adverse drug reaction is defined by the Food and Drug Administration as "a reaction that is noxious, unintended, and occurs at doses normally used in man for the prophylaxis, diagnosis, or therapy of disease." Under this broad definition various investigators have devised schemes for the classification of the mechanisms involved in adverse drug reactions. A review of such classification schemes indicates that most drug reactions can be grouped into one of two major categories. The first includes hypersensitivity or allergic reactions (reactions due to a patient's immune response) and idiosyncratic reactions (responses characterized by inordinate or exaggerated responses to normal doses of drug). Drawing data from previously mentioned surveys, it becomes apparent that drug reactions included in this category account for only 20 to 30% of reactions and are largely unpredictable and unavoidable. By contrast, the *remaining 70 to 80% of reactions*, including overdosage or extension of pharmacologic effects, side effects, toxic reactions, and drug interactions, *are considered to be for the most part predictable and preventable*.

Why do so many adverse reactions occur? To answer adequately this question would require a lengthy essay. It is useful, nevertheless, to review briefly a number of factors which contribute to the problem. Overuse and misuse of prescription and nonprescription medications are probably the most important factors. We live in an over-medicated society, evidenced by the fact that physicians write prescriptions for about 75% of all their patients and by the encouragement via television and radio to over-medicate. Marketing research data indicate that most physicians will issue one or more prescriptions to a patient diagnosed as having a "common cold," with almost 60% of these prescriptions being for antibiotics. Other flagrant examples of inappropriate overprescribing or self-medication are easily found in the literature.

Today's potent medicines, when appropriately and judiciously prescribed, remain double-edged swords. Properly used they are extremely valuable and may even be lifesaving; overused or abused they cause untold suffering and may even take life. Failure of the physician to set a therapeutic endpoint contributes to the number of adverse reactions which occur. The propensity to push to toxicity digitalis, diuretics, corticosteroids, etc, provides heroic examples of poor therapeutics destined to lead to drug toxicity.

In addition to the above, faulty dispensing, medication administration errors, lack of compliance with prescribed medication regimens, and inappropriate prescription-writing practices contribute to the enhancement of drug-toxicity risks.

The lack of uniform bioavailability between different brands or formulations of a therapeutic agent poses a pharmacotherapy hazard. Differences in the bioavailability of various brands of digoxin, oxytetracycline, phenytoin, and other drugs have resulted in variable therapeutic effects, sometimes resulting in toxicity. This subject is considered elsewhere in this text (see Chapter 77).

Physicians and pharmacists are becoming increasingly aware of the adverse consequences which may result from the interaction of certain drugs with other drugs, foods, or environmental factors (see also Chapter 102).

Predispositions

Many factors have been described which appear to predispose patients to the development of drug toxicity. Studies have shown that there is a direct relationship between the number of drugs administered and reaction incidence. While not fully understood, it appears as if patients who have suffered an adverse reaction are predisposed to development of second and third reactions.

Physiologic factors in health and disease influence drug effects (both beneficial and adverse). The response to many drug classes differs in pediatric and geriatric patients as compared to the "usual adult." The incidence of drug toxicity in many series has been shown to be the highest in the very young and very old. Pharmacokinetic principles often can be used to explain drug metabolic and excretory differences as they relate to age. Body weight, sex, racial/genetic characteristics may influence the absorption, distribution, metabolism and excretion (and thus toxicity) of some drugs.

Disease states modify drug response. Compromised renal function and hepatic function influence metabolism and excretion of many drug substances. Toxicity often results in patients who accumulate high serum or tissue levels of medications because of impaired excretory function.

Atopic patients may be reactive to a number of drug substances. The inherited absence or deficiency of certain specific enzyme systems revealed by drug exposure may result in reduced or exaggerated drug effects. Pharmacogenetics is that discipline of study of inherited variations in drug handling and responses. Certain pharmacogenetic conditions

will be described in the following sections (see also Chapter 70).

Drug-Induced Diseases by Systems

This section is intended to provide a broad overview of "drug-induced diseases." The reader interested in a more detailed discussion of such diseases is referred to the excellent books listed in the *Bibliography*. This presentation will highlight only a few specific areas of the subject. Reference is made to recent reviews to enable the reader access to the literature.

Dermatologic Reactions

As new drugs are introduced into clinical medicine the list of those capable of causing dermatologic adverse reactions will undoubtedly expand. It is said that almost any drug can produce some type of drug eruption. For the purposes of this review well-defined and potentially life-threatening reactions will be discussed; it should be pointed out, however, that the majority of adverse dermatologic reactions to drugs are neither well-defined nor life-threatening. The mechanisms of most cutaneous reactions are unknown. Most are believed to occur as an immunological manifestation, yet this assumption is based largely on circumstantial evidence.

Drugs which are commonly considered to rank highest as to their potential for allergic skin reactions include: ampicillin, penicillin G, other semisynthetic penicillins, cephalosporins, sulfonamides, quinidine, phenytoin, aspirin and many, many others.[13] Most dermatologic reactions are reversible when the offending compound is identified and withdrawn. Intervention may be required in the more serious drug-induced dermatologic syndromes. Scarlatiniform or morbilliform exanthematic eruptions are by far the most frequent manifestations of cutaneous reaction to drugs. Urticarial or "hive-like" eruptions occur frequently and are often the sole indication of a generalized allergic reaction after drug exposure.

Toxic *epidermal necrolysis* or Lyell's syndrome or the scalded-skin syndrome is a life-threatening adverse dermatologic reaction which may be induced by drugs or infection. Symptoms of the drug-induced disease include malaise, lethargy, fever, and sore throat. In the initial stages of the disease, the skin is erythematous and tender; this is followed by the appearance of large flaccid bullae which easily rupture. The skin appears scalded. Thirty percent of patients affected will succumb, often within a week after blisters appear. Death results from infection complicated by fluid and electrolyte derangements. Patients who recover usually show no permanent scarring despite the grave appearance of the skin. Aminopyrine, phenylbutazone, penicillin, phenolphthalein, sulfonamides, allopurinol, and phenytoin have all been implicated in the production of toxic epidermal necrolysis.

As the name implies, the manifestations of drug-induced *erythema multiforme* can take many forms. The lesions may appear as bright or dark red macules, papules, vesicles, or bullae. This reaction occurs more frequently in children or young adults. Malaise and fever may accompany the skin eruption. In addition to drugs, etiologic factors associated with the production of erythema multiforme may include foods, neoplasms, and infections. Drugs implicated in the syndrome are furosemide, chlorpropamide, propranolol, aminosalicylic acid, sulfonamides, phenylbutazone, chlordiazepoxide, tetracycline, penicillin, ampicillin, phenobarbital, chlorpromazine, and others. There is lack of agreement as to the causal relationship between long-acting sulfonamides and this adverse effect, although continuing reports suggest these compounds are primary offenders.

Stevens-Johnson syndrome is classified as a serious variant of *bullous erythema multiforme.* In addition to the symptoms described for erythema multiforme, this syndrome usually involves the mucous membranes. The skin becomes hemorrhagic, and serious ocular involvement is common. The duration of illness is usually 4 to 6 weeks; mortality has been estimated at 5 to 20%. Drugs associated with the development of the Stevens-Johnson syndrome are: sulfonamides, phenytoin, penicillins, chlorpropamide, phensuximide, phenobarbital, phenolphthalein, meprobamate, and others.

Exfoliative dermatitis is characterized by large areas of the skin becoming scaly, erythematous, and then sloughing. Secondary bacterial infection may occur and may be responsible for a fatal outcome. Exfoliative dermatitis may also develop after other skin diseases including psoriasis, contact and atopic dermatitis. Exfoliative dermatitis may develop or follow a less severe drug eruption. After withdrawal of the offending agent, this reaction may take months to resolve. Aminosalicylic acid, phenytoin, griseofulvin, phenylbutazone, and sulfonamides are common causative agents. For an assessment of treatment regimens for life-threatening drug eruptions, the interested reader is referred to the article by Cram.[14]

Photosensitivity eruptions appear after exposure to ultraviolet light rays of areas of the skin in which a drug or a drug metabolite is present. Photosensitivity eruptions are divided into two types, *phototoxic* and *photoallergic* reactions. Phototoxic reactions are those that can be elicited in almost everyone if the appropriate concentration of drug is taken systemically or is topically applied and if enough exposure to light of appropriate wavelength is received. Phototoxic eruptions may occur after the first drug exposure, are dose-related, do not display cross-sensitivity, and are generally manifested as an exaggerated sunburn-like reaction. Hexachlorophene, tetracyclines (especially demeclocycline), and phenothiazines are considered the worst offenders. Photoallergic reactions are believed to result from light energy acting on or altering drug and skin proteins in such a manner as to form an antigen. These eruptions require previous contact with the offending substance, are generally not dose-related, and exhibit cross-sensitivity with chemically related compounds. The clinical manifestations of drug-induced photoallergic reactions are variable. Lesions may be eczematous or papular, or may be evidenced as urticaria, bullae, or exaggerated sunburn. In contrast to phototoxic eruptions, the lesions are not localized just at sites of light exposure but may extend beyond areas exposed to light. Sometimes a drug produces both photoallergic and phototoxic reactions. Compounds included in soaps as deodorants and bacteriostatic agents of the halogenated salicylanilide classes are known contact photosensitizers capable of eliciting both phototoxic and photoallergic reactions. Sulfonamides, thiazides, griseofulvin, and promethazine are examples of drugs implicated in producing photoallergic reactions.

Hepatic Diseases

A useful scheme for classifying drugs capable of producing liver injury is that offered by Zimmerman.[15] In essence, *hepatotoxins* can be grouped either as compounds which have *intrinsic* property of being able to produce liver injury or as compounds able to produce *liver damage* through host *hypersensitivity.* The former group of drugs produce liver damage as an effect of their particular chemical structure; they elicit a predictable and dose-dependent effect on liver cells or a specific interference with metabolism. Examples of hepatotoxins in this category include methotrexate, acetaminophen (when taken in overdose), isoniazid, aspirin, tetracycline, methyltestosterone, and C-17 substituted steroids. Hepatic necrosis resulting from acetaminophen overdoses has become a much discussed toxicologic problem.[16] In severe

intoxication, fatal hepatic necrosis may develop in a few days after ingestion. A toxic metabolite of acetaminophen is considered responsible for the production of liver necrosis. Once formed this metabolite binds to liver macromolecules and results in cell death. Normally liver glutathione protects liver cells from metabolites. In large overdoses, glutathione stores are depleted making the liver susceptible to necrosis. Specific antidotes are currently being studied to block development of toxicity. Recently cases of hepatitis have been reported in patients receiving acetaminophen chronically in recommended dose ranges.

The ability of isoniazid to produce hepatitis has been appreciated for quite some time. Allergic mechanisms were previously thought to be responsible in the one percent of isoniazid recipients who developed overt hepatitis. It has been shown that the risk of developing "INH-hepatitis" increases with age ("no" risk in persons under 20 years of age up to a 2.3% incidence in persons from 50 to 64 years of age). Isoniazid-hepatitis may be considered a "pharmacogenetic condition" in that it has been recently shown that this toxicity (hepatitis) occurs more commonly in patients who rapidly metabolize (acetylate) isoniazid. "Rapid acetylators" may produce higher levels of a toxic metabolite capable of binding to liver cells. Those with the genetically determined "slow acetylator" status may be more susceptible to development of polyneuropathy, an effect presumed to be due to high body levels of isoniazid.

After decades of use, aspirin has been incriminated as a significant hepatotoxin. Hepatocellular damage due to aspirin has been noted to occur in patients receiving high doses for connective tissue disease.

MacFarlaine and McCarron[17] have summarized 44 reported cases of fatty metamorphosis of the liver occurring after intravenous tetracycline therapy. Intravenous doses of 2 g or more per day of tetracycline have been associated with a specific fatty change in the liver. In most patients with this complication, renal function is also depressed.

Hypersensitivity-type hepatic drug reactions are more common and less understood. These reactions are unpredictable and are not reproducible in experimental animals. Only a small fraction of exposed individuals is susceptible to this type of hepatic injury. The reactions are unrelated to dose, and the onset is usually delayed. Often the hepatotoxic reaction is accompanied by other hypersensitivity phenomena, such as rash, arthralgia, fever, and eosinophilia. Hypersensitivity-type hepatic drug reactions are usually divided into hepatitis-like and cholestatic reactions but often are of mixed histopathology. An extensive list of agents implicated in the production of hepatic damage of both direct and hypersensitivity types has been compiled by Zimmerman.[15]

Hypersensitivity hepatic reactions of the cholestatic type are particularly associated with the phenothiazines. Chlorpromazine is useful as an example. The incidence of intrahepatic cholestasis secondary to chlorpromazine administration is estimated to be 0.5 to 3% of exposed persons. The reaction is not related to dose and most often occurs in the first month of therapy; its onset is insidious and characterized by malaise, anorexia, low-grade fever, and jaundice. Recovery is usually complete and occurs 1 to 4 weeks after onset of symptoms. If patients are rechallenged, it is said 40% will redevelop the reaction. Other phenothiazines, tricyclic antidepressants, chlorpropamide, hydrochlorothiazide, methyldopa, erythromycin estolate, and many other drugs have been implicated in this reaction.

Hepatitis-like hypersensitivity reactions are associated with a wide variety of drugs, including halothane, sulfonamides, phenytoin, aminosalicylic acid, ethionamide, monoamine oxidase inhibitors, oxyphenisatin, and others. The term *halothane hepatitis* reflects the familiarity of the medical profession with this hepatotoxic reaction. Halothane hepatitis has been the subject of numerous case reports, retrospective surveys, and a large retrospective controlled trial conducted by the National Academy of Sciences-National Research Council.

Hepatocellular necrosis (acute and chronic) has recently been attributed to the irritant cathartic oxyphenisatin. This adverse effect prompted its removal from combination tablet laxative preparations. The potential for methyldopa to produce hepatitis has been only recently described. Currently the incidence of this reaction is estimated to be 1%. Symptoms become apparent usually between 1 and 4 weeks after therapy is started and include nausea, vomiting, malaise, anorexia, fever, rash, and pruritus. Deaths have been reported from methyldopa-induced fulminant hepatic necrosis. Transaminase tests should be performed at the start of treatment and repeated at 4 weeks.

McAvoy et al[18] surveyed the literature and characterized 33 cases of benign hepatic tumors associated with oral contraceptive use. These lesions have been shown to be histologically benign but can be complicated by rupture, bleeding, hemoperitoneum, and shock.

Gastrointestinal Diseases

Acute ulceration of the upper gastrointestinal tract caused by drugs continues to be a prominent iatrogenic disease. There are many drugs in the rheumatologist's armamentarium which are thought to be able to erode the gastrointestinal tract; these include salicylates, other nonsteroidal anti-inflammatory agents, and possibly the glucorcorticoids.

Cooke[19] has reviewed the pathogenesis of aspirin-induced gastrointestinal erosions and hemorrhage and has drawn the following conclusions: (1) When aspirin is in a soluble and alkaline buffered form, so that gastric acid is neutralized, it does not change mucosal permeability or cause stomach damage. (2) Reduction of gastric acid by antacids reduces or abolishes gastric damage by aspirin. (3) The site of adverse action is probably the mucosal cell. Cooke's conclusions are in agreement with earlier observations by Leonards and Levy.[20] These investigators were able to minimize gastrointestinal blood loss by administering aspirin in a highly buffered solution as the acetylsalicylate or as highly buffered, rapidly dissolving tablets. Epidemiologic study by the BCDSP[21] indicated that heavy regular aspirin use by outpatients was associated with hospital admissions for gastric ulcer and bleeding from gastric ulcer.

The association between gastric ulceration and corticosteroid administration is well accepted by most practitioners. The BCDSP has presented a surprising finding relating to this adverse effect.[22] In a series of 82 patients identified as experiencing an acute reaction to prednisone, 32 had an adverse gastrointestinal reaction. Twenty-five of these patients showed evidence of gastrointestinal bleeding (18 required transfusion). *There was no correlation between the daily dose of prednisone and acute gastrointestinal reactions.* After an extensive review of literature reports on corticosteroid management, Conn and Blitzer[23] were not able to demonstrate that the frequency of peptic ulceration was increased by treatment with corticosteroids. These authors state "The steroid-ulcer myth arose from anecdotal reports during the earliest use of ACTH and adrenocorticosteroids when these remarkable agents were viewed with awe and suspicion."

Within the past several years, antibiotic-induced diarrhea and colitis has become a prominent drug-induced gastrointestinal disease. Antibiotic-induced diarrhea may range in severity from a mild, self-limiting process to a severe, fulminant condition which may require colectomy or which may even be fatal. Antibiotics most commonly implicated are lincomycin, clindamycin, ampicillin, and tetracycline. Evidence currently exists which indicates that diarrhea/colitis may result from antibiotic upset of the fecal flora with subsequent proliferation of enterotoxin-producing microorganisms. Specific treatment approaches are now being studied.

To finalize this subsection, it should be mentioned that drugs have the capacity to induce pancreatitis and to induce various malabsorption syndromes.

Hematologic Disorders

Of all the areas of drug-induced disease, the literature on hematologic disorders is the most prodigious. In 1954 the American Medical Association established its Registry on Blood Dyscrasias which later (1961) was expanded to the more comprehensive Registry on Adverse Reactions. Although the Registry was phased out in 1971, information gathered from the single-case reports submitted to the program provided an index of suspicion of those drugs with a high propensity for causing hematologic diseases. The early lists of drugs most often associated with blood dyscrasias have been confirmed in large part by subsequent investigators. The reference text by Swanson and Cook (listed in the bibliography) is the most comprehensive available in this area.

Chloramphenicol, sulfonamides, phenylbutazone, oxyphenbutazone, phenytoin, mephenytoin, meprobamate, and gold have been cited as responsible in one series of 51 patients with the diagnosis of drug-induced aplastic anemia.[24] Chloramphenicol was responsible in 35 of 51 instances of total bone-marrow suppression caused by drugs; sulfonamides were implicated in 8 patients; phenylbutazone and oxyphenbutazone in 3; phenytoin in 2; the other drugs were charged with 1 case apiece. Exposure to a diverse group of other drugs, solvents, and insecticides is also implicated in the production of aplastic anemia.

The first clinical manifestations of aplastic anemia are usually related to bleeding (ecchymoses, epistaxis, and petechiae). Pancytopenia is observed in the majority of the patients on initial examination, and a hypocellular bone-marrow biopsy may be obtained at some time in the course of the illness. Drug-induced aplastic anemia is a serious disorder. Therapy is primarily supportive. "Specific therapy" includes splenectomy, corticosteroids, androgenic steroids, and bone-marrow transplantation. The value of splenectomy and corticosteroids is denied by most authorities, and controversy exists as to the marrow-stimulating effect of androgens. In a few centers marrow transplants have been successful in young patients who were transplanted early in the course of their illness. Mortality remains at about 70%.

Yunis[25] has reviewed the types of bone-marrow suppression which develop secondary to chloramphenicol administration. It is clear that chloramphenicol produces two types of bone-marrow toxicity. One is a fairly common, dose-related, reversible suppression involving primarily the erythroid series of cells. This is a pharmacological effect of the drug resulting from the inhibition of mitochondrial protein synthesis. The other is a rare, devastating bone-marrow aplasia; it has a delayed onset and is not dose-related. The occurrence rate of this form of serious marrow toxicity has been estimated as from 1 in 150,000 to 1 in 25,000 courses of therapy. Even though this toxicity can be considered rare, prescribing of chloramphenicol for trivial infections cannot be condoned. Blood monitoring for early signs of aplastic anemia is of no value.

Drug-induced agranulocytosis is believed to be produced by two basic mechanisms of action. One of these involves a precipitous decline in leukocytes that occurs only a short time after ingestion of a small amount of drug by a patient who has become sensitized by prior administration of the drug. Such an effect suggests destruction of leukocytes in the peripheral circulation and is exemplified by aminopyrine, sulfonamides, oral hypoglycemics, and antithyroid drugs. The other type of reaction exemplified by the phenothiazine drugs occurs several weeks after initiating continuous treatment, during which time large doses of drug are usually given. It is associated with arrest of the production of polymorphonuclear leukocytes in the marrow. In fully developed agranulocytosis the total leukocyte count falls below 3000/cu mm and the absolute number of "polys" may decline to zero. If the diagnosis of drug-induced agranulocytosis is made early and the offending drug is discontinued, recovery is usually expected so long as the patient can avoid overwhelming infection.

Phenothiazines have been implicated in agranulocytosis far more frequently than any other class of drugs. Middle-aged or elderly white women have shown a higher incidence than any other group. Estimates as to the actual incidence are reported as one case in about 1250 recipients when phenothiazines are administered for psychoses. In one of three patients exposed, a transient leukopenia develops during early therapy. A normal blood count returns in these patients without cessation of therapy. Symptoms of chills, fever, and sore throat in patients ingesting phenothiazines should alert prescribers to the potential for drug-induced disease. Agranulocytosis produced by phenothiazines commonly develops after a latent period of 20 to 40 days and after a cumulative dose of 10 to 20 g of drug. These factors support the postulate of a direct effect on developing granulocytes in the marrow. The mechanism of phenothiazine agranulocytosis can readily be differentiated from the immediate reactions of aminopyrine agranulocytosis, quinidine-induced thrombocytopenia, or the delayed and continuous reaction of chloramphenicol-induced aplastic anemia.

Thrombocytopenia can arise by mechanisms involving *bone marrow suppression* and *peripheral platelet destruction*. Antineoplastic agents, because of their known pharmacologic effects, are capable of marrow suppression, with resultant development of thrombocytopenia as well as other cytopenias. Other drugs which have marrow effects in certain individuals (anticonvulsants, chloramphenicol, sulfonamides, phenothiazines, antirheumatics, etc) also are capable of producing "toxic" thrombocytopenia.

Peripheral platelet destruction results from an immunologic mechanism whereby the drug, acting as a hapten, combines with proteins to form an antigen. Antibody production is stimulated and antigen-antibody complexes fix to specific sites on the platelet, inducing complement fixation, agglutination, and platelet damage. Thrombocytopenia is believed to be produced by the elimination of damaged platelets within the reticuloendothelial system. Many drugs have been implicated in causing immune complex thrombocytopenia; examples include quinidine, thiazides, methyldopa, heparin, gold salts, aspirin, cephalothin, sulfonamides, penicillins, antituberculars, and many others. Patients with allergic drug-induced thrombocytopenia usually develop an acute hemorrhagic syndrome. Rechallenge with the suspected causative agent is never indicated because of the potential to precipitate rapidly a life-endangering bleeding episode.

Drugs induce *hemolysis* by two major mechanisms: (1) injury to erythrocytes with defective enzyme systems, and (2) immune drug-induced hemolysis.

The classical example of the first mechanism is the pharmacogenetic condition in which hemolytic anemia is provoked by ingestion of certain oxidant drugs. Hemolysis is seen only in patients with a genetically determined deficiency of the enzyme glucose 6-phosphate dehydrogenase (G6-PD). A wide variety of drugs, including antimalarials, nitrofurantoin, sulfonamides, sulfones, aminosalicylic acid, aspirin, probenecid, and quinidine have the ability to induce hemolysis in sensitive patients. Sensitivity to oxidant drugs is a relative condition. Over 100 variants of G6-PD deficiency are described. American Blacks usually have the "A-" mutation

in which G6-PD is synthesized in normal quantities, but its intra-erythrocyte decay is accelerated as the cell ages. "G6-PD Mediterranean" is the variant most commonly found in caucasians. Extremely low G6-PD activity may be found in these patients who are susceptible to severe, brisk, hemolysis.

Immune drug-induced hemolysis can be classified into two types: (1) immune hemolytic anemia, in which antibodies are directed against the drug and cannot be detected in serum with normal red blood cells unless the drug is also present, and (2) autoimmune hemolytic anemia, in which antibodies are probably directed against intrinsic red-cell antigens and can be detected with normal red cells and are not affected by presence of the drug.

Immune drug-induced hemolytic anemia also can be divided into two groups, depending on the type of antibody produced and its mechanism of attachment to RBC membranes. In the penicillin (or hapten) type, IgG reacts with the RBC-penicillin complex. Penicillin adsorption to the RBC occurs usually after two to three weeks of high-dose therapy. Quinidine, aminosalicylic acid, phenacetin, sulfonamides, oral hypoglycemics, and rifampin bind weakly with red cells. The hemolytic anemia produced by these agents is termed the "innocent bystander" type. In this reaction it is postulated that drug-antibody (IgM) complexes are attracted to the RBC and lead to rapid intravascular hemolysis by activating the complement sequence.

In drug-induced autoimmune hemolytic anemia the antigen is normally present on the surface of the RBC. Antibodies provoked by methyldopa, levodopa, or mefenamic acid react directly with the RBC antigen, probably Rhesus antigen, with resultant hemolysis. Twenty percent of patients taking methyldopa develop a positive direct Coombs' test, indicating antierythrocyte antibodies. Under 1% develop overt hemolysis. How methyldopa, mefenamic acid, and levodopa provoke autoantibody formation is completely unknown.

The symptoms of immune drug-induced hemolytic anemia usually return to normal fairly rapidly, once the offending drug has been discontinued. The direct Coombs' test may take several years to become completely negative.

Drugs have the ability to induce *megaloblastic anemia*. This effect should be anticipated when prescribing agents capable of blocking DNA synthesis. Purine and pyrimidine analogues or folic-acid antagonists are obvious inhibitors. Megaloblastic anemia may develop after administering other agents capable of producing vitamin B_{12} or folate deficiency, such as phenytoin and isoniazid.

Hypersensitivity Phenomena

To the reader of the preceding sections of this chapter dealing with drug-induced dermatologic, hepatic, gastrointestinal, and hematologic diseases, it should be obvious that hypersensitivity or immunologic mechanisms play an important role in adverse drug effects. It has been estimated that up to 20% of adverse drug reactions are due to hypersensitivity, allergic, or immunologic mechanisms. (For purposes of our discussion, these terms are considered synonymous.)

Hypersensitivity drug reactions are the result of allergic sensitization in which antibodies (or immunologically active lymphocytes) to the drug or its metabolic products are formed. Most drugs are relatively simple chemicals in that their molecular weight is below 1000. Such chemicals are usually poor antigens and are not able to cause antibody formation. To produce sensitization small drug molecules must bind covalently with protein molecules to form an antigen. Once sensitization has taken place its duration is largely unpredictable and sensitivity to a particular compound or structurally related compound may never be lost.

Parker[26] has summarized current understanding of allergic adverse drug reactions. His review deals with antigen formation and processing, antibody formation and cell-mediated immunity, cross-allergenicity, and clinical manifestations of drug hypersensitivity reactions. For the purposes of this discussion, only a few classic hypersensitivity drug reactions will be mentioned.

Allergic reactions to penicillin are of particular interest, for it is estimated that between 20 and 50 tons of the antibiotic are sold annually in the United States and that 1 of every 4 persons receives treatment with it. Possibly as much as 90% of the drug is wasted in being prescribed when it is not indicated. Such prescribing contributes materially to the rising numbers of adverse reactions by facilitating sensitization.

The exact incidence of hypersensitivity to penicillins is not known. After exposure, the majority of the population will develop antibodies to penicillin. Most studies indicate that 1 to 10% of patients exposed to penicillin develop some type of clinical allergic reaction. One investigator reports that anaphylactic shock occurs in 0.1 to 0.3% of patients treated with penicillin and that fatal anaphylaxis occurs in 1 of about 50,000 patients.[27] It is frequently quoted that 300 people die in the United States each year because of penicillin anaphylaxis.

Ampicillin is a unique penicillin in that its propensity to cause drug rash is significantly higher than for other penicillins. Whether all ampicillin-induced rashes are immunologically mediated is not yet clear. Data from the BCDSP indicate that ampicillin-induced rash occurs in 5 to 9% of recipients, whereas rash due to other penicillins occurs in about 3% of recipients. Ampicillin rash may also be delayed, occurring after the first week of therapy.

Allergic reactions to penicillins vary from fever to fatal anaphylaxis. Between these extremes, the penicillins can induce the following reactions believed to be allergic in etiology: urticaria, asthma, angioedema, bullous eruptions, exfoliative dermatitis, erythema multiforme, Stevens-Johnson syndrome, fixed drug eruptions, hemolytic anemia, thrombocytopenia, lupus erythematosus-like syndrome, vasculitis, and others.

There is as yet no completely reliable and safe test to screen for patients who are susceptible to anaphylactic responses to penicillin. Much study has been directed to the development of intradermal tests utilizing penicillin's antigenic determinants. Skin patch or intradermal testing to identify allergy to other medications for the most part is of little to no value. Identification of patients with drug allergy rests with accurate history taking.

Idiopathic systemic lupus erythematosus (SLE) is an immunologic syndrome characterized by the deposition of immune complexes in small blood vessels in affected organs. Complex deposition and activation of complement results in inflammation and organ injury. Drug use has been associated with the development of SLE syndromes. Those drugs associated with SLE may be categorized into two groups. Procainamide, hydralazine, isoniazid, and the anticonvulsants are agents able to induce the clinical syndrome through some undetermined pharmacological property. These agents have produced SLE in a large number of cases and in most instances the syndrome developed after prolonged administration of large doses. The development of hydralazine-associated SLE is much more common in patients who are slow acetylators. Griseofulvin, oral contraceptives, penicillin, penicillamine, phenothiazines, thiouracils, and sulfonamides are examples of the second group of drugs which cause an allergic reaction and the development of autoantibodies usually without clinical symptoms. Only very few cases of clinical SLE have been reported for each drug in the second group. In drug-induced lupus syndromes, it is not clear if drugs alter host antigens or if alterations in the immune response are responsible for the serologic and clinical findings.

Ototoxicity Due to Drugs

A number of drugs are known to be *ototoxins*. Ototoxicity due to drugs may be manifested in two ways, depending on the portion of the inner ear affected. *Hearing loss* usually results from drugs affecting the *cochlea*, whereas *balance* may be affected by drug toxicity occurring in the *vestibular apparatus* of the inner ear. Manifestations of ototoxicity may range from mild tinnitus or dizziness to total bilateral irreversible hearing loss or permanent disabling vertigo. Drugs capable of producing permanent ototoxic changes usually produce neuroepithelium end-organ damage as contrasted to drugs which produce reversible impairment by transiently affecting inner-ear blood supply.

Of the drugs which cause permanent damage, the aminoglycoside antibiotics are the most hazardous. These agents (eg, neomycin) destroy the outer hair cells in the neuroepithelium of the cochlea in such a way that high-frequency hearing loss occurs first. Lower and mid-range frequencies or conversational tones are affected later. This phenomenon illustrates the benefits of audiometric testing as a routine monitoring tool, since measurable hearing loss could occur in many patients before they are aware of it.

Factors influencing development of ototoxicity secondary to the administration of aminoglycosides include: (1) dosage, (2) renal function, (3) age (older patients appear more susceptible, probably due to declining renal function), (4) route of administration (parenteral route usually required), and (5) simultaneous use of other ototoxins.

The ototoxic effects of streptomycin are primarily vestibular. Streptomycin destroys the neuroepithelium of the cristae of the semicircular canals. Balance abnormalities are said to occur in up to 90% of patients receiving 2 g daily for 1 month. Streptomycin is not as frequently employed in the treatment of tuberculosis as it once was. When used, dosages are reduced to one-half or less of known ototoxic doses. Careful monitoring of vestibular and renal function during therapy is essential.

Neomycin is the most ototoxic and nephrotoxic aminoglycoside antibiotic. Because of these toxicities and the availability of other agents, its systemic use is never indicated. Neomycin is partially absorbed after topical administration and poorly absorbed from the gastrointestinal tract. Absorption, however poor, does occur and in patients with compromised renal function the drug accumulates in the serum placing patients at risk of developing ototoxicity and additional renal injury. Ototoxicity is expressed as an auditory disturbance. Deafness is usually not reversible.

Kanamycin and viomycin are both ototoxic and nephrotoxic. Gentamicin differs from these agents in that its ototoxicity is primarily vestibular. Precautions as to dose, renal function, and concomitant therapy with other ototoxins must be observed when these agents are prescribed. Tobramycin may be less toxic to the inner ear than gentamicin. Clinical data developed thus far on amikacin indicate its ototoxic potential is equivalent to that of gentamicin.

The diuretic ethacrynic acid has been reported to produce both transient and permanent bilateral deafness. The toxic effect appears to be blood-level related and has usually been reported in patients with reduced renal function. Oral administration does not appear to produce blood levels high enough to induce such toxicity. Some reports describe enhanced ototoxicity when ethacrynic acid was administered with aminoglycoside antibiotics. Furosemide, administered in large intravenous doses, has produced hearing loss in azotemic patients. Peak serum levels have been correlated with development of toxicity and current dosing guidelines were prepared to avoid such effects.

Tinnitus or head noises is a well-known side effect of therapy with salicylates. Tinnitus is dose-related, with symptoms appearing at a serum level of 20 mg % or higher. These levels are in the therapeutic range for treating rheumatoid arthritis; many practitioners employ the development of auditory toxicity as a signal of appropriate drug dose. This may represent faulty technique in that some elderly patients, because of preexisting hearing deficiency, may not be able to hear tinnitus. *Bilateral hearing loss* may also occur in patients treated with salicylates. It is said to be a uniform finding at a salicylate serum level of 40 mg %. Aspirin- or salicylate-induced hearing loss is almost always completely reversible. Hearing returns within 24 to 72 hours after the drug is withdrawn. Reversibility of salicylate-induced hearing deficit supports the postulate that these compounds produce a mechanical disturbance of the blood supply in the cochlear system.

Oral contraceptives, nitrogen mustard, chloroquine, quinine, quinidine, and phenylbutazone are either suspect or proven to be ototoxic.

The BCDSP[28] has gathered at-risk data on the potential of hospitalized patients to suffer from drug-induced ototoxicity. In their series of over 11,000 monitored patients, 0.3% developed deafness attributed to drugs administered in the hospital. The causative drugs were aspirin, the aminoglycoside antibiotics, ethacrynic acid, and quinidine. Over 1% of patients exposed to aspirin developed transitory deafness (4.9% of patients receiving aspirin for rheumatoid arthritis developed ototoxicity); the mean plasma salicylate level at onset of deafness was 31 mg %. Four of 243 patients on kanamycin therapy developed deafness: 3 of the 4 patients had evidence of renal insufficiency. Two of 160 patients on gentamicin developed deafness, one had renal impairment and the other received topical gentamicin treatment for 21 days for extensive skin lesions. Six of 495 neomycin recipients developed deafness; all six suffered from advanced hepatic cirrhosis and four had evidence of renal compromise. Two of 165 patients receiving ethacrynic acid intravenously became deaf immediately after injection; in both cases the deafness lasted several hours before being completely resolved. Both patients had renal impairment. While drug-induced deafness could be considered a rare event in the total hospitalized population, subgroups of patients are at considerable risk, especially those receiving high doses of aspirin for rheumatoid arthritis and those with renal impairment receiving aminoglycoside antibiotics.

Ocular Toxicity Due to Drugs

Unfortunately the list of drugs toxic to the eye is impressively long. Such a list has been compiled[29] to remind prescribers of the propensity of both topically applied drugs and systemic medications to cause adverse ocular reactions. A list of "worst offenders" would include: anti-inflammatory agents of the aminoquinoline family (eg, chloroquine), phenothiazine tranquilizers (eg, chlorpromazine, thioridazine), and corticosteroids. The ocular toxicity of each of these will be briefly mentioned here.

Large numbers of military personnel and civilians have taken chloroquine for malaria therapy over the years. Ocular toxicity is not known to occur in this population receiving prophylactic or acute-treatment dosage therapy. Patients receiving chloroquine or related aminoquinolines for diseases such as systemic lupus erythematosus and rheumatoid arthritis take higher doses for prolonged periods and are at risk of developing ocular toxicity.

A few months of chloroquine therapy has been shown to produce corneal changes. Corneal deposits in a whorl-like pattern may be observed in patients who may be asymptomatic. Patients who have visual complaints may see halos around lights or may experience photophobia. Presence of corneal deposits is not an indication to stop chloroquine therapy for these changes completely disappear after the drug is stopped.

Retinal damage associated with chloroquine administration is the most severe manifestation of ocular toxicity induced by this agent. Chloroquine retinopathy, except if diagnosed in the earliest stages, is not reversible. Hundreds of cases of retinopathy associated with chloroquine therapy have been reported. Of major importance is that chloroquine-induced retinopathy at times can be objectively measured before symptoms appear, but in this asymptomatic stage the retinopathy may already be irreversible. In some cases retinopathy has been delayed, occurring after the drug is discontinued.

It is estimated that a total dose of more than 100 g during a period of one year must be taken for retinopathy to develop. The basic change is that of a pigmentary disturbance or alteration in the background pigmentation of the macular areas. Central vision and night vision are impaired in early stages.

In those rare instances where chloroquine or related agents would be considered useful for trial as anti-inflammatory therapy, a prerequisite before initiating therapy would be thorough base-line ophthalmic study with colored photograph of the retina. Similar evaluation must be made every 6 months in order to identify the earliest evidence of pigmentary disturbance.

Phenothiazine antipsychotic medications were first introduced in 1953. Many ocular side effects were readily recognized, including diplopia, myopia, and oculogyric crisis. These effects are dose-related and rapidly reverse on discontinuing therapy or reducing dosage. The long-term hazards of phenothiazines did not become appreciated until about 10 years after their introduction. The delay in recognizing ocular toxicity was probably due to the limitation of adequate examination of psychiatric patients and to the fact that ocular toxicity is related to the dose and the duration of therapy.

Corneal and lens opacities were first observed in institutionalized patients receiving usually over 300 mg of chlorpromazine daily for periods of 3 or more years. The sites of the lesions are the anterior lens and posterior cornea. This leads to the strong suggestion that phenothiazines or their metabolites accumulate in the anterior chamber and are responsible for the changes. Lenticular opacities may progress to form cataracts which can increase in size despite discontinuance of therapy.

In a few cases chlorpromazine has been reported to cause a retinal toxic effect; the doses in each instance were of the magnitude of 2.5 g daily for two or more years. Thioridazine, on the other hand, is associated with significant retinotoxicity; it (as well as other phenothiazines) accumulates in the choroid and retina. The high concentration of drug in the pigment cells presumably offers an explanation for the ocular toxic effect, and also suggests that the reason for the irreversibility of the lesion is the persistence of the drug in the retina. Markedly decreased visual acuity and impaired dark adaptation are early manifestations. Doses of thioridazine below 800 mg daily are considered low enough to avoid irreversible retinal toxicity.

Conjunctival pigmentation in the form of grayish brown discoloration is a dose-related adverse effect seen in conjunction with other phototoxic effects of phenothiazines.

Question has been raised as to whether or not there is an increased incidence of neuroophthalmological and occlusive vascular conditions in users of oral contraceptives. A causal relationship has not yet been confirmed even though there are some 80 reports in the literature discussing these effects.

Current labeling reads as follows: "Discontinue medication pending examination if there is a gradual or sudden, partial or complete loss of vision, or if there is a sudden onset of proptosis, diplopia, or migraine. If examination reveals papilledema or retinal vascular lesions, medication should be withdrawn."

A well-documented adverse effect of topically administered anti-inflammatory corticosteroids is their potential for increasing intraocular pressure. Intraocular pressure may increase after systemic therapy but this effect is much less common. Pressure increases occur in a matter of weeks after topical administration or, when they occur, in a matter of months after systemic therapy. Corticosteroid-induced glaucoma develops more commonly in families with histories of glaucoma. The increase in intraocular pressure reverses in the majority of patients on withdrawing the drug. If the pressure increases go unrecognized, irreversible damage identical to that produced by open-angle glaucoma can occur. Increased resistance to outflow of aqueous humor is probably the mechanism by which corticosteroids produce pressure rises. Efforts have been made to synthesize anti-inflammatory compounds which will not increase pressure, eg, fluorometholone and medrysone. These compounds do not cause the same degree of pressure increase as does dexamethasone. The extent of penetration of these drugs into ocular tissue is lessened and presumably this, as well as their decreased anti-inflammatory efficacy, accounts for the decreased pressure effect.

Posterior subcapsular cataract formation is a known complication of long-term high-dose systemic administration of corticosteroids. Generally, high doses for a period of a year or more are required for cataract production. Vision is not usually impaired initially. Regression of the cataract is not always noted when therapy is discontinued.

Chloramphenicol can produce *optic neuritis*. This effect was first observed in children with cystic fibrosis on large doses of chloramphenicol for periods up to two years. Peripheral neuritis, characterized by numbness and cramps of the feet and toes, may precede the optic neuritis by a week or two. Acute bilateral loss of visual acuity, with field constriction, are early symptoms. After therapy is discontinued, the prognosis for return of normal visual function is variable.

Optic neuritis and atrophy can occur after exposure to ethambutol which is used in the chemotherapy of tuberculosis. Decrease in visual acuity, central scotoma, and green-color blindness is seen at high doses, eg, 25 mg/kg/day.

The warning that anticholinergic drugs are contraindicated in glaucoma patients is considered valid by most clinicians and is present in all package inserts for such drugs. This conclusion appears to be based on the premise that these agents may induce increases in intraocular pressure of such magnitude as to be harmful to the eyes. Many reports have attempted to dispel these beliefs. Systemically administered anticholinergics have little effect on intraocular pressure in the nondiseased eye. In patients with open-angle glaucoma, rises in intraocular pressure are seen when patients ingest anticholinergics while not taking topical glaucoma medications. Reinstatement of topical therapy returns pressures to near-normal. Thus, anticholinergic therapy should not be withdrawn from patients with open-angle glaucoma who are being adequately treated for their disease. Patients with narrow filtration angles (ie, those with a predisposition for an attack of acute glaucoma) may have an attack of acute-angle closure glaucoma precipitated by doses of anticholinergic medications which are large enough to produce sustained wide mydriasis.

A comprehensive summary of the side effects of drugs in ophthalmology has been prepared by Fraunfelder[30] and should be consulted as further reading.

Pulmonary Diseases

Drug-induced lung disease may originate by direct actions of drugs or by indirect mechanisms. The latter include: (1) pulmonary edema caused by fluid overload, drugs containing substantial quantities of sodium, or drugs which decrease cardiac output; (2) oversedation resulting in hypoventilation or aspiration; (3) intravenous fluids and medications resulting in thrombophlebitis and pulmonary embolism; (4) agents capable of inciting anaphylactic responses causing bronchospasm. Pulmonary edema secondary to over-vigorous fluid therapy was reported to be one of the most common causes of death in hospitalized patients which could be attributed to drugs.

A relatively small list of agents are capable of causing *direct pulmonary toxicity*. Cytotoxic drugs head this list and are considered in the following: "Busulfan lung" is a syndrome of diffuse pulmonary fibrosis associated with long-term busulfan administration. Busulfan is agent of choice in the treatment of chronic myelogenous leukemia, in which prolonged maintenance therapy may be required. Usually 3 to 4 years of therapy is required before insidious onset of symptoms, such as cough, dyspnea, and fever are seen. Chest x-rays reveal diffuse interstitial and intra-alveolar fibrosis. The basic pathologic process is believed to be a chemical alveolitis with proliferation of surfactant-secreting cells followed by fibrosis. Fibrosis induced by busulfan is partially reversible on discontinuing the drug. A similar syndrome has been observed after cyclophosphamide therapy. Azathioprine has also been implicated.

Contrasted to the insidious and delayed onset of pulmonary symptoms associated with busulfan, methotrexate therapy may induce acute or subacute symptoms of fever, cough, and dyspnea. Bilateral diffuse and patchy infiltrates can occur days to months after initiating methotrexate therapy. The illness usually remits on cessation of therapy.

Bleomycin, a chemotherapeutic agent which is not toxic to bone marrow, has been associated with serious pulmonary side effects which develop in a high percentage of treated patients. The most frequent manifestation is pneumonitis, which occasionally progresses to pulmonary fibrosis which may result in death. Approximately 1% of patients treated during the clinical trials of the drug died of pulmonary fibrosis. Pulmonary toxicity is dose- and age-related; it is more common in patients over 70 years of age receiving over 400 mg of bleomycin as a total cumulative dose.

The triad of aspirin intolerance, asthma (bronchoconstriction), and nasal polyps is a well-known syndrome. Asthmatics sensitive to aspirin may comprise a unique group. These patients have usually suffered with nasal polyps and rhinitis before the onset of asthma; asthma begins in middle-life, and usually months or years pass before aspirin intolerance develops. Sodium salicylate does not show this effect. A similar syndrome has occurred with indomethacin and other nonsteroidal anti-inflammatory agents. The pharmaceutical dye tartrazine is also able to produce wheezing in this population. Currently it is suggested that aspirin and other prostaglandin synthesis inhibitors upset the natural balance of prostaglandins in the lung in favor of the F series which are bronchoconstrictors.

Nitrofurantoin is probably the most frequently reported agent implicated in lung disease. The drug can produce an acute pleural effusion associated with an eosinophilia. Characteristically, this reaction occurs 2 hours to 10 days after initiating therapy and is manifested by fever, chills, and dyspnea. A diffuse alveolar or alveolar-interstitial infiltrate is seen on chest X-ray; this usually clears 24 to 48 hours after withdrawing the drug. After chronic administration of nitrofurantoin, a much less common and distinct pulmonary reaction has been observed. This chronic toxicity begins insidiously with cough and dyspnea. Chest films reveal a diffuse interstitial fibrosis which may be partially reversible on discontinuing the drug.

Aminoglycoside antibiotics can induce neuromuscular blockade with subsequent respiratory muscle paralysis under the following conditions: (1) with increased blood levels secondary to renal compromise; (2) with simultaneous use of other skeletal-muscle relaxing agents; (3) with intravenous, intraperitoneal or intrapleural administration; (4) after accidental overdosage; (5) in patients with neuromuscular disease, such as myasthenia gravis.

Isoproterenol, when inhaled for its bronchiolar-relaxant effects, has been shown to increase paradoxically airway resistance in rare situations; the mechanism of this effect is unknown. It appears unrelated to tachyphylaxis and occurs most frequently in patients using aerosol preparations. The reaction may be allergic or may be due to conversion of isoproterenol to a metabolite with beta-adrenergic blocking properties.

Other agents known to produce pulmonary fibrosis include ganglionic blocking drugs, such as hexamethonium, which once enjoyed frequent use as an antihypertensive. Methysergide as well is known to be associated with pulmonary and pleural fibrosis.

Renal Diseases

A large and diverse group of chemicals can produce *kidney injury. Toxic nephropathy* or *drug-induced renal disease* is not rare. The kidney is particularly susceptible to the toxic effects of drugs and chemicals. The reasons for this susceptibility become obvious when one recalls that the kidneys comprise about 4% of body weight yet receive 25% of the cardiac output. This large blood supply exposes the kidney to high concentrations of toxic products. The kidneys are concentrating organs responsible for filtration, secretion, and excretion of body water and ingested chemical substances. Having a large endothelial surface area makes the kidney especially susceptible to deposition of antigen-antibody complexes.

Schreiner[31] classified drugs which induce toxic nephropathy as follows: *Class 1*, drugs exerting a direct, morphologically identifiable effect, eg, mercury compounds. *Class 2*, drugs producing a hypersensitivity reaction observable as the nephrotic syndrome, eg, penicillamine and trimethadione. *Class 3*, drugs producing a hypersensitivity reaction of the vasculitis type involving the kidney, eg, sulfonamides. *Class 4*, drugs which may produce chronic nephrotoxicity after months or years of exposure, eg, analgesic nephropathy. *Class 5*, drugs capable of aggravating preexisting renal disease, eg, diuretics.

Metallic mercury and mercurial diuretics are well-known tubular toxins. Other heavy metals, including lead, bismuth, and gold salts, are also nephrotoxic. While the clinical use of mercurial diuretics has declined due to the advent of more effective and less toxic compounds, the use of gold salts has again gained popularity in the treatment of rheumatoid arthritis. Gold salts rarely produce direct tubular toxicity. More commonly, presumably by immunologic mechanisms, gold therapy may produce the nephrotic syndrome. Lithium administered in the treatment of manic depressive disorders has been reported to produce a nephrogenic diabetes insipidus-like syndrome. Heavy metal antagonists (EDTA and penicillamine) are known renal toxins. Twenty percent of penicillamine recipients are said to develop a nephrotic syndrome during therapy.

The largest single grouping of therapeutic agents capable of producing renal disease are the antibiotics. The relative toxicities of antibiotic drugs capable of inducing renal diseases have been summarized.[32] Penicillins are among the least

nephrotoxic antibiotics in use today. The relatively few cases of renal toxicity due to penicillins described in the literature are characterized by polyarteritis and glomerulonephritis.

Nephropathy due to methicillin is well documented yet, considering the large amounts used since its introduction in 1961, this reaction must be considered as rare. Methicillin and other semisynthetic penicillins including ampicillin, nafcillin, oxacillin, and carbenicillin, are capable of producing interstitial nephritis and tubular damage with an interstitial inflammatory reaction consisting of mononuclear cells and eosinophils. The major hapten of methicillin and IgG has been demonstrated on the tubular basement membrane. Methicillin-induced interstitial nephritis is associated with daily doses in excess of 6 g for several weeks. Recovery usually occurs after therapy is stopped.

From the ever-increasing list of cephalosporin/cephamycin antibiotics, cephaloridine is generally recognized as the cephalosporin with the most significant nephrotoxicity. In patients with normal renal function, doses of cephaloridine in excess of 4 g per day can lead to renal insufficiency. Toxicity is manifested as proximal tubular cell necrosis. Additive toxicity may be produced when cephaloridine is administered with furosemide or ethacrynic acid. For these reasons, cephaloridine has fallen out of use. Some reports suggest that cephalothin may enhance the toxicity of aminoglycoside antibiotics. If cephalothin has nephrotoxic potential when used alone, the incidence of this toxicity must be extremely low. Cephalexin (an oral cephalosporin) has only rarely been implicated in renal disease. Cefazolin, cephapirin, cephamandole, and cefoxitin have not yet been implicated as being able to produce kidney damage in man.

The aminoglycoside and polymyxin antibiotics are capable of producing a significant incidence of nephrotoxicity when given at normal dose levels. Certain generalities may be made relative to each member of these classes of compounds. All are absorbed poorly from the gastrointestinal tract, and clinical use is confined (except for local gastrointestinal effects) to parenteral administration for severe gram-negative infections. Excretion is primarily via the kidney and dosage modifications are required when they are used in patients with renal compromise. Nephrotoxicity is observable as proximal tubular necrosis.

Several patient or therapy variables have been associated with the development of gentamicin-induced renal damage. These are: prolonged duration of therapy, reduced renal function, advanced age, presence of persistent valley serum concentrations greater than 2 μg/mL, combined use with other nephrotoxins, persistent peak serum levels greater than 10 to 12 μg/mL, reduced hematocrit, low serum-protein levels, and metabolic acidosis. While some of these factors implicated in the causation of gentamicin-induced renal disease are debated, they are useful to demonstrate the common complexity of clinical situations which surround this side effect. Considerable debate exists as to the relative nephrotoxic potential of gentamicin, tobramycin, and amikacin.

Many schemes have been published to assist in the adjustment of drug dosage in patients with impaired renal function. While these sources provide useful information, it is best to adjust the dose of antibiotics on the basis of serum-antibiotic level monitoring when possible.

Amphotericin B is a lifesaving drug but a potent nephrotoxin. It is estimated that over 80% of patients receiving intravenous amphotericin B for systemic fungal infections develop decreased renal function. Amphotericin B has the ability to produce renal vasoconstriction and is also a tubular toxin. Nephrotoxicity is dose-related.

There is still lack of agreement concerning the precise etiology of the disease process first described in 1953 and now termed *analgesic abuse nephropathy*. Controversy revolves around factors such as the primary causative agent or agents,

DRUG EXPERIENCE REPORT
(IN CONFIDENCE)

Form Approved
OMB No. 57 - R0071

PATIENT INITIALS (Optional)	AGE	SEX	DATE OF REACTION ONSET
		☐ M ☐ F	

SUSPECTED REACTION(S) (We have particular interest in serious, rare and unusual reactions.)

SUSPECTED DRUG(S); TRADE/GENERIC NAME (Manufacturer's name, if possible)

DISORDER OR REASON FOR USE OF DRUG(S) (Optional)	ROUTE	TOTAL DAILY DOSE	DATES OF ADMINISTRATION

OTHER DRUGS TAKEN CONCOMITANTLY

COMMENTS (Optional)

PHYSICIAN'S NAME, ADDRESS, AND ZIP CODE

FORM FD 1639a (6/74)   PREVIOUS EDITION MAY BE USED.

Fig 69-1

the reasons for a particular geographical distribution of cases, the mechanism by which toxicity is produced, etc. The interested reader is referred to reviews for a comprehensive assessment of analgesic-induced nephrotoxicity.[33-35]

There is much epidemiologic, experimental, and clinical evidence which suggests a causal relationship between prolonged consumption of analgesics and renal disease. The analgesics most commonly incriminated are phenacetin (hence the term phenacetin nephropathy), aspirin, caffeine, and codeine. Widespread consumption of mixtures of these compounds, often for obscure or nonmedical reasons, has fostered the development of the term "analgesic abuse." The dose of analgesic mixtures needed before one can be considered an "analgesic-abuser," and therefore be at risk of developing analgesic nephropathy, is unknown. Estimates of 1 g daily for 1 year of salicylates, phenacetin, or mixtures, or 1 kg of these compounds ingested over any period of time, have been offered as borderline doses.

The type of renal disease associated with excessive analgesic consumption is renal papillary necrosis with cortical changes of chronic interstitial nephritis occurring secondarily. The mechanism by which analgesics produce damage is not understood. Cellular oxidative damage from salicylate inhibition of G-6-PD is being considered. In the US, analgesic abuse was thought to be a rare cause of renal damage. Evidence that 5% of all cases of chronic renal failure is due to

analgesic abuse has been reported in the US. In countries which have limited the sale of analgesic mixtures, the incidence of renal disease has appeared to decline.

Radiopaque contrast media, trimethadione, paramethadione, methoxyflurane, acetazolamide, and platinum should be included in a list of agents with recognized nephrotoxic potential.

Teratogenic Drugs

The present status of drugs as teratogens has been summarized by Hollingsworth[36] and O'Brien and McManus.[37] Several epidemiologic investigations have documented a continuing large exposure to drug substances during pregnancy. While drug effects in the fetus can include growth retardation or behavior retardation, this discussion will emphasize structural malformations induced by drugs.

It should be appreciated that for a drug to produce a teratogenic response it must be given during the period of organogenesis. This organ-forming period, from 13 to 56 days, is the period of susceptibility. Exposure earlier can result in embryocidal effects. A single teratogen can produce multiple malformations and a single malformation may be induced by a number of teratogens. Drug-induced malformations are the same as those which occur spontaneously (ie, drugs do not produce unique birth defects).

DEPARTMENT OF HEALTH AND HUMAN SERVICES
PUBLIC HEALTH SERVICE
FOOD AND DRUG ADMINISTRATION
ROCKVILLE' MD 20857

DRUG EXPERIENCE REPORT

FORM APPROVED: OMB NO. 0910-0002
Use of this form is prohibited after 12/31/84.

FDA CONTROL NO.

ACCESSION NO.

I.   REACTION INFORMATION

1. PATIENT ID/INITIALS (In Confidence)	2. AGE	3. SEX	4. WGT.	5. HT.	6. REPORTING DATE			7. REACTION ONSET DATE		
					MO	DA	YR	MO	DA	YR

8. DESCRIBE SUSPECTED REACTION(S)

9. OUTCOME OF REACTION TO DATE

☐ Alive with sequelae
☐ Recovered
☐ Still under treatment for reaction
☐ Died (Give cause/date)

10. TESTS/LABORATORY DATA CONFIRMING REACTION (Include biopsy and/or autopsy results)

11. WAS OUTPATIENT TREATMENT FOR REACTION REQUIRED?
☐ Yes   ☐ No

12. WAS HOSPITAL TREATMENT FOR REACTION REQUIRED?
☐ Yes   ☐ No

II.   SUSPECT DRUG(S) INFORMATION

13. SUSPECT DRUG(S) - TRADE/GENERIC NAME(S), MANUFACTURER, IND/NDA NO.

14. TOTAL DAILY DOSE

15. ROUTE OF ADMINISTRATION

16. INDICATION(S) FOR USE

17. THERAPY DATES *(From/To)*

18. THERAPY DURATION

19a. WAS TREATMENT WITH SUSPECTED DRUG REDUCED IN DOSAGE?	19b. DID REACTION ABATE?	20a. WAS DRUG REINTRODUCED OR DOSE INCREASED?	20b. DID REACTION REAPPEAR?
☐ Yes ☐ No			
OR: ☐ Discontinued	☐ Yes ☐ No	☐ Yes ☐ No	☐ Yes ☐ No

III.   RECENT/CONCOMITANT DRUGS AND MEDICAL PROBLEMS

21. OTHER DRUGS	TOTAL DAILY DOSE	ROUTE	DATES/DURATION OF ADMINISTRATION	INDICATIONS

22. DESCRIBE OTHER RELEVANT MEDICAL HISTORY (i.e., allergies, environmental or occupational exposure, previous drug reactions, pregnancy with gravidity/parity, ethnic origin.)

Your cooperation is needed to insure comprehensive, accurate, and timely use and interpretation of these data.

23. MFR NAME/ADDRESS	24. Check one	25. REPORTER'S NAME AND ADDRESS (In confidence)
	☐ Initial Report	
MFR CONTROL NO. DATE SENT TO FDA	☐ Follow-up Report	

NOTE: *Required of manufacturers by 21 CFR 310.300, 310.301 and 431.60. Manufacturers may attach additional clinical material and product analyses at their discretion.*

26. MAY THE SOURCE OF THIS REPORT BE RELEASED TO THE ARMED FORCES INSTITUTE OF PATHOLOGY? ☐ Yes ☐ No

FORM FDA 1639 (1/82)   PREVIOUS EDITIONS ARE OBSOLETE.

Fig 69-1   (contd)

Fetal exposure to drugs occurs by passage of drug substances through the maternal placental-fetal unit. It was once thought that a barrier existed to the passage of a large number of drug substances. The "barrier" is best thought of as a "coarse sieve."

Thalidomide is the best recognized teratogen. Thirty to

INSTRUCTIONS FOR COMPLETING FORM FDA 1639

Use a separate report form for each case. If more space is needed, additional pages may be attached.

I. Patient/Reaction Information (Items 1-12)

1. Patient ID/Initials: Record **patient's** identification (i.e. medical record number, initials, etc). *(This information is kept in confidence by the FDA.)*

2. Age: Record the age of the patient. When reporting a congenital malformation, record the age of the **mother.**

3. Sex: Record the sex of the patient. When reporting a congenital malformation, record the sex of the **baby.**

4. Weight: Record the weight of the patient in pounds. When reporting a congenital malformation, record the weight of the **mother.**

5. Height: Record the height of the patient in inches. When reporting a congenital malformation, record the height of the **mother.**

6. Reporting Date: Record the date when the report was initially communicated to the manufacturer.

7. Reaction Onset Date: Record the date on which the reaction was first observed or detected.

8. Suspected Reaction(s): Describe the signs, symptoms and course of the drug related event in the terminology used by the original observer of the reaction. (**Coding terms** e.g. COSTART, SNOMED, etc. may also be noted, but only **in addition** to original description.)

9. Outcome of Reaction: Indicate the status of the patient as of date indicated in Item 23. If the patient died, give the cause and date of death. Include discharge summary and/or autopsy findings, if available.

10. Tests/Laboratory Data: Describe the results of **all** diagnostic tests and exams (e.g. biochemical tests, x-rays, endoscopy, biopsy, etc.) which were done as a result of the event described in Item 8. Pertinent base line values and laboratory normals should be included with each test or exam reported. If this information is not available at the time of the initial report, a follow up report should be submitted.

11. Treatment Required: If "yes", a short description of treatment should be included in Item 8.

12. Hospitalization Required: If "yes", a short description of the treatment should be included in Item 8.

II. Suspect Drug Information (Items 13-20)

13. Suspect Drug(s): Record the trade name. The generic name should be used only when the trade name is not known. Include IND/NDA number of the drug as well as the lot number, when available.

14. Total Daily Dose: Record the total daily dose as of the date recorded in Item 7. If drug(s) was given in a different dose or form on a previous occasion, include dates and total daily dose for each drug exposure.

15. Route of Administration: Record the route of administration (i.e. po, IM, IV) as of the date recorded in Item 7.

16. Indication(s) for use: Record intended use in accepted medical terminology.

17. Therapy Dates: Give starting and stopping dates of administration for each drug listed in Item 13.

18. Therapy Duration: Give duration of therapy in days.

19. Dechallenge:
    (a) Applicable if the suspect drug(s) was either reduced in dosage or discontinued.
    (b) If 19(a) is checked, indicate whether the reaction subsided upon reduced dosage or discontinuation of the drug.

20. Rechallenge:
    (a) Applicable if the suspect drug was reintroduced to the patient's therapy after dechallenge.
    (b) If 20(a) is "yes", indicate whether or not the reaction reappeared upon rechallenge with the drug.

III. Recent/Concomitant Drugs and Medical Problems (Items 21-22)

21. List all recent or concomitant drugs. Include the total daily dose(s), indication(s) for use, route(s) of administration and dates of administration and/or duration of therapy for each drug.

22. Describe other relevant medical conditions or problems which could have contributed to the reaction. Include pertinent medical history such as allergies, occupation, industrial hazards, diet, smoking, climate, ethnic origin, cosmetics and biologicals. When reporting a congenital malformation, include the date of the last menstrual period of the mother, gravidity, parity and previous abortions.

IV. Other Information (Items 23-26)

23. Manufacturers Information: Include manufacturer's name, address, control number and date report is sent to FDA. This control number is the identifying number assigned by the manufacturer to the report for internal record control.

24. Indicate if this is an initial submission to FDA or a follow-up of a previously submitted Form FDA 1639. If this is a follow-up attach copy of initial report.

25. Record the name, title and address of the practitioner originating the report. *(This information is kept in confidence by the FDA.)*

26. Check "yes" or "no", if the source of this report may or may not be released to the Armed Forces Institute of Pathology for further study and follow-up. This is encouraged whenever possible.

Fig 69-1   (contd)

forty percent of mothers who ingested this drug during the critical period of their pregnancies bore defective babies. Thalidomide primarily produced phocomelia which is a term describing the absence or deformity of limbs.

The sex steroid hormones are teratogens in man. Masculinization of the female fetus can result after *in utero* exposure to androgens and some synthetic progestins. Inadvertent use of combination oral contraceptive hormones in early pregnancy has recently been associated with an increase in the number of children born with cardiovascular defects.

The association between maternal ingestion of the non-steroidal estrogen diethylstilbestrol during pregnancy and the development of adenocarcinoma of the vagina in female offspring is not strictly speaking a teratogenic effect yet it raises questions about the relationship of chemical teratogenesis and chemical carcinogenesis. A high percentage of women exposed to diethylstilbestrol *in utero* have readily recognizable vaginal tract abnormalities. Cytotoxic drugs, as expected, are toxic to the developing embryo and fetus. It has recently come to light that moderate alcohol ingestion during pregnancy can lead to what is now termed the "fetal alcohol syndrome." Features include failure of intrauterine growth, postnatal growth deficiency, mental retardation, and structural deformities of the eyes, face and heart.

Certain anticonvulsants are recognized teratogens. Children have been born with the "hydantoin syndrome" and "trimethadione syndrome."

Conflicting reports implicate the amphetamine-like anorexigenic agents as a cause of congenital heart malformations and other defects. No justification exists for use of these compounds in pregnancy. Minor tranquilizers of the benzodiazepine class and meprobamate have been associated with the production of oral clefts in children so exposed. Their use in pregnancy cannot be condoned.

Many, many other compounds including aspirin, gaseous anesthetics, barbiturates, imipramine, haloperidol, quinine, warfarin, and antithyroid medications are currently considered to have teratogenic potential.

A perinatal pharmacology text provides the interested reader further insight into this important area of therapeutics.[38] Also, a computerized compilation of drug monographs, dealing with the teratogenic potential of drugs, has been prepared; this catalog will be revised frequently to assist those interested in obtaining the latest information on drugs associated with congenital anomalies in animals and in humans.[39]

Voluntary Adverse Reaction Reporting

The spontaneous reporting of adverse drug reactions by the practicing physician to the Food and Drug Administration has not been effective. Fewer than 300 reports from individual practitioners were submitted to FDA in 1972. Often the reports submitted contained incomplete data, necessitating follow-up by FDA officials.

In January of 1973, a new drug-experience form was introduced by the FDA through its Division of Drug Experience, with the hope of increasing compliance with the Administration's adverse drug-monitoring program. This new form (FD-1639A) was widely publicized and distributed to practitioners nationwide (see Fig 69-1). By using this much-abbreviated form, it was hoped that marked increases in the quantity and quality of adverse-reaction information will be compiled. When a report is submitted, it is acknowledged and a replacement form is promptly mailed to the reporter. Each report is evaluated by the medical staff in the Division of Drug Experience. If additional information is required, appropriate follow-up is initiated. All reports are entered into a computer system for subsequent retrieval and analysis. This new program apparently has been received with renewed enthusiasm since increased participation in reporting has been noted. FDA's long form (FD-1639) is still preferred for institutional (or manufacturer, mandatory) reporting. Note that the form shown in Fig 69-2 and 69-3 will be void after 12/31/84.

As discussed earlier, spontaneous reporting mechanisms cannot alone solve the problems associated with drug use. These programs will not provide an adequate determination of reaction incidence, nor an estimate of the population at risk. There remains, however, no better way of identifying a rarely occurring adverse event that may pose a major threat to public health. Health practitioners should be encouraged to participate in this program to the fullest extent possible.

Aside from the voluntary reporting system, FDA uses four other sources for monitoring adverse drug effects. These include contract intensive drug monitoring studies (eg, the BCDSP), special epidemiologic studies, communications with the WHO and other national drug-monitoring centers, and screening published literature.

Role of the Pharmacist

The role of the pharmacist continues to change dramatically. In many settings the pharmacist has a profound influence on drug product selection and drug administration. Through efforts in designing and implementing safe drug-delivery systems, the pharmacist has made great strides in reducing medication errors. Many new systems are especially designed to provide for therapy monitoring for beneficial and adverse drug effects. In the institutional setting, many pharmacists participate directly in the evaluation of new drugs to assure that only those drugs which are most effective and least toxic are included in institutional formularies. The responsibility of providing accurate, unbiased drug information has long been recognized as an important role of both community and hospital pharamcists. Questions concerning adverse effects of drugs comprise a major portion of drug information requested of many pharmacists involved in institutional and community patient care. Another very important role for the pharmacist is in improving patient understanding of prescribed medication regimens so that appropriate and safe compliance will be assured. Drug-audit and drug-utilization review programs to effect quality patient care are being designed for use in many settings. The role of the pharmacist in the detection, evaluation, and prevention of adverse reactions has become a major part of the routine of many pharmacists involved in both institutionalized and ambulatory patient care.

The concerned pharmacist knowledgeable in the area of adverse drug effects will have ever expanded opportunities in the future to become increasingly involved in programs which will help to reduce the patient care and economic consequences of this therapeutic dilemma.

Role of the Physician

Today, physicians have the ultimate responsibility of maintaining sound pharmacological knowledge as a requisite to assuring safe and effective therapeutics. Before pen is placed on the prescription blank or order sheet, specific objectives of the anticipated therapy must be reviewed and benefit-to-risk ratio considered for all drugs prescribed. The practice of polypharmacy contributes to high incidence of reaction rates. The urge to supply pharmacological agents to remedy all situations must be subdued.

References

1. Jick H: *New Engl J Med 291:* 824, 1974.
2. Schimmel EM: *Ann Int Med 60:* 100, 1964.
3. Cluff LE, *et al: J Am Med Assoc 188:* 144, 1964.
4. Karch FE, Lasagna L: *J Am Med Assoc 234:* 1236, 1975.
5. Miller RR: *Am J Hosp Pharm 30:* 584, 1973.
6. Cohen MR: *Hosp Pharm 12:* 455, 1977.
7. Miller RR, Greenblatt DJ: *Drug Effects in Hospitalized Patients*, Wiley, New York, 1976.
8. Slone D, *et al: Ibid. 209:* 1668, 1969.
9. Porter J, Jick H: *J Am Med Assoc 237:* 879, 1977.
10. Caranosos GJ, *et al: Arch Int Med 136:* 872, 1976.
11. Miller RR: *Arch Int Med 134:* 219, 1974.
12. Caranosos GJ, *et al: J Am Med Assoc 228:* 713, 1974.
13. Arndt KA, Jick H: *J Am Med Assoc 235:* 918, 1976.
14. Cram DL: *Drug Therap 3:* 31, 1973.
15. Zimmerman HJ: *Med Clin N Am 59:* 897, 1975.
16. *Medical Letter 20:* 61, 1978.
17. MacFarlaine MD, McCarron MM: *Drug Intel 6:* 310, 1972.
18. McAvoy JM, Tompkins RK, Longmire WP: *Arch Surg 111:* 761, 1976.
19. Cooke AR: *Drugs 11:* 36, 1976.

20. Leonards JR, Levy G: *Arch Int Med 129:* 457, 1972.
21. Levy M: *New Eng J Med 290:* 1158, 1974.
22. *BCDSP Clin Pharm Therap 13:* 694, 1972.
23. Conn HO, Blitzer BL: *New Eng J Med 294:* 473, 1976.
24. Williams DM, *et al: Sem Hematol 10:* 195, 1973.
25. Yunis AA: *Ibid. 10:* 225, 1973.
26. Parker CW: *New Eng J Med 292:* 512, *292:* 732, *292:* 957, 1975.
27. Isbister JP: *Med J Aus 1* (part 2): 1067, 1971.
28. BCDSP, *J Am Med Assoc 224:* 515, 1973.
29. *Medical Letter 18:* 63, 1976.
30. Fraunfelder FF: *Drug-Induced Ocular Side Effects and Drug Interactions*, Lea and Febiger, Philadelphia, 1976.
31. Schreiner GE: *Progr Biochem Pharmacol 7:* 248, 1972.
32. Appel GB, New HC: *New Eng J Med 296:* 663, *296:* 722, *296:* 784, 1977.
33. Goldberg M, Murray TG: *New Eng J Med 299:* 716, 1978.
34. Brad J, *et al: Nephron 19:* 311, 1977.
35. Kincaid-Smith P, *et al: Kidney Int 13:* 1, 1978.
36. Hollingsworth M: *Clin Ob Gyn 4:* 503, 1977.
37. O'Brien TE, McManus CE: *US Pharm 2:* 36, 1977.
38. Mirkin BL: *Perinatal Pharmacology and Therapeutics*, Academic Press, New York, 1976.
39. Shepard TH: *Catalog of Teratogenic Agents*, 2nd ed, Johns Hopkins Press, Baltimore, 1976.

Bibliography

Miller RR, Greenblatt DJ: *Drug Effects in Hospitalized Patients*, Wiley, New York, 1976.

Cluff LE, *et al: Clinical Problems with Drugs*, Saunders, Philadelphia, 1975.

Melman KL, Morrelli HF: *Clinical Pharmacology*, Chapter 20, Macmillan, New York, 1978.

Swanson M, Cook R: *Drugs, Chemicals and Blood Dyscrasias*, Drug Intelligence, Hamilton, IL, 1977.

Dukes MNG: *Meyler's Side Effects of Drugs*, Excerpta Medica, Amsterdam, 1975.

Dukes MNG: *Side Effects of Drugs*, Annual I, Excerpta Medica, Amsterdam, 1977 (and subsequent editions).

Davies DM: *Textbook of Adverse Drug Reactions*, Oxford University Press, Oxford, 1977.

CHAPTER 70

Pharmacogenetics

John P Tischio, PhD

Director of Clinical Testing
Pragma Bio-Tech, Inc
Bloomfield, NJ 07003

Perhaps the most fascinating dimension in drug reactions was the identification of a relationship between enzyme systems and drug effects. Large interindividual differences that occur in the disposition of many drugs are controlled in part by genetic factors. Genetic variations that reflect themselves in different rates of drug elimination from the body among normal subjects help to explain the markedly different dosage requirements in many patients. Thus, there is an apparent need to individualize doses of commonly used medication. In 1959 Vogel introduced the term pharmacogenetics into clinical medicine. This was defined as "the study of genetically determined variations that are revealed solely by the effects of drugs." The genetic aberration results in the absence or insufficiency of certain specific enzyme systems. [Terms used throughout this chapter are defined in the glossary (Table I) in this chapter.]

The phenomenon of *polymorphism* is directly involved in pharmacogenetics. This phenomenon recognizes the coexistence of individuals with obviously distinct qualities as normal members of a population. Since individuals are heterozygous at many genetic loci (heterogeneous alleles) the implication that genetics is responsible in part for the varied responses observed to drugs is reasonable. Classically, recognition of a polymorphic condition has been achieved by demonstrating electrophoretic differences among the enzymes under consideration. Pharmacogenetics demonstrates a polymorphic condition by revealing sharply distinct responses to drugs.

In general, if the blood level of a drug is measured at a predetermined time after administration of a standard dose to many individuals, a single, bell-shaped curve (unimodal distribution) is usually observed (Fig 70-1A). This distribution is a result in part of the heterogeneous kinetic nature of the enzymes involved in the biotransformation of the drug among the population. Some people will metabolize the drug faster (exhibiting lower blood levels of drug), some slower (exhibiting higher blood levels of drug), and the majority of the population will metabolize the drug at an "average" rate (exhibiting "average" blood levels of drug). This small variation effect reflects the heterozygosity of the genes in the population.

In contrast, if instead of a unimodal distribution a bimodal or trimodal (two or three bell-shaped curves, respectively) distribution is observed (Fig 70-1B and C, respectively) then a more remarkable variation among the genes responsible for the enzymes metabolizing the drug in the population is implied. These larger, more demonstrable, genetic variations have played a major role in directing the recognition of pharmacogenetics as a factor in the varied responses and adverse effects observed with drugs.

The phenomenon of pharmacogenetics has been cited as one major manifestation of the extraordinary human variability in response to conventional doses of common drugs. Among many situations that may be considered and questions raised, if Drug A is given to a patient with a congenital disorder of specific enzymes, what might happen if that drug inhibits or stimulates enzymes responsible for the metabolism of Drug B given concurrently? To provide a better understanding of such situations, a summary of some notable examples of pharmacogenetic conditions with their apparent enzyme deficiencies, modes of inheritance, frequency, and drug sensitivities is given in Table II. Some of these disorders, and also others, are discussed below.

The historical and classical prototype of a pharmacogenetic disease is the *hemolytic anemia* suffered by some members of certain ethnic groups—specifically, Mediterranean-basin dwellers, rarely Scandinavians, and Negroes, who have a

Table I—Glossary of Terms

Allele: One of two or more alternative forms of a gene at the same site in a chromosome that determines alternative characteristics in inheritance.

Autosome: One of 22 pairs of chromosomes not connected with the determination of the sex of the individual.

Autosomal dominant: A trait that is expressed in the heterozygous state.

Autosomal recessive: A trait that is expressed only in the homozygous state.

Enzyme: A polypeptide or protein with catalytic properties.

Gene: A DNA segment in a chromosome that carries the information necessary to direct the synthesis of a single polypeptide chain.

Heterozygous: Having different alleles at the genetic locus determining a given character.

Homozygous: Having identical alleles at the genetic locus determining a given character.

Isoenzyme: Electrophoretically distinct forms of an enzyme with identical function.

Phenotype: The visible or noticeable expression of a gene.

Polymorphism: The coexistence of individuals with distinct qualities as normal members of a population.

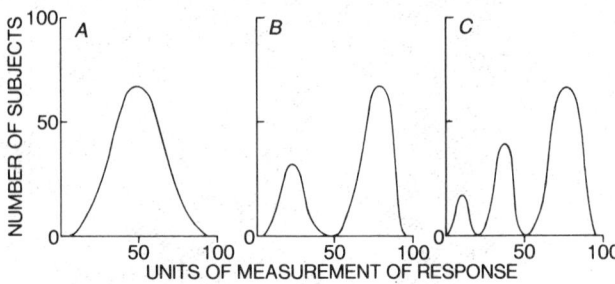

Fig 70-1. Three genetically distinct distribution curves for response to a drug by individuals in a population: *A* unimodal; *B* bimodal; *C* trimodal.

quantitative or qualitative deficiency of glucose 6-phosphate dehydrogenase. Brisk hemolysis may follow exposure to many common therapeutic agents (among these are the 4-aminoquinolines, certain sulfonamides, aspirin, nitrofurantoins, sulfones, aminosalicylic acid, phenacetin, acetanilid, propantheline, and the water-soluble analogues of vitamin K).

The cause of this hemolysis is a genetically transmitted defect that results in varying degrees of deficiency (quantitative or qualitative) of this intraerythrocytic enzyme. The sequence of amino acids of this enzyme is specified by a gene on the X chromosome.[1] At least 80 different mutations affecting the activity of this enzyme have been identified, most of the work having been focused on the deficiencies found in the African and Mediterranean populations. Such patients are normal clinically; they have no morphologic or physiologic abnormality of their red cells, until one of the provocative drugs is given. Then brisk hemolysis occurs. Parenthetically, deficiency of glucose 6-phosphate dehydrogenase has been cited as one cause of neonatal jaundice.

Glucose 6-phosphate dehydrogenase was somewhat of a problem in the chloroquine-primaquine antimalarial prophylaxis program in Southeast Asia. Soldiers known to suffer clinical manifestations of this disorder were restricted from duty in endemic malarious areas.

"Blue soldiers" suffer from congenital intraerythrocytic enzyme insufficiency. It was discovered that congenital heterologous methemoglobin reductase insufficiency can cause significant methemoglobinemia when such individuals are given routine antimalarial prophylaxis with chloroquine, primaquine, and dapsone (DDS), among other drugs. In addition, there is a phenacetin-induced methemoglobinemia condition which appears to be due to a deficiency of a microsomal enzyme system that de-ethylates the drug.[2]

If a certain Swiss family had not been given sulfonamide drugs, it is quite likely that an abnormal hemoglobin disease, *Hemoglobin Zurich* would have continued to escape detection. A frank hemolytic anemia developed after administration of sulfadimethoxine and sulfamethoxypyridazine to family members. A unique hemoglobin with electrophoretic mobility between A and S was identified.

Patients with Hemoglobin H Disease (an alpha-thalassemia variant) have hemoglobin which is a tetramer of four beta-chains. Their erythrocytes appear normal until they are given sulfisoxazole; then an acute hemolytic anemia may develop.

Other red-cell enzyme deficiencies of great subtlety have begun to emerge; these include aldolase, catalase, hexokinase, glutathione reductase, phosphoglucomutase, pyruvate kinase, triose phosphatases, and isomerases. Almost every enzyme involved in the Emden-Meyerhof (anaerobic) glycolytic pathway has come under scrutiny in the evaluation of the role of drugs capable of precipitating clinically significant hemolysis.

In a similar vein, one cause of *kernicterus* in the premature infant is related to immaturity of the neonatal liver. This organ is deficient in glucuronyl transferase and therefore feeble in its effort to conjugate bilirubin. Administration of sulfisoxazole or vitamin K analogues exaggerates this reaction. Novobiocin may provoke jaundice in the newborn (and rarely in adults) by direct inhibition of glucuronyl transferase. The "gray syndrome" of neonates may be related to a defect in chloramphenicol metabolism due to immaturity of hepatic microsomal enzymes.

It is known that there is a variation in the ability of certain patients to metabolize isoniazid (INH), sulfamethoxazole, and hydralazine. Such individuals are classified into phenotypes on the basis of their ability to acetylate these drugs. "Slow acetylators" have a deficiency of hepatic acetyl transferase. They maintain higher concentrations of unacetylated drugs for longer periods in body fluids than "rapid acetylators."

The variation of frequency of this disorder in different populations is very interesting although the significance of its prevalence remains obscure.[3] The incidence of slow acetylators among Canadian Eskimos is about 5% of the population whereas Egyptians rank highest with 83% of their population affected. Most European-origin populations, including Americans, have a 50% chance of having this condition.

In the case of isoniazid it is not surprising that "slow acetylators" suffer a greater incidence of adverse drug reactions due to isoniazid than do the other group. Unduly sustained and elevated blood levels of isoniazid is the current explanation for the initiation of the sequence of events that causes the CNS-damage and polyneuropathy found in slow acetylators of isoniazid. Fortunately, there is no difference in therapeutic responsiveness, and the development of resistance by the tubercle bacillus to isoniazid is similar in both phenotypes.

In another study, investigation of the monoamine-oxidase-inhibitor antidepressant phenelzine revealed that significantly more severe adverse drug reactions were observed in a group of "slow acetylators" than in a group of "rapid acetylators." Adverse drug reactions consisted of drowsiness, nausea, dizziness, and constipation—again related to sustained levels due to slow acetylation.

Other drugs metabolised by the enzyme N-acetyl transferase are also associated with severe side-effects. For example, lupus erythmatous-like reactions to hydralazine are observed mainly in slow acetylators. On the other hand, with procainamide, the same syndrome seems to be more prevalent in rapid acetylators, suggesting that the acetylated metabolite of procainamide is responsible for this adverse effect.

Plasma cholinesterase is required to metabolize succinylcholine. Without this enzyme, unanticipated high serum levels of the drug will persist, with paralysis of the muscles of respiration. Several abnormal forms of thioenzyme (pseudocholinesterase) have been found which account for the inability of these variants to hydrolyze succinylcholine.[1] The genetic determinants for this enzyme have been identified and it appears that there are four allelic genes (one normal and three abnormal) that are responsible for the various types of this enzyme. The abnormal alleles have been identified as atypical (dibucaine-resistant), fluoride-resistant and silent (negligible activity) where the atypical variant accounts for the majority of the incidence of this condition. Approximately 4% of the population are heterozygous for the atypical type and about one out of 2,500 individuals is homozygous and expresses this disorder. This malady will remain asymptomatic and undetected unless the patient is challenged with succinylcholine, usually on induction of anesthesia preparatory to surgery. The response is dramatic; a 2- to 3-min period of apnea will ensue.

The disorder *malignant hyperthermia* is characterized by dramatic muscle rigidity and a rapid rise in body temperature after administering a general anesthetic such as halothane or succinylcholine.[4] Although this condition is thought to be autosomal dominant there is a greater incidence in males as age increases. Statistics show that one out of 20,000 individuals who are given anesthesia have this disorder and that two out of three affected die.

Other pharmacogenetic maladies which are extremely rare include phenytoin toxicity due to a defect in a hepatic para-hydroxylation enzyme system for phenytoin, warfarin resistance due to a vitamin-K sensitive enzyme or receptor in liver, and dicumarol sensitivity also due to an abnormal liver hydroxylase system for the drug.

Oxidative reactions in drug metabolism involving benzylic hydroxylation of debrisoquine, N-oxidation of sparteine, C-hydroxylation of tolbutamide, O-deethylation of phenacetin, p-hydroxylation of phenytoin and mephenytoin, and N-glucosidation of amylobarbitone have been described. The incidence of these various conditions varies between 2–9% of

Table II—Some Pharmacogenetic Conditions[5,9]

	Condition	Aberrant enzyme and location	Mode of inheritance	Frequency	Drugs producing abnormal response
1.	Glucose 6-phosphate dehydrogenase deficiency, favism or drug-induced	Glucose 6-phosphate dehydrogenase	X-linked incomplete codominant	Approximately 100,000,000 affected in world; occurs in high frequency where malaria is endemic; 80 biochemically distinct mutations	A variety of analgesics (acetanilid, aspirin, phenacetin, antipyrine, aminopyrine), sulfonamides and sulfones, antimalarials, nonsulfonamide antibacterial agents (furazolidone, nitrofurantoin, chloramphenicol, aminosalicylic acid), miscellaneous drugs (vitamin K, probenecid, methylene blue, dimercaprol, phenylhydrazine, quinine, quinidine)
2.	Phenacetin-induced methemoglobinemia	?Mixed function oxidase in liver microsomes that de-ethylates phenacetin	Autosomal recessive	Only 1 small pedigree	Phenacetin
3.	Drug-sensitive hemoglobins a) Hemoglobin Zurich	Arginine substitution for histidine at 63d position of β-chain of hemoglobin	Autosomal dominant	2 small pedigrees	Sulfonamides
	b) Hemoglobin M (H-disease)	Hemoglobin composed of 4 β-chains	Autosomal dominant	Approximately 150 cases	Sulfisoxazole
4.	Acatalasia	Catalase in erythrocytes	Autosomal recessive	Mainly in Japan and Switzerland, reaching 1% in certain small areas of Japan	Hydrogen peroxide
5.	Slow inactivation of isoniazid	Isoniazid acetylase in liver	Autosomal recessive	Approximately 50% of US population	Isoniazid, sulfamethazine, sulfamaprine, phenelzine, dapsone, hydralazine
6.	Succinylcholine sensitivity or atypical pseudo-cholinesterase	Pseudocholinesterase in plasma	Autosomal recessive	Several aberrant alleles; most common disorder occurs in 1:2500	Succinylcholine
7.	Malignant hyperthermia with muscular rigidity	Unknown	Autosomal dominant	Approximately 1:20,000 anesthetized patients	Anesthetics such as halothane, methoxyflurane, ether, cyclopropane; also succinylcholine
8.	Diphenylhydantoin toxicity due to deficient para-hydroxylation	?Mixed function oxidase in liver microsomes that para-hydroxylates diphenylhydantoin	Autosomal or X-linked dominant	Only 1 small pedigree	Diphenylhydantoin (phenytoin)
9.	Warfarin resistance	?Altered receptor or enzyme in liver with increased affinity for vitamin K	Autosomal dominant	2 large pedigrees	Warfarin
10.	Dicumarol sensitivity	?Mixed function oxidase in liver microsomes that hydroxylates dicumarol	Unknown	Only 1 small pedigree	Dicumarol
11.	Inability to taste phenylthiourea or phenylthiocarbamide	Unknown	Autosomal recessive	Approximately 30% of Caucasians	Drugs containing —N—C≡S group such as phenylthiourea, methyl propylthiouracil
12.	Glaucoma due to abnormal response of intraocular pressure to steroids	Unknown	Autosomal recessive	Approximately 5% of US population	Corticosteroids
13.	Methemoglobin reductase deficiency	Methemoglobin reductase	Autosomal recessive heterozygous carriers affected	Approximately 1 in 100 are heterozygous carriers	Same drugs as listed for glucose 6-phosphate dehydrogenase deficiency

Table II—continued

	Condition	Abberant enzyme and location	Mode of inheritance	Frequency	Drugs producing abnormal response
14.	Debrisoquine induced hypotension	Aromatic hydroxylase	Autosomal recessive	1.5 to 9% with a large interethnic variation	Debrisoquine
15.	Sparteine induced diplopia, blurred vision, overstimulated uterus	N-oxidation enzyme (aminoxydase)	Autosomal recessive	5%	Sparteine
16.	Tolbutamide induced cardiovascular death	Mixed function oxidase	Autosomal recessive	25%	Tolbutamide

the population. The best studied example of these conditions are the oxidation of debrisoquine and sparteine. In population studies the metabolic processes responsible for removing most of the respective drug from the body were impaired or nearly absent in some subjects. These subjects were designated poor metabolizers (debrisoquine) or non-metabolizers (sparteine). The frequency of the poor metabolizer phenotype of debrisoquine is 8.9% in the white British population, and the non-metabolizer phenotype of sparteine occurs in 5% of the German population. For both drugs, 4-hydroxylation of debrisoquine and N-oxidation of sparteine are determined by two allelic genes at a single gene locus and follow autosomal recessive inheritance. Poor and non-metabolizer subjects are at higher risk of developing drug related side effects when standard doses of these drugs are administered. Since non-metabolizers of sparteine are poor metabolizers of debrisoquine the respective metabolic deficiency appear to be controlled by the same or very similar gene locus. In these subjects the impaired metabolism is not restricted to these two drugs. Poor metabolizers of debrisoquine exhibited an impaired capacity to effect O-deethylation of phenacetin, aromatic hydroxylation of quanoxan, p-hydroxylation of phenytoin and phenformin, and benzylic hydroxylation of nortriptyline.[5]

The genetic control of tolbutamide disposition in humans was studied to provide insight into the potential for high blood levels in individuals receiving fixed dosage regimens. Tolbutamide was administered intravenously to 42 nondiabetic subjects, eight of their relatives, and to five sets of twins. A ninefold variation in the rate of tolbutamide disappearance from plasma was found. This variation was characterized by a trimodal frequency distribution, suggestive of monogenic inheritance and consistent with pedigree analysis, indicating autosomal transmission of rapid and slow inactivation of tolbutamide. Analysis of the metabolites of tolbutamide in urine samples provided evidence for the microsomal oxidation of the drug to hydroxy tolbutamide as the primary site of genetic control. The results suggest that fixed-dosage regimens of this drug might lead to higher accrued blood levels in slow inactivators.[6]

Another curious interplay between drugs and enzymes exists in gout. It is known that certain uric acid overproducers (as opposed to underexcretors) lack the enzyme hypoxanthine-guanine phosphoriboxyl transferase (HGPTase). This is the basic lesion of the Nyhan-Lesch syndrome. Without delving into the complex function of this salvage enzyme, it seems that a significant factor in the anti-uric acid effect of allopurinol depends on a plentiful supply of HGPTase.

Allopurinol appears to decrease the rate of *de novo* biosynthesis of purine. This function apparently is distinct from its better known action, which is to inhibit hypoxanthine oxidase, an enzyme which catalyzes the oxidation of hypoxanthine to xanthine and xanthine to uric acid. Apparently the influence exerted by allopurinol in depressing purine biosynthesis contributes to its effectiveness in decreasing uric acid serum levels.

In patients who suffer a relative deficiency of HGPTase,

allopurinol will not decrease purine biosynthesis. It seems that HGPTase activity is necessary for allopurinol to exert its suppressive effect on purine synthesis. However, this effect of allopurinol is erratic; it did not suppress purine synthesis in several gouty patients who had normal uric acid production and normal HGPTase activity (underexcretors).

There are other inborn errors of metabolism which may alter the ability of afflicted individuals to effectively utilize or eliminate certain drugs. Hypophosphatemic vitamin-D-refractory rickets may be related to a defective receptor enzyme which has poor affinity for vitamin D. This may interfere with transfer of vitamin D across the intestinal mucosa.

At the other extreme, patients who suffer excessive responses to conventional doses of vitamin D, with resultant hypercalcemia and its nefarious sequelae, are suspected of having some other aberration of enzyme-transport mechanisms.

Variations in pyridoxine responsiveness resulting in *hypochromic microcytic anemia* are suspected of being enzyme-insufficiency states. The porphyrin-uric reactions to barbiturates are due to failure of regulatory mechanisms which result in overproduction of alpha-aminolevulenic acid synthetase. This in turn causes an excessive production of porphyrins which exceeds the ability of the marrow to employ them in the synthesis of heme. Porphyrins accumulate in the blood and can cause an exacerbation of acute intermittent porphyria.

Similarly, certain naturally occurring steroids have been shown to be associated with *acute intermittent porphyria*.[7] It appears that in patients with this disease there is also a deficiency in a Δ^4-5α-steroid reductase activity which promotes the production of the 5β H-steroid isomer. The latter is an inducer for delta-aminolevulinate synthetase and consequently porphyrin synthesis. The basis for this relationship of the steroid reductase in acute intermittent porphyria remains obscure and requires further investigation.

Drug-induced acute intermittent porphyrinuria has also been related to sulfonamides, chloramphenicol, quinine, anticoagulants, tranquilizers, diethylstilbestrol, and oral contraceptives.

It is suspected that increased susceptibility to dyskinesias subsequent to phenothiazine administration may be related to congenital enzyme insufficiencies.

One could speculate on Wilson's disease characterized by defective or deficient ceruloplasmin, or hemochromatosis in which a defect permits excessive iron to pass through the small intestine into the blood. Both of these diseases may be related to enzymatic or carrier-protein abnormalities. One might also wonder about the effect of drugs on other enzyme insufficiencies, such as lactase in the small intestine, hydroxylase in the adrenal glands, and others.

Convincing evidence is accumulating that relates a predisposition to alcoholism to genetic factors.[8] Curiously, the biosynthesis of human alcohol dehydrogenase (ADH) is controlled by three separate alleles (ADH_1, ADH_2, and ADH_3), each of which gives rise to the formation of a polypeptide (α,

β, and γ, respectively). Homodimers (e.g., $\alpha\alpha$, $\beta\beta$, and/or $\gamma\gamma$) and heterodimers (e.g., $\alpha\beta$, $\beta\gamma$, etc.) are isoenzymes that have been recognized in human tissues. However, electrophoretic studies have identified a polymorphism involving the ADH_2 allele. The corresponding β-polypeptide has been termed "atypical" (β^2). Heterodimeric isoenzymes containing β^2 have been identified ($\alpha\beta^2$, $\beta^2\gamma^1$, and $\beta^2\gamma^2$) but as yet a homodimer of β^2 has not been found.

The "atypical" ADH enzyme(s) has been shown to be quite different from the normal enzyme(s) (ie, β^2 enzymes are more active under physiological conditions, have different substrate specificities, and have a different sensitivity to thiourea inhibition than have the β enzymes). The actual biological significance of this genetic polymorphism in metabolizing alcohols (not limited to ethanol metabolism) has not yet been determined.

If one reflects on the multitude of known enzyme systems, as well as those suspected as latent or subclinical but not yet identified, it may be that many reactions now classified as idiosyncratic or even allergic will eventually be recognized as pharmacogenetic disorders or acquired enzyme insufficiencies.

References

1. Motulsky AG: *Fed Proc 31:* 1286, 1972.
2. Vesell ES: *Ibid* 1253.
3. LaDu BN: *Ibid* 1276.
4. Kalow W: *Ibid* 1270.
5. Eichelbaum M: *Clinical Pharmaco Kinetics 7:* 1–22, 1982.
6. Scott J and Poffenbarger PL: *Diabetes 28:* 41–51, 1979.
7. Kappas A, *et al: Ibid* 1293.
8. Evans DAP: *Human Pharmacogenetics*, pages 369–391, in *Drug Metabolism-From Microbe to Man*, by Parke DV, Smith RL, eds, Taylor and Francis Ltd. London, 1977.
9. Vesell ES: In *Drug Interactions*, Grahame-Smith DG, ed, Chapter 10, University Park Press, Baltimore, 1977.

Bibliography

Fed Proc 31: 1253–1330, 1972.
Vesell ES: *New Engl J Med 287:* 904, 1972.
Kalow W: *Pharmacogenetics: Heredity and the Response to Drugs*, Saunders, Philadelphia, 1962.
Eichelbaum M: *Clinical Pharmacokinetics 7:* 1, 1982.

CHAPTER 71

Pharmacological Aspects of Drug Abuse

Frederick J Goldstein, PhD
Professor of Pharmacology

G Victor Rossi, PhD
Vice President of Academic Affairs and Professor of Pharmacology

Philadelphia College of Pharmacy and Science
Philadelphia, PA 19104

Drug abuse may originate with the *physician*, the *patient* seeking medical treatment, or with the *adolescent* drug experimenter. Physician-generated misuse may result when there is insufficient concern or time to adequately evaluate the patient as a candidate for psychoactive drug therapy. Treatment is all too often directed toward the alleviation of symptoms without a concerted effort to identify possible deep-seated causes and to respond to the emotional as well as the medical needs of the patient. Overprescribing of mood-altering drugs involves potential harm not just to the individual but to society at large. While physician-generated drug misuse represents a relatively small percentage of the overall problem, it is especially regrettable that any negative contribution arises from the actions or inactions of health professionals.

Patient-originated abuse encompasses a larger aspect and persists despite significant efforts by the majority of physicians and pharmacists to restrict the dispensing of psychoactive agents. Some patients will visit several physicians, obtain a number of prescriptions for barbiturates, tranquilizers, stimulants, and/or narcotics and present each prescription to a different pharmacy. Thus the patient may accumulate substantial quantities of controlled substances either for personal use or for resale. This generally middle-aged middle-class drug abuser has only recently been characterized and attempts to thwart such patterns of drug acquisition have, thus far, been unsuccessful.

Peer pressure, alienation, hedonism, mass media advertising, affluence, and boredom are among the factors most frequently cited as those leading to misuse of drugs by the adolescent group. Consumption of alcoholic beverages, cigarette smoking, and liberal use of sedatives, tranquilizers, and central nervous system (CNS) stimulants by adults, particularly members of the family, foster development of a cavalier attitude toward drugs, and increase the likelihood of drug-taking among adolescents. Three basic stages of adolescent drug usage have been defined: 1) initial experimental phase, 2) periodic recreational phase, and 3) compulsive (chronic) pattern. That many young people resist involvement with drugs or do not progress to chronic or serious patterns of abuse emphasizes the importance of personality traits in the genesis of drug dependency. Persons of any age who have a low frustration tolerance, cannot cope with the daily pressures of life, require instantaneous gratification, and who have unfulfilled dependency needs and serious problems of socialization may come to rely on drug use in order to escape, albeit temporarily, from a psychological environment which is bleak, joyless and/or filled with anxiety.

Although drug abuse in the United States has been a continuously expanding problem for the past 20 years, certain recent data suggest that a reversal may be underway. According to an annual National Institute of Drug Abuse (NIDA) survey of high school seniors throughout the country, a re-duction in use of many psychoactive substances occurred from 1979 to 1982[1]. These data (Tables I and II) show that consumption of alcohol, marijuana/hashish, cigarettes, phencyclidine (*PCP; Angel Dust*) and others has either declined or remained constant during this three year interval (CNS stimulant abuse has increased from 1979 but is down from 1981).

As stated earlier, many factors are involved in the process by which an individual ultimately selects the pharmacological

Table I—National Survey of High School Seniors: Use of Psychoactive Substances at Least Once During Month Preceding Survey[1] (National Institute on Drug Abuse)

		1979	1982
Decrease	Alcohol	71.8[a]	69.7
	Marijuana/Hashish	36.5	28.5
	Cigarettes	34.4	30.0
	Cocaine	5.7	5.0
	Tranquilizers	3.7	2.4
	Barbiturates	3.2	2.0
	PCP	2.4	1.0
	Amyl (& Butyl) Nitrite	2.4	1.1
	Opiates except heroin	2.4	1.8
No change	Heroin	0.2	0.2
	LSD	2.4	2.4
Increase	Stimulants except cocaine	9.9	13.7
	Methaqualone	2.3	2.4

[a] Data are reported as % of high school seniors surveyed (1979—16,662 students; 1982—18,661 students).

Table II—National Survey of High School Seniors: Daily Use of Psychoactive Substances[1] (National Institute on Drug Abuse)

		1979	1982
Decrease	Cigarettes	25.4[a]	21.1
	Marijuana/Hashish	10.3	6.3
	Alcohol	6.9	5.7
No change	Cocaine	0.2	0.2
	Tranquilizers	0.1	0.1
	PCP	0.1	0.1
	Amyl (& Butyl) Nitrite	0.0	0.0
	Heroin	0.0	0.0
	LSD	0.0	0.0
Increase	Stimulants except cocaine	0.6	1.1
	Barbiturates	0.0	0.1
	Opiates except heroin	0.0	0.1
	Methaqualone	0.0	0.1

[a] Data are reported as % of high school seniors surveyed (1979—16,662 students; 1982—18,661 students).

route of escape from stress. However, it is quite clear that some potential addicts can resist entering this pathway if they become aware of the toxicological consequences of drug abuse. Many school, religious, and community organizations have, in fact, made substantial efforts to present educational programs devoted to acute and chronic toxicities produced by psychoactive substances. Pharmacists should expand their participation in these programs and, to this end, the following information can be of assistance.

Central Nervous System Depressants

Narcotics

Heroin is the narcotic most often abused. Preference for heroin is not based on unique euphoric properties but is largely a matter of economics; heroin is the most potent of the narcotics, thus providing maximum profit per kilogram to those engaged in illicit traffic.

Early in the course of heroin use, intravenous injection is followed quickly by a sense of exquisite visceral pleasure which is similar to sexual orgasm (the *rush*), an enveloping feeling of contentment, and the receding of internal conflicts. Taken orally, heroin also produces relaxation, euphoria, and indifference to pain and stress but not the "rush." In the susceptible individual, the intense desire to recapture this drug experience contributes to the establishment of an emotional or psychic dependency.

With frequently repeated administration the individual becomes progressively less responsive to the drug, thus ever-increasing doses are sought in an attempt to duplicate the characteristic effects. Chronic suppression of central nervous system function results in a dependent state in which the drug must be taken on a regular basis to maintain a reasonable semblance of well-being and equilibrium and to prevent the anguish of the abstinence syndrome. Thus narcotic addicts soon find themselves taking heroin not for the pleasurable effects but primarily to prevent withdrawal.

Tolerance to narcotics does not develop uniformly. For example, addicts experience, during chronic use, lessened respiratory depressant, analgesic, sedative, emetic, and euphoric effects; some may show decreased miosis while most suffer chronically from the constipating effects of the drug. Drug tolerance is always relative, never absolute; a dose always exists that is capable of causing death from respiratory paralysis and overdosage is a common cause of fatalities among narcotic addicts. Although death associated with heroin use has routinely been attributed to overdosage, other factors may sometimes be involved. Quinine is frequently employed by "dealers" to dilute pure heroin because, like the narcotic, it is bitter and produces vasodilation simulating the *rush*. Thus, addicts cannot readily detect adulteration and may unknowingly inject themselves with large quantitites of quinine which may produce significant myocardial depression. Codeine, while significantly less potent than heroin, can also produce death from overdosage.

Withdrawal symptoms usually reach maximum intensity 36 to 72 hours after the last dose of heroin and subside gradually within 7 to 10 days. The severity of the abstinence syndrome is determined largely by the degree of acquired physical dependence. Signs and symptoms of narcotic withdrawal include yawning, sneezing, lacrimation, restlessness, anxiety, insomnia, nausea, vomiting, gastrointestinal cramps and diarrhea, sweating, gooseflesh, generalized body aches, fever, tremors, muscle spasms, and jerking movements. Excessive perspiration, vomiting, and diarrhea combined with diminished food and fluid intake may result in dehydration, acid-base disturbances, and ketosis. Occasionally cardiovascular collapse occurs. Withdrawal symptoms can be suppressed either by administering the drug of dependence

or another narcotic. If a narcotic, such as methadone, is given initially in a stabilizing amount and then the dosage is reduced gradually, the intensity of the abstinence syndrome may be lessened appreciably.

The narcotic addict is subject to risks arising out of indifference to minimal nutritional and hygienic requirements with consequent high incidence of viral hepatitis, bacterial endocarditis, tetanus, pulmonary infection, pulmonary edema, and thrombophlebitis. Use of nonsterile injection equipment and intravascular introduction of cotton fibers and adulterants such as lactose and talc all contribute to the development of local and systemic infectious disorders and pulmonary granulomatosis. Hyperamylasemia is often observed during the acute phase of heroin-induced pulmonary disturbances. Increased serum immunoglobulin levels are commonly encountered in addicts. Although the clinical consequences of this finding are incompletely understood, serologic tests for syphilis are false-positive in a significant proportion of such individuals. Noninfectious complications of narcotic addiction include transverse myelitis, rhabdomyolysis with cardiac involvement and myoglobinuria, and Horner's syndrome. Quinine contained in *street* heroin preparations produce amblyopia and thrombocytopenia. An aqueous mixture consisting of crushed tablets of pentazocine (Talwin) and tripelennamine (Pyribenzamine), with the street name of 'T's and Blues', has been used intravenously by addicts; effects are reported to be similar to the heroin *rush*. Toxic reactions can be serious and include tonic-clonic seizures and acute respiratory distress with hypoxia; the latter effects apparently result from deposition of insoluble ingredients of this mixture, eg, talc, in lung tissue forming pulmonary granulomas.

Women who persist in the use of heroin during pregnancy give birth to narcotic-dependent offspring. Signs of withdrawal in the newborn appear within several hours to several days and include high-pitched crying, sleeplessness, irritability, tremor, vomiting, and diarrhea; the latter may result in severe dehydration. Narcotic-dependent infants are born smaller and exhibit an uncoordinated and ineffectual sucking reflex which reduces nutritive consumption. Phenobarbital, diazepam, paregoric, and chlorpromazine have been used to alleviate narcotic withdrawal in neonates.

Approaches to treatment of the adult addict involve medical as well as psychiatric and social aspects. A basic obstacle in any approach to the treatment of narcotic addiction is the characteristic high rate of recidivism.

Methadone maintenance, currently one of the most widely employed techniques in the management of narcotic addiction, involves stabilizing the patient on a regular daily oral dose of methadone, preferably in conjunction with supportive psychological or psychiatric counseling. In this context the maintenance drug does not provide true pharmacologic blockade; rather, regular administration results in the development of tolerance to methadone and cross-tolerance to heroin. Thus, the addict will not experience the heroin-induced "rush" and euphoria unless doses substantially higher than usual are injected. Theoretically, when unburdened by these factors which motivate addiction, methadone may be gradually withdrawn. However, many former narcotic abusers cannot maintain a drug-free state and either reestablish their addiction to heroin or request continued methadone therapy. In contrast, some addicts refuse to enter a methadone maintenance program. Reasons for this decision include: 1) the claim by some narcotic abusers that methadone is just another type of drug dependence and one which is more difficult to surrender than heroin use—in fact, methadone withdrawal can be more intense and painful than heroin detoxification; 2) methadone significantly impairs human reproductive capacity by decreasing both ejaculate volume and sperm motility (heroin produces a lesser effect upon fertility);

3) family members may be endangered—a number of children have died after ingesting the liquid methadone preparations used by their parents.

An alternative approach, based on the conditioning theory of opiate dependence, employs narcotic antagonists to extinguish drug-seeking behavior by blocking the euphoric effects of heroin. Nalorphine was first suggested for this purpose but its limited duration of action and high incidence of hallucinogenic reactions made its use impractical. Cyclazocine is effective orally and provides blockage for up to 24 hours but, like nalorphine, is an active analgesic and is associated with a variety of disturbing psychotomimetic reactions. Naloxone, a "pure" narcotic antagonist (ie, possesses no agonist properties), produces fewer unpleasant effects but is relatively short-acting. Attempts have been made to develop longer-acting derivatives, eg, naloxone pamoate. Naltrexone (structurally related to oxymorphone) is currently being tested; a major problem observed during clinical trials is a high rate of recidivism. At present, narcotic antagonists represent a treatment modality whose ultimate role in the therapy of narcotic addiction remains to be established.

Therapeutic communities, staffed by health professionals as well as former addicts, provide both individualized and group psychotherapy. Dramatic positive changes have been observed in some individuals as a result of the rehabilitative process and evidence exists that behavioral and attitudinal alterations can assist addicts in extrication from their drug dependency state. However, most residency programs have restricted facilities and personnel and cannot admit all addicts desiring entrance. In addition, the cost per patient is extremely high. Therefore, while gratifying individual gains have been demonstrated, the impact of the therapeutic community approach on the overall drug abuse situation is limited.

Barbiturates

Clinical utilization of barbiturates has declined substantially in recent years. Benzodiazepines, while not free of adverse reactions, are safer and have supplanted barbiturates in treatment of anxiety and insomnia. It is clear that, in general, hypnotics (barbiturates and nonbarbiturates) should not be prescribed for more than a 14–28 day period; beyond this time efficacy decreases (a decline in hypnotic activity may begin after only seven days of continuous therapy). Pharmacists should monitor these prescriptions very closely, consulting with both patient and physician in order to insure proper use and to prevent dependency problems.

Hazards encountered in the use of barbiturates include occasional unanticipated idiosyncratic or hypersensitivity reactions and accidental overdosage as may occur in young children unaware of the potential danger or in adults during a hypnotic drug-induced semistuporous state of "automatism." For most persons, sleep provides only a temporary respite but, all too frequently, intentional overdosage with easily accessible sleep-inducing drugs provides an avenue of permanent escape from the pressures of reality.

Barbiturates reduce the amount of time spent in the REM (rapid eye movement) phase of sleep. Reduction of REM sleep for a period of several days may cause the individual to become irritable or to evidence disturbances in personality and rationality. When the hypnotic is withdrawn abruptly, there is a rebound increase in the REM phase often associated with nightmares, a feeling of having slept poorly, or actual insomnia. "Rebound" REM makes it difficult for the patient to give up the drug and contributes to the development of drug dependency.

The signs and symptoms of barbiturate and of alcohol intoxication are strikingly similar. Visual perception, recall, reaction-time coordination, and other indexes of psychomotor functioning are affected, the degree of impairment being largely dependent on the concentration of drug in the brain. Intoxication either with alcohol or with a barbiturate is characterized by difficulty in thinking, reduction of ego controls, poor judgment, confusion, and emotional instability. Neurological impairment and muscular incoordination are major factors in the personal injuries and involvement in vehicular accidents which are common occurrences during the course of intoxication with these drugs. The central nervous system suppressant effects of alcohol, barbiturates, and opiates such as heroin are mutually reinforcing; extemporaneous combinations of these depressants may result in unpredictably abrupt and severe incapacitation.

Low doses of barbiturates (as employed for daytime sedation, nighttime sleep induction, or the control of epilepsy) are often taken for indefinite periods without eliciting tolerance or physical dependence. These phenomena generally occur only with doses considerably in excess of those customarily employed in medical practice. To illustrate, the usual oral hypnotic dose of pentobarbital sodium or secobarbital sodium is 100 to 200 mg, whereas oral doses of these barbiturates in excess of 400 mg/day (and generally in the range of 600 to 800 mg/day) for approximately 1 month are required to induce clinically significant tolerance and physical dependence. Parenteral (subcutaneous or intravenous) administration of barbiturates may lead to physical dependency at lower dose levels and within a shorter period of time.

The amount of barbiturate that may be consumed by the compulsive abuser varies considerably, but average daily doses of 1 to 1.5 g of short-acting derivatives are not uncommon, and some individuals may use as much as 2.5 g/day over prolonged periods of time.

Withdrawal reactions, which in some cases may be more hazardous than the narcotic abstinence syndrome, develop upon abrupt cessation of chronic barbiturate overuse. Mild to moderate withdrawal reactions include anorexia, apprehension, tremulousness, muscular weakness, mental confusion, and postural hypotension. A severe barbiturate withdrawal syndrome may involve profound disorientation, delirium and hallucinations, and convulsive seizures of an episodic or protracted nature. Most individuals who have ingested eight or more hypnotic doses of a barbiturate per day over an extended period will experience convulsions during withdrawal. In extreme cases the barbiturate abstinence syndrome may terminate in cardiovascular collapse and death. With the longer-acting barbiturates, withdrawal symptoms are slower in onset and less severe than those encountered with the shorter-acting derivatives.

Pharmacologic treatment of barbiturate dependency is generally approached by replacement with either pentobarbital or phenobarbital at an initial dose sufficient for stabilization; the dose is then reduced gradually over a period of several days to weeks depending on the individual patient response.

Nonbarbiturate Sedative/Hypnotics

Neurological impairment, psychological and physical dependence, and an abstinence syndrome similar to that associated with barbiturate abuse may result from excessive use of many nonbarbiturate sedative-hypnotic and antianxiety agents, including chloral hydrate, glutethimide, methyprylon, methaqualone, meprobamate, chlordiazepoxide, and diazepam.

Methaqualone ranks currently among the "street" drugs of choice. Although claims have been made that methaqualone and other nonbarbiturate hypnotics (e.g., chloral hydrate, triclofos) produce little or no effect on REM sleep, other reports challenge this distinction and a final conclusion has not yet been advanced. Acroparesthesia (tingling and numbness in the extremities) may occur prior to the onset of hypnotic activity, particularly when sleep does not ensue rapidly, and this sensation is experienced by many methaqualone abusers. Increased muscle tone is often evident; it may even be observed while the patient is in a deep coma and may last for several days. Acute toxicity differs from that of the barbiturates in that marked respiratory and cardiovascular depression are generally not seen after large doses of methaqualone. Psychological dependence and tolerance to methaqualone have been observed but the results of studies on the development of physical dependence are equivocal. Apparent withdrawal symptoms, such as headache, anorexia, nausea, abdominal cramps, and interference with sleep, have been noted in those investigations reporting physical dependency. These relatively minor symptoms may occur during abstinence in the individual who had been taking five hypnotic doses of methaqualone daily for several months. Severe reactions which may occasionally be encountered during methaqualone withdrawal include convulsions and toxic psychoses. Ingesting alcohol with methaqualone is very dangerous, leading to serious impairment of judgment and psychomotor coordination. At least one state reports a high death rate from injuries sustained in car accidents where the drivers, passengers and/or pedestrians used this drug combination.

Mandrax, a combination of methaqualone (250 mg) and diphenhydramine (25 mg), has been abused by addicts in Great Britain, Canada, and Australia. Reactions due to overdosage with this drug combination are similar to those of methaqualone but are potentially more severe since diphenhydramine, which possesses central anticholinergic activity, may produce psychological disturbances, excitation, ataxia, and convulsive seizures.

Meprobamate produces sedation and relaxation comparable to that of barbiturates although the clinically effective dose of meprobamate is higher. Psychological activity may be compromised by chronic oral doses of 800 mg of meprobamate/day, while at daily doses of more than 1600 mg psychomotor performance may be reduced significantly. Psychic dependence and tolerance occur with prolonged high-dose administration and physical dependency develops after consumption of 3 g or more/day for several weeks. Depending on the dosage and duration of use, meprobamate withdrawal reactions may range from anxiety, insomnia, and tremors to hallucinations, convulsions, coma, and death.

Chlordiazepoxide, taken in doses of 300 to 600 mg daily for several months, may result in physical dependence resembling that observed with the barbiturates and meprobamate. However, withdrawal symptoms may be delayed for several days after chlordiazepoxide usage is terminated, due possibly to slow elimination of the drug. Agitation, insomnia, anorexia, depression, psychological disturbances, and convulsions are among the reactions which follow cessation of prolonged administration of high doses of chlordiazepoxide.

Diazepam, the most widely prescribed benzodiazepine derivative, may also induce physical dependence. Patients receiving 15 mg daily for four to six months or higher doses (60–120 mg) for about two months may, upon withdrawal, experience gastric cramps, sweating, agitation, tremors, insomnia, confusion, disorientation, auditory and visual hallucinations, delusions, paranoia, and depression. Serious acute intoxication may occur when benzodiazepines are combined with other depressants, eg, ethanol, narcotics, other sedative-hypnotics, tricyclic antidepressants or antipsychotic agents. Simultaneous ingestion of ethanol and diazepam is particularly dangerous; in addition to the expected additive CNS-depressant effects, in the presence of ethanol, diazepam blood levels are elevated compared to diazepam taken alone. Some reports suggest the possibility of teratogenicity resulting from administration of meprobamate or certain benzodiazepines during the first trimester. In the interest of caution, use of these antianxiety agents should be restricted during this critical period of pregnancy.

The medical and pharmaceutical professions bear a grave responsibility in the prescribing and dispensing of barbiturates, benzodiazepines, and pharmacologically related agents. Physicians, pharmacists, and nurses often fail to convey adequately to the patient the potential of these drugs for ensnarement in a vicious web of emotional need, often progressing to escalated consumption and, ultimately, the development of a dangerous degree of psychological and physiological dependency. Although only a limited number of drugs were discussed in the above sections, it is important to note that *any* substance causing acute central nervous system depression is capable of producing psychological and/or physical dependence during chronic use.

The legitimate application of drugs should not be jeopardized by irrational fears arising from situations created by their uncontrolled use; however, it is equally important to recognize that certain drugs by virtue of their ability to elicit profound changes in mood and feeling may, in the emotionally predisposed person, lead to a degree of psychic dependency and compulsive use detrimental to the individual and to society.

Alcohol

Although greater publicity is accorded usually to marijuana, hallucinogens, and narcotics, alcohol remains the major drug of abuse in the US. It is a recent but necessary shift in official government policy to place emphasis on the diagnosis, treatment, and prevention of alcoholism.

Alcoholic intoxication spans a range of blood-ethanol concentrations from 50 mg%, at which level some impairment of judgment occurs, to above 400 mg%, associated with profound depression of vital physiologic functions. Concentrations in excess of 600 mg% are usually fatal. Although many states regard an individual as being "legally drunk" at levels above 100 mg%, controlled studies have repeatedly demonstrated functional deficits such as impaired adaptation to light, reduced psychomotor performance with prolonged reaction times, and generalized deterioration of simulated driving skills at blood-alcohol concentrations of 80 mg%. Thus individuals with blood-alcohol levels below those required for legal classification as intoxicated may, nevertheless, be dangerous drivers. Compelling statistics compiled over many years implicate alcohol as a principal contributor to motor vehicle accidents with consequent injuries and fatalities. Public outrage by groups such as *Mothers Against Drunk Drivers* (*MADD*) has been directed recently toward the legislative and judicial systems for their minimal penalization of drunk drivers, particularly the repeat offender. As a result, many states now have passed stricter laws with more severe penalties. Two-day jail terms for first offenses and quicker suspension of the operator's license now are routine aspects of punishment. However, none of these statutes can restore the lives of innocent children and adults who have been killed by intoxicated drivers. Prevention of alcohol abuse through educational and other methods remains the approach most likely to reduce deaths. Many airline pilots and railroad engineers currently are involved in such programs.

Severe alcoholic intoxication may result in forms of amnesia characterized as "state-dependent learning" or as a "blackout." In the former, an individual can recall what transpired under the influence of alcohol only if again subjected to an intoxicated state. Generally, information acquired while under the effects of alcohol is poorly remembered or not retained in the nondrug condition. "Blackout" refers to a severe short-term memory deficit; subjects cannot recall what occurred while intoxicated even if they again become inebriated. Assaultive or destructive behavior (eg, suicide, attempted suicide, and homicide) associated with drinking frequently takes place during an amnesic state.

Estimates of the number of alcoholics in any society are very imprecise; the number of individuals in the US alone whose lives are inextricably involved with alcohol is numbered conservatively in the several millions. The cost in terms of lost productivity, accidents, crimes, self-degradation, disruption of family, business, and social bonds is beyond computation. Chronic abuse leads to debilitating pathologic alterations which seriously impair the alcoholic's health and diminish life expectancy; these effects may be summarized as follows:

1. *Mortality*
    The probability of premature death is approximately three times that of the general population, in addition to a greater frequency of fatal accidents and suicides, pathological changes are contributory.
2. *Cardiovascular*
    While several clinical studies show a reduced incidence of heart disease (possibly due to elevation in protective serum high density lipoproteins) among persons who consume an average of two ounces or less of alcohol per day, heavy drinkers (more than two ounces daily) are at greater risk of developing various cardiovascular disorders which include:
    a. permanent dilation of peripheral blood vessels around nose and eyes
    b. hypertension
    c. artherosclerotic heart disease
    d. congestive heart failure
    e. peripheral vascular disease
    f. cerebrovascular disease
3. *Neurological*
    Observed clinical changes may occur as:
    a. cerebellar ataxia (motor incoordination)
    b. decreased ability to perform cognitive tasks (eg, verbal and non-verbal tests)
    c. polyneuropathy
    d. nystagmus
    e. Korsakoff psychosis
    f. Wernike encephalopathy (may include some or all of above, ie, 3a–3e)
    Cerebral atrophy, documented by computerized axial tomography, can be extensive and has been linked to functional neurological deficits. Of particular interest is a report which suggests loss of cognitive skills may be related more to consumption of substantial amounts of alcohol per drinking episode than to frequent use of limited quantities. Partial recovery may occur with total abstinence.
4. *Hepatic*
    Degenerative alterations in liver morphology and function appear during chronic alcoholism and progressively develop in the following order (includes sequelae):
    a. alcoholic fatty liver (hepatic pain and tenderness)
    b. alcoholic hepatitis (nausea, vomiting, anorexia, weight loss, abdominal pain)
    c. cirrhosis (jaundice, encephalopathy)
    As with alcohol-induced neurological changes, cessation of drinking usually prevents further deterioration.
5. *Gastrointestinal*
    Ulcer formation and extensive gastrointestinal bleeding are frequently seen in addition to:
    a. esophagitis
    b. gastritis
    c. intestinal malabsorption (of, for example, fat, folic acid, thiamine, vitamin B_{12})
    d. chronic diarrhea
    e. steatorrhea
6. *Pancreatic*
    Chronic pancreatitis is often observed after approximately seven years of heavy alcohol use (usually appears before cirrhosis). Pancreatic failure may produce insulin-dependent diabetes mellitus.
7. *Hematologic*
    Anemia may be caused by deficiencies of folic acid and/or iron; other disorders are:
    a. thrombocytopenia
    b. granulocytopenia
8. *Endocrine*
    a. diabetes mellitus
    b. pseudo-Cushing's syndrome
    c. hypogonadism
        1) female: amenorrhea
        2) male: low plasma testosterone levels, impotence, infertility, testicular atrophy
9. *Infection*
    a. bacteremia
    b. bacterial peritonitis
    c. pneumonia
    d. tuberculosis
10. *Cancer*
    a. esophageal
    b. hepatic
    c. laryngeal
    d. pharyngeal
    e. mouth

Although alcoholic beverages constitute an appreciable source of calories, they provide no vitamins, minerals, or proteins; nutritional deficiencies associated with long-term heavy drinking may constitute major factors in the development of polyneuritis and cirrhosis of the liver. However, evidence suggests that liver damage results from the direct hepatotoxic effect of alcohol and/or its metabolites and that cirrhosis may occur independently of nutritional status.

Alcohol passes readily from the maternal to the fetal circulation; frequent consumption of alcohol during pregnancy creates an unnatural intrauterine environment for the developing fetus. Infants born to alcoholic mothers are usually underdeveloped and exhibit a slow growth rate and mental retardation. Current evidence suggests that these effects may be permanent. Cardiovascular aberrations, including systolic murmurs (due to possible ventricular septal defects) and congestive heart failure (resulting from possible atrial septal defects), and craniofacial abnormalities, such as short palpebral fissures and maxillary hypoplasia, have been documented as patterns of malformation in infants born to chronic alcoholic women. This dysmorphic pattern has been classified as the Fetal Alcohol Syndrome (FAS) and is most likely to occur when maternal consumption is equivalent to 90 mL (or more) of absolute alcohol per day.

Chronic ingestion of alcohol results in pharmacodynamic and drug disposition tolerance; however, the degree of tolerance is not as great as that which occurs with morphine. Physical dependence, similar to that observed with barbiturates and narcotics, develops to alcohol. The severity of the alcohol abstinence syndrome can be correlated with the degree of intoxication and its duration. A relatively short period of heavy drinking may be followed by headache, nausea and vomiting, general malaise, and slight tremulousness during the drying-out period. Abrupt cessation of alcohol consumption after 1 or more weeks of intoxication may further be associated with anxiety, insomnia, confusion, tremors, and hallucinations. Long periods of intense intoxication may, upon withdrawal, result in delirium tremens, a syndrome characterized by increased autonomic activity (eg, fever, sweating, and tachycardia), agitation, disorientation, severe tremors or convulsive seizures, and frightening hallucinations usually of a visual form.

Hereditary predisposition, endocrine abnormalities, psychological defects, susceptible personality structure, and sociocultural and economic impacts are among the many factors that have been considered as interacting in the causation of alcohol addiction. Because of the many conflicting theories on the etiology of alcoholism there is no standard approach to therapy. There is a general agreement, however, that a prerequisite for successful therapy is *total* abstinence from alcohol and, for all practical purposes, this represents the only viable solution for the individual alcoholic. Efforts to correct the drinking habit almost invariably fail if the patient attempts merely to reduce his consumption of alcohol. Indeed, failure of the alcoholic to accept the realization that he is incapable of drinking in moderation is regarded as a primary obstacle to ultimate resolution of the problem.

Some alcoholics stop drinking of their own volition, others are able to discontinue the habit with the aid of professional or peer group counseling, and still others continue to relapse despite repeated and intensive rehabilitative efforts. Therapeutic measures employed, with varying degrees of success, in the long-term management of the alcoholic patient include participation in supportive social organizations for combating alcoholism (eg, Alcoholics Anonymous), psychiatric therapy, and the use of neuroleptic or antianxiety agents, although the latter may result in substitution of one form of drug dependency for another. The unpleasant interaction between alcohol and disulfiram may be used both as a deconditioning device and as a deterrent.

Volatile Hydrocarbons

Volatile hydrocarbons (eg, glue, carbon tetrachloride, gasoline, nail polish remover, lighter fluid, paint, lacquer, varnish thinner) are most frequently abused by young individuals between 10 and 15 years of age. These liquids are usually deposited in a handkerchief, rag, or bag which is then placed over the nose and mouth and the vapors inhaled, a process known as "huffing." Initial exhilaration and excitation of the central nervous system may occur with blurring of vision, ringing in the ears, slurred speech, and staggering gait. These effects generally last from 30 to 45 min after inhalation. Depending upon the quantity of vapor inhaled, drowsiness, stupor, and unconsciousness may result. Occasionally, volatile hydrocarbon abuse precipitates psychotic behavior but susceptible individuals are apparently those who manifest personality disturbances antecedent to drug use. Amnesia often follows recovery. In extreme cases of intoxication death due to respiratory paralysis may occur.

Psychological dependence can develop and although physical dependence does not, this latter situation is probably attributable primarily to the limited duration of volatile hydrocarbon use rather than to the pharmacologic properties of these chemicals. If volatile hydrocarbons were abused frequently and for a sufficiently long period, physical dependence might be established as is the case with other potent central nervous system depressants, eg, barbiturates and narcotics.

Physical signs associated with the use of volatile hydrocarbons include characteristic odors, irritation of mucous membranes, and elevated pulse rate. Chronic abuse may produce damage to the kidneys, liver, heart, and brain. In glue sniffers with sickle-cell disease severe anemia has been observed, possibly as a result of bone-marrow depression. Chromosome damage in glue sniffers has been reported but this adverse reaction remains to be definitely established.

Butyl nitrite, an industrial chemical with no recognized therapeutic utility, is another abused volatile substance. Immediate effects of inhalation, related both to dose and duration of exposure, include light-headedness, delirium, headaches, cutaneous flushing, hypotension and elevated intraocular pressure; there is considerable similarity to amyl nitrite inhalation. Chronic toxicity is largely unknown but may involve methemoglobinemia.

Aerosol Propellants

More than two billion aerosol spray cans are produced each year for such diverse applications as household cleaners, furniture waxes, insecticides, hair sprays, antitussives, paints, antisticking coatings for cookware, deodorizers and disinfectants, and cocktail glass chillers. Many of these aerosols are also widely abused by youthful drug experimenters, primarily those in the teenage years.

Effects which result from "huffing" aerosols generally are similar to those described for volatile hydrocarbons. Beginning in the mid-1960s, reports in the medical literature have described several cases of collapse and death of young persons within a very short time after deliberate inhalation of the contents of various aerosol containers. This phenomenon has been designated "sudden sniffing death" (SSD); the appellation implies a greater degree of specificity than may, however, be warranted. The mechanisms involved in SSD have yet to be elucidated. Autopsy findings have been negative in that no anatomical cause of death has been established. Suffocation, frozen vocal cords, and respiratory failure may accompany SSD but do not appear to be the primary factors since death occurs so rapidly.

Considerable attention has been directed to the fluoroalkane propellant gases (most often Freons) as possible causative agents of SSD. Data provided by some experimental animal studies suggest that fluoroalkanes are capable of producing direct myocardial depression, bradycardia, atrioventricular block, and ventricular dysrhythmias. Other studies conducted with these chemicals have not, however, revealed significant direct cardiotoxicity. Fluoroalkane propellants and volatile hydrocarbon solvents may also have an indirect action on the heart, ie, sensitization of myocardial tissue to the arrhythmogenic effect of the catecholamines. Thus in individuals exposed to inordinate concentrations of these materials, endogenous epinephrine released during severe stress or physical activity might be expected to produce a markedly deleterious effect on cardiac function. Hypercapnia, as would result from rebreathing the air in a small closed environment (eg, bag sniffing) may further potentiate the cardiotoxicity of catecholamine and fluoroalkane or volatile hydrocarbon combinations.

Asthmatic patients have been found dead surrounded by one or more bronchodilator aerosol containers, the contents of which have been expended. Investigations into the nature of such fatalities indicate that a severe asthmatic attack itself may be the major cause of death. However, it has also been suggested that fluoroalkane propellants combined with epinephrine or isoproterenol may produce lethal cardiac arrhythmias if the recommended dose of inhalant is exceeded.

Isolated reports have linked the appearance of sarcoid-like lesions in the lungs and premalignant pulmonary lesions to the increased use of aerosol preparations; however, the validity of the presumed association remains to be confirmed.

Deaths related to aerosol propellant abuse have declined during the past few years. This trend is apparently due to elimination of Freons from spray cans in order to prevent environmental damage (eg, destruction of ozone layer in upper atmosphere).

Nitrous Oxide

Inhaling nitrous oxide for non-medical purposes, i.e., to induce a "high," remains a current national problem which is not confined to teenagers. Students at both the undergraduate and health professional level, as well as licensed practitioners, are known to be among the abusers. Supplies of nitrous oxide have been obtained through theft of large cylinders (eg, as utilized in hospitals) or by purchase of whipped cream cartridges which contain approximately 3 L of nitrous oxide.

Acute, uncontrolled exposure can be lethal by promoting unconsciousness in the user who then collapses into a body position which could be suffocating. At least one death has occurred in this manner. Other fatalities are known and the Drug Enforcement Administration estimates that nitrous oxide-related deaths are under-reported.

Chronic toxicity develops not only in abusers but also in health professionals who employ nitrous oxide for legitimate purposes. An extensive survey of dentists and dental assistants found that when exposure was "heavy," ie, more than 3000 hours over a ten year period (six hours per week), the number of reported adverse effects was four times greater than those experiencing "light" exposure, ie, less than 3000 hours per ten years. Initial signs and symptoms of nerve damage occur as numbness and paresthesias (unusual feelings in limbs described as burning and/or tingling). Later, muscle weakness and gait disturbances may develop. In abusers, this polyneuropathy could become permanent. Other effects of prolonged use which are less firmly linked include headaches, nephrotoxicity, hepatotoxicity, neoplastic disease, spontaneous abortions (higher than normal rate), and teratogenicity.

Marijuana (Marihuana)

Marijuana is obtained from one of man's oldest cultivated plants, *Cannabis sativa*. The biologically active principles of cannabis are concentrated in the resinous exudate of the flower clusters. Traditionally, the female plants have been harvested for their high resin yield. Chemical analyses have indicated, however, that the cannabinoid content of the resin does not differ significantly between the male and female plants. The potency of preparations derived from cannabis varies enormously depending on their composition and method of formulation; *hashish*, the unadulterated resin from the flowering tops of cultivated female plants, is a most potent form. By legal definition (US Federal Statutes), the term *marijuana* embraces all parts, extracts, derivatives, or preparations of cannabis, including the pure resin. However, as usually encountered in the Western hemisphere, marijuana constitutes a mixture of the leaves, flowering tops, and other structural parts of the cannabis plant, generally dried, chopped and incorporated in a form for smoking.

Although Δ^9-tetrahydrocannabinol (THC) appears to be the major active constituent of marijuana, biological activity may be largely attributable to the 11-hydroxy metabolite. Marijuana cigarettes ordinarily obtainable in the US contain about 1 to 2% THC; based on an average cigarette weight of approximately 500 mg, the amount of available THC ranges from 5 to 10 mg. Stronger products, ie, those with 3–5% THC, are currently available in the American 'market.'

Depending on potency, a marijuana cigarette will produce moderate to intense psychopharmacologic effects which reach a peak within 15 min and persist for 1 to 4 hours. As compared to smoking, marijuana consumed orally is about ⅓ as potent; the onset of activity is delayed but markedly prolonged.

One of the most consistently demonstrable effects of marijuana in humans is elevation of the pulse rate; the rate may rise by 50% or more above the preexposure level and increases may be sustained for several hours. Within limits, the intensity of this response appears to be related to the amount of drug consumed. Blockade by propranolol implicates β-adrenergic receptor activation in the mechanism of THC-induced tachycardia; however, that the increase in heart rate occurs without a simultaneous increase in left ventricular performance suggests the operation of an antivagal mecha-

nism by THC. Smoking marijuana when taking other drugs known to produce tachycardia, eg, nortriptyline, can result in a very substantial elevation of heart rate.

Blood pressure changes are variable; slight elevations and reductions of systolic and diastolic pressure have been noted. Continuous electrocardiographic monitoring of subjects who smoked cigarettes calibrated to contain 20 mg of THC revealed no ECG alterations that could be attributed definitely to marijuana intoxication. In contrast to the increased heart rate observed in humans, THC produces bradycardia in several animal species, eg, rat, cat, and dog.

Reddening of the conjunctiva (conjunctival congestion) is another consistent response to marijuana; that reddening also occurs after oral administration of THC indicates that this is not an artifact produced by irritation from smoke. Despite a belief long associated with marijuana, significant changes in pupillary diameter are not observed. Although marijuana does not elevate the respiratory rate, oral administration may produce airway dilation, probably by direct relaxation of bronchial musculature, for a period of several hours. Appetite is stimulated in human and subhuman species but without concurrent alteration of the blood glucose level. Weight gain, which often occurs during prolonged use of marijuana, is probably related more to increased caloric intake than to excessive fluid retention. Disturbances of equilibrium and muscular coordination as well as hyperreflexia during marijuana intoxication have been reported. Other physiologic changes noted with marijuana include dryness of the mouth and throat, irritation of the oropharyngeal mucosa, nausea and occasional vomiting, tinnitus, and paresthesias.

The marijuana-induced state is characteristically a hypersuggestible state; psychologic and perceptual effects are influenced markedly by the mental attitude, mood, and expectations of the user as well as by the setting and circumstances attending its use. Typically there is a sense of relaxation, inner contentment, euphoria, or even elation; thoughts flow in disconnected fashion in a dream-like state; time and space orientation are impaired; body image is distorted; perception of colors and sounds is altered, usually intensified; and laughter comes easily and may be uncontrollable but sometimes mood is subdued or depressed. The subjective responses to marijuana generally correlate with the onset and duration of tachycardia and conjunctival vascular congestion. EEG changes have been recorded in THC-treated animals, and it has been suggested that activation of septal areas associated with pleasure and emotion may play a role in certain of the observed psychological alterations.

Short-term memory is frequently impaired and information learned while under the influence of marijuana is recalled effectively only when the individual is again subjected to the drug effect, ie, state-dependent learning. Intense depersonalization, loss of insight, disorganized thinking and speech, and grossly distorted perception occur with high doses but true hallucinations are rarely experienced except at toxic levels; this contrasts with the hallucinogenic drugs (eg, LSD, DMT) which induce organized visual illusions and hallucinations at subtoxic doses.

Performance in psychometric tests is variably affected, depending on the nature of the task, its complexity and the dose of marijuana. Generally, marijuana produces a dose-related psychomotor performance decrement. In tests of driving skills, speedometer errors were increased but braking, signaling, and steering responses were essentially unimpaired. There is, however, a significant delay in light adaptation which may seriously impair driving at night. Marijuana prolongs the time needed to regain normal vision after exposure to bright light as, for example, from the headlights of an oncoming automobile. This effect is dose-related and may persist for two hours after marijuana use. That deficiencies in these responses may contribute to automobile accidents is suggested by the finding of measurable blood levels of THC in some motorists involved in traffic violations. In a recent study, subjects with plasma THC levels above 25–30 ng/mL failed coordination tests routinely given to drivers to assess the severity of alcohol intoxication. However, the temporal correlation between plasma THC levels and degree of incoordination was not as accurate as with alcohol.

Adverse reactions to marijuana occur relatively infrequently; they have been classified by Weil[2] as follows:

1. Normal population.
    Simple depressive reactions—occur in neophyte users; terminate spontaneously.
    Panic reactions—occur mainly in individuals who have inhibitions regarding use of psychoactive drugs; patient may be anxious, depressed, fearful, withdrawn, or agitated but, generally, is panicked due to physiological and/or psychological effects which are misinterpreted as life-threatening.
    Toxic psychoses—serious, temporary disturbance of normal brain activity; patients are disoriented and frequently experience hallucinations.
2. Persons who have previously taken hallucinogenic drugs.
    Precipitation of "flashbacks"—marijuana may induce recurrences of a "trip" which originally developed from previous consumption of a hallucinogenic drug.
    Precipitation of delayed psychotic reactions to hallucinogenic drugs—hallucinogens occasionally produce psychotic reactions several months after use—marijuana may have been the triggering factor but this cannot be definitely established.
3. Persons with a history of psychoses.
    Many individuals who have unpleasant experiences with marijuana are ambulant schizophrenics—in some of these cases marijuana may precipitate true psychotic reactions.

Death in humans resulting directly from marijuana toxicity appears to be a rare phenomenon. Acute toxicity determinations in animals reveal that extremely large amounts are necessary to cause lethality and that the median lethal dose-to-median effective dose ratio (ie, LD50/ED50) for marijuana is many times greater than that obtained with either the barbiturates or alcohol. Children who accidently ate marijunana-containing cookies became intoxicated and presented with varying degrees of effects routinely observed in adults, eg, tachycardia, bilateral conjunctival hyperemia (congestion), ataxia and nystagmus; recovery was uneventful and occurred within 6 hours.

Continued use of marijuana may result in psychological dependence, and tolerance may develop to psychological (characteristic "high" time estimation), physiological (tachycardia), and combined (psychomotor coordination) effects of marijuana. Evidence for psychological tolerance accrues, in part, from the observation that chronic users tend to increase the amount consumed or resort to a more potent variety in order to experience altered states of consciousness; clinical laboratory studies provide data to support the other forms of tolerance. Mechanisms involved in tolerance to marijuana may include cellular adaptation, particularly within the central nervous system, and an increased biotransformation capacity.

Conversely, the phenomenon of "reverse tolerance" or sensitization to marijuana has been reported. This may be attributable to psychological or to metabolic factors, or to a combination of both. Experience undoubtedly plays a role in the user's awareness and enjoyment of a marijuana-induced "high," and with repeated conditioning less of a stimulus is necessary to trigger the anticipated subjective effects. In addition, long-term smokers appear to be more efficient, inhaling and retaining more smoke per puff than the novice. THC and, possibly, active metabolites of this molecule are eliminated slowly from the body. Some chronic users continue to excrete THC in the urine for 20–30 days after terminating all marijuana smoking and/or ingestion. Frequent use of marijuana may therefore result in significant *in vivo* accumulation with a consequent reduction in the amount of drug

needed to exceed a psychoactive threshold in the brain. Such accumulation has been reported to occur in volunteer subjects who claim having had no prior exposure to marijuana. Approximately 50% of a standardized dose of THC was present in the plasma of naive subjects 56 hours after administration. Factors possibly contributing to this prolonged retention include an enterohepatic recirculation of THC and/or active metabolites, binding to plasma proteins, and sequestration in adipose tissue with delayed metabolism. In chronic marijuana smokers the biologic half-time of THC was reduced appreciably (ie, $t_{1/2} = 28$ hours) but this period is still sufficiently long to result in accumulation if marijuana is used daily or more frequently.

Physical dependence may occur, since after one week of THC administration, a withdrawal syndrome has been observed which consisted of anorexia, nausea, insomnia, sweating, hyperthermia and tremor. The mildness of these responses is probably due to the slow elimination of THC from the body which allows physiological and psychological systems to gradually adjust to a drug-free state.

Under experimental conditions employing male animals, and in human smokers, marijuana decreased testosterone blood levels, testicular size and weight, spermatogenesis and sexual potency. Inhibition of the release of luteinizing hormone (LH) from the pituitary gland, and the testicular responses to LH stimulation have been cited as possible mechanisms. However, THC also has weak estrogenic activity, as demonstrated by animal studies and clinical examination (including biopsy) of young males who developed gynecomastia during heavy marijuana use. THC inhibits ovulation in rats, rabbits and monkeys. Disruption of menstrual cycles has occurred in women who smoke marijuana on a regular basis.

Studies conducted with laboratory animals have shown that prolonged administration of THC may inhibit growth, impair lactation, promote thyroid hyperplasia, and elevate plasma corticosteroid levels. These physiologic alterations appear to reflect primarily actions of THC on the pituitary gland. High doses of THC in animals have been reported to induce hyperactivity and convulsive seizures indicative of neurotoxicity. Lacking comparable data in humans the significance of these studies must be interpreted cautiously.

Prolonged marijuana use may lead to serious pulmonary toxicity. *In vitro* tests employing lung explants demonstrated that marijuana smoke can induce premalignant and malignant cellular changes. Chronic exposure of animals to marijuana smoke led to severe bronchiolitis and squamous metaplasia of the tracheal mucosa; fatal respiratory complications occurred in some cases. Bronchial biopsies in humans who were long-term marijuana smokers also revealed squamous metaplasia. Substantial respiratory impairment, indicated by a significant increase in resistance to air flow (suggestive of obstructive lung disease), and high carboxyhemoglobin levels have also been observed in these individuals; both abnormalities are comparable to those associated with chronic tobacco smoking. Although extensive epidemiological studies are needed to confirm these findings, pulmonary toxicity should be considered a probable consequence of chronic marijuana smoking.

Suppression of cellular-mediated immune responsiveness has been demonstrated in young chronic marijuana smokers as well as in animals administered THC. The lymphocytic response observed in marijuana smokers was similar to that of patients in whom impairment of T (thymus-derived) cell immunity is known to occur. Some clinical studies have shown no significant suppression of lymphocyte function. Significant impairment of immune responsiveness, if corroborated by further studies documenting increased rates of infection or malignancy, should lead to a serious reappraisal of the risks of marijuana smoking.

Personality, attitudinal and behavioral changes are frequently associated with chronic marijuana smoking. There is characteristically a reduction in motivation, the desire to be productive, creative, or contributive, and the individual may experience acute feelings of insecurity. Although elements of this syndrome are typical of normal adolescent turmoil, compulsive involvement with marijuana may accelerate projection into, intensify, and delay emergence from this ambivalent phase of life. Marijuana may foster similar disruptions in older persons but evidence also exists that individuals can continue to function effectively in artistic and other creative areas while indulging in frequent but moderate use of the drug.

The LaGuardia Report (Mayor's Committee on Marijuana, New York City, 1944) stated that "marijuana will not produce a psychosis *de novo* in a well-integrated stable person." Judging from the medical literature published subsequent to this report, primary marijuana psychosis is relatively rare in the US. The precipitation of serious psychological problems appears to occur primarily in persons with preexisting personality or emotional disturbances. Use of marijuana by schizophrenic patients, including those being treated with antipsychotic agents, may result in rapid and serious deterioration of their mental state necessitating re-hospitalization in some cases.

Some studies have demonstrated a positive correlation between marijuana dosage and birth defects; however, other investigations have failed to provide evidence that marijuana possesses teratogenic activity. THC administered to pregnant rats and dogs is transferred rapidly to fetal tissue and results in a higher than expected incidence of abnormal pregnancies and stillborn offspring. Malformations observed include cleft palate, accessory ribs, fused ribs, and asynchronous and retarded vertebral ossification. Women who smoke marijuana while pregnant experience a longer period of labor and their newborn weigh less than normal and have altered central nervous system activity. THC is lipid-soluble and passes into the milk of the lactating female; thus marijuana should specifically be avoided by women who are breast feeding their newborn.

While primary attention has been directed to the adverse physiologic and social effects of marijuana, there are several indications that the tetrahydrocannabinols may possess clinically useful properties. When administered to patients with advanced cancer, oral doses of THC (capsules containing 7 to 10 mg in sesame oil) elicited mild analgesic, antidepressant, tranquilizing and antiemetic effects. However, a rapid development of tolerance, sometimes by the third dose, has limited THC utilization in these patients. Further, at these doses, and more frequently at a higher (20 mg) dose, disturbing side effects, eg, dizziness, ataxia, blurred vision and excessive sedation, were observed. Although it often stimulates appetite, marijuana is not useful in treatment of anorexia nervosa. In fact, it probably should be contraindicated since persons with this disorder possess some underlying psychological abnormality which can be exacerbated by oral THC administration, ie, some patients receiving this therapy have presented with significant dysphoria manifest as paranoia and loss of self control. Other investigations have demonstrated significant and prolonged reduction of intraocular pressure by marijuana in glaucoma patients. Proposed anti-inflammatory and anticonvulsant activities of THC await further clinical evaluation.

Although much remains to be developed there is beginning to emerge a reasonably clear picture of the acute pharmacologic and toxicologic effects of marijuana. While it will take longer to identify chronic toxic effects the current deficiency of such observations should not, therefore, be misinterpreted.

Cigarettes

Cigarette smoking is sanctioned in most social groups despite continued warnings regarding associated adverse effects. Many individuals continue to smoke in the belief that they will readily abandon the habit upon the development of any adverse reaction. However, with the passage of time the habit becomes deeply ingrained, the pathophysiologic changes consequent to cigarette smoking develop insidiously, and the human is inordinately prone to rationalizing his behavior. Incipient changes in pulmonary function have been detected in teenagers within a relatively short time after the initiation of cigarette smoking. Excessive coughing and sputum production and shortness of breath develop early in the course of cigarette smoking, with the eventual possibility of permanent alterations in lung structure. Emphysema is often detectable at approximately 30 years of age in persons who began smoking in their teens, but most individuals do not seek medical assistance until they experience serious dysfunction and at this point many established changes are irreversible. A reasonable correlation exists between the incidence of emphysema and the average number of cigarettes smoked per day; autopsy reports reveal that emphysema is present three times as frequently in heavy smokers as in nonsmokers.

Cigarette smoking accounts for approximately $\frac{1}{3}$ of all cancer deaths in this country and is the leading single cause of such mortality. Lung cancer and cigarette smoking have been linked convincingly by numerous clinical studies. There is a similar, though less frequent, association with pipe and cigar smoking. Current evidence clearly shows that lung cancer deaths among women has increased substantially over the past 30 years—from 4.6/100,000 in 1950 to 17.5/100,000 in 1978; the projected rate for 1982 is 20.9/100,000. This greater mortality is associated with a proportional increase in the rate of women who have become cigarette smokers. Further evidence of this correlation is found in data from two states. In Washington, over a recent 10 year period, the lung cancer death rate in women increased by more than 100% but the breast cancer death rate did not change significantly. In Utah, where a strong anti-smoking attitude prevails, the lung cancer death rate among women is less than 50% of the breast cancer death rate. All smokers should be encouraged to stop since after several years of non-smoking the risk of developing bronchogenic carcinoma approaches that of non-smokers. Smokers also have a higher incidence of both periodontal disease and cancer of the oral cavity than nonsmokers; bladder carcinoma, manifest both before and after the appearance of lung cancer, is another risk as is cervical cancer. Switching to 'low tar, low nicotine' products may not be an improvement since clinical studies show that smokers take more frequent and deeper puffs of these cigarettes than of regular ones in order to maintain their usual plasma levels of nicotine. Bronchitis and respiratory tract disorders in general are more prevalent not only in smokers but among their family members as well since exposure to cigarette smoke is often inescapable in the relatively closed atmosphere of a house or apartment.

Cardiovascular disorders occur more frequently, and the risk of death from coronary heart disease is significantly greater in smokers than in nonsmokers. In patients with hypertension, hypercholesterolemia, or diabetes the risk of coronary heart disease is further increased by cigarette smoking. Peripheral vascular disease and cerebrovascular insufficiency are also encountered more often in smokers. A common link to these cardiovascular diseases appears to be the damage to blood vessel (eg, coronary artery) walls which occurs more frequently among smokers and which serves to promote formation of atherosclerotic plaques. Myocardial infarction is a relatively rare complication in premenopausal females; however, cigarette smoking progressively increases the incidence of myocardial infarction to as much as 20-fold among women smoking 35 or more cigarettes per day. Since female hormones may be a factor in the lower rates of cardiovascular disease in women as compared to men, it is pertinent to note that menopause often occurs at an earlier age in women smokers.

Smokers have elevated carboxyhemoglobin (COHb) levels due to inhalation of excess carbon monoxide from the combustion of tobacco. Significant carboxyhemoglobinemia reduces oxygen transport by the circulatory system. Environmental conditions result in the formation of COHb equivalent to approximately 0.5% of total hemoglobin in the nonsmoker. Smoking one pack of cigarettes per day may produce COHb in the range of 6% or more, a level which may result in interference with subtle central nervous system processes, eg, judgment as utilized in automobile driving. Heavy smokers may show COHb levels of up to 20% of total hemoglobin, which places substantial strain on the cardiovascular system. Such alterations in oxygen transport have led to consideration of possible restrictions on utilizing smokers' blood for transfusions. An additional consequence of high carbon monoxide levels is secondary polycythemia, ie, tissue hypoxia due to prolonged exposure to carbon monoxide results in increased red cell mass.

Gastrointestinal disturbances associated with smoking include epigastric discomfort, gastritis, and, possibly, gastric and duodenal ulceration. An increase in gastric acid regurgitation into the esophagus apparently accounts for cigarette-induced heartburn which is frequently painful in heavy smokers. Pyloric incompetence and subsequent reflux of duodenal juices may be a contributory factor in the gastritis and gastric ulceration since bile injures the gastric mucosa, particularly in the absence of food in the stomach. In addition, nicotine may cause localized areas of ischemia in the gastrointestinal tract and may reduce pancreatic buffering secretions, thus peptic ulceration may occur in the presence of even normal rates of gastric acid secretion.

Continued cigarette smoking during anti-ulcer therapy diminishes the probability of successful treatment.

In regard to influenza, several studies show that compared to nonsmokers, smokers contract this disease at a higher rate and experience a greater degree of incapacitation (ie, more lost work days).

Considerable data show that smoking during pregnancy is associated with higher than normal rates of miscarriage, spontaneous abortion, prenatal mortality, and premature birth. The newborn of women who smoke during pregnancy are more likely to be underweight, short in stature, and have a smaller head. These effects are dose-related, ie, the incidence increases in proportion to the number of cigarettes smoked per day. Weight, height, and head circumference decrements persist four to seven years after birth.

In 1964 a report on Smoking and Health was issued by the Surgeon General of the Public Health Service; this report included the following statements:

Cigarette smoking is the most important of the causes of chronic bronchitis in the United States and increases the risk of dying from chronic bronchitis . . . The smoking of cigarettes is associated with an increased risk of dying from pulmonary emphysema . . . Cigarette smoking is causally related to lung cancer in men; the magnitude of the effect of cigarette smoking far outweighs all other factors. The data for women, though less extensive, point in the same direction . . . Male cigarette smokers have a higher death rate from coronary artery disease than non-smoking males, but it is not clear that the association has causal significance.

In 1979 a second report issued by the Surgeon General reaffirmed and expanded the health hazards of cigarette smoking; it emphasized more recently accumulated data indicating that women who smoke are at similar risk with men who smoke relative to cancer, heart disease and other illnesses. Further, the report cited disturbing evidence of the rapid development of respiratory problems and lung damage among teen-age cigarette smokers.

Central Nervous System Stimulants

Amphetamines

The term *amphetamine* properly applies to racemic (DL) β-phenylisopropylamine; however, the designation *amphetamines* has come to embrace not only the former chemical entity, the dextrorotatory isomer, *dextroamphetamine*, the N-methyl homologue, *methamphetamine*, but in its broadest context, a large number of structurally and pharmacologically related substances. Listings of drugs of abuse frequently include anorexiants (ie, sympathomimetic amines intended for use as appetite suppressants) under the general classification of *amphetamines* or *amphetamine-like* agents. Other synthetic phenylisopropylamine derivatives, such as trimethoxyamphetamine (TMA) and dimethoxymethylamphetamine (DOM or STP), are considered briefly in the section on *psychotomimetics*.

Clinical indications for amphetamines include (1) the management of certain behavioral disturbances in children, eg, hyperkinetic syndrome associated with minimal brain dysfunction, (2) the symptomatic control of narcolepsy and (3) the treatment of exogenous obesity, as short-term (ie, a few weeks) adjuncts in a regimen of weight reduction based on caloric restriction. Benzphetamine, chlorphentermine, clortermine, diethylpropion, phendimetrazine, and phentermine, alternatives to amphetamines in weight reduction programs, are also subject to misuse and abuse. These compounds are related chemically and pharmacologically to the amphetamines, but possess a somewhat higher ratio of anorexiant to central stimulant and peripheral sympathomimetic activity.

Misuse encompasses the episodic ingestion of amphetamines to suppress fatigue, prolong wakefulness and alertness, thus enabling the individual to continue mental or physical activity beyond his or her usual limit of endurance. Teachers are frequently witness to the futility of hyperamphetaminization—in the form of the tense, distraught student whose effective functioning is precluded by disorientation and mental short-circuiting or in the form of the exhausted and depressed student whose chemical props have collapsed. Despite the hazards involved, long-distance truck drivers similarly use amphetamines to dispel monotony and boredom. Although the practice is overtly pernicious, administration of amphetamines prior to engaging in athletic activity (eg, swimming, running, weight throwing) may improve performance to a degree that could be decisive in competition.

There remains a significant "gray area" of misuse—the prescribing of amphetamines and amphetamine-like drugs for unjustifiable reasons or, at best, in cases where the therapeutic rationale is borderline. To the busy medical practitioner, central nervous system stimulant and depressant drugs may provide an expedient if less than ideal means of helping his patients cope with the pressures and frustrations of everyday life. In the treatment of obesity these drugs provide a questionably effective and often self-deceptive approach to a complex biomedical problem. Clearly, those engaged in prescribing and dispensing drugs must exercise skilled judgment in eliminating as candidates for amphetamine therapy those patients so emotionally predisposed as to explore the secondary values in their anorexiants, ie, the mental lift, the elan, the psychic crutch upon which they may increasingly depend to cope with crises, real or imaginary.

Amphetamine abuse relates primarily to the nonsupervised ingestion or injection of large doses of amphetamine or its many chemical derivatives to experience the drug-induced psychic excitation, euphoria or "high," and the physical maelstrom of restless energy. Methamphetamine (methedrine, "speed") is a favored congener among habitual amphetamine users who generally inject the drug into a vein; this provides an almost instantaneous onset of the euphoric effect (the "flash" or "rush") which is ineffable and ecstatic.

A marked degree of tolerance to the amphetamines may be acquired; eventually several grams of drug per day may be consumed. There have been reports of the use of more than 10 g of methamphetamine intravenously over a 24-hour period. Tolerance does not develop uniformly to all the central nervous system effects; the compulsive user may evidence increased nervousness, anxiety, and persistent insomnia as the dose is increased. In a typical pattern of abuse immense doses of amphetamines are injected every few hours around the clock. These "runs," during which the individual remains continuously awake, generally last 3 to 6 days but may be prolonged to weeks if the user is able to sleep even as little as 1 hour a day. Appetite for food is suppressed and there is a feeling of unbridled energy and a compulsion for constant activity. Intravenous injection of enormous doses of amphetamines elicits a "chemically generated trauma" which appears linked inseparably to the acquired psychological dependency. The intense psychotoxic syndrome ultimately forces interruption of drug use and the individual lapses into a protracted period of deep sleep (the "crash").

Although it is generally considered that the amphetamines do not induce a physical dependence, abrupt withdrawal is characterized by lethargy and profound depression, both psychic and physical, which reinforces the drive to resume their use. Massive abuse of amphetamines frequently leads to considerable mental and physical deterioration. Intravenous injection of large doses is extremely disabling, socially and psychologically, and has resulted in psychiatric complications ranging from subtle personality changes to paranoid psychoses. Harm to the individual and to society often arises during psychotoxic episodes. In contrast to the decreased psychological drives of the opiate user, the compulsive user of central nervous system stimulants has exaggerated drives. Analyzing personality factors which underlie the preferential abuse of central stimulants vs narcotics, it has been postulated that the amphetamine abuser utilizes the stimulant as one of a variety of compensatory maneuvers to maintain a posture of active confrontation with the environment. In contrast, the heroin abuser reduces anxiety via repression and withdrawal. The hyperactivity, the compulsivity, the feeling of great muscular strength, the paranoid delusions, and the auditory and visual hallucinations may combine to make the amphetamine or cocaine user capable of committing serious antisocial acts. Chronic users of stimulant drugs are also accident-prone, since they are unaware of their fatigue until it overcomes them at an inopportune time.

As in any situation in which hypodermic equipment is shared without proper sterilization, there exists a risk of blood-borne infection, notably viral hepatitis. Among amphetamine abusers, evidence has been noted of hepatic damage so common as to suggest the possibility of a direct toxic effect on the liver.

Parenteral administration of large doses of sympathomimetic amines may result in morbidity or mortality due to intracranial hemorrhage or cardiac arrhythmias secondary to severe hypertension. Necrotizing angiitis was observed in Rhesus monkeys given repeated injections of methamphetamine for a 2-week period, and clinical descriptions of cerebral vasculitis and hemorrhage following injection of this sympathomimetic amine have been reported. Intravenous injection of amphetamines may result in a syndrome characterized by fever, leukemoid reaction, disseminated intravascular coagulation and rhabdomyolysis; these factors may be responsible for the development of acute renal failure in certain amphetamine abusers.

Cocaine

Cocaine, as extracted by chewing leaves of the coca plant (*Erythroxylon coca*), has dispelled hunger, provided a sense of well-being, and enhanced the physical endurance of Andean Indians since before the Conquistadors. Even today in the Andean regions of South America the chewing of coca leaves is regarded as no more a deviant practice than the smoking of tobacco leaves by persons in other parts of the world.

Although the pharmacologic spectrums of cocaine and the amphetamines differ in many respects, their subjective effects, toxicity, and present-day patterns of abuse are remarkably similar. Until recently, cocaine was very expensive when purchased from illicit sources. However, larger amounts are now being successfully smuggled into the United States leading to reductions of the 'street' price. This lower cost of acquisition, in the presence of a more plentiful supply, has resulted in a greater number of citizens becoming cocaine addicts. When cocaine is unavailable, abusers often resort to amphetamine. Extemporaneous mixtures of cocaine and amphetamine or heroin are common in the contemporary drug scene.

Regardless of the route of administration of cocaine (oral, nasal insufflation, intravenous), there is good correlation between the appearance of certain physical effects (tachycardia, elevated blood pressure) and psychological alterations ("high," pleasantness, anorexia). Prolonged use may be associated with weight loss, insomnia, anxiety, paranoia, sensations of insects crawling under the skin ("cocaine bugs"), and hallucinations (primarily visual—flashes of light or "snow lights"; may also be tactile, olfactory, and auditory). Ulceration and perforation of the nasal septum may also occur. In one reported case of chronic cocaine sniffing, the patient presented with a continuous nasal discharge that was not mucous. Instead, it was shown to be cerebrospinal fluid leaking from the central nervous system area due to extensive cocaine-induced local tissue and nerve (olfactory) damage. Large doses of cocaine may result in tremors, convulsions, and delirium. Deaths have been reported following every route of cocaine administration, including nasal insufflation. Unusual fatalities have occurred in drug dealers who, to avoid detection, swallowed prophylactics filled with cocaine; upon rupture of several condoms in the gastrointestinal tract, lethal concentrations of cocaine were absorbed.

The frequency of administration and extremely large amounts of cocaine which may be taken daily by the habitué reflect primarily its rapid inactivation in the liver and consequent short-lived effect rather than the development of significant tolerance to the alkaloid. Cocaine does not induce physical dependence; thus no characteristic abstinence syndrome is manifest on abrupt withdrawal. Development of physical dependence is not linked inextricably to compulsive drug use. Cocaine is probably the best example of a drug that induces neither tolerance nor physical dependence. However, the intense psychological dependence produced by cocaine can lead to a degrading and dangerous type of drug abuse. Jaffe[3] has defined *addiction* as "a behavioral pattern of compulsive drug abuse, characterized by overwhelming involvement with the use of a drug, the securing of its supply, and a high tendency to relapse after withdrawal." He further states that in this frame of reference the compulsive user of amphetamine or cocaine is an *addict*.

Psychotomimetics

Psychotomimetics constitute a structurally diverse group of naturally occurring and synthetic molecules. Interest in these compounds resides more in their misuse than in their legitimate medical use. They are of value as research tools in experimental psychiatry and in the exploration of central neurochemical mechanisms but their therapeutic application remains limited and highly controversial.

At high dosage levels many drugs may disorganize mental function with resulting confusion, delirium, hallucinations, and, frequently, memory loss or amnesia. Such drugs include atropine, scopolamine, and related centrally acting anticholinergics, quinine and quinidine, digitalis glycosides, mecamylamine, adrenocorticosteroids, nalorphine, disulfiram, bromides, and certain heavy metals. The *toxic psychoses* produced by these drugs are due primarily to generalized metabolic disruption of both neural and extraneural systems rather than to discrete neurophysiologic perturbations.

Certain chemicals, however, are uniquely capable of inducing dramatic changes in psychic processes (ie, perception, thought, feeling, mood, and behavior) in doses which do not produce generalized metabolic disruption and which do not cause marked disturbances in sensorimotor or autonomic functioning. These compounds are generally classified as *psychotomimetics*, although the extent to which they mimic spontaneously occurring psychotic states is inconsistent and incomplete. Other imaginative designations for such substances include *psychosomimetics, psychotogenics, psychodysleptics, psychedelics, hallucinogenics, mysticomimetics*, and *phantasticants*.

On a structural basis, psychotogenic chemicals may be classified into three major groups: (1) substituted *indole alkylamines*, eg, dimethyltryptamine, psilocybin, and lysergic acid diethylamide, (2) substituted *phenyl alkylamines*, eg, mescaline and dimethoxymethylamphetamine, and (3) a structurally *heterogeneous* group, including the glycolate ester ditran, and the piperidine derivative phencyclidine. With the exception of lysergic acid diethylamide, the chemical nature and pharmacologic properties of the various psychotomimetics will be considered only briefly. The interested reader is referred to several comprehensive reviews on this extensive and complex category of psychoactive agents (refer to *Bibliography*).

Dimethyltryptamine

Hallucinogenic activity is characteristic of a large series of *N*-alkylated tryptamines. Structurally, the simplest of these is *N*,*N*-dimethyltryptamine (DMT). This compound occurs naturally in the seeds of *Piptadenia peregrina;* a powder prepared from these seeds, and referred to as *cohaba snuff*, is used by Haitian natives to induce mystical states of consciousness. DMT is not effective when taken orally; perceptual and mood changes result when the compound is inhaled (snuffed), smoked, or introduced parenterally. Effects are rapid in onset and limited in duration, (few hours), irrespective of route of administration. Synthetic higher homologues of DMT, ie, diethyltryptamine (DET) and dipropyltryptamine (DPT), produce qualitatively similar psychological effects which are, however, considerably longer-lasting; further increases in the size of the *N*-alkyl substituent decrease hallucinogenic activity, eg, the *N*-dihexyl derivative is essentially inactive.

Psilocybin and Psilocin

Psilocybin, the phosphate ester of 4-hydroxy-DMT occurs to the extent of about 0.3% in the Mexican mushroom, *Psilocybe mexicana*. Dephosphorylation *in vivo* by alkaline phosphatase converts psilocybin to psilocin (4-hydroxy-DMT). Loss of the phosphoric acid radical reduces the polarity of the molecule, enabling more efficient penetration of the blood-brain barrier, which may account for the relatively greater hallucinogenic potency of psilocin as compared to psilocybin. Although psilocin is less potent than LSD (ie, approximately $1/100$ as active on a milligram basis) and pro-

duces a less persistent psychedelic state, when equivalent doses are administered blind it is generally impossible for subjects acquainted with the LSD phenomenon to differentiate between the two drugs.

Mescaline

One of the first phenyl alkylamine hallucinogens to be identified was mescaline (3,4,5-trimethoxyphenethylamine), isolated originally from "mescal buttons," the flowering heads of the peyote cactus, *Lophophora williamsii*. This plant material has long been used by the Mescalero Apaches of the Southwest American plains in their quasi-religious ceremonies of peyotism. Mescaline is not a particularly potent psychotomimetic; the equivalent oral dose of mescaline (usually 5 mg/kg in humans) is approximately 4000 times larger than that of LSD. Following oral administration, mescaline produces a characteristic syndrome of sympathomimetic effects, anxiety, hyperreflexia, static tremors, and psychic perturbations including vivid hallucinations, usually of a visual nature. In man, mescaline has a biologic half-life of about 6 hours; it is excreted in the urine principally in the form of the unaltered drug and the inert metabolite 3,4,5-trimethoxyphenylacetic acid.

Addition of an alpha-methyl substituent to mescaline produces 3,4,5-trimethoxyamphetamine (TMA), a psychotogen approximately twice as potent as mescaline. Its enhanced potency is due presumably to a decreased susceptibility to oxidative deamination provided by alkylation of the alpha-carbon. Rearrangement of the three methoxy groups on the benzene ring yields six isomers of TMA, ranging from the weakly active compound 2,3,4-TMA to the 2,4,5-configuration which is about 18 times more active than mescaline.

The TMA analogue, 2,5-dimethoxy-4-methylamphetamine (DOM), is a potent psychedelic agent employed extensively by certain drug abusers and designated by them as STP (an acronym derived ostensibly from the terms "serenity, tranquility, peace"). Hydroxylation at C-4 with subsequent conjugation, forming inactive polar metabolites, constitutes a major pathway for biotransformation of the amphetamines. Introduction of a methyl group at C-4, as in DOM, blocks *p*-hydroxylation and thus markedly prolongs biological activity. DOM, in doses of 5 mg or more, produces intense and relatively long-lasting emotional changes and perceptual distortions. Cases have been reported of individuals actively hallucinating for several days following a single oral dose of DOM.

Consideration of the pharmacology and structure-activity relationships of the numerous synthetic dimethoxyamphetamines, trimethoxyamphetamines, and methoxymethylenedioxyamphetamines is beyond the scope of this presentation; this area has been reviewed extensively by Shulgin *et al.*[4] and Snyder and Richelson.[5]

Lysergic Acid Diethylamide

The dextrorotatory isomer of lysergic acid diethylamide (LSD), synthesized by Hofmann in 1938, remains the most potent psychotogenic agent either of natural or synthetic origin discovered to date. Although as little as 25 µg of LSD may produce subjective effects, intense depersonalization usually requires doses in the range of 100 to 250 µg. Structurally, LSD is related to the ergot alkaloids, notably ergonovine. This structural resemblance may account for certain pharmacologic and toxicologic similarities among LSD and the lysergic acid alkaloids of ergot.

Metabolism—Following oral administration, LSD is rapidly absorbed and widely but not uniformly distributed throughout the body. It is strongly bound to plasma proteins; highest concentrations are found in the liver, kidneys and lungs. Considerably less than 1% of an orally administered dose penetrates into the CNS; however, intense psychic changes occur at levels of less than 3 nano-g of LSD/g of brain tissue. Autoradiographic analyses of brain samples obtained from animals injected with ^{14}C-labeled LSD revealed relatively high concentrations in the pituitary and pineal glands, the hypothalamus and limbic system, and the auditory and visual reflex areas. While the distribution of LSD within the brain would appear to suggest the functional involvement of specific neural areas in the psychotogenic phenomenon, there is an imperfect correlation between drug localization and sites of drug action.

In humans the biologic half-life of LSD is approximately 3.5 hours; this corresponds roughly with the duration of the peak psychosensory effects which then gradually subside over an 8- to 12-hour period. LSD is converted, largely in the liver, to 2-oxy-LSD; this inactive metabolite together with glucuronic acid conjugates is excreted primarily in the urine.

Pharmacologic Effects—LSD possesses considerable CNS-stimulant activity. It produces an EEG pattern characteristic of central activation, alertness, or arousal and causes insomnia in laboratory animals and humans. LSD counteracts the central depressant effect of barbiturates and is antagonized by such suppressants as chlorpromazine.

LSD produces a sequential though somewhat overlapping pattern of physiological and behavioral changes, the intensity and duration of which are largely dose-dependent. Pupillary dilation, tachycardia, tremulousness, hyperthermia, and elevated blood glucose and free fatty acid levels, indicative of adrenergic activation are frequently manifest during early phases of the LSD response. These physiological alterations may be attributed both to primary LSD effects and to nonspecific stress-anxiety reactions.

Controlled studies of individuals under the influence of LSD uniformly reveal a generalized impairment of objective indexes of adaptive behavior and psychomotor performance, especially those processes and procedures that require critical judgment and coordination. It is likely that intellectual and motor decrements are due to attenuation of attention and motivation as well as to sensory-cognitive disturbances.

Perceptual alterations constitute the most dramatic effects of LSD; their kaleidoscopic patterns defy brief description. Illusions and pseudohallucinations, mostly of a visual or tactile nature, are commonly experienced, whereas true hallucinations are relatively infrequent. Synesthesia, the cross-over from one sensory modality to another, is an often-encountered LSD phenomenon. Colors may be "heard" and music may become "palpable." Moods and emotions may range from euphoria, elation, and ecstasy to dysphoria, depression, and despair. The psychological state produced by LSD cannot be generalized with precision; as with other psychotropic drugs, the response depends on many variables, including the dose administered, the personality and expectations of the individual as well as environmental influences.

Mechanisms of Action—The neurophysiologic correlates of LSD-induced alterations in behavior are incompletely understood. The effect of LSD upon raphe neurons resembles that of an excess of serotonin at postsynaptic receptor sites. It has also been shown that LSD facilitates neuronal activity in the ventral tegmental nucleus, which is generally considered to function as a gating device for the organization of sensory experience. While these experiments suggest that LSD may affect synaptic processes involved in the filtration and integration of sensory information within the brain, one cannot project unreservedly these observations in animals to the behavioral effects of LSD in man.

Experimental and Therapeutic Uses—LSD has been employed extensively to induce experimental psychoses for the primary purpose of studying aberrant mental states under controlled conditions. Despite prodigious efforts, the LSD model has not yielded pertinent clues to the biochemical etiology of schizophrenia.

Several investigators have proposed LSD as an adjunct to conventional psychotherapy and as an aid in treatment of chronic alcoholism. LSD has also been reported to provide long-lasting "euphor-analgesia" in patients with terminal cancer. The feasibility and effectiveness of LSD for these purposes remain unestablished and controversial. LSD has no approved therapeutic uses; it is currently an investigational drug subject to rigid state and federal regulations.

Dependence Liability—Marked psychological dependence on LSD is rarely observed; usage tends to be occasional or sporadic rather than frequent or compulsive. A high degree of tolerance to the physiological and behavioral effects of LSD develops after three or four doses taken within a relatively short period of time; this acquired resistance disappears rapidly if drug intake is terminated. There is considerable cross-tolerance among LSD, mescaline, and psilocybin but this phenomenon has not been demonstrated between LSD and either amphetamine or Δ^9-THC. Physical dependence on LSD does not develop; thus there is no characteristic abstinence syndrome upon abrupt discontinuation.

Toxicity—Despite its extreme psychotogenic potency the acute toxicity of LSD is remarkably low. Medical literature records no verified case of death in man attributable to the direct toxic effects of the drug, although fatal accidents and suicides have occurred during states of LSD intoxication. Homicides committed by persons apparently under the influence of LSD have been reported relatively infrequently. Most of the individuals involved evidenced premorbid psychopathologic tendencies and thus the role of LSD in violent and assaultive behavior is equivocal.

LSD-induced feelings of depersonalization and affective, perceptual, and cognitive distortions may on occasion result in disorientation, confusion, and acute panic reactions characterized by anxiety, fear, and a sense of helplessness and loss of control. "Bad trips" generally follow ingestion of high doses of LSD by nontolerant persons; they are also likely to occur in inexperienced users, in those with ambivalent attitudes toward the drug experience, or in disturbing or threatening surroundings. Reequilibration usually takes place within 24 to 48 hours.

Recurrences of perceptual distortions may be experienced in the postdrug state by a relatively high percentage of LSD users. These "flashbacks," which vary in length from a few seconds to several minutes, may occur up to five years after the drug was last taken. Flashbacks may be spontaneous but are often triggered by periods of emotional stress or anxiety or by other psychotropic drugs such as marijuana. The mechanism of recurrent hallucinosis is unknown but may reflect a persistent disruption of psychological defense mechanisms with periodic emergence of repressed fears or conflicts.

Chronic disruptive states associated with anxiety, depression, somatic disturbances, and difficulty in functioning, and which are relatively resistant to psychotherapy, not uncommonly follow LSD usage. Protracted schizophreniform psychotic states with paranoid behavior represent infrequently occurring but tragic psychological consequences of LSD. Most, but possibly not all, such cases involve unstable individuals with prepsychotic or premorbid personality traits. An unfavorable prognosis is indicated by motor retardation, withdrawal, blunt affect, anergy and suicidal ideation during the initial hospitalization period. Treatment varies but lithium has been proven effective for alleviation of LSD-induced psychosis.

There are several reports of inflammatory fibrosis occurring in individuals who have consumed LSD. This complication has previously been recorded with other lysergic acid derivatives, notably methysergide. Arteriospasm resulting in obstruction of the internal carotid artery, and the development of peripheral gangrene necessitating partial amputation of the extremities constitute isolated case reports indicating that LSD shares the vasoconstrictor activity of other ergot alkaloids.

In 1967 investigators first reported chromosome damage in human leukocytes cultured *in vitro* with LSD. Although the clinical significance of this finding was grossly exaggerated in the public news media, the widespread publicity may have contributed to a significant downturn in the abuse of LSD. The possibility of affecting generations yet unborn apparently struck a chord of moral responsibility in many who were convinced of their personal ability to maintain psychic control but who were unwilling to "pollute the genetic stream."

Genetic studies conducted with LSD have been critically reviewed by Dishotsky *et al.*[6] Although the relationships between LSD and chromosomal damage, leukemogenicity, and teratogenicity remain unresolved, certain tentative conclusions appear warranted:

Data supporting a positive relationship between LSD and chromosomal aberrations have been obtained primarily with individuals reported to have taken LSD obtained in the black market. In most instances, the amount of LSD consumed cannot be ascertained or can only be approximated; the reputed LSD samples may contain other drugs or contaminants either added or incompletely separated during the process of illicit synthesis. The population under study frequently extemporize with barbiturates, amphetamines, opiates, cocaine, marijuana, and other psychotogens, in addition to LSD.

Chemically pure LSD administered under controlled conditions has in several studies failed to produce detectable damage to chromosomes or has produced transient chromosomal aberrations in peripheral leukocytes but these defects were no longer evident several months after LSD administration. Transient chromosomal breaks in white blood cells occur spontaneously; they can be increased by certain antibiotics and antineoplastic agents and even by commonly employed drugs such as aspirin and caffeine. Viral infections are associated with an increased rate of chromosomal disruption. Hepatitis, gastrointestinal, and upper respiratory viral infections are common among chronic drug abusers. Thus it appears that chromosomal damage, when found, is related to a history of drug abuse in general and not to LSD specifically.

The pathological significance of chromosomal aberrations in continuously replenished peripheral leukocytes is equivocal. Testicular and bone-marrow biopsies in rhesus monkeys given repeated oral doses of LSD have not revealed significant chromosomal alterations in gametogenic and hemopoietic tissues.

Two cases of acute leukemia developing subsequent to the use of LSD are recorded. Although a causal relationship has not been established it may be premature to dismiss the association as merely coincidental.

Some studies suggest a higher incidence of spontaneous abortion among pregnant women who reportedly took LSD prior to or after conception, and a greater number of congenital anomalies among live infants born to mothers exposed to this drug; however, several complicating factors preclude a definitive correlation of increased reproductive risk with LSD ingestion. Among these are the indeterminate nature of purported LSD samples obtained "on the street," a common history of multiple usage of illicit drugs, a high incidence of infectious diseases, especially viral illnesses, and marginal maternal nutrition. Although the effect of LSD on human pregnancy and fetal malformations remains uncertain, discretion dictates avoidance of this drug by women of childbearing age.

Phencyclidine

Phencyclidine (PCP, "angel dust"), chemically and pharmacologically similar to ketamine (Ketalar) used to induce "dissociative anesthesia," is probably the most dangerous substance abused in the United States. There is no consensus as to the precise pharmacologic classification of PCP; the compound may, depending on the dose and other circumstances of use, exhibit stimulant, depressant, analgesic and hallucinogenic properties. In "street" form, PCP is often adulterated and frequently misrepresented as THC, mescaline, LSD, amphetamine, cocaine and many other psychoactive agents.

Although occasionally ingested orally or injected intravenously, PCP is most commonly smoked (after placing it on marijuana or dried parsley leaves in a "joint") or "snorted" (nasal insufflation). By smoking, the experienced user can limit the dose of PCP (self-titrate) to a level with which he or she is comfortable and is less likely to overdose than when the drug is taken orally.

While PCP ingestion can produce euphoria, adverse reactions are more commonly observed, particularly in naive users. An excellent classification of PCP effects has been developed by Rappolt *et al*[7] based upon their treatment of more than 250 cases. Tachycardia and elevated blood pressure are consistent findings and appear, in varying degrees, within each of the following categories:

Stage I: 2–5 mg PCP (serum concentration of 25–90 ng/mL)
Subjects are disoriented, combative and violent; they also experience ataxia, alterations in perception of visual, auditory and tactile sensations, excessive sweating and salivation, and analgesia (may injure themselves unknowingly due to this analgetic property).
Deaths occurred when subjects lost control of motor function yet attempted activities which require significant physical skill, eg, some tried to swim but subsequently drowned. Other fatalities happened after abusers engaged in violent fights or fell asleep in the middle of a street (and were crushed by a motor vehicle).

Stage II: 5–25 mg PCP (serum concentration of 90–300 ng/mL)
The patient presents with coma and does not respond to verbal communication; reactions to painful stimuli will occur, however. Muscle spasms and severe hyperthermia may also be present.

Stage III: Above 25 mg PCP (serum concentrations above 300 ng/mL)
Deep coma is observed with patients showing no response to extremely painful stimuli. Seizures are also likely and may develop into status epileptics.

Although the data are more difficult to interpret, it appears that a number of deaths are solely and directly related to excessive blood levels of PCP. Cerebral hypoxia due to severe spasm of cerebral blood vessels may be a mechanism of lethality.

Delayed psychological reactions (delirium, psychosis and/or agitation) occurring approximately one week after consumption of high doses of PCP have been observed; this may be due to the high lipid-solubility of the drug resulting in accumulation in, and slow release from, adipose tissue. On occasion, patients hospitalized for psychiatric examination have their blood analyzed for PCP levels. In some of these cases, a result showing an absence of PCP may be incorrect. Methods of analysis utilizing high performance liquid chromatography (HPLC), gas chromatography with flame ionic detection (GC-FID), or radioimmunoassay (RIA) are accurate only down to levels of 100–200 ng/mL. However, as presented above, serum PCP concentrations between 25–90 ng/mL are sufficient to induce aberrant behavior. A recent study employing a more sensitive assay procedure, a glass capillary-gas chromatography thermionic specific (nitrogen) detector (GC^2-N) capable of measuring levels as low as 5 pg/mL, reported that of 135 patients admitted for psychiatric evaluation, 78 had PCP levels between 1 and 50 ng/mL. This is a significant observation since it can assist physicians in determining the correct treatment.

Tolerance from two to four times the original amounts develops if PCP is administered chronically to laboratory animals; however, experiments performed to date do not suggest that PCP produces physical dependence comparable to that which develops to the opiates or other CNS depressants.

In normal volunteers, PCP induces a schizophrenic-like state. Thus, as is the situation with marijuana, individuals with psychoses (diagnosed or undiagnosed) are particularly vulnerable to PCP. Schizophrenics experience a deterioration of their condition, possibly culminating in stuporous or excitatory catatonia or paranoia accompanied by auditory hallucinations.

Rhabdomyolysis (skeletal muscle degeneration), myoglobinuria and renal failure have developed after acute large doses of PCP, whereas chronic use is associated with both psychological and physical dependence, and alterations in memory, speech and vision; these latter changes are suggestive of organic brain damage.

Treatment of Acute Drug Overdosage

A major problem in treating incoherent drug-overdosed patients, ranging from comatose to delirious, is the absence of definitive data regarding the substance(s) responsible for the intoxication. Upon admission to an emergency center it is imperative that staff members consult persons on the scene or the patient's friends in an attempt to obtain as much information as possible about the drug(s), amounts and modes of administration, circumstances leading to the overdosage, and pertinent aspects of the patient's medical history, eg, does the patient have diabetes or epilepsy? Due, however, to extensive adulteration of "street" drugs, the information obtained on drug identity and quantity must be evaluated with caution. Symptomatic treatment is advisable until a definitive diagnosis can be established. The following is a limited presentation of options available for treating adverse reactions to psychoactive substances.

Volatile Hydrocarbons—Treatment of acute intoxication with volatile hydrocarbons is similar to that employed for barbiturate overdosage. If the vapors are inhaled, oxygen (or a 95% O_2 and 5% CO_2 gas mixture) may be administered. When volatile hydrocarbons are swallowed, gastric lavage rather than an emetic should be utilized. Injection of epinephrine or other sympathomimetic amines should be avoided due to the possibility of myocardial sensitization and precipitation of cardiac arrhythmias.

Narcotics—Naloxone remains the drug-of-choice in countering narcotic analgetic overdosage. This narcotic antagonist, which possesses little or no agonistic activity, may be administered to the unconscious patient in the absence of a definitive diagnosis of narcotic overdosage. Naloxone will not produce additional CNS-depressant effects in the event that acute poisoning is due to barbiturates or other non-narcotic depressants.

Psychotomimetics—In cases of adverse psychological reactions to hallucinogens ("bad trips"), patients should be maintained in a supportive and non-threatening environment. Verbal contact should be established for reality defining and reassurance ("talk-down") that the episode will eventually terminate. If pharmacologic intervention appears indicated, use of diazepam (or a related benzodiazepine derivative) avoids the hazards which may be encountered with a phenothiazine in an unsuspected case of anticholinergic drug intoxication or in an individual with a history of convulsive disorders. When known anticholinergic agents are taken in excessive quantities, physostigmine, which antagonizes both central and peripheral atropine-like effects, is the drug treatment of choice.

Phencyclidine—Treatment of PCP overdosage differs from that associated with hallucinogens; intoxicated patients should not be engaged in an extended "talk-down" process. Isolation, with periodic observation, is beneficial as in relieving symptoms of acute schizophrenic reactions. Diazepam may control severe agitation; acidification of the urine with ascorbic acid or cranberry juice (avoid ammonium chloride and orange juice) accelerates excretion of PCP and may reduce the incidence of delayed reactions.

Cocaine—Adverse reactions to cocaine are usually of short duration and may terminate before treatment is initiated. Propranolol may be employed to attenuate the cardiovascular disturbances in cases of moderate cocaine overdosage. Diazepam may suppress the CNS excitation, although the possibility of adding to subsequent cocaine-induced respiratory depression must be considered.

Amphetamines—Disturbances of the sympathetic nervous system observed in amphetamine toxicity should be treated if they threaten the patient; acidification of the urine (avoid ammonium chloride and orange juice) can significantly shorten the duration of attendant psychoses. In the presence of acute renal failure accompanying shock and rhabdomyolysis associated with amphetamine intoxication, substantial fluid replacement is indicated.

* * * *

Pharmacists can participate in the early management of acute drug poisoning by advising the utilization of ipecac *syrup* (not the fluidextract) in appropriate situations. If the subject has ingested a potentially harmful quantity of drugs and is conscious, *syrup of ipecac* may be employed in the following oral doses: patient under 1 year old—10 mL; 1–12 years old—15 mL; over 12 years old—30 mL. Subsequently, 250–500 mL of liquid should be given. Vomiting within 30 minutes occurs in approximately 90% of patients receiving this regimen. If emesis does not ensue within 30 minutes, the recommended dose, with additional fluids, may be repeated. Syrup of ipecac is less useful if more than 60 minutes have elapsed since consumption of the drug overdose. If the patient does not vomit after two doses of the ipecac, the dosage should be recovered by gastric lavage.

References

1. Johnston LD, *et al:* National Institute on Drug Abuse, DHSS Publication No (ADM) 83-1260, 1982.
2. Weil AT: *New Engl J Med 282:* 997, 1970.
3. Jaffe JH, in Goodman LS, Gilman A, eds: *The Pharmacological Basis of Therapeutics,* 5th ed, Macmillan, New York, 284, 1975.
4. Shulgin AT, *et al: Nature 221:* 537, 1969.
5. Snyder SH, Richelson E, in Efron DH, ed: *Psychotomimetic Drugs,* Raven, New York, 43, 1970.
6. Dishotsky NI, *et al: Science 172:* 431, 1971.
7. Rappolt RT, *et al: Clin Tox 16:* 509, 1980.

Bibliography

Narcotics

Christie DJ, *et al: Arch Int Med 143:* 1174, 1983.
Cushman P, Grieco MH: *Am J Med 54:* 320, 1973.
D'Agostino and Arnett EN: *J Am Med Assoc 241:* 277, 1979.
Lupovich P, *et al: J Am Med Assoc 212:* 1216, 1970.
Nathenson G, *et al: J Pediat 81:* 899, 1972.
Pearson MA, *et al: Clin Tox 15:* 267, 1979.
Soin JS, *et al: J Am Med Assoc 224:* 1717, 1973.

Barbiturates

Kay DC, *et al: Clin Pharmacol Ther 13:* 221, 1972.
Smith DE, Wesson DR: *J Am Med Assoc 213:* 294, 1970.
Solomon F, *et al: New Engl J Med 300:* 803, 1979.

Nonbarbiturate Depressants

Faulkner TP, *et al: Clin Tox 15:* 23, 1979.
Gerald MC, Schwirian PM: *Arch Gen Psychiat 28:* 627, 1973.
Schnoll SH, Fishkin R: *J Psychedel Drugs 5:* 79, 1972.

Alcohol

Agarwal BN, *et al: New York J Med 73:* 1331, 1973.
Becker JT, *et al: Alcohol: Clin Exper Res 7:* 213, 1983.
Hammond KB, *et al: J Am Med Assoc 226:* 63, 1973.
Jones KL, *et al: Lancet 1:* 1267, 1973.
Jones RJ, *et al: J Am Med Assoc 249:* 2517, 1983.
Myers RD: *Ann Rev Pharmacol Toxicol 18:* 125, 1978.
Slavney PR, Gran G: *J Clin Psychiatry 39:* 782, 1978.

Volatile Hydrocarbons

Hayden JW, *et al: Clin Tox 11:* 549, 1977.
Sigell LT, *et al: Am J Psychiatry 135:* 1216, 1978.

Aerosols

Harris WS: *Arch Intern Med 131:* 162, 1973.
Kilen SM, Harris WS: *J Pharmacol Exp Ther 183:* 245, 1973.
Sharp CW, Brehm ML, eds: NIDA Research Monograph 15: October, 1977.

Marijuana

Bowman M, Pihl RO: *Psychopharmacologia 29:* 159, 1973.
Braude MC, Szara S, eds: NIDA Monograph, 2 vol., 1976.
Dalterio S, *et al: Pharmacol Biochem & Behavior 8:* 673, 1978.
Dornbush RL, *et al: Ann NY Acad Sci 282:* 1, 1976.
Gross H, *et al: J Clin Psychopharm 3:* 165, 1983.
Hollister LE, Tinklenberg JR: *Psychopharmacologia 29:* 247, 1973.
Lemberger L, Rubin A: *Drug Metab Rev 8:* 59, 1978.
Paton WDM: *Ann Rev Pharmacol 15:* 191, 1975.
Reeve VC *et al: Drug and Alcohol Depend 11:* 167, 1983.
Tashkin DD, *et al: Annal Intern Med 89:* 539, 1978.
Thompson GR, *et al: Toxicol Appl Pharmacol 25:* 373, 1973.
Treffert DA: *Am J Psychiat 135:* 1213, 1978.
Vardaris RM, *et al: Pharmacol Biochem Behavior 4:* 249, 1976.
Weinberg D, *et al: Pediatrics 71:* 848, 1983.

Cigarettes

Edwards TA: *Brit Med J 1:* 637, 1977.
Fielding JE: *New Engl J Med 298:* 337, 1978.
Grimes DS, Goddard J: *Brit Med J 2:* 460, 1978.
Jick H, *et al: Lancet 1:* 1354, 1977.
Kline J, *et al: New Engl J Med 297:* 793, 1977.

Read NW, Grech P: *Brit Med J 3:* 313, 1973.
Rose G: *Am Heart J 85:* 838, 1973.
Slone O, *et al: New Engl J Med 298:* 1273, 1978.
Stolley PD: *New Engl J Med 309:* 428, 1983.
Trevathan E, *et al: J Am Med Assoc 250:* 499, 1983.
Wasserman LR: *J Am Med Assoc 224:* 1654, 1973.

Central Nervous System Stimulants

Cohen S: *J Am Med Assoc 231:* 74, 1975.
Finkle B, McCloskey KL: *J Forensic Sci 23:* 173, 1978.
Resnick RB, Kestenbaum RS: *Science 195:* 696, 1977.
Sawicka EH and Trosser A: *Brit Med J 286:* 1476, 1983.
Siegl RK: *Am J Psychiatry 135:* 309, 1978.
Suarez CA, *et al: J Am Med Assoc 238:* 1391, 1977.

Psychotomimetics

Brawley P, Duffield JC: *Pharmacol Rev 24:* 31, 1972.
Efron DH, ed: *Psychotomimetic Drugs*, Raven, New York, 1970.
Lake CR, *et al: Am J Psychiatry 138:* 1508, 1981.
Lipton MA, *et al*, eds: *Psychopharmacology: A Generation of Progress*, Raven Press, NY, 1978.
Smythies JR, in: Neurosciences Research Symposium Summaries, MIT Press, Cambridge, MA, 1971.
Usdin E, Forrest IS, eds: *Psychotherapeutic Drugs*, Dekker, NY, 1976–77.

Phencyclidine

Allen RM, Young SJ: *Am J Psychiat 135:* 1081, 1978.
Aniline D, *et al: Biol Psychiat 15:* 813, 1980.
Burns RS, *et al: West J Med 125:* 345, 1975.
Burns RS, Lerner SE: *Clin Tox 12:* 463, 1978.
Cohen S: *J Am Med Assoc 238:* 515, 1977.
Hoogwerf B, *et al: Clin Tox 14:* 47, 1979.
James SH, Schnoll SH: *Clin Tox 9:* 573, 1976.
Peterson RC, Stillman RC, eds: NIDA Research Monograph 21: August, 1978.

Treatment of Acute Drug Overdosage

Kline NS, *et al*, eds: *Psychotropic Drugs: A Manual for Emergency Management of Overdose*, Medical Economics, 1974.
Veltri JC, Temple AR: *Clin Tox 9:* 407, 1976.

CHAPTER 72

Introduction of New Drugs

Ewart A Swinyard, PhD, DSc (Hon)
Professor Emeritus of Pharmacology
College of Pharmacy and School of Medicine, University of Utah
Salt Lake City, UT 84112

Most drugs used in primitive medicine were obtained from plants. These naturally occurring substances were employed in the form of infusions, decoctions, or poultices, and came into medicine by way of an accident or the herb doctor. The plants used as drugs were fairly innocuous and relatively free from toxic effects or were so toxic that their lethal effects were well known.

Drugs used in 19th-century medicine were naturally occurring substances extracted ready-made from plants, animals, or minerals. The active principles were isolated and came into medicine largely on an empirical basis. For example, opium and morphine were used in the control of pain, digitalis and other cardiac glycosides in the management of cardiac failure and edema, and quinine in the treatment of malaria. Although these agents, or some synthetic derivative of them, are still used today, they were first used in man without prior laboratory evaluation.

With the development of new methods of organic chemistry in the last decades of the past century and the first decades of the present century, it became possible to elucidate the structures of the pharmacologically active natural products and to synthesize either the active principle or a modified molecule which retained the pharmacological properties of the parent substance. Subsequently, efforts were directed toward the synthesis of molecules in which the pharmacologic properties of the original natural product were preserved or present to a more pronounced degree, while toxic side effects were reduced. This led to the synthesis of agents with novel structures, the pharmacologic properties of which were determined by study in laboratory animals.

This approach proved very fruitful and led to thousands of new and potent synthetic drugs. The discovery of aspirin as an analgesic was the result of attempts to improve on the properties of the plant constituent salicylic acid. The local anesthetic procaine evolved from attempts to synthesize a simple molecule retaining the structural features of the alkaloid cocaine.

Numerous analgesics were discovered in attempts to synthesize simple compounds structurally related in various ways to the alkaloid morphine. Efforts to find a substitute for quinine in the treatment of malaria led to the discovery of atabrine and a number of other effective antiplasmodial compounds. The study of the pharmacologic properties of synthetic antimalarials led unexpectedly to the antihistamines and, eventually, to the discovery of an entirely novel kind of drug, the tranquilizers. Thus, two important modern drug discoveries, antihistamines and tranquilizers, really stem from an old traditional remedy, quinine.

Drug Legislation

The original Food and Drugs Act of 1906 contained no control over the introduction of new drugs. It merely provided that drugs moving in interstate commerce were not to be adulterated or misbranded. It was the pharmaceutical industry which initiated the preclinical testing of candidate drugs in laboratory animals. Over a period of years the laboratory tests employed for efficacy and toxicity were consistently improved.

The first specific legislation directed at drug safety was triggered by a tragedy—the marketing of a sulfanilamide elixir in diethylene glycol. This resulted in a modification of the Food, Drug and Cosmetic Act in 1938 to require firms planning to market a new drug product to submit a *New Drug Application* (NDA). This act provided that, before a drug could be approved for marketing, it must be shown to be safe when used as directed on the label. It was not necessary to show that the claims for efficacy were valid.

From 1938 until the early 1960s drugs were introduced into medicine in ever increasing numbers. Many of these manmade drugs were highly selective in their effects and altered body physiology in very discrete ways. The pharmaceutical industry recognized the remarkable selectivity contained within many of these agents and developed innumerable ingenious pharmacological tests to reveal their profile of action prior to their first clinical use in man. Despite these advances, another drug tragedy—the thalidomide affair—led to the enactment by Congress in 1962 of the Kefauver-Harris amendments to the Food, Drug and Cosmetic Act.

The most significant provisions of the Kefauver-Harris Amendments of 1962 were those which require that all drugs be proved effective as well as safe for their intended uses. To accomplish this the new legislation made four basic changes in the Food, Drug and Cosmetic Act.[1]

1. Subjects participating in investigational drug research must give their informed consent.
2. All clinical investigational drug studies must be registered in the form of a *"Notice of Claimed Investigational Exemption for a New Drug"* (IND).
3. Manufacturers must submit data in a *New Drug Application* (*NDA*) format supporting efficacy of the product as well as safety.
4. The standard of scientific evidence acceptable for demonstrating effectiveness shall be "adequate and well controlled investigations, conducted by experts qualified by scientific training and experience to evaluate the effectiveness of the drug involved."

In addition to these four basic changes, the amendments also provided that drugs introduced between 1938 and 1962 on the basis of safety alone must be reevaluated to determine if clinical evidence supports the manufacturers' claims for clinical effectiveness. In order to accomplish this task the FDA solicited the aid of the National Academy of Sciences–National Research Council (NAS–NCR) to conduct this review. The actual evaluation was conducted by 27 panels of experts, the membership of which was known only to their colleagues. Approximately 3600 drug formulations submitted by 237 pharmaceutical firms were considered.

The recommended therapeutic indication for each formulation was reviewed by the panels (a few drugs were reviewed by as many as 10 or 15 panels) and the product classified as follows: "effective," "probably effective," "possibly effective," and "ineffective." In some cases a fifth category was employed: "effective, or probably effective, but —."

Over 10,000 independent judgments were required to

complete the task. These recommendations were then forwarded to the FDA for review. Subsequently, they were transmitted to the manufacturers involved with the New Drug Applications. At the same time, an announcement was published in the *Federal Register* inviting interested parties to a meeting to discuss the FDA's position on the NAS–NRC recommendations.

The 1962 Kefauver-Harris Amendments were designed to safeguard the public and to prevent another drug tragedy. In order to achieve this objective, the FDA required that new chemical entities (NCE) be subjected to more preclinical tests (eg, mutagenicity, teratogenicity, and long-term carcinogenicity and toxicity tests), and, more importantly, that the clinical studies provide a great deal more detail, controls, and documentation of the results. Moreover, continued congressional and FDA pressures led to the development of the *Good Laboratory Practice Regulations*, first proposed in 1976[2] and made final in June of 1979.

Implementation of the 1962 amendment was followed by dramatic increases in the time required to complete the preclinical phase (1.5 to 3.5 years) and clinical phase (2.5 to 6.0 years). Total development time from synthesis to NDA approval nearly doubled (6 to 12 years).[3] Consequently, effective patent life for NCE dropped from 16.3 years in 1960 to 6.8 years in 1981. Simultaneously, there was a 60% decrease in the average number of NCE submitted to FDA each year (89 to 35) and a 64% decrease in the average number of NCE-NDA approved for marketing (36 to 14).[4] Although the precise reasons for these changes are difficult to define, economic factors (costs of research vs expected return on investment), over regulation, and scientific demands on the state-of-the-art are important considerations.

In order to reverse this "drug lag," the FDA has revised its regulations governing approval of new drugs for human use.[5] The seven main categories of change[4] include: (1) *Data required for submission.* Summary tabulations will replace individual clinical use reports. This will reduce the bulk of the application by 70% (average application in 1982 about 100,000 pages). (2) *The format of the application will be changed.* Technical data will be presented in a 50- to 200-page summary in manuscript form. (3) *Improved communication with drug sponsors* and a new automatic appeals process for promptly resolving scientific disagreements. (4) *New policy on foreign data.* Quality studies by recognized clinical investigators will be accepted if applicable to the US population. (5) *Clarify time frame for FDA decisions.* The agency will determine within 60 days whether application is complete. Action letter (approved, approvable, denied) will be provided the sponsor within 180 days. (6) *Requirements for supplemental applications.* Preclearance by FDA will be required only for those changes which affect safety or effectiveness of the drug. (7) *Maintain vigilant reporting of adverse drug experiences after drug is on the market.* This includes adverse effects; reactions from overdoses, drug abuse, or withdrawal; and failure of expected pharmacological action for the drug.

	Days From Submission	Days From Filing
1. FDA receipt of application	0	—
2. Filing	60	0
3. Action letter issues	180	120
4. Applicants request NOOH*	190	130
5. NOOH issues	240	180

* Notice of Opportunity for Hearing

These "NDA Rewrite" changes represent the most significant revisions of the NDA regulations since passage of the 1962 Drug Amendments. Benefits from these changes include conservation of time, money, and resources. More importantly, some 200,000 persons will benefit each year from significant new drugs which will become available sooner than they would under previous rules and regulations.

The above historical review points up the evolution which has taken place in drug legislation. It also provides a background for the consideration of how new drugs are marketed today.

Development of New Drugs

The discovery, development, and marketing of a new drug is a time-consuming, costly procedure. On the average, 8 years may elapse and $54 million expended between the synthesis of a new chemical entity and final FDA approval.[7] The various steps which must be followed in the development of a new drug have been the subject of a number of reviews[8–11] and are illustrated in Fig 72-1.

Selection of Area—The development of a new drug usually begins with a decision made by the Scientific Advisory Board of a pharmaceutical company. This decision is based on numerous scientific and economic factors, including the need for a drug in a particular illness, the potential market for the drug, the scientific data which justify exploratory research, and the scientific aptitude of the company's research staff.

When the decision is made to create a drug for use in a particular disease state, virtually all departments within the company become involved in its development, including biological research (pharmacology and toxicology), chemical research, quality control, pharmaceutical product development, research administration and legal departments. This multifaceted approach is so complex that computer facilities are required to control and process the vast amount of data

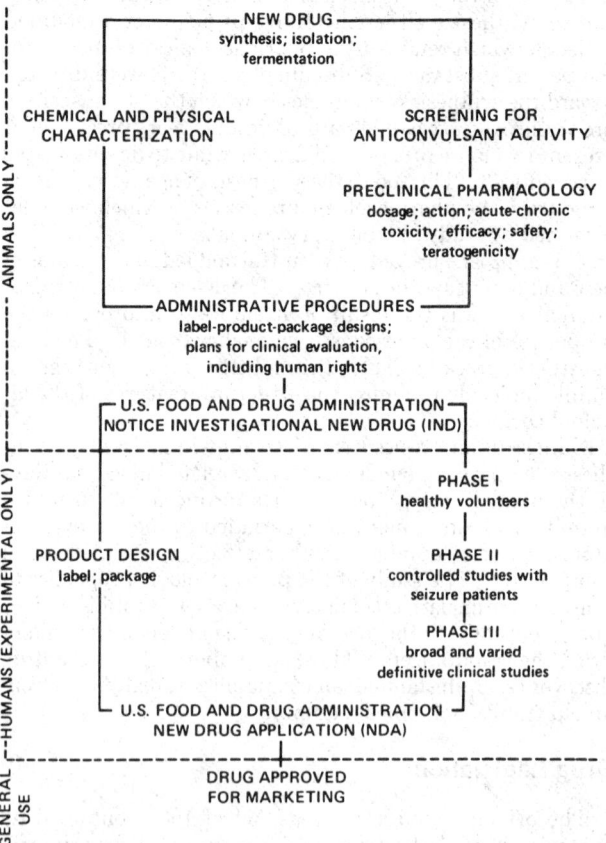

Fig 72-1. Major steps involved in developing a new drug. Determination to return to a previous step or to terminate development may occur at any step.[12]

accumulated during drug development. For this reason this discussion will largely be restricted to the chemical, biological, and clinical aspects of drug development. Little mention will be made of the many legal problems or those associated with product formulation and product, package, and label design. Those interested in the latter are referred to the excellent article entitled "Guidelines: Manufacturing and Controls for IND's and NDA's."[13]

Source and Characterization of New Drugs—Thousands of substances may be made in an effort to find a new agent. For example in 1970, 126,060 chemicals or substances were created by chemical synthesis, fermentation processes, or isolation from natural products for medical research purposes. After discovery of a new material with potential drug activity, isolation and purification of the active principle must be accomplished prior to initial chemical, physical, and biological characterization.

Chemical and physical characterization of a new purified substance is greatly facilitated by the many sophisticated instruments that are now available to the chemist. Instruments and techniques such as infrared, ultraviolet, and nuclear magnetic resonance spectrometry, X-ray diffraction, optical rotatory dispersion, high-performance liquid chromatography, mass spectrometry, polarography, titrimetry, and other technological advances have tremendously improved the exactness and speed with which structural formulas can be determined. Structural formulas which 25 years ago required the combined efforts of four or five chemists and their associates for three or four years can now be revealed in a few days or weeks.

Chemical and physical characterization of substances isolated from natural sources may stimulate chemists to synthesize the naturally occurring materials. This leads to the possibility of synthesizing other substances chemically related to the isolated material.

When an adequate amount of material has been characterized and its purity assured, it is subjected to a series of biological tests designed to detect therapeutic activity in a number of areas. Most of these screening procedures are conducted in the intact animal. However, *in vitro* tests are employed to detect receptor binding, antibiotic activity, and antitumor or antiviral activity.

Many "screening procedures" are employed by the pharmacologist in his search for new drugs. Such procedures usually provide the first clue that a particular compound has some therapeutic activity. Thousands of compounds are screened routinely but only a very small number of encouraging leads are discovered. Those which exhibit some favorable activity are administered in varying amounts and in various forms to selected species of laboratory animals to ascertain their median effective dose (ED50) for the particular activity and their median minimal neurotoxic dose (TD50). The ratio between these values (TD50/ED50) provides the first indication of "margin of safety" or "therapeutic ratio" of the drug. Useful drugs should exert a therapeutic effect in a dose range which is devoid of toxic effects and has little influence on normal body processes. A large margin of safety in experimental animals is a desirable property since it suggests the drug may be safely used in man.

The data accumulated are reviewed at appropriate intervals by the company's Scientific Advisory Board. Based on such review the most promising agent is recommended for more definitive biological study.

At this point, a safety assessment of the candidate drug is initiated. The safety assessment guides the clinical investigator to dosages which he might use cautiously in man. The toxicological assessment reveals what the clinician might expect when the dosage has exceeded the bounds of caution, or what might happen to the occasional patient unusually sensitive to the agent. The safety assessment begins with the

determination of the profile of toxicity and the LD50 (lethal dose to 50% of animals). Thus, the overt toxic manifestations induced by the injection of multiple TD50's (usually 1TD50, 2TD50's and 4TD50's) are carefully recorded and the time for recovery noted. This procedure not only provides a profile of the acute toxic effects induced between the minimal toxic dose and the lethal dose, but also leads to the determination of the median hypnotic dose (HD50). The ratio between the HD50 and the previously determined ED50 (HD50/ED50) provides another measure of the "margin of safety" of the drug.

It is a well accepted premise that drug-induced false cell mutation will lead to death of the cell involved or to tumor production. Consequently, it is a common practice to assess mutagenesis (as well as teratogenesis and carcinogenesis) at the time the subacute toxicity studies are initiated. A positive mutagenic test usually results in termination of further work on the substance under investigation. Subacute toxicity studies are designed to determine the dose range which can be employed when the drug is administered chronically and to reveal possible effects on growth rate and organ function. Any deviation from the growth rate in control animals is considered an undesirable feature. Likewise, adverse effects on renal, hepatic, or bone-marrow function may terminate further investigation of the drug. Some animals are usually sacrificed at the end of 30 days' drug administration and their tissues subjected to careful microscopic examination by a trained pathologist. Metabolic studies may be conducted simultaneously in order to ascertain the mechanism of action and the fate of the drug in animals.

An important part of pharmacology is the pharmacokinetic studies on drug absorption, distribution and excretion. The distribution and concentration of the drug in various organs must be determined. The ultimate fate of the drug must also be ascertained. It is important to know the route by which the drug is excreted and whether it is eliminated from the body unchanged or is changed into some other form. Such studies will often reveal clues as to what might be expected when the drug is used in patients on other medication. This subject is treated more fully in Chapter 37.

Application to the FDA

Upon completion of the screening procedures, acute and subacute toxicity studies, and preliminary metabolic experiments, the company's Scientific Advisory Board again reviews all experimental data and decides whether the drug is sufficiently promising to warrant clinical trial. If an affirmative decision is made, application to do so must then be made to the FDA. In addition, arrangements are made to initiate the chronic toxicity studies. The chronic toxicity studies usually run concurrently with the clinical trial, but must be started *at least* 13 weeks in advance of protracted clinical trials (Phase III). Chronic toxicity studies usually involve two species (rats and dogs) and may continue for 2 years or longer, depending on the contemplated use of the drug. Enough animals must be included in the studies to permit sacrificing a portion of the animals after 6 and 12 months for gross and histomorphic examination of various tissues in addition to the periodic chemical and hematological studies and daily observations. At the end of the required experimental period, the animals are sacrificed and their internal organs examined both grossly and microscopically.

Investigational New Drug Application—This is submitted to the FDA on a special form (FDA form 1571). The compilation of the data required for this form, a "Notice of Claimed Investigational Exemption for a New Drug" (IND), is a time-consuming procedure. The filing of the IND informs the FDA that studies of the efficacy and safety of the drug in man will be initiated. The IND is a very important communication between the pharmaceutical manufacturer and the FDA and should include the following information:

1. A description of the chemistry and the biologic activity (toxicology in animals and pharmacological actions) of the drug.
2. Specifications of the dosage form to be given to man.
3. Details of all quality control measures employed to assure exact reproducibility of manufacture and identification of all ingredients, qualitatively and quantitatively.
4. A description of all manufacturing equipment, manufacturing facilities, and manufacturing procedures employed.
5. The names and qualifications of, and the facilities available to, each investigator who will participate in the initial studies (Phase I).
6. A statement (FDA form 1572) signed by each investigator which (a) confirms his understanding of the nature of the drug he will study; (b) guarantees supervision of every aspect of the study by himself or one or more named associates who are directly responsible to him; (c) describes the facilities available to him; and (d) confirms his understanding that the drug will be administered only to volunteers or patients to whom a full disclosure has been made of the actions of the drug, the purpose of administering it, and the benefits to be derived from the study, and from whom an informed written consent has been obtained for the administration of the drug.
7. Protocols of the doses of the drug to be administered per day, the route and duration of its administration, and the specific clinical observations and laboratory examinations to be performed.
8. A copy of the detailed data sheet supplied to each investigator prior to his initiation of the study.

It should be noted that the major portion of the information required in the IND relates to clinical investigations in man. The FDA, with the assistance of the pharmaceutical industry, developed a set of guidelines for the planning of an "adequate and well-controlled clinical investigation." For example, 16 such guidelines are now available including "General Considerations for the Clinical Evaluation of Drugs" (FDA 77-3040) and "General Considerations for the Evaluation of Drugs in Infants and Children" (FDA 77-3041); similar guidelines are available for antidepressant drugs (FDA 77-3042), antianxiety drugs (FDA 77-3043), radiopharmaceutical drugs (FDA 77-3044), anticonvulsant drugs (FDA 77-3045), anti-infective drugs (FDA 77-3046), anti-anginal drugs (FDA 78-3047), anti-arrhythmic drugs (FDA 78-3048), antidiarrheal drugs (FDA 78-3049), gastric secretory depressant drugs (FDA 78-3050), hypnotic drugs (FDA 78-3051), general anesthetics (FDA 78-3052), local anesthetics (FDA 78-3053), anti-inflammatory drugs (FDA 78-3054), and psychoactive drugs in infants and children (FDA 78-3055). These guidelines have not only standardized the approach to clinical investigations, but have also enhanced their reliability. Indeed, they are recognized by the scientific community as a useful basis for the determination as to whether there is "substantial evidence" to support the claims of effectiveness for "new drugs."

The pertinent principles concerning institutional review, informed consent, and the design of clinical pharmacology and clinical investigational studies are summarized below.

(a) The plan or protocol for the study and the report of the results of the effectiveness study must include the following:[13]
(1) A clear statement of the objectives of the study.
(2) A method of selection of the subjects that—
(i) Provides adequate assurance that they are suitable for the purposes of the study, diagnostic criteria of the condition to be treated or diagnosed, confirmatory laboratory tests where appropriate, and, in the case of prophylactic agents, evidence of susceptibility and exposure to the condition against which prophylaxis is desired.
(ii) Assigns the subjects to test groups in such a way as to minimize bias.
(iii) Assures comparability in test and control groups of pertinent variables, such as age, sex, severity, or duration of disease, and use of drugs other than the test drug.
(3) Explains the methods of observation and recording of results, including the variables measured, quantitation, assessment of any subjective response, and steps taken to minimize bias on the part of the subject and observer.
(4) Provides a comparison of the results of treatment or diagnosis with a control in such a fashion as to permit quantitative evaluation. The precise nature of the control must be stated and an explanation given of the methods used to minimize bias on the part of the observers and the

analysts of the data. Level and methods of "blinding," if used, are to be documented. Generally, four types of comparison are recognized:
(i) No treatment: Where objective measurements of effectiveness are available and placebo effect is negligible, comparison of the objective results in comparable groups of treated and untreated patients.
(ii) Placebo control: Comparison of the results of use of the new drug entity with an inactive preparation designed to resemble the test drug as far as possible.
(iii) Active treatment control: An effective regimen of therapy may be used for comparison, eg, where the condition treated is such that no treatment or administration of a placebo would be contrary to the interest of the patient.
(iv) Historical control: In certain circumstances, such as those involving diseases with high and predictable mortality (acute leukemia of childhood), with signs and symptoms of predictable duration or severity (fever in certain infections), or, in case of prophylaxis, where morbidity is predictable, the results of use of a new drug entity may be compared quantitatively with prior experience historically derived from the adequately documented natural history of the disease or condition in comparable patients or populations with no treatment or with a regimen (therapeutic, diagnostic, prophylactic) the effectiveness of which is established.
(5) A summary of the methods of analysis and an evaluation of data derived from the study, including any appropriate statistical methods. *Provided, however*, that any of the above criteria may be waived in whole or in part, either prior to the investigation or in the evaluation of a completed study, by the Director of the Bureau of Drugs with respect to a specific clinical investigation; a petition for such a waiver may be filed by any person who would be adversely affected by the application of the criteria to a particular clinical investigation; the petition should show that some or all of the criteria are not reasonably applicable to the investigation and that alternative procedures can be, or have been, followed, the results of which will or have yielded data that can and should be accepted as substantial evidence of the drug's effectiveness. A petition for a waiver shall set forth clearly and concisely the specific provision or provisions in the criteria from which waiver is sought, why the criteria are not reasonably applicable to the particular clinical investigation, what alternative procedures, if any, are to be, or have been, employed, what results have been obtained, and the basis on which it can be, or has been, concluded that the clinical investigation will or has yielded substantial evidence of effectiveness, notwithstanding nonconformance with the criteria for which waiver is requested.
(b) For such an investigation to be considered adequate for approval of a new drug, it is required that the test drug be standardized as to identity, strength, quality, purity, and dosage form to give significance to the results of the investigation.
(c) Uncontrolled studies or partially controlled studies are not acceptable as the sole basis for the approval of claims of effectiveness. Such studies, carefully conducted and documented, may provide corroborative support of well-controlled studies regarding efficacy and may yield valuable data regarding safety of the test drug. Such studies will be considered on their merits in the light of the principles listed here, with the exception of the requirement for the comparison of the treated subjects with controls. Isolated case reports, random experience, and reports lacking the details which permit scientific evaluation will not be considered . . . .[13]

Clinical studies of a new drug in man are usually divided into four phases: Phase I, *clinical pharmacology*, is the initial cautious trial in normal man; Phase II, *clinical investigation*, deals with more detailed observations of drug effects in normal patients and initial trials in disease states; and Phase III, *clinical trials*, consists of broad clinical trials designed to ascertain whether the drug is of clinical benefit in the disease state or syndrome for which effectiveness is to be claimed. Phase IV, *post-marketing clinical trials* are conducted only *after* the NDA has been approved by the FDA. These are long-term studies (10 years or more) and are directed by physicians within the pharmaceutical company. Clinical pharmacologists generally direct Phase I and II studies within a hospital setting, whereas Phase III studies, which usually overlap the latter part of Phase II, are directed by physicians within the pharmaceutical company and utilize the services of clinicians who have specialized in the particular illness and are attached to a university medical center, teaching hospital, or private clinic. Phase IV, *post-marketing clinical trials* involve many clinicians throughout the approved marketing area. In addition to continually updating the clinical data relative to safety and efficacy, they are designed to elucidate the incidence of adverse reactions, explore a specific pharmacologic effect, or obtain more discrete information; they also include large-scale, long-term studies to determine the effect of the drug on morbidity and mortality; studies to supplement Phase III trials; clinical trials in specific patient populations (children); and clinical trials for other possible indications.

Phase I, *clinical pharmacology*, studies involve a comparatively small number of normal human volunteers (20 to 80) and is primarily concerned with the determination of the pharmacokinetic activity (absorption, distribution, blood levels, biotransformation, and excretion) in man and effects on such target organ systems as the liver, kidney, bone marrow, and heart. These are performed to ascertain the manner in which the drug is handled metabolically by human subjects, as well as the amount and kind of excretion products produced as a consequence of this metabolism. (Such metabolism studies in humans can be utilized in the intelligent selection of proper animal species for the chronic toxicity studies which may be needed if the drug is subjected to Phase III studies.) Dosage-range studies are also initiated in Phase I, but the determination of safe dosage range may continue over into the Phase II part of the clinical trial.

Phase I studies may be of relatively short duration for new drugs which are related chemically and biologically to drugs of known activity in man. On the other hand, these studies may be quite extensive when completely unrelated novel drugs are under investigation.

Phase II, *clinical investigation*, studies are extended to include the initial therapeutic trials on a limited number of patients (100 to 200) suffering from the disease entity or syndrome for which the drug is expected to be useful. Clinical protocols are constructed setting forth the duration of drug administration, the clinical observations, and the results of any laboratory determinations which were done. These initial observations are critical in the development of a new drug. The data obtained from this small number of patients, and those obtained in the Phase I studies are evaluated by the company's Scientific Advisory Board and a decision is made relative to the advisability of subjecting the drug to the more intensive and expensive studies required in Phase III.

If the data suggest that the drug should be subjected to Phase III studies, the long-term chronic toxicity studies in laboratory animals already underway (see page 1359) are carefully reviewed, a final dosage form is selected, and plans are made to carry out a broad clinical trial. The FDA expects that the duration of chronic toxicity studies in laboratory animals (one rodent and one non-rodent species) be as long as the contemplated duration of administration to man.

The data obtained in these procedures are analyzed and presented for review to the FDA. At this time special animal studies are initiated to determine the effect of the new drug upon the reproductive and fertility processes, as well as its potential for inducing abnormalities in the developing fetus. Many drug firms do these studies at the time the drug is tested for mutagenic properties (see page 1359). Once again the decision must be made whether to proceed further with studies of the drug.

During the early clinical studies in man the chemical manufacturing, quality control, and pharmaceutical research divisions have usually completed their assessments of dosage forms and stability of the drug under investigation. At this point, immediately preceding the initiation of broad clinical trials (Phase III), the final dosage form is selected.

The monitor of the clinical trial (usually a physician employed by the pharmaceutical company) now prepares a new clinical data sheet which incorporates the information obtained to date and develops new protocols for the desired additional investigations. He also selects those clinical investigators who will be invited to participate in the study. Since the data presented in the NDA pertain to the specific formulation of the drug used in the Phase III trials and for which approval for marketing is being sought, the complete

manufacturing process for the drug substance, as well as for the various dosage forms, must be fixed at this time.

In Phase III, *clinical trials*, the study is broadened to include outpatients under treatment by a number of physicians specializing in the particular disease entity. The construction of the clinical protocol, the selection of patients, the treatment regimen to be followed, and the measurements to be made should be designed to satisfy two judgments: is the drug safe and is the drug effective? The word "safe" in this connotation cannot mean absolutely safe; otherwise, there would be few if any new drugs marketed.

The adverse effects must be weighed against the therapeutic benefits. If it is a lifesaving agent or is palliative in a serious condition for which there is no effective remedy, a definite hazard is tolerable, certainly much beyond the degree which would be acceptable for a drug useful only for controlling a symptom amenable to other drugs. Thus, each drug presents an individual problem involving a variety of factors.

It is well known that infants and children react differently to drugs than adults. The incompletely developed enzyme systems of the infant may result in an altered metabolism of drugs or, conversely, drugs may have a greater effect on the incompletely developed enzymatic processes of the infant than of the adult. Therefore, if the new drug has a therapeutic application in infants and children, Phase III studies must be designed to show safety and effectiveness in the various age groups.

It is impossible to predict in advance the number of clinical case reports which may be necessary to demonstrate that the test drug is safe and effective for the proposed indications. In some instances only a few well-controlled detailed case reports may suffice, whereas in others several thousand may be required. Again, this is governed by the disease state for which efficacy is claimed and the nature of the claims for the drug under investigation.

New Drug Application—Upon the completion of all the pharmacology studies (long-term toxicity, effects on fertility and reproduction, and special studies in immature animals) and all three phases of the clinical studies, the company's Scientific Advisory Board must make a decision as to whether the data have satisfactorily demonstrated safety and efficacy of the test drug when used under the recommended conditions. If it is believed safety and efficacy have been demonstrated, the company then submits to the Food and Drug Administration a New Drug Application (NDA). This was formerly an extensive document; many submissions contained over 100 two-inch volumes of material. However, the data are now presented in summary form and are presented in 50 to 200 pages (see page 1360).

On the basis of information provided in the NDA, the safety and effectiveness of the drug are evaluated by the FDA staff. If the studies are adequate in number, well conducted, and clearly reported, the FDA should have all the necessary information for prompt approval of the NDA. (See table page 1363). Supplementary laboratory and clinical studies and frequent conferences between representatives of the pharmaceutical company and the FDA are often necessary before the NDA is approved. Once approved, however, the manufacturer can proceed to make this new drug available through the normal channels of distribution for prescription drugs.

Obstacles to the Evaluation of Drugs

The definitive evaluation of candidate new drugs is compromised by a number of obstacles; the major ones include the limitations of both laboratory screening procedures and animal toxicity tests, the extrapolation of laboratory data to man, and the powerful placebo and its effect.

Limitations of Screening Procedures—The ultimate objective of the routine screening of chemical agents in animals is to sort out those drugs which may prove valuable in the prevention or treatment of specific disease entities. The prediction of possible clinical usefulness is based on the ability of the candidate drug to alter, in laboratory animals, the experimentally induced or naturally occurring counterpart of the particular disease entity, or to modify *normal* tissue or organ function in such a way as to suggest an effect of value in human pathological states. Unfortunately, experimental pharmacology has not yet reached the point where the majority of the principal diseases which occur in man can be simulated reliably in animals.

Even the most dependable laboratory tests, such as the analgesic and antiepileptic screening devices, have inherent weaknesses which are occasionally revealed when candidate drugs with novel chemical structures are subjected to clinical trial. The inadequacies of present techniques are emphasized by the fact that many of the drugs widely employed in neurology and psychiatry today did not originate as a result of correct predictions from planned laboratory investigations but were "discovered" only after they had been tried clinically for some other reason. A number of publications[14,15] have emphasized the need for more reliable screening techniques.

What is the best method for screening drugs for a particular activity? This is a frequent question for which there is no definitive answer; nevertheless, it is of sufficient importance to warrant some consideration. Drug effects can be studied in the test tube, on isolated cells, tissues, and organs, as well as on intact animals.

Many basic pharmacologic problems can be approached at several biologic levels, whereas others can be studied more directly. For example, blood pressure is the sum of numerous factors and drugs which lower blood pressure can be studied at various biologic levels: central nervous system, autonomic ganglia, sympathetic neuroeffector cells, carotid sinus, peripheral blood vessels, or intact normal animals. On the other hand, anti-infective agents can be studied more directly; drugs which inhibit streptococcus *in vitro* will usually inhibit the organism *in vivo*. When the drug effect can be studied at several biologic levels, the particular preparation and screening procedures selected, more often than not, are determined by the skills and prejudices of the experimenter. Be that as it may, there are several criteria which characterize an ideal screening procedure and by which one might evaluate the usefulness of a particular procedure.

Ideally, a drug screen should discern potent new agents. It is one thing to choose a screen because of its theoretical significance or because it may reveal some basic information about a disease entity; it is quite another to select a screen on actual ability to uncover useful new drugs. An ideal screen is simple, rapid, and sorts out potent compounds which have the same order of potency in humans. A screening procedure which yields a high percent of false positives—ie, selects compounds which are active in the laboratory but inactive in the clinic—is a useless screen. Likewise, a screening procedure which yields a high percent of false negatives—ie, fails to detect compounds in the laboratory which are subsequently shown to be active in the clinic—is a useless screen.

An ideal screen is efficient, reveals a minimum number of false positives and false negatives and accurately ranks active agents. These criteria suggest that it might be worthwhile to test an occasional discard clinically in order to see whether the screen is completely dependable. Indeed, one wonders how many active compounds have been "missed" through the use of screening procedures which are not completely reliable.

What are some of the major obstacles to the routine screening of drugs?

1. The etiology of many diseases for which drug treatment is sought is not completely understood. For example, knowledge of the cause of epilepsy is still incomplete and is largely classified on the basis of the electrical activity of the brain and overt symptoms. Therefore, therapy on the basis of etiology is not yet possible. Yet the fact that this disorder is characterized by certain functional disturbances which can be reproduced in animals allows for a reasonable approach to the symptomatic therapy of this disorder, and drug treatment is directed toward control of the seizures rather than removal of the cause.

Useful antiepileptic agents can be detected on the basis of their anticonvulsant properties in animals, despite the fact that the mechanisms of the various forms of experimentally induced seizures in laboratory animals may have little in common with the causes of epilepsy in man. Therefore, even when the etiology of a particular human disease is unknown, one attempts to induce alterations in laboratory animals which simulate the primary functional disturbance of the disorder in order to devise a screening test for detecting agents which might prove useful in the symptomatic control of the disease in man.

2. It is difficult to produce the exact counterpart of many human disabilities in laboratory animals, even when the causes are known. For example, in the field of pain, the reflex response to a noxious stimulus, commonly used in the measurement of experimental pain variously evoked in laboratory animals, is quite different from the pathologic pain in man with its associated psychic components. Although some investigators have devised screening techniques for analgesics which combine anxiety or fear with experimental pain, it is quite unlikely that this contrived situation approximates the real state which arises when pathologic pain or trauma is experienced in man.

This very familiar example serves to illustrate the fact that it is rarely possible to duplicate accurately in laboratory animals a particular human syndrome or disease. Hence the experimental pharmacologist is frequently forced to adopt another line of action. He can adopt as a model a drug that is already successful in clinical therapeutics and then attempt to duplicate, in other chemical structures, the profile of pharmacologic effects of the model. The objective of this type of screening is not to find a novel therapeutic agent but to find a drug that will be preferable to the model compound, for any of a number of well-known reasons, including safety, potency, duration of action, minimal side effects, patient acceptability, cost, etc.

This approach prompts many investigators to emphasize the importance of a battery of tests and profiles of action rather than a single procedure. Although such an approach is essential, it is limited in that it is not directed toward the challenging new fields of therapy for which novel drugs are not yet available.

3. The goals of drug therapy for many diseases have not been clearly defined. This is particularly true in the case of mental diseases such as schizophrenia. Thus, it is difficult to obtain a clear picture of the nature of the behavioral effects which the ideal "psychotherapeutic" drug should produce. Even if the pharmacologist's armamentarium included a wide range of tests which could be used reliably to select drugs with various specific behaviorial effects, it would still be difficult to decide which of these drugs might be beneficial in schizophrenia. Progress in this area might be made, however, by defining the goals of therapy in the same manner as in other fields of experimental therapeutics.

Once the primary behavioral disorders which characterize schizophrenia are sorted out, therapy can then be directed toward their amelioration. Until the primary functional disturbances in schizophrenia and in other mental diseases have been disclosed with certainty, progress in this area will be slow. However, the value of basic neuropharmacologic techniques should not be overlooked. For example, not a single phrenotropic drug known today is devoid of some classical effect on the nervous system, such as analgesic, anticonvulsant, sedative, potentiative, skeletal muscle relaxant, central hypotensive, or antiemetic. Whether these pharmacologic effects are merely side reactions or whether they are related to the primary desiderata of drug action against clinical psychoses has yet to be established. Nevertheless, a battery of tests based on these classical neuropharmacologic actions has proven a valuable adjunct to the laboratory detection of more effective agents.

4. This concerns the experimental design used in the laboratory tests. This obstacle usually results from failure to devote sufficient time to the proposed experiment to assure that the profile of action of the candidate drug is covered in its entirety. Thus, some workers confine their observations to the effect of a single dose for a particular end point. On the other hand, many drugs exhibit their characteristic effects in human patients only after a period of chronic administration. Therefore, it would appear equally important to screen drugs for pharmacologic activity after chronic administration. This suggestion is supported by the fact that some clinically useful agents, for example, many vitamins and hormones, exert little useful effect when administered in a single dose; whereas other drugs (eg, morphine) become less effective when administered frequently. Therefore, it would appear desirable to study in laboratory animals the pharmacologic effects induced by the chronic administration of the drug.

Chronic studies, in addition to revealing valuable information on tolerance and cumulative potentialities of the drug, might reveal valuable therapeutic agents which otherwise would be missed.

5. This is concerned with the proper laboratory evaluation of drug mixtures. Despite the attention given drug mixtures by drug manufacturers and clinicians, comparatively few of them have been subjected to

laboratory study prior to clinical use. The mixtures and doses employed are selected on the basis of trial and error or on the basis of impressions gained from previous clinical experience with the individual agents. This potentially dangerous procedure is encouraged by the complex nature of the problem and the lack of a simple and reliable laboratory method for the evaluation of combined drug effects. For those interested in the theory of drug interactions and the difficulties encountered in the laboratory testing of drug mixtures, the scholarly review by Loewe[16] is recommended.

Limitations of Animal Toxicity Tests—There is no sharp line of demarcation between drug screening and the determination of drug toxicity. Indeed, the initial acute toxicity studies on a candidate drug usually either precede or progress simultaneously with the search for pharmacologic activity. On the other hand, the subacute and long-term toxicity studies are initiated only after the agent has been demonstrated to possess desirable properties in man.

All laboratory toxicity studies and associated pathologic observations are directed toward a single objective: the safe use of the candidate drug in man. According to Beyer,[11] "to assure (drug) safety for all is to deny therapy to any." This statement brings into sharp focus the realistic attitude about the safety assessment of a new drug. People differ qualitatively and/or quantitatively in their reactivity to drugs. Trying to assure safety for everybody would be a little like trying to tailor a pair of trousers to fit exactly all men (and women) over the age of 21.[11] Nevertheless, the reliability of laboratory toxicity tests can be improved if careful attention is directed to three factors:

1. The results of acute toxicity experiments are often incorrectly related to man.
2. Available laboratory tests are either not generally reliable or are incapable of detecting certain types of toxicity.
3. Several laboratory tests which can demonstrate particular types of toxicity when conducted in a particular species are frequently carried out in the wrong laboratory animal.

Each one of these topics is worthy of extensive development, but this discussion will be limited to a few pertinent examples.

It is now generally recognized that the 24-hour LD50 determined in laboratory animals contributes very little to the overall pharmacological and toxicological evaluation of a potentially useful candidate drug.[6] Indeed, it is impossible to relate a 24-hour LD50 determined in laboratory animals to a similar endpoint in man. It is much more meaningful to determine the median minimal toxic dose (TD50), the profile of toxicity induced by multiples of the TD50 (1TD50, 2TD50's, and 4TD50's), and the median hypnotic dose (HD50). Such toxicity studies not only reveal the kinds of overt toxicity that may be induced in man, but also provide two estimates of the margin of safety of the candidate substance (TD50/ED50 and HD50/ED50). For these reasons the 24-hour LD50 is not included in this treatise.

It is well known that even routine toxicity studies may give highly variable results when conducted under certain environmental situations. For example, when mice are employed as test animals for certain sympathomimetic amines, it has been shown that the TD50 is several times higher for singly confined animals than for aggregated mice. This observation has been confirmed by many investigators and emphasizes the fact that even rodents are responsive to their social environment. It also suggests that certain types of acute toxicity studies should be done both with individually isolated animals and with uniform groups of animals housed together under similar conditions.

It should be mentioned that interpretations based on the slope of the dosage–toxicity curves are frequently neglected or ignored. The slope of the dosage–toxicity curve is a measure of the change in the incidence and/or severity of toxicity which occurs with a change of dosage. Very "flat" curves indicate that occasional instances of extreme susceptibility

to the chemical may be expected, perhaps even at the levels of proposed use. On the other hand, a "steep" curve indicates little variability and consequently permits a better estimate of safe dosage.

In general, compounds which have a flat dose–response curve and/or a marked delay in the onset of symptoms are frequently quite toxic upon long-term ingestion. For example, diethylene glycol is a substance which in most species of animals gives rise to a "flat" dose–response curve. This flatness was reflected in the human-poisoning cases with diethylene glycol in which some individuals died from relatively small doses, whereas others survived comparatively large doses. In contrast to diethylene glycol, the dose–response curve of gonyaulax toxin, a toxin occurring occasionally in clams and mussels, is so "steep" that a quarter of the LD50 can be eaten with almost no risk or fatality. These observations point up the weaknesses which occur when even routine toxicity measurements are used merely as tools for estimating the median toxic dose (TD50).

Available laboratory tests are incapable of detecting certain types of toxic manifestations which occur in man. This is emphasized by the data of Zbinden shown in Table I. This table shows that at least 22 of the 45 most frequently recorded untoward effects are unlikely to be recognized in an animal experiment. In addition, available laboratory tests are either weak or entirely lack the ability to reveal the potentiality of the candidate drug for causing serious skin disorders and liver and bone-marrow disturbances. It is possible but not definitely proven that these toxicities are hypersensitivity reactions peculiar to man and cannot be induced in laboratory animals.

Some types of toxicity which can be detected if the drug is administered to a particular species may be missed if the experiment is conducted in the wrong laboratory animals. For example, it is well known that methemoglobin is not readily induced in monkeys, rats, and rabbits; suspect candidate drugs should be tested in the cat or dog, species known to produce this response similar to man.

The data in Table I and the examples cited above indicate that available toxicity tests leave much to be desired. Even

Table I—The Most Frequent Untoward Reactions to Drugs[a,b]

Side effect[c]	No.	Side effect[c]	No.
Drowsiness	426	*Skin rash*	29
Nausea	211	Anorexia	23
Dizziness	198	*Depression*	23
Sedation	176	Increased appetite	21
Dry mouth	133	Tremor	21
Nervousness	98	Perspiration	21
Epigastric distress	98	*Dermatitis*	19
Headache	91	*Increased energy*	18
Vomiting	83	*Vertigo*	16
Weakness	61	Palpitations	16
Nasal stuffiness	57	Blurred vision	16
Hypertension	57	*Lethargy*	15
Insomnia	56	*Nocturia*	15
Fatigue	55	Excitation	14
Constipation	54	*Abdominal distention*	14
Tinnitus	49	Frequent bowel	14
Weight gain	39	movement	
Hypotension	38	Flatulence	14
Dryness of nasopharynx	38	*Stiffness*	13
Heartburn	38	*Urticaria*	13
Diarrhea	30	Tachycardia	13

[a] From Zbinden G: *J New Drugs* 6: 1, 1966.
[b] Observed in 11,115 patients treated with 77 different drugs or drug combinations; summarized from 86 recent drug-evaluation papers.
[c] Side effects for the detection of which there is no satisfactory animal model available are shown in *italics*.

multiple determinations of the minimal toxic dose in several animal species cannot always be relied upon to estimate the minimal toxic dose in man. The effect of environment on toxicity is frequently neglected and little attention is given to the implications of the slope of dose–toxicity curves on toxicity. Many of the commonly encountered untoward effects in man cannot be detected with available laboratory techniques, and certain types of toxicity may be missed if the drug is tested in the wrong animal species.

Extrapolation of Laboratory Data to Man—There is often a large measure of uncertainty when one attempts to project to man the results obtained in laboratory animals. The extent of uncertainty is often inversely proportional to our understanding of the mechanisms involved. It is generally agreed that in certain pharmacologic areas results obtained in laboratory animals can be used reliably to predict the pharmacologic effect in man. Such areas include the effect of drugs on neuromuscular transmission, impulse conduction in nerves, diuresis, blood pressure, etc.

The high reliability with which extrapolations between phylogenetic levels can be made in the case of the above discrete examples results from the fact that a great deal is known concerning the functional basis of the observed effects; consequently, tests used to identify drugs effective in these areas have become highly selective. On the other hand, extrapolations from animal to man in less clearly defined areas of pharmacology are more difficult. To cite an extreme example, extrapolation based on the effects of drugs on more complex and less understood functions in laboratory animals, such as behavior, are less reliable than those based on the actions of drugs on an identifiable enzyme system at the cellular level.

Many examples could be cited to illustrate the difficulties encountered when extrapolating animal data to man. Limitations of space dictate that this discussion be restricted to a brief consideration of the problems encountered when relating animal teratogenic and toxicity studies to human patients.

The major obstacle to the clinical interpretation of teratogenic studies in laboratory animals is the large number of false-positive results obtained with many well-established medications, such as aminophylline, insulin, phenobarbital, salicylates, thyroxine, and others.[30] It has even been shown that nicotine and caffeine are teratogenic in animals.[30] In most instances, enormous doses of the test drug have been used. If these studies are to have relevance in man, the dose levels used must be comparable to those employed in man. For this reason it has been suggested that more attention should be given to the effect of the candidate drug on fetal mortality. In general, agents which kill the fetus at doses tolerated by the mother will also tend to deform the offspring if given in a lower dose. The reliability of extrapolating this observation to man remains to be established.

The extrapolation of chronic toxicity results to man appears to be compromised by at least two major factors: (1) nonspecific consequences of the experimental procedure and (2) species differences. Three dose levels are required in chronic toxicity experiments: a high dose which is expected to produce obvious signs of toxicity; a low dose which will be tolerated without obvious toxic effects; and an intermediate dose. It has been pointed out that the toxicologist must distinguish between the toxic manifestations of the drug and those tissue changes which are nonspecific consequences of the experimental procedure.

Organ functions are limited in their ability to respond to noxious stimuli, and organ change due to general overloading with the drug is not uncommon. Such overloading is frequently accompanied by malnutrition which is known to induce a variety of organ changes, particularly of the hemopoietic system, lymphatic system, adrenals, liver, kidney, and reproductive system. These changes are frequently indistinguishable from those directly related to the drug and complicate extrapolation of such data to man.

Species differences account for many of the limitations of animal toxicity studies. In many cases species differences can be explained by differences in metabolism. It is important to remember that drug absorption, distribution, and penetration through membranes depend on the physicochemical properties of the agent and therefore are essentially the same in various species. Important differences are known to occur in the pathway of metabolism and rate of inactivation. Therefore, drug metabolism studies should be instituted at an early stage of drug investigations and chronic toxicity studies done in animal species which metabolize the drug similar to man.

These examples emphasize the importance of a thorough understanding of the comparative functional biology of both laboratory animals and man. They also suggest that when possible, new drugs should be tested in laboratory animals which respond to the drug in a manner similar to man. It is clearly evident that the pharmacologic, teratogenic, mutagenic, carcinogenic, and toxicologic properties of drugs as determined in laboratory animals can be applied reliably only to those clinical situations which clearly correspond.

The Powerful Placebo—Drug administration is more than the introduction of a drug into the body. It represents the culmination of the physician–patient relationship. The physician prescribes a drug in anticipation that it will induce the expected salutary effect. The patient desperately desires the drug to be effective and shares the physician's expectation that it will produce the desired effect. Thus, drug administration takes place under circumstances characterized by biased expectations and enhanced suggestibility on the part of both physician and patient.

Health and disease are greatly influenced by psychic and emotional factors. Symptoms of psychosomatic origin are just as "real" as those resulting from minor, organic causes. Similarly, psychic responses to drugs and psychic modifications of drug action represent real phenomena.

All reactions to drug administration that arise from the act of taking the drug and that are unrelated to the pharmacologic actions of the drug are known as *placebo effects*. An inert chemical substance used as a drug is called a *placebo* (Latin "I shall please"). Thus, any and every drug administered to a conscious patient elicits a placebo effect superimposed on a pharmacologic effect. This complicates drug evaluation in man and dictates that all clinical studies be designed to enable the clinical pharmacologist to distinguish between the placebo and pharmacologic effects of drugs.

The placebo effect is powerful, universal, either desirable or undesirable, consistent yet variable, and capable of mimicking drug effects. Few would deny the ability of the placebo to influence pain, anxiety, or other "subjective" effects in certain individuals. The ability of placebos to affect "objective" phenomena, such as vomiting, or to produce unwanted side effects is also recognized. Lesser known, however, is the fact that placebos can mimic certain pharmacologic aspects of active drugs, such as time course, cumulative effect, carry-over effect, and efficacy dependent upon the severity of the symptom. Examples will be cited to illustrate three of the more important of these effects.

1. This example illustrates the effect of suggestion. If a physician warns a patient that certain toxic manifestations may occur following drug administration or if the patient has heard about untoward actions occurring from this medication, the patient may then anticipate effects other than the beneficial ones for which the drug is given. This is illustrated by the report of Pincus[17] on the side effects produced by oral contraceptive agents. In order to determine the cause of a number of annoying symptoms such as headache, nausea, dizziness, and abdominal pain, Pincus administered the contraceptive pill to three groups of Puerto Rican women.

Table II—Placebo Side Effects in the Trial of an Oral Contraceptive[17]

Group	No. of patients	Cycles Reactions[a] No.	Cycles Reactions[a] %
No admonition, drug	15	48	6.3
Admonition, drug	13	30	23.3
Admonition, placebo	15	41	17.1

[a] Includes complaints of physical ill-being, such as nausea, vomiting, headache, vertigo, gastrointestinal distress, and malaise.

A group of women using conventional methods of birth control was selected from the same native population and divided into two subgroups. One group received placebo pills, the other received contraceptive pills. Both groups were advised to continue with the same contraceptive practices they had been using but were admonished to note any adverse effects. They were told that the pills had to be tested to see if they were suitable for continued use. A third group of women, selected from a different town, were given the contraceptive pills without any admonition. Table II shows the results of this experiment. It may be seen that the side effects noted were due to the admonition and not to the drug. The study further demonstrated that the incidence of side effects declined to a very low level with continued use of the drug in large groups of women.

2. This example reflects the fact that a placebo has a time–effect relationship. Lasagna and co-workers[18] studied the effects of aspirin or a placebo on postpartum pain; 128 patients were studied in an obstetrical ward during the five-day period after delivery. Identical-appearing capsules of aspirin or a placebo were administered at random to any patients requesting medication for pain. All patients were interviewed by the same technician under double-blind conditions immediately prior to medication, and $\frac{1}{2}$, 1, 2, and 3 hours after medication.

Four arbitrary categories of pain were employed and each patient given a pain relief score for each interview after medication. The sum of all scores for all patients at a given interview point was then divided by the number of patients to give a mean pain relief score for each time interval after medication.

The data obtained are shown in Fig 72-2 from which it may be seen that there is a similarity in the shape of the curves for those patients receiving aspirin and for those receiving a placebo. The two treatments differed considerably in efficacy. The mean total pain relief score for aspirin the first 3 hours after medication was $5.91 \pm$ SE of 0.35; for the placebo it was 3.45 ± 0.44. This difference was found to be significant at the 0.01 level. At least two important points are illustrated by these data: (1) placebo medication elicits a time–effect relationship and (2) the placebo itself relieved pain in a significant number of patients.

3. The final example illustrates that efficacy is inversely related to the severity of a given complaint. In the previously described postpartum-pain study, Lasagna and co-workers[18] plotted the percent of patients completely relieved of slight to moderate pain or severe to very severe pain by placebo medication against time. The results are shown in Fig 72-3. The percentage of patients reporting complete relief of pain at some time during the 3-hour test period was 57% and 21% for the slight-moderate group and severe-very severe group, respectively. This difference is significant at the 0.01 level. The aspirin data were similarly analyzed and also indicate a lessened efficacy in patients with greater pain. Thus the efficacy of placebos, like the efficacy of active drugs, is inversely related to the intensity of the symptom.

There are certain implications in these examples as regards the evaluation of new drugs.

1. Placebo controls are not always necessary or desirable. If a useful drug is already available, and the question is whether or not a new drug

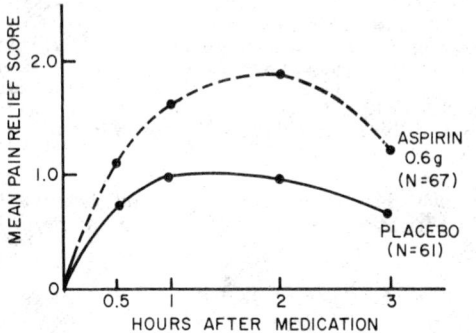

Fig 72-2.   Mean pain relief scores after placebo or aspirin in patients suffering from postpartum pain.[12]

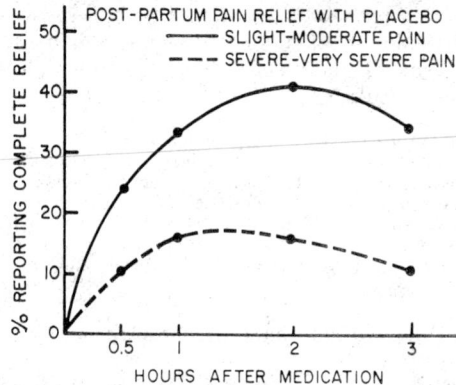

Fig 72-3.   Relationship between reported severity of pain and analgesic efficacy of placebo.[18]

is superior, a placebo control is inappropriate; the clinical study should be designed to compare the toxicity and efficacy of the old drug and the new. On the other hand, if the new drug is to be tested for a clinical condition for which there is no known therapy, a placebo control is indispensable.

2. Uncontrolled studies that claim therapeutic benefit because of "peak effects," "cumulative effects," or persistent benefit after cessation of treatment should be interpreted cautiously.

3. The placebo effect is not an "all or none" phenomenon.

4. The placebo time–effect relationship should be taken into consideration when deciding upon times when data are to be collected in controlled clinical trials.

5. Selection of patients presenting severe therapeutic challenges may lessen the necessity for or the importance of placebo controls.

Adherence to these and other principles enables the clinical pharmacologist to distinguish between the placebo and pharmacological effects of new drugs.

Problems of Drug Selection

Every new drug introduced into medicine further complicates the unique and difficult position assumed by the physician when he selects the best drug to treat a particular illness. His position is unique in that he assumes the responsibility of selecting the least toxic and most efficacious agent for the patient's condition with the full knowledge that it will ultimately be the patient who will pay for this medication. His position is difficult in that he must select one agent from among the several thousand that are available to him.

In addition to the usual routine pharmacological knowledge of the agent, it is the physician's responsibility to know how the medication selected will interact with other medication that might be indicated or with medication the patient might already be taking. The task of drug selection is further complicated by a number of general problems only four of which, namely, drug names, generic equivalency, drug combinations, and drug-induced diseases, will be mentioned here.

Drug Names—By the time a new drug becomes generally available to the physician, it already has several names. A "drug" refers to the active ingredient in a "drug product," such as a tablet, capsule, or other dosage form that is administered to the patient.

First, a drug is given a *chemical name* which describes its structure by standard chemical nomenclature.

Second, a *code number* is assigned to the chemical for use during chemical, biological, and early clinical studies.

Third, it receives a *nonproprietary name* (frequently incorrectly referred to as a generic name) which is often a contraction of the chemical name but which may also indicate the chemical class of drug to which it belongs. The US Adopted Names (USAN) Council, composed of representatives from the AMA, USP, APhA, and FDA, recommends nonproprietary names of all new drugs. The USAN is developed according to a number of guiding principles, which are broken down into general and specific rules. The general rules say that a name should be:

1. Useful primarily to health practitioners.
2. Short, easy to pronounce, easy to recognize and recall.
3. Such that it reflects pharmacologic, chemical, or other characteristics and relationships of actual practical value to the user.
4. Free of conflict with other drug names and neither confusing nor misleading.
5. A name of established usage if it conforms reasonably well to the other guiding principles.

Since 1962 the FDA must approve all nonproprietary names (See Chapt 26).

Fourth, the drug is given a *trademarked name* (brand name) designated by a superscript® at the end of the name, indicating that this name has been registered with the US Patent Office. Only the registrant may use the trademarked name for the particular drug; it is this name which distinguishes a particular product from those of competitors.

Considerable confusion results from the common practice of granting multiple brand names for a single chemical entity. Random selection of a few commonly used drugs from the *American Drug Index* (26th ed, 1982) shows the number of brand names as follows: diphenhydramine, 23; chlorpheniramine maleate, 28; meprobamate, 12; phenobarbital, 12; prednisone, 14; vitamin B_{12}, 18. The possibilities for confusion and misunderstanding among all members of the health profession are readily apparent. For example, instead of using the name "prednisone" the physician may use a word such as Deltasone, Fernisone, Keysone, Lisacort, Maso-Pred, Meticortin, Orasone, Panasol, Pan-Sone, Pred-5, Prednicen M, Ropred, Sarogesic, Sterapred, and others.

To avoid such confusion most authorities recommend that physicians prescribe by nonproprietary name and indicate in parenthesis the manufacturer of the product desired. This procedure has a number of factors in its favor: it encourages accurate recognition of the drug; it uses the name which is employed in current medical literature; it eliminates the burden of memorizing multiple names; and it circumvents the problem sometimes encountered where different names are used for the same drug promoted for different uses. For example, Benadryl is promoted as an antihistaminic, whereas Dramamine is the name used for the same active agent promoted as an anti-motion-sickness remedy. Finally, it should be emphasized that prescribing by nonproprietary name and designating the manufacturer in parentheses still leaves the choice of the particular agent in the hands of the physician.

Generic Equivalency—The several years required to develop a new drug for market drastically reduces the profitable patent life of the agent. Furthermore, as soon as the patent has expired, other companies are free to produce this same drug under their own trade name. The availability of drugs under both a nonproprietary (generic or branded generic) name and a variety of tradenames focused attention on the price differential between products supposedly containing the same chemical entity. This price differential has been brought out repeatedly in government drug hearings which revealed that in some instances the pharmacist paid several hundred percent more for a particular item than the government or a hospital. Numerous instances have been cited showing a similar price differential in favor of products available by generic name.

The original Food and Drugs Act of 1906 charged the USP and the NF with the responsibility of establishing standards for drugs; therefore, it was a logical next step to assume that generic products were also equivalent in efficacy.

Many of the factors in the formulation and manufacture of dosage forms which affect the efficacy of the product have been reviewed in detail. To cite but three examples, a commonly used filler, dicalcium phosphate, was found to depress the blood concentration of tetracycline; particle size has been reported to affect the absorption of the sulfa drugs, griseofulvin, and insulin; tablet hardness has been shown to be inversely related to absorption. Isolated clinical reports also indicate that results obtained with certain nonproprietary products are inferior to those obtained with a trademarked product. For example, clinical results with various nonproprietary brands of prednisone, cortisone, tolbutamide, and phenylbutazone have been reported to be inferior in certain respects to results obtained with the respective trademarked product.

The now classical chloramphenicol studies done by Parke, Davis & Co brought this controversy into sharp focus. These data showed the first nonproprietary brands of chloramphenicol, sampled on the US market after certification by government laboratories, were not clinically equivalent to Chloromycetin. Another potent argument against prescribing by nonproprietary name is the new labeling requirements for phenytoin which advise physicians to keep patients on one dosage form and one manufacturer's product.[19] These observations suggested that some drugs may be "generically equivalent" but "therapeutically nonequivalent." The pros and cons of this interpretation have been discussed in a number of publications.[20-22] For an extensive list of references, the interested reader is referred to the *Bibliography on Biopharmaceutics.*[20]

There is a tendency to minimize the importance of variations in therapeutic equivalence among drug products. For example, the FDA has identified only 110 such drugs out of a total of perhaps 3000 single entities in general use today.[23]

The absolute number of drugs that are known to be "therapeutically nonequivalent" is of little importance, since the number of suspect drugs may vary enormously as newer methods of study are developed and information on this important subject is accumulated.

It is important, however, to recognize that such a phenomenon does occur and to design tests to verify therapeutic availability of formulated products prior to marketing. This demands increased information not only on the pharmacology and toxicology of drugs *per se*, but also on the biologic availability and rate of *in vivo* release of the active ingredient from the drug formulations to be used in man. Beckett and Tucker[22] have devised an *in vivo* test based on urinary excretion data to determine the degree to which a formulation becomes biologically available. These workers[24] have also suggested the following guidelines be observed when testing biologic availability:

1. Use a panel of closely supervised human subjects, acting as their own controls, for comparative tests on drugs and drug formulations. (Animal data and/or *in vitro* tests are not acceptable as sole evidence for the efficacy of a product in humans.)
2. Compare the performance of the product in humans with that of a single and identical dose of the drug in a nonformulated form, preferably in aqueous solution. Estimate the variability of drug release relative to normal biologic variation in response to the drug.
3. Determine the total availability of the drug and the rate at which it becomes available from the preparation to the biologic system.
4. Determine the effects of storage and batch-to-batch variation of the product, not only on the chemical stability of the drug but also on the biologic availability and rate of release of the drug from the formulated product to the biologic system.

In the case of prolonged or sustained-release preparations these investigators suggested an additional requirement, namely:

5. Compare the performance of the product with that of a divided but identical total dose of the drug in a nonformulated form.

The ultimate proof of equivalent efficacy must come from clinical results. However, much can be learned from *in vivo* studies in healthy human subjects. Ideally, target-tissue concentration would be more indicative of therapeutic equivalency. Since such studies are virtually impossible in healthy human subjects, blood and urine level data are generally equated with therapeutic efficacy. Thus, if two preparations are generically equivalent and yield similar blood absorption and urinary excretion curves for the active ingredient after administration, they are assumed to be therapeutically equivalent and to elicit similar pharmacologic effects. Until such tests have been conducted and the information made available, the physician would be well advised to restrict his prescribing of suspect drugs to brands which have survived the test of time.

Drug Combinations—Many effective new drugs are eventually made available in combination with one or more other drugs. A national prescription audit in 1983 indicated that 200 prescription drugs accounted for 69% of all new prescription orders filled. Of these 200 most frequently prescribed drugs, 27.5% (55) were mixtures of two or more drugs.

There are few rational reasons for the administration of two or more drugs in a fixed-dose combination (see also Chapter 36). Physicians who prescribe this kind of medication sacrifice the ability to individualize the dosage of each ingredient to the specific needs of the patient in favor of a supposedly economic factor; ie, a price advantage from two or more ingredients in a single formulation. This is more theoretical than practical, since most drug mixtures are trademarked products, are based on empiricism rather than clinical confirmation, and have not been subjected to an *in vivo* study of drug interaction.

Drug-Induced Diseases—The introduction of hundreds of new proprietary and prescription drugs has undoubtedly made people in the US the most medicated population in the world. Expenditures for proprietary home remedies in 1983 amounted to nearly $3.271 billion, and 1.406 billion new and refill prescription orders were filled in 1980. All this medication is for a population of only a little over 215 million people. Hospital studies show that patients receive an average of 10 potent drugs per stay—some receive as many as 20 or more. There are many reasons to believe that such multiple drug use is as great or even greater on an outpatient basis.

Excessive self-medication is responsible for many ills. It is questionable whether the benefits derived from self-medication with proprietary home remedies outweigh the potential harm they do. They are responsible for many poisonings (by accident or suicidal intent), they cause allergic and other adverse reactions, and their use often delays proper medical attention to serious illness.

The excessive use of prescription drugs also presents a real problem. It is not unusual for a patient to see several medical specialists for wholly unrelated reasons. Likewise, it is not uncommon for a patient to save a drug prescribed for one illness and use it on another occasion or by another member of the family. The seriousness of this situation is reflected by a study in three Boston hospitals covering 13,868 consecutive uses of drugs among 1,400 patients.[25] About 6% (900 reports) of all drugs administered resulted in adverse drug reactions. Adverse drug reactions were believed to be directly responsible for eight deaths and to be a major factor but not the specific cause of the death of 26 others. For more information on this problem the interested reader is referred to the report of the Boston Collaborative Drug Surveillance Program[26] and the study by Talley and Laventurier.[27] (See also Chapter 69, on *Adverse Effects of Drugs*.)

It is experiences of this kind which have led health scientists to speak of "drug-induced diseases" and "iatrogenic diseases." Iatrogenic diseases (Gk *iatros* = physician) are those caused by physicians prescribing drugs irrationally and for trivia.

The magnitude of this problem is not known. However, the high frequency of adverse drug reactions suggests that the problem may be far more extensive than is presently recognized.

What does all this mean? It means that no drug in use today is completely and thoroughly understood. Consequently, physicians are obliged to use drugs about which additional, pertinent information is needed. There are inherent risks in doing so but these are risks which must be taken in order to obtain the benefits afforded by modern drugs. It means also that the pharmacist of today is obliged to keep drug records on his patients. He should record not only all drugs they receive, but also instances of known drug sensitivities, idiosyncrasies, and other unusual responses. Such information, passed on to the physician at the appropriate time, might save a life.

Drug Obsolescence

The introduction of a new prescription drug is usually received by an overly enthusiastic response by prescribing physicians. Hopeful of providing their patients with the latest medication and perhaps of helping patients who are not doing as well as might be expected on existing medication, physicians accept at face value claims for new drugs and prescribe them freely. The widespread clinical use of such new agents naturally results in reports of untoward effects and limitations which had either not been observed or occur so infrequently as to escape detection in early limited clinical trials. Thus, the initial enthusiasm is replaced by a skeptical attitude toward the safety and efficacy of the new agent. As more detailed clinical information accumulates, however, the new drug either falls into obscurity or assumes its well-earned place in the physician's armamentarium.

The pharmaceutical industry spent $1,155 million in 1976 for research and development of new drugs.[28] This expenditure, by function, was as follows: clinical evaluation, (Phases I, II, III), 20.2%; biological screening and pharmacological testing, 19.5%; synthesis, 16.6%; process development for manufacturing, 9.5%; dosage formulation, 9.1%; toxicology and safety testing, 8.9%; IND and NDA preparation, 3.3%; clinical evaluation (Phase IV), 3.2%; bioavailability studies, 2.2%; and other, 7.5%. The research was directed toward the improvement of existing drugs, the development of more effective drugs than those now available, and the discovery of new agents for illnesses for which there are no effective drugs. Such highly competitive research efforts and the time lag between IND submission and NDA approval (96 months) markedly shorten the potential life of new drugs. Indeed, the average effective patent life was 16.3 years in 1960, 10.5 years in 1975, and 6.8 years in 1981.[4,29]

Despite the numerous problems confronting the pharmaceutical industry in the development of new drugs and the numerous unsolved problems in the health sciences, the effect of concerted efforts toward improving the general health of the nation is readily apparent. Today the standard of health care in the US is one of the highest in the world. Statistics indicate that in 1977 the death rate of newborns was the lowest in history (14/1000 live births) and that life expectancy reached 73 years, the highest ever attained in this country. This represents an increase of twelve full years in life expectancy over what existed in 1937.

The pharmaceutical industry tests pharmacologically approximately 8,000 candidate drugs for every one which ultimately reaches the market. In 1977, 17 new chemical entities were approved for use as prescription drugs. Thus, some 136,000 drugs were submitted to pharmacological evaluation. Many of these were for illnesses and conditions for which no effective drug is currently available. This tremendous effort is even more remarkable when it is noted that from 1967 to

1975 the price of prescription drugs increased 8%, whereas during this same period of time medical care and all consumer items increased an average of 61%.[28]

It is generally agreed that these advances resulted from medical and drug research supported by voluntary health agencies, the National Institutes of Health of the US Public Health Service, and the pharmaceutical industry. It is to be hoped that an equal amount of progress and support will be forthcoming in the future.

References

1. Crout, J Richard: The Nature of Regulatory Choices. The Center for the Study of Drug Development, PS 7812, January 1978.
2. *Federal Register:* Part II, November 19, 1976.
3. Wardell, WM and Sheck, LE: Is Pharmaceutical Innovation Declining?: Interpreting Measures of Pharmaceutical Innovation and Regulatory Impact in the USA, 1950–1980. *Rational Drug Therapy*, V 17, No. 1, January 1983.
4. Schweiker, RS: The Drug Application Review Process: Close The Drug Lag. *Vital Speeches of the Day*, 48, 646–648, 1982.
5. Food and Drug Administration, Department of Health and Human Services: *Federal Register 47*, No 202, 46622–46666, 1982.
6. Zbinden, G and Flury-Roversi: Significance of the LD50 Test for the Toxicological Evaluation of Chemical Substances. *Arch Toxicol*, 47, 77–99, 1981.
7. Lasagna L: *Science 200:* 871, 1978.
8. Clinical testing: Symposia on the new drug regulations. *FDA Papers 1 (Mar):* 21, 1967.
9. Anello C: *Ibid 5 (June):* 14, 1970.
10. *Tile and Till 54 (1–4):* 1968.
11. Beyer KH: *Discovery, Development and Delivery of New Drugs,* SP Medical and Scientific Books, 1978.
12. Woodbury DM, *et al,* eds: *Antiepileptic Drugs,* Raven Press, New York, 144 (Fig. 9-1), 1982.
13. *FDA Papers 5:* 4, 1971. 7a. *Federal Register 35* (May 8): 1255, 1970.
14. Tedeschi DH, Tedeschi RE: *Importance of Fundamental Principles in Drug Evaluation,* Raven Press, New York, 1968.
15. Purpura DP, *et al,* eds: *Experimental Models of Epilepsy,* Raven Press, New York, 1972.
16. Loewe S: *Arznei-Forsch 3:* 285, 1953.
17. Pincus G: *Science 153:* 493, 1966.
18. Lasagna L, *et al:* *J Clin Invest 37:* 533, 1958.
19. *Food and Drug Administration*, FDA Drug Bull 8: 27, 1978.
20. *Bibliography on Biopharmaceutics*, Pharm Mfg Assoc, 1155 15th St., Washington, DC 20005.
21. Reese KM: *Chem Eng News 46 (Jan. 29):* 61, 1968.
22. Beckett AH, Tucker GT: *J Pharm Pharmacol S18:* 72, 1966.
23. *Food and Drug Administration*, Federal Register, *42*, No. 5, 1649, 1977.
24. Beckett AH, Tucker GT: Symposium, the influence of formulation on the absorption of drugs. *27th Int Congr Pharm Sci*, Montpelier, France 1967.
25. Stone FL, Brown JHU: *J APhA NS8:* 438, 1968.
26. Boston collaborative drug program. *J Am Med Assoc 220:* 1238, 1972.
27. Talley RB, Laventurier MF: *The incidence of drug-drug interactions in a Medi-Cal population.* Presented to the Am Coll of Physicians, Atlantic City, N.J., April 20, 1972.
28. *Factbook '76. Pharmaceutical Manufacturers*, Washington, DC, 1976.
29. Roll GF: *Center for the Study of Drug Development*, Series PS-7701, 1977.
30. Shepard TH: *Catalog of Teratogenic Agents.* The Johns Hopkins University Press, 1973.

PART 7

Biological Products

Gilbert L Zink, PhD

Associate Professor of Biology
Philadelphia College of Pharmacy and Science
Philadelphia, PA 19104

CHAPTER 73

Principles of Immunology

Gilbert L Zink, PhD
Associate Professor of Biology and Chairman, Dept of Biology
Philadelphia College of Pharmacy and Science
Philadelphia, PA 19104

The science of immunology is concerned with the specific mechanisms by which living tissues react to foreign biological materials (including invading microorganisms) so that resistance or immunity develops. The integrity of the defense system of the host, and its ability to react to and overcome invasion by microorganisms, is of vital importance for the survival of the individual.

Antigens

The antigen (also called *immunogen*) is considered the afferent branch of the immune system (Fig 73-1), and is any substance that will provoke an immune response (production of antibodies and/or sensitization of lymphoid cells) in an immunologically competent individual. In general, antigens must be larger than 10,000 in molecular weight, be protein, carbohydrate or glycoprotein, and be foreign to the individual into whom they have been introduced. Smaller, less rigid, molecules that are not normally antigenic in pure form can be made so by linking them to larger molecules; such smaller molecules are called *haptens* while the larger molecules are called *carriers*.

The practice of administering antigens for the express purpose of stimulating a protective immune response is called immunization. Vaccination is a form of immunization in which the antigen (infectious agent, rendered non-pathogenic whole or in part) is placed in suspension (vaccine) and then administered to the patient.

The antigens may be administered directly to a primary host (man or other host) to induce the desired immune response ("active" acquired immunity), or they may be administered to a secondary host (eg, horse or goat). In the latter case, antibodies so produced are processed from serum, stored indefinitely, and administered to a threatened individual for immediate protection ("passive" acquired immunity). An example of an alternative possibility is to consider an unprotected person who may develop tetanus if exposed to *Clostridium tetani*. This disease, which is caused by a neurotoxin, can be prevented if a person is given active immunity through prophylactic immunization with a series of tetanus toxoid* injections. Once a person has been protected with primary immunizations his immunity may be enhanced by the periodic administration of a "booster" dose of the toxoid. On the other hand, if the subject has not received prior primary immunizations, immediate protection against the effects of *Clostridium* neurotoxin can only be provided by the administration of preformed tetanus antitoxin obtained from a secondary host. For more information on active and passive acquired immunity see Chapter 74.

Examples of innate antigens are the human blood group ABO and Rh isoantigens. Blood group antigens are those characteristic of, but not limited to, erythrocytes. The ABO antigens were discovered by Landsteiner in 1900, a discovery that led to the founding of the science of serology. Rh antigens are well known for their involvement in erythroblastosis fetalis, and together with the ABO antigens and many others identified over the years (eg Lewis, Kell, Duffy, MNS, P, and I), are very important in blood transfusion procedures. The transplantation antigens found on leukocytes and most other body cells are also of major significance. The human leukocyte antigens (HLA) are the most widely known and of special importance in tissue grafting. Antigenic structures—found on the surface of blood cells, organ cells, bacteria, viruses, and many kinds of large independent molecules—enable the vertebrate body to distinguish between its own cells and those of another creature and to destroy the foreign cells before the body's integrity is altered.

Immune Systems

The generation of an immune response is dependent upon the interaction of the three components of the immune mechanism, as illustrated in Fig 73-1. The antigen is called the afferent branch, and stimulates the central or intermediate parts to produce antibody molecules or sensitized lymphocytes (efferent branch), depending on the nature of the stimulating antigen.

Humoral Immunity

The production of antibodies is the function of the humoral division of the immune mechanism. In general, antibodies are directed against antigens that gain access to the blood. Examples of such antigens are transfused blood cells and many kinds of bacteria and viruses.

Antibodies are immunoglobulin molecules (serum proteins), of which there are several classes, designated IgG, IgM, IgA, IgD, and IgE. Each class has characteristic molecular size, electrophoretic migration velocity, carbohydrate content, number of antigen combining sites, etc.

Immunoglobulins of the IgG class are transmitted via placental circulation from the mother to the fetus. Newborn infants therefore have passively acquired temporary immunity to certain diseases, depending on the mother's past exposure to microorganisms or their products.

---

* A toxoid is prepared by treating the exotoxin with substances such as formaldehyde to reduce toxicity while maintaining immunogenicity. However, immunogenicity may be enhanced by combining the toxoid with an adjuvant such as alum or aluminum phosphate. Such products are called adsorbed toxoids.

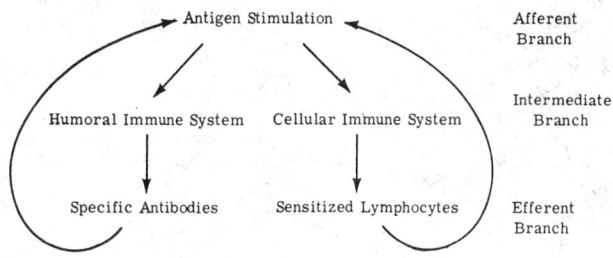

Fig 73-1. The immune mechanism.

This passively acquired immunity affords the infant protection against certain bacterial infections for 1 to 2 months and against viral infections such as measles for approximately 5 to 8 months. Consequently, primary immunizations during the first few weeks of life are avoided because they are unnecessary. Furthermore, better antibody responses are achieved if the immunizing agents are administered later as the passively acquired levels of antibodies are declining.

Antibody molecules are produced by plasma cells which are differentiated from B cells. B cells are lymphocytes produced from stem cells in the bone marrow. B cells are concentrated in the spleen and regional lymph nodes where they await contact by the foreign antigen and conversion into plasma cells.

Antibody production occurs, as believed by most investigators, by some modification of the clonal selection theory. According to this theory, man is born with enough different kinds of antibody-forming cell precursors (B cells) to enable him to defend himself against all possible antibody-stimulating antigens that may be encountered throughout life. To accommodate the millions of possible antigens in existence, each B cell will interact with several antigens of a certain type or group; the resulting antibody, however, is specific only for the stimulating antigen. Thus the number of B cells can be kept to a reasonable number, which might approximate the total number of groups of antigens to which a person may need to respond. It is not known how antigens are grouped or classed to accommodate this theory.

By the modified clonal selection theory, antibodies may be considered to be produced in the following manner (see Fig 73-2). The presence of the antigen is detected by an antigen-reactive cell (ARC) which may possibly be a type of T cell referred to as a T initiator (T_I) cell. The T_I cell (via protein synthesis) stimulates macrophages which partially phagocytizes the antigen cell or molecule, and on some occasions, adds RNA to the antigen. The resulting antigen-RNA complex is believed to be more immunogenic than the unaltered antigen. The antigen-RNA complex is then passed on to a pleuripotential T helper cell (T_H) possessing on its membrane an antigen receptor site specific for the type or group of antigen present. The nature of the contact between helper T cells and antigen-RNA complex is such as to initiate chemical reactions which recruit the proper B cells from all over the body to the spleen or regional lymph node handling the antigen. While the recruitment process is in progress, the antigen-RNA complex is transferred to the membrane surface of stationary macrophages to await contact by recruited B cells. As the recruited B cells arrive specific contact is made with the antigen-RNA complex, the exact nature of which dictates a series of chemical reactions between the cell membrane and the nucleus such that cell duplication, differentiation into plasma cells (actual antibody producers) and proliferation takes place. The result is a large homogeneous population of cells (clone), each of which will produce antibodies specific for the same inciting antigen. Antibody molecules will be synthesized in large numbers by the clone of plasma cells over a period of several days from the time of initial contact between the antigen-RNA complex and the original B cell. In the last few years cell biologists have learned how to remove and isolate sensitized B cells from the spleens of immunized laboratory animals, and culture the cells so that clones of plasma cells result which produce antibodies of identical specificity. Furthermore, these plasma cells can be cultured indefinitely or frozen and stored for years, thawed and recultured. The ability to utilize immunocompetent cells in this fashion provides scientists with an endless supply of antibodies of a particular specificity. This is the monoclonal antibody technique and is now widely used to produce large quantities of antibody of a selected specificity for research, diagnostic testing and passive immunization. The application of this technique extends beyond immunology to genetics, biochemistry, molecular biology, and many other areas of science. The development of the monoclonal antibody technique may be one of the major advancements of science in this century.

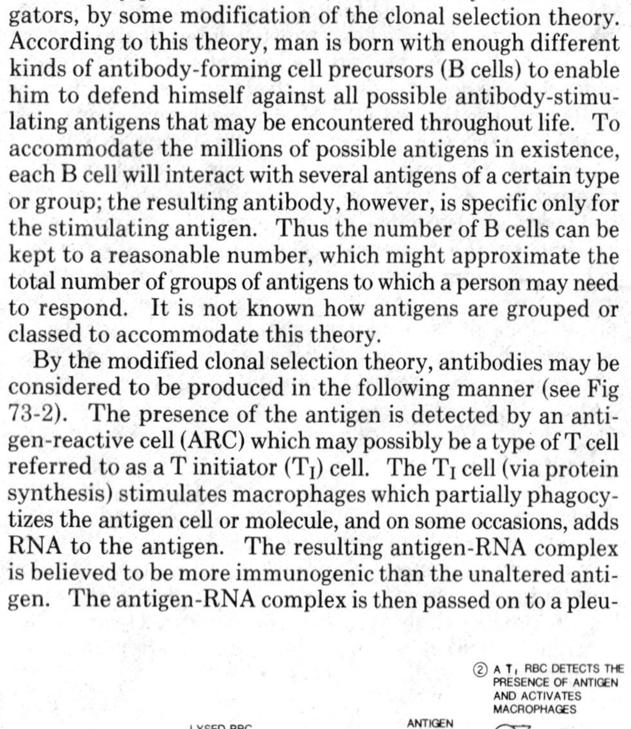

The mechanisms of communication between the different kinds of cells participating in the humoral response is not completely understood but is, at least in part, due to proteins produced by the respective cells. For example, the T_I cells activate macrophages by producing an macrophage activation factor (MAF); the macrophages activate the T_H cells by producing interlukin, I(IL-1), the T_H cells then recruit and cause the proliferation of B cells by producing B cell growth factor. In addition to these proteins, and perhaps several others not yet identified, specific genetically controlled surface receptors are also known to be required in the communication process.

Specific antibody migrates through the circulatory system combining with the prescribed antigen, which is then destroyed by the body in a variety of ways. If the antigen is on red blood cells or certain kinds of bacteria, the resulting antigen-antibody complex triggers complement fixation which results in lysis (rupture) of the cell possessing the antigen. It is then removed by the liver or spleen. Complement, which is comprised of a series of plasma proteins (at least 11), combines with the antigen-antibody complex in the prescribed order (complement fixation) so that the integrity of the cell membrane possessing the antigen is destroyed. This reaction results in cell destruction. The cell possessing the antigen can also be destroyed if the antibody is one that enhances phagocytosis (consumption) of the cell by macrophages; this is called *opsonization*, and is particularly important in resistance against infection caused by encapsulated pneumococci. It is also possible for an antibody (antitoxin) to neutralize a cell product (toxin) and prevent it from reacting with its biochemical target. Eventually the cell producing the toxin is destroyed, usually by phagocytosis.

The different initial (primary) antibody responses just

Fig 73-2.   Humoral immunity.

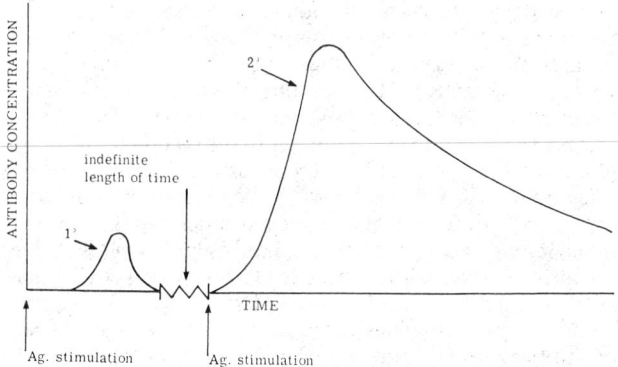

Fig 73-3.   Primary and secondary antibody response.

discussed are usually accompanied by the production of "memory cells." These cells provide the body with an immediate immune response against that antigen if it is ever encountered again. The second and all subsequent reactions against that antigen are more rapid, intense, and prolonged, thus giving the body stronger, more permanent protection against almost any antigen with which it comes in contact more than once (Fig 73-3).

A discussion of humoral immunity is not complete without mentioning those types of hypersensitivity (allergies) involving antibodies. As classified by Gell and Coombs, these kinds of hypersensitivity are generally called "immediate" and are grouped into three categories.

Type I includes anaphylaxis, allergic asthma, urticaria, hay fever and possibly infantile eczema. These conditions are characterized by IgE antibodies (reagins) from prior antigen stimulation. IgE molecules are unique among antibodies because they are cytophilic (non-antigen-antibody type reaction) for the surface of host mast cells, basophils, and possibly other polymorphonuclear cells. Once attached to the cell surface, IgE molecules will remain for the life of the cell. When the stimulating antigens are again present, they bind to the reagins. The resulting antigen-antibody interaction stimulates the mast cells to produce histamine and other substances that cause the allergic reaction.

Type II immediate hypersensitivity includes blood transfusion reactions, hemolytic diseases of the newborn, rejection of homografts from a second donor sharing antigens identical with the first, and lesions produced in tissues by the action of antibody and complement as often occurs in autoallergic diseases. These reactions are characterized by IgG or IgM antibodies binding to soluble antigens or haptens that have become firmly attached to the cells. The way the cells are destroyed varies accordingly to the type of cell, the type of antibody, and whether complement is involved.

Type III immediate hypersensitivity includes allergies characterized by cell destruction caused by toxic antigen-antibody complexes. Soluble antigens in and around small vessels within local tissues react with precipitating antibodies. This is called the *Arthus reaction*. If excess antigen in the blood stream reacts with antibody resulting in soluble circulating complexes which are deposited in blood-vessel walls, the condition is called *serum sickness*. Both situations result in local inflammation.

Type IV hypersensitivity is also described by Gell and Coombs and is classified as delayed. Unlike immediate types, it involves sensitized lymphocytes instead of antibodies. Examples are the tuberculin response and allergic contact dermatitis. Approximately 48 hours after an individual is injected with diluted tuberculin a reading is made. Redness, edema, and possibly slight necrosis of the skin at the site of injection constitute a positive test and indicate that somewhere in the body there is tissue infected with tubercle bacilli.

Allergic contact dermatitis is a common condition experienced by many individuals sensitive to one or more ingredients in detergents or cosmetics.

Cellular Immunity

Cellular immunity involves the system responsible for rejection of organ transplants or skin grafts as well as the defense mechanisms against many types of microorganisms and endogenous neoplastic (tumor) growths. This division of the immune system, like humoral immunity, relies on antigen stimulation for its activation.

The cells (T cells) responsible for cellular immunity originate from precursor cells (stem cells) produced in bone marrow, as is the case with antibody-forming cells in humoral immunity. In cellular immunity, however, the T cells must complete the differentiation process in the thymus before traveling to the spleen and regional lymph nodes or circulating freely in the vascular network. These differentiated cells are of different types. The actual cellular immune response is handled by "effector T cells" which are assisted by "helper T cells" in much the same way as in humoral immunity. In addition, "suppressor" T cells serve to regulate both the humoral and cell mediated responses so that excessive immune reactions do not occur.

If the thymus is removed from neonatal mice, the result is severe impairment of their ability to express cellular immunity; humoral immunity, however, is impaired to a lesser degree. In humans a congenital condition called DiGeorge's pharyngeal pouch syndrome results in the birth of infants without a thymus gland. There is total lack of cellular immunity in these infants, and the condition parallels that in thymectomized mice. There is severe lymphopenia and drastic reduction in small lymphocytes in the lymph nodes and spleen. In contrast, humoral immunity is unimpaired or nearly so.

In cellular immunity (see Fig 73-4) the small lymphocytes mediating antigen recognition are specifically sensitized to the antigen by prior contact with it. The exact nature of the sensitizing phenomenon is not understood. In thymectomized mice or in humans suffering from DiGeorge's syndrome lymphocytes suitable for sensitization are not present. However, if an immediate postnatal implant of viable thymus tissue from an abortus is made into an individual with DiGeorge's syndrome, at least partial and often complete restitution is made in the infant's ability to produce immunologically competent small lymphocytes.

When a T lymphocyte makes contact with its target antigen, a series of chemical reactions takes place within the lymphocyte which results in an immune reaction called cell mediated immunity (CMI). Several physiologically active substances are synthesized within the newly sensitized lymphocyte and released into the surrounding area. Some of these cellular products have been identified and will be mentioned according to type.

One such group of substances is called macrophage affecting factors. Substances in this group regulate macrophage activity according to immunological needs. Representatives of this group include migration inhibiting factor, macrophage aggregating factor and macrophage stimulating factor. A second group of factors are products which are chemotactic to leukocytes or mononuclear phagocytes. These materials attract leukocytes to the area of antigen contact by a chemical concentration gradient caused by the substances themselves. A third group are the growth stimulating factors. These materials enhance proliferation of chemotactically recruited cells. Examples of such materials include mitogenic factor, lymphocyte activation factor, interlukin-2 and interferon. These substances exert a stimulating effect on nonsensitized lymphocytes (blast cells), inducing them to undergo mitotic

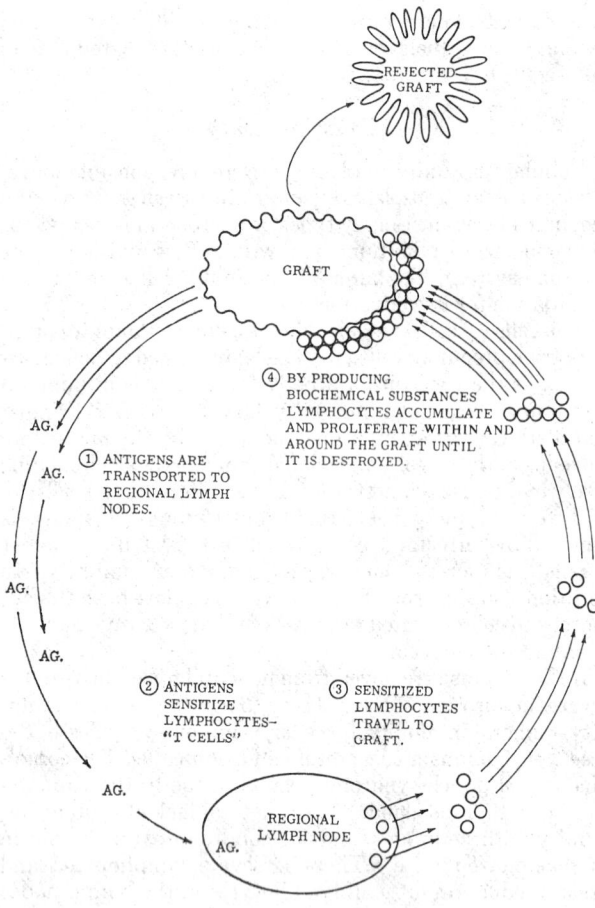

Fig 73-4. Cellular immunity.

① ANTIGENS ARE
TRANSPORTED TO
REGIONAL LYMPH
NODES.

④ BY PRODUCING
BIOCHEMICAL SUBSTANCES
LYMPHOCYTES ACCUMULATE
AND PROLIFERATE WITHIN AND
AROUND THE GRAFT UNTIL
IT IS DESTROYED.

② ANTIGENS
SENSITIZE
LYMPHOCYTES—
"T CELLS"

③ SENSITIZED
LYMPHOCYTES
TRAVEL TO
GRAFT.

REGIONAL
LYMPH NODE

GRAFT

REJECTED
GRAFT

proliferation for the purpose of producing large quantities of the fourth group of substances. These substances are cytotoxic and growth inhibiting molecules which are the actual destructive agents. They inhibit cell proliferation and cause the death of the target cells. Along with the production and release of at least four types of biologically active materials, the sensitized lymphocyte undergoes proliferation itself.

In summary, the general pattern of events is thought to be as follows: The presence of an antigen enables presensitized small-to-medium T lymphocytes to become activated, and then produce and release physiologically active substances into the surrounding area. These effectors cause accumulation of macrophages, monocytes, polymorphonuclear cells, and probably other nonsensitized leukocytes into the area of antigen contact. The unsensitized cells are transformed into blast cells, which mature to produce and release more physiologically active materials. Thus the initial effect is amplified until the invading antigen is destroyed. This typical example of CMI is observed in cases of grafting and organ transplantation. However, the methods by which skin grafts and organ transplants are rejected differ to some degree.

With skin grafts the initial rejection (first-set rejection), equivalent to the primary response in humoral immunity, begins with the appearance of sensitized lymphocytes in the regional lymph nodes that drain the graft area. These sensitized lymphocytes are the result of stimulation of antigens from the graft entering the lymphatic system and traveling to the nearest nodes. The sensitized cells appear approximately 6 to 10 days after the graft has been made. The delay is due to the fact that vascularization must first be established before the antigens can leave the graft. Approximately 10 to 14 days after grafting the first clinical signs of rejection appear. There is an accumulation of sensitized lymphocytes in the area of the graft. These cells from the regional nodes infiltrate the

graft bed, where they are found in increasing numbers. This results in graft destruction caused by vascular damage which leads to thrombosis and compromised blood circulation.

If a second graft containing the same antigens is placed on the same host, accelerated rejection is observed. This is called second-set rejection and is similar to the secondary response of humoral immunity. The second and succeeding grafts are rejected more quickly because the body has been sensitized by the first graft; thus the sensitized small-to-medium lymphocytes are already present and need only to be activated by the antigen. In addition, usually after the first-set rejection, antibodies are produced and remain free in the body's circulation. These antibodies play no part in first-set rejection and most often are formed only after the graft is rejected. On second stimulation by the same antigen, however, the cytotoxic antibodies combine with the graft. The graft cells, coated with antibody, become the target of a special T cell called a killer (K) cell which contacts the graft cells, via the antibody molecules, and kills them. This type of CMI is called antibody-dependent cellular cytotoxicity (ADCC). The mechanism by which the K cell kills the target cells is not understood. This immune response is effective in destroying viral infected host cells that are coated with antiviral antibodies.

In the case of organ transplants, eg, heart or kidney, rejection is basically the same as with skin grafts, except that the surgeon makes the vascular connection. Thus the delay seen with skin graft rejection does not occur since the waiting period for vascularization is not required. As with skin grafts, antibodies are an important factor in second-set rejection of a second organ transplant possessing the same antigen. For these reasons it is extremely important that donors and recipients be properly screened before a transplant is attempted. If the recipient has ever received blood transfusions containing leukocytes (a type of transplant), he may have a high titer of antibodies that can bring about destruction of the transplanted organ within minutes or hours.

In recent years many immunosuppressive drugs have been employed to prolong the life of a transplanted organ. However, none has been permanently satisfactory. When small doses of immunosuppressive drugs are used the recipient's immune system overcomes the drug and rejection is indicated by gradual loss of organ function. The most common symptom of rejection, regardless of the organ, is fibrous thickening of the innermost small arteries of the transplant.

The other extreme alternative is to administer large doses of immunosuppressive drugs, in which the result is complete arrest of the recipient's immune system; the recipient usually dies of a common infection he would normally be able to overcome without medical aid.

Another method of immune system control is to administer *antilymphocyte serum* (ALS), based on a pioneer concept of Elie Metchnikoff around 1900. The serum contains antibodies against lymphocytes and when injected into an individual induces complement fixation that results in lysis of lymphocytes and impairment of cellular immunity; humoral immunity, however, is not severely affected.

At this time one of the best immunosuppressants for prolonging rejection of organ transplants is cyclosporin A. It acts as a specific suppressor of T_H cells by preventing these cells from responding to interlukin-I. Thus, the immune reaction against the graft is inhibited because the necessary helper step is prevented. Unfortunately, cyclosporin A will suppress reaction against any foreign material which induces this same immune mechanism. Furthermore, it has been known to induce B cell lymphomas and may be toxic to kidneys. The massive problems associated with control of the immune system of transplant recipients emphasize the necessity of accurate and detailed tissue and blood typing prior to operation.

Privileged Graft Sites—Problems of graft rejection are not encountered in all cases. There are some parts of the human body which readily accept foreign tissue with little or no rejection in almost all attempts at transplantation. These areas are called immunologically privileged graft sites. One such site is the cornea of the eye. Transplants are almost always successful, for the reason that the vascular supply to that area is minimal. Antigens from a transplanted cornea virtually never reach a lymph node where they can sensitize lymphocytes.

For many years the human uterus was thought to be a privileged site. However, vascularization is abundant at the site and it is now known that the nonpregnant uterus rejects foreign tissue as readily as most other parts of the body. Why then is the fetus usually not rejected? Several factors are believed responsible for the survival of the fetus including several local immunosuppressants native to the fetus and placenta, suppressor cells produced by the mother in response to fetal antigens, and trophoblastic tissue. The trophoblast is that part of the placenta in closest contact with maternal tissue. Trophoblast cells are covered by a layer of mucoprotein that is a potent local immunosuppressor. It must be emphasized that the immunosuppression associated with pregnancy is local and not systemic. Pregnant females have only a minor immunodeficiency in CMI to non-fetal antigens.

Graft vs Host Reaction—In addition to the usual situation where the recipient rejects the donor graft, the reverse may occur when the graft contains immunocompetent cells. This phenomenon is termed graft vs host reaction and is characterized by the graft immunologically rejecting the host.

In theory, three conditions must exist before graft vs host reactions are possible: (1) the graft must contain immunologically competent cells; (2) the host must possess transplantation antigens that are lacking in the graft; and (3) the host must be incapable of immunologically reacting against the graft. Thus, according to the last criterion, a recipient is either immunologically immature or deficient, or both.

Runt disease, a condition characterized by stunted growth of infants, is a graft vs host reaction. When a baby suffering from thymic alymphoplasia is given a transfusion of blood the lymphocytes in the transfused blood react with the infant's tissues which are vulnerable because of thymus deficiency. The condition is often fatal, and babies that do survive suffer from serious growth and developmental problems.

When adults are rendered immunologically incompetent by x-irradiation or immunosuppressive drug therapy, they can be severely or fatally injured by graft transplants containing immunocompetent cells. The condition is called "secondary disease" or "wasting disease" because the individual appears to progressively deteriorate or waste away. The usual result, if not treated, is death. This situation is carefully monitored in bone marrow graft recipients which are becoming more common as a means of correcting some kinds of immune deficiencies.

The Recognition of Self

How does a normal vertebrate distinguish between its own antigens which it does not attack and antigens from a nonidentical twin which it destroys? The answer to the question is uncertain. Through investigations of nonidentical cattle twins it is recognized that quite often each twin possesses not only its own type of red blood cells but also the type of its twin as a result of intrauterine blood exchange between the fetuses. Also, each twin will accept a skin graft from the other, at least temporarily and often permanently. This discovery indicated that the recognition of one's own antigens occurs *in utero* or in neonatal life while the immune system is still immature. Current opinion is that immunologic tolerance of one's own

antigens is not genetically determined as once thought, but is acquired by direct exposure of antigens to potential lymphocytes and immunocytes during the period of immunological immaturity.

As with most biological phenomena, there are exceptions. There are some parts of the body that do not have ready access to lymphocytes, and thus are not recognized as being self-antigens. These are called *occult antigens;* when they are recovered from an individual and later reinjected into the original donor, antibodies are produced against its own tissues. Such antibodies are called *autoantibodies.* Tissues possessing such antigens are the eye lens and certain parts of the brain. Autoantibodies can be produced experimentally, and can arise naturally if any one or more of the following events occur: (1) accidental failure of the neonate to identify accessible antigens; (2) if occult antigens somehow gain access to the circulation and reach antibody-forming tissues, perhaps due to injury; (3) foreign antigens may cross-react with one's own antigens; and (4) if self-antigens become altered in some way, possibly as a result of mutation. When any one of these circumstances develops, a variety of autoimmune diseases, most of which are serious, can result. Examples of such diseases include rheumatic fever, a disease characterized by antibodies directed against group A streptococci, and also able to react with human heart muscle; and autoimmune hemolytic anemia, a condition characterized by the destruction of one's own erythrocytes. In addition, viruses may cause autoimmune diseases by stimulating the production of viral antigens on the surface of host cells they infect.

Tolerance

In addition to being immunologically tolerant of his own cells, it is also possible for a normal individual to be tolerant toward foreign antigens. Immunological tolerance is defined as the condition where an immunologically competent individual is unresponsive to a given antigen while reaction to other antigens is unimpaired. Thus tolerance is specific for a given antigen. In addition to naturally acquired tolerance of one's own antigens, a mother often acquires some degree of tolerance toward grafts from her newborn infant because of transplantation antigens crossing the placental barrier.

Immunological tolerance can also be acquired artificially. If first trimester human embryos are exposed to a foreign antigen, they may become tolerant to it; they recognize it as self. In postnatal individuals tolerance can also be induced when massive doses of an antigen are given. In either case the immunocytes responsible for resisting the antigen become overwhelmed. Also, in both cases subsequent injections of the antigen are required if the tolerant state is to be maintained. Neither of these methods has any current practical application with regard to human medicine.

Intravenous or intramuscular administration of low doses of purified antigen has some practical applicability. Initiation of low-dose tolerance has been used successfully to prolong graft survival in laboratory animals. The principle of low dose tolerance is also used to desensitize humans against many antigens responsible for a variety of allergy syndromes.

If necessary, tolerance can be broken by very precise doses of X-irradiation which kills the unresponsive lymphoid cells, and results in their replacement with a new crop of inducible cells from surviving bone marrow. Another method is to inject a cross-reacting antigen. If a laboratory animal demonstrates tolerance against bovine serum albumin (BSA), the tolerant state may be broken by injecting horse serum albumin (HSA).

Our present state of knowledge indicates in some tolerance conditions, over-reactive suppressor T cells (T_s) may be preventing the immune system from functioning against the antigen in question. If the mechanisms of tolerance can be discovered, organ transplants can become a common and permanent operation. If an individual could be made tolerant toward the antigens of the new organ, immunosuppressive procedures as we know them today would not be necessary, and the entire immune system would not be paralyzed or impaired as often happens. Thus, an organ recipient could live a normal life and defend himself fully against the common infections that claim the lives of many recipients or lead to rejection of the new organ.

Enhancement

This is a phenomenon similar to tolerance in one respect, yet quite different in another. Enhancement is the prolongation of graft survival or promotion of tumor or virus growth induced by blocking antibodies. Its similarity to tolerance stems from the fact that the life of grafts or transplants is prolonged (enhanced), but is different in that immunological responsiveness of the recipient is not impaired. This is because the specific effectors of graft rejection are prohibited from carrying out their designated function. The mechanisms of enhancement are not well understood at present but several theories have experimental evidence to substantiate them. One theory states that noncomplement-fixing (noncytotoxic) antibodies are produced in response to the graft. These are called *blocking antibodies*, and may bind with the graft antigens to coat them so that sensitized lymphocytes are unable to make direct contact. It is also theorized that blocking antibodies may prevent formation of immune cells by a negative feedback mechanism.

In the laboratory, enhancement can be demonstrated by transferring tumors from one donor to two groups of histoincompatible recipients. In one group only tumor is transferred while in the other group tumor transfer is accompanied by an injection of antibodies against the tumor obtained from rabbits. Recipients receiving the rabbit antibodies maintain the tumor much longer than the control group.

The principal of immunological enhancement has been put to practical use in human medicine. Rh-negative mothers who have given birth to their first Rh-positive baby are given an injection of Rh antibody shortly after delivery. The Rh antiserum prevents production of antibodies against the Rh-positive cells of the infant, which have almost certainly entered the mother's circulation during delivery. Thus the mother is not sensitized against future Rh-positive pregnancies because the unrecognized Rh antigens have been removed from the body in the normal manner.

Tumor Immunology

It has been known for several years that carcinogenic agents include a wide range of chemicals, electromagnetic radiation, and viruses. All of these materials cause a change in the genome of the cell. In some cases, such as viruses, the imposed change on the infected cell is consistent from host to host. In the case of chemical and radiation carcinogens, the genetic change is random and inconsistent from host to host. These changes, consistent or not, result in basic cellular alterations that convert healthy cells into neoplastic cells. Accompanying these alterations is the creation of a change in the antigenic density of the cell surface or the creation of new tumor specific transplantation antigens (TSTA) which supposedly identify the abnormal cell and pave the way for its destruction by the immune system.

Recently the understanding of these genetic changes has improved. Molecular biologists have been able to extract from human cancer cells portions of DNA which transform healthy cells into cancer cells. These gene segments are called

oncogenes (cancer genes) and have been found in healthy cells as well. Further evidence indicates that these oncogenes undergo transposition within the genome of the cell as a normal act of cell physiology or induced by a carcinogen. In either case the gene is activated and thus dictates the conversion of the healthy cell into a cancer cell.

The gene transposition event just described is considered normal and probably occurs thousands of times each day in a healthy individual. The resulting abnormal cell(s) are detected by the new TSTA and destroyed by phagocytosis or some branch of the immune system.

The defense mechanisms of the body against cancer development are rather formidable and comprehensive. The attack is led by natural killer (NK) cells; defense cells directed against any abnormal host cell. They make direct contact with the abnormal cell and destroy it by a cytotoxic mechanism not yet understood. If for some reason NK cells fail to identify and destroy the abnormal cell, it is likely that a normal immune response will be mounted. The response will be cell mediated in nature with the target cell being destroyed by one or more lymphokines. If this approach is not totally successful, the number of abnormal cells will increase to a point that antibody production will be induced. The first antibodies produced will bind to the abnormal cells to pave the way for killer (K) cells. These cells destroy host cells which are coated with antibody. If the abnormal cells are still not destroyed, later antibodies will be complement fixing and when they attach to the target cells they will activate the complement system which will destroy the abnormal cells by lysis.

This comprehensive approach to cancer prevention obviously works because all humans produce numerous abnormal cells each day and most individuals do not suffer from cancer. To the contrary, there obviously are weaknesses in the system because cancer in general is a monumental health problem.

In those individuals where the immune system fails to destroy the abnormal cells and thus a tumor results, something obviously has rendered the immune system ineffective. Perhaps the major question in cancer research today is not "what causes cancer," but "why does the immune system fail to destroy the unwanted cells?" Several theories have been proposed in recent years, all with some evidence for support.

One possibility for ineffective immune response is that tumor cells have a lower than normal density of antigenic determinants (TSTA) or an altered ratio of normal determinants. In either case the immunocompetent cells may not be able to recognize the cell as unusual and thus will not attempt to destroy it before it has replicated several times. When a large enough mass of cells has accumulated, a humoral immune response may be generated, but because the defense system is playing "catch-up," the antibodies that are produced are incomplete in some way and are not able to induce their physiological function after binding to the surface of the tumor. These antibodies block the attachment of NK cells and lymphocytes to the surface of the mass and thus CMI is not effective. These antibodies are called blocking or enhancement antibodies because they enhance the growth of the tumor.

Another possibility for an ineffective immune response is that at least some, and perhaps all, tumor cells produce an outer protective covering which camouflages the antigenic structures so that the immune system can not recognize the cells. Furthermore, there is evidence to show that cancerous cells produce a substance which may induce some degree of immune deficiency. It is a well documented statistic that cancer patients demonstrate some degree of immune deficiency. For many years it was assumed that people developed cancer because they were immunodeficient. Today it is believed that the cancer causes the immune deficiency. The most likely target of the cancer cell product appears to be the macrophage; a cell that not only phagocytizes unfriendly cells but also activates the cell mediated and humoral immune responses.

As a result of all the recent progress in cancer research, several approaches to cancer detection, control, and cure are being investigated; some are old, some are new. One of the oldest attempts to control, cure or prevent cancer is the development of a vaccine against a particular type of cancer. The major problem is that human tumors, even within a given category, are very inconsistent in their expression of cell surface antigens from patient to patient. A vaccine that may be effective for one individual with cancer of the colon will have no effect in most other patients with the same type of cancer. To the contrary, some investigators believe there may be enough antigenic consistency among similar tumors if the protective covering can be removed from the immunizing cells. Most studies to date indicate that the protective coating contains N-acetylneuraminic acid. Therefore, if cancer cells can be treated with neuraminidase, the TSTA under the coating will be exposed. These cells can then be killed and used as the antigenic material in a vaccine preparation. Whether this approach proves fruitful is yet to be determined.

Another approach to the utilization of TSTA is to continue to search for an antigenic structure characteristic of a particular type of tumor which may be expressed on the cell membrane of a new cancer cell, but before the protective coating is produced. If there is such an antigen structure, there should be some exposed membrane at all times as the cells of a tumor are rapidly proliferating. Such identified antigen structures can be utilized in two obvious ways; as the target of labelled antibodies used to diagnose and locate a tumor, and as the target of antibodies bound to therapeutic levels of radiated particles. In the latter case it is hoped that therapeutic radiation can be carried by injected antibodies directly into the tumor without the customary side effects of current radiation therapy.

Another immunological approach to cancer control is the isolation of pure tumor antigens from blood samples or biopsy for injection back into the patient. The intent is to boost the CMI response to be aggressive towards the new cells expressing the same antigenic specificities.

Perhaps the most promising immunological approaches include the administration of interferon and the injection of a highly immunogenic microorganism in the close proximity of a tumor. Interferon in pure form has the potential to stimulate NK cells and macrophages; the cells that may be responsible for the abnormal cells getting out of control because they may be the target of a suppressive substance produced by the abnormal cells. Now that interferon can be made in large quantities through the techniques of gene recombination, the major obstacle remaining to a broader use is one of purification of the synthesized material.

Promising results have also been obtained from the injection of an organism like Bacillus Calmette-Guerin (BCG) at the site of a non-metastasized tumor. In the human BCG is a highly immunogenic but non-pathogenic bacterium which enhances the performance of NK cells and other lymphocytes responsible for the CMI response. Both immune mechanisms are non-specific in action, so once initiated against the BCG organisms, they will be equally effective against the nearby tumor.

Much has been learned in the last few years with regard to the cause and development of cancer and the nature of the normal immune responses which usually prevent cancers from developing. The current approaches in cancer research reflect the new knowledge which will most certainly take us closer to detection, prevention and cure.

Immunogenetics

Genetics is a biological discipline closely associated with immunology. The combined discipline, immunogenetics, is concerned with phenomena such as antibody class structure and specificity; the degree of cellular or humoral response possible against a particular antigen, erythrocyte and tissue antigen expression, and most types of immune deficiency conditions. Limiting our interest to the area of human transplantation, the following discussion will include only general aspects of immunogenetics and their application to red blood cell and tissue genetics, and also of some immunological abnormalities found in humans.

The science of immunogenetics had its beginning shortly after the start of the 20th century. Around 1903 Jensen passed cells of living spontaneous mouse tumors through 19 different hosts. He observed that mice of different ancestry were not equally susceptible to the growth of the tumors he studied; some type of resistance existed in some groups of mice that was not present in other groups. It was not until 1914 that Little postulated that acceptance or rejection of tumor grafts depends on a large number of genetically controlled factors. The greater the number of factors that are identical in donor and host, the better the chance that the graft will be accepted. After much study by many investigators, Gorer in 1938 restated the hypothesis of Little to the effect that normal and tumorous tissues contain antigens that are genetically determined. Antigens present in donor tissue but absent in the host are capable of causing a response which may lead to destruction of a graft.

Similar lines of evidence for genetic control of immunological response were obtained in the period of the 1920s through the 1950s concerning the exchange of normal skin between humans. As a result of decades of research, some general principles of transplantation immunogenetics have been defined, notably:

1. Graft acceptance or rejection is controlled by the presence or absence on the graft of genetically determined antigens called *transplantation antigens*. The genes responsible for the development of these antigens are called *histocompatibility genes* and are found at *histocompatibility loci* on the chromosomes. At each locus a family of alternative genes, called *alleles*, may occur.
2. Histocompatibility alleles are codominant. Thus each of the two alleles present in every individual is always expressed. Such is the case of a human who is of blood type AB.
3. Grafts between identical twins are always accepted because the donor and recipient have the same genetic constitution.
4. Grafts between related individuals (not identical twins) are more likely to be accepted than grafts between unrelated individuals because related subjects will probably share more transplantation antigens than those who are unrelated.

In the human two major antigen systems are known and a large number of minor ones have been investigated. Only the major systems will be discussed here—the blood group ABO system characteristic of erythrocytes and the HLA system (human leukocyte antigens) characteristic of most other body tissues.

For many years the influence of the ABO system with regard to blood transfusions has been known. It is also known that the ABO system is important in tissue grafting, particularly of skin and kidney transplants. Even kidneys that have been flushed free of erythrocytes and leukocytes (which also carry ABO antigens) are rejected much faster if grafted between ABO-incompatible individuals (see Table I for a review of the characteristics of the ABO system as presently understood).

The major histocompatibility system in man is not found on mature red blood cells, but rather on almost all nucleated cells. As social and ethical problems involved with human research prohibit planned mating, knowledge about the inheritance of the HLA and other histocompatibility systems has been difficult to obtain. Complicating the problem is the

Table I—Characteristics of the Human ABO Blood Group System

Blood groups	Antigens present		Antibodies present		Frequencies in Caucasians, %
	A	B	Anti A	Anti B	
O	–	–	+	+	40
A	+	–	–	+	44
B	–	+	+	–	12
AB	+	+	–	–	4

Table II—Some HL-A and Disease Associations

Disease	HL-A Antigen
Ankylosing spondylitis	B27
Reiter's syndrome	B27
Celiac disease	Dw3
Dermatitis herpetiformis	Dw3
Psoriasis vulgaris	B13
Pemphigus	Dw4
Pernicious anemia	Dw5
Idiopathic hemochromatosis	A3
Multiple sclerosis	Dw2
Addison's disease	Dw3

fact that many different alleles can be controlled by each histocompatibility locus. Furthermore, in the case of the HLA system, and possibly others, each allele may code for 12 or more antigenic determinants.

In spite of these complexities, much has been discovered through techniques of leukocyte typing and family studies. Leukocyte typing provides a very comprehensive determination of the body's tissue antigens because almost all antigens characteristic of the organism are believed to be represented on leukocytes. Family studies require erythrocyte and leukocyte typing of each member of a family, preferably a large one. By identifying the blood and tissue antigenic structures of children in a large family, the pattern of inheritance of these structures can be determined in the parents.

Some of the many things that have been learned by leukocyte typing and family studies are that certain histocompatibility antigens occur more frequently than others, and some are much more immunogenic than others. Some antigens are even characteristic of a given race. Family studies have also enabled researchers to make estimates as to the number of alleles present in each system and the number of antigenic determinants controlled by each allele. There may be as few as one or two, or more than 30 alleles in each system, with each allele controlling from one to 12 or more antigenic determinants.

Investigations into the complexity of the histocompatibility antigen systems have revealed the presence of genes that control the degree to which we can respond to a foreign antigen (*Immune Response Genes*). Furthermore, the intensity of our immune response is antigen-specific. We can respond well to some antigens, poorly to others and intermediately to others. The variation in response also differs among individuals. Subject "A" may have a friend or relative who never has a cold, while "A" has one most of the time. This may be because the friend has inherited the ability to produce more and better antibodies or sensitized lymphocytes against cold viruses than "A" did. To the contrary, the friend may succumb to flu viruses very easily, while "A" never gets the flu. In this instance "A" has the more intensive and efficient immune response toward the invading antigen.

Histocompatibility antigens also appear to be associated with the frequency of various diseases within the population. The HLA system consists of four different loci referred to as HLA-A, HLA-B, HLA-C and HLA-D. Each locus has several alleles (gene alternatives) and each allele will control the expression of a different HLA antigen. Each antigen is indicated by a number (A1, B27, C5, D2 etc). In many instances there is a strong association between the frequency of appearance of a certain antigen and the occurrence of a specific disease. Exactly what the connection is between the expression of the antigen and susceptibility or resistance to a given disease is not known. Since histocompatibility-typing can be done routinely by many clinical laboratories, it is expected that this kind of information may some day be used diagnostically or as a screening device to indicate the probable development of a certain disease or condition at some future

time in a patient's life. This has tremendous implications at a time when there is concern about preventive medicine and health maintenance.

Some currently recognized associations between various histocompatibility antigens and specific diseases are illustrated in Table II. When reviewing this table it must be remembered that the various associations are not absolute. Not everyone with antigen B27 will become afflicted with ankylosing spondylitis or Reiter's syndrome; these recognized associations indicate only that people with B27 antigens have one of these diseases more frequently than would be expected purely by chance.

Knowledge gained from the exhaustive research in immunogenetics has several additional applications. An understanding of the genetics of the ABO and other blood group systems has been very useful in reducing the risk of death from blood transfusions. Knowledge of blood grouping has limited application in paternity cases. Immunogenetics can also be useful in the study of fetal and neonatal development for the purpose of investigating birth defects, and even birth control. The most exciting and perhaps rewarding use of immunogenetics is in the selection and screening of organ transplant donors and recipients. As techniques for preservation and storage of viable organs improve, the time may come when a large bank of various organs can be maintained so that donor organs may be matched with recipients almost perfectly. Perhaps equally as exciting is the potential for diagnosis and treatment of immunological deficiencies which are genetically controlled.

Immunological Deficiencies

Within the scope of this chapter it is appropriate to discuss briefly several immunological deficiencies known to exist in humans.

The first genetically controlled immunological defect was discovered by Bruton in 1952 and is called Bruton's agammaglobulinemia, a sex-linked disease occurring only in males. It is evident during the sixth to the twelfth month of life, after the antibodies received from the mother are expended. Individuals suffering from Bruton's syndrome are unable to produce antibodies, but their cellular response is normal. The probable site of the defect is a lack of plasma cells differentiated for humoral immunity by the bone marrow.

The opposite condition is called DiGeorge's syndrome and is characterized by thymic aplasia caused by an embryonic failure of development of the third and fourth pharyngeal pouches, which results in absence of parathyroid and thymus glands or at best, a severely hypoplastic thymus. There is a deficiency of T cells in the cortical areas of the lymph nodes, in consequence of which cellular immunity is absent although humoral immunity against many antigens is normal. Unlike Bruton's syndrome, DiGeorge's syndrome is not believed to be a genetic disorder, but rather a problem encountered *in utero*. In some cases a thymus transplant is helpful. This is possible because the thymus itself does not possess cells capable of producing an immune response, thus avoiding a graft vs host reaction.

The Wiskott-Aldrich syndrome is a condition characterized by a depression of cellular immunity as well as a lack of IgM antibodies in humoral immunity. The severity of the conditions varies considerably and a single cure or type of treatment is not possible.

Reticular dysgenesis or congenital aleukocytosis is a fatal condition found in infants. An abnormality exists in the development of all white cells, and this leads to a variety of simultaneous immunological problems. The T and B precursors fail to develop and thus cellular and humoral immunity are both lacking. All lymphoid tissue, including the thymus, is hypoplastic. Until recently this sex-linked recessive and autosomal recessive (two genotype patterns exist) condition has been fatal, although a few cases have been successfully treated with bone marrow grafts from HLA matched or related individuals.

A final example of genetically controlled immune deficiency is adult hypogammaglobulinemia; probably an autosomal recessive. Serum immunoglobulin levels drop to 10% or less of normal, and late in the disease variable cellular immune defects occur. This was the first example of an inherited condition involving the immune system becoming manifest in adult life.

Current research and diagnostic techniques have identified a long list of genetically controlled immune deficiencies and the list promises to continue to grow. However, the immune deficiency receiving the most attention is not genetically controlled but is acquired. Acquired Immune Deficiency Syndrome (AIDS) is the most feared and currently one of the least understood diseases of all of mankind. It is a transmittable condition with a long incubation period and appears to have a fatality rate of 100%. The number of cases are doubling every six months with no causative agent as yet identified. The disease is most frequent in promiscuous homosexual males, intravenous drug users, Haitian males and type A hemophiliacs. However, it is feared that individuals in the general population will eventually acquire the disease. As deadly and feared as is the disease, immunologists believe that as the AIDS puzzle is unraveled there will be an explosion of knowledge to come forth that will answer many questions about the function of the immune system.

Drug Allergies

A problem of increasing significance in the use of therapeutic drugs is the occurrence of drug allergies. These are not reactions due to drug interactions, toxicity or overdose; rather they are the result of an immunological response initiated by a drug metabolite. Such reactions ultimately reduce a drug's effectiveness and cause new problems for the patient.

An explanation of drug allergies may be as follows. Many drugs or their metabolites are very small, structurally simple, molecules that are harmless from an immunological standpoint. Immunologists call them *haptens*, because by themselves they are unable to induce an immune response. However, if a drug metabolite binds to a patient's plasma proteins or similar structures it can acquire sufficient size and complexity to make it immunologically active. It induces the patient to produce antibodies which bind to the metabolite and thus impede its pharmacological effectiveness. More importantly, when the metabolite is conjugated to the plasma protein the structure of the protein may be altered slightly and

thus appear different or "foreign" to the patient's immune system. The patient may actually produce antibodies against his own proteins that may lead to their destruction; this is called *autoimmune disease* and is usually quite serious.

Drug allergies are very difficult to investigate because of several built-in complexities: (1) Drugs are degraded through a variety of enzymatic pathways, many of which are not known; (2) many medicinal agents are converted to a number of metabolites, each with slightly different characteristics; (3) in some cases a tiny amount of any one metabolite is all that is needed to initiate an immune response, and that amount may be so small that the metabolite may never have been identified in laboratory studies. The investigation of drug allergies becomes especially difficult when it has not been possible to identify and isolate the metabolites(s) responsible for the immunological reaction. Furthermore, the immunological reaction may take a variety of forms in addition to that of some type of autoimmune mechanism. Thus, the patient may develop fever, vasculitis, kidney disease, rash, serum sickness, anaphylaxis or any variation or combination of these reactions.

The likelihood of occurrence of drug allergies is influenced by many factors. The duration and number of courses of therapy, occurrence of diseases that interfere with drug biotransformation or excretion, drugs that are taken sporadically or from different lots, and existing allergies all tend to increase the onset of a drug allergy. Adults are more likely to have a drug allergy than are children. Sensitivity toward a drug usually diminishes after exposure has been discontinued.

Since laboratory testing for drug allergies is very difficult, little can be done to prevent development of such conditions. However, once a drug allergy is suspected, several things can be done through cooperation of the physician and pharmacist to minimize the patient's problem. Precise records, including properly labeled charts, pertaining to use of medication are essential. Whenever possible, other drugs of similar therapeutic effect should be used. A medication that can be given orally should be administered because oral dosage is less likely to induce an immune response.

The structural complexity of many modern medicines magnifies a problem that in the past has been relatively minor. Moreover, until scientists are able to identify all metabolites of a medicinal agent, determine how the body handles each metabolite, and isolate or synthesize each in pure form for laboratory investigation, drug allergies likely will continue to be an increasingly significant problem in therapeutics.

As this chapter concludes it should be obvious that immunology is a rapidly changing area. The surface of some topics has been skimmed and many others omitted because of space constraints. Therefore, the reader is referred to any one or combination of the following books for more information.

Bibliography

Barrett JT: *Textbook of Immunology*, 4th ed, Mosby, St Louis, 1983.

Myrvik QN, Weiser RS: *Fundamentals of Immunology*, 2nd ed, Lea & Febiger, Philadelphia, 1984.

Pittiglio OH: *Modern Blood Banking and Transfusion Practices*, Davis, Philadelphia, 1983.

Richter MA: *Clinical Immunology, A Physician's Guide*, 2nd ed, Williams & Wilkins, Baltimore, 1982.

Tizard IR: *Immunology: An Introduction*, Saunders, Philadelphia, 1984.

Zaleski MB, *et al*: *Immunogenetics*, Pitman, Boston, 1983.

CHAPTER 74

Immunizing Agents and Diagnostic Skin Antigens

Frank Roia, PhD

Professor of Biology
Philadelphia College of Pharmacy and Science
Philadelphia, PA 19104

The Food and Drug Administration refers to immunizing agents as *biologics* (*biologicals*, *biological products*); whereas the Advisory Committee on Immunization Practices (ACIP) refers to immunizing agents as *immunobiologics*. The term *biologic* will be used in this discussion. In its broadest meaning, a biologic refers to something produced from a living source and thus would include: hormones, vitamins, antibiotics, enzymes and so forth; however, according to the Public Health Service Act, a biologic includes only those preparations primarily designed to develop a type of immunity or is concerned with immunity. *Immunity* in the most general sense may be defined simply as natural or acquired resistance to disease.

Providing immunity by using any type of biologic is termed *immunization*. Immunization often is used interchangeably with vaccination. Originally the term *vaccination* meant the inoculation of vaccinia (cowpox) virus in order to render an individual immune to smallpox. Although some sources prefer that the word vaccination be limited to this original meaning, other sources use vaccination as a more general term to indicate the administration of a biologic such as a vaccine for active immunity (see following discussion) without any consideration as to whether or not it confers immunity.

ACIP in its statements of recommendation uses the two terms interchangeably when referring to active immunization. ACIP, however, points out that whichever term is used, one should not equate automatically the administration of a biologic with the development of adequate immunity because of a variety of specific factors that might interfere with the immune response.

Types of Immunity

Before discussing biologics, it is important to have an understanding of the different types of immunity. The scheme below illustrates the main categories into which the various kinds of natural and acquired immunity may be classified arbitrarily;

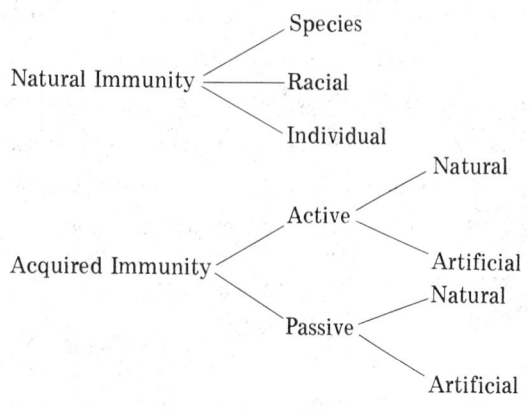

The following discussion is intended to be an overview of the above scheme and is in no way intended to be a comprehensive treatment. Note: for information on cellular immunity see Chapter 73.

Natural Immunity

Species Immunity—It is well known that humans are resistant to a variety of infections of lower animals including canine distemper, hog cholera and cattle plague. In a similar manner lower animals exhibit a *nonsusceptibility* to certain human infections such as gonorrhea, measles, bacillary dysentery and smallpox. In fact, an important reason why smallpox was able to be eradicated (the last case recorded was in Somalia in 1977) was that man was the only host and there were no lower animals to serve as reservoirs for the infection. On the other hand there are some ninety diseases, like tuberculosis, anthrax, ornithosis, and rabies which occur in both man and lower animals alike.

Not all factors involved in species immunity are known, but in part, species immunity is determined by the anatomy and physiology of the particular animal species. There is evidence, for example, that certain microorganisms are able to penetrate the epithelial barrier or other tissue barriers of one species and not another. It also has been shown that certain species are resistant to specific infections because they possess *natural antibodies* which as far as is known are present without obvious external stimuli.

Racial Immunity—Certain races are more resistant or susceptible to specific diseases; for example, certain races are more resistant to yellow fever, whereas others are more susceptible to tuberculosis.

Like species immunity, the factors which determine racial immunity are not all known. Some, like resistance to malaria, have some physiologic basis in that resistance to malaria is highest in persons carrying the sickle cell trait. Some racial immunity, however, may be the result of resistance to infection among individuals in a given community due to the degree of acquired immunity and to such factors as nutrition, fatigue and genetic constitution (Chapter 73).

Individual Immunity—Individuals in good health are endowed with a high level of natural immunity without having had an opportunity to generate specific antibodies as a result of a previous infection (Chapter 73). General good health also implies healthy body tissues, skin and mucous membranes (all important bacterial barriers) of good quality, leukocytes in plentiful supply and properly active, and so forth. Also involved in individual resistance is the kind and quality of the resident bacterial flora in the large intestine, in the upper respiratory tract, including the oral cavity, and in other parts of the body. Undoubtedly, the resident flora play a part in resisting invasion by other species of microorganisms capable of producing infection. Similarly, the gastric juice, as a result of acidic properties, is to a marked degree bactericidal and capable of destroying many species of harmful bacteria and viruses which may be ingested during eating and drinking. In addition, the intestinal enzymes help to set up a valuable secondary defense mechanism.

Active Acquired Immunity

Active acquired immunity occurs when the stimulus introduced is an antigen (immunogen) which elicits an immune response (Chapter 73); thus, the host (human or lower animal) is "actively" involved in the production of protecting antibodies (immunoglobulins).

Active acquired immunity may be acquired in one of two general ways: natural or artificial.

Naturally Acquired Active Immunity—This occurs when the introduction of a *virulent antigen* results in a disease state in its recognizable clinical presentation. However, in some individuals, either because of increased host resistance, moderate exposure to the antigen or decreased virulence of the antigen, the disease may be so mild that it never reaches the clinical stage (*subclinical infection*). Antibodies, however, may be produced in sufficient amount to protect the individual from possible future infections by the same species of microorganism. Infections such as polio and rubella, for example, often occur subclinically and are detected, along with protective antibodies to a variety of other infections, in routine immunological studies in individuals who never have had a clinically recognizable case of the disease in question.

It must be kept in mind that the degree of immunity possessed is the determining factor in successful resistance against future exposures. It is known that a level of immunity can be entirely effective against a moderate contact with a given disease, yet become ineffective in the event of exposure to an overwhelming dose of infective organisms.

The outcome of any infection, therefore, is determined not only by the degree of acquired immunity but also by several complex inter-reacting factors including the virulence of the invading microorganism, the level of resistance offered by body tissues and cells and by the general level of health in the host.

Artificially Acquired Active Immunity—This involves the use of *avirulent antigens* in the form of biologics such as *vaccines* and *toxoids* (Table I). Vaccines and toxoids contain antigens that are so modified as to be incapable of producing the disease state, yet at the same time modified so slightly that when introduced in the body will elicit the production of specific protective antibodies against the disease.

The duration of active acquired immunity, both natural and artificial, is variable. In some cases it is rather brief; but usually protection lasts many years, and in some diseases for life. For most vaccines and toxoids secondary stimuli or *boosters* are required at periodic intervals of months to years if the acquired immunity is to be maintained.

Passive Acquired Immunity

In passive acquired immunity, the antibodies are produced in another individual (human or lower animal). Thus immunity is acquired by the introduction of these antibodies and the host is not "actively" involved in antibody production but is "passively" receiving antibodies. Passive acquired immunity like active acquired immunity may be classified as natural or artificial.

Naturally Acquired Passive Immunity—This occurs by placental transmission of immunoglobulin G (IgG) from mother to fetus (Chapter 73). The infant may have passive immunity for the first four to six months of life to diphtheria, tetanus, measles, mumps and other infections because of the transfer of these antibodies.

Artificially Acquired Passive Immunity—Several biologics (Table I) are involved in providing antibodies including antitoxins and sera of animal origin, and immune globulin and hyperimmune sera derived from human plasma. In this category also would be placed antivenins used for the treatment of the bites of poisonous snakes and spiders.

Biologics for passive immunity are limited to temporary prophylaxis of susceptible individuals, for example during an epidemic, and to supplying immediate antibodies for the treatment of infections and toxicities.

The immunity provided by these means is not long-lasting, and such antibodies leave the body tissues and fluids of the host within a comparatively short time (usually 1 or 2 weeks). Thus the administration of diphtheria antitoxin to a susceptible patient exposed to diphtheria will offer protection during the critical period when help is most urgently needed, but will not be permanent because the injected antibodies will be utilized either by binding to the pathogen as needed or metabolized by the body (because the antibodies are foreign) if not needed for immunological purposes.

Table I—Types of Biologics

Biologics for Active Immunity

    Vaccine—a suspension of attenuated (live) or inactivated (killed) microorganisms or fractions thereof administered to induce immunity and thus prevent infectious disease.

    Toxoid—a modified bacterial toxin (exotoxin) that has been rendered nontoxic (detoxified) but retains the ability to stimulate the formation of antitoxin and thus prevent bacterial toxicities.

Biologics for Passive Immunity

  Human Immune Sera (Homologous Sera)[a]

    Immune Globulin—A solution containing antibodies from the pooled plasmas of not less than 1,000 normal individuals. It is used primarily for routine maintenance of certain immunodeficient persons and for passive immunization against measles and hepatitis A.

    Hyperimmune Serum (Specific immune globulin)—a special preparation obtained from human donor pools selected for high antibody titer against a specific disease, eg, hepatitis B immune globulin (HBIG) and rabies immune globulin (RIG).

  Animal Immune Serum (Heterologous Sera)

    Antitoxin—a solution of antibodies derived from the serum of animals (usually a horse) immunized with specific toxins (toxoids) eg, botulism diphtheria and tetanus used to achieve passive immunity or to effect a treatment.

    Antiviral Serum—a solution of antibodies derived from the serum of animals (usually a horse) immunized with a specific viral vaccine. There is only one commercially important biologic available, antirabies serum (equine).

    Antivenin—a preparation of antibodies derived from the serum of animals (usually horses) immunized with specific venoms, eg, rattle snakes, coral snake and black widow spider, used to neutralize the venoms produced by the specific organisms.

---

[a] There are also preparations of whole human plasma that contain antibodies against specific infections. These are available from CDC on an emergency basis and include immune plasma for African hemorrhagic fever, California encephalitis, eastern equine encephalitis, herpes simian B, junin (Argentinian hemorrhagic fever), lassa fever, muchupo (Bolivian hemorrhagic fever), Marburg (green monkey disease), monkey B, Russian spring summer encephalitis, St Louis encephalitis, western equine encephalitis.

Hypersensitivity to Biologics

Hypersensitivity reactions (Chapter 73) primarily are associated with three general types of biologics.

1. *Antisera or Antitoxins of animal origin (usually equine).*
2. *Viral vaccines grown in embryonic egg.*
3. *Biologics (mainly viral vaccines) with antibiotics.*

Antisera or Antitoxins of Animal Origin

Antivenins, antirabies serum (equine) and antitoxins such as botulism, diphtheria and tetanus are prepared from horse sera which are proteinaceous and foreign to the recipient and thus may be immunogenic in their own right (Chapter 73).

Before the administration of any product containing horse serum, it is customary for the physician to inquire into the history of the patient to determine whether or not antitoxins may have been given some time earlier. It also is important to ascertain whether the patient has a history of asthma or any allergy and particularly whether the patient suffers distress when in proximity to horses. Patients with such a history may develop serious systemic reactions.

Sensitiveness can be determined readily by a conjunctival and an intracutaneous skin test using small quantities of a dilution of the product to be administered. In fact it is recommended that all patients regardless of history be tested by these two tests before the injection of the biologic. If the patient is sensitive, positive reactions will occur within 30 minutes. In the case of the skin test a positive reaction is a wheal with a hyperaemic aerola and in the conjunctival test it is lacrimation and conjunctivitis.

A negative sensitivity test usually is considered reliable; but does not entirely preclude the possibility of the occurrence of systemic reactions. If the sensitivity test is positive, the biologic may still be administered to the patient but with *extreme* caution. This is accomplished by following a *desensitization* schedule which involves a series of injections, beginning with a very small dose of diluted antitoxin given *subcutaneously* and increased at 15–20 minutes until the biologic is eventually given undiluted *intramuscularly* and the required therapeutic dose has been administered. The various manufacturers' package inserts may vary somewhat and therefore should be consulted before using a specific product.

It should be noted that it is exceedingly dangerous to readminister any animal antiserum of the same animal origin. In such cases serious systemic reactions are a real possibility.

Fortunately there currently is little need for use of immunizing agents from animal sera. With proper utilization of diphtheria and tetanus toxoids for active immunization, the use of antitoxins for these two diseases can be avoided. In addition with the availability of human tetanus immune globulin and rabies immune globulin, use of antisera of animal origin should be avoided whenever possible. Only lifesaving antisera such as botulism antitoxin and the antivenins must be used occasionally.

Viral Vaccines Grown in Embryonic Egg

Vaccines propagated in embryonic egg may cause hypersensitivity reactions including anaphylaxis especially when there is a substantial amount of egg protein in the final product as is the case with yellow fever vaccine. Yellow fever vaccine, therefore, should not be administered to an individual with a proved sensitivity to egg or chicken embryo protein. If there is any question, an intracutaneous sensitivity skin test should be performed. The vaccine is contraindicated if the sensitivity test is positive.

Measles, mumps, and influenza vaccines also are propa-

gated in egg; but can be given safely to individuals sensitive to chicken protein provided that the allergies are not manifested by anaphylactic symptoms. Influenza vaccines, both whole and split, are highly purified during preparation and have been reported only rarely to be associated with hypersensitivity reactions.

Screening persons by a history of ability to eat eggs without adverse effects is usually sufficient to identify those individuals at possible risk from receiving measles, mumps and influenza vaccines. The vaccines should not be given to those individuals who have demonstrated anaphylactic hypersensitivity.

Biologics with Antibiotics

Viral vaccines such as rubella that are propagated on human tissue culture are essentially devoid of any potential hypersensitivity related to host tissue; but they may contain trace amounts of antibiotics, eg neomycin to which patients occasionally may be hypersensitive. Patients also very rarely may be hypersensitive to other additives and preservatives in biologics, eg thimerosal, a common preservative of many biologics.

Health personnel administering these biologics should review carefully the information provided with the package insert before deciding whether a person with a known hypersensitivity to such ingredients be administered the biologic.

Note: no currently recommended biologic contains penicillin or its derivatives.

Other Reactions

All biologics can cause a variety of local and systemic adverse reactions which do not appear to be allergic. These reactions range from frequent minor local reactions such as redness, tenderness and induration surrounding the injection site to systemic manifestations including malaise, generalized aches and pains and fever. In extremely rare situations there have been severe, systemic illness, such as paralysis associated with oral polio vaccine.

Generally, the risk of serious reaction is far outweighed by the lifesaving benefits derived by prudent use of these agents. The relative balance of benefits and risks may change as diseases are brought under control or eradicated. This is best exemplified by smallpox vaccination. Since smallpox has been eradicated the very small risk from receiving smallpox vaccine now exceeds the risk of smallpox itself; thus smallpox vaccination of civilians is limited to laboratory personnel directly involved with smallpox or closely related orthopox viruses. *Note: There, however, have been a few reported cases of contact spread of vaccinia from recently vaccinated persons.*

The vaccines for cholera, plague and typhoid fever and even DTP (diphtheria and tetanus toxoids and pertussis vaccine) are frequently associated with local and systemic adverse effects. It is not possible to discuss these specific reactions here, although as is mentioned in the discussions of individual products, some of the recommendations for their use is based upon minimizing potential adverse reactions.

Federal Control of Biologics

Interstate shipment and the export or import of biologic products were originally subject to Federal control under the provisions of the "Act of July 1, 1902," (32 Stat 728, 729). On July 1, 1944, this authority was consolidated with other laws relating to the Public Health Service by enactment of "An Act to consolidate and revise the laws relating to the Public Health Service, and for other purposes" (Public Law 410, 78th Congress; 58 Stat. 682).

Section 351 (a) of that Act provides that:

No person shall sell, barter, or exchange, or offer for sale, barter, or exchange in the District of Columbia, or send, carry, or bring for sale, barter, or exchange from any State or possession into any other State or possession or into any foreign country, or from any foreign country into any State or possession, any virus, therapeutic serum, toxin, antitoxin, vaccine, blood, blood component or derivative, allergenic product, or analogous product, or arsphenamine or its derivatives (or any other trivalent organic arsenic compound), applicable to the prevention, treatment, or cure of diseases, or injuries of man, unless (1) such virus, serum, toxin, antitoxin, vaccine, blood, blood component or derivative, allergenic product, or other product has been propagated or manufactured and prepared at an establishment holding an unsuspended and unrevoked license, issued by the Secretary as hereinafter authorized, to propagate or manufacture, and prepare such virus, serum, toxin, antitoxin, vaccine, blood, blood component or derivative, allergenic product, or other product for sale in the District of Columbia, or for sending, bringing, or carrying from place to place aforesaid; and (2) each package of such virus, serum, toxin, antitoxin, vaccine, blood, blood component or derivative, allergenic product, or other product is plainly marked with the proper name of the article contained therein, the name, address, and license number of the manufacturer, and the date beyond which the contents cannot be expected beyond reasonable doubt to yield their specific results. The suspension or revocation of any license shall not prevent the sale, barter, or exchange of any virus, serum, toxin, antitoxin, vaccine, blood, blood component or derivative, allergenic product, or other product aforesaid which has been sold and delivered by the licensee prior to such suspension or revocation, unless the owner or custodian of such virus, serum, toxin, antitoxin, vaccine, blood, blood component or derivative, allergenic product, or other product aforesaid has been notified by the Secretary not to sell, barter, or exchange the same.

The Act also provides that standards, designed to insure the continued *safety*, *purity*, and *potency* of licensed products, shall be prescribed in regulations issued by the Surgeon General of the Public Health Service and approved by the Secretary of the Department of Health, Education and Welfare.

Reorganization Plan No. 1, 1953 (67 Stat 613), transferred the Public Health Service to the Department of Health, Education, and Welfare. By reorganization orders of March 13, 1968 (33 FR 4894), and April 1, 1968 (33 FR 5246), the Acting Secretary of Health, Education, and Welfare ordered the reorganization of certain health functions of the Department. One of the results of this reorganization was to place under the Director of the National Institutes of Health all functions relating to licensing and control of biological products previously vested in the Surgeon General. The division responsible for these activities was known as the Division of Biologics Standards. Veterinary biological products are regulated by the US Dept. of Agriculture.

Although biological products were subject to regulation and licensing under Section 351 of the 1944 Public Health Service Act, the Act contains no explicit requirement for demonstration of effectiveness. The legislative history of both the Public Health Service Act and the 1962 Amendments to the Federal Food, Drug, and Cosmetic Act of 1938 was that in the former an effectiveness requirement for biologicals was deleted and in the latter a section on biologicals that included requirements for their effectiveness was also deleted. Nevertheless, the National Institutes of Health in 1962 began asking for a demonstration of effectiveness for new types of biological products being developed. This was done through a liberal interpretation of the potency requirements authorized under Section 351, even though potency is not synonymous with effectiveness.

Section 351 also lacked a provision for removal of ineffective products from the market as was provided for pharmaceuticals in the 1962 Amendments to the Food, Drug, and Cosmetic Act. The National Institutes of Health asked Congress to amend the Public Health Service Act to require effectiveness, but no action was taken. In 1972 the Secretary of the Department of Health, Education, and Welfare decided to delegate authority to the National Institutes of Health to invoke the Food, Drug, and Cosmetic Act to remove ineffective products, and

NIH shortly afterward announced that it would conduct a review of biological products. The Secretary also moved to transfer the Division of Biologics Standards to the FDA; the transfer became effective July 1, 1972. The new FDA bureau is now known as the Bureau of Biologics, and has authority to administer the pertinent parts of both statutes to biological products. A thorough review of all biological products licensed under preexisting regulations has been undertaken by special panels of experts from various medical and scientific organizations.

The complete text of regulations pertaining to the development, testing, labeling, sale, and other aspects of biological products, formerly known as Part 73 of Title 42 of the Code of Federal Regulations, was transferred to the newly established Part 273 (more recently renumbered Part 600) of Title 21 of the Code of Federal Regulations to reflect the organizational changes described above. The interested reader is referred to this document for details.

Licensees—A listing of manufacturers licensed to produce biologicals, *Establishments and Products*, is revised annually and is available from the Bureau of Biologics, FDA, Rockville, MD 20852.

The production and distribution of biological products are subject to federal regulations.

Compendial Standards—The USP indicates that the antitoxins, antivenins, blood derivatives, immune serums, immunologic diagnostic aids, toxoids, vaccines, and related articles that are produced under license in accordance with the terms of the federal Public Health Service Act of 1944, as amended have long been known as biologics. However, in Title III, Part F, of the Act, the term "biological products" is applied to the group of licensed products as a whole. For Pharmacopeial purposes, the term "biologics" refers to those products that must be licensed under the Act and comply with Parts 600–680 of Title 21 of the Code of Federal Regulations, pertaining to federal control of these products, as administered by the Bureau of Biologics of the FDA. The USP standards for "biologics" conform to Parts 600–680 of Title 21 of the Code of Federal Regulations in covering those aspects of identity, purity, potency, and packaging and storage that are of particular interest to pharmacists and physicians responsible for the purchase, storage, and use of biologics.

Care in Dispensing—In dispensing biologics the pharmacist must recognize that he is dealing with preparations most of which are intended for injection subcutaneously, intramuscularly, intravenously, or by some other parenteral route. It is, therefore, of paramount importance that the sterility and potency of the preparations be maintained until they are actually injected. Sterility is assured by the processes used in manufacturing establishments, and no product is released until repeated tests have shown it to be safe in this respect. The pharmacist contributes to the maintenance of potency of the product and insures safety to the patient by observing specified requirements. The label should be carefully examined for specific instructions as to the temperature at which the product should be maintained, the expiration date, and other essential information pertaining not only to the product but also to the particular lot. All products must be dispensed in the unopened containers in which they were placed by the manufacturer. Freezing temperatures should be avoided, unless otherwise directed on the labeling. The risk of damage from freezing may be greatest for the aqueous diluents frequently packaged with biologics.

Sources of Information

The information presented in this chapter is derived primarily from the following:
(1) Morbidity and Mortality Weekly Report (MMWR)

This report is published weekly by CDC and contains recommendations on biologics, reports on specific disease activity, policy statements and the regular and special recommendations of the Advisory Committee of Immunization Practices (ACIP).

(2) Manufacturer's Package Inserts

In addition to the type of information discussed in this chapter, the package insert contains data on contraindications, warnings, precautions, adverse reactions, clinical pharmacology, storage requirements, references, and so forth.

(3) United States Pharmacopeia

This compendium contains the official monographs for most of the biologics described in this chapter. These monographs contain standards of preparation and potency, storage requirements, expiration data and so forth.

(4) Federal Code of Regulations, 1983

Chapter 1, Subchapter F-Biologics, Parts 600–680 contains federal regulations pertaining to licensing, good manufacturing practices, general biological products standards, and additional standards on specific biologics.

Biologics for Active Immunization

Bacterial Vaccines

Preparation—The organisms are grown in suitable broth medium under controlled conditions of temperature, pH, oxygen tension and so forth. Whenever possible the medium consists of chemically defined ingredients to reduce the potential for hypersensitivity reactions of the finished product. The incubation period is usually 24 hours; but may be extended to 48 to 72 hours or longer for slower growing bacteria.

Following a suitable amount of growth, the culture is then processed in two main steps:

(1) If the vaccine is killed, the organisms are *inactivated* with formaldehyde or phenol. Typhoid fever vaccine is inactivated with heat and phenol.

(2) The organisms are then separated from the medium by means of centrifugation and resuspended in sterile saline or sterile water for injection. The cells may be purified further by several methods including additional centrifugation and/or dialysis.

In the preparation of anthrax vaccine, the culture is filtered and the filtrate, not the organism, is further processed and used as the source of the antigen.

Product Form—In cholera, pertussis, plague and typhoid fever vaccines, the resuspended cells are standardized (see Strength) and the final vaccine is in the form of a suspension of cells. Anthrax vaccine as mentioned is a liquid filtrate and the filtrate is adsorbed onto aluminum hydroxide. Aluminum hydroxide is an *adjuvant* which is used to enhance the immune response. For the preparation of BCG vaccine, the purified cells are lyophilized (freeze-dried) and the vaccine is reconstituted as directed with a diluent before use.

Meningococcal and pneumococcal vaccines are prepared by further processing the suspended cells in a series of steps including, lyses and differential centrifugation in order to extract the polysaccharide capsular antigens. The pneumococcal vaccine contains a mixture of polysaccharide antigens in a liquid form; whereas the meningococcal vaccine is a lyophilized product.

The final vaccine product may contain a single antigen (*monovalent*), eg, typhoid fever vaccine or it may contain multiple antigens (*polyvalent*, *trivalent* etc) to elicit immunity against the same disease state, eg, cholera vaccine (has two serotypes of the cholera vibrio).

In addition the product may be in the form of a mixed vaccine or a mixed biologic. A *mixed vaccine* such as measles, mumps and rubella vaccines (MMR) is a single product with three antigens for three different disease states. A *mixed biologic*, on the other hand has a combination of a vaccine and toxoid(s) in the same preparation, eg, DTP.

Strength—The strength of a bacterial vaccine may be expressed in terms of total (1) organisms (or colony forming units as with BCG vaccine), (2) protective units or (3) μg of antigen, found in each mL or in each dose of vaccine.

(1) When total number of organisms is used to designate strength, the potency of that number of organisms usually is verified by an animal protection test as compared to a US Reference Vaccine for that organism. For example, the number of vaccine organisms when injected into a specified laboratory animal should stimulate enough antibodies to protect the animal from a specific challenge with the corresponding pathogenic organism.

(2) For some vaccines the strength is directly expressed as protective units per mL or dose rather than a specified number of organisms. Pertussis vaccine, for example, contains four protective units. One protective unit of pertussis vaccine is the amount of vaccine needed to protect a mouse against a lethal intracerebral challenge with *Bordetella pertussis*.

(3) The strength of a vaccine composed of extracts of cellular components is expressed in μg of antigen per mL or per dose. For example, meningococcal vaccine contains 50 μg of polysaccharide antigen in each 0.5 mL dose, an amount which when injected into no less than 25 volunteers will show a four fold or greater rise in antibody titer in not less than 90% of the volunteers.

It is important to note that the strengths of these vaccines (and other biologics), regardless of how they are expressed, are correlated with the dosage schedule and are based upon theoretical considerations, experimental trials and clinical experience.

Anthrax Vaccine Adsorbed

A sterile slightly opaque liquid derived from a microaerophilic culture of an avirulent, nonencapsulated strain of *Bacillus anthracis*. A sterile filtrate of the culture is obtained and the filtrate then is adsorbed on sterile aluminum hydroxide. The potency is determined by a guinea pig protection test compared to a US Reference Anthrax Vaccine. Benzethonium chloride (0.0025%) is added as a preservative.

Uses—Recommended for active immunization of individuals who come in contact with imported animal hides, furs, bonemeal, wool, hair (especially goat hair) and bristles; for all personnel in factories handling these materials and for individuals contemplating investigational studies involving *Bacillus anthracis*.

Dose—*Subcutaneous*, 3 injections of **0.5 mL** 2 weeks apart, followed by **3 more 0.5 mL** doses 6, 12 and 18 months after the initial injection.

Booster—0.5 mL at 1 year intervals.

Dosage Form—5 mL (available from CDC).

BCG Vaccine

A lyophilized living culture of Danish substrain 1077 of the bacillus Calmette-Guérin strain of *Mycobacterium tuberculosis* var *bovis*. The vaccine when reconstituted as directed contains not less than 8 million and not more than 26 million colony-forming units per mL so that inoculation of tuberculin-negative persons with the recommended dose results in an acceptable tuberculin conversion rate. BCG vaccine is free from other living organisms and contains no preservative.

Uses—The Advisory Committee on Immunization Practices recommends that BCG vaccine be seriously considered for persons who have negative tuberculin skin tests and repeated exposure to persistently untreated or ineffectively treated sputum-positive cases of pulmonary tuberculosis. Vaccination also should be considered for well-defined communities or groups if an excessive rate of new infections can be demonstrated and the usual surveillance and treatment programs have failed or have been shown not to be applicable.

Dose—*Usual, Intradermal,* **0.1 mL** of reconstituted vaccine. A **0.05 mL** dose may be given to infants under 28 days of age. *Note:* for BCG Vaccine for percutaneous use, see *Other Bacterial Vaccines.*

Booster—Protection from tuberculosis by BCG vaccination is only relative and is not permanent or entirely predictable. If the tuberculin test again becomes negative and the risk of infection continues, then a booster shot may need to be given.

Dosage Form—1 mL.

Cholera Vaccine

A sterile whitish suspension of equal parts of phenol killed Ogawa and Inaba serotypes of *Vibrio cholerae.* These strains are selected for high antigenetic efficiency. Each mL contains not more than 4,000 million (8 units) of each serotype based on a mouse protection test compared to a US Reference Cholera Vaccine for each respective serotype. Phenol (0.5%) is added as a preservative.

Uses—Indicated in the US to facilitate foreign travel to certain countries in Asia, the Middle East and Africa. It has limited usefulness and protects only about 60% of those immunized for a period of 3 to 6 months. In addition it does not prevent transmission of the disease.

Dose—*Subcutaneous* or *Intramuscular,* 2 injections of **0.5 mL,** 1 week to 1 month or more apart. For dosage schedules for children 10 years of age and younger, see manufacturer's package insert.

Booster—**0.5 mL** reinforcing dose repeated every 6 months if necessary (adult booster).

Dosage Forms—1, 1.5 and 20 mL.

Meningococcal Polysaccharide Vaccine
Groups A and C Combined; Groups A, C, Y and W-135 Combined

A sterile lyophilized extract of the group specified polysaccharide capsular antigens from *Neisseria meningitidis.* The capsular antigens from each bacterial type are purified separately and then pooled either as a combination of Groups A and C or as a combination of Groups A, C, Y and W-135. After reconstitution as directed, each 0.5 mL dose contains 50 μg of each polysaccharide antigen. Potency is based on a gel-permeation chromatography determination and on immunization of not less than 25 healthy adult human subjects, in whom the antibody titers of the sera from no less than 90% of the subjects show a fourfold or greater rise after immunization. After reconstitution the vaccine contains thimerosal (1:10,000).

Uses—The A/C combination is indicated primarily for active immunization of children 2 years of age and older and the adult population at risk in epidemic or highly endemic areas. Immunization of infants under 2 years of age is not recommended as efficacy of Group C component has not been established in this age group. The A/C/Y/W-135 combination is indicated primarily for active immunization of adults 18 years of age and older at risk in epidemic or highly endemic areas. Immunization of individuals less than 18 years of age is not recommended as efficacy of Groups Y and W-135 components has not been established in this group. For more detailed information on use, see manufacturer's package inserts.

Dose—*Subcutaneous,* 1 injection of **0.5 mL** of reconstituted vaccine.

Booster—Length of immunity not known.

Dosage Forms—10 mL; 50 mL *for jet injector use only.*

Pertussis Vaccine

A sterile whitish suspension of a formalin killed strain of Phase I *Bordetella pertussis.* Each 0.5 mL dose contains 4 protective units of pertussis vaccine based on a mouse protection test compared to a US Reference Pertussis Vaccine. Thimerosal (1:10,000) is added as a preservative.

Uses—Available in the multiple antigen form of Diphtheria and Tetanus Toxoids and Pertussis Vaccine Adsorbed (DTP) which is recommended for active immunization of infants and children through 6 years of age against diphtheria, tetanus and pertussis simultaneously. Injections should be completed no later than the age of 6 years. Note: *Pertussis Vaccine is not recommended for immunizing persons 7 years of age and older because the severity of adverse reactions to pertussis vaccine increases with age, whereas the severity of pertussis infection decreases.*

Dose—*Intramuscular,* 3 injections of **0.5 mL** given 4 to 8 weeks apart followed by a fourth reinforcing dose of **0.5 mL** 1 year later. Primary immunization cannot be considered complete without the fourth reinforcing dose being given since this dose is an integral part of the basic immunizing course.

Booster—**0.5 mL** between 4 and 6 years of age (preferably at time of entrance to school).

Dosage Forms—(For DTP) 0.5 and 7.5 mL.

Pertussis Vaccine Adsorbed

A sterile, whitish suspension of formalin-killed *Bordetella pertussis* which has been adsorbed by the addition of aluminum phosphate. Each 0.5 mL dose contains 4 protective units of pertussis vaccine based on a mouse protection test compared to a US Reference Pertussis Vaccine. Thimerosal (1:10,000) is added as a preservative.

Uses—Indicated for active immunization of children against pertussis especially when the commonly used multiple antigen form Diphtheria and Tetanus Toxoids and Pertussis Vaccine Adsorbed (DTP) causes untoward reaction or is contraindicated. *Note: Pertussis Vaccine Adsorbed is not recommended for immunizing persons 7 years of age and older because the severity of adverse reactions to pertussis vaccine increases with age, whereas the severity of pertussis infection decreases.*

Dose—*Intramuscular,* 3 injections of **0.5 mL** given 4 to 8 weeks apart followed by a fourth reinforcing dose of **0.5 mL** 1 year later. Primary immunization cannot be considered complete without the fourth reinforcing dose being given since this dose is an integral part of the basic immunizing course.

Booster—**0.5 mL** between 4 and 6 years of age (preferably at time of entrance to school).

Dosage Form—5 mL.

Plague Vaccine

A sterile, whitish suspension of formaldehyde-killed *Yersinia pestis.* Each mL contains 2×10^9 organisms based on a mouse protection test compared to a US Reference Plague Vaccine. Phenol (0.5%) is added as a preservative.

Uses—Indicated for active immunization of persons at particularly high risk to plague including persons engaged in laboratory and field work involving *Y pestis* organisms and those involved in natural disasters or in situations when regular sanitary practices are interrupted. Routine vaccination is not necessary for travelers in countries where cases have been reported particularly if travel is limited to urban areas. For more detailed information, see manufacturer's package insert.

Dose—*Intramuscular,* for adults and children over 10 years of age, 2 injections **1.0 mL** followed by **0.2 mL** 1 to 3 months later. A third injection of **0.2 mL** 3 to 6 months after the second injection is strongly recommended. For children less than 10 years old, see manufacturer's package insert.

Booster—1 injection (**0.1 to 0.2 mL**) every 6 months for individuals remaining in a known plague area. The smaller dose should be approached as the total number of such injections increases.

Dosage Form—20 mL.

Pneumococcal Vaccine Polyvalent

A sterile liquid consisting of a mixture of purified capsular polysaccharide antigens from 23 types of *Streptococcus pneumoniae.* For specific capsular antigens, see manufacturer's package insert. The capsular antigens from each bacterial type are purified separately and then pooled so that each dose of vaccine contains 25 μg of each polysaccharide antigen. The preservative used is phenol (0.25%) or thimerosal (1:10,000).

Uses—Indicated for persons over 2 years of age for selective immunization against infections caused by the 23 most prevalent types of pneumococci responsible for approximately 90% of serious pneumococcal disease in the US and the rest of the world. Examples of persons for whom the vaccine is intended include: (1) persons with chronic illnesses in which there is an increased risk of experiencing more severe pneumococcal diseases, such as alcoholism or coexisting diseases including diabetes mellitus, and functional impairment of cardiorespiratory, hepatic and renal systems; (2) persons who have anatomical asplenia or who have splenic dysfunction due to sickle cell disease or other causes; (3) persons 50 years of age or older; and (4) persons about to undergo immunosuppressive therapy.

Dose—*Subcutaneous* or *Intramuscular*, 1 injection of **0.5 mL.**
Booster—Not recommended.
Dosage Forms—0.5 and 2.5 mL.

Typhoid Vaccine

A sterile milky suspension of phenol and heat killed *Salmonella typhi* (Ty-2 strain). The vaccine contains not more than 10^9 organisms per mL based on a potency of 8 units per mL determined by the mouse protection test compared to a US Reference Typhoid Fever Vaccine. Phenol (0.5%) is added as a preservative.

Uses—Indicated for active immunization against typhoid fever in selective situations including intimate exposure to a known typhoid carrier and foreign travel to areas where typhoid fever is endemic. The vaccine is estimated to be 70% or more effective in preventing typhoid fever depending in part on the degree of exposure.

Dose—*Subcutaneous*, adults and children over 10 years old, **2** injections of **0.5 mL** at least 4 weeks apart. For children less than 10 years old, **2** injections of **0.25 mL** at least 4 weeks apart.

Booster—Under conditions of continued or repeated exposure, a single booster injection of **0.5 mL** or **0.25 mL** (according to age) every three years.

Dosage Forms—5, 10, and 20 mL.

Other Bacterial Vaccines

There are other bacterial vaccines which have not been mentioned in the foregoing. These are either non-licensed or not readily available and include:

BCG Vaccine for Percutaneous Use

A live lyophilized preparation of *Mycobacterium tuberculosis* var *bovis* which has an immunizing dose of 0.02 to 0.03 mL by a multipuncture technique.

Mixed Respiratory Vaccine*

A killed vaccine containing *Staphylococcus aureus*, *Streptococcus viridans* (non hemolytic), *Streptococcus pneumoniae*, *Branhamella catarrhalis*, *Klebsiella pneumoniae* and *Haemophilus influenzae*.

Staphylococcus Aureus Vaccine*

A preparation of lysed cultures of *Staphylococcus aureus* Types I and III.

Tularemia Vaccine

This is an Investigational New Drug (IND) from CDC. It is available for nonemergency, high laboratory risk immunization.

___

* *Based on a review by the Panel on Bacterial Vaccines and Bacterial Antigens with no US Standard of Potency and other information, the Food and Drug Administration has directd that further investigation be considered before these two products (Mixed Respiratory Vaccine and Staphylococcus Aureus Vaccine) are determined fully effective for the labeled indication(s).*

Viral Vaccines

Preparation—Viruses are intracellular obligate parasites that cannot be grown on inanimate media used for cultivating bacteria and must be propagated on one of several types of *animate media* including: (1) *embryonic egg* (viruses of influenza, measles, mumps and yellow fever), (2) *human diploid cell culture* (viruses of rubella and rabies), (3) *monkey cell culture* (viruses of polio in both inactivated and live polio vaccines), (4) the *skin of living calves* (smallpox virus) and (5) for hepatitis B vaccine, the *plasma* of *human volunteers* is used as a source of the surface antigen.

Following growth, various techniques including disintegration, column filtration, differential centrifugation and so forth, are used to separate the virus from its host cell. The purification steps reduce the incidence of possible hypersensitivity due to the animate media, especially embryonic egg.

Influenza and rabies vaccines may remain as the *whole virion* or be further processed chemically and be split into subunit particles (subvirion vaccines). Hepatitis B, also a subunit vaccine since it contains only the surface antigen, contains an adjuvant (alum) for prolonged stimulation of antibodies.

Most viral vaccines are living and have the advantage of being able to continue to multiply in the body of the immunized individual; thus exerting a prolonged and increasingly strong stimulation to the host to produce antibodies. Some viral vaccines (hepatitis B, influenza and polio for injection) are inactivated with formaldehyde; whereas the vaccine for rabies is inactivated with beta-propiolactone (BPL).

Product Form—Many viral vaccines occur as a lyophilized (freeze-dried) final product that must be reconstituted before injection with the diluent provided. Inactivated vaccines like hepatitis B, influenza, and poliovirus occur as suspensions for injection; whereas living polio vaccine is in a liquid drop form for oral use.

As with bacterial vaccines, the final viral vaccine product may contain a single antigen (monovalent), eg, measles vaccine or it may contain multiple antigens (polyvalent, trivalent, etc) to elicit immunity against the same disease state, eg, trivalent influenza vaccine and trivalent polio vaccines. In addition there is the mixed vaccine (measles, mumps and rubella) which is a single product with three antigens for three different disease states.

Strength—The strength of a viral vaccine is expressed most commonly in terms of (1) tissue culture infectious dose ($TCID_{50}$), which is the quantity of virus estimated to infect 50% of inoculated cultures. Rubella vaccine, for example contains 1,000 $TCID_{50}$ or 1,000 times the amount of virus present in one tissue culture infectious dose.

Other forms of expressing strength include (2) μg of antigen present (hepatitis B and influenza vaccines), (3) number of organisms per mL (small pox vaccine), (4) International units (rabies vaccine, based on mouse potency tests) and (5) LD_{50} (lethal dose). For yellow fever vaccine, one LD_{50} is the quantity of virus estimated to produce fatal specific encephalitis in 50% of the mice employed in the test.

Hepatitis B Vaccine

A sterile white suspension of formalin-inactivated surface antigen (HBsAg or Australia antigen) of hepatitis B virus. The antigen is harvested and purified from the plasma of human carriers of hepatitis B virus. Each 1.0 mL dose contains 20 μg of hepatitis B antigen (alum precipitated). Thimerosal (1:20,000) is added as a preservative.

Uses—Recommended for immunization against infection caused by all known subtypes of hepatitis B virus especially for persons who are or will be at increased risk of infection with hepatitis B. These higher risk groups include immigrants from areas of high hepatitis B virus endemicity, homosexually active males, users of illicit drugs and clients in institutions for the mentally retarded. For more detailed information see manufacturer's package insert.

Dose—*Intramuscular*, 3 injections of **1.0 mL** with the second and third injections given 1 month and 6 months after the first dose. The volume for younger children (birth to 10 years of age) is **0.5 mL** and that for dialysis patients and immunocompromised patients **2.0 mL** (2-1.0 mL doses given at different sites). *Note: hepatitis B vaccine may be administered subcutaneously to persons at risk of hemorrhage following intramuscular injections.*

Booster—The duration of the protective effect of the vaccine is not known at present. Available data suggest that immunity will last approximately 5 years in patients who have received all 3 doses. Thus a single booster may be necessary every five years.

Dosage Form—3 mL.

Influenza Virus Vaccine

A sterile, slightly opalescent suspension of the formaldehyde inactivated influenza virus types A and B which are harvested from allantoic fluids of chicken embryos infected with the specific influenza virus. The virus may be used whole (whole virion vaccine) or may be in the form of a split virus (subvirion vaccine) prepared by chemically disrupting the virus into subunit particles. There are several methods employed for concentrating and purifying the virus including: column chromatography, ultracentrifugation, zonal centrifugation, and continuous flow centrifugation. For more detailed information see individual manufacturer's package inserts.

The vaccine is standardized each year according to USPHS requirements; eg, the vaccine for the 1983–84 influenza season was *Influenza Virus Vaccine Trivalent Types A and B* and contained 45 μg hemagglutinin (HA) per 0.5 mL dose, in the recommended ratio of 15 μg HA each, representative of the following three prototype strains: A/Brazil/11/78 (H1N1), A/Philippines/2/82 (H3N2) and B/Singapore/222/79. *Note: because of antigenic variation (drift), the antigenic characteristics of influenza vaccine may vary from year to year.* Thimerosal (1:10,000) is added as a preservative (no antibiotics are used in the manufacture of the vaccine).

Uses—Indicated only for immunization against those strains of viruses from which the vaccine is prepared or against closely related strains. Annual routine immunization is recommended only for persons, children and adults, who are at increased risk of adverse consequences from influenza infection. These include: (1) all older persons, particularly those over 65; (2) all adults and children with preexisting medical conditions including: (a) acquired or congenital heart disease with actually or potentially altered circulatory dynamics, (b) any chronic disorder or condition which compromises pulmonary function such as heavy smoking, tuberculosis, severe asthma etc, (c) chronic renal disease with azotemia or nephrotic syndrome, (d) diabetes mellitus or other metabolic diseases, (e) chronic, severe anemia such as sickle cell disease, (f) conditions which compromise the immune mechanism, including certain malignancies and immunosuppressive therapy. For further information, see manufacturer's package insert.

Dose—*Intramuscular or subcutaneous* (although intramuscular preferred), 1 injection of **0.5 mL**. See manufacturer's package insert for dosage for persons under 13 years of age. *Note: because the split vaccine has been shown to be less reactogenic than whole-virus vaccines, particularly in the younger age groups, it is recommended that only the subvirion vaccine be given to those persons under 13 years of age.*

Booster—A single yearly dose for high risk individuals.

Dosage Forms—0.5 and 5 mL; 25 mL *for jet injector use only.*

Measles Virus Vaccine Live

Measles Virus Vaccine Live, Attenuated

A bacterially sterile lyophilized preparation of a more attenuated line of live measles virus derived from Enders' attenuated Edmonston strain prepared in cell cultures of chick embryo. When reconstituted as directed each dose of vaccine meets the requirements of not less than 1,000 TCID$_{50}$ (tissue culture infectious doses) of measles virus vaccine when tested in parallel with a US Reference Measles Virus,

Live, Attenuated. The reconstituted vaccine is yellow and clear and each dose contains approximately 25 μg of neomycin.

Uses—Recommended for active immunization against measles (rubeola) in children 15 months of age or older, especially when the commonly used mixed vaccine form of Measles, Mumps and Rubella Virus Vaccine, Live (MMR) causes untoward reaction or is contraindicated. Since most adults are immune to measles they need not be immunized. However, vaccination may be advisable for high school and college persons in epidemic situations and for adults in isolated communities where measles is not endemic. The vaccine may provide some protection if given within 72 hours after exposure to natural measles. However, better protection may be provided if the vaccine is given a few days before exposure.

Dose—*Subcutaneous*, 1 injection of reconstituted vaccine.

Booster—Not needed.

Dosage Form—Single dose vial.

Mumps Virus Vaccine Live

A bacterially sterile lyophilized preparation of the Jeryl Lynn (B level) strain of live mumps virus grown in cell cultures of chick embryos. When reconstituted as directed each dose of vaccine meets the requirements of not less than 5,000 TCID$_{50}$ (tissue culture infectious doses) of mumps virus vaccine when tested in parallel with the US Reference Mumps Virus, Live. The reconstituted vaccine is yellow and each dose contains approximately 25 μg of neomycin.

Uses—Recommended for active immunization against mumps in children 12 months of age or older and adults especially when the commonly used mixed vaccine form of Measles, Mumps, and Rubella Virus Vaccine, Live (MMR) causes untoward reaction or is contraindicated or when it is advantageous to begin immunization against mumps before 18 months of age (the recommended starting age for MMR). The vaccine will not offer protection after exposure to natural mumps.

Dose—*Subcutaneous*, 1 injection of reconstituted vaccine.

Booster—Not needed.

Dosage Form—Single dose vial.

Poliovirus Vaccine Inactivated

Inactivated Polio Vaccine (IPV), Poliomyelitis Vaccine, Salk Polio Vaccine

A sterile suspension of three types of poliovirus, type 1 (Mahoney), Type 2 (MEF 1) and Type 3 (Saukett). The virus strains are grown separately in primary cell cultures of monkey kidney tissue, and filtered or clarified. From a virus titer of not less than $10^{6.5}$ TCID$_{50}$ (tissue culture infectious doses) measured in comparison with the US Reference Poliovirus of the corresponding type, the strains are then inactivated with formaldehyde so as to reduce the virus titer by a factor of 10^{-8}, and after inactivation, are combined in suitable proportions. The final preparation contains in each 1.0 mL dose, 2-phenoxyethanol (0.375%) as a preservative and not more than 200 μg of streptomycin and 7 μg of neomycin. It is perfectly clear and cherry-red in color due to the presence of a small amount of phenol red indicator.

Uses—Poliovirus Vaccine Inactivated (IPV) has been largely replaced by Poliovirus Vaccine Live Oral (OPV) in the US. IPV is used for adult immunization because there is less risk of vaccine-associated paralysis than with OPV for adults. IPV is likewise safer to administer to immune-deficient persons. Current recommendations of the Immunization Practices Advisory Committee (ACIP), however, indicate that routine primary polio vaccination of adults (passed the 18th birthday) residing in the US is not necessary. For more details refer to manufacturer's package insert.

Dose—*Subcutaneous*, 3 injections of **1.0 mL** at intervals of 4 to 8 weeks, followed by a reinforcing dose of **1.0 mL** 6 to 12 months after the third dose. The third reinforcing dose is considered an integral part of the primary stimulus.

Booster—Children receiving the initial four doses in early childhood should be given a booster dose of **1.0 mL** before entering school. Further booster doses of **1.0 mL** should be given every 5 years until age 18.

Dosage Forms—1 mL and 10 mL.

Poliovirus Vaccine Live Oral

Trivalent Oral Polio Vaccine (TOPV), Sabin Vaccine

A mixture of three types of live, attenuated polioviruses which have been propagated separately in cercopithecus monkey kidney cell culture. The potency is expressed in terms of the amount of virus contained in the recommended dose as $TCID_{50}$ (tissue culture infectious doses). Each dose contains infectivity titers of $10^{5.4}$ to $10^{6.4}$ for Type 1, $10^{4.5}$ to $10^{5.5}$ for Type 2, and $10^{5.2}$ to $10^{6.2}$ for Type 3. The vaccine is free from any known microbial agent other than the attenuated polioviruses listed. Each 0.5 mL dose, dosage form, contains less than 25 μg of each of the antibiotics, streptomycin and neomycin. Each 2 drop dose (0.1 mL) contains less than 5 μg of each of the antibiotics, streptomycin and neomycin. The usual color of the vaccine is pink and clear because of the phenol red pH indicator. However, some containers of vaccine shipped in ice may exhibit a yellow color due to very low temperature or the possible absorption of carbon dioxide.

Uses—Indicated for active immunization against infections of poliomyelitis caused by Poliovirus Types 1, 2 and 3 in infants starting at 6 to 12 weeks of age and all unimmunized children and adolescents through age 18. Poliovirus Vaccine Live Oral (OPV) is considered by the Advisory Committee on Immunization Practices to be the vaccine of choice for primary immunization of children. Because of the potential risk of developing vaccine-associated paralysis with OPV in adults, adults over 18 should be administered Poliovirus Vaccine Inactivated; however, it is recommended that routine primary polio vaccination of adults (passed the 18th birthday) residing in the US is not necessary. For further information see manufacturer's package insert.

Dose—*Oral*, 2 doses 6 to 8 weeks apart, followed by a **third** dose 8 to 12 months later.

Booster—Oral dose upon entering elementary school.

Dosage Forms—2 drop dose: 10 dose vial with dropper; 0.5 mL dose: 10 and 50 dose (each dose in a disposable pipette).

Rabies Vaccine

A sterile lyophilized preparation of the whole or subvirion rabies virus. The *whole virion vaccine* is prepared from Wistar rabies virus strain PM-1503-3M which has been grown on human diploid cell cultures and inactivated with beta-propiolactone (BPL). When reconstituted as directed each 1.0 mL dose contains less than 150 μg of neomycin. The *subvirion vaccine* is prepared from the Pasteur-derived Pitman-Moore virus grown on human diploid cell cultures and split with tri-n-butylphosphate and Polysorbate 80 with further inactivation by treatment with BPL. The vaccine is preserved with thimerosal (1:10,000) and after reconstitution each 1.0 mL dose contains not more than 50 μg neomycin, 2.5 μg amphotericin and 50 μg gentamicin.

Both vaccines after reconstitution are pink in color and each 1.0 mL dose contains at least 2.5 International Units (IU) of rabies antigen. An International Unit is established by tests in parallel with the Standard Rabies Vaccine in the NIH mouse potency test as required by the Bureau of Biologics, Food and Drug Administration.

Uses—Indicated for active immunization in pre-exposure situations for veterinarians, animal handlers, researchers and other similar personnel working in laboratories, hospitals etc. who are concerned with the treatment of rabid animals or with the handling of rabies virus or potentially contaminated material. The vaccine also is recommended for post-exposure treatment of animal bites with a potential risk of rabies. For more detailed information on both pre-exposure immunization and the rationale of post-exposure treatment, see manufacturer's package insert. The Human Diploid Cell Rabies Vaccine has completely replaced Rabies Duck Embryo Vaccine whose sales were discontinued in the US 11-30-81.

Dose—*Intramuscular*, Pre-exposure: 3 injections of **1.0 mL** of reconstituted vaccine on each of days 0, 7 and 21 or 28; *Post-exposure:* 5 injections of **1.0 mL** of reconstituted vaccine on each of days 0, 3, 7, 14 and 28 in conjunction with Rabies Immune Globulin (RIG) on day 0. This dosage schedule is recommended by the CDC. For World Health Organization recommendations and further information, see manufacturer's package insert.

Booster—Given selectively every two years to persons with continuing risk of exposure, or titers are checked every two years, and if the titer is inadequate a booster is given. Persons working with the live virus in research laboratories or vaccine production facilities should have rabies antibody titers checked every six months and boosters given as needed. For further information see manufacturer's package insert.

Dosage Form—Single dose vial.

Rubella Virus Vaccine Live

A bacterially sterile lyophilized preparation of the Wistar Institute RA 27/3 strain of live attenuated rubella virus propagated in human diploid cell culture. When reconstituted each 0.5 mL dose meets the requirements of not less than 1,000 $TCID_{50}$ (tissue culture infectious doses) of rubella virus vaccine when tested in parallel with the US Reference Rubella Virus, Live. The reconstituted vaccine is yellow and each 0.5 mL dose contains approximately 25 μg of neomycin.

Uses—Indicated for active immunization against rubella (German measles) in children from 12 months of age to puberty especially when the commonly used mixed vaccine form of Measles, Mumps and Rubella Virus Vaccine, Live (MMR) causes untoward reaction or is contraindicated or when it is advantageous to begin immunization against rubella before 18 months of age (the recommended starting age for MMR). Increased emphasis should be placed on immunizing susceptible non-pregnant adolescent and adult females of childbearing age to protect against subsequently acquiring rubella infection during pregnancy, which in turn prevents infection of the fetus and consequent congenital rubella injury. For more detailed information on usage see manufacturer's package insert.

Dose—*Subcutaneous*, **1–0.5 mL** injection of reconstituted vaccine.

Booster—Not needed.

Dosage Form—0.5 mL.

Smallpox Vaccine

A bacterially sterile lyophilized preparation of the live vaccinia virus grown on calf lymph. Each mL of the reconstituted product meets the requirements of not more than 200 organisms (pox forming units) per mL calculated from the number of lesions produced on membranes from living embryonated chicken eggs run in parallel with the US Reference Smallpox Vaccine. During processing, not more than 100 units of polymyxin B, 200 μg of dihydrostreptomycin, 200 μg of chlortetracycline and 100 μg of neomycin per mL are added, and trace amounts of these antibiotics may be present in the reconstituted product. The reconstituted product is slightly greenish due to the presence of brilliant green indicator (0.005%).

Uses—Recommended for protection of civilian laboratory personnel exposed to orthopox viruses (particularly variola (smallpox) and vaccinia viruses) and for civilian persons involved in producing or testing smallpox vaccine. Production of smallpox vaccine for general use was discontinued in 1982 and in May, 1983 distribution of the vaccine to civilians was discontinued. *The only source of the vaccine to civilians is CDC. The vaccine will be provided only to laboratories meeting the sole remaining indications.* These developments have occurred because of world-wide efforts to eradicate smallpox by judicious use of smallpox vaccine. The last case reported was in Somalia in 1977. At the World Health Assembly in May 1980, the World Health Organization (WHO) declared the world free of smallpox. *There, however, have been a few reported cases of contact spread of vaccinia from recently vaccinated persons.*

Dose—*Percutaneous*, **2 to 3 needle punctures** or pressures of reconstituted vaccine. Each needle puncture contains a drop of vaccine. For revaccination **15 needle punctures** are necessary. For interpretation of responses and more detailed information see manufacturer's package insert.

Booster—Approximately every 3 years for special risk categories.

Dosage Form—Enough for 25 vaccinations (approximately 0.15 mL) and enough for 100 vaccinations (approximately 0.25 mL).

Yellow Fever Vaccine

A bacterially sterile, light orange lyophilized preparation of the live 17D strain of yellow fever virus prepared in chicken embryos. When reconstituted as directed each 0.5 mL dose contains not less than 7,500 mouse LD_{50} (lethal doses) units. There is no preservative added.

Uses—For active immunization of travelers planning a trip to countries primarily in Africa and South America which require a certificate of vaccination against yellow fever. Certificates are required of children 6 months of age or older and are valid for a period of 10 years commencing 10 days after initial vaccination or revaccination. Yellow Fever Vaccine is supplied in the US to designated authorized Yellow Fever Vaccination Centers only. Location of the nearest Centers may be obtained from the CDC.

Dose—*Subcutaneous*, 1 injection of **0.5 mL** of reconstituted vaccine.

Booster—Every 10 years.

Dosage Forms—1, 5 and 20 dose; 100 dose for *jet injector use only*. The 20 dose vial may be administered with needle and syringe or jet injector use.

Mixed Vaccines

There are three commonly used mixed viral vaccines that contain multiple antigens for different viral infections. These combinations provide a broad immunization coverage with a reduced number of injections.

Measles, Mumps, and Rubella Virus Vaccine Live

MMR Vaccine

A bacterially sterile lyophilized preparation of a combination of Measles Virus Vaccine Live, Attenuated; Mumps Virus Vaccine Live and Rubella Virus Vaccine Live. The three viruses are mixed before being lyophilized. When reconstituted as directed each 0.5 mL dose contains not less than 1,000 $TCID_{50}$ (tissue culture infectious doses) of Measles Virus Vaccine Live, Attenuated; 5,000 $TCID_{50}$ of Mumps Virus Vaccine, Live; and 1,000 $TCID_{50}$ of Rubella Virus Vaccine, Live, expressed in terms of the assigned titer of the US Reference Measles, Mumps and Rubella Viruses. The reconstituted vaccine is yellow and each 0.5 mL dose contains approximately 25 μg of neomycin.

Uses—Indicated for simultaneous active immunization against measles (rubeola), mumps and rubella (German measles) in children 15 months of age or older, and in adults. For other recommendations see manufacturer's package insert.

Dose—*Subcutaneous*, 1 injection of **0.5 mL** of reconstituted vaccine.

Booster—Not needed.

Dosage Form—Single dose.

Measles and Rubella Virus Vaccine Live

MR Vaccine

A bacterially sterile lyophilized preparation of a combination of Measles Virus Vaccine Live, Attenuated, and Rubella Virus Vaccine Live. The two viruses are mixed before being lyophilized. When reconstituted as directed each 0.5 mL dose contains not less than 1,000 $TCID_{50}$ of Measles Virus Vaccine Live, Attenuated and 1,000 $TCID_{50}$

of Rubella Virus Vaccine Live expressed in terms of the assigned titer of the US Reference Measles and Rubella Viruses. The reconstituted vaccine is yellow and each 0.5 mL dose contains approximately 25 μg of neomycin.

Uses—Indicated for simultaneous active immunization against measles (rubeola) and rubella (German measles) in children 15 months of age or older and adults. For other recommendations see manufacturer's package insert.

Dose—*Subcutaneous*, 1 injection of **0.5 mL** of reconstituted vaccine.

Booster—Not needed.

Dosage Form—Single dose.

Rubella and Mumps Virus Vaccine Live

RM Vaccine

A bacterially sterile lyophilized preparation of a combination of Measles Virus Vaccine Live and Rubella Virus Vaccine Live. The two viruses are mixed before being lyophilized. When reconstituted as directed each 0.5 mL dose contains not less than 1,000 $TCID_{50}$ of Rubella Virus Vaccine Live and 5,000 $TCID_{50}$ of Mumps Virus Vaccine Live, expressed in terms of the assigned titer of the US Reference Rubella and Mumps Viruses. The reconstituted vaccine is yellow and each 0.5 mL dose contains approximately 25 μg of neomycin.

Uses—Indicated for simultaneous active immunization against rubella (German measles) and mumps in children 12 months of age or older and adults. For other recommendations see manufacturer's package insert.

Dose—*Subcutaneous*, 1 injection of **0.5 mL** of reconstituted vaccine.

Booster—Not needed.

Dosage Form—Single dose.

Other Viral Vaccines

There are other viral vaccines which have not been listed in the foregoing. These are all Investigational New Drugs (IND) available from CDC. The vaccines include:

Eastern Equine Encephalitis (EEE) Vaccine
Japanese Equine Encephalitis Vaccine
Venezuelan Equine Encephalitis (VEE) Vaccine
Western Equine Encephalitis (WEE) Vaccine

These are for nonemergency, high laboratory risk immunization.

Toxoids

Preparation—Bacteria are propagated in a similar manner as for a bacterial vaccine, and after the required growth is attained, the culture is filtered through a sterilizing membrane filter. Then the filtrate containing the toxin (exotoxin) is usually processed as follows: (1) a concentrated salt solution is added to precipitate the toxin from the filtrate, (2) the precipitated toxin is washed and purified by dialysis and (3) the toxin is detoxified with formaldehyde.

The detoxified toxin (toxoid) may be *plain* or may contain an *adjuvant* such as alum, aluminum hydroxide or aluminum phosphate. These adjuvants are insoluble materials which act to keep the antigens (toxoids) in tissue for longer periods and thus cause a prolonged antibody stimulation.

Product Form—As with both bacterial and viral vaccines, the final preparation may contain single, multiple or mixed antigens. If the toxoid is adsorbed, it is in the form of a liquid suspension and if plain, a slightly cloudy solution.

Strength—The strength of a toxoid is expressed in terms of flocculating units (Lf). A flocculating unit is the smallest amount of toxin which flocculates (a modified precipitation) most rapidly one unit of standard antitoxin in a series of mixtures containing fixed amounts of antitoxin and varying amounts of toxin.

Diphtheria Toxoid Adsorbed
(For Pediatric Use)

A sterile white, slightly gray or slightly pink suspension of purified diphtheria toxoid (formaldehyde treated toxin of *Corynebacterium diphtheriae*) adsorbed onto aluminum hydroxide. Each 0.5 mL dose contains 15 Lf Units of diphtheria toxoid (determined prior to adsorption onto aluminum hydroxide). Thimerosal (0.01%) is added as a preservative.

Uses—Recommended for active immunization against diphtheria in infants and children under 6 years of age for whom products containing tetanus toxoid and/or pertussis vaccine would not be advisable.

Dose—*Intramuscular*, **2** injections of **0.5 mL** 6 to 8 weeks apart, and a third reinforcing dose of **0.5 mL** approximately one year later.

Booster—1 injection at 5 to 10 year intervals. For adults and children 6 years and older, products containing diphtheria toxoid with a suitable composition for adults are recommended.

Dosage Form—5 mL.

Tetanus Toxoid

Tetanus Toxoid Fluid; Tetanus Toxoid Plain

A clear or slightly turbid brownish yellow sterile solution of fluid tetanus toxoid (formaldehyde treated toxin of *Clostridium tetani*).

Products of different manufacturers may vary in potency from 4 to 5 Lf Units per 0.5 mL dose. Thimerosal (0.01%) is added as a preservative.

Uses—May be used for active immunization against tetanus. However, Tetanus Toxoid Adsorbed is preferred for all basic immunizing and recall reactions because of more persistent antitoxin titer induction.

Dose—*Intramuscular* or *Subcutaneous*, 3 injections of **0.5 mL** 4 to 8 weeks apart, followed by a fourth reinforcing dose of **0.5 mL** 6 to 12 months later. (Primary immunization cannot be considered complete without the fourth reinforcing dose being given since this dose is an integral part of the basic immunizing course.)

Booster—**0.5 mL** every 10 years. For additional information on wound management see manufacturer's package insert.

Dosage Forms—0.5, 1.5 and 7.5 mL.

Tetanus Toxoid Adsorbed

A sterile white, slightly gray or slightly pink suspension of purified tetanus toxoid (formaldehyde treated toxin of *Clostridium tetani*) alum precipitated or adsorbed onto aluminum hydroxide or aluminum phosphate. Products of different manufacturers may vary in potency from 5 to 10 Lf Units per 0.5 mL dose. Thimerosal (0.01%) is added as a preservative.

Uses—For active immunization against tetanus. Commonly administered in the form of Diphtheria and Tetanus Toxoids and Pertussis Vaccine Adsorbed (DTP) to children under 7 years of age or as Tetanus and Diphtheria Toxoids Adsorbed (Td) For Adult Use for adults and children 7 years of age and older.

Dose—*Intramuscular*, 2 injections of **0.5 mL** 4 to 8 weeks apart, followed by a third reinforcing dose of 0.5 mL approximately 12 months later. Primary immunization cannot be considered complete without the fourth reinforcing dose being given since this dose is an integral part of the basic immunizing course.

Booster—**0.5 mL** every 10 years. For additional information on wound management see manufacturer's package insert.

Dosage Forms—0.5, 1 and 5 mL.

Mixed Toxoids and Mixed Biologics

A mixed toxoid such as Tetanus and Diphtheria Toxoids Adsorbed for Adult Use contains two or more toxoids in a single preparation for active immunization of *different toxicities*.

A mixed biologic has *toxoids and vaccines* in a single dose form for active immunization of different *toxicities and infections*. The only common example of a mixed biologic is Diphtheria and Tetanus Toxoids and Pertussis Vaccine Adsorbed.

These two types of biologics differ from *polyvalent* products which are used for different strains of the same toxicity or infection, eg, Botulism Antitoxin Trivalent (for passive immunization) and Pneumococcal Vaccine Polyvalent.

Mixed toxoids and biologics have the obvious advantage of providing broad immunization coverage with a reduced number of injections.

Diphtheria and Tetanus Toxoids Adsorbed
(For Pediatric Use)

A sterile white, slightly gray or slightly pink suspension of purified diphtheria and tetanus toxoids adsorbed onto aluminum hydroxide or aluminum phosphate. Products of different manufacturers may vary in potency from 10 to 15 Lf Units of diphtheria toxoid and from 5 to 10 Lf Units of tetanus toxoid per 0.5 mL dose. Thimerosal (0.01%) is added as a preservative.

Uses—Recommended for active immunization against diphtheria and tetanus in infants and children through 6 years of age when it is unadvisable or contraindicated to give a triple antigen (DTP) containing the pertussis component.

Dose—*Intramuscular*, 2 injections of **0.5 mL** 4 to 8 weeks apart, followed by a third reinforcing dose of **0.5 mL** approximately 1 year

later. Primary immunization cannot be considered complete without the third reinforcing dose being given since this dose is an integral part of the basic immunizing course.

Booster—If active immunization is initiated during the first year of life, a booster dose of 0.5 mL is given at 4 to 6 years of age. Over age 6, Tetanus and Diphtheria Toxoids Adsorbed (For Adult Use) is recommended every 10 years.

Dosage Forms—0.5 and 5 mL.

Tetanus and Diphtheria Toxoids Adsorbed For Adult Use

A sterile white, slightly gray or cream colored suspension of purified diphtheria and tetanus toxoids alum precipitated or adsorbed onto aluminum hydroxide or aluminum phosphate. Products of different manufacturers may vary from 5 to 10 Lf Units of tetanus toxoid per 0.5 mL. Each 0.5 mL contains not more than 2 Lf Units of diphtheria toxoid. Thimerosal (0.01%) is added as a preservative.

Uses—For active immunization of adults and children 7 years of age and older. The small amount of diphtheria toxoid in the product minimizes sensitivity reactions.

Dose—*Intramuscular*, 2 injections of **0.5 mL** 4 to 8 weeks apart, followed by a third reinforcing dose of **0.5 mL** approximately 1 year later. Primary immunization cannot be considered complete without the third reinforcing dose being given since this dose is an integral part of the basic immunizing course.

Booster—0.5 mL every 10 years. For additional information on wound management see manufacturer's package insert.

Dosage Forms—0.5 and 5 mL; 30 mL *for jet injector use only*.

Diphtheria and Tetanus Toxoids and Pertussis Vaccine Adsorbed
(For Pediatric Use)

A sterile whitish to light yellowish or brownish suspension of purified diphtheria and tetanus toxoids alum precipitated or aluminum phosphate adsorbed and phase 1 pertussis vaccine. Each 0.5 mL dose contains from 6.7 to 12.5 Lf Units of diphtheria toxoid, 5 Lf Units of tetanus toxoid and 4 protective units of pertussis vaccine. Thimerosal (0.01%) is added as a preservative.

Uses—For active immunization of infants and children through 6 years of age against diphtheria, tetanus and pertussis simultaneously. Injections should be started at 2 to 3 months of age and be completed no later than the age of 6 years.

Dose—*Intramuscular*, 3 injections of **0.5 mL** 4 to 8 weeks apart, followed by a fourth reinforcing dose of **0.5 mL** 1 year later. (Primary immunization cannot be considered complete without the fourth reinforcing dose being given since this dose is an integral part of the basic immunizing course.)

Booster—For children between 4 and 6 years of age (preferably at time of entrance to school), **0.5 mL**. For persons 7 years of age and older, Tetanus and Diphtheria Toxoids Adsorbed for Adult Use is recommended every 10 years. DTP is not used after 6 years of age because of the increased possibility of severe reactions, most often attributed to the pediatric levels of diphtheria toxoid, and moreover, because the incidence, severity and fatality of pertussis decrease with age.

Dosage Forms—0.5 and 7.5 mL.

Other Toxoids

There are certain toxoids that have not been described in the foregoing. These include plain or fluid forms such as Diphtheria Toxoid, Diphtheria and Tetanus Toxoids and Diphtheria and Tetanus Toxoids and Pertussis Vaccines which all have been replaced by the respective adsorbed forms.

Another toxoid not mentioned is:

Botulinum Toxoid pentavalent (ABCDE)

This is an Investigational New Drug (IND) available from CDC for nonemergency, high laboratory risk immunization.

Biologics for Passive Immunization

Human Immune Sera

(Homologous Sera)

Human immune sera or homologous sera include immune globulin and hyperimmune sera (including $Rh_0(D)$ immune globulin) for specific diseases (Table I).

An homologous serum has less potential for hypersensitivity reactions and a longer half-life than does the more foreign heterologous serum of animal origin. The half-life of an homologous serum such as tetanus immune globulin (TIG) is approximately 26 to 30 days and that for tetanus antitoxin an heterologous serum is approximately 7 days. Thus not only does TIG have less potential for hypersensitivity reactions but it can be administered in a smaller dose, since it is capable of remaining in the body longer.

The source of homologous sera is the pooled plasma (free of hepatitis B antigen) of adult donors either from the general population (for immune globulin) or from hyperimmunized donors (for immune globulins for specific diseases). The plasma is then precipitated fractionally, usually with ethanol, under rigorous controls of pH and ionic strength. Different manufacturers may modify the precipitation procedure to increase the yield.

The precipitated immunoglobulins are further purified and the finished biologic is a solution usually containing not less than 15% and not more than 18% protein. Hepatitis B, $Rh_0(D)$ and varicella-zoster immune globulins contain not less than 10% protein.

Immune sera are intended for *intramuscular* use only and should not be given *intravenously*. However, one product, immune globulin intravenous 5%, is intended for intravenous use. It contains less protein and is prepared in a manner that makes it suitable for intravenous administration.

Immune Globulin

Immune Serum Globulin Human, Gamma Globulin

A sterile, transparent or slightly opalescent and colorless, non-pyrogenic solution of globulins that contain many antibodies normally present in adult human blood. The product is prepared by pooling approximately equal amounts of material (source blood, serum or placentas) from not less than 1000 donors. It contains 15% to 18% protein and meets the potency requirements of certain antibodies as determined by the FDA. Thimerosal (1:10,000) is added as a preservative. *Note: the product is prepared from human plasma that was not reactive when tested for hepatitis B surface antigen.*

Uses—Recommended for the passive prevention or modification of measles (rubeola) and viral hepatitis A and for the routine maintenance of certain immunodeficient persons. It also may be used when hepatitis B immune globulin is indicated but not available. *There are no other currently recommended uses.*

Dose—*Intramuscular* only. For doses and frequency of administration for various uses and other essential information see manufacturer's package insert.

Dosage Forms—2 and 10 mL.

Hepatitis B Immune Globulin (Human)

A sterile, slightly amber, non-pyrogenic solution consisting of the globulins derived from blood plasma of human donors who have high titers of antibodies against hepatitis B surface antigen. Each vial contains anti-HBs antibody equivalent to or exceeding the potency of anti-HBs in a US Reference Hepatitis B Immune Globulin (Bureau of Biologics, FDA). Thimerosal (1:10,000) is added as a preservative. *Note: the product is prepared from human plasma that was not reactive when tested for hepatitis B surface antigen.*

Uses—Indicated for post-exposure passive immunization following either parenteral exposure, direct mucous membrane contact or oral ingestion involving HBsAg-positive materials such as blood, plasma or serum. The product is also recommended for passive immuniza-

tion of infants born to HBsAg-positive mothers. For more complete information on uses see manufacturer's package insert.

Dose—*Intramuscular*, Adult, **0.06 mL/kg** of body weight, preferably administered within 7 days of exposure and repeated 28–30 days after initial dose. For dosage for newborns see manufacturer's package insert.

Dosage Forms—1, 4 and 5 mL.

Pertussis Immune Globulin (Human)

A sterile, transparent or slightly opalescent, nearly colorless non-pyrogenic solution of globulins derived from the blood plasma of adult human donors who have been immunized with pertussis vaccine. Each 1.25 mL contains not less than the amount of immune globulin to be equivalent to 25 mL of human hyperimmune serum. Thimerosal (1:10,000) is added as a preservative. *Note: the product is prepared from human plasma that was not reactive when tested for hepatitis B surface antigen.*

Uses—Indicated for the passive prevention or attenuation and treatment of pertussis.

Dose—*Intramuscular*, Prophylactic, **1.25 to 2.5 mL** depending on age of child, 1 or 2 times at 1 to 2 week intervals.

Intramuscular, Therapeutic, **1.25 to 2.5 mL** depending on severity of disease, repeated 1 or 2 times at 1 to 2 day intervals depending on the clinical response.

Dosage Form—1.25 mL.

Rabies Immune Globulin (Human)

A sterile, transparent or slightly opalescent, nearly colorless non-pyrogenic solution of globulins derived from the blood plasma of individuals immunized with rabies vaccine. Each mL contains 150 International Units (IU) based on the US Standard Rabies Immune Globulin and using the CVS Virus Challenge by neutralization test in mice or tissue culture. The US unit of potency is equivalent to the International Unit for rabies antibody. Thimerosal (1:10,000) is added as a preservative. *Note: the product is prepared from human plasma that was found not reactive when tested for hepatitis B surface antigen.*

Uses—Indicated for individuals suspected of exposure to rabies, particularly severe exposure, with the exception of persons who have been previously immunized with rabies vaccine and have confirmed adequate antibody titers. For more complete information see manufacturer's package insert.

Dose—*Intramuscular*, **20 IU/kg** of body weight at the time of administration of the first vaccine dose. If possible up to half the dose should be used to *infiltrate* the wound and the rest administered *intramuscularly*, preferably in the gluteal or deltoid region.

Dosage Forms—2 mL pediatric vial (300 IU), 10 mL adult vial (1,500 IU).

$Rh_0(D)$ Immune Globulin (Human)

A sterile, transparent or slightly opalescent and practically clear, non-pyrogenic solution of globulins derived from human blood plasma containing antibody to the erythrocyte factor $Rh_0(D)$. The $Rh_0(D)$ antibody level in each single dose vial is equal to or greater than that of the Bureau of Biologic Reference $Rh_0(D)$ Immune Globulin (Human). This dose has been shown to effectively inhibit the immunizing potential of up to 15 mL of Rh-positive packed red blood cells. Thimerosal (1:10,000) is added as a preservative. *Note: the product is prepared from human plasma that was not reactive when tested for hepatitis B surface antigen.*

Uses—Indicated for an Rh negative female who delivers an $Rh_0(D)$ positive baby or for an Rh negative female after abortion or ectopic pregnancy unless the products of conception or the father are conclusively shown to be Rh negative. The product also is indicated for amniocentesis and other abdominal trauma resulting in fetal cells entering the maternal circulation. Administration of $Rh_0(D)$ immune globulin within 72 hours reduces the incidence of Rh isoimmunization from 12–13% to 1–2%, thus offering protection to the next infant if born $Rh_0(D)$ positive.

Dose—*Intramuscular*, 1 **vial.**

Dosage Form—Single dose vial. *Note: a "micro" or "mini" dose form is available which contains approximately $^1/_6$ the quantity of $Rh_0(D)$ antibody contained in a standard dose of $Rh_0(D)$ immune globulin. The "micro" or "mini" dose form is for use only after abortion or miscarriage up to 12 weeks gestation.*

Tetanus Immune Globulin (Human)

TIG

A sterile, transparent or slightly opalescent and practically clear, non-pyrogenic solution of globulins derived from the blood plasma of adult human donors who have been immunized with tetanus toxoid. Each mL has not less than 50 antitoxin units based on the US Standard Tetanus Antitoxin and the US Control Tetanus Test Toxin tested in guinea pigs. Thimerosal (1:10,000) is added as a preservative. *Note: the product is prepared from human plasma that was not reactive when tested for hepatitis B surface antigen.*

Uses—Indicated for immediate immunization against tetanus toxin, especially individuals who have little or no active immunity against it. It also is used in the regimen of treatment of active cases of tetanus. For more complete information see manufacturer's package insert.

Dose—*Intramuscular*, Prophylactic, **250 units.** For severe wounds, **500 units.**

Intramuscular, Therapeutic, **3,000 to 6,000 units;** however, the optimum therapeutic dose has not yet been established and no claim can be made for the therapeutic effectiveness of the recommended dose.

Dosage Form—250 unit vial.

Varicella-Zoster Immune Globulin (Human)

A sterile 10.0 to 18.0% solution of globulins (primarily IgG) derived from the blood plasmas of adult human volunteers selected for high titers of varicella-zoster antibodies. Each dose contains 125 units of antibody to varicella-zoster virus. Thimerosal (1:10,000) is added as a preservative. *Note: the product is prepared from human plasma that was not reactive when tested for hepatitis B surface antigen.*

Uses—For passive immunization of susceptible immunodeficient children following exposure to varicella. These children include: (1) those with primary immune deficiency disorders or neoplastic diseases, (2) recipients of immunosuppressive doses of steroids, antimetabolites or other immunosuppressive treatment regimens and

(3) newborns of mothers with recent chickenpox less than five days before birth or 48 hours after birth.

Dose—*Intramuscular*, **1 to 5 vials** depending upon body weight. For more detailed information see manufacturer's package insert. The proposed dosage, if given within 96 hours after exposure, was found to be effective in modifying significantly the expected severity of chickenpox and reducing the observed frequency of death, pneumonia and encephalitis to less than 25% of the expected rate without treatment.

The value of varicella-zoster immune globulin (VZIG) given after 96 hours of exposure is uncertain and there is no evidence that it can modify an established varicella infection. In addition, VZIG is not recommended for non-immunodeficient patients. For more information, see manufacturer's package insert.

Dosage Form—Single dose vial in a volume of 2.5 mL or less. Distributed by CDC through various regional distribution centers.

Other Human Immune Sera

There are other human immune sera which have not been listed in the foregoing. These include:

Immune Globulin Intravenous (IGIV) 5%

This preparation contains less protein than Immune Globulin for Intramuscular use which has 15% to 18%. IGIV also differs in that it has been selectively reduced under controlled conditions using dithiothreitol and alkylated with iodoacetamide to render it suitable for intravenous use. It is indicated for the maintenance treatment of patients who are unable to produce sufficient amounts of IgG antibodies, especially when an immediate rise in antibodies is required. For more detailed information see manufacturer's package insert.

Vaccinia Immune Globulin (VIG)

VIG is used to treat complications of smallpox vaccination. It is available from the CDC and is of limited value since the eradication of smallpox and the limited use of the vaccine.

Western Equine Encephalitis (WEE) Immune Globulin

This is an Investigational New Drug available from CDC.

Animal Immune Sera

(Heterologous Sera)

Animal immune sera or heterologous sera include antitoxins, an antiviral serum and antivenins (Table I).

These preparations are obtained from the plasma of horses that have been immunized against the specific antigen (toxin, virus, or venom). The refining and concentration of the immunoglobulins from the plasma may vary with the manufacturer and the particular biologic. In general, however, the plasma is diluted with water and briefly digested with pepsin which splits the protein molecules into *immunologically active* fragments (immunoglobulins) and *immunologically inactive* fragments (albumins and fibrinogen). These latter two fragments are then separated by fractional precipitation using ammonium sulfate, for example. The precipitated immunoglobulin fraction is then dialyzed to remove the salt.

The finished biologic is usually in the form of a solution or if an antivenin, lyophilized.

As previously indicated, these products have potential for hypersensitivity reactions and the precautions mentioned previously should be followed.

Antitoxins (Equine)

Botulism Antitoxin (Equine)

Botulism Antitoxin Trivalent (Equine)

A sterile, transparent or slightly opalescent, nearly colorless, non-pyrogenic solution containing refined and concentrated antitoxic antibodies, chiefly globulins, obtained from the blood of healthy horses that have been immunized against the toxins produced by type A, type B and type E strains of *Clostridium botulinum*. Each vial contains: type A, 7,500 International Units (IU) equivalent to 2,381 US units; type B, 5,500 IU equivalent to 1,839 US units and type E, 8,500 IU equivalent to 8,500 US units. The potency is determined with the US Standard Botulism Antitoxin of relevant type, tested by neutralizing activity in mice of the corresponding US Control Botulism Test Toxin. The product contains 0.4% phenol as a preservative.

Uses—Indicated for the passive prevention and treatment of botulism known or suspected to be produced by *Clostridium botulinum*, type A, B or E. The antitoxin will only neutralize circulating toxin and will not counteract the effect of toxin already bound to receptor cells in tissue, hence it will not be effective unless administered before extensive binding of toxin has occurred. *Note: serum reactions to horse protein have an incidence of 15–20%.*

Dose—Prophylactic, *Intramuscular*, $\frac{1}{5}$ **to 1 vial** depending upon the amount of food eaten. A second injection of **1 vial** may be given in 12 to 24 hours if any signs of botulism appear.

Therapeutic, *Intravenous* and *Intramuscular*, **1 vial** *Intravenously* diluted 1:10 followed by **1 vial** *Intramuscularly* (to provide reservoir of antitoxin). Further doses may be indicated in 2 to 4 hours if signs and symptoms worsen.

Dosage Forms—Vial containing type A 7,500 IU, type B 5,500 IU and type E 8,500 IU. (Distributed by the CDC).

Diphtheria Antitoxin (Equine)

A sterile, transparent or slightly opalescent, nearly colorless, non-pyrogenic solution containing refined and concentrated antibodies chiefly globulins obtained from the blood of healthy horses that have been immunized against diphtheria toxin or toxoid (produced by *Corynebacterium diphtheriae*). It has a potency of not less than 500 antitoxin units per mL based on the US Standard Diphtheria Antitoxin, and a diphtheria test toxin, tested in guinea pigs. The preparation contains tricresol (0.4%) or *m*-cresol (0.3%) as a preservative.

Uses—Indicated for passive prevention and treatment of diphtheria. Prevention should be given to contacts intimately exposed and not previously immunized with toxoid.

Dose—Prophylactic, *Intramuscular*, **10,000 units** (varies with exposure, etc). For more details see manufacturer's package insert.

Therapeutic, *Intramuscular* or *Intravenous*, **20,000 to 120,000** units IM or slow IV depending upon severity (at least $\frac{1}{2}$ of the dose should be preferably IV). For more details see manufacturer's package insert.

Note: the incidence of serum sickness with prophylactic doses is generally below 10%; with therapeutic dosage a higher incidence should be anticipated, depending upon the amount administered.

Dosage Forms—10,000 and 20,000 units. (Distributed by CDC).

Tetanus Antitoxin (Equine)

TAT

A sterile, transparent or slightly opalescent, faint brownish, yellowish or greenish, non-pyrogenic solution containing the refined and concentrated antitoxic antibodies, obtained from the blood of healthy horses that have been immunized against tetanus toxin or toxoid (produced by *Clostridium tetani*). It has a potency of not less than 400 antitoxin units per mL based on the US Standard Tetanus Antitoxin and the US Control Tetanus Test Toxin, tested in guinea pigs. The product contains *m*-cresol (0.3%) as a preservative.

Uses—Indicated for passive prevention and treatment of tetanus when Tetanus Immune Globulin (TIG) is not available. For more detailed information see manufacturer's package insert.

Dose—Prophylactic, *Intramuscular* or *Subcutaneous*, **1,500 to 5,000 units** according to body weight. 1,500 units up to 65 pounds and 3,000 to 5,000 units over this weight.

Therapeutic, *Intramuscular* and *Intravenous*, **50,000 to 100,000 units.** At least part of this dose should preferably be given *intravenously*, the rest *intramuscularly*. Antitoxin treatment should be instituted as early as possible.

Dosage Forms—1,500 units, 3,000 units, 5,000 units and 20,000 units.

Antiviral Serum (Equine)

Antirabies Serum
(Equine)

A sterile, transparent or slightly opalescent, faint brownish, yellowish or greenish, non-pyrogenic solution containing the antiviral substances obtained from the blood plasma of healthy horses that have been immunized against rabies by means of vaccine. Each mL contains 125 units. The potency is determined in mice, in comparison with the US Standard Antirabies Serum by neutralization of the CVS

strain of virus. The product contains *m*-cresol (0.3%) as a preservative.

Uses—Used in conjunction with the first dose of Rabies Vaccine when Rabies Immune Globulin (RIG) is not available. For detailed information on the rationale of post-exposure treatment, see manufacturer's package insert.

Dose—*Intramuscular*, Post-exposure, Prophylactic, at least **1,000 units** per 55 pounds of body weight. A portion (up to 50%) is used to *infiltrate* the wound and the remainder is given *intramuscularly.*

Dosage Form—8 mL (1000 units).

Antivenins (Equine)

Antivenin (*Crotalidae*) Polyvalent
(Equine)

A sterile, non-pyrogenic lyophilized preparation containing concentrated serum globulins obtained by fractionating plasma from healthy horses immunized with the venoms of the following four species of crotalids (pit vipers): *Crotalus adamanteus* (eastern diamond rattlesnake), *C atrox* (western diamond rattlesnake), *C durissus terrificus* (tropical rattlesnake, Cascabel), and *Bothrops atrox* ("Fer-de-lance"). The potency is determined by a mouse protection test. Phenol (0.25%) and thimerosal (0.005%) are added as preservatives to the lyophilized preparation and phenylmercuric nitrate (0.001%) is added as a preservative to the diluent (Bacteriostatic Water for Injection, USP).

Uses—Indicated only for the treatment of envenomation caused by the bites of the four pit vipers mentioned above and for other pit vipers native to North, Central and South America, as described in the manufacturer's package insert.

Dose—*Intravenous* (preferred), initial dose **20 mL to 150 mL** or more of reconstituted antivenin depending upon an estimate of the severity of the envenomation. The administration of additional antivenin is based upon the clinical response to the initial dose and continuing assessment of the severity of poisoning. For complete information, see manufacturer's package insert.

Dosage Form—Vial of lyophilized serum and 10 mL vial of diluent.

Antivenin (*Latrodectus Mactans*)
(Equine)

Black Widow Spider Antivenin

A sterile lyophilized product prepared from the blood serum of horses immunized with the venom of the black widow spider (*Latrodectus mactans*). Each vial contains not less than 6,000 Antivenin units based on a mouse protection test. One unit of Antivenin will neutralize one average mouse lethal dose of black widow spider venom when the Antivenin and the venom are injected simultaneously. Thimerosal (1:10,000) is added as a preservative.

Uses—Indicated only for the treatment of symptoms due to bites by the black widow spider.

Dose—*Intramuscular*, **1 vial** of reconstituted Antivenin. A second dose may be necessary in some cases.

Intravenous, for severe cases, or when the patient is under 12, or in shock, 1 vial of reconstituted Antivenin in 10 to 50 mL of saline solution over a 15 minute period.

Dosage Form—vial of lyophilized serum and a 2.5 mL vial of sterile diluent. (A 1 mL vial of normal horse serum (1:10 dilution) also is supplied for sensitivity testing.)

Antivenin (*Micrurus Fulvius*)
Equine

North American Coral Snake Antivenin

A sterile, non-pyrogenic lyophilized preparation containing concentrated serum globulins obtained by fractionating blood from healthy horses immunized with the venom of eastern coral snake (*Micrurus fulvius fulvius*). Each 10 mL of reconstituted product will neutralize approximately 250 mouse LD_{50} (lethal doses) or approximately 2 mg of *M fulvius fulvius* venom. Phenol (0.25%) and thimerosal (0.005%) are added as preservatives prior to lyophilization. Phenylmercuric nitrate (1:100,000) is added to the diluent as a preservative.

Uses—Indicated only for neutralization of the venom of North American coral snake and the venom of *M fulvius tenere* (Texas coral snake). It will not neutralize the venom of *Micruroides euryxanthus* (Arizona or Sonoran coral snake).

Dose—*Intravenous infusion*, **3** to **5 vials** of reconstituted product administered as directed in the manufacturer's package insert. Some patients may require administration of the contents of **10** or more vials if the entire venom load were delivered by the bite(s).

Dosage Form—vial of lyophilized serum and 10 mL vial of diluent.

Diagnostic Skin Antigens

In certain instances antigens may be used as *in vivo* diagnostic aids when injected intradermally into the patient. These diagnostic skin tests are based upon one of two mechanisms: (1) lack of antibodies or (2) hypersensitivity.

Lack of Antibodies—The Schick Test for diphtheria is the common example of this type of skin test. A positive reaction (at the "toxin" injection site only) signifies that the injected toxin was not neutralized and therefore, the individual possesses little or no antitoxin antibodies and is probably susceptible to diphtheria.

Hypersensitivity—The classical illustration of a skin test based upon hypersensitivity is the Tuberculin Skin Test for tuberculosis. The Coccidioidin, Mumps Skin Test Antigen and Histoplasmin diagnostic tests also are based upon hypersensitivity. A positive reaction in these tests indicates sensitivity to the antigen and therefore, the presence of antibodies due either to a present or past infection with the particular organism.

Hypersensitivity skin tests also may be used for the assessment of immunocompetency in individuals with possible cell-mediated immune deficiency diseases (see *Mumps Skin Test Antigen* and *Other Diagnostic Skin Biologics*).

The number of diagnostic skin biologics is relatively small. Several of them were removed from the market as a result of the study made by the FDA Panel on Review of Skin Test Antigens whose principle conclusions and recommendations were reported in the FDA *Drug Bulletin*, March–April, 1978.

Coccidioidin

A clear sterile filtrate prepared from spherules of *Coccidioides immitis*, grown in liquid synthetic medium. The product may be either in the form of the usual skin test strength or the high skin test strength. The usual skin test strength is tested in known positive subjects and is prepared to be bioequivalent in potency to the US Reference Standard Coccidioidin 1:100. The high test strength (1:10 dilution) is to be used only on persons who are negative to the usual skin test strength. Thimerosal (1:10,000) is added as a preservative.

Uses—Used as an aid in the diagnosis of coccidioidomycosis and in the differentiation of this disease from sarcoidosis, histoplasmosis and other mycotic and bacterial infections.

Dose—*Intradermal*, **0.1 mL** on the flexor surface of the forearm.

Interpretation—A positive reaction consists of the development of induration measuring 5 mm or more in diameter. Readings should be made at both 24 and 48 hours. A positive skin test is indicative of a present or past infection with *C immitis*. A negative reaction may indicate either that the patient has never been sensitized or has lost sensitivity.

Dosage Forms—1 mL (usual test strength 1:100) and 0.5 mL (high test strength 1:10).

Diphtheria Toxin For Schick Test

A sterile solution of the diluted, standardized toxic products of growth of the diphtheria bacillus (*Corynebacterium diphtheriae*) of which the parent toxin contains not less than 400 MLD (minimum lethal doses) per mL or 400,000 MRD (minimum skin reaction doses) per mL in guinea pigs. Its potency is determined in terms of the US Standard Diphtheria Toxin for Schick Test, tested in guinea pigs. Thimerosal (1:30,000) is added as a preservative.

Uses—Indicated for the determination of serologic immunity to diphtheria. It may be used to evaluate the current capacity of an immunocompromised individual to display the expected evidence of prior successful immunization against diphtheria.

Dose—*Intradermal*, **0.1 mL** into the right arm (**0.1 mL** of the "Schick Control" should be injected into the left arm).

Interpretation—A positive test (reaction at the "toxin" site only) is characterized by a circumscribed area of redness and slight infiltration which measures 1 cm or more in diameter. The results of the test should be observed on the fourth or fifth day. A positive test indicates that the individual possesses little or no antitoxin and is probably susceptible to diphtheria.

A negative reaction (no reaction at "toxin" site) almost always indicates a circulating serum antitoxin titer of not less than 0.005 units per mL.

A combined reaction (reactions at both "toxin" and "control" sites, with the "toxin" site reaction larger at the end of four days and more persistent than at the "control" site) signifies possible susceptibility to diphtheria and a sensitivity to the diphtheria bacillus proteins, suggesting that caution should be exercised in administration of diphtheria toxoid.

A pseudo reaction (reactions of similar course that reach a maximum intensity by the third day on both the "toxin" and "control" sites) indicates that the individual is hypersensitive to the diphtheria bacillus protein and may have measurable amounts of antitoxin.

Dosage Form—5 mL (50 doses).

Schick Test Control

Diphtheria Toxoid-Schick Test Control

A sterile solution of Diphtheria Toxin for Schick Test that has been inactivated by heat for use as control for the Schick Test. It contains 0.008 Lf of diphtheria toxoid per dose and meets the specific guinea pig test for inactivation. Thimerosal (1:30,000) is added as a preservative.

Uses—Used as a control for the Schick Test. Because of the frequency of pseudo reactions due to sensitivity to diphtheria bacillus protein, it is advisable to run a control.

Dose—*Intradermal*, **0.1 mL** in the left arm.

Interpretation—see the foregoing description under Diphtheria Toxin for Schick Test.

Dosage Form—5 mL (50 doses), available only with vials of Diphtheria Toxin for Schick Test.

Histoplasmin

A sterile colorless solution containing standardized culture filtrates of *Histoplasma capsulatum* grown on liquid synthetic medium. The product is standardized to be clinically equivalent in potency to the US Reference Standard Histoplasmin H-42, 1:100. Phenol (0.4% or 0.5%) is added as a preservative.

Uses—Used to detect delayed hypersensitivity of *H capsulatum* and is employed as an aid in the diagnosis of histoplasmosis. It also may be helpful in the differentiation of histoplasmosis from coccidioidomycosis, sarcoidosis and other mycotic or bacterial infections. However, many authorities consider the skin test of little diagnostic or prognostic value except in cases of disseminated disease, in which absence of reactivity denotes anergy, or in very early infections, in which the test also may be negative. In addition, the skin test may evoke a false rise in the complement fixation titer for histoplasmosis. For other possible uses, see manufacturer's package insert.

Dose—*Intradermal*, **0.1 mL** into the flexor surface of the forearm.

Interpretation—The reaction should be described and measured in terms of mms of induration and degree of reaction from slight induration to vesiculation and necrosis. In many studies reported in the literature a positive reaction is considered to be an induration of 5 mm or greater. A positive reaction may be indicative of a past infection with *H capsulatum* or related organisms such as *Blastomyces* or *Coccidioides* species. The reaction should be read 48 to 72 hours after injection. For further information on interpretation, see manufacturer's package insert.

Dosage Forms—1 and 1.3 mL.

Mumps Skin Test Antigen

A sterile suspension of formaldehyde inactivated mumps virus prepared from the extraembryonic fluid of mumps virus-infected chicken embryo, concentrated and purified by differential centrifugation. Each mL of the skin test antigen contains at least 20 complement-fixing units. Thimerosal (1:10,000) is added as a preservative.

Uses—Has been used for the assessment of immunocompetency. Most of the population (except for the very young) have had contact or infection with mumps virus and therefore usually demonstrate a delayed cutaneous hypersensitivity to mumps skin test antigen if the immune system is intact. *Mumps skin test antigen is not recommended for immunization, diagnosis or treatment of mumps, nor for the diagnosis of immunity to mumps. Based on a review by the Panel on Review of Skin Test Antigens and other information, the Food and Drug Administration has directed that further investigation be conducted before this product is determined to be fully effective for labeled indications.*

Dose—*Intradermal,* 0.1 mL on the inner surface of the forearm.

Interpretation—A positive reaction (sensitivity to the antigen) is indicated by an area of erythema of 1.5 cm or more in diameter, with or without induration. A negative reaction (if the test dose has been given correctly) probably indicates either anergy or nonsensitivity. Pseudopositive reactions may develop in persons sensitive to egg protein. Readings should be made at 24 and 48 hours.

Dosage Form—1 mL (10 tests).

Tuberculin (Old Tuberculin)

OT

A sterile solution derived from the concentrated soluble products of the tubercle bacillus (*Mycobacterium tuberculosis* or *Mycobacterium bovis*). Old tuberculin is a culture filtrate that has been standardized by clinical evaluation in human subjects to give reactions equivalent to or more potent than 5 TU. [US (International) tuberculin units] of standard old tuberculin administered intradermally in the Mantoux test. No preservative is added.

Uses—Indicated for use with multipuncture devices as a screening test for the detection of tuberculin-sensitive individuals. It also is useful in programs to determine priorities for additional testing (ie, chest x-rays) and in epidemiological surveys to determine areas having high levels of infection.

Dose—*Intradermal,* multipuncture technique, **5 TU.**

Interpretation—a positive reaction is read after 48 to 96 hours and is determined by vesiculation or the extent of induration; erythema without induration is of no significance. If vesiculation is present, the test may be interpreted as positive, in which case the management of the patient is the same as that for one classified as positive to the Mantoux test. See the following discussion on Tuberculin (Purified Protein Derivative). If induration is 1 to 2 mm or greater, the test may be considered positive but further diagnostic procedures must be considered, including chest X-ray, microbiologic examination of sputa and other specimens and confirmation of a positive test reaction by using the Mantoux method. A negative reaction is the absence of induration or induration of 1 to 2 mm or less and indicates that there is no need to retest unless the person is a contact of a patient with tuberculosis or there is clinical evidence suggestive of the disease.

Dosage Forms—Individual disposable units with 4 stainless steel tongs or prines (Tine Test) in containers of 25, 100, or 250 individual tests. Individual disposable units with a 9 point plastic scarifier (Mono-Vac) in boxes of 25 tests.

Tuberculin (Purified Protein Derivative)

PPD

A sterile solution derived from a further purified protein fraction of culture filtrates obtained from a human strain of *Mycobacterium*

tuberculosis grown on a protein-free synthetic medium. It is standardized with the US Standard Tuberculin, PPD and the potency is tested by comparison with the corresponding US Standard Tuberculin on sensitized guinea pigs. Phenol (0.28% to 0.5%) or Quinosol (0.01%) are used as preservatives.

Uses—Indicated for (1) use with multipuncture devices as a screening test for the detection of tuberculin-sensitive individuals or for (2) use in the more sensitive intradermal Mantoux test which is recommended as the standard tuberculin test.

Dose—*Intradermal,* multipuncture screening technique, **5 tuberculin units** (TU). (There is a concentrated solution for the Heaf test containing the equivalent to 100,000 units of the US Standard Tuberculin, PPD in 1 mL which is enough for 150 tests.)

Intradermal, Mantoux test, customary initial dose, **0.1 mL containing 5 TU.** There are two other strengths available: 1 TU per 0.1 mL and 250 TU per 0.1 mL. The 1 TU dose is recommended as the initial dose for individuals suspected of being highly sensitized , since larger initial doses may result in severe skin reactions. The 250 TU strength is used exclusively for testing individuals who fail to react to a previous injection of either 1 TU and/or 5 TU and *under no circumstances should be used for the initial injection.*

Interpretation—For the multipuncture screening test, see the discussion for Interpretation of Old Tuberculin reactions. For more specific information, see manufacturer's package insert.

The Mantoux test should be read at 48 to 72 hours after administration. A positive test (an induration measuring 10 mm or more) indicates hypersensitivity and is interpreted as positive for past or present infection with *M tuberculosis.* An induration measuring 5 to 9 mm indicates a doubtful reaction and should be repeated in a different site. In the case of known contacts, an induration of 5 to 9 mm should be interpreted as positive. A negative reaction (an induration of less than 5 mm) indicates lack of sensitivity and tuberculosis infection is highly unlikely.

Dosage Forms—Individual disposable units for multipuncture screening tests in multidose packets containing from 2 to 250 tests. The concentrated solution for the Heaf test is supplied in 1 mL (for 150 tests) vial. PPD for the Mantoux test is supplied as follows: 5 TU (10 and 50 test vials); 1 TU and 250 TU (10 test vials).

Other Diagnostic Skin Biologics

In addition to Diphtheria Toxin For Schick Test and Mumps Skin Test Antigen, there are other antigens that can be used as components of a battery of skin tests to screen for detection of anergy (non-responsiveness to antigens) in immunocompromised individuals. These include:

Candida Extract

Prepared from a filtrate of a 21 day maltose broth culture of *Candida albicans.*

Trichophyton Extract

Prepared from the filtrates of mixtures of 21 day maltose broth cultures of *Trichophyton mentagrophytes, T rubrum* and *T tonsurans.*

Multitest CMI

An 8 test applicator system consisting of: (1) Tetanus Toxoid Antigen, (2) Diphtheria Toxoid Antigen, (3) Streptococcus Antigen, (4) Tuberculin, Old, (5) Glycerin Negative Control, (6) Candida Antigen, (7) Trichophyton Antigen and (8) Proteus Antigen.

CHAPTER 75

Allergenic Extracts

H Richard Shough, PhD

Associate Dean and Professor
University of Oklahoma, Health Sciences Center
College of Pharmacy
Oklahoma City, OK 73190

Allergenic extracts comprise a large group of products that are unique compared to other biologicals and conventional pharmaceuticals. A specific license is required for their manufacture and they are available mainly from specialty companies. In spite of nearly seventy years of clinical use for the diagnosis and treatment of allergy, allergenic extracts are relatively crude drugs by contemporary standards. Their composition is heterogeneous and ill-defined, their mechanism of action is poorly understood, and to date there is no totally reliable standard of potency. Allergenic extracts are employed primarily in the allergist's office and, with few exceptions, these drugs do not enter conventional pharmaceutical distribution systems.

Common allergies are estimated to affect routinely 10 to 20% of the population and allergenic extracts, despite their shortcomings, are mainstays in the control of these diseases.

Every pharmacist should have a fundamental understanding of allergenic extracts and some clinical, institutional, and industrial specialists require expertise. In recent years allergy research has intensified but an unfortunately small number of pharmaceutical scientists have entered the field.

Because of the complexity and large number of allergenic extracts only the fundamental terminology, principles, properties, and types of products are included in this chapter. The reader desiring detailed information on allergy and allergenic extracts may consult the references in the *Bibliography*. More information on the products as well as specialty supplies and services employed in allergy is also available from the manufacturers. The *Panel on Review of Allergenic Extracts—Final Report* (March 1981) is an excellent review and the Food and Drug Administration has maintained the Panel for continuing examination of these products.

Allergy

Allergy (*hypersensitivity*) may be defined as an *untoward immunological reaction* to an antigen called the *allergen*. The phenomenon is not a simple cause-effect relationship, however, for exposure to an allergen results in disease only in a small portion of the population. The occurrence of allergic disease is determined by the characteristics of the individual as well as those of the allergen and even the conditions of exposure. Disease occurs only in those previously *sensitized* by exposure to the allergen and the ability to become sensitized is, at least sometimes, genetically determined (*cf*, *Atopy*). Sensitization may also vary with the age of the individual, nature of the allergen, route and degree of exposure, and many other factors.

The immunological processes involved in allergy result in tissue damage but otherwise do not differ fundamentally from those seen in the normal immune response (Chapter 73). Allergy can be divided into four types on the basis of the immune effectors, mediators, and cells involved in the reaction (Table I). While this classification is not totally reflective of the clinical situation, it is a very useful frame of reference providing one recognizes its limitations (eg, similar manifestations by different mechanisms).

Most of the common allergies to environmental allergens involve mainly the type I immediate reactions. It is for this group that sensitivity testing and immunotherapy with allergenic extracts is most useful. Type II and III reactions are more prominent in autoimmune and alloimmune diseases (Chapter 73) and are not as important in the present context. Common *contactant allergens* (eg, poison ivy) produce dermatitis by the cellular-mediated type IV processes and the *patch-testing materials* described later are used to detect this type of sensitivity.

Atopy

The term atopy was coined by allergists early in the century to describe a set of common allergies which appeared to correlate well with positive skin tests to specific allergens. The meaning of the term has changed somewhat over the years and today atopy generally implies an *inherited tendency* to develop these common allergies. The *atopic diseases* include allergic rhinitis (*hay fever*), allergic asthma, allergic urticaria (*hives*), and atopic eczema (*atopic dermatitis*).

The atopic individual frequently has a family history of allergy and typically is allergic to multiple allergens. Serum IgE is usually elevated and the diseases appear to involve mainly the type I mechanism. The nature of the heritable defect in atopy is unknown but certainly involves more than the tendency to form excessive IgE. It has been suggested that atopy may involve a defect or imbalance in cellular-mediated immunity in addition to the IgE.

Atopic individuals may be more prone to develop immediate-type hypersensitivities to certain drugs (eg, penicillins) but this point is controversial at present. It is important that pharmacists recognize atopic patients and have as much information as possible on their specific allergies in the patient profiles.

Allergens

Allergens are the inciting agents of allergy. It is common to speak of substances such as pollens, danders, dusts, etc, as *allergens* when, in fact, the true allergens comprise only a small part of these materials. The chemical identity of most allergens is unknown at present. However, known allergens are usually *proteins* or *glycoproteins* and do not appear to differ much from other antigens except perhaps being somewhat smaller (mol wt 5,000 to 40,000). Most allergenic substances contain multiple allergens which vary in their allergenic potency, ie, "major" and "minor" allergens. Allergens from related sources are often chemically similar and *cross-allergenic*. The number and diversity of potential allergens in the environment is great which provides a major complication in the control of allergy.

Table I—Mechanisms and Manifestations of Allergy [a]

	Type I	Type II	Type III	Type IV
Name(s)	Immediate Reagin-mediated	Cytotoxic	Immune complex Arthus type	Delayed cellular-mediated tuberculin-type
Immune effectors	IgE	IgG; IgM	IgG (IgM)	"sensitized lymphocytes"
Cells involved in inflammation	Mast cells Basophils	Macrophages (cell-mediated lysis) or	Neutrophils	Macrophages Lymphocytes
Mediators	Histamine SRS-A	Complement (C'-mediated lysis)	Lysosomal enzymes	Lymphokines
Time of onset in sensitized individuals	0–30 min	Immediate but may not be apparent for some time	2–24 hr	6–24 hr
Manifestations	Rhinitis Urticaria Angioedema Asthma Anaphylaxis	Hemolytic anemia Neutropenia Thrombocytopenia	Serum sickness Vasculitis Glomerulonephritis Extrinsic alveolitis	Contact dermatitis Allergy of many infections

[a] Based on classification of Coombs and Gell, *Classification of Allergic Reactions Responsible for Clinical Hypersensitivity and Disease*, in Gell PGH, Coombs RRA, Lachmann PJ (eds): *Clinical Aspects of Immunology*, Blackwell, London, 1975.

A variety of low molecular weight chemicals may serve as *allergenic haptens* (partial antigens) and induce allergy after combining covalently with a suitable protein carrier. While this is an important process in *drug allergy*, most common environmental allergens appear to be complete antigens. A notable exception is the case of common *allergic contact dermatitis* caused by a variety of plants, drugs, clothing additives, and other substances. The plants most responsible for contact dermatitis in North America belong to the Anacardiaceae family, primarily the genus *Toxicodendron (Rhus)*, and include poison ivy, oak, and sumac. The allergenic components of these plants, called *urushiols*, are found in the oleoresin fraction and are derivatives of pentadecylcatechol or heptadecylcatechol. Many plants of the Compositae family, which includes the ragweeds, also cause contact dermatitis and the allergens have been identified as sesquiterpenoid lactones.

The chemical differences between the common *atopic* and *contactant allergens* is of significance in the preparation of allergenic extracts. The plant oleoresins containing the contactants are usually removed during the defatting process and are not present in the aqueous allergenic extracts. The ether-soluble fraction on the other hand can be used for the preparation of patch-testing materials.

Diagnosis of Allergy

The diagnosis of an allergic disease requires first the determination of allergic etiology and second the identification of the specific allergen(s). *Physical diagnosis*, while important, is not sufficient to establish allergic etiology since the symptoms of allergic diseases can result from other causes. Important in this respect are the *intrinsic* (non-allergic) diseases of asthma, rhinitis, and urticaria which must be distinguished from the *extrinsic* (allergic) diseases. This distinction between allergy and intrinsic diseases is not always clear and some clinical conditions likely involve both. It is important, however, since a number of *drug idiosyncrasies* are associated with intrinsic disease and may be mistaken for allergy.

A *detailed history* is one of the most important steps both in determining whether the condition is an allergy as well as suggesting possible allergens. This should include consideration of the patient's symptoms in relation to familial, seasonal, home environment, occupational, medication, and related personal factors.

Clinical laboratory tests are assuming greater importance in the diagnosis of allergy. Diagnostic testing services are available to measure total serum IgE and antigen-specific IgE for many allergens. These tests can be used in conjunction with sensitivity tests and in those with dermographia, very young patients, or others where skin testing may be unreliable. Determinatioin of IgG, IgA, and IgM may be helpful in differentiating various autoimmune, infectious, or other diseases that may mimic allergies. These and related tests may also be used to monitor immunotherapy. In spite of these developments, *sensitivity testing* with allergenic extracts is still the principal method of determining specific allergic etiology.

Sensitivity Testing

Sensitivity testing with allergenic extracts has been used since the early part of the century for the diagnosis of allergy. A variety of different test methods may be employed but all involve the administration of a small amount of allergen to the patient who is observed for reactions suggestive of allergy. While simple in principle, both the administration and interpretation of sensitivity tests require a great deal of expertise and should only be conducted by qualified individuals. Also, since sensitivity testing is an expensive, discomforting, and time-consuming procedure, it is impractical to test the patient for all possible allergens. A careful history provides the main basis for selection of the specific tests to be performed.

Intradermal Tests—These are the most sensitive of the direct skin tests and are accomplished by injecting allergenic extracts directly into the skin on the volar surface of the lower or upper arm. The back, which may be used in scratch testing, should not be used because of the difficulty in dealing with systemic reactions. Multiple extracts can be tested at one time using sites two to three inches apart and marked with an appropriate code. The tests are inspected after 15 minutes or again at 30 minutes if the characteristic *wheal and flare reactions* are not fully developed. The tests are graded from 0 to 4+ depending upon the size of the wheal although the specific grading systems vary extensively. *Histamine controls* are used to eliminate false negative reactions by confirming the wheal/flare reaction of the skin and quality of the technique. *Diluent controls* are used to detect the rare dermographic individual that gives positive tests to the skin trauma. Although a single concentration of allergenic extract is often used for testing, more information can be obtained by a *threshold dilution titration* using a tenfold dilution series. Generalized allergic reactions are relatively uncommon but a rubber tourniquet and epinephrine (1:1000) should always be available when tests are performed.

Prick or Scratch Tests—These tests are simpler and somewhat safer than intradermal tests. They are also less sensitive which some feel is an advantage that provides better correlation with clinical allergy. Many allergists employ a combination of the two methods, using the scratch tests for preliminary screening purposes. The skin is abraded with a sharp needle (prick test) or scarifier (scratch test) either before or after application of one drop of allergenic extract. Much more concentrated extracts are employed since these tests require up to one thousand-fold higher concentration to elicit an equivalent reaction to the intradermal test. The test sites, grading of reactions, and precautions are similar to those for the intradermal test.

Challenge Tests—These tests involve the application of allergenic extracts directly to mucous membranes and may be used occasionally when skin tests are impractical or to obtain some additional information. *Bronchial challenge* as well as *nasal* and *ophthalmic tests* may be employed in these special situations. They are all more hazardous than skin tests.

Passive Transfer Tests—These tests are performed only in rare patients with generalized skin eruptions or severe dermographia where direct skin tests cannot be interpreted. Passive transfer testing requires a second individual, usually a relative, who receives an intradermal injection of the patient's serum. After one or two days, during which time the patient's IgE can affix to the recipient's cells, allergenic extract is injected precisely into the transfer site(s). The skin is then observed for the characteristic wheal and flare reactions which are graded as in the direct tests.

Patch Testing—This is presently the only routine method for demonstrating allergic contact dermatitis. The procedure usually involves application of the test substance to a piece of cloth or soft paper placed on the outer arm or upper back, covered with an impermeable substance and taped in place. After 24 to 48 hours the patch is removed and the test site examined for presence of the characteristic rash. The specific test procedures used over the years have varied considerably and only recently has there been an attempt to standardize patch testing. The International Contact Dermatitis Research Group has recommended a set of standardized patch test procedures and patch test material concentrations (Fregert and Bandman, 1975).

Effect of Drugs on Tests—A variety of drugs may interfere with sensitivity tests. Antihistamines, especially hydroxyzine, and sympathomimetic amines (eg, ephedrine, isoproterenol, phenylephrine) depress the immediate skin test reactions and aminophylline, iodides, and calcium gluconate may have an effect in some patients. These drugs should be discontinued 24 to 48 hours before testing. Corticosteroids have little effect on the immediate skin tests but may depress the cellular-mediated reactions in patch-testing.

Antihistamines may be administered during immunotherapy but steroids generally should not since they may interfere with IgG blocking antibody formation (see *Immunotherapy*).

Treatment of Allergy

The types, causes, and contributing factors of allergy are numerous. Therapy is thus complex and variable but can be divided into three main types. *Environmental controls* are designed to eliminate or at least minimize exposure to the allergen. Avoidance of an allergen is relatively simple and effective in some instances but most allergens cannot be eliminated totally from the environment. However, minimizing exposure to the allergen nearly always enhances the effectiveness of other measures. *Symptomatic drug therapy*

is required in the control of most common allergies. The many drugs used for this purpose include the antihistamines (Chapter 61), corticosteroids (Chapter 52), and sympathomimetics (Chapter 45). Specific *immunotherapy* may be employed for certain allergies as described below.

Immunotherapy

The immunotherapy of allergy is accomplished by administration of gradually increasing doses of allergen over a period of months or years with the anticipation of the patient developing increasing tolerance to the allergen. This is commonly called *desensitization* or *hyposensitization* but these terms tend to imply unconfirmed mechanisms and may be confused with other clinical procedures. For example, in some special cases of penicillin or horse-serum allergy the patient may be desensitized by administering the antigen in sufficient speed and quantity to effectively neutralize the IgE present. The exact mechanism of immunotherapy is poorly understood but is often attributed to the formation of IgG *blocking antibodies* which neutralize the allergen before it can contact the cell-bound IgE. However, other things, such as reduction of serum IgE, inhibition of the secondary IgE response, and decreased cell responsiveness may also play a part in successful immunotherapy.

The efficacy of immunotherapy is difficult to judge. There have been many controlled clinical trials but most of these have considered only allergic rhinitis and asthma caused by common aeroallergens (eg, ragweed pollens, certain grass and tree pollens, house dust). Immunotherapy is commonly recommended and appears to be effective for these conditions when properly employed. The treatment of hay fever and asthma due to other aeroallergens (eg, molds) is also fairly common but based mainly upon experience with the common allergens. Immunotherapy is rarely recommended for food allergies which are best treated by elimination diets or for dander allergies except in rare instances where avoidance is impossible (eg, veterinarians). It is commonly recommended for the serious stinging insect allergy and the newer purified venom extracts appear to be most effective for this purpose. Information on the use of immunotherapy for other allergic diseases is either scanty or contradictory (eg, atopic dermatitis).

Whether the immunotherapy of allergy is worthwhile in terms of cost, time, inconvenience, and risk when compared to other forms of therapy is difficult to determine. At present this judgment is best made by the experienced clinician and informed patient in each individual situation. However, as noted previously, improved analytical techniques are expected to enable both the better monitoring of patient reponse to immunotherapy and development of products of greater efficacy.

Three main techniques are used for the immunotherapy of allergic rhinitis and asthma due to the common aeroallergens. *Coseasonal therapy* is not generally recommended but may be employed when the patient is first seen during the allergy season. *Preseasonal treatment* is used in some instances and consists of administering the allergen for 3 to 6 months prior to the allergy season at 4- to 7-day intervals. *Perennial treatment* is considered by most to provide maximum therapeutic benefit. Typically the allergenic extract is administered weekly by subcutaneous injection in the upper arm; intradermal injections often result in severe local reactions, intramuscular injections are painful, and intravenous injections may result in serious systemic reactions. The dose is gradually increased up to maximum tolerated levels and the frequency of maintenance doses may sometimes be reduced to every 2 to 4 weeks with amelioration of symptoms. The optimum duration of therapy is variable but most continue until the patient is symptom-free for one year and the average course of therapy is some 3 to 5 years. Success is often relative but some patients remain free of symptoms for extended periods. In others there is sufficient reduction of symptoms that symptomatic therapy alone can be employed but some patients require resumption of immunotherapy.

Immunotherapy is not without risk. Most patients develop some swelling and redness at the injection site but reactions that persist for more than 24 hours are a signal to proceed cautiously. Particularly uncomfortable local reactions may be treated with oral antihistamines and cold compresses. The possibility of serious generalized allergic reactions is always present. The patient should remain in the physician's office for at least thirty minutes after each course of therapy and the clinician should be prepared to deal with such reactions.

During pregnancy there is no evidence of major adverse effects of allergenic extracts on the fetus but uterine contractions may occur as part of a generalized allergic reaction. It is generally recommended that immunotherapy not be started during pregnancy and that slight reduction of the maintenance dose be considered for those who become pregnant during therapy.

Immunotherapy should not be continued indefinitely in the absence of clinical improvement. Treatment failures may result from improper selection of allergens, development of new sensitivities, improper use of environmental controls, and various problems associated with the allergenic extracts. The characteristics of these products are discussed in the next section.

Allergenic Extracts

Allergenic extracts are concentrated solutions or suspensions of allergens used for the diagnosis and treatment of allergic diseases. Most are injectable products administered in the physician's office and for many years they were prepared by the individual users. Commercial preparations are used mainly today and these are produced largely by companies specializing in the manufacture of allergy products. Because of the large number of allergenic extracts on the market only the general characteristics of the products are described here. Additional information on these and related products may be obtained from the licensed manufacturers listed in Table II.

Federal Licensure

The manufacture of allergenic extracts intended for interstate sale, export, or import must be carried out in laboratories that have been licensed as required by section 351 of the Public Health Services Act (see *Federal Control of Biological Products*, Chapter 74). The provisions of this act do not prohibit compounding of allergenics dispensed on a prescription when dispensing and patient-use are within the state of origin of the prescription order.

Types

Allergenic extracts are usually designated as being *aqueous* or *glycerinated* products. Normal saline or similar isotonic electrolyte solution is the diluent for the former while the latter contain 50% glycerin in the diluent. The preparations are normally buffered to pH 8 and contain phenol (0.4%) as a preservative. *Stock extracts* are prepared from a single allergen source although these do contain multiple allergens.

Table II—Licensed Manufacturers of Allergenic Extracts[a]

Allergy Laboratories, Inc.
Allergy Laboratories of Ohio, Inc.
Allermed Laboratories, Inc.
Antigen Laboratories, Inc.
Barry Laboratories, Inc.
Berkely Biologicals, Inc.
Center Laboratories, Inc.
    Division of EM Industries, Inc.
Dome Laboratories
    Division of Miles Laboratories, Inc.
Greer Laboratories, Inc.
Hollister-Stier Laboratories
    Division of Miles Laboratories, Inc.
Iatric Corporation
Meridian Bio-Medical, Inc.
Nelco Laboratories, Inc.
Pharmacia Diagnostics
    Division of Pharmacia, Inc.

[a] *Establishments and Products Licensed under section 351 of the Public Health Service Act.* 1982. HEW Publication No. (FDA) 82-9003.

Diagnostic mixtures are commercially available and since many patients have multiple allergies *custom treatment mixtures* are commonly employed. The formulation of these requires a great deal of expertise and should be done only under the direction of the attending physician. Six or seven allergen sources (less according to some) is the maximum that should be included in any therapeutic mixture and it is recommended that allergens to which a patient is particularly sensitive be administered separately.

Scratch-testing extracts are glycerinated products supplied in 1- to 5-mL dropper vials. They are relatively concentrated solutions, usually in strengths of 1:5 to 1:20, depending on the allergen (see *Standardization* below). *Intradermal-test extracts* are aqueous solutions supplied in 1- to 5-mL multiple dose vials and are more dilute (1:500 to 1:5000). *Therapeutic extracts*, both aqueous and glycerinated, are supplied in multiple-dose vials in a variety of sizes (5 to 100 mL) and dilutions (1:10 to 1:100). Since these extracts are diluted before use, most companies provide a variety of *dilution vials* which contain a volume of diluent that facilitates preparation of ten-fold dilutions. Standard and custom *diagnostic and therapeutic sets and mixtures* are also available as are a variety of auxiliary supplies used in allergy practice. *Autogenous extracts* are sometimes prepared from allergenic substances collected from the individual patient's environment.

Repository extracts of various types have been used for years in an attempt to delay absorption and enhance the blocking antibody response of the allergen but it is still controversial as to whether these products offer any major advantages. Water-in-oil *emulsions* were formerly quite popular but these resulted in more local reactions and controlled studies failed to demonstrate increased efficacy. None of these are licensed at the present time. Two series of therapeutic *adjuvant extracts* are currently marketed—the alum-precipitated Center-Al* line (*Center Laboratories*) and the pyridine-extracted, alum-precipitated Allpyral* products (*Dome*). It is claimed that these products have the advantage of requiring fewer doses and reduced systemic side effects. However, delayed local reactions appear to be more common with these adjuvant products. Alum precipitation does not generally alter the antigenicity of allergens but there is some evidence that alkaline-pyridine extraction may. Additional study is required to determine completely the advantages and disadvantages of the adjuvant preparations.

Many efforts are being made to improve allergenic extracts by the use of *purified* and/or better *standardized allergens* (eg, antigen E of short ragweed). Several procedures have been used in attempts to reduce allergenicity without affecting the immunogenicity of allergens. These include the preparation of formalin-treated *allergoids*, polymerization of allergens with glutaraldehyde, and photoinactivation of allergens. Most of these products are still investigational but continued improvements in immunological analytical techniques can be expected to facilitate evaluation of the efficacy of these as well as the older products.

Preparation

The preparation of allergenic extracts involves the same general procedures and precautions employed with all parenteral products (Chapter 85). In addition to the usual aseptic procedures the extraction process should be carried out in a cold room. The extracts are thermolabile and must be sterilized by filtration (Chapter 79) and sterility tests for both aerobic and anaerobic microorganisms must be performed on the finished product. Toxicity testing is usually performed in guinea pigs and particularly recommended for autogenous extracts where unknown toxic constituents may be present. Recent concerns for possible mycotoxin contaminants in mold extracts or from mold contamination of other substances have resulted in more intensive efforts to detect and eliminate these toxins. The general procedures used for the preparation of other extractives (Chapter 84) are employed and only those unique for allergenic extracts are included below.

Materials—The allergenic substances to be extracted are obtained mainly from commercial suppliers and only the most reliable sources should be used. For example, pollens are obtained from botanical supply houses that specialize in pollen collection. Samples must be properly identified, free of other pollens, and contain no more than 1% extraneous foreign matter. Prompt and proper dehydration is important to prevent alteration of the allergens and microbial contamination. In spite of these and other precautions one can expect lot-to-lot variation in the allergenicity of pollens due to climatic, geographical, and other factors. Such variation in the original allergenic substances is largely uncontrollable at present and is unquestionably a major source of the variation ultimately seen in the final products.

Grinding—The material to be extracted must be ground or subdivided in order to effect efficient extraction of the allergens. Household blenders or small plant mills can be used for dried materials while juicers or food grinders can be used for those containing much moisture. Materials such as hairs, feathers, and textiles should be finely divided with shears.

Defatting—Many allergenic substances including all pollens should be defatted before final extraction. Ether and petroleum ether are most commonly used for this purpose but alcohols may occasionally be included in the menstruum. Defatting provides a clearer final extract and also removes irritants found in large amounts in some substances, eg, coffee, tea, cocoa, cottonseed, pepper, mustard, ginger. The extract obtained in the defatting process may be used in the preparation of some patch testing substances.

Extraction—The extraction procedures in current use are based upon the assumption that allergens are water-soluble proteins or glycoproteins although the identity of only a few is known. Extraction is normally carried out for 24 to 72 hours in a cold room using sterile, pyrogen-free buffered saline, Coca's solution, or similar aqueous menstruum of pH 8.

Buffered Saline

Sodium Chloride	5	g
Monobasic Potassium Phosphate	0.36	g
Dibasic Sodium Phosphate, anhydrous	7	g
Phenol Crystals	4	g
Water for Injection USP, to make	1000	mL

Coca's Solution

Sodium Chloride	5	g
Phenol Crystals	5	g
Sodium Bicarbonate	2.5	g
Water for Injection USP, to make	1000	mL

After extraction the mixture is clarified by coarse filtration. Some extracts are dialyzed against saline or running tap water to remove irritants or coloring agents. Most pollens require no dialysis but some substances (eg, house dust, mustard, potato, spinach, beets) give nearly universally positive reactions unless dialyzed. Concentration of the extract where required may be achieved by a number of methods but care should be taken not to alter the allergens. The processed extract is sterilized by filtration, usually through a cellulose-membrane filter. Prefilters are usually required but asbestos should not be used since it may adsorb some antigens and may be carcinogenic.

Freeze-dried pollen extracts are prepared essentially as described above except that water rather than electrolyte solution is used as the extracting medium. The lyophilized products are reconstituted with buffered saline at time of use.

Standardization—Allergenic extracts are standardized by several different systems: pollen units, Freeman-Noon units, weight/volume (w/v), protein nitrogen units (PNU), nitrogen units, and milligrams total nitrogen (Table III). *Weight/volume* is the most common measure of allergen concentration and expresses the weight of allergenic substance per volume of extracting fluid. For example, a 1:50 extract is prepared by extracting 1 g of substance with 50 mL of solvent and decimal dilutions of this extract would provide 1:500, 1:5000, etc. concentrations. The potency of commercial allergenic extracts is usually also expressed in terms of *protein nitrogen units* (1 mg protein nitrogen equals 100,000 PNU). However, the allergenic protein is but a small part of the total extractable protein and neither the PNU nor weight/volume standards correlate consistently with each other or clinical potency.

Because allergenic extracts cannot be reliably standardized the appropriate dosage for immunotherapy must be determined clinically. The initial dilution of extract, starting dose, and progression of dosage must be carefully determined on the basis of the patient's history and sensitivity tests. Because dilute extracts tend to lose activity more rapidly, the first dose from a more concentrated vial should generally be the same or less than the previous dose. Also, it is common to reduce the dose whenever a new lot of extract is started and then build the dose back to the maintenance level over a period of several weeks.

Much recent work on allergenic extracts has been concerned with improved methods of standardization such as the *radioallergoadsorbent test* (RAST). RAST tests have been widely used to measure total serum IgE and antigen specific IgE but can easily be modified as a quantitative test for specific allergens.

A number of other methods have been used to measure the content and/or potency of allergenic extracts, including *quantitative skin testing*, the *histamine-release test*, and *gel-diffusion techniques* (eg, radial immunodiffusion). Commercial Short Ragweed Allergenic Extract assayed for Antigen E by radial immunodiffusion is now available and the Food and Drug Administration expects to have suitable reference standards for several allergens soon. A desirable but challenging goal is that all allergenic extracts will some day be standardized to contain measured quantities of known

Table III—Equivalent Standards for Allergenic Extracts[a]

Weight/Volume (w/v)	1 mL of 1:50
Pollen Units	20,000
Freeman-Noon Units	20,000
Protein Nitrogen Units (PNU)	10,000
Total Nitrogen Units	26,000
Total Nitrogen	0.26 mg

[a] These are only approximate equivalents for pollen extracts.

allergens which correlate with clinical potency.

Stability and Storage

Allergenic extracts tend to show reduced potency within a matter of weeks or months after their preparation but there have been few detailed studies on the stability of these products. Both high temperatures and freezing usually have deleterious effects and the latter may cause agglomeration of adjuvant extracts. Some extracts also contain proteolytic enzymes and these may contribute to decomposition of the allergens. Both glycerinated and lyophilized products are more stable than aqueous extracts. Very dilute extracts tend to lose potency by adsorption to the surfaces of containers and syringes and thus are usually prepared close to the time of use. Several studies have shown that the inclusion of Tween 80, Tween 20, or human serum albumin reduces sorption but more complete investigation of this problem is required. The adjuvant extracts should not be diluted with either phosphate buffered saline or Coca's solution since these may cause partial release of allergen; normal saline containing 0.4% phenol is a satisfactory diluent. The adjuvant extracts may be mixed with one another but should not be mixed with other types of extracts.

All allergenic extracts should be refrigerated at 2 to 8° and freezing should be avoided. The expiration date for aqueous extracts is usually 18 months, while that for glycerinated scratch-test and bulk extracts is usually 3 years. Lyophilized products have an expiration date of 4 years or 18 months after reconstitution, as long as the time falls within the original 4 years. Care must be exercised in changing to new lots or different dilutions of extracts because of possible variations in potency. It is generally recommended that quantities of extract sufficient to last the patient for one year be prepared to avoid frequent changes in extracts.

Role of the Pharmacist

Few pharmacists are called on today to prepare allergenic extracts or to fill prescriptions for these products. Some pharmacies, particularly in hospitals, may stock allergenic extracts and related supplies for allergists. Actually the training of a pharmacist is suited uniquely to many of the services required in the allergy clinic and it is unfortunate that more pharmacists have not become involved in this area.

In a few institutions allergenic extracts are provided by the pharmacist on prescription order. Some patients require only a single extract but even in these cases appropriate dilutions must be prepared. More frequently patients are allergic to multiple allergens and extract mixtures are required. The basic techniques and facilities required for this service are essentially the same as those used in a typical IV additive program but the pharmacist should have some additional training and experience in handling allergenic extracts. There is an opportunity to provide a variety of product services to the allergist. For example, some clinicians prefer to use color-coding to represent different dilutions of extracts. This can be accomplished by using different colored rubber stoppers or anodized-aluminum foil closures.

In addition to assuming responsibility for the preparation and control of allergenic extracts, the pharmacist may also provide a variety of patient-oriented services in the allergy clinic (Hunter and Osterberger, 1975). These services include the obtaining of patient histories, performing allergy testing procedures, and patient consultation.

Common allergic diseases are found in 10 to 20% of the population and patients with these ailments obtain a variety of drugs and medical supplies from community pharmacies. Thus there are many opportunities for pharmacists to be of service to the allergy patient in traditional practice sites as well

as the allergy clinic. To accomplish this effectively pharmacists must have a fundamental understanding of allergy and the products used in the control of allergic diseases.

Products

This section contains a summary of the principal allergenic extracts available today. It is impractical to provide an individual monograph for each product and they have been grouped according to the type of allergenic substance (eg, pollens, dusts, etc). This classification is not perfect but was chosen in part because the extracts are listed this way in manufacturers' literature. It is also found to have some merit when considering both the product characteristics and clinical allergy. These are briefly described for each group with emphasis on the following: clinical significance of the allergen group; most common offenders of the group; and general usefulness and limitations of the extracts.

The lists of allergenic extracts are intended to be reasonably comprehensive but there have been some intentional omissions. Only one name—usually the common one—is given for each extract while in practice a number of both common and scientific names may be used. Similarly, individual extracts are usually derived from a single species of plant, animal, or microorganism but only the genus is given in the list; however, extracts of most of the common allergenic species are commercially available. Extracts containing allergens from more than one source are designated as *mixtures* and, while many are commercially available, only a few are listed. Not all manufacturers produce all of the extracts and it should be recognized that different companies may employ significantly different source materials and processes in preparing products of the same name. As noted previously, none of these products can be considered to be standardized in terms of either allergenic content or potency.

Most of the products listed are provided as *diagnostic extracts* for both scratch and intradermal testing but *therapeutic extracts* may or may not be routinely available. Similarly, the availability of both lyophilized and adjuvant products is limited. Many of the extracts are also available in diagnostic *test sets*. These are not listed but include various regional, pollen, food, mold, pediatric, titration, and other test sets. Manufacturing services for *custom therapeutic mixtures* and *autogenous* extracts are also available. The individual manufacturers should be contacted for more specific information on their products and services.

FDA Panel on Review of Allergenic Extracts

The Food and Drug Administration *Panel on Review of Allergenic Extracts* presented its final report on a five year study of the safety and efficacy of allergenic extracts in 1981. The panel considered allergenic extracts on both a generic and individual product basis and recommended classification into one of the following categories:

1. Category I: Products determined to be safe, effective, and not misbranded.

2. Category II: Products determined to be unsafe, ineffective, or misbranded.

3. Category III: Products for which data is insufficient for classification and further testing is required. Category III A Products are recommended for continued licensing and Category III B not recommended for continued licensing during the period of further testing on the basis of available data concerning potential benefits and risks.

The Panel considered nearly 1600 generic varieties of commercially available allergenic extracts. A small number were generically classified in category I and another group in category II or III B. The vast majority (ca 1300) of the products were classified in Category III A. These are largely extracts of materials known or highly suspected to be allergenic but for which there is little published data to establish efficacy.

The FDA has charged the Panel with reexamination of these products classified in Category III A with the purpose of eliminating this category and classifying all products in Categories I or II. Those products which meet the standards of safety and effectiveness consistent with "state-of-the-art" methodology would be placed in Category I. Category II products determined to be "safe and presumptively effective" and for which there is a "compelling medical need with no suitable alternative" would also be permitted to remain on the market pending completion of further studies.

The reader should consult the Panel Reports for a more detailed review of the safety and efficacy of these products.

Pollen Extracts

Pollens are the most common cause of the atopic diseases and, in fact, hay fever is sometimes called "pollinosis." Pollens are produced only by seed-bearing plants and not by algae, fungi, mosses, and ferns. Not all pollens are of equal clinical significance for there is variation in both allergenicity and degree of exposure. Allergy usually results from *anemophilous* (wind-borne) rather than *entomophilous* (insect-borne) pollens. Conifers such as the pines are copious pollen producers but the pollens, with few exceptions, are hypoallergenic.

Pollen allergy is largely a problem of *temperate climates*. In arctic and alpine regions where summers are short, plants generally reproduce vegetatively (asexually) and most subarctic plants are conifers. In the tropics there tends to be a proliferation of species with a small number of individual plants so that exposure to a specific pollen is minimized. Anemophilous plants also tend to be less common in regions of extremely high humidity.

Seasonal and geographical variation is more pronounced with pollen allergy than other types. Pollen seasons vary with both the plant and locale but the following generalizations can be made: trees from late winter to spring; grasses from spring to early summer; and weeds from late summer to fall. Pollen allergy is a significant problem in most parts of this country but the allergens vary somewhat with the region and are best determined by consulting one of the published guides (eg, Nelson, 1975). Perhaps 100 of the approximately 300 pollens represented in commercial extracts are fairly common offenders.

Allergenic extracts prepared from some of the common pollens (eg, ragweed, several grass and tree) have been among the most widely studied. Controlled studies have generally shown these products to be reliable for both diagnosis and, in several cases, for therapy when properly prepared and employed. Many of the products listed below have not been extensively studied but their reliability often is assumed based on extrapolation of the data on the common pollens. (Table IV).

Dust Extracts

House dust is probably the most common non-pollen inhalant allergen. The allergens in house dust are not related to the inorganic dirt from outside but to the products of aging and decomposition of materials around the home. Whether there is a specific dust-associated allergen is not known for sure but dust contains mold spores, feathers, hairs, food, cleaning-agent residues, danders, etc, and the composition may vary considerably with the source. The dust for commercial extracts is usually obtained from house cleaning or rug cleaning firms and is pooled to obtain some homogeneity.

A great deal of attention has been focused on the *dust mite*

Table IV—Pollen Extracts

Trees

Acacia	Elderberry	Orange
Alder[a]	Elm[a]	Osage Orange
Almond	Eucalyptus	Palm
Apple	Fir	Palo Verde
Apricot	Hackberry	Peach
Arbor vitae	Hazelnut	Pear
Ash[a]	Hemlock	Pecan
Aspen	Hickory[a]	Pepper Tree
Bayberry	Hop-Hornbean	Pine
Beech	Hickory/Pecan	Plum
Birch[a]	Ironwood	Poplar
Blue Beech	Juniper	Privet
Bottle Brush Beech	Lilac	Redwood
Box Elder	Locust	Russian Olive
Butternut	Maple	Spruce
Carob Tree	Melaleuca	Sweet Gum
Cedar[a]	Mesquite	Sycamore[a]
Cherry	Mock Orange	Tamarack
Chestnut	Mulberry	Tree of Heaven
Cottonwood[a]	Oak[a]	Walnut[a]
Cypress[a]	Olive	Willow

Grasses

Bahia	Corn	Redtop[a]
Barley	Fescue	Ryegrass
Beach	Fingergrass	Salt
Bent	Grama	Sorghum
Bermuda[a]	Johnson	Sudan
Bluegrass	Koeler's[a]	Sweet Vernal[a]
Brome	Lovegrass	Timothy[a]
Bunch	Oats	Velvetgrass
Canarygrass	Orchard[a]	Wheat
Chess	Quack	Wheatgrass

Weeds & Garden Plants

Alfalfa	Dog Fennel	Povertyweed
Amaranth[a]	Fireweed	Quailbush
Aster	Gladiolus	Ragweed[a]
Balsam Root	Goldenrod	Rose
Bassia	Greasewood	Russian Thistle[a]
Beach Bar	Hemp	Sagebrush[a]
Broomweed	Honeysuckle	Saltbrush[a]
Bulrush	Hops	Scale
Burrow Brush	Iodine Bush	Scotch Broom
Careless Weed	Jerusalem Oak	Sea Blight
Castor Bean	Kochia[a]	Sedge
Cattail	Lamb's Quarters	Sheep Fat
Chamise	Lily	Sheep Sorrel
Clover	Marigold	Snapdragon
Cocklebur	Marshelder[a]	Sugar Beet
Coreopsis	Mexican Tea	Sunflower
Cosmos	Mustard	Western Water Hemp
Daffodil	Nettle	Winter Fat
Dahlia	Pickleweed	Wormseed
Daisy	Pigweed	Wormwood
Dandelion	Plantain[a]	
Dock	Poppy	

[a] Most common offenders

(*Dermatophagoides* spp) as a possible source of a common allergen in dusts. The dust mite appears to be virtually universally distributed and is usually found in furnishings stuffed with vegetable fibers (eg, cotton) used by humans. While many feel that mite allergens are responsible for most dust allergy this is not a complete explanation of the phenomenon. Some individuals are allergic to dust but not the mite and it is not found in some dusts.

House-dust sensitivity differs from pollen allergy in several respects and is particularly suspected when the patient's history includes one or more of the following factors: perennial symptoms that worsen when the patient remains indoors; increased nocturnal symptoms; increased symptoms when performing household chores; and increased symptoms associated with turning on of heating or air conditioning systems.

House dust is a ubiquitous allergen and its total elimination is virtually impossible. However, it is important that the patient maintain as *dust-free* an *environment* as possible, particularly in the bedroom. Instructions for preparation of

Table V—Dust Extracts

Mixtures	House Dusts	
	Mattress	Upholstery
	Wood Dusts	
Cedar/Juniper	Maple	Sawdust/Mixture
Fir/Hemlock	Oak Mix	Spruce
Gum	Pine Mix	Walnut
Mahogany	Redwood	
	Grain Dusts	
Alfalfa	Oat	Rye
Barley	Pea	Sorghum
Corn	Prairie Hay	Soybean
Grain Mill	Rice	Wheat

Table VI—Fungal Extracts

Molds		
Alternaria	Gliocladium	Phoma
Aspergillus	Helminthosporium	Pullularia
Botrytis	Hormodendrom	Rhizopus
Candida	Microsporum	Rhodotorula
Cephalosporium	Monatospora	Saccharomyces
Cephalothecium	Monilia	Scopulariopsis
Chaetomium	Mucor	Spondylocladium
Curvularia	Mycogone	Sporotrichum
Epicoccum	Neurospora	Stemphylium
Epidermophyton	Nigraspora	Streptomyces
Fusarium	Oidiodendrum	Trichoderma
Gelasinospora	Paecilomyces	Trichophyton
Geotrichum	Penicillium	Verticullium
	Smuts	
Barley Smut	Foxtail Smut	Sorghum Smut
Bermuda Smut	Johnson Grass Smut	Wheat Smut
Corn Smut	Oat Smut	

dust-free rooms and products to minimize the circulation of dust (Allergex, *Hollister-Stier*) are available.

Allergy to house dust is probably the most common immediate hypersensitivity observed in clinical sensitivity testing. House dust extracts have been extensively investigated and in some study groups 75% or more of allergic patients have shown positive reactions. However, significant numbers of non-allergic individuals also show positive reactions and it is indeed difficult to evaluate the efficacy of these heterogeneous products. Predictably, the effectiveness of house dust extracts in therapy has not been established but there have been claims of success. Also, some clinicians choose to attempt desensitization of seriously allergic individuals with *autogenous extracts* when they fail to respond to stock extracts. The control of common house-dust allergy should improve greatly with better knowledge of the allergenic composition of this complex mixture (see Table V).

Relatively little information is available on other dust extracts. These are generally less common allergens and many are associated with occupational allergies. Some of these may also be involved in the *extrinsic allergic alveolitis* described under *Fungal Extracts*.

Fungal Extracts

The fungi are a large group of organisms that may be involved in many types of diseases, including intoxications, infections, and allergy. Most fungi are saprophytes and compared to bacteria are relatively uncommon causes of infectious disease. *Mycotoxins* are of great concern in several areas of health including as possible contaminants of allergic extracts. A number of fungi have been increasingly implicated as important causes of several types of allergic disease.

Molds are one of the major causes of non-pollen atopic allergies. Asthma and rhinitis as well as various cutaneous reactions can be precipitated by inhalation of mold spores or mycelial fragments in sensitive individuals. Fungi are ubiquitous and may be found in the home on textiles, leather goods, upholstered furniture, food, and plants. Damp warm places such as basements and closets tend to favor mold growth, which is often encountered as common "mildew" that is most often *Aspergillus* or *Penicillium* spp. Fungal allergy resulting from indoor exposure tends to be perennial. That from outdoor exposure shows more distinctive seasonal and geographical patterns but these are less pronounced than in pollen allergy. Fungal allergy is also more likely to be associated with occupation or hobby.

Sensitivity testing for fungal allergens appears to be generally reliable. It is also useful at times to identify the specific fungi in the patient's environment and fungal identification services are available. Therapy should include efforts to create a *mold-free environment* but this is difficult to accomplish completely. Several studies indicate that immunotherapy may be of value for some patients. One problem is that the allergenic extracts are variously prepared from

mycelium, medium, or both but too little is known about the fungal allergens to know the most appropriate method.

Fungi, along with a variety of organic dusts, have been found to be important causes of another respiratory allergy, *extrinsic allergic alveolitis* (hypersensitivity pneumonitis). Many names related to either the allergen or affected individuals have been applied to this condition; eg, farmer's lung, mushroom-workers disease, wood-dust asthma, etc. The disease shows no relationship to atopy but can usually be related to recent high-level exposures to the offending inhalant. Extrinsic allergic alveolitis appears to result from the formation of IgG immune complexes in the lung (type III reaction) but may involve cellular-mediated (type IV) reactions also. Diagnosis is based mainly on a detailed personal history but the demonstration of specific *precipitins* in the serum of the patient provides supporting evidence. Commercial tests and testing services are available for this purpose. Both type III and IV allergies may provide cutaneous reactions on allergen challenge but they differ in time-course and type from the immediate skin-test reactions. The products listed in Table VI are not useful in the diagnosis of extrinsic allergic alveolitis; effective therapy depends mainly on avoidance of the allergen.

Miscellaneous Inhalant Extracts

Atopic allergies may be caused by a variety of inhalant allergens other than pollens, dusts, and molds. The epidermals from domestic animals (cat, dog, horse) are the best known but the variety of inhalant allergens is remarkable. Exposure of an average individual to some of the substances listed below might appear unlikely but this is not necessarily the case. Probably few people recognize that orris root is a common component of cosmetics, including many dusting powders; that camel hair may be found in imported textiles and rugs; that the plant gums acacia, karaya, and tragacanth are present in hundreds of food, cosmetic and drug products; and that pyrethrum is an active constituent of many household insecticides. Many of these substances are also ingestant (see *Food Extracts*) and contactant (see *Patch-Testing Materials*) as well as inhalant allergens.

Sensitivity testing with many of the extracts listed in Table VII is fairly common but based largely on experience with common aeroallergen extracts. Little information is available on the use of these products for immunotherapy. Avoidance of the allergen is preferred and can usually be achieved although at times only with great effort.

Insect Allergy

Insect allergy is a term rather loosely applied to describe allergy from both insects and arthropods such as spiders and

Table VII— Miscellaneous Inhalant Extracts

Epidermals

Camel Hair	Goat Hair and Dander	Mohair
Cat Hair and Dander	Guinea Pig Hair	Monkey Hair
Cattle Hair and	Hamster Hair	Mouse Hair
Dander	Hog Hair and Dander	Rabbit Fur
Deer Hair	Horse Hair and	Rat Hair
Dog Hair and Dander	Dander	Seal Fur
Fox Fur	Human Hair	Wool
Gerbil Hair and	Mink Fur	
Dander		

Feathers

Canary	Duck	Pigeon
Chicken	Goose	Turkey
	Parakeet	

Miscellaneous

Acacia Gum	Glue, Animal	Lycopodium
Alfalfa Hay	Glue, Fish	Orris Root
Algae	Guar Gum	Paper Mixture
Carragheen Gum	Hay Dust	Pyrethrum
Coconut Fiber	Hemp	Quince Seed
Cotton Linters	Henna	Silk
Cottonseed	Jute	Sisal
Fern Spores	Kafir Dust	Timothy Hay
Flax Fiber	Kapok	Tobacco
Flaxseed	Karaya Gum	Tragacanth Gum

Table VIII—Insect Allergen Extracts

Insects

Ant, Black	Butterfly	Horse Fly
Ant, Carpenter	Caddis Fly	House Fly
Ant, Fire	Cockroach	May Fly
Ant, Red	Cricket	Mites
Aphid	Deerfly	Mosquitoes
Bee, Bumble	Fleas	Moth/Miller
Bee, Honey	Fruit Fly	Wasps
Bee, Sweat	Gnats	Yellow Jacket
Blackfly	Hornet	Stinging Insect Mixt

Venoms

Honeybee	Wasp Protein	Yellow Hornet Protein
Mixed Vespid Protein	White-Faced Hornet	Yellow Jacket Protein
	Protein	

mites. Allergy may result from inhalation of body emanations but most often occurs following a sting or bite.

Allergy to stinging insects of the order *Hymenoptera* is of greatest clinical significance and has been most widely studied. The honeybee is the most common offender but the bumblebee, wasp, hornet, and yellow jacket may also cause reactions. Hymenoptera sensitivity is estimated to result in 40 deaths annually in this country and the incidence of serious allergy is estimated at 1 to 10:100,000. Allergy with few exceptions involves type I reactions and may be manifest as urticaria, angioedema, asthma, or systemic anaphylaxis. Death usually results from cardiovascular collapse and/or respiratory failure and typically occurs within *one hour* following the sting.

Atopic individuals appear more likely to develop hymenoptera sensitivity but the majority of reactions are seen in those without atopy. Serious reactions may occur in individuals without a history of sensitization but they are more common in those who have previously exhibited an exaggerated local or systemic reaction following a sting. It is of the utmost importance that sensitive individuals be aware of their problem and understand preventive measures and emergency procedures. *Emergency kits* are available for the treatment of hymenoptera sensitivity in the field. These and the services that can be rendered by the community pharmacist are discussed by Sadik and Delafuente (1982).

Diagnosis of insect allergy is usually self-evident but problems may arise in identifying the insect. *Cross-sensitivity* among hymenoptera is common but by no means absolute and species-specific allergens are important. Very little is known about the chemistry of hymenoptera allergens but it has been suggested that phospholipase A may be a major allergen of honeybee venom.

Both sensitivity testing and immunotherapy have been commonly recommended and employed in the control of hymenoptera sensitivity. Unfortunately, the products used have nearly always been *whole-body extracts* and the reliability of these is now being seriously questioned. The newer venom preparations appear to be a definite improvement for both diagnosis and therapy but even here additional work is required to develop reliable methods of standardization.

Fire-ant allergy is being reported with increasing frequency. The fire ant has now spread over thirteen southern states and is particularly a problem along the Gulf coast. It is a member of the hymenoptera and causes similar allergic reactions but its allergens appear to differ considerably from those of other stinging insects. Skin-testing with whole-body extracts appears to be reliable for the determination of sensitivity and early reports on immunotherapy are encouraging.

Allergic reactions have been attributed to many *biting insects* including the mosquito, chigger, flea, louse, bedbug, kissing bug, and many flies. The majority of the reactions have been localized, with both the immediate- and delayed-types been reported. The pathogenesis of most of these sensitivities remains to be verified but since many appear to be cellular-mediated type IV reactions it is not surprising that the limited information on sensitivity testing and immunotherapy is contradictory.

Allergic rhinitis and asthma can develop after *inhalation* of scales, hairs, or other emanations of various insects. This is analogous to the allergy seen with common inhalants but most often is seen in individuals who by reason of occupation or hobby are exposed to large numbers of insects. The caddis fly, mayfly, and aphid occur in large numbers in some locales and have been most frequently implicated. Allergenic extracts for a number of these have proven to be effective for skin test diagnosis and may be of value for immunotherapy (see Table VIII).

Food Extracts

Various food products are the most common *ingestant allergens*. Food allergy may seem simple but, in fact, is an extremely complex clinical entity. One problem stems from the tendency of many to attribute virtually any gastrointestinal disturbance of unknown etiology to "food allergy." Gastrointestinal disturbance may arise from many causes, including enzyme deficiencies (lactose intolerance), intoxications, infections, and others. Also, food allergy may and often is manifest outside the GI tract. The indiscriminate use of the term "food allergy" is to be strongly condemned.

Food allergy may occur at any age but is most common in infancy and may be related to an underdeveloped GI system. Most individuals may eventually "outgrow" the allergy and only occasionally does it persist into adult life. This transitory nature of food allergy makes it difficult to assess therapy. The overall incidence is hard to estimate but allergy to cow's milk is probably most common and occurs in less than 1% of infants. Food allergy may be responsible for an amazing array of symptoms including rhinitis, urticaria, asthma, systemic anaphylaxis, GI disturbances, headache, and others.

The nature of most food allergens is unknown but it is clear that many may not be present in fresh foods but are products of digestion or food processing. Allergenic extracts are usually prepared from fresh or freeze-dried foods and many contain primary irritants which are not easily removed. Because of the many variables in food allergy it is difficult to generalize on the efficacy of food extracts for diagnosis. Some are of proven efficacy while others are ineffective and many are of uncertain status. In any case diagnosis does depend heavily upon a detailed history along with the use of *elimination* and *challenge test diets*. While simple in principle, test diets require much patient education and cooperation and are often difficult to design and interpret.

The therapy of food allergy is often more difficult than the diagnosis. Elimination of the offending food(s) is about the only effective therapy but it is often hard to design a nutritious and palatable diet when multiple and/or common allergens are involved (eg, corn, milk, eggs, wheat). Immunotherapy is very difficult to assess for reasons noted above and therapeutic food extracts are not used as routinely as those of inhalant allergens.

Food allergy may involve food additives in addition to the natural allergens. Tartrazine dye (FDC Yellow No 5) is perhaps the best known food (and drug) additive that may cause rhinitis, urticaria, asthma and anaphylaxis. In spite of these typically allergic manifestations this appears to be a *pharmacologic response* related to intolerance to aspirin and nonsteroidal anti-inflammatory drugs. *Idiosyncrasy* to these compounds is seen mainly in individuals with *intrinsic* rhinitis, asthma or urticaria, rather than in atopics. It is also interesting that these individuals may occasionally be intolerant to *natural salicylates* and *benzoates* which occur in many foods, especially fruits. Under the circumstances it is quite understandable that these idiosyncrasies are mistaken for allergies but the distinction between the two fundamentally different mechanisms has important implications in the control of these reactions.

Of all of the allergies to environmental substances, food allergy is probably the most similar to *drug allergy*. Foods and drugs are the most common *ingestants* and may, in fact, share common allergens (eg, flavoring agents, preservatives, dyes, etc). It is clear that the pharmacist must be concerned with more than simply the patient's drug regimen.

Table IX—Food Allergen Extracts

Dairy

Casein	Lactalbumin	Milk, Goat
Cheese (9)	Milk, Cow	Whey (Cow)

Meats

Beef	Liver, Beef	Rabbit
Lamb	Pork	Venison

Poultry

Chicken	Egg, Whole	Goose
Duck	Egg, White	Turkey
	Egg, Yolk	

Fruits & Vegetables

Apple	Fig	Pear
Apricot	Grape	Pepper
Artichoke	Grapefruit	Pepper, Cayenne
Asparagus	Horseradish	Pepper, Bell
Avacado	Leek	Pineapple
Banana	Lemon	Plum/Prune
Beans (7)	Lentil	Potatoes (3)
Beet	Lettuce	Pumpkin
Berries (9)	Lime	Radish
Black-eyed Peas	Mangoes	Rhubarb
Cabbage Family (4)	Melons (5)	Rutabaga
Carrot	Nuts (10)	Spices (29)
Celery	Okra	Spinach
Cherry	Olive	Squash Mixtures
Coconut	Onion	Tangerine
Cranberry	Orange (3)	Tomato
Cucumbers	Papaya	Turnip
Date	Pea	Watercress
Eggplant	Peach	Watermelon
Endive	Peanut	

Miscellaneous

Arrowroot	Coffee	Sugar, Beet
Cascara Bark	Gelatin	Sugar, Cane
Chewing Gum Base	Honey	Tapioca
Chicory	Licorice	Tea
Chocolate	Maple Syrup/Sugar	Vanilla
Cola	Mushroom	Yeast (3)
	Psyllium Seed	

The products listed in Table IX illustrate the wide variety of foods that may be implicated in allergic disease. Because of the large number of individual extracts available, the list has been abbreviated by simply listing the number of products in several major groups (numbers in parenthesis following a food group).

Patch-Testing Materials

Contact dermatitis is a term that has been used in two main ways: first, to describe any rash resulting from a substance touching the skin and second, as a synonym for *allergic contact dermatitis*. The latter is used in present context and refers to eczematous lesions resulting from cellular-mediated type IV reactions analogous to tuberculin sensitivity (Chapter 73). Similar clinical manifestations may occur by other mechanisms: *primary irritant dermatitis*, from direct chemical irritation; *photocontact (phototoxic) dermatitis*, which requires light to generate the irritant; and *photoallergic dermatitis*, which requires light to generate the allergen. These are not necessarily independent for a number of contact allergens may also be irritants but allergic reactions generally occur with lower concentrations of the offending agent. A variety of other conditions must also be differentiated from contact dermatitis (eg, atopic dermatitis, dermatomycoses) and virtually any disease of the skin may result in increased response to both contact irritants and allergens.

Contact sensitivity is a common problem but the incidence and causes vary in different populations. The overall socioeconomic impact is great for it is a leading cause of *industrial illness*. The list of common contact allergens below illustrates the problem of contact sensitivity. Particularly notable are the *drugs and drug additives* which laymen may not recognize as constituents of drug products. The pharmacist should assist the sensitive patient with both drug selection and avoidance.

The likelihood of developing contact sensitivity depends on both the characteristics of the allergen and the individual. Dinitrochlorobenzene (DNCB), for example, will induce sensitivity in nearly everyone and has been used to evaluate the status of cellular-mediated immunity. The oleoresins of poison ivy are also strong sensitizers. However, sensitization is in part genetically determined for about 5% of the population cannot be sensitized to DNCB and others are easily sensitized even to weak allergens. This susceptibility is not related to atopy although atopic individuals are more likely to show topical sensitization of the immediate type. Also, individuals with atopic dermatitis or other skin conditions may be more readily sensitized and exhibit more pronounced reactions. This should be kept in mind when recommending topical medications.

The diagnosis of contact dermatitis depends mainly on a detailed history and complete physical examination. The area of the body affected is suggestive of the contactant and other factors (eg, light, dermatophytes). The patch test is presently the only practical way to demonstrate contact sensitivity (see *Sensitivity Testing*). The patch test may be used for the following purposes: to verify clinically diagnosed contact sensitivity; to determine the specific allergens including those that may not have been clinically suspected; as a predictive test to determine what the patient can safely tolerate; and to exclude contact dermatitis in puzzling clinical situations.

The therapy of contact dermatitis involves most importantly avoidance of the contactant. Cool compresses and topical steroids are the mainstay of therapy but systemic steroids may be employed for serious cases. Other topical medications should be avoided since they may contain irritants or sensitizers.

Immunotherapy has been often attempted for contact dermatitis and other delayed hypersensitivities. Oral im-

Table X—Patch-Testing Products

Plant Oleoresins

Bermuda Grass	Dog Fennel	Ragweed, Giant & Short
Birch	Douglas Fir/Hemlock	1:20
Burweed Marshelder	English Ivy	Redwood
1:20	Fleabane	Sagebrush
Carrot	Geranium	Sneezeweed 1:20
Cedar/Juniper	Goldenrod	Spruce
Cedar Mix	Jonquil/Daffodil	Sweet Clover
Celery	Lettuce	Sweetgum
Chicory	Mahogany, Honduras	Tansy
Chrysanthemum	Maple, Hard	Timothy Grass
Cocklebur	Oak Mix	Tomato
Crabgrass	Pine Mix	Walnut, Black
Dahlia	Poison Ivy/Oak Mix	Wild Feverfew 1:20
Dandelion	1:50	Yarrow
	Ragweed, False 1:20	

Chemicals Test Set

Acrylic Monomer 10%	Naphthyl Mix (Rubber)
Balsam of Peru 25%	Neomycin Sulfate 20%
Benzocaine 5%	Nickel Sulfate 2.5%
Benzyl Alcohol 5%	Nitrofurazone 0.2%
Caine Screening Mix	Paraben, Benzyl 3%
Captan 1%	Paraben, Butyl 3%
Cinnamic Alcohol 5%	Paraben, Ethyl 3%
Cinnamic Aldehyde 2%	Paraben, Methyl 3%
Coal Tar 5%	Paraben, Propyl 3%
Cobalt Sulfate 2.3%	Paraben Screening Mix
Diaminodiphenylmethane 0.5%	p-Chlor-m-xylenol (PCMX) 2%
Dibucaine Hydrochloride 1%	Potassium Dichromate 0.5%
Dichlorophen 1%	PPD Mix (Black Rubber Mix)
Epoxy Resin 1%	p-Phenylenediamine 1%
Ethylenediamine Dihydrochloride	p-$tert$-butylphenol 2%
1%	Quaternium-15 2%
Formaldehyde 2%	Rubber Screening Mix
Hexachlorophene 1%	Tetramethylthiuram Disulfide 2%
Hydroxycitronellal 4%	3,4,4'–TCC 1%
Imidazolidnyl Urea 2%	Thiuram Mix (Rubber)
Iodochlorohydroxyquin 3%	Tribrominated Salicylanilide 1%
Lanolin 100%	Triethylenetetramine 0.5%
Meda Screening Mix	Tripelennamine Hydrochloride 2%
Mercaptobenzothiazole 2%	Turpentine 10%
Mercapto Mix (Rubber)	Wool Wax Alcohols 30%
Mercuric Chloride, Ammoniated	Petrolatum Control
1%	
Methapyrilene Hydrochloride 1%	

Vehicle Sensitivity Series

Benzalkonium Chloride 0.01%	Paraben Mix 15% (3% ea Ethyl,
2-Bromo-2-Nitropropane-1,3-Diol	Methyl, Butyl, Benzyl, Propyl)
0.25%	p-Chloro-m-Xylenol (PCMX) 2%
Chlorocresol 2%	Phenylmeruric Acetate 0.05%
Dichlorophen 1%	Propylene Glycol 10%
Ethylenediamine Dihydrochloride	Quaterium-15 2%
1%	Sorbic Acid 5%
Formaldehyde 2%	Thimerosal 0.1%
Hexachlorophene 1%	Tincture of Benzoin 10%
Imidazolidinyl Urea 2%	Wool Wax Alcohols 30%
Isopropyl Myristate 2%	Petrolatum Control
Lanolin 100%	

munotherapy appears to be effective for poison ivy and several other plant oleoresins but injection therapy is not recommended because of frequent adverse reactions. When desensitization is achieved it is nearly always partial and temporary. Several products are available for the immunotherapy of *rhus dermatitis* (poison ivy, oak, sumac) and other plant oleoresins for treatment may be special-ordered. The following should be considered in the use of these products: avoidance is the treatment and immunotherapy should be attempted only in severe cases when exposure is unavoidable; hyposensitization requires several months, is only partial, and lasts only several months; patients with active dermatitis should not be treated; and immunotherapy is not without risk

of both local and systemic reactions. These products for delayed hypersensitivity differ from other allergenic extracts both in route of administration (oral or IM) and vehicle (fixed oil or alcohol).

The following plant oleoresins and chemicals for patch-testing (Table X) are available from Hollister-Stier Laboratories. The products are supplied in a petrolatum vehicle and the plant oleoresins are 1:10 dilutions except where noted otherwise.

Veterinary Allergenic Products

Veterinary allergy is an emerging field and pharmacists involved in animal health can expect increasing activity in this area. The general principles of immunology and allergy noted earlier apply for the most part to animals as well. Veterinary pharmaceuticals are controlled by the US Department of Agriculture (USDA) but the products are essentially analogous to the human products described in this chapter.

Canine Allergic Inhalant Dermatitis is one of the most common and widely studied of the animal allergies. It is a IgE-mediated immediate (type I) hypersensitivity which is illustrative of the close relationship of animal and human allergy. Canine Inhalant Dermatitis is a hereditary hypersensitivity to environmental allergens such as pollens (tree, grass, weed), molds, epidermals, house dust, etc. Symptoms may be seasonal or perennial and include primarily *pruritis* with associated scratching, footlicking, and face rubbing. Sneezing, rhinitis, and conjunctivitis may be present.

Canine Inhalant Dermatitis usually appears at one to three years of age and diagnosis is similar to that of human allergies including intradermal skin testing with allergenic extracts. The symptoms respond to corticosteroids. Immunotherapy is claimed to control the disease without steroids in up to 50% of the afflicted animals and to permit steroid dosage reduction in others. Unfortunately about 25% are reported to be unresponsive to immunotherapy. However, the reader is reminded that the evaluation of the safety and effectiveness of veterinary allergenic extracts is subject to similar problems as that of human products.

Bibliography

Food and Drug Administration: Licensing; Reclassification Procedures to Determine That License Biologicals are Safe, Effective, and Not Misbranded Under Prescribed Recommended or Suggested Conditions of Use, *Federal Register 47*: 44062, 1982.

Fregert S, Bandman HJ: *Patch Testing*, Springer Verlag, New York, 1975.

Fudenberg HH, *et al*: *Basic and Clinical Immunology*, Lange, Los Altos, CA, 1982.

Hunter RB, Osterberger DJ: Role of the Pharmacist in an Allergy Clinic, *Am J Hosp Pharm 32*: 392, 1975.

Marsh DG: Allergens and the Genetics of Allergy, in Sela M, ed: *The Antigens*, vol 3, Academic Press, New York, 1975.

Middleton E, *et al*, eds: *Allergy: Principles and Practice*, 2 vols, Mosby, St. Louis, 1978.

Nelson R: *Pollen Guide for Allergy*, Hollister-Stier Labs, Spokane, WA, 1975.

Nesbit, GH: Canine Allergic Inhalent Dermatitis: A Review of 230 Cases, J AM Vet Med Assoc 172: 55, 1978.

Panel on Review of Allergenic Extracts, *Final Report*, Publication No. PB-81-182115, US Department of Commerce National Technical Information Service, Springfield, VA, 13 March 1981.

Rose NR, Friedman H, eds: *Manual of Clinical Immunology*, Am Soc for Microbiol, Washington, DC, 1976.

Sadik F: Insect Sting and Bite Products, in *Handbook of Nonprescription Products*, APhA, Washington, DC, 1977.

Samter M, ed: *Hypersensitivity to Drugs*, International Encyclopedia of Pharmacology and Therapeutics, vol 1, Pergamon Press, New York, 1972.

PART 8

Pharmaceutical Preparations and Their Manufacture

Robert E King, PhD

Professor of Industrial Pharmacy
Philadelphia College of Pharmacy and Science
Philadelphia, PA 19104

CHAPTER 76

Preformulation

Louis J Ravin, PhD

Assistant Director, Pharmaceutics Department, SmithKline Beckman Corporation
Philadelphia, PA 19101

The attention presently being given to multi-sourced pharmaceutical products regarding their equivalency places much emphasis on the formulation of these products. In some instances, the bioavailability of a drug formulation represents a quality parameter of enormous proportions. It is a matter of record that with certain drugs, depending on the formulation, the rate at which the drug substance becomes available can vary significantly from very high to none at all. As a result, the effectiveness of these formulations will range dramatically from that expected to no effect. Unfortunately, most examples are less dramatic and fall somewhere in between. The difference in the bioavailability of these drug products is less readily discernible, but none the less real. This has led to a great deal of confusion and information which, though understood by the scientist, is unclear and jumbled to the practitioner. That information which is available also has been interpreted differently by different individuals or groups, depending very often on the motivation, viewpoint, and attitude of the interpreter.

The fact of the matter is that drug products do indeed vary in their bioavailability characteristics and this variation, in most instances, is related directly to formulation considerations. To optimize the performance of drug products it is necessary to have a complete understanding of the physical-chemical properties of drug substances prior to formulating them into drug products. The development of an optimum formulation is not an easy task and many factors readily influence formulation properties. Drug substances are rarely administered as chemical entities, but are almost always given in some kind of formulation. These may vary from a simple solution to a very complex drug delivery system. The complexity usually is not intentional, but rather is determined by the properties that are expected from or built into the dosage form and by the resulting composition that is required to achieve these qualities.

The high degree of uniformity, the physiological availability, and the therapeutic quality expected of modern medicinal products usually are the results of considerable effort and expertise on the part of the formulating pharmacist. These qualities are attained by careful selection and control of the quality of the various ingredients employed, by appropriate manufacturing according to well-defined processes and, most important, by adequate consideration of the many variables that may influence the composition, stability, and utility of the product. In dealing with the formulation of new products it has become necessary to apply the best research methods and tools in order to develop, produce, and control the potent, stable, and effective dosage forms which make up our modern medical armamentarium.

The pharmaceutical formulator has need for specialized areas of science in order to acquire scientific information about the drug substance which is necessary to develop an optimum dosage form. We are in an era in the pharmaceutical industry where we can no longer rely on past experience to formulate. We must have a thorough understanding of the physical-chemical properties as well as the pharmacokinetic and biopharmaceutical behavior of each drug substance being de-

veloped. In short, we must learn as much as possible about the drug substance very early in its development. This requires an interdisciplinary approach at the preformulation stage of development. Fig 76-1 depicts a schematic diagram which indicates that the development of any drug product requires a multidisciplinary approach involving basic science during the preformulation stage followed by applied science during the development stage.

This chapter will discuss the physical-chemical evaluation that takes place during the preformulation stage of development. In addition, consideration will be given to some specialized formulation ingredients that may require discretion in their selection.

Preformulation may be described as a stage of development during which the physical pharmacist characterizes the physical-chemical properties of the drug substance in question which are considered important in the formulation of a stable, effective, and safe dosage form. Such parameters as crystal size and shape, pH-solubility profile, pH-stability profile, polymorphism, partitioning effect, drug permeability, and dissolution behavior are evaluated. During this evaluation possible interactions with various inert ingredients intended for use in the final dosage form are also considered. The data obtained from this evaluation are integrated with data obtained from the preliminary pharmacologic and biochemical studies and provide the formulating pharmacist with information that permits selection of the optimum dosage form containing the most desirable inert ingredients for use in its development.

Preformulation work is usually initiated after a compound has shown sufficient activity to merit further testing in humans. When this decision is made, the various disciplines begin to generate data essential for properly evaluating the performance of the drug substance. A stability-indicating analytical assay method is very important. Since this often takes considerable time, it is sometimes necessary to rely on thin-layer chromatographic procedures to determine if a drug molecule is degrading. Accelerated testing procedures are utilized to promote breakdown of the compound being tested. Attempts are made to isolate and characterize the breakdown products in order to identify the mechanism of breakdown.

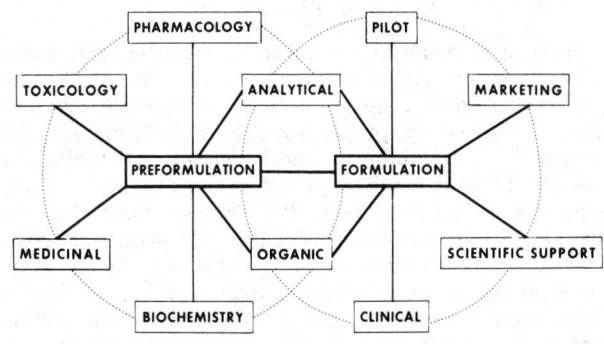

Fig 76-1. The wheels of product development.

This information provides a lead to the development pharmacist in his efforts to formulate the product.

During a preformulation study it is necessary to maintain some degree of flexibility. Problem areas must be identified early. For example, selection of a suitable salt form is critical. Toxicity studies are usually scheduled early. Consequently, if the salt form under consideration has some deficiencies they should be pointed out so that alternate salts may be prepared and evaluated prior to beginning toxicity studies.

When preformulation studies are initiated, the chemical is usually in short supply. Twenty-five grams of chemical is an ample supply, but many preliminary evaluations have been done with less. The initial supply usually originates as excess from batches prepared by the medicinal chemists. They usually have preliminary data such as melting point, spectral data, and structure of the compound. The direction taken for the evaluation is determined by the structure and the intended dosage forms to be developed. For example, one would not waste time determining the stability of a solution of a compound if there was no interest in a liquid dosage form. Many areas must be critically evaluated for each compound, and it is essential that problem areas be identified early, otherwise delays could occur if a problem surfaced during the development phase for the compound. Some consequences of poor preformulation work are: (1) possible use of unsatisfactory salt form; (2) poor stability of the active ingredient; (3) testing compound of marginal activity; (4) increased development costs; (5) increased development time. When preformulation studies are completed, the data are compiled and transferred to the development pharmacist, who, in turn, utilizes this information to plan his development work on the finished dosage forms.

Physical Properties

Description

Since chemical is in short supply at the outset of most preliminary evaluations, it is extremely important to note the general appearance, color, and odor of the compound. These characteristics provide a basis for comparison with future lots. During the preparation of scale-up lots the chemist usually refines or alters the original chemical synthetic route. This sometimes results in a change in some of the physical properties. When this takes place, comparisons can be made with earlier lots and decisions made regarding solvents for recrystallization.

Taste usually warrants some consideration, especially if the drug is intended for oral use in pediatric dosage forms. In such cases consideration should be given to the preparation of alternate salt forms or possible evaluation of excipients that mask the undesirable taste.

Microscopic Examination

Each lot of chemical, regardless of size, is examined microscopically and a photomicrograph taken. The microscopic examination gives a gross indication of particle size and characteristic crystal properties. These photomicrographs are useful in determining the consistency of particle size and crystal habit from batch to batch, especially during the early periods of chemical synthesis. If a synthesis step is changed, they also give an indication of any effect the change may have on crystal habit. One must keep in mind that the photomicrograph only gives a qualitative indication of particle size distribution; it is always necessary to do a particle size analysis for a more accurate picture of the distribution of particles in any particular batch of chemical.

Particle Size

The uses of pharmaceutical products in a finely divided form are diverse. From knowledge of their particle size, such drugs as griseofulvin, nitrofurantoin, spironolactone, procaine penicillin, and phenobarbital have been formulated so as to optimize activity. Other drugs, formulated in suspension or emulsion systems, in inhalation aerosols, and in oral dosage forms, may contain finely divided material as an essential component. One of the basic physical properties common to all these finely divided substances is the particle size distribution, ie, the frequency of occurrence of particles of every size. What is of practical interest is usually not the characteristics of single particles but rather the mean characteristics of a large number of particles. It must be emphasized, however, that knowledge of size characteristics is of no value unless adequate correlation has been established with functional properties of specific interest in the drug formulation. Many investigations demonstrating the significance of particle size are reported in the literature. It has been shown that dissolution rate, absorption rate, content uniformity, color, taste, texture, and stability are dependent to varying degrees on particle size and distribution. In preformulation work it is important that the significance of particle size in relation to formulation be established early. Preliminary physical observations can sometimes detect subtle differences in color. If this can be attributed to differences in particle size distribution it is important to define this distribution and recommend that more attention be given to particle size in preparing future batches of chemical. This effect is also evident when preparing suspensions of poorly soluble materials. One may observe batch-to-batch differences in the color of a suspension which can be related to differences in particle size. Sometimes, when small particles tend to agglomerate, a subtle change in color or texture may be evident.

Sedimentation and flocculation rates in suspensions are in part governed by particle size. In concentrated deflocculated suspensions the larger particles exhibit hindered settling and the smaller particles settle more rapidly. In flocculated suspensions, the particles are linked together into flocs which settle according to the size of the floc and porosity of the aggregated mass. Flocculated suspensions are preferred since they have less tendency to cake and are more rapidly dispersible. Thus it is apparent that the ultimate height, H_u, of sediment as a suspension settles depends on particle size. The ratio H_u/H_o or the degree of suspendibility as affected by particle size is valuable information for the formulator in order to prepare a satisfactory dosage form.

The rate of dissolution of small particles is usually faster than that of larger ones because rate of dissolution is dependent on the specific surface area in contact with the liquid medium. This is usually described by the modified Noyes-Whitney equation for dissolution rate dA/dt.

$$\frac{dA}{dt} = KS(C_s - C)$$

where A is the amount of drug in solution, K is the intrinsic dissolution rate constant, S is the surface area, C_s the concentration of a saturated solution of the drug, and C is the drug concentration at time t. The surface area of an object, regardless of shape, varies inversely with its diameter and confirms the above effect of particle size on dissolution rate. Solubility has also been observed to be dependent on particle size. Dittert et al[1] reported data for an experimental drug, 4-acetamidophenyl 2,2,2-trichloroethyl carbonate, which demonstrated that the dissolution rate and in turn bioavailability were affected by particle size. Although the ultimate amount of drug in solution may not be significant with respect to the dose administered, the formulator should be aware of this potential. With poorly soluble drugs it is extremely important that these factors be taken into account during the design of the dosage form.

Flow properties of drugs can be influenced by particle size, and particle size reduction to extremely small sizes (less than 10 μm) may be inadvisable for some drug substances. Entrapped air adsorbed on the surface of the particles and/or surface electrical charges sometimes impart undesirable properties to the drug. For example, adsorbed air at the drug-particle surface may prevent wetting of the drug by surrounding fluid, and electrically induced agglomeration of fine particles may decrease exposure of the drug surface to surrounding dissolution medium. Such effects act as dissolution rate-limiting steps since they minimize maximum drug surface-liquid contact.

Crystal growth is also a function of particle size. Finer particles tend to dissolve and subsequently recrystallize and adhere to larger particles. This phenomenon is referred to as *Ostwald ripening*. Protective colloid systems can be utilized to suppress this nucleation. Preformulators can generate information concerning the effectiveness of different colloids that is extremely important to the formulator when he is given the task of preparing a suspension dosage form.

Particle size reduction may be deleterious for some drug substances. Increasing surface area by milling or other methods may lead to rapid degradation of a compound. Drug substances may also undergo polymorphic transformation during the milling process. The preformulator must always be cognizant of these potential problems and whenever the decision is made to reduce particle size, the conditions must be controlled and the stability profile evaluated. If a problem does arise, it is the responsibility of the preformulator to note it and attempt to resolve it prior to turning the drug substance over to the formulating pharmacist.

Gastrointestinal absorption of a poorly soluble drug may be affected by the particle size distribution. If the dissolution rate of the drug is less than the diffusion rate to the site of absorption and the absorption rate itself, then the particle size of the drug is of great importance. Smaller particles should increase dissolution rate and thus bring about more rapid gastrointestinal absorption. One of the first observations of this phenomenon was made with sulfadiazine. Blood-level determinations showed that the drug in suspension containing particles 1 to 3 μm in size was absorbed more rapidly and more efficiently than from a suspension containing particles 7 times larger. Maximum blood levels were about 40% higher and occurred 2 hours earlier. Increased bioavailability with particle size reduction has also been observed with griseofulvin. The extent of absorption of an oral dose increased 2.5 times when the surface area was increased approximately six-fold. Micronized griseofulvin permits a 50% decrease in dosage to obtain a satisfactory clinical response.

On the other hand it was found that with nitrofurantoin there was an optimal average particle size that minimized side effects without affecting therapeutic response. In fact a commercial product containing large particles is available. For chloramphenicol, particle size has virtually no effect on total absorption but it significantly affects the rate of appearance of peak blood-levels of the drug. After administration of 50-μm particles, as well as 200-μm particles, peak levels occurred in 1 hour; with 400-μm particles peak levels occurred in 2 hours; with 800-μm particles peak levels occurred in 3 hours. All four preparations had the same physiological availability, which implies that the absorption of chloramphenicol occurs uniformly over a major portion of the intestinal tract.

Reduction of particle size may also create adverse responses. For example, fine particles of the prodrug trichloroethyl carbonate were more toxic in mice than regular and coarse particles.[2] Increasing the surface area for water-soluble drugs and possibly for weakly basic drugs appears to be of little

value. Absorption of weak bases is usually rate-limited by stomach emptying time rather than by dissolution. As previously mentioned, particle size is of importance only when the absorption process is rate-limited by the dissolution rate in gastrointestinal fluids.

We have been discussing the effect of particle size of the drug substance and its relationship to formulation. The particle size of the inert ingredients merits some attention. When one is concerned with particle size all ingredients utilized in preparing the dosage form should be evaluated and some recommendation regarding their control should be made prior to full-scale development of a dosage form. It is highly recommended that particle size and its distribution be determined, optimized, monitored, and controlled when applicable, particularly during early preformulation studies when the decision is made with regard to a suitable dosage form. The more common methods of determining particle size of powders used in the pharmaceutical industry include sieving, microscopy, sedimentation, and stream scanning.

Sieving or Screening—Sieving or screening is probably one of the oldest methods of sizing particles and is still commonly using to determine the size distribution of powders in the size range of 325 mesh (44 μm) and greater. These data usually serve as a rough guideline in evaluating raw materials with regard to the need for milling. The basic disadvantages of screen analysis are the large sample size required and the tendency for blinding of the screens due to static change or mechanical clogging. The advantages include simplicity, low cost, and little skill requirement.

Microscopy—Microscopy is the most universally accepted and direct method of determining particle-size distribution of powders in the subsieve range. The method is tedious and time-consuming. The preparation of the slide for counting particles is important because the sample must represent the particle size distribution of the bulk sample. Extreme care must be taken in obtaining a truly representative sample from the bulk chemical. The cone and quartering technique usually gives a satisfactory sample. The sample should be properly suspended, dispersed, and thoroughly mixed in a liquid which has a different refractive index from the particles being counted. A representative sample is mounted on a slide having a calibrated grid. For counting, random fields are selected on the slide and the particles are sized and counted. Between 500 and 1000 particles should be counted to make statistical treatment of the data meaningful.

Sedimentation—Sedimentation techniques utilize the dependence of velocity of fall of particles on their size. Application is made of the Stokes equation (see page 314) which describes a relationship between the rate at which a particle settles in a fluid medium to the size of that particle. Although the equation is based on spherical-shaped particles, it is widely used to determine the weight-size distribution of irregularly-shaped particles. Data obtained by this procedure are usually reliable; however, the result may not agree with those obtained by other methods because of the limitations of the shape factor.

The *Andreasen Pipette Method* is most commonly used for sedimentation studies. Exact volumes are withdrawn at prescribed times and at a specified liquid depth. The liquid is evaporated and the residue of powder is weighed. The data are utilized in the Stokes equation and a weight-size distribution is calculated. Precautions must be observed with this method. Proper dispersion, consistent sampling, temperature control of the suspending medium, and concentration should be achieved in order to obtain consistent results.

Stream Scanning—Stream scanning is a technique in which a fluid suspension passes through a sensing zone where the individual particles are electronically sized, counted, and tabulated. The great advantage of this technique is that data can be generated in relatively short periods of time with rea-

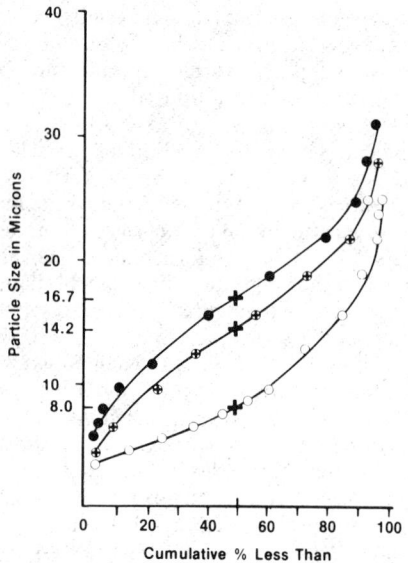

Fig 76-2.   Particle size distribution of NBS glass beads expressed in terms of O = number of particles; ● = weight of particles; ⊗ = surface area of particles.

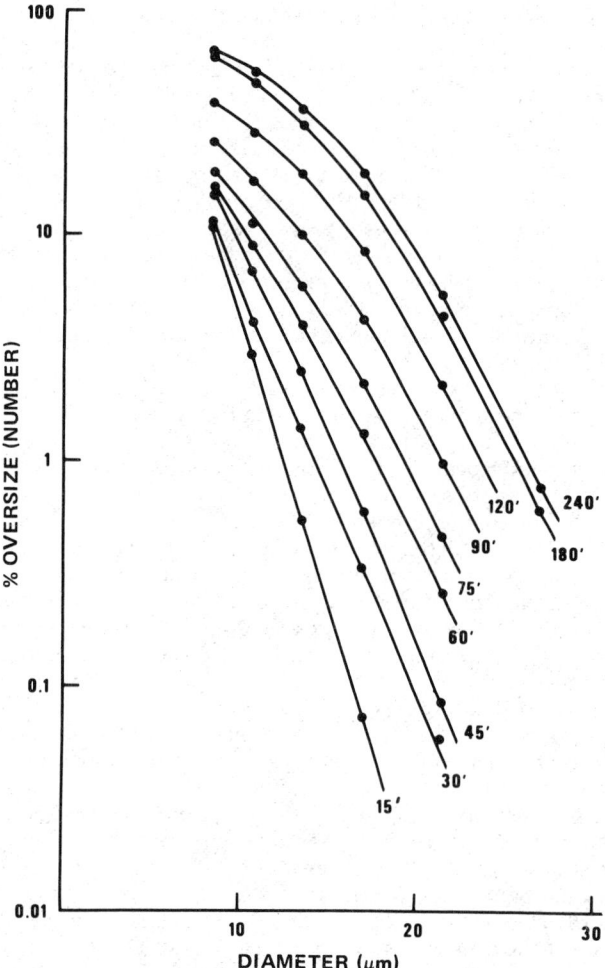

Fig 76-3.   Change in particle size with time for an aqueous suspension of Form I of experimental drug.

sonable accuracy. Literally thousands of particles can be counted in seconds and used in determining the size distribution curve. The data are in a number of particles per class interval and can be expressed mathematically as the arithmetic mean diameter and graphed accordingly. Fig 76-2 illustrates a plot of typical data obtained for NBS Standard Reference Material No 1003.

The *Coulter Counter* and the *HIAC Counter* are widely used in the field of particle size analysis in the pharmaceutical industry. They can be used to follow crystal growth in suspensions very effectively. Fig 76-3 shows the change in particle size with time for an aqueous suspension of Form I of an experimental drug. It appears that the growth of the particles decreases significantly after six hours. The photomicrograph shown in Fig 76-4 depicts the significant increase in particle size after six hours. Further treatment of the data as shown in Fig 76-5 enables one to establish rates of growth for suspended particles. Simply reading off the intercepts at the 1%, 2% or 3% oversize and plotting this increase in diameter with time enables one to calculate the rate of growth of particles in a suspension. This is shown in Fig 76-6.

Partitioning Effect

If an excess of liquid or solid is added to a mixture of two immiscible liquids, it will distribute itself between the two phases so that each becomes saturated. If the substance is added to the immiscible solvents in an amount insufficient to saturate the solutions it will still distribute between the two layers in a definite concentration ratio. If C_1 and C_2 are the equilibrium concentrations of the substance in solvent 1 and solvent 2 the equilibrium expression becomes

$$\frac{C_1}{C_2} = k$$

The equilibrium constant k is known as the distribution ratio or partition coefficient. Biologically, in order for a pharmacological response to occur it is necessary that the drug molecule cross a biological membrane. The membrane, consisting of protein and lipid material, acts as a lipophilic barrier to most drugs. The resistance of this barrier to drug transfer is related to the lipophilic nature of the molecule involved. (See Chapter 37, on *Drug Absorption, Action, and Disposition*.)

Understanding the partitioning effect and the dissociation constant enables one to estimate the site of absorption of a new chemical entity. If one assumes the stomach to have a pH range of 1.0 to 3.0 and the small intestines to have a pH range from 5 to 8, in most cases acidic drugs (pK_a 3) will be more rapidly absorbed in the stomach while more basic drugs (pK_a 8) will be absorbed more rapidly in the intestinal tract. There are, however, exceptions. Some compounds have low partition coefficients and/or are highly ionized over the entire physiological pH range, but still show good bioavailability.

Polymorphism

A polymorph is a solid crystalline phase of a given compound resulting from the possibility of at least two different arrangements of the molecules of the compound in the solid state. The molecule itself may be of different shape in the two polymorphs, but that is not necessary and indeed, certain changes in shape involve formation of different molecules and hence do not constitute polymorphism. Geometric isomers or tautomers, even though interconvertible and reversibly so, cannot be called polymorphs although they may behave in a confusingly similar manner.

A safe criterion for classification of a system as polymorphic is the following: Two polymorphs will be different in crystal structure but identical in the liquid or vapor states. Dynamic isomers will melt at different temperatures, as do polymorphs, but will give melts of different composition. In time each of these melts changes to an equilibrium mixture of the two isomers with temperature-dependent compositions. Some reported cases of polymorphism are undoubtedly dynamic isomerism, since the two behave quite similarly.

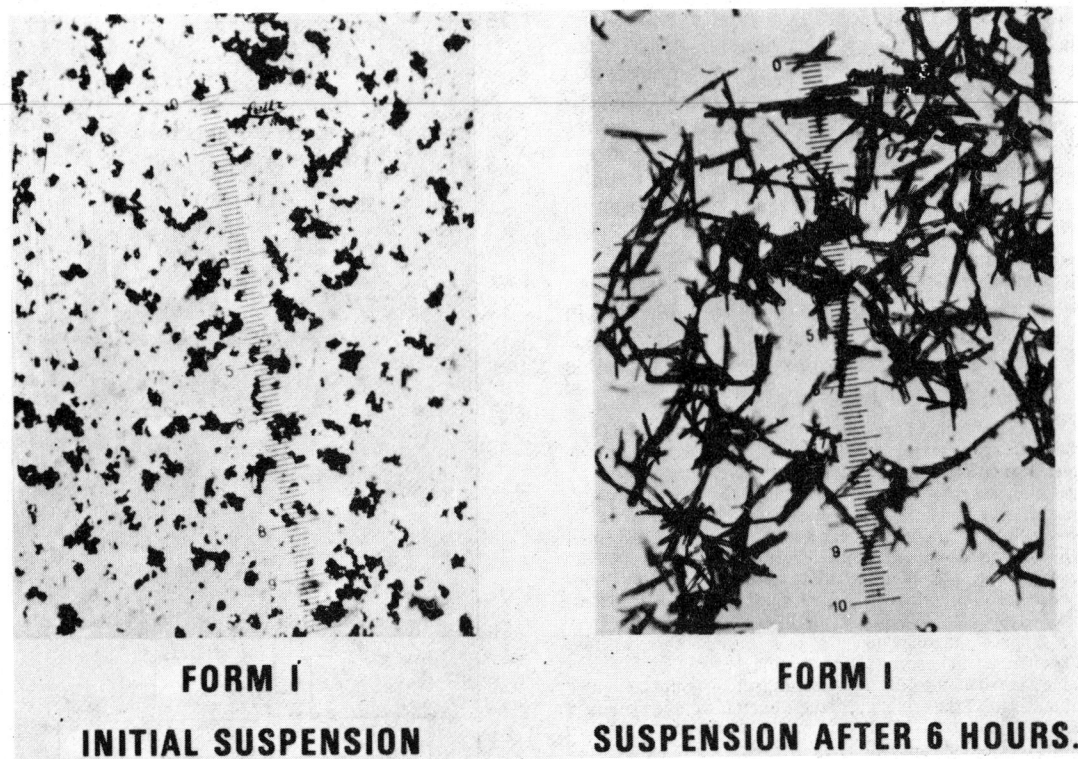

FORM I
INITIAL SUSPENSION

FORM I
SUSPENSION AFTER 6 HOURS.

Fig 76-4.   Photomicrographs showing change in crystal size for a suspension of Form I of experimental drug.

Polymorphism is the ability of any element or compound to crystallize as more than one distinct crystalline species, eg, carbon as a cubic diamond or hexagonal graphite. Different polymorphs of a given compound are, in general, as different in structure and properties as the crystals of two different compounds. Solubility, melting point, density, hardness, crystal shape, optical and electrical properties, vapor pressure, stability, etc. all vary with the polymorphic form. In general, it should be possible to obtain different crystal forms of a drug substance and thus modify the performance properties for that compound. To do so requires a knowledge of the behavior of polymorphs. There are numerous reviews on the subject of polymorphism. In addition, numerous indications of the importance of polymorphism in pharmaceuticals are reported in the literature. The work of Kuhnert-Brandstatter *et al* with steroids, barbiturates, and antihistamines probably represents the most intensive study of polymorphism and drugs. In England, Mesley et al, using infrared spectroscopy described the polymorphism of steroids, barbiturates, and

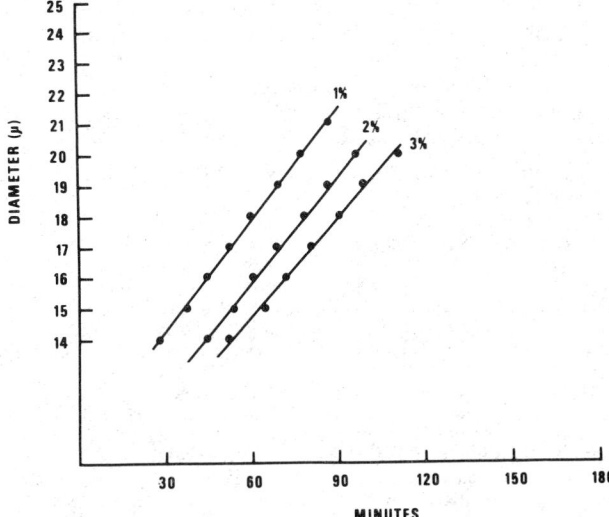

Fig 76-5.   Change in cumulative count with time for an aqueous suspension of Form I of experimental drug.

Fig 76-6.   Rate of growth of Form I of experimental drug in aqueous suspension.

sulfonamides. Preformulation studies usually include rigorous studies to determine the presence of polymorphs in new drug substances being prepared for preliminary investigation in test animals. Some of the parameters routinely investigated are the number of polymorphs that exist, relative degree of stability of the various polymorphs, presence of a glassy state, stabilization of metastable forms, temperature stability ranges for each polymorph, solubilities, method of preparation of each form, effect of micronization or tableting, and interaction with formulation ingredients.

The initial task of the preformulator is to determine whether or not the drug substance being evaluated exists in more than one crystalline form. The following procedures are usually followed to cause crystallization of a metastable form:[3]

(a) Melt completely a small amount of the compound on a slide and observe the solidification between crossed polars. If, after spontaneous freezing, a transformation occurs spontaneously or can be induced by seeding or scratching, the compound probably exists in at least two polymorphic forms. It is essential to prevent nucleation of the stable form by inducing supercooling. Supercooling can be induced by using a small sample size, by holding the melt for approximately 30 seconds about 10° above the melting point; by carefully setting aside the compound without physical shock before observing it; and by rapid cooling of the compound.

(b) Heat a sample of the compound on a hot stage and observe whether a solid–solid transformation occurs during heating.

(c) Sublime a small amount of the compound and attempt to induce a transformation between the sublimate and the original sample by mixing the two in a drop of saturated solution of one of them. If the two are polymorphs, the more stable one will be more insoluble and will grow at the expense of the more soluble metastable form. This process will continue until the metastable form is completely transformed to the stable form. If the samples are not polymorphs, one may dissolve but the other will not grow. If the two are identical forms nothing will occur.

(d) Maintain an excess of the compound in a small amount of solvent held near the melting point of the compound. Isolate the suspended solid. Care should be taken to maintain the temperature during this step. Test the isolated material with an original sample using the procedure outlined in (c).

(e) Recrystallize the compound from solution by shock-cooling, and observe a portion of the precipitated material suspended in a drop of the mother liquor. The drop may then be seeded with the original compound to check for solution phase transformation. If the precipitate is a different polymorph, a solution phase transformation should take place.

Once it has been established that polymorphism occurs there are procedures which enable the preformulator to prepare the various forms in larger quantities for further evaluation and suitability for incorporation into dosage forms.

Once a compound has been shown to exist in more than one crystalline form, a number of techniques are available to identify the different polymorphic phases present. Each of these techniques could be successful in identifying the phase, but a combination of methods provides a means for isolation and identification of each crystalline modification. In order to confirm the presence of more than one crystalline form of a compound it is advisable to identify the modifications present by more than one method. Using only one method for confirming the presence of polymorphs may sometimes be misleading.

Microscopy—Optical crystallography is used in the identification of polymorphs. Biles in his review of crystallography discusses this application. Crystals exist in isotropic and anisotropic forms. When isotropic crystals are present the velocity of light is the same in all directions while anisotropic crystals have two or three different light velocities or refractive indices. This method requires the services of a trained crystallographer.

Hot-Stage Methods—The polarizing microscope fitted with a hot or cold stage is very useful for investigating polymorphs. An experienced microscopist can quickly tell whether polymorphs exist; the degree of stability of the metastable forms; transition temperatures and melting points; rates of transition under various thermal and physical conditions and whether to pursue polymorphism as a route to an improved dosage form. Kodlers and McCrone discuss these methods in detail.

X-Ray Powder Diffraction—Crystalline materials in powder form give characteristic X-ray diffraction patterns made up of peaks in certain positions and varying intensities. Each powder pattern of the crystal

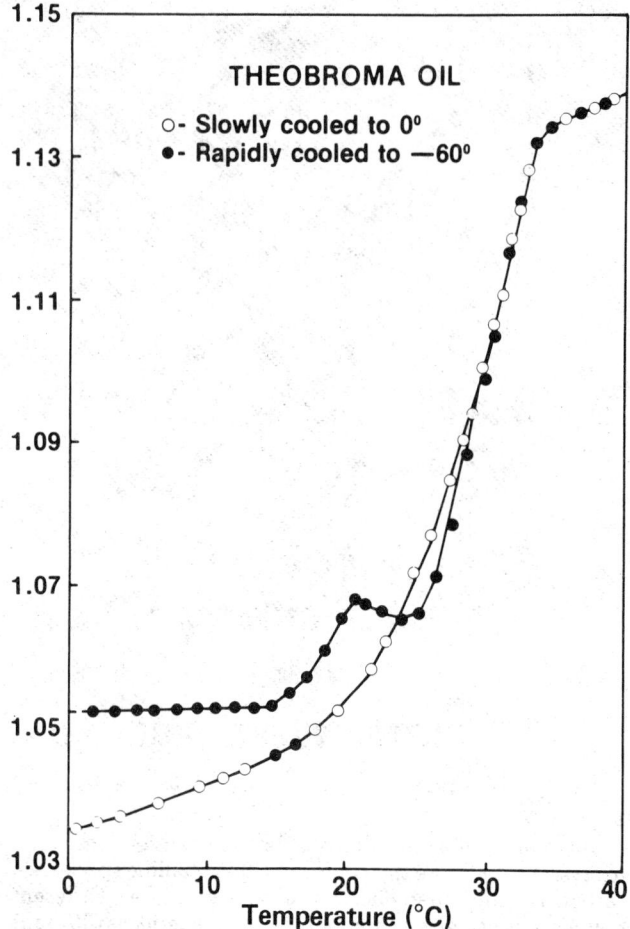

Fig 76-7. Dilatometric curves, theobroma oil, slowly and rapidly cooled.

lattice is characteristic for a given polymorph. This method has the advantage over other identification techniques in that the sample is examined as presented. Some care should be exercised in reducing and maintaining particle size control. A very small sample size is needed and the method is nondestructive. This method has been used by several investigators in identifying polymorphs in pharmaceuticals.

Infrared Spectroscopy—This procedure is useful in identification of polymorphs. Solid samples must be used since polymorphs of a compound have identical spectra in solution. The technique can be used for both qualitative and quantitative identification.

Thermal Methods—Differential scanning calorimetry and differential thermal analysis have been used extensively to identify polymorphs. In both methods, the heat loss or gain resulting from physical or chemical changes occurring in a sample is recorded as a function of temperature as the substance is heated at a uniform rate. Enthalpic changes, both endothermic and exothermic, are caused by phase transitions. For example, fusion, sublimation, solid–solid transition, and water loss generally produce endothermic effects while crystallization produces exothermic effects. Thermal analysis enables one to calculate the thermodynamic parameters for the systems being evaluated. Guillory obtained the heats of fusion for sulfathiazole and methylprednisolone. Ravin et al. utilized differential scanning calorimetry to follow the rate of conversion of sulfathiazole polymorphs.

Dilatometry—Dilatometry measures the change in volume caused by thermal or chemical effects. Ravin and Higuchi[4] utilized dilatometry to follow the melting behavior of theobroma oil by measuring the specific volume of both rapidly and slowly cooled theobroma oil as a function of increasing temperature. The presence of the metastable form was shown by a contraction in the temperature range of 20° to 24°. This is illustrated in Fig 76-7. Dilatometry is extremely accurate; however, it is extremely tedious and time-consuming. It is not widely used.

Proton magnetic resonance, nuclear magnetic resonance and electron microscopy are sometimes used to study polymorphism.

Polymorphs can be classified into one of two types: (1) Enantiotropic—one polymorphic form can be reversibly

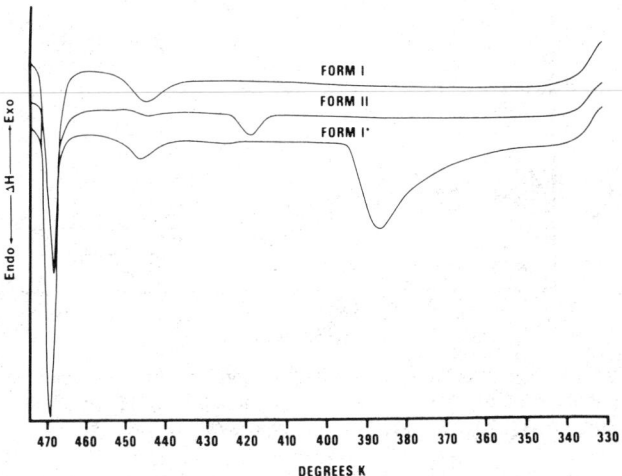

Fig 76-8.   Thermograms for Forms I, I* and II of SK&F 30097.

changed into another one by varying the temperature or pressure, eg, sulfur. (2) Monotropic—one polymorphic form is unstable at all temperatures and pressures, eg, glyceryl stearates. At a specified temperature and pressure only one polymorphic form will be thermodynamically stable. However, other metastable forms may exist under the same conditions. These metastable forms will convert to the stable lattice structures with time. The first indication of the significance of a polymorphic transformation in a pharmaceutical system was noted with novobiocin. The amorphous form of novobiocin was found to be well absorbed; however, when formulated into a suspension a reversion of the metastable form to the more stable crystalline form occurred resulting in poor absorption.

After it has been determined that a drug substance does exist in more than one crystalline form, the conditions under which each can be produced should be established. In this manner, proper crystallizing conditions can be maintained from batch to batch to ensure a uniform and acceptable raw material. Recrystallization solvent, rate of crystallization, and other factors may cause one crystal form to dominate. During the preliminary investigation to establish these conditions it is necessary to monitor the forms prepared. For example, during the preliminary work with an indole derivative, differential scanning calorimetry, X-ray analysis, and infrared analysis were utilized to establish that polymorphs were present and that they could be prepared satisfactorily. Figs 76-8, 76-9, and 76-10 show the respective data for this conclusion. When polymorphs are shown to be present, experiments should be designed to determine whether or not the properties differ sufficiently to alter their pharmaceutical or biological behavior.

Dissolution tests can be utilized initially to show differences in apparent equilibrium solubilities provided a discriminating solvent system is utilized. Fig 76-11 illustrates dissolution data for two polymorphs of an indole derivative which had similar dissolution in the medium used; however, when a more discriminating dissolution medium was used it was possible to show differences in their dissolution characteristics. This is illustrated in Fig 76-12. From the data presented for the indole derivative it was concluded that there would be no appreciable difference in the availability of the two forms if they were to be administered orally in a solid dosage form. Subsequent testing in animals confirmed this. The Nernst equation relates the rate of concentration increase to the solubility of a dissolving solid and is commonly written as:

$$\frac{dc}{dt} = \frac{AD}{Vh}(C_s - C_t)$$

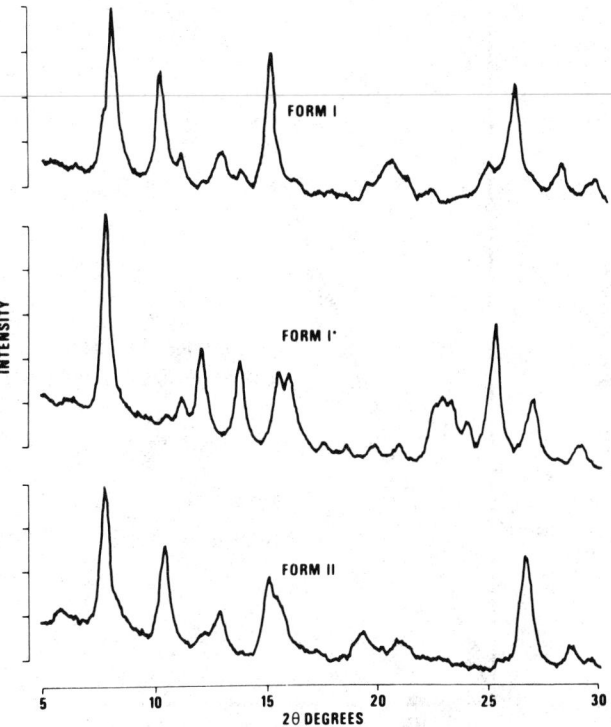

Fig 76-9.   X-Ray diffractograms for Forms I, I* and II of SK&F 30097.

where A is the area of the dissolving interface of the solid, D is the diffusion coefficient of the solute in the solvent, V is the volume of the solvent, h is the thickness of the diffusion layer and C_s and C_t are concentration of the solute at saturation and at time t respectively. The equation reduces to:

$$\frac{dc}{dt} = \frac{AD}{Vh}C_s$$

for the experimental conditions where $C_s > C_t$. Since D is a property of the solute molecule and the solvent, it is independent of the solid state form. The experimental conditions can be selected such that A, V and h can be maintained constant in measuring the dissolution rates of different polymorphic forms. The dissolution rate is then directly pro-

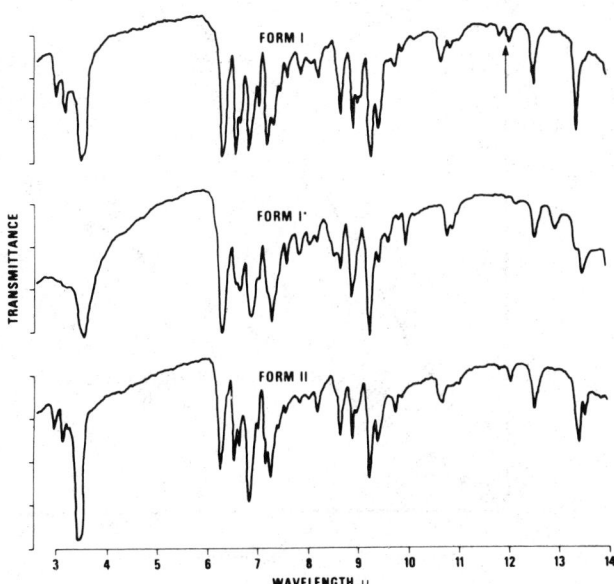

Fig 76-10.   Infrared spectra of Forms I, I* and II of SK&F 30097.

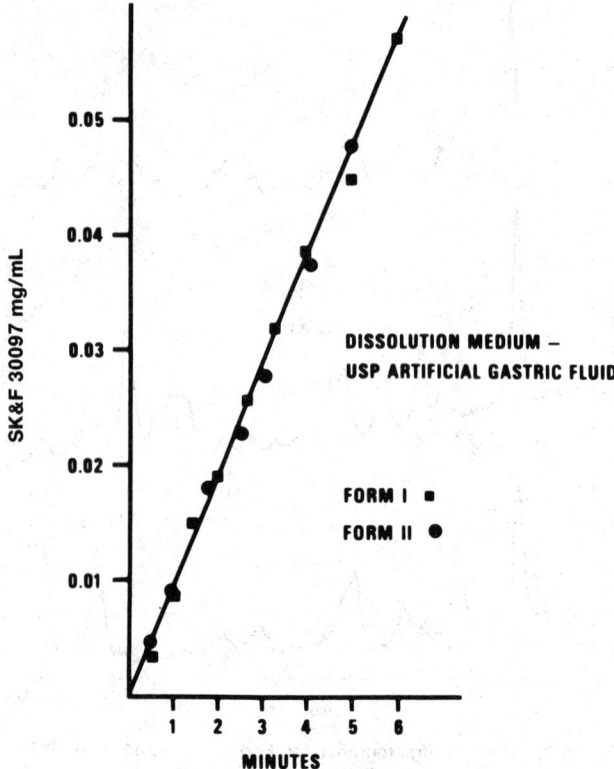

Fig 76-11.   Dissolution behavior of Forms I and II of SK&F 30097 in artificial gastric fluid.

portional to C_s, the saturation solubility and the differences in the solubilities can be related to their free energies.

The solubility and dissolution behavior of several polymorphs of chloramphenicol palmitate have been determined. Figs 76-13 and 76-14 illustrate the data obtained at several temperatures.   It is apparent from the dissolution behavior

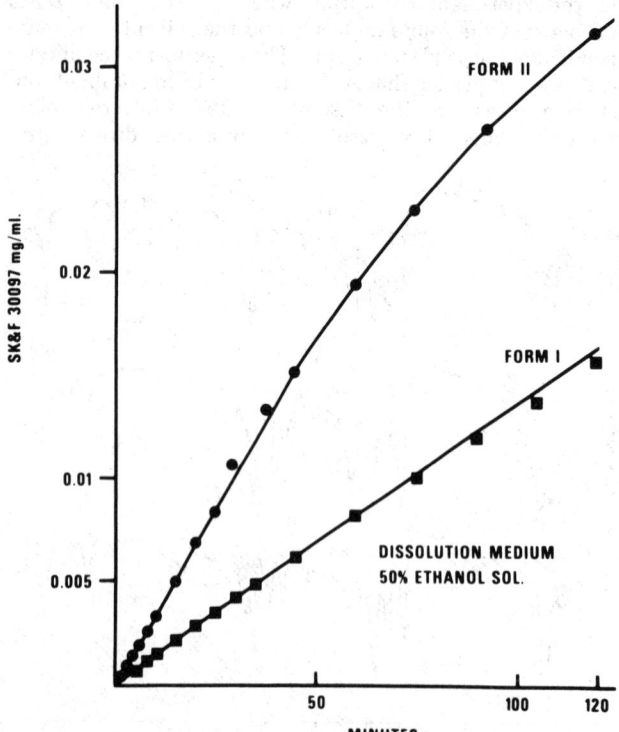

Fig 76-12.   Dissolution behavior of Forms I and II of SK&F 30097 in 50% ethanol solution.

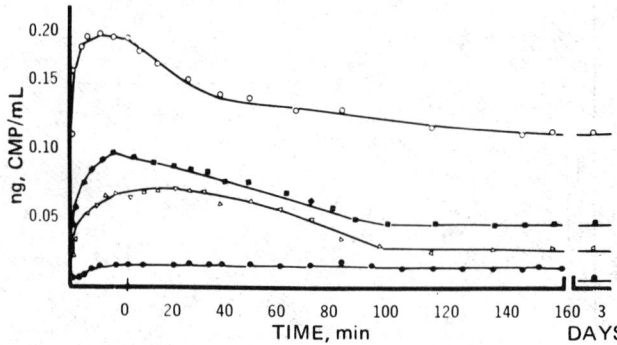

Fig 76-13.   Dissolution curves for Polymorph C of chloramphenicol palmitate in 35% t-butyl alcohol and water at 30, 20, 15 and 6°. Key: 30°, O—O; 20°, ■—■; 15°, Δ—Δ; 6°, ●—●.

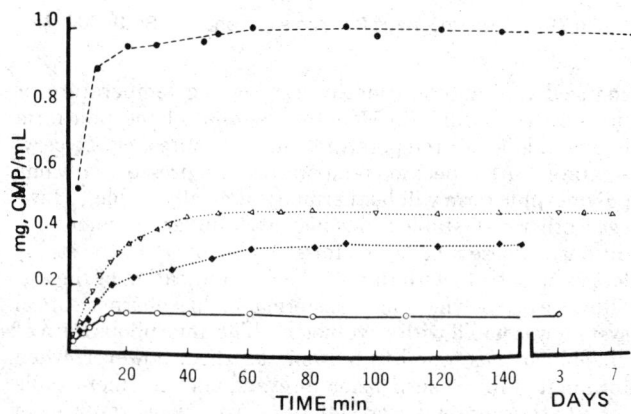

Fig 76-14.   Dissolution curves for Polymorphs A and B of chloramphenicol palmitate in 35% t-butyl alcohol and water at 30 and 38°. Key: Polymorph A, 30°, O—O: Polymorph B, 30°, Δ...Δ; Polymorph A, 38°, ◆- - -◆: Polymorph B, 38° ●- - -●.

that the maximum values obtained were good approximations of the solubility of the various forms.   Therefore obtaining data at several temperatures would enable one to calculate the thermodynamic quantities involved in the transition from the metastable to the stable form.   A plot of the solubility data as a function of temperature in a typical van't Hoff fashion is shown in Fig 76-15.   The straight-line relationship enables one to calculate the heats of solution for the various forms and also by extrapolation to approximate the transition temperatures for the various forms.   These values are shown in Table I.[5]

At constant temperature and pressure, the free energy differences between the polymorphs can be calculated by:

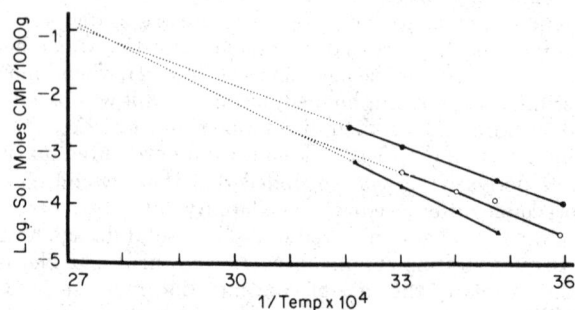

Fig 76-15.   The van't Hoff type plot for Polymorphs A, B, and C of chloramphenicol palmitate.   Key: Polymorphs A →; B ●—●; and C O—O.

Table I—Thermodynamic Values Calculated for Polymorphs A, B, and C of Chloramphenicol Palmitate

Poly- morph	Transi- tion Temp. (°C.) to Form A	Heat of Solution, kcal./mole	ΔG_T, cal./mole[a]	ΔS_{303} e.s.u.	ΔS_{trans} e.s.u.[a]
A	—	21.8	—	—	—
B	88	15.4	−774	−18	−17
C	50	17.2	−465	−13	−14

[a] Calculated for the conversion to Polymorph A.

$$\Delta G_t = RT \ln \frac{C_s \text{ Polymorph A}}{C_s \text{ Polymorph B}}$$

This equation relates the solubility, C_s, of the polymorphic forms at a particular temperature, T, to the free energy differences, ΔG_t. Table I also contains the free energy differences calculated for the polymorphs. The enthalpy changes can also be determined for the various transitions by subtracting the heat of solution derived for the stable form from that of the metastable form. Also at any particular temperature, T, the entropy for the transition of polymorphs can be evaluated by the following relationship:

$$\Delta S_t = \frac{\Delta H_{B \rightarrow A} - \Delta G_t}{T}$$

The values computed for the transitions are also included in Table I. At the transition temperature the ΔG_t is equal to zero and the entropy can be calculated neglecting the free energy term in the above equation.

The thermodynamic relationships discussed are based on the assumption that Henry's Law is obeyed. Knowledge of these thermodynamic relationships enables the preformulator to select more rationally the more energetic polymorphic form of the drug being investigated for further pharmacological studies and also to have a preliminary assessment of its probable stability.

When a preformulation group inadequately investigates polymorphic drug forms, problems may develop during the development stage. Crystal growth in suspensions resulting in poor uniformity, poor appearance, poor bioavailability, transformation occurring during milling or granulation resulting in changes in the physical and biological characteristics, inadequate pharmacologic response, and poor chemical stability are typical problems that will become evident.

Solubility

In dealing with new drug substances, it is extremely important to know something about their solubility characteristics, especially in aqueous systems since they must possess some limited aqueous solubility to elicit a therapeutic response. When a drug substance has an aqueous solubility less than 1 mg/mL in the physiologic pH range (1–7), a potential bioavailability problem may exist and preformulation studies should be initiated to alleviate the problem. Equilibrium solubility of the drug substance should be determined in a solvent or solvent system which does not have any toxic effects on the test animal. This is done by placing an excess of drug in a vial with the solvent. The vial is agitated at constant temperature and the amount of drug determined periodically by analysis of the supernatant fluid. Equilibrium is not achieved until at least two successive samples have the same result. Experience with solubility determinations would indicate that equilibrium is usually attained by agitating overnight (approximately 24 hours). Solubility determinations

can be conducted at several temperatures since the resultant drug products will ultimately be subjected to a wide variation in temperature.

If the solubility of the drug substance is less than the required concentration necessary for the recommended dose, steps must be taken to improve its solubility. The approach taken will usually depend on the chemical nature of the drug substance and the type of drug product desired. If the drug substance is acidic or basic, its solubility can be influenced by pH. Through the application of the Law of Mass Action, the solubility of weakly acidic and basic drug substances can be predicted as a function of pH with a considerable degree of accuracy, utilizing the following equations for the weakly acidic and basic drugs.

Weak Acid

$$S_t = K_s \left(1 + \frac{K_a}{[H^+]}\right)$$

Weak Base

$$S_t = K_s \left(1 + \frac{[H^+]}{K_a}\right)$$

There are many drug substances for which pH adjustment does not provide an appropriate means for effecting solution. Very weakly acidic or basic drugs may require a pH that may be outside the accepted tolerable physiological range or may cause stability problems with formulation ingredients. For example, an experimental indole had an equilibrium solubility at pH 1.2 of approximately 50 mg/mL. However, when the pH of this system was increased to approximately 2.0 the solubility decreased to less than 0.1 mg/mL. In cases like this one or with nonelectrolytes, it is necessary to utilize some other means of achieving better solubility.

Cosolvent systems have been utilized quite effectively to achieve solubility for poorly soluble drug substances under investigation. Propylene glycol, glycerin, sorbitol, and polyethylene glycols have enjoyed a wide range of success in this area. They have been very useful and generally acceptable for improving solubility. Additional solvents, such as glyceryl formal, glycofurol, ethyl carbonate, ethyl lactate, and dimethylacetamide have been cited in a review article by Spiegel and Noseworthy,[6] however, it must be emphasized that with the possible exception of dimethylacetamide all of these solvents have not been utilized in oral products and their acceptability may be doubtful. The number of vehicles readily available to improve solubility is rather limited yet the frequency of their use is rather high. Solubilizing a new drug substance can improve its availability. For example, when a triazinoindole was administered in a 0.02% solution it showed an equivalent response in antiviral activity to a 2.5% suspension. Information generated early in the preformulation stage can result in a refinement of the dosage regimen and allow for a more accurate estimation of the effective dose.

Cosolvents usually serve a two-fold purpose in many pharmaceutical liquid products. Not only do they effect solution of the drug substance but also they improve the solubility of flavoring constituents added to the product. Ideally in determining the appropriate ratio of cosolvents to achieve the concentration one must achieve, it is recommended to effect solution at the concentration desired and then place the solution at 5° and allow it to equilibrate. If precipitation occurs under these conditions it may be necessary to alter the cosolvent ratio.

Use of surfactants of various types—nonionic, cationic, anionic—as solubilizing agents for medicinal substances is widespread (see Chapter 20, on *Colloidal Dispersions*, page 297, for illustrations of specific uses). The effect of Triton WR-1339 in solubilizing several steroids is shown in Fig 76-16.[7] The effect of an anionic, a cationic, and a nonionic surfactant on the solubility of an antianginal compound being considered for clinical trials is shown in Fig 76-17. From such data investigators may be guided in selecting solubilizing

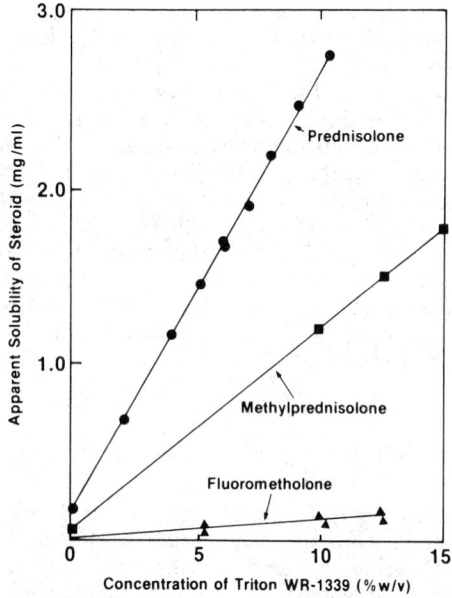

Fig 76-16.   The effect of varying concentrations of Triton WR-1339 in water on the solubility of some anti-inflammatory steroids.

agents for use in preparations to be studied in humans, but it must be emphasized that the acceptability of a particular solubilizing agent is dependent also on other factors that determine its suitability for the intended use. For example, surfactants are known to interact with some preservatives and thereby decrease preservative action, for which reason the preformulator should always recommend some type of biological test to demonstrate that the activity of the drug substance being studied is not reduced when it is solubilized by a surfactant.

Complexation phenomena can sometimes be utilized to impart better solubility characteristics. However, the degree of association and the extent to which solubility can be increased is generally not adequate for use in pharmaceutical

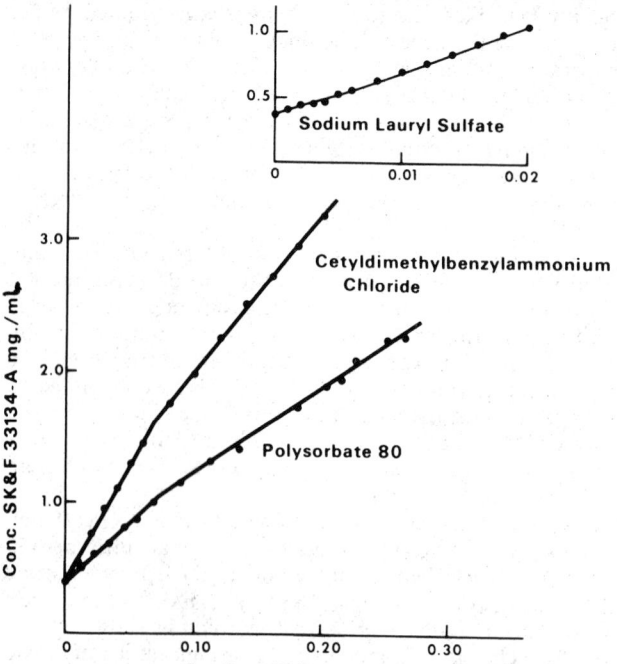

Fig 76-17.   Effect of surfactant concentration on the solubility of SK&F 33134-A.

products. In addition, many complexing agents have physiological activity. The most noteworthy example of the utility of complexation to enhance solubility is the PVP-iodine complex. Hydrotropy can sometimes be utilized to enhance solubility. High concentrations of urea, salicylates, and xanthines have been used successfully on several occasions. Again, the concept is available but the increase in solubility normally observed is not adequate for use in pharmaceutical products.

Salt Formation

Salt-forming agents are often chosen empirically by the pharmaceutical chemist primarily on the basis of the cost of raw materials, the ease of recrystallization, and the percentage yield. Unfortunately there is no reliable way of predicting the influence of a particular salt species on the behavior of the parent compound in dosage forms. Furthermore, even when many salts of the basic compound have been prepared there are no effective screening techniques which make the selection process of the salt an easier task for the pharmacist. The basic considerations which may have some influence on salt selection are physical and chemical stability, hygroscopicity, flowability, and solubility.

The number of salt forms available to the chemist is large. Table II lists the cations and anions present in FDA-approved

Table II—FDA-Approved Commercially Marketed Salts.

Anion	Percent[a]	Anion	Percent[a]
Acetate	1.26	Iodide	2.02
Benzenesulfonate	0.25	Isethionate[i]	0.88
Benzoate	0.51	Lactate	0.76
Bicarbonate	0.13	Lactobionate	0.13
Bitartrate	0.63	Malate	0.13
Bromide	4.68	Maleate	3.03
Calcium edetate	0.25	Mandelate	0.38
Camsylate[b]	0.25	Mesylate	2.02
Carbonate	0.38	Methylbromide	0.76
Chloride	4.17	Methylnitrate	0.38
Citrate	3.03	Methylsulfate	0.88
Dihydrochloride	0.51	Mucate	0.13
Edetate	0.25	Napsylate	0.25
Edisylate[c]	0.38	Nitrate	0.64
Estolate[d]	0.13	Pamoate (Embonate)	1.01
Esylate[e]	0.13	Pantothenate	0.25
Fumarate	0.25	Phosphate/diphosphate	3.16
Gluceptate[f]	0.18	Polygalacturonate	0.13
Gluconate	0.51	Salicylate	0.88
Glutamate	0.25	Stearate	0.25
Glycollylarsanilate[g]	0.13	Subacetate	0.38
Hexylresorcinate	0.13	Succinate	0.38
Hydrabamine[h]	0.25	Sulfate	7.46
Hydrobromide	1.90	Tannate	0.88
Hydrochloride	42.98	Tartrate	3.54
Hydroxynaphthoate	0.25	Teoclate[j]	0.13
		Triethiodide	0.13

Cation	Percent[a]	Cation	Percent[a]
Organic:		Metallic:	
Benzathine[k]	0.66	Aluminum	0.66
Chloroprocaine	0.33	Calcium	10.49
Choline	0.33	Lithium	1.64
Diethanolamine	0.98	Magnesium	1.31
Ethylenediamine	0.66	Potassium	10.82
Meglumine[l]	2.29	Sodium	61.97
Procaine	0.66	Zinc	2.95

[a] Percent is based on total number of anionic or cationic salts in use through 1974.   [b] Camphorsulfonate.   [c] 1,2-Ethanedisulfonate.   [d] Lauryl sulfate.   [e] Ethanesulfonate.   [f] Glucoheptonate.   [g] p-Glycollamidophenylarsonate.   [h] N,N′-Di(dehydroabietyl)ethylenediamine.   [i] 2-Hydroxyethanesulfonate.   [j] 8-Chlorotheophyllinate.   [k] N,N′-Dibenzylethylenediamine.   [l] N-Methylglucamine.

commercially marketed salts of pharmaceutical agents.[8] The monoprotic hydrochlorides have been the most frequent choice of the available anionic salt-forming radicals, while sodium has been the most predominant cation. During preformulation evaluation it is extremely important to establish that the particular salt form in question will have properties that will result in a minimum of problems during the development of the dosage forms. Since toxicity studies are usually initiated soon after a compound has been designated for further studies in man it is important that the salt form selected has been given a critical evaluation to determine whether or not its properties are suitable.

Since physical and chemical stability are vital to any pharmaceutical product it is imperative that the preformulator evaluate both parameters. A systematic determination of the thermal stability, solution stability (at several pH's) and light sensitivity of the drug substance provides essential input toward the selection of the most suitable derivative. Studies are usually initiated early to identify problems. Samples of the salts in question are usually placed under exaggerated conditions of heat and light in the presence and absence of moisture and subsequently analyzed to determine the amount of breakdown. In many instances stability-indicating analytical methods may not be available. In these cases it is necessary to resort to thin-layer chromatography to establish a qualitative assessment of stability. At the same time samples are placed under high-humidity conditions and weighed periodically to determine the degree of hygroscopicity of the compounds. Compounds that have a tendency to adsorb or absorb moisture may present flowability problems during encapsulation.

Solubility characteristics are also evaluated. When a particular salt form has very good solubility (greater than 10%) it is sometimes difficult to prepare a suitable granulation using an aqueous granulating fluid, especially for high doses. Granulations prepared by these methods will not dry satisfactorily or the granulation will not flow uniformly from the hopper, resulting in large weight variation during the compression stage. A critical evaluation of this type with different salt forms has been proven quite effective in enabling the preformulator to make the selection of the salt form of choice for further development.

Chemical Properties

The evaluation of the physical and chemical stability of a new drug substance is an important function of the preformulation group. The initial work should be designed to identify those factors that may result in an alteration of the drug substance under study. The physical pharmacist can initially anticipate the possible type of breakdown that a compound will be subjected to by examination of the chemical structure of the compound. For example, esters and amides are sensitive to hydrolytic degradation while acridanes and catecholamines are sensitive to oxidation degradation. With this preliminary knowledge he can more effectively design his studies to identify the problems early. At this point the primary concern is not the pathway or mechanism of degradation. A stability-indicating method of analysis is usually not available early in the preformulation phase. Techniques such as thin-layer chromatography, diffuse reflectance, and thermal analysis can be utilized to provide data to assess preliminary stability. Sometimes the preliminary evaluation is complicated by the presence of impurities. It is essential that the drug under study be pure before any stability tests are undertaken. The presence of impurities can lead to erroneous conclusions in the preformulation evaluation.

Drug Substance Stability—It is extremely important to determine the stability of the bulk chemical as early as possible. One would hardly expect to prepare stable dosage

forms with a chemical substance that was not stable in the pure state. Samples of the chemical are usually subjected to various conditions of light, heat, and moisture in the presence and absence of oxygen. The chemical is placed in sealed vials with and without moisture and stored at various elevated temperatures which may vary to some degree from laboratory to laboratory. Light sensitivity is measured by exposing the surface of the compound to light. Sunlamps are sometimes used to exaggerate light conditions. Hygroscopicity is evaluated by placing the chemical in open petri dishes at relative humidities from 30 to 100%. The samples are monitored regularly for physical changes, moisture pick-up and chemical degradation.

Most drug substances are either stable at all conditions, or stable under special conditions of handling, or unstable with special handling, or unstable. When drug substances are found to have some stability problems, then it may be important to define the pathway of degradation and initiate studies to stabilize the compound with appropriate additives.

At this point it may be advisable to consider some of the more prominent reactions accounting for instability of new drug substances. Obviously, some compounds will not undergo any appreciable decomposition if kept dry and away from air in a sealed container. We must always assume that the new drug substance is in some kind of formulation environment that may lead to instability problems.

Hydrolytic Degradation—Hydrolysis is probably the degradative process most frequently encountered in the formulation of new drugs. It is safe to assume that most new drugs will be exposed to water at some stage during processing or during storage; hence, hydrolysis may occur unless the conditions are optimum. Hydrolysis occurs with esters, amides, salts of weak acids and strong bases, and thioesters among others. A few drug compounds that undergo hydrolytic degradation are procaine, penicillin, aspirin, and chlorothiazide.

From a kinetic standpoint hydrolysis reactions are second-order reactions because the rate is proportional to the concentration of two reactants. However, in aqueous solutions since water is usually present in excess and at relatively constant concentration, the reactions are treated experimentally as monomolecular or first-order reactions. This simplification permits calculations of the extent of decomposition under precise experimental conditions by less complicated means. Extrapolation of the exaggerated rates to room temperature makes it possible to more expeditiously establish shelf-life stability of potential new drug products.

The rate of hydrolysis can be affected by temperature and by hydrogen or hydroxyl ion concentration when the hydrolytic process is dependent on pH. Fig 76-18 shows the

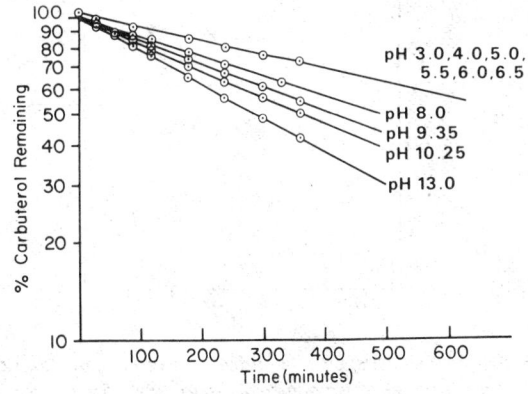

Fig 76-18. Effect of pH on carbuterol degradation at 85° (μ = 0.5).

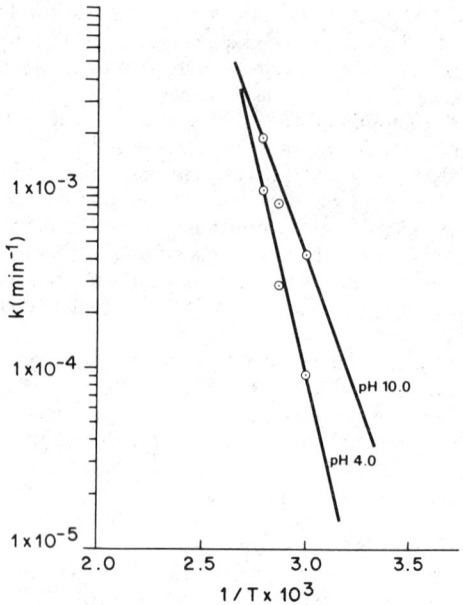

Fig 76-19.   Typical Arrhenius-type plot depicting the temperature dependency of carbuterol hydrolysis at pH 4.0 and 10.0.

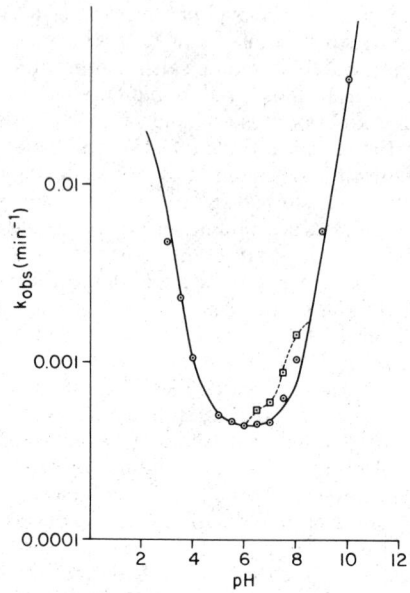

Fig 76-21.   pH-Rate profile of cefazolin degradation in aqueous solution at 60° ($\mu = 0.5$). Solid line: theoretical profile; circles: experimental profile; squares: rates uncorrected for buffer effect.

pseudo-first-order behavior as a function of pH for carbuterol in aqueous solution at constant ionic strength at 85°. The effect of temperature is illustrated in Fig 76-19 for carbuterol at pH 4.0 and 10.0 respectively.[9] When we are concerned with solids, the amount of moisture present is minimal. When a physical pharmacist has a drug substance that undergoes hydrolytic degradation, he usually designs studies to establish the conditions of pH and buffer concentration where minimum decomposition occurs. There is sometimes a wide range of pH adjustment that a drug substance can tolerate. For example, idoxuridine was shown to have maximum stability over a pH range from 2 to 6. Fig 76-20 shows the pH-stability profile.[10] Another drug substance, carbuterol, hydrolyzed by an intra-molecular process showed maximum stability over a wide pH range. Even though these compounds had a wide range of pH for optimum stability in aqueous solution they could not be formulated and provide products with satisfactory shelf lives without special cosolvent systems and/or

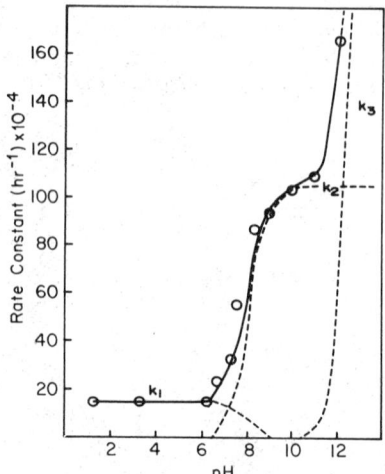

Fig 76-20.   Plot showing pH-rate profile for hydrolysis of idoxuridine at 60°.   Circles represent experimental results.   Solid line corresponds to theoretical pH-rate profile.   Broken line designates contribution of k_1, k_2, and k_3 at any pH value.

special storage conditions. Cefazolin was shown to have a narrow pH range for maximum stability as indicated in Fig 76-21.[11] Buffering aqueous solutions to provide a pH for optimum stability can lead to stability problems. Stability is sometimes affected by buffer concentration, for example, carbuterol stability was shown to be affected by phosphate buffer concentration.

Another manner in which the physical pharmacist can overcome an instability due to hydrolysis is to recommend the preparation of an insoluble salt form or to prepare a solid dosage form. Insoluble chlorothiazide is stable in neutral aqueous suspensions but solutions of the sodium salt at relatively high pH's decompose rapidly. Frequently the replacement of water by some other solvent such as alcohol or the polyhydroxy solvents reduces the hydrolytic rate of degradation for some systems. Acetylsalicylic acid suspensions containing high concentrations of sorbitol improved stability. Ampicillin was also shown to be more stable when the concentration of alcohol was increased. Higuchi and his associates greatly reduced the hydrolytic rate of degradation for aromatic esters by forming molecular complexes.

It has also recently been shown that stability of some compounds may vary depending on whether or not they exist in the micellar or nonmicellar state. Recently Kostenbauder showed a difference in the chemical stability of penicillin that existed in the micellar state from that in the monomeric state.

Oxidation—Oxidative degradation is as important as hydrolysis in the preliminary stability evaluation of new drug substances. Studies should be initiated to establish the oxidative route, then steps should be taken to determine what additives can minimize the degradation. Oxidative degradation is common with many drug compounds. Ascorbic acid, epinephrine, vitamin A, chlorpromazine, isoproterenol, morphine, resorcinol, and unsaturated fats and oils are subject to oxidative degradation. The oxidation reaction depends on several factors, including temperature, oxygen concentration in the liquid, impurities present, and the concentration of the oxidizable component. The temperature effect in solutions is usually minimal; however, in the dry state it is more pronounced since other factors such as moisture dictate its stability behavior.

Initially it is important to establish that oxidation is taking place. Solutions of the drug substance in question are exposed to various exaggerated conditions of light and oxygen tension in amber and flint-glass containers. Samples are analyzed for degradation. When it has been established that the oxidative route is the principal pathway for degradation, appropriate additives are utilized to determine what effect they might have on the stability. pH sometimes is critical since a great number of oxidation-reduction processes depend on the concentration of hydrogen or hydroxyl ions. Light usually accelerates the degradation, thus the storage of products in dark containers does much to preserve stability. Photochemical changes many times involve the formation of other reactive compounds or free radicals which function to propagate the decomposition, once started. Auto-oxidation may occur in the absence of light when susceptible materials such as fats and oils are stored in the presence of air. The auto-oxidation of phenolic compounds is of special significance since compounds such as epinephrine and isoproterenol degrade in this manner. Heavy metal ions, eg, cupric and ferric, accelerate the oxidation of ascorbic acid and the phenothiazines. Frequently only trace quantities of these ions occurring as impurities may be sufficient to cause an increased rate of decomposition. This can be a consistent problem since many of the so-called inert ingredients may have heavy metal contaminants.

The oxygen concentration in solution is a factor in many cases and often depends upon the temperature of storage or the solvent employed. Oxygen is more soluble in water at lower temperatures so that oxygen-dependent reactions can sometimes proceed more rapidly at the lower temperatures. Ascorbic acid is more stable in 90% propylene glycol or in USP syrup than in water, presumably because of the lower oxygen concentration in these vehicles. Oxidative degradation is an extremely complex process since the overall rate is dependent upon several factors. Preparations sensitive to oxidation are sometimes stabilized by effectively removing the oxygen and by the addition of suitable additives. Nitrogen flushing has been utilized successfully for this purpose. A wide variety of reducing agents and compounds to sequester metals and inhibit chain reactions have been employed for stabilization, but relatively few are acceptable for parenteral products. Oftentimes it is necessary to combine ingredients and adjust pH to maximize stability. Detailed kinetic studies have been reported for the oxidative decomposition of prednisolone.

The physical pharmacist has a difficult task with oxidative degradation. He must design experiments initially that will encompass many variables. Preparing samples at several concentrations containing antioxidants plus sequestering agents at several pH levels and placing them in flint or amber containers with and without nitrogen is commonplace procedure. The subsequent evaluation of these limited data is critical. Light-sensitivity studies with several formulations of prochlorperazine resulted in the selection of a stable formula. In a study with idoxuridine it was shown that placing the aqueous solution in an amber container was sufficient to protect the product from oxidative degradation.

Drug Substance–Excipient Interaction—Drug substance–excipient studies are designed to determine a list of excipients that can be used routinely in the final dosage forms. Lactose, sucrose, calcium sulfate, dicalcium phosphate, starch, and magnesium stearate are some of the substances routinely tested in combinations. Some basic observations with the drug substance and/or its salt form can sometimes dictate what excipients can be used. For example, one would not consider using sucrose or lactose if the drug substance being considered is a primary amine. This system has the potential for interaction to form a colored compound readily detected by a color change.

Various means have been utilized for detecting potential interactions and incompatibilities. Diffuse reflectance techniques have been used to detect interactions. This has been done by comparing the spectra obtained initially with those obtained after storage at exaggerated conditions. A shift in absorption has been interpreted as an interaction. Thin-layer chromatography has also been used. When excipients are present it is usually advisable to set a mixture of the excipients at the same conditions as the active mixtures. This will give a comparison of the thin layer of both systems. If any new degradation products are present the source can more easily be determined.

Mixtures containing at least two levels of drug concentration with excipients are sealed in vials containing 5% water in half of the samples. These vials are stored under exaggerated conditions of light and heat for various time periods. The resultant samples are observed physically and analyzed by an appropriate technique to get a qualitative determination. At this point in the stability evaluation, which is a preliminary screening process, it is not necessary to know exactly how much has degraded. It is an all-or-none type effect. The search is for the excipients that have no effect on the stability of the active ingredient.

When solution interactions are being investigated and no incompatibilities are evident, it is wise to recommend an *in vivo* experiment to evaluate availability. On occasion interaction may occur in solution that is not detectable with routine procedures. For example, clindamycin was found to interact with cyclamates and interfere with the absorption of the drug.

Other Changes—Optically active substances may lose their optical activity without a structural change. If the entiomorphic compounds possess different degrees of physiologic action, such changes may result in reduced therapeutic effects. Epinephrine has been shown to undergo racemization under various acidic and basic conditions. Although the potential for this to become evident during a preformulation evaluation is rare, one should always be aware of this possibility. Polymerization is also a remote possibility. Darkening of glucose solution is attributed to polymerization of the breakdown product, 5-hydroxymethylfurfural. Isomerization, which is the process involving the change of one structure into another having the same empirical formula but with different properties in one or more respects, can also occur. Again, the occurrence is rare. Deamination and decarboxylation can sometimes occur. This type of change would be easily detected since the resultant degradation products would have completely different properties.

Permeability

A preformulation evaluation should include studies to assess the passage of drug molecules across biological membranes. These membranes act as lipid barriers to most drugs and permit the absorption of lipid-soluble substances by passive diffusion. Lipid-insoluble substances can cross the barrier only with considerable difficulty. The pH-partition theory explains the interrelationship of the dissociation constant, lipid solubility, pH at the absorption site, and the absorption characteristics of drugs across membranes. The theory has evolved following a series of investigations in laboratory animals and man and is the basis of much of the current understanding of absorption of drugs.

Data obtained from basic physical-chemical studies described earlier may give the preformulation scientist an indication of possible absorption difficulties. Experimental techniques are available that can be utilized to give a more accurate assessment of absorption problems. An *in vitro* system that has been used extensively consists of an aqueous/organic solvent/aqueous system which has the advantage of being simple, allows for accurate pH control, membrane thickness, and other variables. It can be described mathematically in precise terms. However, the interpretation and correlation of data are limited when applied to biological systems.

Another *in vitro* procedure, the everted sac technique, is a simple and reproducible method for determining the absorption characteristics of drugs. Isolated segments of rat small intestines are everted and filled with a solution of the drug being evaluated and the passage of drug through the membrane is determined. This technique has been used to measure the permeability of a number of drug substances.[12] It can also evaluate both passive and active transport of drugs. The fact that the preparation has been removed from the animal and its normal blood supply is a distinct disadvantage.

The *in situ* technique developed by Doluisio, et al[13] for the study of membrane permeability appears to overcome the disadvantages of the everted sac technique. Since the intestine is not removed from its blood supply the results would be expected to be similar to those obtained in intact animals. A disadvantage of the technique is that the procedure does not account for the loss of fluid from the solution by absorption in the intestine. Nonabsorbable markers, ie, phenol red, can be added to the drug solution to solve this problem.

The techniques described can give the preformulation scientist an indication of possible absorption problems or suggest that little or no difficulty will be observed in the passage of a particular drug product throught the biological membranes. This information, along with eventual studies in man, serves to establish possible *in vitro/in vivo* correlation for dissolution and bioavailability. These data are important in establishing quality control specifications for the products which will ensure consistent biological performance from subsequent lots.

Formulation Ingredients

Although preliminary screening of commonly used excipients with new drug substances has become routine in preformulation studies, there are occasions when problems arise because of the interaction with additives such as preservatives, stabilizers, dyes, and possibly flavors. A discussion of some problems that have risen is in order to make formulators aware that they should be concerned about the potential for interaction whenever another ingredient is added to a formulation.

Preservatives—Each time a liquid or semisolid pharmaceutical dosage form is prepared it is necessary to include a preservative in the formulation. Such preservatives as sodium benzoate, sorbic acid and the methyl and propyl esters of *p*-hydroxybenzoic acid have been utilized in these systems for many years. There have been reports that the parabens have been inactivated when used in the presence of various surface-active agents and vegetable gums. This loss of activity might be due to the formation of complexes between the preservative and the surfactant. Kostenbauder utilized a dialysis technique to demonstrate an interaction between polysorbate 80 and the methyl and propyl esters of *p*-hydroxybenzoic acid. This observation becomes critical if the level of preservative added is borderline with respect to the preservative activity threshold. The desired preservative effect may not be achieved unless an excess of the preservative is added to compensate for that which is complexed. It has also been shown that molecular complexes form when the *p*-hydroxybenzoates are mixed with polyethylene glycol, methylcellulose, polyvinylpyrrolidone, and gelatin. The degree of binding was less than that observed with polysorbate 80. Sorbic acid also interacts with the polysorbates but does not interact with the polyethylene glycols. The quaternary ammonium compounds are also bound by polysorbate 80 to

reduce their preservative activity. Benzyl alcohol was also shown to be adsorbed by certain types of rubber stoppers. Subsequent work has shown that butyl rubber does not interact with benzyl alcohol.

Antioxidants—During the preformulation evaluation of compounds that are sensitive to oxidation it is often commonplace to add several levels of antioxidant concentrations to aqueous systems in order to determine the relative effectiveness of the antioxidants. Sodium bisulfite and ascorbic acid are two antioxidants that enjoy widespread usage in pharmaceutical systems. Sodium bisulfite yields a colorless water-soluble salt when it is oxidized. It is also a very reactive ion. It will add to double bonds, react with aldehydes and certain ketones and contributes in bisulfite cleavage reactions. Many of the reactions with bisulfite are irreversible and the resulting sulfonic acids frequently are biologically inactive. Epinephrine has been shown to interact with bisulfite to form a bisulfite addition product. Other sympathomimetic drugs, principally the ortho- or para-hydroxybenzyl alcohol derivatives, also react with bisulfite in a similar manner. The meta-hydroxy alcohol did not react. Sometimes these interactions are reversible as in the case with the adrenocorticosteroid molecules.

Ascorbic acid on the other hand is relatively nonreactive. However, when mixed with compounds having a primary amine nucleus there is the tendency for interaction to form a highly colored Schiff base. One must be aware of this possibility when selecting a suitable antioxidant.

Suspending Agents—Occasionally it will be necessary to consider use of a suspending agent to prepare some preliminary suspension preparations for stability evaluation prior to starting toxicity testing. The physical pharmacist should be aware of the potential for these additives to react with the drug substance being evaluated. Anionic water-soluble compounds such as sodium carboxymethylcellulose, alginic acid, carrageenin and other hydrocolloids, although generally considered inert, frequently interact in solution with drug compounds. Carboxymethylcellulose and carrageenin form complexes or possibly salts with many medicinal agents including procaine, chlorpromazine, benadryl, quinine, chlorpheniramine, neomycin, and kanamycin. In some instances the formation of the complex imparted better stability to the system. When this problem is suspect it is important to conduct appropriate tests to insure that an interaction does not take place in the system being evaluated.

Dyes—Although preformulation tests are usually conducted long before any consideration of coloring the intended dosage forms, they should not be overlooked. Dyes are chemical in nature and contain reactive sites capable of causing incompatibilities. Several studies have demonstrated that certified dyes do react with drug substances. Sugars such as dextrose, lactose and sucrose were found to increase the rate of fading of FD&C Blue #2. Insoluble complexes were also formed when quaternary ammonium compounds were formulated with FD&C Red #1 and Blue #1.

Summary

The preformulation evaluation of new drug substances has become an integral part of the development process. A thorough understanding of the physical-chemical properties of the new drug substance under study provides the development pharmacist with data that are essential in designing stable and efficacious dosage forms. Many of the problems discussed and the solutions offered in this chapter resulted from application of scientific training of present-day pharmaceutical scientists. Their diverse skills, creative aptitudes, and initiative provide the pharmaceutical industry with the essential ingredients to develop drug products that help maintain the health-care process at its highest level of excellence.

References

1. Dittert LW, *et al: J Pharm Sci 57:* 1146, 1968.
2. Dittert LW, *et al: J Pharm Sci 57:* 1269, 1968.
3. Haleblian H, McCrone W: *J Pharm Sci 58:* 911, 1969.
4. Ravin LJ, Higuchi T: *J APhA, Sci Ed 46:* 732, 1957.
5. Aguiar AJ, Zelmer JE: *J Pharm Sci 58:* 983, 1969.
6. Spiegel AJ, Noseworthy MM: *J Pharm Sci 52:* 917, 1963.
7. Guttman DE, *et al: J Pharm Sci 50:* 305, 1961.
8. Berge SM, *et al: J Pharm Sci 66:* 1, 1977.
9. Ravin LJ, *et al: J Pharm Sci 67:* 1523, 1978.
10. Ravin LJ, *et al: J Pharm Sci 53:* 1064, 1964.
11. Rattie ES, Guttman DE, Ravin LJ: *Arzneim Forsch 28:* 944, 1978.
12. Kaplan SA, Cotler S: *J Pharm Sci 61:* 1361, 1972.
13. Doluisio JT, Billups NF, Dittert LW, Sugita ET, Swintosky JV: *J Pharm Sci 58:* 1196, 1969.

Bibliography

Shami EG, *et al: The Theory and Practice of Industrial Pharmacy*, Lea and Febiger, Philadelphia, Chap 1, 1976.

Macek TJ: *Remington's Pharmaceutical Sciences*, Mack Publishing Company, Easton, PA, Chap 75, 1975.

Carstensen JT: *Pharmaceutics of Solids and Solid Dosage Forms*, Wiley, New York, 1977.

Greene DS: *Modern Pharmaceutics*, Marcel Dekker, New York, Chap 6, 1979.

Poole JW: *FMC Problem Solver and Reference Manual*, FMC Corp, Philadelphia, PA, Section 5, 1982.

CHAPTER 77

Bioavailability and Bioequivalency Testing

Anthony R DiSanto, PhD

Director, Clinical Biopharmaceutics/New Formulation Development
The Upjohn Company
Kalamazoo, MI 49001

Pharmacy is a profession that requires utilization of a number of scientific disciplines as well as the individual professional experience of its practitioners. Compounding of medications has become a small part of the pharmacist's practice, now largely replaced by his major role and responsibility for safeguarding drug-product quality through proper selection of multisource drug products. One need not embroil oneself in the controversy of brand-name vs generic products, for this is not the issue. The problem is one of discriminate selection of a drug product available from different manufacturers—often of substitution of one product for another, whether it involves a brand-to-generic, generic-to-brand, or generic-to-generic change. For the pharmacist to accept such responsibility, he must be reasonably knowledgeable in biopharmaceutics, with particular emphasis on drug bioavailability and bioequivalence. Variable clinical response to the same dosage form of a drug product supplied by two or more drug manufacturers is well recognized. In this chapter only bioavailability problems will be discussed. Chemical equivalence, lot-to-lot uniformity of physicochemical characteristics, and stability equivalence are but a few of the other factors that are important, as they too can affect a patient's ultimate clinical response to a drug.

One must not be led to a feeling of overconfidence in the simplicity of product selection because the Food and Drug Administration promulgated bioavailability regulations. Even for the limited number of multisource drug products that require some type of bioequivalence testing, it should be recognized that the testing is only on one lot of the product. Similarly, where only *in vitro* assessment is required, data provided are limited to one to three lots. The question of *continued* assurance of bioequivalence and chemical equivalence must, therefore, be posed by the pharmacist. This is where the challenge lies, and the pharmacist has to call on both his technical training and his experience to make appropriate drug-product selection decisions.

Bioavailability

In any discussion of bioavailability and bioequivalency testing, it is perhaps best to start with the basic concepts and factors that can affect the bioavailability of a drug and consider how these can affect bioequivalency and the clinical outcome of drug treatment. At the outset, the terms used in this chapter require careful definition since, as in any area, some terms have been used in many different contexts by different authors.

Bioavailability is an absolute term that indicates measurement of both the true rate and total amount (extent) of drug that reaches the general circulation from an administered dosage form.

Equivalence is more a relative term that compares one drug product with another or with a set of established standards. Equivalence may be defined in several ways:

1. *Chemical equivalence* indicates that two or more dosage forms contain the labeled quantities (plus or minus specified range limits) of the drug.
2. *Clinical equivalence* occurs when the same drug from two or more dosage forms gives identical *in vivo* effects as measured by a pharmacological response or by control of a symptom or disease.
3. *Therapeutic equivalence* implies that one structurally different chemical can yield the same clinical result as another chemical.
4. *Bioequivalence* indicates that a drug in two or more similar dosage forms reaches the general circulation at the same *relative* rate and the same *relative* extent, ie, that the plasma (blood or serum) level profiles of the drug obtained using the two dosage forms are, within reason, "superimposable."

Dosage Forms—In the dose titration of any patient the objective is, in conceptual terms, to attain and maintain a blood level which exceeds the minimum effective level required for response, but which does not exceed the minimum toxic (side-effect) level. This is shown graphically in Fig 77-1. There are three major absorption factors which can affect the general shape of this blood level curve and thus drug response.

1. The dose of the drug administered, ie, the blood levels will rise and fall in proportion to the dose administered.
2. The same as the first but brought about by a different process, is the amount of drug absorbed from a given dosage form. The effect of having only ½ the drug absorbed from a dosage form is equivalent to lowering the dose (Fig 77-2).
3. The rate of absorption of the drug. If absorption from the dosage form is more rapid than the rate of absorption which gave the profile in Fig 77-1, toxic (side-effect) levels can be exceeded. If absorption from the dosage form is sufficiently slow, minimum effective levels may never be attained (Fig 77-3).

A combination of these last two factors is also possible (Fig 77-4) and is probably the most likely result in real life.

In any of the above three instances, we have altered the time course and extent of clinical response to the drug.

Both factors, extent and rate of drug absorption, can be affected by the dosage form in which the drug is contained. The effect may be intentional, as in sustained-release medi-

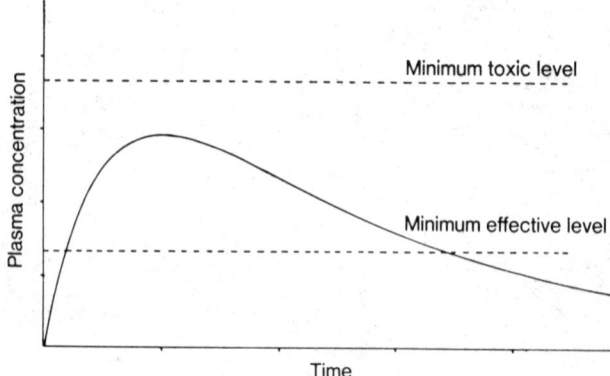

Fig 77-1. Typical plasma-level curve of a drug with effective and toxic (side-effect) levels defined.

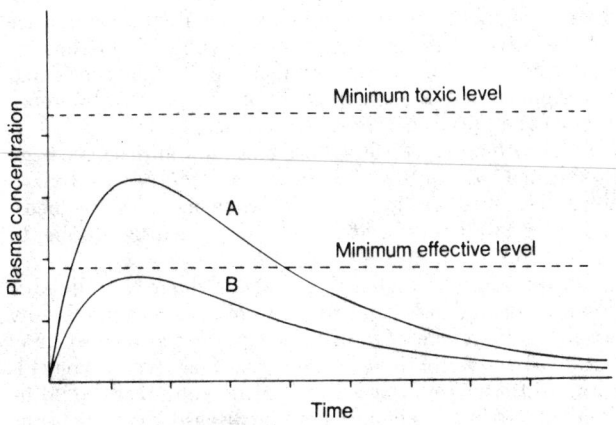

Fig 77-2.   Effect of the extent of drug absorption from a dosage form on drug-plasma levels and efficacy.   The extent of absorption from Dosage Form B is 50% of that from Dosage Form A.

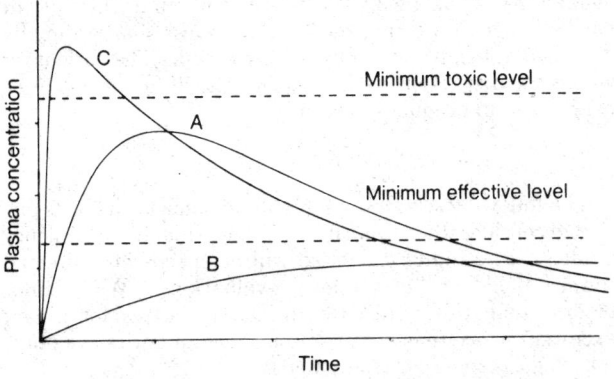

Fig 77-3.   Effect of rate of drug absorption from a dosage form on the plasma-level profile and efficacy.   The rates of absorption from Dosage Forms B and C are $\frac{1}{10}$ and 10 times that from Dosage Form A.

cation, or unintentional, as brought about by a change in the composition and/or method of manufacture of the dosage form.

It is important to remember that in most dosage forms the only ingredient regulated by law is the active drug.   The choice of the other materials (adjuvants) used to prepare a satisfactory dosage form is up to the individual manufacturer.   It is through these changes, in composition and manufacturing technique, that unintended changes in bioavailability and bioequivalency may occur.   A description of the formulation of dosage forms and the factors which must be considered by the formulating pharmacist is given in Chapter 76.

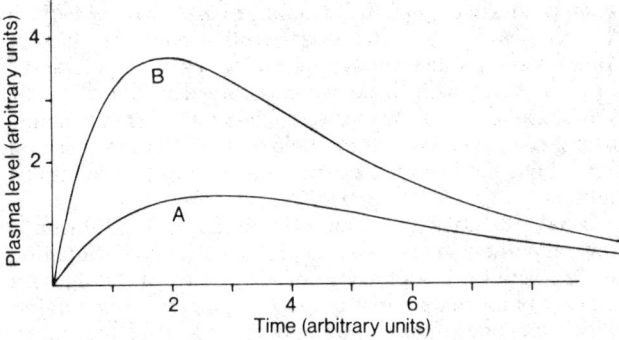

Fig 77-4.   Computer simulation of the plasma-level curves for two dosage forms of the same drug assuming that the rate and extent of drug absorption for Dosage Form A were 50% and 50%, respectively, those for Dosage Form B.

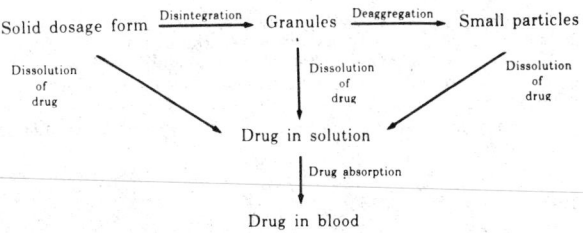

Fig 77-5.   Sequence of events involved in the dissolution and absorption of a drug from a tablet dosage form.

Dissolution Rate—For any drug to be absorbed, it must first go into solution.   In Fig 77-5, the steps in the dissolution and absorption of a tablet or capsule dosage form are outlined.   Similar profiles could be developed for any solid or semisolid dosage form, ie, oral suspensions, parenteral suspensions, or suppositories.   The theory and mechanics of drug dissolution rate are described in detail in Chapter 35.   Suffice it to say that the physical characteristics of the drug and the composition of the tablet (dosage form) can have an effect on the rates of disintegration, deaggregation, and dissolution of the drug.   As such, these can affect the rate of absorption and resultant blood levels of the drug.

Properties of the Drug—Physical characteristics of the drug which can alter bioavailability are discussed in Chapters 37 and 76 and consist of the following: the polymorphic crystal form, the choice of the salt form, the particle size, the use of the hydrated or anhydrous form, and wettability and solubility of the drug.   Chapter 76 also discusses several other properties of the drug which can adversely affect drug product quality.   Many of these factors should be discovered during the chemical testing of the drug product prior to sale of the dosage form and should not, therefore, affect, unknowingly, the bioavailability of the drug product.

Properties of the Dosage Form—The various components of the solid or semisolid dosage form, other than the active ingredient, are discussed in Chapter 90.   Only an overview, for tablet dosage forms, will be given here.   In addition to the active ingredient, a tablet product will usually contain:

Binder is used to provide a free-flowing powder from the mix of tablet ingredients so that the material will flow when used on a tablet machine. The binder also provides a cohesiveness to the tablet.   Too little binder will give flow problems and tablets which do not maintain their integrity. Too much may adversely affect the release (dissolution rate) of the drug from the tablet.

Filler is used to give the powder bulk so that an acceptable size tablet is produced.   Most commercial tablets weigh from 100 to 500 mg so it is obvious that for many potent drugs the filler comprises a large portion of the tablet.   Binding of drug to the filler may occur and affect bioavailability.

Disintegrant is used to cause the tablets to disintegrate when exposed to an aqueous environment.   Too much will produce tablets which may disintegrate in the bottle due to atmospheric moisture.   Too little may be insufficient for disintegration to occur and may thus alter the rate and extent of release of the drug from the dosage form.

Lubricant is used to enhance the flow of the powder to the tablet machine and to prevent sticking of the tablet in the die of the tablet machine after the tablet is compressed.   Lubricants are usually hydrophobic materials such as stearic acid or magnesium or calcium stearate.   Too little lubricant will not permit satisfactory tablets to be made and too much may produce a tablet with a water-impervious hydrophobic coat.   This impervious coat can inhibit disintegration of the tablet and dissolution of the drug.

Integrity of the Manufacturer is not a true physical ingredient of the tablet, but can have an effect on the clinical performance of the dosage form.   Many of the problems which arise here are related to, and detectable by, the physical and chemical quality controls the manufacturer applies to his product (see Chapter 83).   For example, with low-dose potent drugs the determination that all the active ingredient is present, on the average, in the dosage form must be complemented by the determination that each tablet contains the specified dose.   It is quite possible with potent drugs that the assay of combined tablets (10 to 20) may be within compendial limits while the drug contents of individual tablets may far exceed these limits in both positive and negative directions.   Such variations in dose, and thus bioavailability, are detectable and controllable via chemical assay of the tablets. However, these assays and other determinations may not always be done by manufacturers of low integrity. This defect may be out of ignorance of the law or intentional disregard for it. The existence of laws and federal regulations does not mean that everyone, at any given point in time, is complying with such laws and regulations.

Bioequivalency Testing

Awareness of the potential for clinical differences between otherwise chemically equivalent drug products has been brought about by a multiplicity of factors which include, among others, better methods for clinical efficacy evaluation; development of techniques to measure microgram or nanogram quantities of drugs in biological fluids; improvements in the technology of dosage-form formulation and physical testing; awareness of a significant number of reported clinical inequivalencies in the literature; increased costs of classical clinical evaluation; the objective, quantitative nature of bioavailability tests; and last, but by no means least, the increase in the number of chemically equivalent products on the market due to patent expirations on the wonder drugs of the 1950s and 1960s. The increase in the number of similar products from multiple sources has frequently placed people involved in the delivery of health care in the position of having to select one product from among several apparently equivalent products. As with any decision, the more pertinent the data available, the more comfortable one is in arriving at the final decision. The need to make these choices, in light of the potential for *in vivo* inequivalency among products, has increased the demand for quantitative data on the clinical equivalence of similar drug products. Bioequivalency testing represents one alternative solution to clinical testing for efficacy.

Requirements for bioavailability data on drug products should not be applied indiscriminately. For example, with single-supplier drugs, for which clinical efficacy has been established, proof of bioavailability is not essential. In this context the *raison d'etre* for bioequivalence testing should not be forgotten, ie, bioequivalence testing has been developed to substitute, where applicable, for clinical evaluation of drug products. Bioequivalence data should obviously not be required if *adequate* tests of relative clinical efficacy are available. However, in many instances bioavailability testing will provide a more sensitive, objective evaluation of a product's *potential* for clinical equivalency than will clinical testing.

Pharmacokinetic evaluation of bioavailability data is not necessary to show bioequivalence of two drug products. Pharmacokinetics has its major utility in the prediction or projection of dosage regimens and/or in providing a better understanding of observed drug reactions or interactions which result from buildup of drug in some specific site, tissue, or "compartment" of the body. The basis of all statements that two drug products are bioequivalent must be that the responses observed (blood, serum, or plasma level, urinary excretion, or pharmacologic response) for one drug product are essentially superimposable on the responses observed for the second drug product.

The term "essentially superimposable" must be consistent with the clinical realities of the situation. The easy, but relatively rare, decisions in the evaluation of the bioequivalence of two drug products are those where the two products are exactly superimposable (definitely bioequivalent) and those where the two products differ in their bioequivalence parameters by 50% or more (definitely *bioinequivalent*). The demonstration of absolute differences of 10% or less in the bioavailability of two dosage forms is an assignment which is frequently not possible with today's analytical tools and clinical facilities. In the area of 10–20% or even 30% differences between two dosage forms in bioequivalence parameters,

clinical judgment must be applied to evaluate the significance of these differences. The effect of a possible 10–30% change in dose on the patient's response must be carefully considered before one decides that an apparent or possible 30% difference in bioavailability is acceptable *or* unacceptable.

Even with dosage forms whose bioavailabilities have been established (within 10–20%), there is a potential for undesirable, unexpected clinical response when changing the medication for a well-stabilized patient from one drug supplier to another.

It is important to realize that a 10–20% bioavailability difference observed in normal, healthy volunteers cannot be any less in a patient where factors affecting drug absorption may already be compromised. These relatively small bioavailability differences observed in healthy volunteers could be doubled or tripled depending on the disease, the state of the disease, the age of the patient, whether the patient is bedridden, has achlorhydria, has hypermotility or hypomobility, etc. Variables associated with the patient are in general unreconcilable and their individual cumulative effect on bioavailability is unknown. When one compounds this patient variability with a drug product that is less than optimally absorbed, the outcome cannot be predicted. The patient for whom the drug is prescribed is the critical factor not to be overlooked in product selection.

Evaluation of Bioequivalence Data

The following sections will highlight some of the tests one should consider when evaluating the data from bioequivalency studies. The topics discussed will be specifically directed toward blood or plasma level evaluations. With minor modifications, the approaches outlined can be used for urinary excretion measurements or for suitable, quantitative pharmacologic response measurements.

General Study Design—Bioavailability studies are usually conducted in normal, healthy adults under standardized conditions. Usually single doses of the test and reference product will be evaluated: however, in selected cases, multiple-dose regimens must be used, eg, acid-labile drugs. The goal of the studies is to evaluate the performance of the dosage forms under standardized conditions. The assumption that any change in conditions or subject health will affect both dosage forms in a similar fashion is not valid and separate tests should be performed.

The protocol should define the acceptable age and weight range for the subjects to be used. It should define the clinical parameters which will be used to characterize a normal, healthy adult; eg, physical examination observations and clinical chemistry and hematologic evaluations. The subjects should have been drug-free for at least 2 weeks prior to testing to eliminate possible drug-induced influences on liver enzyme systems. Normally, the subjects will fast overnight prior to dosing and will not eat until a standard meal is provided 2 to 4 hours postdosing. The dosage forms should be given to subjects in a randomized manner using a suitable crossover design so that possible daily variations are distributed equally between all dosage forms tested. The protocol should define sample collection times and techniques to collect the biological fluid. The method of storage of the samples should also be defined.

Bioavailability Assessment and Data Evaluation—Several parameters are used to provide a general evaluation of the overall rate and extent of absorption of a drug. An analysis of all characteristics is required before one can implicate any one factor or parameter as indicating bioequivalence or a lack of bioequivalence.

The blood (or serum or plasma) concentration-time curve is the focal point of bioavailability assessment and is obtained when serial blood samples taken after drug administration are

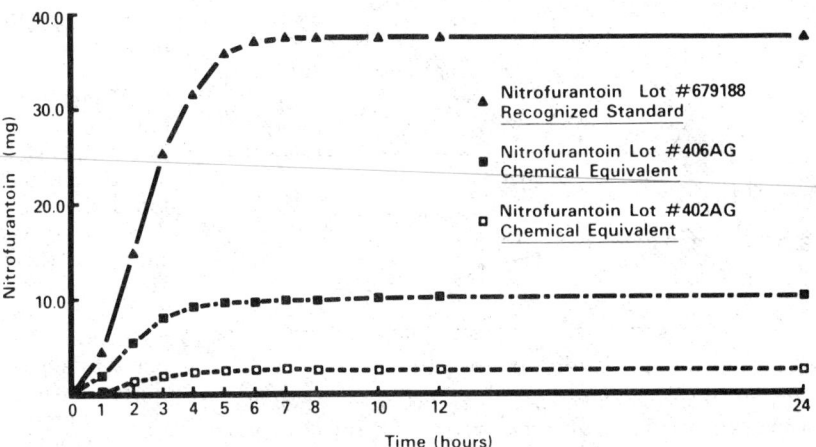

Fig 77-6.   Average cumulative amounts of nitrofurantoin excreted from three lots of two commercially available products after a single oral dose of 100 mg nitrofurantoin.

analyzed for drug concentration. The concentrations are plotted on graph paper on the ordinate (or y) axis and the times after drug administration that the samples were obtained on the abscissa (or x) axis.

A drug product is administered orally at time zero, and the blood drug concentration at this time clearly should be zero. As the product passes through the gastrointestinal system (stomach, intestine) it must go through the sequence of events depicted in Fig 77-5. As drug is absorbed, increasing concentrations of drug are observed in successive samples until the maximum concentration is achieved. This point of maximum concentration is called the peak of the concentration-time curve. It represents approximately the point in time when absorption and elimination of the drug have equalized. The section of the curve to the left of the peak represents the absorption phase, during which the rate of absorption exceeds the rate of elimination. The section of the curve to the right of the peak is called the elimination phase, during which the rate of elimination exceeds the rate of absorption. It should be understood that elimination begins as soon as drug appears in the blood stream and continues until all drug has been eliminated. Absorption continues too for some period of time into the elimination phase. One must recognize that elimination of the drug includes all processes of elimination, urinary excretion as well as metabolism of the drug by various tissues and organs. The "efficiency" of metabolism and urinary excretion will determine the shape of the elimination phase of the curve.

Bioavailability studies are performed in healthy, adult volunteers under rigid conditions of fasting and activity because the objective is to obtain *quantitative* information on the influence of pharmaceutical formulation variables on the drug product's absorption. Drug blood-level profiles, therefore, allow quantitations of the *rate* and *extent* of drug absorption and are critical in establishing the *efficiency* of the drug product in delivering the drug to the systemic circulation. Arguments that bioavailability testing should be done in a "disease-state population" are not tenable if the object of the study is to assess drug formulations. If, on the other hand, the purpose is to determine the effect of "disease" on the efficiency of absorption from the drug product(s), then one must use the "disease-state population." The reasoning is obvious. In order to assure that any differences observed in the drug blood-level profiles are attributable to formulation factors, one must hold all other variables constant, ie, food, activity, state of disease, etc.

One need not be limited to drug blood-level profiles, but in a similar manner many obtain cumulative urinary drug amount-time profiles. Drug *concentration* is determined in the urine at specified time intervals and the *amount* excreted per interval determined by multiplying the concentration by

the volume of urine obtained in that interval. The amounts per interval are then cumulated and ultimately the maximum amount excreted in the urine is obtained. This value is analogous to the area under the blood concentration-time curve. A typical cumulative urinary drug amount-time profile for several nitrofurantoin products is presented in Fig 77-6.

In assessing the bioequivalence of drug products one must quantitate the *rate* and *extent* of absorption. The factors of rate and extent of absorption can be determined by evaluating three parameters of a blood level concentration-time profile. Three parameters describing a blood level curve are considered important in evaluating the bioequivalency of two or more formulations of the same drug; these are (1) the peak height concentration; (2) the time of the peak concentration and; (3) the area under the blood (serum or plasma) concentration-time curve.

Peak Height Concentration—The height of the peak of the blood level-time curve obviously represents the highest drug concentration achieved after oral administration. It is reported as an amount per volume measurement, eg, micrograms/mL or units/mL or grams/100 mL, etc. The importance of this parameter is illustrated in Fig 77-7 where the blood concentration-time curves of two different formulations of a drug are represented. A line has been drawn across the curve at 4 µg/mL. Suppose the drug is an analgesic and 4 µg/mL is the minimum effective concentration (MEC) of the drug in blood. If, then, the blood concentration curves in Fig 77-7 represent the blood levels obtained after administration of equal doses of two formulations of the drug and it is known that analgesia would not be produced unless the minimum effective concentration was achieved or exceeded, it becomes

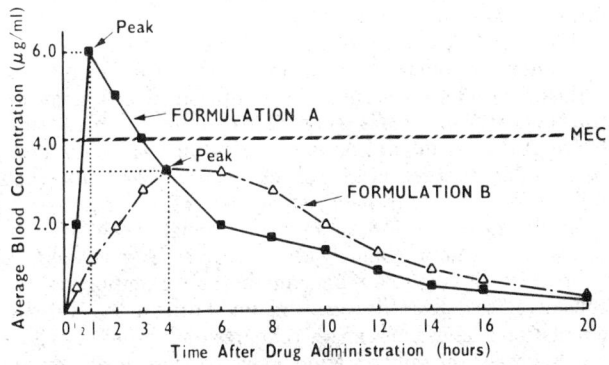

Fig 77-7.   Blood concentration-time curves obtained for two different formulations of the same drug demonstrating relationship of the profiles to the Minimum Effective Concentration (MEC).

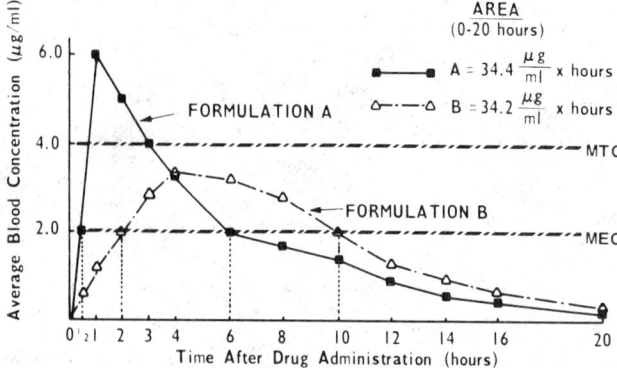

Fig 77-8.   Blood concentration-time curves obtained for two different formulations of same the drug demonstrating relationship of the profiles to the Minimum Toxic Concentration (MTC) and the Minimum Effective Concentration (MEC).

clear that formulation A should produce pain relief while formulation B, even though it seemed well absorbed, would not produce the desired pharmacologic effect and would be ineffective in producing analgesia.

On the other hand, if the two curves represent blood concentrations following equal doses of two different formulations of the same cardiac glycoside, and 4 μg/mL now represents the minimum toxic concentration (MTC) and 2 μg/mL represents the minimum effective concentration (Fig 77-8) then formulation A, although effective, may also be toxic, while formulation B produces concentrations well above the minimum effective concentration but never achieves toxic levels.

Time of Peak Concentration—The second parameter of importance is the measurement of the length of time necessary to achieve the maximum concentration after drug administration. This time is called the time of peak blood concentration. In Fig 77-7, for formulation A the time necessary to achieve peak blood concentration is 1 hour; for formulation B it is 4 hours. This parameter is closely related to the rate of absorption of the drug from a formulation and may be used as a simple measure of rate of absorption.

To illustrate its importance, suppose the two curves in Fig 77-8 now represent two formulations of an analgesic and that in this case the minimum effective concentration is 2 μg/mL. Formulation A will achieve the minimum effective concentration in 30 minutes; formulation B does not achieve that concentration until 2 hours. Obviously, formulation A would then produce analgesia much more rapidly than formulation B and would probably be preferable as an analgesic agent. On the other hand, if one were more interested in the duration of the analgesic effect than on the time of onset, formulation B would present more sustained activity, maintaining serum concentrations above the MEC for a longer time (8 hours) than formulation A (5½ hours).

Area Under the Concentration-Time Curve—The third, and sometimes the most important parameter for evaluation, is the area under the serum, blood or plasma concentration-time curve. This area is reported in amount/volume × time (eg, μg/mL × hours or grams/100 mL × hours, etc) and can be considered representative of the amount of drug absorbed following administration of a single dose of the drug.

Returning to Fig 77-8, the curves, although much different in shape, have approximately the same areas (A = 34.4 μg/mL × hrs.; B = 34.2 μg/mL × hrs.) and both formulations can be considered to deliver the same amount of drug to the systemic circulation. Thus, one can see that area under the curve does not represent the only criterion on which bioequivalency can be judged. All the results, as a composite, must be utilized in reaching a decision as to bioequivalency; no one parameter suffices this purpose.

Statistical Sense and Nonsense—When statistical evaluations are employed in bioequivalency testing one must be careful not to assume, from a statement that "no statistically significant differences were detected," that two drug products are, therefore, bioequivalent. The basis of most tests for statistically significant differences is that the two products are assumed to be the same until proven otherwise. Therefore, if the data presented are highly variable (large standard deviation, ie, wide range of values), it would be possible to show that there was no statistically significant difference between an area underneath the curve (AUC) of 100 units (%) vs an AUC of 40 units (%). In this case the statistical test does not indicate that the AUC's are truly similar; it simply means that the data were too variable from patient to patient for the statistics to be able to detect a 60-unit (%) difference in areas, even if it existed.

There are two types of errors associated with any statistical test. These are:

1. *Alpha Error*—This is the error with which most people are familiar and is the error associated with the statement, "The data have been analyzed statistically." Alpha error is the probability (defined by the "p" value) by saying the two treatments are different when in fact they are the same. It should be noted that while highly significant "p" values reduce the alpha error, they provide no indication of the possibility that the two treatments being called the same when in fact they are different.

2. *Beta Error*—This is the error associated with the possibility of calling two treatments the same when in fact they are different. As the maximum percent difference between means which can be detected with an alpha error of p $\leq$ 0.05 is reduced, the beta error is also reduced. This increase in statistical sensitivity (reduced alpha and beta error) is obtained by reducing the variability of the data. Variability is usually reduced by increasing the number of data points (subjects) in a bioavailability study.

The objective of statistical testing for bioavailability evaluation should be to minimize both the alpha and the beta error. Since both errors are mathematically related to the variability of the data collected, the solution is relatively simple. Sufficient data should be gathered so that the general statistical test (alpha error test) would detect, if it existed, a predetermined percent difference (20% for example) between the two dosage forms. If, for example, the two treatments are found not to be statistically (p $\leq$ 0.05) significantly different, then the results indicate that there is only 1 chance in 20 that the treatments are claimed to be different when in fact they are the same. If there were 18 subjects in the above example and a 20% difference would have been statistically significantly different, there would be a beta error of 4 chances in 20 that a 25% difference between means was not detected (ie, that treatments which differed by more than 25% were claimed to be the same when in fact they were different). The level of statistical sensitivity which one feels is adequate (20% as a rule of thumb) must be reevaluated for each drug product tested based on the clinical performance of the drug.

Statistical analysis can also go to the other extreme. For example, tests might show that an AUC of 100 units (100%) was statistically significantly different from an AUC of 90 units (90%). If the clinical impression of the drug being evaluated was that a 20% difference in dose (plasma levels) would not be clinically significant, then in this example we must conclude that the statistical test is too sensitive and the difference observed, even if real, is not clinically significant. Therefore, the drug products are bioequivalent in spite of the statistical findings.

Statistics should be used, in bioavailability testing, as a tool to determine if sufficient subjects have been included to minimize the effect of patient-to-patient variability in the data analysis. The results of statistical testing should not be used *as the decision;* they should be used to help *make the decision.* One must apply some statistical sense in order to avoid statistical nonsense.

A Common Pitfall: Cross-Study Comparisons—Per-

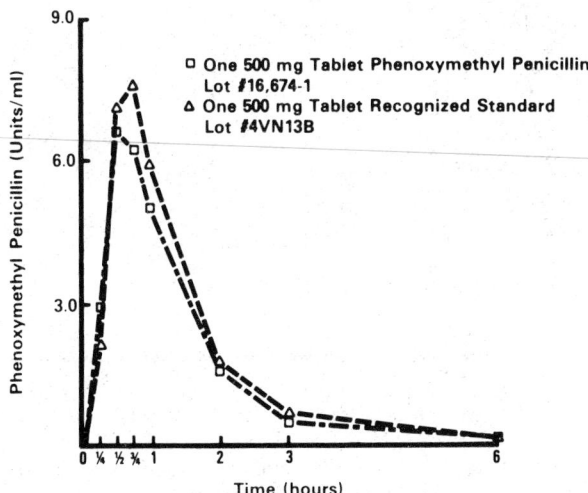

Fig 77-9.   Average serum concentration of phenoxymethyl penicillin following oral administration of 500 mg given as one tablet of Recognized Standard, or of Test Product, Research Lot.

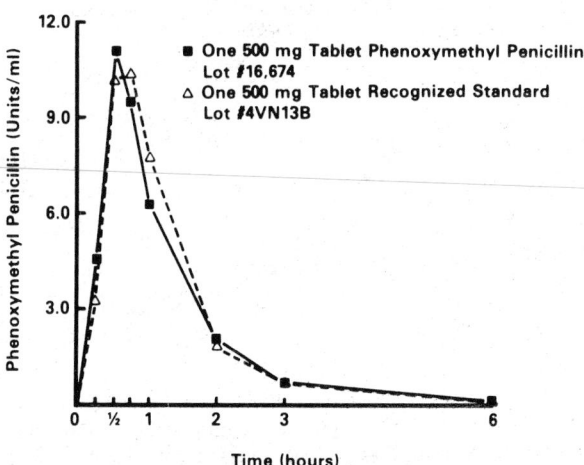

Fig 77-10.   Average serum concentration of phenoxymethyl penicillin following oral administration of 500 mg given as one tablet of Recognized Standard, or of Test Product, Full Mfg. Lot.

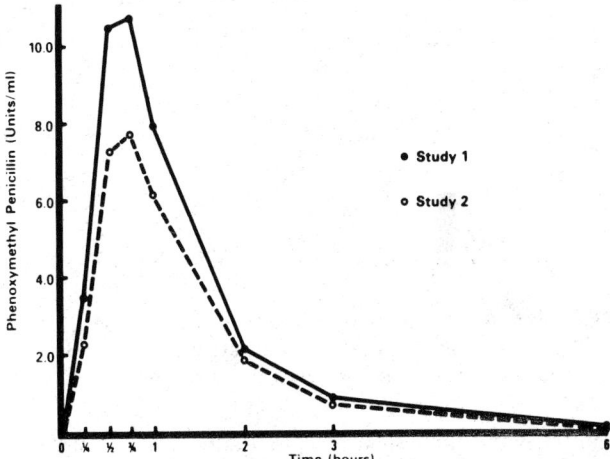

Fig 77-11.   Average serum concentration of phenoxymethyl penicillin following a single oral 500-mg dose of Recognized Standard, in two different subject populations.

haps the single most common error made in interpreting bioavailability data is that of *cross-study comparison*. This occurs when the blood concentration-time curve of a drug product in one study is compared with the blood concentration-time curve of that drug product in another study. There are three reasons why such cross-study comparisons are dangerous and can lead to false conclusions. The following examples used to illustrate the three points are taken from actual bioavailability data.

Different Subject Population—In Fig 77-9, a research lot of potassium phenoxymethyl penicillin was compared with the appropriate reference standard for that product. The research lot drug was found to be bioequivalent, with average peak-serum concentrations differing by 8% and the area differing by only 9%. In another study conducted with a full-manufacture lot of the test product, the same lot of the reference standard potassium phenoxymethyl penicillin was utilized. The results of this study are shown in Fig 77-10. Again, the two products were found to be bioequivalent as the peak and area parameters differed by less than 5%. In these two studies, identical test conditions were used and the same analytical procedure and laboratory was employed. However, if one compares the serum levels for the reference standard lot found in Fig 77-9, with the levels for the same lot of tablets in the study in Fig 77-10, then sizable differences in blood levels are found as shown in Fig 77-11.

The average peak serum levels for this lot of tablets were found to be 8.5 units/mL and 12.5 units/mL in the two respective studies; a difference of approximately 31%. Likewise, the average area under the curve was found to differ by approximately 21%. Such differences are the sole result of cross-study comparisons and are not due to differences in actual bioavailability.

The same lot of reference standard tablets was used in both studies. Hence, the difference must be due to the experimental variables which normally occur from study to study. The major difference between the two studies was the subject population involved. In the first study, healthy, adult, male, prison volunteers were used, whereas in the second study, there were 17 females and 7 males in a hospital clinic also described as normal, healthy volunteers. An appreciable difference in sex distribution was obvious when comparing these studies. Adjustments for body weight and surface area alone did not correct for the apparent discrepancies in peak concentration or area under the blood level curve. It is difficult to determine the exact factors which caused the observed differences. This example should serve as a note of

caution in comparing absolute bioavailability values of peak concentration and area under the curve from different studies.

Different Study Conditions—Parameters such as the food or fluid intake of the subject before, during and after drug administration can have dramatic effects on the absorption of certain drugs. Fig 77-12 shows the results of a three-way crossover test where the subjects were fasted 12 hours overnight and two hours after drug administration of (1) an uncoated tablet, (2) a film-coated tablet and (3) an enteric-coated tablet of erythromycin. The results of this study suggest that the unprotected tablet is superior to both the film-coated and enteric-coated tablets in terms of blood level performance. These results also suggest that neither film-coating nor enteric-coating is necessary for optimal blood level performance. Fig 77-13 shows results with the same tablets when the study conditions were changed to only a two-hour pre-administration fast with two hours fasting post-administration. In this case, the blood levels of the uncoated tablet were markedly depressed while the film-coated and enteric-coated tablets showed relatively little difference in blood levels. From this second study, it might be concluded that film-coating appears to impart the same degree of acid stability as an enteric coating. This might be acceptable if only one dose of the antibiotic were required. However, Fig 77-14 shows the results of a multiple-dose study in which the enteric-coated

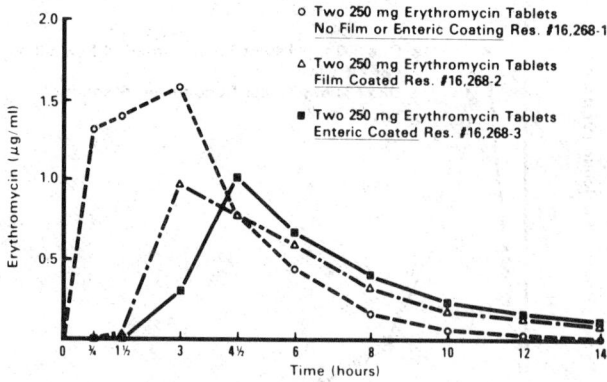

Fig 77-12. Average serum erythromycin concentration administered in 500-mg doses as three different tablet dosage forms. The results were obtained from 21 healthy adult subjects following an overnight fast of 12 hours before and 2 hours after drug administration.

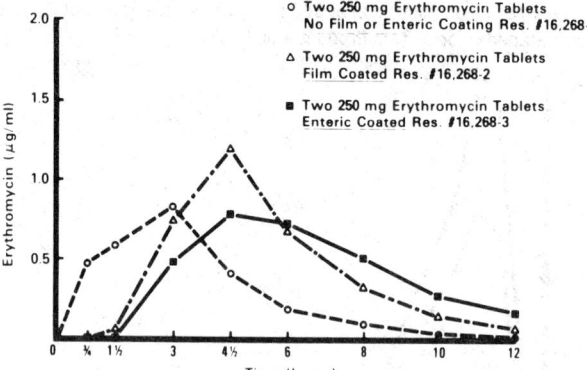

Fig 77-13. Average serum erythromycin concentration administered in 500-mg doses as three different tablet dosage forms. The results were obtained from 12 healthy adult subjects with only a 2-hour fast before drug administration.

tablet and the film-coated tablet were administered four times a day immediately after meals. The results show that the film coating does not impart the degree of acid stability the enteric coating does when the tablets are administered immediately after food in a typical clinical situation.

Different Assay Methodology—Depending on the drug

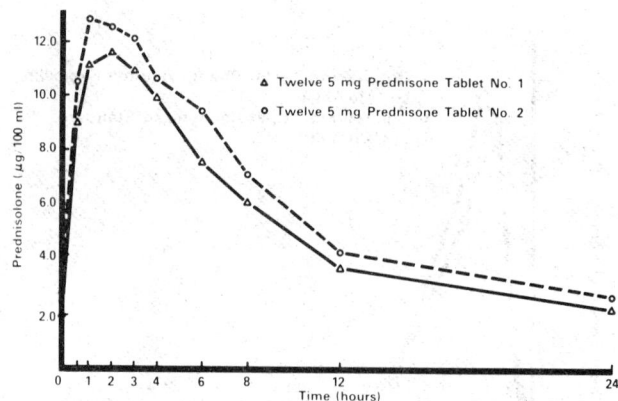

Fig 77-15. Average plasma prednisolone levels following 60 mg of prednisone administered to 24 normal adults as a single oral dose of twelve 5-mg prednisone tablets from two different manufacturers. Plasma levels were determined by a competitive protein-binding assay.

under study, there may be more than one assay method available. For example, some steroids can be assayed by a radioimmunoassay, competitive protein-binding, gas-liquid chromatograph or indirectly by a 17-hydroxycorticosteroid assay. Fig 77-15 and 77-16 show the results of a comparison of prednisone tablets using a competitive protein-binding method and a radioimmunoassay, respectively. The serum concentration-time curves resulting from each method lead to the same conclusion, that the products are bioequivalent. However, Fig 77-17 shows a comparison of the absolute values obtained by the two assay methods with the same product. Obviously, the wrong conclusion would have been reached if one product had been assayed by one method and the other product by the other method and the results had been compared. Even in cases where only one assay method is employed, there are numerous modifications with respect to technique among laboratories which could make direct comparisons hazardous.

The backbone of any bioavailability study involving plasma (or urine) levels of drug, in addition to good study design and subject controls, is the analytical methodology used to determine the levels of drug. In most cases one can *probably* assume that the precision and reliability of the method em-

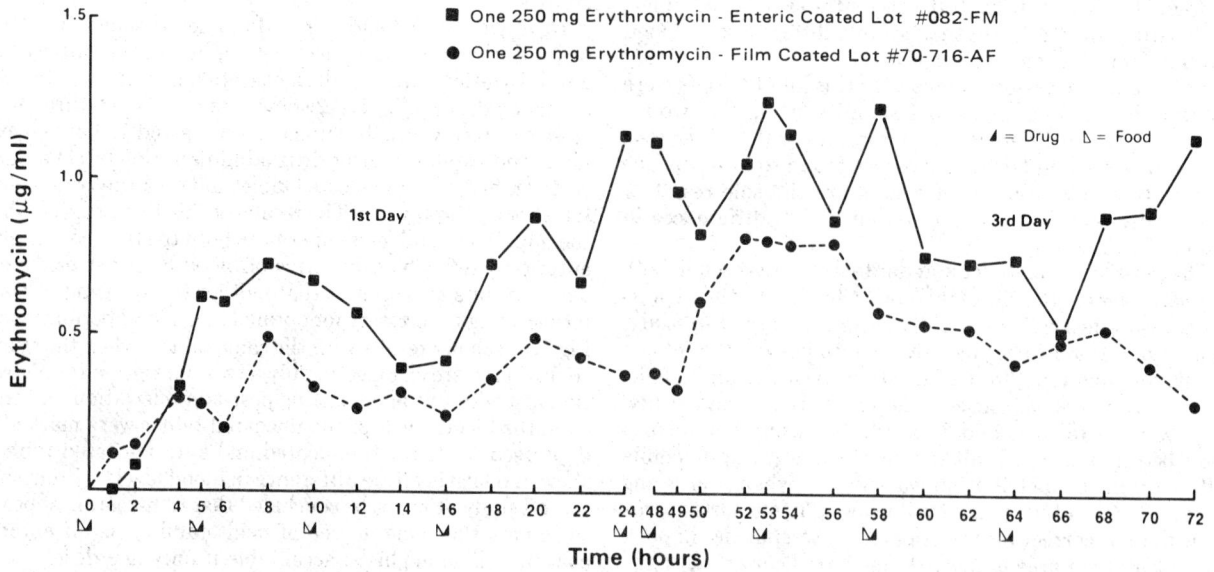

Fig 77-14. Average serum erythromycin concentration-time profiles administered in two different tablet dosage forms. The results were obtained from 24 healthy adult subjects following administration of 250 mg qid, with meals and at bedtime.

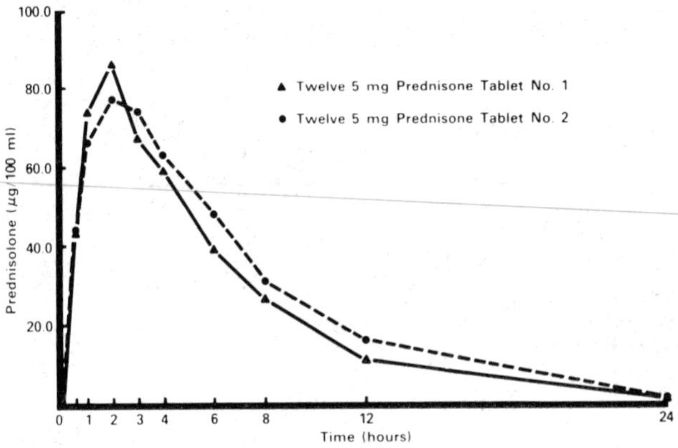

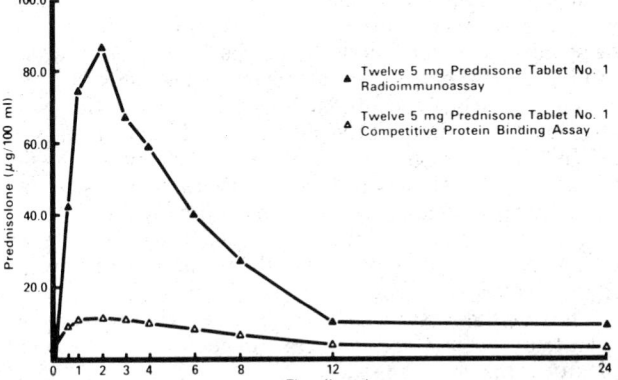

Fig 77-16.   Average plasma prednisolone levels following 60 mg of prednisone administered to 24 normal adults as a single oral dose of twelve 5-mg prednisone tablets from two different manufacturers. Plasma levels were determined by a radioimmunoassay procedure.

Fig 77-17.   Average plasma prednisolone profiles administered as a single 60-mg dose to 24 normal adults.   Plasma levels were determined by both a competitive protein binding assay and a radioimmunoassay.

ployed in a given study have been established to a sufficient degree to make the results of the study internally consistent. As demonstrated, major problems arise when, without careful evaluation of the analytical methodology employed, one attempts to compare the data of studies from different laboratories.   Even with similar analytical methodology performed by the same laboratory, it would be unreasonable to expect agreement, using the same dosage form, of closer than 20–25% for plasma levels, AUC's, etc, from one study to the next. Under the *best* conditions, cross-study comparisons are relatively insensitive, and at worst they can be misleading. Cross-study comparisons certainly cannot be used to make decisions or estimations of differences in drug products with the generally acceptable sensitivity of difference detection of 20% or less.

With insufficient data on the correlation of plasma levels with clinical response, it is difficult to decide if it is the peak plasma level or the total body load of a drug that is important. Changes in rate of absorption require changes in the dose given (body load) for maintenance of similar peak plasma levels.   Decisions as to which is more important, body load or peak level, are made with difficulty and tend to reduce the objective quantitation sought in bioavailability testing.

Summary—It is hoped that this chapter has placed bioavailability testing in perspective in the minds of the reader. Such testing is an extremely useful tool for attempting to quantitate the potential clinical equivalence of drug products. However, as with any evaluation that is a function of a wide variety of complex and often interacting variables, one should be careful that oversimplification of data evaluation does not lead to distortion of facts.

Bibliography

Chodos DJ, DiSanto AR: *Basics of Bioavailability*, The Upjohn Company, Kalamazoo, 1973.
Dittert LW, DiSanto AR: *J APhA NS13:* August 1973.
DiSanto AR, *et al: Int J Clin Pharmacol 13:* 220–227, 1976.

CHAPTER 78

Separation

Adelbert M Knevel, PhD

Professor of Medicinal Chemistry and Associate Dean
School of Pharmacy and Pharmacal Sciences
Purdue University
West Lafayette, IN 47907

Separation may be defined as an operation that brings about isolation and/or purification of a single chemical constituent or a group of chemically related substances. Most medicinal agents require some degree of purification before being incorporated into desirable dosage forms. The analysis of pharmaceutical preparations many times requires separation of the chief constituent from other formulation constituents before quantitative measurement can be made.

While the problems of separation are the concern chiefly of pharmaceutical manufacturers, at times they may be encountered also by the pharmacist in the prescription laboratory; hence, all pharmacy practitioners should have knowledge of the principles underlying, and the techniques employed, in the basic processes of separation.

The processes of separation may be divided into two general categories—simple and complex—depending on the complexity of the method used.

Simple processes bring about separation of constituents through a single mechanical manipulation. Some examples of this type are the use of (1) a separatory funnel or pipette to separate two immiscible liquids such as water and ether; (2) a distillation process to separate two miscible liquids such as benzene and chloroform; (3) a garbling process to separate solids; and (4) centrifugation, filtration, and expression processes to separate solids from liquids. Processes in this category are limited usually to separations of relatively simple mixtures or solutions.

Complex processes usually require formation of a second phase by addition of either a solid, liquid, or gas plus mechanical manipulation in order to bring about effective separation. One example is the separation of acetylsalicylic acid from salicylic acid. In this mixture, salicylic acid is considered to be an impurity and, in order to separate the impurity from the desired constituent, a suitable solvent is added to the mixture for the purpose of recrystallizing only the acetylsalicylic acid. The contaminant remains in solution and is removed in the filtrate during the filtration process.

Only selected processes involving separations will be covered in this chapter. Other methods are discussed in such chapters as *Complexation, Colloidal Dispersions,* and *Chromatography.*

Countercurrent Distribution

Countercurrent distribution (CCD) may be defined as a series of liquid–liquid extractions (immiscible solvents) conducted in a multiple-tube apparatus in which one phase is permitted to advance to the next tube in the series independently of the other phase.[1] The separation of the components in the mixture depends upon the distribution coefficients of each of the components, volume of the solvents used, and the number of transfers taken.

Some important applications of CCD in the pharmaceutical sciences are (1) the isolation and purification of chemicals and biochemicals which might otherwise be damaged by the ex-

tremes of temperature or pH which occur during the separation processes, (2) the separation of a crude plant extract into its various chemically related fractions as a preparative step, (3) the determination of purity and homogeneity of chemicals and medicinal agents, and (4) the characterization of substances extracted from biochemical systems in studies determining the metabolic or biologic disposition of drugs.

Separation using CCD is based on Nernst's Law. According to this law, when two practically immiscible solvents are in contact with each other and a substance which is soluble in each is added, the substance distributes itself in such a way that at equilibrium and at a given temperature the ratio of the concentrations of the two solutions is a constant. Strictly speaking, it is the activity ratio rather than the concentration ratio which remains constant. For most purposes, however, concentration values give satisfactory approximations.

When the ratio of concentrations expresses a distribution value for a single chemical species, the constant is designated as a partition coefficient or distribution coefficient, K, and may be expressed mathematically as

$$K = C_u/C_l \qquad (1)$$

In this expression C_u and C_l represent concentrations in the upper and lower phases, respectively. There is no accepted convention to date and the distribution coefficient could just as well be expressed as the reciprocal of Eq 1, C_l/C_u.

In actual practice one deals with and measures total analytical concentrations and hence more than one chemical species is usually present in each phase. This type of distribution between solvents is called the partition ratio and is defined mathematically as $K_p = C_u/C_l$, where C_u and C_l represent total analytical concentrations of the chemical in the upper and lower phases, respectively. An example would be the distribution of benzoic acid between benzene and water. In the aqueous phase, benzoic acid would be present both in the ionized (A^-) and un-ionized form (HA). In benzene, benzoic acid would be present in the un-ionized form (HA) and in the dimerized form $(HA)_2$. The ratio expressing total benzoic acid in the organic phase and total benzoic acid in the aqueous phase is the partition ratio or the apparent distribution coefficient, K_p.

Although the purpose of using CCD is to bring about the separation of two or more substances, the basic principles of operation are best introduced by first considering the distribution pattern of a single solute in the two immiscible solvents.

First, assume that the solute under consideration has a distribution coefficient of unity when distributed between chloroform and buffer solution and that there are no deviations from Nernst's law of distribution due to molecular association, dissociation, ionization, or chemical reactions.

Next, consider six containers such as 250-mL glass-stoppered Erlenmeyer flasks, each holding 50 mL of chloroform (lower phase) as shown in Fig 78-1 (Row A). Add to container No 0,100 mg of solute under consideration dissolved in 50 mL

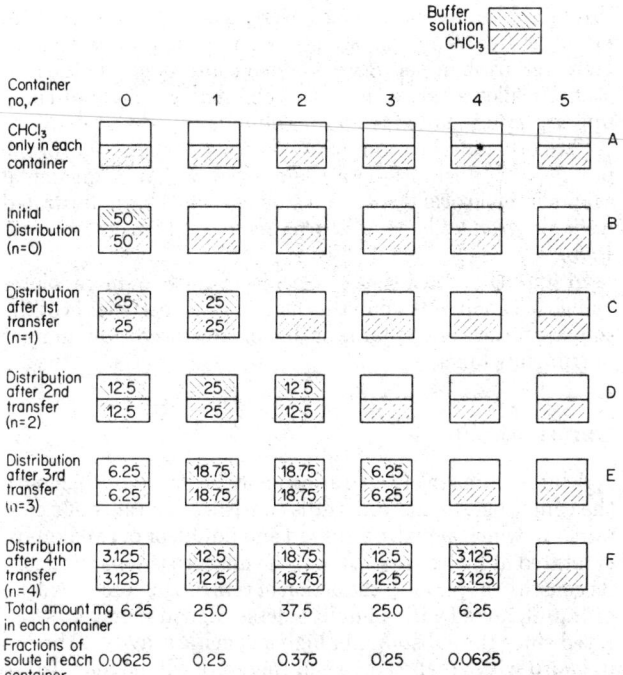

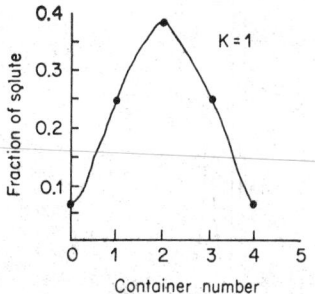

Fig 78-2.   Distribution of solute after four transfers.

Fig 78-1.   Theoretical distribution of solute after varying numbers of transfer.

of buffer solution, and shake until equilibrium has been established. Because equal volumes of solvent are used and the distribution coefficient of solute in these two solvents is unity, the solute at equilibrium will distribute itself in such a way that one-half is found in each of the upper and lower phases (Row B). Since 100 mg was originally present, 50 mg will be found in both layers of Container 0 (Row B).

Now, transfer the upper phase of Container 0 holding 50 mg of solute to Container 1 (Row B) and add fresh buffer solution to Container 0 (Row B). Shake both containers until equilibrium has been established. At equilibrium the quantity of solute in each phase of Containers 0 and 1 (Row C) will be 25 mg.

Next, transfer the upper phase of Container 1 (Row C) to Container 2 (Row C), and the upper phase of Container 0 (Row C) to Container 1. Add fresh buffer solution to Container 0 (Row C) and shake all three containers until equilibrium has been established. At equilibrium the quantity of solute (25 mg) in Container 2 (Row D) will have distributed itself so that one-half (12.5 mg) is in the upper phase and one-half (12.5 mg) is in the lower phase. Since 25 mg of solute was transferred to Container 1 from Container 0, 25 mg of solute will be present in each phase of Container 1 (Row D). The quantity (25 mg) of solute in Container 0 will distribute itself between the chloroform layer and freshly added buffer solution so that one-half (12.5 mg) will be present in each layer (Row D).

Continue this general procedure of transferring the upper phases of Containers 0, 1, and 2 to Containers 1, 2, and 3, respectively; then add fresh buffer to Container 0. Shake the four flasks until equilibrium is established. A distribution is obtained as shown in Row E. Continuing in a like manner will give a distribution as shown in Row F. A plot of the fraction of solute in each container vs container number is shown in Fig 78-2. The significance of this curve is that the distribution of the solute shows a peak in which the maximum is located in a specific container and the location of the peak container is a function of the partition coefficient. Hence it can be seen that two or more solutes with different K values can be effectively separated after the passage of a mixture

through many tubes (usually 25 or more depending upon K values) in a CCD apparatus.

Fig 78-2 illustrates the distribution of a solute after only four transfers. In actual practice between 8 and 2000 containers or tubes are usually used in multiple extractions of this kind. The tubes are connected in series in a train and are rocked simultaneously rather than individually in order to bring about distribution of solutes between the two phases. The device also permits the transfer of upper phases to the next tube in series in one operation. A device of this type is called a countercurrent distribution apparatus.

To study the fraction of a given solute present in each tube r, after n number of transfers, it is convenient to use Eq 2. The complete derivation of Eq 2 appears in *Remington's Pharmaceutical Sciences*, 14th ed, 374, 1970.

$$f_{n,r} = \frac{n!}{r!\,(n-r)!}\left(\frac{1}{1+KR}\right)^n (KR)^r \qquad (2)$$

where K is defined as the partition coefficient, and R is defined as the ratio of the volume of the upper phase to the volume of the lower phase, (V_u/V_l).

The use of Eq 2 is illustrated as follows: Calculate the fraction of solute in tubes no 0, 1, 2, 3, and 4 after four transfers are made in a CCD apparatus using equal volumes of upper and lower phases. The K value for the solute in the solvent system is assumed to be 1.0 in this example.

For tube no 3:

$$f_{4,3} = \frac{4!}{3!\,(4-3)!}\left(\frac{1}{1+1}\right)^4 (1)^3 = 0.25$$

By similar calculations the fraction of solutes in Tube 0, 1, 2, and 4 are found to equal:

$$f_{4,0} = 0.0625; \quad f_{4,1} = 0.25; \quad f_{4,2} = 0.375; \quad f_{4,4} = 0.0625$$

The distribution of solute using Eq 2 is shown in Fig 78.2.

When a large number of transfers (>50) are made and K is near unity it is more convenient to use a Gaussian treatment[2] to calculate the fraction of solute in a particular tube. The appropriate equations are:

$$y_x = \frac{1.00}{\sqrt{2\pi nKR/(KR+1)^2}}\,\exp\left\{-\left(\frac{x^2}{2nKR/(KR+1)^2}\right)\right\} \qquad (3)$$

$$r_{max} = \frac{nKR}{KR+1} \qquad (4)$$

where y_x represents the fraction of solute with distribution coefficient K in the tube that is x distant from the peak tube; exp is the exponent of the base e, ex, $\exp\{2\} = e^2$; $\pi = 3.14$; K, R, and n are terms which have been previously defined; and r_{max} represents the number of the tube containing the maximum amount of solute.

The use of these equations has been illustrated in *Remington's Pharmaceutical Sciences*, 14th ed, 375, 1970.

Distribution curves may be prepared from hypothetical

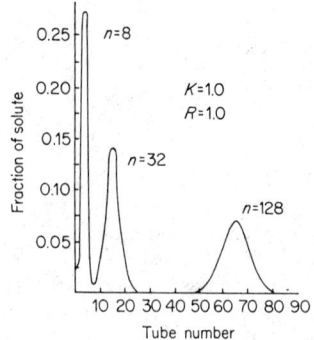

Fig 78-3. Distribution of solute after varying number of transfers.

data using Eqs 3 and 4 or from a computer program utilizing these equations. Fig 78-3 illustrates a series of curves for a solute in which $K = 1.0$ and $R = 1.0$ following 8, 32, and 128 transfers. It is interesting to observe that as the number of transfers increases, the amplitude of the curve decreases and the solute spreads through more and more tubes. At first thought, this would seem undesirable, but the significant point is that the fraction of vessels containing solute after 128 transfers is now much less than after 10 transfers. Therefore, two solutes with different but similar K values can be separated in 128 transfers because each solute occupies a smaller fraction of total tubes. If this separation were attempted with 10 to 20 transfers, both solutes would occupy nearly all of the tubes and no separation would be obtained.

Fig 78-4 illustrates the distribution patterns obtained in a 16-transfer experiment for solutes having distribution coefficients which differ by one order of magnitude. Under no circumstances can a separation be obtained if the distribution coefficients of the solutes are equal.

The procedure of operation which has been considered thus far is known as the *fundamental procedure*. Here the solute is distributed through a specified number of tubes and nothing is withdrawn from the system until the entire operation is completed. Then the tube contents are withdrawn and analyzed for the purpose of determining solute concentrations or the solutes are withdrawn simply for the purpose of isolating them from a mixture.

Another procedure of operation which is of interest primarily due to its analogy to elution chromatography is known as *end withdrawal*. In this operation the fundamental procedure is followed for a predetermined number of transfers as previously described. Then the upper phase only of the last tube in the train is collected. All other upper phases are advanced to the next tube in succession and after equilibration the upper phase of the last tube, n, is again collected. This process is continued until all upper phases have passed

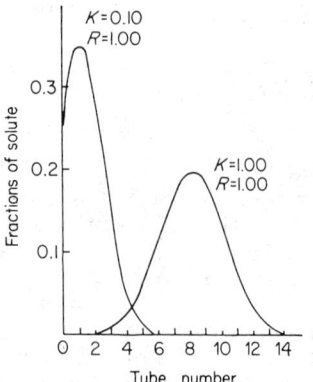

Fig 78-4. Distribution of two solutes with different K values.

through n tubes containing lower phase. In elution chromatography, as previously stated, the analogy is similar. However, fresh upper phase is added continuously to the first "tube" (called a "plate" in elution chromatography) until only upper phase is eluted from the column.

Two other applications of CCD—the determination of the purity of a substance, and the determination of medicinal agents in biological disposition studies—have been illustrated in *Remington's Pharmaceutical Sciences*, 14th ed, 375–377, 1970.

In summary, the degree of separation of two or more solutes using CCD depends upon the distribution coefficients of the solutes, nature and volume of the solvents used, and number of transfers taken.

Centrifugation

A large number of separations may be accomplished with the centrifuge. This apparatus consists essentially of a container in which a mixture of solid and liquid, or of two liquids, is rotated at high speeds so that the mixture is separated into its constituent parts by the action of centrifugal force. A solid or liquid, mixed with a liquid of lesser density, may be separated since the substance of higher specific gravity is thrown outward with greater force and therefore will be impelled to the bottom of the container leaving a clear supernatant layer of pure liquid.

Centrifugation is particularly useful when separation by ordinary filtration is difficult, eg, in separating a highly viscous mixture. Separations may be accompanied more rapidly in a centrifuge than under the action of gravity. In addition, the degree of separation which is attainable may be greater since the forces available are of a far higher order of magnitude. The centrifuge has become a valuable analytical tool, particularly in biochemical and microbiological research. It has wide application in pharmaceutical laboratories and its use as a means of predicting emulsion stability has been suggested.

Two basic types of centrifuges are available: *sedimentation* and *filtration*. The *sedimentation type* of centrifuge depends on differences in the densities of the two or more phases comprising the mixture. This instrument is capable of separating both solid–liquid and liquid–liquid mixtures. *Filtration centrifuges*, however, are limited to the separation of solid–liquid mixtures only.

Sedimentation Centrifuges

The design of the bottle centrifuge and the disc centrifuge are based on the sedimentation principle (ie, separation by density difference).

Bottle Centrifuge—This type of centrifuge consists of a vertical spindle that rotates the containers in a horizontal plane and is commonly used to separate materials of different densities. Separation in a centrifugal field is brought about because denser particles in a mixture require greater forces to hold them in a circular path of a given radius than lighter particles. Thus, the lighter particles are displaced toward the axis of the centrifuge by the heavier particles. During the centrifugation of blood, for example, a speed of 3000 rpm is required to separate blood corpuscles from serum. If the radius of the centrifuge is assumed to be 10 cm, the acceleration, a, acting on a particle can be approximated to be 10^6 cm/sec^2; or about 1000 times the acceleration due to gravity (g):

$$a = 4\pi^2 N^2 r = \frac{4(3.14)^2(3000)^2(10)}{3600} = 10^6 \text{ cm/sec}^2$$

N = revolutions/sec; r = radius in cm

$$\frac{10^6 \text{ cm/sec}^2}{10^3 \text{ cm/sec}^2} = 1000 \ (g)$$

10^3 cm/sec^2 = approximate acceleration due to gravity

Under these conditions the blood corpuscles eventually migrate under the influence of centrifugal force to the tip of the centrifuge tube.

The separation of particles in a liquid medium also depends on the nature of the medium. A solid particle settling under the influence of acceleration due to gravity in a liquid phase accelerates until a constant terminal velocity is reached. The terminal velocity is known as the settling velocity of the particle and is described mathematically by Stokes' Law. It can be shown that Stokes' Law can be extended to those cases where settling takes place in a centrifugal field:

$$v_s = v_g \frac{\omega^2 r}{g} \qquad (5)$$

where v_s is the settling velocity of a particle in a centrifugal field, v_g is the settling velocity of a particle in a gravitational field (Stokes' Law), ω is the angular velocity of the particle in the settling zone, and r is the radius at which the settling velocity is determined.

Consider a solid particle at an initial position in a liquid medium and a distance r from the axis of rotation. Under these conditions

$$v_s = dr/dt \qquad (6)$$

Substituting Eq 6 into Eq 5 gives

$$dr/dt = v_g \frac{\omega^2 r}{g} \qquad (7)$$

Rearranging and integrating between limits gives

$$\int_r^{r_c} \frac{dr}{r} = \int_0^t v_g \frac{\omega^2 r}{g} \, dt \qquad (8)$$

$$\ln \frac{r_c}{r} = v_g \frac{\omega^2 t}{g} \qquad (9)$$

where r_c is the distance between the surface of the sedimented cake in the tip of the tube and the axis of rotation and t is the time during which the particle is subjected to centrifugal acceleration while the particle travels the distance from r to r_c. Eq. 9 shows that if centrifuging conditions for a given suspension are to be compared in different centrifuges, the speed, bottle size, centrifuge dimensions, and centrifuging time must be taken into consideration. Ambler and Keith[3] and Lavanchy and Keith[4] describe mathematically approaches which should be taken for this purpose.

The Ultracentrifuge—When extremely fine solid matter must be separated from a liquid, eg, in colloid or biological research, the ultracentrifuge is employed. In this instrument a relatively small rotor is operated at speeds exceeding 100,000 rpm and forces up to one million times gravity are exerted. High speeds are attained with air or oil turbines and bearings lubricated with a film of compressed air. Friction heat may be minimized by the use of high vacuum.

By placing the samples in specially constructed cells and spinning them in the ultracentrifuge, it is possible to separate the dispersed phase from the continuous phase rather rapidly. To aid the investigator, optical attachments may be employed to photograph the settling while the centrifuge is in operation.

Only small batches of material can be handled in these instruments during a single run. Ultracentrifuges are employed in the determination of particle size and molecular weight of polymeric and other high-molecular-weight materials such as proteins and nucleic acids by direct or indirect observation of the rate of separation of particles in solution or suspension.

Description and use of other types of sedimentation centrifuges, such as the Disc Centrifuge and the Tubular Centrifuge, are given in *Remington's Pharmaceutical Sciences*, 14th ed, 378–379, 1970.

Filtration Methods

The filtration centrifuge is restricted to the separation of solid–liquid mixtures. It is similar in principle to the sedimentation type but rather than containers it possesses a porous wall through which the liquid phase may pass but upon which the solid phase is retained. Analogous to filtration, this process requires consideration of the flow of liquid through the solid bed which accumulates on the porous plate.

Filtration

Filtration is the process of separating liquids from solids with the purpose of obtaining optically transparent liquids. This is accomplished by the intervention of a porous substance, called the *filter* or the *filtering medium*. The liquid which has passed through the filter is called the *filtrate*.

Mathematics of Filtration

In 1842 Poiseuille proposed a relationship for streamlined flow of liquids under pressure through capillaries. This equation in its simplified form is represented by

$$V = \frac{\pi \Delta p r^4}{8L\eta}$$

where V = flow velocity, r = capillary radius, L = capillary length, η = viscosity of the fluid, and Δp = pressure differential at the two ends of the capillary.

The modified Poiseuille equation has been shown to be valid for liquid flow through sand, glass beads, and various porous media. It represents the foundation for all mathematical models of filtration which were subsequently developed. Of critical importance in this equation is the powerful effect of capillary radius, ie, by reducing it to $\frac{1}{8}$ its size, the pressure differential must be increased more than 4000 times in order to obtain the same flow velocity, all other factors remaining constant.

On the basis of the Poiseuille formula, the Kozeny–Carman relationship was established. This may be expressed as

$$V = \left[\frac{e^3}{KS^2(1-e)^2}\right]\left[\frac{A \Delta pg}{\eta L}\right]$$

where A = cross-sectional area of porous bed (filter medium), e = porosity of bed, S = surface area of medium, K = constant, and the remaining symbols are the same as in the Poiseuille equation.

The Kozeny–Carman relationship, like Poiseuille's law, states that the rate of flow is directly proportional to the pressure drop across the medium and to the area of the bed, and inversely proportional to the viscosity of the liquid and the thickness of the bed. To characterize the material composing the bed, two new quantities, e and S, are introduced, replacing capillary radius.

The use of a nondefinite constant, K, rather than the definite constant in Poiseuille's equation, $\pi/8$, offers greater utility in the use of this equation in accounting for the geometry of the medium. The constant, K, generally ranges in value from 3 to 6. The Kozeny–Carman equation finds its greatest limitation in complex systems such as filter paper but provides excellent correlation in filter beds composed of porous material.

In applying Poiseuille's law to filtration processes, one must recognize that the capillaries found in the filter bed are highly irregular and nonuniform. Therefore, if the length of a capillary is taken as the thickness of the bed or medium and the correction factor for the radius is applied, the flow rate is more closely approximated. These factors have been taken into account in the formulation of the Darcy equation:

$$V = \frac{k\,\Delta p}{L\eta}$$

where k = the permeability coefficient and is dependent on the nature of the precipitate to be filtered and the filter medium itself.

Recently, computer assisted design of microfiltration systems has been reported.[5] This technique is used to design an optimum filtration system from actual filtration data, and thereby, predict its performance with any given fluid.

In considering the nature of the precipitate it is known that large particles are easier to filter than are small particles because of the tendency of the latter to enter into and occlude the pores of the bed, thus hindering the passage of the filtrate. In addition, the buildup of small particles on the filter tends to form a nonporous, densely packed bed which also resists passage of the filtrate.

Filtering Media

The filtering medium, whether a filter paper, synthetic fiber, or porous bed of glass, sand, or stone, is composed of countless channels which impart *porosity* to the medium. Almost without exception these channels or pores are non-uniform and possess a rather tortuous nature.

The mechanism of filtration basically involves a two-step process: (1) the filter medium itself resists the flow of solid material while permitting the passage of liquid and (2) during the course of the filtration the suspended, solid material builds up on the filter medium and thereby forms a *filter bed* which acts as a second, and often more efficient, filter medium.

The ability of a filter medium to eliminate solid matter from a liquid is termed *retention*. It must be borne in mind that the filtration process must compromise retention with filtration rate, i.e., the speed at which the purified liquid (the filtrate) is recovered. To illustrate this point, it will be noted that a slab of marble will most effectively retain the solid material contained in a suspension; unfortunately, it would require a few centuries to collect the purified filtrate.

Both the retentive ability of a filter medium and filtration rate of a liquid through the medium are dependent on the porosity of the medium. Each factor, however, is influenced significantly by the following: (1) the viscosity of the liquid, (2) the proportion of solid matter in the liquid, and (3) the size, shape, and physical nature of the suspended solids.

The flow of a liquid through a filter bed follows the same basic rules that govern the flow of any liquid through a medium offering resistance. The flow rate through the medium will vary directly with the area of the medium, as well as the pressure drop or driving force across the bed.

$$\text{Rate of flow} \propto \frac{(\text{driving force})(\text{cross-sectional area})}{\text{resistance}}$$

The flow rate is retarded by the viscosity of the liquid being filtered and by any obstruction to flow. These obstructions include the resistance of the filter medium itself and the second filter bed or filter cake which builds up on the medium at a rate dependent on the solids content of the liquid. The resistance offered by the medium itself will not vary significantly during the filtration process. It is dependent on the thickness of the medium as well as its porosity. The resistance of the filter cake, on the other hand, is not constant and generally increases continuously during the operation. The resistance offered by the cake is dependent both on its thickness and physical nature. The thickness of the cake is

dictated by the amount of filtrate passing through the filter and on the solids content of the liquid. The physical nature of the cake, ie, whether it is loose, compacted, coarse, fine, granular or gelatinous, determines whether or not it will readily allow the flow of liquid.

Filter Paper—Filter paper is most frequently employed in clarification processes required of the pharmacy practitioner. Only high-quality filter paper should be used to assure maximum filtering efficiency. When possible the first few milliliters of filtrate should be discarded in order to eliminate in so far as possible contamination of the pharmaceutical product by free fibers associated with most filter paper. This is especially true in the preparation of ophthalmic solutions. Methods of folding filter paper are found in *Remington's Pharmaceutical Sciences*, 14th ed, 381, 1970.

Membrane Filters—These filter media are produced from pure cellulose, cellulose derivatives, and polymeric materials. All have an extremely uniform micropore structure as well as an exceptionally smooth surface. The integral structure contains no fibers or particles which can work loose and contaminate a filtrate. This is a particular advantage in the filtration of ophthalmic solutions. The presence of these fibers is difficult to prevent when using many other filter media, including paper filters.

The efficiency of membrane filters is due to the uniform pore system which functions like a highly effective sieve. The pore size, of different types of these filters, ranges from 10 nm to 10 μm. All particles in liquids or gases which are larger than the pore of a given filter are retained on the surface. The thickness of these membrane filters ranges from 50 to 200 μm.

The pores which penetrate these filters pass directly through the entire thickness of the membrane, with a minimum of crosslinkage. Porosity or pore volume is estimated as 80% of the total filter volume. The high porosity of these filters, coupled with the "straight-through" configuration of the pores, results in flow rates through membrane filters which are at least 40 times faster than flow rates through conventional filter media which possess the same particle size retention capabilities.

Major producers of these filters include the Millipore Filter Corp., Bedford, MA; Gelman Instrument Corp, Ann Arbor, MI; Pall Corp, Glen Cove, NY; Nuclepore Corp, Pleasanton, CA; and Carl Schleicher & Schuell Co, Keene, NH. The membrane filters are available as circular discs of varying diameter. Different types are available for use in the filtration of either aqueous or nonaqueous liquids. The discs are generally used in conjunction with specialized holders of either metal or glass composition. With small volumes (i.e., less than 500 mL), solutions are usually filtered using vacuum techniques. Larger volumes require filtration under pressure provided by an inert gas such as nitrogen.

In addition to their obvious utility in routine filtration processes on both a laboratory and industrial scale, these filters have been used for a wide range of purposes, including chemical analysis, microbiological analysis, and bacterial filtration. The latter process provides an economical and rapid method for sterilizing heat-labile material (see the chapter on *Sterilization*).

Other Filtering Media—Many devices have been advanced to replace filter paper, which has many disadvantages, particularly for large-scale operations. A great many variations of filtering processes, each designed to fit the needs of special cases, are found in the modern pharmaceutical laboratory. The filter press, the centrifugal filter, the vacuum filter, the sand-bed filter, the charcoal filter, paper–pulp filter, and porous porcelain filter, are all examples of specialized filtration methods. Each one of these possesses some advantageous quality, and it is the experience of the laboratory operators that guides them in their selection of appropriate filtering devices. Reference is made later in the text to many of these special-scale filters.

However, it would not be inappropriate to refer briefly to special filtering devices which may be useful in the prescription or research laboratory.

Cotton Filters—A small pledget of absorbent cotton, loosely inserted in the neck of a funnel, adequately serves to remove large particles of extraneous material from a clear liquid. Although this properly might be termed colation, the cotton can also be used to serve as a fairly efficient filter. It is sometimes necessary to return the liquid a number of times to secure perfect transparency. This should be remembered in filtering ophthalmic solutions through cotton, when small detached filaments are carried through on initial filtration.

Glass-Wool Filters—When solutions of highly reactive chemicals, such as strong acids, are to be filtered, filter paper cannot be used. In its place glass wool may be used as one uses absorbent cotton for filtering. This material is resistant to ordinary chemical action and when properly packed into the neck of a funnel constitutes a very effective filtering medium.

Sintered Glass Filters—These filters have as the filtering medium a flat or convex plate consisting of particles of Jena glass powdered and sifted to produce granules of uniform size which are molded together. The plates can be fused into glass apparatus of any required shape (Fig 78-5). These filters vary in porosity, depending on the size of the granules used in the plate. They are very useful in the filtration of solutions such as those intended for parenteral injection. A vacuum attachment is necessary to facilitate the passage of the liquid through the filter plate (see the chapter on *Sterilization*).

Funnels

Funnels are conical-shaped utensils intended to facilitate the pouring of liquids into narrow-mouthed vessels. They are also widely used in pharmacy for supporting filter media. Funnels may be made of glass, polyethylene, metal, or any other material which serves a specific purpose. The community pharmacist will find the glass funnel to be quite adequate for all processes of clarification in prescription practice.

Most funnels used by the pharmacy practitioner are conical in shape and may be fluted, grooved, or ribbed for the purpose of facilitating the downward flow of the filtrate.

The *Büchner* type of funnel is largely used today in pharmaceutical laboratories. A piece of round filter paper is laid on the perforated porcelain diaphragm and the filtration conducted. This funnel is especially applicable to vacuum filtration (see *Vacuum Filtration*).

Filtration of Volatile Liquids—It is evident that the ordinary methods of filtering liquids will not be practical for very volatile liquids because of the loss through evaporation and the liability to explosion, in the case of flammable volatile liquids. Funnels must be covered, the receiving vessel must be closed, and provision made for the escape of the confined air in the receiving vessel. The following method is quite useful. A rubber cover, perforated to admit a tube, is placed on top of the funnel, and connection between the bottle and funnel is effected as shown in Fig 78-6.

Aids to Filtration—It has long been known that addition of an insoluble adsorbent powder to a liquid prior to its filtration greatly increases the efficiency of the process. Purified talc, siliceous earth (kieselguhr), clays, charcoal, paper pulp, chalk, magnesium carbonate, bentonite, silica gel, etc, have been used for this purpose.

It must not be overlooked, however, that powdered substances employed for such purposes must be insoluble and inert and not all of those in the foregoing list are applicable for general filtration.

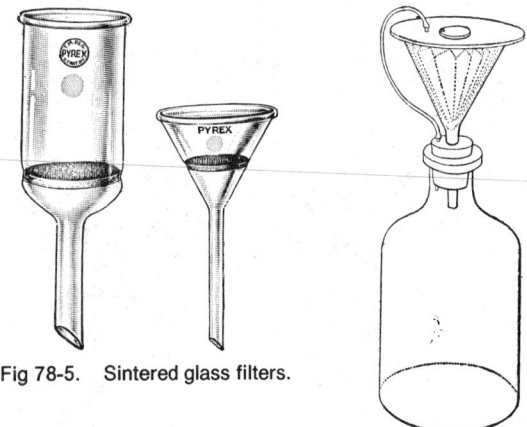

Fig 78-5.   Sintered glass filters.

Fig 78-6.   Filtration of volatile liquids.

Talc is nonadsorbent to materials in solution and is a chemically inert medium for filtering any liquid, provided it has been purified for this purpose and it is not the impalpably fine variety which will pass through the filter paper.

Kieselguhr is almost pure silica (SiO_2). It is as applicable as talc for general filtration purposes, with no danger of removing active constituents by adsorption.

Siliceous earths or *clays*, such as fuller's earth or kaolin in the hydrated form that is produced when they are brought into contact with aqueous liquids, are safe for general use only in filtering fixed oils. Liquids containing coloring matter or alkaloidal principles must not be filtered through these media, for adsorption of both color and alkaloids occurs and the filtrate is altered in comparison.

Charcoals, as a rule, possess adsorptive properties not only toward color but for many active constituents of medicinal preparations, eg, alkaloids and glycosides. Consequently, charcoal should never be used as a filtering medium unless the removal of such constituents is desirable.

Chalk and *magnesium carbonate* readily react with acids and possess a finite solubility in water and aqueous fluids, with the production of alkalinity in the filtrate. This is particularly true of magnesium carbonate; the degree of alkalinity imparted to the filtrate is sufficiently great to cause precipitation of alkaloids. Either of these media, when added to an alkaloidal preparation prior to filtration, will precipitate and remove all of the alkaloidal constituents. Neither is suitable for general use.

Rapid Filtering Apparatus—Much attention has been given to methods for increasing the rapidity of filtration. This may be accomplished by applying pressure on the filter or by creating a vacuum in the receiving vessel.

Vacuum Filtration—One of the first practical efforts made to create a vacuum to aid filtration was by means of the Bunsen pump. Its action depends on the principle that a column of water descending through a tube from a height is capable of carrying with it the air contained in a lateral tube, if the latter is properly placed. This form of aspirator is practicable where water pressure is available.

Pumps Acting by Water Pressure—The variety of aspirator or vacuum pumps which operate under the influence of water pressure are all based on the same principle. The following are selected for illustration from the great variety in use. Fig 78-7 shows Chapman's vacuum pump. Valve *a* prevents the water from flowing into the bottle which carries the filter when the pressure of water ceases or is reduced.

On a larger scale the vacuum for filtration is produced by one of the many types of vacuum pumps now available. The pump should be protected from vapors by placing a suitable vapor trap between the filter unit and the pump. The trap

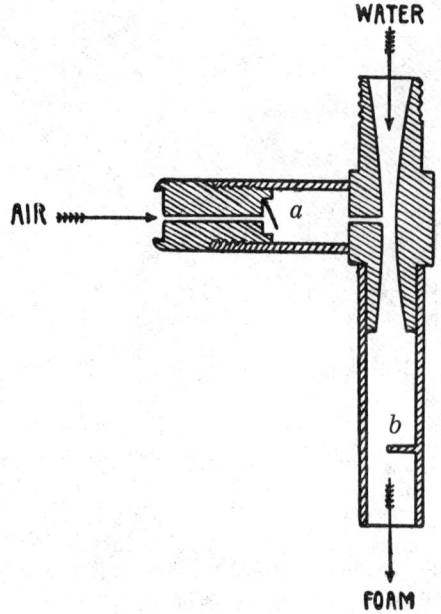

Fig 78-7. Chapman's pump.

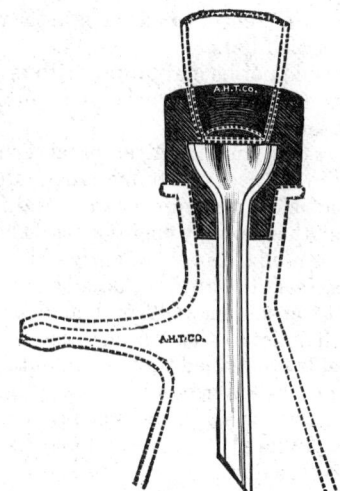

Fig 78-8. Gooch crucible arranged for vacuum filtration (courtesy, Thomas).

is usually cooled to very low temperatures by means of dry ice and acetone when very high vacuum is needed.

In assembling a filtering apparatus using the vacuum principle, it is necessary that there be no leaks in the connections from the filter to the aspirator. If filter paper is used in connection therewith, a plainly folded paper must be used and its tip must be protected against breakage by reinforcing it with a filter paper support or some other device. A Büchner filter may also be used employing a specially strong filter paper.

In analytical work it is customary to use the Gooch crucible and flask (Fig 78-8) for rapid filtration. The flask, of especially thick glass, is provided with a side tube which is connected to a water aspirator pump. The perforated crucible bottom is converted into a filter bed of the required thickness by means of a filter mat placed over the perforations in the porcelain base.

Filtration under Pressure—Fig 78-9 illustrates a sectional drawing of a plate-and-frame filter press. Material to be filtered enters the apparatus under pressure through a pipe at the bottom and is forced into one of the many chambers. A filter cloth is positioned on both sides of each chamber. As the material passes through the filtering cloths, solids remain behind in the chamber and the clear filtrate passes through and out of an opening located on top of the apparatus.

Rotary-drum vacuum filters are widely used in the pharmaceutical industry, especially in the preparation of antibiotics by the fermentation process. In this type of filtration a perforated drum, wrapped with a cloth or other suitable substance holding a filter medium, is partially immersed in a tank holding the material to be filtered (Fig 78-10).

The drum is rotated through the slurry of material and a vacuum within the drum draws the material into and through

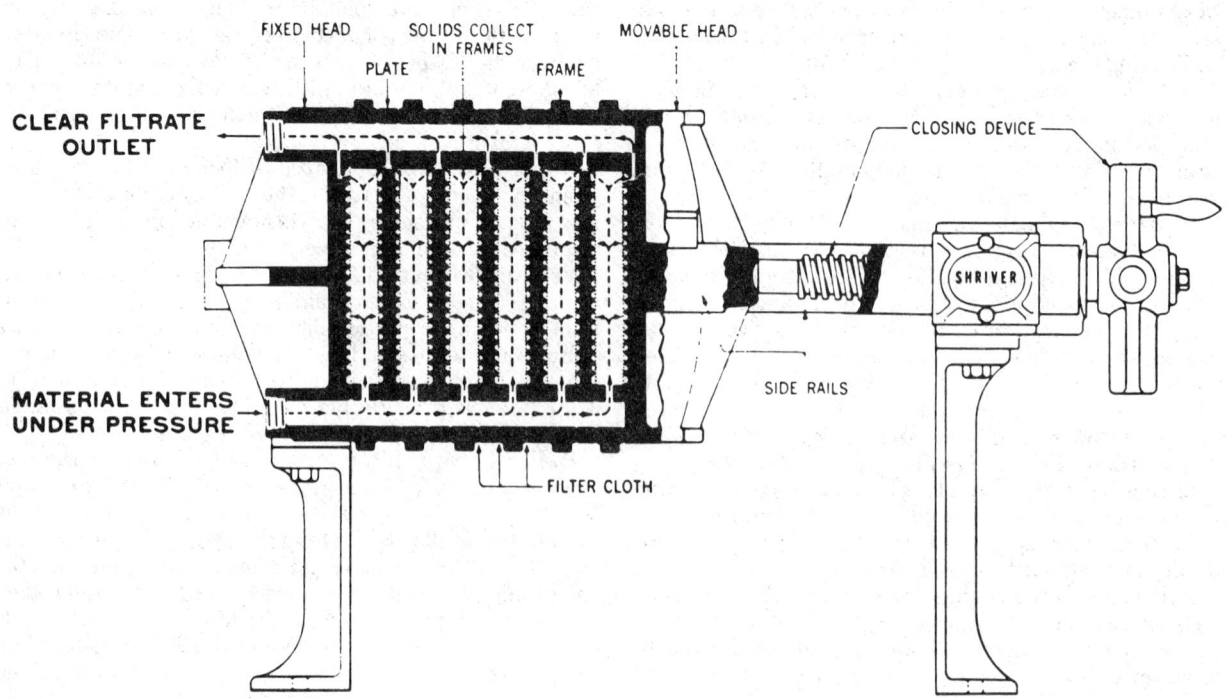

Fig 78-9. A plate-and-frame filter press (courtesy, Shriver).

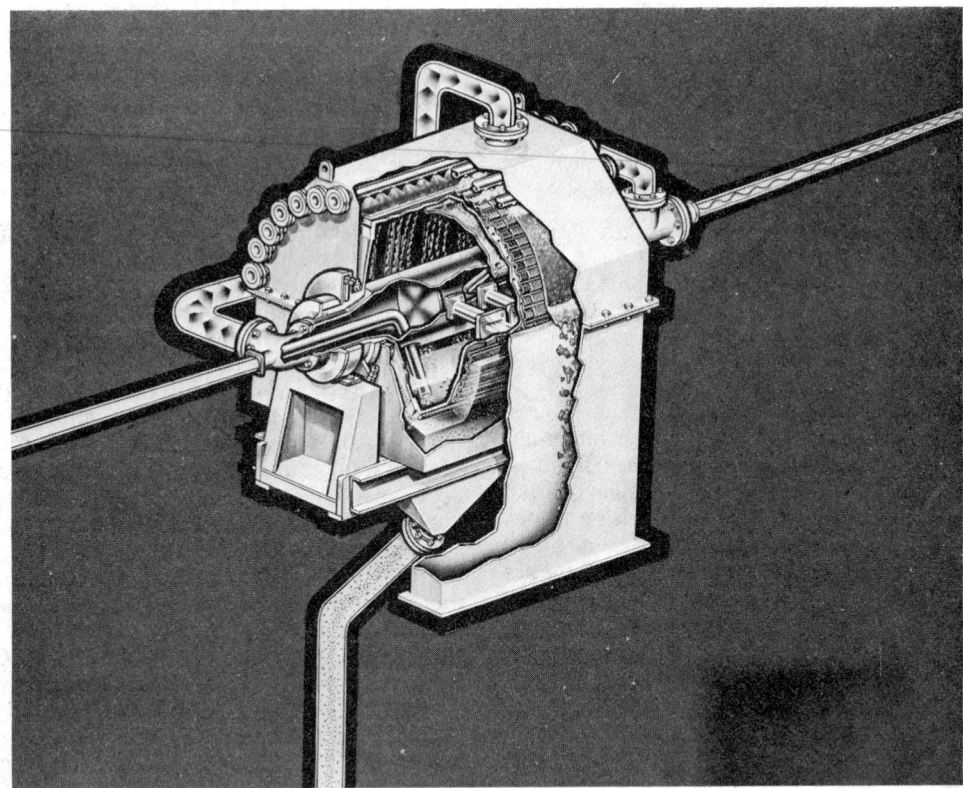

Fig 78-10.   Rotary filter (courtesy Bird Machine).

the filter medium. During this step of the process the filtrate is taken into the drum and collected, while the solid material remains deposited on the outer surface of the drum. This material is then removed by a scraper in the last step of the operating cycle, just before the rotating drum repeats another cycle.

Clarification and Decoloration

Clarification

Clarification is the process by which finely divided solids and colloidal materials are separated from liquids without the use of filters. The process is employed to remove suspended oil from aqueous solutions, eg, as in aromatic waters, and for the removal of undesirable solids which interfere with the transparency of such natural products as honey and fruit juices.

Clarification is generally resorted to when the contaminating material is finely subdivided, amorphous, or colloidal in nature and tends to plug a filtration medium rapidly. A number of methods are available to handle this difficult problem.

When the solids are not of a granular or free-filtering nature, it may be possible to improve the characteristics of the suspended solids. This may involve varying the temperature or pH of the medium. When a viscid liquid is heated, its viscosity and specific gravity are decreased and particles which are suspended in it will separate. Those particles which are more dense than the liquid will fall to the bottom, while those which are less dense will rise to the surface. In the latter case the minute bubbles of steam formed in the heating process become enveloped in the viscid particles, rise through their buoyancy, and a scum is formed which may be separated readily.

The dewaxing of oils at a reduced temperature offers a further example of the possibilities of contaminant modification. Oil which is rapidly chilled often produces an amorphous wax which will plug a straining medium. Slow chilling, on the other hand, produces a wax with a more crystalline nature which has good filtration characteristics.

The simplest method of clarification, although not always feasible, is gravitational sedimentation. This method involves the least amount of labor and expense and is used frequently, particularly on a large scale, when haste is unnecessary. The deposit formed is called a *sediment* or *sludge*. These terms are not synonymous with *precipitate*. A sediment is solid matter separated merely by the action of gravity from a liquid in which it has been suspended. A precipitate, on the other hand, is solid matter separated from a previously clear solution by physical or chemical change. Fixed oils are usually clarified by gravitational sedimentation; in vegetable oils the sediment consists principally of albuminous and gummy substances, cellular tissue, and water, all of which have been separated with the oil during the expression process.

The clarification process is generally carried out by adding a clarifying agent such as paper, pulp, talc, infusorial earth, as well as a number of other materials to the turbid liquid. These agents usually act to reduce turbidity by physical adsorption of the contaminating material, although a large number of specific, physical–chemical coagulants are also in use. After the addition of the clarifying agent the mixture is agitated and the agents, along with the adsorbed impurities, are removed by filtration or any other suitable means. Albumin and gelatin are examples of clarifying agents obtained from natural sources. Substances of a synthetic nature, such as polyamines, are also used for this purpose. Additional information describing use of these materials as clarifying agents may be found in RPS-15: 1384–1385, 1975.

Decoloration

Decoloration or decolorization, as it is sometimes called, is the process of depriving solutions of color by use of an appropriate adsorptive medium. In many respects it is closely related to the clarification process. Decoloration is used for

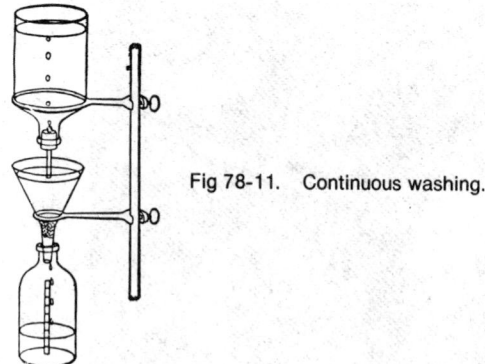

Fig 78-11.   Continuous washing.

removal of coloring matter from a number of raw materials, both natural and synthetic, and from many finished products. Animal charcoal (also called bone black), wood charcoal, and activated charcoal are frequently used as decolorizing agents. Clays such as bentonite, kaolin, and fuller's earth are also used for this purpose. For further information on this topic see RPS 15: 1385, 1975.

Lotion, Decantation, and Colation

Lotion

Lotion (displacement washing) is the process by which soluble impurities are removed from insoluble material by the addition of a suitable washing solvent. The wash liquid is usually separated from the purified solid by decantation or filtration. An expedient method of adding the washing solvent to the solid in a fine, controlled spray is by the use of wash bottles.

Continuous Washing—The use of the wash bottle is limited to small operations. A simple method of automatically supplying the wash liquid in larger quantities is shown in Fig 78-11. This requires attention from the operator only at the beginning of the operation. The inverted bottle containing the washing solvent is furnished with a perforated stopper and a short glass tube. All that is necessary is to fill the bottle and adjust it over the funnel so that the end of the tube is at the height at which the level of liquid in the funnel is to be maintained. On tilting the bottle slightly (if the tube selected is not too narrow in diameter) the liquid runs into the funnel until it rises to the orifice of the tube, whereupon the flow ceases. As the liquid gradually passes through the solid substance in the funnel, the level falls below the orifice, bubbles of air pass through the tube into the bottle, the liquid once more flows, and the operation continues until the upper bottle is empty. Many elaborate methods of continuous washing have been suggested, but the simple apparatus just described is quite satisfactory if a tube of proper diameter has been selected, that is, one of such size that the force of capillary attraction will not be strong enough to prevent the passage of air.

Decantation

The simplest method available for the separation of a solid from its soluble impurities is the technique of decantation. This method involves the following steps: (1) washing and subsequent agitation of the solid with an appropriate solvent, (2) allowing the solid to settle, and (3) removing the supernatant solvent. These three steps are repeated as often as required to attain the desired purity of the solid. This method is also applicable to the simple separation of solids and liquids, eg, after precipitation of a material from a mother liquor. Decantation provides an efficient method for washing magmas and other gelatinous products.

Some degree of skill is required to effectively decant liquids. It is most convenient to decant from a lipped vessel which is not filled to capacity. In addition, the use of a stirring rod is suggested as a guide to steady the hand of the operator.

Colation

Colation, or straining (L, *colare*, to strain), is the process of separating a solid from a fluid by pouring the mixture on a cloth or porous substance which will permit the fluid to pass through, but will retain the solid. This operation is frequently used for separating sediment or mechanical impurities of various kinds from liquids.

Colation should not be considered as a separate process but simply as a crude form of filtration, with larger pores in the straining medium than are usually employed for filtration.

The essential apparatus is a straining medium and a strainer support or frame. The straining medium is usually a cloth material such as flannel, muslin, wool, or cheesecloth. The material should be colorless and washed before use.

Fabrics, particularly those of cotton, are usually treated or impregnated with a material called *sizing* to improve their appearance and quality for certain purposes. For use as a strainer, the fabric must be free of sizing as it causes contamination. Many different substances are used for sizing, some being soluble in cold water, others only in hot water. The proper method for their removal, therefore, is first to soak the fabric for a few hours in cold *distilled water*, rinse thoroughly and cover with *distilled water*, boil for a few minutes, finally rinsing well in distilled water to remove the last traces of the gelatin, albumin, glue, or starch which may have been present in the sizing.

Expression

Expression is a process of *forcibly* separating liquids from solids. A number of mechanical principles have been recognized in the operation of expression: namely, the use of the spiral twist press, the screw press, the roller press, the filter press, and the hydraulic press.

Spiral Twist Press—The principle of this press is best and most practically illustrated in the usual process of manually expressing a substance contained in a cloth.

Roller Press—This is used for large-scale pressing of oily seeds, fatty substances, etc. Care must be taken to apply the force gradually to the bag containing the material to be pressed, and not to use it on substances which will be corrosive to the rubber rollers.

Hydrostatic or Hydraulic Press—Of the presses heretofore mentioned, each has some special advantage of use, but each also has some objectionable feature. The spiral twist is not powerful and its action is limited. The screw presses have friction with which to contend. The friction of a screw increases with the intensity of the pressure applied, and when a certain limit is reached all further force applied is wasted, and if continued may result in destruction of the press. The roller press is very limited in its action. The hydraulic press is expensive, but after the first cost it is the most economical because the greatest power is obtained at the expense of the least labor. The principle of a hydraulic press is based on the fact that pressure exerted upon an enclosed liquid is transmitted equally in all directions. Tremendous pressures can be developed with hydraulic presses.

Precipitation

Precipitation is the process of separating solid particles from a previously clear liquid, ie, a solution, by physical or chemical changes. The separated solid is termed a *precipitate;* the cause of precipitation, the *precipitant;* and the liquid which remains in the vessel above the precipitate, the supernatant liquid.

In pharmacy, precipitation may be useful for many purposes. It provides a convenient method of obtaining solid substances in the form of fine particles, eg, the precipitation of calcium carbonate (precipitated chalk). White Lotion is an example of a preparation prepared by precipitation, ie, by mixing aqueous solutions of zinc sulfate and sulfurated potash to form an insoluble, finely divided zinc sulfide, free sulfur, and various polysulfides.

One of the most important uses of precipitation is in the purification of solids. The process as applied to purification is termed *recrystallization*. The impure solid is usually dissolved in a suitable solvent at elevated temperatures. On cooling, the bulk of the impurities remain solubilized while the purified solid product precipitates. This procedure is repeated as many times as necessary, utilizing a number of solvents if required.

Separation of Immiscible Liquids

Separation of liquids that are mutually soluble is usually effected by distillation, if one or both of the liquids are volatile. Separation of liquids that are immiscible is generally a simpler process.

Separations of this kind are necessary in (1) analytical procedures, (2) manufacturing operations, (3) distillation of volatile oils, and (4) accidental contaminations and admixtures, and are usually best made using a separatory funnel. When very small amounts of liquids are floating on the surface of another liquid, separation is most easily accomplished by using a pipet, medicine dropper, or a glass syringe with an attached needle.

Florentine Receiver—The separation of volatile oils from the water which accompanies them during steam distillation is a very important part of their manufacturing process. Where the volatile oil is lighter than water, the principle shown in Fig 78-12 may be used. The oil and water collect in the glass receiver during distillation, the oil floating on the top, while the water ascends the bent tube from the bottom; further addition of distillate causes the water to overflow from the side tube. The reverse action is produced in the receiver for light or heavy oils (Fig 78-13), in which either a lighter or a heavier fraction may be collected continuously.

Specialized Separation Techniques

Diffusion Phenomena

Diffusion is the spontaneous penetration of one substance into another under the potential of concentration gradient. Simply stated, material will tend to move from a region of higher concentration to one of lower concentration. The driving force or potential of such a process may be enhanced by the application of an electric field.

If the two regions of concentration noted are separated by a selective membrane, certain species will diffuse through the membrane, while other molecular species will be held back. When this selectivity is dictated by the porosity of the membrane, the process is termed *dialysis*. Dialysis is used principally for the separation of small molecules and ions contained in a mixture with colloidal material. The latter substances diffuse with difficulty or not at all. Materials such as gums, starch, albumin, and proteins fall into this colloidal, nondiffusible category.

The rate of diffusion across a semipermeable membrane is directly proportional to the concentration gradient between the two surfaces of the membrane and to the area of the membrane but inversely proportional to the membrane thickness. These factors are expressed in Fick's law of diffusion:

$$\frac{dS}{dt} = \frac{kA(C_i - C_0)}{h}$$

where S = the amount of substance diffused at time t, k = a permeability constant, A = the membrane area, h = the membrane thickness, dS/dt = the diffusion rate, C_i = concentration on one side, and C_0 = concentration on the other side of the membrane.

Gel Filtration

Gel filtration is defined as a fractionation procedure in which separation is based on molecular size. The phenomenon of "molecular sieving" is an essential factor in gel filtration. The major breakthrough in this field was the introduction of cross-linked dextran gels.

The principle by which dextran gels (*Sephadex*) operate as molecular sieves is rather complex. The gel-forming particles are allowed to hydrate and swell in an aqueous solvent. Solute molecules penetrate the gel matrix to an extent which is dependent on the steric relationship existing between the molecular structure of the gel itself and that of the solute. Therefore, the shape and size of the solute molecules largely dictate their distribution between the gel particles and the interstitial solvent between the particles.

The following procedure is generally prescribed for the use of dextran gels. The solution containing the solutes to be separated is allowed to enter one end of a column packed with dextran gel which has been allowed to hydrate and swell in a suitable solvent. On washing the column with a solvent, the components of the mixture migrate at different rates and eventually appear in the filtrate in the order of decreasing molecular size.

Reverse Osmosis

A relatively new separation process which in principle may be applied to the separation, concentration, and fractionation of inorganic or organic substances in aqueous or nonaqueous solutions in the liquid or the gaseous phase is known as reverse osmosis (RO). (Related techniques are ultrafiltration and hyperfiltration.) Presently, the major thrust to research development of reverse osmosis is in the field of water treatment with emphasis given to the conversion of saline water to an acceptable quality of drinking water. It is recognized by the USP as an acceptable method to prepare Water for Injection.

Although the mechanism of reverse osmosis is still an open question, under certain conditions solute separation is brought about by a process closely resembling osmosis in reverse. The term osmosis is generally used to describe the spontaneous flow of pure water from a less to a more concentrated aqueous solution when separated by a suitable membrane (Figure 78-14 a and b). In the reverse osmosis process, a pressure is applied to the saline water compartment which is greater than the osmotic pressure acting in the opposite direction. The

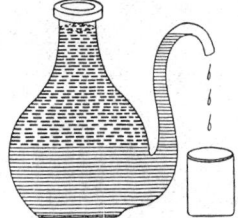

Fig 78-12.   Florentine receiver.

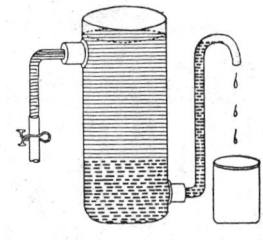

Fig 78-13.   Receiver for light or heavy oils.

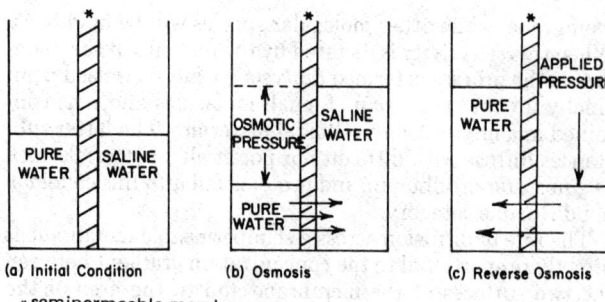

(a) Initial Condition   (b) Osmosis   (c) Reverse Osmosis

*semipermeable membrane

Fig 78-14.   Principles of reverse osmosis.

additional pressure forces water to move from the saline water to the pure water compartment thereby bringing about a separation and in this case purification of water. In practice a source of feed water (or solution) is forced over the surface of the membrane. As the solution flows across the membrane, water (solvent) is forced through the membrane by a suitable mechanical device and water (solvent) is collected on the pure water (solvent) side of the membrane. Impurities (solutes) are concentrated in the solution and carried out of the unit.

The mechanism of separation in the reverse osmosis process involves repulsion of ions and the sieving of uncharged organic chemical species by the membrane separating the two solutions. In other words, the membrane repels ions and sieves organic substances thereby allowing water (solvent) to pass through the micropores in the membrane surface. Hence, the reverse osmosis membrane removes nearly all organic substances with molecular weights greater than 200 including bacteria, viruses, and pyrogens. The substances with molecular weights under 200 will pass through the membrane to varying degrees depending upon the physical size and shape of the molecule. Because of the low molecular weight of the formaldehyde molecule, this substance has the ability to pass through the membrane both on the feed water side and on the pure water side of the apparatus. Hence, the RO equipment may be conveniently sterilized with one flushing of a solution of formaldehyde. For patients using RO as a means of purifying water for dialysis purposes, the sterilizing property of formaldehyde is very important, because it provides a simple, effective and rapid means of sterilizing RO equipment.

Other applications of this technique in the separation of solutes from solvents are found in the reference on *Membranes in Separation* listed at the end of this chapter.

References

1.   Craig LC, Craig D, in Weissberger A: *Technique of Organic Chemistry*, vol III, part 1, 2nd ed, Interscience, New York, Chap. II, 1956.
2.   Rogers LB, in Kolthoff IM, Elving PJ: *Treatise on Analytical Chemistry*, vol 2, part 1, Interscience, New York, Chap. 22, 1961.
3.   Weissberger A: *loc cit*, Chap IV.
4.   Mark HF, *et al: Kirk-Othmer Encyclopedia of Chemical Technology*, vol 4, 2nd ed, Interscience, New York, 710–758, 1964.
5.   Weyand J, in Shoemaker W. *What the filterman needs to know about filtration*. AIChE Symposium Series no 171 vol 73, American Institute of Chemical Engineers, New York, 1977.

Bibliography

Perry JH, *et al: Chemical Engineer's Handbook*, 5th ed, McGraw-Hill, New York, 1973.
Lachman L, *et al: The Theory and Practice of Industrial Pharmacy*, 2nd ed, Lea & Febiger, Philadelphia, Chap. 18, 1976.
Perry ES, Weissberger, A: *Technique of Chemistry*, vol XII, 3rd ed, Wiley-Interscience, New York, 1978.
Hwang ST, Kammermeyer K: *Membranes in Separations*, vol VII, Wiley-Interscience, New York, 1975.
Kolthoff IM, Elving PJ: *Treatise on Analytical Chemistry*, vol 5, part 1, Interscience Publication, New York, 1982.

CHAPTER 79

Sterilization

G Briggs Phillips, PhD

Senior Vice President for Scientific Affairs
Health Industries Manufacturers Association
Washington, DC 20005

Frank E Halleck, PhD

Corporate Director for Scientific Affairs
American Sterilizer Company
Erie, PA 16512

The objective of a sterilization process is to destroy all microorganisms in or on an object or preparation and to assure that it is free of infectious hazards. Since the variety and amounts of sterile materials required for health care have increased in recent years, sterilization techniques have become increasingly important. An essential element, therefore, in the practice of modern-day pharmacy is that of sterilizing pharmaceuticals and other materials and verifying that they are sterile.

Sterilization technology is not stagnant; new and improved techniques constantly evolve. Changes in the method of delivering health care services, differences in the types of medical products requiring sterilization, and new guidelines and requirements issued by the regulatory agencies also change practices used for product sterilization.

Unlike industrial sterilization practices, where similar products will be sterilized in the same apparatus with great uniformity and under consistent control, the pharmacist has the unique problem of handling many different products, sterilized in multipurpose equipment on a small scale. Furthermore, his employees may be relatively inexperienced. Hospitals traditionally have not used control and sterility validation methods to the same extent as industry.

The purpose of this chapter is to provide a basic understanding of sterilization methods and sterility verification that will be of use in the practice of pharmaceutical science. This chapter is also intended to provide the pharmacist with some understanding of sterilization methods used by industrial firms because he increasingly deals with sterile prepackaged items.

Definitions

From the point of view of the pharmacist or the pharmaceutical manufacturer, terms related to sterility, asepsis, etc, must be clearly understood:

Antiseptic: A substance that arrests or prevents the growth of microorganisms by inhibiting their activity without necessarily destroying them.
Bactericide: Anything that kills bacteria.
Bacteriostat: Anything that arrests or retards the growth of bacteria.
Disinfection: A process that removes infection potential by destroying microorganisms but not ordinarily bacterial spores. The term is usually used to designate the results of the application of chemical agents to inanimate objects.
Germicide: A substance that kills disease microorganisms but not necessarily bacterial spores.
Sterility: The absence of viable microorganisms.
Sterilization: A process by which all viable forms of microorganisms are removed or destroyed, based on a probability function.
Viricide: A substance that kills viruses.

Sterility as a Total System

The task of providing sterile pharmaceuticals and hospital goods can be perceived as a system comprised of a number of essential elements.

1. Selection of raw materials, and compounding or preparation of the material in such a way that the microbial load (the types and amounts of microbial contamination to be inactivated by the sterilization process) is minimal.
2. Selection of packaging that is compatible with the sterilization process and will maintain sterility after sterilization.
3. Application of an adequate sterilization treatment that is compatible with the materials and packaging being sterilized.
4. Verification of sterilization.
5. Proper storage of sterile goods.
6. Delivering, opening, and use of sterile materials without recontamination.

Attention to each of these essential elements provides maximum assurance that materials will not be contaminated at the time of use.

Contamination

Certain facts about microorganisms must be kept in mind when preparing sterile products. Some microbes (bacteria, molds, etc) multiply in the refrigerator, others at temperatures as high as 60°. Microbes vary in their oxygen requirements from the strict anaerobes that cannot tolerate oxygen to aerobes that demand it. Slightly alkaline growth media will support the multiplication of many microorganisms while others flourish in acidic environments. Some microorganisms have the ability to utilize nitrogen and carbon dioxide from the air and thus can actually multiply in distilled water. In general, however, most pathogenic bacteria have rather selective cultural requirements, with optimum temperatures of 30–37° and a pH of 7.0. Contaminating yeasts and molds can develop readily in glucose and other sugar solutions.

Actively growing microbes are, for the most part, vegetative forms with little resistance to heat and disinfectants. However, some forms of bacteria—among them are the bacteria that cause anthrax, tetanus, and gas gangrene—have ability to assume a spore state which is very resistant to heat as well as to many disinfectants. For this reason, an excellent measure of successful sterilization is whether the highly resistant spore forms of nonpathogenic bacteria have been killed.

The nature of expected contamination is important to the pharmacist preparing materials to be sterilized. The raw materials he works with will rarely be sterile and improper storage may increase the microbial content. Because the pharmacist seldom handles all raw materials in a sterile or protected environment, the environmental elements of the pharmacy (air, surfaces, water, etc) can be expected to contribute to the contamination of a preparation. Likewise, the container or packaging material is rarely sterile and will contribute to the total microbial load.

Understanding the nature of contaminants prior to sterilization and application of methods for minimizing such contamination will assist in preparing successful pharmaceutical sterilization. Examples of such methods include:

1. Maintenance of a hygienic laboratory.
2. Frequent disinfection of floors and surfaces.
3. Minimization traffic in and out of the pharmacy.
4. Refrigerated storage of raw materials and preparations which support microbial growth.

5. Use of laminar airflow devices (see page 1451) for certain critical operations.

6. Use of water that is relatively free of microbial contamination.

Methods

General

The procedure to be used for sterilizing a drug, a pharmaceutical preparation, or a medical device is determined to a large extent by the nature of the product. Methods of inactivating microorganisms may be classified as either physical or chemical. Physical methods include moist heat, dry heat, and irradiation. Sterile filtration is another process, but it only removes, not inactivates, microorganisms. Chemical methods include the use of either gaseous or liquid sterilants.

Each sterilization method can be evaluated by experimentally derived values representing the general reaction rates of the process. For example, a death rate or survivor curve for a standardized species can be diagrammed for different sterilization methods. This is done by plotting the logarithm of surviving organisms against time of exposure. In most instances, these data show a linear relationship, typical of first-order kinetics and suggest that a constant proportion of a contaminant population is inactivated in any given time interval. Based on such inactivation curves, it is possible to derive values that represent the general reaction rates of the process. For example, based on such data, it has become common to derive a decimal reduction time or D value, which represents the time under a stated set of exposure conditions required to reduce a surviving microbial population by a factor of 90%.

D values, or other expressions of sterilization process rates, provide a means of establishing dependable sterilization cycles. Obviously, the initial microbial load on a product to be sterilized becomes an important consideration. Beyond this, however, kinetic data also can be used to provide a statistical basis for the success of sterilization cycles. A simple example will suffice (Fig 79-1). When the initial microbial contamination level is assumed to be 10^6 and if the D value of the sterilization process is 7 min, complete kill is approached by application of 6 D values (42 min). However, at this point reliable sterilization would not be assured because a few abnormally resistant members of the population may remain. In this example, by extending the process to include an additional 6 D values, most of the remaining population is inactivated, reducing the probability of one organism surviving is one in one million.

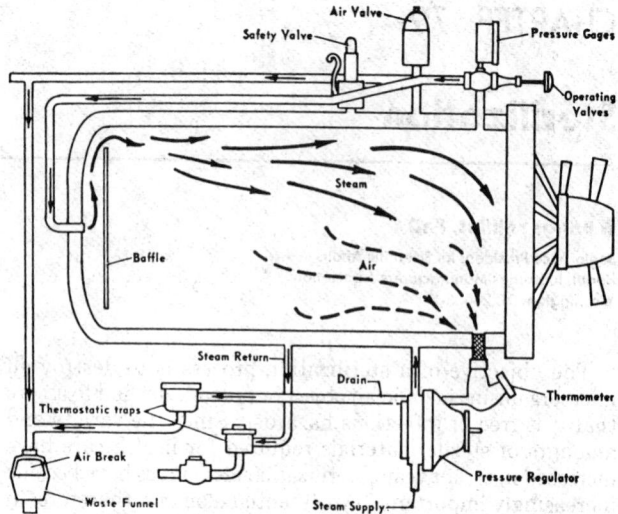

Fig 79-2. Longitudinal cross-section of a downward displacement sterilizer showing essential parts and a flow pattern for the movement of steam and air (courtesy, Castle).

Steam Sterilization

Moist heat in the form of saturated steam under pressure is the most dependable and widely used method for sterilization. The cause of death in moist heat sterilization is different from that by dry heat; death by moist heat is the result of coagulation of cellular protein whereas dry heat causes death primarily by an oxidation process.[1]

The USP defines steam sterilization as employing saturated steam under pressure for at least 15 min at a minimum temperature of 121°C in a pressurized vessel. The simplest form of an autoclave is the home pressure cooker. Such a device, however, is not recommended for the sterilization of pharmaceuticals because it lacks suitable pressure and temperature recording devices and does not have efficient means of displacing entrapped air.

A gravity or downward displacement autoclave (Fig 79-2) depends on the difference in density between air and steam. Air, being heavier, is displaced to the bottom of the chamber and exits while the steam is admitted at the top of the chamber. The temperature is usually measured at the drain point to assure that air has been adequately exhausted from the chamber. Other steam sterilizers utilize vacuum pumps and other devices to remove air rapidly from the chamber and these types of sterilizers employ prevacuum sterilization cycles or processes. Rapid air removal considerably reduces the sterilization process time. Specialized steam sterilizers are also available for hermetic and nonhermetic sealed products where conventional steam sterilizers cannot be utilized because of product, package, or seal retention integrity problems. Modern-day hospital autoclaves are available in a wide range of sizes, from about 12 in in diameter to 6 ft or larger in diameter (Fig 79-3).

The importance of removing all air from steam sterilizers, as steam is introduced, cannot be overemphasized. Mixtures of air and steam result in slower heating times for the chamber as well as lower final temperatures. Fig 79-4 illustrates the effect on temperatures of several air-steam mixtures as contrasted with pure steam. Sterilizer operators cannot depend on pressure readings to assure sterilization, but rather temperature readings. In this way adequate cycles are assured and failures of air exhaust systems can be detected.

A deterrent to maximizing the efficiency of steam sterilizers has been the difficulty in removing all of the entrained and entrapped air. Recent developments, however, have greatly improved this situation by providing a variety of prevacuum

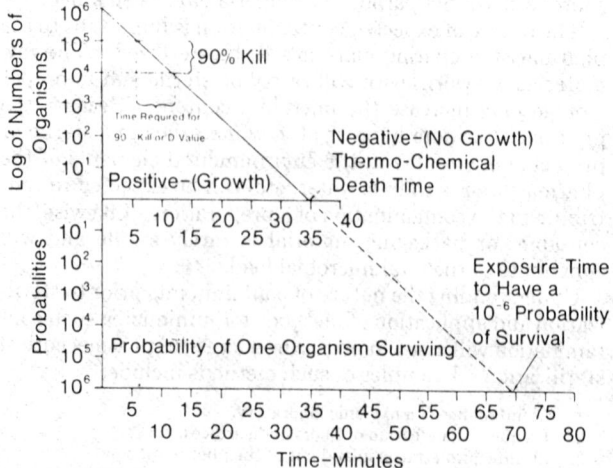

Fig 79-1. Sterilization model using D values.

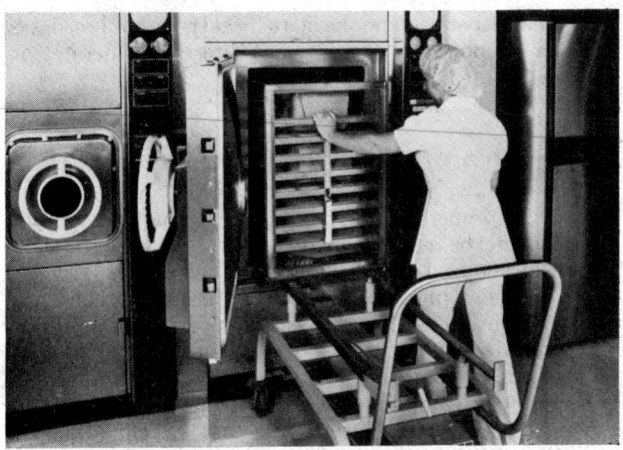

Fig 79-3.   Hospital sterilizer with automatic controls showing shelves for loading (courtesy, American Sterilizer).

Table I—Steam Sterilization of Liquids—Effect of Volume per Container (Erlenmeyer Flasks) on Time Required to Reach 121°C (Single Container Load)[5]

Size of container (mL)	Ml of liquid per container	Chamber temp (C) at initiation of cycle	Liquid temp (C) at initiation of cycle	Mins for chamber to reach 121°	Mins for center of liquid to reach 121°	Total time of cycle (mins)
50	25	110	25	2	4	14
125	75	110	25	2	5	15
200	150	110	25	3	7	17
500	400	110	25	3	10	20
1000	800	110	25	3	14	24
2000	1500	110	25	6	19	29
3000	2500	110	25	7	25	35
5000	4500	110	25	8	33	43
6000	5500	110	25	8	44	54

and pulsing sterilizer cycle systems. Systems of pulsing for vacuum and steam apply more specifically to the removal of air from packs of material in the chamber rather than from the chamber itself.

The prevacuum steam sterilization method involves the rapid evacuation of a chamber to 15 torr before the steam is added. Other modifications use rapid removal of air, followed by higher steam pressures and thus by higher temperatures. This can substantially reduce the required sterilization exposure time. With a prevacuum high-pressure cycle one can, for example, use 134°C (270°F) for 3 min instead of 121°C (250°F) for 15 min.

In addition to eliminating air from the chamber and establishing correct sterilization temperatures, it is necessary to consider how long it will take for the material to reach the correct temperature and how long after reaching the required temperature it should be held to achieve sterility. For small volumes (up to 250-mL flasks), the time required to reach

thermal equilibrium is short. However, larger volumes will often require a longer heating period before all of the solution has reached 121°C. As long as 55 min at 121°C may be required for the solution (8 liters in a standard Pyrex bottle) to be sterilized. Tables I and II exemplify the need to lengthen the sterilization cycle time when container size or number of containers per load are increased.

Regardless of the type of autoclave, the arrangement of the load in the chamber is of paramount importance. All products should be arranged loosely to allow direct steam penetration and contact. All packages containing glass or metal vessels should be placed on their side so that a path is provided for the escape of the heavier air. Automatically controlled sterilizers are most desirable, when equipped with thermocouples for measuring temperatures in various locations in the chamber and product control and with automatic timers that time sterilization, beginning when the appropriate temperature is reached. Such autoclaves automatically turn off at the end of the sterilizing period. The jackets of some large sterilizers used for sterilizing liquids and solutions may be equipped with a cold water spray cycle that will rapidly cool the load to expedite removal from the chamber.

A specific precaution should be exercised in sterilization of fluids in containers. When a flask or bottle with a loose-

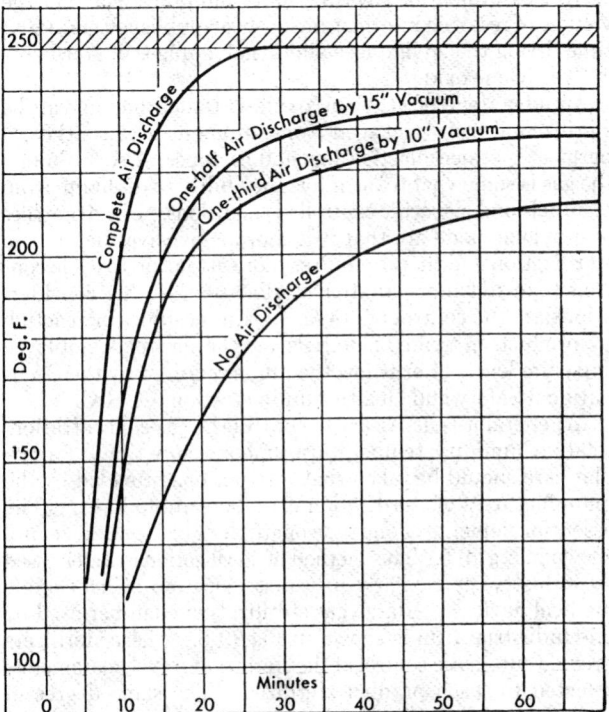

Fig 79-4.   The temperatures resulting from complete and partial air discharge from a sterilizing chamber operated at 15 lb pressure.[2]

Table II—Steam Sterilization of Liquids—Effect of Volume per Container and Number of Containers on Time Required for Liquid to Reach 121°C[3, a]

Liquid per container (liter)	No. of containers per load	Chamber temp (C) at initiation of cycle	Liquid temp (C) at initiation of cycle	Mins for chamber to reach 121°	Mins for center of liquid to reach 121°	Total time of cycle (mins)
0.5	30	27	29	10	19	29
1.0	20	27	26	12	34	44
1.5	15	56	26	12	36	46
2.0	10	46	27	13	37	47
2.5	10	66	26	15	40	50
3.0	8	46	26	15	43	53
3.5	6	46	26	12	50	60
4.0	5	43	26	12	52	62
4.5	5	44	26	14	58	68
5.0	5	46	26	15	60	70
5.5	5	42	26	17	60	70
6.0	4	42	26	15	62	72

[a] Chart or external thermometer readings reflect the temperature of the chamber, not the load. Variations in load and equipment necessitate the use of a temperature sensing device in the center of the load. Consequently a thermocouple and potentiometer or similar device shall be used to determine the sterilization cycle. Once the cycle has been established there is no need to use thermocouples for daily use. It is recommended, however, that the cycle be checked once every 2 wk.

fitting closure (to allow air removal and steam penetration and prevent breakage) is sterilized and then removed, a vacuum may result upon cooling. If the closure fails or if conditions are not otherwise controlled, contamination can be drawn into the container. Special precautions must be utilized to insure the safety of the sterilizer operator.

Dry Heat

Some materials cannot withstand steam sterilization and are best sterilized by dry heat. Examples include petroleum jelly, mineral oils, greases, waxes, and talcum powder. Because dry heat is less efficient than moist heat, longer exposure times and higher temperatures are required. Although dry-heat sterilization is one of the oldest known methods, establishing exact and correct time-temperature cycles is not routine. A wide range of inactivation times at various temperatures has been established based on the type of sterility indicators used, the humidity conditions, and other factors. The amount of water in a microbial cell is known to influence its resistance to dry-heat destruction. Although it has been generally accepted that microbial cells in an extremely dry state exhibit increased resistance to dry-heat inactivation, recent research has demonstrated that the influence of moisture in the dry-heat process is considerably more complicated than previously anticipated. It is clear, however, that care should be taken in the design of dry-heat sterilization cycles for hospital products and that systematic validation of sterility by some accepted standardized method should be practiced.

Ovens used for dry-heat sterilization are usually thermostatically controlled and may be either gas- or electric-heated. They should be constructed to provide proper circulation of air to avoid the layering of hot air that could cause overheating in some areas and less than sterilizing temperatures in others. In some models fans are employed to circulate the hot air, while in others uniform heat distribution is accomplished by using baffling devices. Because of the varied nature of the products sterilized by dry heat and other uncertainties, it is impractical to establish a single time-temperature relationship for pharmaceutical and hospital materials. However, some time-temperature figures commonly mentioned for the dry-heat sterilization of hospital supplies are as follows:

170°C (340°F)—1 hour
160°C (320°F)—2 hours
150°C (300°F)—2.5 hours
140°C (285°F)—3 hours

Many pharmaceutical preparations, however, cannot be subjected to such temperatures. Therefore, other dry-heat sterilization cycles have been established. The chemotherapeutic agents, powders with low melting points, certain liquids in oil (for example, dimercaprol) and a variety of other substances require specially designed cycles utilizing lower temperatures for longer times.

The most important point, however, is that any method for dry-heat sterilization should be systemically tested using suitable biological indicators to validate that the procedure does in fact consistently sterilize the product. To accomplish this, adequate numbers of test samples identified with specific positions within the oven and containing known adequate numbers of appropriate biological indicators be used and that the resulting tests on the indicators show consistently the absence of contamination. The use of the statistical methods such as those of Bruch[4] and Pflug[5] are recommended in such procedures.

Finally, it should be pointed out that the heating of an object over a direct flame is a method of sterilization that is often used and is satisfactory for instruments such as forceps,

loops, metal spatulas, and the lips of beakers, test tubes, flasks, and similar objects. This process directly incinerates organisms on the instrument.

Ethylene Oxide

Although a variety of gases have been shown to possess germicidal properties (ethylene oxide, formaldehyde, propylene oxide, beta-propiolactone, ozone, chloropicrin, peracetic acid, and methyl bromide), only ethylene oxide is widely used for medical product sterilization. Its use has come about because many medical products are damaged or destroyed by other sterilization methods.

The proper application of any type of gaseous sterilization process is considerably more difficult than that of steam or dry-heat because more parameters must be controlled. For example, chambers designed for sterilization with gases require control of temperature, humidity, gas concentration, and exposure time. The gas must be evenly distributed within the chamber and the packaging material must be permeable enough to allow the penetration of moisture, heat and the gas itself but at the same time adequately protecting the sterile package after treatment.

Ethylene Oxide—Ethylene oxide, the simplest epoxy compound, has the formula

$$H_2C\underset{O}{\overset{}{\diagdown\diagup}}CH_2$$

A very reactive, flammable, colorless gas (the boiling point of the liquid is 10.8° under atmospheric pressure), ethylene oxide is used in the chemical industry for the synthesis of organic polymers. For sterilization purposes it is available as a pure liquid, as a 10% mixture with carbon dioxide, or as a 12% mixture with chlorofluorocarbons. The pure gas is highly explosive; its range of flammability as a mixture with air extends from 3.6% to 100% by volume. Dilution of the gas with carbon dioxide or chlorofluorocarbons provides a nonflammable mixture.

The use of ethylene oxide as a sterilant derives from the early basic evaluations by Kaye and Phillips in 1949. A large volume of research information has been published since that time listing the advantages and disadvantages of sterilizing with ethylene oxide.

An advantage of ethylene oxide is that products can be sterilized already packaged from shipment because the gas permeates sealed plastic films and cartons. Also, although the gas is somewhat toxic, it has the ability to dissipate from materials under specific controlled conditions. Disadvantages of ethylene oxide are that it is more expensive than steam sterilization and that it requires more attention to cycle controls than steam or radiation sterilization. Other considerations are the control of ethylene oxide residues or reaction by-products in treated materials and the control of employee exposure levels to or below the limits required by the Occupational Safety and Health Administration (OSHA).

In general it is necessary to control the gas concentration, relative humidity, temperature, and exposure time. Particular care should be taken that instructions provided by the manufacturers of sterilization chambers are followed. The essential elements of one type of ethylene oxide sterilizer are shown in Fig 79-5. This method of sterilization is widely used by industry, particularly in the sterilization of heat-labile medical devices. A large gas sterilization chamber used by one industrial firm is shown in Fig 79-6. These sterilizers provide automatic control of the sterilization cycle parameters selected for each product sterilized. The same degree of control can be achieved with many units suitable for use in hospitals and by hospital pharmacists. As a minimum, the instrumentation should provide control over the parameters

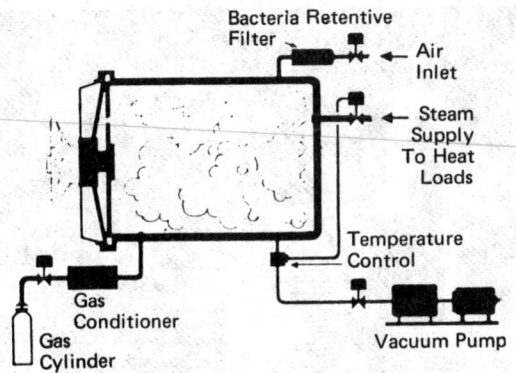

Fig 79-5.   The essential systems of a gas sterilizer.

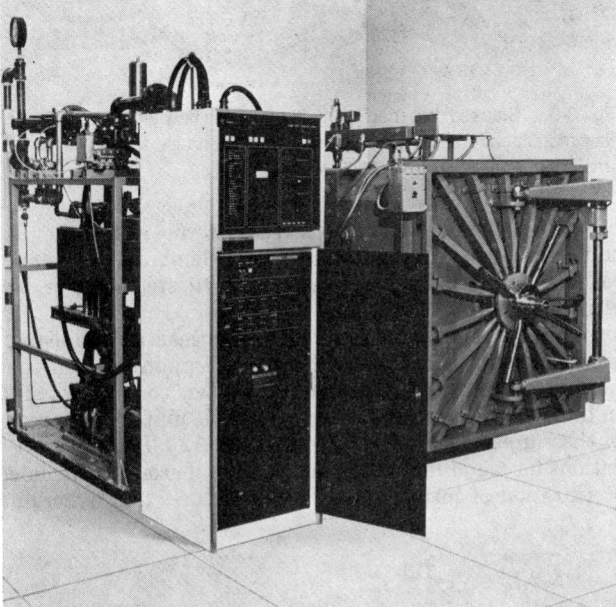

Fig 79-6.   Large ethylene oxide sterilizer with automatically controls (courtesy, American Sterilizer).

mentioned above and allow for the dissipation of ethylene oxide residues in the chamber and packaged products. The ethylene oxide products will require additional aeration to remove sterilant residues. This is best performed by the use of a heated chamber called an aerator.

The effectiveness of ethylene oxide sterilization is increased by an increase in temperature, as shown by Ernst (Fig 79-7). For efficient sterilization the materials should be maintained in an environment with relative humidity in excess of 40%. Most modern sterilizers provide a prehumidification stage at the beginning of the cycle, which is considered essential. A vacuum pump is usually used to remove most of the air in the chamber. Following this preparation ethylene oxide gas or a gas mixture enters the chamber via a conditioning unit to assure proper vaporization of the gas. Some large sterilizers provide the automatic admission of makeup gas during the exposure period. At the end of a cycle the vacuum is again used to purge the chamber and to reduce gas adsorbed into the product. Obviously, only container and wrapping materials which provide good and rapid permeation to moisture, air, and gas should be used in ethylene oxide sterilization chambers. Fig 79-8 shows a typical ethylene oxide cycle.

Filtration

Filtration is the removal of particulate matter from a fluid stream. Sterilizing filtration is a process which removes but

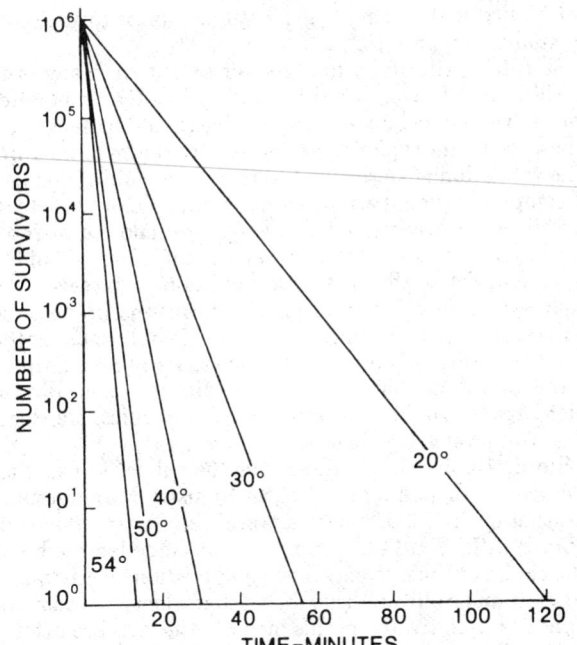

Fig 79-7.   Inactivation rates at various temperatures for *Bacillus subtilis* var *niger* spores on paper strips in gaseous ethylene oxide at 1200 mg/liter and 40% relative humidity.

does not destroy, microorganisms. Filtration, one of the oldest methods of sterilization, is the method of choice for solutions that are unstable to other types of sterilizing processes.

Pasteur, Chamberland, Seitz and Berkfeld filters have been used in the past to sterilize pharmaceutical products. These types of filters were composed of various materials such as sintered glass, porcelain or fibrous materials, ie, asbestos or cellulose. The filtration mechanism of these depth filters is random adsorption or entrapment in the filter matrix. The disadvantages of these filters are low flow rates, difficulty in cleaning, and media migration into the filtrate. Fiber-releasing and asbestos filters are now prohibited by the Food and Drug Administration for the filtration of parenteral products.[6,7]

Over the past thirty years, membrane filters have become the method of choice for the sterilization of heat-labile parenteral products. Membrane filters are thin, rigid, and homogenous polymeric structures. Microorganisms, present in fluids, are removed by a process of physical sieving and are retained on or near the membrane surface. Membrane filters of 0.22 μm pore size are commonly employed as sterilizing filters. However, 0.45 μm pore size filters are used to sterilize

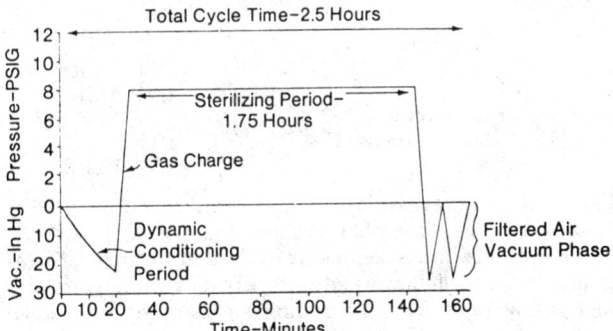

Fig 79-8.   Typical ethylene oxide sterilization cycle showing initial chamber evacuation and preconditioning and evacuation at the end of the cycle.

antibiotics or steroids in organic vehicles prior to an aseptic crystallization process.*

Sterilizing filtration, to a greater extent than any other sterilization process, should be validated. Membrane filters can be validated by a destructive bacterial challenge test. These tests are typically performed by the manufacturer. The validation of sterilizing filters poses an additional level of complexity since performance is a function of the filter to be validated, the choice of the test organism, and the operating conditions. The validation protocol, therefore, should be representative of the worst case condition. The severity of such test assures that the degree of sterility assurance associated with sterilizing filtration is equivalent to that in other types of sterilizing processes. Unique to membrane filtration is the condition that beyond a certain challenge level of microorganisms, the filter will clog. For a typical sterilizing filter this level is 10^9 organisms per cm^2.

Sterilizing membrane filters may be validated using the protocol developed by the Health Industry Manufacturers Association (HIMA).[8] In this procedure, *Pseudomonas diminuta* (ATTC 19146) is cultivated in saline lactose broth. The choice of the microorganism and medium is critical.

Leahy and Sullivan[9] have shown that when *Pseudomonas diminuta* is cultivated in this medium the cells are discrete and small (approximately 0.3 μm in diameter)—a range recommended for sterilizing filtration with 0.22 μm filters. Each cm^2 of the filter to be validated is challenged with 10^7 microorganisms at a differential pressure of 30 psig. The entire filtrate is collected and tested for viable microorganisms. The retention efficiency (log reduction value) of the membrane filter may be calculated using the procedure described in the HIMA protocol. Dawson *et al*[10] have demonstrated that the probability of a nonsterile filtration with a properly validated membrane filter is approximately 10^{-6}.

Once the performance of the membrane filter has been validated, a non-destructive integrity test that has been correlated to the bacterial challenge test (the bubble point or diffusion test) can be routinely used prior to and after a sterilizing filtration to assure that the membrane filter is integral.[11,12]

Process Filtration—Until recently, membrane filters were available only in disc configuration. Advances in membrane technology have provided filters in both stacked disc and pleated cartridge configurations. These advances have provided larger surface areas and higher flow rate capabilities. Fig 79-9 is an example of these larger surface area filters.

Membrane filters are manufactured from a variety of polymers; cellulosic esters (MCE), polyvinylidiene fluoride (PVF), polytetrafluoroethylene (PTTE), etc. The type of fluid to be sterilized will dictate the polymer to be used. The listing below is intended to serve only as a guide for the selection of membrane filters for a particular application. The filter manufacturer should be consulted before making a final choice.

Fluid	Polymer
Aqueous	PVF, MCE
Oil	PVF, MCE
Organic Solvents	PVF, PTFE
Aqueous, extreme pH	PVF
Gases	PVF, PTFE

Fig 79-10 is an example of a sterilizing filtration system commonly used in the pharmaceutical industry.

Positive pressure is commonly utilized in sterilizing filtrations. It has the following advantages over vacuum; provides higher flow rates, integrity testing is easier, and it avoids a

---

* The authors gratefully acknowledge the assistance of Fred Dawson, Millipore Corporation, in preparation information on filtration sterilization.

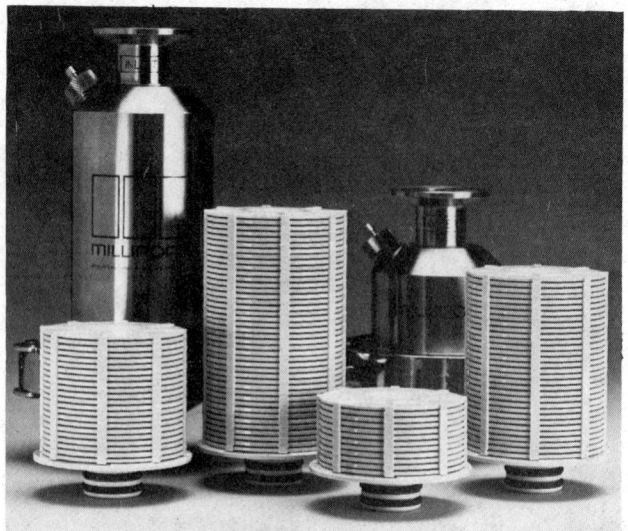

Fig 79-9. Stacked disc membrane filters. This new technology allows filter manufacturers to supply filters with large surface area in relatively small packages (courtesy, Millipore Corp).

negative pressure on the downstream (sterile) side of the filtrate thus precluding contamination. Membrane filters are readily sterilized by autoclaving, *in-situ* steaming, or by ethylene oxide sterilization.

In addition to their use in the pharmaceutical industry, membrane filters are utilized in many applications in the hospital pharmacy. The membrane filters commonly used in these applications are small disposable units. Examples of these are shown in Figs 79-11 and 79-12. Typical applications for membrane filters in hospital pharmacies include sterilization of intravenous (IV) admixtures and hyperali-

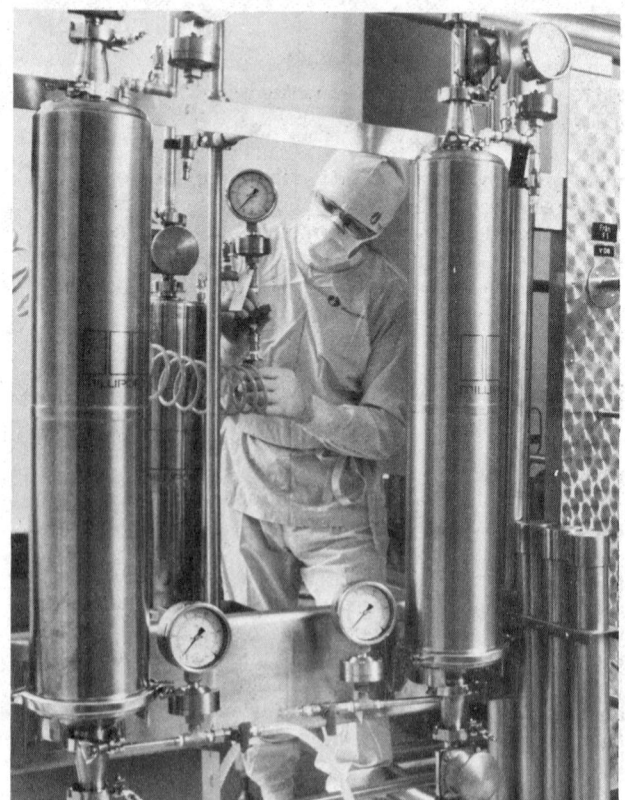

Fig 79-10. An example of a process filtration system in a pharmaceutical plant (courtesy, Millipore Corp).

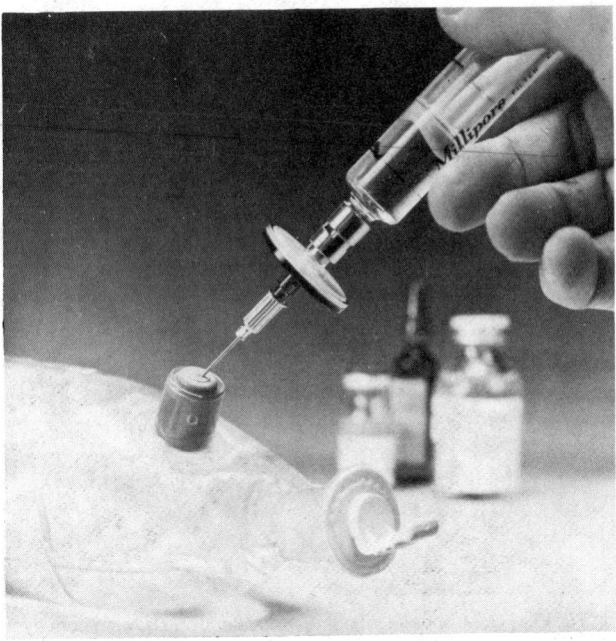

Fig 79-11.   IV additive filtration using a small disposable membrane filter (courtesy, Millipore Corp).

mentation solutions, sterilization of extemporaneously compounded preparations, sterility testing of admixtures as well as in direct patient care.   (See Chapter 86.)

Radiation

Sterilization by radiation may employ either electromagnetic radiation or particulate radiation.   Electromagnetic radiation, comprised of photons of energy, includes ultraviolet, gamma, X-, and cosmic radiation.   Particulate or corpuscular radiation includes a formidable list of particles.   The pharmacist probably has little use for radiation sterilization in hospital and laboratory applications.   However, because many industrial sterilization procedures use radiation, a short discussion is included.   Some information on the sterilizing effects of ultraviolet radiation is also presented.

The principles of sterilization by irradiation have been known since the early 1940s.   Basically, the interaction of charged particles with matter causes both ionizations and excitations.   Ionization results in the formation of ion pairs, comprised of ejected orbital electrons (negatively charged) and their counterparts (positively charged).

Charged particles such as electrons interact directly with matter causing ionization, whereas electromagnetic radiation causes ionization through various mechanisms that result in the ejection of an orbital electron with a specific amount of energy transferred from the incident gamma ray.   These ejected electrons then behave similarly to beta particles in ionization reactions.   Thus, both corpuscular and electromagnetic radiation (ie, high-energy gamma and X-rays) are considered as ionizing radiation and differ from ultraviolet radiation in this respect.

Sterilization by ionizing radiation requires consideration of: the dose, or the amount of radiation that is absorbed by the material; the energy level available (which along with the bulk density of the material will determine the thickness of penetration); and the power output available (which determines the rate at which the dose can be applied).

The unit of radiation dosage in widest use is the rad which is defined as the absorption of 100 ergs/g, independent of the nature of the irradiated substance.   Sterilization doses, for convenience, are usually expressed in megarads (Mrad).

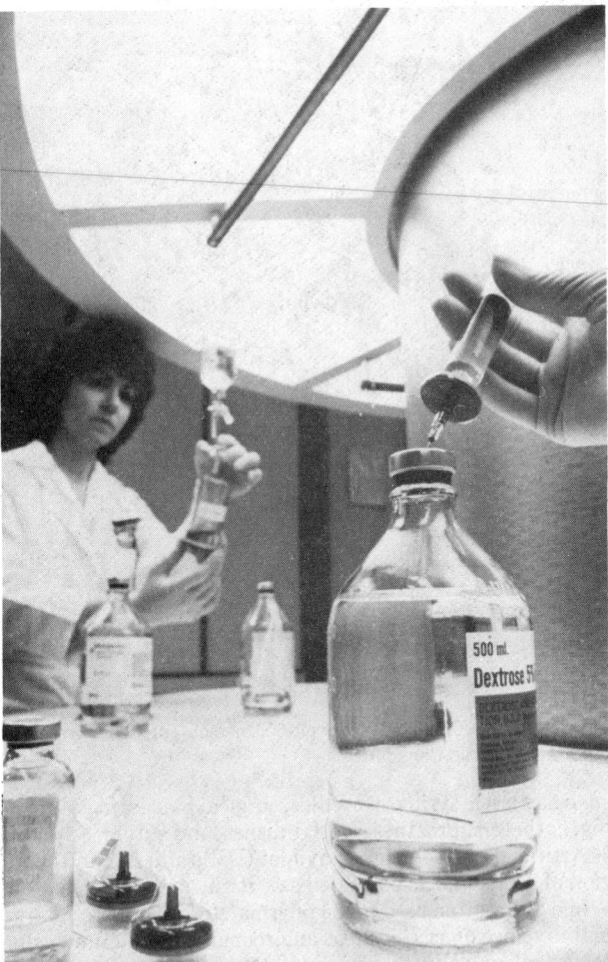

Fig 79-12.   IV additive filtration and sterility testing.   Both procedures utilize membrane filtration (courtesy, Millipore Corp).

Many investigators have studied the relative resistance of microorganisms to sterilization by radiation.   The consensus is that vegetative forms are most sensitive, followed by molds, yeasts, spore formers, and viruses.   It is generally agreed that under most conditions radiation doses of 1.5 to 2.5 Mrad are sufficient to kill the most resistant microorganisms with an adequate safety factor.

The source of gamma rays used for radiosterilization is cobalt 60.   Modern sterilization facilities used by pharmaceutical and medical device firms generally hold up to 2,000,000 curies of radioactive source material.   Fig 79-13 shows a schematic of a modern cobalt-60 radiosterilization facility and Fig 79-14 is a diagram of the source pass mechanism in a sterilization plant.

Electron accelerators may be of the electrostatic type such as the van der Graaff accelerator in which negative electricity is carried by a continuous belt to a hollow dome where the electrons are removed and accumulated.   The electrons are then discharged through a vacuum column where they are accelerated by a series of magnetic fields.   The electron beam is then spread over the conveyor carrying the product to be sterilized.   In the linear accelerator, electrons are emitted from a cathode source at the top of the column.   The electrons are accelerated by means of microwaves traveling down the accelerator tube.   Fig 79-15 shows the control panel of a linear accelerator.

Ionizing radiation is used for the industrial sterilization of such items as hospital supplies, vitamins, antibiotics, steroids, hormones, bone and tissue transplants, and medical devices

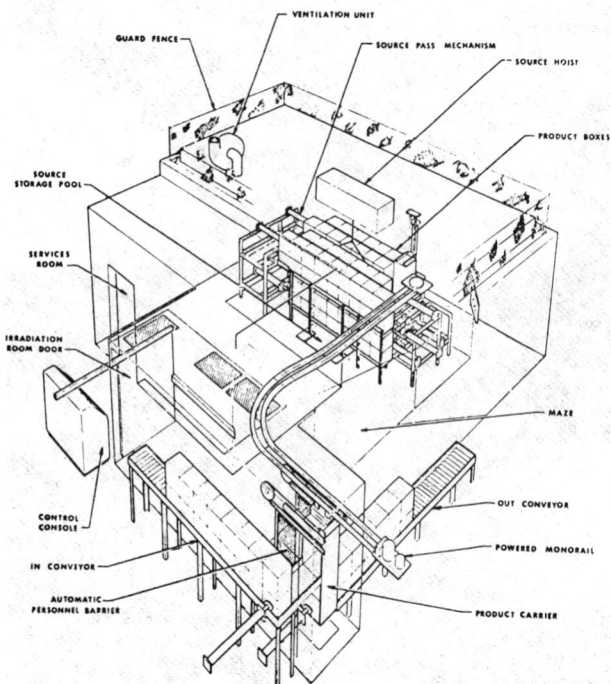

Fig 79-13. 500,000-curie cobalt-60 medical products irradiator (courtesy, Atomic-Canada).

such as plastic syringes, needles, surgical blades, plastic tubing, catheters, prostheses, petri dishes, and sutures.

Artificially produced ultraviolet (UV) radiation in the region of 253.7 nm has been used as a germicide for many years. While UV is often used in the pharmaceutical industry for the maintenance of aseptic areas and rooms, it is of limited value as a sterilizing agent.

Inactivation of microorganisms by UV is principally a function of radiant energy dose, which varies widely for different microorganisms. Vegetative bacteria are most susceptible while bacterial spores appear to be 3–10 times as resistant to inactivation and fungal spores may be 100 to 1,000 times more resistant. Bacterial spores on stainless steel surfaces require approximately 800 μw min/cm^2 for inacti-

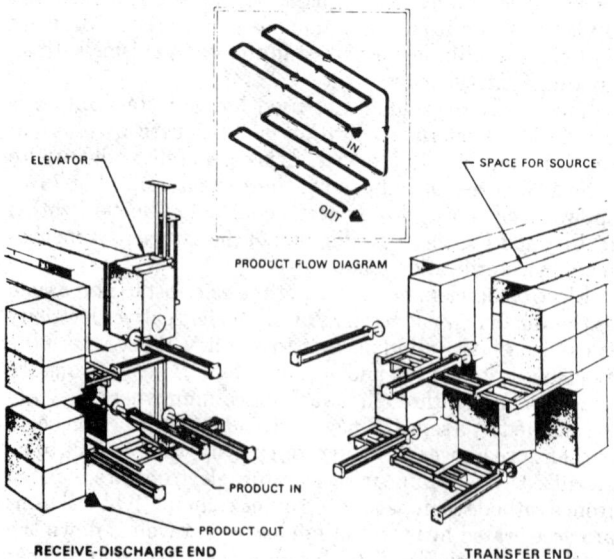

SOURCE PASS MECHANISM

Fig 79-14. Mechanisms for passing medical articles through the cobalt-60 irradiator (courtesy, Atomic-Canada).

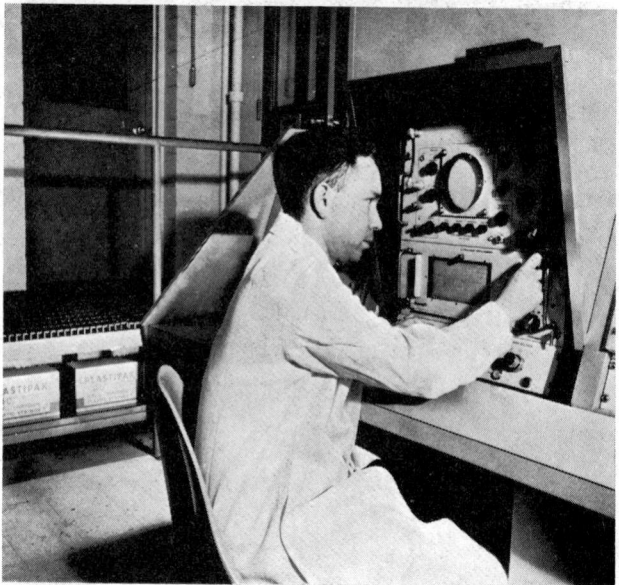

Fig 79-15. Control panel of a linear accelerator, showing conveyor carrying products to be sterilized to the shielded target area (courtesy, BD & Co).

vation. By comparison, the black spores of *Aspergillus niger* require an exposure of over 5,000 μw min/cm^2. Even with adequate dose, however, the requirements for proper application of germicidal UV in most pharmaceutical situations are such as to discourage its use for *sterilization* purposes. On the other hand, as an ancillary germicidal agent, UV can be useful.

When using UV, it is very important that lamps be cleaned periodically with alcohol and tested for output. Also, the use of UV requires that personnel be properly protected. Eye protection is particularly important.

The principal disadvantage to the use of germicidal UV is its limited penetration—its 253.7 nm wavelength is screened out by most materials, allowing clumps of organisms, and those protected by dust or debris to escape the lethal action. The use of UV as a sterilizing agent is not recommended unless the material to be irradiated is very clean and free of crevices that can protect microorganisms.

Aseptic Handling—Although not actually a sterilization process, aseptic handling is a technique frequently used in the compounding of prescriptions that will not withstand sterilization but in which all of the ingredients are sterile. In such cases sterility must be maintained by using sterile materials and a controlled working environment. All containers and apparatus used should be sterilized by one of the previously mentioned processes and such work should be conducted only by an operator fully versed in the control of contamination. The use of laminar airflow devices for aseptic handling is essential.

With the availability of sterile bulk drugs and sterilized syringe parts from manufacturers, the purchase of several pieces of equipment permits pharmacies to produce filled sterile unit-dose syringes with minimum effort. The equipment needs have been described in a paper by Patel *et al.*[13] Fig 79-16 illustrates this system.

Effects

In selecting the procedure for sterilizing medical materials, it is important to remember that the same sterilization technique cannot be universally applied because the unique properties of some materials may result in their destruction or modification. Some of the more important effects of par-

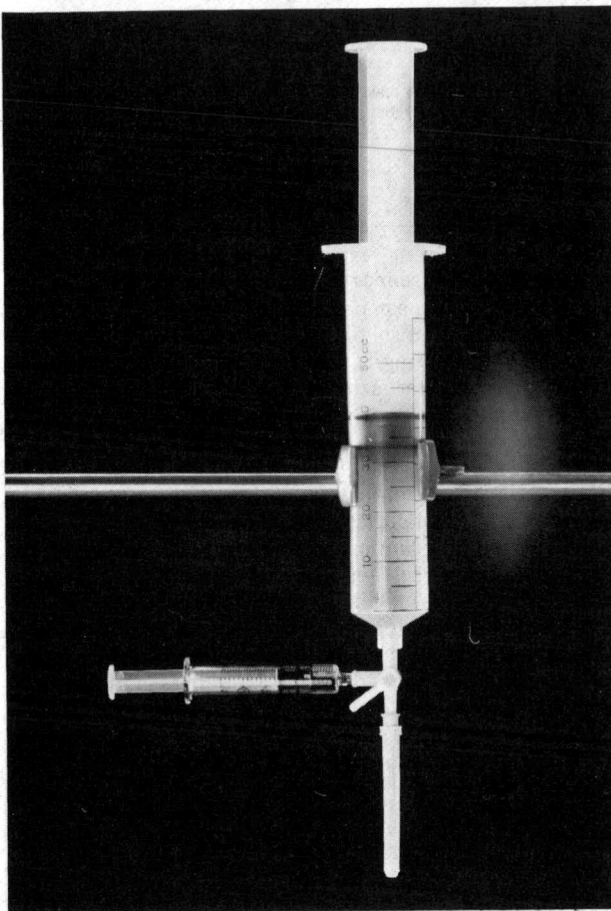

Fig 79-16.   Unit-of-use system for sterile injectable medication.[13]

ticular sterilization approaches are summarized in the following paragraphs.

Although steam sterilization is considered the most effective and efficient sterilization procedure, many heat-sensitive substances, particularly biochemicals and certain plastics, are seriously modified by exposure to temperatures of 110 to 130°. These materials must, therefore, be sterilized by temperatures of generally less than 60° utilizing such methods as ionizing radiation or exposure to ethylene oxide.

Conversely, the use of ionizing radiation and ethylene oxide has certain disadvantages. Ionizing radiation can produce changes in organic molecules which will affect efficacy of the preparations and may induce toxicity. Ethylene oxide exposure occasionally produces undersirable residues, including ethylene chlorohydrin and ethylene glycol. Some types of plastics, fibers, and rubber products will absorb gases that may cause dermal injury. The greatest hazards from these residues occur in small laboratories and hospitals where materials are used soon after sterilization and inadequate aeration. Industrial practices, on the other hand, generally lower the hazard because several days or weeks pass pass before products reach the market. Ideally, for sufficient degassing of ethylene oxide-treated products, they should remain at room temperature for seven days or be subjected to specially designed aerators for times recommended by the manufacturer.

Packaging

Following exposure of a product to a well-controlled sterilization treatment, the packaging material of the product is expected to maintain sterility until time of use. Packaging must be durable, provide for permanent-seal integrity, and have pore sizes small enough to prevent entry of contaminants.

Obviously, the packaging must be compatible with the method of sterilization.

The package design is important if the contents are to be removed without recontamination. Tearing of plastics or paper can be tempered by coatings and sealed containers should be carefully tested to assure retention of sterility at time of use.

If sterile material passes through many hands, it is important to provide a tamper-proof closure to indicate if the container has been inadvertently opened. These four features—compatibility with sterilization, proven storage protection, ease of opening, tamper proofing—are highly desirable characteristics of medical packaging.

A review of the principles of sterile material packaging by Powell[14] discusses suitability of packaging materials for various sterilization methods, including resistance to bacteria, types of openings, strength of packaging, testing of packaging, and types of packaging. These topics are also discussed in Chapter 81.

Laminar Airflow

Laminar airflow equipment is essential for proper performance of sterility tests and aseptic filling or assembling operations. These procedures require exact control over the working environment, but while many techniques and different types of equipment for performing these operations have been used over the years, laminar airflow devices are superior to all other environmental controls. In this chapter, therefore, we will consider laminar airflow devices as essential to these operations and avoid discussion of older methods employed.

The laminar airflow procedure for producing very clean and dust-free areas was developed in 1961. In a laminar airflow device the entire body of air within a confined area moves with uniform velocity along parallel flow lines. By employing prefilters and high-efficiency bacterial filters, the air delivered to the area is essentially sterile and sweeps all dust and airborne particles from the chamber through the open side. The velocity of the air used in such devices is generally 90 ± 20 fpm. Laminar airflow devices that deliver the clean air in a vertical, horizontal, or curvilinear fashion are available. The devices can be in the form of rooms, cabinets, or benches. For a comprehensive discussion of the biomedical application of laminar airflow the reader is referred to Phillips and Runkle.[15]

For sterility testing and aseptic assembly operations, laminar airflow cabinets or benches are recommended. If possible, each cabinet or bench should be located in a separate, small, clean room having a filtered air supply. The selection of the type of cabinet will depend on the operation itself. For most sterility testing operations, horizontal laminar airflow units appear to be superior to vertical flow hoods because the air movement is less likely to wash organisms from the operator's hands or equipment into the sterility test media. Fig 79-17 shows the sterility testing of syringes in a horizontal laminar airflow hood. Fig 79-18 shows an outward convergent flow hood, called the *Mini-Bench*, that is convenient for many pharmaceutical uses and for sterility testing.

The major disadvantage of the horizontal laminar airflow units is that any airborne particulate matter generated in the units is blown directly into the room and against the working personnel. In situations where infectious material is involved or where one must prevent contamination of the environment with a powder or drug, use of specifically designed laminar *down-flow* units is recommended. Downflow units have recently become available that do an excellent job of providing both product and personnel protection. Such a unit is shown in Fig 79-19.

To achieve maximum benefit from laminar airflow it is

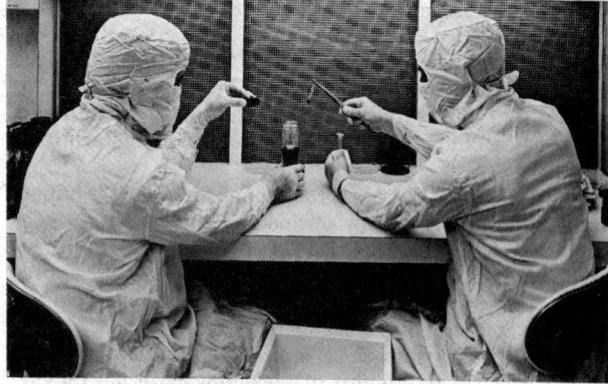

Fig 79-17.   Sterility testing of plastic disposable syringes in a horizontal laminar air flow bench (courtesy, BD & Co).

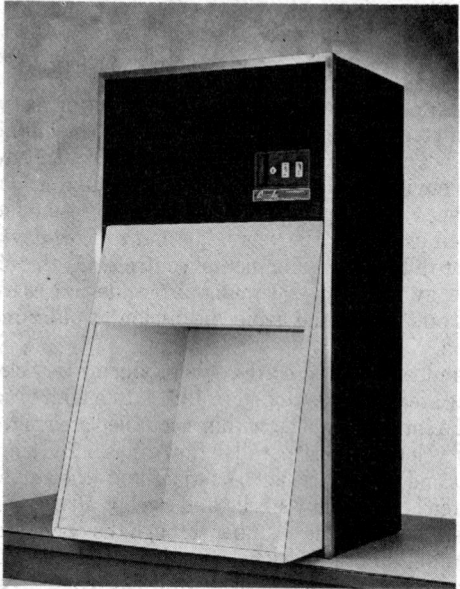

Fig 79-18.   Convergent laminar airflow Minibench for sterility testing and aseptic assembly operations (courtesy, BD & Co).

important to first realize that the filtered airflow does not it-self remove microbial contamination from the surface of objects. Thus, to avoid positive results, it is necessary to re-duce the microbial load on the outside of materials used in sterility testing. Laminar flow will do an excellent job of maintaining the sterility of an article bathed in the airflow; however, to be accurate, the sterility testing procedure must create the least possible turbulence within the unit. More-over, an awareness of the turbulent air patterns created by the operation is necessary to avoid critical operations in turbulent zones. To illustrate how effectively airborne particles are washed from an environment by laminar airflow, Fig 79-20 shows the distance various size particles will travel horizon-tally before falling 5 ft in a cross-flow of air moving at 50 fpm.

Laminar flow clean benches should supply Class 100 air as defined in Federal Standard 209B.[16] They should be certified to this standard when installed and tested periodically. An air velometer should be used at regular intervals to check the airflow rates across the face of the filter; smoke tests are useful in visualizing airflow patterns; and a particle analyzer can be used to check the quality of the air. The filters of each lam-inar airflow device should be tested at the time of installation and annually thereafter. The dioctyl phthalate (DOP) test is generally employed to check filter efficiency. This standard

Table III—False Positives Occurring in a Laminar Flow Hood[13]

Product	No. of units sterility tested	No. of false positives	% false positives
Syringes	9793	2	0.02
Needles	4676	2	0.04
Misc.	306	0	0

acceptance test determines the validity of the filter and its seal using DOP smoke (mean particulate diameter of 0.3 μm) and a light scattering aerosol photometer. The smoke, at a con-centration of 80–100 mg/L, is introduced to the plenum of the unit and the entire perimeter of the filter face is scanned with the photometer probe at a sampling rate of 1 ft^3/min. A reading of 0.01% of the upstream smoke concentration is considered a leak.

In addition to the routine airflow measurements and filter efficiency testing, biological testing may be done to monitor the effectiveness of laminar airflow systems. Microbial air sampling and agar settling plates are useful in monitoring these environments. Phillips evaluated horizontal laminar flow hoods by tabulating the number of "false positives" ap-pearing in sterility test media over a period of time. These results (Table III) showed very low numbers of "false posi-tives."

Testing

After sterilization, there are several techniques for deter-mining whether or not the particular lot of material is sterile. The only method for determining sterility with 100% assur-ance would be to run a total sterility test; ie, to test every item in the lot.

Representative probabilities are shown in Tables IV and V to illustrate more specifically how low levels of contami-nation in treated lots of medical articles may escape detection by the usual sterility test procedures. The data are calculated by binomial expansion, employing certain assumed values of percent contamination with large lot sizes (greater than 5000) and including standard assumptions with regard to the effi-ciency of recovery media, etc.

Table IV—Probabilities for Sterility Testing of Articles with Assumed Levels of Contamination

"True" % Contamination	Probability of designated positives out of 10 samples tested			
	0	1	5	10
0.1	0.990	(Total = 0.010)		
1.0	0.904	0.091		
5.0	0.599	0.315		
10.0	0.349	0.387	0.001	
30.0	0.028	0.121	0.103	
50.0	0.001	0.010	0.246	0.001

Table V—Relationship of Probabilities of Acceptance of Lots of Varying Assumed Degrees of Contamination to Sample Size

Number of samples tested (n)	Probability of no positive growth "True" % contamination of lot					
	0.1	1	5	10	15	20
10	0.99	0.91	0.60	0.35	0.20	0.11
20	0.98	0.82	0.36	0.12	0.04	0.01
50	0.95	0.61	0.08	0.007		
100	0.91	0.37	0.01	0.00		
300	0.74	0.05				
500	0.61	0.01				

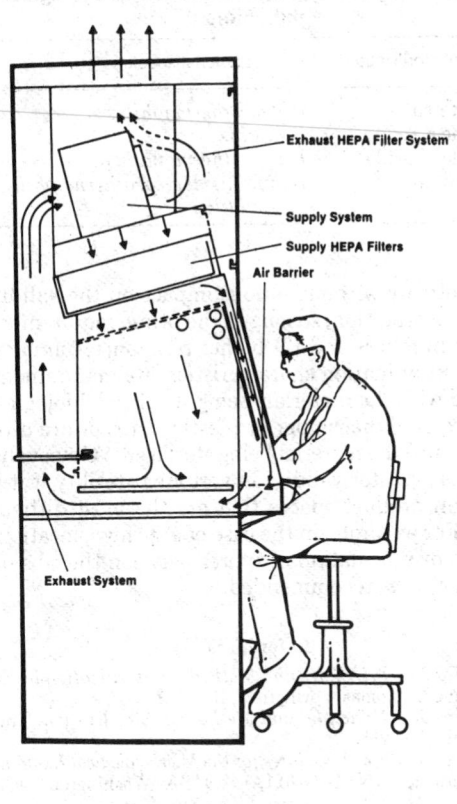

Exhaust HEPA Filter System

Supply System

Supply HEPA Filters

Air Barrier

Exhaust System

BioQuest Biological Cabinet
Air Flow Patterns

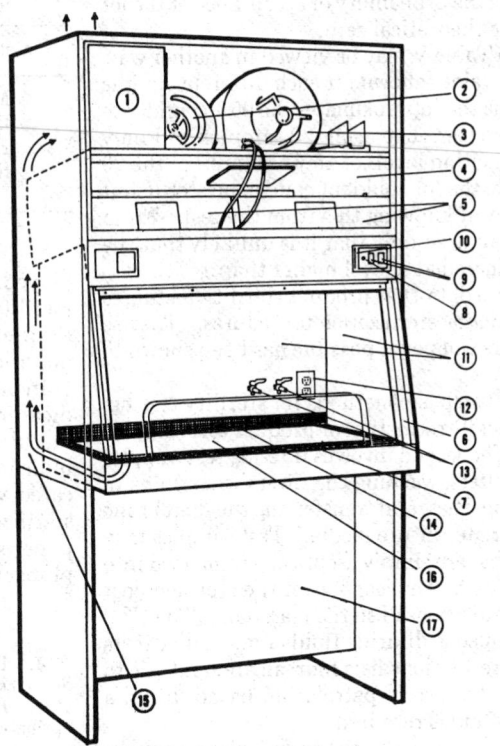

1. Exhaust HEPA filter
2. Exhaust Blower
3. Supply Blower
4. Supply Plenum
5. Supply HEPA filters
6. Polycarbonate View
   Screen (Air Curtain)
7. Front Return Grill
8. Air Velocity Control
9. Control Switches
10. Air Velocity Indicator
11. Stainless Steel Interior Sides
12. 115 Volt AC Duplex Outlet
13. Gas, Air/Vacuum Fixtures
14. Rear Return Grill
15. Return Plenum
16. Solid Work Surface
17. Base Support

BioQuest Biological Cabinet
Special Features

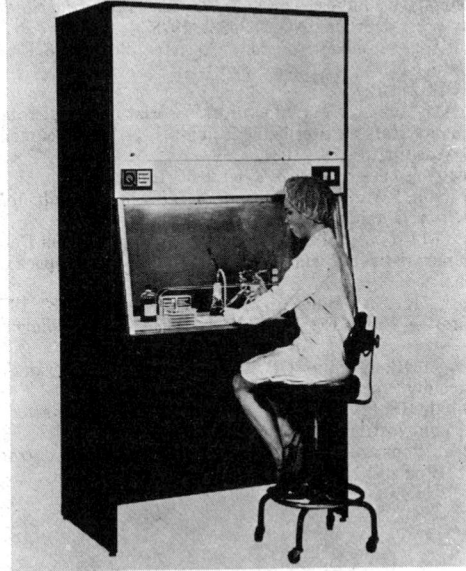

Fig 79-19.   Sketch (*above*) and photograph (*left*) of a biological cabinet with vertical, recirculating laminar flow cabinet and HEPA-filtered exhaust.   HEPA-filtered air is supplied to the work area at 90 ± 20 fpm. Airflow patterns in combination with a high-velocity curtain of air form a barrier at the front access opening which protects both the work and the worker from airborne contamination (courtesy, BioQuest).

In Table IV the probability data are calculated for lots with various degrees of assumed contamination when 10 random samples per lot are tested.   For example, a lot that has one in each 1000 items contaminated (0.1% contamination) could be passed as satisfactory (by showing no positive samples from 10 tested) in 99 tests out of 100.   Even at the 10% contamination level, contamination would be detected only two out of three times.

Table V shows the difficulty in attempting to improve the reliability of sterility tests by increasing sample size.   For contamination levels as low as 0.1%, increasing the sample size from 10 to 100 has a relatively small effect in improving the probability of accepting lots.   Even a sample size of 500 would result in erroneously accepting a lot six times out of ten.   On

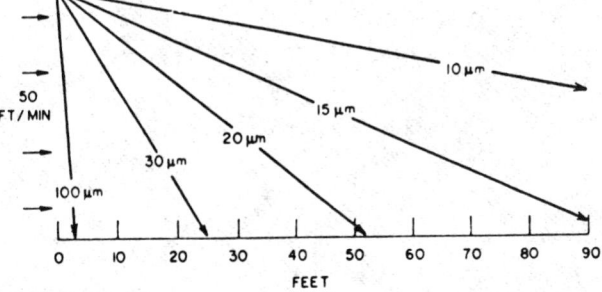

Fig 79-20.   Distance traveled by particles settling from a height of 5 ft.

the other hand, with a lot contaminated to the extent of 10%, by testing 100 samples the probability of acceptance of the lot would be reduced to a theoretical zero.

The information in Table V may be viewed in another way. If, for the probability values shown for each different sample size, we select the value that approximates the 95% confidence level (P = 0.05), it is clear that using 20 samples will only discriminate contamination levels of 15% or more. If the 20 tubes show no growth, the lot could, of course, be sterile but there would be no way of knowing this from the test. From such a test it could be stated only that it is unlikely that the lot would be contaminated at a level higher than 15%.

It is clear from these data that product sterility testing is a poor method of validating sterilization procedures. The use of biological indicators whenever possible has been shown to better verify sterility.

The USP provides two basic methods for sterility testing. One involves the direct introduction of product test samples into culture media. The second involves filtering test samples through membrane filters, washing the filters with fluids to remove inhibitory properties, and transferring the membrane aseptically to appropriate culture media. Test samples may be sterilized devices that are simply aseptically immersed into the appropriate culture broth washings of the sterile object with sterile diluent, or dilutions of sterile materials. The USP recommends three aqueous diluting fluids for sterility tests while the Antibiotic Regulations lists four; all are nontoxic to microorganisms. In the case of petrolatum-based drugs, a nonaqueous diluting fluid is required.

Many studies have been conducted to find the minimum number of culture media that will provide greatest sensitivity in detecting contamination. Internationally recognized experts and bodies now recommend the use of two culture media: Soybean-Casein Digest Medium, incubated at 20–25°, and Fluid Thioglycollate Medium, incubated at 30–35°. The time of incubation specified usually is 7 days for the membrane filtration method and 7–14 days for the direct inoculation method depending on the method of sterilization. The requirements are described in detail in the USP.

The preferred method of verifying sterility is not by testing sterilized materials but by the use of biological indicators. This is not possible, however, when products are sterilized by filtration and aseptically filled into their final containers, as is the case with such important drugs as antibiotics, insulin, and hormones. The indicators are generally highly resistant bacterial spores present in greater numbers than the normal contamination of the product and with equal or greater resistance than normal microbial flora in the products being sterilized. Various properties of commercially available bacterial spores have been recommended for specific methods of sterilization based on unique resistance characteristics. Commonly accepted species of bacteria used for biological indicators are shown in Table VI. Other species can be em-

Table VI—Species of Bacteria Used as Biological Indicators

Method of sterilization	Bacterial species
Moist heat	B stearothermophilus
Dry heat	B subtilis
Ethylene oxide	B stearothermophilus
Radiation	B pumilus, B stearothermophilus, B subtilis

ployed, probably without serious impact on the validity of sterility interpretation, so long as the prime requirements of (1) greater numbers and (2) higher resistance compared to material contamination characteristics, are maintained.

Included with the materials being sterilized, biological indicators are on either paper or plastic strips or are directly inoculated onto the material being sterilized. Obviously, the indicator has greater validity in verifying sterility if it is located within product spaces that are the most difficult to sterilize. For example, in the case of a syringe, location of a paper strip or inoculation of spores between the ribs of the plunger stopper is recommended.

References

1. Perkins JJ: *Principles and Methods of Sterilization in Health Sciences*, 2nd ed, Thomas, Springfield, IL, 1969.
2. Perkins JJ: *Principles and Methods of Sterilization*, Thomas, Springfield, IL, 55, 1965.
3. *NASA Standard Procedures for the Microbiological Examination of Space Hardware* (NHB 5340.1A). NASA, Washington, DC, Oct. 1968.
4. Bruch CA: *Proceedings of the First National Conference on Spacecraft Sterilization Technology* (Publ. SP-108), NASA, Washington, DC, 207–229, 1965.
5. Pflug IJ, in Phillips GB, Miller WS, eds: *Industrial Sterilization*, Duke Univ Press, Durham, NC, 239–282, 1973.
6. National Archives: *Federal Register*, 40: 11865 (March 14, 1975).
7. 21CFR211.72.
8. Health Industry Manufacturers Association: "Microbiological Evaluation of Filters for Sterilizing Liquids." HIMA Document No. 3, Volume 4, Washington, DC, 1981.
9. Leahy, TJ *et al: Pharm Tech 2*: 65, 1978.
10. Dawson, FW *et al: Nordiska Föreningen för Renlighelsteknik och Rena Rum*, Göteborg, Sweden: 5, 1981.
11. ASTM Proposed Tentative Test Method: "Test for Determination of Characteristics of Membrane Filters for Use in Aerospace Liquids." June, 1965.
12. Reti, AR *et al:* Bull Parenteral Drug Assoc. *31:* 187, 1977.
13. Patel JA, Curtis EG, Phillips GL. *Amer J Hosp Pharm 29:* 947, 1972.
14. Powell DB, in Philips GB, Miller WS, eds: *Industrial Sterilization*, Duke Univ Press, Durham, NC, 79–99, 1973.
15. Runkle RS, Phillips GB, eds. *Microbial Contamination Control Facilities*, Van Nostrand-Reinhold, New York, 1969.
16. *Clean Room and Work Station Requirements: Controlled Environment*, (Fed Std No 209B), USGPO, Washington, DC, 4, April 24, 1973.

CHAPTER 80

Tonicity, Osmoticity, Osmolality, and Osmolarity

Frederick P Siegel, PhD

Professor of Pharmaceutics
College of Pharmacy, University of Illinois
Chicago, IL 60612

It is generally accepted that osmotic effects have a major place in the maintenance of homeostasis (the state of equilibrium in the living body with respect to various functions and to the chemical composition of the fluids and tissues, eg, temperature, heart rate, blood pressure, water content, blood sugar, etc). To a great extent these effects occur within or between cells and tissues where they cannot be measured. One of the most troublesome problems in clinical medicine is the maintenance of adequate body fluids and proper balance between extracellular and intracellular fluid volumes in seriously ill patients. It should be kept in mind, however, that fluid and electrolyte abnormalities are not diseases, but are the manifestations of disease.

The physiologic mechanisms which control water intake and output appear to respond primarily to serum osmoticity. Renal regulation of output is influenced by variation in rate of release of pituitary antidiuretic hormone (ADH) and other factors in response to changes in serum osmoticity. Osmotic changes also serve as a stimulus to moderate thirst. This mechanism is sufficiently sensitive to limit variations in osmoticity in the normal individual to less than about 1%. Body fluid continually oscillates within this narrow range. An increase of plasma osmoticity of 1% will stimulate ADH release, result in reduction of urine flow, and at the same time stimulate thirst that results in increased water intake. Both the increased renal reabsorption of water (without solute) stimulated by circulating ADH and the increased water intake tend to lower serum osmoticity.

The transfer of water through the cell membrane occurs so rapidly that any lack of osmotic equilibrium between the two fluid compartments in any given tissue is usually corrected within a few seconds, and at most within a minute or so. However, this rapid transfer of water does not mean that complete equilibration occurs between the extracellular and intracellular compartments throughout the whole body within this same short period of time. The reason for this is that fluid usually enters the body through the gut and must then be transported by the circulatory system to all tissues before complete equilibration can occur. In the normal person it may require 30–60 minutes to achieve reasonably good equilibration throughout the body after drinking water. Osmoticity is the property that largely determines the physiologic acceptability of a variety of solutions used for therapeutic and nutritional purposes.

Pharmaceutical and therapeutic consideration of osmotic effects has been to a great extent directed toward the side effects of ophthalmic and parenteral medicinals due to abnormal osmoticity, and to either formulating to avoid the side effects or finding methods of administration to minimize them. More recently this consideration has been extended to total (central) parenteral nutrition, to enteral hyperalimentation ("tube" feeding), and to concentrated-fluid infant formulas.[1] Also, in recent years the importance of osmometry of serum and urine in the diagnosis of many pathological conditions has been recognized.

There are a number of examples of the direct therapeutic effect of osmotic action, such as the intravenous use of mannitol as a diuretic which is filtered at the glomeruli and thus increases the osmotic pressure of tubular urine. Water must then be reabsorbed against a higher osmotic gradient than otherwise, so reabsorption is slower and diuresis is observed. The same fundamental principle applies to the intravenous administration of 30% urea used to affect intracranial pressure in the control of cerebral edema. Peritoneal dialysis fluids tend to be somewhat hyperosmotic to withdraw water and nitrogenous metabolites. Two to five percent sodium chloride solutions and a 40% glucose ointment are used topically for corneal edema. Ophthalgan (*Ayerst*) is ophthalmic glycerin employed for its osmotic effect to clear edematous cornea to facilitate an ophthalmoscopic or genioscopic examination. Glycerin solutions in 50–75% concentrations [Glyrol (*Cooper Vision*), Osmoglyn (*Alcon*)] and isosorbide solution [Ismotic (*Alcon*)] are oral osmotic agents for reducing intraocular pressure. The osmotic principle also applies to plasma extenders such as polyvinylpyrrolidone and to saline laxatives such as magnesium sulfate, magnesium citrate solution, magnesium hydroxide (via gastric neutralization), sodium sulfate, sodium phosphate and sodium biphosphate oral solution and enema (*Fleet*).

An interesting osmotic laxative which is a nonelectrolyte is a lactulose solution. Lactulose is a nonabsorbable disaccharide which is colon specific, wherein colonic bacteria degrade some of the disaccharide to lactic and other simple organic acids. These, *in toto*, lead to an osmotic effect and laxation. An extension of this therapy is illustrated by Cephulic (*Merrell-National*) solution, which uses the acidification of the colon via lactulose degradation to serve as a trap for ammonia migrating from the blood to the colon. The conversion of ammonia of blood to the ammonium ion in the colon is ultimately coupled with the osmotic effect and laxation thus expelling undesirable levels of blood ammonia. This product is employed to prevent and treat frontal systemic encaphalopathy.

Osmotic laxation is known with the oral or rectal use of glycerin and sorbitol. Epsom salt has been used in baths and compresses to reduce edema associated with sprains. A relatively new approach is the indirect application of the osmotic effect in therapy via osmotic pump drug delivery systems.[2]

If a solution is placed in contact with a membrane that is permeable to molecules of the solvent, but not to molecules of the solute, the movement of solvent through the membrane is called osmosis. Such a membrane is often called *semipermeable*. As the several types of membranes of the body vary in their permeability, it is well to note that they are *se-*

The author gratefully acknowledges suggestions received from Dr Dwight L Deardorff, Emeritus Professor of Pharmacy, College of Pharmacy, University of Illinois, who established the framework for this chapter in the 16th edition.

lectively permeable. Most normal living-cell membranes maintain various solute concentration gradients. A selectively permeable membrane may be defined either as one that does not permit free, unhampered diffusion of all the solutes present, or as one that maintains at least one solute concentration gradient across itself. Osmosis then is the diffusion of water through a membrane that maintains at least one solute concentration gradient across itself.

Assume a solution A on one side of the membrane, and a solution B of the same solute but of a higher concentration on the other side; the solvent will tend to pass into the more concentrated solution until equilibrium has been established. The pressure required to prevent this movement is the osmotic pressure. It is defined as the excess pressure, or pressure greater than that above the pure solvent, which must be applied to solution B to prevent passage of solvent through a perfect semipermeable membrane from A to B. The concentration of a solution with respect to effect on osmotic pressure is related to the number of particles (un-ionized molecules, ions, macromolecules, aggregates) of solute(s) in solution and thus is affected by the degree of ionization or aggregation of the solute. See Chapter 16 for review of colligative properties of solutions.

Body fluids, including blood and lacrimal fluid, normally have an osmotic pressure which is often described as corresponding to that of a 0.9% solution of sodium chloride. The body also attempts to keep the osmotic pressure of the contents of the gastrointestinal tract at about this level, but there the normal range is much wider than that of most body fluids. The 0.9% sodium chloride solution is said to be *isoosmotic* with physiologic fluids. The term *isotonic*, meaning equal tone, is in medical usage commonly used interchangeably with isoosmotic. However, terms such as isotonic and tonicity should be used *only* with reference to a physiologic fluid. Isoosmotic is actually a physical term which compares the osmotic pressure (or another colligative property, such as freezing point depression) of two liquids, neither of which may be a physiologic fluid, or which may be a physiologic fluid only under certain circumstances. For example, a solution of boric acid that is isoosmotic with both blood and lacrimal fluid is isotonic only with the lacrimal fluid. This solution causes hemolysis of red blood cells because molecules of boric acid pass freely through the erythrocyte membrane regardless of concentration. Thus isotonicity infers a sense of physiologic compatibility where isoosmoticity need not. As another example, a "chemically defined elemental diet" or enteral nutritional fluid can be isoosmotic with the contents of the gastrointestinal tract, but would not be considered a physiologic fluid, or suitable for parenteral use.

A solution is isotonic with a living cell if there is no net gain or loss of water by the cell, or other change in the cell when it is in contact with that solution. Physiologic solutions with an osmotic pressure lower than that of body fluids, or of 0.9% sodium chloride solution, are commonly referred to as being *hypotonic*. Physiologic solutions having a greater osmotic pressure are termed *hypertonic*.

Such qualitative terms are of limited value, and it has become necessary to state osmotic properties in quantitative terms. To do so a term must be used that will represent all particles that may be present in a given system. The term used is *osmol*. An osmol is defined as the weight in grams of a solute, existing in a solution as molecules (and/or ions, macromolecules, aggregates, etc), that is osmotically equivalent to the gram-molecular-weight of an ideally behaving nonelectrolyte. Thus the osmol-weight of a nonelectrolyte, in a dilute solution, is generally equal to its gram-molecular-weight. A milliosmol, abbreviated mOsm, is the weight stated in milligrams.

If one extrapolates this concept of relating an osmol and a mole of a nonelectrolyte as being equivalent, then one may also define an osmol in these following ways. It is the amount of solute which will provide one Avogadro's number, 6.02×10^{23} particles in solution and it is the amount of solute which on dissolution in one kg of water will result in an osmotic pressure increase of 22.4 atmospheres. This is derived from the gas equation, $PV = nRT$, assuming ideal conditions and standard temperature of 0°. This is equivalent to an increase of 17,000 mm Hg or 19,300 mm Hg at 37°. A milliosmol (mOsm) is one-thousandth of an osmol. For example, one mole of anhydrous dextrose is equal to 180 g. One Osm of this nonelectrolyte is also 180 g. One mOsm would be 180 mg. Thus 180 mg of this solute dissolved in one kg of water will produce an increase in osmotic pressure of 19.3 mm Hg at body temperature.

For a solution of an electrolyte such as sodium chloride, one molecule of sodium chloride represents one sodium and one chloride ion. Hence, one mole will represent 2 osmols of sodium chloride theoretically. Accordingly, one Osm NaCl = 58.5 g/2 or 29.25 g. This quantity represents the sum total of 6.02×10^{23} ions as the total number of particles. Ideal solutions infer very dilute solutions or infinite dilution. However, as concentration is increased, other factors enter. With strong electrolytes, interionic attraction causes a decrease in their effect on colligative properties. In addition, and in opposition, for all solutes, including nonelectrolytes, solvation and possibly other factors operate to intensify their colligative effect. Therefore it is very difficult and often impossible to predict accurately the osmoticity of a solution. It may be possible to do so for a dilute solution of a single, pure and well-characterized solute, but not for most parenteral and enteral medicinal and/or nutritional fluids; experimental determination is likely to be needed.

Osmolality and Osmolarity

It is necessary to use several additional terms to define expressions of concentration in reflecting the osmoticity of solutions. The terms include osmolality, the expression of osmolal concentration, and osmolarity, the expression of osmolar concentration.

Osmolality—A solution has an osmolal concentration of one when it contains one osmol of solute per kilogram of water. A solution has an osmolality of n when it contains n osmols per kilogram of water. Osmolal solutions, like their counterpart molal solutions, reflect a weight to weight relationship between the solute and the solvent. All solutions with the same molal concentrations, irrespective of solute, contain the same mole fraction (f_m) of solute. In water

$$f_m = \frac{\text{moles solute}}{\text{moles solute} + \text{moles solvent}}$$

thus, for a one molal solution

$$f_m = \frac{1 \text{ mole solute}}{1 \text{ mole solute} + 55.5 \text{ moles water per kg}} = \frac{1}{56.5}$$

Since an osmol of any nonelectrolyte is equivalent to one mole of that compound, then a one osmolal solution is synonymous to a one molal solution for a typical nonelectrolyte.

With a typical electrolyte like sodium chloride, one osmol is approximately 0.5 mole of sodium chloride. Thus it follows that a one osmolal solution of sodium chloride is essentially equivalent to a 0.5 molal solution. Recall that one osmolal solutions of dextrose or sodium chloride will each contain the same particle concentration. In the dextrose solution there will be 6.02×10^{23} molecules per kilogram of water and in the sodium chloride solution one will have 6.02×10^{23} total ions per kilogram of water, one-half of which are Na^+ ions and the other half Cl^- ions. The mole fraction in terms of total particles will be the same and hence the same osmotic pressure.

As in molal solutions, osmolal solutions are usually employed where quantitative precision is required, as in the measurement of physical and chemical properties of solutions (ie, colligative properties). The advantage to the weight to weight relationship is that the concentration of the system is not influenced by temperature.

Osmolarity—The relationship that we observed between molality and osmolality is similarly shared between molarity and osmolarity. A solution has an osmolar concentration of one when it contains one osmol of solute per liter of solution. Likewise, a solution has an osmolarity of *n* when it contains *n* osmols per liter of solution. Osmolar solutions, unlike osmolal solutions, reflect a weight in volume relationship between the solute and final solution. A one molar and one osmolar solutions would be synonymous for nonelectrolytes. For sodium chloride a one osmolar solution would contain one osmol of sodium chloride per liter which approximates a 0.5 molar solution. The advantage of employing osmolar concentrations over osmolal concentrations is the ability to relate a specific number of osmols or milliosmols to a volume, such as a liter or mL. Thus the osmolar concept is simpler and more practical. The osmolal concept does not allow for this convenience because of the w/w relationship. Also, additional data such as the density are usually not available. Volumes of solution rather than weights of solution are more practical in the delivery of liquid dosage forms.

Many health professionals do not have a clear understanding of the difference between osmolality and osmolarity. In fact, the terms have been used interchangeably. This is partly due to the circumstance that until recent years most of the systems involved were body fluids in which the difference between the numerical values of the two concentration expressions is small and similar in magnitude to the error involved in their determination. The problem may partly center around the interpretation by some to view one kilogram of water in the osmolal concept as being equivalent to one liter, and more importantly, the interpretation that to make up to volume of one liter as in osmolarity is reasonably the same as plus one liter (a distortion of the osmolal concept). The essential difference resides in the error introduced which revolves around the volume of water occupied by the solute. A one osmolar solution of a solute will always be more concentrated than a one osmolal solution. With dilute solutions the difference may be acceptably small. Nine grams of sodium chloride per liter of aqueous solution is approximately equivalent to 9 g in 996.5 mL of water. This represents an error under one percent when comparing the osmoticity of 0.9% w/v solution to a solution of 9 g plus one kilogram of water. Using dextrose in a parallel comparison, errors range from approximately 3.5% in osmoticity with 50 g dextrose per liter versus 50 g plus one kilogram water to a difference of about 25% in osmoticity with 250 g dextrose per liter versus 250 g plus one kilogram water. The confusion appears to be without cause for concern at this time. However, one should be alerted to the sizeable errors with concentrated solutions or fluids such as those employed in total parenteral nutrition, enteral hyperalimentation, and oral nutritional fluids for infants.

Reference has been made to the terms hypertonic and hypotonic. Analogous terms are hyperosmotic and hypoosmotic. The significance of hyper- and hypo-osmoticity for medicinal and nutritional fluids will be discussed in later sections. The values which correspond to those terms for serum may be approximately visualized from the following example. *Assuming* normal serum osmolality to be *285 mOsm/kg*, as serum osmolality increases due to water *deficit* the following signs and symptoms usually are found to progressively accumulate at approximately these values: 294–298—thirst (if the patient is alert and communicative); 299–313—dry mucous membranes; 314–329—weakness,

doughy skin; above 330—disorientation, postural hypotension, severe weakness, fainting, CNS changes, stupor, coma. As serum osmolality decreases due to water *excess* the following may occur: 275–261—headache; 262–251—drowsiness, weakness; 250–233—disorientation, cramps; below 233—seizures, stupor, coma.

As indicated previously, the body's mechanisms actively combat such major changes by limiting the variation in osmolality for normal individuals to less than about 1% (approximately in the range 282–288 mOsm/kg, based on the above assumption).

The value given for normal serum osmolality above was described as an assumption because of the variety of values found in the references. Serum osmolality is often loosely stated to be about 300 mOsm/L. Apart from that, and more specifically, two references state it as 280–295 mOsm/L; other references give it as 275–300 mOsm/L, 290 mOsm/L, 306 mOsm/L, and 275–295 mOsm/kg. There is a strong tendency to call it *osmolality* but to state it as *mOsm/L* (*not as mOsm/kg*). In the light of these varying values, one may ask about the reproducibility of the experimental measurements, assuming that is their source. It has been stated that most osmometers are accurate to 5 mOsm/L. With that type of reproducibility, the above variations may perhaps be expected. The difference between liter and kilogram is probably insignificant for serum and urine. It is difficult to measure kilograms of water in a solution, and easy to express body fluid quantities in liters. Perhaps no harm has been done to date by this practice for body fluids. However, loose terminology here may lead to loose terminology when dealing with the rather concentrated fluids used at times in parenteral and enteral nutrition.

Reference has been made to confusion in the use of the terms osmolality and osmolarity, a distinction of special importance for nutritional fluids. Awareness of high concentrations of formula should give warning as to possible risks. Unfortunately, the osmoticity of infant formulas, tube feedings, and total parenteral nutrition solutions has not been adequately described either in textbooks or in the literature,[3] and the labels of many commercial nutritional fluids do not in any way state their osmoticity. Only recently have enteral fluids been characterized in terms of osmoticity. Some product lines are now accenting isoosmotic enteral nutritional supplements. Often, when the term osmolarity is used, one cannot discern whether this is simply incorrect terminology, or if osmolarity has actually been calculated from osmolality.

Another current practice that can cause confusion is the use of the terms *normal* and/or *physiological* for isotonic sodium chloride solution (0.9%). The solution is surely isoosmotic. However, as to being physiological, the ions are each of 154 mEq/L concentration while serum contains about 140 mEq of sodium and about 103 mEq of chloride.

The range of mOsm values found for serum raises the question as to what is really meant by the terms hypotonic and hypertonic for medicinal and nutritional fluids. One can find the statement that fluids with an osmolality of 50 mOsm or more above normal are hypertonic, and if 50 mOsm or more below normal are hypotonic. One can also find the statement that peripheral infusions should not have an osmolarity exceeding 700–800 mOsm/L.[4] Examples of osmol concentrations of solutions used in peripheral infusions are: D5W—252 mOsm/L; D10W—505 mOsm/L; Lactated Ringer's 5% Dextrose—525 mOsm/L. When a fluid is hypertonic, undesirable effects can often be decreased by using relatively slow rates of infusion, and/or relatively short periods of infusion. D25W—4.25% Amino Acids is a representative example of a highly osmotic hyperalimentation solution. It has been stated that when osmolal loading is needed, a maximum safe tolerance for a normally hydrated subject would be an approximate increase of 25 mOsm per kg of water over 4 hours.[3]

Computation of Osmolarity

Several methods are used to obtain numerical values of osmolarity. The osmolar concentration sometimes referred to as the "theoretical osmolarity" is calculated from the wt/vol concentration using one of the following equations:

(1) For a nonelectrolyte

$$\frac{\text{grams/liter}}{\text{mol wt}} \times 1000 = \text{mOsm/liter}$$

(2) For a strong electrolyte

$$\frac{\text{grams/liter}}{\text{mol wt}} \times \frac{\text{number of ions}}{\text{formed}} \times 1000 = \text{mOsm/liter}$$

(3) For individual ions, if desired

$$\frac{\text{grams of ion/liter}}{\text{ionic wt}} \times 1000 = \text{mOsm (of ion)/liter}$$

These are simple calculations; however, they omit consideration of factors such as solvation and interionic forces. By this method of calculation 0.9% sodium chloride has an osmolar concentration of 308 mOsm/L.

Two other methods compute osmolarity from values of osmolality. The determination of osmolality will be discussed in a later section. One method has a strong theoretical basis of physical-chemical principles;[5] it uses values of the partial molal volume(s) of the solute(s). A 0.9% sodium chloride solution, found experimentally to have an osmolality of 286 mOsm/kg, was calculated to have an osmolarity of 280 mOsm/L, rather different from the value of 308 mOsm/L calculated as above. The method using partial molal volumes is relatively rigorous, but many systems appear to be too complex and/or too poorly defined to be dealt with by this method.

The other method is based on the following relationship:[6,7] actual osmolarity = measured osmolality × (density − g solute/mL). This expression can be written:

mOsm/L solution = mOsm/1000 g water

× g water/mL solution

The experimental value for the osmolality of 0.9% sodium chloride solution was 292.7 mOsm/kg; the value computed for osmolarity was 291.4 mOsm/L. This method does not have as firm a theoretical basis as the preceding method but it has the advantage that it uses easily obtained values of density of the solution and of its solute content. Apparently it can be used with all systems. For example, the osmolality of a nutritional product was determined by the freezing point depression method to be 625 mOsm/kg;[7] its osmolarity was calculated as 625 × 0.839 = 524 mOsm/L.

The USP requires that labels of pharmacopeial solutions which provide intravenous replenishment of fluid, nutrient(s), or electrolyte(s), as well as of the osmotic diuretic Mannitol Injection, state the osmolar concentration, in milliosmols per liter, except that where the contents are less than 100 mL, or where the label states the article is not for direct injection but is to be diluted before use, the label may alternatively state the total osmolar concentration in milliosmols per mL. This is a reasonable request from several standpoints, and intravenous fluids are being labeled in accordance with this stipulation, as shown in the next section.

An example of the use of the first method described above is the computation of the approximate osmolar concentration ("theoretical osmolarity") of a Lactated Ringer's 5% Dextrose Solution (Travenol Solution), which is labeled to contain, per liter, dextrose (hydrous) 50 g, sodium chloride 6 g, potassium chloride 300 mg, calcium chloride 200 mg, sodium lactate 3.1 g. Also stated is that the total osmolar concentration of the solution is approximately 524 mOsm per liter, in part contributed by 130 mEq of Na$^+$, 109 mEq of Cl$^-$, 4 mEq of K$^+$, 3 mEq of Ca^{2+}, and 28 mEq of lactate ion.

The derivation of the osmolar concentrations from the stated composition of the solution may be verified by calculations using equation (1) above for the nonelectrolyte dextrose, and equation (2) for the electrolytes.

Dextrose

$$\frac{50 \text{ g} \times 1000}{198.17} = 252.3 \text{ mOsm/liter}$$

Sodium Chloride

$$\frac{6 \text{ g} \times 2 \times 1000}{58.44} = 205.33 \text{ mOsm/liter} \begin{cases} (102.66 \text{ mOsm Na}^+) \\ (102.66 \text{ mOsm Cl}^-) \end{cases}$$

Potassium Chloride

$$\frac{0.3 \text{ g} \times 2 \times 1000}{74.55} = 8.04 \text{ mOsm/liter} \begin{cases} (4.02 \text{ mOsm K}^+) \\ (4.02 \text{ mOsm Cl}^-) \end{cases}$$

Calcium Chloride

$$\frac{0.2 \text{ g} \times 3 \times 1000}{110.99} = 5.4 \text{ mOsm/liter} \begin{cases} (1.8 \text{ mOsm Ca}^{2+}) \\ (3.6 \text{ mOsm Cl}^-) \end{cases}$$

Sodium Lactate

$$\frac{3.1 \text{ g} \times 2 \times 1000}{112.06} = 55.32 \text{ mOsm/liter} \begin{cases} (27.66 \text{ mOsm Na}^+) \\ (27.66 \text{ mOsm lactate}) \end{cases}$$

The total osmolar concentration of the five solutes in the solution is 526.4, in good agreement with the labeled total osmolar concentration of approximately 524 mOsm/liter.

The mOsm of sodium in one liter of the solution is the sum of the mOsm of the ion from sodium chloride and sodium lactate, ie, 102.66 + 27.66 = 130.32 mOsm. Chloride ions come from the sodium chloride, potassium chloride, and calcium chloride, the total osmolar concentration being 102.66 + 4.02 + 3.6 = 110.3 mOsm. The mOsm values of potassium, calcium, and lactate are calculated to be 4.02, 1.8, and 27.66, respectively. Thus, with the possible exception of calcium, there is close agreement with the labeled mEq content of each of these ions.

The osmolarity of a mixture of complex composition, such as an enteral hyperalimentation fluid, probably cannot be calculated with any acceptable degree of certainty, and therefore the *osmolality* of such preparations probably should be determined experimentally.

The approximate osmolarity of mixtures of two solutions can be computed from the following relationship (the method is known as *alligation medial*):

$$\text{osm}_{\text{final}} = \frac{\text{osm}_a \times V_a}{V_{\text{final}}} + \frac{\text{osm}_b \times V_b}{V_{\text{final}}}$$

where

V_a = volume of component a
V_b = volume of component b
V_{final} = volume of final solution
osm_a = osmolarity of component a
osm_b = osmolarity of component b
$\text{osm}_{\text{final}}$ = osmolarity of final solution

For example, to calculate the osmolarity of a mixture of 500 mL of a solution of osmolarity 850 and 500 mL of a solution of osmolarity 252:

$$\text{osm}_{\text{final}} = \frac{850 \times 500}{1000} + \frac{252 \times 500}{1000}$$

$$= 425 \text{ mOsm/L} + 126 \text{ mOsm/L} = 551 \text{ mOsm/L}$$

This example illustrates the ease of calculating the osmoticity, by use of osmolarity, when solutions are mixed. Such a calculation would be much less valid if osmolality values were used. From the previous example one can see how to calculate the approximate effect if an additional solute is added.

Undesirable Effects of Abnormal Osmoticity

Ophthalmic Medication—It has been generally accepted that ophthalmic preparations intended for instillation into the cul-de-sac of the eye should, if possible, be approximately isotonic to avoid irritation (see Chapter 87). It has also been stated that abnormal tonicity of contact lens solutions can cause the lens to adhere to the eye and/or cause burning or dryness or photophobia.

Parenteral Medication—Osmoticity is of great importance in parenteral injections, its effects depending on the degree of deviation from tonicity, the concentration, the location of the injection, the volume injected, the speed of the injection, the rapidity of dilution and diffusion, etc. When formulating parenterals, solutions otherwise hypotonic usually have their tonicity adjusted by the addition of dextrose or sodium chloride. Hypertonic parenteral drug solutions cannot be adjusted. Hypotonic and hypertonic solutions are usually administered slowly in small volumes, or into a large vein such as the subclavian, where dilution and distribution occur rapidly. Solutions that differ from the serum in tonicity are generally stated to cause tissue irritation, pain on injection, and electrolyte shifts, the effect depending on the degree of deviation from tonicity.

Excessive infusion of *hypo*tonic fluids may cause swelling of red blood cells, hemolysis, and water invasion of the body's cells in general. When this is beyond the body's tolerance for water, water intoxication results, with convulsions and edema, such as pulmonary edema.

Excessive infusion of *iso*tonic fluids can cause an increase in extracellular fluid volume, which can result in circulatory overload.

Excessive infusion of *hyper*tonic fluids leads to a wide variety of complications. For example, the sequence of events when the body is presented with a large intravenous load of hypertonic fluid, rich in dextrose, is as follows: hyperglycemia, glycosuria and intracellular dehydration, osmotic diuresis, loss of water and electrolytes, dehydration, and coma.

One cause of osmotic diuresis is the infusion of dextrose at a rate faster than the ability of the patient to metabolize it (as greater than perhaps 400–500 mg/kg/hr for an adult on total parenteral nutrition). A heavy load of nonmetabolizable dextrose increases the osmoticity of blood and acts as a diuretic; the increased solute load requires more fluid for excretion, 10–20 mL of water being required to excrete each gram of dextrose. Solutions such as those for total parenteral nutrition should be administered by means of a metered constant-infusion apparatus over a lengthy period (usually more than 24 hours) to avoid sudden hyperosmotic dextrose loads. Such solutions may cause osmotic diuresis; if this occurs, water balance is likely to become negative because of the increased urinary volume and electrolyte depletion may occur because of excretion of sodium and potassium secondary to the osmotic diuresis. If such diuresis is marked, body weight falls abruptly and signs of dehydration appear. Urine should be monitored for signs of osmotic diuresis, such as glycosuria and increased urine volume.

If the intravenous injection rate of hypertonic solution is too rapid, there may be catastrophic effects on the circulatory and respiratory systems. Blood pressure may fall to dangerous levels; cardiac irregularities or arrest may ensue; respiration may become shallow and irregular; there may be heart failure and pulmonary edema. Probably the precipitating factor is a bolus of concentrated solute suddenly reaching the myocardium and the chemoreceptors in the aortic arch and carotid sinus.[3]

Abrupt changes in serum osmoticity can lead to cerebral hemorrhage. It has been shown experimentally that rapid infusions of therapeutic doses of hypertonic saline with osmotic loads produce a sudden rise in cerebrospinal fluid (CSF) and venous pressure (VP) followed by a precipitous fall in CSF pressure. This may be particularly conducive to intracranial hemorrhage, as the rapid infusion produces an increase in plasma volume and venous pressure at the same time the CSF pressure is falling. During the CSF pressure rise, there is a

drop in hemoglobin and hematocrit, reflecting a marked increase in blood volume.

Hyperosmotic medications, such as sodium bicarbonate (osmolarity of 1563 at 1 mEq/mL), that are administered intravenously should be diluted prior to use and should be injected slowly to allow dilution by the circulating blood. Rapid "push" injections may cause a significant increase in blood osmoticity.[5]

As to other possibilities, there may be crenation of red blood cells and general cellular dehydration. Hypertonic dextrose or saline, etc. infused through a peripheral vein with small blood volume may traumatize the vein and cause thrombophlebitis. Infiltration can cause trauma and necrosis of tissues. Safety therefore demands that all intravenous injections, especially highly osmotic solutions, be performed slowly, usually being given preferably over a period not less than required for a complete circulation of the blood, e.g., *one minute*. The exact danger point varies with the state of the patient, the concentration of the solution, the nature of the solute, and the rate of administration.

Hyperosmotic solutions also should not be discontinued suddenly. In dogs, marked increase in levels of intracranial pressure occur when hyperglycemia produced by dextrose infusions is suddenly reversed by stopping the infusion and administering saline. It has also been shown that the CSF pressure in humans rises during treatment of diabetic ketoacidosis in association with fall in the plasma concentration of dextrose and fall in plasma osmolality. These observations may be explained by the different rates of decline in dextrose content of the brain and of plasma. The concentration of dextrose in the brain may fall more slowly than in the plasma, causing a shift of fluid from the extracellular fluid space to the intracellular compartment of the CNS, resulting in increased intracranial pressure.

Osmometry and the Clinical Laboratory

Osmometry is a fairly recent innovation in the clinical laboratory; an article in 1971 had the title: "Osmometry: A New Bedside Laboratory Aid for the Management of Surgical Patients." Serum and urine osmometry may assist in the diagnosis of certain fluid and electrolyte problems. However, osmometry values have little meaning unless the clinical situation is known. Osmometry is used in renal dialysis as a check on the electrolyte composition of the fluid. In the clinical laboratory, as stated above, the term "osmolality" is generally used, but is usually reported as mOsm/L. It may seem unnecessary to mention that osmolality depends not only on the number of solute particles, but also on the quantity of water in which they are dissolved. However, it may help one to understand the statement that the normal range of urine osmolality is 50–1400 mOsm/L, and for a random specimen is 500–800 mOsm/L.

Serum Osmoticity

Sodium is by far the principal solute involved in serum osmoticity. Therefore abnormal serum osmoticity is most likely to be associated with conditions that cause abnormal sodium concentration and/or abnormal water volume.

Thus hyperosmotic serum is likely to be due to an increase in serum sodium and/or loss of water. It may be associated with diabetes insipidus, hypercalcemia, diuresis during severe hyperglycemia, or with early recovery from renal shutdown. Alcohol ingestion is said to be the most common cause of the hyperosmotic state and of coexisting coma and the hyperosmotic state. An example of hyperosmoticity is a comatose diabetic with a serum osmoticity of 365 mOsm/L.

In a somewhat analogous fashion hypoosmotic serum is

likely to be due to decrease in serum sodium and/or excess of water. It may be associated with: (a) the postoperative state (especially with excessive water replacement therapy); (b) treatment with diuretic drugs and low-salt diet (as with patients with heart failure, cirrhosis, etc); (c) adrenal disease (eg, Addison's disease, adrenogenital syndrome); (d) SIADH (syndrome of inappropriate ADH secretion). There are many diseases that cause ADH to be released inappropriately (ie, in spite of the fact that serum osmoticity and volume may have been normal initially). These include oat-cell carcinoma of the lung, bronchogenic carcinoma, congestive heart failure, inflammatory pulmonary lesions, porphyria, severe hypothyroidism, cerebral disease (such as tumor, trauma, infection, vascular abnormalities). It may also be found with some patients with excessive diuretic use. Serum and urine osmoticity are measured when SIADH is suspected. In SIADH there is hypoosmoticity of the blood in association with a relative hyperosmoticity of urine. The usual cause is a malfunction of the normal osmotic response of osmoreceptors, an excess of exogenous vasopressin, or a production of a vasopressin-like hormone that is not under the regular control of serum osmoticity. The diagnosis is made by simultaneous measurement of urine and serum osmolality. The serum osmolality will be lower than normal and much lower than the urine osmolality, indicating inappropriate secretion of a concentrated urine in the presence of a dilute serum.

Cardiac, renal and hepatic disease characteristically reduce the sodium/osmolality ratio, this being partially attributed to the effects of increased blood sugar, urea, or unknown metabolic products. Patients in shock may develop disproportionately elevated measured osmolality compared to calculated osmolality, which points toward the presence of circulating metabolic products.

There are several approximate methods for estimating serum osmolality from clinical laboratory values for sodium ion, etc. They may be of considerable value in an emergency situation.

(a) Serum osmolality may be estimated from the formula:

$$mOsm = (1.86 \times sodium) + \frac{blood\ sugar}{18} + \frac{BUN}{2.8} + 5$$

(Na in mEq/L, blood sugar and BUN in mg/100 mL)

(b) A quick approximation is:

$$mOsm = 2\ Na + \frac{BS}{20} + \frac{BUN}{3}$$

(c) The osmolality is usually, *but not always*, very close to two times the sodium reading plus 10.

Urine Osmoticity

The two main functions of the kidney are glomerular filtration and tubular reabsorption. Clinically, tubular function is best measured by tests that determine the ability of the tubules to concentrate and dilute the urine. Tests of urinary dilution are not as sensitive in the detection of disease as are tests of urinary concentration. As concentration of urine occurs in the renal medulla (interstitial fluids, loops of Henle, capillaries of the medulla, and collecting tubules), the disease processes that disturb the function or structure of the medulla produce early impairment of the concentrating power of the kidney. Such diseases include acute tubular necrosis, obstructive uropathy, pyelonephritis, papillary necrosis, medullary cysts, hypokalemic and hypercalcemic nephropathy, and sickle-cell disease.

Measurement of urine osmolality is an accurate test for the diluting and concentrating ability of the kidneys. In the absence of ADH, the daily urinary output is likely to be 6–8 liters, or more. The normal urine osmolality depends on the clinical setting; normally, with maximum ADH stimulation, it can be as much as 1200 mOsm/kg, and with maximum ADH suppression as little as 50 mOsm/kg. Simultaneous determination of serum and urine osmolality is often valuable in assessing the distal tubular response to circulating ADH. For example, if the patient's serum is hyperosmolal, or in the upper limits of normal ranges, and the patient's urine osmolality measured at the same time is much lower, a decreased responsiveness of the distal tubules to circulating ADH is suggested.

Measurement of urine osmolality during water restriction is an accurate, sensitive test of decreased renal function. For example, under the conditions of one test, normal osmolality would be greater than 800 mOsm/kg. With severe impairment the value would be less than 400 mOsm/kg. Knowledge of urine osmolality may point to a problem even though other tests are normal (eg, the Fishberg concentration test, BUN, PSP excretion, creatinine clearance, IV pyelogram). Knowledge of its value may be especially useful in diabetes mellitus, essential hypertension, and silent pyelonephritis. The urine/serum osmolality ratio should be calculated; it should be equal to or greater than 3.

Osmoticity and Enteral Hyperalimentation

Some aspects of nutrition are discussed briefly here because of the potential major side effects due to abnormal osmoticity of nutritional fluids, and because there exists increasing dialogue on nutrition among pharmacists, dietitians, nurses, and physicians. An example is the professional organization, ASPEN, "The American Society for Parenteral and Enteral Nutrition," with membership open to all of the above health practitioners. It is desirable, therefore, that pharmacists be able to discuss these matters with these other health professionals in terms of nutrition as well as medicine.

Osmoticity has been of special importance in the intravenous infusion of large volumes of highly concentrated nutritional solutions. Their hyperosmoticity has been a major factor in the requirement that they be injected centrally into a large volume of rapidly moving blood, instead of using peripheral infusion. Use of such solutions and knowledge of their value seems to have led more recently to the use of rather similar formulations administered, not parenterally, but by instillation into some part of the gastrointestinal tract, usually, but not necessarily, by gavage. Of course, gavage feeding is not new. This method has given excellent total nutrition, for a period of time, to many patients. It has furnished an important part of their nutrition to others. It obviously avoids some of the problems associated with injections. Many of the reports on this topic refer to the use of a "Chemically Defined Elemental Diet." These are special nutritionally complete formulations that contain protein in so-called "elemental" or "predigested" form (protein hydrolysates or synthetic amino acids), and carbohydrate and fat in simple, easily digestible forms. These diets are necessarily relatively high in osmoticity because their smaller molecules result in more particles per gram than in normal foods. An example is a fluid consisting of: L-amino acids, dextrose oligosaccharides, vitamins (including fat-soluble vitamins), fat as a highly purified safflower oil or soybean oil, electrolytes, trace minerals, and water. As it contains fat, that component is not in solution and therefore should have no direct effect on osmoticity. However, the potential for interactions can cause some significant changes in total particle concentration and indirectly affect the osmoticity.[8]

Although easily digested, dextrose contributes more particles than most other carbohydrate sources, such as starch, and is more likely to cause osmotic diarrhea, especially with bolus feeding. Osmoticity is improved (decreased) in the above formula by replacing dextrose with dextrose oligosaccharides (carbohydrates that yield on hydrolysis 2 to 10 monosaccharides). Flavoring also increases the osmoticity of a product, different flavors cause varying increases.

Commercial diets of this type are packaged as fluids or as powders for reconstitution. Reconstitution is usually with water. The labels of some preparations state the osmolality or osmolarity of the fluid obtained at standard dilution. However, the labels of many products do not state either their osmolality or osmolarity (or their osmoticity in any way). Often, as stated above, when the term osmolarity *is* used, one cannot discern whether this is simply incorrect terminology, or whether the osmolarity has actually been calculated from the osmolality. With concentrated infant formulas or tube feedings, the osmolarity may be only 80% of the osmolality. As mentioned earlier, the osmoticity (osmolality, etc.) of infant formulas, tube feedings, and total parenteral nutrition solutions are not adequately described either in textbooks or in the literature.

There are other areas of concern. A wide variation in osmolality was found when powdered samples from different containers were reconstituted in the same manner. This difference was found both within and among different lots of the same product. In addition, reconstitution of some powdered enteral formulas using the scoops supplied by the manufacturer gave formulas that had almost twice the osmolality of the same product when reconstituted accurately by weight.

This form of nutrition has been called, somewhat inaccurately, "Enteral Hyperalimentation."[1] It should be distinguished from (a) "Central Parenteral Nutrition" (which has also been called "Hyperalimentation," "Total Parenteral Nutrition" (TPN), and "Parenteral Hyperalimentation"); and from (b) the more recently reported "Peripheral Hyperalimentation." The terminology is in a state of flux due to the recent rapid progress in the forms of metabolic support.

The enteric route for hyperalimentation is frequently overlooked in many diseases or post-trauma states, if the patient is not readily responsive to traditional oral feedings. Poor appetite, chronic nausea, general apathy, and a degree of somnolence or sedation are common concomitants of serious disease. This frequently prevents adequate oral alimentation and results in progressive energy and nutrient deficits. Often, supplementary feedings of a highly nutritious formula are taken poorly or refused entirely. However, the digestive and absorptive capabilities of the gastrointestinal tract are frequently intact and, when challenged with appropriate nutrient fluids, can be effectively used. By using an intact GI tract for proper alimentation, the major problems of sepsis and metabolic derangement which relate to intravenous hyperalimentation are largely obviated, and adequate nutritional support is greatly simplified. Because of this increased safety and ease of administration, the enteric route for hyperalimentation should be used whenever possible.[9]

When ingested in large amounts or concentrated fluids, the osmotic characteristics of certain foods can cause an upset in the normal water balance within the body. For a given weight of solute the osmolality of the solution is inversely proportional to the size of the particles. Nutritional components can be listed in an approximate order of decreasing osmotic effect per gram, as follows:[10]

1. Electrolytes such as sodium chloride
2. Relatively small organic molecules such as dextrose (glucose) and amino acids
3. Dextrose oligosaccharides
4. Starches
5. Proteins
6. Fats (as fats are not water-soluble they have no osmotic effect)

Thus, in foods, high proportions of electrolytes, amino acids, and simple sugars have the greatest effect on osmolality,

and as a result, on tolerance. The approximate osmolality of a few common foods and beverages is as follows:

	mOsm/kg
Whole milk	295
Tomato juice	595
Orange juice	935
Ice cream	1150

When nutrition of high osmoticity is ingested, large amounts of water will transfer to the stomach and intestines from the fluid surrounding those organs in an attempt to lower the osmoticity. The higher the osmoticity, the larger the amount of water required; a large amount of water in the GI tract can cause distention, cramps, nausea, vomiting, hypermotility, and shock. The food may move through the tract too rapidly for the water to be reabsorbed, and result in diarrhea; severe diarrhea can cause dehydration. Thus there is some analogy to the effect of hyperosmotic intravenous infusions.

Hyperosmotic feedings may result in mucosal damage in the GI tract. Rats given hyperosmotic feedings showed transient decrease in disaccharidase activities, and an increase in alkaline phosphatase activities. They also showed morphologic alterations in the microvilli of the small intestines. After a period of severe gastroenteritis, the bowel may be unusually susceptible to highly osmotic formulas, and their use may increase the diarrhea. Infant formulas that are hyperosmotic may affect preterm infants adversely during the early neonatal period, and they may produce or predispose neonates to necrotizing enterocolitis when delivered to the jejunum through a nasogastric tube.

The body attempts to keep the osmoticity of contents of the stomach and intestines at approximately the same level as that of the fluid surrounding them. As a fluid of lower osmoticity requires the transfer of less water to dilute it, it should be better tolerated than one of higher osmoticity. As to tolerance, there is a great variation from one individual to another in sensitivity to osmoticity of foods. The majority of patients receiving nutritional formulas, either orally or by tube, are able to tolerate feedings with a wide range of osmoticities if administered slowly and if adequate additional fluids are given. However, certain patients are more likely to develop symptoms of intolerance when receiving fluids of high osmoticity. These include debilitated patients, patients with GI disorders, pre- and post-operative patients, gastrostomy- and jejunostomy-fed patients, and patients whose GI tracts have not been challenged for an extended period of time. Thus osmoticity should always be considered in the selection of the formula for each individual patient. With all products, additional fluid intake may be indicated for individuals with certain clinical conditions. Frequent feedings of small volume or a continual instillation (pumped) may be of benefit initially in establishing tolerance to a formula. For other than isoosmotic formulas, feedings of reduced concentration (osmolality less than 400 mOsm/kg) may also be helpful initially if tolerance problems arise in sensitive individuals. Concentration and size of feeding can then be gradually increased to normal as tolerance is established.

A common disturbance of intake encountered in elderly individuals relates to excess solid intake rather than to reduced water intake. For example, an elderly victim of a cerebral vascular accident who is being fed by nasogastric tube may be given a formula whose solute load requires a greatly increased water intake. Thus, tube feeding containing 120 g of protein and 10 g of salt will result in the excretion of more than 1000 mOsm of solute. This requires the obligatory excretion of a volume of urine between 1200 and 1500 mL when the kidney is capable of concentration normally. As elderly individuals often have significant impairment in renal concentration ability, water loss as urine may exceed 2000–2500 mL per day. Such an individual would require 3–4 liters of water per day simply to meet the increased demand created by this high solute intake. Failure of the physician to provide such a patient with the increased water intake needed will result in a progressive water deficit that may rapidly become critical. The importance of knowing the complete composition of the tube feeding formulas used for incapacitated patients cannot be overemphasized.

Osmolality Determination

The need for experimental determination of osmolality has been established. In regard to this there are four properties of solutions that depend only on the number of "particles" in the solution. They are: osmotic pressure elevation, boiling point elevation, vapor pressure depression, and freezing point depression. These are called colligative properties and if one of them is known, the others can be calculated from its value. Osmotic pressure elevation is the most difficult to measure satisfactorily. The boiling point elevation may be determined but the readings are rather sensitive to changes in barometric pressure. Also, for an aqueous solution the molal boiling point elevation is considerably less than the freezing point depression. Thus it is less accurate than the freezing point method. Determinations of vapor pressure lowering have been considered to be impractical because of the elaborate apparatus required. However Zenk and Huxtable used a vapor pressure osmometer and state that it has much to recommend it for most of the systems under consideration here.[3] The method usually used is that of freezing point depression, which can be measured quite readily with a fair degree of accuracy (see *Freezing Point Depression*, Chapter 16). It should be noted that the data in Appendix A can be readily converted to vapor pressure lowering if desired.

Semiautomatic, high sensitivity osmometers that measure freezing point depression provide digital readouts or computer printouts of the results expressed in milliosmol units.

The results of investigations by Lund and coworkers[11] indicate that the freezing point of normal, healthy human blood is −0.52° and not −0.56°, as previously assumed.* Inasmuch as water is the medium in which the various constituents of blood are either suspended or dissolved in this method, it is assumed that *any aqueous solution* freezing at −0.52° is *isotonic with blood.* Now it is only rarely that a simple aqueous solution of the therapeutic agent to be injected parenterally has a freezing point of −0.52°, and to obtain this freezing point it is necessary either to add some other therapeutically inactive solute if the solution is hypotonic (freezing point above −0.52°) or to dilute the solution if it is hypertonic (freezing point below −0.52°). The usual practice is to add either sodium chloride or dextrose to adjust hypotonic parenteral solutions to isotonicity. Certain solutes, including ammonium chloride, boric acid, urea, glycerin, and propylene glycol, cause hemolysis even when they are present in a concentration that is isoosmotic; such solutions obviously are not isotonic. See Appendix A.

In a similar manner solutions intended for ophthalmic use may be adjusted to have a freezing point identical with that of lacrimal fluid, namely, −0.52°.* Ophthalmic solutions with higher freezing points are usually made isotonic by the addition of boric acid or sodium chloride.

In laboratories where the necessary equipment is available, the method usually followed for adjusting hypotonic solutions is to determine the freezing point depression produced by the ingredients of a given prescription or formula, and then to add a quantity of a suitable inert solute calculated to lower the freezing point to −0.52°, whether the solution is for parenteral injection or ophthalmic application. A final determination of the freezing point depression may be made to verify the

---

* See discussion of Reliability of Data in this chapter.

accuracy of the calculation. If the solution is hypertonic, it must be diluted if an isotonic solution is to be prepared, but it must be remembered that some solutions cannot be diluted without impairing their therapeutic activity. For example, solutions to be used for treating varicose veins require a high concentration of the active ingredient (solute) to make the solution effective. Dilution to isotonic concentration is not indicated in such cases.

Freezing-Point Calculations

As explained in the preceding section, freezing point data often may be employed in solving problems of isotonicity adjustment. Obviously, the utility of such data is limited to those solutions where the solute does not penetrate the membrane of the tissue, eg, red blood cells, with which it is in contact. In such cases, Appendix A, giving the freezing point depression of solutions of different concentrations of various substances, provides information essential for solving the problem.

For most substances listed in the table the concentration of an isotonic solution, ie, one that has a freezing point of −0.52°, is given. If this is not listed in the table, it may be determined with sufficient accuracy by simple proportion using, as the basis for calculation, that figure which most nearly produces an isotonic solution. Actually the depression of the freezing point of a solution of an electrolyte is not absolutely proportional to the concentration but varies according to dilution; for example, a solution containing 1 g of procaine hydrochloride in 100 mL has a freezing point depression of 0.12°, whereas a solution containing 3 g of the same salt in 100 mL has a freezing point depression of 0.33°, *not* 0.36° (3 × 0.12°). Since the adjustment to isotonicity need not be absolutely exact, approximations may be made. When it is recalled that for many years an 0.85% solution of sodium chloride, rather than the presently employed 0.90% concentration, was widely accepted and proved to be eminently satisfactory as the isotonic equivalent of blood serum, it is apparent that minor deviations are not of great concern. Also, formerly a 1.4% solution of sodium chloride was considered to be isotonic with lacrimal fluid and found to be relatively tolerable when applied to the eye. Nevertheless, adjustments to isotonicity should be as exact as practicable.

As a specific illustration of the manner in which the data in the table may be used, suppose it is required to calculate the quantity of sodium chloride needed to make 100 mL of a 1% solution of calcium disodium edetate isoosmotic with blood serum. Reference to the table indicates that the 1% solution provides for 0.12° of the necessary 0.52° of freezing point depression required of an isoosmotic solution, thus leaving 0.40° to be supplied by the sodium chloride. Again referring to the table, 0.52° is found to be the freezing point depression of a 0.9% solution of sodium chloride and by simple proportion it is calculated that a 0.69% solution will have a freezing point depression of 0.40°. Assuming additivity of the freezing point depressions, a solution of 0.69 g of sodium chloride and 1 g of calcium disodium edetate in sufficient water to make 100 mL will be isoosmotic with blood serum.

Likewise, to render a 1% solution of boric acid isotonic with lacrimal fluid by the addition of sodium chloride, one would proceed with the calculation as follows:

Freezing point depression of lacrimal fluid	0.52°
Freezing point depression of 1% boric acid solution	0.29°
Freezing point depression to be supplied by sodium chloride	0.23°
Freezing point depression of a 0.9% solution of sodium chloride	0.52°

Therefore

$$0.52 : 0.9 = 0.23 : x$$
$$0.52x = 0.207$$

x = 0.4% sodium chloride to be incorporated with 1% boric acid to produce a solution which will be isotonic with lacrimal fluid.

Similarly, should a solution contain more than one ingredient, the sum of the respective freezing points of each ingredient would be determined and the difference between this sum and the required freezing point would represent the freezing point to be supplied by the added substance.

The preceding calculation can be expressed in the form of an equation, as follows:

$$x = \frac{(0.52° - a) \times c}{b}$$

where

x   = g of adjusting solute required for each 100 mL of solution.

0.52°   = Freezing point depression of blood serum or lacrimal fluid.

a   = Freezing point depression of given ingredients in 100 mL of solution.

b   = Freezing point depression of c g of adjusting substance per 100 mL.

c   = g of adjusting solute per 100 mL, producing a freezing point depression of b.

L Values—In dilute solutions, the expression for freezing-point depression may be written as:

$$\Delta T_f = Lc$$

in which ΔT_f is the freezing-point depression in °C, L is a constant, and c is the molar concentration of the drug. L_{iso} is defined as the specific value of L at a concentration of drug which is isotonic with blood or lacrimal fluid.

For a more complete discussion of the use of L values, the reader is referred to RPS-14, page 1560.

Effect of Solvents—Besides water, certain other solvents are frequently employed in nose drops, ear drops, and other preparations to be used in various parts of the body. Liquids such as glycerin, propylene glycol, or alcohol may compose part of the solvent. In solving isotonicity adjustment problems for such solutions it should be kept in mind that while these solvent components contribute to the freezing-point depression they may or may not have an effect on the "tone" of the tissue to which they are applied, ie, an *isoosmotic* solution may not be *isotonic*. It is apparent that in such cases, the utility of the methods described above or, for that matter, of any other method of evaluating "tonicity" is questionable.

Reliability of Data—While the freezing point of blood was formerly assumed to be −0.56°, later investigators[11] reported that in consequence of ice being disengaged in freezing-point determinations as ordinarily performed the observed freezing point of blood is low; according to them the correct freezing point is −0.52°. The same investigators found the freezing point of a 0.9% solution of sodium chloride to be correspondingly low; the correct freezing point in this case is also −0.52°. Presumably all solutions commonly considered to be isotonic with blood will freeze, when a correction for disengaged ice is applied, at −0.52°. It is apparent, therefore, that there is no need to change the isotonic concentration, if the reference temperature for both blood and the solution under consideration is always the same, and provided that the *method* of determining the freezing point is the same. Also, there appears to be no objection to using freezing-point data for solutions of other than isotonic concentration if the method of determining the freezing point is the same in all cases, since any differences that may be obtained when another method is used (such as that of Lund *et al*[11]), will probably be proportional to concentration.

In a discussion of the significance of freezing point data it is to be noted that there are some discrepancies in the literature concerning freezing points of solutions. An *exact* determination of freezing point is actually a difficult experiment, one which calls for the control of several variables that are commonly neglected, of which disengagement of ice is one. It is not possible at this time to select unequivocal freezing point data for most of the solutions listed in Appendix A included in this chapter. The comprehensive and valuable data of Lund, *et al*[11] referred to above, actually represent in most instances measurements of vapor pressure which have been *calculated* to corresponding freezing point depressions; it would seem to be desirable to have confirmatory evidence based on actual measurements of freezing point, determined more accurately than has generally been the case, before revisions of existing data are made. In the case of boric acid, which enters into the composition of many collyria, there is the further variable that a sterilized solution freezes at a higher temperature than a freshly prepared, unsterilized solution of the same strength; specifically, a freshly prepared solution containing 2.85% of boric acid was found to freeze at the same temperature (−0.82°) as a 3.1% solution which had been sterilized under pressure.

Earlier in this section it was stated that at one time lacrimal fluid was considered to have the same osmotic pressure as a 1.4% solution of sodium chloride, the freezing point of which was found to be, by the usual method of determination, −0.80°. The experiments of Krogh, *et al*[12] have indicated that lacrimal fluid has the same osmotic pressure as blood and that instead of assuming that the freezing point of solutions isotonic with lacrimal fluid is −0.80° it should be the same as that of blood, namely, −0.52°. Accordingly, the procedure for adjusting solutions to isotonicity with lacrimal fluid is qualitatively and quantitatively the same as the procedure for adjusting solutions to isotonicity with blood.

Tonicity Testing by Observing Erythrocyte Changes

Observation of the behavior of human erythrocytes when suspended in a solution is the ultimate and direct procedure for determining whether the solution is isotonic, hypotonic, or hypertonic. If hemolysis or marked change in the appearance of the erythrocytes occurs, the solution is not isotonic with the cells; if the cells retain their normal characteristics, the solution is isotonic.

Hemolysis may occur when the osmotic pressure of the fluid in the erythrocytes is greater than that of the solution in which the cells are suspended, but the specific chemical reactivity of the solute in the solution is often far more important in producing hemolysis than is the osmotic effect. There is no certain evidence that any single mechanism of action causes hemolysis; the process appears to involve such factors as pH, lipid solubility, molecular and ionic sizes of solute particles, and possibly inhibition of cholinesterase in cell membranes and denaturing action on plasma membrane protein.

Some investigators test the tonicity of injectable solutions by observing variations of red cell volume produced by the solutions. This method appears to be more sensitive to small differences in tonicity than are methods based on observation of a hemolytic effect. Much useful information concerning the effect of various solutes on erythrocytes has been obtained by this procedure; a summary of many of these data is given in RPS-14, page 1562.

Other Methods of Adjusting Tonicity

Several methods for adjusting tonicity, other than those already described, are used.

Sodium Chloride Equivalent Methods—Sodium chloride equivalent is defined as the weight of sodium chloride that will produce the same osmotic effect as 1 g of the drug which is to be prepared as an isotonic solution. Appendix A lists the sodium chloride equivalents for many drugs; some of the equivalents vary with the concentration of the drug (in certain cases because of changes of interionic attraction at different concentrations) but in every case the equivalent is for 1 g of drug. As an example of the use of these data, if the sodium chloride equivalent of boric acid is 0.5 at 1% concentration, this is interpreted to mean that 1 g of boric acid in solution will produce the same freezing-point depression as 0.5 g of sodium chloride, or that a 1% boric acid solution is equivalent in its colligative properties to a 0.5% solution of sodium chloride. From Appendix A it is found that for a 1.9% boric acid solution (ie, at isotonicity) the sodium chloride equivalent is 0.47, corresponding to a 0.9% sodium chloride solution (1.9 × 0.47).

Examples illustrating use of the sodium chloride equivalent method to adjust collyria to isotonicity follow. The same type of calculation may be used for other solutions that are to be made isotonic.

Example 1:

Homatropine Hydrobromide 1%
to make collyr isotonic .... 60 mL

0.6 g of homatropine hydrobromide is required. 1 g or 1% of the drug is equivalent in osmotic effect to 0.17 g or 0.17% of sodium chloride.

$$0.17 \times 0.6 = 0.102 \text{ g (sodium chloride)}$$

60 mL of an isotonic sodium chloride
  solution contains   0.54   g sodium chloride
0.6 g homatropine hydrobromide is
  equivalent to   0.102 g sodium chloride
         0.438 g sodium chloride

Therefore, 0.438 g of sodium chloride must be added to make 60 mL of a 1% homatropine hydrobromide solution isotonic with tear fluid. The same calculations may be made using percentage calculations. 1% of homatropine hydrobromide corresponds to 0.17% sodium chloride in colligative properties.

Thus, 0.9% minus 0.17% = 0.73% must be added, 0.73% of 60 mL = 0.438 g of sodium chloride to be added.

If boric acid is to be used as the adjusting substance the calculations have to be carried one step further. There is no "boric acid equivalent," but the sodium chloride equivalent of boric acid at 1% concentration is 0.5, meaning that 1 g of boric acid (or 1%) corresponds in colligative properties to 0.5 g sodium chloride (or 0.5%). Using the result obtained above, which was 0.438 g of sodium chloride to be added, it now follows that the sodium chloride equivalent of boric acid must be divided into the amount of sodium chloride or expressed as an equation:

$$1 \text{ g boric acid}: 0.5 \text{ g sodium chloride} = x \text{ g}: 0.438 \text{ g}$$
$$x = 0.876 \text{ g boric acid to be added}$$

For a prescription containing more than one active drug, the calculations for sodium chloride are carried out separately, the obtained quantities are added, and then the total is deducted from the 0.9% amount.

Example 2:

Epinephrine Hydrochloride 0.5%
Zinc Sulfate 0.3%
Sterile Preserved Water qs, to make 30   mL

M Ft Collyr isotonic SA

Sodium chloride equivalent of epinephrine HCl is 0.29
Sodium chloride equivalent of zinc sulfate is   0.15
  150 mg epinephrine hydrochloride   ~43.5 mg sodium chloride
  90 mg zinc sulfate   ~13.5 mg sodium chloride
  Total ingredients are equivalent to   ~57   mg sodium chloride

  0.9% of 30 mL   270 mg sodium chloride
         57 mg
         213 mg

213 mg of sodium chloride must be added to make this solution isotonic with tear fluid. Since boric acid is the adjusting substance of choice for the solution 426 mg should be used (0.5 divided into 213 mg).

Isotonic Solution V-Values—These are the volumes of sterile water to be added to a specified weight of drug (often 0.3 g but sometimes 1 g) to prepare an isotonic solution. Appendix B gives such values for some commonly used drugs. The reason for providing data for 0.3 g drug is only that of convenience in preparing 30 mL (1 fl oz) of solution, as is often

prescribed; if values for 100 mL of final solution are desired, the data in Appendix B should be multiplied by 100/30. The basic principle underlying the use of these values is to prepare an isotonic solution of the prescribed drug in sterile water and then dilute this solution to the required final volume with a suitable isotonic vehicle. For example, if 0.3 g of a drug is specified to be used (as in preparing 30 mL of 1% solution of the drug), it is first dissolved in the volume of sterile water stated in Appendix B and then diluted to 30 mL with a suitable isotonic vehicle. Isotonic solution values can be used, of course, for calculating tonicity-adjusting data for concentrations of drugs other than 1% and for volumes other than 30 mL. How this is done is illustrated in the following examples.

Example 1:

A prescription calls for:

Atropine Sulfate .... 0.3 g
Sterile Preserved Water qs 60   mL

M Ft Collyr isotonic and buffered SA
Sig: For Office Use.

This order is for a 0.5% solution of atropine sulfate. According to Appendix B, 0.3 g of atropine sulfate dissolved in 4.3 mL of sterile preserved water will produce a 1% isotonic solution when diluted to 30 mL with an isotonic vehicle. For 30 mL of 0.5% solution, half the quantities of atropine sulfate and sterile preserved water would be used, but for 60 mL of 0.5% solution the same quantities as for 30 mL of 1% solution are required.

Therefore, to fill this prescription order, 0.3 g of atropine sulfate should be dissolved in 4.3 mL of sterile preserved water and diluted with isotonic preserved Sørensen's pH 6.8 phosphate buffer to 60 mL.

* * * *

For more than one active ingredient in solution the quantity of water to be used is calculated for each ingredient separately. The values thus obtained are added, the total amount of sterile preserved water is then used to dissolve the active ingredients, and finally sufficient isotonic, buffered solution (diluting solution) is used to make the required volume.

Example 2:

A prescription calls for:

Epinephrine Hydrochloride 0.5%
Zinc Sulfate 0.3%
Sterile Preserved Water qs to make 30   mL

M Ft Collyr isotonic

In this example the active ingredients are given in percentage. The ideal vehicle is 1.9% boric acid solution. Reference to the table for isotonic solution values shows the following:

Epinephrine hydrochloride 0.3 g (1%) will make 9.7 mL of an isotonic solution when dissolved in sterile preserved water. Zinc sulfate 0.3 g will make 5 mL of an isotonic solution with sterile water.

Therefore, the quantities called for in this prescription will make 4.85 mL and 1.5 mL of isotonic solutions, respectively. Dissolve the salts in sufficient sterile preserved water to make 6.35 mL and add sufficient 1.9% preserved boric acid solution to make 30 mL. The resulting solution is isotonic.

Since it is practically impossible to measure the required volumes accurately, it is feasible, in this instance, to use 6.35 mL of sterile preserved water as the total solvent for these two drugs. Graduated pipets, previously sterilized, are necessary for this work.

References

1. Kaminski MV: *Surg Gyn Obst 143:* 12, 1976.
2. Theeuwes F: *J Pharm Sci 64:* 1987, 1975.
3. Zenk K, Huxtable RF: *Hosp Pharm 13:* 577, 1978.
4. McDuffee L: *Illinois Council of Hospital Pharmacy Drug Information Newsletter 8:* Oct–Nov, 1978.
5. Streng WH, et al.: *J Pharm Sci 67:* 384, 1978.
6. Murty BSR, et al: *Am J Hosp Pharm 33:* 546, 1976.
7. Bray AJ: Personal Communication, Mead Johnson Nutritional Division, Evansville, IN, 1978.
8. Andrassy RJ, et al: *Surg 82:* 205, 1977.
9. Dobbie RP, Hoffmeister JA: *Surg Gyn Obst 143:* 273, 1976.
10. Anon. Osmolality: Doyle Pharmaceutical Co, Minneapolis, 1978.
11. Lund CG, et al: *The Preparation of Solutions Iso-osmotic with Blood, Tears, and Tissue.* Danish Pharmacopoeial Commission, Einar Munksgaard, Copenhagen, 1947.
12. Krogh A, et al: *Acta Physiol Scand 10:* 88, 1945.

13. Hammarlund ER, *et al: J Pharm Sci 54:* 160, 1965.
14. Hammarlund ER, Pedersen-Bjergaard K: *J APhA Sci Ed 47:* 107, 1958.
15. Hammarlund ER, Pedersen-Bjergaard K: *J Pharm Sci 50:* 24, 1961.
16. Hammarlund ER, Van Pevenage GL: *J Pharm Sci 55:* 1448, 1966.
17. Fassett WE, *et al: J Pharm Sci 58:* 1540, 1969.
18. Sapp C, *et al: J Pharm Sci 64:* 1884, 1975.
19. *British Pharmaceutical Codex*, Pharmaceutical Press, London, 1973.
20. Kogan DG, Kinsey VE: *Arch Ophthalmol 27:* 696, 1942.

Bibliography

Alberty RA, Daniels F: *Physical Chemistry*, 5th ed, Wiley, New York, 1979.
Anthony CP, Kolthoff NJ: *Textbook of Anatomy and Physiology*, Mosby, St. Louis, 1971.

Cowan G, Scheetz W, eds: *Intravenous Hyperalimentation*, Lea & Febiger, Philadelphia, 1972.
Garb S: *Laboratory Tests*, 6th ed, Springer, New York, 1976.
Hall WE: *Am J Pharm Educ 34:* 204, 1970.
Harvey AM, Johns RJ, Owens AH, Ross RS: *The Principles and Practice of Medicine*, 18th ed, Appleton-Century-Crofts, New York, 1972.
Martin AN, Swarbrick J, Cammarata A: *Physical Pharmacy*, 2nd ed, Lea & Febiger, Philadelphia, 1969.
Plumer AL: *Principles and Practice of Intravenous Therapy*, 2nd ed, Little, Brown, Boston, 1975.
Ravel R: *Clinical Laboratory Medicine*, 2nd ed, Year Book Medical Publishers, Chicago, 1973.
Tilkian SM, Conover MH: *Clinical Implications of Laboratory Tests*, Mosby, St Louis, 1975.
Turco S, King RE: *Sterile Dosage Forms*, 2nd ed, Lea & Febiger, Philadelphia, 1974.
Wallach J: *Interpretation of Diagnostic Tests*, 3rd ed, Little, Brown, Boston, 1978.

Appendix A—Sodium Chloride Equivalents, Freezing-Point Depressions, and Hemolytic Effects of Certain Medicinals in Aqueous Solution

	0.5% E	0.5% D	1% E	1% D	2% E	2% D	3% E	3% D	5% E	5% D	Isoosmotic %	Isoosmotic E	Isoosmotic D	Isoosmotic H	pH
Acetrizoate methylglucamine	0.09		0.08		0.08		0.08		0.08		12.12	0.07		0	7.1
Acetrizoate sodium	0.10	0.027	0.10	0.055	0.10	0.109	0.10	0.163	0.10	0.273	9.64	0.09	0.52	0	6.9[†]
Acetylcysteine	0.20	0.055	0.20	0.113	0.20	0.227	0.20	0.341			4.58	0.20	0.52	100*	2.0
Adrenaline HCl											4.24			68	4.5
Alphaprodine HCl	0.19	0.053	0.19	0.105	0.18	0.212	0.18	0.315			4.98	0.18	0.52	100	5.3
Alum (potassium)			0.18				0.15		0.15		6.35	0.14		24*	3.4
Amantadine HCl	0.31	0.090	0.31	0.180	0.31	0.354					2.95	0.31	0.52	91	5.7
Aminoacetic acid	0.42	0.119	0.41	0.235	0.41	0.470					2.20	0.41	0.52	0*	6.2
Aminohippuric acid	0.13	0.035	0.13	0.075											
Aminophylline				0.098[c]											
Ammonium carbonate	0.70	0.202	0.70	0.405							1.29	0.70	0.52	97	7.7
Ammonium chloride			1.12								0.8	1.12	0.52	93	5.0
Ammonium lactate	0.33	0.093	0.33	0.185	0.33	0.370					2.76	0.33	0.52	98	5.9
Ammonium nitrate	0.69	0.200	0.69	0.400							1.30	0.69	0.52	91	5.3
Ammonium phosphate, dibasic	0.58	0.165	0.55	0.315							1.76	0.51	0.52	0	7.9
Ammonium sulfate	0.55	0.158	0.55	0.315							1.68	0.54	0.52	0	5.3
Amobarbital sodium			0.25	0.143[c]			0.25				3.6	0.25	0.52	0	9.3
d-Amphetamine HCl											2.64			98	5.7
Amphetamine phosphate			0.34	0.20			0.27	0.47			3.47	0.26	0.52	0	4.5
Amphetamine sulfate			0.22	0.129[c]			0.21	0.36			4.23	0.21	0.52	0	5.9
Amprotropine phosphate											5.90			0	4.2
Amylcaine HCl			0.22				0.19				4.98	0.18		100	5.6
Anileridine HCl	0.19	0.052	0.19	0.104	0.19	0.212	0.18	0.316	0.18	0.509	5.13	0.18	0.52	12	2.6
Antazoline phosphate											6.05			90	4.0
Antimony potassium tartrate			0.18				0.13		0.10						
Antipyrine			0.17	0.10			0.14	0.24	0.14	0.40	6.81	0.13	0.52	100	6.1
Apomorphine HCl			0.14	0.080[c]											
Arginine glutamate	0.17	0.048	0.17	0.097	0.17	0.195	0.17	0.292	0.17	0.487	5.37	0.17	0.52	0	6.9
Ascorbic acid				0.105[c]							5.05		0.52[b]	100*	2.2
Atropine methylbromide			0.14				0.13		0.13		7.03	0.13			
Atropine methylnitrate											6.52			0	5.2
Atropine sulfate			0.13	0.075			0.11	0.19	0.11	0.32	8.85	0.10	0.52	0	5.0
Bacitracin			0.05	0.03			0.04	0.07	0.04	0.12					
Barbital sodium			0.30	0.171[c]			0.29	0.50			3.12	0.29	0.52	0	9.8
Benzalkonium chloride			0.16				0.14		0.13						
Benztropine mesylate	0.26	0.073	0.21	0.115	0.15	0.170	0.12	0.203	0.09	0.242					
Benzyl alcohol			0.17	0.09[c]			0.15								
Bethanechol chloride	0.50	0.140	0.39	0.225	0.32	0.368	0.30	0.512			3.05	0.30		0	6.0
Bismuth potassium tartrate			0.09				0.06		0.05						
Bismuth sodium tartrate			0.13				0.12		0.11		8.91	0.10		0	6.1
Boric acid			0.50	0.288[c]							1.9	0.47	0.52	100	4.6
Brompheniramine maleate	0.10	0.026	0.09	0.050	0.08	0.084									
Bupivacaine HCl	0.17	0.048	0.17	0.096	0.17	0.193	0.17	0.290	0.17	0.484	5.38	0.17	0.52	83	6.8

Appendix A—Continued

	0.5%		1%		2%		3%		5%		Isoosmotic concentration[e]				
	E	D	E	D	E	D	E	D	E	D	%	E	D	H	pH
Butabarbital sodium	0.27	0.078	0.27	0.155	0.27	0.313	0.27	0.470			3.33	0.27	0.52	0	6.8
Butacaine sulfate			0.20	0.12			0.13	0.23	0.10	0.29					
Caffeine and sodium benzoate			0.26	0.15			0.23	0.40			3.92	0.23	0.52	0	7.0
Caffeine and sodium salicylate			0.12	0.12			0.17	0.295	0.16	0.46	5.77	0.16	0.52	0	6.8
Calcium aminosalicylate											4.80			0	6.0
Calcium chloride			0.51	0.298[c]							1.70	0.53	0.52	0	5.6
Calcium chloride (6 H$_2$O)			0.35	0.20							2.5	0.36	0.52	0	5.7
Calcium chloride, anhydrous			0.68	0.39							1.3	0.69	0.52	0	5.6
Calcium disodium edetate	0.21	0.061	0.21	0.120	0.21	0.240	0.20	0.357			4.50	0.20	0.52	0	6.1
Calcium gluconate			0.16	0.091[c]			0.14	0.24							
Calcium lactate			0.23	0.13			0.12	0.36			4.5	0.20	0.52	0	6.7
Calcium lactobionate	0.08	0.022	0.08	0.043	0.08	0.085	0.07	0.126	0.07	0.197					
Calcium levulinate			0.27	0.16			0.25	0.43			3.58			0	7.2
Calcium pantothenate											5.50			0	7.4
Camphor			0.12[d]												
Capreomycin sulfate	0.04	0.011	0.04	0.020	0.04	0.042	0.04	0.063	0.04	0.106					
Carbachol			0.205[c]								2.82			0	5.9
Carbenicillin sodium	0.20	0.059	0.20	0.118	0.20	0.236	0.20	0.355			4.40	0.20	0.52	0	6.6
Carboxymethylcellulose sodium	0.03	0.007	0.03	0.017											
Cephaloridine	0.09	0.023	0.07	0.041	0.06	0.074	0.06	0.106	0.05	0.145					
Chloramine-T											4.10			100*	9.1
Chloramphenicol			0.06[d]												
Chloramphenicol sodium succinate	0.14	0.038	0.14	0.078	0.14	0.154	0.13	0.230	0.13	0.382	6.83	0.13	0.52	Partial	6.1
Chlordiazepoxide HCl	0.24	0.068	0.22	0.125	0.19	0.220	0.18	0.315	0.17	0.487	5.50	0.16	0.52	66	2.7
Chlorobutanol (hydrated)			0.24	0.14											
Chloroprocaine HCl	0.20	0.054	0.20	0.108	0.18	0.210									
Chloroquine phosphate	0.14	0.039	0.14	0.082	0.14	0.162	0.14	0.242	0.13	0.379	7.15	0.13	0.52	0	4.3
Chloroquine sulfate	0.10	0.028	0.09	0.050	0.08	0.090	0.07	0.127	0.07	0.195					
Chlorpheniramine maleate	0.17	0.048	0.15	0.085	0.14	0.165	0.13	0.220	0.09	0.265					
Chlortetracycline HCl	0.10	0.030	0.10	0.061	0.10	0.121									
Chlortetracycline sulfate			0.13	0.08			0.10	0.17							
Citric acid			0.18	0.10			0.17	0.295	0.16	0.46	5.52	0.16	0.52	100*	1.8
Clindamycin phosphate	0.08	0.022	0.08	0.046	0.08	0.095	0.08	0.144	0.08	0.242	10.73	0.08	0.52	58*	6.8
Cocaine HCl			0.16	0.090[c]			0.15	0.26	0.14	0.40	6.33	0.14	0.52	47	4.4
Codeine phosphate			0.14	0.080[c]			0.13	0.23	0.13	0.38	7.29	0.12	0.52	0	4.4
Colistimethate sodium	0.15	0.045	0.15	0.085	0.15	0.170	0.15	0.253	0.14	0.411	6.73	0.13	0.52	0	7.6
Cupric sulfate			0.18	0.100[c]			0.15		0.14		6.85	0.13		trace*	3.9
Cyclizine HCl	0.20	0.060													
Cyclophosphamide	0.10	0.031	0.10	0.061	0.10	0.125									
Cytarabine	0.11	0.034	0.11	0.066	0.11	0.134	0.11	0.198	0.11	0.317	8.92	0.10	0.52	0	8.0
Deferoxamine mesylate	0.09	0.023	0.09	0.047	0.09	0.093	0.09	0.142	0.09	0.241					
Demecarium bromide	0.14	0.038	0.12	0.069	0.10	0.108	0.08	0.139	0.07	0.192					
Dexamethasone sodium phosphate	0.18	0.050	0.17	0.095	0.16	0.180	0.15	0.260	0.14	0.410	6.75	0.13	0.52	0	8.9
Dextroamphetamine HCl	0.34	0.097	0.34	0.196	0.34	0.392					2.64	0.34	0.52		
Dextroamphetamine phosphate			0.25	0.14			0.25	0.44			3.62	0.25	0.52	0	4.7
Dextroamphetamine sulfate	0.24	0.069	0.23	0.134	0.22	0.259	0.22	0.380			4.16	0.22	0.52	0	5.9
Dextrose			0.16	0.091[c]			0.16	0.28	0.16	0.46	5.51	0.16	0.52	0	5.9
Dextrose (anhydrous)			0.18	0.101[c]			0.18	0.31			5.05	0.18	0.52	0	6.0
Diatrizoate sodium	0.10	0.025	0.09	0.049	0.09	0.098	0.09	0.149	0.09	0.248	10.55	0.09	0.52	0	7.9
Dibucaine HCl			0.074[c]												
Dicloxacillin sodium (1 H$_2$O)	0.10	0.030	0.10	0.061	0.10	0.122	0.10	0.182							
Diethanolamine	0.31	0.089	0.31	0.177	0.31	0.358					2.90	0.31	0.52	100	11.3
Dihydrostreptomycin sulfate			0.06	0.03			0.05	0.09	0.05	0.14	19.4	0.05	0.52	0	6.1

Appendix A—Continued

	0.5%		1%		2%		3%		5%		Isoosmotic concentration[e]				
	E	D	E	D	E	D	E	D	E	D	%	E	D	H	pH
Dimethpyrindene maleate	0.13	0.039	0.12	0.070	0.11	0.120									
Dimethyl sulfoxide	0.42	0.122	0.42	0.245	0.42	0.480					2.16	0.42	0.52	100	7.6
Diperodon HCl	0.15	0.045	0.14	0.079	0.13	0.141									
Diphenhydramine HCl				0.161[c]							5.70			88*	5.5
Diphenidol HCl	0.16	0.045	0.16	0.09	0.16	0.180									
Doxapram HCl	0.12	0.035	0.12	0.070	0.12	0.140	0.12	0.210							
Doxycycline hyclate	0.12	0.035	0.12	0.072	0.12	0.134	0.11	0.186	0.09	0.264					
Dyphylline	0.10	0.025	0.10	0.052	0.09	0.104	0.09	0.155	0.08	0.245					
Echothiophate iodide	0.16	0.045	0.16	0.090	0.16	0.179									
Edetate disodium	0.24	0.070	0.23	0.132	0.22	0.248	0.21	0.360			4.44	0.20	0.52	0	4.7
Edetate trisodium monohydrate	0.29	0.079	0.29	0.158	0.28	0.316	0.27	0.472			3.31	0.27	0.52	0	8.0
Emetine HCl				0.058[c]				0.17		0.29					
Ephedrine HCl			0.30	0.165[c]			0.28				3.2	0.28		96	5.9
Ephedrine sulfate			0.23	0.13			0.20	0.35			4.54	0.20	0.52	0	5.7
Epinephrine bitartrate			0.18	0.104			0.16	0.28	0.16	0.462	5.7	0.16	0.52	100*	3.4
Epinephrine hydrochloride			0.29	0.16[b]			0.26				3.47	0.26			
Ergonovine maleate				0.089[c]											
Erythromycin lactobionate	0.08	0.020	0.07	0.040	0.07	0.078	0.07	0.115	0.06	0.187					
Ethyl alcohol											1.39			100	6.0
Ethylenediamine				0.253[c]							2.08			100*	11.4
Ethylmorphine HCl			0.16	0.088[c]			0.15	0.26	0.15	0.43	6.18	0.15	0.52	38	4.7
Eucatropine HCl				0.11[d]											
Ferric ammonium citrate (green)											6.83			0	5.2
Floxuridine	0.14	0.040	0.13	0.076	0.13	0.147	0.12	0.213	0.12	0.335	8.47	0.12	0.52	3*	4.5
Fluorescein sodium			0.31	0.181[c]			0.27	0.47			3.34	0.27	0.52	0	8.7
Fluphenazine di-HCl	0.14	0.041	0.14	0.082	0.12	0.145	0.09	0.155							
d-Fructose											5.05			0*	5.9
Furtrethonium iodide	0.24	0.070	0.24	0.133	0.22	0.250	0.21	0.360			4.44	0.20	0.52	0	5.4
Galactose											4.92			0	5.9
Gentamicin sulfate	0.05	0.015	0.05	0.030	0.05	0.060	0.05	0.093	0.05	0.153					
D-Glucuronic acid											5.02			48*	1.6
Glycerin				0.203[c]							2.6			100	5.9
Glycopyrrolate	0.15	0.042	0.15	0.084	0.15	0.166	0.14	0.242	0.13	0.381	7.22	0.12	0.52	92*	4.0
Gold sodium thiomalate	0.10	0.032	0.10	0.061	0.10	0.111	0.09	0.159	0.09	0.250					
Hetacillin potassium	0.17	0.048	0.17	0.095	0.17	0.190	0.17	0.284	0.17	0.474	5.50	0.17	0.52	0	6.3
Hexafluorenium bromide	0.12	0.033	0.11	0.065											
Hexamethonium tartrate	0.16	0.045	0.16	0.089	0.16	0.181	0.16	0.271	0.16	0.456	5.68	0.16	0.52		
Hexamethylene sodium acetaminosalicylate	0.18	0.049	0.18	0.099	0.17	0.199	0.17	0.297	0.16	0.485	5.48	0.16	0.52	0*	4.0
Hexobarbital sodium				0.15[c]											—
Hexylcaine HCl											4.30			100	4.8
Histamine 2HCl	0.40	0.115	0.40	0.233	0.40	0.466					2.24	0.40	0.52	79*	3.7
Histamine phosphate				0.149[c]							4.10			0	4.6
Histidine HCl											3.45			40	3.9
Holocaine HCl			0.20	0.12											
Homatropine hydrobromide			0.17	0.097[c]			0.16	0.28	0.16	0.46	5.67	0.16	0.52	92	5.0
Homatropine methylbromide			0.19	0.11			0.15	0.26	0.13	0.38					
4-Homosulfanilamide HCl											3.69			0	4.9
Hyaluronidase	0.01	0.004	0.01	0.007	0.01	0.013	0.01	0.020	0.01	0.033					
Hydromorphone HCl											6.39			64	5.6
Hydroxyamphetamine HBr				0.15[d]							3.71			92	5.0
8-Hydroxyquinoline sulfate											9.75			59*	2.5
Hydroxystilbamidine isethionate	0.20	0.060	0.16	0.090	0.12	0.137	0.10	0.170	0.07	0.216					
Hyoscyamine hydrobromide											6.53			68	5.9
Imipramine HCl	0.20	0.058	0.20	0.110	0.13	0.143									

Appendix A—Continued

	0.5% E	0.5% D	1% E	1% D	2% E	2% D	3% E	3% D	5% E	5% D	Isoosmotic concentration[e] %	E	D	H	pH
Indigotindisulfonate sodium	0.30	0.085	0.30	0.172											
Intracaine HCl											4.97			85	5.0
Iodophthalein sodium				0.07[c]							9.58			100	9.4
Isometheptene mucate	0.18	0.048	0.18	0.095	0.18	0.196	0.18	0.302			4.95	0.18	0.52	0	6.2
Isoproterenol sulfate	0.14	0.039	0.14	0.078	0.14	0.156	0.14	0.234	0.14	0.389	6.65	0.14	0.52	trace	4.5
Kanamycin sulfate	0.08	0.021	0.07	0.041	0.07	0.083	0.07	0.125	0.07	0.210					
Lactic acid				0.239[c]							2.30			100*	2.1
Lactose			0.07	0.040[c]			0.08		0.09		9.75	0.09		0*	5.8
Levallorphan tartrate	0.13	0.036	0.13	0.073	0.13	0.143	0.12	0.210	0.12	0.329	9.40	0.10	0.52	59*	6.9
Levorphanol tartrate	0.12	0.033	0.12	0.067	0.12	0.136	0.12	0.203							
Lidocaine HCl				0.13[c]							4.42			85	4.3
Lincomycin HCl	0.16	0.045	0.16	0.090	0.15	0.170	0.14	0.247	0.14	0.400	6.60	0.14	0.52	0	4.5
Lobeline HCl				0.09[b]											
Lyapolate sodium	0.10	0.025	0.09	0.051	0.09	0.103	0.09	0.157	0.09	0.263	9.96	0.09	0.52	0	6.5†
Magnesium chloride				0.45							2.02	0.45		0	6.3
Magnesium sulfate			0.17	0.094[c]			0.15	0.26	0.15	0.43	6.3	0.14	0.52	0	6.2
Magnesium sulfate, anhydrous	0.34	0.093	0.32	0.184	0.30	0.345	0.29	0.495			3.18	0.28	0.52	0	7.0
Mannitol				0.098[c]							5.07			0*	6.2
Maphenide HCl	0.27	0.075	0.27	0.153	0.27	0.303	0.26	0.448			3.55	0.25	0.52		
Menadiol sodium diphosphate											4.36			0	8.2
Menadione sodium bisulfite											5.07			0	5.3
Menthol				0.12[d]											
Meperidine HCl				0.125[c]							4.80			98	5.0
Mepivacaine HCl	0.21	0.060	0.21	0.116	0.20	0.230	0.20	0.342			4.60	0.20	0.52	45	4.5
Merbromin				0.08[b]											
Mercuric cyanide			0.15				0.14		0.13						
Mersalyl				0.06[b]											
Mesoridazine besylate	0.10	0.024	0.07	0.040	0.05	0.058	0.04	0.071	0.03	0.087					
Metaraminol bitartrate	0.20	0.060	0.20	0.112	0.19	0.210	0.18	0.308	0.17	0.505	5.17	0.17	0.52	59	3.8
Methacholine chloride				0.184[c]							3.21			0	4.5
Methadone HCl				0.101[c]							8.59			100*	5.0
Methamphetamine HCl				0.213[c]							2.75			97	5.9
Methdilazine HCl	0.12	0.035	0.10	0.056	0.08	0.080	0.06	0.093	0.04	0.112					
Methenamine			0.23				0.24				3.68	0.25		100	8.4
Methiodal sodium	0.24	0.068	0.24	0.136	0.24	0.274	0.24	0.410			3.81	0.24	0.52	0	5.9
Methitural sodium	0.26	0.074	0.25	0.142	0.24	0.275	0.23	0.407			3.85	0.23	0.52	78	9.8
Methocarbamol	0.10	0.030	0.10	0.060											
Methotrimeprazine HCl	0.12	0.034	0.10	0.060	0.07	0.077	0.06	0.094	0.04	0.125					
Methoxyphenamine HCl	0.26	0.075	0.26	0.150	0.26	0.300	0.26	0.450			3.47	0.26	0.52	96	5.4
p-Methylaminoethanolphenol tartrate	0.18	0.048	0.17	0.095	0.16	0.190	0.16	0.282	0.16	0.453	5.83	0.16	0.52	0	6.2
Methyldopate HCl	0.21	0.063	0.21	0.122	0.21	0.244	0.21	0.365			4.28	0.21	0.52	Partial	3.0
Methylergonovine maleate	0.10	0.028	0.10	0.056											
N-Methylglucamine	0.20	0.057	0.20	0.111	0.18	0.214	0.18	0.315	0.18	0.517	5.02	0.18	0.52	4	11.3
Methylphenidate HCl	0.22	0.065	0.22	0.127	0.22	0.258	0.22	0.388			4.07	0.22	0.52	66	4.3
Methylprednisolone Na succinate	0.10	0.025	0.09	0.051	0.09	0.102	0.08	0.143	0.07	0.200					
Minocycline HCl	0.10	0.030	0.10	0.058	0.09	0.107	0.08	0.146							
Monoethanolamine	0.53	0.154	0.53	0.306							1.70	0.53	0.52	100	11.4
Morphine HCl			0.15	0.086[c]			0.14								
Morphine sulfate			0.14	0.079[c]			0.11	0.19	0.09	0.26					
Nalorphine HCl	0.24	0.070	0.21	0.121	0.18	0.210	0.17	0.288	0.15	0.434	6.36	0.14	0.52	63	4.1
Naloxone HCl	0.14	0.042	0.14	0.083	0.14	0.158	0.13	0.230	0.13	0.367	8.07	0.11	0.52	35	5.2
Naphazoline HCl			0.27	0.14[d]			0.24				3.99	0.22		100	5.3
Neoarsphenamine											2.32			17	7.8
Neomycin sulfate			0.11	0.063[c]			0.09	0.16	0.08	0.232					
Neostigmine bromide			0.22	0.127[c]			0.19				4.98			0	4.6
Neostigmine methylsulfate			0.20	0.115[c]			0.18		0.17		5.22	0.17			
Nicotinamide			0.26	0.148[c]			0.21	0.36			4.49	0.20	0.52	100	7.0
Nicotinic acid			0.25	0.144[c]											
Nikethamide				0.100[c]							5.94			100	6.9
Novobiocin sodium	0.12	0.033	0.10	0.057	0.07	0.073									

Appendix A—Continued

	0.5%		1%		2%		3%		5%		Isoosmotic concentration[c]				
	E	D	E	D	E	D	E	D	E	D	%	E	D	H	pH
Oleandomycin phosphate	0.08	0.017	0.08	0.038	0.08	0.084	0.08	0.129	0.08	0.255	10.82	0.08	0.52	0	5.0
Orphenadrine citrate	0.13	0.037	0.13	0.074	0.13	0.144	0.12	0.204	0.10	0.285					
Oxophenarsine HCl											3.67			trace*	2.3
Oxymetazoline HCl	0.22	0.063	0.22	0.124	0.20	0.232	0.19	0.335			4.92	0.18	0.52	86	5.7
Oxyquinoline sulfate	0.24	0.068	0.21	0.113	0.16	0.182	0.14	0.236	0.11	0.315					
d-Pantothenyl alcohol	0.20	0.053	0.18	0.100	0.17	0.193	0.17	0.283	0.16	0.468	5.60	0.16	0.52	92	6.8
Papaverine HCl			0.10	0.061[c]											
Paraldehyde	0.25	0.071	0.25	0.142	0.25	0.288	0.25	0.430			3.65	0.25	0.52	97	5.3
Pargyline HCl	0.30	0.083	0.29	0.165	0.29	0.327	0.28	0.491			3.18	0.28	0.52	91	3.8
Penicillin G, potassium			0.18	0.102[c]			0.17	0.29	0.16	0.46	5.48	0.16	0.52	0	6.2
Penicillin G, procaine				0.06[d]											
Penicillin G, sodium			0.18	0.100[c]			0.16	0.28	0.16	0.46	5.90			18	5.2
Pentazocine lactate	0.15	0.042	0.15	0.085	0.15	0.169	0.15	0.253	0.15	0.420					
Pentobarbital sodium				0.145[c]							4.07			0	9.9
Pentolinium tartrate											5.95			55*	3.4
Phenacaine HCl				0.09[d]											
Pheniramine maleate				0.09[d]											
Phenobarbital sodium			0.24	0.135[c]			0.23	0.40			3.95	0.23	0.52	0	9.2
Phenol			0.35	0.20							2.8	0.32	0.52	0*	5.6
Phentolamine mesylate	0.18	0.052	0.17	0.096	0.16	0.173	0.14	0.244	0.13	0.364	8.23	0.11	0.52	83	3.5
Phenylephrine HCl			0.32	0.184[c]			0.30				3.0	0.30		0	4.5
Phenylephrine tartrate											5.90			58*	5.4
Phenylethyl alcohol	0.25	0.070	0.25	0.141	0.25	0.283									
Phenylpropanolamine HCl			0.38	0.219[c]							2.6	0.35		95	5.3
Physostigmine salicylate			0.16	0.090[c]											
Physostigmine sulfate				0.074[c]											
Pilocarpine HCl			0.24	0.138[c]			0.22	0.38			4.08	0.22	0.52	89	4.0
Pilocarpine nitrate			0.23	0.132[c]			0.20	0.35			4.84	0.20	0.52	88	3.9
Piperocaine HCl				0.12[d]							5.22			65	5.7
Polyethylene glycol 300	0.12	0.034	0.12	0.069	0.12	0.141	0.12	0.216	0.13	0.378	6.73	0.13	0.52	53	3.8
Polyethylene glycol 400	0.08	0.022	0.08	0.047	0.09	0.098	0.09	0.153	0.09	0.272	8.50	0.11	0.52	0	4.4
Polyethylene glycol 1500	0.06	0.015	0.06	0.036	0.07	0.078	0.07	0.120	0.07	0.215	10.00	0.09	0.52	4	4.1
Polyethylene glycol 1540	0.02	0.005	0.02	0.012	0.02	0.028	0.03	0.047	0.03	0.094					
Polyethylene glycol 4000	0.02	0.004	0.02	0.008	0.02	0.020	0.02	0.033	0.02	0.067					
Polymyxin B sulfate			0.09	0.052[c]			0.06	0.10	0.04	0.12					
Polysorbate 80	0.02	0.005	0.02	0.010	0.02	0.020	0.02	0.032	0.02	0.055					
Polyvinyl alcohol (99% hydrol.)	0.02	0.004	0.02	0.008	0.02	0.020	0.02	0.035	0.03	0.075					
Polyvinylpyrrolidone	0.01	0.003	0.01	0.006	0.01	0.010	0.01	0.017	0.01	0.035					
Potassium acetate	0.59	0.172	0.59	0.342							1.53	0.59	0.52	0	7.6
Potassium chlorate											1.88			0	6.9
Potassium chloride			0.76	0.439[c]							1.19	0.76	0.52	0	5.9
Potassium iodide			0.34	0.196[c]							2.59	0.34	0.52	0	7.0
Potassium nitrate			0.56	0.324[c]							1.62	0.56		0	5.9
Potassium phosphate			0.46	0.27							2.08	0.43	0.52	0	8.4
Potassium phosphate, monobasic			0.44	0.25							2.18	0.41	0.52	0	4.4
Potassium sulfate			0.44								2.11	0.43		0	6.6
Pralidoxime chloride	0.32	0.092	0.32	0.183	0.32	0.364					2.87	0.32	0.52	0	4.6
Prilocaine HCl	0.22	0.062	0.22	0.125	0.22	0.250	0.22	0.375			4.18	0.22	0.52	45	4.6
Procainamide HCl			0.22	0.13			0.19	0.33	0.17	0.49					
Procaine HCl			0.21	0.122[c]			0.19	0.33	0.18		5.05	0.18	0.52	91	5.6
Prochlorperazine edisylate	0.08	0.020	0.06	0.033	0.05	0.048	0.03	0.056	0.02	0.065					
Promazine HCl	0.18	0.050	0.13	0.077	0.09	0.102	0.07	0.112	0.05	0.137					
Proparacaine HCl	0.16	0.044	0.15	0.086	0.15	0.169	0.14	0.247	0.13	0.380	7.46	0.12	0.52		
Propiomazine HCl	0.18	0.050	0.15	0.084	0.12	0.133	0.10	0.165	0.08	0.215					
Propoxycaine HCl											6.40			16	5.3
Propylene glycol											2.00			100	5.5
Pyrathiazine HCl	0.22	0.065	0.17	0.095	0.11	0.123	0.08	0.140	0.06	0.170					
Pyridostigmine bromide	0.22	0.062	0.22	0.125	0.22	0.250	0.22	0.377			4.13	0.22	0.52	0	7.2
Pyridoxine HCl											3.05			31*	3.2

Appendix A—Continued

	0.5%		1%		2%		3%		5%		Isoosmotic concentration[e]				
	E	D	E	D	E	D	E	D	E	D	%	E	D	H	pH
Quinacrine methanesulfonate				0.06[c]											
Quinine bisulfate			0.09	0.05			0.09	0.16							
Quinine dihydrochloride			0.23	0.130[c]			0.19	0.33	0.18		5.07	0.18	0.52	trace*	2.5
Quinine hydrochloride			0.14	0.077[c]			0.11	0.19							
Quinine and urea HCl			0.23	0.13			0.21	0.36			4.5	0.20	0.52	64	2.9
Resorcinol				0.161[c]							3.30			96	5.0
Rolitetracycline	0.11	0.032	0.11	0.064	0.10	0.113	0.09	0.158	0.07	0.204					
Rose Bengal	0.08	0.020	0.07	0.040	0.07	0.083	0.07	0.124	0.07	0.198	14.9	0.06	0.52		
Rose Bengal B	0.08	0.022	0.08	0.044	0.08	0.087	0.08	0.131	0.08	0.218					
Scopolamine HBr			0.12	0.07			0.12	0.21	0.12	0.35	7.85	0.11	0.52	8	4.8
Scopolamine methylnitrate			0.16				0.14			0.13	6.95	0.13		0	6.0
Secobarbital sodium			0.24	0.14			0.23	0.40			3.9	0.23	0.52	trace	9.8
Silver nitrate			0.33	0.190[c]							2.74	0.33	0.52	0*	5.0
Silver protein, mild			0.17	0.10			0.17	0.29	0.16	0.46	5.51	0.16	0.52	0	9.0
Silver protein, strong				0.06[d]											
Sodium acetate			0.46	0.267							2.0	0.45	0.52		
Sodium acetazolamide	0.24	0.068	0.23	0.135	0.23	0.271	0.23	0.406			3.85	0.23	0.52		
Sodium aminosalicylate				0.170[c]							3.27			0	7.3
Sodium ampicillin	0.16	0.045	0.16	0.090	0.16	0.181	0.16	0.072	0.16	0.451	5.78	0.16	0.52	0	8.5
Sodium ascorbate											3.00			0	6.9
Sodium benzoate			0.40	0.230[c]							2.25	0.40	0.52	0	7.5
Sodium bicarbonate			0.65	0.375							1.39	0.65	0.52	0	8.3
Sodium biphosphate (H_2O)			0.40	0.23							2.45	0.37	0.52	0	4.1
Sodium biphosphate (2 H_2O)			0.36								2.77	0.32	0.52	0	4.0
Sodium bismuth thioglycollate	0.20	0.055	0.19	0.107	0.18	0.208	0.18	0.303	0.17	0.493	5.29			0	8.3
Sodium bisulfite			0.61	0.35							1.5	0.61	0.52	0*	3.0
Sodium borate			0.42	0.241[c]							2.6	0.35	0.52	0	9.2
Sodium bromide											1.60			0	6.1
Sodium cacodylate			0.32				0.28				3.3	0.27	0.52	0	8.0
Sodium carbonate, monohydrated			0.60	0.346							1.56	0.58	0.52	100	11.1
Sodium cephalothin	0.18	0.050	0.17	0.095	0.16	0.179	0.15	0.259	0.14	0.400	6.80	0.13	0.52	Par-tial	8.5
Sodium chloride			1.00	0.576[c]			1.00	1.73	1.00	2.88	0.9	1.00	0.52	0	6.7
Sodium citrate			0.31	0.178[c]			0.30	0.52			3.02	0.30	0.52	0	7.8
Sodium colistimethate	0.16	0.045	0.15	0.087	0.14	0.161	0.14	0.235	0.13	0.383	6.85	0.13	0.52	0	8.4
Sodium hypophosphite											1.60			0	7.3
Sodium iodide			0.39	0.222[c]							2.37	0.38	0.52	0	6.9
Sodium iodohippurate											5.92			0	7.3
Sodium lactate											1.72			0	6.5
Sodium lauryl sulfate	0.10	0.029	0.08	0.046	0.07	0.068	0.05	0.086							
Sodium mercaptomerin											5.30			0	8.4
Sodium metabisulfite			0.67	0.386[c]							1.38	0.65	0.52	5*	4.5
Sodium methicillin	0.18	0.050	0.18	0.099	0.17	0.192	0.16	0.281	0.15	0.445	6.00	0.15	0.52	0	5.8
Sodium nafcillin	0.14	0.039	0.14	0.078	0.14	0.158	0.13	0.219	0.10	0.285					
Sodium nitrate			0.68								1.36	0.66	0.52	0	6.0
Sodium nitrite			0.84	0.480[c]							1.08	0.83	0.52	0*	8.5
Sodium oxacillin	0.18	0.050	0.17	0.095	0.16	0.177	0.15	0.257	0.14	0.408	6.64	0.14	0.52	0	6.0
Sodium phenylbutazone	0.19	0.054	0.18	0.104	0.17	0.202	0.17	0.298	0.17	0.488	5.34	0.17	0.52		
Sodium phosphate			0.29	0.168			0.27	0.47			3.33	0.27	0.52	0	9.2
Sodium phosphate, dibasic (2 H_2O)			0.42	0.24							2.23	0.40	0.52	0	9.2
Sodium phosphate, dibasic (12 H_2O)			0.22				0.21				4.45	0.20	0.52	0	9.2
Sodium propionate			0.61	0.35							1.47	0.61	0.52	0	7.8
Sodium salicylate			0.36	0.210[c]							2.53	0.36	0.52	0	6.7
Sodium succinate	0.32	0.092	0.32	0.184	0.31	0.361					2.90	0.31	0.52	0	8.5
Sodium sulfate, anhydrous			0.58	0.34							1.61	0.56	0.52	0	6.2
Sodium sulfite, exsiccated			0.65	0.38							1.45			0	9.6
Sodium sulfobromophthalein	0.07	0.019	0.06	0.034	0.05	0.060	0.05	0.084	0.04	0.123					

Appendix A—Continued

	0.5% E	0.5% D	1% E	1% D	2% E	2% D	3% E	3% D	5% E	5% D	Isoosmotic concentration[e] %	E	D	H	pH
Sodium tartrate	0.33	0.098	0.33	0.193	0.33	0.385					2.72	0.33	0.52	0	7.3
Sodium thiosulfate			0.31	0.181[c]							2.98	0.30	0.52	0	7.4
Sodium warfarin	0.18	0.049	0.17	0.095	0.16	0.181	0.15	0.264	0.15	0.430	6.10	0.15	0.52	0	8.1
Sorbitol (½ H₂O)											5.48			0	5.9
Sparteine sulfate	0.10	0.030	0.10	0.056	0.10	0.111	0.10	0.167	0.10	0.277	9.46	0.10	0.52	19*	3.5
Spectinomycin HCl	0.16	0.045	0.16	0.092	0.16	0.185	0.16	0.280	0.16	0.460	5.66	0.16	0.52	3	4.4
Streptomycin HCl			0.17	0.10[c]			0.16		0.16						
Streptomycin sulfate			0.07	0.036[c]			0.06	0.10	0.06	0.17					
Sucrose			0.08	0.047[c]			0.09	0.16	0.09	0.26	9.25	0.10	0.52	0	6.4
Sulfacetamide sodium			0.23	0.132[c]			0.23	0.40			3.85	0.23	0.52	0	8.7
Sulfadiazine sodium			0.24	0.14			0.24	0.38			4.24	0.21	0.52	0	9.5
Sulfamerazine sodium			0.23	0.13			0.21	0.36			4.53	0.20	0.52	0	9.8
Sulfapyridine sodium			0.23	0.13			0.21	0.36			4.55	0.20	0.52	5	10.4
Sulfathiazole sodium			0.22	0.13			0.20	0.35			4.82	0.19	0.52	0	9.9
Tartaric acid			0.15	0.143[c]							3.90			75*	1.7
Tetracaine HCl			0.18	0.109[c]			0.15	0.26	0.12	0.35					
Tetracycline HCl			0.14	0.081[c]			0.10								
Tetrahydrozoline HCl											4.10			60*	6.7
Theophylline				0.02[b]											
Theophylline sodium glycinate											2.94			0	8.9
Thiamine HCl				0.139[c]							4.24			87*	3.0
Thiethylperazine maleate	0.10	0.030	0.09	0.050	0.08	0.089	0.07	0.119	0.05	0.153					
Thiopental sodium				0.155[c]							3.50			74	10.3
Thiopropazate diHCl	0.20	0.053	0.16	0.090	0.12	0.137	0.10	0.170	0.08	0.222					
Thioridazine HCl	0.06	0.015	0.05	0.025	0.04	0.042	0.03	0.055	0.03	0.075					
Thiotepa	0.16	0.045	0.16	0.090	0.16	0.182	0.16	0.278	0.16	0.460	5.67	0.16	0.52	10*	8.2
Tridihexethyl chloride	0.16	0.047	0.16	0.096	0.16	0.191	0.16	0.280	0.16	0.463	5.62	0.16	0.52	97	5.4
Triethanolamine	0.20	0.058	0.21	0.121	0.22	0.252	0.22	0.383			4.05	0.22	0.52	100	10.7
Trifluoperazine diHCl	0.18	0.052	0.18	0.100	0.13	0.144									
Triflupromazine HCl	0.10	0.031	0.09	0.051	0.05	0.061	0.04	0.073	0.03	0.092					
Trimeprazine tartrate	0.10	0.023	0.06	0.035	0.04	0.045	0.03	0.052	0.02	0.061					
Trimethadione	0.23	0.069	0.23	0.133	0.22	0.257	0.22	0.378			4.22	0.21	0.52	100	6.0
Trimethobenzamide HCl	0.12	0.033	0.10	0.062	0.10	0.108	0.09	0.153	0.08	0.232					
Tripelennamine HCl				0.13[d]							5.50			100	6.3
Tromethamine	0.26	0.074	0.26	0.150	0.26	0.300	0.26	0.450			3.45	0.26	0.52	0	10.2
Tropicamide	0.10	0.030	0.09	0.050											
Trypan blue	0.26	0.075	0.26	0.150											
Tryparsamide				0.11[c]											
Tubocurarine chloride				0.076[c]											
Urea			0.59	0.34							1.63	0.55	0.52	100	6.6
Urethan				0.18[b]							2.93			100	6.3
Uridine	0.12	0.035	0.12	0.069	0.12	0.138	0.12	0.208	0.12	0.333	8.18	0.11	0.52	0*	6.1
Valethamate bromide	0.16	0.044	0.15	0.085	0.15	0.168	0.14	0.238	0.11	0.324					
Vancomycin sulfate	0.06	0.015	0.05	0.028	0.04	0.049	0.04	0.066	0.04	0.098					
Viomycin sulfate			0.08	0.05			0.07	0.12	0.07	0.20					
Xylometazoline HCl	0.22	0.065	0.21	0.121	0.20	0.232	0.20	0.342			4.68	0.19	0.52	88	5.0
Zinc phenolsulfonate											5.40			0*	5.4
Zinc sulfate			0.15	0.086[c]			0.13	0.23	0.12	0.35	7.65	0.12	0.52		

[a] The unmarked values were taken from Hammarlund and co-workers,[13–16] and Sapp *et al.*[18]

[b] Adapted from Lund, *et al.*[11]

[c] Adapted from BPC.[19]

[d] Obtained from several sources.

[e] E: sodium chloride equivalents; D: freezing-point depression, °C; H: hemolysis, %, at the concentration which is isoosmotic with 0.9% NaCl, based on freezing-point determination or equivalent test; pH: approximate pH of solution studied for hemolytic action; *: change in appearance of erythrocytes and/or solution[17–19]; †: pH determined after addition of blood.

Appendix B—Volumes of Water for Isotonicity[20,a]

Drug (0.3 g)	Water needed for isotonicity, mL	Drug (0.3 g)	Water needed for isotonicity, mL	Drug (0.3 g)	Water needed for isotonicity, mL
Alcohol	21.7	Apomorphine hydrochloride	4.7	Bismuth potassium tartrate	3.0
Ammonium chloride	37.3	Ascorbic acid	6.0	Boric acid	16.7
Amobarbital sodium	8.3	Atropine methylbromide	4.7	Butacaine sulfate	6.7
Amphetamine phosphate	11.3	Atropine sulfate	4.3	Caffeine and sodium benzoate	8.7
Amphetamine sulfate	7.3	Bacitracin	1.7	Calcium chloride	17.0
Antipyrine	5.7	Barbital sodium	10.0	Calcium chloride (6 H₂O)	11.7

Appendix B—Continued

Drug (0.3 g)	Water needed for isotonicity, mL	Drug (0.3 g)	Water needed for isotonicity, mL	Drug (0.3 g)	Water needed for isotonicity, mL
Chlorobutanol (hydrated)	8.0	Pentobarbital sodium	8.3	Sodium biphosphate	13.3
Chlortetracycline sulfate	4.3	Phenobarbital sodium	8.0	Sodium bisulfite	20.3
Cocaine hydrochloride	5.3	Physostigmine salicylate	5.3	Sodium borate	14.0
Cupric sulfate	6.0	Pilocarpine hydrochloride	8.0	Sodium iodide	13.0
Dextrose, anhydrous	6.0	Pilocarpine nitrate	7.7	Sodium metabisulfite	22.3
Dibucaine hydrochloride	4.3	Piperocaine hydrochloride	7.0	Sodium nitrate	22.7
Dihydrostreptomycin sulfate	2.0	Polymyxin B sulfate	3.0	Sodium phosphate	9.7
Ephedrine hydrochloride	10.0	Potassium chloride	25.3	Sodium propionate	20.3
Ephedrine sulfate	7.7	Potassium nitrate	18.7	Sodium sulfite, exsiccated	21.7
Epinephrine bitartrate	6.0	Potassium phosphate, monobasic	14.7	Sodium thiosulfate	10.3
Epinephrine hydrochloride	9.7			Streptomycin sulfate	2.3
Ethylmorphine hydrochloride	5.3	Procainamide hydrochloride	7.3	Sulfacetamide sodium	7.7
Fluorescein sodium	10.3	Procaine hydrochloride	7.0	Sulfadiazine sodium	8.0
Glycerin	11.7	Scopolamine hydrobromide	4.0	Sulfamerazine sodium	7.7
Holocaine hydrochloride	6.7	Scopolamine methylnitrate	5.3	Sulfapyridine sodium	7.7
Homatropine hydrobromide	5.7	Secobarbital sodium	8.0	Sulfathiazole sodium	7.3
Homatropine methylbromide	6.3	Silver nitrate	11.0	Tetracaine hydrochloride	6.0
Hyoscyamine sulfate	4.7	Silver protein, mild	5.7	Tetracycline hydrochloride	4.7
Neomycin sulfate	3.7	Sodium acetate	15.3	Viomycin sulfate	2.7
Oxytetracycline hydrochloride	4.3	Sodium bicarbonate	21.7	Zinc chloride	20.3
Penicillin G, potassium	6.0	Sodium biphosphate, anhydrous	15.3	Zinc sulfate	5.0
Penicillin G, sodium	6.0				

[a] Table of "Isotonic Solution Values" showing volumes in mL of solution that can be prepared by dissolving 300 mg of the specified drug in sterile water. The addition of an isotonic vehicle (commonly referred to as diluting solution) to make 30 mL yields a 1% solution. Solutions prepared as directed above are isoosmotic with 0.9% sodium chloride solution but may not be isotonic with blood (see Appendix A for hemolysis data).

CHAPTER 81

Plastic Packaging Materials

Robert L Giles, BA

Vice President & General Manager
Glenn Beall Engineering, Inc
Gurnee, IL 60031

Richard W Pecina, PhD

President
Richard W Pecina & Associates
Waukegan, IL 60087

As defined by the American Society for Testing and Materials (ASTM):

A plastic is a material that contains as an essential ingredient one or more polymeric organic substances of large molecular weight, is solid in its finished state and at some stage in its manufacture or processing into finished articles can be shaped by flow.

The large-molecular-weight organic substance is called a polymer. The use of plastics in the health care industry has grown at a very rapid rate during the last two decades. This phenomenal growth is primarily due to the wide flexibility in choice of properties offered by plastics. However, because of the wide range of properties of plastics, judicious selection must be made for the intended application.

Prior to the recognition of the potential use of plastics in health care practice, glass was the predominate material used in the primary packaging of pharmaceutical products. One reason for this is that glass has a definite advantage in being a relatively unreactive and inert substance. As such, it can be used in contact with many critical products, both dry or liquid in nature. Additionally, it provides excellent protection against water vapor and gas permeation. Another advantage is its ability to withstand steam sterilization (autoclaving) without resulting in physical distortion. Two definite disadvantages of glass in the field of packaging, however, are its fragility and weight. Due to these negative aspects, coupled with the many positive attributes of plastics, significant inroads for the use of plastic in pharmaceutical packaging have been made. Today, for example, plastics are being used in the following primary packaging areas where 25 years ago only glass could be considered: syringes, bottles, vials, and ampuls.

There are many other significant medical uses which, without the use of plastics, would never have been technically feasible. A few examples include indwelling catheters, prosthetic devices, tracheotomy tubes, flexible blood collection containers, and semirigid and flexible containers for intravenous, irrigation, and inhalation solutions. An additional area for the use of plastics is in secondary container packaging; this is defined as packaging that is not in direct contact with the product itself. This particular kind of use normally involves plastic films of various types and thicknesses used for tamper proof overwrapping, whereas the previously mentioned devices are normally fabricated by molding or extrusion of the finished part.

The rapid adoption of plastics for health care uses has raised many questions concerning their safety and adequacy of application. The chemical makeup of plastic formulations can be quite complex, and prior to the use of a device or package fabricated from plastics considerable testing must be conducted.

In the case of plastics used in direct contact with a product—either in dry or liquid form—the length of time that the medication and the container are in contact may determine whether problems such as discoloration, leaching, and absorption or adsorption of a constituent of the product may arise. It is possible that both the product and the package containing it could change significantly from the time of manufacture. Other factors that may affect the plastic packaging and/or the product are product storage conditions, pH, temperature and/or time, surface treatment of the plastic, container configuration, type of polymer used, method of package preparation, light transmission, and means of assembly or sterilization.

Classifications

There are over 100 different polymer types available for use which can be further classified into two subcategories. These are identified as *Thermoplastics* and *Thermosets*. The thermoplastics family consists of those plastics which normally are rigid at operating temperatures, but can be remelted and reprocessed. The thermosetting family consists of those plastics which, when subjected to heat, will normally become infusible or insoluble, and as such cannot be remelted.

Additives

Thermoplastics can be greatly modified and their properties enhanced by the addition of specific additives. As chemicals may act synergistically, any two safe additives may have the potential to produce undesirable effects when combined. For these reasons, the Food and Drug Administration (FDA) requires that these blends or combinations be totally evaluated, prior to marketing in product form. Chemical, pharmacological, and biological tests should be conducted in order to establish safety. The following types of additives are routinely used in thermoplastic formulations:

Lubricants are used to assist processing of the plastic during the molding or extrusion operation. A commonly used lubricant in the case of polyethylene is zinc stearate. The quantities employed vary from formulation to formulation.

Stabilizers are used to retard or prevent degradation of the polymer by heat and light, as well as to improve its aging characteristics. Stabilizers, however, are not without problems, for some have a tendency to migrate to the surface of the molded part during storage. Some have limited solubility in aqueous media and consequently could be extracted into the product itself. Common stabilizer families include organometallic compounds, fatty acid salts, and inorganic oxides.

Plasticizers are used in order to achieve softness and flexibility. They are commonly used in plastic materials such as vinyls, cellulosics, and propionates. As with stabilizers, plasticizers can easily migrate to the surface of the polymer and potentially be extracted by the product. Therefore, appropriate selection of plasticizers is imperative.

Antioxidants are a special type of stabilizer used primarily to assist in retarding oxidation. Under certain environmental conditions, these materials too can migrate to the surface of the polymer. Also, combinations of antioxidants with other additives may result in undesirable chemical reactions.

Antistatic agents are used to prevent the buildup of static charges on the plastic surface.

Slip agents are added primarily to polyolefins (polyethylene and polypropylene) in order to reduce the coefficient of friction of the material. These particular chemicals result in antitack and antiblock characteristics in the end product.

Dyes and pigments are added to impart color to plastics. As with many other additives, both dyes and pigments may be leached or solubilized into the product.

Thus there are a number of additives used in the preparation of plastic packaging materials, and it is quite possible and probable that an additive could be extracted during use. Therefore, it is essential that the final product/package be evaluated for safety and stability. Evaluations should be conducted with the product under various time and storage conditions. Wherever possible, conditions simulating those to which the product is expected to be subjected should be evaluated. Evaluations under varying storage conditions should take into consideration not only the chemical compatibility of the product with the package but should also include an investigation of the compatibility of the primary plastic container with its secondary packaging (since it is possible that although the product could be compatible with its immediate container, incompatibilities could exist between the primary and secondary packaging, thereby resulting in an incompatible substance in the final product). Crazing and stress-cracking of plastic packaging, which could arise due to product and/or environmental attack, should also be considered. Prolonged exposure to ultraviolet light has been shown to enhance the migration of certain additives, which in turn can accelerate the aging characteristics of the plastic, and decrease the shelf life of the product. In some instances, incompatibilities that might occur can readily be detected visually; in others, sophisticated extraction techniques must be followed in order to ascertain the effects storage conditions may have had. For this reason, well-planned stability studies (ie, time and temperature of storage) need to be established.

Processing

As already stated, additives are used to modify the properties of a plastic. In addition, the manner in which a plastic is formed into the desired configuration can affect the end properties. It is important that process parameters such as temperature, pressure, and time be rigidly controlled to insure batch-to-batch uniformity for plastic objects. If process parameters are not adequately controlled, such deleterious effects on plastic properties as thermal degradation, piece-part stresses, and incorrect physical dimensions may result. Process thermal degradation of a plastic (or additive modified plastic formulation) can affect the leaching characteristics of the plastic object, its permeation characteristics, and its long-term stability during the shelf life of the pharmaceutical product. Piece-part stresses may relieve when the pharmaceutical package is subjected to certain environmental conditions resulting in package failure during the shelf life of the product.

The more common plastic processing methods employed for pharmaceutical packaging components follow.

Injection Molding

Injection molding is an intermittent process, the plastic being heated to a melted or viscous state, and then forced into a cavity (mold) at high pressure. The melted material cools in the cavity and solidifies. The mold is then opened and the part removed. A wide range of thermoplastic and several thermosetting materials can be injection molded. Very in-tricate configurations can be obtained by injection molding of plastics.

Extrusion

Extrusion is a continuous process, the plastic being heated to a melted or viscous state, and forced under pressure through a die, resulting in a configuration of desired shape. The extruded profile is cooled to a solid state, generally by spraying with water, by immersion in water, or by use of chilled rolls for film material. A wide range of thermoplastic materials can be extruded. Typical extruded profiles utilized by the pharmaceutical industry are packaging films and medical tubing. Plastic packaging film is also formed by blow extrusion, an extruded tube being blown into a large cylinder and then slit after cooling.

Blow Molding

The plastic is heated to a melted or viscous state and formed into a hollow cylinder (parison). The parison is generally extruded, but may be injection molded. If extruded, the parison is cut to the required length and transferred to the blowing cavity (mold). The bottom of the parison is pinched off by the mold and air is blown into the parison, expanding the viscous plastic to the walls of the cavity, thus forming the desired shape of the container. The melted material cools in the cavity and solidifies. The mold is opened and the container removed. Pharmaceutical bottles are blow-molded from a wide range of thermoplastic materials, of which polyethylene and polypropylene are predominantly used.

Compression Molding

Compression molding is used for thermosetting materials, and is an intermittent process. The thermosetting material (powder or a tablet preform) is placed into a heated cavity (mold). The material melts and flows to fill the cavity. The mold is held under pressure until the thermosetting material cures, after which the mold is opened and the part removed. As with injection molding, very intricate configurations can be obtained by compression molding of thermosetting materials.

Types and Uses

The following types of plastics are commonly used in health care practice; several of their properties and end uses are indicated.

Thermoplastics

The following are commonly used in injection molding, blow molding, extrusion, and fabricated sheeting.

Acrylics—This class includes the polymethacrylates, polyacrylates, and copolymers of acrylonitrile. There are many variations in this class, mainly concerned with the combinations of methacrylate and acrylate esters, as well as acrylonitrile. These plastics are characterized by clarity and unusual optical properties, low water absorption, good electrical resistivity, excellent weatherability, and fair tensile strength. Their heat resistance is low and care should be taken to keep them below temperatures of 200°F, at which they tend to soften. Acrylics find considerable use in a multiplicity of devices employed in today's hospitals and clinics. A specific application is in the adapters used in solution administration sets and blood collection sets.

Cellulosics—The members of this class are available in a very wide range of physical characteristics. Cellulose acetate propionate and cellulose acetate butyrate are important examples of cellulosics. Plasticizers frequently used with cellulose acetate butyrate include butyl and higher phthalate esters, and also esters of adipic, azelaic, and sebacic acids. This family of compounds is used in such medical articles as tubing, and special trays for use in urology or spinal procedures.

Nylons—Nylon is the generic designation for a class of polyamides containing repeating amide groups (—CONH—) connected to methylene units (—CH$_2$—) in the structure of the polymer. Other types of polyamides are derived from the ureas, melamines, casein and other natural protein substances which contain the amide groups. The latter types are composed of more complex polymer structures and have properties different from the nylons.

Nylons are characterized by good chemical resistance to most solvents and chemicals, with the exception of strong solutions of certain mineral acids, phenolic compounds, and strong oxidizers. Nylons can be used in the fabrication of adapters for devices and equipment, as well as in the manufacture of packaging films and laminates. Nylon provides a relatively clear film and imparts excellent resistance to puncture and abrasion.

Polyethylene—The properties of polyethylene vary according to molecular weight and type: low-density or branched, and high-density or linear. The linear type is more crystalline, more heat-resistant, and stiffer than the low-density or conventional type. Both have low water absorption, excellent electrical resistance, high resistance to most solvents and chemicals, and are tasteless and odorless. They are thus well suited to many applications where only moderate to low heat exposure will be encountered. Due to their excellent properties, the polyethylenes have been of tremendous value in the pharmaceutical industry and in hospitals. Their use ranges from containers for liquid or dry products, to films for sterile device packaging, and to molded parts for a variety of devices and equipment.

Polypropylene—The polymer of propylene is lighter than polyethylene, yet it is much stiffer and more heat-resistant with the same chemical and electrical resistance properties. This material is available as the highly crystalline, isotactic polypropylene and the higher impact grades of atactic and syndiotactic types. *Isotactic* refers to a plastic with the organic groups (R) being on the same side of the polymer chain, whereas *syndiotactic* refers to the alternation of organic groups above and below the polymer chain, and *atactic* signifies no regular sequences of the groups.

Like polyethylene, polypropylenes have numerous uses. This particular family of plastics can be used in almost every application that polyethylene can. Devices made of this material can be autoclaved for sterilization.

Polystyrene—This polymer is one of the oldest and most widely used plastics. In pharmaceutics and therapeutics it has enjoyed wide use for fabrication of containers and syringes. Polystyrene has relatively low heat resistance and is attacked by a number of chemical agents. There is a continuing increase in the use of the impact type made with the copolymers containing acrylonitrile and butadiene.

Vinyl Plastics—The term vinyl comes from the radical (CH$_2$=CH—), which has many derivatives. The versatile vinyl plastics are used to prepare materials ranging from soft, flexible sheeting to rigid, hard tubing. Several derivatives of the (CH$_2$=CH—) radical are employed such as vinyl chloride (CH$_2$=CHCl) and vinyl acetate (CH$_2$=CHOCOCH$_3$). In the polymer forms, there are two other derivatives, polyvinyl alcohol and polyvinyl acetals. Still another member of the family is vinylidene chloride (CH$_2$=CCl$_2$). With this group of vinyl compounds, a great many polymers are made as homopolymers of themselves or as copolymers with other vinyl derivatives or other monomeric materials. The copolymers of vinyl chloride with vinyl acetate are the most common. Polyvinyl acetals are made by condensation of the polyvinyl

alcohol with aldehydes, eg, formaldehyde or butyraldehyde.

The polyvinylidene chloride resins are for the most part copolymers of vinylidene chloride with vinyl chloride, acrylonitrile, and acrylate esters. These polymers are characterized by high temperature resistance, with softening points ranging from 70 to 180°C or higher. Other outstanding characteristics are high solvent and chemical resistance, low water absorption and moisture permeability, and nonflammability. They are also odorless and tasteless.

The high concentration of additives found in the polyvinyl chloride formulations may cause problems of leaching from the material when in contact with drugs or tissues. However, most tubings in use today in therapeutic procedures are of the vinyl plastics class.

The great variety of polyvinyl chloride resins, with their wide range of physical properties, had led to the development of many applications of this material in the fields of pharmacy and medicine, as in the manufacture of blood bags and, more recently, of intravenous solution containers. An unplasticized form is used in the fabrication of rigid parts for devices and administration equipment.

Polycarbonates are formed by condensation of polyphenols such as Bisphenol-A with phosgene. The polymers are transparent thermoplastics, with high strengths and high temperature resistance. They can be heat- or solvent-sealed, facilitating fabrication procedures. The polycarbonates have hardness properties similar to those of metals and are being used to replace metals in numerous industrial applications. Containers requiring clarity are produced from polycarbonates.

Thermosetting Plastics

The following are some of the commonly used compression-molded thermosetting compounds. These plastics are used when good dimensional and temperature stability are required. Parts are fabricated by means of compression molding techniques. The formaldehyde plastics are obtained by condensation reactions between formaldehyde and substances such as melamine, phenol, and urea.

Melamine Formaldehyde—This family of plastics exhibits good to excellent dimensional stability. When used in the manufacture of closures, high torque strength and good impact strength are obtained. These plastics also exhibit good resistance to oils, grease, and many organic solvents.

Phenol Formaldehyde—This type of plastic provides good scratch-resistant parts. It exhibits very low shrinkage, and low water-absorption properties. It is, however, a relatively brittle plastic.

Urea Formaldehyde—This plastic exhibits good dimensional stability as well as good strength properties. Articles produced from this material are highly rigid and provide good resistance to alcohols, oils, grease, and some of the weaker acids.

As a family, the formaldehydes have been found to be of most use in the pharmaceutical industry, as closures for glass and/or plastic containers. By virtue of high resistance to heat, they are used in specific applications where the molded part requires sterilization by steam.

Evaluation Procedures

Numerous testing procedures must be followed in order to insure the safety of use of any plastic. Among these are biological, chemical, physical, and pharmacological procedures. Use of the various polymers in the field of health care can be divided into three major categories as (1) containers, (2) tubings and devices, and (3) secondary packing. The second category includes also medical devices that are left intact in the human body for prolonged periods of time; such devices are vascular grafts, supportive cartilage replacements, pacemakers, and prosthetics. It is essential, therefore, that their reactivity and degree of safety and toxicity be determined. In all cases, it is imperative that the plastic and its processing procedure provide a nonreactive and nontoxic end product.

The official compendia provide procedures for performing certain biological and physicochemical tests on plastic containers, for the details of which the USP should be consulted. The principles of these tests are described in the following sections.

Biological Test Procedures

The official biological procedures are designed to determine the suitability of plastic materials intended for use in fabricating containers or accessories thereto for parenteral preparations and for ophthalmic preparations. The procedures for the former determine the reaction of living animal tissues and of normal animals to implanted portions of the plastic or of injected extracts prepared from it by use of sodium chloride injection, 1 in 20 solution of alcohol in sodium chloride injection, polyethylene glycol 400, and sesame or cottonseed oil as extracting media at 50° for 72 hours, 70° for 24 hours, or 121° for 1 hour (the temperature depending on the plastic used). In the implantation test, strips of the plastic are inserted into the paravertebral muscles of rabbits, along with strips of Negative Control Plastic Reference Standard; after not less than 72 hours the reaction of the tissue surrounding the implants is observed. The requirement of the test is that the reaction to three of four strips of the sample is not significantly greater than to the control strips.

In the tests with extracts, specified doses of the various extracts are injected intravenously, intracutaneously, or intraperitoneally into mice or rabbits, as directed, to observe any evidence of systemic toxicity or local tissue reaction. In these tests none of the animals injected with an extract of the sample should show significantly greater reaction than that observed in animals injected with a blank.

The biological test procedures for ophthalmic preparation containers consist of (1) an Acute Systemic Toxicity Test, in which extracts of the plastic prepared with sodium chloride injection and cottonseed oil, respectively, at one of the temperatures given above, are injected intravenously (in the case of the aqueous extract) or intraperitoneally (in the case of the oil extract) into mice, and (2) an Eye Irritation Test on rabbits using the same extracts as in Test 1. The requirement in Test 1 is that none of the animals treated with the sample should show significant reaction above that of the blank animals during the observation period; the requirement in Test 2 is that no animal treated with the sample should show significant irritation over that produced by the blank during the observation period.

Depending on the use of the plastic, other biological tests may be performed, such as freedom from pyrogenic effects, compatibility with blood, absence of antigenicity, suitability for use in cardiovascular devices, embryological reaction, and tissue toxicity testing.

Physicochemical Test Procedures

Many chemical and physical tests are applied to plastics, the particular ones used depending on the intended applications of the substances. The physicochemical procedures utilized by the USP are designed to determine the physical and chemical properties of plastics used as containers, based on tests with extracts prepared by heating samples with water for injection at 70° for 24 hr. Portions of extract are used to determine Nonvolatile Residue, Residue on Ignition, Heavy Metals, and Buffering Capacity or Reaction, official limits for each of which are specified. Also described is a procedure for

determining the light transmission of plastics, with limits for maximum transmission.

Mass Transfer Aspects

Unlike glass, plastics are not impermeable. Many pharmaceutical preparations must be adequately protected from oxygen, water vapor, carbon dioxide, and many other permeants. In addition, components of the product can permeate through the package. Examples include parabens, flavorants, water vapor, and oils. Permeation through a plastic barrier depends on the composition of the plastic, the permeation area, the thickness of the barrier, the partial pressure differential of the permeant across the barrier, and time. Permeation through a plastic can also be greatly affected by additives and the crystalline structure of the plastic. Specific additives, primarily plasticizers, can greatly increase the permeation rate. Highly crystalline plastics (such as polypropylene) generally exhibit low water permeation rates.

Adequate stability studies should be conducted to insure that the product is protected from undesirable permeants and that loss of any product component is within specified limits for the intended shelf life of the product.

As a guide, the approximate relative permeation rates for water vapor, oxygen, and carbon dioxide through the more commonly used plastics in packaging are given in Table I.

Chemical Attack

Chemical reactions between the plastic and the drug in contact with it generally require prolonged periods of time for significant change to occur. Lack of visual indication of a reaction at the onset of a stability study does not imply that the reaction(s) was not occurring during the early stages of storage. In certain instances, a specific set of storage parameters must exist before a reaction is initiated. The higher the temperature and humidity in the storage area, the more rapid the chemical attack.

Incompatibilities that may occur can manifest themselves in a number of ways. The product may undergo changes in

Table I—Permeability Rates of Selective Plastic Packaging Materials[a]

Plastic	g/100 in²/ 24 hr/mil @ 37.8°C water vapor	cc/100 in²/mil/ 24 hr/atm @ 25°C	
		Oxygen	Carbon dioxide
Nylon			
Type 6	16–22	2.6	10–12
Type 12	4	34–92	156–336
Polyethylene			
Low density	1.0–1.5	500	2700
Medium density	0.7	250–535	1000–2500
High density	0.3	185	580
Polypropylene	0.7	150–240	500–800
Polystyrene	7–10	250–350	900
Vinyl			
Non-plasticized	2–5	4–30	4–30
Plasticized	30	300–600	3000–6000
Vinyl chloride-acetate copolymer			
Non-plasticized	4	15–20	40–70
Plasticized	5–8	20–150	70–800
Polyvinylidene chloride	0.2–0.6	0.8–6.9	3.8–44
Polycarbonate	11	300	1075

[a] Data obtained from *Modern Plastics Encyclopedia*, pp 540–544 (see *Bibliography*).

color, viscosity, or potency. Also, a haze or precipitate may develop in the solution. Such phenomena have been known to occur even in a short period of time. A notable change in aqueous products is a variation in pH.

The plastic itself can be physically affected by a chemical reaction. Stress cracking of the part (as in the case of a molded article) is one way in which chemicals can affect plastics. Surface-active agents or external mold-release agents have demonstrated this ability. In the case of solvent-bonding of plastic components, the solvent can cause the article to craze or crack in time.

Iodine-containing liquids permanently stain many polyolefin compounds after a brief exposure. In many instances pigmentation used in the plastic is chemically attacked and leached by the product. In either case the product is no longer as it was originally intended to be.

Sterilization

In recent years, the subject of plastic sterilization techniques has become a prominent topic of discussion in the health care professions. For plastic medical devices and packaging materials, a number of sterilizing agents have been used, these including (1) steam, (2) dry heat, (3) gas, and (4) irradiation (cobalt and electron discharge). Of these agents, steam can be used only on a few polymers due to their inability to withstand heat without distortion. The following commonly used plastic types can generally withstand steam sterilization at temperatures of 121°: polypropylene, high-density polyethylene, polycarbonate, and all thermosets. Dry heat sterilization has the potential disadvantage of requiring long periods of exposure and may also result in product deformation.

The most commonly used procedure for sterilizing plastic devices is that of gas sterilization. Several gas mixtures can be and are being used daily in commercial, academic, and hospital sterilization processes. Some of the gases available are (1) 100% ethylene oxide, (2) 88%/12% mixtures of Freon and ethylene oxide, and (3) 80%/20% and 90%/10% mixtures of carbon dioxide and ethylene oxide.

Although the acceptance of gas sterilization for plastic medical devices and packaging has been overwhelming, gas sterilization is not without problems. Thus, gas sterilization cannot be used for aqueous products because side reaction products such as ethylene glycol and 2-chloroethanol are known to be formed. There also remain many unanswered questions about the effect of residual ethylene oxide gas on the various plastic packaging materials, and the chemicals used to produce them. See the chapter on *Sterilization*.

Numerous experiments have been conducted with plastics and their absorptive and adsorptive characteristics as related to ethylene oxide. It has been shown that toxicity or tissue sensitivity reactions, when the plastic is not adequately degassed, can take place by either direct contact with plastic materials or product with tissue, or indirect contact with tissue via injection or application of a solution which had previously been in contact with a plastic (ie, administration of an intravenous solution through a gas-sterilized device).

Studies have demonstrated that improperly selected or degassed plastics can and do result in tissue reactions. Unfortunately, no two polymers behave in the same manner with regard to time required for degassing. To complicate matters further, as a plastic (for which degassing data might exist) is molded into a part, its degassing properties may change substantially. This change is the result of several factors, of which the geometry, heat-history, storage conditions, contact with other plastics, and type of secondary packages used are but a few. The only certain method of having a safe product for use is to test it subsequent to sterilization and prior to use.

A survey of the literature shows that most investigators recommend that an adequate degassing time be allowed for plastic articles, and it may be concluded from the survey that a degassing time of 7 days at ambient conditions is sufficient to insure that the level of residual ethylene oxide is safe for all of the commonly used plastics.

Plastics Quality Control Considerations

As important as is the selection and approval of a polymer type (and a specific compound within that type), is the need to check it routinely against the criteria used in its selection. The following basic areas of control and/or procedures are recommended as relating to an ongoing quality control program.

1. Tissue-cell toxicity testing (or a similar toxicity test) should be conducted in order to provide assurance that the material being used is nontoxic or falls within the toxicity range originally specified.
2. Characterization analysis should be conducted in order to provide assurances that the proper polymer type is used and that the physical parameters have not been altered, which in turn could affect the function of the product/package. Such techniques as infrared spectrometric analysis, density, and melt flow can assist in providing the necessary assurances.
3. Any plastic part or package should routinely be inspected on an incoming basis for dimensional and attribute variables against statistically accepted sampling plans such as MIL-STD-105D.

Summary

Before the selection of a plastic is made, it must demonstrate physical and chemical stability. It should also demonstrate physical and chemical compatibility with the product or packaging with which it will be in contact, the compatibility lasting for the anticipated shelf life of the product. Additionally, the plastic should be shown to be nontoxic and satisfactory for its intended end use. Proper sterilization procedures, including adequate degassing, must be identified in order to obtain a sterile product that is nontoxic.

As the field of plastics utilization in packaging is so vast, it is virtually impossible to present a detailed overview which will address itself to the needs and interests of the many disciplines concerned. It is recommended that for more specific and in-depth information the *Bibliography* be consulted.

Bibliography

Eaborn C: *Organosilicon Compounds*, Butterworths, London, 1960.

Modern Packaging Encyclopedia and Planning Guide, McGraw-Hill, New York, 1973.

Dubois HJ, John F: *Plastics*, Reinhold, New York, 1967.

Haslam J, Willis H: *Identification and Analysis of Plastics*, Butterworths, London, 1965.

Modern Plastics Encyclopedia, McGraw-Hill, New York, vol 58, no. 10A, 1981–82.

CHAPTER 82

Stability of Pharmaceutical Products

Carl J Lintner, PhD

Lintner Associates
Kalamazoo, MI 49008

The use of kinetic and predictive studies for establishing credible expiration dates for pharmaceutical products is now accepted worldwide. However, prior to 1950 only qualitative or semiquantitative methods and procedures were used in pharmaceutical studies. As these rule-of-thumb methods are deficient; they have been replaced by rigorous, scientifically designed studies using reliable, meaningful, and specific stability-indicating assays, appropriate statistical concepts, and a computer to analyze the resulting data. In this way the maximum amount of valid information is obtained to establish a reliable, defendable expiration date for each formulation.

Stability information is ubiquitous. It may be in a well-planned rigorous kinetic study, in an obscure journal footnote, in a package insert, or label copy, or in a monograph in a book such as *The Merck Index* or *Physicians' Desk Reference*. Various journals periodically publish digests of compatibility studies. A comprehensive treatment of all aspects of pharmaceutical product stability has been published by Lintner.[1]

The main purpose of a quality assurance program is to devise and implement systems and procedures that provide a high probability that each dose or package of a pharmaceutical product will have homogeneous characteristics and properties (within reasonably acceptable limits) to insure both clinical safety and efficacy of the formulation. A broad, well-designed stability testing plan is an essential and pertinent expansion of the quality assurance program. The assigned expiration date is a direct application and interpretation of the knowledge gained from the stability study.

Stability of a pharmaceutical product may be defined as the capability of a particular formulation, in a specific container/closure system to remain within its physical, chemical, microbiological, therapeutic, and toxicological specifications. Assurances that the packaged product will be stable for its anticipated shelf life must come from an accumulation of valid data on the drug in its commercial package. These stability data involve selected parameters which, taken together, form the stability profile.

Stability of a drug can also be defined as the time from the date of manufacture and packaging of the formulation until its chemical or biological activity is not less than a predetermined level of labeled potency and its physical characteristics have not changed appreciably or deleteriously. Although there are exceptions, 90% of labeled potency is generally recognized as the minimum acceptable potency level. Expiration dating is then defined as the time in which the preparation will remain stable when stored under recommended conditions.

An expiration date, which is expressed traditionally in terms of month and year, denotes the last day of the month. The expiration date should appear on the immediate container and the outer retail package. However, when single-dose containers are packaged in individual cartons, the expiration date may be placed on the individual carton instead of the immediate product container. If a dry product is to be reconstituted at the time of dispensing, expiration dates are assigned to both the dry mixture and the reconstituted product. Tamper resistant packaging is to be used where applicable.

A second quality assurance goal is drug or clinical safety and it, too, is closely related to pharmaceutical stability. Drug or clinical safety (ie, the nonoccurrence of harm), however, cannot be studied by itself. Rather, it is a negative concept which cannot be proven and must be expressed only in terms of the nonoccurrence of some harmful event. The latter probability, in turn, can be estimated only when the probability occurrence of the harmful event is known.

One type of time-related harmful event is a decrease in therapeutic activity of the preparation to below some arbitrary labeled content. A second type of harmful event is the appearance of a toxic substance, formed as a degradation product upon storage of the formulation. The number of published cases reflecting this second type is fortunately quite small. However, it is possible, though remote, for both types of harmful events to occur simultaneously within the same pharmaceutical product. Thus, the use of stability studies with the resulting application of expiration dating to pharmaceuticals is an attempt to predict the approximate time at which the probability of occurrence of a harmful event may reach an intolerable level. This estimate is subject to the usual Type 1 or alpha error (setting the expiration too early so that the product will be destroyed or recalled from the market at an appreciably earlier time than is actually necessary) and the Type 2 or beta error (setting the date too late so that the harmful event occurs in an unacceptably large proportion of cases). Thus, it is obligatory that the manufacturer clearly and succinctly define the method for determining the degree of change in a formulation and the statistical approach to be used in making the shelf-life prediction. An intrinsic part of the statistical methodology must be the statements of value for the two types of error. For the safety of the patient a Type 1 error can be accepted, but not a Type 2 error.

Requirements

Stability study requirements and expiration dating are covered in the Good Manufacturing Practices (GMPs), and the USP.

Good Manufacturing Practices—The GMPs[2] state that there shall be a written testing program designed to assess the stability characteristics of drug products. The results of such stability testing shall be used to determine appropriate storage conditions and expiration dating. The latter is to assure that the pharmaceutical product meets applicable standards of identity, strength, quality, and purity at time of use. These regulations, which apply to both human and veterinary drugs, are updated periodically in light of current knowledge and technology.

Compendiums—The compendiums also contain extensive stability and expiration dating information. Included are a discussion of stability considerations in dispensing practices and the responsibilities of both the pharmaceutical manufacturer and the dispensing pharmacist. It is now required that product labeling of official articles provide recommended storage conditions and an expiration date assigned to the specific formulation and package. Official storage conditions are defined as follows: "Cold" is any temperature not exceeding 8°, and "refrigerator" is a cold place where the temperature is maintained thermostatically between 2° and 8°; a "freezer" is a cold place maintained between −20° and −10°. "Cool" is defined as any temperature between 8° and 15°, and "room temperature" is that temperature prevailing in a working area. "Controlled room temperature" is that temperature maintained thermostatically between 15° and 30°. "Warm" is any temperature between 30° and

40°, while "excessive heat" is any heat above 40°. Should freezing subject a product to a loss of potency or to destructive alteration of the dosage form, the container label should bear appropriate instructions to protect the product from freezing. Bulk packages are exempt from storage requirements if the products are intended for manufacture or repacking for dispensing or distribution. Where no specific storage instructions are given in a monograph, it is understood that the product's storage conditions shall include protection from moisture, freezing, and excessive heat.

Product Stability

Many factors affect the stability of a pharmaceutical product, including the stability of the active ingredient(s), the potential interaction between active and inactive ingredients, the manufacturing process, the dosage form, the container-liner-closure system, the environmental conditions encountered during shipment, storage, handling, and length of time between manufacture and usage.

Classically, pharmaceutical product stability evaluations have been separated into studies of chemical, including biochemical, and physical stability of formulations. Realistically, there is no absolute division between these two arbitrary divisions. Physical factors—such as heat, light, and moisture—may initiate or accelerate chemical reactions, while every time a measurement is made on a chemical compound, physical dimensions are included in the study.

In this treatment, physical and chemical stability will be discussed along with those dosage form properties which can be measured and are useful in predicting shelf life. The effect of various physical and chemical phenomena of pharmaceuticals will also be treated.

Knowledge of the physical stability of a formulation is very important for three primary reasons. First, a pharmaceutical product must appear fresh, elegant, and professional, so long as it remains on the shelf. Any changes in physical appearance such as color fading or haziness can cause the patient or consumer to lose confidence in the product. Second, since some products are dispensed in multiple-dose containers, uniformity of dose content of the active ingredient over time must be assured. A cloudy solution or a broken emulsion can lead to a nonuniform dosage pattern. Third, the active ingredient must be available to the patient throughout the expected shelf life of the preparation. A breakdown in the physical system can lead to nonavailability of the medicament to the patient.

The chemical causes of drug deterioration have been classified into incompatibility, oxidation, reduction, hydrolysis, racemization, and others. In the latter category decarboxylation, deterioration of hydrogen peroxide and hypochlorites, and the formation of precipitates have been included.

Galenical Dosage Forms

As the various galenical dosage forms present unique stability problems, they will be discussed separately in the following section.

Suspensions—A stable suspension can be homogeneously redispersed with moderate shaking and can be easily poured throughout its shelf life, with neither the particle-size distribution, the crystal form, nor the physiological availability of the suspended active ingredient changing appreciably with time.

Most stable pharmaceutical suspensions are flocculated; that is, the suspended particles are physically bonded together to form a loose, semirigid structure. The particles are said to uphold each other while exerting no significant force on the liquid. Sedimented particles of a flocculated suspension can be easily redispersed at any time with only moderate shaking.

In nonflocculated suspensions, the particles remain as individuals unaffected by neighboring particles and are affected only by the suspension vehicle. These particles, which are smaller and lighter, settle slowly, but once they have settled, often form a rock-hard, difficult-to-disperse sediment. Nonflocculated suspensions can be made acceptable by decreasing the particle size of the suspended material or by increasing the density and viscosity of the vehicle.

When studying the stability of a suspension, first determine with a differential manometer if the suspension is flocculated. If the suspension is flocculated, the liquid will travel the same distance in the two side arms. With nonflocculated suspensions, the hydrostatic pressures in the two arms are unequal; hence the liquids will be at different levels.

The history of settling of the particles of a suspension may be followed by a Brookfield viscometer fitted with a Helipath attachment. This instrument consists of a rotating T-bar spindle which descends slowly into the suspension as it rotates. The dial reading on the viscometer is a measure of the resistance that the spindle encounters at various levels of the sedimented suspension. This test must be run only on fresh, undisturbed samples (see Chapter 22).

An electronic particle counter and sizer, such as a Coulter counter, or a microscope may be used to determine changes in particle-size distribution. Crystal form alterations can be detected by x-ray diffraction or by a microscopic examination.

All suspensions should be subjected to cycling temperature conditions to determine the tendency for crystal growth to occur within a suspension. Shipping tests, ie, transporting bottles across the country by rail or truck, are also used advantageously to study the stability of suspensions.

Emulsions—A stable emulsion can be homogeneously redispersed to its original state with moderate shaking and can be poured at any stage of its shelf life. Although most of the important pharmaceutical emulsions are of the O/W type, many stability test methods can be applied to either an O/W or a W/O emulsion.

Two simple tests are used to screen emulsion formulations. First, the stability of an emulsion can be determined by heating it to 50–70° and its gross physical stability observed visually or checked by turbidimetric measurements. Usually the emulsion that is the most stable to heat is the one most stable at room temperature. However, this may not always be true because an emulsion at 60° may not be the same as it is at room temperature. Second, the stability of the emulsion can be estimated by the "coalescence time" test. Although this is only a rough quantitative test, it is useful for detecting gross differences in emulsion stability at room temperature.

Emulsions should also be subjected to refrigeration temperatures. An emulsion stable at room temperature has been found to be unstable at 4°. It was reasoned that an oil-soluble emulsifier precipitated at the lower temperature and disrupted the system. An emulsion chilled to the extent that the aqueous base crystallizes is irreversibly damaged.

The ultracentrifuge is also used to determine emulsion stability. When the amount of separated oil is plotted against the time of centrifugation, a plateau curve is obtained. A linear graph results when the oil flotation (creaming) rate is plotted vs the square of the number of centrifuge revolutions per minute. The flotation rate is represented by the slope of the line resulting when the log distance of emulsion-water boundary from the rotor center is plotted against time for each resolution per minute.

For stability studies, two batches of an emulsion should be made at one time on production size equipment. One should be a bench-size lot and the other a larger, preferably production-size, batch. Different types of homogenizers produce different results and different sizes of the same kind of homogenizer can yield emulsions with different characteristics.

Solutions—A stable solution retains its original clarity, color, and odor throughout its shelf life. Retention of clarity of a solution is a main concern of a physical stability program. As visual observation alone under ordinary light is a poor test of clarity, a microscope light should be projected through a diaphragm into the solution. Undissolved particles will scatter the light and the solution will appear hazy. While the Coulter counter can also be used, light-scattering instruments are the most sensitive means of following solution clarity.

Solutions should remain clear over a relatively wide temperature range such as 4–47°. At the lower range an ingredient may precipitate due to its lower solubility at that temperature while at the higher temperature homogeneity may be destroyed by the flaking of particles from the glass containers or rubber closures. Thus, solutions should be subjected to cycling temperature conditions.

The stability program for solutions should also include the study of pH changes, especially when the active ingredients are soluble salts of insoluble acids or bases. Among other tests are observations for changes in odor, appearance, color, taste, light-stability, redispersibility, suspendibility, pourability, viscosity, isotonicity, gas evolution, microbial stability, specific gravity, surface tension, and pyrogen content in the case of parenteral products.

When solutions are filtered, the filter media may absorb some of the ingredients from the solution. Thus, the same type of filter should be used for preparing the stability samples as will be used to prepare the production-size batches.

For dry-packaged formulations intended to be reconstituted prior to use, the visual appearance should be observed on both the original dry material and on the reconstituted preparation. The color and odor of the cake, the color and odor of the solution, the moisture content of the cake, and the rate of reconstitution should be followed as a part of its stability profile.

Tablets—Stable tablets retain their original size, shape, weight, and color under normal handling and storage conditions throughout their shelf life. In addition, the *in vitro* availability of the active ingredients should not change appreciably with time.

Excessive powder or solid particles at the bottom of the container, cracks or chips on the face of a tablet, or appearance of crystals on the surface of tablets or on container walls are indications of physical instability of uncoated tablets. Hence, the effect of mild, uniform, and reproducible shaking and tumbling of tablets should be studied. After visual observation of the tablets for chips, cracks, and splits, the intact tablets are sorted and weighed to determine the amount of material worn away by abrasion. The results of these tests are comparative rather than absolute and should be correlated with actual stress experience. Packaged tablets should also be subjected to cross-country shipping tests as well as to various "drop tests."

Tablet hardness (or resistance to crushing or fracturing) can be followed by the commercially available hardness testers. As results will vary with the specific make of the test apparatus used, direct comparison of results obtained on different instruments cannot be made. Thus, the same instrument should be used consistently throughout a particular study.

Color stability of tablets can be followed by an appropriate colorimeter or reflectometer with heat, sunlight, and intense artificial light employed to accelerate the color deterioration. Caution must be used in interpreting the elevated temperature data as the system at that temperature may be different from that at a lower temperature. It is not always proper to assume that the same changes will occur at elevated temperatures as will happen later at room temperature. Evidence of instability of coated tablets is also indicated by cracks, mottling or tackiness of the coating.

For the more insoluble tableted active ingredients, the results of dissolution tests are more meaningful than disintegration results for making availability predictions. Dissolution rate tests should be run in an appropriate medium such as artificial gastric and/or intestinal juice at 37° (see Chapter 35). When no significant change (such as a change in the polymorphic form of the crystal) has occurred, an unaltered dissolution rate profile of a tablet formulation usually indicates constant *in vivo* availability.

Disintegration tests may be used to detect periodic gross changes in the physical characteristics of a tablet, but these tests must be correlated with the dissolution rate study of a particular tableted product. When there is no such correlation, *in vivo* tests must be run. The release pattern of sustained-release formulations should be determined periodically during the stability test period.

Uniformity of weight, odor, texture, drug and moisture contents, and humidity effect are also studied during a tablet stability test.

Gelatin Capsules—When stored under adverse conditions, capsule shells may soften and stick together or harden and crack under slight pressure. They should be protected from sources of microbial contamination. The shell of soft gelatin capsules should contain a preservative to prevent growth of fungi. Encapsulated products, like all other dosage forms, must be properly packaged.

Ointments—Ointments have been defined as high-viscosity suspensions of active ingredients in a nonreacting vehicle. A stable ointment is one which retains its homogeneity throughout its shelf-life period. The main stability problems seen in ointments are "bleeding" and changes in consistency due to aging or changes in temperature. When fluid components such as mineral oil separate at the top of an ointment, the phenomenon is known as "bleeding" and can be observed visually. Unfortunately, as there is no known way to accelerate this event, the tendency to "bleed" cannot be predicted.

An ointment which is too soft is messy to use while one which is very stiff is difficult to extrude and apply. Hence, it is important to be able to define quantitatively an ointment's consistency. This may be done with a penetrometer, an apparatus which allows a pointed weight to penetrate into the sample under a measurable force. The depth of the penetration is a measure of the consistency of an ointment. Consistency can also be measured by the Helipath attachment to a high viscosity viscometer or by a Burrell Severs rheometer. In the latter instrument the ointment is loaded into a cylinder and extruded with a measured force. The amount extruded is a measure of the consistency of the ointment.

Ointments have a considerable degree of structure which requires a minimum of 48 hours to develop after preparation. As rheological data on a freshly made ointment may be erroneous, such tests should be performed only after the ointment has achieved equilibrium.

Slight changes in temperature (1 or 2°) can greatly affect an ointment's consistency; hence rheological studies on ointments must be performed only at constant and controlled temperatures.

Among the other tests performed during the stability study of an ointment are a check of visual appearance, color, odor, viscosity, softening range, consistency, homogeneity, particle-size distribution, and sterility.

Undissolved components of an ointment may change in crystal form or in size with time. Microscopic examination or an X-ray diffraction measurement may be used to monitor these parameters.

In some instances it is necessary to use an ointment base that is less than ideal in order to achieve the stability required. For example, drugs that hydrolyze rapidly are more stable in a hydrocarbon base than in a base containing water, even though they may be more effective in the latter.

Incompatibility

Obvious sources of pharmaceutical instability include the incompatibility of various ingredients within a formulation. Numerous examples are described in other sections of this book and the literature is replete with illustrations. Thus the subject need not be treated in detail here.

While undesirable reactions between two or more drugs are said to result in a "physical," "chemical," or "therapeutic" incompatibility, physical incompatibility is somewhat of a misnomer. It has been defined as a physical or chemical interaction between two or more ingredients which leads to a visible recognizable change. The latter may be in the form of a gross precipitate, haze, or color change.

On the other hand, a chemical incompatibility is classified as a reaction in which a visible change does not occur. Since there is no visible evidence of deterioration, this type of incompatibility requires trained, knowledgeable personnel to recognize it, should it occur.

A therapeutic incompatibility has been defined as an undesirable pharmacological interaction between two or more ingredients which leads to (1) potentiation of the therapeutic effects of the ingredients, (2) destruction of the effectiveness of one or more of the ingredients, or (3) occurrence of a toxic manifestation within the patient.

Oxidation-Reduction

Oxidation is a prime cause of product instability and often, but not always, the addition of oxygen or the removal of hydrogen is involved. When molecular oxygen is involved, the reaction is known as autooxidation because it occurs spontaneously, though slowly, at room temperature.

Oxidation, or the loss of electrons from an atom, frequently involves free radicals and subsequent chain reactions. Only a very small amount of oxygen is required to initiate a chain reaction. In practice, it is easy to remove most of the oxygen from a container, but very difficult to remove all. Hence, nitrogen and carbon dioxide are frequently used to displace the headspace air in pharmaceutical containers to help minimize deterioration by oxidation.

As an oxidation reaction is complicated, it is difficult to perform a kinetic study on oxidative processes within a general stability program. The redox potential, which is constant and relatively easy to determine, can, however, provide valuable predictive information. In many oxidative reactions, the rate is proportional to the concentration of the oxidizing species but may be independent of the concentration of the oxygen present. The rate is influenced by temperature, radiation and the presence of a catalyst. An increase in temperature leads to an acceleration in the rate of oxidation. If the storage temperature of a preparation can be reduced to 0–5°, it can usually be assumed that the rate of oxidation will be at least halved.

Trace amounts of heavy metals such as cupric, chromic, ferrous, and ferric ions catalyze oxidation reactions. As little as 0.2 mg of copper ion/liter considerably reduces the stability of penicillin. Similar examples include the deterioration of epinephrine, phenylephrine, lincomycin, isoprenaline, and procaine hydrochloride. Adding chelating agents to water which is free of heavy metals and working in special manufacturing equipment (eg, glass) are some means used to reduce the influence of heavy metals on a formulation. Parenteral formulations should not come in contact with heavy metal ions during their manufacture, packaging, or storage.

Hydronium and hydroxyl ions catalyze oxidative reactions. The rate of decomposition for epinephrine, for example, is more rapid in a neutral or alkaline solution with maximum stability (minimum oxidative decomposition) at pH 3.4. There is a pH range for maximum stability for any antibiotic and vitamin preparation which can usually be achieved by adding an acid, alkali or buffer.

Oxidation may be inhibited by the use of antioxidants, called negative catalysts. They are very effective in stabilizing pharmaceutical products undergoing a free-radical-mediated chain reaction. These substances, which are easily oxidizable, act by possessing lower oxidation potentials than the active ingredient. Thus they undergo preferential degradation or act as chain inhibitors of free radicals by providing an electron and receiving the excess energy possessed by the activated molecule.

The ideal antioxidant should be stable and effective over a wide pH range, soluble in its oxidized form, colorless, nontoxic, nonvolatile, nonirritating, effective in low concentrations, thermostable, and compatible with the container-closure system and formulation ingredients.

The commonly used antioxidants for aqueous systems include sodium sulfite, sodium metabisulfite, sodium bisulfite, sodium thiosulfate, and ascorbic acid. For oil systems, ascorbyl palmitate, hydroquinone, propyl gallate, nordihydroguaiaretic acid, butylated hydroxytoluene, butylated hydroxyanisole, and alpha tocopherol are employed.

Synergists, which increase the activity of antioxidants, are generally organic compounds that complex small amounts of heavy metal ions (see Chapter 14). These include the ethylenediamine tetraacetic acid (EDTA) derivatives, dihydroethylglycine, and citric, tartaric, gluconic, and saccharic acids. EDTA has been used to stabilize ascorbic acid, oxytetracycline, penicillin, epinephrine, and prednisolone.

Reduction reactions are much less common than oxidative processes in pharmaceutical practice. Examples include the reduction of gold, silver, and mercury salts by light to form the corresponding free metal.

Hydrolysis

Drugs containing an ester or amide linkage are prone to hydrolysis. Some examples include cocaine, physostigmine, procaine, tetracaine, thiamine, and benzylpenicillin.

The rate of hydrolysis depends on the temperature and the pH of the solution. A much quoted rule-of-thumb is that for each 10° rise in storage temperature, the rate of reaction doubles or triples. As this is an empiricism, it is not always applicable.

When hydrolysis occurs, the concentration of the active ingredient decreases while the concentration of the decomposition products increases. The effect of this change on the rate of the reaction depends on the order of the reaction. With zero-order reactions the rate of decomposition is independent of concentration of the ingredient. Although weak solutions decompose at the same absolute rate as stronger ones, the weaker the solution, the greater the proportion of active ingredient destroyed in a given time, ie, the percentage of decomposition is greater in weaker solutions. Increasing the concentration of an active ingredient which is hydrolyzing by zero-order kinetics will slow the percentage decomposition.

With first-order reactions, which occur frequently in the hydrolysis of drugs, the rate of change is directly proportional to the concentration of the reactive substance. Thus changes in the concentration of the active ingredient have no influence on the percentage decomposition.

As many hydrolytic reactions are catalyzed by both hydronium and hydroxyl ions, pH is an important factor in determining the rate of a reaction. The pH range of minimum decomposition (or maximum stability) depends on the ion having the greatest effect on the reaction. If the minimum occurs at about pH 7, the two ions are of equal effect. A shift of the minimum toward the acid side indicates that the hydroxyl ion has the stronger catalytic effect and vice-versa in the case of a shift toward the alkaline side. In general, hydroxyl ions have the stronger effect. Thus, the minimum is often found between pH 3 and 4.

Sometimes it is necessary to compromise between the optimum pH for stability and that for pharmacologic activity. For example, several local anesthetics are most stable at a distinctly acid pH, whereas for maximum activity they should be neutral or slightly alkaline.

Small amounts of acids, alkalies, or buffers are used to adjust the pH of a formulation. Buffers are used when small changes in pH are likely to cause major degradation of the active ingredient.

Obviously, the amount of water present can have profound effect on the rate of a hydrolysis reaction. When the reaction takes place fairly rapidly in water, other solvents can sometimes be substituted. For example, barbiturates are much more stable at room temperature in propylene glycol-water than in water alone.

Modification of chemical structure may be used to retard hydrolysis. In general, as it is only the fraction of the drug in solution that hydrolyzes, a compound may be stabilized by reducing its solubility. This can be done by adding various substituents to the alkyl or acyl chain of aliphatic or aromatic esters or to the ring of an aromatic ester. In some cases less-soluble salts or esters of the parent compound have been found to aid product stability. Steric and polar complexation have also been employed to alter the rate of hydrolysis. Caffeine complexes with local anesthetics such as benzocaine, procaine, and tetracaine to reduce their rate of hydrolysis and thus promotes stability.

Surfactants may also be used to stabilize drugs. For example, the half-life of benzocaine was increased 18 times by the addition of sodium lauryl sulfate.

Decarboxylation

Pyrolytic solid-state degradation through decarboxylation is not usually encountered in pharmacy as relatively high heats of activation (25 to 30 kcal) are required for the reaction. However, solid p-aminosalicylic acid undergoes pyrolytic degradation to m-aminophenol and carbon dioxide. The reaction, which follows first-order kinetics, is highly pH-dependent and is catalyzed by hydronium ions. The decarboxylation of p-aminobenzoic acid occurs only at extremely low pH values and at high temperatures.

Racemization

Racemization or the action or process of changing from an optically active compound into a racemic compound or an optically inactive mixture of corresponding dextro (d-) and levo (l-) forms is a major factor in pharmaceutical stability. Frequently, the l-form is more pharmacologically active than the d-form. For example, l-epinephrine is 15–20 times more active than its d-counterpart, while the activity of the racemic mixture is just over half that of the l-form. Current nomenclature practice uses (+) for d- and (−) for l-, therefore, l-epinephrine would be named (−)-epinephrine, etc.

In general, racemization follows first-order kinetics and depends on temperature, solvent, catalyst, and the presence or absence of light. Racemization appears to depend on the functional group bound to the asymmetric carbon atom, with aromatic groups tending to accelerate the process.

Photochemical

Photolytic degradation can be an important limiting factor in the stability of pharmaceuticals.

A drug can be chemically affected by radiation of a particular wavelength only if (1) it absorbs radiation at that wavelength and (2) the energy exceeds a threshold. Ultraviolet radiation, which has a large energy level, is the cause of many degradation reactions.

If the absorbing molecule reacts, the reaction is said to be photochemical in nature. Where the absorbing molecules do not participate directly in the reaction, but pass their energy to other reacting molecules, the absorbing substance is said to be a photosensitizer.

As many variables may be involved in a photochemical reaction, the kinetics may be quite complex. The intensity and wavelength of the light, the size, shape, composition, and color of the container may affect the velocity of the reaction.

The photodegradation of chlorpromazine through a semi-quinone free-radical intermediate follows zero order kinetics. On the other hand, alcoholic solutions of hydrocortisone, prednisolone, and methylprednisolone degrade by reactions following first-order kinetics.

Colored-glass containers are most commonly used to protect light-sensitive formulations. Yellow-green glass gives the best protection in the ultraviolet region while amber confers considerable protection from ultraviolet radiation but little from infrared. Riboflavin is best protected by a stabilizer which has a hydroxyl group attached to or near the aromatic ring. The photodegradation of sulfacetamide solutions may be inhibited by an antioxidant such as sodium thiosulfate or metabisulfite.

Ultrasonic Energy

Ultrasonic energy, which consists of vibrations and waves with frequencies greater than 20,000/sec, promotes the formation of free radicals and alters drug molecules.

Changes in prednisolone, prednisone acetate, and deoxycorticosterone acetate suspensions in an ultrasonic field have been observed spectrophotometrically in the side chain at C-17 and in the oxo group of the A ring. With sodium alginate in an ultrasonic field, it has been reported that above a minimum power output, degradation increased linearly with increased power.

Ionizing Radiation

Ionizing radiation, particularly the gamma rays, has been used for the sterilization of certain pharmaceutical products. At the usual sterilizing dose, 2.5 Mrad, it seldom causes appreciable chemical degradation. In general, formulations which are in the solid or frozen state are more resistant to degradation from ionizing radiation than are those in liquid form. For example, many of the vitamins are little affected by irradiation in the solid state, but are appreciably decomposed in solution. On the other hand, both the liquid- and solid-state forms of atropine sulfate are seriously affected by radiation.

Predicting Shelf Life

The technique of estimating the shelf life of a formulation from its accumulated stability data has evolved from examining the data and making an educated guess through plotting the time-temperature points on appropriate graph paper and crudely extrapolating a regression line to the application of rigorous physical chemical laws, statistical concepts, and computers to obtain meaningful, reliable estimates.

A simple means of estimating shelf life from a set of computer-prepared tables has been described by Lintner, et al.[3] This system was developed to (1) select the best prototype formulation based on short-term stability data and (2) predict both estimated and minimum shelf-life values for the formulation. It is a middle-ground approach between the empirical methods and the modern, rigorous statistical concepts. All calculations can be made readily by hand and the estimated values can be obtained easily from appropriate tables. The system assumes that:

1. Shelf-life predictions can be made satisfactorily for lower temperatures using the classical Arrhenius model from data obtained at higher temperatures.
2. The energy of activation of the degradation reaction is between 10 to 20 kcal/mole (this is a safe assumption as Kennon[4] has noted that rarely are drugs with energies of activation of less than 10 kcal/mole used in pharmacy and for values as high as 20 kcal/mole the error in the shelf-life prediction will be on the conservative side).
3. The rate of decomposition will not increase beyond that already observed.
4. The standard deviation of the replicated assays is known or can be estimated from the analytical data.

This concept further assumes that the degradation reaction follows zero or pseudo zero order kinetics. As shown in Fig 82-1, this is an excellent assumption. For data corresponding to a zero, first, or second order degradation pattern, it is impossible to distinguish one order from another with usual analytical procedures where the total degraded material is not large. In addition, shelf-life calculations assuming zero order kinetics are more conservative than those for higher orders.

This middle-ground system is useful in creating the experimental design for the stability study. The formulator has the opportunity to study various combinations of parameters to try to optimize the physical-statistical model. One can check the effect of improving the assay standard deviation, of running additional replicates, of using different time points, and of assuming various degradation rates and energies of activation on the stability of the test formulation.

McMinn and Lintner later developed and reported on an information processing system for handling product stability data.[5] This system saves the time of formulators in analyzing and interpreting their product stability data in addition to minimizing the amount of clerical help needed to handle an ever-increasing assay load. For products such as those of vitamins, for example, where large overages are required, the statistical portions of this advanced technique aid the manufacturer to tailor the formula composition to obtain the desired and most economical expiration dating.

This system stores both physical and chemical data, retrieves the information in three different formats (one of which was designed specifically for submitting to regulatory agencies), analyzes single-temperature data statistically by analysis of covariance and regression or multiple temperature data by weighted or unweighted analysis using the Arrhenius relationship, and provides estimates of the shelf life of the preparation with the appropriate confidence intervals, preprints the assay request cards which are used to record the results of the respective assay procedures and to enter the data into the system and produces a 5-year master-stability schedule as well as periodic 14-day schedules of upcoming assays.

As mentioned above, a portion of the advanced system analyzes the stability data obtained at a single temperature by analysis of covariance and regression. This analysis is based on the linear (zero-order) model

$$Y_{ij} = \beta_i X_{ij} + \alpha_i + \epsilon_{ij}$$

where Y_{ij} is the percent of label of the jth stability assay of the ith lot, X_{ij} is the time in months at which Y_{ij} was observed, β_i and α_i are the slope and intercept respectively of the regression line of the ith lot and ϵ_{ij} is a random error associated with Y_{ij}. The random errors are assumed to be identically and independently distributed normal variables with a zero mean and a common variance, σ^2.

A summary of the regression analysis for each individual lot and for the combination of these lots plus a summary of the analyses of covariance and deviation from regression are prepared by the computer.

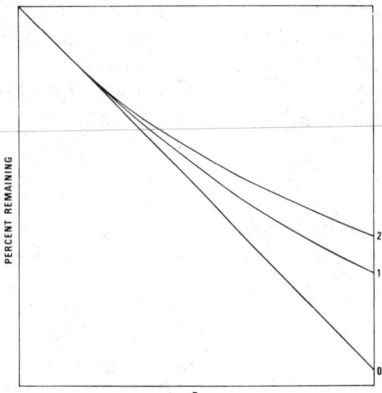

Fig 82-1. Zero order plots for reactions which are zero, first, and second order.

Because the computer combines or pools the stability data from the individual lots, irrespective of the statistical integrity of this step, the pooled data are examined for validity by the F test. The mean square of the regression coefficient (slope) is divided by the mean square of the deviation within lots, and similarly, the adjusted mean (y intercept) is divided by the common mean square to give the respective F ratios. The latter values are then compared to the critical 5% F values. When the calculated F values are smaller than the critical F values, the data may be combined and the pooled data analyzed.

A print-out for the combined lots as well as for each individual lot provides the estimated rate of degradation and its standard error in percent per month for each ingredient. The student t value is calculated from these estimates and tested for significance from zero. When the t value is significant, the print-out contains an estimate of the shelf life with the appropriate confidence interval. When the t value is not significantly different from zero, estimates of the minimum and projected shelf-life values are made. In addition, coordinates of the calculated least squares regression line with appropriate confidence limits for the mean and individual predicted assays are printed.

Plots of the resulting least squares line containing the individual data points are also printed by the computer. For the calculation of X_0, $\hat{Y}$ equals $\overline{Y} + \hat{\beta}(X_0 - \overline{X}..)$ where $\hat{\beta}$ is the least-squares estimate of the slope and $\overline{X}..$ is the mean time of assay.

The sample variance for this estimate, $S^2(\hat{Y})$, is equal to

$$S^2_{Y \cdot X} \left[\frac{1}{N} + \frac{(X_0 - \overline{X}..)^2}{\Sigma(X_{ij} - \overline{X}..)^2} \right]$$

where N is the number of assays. The 95% confidence interval is equal to $\hat{Y} \pm t_{0.05} S(\hat{Y})$.

For the cases where the slope of the best fitting line is positive and significantly different from zero (resulting, for example, from solvent evaporation), the statement "no degradation has been detected and hence no shelf-life estimate is made" is printed. Where the computed line has a positive slope but not significantly different from zero, only the minimum shelf-life value is calculated.

Traditionally, extensive stability data are collected at the recommended storage temperatures (usually refrigerator and/or room temperature) to be placed on the label of the package. However, elevated temperature data are very valuable in determining the shelf life of a product. In practice, multiple levels of thermal stress are applied to the formulation so that appropriate shelf-life estimates can be made for normally expected marketing conditions. In cases where data from accelerated studies are used to project a tentative expiration date that is beyond the date supported by actual shelf-life studies, testing must continue until the tentative expiration date is verified.

It was noted in Chapter 18 that the effect of temperature variation on the rate of a reaction can be expressed by the Arrhenius equation

$$k = se^{-E_A/RT}$$

where k is the velocity or rate constant, s is the frequency factor, E_A is the activation energy, R is the gas constant, and T is the absolute temperature.

This relationship may be written in logarithmic form

$$\ln k = \ln s - \frac{E_A}{RT}$$

which on differentiation becomes

$$\frac{d \ln k}{dT} = \frac{E_A}{RT^2}$$

This can be integrated between the limits k_1 and k_2, and T_1 and T_2, and on subsequent transforming to the base 10 becomes

$$\log \frac{k_2}{k_1} = \frac{E_A}{2.303R} \left(\frac{T_2 - T_1}{T_2 \cdot T_1} \right)$$

A weighted modification of this model has been incorporated into the previously described computerized system. Each print-out contains a statement concerning the acceptability of the Arrhenius assumption with its appropriate probability level, the slope and intercept for the Arrhenius line, the estimated apparent energy of activation with its 95% confidence limits, plus estimated shelf-life values at selected temperatures.

The analysis of first-order stability data is based on the linear model

$$Y_{ij} = \alpha_i + \beta_i X_{ij} + \epsilon_{ij}$$

where Y_{ij} is the natural logarithm of the assay value for the jth observation of the ith temperature, X_{ij} is the elapsed time in months for the assay sample for the ith temperature, β_i and α_i are the slope and intercept respectively, and ϵ_{ij} is a random error associated with Y_{ij}. The errors are assumed to be identically and independently normally distributed with a zero mean and variance σ^2.

For orders other than first, Y_{ij}, represents the concentration raised to the power of 1 minus the order.

The estimated rate constant (ie, the negative slope) is

$$-b_i = - \sum_j (Y_{ij} - Y_{i.})(X_{ij} - X_{i.}) \Big/ \sum_j (X_{ij} - X_{i.})^2$$

The standard error of the estimated rate constant is

$$S_{-b_i} = \frac{S(Y/X)}{[\Sigma(X_{ij} - X_{i.})^2]^{1/2}}$$

where $S(Y/X)$, the residual standard error, is equal to

$$S(Y/X) = \left\{ \frac{1}{N-2} \left[\sum_{j=1}^{12} (Y_{ij} - Y_{1.})^2 - \frac{[\Sigma(X_{ij} - X_{i.})(Y_{ij} - Y_{i.})]^2}{\Sigma(X_{ij} - X_{i.})^2} \right] \right\}^{1/2}$$

According to the Arrhenius relationship, faster degradation occurs at the higher temperatures; hence assays for the high-temperature data are usually run more often but for a shorter period of time. The effect of simple least-squares analysis of this type of data is to force the Arrhenius equation through the low temperature data and essentially ignore the high temperature information. Thus much more credence is placed in the point estimates of the low temperature than is warranted. In addition, the usual confidence limits on

extrapolated degradation rates at refrigerator or room temperature cannot validly be made. For these reasons, Bentley[6] presented a method based on weighted least-squares analysis to replace the unweighted approximation. He also developed a statistical test for the validity of the Arrhenius assumption which is easily computed from the results of the unweighted method.

To make shelf-life estimates from elevated temperature data, two storage temperatures are obviously the minimum. As the accuracy of the extrapolation is enhanced by using additional temperatures, a minimum of four different temperatures is recommended for most product stability studies. With the current use of computers to do the bulk of stability calculations, including weighted least-squares analysis, the temperatures and storage conditions need not be selected for arithmetic convenience.

It is not necessary to determine the mechanism of the degradation reaction. In most cases, it is necessary only to follow some property of degradation and to linearize this function. Either the amount of undegraded drug or the amount of a formed decomposition product may be followed. It is usually impractical to determine the exact order of the reaction. With assay errors in the range of 2 to 5%, at least 50% decomposition must occur before the reaction order can be determined. As the loss with pharmaceuticals is generally less, zero-order kinetics should be assumed unless the reaction order is known from previous work. In any case, replication of stability assays is advisable.

The batches of drugs used for a stability study should be representative of production run material or at least of a known degree of purity. The quality of the excipients should also be known as their impurities or even their moisture content can deleteriously affect product stability. Likewise, the samples of the formulation taken for the stability study must be representative of the lot.

Specific assay methods must be used when at all possible. In any case, the reliability and specificity of the test method on the intact molecule and on the degradation products must be determined.

Addition of Overage

The problem of declining potency in an unstable preparation can be ameliorated by the addition of an excess or overage of the active ingredient. Overages, then, are added to pharmaceutical formulations to keep the content of the active ingredient within the limits compatible with therapeutic requirements for a predetermined period of time.

The amount of the overage depends upon the specific ingredient and the galenical dosage form. The International Pharmaceutical Federation has recommended that overages be limited to a maximum of 30% over the labeled potency of an ingredient.

Pharmaceutical Containers

Unless otherwise indicated in a compendial monograph, the official standards for containers apply to articles packaged either by the pharmaceutical manufacturer or the dispensing pharmacist. In general, repackaging of pharmaceuticals is inadvisable. However, if repackaging is necessary, the manufacturer of the product should be consulted for potential stability problems.

A pharmaceutical container has been defined as a device which holds the drug and is or may be in direct contact with the preparation. The immediate container is described as that which is in direct contact with the drug at all times. The liner and closure have traditionally been considered to be part of the container system. The container should not interact physically or chemically with the formulation so as to alter the strength, quality, or purity of its contents beyond permissible limits.

The choice of containers and closures can have a profound effect on the stability of many pharmaceuticals. Now that a large variety of glass, plastics, rubber closures, tubes, tube liners, etc. are available, the possibilities for interaction between the packaging components and the formulation ingredients are immense. Some of the packaging elements themselves are subject to physical and chemical changes that may be time-temperature dependent.

Frequently it is necessary to use a well-closed or a tight container to protect a pharmaceutical product. A *well-closed container* is used to protect its contents from extraneous solids or a loss in potency of the active ingredient under normal commercial conditions. A *tight container* protects the contents from contamination by extraneous materials, loss of contents, and from efflorescence, deliquescence, or evaporation, and is capable of tight reclosure. When the packaging and storage of an official article in a well-closed or tight container is specified, water permeation tests should be performed on the selected container.

In a stability program, the appearance of the container with special emphasis on the inner walls, the migration of ingredients onto/into the plastic or into the rubber closure, the migration of plasticizer or components from the rubber closure into the formulation, the possibility of two-way moisture penetration through the container walls, the integrity of the tac-seal, and the back-off torque of the cap must be studied.

Glass, plastics, and metals are the commonly used components of pharmaceutical containers.

Traditionally, glass has been the most widely used container for pharmaceutical products to insure inertness, visibility, strength, rigidity, moisture protection, ease of reclosure, and economy of packaging. While glass has some disadvantages such as the leaching of alkali and insoluble flakes into the formulation, these can be offset by the choice of an appropriate glass. As the composition of glass formulations may be varied by the amounts and types of sand and silica added and the heat treatment conditions used, the proper container for any formulation can be selected.

New, unused glass containers are tested for resistance to attack by high-purity water using a sulfuric acid titration to determine the amount of released alkali. Both glass and plastic containers are used to protect light-sensitive formulations from degradation. The amount of transmitted light is measured using a spectrometer of suitable sensitivity and accuracy.

Glass is generally available in flint, amber, blue, emerald green, and certain light-resistant green and opal colors. The blue-, green-, and flint-colored glasses, which transmit ultraviolet and violet light rays, do not meet the official specifications for light-resistant containers.

Colored glass is not usually used for injectable preparations since it is difficult to detect the presence of discoloration, glass particles, and particulate matter in the formulations. Light-sensitive drugs for parenteral use are usually sealed in flint ampuls and placed in a box. Multiple-dose vials should be stored in a dark place.

Manufacturers of prescription drug products should include sufficient information on their product labels to inform the pharmacist of the type of dispensing container needed to maintain the identity, strength, quality, and purity of the product. This brief description of the proper container, eg, light-resistant, well-closed or tight, may be omitted for those products dispensed in the manufacturer's original container.

Plastics—Plastic containers have become very popular for storing pharmaceutical products. Polyethylene, polystyrene, polyvinyl chloride, and polypropylene are used to prepare plastic containers of various densities to fit specific formulation needs.

Factors such as plastic composition, processing and cleaning procedures, contacting media, inks, adhesives, absorption, adsorption, and permeability of preservatives also affect the suitability of a plastic for pharmaceutical use. Hence, biological test procedures are used to determine the suitability of a plastic for packaging products intended for parenteral use and for polymers intended for use in implants and medical devices. Systemic injection, intracutaneous, and implantation tests are employed. In addition, tests for nonvolatile residue, residue on ignition, heavy metals, and buffering capacity, were designed to determine the physical and chemical properties of plastics and their extracts.

The high-density polyethylene containers, which are used for packaging capsules and tablets, possess characteristic thermal properties, a distinctive infrared absorption spectrum and a density between 0.941 and 0.965 g/cm^3. In addition, these containers are tested for light transmission, water vapor permeation, extractable substances, nonvolatile residue, and heavy metals. Where a stability study has been performed to establish the expiration date for a dosage form in an acceptable high-density polyethylene container, any other high-density polyethylene container may be substituted provided that it, too, meets compendial standards and that the stability program is expanded to include the alternate container.

Materials from the plastic itself can leach into the formulation, and materials from the latter can be absorbed onto, into, or through the container wall. Various pharmaceutical preservatives are bound by the barrels of some plastic syringes. However, changing the composition of the syringe barrel from nylon to polyethylene or polystyrene has eliminated the binding in some cases.

A major disadvantage of plastic containers is the two-way permeation of "breathing" through the container walls. Volatile oils and flavoring and perfume agents are permeable through plastics to varying degrees. Components of emulsions and creams have been reported to migrate through the walls of some plastics causing either a deleterious change in the formulation or collapse of the container. Loss of moisture from a formulation is common. Gases, such as oxygen or carbon dioxide in the air, have been known to migrate through container walls and to affect a preparation.

Solid dosage forms, such as penicillin tablets, when stored in some plastics, are deleteriously affected by moisture penetration from the atmosphere into the container.

Metals—The pharmaceutical industry was, and to a degree still is, a tin stronghold. However, as the price of tin constantly varies, more aluminum tubes are being used. Lead tubes tend to have pinholes and are little used in the industry.

A variety of internal linings and closure or fold seals are available for both tin and aluminum tubes. Tin tubes can be coated with wax or with vinyl linings. Aluminum tubes are available with epoxy or phenolic resin, wax, vinyl, or a combination of epoxy or phenolic resin with wax. As aluminum is able to withstand the high temperatures required to cure adequately epoxy and phenolic resins, tubes made from this metal presently offer the widest range of lining possibilities.

Closure foldseals may consist of unmodified vinyl resin or plasticized cellulose and resin with or without added color.

Collapsible tubes are available in many combinations of diameters, lengths, openings, and caps. Custom-use tips for ophthalmic, nasal, mastitis, and rectal applications are also available. Only a limited number of internal liners and closure seals are available for tubes fitted with these special-use tips.

Lined tubes from different manufacturers are not necessarily interchangeable. While some converted resin liners may be composed of the same base resin, the actual liner may have been modified to achieve better adhesion, flow properties, drying qualities, or flexibility. These modifications may have been necessitated by the method of applying the liner, the curing procedure, or finally by the nature of the liner itself.

Closures

The closures for the formulations must also be studied as a portion of the overall stability program. While the closure must form an effective seal for the container, the closure must not react chemically or physically with the product. It must not absorb materials from the formulation or leach its ingredients into the contents.

The integrity of the seal between the closure and container depends on the geometry of the two, the materials used in their construction, the composition of the cap liner, and the tightness with which the cap has been applied. Torque is a measure of the circular force, measured in inch-pounds, which must be applied to open or close a container. When pharmaceutical products are set up on a stability study, the formulation must be in the proposed market package. Thus they should be capped with essentially the same torque to be used in the manufacturing step.

Rubber is a common component of stoppers, cap liners, and parts of dropper assemblies. Sorption of the active ingredient, preservative, or other formulation ingredients into the rubber and the extraction of one or more components of the rubber into the formulation are common problems.

The application of an epoxy lining to the rubber closure reduces the amount of leached extractives but has essentially no effect on the sorption of the preservative from the solution. Teflon-coated rubber stoppers may prevent most of the sorption and leaching.

References

1. Lintner CJ: *Quality Control in the Pharmaceutical Industry*, vol 2, Academic, New York, 141, 1973.
2. *Current Good Manufacturing Practice*, Code of Federal Regulations, Title 21, Food and Drugs, Part 211, 1980.
3. Lintner CJ: *et al: Am Perfum Cosmet 85 (Dec.):* 31, 1970.
4. Kennon L: *J Pharm Sci 53:* 815, 1964.
5. McMinn CS, Lintner CJ (oral presentation), APhA Acad. Pharm. Sci Mtg, Ind Pharm Tech Sect, Chicago, IL, May 14, 1973.
6. Bentley DL: *J Pharm Sci 59:* 464, 1970.

Bibliography

Windheuser JJ, ed: *The Dating of Pharmaceuticals*, Univ. Extension, Univ. Wisconsin, Madison, WI, 1970.
Wagner JG, ed: *Biopharmaceutics and Relevant Pharmacokinetics*, Hamilton Press, Hamilton, IL, 1971.
Lachman L, *et al: The Theory and Practice of Industrial Pharmacy*, 2nd ed, Lea & Febiger, Philadelphia, 1976.

CHAPTER 83

Quality Assurance and Control

Clyde R Erskine, Jr

Director, Corporate Quality Assurance
SmithKline Beckman Corporation
One Franklin Plaza, PO Box 7929
Philadelphia, PA 19101

The Pharmaceutical Industry continues as a vital segment of the health care cycle in conducting research and manufacturing products which are life maintaining and life restoring. The last decade has seen an evolution in the concepts relating to the Quality Assurance and Control of these products.

The changes brought about in assuring the safety and therapeutic efficacy of drug products have resulted from a number of factors which are either internal or external to the industry. Internally are the self-designed guidelines the industry has imposed on themselves, exemplified by a document prepared in 1967 by the Pharmaceutical Manufacturers Association titled "General Principles of Total Quality Control in the Drug Industry." This PMA document became the basis for later regulatory Guidelines prepared by the Food and Drug Administration titled "Current Good Manufacturing Practice in Manufacture, Processing, Packing or Holding of Human and Veterinary Drugs." These CGMP's, as they are commonly referred to, have become the primary external guidelines used by industry and the Food and Drug Administration in the control and inspections of manufacturing facilities.

Quality Control and Assurance Organization

Although the terms Quality Control and Quality Assurance are often used interchangeably, depending on the structure of a specific company, there is a continuing trend to separate and define their functional responsibilities.

Quality Control can be broadly defined as the day-to-day control of quality within a company, a department staffed with scientists and technicians responsible for the acceptance or rejection of incoming raw materials and packaging components, for the myriad of in-process tests and inspections, to assure that systems are being controlled and monitored and, finally, for the approval or rejection of completed dosage forms.

Quality Control therefore includes not only the analytical testing of the finished product, but also the assessment of all operations beginning with the receipt of raw materials and continuing throughout the production and packaging operations, finished product testing, documentation, surveillance and distribution.

Quality Assurance may be defined as the responsibility of an organization to determine that systems, facilities and written procedures are both adequate and followed in order to assure that products are controlled and will meet, in the final dosage form, all the applicable specifications. Quality Assurance naturally then becomes an oversight function, often auditing operations to determine that procedures and systems are suitable and, if not, to recommend the required changes. Higher management looks toward the Quality Assurance unit in order to develop some level of "comfort" as to how well they are doing in meeting company standards and applicable government regulations.

Total Quality Control

The high quality of pharmaceutical products results from meticulous adherence to written procedures in carrying out all operations, beginning with research. It is at this early point that the quality begins to be designed into a product. Raw materials must be characterized and purchased from reputable suppliers so that uniform, stable products will result when these materials are incorporated into the finished dosage form. Facilities must be designed and the proper equipment selected so that the potential for cross contamination of one product by another is eliminated, that material flow and personnel movements are planned to reduce the potential for product mix-ups and that the air and water which is being provided to production is adequate in amount and quality for the particular operations being performed.

Production personnel must be properly trained to perform their jobs, and the directions they follow must be written, approved by responsible individuals and adhered to strictly.

Shipping departments are responsible for seeing that the products are protected from adverse handling and environmental conditions while in transit to distribution points and customers.

Quality Control is ever present, overseeing each of these operations and giving the final release approval for distribution only after assessing and being satisfied that each step in this process has been completed correctly.

These principles were all highlighted in that original PMA document from which the following excerpt is taken:

"The quality of a product is its degree of possession of those characteristics designed and manufactured into it which contribute to the performance of an intended function when the product is used as directed. The quality of medicinal and related products is the sum of all factors which contribute directly or indirectly to the safety, effectiveness and acceptability of the product. Quality must be built into the product during research, development and production.

"Total control of quality as it applies to the drug industry is the organized effort within an entire establishment to design, produce, maintain and assure the specified quality in each unit of product distributed. The effort should not only establish specifications for product acceptance but should provide procedures and methods for achieving conformance with such specifications.

"The large variety of substances used in this industry, the complexity of its products and the various types of company organization make it impossible to design in detail a single universally applicable system for the total control of quality.

"The ultimate objective of a program for the total control of quality in a drug company is the attainment of perfection in meeting specifications for a product of high quality. It is a program designed to assure the professional user or ultimate consumer that every lot of a product conforms to specifications and that each dose distributed will fulfill the representations made in the labeling and will meet all legal requirements and such additional standards as the management of a firm may adopt.

"Total control of quality is a plantwide activity and represents the aggregate responsibility of all segments of a company. The responsibility for auditing the control system and for evaluating product quality is that of a specific group referred to in this statement as Quality Control. The head of Quality Control should have the authority to release satisfactory lots of products, to reject unsuitable lots and to recommend the recall from distribution of any lots subsequently found to be unsuitable. He should be responsible to a level of management which enables him to exercise independent judgment. His responsibility and authority should be clearly defined by management."

It becomes readily apparent that quality must be built into a product and that it cannot be inspected or tested into a product. Quality results from teamwork, an association which is becoming increasingly important as the industry advances in new technologies which themselves are becoming more complex and demanding.

Quality Control and Assurance Functions

The head of Quality Control, who is ultimately responsible for decisions relating to the acceptability of finished product, should report to someone other than the person directly responsible for producing the product. Often in current organizational structures, the persons in charge of both quality control and production will report to some higher level of authority. This may be the same or different individuals, but it does allow the independent operations of both functions without direct conflicts arising when reaching the ultimate decision on the acceptability of product. The Quality Control function in an organization normally consists of at least two primary units, analytical control and inspection control.

Analytical Control

The Analytical Control Laboratory is responsible for testing and approving raw materials, work in-process and finished product. The Laboratory must be staffed with persons who are trained both academically and by experience to perform the often complex analyses required to evaluate the acceptability of a product. Proper personnel is not the only necessity in the laboratory. Equipment also is required which will allow timely and accurate analysis. This equipment continues to become more sophisticated, providing more information about compounds than previously known and has led to a level of accuracy and detectability heretofore unknown.

Detailed specifications must also be available, as well as the test methods against which the products are measured. The specifications include the criteria against which the product will be evaluated and the limits for acceptance or rejection for each critical parameter.

The testing and acceptance of only high quality raw materials is essential in the preparation of products. Part of this acceptance is to purchase raw materials only from known reputable suppliers. In order to assure this condition, it is essential that Quality Control be part of a pre-approval program of all potential suppliers. This approval always includes testing the material and in many cases will necessitate an inspection of the supplier's facility to determine its suitability and degree of compliance with GMP's. At various critical in-process production or intermediate steps it may be necessary to sample and test the materials against criteria previously established for that particular step in the process.

Often in-process alert or action levels will be identified at the critical operational steps as a means of process control. These alert or action levels are limits or specifications which are more restrictive than the final acceptance limits, but serve as in-process controls by giving early warnings of conditions which could lead to an out-of-control situation and allow timely corrective action to be taken before this occurs. Thus materials reaching the alert or action level criteria are acceptable, since they have not exceeded a rejection or unacceptable level.

In-process critical testing will vary depending on the dosage form being manufactured. Sterile parenteral products probably receive the most critical in-process control and testing in order to insure a finished product which is sterile and free of microbial contamination and particulate matter. With sterile products the end product sterility testing cannot be relied upon to insure that each and every container in a lot of an injectable product is sterile and dependence is placed on in-process controls. These in-process controls must have been developed following a prescribed protocol which defines operating conditions and parameters. Only after a series of successful production runs, using the prescribed parameters, can a process be judged to have been validated. Validation of processes is a critical step in the quality assurance of both sterile and nonsterile products. Validation may be defined as "assurance that production processes are controlled in such a manner that they will routinely perform in the manner in which they are purported to."

Testing of the completed lot of a dosage form, in order to measure its conformance with predetermined specifications and appropriate acceptance criteria, is always desirable before releasing the lot for shipment. However, the use of a properly validated manufacturing process is more critical to the quality of a product. End product testing suffers due to the normal variations that arise in the statistical sampling of a lot in assuring that a sample is homogeneous and representative of the lot.

Tests and specifications may be found in several sources. The *United States Pharmacopeia/National Formulary* (USP) is published on a five-year cycle program by the United States Pharmacopeial Convention. The standards established by and published in the USP have been recognized as being official by the Congress of the United States and are recognized in the Federal Food, Drug and Cosmetic Act. These standards are prepared and reviewed so that through regular revision, entirely or in part, they remain current. The reviewing body known as the Committee of Revision represents medical, academe, industrial and other scientific experts. The primary purpose of the Committee is "to provide authoritative standards for materials and substances and their preparations that are used in the healing arts." They establish titles, definitions, descriptions and standards for the identity, quality, strength, purity and, where practical, methods for their examination and formulas for their manufacture.

In addition to the procedures defined in the USP, companies often will prepare their own test specifications when the products are not "official" (listed in the USP). These tests and specifications form a necessary part of the Control Sections of New Drug Applications submitted to the federal government and which, following careful review by the Food and Drug Administration, may be approved. Finally, there are test procedures for unofficial products (not in the USP) which do not require the submission of a New Drug Application. Companies in these cases prepare their own in-house test procedures for controlling the products they produce.

Inspection Control

Many responsibilities assumed by Quality Control are ancillary to the analytical testing. These include the sampling of incoming raw materials, packaging and labeling components; the physical inspection of product at various intermediate stages; packaging line inspection and the control of shipping inventory within the distribution cycle. Depending on the organizational structure, additional or different responsibilities will be assigned to this unit.

Documentation

During the course of producing a pharmaceutical product, numerous documents and records are generated. Each batch is assigned a specific code or lot number. All documentation relating to a specific code is referred to as a "batch record," which will include data on each significant phase of production, control and distribution. The batch record provides a historical blueprint of every step, beginning with the receipt of chemical raw materials and packaging components and continuing through each in-process stage. Recording charts or computer printouts of significant operations such as autoclaving, drying, air particulate monitoring, lyophylizing, etc, all become part of this batch history. After the batch has been completed, including final analytical and physical testing, one additional step should be completed prior to approving the lot for distribution. All documents and records relating to the specific batch are given a final review. Each required document in the batch record must be checked for completeness and accuracy. Any discrepancy must be immediately investigated and answered. Only after this review has been completed satisfactorily may the batch be released for distribution.

When the batch has been released, accurate shipping records must be maintained showing the batch distribution. With these records it is then possible to trace the batch to the market place which will facilitate, if the need arose, recalling the product (batch) from the market place.

Quality Assurance

Total control of quality not only requires the assignments described above, but should include a monitoring or audit function as well. The responsibility for this function is normally separate from both the production and control operations, thus allowing an independent oversight of all operations. Although the function may be separated, the audit responsibilities are often shared by a team representing both the production and control disciplines. It is the duty of this individual (team) through review and inspection to assure that written procedures and policies are available for each significant production and control operation. Normally, standard operating procedures (SOP's) are developed which, when followed by properly trained operators, will help to assure the quality and integrity of the product. Thus the QA review function not only determines that the procedures are current and correct, but that they are being followed. Combining a review of SOP's with an audit of facilities and operations following the applicable CGMP regulations will give a company an "inside" report on its level of compliance and will allow necessary changes and or corrections to be made prior to either causing a product failure or being observed during an inspection by an FDA investigator.

Production is responsible for following prescribed procedures to produce acceptable products. The system of total quality management becomes the joint responsibility of quality control and quality assurance.

Quality depends to a major degree upon the employees engaged in the production operations. They are responsible for following the prescribed procedures and, along with their training and experience are able to produce uniformly acceptable products. GMP's properly organized and followed afford the only mechanism for preventing human error, the potential for which is especially great in this industry.

New Advances

The use of statistics and trend analysis are tools already used by the pharmaceutical industry in determining the proper sample size required for testing, for measuring the uniformity of solid dosage forms and for plotting trends of significant factors in order to correct out-of-control situations before unacceptable product results.

Electronic data processing has become another useful tool for assessing process and test parameters and for analyzing the data collected during production. The control of many operations by computers and microprocessors is providing the capability for producing products of further improved uniform quality. These systems have challenged the older ones, resulting in new approaches to in-process controls, collection and analysis of data and to the entire system of quality control.

Environmental Control

Along with the many other advances in the total control of quality is the growing recognition that the environment and the systems used for its control can have a significant effect on the finished product quality. It is well recognized that parenteral or sterile ophthalmic products must be produced in a manner which will insure their sterility; therefore, control of the areas in which they are manufactured is essential.

Microbiological monitoring of air and water to control the level of particulate and microbial matter in these production areas is necessary. Several levels of "clean" areas are described in Federal Government Standard 209B, "Clean Room and Work Station Requirements, Controlled Environment." The industry commonly uses the specifications described which classify air cleanliness based on the number of particles (of a given size) per cubic foot of air. Generally, conditions listed as "Class 100" are maintained in areas where parenteral products are filled into sterile containers. Class 100 is defined as an area which can be maintained at less than 100 particles per cubic foot of air 0.5 μm and larger.

Another essential control procedure is microbiological monitoring of the environment in which nonsterile products are manufactured. The objective of this monitoring is to first determine particulate and microbial levels within an area to assure that they are reasonable. If found to be excessive, steps must be taken to bring the levels to within acceptable limits. Once this base has been developed, regular monitoring will indicate if operations are continuing under acceptable limits. If not, immediate corrective action should be taken.

The monitoring and control of particulate and microbial matter will further assure the final quality and stability of the product because the environment has been controlled and the product has not been challenged by an unacceptable level of particulate generated by an out-of-control situation.

Good Manufacturing Practice Regulations

In June, 1963, the Food and Drug Administration first issued regulations describing the current good manufacturing practice to be followed in the manufacture, packaging and holding of finished pharmaceuticals. The regulations underwent significant revision and updating in 1978 and became official in March, 1979. These regulations present the minimum requirements to be met by industry when manufacturing, processing, packaging and holding of human and veterinary drugs. Under the Federal Food, Drug and Cosmetic Act, a drug is deemed to be adulterated unless the methods used in its manufacture, processing, packing and holding, as well as the facilities and controls used, conform to current good manufacturing practice so that the drug meets the safety requirements of the Act and has the identity and strength to meet the quality and purity characteristics that it is represented to have. In the preamble to the regulations, the FDA Commissioner answers the comments received from interested persons who responded when the proposed rules were first issued. The preamble provides interesting background information as to why specific sections of the regulations were believed to be necessary and their interpretation.

In July, 1978, the FDA issued regulations establishing similar Good Manufacturing Practices for the Manufacture, Packing, Storage and Installation of Medical Devices. These were published following an amendment to the Food, Drug and Cosmetic Act of 1976, which provided the FDA with the authority to prescribe regulations pertaining to medical devices. In December, 1978, regulations concerning Good Laboratory Practices for the control and conducting of clinical studies were issued and for the first time came under FDA inspectional authority.

The Food and Drug Administration proposed, in June 1978, regulations covering the GMP's relating to the manufacture and control of large volume parenteral products. These regulations, although never officially issued, have become the guideline used by the industry and FDA in the manufacture, control and inspection of large volume parenteral production. Due to the similarity of the controls required for the production of small volume parenterals, the guidelines have also been used to assess the adequacy of the manufacture and controls used with these products.

A number of other "guidelines" or "concept" papers have been prepared by various organizations within the industry itself, such as the Pharmaceutical Manufacturers Association and the Parenteral Drug Association. A partial listing is provided at the end of this section.

The current Good Manufacturing Practice Regulations should be read and thoroughly understood by those involved in or interested in pursuing quality control or quality assurance responsibilities. The scope of the present regulations is given in the following outline, along with a brief interpretation of each section.

References

1. *Human and Veterinary Drugs—Current Good Manufacturing Practice in Manufacture, Processing, Packing or Holding.* Code of Federal Regulations Title 21, Part 211, Washington, DC, General Services Administration, 1982.

2. *General Principles of Total Quality Control in the Drug Industry.* Pharmaceutical Manufacturers Association, 1100 15th Street NW, Washington, DC 20005, June, 1967.

3. *Clean Room and Work Station Requirements, Controlled Environment.* Federal Standard 209B, Washington, DC, General Services Administration, April 1973.

4. *Good Manufacturing Practice for Medical Devices, General.* Code of Federal Regulations Title 21, Part 820, Washington, DC, General Services Administration, April, 1982.

5. *Good Laboratory Practice for Non-Clinical Laboratory Studies.* Code of Federal Regulations Title 21, Part 58, Washington, DC, General Services Administration, April, 1982.

6. *Human Drugs—Current Good Manufacturing Practice in Manufacture, Processing, Packing or Holding of Large Volume Parenterals.* Federal Register, Volume 41, No 106, Tuesday, June 1, 1976.

7. *The Pharmacopeia of the United States XX, National Formulary XV.* United States Pharmacopeial Convention, Inc, 12601 Twinbrook Parkway, Rockville, MD 20852, July 1, 1980.

8. *Validation of Steam Sterilization Cycles.* Technical Monograph No. 1, Parenteral Drug Association, Inc, 1346 Chestnut Street, Philadelphia, PA 19107, 1978.

9. *Validation of Asceptic Filling for Solution Drug Products.* Technical Monograph No 2, Parenteral Drug Association, Inc, 1346 Chestnut Street, Philadelphia, PA 19107, 1980.

10. *Validation of Dry Heat Processes Used for Sterilization and Depyrogenation.* Technical Monograph No 3, Parenteral Drug Association, Inc, 1346 Chestnut Street, Philadelphia, PA 19107, 1981.

11. *Proceedings of the PMA Seminar Program on Validation of Solid Dosage Form Processes.* Pharmaceutical Manufacturers Association, 1100 15th Street NW, Washington, DC 20005, May 1980.

12. *Validation of Sterilization of Large Volume Parenterals—Current Concepts.* Pharmaceutical Manufacturers Association, 1100 15th Street NW, Washington, DC 20005, February, 1979.

PART 211—CURRENT GOOD MANUFACTURING PRACTICE IN MANUFACTURE, PROCESSING, PACKING OR HOLDING—HUMAN AND VETERINARY DRUGS

		Interpretation
Subpart A—General Provisions		
211.3	Definitions	The scope of the regulations are explained for human prescription and OTC drug products including biological products.
		Reference is made to Part 210.3 of the chapter which gives definitions for all significant terms used in the regulations.
Subpart B—Organization and Personnel		
211.22	Responsibilities of quality control unit	Highlighted here is the assignment to the quality control unit total responsibility for ensuring that adequate systems and procedures exist and are followed to assure product quality.
211.25	Personnel qualifications	Personnel, either supervisory or operational, must be qualified by training and experience to perform their assigned tasks.
211.28	Personnel responsibilities	The obligations of personnel engaged in the manufacture of drug products concerning their personal hygiene, clothing and medical status are defined.
211.34	Consultants	The qualifications of consultants must be approved by Quality Control.
Subpart C—Buildings and Facilities		
211.42	Design and construction features	Buildings and facilities can be considered acceptable only if they are suitable for their intended purpose and can be maintained. Construction concepts, such as air handling systems, lighting, eating facilities and plumbing systems including water, sewage and toilet facilities, are outlined.
211.44	Lighting	
211.46	Ventilation, air filtration, air heating and cooling	
211.48	Plumbing	
211.50	Sewage and refuse	
211.52	Washing and toilet facilities	
211.56	Sanitation	
211.58	Maintenance	
Subpart D—Equipment		
211.63	Equipment design, size and location	Equipment must be designed, constructed, of adequate size, suitably located and able to be maintained in order to be considered suitable for its intended use.
211.65	Equipment construction	
211.67	Equipment cleaning and maintenance	
211.68	Automatic, mechanical and electronic equipment	Reference is made to the use of automatic equipment, data processors and computers highlighting the need to verify output versus input and for proper calibration of recorders, counters, and other electrical or mechanical devices.
211.72	Filters	Special note is made that only filters are to be used which do not release fibers into products.
Subpart E—Control of Components and Drug Product Containers and Closures		
211.80	General requirements	Written procedures must be available which describe the receipt, identification, storage, handling, sampling, testing and approval or rejection of components (raw materials) and drug products.
211.82	Receipt and storage of untested components, drug product containers and closures	
211.84	Testing and approval or rejection of components, drug product containers and closures	Once approved or rejected, these materials must be so identified and stored. If approved, they must be inventoried in a manner to assure that the oldest approved stock is used first (FIFO). Materials which are subject to deterioration during storage should be retested at an appropriate time based on stability profiles.
211.86	Use of approved components, drug product containers and closures	
211.87	Retesting of approved components, drug product containers and closures	

211.89 Rejected components, drug product containers and closures
211.94 Drug product containers and closures

Containers and closures (product contact materials) must be non-reactive with or additive to the product.

Subpart F—Production and Process Controls
211.100 Written procedures; deviations

Written standard operating procedures (SOP's) for each production process and control procedure are necessary. Any deviation to a SOP must be investigated, recorded and approved prior to final product acceptance.

211.101 Charge-in of components
211.103 Calculation of yield
211.105 Equipment identification

All products are to be formulated to provide not less than 100% of the required amount of active ingredient. Records are to be maintained of each component and the quantity which is incorporated into a batch.

211.110 Sampling and testing of in-process materials and drug products

Significant in-process steps are to be identified and appropriate sampling, testing and approvals obtained before proceeding further in the production cycle. If required, time limitations will be placed on in-process steps.

211.111 Time limitations on production
211.113 Control of microbiological contamination

Appropriate procedures are to be prepared for testing components, products and the environment in order to establish that a product is not microbiologically contaminated.

211.115 Reprocessing

Reprocessing of product is allowed providing there are written procedures covering the methods to be used and approved by quality control. Additional testing of the reprocessed batch may be required to assure conformity with specifications.

Subpart G—Packaging and Labeling Control
211.122 Materials examination and usage criteria

Labeling & packaging materials are to be received, identified, stored, sampled and tested following detailed written procedures.

211.125 Labeling issuance
211.130 Packaging and labeling operations
211.134 Drug product inspection
211.137 Expiration dating

Special controls must be exercised over labeling to assure that only the correct labels are issued to packaging for a specific product and that the quantities used are reconciled with the quantity issued.

Following appropriate stability studies at prescribed temperature conditions, products on the market shall bear an expiration date to assure that they are used within their expected shelf life.

Subpart H—Holding and Distribution
211.142 Warehousing procedures
211.150 Distribution procedures

Describes the requirements for warehousing and distribution of products and their holding under appropriate conditions of light, temperature and humidity.

Subpart I—Laboratory Controls
211.160 General requirements
211.165 Testing and release for distribution

Concerns written procedures in the form of specifications, standards, sampling plans, and test procedures which are used in a laboratory for controlling components and finished drug products. Acceptance criteria for sampling and approval shall be adequate for support release of product to distribution.

211.166 Stability testing
211.167 Special testing requirements
211.170 Reserve samples

A stability testing program will be followed in order to assess the stability characteristics of drug products. The results of this testing shall be used in assigning appropriate storage conditions and expiration dates.

211.173 Laboratory animals

Animals used in any testing shall be maintained and controlled in a manner suitable for use.

211.176 Penicillin contamination

Drug products cannot be marketed if, when tested by a prescribed procedure, found to contain any detectable levels of penicillin.

Subpart J—Records and Reports
211.180 General requirements
211.182 Equipment cleaning and use log
211.184 Component, drug product container, closure and labeling records

Details the various records and documents which should be generated during the manufacture of drug products and which are to be available for review.

211.186 Master production and control records
211.188 Batch production and control records
211.192 Production record review
211.194 Laboratory records
211.196 Distribution records

A master production record must be prepared for each drug product, describing all aspects of its manufacture, packaging and control. Individual batch records are derived from this approved master.

Distribution records include warehouse shipping logs, invoices, bills of lading and all documents associated with distribution. These records should provide all the information necessary to trace lot distribution in order to facilitate product retrieval if necessary.

211.198 Complaint files

Records of complaints received from consumers and professionals are to be maintained along with the report of their investigation and response.

Subpart K—Returned and Salvaged Drug Products
211.204 Returned drug products

Records are to be maintained of drug products returned from distribution channels and the reason for their return. This data can be used as part of the total lot accountability, should the need arise, to trace its distribution and/or for its recall.

211.208 Drug product salvaging

Drug products that have been improperly stored are not to be salvaged.

CHAPTER 84

Solutions, Emulsions, Suspensions and Extractives

J G Nairn, PhD

Professor of Pharmacy
Faculty of Pharmacy, University of Toronto
Toronto, Canada M5S 1A1

The dosage forms described in this chapter may be prepared by dissolving the active ingredient(s) in an aqueous or non-aqueous solvent, by suspending the drug (if it is insoluble in pharmaceutically or therapeutically acceptable solvents) in an appropriate medium, or by incorporating the medicinal agent into one of the two phases of an oil and water system. Such solutions, suspensions, and emulsions are further defined in subsequent paragraphs but some, with similar properties, are considered elsewhere. These dosage forms are useful for a number of reasons. They can be formulated for different routes of administration: oral use, introduction into body cavities or applied externally. The dose easily can be adjusted by dilution, and the oral liquid form readily can be administered to children or people unable to swallow tablets or capsules. Extracts eliminate the need to isolate the drug in pure form, allow several ingredients to be administered from a single source, eg, pancreatic extract, and permit the preliminary study of drugs from natural sources. Occasionally solutions of drugs such as potassium chloride are used to minimize adverse effects in the gastrointestinal tract.

The preparation of these dosage forms involves several considerations on the part of the pharmacist: purpose of the drug, internal or external use, concentration of the drug, selection of the liquid vehicle, physical and chemical stability of the drug, the preservation of the preparation, use of the appropriate excipients such as: buffers, solubilizers, suspending agents, emulsifying agents, viscosity controlling agents, colors, and flavors. The appropriate chapters (see the index) should be consulted for information on the preparation and characteristics of those liquid preparations that are intended for ophthalmic or parenteral use.

Much has been written during the past decade about the biopharmaceutical properties of, in particular, the solid dosage forms. In assessing the bioavailability of drugs in tablets and capsules, many researchers have first studied the absorption of drugs administered in solution. Since drugs are absorbed in their dissolved state, frequently it is found that the absorption rate of oral dosage forms decreases in the following order: aqueous solution > aqueous suspension > tablets or capsules. The bioavailability of a medicament, for oral ingestion and absorption, should be such that eventually all of the drug is absorbed as it passes through the gastrointestinal tract, regardless of the dosage form. There are a number of reasons for formulating drugs in forms in which the drug is not in the molecular state. These are: (a) improved stability, (b) improved taste, (c) low water solubility, (d) palatability, and (e) ease of administration. It becomes apparent, then, that each dosage form will have advantages and disadvantages.

The pharmacist handles liquid preparations in one of three ways. First, he may dispense the product in its original container. Secondly, he may buy the product in bulk and repackage it at the time a prescription is presented by the patient. Lastly, he may compound the solution, suspension, or emulsion in the dispensary. Compounding may involve nothing more than mixing two marketed products in the manner indicated on the prescription or, in specific instances, may require the incorporation of active ingredients in a logical and pharmaceutically acceptable manner into the aqueous or nonaqueous solvents which will form the bulk of the product.

The pharmacist, in the first instance, depends on the manufacturer to produce a product that is effective, elegant, and stable when stored under reasonably adverse conditions. Most drug manufacturers attempt to guarantee efficacy by evaluating their products in a scientifically acceptable manner but, in some instances, such efficacy is relative. For example, cough mixtures marketed by two different manufacturers may contain active ingredients in the same therapeutic class and it becomes difficult to assess the relative merits of the two products. In such instances the commercial advantage gained by one over the other may be based on product elegance. Thus, color, odor, taste, pourability, and homogeneity are important pharmaceutical properties.

The stability of the active ingredient in the final product is of prime concern to the formulator. In general, drug substances are less stable in aqueous media than in the solid dosage form and it is important, therefore, to properly buffer, stabilize, or preserve, in particular, those solutions, suspensions, and emulsions that contain water. Certain simple chemical reactions can occur in these products. These may involve an ingredient-ingredient interaction (which implies a poor formulation), a container-product interaction (which may alter product pH and thus, for pH-sensitive ingredients, be responsible for the subsequent formation of precipitates), or a direct reaction with water (ie, hydrolysis). The stability of pharmaceutical products is discussed in Chapter 82. The more complicated reactions usually involve oxygen. Vitamins, essential oils, and almost all fats and oils can be oxidized. Formulators usually use the word *autoxidation* when the ingredient(s) in the product react with oxygen but without drastic external interference. Such reactions must be first initiated by heat, light (including ultraviolet radiant energy), peroxides or other labile compounds, or heavy metals such as copper or iron. This initiation step results in the formation of a free radical (R*) which then reacts with oxygen.

$$R^* + O_2 \rightarrow RO_2^* \text{ (peroxy radical)}$$

$$RO_2^* + RH \rightarrow ROOH + R^*$$

The free radical is thus regenerated and reacts with more oxygen. This propagation step is followed by the termination reactions.

$$RO_2^* + RO_2^* \rightarrow \text{inactive product}$$

$$RO_2^* + R^* \rightarrow \text{inactive product}$$

$$R^* + R^* \rightarrow \text{inactive product}$$

The effect of trace metals can be minimized by the use of citric acid or EDTA (ie, by use of sequestering agents). Antioxidants, on the other hand, may retard or delay oxidation by reacting with the free radicals formed in the product. Examples of antioxidants are the propyl, octyl, and dodecyl esters of gallic acid, butylated hydroxyanisole (BHA), and the tocopherols or vitamin E. For a more detailed approach to the prevention of oxidative deterioration in pharmaceuticals, the papers by Ostendorf[1] and Chalmers,[2] should be consulted. A description of many antioxidants is given in Chapter 68.

The problem of drug stability has been well defined by pharmaceutical scientists but, during the past few years, a secondary and, in some respects, more serious problem has confronted the manufacturer of liquid preparations. Such pharmaceutically diverse products as baby lotions and milk of magnesia have been recalled from the market because of microbial contamination. In a survey of retail packages of liquid antacid preparations containing magnesium hydroxide, it was found that 30.5% of the finished bottles were contaminated with *Pseudomonas aeruginosa.* The aerobic plate count ranged from less than 100 to 9,300,000 organisms/gram. Other examples could be cited but the range of microorganisms which can contaminate the liquid preparation includes the *Salmonella* sp, *E coli*, certain *Pseudomonas* sp, including *P aeruginosa* and *Staphylococcus aureus.* Bruch[3] describes the types of microorganisms found in various products and attempts to evaluate the hazards associated with the use of nonsterile pharmaceuticals. Coates[4] in a series of papers describes various interactions which must be considered when preservatives are selected.

The USP recommends that certain classes of products be routinely tested for microbial contamination, eg, natural plant and animal products, for freedom from *Salmonella* species; oral solutions and suspensions, for freedom from *E coli*; articles applied topically, for freedom from *P aeruginosa* and *S aureus*; articles for rectal, urethral or vaginal administration, for total microbial count.

Products may become contaminated for a number of reasons. First, the raw materials used in the manufacture of solutions, suspensions, and emulsions are excellent growth media for bacteria. Water, in particular, must be handled with care but substances such as gums, dispersing agents, surfactants, sugars, and flavors can be the carriers of bacteria which ultimately contaminate the product. A second source of contamination is equipment. Bacteria grow well in the nooks and crevices of pharmaceutical equipment (and in the simple equipment used in the dispensary). Such equipment should be thoroughly cleaned prior to use. Environment and personnel can contribute to product contamination. Hands and hair are the most important carriers of contaminants. General cleanliness is thus vital. Head coverings must be used by those involved in the manufacturing process and face masks should be used by those individuals suffering from colds, coughs, hay fever, and other allergic manifestations. Finally, packaging should be selected so that it will not contaminate the product and also will protect it from the environment.

The factors cited above relate to good manufacturing practice. However, the formulator can add a preservative to the product and decrease the probability of product contamination. If the product contains water, it is almost mandatory to include a preservative in the formulation. It must be stressed that this in no way replaces good in-plant control but merely provides further assurance that the product will retain its pharmaceutically acceptable characteristics to the patient level.

The major criteria that should be considered in selecting a preservative are: (a) it should be effective against a wide spectrum of microorganisms; (b) it should be stable for the shelf life of the product; (c) it should be nontoxic; (d) it should be nonsensitizing (e) it should be compatible with the ingredients in the dosage form; (f) it should be relatively free of taste and odor.

Preservatives may be used alone or in combination with each other to prevent the growth of microorganisms. Ethanol is a highly effective preservative. It is used at the 15% level in acidic media and at the 18% level in neutral or slightly alkaline media. Isopropyl alcohol is a fairly effective agent but it can be used only in topical preparations. Propylene glycol, a dihydric alcohol, has germicidal activity similar to that of ethanol. It is normally used at the 10% concentration level.

A 0.5% solution of phenol is a good preservative but it is toxic, has its own characteristic odor, and reacts chemically with many of the drugs and adjuvants which are incorporated into liquid preparations.

The use of hexachlorophene, a germicidal agent which is mainly effective against gram-positive organisms, is restricted to those preparations which are intended for external use only. Several years ago, an incorrectly formulated baby powder (which was found to contain 6.5% hexachlorophene) was responsible for the deaths of 30 French infants. Because of this and other evidence, this substance can be used as a preservative only if its concentration in the final product is 0.1% or less. However, certain liquid preparations (eg, Hexachlorophene Liquid Soap USP) are available. The hexachlorophene content is usually 0.25% in the USP product.

Organic mercury compounds are powerful biostatic agents. Their activity may be reduced in the presence of anionic emulsifying or suspending agents. They are not suitable for oral consumption but are used at the 0.005% concentration level in ophthalmic, nasal, and topical preparations.

Benzoic acid is effective only at pH 4 or less. Its solubility in certain aqueous preparations is poor and, in those instances, sodium benzoate may be utilized. Sorbic acid has a broad range of antimycotic activity but its antibacterial properties are more limited. It is effective only at a pH of less than 5.

Quaternary ammonium surface-active agents, eg, benzalkonium chloride, exhibit an objectionable off-taste and have been reported to be incompatible with a number of anionic substances. In concentrations of 1:5000 to 1:20,000 they are used in ophthalmic preparations.

3-Phenylpropan-1-ol (hydrocinnamyl alcohol) is claimed to be more effective than 2-phenylethanol and benzyl alcohol in inhibiting the growth of *P aeruginosa*, and it has been suggested that this substance may be a suitable preservative for oral suspensions and mixtures.

The methyl and propyl esters of para-hydroxybenzoic acid (the parabens) are widely used in the pharmaceutical industry. They are effective over a wide pH range (from about 3 to 9) and are used at up to about the 0.2% concentration level. The two esters are often used in combination in the same preparation. This achieves a higher total concentration and the mixture is active against a wide range of organisms. The hydroxybenzoates are effective against most organisms; however, their activity may be reduced in the presence of nonionic surface-active agents because of binding.

It should now be obvious that when the pharmacist dispenses or compounds the various liquid preparations he assumes responsibility, with the manufacturer, for the maintenance of product stability. The USP includes a section on stability considerations in dispensing practice. This section of the compendium should be studied in detail. Certain points are self-evident. Stock should be rotated and replaced if expiration dates on the label so indicate. Products should be stored in the manner indicated in the compendium; eg, in a cool place, a tight, light-resistant container, etc. Further, products should be checked for evidence of instability. With respect to solutions, elixirs, and syrups, precipitation and evidence of microbial or chemical gas formation are the two major signs of instability. Emulsions may cream but if they break (ie, there is a separation of an oil phase) the product is considered to be unstable. Caking is a primary indication of instability in suspensions. The presence of large particles may mean that excessive crystal growth has occurred.

The USP states that repackaging is inadvisable. However, if the product must be repackaged, care and the container specified by the compendium must be used. For example, a plastic container should never be used if a light-resistant container is specified by the compendium. If a product is diluted, or where two products are mixed, the pharmacist should utilize his knowledge to guard against incompatibility and instability. Oral antibiotic preparations constituted into liquid form should never be mixed with other products. Since the chemical stability of extemporaneously prepared liquid preparations is often an unknown, their use should be minimized and every care taken to insure that product characteristics will not change during the time it must be used by the patient.

Aqueous Solutions

A solution is a homogeneous mixture that is prepared by dissolving a solid, liquid, or gas in another liquid and represents a group of preparations in which the molecules of the solute or dissolved substance are dispersed among those of the solvent. Solutions may also be classified on the basis of physical or chemical properties, method of preparation, use, physical state, number of ingredients, and particle size. The narrower definition herein limits the solvent to water and excludes those preparations that are sweet and/or viscid in character. This section includes, therefore, those pharmaceutical forms that are designated as *Waters*, *Aqueous Acids*, *Solutions*, *Douches*, *Enemas*, *Gargles*, *Mouthwashes*, *Juices*, *Nasal Solutions*, and *Otic Solutions*.

This section, and the chapter as a whole, must be considered as part of a broad subject that is based on principles presented in several chapters of Part 2, Pharmaceutics.

Water

The major ingredient in most of the dosage forms described herein is water. Water is used both as a vehicle and as a solvent for the desired flavoring or medicinal ingredients. Its tastelessness, freedom from irritating qualities, and lack of pharmacological activity make it ideal for such purposes. There is, however, a tendency to assume that its purity is constant and that it can be stored, handled, and used with a minimum of care. While it is true that municipal supplies must comply with Environmental Protection Agency regulations (or comparable regulations in other countries), drinking water *must* be repurified before it can be used in pharmaceuticals. For further information on water as H_2O, see Chapter 23.

Five of the six solvent waters described in the USP are used in the preparation of parenterals, irrigations, or inhalations. *Purified water* must be used for all other pharmaceutical operations and, as needed, in all the tests and assays of the compendia. Purified water must meet rigid specifications for chemical purity. Such water may be prepared by distillation, by use of ion-exchange resins, or by reverse osmosis.

A wide variety of commercially available stills are used to produce distilled water. The end use of the product dictates the size of the still and extent of pretreatment of the drinking water introduced into the system. A description of stills is provided in Chapter 85. Such water may be sterile provided the condenser is sterile, but to be called sterile, it must be subjected to a satisfactory sterilization process. However, it has been shown that *P aeruginosa* (and other microorganisms) can grow in the distilled water produced in hospitals. The implications of this are obvious. Sterile water may be sterile at the time of production but may lose this characteristic if it is improperly stored. Hickman *et al*,[5] by regrouping the components of conventional distillation equipment, have described a method for the continuous supply of sterile, ultrapure water.

The major impurities in water are calcium, iron, magnesium, manganese, silica, and sodium. The cations are usually combined with the bicarbonate, sulfate, or chloride anions. "Hard" waters are those that contain the calcium and magnesium cations. Bicarbonates are the major impurity in the "alkaline" waters.

Ion-exchange (deionization, demineralization) processes will efficiently and economically remove most of the major impurities in water. A cation exchanger, H_2R, first converts bicarbonates, sulfates, and chlorides to their respective acids.

$$\left.\begin{array}{l} CaSO_4 \\ MgSO_4 \\ Na_2SO_4 \end{array}\right| + H_2R \rightarrow \left.\begin{array}{l} Ca \\ Mg \\ Na_2 \end{array}\right| R + H_2SO_4$$

$$\left.\begin{array}{l} Ca(HCO_3)_2 \\ Mg(HCO_3)_2 \\ 2NaHCO_3 \end{array}\right| + H_2R \rightarrow \left.\begin{array}{l} Ca \\ Mg \\ Na_2 \end{array}\right| R + 2H_2CO_3$$

Carbonic acid decomposes to carbon dioxide (which is removed by aeration in the decarbonator) and water.

The anion exchanger unit may contain either a weakly basic or a strongly basic anion resin. These resins adsorb sulfuric, hydrochloric, and nitric acids. Chemical reactions may involve complete adsorption or an exchange with some other anion.

$$H_2SO_4 + A \rightarrow A \cdot H_2SO_4$$

If the resin contains a hydroxyl radical, water is formed during the purification process.

$$H_2SO_4 + 2AOH \rightarrow A_2SO_4 + 2H_2O$$

Weakly dissociated carbonic and silicic acids can be removed only by strongly basic anion resins.

$$H_2SiO_3 + 2AOH \rightarrow A_2SiO_2 + 2H_2O$$

Unit capacity varies with the nature of the installation but it is possible to process as much as 15,000 gal of water/min.

Deionization processes do not necessarily produce *Purified Water* which will comply with US EPA requirements for drinking water. Resin columns retain phosphates and organic debris. Either alone or in combination, these substances can act as growth media for microorganisms. Observations have shown that deionized water containing 90 organisms/mL contained, after 24 hours storage, 10^6 organisms/mL. Columns can be partially cleaned of pseudomonads by recharging but a 0.25% solution of formaldehyde will destroy most bacteria. The column must be thoroughly washed and checked for the absence of aldehyde (by use of Schiffs Reagent) before it can be used to generate deionized water.

Ultraviolet radiant energy (240–280 nm), heat, or filtration can be used to limit the growth, to kill or to remove microorganisms in water. The latter method employs membrane filters and can be used to remove bacteria from heat labile materials as described under membrane filters in Chapter 79.

The phenomenon of osmosis involves the passage of water from a dilute solution across a semipermeable membrane to a more concentrated solution. Flow of water can be stopped by applying pressure, equal to the osmotic pressure, to the concentrated solution. The flow of water can be reversed by applying a pressure, greater than the osmotic pressure. The process of reverse osmosis utilizes the latter principle; by applying pressure, greater than the osmotic pressure, to the concentrated solution, eg, tap water, pure water may be obtained (see *Reverse Osmosis* in Chapter 78).

Cellulose acetate is used in the manufacture of semipermeable membranes for purifying water by reverse osmosis. This polymer has functional groups that can hydrogen-bond to water or other substances such as alcohol. The water molecules which enter the polymer are transported from one bonding site to the next under pressure. Because of the thin layer of pure water strongly adsorbed at the surface of the membrane, salts, to a large extent, are repelled from the surface, the higher-valent ions being repelled to a greater extent, thus causing a separation of ions from the water. Organic molecules are rejected on the basis of a sieve mechanism related to their size and shape. Small organic molecules, with a molecular weight smaller than approximately 200, will pass through the membrane material. Since there are few organic molecules with a molecular weight of less than 200 in the municipal water supply, reverse osmosis is usually sufficient for the removal of organic material. The pore sizes of the selectively permeable reverse osmosis membranes are between 5 Å and 100 Å. Viruses and bacteria larger than 100 Å are rejected if no imperfections exist in the membrane. The membranes have and do develop openings which permit the passage of microorganisms. Because of the semistatic conditions, bacteria can grow both upstream and downstream of the membrane. Improvements are continually being made in the kind and manufacture of membranes, for example polyamide materials. It is expected that the preparation of water with negligible or no bacteria present will be achieved by this process.

The selection of water treatment equipment depends upon the quality of water to be tested, the quality of water required and the specific pharmaceutical purpose of the water. Frequently two or more methods are used to produce the water desired, for example, filtration and distillation, or filtration, reverse osmosis, and ion-exchange.

Aromatic Waters

Aromatic waters, known also as medicated waters, are clear, saturated aqueous solutions of volatile oils or other aromatic or volatile substances. Their odors and tastes are similar to those of the drugs or volatile substances from which they are prepared, and the preparations should be free from empyreumatic (smoke-like) and other foreign odors. They are used principally as flavored or perfumed vehicles. The volatile substances from which aromatic waters are to be made should be of pharmacopeial quality or, in the case of nonofficial preparations, of the best quality if the finest flavors are to be obtained.

Aromatic waters may be prepared by one of two official processes.

Distillation—Distillation represents the most ancient and frequently the most satisfactory method for making this class of preparations. However, it is the slowest and the more expensive of the two methods.

Different authorities give different directions for the preparation of aromatic waters by distillation. For fresh drugs the proportions range from one part of drug to two of distillate, to two parts of drug to one part of distillate. For dried drugs such as cinnamon, anise, dill, caraway, and fennel the proportion is one part of drug to ten parts of distillate. In the case of dried leaf drugs such as peppermint, the proportion is three parts of drug to ten parts of distillate. Metallic distillation apparatus is usually employed, sometimes using a current of steam passed through the still. The drug should be contused or coarsely ground and combined with a sufficient quantity of *Purified Water*. On completion of the distillation process, any excess of oil in the distillate is removed and, if necessary, the clear water portion is filtered. Most distilled aromatic waters acquire an unpleasant empyreumatic odor as soon as they are distilled. This passes off gradually on exposure to air, if care has been taken not to expose the drug to direct heat during distillation. If precautions are not taken to protect the drug from partial burning, the odor of the carbonized substance will be noticeable in the distilled aromatic water. To avoid this difficulty, the drug should be placed in a partially filled round-bottomed copper wire cage, which is placed in the still to thus avoid any contact of the substance with the heated surface. The meshes of the cage are coarse enough to permit free passage of vapors and boiling water. If the volatile principles in the water are delicate and present in small quantities (eg, as in orange flower and rose waters), the distillate is returned several times to the still with fresh portions of flowers, thus giving rise to the commercial terms *double distilled*, *triple distilled*, or *quadruple distilled*, according to the number of redistillations. This process is called *cohobation*.

Stronger Rose Water is an example of an aromatic water prepared by distillation. It acquires a musty odor when stored in tightly closed containers over long periods of time. The odor of this water is best preserved by allowing limited access of fresh air to the container. Cotton plugs exclude foreign matter but, at the same time, permit air to enter the container. Stronger Rose Water, diluted with an equal volume of purified water, may be used when *Rose Water* is specified in a formulation.

Solution—Aromatic waters may be prepared by repeatedly shaking 2 g or 2 mL (if a liquid) of the volatile substance with 1000 mL of purified water over a period of 15 minutes. The mixture is set aside for 12 hours, filtered through wetted filter paper, and made to volume (1000 mL) by adding purified water through the filter. Peppermint Water USP can be prepared by either of the two official methods.

In terms of time and equipment this method is more convenient than that described above. However, making medicated waters by agitation with an excess of volatile oil, permitting the excess to remain and drawing off the water as required, is not recommended. Volatile oils may deteriorate through exposure to light and air and, because of this, may yield unsatisfactory aromatic waters.

Certain waters are prepared by dissolving well-defined substances in purified water. Camphor water is a saturated solution of camphor in purified water. Chloroform water is prepared by adding enough chloroform to purified water (in a dark amber-colored bottle) to maintain a slight excess after the mixture has been thoroughly agitated. The latter water has been used as a sedative in cough, asthma, and colic mixtures and as a vehicle for administering active ingredients.

Aromatic waters may also be prepared by thoroughly incorporating the volatile oil with 15 g of talc or with a sufficient quantity of purified siliceous earth or pulped filter paper.

Purified water (1000 mL) is added and the mixture is agitated for 10 min. The water is then filtered (and, if necessary, re-filtered) and its volume adjusted to 1000 mL by passing purified water through the filter.

This is the process most frequently employed since the water can be prepared promptly, only 10 min of agitation being required. The use of talc, purified siliceous earth, or pulped filter paper greatly increases the surface of the volatile substance, insuring more rapid saturation of the water. These dispersing substances also form an efficient filter bed which produces a clear solution. They are also unreactive.

Other methods have been suggested for the preparation of aromatic waters. These are based on use of soluble concentrates or on incorporation of solubilizing agents such as polysorbate 20 (Tween 20, *Atlas*). However, such preparations are susceptible to mold growth and, in concentrations higher than 2%, impart an objectionable oily taste.

Concentrated waters (eg, peppermint, dill, cinnamon, caraway, and anise) may be prepared in the following manner.

Dissolve 20 mL of the volatile oil in 600 mL of 90% ethanol. Add sufficient purified water in successive small portions to produce 1000 mL solution. Shake vigorously after each addition. Add 50 g of sterilized purified talc, shake occasionally for several hours, and filter.

If anise concentrate is being prepared, the volume of ethanol must be increased to 700 mL.

The aromatic water is prepared by diluting the concentrate with 39 times its volume of water. In general, these methods yield aromatic waters that are slightly inferior in quality to those prepared by distillation or solution.

The chemical composition of many of the volatile oils used in the preparation of pharmaceuticals and cosmetics is now known. Similarly, many synthetic aromatic substances have a characteristic odor. For example, geranyl phenyl acetate has a honey odor. Such substances, either alone or in combination, can be used in nonofficial preparations and, by combining them in definite proportions, it is possible to produce substitutes for the officially recognized oil. Imitation Otto Rose (which contains phenylethyl alcohol, rhodinol, citronellol, and other ingredients) is an example of the types of substitutes which are now available.

Incompatibilities—The principal difficulty experienced in the compounding of prescriptions containing aromatic waters is due to a "salting out" action of certain ingredients, such as very soluble salts, on the volatile principle of the aromatic water. A replacement of part of the aromatic water with purified water is permissible when no other function is being served than that of a vehicle. Otherwise a dilution of the product with a suitable increase in dosage is indicated.

Preservation—Aromatic waters will deteriorate with time and should, therefore, be made in small quantities and protected from intense light and excessive heat, and stored in airtight, light-resistant containers. Deterioration may be due to volatilization, decomposition, or mold growth and will produce solutions that are cloudy and have lost all traces of their agreeable odor. Distilled water is usually contaminated with mold-producing organisms. *Recently* distilled and boiled water should, therefore, be used in the preparation of medicated waters. No preservative should be added to medicated waters. If they become cloudy or otherwise deteriorate, they should be discarded.

Aqueous Acids

The official inorganic acids and certain organic acids, although of minor significance as therapeutic agents, are of great importance in chemical and pharmaceutical manufacturing. This is especially true of acetic, hydrochloric, and nitric acids. The two latter acids, because of their relative completeness

of ionization, are termed strong acids. These acids, and especially the last is very caustic and corrosive.

The inorganic acids are generally divided into two groups: (1) the *hydracids*, which contain no oxygen, eg, hydriodic, hydrobromic, hydrochloric, and hydrofluoric acids and (2) the oxygen-containing acids, eg, hypophosphorous, nitric, phosphoric, and sulfuric acids.

Percentage Strengths—Many of the more important inorganic acids are available commercially in the form of concentrated aqueous solutions. The percentage strength varies from one acid to another and depends on the solubility and stability of the solute in water and on the manufacturing process. Thus, the official Hydrochloric Acid contains from 36.5 to 38% by weight of HCl, whereas Nitric Acid contains from 69 to 71% by weight of HNO_3.

Because the strengths of these concentrated acids are stated in terms of % by weight, it is essential that specific gravities also be provided if one is to be able to calculate conveniently the amount of absolute acid contained in a unit volume of the solution as purchased. The mathematical relationship involved is given by the equation $M = V \times S \times F$, wherein M is the mass in g of absolute acid contained in V mL of solution having a specific gravity S and a fractional percentage strength F. As an example, Hydrochloric Acid containing 36.93% by weight of HCl has a specific gravity of 1.1875. Therefore, the amount of absolute HCl supplied by 100 mL of this hydrochloric acid solution is given by:

$$M = 100 \times 1.1875 \times 0.3693 = 43.85 \text{ g HCl}$$

Incompatibilities—Although many of the reactions characteristic of acids offer opportunities for incompatibilities, only a few are of sufficient importance to require more than casual mention. Acids and acid salts decompose carbonates with liberation of carbon dioxide and, in a closed container, sufficient pressure may be developed to produce an explosion. Inorganic acids react with salts of organic acids to produce the free organic acid and a salt of the inorganic acid. If insoluble, the organic acid will be precipitated. Thus, salicylic acid and benzoic acid are precipitated from solutions of salicylates and benzoates. Boric acid is likewise precipitated from concentrated solutions of borates. By a similar reaction, certain soluble organic compounds are converted into an insoluble form. Sodium phenobarbital, for example, is converted into phenobarbital which in aqueous solution will precipitate.

The ability of acids to combine with alkaloids and other organic compounds containing a basic nitrogen atom is utilized in preparing soluble salts of these substances.

It should be borne in mind that certain solutions, syrups, elixirs, and other pharmaceutical preparations may contain free acid which causes these preparations to exhibit the incompatibilities of the acid.

Acids also possess the incompatibilities of the anions which they contain, and in the case of organic acids, these are frequently of prime importance. These are discussed under the specific anions.

Diluted Acids—The diluted acids in the US are aqueous solutions of acids, of a suitable strength (usually 10% *w/v* but Diluted Acetic Acid is 6% *w/v*) for internal administration or for the manufacture of other preparations.

The strengths of the official undiluted acids are expressed as percentages weight in weight whereas the strengths of the official diluted acids are expressed as percentages weight in volume. It therefore becomes necessary to consider the specific gravities of the concentrated acids when calculating the volume required to make a given quantity of diluted acid. The following equation will give the number of mL required to make 1000 mL of diluted acid:

$$\frac{\text{Strength of diluted acid} \times 1000}{\text{Strength of undiluted acid} \times \text{sp gr of undiluted acid}}$$

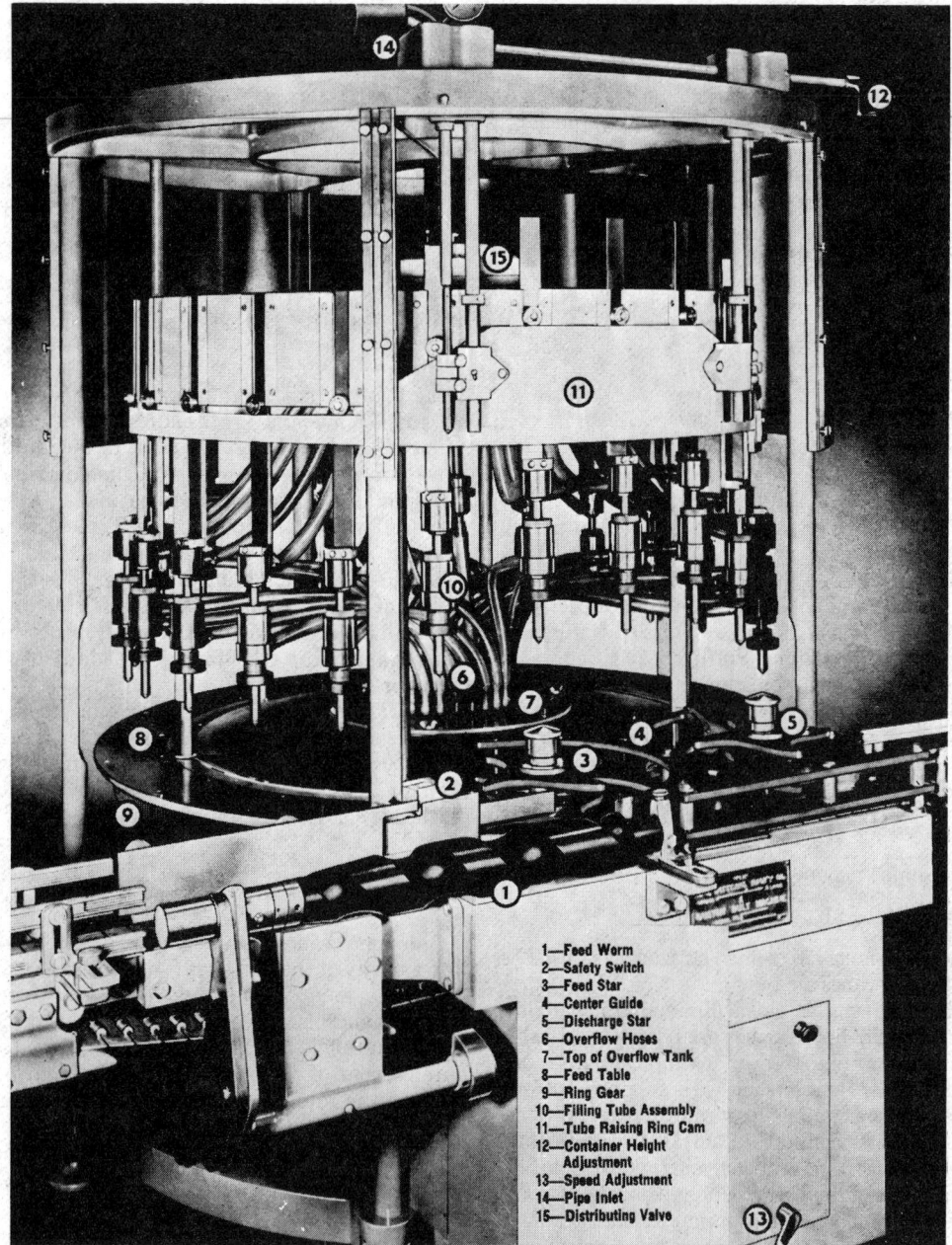

1—Feed Worm
2—Safety Switch
3—Feed Star
4—Center Guide
5—Discharge Star
6—Overflow Hoses
7—Top of Overflow Tank
8—Feed Table
9—Ring Gear
10—Filling Tube Assembly
11—Tube Raising Ring Cam
12—Container Height
       Adjustment
13—Speed Adjustment
14—Pipe Inlet
15—Distributing Valve

Fig 84-1.   A rotary gravity bottle filler (courtesy, US Bottlers).

Thus, if one wishes to make 1000 mL of Diluted Hydrochloric Acid USP using Hydrochloric Acid which assays 37.5% HCl (sp gr 1.18), the amount required is

$$\frac{10 \times 1000}{37.5 \times 1.18} = 226 \text{ mL}$$

One of these diluted acids, Diluted Hydrochloric Acid USP is used in the treatment of achlorhydria. However, it may irritate the mucous membrane of the mouth and attack the enamel of the teeth. The usual dose is 5 mL, well diluted with water. In the treatment of achlorhydria no attempt is made to administer more than a relief-producing dose. The normal pH of the gastric juice is 0.9 to 1.5 and, in order to attain this level, particularly in severe cases of gastric malfunction, somewhat larger doses of the acid would be required.

Solutions

A solution is a liquid preparation that contains one or more soluble chemical substances dissolved in water. The solute is usually nonvolatile. Solutions are used for the specific therapeutic effect of the solute, either internally or externally. Although the emphasis here is on the aqueous solution, certain preparations of this type (syrups, infusions, and decoctions) have distinctive characteristics and are, therefore, described later in the chapter.

Solvents, solubility, and general methods for the incorporation of a solute in a solvent are discussed in Chapter 16. Solutions are usually bottled automatically by utilizing equipment of the type shown in Fig 84-1.

Preparation—A specific method of preparation is given in the compendia for most solutions. These procedures fall into three main categories.

Simple Solutions—Solutions of this type are prepared by dissolving the solute in a suitable solvent. The solvent may contain other ingredients which stabilize or solubilize the active ingredient. Calcium Hydroxide Topical Solution (Lime Water), Sodium Phosphates Oral Solution, and Strong Iodine Solution are examples of solutions that are prepared in this way.

Calcium Hydroxide Topical Solution contains, in each 100 mL, not less than 140 mg of $Ca(OH)_2$. The solution is prepared by vigorously agitating 3 g of calcium hydroxide with 1000 mL cool, purified water. Excess calcium hydroxide is allowed to settle out and the clear, supernatant liquid is dispensed.

An increase in solvent temperature usually implies an increase in solute solubility. This rule does not apply, however, to the solubility of calcium hydroxide in water, which decreases with increase in temperature. The official solution is prepared at a temperature of 25°.

Solutions containing hydroxides react with the carbon dioxide in the atmosphere.

$$OH^- + CO_2 \rightarrow HCO_3^-$$

$$OH^- + HCO_3^- \rightarrow CO_3^{2-} + H_2O$$

$$Ca^{2+} + CO_3^{2-} \rightarrow CaCO_3$$

Calcium Hydroxide Topical Solution should, therefore, be preserved in well-filled, tight containers, at a temperature not exceeding 25°.

Strong Iodine Solution contains, in each 100 mL, 4.5–5.5 g of iodine, and 9.5–10.5 g of potassium iodide. It is prepared by dissolving 50 g of iodine in 100 mL of purified water containing 100 g of potassium iodide. Sufficient purified water is then added to make 1000 mL of solution.

One g of iodine dissolves in 2950 mL of water. However, solutions of iodides dissolve large quantities of iodine. Strong Iodine Solution is, therefore, a solution of polyiodides in excess iodide.

$$I^- + nI_2 \rightarrow I^-_{(2n+1)}$$

Doubly charged anions may be found also

$$2I^- + nI_2 \rightarrow I^{2-}_{(2n+2)}$$

Strong Iodine Solution is classified as an antigoitrogenic. The usual dose is 0.3 mL 3 times a day.

Several antibiotics, such as cloxacillin sodium, nafcillin sodium, and vancomycin, because they are relatively unstable in aqueous solution, are prepared by manufacturers as dry powders or granules in combination with suitable buffers, colors, diluents, dispersants, flavors and/or preservatives. These preparations, Cloxacillin Sodium for Oral Solution, Nafcillin for Oral Solution and Vancomycin for Oral Solution meet the requirements of the USP. Upon dispensing for the patient, the pharmacist adds the appropriate amount of water. The products are stable for a period of up to 14 days when stored under refrigeration. This period usually provides sufficient time for the patient to complete the administration of all the medication.

Solution by Chemical Reaction—These solutions are prepared by reacting two or more solutes with each other in a suitable solvent. An example of a solution of this type is Aluminum Subacetate Topical Solution.

Aluminum sulfate (145 g) is dissolved in 600 mL of cold water. The solution is filtered and precipitated calcium carbonate (70 g) is added, in several portions, with constant stirring. Acetic acid (160 mL) is slowly added and the mixture is set aside for 24 hr. The product is filtered and the magma on the Büchner filter is washed with cold water until the total filtrate measures 1000 mL.

The solution contains pentaquohydroxo- and tetraquo-dihydroxoaluminum (III) acetates and sulfates dissolved in an aqueous medium saturated with calcium sulfate. The solution contains a small amount of acetic acid. It is stabilized by the addition of not more than 0.9% boric acid.

The reactions involved in the preparation of the solution are given below. The hexaquo aluminum cations are first converted to the nonirritating $[Al(H_2O)_5(OH)]^{2+}$ and

$[Al(H_2O)_4(OH)_2]^+$ cations.

$$[Al(H_2O)_6]^{3+} + CO_3^{2-} \rightarrow [Al(H_2O)_5(OH)]^{2+} + HCO_3^-$$

$$[Al(H_2O)_6]^{3+} + HCO_3^- \rightarrow [Al(H_2O)_5(OH)]^{2+}$$
$$+ H_2O + CO_2$$

As the concentration of the hexaquo cations decreases, secondary reactions involving carbonate and bicarbonate occur.

$$[Al(H_2O)_5(OH)]^{2+} + CO_3^{2-} \rightarrow [Al(H_2O)_4(OH)_2]^+ + HCO_3^-$$

$$[Al(H_2O)_5(OH)]^{2+} + HCO_3^- \rightarrow [Al(H_2O)_4(OH)_2]^+$$
$$+ H_2CO_3$$

The pH of the solution now favors the precipitation of dissolved calcium ions as the insoluble sulfate. Acetic acid is now added. The bicarbonate which is formed in the final stages of the procedure is removed as carbon dioxide.

Aluminum Subacetate Topical Solution is used in the preparation of Aluminum Acetate Topical Solution (Burow's Solution). The latter solution contains 15 mL of glacial acetic acid, 545 mL of Aluminum Subacetate Topical Solution, and sufficient water to make 1000 mL. It is defined as a solution of aluminum acetate in approximately 5%, by weight, of acetic acid in water. It is stabilized by the addition of not more than 0.6% boric acid.

Solution by Extraction—Drugs or pharmaceutical necessities of vegetable or animal origin are often extracted with water or with water containing other substances. Preparations of this type may be classified as solutions but, more often, are classified as extracts.

Douches

A douche is an aqueous solution directed against a part or into a cavity of the body. It functions as a cleansing agent or antiseptic agent. An *eye douche*, used to remove foreign particles and discharges from the eyes, is directed gently at an oblique angle and is allowed to run from the inner to the outer corner of the eye. *Pharyngeal douches* are used to prepare the interior of the throat for an operation and to cleanse it in suppurative conditions. Similarly, there are *nasal douches* and *vaginal douches*. Douches are usually directed to the appropriate body part by using bulb syringes. These are described in Chapter 104.

Douches are most frequently dispensed in the form of a powder with directions for dissolving in a specified quantity of water, usually warm. However, tablets for preparing solutions are available (eg, Dobell's Solution Tablets) or the solution may be prepared by the pharmacist. If powders or tablets are supplied, they must be free from insoluble material, in order to produce a clear solution. Tablets are produced by the usual processes but any lubricants or diluents used must be readily soluble in water. Boric acid may be used as a lubricant and sodium chloride is normally used as a diluent. Tablets deteriorate on exposure to moist air and should be stored in airtight containers.

Preparations of this type may contain alum, zinc sulfate, boric acid, phenol, or sodium borate. The ingredients in one douche are alum (4 g), zinc sulfate (4 g), liquefied phenol (5 mL), glycerin (125 mL), and water (a sufficient quantity to make 1000 mL of solution). Sodium borate (borax, sodium tetraborate) is used in the preparation of Compound Sodium Borate Solution NF XI (Dobell's Solution). A solution of sodium borate in water is alkaline to litmus paper. In the presence of water, sodium metaborate, boric acid, and sodium hydroxide are formed.

$$Na_2B_4O_7 + 3H_2O \rightarrow 2NaBO_2 + 2H_3BO_3$$

$$NaBO_2 + 2H_2O \rightarrow NaOH + H_3BO_3$$

The official solution contains sodium borate, sodium bicarbonate, liquefied phenol, and glycerin. The reaction between boric acid and glycerin is given in the section on *Mouthwashes*. See also the section on *Honeys* for a discussion on the toxic manifestations associated with the topical application of boric acid and borax.

Douches are not official as a class of preparations but several substances in the compendia are frequently employed as such in weak solutions, eg, Benzalkonium Chloride is used in various douches and Compound Sodium Borate Solution is used as a nasal or pharyngeal douche. A sodium bicarbonate vaginal douche has been used to improve the postcoital test.

Vaginal or urethral douches are occasionally referred to as Irrigations. These solutions may have an antiseptic, astringent, or soothing action and are prepared immediately before use by dissolving the medicament in the required amount of water. One example of such a preparation is Irrigation of Lactic Acid BPC 1963. This solution contains 3.75 mL of lactic acid in every 600 mL of aqueous product. There are a number of irrigations described in the USP: Acetic Acid Irrigation for bladder irrigation, Aminoacetic Acid Irrigation for urethral surgery, and Sodium Chloride Irrigation for washing wounds. These solutions are sterile and meet the same stringent standards used for parenteral preparations because they are used in areas of the body where it is essential that no microorganisms be introduced.

Enemas

Evacuation enemas are rectal injections employed to evacuate the bowel, retention enemas to influence the general system by absorption, or to affect locally the seat of disease. They may possess anthelmintic, nutritive, sedative, or stimulating properties, or they may contain radiopaque substances for roentgenographic examination of the lower bowel. Some official enemas are those of aminophylline, hydrocortisone, and methylprednisolone acetate. Enemas are usually given at body temperature in quantities of 1 to 2 pt injected slowly with a syringe. If they are to be retained in the intestine, they should not be used in larger quantities than 6 fluid ounces for an adult.

Starch enema may be used either by itself or as a vehicle for other forms of medication. A thin paste is made by triturating 30 g of powdered starch with 200 mL of cold water. Sufficient boiling water is added to make 1000 mL of enema. The preparation is then reheated to obtain a transparent liquid.

Barium sulfate enema contains 120 g of barium sulfate, 100 mL of acacia mucilage, and sufficient starch enema to make 500 mL.

Sodium chloride, sodium bicarbonate, sodium monohydrogen phosphate, and sodium dihydrogen phosphate are used in enemas. These substances may be used alone, in combination with each other, or in combination with irritants such as soap. Enema of Soap BPC 1963 is prepared by dissolving 50 g of soft soap in sufficient purified water to make 1000 mL of enema. Fleet Enema, a commercially available enema containing 16 g of sodium acid phosphate and 6 g of sodium phosphate in 100 mL, is marketed as a single-dose disposable unit. Sulfasalazine rectal enema has been administered for the treatment of ulcerative colitis and may be prepared by dispersing the tablets (1 g strength) in 250 mL water.

Gargles

Gargles are aqueous solutions used for treating the pharynx and nasopharynx by forcing air from the lungs through the gargle which is held in the throat. Many gargles must be diluted with water prior to use. Although mouthwashes are considered as a separate class of pharmaceuticals, many are used as gargles, either as is or diluted with water.

Phenol Gargle, and Potassium Chlorate and Phenol Gargle are official in the BPC. The former gargle contains 50 mL of phenol glycerin (16% *w/w* phenol and 84% *w/w* glycerin), 10 mL of amaranth solution (1% *w/v* in chloroform water), and water to make 1000 mL. This gargle should be diluted with an equal volume of warm water before use. The product should be so labeled that it cannot be mistaken for preparations intended for internal administration.

A flavored solution containing 1% povidone-iodine USP and 8% alcohol is commercially available as a mouthwash or gargle.

Mouthwashes

A mouthwash is an aqueous solution which is most often used for its deodorant, refreshing, or antiseptic effect. It may contain alcohol, glycerin, synthetic sweeteners, and surface-active, flavoring, and coloring agents. Commercial preparations contain such local anti-infective agents as hexetidine and cetylpyridinium chloride. They may be either acidic or basic in reaction and, in some instances, are fairly effective in reducing bacterial concentrations and odors in the mouth for short periods of time.

The products of commerce (eg, Cepacol, Listerine, Micrin, Scope, etc) vary widely in composition. Compound Sodium Borate Solution NF XI (Dobell's Solution) is used as an antiseptic mouthwash and gargle. Antiseptic Solution and Mouthwash are described in NF XII. The latter wash contains sodium borate, glycerin, and potassium bicarbonate. The reactions which take place when these substances are dissolved in water are given below.

$$2\underset{\substack{|\\CH_2OH}}{\overset{\substack{CH_2OH\\|}}{CHOH}} + B(OH)_3 \rightarrow \left[\begin{array}{cc} CH_2OH & HOCH_2 \\ | & | \\ CH\!-\!O \quad\quad O\!-\!CH \\ \diagdown \quad \diagup \\ B \\ \diagup \quad \diagdown \\ CH_2\!-\!O \quad\quad O\!-\!CH_2 \\ | & | \end{array}\right]^- H^+ + 3H_2O$$

$$\left[\begin{array}{cc} CH_2OH & HOCH_2 \\ | & | \\ CH\!-\!O \quad\quad O\!-\!CH \\ \diagdown \quad \diagup \\ B \\ \diagup \quad \diagdown \\ CH_2O \quad\quad O\!-\!CH_2 \\ | & | \end{array}\right]^- K^+ \leftarrow \overset{KHCO_3}{\underset{}{}}$$
$$+ H_2O + CO_2$$

Compound Sodium Chloride Mouthwash, and Zinc Sulphate and Zinc Chloride Mouthwash are described in the BPC. The former wash contains sodium chloride, sodium bicarbonate, concentrated peppermint emulsion, and double-strength chloroform water; the latter, zinc sulfate, and amaranth solution.

Mouthwashes may be used for a number of purposes: for example, cetylpyridinum chloride and dibucaine hydrochloride mouthwashes provide satisfactory relief of pain in patients with ulcerative lesions of the mouth, mouthwashes or creams containing carbenoxolone are highly effective dosage forms for the treatment of orofacial herpes simplex infections, and undetected oral cancer has been detected using toluidine blue in the form of a mouth rinse.

Juices

A juice is prepared from fresh ripe fruit, is aqueous in character, and is used in making syrups which are employed as vehicles. The freshly expressed juice is preserved with benzoic acid, and is allowed to stand at room temperature for several days, until the pectins which are naturally present are destroyed by enzymatic action, as indicated by the filtered juice yielding a clear solution with alcohol. Pectins, if allowed to remain, would cause precipitation in the final syrup.

Cherry Juice is described in the USP, and Raspberry Juice in USP XVIII. Concentrated Raspberry Juice BPC is prepared from the clarified juice of raspberries. Pectinase is stirred into pulped raspberries and the mixture is allowed to stand for 12 hours. The pulp is pressed, the juice is clarified, and sufficient sucrose is added to adjust the weight per mL at 20° to 1.050–1.060 g. The juice is then concentrated to one-sixth of its original volume. Sufficient sulfurous acid or sodium metabisulfite is added to preserve the juice.

Artificial flavors have now replaced many of the natural fruit juices. Although they lack the flavor of the natural juice, they are more stable and are easier to incorporate into the final pharmaceutical form.

Recent information on cranberry juice indicates that it may be effective in controlling some urinary tract infections and urolithiosis.

Nasal Solutions

Nasal solutions are usually aqueous solutions which are designed to be administered to the nasal passages in drops or spray form. While many of the drugs are administered for their local sympathomimetic effect such as Ephedrine Sulfate or Naphazoline Hydrochloride Nasal Solution, to reduce nasal congestion, a few other official preparations, Lypressin Nasal Solution and Oxytocin Nasal Solution are administered in spray form for systemic effect for the treatment of diabetes insipidus and *milk let down* prior to breast feeding, respectively.

Nasal solutions are prepared in such a way that they are similar in many respects to nasal secretions so that normal ciliary action is maintained. Thus the aqueous nasal solutions are usually isotonic and slightly buffered to maintain a pH of 5.5 to 6.5. In addition, antimicrobial preservatives similar to those used in ophthalmic preparations, and appropriate drug stabilizers, if required, are included in the formulation.

Commercial nasal preparations, in addition to the drugs listed above also include antibiotics, antihistamines and drugs for asthma prophylaxis.

A formula for Ephedrine Nasal Drops BPC is:

Ephedrine Hydrochloride	0.5 g
Chlorobutanol	0.5 g
Sodium Chloride	0.5 g
Water for preparations	to 100 mL

Otic Solutions

These solutions are occasionally referred to as aural preparations. Other otic preparations also often include formulations such as suspensions and ointments for topical application in the ear.

The main classes of drugs used for topical administration to the ear include analgesics, eg, benzocaine; antibiotics, eg, neomycin, and anti-inflammatory agents, eg, cortisone. The USP preparations include Glycerin Otic Solution which incorporates the drugs antipyrine and benzocaine in a glycerin solvent. The Neomycin and Polymyxin B Sulfates and Cortisol Otic Solutions contain appropriate buffers, dispersants usually in an aqueous solution. These otic preparations include the main types of solvents used, namely glycerin or water. The viscous glycerin vehicle, permits the drug to remain in the ear for a long time. Anhydrous glycerin being hygroscopic tends to remove moisture from surrounding tissues thus reducing swelling.

In order to provide sufficient time for aqueous preparations to act, it is necessary for the patient to remain on his side for a few minutes so the drops do not run out of the ear. Otic preparations are dispensed in a container which permits the administration of drops.

Sweet or Other Viscid Aqueous Solutions

Solutions which are sweet or viscid include Syrups, Honeys, Mucilages, and Jellies. All of these preparations are viscous liquids or semisolids. The basic sweet or viscid substances giving body to these preparations are sugars, polyols, or polysaccharides (gums).

Syrups

Syrups are concentrated solutions of a sugar such as sucrose in water or other aqueous liquid. When Purified Water alone is used in making the solution of sucrose, the preparation is known as *Syrup,* or *simple syrup*. In addition to sucrose, certain other polyols, such as glycerin or sorbitol, may be added to retard crystallization of sucrose or to increase the solubility of added ingredients. Alcohol is often included as a preservative and also as a solvent for flavors; further resistance to microbial attack can be enhanced by incorporating antimicrobial agents. When the aqueous preparation contains some added medicinal substance, the syrup is called a *medicated* syrup. A *flavored* syrup is one which is usually not medicated, but which contains various aromatic or pleasantly flavored substances and is intended to be used as a vehicle or flavor for prescriptions.

Flavored syrups offer unusual opportunities as vehicles in extemporaneous compounding and are readily accepted by both children and adults. Because they contain no or very little alcohol, they are vehicles of choice for many of the drugs that are prescribed by pediatricians. Their lack of alcohol makes them superior solvents for water-soluble substances. However sucrose based medicines continuously administered to children apparently cause an increase in dental caries and gingivitis; consequently, alternate formulations of the drug either unsweetened or sweetened with non-cariogenic substances should be considered. A knowledge of the sugar content of liquid medicines is useful for patients who are on a restricted calorie intake; such a list may be found in the literature[6].

Syrups possess remarkable masking properties for bitter and saline drugs. Glycyrrhiza Syrup has been recommended for disguising the salty taste of bromides, iodides, and chlorides. This has been attributed to its colloidal character and to its double sweetness—the immediate sweetness of the sugar and the lingering sweetness of the glycyrrhizin. This syrup is also of value in masking bitterness in preparations containing the B complex vitamins. Acacia Syrup, because of its colloidal character, is of particular value as a vehicle for masking the disagreeable taste of many medicaments. Raspberry Syrup is one of the most efficient flavoring agents and is especially useful in masking the taste of bitter drugs. Many factors, however, enter into the choice of a suitable flavoring agent. Literature reports are often contradictory and there appears to be no substitute for the taste panel. The literature on this subject has been reviewed by Meer,[7] and this reference and Chapter 68 should be consulted for further information on the flavoring of pharmaceuticals and the preparation of a number of official syrups. A series of papers is available in improving the palatability of bulk compounded products using flavoring and sweetening agents.[8]

In manufacturing syrups the sucrose must be carefully selected and a purified water, free from foreign substances, and clean vessels and containers must be used. The operation must be conducted with care so as to avoid contamination, if the products are to be stable preparations.

It is important that the concentration of sucrose approach but not quite reach the saturation point. In dilute solutions sucrose provides an excellent nutrient for molds, yeasts, and other microorganisms. In concentrations of 65% by weight or more, the solution will retard the growth of such microorganisms. However, a saturated solution may lead to crystallization of a part of the sucrose under conditions of changing temperature.

When heat is used in the preparation of syrups, there is almost certain to be an inversion of a slight portion of the sucrose.

$$C_{12}H_{22}O_{11} + H_2O \rightarrow 2C_6H_{12}O_6$$
$$\underset{\text{Sucrose}}{} \qquad \underset{\text{Invert sugar}}{}$$

Sucrose solutions rotate polarized light to the right but, as hydrolysis proceeds, the optical rotation decreases and becomes negative when the reaction is complete. This reaction is termed *inversion* because *invert sugar* (dextrose plus levulose) is formed. The speed of inversion is greatly increased by the presence of acids; the hydrogen ion acts as a catalyst in this hydrolytic reaction. Invert sugar is more readily fermentable than sucrose and tends to darken in color. Nevertheless its two reducing sugars are of value in retarding the oxidation of other substances.

Invert Syrup is described in the BPC. The syrup is prepared by hydrolyzing sucrose with hydrochloric acid and neutralizing the solution with calcium or sodium carbonate. The sucrose in the 66.7% *w/w* solution must be at least 95% inverted. The monograph states that invert syrup, when mixed in suitable proportions with syrup, prevents the deposition of crystals of sucrose under most conditions of storage.

The levulose formed during inversion is sweeter than sucrose and therefore the resulting syrup is sweeter than the original syrup. The relative sweetness of levulose, sucrose, and dextrose is in the ratio 173:100:74. Thus invert sugar is $1/100 (173 + 74)^{1/2} = 1.23$ times as sweet as sucrose. The levulose formed during the hydrolysis is also responsible for the darkening of syrup. It is sensitive to heat and darkens readily, particularly in solution. When syrup or sucrose is overheated, it caramelizes. See *Caramel* (page 1282). Occasionally it is appropriate to use a sugar free liquid preparation, a list of these has recently been published.[9]

Preparation—Syrups are prepared in various ways, the choice of the proper method depending on the physical and chemical characteristics of the substances entering into the preparation. Four methods which are employed may be summarized as follows: (1) solution with heat; (2) agitation without heat; (3) addition of a medicating liquid to syrup; and (4) percolation.

Solution with Heat—This is the usual method of making syrups when the valuable constituent is neither volatile nor injured by heat, and when it is desirable to make the syrup rapidly. The sucrose is usually added to the purified water or aqueous solution and heated until solution is effected, then strained, and sufficient purified water added to make the desired weight or volume. If the syrup is made from an infusion, a decoction, or an aqueous solution containing organic matter, it is usually proper to heat the syrup to the boiling point to coagulate albuminous matter; this is separated subsequently by straining. If the albumin or other impurities were permitted to remain in the syrup, fermentation would probably be induced in warm weather. Saccharometers are very useful in making syrups by the hot process in cases where the proper specific gravity of the finished syrup is known. The saccharometer may be floated in the syrup while boiling, and thus the exact degree of concentration determined without waiting to cool the syrup and having to heat it again to concentrate it further. When taking a reading of the specific gravity of the hot syrup allowance must be made for the variation from the official temperature (specific gravities in the USP are taken at 25°).

Excessive heating of syrups at the boiling temperature is undesirable since more or less inversion of the sucrose occurs with an increased tendency to ferment. Syrups cannot be sterilized in an autoclave without some caramelization. This is indicated by a yellowish or brownish color resulting from the formation of caramel, by the action of heat upon sucrose.

The formula and procedure given for Acacia Syrup (page 1293) illustrate this method of preparation.

Agitation without Heat—This process is used in those cases where heat would cause the loss of valuable volatile constituents. In making quantities up to 2000 mL the sucrose should be added to the aqueous solution in a bottle of about twice the size required for the syrup. This permits active agitation and rapid solution. Stoppering of the bottle is important, as it prevents contamination and loss during the process. The bottle should be allowed to lie on its side when not being agitated. Glass-lined tanks with mechanical agitators, especially adapted to dissolving of sucrose, are used for making syrups in large quantities.

This method and that previously described are used for the preparation of a wide variety of preparations that are popularly described as syrups. Most cough syrups, for example, contain sucrose and one or more active ingredients. However, the exact composition of such products is not given on the label. Furthermore, some of these products are listed in the compendium but no directions are given for their preparation. For example, Guaifenesin Syrup (glyceryl guaiacolate syrup) is official but the only known ingredients are guaifenesin (glyceryl guaiacolate) and ethanol (not less than 3% or more than 4%).

The BPC, on the other hand, gives a method for the preparation of Codeine Phosphate Syrup. This product contains codeine phosphate (5 g), purified water (15 mL), chloroform spirit (25 mL), and sufficient syrup to make 1000 mL. It can be used for the relief of cough but the official cough syrup in the BPC is Codeine Linctus. This linctus is really a medicated syrup which possesses demulcent, expectorant, or sedative properties. Unlike the syrup, it is colored and flavored. The formula for Codeine Linctus BPC is:

Codeine Phosphate	3 g
Compound Tartrazine Solution	10 mL
Benzoic Acid Solution	20 mL
Chloroform Spirit	20 mL
Water	20 mL
Lemon Syrup	200 mL
Syrup	to 1000 mL

Dissolve the codeine phosphate in the water, add 500 mL of the syrup, and mix. Add the other ingredients and sufficient syrup to produce 1000 mL.

For pediatric use, 200 mL of this linctus is diluted with sufficient syrup to make 1000 mL. If sugar is contraindicated in the diet, Diabetic Codeine Linctus can be used:

Codeine Phosphate	3 g
Citric Acid	5 g
Lemon Spirit	1 mL
Compound Tartrazine Solution	10 mL
Benzoic Acid Solution	20 mL
Chloroform Spirit	20 mL
Water	20 mL
Sorbitol Solution	to 1000 mL

Dissolve the codeine phosphate and the citric acid in the water, add 750 mL of the sorbitol solution, and mix. Add the other ingredients and sufficient sorbitol solution to produce 1000 mL.

Sorbitol Solution is the sweetening agent and contains 70% *w/w* of total solids, consisting mainly of D-sorbitol. It has about half the sweetening power of syrup.[10]

Basic formulations can easily be varied to produce the highly advertised articles of commerce. The prescription-only drug (eg, codeine phosphate, methadone, etc) must, of course, be omitted from the formulation but, in certain countries, such as Canada, a decreased quantity of codeine phosphate is permitted in the OTC cough syrup. In addition to the ingredients cited or listed in the official compendia (eg, tolu, squill, ipecacuanha, etc), many cough syrups contain an antihistamine.

Many other active ingredients (eg, ephedrine sulfate, dicyclomine hydrochloride, chloral hydrate, chlorpromazine hydrochloride, etc) are marketed as syrups. Like the cough syrups, these preparations are flavored and colored and are recommended in those instances where the patient cannot swallow the solid dosage form. An example of such a preparation is Ephedrine Sulfate Syrup USP XVIII. Besides the active ingredient, the syrup contains citric acid, amaranth solution, caramel, lemon and orange oils, benzaldehyde, vanillin, ethanol, and sucrose. Amaranth has been banned as an ingredient in manufactured products in a number of countries, including the US.

Addition of a Medicating Liquid to Syrup—This method is resorted to in those cases in which fluidextracts, tinctures, or other liquids are added to syrup to medicate it. Syrups made in this way usually develop precipitates since alcohol is often an ingredient of the liquids thus used, and the resinous and oily substances dissolved by the alcohol precipitate when mixed with the syrup, producing unsightly preparations. A modification of this process, frequently adopted, consists of mixing the fluidextract or tincture with the water, allowing the mixture to stand to permit the separation of insoluble constituents, filtering, and then dissolving the sucrose in the filtrate. It is obvious that this procedure is not permissible when the precipitated ingredients are the valuable medicinal agents.

The formula and procedure given for Aromatic Eriodictyon Syrup (page 1293) illustrate this method of preparation.

Percolation—In this procedure, purified water or an aqueous solution is permitted to pass slowly through a bed of crystalline sucrose, thus dissolving it and forming a syrup. A pledget of cotton is placed in the neck of the percolator and the water or aqueous solution added. By means of a suitable stopcock the flow is regulated so that drops appear in rapid succession. If necessary, a portion of the liquid is repassed through the percolator to dissolve all of the sucrose. Finally, sufficient purified water is passed through the cotton to make the required volume.

To be successful in using this process, care in several particulars must be exercised: (1) the percolator used should be cylindrical or semicylindrical, and cone-shaped as it nears the lower orifice; (2) a coarse granular sugar must be used, otherwise it will form into a compact mass, which the liquid cannot permeate; (3) the purified cotton must be introduced with care. If pressed in too tightly, it will effectually stop the process; if inserted too loosely, the liquid will pass through the cotton rapidly and the filtrate will be weak and turbid (from imperfect filtration); it should be inserted completely within the neck of the percolator, since a protruding end, inside the percolator, up through the sucrose, will permit the last portions of water to pass out at the lower orifice without dissolving all of the sucrose. For specific directions see *Syrup* (page 1500). The process of percolation is applied on a commercial scale for the making of official syrups as well as those for confectionary use.

Percolation is the preferred method for the preparation of Syrup USP (page 1293). The sucrose, in this instance, is placed in the percolator. However, a slightly modified approach must be used if a drug of vegetable origin is to be incorporated into the syrup. For example, wild cherry bark is first percolated with water; the collection vessel contains sucrose (800 g) and glycerol (50 mL). When the total volume is 1000 mL, the percolate is agitated to produce Wild Cherry Syrup BPC.

Preservation—Syrups should not be made in larger quantities than can be used within a few months, except in those cases where special facilities can be employed for their preservation. A low temperature is the best method of preservation for syrups. The USP indicates that syrups not be exposed to excessive heat. Concentration without supersaturation is also a condition favorable to preservation. The USP states that syrups may contain preservatives to prevent bacterial and mold growth. Preservatives such as glycerin, methylparaben, benzoic acid, and sodium benzoate may be added, particularly when the concentration of sucrose in the syrup is low. Combinations of alkyl esters of *p*-hydroxybenzoic acid are effective inhibitors of yeasts which have been implicated in the contamination of commercial syrups.[11] Any attempt to restore syrups which have been spoiled through fermentation by heating them and "working them over" is reprehensible.

The official syrups should be preserved in well-dried bottles, preferably those which have been sterilized. These bottles should not hold more than is likely to be required during four to six weeks and should be completely filled, carefully stoppered, and stored in a cool, dark place.

Syrups Prepared from Juices

Blackberry syrup, pineapple syrup, and strawberry syrup may be prepared by following the directions given in the BPC for Raspberry Syrup. One volume of the concentrated raspberry juice is diluted with 11 volumes of syrup. Syrup of Black Currant BPC is prepared in a similar manner but with certain modifications. The pectin in the juice is destroyed with pectinase. The syrup is prepared from 700 g of sucrose and 560 mL of clarified juice and is preserved with sulfurous acid or sodium metabisulfite. The addition of a dye is permitted, provided it complies with the pertinent government regulations. Cherry Syrup USP is prepared from cherry juice by the addition of alcohol, sucrose, and water (page 1293).

Honeys

Honeys are thick liquid preparations somewhat allied to the syrups, differing in the use of honey, instead of syrup, as a base. They are unimportant as a class of preparations today but at one time, before sugar was available and honey was the most common sweetening agent, they were widely used. BPC lists two preparations containing honey. The first, Oxymel, or "acid honey," is a mixture of acetic acid (150 mL), purified water (150 mL), and honey (sufficient to produce 1000 mL of product). Squill Oxymel contains squill, water, acetic acid, and honey and is prepared by a maceration process.

One nonofficial preparation contains borax (10.5 g), glycerin (5.25 g), and sufficient honey to make 1000 g. It has been indicated that this type of product can cause serious boric acid intoxication in babies. It should not be used in pharmaceutical practice.

Mucilages

The official mucilages are thick, viscid, adhesive liquids, produced by dispersing gum in water, or by extracting with water the mucilaginous principles from vegetable substances. The mucilages are all prone to decomposition, showing appreciable decrease in viscosity on storage; they should never be made in larger quantities than can be used immediately, unless a preservative is added. Acacia Mucilage NF XII contains benzoic acid and Tragacanth Mucilage BPC (1973) contains alcohol and chloroform water. Chloroform in manufactured products for internal use is banned in some countries.

The former mucilage may be prepared by placing 350 g of acacia in a graduated bottle, washing the drug with cold purified water, allowing it to drain, and adding enough warm purified water, in which 2 g of benzoic acid has been dissolved, to make the product measure 1000 mL. The bottle is then stoppered, placed on its side, rotated occasionally, and the product is strained when the acacia has dissolved.

Tragacanth Mucilage BPC (1973) is prepared by mixing 12.5 g of tragacanth with 25 mL alcohol (90%) in a dry bottle and then adding quickly sufficient chloroform water to 1000 mL and shaking vigorously. The alcohol is used to disperse the gum to prevent agglomeration on addition of the water.

Mucilages are used primarily to aid in suspending insoluble substances in liquids; their colloidal character and viscosity help them prevent immediate sedimentation. Examples include sulfur in lotions, resin in mixtures, and oils in emulsions. Both tragacanth and acacia are either partially or completely insoluble in alcohol. Tragacanth is precipitated from solution by alcohol, but acacia, on the other hand, is soluble in diluted alcoholic solutions. A 60% solution of acacia may be prepared with 20% alcohol, and a 4% solution of acacia may be prepared even with 50% alcohol.

The viscosity of tragacanth mucilage is reduced by acid, alkali, and sodium chloride, particularly if the mucilage is heated. It shows maximum viscosity at a pH of 5. Acacia is hydrolyzed by dilute mineral acids to arabinose, galactose, aldobionic and galacturonic acids. Its viscosity is low but is maintained over a wide pH range.

Several synthetic mucilage-like substances such as *polyvinyl alcohol*, *methylcellulose*, *carboxymethylcellulose*, and related substances, as described in Chapter 68, are used as mucilage substitutes, emulsifying and suspending agents. Methylcellulose (page 1297) is widely used as a bulk laxative since it absorbs water and swells to a hydrogel in the intestine in much the same manner as *psyllium* or *karaya gum*. Methylcellulose Oral Solution is a flavored solution of the agent. The solution may be prepared by slowly adding the methylcellulose to about one-third the amount of water, boiling, with stirring until it is thoroughly wetted. Cold water should then be added and the wetted material allowed to dissolve while stirring. The viscosity of the solution will depend upon the concentration and the specifications of the methylcellulose. The synthetic gums are nonglycogenetic and may be used in the preparation of diabetic syrups. Several formulas for such syrups, based on sodium carboxymethylcellulose, have been proposed.

Jellies

Jellies are a class of gels in which the structural coherent matrix contains a high portion of liquid, usually water. They are similar to mucilages, in that they may be prepared from gums similar to those used for mucilage, but they differ from the latter in having a jelly-like consistency. A whole gum of the best quality rather than a powdered gum is desirable in order to obtain a clear preparation of uniform consistency. Tragacanth is the gum used in the preparation of Ephedrine Sulfate Jelly NF XII. These preparations may also be formulated from acacia, chondrus, gelatin, carboxymethylcellulose, and similar substances, with water.

Jellies are used as lubricants for surgical gloves, catheters, and rectal thermometers. Lidocaine Hydrochloride Jelly USP is used as a topical anesthetic. Therapeutic vaginal jellies are available and certain jelly-like preparations are used for contraceptive purposes. The latter preparations often contain surface-active agents to enhance the spermatocidal properties of the jelly. Aromatics, such as methyl salicylate and eucalyptol, are often added to give the preparation a desirable odor.

Jellies are prone to microbial contamination and therefore contain preservatives, eg, methyl *p*-hydroxybenzoate is used as a preservative in a base for medicated jellies. This base contains sodium alginate, glycerin, calcium gluconate, and water. The calcium ions cause a cross-linking with sodium alginate to form a gel of firmer consistency.[12] A discussion of gels is provided later in the chapter.

Nonaqueous Solutions

It is difficult to evaluate fairly the importance of nonaqueous solvents in pharmaceutical processes. That they are important in the manufacture of pharmaceuticals is an understatement. However, pharmaceutical preparations, and, in particular, those intended for internal use, rarely contain more than minor quantities of the organic solvents that are common to the manufacturing or analytical operation. For example, industry uses large quantities of chloroform in some operations but the solvent is of only minor importance with respect to the final product. One mL of chloroform dissolves in about 200 mL of water and the solution so formed finds some use as a vehicle (see the section on *Aromatic Waters*). Chloroform has been an ingredient in a number of cough syrups but in some countries it has been banned in manufactured products intended for internal use. Solvents such as acetone, benzene, and petroleum ether should not be ingredients in preparations intended for internal use.

Products of commerce may contain solvents such as ethanol, glycerin, propylene glycol, certain oils, and liquid paraffin. Preparations intended for external use may contain ethanol, methanol, isopropyl alcohol, polyethylene glycols, various ethers, and certain esters. A good example of preparations of this type are the rubefacient rubbing alcohols. Rubbing Alcohol must be manufactured in accordance with the requirements of the Bureau of Alcohol, Tobacco, and Firearms, US Treasury Dept., using Formula 23-H. This mixture contains 8 parts by volume of acetone, 1.5 parts by volume of methyl isobutyl ketone, and 100 parts by volume of ethanol. Besides the alcohol in the Rubbing Alcohol, the final product must contain water, sucrose octaacetate or denatonium benzoate and may contain color additives, perfume oils, and a suitable stabilizer. The alcohol content, by volume, is not less than 68.5% and not more than 71.5%. The isopropyl alcohol content in Isopropyl Rubbing Alcohol can vary from 68.0% to 72.0% and the finished product may contain color additives, perfume oils, and suitable stabilizers.

Although the lines between aqueous and nonaqueous preparations tend to blur in those cases where the solvent is water-soluble, it is possible to categorize a number of products as nonaqueous. This section is, therefore, devoted to five groups of nonaqueous solutions; the first includes the alcoholic or hydroalcoholic solutions, examples of these being elixirs and spirits; the second, the ethereal solutions, an example being the collodions; the third, the glycerin solutions, as exemplified by the glycerins; the oleaginous solutions, as represented by the liniments, oleovitamins, toothache drops, inhalations, and inhalants.

Although the above list is self-limiting, a wide variety of solvents are used in various pharmaceutical preparations. Solvents such as glycerol formal, dimethylacetamide, and glycerol dimethylketal have been recommended for many of the products produced by the industry. However, the toxicity of many of these solvents is not well established and, for this reason, careful clinical studies should be carried out on the formulated product before it is released to the marketplace.

Collodions

Collodions are liquid preparations containing pyroxylin (a nitrocellulose) in a mixture of ethyl ether and ethanol. They are applied to the skin by means of a soft brush or other suitable applicator and, when the ether and ethanol have evaporated, leave a film of pyroxylin on the surface. The official medicated collodion, Salicylic Acid Collodion USP, contains 10% w/v of salicylic acid in Flexible Collodion USP and is used as a keratolytic agent in the treatment of corns and warts. Collodion USP and Flexible Collodion USP are water-repellent protectives for minor cuts and scratches. Collodion is made flexible by the addition of castor oil and camphor. Collodion has been used to reduce or eliminate the side effects of fluorouracil treatment of solar keratoses.

Elixirs

Elixirs are clear, pleasantly flavored, sweetened hydroalcoholic liquids intended for oral use. They are used as flavors and vehicles such as Aromatic Elixir (page 1294) for drug substances and, when such substances are incorporated into the specified solvents, they are classified as medicated elixirs, eg, Dexamethasone Elixir USP and Phenobarbital Elixir USP. The main ingredients in the elixir are ethanol and water but glycerin, sorbitol, propylene glycol, flavoring agents, preservatives, and syrups are often used in the preparation of the final product.

The distinction between some of the medicated syrups and elixirs is not always clear. For example, Ephedrine Sulfate Syrup USP contains between 20 and 40 mL of alcohol in 1000 mL of product. Ephedrine Elixir BPC contains syrup and 100 mL of ethanol in the same final volume. Definitions are, therefore, inconsistent and, in some instances, not too important with respect to the naming of the articles of commerce. The exact composition must, however, be known if the presence or absence of an ingredient (eg, sucrose) is of therapeutic significance or when an additional ingredient must be incorporated in the product.

Elixirs contain ethyl alcohol. However, the alcoholic content will vary greatly, from elixirs containing only a small quantity, to those that contain a considerable portion as a necessary aid to solubility. For example, Aromatic Elixir USP contains 21 to 23% C_2H_5OH; Compound Benzaldehyde Elixir, on the other hand, contains 3 to 5% C_2H_5OH.

Elixirs may also contain glycerin and syrup. These may be added to increase the solubility of the medicinal agent or for sweetening purposes. Some elixirs contain propylene glycol. Claims have been made that this solvent is a satisfactory substitute for both glycerin and alcohol. Sumner,[13] in his paper on terpin hydrate preparations, summarized the advantages and disadvantages of this solvent and suggested several formulations with therapeutic characteristics superior to those of the elixir described in NF XIII.

One usual dose of the elixir (5 mL) contains 85 mg of terpin hydrate. This substance is used in bronchitis in doses of 125 to 300 mg as an expectorant. The elixir is, therefore, ineffective for the treatment of bronchitis. However, the elixir is used as a vehicle for the drugs in many commercially available cough syrups. These may contain dextromethorphan hydrobromide, codeine phosphate, chlorpheniramine maleate, pyrilamine maleate, ammonium chloride, creosote, chloroform, and a wide variety of other drugs with expectorant and antitussive properties.

One of the four formulations described in Sumner's paper is given below:

Terpin Hydrate	6.0 g
Orange Oil	0.1 mL
Benzaldehyde	0.005 mL
Sorbitol Solution USP	10.0 mL
Propylene Glycol	40.0 mL
Alcohol	43.0 mL
Purified Water, a sufficient quantity, to make	100.0 mL

Dissolve the terpin hydrate in the propylene glycol and sorbitol solution which have been heated to 50°. Add the oil and the benzaldehyde to the alcohol and mix with the terpin hydrate solution at 25°. Add sufficient purified water to make the product measure 100 mL.

The elixir contains 300 mg of terpin hydrate/5 mL, a minimal quantity of alcohol, and flavoring agents which adequately mask the taste of propylene glycol.

Although alcohol is an excellent solvent for some drugs, it does accentuate the saline taste of bromides and similar salts. It is often desirable, therefore, to substitute some other solvent that is more effective in masking such tastes for part of the alcohol in the formula. In general, if taste is a consideration, the formulator is more prone to utilize a syrup rather than a hydroalcoholic vehicle.

An elixir may contain water and alcohol soluble ingredients. If such is the case, the following procedure is indicated:

Dissolve the water-soluble ingredients in part of the water. Add and solubilize the sucrose in the aqueous solution. Prepare an alcoholic solution containing the other ingredients. Add the aqueous phase to the alcoholic solution, filter, and make to volume with water.

Sucrose increases viscosity and decreases the solubilizing properties of water and so must be added after primary solution has been carried out. A high alcoholic content is maintained during preparation by adding the aqueous phase to the alcoholic solution. Elixirs should always be brilliantly clear. They may be strained or filtered and, if necessary, subjected to the clarifying action of purified talc or siliceous earth.

One of the official elixirs, Iso-Alcoholic Elixir (page 1319), is actually a combination of two solutions, one containing 8 to 10% ethanol and the other containing 73 to 78% ethanol. The elixir is used as a vehicle for various medicaments that require solvents of different alcohol strengths. For example, the alcohol strength of the elixir to be used with a single liquid galenical is approximately the same as that of the galenical. When different alcohol strengths are used in the same prescription, the elixir to be used is the one that produces the best solution. This is usually the average of the alcohol strengths of the several ingredients. For nonextractive substances, the lowest alcohol strength of elixir that will produce a clear solution should be used.

The formula for High-Alcoholic Elixir is:

Compound Orange Spirit	4 mL
Saccharin	3 g
Glycerin	200 mL
Alcohol, a sufficient quantity, to make	1000 mL

This elixir and many other liquid preparations intended for internal use (eg, the diabetic syrups thickened with sodium carboxymethylcellulose or similar substances) contain saccharin. During the past few years, scientists have been studying the toxic effects of this sweetening agent and of the cyclamates. The cyclamate studies showed that the sweetener could produce cancer in animals and, as a result, this substance was removed from a wide variety of products. Similar studies have been carried out on saccharin.

Cyclamates and saccharin have been banned in some countries as ingredients in manufactured products. However, these substances may still be purchased as OTC products themselves. Much research has been done to find a safe synthetic substitute for sucrose. As a result aspartame (methyl N-L-α-aspartyl-L-phenylalaninate), which is about 200 times sweeter than sucrose, is now being used in many commercial preparations as the sweetening agent. It is sparingly soluble in water and is most stable at a pH of 4.3. This compound will likely be used in a number of pharmaceutical formulations in the near future.[14]

Incompatibilities—Since elixirs contain alcohol, incompatibilities of this solvent are an important consideration during the formulation phase. Alcohol precipitates tragacanth, acacia, and agar from aqueous solutions. Similarly, it will precipitate many inorganic salts from similar solutions. The implication here is that such substances should be absent from the aqueous phase or should be present in such concentrations that there is no danger of precipitation on standing.

If an aqueous solution is added to an elixir, a partial precipitation of ingredients may occur. This is due to the reduced alcohol content of the final preparation. Usually, however, the alcohol content of the mixture is not sufficiently high to cause separation. As vehicles for tinctures and fluidextracts, the elixirs generally cause a separation of extractive matter from these products due to a reduction of the alcohol content.

Many of the incompatibilities between elixirs and the substances combined with them are due to the chemical characteristics of the elixir *per se* or of the ingredients in the final preparation. Thus certain elixirs are acid in reaction while others may be alkaline and will, therefore, behave accordingly.

Glycerins

Glycerins or glycerites are solutions or mixtures of medicinal substances in not less than 50% by weight of glycerin. Most of the glycerins are extremely viscous and some of them are of a jelly-like consistency. Few of the glycerins are extensively used.

Glycerin is a valuable pharmaceutical solvent forming permanent and concentrated solutions not otherwise obtainable. Some of these solutions are used in their original form as medicinal agents while others are used to prepare aqueous and alcoholic dilutions of substances which are not readily soluble in water or alcohol. Glycerin Otic Solution of the USP is discussed previously under Otic solutions. One of the glycerins, Phenol Glycerin BPC is diluted with glycerin to form the pharmaceutical preparation, Phenol Ear-Drops BPC.

Phenol Glycerin BPC

Phenol	160 g
Glycerin	840 g

Dissolve the phenol in the glycerin.

Phenol Ear-Drops BPC

Phenol Glycerin	40 mL
Glycerin, a sufficient quantity, to make	100 mL

Add the glycerin to the glycerite.

Water must not be added to this preparation. It reacts with the phenol to produce a preparation which is caustic and, consequently, damaging to the area of application.

Although not within the context of the definitions given in this section, certain aqueous and nonaqueous preparations are used to remove wax (cerumen) from the ear. One commercially available preparation contains benzocaine, chlorbutol, p-dichlorobenzene, and turpentine; others contain olive oil, dioctyl sodium sulfosuccinate, or triethanolamine polypeptide oleate-condensate. Sodium Bicarbonate Ear-Drops BPC should be used if wax is to be removed from the ear. This preparation contains sodium bicarbonate (5 g), glycerin (30 mL), and purified water (a sufficient quantity to make 100 mL).

Starch Glycerin, an emollient, contains starch (100 g), benzoic acid (2 g), purified water (200 mL), and glycerin (700 mL).

Glycerins are hygroscopic and should be stored in tightly closed containers.

Inhalations and Inhalants

Inhalations

These preparations are so used or designed that the drug is carried into the respiratory tree of the patient. The vapor or mist reaches the affected area and gives prompt relief from the symptoms of bronchial and nasal congestion. The USP defines Inhalations in the following way:

Inhalations are drugs or solutions of drugs administered by the nasal or oral respiratory route for local or systemic effect. Examples in this Pharmacopeia are Epinephrine Inhalation and Isoproterenol Hydrochloride Inhalation. Nebulizers are suitable for the administration of inhalation solutions only if they give droplets sufficiently fine and uniform in size so that the mist reaches the bronchioles.

Another group of products, also known as inhalations and sometimes called insufflations, consists of finely powdered or liquid drugs that are carried into the respiratory passages by the use of special delivery systems such as pharmaceutical aerosols that hold a solution or suspension of the drug in a liquefied gas propellant (see Aerosols). When released through a suitable valve and oral adapter, a metered dose of the inhalation is propelled into the respiratory tract of the patient. Powders may also be administered by mechanical devices that require a manually produced pressure or a deep inspiration by the patient, eg, *Cromolyn Sodium*.

Solutions may be nebulized by use of inert gases. Nebulized solutions may be breathed directly from the nebulizer, or the nebulizer may be attached to a plastic face mask, tent, or intermittent positive-pressure breathing (IPPB) machine.

As stated in the pharmacopeia, particle size is of major importance in the administration of this type of preparation. The various types of mechanical devices that are used in conjunction with inhalations are described in some detail in Chapter 104. It has been reported in the literature that the optimum particle size for penetration into the pulmonary cavity is of the order of $\frac{1}{2}$ to 7 μm. Fine mists are produced by pressurized aerosols and hence possess basic advantages over the older nebulizers. In addition to this, metered aerosols deliver more uniform doses than those obtained with the older mechanical devices. Chapter 93 should be consulted for further details on this subject.

The term *Inhalation* is used commonly by the layman to represent preparations intended to be vaporized with the aid of heat, usually steam, and inhaled. Benzoin Inhalation BPC contains benzoin, storax, and alcohol. The vapors from a preparation containing 1 teaspoonful of the tincture and 1 qt of boiling water may be inhaled. The device known as a *vaporizer* is used with a number of commercially available preparations of this type.

Epinephrine Inhalation and Isoproterenol Hydrochloride Inhalation are described in USP.

Inhalants

The USP defines inhalants as follows:

A special class of inhalations termed "inhalants" consists of drugs or combinations of drugs that, by virtue of their high vapor pressure, can be carried by an air current into the nasal passage where they exert their effect. The container from which the inhalant is administered is known as an inhaler.

Propylhexedrine Inhalant and Tuaminoheptane Inhalant are described as consisting of cylindrical rolls of suitable fibrous material impregnated with propylhexedrine or tuaminoheptane (as carbonate) usually aromatized, and contained in a suitable inhaler. Propylhexedrine is the active ingredient in the widely used Benzedrex Inhaler. Both of these drugs are vasoconstrictors and are used to relieve nasal congestion.

The other inhalant in the USP is Amyl Nitrite which is very flammable and should not be used where it may be ignited. It is packaged in sealed glass vials in a protective gauze. Upon breaking the vial, the gauze absorbs the drug which is then inhaled for the treatment of anginal pain.

Liniments

Liniments are solutions or mixtures of various substances in oil, alcoholic solutions of soap, or emulsions. They are intended for external application and should be so labeled. They are applied with rubbing to the affected area and, because of this, were once called *embrocations*. Dental liniments, which are no longer official, are solutions of active substances and are rubbed into the gums. Most dentists question their usefulness and, consequently, this type of preparation is relatively unimportant as a pharmaceutical form.

Liniments are usually applied with friction and rubbing of the skin, the oil or soap base providing for ease of application and massage. Alcoholic liniments are used generally for their rubefacient, counterirritant, mildly astringent, and penetrating effects. Such liniments penetrate the skin more readily than do those with an oil base. The oily liniments, therefore, are milder in their action but are more useful when massage is required. Depending on the ingredients in the preparation, such liniments may function solely as protective coatings. Liniments should not be applied to skin areas that are bruised or broken.

Many of the marketed "white" liniments are based on the formulation below or variations thereof.

White Liniment BPC

Ammonium Chloride	12.5 g
Dilute Ammonia Solution	45 mL
Oleic Acid	85 mL
Turpentine Oil	250 mL
Water	625 mL

Mix the oleic acid with the turpentine oil. Add the dilute ammonia solution mixed with 45 mL of previously warmed water. Shake. Dissolve the ammonium chloride in the remainder of the water, add to the emulsion, and mix.

Other liniments contain antipruritics, astringents, emollients, and analgesics and are classified on the basis of the active ingredient in the formulation. An example of a liniment in this category is:

Compound Calamine Application BPC
(Compound Calamine Liniment)

Calamine	100 g
Zinc Oxide	50 g
Wool Fat	25 g
Zinc Stearate	25 g
Yellow Soft Paraffin	250 g
Liquid Paraffin	550 g

The powders are triturated to a smooth paste with some of the liquid paraffin (Liquid Petrolatum). The wool fat, zinc stearate, and yellow soft paraffin (Petrolatum) are melted and then mixed with some of the liquid paraffin, this mixture is incorporated with the triturated powders, the rest of the liquid paraffin is added with mixing.

Dermatologists prescribe products of this type but only those containing the rubefacients are extensively advertised and used by consumers for treatment of minor muscular aches and pains.

Because of the confusion of camphorated oil (camphor liniment) with castor oil resulting in ingestion and leading to poisoning, camphorated oil has been banned from the market. It is essential that these applications be clearly marked for external use only. (Camphorated Oil is presently classified as a new drug by the Food and Drug Administration).

Oleovitamins

Oleovitamins are fish liver oils diluted with edible vegetable oil or solutions of the indicated vitamins or vitamin concentrates (usually vitamins A and D) in fish liver oil. The definition is sufficiently broad to include a wide variety of marketed products.

Oleovitamin A and D is official. The vitamin D in the oleovitamin may be present as ergocalciferol or cholecalciferol obtained by the activation of ergosterol or 7-dehydrocholesterol or may be obtained from natural sources. Synthetic vitamin A or a concentrate may be used to prepare oleovitamin A. The starting material for the concentrate is a fish liver oil, the active ingredient being isolated by molecular distillation or by a saponification and extraction procedure. The latter procedure is described in detail in the monograph for Concentrated Vitamin A Solution BPC.

The indicated vitamins are unstable in the presence of rancid oils and, therefore, these preparations, and in particular, Oleovitamin A, should be stored in small, tight containers, preferably under vacuum or under an atmosphere of an inert gas, protected from light.

Spirits

Spirits, popularly known as essences, are alcoholic or hydroalcoholic solutions of volatile substances. Like the aromatic waters, the active ingredient in the spirit may be a solid, liquid, or gas. The genealogical tree for this class of preparations begins with the distinguished pair of products, Brandy (*Spiritus Vini Vitis*) and Whisky (*Spiritis Frumenti*), and ends with a wide variety of products that comply with the definition given above. Physicians have debated the therapeutic value of the former products and these are no longer official in the compendia.

Some of these spirits are used internally for their medicinal value, a few are used medicinally by inhalation, while a large number are used as flavoring agents. The latter group provides a convenient and ready means of obtaining the volatile oil in the proper quantity. For example, a spirit or spirit-like preparation may be used in the formulation of aromatic waters or other pharmaceuticals that require a distinctive flavor.

Spirits should be stored in tight, light-resistant containers, and in a cool place. This prevents evaporation and volatilization of either the alcohol or the active principle.

Preparation—There are four classic methods for the preparation of this official group: These are *simple solution*, *solution with maceration*, *chemical reaction*, and *distillation*.

Simple Solution—This is the method by which the majority of spirits are prepared. The formula and procedure given for Aromatic Ammonia Spirit illustrate this method of preparation.

Aromatic Ammonia Spirit

Ammonium Carbonate, in translucent pieces	**34 g**
Strong Ammonia Solution	**36 mL**
Lemon Oil	**10 mL**
Lavender Oil	**1 mL**
Nutmeg Oil	**1 mL**
Alcohol	**700 mL**
Purified Water, a sufficient quantity to make	**1000 mL**

Dissolve the ammonium carbonate in the strong ammonia solution and 195 mL of purified water by gentle agitation, and allow the solution to stand for 12 hours. Dissolve the oils in the alcohol, contained in a graduated bottle or cylinder, and gradually add the ammonium carbonate solution and enough purified water to make the product measure 1000 mL. Set the mixture aside in a cool place for 24 hours, occasionally agitating it, and then filter, using a covered funnel.

The spirit is a respiratory stimulant and is administered by inhalation of the vapor as required. It is marketed in suitable tight, light-resistant containers but is also available in a single-dose glass vial wrapped in a soft cotton envelope. The vial is easily broken; the cotton acts as a sponge for the spirit.

Ammonium carbonate is a mixture of ammonium bicarbonate and ammonium carbamate (NH_2COONH_4). The carbamate reacts with water to form the carbonate.

$$NH_2COONH_4 + H_2O \rightarrow (NH_4)_2CO_3$$

An ammonium carbonate solution is, therefore, a solution of ammonium bicarbonate and ammonium carbonate in water. However, it decomposes in water, the decomposition products being ammonia, carbon dioxide, and water. The stability of the spirit is improved by the addition of strong ammonia solution. This represses the hydrolysis of ammonium carbonate and, in this way, decreases the loss of dissolved gases.

Solution with Maceration—In this procedure, leaves of the drug are macerated in purified water to extract water-soluble matter. They are then expressed, and the moist macerated leaves are added to a prescribed quantity of alcohol. The volatile oil is added to the filtered liquid. Peppermint Spirit is made by this process. Peppermint Spirit BPC differs from the official product in that it is a solution of the volatile oil in alcohol only. The concentration of volatile oil in the final product is about the same but the official preparation possesses a green color. The ready availability of soluble chlorophyll and other coloring agents has led to the frequent suggestion that a more uniform product could be obtained

through their use. However, these agents cannot be used in preparing the official article.

The formula and procedure for Peppermint Spirit (page 814) illustrate this method of preparation.

Chemical Reaction—No official spirits are prepared by this process. Ethyl nitrite is made by the action of sodium nitrite on a mixture of alcohol and sulfuric acid in the cold. This substance is then used to prepare Ethyl Nitrite Spirit, a product no longer official.

Distillation—Brandy and Whisky are made by distillation. The latter is derived from the fermented mash of wholly or partially germinated malted cereal grains and the former from the fermented juice of ripe grapes.

Incompatibilities—Spirits are, for the most part, preparations of high alcoholic strength and do not lend themselves well to dilution with aqueous solutions or liquids of low alcoholic content. The addition of such a solution invariably causes separation of some of the material dissolved in the spirit, evidenced by a turbidity which, in time, may disappear as distinct layering occurs. Salts may be precipitated from their aqueous solutions by addition of spirits due to lesser solubility in alcoholic liquids.

Some spirits show incompatibilities characteristic of the ingredients which they contain. For example, Aromatic Ammonia Spirit cannot be mixed with aqueous preparations containing alkaloids (eg, codeine phosphate). An acid-base reaction (ammonia-phosphate) occurs and, if the alcohol content of the final mixture is too low, codeine will precipitate.

Toothache Drops

Toothache drops are preparations used for temporary relief of toothache by application of a small pledget of cotton saturated with the product into the tooth cavity. Anesthetic compounds include clove oil, eugenol, and benzocaine; other ingredients include camphor, creosote, menthol, and alcohol.

These preparations are no longer officially recognized. Furthermore, dentists do not recommend use of toothache drops if the patient has ready access to adequate dental services. The preparations may damage the gums and produce complications more severe than the original toothache. However, many areas do not have adequate dental services and the pharmacist will, of necessity, handle these preparations. If such is the case, the pharmacist should warn the patient of possible hazards associated with the use of these products.

Toothache Drops NF XI contain 25 g of chlorobutanol in sufficient clove oil to make the product measure 100 mL. Another formulation contains creosote, clove oil, benzocaine, and alcohol in a flexible collodion base.

Emulsions

An emulsion is a two-phase system prepared by combining two immiscible liquids, one of which is uniformly dispersed throughout the other and consists of globules that have diameters equal to or greater than those of the largest colloidal particles. The globule size is, of course, critical and must be such that the system achieves maximum stability. However, even under the best of conditions, separation of the two phases will occur unless a third substance, an *emulsifying agent*, is incorporated. The basic emulsion must, therefore, contain three components but the products of commerce may consist of a number of therapeutic agents dissolved in either of the two phases of the preparation.

Most emulsions are so prepared as to incorporate an aqueous phase into a nonaqueous phase (or *vice versa*). However, it is possible to prepare emulsions that are basically nonaqueous. For example, investigations of the emulsifying effects of anionic and cationic surfactants on the nonaqueous immiscible system, glycerin and olive oil, have shown that certain amines and three cationic agents produced stable emulsions. This broadening of the basic definition for the term *emulsion* is recognized in the USP.

An emulsion is a two-phase system in which one liquid is dispersed in the form of small droplets throughout another liquid. The dispersed liquid is known as the internal or discontinuous phase, whereas the dispersion medium is known as the external or continuous phase. Where oil is the dispersed phase and an aqueous solution is the continuous phase, the system is designated as an oil-in-water (O/W) emulsion and this can be easily and uniformly diluted with water. Conversely, where water or an aqueous solution is the dispersed phase and oil or oleaginous material is the continuous phase, the system is designated as a water-in-oil (W/O) emulsion.

Many emulsifying agents are available for use in preparing emulsions, among them the following:

Natural Emulsifying Agents—These substances may be derived from either animal or vegetable sources. Examples of those obtained from the former source are gelatin, egg yolk, casein, wool fat, and cholesterol. Acacia, tragacanth, chondrus, and pectin are representative of those obtained from vegetable sources. Various cellulose derivatives, eg, methylcellulose and carboxymethylcellulose, are used to increase viscosity of the aqueous phase and thereby enhance emulsion stability.

Finely Divided Solids—Examples of emulsifying agents of this type are bentonite, magnesium hydroxide, aluminum hydroxide, and magnesium trisilicate.

Synthetic Emulsifying Agents—This group may be further subdivided into the anionic, cationic, and nonionic agents. Examples of these three types of emulsifying agents are, in order of presentation, sodium lauryl sulfate, benzalkonium chloride, and polyethylene glycol 400 monostearate.

Many of these emulsifying agents are described in greater detail in Chapter 68.

NF XIII suggested that only O/W emulsions are suitable for oral use because these are water-miscible and thus their oiliness is masked. This compendium gave specific directions for the preparation of emulsions utilizing gelatin as an emulsifying agent. These preparations are based on either type A or type B gelatin. Type A gelatin is prepared from acid-treated precursors and is used at a pH of about 3.2. It is incompatible with anionic emulsifying agents such as the vegetable gums. The following formula was recommended:

Gelatin (Type A)	8	g
Tartaric Acid	0.6	g
Flavor as desired		
Alcohol	60	mL
Oil	500	mL
Purified Water, to make	1000	mL

Add the gelatin and the tartaric acid to about 300 mL of purified water, allow to stand for a few minutes, heat until the gelatin is dissolved, then raise the temperature to about 98°, and maintain this temperature for about 20 min. Cool to 50°, and add the flavor, the alcohol, and sufficient purified water to make 500 mL. Add the oil, agitate the mixture thoroughly, and pass it through a homogenizer or a colloid mill until the oil is completely and uniformly dispersed.

This emulsion cannot be prepared by trituration or by the use of the usual stirring devices.

Type B gelatin is prepared from alkali-treated precursors and is used at a pH of about 8.0. It may be used with other anionic emulsifying agents but is incompatible with cationic types. If the emulsion contains 50% oil, 5 g of Type B gelatin, 2.5 g of sodium bicarbonate, and sufficient tragacanth or agar should be incorporated into the aqueous phase so as to yield 1000 mL of product of the required viscosity.

The emulsion type (O/W or W/O) is of lesser significance if the final preparation is to be applied to the skin. If there are no breaks in the skin, a W/O emulsion can be applied more evenly since the skin is covered with a thin film of sebum. The latter substance favors the oily phase and contributes to the ease of application. The choice of emulsion type will, however, depend on many other factors. This is particularly true for those preparations which have basic cosmetic characteristics. It may be advantageous to formulate an O/W emulsion if ease of removal is an important consideration to the patient.

An emulsion that may be prepared by the mortar and pestle method is the following Mineral Oil Emulsion USP.

Mineral Oil	500	mL
Acacia, very fine powder	125	g
Syrup	100	mL
Vanillin	40	mg
Alcohol	60	mL
Purified Water, to make	1000	mL

The mineral oil and acacia are mixed in a dry Wedgwood mortar. Water (250 mL) is added and the mixture is triturated vigorously until an emulsion is formed. A mixture of the syrup, 50 mL of purified water and the vanillin dissolved in alcohol is added in divided portions with trituration; sufficient purified water is then added to the proper volume. The mixture is mixed well and homogenized.

Very few emulsions are now included in the official compendia. The BPC states that the term "emulsion" should be restricted to oil-in-water preparations intended for internal use and lists the following: Liquid Paraffin Emulsion, Liquid Paraffin and Magnesium Hydroxide Emulsion, Liquid Paraffin and Phenolphthalein Emulsion, and Concentrated Peppermint Emulsion.

This, however, should not lead the student to the conclusion that emulsions are a relatively unimportant class of pharmaceuticals. While it is true that few preparations carry the term *emulsion* in their titles, they are of great significance as bases for other types of preparations, particularly in the dermatological and cosmetic areas. Academically, they illustrate the importance of the relationship between the theory and practice of emulsion technology and, practically, they possess a number of important advantages over other liquid forms. These may be summarized in the following way:

1. In an emulsion, the therapeutic properties and the spreading ability of the constituents are increased.
2. The unpleasant taste or odor of the oil can be partially or wholly masked by the process of emulsification. Secondary masking techniques are available to the formulator but these must be used with caution. If flavors and sweetening agents are added to the emulsion, only minimal amounts should be used in order to prevent the nausea or gastric distress that results on ingestion of larger quantities of these formulation aids.
3. The absorption and penetration of medicaments are more easily controlled if they are incorporated into an emulsion.
4. Emulsion action is more prolonged and the emollient effect is greater than that observed with comparable preparations.
5. Water is not only an inexpensive diluent but is a good solvent for the many drugs and flavors that are incorporated into the emulsion.

The aqueous phase of the emulsion favors the growth of microorganisms and, because of this, a preservative is usually added to the product. Some of the preservatives that have been used in emulsions include chlorocresol, chlorobutanol, mercurial preparations, salicylic acid, the esters of p-hydroxybenzoic acid, benzoic acid, sodium benzoate, and sorbic acid. The preservative should be selected having regard for the use of the preparation and possible incompatibilities between the preservative and the ingredients in the emulsion, eg, binding between the surface-active agent and the preservative.

Most emulsions consist of an oil phase and a water phase, thus some of the preservative may pass into the oil phase and be removed from the aqueous phase. It is in the aqueous phase that microorganisms tend to grow. As a result, water-soluble preservatives are more effective since the concentration of the unbound preservative in the water phase assumes a great deal of importance in inhibiting the microbial growth. Esters of p-hydroxybenzoic acid appear to be the most satisfactory preservatives for emulsions. Many mathematical models have been used in determining availability of preservatives in emulsified systems. However, because of the number of factors which reduce the effectiveness of the preservative, a final microbiological evaluation of the emulsion should be performed.

While emphasis concerning preservation of emulsions deals with the aqueous phase, microorganisms can reside also in the lipid (oil) phase. Consequently, it has been recommended that pairs of preservatives be used to ensure adequate concentration in both phases.[15] Esters of p-hydroxybenzoic acid can be used to ensure appropriate concentrations in both phases because of their difference in oil and water solubilities.

An emulsion can be diluted with the liquid that constitutes or is miscible with the external phase. The diluting liquid will, however, decrease the viscosity of the preparation and, in certain instances, will invert the emulsion. The latter phenomena may occur if the emulsifier-in-water method (see below) is used to prepare the emulsion.

Preparation

The theory of emulsion preparation is discussed in Chapter 21. The following procedures are those suggested by Griffin et al.[16]

The formulator must first determine the physical and chemical characteristics of the active ingredient. He must know the following:

1. Structural formula
2. Melting point
3. Solubility
4. Stability
5. Dose
6. Specific chemical incompatibilities

It is also necessary, at this stage, to decide on the type of emulsion required. Washable emulsions are of the O/W type; nonwashable, the W/O type. In general, O/W emulsions contain over 70% water. W/O emulsions will usually contain higher concentrations of oils and waxes. The preparation of cream and ointment emulsions for topical use is given in Chapter 88.

Experimental formulations may be prepared by the following procedure:

1. Group the ingredients on the basis of their solubilities in the aqueous and nonaqueous phases.
2. Determine the type of emulsion required and calculate an approximate HLB value.
3. Blend a low HLB emulsifier and a high HLB emulsifer to the calculated value. For experimental formulations, use a higher concentration of emulsifier (eg, 10–30% of the oil phase) than that required to produce a satisfactory product. Emulsifiers should, in general, be chemically stable, nontoxic, and suitably low in color, odor, and taste. The emulsifier is selected on the basis of these characteristics, on the type of equipment being used to blend the ingredients, and on the stability characteristics of the final product. Emulsions should not coalesce at room temperature, when frozen and thawed repeatedly, and at elevated temperatures of up to 50°. Mechanical energy input varies with the type of equipment used to prepare the emulsion. The more the energy input, the less the demand on the emulsifier. Both process and formulation variables can affect the stability of an emulsion.
4. Dissolve the oil-soluble ingredients and the emulsifiers in the oil. Heat, if necessary, to approximately 5° to 10° over the melting point of the highest melting ingredient or to a maximum temperature of 70° to 80°.
5. Dissolve the water-soluble ingredients (except acids and salts) in a sufficient quantity of water.
6. Heat the aqueous phase to a temperature which is 3° to 5° higher than that of the oil phase.
7. Add the aqueous phase to the oily phase with suitable agitation.
8. If acids or salts are employed, dissolve them in water and add the solution to the cold emulsion.
9. Examine the emulsion and make adjustments in the formulation if the product is unstable. It may be necessary to add more emulsifier, to change to an emulsifier with a slightly higher or lower HLB value, or to use an emulsifier with different chemical characteristics.

The technique of emulsification of pharmaceutical preparations has been described by White.[17] The preparation of an emulsion requires work to reduce the internal phase into small droplets and disperse them through the external phase: this can be accomplished by a mortar and pestle or a high speed emulsifier. The addition of emulsifying agents not only reduces this work but also stabilizes the final emulsion. Emulsions may be prepared by four principle methods.

Addition of Internal Phase to External Phase—This is usually the most satisfactory method for preparing emulsions since there is always an excess of the external phase present which promotes the type of emulsion desired. If the external phase is water and the internal phase is oil, the water soluble substances are dissolved in the water and the oil-soluble substances mixed thoroughly in the oil. The oil mixture is added in portions to the aqueous preparation with agitation. Sometimes, in order to give a better shearing action during the preparation all of the water is not mixed with the emulsifying agent, until the primary emulsion with the oil is formed, subsequently the remainder of the water is added. An example using gelatin Type A is given above.

Addition of the External Phase to the Internal Phase—Using an oil-in-water emulsion as an example, the addition of the water (external phase) to the oil (internal phase) will promote the formation of a water-in-oil emulsion due to the preponderance of the oil phase. After further addition of the water, phase inversion to an oil-in-water emulsion should take place. This method is especially useful and successful when hydrophilic agents such as acacia, tragacanth, and methylcellulose which are first mixed with the oil, effecting dispersion without wetting. Water is added and eventually an oil-in-water emulsion is formed. This "dry gum" method is a rapid method for preparing small quantities of emulsion. The ratio 4 parts of oil, 2 parts of water, and 1 part of gum provides maximum shearing action on the oil globules in the mortar. The emulsion can then be diluted and triturated with water to the appropriate concentrations. The preparation of Mineral Oil Emulsions described above is an example of this method.

Mixing Both Phases after Warming Each—This method is used when waxes or other substances which require melting are used. The oil-soluble emulsifying agents, oils, and waxes are melted and thoroughly mixed. The water-soluble ingredients dissolved in the water are warmed to a temperature slightly higher than the oil phase. The two phases are then mixed and stirred until cold. For convenience, but not necessary, the aqueous solution is added to the oil mixture. This method is frequently used in the preparation of ointments and creams.

Alternate Addition of the Two Phases to the Emulsifying Agent—A portion of the oil, if an oil-in-water emulsion is being prepared is added to all of the oil-soluble emulsifying agent with mixing, then an equal quantity of water containing all the water-soluble emulsifying agents is added with stirring until the emulsion is formed. Further portions of the oil and water are added alternately until the final product is formed. The high concentration of the emulsifying agent in the original emulsion makes the initial emulsification more likely and the high viscosity provides effective shearing action leading to small droplets in the emulsion. This method is often successfully used with soaps.

A recent innovation in emulsion technology is the development of multiple emulsions. The dispersed phase of these emulsions contains even smaller droplets which are miscible with the continuous phase. Thus the multiple emulsion may be O/W/O where the aqueous phase is between two oil phases, or W/O/W where the internal and external aqueous phases are separated by an oil phase. While the technique of preparing these emulsions is more complicated, recent research indicates potential use of these emulsions for prolonged action, more effective dosage forms, parenteral preparations, protection against the external environment, and enzyme entrapment.[18]

Equipment

When emulsions are prepared, energy must be expended to form an interface between the oily and aqueous phases. Emulsification equipment includes, therefore, a wide variety of agitators, homogenizers, colloid mills, and ultrasonic devices. Griffin, et al,[16] Becher,[19] and Peck, et al,[20] have evaluated the emulsification equipment used by pharmacists and drug manufacturers. These publications should be consulted for further details on the use of such apparatus for the preparation of emulsions and related products.

The preparation of emulsions on a large scale usually requires the expenditure of considerable amounts of energy for heating and mixing. Careful consideration of these processes has led to the development of low energy emulsification by using an appropriate emulsification temperature and selective heating of the ingredients. This process involves the preparation of an emulsion concentrate subsequently diluted with the external phase at room temperature.[21]

Agitators—Ordinary agitation or shaking may be used to prepare the emulsion. This method is frequently employed

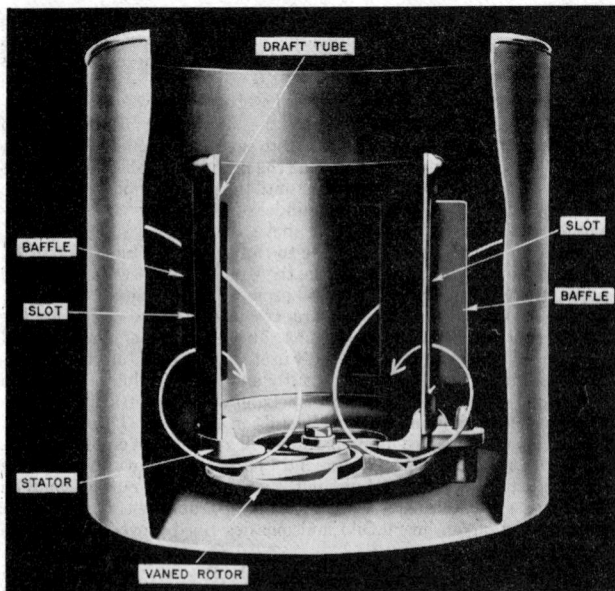

Fig 84-2. Standard slurry-type dispersall mixer with vaned-rotor "mixing" element and slotted draft-tube circulating element (courtesy, Abbe Eng).

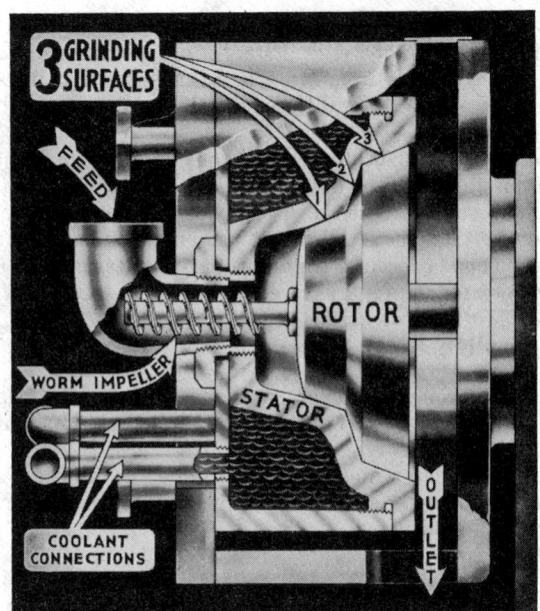

Fig 84-4. A colloid mill shown in cross section (courtesy, Tri-Homo).

by the pharmacist, particularly in the emulsification of easily dispersed, low-viscosity oils. Under certain conditions, intermittent shaking is considerably more effective than ordinary continuous shaking. Continuous shaking tends to break up not only the phase to be dispersed but also the dispersion medium and, in this way, impairs ease of emulsification. Laboratory shaking devices may be used for small-scale production of emulsions.

The mortar and pestle are widely used by the prescription pharmacist in extemporaneous preparation of emulsions. This equipment has very definite limitations because its usefulness depends largely on the viscosity of the emulsifying agent. A mortar and pestle cannot be used to prepare an

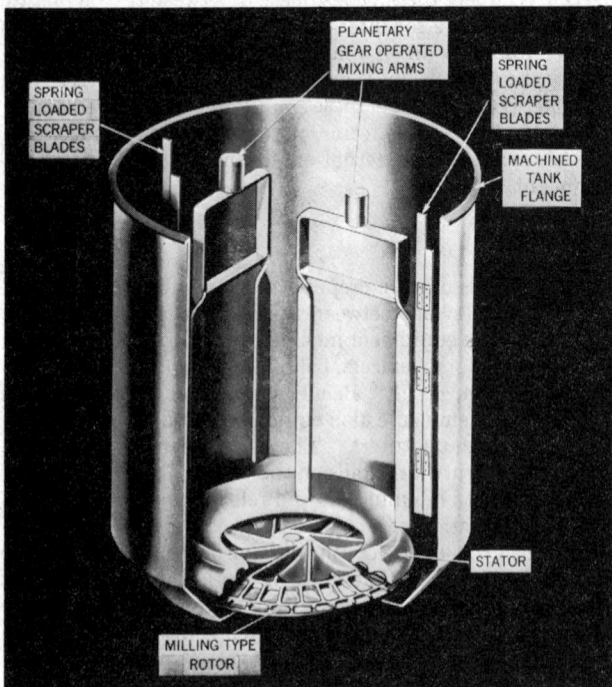

Fig 84-3. Standard paste-type dispersall mixer with "cupped-rotor" milling element and double-rotating mixing arm circulating element (courtesy, Abbe Eng).

emulsion if the emulsifying agent lacks viscidity (eg, gelatin solutions). These emulsifying agents will produce stable emulsions only if other types of equipment are used to mix the ingredients and the agent together.

Small electric mixers may be used to prepare emulsions at the prescription counter. These mixers will save time and energy and produce satisfactory emulsions when the emulsifying agent is acacia or agar. However, the mixers cannot be used if the emulsifying agent is gelatin.

The commercially available *Waring Blendor* disperses efficiently by means of the shearing action of rapidly rotating blades. This mixer transfers large amounts of energy and incorporates air into the emulsion. If an emulsion is first produced by using a blender of this type, the formulator must remember that the emulsion characteristics obtained in the laboratory will not necessarily be duplicated by the production-size agitators.

Production-size agitators include high-powered propeller shaft stirrers immersed in a tank or self-contained units with propeller and paddle systems. The latter units are usually so constructed that the contents of the tank may be either heated or cooled during the production process. Baffles are often built into a tank and these increase the efficiency of agitation. Two mixers manufactured by the same company are shown in Figs 84-2 and 84-3.

Colloid Mills—The principle of operation of the colloid mill is the passage of the mixed phases of an emulsion formula between a stator and a high-speed rotor revolving at speeds of 2000–18,000 rpm. The clearance between the rotor and the stator is adjustable, usually from 0.001 in. upward. The emulsion mixture, in passing between the rotor and stator, is subjected to a tremendous shearing action which effects a fine dispersion. Two of the many types of colloid mills on the market are shown in Figs 84-4 and 84-5. The operating principle is the same for all but each manufacturer incorporates specific features which result in changes in operating efficiency. The shearing forces applied in the colloid mill may result in a temperature increase within the emulsion. It may be necessary, therefore, to cool the equipment when the emulsion is being produced.

Homogenizers and Viscolizers—In the viscolizer and the homogenizer, the mixed phases are passed between a finely ground valve and seat under high pressure. This, in effect,

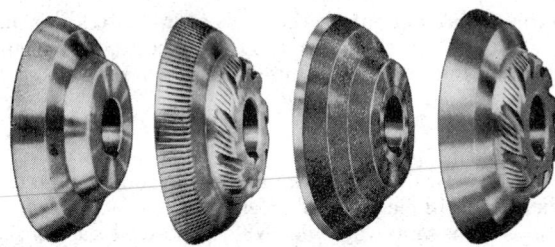

Fig 84-5.   Types of rotors used in colloid mills.   These may be smooth (for emulsification of most emulsions), serrated (for the emulsification of ointments and very viscous products), or of vitrified stone (for the emulsifications of paints and pigment dispersions) (courtesy, Tri-Homo).

produces an atomization which is enhanced by the impact received by the atomized mixture as it strikes the valve head. This type of apparatus operates at pressures of 1000–5000 lb/sq in. and produces some of the finest dispersions obtainable in an emulsion.

Homogenizers may be used in one of two ways: (1) the ingredients in the emulsion are mixed and then passed through the homogenizer to produce the final product; or (2) an emulsion is prepared in some other way and is then passed through a homogenizer for the purpose of decreasing the particle size and obtaining a greater degree of uniformity and stability.

Two-stage homogenizers are so constructed that the emulsion, after treatment in the first valve system, is conducted directly to another where it receives a second treatment.   A single homogenization may produce an emulsion which, although its particle size is small, has a tendency to clump or form clusters.   Emulsions of this type exhibit increased creaming tendencies.   This is corrected by passing the emulsion through the first stage of homogenization at a high pressure (eg, 3000–5000 lb/sq in) and then through the second stage at a greatly reduced pressure (eg, 1000 lb/sq in). This breaks down any clusters formed in the first step.

For small-scale extemporaneous preparation of emulsions, the inexpensive *hand homogenizer* (available from *Med. Times*) is particularly useful.   It is probably the most efficient emulsifying apparatus available to the prescription pharmacist.   The two phases, previously mixed in a bottle, are hand pumped through the apparatus.   Recirculation of the emulsion through the apparatus will improve its quality.

A homogenizer does not incorporate air into the final product.   Air may ruin an emulsion because the emulsifying agent is preferentially adsorbed at the air/water interface. This is followed by an irreversible precipitation termed *denaturization*.   This is particularly prone to occur with protein emulsifying agents.

Homogenization may spoil an emulsion if the concentration of emulsifying agent in the formulation is less than that re-quired to take care of the increase in surface area produced by the process.

The temperature rise during homogenization is not very large.   However, temperature does play an important role in the emulsification process.   An increase in temperature will reduce the viscosity and, in certain instances, the interfacial tension between the oil and the water.   There are, however, many instances, particularly in the manufacturing of cosmetic creams and ointments, where the ingredients will fail to emulsify properly if they are processed at too high a temperature.   Emulsions of this type are first processed at an elevated temperature and then homogenized at a temperature not exceeding 40°.

The Marco Flow-Master Kom-bi-nator employs a number of different actions, each of which takes the ingredients a little further along in the process of subdividing droplets until complete homogenization results.   The machine is equipped with a pump which carries the liquid through the various stages of the process.   In the first stage, the ingredients are forced between two specially designed rotors (gears) which shoot the liquid in opposite directions in a small chamber and, in this way, mixed thoroughly.   These rotors also set up a swirling action in the next chamber into which the liquid is forced and swirled back and forth in eddies and cross currents. The second stage is a pulsing or vibrating action at rapid frequency.   The product then leaves this chamber, goes through a small valve opening, and is dashed against the wall of the homogenizing chamber.   Pressure is applied but is not as great as that used in other types of homogenizers.   Pressure is accurately controlled by adjusting devices on the front of the machine, and temperature is controlled by passing coolants through the stators.

Ultrasonic Devices—The preparation of emulsions by the use of ultrasonic vibrations is also possible.   An oscillator of high frequency (100,000–500,000/sec) is connected to two electrodes between which is placed a piezoelectric quartz plate. The quartz plate and electrodes are immersed in an oil bath and, when the oscillator is operating, high-frequency waves flow through the fluid.   Emulsification is accomplished by simply immersing a tube containing the emulsion ingredients into this oil bath.   Considerable research has been done on ultrasonic emulsification, particularly with regard to the mechanism of emulsion formation by this method.   Limited data indicate that these devices will produce stable emulsions only with liquids of low viscosity.   The method is not, however, practical for large-scale production of emulsions.

Special techniques and equipment will, in certain instances, produce superior emulsions, including rapid cooling, reduction in particle size, ultrasonic devices, etc.   A wide selection of equipment for processing both emulsions and suspensions has been recently described[22].   A number of improvements have been made to make the various processes more effective and energy efficient.

Suspensions

The physical chemist defines the word "suspension" as a two-phase system consisting of a finely divided solid dispersed in a solid, liquid, or gas.   The pharmacist accepts this definition and can show that a variety of dosage forms fall within the scope of the preceding statement.   There is, however, a reluctance to be all-inclusive and it is for this reason that the main emphasis is placed on solids dispersed in liquids.   In addition to this, and because there is a need for more specific terminology, the pharmaceutical scientist differentiates between such preparations as Suspensions, Mixtures, Magmas, Gels, and Lotions.   In a general sense, each of these prepa-rations represents a suspension but the state of subdivision of the insoluble solid varies from particles which gradually subside on standing to particles which are colloidal in nature. The lower limit of particle size is approximately 0.1 μm and it is the preparations containing dispersed solids of this magnitude or greater that are pharmaceutically defined as suspensions.

Certain authors also include liniments and the newer sustained-release suspensions in any discussion of this particular subject.   The former preparations are now usually considered as solutions although a number of older liniments were, in fact, suspensions. The sustained-release suspensions represent a very specialized class of preparation, and as such, are discussed in more detail in Chapter 92. Some insoluble drugs are also administered in aerosol form. One example of such a preparation is dexamethasone phosphate suspended in a propellant mixture of fluorochlorocarbons. More detail on aerosols is available in Chapter 93.

Suspension formulation and control is based on the principles outlined in Chapters 19 to 22. Formulation involves more than suspending a solid in a liquid. A knowledge of the behavior of particles in liquids, of suspending agents, and of flavors and colors is required to produce a satisfactory suspension.

Briefly, the preparation of a stable suspension depends upon the appropriate dispersion of the drug in the suspending medium. To ensure that the particles are wetted by the dispersion medium a surface-active agent should be used, especially if the dispersed phase is hydrophobic. The suspending agent in the aqueous medium can then be added. Alternatively, the dry suspending agent can be thoroughly mixed with the drug particles and then triturated with the diluent. Other approaches to suspension preparation include the formation of a flocculated suspension and also a flocculated preparation in a suspending vehicle. Details of these procedures are given in Chapter 21.

The most efficient method of producing fine particles is by dry milling prior to suspension. Suspension equipment such as colloid mills or homogenizers are normally used in wet milling finished suspensions to reduce particle agglomerates. These machines (Fig 84-4) usually have a stator and a rotor which effects the dispersion action. Several methods of producing small uniform dry particles are: micropulverization fluid energy grinding, spray drying, and controlled precipitation with ultrasound.[23]

The choice of an appropriate suspending agent depends upon the use of the products, external or internal, facilities for preparation, and the duration of product storage.

Preparations made extemporaneously for internal use may include as suspending agents: acacia, methylcellulose and other cellulose derivatives, sodium alginate, and tragacanth. Agents suitable for external use include bentonite, methylcellulose and other cellulose derivatives, sodium alginate, and tragacanth. Agents which may require high speed equipment and which are suitable for internal or external use include aluminum magnesium silicates and carbomer.[24]

Preparations such as those mentioned above possess certain advantages over other dosage forms. Some drugs are insoluble in all acceptable media and must, therefore, be administered as a tablet, capsule, etc, or as a suspension. Because of its liquid character, the last preparation insures some uniformity of dosage but does present some problems in maintenance of a consistent dosage regimen. Disagreeable tastes can be covered by use of a suspension of the drug or a derivative of the drug, an example of the latter being the drug chloramphenicol palmitate. Suspensions are also chemically more stable than solutions. This is particularly important with certain antibiotics and the pharmacist is often called on to prepare such a suspension just prior to the dispensing of the preparation. In addition to this, a suspension is an ideal dosage form for patients who have difficulty swallowing tablets or capsules. This factor is of particular importance in administration of drugs to children.

Suspensions should possess certain basic properties. The dispersed phase should settle slowly and should be readily redispersed on shaking. They should not cake on settling and the viscosity should be such that the preparation pours easily. As with all dosage forms, there should be no question as to the chemical stability of the suspension. Appropriate preservatives should be incorporated in order to minimize microbiological contamination. Lastly, the suspension must be acceptable to the patient on the basis of its taste, color, and cosmetic qualities, the latter two factors being of particular importance in preparations intended for external use.

Gels

Pharmaceutical terminology is, at best, confusing and no two authors will classify Gels, Jellies, Magmas, Milks, and Mixtures in the same way. The NF described Gels as a special class of pharmaceutical preparations but considered Jellies under the same heading. The latter preparations usually contain water-soluble active ingredients and are, therefore, considered in another part of this chapter. The USP definition for Gels is given below.

Gels are semisolid systems of either suspensions made up of small inorganic particles or large organic molecules interpenetrated by a liquid. Where the gel mass consists of a network of small discrete particles, the gel is classified as a two-phase system (eg, Aluminum Hydroxide Gel). In a two-phase system, if the particle size of the dispersed phase is relatively large, the gel mass is sometimes referred to as a magma (eg Bentonite Magma). Both gels and magmas may be thixotropic, forming semisolids on standing and becoming liquid on agitation. They should be shaken before use to ensure homogeneity and should be labeled to that effect.

Single-phase gels consist of organic macromolecules uniformly distributed throughout a liquid in such a manner that no apparent boundaries exist between the dispersed macromolecules and the liquid. Single-phase gels may be made from synthetic macromolecules (eg, Carbomer) or from natural gums (eg, Tragacanth). The latter preparations are also called mucilages. Although these gels are commonly aqueous, alcohol and oils may be used as the continuous phase. For example, mineral oil can be combined with a polyethylene resin to form an oleaginous ointment base.

The USP states that each 100 g of Aluminum Hydroxide Gel contains the equivalent of not less than 3.6 and not more than 4.4 g of aluminum oxide (Al_2O_3), in the form of aluminum hydroxide and hydrated oxide, and it may contain varying quantities of basic aluminum carbonate and bicarbonate. The gel itself is usually prepared by the interaction of a soluble aluminum salt, such as a chloride or sulfate, with ammonia solution, sodium carbonate or bicarbonate. The reactions which occur during the preparation are:

$$3CO_3^{2-} + 3H_2O \rightarrow 3HCO_3^- + 3OH^-$$

$$[Al(H_2O)_6]^{3+} + 3OH^- \rightarrow [Al(H_2O)_3(OH)_3] + 3H_2O$$

$$2HCO_3^- \rightarrow CO_3^{2-} + H_2O + CO_2$$

The physical and chemical properties of the gel will be affected by the order of addition of reactants, pH of precipitation, temperature of precipitation, concentration of the reactants, the reactants used, and the conditions of aging of the precipitated gel.

Aluminum Hydroxide Gel is soluble in acidic (or very strongly basic) media. The mechanism in acidic media is:

$$Aluminum\ Hydroxide\ Gel + 3H_2O \rightarrow [Al(H_2O)_3(OH)_3]^\circ$$

$$[Al(H_2O)_3]^\circ + H_3O^+ \rightarrow [Al(H_2O)_4(OH)_2]^+ + H_2O$$

$$[Al(H_2O)_4(OH)_2]^+ + H_3O^+ \rightarrow [Al(H_2O)_5(OH)^{2+} + H_2O$$

$$[Al(H_2O)_5(OH)]^{2+} + H_3O^+ \rightarrow [Al(H_2O)_6^{3+} + H_2O$$

It is unlikely that the last reaction given proceeds to completion. Since the activity of the gel is controlled by its insolubility (solution will decrease with an increase in the pH of the gastric media), there is no acid rebound. Further, since a certain quantity of insoluble gel is always available, the neutralizing capability of the gel extends over a considerable period of time.

Aluminum hydroxide gels may also contain peppermint oil, glycerin, sorbitol, sucrose, saccharin, and various preservatives. Sorbitol improves the acid-consuming capacity, apparently by inhibiting a secondary polymerization that takes place on aging. In addition polyols such as mannitol, sorbitol, and inositol have been shown to improve the stability of aluminum hydroxide and aluminum hydroxycarbonate gels.

Aluminum Hydroxide and Belladonna Mixture BPC

Belladonna Tincture	100 mL
Chloroform Spirit	50 mL
Aluminum Hydroxide Gel to	1000 mL

It should be noted, however, that the addition of other drugs (e.g., antibiotics) to the gel may result in a loss of the activity anticipated for that active ingredient.

Generally, if left undisturbed for some time, gels may become semisolid or gelatinous. With some gels, small amounts of water may separate on standing.

The single phase gels are being used more frequently in pharmacy and cosmetics because of several properties: semi-solid state, high degree of clarity, ease of application, ease of removal, and use. The gels often provide a faster release of drug substance, independent of the water solubility of the drug, as compared to creams and ointments. Some drugs used in medication gels include: urea, hydrogen peroxide, ephedrine sulphate, erythromycin, and povidone iodine.

The gels may be used as lubricants for catheters, bases for patch testing, sodium chloride gels for electrocardiography, fluoride gels for topical dental use, and prostaglandin-E_2 gel for intravaginal administration.

The gels can be prepared from a number of pharmaceutical agents such as tragacanth 2–5%, sodium alginate 2–10%, gelatin 2–15%, methylcellulose 2–4%, sodium carboxymethylcellulose 2–5%, carbomer 0.3–5%, polyvinyl alcohols 10–20%.[25] The percentages indicate the concentration ranges of the gelling agent. The lower percentage preparations may be used as lubricants and the higher percentage preparations are used as dermatological bases. Some of the gelling agents are available in different grades indicating the viscosity at a definite concentration. In general, high viscosity grades result in gels at lower concentrations.

Preservatives should be incorporated into the gels, especially those prepared from natural sources. Appropriate preservatives depending upon use and the gelling agent include: the parabens at about 0.2%, benzoic acid 0.2% if the product is acidic, and chlorocresol 0.1%.

The preparation of a few gel bases is given below:

Sodium Alginate Gel Base

Sodium Alginate	2–10 g
Glycerin	2–10 g
Methyl Hydroxybenzoate	0.2 g
a soluble calcium salt	
(calcium or gluconate	0.5 g
Purified Water, to make	100 mL

The sodium alginate is wetted with glycerin, which aids the dispersion, in a mortar. The preservative is dissolved in about 80 mL of water with the aid of heat and allowed to cool, the calcium salt is then added, which will increase the viscosity of the preparation. This solution is stirred in a high speed stirrer and then the sodium alginate-glycerin mixture is slowly added while stirring until the preparation is homogeneous. The preparation should be stored in a tightly sealed container in a wide mouth jar or tube.

Carbomer Jelly

Carbopol 934	2 g
Triethanolamine	1.65 mL
Parabens	0.2 g
Purified Water, to make	100 mL

The parabens are dissolved in 95 mL of water with the aid of heat and allowed to cool, the Carbopol 934, a commercial grade of carbomer, is added in small amounts to the solution in a high speed stirrer, after a smooth dispersion is obtained, the preparation is allowed to stand permitting entrapped air to separate. Then triethanolamine, the gelling agent, is added, dropwise, stirring with a plastic spatula to avoid entrapping air and the remaining water incorporated.

The USP lists a number of gels: Sodium Fluoride and Phosphoric Acid Gel for application to the teeth to reduce cavities, Betamethasone Benzoate Gel and Fluocinonide Gel, anti-inflammatory corticosteroids, Tolnaftate Gel, an antifungal agent, and Tretinoin Gel for acne treatment.

Lotions

Lotions are usually liquid suspensions or dispersions intended for external application to the body. They may be prepared by triturating the ingredients to a smooth paste and then cautiously adding the remaining liquid phase. High-speed mixers or homogenizers produce better dispersions and are, therefore, the tools of choice in the preparation of larger quantities of lotion. Calamine Lotion USP is the classical example of this type of preparation and consists of finely powdered, insoluble solids held in more or less permanent suspension by the presence of suspending agents and/or surface-active agents. Many investigators have studied Calamine Lotion and this had led to the publication of many formulations, each possessing certain advantages over the others but none satisfying the collective needs of all dermatologists. The formula for the official lotion is given on page 779.

Phenolated Calamine Lotion USP (page 780) contains 10 mL of liquefied phenol in sufficient calamine lotion to make the product measure 1000 mL. Formulations containing Avicel R (hydrated microcrystalline cellulose, *FMC Corp.*) and carboxymethylcellulose settle less than do the official preparations.

Calamine Lotion

Calamine	8 g
Zinc Oxide	8 g
Glycerin	2 mL
Avicel R Gel	2 g
Carboxymethylcellulose	2 g
Calcium Hydroxide Solution, a sufficient quantity, to make	100 mL

Phenolated Calamine Lotion

Calamine	8 g
Zinc Oxide	8 g
Glycerin	2 mL
Avicel R Gel	2 g
Carboxymethylcellulose	2 g
Liquefied Phenol	1 mL
Calcium Hydroxide Solution, a sufficient quantity, to make	100 mL

Mix 45 g of Avicel R with 55 g of water in a suitable electric mixer. This gel is used in the preparation of the calamine lotion. Mix the calamine and the zinc oxide with the glycerin, the gel and the carboxymethylcellulose. Add sufficient calcium hydroxide solution to make the product measure 100 mL.

Suspensions may also be formed by chemical interaction in the liquid. White Lotion is an example of this type of preparation.

White Lotion

Zinc Sulfate	40 g
Sulfurated Potash	40 g
Purified Water, a sufficient quantity to make	1000 mL

Dissolve the zinc sulfate and the sulfurated potash separately, each in 450 mL of purified water, and filter each solution. Add slowly the sulfurated potash solution to the zinc sulfate solution with constant stirring. Then add the required amount of purified water, and mix.

Sulfurated potash is a solid of variable composition but is usually described as $K_2S_3 \cdot K_2S_2O_3$. The chemical reaction which occurs when sulfurated potash solution is added to the zinc sulfate solution is given below.

$$ZnSO_4 \cdot 7H_2O + K_2S_3 \cdot K_2S_2O_3 \rightarrow ZnS + S_2$$
$$+ K_2SO_4 + K_2S_2O_3 + 7H_2O$$

This lotion must be freshly prepared and does not contain a suspending agent. Bentonite Magma has been used in some formulations. Coffman and Huyck[26] include a detailed discussion of the chemistry and the problems involved in the preparation of a suitable product.

The USP recognizes a second type of lotion. These are emulsions of the O/W type stabilized by a surface-active agent. Benzyl Benzoate Lotion is an example of this type of preparation. Lastly, some lotions are clear solutions and, in fact, the active ingredient of one official lotion, Dimethisoquin Hydrochloride Lotion, is a water-soluble substance. However, one unofficial formulation for this lotion lists dimethisoquin hydrochloride, menthol, and zinc oxide as active ingredients and the preparation thus becomes a suspension. Several lotions are listed in the USP and contain for example: antibiotics, steroids, keratolytics, and scabicides.

A formula for hydrocortisone lotion is given in the BPC 1973:

Hydrocortisone, finely powdered	**10.0 g**
Chlorocresol	**0.5 g**
Glyceryl Monostearate, self-emulsifying	**40.0 g**
Glycerin	**63.0 g**
Purified Water, to make	**1000.0 g**

The chlorocresol is dissolved in 850 mL of water with the aid of gentle heat, the glyceryl monostearate, self-emulsifying, is added and the mixture heated to 60° with stirring until completely dispersed. The hydrocortisone is triturated with the glycerin which is then incorporated with stirring into the warm base, allowed to cool while stirring, then add the remainder of the water and mix.

Lotions are usually applied without friction. Even so, the insoluble matter should be very finely divided. Particles approaching colloidal dimensions are more soothing to inflamed areas and are more effective in contact with infected surfaces. A wide variety of ingredients may be added to the preparation to produce better dispersions or to accentuate the cooling, soothing, drying, or protective properties of the lotion. Bentonite is a good example of a suspending agent used in the preparation of lotions. Methylcellulose or sodium carboxymethylcellulose will localize and hold the active ingredient in contact with the affected site. A formulation containing glycerin will keep the skin moist for a considerable period of time. The drying and cooling effect may be accentuated by the addition of alcohol to the formula.

Dermatologists frequently prescribe lotions containing anesthetics, antiseptics, astringents, germicides, protectives, or screening agents, to be used in treating or preventing various types of skin diseases and dermatitis. Antihistamines, benzocaine, calamine, resorcin, steroids, sulfur, zinc oxide, and zirconium oxide are common ingredients in unofficial lotions. In many instances the cosmetic aspects of the lotion are of great importance. Many lotions compare badly with cosmetic preparations of a similar nature. The manufacture of fine lotions to meet the specialized needs of the dermatologist provides the pharmacist with an excellent opportunity to demonstrate his professional competence. Recent extensive studies on lotions will assist the pharmacist to gain this goal.[27]

Lotions tend to separate or stratify on long standing, and they require a label directing that they be shaken well before

each use. All lotions should be labeled "For External Use Only."

Microorganisms may grow in certain lotions if no preservative is included in the preparation. Care should be taken to avoid contaminating the lotion during preparation, even if a preservative is present.

Magmas and Milks

Magmas and milks are aqueous suspensions of insoluble, inorganic drugs and differ from gels mainly in that the suspended particles are larger. When prepared, they are thick and viscous, and because of this, there is no need to add a suspending agent to the preparation.

Bentonite Magma USP (page 1297) is prepared by simple hydration. Two procedures are given in the compendium for the preparation of this product.

Magmas may also be prepared by chemical reaction. Magnesium hydroxide is prepared by the hydration of magnesium oxide.

$$MgO + H_2O \rightarrow Mg(OH)_2$$

Milk of Magnesia USP (page 795) is a suspension of magnesium hydroxide containing 7.0–8.5% $Mg(OH)_2$. It has an unpleasant alkaline taste. This taste can be masked with 0.1% citric acid and 0.05% of a volatile oil or a blend of volatile oils. The citric acid reduces the alkalinity of the preparation.

Milk of Bismuth (page 797) contains bismuth hydroxide and basic bismuth carbonate in suspension in water. The Magma is prepared by reacting bismuth subnitrate with nitric acid and ammonium carbonate with ammonia solution and then mixing the resulting two solutions.

The following reactions occur during the preparation of the magma.

$$(NH_4)_2CO_3 \rightarrow 2NH_4^+ + CO_3^{2-}$$

$$NH_3 + H_2O \rightarrow NH_4^+ + OH^-$$

$$2BiO^+ + CO_3^{2-} \rightarrow (BiO)_2CO_3$$

$$BiO^+ + OH^- \rightarrow BiO(OH)$$

If the insoluble substance is freshly precipitated by mixing hot, dilute solutions, there is only slight sedimentation on standing. This characteristic of magmas is sometimes enhanced by passing the product through a colloid mill.

For the most part, magmas and milks are intended for internal use, although Bentonite Magma is used primarily as a suspending eg, Milk of Magnesia USP and Dihydroxy Aluminum Aminoacetate Magma USP, agent for insoluble substances either for local application or for internal use. All magmas require a label directing that they be shaken well before use. Freezing must be avoided.

Mixtures

The official mixtures are aqueous liquid preparations which contain suspended, insoluble, solid substances and are intended for internal use. The insoluble substance does not make the mixture very viscous and the particles may be held in suspension by the use of suitable suspending or thickening agents. This class was originally introduced to secure uniformity in the formulas of certain well-known and largely used preparations. Frequently the term *mixture* is applied loosely to aqueous preparations of every description. The term *shake mixture* is often used for liquid preparations which contain insoluble ingredients and must, therefore, be shaken before use. The USP does not recognize the term. The term *suspension* is now used to describe a number of similar preparations. The BPC uses the term *mixtures* and includes suspensions in this category, for example:

Ammonium Chloride Mixture BPC

Ammonium Chloride	100 g
Aromatic Ammonia Solution	50 mL
Liquorice Liquid Extract	100 mL
Purified Water, to make	1000 mL

It should be recently prepared.

The term mixture occurs in the expression dry mixture which may be used to describe many official USP products, in particular antibiotic powders for oral solutions which have been previously described on page 1498.

The pectin and the tragacanth in Kaolin Mixture with Pectin (page 812) act as suspending agents. An alternate formula, based on Veegum (*Vanderbilt*) and sodium carboxymethylcellulose, has been proposed.[28]

Kaolin Mixture with Pectin

Veegum	0.88 g
Sodium Carboxymethylcellulose	0.22 g
Purified Water	79.12 g
Kaolin	17.50 g
Pectin	0.44 g
Saccharin	0.09 g
Glycerin	1.75 g

Add the Veegum and the sodium carboxymethylcellulose to the water with continuous stirring. Add, with mixing, the kaolin. Mix the pectin, the saccharin, and the glycerin and add to the suspension. A preservative and a flavoring agent may be added to the product.

The insoluble material in mixtures must be in a very finely divided state and it must be uniformly distributed throughout the preparation. This is accomplished by the use of colloid mills, special methods of precipitation, and suspending agents. There are three main reasons for having the insoluble substances in as fine a state of subdivision as possible.

1. The more nearly the colloidal state is approached by protectives, such as kaolin, magnesium trisilicate, and magnesium phosphate, the more active they become as adsorbents and protectives when in contact with inflamed surfaces.
2. Finely divided particles are suspended more readily and settle out much more slowly than large particles, thus enabling the patient to obtain uniform doses of suspended substances. Homogeneous mixtures are especially desirable when administering medication to form an evenly distributed, protective coating on the gastrointestinal tract.
3. The palatability of many preparations is enhanced by the use of colloidal suspending agents.

Mixtures containing suspended material should have a "Shake Well" label affixed to the container in which they are dispensed.

Mixtures, including suspensions, are subject to contamination by microorganisms that remain viable and are a potential health hazard during the period of use of the products. Survival times of organisms depend on the preservative used in the formulation. A kaolin pediatric mixture that contains benzoic acid kills organisms rapidly, whereas organisms survived for more than a week in a magnesium trisilicate mixture that contained no more than a trace of peppermint oil.[29]

Occasionally it is necessary to prepare suspensions from crushed tablets. A general formula for this purpose is given.[24]

Methylcellulose 20	0.75
Parabens	0.1
Purified Water	60.0
Propylene Glycol	2.0
Simple Syrup, to make	100.0

An extemporaneous suspension of cimetidine tablets which retained its potency at 40° over 14 days is:

Cimetidine 300 mg tablets	24 (7,200 mg)
Glycerin	10 mL
Simple Syrup, to make	120 mL

The tablets are triturated using a mortar to a fine powder, the mixture is levigated with the glycerin, the simple syrup is added and mixed well. The mixture is placed in a blender until smooth and is then refrigerated.[30]

Official Suspensions

The USP places particular emphasis on the term suspension by providing specific definitions for a variety of oral, parenteral, and ophthalmic preparations formulated in such a way that an insoluble substance is suspended in a liquid at some stage of the manufacturing or dispensing process. The USP definition begins as follows:

Suspensions are preparations of finely divided, undissolved drugs dispersed in liquid vehicles. Powders for suspension are preparations of finely powdered drugs intended for suspension in liquid vehicles. An example of the ready-to-use type is *Trisulfapyrimidines Oral Suspension*, in which the three sulfapyrimidines are already suspended in a liquid, flavored vehicle in a form suitable for oral administration. *Tetracycline for Oral Suspension* is finely divided tetracycline mixed with suspending and dispersing agents. It is intended to be constituted with the prescribed volume of purified water and mixed before it is dispensed by the pharmacist for oral administration to the patient.

Neither this definition nor the monographs give specific directions for the preparation of the suspension although pharmacopeias usually permit the addition of suitable flavoring agents, suspending agents, preservatives, and certified color additives. One procedure for the preparation of the commonly used *Trisulfapyrimidines Oral Suspension* is given below.

Trisulfapyrimidines Oral Suspension

Veegum	1.00 g
Syrup USP	90.60 g
Sodium Citrate	0.78 g
Sulfadiazine	2.54 g
Sulfamerazine	2.54 g
Sulfamethazine	2.54 g

Add the Veegum, slowly and with continuous stirring, to the syrup. Incorporate the sodium citrate into the Veegum-syrup mixture. Premix the sulfa drugs and add to the syrup. Stir and homogenize. Add sufficient 5% citric acid to adjust the pH of the product to 5.6. A preservative and a flavoring agent may be added to the product.

Methods of preparation for those formulations which contain several active ingredients and are produced in large quantities tend to be more complex than that given above.

Many formulations for suspensions are given in the BPC under the heading of *mixtures*. A properly prepared suspension has a number of desirable properties: (a) the suspended material should not settle rapidly; (b) particles that do settle should not form a hard cake and should easily be uniformly resuspended on shaking; (c) the suspension should pour freely from the container. Insoluble powders that do not disperse evenly throughout the suspending medium, when shaken, should be finely powdered and levigated with a small amount of an agent such as glycerin or alcohol or a portion of the dispersion of the suspending agent. The other ingredients are incorporated and the remainder of the dispersion of the suspending agent is gradually incorporated by trituration to produce the appropriate volume.

Suspensions intended for parenteral or ophthalmic use are also described in the USP. For a discussion of these suspensions, reference should be made to Chapters 85 and 87.

Extraction

Extraction, as the term is used pharmaceutically, involves the separation of medicinally active portions of plant or animal tissues from the inactive or inert components by use of selective solvents in standard extraction procedures. The products so obtained from plants are relatively impure liquids, semisolids, or powders, intended only for oral or external use; they include classes of preparations known as decoctions, infusions, fluidextracts, tinctures, pilular (semisolid) extracts and powdered extracts. Such preparations have been popularly called galenicals, after Galen, the 2nd century Greek physician. For additional information concerning extraction and extractives, which are briefly discussed in the following, see RPS 15, Chapter 86.

In this discussion we are concerned primarily with basic extraction procedures for crude drugs to obtain the therapeutically desirable portion and eliminate the inert material by treatment with a selective solvent, known as the menstruum. Extraction differs from solution in that the presence of insoluble matter is implied in the former process. The principal methods of extraction are: (1) maceration, (2) percolation, (3) digestion, (4) infusion, and (5) decoction.

The processes of particular importance, insofar as the USP is concerned, are those of maceration and percolation; most pharmacopeias refer to such processes for extraction of active principles from crude drugs.

Maceration—In this process the solid ingredients are placed in a stoppered container with the whole of the solvent and allowed to stand for a period of at least three days (until soluble matter is dissolved), with frequent agitation. The mixture is then strained, the marc (the damp solid material) pressed, and the combined liquids are clarified by filtration or by decantation after standing.

Percolation—This is the procedure most frequently used to extract the active ingredients in the preparation of tinctures and fluidextracts. Certain specific procedural details are provided in USP, which should be consulted for such information. In the BPC general procedure, a percolator (a narrow cone-shaped vessel open at both ends) is used. The solid ingredient(s) are moistened with an appropriate amount of specified menstruum and allowed to stand for approximately four hours in a well-closed container, after which the drug mass is packed into the percolator. Sufficient menstruum is added to saturate the mass and the top of the percolator is closed. When the liquid is about to drip from the neck (bottom) of the percolator, the outlet is closed. Additional menstruum is added to give a shallow layer above the mass and the mixture is allowed to macerate in the closed percolator for 24 hours. The outlet of the percolator is then opened and the liquid contained therein is allowed to drip slowly, additional menstruum being added as required, until the percolate measures about three-quarters of the required volume of the finished product. The marc is pressed and the expressed liquid is added to the percolate. Sufficient menstruum is added to produce the required volume, and the mixed liquid is clarified by filtration or by allowing it to stand and then decanting.

For a detailed discussion of various aspects of percolation see RPS 15, Chapter 86.

Digestion—This is a form of maceration in which *gentle heat* is used during the process of extraction. It is used when moderately elevated temperature is not objectionable and the solvent efficiency of the menstruum is increased thereby.

Infusion—An infusion is a dilute solution of the readily soluble constituents of crude drugs. Fresh infusions are prepared by macerating the drugs for a short period of time with either cold or boiling water. US official compendia have not included infusions for some time. An example is Concentrated Compound Gentian Infusion BP 1973.

Decoction—This once-popular process extracts water-soluble and heat-stable constituents from crude drugs by boiling in water for 15 minutes, cooling, straining, and passing sufficient cold water through the drug to produce the required volume.

Extracts

After a solution of the active constituents of a crude drug is obtained by maceration or percolation, it may be ready for use as a medicinal agent, as with certain tinctures or fluidextracts, or it may be further processed to produce a solid or semisolid extract. Information concerning these three classes of extractive preparations follows.*

Tinctures—Tinctures are defined in the USP as being alcoholic or hydroalcoholic solutions prepared from vegetable materials or from chemical substances, an example of the latter being Iodine Tincture. Traditionally, tinctures of potent vegetable drugs essentially represent the activity of 10 g of the drug in each 100 mL of tincture, the potency being adjusted following assay. Most other tinctures of vegetable drugs represent the extractive from 20 g of the drug in 100 mL of tincture.

The USP specifically describes two general processes for preparing tinctures, one by percolation designated as Process P, and the other by maceration designated as Process M. These utilize the methods described above, on this page. Process P includes a modification so that tinctures that require assay for adjustment to specified potency may be thus tested before dilution to final volume. A tincture prepared by Process P as modified for assayed tinctures is Belladonna Tincture. Examples of tinctures prepared by Process M are Compound Benzoin Tincture and Sweet Orange Peel Tincture (the latter contains the extractive from 50 g of sweet orange peel in 100 mL of tincture).

Fluidextracts—The USP defines fluidextracts as being liquid preparations of vegetable drugs, containing alcohol as a solvent or as a preservative, or both, so made that each mL contains the therapeutic constituents of 1 g of the standard drug that it represents. While the USP states that pharmacopeial fluidextracts are made by percolation, the official compendia have previously described general procedures for three percolation methods used in making fluidextracts. Process A is a percolation method that can be modified for fluidextracts that must be assayed. Process E is an alternative for Process A in which percolation is conducted on a column of drug much greater in length than in diameter. Process D is used for preparing fluidextracts with boiling water as the menstruum, alcohol being added as a preservative to the concentrated percolate; this is the procedure used for preparing Cascara Sagrada Fluidextract.

The BP and BPC use the designation *Liquid Extracts* for the category of fluidextracts.

---

* For a discussion of *resins* and *oleoresins* obtained by solvent extraction of plant exudates see Chapter 25, under *Plant Exudates*.

Extracts—Extracts are defined by USP as concentrated preparations of vegetable or animal drugs obtained by removal of the active constituents of the respective drugs with suitable menstrua, evaporation of all or nearly all of the solvent, and adjustment of the residual masses or powders to the prescribed standards.

Three forms of extracts are recognized: semiliquids or liquids of syrupy consistency; plastic masses, known as *pilular* or *solid extracts*; and dry powders, known as *powdered extracts*. Extracts, as concentrated forms of the drugs from which they are prepared, are used in a variety of solid or semisolid dosage forms. The USP states that pilular extracts and powdered extracts of any one drug are interchangeable medicinally, but each has its own pharmaceutical advantages. Pilular extracts, so-called because they are of a consistency that they could be used in pill masses and made into pills, are especially suited for use in ointments and suppositories; powdered extracts are better suited for incorporation into a powdered formulation, as in capsules, powders, or tablets. Semiliquid extracts or extracts of a syrupy consistency may be used in the manufacture of some pharmaceutical preparations.

Most extracts are prepared by extracting the drug by percolation. The percolate is concentrated, generally by distillation under reduced pressure; use of heat is avoided where possible because of potential injurious effect on active constituents. Powdered extracts that are made from drugs that contain inactive oily or fatty matter may have to be defatted or prepared from defatted drug. For diluents that may be used to adjust an extract to prescribed standards, see the USP.

Pure Glycyrrhiza Extract USP is an example of a pilular extract; Belladonna Extract USP and Hyoscyamus Extract BPC are examples of powdered extracts (the former is prepared also as a pilular extract and the latter as a liquid extract).

References

1. Ostendorf JP: *J Soc Cosmet Chem 16:* 203, 1965.
2. Chalmers L: *Soap Perfum Cosmet 44:* Jan. 29, 1971.
3. Bruch CW: *Drug Cosmetic Ind 111:* Oct. 51, 1972.
4. Coates D: *Manuf Chem Aerosol News 44:* June 35, Aug 41, Oct 34, Dec 19, 1973; *45:* Jan 19, 1974.
5. Hickman K, *et al: Science 180:* 15, 1973.
6. Bergen A: *Can J Hosp Pharm 30:* July–Aug. 109, 1977.
7. Meer T: *Flavoring Pharmaceutical Preparations* (SK&F Selected Pharm Res Refs No 4) SK&F, Philadelphia, Feb 11, 1957.
8. Schumacher GE: *Am J Hosp Pharm 24:* 588, 713, 1967: *25:* 154, 1968.
9. *Am Drug 175:* May 24, 1977.
10. Daoust RG, Lynch MJ: *Drug Cosmetic Ind 90:* 689, 1962.
11. Boehm EE, Maddox DN: *Manuf Chem Aerosol News 43:* Aug. 21, 1972.
12. Hutchins HH, Singiser RE: *J Am Pharm Assoc Pract Pharm Ed 16:* 226, 1955.
13. Sumner ED: *J Am Pharm Assoc NS8:* 250, 1968.
14. Reynolds JEF ed: "*Martindale The Extra Pharmacopoeia,*" 28th ed., The Pharmaceutical Press, London, 425, 1982.
15. Ecker V, Fisher E: *Harokeach Haivri 13:* 350, 1969, through *Inter Pharm Abstr 7:* 4241, 1970.
16. Griffin WC, *et al: Drug Cosmetic Ind 101:* Oct 41, Nov 52, 1967.
17. White RF: "*Pharmaceutical Emulsions and Emulsifying Agents,*" 4th ed, The Chemist and Druggist, London, 1964.
18. Whitehill D: *Chem Drug 213:* Jan 130, 1980.
19. Becher P: *Emulsions: Theory and Practice,* Reinhold, New York, 267, 1965.
20. Peck GE, *et al: J Am Pharm Assoc Sci Ed 49:* 75, 1960.
21. Lin TJ: *J Soc Cosmetic Chem 29:* 117, 1978.
22. Eisberg N: *Manuf Chem 53:* Jan. 27, 1982.
23. Nash RA: *Drug and Cosmetic Ind 97:* 843, 1965: *98:* 39, 1966.
24. See Ref 14, 947, 948.
25. Carter SJ: "*Cooper and Gunn's Dispensing for Pharmaceutical Students,*" 12th ed, Pitman Medical, London 214, 1975.
26. Coffman HL, Huyck CL: *Am J Hosp Pharm 20:* 132, 1963.
27. Harb NSA: *Cosmet Perfum 89:* April 67, 1974 through *Inter Pharm Abstr 11:* 3304, 1974.
28. Kalish J: *Drug Cosmet Ind 94:* 276, 1964.
29. Westwood N: *Pharm J 208:* 153, 1972.
30. Tortorici MP: *Am J Hosp Pharm 36:* 22, 1979.

CHAPTER 85

Parenteral Preparations

Kenneth E Avis, DSc

Goodman Professor and Chairman, Department of Pharmaceutics
College of Pharmacy, University of Tennessee Center for the Health Sciences
Memphis, TN 38163

The term parenteral (Gk, *para enteron* = beside the intestine) refers to the route of administration of drugs by injection under or through one or more layers of skin or mucous membrane. Since this route circumvents the highly efficient protective barriers of the human body, the skin and mucous membranes, exceptional purity of the dosage form must be achieved. The processes utilized in preparing the dosage form must embody good manufacturing practices that will produce and maintain the required quality of the product. New developments in process technology and quality control should be adopted as soon as their value and reliability have been established as a means for further improving the quality of the product.

History[1]

One of the most significant events in the beginnings of parenteral therapy was the first recorded injection of drugs into the veins of living animals, in about the year 1657, by the architect Sir Christopher Wren. From such a very crude beginning, the technique for intravenous injection and knowledge of the implications thereof developed slowly during the next century and a half. In 1855 Dr Alexander Wood of Edinburgh described what was probably the first subcutaneous injection of drugs for therapeutic purposes using a true hypodermic syringe.

The latter half of the 19th century brought increasing concern for safety in the administration of parenteral solutions, largely because of the work of Robert Koch and Louis Pasteur. While Charles Chamberland was developing both hot-air and steam sterilization techniques and the first bacteria-retaining filter (made of unglazed porcelain), Stanislaus Limousin was developing a suitable container, the all-glass ampul. In the middle 1920s Dr. Florence Seibert provided proof that the disturbing chills and fever which often followed the intravenous injection of drugs was caused by potent products of microbial growth, pyrogens, which could be eliminated from water by distillation and from glassware by heating at elevated temperatures.

Of the recent developments that have contributed to the high quality standards currently achievable in the preparation of parenteral dosage forms, the two that have probably contributed most are the development of HEPA-filtered laminar air flow and the development of membrane microfiltration for solutions. The former has made it possible to achieve ultraclean environmental conditions for the processing of sterile products, and the latter has made it possible to remove from solutions by filtration both viable and nonviable particles of microbial size and smaller. However, many other developments in recent years have produced an impressive advance in the technology associated with the safe and reliable preparation of parenteral dosage forms. The following list identifies a few of the events which have contributed to that development.

1926—Parenterals were accepted for inclusion in the fifth edition of the *National Formulary.*

1933—The practical application of freeze-drying to clinical materials was accomplished by a team of scientists at the University of Pennsylvania.

1938—The Food, Drug and Cosmetic Act was passed by Congress, establishing the Food and Drug Administration (FDA).

1944—The sterilant ethylene oxide was discovered.

1946—The Parenteral Drug Association was organized.

1961—The concept of laminar airflow was developed by WJ Whitfield.

1962—The FDA was authorized by Congress to establish current good manufacturing practices (CGMP) regulations.

1965—Total parenteral nutrition (TPN) was developed by SJ Dudrick.

1972—The Limulus Amebocyte Lysate test for pyrogens in parenteral products was developed by JF Cooper.

Administration

Injections may be classified in five general categories: (1) solutions ready for injection, (2) dry, soluble products ready to be combined with a solvent just prior to use, (3) suspensions ready for injection, (4) dry, insoluble products ready to be combined with a vehicle just prior to use, and (5) emulsions. These injections may be administered by such routes as intravenous, subcutaneous, intradermal, intramuscular, intraspinal, intracisternal, and intrathecal. The nature of the product will determine the particular route of administration that may be employed. Conversely, the desired route of administration will place requirements on the formulation. For example, suspensions would not be administered directly into the blood stream because of the danger of insoluble particles blocking capillaries. Solutions to be administered subcutaneously would require strict attention to tonicity adjustment, otherwise irritation of the plentiful supply of nerve endings in this anatomical area would give rise to pronounced pain. Injections intended for intraocular, intraspinal, intracisternal, and intrathecal administration require the highest purity standards because of the sensitivity of nerve tissue to irritant and toxic substances.

When compared with other dosage forms, injections possess select advantages. If immediate physiological action is needed from a drug, it usually can be provided by intravenous injection of an aqueous solution. Modification of the formulation or another route of injection can be used to slow the onset and prolong the action of the drug. The therapeutic response of a drug is more readily controlled by parenteral administration since the irregularities of intestinal absorption are circumvented. Also, since the drug normally is administered by a professionally trained person, it may be confidently expected that the dose was actually and accurately administered. Drugs can be administered parenterally when they cannot be given orally because of the unconscious or uncooperative state of the patient, or because of inactivation or lack of absorption in the intestinal tract. Among the disadvantages of this dosage form are the requirement of asepsis at administration, the risk of tissue toxicity from local irritation, the real or psychological pain factor, and the difficulty in correcting an error, should one be made. In the latter situation, unless a direct pharmacological antagonist is immediately available, correction of an error may be impossible. One other disadvantage is that daily or frequent administration poses difficulties, either for the patient to visit a professionally trained person or to learn to inject oneself.

Parenteral Combinations

Since there is a degree of discomfort for the patient with each injection, a physician will frequently seek to reduce this discomfort by combining more than one drug in one injection. This is most commonly encountered when therapeutic agents are added to large-volume solutions of electrolytes or nutrients, commonly called "IV additives," during intravenous administration. Since these preparations would be aqueous solutions, there is a high potential for chemical and physical interactions to occur. See Chapter 101. The pharmacist is the professional best qualified to cope with these incompatibilities. However, in the past, these have been handled largely at the patient's bedside by the nurse and physician. Only recently has it been recognized that this professional area is the proper function of a pharmacist and has been so stated by the Joint Commission on Accreditation of Hospitals.[2]

As pharmacists have assumed increasing responsibility in this area, awareness has gradually developed of the widespread occurrence of visible, as well as invisible, physical, chemical, and therapeutic incompatibilities when certain drugs are combined or added to intravenous fluids.

Development of a precipitate or a color change when preparations are combined is an immediate warning that an alteration has occurred. Such a combination should not be administered to the patient because the solid particles may occlude the blood vessels, the therapeutic agent may not be available for absorption, or the drug may have been degraded into toxic substances. Moreover, in other instances changes not visually apparent may have occurred which could be equally or more dangerous to the welfare of the patient.

The almost innumerable potential combinations present a complex situation even for the pharmacist. In an attempt to organize the information available and to aid the pharmacist in making rapid decisions concerning potential problems, a number of charts have been compiled based on the visible changes that may be observed when two or more preparations are combined. The value of such charts is limited by such factors as frequent changes in commercial products, variations in order of mixing or the proportions in the mixture, differences in concentration of each ingredient, or variations in the period of time that the combination is held before use.

As studies have been undertaken and more information has been gained, it has been shown that knowledge of variable factors such as pH and the ionic character of the active constituents aids substantially in understanding and predicting potential incompatibilities. Kinetic studies of reaction rates may be utilized to describe or predict the extent of degradation. Ultimately, a thorough study should be undertaken of each therapeutic agent in combination with other drugs and intravenous fluids, not only of generic but of commercial preparations, from the physical, chemical, and therapeutic aspects. Such studies are being undertaken and some have been reported.

Ideally, no parenteral combination should be administered unless it has been thoroughly studied to determine the effect of the combination on the therapeutic value and the safety of each such combination. However, such an ideal situation does not and may never exist. Therefore, it is the responsibility of the pharmacist to be as familiar as possible with the phys-

ical, chemical, and therapeutic aspects of parenteral combinations and to exercise the best possible judgment as to whether or not the specific combination extemporaneously prescribed is suitable for use in a patient. A service to pharmacists has been provided through reviews of this subject area.[3]

General Requirements

An inherent requirement for parenteral preparations is that they be of the very best quality and provide the maximum safety for the patient. Therefore, the pharmacist, being responsible for their preparation, must utilize skills and resourcefulness at the highest level of efficiency to achieve this end. Among the areas requiring dedicated attention are the following:

1. Possession and application of high moral and professional ethics. Even the thought of using inferior techniques or ingredients in a manufacturing process must not be countenanced by the pharmacist. The proper attitude of the person responsible for the preparation of the product is its most vital ingredient.
2. The pharmaceutical training received must be utilized to the fullest measure. The challenges to this knowledge bank will be many and varied.
3. Specialized techniques will be required for the manufacture of sterile preparations, employing them with alertness and sound judgment. These techniques must be subjected to continuous critical review for faults, omissions, and improvements.
4. Ingredients of the highest quality obtainable must be utilized. At times ingredients may require special purification beyond that of the commercial supply. This will normally require that cost factors be given second place in importance.
5. The stability and effectiveness of the product must be established with substantiating data, either from original or published sources. This must take into account process variations and differences in ingredient specifications from plant to plant.
6. A well-defined and controlled program must be established to assure the quality of the product and the repetition of valid production procedures. This involves evaluation of all ingredients, vigilant controls of all steps in the production procedures, and careful evaluation of the finished product.

Injections or other sterile products are rarely prepared in the community pharmacy because of the lack of adequate facilities necessary to prepare a reliable and safe product.

In some hospital pharmacies injections or irrigating fluids are manufactured, but in an increasing number aseptic processing is utilized primarily in the addition of various drugs to intravenous solutions for the individual patient. The vast majority of injectable products used clinically are prepared by the pharmaceutical industry.

General Process

The preparation of a parenteral product may be considered to encompass four general areas as follows: (1) procurement and selection of the components, (2) production facilities and procedures, (3) control of quality, and (4) packaging and labeling. The components of the product to be procured include vehicles, solutes, containers, and closures. The steps constituting production include the maintenance of facilities and equipment, preparing and controlling the environment, cleaning the containers and equipment, preparing the product, filtering the solution, filling containers with the product, sealing the containers, and sterilizing the product. Control of quality includes the evaluation of the components, validation of equipment and processes, determination that the production has been executed within prescribed requirements, and performance of necessary evaluative tests on the finished product. The final area of packaging and labeling includes all steps necessary to identify the finished product and enclose it in such manner that it is safely and properly prepared for sale and delivery to the user. In the following sections, these four areas and appropriate subtopics will be discussed in detail.

Components and Containers

Establishing specifications to insure the quality of each of the components of an injection is of vital importance. These specifications will be coordinated with the requirements of the specific formulation and will not necessarily be identical for a particular component if used in several different formulations.

The most stringent requirements normally will be encountered with aqueous solutions, particularly if the product is to be sterilized at an elevated temperature where reaction rates will be greatly accelerated. Modification of aqueous vehicles to include a glycol, or replacement with a nonaqueous vehicle, will usually reduce reaction rates. Dry preparations pose relatively few reaction problems but may require definitive physical specifications for ingredients that must have certain solution or dispersion characteristics when a vehicle is added.

Containers and closures are herein considered components of the product because they are in prolonged, intimate contact with the product and may release substances or remove ingredients from the product. While not usually considered a part of a container, administration devices are a part of a container system and their effect upon the product must be assessed even though the contact period is usually brief.

Vehicles

Since most liquid injections are quite dilute, the component present in the highest proportion is the vehicle. A vehicle normally has no therapeutic activity and is nontoxic. However, it is of great importance in the formulation since it presents to body tissues the form of the active constituent for absorption. Absorption normally occurs most rapidly and completely when a drug is presented as an aqueous solution. Modification of the vehicle with water-miscible liquids or substitution with water-immiscible liquids normally decreases the rate of absorption. Absorption from a suspension may be affected by such factors as the viscosity of the vehicle, its capacity for wetting the solid particles, the solubility equilibrium produced by the vehicle, and the distribution coefficient between the vehicle and aqueous body systems.

The vehicle of greatest importance for parenteral products is water. Water of suitable quality for parenteral administration must be prepared either by distillation or by reverse osmosis. Only by these means is it possible to separate adequately various liquid, gas and solid contaminating substances from water.

Preparation of Water

In general, a conventional still consists of a boiler (evaporator) containing raw water (distilland), a source of heat to vaporize the water in the evaporator, a headspace above the level of distilland with condensing surfaces for refluxing the vapor and thereby returning nonvolatile impurities to the distilland, a means for eliminating volatile impurities before the hot water vapor is condensed, and a condenser for removing the heat of vaporization, thereby converting the water vapor to a liquid distillate.

It should be apparent that the specific construction features of a still and the process specifications will markedly affect the quality of distillate obtained from a still. Those required for producing high-purity water, such as Water for Injection USP, must be considerably more stringent than those required for Purified Water USP. Among the factors that must be considered are:

1. The quality of the raw water will affect the quality of the distillate. It may be necessary that the raw water be first softened, deionized, or treated by reverse osmosis to obtain a final distillate of adequate quality.

2. The size of the evaporator will affect the efficiency. The evaporator should be large enough to provide a low vapor velocity, thus reducing entrainment of distilland either as a film on vapor bubbles or as separate droplets.

3. The baffles (condensing surfaces) determine the effectiveness of refluxing. They should be designed to efficiently remove entrainment at optimal vapor velocity, collecting and returning the heavier droplets contaminated with distilland.

4. Redissolving of volatile impurities in the distillate reduces purity. Therefore, volatile impurities should be separated efficiently from the hot water vapor and eliminated by aspirating to the drain or venting to the atmosphere.

5. Contamination of the vapor and distillate from the metal parts of the still can occur. Present standards for high-purity stills are that all parts contacted by the vapor or distillate should be constructed of metal coated with pure tin, of 304 or 316 stainless steel, or of chemically resistant glass.

Design features of a still also influence its efficiency of operation, relative freedom from maintenance problems, or the extent of automatic operation. Stills may be constructed of varying size, rated according to the volume of distillate that can be produced per hour of operation under optimum conditions. Only stills designed to produce high-purity water may be considered for use in the production of Water for Injection (WFI).

Conventional commercial stills designed for the production of high-purity water, such as shown in Fig 85-1, are available from several suppliers.*

Compression Distillation—The vapor compression still, primarily designed for the production of large volumes of high purity distillate with low consumption of energy and water,

_____
* *Am Sterilizer, Barnstead, Consolidated, Corning, Finn-Aqua.*

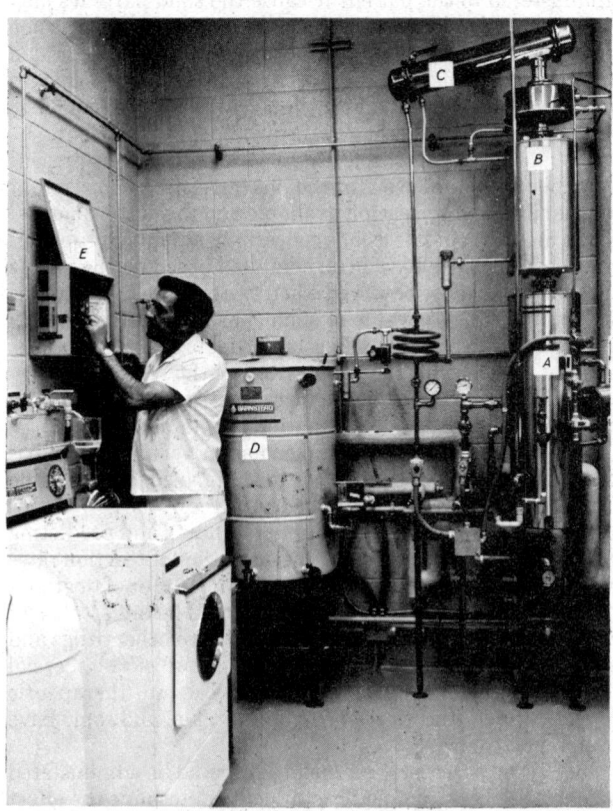

Fig. 85-1. High-purity still and sealed water storage system. *A:* Evaporator; *B:* high-purity baffle unit; *C:* condenser; *D:* storage tank with ultraviolet lamp; *E:* control panel (courtesy, Ciba-Geigy).

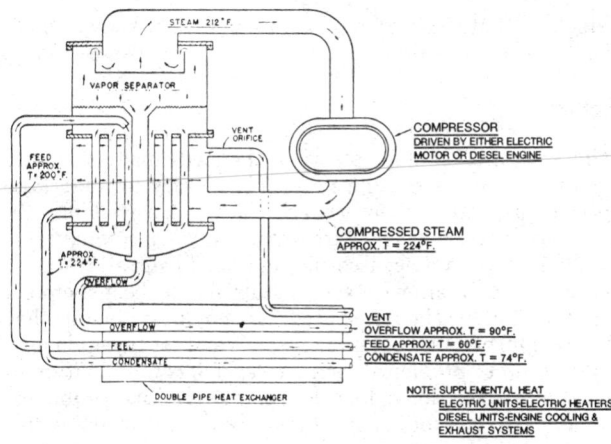

Fig. 85-2.   Vapor compression still.

is illustrated diagrammatically in Fig 85-2. To start, the feed water is heated in the evaporator to boiling. The vapor produced in the tubes is separated from entrained distilland in the separator and conveyed to a compressor which compresses the vapor and raises its temperature to approximately 224°F. It then flows to the steam chest where it condenses on the outer surfaces of the tubes containing distilland; thereby the vapor is condensed and drawn off as distillate while giving up its heat to bring the distilland in the tubes to the boiling point.

Vapor compression stills are available in capacities from 50 to 2800 gal/hour (*Aqua-Chem, Barnstead, Meco*).

Multiple-Effect Stills—The multiple-effect still also is designed to conserve energy and water usage. In principle, this still is simply a series of single effect stills running at differing pressures. A series of up to seven effects may be used, with the first effect operated at the highest pressure and the last effect at atmospheric pressure. Steam from an external source is used in the first effect to generate steam from raw water. The generated steam is under pressure and is used as the power source to drive the second effect. The steam used to drive the second effect condenses as it gives up its heat of vaporization and forms distillate. This process continues until the last effect when the steam is at atmospheric pressure and must be condensed in a heat exchanger.

The capacity of a multiple-effect still can be increased by adding effects. The quality of distillate also will be affected by the inlet steam pressure, thus a 600 gallon per hour unit designed to operate at 115 psig steam pressure could be run at approximately 55 psig and would deliver about 400 gallons per hour. These stills have no moving parts and operate quietly. They are available in capacities from about 50 to 7,000 gallons per hour (*AMSCO, Barnstead, Finn-Aqua*).

Reverse Osmosis—Reverse osmosis has recently been added by the USP as a method suitable for preparation of Water for Injection. As the name suggests, the natural process of selective permeation of molecules through a semipermeable membrane separating two aqueous solutions of different concentrations is reversed. Pressure, usually between 200 and 400 psig, is applied to overcome osmotic pressure and force pure water to permeate through the membrane. Membranes, usually composed of cellulose esters or polyamides, are selected to provide an efficient rejection of contaminant molecules in raw water. The molecules most difficult to remove are small inorganic molecules such as sodium chloride. Passage through two membranes in series is sometimes utilized to increase the efficiency of removal of these small molecules and to decrease the risk of structural failure of a membrane to remove other contaminants, such as bacteria and pyrogens (for additional information concerning

reverse osmosis see under this title in Chapter 78, and Fig. 78-21, in that chapter; also the discussion under *Water* in Chapter 84).

Currently, extensive validation is being undertaken to determine whether, in fact, this method is capable of consistently producing high-purity water of a quality equal or superior to that producible by distillation.

Water for Injection USP

This is a high-purity water intended to be used as a vehicle for injectable preparations. Sterile Water for Injection USP is described in a separate monograph and differs in that it is intended as a packaged and sterilized product.

Storage—If WFI cannot be used immediately after it is produced, the USP permits storage at room temperature for a period not exceeding 24 hours or for longer periods at a temperature too high or too low for microbial growth to occur. Therefore, WFI usually is collected directly from the reverse osmosis unit or a still in a closed system designed to prevent recontamination of the water and to hold it at a constant temperature of 60–80°C. The system may range from a relatively small single storage tank with a draw-off spout (Figure 85-1) to a very large system holding several thousand gallons of water. The stainless steel tank in such a system is usually connected to a welded stainless steel distribution loop supplying the various use sites with a continuously circulating water supply. The tank would be provided with a hydrophobic membrane vent filter capable of excluding bacteria and nonviable particulate matter. Such a vent filter is necessary to permit changes in pressure during filling and emptying of the tank. The material of construction for the tank and connecting lines is usually electropolished 316L stainless steel with heliarc welded pipe. The tanks also may be lined with glass or a coating of pure tin. Such systems are very carefully designed and constructed and often constitute the most costly installation within the plant.

When the water cannot be used at 80°C, heat exchangers must be installed to reduce the temperature at the point of use. Bacterial retentive filters should not be installed in such systems because of the risk of bacterial build-up on the filters and the consequential release of pyrogenic substances.

Purity—The USP monographs provide standards of purity for Water for Injection (WFI) and for Sterile Water for Injection (SWFI). A few of these standards require comment.

SWFI must meet the requirements of the USP Sterility Test, but WFI need not since it is to be used in a product which will be sterilized. Both must meet the requirements of the USP Pyrogen Test (page 558).

The limits for total solids varies in the two monographs. The larger the surface area of the glass container per unit volume of water, the greater the amount of glass constituents that may be leached into the water, particularly during the elevated temperature of steam sterilization.

The WFI monograph stipulates a maximum of 10 ppm of total solids. This is generally considered to be much too high to assure a quality of water that would permit stable formulation of many drugs. A relatively few metallic ions present can often render a formulation unstable. Therefore, it is common practice to set a limit of 0.1 ppm or less of ionic contaminants expressed as sodium chloride.

Ionic contaminant level is not the same as total solids, the former being a measurement of only the ionic content, while the latter is a measurement of undissociated constituents as well. The ionic content of water can be measured very easily by means of a conductivity meter, and is frequently used as an indication of the purity. The results are expressed in one of three terms; namely, as sodium chloride ions, as resistance in ohms or megohms, or as conductance in micromhos. Ohms and mhos have a reciprocal relationship to each other, but they are related to ppm sodium chloride by an experimentally determined curve. To give one point of comparison, 0.1 ppm sodium chloride is equal to approximately 1.01 megohms and 0.99 micromhos. It should be mentioned that conductivity measurements give no direct indication of pyrogen content of water since pyrogens are undissociated organic compounds.

WFI may not contain an added substance. SWFI may contain a bacteriostatic agent when in containers of 30-mL capacity or smaller. This restriction is designed to prevent the administration of a large quantity of a bacteriostatic agent that probably would be toxic in the accumulated amount of a large volume of solution, even though the concentration was low.

Types of Vehicles

Aqueous Vehicles—Certain aqueous vehicles are recognized officially because of their valid use in parenteral formulations. Often they are used as isotonic vehicles to which a drug may be added at the time of administration. The additional osmotic effect of the drug may not be enough to produce any discomfort when administered. These vehicles include: Sodium Chloride Injection, Ringer's Injection, Dextrose Injection, Dextrose and Sodium Chloride Injection, and Lactated Ringer's Injection.

Water-Miscible Vehicles—A number of solvents that are miscible with water have been used as a portion of the vehicle in the formulation of parenterals. These solvents are used primarily to effect solubility of certain drugs and to reduce hydrolysis. The most important solvents in this group are ethyl alcohol, polyethylene glycol of the liquid series, and propylene glycol. Ethyl alcohol is used particularly in the preparation of solutions of cardiac glycosides and the glycols in solutions of barbiturates, certain alkaloids, and certain antibiotics. Such preparations are usually given intramuscularly.

These solvents, as well as nonaqueous vehicles, have been reviewed by Spiegel and Noseworthy.[4]

Nonaqueous Vehicles—The most important group of nonaqueous vehicles are the fixed oils. The USP provides specifications for such vehicles. A few of these requirements need to be discussed. The fixed oils must be of vegetable origin in order that they may be metabolized, will be liquid at room temperature, and will not become rancid rapidly. The first specification eliminates oils of mineral origin and the latter two, those of animal origin. To be liquid at room temperature, a fixed oil must contain esters of unsaturated fatty acids. However, excessive unsaturation will produce tissue irritation. Therefore, the USP stipulates upper and lower limits to the iodine value for the oil. The development of rancidity must be prevented by the inclusion of antioxidants such as tocopherol, a natural constituent of many fixed oils. The USP also prescribes an upper limit for free fatty acids in order to minimize the degree of tissue irritation. Other specifications are included primarily to detect adulteration. The oils most commonly used are corn oil, cottonseed oil, peanut oil, and sesame oil. It should be noted that the official monographs for some of these oils provide for greater latitude than the specifications required for the use of the oil as a vehicle for a parenteral. Therefore, parenteral vehicle oils must be select oils or specially purified to meet the more stringent requirements. Fixed oils are used particularly as vehicles for certain hormone preparations. These and other nonaqueous vehicles, such as ethyl oleate, isopropyl myristate, and benzyl benzoate, may be used provided they are safe in the volume administered and do not interfere with the therapeutic efficacy of the preparation or with its response to prescribed assays and tests. The label also must state the name of the vehicle so that the user may beware in case of known sensitivity or other reactions to it.

Solutes

The requirements for purity of the medicinal compound used in an injection often make it necessary to undertake special purification of the usual chemical grade available. In a few instances, a special parenteral grade of a compound is available, for example, ascorbic acid freed from all traces of copper contamination. As a general rule, the best chemical grade obtainable should be used. It should be obvious that if a few ppm of ionic contaminants in Water for Injection may cause stability problems, a similar level of contamination in the solute itself may, likewise, cause stability problems. Metallic catalysis of chemical reactions is one which is frequently encountered.

Other factors to be considered with respect to the quality of solutes include: the level of microbial and pyrogenic contamination, solubility characteristics as determined by the chemical or physical form of the compound, and freedom from gross dirt.

Added Substances—The USP includes in this category all substances added to a preparation to improve or safeguard the quality of the product. An added substance may effect solubility, as does sodium benzoate in Caffeine and Sodium Benzoate Injection, or provide patient comfort, as do substances added to make a solution isotonic. They may enhance the chemical stability of a solution, as do antioxidants, inert gases, chelating agents, and buffers, or they may preserve a preparation against the growth of microorganisms. The term "preservative" is sometimes applied only to those substances which prevent the growth of microorganisms in a preparation. However, such limited use is inappropriate, being better used for all substances that act to retard or prevent the chemical, physical, or biological degradation of a preparation.

While added substances may prevent a certain reaction from taking place, they may induce others. Not only may visible incompatibilities occur, but hydrolysis, complexation, oxidation, and other invisible reactions may decompose or otherwise inactivate the therapeutic agent. Therefore, added substances must be selected with due consideration and investigation of the effect of the substance on the total formulation.

Antimicrobial Agents—The USP states that antimicrobial agents in bacteriostatic or fungistatic concentrations must be added to preparations contained in multiple-dose containers. They must be present in adequate concentration at the time of use to prevent the multiplication of microorganisms inadvertently introduced into the preparation while withdrawing a portion of the contents with a hypodermic needle and syringe. Among the compounds most frequently employed, with the concentration limit prescribed by the USP, are: phenylmercuric nitrate and thimerosal 0.01%, benzethonium chloride and benzalkonium chloride 0.01%, phenol or cresol 0.5%, and chlorobutanol 0.5%. The above limit is rarely used for phenylmercuric nitrate, being most frequently employed in a concentration of 0.002%. Methyl p-hydroxybenzoate 0.18% and propyl p-hydroxybenzoate 0.02% in combination, and benzyl alcohol 2% are also frequently used. In oleaginous preparations, no antibacterial agent commonly employed appears to be effective. However, it has been reported that hexylresorcinol 0.5% and phenylmercuric benzoate 0.1% are moderately bactericidal.

Antimicrobial agents must be studied with respect to compatibility with all other components of the formula. In addition, their activity must be evaluated in the total formula. It is not uncommon to find that a particular agent will be effective in one formulation but ineffective in another. This may be due to the effect of various components of the formula on the biological activity or availability of the compound; for example, the binding and inactivation of esters of *p*-hydroxybenzoic acid by macromolecules such as Polysorbate 80 or the reduction of phenylmercuric nitrate by sulfide residues in rubber closures. A physical reaction encountered is that bacteriostatic agents are sometimes removed from solution by rubber closures. These facts establish the principle that antimicrobial agents must be evaluated for their activity in the total formula to assure their activity when needed, normally at the time of use.

Buffers—Buffers are used primarily to stabilize a solution against the chemical degradation that might occur if the pH changed appreciably. Buffer systems employed should normally have as low a buffer capacity as feasible in order not to disturb significantly the body buffer systems when injected. In addition, the buffer range and the effect of the buffer on the activity of the product must be evaluated carefully. The acid salts most frequently employed as buffers are citrates, acetates, and phosphates.

Antioxidants—Antioxidants are frequently required to preserve products because of the ease with which many drugs are oxidized. Sodium bisulfite 0.1% is most frequently used. The use of sulfites as antioxidants has been reviewed by Schroeter[5]. Acetone sodium bisulfite, sodium formaldehyde sulfoxylate, and thiourea are also sometimes used. The sodium salt of ethylenediaminetetraacetic acid has been found to enhance the activity of antioxidants in some cases, apparently by chelating metallic ions that would otherwise catalyze the oxidation reaction.

Pyrogens

Pyrogens may be anticipated contaminants in crude drugs, such as antibiotics produced by fermentation, or they may be present as unexpected and unwanted contaminants in a finished product as a result of inadvertent contamination during processing. In the former instance, they must be eliminated during the purification steps of the drug. In the latter instance, they can best be eliminated by preventing their introduction during the process. In general, the presence of pyrogens in a finished product is indicative of a product prepared under inadequately controlled clean conditions.

Pyrogens cause a febrile reaction in human beings. Other symptoms include chills, pains in back and legs, and malaise. While pyrogenic substances are rarely fatal, they produce significant discomfort for the patient. On the other hand, pyrogens have been shown to induce a general'nonspecific resistance to microorganisms and, on this basis, have been used therapeutically.

Pyrogens are products of the growth of microorganisms. The most potent pyrogenic substances are produced by Gram-negative bacteria, but Gram-positive bacteria and fungi also produce pyrogenic substances. The potency varies with the species producing it. Chemically, pyrogenic material has been shown to be lipid in nature, sometimes containing phosphorus, and is attached to a polysaccharide or a protein or both. When so complexed, it is a weak antigen. A temporary tolerance to pyrogens will develop in man and susceptible animals.

Pyrogens can be destroyed by heating at high temperatures. The recommended procedure for depyrogenation of glassware and equipment is heating at a temperature of 250°C for 45 min. It has been reported that 650°C for 1 min or 180°C for 4 hours likewise will destroy pyrogens. The usual autoclaving cycle will not do so. Heating with strong alkali or oxidizing solutions will destroy pyrogens. It has been claimed that thorough washing with detergent treatment will render glassware pyrogen-free if it has been protected during manufacture and storage from heavy pyrogenic contamination. Likewise, plastic containers and devices must be protected from pyrogenic contamination during manufacture and storage since known ways to destroy pyrogens will adversely affect the plastic. It has been reported that anion exchange resins will adsorb pyrogens from water and reverse osmosis will eliminate them. However, the most reliable method for the elimination of these substances from water is distillation. Pyrogenic substances are not volatile and thus will remain in the distilland.

A method that has been used for the removal of pyrogens from solutions is adsorption on adsorptive agents. However, since the adsorption phenomenon may also cause selective removal of chemical substances from the solution and the filtrate may be contaminated with the agent, this method has limited application. Other in-process methods for the destruction or elimination of pyrogens include selective extraction procedures and careful heating with dilute alkali, dilute acid, or mild oxidizing agents. In each instance, the method must be thoroughly studied to be sure it will not have an adverse effect on the constituents of the product. New developments in ultrafiltration have made possible pyrogen separation on a molecular weight basis but, currently, this is not a feasible method for large scale processing.

Sources of Pyrogens—Pyrogens may enter a preparation by any means that will introduce living or dead microorganisms or the products of their growth. Perhaps the greatest potential source of such contamination is the water used in products. Although proper distillation will provide pyrogen-free water, storage conditions must be such that microorganisms are not introduced and subsequent growth is prevented.

Another potential source of contamination is equipment. Pyrogenic materials adhere strongly to glass and other surfaces. Reusing containers, as is sometimes practiced in hospitals, may be a significant source of pyrogenic contamination. Residues of solutions in used bottles often become bacterial cultures from septic patients or the environment. Such bottles will be heavily contaminated with pyrogens. Even washed bottles left wet and exposed to the atmosphere may contain sufficient nutrients for microorganisms to grow. Since drying does not destroy pyrogens, they may remain in equipment for long periods of time. Adequate washing accompanied by dry-heat depyrogenation will render contaminated equipment suitable for use.

The solute also may be a source of pyrogens. Solutes may be crystallized or precipitated from aqueous liquids containing pyrogenic contamination. In the process pyrogens may be trapped within the particle layers. In such cases the solute must be purified by recrystallization, precipitate washing, or other means to eliminate the pyrogens.

The manufacturing process also must be carried out with great care and as rapidly as possible to minimize the risk of microbial contamination. Preferably, no more product should be prepared than can be completely processed within one working day, including sterilization.

Containers

Containers are an integral part of the formulation of an injection and may be considered a component, for there is no container that is totally insoluble or does not in some way affect the liquid it contains, particularly if the liquid is aqueous. Therefore, the selection of a container for a particular injection must be based on a consideration of the composition of the container, as well as of the solution, and the treatment to which it will be subjected.

Plastic

Thermoplastic polymers are increasingly being used as packaging materials for sterile preparations such as large-volume parenterals and ophthalmic solutions. For this to be acceptable, an understanding of the characteristics, potential problems, and advantages for use must be developed. One thorough review of these factors relative to pharmaceuticals has been prepared by Autian.[6] He stated that three principal problem areas exist in utilization of these materials, namely, (1) permeation of vapors and other molecules in either direction through the wall of the plastic container, (2) leaching of constituents from the plastic into the product, and (3) sorption (absorption and/or adsorption) of drug molecules or ions on the plastic material. Permeation, the most extensive problem, may be troublesome by permitting volatile constituents or selected drug molecules to migrate through the wall of the container to the outside and thereby be lost. The reverse of this also may occur by which oxygen or other molecules may permeate to the inside of the container and cause oxidative or other degradation of susceptible constituents. Leaching may be a problem when certain constituents of the plastic material migrate into the product. This potential problem often may be controlled by careful formulation of the polymer mixture with a minimum of additives. Sorption seems to be a limited problem in the packaging of parenterals and is found most commonly in association with polyamides such as nylon.

In the use of plastic packaging materials, one of the principal advantages is that such materials are not breakable as is glass. In addition, there is a substantial reduction in weight. The flexibility of the low-density polyethylene polymer, for ophthalmic preparations, makes it possible to squeeze the side wall of the container and discharge one or more drops without introducing contamination into the remainder of the preparation. The flexible bags of polyvinyl chloride or select polyolefins, currently in use for large-volume intravenous fluids, have the added advantage that no air interchange is required; the flexible wall of the bag simply collapses as the solution flows out of the bag.

Most plastic materials have the disadvantage that they are not as clear as glass and, therefore, inspection of the contents is impeded. In addition, many of these materials will soften or melt under the conditions of thermal sterilization. However, careful selection of the plastic utilized and control of the autoclave cycle has made thermal sterilization of some products possible, large volume parenterals in particular. Ethylene oxide sterilization may be employed for the empty container with subsequent aseptic filling of the product. However, careful evaluation of the residues from ethylene oxide and their potential toxic effect must be undertaken.

Because of the relatively new use of plastic materials for packaging sterile preparations, considerable investigation is still required concerning potential interactions and other problems that may be encountered. For further details see Chapter 81.

Glass

Glass is employed as the container material of choice for most injections. It is composed principally of silicon dioxide with varying amounts of other oxides such as those of sodium, potassium, calcium, magnesium, aluminum, boron, and iron. The basic structural network of glass is formed by the silicon oxide tetrahedron.[7] Boric oxide will enter into this structure, but most of the other oxides do not. The latter are only loosely bound, are present in the network interstices, and are relatively free to migrate. These migratory oxides may be leached into a solution in contact with the glass, particularly during the increased reactivity of thermal sterilization. The oxides thus dissolved may hydrolyze to raise the pH of the solution, catalyze reactions, or enter into reactions. In a manner as yet uncertain, some glass compounds will be attacked by solutions and, in time, dislodge glass flakes into the

solution. Disturbing reactions such as these can, however, be minimized by the proper selection of the glass composition.

Types—The USP has aided in this selection by providing a classification of glass; namely, Type I, a borosilicate glass; Type II, a soda-lime treated glass; Type III, a soda-lime glass; and NP, a soda-lime glass not suitable for containers for parenterals. Type I glass is composed principally of silicon dioxide and boric oxide, with low levels of the nonnetwork-forming oxides. It is a chemically resistant glass (low leachability) also having a low thermal coefficient of expansion. Type II and Type III glass compounds are composed of relatively high proportions of sodium oxide and calcium oxide. This makes the glass chemically less resistant. Both of these types melt at a lower temperature, are easier to mold into various shapes, and have a higher thermal coefficient of expansion than Type I. While there is no one standard formulation for glass among manufacturers of these USP type categories, Type II glass usually has a lower concentration of the migratory oxides than Type III. In addition, Type II glass has been treated under controlled temperature and humidity conditions with sulfur dioxide to dealkalize the internal surface of the container. While it remains intact, this surface will substantially increase the chemical resistance of the glass. However, repeated exposures to sterilization procedures and to alkaline detergents will break down this dealkalized surface and expose the soda-lime compound. Therefore, Type II glass containers may be considered to be of relatively good chemical resistance for only one use.

The glass types are determined from the results of two tests provided by the USP, the Powdered Glass Test and the Water Attack Test. The latter is used only for Type II glass and is performed on the whole container, because of the dealkalized surface. The former test is performed on powdered glass, which exposes internal surfaces of the glass compound. The results are based upon the amount of alkali titrated by 0.02 N sulfuric acid after an autoclaving cycle with the glass sample in contact with a high-purity distilled water.

Care must be used in selecting the glass type to be used for a particular injectable product. In general, Type I glass will be suitable for all products, although sulfur dioxide treatment is sometimes used for a further increase in resistance. Because cost must be considered, one of the other less expensive types may be acceptable. Type II glass may be suitable, for example, for a solution which is buffered, has a pH below 7, or is not reactive with the glass. Type III glass will usually be suitable principally for anhydrous liquids or dry substances.

Physical Characteristics—Examples of the physical shape of glass ampuls and vials are illustrated in Fig 85-3. Commercially available containers vary in size from 0.5 to 1000 mL. Sizes up to 100 mL may be obtained as ampuls and vials, and larger sizes as bottles. The latter are used mostly for intravenous and irrigating solutions. Smaller sizes are also available as cartridges. Ampuls and cartridges are made by being drawn from glass tubing. The smaller size vials, drawn from tubing, have recently become obtainable. The making of tubing is illustrated in Fig 85-4. Other vials and bottles are made by molding. Containers made by drawing from tubing are generally optically clearer and have a thinner wall than molded containers (see Fig 85-3). Molded containers are more uniform in external dimensions and are stronger. Therefore, larger containers are made by molding.

Easy-opening ampuls that permit the user to break off the tip of the ampul at the neck constriction without the use of a file are marketed under the names Color-Break (*Kimble*) and Score-Break (*Wheaton*). An example of a modification of container design to meet a particular need is the double-chambered vial, under the name Univial (*Univial*), designed to contain a freeze-dried product in one chamber and solvent

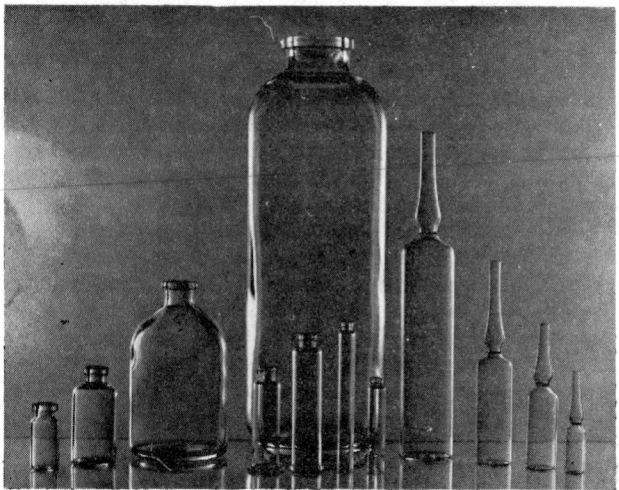

Fig. 85-3.   Various types of ampuls and multiple-dose vials for parenterals (courtesy, Kimble).

in the other. Other examples are wide-mouth ampuls with flat or rounded bottoms to facilitate filling with dry materials or suspensions, and various modifications of the cartridge for use with disposable dosage units.

Glass containers must be strong enough to withstand the physical shocks of handling and shipping and the pressure differentials that develop, particularly during the autoclave sterilization cycle. They must be able to withstand the thermal shock resulting from large temperature changes during processing, for example, when the hot bottle and contents are exposed to room air at the end of the sterilization cycle. Therefore, a glass having a low coefficient of thermal expansion is necessary. The glass container also must be transparent to permit inspection of the contents. Preparations which are light-sensitive must be protected by placing them in amber glass containers or by enclosing flint glass containers in opaque cartons labeled to remain on the container during the period of use. Silicone coatings are sometimes applied to containers to produce a hydrophobic surface as a means of reducing adherence of a heavy, costly suspension or the friction of a rubber-tip of a syringe plunger.

The size of single-dose containers is limited to 1000 mL by the USP and multiple-dose containers to 30 mL, unless stated otherwise in a particular monograph. Multiple-dose vials are limited in size to reduce the number of punctures for withdrawing doses and the accompanying risk of contamination of the contents. As the name implies, single-dose containers are opened with aseptic care and the contents used at one time. These may range in size from 1000-mL bottles to 1-mL or less ampuls, vials or syringes. The integrity of the container is destroyed when opened so that the container cannot be closed again. A multiple-dose container is designed so that more than one dose can be withdrawn at different times, the container maintaining a seal between uses. It should be evident that with full aseptic precautions, including sterile syringe and needle for withdrawing the dose and disinfection of the exposed surface of the closure, there is still a substantial risk of introducing contaminating microorganisms and viruses into the contents of the vial. Because of this risk, the USP requires that all multiple-dose vials must contain an antibacterial agent. However, there is no effective antiviral agent available for such use. Therefore, in spite of the advantage of flexibility of dosage provided the physician by a multiple-dose vial, the greater safety of single-dose, disposable administration units has caused their use to increase rapidly during recent years.

Rubber Closures

In order to permit introduction of a needle from a hypodermic syringe into a multiple-dose vial and provide for resealing of the vial as soon as the needle is withdrawn, each vial is sealed with a rubber closure held in place by an aluminum band. Fig 85-5 illustrates how this is done. This principle is also followed for single-dose containers of the cartridge type, except that there is only a single introduction of the needle to make possible the withdrawal or expulsion of the contents.

Rubber closures are composed of several ingredients, the

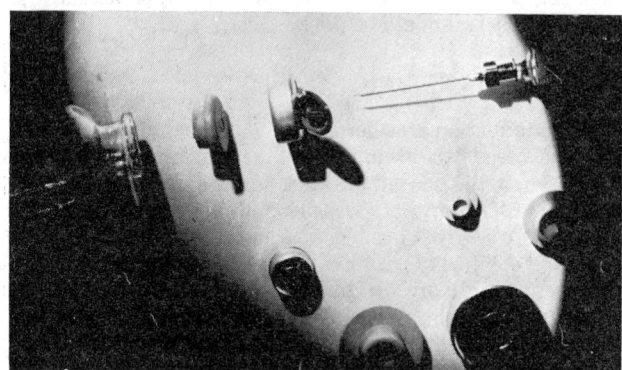

Fig. 85-5.   Extended view of sealing components for a multiple-dose vial (courtesy, West).

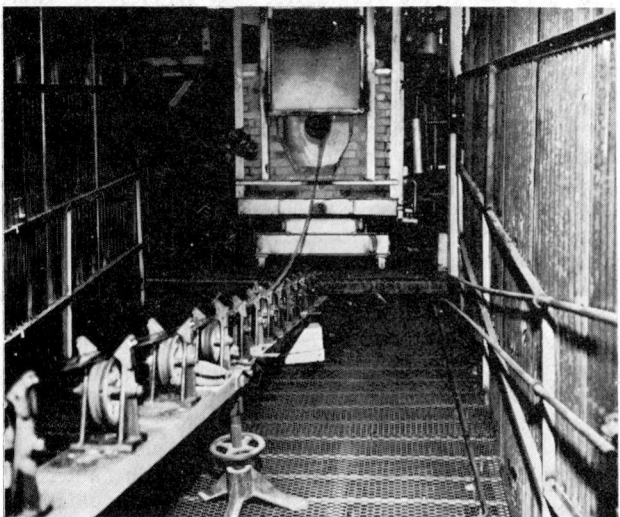

Fig. 85-4.   Tubing being formed from molten glass in brick tank (courtesy, Wheaton).

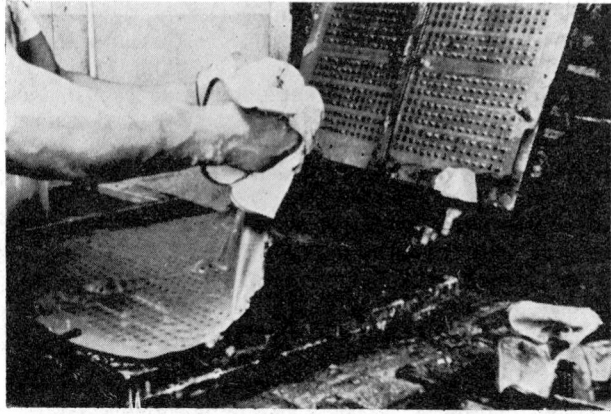

Fig. 85-6.   Removing a sheet of rubber closures from a mold.

primary ones being natural rubber (latex), a synthetic polymer, or a combination of natural rubber and a synthetic polymer. Other ingredients include a vulcanizing agent, usually sulfur; an accelerator, one of several active organic compounds such as 2-mercaptobenzothiazole; an activator, usually zinc oxide; fillers, such as carbon black or limestone; and various other ingredients such as antioxidants and lubricants. These ingredients are compounded together and then vulcanized in the desired shape, making use of molds under high pressure and temperature. Fig 85-6 shows the molding of rubber closures.

Rubber closures must have sufficient elasticity to provide a snug fit between the closure and the lip and neck of the vial and must spring back to close the hole made by the needle immediately on withdrawal. They must not be so hard that they are highly resistant to the insertion of the needle, and they must not fragment as the hollow needle passes through them. Ideally, they should be completely nonreactive with the solution and its ingredients and should provide a complete barrier to vapor transfer. These qualities are not perfectly met by any rubber compound now available. It is, therefore, essential to determine the compatibility of the rubber compound with each preparation with which it is to be used.[8] In addition to the physical tests of elasticity, hardness, fragmentation, and vapor transfer, the closures should be exposed to the product for prescribed periods of time at designated temperature and humidity conditions. The effect on the product of extractives from the rubber compound or loss of ingredients from the product to the closure should be determined analytically. Physicochemical and toxicological tests for evaluating rubber closures are officially described.

The physical shape of some typical closures may be seen in Fig 85-5. Most closures have a lip and a protruding flange that extends into the neck of the vial or bottle. Many disk closures are now being used, particularly in the high-speed packaging of antibiotics. Slotted closures are used on freeze-dried products to make it possible to insert the closure part way into the neck of the vial during the drying phase of the cycle. Partial insertion provides protection from contamination while permitting escape of water vapor from the drying product. The plunger type is used to seal one end of a cartridge. At the time of use, the plunger expels the product by a needle inserted through the closure at the distal end of the cartridge. Intravenous solution closures often have permanent holes for adapters of administration sets; irrigating solution closures usually are designed for pouring.

Production Facilities

A product having components of the best quality quickly may become totally unacceptable if the environment in which it is processed is contaminated or if the manufacturing procedure is not carried out properly. Therefore, the production facilities and the procedure used in processing the product must meet standards adequate for the task to be accomplished. The nearer these standards approach perfection, the better and safer should be the product.

Arrangement of Area

The production area normally should be divided into five sectional areas: the clean-up area, the compounding area, the aseptic area, the quarantine area, and the finishing or packaging area. All of these areas should be designed and constructed for ease of cleaning, efficient operation, attractiveness, and comfort of personnel. The extra requirements for the aseptic area are designed to provide an environment where, for example, an injection may be exposed to the environment for only brief periods during subdivision from a bulk container to the individual dose containers without becoming contaminated. Contaminants such as dust, lint, and microorganisms are normally found floating in the air, lying on counters and other surfaces, on clothing and body surfaces of personnel, in the exhaled breath of personnel, and deposited on the floor. The design and control of an aseptic area is directed toward so reducing the presence of these contaminants that they are no longer a hazard to aseptic filling. Although the aseptic area must be adjacent to support areas so that an efficient flow of components may be achieved, barriers must be provided to minimize ingress of contaminants to the aseptic area. Such barriers may be sealed partitions, often glass-paneled for greater visibility and light. Another type of barrier is an entrance way through security doors that require passage through an airlock so designed that both doors cannot be opened at the same time. Fig 85-7 shows an arrangement of an aseptic area modified to provide a service area for the areas of maximum security, the aseptic filling rooms.

Flow Plan—In general, the components for a parenteral product will flow from the stockroom, either: (1) to the compounding area, as for ingredients of the formula, or (2) to the clean-up area, as for containers and equipment. See Fig 85-8 for a process flow diagram. After proper processing in these areas, the components will flow into the security of the aseptic area for filling of the product in appropriate containers. From there the product will pass into the quarantine area where it will be held until all necessary tests have been performed. If the product is to be sterilized in its final container, the passage normally will be interrupted after the product leaves the aseptic area for subjection to the sterilization process. After the results from all tests are known and the product has been found effective and safe, it will pass to the finishing area for final labeling and packaging. There are sometimes variations from this flow plan to meet the specific needs of an individual product or to conform to available facilities.

Clean-Up Area—The clean-up area will be constructed to withstand moisture, steam, and detergents. The ceiling, walls, and floor should be constructed of impervious materials so that moisture will run off and not be held. One of the "spray-on-tile" finishes with a vinyl or epoxy sealing coat provides a continuous surface free from all holes or crevices. All such surfaces can be washed at regular intervals to keep them thoroughly clean. These areas should be exhausted adequately so that the heat and humidity will be removed for the comfort of personnel. Precautions must be taken to prevent the accumulation of dirt and the growth of microorganisms, especially in the presence of high humidity and heat. In this area preparation for the filling operation, such as assembling equipment is undertaken. Adequate sink and counter space must be provided. While this area does not need to be aseptic, it must be cleanable and kept clean and the microbial load must be monitored and controlled. Precautions also must be taken to prevent deposit of particles or other contaminants on clean containers and equipment.

Compounding Area—In the compounding area the formula is compounded. Although it is not essential that this area be aseptic, control over it should be more stringent than in the clean-up area. For example, means may need to be provided to control dust generated from weighing and compounding operations. Cabinets and counters should, preferably, be constructed of stainless steel. They should fit snugly to walls and other furniture so that there are no catch areas for dirt to accumulate. Ceiling, walls, and floor should

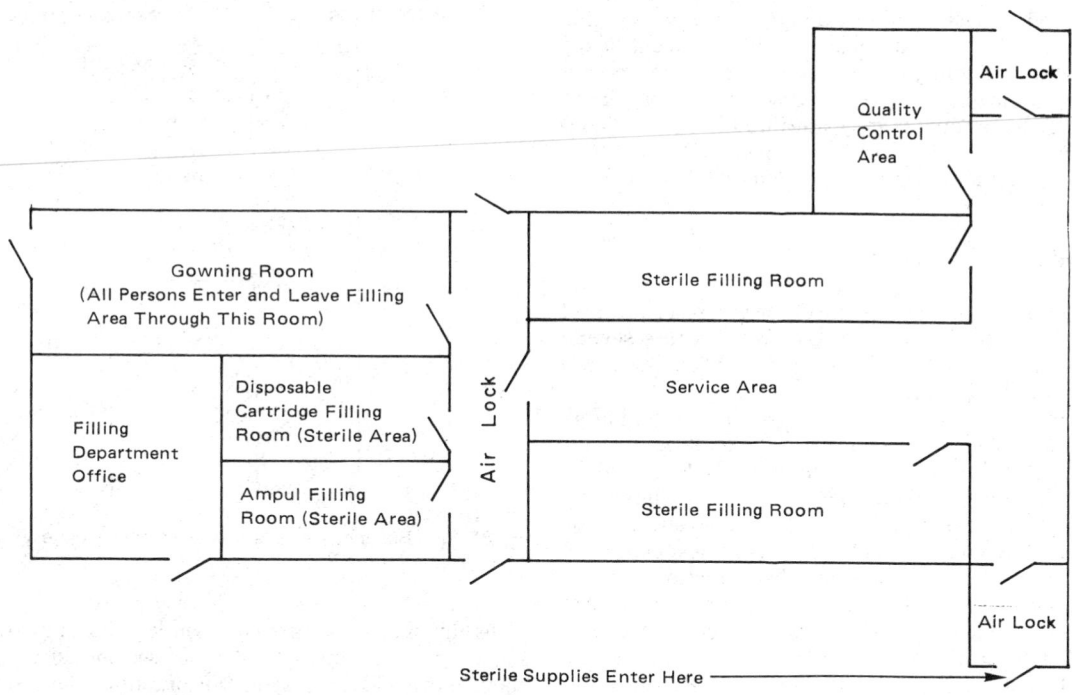

Fig 85-7.   Floor plan of an aseptic filling area with its service area (courtesy, Wyeth).

be constructed similar to those for the clean-up area. Fig 85-9 illustrates such an area located adjacent to an aseptic filling area.

Aseptic Area

The aseptic area requires construction features which have been designed for maximum security. The ceiling, walls, and floor must be sealed so that they may be washed and sanitized

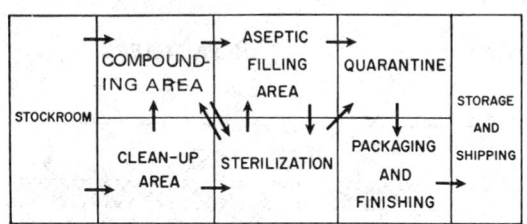

Fig 85-8.   Process flow diagram.

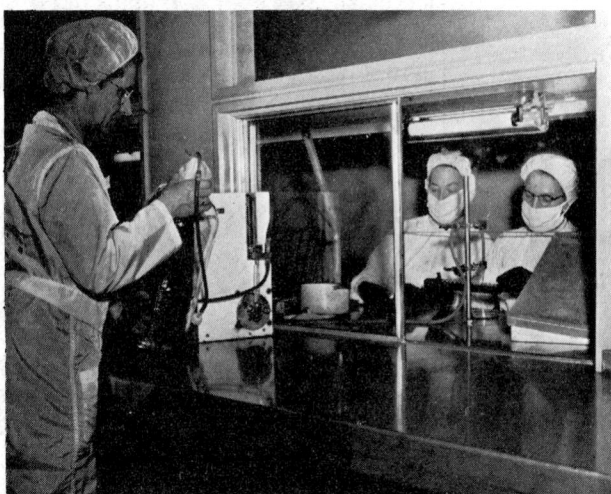

Fig 85-9.   View from service area with pipetting machine and stock bottle retained outside of aseptic filling area (courtesy, Wyeth).

with a disinfectant, as needed. All counters should be constructed of stainless steel and hung from the wall so that there are no legs to accumulate dirt where they rest on the floor. All light fixtures, utility service lines, and ventilation fixtures should be recessed in the walls or ceiling to eliminate ledges, joints, and other locations for the accumulation of dust and dirt. As much as possible, tanks containing the compounded product should remain outside the aseptic filling area and the product fed into the area through hose lines. Fig 85-10 shows such an arrangement. Mechanical equipment that must be located in the aseptic area should be housed as completely as possible within a stainless steel cabinet in order to seal the operating parts and their dirt-producing and accumulating tendencies from the aseptic environment. Mechanical parts that will contact the parenteral product should be demountable so that they can be sterilized.

Personnel entering the aseptic area should enter only through an airlock. They should be attired in sterile coveralls

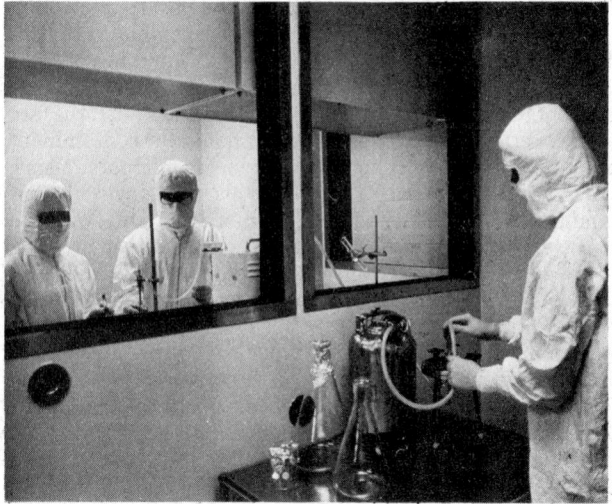

Fig 85-10.   Filtration of product from aseptic staging room through port into aseptic filling room (courtesy, The University of Tennessee College of Pharmacy).

with sterile hats, masks, and foot covers. Movement within the room should be minimal and in-and-out movement rigidly restricted during a filling procedure. The requirements for preparation of the room and for the personnel may be relaxed somewhat if the product is to be sterilized in a sealed container. Some are convinced, however, that it is better to have one standard procedure meeting the most rigid requirements.

Air Cleaning

The air in these areas can be one of the greatest sources of contamination. It need not be, however, because several methods are available for providing clean air that is essentially free from dirt particles and microorganisms.

To provide such air, it must be thoroughly cleaned of all contaminants. This may be done by a series of treatments. Air from the outside is first passed through a prefilter, usually of glass wool, cloth, or shredded plastic, to remove large particles. Then it is treated by passage through an electrostatic precipitator.* Such a unit induces an electrical charge on particles in the air and removes them by attraction to oppositely charged plates. The air then passes through the most efficient cleaning device, a HEPA (high efficiency particulate air) filter having an efficiency of at least 99.97% in removing particles of 0.3 μm and larger, based on the DOP test.[†]

For the comfort of personnel, air conditioning and humidity control should be incorporated into the system. Another available system, the Kathabar system (*Surface Combustion*), cleans the air of dirt and microorganisms by washing it in an antiseptic solution and, at the same time, controls the humidity. The clean, aseptic air is introduced into the aseptic area under positive pressure, which prevents outside air from rushing into the aseptic area through cracks, temporarily open doors, or other openings.

Laminar-Flow Environments—Marked improvement in the environmental control of aseptic areas has been made possible by the development of laminar-flow enclosures. Laminar airflow provides a total sweep of a confined area because the entire body of air moves with uniform velocity along parallel lines, originating through a HEPA filter occupying one entire side of the confined area. Therefore, it bathes the total area with very clean air, sweeping away contaminants.

The arrangement for the direction of airflow can be horizontal (see Fig 85-11) or vertical (see Fig 85-12), and may involve a limited area such as a workbench or an entire room. The effective air velocity is considered to be 90 ± 20 ft/min.

It must be borne in mind that any contamination introduced upstream by equipment, arms of the operator, or leaks in the filter will be blown downstream. In the instance of horizontal flow this may be to the critical working site, the face of the operator, or across the room. Should the contaminant be, for example, penicillin powder or viable microorganisms, the danger is apparent. For operations involving such contaminants a vertical system is much more desirable, with the air flowing through perforations in the counter top or along the edge of the counter where it can be directed for decontamination. Vertical flow has been recommended for sterility-testing procedures.

Laminar-flow environments provide well-controlled work areas only if proper precautions are observed. Any air currents or movements exceeding the velocity of the HEPA-filtered air flow may introduce contamination, as may coughing, reaching, or other manipulations of operators.

Therefore, laminar-flow work areas should be protected by being located within controlled environments. Personnel

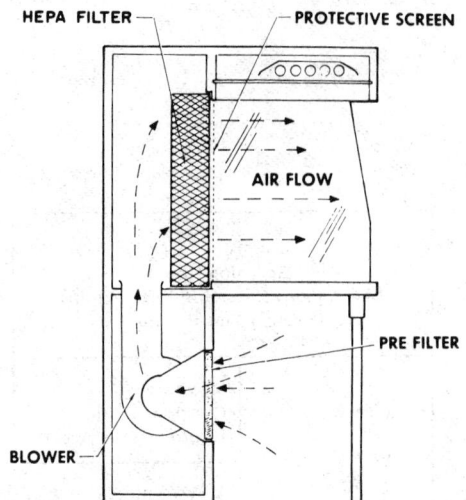

Fig. 85-11. Horizontal laminar flow workbench (courtesy, adaptation, Sandia).

preferably should be attired for aseptic processing as described above. All movements and processes should be carefully planned to avoid the introduction of contamination upstream of the critical work area. Checks of the air stream should be performed initially and at regular intervals to be sure no leaks have developed through or around the HEPA filters. This can be done most effectively with electronic particle counters.[‡]

In the manufacture of parenterals, conventional clean room facilities are frequently supplemented by vertical laminar airflow modules suspended above critical sites, such as filling lines. These critical operations are thereby bathed with

---

[‡] Suppliers: *Air Techniques, Bausch & Lomb, Climet, Dynac, Met One, Royco.*

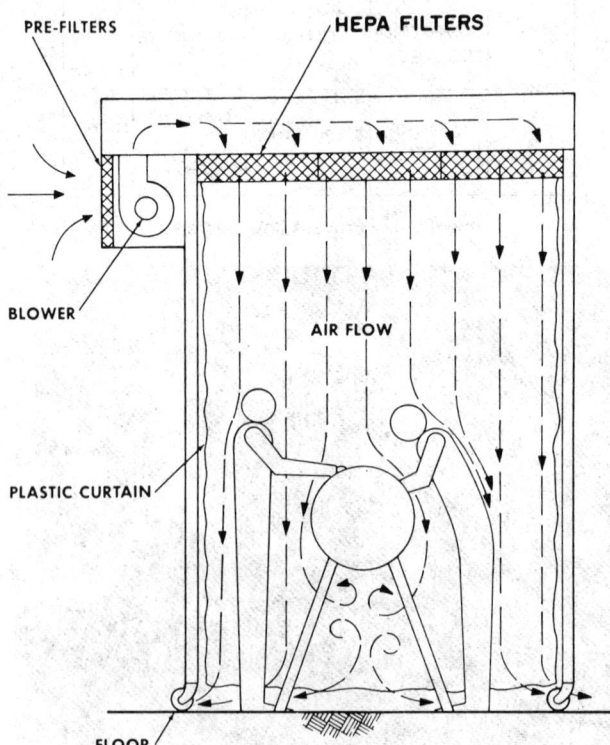

Fig 85-12. Vertical laminar flow portable room with equipment and operators (courtesy, adaptation, Sandia).

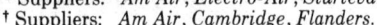

* Suppliers: *Am Air, Electro-Air, Sturtevant.*
[†] Suppliers: *Am Air, Cambridge, Flanders.*

HEPA-filtered air to provide extra protection for the product.

Laminar flow of HEPA-filtered air should meet the standard for a Class 100 clean room as defined by Federal Standard 209b,[9] which states that such an environment contains no more than 100 particles per cu ft of 0.5 μm and larger size. Conventional clean rooms would be of a lesser degree of cleanliness, such as Class 10,000, defined on the same basis. This standard has brought order into defining clean rooms and provided a common basis for their description.

Work benches and other types of laminar-flow enclosures are available from several commercial sources.[§]

Ultraviolet Radiation

Ultraviolet (UV) light rays have an antibacterial action, thereby producing a disinfectant action on directly irradiated surfaces. Since these rays cannot penetrate most materials, only a surface effect is produced, with the principal exception being limited penetration through air and pure water. UV light rays travel in straight lines only; therefore, objects in the path of the light beam will cast shadows with a resultant lack of irradiation in the shadow area.

UV rays are irritating to the skin and, particularly, the eyes of human beings. Therefore, personnel in the area of irradiation must be protected from direct exposure.

UV lamps may be installed so as to provide either direct or indirect radiation. Direct irradiation of a room when personnel are not present is a valuable means of reducing bacterial count on working surfaces and floors. Lamps installed above head level, so that personnel present would not be irradiated, can irradiate circulating air to reduce the microbial level continuously during processing.

Local irradiation may be useful in hood-type fixtures, over filling and other process operations, within large storage tanks, or in any place where additional protection from contamination is needed, provided any product present is not adversely affected by UV rays. Ultraviolet lamps usually are not employed in conjunction with laminar-flow facilities because the HEPA-filtered air sweeps exposed surfaces clean and because the air itself flows too fast for adequate lethal irradiation of microorganisms being carried in the air stream.

The best practical source of UV light rays is the cold-cathode mercury vapor lamp. This lamp emits a high proportion of radiation at the 253.7 nm wavelength. A special glass is used for the tube so that the rays will pass to the outside. This glass will gradually change in crystal structure with use so that passage of the rays is gradually reduced. Such lamps, therefore, rarely burn out as do visible light lamps but gradually reach an emission level which is ineffective. These lamps also must be kept clean, for dust and grease will drastically lower the effective emission. It is generally stated that an irradiation intensity of 20 μw/cm^2 is required for effective antibacterial activity.

Maintenance of the Aseptic Area

One of the most important aspects in the control of environmental contamination in the aseptic area is the care and maintenance. This work should not be done in a haphazard manner by the general maintenance crews, but rather by crews given special instruction and under the supervision of personnel trained in the care of aseptic areas. In general, the cleaning and maintenance should be done after the completion of the day's work with an interval of quietude before the beginning of another aseptic operation. With the advent of

laminar flow of HEPA-filtered air the rigors of cleaning have been reduced since the clean air flow keeps a clean area "swept" clean once it has been cleaned. All maintenance equipment should be selected for its effectiveness and freedom from lint-producing tendencies and should be reserved for use in the aseptic areas only.

Personnel

Personnel selected to work on the preparation of a parenteral product must be neat, orderly, and reliable. They should be in good health and free from dermatological conditions that might increase the microbial load. If they show symptoms of a head cold or other illness, they should not be permitted in the aseptic area until recovery is complete. They must receive intensive instruction in the principles of aseptic processes. They also must be made to appreciate the vital part that every movement they make has in determining the reliability of the final product. Supervisors should be selected with particular care. They must be individuals who understand the particular requirements of aseptic procedures and who are able to obtain the full participation of other employees in fulfilling these exacting requirements.

The attire prescribed for personnel varies from one manufacturing facility to another. However, uniforms should be freshly laundered for each day. For use in the aseptic area, it is generally agreed that uniforms should be sterile. This means that fresh, sterile uniforms should be used after every break period, or whenever the individual returns to the aseptic area. In some plants this is not required if the product is to be sterilized in its final container. The uniform usually consists of coveralls for both men and women, hoods to completely cover the hair, face masks, and cloth or plastic boots (Fig 85-13). Sterile rubber gloves also may be required for most aseptic operations, preceded by thorough scrubbing of the hands with a disinfectant soap. In addition, goggles may be required to complete the coverage of all skin areas. The uniform is designed to confine the contaminants discharged

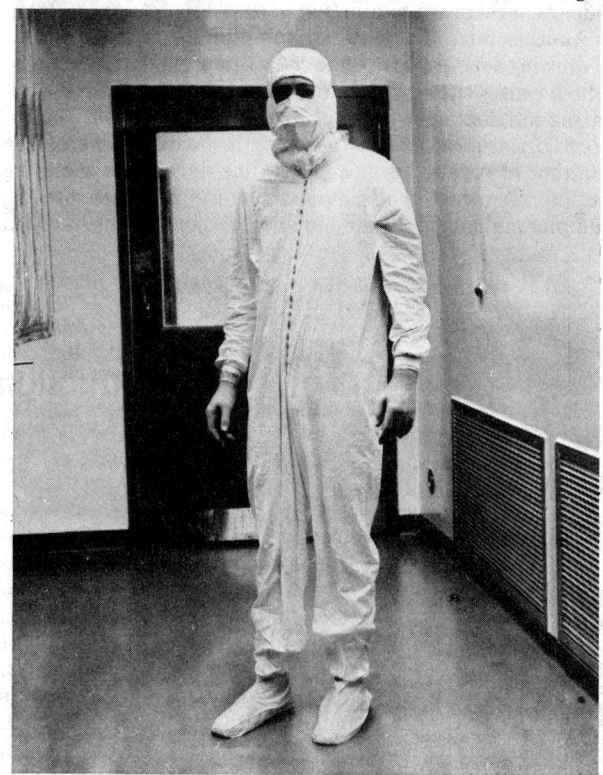

Fig 85-13.   Appropriate uniform for operators entering aseptic filling room (courtesy, Abbott).

from the body of the operator, thereby preventing their ingress into the product.

Lint is also a problem in these areas. Although cotton uniforms are usually more comfortable, Dacron or Tyvek uniforms are essentially lint-free and are reasonably comfortable. Air showers are sometimes directed on personnel entering the processing area to blow loose lint from the uniforms.

Environmental Control Tests

In spite of the elaborate precautions taken by pharmaceutical manufacturers to provide satisfactory conditions for the proper processing of parenterals, the air may become laden with bacteria or other particles with subsequent contamination of the product. To monitor this condition suitable environmental control tests should be performed at regular intervals.

One air-sampling technique employed involves the collection of particulate matter from the air by drawing a sample of the air through a clean, sterile membrane filter of bacterial retentive porosity. The filter is placed in a holder* designed to hold the filter flat and to prevent leakage. An accurately measured, predetermined volume of air is drawn through the filter. Planned locations for sampling should be chosen to reveal potential contamination levels at such places as the filling and sealing area, beside personnel, next to moving equipment, and near doorways or other openings. A new filter should be used at each location. The filters then may be examined microscopically for particulate matter, such as lint and dust, or placed on culture media and incubated for the detection of microorganisms.

To eliminate the dehydrating effect on microorganisms, the air sample may be drawn into a measured volume of nutrient broth in an impinger. Organisms in the broth then may be collected by filtration on a membrane filter and incubated. In order to be meaningful, such a test must be conducted at planned intervals, with standards set from experience to decide the level of contamination permissible.

Another microbiological air-sampling technique consists of drawing a measured volume of air through a narrow opening which causes the air to impinge on the surface of a slowly rotating nutrient agar plate, a slit sampler (*Mattson-Garvin, New Brunswick*). This provides a measurement of the number of organisms at a given time during the sampling period. A centrifugal sampler (*Biotest*) pulls air into the sampler and slings the air and any microorganisms outward to a nutrient agar strip. This sampler is portable and can be disinfected and hand-carried wherever needed.

Probably the most widely used method involves the exposure of nutrient agar culture plates to the settling of microorganisms from the air. If pathogenic microorganisms are particularly of interest, blood agar plates may be needed. With this method also, the locations for the collection of the samples should be planned carefully. The exposure period should be planned and should be uniform each time in order that comparisons may be meaningful. The exposure period may vary as deemed needful for given circumstances, but even a period of one hour may not collect one microorganism under conditions of use in a well-controlled aseptic area.

Samples of the level of microorganisms on surfaces can be determined with specially designed nutrient agar plates having a convex surface (*Rodac Plates*). With these plates it is possible to roll the raised agar surface over flat or irregular surfaces to be tested. Organisms will be picked up on the agar and will grow during subsequent incubation.

Results from these tests are very valuable to keep cleaning, production, and quality control personnel apprised of the level of contamination in a given area. The results may also serve to detect environmental control defects such as failure in air-cleaning equipment or the presence of personnel who may be disseminating large numbers of bacteria without apparent physical ill effects.

Another test which is much more stringent is to fill and seal sterile fluid thioglycollate medium or trypticase soy broth in sterile containers under the same conditions used for an aseptic fill of a product. The entire lot is then incubated and examined subsequently for the appearance of growth of microorganisms. Such growth is indicative of contamination from the environment, including the equipment. It also may be used as a measure of the efficiency of a particular operator. Since this is a total sterility test, it is the best indication of the efficiency of the aseptic filling process.

Several instrumental methods are currently being utilized to obtain particle counts from a measured volume of air as a means of indicating the level of particle contamination in the environment. These instruments operate on the principle of the measurement of light scattered from particles passed through the optical system.[†] They can be adjusted to measure particles of a broad or narrow range of particle size. Difficulty has been experienced in obtaining consistent results, but their automatic features and immediate results make them useful for routine monitoring of an environment.

---

* Suppliers: *Gelman, Millipore, Nuclepore, Sartorius.*

† Suppliers: *ATI, Bausch & Lomb, Climet, Dynac, Particle Tech, Royco.*

Production Procedures

Cleaning Containers and Equipment

Containers and equipment coming in contact with parenteral preparations must be meticulously cleaned. It is obvious that if this were not so, all other precautions to prevent contamination of the product would be useless. It also should be obvious that even new, unused containers and equipment will be contaminated with such debris as dust, fibers, chemical films, and other materials arising from such sources as the atmosphere, cartons, the manufacturing process, and human hands. Much greater contamination must be removed from previously used containers and equipment before they will be suitable for reuse. Equipment should be rigidly reserved for use only with parenteral preparations and, where conditions dictate, only for one type product in order to reduce the risk of contamination.

A variety of machines are available for the cleaning of containers for parenteral products. These vary in complexity from a single jet tube for rinsing by hand one inverted container at a time with distilled water, to complex, automatic washers capable of processing several thousand containers an hour. The selection of the particular type to be used will be determined largely by the physical type of containers, their condition with respect to contamination, and the number of containers to be processed in a given period of time.

Characteristics of Machinery—Regardless of the type of cleaning machine selected, certain fundamental characteristics are usually required.

1. The liquid or air treatment must be introduced in such a manner that it will strike the bottom of the inside of the inverted container, spread in all directions, and smoothly flow down the walls and out the opening with a sweeping action. The pressure of the jet stream should be such that there is minimal splashing, and the flow should be such that it can leave the container opening without accumulating and producing turbulence inside. Splashing may prevent cleaning all areas and turbulence may redeposit loosened debris. Therefore, direct introduction of the jet stream within the container with control of the flow of the jet stream is required.

2. The container must receive a concurrent outside rinse.

3. The cycle of treatment should provide for a planned sequence with alternation of very hot and cool treatments. The final treatment should be an effective rinse with water of a quality equivalent to Water for Injection.

4. All metal parts coming in contact with the containers and with the treatments should be constructed of stainless steel or some other noncorroding and noncontaminating material.

Treatment Cycle—The cycle of treatments to be employed will vary with the condition of the containers to be cleaned. In general, loose dirt can be removed by vigorous rinsing with water. Detergents are rarely used for new containers because of the risk of leaving detergent residues. However, a thermal-shock sequence in the cycle is usually employed to aid, by expansion and contraction, loosening of debris that may be adhering to the container wall. Sometimes only an air rinse is used for new containers, particularly if used for a dry powder. In all instances the final rinse, whether air or Water for Injection, must be ultraclean so that no particulate residues are left by the rinsing agent.

Containers previously used cannot be reliably cleaned and the cost of attempting to do so is prohibitive. Therefore, normally, only new containers are used for parenterals. Improvements have been made in maintaining their cleanliness during shipment from the manufacturer through tight, low-shedding packaging, including plastic blister packs.

Machinery for Containers—The machinery available for cleaning large numbers of containers embodies the above principles but varies in the mechanics by which it is accomplished. In one approach, the jet tubes are arranged on arms like the spokes of a wheel, which rotate around a center post through which the treatments are introduced. An operator places the unclean containers on the jet tubes as they pass the loading point and removes the clean containers as they complete one rotation. Such a machine is pictured in Fig 85-14. Another machine has a row of jet tubes across a conveyor belt. The belt moves the row of containers past the treatment stations and discharges the clean containers on the opposite end of the machine, preferably through a wall into a clean room. Two operators are required for this machine (Fig 85-15). A cabinet-type washer permits loading the containers on a rack

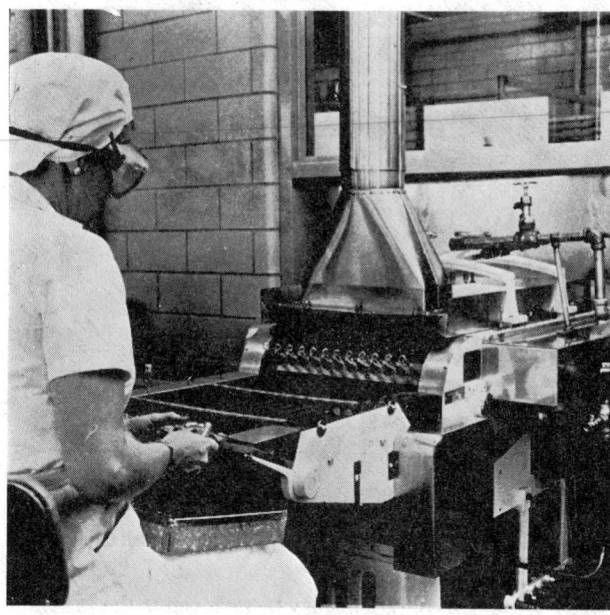

Fig 85-15. Conveyor rinser discharging clean vials in preparation area (courtesy, Schering).

of jet tubes. The rack is pushed inside the cabinet during the cleaning cycle. This type of machine permits handling a variety of sizes and types of containers quite easily, but the number of containers handled in a given period of time is relatively small. Fig 85-16 shows a machine of this type. A machine designed to process a large number of containers, particularly bottles and larger size containers, employs a conveyor chain to draw rows of jet tubes through a long tunnel where the treatments are introduced. The clean containers are returned to the loading point for removal (*Better Built*).

The disadvantage common to all of the above types of machines is that they require the individual handling of each container for loading and unloading. A type which overcomes this disadvantage is the rack-loading washer. Racks are prepared to fit over the open ends of ampuls or vials as they are found in shipping cartons. Inverting the carton permits the containers to be transferred from the carton to the washer without handling the individual containers. A battery of jet tubes is arranged to enter each container positioned in the

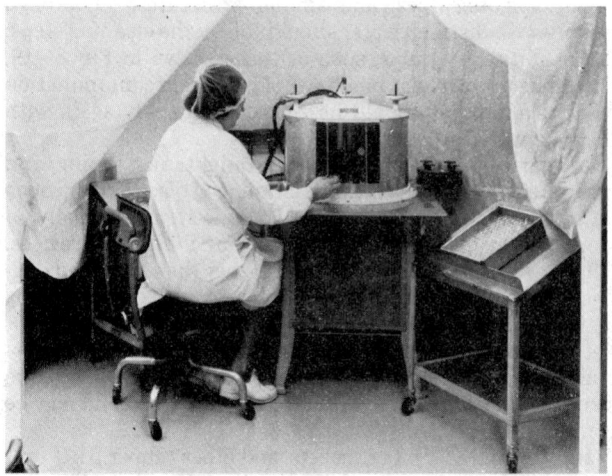

Fig 85-14. Rotary rinser in clean environment provided by vertical laminar air flow within curtained enclosure (courtesy, Ciba-Geigy).

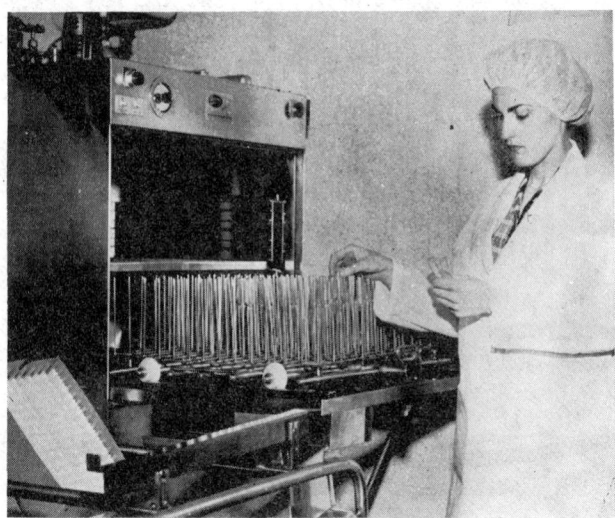

Fig 85-16. Cabinet washer being loaded with ampuls (courtesy, The University of Tennessee College of Pharmacy).

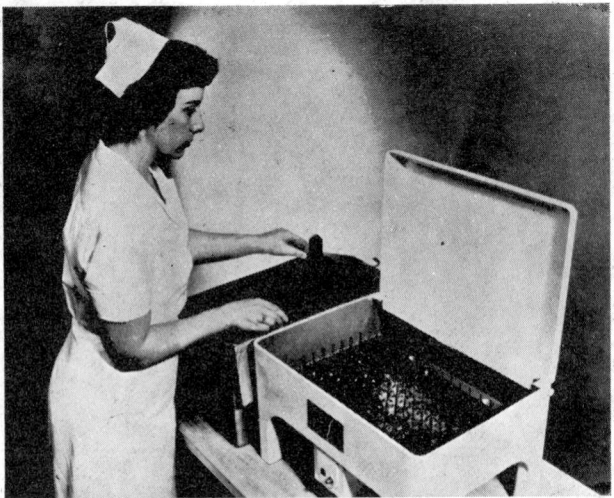

Fig 85-17.   Metromatic rack-loader washer being loaded directly from container carton (courtesy, Price).

rack. The clean containers may be removed in the rack and transferred to a box for dry-heat sterilization and storage (see Fig 85-17). More details of the industrial washing of glassware have been given by Anschel.[10]

Handling after Cleaning—The wet, clean containers must be handled in such a way that contamination will not be reintroduced. A wet surface will much more readily collect contaminants than will a dry surface. For this reason wet, rinsed containers should be protected, such as by a laminar flow of clean air until covered, as within a stainless steel box. (See Figs 85-14 and 85-18.) In addition, microorganisms are more likely to grow in the presence of moisture. Therefore, it is preferable, if not required, that containers be dry-heat sterilized in a stainless steel box that will protect the containers from contamination during storage after sterilization. Doubling the heating period has been generally considered to be adequate also to destroy pyrogens, but the actual time-temperature conditions required must be validated. If it is proved that sterilization is not essential, the containers should be filled immediately with product or dried and stored where they will be protected from contamination until used. Immediate filling eliminates the need for storage of the clean containers, but it also eliminates the sterilizing and depyrogenating step of the dry-heat treatment, often a vital step.

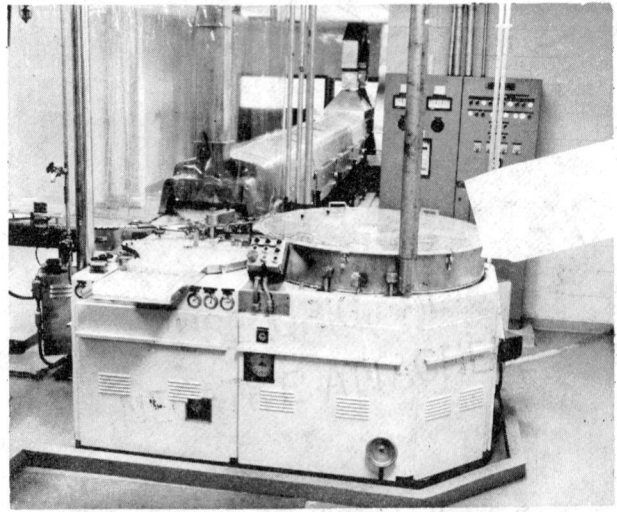

Fig 85-18.   Continuous automatic line operation for vials from rotary rinser through sterilizing tunnel with vertical laminar air flow protection of clean vials (courtesy, Abbott).

Therefore, it should be used only where a sterile pyrogen-free container is not essential.

Increases in process rates have necessitated the development of continuous-line processing with a minimum of individual handling, still maintaining adequate control of the cleaning and handling of the containers. Fig 85-18 shows a continuous automatic-line operation from feeding the unwashed container into the rotary rinser to passage through the drying and sterilizing tunnel. The clean, wet containers are protected by filtered laminar-flow air from the rinser through the tunnel and are then delivered to the filling line.

Closures—Rubber closures are coated with lubricant from the molding operation. In addition, the rough surface and electrostatic attraction tend to hold debris. Also, the surface "bloom" from migrated inorganic constituents of the compound must be removed. The recommended procedure calls for gentle agitation in a hot solution of a water softener such as 0.5% sodium pyrophosphate. The closures are removed from the solution and rinsed several times, or continuously for a prolonged period, with water and finally with filtered WFI. The rinsing is to be done in a manner which will flush away loosened debris. The wet closures are then usually sterilized by autoclaving and stored in closed containers until ready for use. At times this step is carried out in a solution of the bacteriostatic agent to be used in the product, in order to equilibrate the rubber closure with the agent. Subsequent loss of the agent from the solution to the closure is then less likely to occur. If the closures were immersed during autoclaving, to reduce hydration of the rubber compound the solution is drained off before storage. If the closures must be dry for use, they may be subjected to vacuum drying at a temperature in the vicinity of 100°C.

The equipment used for washing large numbers of closures is usually an agitator or horizontal basket-type automatic washing machine. Because of particulate generation from the abrading action of these machines, some heat the closures in kettles in detergent solution and follow with prolonged flush rinsing. The final rinse always should be ultraclean WFI.

Equipment—Details of certain prescribed techniques for the cleaning and preparation of equipment, as well as of containers and closures, have been presented elsewhere.[11] Here, a few points will be emphasized.

All equipment should be disassembled as much as possible to provide access to internal structures. For thorough cleaning, surfaces should be scrubbed thoroughly with a stiff brush using an effective detergent, paying particular attention to joints, crevices, screw threads, and other structures where debris is apt to collect. Exposure to a stream of clean steam will aid in dislodging residues from the walls of stationary tanks, spigots, pipes, and similar structures. Thorough rinsing with distilled water should follow the cleaning steps. Large stationary tanks, such as those shown in Fig 85-19, should be protected as much as possible from contamination after cleaning but should be rinsed thoroughly again with distilled water prior to reuse.

A relatively new concept for cleaning tanks, piping, and associated attachments is called cleaning in place (CIP). Such an approach involves designing the system, normally of stainless steel, with smooth surfaces and without crevices. That is, for example, with welded rather than threaded connections. The cleaning is accomplished with the scrubbing action of high pressure spray balls or nozzles delivering hot detergent solution from tanks captive to the system. Thorough rinsing with WFI follows and is accomplished within the same system. Such a process is often automated and may be computer-controlled.[12]

Rubber tubing, rubber gaskets, and other rubber parts may be washed in a manner such as described for rubber closures. Thorough rinsing of tubing must be done by passing distilled water through it. However, due to the relatively porous na-

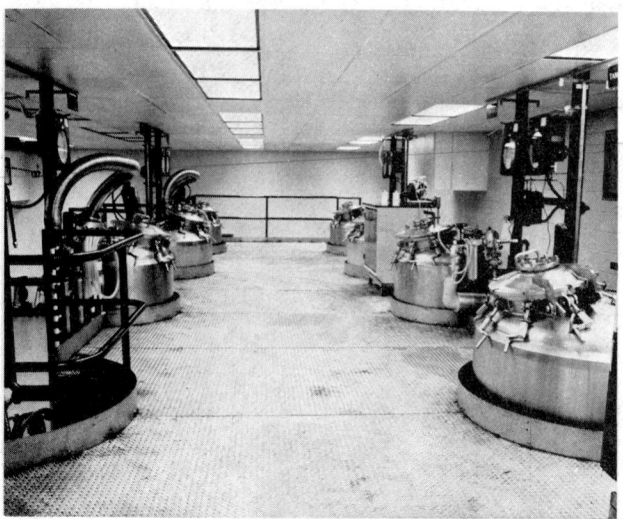

Fig. 85-19. Large stainless steel tanks for product preparation showing mezzanine level for access (courtesy, Abbott).

ture of rubber compounds and the difficulty in removing all traces of chemicals from previous use, it is considered by some inadvisable to reuse rubber tubing. Rubber tubing must be left wet when preparing for sterilization by autoclaving.

Product Preparation

The basic principles employed in the compounding of the product do not vary from those used routinely by qualified pharmacists. However, selected aspects will be mentioned for emphasis. All measurements should be made as accurately as possible and should be checked by a second qualified person. Although most liquid preparations are made by volume, where possible they should be made by weight, with the weight experimentally determined from a prescribed volume. This method is more accurate since no consideration need be given to the temperature of the components. In addition, measurements by weight normally can be performed more accurately than those by volume.

Care must be taken that equipment is not wet enough to significantly dilute the product or, in the case of anhydrous products, to cause a physical incompatibility. The order of mixing of ingredients may significantly affect the product, particularly those of large volume where attaining homogeneity requires considerable mixing time. For example, adjustment of pH by addition of a dilute acid may cause excessive local reduction in the pH of the product so that adverse effects are produced before the acid can be dispersed throughout the entire volume of product.

Parenteral dispersions, including colloids, emulsions, and suspensions, provide particular problems. These have been reviewed by Macek[13] and by Nash.[14] In addition to the problems of achieving and maintaining proper reduction in particle size under aseptic conditions, the dispersion must be kept in a uniform state of suspension throughout preparative, transfer, and subdividing operations.

The formulation of a stable product is of paramount importance. Certain aspects of this have been mentioned in the discussion of components of the product. Exhaustive coverage of the topic is not possible within the limits of this text, but further coverage is provided in Chapter 76. It should be mentioned here, however, that thermal sterilization of parenteral products increases the possibility of chemical reactions. Such reactions may progress to completion during the period of elevated temperature in the autoclave, or be initiated at this time but continue during subsequent storage. As-

surance of attainment of stability in a product requires a high order of pharmaceutical knowledge and responsibility.

Filtration

After a product has been compounded, if it is a solution it must be filtered. The primary objective of filtration is to clarify a solution. A high degree of clarification is termed "polishing" a solution. This term is applied when particulate matter down to approximately 2 μm in size is removed. A further step, removing particulate matter down to 0.2 μm in size, would eliminate microorganisms and would accomplish "cold" sterilization. A solution having a high degree of clarity conveys the impression of high quality and purity, desirable characteristics for a parenteral solution.

Filters are thought to function by one or, usually, a combination of the following: (1) sieving or screening, (2) entrapment or impaction, and (3) electrostatic attraction. When a filter retains particles by sieving, the particles are retained on the surface of the filter. Entrapment occurs when a particle, smaller than the dimensions of the passageway (pore), becomes lodged in a turn or impacted on the surface of the passageway. Electrostatic attraction causes particles opposite in charge to that of the surface of the filter pore to be held or adsorbed to the surface. It should be noted that increasing, prolonging, or varying the force behind the solution may tend to sweep particles initially held by entrapment or electrostatic charge through the pores and into the filtrate.

Today, membrane filters are used almost exclusively for filtration of parenteral solutions. Their particle retention effectiveness, flow rate, nonreactivity, and disposable characteristics have justified their use to the exclusion of most other types. The most common membranes are composed of cellulose ester*, polysulfone,† or polycarbonate‡ but other materials are being used, including Teflon and other plastic polymers. They are available as flat membranes or pleated into cylinders to increase surface area and, thus, flow rate. Each filter in its holder should be tested for integrity before and after use, particularly if being used to eliminate microorganisms. While membrane filters are disposable, and thus discarded after use, the holders must be thoroughly cleaned between uses. Increasingly, clean, sterile, pretested, disposable assemblies for small as well as relatively large volumes of solutions are becoming commercially available. Other characteristics of these filters, important for a full understanding of their use, are given in Chapter 79.

Filling

During the filling of containers with a product, the most stringent requirements must be exercised to prevent contamination, particularly if the product has been sterilized by filtration and will not be sterilized in the final container. Under the latter conditions the process is usually called an "aseptic fill." During the filling operation, the product must be transferred from a bulk container and subdivided into dose containers. This operation exposes the product to the environment, equipment, and manipulative technique of the operator until it can be sealed in the dose container. Therefore, this operation is carried out in the aseptic filling area where maximum protection is provided. Additional protection may be provided by filling under a blanket of HEPA-filtered laminar-flow air within the aseptic area.

Normally, the compounded product is in the form of either a liquid or a solid. A liquid is more readily subdivided uniformly and introduced into a container having a narrow mouth

---

* Suppliers: *AMF Cuno, Gelman, Millipore, Pall, Sartorius, Schleicher.*
† Supplier: *Gelman.*
‡ Supplier: *Nuclepore.*

than is a solid. Mobile, nonsticking liquids are considerably easier to transfer and subdivide than viscous, sticky liquids. The latter require heavy-duty machinery for rapid production filling.

Although many devices are available for filling containers with liquids, certain characteristics are fundamental to them all. A means is provided for repetitively forcing a measured volume of the liquid through the orifice of a delivery tube which is introduced into the container. The size of the delivery tube will vary from that of about a 20-gauge hypodermic needle to a tube ½ in. or more in diameter. The size required is determined by the physical characteristics of the liquid, the speed of delivery desired, and the inside diameter of the neck of the container. The tube must enter the neck of the container and deliver the liquid well into the neck to eliminate spillage, allowing sufficient clearance to permit air to leave the container as the liquid enters. The delivery tube should be as large as possible in diameter in order to reduce the resistance to the flow of the liquid. For smaller volumes of liquids, the delivery is usually obtained from the stroke of the plunger of a syringe, forcing the liquid through a two-way valve providing for alternate filling of the syringe and delivery of mobile liquids. A sliding piston valve would be used for heavy, viscous liquids. Other mechanisms include the turn of an auger in the neck of a funnel or the oscillation of a rubber diaphragm. For large volumes the quantity delivered is usually measured in the container by the level of fill in the container, the force required to transfer the liquid being provided by gravity, a pressure pump, or a vacuum pump.

The narrow neck of an ampul limits the clearance possible between the delivery tube and the inside of the neck. Since a drop of liquid normally hangs at the tip of the delivery tube after a delivery, the neck of an ampul will be wet as the delivery tube is withdrawn, unless the drop is retracted. Therefore, filling machines should have a mechanism by which this drop can be drawn back into the lumen of the tube.

Since the liquid will be in intimate contact with the parts of the machine through which it flows, these parts must be constructed of nonreactive materials such as borosilicate glass or stainless steel. In addition, these parts should be easily demountable for cleaning and for sterilization.

Because of the increased concern for particulate matter in injectable preparations, a final filter is often inserted in the system between the filler and the delivery tube. Most frequently this is a membrane filter, having a porosity of approximately 1 µm and treated to have a hydrophobic edge. The latter is necessary to reduce the risk of rupture of the membrane due to filling pulsations. It should be noted that the insertion of the filter at this point should collect all particulate matter generated during the process, only that which may be found in inadequately cleaned containers or picked up from exposure to the environment after passage through the final filter potentially remaining as contaminants. However, the filter does cushion liquid flow and reduces the efficiency of drop retraction from the end of the delivery tube, sometimes making it difficult to control delivery volume as precisely as would be possible without the filter.

Liquids—The filling of a small number of containers may be accomplished with a hypodermic syringe and needle, the liquid being drawn into the syringe and forced through the needle into the container. A device for providing greater speed of filling is the Cornwall Pipet (*BD & Co*). This device has a two-way valve between the syringe and the needle and a means for setting the stroke of the syringe so that the same volume will be delivered each time. Clean, sterile, disposable assemblies* operating on the same principle are available and have particular usefulness in hospital pharmacy operations.

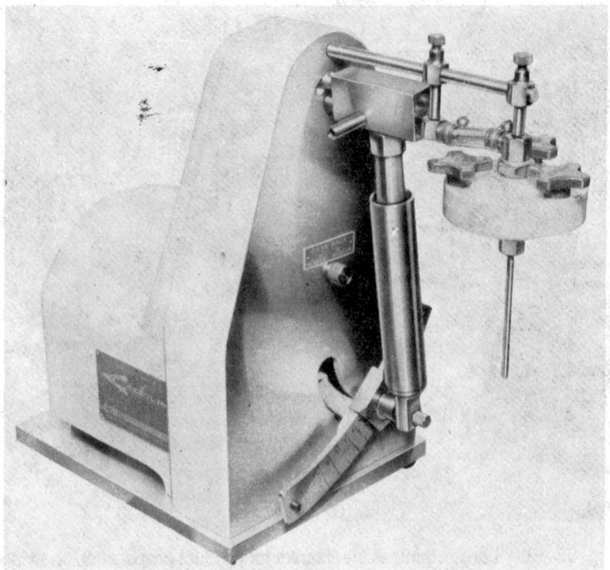

---

* Suppliers: *Burron, Pharmaseal.*

Fig. 85-20.   Filling machine employing piston valve and stainless steel syringe (courtesy, Cozzoli).

Mechanically operated instruments substitute a motor for the operator's hand in the previous devices described. Thereby, a much faster filling rate can be achieved. By careful engineering, the stroke of the syringe can be repeated precisely; and so, once a particular setting has been calibrated to the delivery, high delivery precision is possible. However, the speed of delivery, the expansion of rubber tubing connecting the valve with the delivery tube, and the rapidity of action of the valves can affect the precision of delivery. A filling machine employing a two-way valve assembly is shown in operation in Fig 85-9. One employing a piston valve is shown in Fig 85-20. Stainless steel syringes are required with viscous liquids because glass syringes are not strong enough to withstand the high pressures developed during delivery.

When high-speed filling rates are desired but accuracy and precision must be maintained, multiple filling units are often joined together in an electronically coordinated machine, such as shown in Fig 85-21.

Most high-speed fillers for large volume solutions utilize the bottle as the measuring device, transferring the liquid either by vacuum or positive pressure from the bulk reservoir to the individual unit containers. Therefore, a high accuracy of fill is not achievable.

The USP indicates that each container should be filled with

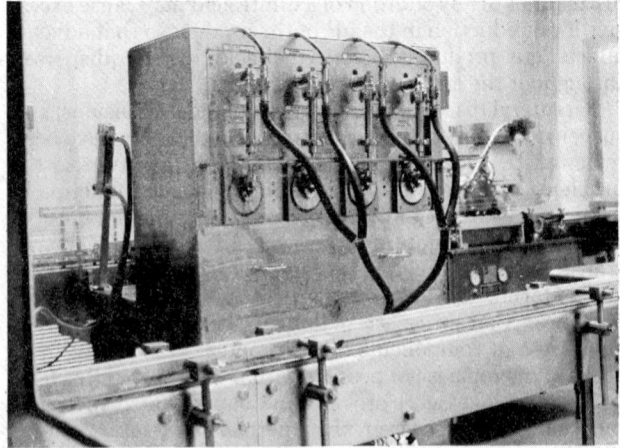

Fig. 85-21.   Four-pump liquid filler, with conveyor line for vials protected by vertical laminar air flow and plastic curtain; note automatic stoppering machine on right within curtain (courtesy, Abbott).

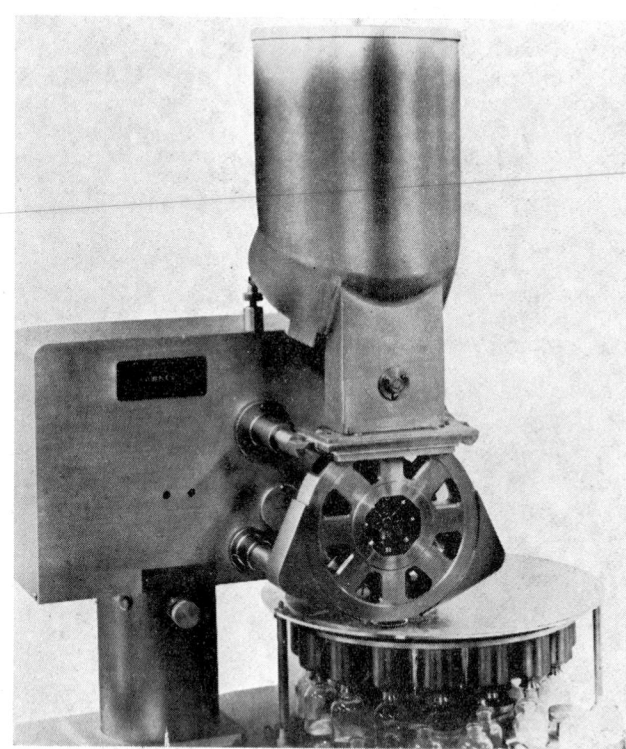

Fig 85-22.   Accofil vacuum powder filler (courtesy, Perry).

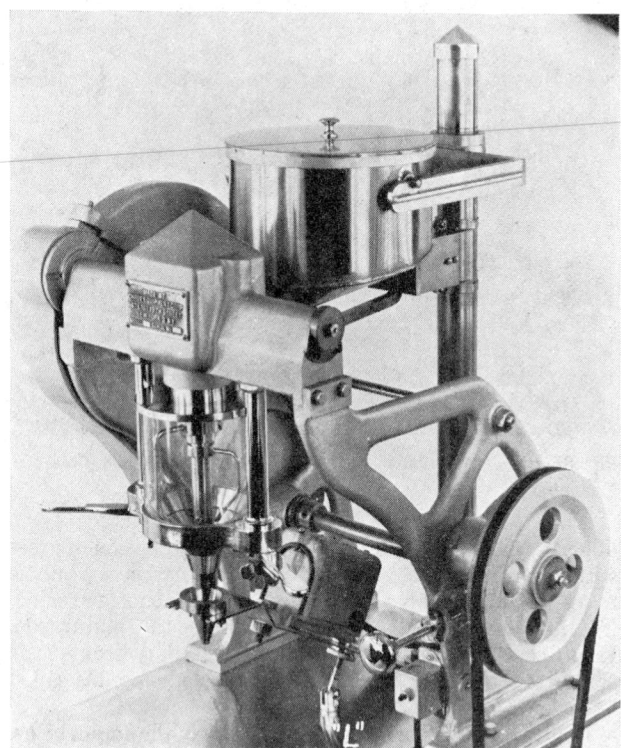

Fig 85-23.   Auger-type powder filler (courtesy, Chase-Logeman).

a slight excess of volume and gives a table of such suggested excess.

Solids—Sterile solids, such as antibiotics, are more difficult to subdivide evenly into containers than are liquids. The rate of flow of solid material is slow and irregular. Even though a container with a larger diameter opening is used to facilitate filling, it is difficult to introduce the solid particles, and the risk of spillage is ever present. The accuracy of the quantity delivered cannot be controlled as well as with liquids. Because of these factors, the tolerances permitted for the content of such containers must be relatively large. Suggested tolerances will be found in the USP.

Some sterile solids are subdivided into containers by individual weighing. A scoop is usually provided to aid in approximating the quantity required, but the quantity filled into the container is finally weighed on a balance. This is a slow process. When the solid is obtainable in a granular form so that it will flow more freely, other methods of filling may be employed. In general, these methods involve the measurement and delivery of a volume of the granular material which has been calibrated in terms of the weight desired. In a machine, shown in Fig 85-22, an adjustable cavity in the rim of a wheel is filled by vacuum and the contents held by vacuum until the cavity is inverted over the container. The solid material is then discharged into the container by the use of sterile air. Another machine employs an auger in the stem of a funnel at the bottom of a hopper. The granular material is placed in the hopper. By controlling the size of the auger and its rotation, a regulated volume of granular material can be delivered from the funnel stem into the container. Such a machine is shown in Fig 85-23.

Sealing

Ampuls—Filled containers should be sealed as soon as possible to prevent the contents from being contaminated by the environment. Ampuls are sealed by melting a portion of the glass neck. Two types of seals are normally employed, either tip-seals (bead-seals) or pull-seals. Tip-seals are made

by melting enough glass at the tip of the neck of an ampul to form a bead and close the opening. Such seals can be made rapidly in a high-temperature gas–oxygen flame. To produce a uniform bead, the ampul neck must be heated evenly on all sides. This may be accomplished by means of burners on opposite sides of stationary ampuls (see Fig 85-24) or by rotating the ampul in a single flame. Care must be taken to properly adjust the flame temperature and the interval of heating to obtain complete closing of the opening with a bead

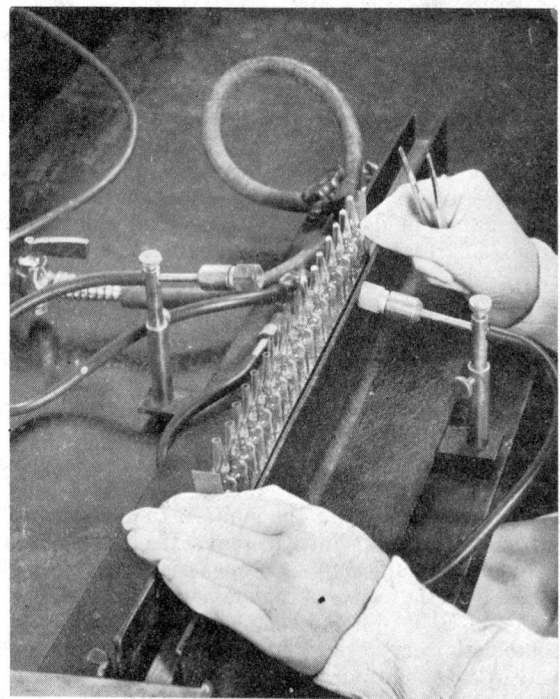

Fig 85-24.   Ampuls being sealed in a crossfire of a Bunsen burner (courtesy, Hynson).

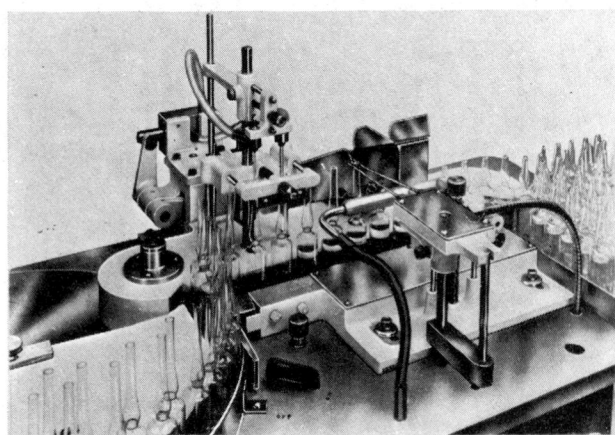

Fig. 85-25.   Automatic filling and pull-sealing of ampuls (courtesy, Cozzoli).

of glass. Excessive heating will result in expansion of gases within the ampul against the soft bead seal and cause a bubble to form. If the bubble bursts, the ampul is no longer sealed; if it does not, the wall of the bubble will be thin and fragile. Insufficient heating will leave an open capillary through the center of the bead. An incompletely sealed ampul is called a "leaker."

Pull-seals are made by heating the neck of the ampul below the tip, leaving enough of the tip for grasping with forceps or other mechanical devices. The ampul is rotated in the flame from a single burner. When the glass has softened, the tip is grasped firmly and pulled quickly away from the body of the ampul, which continues to rotate. The small capillary tube thus formed is twisted closed. Pull-sealing is slower, but the seals are more sure than tip-sealing. Fig 85-25 shows a machine combining the steps of filling and pull-sealing ampuls.

Powder ampuls or other types having a wide opening must be sealed by pull-sealing. Were these ampuls sealed by bead-sealing, the very large bead produced would induce glass strain with subsequent fracture at the juncture of the bead and neck wall. Fracture of the neck of ampuls during sealing also may occur if wetting of the necks occurred at the time of filling. Also, wet necks increase the frequency of bubble formation. If the product in the ampul is organic in nature, wet necks also will result in unsightly carbon deposits from the heat of sealing.

In order to prevent decomposition of a product, it is sometimes necessary to displace the air in the space above the product in the ampul with an inert gas. This is done by introducing a stream of the gas, such as nitrogen or carbon dioxide, during or after filling with the product. Immediately thereafter the ampul is sealed before the gas can diffuse to the outside.

Vials and Bottles—These are sealed by closing the opening with a rubber closure (stopper). This must be accomplished as rapidly as possible after filling and with reasoned care to prevent contamination of the contents. The large opening makes the introduction of contamination much easier than with ampuls. Therefore, a covering should be provided for such containers except for the minimal time required for filling and for the actual introduction of the rubber closure. During the latter critical time the open containers should be protected from the ingress of contamination, preferably with a blanket of HEPA-filtered laminar air flow. In Fig 85-21 the automatic conveyorized procedure is being performed under vertical laminar air flow within plastic side curtains.

The closure must fit the mouth of the container snugly enough so that its elasticity will permit adjustment to slight irregularities in the lip and neck of the container. However,

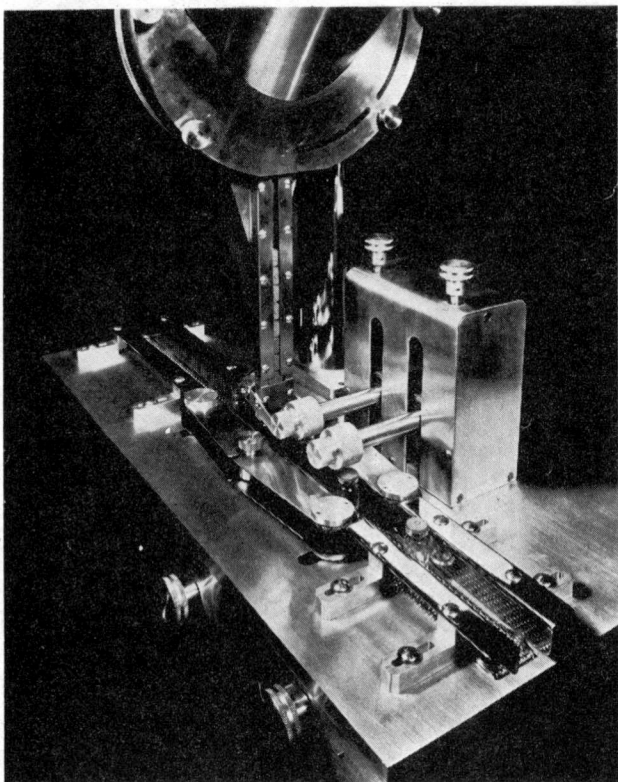

Fig 85-26.   Mechanical device for inserting rubber closures in vials (courtesy, Perry).

it must not fit so snugly that it is difficult to introduce into the neck of the container. When rubber closures are to be inserted mechanically, the surface of the closure is often halogenated or treated with silicone to give it less friction. Thus, it is possible to convey the closure through a shute to the place where it is positioned over a vial and then inserted by a plunger or some other pressure device. Mechanical stoppering has been developed to meet the need for high-speed production. An example of such a mechanical device is shown in Fig 85-26. Closures may also be inserted aseptically with sterile forceps or directly with hands encased in sterile rubber gloves. In a modification of this technique, rubber closures may be picked up and then inserted into a vial by means of a tool connected to a vacuum line.

Rubber closures are held in place by means of aluminum caps. The aluminum cap covers the closure and is crimped under the lip of the vial or bottle to hold the closure in place (see Fig 85-5). The closure cannot be removed without destroying the aluminum cap. Therefore, an intact aluminum cap is proof that the closure has not been intentionally or unintentionally removed. Such confirmation is necessary to assure the integrity of the contents as to sterility and other aspects of quality. The aluminum caps are so designed that the outer layer of double-layered caps, or the center of single-layered caps, can be removed to expose the center of the rubber closure without disturbing the band which holds the closure in the container. Rubber closures for use with intravenous administration sets often have a permanent hole through the closure. In such cases, a thin rubber disk overlayed with a solid aluminum disk is placed between an inner and outer aluminum cap. A seal of the hole through the closure is thereby provided. These are called triple-layered aluminum caps.

Single-layered aluminum caps may be applied by means of a hand crimper known as the Fermpress.* Double- or tri-

* Suppliers: *West, Wheaton.*

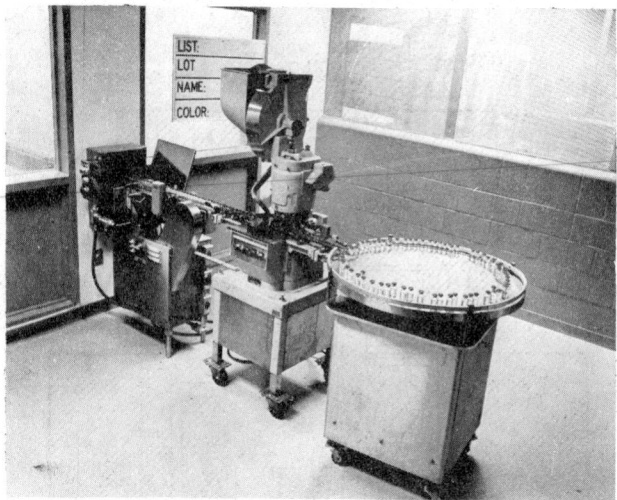

Fig 85-27.   Applying aluminum caps to vials at end of process line (courtesy, Abbott).

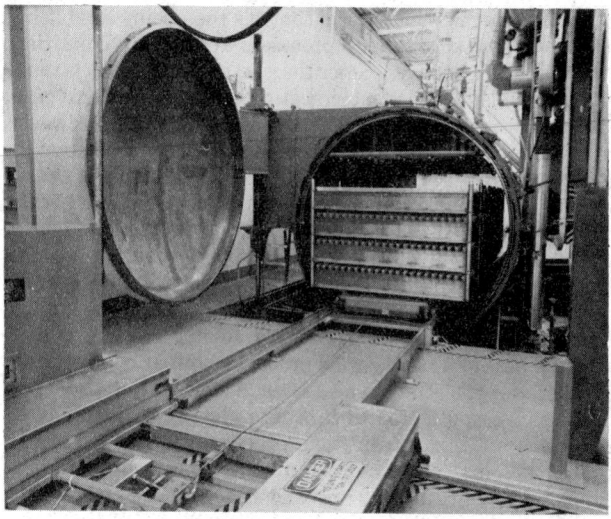

Fig 85-28.   A large autoclave being loaded with liter bottles of parenteral solutions (courtesy, Abbott).

ple-layered caps require greater force for crimping; therefore, heavy-duty mechanical crimpers are required,[†] as shown in Fig 85-27.

Sterilization

Whenever possible, the parenteral product should be sterilized after being sealed in its final container and within as short a time as possible after the filling and sealing have been completed. Since this usually involves a thermal process, due consideration must be given to the effect of the elevated temperature upon the stability of the product. Many products, both pharmaceutical and biological, will be adversely affected by the elevated temperatures required for thermal sterilization. Such products must, therefore, be sterilized by a nonthermal method. Most thermolabile solutions may be sterilized by filtration through bacteria-retaining filters. Subsequently, all operations must be carried out in an aseptic manner so that contamination will not be introduced into the filtrate. To perform such an aseptic procedure is difficult, and the degree of its accomplishment is always uncertain. Colloids, oleaginous solutions, suspensions, and emulsions that are thermolabile may require a process in which each component is sterilized and the product is formulated and processed under aseptic conditions. Because of the ever-present risk of a momentary or prolonged lapse in aseptic control during an aseptic process, and the dangerous condition that could result, sterilization of a product in its final container (terminal sterilization) is preferred, if possible.

Some of the newer nonthermal methods of sterilization are finding important application to components of injections and to administration devices. Certain dry solids such as penicillin, streptomycin, polyvitamins, and certain hormones are being effectively sterilized by ionized radiations without adverse effects. Catgut sutures are now being routinely sterilized in the final package by this method. Administration sets, disposable needles and syringes, and other plastic and stainless steel equipment and components are being sterilized by ionizing radiations and by gaseous ethylene oxide sterilization. Generally speaking, however, neither of these methods may be used for liquid preparations without adverse effects on the product, and gaseous sterilization cannot be used where a glass container or other impervious barrier prevents the gas from permeating the material.

[†] Suppliers: *Alcoa, United Machinery, West, Wheaton.*

Dry-heat sterilization may be employed for a few dry solids that are not adversely affected by the high temperatures and for the relatively long heating period required. This method is most effectively applied to the sterilization of glassware and metalware. After sterilization, the equipment will be sterile, dry, and, if the sterilization period is long enough, pyrogen-free.

Saturated steam under pressure (autoclaving) is the most commonly used and the most effective method for the sterilization of aqueous liquids or substances that can be reached or penetrated by steam.

Fig 85-28 shows liter containers of solution being loaded into an autoclave for sterilization. It is ineffective in anhydrous conditions, such as within a sealed ampul containing a dry solid or an anhydrous oil. Since the temperature employed in an autoclave is lower than that for dry-heat sterilization, equipment made of materials such as rubber and polypropylene may be sterilized if the time and temperature are carefully controlled. As mentioned previously, some injections will be adversely affected by the elevated temperature required for autoclaving. For some products, such as Dextrose Injection, the use of an autoclave designed to permit a rapid rise to sterilizing temperature and rapid cooling with water spray after the sterilizing hold-period will make it possible to use this method. Other products that will not withstand autoclaving temperatures may withstand marginal thermal methods such as tyndallization or inspissation. These methods may be rendered more effective for some injections by the inclusion of a bacteriostatic agent in the product.

It should be obvious that all materials subjected to sterilization must be protected from subsequent contamination to maintain their sterile state. Therefore, materials subjected to autoclaving must be wrapped or covered so that microorganisms may not gain access when removed from the autoclave. Equipment and supplies are most frequently wrapped with paper and tied or sealed with special autoclave tape. The wrapping must permit penetration of steam during autoclaving but screen out microorganisms when dry. A double wrapping with lint-free parchment paper designed for such use is probably best. Synthetic fiber cloth such as nylon or Dacron also may be used for the inner wrapping. The openings of equipment subjected to dry-heat sterilization are often covered with silver–aluminum foil or with metal or glass covers. Cellulose wrapping materials are adversely affected by the high temperatures of dry-heat sterilization.

The effectiveness of any sterilization technique must be

proved before it is employed; controls then being established to show that subsequent processes repeat the conditions proven to be effective. Since the goal of sterilization is to kill microorganisms, the ideal indicator to prove the effectiveness of the process is a biological one, resistant spores. However, many feel considerable hesitation about using biological indicators during the processing of products because of the inherent risk of inadvertent contamination of the product or the environment. Also, it has been found that the resistance of spores varies from lot to lot, thereby possibly giving false indications of reliability when used as a biological indicator for a sterilization procedure. However, others feel as strongly that biological indicators should be used, not only to prove the effectiveness of a sterilization procedure but as confirmatory evidence for the effectiveness of each sterilization process.

It also is essential to utilize other indicators to confirm the reliability of the sterilization process, such as recording thermocouples, color-change indicators, and melting indicators. Such confirmatory evidence is an essential part of the sterilization record for a product.

Further details concerning methods of sterilization and their application will be found in Chapter 79. In addition, the USP provides suggestions concerning the sterilization of injections and related materials.

Freeze-Drying

Freeze-drying (lyophilization) is a process of drying in which water is sublimed from the product after it is frozen.[15]

The particular advantages of this process are that biologicals and pharmaceuticals which are relatively unstable in aqueous solution can be processed and filled into dosage containers in the liquid state, taking advantage of the relative ease of processing a liquid; dried without elevated temperatures, thereby eliminating adverse thermal effects; and then stored in the dry state in which there are relatively few stability problems.

Further advantages include the fact that freeze-dried products are often more soluble and/or more rapidly soluble, dispersions are stabilized throughout the shelf life of the product, and products subject to degradation by oxidation have enhanced stability because the process is carried out in a vacuum.

However, the increased time and handling required for processing and the cost of the equipment limit the use of this process to those products which have significantly enhanced stability if stored in the dry state.

The fact that ice will sublime at pressures below 3 mm Hg has been a long-established laboratory principle. The extensive program for the freeze-drying of human plasma during World War II provided the impetus for the rapid development of the process.

Freeze-drying essentially consists of the following:

1. Freezing an aqueous product at a temperature below its eutectic temperature.
2. Evacuating the chamber, usually below 0.1 torr (100 μm Hg).
3. Subliming ice on a cold condensing surface at a temperature below that of the product, the condensing surface being within the chamber or in a connecting chamber.
4. Introducing heat to the product under controlled conditions, thereby providing energy for sublimation at a rate designed to keep the product temperature below its eutectic temperature.

Fig 85-29 shows such a system. The product may be frozen on the shelf in the chamber by circulating refrigerant (usually Freon, ammonia, or ethylene glycol) from the compressor through pipes within the shelf. After freezing is complete, which may require several hours, the chamber and condenser are evacuated by the vacuum pump, the condenser surface having been previously chilled by circulating refrigerant from the large compressor.

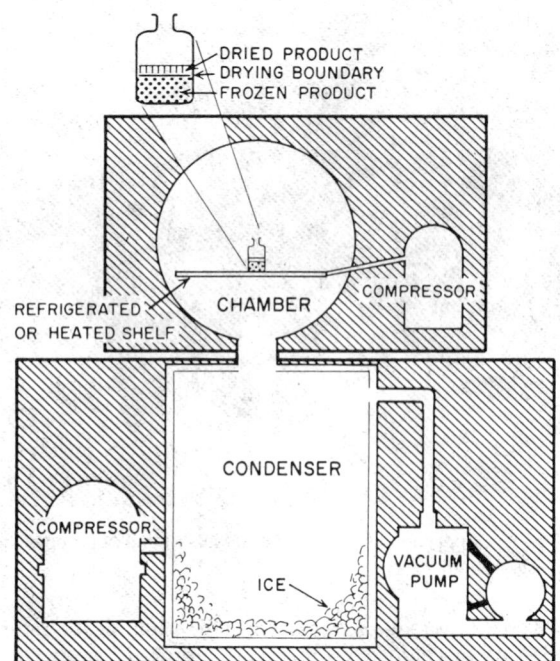

Fig 85-29. Essential components of a freeze-drying system.

Heat is then introduced from the shelf to the product by electric resistance coils or by circulating hot water, silicone, or glycol. The process continues until the product is dry (usually 1% or less moisture), leaving a sponge-like matrix of the solids originally present in the product, the input of heat being controlled so as not to degrade the product.

For most pharmaceuticals and biologicals the liquid product is sterilized by filtration and then filled into the dosage container aseptically. The containers must remain open during the drying process; therefore, they must be protected from contamination during transfer from the filling area to the freeze-drying chamber, while in the freeze-drying chamber, and at the end of the drying process until sealed.

Chambers may be equipped with hydraulic or rubber diaphragm internal-stoppering devices designed to push slotted rubber closures into the vials to be sealed while the chamber is still evacuated, the closures having been partially inserted immediately after filling so that the slots were open to the outside.

If internal stoppering is not available or containers such as ampuls are used, filtered dry air or nitrogen must be introduced to the chamber at the end of the process to establish atmospheric pressure. Then the containers must be removed and sealed under aseptic conditions. If the product is very sensitive to moisture, the environmental humidity also must be controlled until it is sealed.

Factors Affecting the Process Rate—The greater the depth of the product in the container, the longer will be the drying process. Therefore, a product to be frozen by placing the container on a refrigerated shelf (plug freezing) should be filled to a planned, limited depth. If a large volume of solution must be processed, the surface area may be increased and the depth decreased by freezing the solution on a slant or while rotating the container on an angle (shell freezing) in a liquid refrigerant bath, such as dry ice and alcohol.

The actual driving force for the process is the vapor pressure differential between the vapor at the surface where drying of the product is occurring (the drying boundary) and the vapor pressure at the surface of the ice on the condenser. The latter is determined by the temperature of the condenser as modified by the insulating effect of the accumulated ice. The former is determined by a number of factors, including:

1. The rate of heat conduction through the container and the frozen material, both usually relatively poor thermal conductors, to the drying boundary while maintaining all of the product below its eutectic temperature.

2. The impeding effect of the increasing depth of dried porous product above the drying boundary.

3. The temperature and heat capacity of the shelf itself.

This may be visualized by referring to Fig 85-29.

The passageways between the product surface and the condenser surface must be wide open and direct for effective operation. Therefore, the condensing surfaces in large freeze-driers are usually in the same chamber as the product. Evacuation of the system is necessary to reduce the impeding effect that collisions with air molecules would have on the passage of water molecules. However, the residual pressure in the system must be greater than the vapor pressure of the ice on the condenser or the ice will be vaporized and pulled into the pump, an event detrimental to most pumps.

The amount of solids in the product, their particle size, and their thermal conductance will affect the rate of drying. The more solids present, the more impediment will be provided to the escape of the water vapor. The smaller the particle size, particularly the crystal size of the ice, the faster the drying generally will be. The poorer the thermal conducting properties of the solids in the product, the slower will be the rate of transfer of heat through the frozen material to the drying boundary.

The rate of drying is essentially slow, most often requiring 24 hours or longer for completion. The actual time required, the rate of heat input, and the product temperatures that may be utilized must be determined for each product and then carefully reproduced with successive processes.

Factors Affecting Formulation—The active constituent of many pharmaceutical products is present in such a small quantity that if freeze-dried alone its presence would be hard to detect visually. Therefore, excipients are often added to increase the amount of solids present.

Some consider it ideal for the dried product plug to occupy essentially the same volume as that of the original solution. To achieve this, the solids content of the original product must be between approximately 5 and 25%. Among the substances found most useful for this purpose, usually as a combination, are sodium or potassium phosphates, citric acid, tartaric acid, gelatin, and carbohydrates such as dextrose, mannitol, and dextran.

Each of these substances contributes appearance characteristics to the plug, such as whether dull and spongy or sparkling and crystalline, firm or friable, expanded or shrunken, and uniform or striated. Therefore, the formulation of a product to be freeze-dried must include consideration not only of the nature and stability characteristics required during the liquid state, both freshly prepared and when reconstituted before use, but the characteristics desired in the dried plug.

Modifications in the Process and Equipment—In some

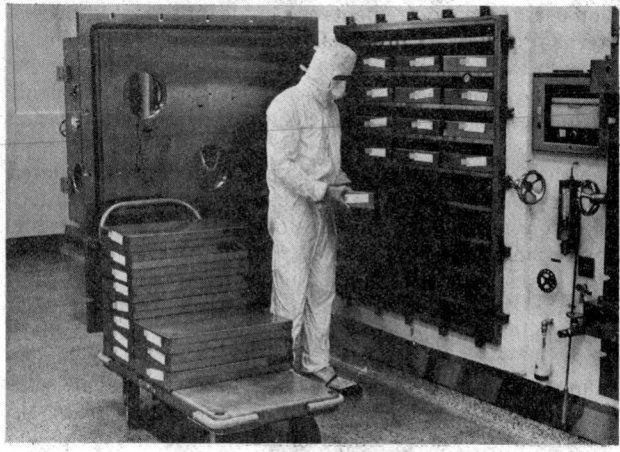

Fig 85-30. Aseptic loading of freeze-drier (courtesy, Upjohn).

instances a product may be frozen in a bulk container or in trays rather than in the final container and then handled as a dry solid. This may be desirable when large volumes of a product are processed.

Heat may be introduced to all sides of the product by radiation from infrared sources, rather than only from the bottom as with conductive heating. While this generally increases the rate of drying, there are at least two major disadvantages to radiant heating of pharmaceuticals; these are (1) multiple containers produce shadowing with resultant blockage of the radiations and (2) the dried material on the outside of the frozen product may be scorched easily by the heat as drying progresses.

When large quantities of material are processed it may be desirable to utilize ejection pumps in the equipment system. These draw the vapor into the pump and eject it to the outside, thereby eliminating the need for a condensing surface. Such pumps are expensive and usually practical only in large installations.

Available freeze-driers* range in size from small laboratory units to large industrial models such as the one shown in Fig 85-30. Their selection requires consideration of such factors as tray area required, volume of water to be removed, whether or not aseptic processing will be involved, is internal stoppering required, will separate freezers be used for initial freezing of the product, and the degree of automatic operation desired. Further factors involved in the selection and use of equipment are considered in the literature.[16]

Freeze-drying is now being utilized for research in the preservation of human tissue and is finding increasing application in the food industry. Progress on new developments is being made in both the process and the equipment.

---

* Suppliers: *Hull, Industrial Dynamics, NRC, Repp, Stokes, Thermovac, Virtis.*

Quality Control

The importance of undertaking every possible means to be assured of the quality of the finished product cannot be overemphasized. Every component and every step of the manufacturing process must be subjected to intense scrutiny to be confident that quality is attained in the finished product. The responsibility for supervising this is a grave one, and lapses of requirements or short cuts in procedure may not be permitted. Such responsibility applies wherever parenteral preparations are manufactured.

The principles of quality control are basically the same for the manufacture of any pharmaceutical. These are discussed in Chapter 83. During the discussion of the preparation of injections, mention was made of numerous quality requirements for components and manufacturing processes. Here, only certain tests characteristically applicable to the finished parenteral products will be discussed.

Sterility Test

All lots of injections in their final containers must be tested for sterility. The USP prescribes the requirements for this test for official injections. The Food and Drug Administration uses these requirements as a guide for testing unofficial sterile products. The official test has acknowledged limitations in the information that it can provide. Therefore, it should be noted that this test is not intended as a thoroughly evaluative test for a product subjected to a sterilization method of unknown effectiveness. It is intended primarily as a check test on the probability that a previously validated sterilization procedure has been repeated, or to give assurance of its continued effectiveness. A discussion of sterility testing is given in Chapter 79.

It should be noted that a "lot" with respect to sterility testing is that group of product containers which has been subjected to the same sterilization procedure. For containers of a product which have been sterilized by autoclaving, for example, a lot would constitute those processed in a particular sterilizer cycle. For an aseptic filling operation, a lot would constitute all of those product containers filled during a period when there was no change in the filling assembly or equipment and which is no longer than one working day or shift.

Pyrogen Test

The presence of pyrogens in parenteral preparations is evaluated by a qualitative fever response test in rabbits. The USP test is described in Chapter 31. Rabbits are used as test animals because they show physiologic response to pyrogenic substances similar to that by man. While a minimum pyrogenic dose (MPD), the amount just sufficient to cause a positive USP Pyrogen Test response, may sometimes produce uncertain test results, a content equal to a few times the MPD will leave no uncertainty. Therefore, the test is valid and has continued in use since introduced by Seibert in 1923. It should be understood that not all injections may be subjected to the rabbit test since the medicinal agent may have a physiologic effect on the test animal such that any fever response would be masked. Therefore, the pyrogen test is performed primarily on vehicles.

A new test for pyrogens has recently been accepted, not only for in-process control for pharmaceutical products, but for release testing of such products and for devices. It is an *in vitro* test based on the gelling or color development of a pyrogenic preparation in the presence of the lysate of the amebocytes of the horseshoe crab (*Limulus polyphemus*). The Limulus Test, as it is called, is simpler, more rapid, and of greater sensitivity than the rabbit test.[17] Although it detects only the endotoxic pyrogens of Gram-negative bacteria, this probably will not significantly limit its use since most environmental contaminants gaining entrance to sterile products are Gram-negative. The test has gained in stature to the point that automated techniques have been developed.[18]

Clarity Tests

The USP does not provide specifications for a clarity test. It contains only the statement that good manufacturing practice requires that each final container of an injection should be subjected individually to a visual inspection. The development of test procedures to meet this general requirement is the responsibility of the manufacturer.

The objective of the clarity inspection is to prevent the distribution and use of parenterals which contain particulate matter that may be psychologically or actually harmful to the recipient. Solutions to be introduced intravenously require the most critical evaluation.

Concern about particulate matter in parenteral solutions must not be limited to the psychological effect that the presence of visible "dirt" would suggest that the product was of inferior quality. Recent investigations have caused a new assessment of the significance of particles in solution to be introduced into the blood stream. While data defining the extent and risk of toxic effects are still limited, it has been shown that particles of lint, rubber, insoluble chemicals, and other foreign particulate matter can produce emboli in vital organs of animals and man.[19] Another study suggests that an adverse physiologic effect may be related to the presence of particulate matter in intravenous fluids, namely, the development of infusion phlebitis.[20]

A study of the size distribution of particulate matter in commercial intravenous solutions showed that the number of particles increased approximately logarithmically with decreasing size. This finding would suggest that a count made at an arbitrarily chosen size could be used to predict the number of particles at another size. The counts were made with a Coulter Counter, a resistance-type counter. Other electronic counters utilize the light-scattering* or light-shadowing† principle to count particles in a liquid sample. Particles may also be counted and examined microscopically by collection on the surface of a membrane filter, a method used by the USP that permits identification of the particles as well as a count. Such methods cannot be utilized for the in-line evaluation of every container produced commercially, but may be used for quality-control sampling of the process.

The particle size that should be of particular concern has not been determined but it has been suggested that, since erythrocytes have a diameter of approximately 4.5 μm, particles of more than 5 μm should be the basis for evaluation. This is a considerably smaller particle than can be seen with the unaided eye; approximately 50 μm is the lower limit unless the Tyndall effect is utilized, whereby particles as small as 10 μm may be seen by the light scattered from them.

Meanwhile, all the product units from the production line are being inspected individually by human inspectors under a good light, baffled against reflection into the eye, against a black and a white background. Although this inspection is subject to the limitations in the size of particles that can be seen, the variation in visual acuity from inspector to inspector, the emotional state of the inspector, eye strain and fatigue, and other personal factors that will affect what the inspector sees, it does provide a means for eliminating the normally few units which contain visible particles and it is a check on the repetition of the standard clean processing procedure established for that product.

This concern over the presence of particulate matter in parenteral products, particularly those given intravenously, has brought about a dramatic improvement through the voluntary effort of the pharmaceutical industry. One study[21] clearly shows a reduced particulate content of commercially prepared intravenous infusion fluids, as compared with earlier products. Also, it has been shown that additives and administration sets may introduce a substantial amount of particulate matter to an otherwise relatively clean solution. In addition, the technique utilized in the hospital for the preparation and administration of the intravenous infusion fluid must be carefully controlled to avoid the introduction of particulate matter. Therefore, the pharmaceutical manufacturer, the administration set manufacturer, the hospital pharmacist, the nurse, and the physician must share responsibility for making sure that the patient receives a clean intravenous injection.

Leaker Test

Ampuls that have been sealed by fusion must be subjected to a test to determine whether or not a passageway remains to the outside. If such a passageway remains, all or a part of

---

* Suppliers: *Climet, Royco.*
† Supplier: *HIAC.*

the contents of the ampul may leak to the outside and spoil the package, or microorganisms or other contaminants may enter. Changes in temperature during storage cause expansion and contraction of the ampul and contents, and will accentuate interchange if a passageway exists, even if microscopic in size.

A leaker test is usually performed by producing a negative pressure within an incompletely sealed ampul while the ampul is entirely submerged in a deeply colored dye solution. Most often, approximately a 1% methylene blue solution is employed. The test may be performed by subjecting the ampuls to a vacuum in a vacuum chamber, the ampuls being submerged in a dye bath throughout the process. Another procedure frequently employed is to simply autoclave the ampuls in a dye bath. A modification of this is to remove them from the autoclave while hot and quickly submerge them in a cool bath of dye solution. After carefully rinsing the dye solution from the outside, color from the dye will be visible within a leaker. Leakers are, of course, discarded.

Vials and bottles are not subjected to a leaker test because the sealing material (rubber stoppers) is not rigid. Therefore, results from such a test would be meaningless. However, evacuated bottles containing a liquid may be checked for a sharp "click" sound produced when struck with an implement such as a rubber mallet.

Safety Test

The National Institutes of Health requires of most biological products routine safety testing in animals. Under the Kefauver-Harris Amendments to the Federal Food, Drug, and Cosmetic Act, most pharmaceutical preparations are now required to be tested for safety. Because it is entirely possible for a parenteral product to pass the routine sterility test, pyrogen test, and chemical analyses and still cause unfavorable reactions when injected, a safety test in animals is essential to provide additional assurance that the product does not have unexpected toxic properties. Safety tests in animals are discussed in detail in the USP.

Packaging and Labeling

A full discussion of the packaging of parenteral preparations is beyond the scope of this text. It is essential, of course, that the packaging should provide ample protection for the product against physical damage from shipping, handling, and storage and should protect light-sensitive materials from ultraviolet radiation.

Packaging—The USP includes certain requirements for the packaging and storage of injections, as follows:

1. The volume of injection in single-dose containers is defined as that which is specified for parenteral administration at one time and is limited to a volume of 1 L.
2. Parenterals intended for intraspinal, intracisternal, or peridural administration are packaged only in single-dose containers.
3. Unless an individual monograph specifies otherwise, no multiple-dose container shall contain a volume of injection more than sufficient to permit the withdrawal and administration of 30 mL.
4. Injections packaged for use as irrigation solutions or for hemofiltration or dialysis are exempt from foregoing requirements relating to packaging. Containers for injections packaged for use as hemofiltration or irrigation solutions may be designed to empty rapidly and may contain a volume in excess of 1 L.
5. Injections intended for veterinary use are exempt from the packaging and storage requirements concerning the limitation to single-dose containers and to volume of multiple-dose containers.

Labeling—The labeling of an injection must provide the physician or other user with all of the information needed to assure the safe and proper use of the therapeutic agent. Since all of this information cannot be placed on the immediate container and be legible, it may be provided on accompanying printed matter. General labeling requirements for drugs are discussed in Chapter 107.

A restatement of the labeling definitions and requirements of the USP for Injections is as follows:

The term "labeling" designates all labels and other written, printed, or graphic matter upon an immediate container or upon, or in, any package or wrapper in which it is enclosed, with the exception of the outer shipping container. The term "label" designates that part of the labeling upon the immediate container.

The label states the name of the preparation, the percentage content of drug of a liquid preparation, the amount of active ingredient of a dry preparation, the volume of liquid to be added to prepare an injection or suspension from a dry preparation, the route of administration, a statement of storage conditions, and an expiration date. Also, the label must indicate the name of the manufacturer or distributor and carry an identifying lot number. The lot number is capable of providing access to the complete manufacturing history of the specific package, including each single manufacturing step.

The container label is so arranged that a sufficient area of the container remains uncovered for its full length or circumference to permit inspection of the contents.

The label must state the name of the vehicle and the proportions of each constituent, if it is a mixture; the names and proportions of all substances added to increase stability or usefulness; and the expiration date where required by the individual monograph.

Preparations labeled for use as dialysis, hemofiltration, or irrigation solutions must meet the requirements for Injections other than those relating to volume and also must bear on the label statements that they are not intended for intravenous injection.

Injections intended for veterinary use are so labeled.

References

1. Griffenhagen GB: *Bull Parenteral Drug Assoc 16*(2): 12, 1962.
2. Tousignaut DR: *Am J Hosp Pharm 34:* 943, 1977.
3. Bergman DH: *Drug Intel Clin Pharm 11:* 345, 1977.
4. Spiegel AJ, Noseworthy MM: *J Pharm Sci 52:* 917, 1963.
5. Schroeter LC: *J Pharm Sci 50:* 891, 1961.
6. Autian J: *Bull Parenteral Drug Assoc 22:* 276, 1968.
7. Subrahmanyam SV, Majeske JP: *Am J Pharm 129:* 222, 1957.
8. Hopkins GH: *J Pharm Sci 54:* 138, 1965.
9. Federal Std No. 209b, GSA, Washington, DC 20407, April 24, 1973.
10. Anschel J: *Bull Parenteral Drug Assoc 31:* 47, 1977.
11. Grimes TL, Fonner DE, *et al: Bull Parenteral Drug Assoc 31:* 179, 1977.
12. Myers T, Chrai S: *J Parenteral Sci Tech 35:* 8, 1981.
13. Macek TJ: *J Pharm Sci 52:* 694, 1963.
14. Nash RA: *Drug Cosmet Ind 97:* 843, 1965; *98:* 39, 1966.
15. *Ann NY Acad Sci, 85:* 501–734, 1965.
16. Morgan SL, Spotts MR: *Pharm Technol 3:* 94–101, 114, 1979.
17. Cooper JF: *Bull Parenteral Drug Assoc 29:* 122, 1975.
18. Novitsky TJ, Ryther SS, et al: *J Parenteral Sci Tech 36:* 11, 1982.
19. Garvan JM, Gunner BW: *Med J Austral 2:* 1(July 4) 1964.
20. Deluca P et al: *Am J Hosp Pharm 32:* 1001, 1975.
21. Turco SJ, Davis NM: *Am J Hosp Pharm 30:* 557, 1973.

Bibliography

Martin EW, *et al: Techniques of Medication*, Lippincott, Philadelphia, 1969.

Avis KE, Miller WA, in Hoover JE, ed: *Dispensing of Medication*, 8th ed, Mack Publ Co, Easton, PA, Chap 10, 1976.

Avis KE, in Lachman L, *et al: The Theory and Practice of Industrial Pharmacy*, 2nd ed, Lea & Febiger, Philadelphia, Chaps. 20 and 21, 1976.

Turco S, King RE: *Sterile Dosage Forms*, 2nd ed, Lea & Febiger, Philadelphia, 1979.

Avis KE, *et al: Parenteral Dosage Forms—An Annotated Bibliography*, 5 vols, (1959–63, 1964–67, 1968–70, 1971–72, 1973). Parenteral Drug Assoc, Philadelphia.

Useller JW: *Clean Room Technology* (NASA SP-5074), USGPO, Washington, DC, 1969.

Perkins JJ: *Principles and Methods of Sterilization in Health Sciences*, 2nd ed, Thomas, Springfield, IL, 1969.

Block SS, ed: *Disinfection, Sterilization and Preservation*, 3rd ed, Lea and Febiger, Philadelphia, 1983.

Phillips GB, Miller WS, eds: *Industrial Sterilization*, Duke Univ. Press, Durham, NC, 1973.

Gaughran ERL, Kereluk K, eds: *Sterilization of Medical Products*, Johnson & Johnson, New Brunswick, NJ, 1977.

Meryman HT, ed: *Cryobiology*, Academic, New York, 1966.

CHAPTER 86

Intravenous Admixtures

Salvatore J Turco, PharmD

Professor of Pharmacy
Temple University School of Pharmacy
Philadelphia, PA 19140

Robert E King, PhD

Professor of Industrial Pharmacy
Philadelphia College of Pharmacy and Science
Philadelphia, PA 19104

It has been estimated that 40% of all drugs administered in hospitals are given in the form of injections and their use is increasing. Part of this increase in parenteral therapy is due to the wider utilization of intravenous fluids (IV fluids). In the last decade the use of IV fluids has doubled, increasing from 150 million units to 300 million units annually. Not only do IV fluids continue to serve as the means for fluid replacement, electrolyte-balance restoration, and supplementary nutrition, but they are also playing major roles as vehicles for other drug substances and in total parenteral nutrition. Intravenous fluids are finding greater use as the means of administering other drugs because of convenience, the means of reducing the irritation potential of the drugs, and the desirability for continuous and intermittent drug therapy. The techniques for providing total parenteral nutrition parenterally have improved steadily in the last decade and such use is increasing at the rate of 40% annually. The use of IV fluids for these purposes requires the compounding of specific intravenous admixtures (parenteral prescriptions) to meet the clinical needs of a given patient. However, the combination of drug substances in an intravenous fluid can promote parenteral incompatibilities and give rise to conditions not favorable for drug stability. A new area of specialization has been created for hospital pharmacists who can develop the expertise to prepare these solutions, recognizing their compatibility and stability problems and the potential for contamination, and to participate in the administration of the solutions. The complex compounding of an order for total parenteral nutrition requires knowledgeable personnel capable of making accurate calculations, compounding, and having perfect aseptic technique. The parenteral prescription is becoming increasingly important in hospitals. Centralized admixture programs are now found in 70% of the nation's hospitals having 300 beds or more. Equipment available for administering intravenous fluids has become more sophisticated, and has made possible increased accuracy of dosage and led to the development of new concepts and methods of nutrition and drug treatment.

Intravenous Fluids

Large-volume injections intended to be administered by intravenous infusion are commonly called IV fluids and are included in the group of sterile products referred to as large-volume parenterals. Large-volume parenterals consist of single-dose injections having a volume of 100 mL or more and containing no added substances. Intravenous fluids are packaged in containers having a capacity of 150 mL to 1000 mL. Minitype infusion containers of 250-mL capacity are available with 50- and 100-mL partial fills for solution of drugs when used in the "piggyback" technique. This technique refers to the administration of a second solution through a Y-tube or gum-rubber connection in the administration set of the first intravenous fluid, thus avoiding the need for another injection site. In addition to the IV fluids, the group also includes irrigation solutions and solutions for dialysis.

Intravenous fluids are sterile solutions of simple chemicals such as sugars, amino acids, or electrolytes—materials which can easily be carried by the circulatory system and assimilated. Prepared with Water for Injection USP, the solutions are pyrogen-free. Because of the large volumes administered intravenously, the absence of particulate matter assumes a more significant role in view of possible biological hazards resulting from particulate matter. Absence of particulate matter or clarity of IV fluids is as important at the time of administration following their manipulation in the hospital as it is at the time of injection manufacture.

Limits for particulate matter occurring in IV fluids, or large-volume injections used for single-dose infusion, have been defined in the USP. This represents the first regulatory attempt to define limits for particulate matter in parenterals. These limits do not apply to multiple-dose injections, small-volume injections, or injections prepared by reconstitution from sterile solids. The USP defines particulate matter as extraneous, mobile, undissolved substances, other than gas bubbles, unintentionally present in parenteral solutions. The microscopic membrane method is used for determining the presence and size distribution of the particles observed. The determination is carried out in a laminar airflow hood using ultraclean equipment. The IV fluid sample is placed in an ultraclean funnel containing an ultraclean grid membrane through which the sample passes. After the particulate matter is collected on the membrane, the membrane is rinsed and dried within the hood. The entire surface of the membrane is examined within the hood, using a suitable microscope under 100× magnification. The total numbers of particles having effective linear dimensions equal to or larger than 10 μm and larger than 25 μm are counted. The IV fluid meets the requirement of the test if it contains not more than 50 particles per mL that are equal to or larger than 10 μm, and not more than 5 particles per mL that are equal to or larger than 25 μm in linear dimensions.

Intravenous fluids are commonly used for a number of clinical conditions. These include: (1) correction of disturbances in electrolyte balance; (2) correction of disturbances in body fluids (fluid replacement); (3) the means of providing basic nutrition; (4) the basis for the practice of providing total parenteral nutrition (TPN) or parenteral hyperalimentation; and (5) use as vehicles for other drug substances. In both of

Table I—IV Fluids Commonly Used For Intravenous Admixtures

Injection	Concentration	pH	Therapeutic Use
Amino Acid (Synthetic)			Fluid and nutrient replenisher
Aminosyn (Abbott)	3.5%; 7%	5.25	
FreAmine II (McGaw)	8.5%	6.6	
Travasol (Travenol)	5.5%; 8.5%	6.0	
Dextrose (Glucose, D5/W)	2.5%–50%	3.5–6.5	Fluid and nutrient replenisher
Dextrose and Sodium Chloride	Varying concn of dextrose from 5%–20% with varying concn of sodium chloride from 0.11%–0.9%	3.5–6.5	Fluid, nutrient, and electrolyte replenisher
Fructose (Levulose)	10%	3.0–6.0	Fluid and nutrient replenisher
Fructose and Sodium Chloride	10% 0.9%	3.0–6.0	Fluid, nutrient, and electrolyte replenisher
Invert Sugar	5%, 10%	4.0	Fluid and nutrient replenisher
Lactated Ringer's (Hartmann's)		6.0–7.5	Systemic alkalizer; fluid and electrolyte replenisher
NaCl	0.6%		
KCl	0.03%		
$CaCl_2$	0.02%		
Na Lactate	0.3%		
Protein Hydrolysate	5% from either casein or fibrin	5.0–7.0	Fluid and nutrient replenisher
Amigen (Travenol) Aminosol (Abbott) Hyprotigen (McGaw)			
Ringer's		5.0–7.5	Fluid and electrolyte replenisher
NaCl	0.86%		
KCl	0.03%		
$CaCl_2$	0.033%		
Sodium Chloride	0.45%; 0.9%; 3%; 5%	4.5–7.0	Fluid and electrolyte replenisher
Sodium Lactate	1/6 M	6.3–7.3	Fluid and electrolyte replenisher

the latter two cases it has become common practice to add other drugs to certain IV fluids to meet the clinical needs of the patient. Using IV fluids as vehicles offers the advantages of convenience, the means of reducing the irritation potential of the drug, and provides a method for continuous drug therapy. However, the practice requires that careful consideration be given to the stability and compatibility of additives present in the IV fluids serving as vehicles. This approach also demands strict adherence to aseptic techniques in adding the drugs, as well as in the administration of the IV fluids. These procedures are discussed later in the chapter. The IV fluids commonly used for parenteral admixtures are shown in Table I.

Many disease states result in electrolyte depletion and loss. Proper electrolyte concentration and balance in plasma and tissues are critical for proper body function. Electrolyte restoration and balance are most rapidly achieved through administration of IV fluids. Required electrolytes include sodium and chloride ions, which in normal saline more closely approximate the composition of the extracellular fluid than solutions of any other single salt; potassium, the principal intracellular cation of most body tissues and an essential for the functioning of the nervous and muscular systems as well as the heart; magnesium, as a nutritional supplement especially in hyperalimentation solutions; and phosphate ion, important in a variety of biochemical reactions. In addition to the number of standard electrolyte fluids shown in Table I, a large number of combinations of electrolytes in varying concentrations are available commercially. Some of these electrolyte fluids also contain dextrose and vitamins.

Dextrose Injection 5% is the most frequently used IV fluid, either for nutrition or fluid replacement. It is isotonic and administered intravenously into a peripheral vein. One gram of dextrose provides 3.4 Calories and a L of Dextrose Injection 5% supplies 170 Calories. The body utilizes dextrose at a rate of 0.5 g per kilogram of body weight per hour. More rapid administration can result in glycosuria. Therefore a L of Dextrose Injection 5% requires one and one-half hours for assimilation. The pH range of Dextrose Injection 5% can vary from 3.5 to 6.5. The wide range permitted is due to the free sugar acids present and formed during the sterilization and storage of the injection. To avoid incompatibilities when other drug substances are added to Dextrose Injection, the possible low pH should be considered in using it as a vehicle. More concentrated solutions of dextrose are available and provide increased calorie intake with less fluid volume. Being hypertonic, the more concentrated solutions may be irritating to peripheral veins. Highly concentrated solutions are administered only in a larger central vein. Other IV fluids used for intravenous admixtures and providing calories include solutions of fructose (levulose) and those containing invert sugar. There is some evidence that fructose, unlike dextrose, may be used in diabetic patients; the 10% injection is hypertonic and provides 375 calories per L. Invert sugar consists of equal parts of dextrose and levulose; it is claimed that the presence of levulose promotes more rapid utilization of dextrose.

Intravenous fluids containing crystalline amino acids or low-molecular-weight peptides hydrolyzed from casein or fibrin can provide biologically utilizable amino acids for protein synthesis (Chapter 53). Protein contributes to tissue growth, wound repair, and resistance to infection. The protein requirement for the normal adult is 1 g per kilogram of body weight per day; children and patients under stress require greater amounts. Attempts are made to maintain a positive nitrogen balance, indicating that the protein administered is being properly utilized and not broken down and eliminated through the urine as creatinine and urea, which are normal waste products. In positive nitrogen balance the patient is taking in more nitrogen than he is eliminating. In negative nitrogen balance there is more nitrogen being eliminated through the urine regularly than is being administered intravenously. This means that tissues are continuing to be torn down and repair is not necessarily taking place. Protein Hydrolysate Injection and Amino Acid Injection can afford the total body requirements for proteins by the procedure known as total parenteral nutrition (discussed below), or be used for supplemental nutrition by peripheral administration. In addition to the amino acids or peptides, these nutritional injections may also contain dextrose, electrolytes, vitamins, and insulin. Fat emulsion (*Intralipid*, Cutter; *Liposyn*, Abbott) is sometimes used concurrently but usually administered at another site.

Packaging Systems

Containers for intravenous fluids must be designed to maintain solution sterility, clarity (freedom from particulate matter), and nonpyrogenicity from the time of preparation, through storage, and during clinical administration. Container closures must be designed to facilitate insertion of administration sets through which the injections are administered at a regulated flow-rate into suitable veins. IV fluids are available in glass and plastic containers; the latter may be made from either a flexible or semirigid plastic material. IV fluids are supplied in 1000-mL, 500-mL, and 250-mL sizes in addition to 250-mL capacity containers packaged with 50 or 100 mL of Dextrose Injection 5% or Sodium Chloride Injection for piggyback use. IV fluids in glass containers are packaged under vacuum, which must be dissipated prior to use. For fluid to leave the IV glass container and flow through the administration set, some mechanism is necessary to permit air to enter the container. Current flexible plastic systems do not require air introduction in order to function. Atmospheric pressure pressing on the container forces the fluid to flow.

All glass and plastic containers are single-dose and should be discarded if not used after opening. Intravenous fluids are packaged with approximately 3% excess fill to allow for removal of air from the administration set and permit the labeled volume to be delivered from the container. The containers are graduated at 20-mL increments on scales that permit the volume in container to be determined either from an upright or inverted position. Glass containers have aluminum and plastic bands for hanging while plastic containers have eyelet openings or plastic straps for attachment to IV poles.

Fluids for IV use are available from three sources. All provide both glass and plastic containers. The glass-container systems of Travenol/Baxter and McGaw are similar. The characteristics of current packaging systems are summarized in Table II.

Administration Sets

Administration sets used to deliver fluids intravenously are sterile, pyrogen-free, and disposable. Although these sets are supplied by different manufacturers, each for its own system, they have certain basic components. These include a plastic spike to pierce the rubber closure or plastic seal on the IV container; a drip (sight) chamber to trap air and to permit

Table II—IV Fluid Systems

Source	Container	Characteristics
Travenol/Baxter	Glass	Vacuum Air tube
Travenol/Baxter (Viaflex®)	Plastic	Polyvinyl chloride Flexible Non-vented
McGaw	Glass	Vacuum Air tube
McGaw (Accumed®)	Plastic	Polyolefin Semirigid Non-vented
Abbott	Glass	Vacuum Air filter[a]
Abbott (Lifecare®)	Plastic	Polyvinyl chloride Flexible Non-vented

[a] Part of administration set.

adjustment of flow rate; and a length (150 to 450 cm) of polyvinyl chloride tubing terminating in a gum-rubber injection port. At the tip of the port is a rigid needle or catheter adapter. An adjustable clamp (screw or roller type) on the tubing pinches the tubing to regulate flow. Since the gum-rubber port is self-sealing, additional medication can be added to the IV system at these ports of entry. Glass containers that have no air tubes require air-inlet filters designed as part of the administration set (Abbott). See Figs 86-1 to 86-5.

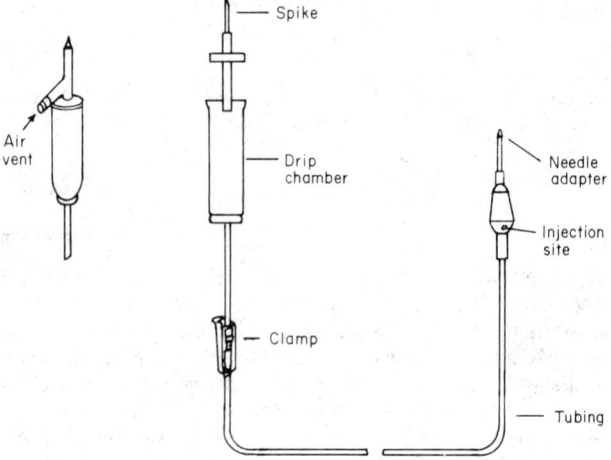

Fig 86-1. Parts of basic administration sets.

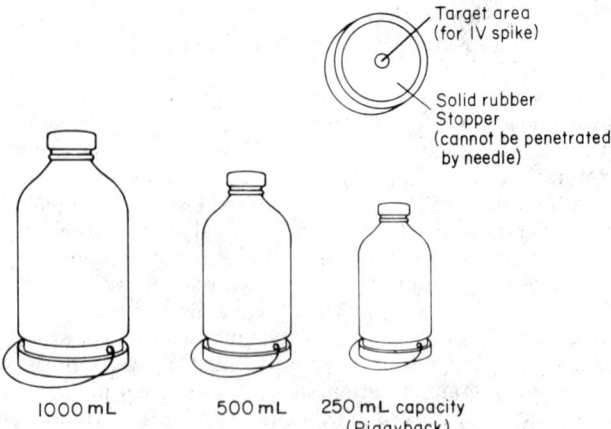

Fig 86-2. Abbott and Cutter IV glass container. The air venting is provided through the air filter located in the spike of the administration set. See Fig 86-1.

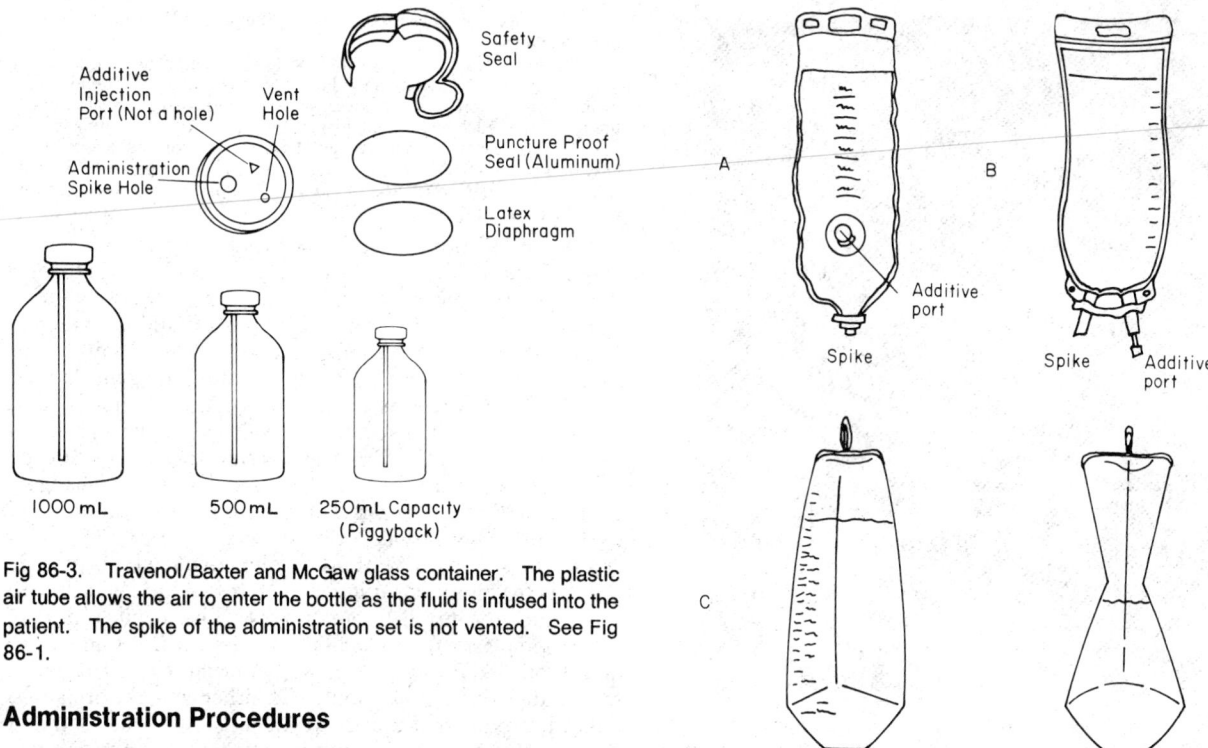

Fig 86-3. Travenol/Baxter and McGaw glass container. The plastic air tube allows the air to enter the bottle as the fluid is infused into the patient. The spike of the administration set is not vented. See Fig 86-1.

Administration Procedures

In the administration of IV fluids, the primary IV container provides for fluid replacement, electrolyte replenishment, drug therapy, or nutrition; the fluid can be infused over a 4- to 8-hour period. In some cases an IV fluid is slowly infused for the purpose of keeping the vein open (KVO). This will allow additional drugs to be administered when required. The primary IV fluid can also serve as a vehicle for other drugs to be administered. This would then become an intravenous

Fig 86-4. (A) Abbott (Lifecare®) polyvinyl chloride flexible container; (B) Travenol/Baxter (Viaflex®) polyvinyl chloride flexible container; McGaw (Accumed®) polyolefin semirigid container, front and side views. These containers take non-vented administration sets. See Fig 86-1.

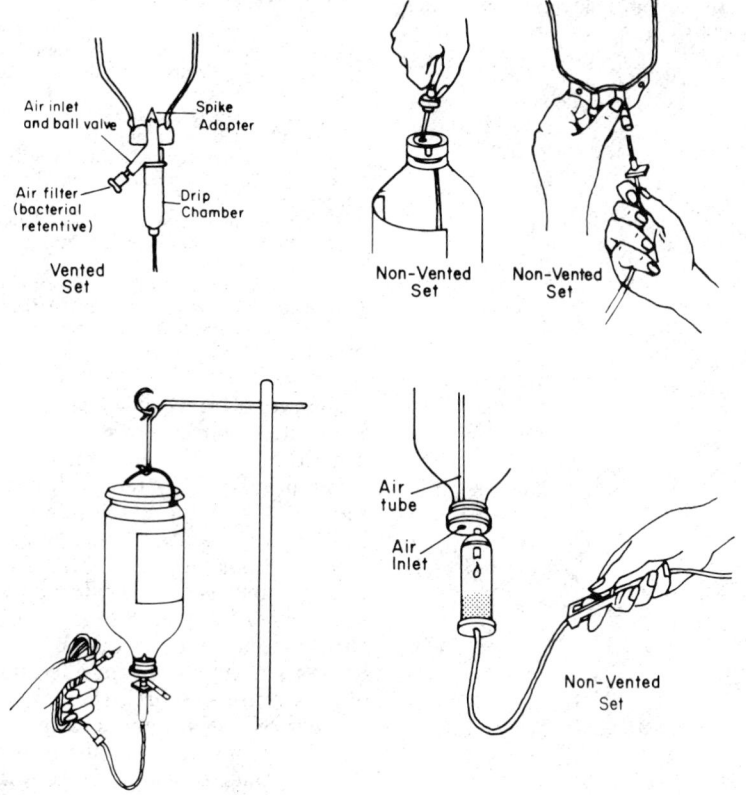

Fig 86-5. Setting up primary IV fluid for administration.

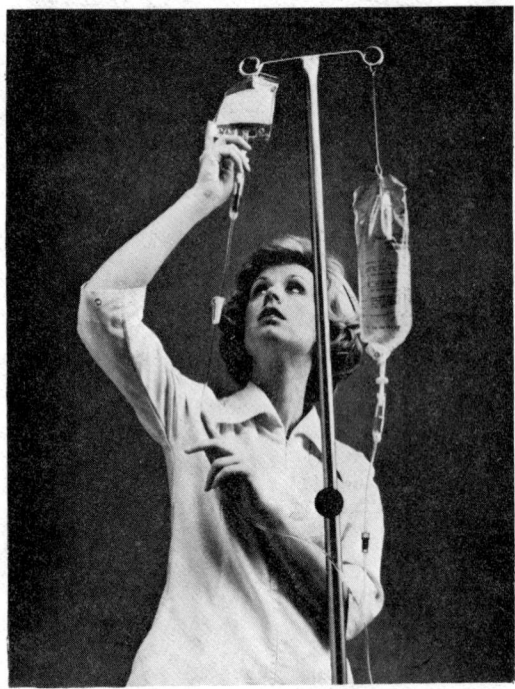

Fig 86-6.   Piggyback method: the intermittent administration of a second solution through the venipuncture site of an established primary IV system.

admixture (IV drip) and results in continuous blood levels of added drugs once the steady-state has been reached.

In preparing an IV fluid for administration, the following procedure is used.

1.   The spike adapter of the administration set is inserted into stopper or seal of the IV container.   Fig 86-5.
2.   The IV fluid is hung on a stand at bedside and air is purged from the administration set by opening clamp until fluid comes out of needle. The tubing is then clamped off.   Fig 86-5.

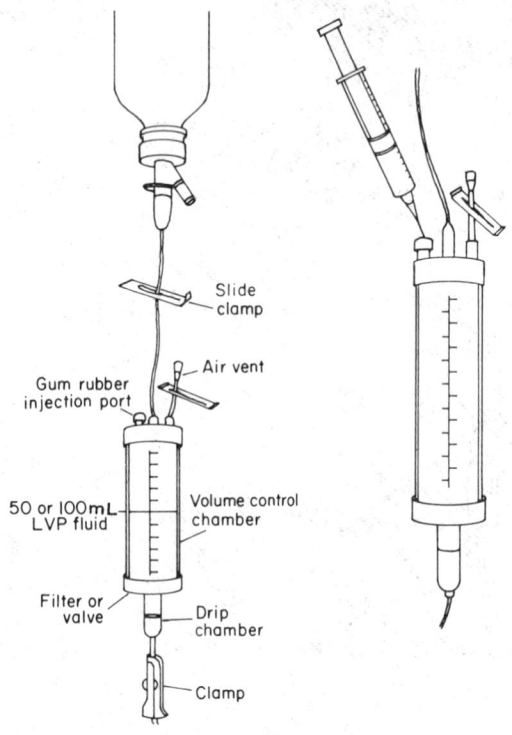

Fig 86-7.   Volume control set.

3.   The venipuncture is made by member of the IV team, floor nurse or physician.
4.   The infusion rate is adjusted by slowly opening and closing clamp until the desired drop rate, viewed in the drip chamber, is obtained.   The usual running time is 4 to 8 hours (usually 125 mL are delivered in one hour).   Drugs such as heparin, insulin, lidocaine, and dopamine may be present in the IV drip.   When potent drugs are present, the flow-rates will vary and be dependent on the clinical condition of the patient.   Sets are calculated to deliver 10, 15, 20, 50 or 60 drops per mL depending on manufacturer.   Fig 86-5.

Intermittent administration of an antibiotic and other drugs can be achieved by any of three methods.   These are by (1) direct intravenous injection (IV bolus or push), (2) addition of the drug to a predetermined volume of fluid in a volume-control device, or (3) use of a second container (minibottle, minibag) with an already hanging IV fluid (piggybacking).

Direct Intravenous Injection—Small volumes (1 to 50 mL) of drugs are injected into the vein over a short period of time (1 to 5 minutes).   The injection can also be made through a resealable gum-rubber injection site of an already hanging IV fluid.   This method is suitable for a limited number of drugs but too hazardous for most drugs.

Volume-Control Method—Volume-control sets provide a means for intermittent infusion of drug solutions in precise quantities, at controlled rates of flow.   These units consist of calibrated plastic fluid-chambers placed in a direct line under an established primary IV container or more often attached to an independent fluid supply.   In either case, the drug to be administered is first reconstituted if it is a sterile solid and injected into the gum-rubber injection port of the volume-control unit.   It is then further diluted to 50 to 150 mL with the primary fluid or the separate fluid reservoir.   Administration of the total drug-containing solution requires 30 to 60 minutes and produces a peak concentration in the blood followed by a valley if the dosage is discontinued.   The following volume control sets are available commercially: *Soluset®*, Abbott;   *Buretrol®*, Travenol/Baxter;   and   *Metriset®*, McGaw.

The procedure for setting up an intermittent IV infusion with a volume-control set is as follows:

1.   Using aseptic technique, the spike of the volume control set is inserted into the primary IV fluid or a separate fluid container.   See Fig 86-7.
2.   Air is purged from tubing of the volume control set by opening clamps until fluid comes through.
3.   The clamp is opened above the calibrated chamber and it is filled with 25 to 50 mL fluid from the primary IV container or separate fluid container.
4.   The clamp is closed above the chamber.
5.   The medication is injected through the gum-rubber port of the volume-control unit.
6.   The clamp above the chamber is opened to complete the dilution to the desired volume (50 to 150 mL), then closed.
7.   Flow commences when clamp below volume-control unit is opened.

Piggyback Method—The piggyback method refers to the intermittent intravenous drip of a second solution, the reconstituted drug, through the venipuncture site of an established primary IV system.   With this setup the drug can be thought of as entering the vein on "top" of the primary IV fluid, hence the designation "piggyback."   The piggyback technique not only eliminates the need for another venipuncture, but also achieves drug dilution and peak blood levels within a relatively short time span, usually 30 to 60 minutes. Drug dilution helps to reduce irritation, and early high serum levels are an important consideration in serious infection requiring aggressive drug therapy.   These advantages have popularized the piggyback method of IV therapy, especially for the intermittent administration of antibiotics.   In using the piggyback technique, the secondary unit is purged of air and its needle inserted into a Y-injection site of the primary set or into the injection site at the end of the primary set.   The

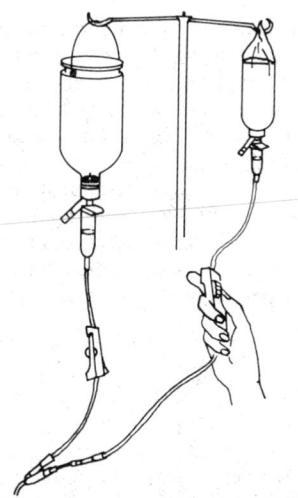

Fig 86-8. Piggyback administration setup.

piggyback infusion is then started. Once it is completed, the primary fluid infusion will be restarted. See Fig 86-8.

Primary IV administration sets are available that have a built-in checkvalve for use in piggyback administration. When the piggyback is connected to one of these sets and started, the checkvalve automatically closes off the primary infusion. When the piggyback runs out, the check valve automatically opens, thereby restarting the primary infusion. The checkvalve works because of pressure differences. To achieve this difference, the primary container is hung lower than the secondary bottle by means of an extension hanger. See Fig 86-9.

Several manufacturers have introduced minibottles prefilled with various antibiotic products; each container is provided with a plastic hanger for direct suspension from an IV pole as the piggyback solution is administered through the resealable gum-rubber injection site or Y-type facility of an existing IV system. Reconstitution of piggyback units requires only the addition of a small volume of compatible diluent. Since reconstitution and administration proceed from the same bottle, no drug transfer is involved, so transfer syringes and additional IV containers are not necessary. Pre-

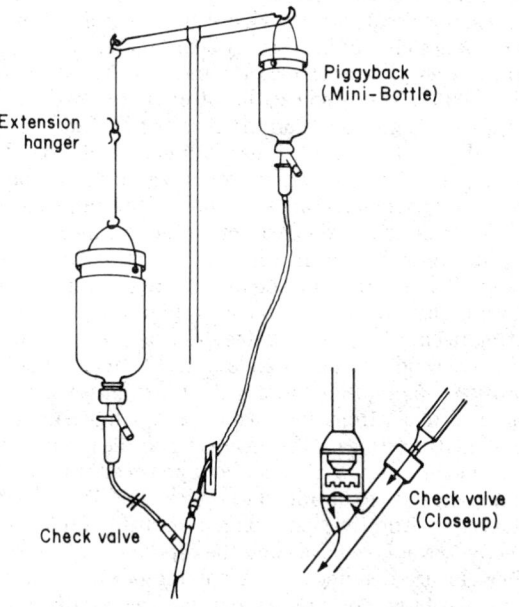

Fig 86-9. Piggyback administration setup with check valve in primary set.

filled drug containers offer significant advantages to hospitals. Time-saving, less potential for error and contamination, and convenience are outstanding qualities of this type of packaging. The need exists in hospitals for these types of innovative packaging to help alleviate the critical nursing shortage and to reduce the error potential. It is a significant event that drug manufacturers and intravenous fluid manufacturers have combined efforts to achieve optimal packaging for hospital use.

Partial-fill containers available for piggybacking are 250-mL capacity infusion bottles or bags underfilled with 50 or 100 mL Dextrose Injection, 5% or normal saline. The drug to be administered is first reconstituted in its original parenteral vial and then added by needle and syringe to the partial-fill container. The needle of the piggyback delivery system is inserted into the Y-site or gum-rubber injection port of a hanging primary infusion set. Flow of the primary intravenous fluid is stopped while the drug solution in the partial-fill container is administered (30 to 60 minutes). After the drug solution has been totally infused, the primary fluid flow is reestablished. When the next dose of drug is required, the piggyback procedure is repeated, replacing the prefilled partial-fill container.

Mechanical-Electronic Infusion Devices—Gravity IV administration systems are affected by many variables which tend to alter the accuracy of the system. These include variations in size of drip-chamber orifice, the viscosity of the solution being administered, plastic cold flow, clamp slippage, final filters, variations in the patient's blood pressure and body movements, clot formation, pressure changes in IV containers, rate of flow, temperature of the IV fluid, changes in the needle, and other factors such as kinked tubing, extravasation, and changes in the height of the IV container. The control of flow in traditional gravity IV systems utilizes manual clamps (either screw or roller clamps) which can provide considerable discrepancies in volume delivery. These factors have promoted the development and use of mechanical-electronic infusion devices to control more accurately the administration of IV fluids. This group of devices includes infusion controllers and infusion pumps.

Infusion controllers count drops electronically or extrude volumes of fluid mechanically and electronically. Having no moving components, controllers are less complex than pumps, being usually less expensive and having fewer maintenance problems. Infusion controllers are gravity type systems but the control is regulated automatically rather than manually. In addition to increasing accuracy of delivery, electronic equipment may be able to detect infiltration of air, empty containers, and excess or deficient flow.

Infusion pumps do not depend on gravity to provide the pressure required to infuse the drug. Pressure is provided by an electric motor pump that propels a syringe, a peristaltic or roller device, or a cassette. Most pumps are volumetric in that the delivery is measured in mL rather than drops.

The quality of patient care has improved with the use of infusion devices. Flow rates can be maintained, therefore parenteral and enteral nutrition can be safely conducted. In addition, accurate drug therapy can be accomplished with adults and children and runaways of IV fluid administration can be eliminated.

Final Filter Devices—Particulate matter in intravenous fluids and intravenous admixtures can originate from many sources. It can result from the packaging components of the IV fluid, from admixture incompatibilities, from manipulation in preparing the admixture, and even from the administration set itself. Concern for particulate matter led to the design of final filter devices for attaching to the end of the tubing of the administration set. They afford a final filtration of the IV fluid before it passes through the needle into the vein. The device consists of a plastic chamber containing a membrane or stainless steel filter having porosities varying from 5 to 0.22 μm. Air lock can be a problem with membrane filters. When wet, membranes with a porosity of 0.22 μm and 0.45 μm are impervious to air at normal pressures and air in the system causes blockage. In order to prevent this, the filter housing must be completely purged of air prior to use. Newer device designs have air eliminators. Using final filter devices increases medication cost but reduces the biological hazards associated with particulate matter.

Although considerable information is available concerning the clinical use of membrane filters in entrapping particulate matter and microorganisms, little information exists describing drug absorption by the filter. Literature reports on a limited number of drugs and filter materials indicate that drugs administered in low doses might present a problem with drug bonding to the filter.[1] Solutions containing minute dosages of drugs, 5 mg or less, should not be filtered until sufficient data are available to confirm insignificant absorption. Drugs not recommended to be filtered include all parenteral suspensions, blood and blood products, amphotericin B, digitoxin, insulin, intravenous fat emulsions, mithramycin, nitroglycerin, and vincristine.

Intravenous Admixtures

When one or more sterile products are added to an IV fluid for administration, the resulting combination is known as an intravenous admixture. To maintain the characteristics of sterile products, namely sterility, freedom from particulate matter, and pyrogens, it is imperative that they be manipulated in a suitable environment using aseptic techniques.

Environment—Proper conditions for aseptic handling can be provided by laminar airflow hoods (see Chapters 79, 85). Within a laminar airflow hood, air filtered through a HEPA (high efficiency particulate air) filter moves in a parallel flow configuration at a velocity of 90 ft per minute. HEPA filters remove 99.97% of all particles larger than 0.3 μm. Since microbial contaminants present in air are usually found on other particulates, removal of the latter results in a flow of air free of both microbial contaminants and particulate matter. The movement of the filtered air in a laminar flow configuration at a velocity of 90 ft per minute can maintain the area free of contamination. The flow of air may be either in a horizontal or vertical pattern. In the former case the HEPA filter is located at the back of the hood and the air flows to the front. In vertical flow the air passes through the HEPA filter located in the top of the cabinet and is exhausted through a grated area around the working surface of the hood. Regardless of the type of laminar airflow, the hood must be properly operated and maintained in order to achieve a satisfactory environment for preparing parenteral admixtures.

The hood is best situated in a clean area in which there is little traffic flow past the front of the hood. The inside of the hood is thoroughly wiped down with a suitable disinfectant and allowed to run for at least 30 minutes before starting manipulations. It is important to remember that the laminar flow hood is not a means of sterilization. It only maintains an area free of microbial contaminants and particulate matter when it has been properly prepared, properly maintained, and utilized by operators having proper aseptic techniques.

Before working in a laminar airflow hood the operator washes his hands thoroughly and scrubs them with a suitable disinfectant. Some laboratories may require gowning and use of sterile gloves. Sterile gloves can be an asset but there is always the problem that they can give the operator a false sense of security. Gloved hands can become contaminated as easily as ungloved hands. Additives and IV fluids to be used in the preparation of the admixture, along with suitable syringes, are lined up in the hood in the order they are going to be used. The containers must be clean and dust free. They are inspected for clarity and freedom from cracks. Operators are encouraged to use a lighting device for inspecting IV fluids for particulate matter and cracks. The lighting device should be of the type that permits the container to be viewed against both a light and a dark background during inspection. If the IV fluid is packaged in plastic containers, pressure is applied to assure that they are properly sealed and do not leak. Some laboratories disinfect the containers prior to placing them in the hood.

In working within the hood the operator works in the center of the hood with the space between the point of operation and the filter unobstructed. If the flow of air is blocked, then the validity of the laminar flow is destroyed. Articles are arranged within the hood in a manner to prevent clean air from washing over dirty objects and contaminating other objects that must remain sterile. The working area must be at least six inches from the front edge of the hood. As the operator stands in front of the hood, his body acts as a barrier to the laminar air flow causing it to pass around him and create backflow patterns which can carry room air into the front of the hood.

Laminar flow hoods must be maintained and evaluated periodically to insure that they are functioning properly. The velocity of air flow can be determined routinely using a velometer. Decrease in the air flow usually indicates a clogged HEPA filter. Some laminar flow hoods are equipped with pressure gauges indicating pressure in the plenum behind the filter; in these hoods pressure increase can also indicate a clogged filter. Settling plates can be exposed within the hood for given periods of time to determine the presence of microbial contaminants.

The best way to determine the proper functioning of a HEPA filter is to use the dioctyl phthalate (DOP) test using the vapor at room temperature. DOP vapor (particles of ~ 0.3 μm) is allowed to be taken up by the hood through its intake filter. If the HEPA filter is intact and properly installed, no DOP can be detected in the filtered air stream using a smoke photometer. Certification services are available through commercial laboratories; the HEPA filters within laminar flow hoods should be evaluated every six months.

Additives—The additives are injections packaged in ampuls or vials, or sterile solids; the latter are reconstituted with a suitable diluent before addition to the IV fluid. A fresh, sterile, disposable syringe is used for each additive. Before removing a measured volume from an ampul, the container is wiped with a disinfectant solution. If the ampul is scored, the top can be snapped off; if not scored, an ampul file must be used. A sterile syringe is removed from its protective wrapping. The syringe needle with its cover is separated from the syringe aseptically and may be replaced with a sterile aspirating needle. Aspirating needles are usually made from clear plastic and contain a stainless steel or nylon filter having a porosity of 5 μm. The filter will remove glass particles and other particulates from the injection as it is drawn up from the ampul into the syringe. The aspirating needle is replaced with the regular needle. The exact volume is calibrated and the injection is ready to be added to the IV fluid (see Fig 86-10). In the case of additives packaged in multiple-dose vials, the protective cover is removed and the exposed target area of the rubber closure disinfected. A volume of air, equal to the volume of solution to be removed, is drawn up into the syringe and injected into the air space above the injection within the vial. This will facilitate withdrawal of the injection. The

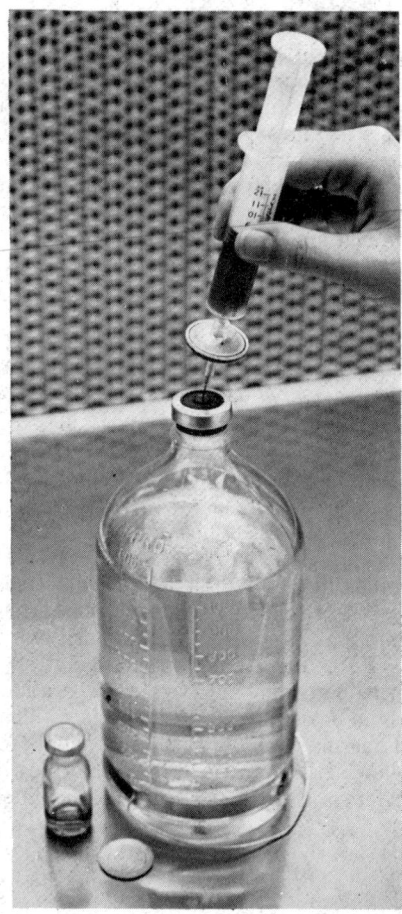

Fig 86-10. Placing an additive into an IV fluid with filtration through a membrane filter (courtesy, Millipore).

solution is drawn into the syringe, the exact dose is measured, and the injection is ready to be added to the IV fluid.

Certain injections are light sensitive and are protected against photolysis by the container packaging. The manufacturer may use amber glass, individual container wrapping, or an amber plastic cover. Many hospital pharmacists utilize aluminum foil as a protective wrap for light-sensitive drugs during their administration.

In the case of drug substances having poor stability in aqueous solution, the drug is packaged as a sterile solid, either dry-filled or lyophilized. The diluent recommended on the labeling is used to reconstitute the powder; the proper quantity of solution is then removed for addition to the IV fluid. When large volumes of diluent are required for reconstitution, as for Keflin 4 g, a sterile needle is placed through the closure to vent the container and facilitate addition of the diluent. In order to increase the efficiency of IV admixture programs, a limited number of hospital pharmacies have found it convenient to freeze reconstituted drugs, particularly antibiotics. The stability of reconstituted drugs is somewhat limited. In some cases stability is limited to only a few hours; in many cases, however, reconstituted solutions can be frozen and thawed at time of use. In the frozen form the stability of the antibiotic solution can be increased. In a number of instances, the stability in the frozen form is known and supplied by the manufacturer. Reports have been published on the frozen stability of certain drugs. However, it is unwise to freeze drug solutions without adequate stability studies for guidance. In those cases where published information is available, close adherence must be observed as to freezing temperature, storage conditions, and packaging.

There is an increasing awareness of the potential hazard to pharmacists handling antineoplastic drugs.[2] Although the evidence is not conclusive, it appears that measures should be taken to minimize unnecessary exposure.[3] These precautions include: the use of vertical laminar flow hoods for the preparation and reconstitution of these agents; the wearing of gloves and masks by the personnel; special labeling of the containers to insure their proper handling and disposal; and periodic blood studies of personnel involved in preparing admixtures of antineoplastic agents.

The procedure for placing an additive in an IV fluid will vary depending on the type of IV fluid packaging system being used by the hospital. The packaging systems have been described in Table II.

Abbott Glass Containers (Fig 86-2)

1. Remove the aluminum tear seal exposing the solid rubber closure with a target circle in the center.
2. Wipe closure with suitable disinfectant.
3. Insert needle of additive syringe through target area. The vacuum within bottle draws in the solution.
4. Gently shake the bottle after each addition.
5. When completed, cover the closure with a plastic protective cap if it is not to be used immediately.

Travenol/Baxter and McGaw Rigid Glass Containers (Fig 86-3)

1. Remove the aluminum tear seal and the aluminum disc covering the latex diaphragm.
2. Upon exposing the latex diaphragm, note that the latex cover is drawn in over the openings in the rubber closure.
3. The larger of the two holes receives the administration set, the other is the air vent. The triangle-shaped indentation can serve as the site for injecting the additives as well as the opening for the administration set.
4. Wipe diaphragm with suitable disinfectant and pierce latex cover to place additive into bottle. The vacuum within bottle will draw additive from the syringe. Do not remove diaphragm or the vacuum will dissipate. It will be removed at the time of administration prior to the insertion of the administration set.
5. Gently shake the bottle after each additive.
6. When completed, cover the bottle with a plastic additive cap if administration set is not to be inserted immediately.

Travenol/Baxter and Abbott Plastic Container (Fig 86-4)

1. Remove additive port protective sleeve and rub gum-rubber plug with suitable disinfectant.
2. Additives are placed in container by piercing gum-rubber cover over the additive port.
3. After each addition, milk the container to insure adequate mixing.
4. Containers do not contain a vacuum, but vacuum chambers are available for use in conjunction with the flexible plastic container.
5. Protective additive caps are available if administration set is not inserted immediately.

McGaw Semirigid Plastic Container (Fig 86-4)

1. Remove additive port protective covering and rub gum-rubber plug with suitable disinfectant.
2. Additives are placed in containers by piercing gum-rubber over the additive port.
3. After each addition, shake the container gently to insure adequate mixing.
4. Containers do not contain a vacuum.

Parenteral Incompatibility—When one or more additives are combined with an IV fluid, their presence together may modify the inherent characteristics of the drug substances present, resulting in a parenteral incompatibility. Parenteral incompatibilities have been arbitrarily divided into three groups: physical, chemical, and therapeutic. The last are the most difficult to observe because the combination results in undesirable antagonistic or synergistic pharmacological activity. For example, the report that penicillin or cortisone antagonizes the effect of heparin and produces a misleading picture of the anticoagulant effect of heparin represents a therapeutic incompatibility. Physical incompatibilities are the most easily observed and can be detected by changes in the appearance of the admixture, such as a change in color, formation of a precipitate, or evolution of a gas. Physical incompatibilities frequently can be predicted by knowing the chemical characteristics of the drugs involved. For example, the sodium salts of weak acids, such as phenytoin sodium or phenobarbital sodium, precipitate as free acids when added to intravenous fluids having an acidic pH. Calcium salts precipitate when added to an alkaline medium. Injections that require a special diluent for solubilization, such as Valium, precipitate when added to aqueous solutions because of their low water-solubility.

Decomposition of drug substances resulting from combination of parenteral dosage forms is called a chemical incompatibility, an arbitrary classification since physical incompatibilities also result from chemical changes. Most chemical incompatibilities result from hydrolysis, oxidation, reduction, or complexation and can be detected only with a suitable analytical method.

An important factor in causing a parenteral incompatibility is a change in the acid-base environment.[4] The solubility and stability of a drug may vary as the pH of the solution changes. A change in the pH of the solution may be an indication in predicting an incompatibility, especially one involving drug stability, since this is not necessarily apparent physically. The effect of pH on stability is illustrated in the case of penicillin. The antibiotic remains active for 24 hr at pH 6.5, but at pH 3.5 it is destroyed in a short time. Potassium penicillin G contains a citrate buffer and is buffered at pH 6.0 to 6.5 when reconstituted with Sterile Water for Injection, Dextrose Injection, or Sodium Chloride Injection. When this reconstituted solution is added to an intravenous fluid such as Dextrose Injection or Sodium Chloride Injection, the normal acid pH of the solution is buffered at pH 6.0 to 6.5, thus assuring the activity of the antibiotic.

While it may be impossible to predict and prevent all parenteral incompatibilities, their occurrence can be minimized. The IV admixture pharmacist should be cognizant of the increasing body of literature concerning parenteral incompatibilities. This includes compatibility guides published by large-volume parenteral manufacturers;[5-7] compatibility studies on individual parenteral products by the manufacturer and published with the product as part of the labeling; the study of the National Coordinating Committee on Large-Volume Parenterals;[8] reference books;[9,10] and literature reports of studies with specific parenteral drugs.[11] The pharmacist should encourage use of as few additives as possible in intravenous fluids since the number of potential problems increases as the number of additives increases. Physicians should be made aware of possible incompatibilities and the pharmacist can suggest alternate approaches to avoid the difficulties. In some instances, incompatibilities can be avoided by selecting another route of administration for one or more of the drugs involved.

Quality Control—Each hospital should have written procedures covering the handling and storage of IV fluids, their use in preparing admixtures, labeling, and transportation to the floors. In-use clarity and sterility tests should be devised to assure that IV admixtures retain the characteristics of sterility and freedom from particulate matter. Training and monitoring personnel involved in preparation of IV admixtures should be done on a regular basis.[12] The efforts of the hospital pharmacy should be no less than those of the industry in following Current Good Manufacturing Practice to assure the safety and efficacy of these compounded medications.

Total Parenteral Nutrition

Intravenous administration of calories, nitrogen, and other nutrients in sufficient quantities to achieve tissue synthesis and anabolism is called total parenteral nutrition (TPN).[13] Originally the term hyperalimentation was used to describe the procedure, but it is being replaced by TPN, the latter being more descriptive for the technique.

The normal calorie requirement for an adult is approximately 2500 per day. If these were to be provided totally by Dextrose Injection 5%, approximately 15 L would be required. Each L contains 50 g dextrose, equivalent to 170 calories. However, it is only possible to administer three or four liters per day without causing fluid overload. To reduce this fluid volume the concentration of dextrose would have to be increased. By increasing the dextrose to 25%, it is possible to administer five times the calories in one-fifth the volume. Dextrose Injection 25% is hypertonic and cannot be administered in large amounts into a peripheral vein without sclerosing the vein.

Dudrick developed the technique for administering fluids for total parenteral nutrition by way of the subclavian vein into the superior vena cava where the solution is rapidly diluted by the large volume of blood available, thus minimizing the hypertonicity of the solution. For administration of the TPN fluids, a catheter is inserted and retained in place in the subclavian vein. TPN is indicated in patients who are unable to ingest food due to carcinoma or extensive burns; patients who refuse to eat, as in the case of depressed geriatrics or young patients suffering from anorexia nervosa; and surgical patients who should not be fed orally.

The preferred source for calories in TPN fluids is the carbohydrate dextrose. Both fat emulsions and alcohol are caloric sources, but they are not used in TPN fluids. In IV fluid

kits commercially available for the preparation of TPN solutions, Dextrose Injection 50% is provided. On dilution with protein hydrolysate or amino acid injection, the resulting dextrose concentration is approximately 25%. It is this concentration that is administered.

The source of nitrogen in TPN fluids is either protein hydrolysates (*Amigen®*—Travenol; *Aminosol®*—Abbott; *Hyprotigen®*—McGaw) or crystalline amino acids (*Aminosyn®*—Abbott; *FreAmine II®*—McGaw; *Travasol®*—Travenol). Protein hydrolysates are obtained from casein or fibrin and contain polypeptides which must be broken down before they can be utilized. Although available at lower cost than crystalline amino acids, they contain higher amounts of ammonia and free chloride. In the case of hydrolysates, the exact amount of protein being administered is not known. The crystalline amino acid injections contain all the essential and nonessential amino acids in the L-form. They are more expensive than the protein hydrolysates but contain less ammonia and free chloride. For optimum utilization of amino acids and for promoting tissue regeneration, the nitrogen-to-calorie ratio should be 1:150. Calories are needed to provide energy for the metabolism of nitrogen.

Electrolyte requirements will vary with the individual patient. The electrolytes present in Protein Hydrolysate Injection or Amino Acid Injection are given on the label and must be taken into consideration in determining the quantities to be added. Usual electrolyte concentrations required to fall within the following ranges: sodium, 100–120 mEq; potassium, 80–120 mEq; magnesium, 8–16 mEq; calcium, 5–10 mEq; chloride, 100–120 mEq; and phosphate, 40–60 mEq. It is better to keep a 1:1 ratio between sodium and chloride ions. In adding potassium, the acetate salt is preferred to the chloride. If the combination of calcium and phosphate ions exceeds 20 mEq, precipitation occurs.

In addition to the electrolytes, the daily requirement for both water-soluble and fat-soluble vitamins may be added, usually in the form of a multivitamin infusion concentrate. Iron, folic acid, and vitamin B_{12} should be administered separately from the TPN fluids. Trace elements such as zinc, copper, manganese, and iodide are a concern only in long-term cases and can be added when required.

The Parenteral Prescription

The physician writes an admixture order or parenteral prescription on a physician's order-form located on the patient's chart. A copy of the order is sent to the pharmacy for compounding. It includes the patient's name, room number, the intravenous fluid wanted, additives and their concentrations, rate of flow, starting time, and length of therapy. The order is taken by the technician, nurse, or pharmacist to the pharmacy. Orders may be telephoned to the pharmacy; verification with the original order is made on delivery of the admixture. IV orders are usually written for a 24-hour therapy period; the patient's chart is reviewed daily and new orders are written on a daily basis. The order may be for multiple containers, in which case the containers are numbered consecutively. Unlike the extemporaneously compounded prescription, additives are added without regard to final volume of IV fluid. The prescription is checked for proper dose, compatibility, drug allergies, and stability. Additives are usually given an expiration period of 24 hours from time of preparation. Drugs such as ampicillin may require shorter expiration periods.

The clerical work for the admixture is prepared. This includes typing of the label and the preparation of the profile work sheet. The profile sheet is filed so that the pharmacist will be alerted when subsequent containers are due for preparation. Charging the patient's account can be done from the profile work sheet. The label includes the patient's name,

Table III—Typical IV Orders (Parenteral Prescriptions)

Prescription	Comment	Prescription	Comment
1. Ṛ NSS 1000 mL 125 mL/hr	Sodium Chloride Injection (Normal Saline Solution) 1000 mL, is to be administered at the flow-rate of 125 mL per hour. It will require approximately eight hours.	7. Ṛ 1000 cc Hyperal (FreAmine) + 40 mEq $NaHCO_3$ + 30 mEq KCl + Vits + 5u Reg Insulin to run 80 cc/hr	One L of the basic TPN solution, FreAmine II, is to be provided with the addition of 40 mEq $NaHCO_3$, 30 mEq potassium chloride, the contents of one container vitamin B complex with vitamin C plus 5 units of regular zinc insulin. It is to be administered at the flow rate of 80 mL per hour (approximately 12 hours).
2. Ṛ 1000 D5 + NSS + Vits 12 hr	Dextrose Injection 5%, 1000 mL, containing 0.9% sodium chloride and container of vitamin B complex with vitamin C is to be administered over a 12-hour period.		
3. Ṛ 500 D5 + ½NSS KVO	Dextrose Injection 5%, 500 mL, containing 0.45% sodium chloride is to be administered at a rate of flow to keep the vein open (KVO). The flow rate will be approximately 10 mL per hour.	8. Ṛ 1000 Hyperal + 40 mEq NaCl + 10 KCl + 10 Insulin + 10 Cal Gluc.	One L of the hospital's basic TPN solution is to be provided with the addition of 40 mEq sodium chloride, 10 mEq potassium chloride, 10 units regular zinc insulin, and 10 mL Calcium Gluconate Injection.
4. Ṛ 1000 cc D5 + ½NSS Add 1 amp Vits to each + 100 mg Thiamine Each to run 6 hr	Dextrose Injection 5%, 1000 mL, containing 0.45% sodium chloride, the contents of one ampul vitamin B complex with vitamin C, and sufficient volume of Thiamine Hydrochloride Injection to give 100 mg thiamine, is to be administered over a 6-hour period (approximately 170 mL per hour). Additional orders of the same can be anticipated.	9. Ṛ Keflin 2 g + 100 mL D_5W q 6 hr	Cephalothin, 2 g, is reconstituted with Sterile Water for Injection and added to a minibottle containing 100 mL Dextrose Injection 5%. This dose is given every 6 hours using a piggyback technique with a flow rate requiring 30 to 60 minutes for delivery.
5. Ṛ 1000 cc D5 + ½ NSS + 20 mEq KCl	Dextrose Injection 5%, 1000 mL, is to be provided containing 0.45% sodium chloride and 20 mEq potassium chloride.	10. Ṛ Gentamicin 80 mg IVPB q 8 hr	Gentamicin, 80 mg, is added to a minibottle containing 100 mL Dextrose Injection 5%. This dose is given every 8 hours using the piggyback technique (IVPB) with a flow-rate requiring at least 80 minutes (not less than 1 mg per minute).
6. Ṛ 1000 Hyperal + 10 NaCl + 10 KCl + 5 $MgSO_4$ + 10 Insulin	One L of the hospital's basic TPN solution is to be provided with the addition of 10 mEq sodium chloride, 10 mEq potassium chloride, 5 mEq magnesium sulfate, and 10 units regular zinc insulin.		

room number, bottle number, preparation date, expiration time and date, intravenous fluid and quantity, additives and quantities, total time for infusion, the milliliters per hour or drops per minute, and space for the name of the nurse who hangs the container. The label will be affixed to the container upside down in order that it can be read when hung.

The admixture is prepared by the pharmacist or a supervised technician. In handling sterile products, aseptic techniques as discussed previously must be observed. When completed, a plastic additive cap is affixed before delivery to the floor. The label is applied and checked with the original order. The empty additive containers are checked to confirm the additives present. The admixture is inspected for any color change or particulate matter.

The completed admixture is delivered to the floor. If it is not to be infused immediately (within one hour), it is stored under refrigeration; if refrigerated, it must be used within 24 hours. The nurse checks for accuracy of patient's name, drug and concentration, IV fluid, expiration date, time started, and clarity. The infusion of admixtures can run ahead or behind schedule, necessitating the pharmacist to modify the preparation of continued orders. Examples of IV orders are shown in Table III.

References

1. Turco SJ: Drug absorption to membrane filters, *Am J IV Ther Clin Nutr 9:* 6, 1982.
2. Zimmerman PF, Randolph KL, Barkley EW, Gallelli JF: Recommendations for the safe handling of injectable antineoplastic drug products, *Am J Hosp Pharm: 38:* 1693, 1981.
3. Gallelli JF: Evaluating the potential hazard of handling antineoplastic drugs, *Am J Hosp Pharm 39:* 1877, 1982.
4. Newton DW: Physicochemical determinants of incompatibility and instability of injectable drug solutions and admixtures. *Am J Hosp Pharm 35:* 1213, 1978.
5. King JC: Guide to Parenteral Admixtures. Cutter Laboratories, Berkeley, CA, 1973.
6. Shoup LK, Goodwin NH: Implementation Guide—Centralized Admixture Program. Travenol Laboratories, Morton Grove, IL, 1977.
7. Good IV Procedures Manual. Abbott Laboratories, North Chicago, IL, 1979.
8. Bergman HD: Incompatibilities in large-volume parenterals. *Drug Intell Clin Pharm 11:* 345, 1977.
9. Trissel LA: *Parenteral Drug Information Guide.* Am Soc Hosp Pharm, Washington, DC, 1974.
10. Trissel LA: *Handbook on Injectable Drugs.* Am Soc Hosp Pharm, Washington, DC, 1977.
11. Kobayashi NH, King JC: Compatibility of common additives in protein hydrolysate/dextrose solutions. *Am J Hosp Pharm 34:* 589, 1977.
12. Sanders SJ, Mabadeje SA, Avis KE, Cruze CA, Martinez DR: Evaluation of compounding accuracy and aseptic techniques for intravenous admixtures. *Am J Hosp Pharm 35:* 531, 1978.
13. Dudrick SJ, Rhoads JE: Total intravenous feeding. *Sci Amer 226:* 73, 1972.

Bibliography

Turco SJ, King RE: *Sterile Dosage Forms: Their Preparation and Clinical Applications*, 2nd ed, Lea & Febiger, Philadelphia, 1979.

Trissel LA: *Handbook on Injectable Drugs*, 3rd ed., Am Soc Hosp Pharm, Washington, DC, 1983.

National Coordinating Committee on Large-Volume Parenterals: Recommended methods for compounding intravenous admixtures in hospitals. *Am J Hosp Pharm 32:* 261, 1975.

Francke DE, ed: *Handbook of IV Additive Reviews*, Drug Intelligence Publications, Hamilton, IL, 1970, 1971, 1972, 1973.

IV Additives and Sterile Technology, Am Soc Hosp Pharm, Washington, DC, 1975.

Avis KE, Akers MJ: *Sterile Preparation for the Hospital Pharmacist*, Ann Arbor Science Publishers, Ann Arbor, MI, 1981.

CHAPTER 87

Ophthalmic Preparations

John D Mullins, PhD
Director Pharmaceutical Sciences
Research and Development
Alcon Laboratories
Fort Worth, TX 76101

Ophthalmic preparations are sterile products essentially free from foreign particles, suitably compounded and packaged for instillation into the eye. Ophthalmic preparations include solutions, suspensions, ointments, and solid dosage forms. The solutions and suspensions are, for the most part, aqueous. Ophthalmic ointments usually contain a white petrolatum-mineral oil base.

Ophthalmic preparations can be broadly grouped into two divisions of major significance to the pharmacist. These include single or multidose prescription products and the category described as OTC or over-the-counter ophthalmic products. The latter group has been subjected to a searching review and analysis by a body of experts as a part of the Food and Drug Administration OTC Drug Review process.

The single dominant factor characteristic of all ophthalmic products is the specification of sterility. Any product intended for use in the eye regardless of form, substance or intent must be sterile. This requirement increases the similarity between ophthalmic and parenteral products, however the physiology of the human eye in many respects imposes more rigid formulation requirements. This will be considered in the following discussion.

Preparations intended for the treatment of eye disorders can be traced to antiquity. Egyptian papyri writings describe eye medications. The Greeks and Romans expanded such uses and gave us the term *collyria*. Collyria refer collectively to materials which were dissolved in water, milk or egg white for use as eyedrops. In the Middle Ages collyria included substances to dilate the pupils of milady's eyes for cosmetic purposes, thus the term belladonna or "beautiful lady."

From the time of belladonna collyria ophthalmic technology progressed at a pharmaceutical snail's pace well into modern times. It was not until after the second World War that the concept of sterility became mandatory for ophthalmic solutions. Prior to World War II and continuing into the 1940's very few ophthalmic preparations were available commercially or were officially described. The USP XIV, official in 1950, included only three ophthalmic preparations and all three were ointments.

Preparations to be used in the eye, either solutions or ointments, were invariably compounded in the community or hospital pharmacy and were intended for immediate (prescription) use. Such preparation and prompt use is reflected in the pharmaceutical literature of the times. The stability of ophthalmic preparations is discussed in terms of days or a few months.

One of the most important attributes of ophthalmic products is the requirement of sterility. Even that, however is a surprisingly recent event. The USP XV in 1955 was the first official compendium to include a sterility requirement for ophthalmic solutions. The Food and Drug Administration in 1953 adopted the position that a nonsterile ophthalmic solution was adulterated. Sterile ophthalmic products were, of course, available prior to the mid 1950's, however the legal requirement of sterility dates only from 1955.

The sterility requirements for ophthalmic ointments appeared first in the USP XVIII, *Third Supplement* (1972). Prior to that date there was no legal requirement for a sterile ophthalmic ointment. This was probably due to the difficulty (at that time) of testing for sterility in such nonaqueous systems and also for the anticipated difficulties in sterilizing and maintaining sterile conditions during the manufacture and filling of ointments on a large scale.

Anatomy and Physiology of the Eye

The human eye is a challenging subject for topical administration of drugs. The basis of this can be found in the anatomical arrangement of the surface tissues and in the permeability of the cornea. The protective operation of the eyelids and lacrimal system is such that there is rapid removal of material instilled into the eye, unless the material is suitably small in volume and chemically and physiologically compatible with surface tissues. Figs 87-2 and 87-3 include pertinent anatomy of the human eye.

Eyelids—The eyelids serve two purposes: mechanical protection of the globe and creation of an optimum milieu for the cornea. The eyelids are lubricated and kept fluid-filled by secretions of the lacrimal glands and other glands. The antechamber has the shape of a narrow cleft directly over the front of the eyeball, with pocket-like extensions upward and downward. The pockets are called the superior and inferior fornix (vault), and the entire space the cul-de-sac. The elliptical opening between the eyelids is called the palpebral fissure.

Eyeball—The wall of the human eyeball (bulbus, globe) is composed of three concentric layers or tunics.

1. The outer fibrous tunic.
2. A middle vascular tunic—the uvea or uveal tract, consisting of the choroid, the ciliary body, and the iris.
3. A nervous tunic—the retina.

The outer tunic is tough, pliable, but only slightly stretchable. In its front portion—the portion facing the outside world—the fine structure of the outer tunic is so regular and the water content so carefully adjusted that it acts as a clear transparent window (the cornea). Over the remaining two-thirds the fibrous coat is opaque (the "white" of the eye) and is called the sclera. It ordinarily contains very few blood vessels.

The eyeball houses an optical apparatus that causes inverted reduced images of the outside world to form on the retina, which is a thin translucent membrane. The optical apparatus consists, in sequence, of the cornea, the pupil, and the crystalline lens, with layers of clear fluid or gel-like material interposed between the solid structures. The pupil, a round centric hole in a contractile membranous partition (called the iris), acts as the variable aperture of the system. The crystalline lens is a refractive element with variable power controlled and supported by a muscle incorporated in the ciliary body. The choroid is the metabolic support for the retina.

The optical function of the eye calls for stability of its dimensions, which is provided partly by the fibrous outer coat; more effective as a stabilizing factor is the intraocular pressure, which is in excess of the pressure prevailing in the surrounding tissues. This intraocular pressure is the result of a steady production of specific fluid, the aqueous humor, which originates from the ciliary processes and leaves the eye by an intricate system of outflow channels. The resistance encountered during this passage and the rate of aqueous production are the principal factors determining the level of the intraocular pressure. In addition to this hydromechanical function, the aqueous humor acts as a carrier of nutrients, substrates, and metabolites for the avascular tissues of the eye.

The bones of the skull join to form an approximately pyramid-shaped housing for the eyeball, called the orbit.

Conjunctiva—The conjunctival membrane covers the outer surface of the white portion of the eye and the inner aspect of the eyelids. In most places it is loosely attached and thereby permits free movement of the eyeball. This makes possible subconjunctival injections. Except for the cornea the conjunctiva is the most exposed portion of the eye.

Lacrimal System—The conjunctival and corneal surfaces are covered and lubricated by a film of fluid secreted by the conjunctival and the lacrimal glands. The secretion of the lacrimal gland, the tears, is delivered through a number of fine ducts into the conjunctival fornix. The secretion is a clear, watery fluid containing 0.7% protein and the enzyme lysozyme. Small accessory lacrimal glands are situated in the conjunctival fornices. Their secretion suffices for lubrication and cleansing under ordinary conditions and for maintaining a thin fluid film covering the cornea and conjunctiva (the precorneal film). The mucin-protein layer of the film is especially important in maintaining the stability of the film. The main lacrimal gland is called into play only on special occasions. The sebaceous glands of the eyelids secrete an oily fluid which helps to prevent overflowing of tears at the lid margin and reduces evaporation from the exposed surfaces of the eye by spreading over the tear film.

Spontaneous blinking replenishes the fluid film by pushing a thin layer of fluid ahead of the lid margins as they come together. The excess fluid is directed into the lacrimal lake—a small triangular area lying in the angle bounded by the innermost portions of the lids. The skin of the eyelids is the thinnest in the body and folds easily, thus permitting rapid opening and closing of the palpebral fissures. The movement of the eyelids includes a narrowing of the palpebral fissues in a zipper-like action from the lateral canthus toward the medial canthus (canthi: the corners where the eyelids meet). This aids the transport or movement of fluid toward the lacrimal lake.

Tears are drained from the lacrimal lake by two small tubes—the lacrimal canaliculi—which lead into the upper part of the nasolacrimal duct, the roomy beginning of which is called the lacrimal sac. The drainage of tears into the nose does not depend merely on gravity. Fluid enters and passes along the lacrimal canaliculi by capillary attraction aided by aspiration caused by contraction of muscle embedded in the eyelids. When the lids close, as in blinking, contraction of the muscle causes dilation of the upper part of the lacrimal sac and compression of its lower portion. Tears are thus aspirated into the sac, and any which have collected in its lower part are forced down the nasolacrimal duct toward its opening into the nose. As the lids open, the muscle relaxes. The upper part of the sac then collapses and forces fluid into the lower part, which at the same time is released from compression. Thus, the act of blinking exerts a suction-force-pump action in removing tears from the lacrimal lake and emptying them into the nasal cavity. Lacrimation is induced reflexly by stimulation of nerve endings of the cornea or conjunctiva. The reflex is abolished by anesthetization of the surface of the eye, and by disorders affecting its nerve components.

The normal cul-de-sac is usually free of pathogenic organisms and often found sterile. The sterility may be due partly to the action of lysozyme in the tears, which normally destroys saprophytic organisms but has little action against pathogens. More effective in producing sterility may be the fact that the secretions, which are normally sterile as they leave the glands, constantly wash the bacteria, dust, etc, down in the nose. In certain diseases the lacrimal gland, like other grandular structures in the body, undergoes involution, with the result that the lacrimal fluid becomes scanty. Furthermore, changes in the conjunctival glands may lead to alteration in the character of the secretion so that quality as well as quantity of tears may be abnormal. This may lead to symptoms of dryness, burning, and general discomfort and may interfere with visual acuity.

Precorneal Film—The cornea must be wet to be an optically adequate surface; when dry, it loses both its regular gloss and its transparency. The precorneal film, part of the tear fluid, provides this important moist surface. Its character depends on the condition of the corneal epithelium.

The film, compatible with both aqueous and lipid ophthalmic preparations, is composed of a thin outer lipid layer, a thicker middle aqueous layer, and a thin inner mucoid layer. It is renewed during each blink and when blinking is suppressed, either by drugs or by mechanical means, it dries in patches. It seems to be unaffected by addition of concentrations of up to 2% sodium chloride to conjunctival fluid. A pH below 4 or above 9 causes derangement of the film.

The film affects the movement of contact lenses and forms more easily on glass than on plastic prostheses.

Cornea—The cornea, from 0.5 to 1 mm thick, consists mainly of the following structures (from the front backwards):

1. Corneal epithelium.
2. Substantia propria (stroma).
3. Corneal endothelium.

The cornea is transparent to ordinary diffuse light, largely because of a special laminar arrangement of the cells and fibers and because of the absence of blood vessels. Cloudiness of the cornea may be due to any one of several factors including: excess pressure in the eyeball as in glaucoma; scar tissue, as due to injury or infection; or deficiency of oxygen or excess hydration such as may occur during the wearing of improperly fitted contact lenses. A wound of the cornea usually heals as an opaque patch which can be a permanent disability unless it is located in the periphery of the cornea.

The chief refraction of light for the eye occurs at the outer surface of the cornea where the index of refraction changes from that of air (1.00) to that of corneal substance (1.38). Any alteration in its shape or transparency interferes with the formation of a clear image, therefore, any pathologic process, however slight, may interfere seriously with the resolving power or visual acuity of the eye.

The normal cornea possesses no blood vessels except at the corneoscleral junction. The cornea, therefore, must derive its nutrition by diffusion and must have certain permeability characteristics; it also receives nourishment from the fluid circulating through the chambers of the eye and from the air. The fact that the normal cornea is devoid of blood vessels is an important feature in surgical grafting. The corneal nerves do not supply all forms of sensation to the cornea. Pain and cold are well supplied. The pain fibers have a very low threshold, which makes the cornea one of the most sensitive portions on the surface of the body. It is now generally agreed that the cornea possesses a true sense of touch; nerve endings supplying the sensation of heat are lacking.

The corneal epithelium provides an efficient barrier against bacterial invasion. Unless its continuity has been broken by an abrasion (a traumatic opening or defect in the epithelium) pathogenic bacteria, as a rule, cannot gain a foothold. Trauma, therefore, plays an important part in most of the infectious diseases of the cornea which occur exogenously. Any foreign body that either scratches the cornea or lodges and becomes imbedded in the cornea is of serious moment because of the role it may play in permitting pyogenic bacteria to gain a foothold.

A means of detecting abrasions on the corneal surface is afforded by staining the cornea with sodium fluorescein. If there is an abrasion on the epithelium, the underlying layer stains a brilliant green, so that even pinpoint abrasions show up quite clearly. Abrasion may occur during tonometry; that is, during the measurement of ocular tension with a tonometer. Care must be used in applying the device to the cornea to avoid abrasion of the cornea. Corneal abrasions sometimes result from wearing contact lenses. Every corneal abrasion is subject to infection.

Bioavailability

Physical Consideration—Under normal conditions the human tear volume averages about 7 µL.[4] The estimated maximum volume of the cul-de-sac is about 30 µL with drainage capacity far exceeding lacrimation rate. The outflow capacity accommodates the sudden large volume resulting from the instillation of an eye drop. Most commercial eye drops range from 50 to 75 µL in volume, however, much in excess of 50 µL is probably unable to enter the cul-de-sac.

Within the rabbit cul-de-sac, drainage rate has been shown to be proportional to the instilled drop volume. Multiple drops administered at intervals produced higher drug concentrations. Ideally a high concentration of drug in a minimum drop volume is desirable. Patton[5] has shown that approximately equal tear film concentrations result from the instillation of 5 µL of 1.61×10^{-2} M pilocarpine nitrate or from 25 µL of 1.0×10^{-2} M solution. The 5 µL contains only 38% as much pilocarpine, yet its bioavailability is greater due to decreased drainage loss.

There is a practical limit or limits to the concept of minimum dosage volume. There is a difficulty in designing and producing a dropper configuration which will deliver small volumes without override. Secondly, the patient often cannot detect the administration of such a small volume. This sensation or lack of sensation is particularly apparent at the 5.0–7.5 µL dose volume range.

The concept of dosage volume drainage and cul-de-sac capacity directly effects the prescribing and administering of separate ophthalmic preparations. The first drug administered may be significantly diluted by the administration of the second. On this basis combination drug products for use in ophthalmology have considerable merit.

Corneal Absorption—Drugs administered by instillation must penetrate the eye and do so primarily through the cornea. Corneal absorption is much more effective than scleral or conjunctival absorption.

Many ophthalmic drugs are weak bases and are applied to the eye as aqueous solutions of their salts. The free base and the salt will be in an equilibrium which will depend on the pH and on the individual characteristics of the compound. To aid in maintaining storage stability and solubility, the medication may be acidic at the moment of instillation but usually the neutralizing action of the lacrimal fluid will convert it rapidly to the physiological pH range (approximately pH 7.4) at which there will be enough free base present to begin penetration of the corneal epithelium. Once inside the epithelium the undissociated free base immediately dissociates to a degree. The dissociated moiety will then tend to penetrate the stroma because it is water-soluble. At the junction of the

stroma and endothelium the same process that took place at the outer surface of the epithelium must again occur. Finally, the dissociated drug leaves the endothelium for the aqueous humor. Here it can readily diffuse to the iris and the ciliary body, the site of its pharmacological action.

The cornea can be penetrated by ions to a small, but measurable, degree. Under comparable conditions, the permeabilities are similar for all ions of small molecular weight, which suggests that the passage is through extracellular spaces. The diameter of the largest particles which can pass across the cellular layers seems to be in the range 10–25 Å. An instilled drug is subject to protein binding in the tear fluid and metabolic degradation by enzymes such as lysozyme, in addition to the losses by simple overflow and lacrimal drainage.

Since the cornea is a membrane including both hydrophilic and liophilic layers, most effective penetration is obtained with drugs having both lipid and hydrophilic properties. Highly water soluble drugs penetrate less readily. As an example highly water soluble steroid phosphate esters penetrate the cornea poorly. Better penetration is achieved with the poorly soluble but more lipophilic steroid alcohol; still greater absorption is seen with the steroid acetate form.

In 1976 Lee and Robinson[6] presented a summary of the factors controlling precorneal pilocarpine disposition and pilocarpine bioavailability in the rabbit eye. Combining experimental work and computer simulation the investigators discussed the mechanisms competing with corneal absorption of pilocarpine. Included were solution drainage, drug induced vasodilation, nonconjunctival loss including uptake by the nictitating membrane, conjunctival absorption, induced lacrimation and normal tear turnover. Subject to experimental conditions the relative effectiveness of the factors involved in precorneal drug removal are drainage ≃ vasodilation > nonconjunctival loss > induced lacrimation ≃ conjunctival absorption > normal tear turnover.

The authors discuss the implications of the mechanisms of precorneal drug loss in the design of ocular drug delivery systems including the effect of instilled drug volume on aqueous humor concentration and the amount of drug available for systemic absorption. On an absolute basis a smaller volume allows more drug to be absorbed. For a given instilled concentration the opposite is true, however, a smaller volume instilled remains more efficient, ie, the fraction of dose absorbed is greater.

Ophthalmic ointments generally produce greater bioavailability than the equivalent aqueous solution. Because of the greater contact time drug levels are prolonged and total drug absorption is increased.

Types of Ophthalmic Products

Administration—The instillation of eye drops remains one of the less precise, yet one of the more accepted means of topical drug delivery. The method of administration is cumbersome at best particularly for the elderly; patients with poor vision who have difficulty seeing without eye glasses and patients with other physical handicaps. Perhaps surprisingly, the majority of patients become quite adept at routine instillation.

The pharmacist should advise each patient to keep the following points in mind to aid in the instillation of eye drops or ointments:

How to Use Eye Drops:

1. Wash hands.
2. With one hand gently pull lower eyelid down.
3. If dropper is separate, squeeze rubber bulb once while dropper is in bottle to bring liquid into dropper.
4. Holding dropper above eye, drop medicine inside lower lid while looking up; do not touch dropper to eye or fingers.

5. Release lower lid. Try to keep eye open and not blink for at least 30 seconds.

6. If dropper is separate, replace on bottle and tighten cap.

• If dropper is separate, always hold it with tip down.

• Never touch dropper to any surface.

• Never rinse dropper.

• When dropper is at the top of bottle, avoid contaminating cap when removed.

• Never use eye drops that have changed color.

• If you have more than one bottle of the same kind of drops, open only one bottle at a time.

• If you are using more than one kind of drop at the same time, wait several minutes before use of other drops.

• It may be helpful in use of the medicine to practice use by positioning yourself in front of a mirror.

• After instillation of drops, do not close eyes tightly and try not to blink more often than usual, as this removes the medicine from the place on the eye where it will be effective.

How to Use Ophthalmic Ointment:

1. Wash hands.

2. Remove cap from tube.

3. With one hand gently pull lower eyelid down.

4. While looking up, squeeze a small amount of ointment (about $1/4$ to $1/2$ inch) inside lower lid. Be careful not to touch tip of tube to eye, eyelid, fingers, etc.

5. Close eye gently and roll eyeball in all directions while eye is closed. Temporary blurring may occur.

6. Replace cap on tube.

• Take care to avoid contaminating cap when removed.

• When opening ointment tube for the first time, squeeze out the first $1/4$ inch of ointment and discard as it may be too dry.

• Never touch tip of tube to any surface.

• If you have more than one tube of the same ointment, open only one at a time.

• If you are using more than one kind of ointment at the same time, wait about 10 minutes before use of another ointment.

• To improve flow of ointment, hold tube in hand several minutes to warm before use.

• It may be helpful in use of the ointment to practice use by positioning yourself in front of a mirror.

Ophthalmic Solutions—This is by far the most common means of administering a drug to the eye. The USP XX describes over 40 ophthalmic solutions. By definition all ingredients are completely in solution, uniformity is not a problem and there is little physical interference with vision. The principal disadvantage of solutions is the relatively brief contact time between the medication and absorbing surfaces. Contact time may be increased to some extent by the inclusion of a viscosity increasing agent such as methylcellulose. Inclusions of this sort are permitted by the USP. A viscosity in the range of 15–25 centipoises is considered optimum for drug retention and visual comfort.

Ophthalmic Suspensions—Suspensions are dispersions of a finely divided, relatively insoluble drug substances in an aqueous vehicle containing suitable suspending and dispersing agents. The vehicle is, among other things, a saturated solution of the drug substance. Because of a tendency of particles to be retained in the cul-de-sac the contact time and duration of action of a suspension probably exceeds that of a solution. The drug is absorbed from solution and the solution concentration is replenished from retained particles. Each of these actions is a function of particle size, with solubility rate being favored by smaller size and retention favored by a larger size, thus optimum activity should result from an optimum particle size.

For aqueous suspensions the parameters of intrinsic solubility and dissolution rate must be considered. The intrinsic solubility determines the amount of drug actually in solution and available for immediate absorption upon instillation of the dose. As the intrinsic solubility of the drug increases, the concentration of the drug in the saturated solution surrounding the suspended drug particle also increases. For this reason, any comparison of different drugs in suspension systems should include their relative intrinsic solubilities. The observed differences in their biological activities may be ascribed wholly or in part to the differences in this physical parameter. As the drug penetrates the cornea and the initial saturated solution becomes depleted, the particles must dissolve to provide a further supply of the drug. The requirement here is that the particles must undergo significant dissolution within the residence time of the dose in the eye if any benefit is to be gained from their presence in the dosing system.

For a drug whose dissolution rate is rapid, the dissolution requirement may present few problems, but for a slowly soluble substance the dissolution rate becomes critical. If the dissolution rate is not sufficiently rapid to supply significant additional dissolved drug, there is the possibility that the slowly soluble substance in suspension provides no more drug to the aqueous humor than does a more dilute suspension or a saturated solution of the substance in a similar vehicle. Obviously, the particle size of the suspended drug affects the surface area available for dissolution. Particle size also plays an important part in the irritation potential of the dosing system. This consideration is important, as irritation produces excessive tearing and rapid drainage of the instilled dose. It has been recommended that particles be less than 10 μm in size to minimize irritation to the eye. It should be kept in mind, however, that in any suspension system, the smallest particles tend to dissolve and the largest particles may become larger. In summary, aqueous suspensions should, in general, give a more extended effect than aqueous solutions.

The pharmacist should be aware of two potential difficulties inherent in suspension dosage forms. In the first instance dosage uniformity nearly always requires brisk shaking to distribute the suspended drug. Adequate shaking is a function of the suitability of the suspension formulation but also and most importantly, patient compliance. Studies have demonstrated that a significant number of patients may not shake the container at all, others may contribute a few trivial shakes. The pharmacist should stress the need of vigorous shaking whenever an ophthalmic suspension is dispensed.

A second and infrequent characteristic of suspensions is the phenomenon of polymorphism or the ability of a substance to exist in several different crystalline forms. A change in crystal structure may occur during storage resulting in an increase (or decrease) in crystal size and alteration in the suspension characteristics causing solubility changes reflected in increased or decreased bioavailability.

Ophthalmic Ointments—Despite disadvantages ophthalmic ointments remain a popular and frequently prescribed dosage form. Dosage variability is probably greater than with solutions (although probably not with suspensions). Ointments will interfere with vision unless use is limited to bedtime instillation.

Ointments do offer the advantage of longer contact time and greater total drug bioavailability albeit with slower onset and time to peak absorption. The relationship describing the availability of finely divided solids dispersed in an ointment base was given by Higuchi where the amount of solid (drug) released in unit time is a function of concentration, solubility in the ointment base and the diffusivity of the drug in the base.

Special precautions must be taken in the preparation of ophthalmic ointments. They are manufactured from sterilized ingredients under rigidly aseptic conditions and meet the requirements of the official sterility tests. If the specific ingredients used in the formulation do not lend themselves to routine sterilization techniques, other ingredients that meet the sterility requirements described under the official sterility tests, along with aseptic manufacture, may be employed.

Ophthalmic ointments must contain a suitable substance or mixture of substances to prevent growth of, or to destroy, microorganisms accidentally introduced when the container is opened during use. The antimicrobial agents currently used are chlorobutanol, the parabens, or one of the organic mercurials. The medicinal agent is added to the ointment base either as a solution or as a micronized powder. The finished ointment must be free from large particles. Most ophthalmic ointments are prepared with a base of white petrolatum and mineral oil, often with anhydrous lanolin. Some contain a polyethylene-mineral oil gel. Whichever base is selected, it must be nonirritating to the eye, permit diffusion of the drug throughout the secretions bathing the eye, and retain the activity of the medicament for a reasonable period of time under proper storage conditions.

It is obligatory that ophthalmic ointments not contain particulate matter that may be harmful to eye tissues. Hence, in preparing such ointments special precautions must be taken to exclude or to minimize contamination with foreign particulate matter, eg, metal particles fragmented from equipment used in preparing ointments and also to reduce the particle size of the active ingredient(s) to impalpability. The official compendium provides tests designed to limit to a level considered to be unobjectionable the number and size of discrete particles that may occur in ophthalmic ointments. In these tests the extruded contents of 10 tubes of ointment, previously melted in flat-bottom Petri dishes and then allowed to solidify, are scanned under a low-power microscope fitted with a micrometer eyepiece for metal particles 50 μm or larger in any dimension. The requirements are met if the total number of metal particles in all 10 tubes does not exceed 50, and if not more than one tube is found to contain eight such particles.

Testing for sterility of products such as ophthalmic ointments has been greatly facilitated by use of sterile bacteria-retaining membranes (those having a nominal porosity of 0.45 or 0.22 μm are commonly used). For ointments soluble in isopropyl myristate (the solvent used in the official test for sterility) a sample of the ointment is dissolved in the sterile test solvent. For ointments insoluble in isopropyl myristate the sample is suspended in a suitable aqueous vehicle that may contain a dispersing agent and tested by the conventional *General Procedure* (see USP for details).

For a long time the technology available for manufacture of ophthalmic ointments was considered inadequate to produce sterile products; indeed it was believed by some to be impossible to operate a tube-filling machine so as to maintain sterility even in a sterile room. In recent years technological advances have made it possible to manufacture sterile ophthalmic ointment units. Major improvement was achieved in the area of filtration technology. Membrane filters have improved the reliability of both sterile filtration procedures and sterility-testing methods. Use of laminar flow of HEPA-filtered air in appropriately designed rooms and hoods has been a major factor in the successful aseptic operation of the roller mill and of devices for filling tubes with ointment. While the ideal method of sterilization is one in which the finished ointment is sterilized in its final container, at present it does not appear feasible to do so by any method with the possible exception of the use of ionizing radiation.

As previously noted, the official compendium directs that ophthalmic ointments be prepared from previously sterilized ingredients, under rigidly aseptic conditions. This is the procedure followed in commercial manufacture as well as in extemporaneous preparation of ophthalmic ointments. In extemporaneous compounding the following information may be helpful: Petrolatum vehicles and many medicaments may be sterilized by heating in a hot air oven; utensils required for compounding may be sterilized by autoclaving. A sterile disposable syringe without a needle may be used to transfer the finished ointment, if it is semifluid, to the ointment tube, or sterile aluminum foil or powder paper may be used for the same purpose. Probability of microbial contamination may be greatly reduced by carrying out selected steps of the procedure in a laminar flow hood.

Ocular Inserts—The use of solid dosage forms in the eye actually dates from the *lamellae* of the British Pharmacopeia of the 1940's. These drug-impregnated wafers were designed to dissolve on insertion beneath the eyelid. Other slowly soluble or erodible matrices were investigated from time to time. Each is characterized by a form of enhanced pulse drug activity. That is, the bioavailability curve of the drug instilled in aqueous solutions was greatly enhanced both in peak absorption and in duration. Drug side effects were concomitantly enhanced as well.

More recently ocular inserts have been developed in which the drug is delivered based on diffusional mechanisms. Such a device delivers an ophthalmic drug at a constant known rate, minimizing side effects by avoiding excessive absorption peaks. The delivery of pilocarpine by such a device is a well-known commercial product (*Ocusert*, Alza).

Ocular inserts are plagued with some of the same manipulative disadvantages as conventional eye drops. The insert must be placed in the eye in a manner similar to the insertion of a contact lens. Additionally the insert, exhausted of its drug content, must be removed from the eye. Such manipulations can be difficult for the elderly patient. Nonetheless such therapeutic inserts represent a notable scientific contribution to ophthalmic therapy.

Intraocular Solutions—Ophthalmic solutions intended for intraocular use are relatively recent additions to the armamentarium of the ophthalmologist surgeon. Surgical procedures such as cataract removal require two types of intraocular solutions. During the surgery the operating site is frequently rinsed with an irrigating solution. Late in the surgical procedure the surgeon may choose to constrict the iris by the use of a miotic solution such as carbachol. Drugs such as the latter are usually used in a unit dose, minimum volume form. Irrigating solutions, in contrast, may be used over a period of hours during surgery and are available in volumes ranging from 15 to 500 mL.

The formulation of intraocular ophthalmic products presents requirements that differ depending on the type product. Medicated solutions such as carbachol or acetylcholine are best formulated in relatively simple isotonic vehicles. Preservatives should not be used and buffers should be avoided if possible. The product pH should be adjusted as close to the physiologic range as possible. Needless to say the product should be sterile and particle free.

Intraocular irrigating solutions present a considerable formulation challenge distinct from the active ingredient solutions described above. Intraocular irrigating solutions are in contact with the delicate internal structures of the eye throughout the course of various surgeries, ie, for time periods measured in hours. The requirements of tonicity, pH, sterility and clarity are obvious; additionally however, such irrigating solutions require a balanced ionic structure to prevent or minimize deleterious effects on structures such as the corneal endothelium. Edelhauser[7] has shown that isotonic sodium chloride can be toxic to corneal epithelial, endothial, iris and conjunctival cells. The same cells in contrast are unchanged after exposure to Ringer's Solution containing glutathione, bicarbonate and adenosine.

The question of particulate matter in intraocular irrigating solutions is particularly important. In view of the volumes used for irrigations in the surgically opened eye any particulates could impair the trabecular meshwork and canals of Schlemm. The latter are vital in the outflow of aqueous humor and help maintain proper intraocular pressure in the intact eye.

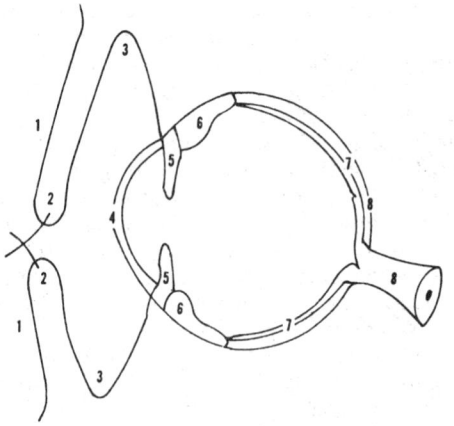

Fig 87-1.   Modes of local therapy in ocular inflammation: *Ointment:*
1–5. Drops: 3–5. Parenteral Injections—subconjunctival: 4–6;
deep sub-tenons: 6–8; retrobulbar: 8.[2]

Other Modes of Administration

Packs—These are sometimes used to give prolonged contact of the solution with the eye. A cotton pledget is saturated with an ophthalmic solution and this pledget is inserted into the superior or inferior fornix. Packs may be used to produce maximal mydriasis. In this case the cotton pledgets can be, for example, saturated with phenylephrine solution.

Intracameral Injections—Injections may be made directly into the anterior chamber (eg, acetylcholine chloride, alpha-chymotrypsin, carbamylcholine chloride, certain antibiotics and steroids), or directly into the vitreous chamber (eg, amphotericin B, gentamicin sulfate, and certain steroids). Injections are not made into the posterior chamber.

Iontophoresis—This procedure keeps the solution in contact with the cornea by means of an eyecup bearing an electrode. Diffusion of the drug (eg, fluorescein sodium, an antibiotic, etc) is effected by difference of electrical potential.

Subconjunctival Injections—Subconjunctival injections (Fig 87-1) are frequently used to introduce medications which, if instilled, either do not penetrate into the anterior segment or penetrate too slowly to attain the concentration required. The drug is injected underneath the conjunctiva and probably passes through the sclera and into the eye by simple diffusion. The most common use of subconjunctival injection is for the administration of antibiotics in infections of the anterior segment of the eye. Subconjunctival injections of mydriatics and cycloplegics are also used to achieve maximal pupillary dilation or relaxation of the ciliary muscle. If the drug is injected underneath the conjunctiva and the underlying Tenon's capsule in the more posterior portion of the eye, effects on the ciliary body, choroid, and retina can be obtained.

Retrobulbar Injections—Drugs administered by retrobulbar injection (Fig 87-1) may enter the globe in essentially the same manner as the medications given subconjunctivally. The orbit is not well vascularized and the possibility of significant via-blood stream effects from these injections is very remote. In general, such injections are given for the purpose of getting medications (eg, antibiotics, local anesthetics, enzymes with local anesthetics, steroids, vasodilators) into the posterior segment of the globe and to affect the nerves and other structures in that space.

Preparation

The preparation of ophthalmic solutions, suspensions or ointments by the community pharmacist or even the hospital pharmacist is becoming less common. The pharmacist may be called upon to prepare a special concentration, particularly of an antibiotic in the hospital setting. However the extemporaneous compounding of ophthalmic prescriptions is becoming rare. In the view of many, the advantages of commercial preparations such as stability, uniformity and sterility outweigh possible disadvantages such as standardization of

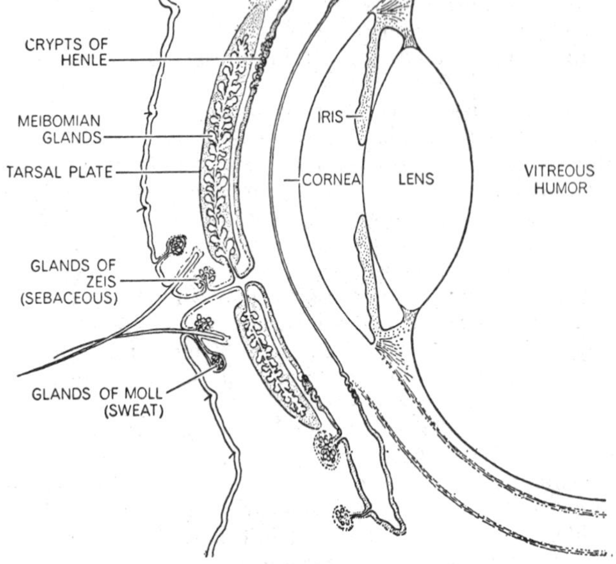

Fig 87-2.   The eye: vertical section.[3]

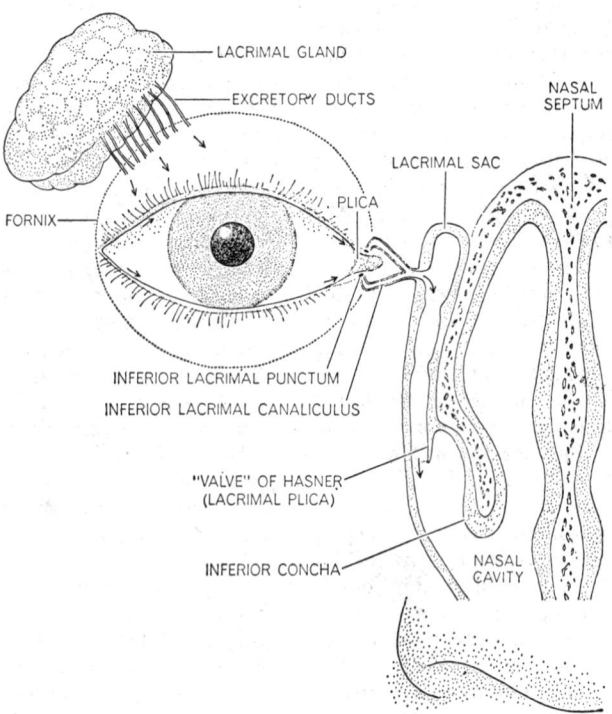

Fig 87-3.   Nasolacrimal duct.[3]

dosage. A general discussion concerning the preparation of ophthalmic solutions is found in the USP.

Vehicles—Sterile isotonic solutions, properly preserved are suitable for preparing ophthalmic solutions. In most cases where the concentration of active ingredient is low, ie, less than 2.5–3.0% of the drug can be dissolved directly in the isotonic vehicle. The finished solutions will be somewhat hypertonic but well within the comfort tolerance of the eye.

Typical stock solutions are as follows:

Isotonic Sodium Chloride Solution

Sodium Chloride, USP	0.9 g
Benzalkonium Chloride	1:10,000
Sterile Distilled Water	qs 100 mL

Boric Acid Solution

Boric Acid, USP	1.9 g
Benzalkonium Chloride	1:10,000
Sterile Distilled Water	qs 100 mL

Boric acid solution at pH 5 is an appropriate vehicle for the following:

Cocaine	Tetracaine
Neostigmine	Zinc Salts
Phenacaine	Piperocaine
Procaine	

Boric acid solution with antioxidant.

For oxygen sensitive drugs such as epinephrine, phenylephrine and physostigmine. The following solution is suggested. Phenylmercuric nitrate replaces benzalkonium chloride.

Boric Acid	1.9 g
Sodium Sulfite Anhydrous	0.1 g
Phenylmercuric nitrate	1:50,000
Sterile Purified Water	qs 100 mL
Sodium Acid Phosphate (NaH_2PO_4) anhydrous	0.56 g
Disodium Phosphate (Na_2HPO_4) anhydrous	0.284
Sodium Chloride	0.5
Disodium Edetate	0.1
Benzalkonium Chloride	1:10,000
Sterile Purified Water	qs 100 mL

These vehicles are suitable for salts of:

Atropine	Homatropine
Ephedrine	Pilocarpine

Sterilization Procedures—Those procedures best suited for the extemporaneous preparation of ophthalmic solutions are as follows:

1. Solutions in Final Container
   a. Place the filtered solution in containers that have been washed and rinsed with distilled water.
   b. Seal dropper bottles with regular screw caps. The dropper assembly should be stapled into a paper envelope.
   c. Sterilize 15 minutes at 15 psi (121°).
   d. Do not assemble until ready to use.
2. Dropper Bottles
   a. Wash container thoroughly and rinse with distilled water.
   b. Loosen caps and place bottles in autoclave.
   c. Autoclave 15 minutes at 15 psi (121°).
   d. Partially cool autoclave.
   e. Remove bottles from autoclave and secure caps.
   f. Store sterilized bottles in a clean, dust-proof cabinet.
3. Glassware and Equipment
   a. Wrap adapters (containing filter), syringes, glassware, spatulas, etc in autoclave paper and secure with masking tape.
   b. Place articles in autoclave and sterilize in the manner described in section 2 above.
   c. Store in separate cabinet until ready to use.
4. Microbiological Filtration
   a. All equipment and glassware as well as stock solutions should be sterile. The prescription should be dispensed in a sterile container.

   b. Unwrap sterile syringe and draw prepared solution into syringe.
   c. Unwrap sterile adapter containing bacterial filter and attach to syringe. These are available as single-filtration, presterilized disposable units and should be utilized whenever possible.
   d. Force solution through filter directly into sterile container (dropper or plastic *Drop-Tainer* type).
   e. By employing an automatic filling outfit, more than one container of the same prescription can be prepared.
   f. Cap container immediately.

The procedures outlined above should be carried out in a clean area equipped with ultraviolet lighting and preferably in a laminar flow hood.

Laminar Flow Principles—A laminar flow work area is a particularly convenient means of preparing sterile, particulate free solutions. Laminar flow is defined as air flow in which the total body of air moves with uniform velocity along parallel lines with a minimum of eddies. Laminar flow minimizes the possibility of airborne microbial contamination by providing air free of viable particles and free of all inert particulates. Laminar flow units are available in a variety of shapes and size and in two broad categories, horizontal and vertical laminar flow.

General Considerations

A number of requirements must be considered in the preparation of ophthalmic solutions, suspensions or ointments. These include sterility, clarity, buffer and pH, tonicity, viscosity, stability, comfort, additives, packaging, and preservatives. Many of these requirements are interrelated and must be considered collectively in the preparation of an ophthalmic product. The buffer system must be considered with tonicity and comfort in mind. Stability can be related to pH, the buffer system, and packaging. Sterilization must be considered in terms of stability and packaging.

Ophthalmic solutions are formulated to be sterile, isotonic and buffered for stability and comfort. A viscosity imparting agent may or may not be present. Solutions must be free from foreign particles. Solution pH must be selected for optimum drug stability. The pH should then be maintained by the inclusion of a buffer system of sufficient capacity to maintain pH throughout the extent of product shelf life.

The proper pH, buffer and buffer capacity often represent a compromise between stability of the drug and comfort in the eye since optimum patient comfort is usually found at the pH of the tear fluid or about 7.4 while optimum stability for many drugs is generally lower, perhaps as low as 5.0. Buffer capacity should be sufficient to maintain pH but minimized to the point where tear fluid can overcome capacity and readjust pH to 7.4 immediately after instillation in the eye.

Sterilization represents the major requirement of eye products and the method or methods employed depend on the active ingredient and product resistance to heat and to the packaging used. More than one means of sterilization may be used. The sterile solution or suspension usually will contain an antimicrobial preservative to prevent inadvertent contamination during use. The preservative should not be depended upon to produce a sterile product and should not be considered as a substitute for sterile techniques and procedures.

Sterilization

Common methods of sterilization include moist heat under pressure (autoclave), dry heat, filtration, gas sterilization, and ionizing radiation.

Dangers of Nonsterile Medications—The possibility of serious ocular infection resulting from the use of contaminated ophthalmic solutions has been amply documented in the literature. Such solutions repeatedly have been the cause of corneal ulcers and loss of eyesight. Contaminated solutions have been found in use in physicians' offices, eye clinics, and industrial infirmaries, and dispensed on prescription in community and hospital pharmacies. The microbe most frequently found as a contaminant is *Pseudomonas aeruginosa* and the solution most often found contaminated is that of sodium fluorescein.

Pseudomonas aeruginosa (B pyocyaneus; Pseudomonas pyocyanea; Blue pus bacillus)—This is a very dangerous and opportunistic organism that grows well on most culture media and produces both toxins and antibacterial products. The latter tend to kill off other contaminants and allow the *P. aeruginosa* to grow in pure culture. This gram-negative bacillus also grows readily in ophthalmic solutions which may become the source of extremely serious infections of the cornea. It can cause complete loss of sight in 24–48 hours. In concentrations tolerated by tissues of the eye, it seems that all the antimicrobial agents discussed in the following sections may be ineffective against some strains of this organism.

A sterile ophthalmic solution in a multiple-dose container can be contaminated in a number of ways unless precautions are taken. For example, if a dropper bottle is used, the tip of the dropper while out of the bottle can touch the surface of a table or shelf if laid down, or it can touch the eyelid or eyelash of the patient during administration. If the "Droptainer" type of bottle is used, the dropper tip can touch an eyelash, or the cap while removed to permit administration, or its edge may touch a table or finger and that edge can touch the dropper tip as the cap is replaced.

The solution may contain an effective antimicrobial but the next use of the contaminated solution may occur before enough time has elapsed for all of the organisms to be killed, and living organisms can find their way through an abrasion into the corneal stroma. Once in the corneal stroma, any residual traces of antimicrobial agents are neutralized by tissue components and the organisms find an excellent culture medium for rapid growth and dissemination through the cornea and the anterior segment of the eye.

Other Organisms—*Bacillus subtilis* may produce a serious abscess when it infects vitreous humor. The pathogenic fungus considered of particular importance in eye solutions is *Aspergillus fumigatus*. Other fungi or molds may be harmful by accelerating deterioration of the active drugs.

With regard to viruses, as many as 42 cases of epidemic keratoconjunctivitis were caused by one bottle of virus-contaminated tetracaine solution. Virus contamination is particularly difficult to control because none of the preservatives now available is virucidal. Moreover, viruses are not removable by filtration. However, they are destroyed by autoclaving. The pharmacist and physician have not been made adequately aware of the dangers of transmitting virus infection via contaminated solutions. This is particularly pertinent to the adenoviruses (Types III and VIII) which are now believed to be the causative agents of viral conjunctivitis such as epidemic keratoconjunctivitis.

Methods of Sterilization

Steam under Pressure—Terminal sterilization by autoclaving is an acceptable, effective method of sterilization, however, the solution or suspension components must be sufficiently heat resistant to survive the procedure. If sterilization is carried out in the final container the container must also be able to survive the heat and pressure. A recent addition to this technique is the so-called air over steam autoclave. This combination allows pressure adjustments to be made during the autoclave cycle. Pressure manipulations permit

the autoclave sterilization of materials which, while heat resistant, tend to deform, ie, polypropylene containers.

Filtration—The USP XX states that sterile membrane filtration under aseptic conditions is the preferred method of sterilization. Membrane filtration offers the substantial advantage of room temperature operation with none of the deleterious effects of exposure to heat or sterilizing gas.

Sterilization by filtration does involve the transfer of the finished sterile product into previously sterilized containers using aseptic techniques. The membrane filtration equipment itself is usually sterilized as an assembly by autoclaving.

The application of filtration procedures to the extemporaneous preparation of sterile ophthalmic solutions has been proposed by several workers. Several types of equipment are available for small-scale work, as described in Chapter 78. Particular interest has been shown in the Swinny adapter fitted on a syringe, and in the Milipore *Swinnex* disposable filter units. Empty sterile plastic "squeeze" containers and sterile plastic filtration units can be purchased directly from the manufacturers; eg, Wheaton (polyethylene containers) and Millipore (Swinnex filter units). They permit extemporaneous preparation of ophthalmic solutions which have a high probability of being sterile if the work is carried out under aseptic conditions. A supplementary device can permit automatic refilling of the syringe. The filter unit must be replaced after use.

Gas Sterilization—Gas sterilization of heat sensitive materials may be carried out by exposure to ethylene oxide gas in the presence of moisture. Ethylene oxide gas for sterilization use is available commercially diluted either with carbon dioxide or halogenated hydrocarbons. Ethylene oxide sterilization requires careful consideration of conditions required to effect sterility. Temperature and pressure conditions are quite nominal in contrast to wet or dry heat however careful control of exposure time, ethylene oxide concentration and moisture is essential.

Gas sterilization requires the use of specialized but not necessarily elaborate equipment. Gas autoclaves may range from very large walk-in units to small laboratory bench scale units suitable for small hospitals, laboratories or pharmacies.

In using gas sterilization the possibility of human toxicity must be kept in mind. Care should be taken to restrict any exposure to ethylene oxide during the loading and venting of the autoclave. Ethylene oxide sterilization produces irritating byproducts which remain as residues in or on the articles sterilized. Residues include ethylene glycol and ethylene chlorohydrin in addition to ethylene oxide itself. To minimize such residues the sterilized articles should be aerated for at least 24 to 48 hours.

Ambient aeration time for sterilized polyethylene bottles should be about 48 hours. Ethylene oxide is recommended for the sterilization of solid materials which will not withstand heat sterilization. The Food and Drug Administration has recommended maximum residues in the parts per million range for ethylene oxide, ethylene glycol and ethylene chlorohydrin.

Radiation—Sterilization by exposure to ionizing radiation is an acceptable procedure for components of ophthalmic preparations or indeed for the total product as in certain ophthalmic ointments. Sources of radiation are two-fold and include linear electron accelerators and radioisotopes. The linear accelerators produce high energy electrons with very little penetrating power. Radioisotopes, particularly ^{60}Co are more widely employed for sterilization. Sterilization by radiation may produce untoward effects such as chemical changes in product components as well as changes in color or physical characteristics of package components.

Clarity—Ophthalmic solutions are by definition free from foreign particles and clarity is normally achieved by filtration. It is, of course, essential that the filtration equipment be clean and well-rinsed so that particulate matter is not contributed to the solution by equipment designed to remove it. Operations performed in clean surroundings, the use of laminar flow hoods and proper nonshedding garb will collectively contribute to the preparation of brilliantly clear solutions free from foreign particles. In many instances clarity and sterility may be achieved in the same filtration step. It is essential to realize that solution clarity is equally a function of the cleanliness of the intended container and closure. Both container and closure must be thoroughly clean, sterile and nonshedding. That is, the container or closure must not contribute particles to the solution during prolonged contact such as shelf life storage. This is normally established by thorough stability testing.

Stability—The stability of a drug in solution, ie, an ophthalmic product, depends on the chemical nature of the drug substance, the product pH, method of preparation (particularly temperature exposure), solution additives, and the type of packaging. Until two or three decades ago the stability of ophthalmic solutions was an exceedingly short term concept, generally it was the time required for a patient to complete the use of 15 or 30 mL of solution. Now of course, the stability of ophthalmic products is expressed in terms of years. However, two to three year stability is often achieved only by virtue of compromise.

Drugs such as pilocarpine and physostigmine are both active and comfortable in the eye at a pH of 6.8, however at this pH chemical stability (or instability) can be measured in days or months. With either drug a substantial loss in chemical stability will occur in less than a year. On the other hand at pH 5 both drugs are stable for a period of several years.

In addition to optimal pH, if oxygen sensitivity is a factor, adequate stability may require the inclusion of an antioxidant. Plastic packaging, ie, the low density polyethylene Droptainer that represents such a patient convenience, may prove detrimental to stability by permitting oxygen permeation resulting in oxidative decomposition of the drug substance.

The attainment of optimum stability most often imposes a series of compromises on the formulator. The optimum pH may be lower than preferable for product comfort, although this effect may be minimized by adjusting pH with a buffer of minimum capacity. Additives such as chelating agents and antioxidants may be required and convenience packaging may diminish shelf life of the product.

It should be stressed that stability refers to total product stability not just the chemical stability of a single product component. That is an oversimplification. A well-planned stability program will consider and evaluate chemical stability of the active ingredient, chemical stability of the preservative substance, the continuing preservative efficacy against selected test organisms, the adequacy of the package as a function of time, ie, does the package protect sterility in addition to various physical measures such as pH, clarity, resuspendability of suspensions and the like. One must also support the thesis that the material on test is representative of all lots of a given product.

Buffer and pH—Ideally ophthalmic preparations should be formulated at a pH equivalent to the tear fluid value of 7.4. Practically this is seldom achieved. The large majority of active ingredients used in ophthalmology are salts of weak bases and are most stable at an acid pH. This can generally be extended to suspensions of insoluble corticosteroids. Such suspensions are usually most stable at an acid pH.

Optimum pH adjustment generally requires a compromise on the part of the formulator. The pH selected should be optimum for stability. The buffer system selected should have a capacity adequate to maintain pH within the stability range for the duration of the product shelf life. Buffer capacity is the key in this situation.

It is generally accepted that a low (acid) pH *per se* will not necessarily cause stinging or discomfort on instillation. If the overall pH of the tears after instillation reverts rapidly to pH 7.4 discomfort is minimal. On the other hand, if the buffer capacity is sufficient to resist adjustment by tear fluid and the overall eye pH remains acid for an appreciable period of time then stinging and discomfort may result. Consequently, buffer capacity should be adequate for stability but minimized sofar as possible to allow the overall pH of the tear fluid to be disrupted only momentarily.

Tonicity—Tonicity refers to the osmotic pressure exerted by salts in aqueous solution. An ophthalmic solution is isotonic with another solution when the magnitudes of the colligative properties of the solutions are equal. An ophthalmic solution is considered isotonic when its tonicity is equal to that of an 0.9% sodium chloride solution.

The calculation of tonicity was at one time stressed rather heavily. The fledging pharmacist was taught in great detail the requirements of and means of achieving exact tonicity sometimes to the detriment of other factors such as sterility and stability.

In actuality the eye is much more tolerant of tonicity variations than was at one time suggested. The eye can usually tolerate solutions equivalent to a range of 0.5% to 1.8% sodium chloride. Given a choice, isotonicity is always desirable and is particularly important in intraocular solutions. It need not, however, be an overriding concern when total product stability is to be considered.

The tonicity of ophthalmic (and parenteral) solutions has been investigated intensively over the years. These studies have resulted in the accumulation and publication of a large number of sodium chloride equivalents which are useful in calculating tonicity values. Such listings are available in the *Merck Index* (10th edition Misc 47), in Remington's *Pharmaceutical Sciences* and in other texts.

Viscosity—The USP permits the use of viscosity increasing agents to prolong contact time in the eye and thus enhance drug absorption and activity. Substances such as methylcellulose, polyvinyl alcohol and hydroxymethyl cellulose are frequently added to increase viscosity.

Various investigators have studied the effect of increased viscosity on contact time in the eye. In general terms viscosity increases up to the 25–50 cps range significantly improve contact time in the eye. Results tend to plateau beyond the 50 centipose range; higher viscosity values offer no significant advantage and have a tendency to leave a noticeable residue on the lid margins.

Additives—The use of various additives in ophthalmic solutions is permissible, however the choices are few in number. An antioxidant, specifically sodium bisulfite or metabisulfite is permitted in concentrations up to 0.3% particularly in solutions containing epinephrine salts. The antioxidant acts in this case as a stabilizer to minimize oxidation of epinephrine.

The use of surfactants in ophthalmic preparations is similarly restricted. Nonionic surfactants, the least toxic class of such compounds, are used in low concentrations particularly in steroid suspensions and as aids in achieving solution clarity. Surfactants may rarely be used as cosolvents to increase solubility.

The use of surfactants particularly in any significant concentration should be tempered by recognition of the sorption characteristics of these compounds. Nonionic surfactants in particular may react by adsorption with antimicrobial preservatives compounds and inactivate much of the preservative system.

Cationic surfactants are used frequently in ophthalmic solutions but almost invariably as antimicrobial preservatives.

Benzalkonium chloride is typical of this class of substances. Concentrations are in the range of 0.01% to 0.02% with toxicity limiting the concentration used. Because of its large molecular weight the benzalkonium cation is easily inactivated by macromolecules of opposite charge or by sorption. Despite such limitations benzalkonium chloride is the preservative used in the large majority of commercial ophthalmic solutions and suspensions.

Packaging

The traditional ophthalmic glass container with accompanying glass dropper has been almost completely supplanted by the low density polyethylene dropper unit called the *Droptainer*. In only a very few instances are glass containers still in use, usually because of stability limitations. Large volume intraocular solutions of 250 and 500 mL have been packaged in glass but even these quasi-parenterals are beginning to be packaged in specially fabricated polyethylene/polypropylene containers.

One should be ever mindful that plastic packaging, usually low density polyethylene, is by no means interchangeable with glass. Plastic packaging is permeable to a variety of substances including light and air. The plastic package may contain a variety of extraneous substances such as mold release agents, antioxidants, reaction quenchers, and the like that may readily leach out of the plastic and into the contained solution. Label glues, inks, and dyes may readily penetrate polyethylene. In the opposite sense volatile materials may permeate from solution into or through plastic containers.

Glass containers remain a convenient package material for extemporaneous preparation of ophthalmic solutions. Type 1 glass should be used. The container should be well-rinsed with sterile distilled water and may be sterilized by autoclaving. Droppers are normally available presterilized and packaged in a convenient blister pack.

Ophthalmic ointments are invariably packaged in tin tubes with an ophthalmic tip. Such tubes are conveniently sterilized by autoclaving or by ethylene oxide. In rare cases of metal reactivity or incompatibility, tubes lined with epoxy or vinyl plastic may be obtained.

Regardless of the form of packaging some type of tamper evident feature must be used for product protection. The common tamper evident feature used on most ophthalmic preparations is the moisture or heat sensitive shrink band. The band should be identified in such a way that its disruption or absence should constitute a warning that tampering, either accidental or purposeful, has occurred.

The eye cup, an ancillary packaging device, fortunately seems to have gone the way of the community drinking cup. An eye cup should not be used. Its use will inevitably spread or aggravate eye infections. The pharmacist should not fail to discourage such use just as he or she should take the time to instruct the patient in the proper use and care of eye medications. While ophthalmic administration may seem simple enough it may be a foreign and difficult task for many people. The suggestions and precautions given on page 1555 may be useful in instructing patients.

Antimicrobial Preservatives

The USP states that ophthalmic solutions may be packaged in multiple-dose containers. Each solution must contain a substance or mixture of substances to prevent the growth of or to destroy microorganisms accidentally introduced when the container is opened during use. The preservative is not intended to be used as a means of preparing a sterile solution. Appropriate techniques discussed elsewhere are to be employed to prepare a sterile solution.

Preservatives are not to be used in solutions intended for intraocular use because of the risk of irritation. Ophthalmic solutions prepared and packaged for a single application, ie, a unit dose need not contain a preservative because it is not intended for reuse.

The need for proper control of ophthalmic solutions to prevent serious contamination was recognized in the 1930's. The first preservative recommended for use in ophthalmics was chlorobutanol. Its use was recommended as an alternative to daily boiling!

The selection of an ophthalmic preservative can be a rather difficult task, in part, because of the relatively small number of suitable candidates. There is of course no such thing as an ideal preservative, however, the following criteria may be useful in preservative selection.

1. The agent should have a broad spectrum, active against gram-positive and gram-negative organisms and against fungi. The agent should exert a rapid bactericidal activity particularly against known virulent organisms such as *P aeruginosa* strains.
2. The agent should be stable over a wide range of conditions including autoclaving temperatures and a wide pH range.
3. Compatibility should be established with other preparation components and with package systems.
4. Lack of toxicity and irritation should be established with a reasonable margin of safety.

Preservative substances must be evaluated as a part of the total ophthalmic preparation in the proposed package. Only in this way can the adequacy of the preservative be established. The USP includes a test for preservative effectiveness; additionally, certain manufacturers have developed a panel of test organisms to further challenge and verify preservative activity.

In addition to preservative effectiveness as an immediate measure, its adequacy or stability as a function of time must also be ascertained. This is often done by measuring both chemical stability and preservative effectiveness over a given period of time and under varying conditions.

Many of these test procedures are of course not completely pertinent to the preparation of an extemporaneous ophthalmic solution. In such a situation the pharmacist must make selections based upon known conditions and physical and chemical characteristics. In such circumstances it would be prudent to prepare minimum volumes for short term patient use.

The choice of preservatives suitable for ophthalmic use is surprisingly narrow. The classes of compounds available for such use are described in Table I. In each case or category there are specific limitations and shortcomings.

Quaternary Ammonium Compounds—Benzalkonium chloride is a typical quaternary ammonium compound and is by far the most common preservative used in ophthalmic preparations. Over 65% of commercial ophthalmic products are preserved with benzalkonium chloride. Despite this broad use the compound has definite limitations. As a cationic surface active material of high molecular weight it is not compatible with anionic compounds. It is incompatible with salicylates and nitrates and may be inactivated by high molecular weight nonionic compounds. Conversely, benzalkonium chloride has excellent chemical stability characteristics and very good antimicrobial characteristics. Given the alternative it would be preferable to modify a formulation to remove the incompatibility rather than include a compatible but less effective preservative.

The literature on benzalkonium chloride is somewhat mixed, however, this is not unexpected given the wide variation in test methods and indeed the chemical variability of benzalkonium chloride itself. The official substance is defined as a mixture of alkyl benzyldimethylammonium chlorides including all or some of the group ranging from n-C_8H_{17} through n-$C_{16}H_{33}$. The n-$C_{12}H_{25}$ homolog content is not less than 40% on an anhydrous basis.

Table I—Ophthalmic Preservatives[8]

Type	Typical Structure	Concentration Range	Incompatibilities
Quaternary Ammonium Compounds	$\left[R_1{-}N{-}R_4 \right] Y^-$ (with R_2, R_3)	0.004%–0.02% 0.01% most common	Soaps Anionic materials Salicylates Nitrates
Organic Mercurials	$SHgC_2H_5$ ... $COONa$	0.001%–0.01%	Certain halides with phenylmercuric acetate
Parahydroxy Benzoates	$COOCH_3$ ... OH	Maximum 0.1%	Adsorption by macromolecules; marginal activity
Chlorobutanol	$CH_3{-}C({-}CCl_3)({-}OH){-}CH_3$	0.5%	Stability is pH-dependent; activity concentration is near solubility maximum
Aromatic Alcohols	CH_2OH (benzyl)	0.5%–0.9%	Low solubility in water; marginal activity

Recent reviews[9] of benzalkonium chloride indicate that benzalkonium is well-suited for use as an ophthalmic preservative. Certain early negative reports have been shown to be quite erroneous; in some cases adverse tissue reactions were attributed to benzalkonium chloride when in fact a totally different compound was used as the test material. Although benzalkonium chloride is by far the most common quaternary preservative others occasionally referred to include benzethonium chloride and cetyl pyridinium chloride. All are official compounds. Refer to RPS-14, page 1571 for a summary of quaternary germicides in ophthalmic drugs.

Organic Mercurials—It is generally stated that phenylmercuric nitrate or phenylmercuric acetate, in 0.002% concentration, should be used instead of benzalkonium chloride as a preservative for salicylates and nitrates and in solutions of salts of physostigmine and epinephrine that contain 0.1% of sodium sulfite. The usual range of concentrations employed is 0.002 to 0.004%. Phenylmercuric borate is sometimes used in place of the nitrate or acetate.

Phenylmercuric nitrate has the advantage over some other organic mercurials in not being precipitated at a slightly acid pH. As with other mercurials it is slow in its bactericidal action, and it also produces sensitization reactions. Phenylmercuric ion is incompatible with halides, with which precipitates are formed.

The effectiveness of phenylmercuric nitrate against *P aeruginosa* is questionable; it has been found that pseudomonal organisms survive after exposure to a concentration of 0.004% for longer than a week.

Development of iatrogenic mercury deposits in the crystalline lens resulting from use of miotic eye drops containing 0.004% phenylmercuric nitrate 3 times daily for periods of 3 to 6 years has been reported. No impairment of vision was found, but the yellowish brown discoloration of the lens capsule is reported to be permanent.

Thimerosal (*Merthiolate*, Lilly) is an organomercurial with bacteriostatic and antifungal activity and is used as an antimicrobial preservative in concentrations of 0.005 to 0.02%. Its action, as with other mercurials, has been reported to be slow.

Parahydroxybenzoic Acid Esters—Mixtures of methylparaben and propylparaben are sometimes used as ophthalmic antimicrobial preservatives; the concentration of methylparaben is in the range of 0.1 to 0.2% while that of propylparaben approaches its solubility in water (approximately 0.04%). They are not considered efficient bacteriostatic agents and are slow in their antimicrobial action. Ocular irritation and stinging have been attributed to their use in ophthalmic preparations. In a review of OTC drugs for use in ophthalmology the FDA expert panel found the parabens unacceptable as ophthalmic solution preservatives.

Substituted Alcohols and Phenols—Chlorobutanol is stated to be effective against both gram-positive and gram-negative organisms, including *P aeruginosa* and some fungi. It is broadly compatible with other ingredients, is usually used in a concentration of 0.5%. Upon hydrolysis, one product is hydrochloric acid, causing a resultant decrease in the pH of its solutions. This decomposition occurs rapidly at high temperatures and slowly at room temperature in unbuffered solutions that were originally neutral or alkaline. Therefore, ophthalmic solutions that contain chlorobutanol should be buffered between pH 5.0 and 5.5. At room temperature it dissolves slowly in water and although it dissolves more rapidly on heating decomposition is accelerated.

A combination of chlorobutanol and phenylethyl alcohol (0.5% of each) has been reported to be more effective against *P aeruginosa*, *S aureus*, and *P vulgaris* than either antimicrobial singly. Also, preliminary solution of the chlorobutanol in phenylethyl alcohol effects solution of the former in water without use of heat.

Ophthalmic Preparations for OTC Use

A comprehensive review of ophthalmic over-the-counter preparations has recently been completed by an expert panel approved by the Food and Drug Administration. The panel review extended over the period 1973 through 1979. The finding of this panel in the form of a proposed rule appeared in the *Federal Register*, Vol 45, No 89, pp 30002–30050, May, 1980.

In a comprehensive assessment the panel considered the following conditions amenable to OTC drug therapy.

a. Tear insufficiency
   Rational formulations used to treat tear insufficiency are aqueous solutions containing demulcent agents, tonicity

agents and pH and buffering agents. Tear insufficiency includes:
1) Keratoconjunctivitis sicca
2) Sjogren's syndrome
3) Dry eye in the elderly
b. Corneal edema
Increased water content in the cornea is usually treated with hypertonic solutions of sodium chloride either 2 or 5%.
c. Inflammation and irritation of the eye
1) Presence of loose foreign material in the eye, commonly treated with an isotonic eye wash properly buffered and preserved.
2) Irritation from airborne pollutants and chlorinated water. Management consists of avoiding the offending allergens and the use of vasoconstrictors, astringents, demulcents and emollients for symptomatic relief.
3) Allergic conjunctivitis
Treatment by topically applied vasoconstrictors and astringents, demulcents, emollients and cold compresses. Only in mild cases where edema and congestion are slight is OTC treatment alone adequate.

In providing such OTC medications, the pharmacist should take the opportunity to point out that unsupervised use of such OTC products should be limited to 72 hours when based on self-diagnosis. If the condition persists or worsens at any time treatment should be discontinued and a physician consulted at once.

Contact Lenses

Contact lenses are optical and/or therapeutic ophthalmic devices divisible into four general categories. The rigid, hydrophobic, so called hard contact lenses, principally PMMA (polymethyl methacrylate); rigid, semihydrophobic; flexible hydrophilic and flexible hydrophobic. Each lens class is accompanied by its support solution products and devices. Solutions used with hard contact lenses are rather conventional compositions usually regarded as OTC products. Conversely, solutions ancillary to the hydrophilic lenses may be classed as new drugs or devices from a regulatory standpoint. Such preparations require great care and considerable pharmaceutical skill to formulate. Lens materials and support products are further classified and identified in Table II.

Hard Contact Lens—Some evidence is available to show that contact lenses were visualized by Leonardo da Vinci in 1508 and later in 1637 by Rene Descartes. In 1827 the British astronomer, Sir John Herschel, described the mathematics of these devices. He speculated on the possibility of filling a glass contact lens with transparent gelatin to correct for corneal irregularities. Not until 1888 was the original concept executed by the artificial eye maker Albert Muller. He made a glass protective shell for the cornea of a lagophthalmic patient who had carcinoma of the upper lid. The patient wore the device for 20 years, and corneal clarity was maintained. Other cases were reported in Europe of glass shells placed on the eye as corneal protective devices.

Until the latter part of the 1940s almost all contact lenses had a portion resting directly on, or arching over, the cornea with a supporting flange resting beyond the limbus on the sclera. Thus they were scleral lenses. However, contact lenses without scleral portions (corneal lenses) were in existence at least as early as 1912, when they were being manufactured by Carl Zeiss.

The glass scleral contact lenses that were made from 1888 to 1938 were fitted by a tedious method of trial and error using a fitting set that might contain more than 1000 lenses. The lenses were heavy and adjustments on them by the fitter were impossible. Their life in the eye was short, because the glass was vigorously attacked by lacrimal fluid; in about 6 months the lenses became too rough to wear or to see through. However, they had the advantage that tears readily wet glass. In 1922 Dallos, in Budapest, perfected a molding technique by which a glass shell could be fabricated to closely approximate the curvature of the globe. With the introduction of the methyl methacrylate plastic molded scleral contact lens in 1938, by Obrig and Muller, the feasibility of using plastic for lens fabrication was demonstrated. Although the optical properties of glass are superior to those of plastic, the relative gain in ruggedness and the reduction in weight to one-third that of glass far offset this disadvantage. Not until polymethyl methacrylate (PMMA) became available was a flush-fitting shell possible. The concept was developed by Ridley in England in 1954. The protective effect is very useful in various conditions characterized by corneal epithelial fragility, and for cosmetic effects.

The "hard" plastic corneal contact lens was introduced by Tuohy in 1948. This was a major development. He specified a lens of smaller diameter that rested within the limbal area of the cornea. The results were poor. Development of a corneal lens was hindered by the fear of traumatizing the cornea with an appliance that fitted directly onto it. The first corneal lens to have any measure of success was developed in the early 1950s by Dickinson, Sohnges, and Neill. Its thickness was about 0.2 mm and is considered to be a fairly thick lens. Thinner lenses, about 0.1 mm, were introduced in the early 1960s.

Scleral bifocal lenses were initially developed in 1936, the corneal type in 1958. Bifocal contact lenses are more difficult to fit, more costly, and in many cases more uncomfortable than single-vision lenses.

Table II—Contact Lens Classes, Characteristics and Support Products

Lens Type	Chemical Classification	Major Characteristics	Typical Support Products
"Hard," rigid, hydrophobic	PMMA (polymethylmethacrylate)	Negligible gas permeability, low water content, medium wettability	Wetting solutions Soaking solutions Cleaning solutions Combination Artificial tears
"Soft," flexible, hydrophilic	HEMA (hydroxyethyl methylmethacrylate)	High water content, low gas permeability, good wettability	Cleaning solutions Disinfection solutions
Flexible hydrophobic	Silicone rubber	Good gas permeability Poor wettability	Wetting solutions Cleaning solutions Soaking solutions
	Silicone vinylpyrollidone	Good gas permeability Good wettability	
Rigid, hydrophilic	CAB (cellulose acetate butyrate)	Good gas permeability Good wettability	Wetting solutions Cleaning solutions Soaking solutions Rewetting solutions

Lens Care Products

Wetting Solutions—Preparations designed to furnish an hydrophilic coating over the characteristically hydrophobic surface of PMMA, silicon rubber and other rigid lens surfaces. Typically wetting solutions include an acceptable viscosity imparting agent, a surfactant, and a preservative. The surface activity and viscosity effect may be obtained from a single compound. Agents commonly used include cellulose derivatives, polyvinyl pyrrolidone, polyvinyl alcohol, and polyethylene glycol derivatives. Preservatives include those acceptable for ophthalmic use. Such solutions are sterile.

Cleaning Solutions—Cleaning solutions are commonly used to remove surface contaminants—lipids, protein and the like. Cleaning is accomplished by the use of surfactants preferably nonionic or amphoteric. Solutions are sterile and properly preserved. Viscosity imparting agents are generally not included.

Adequate cleaning of hydrophilic lenses is a far more complex and challenging problem than hard lens cleaning. Because of their permeability characteristics contaminants penetrate into the lens structure and may easily chemically or physically bind to the HEMA lens material. Contaminants may be surface films or crystals, amorphous aggregates of protein material, cellular debris or insoluble inorganic salts.

Cleaning products are generally specific to the lens material and require FDA approval with proof of cleaning efficacy and safety. Cleaners are based on surface activity, enzyme action or even abradant action in which case the abradant material is softer than the lens itself. Adequate cleaning of hydrophilic lens material is a daily necessary prelude to disinfection.

Disinfecting Systems—Disinfection of the first hydrophilic lens approved by the Food and Drug Association was accomplished using a heating device which generated steam from a saline solution. The latter was either prepared by the user or available from the manufacturer. Subsequent to the so-called thermal systems, disinfection solutions were developed which met the requirements necessary for FDA approval. Because of the sorption characteristics of hydrophilic lens materials many of the accepted ophthalmic preservatives are unsatisfactory for use in soft lens disinfecting systems including the ubiquitous benzalkonium chloride.

In addition to satisfactory disinfecting activity such a preparation must be isotonic, in an acceptable pH range, nonreactive (nonbinding) with lens materials and, over a normal use period induce or bring about no physical, chemical or optical changes in the lens. It is of course sterile and safe for use in the eye even though direct instillation into the eye is not intended.

Soaking Solutions—Soaking or storage solutions as the name suggests are used to store and hydrate hard lenses but most importantly to disinfect such lenses. Disinfection should be rapid and as complete as possible making use once again of acceptable ophthalmic preservative substances. Soaking solutions typically contain chlorhexidine (gluconate) or benzalkonium or cetylpyridinium chloride enhanced by sodium edetate.

Artificial Tears—Solutions intended to rewet hard lenses *in situ* are referred to as rewetting solutions or artificial tears. Such preparations are intended to reinforce the wetting capacity of the normal tear film. Early products of this type tended to be somewhat viscous wetting solutions acceptable for direct installation into the eye. More recent preparations more accurately mimic tears; viscosity is rather low and user acceptability is improved.

Guidelines for Safety and Efficacy Testing—The Food and Drug Administration periodically issues or updates guidelines describing recommended test procedures for contact lens care products other than those used with PMMA lenses and also for typical OTC products used with hard lenses. The reader is advised to review the most recent guidelines for appropriate protocols for non-PMMA products.

Tests for OTC (hard) lens products are divided into those appropriate for products intended for direct instillation in the eye and those not so intended. Products intended for direct instillation require multiple application safety tests in the rabbit eye, preservative efficacy tests, and sterility testing in addition to adequate efficacy tests.

Products not intended for direct instillation require short term evaluation in the rabbit eye and, of course, preservative efficacy and sterility testing.

Soft Contact Lens—In 1960 Wichterle and Lim introduced a new, soft, hydrophilic gel lens synthesized by copolymerization of hydroxyethyl methacrylate (HEMA) with ethylene glycol dimethacrylate (EGDM). Its hydrophilic nature was in marked contrast to the hydrophobic properties of PMMA; its increased permeability to water, oxygen, and other constituents of tears having low molecular weight appears to offer metabolic advantages.

Hydrophilic (gel, hydrogel, soft, flexible) lenses are made of polymerized or copolymerized hydrophilic monomers with a cross-linking agent such as ethylene glycol dimethacrylate (EGDM). The cross-links add stability to the gel lenses and act to decrease the water saturation. The most widely used monomer is 2-hydroxyethyl methacrylate (HEMA) which is usually copolymerized with lesser amounts of polyvinylpyrrolidone (PVP), a more hydrophilic polymer. The copolymer acts to increase the hydration level beyond the maximum 40% potential of homogenous poly-HEMA. Gel lenses of even higher water content can be formed by combining a hydrophilic monomer or polymer (usually PVP) with a relatively hydrophobic monomer (usually methyl methacrylate). Lenses of this type are available with as much as 85% water at equilibrium. In addition, these cross-linked polymers cannot be formed by heat or pressure, thus are usually not harmed by boiling in aqueous solution or by autoclaving.

Hydrophilic lenses are elastic and flexible when hydrated, yet they are brittle when dry. They can absorb and concentrate tear film constituents as well as environmental pollutants, vapors, cosmetic ingredients, water impurities, and antimicrobial preservatives as well as active ingredients in ophthalmic preparations. The refractive index for HEMA is 1.43 when hydrated in normal saline; hydrophilic lenses of greater hydration level have a correspondingly lower refractive index. Depending on the amount of cross-linking and the amount and type of additives, the dimensions can be influenced by such factors as pH, tonicity, and molecular or ionic species.

Advantages and Disadvantages of Soft Contact Lenses— Soft contact lenses have the major advantage of wearer comfort and easy adaptability particularly for the first time lens wearer. Soft lenses are less easily misplaced or lost and allow an easier transition to eye glasses. The typical vision blurring associated with a transition from hard lenses to eye glasses is absent.

Because of the flexibility of soft contact lenses an accurate fit to the eye is more difficult than is the case with hard lenses. Visual clarity is usually less with soft lenses, indeed the long time hard lens wearer may find visual clarity or acuity of soft lenses unacceptable at first wearing.

Soft lenses require far more care than hard. The soft polymers will allow penetration of contaminants deep into the lens body where even simple removal become difficult. Soft lenses may become more or less permanently contaminated by sorption of drug product components in addition to protein fragments of various other debris.

Even with reasonable care soft lenses can be expected to have a wearer life substantially shorter than hard lenses. Eye corrective changes may well occur before hard lenses require replacing because of wear.

Despite the obvious practical disparities the popularity of soft contact lenses is immense and increasing as durability and wearing time are increased. Wearer comfort, easy adaptability and adequacy for most relatively minor visual corrections contribute to soft lens acceptability and popularity.

Therapeutic Uses

The majority of contact lenses are used for reasons of optical acuity, convenience, and/or cosmetic value. However, as far as we know, the first use of such a device, in 1888, was to protect a cornea, and therapeutic usefulness has continued since that time. A major therapeutic advance was made by Ridley, in 1954, using PMMA, at the time that it was replacing glass as the principal material used in making lenses. At the present time we are again seeing a contact lens development of major therapeutic importance in the use of soft lenses in the treatment of very serious pathologic conditions. They are of value in several ways, which are interrelated to the extent it is difficult to give an example which illustrates only one point. The several functions can be listed as follows:

1. As "bandages" (through which one can see) to protect the epithelium of the cornea.
2. While in use as bandages, to permit movement of medicinal fluids through the lens to the eye, as well as under the lens (see below).
3. When so used, to increase the duration of the effect from a given quantity of drug.
4. When so used, to increase the degree of effect from a given amount of drug (see below).

The first two functions have become rather well established in the past few years; the last two have been of less therapeutic value.

Bullous keratopathy is the most severe form of corneal edema. Its treatment is presented as an example of the first two functions of soft contact lenses. The lens acts basically as a simple bandage, but has the added valuable quality that the ophthalmic solutions, used as drops, can pass through the lenses and act on the eye. The pain of bullous keratopathy is usually dramatically relieved by the use of the lens as a protective shield, as similarly accomplished by the earlier hard scleral lenses. Vision may be slightly improved. The pain results mainly from the lids rubbing on the bullae, rupturing them, and exposing corneal nerves. The lenses can be worn fulltime, 24 hr a day for months, except for removal for cleaning. They may need to be cleaned only when protein deposits build up on them. They should be removed and inserted only by a physician. New lenses will be needed as the cornea changes in shape.

Compared with hard lenses, use of the soft lens is much simpler. No moldings of the eye or keratometer readings are needed. The iatrogenic aspects of the hard lens have, to a great extent, been alleviated by the soft lens. Few problems occur on over-wearing the lenses. Usually no abrasions are found. The eyes are white and usually free of conjunctival injection. As to medicinal agents, because of the concomitant iritis, pupils must be dilated with cycloplegics for the first few days, as by use of atropine. Eyelid hygiene techniques are needed. Antibiotics, such as chloramphenicol drops, are used if secondary infection or blepharitis is present. A 5% hypertonic saline solution may be used to improve vision; the patient can use it as often as it is helpful.

The conditions for which the use of soft lenses is apparently very helpful and well established are:

1. Edema
    a. Bullous keratopathy
    b. Aphakic
    c. Secondary to glaucoma
    d. Fuchs' dystrophy
    e. Uveitis, etc
2. Epithelial erosion and defects
    a. Ulcers
    b. Chemical burns
    c. Post-graft

3. Exposure
    a. Neurotropic keratitis
    b. Lid abnormalities
4. Irregular cornea
    a. Scars
    b. Dystrophy
5. Dry eye
    a. Nonprogressive conjunctival cicatrization (Stevens-Johnson syndrome)
    b. Sjögren's syndrome
    c. Trachoma
    d. Pemphigoid

Summary

The progress in ophthalmic pharmaceutics and in lens care pharmaceutics during the last decade must be considered as striking. Very substantial advances have been made in ophthalmic bioavailability and the factors influencing ophthalmic drug absorption. New approaches and new techniques have confirmed (or refuted) many long held tenets of ophthalmic formulation technology. Continuing studies in the general field of ophthalmic pharmaceutics and pharmacokinetics should continue to advance the frontiers of ophthalmic drug therapy and ophthalmic drug delivery.

In the contact lens and lens care field we are confronted with a plethora of new lenses and lens polymers. Wearing time has been lengthened substantially, comfort improved and correctable visual defects increased. By the same token the requirements for lens hygiene have also increased. Advances in this broad field also show no signs of abating.

References

1. Deardorff DL: In *Remington's Pharmaceutical Sciences*, 16th ed, Mack Publ Co, Easton, PA, 1498, 1980.
2. Aronson SD, Elliott JH: *Ocular Inflammation*, Mosby, St. Louis, 899, 1972.
3. Botelho SY: *Sci Am 211:* 80, 1964.
4. Shell JW: *Survey Ophthalmol 26:* 207, 1982.
5. Patton TF: *J Pharm Sci 66:* 1058, 1977.
6. Lee VHL, Robinson JR: *J Pharm Sci 68:* 673, 1979.
7. Edelhauser HF, Van Horn DL, Scholtz RO, Hyndiuk RA: *Am J Ophthalmol 81:* 473, 1976.
7. National Formulary XII. APhA, Washington, DC, 481, 1965.
8. Hoover J: *Dispensing of Medication*, 8th ed, Mack Publishing Co, 237, 1976.
9. Mullen W, Shepherd W and Labovitz J: *Survey Ophthalmol 17:* 469, 1973.

Bibliography

Adler FH: *Physiology of the Eye, Clinical Application*, 7th ed, Mosby, St. Louis, 1981.
Newell FW: *Ophthalmology—Principles and Concepts*, 4th ed, Mosby, St Louis, 1978.
Adler FH: *Textbook of Ophthalmology*, 8th ed, Saunders, Philadelphia, 1969.
Havener WH: *Ocular Pharmacology*, 4th ed, Mosby, St. Louis, 1978.
Handbook of Nonprescription Drugs, 7th ed, pp 417–450, APhA, Washington, DC, 1982.
Hoover J: *Dispensing of Medication*, 8th ed, Mack Publ Co, pp 228–254, 1976.
Banker GS, Rhodes CT: *Modern Pharmaceutics*, vol 7, Dekker, New York, pp 479–564, 1979.
Symposium on Contact Lenses, Mosby, 1973.
Stone J, Phillips A: *Contact Lenses*, 2nd ed, Butterworths, Boston, 1980.

CHAPTER 88

Medicated Applications

Lawrence H Block, PhD
Professor of Pharmaceutics
Duquesne University School of Pharmacy
Pittsburgh, PA 15282

The application of medicinal substances to the skin or to various body orifices is a concept doubtless as old as humanity. The papyrus records of ancient Egypt describe a variety of such medications for external use. Galen described the use in Roman times of a forerunner to today's vanishing creams.

Medications are applied in a variety of forms reflecting the ingenuity and scientific imagination of pharmacists through the centuries. New modes of drug delivery have been developed to remedy the shortcomings of earlier vehicles or, more recently, to optimize drug delivery. Conversely, some ex-

ternal medications have fallen into disuse because of changes in the practice of medicine.

Medications are applied to the skin or inserted into body orifices in liquid, semisolid, or solid form. Ophthalmic ointments and topical aerosol products will not be discussed in this chapter. Ophthalmic use imposes unusual particle size, viscosity, and sterility specifications that require separate, detailed discussion (see Chapter 87). The complexity of pharmaceutical aerosol systems necessitates their inclusion elsewhere (see Chapter 93).

Epidermal and Transdermal Drug Delivery

The Skin

The skin has often been referred to as the largest of the body organs: an average adult's skin has a surface area of about 2 m². It is probably the heaviest organ of the body. Its accessibility and the opportunity it affords to maintain applied preparations intact for a prolonged time have resulted in its increasing use as a route of drug administration, whether for local or systemic effects.

Anatomically, human skin may be described as a stratified organ with three distinct tissue layers: the epidermis, the dermis, and the subcutaneous fat layer (Fig 88-1).

Epidermis, the outermost skin layer, comprises stratified squamous epithelial cells. Keratinized, flattened remnants of these actively dividing epidermal cells accumulate at the skin surface as a relatively thin region (about 10 μm thick) termed the stratum corneum, or horny layer. The horny layer is itself lamellar with the keratinized cells overlapping one another and compressed into about 15 layers. The region behaves as a tough but flexible coherent membrane. The stratum corneum is also markedly hygroscopic—far more so than other keratinous materials such as hair or nails. Immersed in water the isolated stratum corneum swells to about three times its original thickness, absorbing about four to five times its weight in water in the process. The stratum corneum functions as a protective physical and chemical barrier and

is only slightly permeable to water. It retards water loss from underlying tissues, minimizes ultraviolet light penetration, and limits the entrance of microorganisms, medications, and toxic substances from without. The stratum corneum is continuously abraded. Thus, it tends to be thicker in regions more subject to abrasion or the bearing of weight. Its regeneration is provided by rapid cell division in the basal cell layer of the epidermis. Migration or displacement of dividing cells towards the skin surface is accompanied by differentiation of the epidermal cells into layers of flat, laminated plates, as noted above. An acidic film (pH ranging between 4.0 and 6.5, depending on the area tested) made up of emulsified lipids covers the surface of the stratum corneum.

The dermis is apparently a gel structure involving a fibrous protein matrix embedded in an amorphous colloidal ground substance. Protein, including collagen and elastin fibers, is oriented approximately parallel to the epidermis. The dermis supports and interacts with the epidermis facilitating its conformation to underlying muscles and bones. Blood vessels, lymphatics, and nerves are found within the dermis, through only nerve fibers reach beyond the dermal ridges or papillae into the germinative region of the epidermis. Sweat glands and hair follicles extending from the dermis through the epidermis provide discontinuities in an otherwise uniform integument.

The subcutaneous fat layer serves as a cushion for the dermis and epidermis. Collagenous fibers from the dermis thread between the accumulations of fat cells providing a connection between the superficial skin layers and the subcutaneous layer.

Hair Follicles and Sweat Glands—Human skin is liberally sprinkled with surface openings extending well into the dermis. Hair follicles, together with the sebaceous glands that empty into the follicles, make up the pilosebaceous unit. Apocrine and eccrine sweat glands add to the total.

Pilosebaceous Unit—Human hair consists of compacted keratinized cells formed by follicles. Sebaceous glands empty into the follicle sites to form the pilosebaceous unit. The hair follicles are surrounded by sensory nerves; thus an important function of human hair is sensory. Human hair varies enormously within the same individual, even within the same

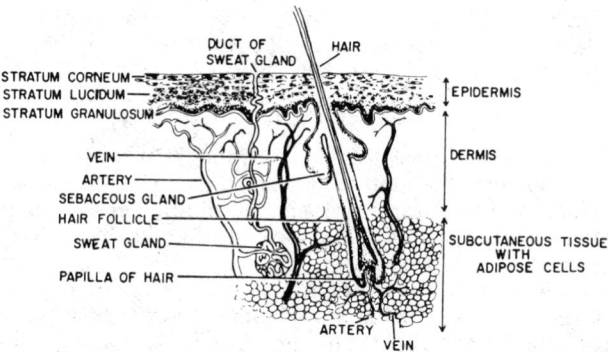

Fig 88-1. Vertical section of human skin.

Table I—Composition of Sebum

Constituents	Percent W/W
Triglycerides	57.5
Wax Esters	26.0
Squalene	12.0
Cholesterol Esters	3.0
Cholesterol	1.5

specific body area. Individual hairs can vary in microscopic appearance, diameter, cuticle appearance, and even presence or absence of medulla.

Sebaceous glands are anatomically and functionally similar but vary in size and activity according to location. Population in the scalp, face and anogenital areas may vary from 400–900 per square centimeter. Fewer than 100 per sq cm are found in other areas. Sebaceous glands are richly supplied with blood vessels.

Sebaceous cells synthesize and accumulate lipid droplets. This accumulation results in enlarged cells which fragment to form sebum. Sebum is made up of a mixture of lipids, approximately as shown in Table I.

The sebaceous gland, containing sebum, cell debris and microorganisms such as *Propionibacterium acnes*, is connected to the pilosebaceous canal by a duct of squamous epithelium. When access to the surface is blocked and bacteria multiply, the result is the comedo of acne.

Sebum presumably functions as an emollient, although Kligman once stated it was useless. Montagna suggests that sebum functions as a pheromone to provide the human with a distinctive aroma.

Sweat Glands—Sweat glands are classified as apocrine and eccrine. Apocrine glands are secretory but are not necessarily responsive to thermal stimulation. Such glands do not produce sweat in the normal sense of the word. Apocrine glands, however, are often associated with eccrine sweat glands particularly in the axilla.

Eccrine sweat glands are coiled secretory glands, equipped with a blood supply, extending from the dermis to the epidermal surface. Eccrine sweat glands function to regulate heat exchange in man. As such they are indispensable to survival.

About 3 million eccrine glands are thought to be distributed over the human body. Distribution varies from less than 100 to more than 300 per square centimeter. Gland counts after thermal stimulation do not always square with anatomical counts.

Drug Effects and the Extent of Percutaneous Drug Delivery

Drugs are applied to the skin to elicit one or more of four general effects: an effect on the skin surface, an effect within the stratum corneum, a more deep-seated effect requiring penetration into the epidermis and dermis, or a systemic effect resulting from delivery of sufficient drug through the epidermis and the dermis to the vasculature to produce therapeutic systemic concentrations.

Surface Effects—An activity on the skin surface may be in the form of a film, an action against surface microorganisms, or a cleansing effect. Film formation on the skin surface may be protective, eg, a zinc oxide cream or a sunscreen. Films may be somewhat occlusive and provide a moisturizing effect by diminishing loss of moisture from the skin surface. In such instances the film or film formation *per se* fulfils the objective of product design. The action of antimicrobials against surface flora requires more than simple delivery to the site. The vehicle must facilitate contact between the surface organisms and the active ingredient. Skin cleansers employ soaps or surfactants to remove expeditiously superficial soil.

Stratum Corneum Effects—Drug effects within the stratum corneum are seen with certain sunscreens; p-aminobenzoic acid is an example of a sunscreening agent which both penetrates and is substantive to stratum corneum cells. Skin moisturization takes place within the stratum corneum. The dry outer cells are hydrated by surface films. The increased moisture results in an apparent softening of the skin. Keratolytic agents such as salicylic acid act within the stratum corneum to cause a breakup or sloughing of stratum corneum cell aggregates. This is particularly important in conditions of abnormal stratum corneum such as psoriasis, a disease characterized by thickened scaly plaques.

The stratum corneum may also serve as a *reservoir phase* or depot wherein topically applied drug accumulates due to partitioning into or binding with skin components. This interaction can limit the subsequent migration of the penetrant unless the interaction capacity of the stratum corneum is surpassed by providing excess drug. Examples of drugs which exhibit significant skin interaction include benzocaine, scopolamine, and corticosteroids.

Epidermal, Dermal, Local, and Systemic Effects—Penetration of a drug into the viable epidermis and dermis may be difficult to achieve, as noted above. But, once transepidermal permeation has occurred, the continued diffusion of drug into the dermis is likely to result in drug transfer into the microcirculation of the dermis and then into general circulation. Nonetheless, it is possible to formulate drug delivery systems which provide substantial localized drug delivery without achieving correspondingly high systemic concentrations. Limited studies in man of topical triethanolamine salicylate demonstrate the potential of this approach.

Unwanted systemic effects stemming from the inadvertent transdermal penetration of drugs have been reported for a wide variety of compounds (eg, hexachlorophene, lindane, corticosteroids) over the years. With the commercial introduction of transdermal drug delivery systems for scopolamine and nitroglycerin, transdermal penetration is being increasingly regarded as an opportunity rather than a nuisance.

Percutaneous Absorption

Percutaneous absorption involves the transfer of drug from the skin surface into the stratum corneum and its subsequent diffusion through the stratum corneum and underlying epidermis, through the dermis, and into the microcirculation. The skin behaves as a passive barrier to diffusing molecules. Evidence for this includes the fact that the impermeability of the skin persists long after the skin has been excised. Furthermore, Fick's Law is obeyed in the vast majority of instances.

Molecular penetration through the various regions of the skin is limited by the diffusional resistances encountered. The total diffusional resistance (R_{skin}) to permeation through the skin has been described by Chien as

$$R_{skin} = R_{sc} + R_e + R_{pd},$$

where R is the diffusional resistance and the subscripts sc, e, and pd refer to the stratum corneum, epidermis, and papillary layer of the dermis, respectively. In addition, resistance to transfer in the microvasculature limits the systemic delivery of drug.

By and large, the greatest resistance to penetration is met in the stratum corneum, ie, diffusion through the stratum corneum tends to be the rate-limiting step in percutaneous absorption.

The role of hair follicles and sweat glands must be considered; however, as a general rule their effect is minimized by the relatively small fractional areas occupied by these appendages. In the very early stages of absorption, transit through the appendages may be comparatively large, particularly for lipid-soluble molecules and those whose permeation through the stratum corneum is relatively low.

The stratum corneum can be regarded as a passive diffusion membrane but not an inert system; it usually has an affinity for the applied substance. The isotherm is frequently linear in dilute concentration ranges. The correlation between external and surface concentrations is given in terms of the solvent membrane distribution coefficient K_m. The integrated form of Fick's Law is given as

$$J_s = \frac{K_m D C_s}{\delta}$$

and

$$K_p = \frac{K_m D}{\delta}$$

where

K_p = permeability coefficient
J_s = steady state flux of solute
C_s = concentration difference of solute across membrane
δ = membrane thickness
$K_m = \dfrac{\text{solute sorbed per cc of tissue}}{\text{solute in solution per cc solvent}} = \dfrac{C_m}{C_s}$
D = average membrane diffusion coefficient for solute.

Permeability experiments have shown that the hydrated stratum corneum has an affinity for both lipophilic and hydrophilic compounds. The bifunctional solubility arises from the filament-matrix ultrastructure of the keratin, which allows aqueous and lipid regions to coexist. Thus attempts to predict permeability constants from oil:water or solvent:water partition coefficients should have limited success.

The effect of regional variation on skin permeability can be marked. Kligman suggests that two species of horny layer be recognized: the palms and soles, adapted for weight-bearing and friction; and the body horny layer, adapted for flexibility, impermeability and sensory discrimination.

Overall, data suggest the following order for diffusion of simple molecules through the skin: plantar > palmar > dorsum of hand > scrotal and postauricular > axillary > scalp > arms, legs, trunk. Electrolytes in solution penetrate the skin poorly. Ionization of a weak electrolyte substantially reduces its permeability, eg, sodium salicylate permeates poorly compared with salicylic acid. Feldmann and Maibach[1] studied the permeability of 16 steroids applied topically, using carbon[14] labeling, and analysis in urine. From their results the authors concluded that active glucocorticoids show the least absorption, while natural androgens showed the greatest absorption.

In Vitro and In Vivo Studies

Classically, percutaneous absorption has been studied *in vivo* using radioactively labeled compounds or by *in vitro* techniques using excised human skin. A diffusion cell frequently used for *in vitro* experiments is shown in Fig 88-2. In this system the intact skin or the epidermis is treated as a semipermeable membrane separating two fluid media. The transport rate of a particular drug is evaluated by introducing the drug in solution on the stratum corneum side of the "membrane," then measuring penetration by periodic sampling and analysis of the fluid across the skin membrane.

More recently investigators have recognized that transport across an immersed, fully hydrated stratum corneum may not

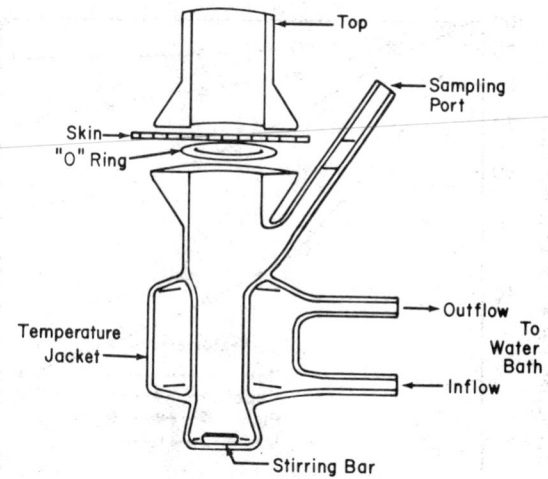

Fig 88-2. Schematic representation of diffusion cell. Top is open to ambient laboratory environment (courtesy, Franz[3]).

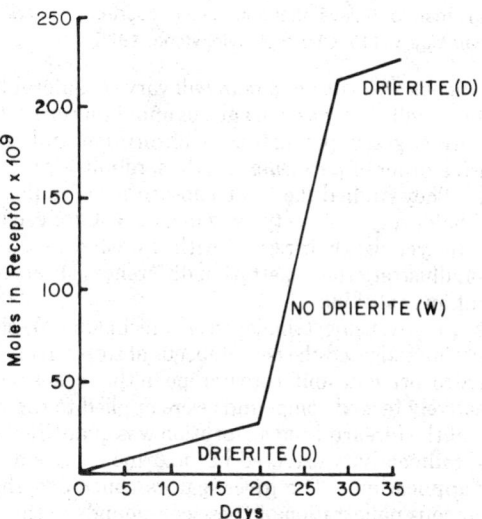

Fig 88-3. Change in cortisone penetration by alternately drying (D) and humidifying (W) the stratum corneum (courtesy, Scheuplein and Ross[2]).

represent the absorption system or rate observed in *in vivo* studies. Percutaneous absorption across a fully hydrated stratum corneum may be an exaggeration; more representative of enhanced absorption that is seen after *in vivo* skin is hydrated by occlusive wrapping.

Using separated epidermal skin mounted in diffusion cells, Scheuplein and Ross[2] varied the atmosphere above the skin strip by use of Drierite to simulate dry conditions and wetted paper strips to simulate the effect of occlusion and observed marked reduction in penetration of cortisone under dry conditions but greatly enhanced penetration on humidifying the stratum corneum (see Fig 88-3).

The studies of Scheuplein and Ross, and of Franz,[3] demonstrate that *in vitro* studies of percutaneous absorption under controlled conditions are relevant to *in vivo* drug penetration. As stated by Franz, "whenever a question is asked requiring only a qualitative or directional answer, the *in vitro* technique appears perfectly adequate."

Relevance of Animal Studies

Any evaluation of a study of percutaneous absorption in animals must take cognizance of species variation. Just as

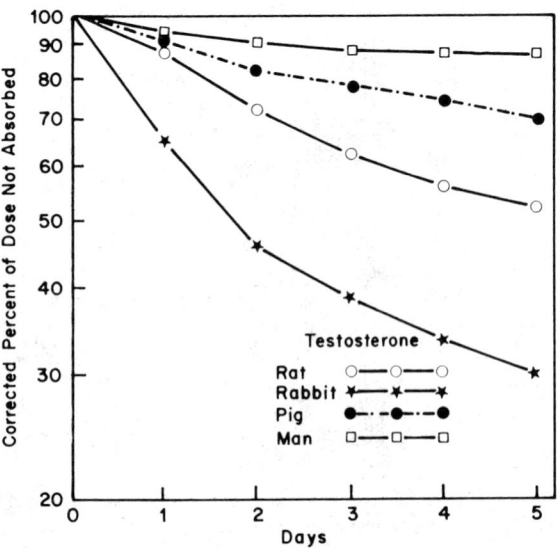

Fig 88-4. Percutaneous absorption of testosterone in rats, rabbits, swine and man for 5 days after application (courtesy, *Animal Models in Dermatology*, p 110, Churchill Livingstone, 1975).

Table II—Relative Potency of Anti-Inflammatory Agents [a]

| Compound | Topical Anti-Inflammatory Potency | |
	Rat Ear Edema Assay	Human Vasoconstrictor Assay
Dexamethasone	73.2 (49.4–110)	10–20
Dexamethasone 21-acetate	117.3 (85.9–106)	10–20
Prednisolone	2.44(1.54–7.76)	1–2
Predniosolone 21-acetate	5.43(4.05–7.70)	3
Betamethasone	97.3 (16.7–141)	3–5
Betamethasone 21-acetate	1072.0 (876–1179)	18–33
Fluorometholone	138.3 (57.9–333)	30–40
Fluorometholone acetate	219.5 (9.15–536)	
Fluprednisolone	31.8 (13.3–76.1)	4–6
Fluprednisolone acetate	61.3 (25.6–147)	
Hydrocortisone	1	1

( ) = 95% confidence limits
[a] From: *Animal Models in Dermatology*, p 221, Churchill Livingstone, 1975.

percutaneous absorption in man will vary considerably with skin site, so will absorption in various animal species. Bartek *et al*[4] investigated percutaneous absorption and found a decreasing order of permeability, thus, rabbit > rat > swine > man. They studied the *in vivo* absorption of radioactively labeled haloprogin, *N*-acetylcysteine, testosterone, caffeine, and butter yellow; their results with testosterone, shown in Fig 88-4, illustrate the penetration differences observed with different animal skins.

Subsequently, using a similar *in vivo* technique, Wester and Maibach[5] investigated the percutaneous absorption of benzoic acid, hydrocortisone and testosterone in the rhesus monkey. Radioactively tagged compounds were applied to the ventral surface of the forearm, and absorption was quantified on the basis of radioactivity excreted in the urine for five days following application. The investigators concluded that the percutaneous penetration of these compounds in the rhesus monkey is similar to that in man, and regarded the data as encouraging because of the similarity.

Stoughton[6] performed *in vitro* studies using animal skins. Using a variety of compounds and a diffusion-cell apparatus he concluded that the skin of the hairless mouse or the baby rat is useful for screening for absorption or epidermal response.

It should again be stressed that percutaneous absorption studies in animals, either *in vivo* or *in vitro*, can only be useful approximations of activity in man. The effect of species variation, site variability (about which little is known in animals), skin condition, experimental variables and, of major importance, the vehicle, must be kept in mind.

Drug Testing in Animals

Drug testing in animals is a characteristic of new-drug development, and the testing of dermatologic products or drugs in animals is no exception. Such testing typically may take three forms: Animals may be used to estimate the safety of a drug product or substance; animal skin may be substituted for human skin for a specific measurement, eg, percutaneous absorption; animal skin may be used as a disease model to simulate an equivalent human condition.

Animals have been used to detect contact sensitization, to measure antimitotic drug activity, to measure phototoxicity, and to evaluate the comedogenic and comedolytic potential of substances. In each of these test procedures, be it a safety

test or assay model, the animal is considered a substitute for man. It is therefore important to realize that the animal is not man, even though man is the ultimate test animal. Animal-testing presents the investigator with unique advantages; lack of appreciation of the variables involved can destroy these advantages.

Mershon and Callahan[7] have recorded and illustrated the considerations involved in selecting an animal test model. They interpreted the rabbit irritancy data of several investigators, and impressively visualized different possible interpretations of the differing response between rabbit and man.

While the ultimate system for establishing therapeutic efficacy is man, there are specific animal test models that are recognized to be valuable as pre-human-use screens predictive of drug activity in humans. For example, the rat-ear assay and the granuloma-pouch procedure in rats are recognized procedures for the estimation of steroid anti-inflammatory activity.

Lorenzetti[8] has tabulated the potency of various topical steroids, comparing the rat-ear-edema assay with potency measured in humans using the vasoconstrictor procedure of Stoughton and McKenzie; the results are given in Table II. Animal assay models of this kind, particularly the steroid anti-inflammatory assays, are most useful as preliminary activity screens. The simplicity, safety and reproducibility of the vasoconstrictor assay in humans recommend it over any corresponding animal procedure.

Dosage Form Design

More than 30 years ago Lane and Blank pointed out that sufficient thought is rarely given to the function which the vehicle performs and to the physicochemical characteristics of the base. These investigators were not discussing optimization of drug activity in today's meaning of the term. They emphasized that the type of skin, application site, lesion type, and physicochemical action of the base are important considerations.

In many (if not most) clinical situations the rate-limiting step is penetration of the drug across the skin barrier, ie, percutaneous penetration through the skin alone. Diffusion of the drug from its vehicle, although dependent on the same diffusion parameters, should not unknowingly be the rate-limiting step in percutaneous absorption. Such a rate limitation or control may, of course, be an objective and the end point of specific drug optimization, but inappropriate formulation can substantially reduce the effectiveness of a topical drug substance.

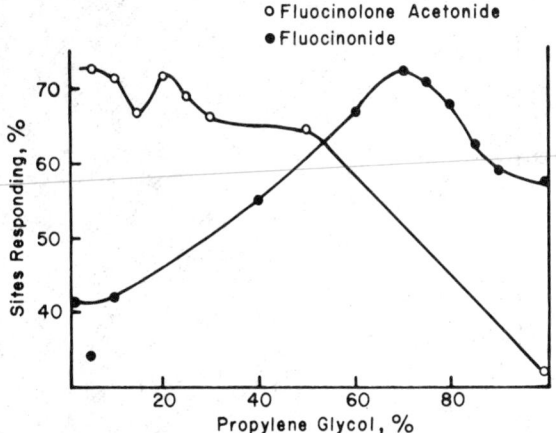

Fig 88-5. *In vivo* response as a function of vehicle composition (24-hour vasoconstriction) (courtesy, Ostrenga *et al* [9]).

In the formulation of a vehicle for topical drug application many factors must be considered. Drug stability, specific product use, site of application, and product type must be combined in a dosage form which will readily release the drug when placed in contact with the skin. Further, the release characteristics of the vehicle are dependent on the physical-chemical properties of the specific drug substance to be delivered to the skin. A vehicle optimized for delivery of hydrocortisone may be quite inappropriate for delivery of a different steroid.

T Higuchi discussed (1960–1961) equations describing the rate of release of solid drugs suspended in ointment bases. More recently Ostrenga and associates, in a series of publications, discussed the significance of vehicle composition on the percutaneous absorption of fluocinolone acetonide and fluocinolone acetonide 21-acetate (fluocinonide) (see Fig 88-5). These investigators used propylene glycol/isopropyl myristate partition coefficients, *in vitro* (human) skin penetration, and finally *in vivo* vasoconstrictor studies to evaluate formulation variables. They concluded that "in general, an efficacious topical gel preparation is one in which (a) the concentration of diffusible drug in the vehicle C for a given labeled strength is optimized by ensuring that all of the drug is in solution, (b) the minimum amount of solvent is used to dissolve the drug completely and yet maintain a favorable partition coefficient and, (c) the vehicle components affect the permeability of the stratum corneum in a favorable manner."

The effect of propylene glycol concentration on *in vivo* vasoconstrictor activity is strikingly illustrated in Fig 88-5, taken from Ostrenga *et al.* [9]

Experimental work of the kind described by Ostrenga *et al.* provides a means of optimizing drug release from a vehicle and penetration of the drug into the skin. This is a beginning. The formulator must proceed to develop a total composition in which the drug is stable and causes no irritation to sensitive skin areas. Safety, stability, and effective preservative efficacy must be combined with optimum drug delivery in the total formulation.

Optimization of drugs other than steroids may be approached by direct *in vivo* assays. Layers of the stratum corneum can be successively removed or stripped away by the repeated application and removal of cellulose adhesive tape strips. The penetration into the skin as well as the effect of additives on *p*-aminobenzoic acid were studied by Lorenzetti through analysis of individual skin strips; the results provided a profile of skin penetration and visualized the effect of additives. Similar experiments have been carried out using benzoyl peroxide. Penetration *per se*, as well as the effect of additives, can be measured by chemical analysis of individual

tape strips following application of a specific quantity of drug or drug product.

Factors Affecting Drug Absorption

In the foregoing we have seen that drug-release from its vehicle is a function of concentration, solubility in the vehicle, and partition coefficient between the vehicle and the receptor site. Percutaneous absorption of a drug can also be enhanced by the use of occlusive techniques or by the use of so-called penetration enhancers.

Skin Hydration and Temperature—Occluding the skin with wraps or impermeable plastic film such as Saran Wrap prevents the loss of surface water from the skin. Since water is readily absorbed by the protein components of the skin the occlusive wrap causes greatly increased levels of hydration in the stratum corneum. The concomitant swelling of the horny layer ostensibly decreases protein network density and the diffusional path length. Occlusion of the skin surface also increases skin temperature (~2–3°) resulting in increased molecular motion and skin permeation.

Hydrocarbon bases which occlude the skin to a degree will bring about an increase in drug penetration; however, this effect is trivial compared with the effects seen with a true occlusive skin wrap. Occlusive techniques are useful in some clinical situations requiring anti-inflammatory activity and it is with steroids that occlusive wrappings are most commonly used. Since steroid activity can be so enormously enhanced by skin occlusion it is possible to depress adrenal function unknowingly. Early in the 1960s McKenzie demonstrated that penetration of steroid could be increased 100-fold by use of occlusion. The Food and Drug Administration requires the following label statement:

If extensive areas are treated or if the occlusive technique is used, the possibility exists of increased systemic absorption of the corticosteroid and suitable precautions should be taken.

Transdermal delivery systems, with their occlusive backing, can effect increased percutaneous absorption as a result of increased skin temperature and hydration.

Penetration Enhancers—This term is used to describe materials that have a direct effect on the permeability of the skin. Increased permeability may result from chemical insult, from increased water content in the stratum corneum, surface tension reduction, or by membrane expansion. In view of its effectiveness, particularly under occlusion, and its safety, water is probably the ultimate penetration enhancer.

Dimethyl sulfoxide (DMSO) can be considered a classic penetration enhancer. This solvent has been studied intensely since its early notoriety as a vehicle. It has been studied thoroughly as a vehicle for the topical application of griseofulvin, and for many other compounds. DMSO apparently functions to enhance penetration by producing structural changes in the stratum corneum and by replacement of water as the continuous membrane phase of the skin barrier. Other penetration enhancers similar to DMSO are dimethyl acetamide (DMA), dimethylformamide (DMFA), and Azone (1-dodecylazacycloheptan-2-one).

With the exception of Azone, solvents such as those indicated above do not function well in dilute solution. In contrast, anionic detergents and soaps enhance permeability in dilute aqueous solution. Scheuplein and Ross[10] reported the effects of surfactants and solvents on the permeability of the epidermis.

Stratum Corneum Barrier Efficacy and Dermal Clearance—Even though *in vitro* studies of percutaneous transport may reflect the resistance of the skin to drug diffusion, there is no way such studies can characterize adequately the transfer of diffusing drug into the microvascu-

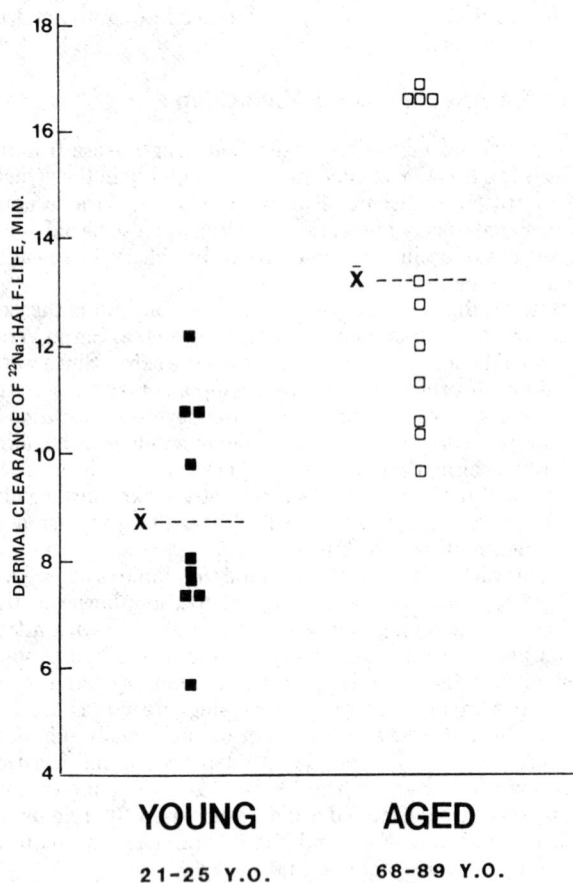

Fig 88-6.   Dermal clearance of ^{22}Na in young and aged subjects after intradermal injection (data from Christophers and Kligman[12]).

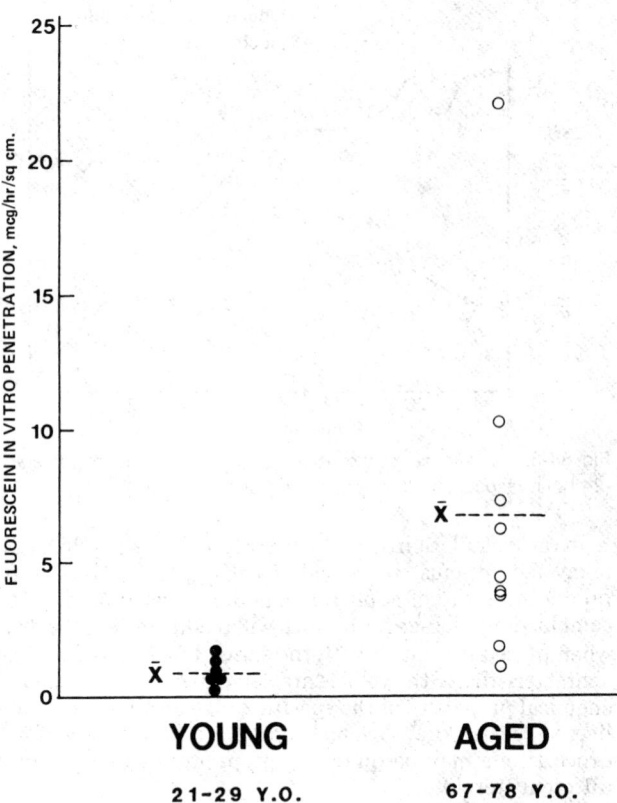

Fig 88-7.   Flux of fluorescein through stratum corneum excised from young and aged subjects (data from Christophers and Kligman[12]).

lature of the dermis and its subsequent transfer into general circulation.

Christophers and Kligman[12] evaluated the dermal "clearance" of ^{22}Na from the midback skin of volunteers following the intradermal injection of ^{22}Na as normal saline solution. The dermal "clearances," expressed in terms of the half-life for disappearance of radioactivity, are plotted in Fig 88-6. Similar results were obtained with disappearance of skin fluorescence after intradermal injection of sodium fluorescein. The data are indicative of markedly delayed dermal clearance in the aged. This may reflect, in part, a decrease in older subjects in dermal capillary loop density, a decrease in the rate and/or extent of dermal blood perfusion, or an increase in resistance to transfer into the capillaries.

On the other hand, Christophers and Kligman[12] demonstrated increased *in vitro* skin permeation by sodium fluorescein in the stratum corneum excised from young and old subjects (Fig 88-7). Thus, the stratum corneum of older subjects may offer less resistance to the penetration of topically applied drugs.

Given the substantial intersubject variations that occur in diffusional resistance and in dermal clearance, it is not surprising that *in vivo* studies of percutaneous absorption often demonstrate marked differences in systemic availability of drugs. Furthermore, the tendency to employ normal, healthy, *young* adults in such studies may not provide data that is indicative of drug permeation through the skin of older subjects or patients. It would seem that more comprehensive studies of percutaneous absorption as a function of age are warranted.

Cutaneous Biotransformation—Catabolic enzyme activity in the viable epidermis is substantial. In fact, the viable epidermis is metabolically more active than the dermis. If the topically applied drug is subject to biotransformation during skin permeation, local and systemic bioavailability can be markedly affected. Enzymatic activity in the skin, or for that matter in systemic fluids and tissues, can be taken advantage of to facilitate percutaneous absorption. Sloan and Bodor,[13] for example, synthesized 7-acyloxymethyl derivatives of theophylline which diffuse through the skin far more efficiently than theophylline itself (Fig 88-8) but which are rapidly biotransformed to theophylline. Thus, theophylline delivery to systemic circulation can be enhanced substantially.

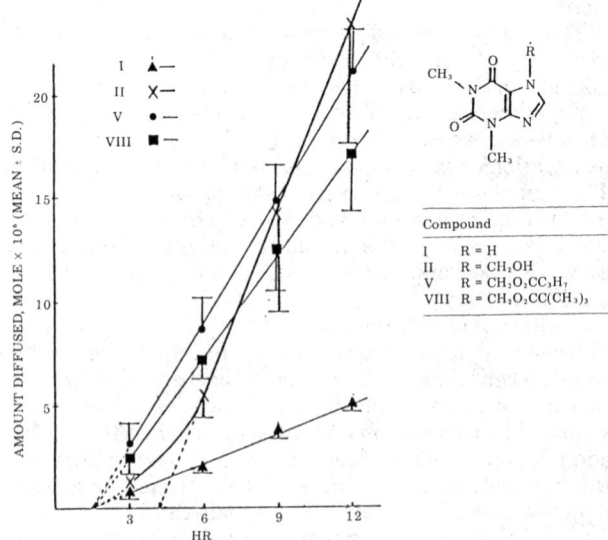

Fig 88-8.   Diffusion of theophylline (I) and its derivatives through hairless mouse skin (from Sloan and Bodor[13]).

Further Considerations for Transdermal Drug Delivery

In order for a drug to qualify as a candidate for systemic delivery after topical application, it must satisfy requirements in addition to exhibiting good skin permeation. Successful candidates for transdermal drug delivery should be non-irri-
tating and non-sensitizing to the skin. Since relatively little drug may reach systemic circulation over a relatively long time, drug candidates should be relatively potent drugs. In addition, the limitation to relatively potent drugs can ease problems of formulation since the amount of drug that can be incorporated in the formulation may be limited by physico-chemical considerations such as solubility.

Ointments

Ointments are semisolid preparations intended for external application to the skin or mucous membranes; usually, but not always, they contain medicinal substances. The types of ointment bases used as vehicles for drugs are selected or designed for optimum delivery of the drugs and also to contribute emolliency or other quasi-medicinal qualities. Ointment properties vary, since they are designed for specific uses, ease of application, or extent of application.

The official definition of ointment in its present form was introduced in the USP XV in 1955. The definition is broad and encompasses petrolatum, ie, oleaginous bases, emulsion bases (either water-in-oil or oil-in-water), and the so-called water-soluble bases.

In unofficial terms, oleaginous bases are described as ointments, but emulsion bases may be termed creams or lotions. Either of these containing large amounts of solids is termed a paste. All of these subclasses are officially defined as ointments.

Pharmaceutical authors have a penchant for defining "ideal" preparations eg, the ideal base, the ideal vehicle, and so on. In practice, of course, there is no such thing. An individual cannot be all things to all people; neither can an ointment base be ideal for all drugs, all situations, or all skins for that matter. An ointment base functioning as a drug vehicle should be optimized for a specific drug and, insofar as possible, for specific disease states or skin conditions.

It is, of course, possible to define certain specific requirements for an ointment base to be used for extemporaneous compounding. Such a base should be nonirritating, easily removable, nonstaining, stable, non-pH-dependent, and widely compatible with a variety of medicaments. When one adds the stipulation that the base must release the same variety of medicaments, the implausibility of such definitions becomes evident.

Classification and Properties of Ointment Bases

The USP recognizes four general classes of ointment bases, hereunder categorized into five classes for the purpose of indicating more definitively some differences in the principal properties of the bases.

Hydrocarbon Bases (Oleaginous)
Example: White Petrolatum
1. Emollient
2. Occlusive
3. Nonwater-washable
4. Hydrophobic
5. Greasy

Absorption Bases (Anhydrous)
Example: Hydrophilic Petrolatum
1. Emollient
2. Occlusive
3. Absorb water
4. Anhydrous
5. Greasy

Emulsion Bases (W/O Type)
Examples: Lanolin, Cold Cream
1. Emollient
2. Occlusive
3. Contain water
4. Some absorb additional water
5. Greasy

Emulsion Bases (O/W Type)
Example: Hydrophilic Ointment
1. Water-washable
2. Nongreasy
3. Can be diluted with water
4. Nonocclusive

Water-Soluble Bases
Example: Polyethylene Glycol Ointment
1. Usually anhydrous
2. Water-soluble and washable
3. Nongreasy
4. Nonocclusive
5. Lipid-free

The selection of the optimum vehicle from the classification above may require compromises so often encountered in drug formulation. For example, stability or drug activity might be superior in a hydrocarbon base, however acceptability is diminished because of the greasy nature of the base. The water-solubility of the polyethylene glycol bases may be attractive, but the glycol(s) may be irritating to traumatized tissue. Drug activity and percutaneous absorption may be superior when using a hydrocarbon base; however, it may be prudent to minimize percutaneous absorption by the use of a less occlusive base.

Ointment Bases

Hydrocarbon Bases

Hydrocarbon bases are usually petrolatum *per se* or petrolatum modified by waxes or liquid petrolatum to change viscosity characteristics. Liquid petrolatum gelled by the addition of a polyethylene resin is also considered a hydrocarbon ointment base, albeit one with unusual viscosity characteristics.

Hydrocarbon ointment bases are classified as oleaginous bases along with bases prepared from vegetable fixed oils or animal fats. Bases of this type include lard, benzoinated lard, olive oil, cottonseed oil, and other oils. Such bases are emollient but generally require addition of antioxidants and other preservatives. They are now largely of historic interest.

Petrolatum USP is a tasteless, odorless, unctuous material with a melting range of 38–60°; its color ranges from amber to white (when decolorized). Petrolatum is often used externally, without modification or added medication, for its emollient qualities.

Petrolatum used as an ointment base has a high degree of compatibility with a variety of medicaments. Bases of this type are occlusive and nearly anhydrous and thus provide optimum stability for medicaments such as antibiotics. The wide melting range permits some latitude in vehicle selection and the USP permits addition of waxy materials as an aid in minimizing temperature effects.

Hydrocarbon bases, being occlusive, increase skin hydration by reducing the rate of loss of surface water. Bases of this kind may be used solely for such a skin-moisturizing effect, eg, white petroleum jelly as noted above. Skin hydration on the other hand may increase drug activity. Studies have indicated that steroids have increased activity, as measured by vasoconstrictor effects, when applied to the skin in a hydrocarbon vehicle. Stoughton consistently found the same steroid more active when applied in a petrolatum vehicle than when applied in a cream (ie, oil-in-water emulsion) vehicle.

A gelled mineral oil vehicle represents a unique addition to this class of bases comprised of refined natural products. Liquid petrolatum may be gelled by addition of a polyethylene. When approximately 5% of low-density polyethylene is added, the mixture heated and then shock-cooled, a soft unctuous, colorless material resembling white petrolatum is produced. The mass maintains unchanged consistency over a wide temperature range. It neither hardens at low temperatures nor melts at reasonably high temperatures. Its useful working range is between −15° and 60°. Excessive heat, ie, above 90°, will destroy the gel structure.

On the basis of *in vitro* studies, drugs may be released faster from the gelled mineral oil vehicle than from conventional petrolatum. This quicker release has been attributed to easier migration of drug particulates through a vehicle which is essentially a liquid, compared with petrolatum.

Despite the advantages hydrocarbon or oleaginous vehicles provide in terms of stability and emolliency such bases have the considerable disadvantage of greasiness. The greasy or oily material may stain clothing and is difficult to remove. In terms of patient acceptance, hydrocarbon bases, ie, ointments, rank well below emulsion bases such as creams and lotions.

Absorption Bases

Absorption bases are hydrophilic, anhydrous materials or hydrous bases that have the ability to absorb additional water. The former are anhydrous bases which absorb water to become water-in-oil emulsions; the latter are water-in-oil emulsions which have the ability to absorb additional water. The word absorption in this connotation refers only to the ability of the base to absorb water. Both types of base are exemplified by Anhydrous Lanolin and Lanolin. The former is converted to the latter by the addition of 30% water. The latter in turn will absorb additional amounts of water.

Hydrophilic Petrolatum USP is an anhydrous absorption base. The water-in-oil emulsifying property is conferred by the inclusion of cholesterol. This composition is a modification of the original formulation which contained anhydrous lanolin. The lanolin was deleted because of reports of allergy; cholesterol was added. Inclusion of stearyl alcohol and wax add to the physical characteristics, particularly firmness and heat stability.

Hydrophilic Petrolatum USP

Cholesterol	30 g
Stearyl Alcohol	30 g
White Wax	80 g
White Petrolatum	860 g
To make	1000 g

Melt the stearyl alcohol and white wax together on a steam bath, then add the cholesterol and stir until it completely dissolves. Add the white petrolatum and mix. Remove from the bath, and stir until the mixture congeals.

Lanolin is a complex mixture of substances. Its ability to absorb water is probably a characteristic of the material rather than a single component. The chemistry of lanolin has been studied in detail. Such studies have resulted in the introduction of a large variety of lanolin derivatives and separated fractions. Available now are lanolin alcohols, dewaxed lanolins, acetylated lanolins, ethoxylated lanolins, hydrogenated lanolins, lanolin esters, and other products. Most of these derivatives have been produced for specific purposes, such as

improved emulsification characteristics or to reduce allergic reactivity.

The specific compounds responsible for lanolin allergy remain unknown; however, the greater portion of lanolin allergens reside in the wool wax alcohols fraction. Thus fractional separation to obtain, for example, the so-called liquid lanolins substantially reduces the incidence of allergic reactions. Given the plethora of lanolin fractions, derivatives, modifications and levels of purity it is quite possible, even likely, that lanolin-sensitive individuals can tolerate specific lanolin products.

Absorption bases, particularly the emulsion bases, impart excellent emolliency and a degree of occlusiveness on application. The anhydrous types can be used when the presence of water would cause stability problems with specific drug substances, eg, antibiotics. Absorption bases are also greasy when applied and are difficult to remove. Both of these properties are, however, less obvious than with hydrocarbon bases.

Commercially available absorption bases include *Aquaphor* (*Beiersdorf*) and *Polysorb* (Fougera). *Nivea Cream* (*Beiersdorf*) is a hydrated emollient base. Absorption bases, either hydrous or anhydrous, are seldom used as vehicles for commercial drug products. The water-in-oil emulsion system is more difficult to deal with than the more conventional oil-in-water systems and there is, of course, reduced patient acceptance because of greasiness.

Water-Removable Bases

Water-washable bases or emulsion bases, commonly referred to as creams, represent the most commonly used type of ointment base. By far the majority of commercial dermatologic drug products are formulated in an emulsion or cream base. Emulsion bases are washable and easily removed from skin or clothing. Emulsion bases can be diluted with water, although such additions are uncommon.

As a result of advances in synthetic cosmetic chemistry the formulator of an emulsion base can be faced with a bewildering variety of selections. Fortunately the emulsion base can be subdivided into three component parts, designated as the oil phase, the emulsifier, and the aqueous phase. The medicinal agent may be included in one of these phases or added to the formed emulsion.

The oil phase, sometimes called the internal phase, is typically made up of petrolatum and/or liquid petrolatum together with one or more of the higher-molecular-weight alcohols, such as cetyl or stearyl alcohol. Stearic acid may be included if the emulsion is to be based on a soap formed *in situ*, eg, triethanolamine stearate. A calculated excess of stearic acid in such a formulation will produce a pearlescent appearance in the finished product.

For drug-delivery vehicles, simplified systems are in order to minimize component interactions, either physical or chemical, and, of course, to minimize cost. Hydrophilic Ointment USP is a typical emulsion base. The composition is as follows:

Hydrophilic Ointment USP

Methylparaben	0.25	g
Propylparaben	0.15	g
Sodium Lauryl Sulfate	10	g
Propylene Glycol	120	g
Stearyl Alcohol	250	g
White Petrolatum	250	g
Purified Water	370	g
To make about	1000	g

Melt the stearyl alcohol and the white petrolatum on a steam bath, and warm to about 75°. Add the other ingredients, previously dissolved in the water and warmed to 75°, and stir the mixture until it congeals.

Stearyl alcohol and petrolatum comprise an oil phase with the proper smoothness and comfort for the skin. Stearyl alcohol also serves as an adjuvant emulsifer. Petrolatum in the oil phase also contributes to the water-holding ability of the overall formulation.

A glance at the cosmetic literature and such volumes as the *Cosmetic Ingredient Dictionary* impresses one with the enormous number and variety of emulsion-base components, particularly oil-phase components. Many of these substances impart subtle but distinct characteristics to cosmetic emulsion systems. While desirable, many of these characteristics are not really necessary in drug dosage forms and delivery systems.

The aqueous phase of an emulsion base usually, but not always, exceeds the oil phase in volume. The aqueous phase contains the preservative materials, the emulsifier or a part of the emulsifier system, and humectant. The last is usually glycerin, propylene glycol, or a polyethylene glycol. The humectant is normally included to minimize water loss in the finished composition. Humectants also add to overall physical product acceptability.

The aqueous phase contains the preservative(s) which are included to control microbial growth. Preservatives in emulsion bases usually include one or more of the following: methylparaben and propylparaben, benzyl alcohol, sorbic acid, or quaternary ammonium compounds. Propylene glycol in sufficient concentration can also function as a preservative. The general subject of preservatives and preservation is discussed elsewhere in this chapter.

The aqueous phase also contains the water-soluble components of the emulsion system, together with any additional stabilizers, antioxidants, buffers, etc. that may be necessary for stability, pH control, or other considerations associated with aqueous systems.

The emulsifier or emulsifier system in a cream formulation is a major consideration. The emulsifier may be nonionic, anionic, cationic or amphoteric.

Anionic Emulsifiers—Sodium lauryl sulfate, the emulsifier in Hydrophilic Ointment USP, is typical of this class. The active portion of the emulsifier is the anion (lauryl sulfate ion). Similar anionic emulsifiers include soaps such as triethanolamine stearate. Soaps, of course, are alkaline and hence incompatible with acids.

Sodium lauryl sulfate and other anionic surfactants of its type are more acid-stable and permit adjustment of the emulsion pH to the desirable acid range of 4.5 to 6.5. As anionic emulsifiers are incompatible with cations, the overall product composition must be kept in mind.

Depending on the chemical type and concentration, anionic surfactants may be irritating in certain situations. It has been reported that percutaneous absorption of certain drugs, notably steroids, may be enhanced by the use of anionic compounds such as sodium lauryl sulfate.

Cationic Emulsifiers—Cationic compounds are highly surface-active but are infrequently used as emulsifiers. The cation portion of the molecule is generally a quaternary ammonium salt including (usually) a fatty acid derivative, eg, dilauryldimethylammonium chloride. Cationics may be irritating to the skin and eyes, and they have a considerable range of incompatibilities, including anionic materials.

The *CTFA Cosmetic Ingredient Dictionary* lists a variety of cationic surfactants under the general title of *Quaternium*. Individual compounds are identified by a numerical suffix, eg, Quaternium-25 is identified as cetylethylmorpholinium ethosulfate.

Nonionic Emulsifiers—Nonionic emulsifiers show no tendency to ionize in solution. This advantage results in excellent pH and electrolyte compatibility in such emulsions. Nonionic emulsifiers range from lipophilic to hydrophilic. The usual emulsifier system may include both a lipophilic and

Table III—Nonionic Emulsifiers[a]

Type	Examples
Polyoxyethylene fatty alcohol ethers	Polyoxyethylene lauryl alcohol
Polyoxypropylene fatty alcohol ethers	Propoxylated oleyl alcohol
Polyoxyethylene fatty acid esters	Polyoxyethylene stearate
Polyoxyethylene sorbitan fatty acid esters	Polyoxyethylene sorbitan monostearate
Sorbitan fatty acid esters	Sorbitan monostearate
Polyoxyethylene glycol fatty acid esters	Polyoxyethylene glycol monostearate
Polyol fatty acid esters	Glyceryl monostearate Propylene glycol monostearate
Ethoxylated lanolin derivatives	Ethoxylated lanolins Ethoxylated cholesterol

[a] From *Cosmetics Science and Technology*, Sec Ed, Vol One, p 205; ed by M S Balsam and Edward Sagarin.

hydrophilic member to produce a so-called hydrophilic-lipophilic balance or HLB.

Many nonionic surfactants are the result of condensation of ethylene oxide groups with a long chain hydrophobic compound. The hydrophilic characteristics of the condensation product are controlled by the number of (usually) oxyethylene groups (OCH_2CH_2). Examples of nonionic surfactants are given in Table III.

Emulsions containing nonionic emulsifiers are usually prepared by dissolving or dispersing the lipophilic component in the oil phase and the hydrophilic component in the aqueous phase. The two phases are then heated separately and combined as described on page 1574. The nonionic emulsifier content of an emulsion may total as much as 10% of total weight or volume. Emulsions based on nonionic emulsifiers are generally low in irritation potential, stable and have excellent compatibility characteristics.

Soaps and detergents, ie, emulsifiers, have, overall, a damaging effect on the skin. Both anionic and cationic surfactants can cause damage to the stratum corneum in direct proportion to concentration and duration of contact. Nonionic surfactants appear to have much less effect on the stratum corneum.

After the proper selection of ingredients the emulsion base is formed by heat and agitation. The oil phase is melted and heated to 75° in a container equipped with a variable speed agitator. The aqueous phase with the emulsifier added is placed in a second container; components are dissolved and the whole heated to 75° or slightly in excess. The aqueous phase is then added slowly with continuous stirring to the oil phase. The first addition should be carried out slowly but continuously with thorough but careful agitation, ie, the emulsion should not be agitated at a rate that incorporates excess air. Progressively slower stirring should be continued during addition of the aqueous phase and until the temperature reaches about 30°. Medicinal agents are usually added after the emulsion has formed and much of the aqueous phase has been added. Drug substances are frequently added as dispersed concentrates in aqueous suspension. Colors and dyes are similarly added as concentrates. Colors are sometimes employed to distinguish different concentrations of the same drug product. Fragrances, if any, are added after the formed emulsion has cooled to about 35°.

Water-Soluble Bases

Soluble ointment bases, as the name implies, are made up of soluble components, or may include gelled aqueous solutions. The latter are often referred to as gels, and in recent years have been formulated specifically to maximize drug availability.

Major components, and in some instances the only components, of water-soluble bases are the polyethylene glycols. These are liquids or waxy solids identified by numbers which are an approximate indication of molecular weight. Polyethylene glycol 400 is a liquid superficially similar to propylene glycol, while polyethylene glycol 4000 is a waxy solid.

Polyethylene glycols have the general chemical formula:

$$HOCH_2(CH_2OCH_2)_n CH_2OH$$

They are nonvolatile, water-soluble or water-miscible compounds, chemically inert, varying in molecular weight from several hundred to several thousand. Patch tests have shown that these compounds are innocuous and continuous use has confirmed their lack of irritation.

Polyethylene glycols of interest as vehicles include the 1500, 1600, 4000, and 6000 products, ranging from soft waxy solids (polyethylene glycol 1500 is similar to petrolatum) to hard waxes. Polyethylene glycol 6000 is a hard wax-like material melting at 58–62°; it is nonhygroscopic.

Polyethylene glycols, particularly 1500, can be used as a vehicle *per se;* however, better results are often obtained by using blends of high- and low-molecular-weight glycols, as in Polyethylene Glycol Ointment USP.

Polyethylene Glycol Ointment USP

Polyethylene Glycol 3350	400 g
Polyethylene Glycol 400	600 g

Heat the two ingredients on a water bath to 65°. Allow to cool and stir until congealed. If a firmer preparation is desired, replace up to 100 g of the polyethylene glycol 400 with an equal amount of polyethylene glycol 3350.

Note—If 6–25% of an aqueous solution is to be incorporated in polyethylene glycol ointment, replace 50 g of the polyethylene glycol 3350 with an equal amount of stearyl alcohol.

The water-solubility of polyethylene glycol vehicles does not insure availability of drugs contained in the vehicle. As hydrated stratum corneum is an important factor in drug penetration, use of polyethylene glycol vehicles which are anhydrous and nonocclusive may actually hinder percutaneous absorption due to dehydration of the stratum corneum.

Aqueous gel vehicles containing water, propylene and/or polyethylene glycol, and gelled with carbopol or a cellulose derivative, are also classed as water-soluble bases. Bases of this kind, sometimes referred to as gels, may be formulated to optimize delivery of a drug, particularly steroids. In such a preparation propylene glycol is used as a steroid solvent as well as an antimicrobial or preservative.

Gelling agents used in these preparations may be nonionic or anionic. Nonionics include cellulose derivatives, such as methylcellulose or hydroxypropyl methylcellulose. These derivatives form gels when dissolved in water but also exhibit the characteristic of reverse solubility. The celluloses are wetted, ie, dispersed in hot water, and then cooled to effect solution. Sodium carboxymethylcellulose is an ionic form of cellulose gelling agent. It is conventionally soluble, and not heat-insoluble.

Carbopol 934 is a white, fluffy, powdered polymeric acid, dispersible but insoluble in water. When the acid dispersion is neutralized with a base a clear, stable gel is formed. Carbopol 934 is physiologically inert and is not a primary irritant or sensitizer.

Another gelling agent is colloidal magnesium aluminum silicate (*Veegum*). It is an inorganic emulsifier and suspending agent, as well as a gelling agent. Veegum dispersions are compatible with alcohols (20–30%), acetone, and glycols. It is frequently employed as a gel stabilizer, rather than as the sole gelling agent.

Sodium alginate and the propylene glycol ester of alginic acid (*Kelcoloid*) are also satisfactory gelling agents. Sodium alginate is a hydrophilic colloid that functions satisfactorily between pH 4.5 and 10; addition of calcium ions will gel fluid solutions of sodium alginate.

Preparation of Ointments

Ointment preparation or manufacture is dependent on the type of vehicle and the quantity to be prepared. The objective is the same, ie, to disperse uniformly throughout the vehicle a finely subdivided or dissolved drug substance(s). Normally the drug materials are in finely powdered form before being dispersed in the vehicle.

Incorporation by Levigation

The preparation of small quantities of ointment by the pharmacist, ie, one to several ounces, can be accomplished by using a spatula and an ointment tile (either porcelain or glass). The finely powdered drug material is thoroughly levigated with a small quantity of the base to form a concentrate. The concentrate is then geometrically diluted with the remainder of the base. Such a procedure is particularly useful with petrolatum or oleaginous bases.

If the drug substance is water-soluble it can be dissolved in water and the resulting solution incorporated into the vehicle using a small quantity of lanolin if the base is oleaginous. Generally speaking, an amount of anhydrous lanolin equal in volume to the amount of water used will suffice.

When ointments are made by incorporation in quantities too large to be handled with a tile and spatula, mechanical mixers are used. Hobart mixers, pony mixers and others of the type are usually used for this purpose. The drug substance in finely divided form is usually added slowly or sifted into the vehicle contained in the rotating mixer. When the ointment is uniform, the finished product may be processed through a roller mill to assure complete dispersion and to reduce any aggregates.

This procedure may be modified by preparing and milling a concentrate of the drug in a portion of the base. The concentrate is then dispersed in the balance of the vehicle, using a mixer of appropriate size. Occasionally the (petrolatum) base may be melted for easier handling and dispersing. In such cases the drug is dispersed and the base slowly cooled using continuous agitation to maintain dispersion.

Preparation of Emulsion Products

Medicated creams and lotions are prepared by means of a two-phase heat system. The oil-phase ingredients are combined in a jacketed tank and heated to about 75°. At this temperature the oil-phase ingredients are liquefied and uniform. In a separate tank the aqueous-phase ingredients, including the emulsifier, are heated together to slightly above 75°. The aqueous phase is then added to the oil phase, slowly and with constant agitation. When the emulsion is formed the mixture is allowed to cool, maintaining slow agitation.

At this stage in the process the medicinal ingredients are usually added as a concentrated slurry, which usually has been milled to reduce any particle aggregates. Volatile or aromatic materials are generally added when the finished emulsion has cooled to about 35°. At this point additional water may be added to compensate for any evaporative losses occurring

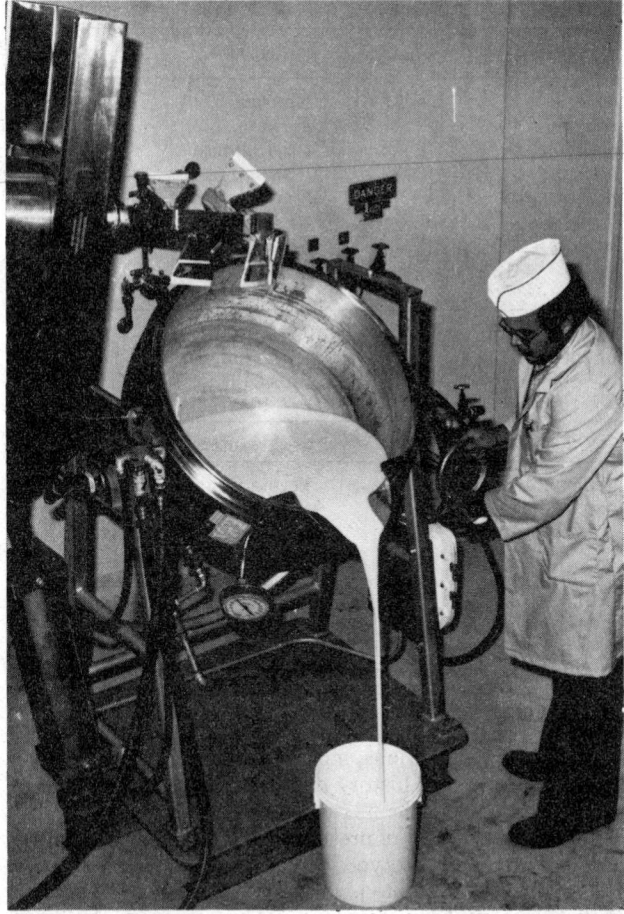

Fig 88-9.   Pilot scale ointment manufacture (courtesy, Alcon Laboratories).

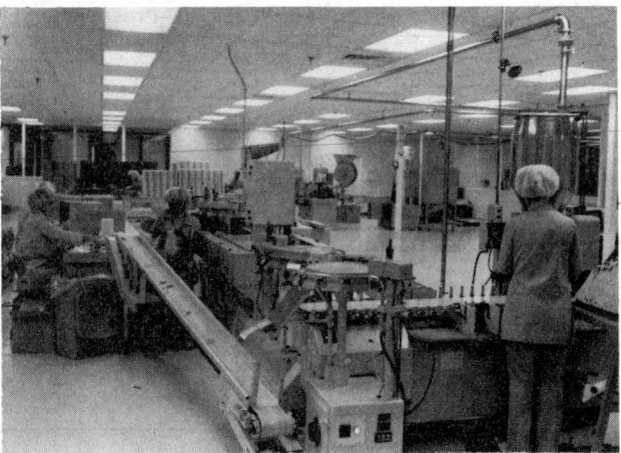

Fig 88-10.   Ointment manufacture and packaging (courtesy, Owen Laboratories).

Preservatives in Ointment Bases

Antimicrobial preservative substances are included in ointment formulations to maintain the potency and integrity of product forms and to protect the health and safety of the consumer.   The USP addresses this subject in its monograph on Microbiological Attributes of Non-Sterile Pharmaceutical Products.   The significance of microorganisms in nonsterile products should be evaluated in terms of the use of the product, the nature of the product and the potential hazard to the user.   The USP suggests that products applied topically should be free from *P aeruginosa* and *S aureus*.

The attributes of an ideal preservative system have been defined by various authors as follows:

1. Effective at relatively low concentrations against a broad spectrum or variety of microorganisms which could cause disease or product deterioration.
2. Soluble in the required concentration.
3. Nontoxic and nonsensitizing at in-use concentrations.
4. Compatible with ingredients of the formulation and package components.
5. Free from objectionable odors and colors.
6. Stable over a wide spectrum of conditions.
7. Inexpensive.

during exposure and transfer at the higher temperatures of emulsion formation.

While the product remains in the tank in bulk, quality-control procedures are carried out, ie, for pH, active ingredients, etc.   If control results are satisfactory the product is filled into the appropriate containers.

Table IV—Topical Preservatives: Benefits and Risks[a]

Preservatives	Limitations Relative to Use in Cosmetic/ Dermatological Formulations
Quaternary ammonium compounds	a) inactivated by numerous ingredients including anionics, nonionics, and proteins
Organic mercurial compounds	a) potentially toxic and may sensitize the skin b) limited use in formulations used near or in the eye
Formaldehyde	a) volatile compound with an objectionable odor b) irritating to the skin c) high chemical reactivity

Halogenated phenols
    hexachlorophene, *p*-chloro-*m*-cresol (PCMC)
    p-chloro-*m*-xylenol (PCMX)
    dichloro-*m*-xylenol (DCMX)
	a) objectionable odor
	b) often inactivated by nonionics, anionics, or proteins
	c) limited gram-negative antibacterial activity

Sorbic acid potassium sorbate	a) pH dependent (can be utilized only in formulations below the pH of 6.5–7.0) b) higher concentrations are oxidized by sunlight resulting in product discoloration c) limited antibacterial activity
Benzoic acid sodium benzoate	a) pH dependent (limited to use in formulations with pH of 5.5 or less) b) replaced by newer antimicrobials because of its limited antimicrobial activity

Dioxin
    Giv-Gard DXN
    (6-acetoxy-2,4-dimethyl-*m*-dioxane)
	a) strong pungent odor which is difficult to mask
	b) may cause darkening or discoloration of protein-containing formulations

[a] From: Lorenzetti OJ, Wernet TC: *Dermatologica 154:* 244, 1977.

Table V—Preservative Effectiveness Test Procedures

	USP XX	CTFA	FDA
Challenge microorganisms	*S aureus* *E coli* *P aeruginosa* *C albicans* *A niger*	*S aureus* *E coli* *P aeruginosa* *C albicans* *A niger* *P luteum* *B subtilis*	*S aureus* *E coli* *P aeruginosa* *P putida* *P multivorans* *Klebsiella* *S marcescens* *C albicans* *A niger*
Inoculum level	1×10^5–1×10^6 cells/mL or gm	1×10^6 cells/mL or gm	0.8–1.2×10^6 cells/mL or gm rechallenge 1–2.0×10^5 vegetative cells
Sampling schedule	0, 7, 14, 21, 28 days	0, 1–2, 7, 14, 28 days	weekly intervals
Standards	Bacteria < 0.1% survival by 14th day. Yeast & molds at or below initial concentration during first 14 days. No increase in organism counts for remainder of 28-day survival	Based on intended use	Vegetative cells < 0.01% survival in 28 days *C albicans* < 1% survival *A niger* < 1% survival Rechallenge 0.1% survival in 28 days

No preservative or preservative system meets these ideal criteria. In fact, preservative substances once considered most acceptable, if not ideal, have recently been questioned. Methylparaben and propylparaben, second and third only to water in frequency of use in cosmetic formulations, have been associated with allergic reactions.

Use of parabens as preservatives in topical products began nearly a half-century ago. Animal testing indicated that they are virtually nontoxic and the compounds, usually in combination, became nearly ubiquitous as preservatives in dermatologic and cosmetic products. In 1968 Schorr was among the first in this country to express concern about contact sensitization to parabens. Other investigators have voiced similar concerns.

The status of parabens was reviewed by Maibach and Marzulli[11] in 1974. These authors stated that on the basis of low index of sensitization by predictive and diagnostic tests as well as clinical impressions, the wide use of parabens, the risk to benefit potential, the low overall toxicity, and new requirements for disclosure labeling, topical parabens do not appear to constitute a significant hazard to the US public.

Maibach and Marzulli made the significant point that "It is hoped that alternatives to the parabens will be carefully studied so that they do not surprise us and prove to be a greater topical or systemic hazard." This statement is particularly pertinent in view of the trend to abandon paraben preservatives in favor of alternatives.

Alternative preservation substances available for use in ointment bases, together with comments on possible limita-tions, are given in Table IV.[14] It is probably sensible to note that, with few exceptions, most of these compounds do not have a half-century history of use nor have had extensive patch-testing experiments carried out.

Following selection of preservative candidates and preparation of product prototypes, the efficacy of the preservative system must be evaluated. A variety of methods to accomplish this have been proposed. The organism challenge procedure is currently the most acceptable. In this procedure the test-product formulation is inoculated with specific levels and types of microorganisms. Preservative efficacy is evaluated on the basis of the number of organisms killed or whose growth is inhibited as determined during a specific sampling schedule. Critical to the organism challenge procedure are the selection of challenge microorganisms, the level of organisms in the inoculum, the sampling schedule, and data interpretation.

Variations of the organism challenge procedure have usually centered around the selection of organisms, the challenge schedule, use of a rechallenge, and standards of effectiveness, ie, cidal activity required rather than static or inhibitory activity.

Given in Table V are the challenge organisms and other criteria used in several preservative challenge procedures.

In addition to efficacy in terms of antimicrobial effects, the preservative system must be assessed in terms of chemical and physical stability as a function of time. This is often done using antimicrobial measurements in addition to chemical analysis.

Safety, Safety Testing, and Toxicity

Safety is defined as the condition of being safe from undergoing (or causing) injury. Safety is not absolute but must be taken in the context of conditions of use. Toxicity refers to a specific substance or product and the adverse effect on a system caused by such a substance or product acting for a given period of time at a specific dose level.

Ointment bases may cause irritant reactions or allergic reactions. Allergic reactions are usually to a specific base component. Irritant reactions are more frequent and more important, hence a number of test procedures have been de-vised to test for irritancy levels, both in the animal and in man. As noted previously, the consequences of species differences and specificity must be included in the evaluation of animal-test results.

Probably the most common irritancy measure is the Draize dermal irritation test in rabbits. In this procedure the test material is applied repeatedly to the clipped skin on the rabbit's back. The test material may be compared with one or more control materials.

End points are dermal erythema and/or edema. By assigning numerical scores for erythema and edema, mathematical and statistical treatment of results is possible.

In the human a variety of test procedures are used to measure irritancy, sensitization potential, and phototoxicity. Among the most common are the following:

21-Day Cumulative Irritation Study

In this test the test compound is applied daily to the same site on the back or volar forearm. Test materials are applied under occlusive tape and scores are read daily. The test application and scoring is repeated daily for 21 days or until irritation produces a predetermined maximum score. Typical erythema scores are as follows:

0 = no visible reaction
1 = mild erythema
2 = intense erythema
3 = intense erythema with edema
4 = intense erythema with edema and vesicular erosion.

Usually 24 subjects are used in this test. Fewer subjects and a shorter application time in days are variants of the test.

Draize-Shelanski Repeat-Insult Patch Test

This test is designed to measure the potential to cause sensitization. The test also provides a measure of irritancy potential. In the usual procedure the test material or a suitable dilution is applied under occlusion to the same site, for 10 alternate-day 24-hour periods. Following a 7-day rest period the test material is again applied to a fresh site for 24 hours. The challenge sites are read on removal of the patch and again 24 hours later. The 0–4 erythema scale is used. A test panel of 100 individuals is common.

Kligman Maximization Test

This test is used to detect the contact sensitizing potential of a product or material. The test material is applied under occlusion to the same site for 48-hour periods. Prior to each exposure the site may be pretreated with a solution of sodium lauryl sulfate under occlusion. Following a 10-day interval the test material is again applied to a different site for 48 hours under occlusion. The challenge site may be treated briefly with a sodium lauryl sulfate solution.

The Maximization test is of shorter duration and makes use of fewer test subjects than the Draize Shelanski test. The use of sodium lauryl sulfate as a pretreatment increases the ability to detect weaker allergens.

The test methods noted above are adequate to detect even weak irritants and weak contact sensitizers. Positive results, however, do not automatically disqualify the use of a substance as unsafe. The actual risk of use depends on concentration, period of use, and skin condition. Benzoyl peroxide in tests such as the Draize Shelanski and Maximization is a potent sensitizer, yet the incidence of sensitization among acne patients is low.

Packaging and Labeling

Ointments are usually packaged in ointment jars or in metal or plastic tubes of a convenient size. Ointment jars are available in one-half to 16-ounce sizes; tubes from 3.5-gram capacity (often ophthalmic) to 4-ounce and on occasion greater capacities.

Ointment Jars—Straight-sided screw cap jars of glass or plastic are available. Clear, amber or opaque glass containers are used; also white, opaque, plastic, usually high-density polyethylene, jars. Metal or composition plastic tops are available, with a variety of inner liners to assure a dust- and air-tight closure. Liners are usually paper or plastic laminates or discs glued or otherwise fitted to the closure.

Ointment jars are filled mechanically to somewhat less than capacity to minimize contact between the ointment and the cap or cap-liner. Ointment jars hand-filled by the pharmacist should also be finished to avoid contact between the ointment and cap. This can be accomplished quite readily by skillful use of a flexible spatula. The spatula is forced across the ointment jar while depressed slightly into the ointment. The result is a conical depression that is esthetically acceptable. Much of the same result can be accomplished by depressing the spatula into the center of the filled jar and gradually rotating the jar against the stationary spatula. Small points perhaps, but time well spent to avoid having part of the ointment-jar contents removed inadvertently by the cap when the patient opens the jar.

Ointment Tubes—Ointment tubes made of tin or aluminum or of an increasing variety of plastic materials are available. The latter are normally polyethylene, polypropylene or other flexible, heat-sealable plastics. Ointment tubes have obvious advantages over jars; use of fingers is minimized, as is dust and air contact, and light exposure.

Depending on the expected shelf life, a number of factors should be considered in selecting an ointment tube. Metal contact and the possibility of metal-ion catalyzed instability must be considered. Conversely, plastic tubes may become stained or discolored by migration of colored materials into the plastic sidewalls of the tube; coal tar in ointment form may cause such discoloration. Tube interactions involving either metal or plastic can be minimized by internal coatings. Such coatings are usually epoxy films that become the primary product contact.

The suitability of ointment containers, either jars or tubes, should be verified by adequate testing prior to use. Compatibility and physical and chemical stability should be established by proper tests before final selection of a jar or tube.

Ointments prepared on prescription can be conveniently filled into a metal ointment tube using the following procedure.

Select an ointment tube of the proper size and remove any lint or dust. Transfer the ointment to a piece of paper of suitable size (use glassine or strong paper). Roll the paper and ointment into a cylinder shape of a diameter slightly less than that of the ointment tube. Insert the rolled paper-ointment cylinder into the ointment tube. The length of the paper cylinder should exceed the tube length. Remove the ointment tube cap and, using a spatula, compress the paper cylinder and tube. Continue compressing the ointment and tube until the ointment appears in the neck-orifice of the open tube. Replace the cap. Using the spatula side as a knife-edge, compress the ointment tube and paper cylinder a reasonable distance from the end of the tube. Holding the spatula firmly in place, the paper cylinder is drawn out, leaving the ointment within the tube.

The ointment tube selected should be of adequate capacity. After compressing the ointment and paper cylinder into the tube the tube should be constricted for cylinder removal at a distance from the end of the tube that will allow at least a double foldover to seal the tube. The fold dimensions are inexact, however, the individual folds on a one-ounce tube are approximately $1/8$ to $3/16$ in. Ointment tube sealing folds can easily be made by folding the tube over on itself using a spatula blade to flatten the tube and to serve as a folding point. Ointment tube clips can be fixed over the tube ends and clamped in place using pliers or a small vise. The sole purpose of folding and clamping is to prevent leakage when routine-use pressure is applied to the tube.

On a larger scale, ointment-tube filling is accomplished using automatic equipment which air-cleans the tubes, fills, folds and crimps the end in one continuous operation. Some equipment will stamp an expiration date onto the crimped surface. In larger scale manufacturing operations plastic tubes are used with increasing frequency. From a filling standpoint plastic tubes are handled much like metal tubes. The final step, however, is a heat seal with no end foldover.

Labeling Ointment Tubes—Attaching labels to ointment tubes is a minor difficulty compounded by the increasing unsightliness characteristic of many ointment tubes during use. The label can become increasingly obliterated, difficult to read and, frequently, lost. As a general rule the label should be attached to itself, ie, it should completely encircle the tube. It should be attached to the tube, affixed close to the neck end.

Given the usual handling of ointment tubes by the patient, it is good practice to dispense the tube in a hinged pasteboard box of convenient size. The box serves to hold and protect the ointment tube as well as to carry the label. The ointment tube is identified with an inked-on prescription number so that both tube and box are identified.

On a manufacturing scale tubes are labeled in a variety of ways. Paper labels may be used, labeling may be silk-screened onto plastic surfaces; expiration dates and code lot numbers may be stamped on as a part of the tube crimping procedure.

Other Medicated Applications

Cataplasms (Poultices)

Poultices represent one of the most ancient classes of pharmaceutical preparations. A poultice, or cataplasm, is a soft moist mass of meal, herbs, seed, etc, usually applied hot in cloth. The consistency is gruel-like, which is probably the origin of the word poultice.

Cataplasms were intended to localize infectious material in the body or to act as counterirritants. The materials tended to be absorptive, which, together with heat accounts for their popular use. None is now official in the Pharmacopeia. The last official product was Kaolin Poultice NF IX.

Pastes

Pastes are concentrates of absorptive powders dispersed (usually) in petrolatum or hydrophilic petrolatum. Pastes are stiff to the point of dryness and reasonably absorptive in view of the petrolatum base. Pastes are often used in the treatment of oozing lesions where they act to absorb serous secretions. Pastes are also used to restrict the area of treatment by acting as an absorbent and physical dam.

Pastes adhere reasonably well to the skin, and are poorly occlusive. For this reason they are suited for application on and around moist lesions. The heavy consistency of pastes imparts a degree of protection and may, in some instances, make the use of bandages unnecessary. Pastes are less macerating than ointments.

Because of their physical properties pastes may be easily removed from the skin by the use of mineral oil or a vegetable oil. This is particularly true when the underlying or surrounding skin is easily traumatized.

An official paste is the conventional Zinc Oxide Paste; another is Triamcinolone Acetonide Dental Paste, for the specialized use the name implies.

Powders

Powders for external use are usually described as dusting powders. Such powders should have a particle size of not more than 150 μm, ie, less than 100-mesh, to avoid any sensation of grittiness which could irritate traumatized skin. Dusting powders usually contain starch, talc, and zinc stearate. Absorbable Dusting Powder USP is comprised of starch treated with epichlorohydrin, with not more than 2.0% mag-nesium oxide added to maintain the modified starch in impalpable powder form; as it is intended for use as a lubricant for surgical gloves it should be sterilized (by autoclaving) and packaged in sealed paper packets.

The fineness of powders is often expressed in terms of mesh size, with impalpable powders generally in the range of 100- to 200-mesh (149–125 μm). Determination of size by mesh analysis becomes increasingly difficult as particle size decreases below 200-mesh.

Dressings

Dressings are external applications resembling ointments usually used as a covering or protection. Petrolatum Gauze is a sterile dressing prepared by adding sterile molten white petrolatum to precut sterile gauze in a ratio of 60 g of petrolatum to 20 g of gauze. Topical antibacterials are available in the form of dressings.

Creams

Creams are viscous liquid or semisolid emulsions of either the oil-in-water or water-in-oil type. Pharmaceutical creams are classified as water-removable bases and are described under Ointments. In addition to ointment bases, creams include a variety of cosmetic-type preparations. Creams of the oil-in-water type include shaving creams, hand creams, foundation creams, etc. Water-in-oil creams include cold creams and emollient creams.

Plasters

Plasters are substances intended for external application made of such materials and of such consistency as to adhere to the skin and attach to a dressing. Plasters are intended to afford protection and support and/or to furnish an occlusive and macerating action and to bring medication into close contact with the skin.

Plasters usually adhere to the skin by means of an adhesive material. The adhesive must bond to the plastic backing and to the skin (or dressing) with proper balance of cohesive strengths. Such a proper balance provides for removal, ie, adhesive breakage at the surface of application thus leaving a clean (skin) surface when the plaster is removed.

Suppositories

Suppositories are solid dosage forms of various weights and shapes, usually medicated, for insertion into the rectum, vagina or the urethra. After insertion, suppositories melt or dissolve in the cavity fluids.

The use of suppositories dates from the distant past, this dosage form being referred to in writings of the early Egyptians, Greeks, and Romans. Suppositories are particularly suited for administration of drugs to the very young and the very old, a notion first recorded by Hippocrates. Despite the antiquity of this dosage form, little was known about drug absorption or drug activity via suppository administration until recent years.

Types

Rectal Suppositories—The USP describes rectal suppositories for adults as tapered at one or both ends and usually weighing about 2 g each. Infant rectal suppositories usually weigh about one-half that of adult suppositories. Drugs having systemic effects, such as sedatives, tranquilizers, and analgesics, are administered by rectal suppository; however, the largest single-use category is probably that of hemorrhoid remedies dispensed over-the-counter. The 2-gram weight for adult rectal suppositories is based on use of cocoa butter as the base; when other bases are used the weights may be greater or less than 2 grams.

Vaginal Suppositories—The USP describes vaginal suppositories as usually globular or oviform and weighing about 5 g each. Vaginal medications are available in a variety of physical forms, eg, creams, gels, liquids, which depart from the classical concept of suppositories. Vaginal tablets, however, do meet the definition, and represent convenience both of administration and manufacture.

Urethral Suppositories—Urethral suppositories are not specifically described in USP, either by weight or dimension. Traditional values, based on use of cocoa butter as base, are as follows for these cylindrical dosage forms: diameter, 5 mm; length, 50 mm female, 125 mm male; weight, 2 g female, 4 g male. Urethral suppositories are an unusual dosage form and are rarely encountered.

Rectal Absorption

Although there are three suppository types, drug absorption for systemic activity is generally limited to rectal administration. As noted previously, the bioavailability of rectally administered drugs is a relatively recent concern. Literature information indicates that rectal drug absorption can be erratic and may be substantially different from absorption following oral administration. With only a few recent exceptions, suppository studies are based on either *in vivo* or *in vitro* data with few attempts to correlate *in vitro* results with *in vivo* studies.

Major factors affecting the absorption of drugs from suppositories administered rectally are the following: anorectal physiology, suppository vehicle, absorption site pH, drug pK_a, degree of ionization, and lipid solubility.

Anorectal Physiology—The rectum is about 150 mm in length, terminating in the anal opening. In the absence of fecal matter the rectum contains a small amount of fluid of low buffering capacity. Fluid pH is said to be about 7.2; because of the low buffer capacity pH will vary with the pH of the drug product or drug dissolved in it. The rectal epithelium is lipoidal in character. The lower, middle and upper hemorrhoidal veins surround the rectum. Only the upper vein passes into the portal system, thus drugs absorbed into the lower and middle hemorrhoidal veins will bypass the liver. Absorption and biological distribution of a drug therefore is modified by its position in the rectum, in the sense that at least a portion of the drug absorbed from the rectum may pass directly into the inferior vena cava, bypassing the liver.

Suppository Vehicle—The ideal suppository base should meet the following general specifications:

1. The base is nontoxic and nonirritating to mucous membranes.
2. The base is compatible with a variety of drugs.
3. The base melts or dissolves in rectal fluids.
4. The base should be stable on storage; it should not bind or otherwise interfere with release and absorption of drug substances.

Absorption Factors—Prior to absorption the administered drug must be in solution. Solution therefore must be preceded by dissolution of the vehicle or melting of the vehicle and subsequent partition of the drug from the vehicle into the rectal fluid.

Rectal suppository bases can be broadly classified into two types. The traditional cocoa butter vehicle is immiscible with aqueous tissue fluids but melts at body temperature. More recently, water-soluble vehicles have been used. Typical of this class is the polyethylene glycol vehicle. Drug absorption from such dissimilar bases can differ substantially. Lowenthal and Borzelleca[15] investigated the absorption of salicylic acid and sodium salicylate administered to dogs. The drugs were formulated in a cocoa butter base and in a base comprised of polyethylene glycol, synthetic glycerides, and a surfactant. Absorption of salicylic acid and sodium salicylate was about equal from the cocoa butter base; however, salicylic acid gave higher plasma levels than sodium salicylate when the glycol base was used.

Parrott[16] compared the absorption of salicylates after rectal and oral administration. Using urinary excretion data both aspirin and sodium salicylate were found to be equally bioavailable orally or rectally. Aspirin was more rapidly released from water-miscible suppositories than from the oily type. Conversely, sodium salicylate was more rapidly released from a cocoa butter vehicle.

Based on available data the bioavailability of a drug from a suppository dosage form is dependent on the physicochemical properties of the drug as well as the composition of the base. The drug dissolution rate and, where appropriate, the partition coefficient between lipid and aqueous phase should be known.

For suppository formulation the relative solubility of the drug in the vehicle is a convenient comparison measure. Lipid-soluble drugs present in low concentration in a cocoa butter base will have little tendency to diffuse into rectal fluids. Drugs that are only slightly soluble in the lipid base will partition readily into the rectal fluid. The partition coefficient between suppository base and rectal fluid thus becomes a useful measure. In water-soluble bases and assuming rapid dissolution, the rate-limiting step in absorption would be transport of the drug through the rectal mucosa.

Clearly the bioavailability of a drug administered rectally depends on the nature of the drug and on the composition of the vehicle or base. The physical properties of the drug can be modified to a degree; so too can the characteristics of the base selected as the delivery system. Preformulation evaluations of physicochemical properties must then be confirmed by *in vivo* studies in animals and ultimately in the primary primate, man.

***In Vivo* Rectal Absorption Studies**—Dogs are probably the animal of choice in evaluating rectal drug availability. (The pig is a closer physiological match but size and manageability argue in favor of the dog.) Blood and urine samples can be obtained from the dog and rectal retention can be accomplished with facility. Smaller animals have been used; rabbits, rats and even mice have been employed but dosing and sampling become progressively more difficult.

Human subjects provide the ultimate measure of drug bioavailability. Subjects are selected on the basis of age, weight, and medical history. Subjects are usually required to fast overnight and evacuate the bowel prior to initiation of the study. Fluid volume and food intake are usually standardized in studies of this kind.

Given the difficulty of standardizing pharmacologic end points the usual measure of rectal drug bioavailability is the concentration of the drug in blood and or urine as a function of time. A control group using oral drug administration provides a convenient means of comparing oral and rectal drug availability. Such a comparison is particularly meaningful in view of uncertainties and conflicts encountered in the literature. While there is general agreement about drug absorption from the rectum there is less agreement on dosage adequacy and the relationship between oral and rectal dosage. This state of affairs argues in favor of adequate studies to establish proper dosage and verify bioavailability.

Suppository Bases

The USP lists the following as usual suppository bases: cocoa butter, glycerinated gelatin, hydrogenated vegetable oils, mixtures of polyethylene glycols of various molecular weights, and fatty acid esters of polyethylene glycol.

Cocoa Butter—Theobroma oil, or cocoa butter, is a naturally occurring triglyceride. About 40% of the fatty acid content is unsaturated. As a natural material there is considerable batch-to-batch variability. A major characteristic of theobroma oil is its polymorphism, ie, its ability to exist in more than one crystal form. While cocoa butter melts quickly at body temperature it is immiscible with body fluids; this may inhibit the diffusion of fat-soluble drugs to the affected sites.

If, in the preparation of suppositories, the theobroma oil is overheated, ie, heated to about 60°, molded and chilled, the suppositories formed will melt below 30°. The fusion treatment of theobroma oil requires maximum temperatures of 40–50° to avoid a change in crystal form and melting point. Theobroma oil, heated to about 60° and cooled rapidly will crystallize in an alpha configuration characterized by a melting point below 30°. The alpha form is metastable and will slowly revert to the beta form with the characteristic melting point approaching 35°. The transition from alpha to beta is slow, taking several days. The use of low heat and slow cooling allows direct crystallization of the more stable beta crystal form.

Certain drugs will depress the melting point of theobroma oil. This involves no polymorphic change although the net effect is similar. Chloral hydrate is the most important of these substances because its rectal hypnotic dose of 0.5 to 1.0 gram will cause a substantial melting-point depression. This effect can be countered by addition of a higher melting wax, such as white wax or synthetic spermaceti. The amount to be added must be determined by temperature measurements. The effect of such additives on bioavailability must also be considered.

Water-soluble or Dispersible Bases—Water-miscible suppository bases are of comparatively recent origin. The majority are comprised of polyethylene glycols or of glycol-surfactant combinations. Water-miscible suppository bases have the substantial advantage of lack of dependence on a melting point approximating body temperature. Problems of handling, storage and shipping are considerably simplified.

Polymers of ethylene glycol are available as polyethylene glycol polymers (Carbowax, polyglycols) of assorted molecular weights. Suppositories of varying melting points and solubility characteristics can be prepared by blending polyethylene glycols of 1000, 4000, or 6000 molecular weight.

Polyethylene glycol suppositories are rather easily prepared by molding. The drug-glycol mixture is prepared by melting and is then cooled to just above the melting point before pouring into dry unlubricated molds. Cooling to near the melting point prevents fissuring caused by crystallization and contraction. Polyethylene glycol suppositories cannot be prepared satisfactorily by hand-rolling.

Water-miscible or water-dispersible suppositories can also be prepared using selected nonionic surfactant materials. Polyoxyl 40 stearate is a white, water-soluble solid melting slightly above body temperature. A polyoxyethylene derivative of sorbitan monostearate is water-insoluble but dispersible. In using surfactant materials the possibility of drug–base interactions must be borne in mind. Interactions caused by macromolecular adsorption may have a significant effect on bioavailability.

Examples of water-miscible suppository bases, devised by Zopf *et al*, are as follows:

Base 1

Polyethylene glycol 1000	96%
Polyethylene glycol 4000	4%

Base 2

Polyethylene glycol 1000	75%
Polyethylene glycol 4000	25%

Base 1 is low-melting and may require refrigeration; Base 2 is more heat-stable. Each is conveniently prepared by molding techniques.

Water-dispersible bases may include polyoxyethylene sorbitan fatty acid esters. These are either soluble (Tween, Myrj) or water-dispersible (Arlacel), used alone or in combination with other wax or fatty materials. Surfactants in suppositories should be used only with recognition of reports that such materials may either increase or decrease drug absorption.

Glycerinated Gelatin—Glycerinated gelatin is usually used as a vehicle for vaginal suppositories. For rectal use a firmer suppository can be obtained by increasing the gelatin content. Glycerinated gelatin suppositories are prepared by dissolving or dispersing the drug substance in enough water to equal 10% of the final suppository weight. Glycerin (70%) is then added and Pharmagel A or B (20%), depending on the drug compatibility requirements. Pharmagel A is acid in reaction, Pharmagel B is alkaline. Glycerinated gelatin suppositories must be formed by molding. The mass cannot be processed by hand-rolling. These suppositories, if not for immediate use, should contain a preservative such as methylparaben and propylparaben.

Preparation of Suppositories

Suppositories are prepared by rolling or hand-shaping, by molding (fusion), and by cold compression.

Rolled (Hand-Shaped) Suppositories—Hand-shaping suppositories is the oldest and the simplest method of preparing this dosage form. The manipulation requires considerable skill, yet avoids the complications of heat and mold preparation.

The general process can be described as follows:

General Process

Take the prescribed quantity of the medicinal substances and a sufficient quantity of grated theobroma oil. In a mortar reduce the medicating ingredients to a fine powder, or, if composed of extracts, soften with diluted alcohol and rub until a smooth paste is formed; the correct amount of grated theobroma oil is then added, and a mass resembling a pill mass is made by thoroughly incorporating the ingredients with a pestle, sometimes with the aid of a small amount of wool fat. When the mass has become plastic under the vigorous kneading of the pestle, it is quickly loosened from the mortar with a spatula, pressed into a roughly shaped mass in the center of the mortar, and then transferred with the spatula to a piece of filter paper which is kept between the mass and the hands during the kneading and rolling procedure. By quick, rotary movements of the hands, the mass is rolled to a ball which is immediately placed on a pill tile. A suppository cylinder is formed by rolling the mass on the tile with a flat board, partially aided by the palm of the other hand, if weather conditions permit. The suppository "pipe" will frequently show a tendency to crack in the center, developing a hollow core. This occurs when the mass has not been kneaded and softened sufficiently, with the result that the pressure of the roller board is not carried uniformly throughout the mass but is exerted primarily on the surface. The length of the cylinder usually corresponds to about four spaces on the pill tile for each suppository, thus making the piece, when cut, practically a finished suppository except for the shaping of the point. When the cylinder has been cut into the proper number of pieces with a spatula, the conical shape is given it by rolling one end on the tile with a spatula, or in some cases even by shaping it with the fingers to produce a rounded point.

Compression-Molded Suppositories—This method of suppository preparation also avoids heat. The suppository mass, such as a mixture of grated theobroma oil and drug, is forced into a mold under pressure, using a wheel-operated press. The mass is forced into mold openings, pressure is then released, the mold removed, opened and replaced. On a large scale cold-compression machines are hydraulically operated, water-jacketed for cooling, and screw-fed. Pressure is applied via a piston to compress the mass into mold openings.

Fusion or Melt Molding—In this method the drug(s) is dispersed or dissolved in the melted suppository base. The mixture is then poured into a suppository mold, allowed to cool, and the finished suppositories removed by opening the mold. Using this procedure one to hundreds of suppositories can be made at one time.

Suppository molds are available for the preparation of various types and sizes of suppositories. Molds are made of aluminum alloy, brass or plastic, and are available with from six to several hundred cavities.

Suppositories are usually formulated on a weight basis so that the medication replaces a portion of the vehicle as a function of specific gravity. If the medicinal substance has a density approximately the same as theobroma oil it will replace an equal weight of oil. If the medication is heavier, it will replace a proportionally smaller amount of theobroma oil.

For instance, tannic acid has a density of 1.6 as compared with cocoa butter (see Table VI). If a suppository is to contain 0.1 g tannic acid, then 0.1 g ÷ 1.6 or 0.062 g cocoa butter should be replaced by 0.1 g of drug. If the blank weight of the suppository is 2.0 g, then 2.0 − 0.062 g or 1.938 g cocoa butter is required per suppository. The suppository will actually weigh 1.938 g + 0.1 g or 2.038 g. Table VI indicates the density factor, or the density as compared with cocoa butter, of many substances used in suppositories.

It is always possible to determine the density of a medicinal substance relative to cocoa butter, if the density factor is not available, by mixing the amount of drug for one or more suppositories with a small quantity of cocoa butter, pouring the mixture into a suppository mold and carefully filling the mold with additional melted cocoa butter. The cooled suppositories are weighed providing data from which a working formula can be calculated as well as the density factor itself.

When using suppository bases other than cocoa butter, such as a polyethylene glycol base, it is necessary to know either the density of the drug relative to the new base or both the densities of the drug and the new base relative to cocoa butter. The density factor for a base other than cocoa butter is simply the ratio of the blank weight of the base and cocoa butter.

For instance, if a suppository is to contain 0.1 g tannic acid in a polyethylene glycol base, then 0.1 g ÷ 1.6 × 1.25 or 0.078 g polyethylene glycol base should be replaced by 0.1 g drug (the polyethylene glycol base is assumed to have a density factor of 1.25). If the blank weight is 1.75 g for the polyethylene glycol base, then 1.75 g − 0.078 g or 1.672 g of base is required per suppository. The final weight will be 1.672 g base + 0.1 g drug or 1.772 g.

When the dosage and mold calibration are complete the drug–base mass should be prepared using minimum heat. A water bath or water jacketing is usually used. The melted mass should be stirred constantly but slowly to avoid air entrapment. The mass should be poured into the mold openings slowly. Prelubrication of the mold will depend on the vehicle.

Table VI—Density Factors for Cocoa Butter Suppositories [a]

Medication	Factor
Acid, boric	1.5
Acid, benzoic	1.5
Acid, gallic	2.0
Acid, salicylic	1.3
Acid, tannic	1.6
Alum	1.7
Aminophylline	1.1
Aminopyrine	1.3
Aspirin	1.3
Barbital	1.2
Belladonna extract	1.3
Bismuth carbonate	4.5
Bismuth salicylate	4.5
Bismuth subgallate	2.7
Bismuth subnitrate	6.0
Castor oil	1.0
Chloral hydrate	1.3
Cocaine hydrochloride	1.3
Digitalis leaf	1.6
Glycerin	1.6
Ichthammol	1.1
Iodoform	4.0
Menthol	0.7
Morphine hydrochloride	1.6
Opium	1.4
Paraffin	1.0
Peruvian Balsam [b]	1.1
Phenobarbital	1.2
Phenol [b]	0.9
Potassium bromide	2.2
Potassium iodide	4.5
Procaine	1.2
Quinine hydrochloride	1.2
Resorcinol	1.4
Sodium bromide	2.3
Spermaceti	1.0
Sulfathiazole	1.6
Tannic acid	1.6
White wax	1.0
Witch hazel fluidextract	1.1
Zinc oxide	4.0
Zinc sulfate	2.8

[a] Davis H: *Bentley's Textbook of Pharmaceutics*, 5th ed, Williams & Wilkins, Baltimore, 1949; Büchi J. *Pharm Acta Helv 20:* 403, 1940.
[b] Density adjusted taking into account white wax in mass.

Mineral oil or tincture of green soap are good lubricants for cocoa butter suppositories. Molds should be dry for polyethylene glycol suppositories.

After pouring into tightly clamped molds the suppositories and mold are allowed to cool thoroughly using refrigeration on a small scale or refrigerated air on a larger scale. After thorough chilling any excess suppository mass should be removed from the mold by scraping, the mold opened and the suppositories removed. It is important to allow cooling time adequate for suppository contraction. This aids in removal and minimizes splitting of the finished suppository.

Packaging and Storage—Suppositories are usually packaged in partitioned boxes which hold the suppositories upright. Glycerin and glycerinated gelatin suppositories are often packaged in tightly closed screw-capped glass containers. Many commercial suppositories are wrapped individually in aluminum foil. In Europe, where suppositories are a more common dosage form, technology has progressed to the point where the final package and the mold are one and the same, formed of non-reactive plastic.

Suppositories with low-melting ingredients are best stored in a cool place. Theobroma oil suppositories in particular should be refrigerated.

In large-scale operations suppositories are wrapped indi-

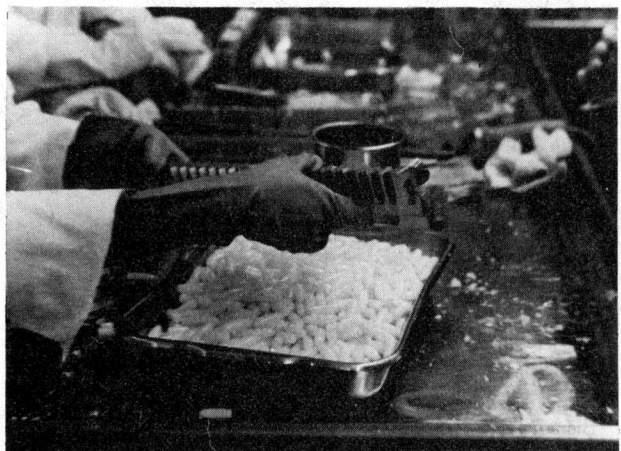

Fig 88-11. Removing cocoa butter suppositories from mold (courtesy, Webcon Division, Alcon Laboratories).

vidually or separated in foil packs. Individual wrapping may vary from the twisted end paper wrap, ie, candy wrapping, to the more familiar aluminum foil or PVC-polyethylene strip packaging.

The most recent innovation in suppository manufacture is the procedure for molding the suppository directly into its primary packaging. In this operation the form into which the suppository mass flows consists of a series of individual molds formed from plastic or foil. After the suppository is poured and cooled the excess is trimmed off and the units are sealed and cut into 3's or 6's as desired. Cooling and final cartoning can then be carried out.

Contraceptives

In the context of this chapter contraceptives are considered in the form of creams, jellies or aerosol foams intended for vaginal use to protect against pregnancy. Contraceptive creams and jellies are designed to melt or spread, following insertion, over the vaginal surfaces. These agents act to immobilize spermatozoa.

Creams and jellies for contraceptive use may contain spermicidal agents such as phenylmercuric nitrate or they may function by a specific pH effect. A pH of 3.5 or less has an appreciable spermicidal effect. It is important to note that a final *in situ* pH of 3.5 or less is required, thus the dilution effect and pH change brought about by vaginal fluids must be considered. To achieve the proper pH effect and control, buffer systems composed of acid and acid salts such as lactates, acetates and citrates are frequently used. The user must, of course, be assured of the safety, lack of irritancy, acceptability, and effectiveness of such products; also, detailed and specific information and instructions should be available to physicians.

References

1. Feldmann RJ, Maibach HI: *J Invest Derm 52:* 89, 1969.
2. Scheuplein RJ, Ross LW: *Ibid. 63:* 353, 1974.
3. Franz TJ: *Ibid. 64:* 191, 1975.
4. Bartek MJ, La Bodde JA, Maibach HI: *Ibid. 58:* 114, 1972.
5. Wester RC, Maibach HI: *Ibid. 67:* 518, 1976.
6. Stoughton RB: In *Animal Models in Dermatology,* edited by Maibach HI, p 121, Churchill Livingstone, Edinburgh, 1975.
7. Mershon MM, Callahan, JF: *Ibid.* p. 36.
8. Lorenzetti OJ: *Ibid* p 212.
9. Ostrenga J, Steinmetz C, Poulsen B: *J Pharm Sci 60:* 1175, 1971.
10. Scheuplein RJ, Ross LW: *J Soc Cos Chem 21:* 853, 1970.
11. Maibach HI, Marzulli FN: *Intl J Derm 13:* 397, 1974.
12. Christophers E, Kligman AM: In *Advances in the Biology of Skin,* vol. 6, edited by Montagna W, p 163, Pergamon Press, Oxford, 1965.
13. Sloan KB, Bodor N: *Int J Pharmaceut 12:* 299, 1982.
14. Lorenzetti OJ, Wernet TC: *Dermatologica 154:* 244, 1977.
15. Lowenthal W, Borzelleca JF: *J Pharm Sci 54:* 1790, 1965.
16. Parrott EL: *J Pharm Sci 60:* 867, 1971.

Bibliography

Montagna W, Parrakkal PF: *The Structure and Function of the Skin,* 3rd ed, Academic Press, New York, 1974.
Cosmetic Ingredient Dictionary, 2nd ed, The Cosmetic, Toiletry and Fragrance Assoc, 1977.
Hoover JE, ed: *Dispensing of Medication,* 8th ed, Mack Publishing Co, Easton, PA, 1976.
Maibach HI: *Animal Models in Dermatology,* Churchill Livingstone, Edinburgh, 1975.
Marples MJ: *The Ecology of the Human Skin,* Charles Thomas, Springfield, IL, 1965.
Frost P, Gomez EC, Zaias N: *Recent Advances in Dermatopharmacology,* Spectrum Publications, New York, 1978.
Mier PD, Cotton DWK: *The Molecular Biology of Skin,* Blackwell Scientific Publications, Oxford.
Chien YW: *Novel Drug Delivery Systems,* Marcel Dekker, New York, 1982.

CHAPTER 89

Powders

Edward G Rippie, PhD

Professor of Pharmaceutics
College of Pharmacy, University of Minnesota
Minneapolis, MN 55455

Powders are encountered in almost every aspect of pharmacy, both in industry and in practice. Drugs and other ingredients, when they occur in the solid state in the course of being processed into a dosage form, usually are in a more or less finely divided condition. Frequently this is a powder whose state of subdivision is critical in determining its behavior both during processing and in the finished dosage form. Apart from their use in the manufacture of tablets, capsules, suspensions, etc, powders also occur as a pharmaceutical dosage form. While use of powders as a dosage form has declined, the properties and behavior of finely divided solids material are of considerable importance in pharmacy.

This chapter is intended to provide an introduction to the fundamentals of powder mechanics and to the primary means of powder production and handling. The relationships of the principles of powder behavior to powders as dosage forms are discussed.

Production Methods

Molecular Aggregation

Precipitation and Crystallization—These two processes are fundamentally similar and depend on achieving three conditions in succession: (1) a state of supersaturation (supercooling in the case of crystallization from a melt), (2) formation of nuclei, and (3) growth of crystals or amorphous particles.

Supersaturation can be achieved through evaporation of solvent from a solution, cooling of the solution if the solute has a positive heat of solution, by production of additional solute as a result of a chemical reaction, or by a change in the solvent medium by addition of various soluble secondary substances. In the absence of seed crystals, significant supersaturation is required to initiate the crystallization process through formation of nuclei. A nucleus is thought to consist of from ten to a few hundred molecules having the spatial arrangement of the crystals that will ultimately be grown from them. Such small particles are shown by the Kelvin equation to be more soluble than large crystals and, therefore, to require supersaturation, relative to large crystals, for their formation and subsequent growth. It is a gross oversimplification to assume that, for a concentration gradient of a given value, the rate of crystallization is the negative of the rate of dissolution. The latter is generally somewhat greater.

Depending on the conditions of crystallization, it is possible to control or modify the nature of the crystals obtained. When polymorphs exist, careful temperature control and seeding with the desired crystal form are often necessary. The habit or shape of a given crystal form is often highly dependent on impurities in solution, pH, rate of stirring, rate of cooling, and the solvent. Very rapid rates of crystallization can result in impurities being included in the crystals by entrapment.

Spray Drying—Atomization of a solution of one or more solids *via* a nozzle, spinning disk, or other device, followed by evaporation of the solvent from the droplets is termed spray drying. The nature of the powder that results is a function of several variables, including the initial solute concentration, size distribution of droplets produced, and rate of solvent removal. The weight of a given particle is determined by the volume of the droplet from which it was derived and by the solute concentration. The particles produced are aggregates of primary particles consisting of crystals and/or amorphous solids, depending on the rate and conditions of solvent removal. This approach to the powdered state provides the opportunity to incorporate multiple solid substances into individual particles at a fixed composition, independent of particle size, and avoiding difficulties that can arise in attempting to obtain a uniform mixture of several powdered ingredients by other procedures.

Particle Size Reduction

Comminution in its broadest sense is the mechanical process of reducing the size of particles or aggregates. Thus, it embraces a wide variety of operations including cutting, chopping, crushing, grinding, milling, micronizing, and trituration, which depend primarily on the type of equipment employed. The selection of equipment in turn is determined by the characteristics of the material, the initial particle size, and the degree of size reduction desired. For example, very large particles may require size reduction in stages simply because the equipment required to produce the final product will not accept the initial feed, as in crushing prior to grinding. In the case of vegetable and other fibrous material, size reduction generally must be, at least initially, accomplished by cutting or chopping. Chemical substances used in pharmaceuticals, in contrast, generally need not be subjected to either crushing or cutting operations prior to reduction to the required particle size. However, these materials do differ considerably in melting point, brittleness, hardness, and moisture content, all of which affect the ease of particle size reduction and dictate the choice of equipment. The heat generated in the mechanical grinding, in particular, presents problems with materials which tend to liquefy or stick together and with the thermolabile products which may degrade unless the heat is dissipated by use of a flowing stream of water or air. The desired particle size, shape, and size distribution must also be considered in the selection of grinding or milling equipment. For example, attrition mills tend to produce spheroidal, more free-flowing particles than do impact-type mills, which yield more irregular-shaped particles.

Fracture Mechanics—Reduction of particle size through fracture requires application of mechanical stress to the material to be crushed or ground. Materials respond to stress by yielding, with consequent generation of strain. Depending on the time course of strain as a function of applied stresses, materials can be classified according to their behavior over a continuous spectrum ranging from brittle to plastic. In the case of a totally brittle substance, complete rebound would occur on release of applied stress at stresses up to the yield point, where fracture would occur. In contrast, a totally plastic material would not rebound nor would it fracture. The vast majority of pharmaceutical solids lie somewhere between these extremes and thus possess both elastic and viscous properties. Linear and, to a lesser extent, nonlinear viscoelastic theory has been well developed to account for quantitatively and explain the simultaneous elastic and viscous deformations produced in solids by applied stresses.

The energy expended by comminution ultimately appears as surface energy associated with newly created particle surfaces, internal free energy associated with lattice changes, and as heat. Most of the energy expressed as heat is consumed in the viscoelastic deformation of particles, friction, and in imparting kinetic energy to particles. Energy is exchanged among these modes and some is, of course, effective in producing fracture. It has been estimated that 1% or less of the total mechanical energy used is associated with newly created surface or with crystal lattice imperfections.

While the grinding process has been described mathematically, the theory of grinding has not been developed to the point where the actual performance of the grinding equipment can be predicted quantitatively. However, three fundamental laws have been advanced:

Kick's Law—The work required to reduce the size of a given quantity of material is constant for the same reduction ratio regardless of the original size of the initial material.

Rittinger's Law—The work used for particulate size reduction is directly proportional to the new surface produced.

Bond's Law—The work used to reduce the particle size is proportional to the square root of the diameter of the particles produced.

In general, however, these laws have been useful only in providing trends and qualitative information on the grinding process. Usually laboratory testing is required to evaluate the performance of particular equipment. A work index, developed from Bond's Law, is a useful way of comparing the efficiency of milling operations.[1] A grindability index, which has been developed for a number of materials, also can be used to evaluate mill performance.[2]

A number of other factors must also be considered in equipment selection. Abrasion or mill wear is an important factor in the grinding of hard materials, particularly in high-speed, close-clearance equipment (eg, hammer mills). In some instances mill wear may be so extensive as to lead to highly contaminated products and excessive maintenance costs that make the milling process uneconomical. Hardness of the material, which is often related to abrasiveness, must also be considered. This is usually measured on the Moh's Scale. Qualitatively, materials from 1 to 3 are considered as soft and from 8 to 10 as hard. Friability (ease of fracture) and fibrousness can be of equal importance in mill selection. Fibrous materials, eg, plant products, require a cutting or chopping action and cannot usually be reduced in size effectively by pressure or impact techniques. A moisture content above about 5% will in most instances also create a problem and can lead to agglomeration or even liquefaction of the milled material. Hydrates will often release their water of hydration under the influence of a high-temperature milling process and thus may require cooling or low-speed processing.

Methods and Equipment—When a narrow particle size distribution with a minimum of fines is desired, closed-circuit milling is advantageous. This technique combines the milling equipment with some type of classifier (see *Particle Size Measurement and Classification*). In the simplest arrangement, a screen is used to make the separation, and the oversize particles are returned to the mill on a continuous basis while the particles of the desired size pass through the screen and out of the grinding chamber. Overmilling, with its subsequent production of fines, is thereby minimized.

In order to avoid contamination or deterioration, the equipment used for pharmaceuticals should be fabricated of

materials which are chemically and mechanically compatible with the substance being processed. The equipment should be readily disassembled for ease in cleaning to prevent cross-contamination. Dust-free operation, durability, simplified construction and operation, and suitable feed and outlet capacities are additional considerations in equipment selection.

While there is no rigid classification of large-scale comminution equipment, it generally is divided into three broad categories based on feed and product size:

1. *Coarse crushers* (eg, jaw; gyratory; roll and impact crushers).
2. *Intermediate grinders* (eg, rotary cutters; disk; hammer, roller, and chaser mills).
3. *Fine grinding mills* (eg, ball, rod, hammer, colloid, and fluid energy mills; high-speed mechanical screen and centrifugal classifier).

Machines in the first category are ordinarily employed where the size of the feed material is relatively large, ranging from $1\frac{1}{2}$ to 60″ in diameter. These are used most frequently in the mineral crushing industry and will not be considered further. The machines in the second category are used for feed materials of relatively small size and provide products which fall between 20- and 200-mesh. Those in the third category produce particles, most of which will pass through a 200-mesh sieve, though, often the particle size of the products from fine grinding mills is well into the micron range.

The comminution effect of any given operation can be described mathematically in terms of a matrix whose elements represent the probabilities of transformation of the various-size particles in the feed material to the particle sizes present in the output. The numerical values of the elements in the transition matrix can be determined experimentally and the matrix serves to characterize the mill. Matrices of this type are frequently a function of feed rate and feed particle size distribution but are useful in predicting mill behavior. Multiplication of the appropriate comminution matrix with the feed size distribution line-matrix yields the predicted output size distribution.

Intermediate and Fine Grinding Mills—The various types of comminuting equipment in this class generally employ one of three basic actions or, more commonly, a combination of these actions.

1. *Attrition*—This involves breaking down of the material by a rubbing action between two surfaces. The procedure is particularly applicable to the grinding of fibrous materials where a tearing action is required to reduce the fibers to powder.
2. *Rolling*—This uses a heavy rolling member to crush and pulverize the material. Theoretically, only a rolling-crushing type of action is involved, but in actual practice some slight attrition takes place between the face of the roller and the bed of the mill.
3. *Impact*—This involves the operation of hammers (or bars) at high speeds. These strike the lumps of material and throw them against each other or against the walls of the containing chamber. The impact causes large particles to split apart, the action continuing until small particles of required size are produced. In some instances high-velocity air or centrifugal force may be utilized to generate high impact velocities.

Roller Mills in their basic form consist of two rollers revolving in the same direction at different rates of speed. This principle, which provides particle size reduction mainly through compression (crushing) and shear has been applied to the development of a wide variety of roller mills. Some use multiple smooth rollers or corrugated, ribbed, or saw-toothed rollers to provide a cutting action. Most allow adjustment of the gap between rollers to control the particle size of the product. The roller mill is quite versatile and can be used to crush a variety of materials.

Hammer Mills consist of a rotating shaft on which are mounted either rigid or swing hammers (beaters). This unit is enclosed with a chamber containing a grid or removable screen through which the material must pass. On the upper part is the feed hopper. As the material enters the chamber, the rapidly rotating hammers strike against it and break it into

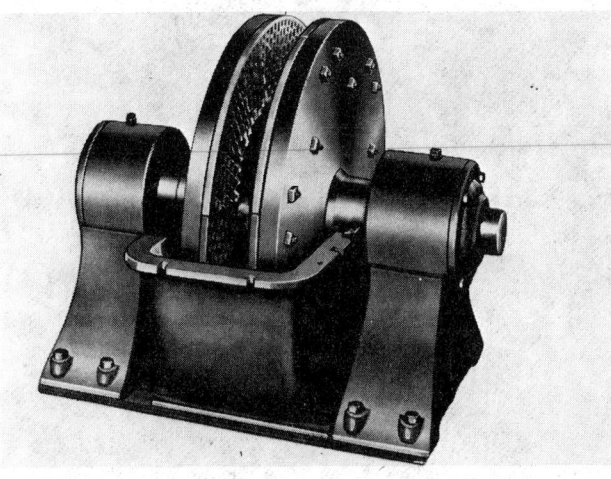

Fig 89-1. Sprout-Waldron double attrition mill.

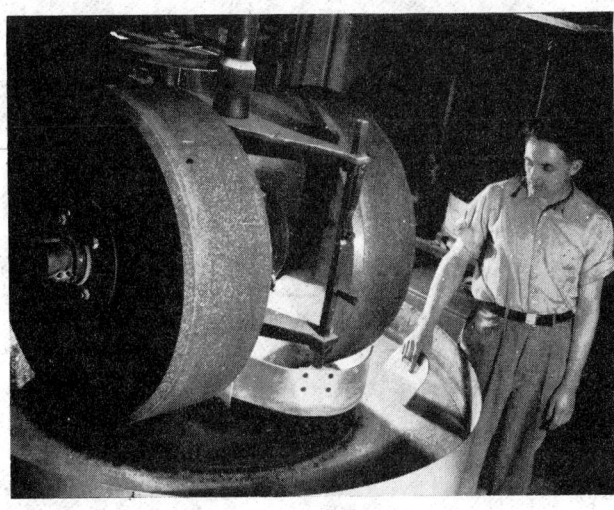

Fig 89-2. Chaser mill (courtesy, MSD).

smaller fragments. These are swept downward against the screen where they undergo additional "hammering" action until they are reduced to a size small enough to pass through the openings and out. Oversize particles are hurled upward into the chamber where they also undergo further blows by the revolving hammers.

These mills operate at high speed and generally with controlled feed rate. Both impact and attrition provide the grinding action. Particle size is regulated by rotor speed, feed rate, type and number of hammers, clearance between hammers and chamber wall, and discharge openings. The higher the speed, the steeper the approach angle of the particle to the screen hole. Thus, for any screen size opening, the higher the blade speed, the smaller the particle obtained. Increasing the screen thickness will have a similar effect. In general flat-edged blades are most effective for pulverizing, while sharp-edged blades will act to chop or cut fibrous materials.

A wide range of particle sizes down to the micron size can be produced by these mills. The particle shape, however, is generally sharper and more irregular than that produced by compression methods. When very fine particles are desired, hammer mills can be operated in conjunction with an air classifier. Under such conditions a narrower particle size distribution and lower grinding temperatures are obtained. Fine pulverizing of plastic material can be accomplished in these mills by embrittlement with liquid N_2 or CO_2 or by jacketing the grinding chamber.

Cutter Mills are useful in reducing the particle size of fibrous material and act by a combined cutting and shearing action. They consist of a horizontal rotor in which are set a series of knives or blades. This rotor turns within a housing into which are set stationary bed knives. The feed is from the top and a perforated plate or screen is set into the bottom of the housing through which the finished product is discharged. The particle size and shape is determined by the plate size, gap between rotor and bed knives, and size of the openings. A number of rotor styles are available to provide different particle shapes and sizes, though cutter mills are normally not designed to produce particles finer than 80 to 100 mesh.

Attrition Mills make use of two stone or steel grinding plates, one or both of which revolve to provide grinding mainly through attrition. These mills are most suitable for friable or medium-hard, free-flowing material.

The Sprout-Waldron double runner attrition mill (Fig 89-1) is an example of a mill which utilizes two rotating disks revolving in opposite directions. The particle size reduction is controlled by varying the speed at which the disks revolve, the space between the disks, and the size and number of ridges and indentations in the face of the disks. By using other plates and shell construction, these mills can be adapted for

coarse granulating, pulverizing, shredding, and cutting. Projecting spikes, when added to the rotating plates to mesh with spikes on the stationary plate, provide a milling action that is similar to that obtained with a hammer mill. By appropriate combination with a classifier, particle sizes ranging from 10 mesh to 20 μm can be obtained by these attrition mills.

Chaser Mills are so called because two heavy granite stones, mounted vertically like wheels and connected by a short horizontal shaft, are made to revolve or *chase* each other upon a granite base (Fig 89-2). In practice chasers are enclosed in a tight box or small room with airtight doors and the substances to be powdered are fed in from the top by an elongated funnel, the spout of which delivers the material in the path of the stones. The height of a curb in the mill may be increased and the fineness of the powder thereby influenced by its height. Revolution of the chasers produces an upward current of air; this carries over the lighter particles, which fall outside the curb and are subsequently collected as a fine powder.

Pebble or Ball Mills, sometimes called "pot mills" or "jar mills," are operated on the principle of attrition and impact, the grinding being effected by placing the substance in jars or cylindrical vessels, lined with porcelain or a similar hard substance and containing "pebbles" or "balls" of flint, porcelain, steel, or stainless steel. These cylindrical vessels revolve horizontally on their long axis and the tumbling of the pebbles or balls over one another and against the sides of the cylinder produces pulverization with a minimum loss of material. Ball milling is a relatively slow process and generally requires many hours to produce material of suitable fineness. In order to keep the grinding time within reasonable limits, coarse material (>10-mesh) should be preground before introduction into a ball mill. Fig 89-3 shows a sectional view of a single jar mill. Rod mills are a modification in which rods about 3" shorter than the length of the mill are used in place of balls. This results in a lower production of fines and a somewhat more granular product.

Vibrating Ball Mills, which also combine attrition and impact, consist of a mill shell containing a charge of balls similar to rotating ball mills. However, in this case the shell is vibrated at some suitable frequency, rather than rotated. These mills offer the advantage of being free of rotating parts, and thus can be integrated readily into a particle classifying system or other ancillary equipment. Furthermore, there have been several studies which have demonstrated that the vibrating ball mill will grind at rates often as high as 20 to 30 times that of the conventional tumbling mill and offer a higher order of grinding rate and efficiency than other prevailing milling procedures.

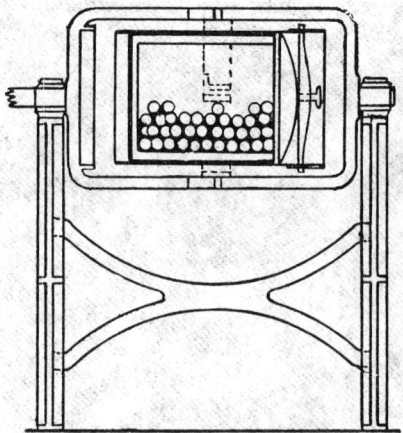

Fig 89-3.   Single jar mill.

Fluid-Energy Mills are used for pulverizing and classifying extremely small particles of many materials. The mills have no moving parts, grinding being achieved by subjecting the solid material to streams of high velocity elastic fluids, usually air, steam or an inert gas. The material to be pulverized is swept into violent turbulence by the sonic and supersonic velocity of the streams. The particles are accelerated to relatively high speeds and when they collide with each other the impact causes violent fracture of the particles.

A schematic representation of one type of fluid-energy mill is shown in Fig 89-4. The elastic grinding fluid is introduced through nozzles in the lower portion of the mill under pressures ranging from 25 to 300 pounds per square inch. In this way, a rapidly circulating flow of gas is generated in the hollow, doughnut-shaped mill. A Venturi feeder introduces the coarse material into the mill and the particles enter into the jet stream of rapidly moving gas. The raw material is quickly pulverized by mutual impact in the reduction chamber. As the fine particles form they are carried upward in the track. Particles are simultaneously ground and classified in this process. The smaller particles are entrapped by the drag of gas leaving the mill and are carried out to a collecting chamber or bag. Centrifugal force at the top of the chamber stratifies the larger, heavy particles and their greater momentum carries them downward and back to the grinding chamber.

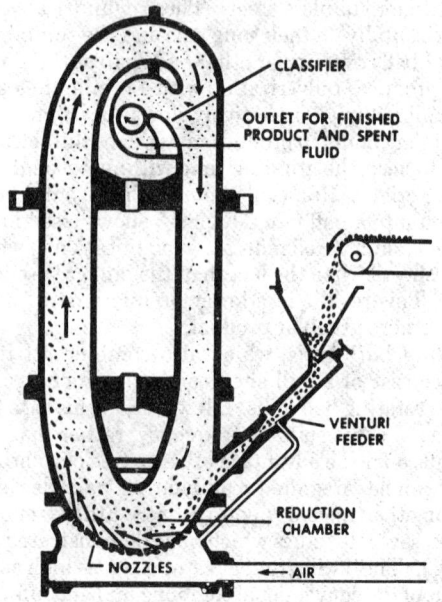

Fig 89-4.   The Jet-O-Mizer fluid energy mill (courtesy, Fluid Energy).

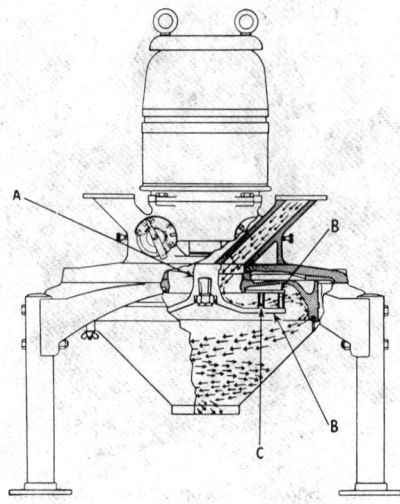

Fig 89-5.   CentriMil, a centrifugal-impact mill, available in models ranging from 2 to 250 hp. A: Spinning rotor; B: rotor hub disks; C: impacters (courtesy, Entoleter).

A major advantage of the fluid-energy mill lies in the fact that the cooling effect of the grinding fluid as it expands in the grinding chamber more than compensates for the moderate heat generated during the grinding process. Another advantage in the use of these mills is the rather narrow range of particle sizes produced. When precise control of particle size is an important factor, the fluid-energy mill produces very narrow ranges of particles with minimum effort.

One major disadvantage is the necessity of controlling the feeding of the coarse, raw material into the jet stream. Often the feeding device becomes clogged by a clump of material, and special feeding devices must be built to produce a uniform rate of feed.

Centrifugal-Impact Pulverizers also have been found to be effective for the reduction of the particle size of a wide variety of materials ranging from very soft organic chemicals to hard abrasive minerals. In addition, this type of mill is well suited for the size reduction of heat-sensitive substances. Basically, in these pulverizers, the material is fed into the center of a spinning rotor which applies a high centrifugal force to the particles. The material, thus accelerated, moves toward the impactor set at the periphery of the rotor. On striking these impactors the material is hurled against the outer casing where final reduction is achieved. Processed material is removed from the bottom of the conical discharge hopper (Fig 89-5). Particle size reduction in the range of 10- to 325-mesh can be obtained with this type of mill with a minimum of fines.

Particle Size Measurement and Classification

Size and Distribution

Statistical Parameters—Monodisperse systems of particles of regular shape, such as perfect cubes or spheres, can be completely described by a single parameter, ie, length of a side or diameter. However, when either nonuniform size distributions or anisometric shapes exist, any single parameter is incapable of totally defining the powder. Measurements must be made over the total range of sizes present. Statistical diameters, for example, are useful measures of central size tendency and are computed from some measured property that is a function of size and related to a linear dimension. For irregular particles the assigned size will be strongly dependent on the method of measurement.

Once a method of assignment of numerical value for the

Table I—Definition of Statistical Diameters*

Type of Mean Diameter	Statistical Definition	Description
Arithmetic	$\Sigma nd/\Sigma n$	Mean diameter weighted by number
Diameter moment	$\Sigma nd^2/\Sigma nd$	Mean diameter weighted by particle diameter
Surface moment	$\Sigma nd^3/\Sigma nd^2$	Mean diameter weighted by particle surface
Volume moment	$\Sigma nd^4/\Sigma nd^3$	Mean diameter weighted by particle volume
Surface	$(\Sigma nd^2/\Sigma n)^{1/2}$	Root mean square
Volume	$(\Sigma nd^3/\Sigma n)^{1/3}$	

* When grouped data are used, n is the number of particles in a size interval characterized by a diameter, d.

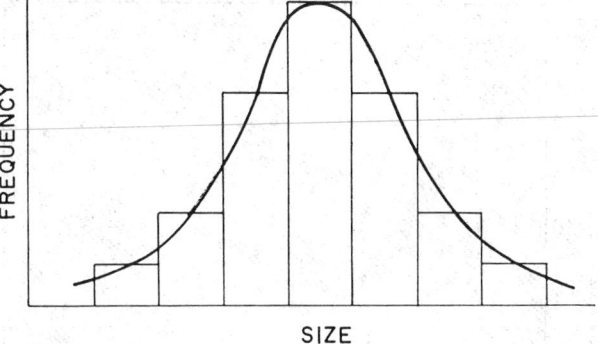

Fig 89-6.   Symmetrical particle size distribution curve.

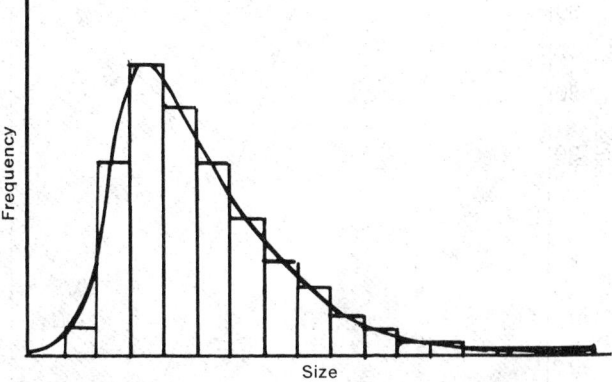

Fig 89-7.   Skewed particle size distribution curve.

diameter, surface area, or other parameter has been established, the average value computed for the parameter is dependent on the weighting given the various sizes. Mean particle diameter is the most important single statistical parameter since, if the proper diameter is chosen, the various other parameters of interest such as specific surface area, number, mean particle weight, etc, often may be calculated. Thus the choice of the mean diameter to be measured or calculated is based on its intended use. For example, specific surface area, which may control drug dissolution, frequently can be related to the root mean square diameter. Depending on the method of measurement, various diameters are obtained; these will be discussed later. The particle diameters most commonly used are listed in Table I.

Size Distributions—As has been pointed out, size distributions are often complex and no single particle size parameter is sufficient to characterize or permit prediction of the many bulk properties of pharmaceutical interest, eg, flow characteristics, packing densities, compressibility, segregation tendencies. Thus, descriptions beyond the central tendency provided by the various mean diameters are needed. These generally take the form of equations or charts that describe in detail the distribution of particle size. In measuring particle size it is important first to select the parameter that is related to the ultimate use of the product, and then select the method that will measure this parameter.

Certainly more useful information would be gained if the particle size of a powder used in a suspension were determined by sedimentation than by microscopy, or if the total surface area of the particles were the critical factor (as in use as an adsorbant) by the more useful method of permeability or gas adsorption.

Particles can be classified by determining the number of particles in successive size ranges. The distribution can be represented by a bar graph or histogram (Fig 89-6), where the widths of the bars represent the size range and the heights represent the frequency of occurrence in each range. A smooth curve drawn through the midpoints of the tops of the bars in this case results in a normal probability size distribution curve. A line drawn through the center of the curve to the abscissa divides the area into two equal parts and represents the mean value. Since a number of other symmetrical distributions could have this same midpoint a term to describe the scatter about the mean value is needed. Standard deviation (the root-mean square deviation about the mean) serves to define the spread of the curve on either side of the midpoint.

Most particulate material cannot, however, be described by a normal distribution curve. The resultant curves are usually skewed as shown in Fig 89-7, making mathematical

analysis complex. In a skewed size distribution the mean value is affected by very large or very small values. In these cases the median (ie, the central value of a series of observations) is a more useful average. In a symmetrical distribution the mean and the median values are the same. Most asymmetrical size distribution curves relating to powders can be converted into symmetrical curves by using the logarithm of the size, ie, Log Normal Distribution curve. The symmetrical shape of the latter curve allows for simplified mathematical analysis.

Cumulative plots are also useful for particle size distribution analysis. Here the cumulative percent of the particles which are finer (or larger) than a given size is plotted against the size. By use of logarithmic–probability paper the median size (geometric mean) and standard deviation (geometric standard deviation) can be readily obtained by graphical solution. The median is the 50% size and the standard deviation is the slope of the line and equal to the ratio 50% size/15.87% size (Fig 89-8).

Size Measurement

Frequently, particle size measurements are made in conjunction with separation of the powder into fractions on the basis of size. Methods that lead primarily to size distribution analysis only are discussed first, followed by methods in which classification by size is a central feature.

The basic processes employed for measurement, classification or fractionation of fine solid particles involve direct and indirect techniques. Direct methods measure the actual dimensions of the particle by use of a calibration scale as in microscopy and sieving. Indirect measurements make use of some characteristic of the particle that can be related to particle size; eg, sedimentation rates, permeability, and optical properties.

Microscopy—Microscopic techniques have been classified as one of the most accurate of *direct* methods. Here, particles

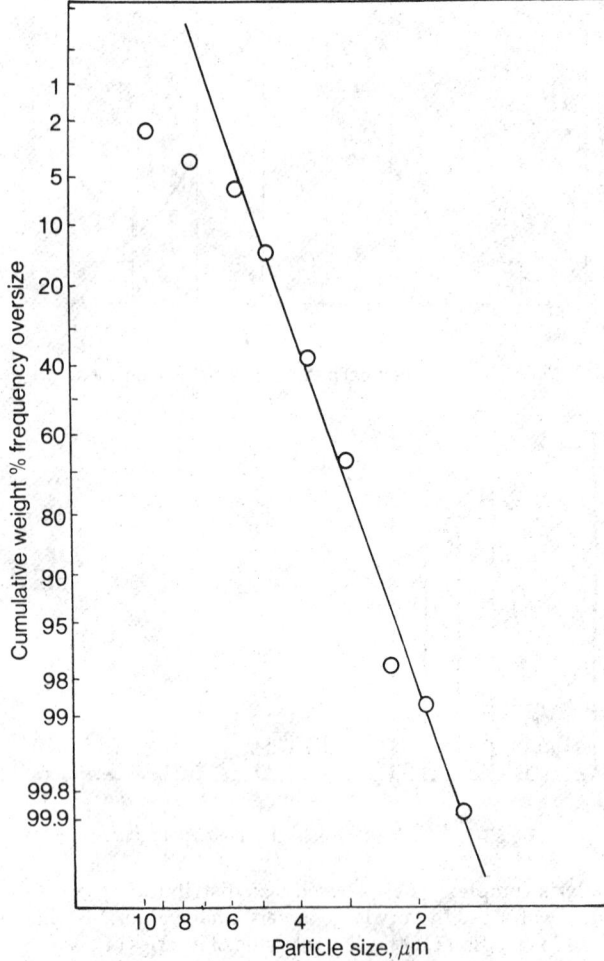

Fig 89-8.   Log-probability plot of particle size vs cumulative weight % frequency oversize.

counting of particles. These are represented by instruments such as the Imanco Quantimet 720 and the πMC System (*Millipore*) which scan the powder image in a manner similar to a TV scanner. The signal obtained is analyzed by a pulse-height analyzer and is expressed as a particle size distribution.

Adsorption of Gases—Adsorption of a solute from solution or of a gas at low temperatures onto powdered material serves as a measure of the particle surface area, generally reported as specific surface (area/unit mass). Common adsorption techniques utilize the adsorption of nitrogen and krypton at low temperatures. The volume of the gas adsorbed by a powdered sample is determined as a function of gas pressure, and an appropriate plot is prepared. The point at which a monomolecular layer of adsorbate occurs is estimated from the discontinuity that shows in the curve. The specific surface area then can be calculated from a knowledge of the volume of gas required to achieve this monolayer, and the area/molecule occupied by the gas, its molecular weight, and density. Frequently, more complex expressions such as the Brunauer, Emmett, and Teller (BET) equation must be used to describe the surface adsorption of some materials, and to determine the volume of gas required to produce an adsorbed monolayer. The surface properties of a number of pharmaceuticals have been investigated by this technique.

Permeability—When a gas or liquid is allowed to flow through a powdered material, the resistance to this flow is found to be a function of such factors as specific surface of the powder, area of the bed, pore space, pressure drop across the bed, and viscosity of the fluid. This resistance can be described and the specific surface calculated by the Kozeny-Carmen equation which relates these factors. This method, while it does not provide a size distribution analysis, does offer a rapid and convenient means of size estimation that is useful for some industrial operations.

Instruments that measure the rate of flow of a gas through a powder bed under controlled pressure differential are available commercially. The Fisher *Sub-Sieve Sizer* permits the reading of average particle size directly. The Blaine *Permeameter* produced by Precision Scientific Company utilizes the principle of filling the void spaces in a powder with mercury and then weighing it. The void fraction is calculated from the known density of mercury at different temperatures.

The calculations involved in permeability techniques are often complicated and yield only an average size of particles. In measuring particles in the subsieve ranges, rather large deviations may be encountered. With larger mesh sizes, some good agreement is found between the results obtained by techniques employing permeability and microscopy, particularly if the powders are made up of spherical or near-spherical particles.

Impaction and Inertial Techniques—The laws that govern the trajectories of particles in fluid streams are utilized in several methods of particle size measurement. Impaction devices are based on the dynamics of deposition of fine particles in a moving air stream when directed past obstacles of defined geometric form, or when forced from a jet device onto a plane surface.

The *cascade impactor*, described by Pilcher and his co-workers,[3] forces particle laden air at a very high speed and fixed rate through a series of jets (each smaller than the preceding one) onto glass slides; impaction takes place in a series of stages. The velocities of the air stream and the particles suspended in it are increased as they advance through the impactor. As a result, the particles are classified by impaction on the different slides, with the larger particles on the top slides and the smaller ones on the downstream slides. Fig 89-9 illustrates the principle of the cascade impactor. The exact size of impacted particles on each slide must subse-

are sized directly and individually, rather than being grouped statistically by some other means of classification. The linear measurement of particles is made by comparison with a calibrated scale usually incorporated into the microscope. For spherical particles the size is defined by the measurement of the diameter. However, for other-shaped particles some other single size designation is generally used; eg, the diameter of a sphere with the same projected area as the nonspheroidal particle being measured. Other characteristic diameters based on various aspects of the projected particle outline as seen through the microscope also have been reported in the literature to describe nonspheroidal particles.

The method is rather tedious and other limitations are found in the techniques required for preparation of the slides and in the maximum resolution which sets the lower limits of particle size measurement using visible light. White light can resolve particles within the range of 0.2 to 100 μm. This lower limit can be decreased to about 0.1 μm by the use of ultraviolet light and to about 0.01 μm by the use of the ultramicroscope. The electron microscope finds its greatest usefulness in particle size measurements in the range of 0.2 to 0.001 μm.

While microscopic methods for particle size determination are time consuming, tedious, and generally require more skill than some of the other techniques, they do offer a number of advantages. They supply information about the shape and thickness that cannot be obtained by other methods and, in addition, supply a permanent record through use of photomicrographs.

A variety of semiautomated procedures have been developed to reduce the fatigue and tedium associated with manual

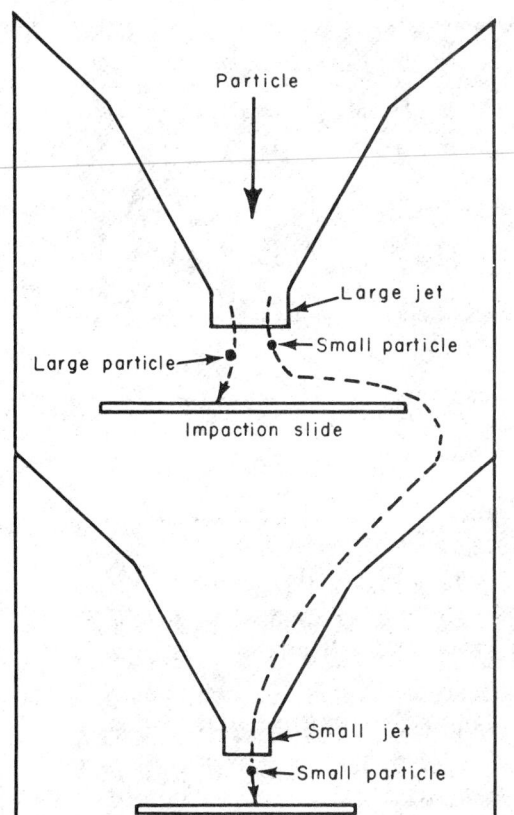

Fig 89-9.   The principle of the cascade impactor.[3]

quently be determined. Size analyses may be obtained directly by theoretical treatment or prior calibration of the instrument.

Tillotson[4] has described an instrument based on inertial principles similar to those of the cascade impactor. This instrument may be adapted for automatic readout of size distribution by means of light-scattering techniques and electronic counters. The method is claimed to provide complete particle size distribution data in a few minutes.

Automatic Particle Size Counters—The Coulter Counter, HIAC Counter, and Gelman Automatic Particle Counter represent three examples of automatic counting equipment.

The *Coulter Counter* will determine the particle volume distribution of material suspended in an electrolyte-containing solution. A table of size ranges of several methods compared with the Coulter principle is shown in Fig 89-10. The principle underlying use of this instrument is described on page 560.

The *HIAC Counter* measures the size distribution of particles suspended in either liquids or gases. The standard models will measure sizes from 2 to 2500 µm at pressures up to 3000 psi. Basically, in this instrument the particles pass

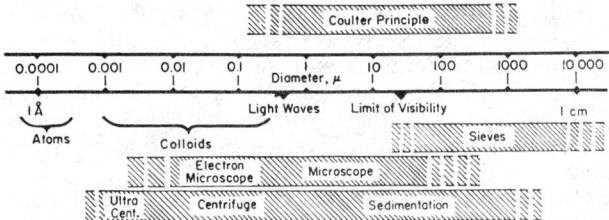

Fig 89-10.   Size range of Coulter method compared with coverage of sieve, sedimentation, and microscopic methods, and overlap of electron microscope and centrifuge ranges (courtesy, Coulter).

a window one-by-one. Each particle as it passes, depending on its size, interrupts some portion of a light beam. This causes an instantaneous reduction in the voltage from a photodetector which is proportional to the size of the particle. Several counting circuits with preset thresholds tally the particles by size.

The *Gelman Counter* uses the principles of light-scattering to count particles in the air in the range of 0.5 µm and larger.

Size Classification

Sieving—This is one of the simplest and probably the most frequently used method for determining particle size distribution. The technique basically involves size classification followed by the determination of the weight of each fraction.

In this technique, particles of a powder mass are placed on a screen made up of uniform apertures. By application of some type of motion to the screen, the particles smaller than the apertures are made to pass through. The sieve motion generally is either (a) horizontal, which tends to loosen the packing of the particles in contact with the screen surface, permitting the entrapped subsieve particles to pass through or (b) vertical, which serves to agitate and mix the particles as well as to bring more of the subsieve particles to the screen surface.

One major difficulty associated with this method is the production of screens with uniform apertures, particularly in the very fine mesh sizes. As a result the practical lower limit for woven-wire mesh screens is about 43 µm (325-mesh). However, with the introduction of electroformed screens, sieves capable of analyzing particles in the 5-µm range are now available. In addition, "blinding" of the openings by oversize or irregular particles and inefficient presentation of the particles to the screen surface are problems associated with this technique. The use of horizontal and vertical screening motions, airjets, sudden periodic reversal of the sieve motion, and continuous cycling all have been used in an attempt to eliminate these problems.

For continuous operations, the screens are attached to mechanical or electromagnetic devices which supply the energy required to shake the particles through the openings in the screen and also prevent accumulation of fines within the openings as this tends to clog them and slow down the operation. The use of an electromagnetic instead of mechanical drive provides a more gentle sieving action with a resultant decrease in sieve wear, blinding, and less machine noise. Sieves may be used either in a sequence of sizes through which the material must pass or singly in the required size.

This apparatus is useful in obtaining size analysis data under controlled conditions. The sample is placed in the top of the nest of standard sieves arranged in a descending order. The length of time and force of vibration to which the sample is subjected may be preset by variable time and voltage controls. The controlled vibration causes the powder particles to pass through the sieves, each fraction coming to rest in the sieve through which it cannot pass. For the purpose of analysis, the weight of each fraction is determined and the percentage calculated.

The Sonic Sifter (*Allen-Bradley* and *ATM*) is a laboratory sifter that utilizes sonic oscillation to classify particles. A mechanical pulse action is used to reduce blinding and agglomeration in the subsieve sizes. This combination of sonic and mechanical agitation permits dry sifting down to 5 µm. US Standard Sieves are available for this unit from 3½- to 400-mesh and in precision electroformed mesh sizes from 150 to 5 µm.

Industrial-size mechanical sieves are varied in design and capacity, and include the gyratory, circular rotatory, vibrating, shaking, and revolving sifters. In gyratory sifters the motion

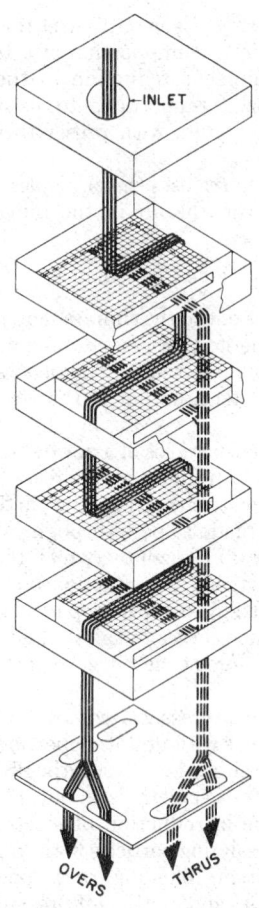

Fig 89-11. Gyro-Whip sifter (courtesy, Sprout-Waldron).

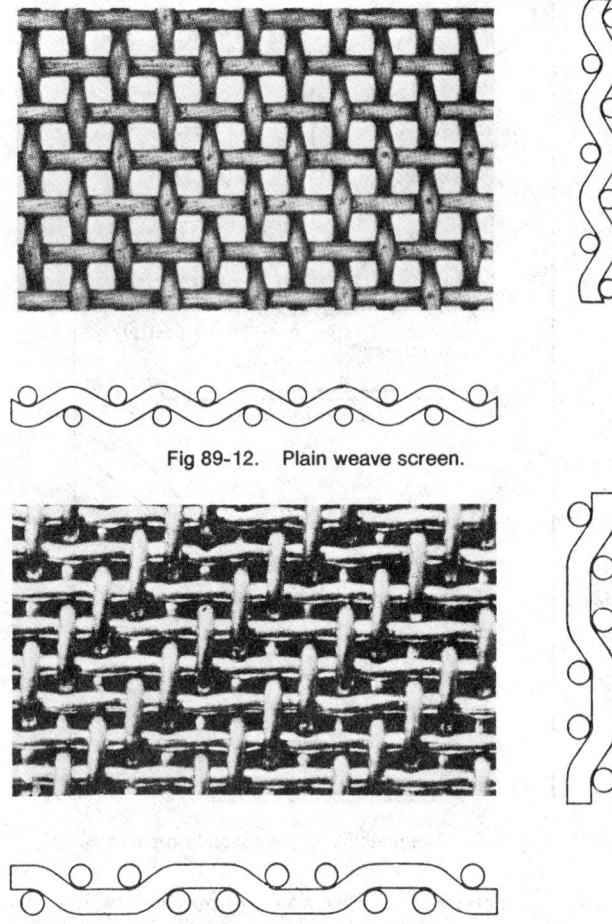

Fig 89-12. Plain weave screen.

Fig 89-13. Twilled weave screen.

is in a single horizontal plane, but may vary from circular to reciprocal from the feed to the discharge end. The circular sifter also confines the screen motion to a horizontal plane, but in this case the total motion applied to the sieve is circular. The Sprout-Waldron *Gyro-Whip* is an example of such a sifter in which the material enters the top and spreads over the first sieve. Some of the finer particles drop through and are discharged into the "throughs" channel. The remaining powder moves to the next sieve in order, the process is repeated until complete separation is accomplished (Fig 89-11).

Centrifugal screening is utilized in the Symons *V-Screen* developed by Nordberg. Here the material is pushed through a spinning vertical wire cloth cylinder. Sharp cuts in particle size can be obtained with this equipment. Downward air flow, instead of shaking and tapping, has been used to move the particles through the screen openings; alternating with a reverse air flow serves to prevent "blinding," particularly with fine-mesh sieves.

Wet Screening—The addition of water is sometimes employed to dissolve out any unwanted binders, remove fines or surface contamination, and to reduce surface forces, particularly in micro-mesh sieves, that oppose the flow of particles through the sieve. Particles that tend to agglomerate or react with oxygen or moisture and thus cannot be dry-sieved often can be handled by wet-sieving. Particles in the 6 to 150-μm range have been classified with good precision using electroformed sieves. Some hydrophobic substances which resist wetting by water may be wet screened by the use of organic liquids such as petroleum ether, acetone, or alcohol. Wet screening may be accomplished by spraying both the screen surface and the material as it is fed onto the screen or by feeding a slurry of material directly onto the screen.

Screening Surfaces—A number of factors must be considered in selecting screening surfaces. Primary consideration is given to the size and shape of the aperture opening, selection of which is determined by the particle size that is to be separated. Screens commonly used in pharmaceutical processing include *woven wire screens*, *bolting cloth*, *closely spaced bars*, and *punched plates*. Punched plates are used for coarse sizing; their holes may be round, oval, square, or rectangular. The plates must be sturdy and withstand rough service. Sizes in common use range upward from $\frac{1}{4}$ inch.

Most screening, however, is accomplished with woven wire screens ranging in size from those with 400 openings to the inch to screens with 4-inch square openings or larger. There are numerous types of woven wire screens, including plain, twilled and braided weave. An example of the plain and twilled weave is shown in Figs 89-12 and 89-13.

In the US, the two common standards are the *Tyler Standard* and *US Standard* sieves. In both these series the sieve number refers to the number of openings per linear inch. For most purposes, screens from the two series are interchangeable, though in a few instances the number designations are different. Since these numbers do not define the size of the openings the Bureau of Standards has established specifications for *Standard Sieves*, as given in Table II. These specifications also establish tolerances for the evenness of weaving, as irregularities from careless weaving might permit much larger particles to pass the sieve than would be indicated. The standard sieves used for pharmaceutical testing are of wire cloth.

Sedimentation—This method employs the settling of particles in a liquid of a relatively low density, under the influence of a gravitational or centrifugal field. In free settling (ie, no particle–particle interference) the particles are supported by hydraulic forces and their fall can be described by

Table II—Nominal Dimensions of Standard Sieves

No	Sieve opening mm	Sieve opening μm	Permissible variation in average opening, %	Permissible variation in maximum opening, %	Wire diameter, mm
2	9.52	9520	±3	+ 5	2.11 to 2.59
4	4.76	4760	±3	+10	1.14 to 1.68
8	2.38	2380	±3	+10	0.74 to 1.10
10	2.00	2000	±3	+10	0.68 to 1.00
20	0.84	840	±5	+15	0.38 to 0.55
30	0.59	590	±5	+15	0.29 to 0.42
40	0.42	420	±5	+25	0.23 to 0.33
50	0.297	297	±5	+25	0.170 to 0.253
60	0.250	250	±5	+25	0.149 to 0.220
70	0.210	210	±5	+25	0.130 to 0.187
80	0.177	177	±6	+40	0.114 to 0.154
100	0.149	149	±6	+40	0.096 to 0.125
120	0.125	125	±6	+40	0.079 to 0.103
200	0.074	74	±7	+60	0.045 to 0.061

Stokes' law. However, in most real situations particle–particle interference, nonuniformity, and turbulence are all present, resulting in more complex settling patterns. The Andreason pipet, which is based on sampling near the bottom of a glass sedimentation chamber, is perhaps the best known of the early instruments. With centrifugation, entrainment of particles in the currents produced by other particles may also interfere with fractionation.

Gravitational settling chambers are often used for large-scale separation of relatively coarse particles in the range of 100 μm. Centrifugal devices are useful for the separation of much smaller particles (5–10 μm).

Sedimentation balances are available which provide a means of directly weighing particles at selected time intervals as they fall in a liquid system. For continuous observations, automatic recording balances are also available. A commercially available instrument called a *Micromerograph* utilizes the principle of sedimentation in an air column. This instrument and others related to it in principle offer more rapid determinations than those which utilize a liquid medium. There are, however, serious uncertainties in the method which must be taken into consideration. Deviations from Stokes' law and impaction of particles against the inner wall of the settling chamber are sources of possible error.

The Carey and Stairmand *photosedimentometer* photographs the tracks of particles as they fall in a dispersion medium. The size determination is derived from the length of the photographic track, which is an indication of the distance traveled by the particles, and the time of exposure of the photograph.

Elutriation—In this process the particles are suspended in a moving fluid, generally water or air. In vertical elutriation at any particular velocity of the fluid, particles of a given size will move upwards with the fluid, while larger particles will settle out under the influence of gravity. In horizontal elutriation a stream of suspended particles is passed over a settling chamber. Particles that leave the stream are collected in the bottom of the chamber. Normally, for all elutriation techniques, both undersize and oversize particles appear in each fraction and recycling is required if a clean cut is desired. By varying the fluid velocities stepwise the sample may be separated into fractions. The amount in each fraction then can be determined and the size limits calculated by the use of the Stokes' equation or measured directly by microscopy. Air elutriation usually will give a sharper fractionation in a shorter time than will water elutriation.

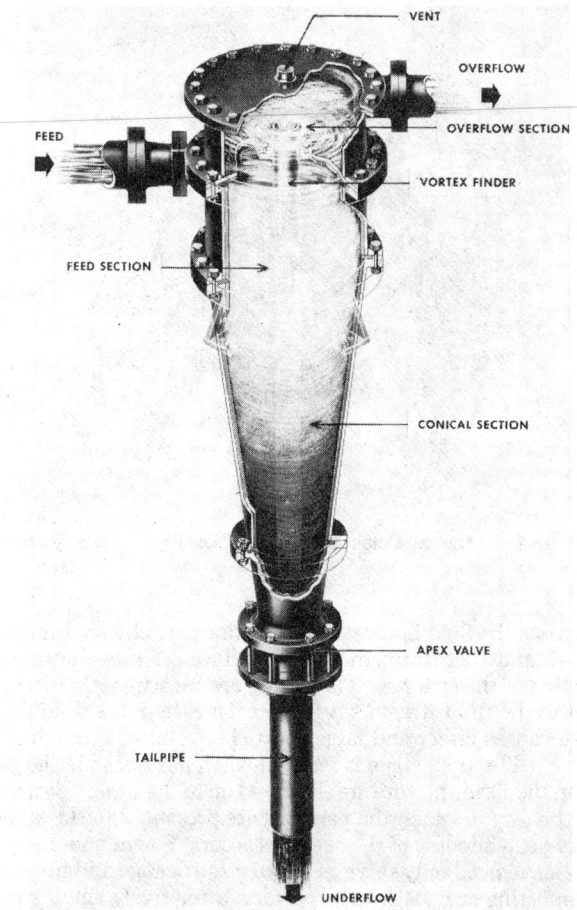

Fig 89-14. DorrClone, a hydrocentrifugal classifier (courtesy, Dorr-Oliver).

Centrifugal elutriation is basically the same process, except in this case the fluid stream is caused to spin so as to impart a high centrifugal force to the suspended particles. Those particles which are too large to follow the direction of flow separate out on the walls or bottom of the elutriator or cyclone. The finer particles escape with the discharge stream. Separation down to about 0.5 μm can be achieved with some centrifugal classifiers.

The DorrClone (*Dorr-Oliver*) shown in Fig 89-14 is an example of a centrifugal type classifier. The feed enters tangentially into the upper section. Centrifugal forces in the vortex throw the coarser particles to the wall where they collect and then drop down and out of the unit. The fine particles move to the inner spiral of the vortex and are displaced upward and finally out of the top of the unit.

The Sharples *Super Classifier* (Fig 89-15) is another example of a centrifugal classifier useful for the high-speed separation of fine particles. It has a capacity of about 250 lb/hr and operates at an air flow of about 100 cu ft/min at a maximum rotor speed of about 15,000 rpm.

The Donaldson air classifier subjects the feed particles to a high degree of dispersion just prior to classification and thus is able to make sharp separations in production quantities as low as 0.5 μm.

Inertial elutriators, which utilize an abrupt change in direction of the fluid stream to produce separation, are effective down to about 200-mesh. However, as with other elutriators a clean cut cannot usually be obtained without recycling.

Felvation is a unique process that combines elutriation and sieving along with a varying fluid flow rate and a turbulent fluidized bed to achieve particle separation. The particles are fluidized within the felvation column. By gradually in-

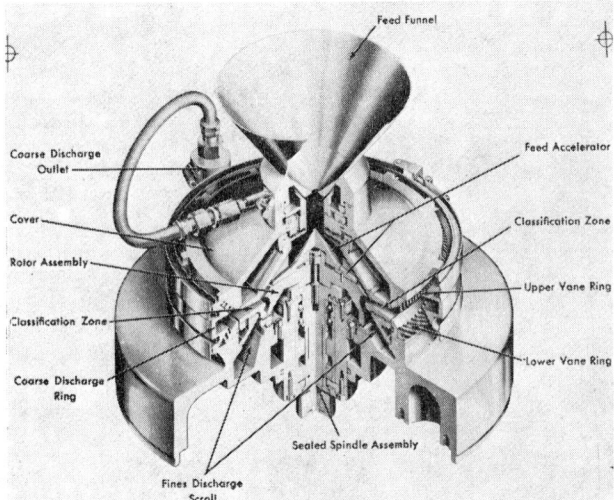

Fig 89-15. The Sharples K-8 Super Classifier (courtesy, Sharples).

creasing the fluid flow rate the very fine particles are brought up to and then through a sieve surface set into the upper section of the column. These fines are subsequently filtered out of the fluid stream. A further increase in the fluid flow rate causes larger and larger particles to move through the sieve. The final stage is reached when particles just larger than the sieve aperture are elutriated up to the sieve. Because of the way in which the particles are presented to the sieve, very little blinding of the openings occur. Furthermore, since the sieve need only serve as a "go, no go" gauge and not as a supporting surface for the powder, a relatively small sieve surface is required. Thus, the more uniform but more expensive electroform sieves, even down to a 10-μm size, can be utilized in this process.

Miscellaneous Methods—Numerous other methods have been applied to particle size determination, including X-ray and electron diffraction, ultrasound, flotation, and electrostatic, magnetic, and dielectrophoretic methods. These techniques either are used principally as research tools or are industrial-scale methods of use outside the pharmaceutical industry. Detailed descriptions of their principles of operation and their applications can be found in the texts listed at the end of this chapter.

Solids Handling

Packing and Bulk Properties

Bulk Density; Angles of Repose—Systems of particulate solids are the most complex physical systems encountered in pharmacy. No two particles in a powder are identical and the nature of momentum and energy exchange between particles defies description except in the most idealized and approximate terms. Bulk properties of powders are determined in part by the chemical and physical properties of their component solids and in part by the manner in which the various components interact. These interactions in turn frequently depend on the past history of the powder bed as well as on the ambient conditions.

The static properties of a particulate bed are dependent on particle–particle interactions and in particular on the way in which applied stresses are distributed through the bed. The number of contacts between particles and hence the average number of interparticulate contact points per particle increases as bed packing increases. Packing may be expressed in terms of porosity, percent voids, or fraction of solids by volume. Packings for regular arrangements of uniform

spheres can be calculated and range in fractional solids from 0.53 for cubic to 0.74 for tetrahedral lattices. Powders comprised of irregular-shaped particles in a distribution of sizes can pack to fractional densities approaching unity.

The manner in which stresses are transmitted through a bed and the bed's response to applied stress are reflected in the various angles of friction and repose. The most commonly used of these is the angle of repose which may be experimentally determined by a number of methods, with slightly differing results. The typical method is to pour the powder in a conical heap on a level flat surface and to measure the included angle with the horizontal. Angles of repose range from 23 degrees for smooth uniform glass beads to 64 degrees for granular limestone. Cohesive materials frequently behave in an anomalous manner yielding values in excess of 90 degrees.

The angle of internal friction is a measure of internal stress distributions and is the angle at which an applied stress diverges as it passes through the bed. This angle together with the angle of slide are useful parameters in the design of storage/discharge bins. The latter angle is defined as the least slope at which a powder will slide down an inclined plane surface. Various other angles are in lesser use and will not be discussed here.

Statics—Powders at rest experience stresses that vary with location throughout their volume and that arise from pressures exerted by the container as well as from the weight of the bed above. Each point within the bed experiences both normal and shear stresses in general. Normal stresses may be either tensile or compressive. The powder bed will remain motionless and no flow will occur unless the normal and/or the shear strength is exceeded at some point within the bed. In general, the yield strengths, both normal and shear, are functions of the normal and shear stresses at the point of interest and depend upon the orientation of the axes of reference and the nature of the powder itself. It is apparent that to understand powder flow it is necessary to understand the conditions under which bed failure occurs and powder flow is initiated and sustained.

Consider the stresses which are applied to the faces of a small cube that is centered about a point chosen at random within a powder bed. Normal stresses are designated σ_i, where the subscript indicates the axis normal to the face and shear stresses are designated τ_{ij}, where the first subscript indicates the face and the second indicates the direction of the applied force. If the cube has an edge length, 1, which is not infinitesimal, and if a stress gradient exists within the region, the corresponding stresses on opposite faces of the cube will not be equal. However, if the cube is made progressively smaller and as 1 approaches zero, the stress values will converge to those at the point of interest. These forces are illustrated in Fig 89-16. It can be seen from this diagram that the state of stress at a point can be described by nine stress components.

If the system is in static equilibrium, and is not being accelerated translationally or rotationally, the forces which would otherwise result in movement must be in balance and have the effect of canceling each other. For example, τ_{xy} must equal τ_{yx} if rotation about the z-axis is not to occur. In a similar manner, shear and normal stresses, which would lead to translational movement along any of the three axes, must also balance.

Because the directions of the mutually perpendicular axes in Fig 89-16 were chosen arbitrarily, any other orientation of the cube corresponding to another set of axes must also result in a balance of forces. However, the distribution of stress among normal and shear components will depend on the particular axes selected. Thus, the stress condition of a powder can be analyzed in terms of the dependence of the normal and shear stresses on the direction chosen for the

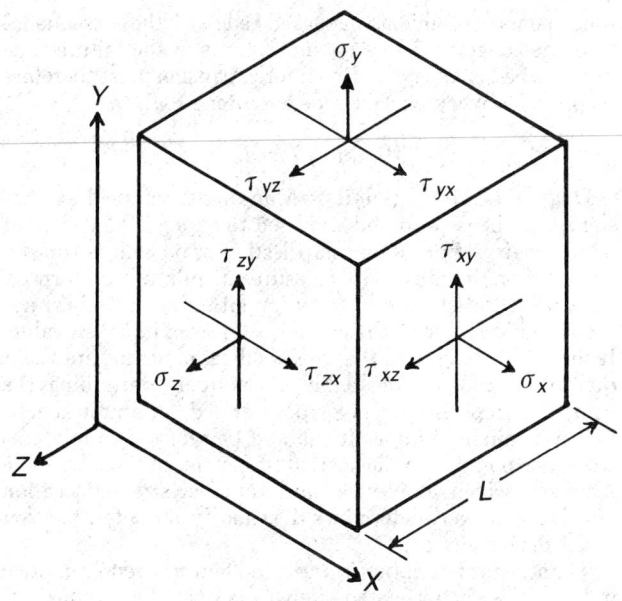

Fig 89-16.

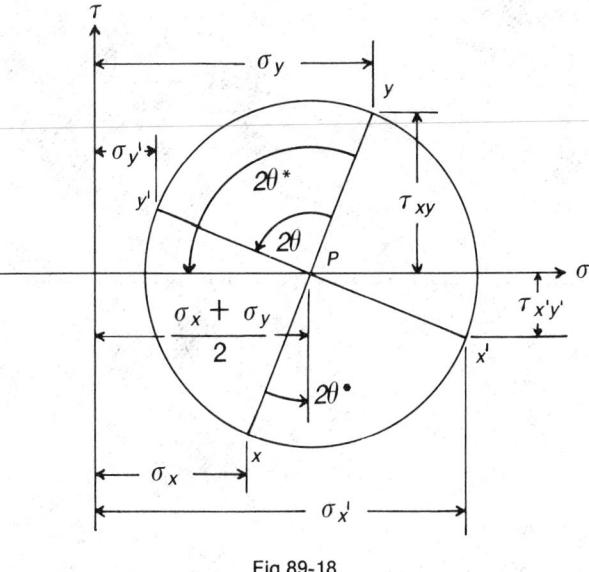

Fig 89-18.

reference axes. This can be done by a method of analysis devised by Mohr, and can be visualized using a Mohr circle diagram. The Mohr diagram permits stresses at any given point within a powder bed to be graphically resolved into normal, σ, and shear, τ, stresses for any arbitrary choice of axes.

For simplicity, assume that stress in the z-direction is not a function of z and that stress gradients exist in the x and y directions only. Stresses then can be analyzed in the xy plane without reference to the z-axis. Fig 89-17 shows the relationship between stresses relative to two xy coordinate systems at an angle θ to each other. If the condition of stress in the powder remains constant and only the angle θ between the two sets of reference axes is allowed to change, the resolution of stress into normal and shear components will be different for each set of axes and will depend on θ. By means of trigonometry, the relationships between these two sets of stresses is shown to be:

$$\sigma_{x'} = \frac{\sigma_x + \sigma_y}{2} + \frac{\sigma_x - \sigma_y}{2}\cos2\theta + \tau_{xy}\sin2\theta$$

$$\sigma_{y'} = \frac{\sigma_x + \sigma_y}{2} - \frac{\sigma_x - \sigma_y}{2}\cos2\theta - \tau_{xy}\sin2\theta$$

$$\tau_{x'y'} = -\frac{\sigma_x - \sigma_y}{2}\sin2\theta - \tau_{xy}\cos2\theta$$

These equations permit the calculation of σ and τ values for any desired set of axes if the values are known for any given set of axes. In particular, if θ is chosen properly, $\tau_{x'y'}$ can be made to vanish and normal stresses only will remain. The set of axes for which this is true are called the *principal axes* of stress and the corresponding σ's are called the *principal stresses*. All points within static beds of powders can be characterized by principal axes and stresses which will, in general, vary from point to point throughout the bed. The principal axes do not necessarily correspond to the orientation of the walls of the powder container.

These concepts can be extended to three dimensions. Thus, it is possible to find a set of three mutually perpendicular planes, on which there are no shear stresses acting, for each location within the powder. The normals to these planes are the principal axes. It is also possible to find a set of planes for which the shear stresses are a maximum and the normal stresses are equal. The associated axes are called the axes of maximum shear. These two sets of axes are important since they represent directions of bed failure were it to occur.

The relationships between stresses, as functions of θ, can be illustrated and determined graphically. Fig 89-18 is an example of a Mohr's circle diagram for stress. Such diagrams are based on the stress equations. This can be seen by comparison of Fig 89-18 with the equations, noting the relationships of the stresses of θ. A Mohr diagram can be constructed for any point within the powder, permitting stresses to be graphically resolved into normal and shear components for any arbitrary choice of axes.

Steps in constructing a diagram are as follows. (1) Plot the center of the circle, p, on the σ axis at the average normal stress, $(\sigma_x + \sigma_y)/2$. (2) Plot point x and y with coordinates (σ_x, τ_{xy}) and (σ_y, τ_{xy}), respectively. Note that these three points lie on a diameter of the circle. (3) Draw a circle with its center at p and passing through points x and y. (4) Locate the $x'y'$ diameter using the angle 2θ. The stress components corresponding to the new axes can be read off the graph. Both

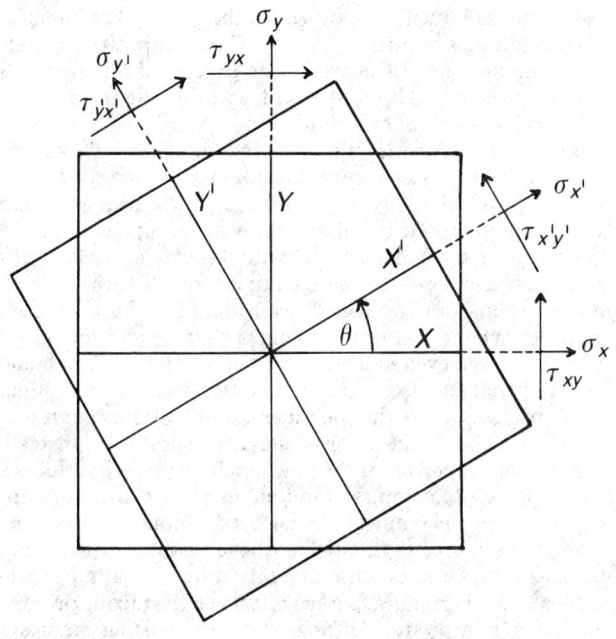

Fig 89-17.

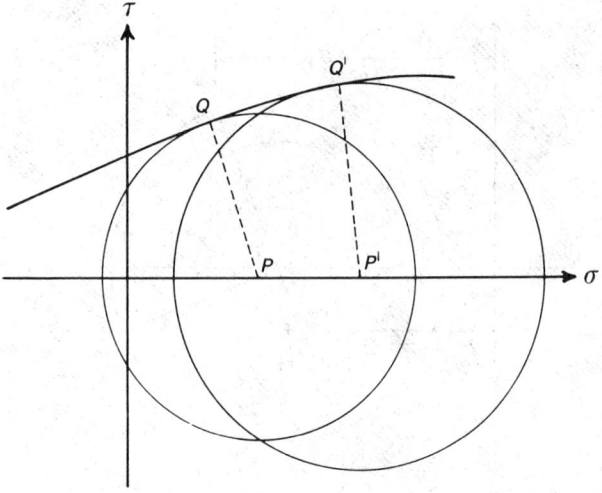

Fig 89-19.

$\sigma_{x'}$ and $\sigma_{y'}$ are read off the same axes on the graph since both are normal stresses.

For the particular case in Fig 89-18, the principal axes lie at an angle of θ^* to the original axes. The axes of maximum shear stress lie at an angle of θ from the original axes since the xy line corresponding to maximum shear is perpendicular to the σ axis. Depending on the state of the powder, it is possible to have negative σ values, where the Mohr circle passes to the left of the τ axis.

The application of stress normal to a plane of shear influences the shear stress at which the powder fails. Because of this, a given powder will fail at various combinations of normal and shear stresses. These combinations can be expressed graphically by a line in the σ,τ plane which separates regions on the graph at which the powder either flows or is stable. This is shown in Fig 89-19 for a typical powder. Various powders will display curves which uniquely define their failure characteristics. Each point on such a curve corresponds to a σ,τ combination at which failure occurs and can be analyzed by constructing a Mohr circle which passes through the point and is centered on the intersection of a line perpendicular to the point, q, and the σ axis. An example is shown in Fig 89-19.

Bulk Properties—In addition to the angles of repose and friction which reflect bulk behavior, tensile and shear strength and dilatancy are of interest. Tensile strength is measured by forming a powder bed on a roughened and split plate. Half of the plate is laterally movable and the force necessary to rupture the bed by pulling the plate halves apart, minus sliding plate friction corrections, represents the bed tensile strength. Various methods of applying force to the movable plate are used, including tipping the plate from the horizontal and allowing it to react to gravity by rolling on steel balls.

Shear strength is determined from the force necessary to shear horizontally a bed of known cross section. The Jenike shear cell is typical of those in use. It permits various loads to be applied normal to the plane of shear, whereby a shear failure locus can be determined. With the desired normal load applied, a steadily increasing shearing force is applied until failure occurs. These measurements are the basis for constructing powder failure curves such as that in Fig 89-19.

When packed powder beds are deformed, local expansion occurs along the failure planes, barring fracture of the particles themselves. This phenomenon is termed dilatancy and is a direct consequence of the micromechanics of interparticulate movement. For one particle to move past another it is necessary for it to move to the side in order to move forward when the particles are in an "interlocked" arrangement. Such ar-

rangements predominate in packed beds with the consequence that the collective sideways movements in the failure zone produce bed expansion. Room for expansion must therefore be provided when packed beds are forced to flow.

Mixing of Powders

Degree of Homogeneity—Many mathematical expressions have been proposed and used to express the degree of homogeneity of powders comprised of two or more components. For the most part measures of mixture uniformity have been statistical and based on either the standard deviation or variance of the composition from its mean value. It should be recognized that these indices of mixing are scalar quantities and are incapable of uniquely describing the composition profile of a given powder bed. A practical definition of mixing uniformity should be selected to relate as closely as possible to the desired properties of the mix. The manner in which samples are taken (number, size, and location of samples) largely determines the validity and interpretation of the derived index.

The standard deviation is presented here as a representative index. It can be estimated solely from a set of n samples. If sample number i has composition x_i, and all samples are of uniform size, then the sample standard deviation is defined in the usual way as:

$$s = \sqrt{\sum_{i=1}^{n} (x_i - \bar{x})^2/(n-1)}$$

where $\bar{x}$ is the mean composition estimated from the samples alone.

In sampling a bed, there should be assurance that the bed is sampled uniformly over its entirety. This can be done either by use of a sampling "thief" designed to probe the bed and collect samples at selected points or serially as the powder is discharged from the mixer.

The "scale of scrutiny" at which the powder is examined for uniformity is determined by the sample size. This should be chosen based on the ultimate use of the powder. For a tablet or capsule formulation the appropriate sample size is that of the dosage form.

Two important concepts related to mixing uniformity have been described by Danckwerts as the scale and the intensity of segregation. Assuming that zones having uniform but differing compositions exist in a powder bed, the scale of segregation is a function of the size of the zones. The intensity of segregation is in turn a function of the composition differences among zones. Generally, the process of mixing tends to reduce the intensity of segregation while the scale of segregation passes through a minimum.

Mechanisms of Mixing and Segregation—Three primary mechanisms are responsible for mixing: (i) convective movement of relatively large portions of the bed, (ii) shear failure which primarily reduces the scale of segregation, and (iii) diffusive movement of individual particles. Most efficient mixers operate to induce mixing by all three mechanisms. Thus, mixing can be considered to be a random shuffling-type operation involving both large and small particle groups and even individual particles. However, it should be noted that the use of random motion to achieve random distribution assumes that no other factors influence this distribution. This is rarely if ever the case in practice. Instead, a variety of properties of the powders being mixed influence this approach to complete randomness. Stickiness or slipperiness of particles must be considered, among other factors. As might be expected, the stickier the material the less readily it mixes and demixes. Electrostatic forces on the particle surface also can produce marked effects on the mixing process, and in fact may produce sufficient particle–particle repulsion to make random mixing impossible.

By enabling particles to undergo movement relative to each other, mixers also provide the conditions necessary for segregation to occur. Any manipulation of a powder bed for purposes of conveying, discharge from a hopper, etc. provides the opportunity for segregation. Thus, many of the so-called mechanisms of segregation are actually conditions under which segregation can happen.

The segregation that occurs in free-flowing solids usually does so as a result of differences in particle size and, to a lesser extent, to differences in particle density and shape. The circumstances leading to segregation can be generalized from a fundamental physical standpoint. The necessary and sufficient conditions for segregation to occur are twofold: (i) that various mixture components exhibit mobilities for interparticulate movement which differ and (ii) that the mixture experience either a field which exerts a directional motive force on the particles or a gradient in a mechanism capable of inducing or modifying interparticulate movement. The combination of these conditions results in asymmetric particle migrations and leads to segregation.

Rates of Mixing and Segregation—Rate expressions analogous to those of chemical kinetics can be derived using any of the various indices of mixing as time dependent variables. When this is done, it is usually found that mixing follows a first-order approach to an equilibrium state of mixedness. More recently, mixing has been described as a stochastic process (by means of stationary and nonstationary Markov chains) in which the probabilities of particle movement from place to place in the bed are determined. When applied to a mixer, this approach is capable of indicating zones of greater and lesser mixing intensity.

Large-Scale Mixing Equipment—The ideal mixer should produce a complete blend rapidly with as gentle as possible a mixing action to avoid product damage. It should be easily cleaned and discharged, be dust-tight, and require low maintenance and low power consumption. All of these assets generally are not found in any single piece of equipment, thus requiring some compromise in the selection of a mixer.

Rotating Shell Mixers—The drum-type, cubical-shaped, double-cone, and twin-shell blenders are all examples of this class of mixers. Drum-type blenders with their axis of rotation horizontal to the center of the drum are used quite commonly. These, however, suffer from poor crossflow along the axis. The addition of baffles or inclining the drum on its axis increases crossflow and improves the mixing action. Cubical- and polyhedron-shaped blenders with the rotating axis set at various angles also are available. However, in the latter, because of their flat surfaces, the powder is subjected more to a sliding than a rolling action, a motion which is not conducive to the most efficient mixing.

Double-cone blenders, an important class of rotating shell or tumbling mixers, were developed in an attempt to overcome some of the shortcomings of the previously discussed mixers. Here, the mixing pattern provides a good crossflow with a rolling rather than a sliding motion. Normally, no baffles are required so that cleaning is simplified. The twin-shell blender is another important tumbling-type blender. This blender combines the efficiency of the inclined drum-type with the intermixing that occurs when two such mixers combine their flow. The Zig-Zag blender, an extension of the twin-shell blender, provides efficient continuous precision blending.

Fixed-Shell Mixers—The ribbon mixer, one of the oldest mechanical solid–solid blending devices, exemplifies this type of mixer. The ribbon mixer consists of a relatively long troughlike shell with a semicircular bottom. The shell is fitted with a shaft on which are mounted spiral ribbons, paddles, or helical screws, alone or in combination. These mixing blades produce a continuous cutting and shuffling of the charge by circulating the powder from end to end of the trough as well as rotationally. The shearing action that develops between

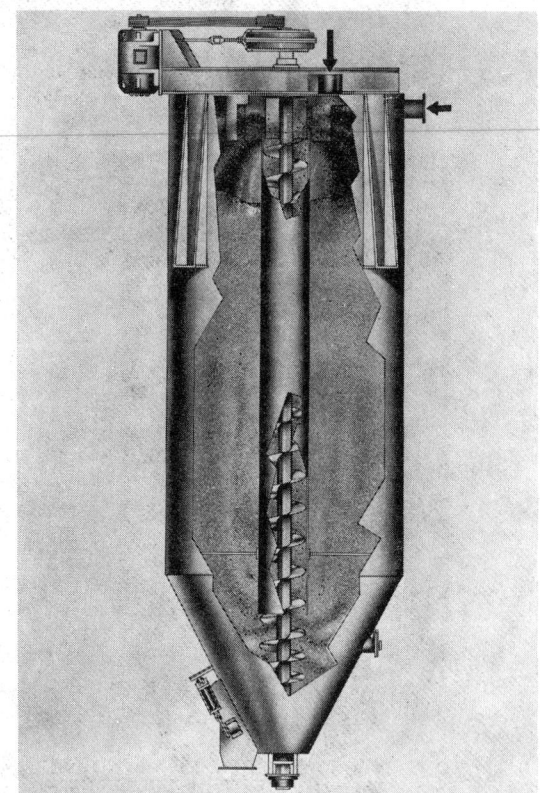

Fig 89-20. Sprout-Waldron vertical mixer.

the moving blade and the trough serves to break down powder agglomerates. However, ribbon mixers are not precision blenders; in addition, they suffer from the disadvantage of being more difficult to clean than the tumbler-type blenders and of having a higher power requirement.

Sigma-Blade and Planetary Paddle Mixers are also used for solid–solid blending, although most generally as a step prior to the introduction of liquids. Mixers with high-speed impeller blades set into the bottom of a vertical or cylindrical shell have been shown to be very efficient blenders. This type of mixer, in addition to its ability to produce precise blends, serves also to break down agglomerates rapidly. The mechanical heat buildup produced by this mixer within the powder mix, and the relatively high power requirement are often drawbacks to the use of this type of mixer.

Muller Mixers are a specialized class of mixers, useful for heavy-duty operations requiring high shearing forces. The mulling action is a shearing mechanism, and is the closest to the type of mixing achieved by the hand-operated mortar and pestle. *Vertical Impeller Mixers*, which have the advantage of requiring little floor space, employ a screw type of impeller which constantly overturns the batch (Fig 89-20). The fluidized mixer is a modification of the vertical impeller type. The impeller is replaced by a rapidly moving stream of air fed into the bottom of the shell. The body of the powder is fluidized and mixing is accomplished by circulation and overtumbling in the bed (Fig 89-21). Generally, when precision solid–solid blending is required, the rotating twin shell or the double cone type blenders are recommended.

Motionless Mixers—These are in-line continuous processing devices with no moving parts. They consist of a series of fixed flow-twisting or flow-splitting elements. The Ross Blendex (*Ross & Son*), designed for blending of free-flowing solids, is constructed to operate in a vertical plane. Four pipes interconnect with successive tetrahedral chambers, the number of chambers needed depending on the quality of mix desired. The powders enter the mixer from overhead hoppers

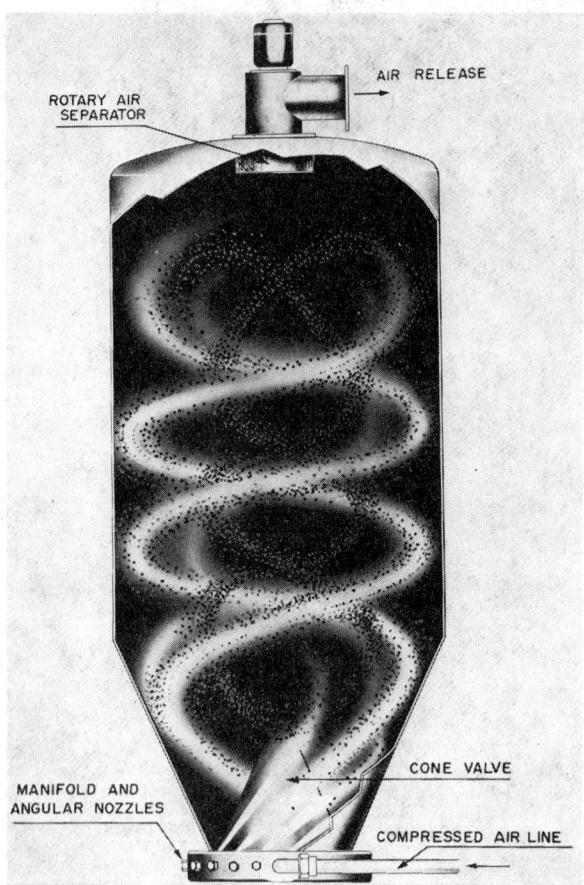

ROTARY AIR
SEPARATOR

AIR RELEASE

MANIFOLD AND
ANGULAR NOZZLES

CONE VALVE

COMPRESSED AIR LINE

Fig 89-21.   Air Mix mixer (courtesy, Sprout-Waldron).

and free fall through the mixer and are mixed by what is described as Interfacial Surface Generation. For two input streams entering this mixer the number of layers, L, emerging from each of the successive chambers, C, is $L = 2(4)^C$. Thus for 10 chambers over 2 million layers are generated. This type of blender provides efficient batch or continuous mixing for a wide variety of solids without particle size reduction or heat generation and essentially no maintenance. Units are available to mix quantities ranging from 100 to 5000 lb/hr.

Small-Scale Mixing Equipment—The pharmacist most generally employs the mortar and pestle for the small-scale mixing usually required for prescription compounding. However, the use of spatulas and sieves also may be utilized on occasion. The mortar and pestle method combines comminution and mixing in a single operation. Thus, it is particularly useful where some degree of particle size reduction as well as mixing is required as in the case of mixtures of crystalline material.

The blending of powders with a spatula on a tile or paper, a relatively inefficient method, is sometimes used for small quantities of powders often as an auxiliary blending technique or when the compaction produced by the mortar and pestle technique is undesirable.

Sieving is usually employed as a pre- or post-mixing method to reduce loosely held agglomerates and to increase the overall effectiveness of a blending process. When used alone as a solid–solid blending technique, several passes through the sieve are required to produce a reasonably homogeneous mix.

Storage and Flow

Flow Patterns—Discharge of powders from large-scale mixers, storage bins, or machine-feed hoppers primarily

generates flow in the form of shear failure. That is, the powder behaves in a manner analogous to a viscous liquid in laminar flow. The analogy ends at that point since conditions are then present in the powder bed conducive to segregation. The overall pattern of discharge from a bin takes the form of either funnel-flow or mass-flow. Bin design characteristics, which take into account the powder's angles of slide and internal friction and its yield locus in terms of normal and shear stresses, determine which flow pattern will occur.

In funnel flow the powder moves in a column down the center of the bin toward the exit orifice at the bottom. Material surrounding this relatively rapidly moving core remains stationary or is slowly drawn into the core. The core is primarily fed from the top where powder moves to the center and then down in the manner of a funnel.

The powder in a mass flow bin moves downward toward the orifice as a coherent mass. When it reaches the tapered section of the bin leading to the orifice it is compressed and flows in shear analogous to a plastic mass being compressed. This type of bin is advantageous for use with powders having a strong tendency to segregate.

The rate of discharge from a hopper varies as a function of the cube of the orifice diameter and is nearly independent of the height of the bed. An arch forms over the orifice which in effect is a boundary between material in essentially free fall and material in the closely packed condition of the powder bed. The rate of mass transport across this constantly renewed surface determines the rate of orifice flow. It has been shown that flow can be substantially increased if gas is pumped through the bed and across the orifice in the direction of solids flow. Flow conditioners are also an important means of improving flow and are discussed in Chapter 21.

Pneumatic Transport—This method of transporting powders is of interest since it can be used to mix powders at the same time as they are being conveyed. The method consists of propelling a solids–gas mixture along a conduit *via* a gas pressure drop. The solids are held in suspension by the turbulence of the gas stream. At low solids concentrations where the particles are relatively small, the solids are uniformly dispersed over the pipe cross-section. However, at higher solids content or with larger particles some stratification will occur in a horizontal pipe and solids will settle out if the pipe is overloaded.

As mentioned before, gas flow must be turbulent so as to suspend the solids; however, the solids behave as in laminar flow. Slippage between gas and solid occurs, particularly in vertical pipes, with the consequence that gas and solids flow rates are not in proportion to flow stream composition. Further, smaller and less dense particles flow more rapidly than large and dense material and a chromatographic-like separation occurs. This is not a problem, however, once steady state is achieved. Because of the industrial importance of this process in many fields it has been extensively investigated and a number of useful theoretical and empirical expressions have been derived and may be used to predict conditions necessary for satisfactory pneumatic transport.

Powders as a Dosage Form

Historically, powders represent one of the oldest dosage forms. They are a natural outgrowth of man's attempt to prepare crude drugs and other natural products in a more conveniently administered form. However, with declining use of crude drugs and increasing use of many highly potent compounds, powders as a dosage form have been replaced largely by capsules and tablets.

In certain situations powders possess advantages and thus still represent a portion (although small) of the solid dosage forms currently being employed. These advantages are flexibility in compounding and relatively good chemical stability. The chief disadvantages of powders as a dosage form are (1) they are time-consuming to prepare and (2) they are not well suited for the dispensing of many unpleasant-tasting, hygroscopic, or deliquescent drugs.

Bulk powders have another serious disadvantage when compared with divided and individually weighed powders—inaccuracy of dose. The dose is influenced by many factors including size of measuring spoon, density of powder, humidity, degree of settling, fluffiness due to agitation, and personal judgment. Not only do patients measure varying amounts of powder when using the same spoon but they often select one differing in size from that specified by their physician.

Extemporaneous Techniques

In both the manufacturing and extemporaneous preparation of powders the general techniques of weighing, measuring, sifting, mixing, etc, as described previously are applied. However, the following procedures should receive special attention.

1. Use of geometric dilution for the incorporation of small amounts of potent drugs.
2. Reduction of particle size of all ingredients to the same range to prevent stratification of large and small particles.
3. Sieving when necessary to achieve mixing or reduction of agglomerates, especially in the preparation of dusting powders or powders into which liquids have been incorporated.
4. Heavy trituration, when applicable, to reduce the bulkiness of a powder.
5. Protection against humidity, air oxidation, and loss of volatile ingredients.

Powders are most commonly prepared either as divided powders and bulk powders which are mixed with water or other suitable material prior to administration, or as dusting powders which are applied locally. They also may be prepared as dentifrices, products for reconstitution, insufflations, aerosols, and other miscellaneous products.

The manually operated procedures usually employed by the prescription pharmacist today are *trituration*, *pulverization by intervention*, and *levigation*.

Trituration—This term refers to the process of reducing substances to fine particles by rubbing them in a mortar with a pestle. The term also designates the process whereby a mixture of fine powders is intimately mixed in a mortar. The circular mixing motion of the pestle on the powders contained in a mortar results in blending them and in also breaking up soft aggregates of powders. By means of the application of pressure on the pestle, crushing or grinding also can be effected.

When granular or crystalline materials are to be incorporated into a powdered product, these materials are comminuted individually and then blended together in the mortar.

Pulverization by Intervention—This is the process of reducing the state of subdivision of solids with the aid of an additional material which can be removed easily after the pulverization has been completed. This technique is often applied to substances which are gummy and tend to reagglomerate or which resist grinding. A prime example is camphor which cannot be pulverized easily by trituration because of its gummy properties. However, on the addition of a small amount of alcohol or other volatile solvent, this compound can be reduced readily to a fine powder. Similarly, iodine crystals may be comminuted with the aid of a small quantity of ether. In both instances the solvent is permitted to evaporate and the powdered material is recovered.

Levigation—In this process a paste is first formed by the addition of a suitable nonsolvent to the solid material. Particle size reduction is then accomplished by rubbing the paste in a mortar with a pestle or on an ointment slab using a spatula. Levigation is generally used by the pharmacist to incorporate solids into dermatologic and ophthalmic ointments and suspensions.

The Mortar and Pestle—These are the most frequently used utensils in small-scale comminution. Mortars made of various materials and in diverse shapes are available and while these are often used interchangeably the different kinds of mortars have specific utility in preparing or grinding different materials.

Modern mortars and pestles are usually prepared from Wedgwood ware, porcelain, or glass. While pharmacists often use different mortars interchangeably, each type has a preferential range of utility which makes its use more efficient. Glass mortars, for example, are designed primarily for use in preparing solutions and suspensions of chemical materials in a liquid. They also are suitable for preparing ointments which require the reduction of soft aggregates of powdered materials or the incorporation of relatively large amounts of liquid. Glass also has the advantage of being comparatively nonporous and of not staining easily and thus is particularly useful when substances such as flavoring oils or highly colored substances are used. Glass cannot be used for comminuting hard solids.

Wedgwood mortars are well suited for comminution of crystalline solids or for the reduction in particle size of most materials used in modern prescription practice. They are capable of adequately powdering most substances which are available only as crystals or hard lumps. However, Wedgwood is relatively porous and will stain quite easily. A Wedgwood mortar is available with a roughened interior which aids in the comminution process but which requires meticulous care in washing since particles of the drugs may be trapped in the rough surface and cause contamination of materials subsequently comminuted in the mortar.

Porcelain mortars are very similar to Wedgwood except that the exterior surface of the former is usually glazed and thus less porous than the Wedgwood mortar. Porcelain mortars may be used for comminution of soft aggregates or crystals but are more generally used for the blending of powders of approximately uniform particle size.

Pestles are made of the same material as the mortar. Pestles for Wedgwood or porcelain mortars are available with hard rubber or wooden handles screwed into the head of the pestle. Also available are one-piece Wedgwood pestles. Pestles made entirely of porcelain are objectionable, because they are easily broken.

Pestles and mortars should not be interchanged. The efficiency of the grinding or mixing operation depends largely on a maximum contact between the surfaces of the head of the pestle and the interior of the mortar. The pestle should have as much bearing on the interior surface of the mortar as its size will permit. A pestle which does not "fit" the mortar will result in a waste of labor.

Divided Powders

Divided powders (*chartula* or *chartulae*) are dispensed in the form of individual doses and are generally dispensed in papers, properly folded. They also may be dispensed in metal foil, small heat-sealed plastic bags, or other containers.

Dividing Powders—After the weighing, comminuting, and mixing of ingredients are completed, the powders must be accurately divided into the prescribed number of doses. In order to achieve accuracy consistent with the other steps in the preparation, *each dose should be weighed individually* and transferred to a powder paper. Following completion of this step the powder papers are folded.

Folding Powders—The operations of folding powder papers are illustrated in Fig 89-22. Care in making the several

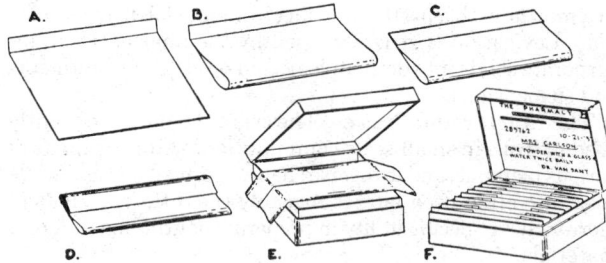

Fig 89-22. Folding powder papers.

folds, and experience gained by repetition, are necessary to obtain uniformity when the powders are finally placed in the box for dispensing. Deviation from any of the three main folds will result in powders of varying height being formed, and variations in the folded ends will likewise be noticeable when the powders are placed side by side.

All of the powder papers for the prescription being filled should be creased by folding down a margin on the top. For a standard 3- by 4-inch powder paper, the fold should be about $\frac{1}{2}$ inch wide; for other powder papers it should be in proportion.

After the powder has been distributed over the papers as described, the additional folds are made as follows. The lower edge of the paper is lifted and folded over until it lies exactly in the crease of the original top fold (Fig 89-22B) which is then pressed down over this lower edge (Fig 89-22C). The top of the paper, as it now appears, is folded toward the operator until it exactly divides the folded paper in the center (Fig 89-22D). The three folds mentioned will so regulate the height of the powders in a low-style powder box that they will just protrude slightly, thus making it possible to pick out one powder with the fingers without disturbing the others. For the old-style boxes having greater depth the final fold should be adjusted to make the powder at least even with the edge of the box.

When the individual powder paper has been folded lengthwise, it is picked up in both hands by the ends and pressed down over the ends of the box so that both ends are turned over exactly the same length. At the same time the end of the box is pressed in slightly so that the powder when finally completed will fit and slide evenly in the box (Fig 89-22E).

The turned ends are simultaneously and firmly pressed between the thumb and finger to complete the folding. The top of the powder paper, at the center, should not be creased with the fingers or with a spatula, as the "roll edge" adds materially to the appearance of the finished box of powders, and creasing may unnecessarily cake the powder. However, where a large number of powders must be placed in a comparatively small box, creasing may help.

When all the powders are folded they may be assembled in one hand, with the lengthwise folds uppermost and toward the operator, and placed in the box. Some pharmacists prefer to alternate the folds, having one forward and one backward, and some even prefer to turn every other powder upside down to lessen the likelihood of the powders springing from the box when a powder is removed. This occurs most frequently when the powder is bulky, and it is possible to adjust this partially by tapping the assembled powders down, first from one side or end and then from the other to effect a more uniform distribution of the powder.

Packaging Divided Powders—Specially manufactured paper and boxes are available for dispensing divided powders.

Powder Papers—Four basic types of powder papers are available.

1. Vegetable parchment, a thin semiopaque moisture-resistant paper.
2. White bond, an opaque paper with no moisture-resistant properties.
3. Glassine, a glazed, transparent moisture-resistant paper.
4. Waxed, a transparent waterproof paper.

Hygroscopic and volatile drugs can be protected best by use of a waxed paper, double-wrapped with a bond paper to improve the appearance of the completed powder. Parchment and glassine papers offer limited protection for these drugs.

A variety of sizes of powder papers are available. The selection of the proper size depends on the bulk of each dose and the dimensions of the powder box required to hold the number of doses prescribed.

Powder Boxes—Various types of boxes are supplied in several sizes for dispensing divided powders. The hinged-shoulder boxes shown in Fig 89-22F are the most popular and have the advantage of preventing the switching of lids with the directions for use when several boxes of the same size are in the same home. The prescription label may be pasted directly on top of the lid or inside the lid. In the latter case the name of the pharmacy is lithographed on top of the lid.

Special Problems

The incorporation of volatile substances, eutectic mixtures, liquids, and hygroscopic or deliquescent substances into powders presents problems that require special treatment.

Volatile Substances—The loss of camphor, menthol, and essential oils by volatilization when incorporated into powders may be prevented or retarded by use of heat-sealed plastic bags or by double wrapping with a waxed or glassine paper inside of bond paper.

Eutectic Mixtures—Liquids result from the combination of phenol, camphor, menthol, thymol, antipyrine, phenacetin, acetanilid, aspirin, salol, and related compounds at ordinary temperatures. These so-called eutectic mixtures may be incorporated into powders by addition of an inert diluent. Magnesium carbonate or light magnesium oxide are commonly used and effective diluents for this purpose, although kaolin, starch, bentonite, and other absorbents have been recommended. Silicic acid prevents eutexia with aspirin, phenyl salicylate, and other troublesome compounds; incorporation of about 20% silicic acid (particle size, 50 μm) prevented liquefaction even under the compression pressures required to form tablets.

In handling this problem each eutectic compound should be first mixed with a portion of the diluent and gently blended together, preferably with a spatula on a sheet of paper. Generally, an amount of diluent equal to the eutectic compounds is sufficient to prevent liquefaction for about two weeks. Deliberate forcing of the formation of the liquid state, by direct trituration, followed by absorption of the moist mass, will also overcome this problem. This technique requires use of more diluent than previously mentioned methods but offers the advantage of extended product stability. Thus the technique is useful for dispensing a large number of doses that normally would not be consumed over a period of one or two weeks.

Liquids—In small amounts, liquids may be incorporated into divided powders. Magnesium carbonate, starch, or lactose may be added to increase the absorbability of the powders if necessary. When the liquid is a solvent for a nonvolatile heat-stable compound, it may be evaporated gently on a water bath. Lactose may be added during the course of the evaporation to increase the rate of solvent loss by increasing the surface area. Some fluidextracts and tinctures may be treated in this manner, although use of an equivalent amount of a powdered extract, when available, is a more desirable technique.

Hygroscopic and Deliquescent Substances—Substances that become moist because of affinity for moisture in the air may be prepared as divided powders by adding inert diluents. Double wrapping is desirable for further protection. Extremely deliquescent compounds cannot be satisfactorily prepared as powders.

Bulk Powders

Bulk powders may be classified as (1) oral powders, (2) dentifrices, (3) douche powders, (4) dusting powders, (5) insufflations, and (6) triturations.

Oral Powders—These are generally supplied as *finely divided powders* or as *effervescent granules*.

The finely divided powders are intended to be suspended or dissolved in water or mixed with soft foods, eg, applesauce, prior to administration. Antacids and laxative powders are frequently administered in this form.

Effervescent granules contain sodium bicarbonate and either citric acid, tartaric acid, or sodium biphosphate in addition to the active ingredients. On solution in water carbon dioxide is released as a result of the acid–base reaction. The effervescence from the release of the carbon dioxide serves to mask the taste of salty or bitter medications.

Granulation is generally accomplished by producing a moist mass, forcing it through a coarse sieve, and drying it in an oven. The moisture necessary for massing the materials is readily obtained by heating them sufficiently to drive off the water of hydration from the uneffloresced citric acid. The completed product must be dispensed in tightly closed glass containers to protect it against the humidity of the air. For a formerly official general formula for preparing effervescent salts see RPS-15, page 1574.

Effervescent powders may be prepared also by adding small amounts of water to the dry salts in order to obtain a workable mass. The mass is dried and ground to yield the powder or granule. Care must be utilized in this procedure to ensure that the reaction which occurs in the presence of water does not proceed too far before it is stopped by the drying process. Should this happen, the effervescent properties of the product will be destroyed.

Other preparative techniques have been reported for effervescent powders such as a fluidized bed procedure in which the powders are blended and then suspended in a stream of air in a Wurster chamber. Water is sprayed into the chamber resulting in a slight reaction and an expansion of the particles to form granules ranging in size from 10- to 30-mesh. This approach apparently offers a number of advantages over the older techniques. The extent of reaction and particle size are controlled during the manufacture. A drying oven, trays, and even grinding devices are not required. Furthermore, the technique lends itself to a continuous as well as a batch operation.

The heat generated from the blending and mixing operation also has been used to mass the powders by causing the release of the water of hydration from the citric acid. The massed materials can be dried and sieved through a coarse sieve. This technique thus eliminates the need of an external heat source or a granulating solution.

Dentifrices—These may be prepared in the form of a bulk powder, generally containing a soap or detergent, mild abrasive, and an anticariogenic agent. These products are considered in more detail in Chapter 109.

Douche Powders—These products are completely soluble and are intended to be dissolved in water prior to use as antiseptics or cleansing agents for a body cavity. They are most commonly intended for vaginal use, although they may be formulated for nasal, otic, or ophthalmic use. Generally, since aromatic oils are included in these powders, they are passed through a No 40 or 60 sieve to eliminate agglomeration and to insure complete mixing. Dispensing in wide-mouth glass jars serves to protect against loss of volatile materials and permits easy access by the patient. Bulk powder boxes may be used for dispensing douche powders, although glass containers are preferred because of the protection afforded by these containers against air and moisture.

Dusting Powders—These are locally applied nontoxic preparations that are intended to have no systemic action. They always should be dispensed in a very fine state of subdivision to enhance effectiveness and minimize irritation. When necessary, they may be micronized or passed through a No 80 or 100 sieve.

Extemporaneously prepared dusting powders should be dispensed in sifter-top packages. Commercial dusting powders are available in sifter-top containers or pressure aerosols. The latter, while generally more expensive than the other containers, offer the advantage of protection from air, moisture, and contamination, as well as convenience of application. Foot powders and talcum powders are currently available as pressure aerosols.

Dusting powders are applied to various parts of the body as lubricants, protectives, absorbents, antiseptics, antipruritics, antibromhidrosis agents, astringents, and antiperspirants.

While in most cases dusting powders are considered nontoxic, absorption of boric acid through large areas of abraded skin has caused toxic reactions in infants. Accidental inhalation of zinc stearate powder has led to pulmonary inflammation of the lungs of infants. The pharmacist should be aware of the possible dangers when the patient uses these compounds as well as other externally applied products. See also Chapter 40.

Insufflations—These are finely divided powders introduced into body cavities such as the ears, nose, throat, tooth sockets, and vagina. An insufflator (powder blower) is usually employed to administer these products. However, the difficulty in obtaining a uniform dose has restricted their general use.

Specialized equipment has been developed for the administration of micronized powders of relatively potent drugs. The Norisodrine Sulfate Aerohaler Cartridge (*Abbott*) is an example of such a product. In the use of this Aerohaler, inhalation by the patient causes a small ball to strike a cartridge containing the drug. The force of the ball shakes the proper amount of the powder free, permitting its inhalation. Another device, the Spinhaler turbo-inhaler (*Fisons*), is a propeller-driven device designed to deposit a mixture of lactose and micronized cromolyn sodium into the lung as an aid in the management of bronchial asthma.

Pressure aerosols have also been employed as a means of administering insufflations, especially for potent drugs. This method offers the advantage of excellent control of dose, through metered valves, as well as product protection.

Triturations—These are dilutions of potent powdered drugs, prepared by intimately mixing them with a suitable diluent in a definite proportion by weight. They were at one time official as 1–10 dilutions. The pharmacist sometimes prepares triturations of poisonous substances, e.g., atropine, in a convenient concentration using lactose as the diluent, for use at the prescription counter. These medicinal substances are more accurately and conveniently weighed by using this method.

The correct procedure for preparing such triturations or any similar dilution of a potent powder medicament, to insure uniform distribution of the latter, is as follows: (1) reduce the drug to a moderately fine powder in a mortar; (2) add about an equal amount of diluent and mix well by thorough trituration in the mortar; (3) successsively add portions of diluent, triturating after each addition, until the entire quantity of diluent has been incorporated. Under no circumstance should the entire quantity of diluent be added at once to the drug that is to be diluted in the expectation that uniform dispersion of the latter will be more expeditiously achieved on brief trituration of the mixture.

References

1.   Parrott EL, in Lachman L, *et al: The Theory and Practice of Industrial Pharmacy*, 2nd ed Lea & Febiger, Philadelphia, 466, 1976.
2.   Perry RH, *et al: Chemical Engineers' Handbook*, 4th ed, McGraw-Hill, New York, 8–8, 1963.
3.   Pilcher JM, *et al: Proc Chem Spec Mfrs Assoc Ann Mfg:* 66, 1956.
4.   Tillotson D: *Aerosol Age 3(5):* 41, 1958.

Bibliography

Irani RR, Callis CF: *Particle Size: Measurement, Interpretation and Application*, Wiley, New York, 1963.

Cadle RD: *Particle Size*, Reinhold, New York, 1965.
Silverman L, *et al: Particle Size Analysis in Industrial Hygiene*, Academic, New York, 1971.
Allen T: *Particle Size Measurement*, Chapman & Hall, London, 1968.
Orr C, Jr, Dalla Valle JM: *Fine Particle Measurement*, Macmillan, New York, 1959.
Martin AN: *Physical Pharmacy*, 3rd ed, Lea & Febiger, Philadelphia, 1983.
Orr C, Jr: *Particulate Technology*, Macmillan, New York, 1966.
Brown RL, Richards JC: *Principles of Powder Mechanics*, Pergamon, Oxford, 1970.
Uhl VW, Gray JW: *Mixing*, Vol II, Academic, New York, 1967.
Stockman JD, Fochtman EG eds: *Particle Size Analysis*, Ann Arbor Science Publishers, Ann Arbor, 1977.
Jelinek IZK: *Particle Size Analysis*, Wiley, New York, 1970.
Sterbacek Z, Tausk P: *Mixing in the Chemical Industry*, Pergamon, Oxford, 1965.
DallaValle JM: *Micromeritics*, 2nd ed, Pitman, New York, 1948.
Parfitt GD, Sing KSW: *Characterization of Powder Surfaces*, Academic, London, 1976.

CHAPTER 90

Oral Solid Dosage Forms

Robert E King, PhD
Professor of Industrial Pharmacy

Joseph B Schwartz, PhD
Professor of Pharmaceutics
Philadelphia College of Pharmacy and Science
Philadelphia, PA 19104

Drug substances are most frequently administered orally by means of solid dosage forms such as tablets and capsules. Large-scale production methods used for their preparation as described later in the chapter require the presence of other materials in addition to the active ingredients. Additives may also be included in the formulations to enhance the physical appearance, improve stability, and aid in disintegration after administration. These supposedly inert ingredients, as well as the production methods employed, have been shown in some cases to influence the release of the drug substances.[1] Therefore care must be taken in the selection and evaluation of additives and preparation methods to ensure that the physiological availability and therapeutic efficacy of the active ingredient will not be diminished.

In a limited number of cases it has been shown that the drug substance's solubility and other physical characteristics have influenced its physiological availability from a solid dosage form. These characteristics include its particle size, whether it is amorphous or crystalline, whether it is solvated or non-solvated, and its polymorphic form. After clinically effective formulations are obtained, variations among dosage units of a given batch, as well as batch-to-batch differences, are reduced to a minimum through proper in-process controls and good manufacturing practices. The recognition of the importance of validation both for equipment and processes has greatly enhanced assurance in the reproducibility of formulations. It is in these areas that significant progress has been made with the realization that large-scale production of a satisfactory tablet or capsule depends not only on the avail-

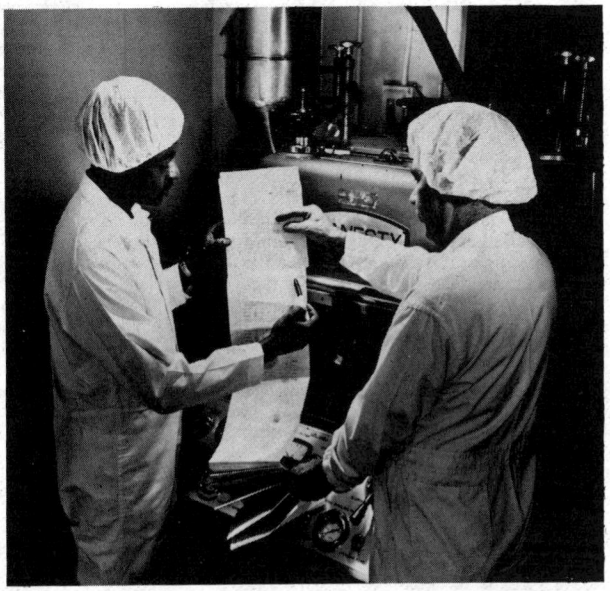

Fig 90-1. Tablet press operators checking batch record in conformance with Current Good Manufacturing Practices (courtesy, Lilly).

ability of a clinically effective formulation but also on the raw materials, facilities, personnel, validated processes and equipment, packaging, and the controls used during and after preparation (Fig 90-1).

Tablets

Tablets may be defined as solid pharmaceutical dosage forms containing drug substances with or without suitable diluents and prepared either by compression or molding methods. They have been in widespread use since the latter part of the 19th century and their popularity continues. The term *compressed tablet* is believed to have been first used by John Wyeth and Brother of Philadelphia. During this same period molded tablets were introduced to be used as "hypodermic" tablets for the extemporaneous preparation of solutions for injection. Tablets remain popular as a dosage form because of the advantages afforded both to the manufacturer (eg, simplicity and economy of preparation, stability, and convenience in packaging, shipping, and dispensing) and the patient (eg, accuracy of dosage, compactness, portability, blandness of taste, and ease of administration).

Although the basic mechanical approach for their manufacture has remained the same, tablet technology has undergone great improvement. Efforts are continually being made to understand more clearly the physical characteristics of tablet compression and the factors affecting the availability of the drug substance from the dosage form after oral ad-

ministration. Compression equipment continues to improve both as to production speed and the uniformity of tablets compressed. Recent advances in tablet technology have been reviewed.[2–5]

Although tablets are more frequently discoid in shape, they also may be round, oval, oblong, cylindrical, or triangular. They may differ greatly in size and weight depending on the amount of drug substance present and the intended method of administration. They are divided into two general classes, whether they are made by compression or molding. Compressed tablets are usually prepared by large-scale production methods while molded tablets generally involve small-scale operations. The various tablet types and abbreviations used in referring to them are listed below.

Compressed Tablets (CT)

These tablets are formed by compression and contain no special coating. They are made from powdered, crystalline, or granular materials, alone or in combination with binders, disintegrants, lubricants, diluents, and in many cases, colorants.

Sugar-Coated Tablets (SCT)—These are compressed tablets containing a sugar coating. Such coatings may be colored and are beneficial in covering up drug substances possessing objectionable tastes or odors, and in protecting materials sensitive to oxidation.

Film-Coated Tablets (FCT)—These are compressed tablets which are covered with a thin layer or film of a water-soluble material. A number of polymeric substances with film-forming properties may be used. Film coating imparts the same general characteristics as sugar coating with the added advantage of a greatly reduced time period required for the coating operation.

Enteric-Coated Tablets (ECT)—These are compressed tablets coated with substances that resist solution in gastric fluid but disintegrate in the intestine. Enteric coatings can be used for tablets containing drug substances which are inactivated or destroyed in the stomach, for those which irritate the mucosa, or as a means of delayed release of the medication.

Multiple Compressed Tablets (MCT)—These are compressed tablets made by more than one compression cycle.

Layered Tablets—Such tablets are prepared by compressing additional tablet granulation on a previously compressed granulation. The operation may be repeated to produce multilayered tablets of two or three layers. Special tablet presses are required to make layered tablets such as the Versa press (*Stokes-Pennwalt*).

Press-Coated Tablets—Such tablets, also referred to as dry-coated, are prepared by feeding previously compressed tablets into a special tableting machine and compressing another granulation layer around the preformed tablets. They have all the advantages of compressed tablets, ie, slotting, monogramming, speed of disintegration, etc, while retaining the attributes of sugar-coated tablets in masking the taste of the drug substance in the core tablets. An example of a press-coated tablet press is the *Manesty* Drycota. Press-coated tablets can also be used to separate incompatible drug substances; in addition, they can provide a means to give an enteric coating to the core tablets. Both types of multiple-compressed tablets have been widely used in the design of prolonged-action dosage forms.

Controlled-Release Tablets—Compressed tablets can be formulated to release the drug substance in a manner to provide medication over a period of time. There are a number of types which include delayed-action tablets in which the release of the drug substance is prevented for an interval of time after administration or until certain physiological conditions exist; repeat-action tablets which periodically release a complete dose of the drug substance to the gastrointestinal fluids; and the extended-release or sustained-release tablets which continuously release increments of the contained drug substance to the gastrointestinal fluids. These tablets are discussed in Chapter 92.

Tablets for Solution—Compressed tablets to be used for preparing solutions or imparting given characteristics to solutions must be labeled to indicate that they are not to be swallowed. Examples of these tablets are Halazone Tablets for Solution and Potassium Permanganate Tablets for Solution.

Effervescent Tablets—In addition to the drug substance, these contain sodium bicarbonate and an organic acid such as tartaric or citric. In the presence of water, these additives react liberating carbon dioxide which acts as a distintegrator and produces effervescence. Except for small quantities of lubricants present, effervescent tablets are soluble.

Compressed Suppositories or Inserts—Occasionally vaginal suppositories, such as Metronidazole Tablets, are prepared by compression. Tablets for this use usually contain lactose as the diluent. In this case, as well as for any tablet intended for administration other than by swallowing, the label must indicate the manner in which it is to be used.

Buccal and Sublingual Tablets—These are small, flat, oval tablets. Tablets intended for buccal administration by inserting into the buccal pouch dissolve or erode slowly, therefore they are formulated and compressed with sufficient pressure to give a hard tablet. Progesterone Tablets may be administered in this way. Sublingual tablets, such as those containing nitroglycerin, isoproterenol hydrochloride, or erythrityl tetranitrate, are placed under the tongue. Sublingual tablets dissolve rapidly and the drug substances are readily absorbed by this form of administration.

Molded Tablets or Tablet Triturates (TT)

Tablet triturates are usually made from moist material using a triturate mold which gives them the shape of cut sections of a cylinder. Such tablets must be completely and rapidly soluble. The problem arising from compression of these tablets is the failure to find a lubricant that is completely water-soluble.

Dispensing Tablets (DT)—These tablets provide a convenient quantity of potent drug that can be incorporated readily into powders and liquids, thus circumventing the necessity to weigh small quantities. These tablets are supplied primarily as a convenience for extemporaneous compounding and should never be dispensed as a dosage form.

Hypodermic Tablets (HT)—Hypodermic tablets are soft, readily soluble tablets and were originally used for the preparation of solutions to be injected. Since stable parenteral solutions are now available for most drug substances, there is no justification for the use of hypodermic tablets for injection. Their use in this manner should be discouraged since the resulting solutions are not sterile. Large quantities of these tablets continue to be made but for oral administration. No hypodermic tablets have ever been recognized by the official compendia.

Compressed Tablets (CT)

In order for medicinal substances, with or without diluents, to be made into solid dosage forms with pressure, using available equipment, it is necessary that the material, either in crystalline or powdered form, possess a number of physical characteristics. These characteristics include the ability to flow freely, cohesiveness, and lubrication. Since most materials have none or only some of these properties, methods of tablet formulation and preparation have been developed to impart these desirable characteristics to the material which is to be compressed into tablets.

The basic mechanical unit in all tablet-compression equipment includes a lower punch which fits into a die from the bottom and an upper punch, having a head of the same shape and dimensions, which enters the die cavity from the top after the tableting material fills the die cavity. See Fig 90-2. The tablet is formed by pressure applied on the punches

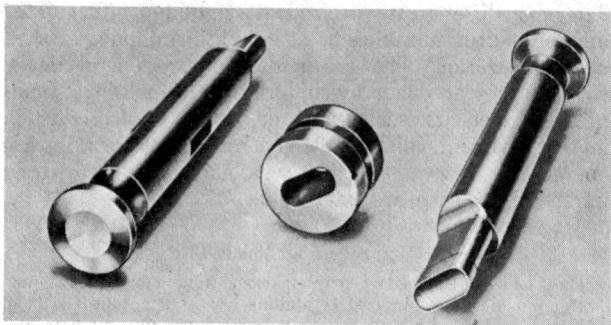

Fig 90-2. Basic mechanical unit for tablet compression: lower punch, die, and upper punch (courtesy, Vector/Colton).

and is subsequently ejected from the die. The weight of the tablet is determined by the volume of the material which fills the die cavity. Therefore, the ability of the granulation to flow freely into the die is important in insuring an uniform fill, as well as the continuous movement of the granulation from the source of supply or feed hopper. If the tablet granulation does not possess cohesive properties, the tablet after compression will crumble and fall apart on handling. As the punches must move freely within the die and the tablet must be readily ejected from the punch faces, the material must have a degree of lubrication to minimize friction and to allow for the removal of the compressed tablets.

There are three general methods of tablet preparation: (1) the wet-granulation method; (2) the dry-granulation method; and (3) direct compression. The method of preparation and the added ingredients are selected in order to give the tablet formulation the desirable physical characteristics allowing the rapid compression of tablets. After compression the tablets must have a number of additional attributes such as appearance, hardness, disintegration ability, appropriate dissolution characteristics, and uniformity which are also influenced both by the method of preparation and by the added materials present in the formulation. In the preparation of compressed tablets the formulator must also be cognizant of the effect which the ingredients and methods of preparation may have on the availability of the active ingredients and hence the therapeutic efficacy of the dosage form. In response to a request by physicians to change a dicumarol tablet in order that it might be more easily broken, a Canadian company reformulated to make a large tablet with a score. Subsequent use of the tablet containing the same amount of drug substance as the previous tablet, resulted in complaints that larger-than-usual doses were needed to produce the same therapeutic response. On the other hand, literature reports indicate that the reformulation of a commercial digoxin tablet resulted in a tablet, although containing the same quantity of drug substance, that gave the desired clinical response at half its original dose. Methods and principles that can be used to assess the effects of excipients and additives on drug absorption have been reviewed.[6,7] See Chapters 38, 76, and 77.

Tablet Ingredients

In addition to the active or therapeutic ingredient, tablets contain a number of inert materials. The latter are known as additives or *excipients*. They may be classified according to the part they play in the finished tablet. The first group contains those which help to impart satisfactory processing and compression characteristics to the formulation. These include (1) diluents, (2) binders, and (3) glidants and lubricants. The second group of added substances helps to give additional desirable physical characteristics to the finished tablet. Included in this group are (1) disintegrants, (2) colors, and in the case of chewable tablets, (3) flavors, and (4) sweetening agents.

Although the term *inert* has been applied to these added materials, it is becoming increasingly apparent that there is an important relationship between the properties of the excipients and the dosage forms containing them. Preformulation studies demonstrate their influence on stability, bioavailability, and the processes by which the dosage forms are prepared. The need for acquiring more information and use standards for excipients has been recognized in a joint venture of the Academy of Pharmaceutical Sciences and the Council of the Pharmaceutical Society of Great Britain. The program is called the Codex of Pharmaceutical Excipient Project and the Academy's Industrial Pharmaceutical Technology Section has undertaken its organization and implementation.

Diluents

Frequently the single dose of the active ingredient is small and an inert substance is added to increase the bulk in order to make the tablet a practical size for compression. Compressed tablets of dexamethasone contain 0.75 mg steroid per tablet, hence it is obvious that another material must be added to make tableting possible. Diluents used for this purpose include dicalcium phosphate, calcium sulfate, lactose, cellulose, kaolin, mannitol, sodium chloride, dry starch, and powdered sugar. Certain diluents, such as mannitol, lactose, sorbitol, sucrose, and inositol, when present in sufficient quantity, can impart properties to some compressed tablets that permit disintegration in the mouth by chewing. Such tablets are commonly called *chewable tablets*. Upon chewing, properly prepared tablets will disintegrate smoothly at a satisfactory rate, have a pleasant taste and feel, and leave no unpleasant aftertaste in the mouth. Diluents used as excipients for direct compression formulas have been subjected to prior processing to give them flowability and compressibility. These are discussed under *Direct Compression*, p 1613.

Most tablet formulators tend to use consistently only one or two diluents selected from the above group in their tablet formulations. Usually these have been selected on the basis of experience and cost factors. However, in the formulation of new therapeutic agents the compatibility of the diluent with the drug must be considered. For example, calcium salts used as diluents for the broad-spectrum antibiotic tetracycline have been shown to interfere with the drug's absorption from the gastrointestinal tract. When drug substances have low water solubility, it is recommended that water-soluble diluents be used to avoid possible bioavailability problems. Highly adsorbent substances, eg, bentonite and kaolin, are to be avoided in making tablets of drugs used clinically in small dosage, such as the cardiac glycosides, alkaloids, and the synthetic estrogens. These drug substances may be adsorbed to the point where they are not completely available after administration. The combination of amine bases with lactose, or amine salts with lactose in the presence of an alkaline lubricant, results in tablets which discolor on aging.

Microcrystalline cellulose (Avicel) is usually used as an excipient in direct compression formulas. However, its presence in 5–15% concentrations in wet granulations has been shown to be beneficial in the granulation and drying processes in minimizing case-hardening of the tablets and in reducing tablet mottling.

Binders

Agents used to impart cohesive qualities to the powdered material are referred to as binders or granulators. They impart a cohesiveness to the tablet formulation which insures the tablet remaining intact after compression, as well as improving the free-flowing qualities by the formulation of granules of desired hardness and size. Materials commonly used as binders include starch, gelatin, and sugars as sucrose, glucose, dextrose, molasses, and lactose. Natural and synthetic gums which have been used include acacia, sodium alginate, extract of Irish moss, panwar gum, ghatti gum, mucilage of isapol husks, carboxymethylcellulose, methylcellulose, polyvinylpyrrolidone, Veegum, and larch arabogalactan. Other agents which may be considered binders under certain circumstances are polyethylene glycol, ethylcellulose, waxes, water, and alcohol.

The quantity of binder used has considerable influence on the characteristics of the compressed tablets. The use of too much binder or too strong a binder will make a hard tablet which will not disintegrate easily and which will cause excessive wear of punches and dies. Differences in binders used for CT Tolbutamide resulted in differences in hypoglycemic effects observed clinically. Materials which have no cohesive qualities of their own will require a stronger binder than those with these qualities. Alcohol and water are not binders in the true sense of the word; but because of their solvent action on some ingredients such as lactose, starch, and celluloses, they change the powdered material to granules and the residual moisture retained enables the materials to adhere together when compressed.

Binders are used both as a solution and in a dry form depending on the other ingredients in the formulation and the method of preparation. The same amount of binder in solution will be more effective than if it were dispersed in a dry form and moistened with the solvent. By the latter procedure the binding agent is not as effective in reaching and wetting each of the particles within the mass of powders. Each of the particles in a powder blend has a coating of adsorbed air on its surface, and it is this film which must be penetrated before the powders can be wetted by the binder solution. Since powders differ with respect to the ease with which they can be wetted, it is preferable to incorporate the binding agent in solution. By this technique it is often possible to gain effective binding with a lower concentration of binder. It should be noted that there are several "pregelatinized" starches available which are intended to be added in the dry form so that water alone can be used as the granulating solution.

The direct compression method for preparing tablets (see page 1613) requires a material that not only is free-flowing but also sufficiently cohesive to act as a binder. This use has been described for a number of materials including microcrystalline cellulose, microcrystalline dextrose, amylose, and polyvinylpyrrolidone. It has been postulated that microcrystalline cellulose is a special form of cellulose fibril in which the individual crystallites are held together largely by hydrogen bonding. The disintegration of tablets containing the cellulose occurs by breaking the intercrystallite bonds by the disintegrating medium.

Starch Paste—Corn starch is widely used as a binder. The concentration may vary from 10 to 20%. It is usually prepared as it is to be used by dispersing corn starch in sufficient cold purified water to make a 10% *w/w* solution and warming in a water bath with continuous stirring until a translucent paste forms.

Gelatin Solution—Gelatin is generally used as a 10–20% solution; gelatin solutions should be freshly prepared as needed and used while warm or they will solidify. The gelatin is added to cold purified water and allowed to stand until it is hydrated. It is then warmed in water bath to dissolve the gelatin and the solution is made up to the final volume on a weight basis to give the concentration desired.

Glucose Solution—Generally a 25–50% solution is used. Glucose does not dry out well and is therefore not suitable where the tablets are subject to humid conditions. These solutions are not true 25 and 50% solutions since the corn syrup contains only approximately 80% solids. To prepare the binder solution, the corn syrup is weighed and dissolved in purified water. Sufficient purified water is added to give the concentration desired on a weight basis. If clarification is desirable, it can be strained through cloth.

Ethylcellulose—This is insoluble in water. It is used effectively as a binder when dissolved in alcohol, or as a dry binder in a granulation which is then wetted with alcohol. As a binder in solution it is usually used as a 5% solution. It is widely used as a binder for moisture-sensitive materials. To make the solution, ethylcellulose is dissolved in anhydrous denatured alcohol and made up to the final volume on a weight basis.

PVP—Polyvinylpyrrolidone can be used as an aqueous or an alcoholic solution and this versatility has increased its popularity. Concentrations range from 2% and vary considerably.

It will be noted that binder solutions are usually made up to weight rather than volume. This is to enable the formulator to determine the weight of the solids which have been added to the tablet granulation in the binding solution. This becomes part of the total weight of the granulation and must be taken into consideration in determining the weight of the compressed tablet which will contain the stated amount of the therapeutic agent.

Lubricants

Lubricants have a number of functions in tablet manufacture. They prevent adhesion of the tablet material to the surface of the dies and punches, reduce interparticle friction, facilitate the ejection of the tablets from the die cavity, and may improve the rate of flow of the tablet granulation. Commonly used lubricants include talc, magnesium stearate, calcium stearate, stearic acid, and hydrogenated vegetable oils. Most lubricants with the exception of talc are used in concentrations less than 1%. When used alone, talc may require concentrations as high as 5%. Lubricants are in most cases hydrophobic materials. Poor selection or excessive amounts can result in "waterproofing" the tablets, resulting in poor tablet disintegration and dissolution of the drug substance.

The addition of the proper lubricant is highly desirable if the material to be tableted tends to stick to the punches and dies. Immediately after compression most tablets have the tendency to expand and will bind and stick to the side of the die. The choice of the proper lubricant will effectively overcome this.

The method of adding a lubricant to a granulation is important if the material is to perform its function satisfactorily. The lubricant should be finely divided by passing it through a 60- to 100-mesh nylon cloth onto the granulation. In production this is called "bolting" the lubricant. After adding the lubricant the granulation is tumbled or mixed gently to distribute the lubricant without coating the particles too well or breaking them down to finer particles.

Prolonged blending of lubricant with a granulation can materially affect the hardness, disintegration time and dissolution performance for the resultant tablets. The quantity of lubricant varies, being as low as 0.1%, and in some cases as high as 5%. Lubricants have been added to the granulating agents in the form of suspensions or emulsions. This technique serves to reduce the number of operational procedures and thus reduce the processing time.

In selecting a lubricant, proper attention must be given to its compatibility with the drug agent. Perhaps the most widely investigated drug is acetylsalicylic acid. Different talcs varied significantly the stability of aspirin. Talc with a high calcium content and a high loss on ignition was associated with increased aspirin decomposition. From a stability standpoint, the relative acceptability of tablet lubricants for combination with aspirin was found to decrease in the following order: hydrogenated vegetable oil, stearic acid, talc, and aluminum stearate.

The primary problem in the preparation of a water-soluble tablet is the selection of a satisfactory lubricant. Soluble lubricants reported to be effective include sodium benzoate, a mixture of sodium benzoate and sodium acetate, sodium chloride, leucine, and Carbowax 4000. However, it has been suggested that formulations used to prepare water-soluble tablets may represent a number of compromises between compression efficiency and water solubility. While magnesium stearate is one of the most widely used lubricants, its hydrophobic properties can retard disintegration and dissolution. To overcome these waterproofing characteristics sodium lauryl sulfate is sometimes included. One compound found to have the lubricating properties of magnesium stearate without its disadvantages is magnesium lauryl sulfate. Its safety for use in pharmaceuticals has not yet been established.

Glidants

A glidant is a substance which improves the flow characteristics of a powder mixture. These materials are always added in the dry state just prior to compression (ie, during the lubrication step). Colloidal silicon dioxide [Cab-o-sil (*Cabot*); Quso (*Phila Quartz*)] is the most commonly used glidant and is generally used in low concentrations of 1% or less. Talc (asbestos-free) is also used and may serve the dual purpose as lubricant/glidant.

Disintegrants

A disintegrant is a substance, or a mixture of substances, added to a tablet to facilitate its breakup or disintegration after administration. The active ingredient must be released from the tablet matrix as efficiently as possible to allow for its rapid dissolution. Materials serving as disintegrants have been chemically classified as starches, clays, celluloses, algins, gums, and crosslinked polymers.

The oldest and still the most popular disintegrants are corn and potato starch which have been well-dried and powdered. Starch has a great affinity for water and swells when moistened, thus facilitating the rupture of the tablet matrix. However, others have suggested that its disintegrating action in tablets is due to capillary action rather than swelling; the spherical shape of the starch grains increases the porosity of the tablet, thus promoting capillary action. Starch, 5%, is suggested, but if more rapid disintegration is desired, this amount may be increased to 10 or 15%. Although it might be expected that disintegration time would decrease as the percentage of starch in the tablet increased, this does not appear to be the case for tolbutamide tablets. In this instance, there appears to be a critical starch concentration for different granulations of the chemical. When their disintegration effect is desired, starches are added to the powder blends in the dry state.

A new group of materials known as "super disintegrants" have recently gained in popularity as disintegrating agents. The name comes from the low levels (2–4%) at which they are completely effective. Croscarmelose, Crospovidone, and sodium starch glycolate represent examples of a crosslinked cellulose, a crosslinked polymer, and a modified starch molecule, respectively.

In addition to the starches a large variety of materials have been used and are reported to be effective as disintegrants. This group includes Veegum HV, methylcellulose, agar, bentonite, cellulose and wood products, natural sponge, cation-exchange resins, alginic acid, guar gum, citrus pulp, and carboxymethylcellulose. Sodium lauryl sulfate in combination with starch also has been demonstrated to be an effective disintegrant. In some cases the apparent effectiveness of surfactants in improving tablet disintegration is postulated as being due to an increase in the rate of wetting.

The disintegrating agent is usually mixed with the active ingredients and diluents prior to granulation. In some cases it may be advantageous to divide the starch into two portions; one part is added to the powdered formula prior to granulation, and the remainder is mixed with the lubricant and added prior to compression. Incorporated in this manner the starch serves a double purpose; the portion added to the lubricant rapidly breaks the tablet down to granules, and the starch mixed with the active ingredients disintegrates the granules into smaller particles. Veegum has been shown to be more effective as a disintegrator in sulfathiazole tablets when most of the quantity is added after granulation and only a small amount before granulation. Likewise, the montmorillonite clays were found to be good tablet disintegrants when added to prepared granulations as powder. They are much less effective as disintegrants when incorporated within the granules.

Factors other than the presence of disintegrants can affect significantly the disintegration time of compressed tablets. The binder, tablet hardness, and the lubricant have been shown to influence the disintegration time. Thus, when the formulator is faced with a problem concerning the disintegration of a compressed tablet, the answer may not lie in the selection and the quantity of the disintegrating agent alone.

The evolution of carbon dioxide is also an effective way to cause the disintegration of compressed tablets. Tablets containing a mixture of sodium bicarbonate and an acidulant such as tartaric or citric acid will effervesce when added to water. Sufficient acid is added to produce a neutral or slightly acidic reaction when disintegration in water is rapid and complete. One drawback to the use of the effervescent type of disintegrator is that such tablets must be kept in a dry atmosphere at all times during manufacture, storage, and packaging. Soluble, effervescent tablets provide a popular form for dispensing aspirin and noncaloric sweetening agents.

Coloring Agents

Colors in compressed tablets serve functions other than making the dosage form more esthetic in appearance. Color helps the manufacturer to control the product during its preparation, as well as serving as a means of identification to the user. The wide diversity in the use of colors in solid dosage forms makes it possible to use color as an important category in the identification code developed by the AMA to establish the identity of an unknown compressed tablet in situations arising from poisoning.

All colorants used in pharmaceuticals must be approved and certified by the FDA. For several decades colorants have been subjected to rigid toxicity standards and as the result a number of colorants have been delisted and several added. The colorants currently approved in the US include the following: FD&C Red No 3, FD&C Red No 40, FD&C Yellow No 5, FD&C Yellow No 6, FD&C Blue No 1, FD&C Blue No 2, FD&C Green No 3, a limited number of D&C colorants, and the iron oxides. Each country has its own list of approved colorants and formulators must consider this in designing products for the international market.

Any of the approved certified water-soluble FD&C dyes, mixtures of the same, or their corresponding lakes may be used to color tablets. A color lake is the combination by adsorption of a water-soluble dye to a hydrous oxide of a heavy metal resulting in an insoluble form of the dye. In some instances multiple dyes are used to give a purposefully heterogeneous coloring in form of speckling to compressed tablets. The dyes available do not meet all the criteria required for the ideal pharmaceutical colorants. The photosensitivity of several of the commonly used colorants and their lakes has been investigated, as well as the protection afforded by a number of glasses used in packaging tablets. Another approach for improving the photostability of dyes has been in the use of ultraviolet-absorbing chemicals in the tablet formulations with the dyes. The Di-Pac line (*Amstar*) is a series of commercially available colored, direct compression sugars.

The most common method of adding color to a tablet formulation is to dissolve the dye in the binding solution prior to the granulating process. Another approach is to adsorb the dye on starch or calcium sulfate from its aqueous solution; the resultant powder is dried and blended with the other ingredients. If the insoluble lakes are used, they may be blended with the other dry ingredients. Frequently during drying, colors in wet granulations migrate, resulting in an uneven distribution of the color in the granulation. After compression the tablets will have a mottled appearance due to the uneven distribution of the color. Migration of colors may be reduced by drying the granulation slowly at low temperatures and stirring the granulation while it is drying. The affinity of several water-soluble anionic certified dyes for natural starches has been demonstrated; in these cases this affinity should aid in preventing color migration. Other additives have been shown to act as dye migration inhibitors. Tragacanth (1%), acacia (3%), attapulgite (5%), and talc (7%) were effective in inhibiting the migration of FD&C Blue No 1 in lactose. In using dye lakes the problem of color migration is avoided since the lakes are insoluble. Prevention of mottling can be helped also by the use of lubricants and other additives which have been colored similarly to the granulation prior to their use. The problem of mottling becomes more pronounced as the concentration of the colorants increases. Color mottling is an undesirable characteristic common to many commercial tablets.

Flavoring Agents

In addition to the sweetness which may be afforded by the diluent of the chewable tablet, eg, mannitol or lactose, artificial sweetening agents may be included. Formerly, the cyclamates, either alone or in combination with saccharin, were widely used. With the banning of the cyclamates and the indefinite status of saccharin new natural sweeteners are being sought. Aspartame (*Searle*), recently made available, may have applications for pharmaceutical formulations. Sweeteners other than the sugars have the advantage of reducing the bulk volume considering the quantity of sucrose required to produce the same degree of sweetness. Being present in small quantities, they do not markedly affect the physical characteristics of the tablet granulation.

Tablet Characteristics

Compressed tablets may be characterized or described by a number of specifications. These include the diameter size, shape, thickness, weight, hardness, disintegration time, and dissolution characteristics. The diameter and shape depend on the die and the punches selected for the compression of the tablet. Generally, tablets are discoid in shape, although they may be oval, oblong, round, cylindrical, or triangular. Their upper and lower surfaces may be flat, round, concave, or convex to various degrees. The concave punches (used to prepare convex tablets) are referred to as shallow, standard, and deep cup, depending on the degree of concavity (see Figs 90-16 and 90-17). The tablets may be scored in halves or quadrants to facilitate breaking if a smaller dose is desired. The top or lower surface may be embossed or engraved with a symbol or letters which serve as an additional means of identifying the source of the tablets. These characteristics along with the color of the tablets tend to make them distinctive and identifiable with the active ingredient which they contain.

The remaining specifications assure the manufacturer that the tablets do not vary from one production lot to another. In the case of new tablet formulations their therapeutic efficacy is demonstrated through clinical trials and it is the manufacturer's aim to reproduce the same tablet with the exact characteristics of the tablets which were used in the clinical evaluation of the dosage form. Therefore, from the control viewpoint these specifications are important for reasons other than physical appearance.

Tablet Hardness

The resistance of the tablet to chipping, abrasion, or breakage under conditions of storage, transportation, and handling before usage depends on its hardness. A commonly used rule of thumb describes a tablet to be of proper hardness if it is firm enough to break with a sharp snap when it is held between the second and third fingers and using the thumb as the fulcrum, yet doesn't break when it falls on the floor. For control purposes a number of attempts have been made to quantitate the degree of hardness.

A small and portable hardness tester was manufactured and introduced in the mid-thirties by the Monsanto Chemical Co. It is now distributed by the Stokes Div (*Pennwalt Corp*) and may be designated as either the Monsanto or Stokes hardness tester. The instrument measures the force required to break the tablet when the force generated by a coil spring is applied diametrically to the tablet. The force is measured in kilograms and when used in production, hardness of 4 kg is considered to be minimum for a satisfactory tablet.

The Strong-Cobb hardness tester introduced in 1950 also measures the diametrically applied force required to break the tablet. In this instrument the force is produced by a manually operated air pump. As the pressure is increased, a plunger is forced against the tablet placed on anvil. The final breaking point is indicated on a dial calibrated into 30 arbitrary units. The hardness values of the Stokes and Strong-Cobb instruments are not equivalent. Values obtained with the Strong-Cobb tester have been found to be 1.6 times those of the Stokes tester.

Another instrument is the Pfizer hardness tester which operates on the same mechanical principle as ordinary pliers.

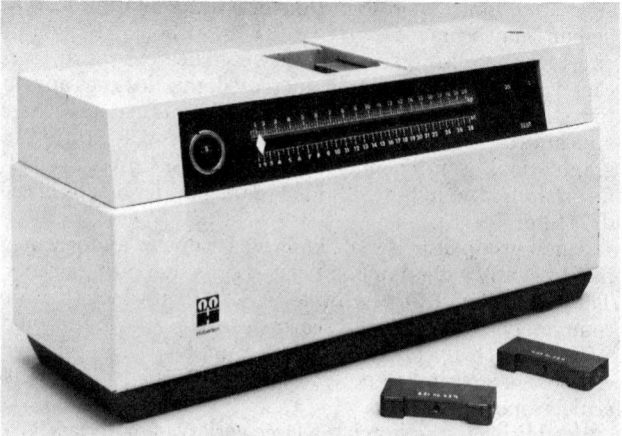

Fig 90-3. The Schleuniger or Heberlein tablet hardness tester shown with calibration blocks (courtesy, Vector).

The force required to break the tablet is recorded on a dial and may be expressed as either kilograms or pounds of force. In an experimental comparison of testers the Pfizer and the Stokes testers were found to check each other fairly well. Again the Strong-Cobb tester was found to give values 1.4–1.7 times the absolute values on the other instruments.

The most widely used apparatus to measure tablet hardness or crushing strength is the Schleuniger apparatus, also known as the Heberlein, distributed by the Vector Corporation. This, and other newer electrically operated test equipment, eliminates the operator variability inherent in the measurements described above. Newer equipment is also available with printers to provide a record of test results. See Fig 90-3.

Hardness determinations are made throughout the tablet runs to determine the need for pressure adjustments on the tableting machine. If the tablet is too hard, it may not disintegrate in the required period of time or meet the dissolution specification; if it is too soft, it will not withstand the handling during subsequent processing such as coating or packaging and shipping operations.

A tablet property related to hardness is tablet *friability*, and the measurement is made by use of the Roche friabilator. Rather than a measure of the force required to crush a tablet, the instrument is designed to evaluate the ability of the tablet to withstand abrasion in packaging, handling, and shipping. A number of tablets are weighed and placed in the tumbling apparatus where they are exposed to rolling and repeated shocks resulting from freefalls within the apparatus. After a given number of rotations the tablets are weighed and the loss in weight indicates the ability of the tablets to withstand this type of wear (Fig 90-4).

A similar approach is taken by many manufacturers when they evaluate a new product in the new market package by sending the package to distant points and back using various methods of transportation. The condition of the product on its return indicates its ability to withstand transportation handling.

Tablet Thickness

The thickness of the tablet from production-run to production-run is carefully controlled. Thickness can vary with no change in weight due to difference in the density of the granulation and the pressure applied to the tablets, as well as the speed of tablet compression. Not only is the tablet thickness important in reproducing tablets identical in appearance but also to insure that every production lot will be usable with selected packaging components. If the tablets

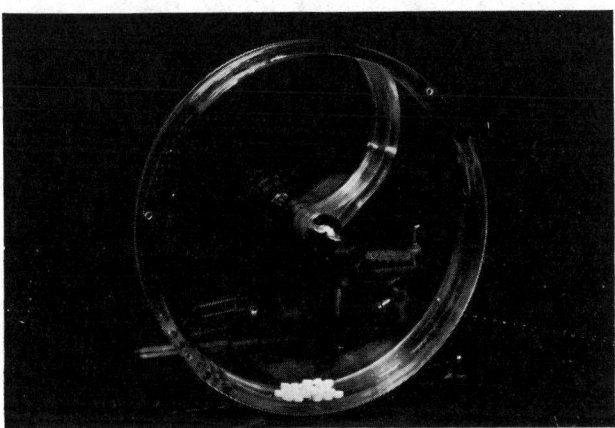

Fig 90-4.   The Roche friabilator (courtesy, Hoffmann-LaRoche).

are thicker than specified, a given number no longer may be contained in the volume of a given size bottle. Tablet thickness also becomes an important characteristic in counting tablets using filling equipment. Some filling equipment utilizes the uniform thickness of the tablets as a counting mechanism. A column containing a known number of tablets is measured for height; filling is then accomplished by continually dropping columns of tablets of the same height into bottles. If thickness varies throughout the lot, the result will be variation in count. Other pieces of filling equipment can malfunction due to variation in tablet thickness since tablets above specified thickness may cause wedging of tablets in previously adjusted depths of the counting slots. Tablet thickness is determined with a caliper or thickness gauge which measures the thickness in millimeters. A plus or minus 5% may be allowed, depending on the size of the tablet.

Uniformity of Dosage Forms

Tablet Weight—The volumetric fill of the die cavity determines the weight of the compressed tablet. In setting up the tablet machine the fill is adjusted to give the desired tablet weight. The weight of the tablet is the quantity of the granulation which contains the labeled amount of the therapeutic ingredient. After the tablet machine is in operation the weights of the tablets are checked routinely either manually or electronically to insure that proper-weight tablets are being made. The USP has provided tolerances for the average weight of uncoated compressed tablets. These are applicable when the tablet contains 50 mg or more of the drug substance or when the latter comprises 50% or more, by weight, of the dosage form. Twenty tablets are weighed individually and the average weight is calculated. The variation from the average weight in the weights of not more than two of the tablets must not differ by more than the percentage listed below; no tablet differs by more than double that percentage. Tablets that are coated are exempt from these requirements but must conform to the test for content uniformity if it is applicable.

Average Weight	Percentage Difference
130 mg or less	10
More than 130 mg through 324 mg	7.5
More than 324 mg	5

Content Uniformity—In order to ensure that every tablet contains the amount of drug substance intended with little variation among tablets within a batch, the USP includes the content uniformity test for certain tablets. Due to the increased awareness of physiological availability, the content

uniformity test has been extended to monographs on all coated and uncoated tablets and all capsules intended for oral administration where the range of sizes of the dosage form available includes a 50 mg or smaller size, in which case the test is applicable to all sizes (50 mg and larger and smaller) of that tablet or capsule. The official compendia can be consulted for the details of the test. Tablet monographs with a content uniformity requirement do not have a weight variation requirement.

Tablet Disintegration

It is generally recognized that the *in vitro* tablet disintegration test does not necessarily bear a relationship to the *in vivo* action of a solid dosage form. To be absorbed, a drug substance must be in solution and the disintegration test is a measure only of the time required under a given set of conditions for a group of tablets to disintegrate into particles. In the present disintegration test the particles are those which will pass through a 10-mesh screen. In a comparison of disintegration times and dissolution rates or initial absorption rates of several brands of aspirin tablets, it was found that the faster absorbed tablets had the longer disintegration time. Regardless of the lack of significance as to *in vivo* action of the tablets, the test provides a means of control in assuring that a given tablet formula is the same as regards disintegration from one production batch to another. The disintegration test is used as a control for tablets intended to be administered by mouth, except where tablets are intended to be chewed before being swallowed or where tablets are designed to release the drug substance over a period of time.

Exact specifications are given for the test apparatus inasmuch as a change in the apparatus can cause a change in the results of the test. The apparatus consists of a basket rack holding six plastic tubes, open at the top and bottom; the bottom of the tubes is covered with 10-mesh screen. See Fig 90-5. The basket rack is immersed in a bath of suitable liquid, held at 37°, preferably in a 1-L beaker. The rack moves up and down in the fluid at a specified rate. The volume of the fluid is such that on the upward stroke the wire mesh remains at least 2.5 cm below the surface of the fluid and descends to not less than 2.5 cm from the bottom on the downward stroke.

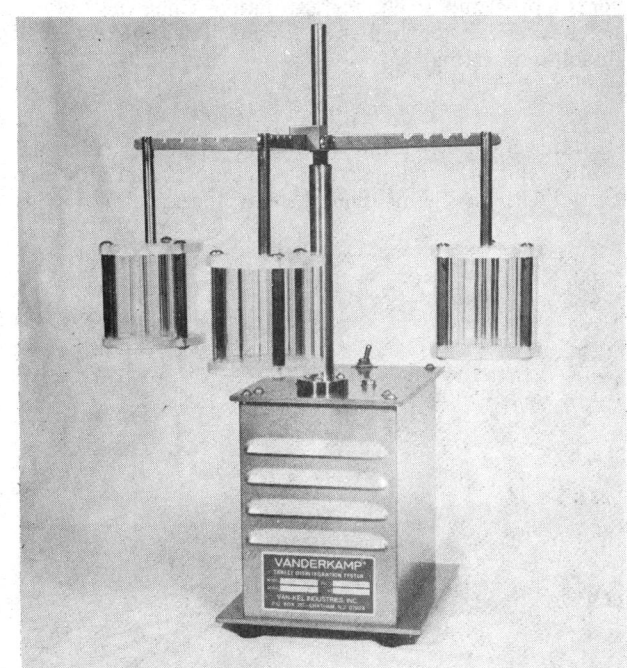

Fig 90-5.   Vanderkamp Tablet Disintegration Tester (courtesy, Van-Kel).

Tablets are placed in each of the six cylinders along with a plastic disk over the tablet unless otherwise directed in the monograph. The end point of the test is indicated when any residue remaining is a soft mass having no palpably soft core. The plastic disks help to force any soft mass which forms through the screen.

For compressed uncoated tablets the testing fluid is usually water at 37°, but in some cases the monographs direct that Simulated Gastric Fluid TS be used. If one or two tablets fail to disintegrate, the test is to be repeated using 12 tablets. Of the 18 tablets then tested, 16 must have disintegrated within the given period of time. The conditions of the test are varied somewhat for coated tablets, buccal tablets, and sublingual tablets. Disintegration times are included in the individual tablet monograph. For most uncoated tablets the period is 30 min although the time for some uncoated tablets varies greatly from this. For coated tablets up to 2 hours may be required, while for sublingual tablets, such as CT Isoproterenol Hydrochloride, the disintegration time is 3 min. For the exact conditions of the test, consult the USP.

Dissolution Test

For certain tablets the monographs direct compliance with limits on dissolution rather than disintegration. Since drug absorption and physiological availability depend on having the drug substance in the dissolved state, suitable dissolution characteristics are an important property of a satisfactory tablet. Like the disintegration test, the dissolution test for measuring the amount of time required for a given percentage of the drug substance in a tablet to go into solution under a specified set of conditions is an *in vitro* test. It is intended to provide a step towards the evaluation of the physiological availability of the drug substance, but as currently described it is not designed to measure the safety or efficacy of the tablet being tested. Both the safety and effectiveness of a specific dosage form must be demonstrated initially by means of appropriate *in vivo* studies and clinical evaluation. Like the disintegration test, the dissolution test does provide a means of control in assuring that a given tablet formulation is the same as regards dissolution as the batch of tablets shown initially to be clinically effective. It also provides an *in vitro* control procedure to eliminate variations among production batches. Refer to Chapter 35 for a complete discussion of dissolution testing.

Validation

In this era of increasing regulatory control of the pharmaceutical industry, manufacturing procedures cannot be discussed without the mention of some process validation ac-

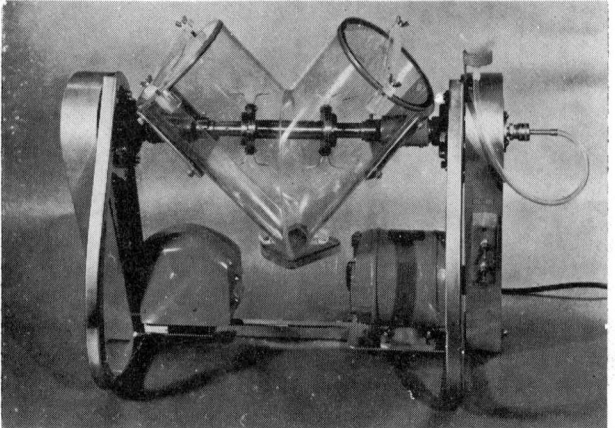

Fig 90-6. Twin-shell blender for solids or liquid–solids blending (courtesy, Patterson-Kelley).

tivity. By way of documentation, product testing, and perhaps in-process testing as well, the manufacturer can demonstrate that his formula and process perform in the manner expected and that it does so reproducibly.

Although the justification for requiring validation is found in the regulations relating to "Current Good Manufacturing Practices for Finished Pharmaceuticals" as well as other sources, there is still much room for interpretation and the process varies from one company to another. General areas of agreement appear to be (1) that the validation activity must begin in R&D and continue through product introduction; (2) that documentation is the key; and (3) that, in general, three batches represent an adequate sample for validation. Until the practice of validation for new products is firmly and universally adopted, retrospective validation (using historical data) for older products is a satisfactory approach.

Methods of Preparation

Wet-Granulation Method

The most widely used and most general method of tablet preparation is the wet-granulation method. Its popularity is due to the greater probability that the granulation will meet all the physical requirements for the compression of good tablets. Its chief disadvantages are the number of separate steps involved, as well as the time and labor necessary to carry out the procedure, especially on the large scale. The steps in the wet method are (1) weighing, (2) mixing, (3) granulation, (4) screening the damp mass, (5) drying, (6) dry screening, (7) lubrication, and (8) compression. The equipment involved depends on the quantity or size of the batch. The active ingredient, diluent, and disintegrant are mixed or blended well. For small batches the ingredients may be mixed in stainless steel bowls or mortars. Small-scale blending also can be carried out on a large piece of paper by holding opposite edges and tumbling the material back and forth. The powder blend may be sifted through a screen of suitable fineness to remove or break up lumps. This screening also affords additional mixing. The screen selected should always be of the same type of wire or cloth that will not affect the potency of the ingredients through interaction. For example, the stability of ascorbic acid is deleteriously affected by even small amounts of copper, thus care must be taken to avoid contact with copper or copper-containing alloys.

For larger quantities of powder the Patterson-Kelley twin-shell blender and the double-cone blender offer means of precision blending and mixing in short periods of time (Fig 90-6). Twin-shell blenders are available in many sizes from laboratory models to large production models. Planetary mixers, eg, the Glen mixer and the Hobart mixer, have served this function in the pharmaceutical industry for many years (Fig 90-7). On a large scale, ribbon blenders are also frequently employed and may be adapted for continuous production procedures. Mass mixers of the sigma-blade type have been widely used in the pharmaceutical industry.

Rapidly increasing in popularity are the high-speed, high-shear mixers such as the Lodige/Littleford, the Diosna, the Fielder, and the Baker-Perkins. For these mixers a full range of sizes are available. Fluid-bed granulation (discussed below) is also gaining wide acceptance in the industry. For both of these types of processing, slight modifications to the following procedures are required.

Solutions of the binding agent are added to the mixed powders with stirring. The powder mass is wetted with the binding solution until the mass has the consistency of damp snow or brown sugar. If the granulation is overwetted, the granules will be hard, requiring considerable pressure to form the tablets, and the resultant tablets may have a mottled appearance. If the powder mixture is not wetted sufficiently,

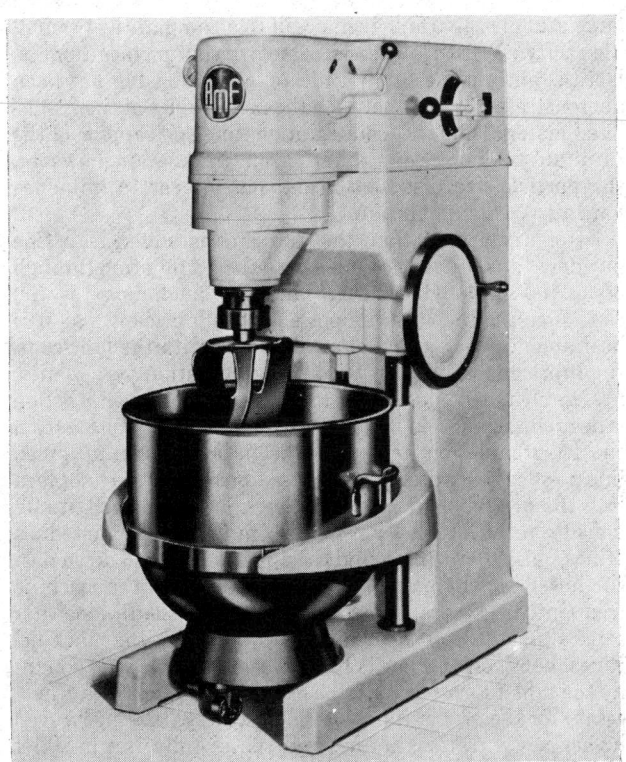

Fig 90-7.   The Glen powder mixer (courtesy, Am Machine).

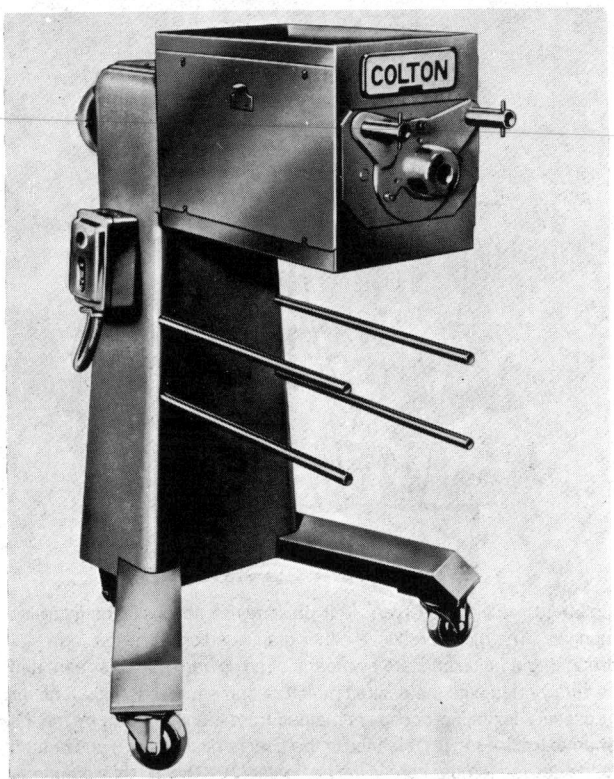

Fig 90-8.   Rotary granulator and sifter (courtesy, Vector/Colton).

the resulting granules will be too soft, breaking down during lubrication and causing difficulty during compression.

The wet granulation is forced through a 6- or 8-mesh screen. Small batches can be forced through by hand using a manual screen. For larger quantities one of several comminuting mills suitable for wet screening can be used. These include the Stokes oscillator, the Colton rotary granulator, the Fitzpatrick comminuting mill, or the Stokes tornado mill. See Fig 90-8. In comminuting mills the granulation is forced through the sieving device by rotating hammers, knives, or oscillating bars. Most high-speed mixers are equipped with a chopper blade which operates independently of the main mixing blades and can replace the wet milling step, ie, can obviate the need for a separate operation.

For tablet formulations where continuous production is justified, extruders such as the Reitz extructor have been adapted for the wet-granulation process. The extruder consists of a screw mixer with a chamber where the powder is mixed with the binding agent and the wet mass is gradually forced through a perforated screen forming threads of the wet granulation. The granulation is then dried by conventional methods. A semiautomatic continuous process using the Reitz extructor has been described for the preparation of the antacid tablet Gelusil (*Warner-Lambert*).

Moist material from the wet milling step is placed on large sheets of paper on shallow wire trays and placed in drying cabinets with a circulating air current and thermostatic heat control. See Fig 90-9. While tray drying was the most widely used method of drying tablet granulations until recently; fluid-bed drying is now equally popular. Notable among the newer methods being introduced are the fluid-bed dryers. In drying tablet granulation by fluidization the material is suspended and agitated in a warm air stream while the granulation is maintained in motion. Drying tests comparing the fluidized bed and a tray dryer for a number of tablet granulations indicated that the former was 15 times faster than the conventional method of tray drying. In addition to the decreased drying time the fluidization method is claimed to have

other advantages such as better control of drying temperatures, decreased handling costs, and the opportunity to blend lubricants and other materials into the dry granulation directly in the fluidized bed. See Fig 90-10.

The application of radio-frequency drying and infrared drying to tablet granulations has been reported as successful for the majority of granulations tried. These methods readily lend themselves to continuous granulation operations. The study of drying methods for tablet granulations led to the development of the Rovac dryer system by Ciba pharmacists and engineers. The dryer is similar in appearance to the cone blender except for the heating jacket and vacuum connections. By excluding oxygen and using the lower drying temperatures made possible by drying in a vacuum, opportunities for degradation of the ingredients during the drying cycle are minimized. A greater uniformity of residual moisture content is achieved because of the moving bed, the controlled temperature, and the controlled time period of the drying cycle. Particle-size distribution can be controlled by varying the speed of rotation and drying temperature as well as by comminuting the granulation to the desired granule size after drying.

In drying granulations it is desirable to maintain a residual amount of moisture in the granulation. This is necessary to

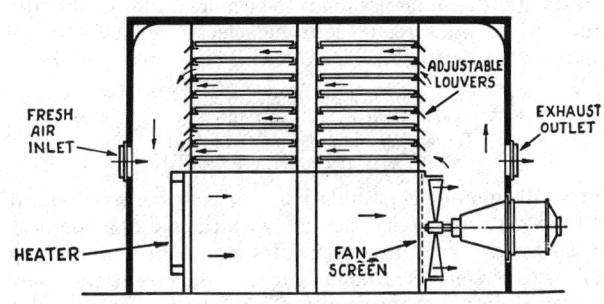

Fig 90-9.   Cross section of tray dryer.

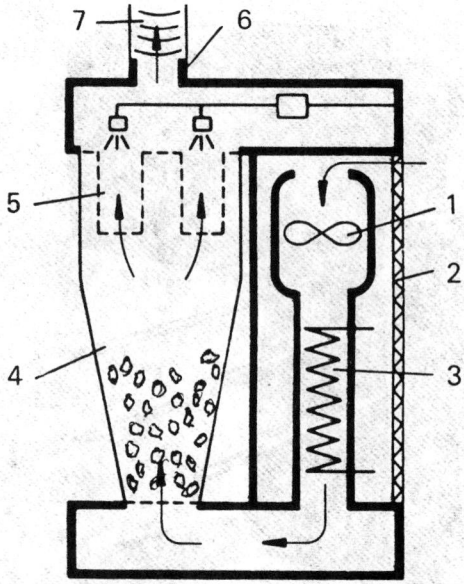

Fig 90-10.   Fluid Bed Dryer. This equipment functions in the following manner. The moist product—either granulated or in powder form—is brought to a fluidized state by means of an upward hot air stream and carefully dried until the desired moisture content is reached. The air necessary for this process is obtained from the work area by means of an extractor fan (1), cleaned in the coarse dust filter (2) and heated to the desired temperature in the air heater (3). The air, thus prepared, now flows upward through the material in the product container (4) soaking up the moisture in the shortest period of time. The filter (5) retains the dust, which is periodically blown off during the process by compressed air. The exhaust air escapes into the open air through the socket (6) and the tube (7) (courtesy, Aeromatic).

maintain the various granulation ingredients such as gums in a hydrated state. Also the residual moisture contributes to the reduction of the static electric charges on the particles. In the selection of any drying process an effort is made to obtain an uniform moisture content. In addition to the importance of moisture content of the granulation in its handling during the manufacturing steps, the stability of the products containing moisture-sensitive active ingredients may be related to the moisture content of the products.

Previously it was indicated that water-soluble colorants can migrate toward the surface of the granulation during the drying process, resulting in mottled tablets after compression. This is also true for water-soluble drug substances, resulting in tablets unsatisfactory as to content uniformity. Migration can be reduced by drying the granulation slowly at low temperatures or using a granulation in which the major diluent is present as granules of large particle size. The presence of microcrystalline cellulose in wet granulations also reduces migration tendencies.

After drying, the granulation is reduced in particle size by passing it through a smaller mesh screen. Following dry screening the granule size tends to be more uniform. For dry granulations the screen size to be selected depends on the diameter of the punch. The following sizes are suggested.

Tablets up to $3/16$ in diam, use 20-mesh
Tablets $7/32$ in to $5/16$ in, use 16-mesh
Tablets $11/32$ in to $13/32$ in, use 14-mesh
Tablets $7/16$ in and larger, use 12-mesh

For small amounts of granulation, hand screens may be used and the material passed through with the aid of a stainless steel spatula. With larger quantities, any of the comminuting mills with screens corresponding to those just mentioned may be used. Note that the smaller the tablet, the finer the dry granulation to enable more uniform filling of the die cavity;

large granules give an irregular fill to a comparatively small die cavity. With compressed tablets of sodium bicarbonate, lactose, and magnesium trisilicate, a relationship has been demonstrated to exist between the particle size of the granulated material and the disintegration time and capping of the resultant tablets. For a sulfathiazole granulation, however, the particle-size distribution did not appear to influence hardness or disintegration.

After dry granulation, the lubricant is added as a fine powder. It is usually screened onto the granulation through 60- or 100-mesh nylon cloth to eliminate small lumps as well as to increase the covering power of the lubricant. As it is desirable for each granule to be covered with the lubricant, the lubricant is blended with the granulation very gently, preferably in a blender using tumbling action. Gentle action is desired to maintain the uniform granule size resulting from the dry-granulation step. It has been claimed that too much fine powder is not desirable because fine powder may not feed into the die evenly; consequently, variations in weight and density result. Fine powders, commonly designated as "fines," also blow out around the upper punch and down past the lower punch, making it necessary to clean the machine frequently. Air trapped in the tablets by the fine powder causes them to split apart after ejection from the machine. Fines, however, at a level of 10–20% are traditionally sought by the tablet formulator. The presence of some fines is necessary for the proper filling of the die cavity. Recently, even higher concentrations of fines were successfully used in tablet manufacture. Some investigators maintain that no general limits exist for the amount of fines that can be present in a granulation but must be determined for each specific formula.

Another approach toward the faster preparation of tablet granulations has come from the utilization of the air-suspension technique developed by Wurster.[8] Both Aeromatic and Glatt fluid-bed granulating equipment are available in a full range of sizes, from laboratory models to the largest production sizes. In this method particles of an inert material, or the active drug, are suspended in a vertical column with a rising air stream; while the particles are suspended, the common granulating materials in solution are sprayed into the column. There is a gradual particle buildup under a controlled set of conditions resulting in a tablet granulation which is ready for compression after addition of the lubricant. An obvious advantage exists since granulating and drying can take place in a single piece of equipment. It should be noted, however, that many of the mixers discussed previously can be supplied with a steam jacket and can provide the same advantage. In addition to its use for the preparation of tablet granulations this technique also has been proposed for the coating of solid particles as a means of improving the flow properties of small particles (see page 1627). Researchers have observed that in general fluid-bed granulation yields a less dense particle than conventional methods and this can affect subsequent compression behavior. A large-scale fluid-bed granulation process has been described for Tylenol (*McNeil*). Methods for the preparation of compressed tablets have been reviewed in the literature.[9]

In the Merck Sharp & Dohme facility at Elkton, Virginia, the entire tablet manufacturing process based on a wet-granulation method is computer-controlled. By means of a computer, the system weighs the ingredients, blends, granulates, dries, and lubricates to prepare a uniform granulation of specified particle size and particle size distribution. The computer directs the compression of the material into tablets having exacting specifications for thickness, weight, and hardness. After compression, the tablets are coated with a water-based film coating. The computer controls and monitors all flow of material. The facility represents an innovation in pharmaceutical manufacturing. See Fig 90-11.

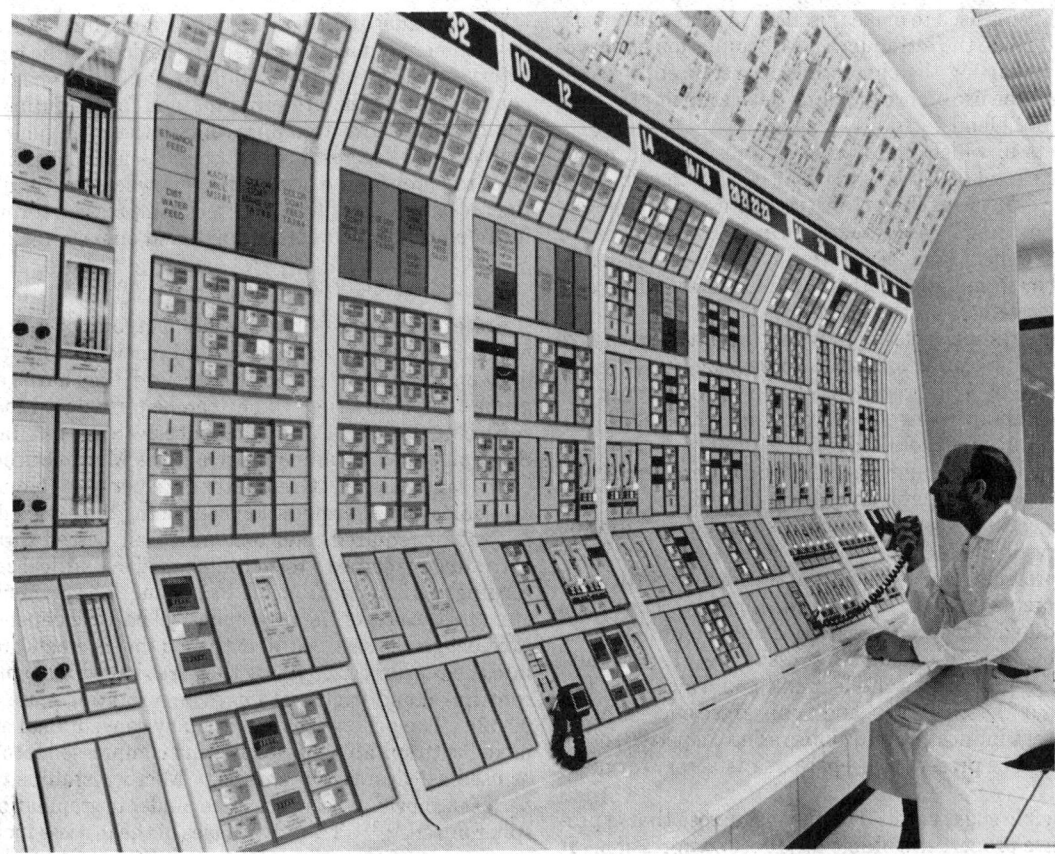

Fig 90-11.   Computer control room for the first large-scale computer-controlled tablet manufacturing facility (courtesy, MSD).

Although the Merck facility represents the most fully automated production operation, there are many others throughout the industry which have parts of the operation (such as a coating, a compressing, or a fluid-bed granulation process) operating under a high degree of sophistication and automation. This is the trend for the future. Equipment suppliers work closely with individual pharmaceutical companies in designing specialized and unique systems.

Dry-Granulation Method

When tablet ingredients are sensitive to moisture or are unable to withstand elevated temperatures during drying, and when the tablet ingredients have sufficient inherent binding or cohesive properties, slugging may be used to form granules. This method is referred to as dry granulation, precompression, or the double-compression method. It eliminates a number of steps but still includes (1) weighing, (2) mixing, (3) slugging, (4) dry screening, (5) lubrication, and (6) compression. The active ingredient, diluent (if one is required), and part of the lubricant are blended. One of the constituents, either the active ingredient or the diluent, must have cohesive properties. Powdered material contains a considerable amount of air; under pressure this air is expelled and a fairly dense piece is formed. The more time allowed for this air to escape, the better the tablet or slug.

When slugging is used, large tablets are made as slugs because fine powders flow better into large cavities. Also, producing large slugs decreases production time; $7/8$ to 1 in. are the most practical sizes for slugs. Sometimes, to obtain the pressure which is desired the slug sizes are reduced to $3/4$ in. The punches should be flat-faced. The compressed slugs are comminuted through the desirable mesh screen either by hand, or for larger quantities through the Fitzpatrick or similar comminuting mill. The lubricant remaining is added to the granulation, blended gently, and the material is com-

pressed into tablets. Aspirin is a good example where slugging is satisfactory. Other materials such as aspirin combinations, acetophenetidin, thiamine hydrochloride, ascorbic acid, magnesium hydroxide, and other antacid compounds may be treated similarly.

Results comparable to those accomplished by the slugging process are also obtained with compacting mills. In the compaction method the powder to be densified passes between high-pressure rollers which compress the powder and remove the air. The densified material is reduced to a uniform granule size and compressed into tablets after the addition of a lubricant. Excessive pressures which may be required to obtain cohesion of certain materials may result in a prolonged dissolution rate. Compaction mills available include the Chilsonator (*Fitzpatrick*), Roller Compactor (*Vector*), and the Compactor Mill (*Allis-Chalmers*).

Direct Compression

As its name implies, direct compression consists of compressing tablets directly from powdered material without modifying the physical nature of the material itself. Formerly, direct compression as a method of tablet manufacture was reserved for a small group of crystalline chemicals having all the physical characteristics required for the formation of a good tablet. This group includes chemicals such as potassium salts (chlorate, chloride, bromide, iodide, nitrate, permanganate), ammonium chloride, and methenamine. These materials possess cohesive and flow properties which make direct compression possible.

Since the pharmaceutical industry is constantly making efforts to increase the efficiency of tableting operations and to reduce costs by utilizing the smallest amount of floor space and labor as possible for a given operation, increasing attention is being given to this method of tablet preparation.

Approaches being used to make this method more universally applicable include the introduction of formulation additives capable of imparting the characteristics required for compression, and the use of force-feeding devices to improve the flow of powder blends.

For tablets in which the drug itself constitutes a major portion of the total tablet weight, it is necessary that the drug possess those physical characteristics required for the formulation to be compressed directly. Direct compression for tablets containing 25% or less of drug substances frequently can be used by formulating with a suitable diluent which acts as a carrier or vehicle for the drug.[10]

Direct-compression vehicles or carriers must have good flow and compressible characteristics. These properties are imparted to them by a preprocessing step such as wet granulation, slugging, spray drying, spheronization, or crystallization. These vehicles include processed forms of most of the common diluents including dicalcium phosphate dihydrate, tricalcium phosphate, calcium sulfate, anhydrous lactose, spray-dried lactose, pregelatinized starch, compressible sugar, mannitol, and microcrystalline cellulose. These commercially available direct compression vehicles may contain small quantities of other ingredients (eg, starch) as processing aids. Dicalcium phosphate dihydrate (*Di-Tab*, Stauffer) in its unmilled form has good flow properties and compressibility. It is a white crystalline agglomerate insoluble in water and alcohol. The chemical is odorless, tasteless, and nonhygroscopic. Since it has no inherent lubricating or disintegrating properties, other additives must be present to prepare a satisfactory formulation.

Compressible sugar consists mainly of sucrose that is processed to have properties suitable for direct compression. It may also contain small quantities of dextrin, starch, or invert sugar. It is a white crystalline powder with a sweet taste and complete water solubility. It requires the incorporation of a suitable lubricant at normal levels for lubricity. The sugar is widely used for chewable vitamin tablets because of its natural sweetness. One commercial source is *Di-Pac* (Amstar) prepared by the co-crystallization of 97% sucrose and 3% dextrins. Some forms of lactose meet the requirements for a direct-compression vehicle. Hydrous lactose does not flow and its use is limited to tablet formulations prepared by the wet granulation method. Both anhydrous lactose and spray-dried lactose have good flowability and compressibility and can be used in direct compression provided a suitable disintegrant and lubricant are present. Mannitol is a popular diluent for chewable tablets due to its pleasant taste and mouthfeel resulting from its negative heat of solution. In its granular form (ICI Americas) it has good flow and compressible qualities. It has a low moisture content and is not hygroscopic.

The excipient that has been studied extensively as a direct compression vehicle is microcrystalline cellulose (*Avicel*, FMC Corp.). This nonfibrous form of cellulose is obtained by spray-drying washed, acid-treated cellulose and is available in several grades which range in average particle size from 20 μm to 100 μm. It is water-insoluble but the material has the ability to draw fluid into a tablet by capillary action; it swells on contact and thus acts as a disintegrating agent. The material flows well and has a degree of self-lubricating qualities, thus requiring a lower level of lubricant as compared to other excipients.

Forced-flow feeders are mechanical devices available from pharmaceutical equipment manufacturers designed to deaerate light and bulky material. Mechanically they maintain a steady flow of powder moving into the die cavities under moderate pressure. They attempt to minimize air entrapment and consequently capping in the finished tablet. By increasing the density of the powder, higher uniformity in tablet weights is obtained. See Fig 90-24.

The gradual improvement of formulation additives and development of mechanical feeding devices for the high-speed rotary tableting machines indicate the acceptance of direct compression as the preferred method for the future. Of all the methods, direct compression is the most adaptable to automation. Interest in direct compression is also stimulating basic research on the flowability of powders with and without the presence of additives. Direct compression formulas are included in the formula section found on page 1622.

Related Granulation Processes

Spheronization—Spheronization, a form of pelletization, refers to the formation of spherical particles from wet granulations. Since the particles are round, they have good flow properties when dried. They can be formulated to contain sufficient binder to impart cohesiveness for tableting. Spheronization equipment such as the Marumerizer (*Luwa Corp*) and the CF-Granulator (*Vector*) is commercially available. A wet granulation containing the drug substance, diluent (if required) and binder, is first passed through an extruding machine to form rod-shaped cylindrical segments ranging in diameter from 0.5 to 12 mm. The segment diameter and the size of the final spherical particle depend on the extruder screen size. After extrusion the segments are placed into the Marumerizer where they are shaped into spheres by centrifugal and frictional forces on a rotating plate (see Fig 90-12). The pellets are then dried by conventional methods, mixed with suitable lubricants, and compressed into tablets, or used as capsule-fill material. Microcrystalline cellulose has been shown to be an effective binder in granulations to be spheronized.[11,12] The advantages of the process include the production of granules, regular in shape, size, and surface characteristics; low friability resulting in fewer fines and dust; and the ability to regulate the size of the spheres within a narrow particle size distribution.

Spheres can also be produced by fluid-bed granulation techniques and by other specialized equipment such as the CF-Granulator (*Vector*). These processes, however, must begin with crystals or nonpareil seeds followed by buildup. Exact results, such as sphere density, are different for the various methods and could be important in product performance.

Spray-Drying—A number of tableting additives suitable for direct compression have been prepared by the drying process known as spray-drying. The method consists of bringing together a highly dispersed liquid and a sufficient volume of hot air to produce evaporation and drying of the liquid droplets. The feed liquid may be a solution, slurry, emulsion, gel, or paste, provided it is pumpable and capable of being atomized. As shown in Fig 90-13, the feed is sprayed into a current of warm filtered air. The air supplies the heat

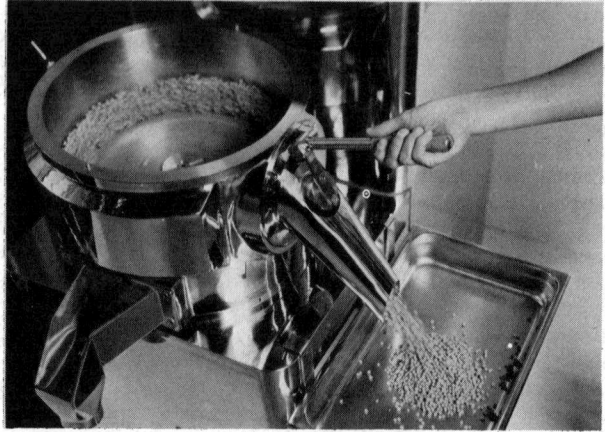

Fig 90-12.   The inside of a QJ-400 Marumerizer (courtesy, Luwa).

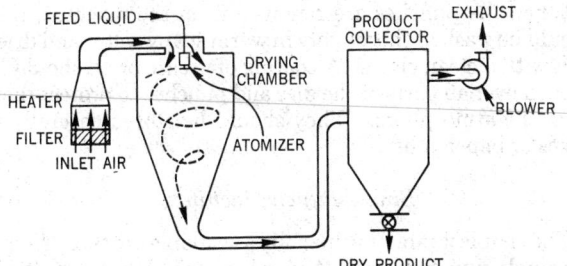

Fig 90-13.   Typical spray-drying system (courtesy, Bowen Eng).

for evaporation and conveys the dried product to the collector; the air is then exhausted with the moisture. As the liquid droplets present a large surface area to the warm air, local heat and transfer coefficients are high.

The spray-dried powder particles are homogeneous, approximately spherical in shape, nearly uniform in size, and frequently hollow. The latter characteristic results in low bulk density with a rapid rate of solution. Being uniform in size and spherical, the particles possess good flowability. The design and operation of the spray-dryer can vary many characteristics of the final product, such as particle size and size distribution, bulk and particle densities, porosity, moisture content, flowability, and friability. Among the spray-dried materials available for direct compression formulas are lactose, mannitol, and flour. Another application of the process in tableting is spray-drying the combination of tablet additives as the diluent, disintegrant, and binder. The spray-dried material is then blended with the active ingredient or drug, lubricated, and compressed directly into tablets.

Since atomization of the feed results in a high surface area, the moisture evaporates rapidly. The evaporation keeps the product cool and as a result the method is applicable for drying heat-sensitive materials. Among heat-sensitive pharmaceuticals successfully spray-dried are the amino acids; antibiotics as aureomycin, bacitracin, penicillin, and streptomycin; ascorbic acid; cascara extracts; liver extracts; pepsin and similar enzymes; protein hydrolysates; and thiamine.[13]

Frequently, spray-drying is more economical than other processes since it produces a dry powder directly from a liquid and eliminates other processing steps as crystallization, precipitation, filtering or drying, particle size reduction, and particle classifying. By the elimination of these steps, labor, equipment costs, space requirements, and possible contamination of the product are reduced. Intrinsic factor concentrate obtained from hog mucosa previously was prepared at Lederle Laboratories using a salt precipitation process, followed by a freeze-drying. By utilizing spray-drying it was possible to manufacture a high-grade material by a continuous process. The spherical particles of the product facilitated its subsequent blending with vitamin B_{12}. Similar efficiencies have been found in processes producing magnesium trisilicate and dihydroxyaluminum sodium carbonate; both chemicals are widely used in antacid preparations.

Encapsulation of chemicals can also be achieved using spray-drying equipment. The process is useful in coating one material on another in order to protect the interior substance or to control the rate of its release. The substance to be coated can either be liquid or solid, but must be insoluble in a solution of the coating material. The oil-soluble vitamins, A and D, can be coated with a variety of materials as acacia gum to prevent their deterioration. Flavoring oils and synthetic flavors are coated to give the so-called dry flavors.

Spray-Congealing—Also called spray-chilling, spray-congealing is a technique similar to spray-drying. It consists of melting solids and reducing them to beads or powder by spraying the molten feed into a stream of air or other gas. The same basic equipment is used as with spray-drying although

no source of heat is required. Either ambient or cooled air is used depending on the freezing point of the product. For example, monoglycerides and similar materials are spray-congealed with air at 50°F. A closed-loop system with refrigeration cools and recycles the air. Using this process, drugs can be dissolved or suspended in a molten wax and spray-congealed; the resultant material then can be adapted for a prolonged-release form of the drug.

Among the carbohydrates used in compressed tablets, mannitol is the only one which possesses high heat stability. Mannitol melts at 167° and either alone or in combination with other carbohydrates can be fused and spray-congealed. Selected drugs have been shown to be soluble in these fused mixtures, and the resultant spray-congealed material possesses excellent flow and compression characteristics.

Tablet Machines

As mentioned previously, the basic mechanical unit in tablet compression involves the operation of two steel punches within a steel die cavity. The tablet is formed by the pressure exerted on the granulation by the punches within the die cavity, or cell. The tablet assumes the size and shape of the punches and die used. See Figs 90-14 and 90-15. While round tablets are more generally used, shapes such as oval, capsule-form, square, triangular, or other irregular shapes may be used. Likewise, the curvature of the faces of the punches determines the curvature of the tablets. The diameters generally found to be satisfactory and frequently referred to as standard are as follows: $\frac{3}{16}$ in, $\frac{7}{32}$ in, $\frac{1}{4}$ in, $\frac{9}{32}$ in, $\frac{5}{16}$ in, $\frac{11}{32}$ in, $\frac{7}{16}$ in, $\frac{1}{2}$ in, $\frac{9}{16}$ in, $\frac{5}{8}$ in, $\frac{11}{16}$ in, and $\frac{3}{4}$ in. Punch faces with ridges are used for compressed tablets scored for breaking into halves or fourths, although it has been indicated that variation among tablet halves is significantly greater than among intact tablets. However, a patented formulation[14] for a tablet scored to form a groove which is one-third to two-thirds the depth of the total tablet thickness is claimed to give equal parts containing substantially equal amounts of the drug substance. Tablets, engraved or embossed with symbols or initials, require punches with faces embossed or engraved with the corresponding designs. See Fig 90-16 and Fig 90-17. The use of the tablet sometimes determines its shape; effervescent tablets are usually large, round, and flat, while vitamin tablets are frequently prepared in capsule-shaped forms. Tablets prepared using deep-cup punches appear to be round and when coated take on the appearance of pills. Veterinary tablets often have a bolus shape and are much larger than those used in medical practice.

The quality-control program for punches and dies, frequently referred to as tooling, instituted by large pharmaceutical companies emphasizes the importance of their care in modern pharmaceutical production. To produce physically perfect compressed tablets, an efficient punch-and-die program must be set up. Provisions for inspection of tooling, parameters for cost-per-product determination, product identification, and tooling specifications must all be considered. A committee of the Industrial and Pharmaceutical Technology Section of the APhA Academy of Pharmaceutical Sciences has established a set of dimensional specifications and tolerances for standard punches and dies.[15]

Regardless of the size of the tableting operation, the at-

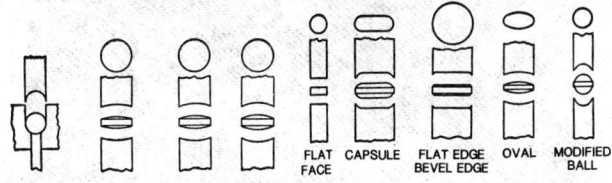

Fig 90-14.   Concave punches.

SPHERICAL   SHALLOW   STANDARD   DEEP

FLAT FACE   CAPSULE   FLAT EDGE BEVEL EDGE   OVAL   MODIFIED BALL

Fig 90-15.   Specially shaped punches.

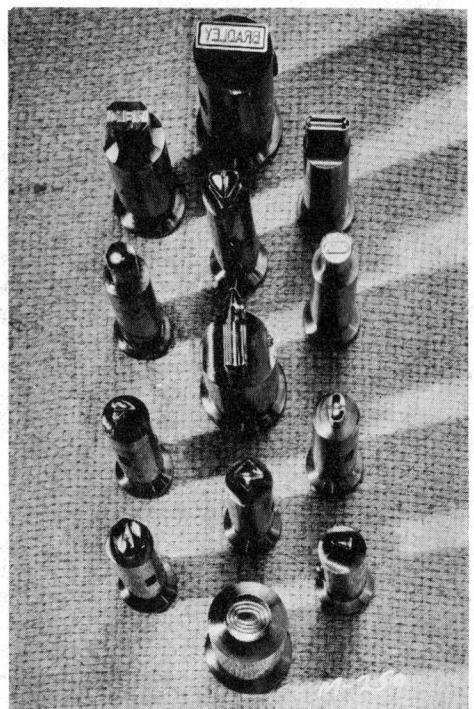

Fig 90-16.   Collection of punches (courtesy, Stokes/Pennwalt).

tention which must be given to the proper care of punches and dies should be noted.   They must be highly polished and kept free from rust and imperfections.   In cases where the material pits or abrades the dies, chromium-plated dies have been used. Dropping the punches on hard surfaces will chip their fine edges.   When the punches are in the machine, the upper and lower punches should not be allowed to contact each other. Otherwise, a curling or flattening of the edges will result which is one of the causes of capping.   This is especially necessary to observe in the case of deep-cup punches.

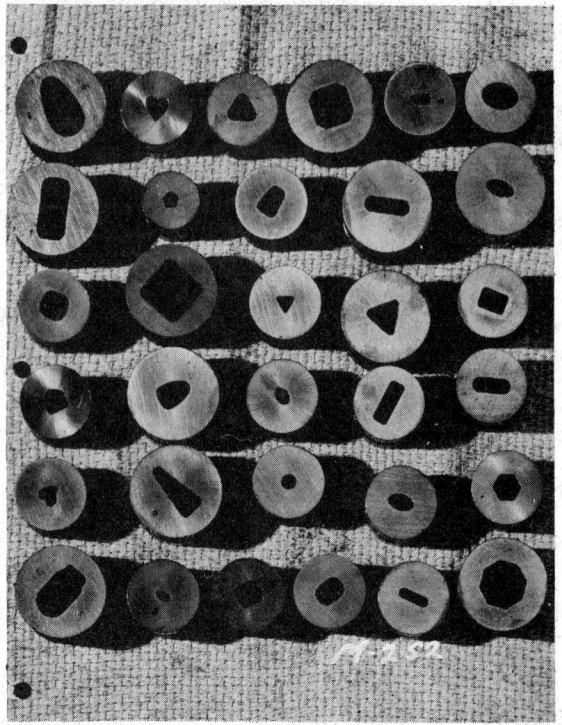

Fig 90-17.   Collection of dies (courtesy, Stokes/Pennwalt).

When the punches are removed from the machine, they should be washed thoroughly in warm soapy water and dried well with a clean cloth.   A coating of grease or oil should be rubbed over all parts of the dies and punches to protect them from the atmosphere.   They should be stored carefully in boxes or paper tubes.

Single-Punch Machines

The simplest tableting machines available are those having the single-punch design.   A number of models are available as outlined in Table I.   While the majority of these are power-driven, several hand-operated models are available. Compression is accomplished on a single-punch machine as shown in Fig 90-18.   The feed shoe filled with the granulation is positioned over the die cavity which then fills.   The feed shoe retracts and scrapes all excess granulation away from the die cavity.   The upper punch lowers to compress the granulation within the die cavity.   The upper punch retracts and the lower punch rises to eject the tablet.   As the feed shoe returns to fill the die cavity, it pushes the compressed tablet from the die platform.   The weight of the tablet is determined by the volume of the die cavity; the lower punch is adjustable to increase or decrease the volume of granulation, thus increasing or decreasing the weight of the tablet.

For tablets having diameters larger than $\frac{1}{2}$ in, sturdier models are required.   This is also true for tablets requiring a high degree of hardness as in the case of compressed lozenges.   The heavier models are capable of much higher pressures and are suitable for slugging.

Operation of Single-Punch Machines

In installing punches and dies in a single-punch machine insert the lower punch first by lining up the notched groove on the punch with the lower punch setscrew and slipping it into the smaller bore in the die table; the setscrew is not tightened as yet.   The lower punch is differentiated from the upper punch in that it has a collar around the punch head.   Slip the die over the punch head so that the notched groove (with the widest area at the top) lines up with the die setscrew.   Tighten the lower punch setscrew after seating the lower punch by pressing on the punch with the thumb.   Tighten the die setscrew, making certain that the surface of the die is flush with the die table.   Insert the upper punch, again lining up the grooved notch with the upper punch setscrew.   To be certain that the upper punch is securely seated, turn the machine over by hand with a block of soft wood or wad of cloth between the upper and lower punches.   When the punch is seated, tighten the upper punch setscrew.   Adjust the pressure so that the upper and lower punches will not come in contact with each other when the machine is turned over.   Adjust the lower punch so that it is flush with the die table at the ejection point.   Install the feed shoe and hopper.

After adding a small amount of granulation to the hopper, turn the machine over by hand and adjust the pressure until a tablet is formed. Adjust the tablet weight until the desired weight is obtained.   The pressure will have to be altered concurrently with the weight adjustments.   It should be remembered that as the fill is increased the lower punch moves further away from the upper punch and more pressure will have to be applied to obtain comparable hardness.   Conversely, when the fill is decreased, the pressure will have to be decreased.   When all the adjustments

Table I—Single-Punch Tablet Machines

Machine model	Maximum tablet diameter (in)	Press speed (tablets/min)	Depth of fill (in)
Stokes-Pennwalt equipment[a]			
511-5	$\frac{1}{2}$	40–75	$\frac{7}{16}$
206-4	$1\frac{3}{4}$	10–40	$1\frac{1}{16}$
530-1	2	12–48	$1\frac{5}{8}$
525-2	3	16–48	2
Manesty equipment (Thomas Eng)			
Hand machine	$\frac{1}{2}$	100	$\frac{7}{16}$
Model F3	$\frac{7}{8}$	85	$\frac{11}{16}$
Model 35T[a]	3	36	$2\frac{1}{4}$

[a] Widely used for veterinary boluses.

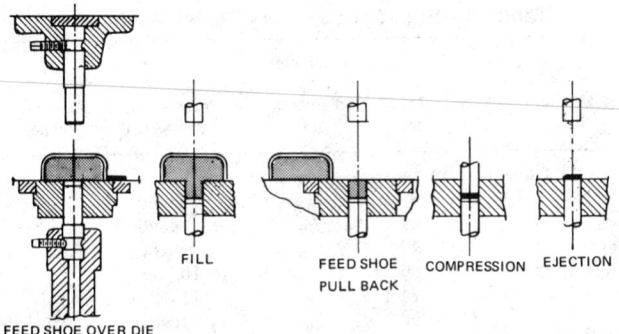

Fig 90-18. Formation of tablet on single-punch machine (courtesy, Vector/Colton).

have been made, fill the hopper with granulation and turn on the motor. Hardness and weight should be checked immediately and suitable adjustments made if necessary. Periodic checks should be made on the tablet hardness and weight during the running of the batch at 15–30 min intervals.

When the batch has been run off, turn off the power and remove loose dust and granulation with the vacuum cleaner. Release the pressure from the punches. Remove the feed hopper and the feed shoe. Remove the upper punch, the lower punch, and the die. Clean all surfaces of the tablet machine and dry well with clean cloth. Cover surfaces with thin coating of grease or oil prior to storage.

As tablets are ejected from the machine after compression, they are usually accompanied with powder and uncompressed granulation. To remove this loose dust, the tablets are passed over a screen, which may be vibrating, and cleaned with a vacuum line.

Rotary Tablet Machines

For increased production rotary machines offer great advantages. A head carrying a number of sets of punches and dies revolves continuously while the tablet granulation runs from the hopper, through a feed frame, and into the dies placed in a large, steel plate revolving under it. This method promotes a uniform fill of the die and therefore an accurate

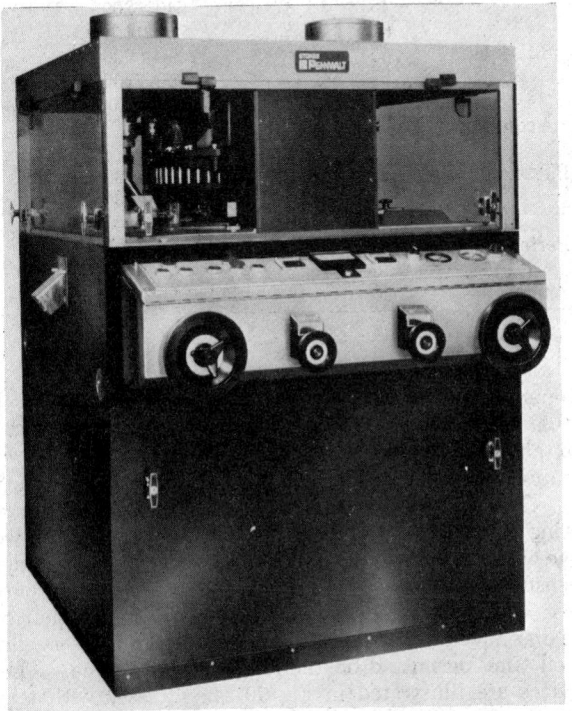

Fig 90-19. Model 747 High Speed Press, double-sided rotary compacting press designed to produce at speeds over 10,000/min (courtesy, Stokes/Pennwalt).

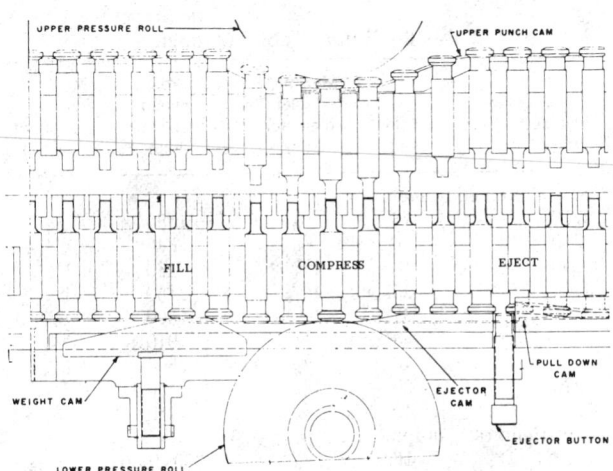

Fig 90-20. Tooling for a 16-station rotary press showing positions of the cycle required to produce 1 tablet/set of tooling (courtesy, Vector/Colton).

weight for the tablet. Compression takes place as the upper and lower punches pass between a pair of rollers. This action produces a slow squeezing effect on the material in the die cavity from the top and bottom and so gives a chance for the entrapped air to escape. The lower punch lifts up and ejects the tablet. Adjustments for tablet weight and hardness can be made without the use of tools while the machine is in operation. Fig 90-20 shows the tooling in a 16-station rotary press in the positions of a complete cycle to produce 1 tablet/set of tooling. One of the factors which contributes to the variation in tablet weight and hardness during compression is the internal flow of the granulation within the feed hopper.

On most rotary machine models there is an excess pressure release which cushions each compression and relieves the machine of all shocks and undue strain. The punches and dies can be readily removed for inspection, cleaning, and for inserting different sets to produce a great variety of sizes and shapes. It is possible to equip the machine with as few punches and dies as the job requires and thus economize on installation costs. For types of rotary machines available, see Table II.

Operation of Rotary Machines

Before inserting punches and dies, make certain that the pressure has been released from the pressure wheel. The die holes should be cleaned thoroughly, making certain that the die seat is completely free of any foreign materials. Back off all die locks and loosely insert dies into the die holes, then tap each die securely into place with a fiber of soft metal rod through the upper punch holes. After all the dies have been tapped into place, tighten each die lockscrew progressively and securely. As each screw is tightened the die is checked to see that it does not project above the die table. Insert the lower punches through the hole made available by removing the punch head. Turn the machine by hand until the punch bore coincides with the plug hole. Insert each lower punch in its place progressively. Insert the upper punches by dropping them into place in the head. Each punch (upper and lower) should be coated with a thin film of mineral oil before inserting them into the machine. Adjust the ejection cam so that the lower punch is flush with the die table at the ejection point.

After insertion of the punches and dies adjust the machine for the tablet weight and hardness. The feed frame should be attached to the machine along with the feed hopper. Add a small amount of the granulation through the hopper and turn over the machine by hand. Increase the pressure by rotating the pressure wheel until a tablet is formed. Check the weight of the tablet and adjust the fill to provide the desired tablet weight. Most likely more than one adjustment of the fill will be necessary before obtaining the acceptable weight. When the fill is decreased, the pressure must be decreased to provide the same hardness in the tablet. Conversely, when the fill is increased, the pressure must be increased to obtain comparable hardness.

Fill the hopper with the granulation and turn on the power. Check tablet weight and hardness immediately after the mechanical operation

Table II—Rotary Tablet Machines

Machine model	Tool sets	Maximum tablet diameter (in)	Press speed (tablets/min)	Depth of fill (in)
Vector-Colton equipment				
2216	16	5/8	1180	3/4
240	16	7/8	640	13/16
250	12	1 1/4	480	1 1/8
260	25	1 3/16	1450	1 3/8
	31	1	1800	1 3/8
	33	15/16	1910	1 3/8
	43	5/8	2500	1 3/8
270	25	1 3/8	450	2 3/4
	42	7/8	750	2 3/4
Stokes-Pennwalt equipment				
512-1	16	5/8	350–1050	11/16
516-1	23	1 3/16	240–720	1 3/8
550-2	16	15/16	365–640	1 1/16
555	45	7/16	1050–4200	11/16
	35	5/8	800–3200	11/16
328-1	45	3/4	1600–4500	11/16
Manesty equipment (Thomas Eng)				
B3B	16	5/8	350–700	11/16
	23	7/16	500–1000	11/16
BB3B	27	5/8	760–1520	11/16
	33	7/16	924–1848	11/16
	35	5/8	1490–2980	11/16
	45	7/16	1913–3826	11/16
D3B	16	1	260–520	13/16
Key equipment				
DC-16	16	15/16	210–510	13/16
BBC	27	5/8	1025–2100	11/16
	35	5/8	1325–2725	11/16
	45	7/16	1700–3500	11/16
Cadpress	37	15/16	850–3500	13/16
	45	5/8	2000–6000	11/16
	55	7/16	2500–7500	11/16
Fette equipment (Raymond Auto)		(mm)		(mm)
Perfecta 1000	28	16	2100	18
	33	13	2475	18
Perfecta 2000	29	25	2175	22
	36	16	3600	18
	43	13	4300	18

Table III—High-Speed Rotary Tablet Machines

Machine model	Tool sets	Maximum tablet diameter (in)	Press speed (tablets/min)	Depth of fill (in)
Vector-Colton equipment				
2247	33	5/8	3480	3/4
	41	7/16	4300	3/4
	49	7/16	5150	3/4
Magna	66	23/32	10,560	3/4
	74	1/2	11,840	3/4
	90	7/16	14,400	3/4
Stokes-Pennwalt equipment				
555-2	35	5/8	800–3200	11/16
328-4	45	3/4	1600–4500	1 3/8
610	65	7/16	3500–10,000	11/16
747	65	7/16	3000–10,000	11/16
	53	5/8	2900–8100	11/16
	41	15/16	2150–6150	11/16
Direct Triple Compression Type				
580-1	45	7/16	525–2100	11/16
580-2	35	5/8	400–1600	11/16
610	65	7/16	3500–10,000	11/16
	53	5/8	2900–8100	11/16
Manesty equipment (Thomas Eng)				
Betapress	16	5/8	600–1500	11/16
	23	7/16	860–2160	11/16
Express	20	1	800–2000	13/16
	25	5/8	1000–2500	11/16
	30	7/16	1200–3000	11/16
Unipress	20	1	970–2420	13/16
	27	5/8	1300–3270	11/16
	34	7/16	1640–4120	11/16
Novapress	37	1	760–3700	13/16
	45	5/8	900–4500	11/16
	61	7/16	1220–6100	11/16
BB3B	35	5/8	1490–2980	11/16
BB4	27	5/8	900–2700	11/16
	35	5/8	1167–3500	11/16
	45	7/16	1500–4500	11/16
Rotapress				
Mark IIA	37	1	710–3550	13/16
	45	5/8	1640–8200	11/16
	61	7/16	2220–11,100	11/16
Mark IV	45	1	2090–6000	13/16
	55	5/8	2550–7330	11/16
	75	7/16	3500–10,000	11/16
Fette equipment (Raymond Auto)		(mm)		(mm)
PT 2080	29	25	435–2900	18
	36	16	540–4100	18
	43	16	645–4900	18
Perfecta 3000	37	25	4400	22
	45	16	6750	18
	55	13	10,500	18

begins and make suitable adjustments, if necessary. Check these properties routinely and regularly at 15–30 min intervals while the machine is in operation. When the batch has been run, turn off the power. Remove the hopper and feed frame from the machine. Remove loose granulation and dust with a vacuum line. Remove all pressure from the wheel. Remove the punches and dies in the reverse order of that used in setting up the machine. First, remove the upper punches individually, then the lower punches, and finally the dies. Wash each punch and die in alcohol and brush with a soft brush to remove adhering material. Dry them with a clean cloth and cover them with a thin coating of grease or oil before storing.

High-Speed Rotary Tablet Machines

The rotary tablet machine has gradually evolved into models capable of compressing tablets at high production rates. See Figs 90-19, 90-21, and 90-22. This has been accomplished by increasing the number of stations, ie, sets of punches and dies, in each revolution of the machine head, improvement in feeding devices, and on some models the installation of dual compression points. In Fig 90-23, the drawing shows a rotary machine having dual compression points. Rotary machines having dual compression points are referred to as double rotary machines, and those with one compression point, single rotary. In the diagram, half of the tablets are produced 180° from the tablet chute. They travel outside the perimeter and discharge with the second tablet production. While these models are mechanically capable of operating at the production rates shown in Table III, the actual speed still depends on the physical characteristics of the tablet granulation and the rate which is consistent with compressed tablets having satisfactory physical characteristics. The main difficulty in rapid machine operation is assuring adequate filling of the dies. With rapid filling, dwell time of the die cavity beneath the feed frame is insufficient to ensure the requirements of uniform flow and packing of the dies. Various methods of force-feeding the granulation into the dies have been devised to refill the dies in the very short dwell time permitted on the high-speed machine. These devices are illustrated in Fig 90-24. Presses with triple compression points (see Table III) permit the partial compaction of material before final compaction. This provides for the partial deaeration and particle orientation of material before final compression. This helps in the direct compacting

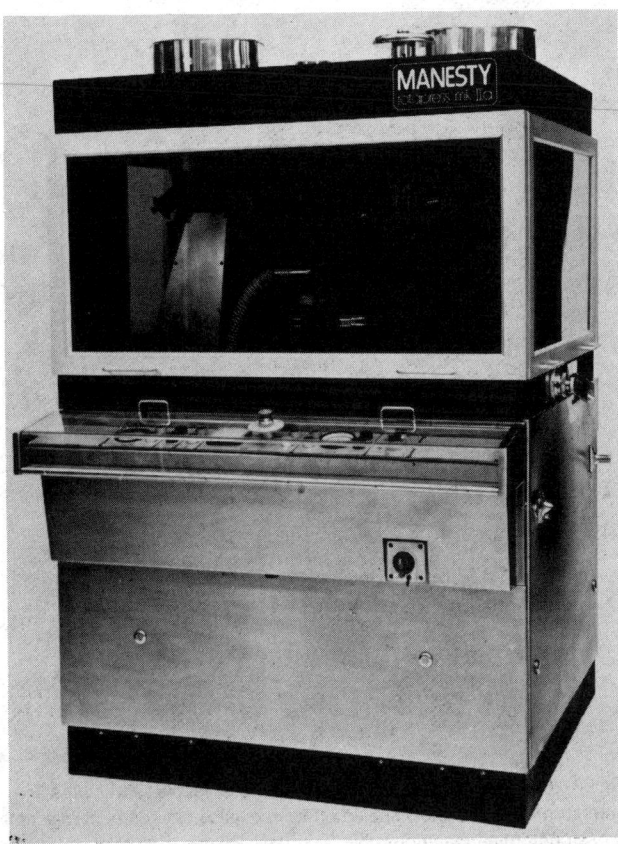

Fig 90-21.   Rotapress Mark IIA; designed for improvements in sound reduction, operator safety, cleanliness, and operational convenience; note control panel on front of machine (courtesy, Thomas/Manesty).

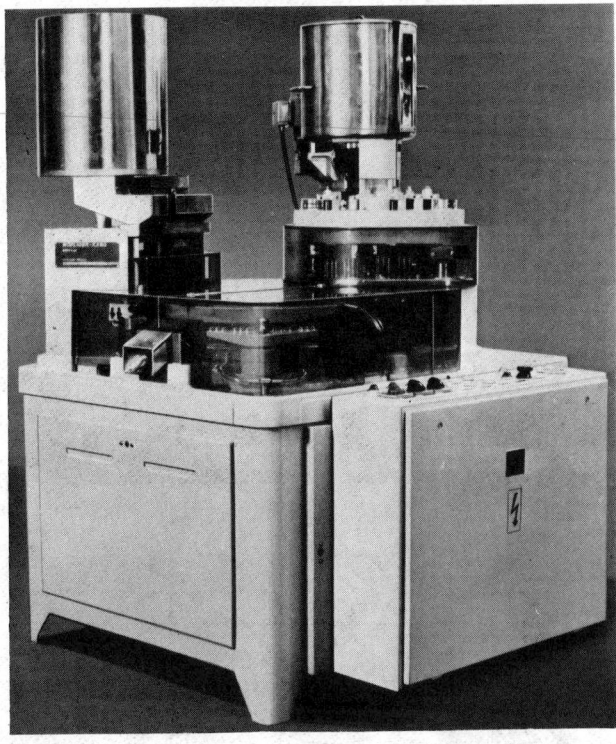

Fig 90-22.   Mark II-A Rotapress with 61 stations to give an output of 11,000 tablets per minute and equipped with remote press control; the Thomas Sentinel II is shown on the left (courtesy, Thomas/Manesty).

of materials and reduces laminating and capping due to entrapped air.

Multilayer Rotary Tablet Machines

The rotary tablet machines also have been developed into models capable of producing multiple-layer tablets; the machines are able to make one-, two-, or three-layer tablets [Versa Press (*Stokes-Pennwalt*)]. Stratified tablets offer a number of advantages. Incompatible drugs can be formed into a single tablet by separating the layers containing them with a layer of inert material. It has permitted the formulation of time-delay medication and offers a wide variety of possibilities in developing color combinations which give the products identity.

Originally the tablets were prepared by a single compression method. The dies were filled with the different granulations in successive layers and the tablet was formed by a single compression stroke. The separation lines of the tablets prepared by this method tended to be irregular. In the machines now available for multilayer production the granulation receives a precompression stroke after the first and second fill, which lightly compacts the granulation and maintains a well-defined surface of separation between each layer. The operator is able to eject either precompressed layer with the machine running at any desired speed for periodic weight and analysis checks.

Other multiple-compression presses can receive previously compressed tablets and compress another granulation around the preformed tablet. An example of a press with this capability is the Manesty Drycota (*Thomas/Manesty*). Press-coated tablets can be used to separate incompatible drug substances and also to give an enteric coating to the core tablets.

Fig 90-23.   The movement of tablets on die table of a double rotary press (courtesy, Vector/Colton).

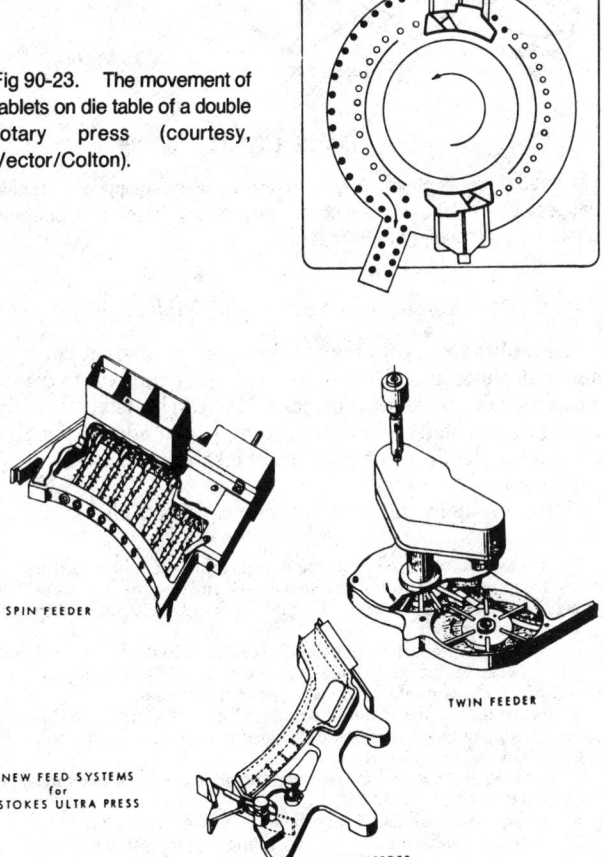

Fig 90-24.   Feeding devices designed to promote flow of granulations for high-speed machines (courtesy, Stokes/Pennwalt).

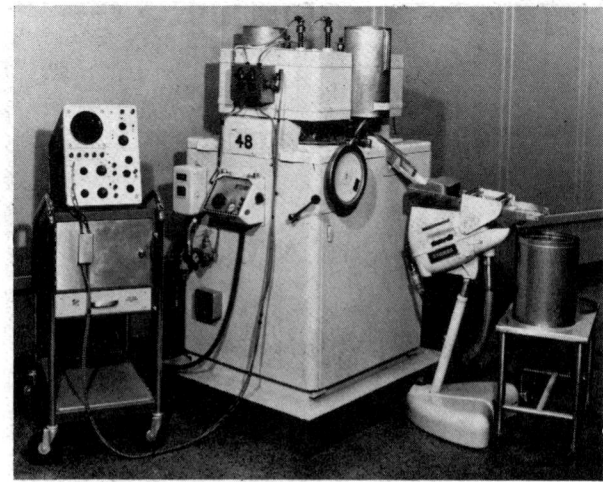

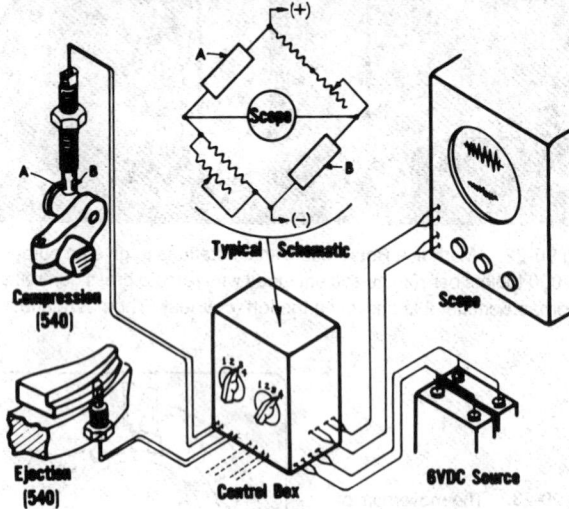

Typical Layout - Rotary

Fig 90-25.   Upper photo: High-speed rotary press equipped with strain gauges; Lower photo: layout showing arrangement of electronic components (courtesy, Upjohn).

Capping and Splitting of Tablets

The splitting or capping of tablets is one of great concern and annoyance in tablet making. It is quite difficult to detect while the tablets are being processed but can be detected easily by vigorously shaking a few in the cupped hands. A slightly chipped tablet does not necessarily mean that the tablet will cap or split.

There are many factors that may cause a tablet to cap or split:

1. Excess "fines" or powder which traps air in the tablet mixture.
2. Deep markings on tablet punches. Many designs or "scores" on punches are too broad and deep. Hairline markings are just as appropriate as deep, heavy markings.
3. Worn and imperfect punches. Punches should be smooth and buffed. Nicked punches will often cause capping. The development of fine feather edges on tablets indicates wear on punches.
4. Worn dies. Dies should be replaced or reversed. Dies that are chrome-plated or have tungsten carbide inserts wear longer and give better results than ordinary steel dies.
5. Too much pressure. By reducing the pressure on the machines the condition may be corrected.
6. Unsuitable formula. It may be necessary to change the formula.
7. Moist and soft granulation. This type of granulation will not flow freely into the dies, thus giving uneven weights and soft or capped tablets.
8. Poorly machined punches. Uneven punches are detrimental to the tablet machine itself and will not produce tablets of accurate weight. One

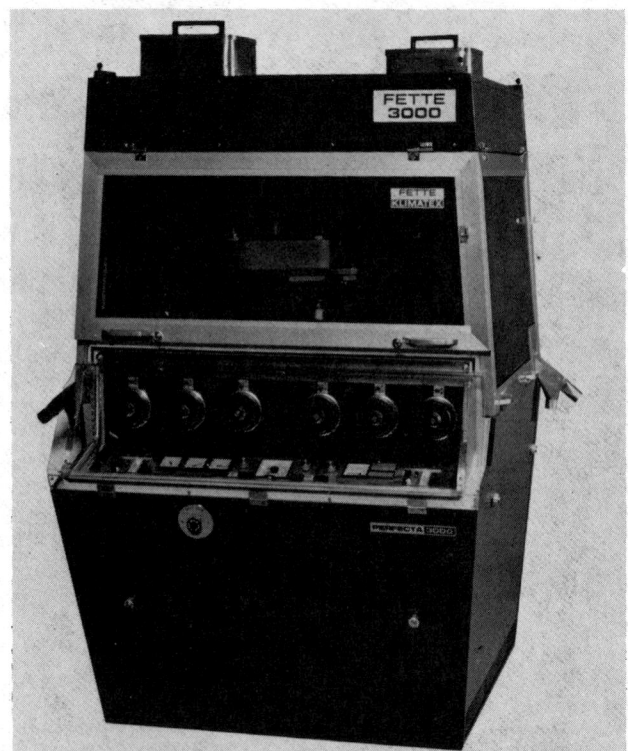

Fig 90-26.   Fette Perfecta 3000 high-speed tablet press with pressing compartment completely sealed off from outside environment making cross contamination impossible (courtesy, Raymond Auto).

punch out of alignment may cause one tablet to split or cap on every revolution.

Instrumented Tablet Presses

Compressional and ejectional forces involved in tablet compression can be studied by attaching strain gauges to the punches and other press components involved in compression. The electrical output of the gauges has been monitored by telemetry or use of a dual beam oscilloscope equipped with camera.[16,17] Instrumentation permits a study of the compaction characteristics of granulations, their flowabilities, and the effect of formulation additives, such as lubricants. Physical characteristics of tablets, such as hardness, friability, disintegration time, and dissolution rate, are influenced not only by the nature of the formulation but by the compressional force as well. Therefore definition of the compressional force giving a satisfactory tablet for a formulation provides an in-process control for obtaining both tablet-to-tablet and lot-to-lot uniformity (see Fig 90-25).

Instrumentation has led to the development of on-line, automatic, electromechanical tablet weight control systems capable of continuously monitoring the weights of tablets as they are produced.   Units are available commercially [Thomas Tablet Sentinel (*Thomas Eng*); Fette Compression Force Monitor (*Raymond Auto*); Vali-Tab (*Stokes-Pennwalt*)] and are applicable to single or rotary tablet machines. When tablet weights vary from preset limits, the monitor will automatically adjust the weight control mechanism to reestablish weights within acceptable limits.   If the difficulty continues, the unit will activate an audible warning signal or an optional shut-down relay on the press (see Fig 90-22). Most production model tablet presses come equipped with complete instrumentation (optional) and with options for statistical analysis and print out of compression/ejection signals. The techniques and applications of press instrumentation have been reviewed.[18,19]

Contamination Control

While good manufacturing practices used by the pharmaceutical industry for many years have stressed the importance of cleanliness of equipment and facilities for the manufacture of drug products, the penicillin contamination problem resulted in renewed emphasis on this aspect of manufacturing. Penicillin, either as an airborne dust or residual quantities remaining in equipment, is believed to have contaminated unrelated products in sufficient concentrations to cause allergic reactions in individuals, hypersensitive to penicillin, who received these products. This resulted in the industry spending thousands of dollars to change or modify buildings, manufacturing processes, equipment, and standard operating procedures to eliminate penicillin contamination.

With this problem has come renewed emphasis on the dust problem, material handling, and equipment cleaning in dealing with drugs, especially potent chemicals. Any process utilizing chemicals in powder form can be a dusty operation; the preparation of compressed tablets and encapsulation falls in this category. In the design of tablet presses attention is being given to the control and elimination of dust generated in the tableting process. In the Perfecta press shown in Fig 90-26, the pressing compartment is completely sealed off from the outside environment, making cross-contamination im-

possible. The pressing compartment can be kept dust-free by the air supply and vacuum equipment developed for the machine. It removes airborne dust and granular particles which have not been compressed, thus keeping the circular pressing compartment and the upper and lower punch guides free of dust.

Drug manufacturers have the responsibility to make certain that microorganisms present in finished products are unlikely to cause harm to the patient and will not be deleterious to the product. An outbreak of *Salmonella* infections in Scandinavian countries was traced to thyroid tablets which had been prepared from contaminated thyroid powder. This concern eventually led to the establishment of microbial limits for raw materials of animal or botanical origin, especially those that readily support microbial growth and are not rendered sterile during subsequent processing. Harmful microorganisms when present in oral products include *Salmonella* sp, *E coli*, certain *Pseudomonas* sp such as *Pseudomonas aeruginosa*, and *Staphylococcus aureus*. The compendia have microbial limits on raw materials such as aluminum hydroxide gel, corn starch, thyroid, acacia, and gelatin.

These represent examples of the industry's efforts to conform with the intent of current good manufacturing practice as defined by the Food and Drug Administration (see page 1489).

Tablet Formulations

Wet Granulation Method

CT Acetaminophen, 300 mg

Ingredients	In each		In 10,000	
Acetaminophen	3000	mg	3000	g
Polyvinylpyrrolidone	22.5	mg	225	g
Lactose	61.75	mg	617.5	g
Alcohol 3A—200 proof	4.5	mL	45	L
Stearic acid	9	mg	90	g
Talc	13.5	mg	135	g
Corn starch	43.25	mg	432.5	g

Blend acetaminophen, polyvinylpyrrolidone, and lactose together; pass through a 40-mesh screen. Add the alcohol slowly and knead well. Screen the wet mass through a 4-mesh screen. Dry granulation at 50°C overnight. Screen the dried granulation through a 20-mesh screen. Bolt the stearic acid, talc, and corn starch through 60-mesh screen prior to mixing by tumbling with the granulation. Compress using $^7/_{16}$-in standard concave punch. 10 tablets should weigh 4.5 g (courtesy, Abbott).

CT Ascorbic Acid USP, 50 mg

Ingredients	In each		In 7000	
Ascorbic Acid USP (powder No. 80)[a]	55	mg	385	g
Lactose	21	mg	147	g
Starch (potato)	13	mg	91	g
Ethylcellulose N 100 (80–105 cps)	16	mg	112	g
Starch (potato)	7	mg	49	g
Talc	6.5	mg	45.5	g
Calcium stearate (impalpable powder)	1	mg	7	g
Weight of granulation			836.5	g

[a] Includes 10% in excess of claim.

Granulate the above first three ingredients with ethylcellulose (5%) dissolved in anhydrous ethyl alcohol adding additional anhydrous alcohol to obtain good wet granules. Wet screen through 8 stainless steel screen and dry at room temperature in an air-conditioned area. Dry screen through 20 stainless steel screen and incorporate the remaining three ingredients. Mix thoroughly and compress. Use a flat beveled, $^1/_4$-in punch. 20 tablets should weigh 2.39 g.

Chewable Antacid Tablets

Ingredients	In each	In 10,000
Magnesium trisilicate	500 mg	5000 g
Aluminum hydroxide, dried gel	250 mg	2500 g
Mannitol	300 mg	3000 g
Sodium saccharin	2 mg	20 g
Starch paste, 5%	qs	qs
Oil of peppermint	1 mg	10 g
Magnesium stearate	10 mg	100 g
Corn starch	10 mg	100 g

Mix the magnesium trisilicate and aluminum hydroxide with the mannitol. Dissolve the sodium saccharin in a small quantity of purified water, then combine this with the starch paste. Granulate the powder blend with the starch paste. Dry at 140°F and screen through 16-mesh screen. Add the flavoring oil, magnesium stearate, and corn starch; mix well. Age the granulation for at least 24 hours and compress using $^5/_8$-in flat-face bevel-edge punch (courtesy, Atlas).

CT Hexavitamin

Ingredients	In each		In 7000	
Ascorbic Acid USP (powder)[a]	82.5	mg	577.5	g
Thiamine Mononitrate USP (powder)[a]	2.4	mg	16.8	g
Riboflavin[a]	3.3	mg	23.1	g
Nicotinamide USP (powder)[a]	22	mg	154	g
Starch	...		97.4	g
Lactose	...		41.2	g
Zein	...		45	g
Vitamin A acetate:	6250	U		
Vitamin D$_2$[a] (use Pfizer crystalets medium granules containing 500,000 U vitamin A acetate and 50,000 U vitamin D$_2$/g).	625	U	87.5	g
Magnesium stearate			7.5	g
Weight of granulation			1050	g

[a] Includes following excess of claim: ascorbic acid 10%, thiamine mononitrate 20%, riboflavin 10%, nicotinamide 10%, and vitamin A acetate–vitamin D$_2$ crystalets 25%.

Thoroughly mix the first six ingredients and granulate with zein (10% in ethyl alcohol, adding additional alcohol if necessary to obtain good wet granules). Wet screen through 8 stainless steel screen and dry at 110–120°F. Dry screen through 20 stainless steel screen and add the vitamin crystalets. Mix thoroughly, lubricate, and compress. 10 tablets should weigh 1.50 g. Coat with syrup.

CT Theobromine–Phenobarbital

Ingredients	In each		In 7000	
Theobromine	325	mg	2275	g
Phenobarbital	33	mg	231	g
Starch	39	mg	273	g
Talc	8	mg	56	g
Acacia (powder)	8	mg	56	g
Stearic acid	0.7	mg	4.9	g
Weight of granulation			2895.9	g

Prepare a paste with the acacia and an equal weight of starch. Use this paste for granulating the theobromine and phenobarbital. Dry and put through a 12-mesh screen, add the remainder of the material, mix thoroughly, and compress into tablets, using a $^{13}/_{32}$-in concave punch. 10 tablets should weigh 4.13 g.

Dry Granulation Method

CT Acetylsalicylic Acid

Ingredients	In each	In 7000
Acetylsalicylic Acid (crystals 20-mesh)	0.325 g	2275 g
Starch		226.8 g
Weight of granulation		2501.8 g

Dry the starch to a moisture content of 10%. Thoroughly mix this with the acetylsalicylic acid. Compress into slugs. Grind the slugs to 14–16 mesh size. Recompress into tablets, using a $^{13}/_{32}$-in punch. 10 tablets should weigh 3.575 g.

CT Sodium Phenobarbital

Ingredients	In each		In 7000	
Phenobarbital sodium	65	mg	455	g
Milk sugar (granular, 12-mesh)	26	mg	182	g
Starch	20	mg	140	g
Talc	20	mg	140	g
Magnesium stearate	0.3	mg	2.1	g
Weight of granulation			919.1	g

Mix all the ingredients thoroughly. Compress into slugs. Grind and screen to 14–16-mesh granules. Recompress into tablets, using a $^9/_{32}$-in concave punch. 10 tablets should weigh 1.3 g.

CT Vitamin B Complex

Ingredients	In each	In 10,000
Thiamine mononitrate[a]	0.733 mg	7.33 g
Riboflavin[a]	0.733 mg	7.33 g
Pyridoxine hydrochloride	0.333 mg	3.33 g
Calcium pantothenate[a]	0.4 mg	4 g
Nicotinamide	5 mg	50 g
Milk sugar (powder)	75.2 mg	752 g
Starch	21.9 mg	219 g
Talc	20 mg	200 g
Stearic acid (powder)	0.701 mg	7.01 g
Weight of granulation		1250 g

[a] Includes 10% in excess of claim.

Mix all the ingredients thoroughly. Compress into slugs. Grind and screen to 14–16-mesh granules. Recompress into tablets, using a $^1/_4$-in concave punch. 10 tablets should weigh 1.25 g.

Sufficient tartaric acid should be used in these tablets to adjust the pH to 4.5.

Direct Compression Method

APC Tablets

Ingredients	In each		In 10,000
Aspirin (40-mesh crystal)	224	mg	2240 g
Phenacetin	160	mg	1600 g
Caffeine (Anhyd. USP gran.)	32	mg	320 g
Compressible sugar (Di-Pac[a])	93.4	mg	934 g
Sterotex	7.8	mg	78 g
Silica gel (Syloid 244[b])	2.8	mg	28 g

[a] Amstar.
[b] Davison Chem.

Blend ingredients in twin-shell blender for 15 minutes and compress on $^{13}/_{32}$-in standard concave punch (courtesy, Amstar).

CT Ascorbic Acid USP, 250 mg

Ingredients	In each	In 10,000
Ascorbic Acid USP (Merck, fine crystals)	255 mg	2550 g
Microcrystalline cellulose[a]	159 gm	1590 g
Stearic acid	9 mg	90 g
Colloidal silica[b]	2 mg	20 g
Weight of granulation		4250 g

[a] Avicel-PH-101.
[b] Cab-O-Sil.

Blend all ingredients in a suitable blender. Compress using $^7/_{16}$-in standard concave punch. 10 tablets should weigh 4.25 g (courtesy, FMC).

Breath Freshener Tablets

Ingredients	In each		In 10,000	
Wintergreen oil	0.6	mg	6	g
Menthol	0.85	mg	8.5	g
Peppermint oil	0.3	mg	3	g
Silica gel (Syloid 244[a])	1	mg	10	g
Sodium saccharin	0.3	mg	3	g
Sodium bicarbonate	14	mg	140	g
Mannitol USP (granular)	180.95	mg	1809.5	g
Calcium stearate	2	mg	20	g

[a] Davison Chem.

Mix the flavor oils and menthol until liquid. Adsorb onto the silica gel. Add the remaining ingredients. Blend and compress on $^5/_{16}$-in flat-face bevel-edge punch to a thickness of 3.1 mm (courtesy, Atlas).

Chewable Antacid Tablets

Ingredients	In each	In 10,000
Aluminum hydroxide and Magnesium carbonate, co-dried gel[a]	325 mg	3250 g
Mannitol USP (granular)	675 mg	6750 g
Microcrystalline cellulose[b]	75 mg	750 g
Corn starch	30 mg	300 g
Calcium stearate	22 mg	220 g
Flavor	qs	qs

[a] Reheis F-MA-11.
[b] Avicel.

Blend all ingredients in a suitable blender. Compress using $^5/_8$-in flat-face bevel-edge punch (courtesy, Atlas).

Chewable Multivitamin Tablets

Ingredients	In each	In 10,000
Vitamin A USP (dry, stabilized form)	5000 USP units	50 million units
Vitamin D (dry, stabilized form)	400 USP units	4 million units
Ascorbic Acid USP	60.0 mg	600 g
Thiamine Hydrochloride USP	1 mg	10 g
Riboflavin USP	1.5 mg	15 g
Pyridoxine Hydrochloride USP	1 mg	10 g
Cyanocobalamin USP	2 μg	20 mg
Calcium Pantothenate USP	3 mg	30 g
Niacinamide USP	10 mg	100 g
Mannitol USP (granular)	236.2 mg	2362 g
Corn starch	16.6 mg	166 g
Sodium Saccharin	1.1 mg	11 g
Magnesium stearate	6.6 mg	66 g
Talc USP	10 mg	100 g
Flavor	qs	qs

Blend all ingredients in a suitable blender. Compress using 3/8-in flat-face bevel-edge punch (courtesy, Atlas).

CT Ferrous Sulfate

Ingredients	In each	In 7000	
Ferrous Sulfate USP (crystalline)	0.325 g	2275	g
Talc		0.975	g
Sterotex		1.95	g
Weight of granulation		2277.93	g

Grind to 12–14-mesh, lubricate, and compress. Coat immediately to avoid oxidation to the ferric state with 0.410 gr of tolu balsam (dissolved in alcohol) and 0.060 gr of salol and chalk. Use a deep concave 11/32-in punch. 10 tablets should weigh 3.25 g.

CT Methenamine

Ingredients	In each, g	In 7000, g
Methenamine (12- to 14-mesh crystals)	0.325	2275
Weight of granulation		2275

Compress directly, using a 7/16-in punch. 10 tablets should weigh 3.25 g.

CT Phenobarbital USP, 30 mg

Ingredients	In each	In 10,000
Phenobarbital	30.59 mg	305.9 g
Microcrystalline cellulose[a]	30.59 mg	305.9 g
Spray-dried lactose	69.16 mg	691.6 g
Colloidal silica[b]	1.33 mg	13.3 g
Stearic acid	1.33 mg	13.3 g
Weight of granulation		1330 g

[a] Avicel-PH-101.
[b] QUSO F-22.

Screen the phenobarbital to break up lumps and blend with microcrystalline cellulose. Add spray-dried lactose and blend. Finally add the stearic acid and colloidal silica; blend to obtain homogeneous mixture. Compress using 9/32-in shallow concave punch. 10 tablets should weigh 1.33 g (courtesy, FMC).

Molded Tablets or Tablet Triturates (TT)

Tablet triturates are small discoid masses of molded powders weighing 30 to 250 mg each. The base consists of lactose, β-lactose, mannitol, dextrose, or other rapidly soluble materials. It is desirable in making tablet triturates to prepare a solid dosage form which is rapidly soluble, and as the result they are generally softer than compressed tablets.

This type of dosage form is selected for a number of drugs because of its rapidly dissolving characteristic. Nitroglycerin in many concentrations is prepared in tablet triturate form since the molded tablet rapidly dissolves when administered by placing under the tongue. Potent alkaloids and highly toxic drugs used in small doses are prepared as tablet triturates which can serve as dispensing tablets to be used as the source of the drug in compounding other formulations or solutions. Narcotics in the form of hypodermic tablets originally were made as tablet triturates because they rapidly dissolve in sterile water for injection prior to administration. Today with stable injections of narcotics available, there is no longer any justification for their use in this manner. Although many hypodermic tablets currently are made, they are used primarily for oral administration.

Tablet triturates are made by forcing a moistened blend of the drug and diluent into a mold, extruding the formed mass, which is allowed to dry. This method is essentially the same as it was when introduced by Fuller in 1878. Hand molds may vary in size but the method of operation is essentially the same. Molds consist of two plates made from polystyrene plastic, hard rubber, nickel-plated brass, or stainless steel. The mold plate contains 50–500 carefully polished perforations. The other plate is fitted with a corresponding number of projecting pegs or punches which fit the perforations in the mold plate. The mold plate is placed on a flat surface, the moistened mass is forced into the perforations, and the excess is scraped from the top surface. The mold plate is placed over the plate with the corresponding pegs and lowered. As the plates come together, the pegs force the tablet triturates from the molds. They remain on the tops of the pegs until dry and they can be handled (see Fig 90-27). In some hand molds, as shown in Fig 90-28, the pegs are forced down onto the plate holding the moist trituration.

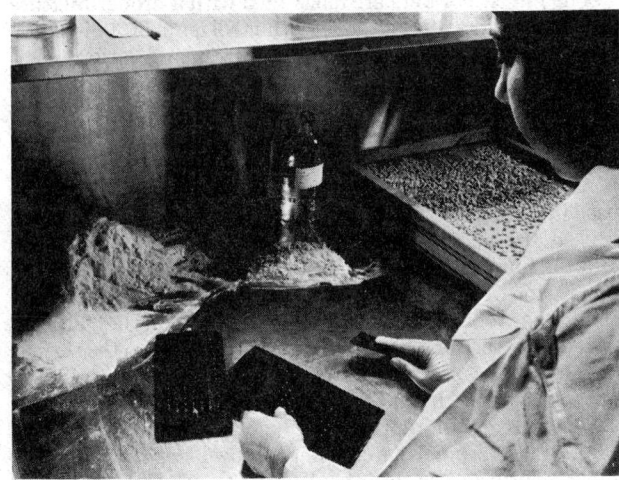

Fig 90-27. Hand molding tablet triturates (courtesy, MSD).

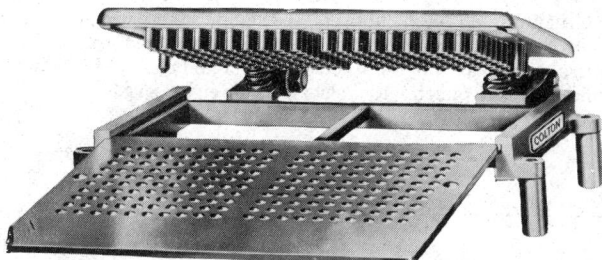

Fig 90-28.   Tablet triturate mold (courtesy, Vector/Colton).

Formulation

In developing a formula it is essential that the blank weight of the mold which is to be used is known. To determine this, the weight of the diluent which exactly fills all the openings in the mold is determined by experiment. This amount of diluent is weighed and placed aside. The total amount of the drug required is determined by multiplying the number of perforations in the plate used in the previous experiment by the amount of drug desired in each tablet. The comparative bulk of this medication is now compared with that of an equal volume of diluent and that quantity of diluent is removed and weighed. The drug and the remaining diluent are mixed by trituration, and the resulting triturate is moistened and forced into the openings of the mold. If the perforations are not completely filled, more diluent is added, its weight noted, and the formula written from the results of the experiments.

It is also permissible in the development of the formula to weigh the quantity of medication needed for the number of tablets represented by the number of perforations in the mold, triturate with a weighed portion (more than $\frac{1}{2}$) of the diluent, moisten the mixture, and press it into the perforations of the mold. An additional quantity of the diluent is immediately moistened and also forced into the perforations in the plate until they are completely filled. All excess diluent is removed, the trial tablets are forced from the mold, then triturated until uniform, moistened again if necessary, and remolded. When these tablets are thoroughly dried and weighed, the difference between their total weight and the weight of medication taken will indicate the amount of diluent required and accordingly supply the formula for future use for that particular tablet triturate.

For proper mixing procedures of the medication with the diluent see Chapter 89.

Preparation

The mixed powders are moistened with a proper mixture of alcohol and water, although other solvents or moistening agents such as acetone, petroleum benzin, and various combinations of these may be used in specific cases; the agent of choice depends on the solvent action which it will exert on the powder mixture. Often the moistening agent is 50% alcohol, but this concentration may be increased or decreased depending on the constituents of the formula. Care must be used in adding the solvent mixture to the powder. If too much is used, the mass will be soggy, will require a long time to dry, and the finished tablet will be hard and slowly soluble; if the mass is too wet, shrinkage will occur in the molded tablets; and finally, a condition known as creeping will be noticed. Creeping is the concentration of the medication on the surface of the tablet caused by capillarity and rapid evaporation of the solvent from the surface. Because molded tablets by their very nature are quite friable, an inaccurate strength in each tablet may result from creeping if powder is lost from the tablet's surface. On the other hand, if an insufficient amount of moistening agent is used, the mass will not have the proper

cohesion to make a firm tablet. The correct amount of moistening agent can only be determined initially by experiment.

Hand-Molding Tablet Triturates

In preparing hand-molded tablets place the mold plate on a glass plate. The properly moistened material is pressed into the perforations of the mold with a broad spatula exerting uniform pressure over each opening. The excess material is removed by passing the spatula at an oblique angle with strong hand pressure over the mold to give a clean, flat surface. The material thus removed should be placed with the remainder of the unmolded material.

The mold with the filled perforations should be reversed and moved to another clean part of the plate where the pressing operation with the spatula is repeated. It may be necessary to add more material to fill the perforations completely and uniformly. The mold should be allowed to stand in a position so that part of the moistening agent will evaporate equally from both faces. While the first plate is drying, another mold can be prepared. As soon as the second mold has been completed, the first mold should be sufficiently surface dried so that the pegs will press the tablets from the mold with a minimum of sticking.

To remove the tablets from the mold, place the mold over the peg plate so that the pegs and the perforations are in juxtaposition. The tablets are released from the mold by hand pressure, which forces the pegs through the perforations. The ejected tablets are spread evenly in single layers on silk trays and dried in a clean, dust-free chamber with warm, circulating air. If only a small quantity of tablet triturates is made and no warm-air oven is available, the tablet triturates may be dried to constant weight at room temperature.

Machine-Molding Tablet Triturates

Tablet triturates also can be made using mechanical equipment. The automatic tablet triturate machine illustrated in Fig 90-29 makes tablet triturates at a rate of 2500/min. For machine-molding, the powder mass need not be as moist as for plate-molding since the time interval between forming the tablets and pressing them is considerably shorter. The moistened mass passes through the funnel of the hopper to the feed plates below. In this feed plate are four holes having the same diameter as the mouth of the funnel. The

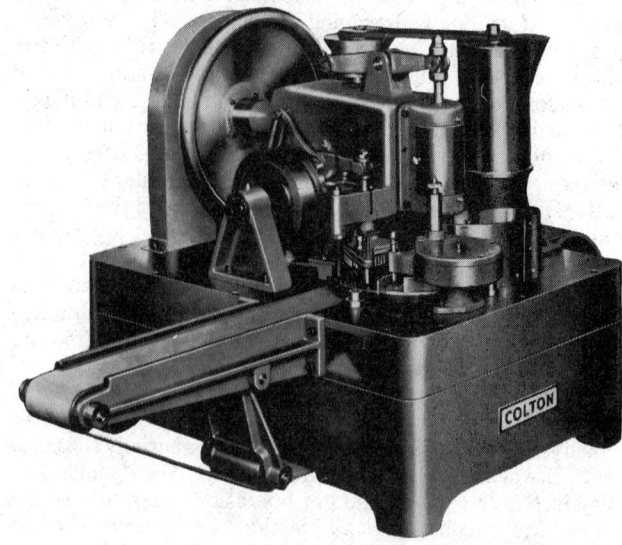

Fig 90-29.   Automatic tablet triturate machine (courtesy, Vector/Colton).

material fills one hole at a time and when filled revolves to a position just over the mold plate. When in position the weighted pressure foot lowers and imprisons the powder. At the same time a spreader in the sole of the pressure foot rubs it into the mold cavities and evens it off so that the triturates are smooth on the surface and are of uniform density. When this operation is completed, the mold passes to the next position, where it registers with a nest of punches or pegs which eject the tablets from the mold plate onto a conveyor belt. The conveyor belt is sometimes extended to a length of 8 or 10 ft under a battery of infrared drying lamps to hasten the setting of the tablets for more rapid handling. This method of drying can be used only if the drug is chemically stable to these drying conditions.

Compressed Tablet Triturates

Frequently, tablet triturates are prepared on compression tablet machines using flat-face punches. When solubility and a clear solution are required, water-soluble lubricants must be used to prevent sticking to the punches. The granulations are prepared as directed for ordinary compressed tablets; lactose is generally used as the diluent. Generally, tablet triturates prepared by this method are not as satisfactory as the molded type regarding their solubility and solution characteristics.

Capsules

Capsules are solid dosage forms in which the drug substance is enclosed in either a hard or soft, soluble container or shell of a suitable form of gelatin. The soft gelatin capsule was invented by Mothes, a French pharmacist in 1833. During the following year DuBlanc obtained a patent for his soft gelatin capsules. In 1848 Murdock patented the two-piece hard gelatin capsule. Although development work has been done on the preparation of capsules from methylcellulose and calcium alginate, gelatin because of its unique properties remains the primary composition material for the manufacture of capsules. The gelatin used in the manufacture of capsules is obtained from collagenous material by hydrolysis. There are two types of gelatin, Type A, derived mainly from pork skins by acid processing, and Type B, obtained from bones and animal skins by alkaline processing. Blends are used to obtain gelatin solutions with the viscosity and bloom strength characteristics desirable for capsule manufacture.[20]

The encapsulation of medicinal agents remains a popular method for administering drugs. Capsules are tasteless, easily administered and easily filled either extemporaneously or in large quantities commercially. In prescription practice the use of hard gelatin capsules permits a choice in prescribing a single drug or a combination of drugs at the exact dosage level considered best for the individual patient. This flexibility is an advantage over tablets. Some patients find it easier to swallow capsules than tablets, therefore preferring to take this form when possible. This preference has prompted pharmaceutical manufacturers to market the product in capsule form even though the product has already been produced in tablet form. While the industry prepares approximately 75% of its solid dosage forms as compressed tablets, 23% as hard gelatin capsules, and 2% as soft elastic capsules, market surveys have indicated a consumer preference of 44.2% for soft elastic capsules, 39.6% for tablets, and 19.4% for hard gelatin capsules.[21]

Hard Gelatin Capsules

The hard gelatin capsule, also referred to as the dry-filled capsule (DFC), consists of two sections, one slipping over the other, thus completely surrounding the drug formulation. The classical capsule shape is illustrated in Fig 90-30. These capsules are filled by introducing the powdered material into the longer end or body of the capsule and then slipping on the cap. Hard gelatin capsules are made largely from gelatin, FD&C colorants, and sometimes an opacifying agent such as titanium dioxide; the USP permits the gelatin for this purpose to contain 0.15% sulfur dioxide to prevent decomposition during manufacture. Hard gelatin capsules contain 12–16% water, but the water content can vary depending on the storage conditions. When the humidity is low, the capsules become brittle; if stored at high humidities, the capsules become flaccid and lose their shape. Storage in high temperature

areas can also affect the quality of hard gelatin capsules. Gelatin capsules do not protect hygroscopic materials from atmospheric water vapor as moisture can diffuse through the gelatin wall.

Companies having equipment for preparing empty hard gelatin capsules include Lilly, Parke-Davis, Scherer Gelatin Corp, and SK&F. The latter's production is mainly for its own use; the others are suppliers to the industry. With this equipment stainless steel pins, set in plates, are dipped into the gelatin solution, which must be maintained at a uniform temperature and an exact degree of fluidity. If the gelatin solution varies in viscosity, it will correspondingly decrease or increase the thickness of the capsule wall. This is important since a slight variation is sufficient to make either a loose or a tight joint. When the pins have been withdrawn from the gelatin solution, they are rotated while being dried in kilns through which a strong blast of filtered air with controlled humidity is forced. Each capsule is stripped, trimmed to uniform length, and joined, the entire process being mechanical. Capsule-making equipment is illustrated in Figs 90-31 and 90-32. These show the stainless steel pins being

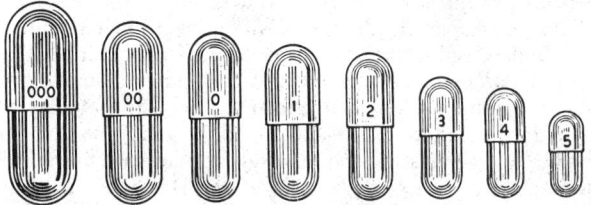

Fig 90-30. Hard gelatin capsules showing relative sizes (courtesy, Parke-Davis).

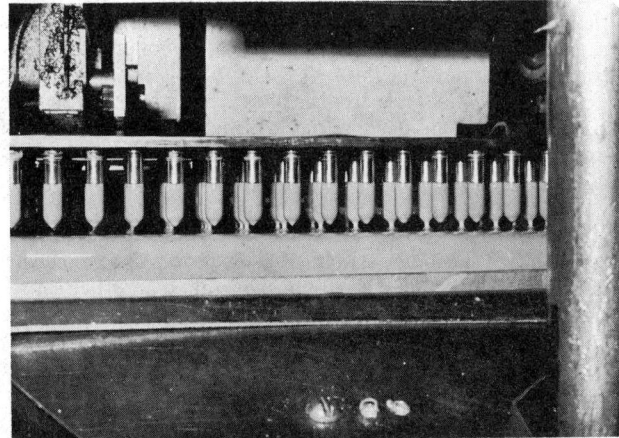

Fig 90-31. Manufacturer of hard gelatin capsules by dipping stainless steel pins into gelatin solutions (courtesy, Lilly).

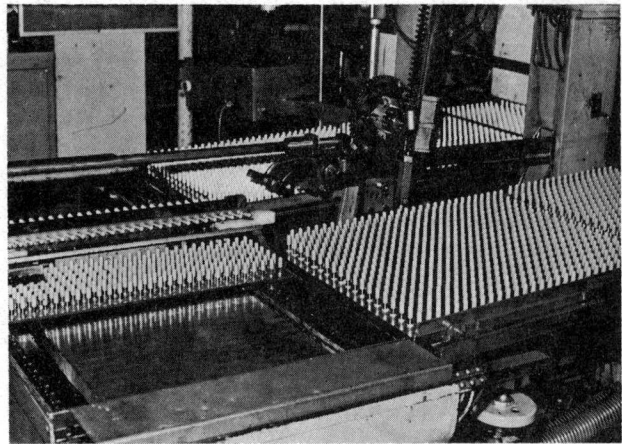

Fig 90-32. Formed capsules being dried by rotating through drying kiln (courtesy, Lilly).

dipped into the gelatin solutions and then being rotated through the drying kiln.

Capsules are supplied in a variety of sizes. The hard, empty capsules (Fig 90-30) are numbered from 000, the largest size which can be swallowed, to 5, which is the smallest. Larger sizes are available for use in veterinary medicine. The approximate capacity for capsules from 000 to 5 ranges from 600 to 30 mg, although this will vary because of the different densities of powdered drug materials.

Commercially filled capsules have the conventional oblong shape illustrated with the exception of capsule products by Lilly and SK&F, which are of distinctive shape. For Lilly products, capsules are used in which the end of the base is tapered to give the capsule a bulletlike shape; products encapsulated in this form are called *Pulvules*. The SK&F capsules differ in that both the ends of the cap and body are angular, rather than round.

After hard gelatin capsules are filled and the cap applied, there are a number of methods used to assure that the capsules will not come apart if subjected to vibration or rough handling as in high-speed counting and packaging equipment. The capsules can be spot-welded by means of a heated metal pin pressed against the cap, fusing it to the body; or they may be banded with molten gelatin laid around the joint in a strip and dried. Colored gelatin bands around capsules have been used for many years as a trade mark by Parke-Davis for their line of capsule products, *Kapseals*. Another approach is used in the *Snap-Fit* and *Coni-Snap* capsules. A pair of matched locking rings are formed into the cap and body portions of the capsule. Prior to filling, these capsules are slightly longer than regular capsules of the same size. When the locking rings are engaged after filling, their length is equivalent to that of the conventional capsule.

It is usually necessary for the pharmacist to determine the size of the capsule needed for a given prescription through experimentation. The experienced pharmacist, having calculated the weight of material to be held by a single capsule, will often select the correct size immediately. If the material is powdered, the base of the capsule is filled and the top is replaced. If the material in the capsule proves to be too heavy after weighing, a smaller size must be taken and the test repeated. If the filled capsule is light, it is possible that more can be forced into it by increasing the pressure or, if necessary, some of the material may be placed in the cap. This is not desirable as it tends to decrease the accuracy of subdivision and it is much better to select another size, the base of which will hold exactly the correct quantity. In prescription filling it is wise to check the weight of each filled capsule.

In addition to the transparent, colorless, hard gelatin cap-

sule, capsules are also available in various transparent colors such as pink, green, reddish-brown, blue, yellow, and black. If they are used, it is important to note the color as well as the capsule size on the prescription so that in the case of renewal the refilled prescription will duplicate the original. Colored capsules have been used chiefly by manufacturers to give a specialty product a distinctive appearance. Titanium dioxide is added to the gelatin to form white capsules, or to make an opaque colored capsule. In addition to color contrasts, many commercial products in capsules are given further identification by markings which may be either the company's name, a symbol on the outer shell of the capsule, or by banding. Some manufacturers mark capsules with special numbers based on a coded system to permit exact identification by the pharmacist or the physician.

Extemporaneous Filling Methods

When filling capsules on prescription, the usual procedure is to mix the ingredients by trituration, reducing them to a fine and uniform powder. The principles and methods for the uniform distribution of an active medicinal agent in a powder mixture are discussed in Chapter 89. Granular powders do not pack readily in capsules and crystalline materials, especially those which consist of a mass of filamentlike crystals as the quinine salts, are not easily fitted into capsules unless powdered. Eutectic mixtures that tend to liquefy may be dispensed in capsules if a suitable absorbent such as magnesium carbonate is used. Potent drugs given in small doses are usually mixed with an inert diluent such as lactose before filling into capsules. When incompatible materials are prescribed together, it is sometimes possible to place one in a smaller capsule and then enclose it with the second drug in a larger capsule.

Usually the powder is placed on paper and flattened with a spatula so that the layer of powder is not greater than about $\frac{1}{3}$ the length of the capsule which is being filled. This helps to keep both the hands and capsules clean. The cap is removed from the selected capsule and held in the left hand; the body is pressed repeatedly into the powder until it is filled. The cap is replaced and the capsule is weighed. In filling the capsule the spatula is helpful in pushing the last quantity of the material into the capsule. If each capsule has not been weighed, there is likely to be an excess or a shortage of material when the specified number of capsules have been packed. This condition is adjusted before dispensing the prescription.

A number of manual filling machines and automatic capsule machines are available for increasing the speed of the capsule filling operation. Fig 90-33 illustrates a capsule filling machine which was formerly known as the Sharp and Dohme machine. This equipment is now available through *Chemi-Pharm*. Many community pharmacists find this a useful piece of apparatus and some pharmaceutical manufacturers use it for small-scale production of specialty items. The machine fills 24 capsules at a time with the possible production of 2000/day. Entire capsules are placed in the machine by hand; the lower plate carries a clamp which holds the capsule bases and makes it possible to remove and replace the caps mechanically. The plate holding the capsule bases is perforated for three sizes of capsules. The powder is packed in the bases; the degree of accuracy depends on the selection of capsule size and the amount of pressure applied in packing. The hand-operated machine (Model 300, *ChemiPharm*) illustrated in Fig 90-34 has a production capacity of 2000 capsules per hour. The machine is made for a single capsule size and cannot be changed over for other sizes. A different machine is required for any additional capsule size. Its principle of operation is similar to that of the Sharp and Dohme machine.

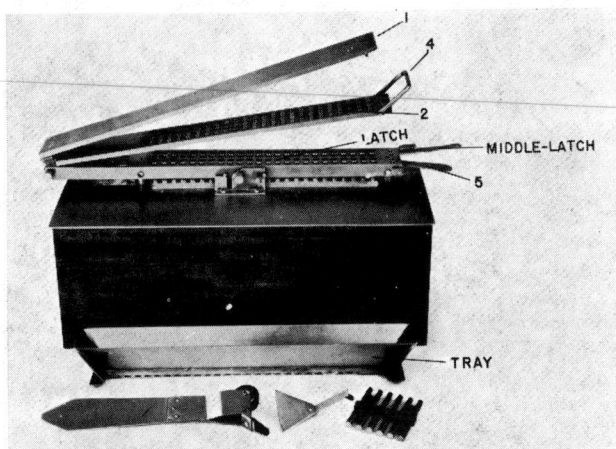

Fig 90-33. Hand-operated capsule machine (courtesy, Chemi-Pharm).

Machine Filling Methods

Large-scale filling equipment for capsules operates on the same principle as the manual machines described above, namely the filling of the base of the capsule. Compared with tablets, powders for filling into hard gelatin capsules require the minimum of formulation efforts. The powders usually contain diluents such as lactose, mannitol, calcium carbonate, or magnesium carbonate. Since the flow of material is of great importance in the rapid and accurate filling of the capsule bodies, lubricants such as the stearates are also frequently used. Because of the absence of numerous additives and manufacturing processing, the capsule form is frequently used to administer new drug substances for evaluation in initial clinical trials. However, it is now realized that the additives present in the capsule formulation, like the compressed tablet, can influence the release of the drug substance from the capsule. Tablets and capsules of a combination product containing triamterene and hydrochlorothiazide in a 2:1 ratio were compared clinically. The tablet caused approximately

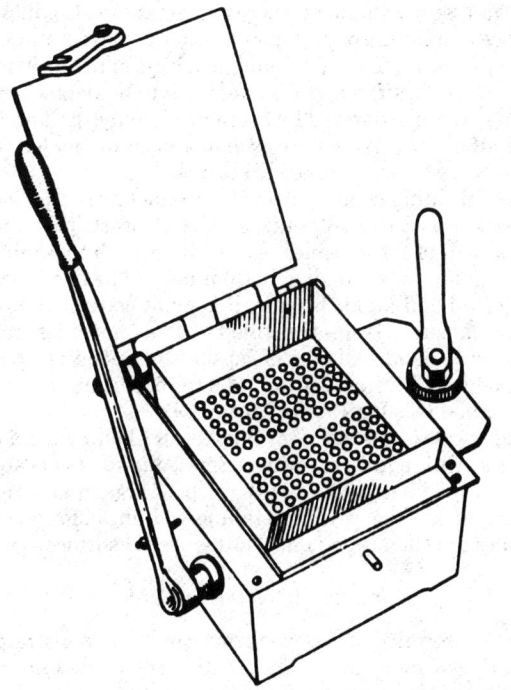

Fig 90-34. Hand-operated capsule machine, Model 300 (courtesy, ChemiPharm).

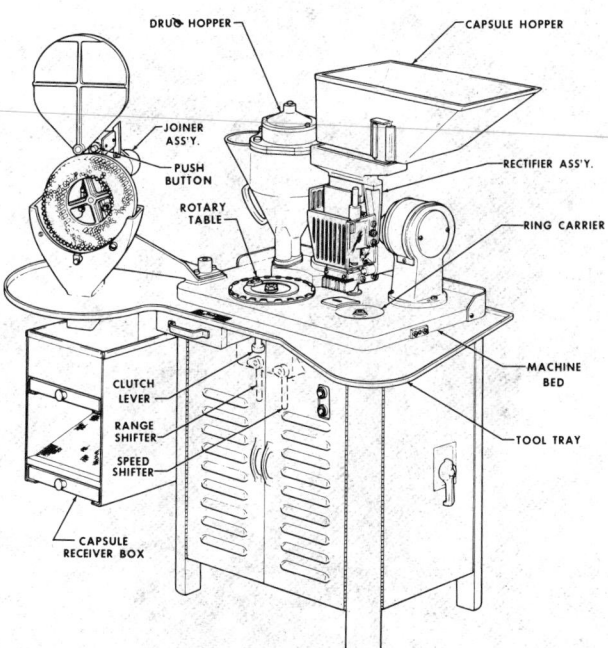

Fig 90-35. Schematic of Type 8 capsule-filling machine (courtesy, Parke-Davis).

twice as much excretion of hydrochlorothiazide and 3 times as much triamterene as the capsule.[22] Most equipment operates on the principle whereby the base of the capsule is filled and the excess is scraped off. Therefore the active ingredient is mixed with sufficient volume of a diluent, usually lactose or mannitol, which will give the desired amount of the drug in the capsule when the base is filled with the powder mixture. The manner of operation of the machine can influence the volume of the powder which will be filled into the base of the capsule; therefore, the weights of the capsules must be checked routinely as they are filled.

Semiautomatic capsule-filling machines manufactured by Parke-Davis and by Lilly are illustrated in Figs 90-35 and 90-36. The Type 8 capsule-filling machine performs mechanically under the same principle as the hand filling of capsules. This includes (1) separation of the cap from the body; (2) filling the body half; and (3) rejoining the cap and body halves.

Empty capsules are taken from the bottom of the capsule hopper into the magazine. The magazine gauge releases one capsule from each tube at the bottom of each stroke of the machine. Leaving the magazine, the capsules drop onto the tracks of the raceway and are pushed forward to the rectifying area with a push blade. The rectifier block descends, turning the capsules in each track, cap up, and drops them into each row of holes in the capsule holding ring assembly.

As the capsules fall into the holding ring, the cap half has a seat on the counter bore in each hole for the top ring. The body half is pulled by vacuum down into the bottom ring. When all rows in the ring assembly are full, the top ring, filled with caps only, is removed and set aside for later assembly. The body halves are now located in the bottom ring, ready for filling.

The ring holding the body halves is rotated at one of 8 speeds on the rotary table. The drug hopper is swung over the rotating ring and the auger forces drug powder into the open body cavities. When the ring has made a complete revolution and the body halves have been filled, the hopper is swung aside. The cap-holding ring is placed over the body holding ring and the assembly is ready for joining. The capsule-holding ring assembly is placed on the joiner and the joiner plate is swung down into position to hold the capsules

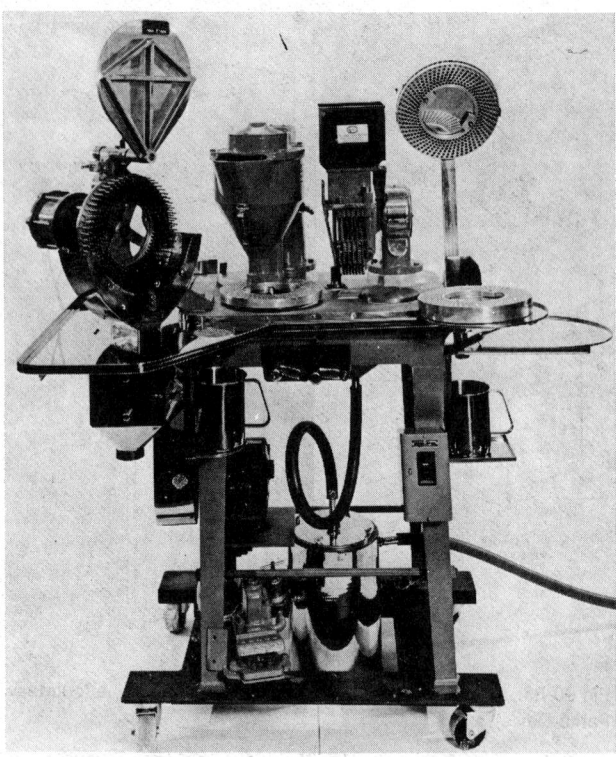

Fig 90-36.   Type 8 capsule-filling machine (courtesy, Lilly).

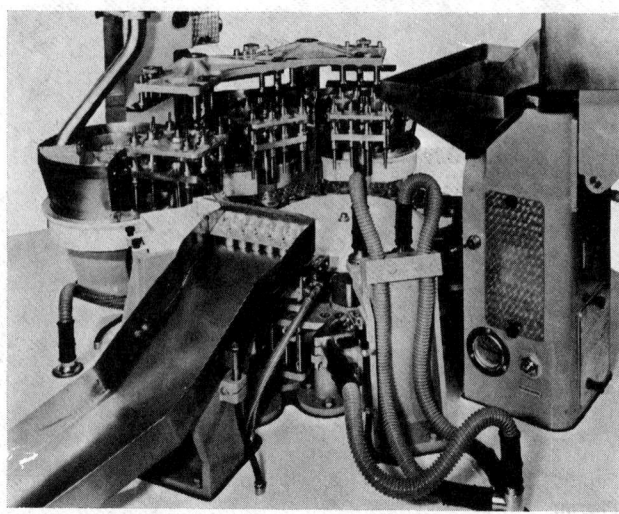

Fig 90-38.   Zanasi automatic filling machine, Model AZ-60.   The set of filling heads shown at the left collects the powder from the hopper, compresses it into a soft slug, and inserts it into the bottom half of the capsule (courtesy, United Machinery).

in the ring. The peg ring pins are entered in the holes of the body holding ring and tapped in place by the air cylinder pushing the body halves back into the cap halves.

The holding ring assembly is now pushed by hand back onto the peg ring away from the joiner plate, thus pushing the capsules out of the holding ring assembly. The joined capsules then fall through the joiner chute into the capsule receiver box. The capsule receiver box screens the excess powder from the capsules and delivers them to any convenient container.

Many companies use the Type 8 capsule-filling equipment because of its ease of operation, low cost, and extreme flexibility. A Type 8 capsule filling machine will produce ap-

proximately 200,000 capsules/day. This, of course, depends upon the operator and the type of material being filled. For this machine, a mathematical model has been developed that describes the effect of selected physical powder properties, as well as mechanical operating conditions on the capsule filling operation. While the Type 8 capsule-filling machine has been in existence for many years, recent modifications have been made to this machine to improve the capsule-filling operations.

There are several pieces of equipment available that are classified as automatic capsule-filling machines. These are automatic in the sense that one operator can handle more than one machine. In this category are the Italian-made Zanasi (*United Machinery*) and MG-2 (*Supermatic*) models plus the West German-made Hoefliger & Karg models (*Bosch*).

Automatic capsule machines are capable of filling either powder or granulated products into hard gelatin capsules. With accessory equipment these machines can also fill pellets or place a tablet into the capsule with the powder or pellets. The capsules are fed at random into a large hopper. They are oriented as required and transferred into holders where the two halves are separated by suction. The top-half and bottom-half of the capsules are each in a separate holder, which at this stage take diverting directions.

A set of filling heads collect the product from the hopper, compresses it into a soft slug, and then inserts this into the bottom half of the capsule. After filling, each top-half is returned to the corresponding bottom-half. The filled capsules are ejected and an air blast at this point separates possible empty capsules from the filled. The machines can be equipped to handle all sizes of capsules. Depending upon the make and model, speeds from 9000 to 150,000 units/hour can be obtained (see Figs 90-37, 38 and 39).

All capsules, whether they have been filled by hand or by machine, will require cleaning. Small quantities of capsules may be wiped individually with cloth. Larger quantities are rotated or shaken with crystalline sodium chloride. The capsules are then rolled on a cloth-covered surface.

Uniformity of Dosage Units

The uniformity of dosage forms can be demonstrated by either of two methods, weight variation or content uniformity. Weight variation may be applied where the product is a liquid-filled soft elastic capsule or where the hard gelatin capsule contains 50 mg or more of a single active ingredient comprising

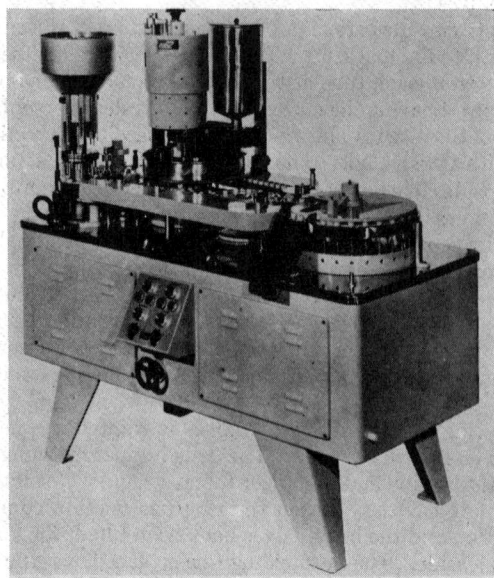

Fig 90-37.   MG-2, automatic capsule-filling machine (courtesy, Supermatic).

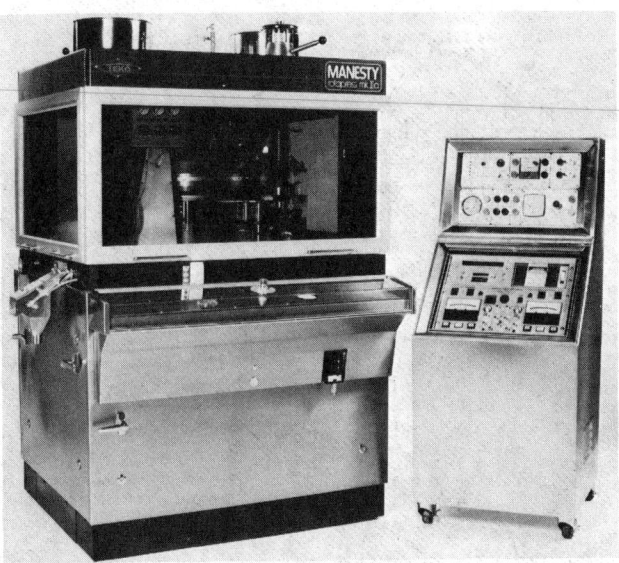

Fig 90-39.   Hoefliger & Karg automatic capsule filling machine, Model GFK 1200 (courtesy, Amaco).

50% or more, by weight, of the dosage form. See the official compendia for details of the procedures.

Disintegration tests are usually not required for capsules unless they have been treated to resist solution in gastric fluid (enteric-coated). In this case they must meet the requirements for disintegration of enteric-coated tablets. For certain capsule dosage forms a dissolution requirement is part of the monograph. Procedures used are similar to those employed in the case of compressed tablets. (See Chap 35).

Soft Elastic Capsules

The soft elastic capsule (SEC) is a soft, globular, gelatin shell somewhat thicker than that of hard gelatin capsules. The gelation is plasticized by the addition of glycerin, sorbitol, or a similar polyol. The soft gelatin shells may contain a preservative to prevent the growth of fungi. Commonly used preservatives are methyl- and propylparabens and sorbic acid. Where the suspending vehicle or solvent can be an oil, soft gelatin capsules provide a convenient and highly acceptable dosage form. Large-scale production methods are generally required for the preparation and filling of soft gelatin capsules. Formerly empty soft gelatin capsules were available to the pharmacist for the extemporaneous compounding of solutions or suspensions in oils. Commercially filled soft gelatin capsules come in a wide choice of sizes and shapes; they may be round, oval, oblong, tube, or suppository shaped. Some sugar-coated tablets are quite similar in appearance to soft gelatin capsules. The essential differences are that the soft gelatin capsule has a seam at the point of closure of the two halves, and the contents can be liquid, paste, or powder. The sugar-coated tablet will not have a seam but will have a compressed core.

Oral SEC dosage forms are generally made so that the heat seam of the gelatin shell opens to release its liquid medication into the stomach less than five minutes after ingestion. Its use is being studied for those drugs poorly soluble in water having bioavailability problems. When used as suppositories, it is the moisture present in the body cavity that causes the capsule to come apart at its heat-sealed seam and to release its contents.

Plate Process

In this method a set of molds is used. A warm sheet of prepared gelatin is laid over the lower plate and the liquid is

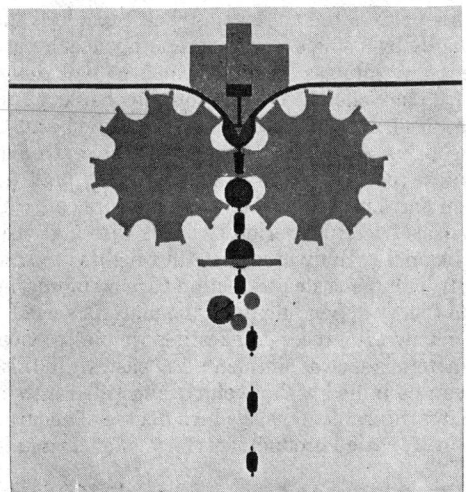

Fig 90-40.   Rotary die elastic capsule filler.

poured on it. A second sheet of gelatin is carefully put in place and this is followed by the top plate of the mold. The set is placed under the press where pressure is applied to form the capsules which are washed off with a volatile solvent to remove any traces of oil from the exterior. This process has been adapted and is used for encapsulation by the Upjohn Co. The sheets of gelatin may have the same color or different colors.

Rotary Die Process

In 1933 the rotary die process for elastic capsules was perfected by Robert P Scherer.[23] This process made it possible to improve the standards of accuracy and uniformity of elastic gelatin capsules and globules.

The rotary die machine is a self-contained unit capable of continuously and automatically producing finished capsules from a supply of gelatin mass and filling material which may be any liquid, semiliquid, or paste that will not dissolve gelatin. Two continuous gelatin ribbons, which the machine forms, are brought into convergence between a pair of revolving dies and an injection wedge. Accurate filling under pressure and sealing of the capsule wall occur as dual and coincident operations; each is delicately timed against the other. Sealing also severs the completed capsule from the net. The principle of operation is shown in Fig 90-40. See also Fig 90-41.

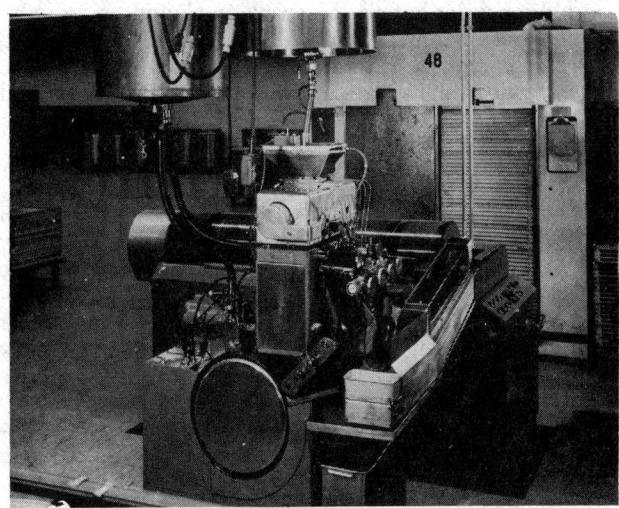

Fig 90-41.   Scherer soft elastic capsule machine (courtesy, Scherer).

By this process the content of each capsule is measured individually by a single stroke of a pump so accurately constructed that plunger travel of 0.025 in will deliver 1 ♏ (apoth). The Scherer machine contains banks of pumps so arranged that many capsules may be formed and filled simultaneously. All pumps are engineered to extremely small mechanical tolerances and to an extremely high degree of precision and similarity. All operations are controlled on a weight basis by actual periodic checks with a group of analytical balances. Individual net-fill weights of capsules resulting from large-scale production vary no more than ±1 to 3% from theory depending upon the materials used.

The rotary die process makes it possible to encapsulate heavy materials such as ointments and pastes. In this manner solids can be milled with a vehicle and filled into capsules. Where it is desirable to have a high degree of accuracy and a hermetically sealed product, this form of enclosure is ideally suited.

The modern and well-equipped capsule plant is completely air conditioned, a practical necessity for fine capsule production. Its facilities and operations include the availability of carbon dioxide at every exposed point of operation for the protection of oxidizable substances before encapsulation. Special ingredients also have been used in the capsule shell to exclude light wavelengths which are destructive to certain drugs.

Norton Capsule Machine

This machine produces capsules completely automatically by leading two films of gelatin between a set of vertical dies. These dies as they close, open, and close, are in effect a continual vertical plate forming row after row of pockets across the gelatin film. These are filled with medicament and, as they progress through the dies, are sealed, shaped, and cut out of the film as capsules which drop into a cooled solvent bath.

Accogel Capsule Machine

Another means of soft gelatin encapsulation utilizes the Accogel machine and process which were developed in the Lederle Laboratories Div of the American Cyanamid Co. The Accogel, or Stern machine, uses a system of rotary dies but is unique in that it is the only machine that can successfully fill dry powder into a soft gelatin capsule. The machine is available to the entire pharmaceutical industry by a lease arrangement and is used in many countries of the world. The machine is extremely versatile, not only producing capsules with dry powder but also encapsulating liquids and combinations of liquids and powders. By means of an attachment, slugs or compressed tablets may be enclosed in a gelatin film. The capsules can be made in a variety of colors, shapes, and sizes.

Microencapsulation

As a technology, microencapsulation is placed in the section on capsules only because of the relationship in terminology to mechanical encapsulation described above. The topic could also have been included in a discussion of coating procedures. Essentially, microencapsulation is a process or technique by which thin coatings can be applied reproducibly to small particles of solids, droplets of liquids, or dispersions, thus forming microcapsules. It can be differentiated readily from other coating methods in the size of the particles involved; these range from several tenths of a μm to 5000 μm in size.

A number of microencapsulation processes have been disclosed in the literature.[24] Some are based on chemical processes and involve a chemical or phase change; others are

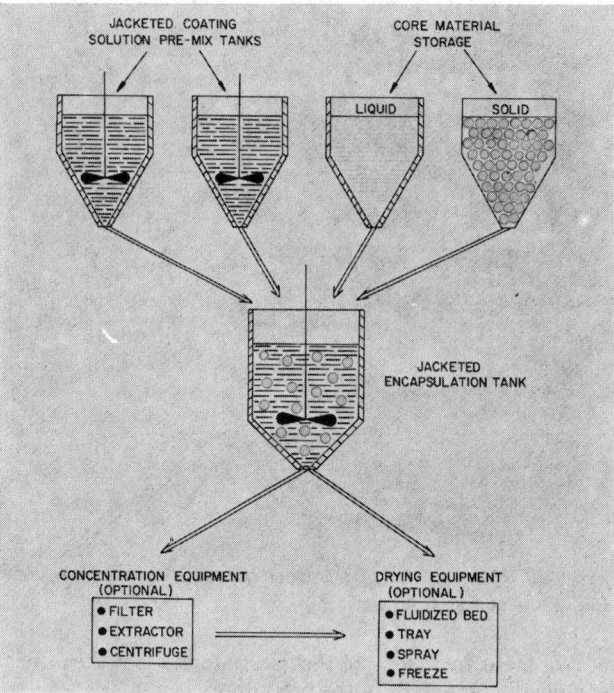

Fig 90-42. Production installation for microencapsulation process (courtesy, NCR).

mechanical and require special equipment to produce the physical change in the systems required.

Among the processes applied to pharmaceutical problems is that developed by the National Cash Register Co (NCR). The NCR process is a chemical operation based on phase separation or coacervation techniques. In colloidal chemistry coacervation refers to the separation of a liquid precipitate, or phase, when solutions of two hydrophilic colloids are mixed under suitable conditions.

The NCR process utilizing phase separation or coacervation techniques consists of three steps: (1) formation of three immiscible phases, a liquid manufacturing phase, a core material phase, and a coating material phase; (2) deposition of the liquid polymer coating on the core material; and (3) rigidizing the coating, usually by thermal, cross-linking or desolvation techniques, to form a microcapsule.

In Step 2, the deposition of the liquid polymer around the core material occurs only if the polymer is absorbed at the interface formed between the core material and the liquid vehicle phase. In many cases physical or chemical changes in the coating polymer solution can be induced so that phase separation (coacervation) of the polymer will occur. Droplets of concentrated polymer solution will form and coalesce to yield a two-phase liquid–liquid system. In cases where the coating material is an immiscible polymer or insoluble liquid polymer, it may be added directly. Also monomers can be dissolved in the liquid vehicle phase and subsequently polymerized at the interface.

Equipment required for microencapsulation by this method is relatively simple; it consists mainly of jacketed tanks with variable speed agitators. Fig 90-42 shows a typical flow diagram of a production installation.

A number of coating materials have been used successfully; examples of these include gelatin, polyvinyl alcohol, ethylcellulose, cellulose acetate phthalate, and styrene maleic anhydride. The film thickness can be varied considerably depending on the surface area of the material to be coated and other physical characteristics of the system. The microcapsules may consist of a single particle or clusters of particles. After isolation from the liquid manufacturing vehicle and drying, the material appears as a free-flowing powder. The powder is suitable for formulation as compressed tablets, hard gelatin capsules, suspensions, and other dosage forms.

The process provides answers for problems such as masking the taste of bitter drugs, a means of formulating prolonged action dosage forms, a means of separating incompatible materials, a method of protecting chemicals against moisture or oxidation, and a means of modifying a material's physical characteristics for ease of handling in formulation and manufacture.

Other Oral Solid Dosage Forms

Pills

Pills are small, round solid dosage forms containing a medicinal agent and are intended for oral administration. Pills were formerly the most extensively used oral dosage form, but they have been largely replaced by compressed tablets and capsules. Substances which are bitter or unpleasant to the taste, if not corrosive or deliquescent, can be administered in this form if the dose is not too large.

Formerly pills were made extemporaneously by the community pharmacist whose skill at pill making became an art. However, the few pills which are now used in pharmacy are prepared on a large scale with mechanical equipment. The pill formulas of the NF were introduced largely for the purpose of establishing standards of strength for the well-known and currently used pills. Hexylresorcinol Pills consist of hexylresorcinol crystals covered with a rupture-resistant coating that is dispersible in the digestive tract. It should be noted that the official hexylresorcinol pills are prepared not by traditional methods but by a patented process, the gelatin coating being sufficiently tough that it can not be readily broken, even when chewed. Therefore the general method for the preparation of pills does not apply to hexylresorcinol pills.

Previous editions of this text should be consulted for methods of pill preparation.

Troches

These forms of oral medication, also known as *lozenges* or *pastilles*, are discoid-shaped solids containing the medicinal agent in a suitably flavored base. The base may be a hard sugar candy, glycerinated gelatin, or the combination of sugar with sufficient mucilage to give it form. Troches are placed in the mouth where they slowly dissolve, liberating the active ingredient. The drug involved can be an antiseptic, local anesthetic, antibiotic, antihistaminic, antitussive, analgesic, or a decongestant.

Formerly troches were prepared extemporaneously by the pharmacist. The mass is formed by adding water slowly to a mixture of the powdered drug, powdered sugar, and a gum until a pliable mass is formed. Powdered acacia in 7% concentration gives sufficient adhesiveness to the mass. The mass is rolled out and the troche pieces cut out using a cutter, or else the mass is rolled into a cylinder and divided. Each piece is shaped and allowed to dry before dispensing.

If the active ingredient is heat stable, it may be prepared in a hard candy base. Syrup is concentrated to the point where it becomes a pliable mass, the active ingredient is added, and the mixture is kneaded while warm to form a homogeneous mass. The mass is gradually worked into a pipe form having the diameter desired for the candy piece and the lozenges cut from the pipe and allowed to cool. This is an entirely mechanical operation with equipment designed for this purpose.

If the active ingredient is heat labile, it may be made into a lozenge preparation by compression. The granulation is prepared in a manner similar to that used for any compressed tablet. The lozenge is made using heavy compression equipment to give a tablet which is harder than usual as it is

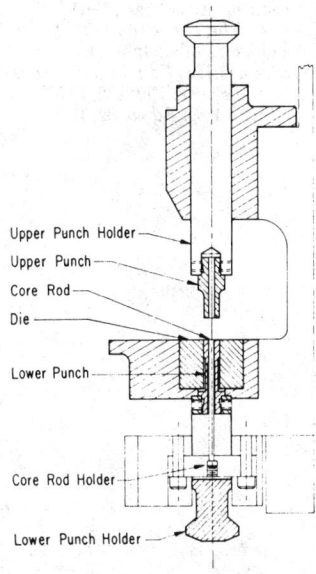

Fig 90-43. Core rod tooling for compressing troches or candy pieces with hole in center (courtesy, Vector/Colton).

desirable for the troche to dissolve or disintegrate slowly in the mouth. In the formulation of the lozenge the ingredients are chosen which will promote its slow-dissolving characteristics. Compression is gaining in popularity as a means of making troches and candy pieces because of the increased speeds of compression equipment. In cases where holes are to be placed in troches or candy pieces, core-rod tooling is used (see Fig 90-43). Core-rod tooling includes a rod centered on the lower punch around which the troche is compressed in the die cavity. The upper punch has an opening in its center for the core rod to enter during compression. It is evident that maximum accuracy is needed to provide alignment as the narrow punches are inserted into the die.

Cachets

Related to capsules, inasmuch as they provide an edible container for the oral administration of solid drugs, cachets were formerly used in pharmacy. They varied in size from $\frac{3}{4}$ to $\frac{1}{8}$ in in diameter and consisted of two concave pieces of wafer made of flour and water. After one section was filled with the prescribed quantity of the medicinal agent, they were tightly sealed by moistening the margins and pressing firmly together. When moistened with water, their character was entirely changed; they became soft, elastic, and slippery. Hence, they could easily be swallowed by floating them on water.

Pellets

The term pellet is now applied to small, sterile cylinders about 3.2 mm in diameter by 8 mm in length, which are formed by compression from medicated masses.[25] Whenever prolonged and continuous absorption of testosterone, estradiol, or desoxycorticosterone is desired, pellets of these potent hormones may be used by implantation.

References

1. Wagner JG: *Fundamentals of Clinical Pharmacokinetics*, Drug Intell Publ, Hamilton, IL, 1975.
2. Lieberman HA, Lachman L, eds: *Pharmaceutical Dosage Forms: Tablets*, *Vol I, II, III*, Marcel Dekker, New York, 1980, 1981, 1982.
3. Evans AJ, Train D: *A Bibliography of the Tableting of Medicinal Substances*, Pharmaceutical Press, London, 1963.
4. Evans AJ: *A Bibliography of the Tableting of Medicinal Substances*, 1st Suppl, Pharmaceutical Press, 1964.
5. Lachman L, *et al*: *The Theory and Practice of Industrial Pharmacy*, 2nd ed, Lea & Febiger, Philadelphia, 1975.
6. Monkhouse DC, Lach JL: *Can J Pharm Sci 7:* 29, 1972.
7. Blanchard J: *Am J Pharm 150:* 132, 1978.
8. Wurster DE: *J APhA Sci Ed 49:* 82, 1960.
9. Mendes RW, Roy SB: *Pharm Tech 2 (Mar):* 35, 1978.
10. Mendes RW, Roy SB: *Pharm Tech 2 (Sept):* 61, 1978.
11. Malinowski HJ, Smith WE: *J Pharm Sci 63:* 285, 1974.
12. Woodruff CW, Nuessle NO: *J Pharm Sci 61:* 787, 1972.
13. Newton JM: *Mfg Chem Aerosol News 37 (Apr):* 33, 1966.
14. US Patent 3,883,647, May 13, 1975.
15. *Tableting Specification Manual*, Am Pharm Assoc, Washington DC, 1981.
16. Knoechel EL, *et al:* *J Pharm Sci 56:* 116, 1967.
17. Wray PE: *Drug Cosmet Ind 105(3):* 53, 1969.
18. Schwartz JB: *Pharm Tech 5(9):* 102, 1981.
19. Marshall K: *Pharm Tech 7(3):* 68, 1983.
20. Jones BE: *Mfg Chem Aerosol News 40 (Feb):* 25, 1969.
21. Delaney R: *Pharm Exec 2 (Mar):* 34, 1982.
22. Tannenbaum PJ, *et al:* *Clin Pharmacol Ther 9:* 598, 1968.
23. Ebert WR: *Pharm Tech 1 (Oct):* 44, 1977.
24. Madan PL: *Pharm Tech 2 (Sept):* 68, 1978.
25. Cox PH, Spanjers F: *Pharm Weekblad 105:* 681, 1970.

CHAPTER 91

Coating of Pharmaceutical Dosage Forms

Stuart C Porter, PhD
Vice President, Research and Development
Colorcon, Inc
West Point, PA 19486

Introduction

Any introduction to tablet coating must be prefaced by an important question—"Why coat tablets?"—since in many instances, the coating is being applied to a dosage form that is already functionally complete. In attempting to answer this question, if one examines the market, it will be immediately obvious that a significant proportion of pharmaceutical solid dosage forms are coated. The reasons for this range from the aesthetic to a desire to control the bioavailability of the drug, and include the following:

1. Protection of the drug from its surrounding environment (particularly air, moisture, and light) with a view to improving stability.

2. Masking of unpleasant taste and odor.

3. Increasing the ease by means of which the product can be ingested by the patient.

4. Improving product identity, from the manufacturing plant, through intermediaries and to the patient.

5. Facilitating handling, particularly in high speed packaging/filling lines, and automated counters in pharmacies, where the coating minimizes cross-contamination due to dust elimination.

6. Improvement in product appearance, particularly where there are noticeable visible differences in tablet core ingredients from batch to batch.

7. Reducing the risk of interaction between incompatible components. This would be achieved by using coated forms of one or more of the offending ingredients (particularly active compounds).

8. Improvement in product mechanical integrity, since coated products are generally more resistant to mishandling (abrasion, attrition, etc).

9. Modification of drug release, as in enteric-coated, repeat-action, and sustained-release products.

Evolution of the Coating Process—Tablet coating is perhaps one of the oldest pharmaceutical processes still in existence, and although a great deal has been written about the materials and methods used, as a process it is still often recognized to be more of an art than a science, a factor which is obviously responsible for many of the problems that can exist. Historically, the literature cites Rhazes (850–932 AD) as being one of the earliest "tablet coaters," having used the mucilage of psyllium seeds to coat pills that had an offending taste. Subsequently, Avicenna[1] was reported to have used gold and silver for pill coating. Since then, there have been many references to the different materials used in "tablet coating." White[2] mentioned the use of finely divided talc in what was at one time popularly known as "pearl coating," while Kremers and Urdang[3] describe the introduction of the gelatin coating of pills by Garot in 1838.

An interesting reference[4] reports the use of waxes to coat poison tablets. These waxes, being insoluble in all parts of the gastrointestinal tract, were intended to prevent accidental poisoning (the contents could be utilized by breaking the tablet prior to use).

A point that must be stressed is that much of the earlier coated products were produced by individuals working in pharmacies, particularly when extemporaneous compounding was the order of the day, and although responsibility for tablet coating has now been assumed by the pharmaceutical industry, skilled individuals still practiced their art until quite recently.

The earliest attempts to apply coatings to pills obviously resulted in variable products, and required the handling of single pills. These would have been mounted on a needle or held with a pair of forceps and literally dipped into the coating fluid, a procedure which would have to be repeated more than once to ensure that the pill was completely coated. Subsequently, the pills were held at the end of a suction tube, dipped and then the process repeated for the other side of the pill. Not surprisingly, these techniques failed to yield a uniformly coated product.[5] Initially, the first sugar coated pills seen in the US were imported from France *circa* 1842[5]; while Warner, a Philadelphia pharmacist, became among the first indigenous manufacturers in 1856.[6]

Methods for the coating of a large number of tablets are essentially derived from those used in the candy industry, where techniques were highly evolved, even in the Middle Ages. Today, most coating pans are fabricated from stainless steel, although early pans were made from copper owing to the fact that drying was effected by means of an externally applied heat source. Current thinking, even with conventional pans, is to dry the coated tablets with a supply of heated air, and to extract the moisture and dust laden air from the vicinity of the pan.

Further evolution in the coating process tended to remain somewhat static until the late 1940's and early 1950's, with the conventional pan being the mainstay of all coating operations up to that time. However, in the last twenty or thirty years there have been some significant advances made in coating technology, advances often pre-empted by a steady evolution in pan design and its associated ancillary equipment.

Interestingly, in the early years of this development, an entirely new form of technology evolved, that of film coating. Recognizing the deficiencies of the sugar coating process, advocates of film coating were achieving success by utilizing coating systems involving highly volatile organic solvents. These circumvented the problems associated with the inefficiency in the drying capabilities of conventional equipment, and enabled production quotas to be met with significant reductions in processing times and materials used. The disadvantage of this approach, however, has always been associated with the solvent system, which often used flammable and toxic materials.

The advances that occurred with equipment design, having begun by the development of the Wurster[7] process and continued by the evolution of side-vented pans, have resulted in the gradual emergence of coating processes where drying efficiency tends to be maximized. Thus, film coating began as a process utilizing inefficient drying equipment, relying on highly volatile coating formulations for success and has evolved into one in which the processing equipment is a major factor. The latter has been largely responsible for the return to an aqueous process.

Obviously, the advances in equipment design have also benefited the sugar coating process, where, because of Good Manufacturing Procedures (GMP) and the need to maintain product uniformity and performance, the trend has been toward fully automated processes. Nonetheless film coating tends to maintain a somewhat dominant position in the area of tablet coating.

Pharmaceutical Coating Processes

Basically, there are four major techniques for applying coatings to pharmaceutical solid dosage forms: (1) Sugar Coating, (2) Film Coating, (3) Microencapsulation and (4) Compression Coating.

Although it could be argued that the use of mucilage of psyllium seed, gelatin, etc, as already discussed was an early form of film coating, sugar coating is regarded as the oldest method for tablet coating, and involves the deposition from aqueous solution of coatings based predominantly on sucrose as a raw material. The large quantities of coating material that are applied and the inherent skill often required of the operators combine to result in a long and tedious process.

Film coating, the deposition of resins as a thin membrane onto the dosage form from solutions that were initially organic-solvent based, but which are beginning to rely more and more on water as the prime solvent, have proven to be a popular alternative to sugar coating.

Microencapsulation is a modified form of film coating, differing from the latter only in the size of the particles (or liquid droplets) to be coated and the methods by which this is accomplished. It is based on either mechanical methods such as pan coating, air suspension techniques, multi-orifice centrifugal techniques, and modified spray drying techniques, or physicochemical ones involving coacervation-phase separation, where the material to be coated is suspended in a solution of the polymer. Phase separation is facilitated by the addition of a nonsolvent, incompatible polymer, inorganic salts, or by altering the temperature of the system.

Compression coating incorporates the use of modified tabletting machines which allow the compaction of a dry coating around the tablet core produced on the same machine. The main advantage of this type of coating is that it eliminates the use of any solvent, whether aqueous or organic in nature. However, the fact that it involves a mechanically complex operation has obviously been a prime factor in limiting its adoption as a popular technique.

The latter two approaches fall outside the scope of this chapter, which will be confined to processes in which liquid systems are applied to the surface of a solid dosage form, no matter how diverse that substrate might be. See Chapter 90.

Sugar Coating of Compressed Tablets

Sugar coating, as the name implies, is a process which relies on the use of two main raw materials, namely sucrose and water. Sugar is a somewhat generic term that lends itself to a whole class of materials. For the purposes of sugar coating, the only material which has stood the test of time is sucrose. The main reason for this, is that based on the techniques evolved, it is probably the only material which has enabled smooth, high quality coatings to be produced, which are essentially dry and tack free at the end of the process.

Although other methods for the coating of solid dosage forms have been and are being evolved, a significant proportion of all coated products are still sugar-coated, and some companies are spending vast amounts of capital to thoroughly

update the process. In spite of certain inherent difficulties associated with the sugar coating process, products which have been expertly sugar coated still remain among the most elegant available.

Since sugar coating is a multi-step process, where success is still measured in terms of the elegance of the final product, it has been, and still is in many companies, highly dependent on the use of skilled manpower. These factors, combined with a certain amount of folklore, are responsible for the process being long and tedious. However, processing times have gradually been improved in the last two decades by the adoption of modern techniques and by the introduction of automation.

The sugar coating process can be subdivided into the following stages: (1) Sealing, (2) Subcoating, (3) Smoothing, (4) Coloring, (5) Polishing, and (6) Printing.

Sealing—The sealing coat is applied directly to the tablet core for the prime purpose of separating the tablet core (and active ingredients contained therein) from the aqueous solutions used in the remainder of the coating process. A secondary function is to strengthen the tablet core. Sealing coats usually consist of alcoholic solutions (approximately 10–30% solids) of resins such as shellac, zein, cellulose acetate phthalate, or polyvinyl acetate phthalate. Historically, shellac has proven to be the most popular material although its use can lead to problems of impaired bioavailability owing to a change in resin properties on storage. A solution to this problem has been to use a shellac-based formulation containing a measured quantity of polyvinylpyrrolidone (PVP).[8]

The quantities of material applied as a sealing coat will obviously depend on the tablet size and pan charge. However, another important factor is the tablet porosity, since highly porous tablets will tend to soak up the first application of solution, thus preventing it from spreading uniformly throughout the whole tablet mass. Thus, one or more further applications of resin solution may be necessary to ensure the cores are sealed.

Since most sealing coats develop a degree of tack at some time during the drying stages, their use is usually accompanied by one or more applications of a dusting powder to prevent tablets from sticking together or to the pan. A common material used as a dusting powder is asbestos-free talc. Overzealous use of this material may cause problems, firstly, by imparting a high degree of slip to the tablets thus preventing them from rolling properly in the pan, and secondly, presenting a surface at the beginning of the subcoating stage which is very difficult to wet, resulting in inadequate subcoat build-up, particularly on the edges. If there is a tendency for either of these problems to occur, one solution is to replace part or all of the talc with some other material such as terra alba, which will form a slightly rougher surface.

If an enteric coated product is desired, it is usually achieved at the seal coat stage by extending the number of applications made, preferably using an enteric coating polymer such as polyvinyl acetate phthalate or cellulose acetate phthalate.

Subcoating—Subcoating is a critical operation in the sugar coating process that can have a marked effect on ultimate tablet quality. Sugar coating is a process which leads to a 50–100% weight increase, and it is at the subcoating stage that most of the build-up occurs, mainly to develop the basis of an elegant tablet profile.

Historically, subcoating has been achieved by the application of a gum-based solution to the sealed tablet cores, and once this has been uniformly distributed throughout the tablet mass, to follow by a liberal dusting of powder which serves to reduce tack and facilitate tablet buildup. This procedure of application of gum solution, spreading, dusting, and drying is continued until the requisite build-up has been achieved. Thus, in this situation, the subcoating is a sandwich of alter-

Table I—Binder Solution Formulations for Subcoating

	A, % w/w	B, % w/w
Gelatin	3.3	6.0
Gum acacia (powdered)	8.7	8.0
Sucrose	55.3	45.0
Water	to 100.0	to 100.0

Table II—Dusting Powder Formulations for Subcoating

	A, % w/w	B, % w/w
Calcium carbonate	40.0	—
Titanium dioxide	5.0	1.0
Talc (asbestos-free)	25.0	61.0
Sucrose (powdered)	28.0	38.0
Gum acacia (powdered)	2.0	—

Table III—Typical Suspension Subcoating Formulation

	% w/w
Distilled water	25.0
Sucrose	40.0
Calcium carbonate	20.0
Talc (asbestos-free)	12.0
Gum acacia (powdered)	2.0
Titanium dioxide	1.0

nate layers of gum and powder. Some examples of binder solutions are shown in Table I, and those of dusting powder formulations in Table II.

This approach has proved to be very effective, particularly where there is difficulty in covering edges, etc. However, if care is not taken, a "lumpy" subcoat will be the result. Also, if the amount of dusting powder applied is not matched to the binding capacity of the gum solution, not only will the ultimate coating be very weak, but also, dust will collect in the back of the pan, a factor which may contribute to ultimate roughness.

An alternative approach which has proved popular, particularly when used in conjunction with an automated dosing system, is the application of a suspension subcoat formulation, in which the powdered materials responsible for coating build-up have been incorporated into a gum-based solution. An example of such a formulation is shown in Table III. Obviously, this approach allows the solids loading to be matched more closely to the binding capacity of the base solution, and often permits the less experienced coater to produce satisfactory subcoats with the minimum of problems.

Smoothing—Depending on how successfully the subcoat was applied, there may be a necessity for further smoothing to be achieved prior to color coating, particularly if the latter is to be accomplished by means of a dye coating process. Smoothing can usually be accomplished by the application of a simple syrup solution (approximately 60–70% sugar solids).

Often the smoothing syrups contain a low percentage of titanium dioxide (1–5%) as an opacifier. This can be particularly useful when following with a dye color coating process since it makes the layer under the color coating more reflective, resulting in a brighter, cleaner ultimate color.

Color Coating—In many ways, color coating is the most important step in the successful completion of a sugar coating process. This is achieved by the multi-step application of simple syrup solutions (60–70% sugar solids) containing the requisite coloring matter. The types of coloring materials used can be divided into two categories: dyes and pigments. The distinction between the two is simply one of solubility in the coating fluid. Since water-soluble dyes behave entirely

differently than water-insoluble pigments, the application procedure used in the color coating of tablets will depend on the type of colorant chosen.

When utilized by a skilled artisan, water-soluble dyes produce the most elegant of sugar-coated tablets, mainly because they yield a much cleaner, brighter color. However, since water-soluble dyes are migratory colorants (that is to say, as the moisture is drawn out of the tablets, this will tend to cause migration of the color, leading to a nonuniform distribution of color), great care must be exercised in their use, particularly when dark shades are required. This involves the application of volumes of coating solution (containing low concentrations of colorant), which are capable of just wetting the entire tablet mass, and then allowing the tablets to dry very slowly to prevent color migration. It is essential that each application is allowed to dry thoroughly before subsequent applications are made, otherwise moisture may become trapped in the coating and may cause the tablets to "sweat" on standing.

Finally, in order to achieve the requisite color uniformity and intensity, it may be necessary to make 60 repeat applications of color solution. This factor, combined with the need to dry each application slowly and thoroughly, results in very long processing times (eg, assuming 50 applications are made which take between 15 and 30 minutes each, the coloring process can extend over a period of up to 25 hours).

Tablet color coating with pigments, as advocated by Tucker et al,[9] can present some significant advantages. First of all, since pigment colors are water insoluble, they present no problems of migration since the colorant remains where it is deposited. In addition, if the pigment is completely opaque, or the system is formulated with an opacifier such as titanium dioxide, the desired color can be developed much more rapidly, thus resulting in a thinner color coat. Since each application can be dried more rapidly, significant savings can be made in processing times.

Although pigment-based color coatings are by no means foolproof, they will permit more abuse than a dye color coating approach, and are more amenable for use by less skilled coaters. Pharmaceutically acceptable pigments can be classified either as inorganic pigments (eg, titanium dioxide, iron oxides) or certified lakes. Certified lakes are produced from water-soluble dyes by means of a process known as "laking" whereby the dye molecule becomes fixed to a suitable insoluble substrate such as aluminum hydroxide.

Certified lakes, particularly when used in conjunction with an opacifier such as titanium dioxide, provide an excellent means of coloring sugar coatings and permit a wide range of shades to be achieved. However, the incorporation of pigments into the syrup solution is not as easy as with water-soluble dyes, since with the former, it is necessary to ensure that all the insoluble matter is completely wetted and dispersed. Thus the use of prepared pigment color concentrates, which are commercially available, is usually beneficial.

Polishing—In order to impart the requisite gloss to the final product, the tablets, when dry, are submitted to a polishing process where wax mixtures (beeswax, carnauba wax, candelilla wax, hard paraffin wax, etc) are applied either as finely divided powder mixtures or as suspensions or solutions in various solvents to the tablets in wax or canvas-lined pans.

Printing—In order to identify sugar-coated tablets apart from shape, size, and color, it is often necessary to submit them to a printing stage, either prior to or subsequent to the polishing stage, using pharmaceutical branding inks by means of the process of *offset rotogravure*.

Sugar Coating Problems—Various problems may be encountered during the sugar coating of tablets. It must be remembered that any process in which tablets are kept constantly tumbling can present difficulties if the tablets are not strong enough to withstand the stress encountered. Tablets which are too soft, or have a tendency to laminate, may break up and the fragments adhere to the surface of otherwise good tablets. Sugar coating pans exhibit inherently poor mixing characteristics. If care is not exercised during the application of the various coating fluids, nonuniform distribution of coating material can occur, resulting in an unacceptable range of sizes of finished tablets within the batch. Overzealous use of dusting powders, particularly during the subcoating stage, may result in a coating being formed in which the solid particulate matter exceeds the capacity of the binder in the formulation, creating soft coatings or those with increased tendency to crack.

Color nonuniformity is a common problem, particularly when water-soluble dyes are used. Since the latter have a tendency to migrate easily, lack of control over the drying phases during the process can result in nonuniform distribution of the coloring material. Rough tablets are obtained either as the result of too rapid drying or lack of uniform distribution of coating fluid after each application. This is particularly troublesome during the color coating stage, when the problem may be highlighted as "marbling" after subsequent polishing.

Film Coating of Solid Dosage Forms

Film coating involves the deposition of a thin, but uniform, membrane onto the surface of the substrate. Unlike sugar coating, the flexibility afforded in film coating allows additional substrates, other than just compressed tablets, to be considered (eg, powder, granules, nonpareils, capsules). Coatings are essentially applied continuously to a moving bed of material, usually by means of a spray technique, although manual application procedures have been used.

Historically, film coating was introduced in the early 1950's in order to combat the shortcomings of the then predominant sugar coating process. That it has proven successful must be attributed to its major advantages which include:

(1) Minimal weight increase (typically 2–3% of tablet core weight)
(2) Significant reduction in processing times
(3) Increased process efficiency and output
(4) Increased flexibility in formulations
(5) Improved resistance to chipping of the coating.

The major process advantages were derived from the greater volatility of the organic solvents used. However, in spite of its success, there has always been an awareness that certain disadvantages could prove ultimately to be a limiting factor.

These disadvantages are mainly attributed to the organic solvents used in the process and include:

(1) Flammability hazards
(2) Toxicity hazards
(3) Concerns over environmental pollution
(4) Cost (either relating to minimizing items 1–3, or to the cost of the solvents themselves).

However, in the interim since its introduction, significant advances have been made in process technology and equipment design. The emphasis has changed from requiring the presence of highly volatile organic solvents so that the product dries rapidly, to achieving the same ultimate effect by designing equipment to have more efficient drying characteristics.

Thus, there has been a transition from conventional pans to side-vented pans and fluid-bed equipment, and consequently from the problematic organic solvent-based process to aqueous systems.

Film Coating Raw Materials—The major components

in any film coating formulation consist of polymer, plasticizer, colorant, and solvent (or vehicle).

A major requirement for the polymer is solubility in a wide range of solvent systems to promote flexibility in formulation. In addition, it must possess an ability to produce coatings which have suitable mechanical properties. Because of the various requirements of the coating, such as being exposed to gastrointestinal fluids, the polymer should meet certain performance characteristics.

Cellulose ethers constitute the majority of polymer types used for film coating; particularly hydroxypropyl methylcellulose. Suitable substitutes are hydroxypropyl cellulose, which may produce slightly tackier coatings, and methylcellulose, although this has been reported to retard drug dissolution.[10] Alternatives to the cellulose ethers are certain acrylics, which are copolymers of methacrylic acid and methyl methacrylate.

Most polymers are employed as solutions in either aqueous or organic solvent based systems. An alternative system utilizes certain water-insoluble polymers such as ethylcellulose and/or some of the acrylics as aqueous dispersions. An additional factor to be considered in the selection of polymers concerns the various molecular weight grades available for each type. Molecular weight may have an important influence on various properties of the coating system and its ultimate performance, such as solution viscosity and mechanical strength and flexibility of the resultant film.

The incorporation of a plasticizer into the formulation lends flexibility to the film, thus better able to withstand stress. This reduces the risk of the film cracking and possibly improves adhesion of the film to the substrate. To ensure that these benefits are achieved, the plasticizer must show a high degree of compatibility with the polymer, and a degree of permanence if the properties of the coating are to be stable on storage. Examples of typical plasticizers include glycerin, propylene glycol, polyethylene glycols, triacetin, acetylated monoglyceride, citrate esters (eg, triethyl citrate) and phthalate esters (eg, diethyl phthalate).

Colorants are usually used to enhance the aesthetic appeal of the product as well as to increase product identification. However, under certain circumstances, they can enhance certain necessary physical properties of the applied film coats. As in the case of sugar coating, colorants can either be classified as water-soluble dyes or insoluble pigments.

The use of water-soluble dyes is precluded with organic solvent based film coating because of lack of solubility in the solvent system. Thus, the use of pigments, particularly the aluminum lakes, provides the most useful means of coloring film coating systems. Obviously, in aqueous film coating there is potential for using water-soluble dyes as colorants, although in fact, pigments still offer some significant advantages for the following reasons:

(1) The tendency of some water-soluble dyes to interfere with bioavailability[11]
(2) The possibility of reduction in permeability of the coating to moisture when pigments are used[12]
(3) Pigments serve as a bulking agent to increase overall solids content in coating system.

The major solvents used in film coating typically belong to one of the following classes: alcohols, ketones, esters, chlorinated hydrocarbons, and water. Solvents serve to perform an important function in the film coating process, since they facilitate the delivery of the film forming materials to the surface of the substrate. Good interaction between solvent and polymer is necessary to ensure that optimal film properties are derived when the coating dries. This initial interaction between solvent and polymer will yield maximum polymer chain extension, producing films having the greatest cohesive strength, and thus, best mechanical properties. An important function of the solvent systems is also to assure a controlled deposition of the polymer onto the surface of the substrate if a coherent and adherent film coat is to be obtained.

Although it is very difficult to give typical examples of film coating formulations, since these will be dependent on the materials used and their various properties, they are usually based on 5–15% (w/w) coating solids in the requisite vehicle (with the higher concentration range preferred for aqueous formulations), of which 60–70% is polymer, 6–7% is plasticizer, and 20–30% is pigment.

Modified Release Film Coatings

Film coatings can be applied to pharmaceutical products in order to modify the release pattern of a drug. One form of coating is used to prevent the release of drugs in, or protect drugs from the effects of, the gastric environment. Such a coating is commonly called an *enteric* coating. Other types of coatings, often called *sustained* or *controlled release* coatings, are primarily used to extend the release of a drug over a long period of time.

Enteric Coatings—By definition, enteric coatings are those which remain intact in the stomach, but will dissolve and release the contents of the dosage form once they arrive at the small intestine. Their purpose is to delay the release of drugs which are inactivated by the stomach contents, (eg, pancreatin, erythromycin) or may cause nausea or bleeding by irritating the gastric mucosa (eg, aspirin, steroids). In addition, they can be used to give a simple repeat-action effect where unprotected drug coated *over* the enteric coat is released in the stomach, while the remainder, being protected by the coating, is released further down the gastrointestinal tract.

The action of enteric coatings results from a difference in composition of the respective gastric and intestinal environments in regard to pH and enzymatic properties. Although there have been repeated attempts to produce coatings which are subject to intestinal enzyme breakdown, this approach is not popular since enzymatic decomposition of the film is rather slow. Thus, many modern enteric coatings are those which remain undissociated in the low pH environment of the stomach, but readily ionize when the pH rises to about 4 or 5. The most effective enteric polymers are polyacids having a pK_a of 3 to 5.

Historically, the earliest enteric coatings utilized formalin-treated gelatin, but this was unreliable since the polymerization of gelatin could not be accurately controlled, and often resulted in failure to release the drug even in the lower intestinal tract. Another early candidate was shellac, but again the main disadvantage was a potential to increase the degree of polymerization on storage, often resulting in failure to release the active contents. Although the pharmaceutical literature has contained references to many potentially suitable polymers, only three or four remain in use.

The most extensively used polymer is cellulose acetate phthalate (CAP) which is capable of functioning effectively as an enteric coating. However, a pH greater than 6 is required for solubility and thus a delay in drug release may ensue. It is also relatively permeable to moisture and gastric juice compared to most enteric polymers, thus susceptible to hydrolytic decomposition. Phthalic and acetic acids can be split off, resulting in a change in polymeric, and therefore enteric, properties. Another useful polymer is polyvinyl acetate phthalate (PVAP) which is less permeable to moisture and gastric juice, more stable to hydrolysis, and able to ionize at a lower pH, resulting in earlier release of actives in the duodenum.

A more recently available polymer is hydroxypropyl methylcellulose phthalate. This has similar stability to PVAP and dissociates in the same pH range. A final example of currently used polymers are those based on methacrylic acid—methacrylic acid ester copolymers with acidic ionizable groups. They have been reported to suffer from the disadvantage of having delayed breakdown even at relatively high pH.[13]

Sustained Release Coatings—The concept of sustained release formulations was developed in order to eliminate the need for multiple dosage regimens, particularly for those drugs requiring reasonably constant blood levels over a long period of time. In addition, it has also been adopted for those drugs which need to be administered in high doses, but where too rapid a release is likely to cause undesirable side effects (eg, the ulceration that occurs when potassium chloride is rapidly released in the gastrointestinal tract).

Formulation methods used to obtain the desired drug availability rate from sustained action dosage forms include:

1. Increasing the particle size of the drug
2. Embedding the drug in a matrix
3. Coating the drug or dosage form containing the drug
4. Forming complexes of the drug with materials such as ion-exchange resins.

Only those methods which involve some form of coating fall within the scope of this chapter.

Materials which have been found suitable for producing sustained release coatings include:

1. Mixtures of waxes (beeswax, carnauba wax, etc) with glyceryl monostearate, stearic acid, palmitic acid, glyceryl monopalmitate, and cetyl alcohol. These provide coatings which are slowly dissolved or decomposed in the gastrointestinal tract.
2. Shellac and zein, polymers which remain intact until the pH of gastrointestinal contents becomes less acidic.
3. Ethylcellulose, which provides a membrane around the particle and remains intact throughout the gastrointestinal tract. However, it does permit water to permeate the film, dissolve the drug, and diffuse out again.
4. Acrylic resins, which behave similarly to ethylcellulose as a diffusion controlled drug release coating material.

Traditionally, the common method of producing a sustained release product has involved one of the following approaches.

A granulation containing the drug which could be *spheronized* prior to drying, if desired, is prepared. Dried granules are coated and then either filled into capsules or compressed into tablets. Alternatively, drugs are applied either in solution or as a suspension, to the surface of sugar *seeds* (nonpareils). These are subsequently coated with the requisite material and usually filled into capsules. In both cases, a fraction of uncoated granules or seeds may be included to provide an initial immediate release of drug.

In another approach, tablets may be coated with a suitable retardant film. A recent example of this approach includes the coating of a tablet core, containing an osmotically active material, in addition to the drug, with a semipermeable membrane. Subsequent to coating, an orifice of predetermined size is made in the coating by means of a laser beam. When such a tablet is swallowed, gastrointestinal fluids permeate the film, causing the contents of the dosage form to dissolve. The osmotic pressure created inside the membrane forces the drug to be diffused through the orifice at a controlled rate, usually following apparent zero-order kinetics. This is, in effect, a very simple form of osmotic pump.

In spite of the various ingenious approaches employed in the creation of oral sustained release dosage forms, the limiting factor in all cases is based on gastrointestinal transit times. One important consideration with any form of modified release coating, since the dose of drug used is often much higher than that used in conventional formulations, is to prevent "dose dumping." This can occur when the integrity of the coating is prematurely broken, either as a result of tablets sticking together during the coating process and becoming subsequently broken apart, or cracking of the coating anytime subsequent to processing.

Film Coating Problems

As with sugar coating, difficulties may develop during, or subsequent to, the film coating process. The tablets being coated may not be sufficiently robust, or may have a tendency to *laminate* while being coated. Since film coats are relatively thin, their ability to hide defects is significantly less than with sugar coating. Hence, tablets which have poor resistance to abrasion (ie, they exhibit high friability characteristics) can be problematic, since the imperfections may be readily apparent after coating. It is very important to identify tablets with suspect properties, whether mechanically or performance related (eg, poor dissolution), prior to a coating process, since subsequent recovery or reworking of tablets may be extremely difficult after a coating has been applied.

Typical process-related problems that can occur during the coating process include *picking*, which is a consequence of the fluid delivery rate exceeding the drying capacity of the process, causing tablets to stick together and subsequently become broken apart, and *orange-peel* or *roughness*. The latter is usually the result of premature drying of atomized droplets of solution, or it may be a consequence of spraying too viscous a coating solution such that effective atomization is difficult.

Mottling, or color nonuniformity, can result from uneven distribution of color in the coating, a problem often related to the use of soluble dyes in aqueous film coating, when color migration can occur either by evolution of residual solvent in the film, or by migration of plasticizer in which the colorant may be soluble. The use of pigments in the film coating process minimizes the incidence of this latter objection considerably. However, uneven color can also result from poor pigment dispersion in the coating solution.

Finally, two significant problems which may occur result from the internal stress that develops within the film as it dries. The first occurs when this stress exceeds the tensile strength of the film, causing it to crack. The second is manifested as "bridging of a logo" (ie, a monogram present in the surface of the tablet core), and occurs when a component of the internal stress is able to overcome the localized forces of attachment of the film to the tablet in the region of the monogram. The film no longer follows the contour of the indented monogram and draws away to bridge the crevices, an unacceptable state.

A fundamental approach to formulation of the coating, in which the behavioral characteristics of materials, particularly the polymer used in the coating, is advocated[14] as providing a solution to such problems resulting from the effects of internal stress.

Coating Procedures and Equipment

Coating Pans—The coating of tablets by means of the sugar coating process has historically involved the manual application of the various coating fluids to a cascading bed of tablets in a conventional coating pan (Fig 91-1), fitted with a means of supplying drying air to the tablets and an exhaust to remove moisture and dust-laden air from the pan.

Typically, after the requisite volume of liquid has been applied, an appropriate amount of time is allowed for the tablets to mix and permit the liquid to be fully dispersed

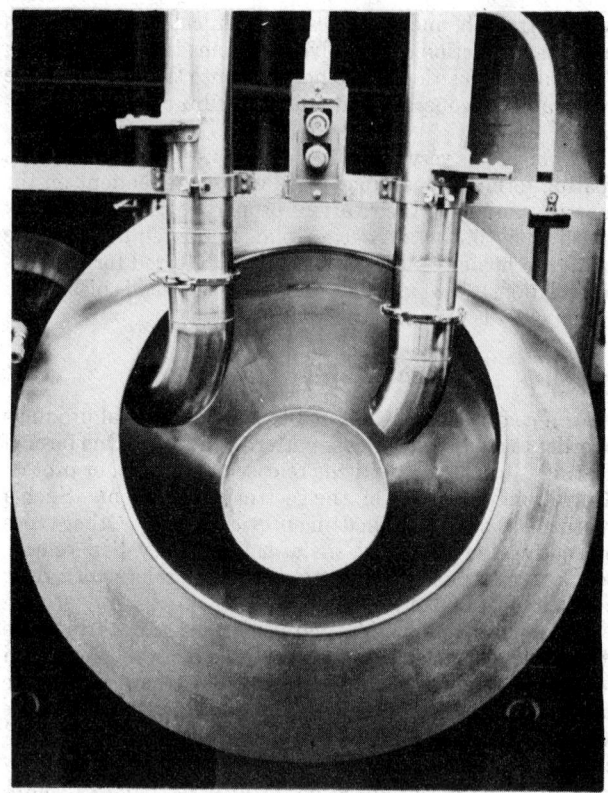

Fig 91-1. Typical equipment set-up for conventional sugar coating.

throughout the batch. To facilitate the uniform transfer of liquid, the tablets are often "stirred" by hand, or in larger pans, by means of a rake, to overcome mixing problems often associated with "dead spots," an inherent feature of conventional pans. Finally, tablets are dried by directing an air supply onto the surface of the tablet bed. Thus, sugar coating is somewhat of a sequential process consisting of consecutive cycles of liquid application, mixing, and drying.

During the early history of film coating, the equipment used was essentially adapted from that already employed for sugar coating. Although the manual application of coating liquids during the film coating process has been practiced, usually the liquid is applied using a spray technique. Spray equipment utilized are essentially of two types:

(1)   Airless (or hydraulic) spray, where coating liquid is pumped under pressure to a spray nozzle, and atomization of the liquid occurs as it emerges from a very small aperture. This is analogous to the effect achieved when one places one's finger over the end of a garden hose.

(2)   Air-spray, whereby liquid which is pumped under little or no pressure to the nozzle is atomized by means of a blast of compressed air that makes contact with the stream of liquid as it passes through the nozzle aperture.

The former is typically used in large-scale film coating operations for organic solvents, while the latter is more efficient in either a small-scale laboratory set-up, or in the currently popular aqueous film coating operations.

The use of spray techniques permits the delivery of finely atomized droplets of a coating solution, to the tablet mass in continual motion, in such a manner as to ensure uniform coverage while preventing adjacent tablets from adhering together as the coating solution rapidly dries. Although all the phases that occur during the spray process occur continuously and concurrently, the overall picture can be simplified and represented in the form of several sequential steps, as shown in Fig 91-2. The spray process can be operated either as an intermittent or continuous one.

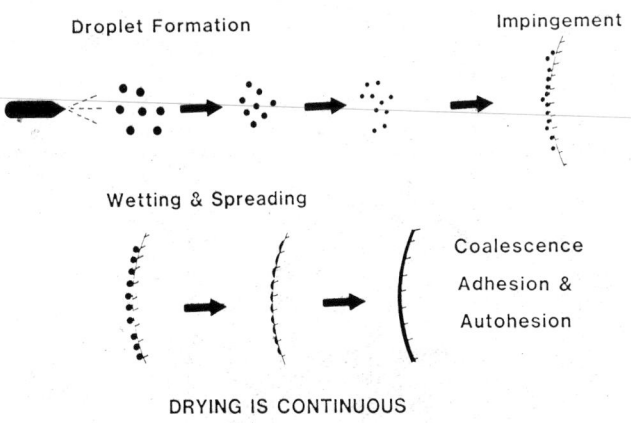

Fig 91-2.   Schematic representation of the film coating process.

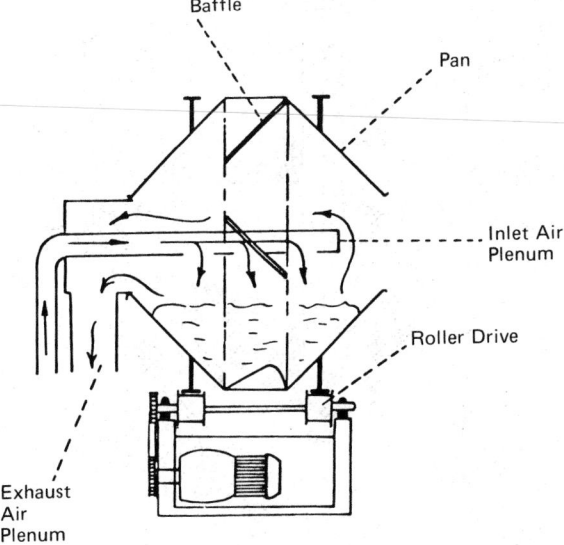

Fig 91-3.   Schematic diagram of a Pellegrini coating pan.

In the early years of film coating, the lack of adequate drying conditions inside the coating apparatus, together with the preference for using airless coating techniques (and their inherently higher delivery rates), with organic solvent based formulations on a production scale, gave rise to an intermittent spray procedure. This allowed excess solvent to be removed during the nonspray part of the cycle, and thus reduced the risk of *picking* and tendency for tablets to stick together. However, in the ensuing years, the improvement in drying capabilities has resulted in a continuous spray procedure being adopted, as this permits a more uniform coating to be developed, usually in a shorter time and simplifies the process. As indicated previously, pan equipment initially was completely conventional in design and, with the exception of the addition of spray application equipment, was similar to that used in sugar coating.

Fortunately, film coating formulations were based on relatively volatile organic solvents, which enabled acceptable processing times to be achieved in spite of the relative deficiencies of the air handling systems. Since the equipment rarely represented a completely enclosed system, it did little to minimize the hazards of using organic solvents. Although conventional pans possessed acceptable properties with regard to mixing of the tablet mass in the sugar coating process (particularly as this could be augmented by manual stirring of the tablets during processing), they were poorly suited to meet the more rigorous demands of the film coating process, even when some simple form of baffle system was installed. In spite of these inadequacies, the use of conventional pans has persisted. The introduction of aqueous film coating in recent years has presented the most serious challenge to this type of equipment. Considering the limitations in both air exchange and mixing capabilities, both must be significantly improved to assure that uniform and high drying rates are available to yield acceptable processing times with minimal risk to product integrity.

Although considerable experimentation has taken place with the geometric design of conventional equipment, the most significant change came with the introduction of the Pellegrini coating pan (Fig 91-3), which is somewhat angular and rotates on a horizontal axis. The geometry of the pan, coupled with the fact that there is an integral baffle system, assures much more uniformity in mixing. Additionally, since the services are introduced through the rear opening, the front can either be left free for inspection purposes, or simply closed off to yield an enclosed coating system. Although drying air is still applied only to the surfaces of the tablet bed, the other advantages derived from the basic over-all design ensure that the Pellegrini pan is more suitable for film coating, including aqueous-based coating solutions, than the conventional equipment previously discussed. Currently, Pellegrini pans are available with capacities ranging from the 10 kg laboratory

scale-up to 1000 kg for high output production. A variant of the Pellegrini pan is the Hush Coater which has extra insulation to reduce the noise level in the pan.

Considering the relative inefficiencies with equipment in which the majority of drying takes place on the surface of the tablet bed, several attempts have been made to improve air exchange, particularly within the tablet bed. The first to be available on a commercial scale was that developed by Strunck, which, by extending the drying air duct so that it is immersed in the tablet bed, creates a submersed void onto the periphery of which coating solution is applied from a spray gun located in the opening of the supply air duct (Fig 91-4). Exhaust air is taken from the pan in a somewhat conventional manner.

A second approach, called the Immersion Sword Process, utilizes a two chamber system situated in the bed of tablets, enabling heated air to be introduced directly into the tablet bed through perforated air chambers. After interacting with the cascading bed of tablets, the air is drawn into a perforated

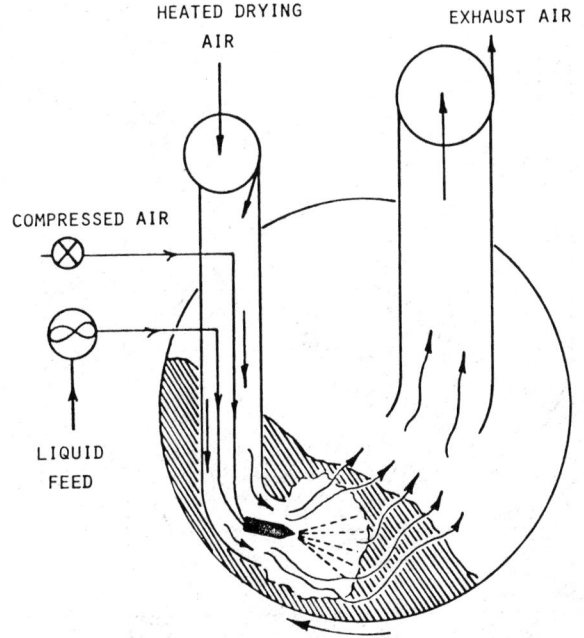

Fig 91-4.   Schematic diagram of Strunck immersed tube coating apparatus.

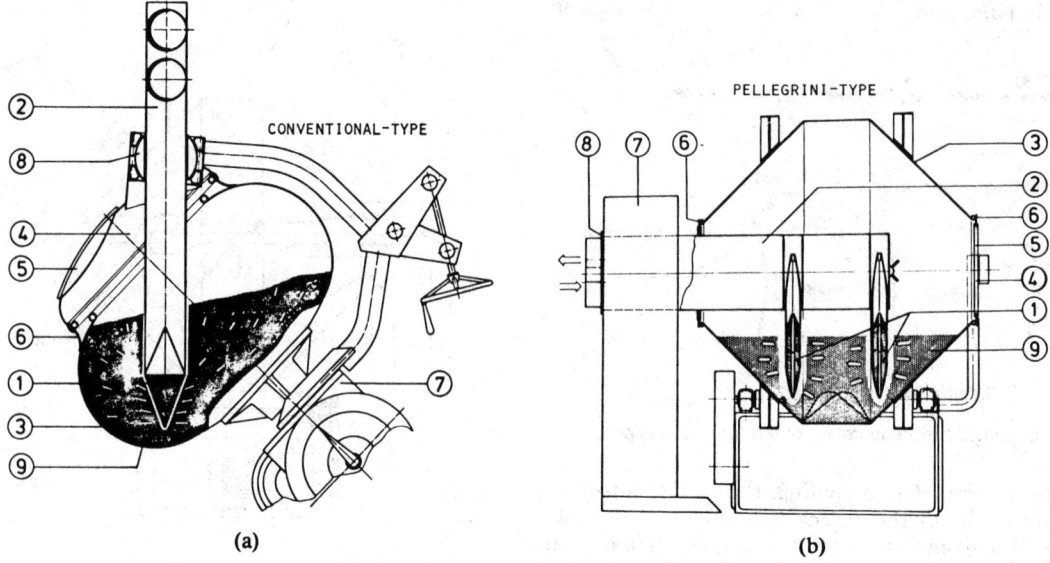

Key: 1. Immersion Sword
2. Coaxial conduit
3. Coating pan
4. Pan cover
5. Clear control cover
6. Silicone seal
7. Stand
8. Coaxial conduit adjustment
9. Coating bed

Fig 91-5.   Schematic diagram of the immersed sword apparatus for use in either (a) a conventional pan or (b) a Pellegrini pan.

exhaust air chamber for venting to the outside. This equipment is currently adaptable to both conventional and Pellegrini type pans (see Fig 91-5). Recently, the manufacturers of the Pellegrini pan have introduced a modification to the inlet air supply which permits drying air to be introduced underneath the tablet bed as well as being applied across the surface. A Pellegrini pan so modified is known as a Fast Dry Coater.

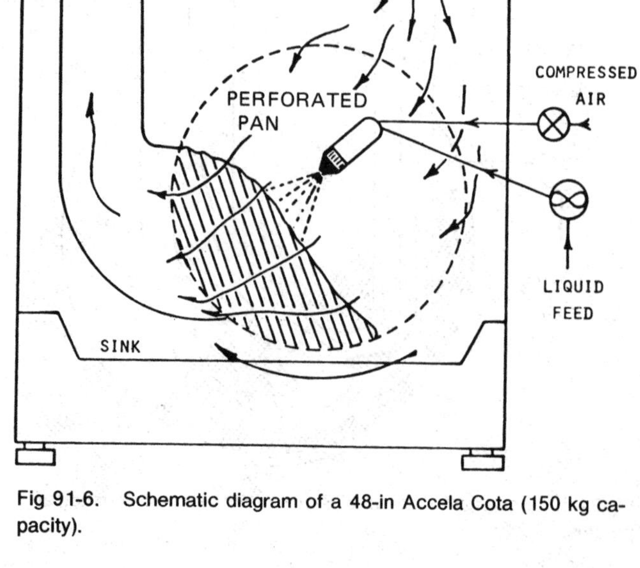

A major contribution to film coating processing technology was made by the introduction of the Accela-Cota, an invention of the Eli Lilly Company. This is also an angular pan rotating on a horizontal axis. The major difference from the Pellegrini pan is that the flat portion of the pan periphery is completely perforated, enabling air of the required volume and temperature to be introduced into the cabinet surrounding the pan from above, and exhausted from a plenum in contact with the pan and positioned directly below the cascading bed of tablets (Fig 91-6). The presence of baffles in the pan augments the high efficiency in air exchange to ensure that processing times can be kept to a minimum. Capacities for this equipment range from the 10–15 kg laboratory scale-up to approximately 700 kg for the 66-in model. On the production scale, unloading is facilitated by the use of the Accela-scoop.

A variation on the concept of side vented pans is afforded by the Hi-Coater. In contrast to the Accela-Cota, the entire perforated area is replaced by four perforated panels linked to air ducts which make contact, at regular intervals during each pan revolution, with an exhaust plenum. Although not immediately obvious, this does permit continuous venting of air from the pan since at least one complete panel, or parts of two of the same, are always in contact with the plenum. Another contrast is evident from the fact that heated air is introduced directly into the front opening of the pan rather than into the cabinet surrounding it (Fig 91-7). Capacities for the Hi-Coater range from a 300 g (mini) to the 700 kg model HCF-200, with unloading in the production equipment being accomplished by means of a port in the pan periphery enabling discharge to be made directly into a bin placed beneath the machine.

Another alternative to pan equipment having rapid drying capabilities is the Driacoater (Fig 91-8), although this utilizes a totally different and somewhat novel approach. Unlike the two previous pieces of equipment, heated air is introduced into

Fig 91-6.   Schematic diagram of a 48-in Accela Cota (150 kg capacity).

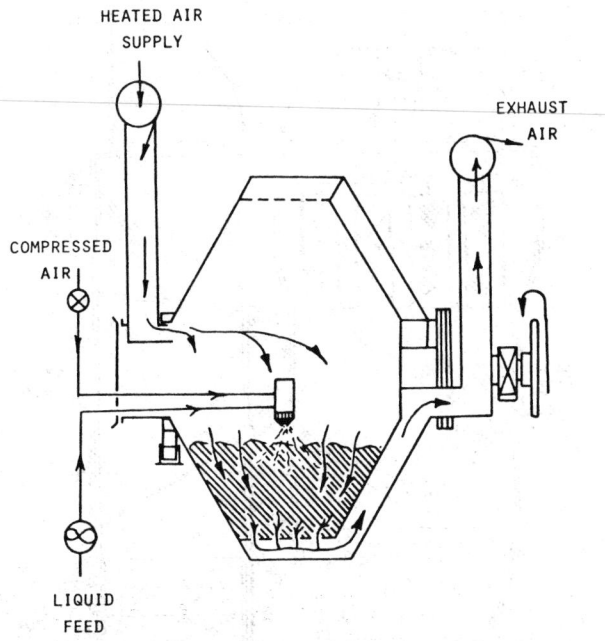

Fig 91-7.   Schematic diagram of the Hi-coater.

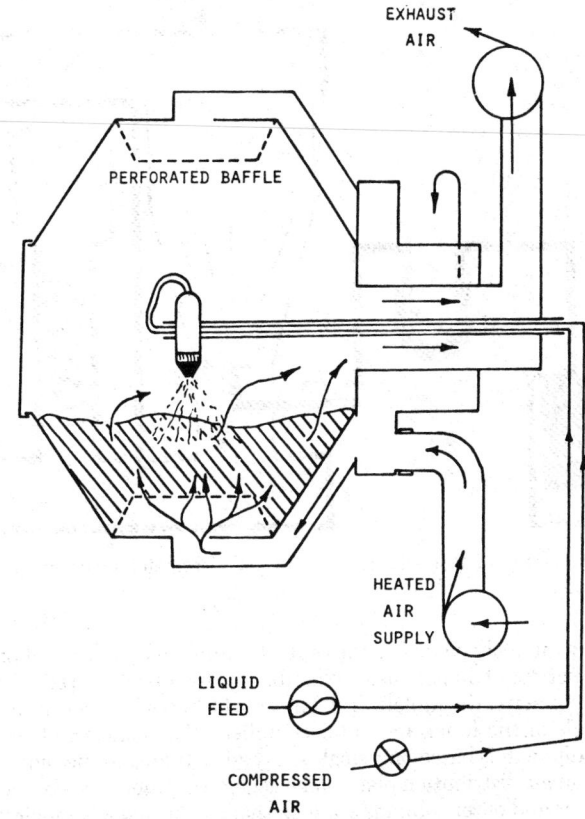

Fig 91-8.   Schematic diagram of the Driacoater.

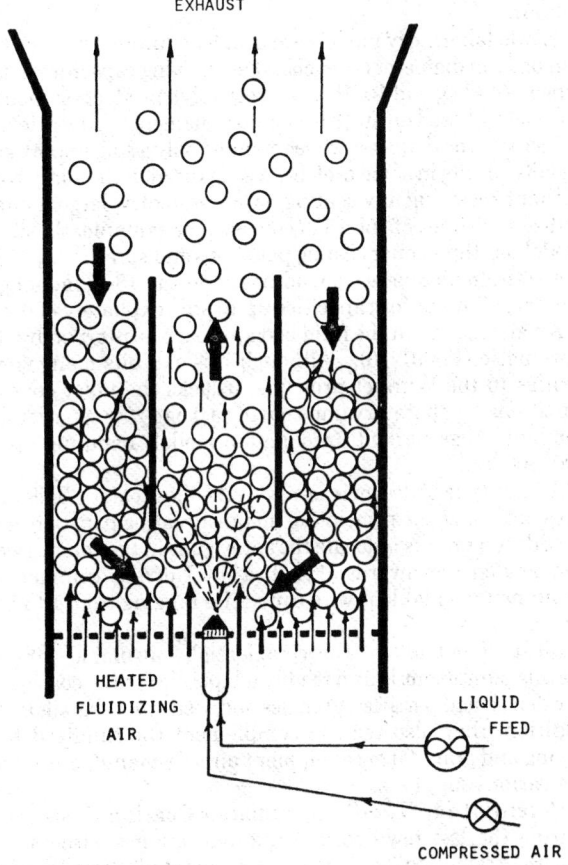

Fig 91-9.   Schematic diagram of the Wurster fluidized bed coater. Perforations in air distribution plate are designed to control direction of particle movement.

the back of the cascading bed of tablets by means of ducts, fixed to the outside of the pan, linked to perforated "baffles" fitted to the inside of the pan. This has the effect of partially lifting the tablets and acts as an aid to mixing. Air is then exhausted from the rear of the pan in a similar manner to that in the Pellegrini. Thus, drying is counter current to the spraying of coating solution. One claim for this equipment, which seems to have been substantiated, is that it tends to be less stressful on the tablets, causing less abrasion. The laboratory model of this equipment holds approximately 5 kg and production models, which are unloaded on reversing the pan via a chute attached to the front of the pan, can handle up to 1000 kg. The list of side-vented pans available was completed recently by the introduction of the Glatt-Coater, having capacities ranging from 25 to 1000 kg.

Because of a growing requirement for coating drug dosage materials smaller in size than conventional tablets (eg, granules and nonpareils), many of the manufacturers of perforated pans offer suitable equipment modifications for this purpose. Although the evolution that has taken place in coating pan design was done expressly to facilitate film coating, particularly when water is the solvent, the advances in processing technology that are derived are readily adaptable to the sugar coating process. Obviously the requirements for in-process drying need not be as rigorous as those for film coating.

Fluidized Bed Coating Equipment—Many exponents of this type of equipment will argue, often justifiably so, that it represents the ultimate in drying efficiency since the tablets are supported on a column of moving air allowing for a high area of contact between the drying medium and the species from which solvent must be removed rapidly. The nature of the fluid-bed process, however, essentially restricts its use to film coating. Tablets film coated by the fluidized bed method are often associated with a higher level of gloss, mainly because the coating solution impinges upon them before much solvent loss has occurred. One possible cause for criticism relates to the potential for more tablet damage to occur owing to the rigorous treatment received. High tablet hardness is not necessarily the major prerequisite here, but low tablet friability.

The earliest fluidized bed coating equipment was based on the Wurster design, (Fig 91-9). A moving bed of tablets

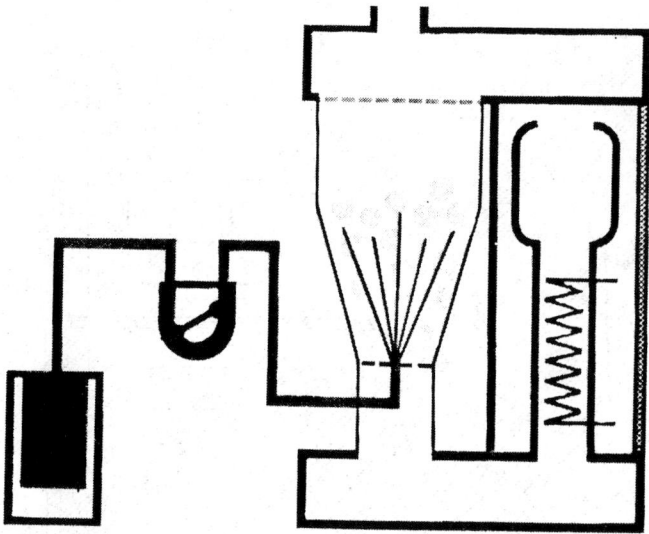

Fig 91-10.   Schematic diagram of an Aeromatic fluidized bed coater.

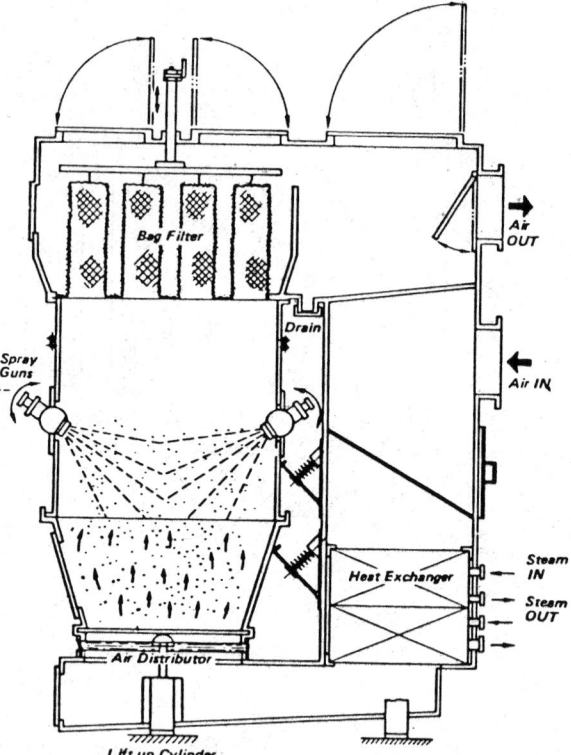

Fig 91-11.   Schematic diagram of the Flo-coater.

continuously passes up the central column and, as a result of the effect of an expansion chamber at the top which reduces air velocity, the tablets drop back to the bottom between the walls of the inner and outer chamber. The concept of the equipment is based on a single spray gun situated in the center of an air distribution plate. The geometric proportions of the inner and outer columns are such that a continuously moving column of tablets passes through the spray path with every tablet capturing some of the coating and at the same time ensuring that little or no solution reaches the wall of the inner column.

While laboratory models are usually equipped with either 6 in or 12 in diameter outer chambers (having capacities in the range of 1–2 kg and 10–15 kg respectively), production models are usually based on an 18 in chamber diameter. Any attempt to increase the diameter while retaining only a single spray gun usually results in some tablets passing through the spray zone without receiving any coating. Consequently, large models utilize multiples of the 18 in concept; for example, the 32-in model has three inner coating partitions and spray guns, while the 46-in model has seven, all based on the 18-in model geometry, allowing for capacities up to approximately 400 kg.

An alternative in the fluid bed approach is afforded by the Aeromatic (Fig 91-10). Although this exhibits many similarities to the Wurster principle, it lacks the inner coating partitions. Laboratory units having a 0.5 to 2 kg capacity are available, together with production models handling up to 100–200 kg.

A third type of design is seen with the Flo-Coater. This also does not utilize the principle of an inner coating partition, and in addition prefers to locate the spray guns in the column wall and angled downwards (Fig 91-11). Current commercial equipment available is with capacities ranging from 1 to 500 kg.

Most, if not all, of the commercially available column coating equipment is also readily adaptable for the coating of powders, small particles, granules and seeds (non-pareils). In addition, they also tend to complement the fluidized bed drying and granulating equipment already manufactured by the various suppliers.

Potential for Totally Automated Coating Systems— During the last few decades, the industry has witnessed a general transition from manually operated sugar coating procedures, requiring total operator involvement, to film coating ones in which operator intervention is infrequent. Increasing familiarity with, and understanding of, tablet

coating as a unit process, and a desire to ensure compliance with GMP's, have increased ultimately the desire for assuring uniformity to design specifications every batch of product made. Obviously, this is difficult for any process where the idiosyncracies of individual operators must have a significant impact.

Total automation of the process can provide a solution to these problems. This involves developing a process where all the important variables and requisite constraints are predetermined. These can then be translated into a form such that ultimate control and monitoring of the various process parameters can be maintained either by a microprocessor or central computer system. However, the system will be only as good as those peripheral devices used to detect various process conditions such as air flow, temperature and humidity, application volumes, and delivery rates, etc.

Since a sugar coating process has always been highly operator dependent, removal of much of the operator intervention could be achieved by automation. Automation has however, been complex because of the various sequences that occur and variety of coating fluids used in a single process. That it has been accomplished is evidenced by the number of commercially available systems that have been introduced.[15] The technology for automated control of sugar coating processes is now being adapted for film coating.

Quality Control of Coated Tablets

The most important aspects of coated tablets which must be assessed from a quality control standpoint are appearance characteristics and drug availiability. From the appearance standpoint, coated tablets must be shown to conform, where applicable, to some color standard, otherwise the dispenser and the consumer may assume that differences have occurred from previous lots signifying a changed or substandard product. In addition, because of the physical abuse that tablets, both in their uncoated and coated forms, receive during the coating process, it is essential to check for defects such as chipped edges, *picking*, etc, and ensure they do not exceed predetermined limits.

Often, in order to identify the products, coated tablets may be imprinted (particularly with sugar-coated tablets) or bear a monogram (commonly seen with tablets that are film coated). The clarity and quality of such identifying features must be assessed. Failure of a batch of coated tablets to comply with such preset standards may result in 100% inspection being required, or the need for the batch to be reworked.

Batch to batch reproducibility for drug availability is of paramount importance, consequently each batch of product should be submitted to some meaningful test such as a dissolution test. Depending on the characteristics of the tablet core to be coated, tablet coatings can modify the drug release profile, even when not intended (unlike the case of enteric or controlled release products). Since this behavior may vary with each batch coated (being dependent, for example, on differences in processing conditions or variability in raw materials used), it is essential that this parameter should be assessed, particularly in products that are typically borderline (Refer to Chapter 90).

Stability Testing of Coated Products

The stability-testing program for coated products will vary depending on the dosage form and its composition. Many stability-testing programs are based on studies which have disclosed the conditions a product may encounter prior to end use. Such conditions are usually referred to as normal, and include ranges in temperature, humidity, light, and handling conditions.

Limits of acceptability are established for each product for qualities such as color, appearance, availability of drug for absorption, and drug content. The time over which the product retains specified properties when tested at normal conditions may be defined as the *shelf life*. The container for the product may be designed to improve the shelf life. For example, if the color in the coating is light-sensitive, the product may be packaged in an amber bottle and/or protected from light through use of a paper carton. When the coating is friable, resilient material such as cotton may be incorporated in both the top and bottom of the container, and if the product is adversely affected by moisture, a moisture-resistant closure may be used and/or a desiccant may be placed in the package. The shelf life of the product is determined in the commercial package tested under normal conditions.

The stability of the product may also be tested at conditions which are exaggerated from the normal. This is usually done for the purpose of accelerating changes so that an early extrapolation can be made concerning the shelf life of the product. Although useful, highly exaggerated conditions of storage can supply misleading data for coated dosage forms. Any change in drug release from the dosage form is measured *in vitro* but an *in vivo* measurement should be used to confirm that drug availability remains within specified limits over its stated shelf life. This confirmation can be obtained by testing the product initially for *in vivo* availability and then repeating at intervals during storage at normal conditions for its estimated shelf life (or longer).

Stability tests are usually conducted on a product at the time of development, during the pilot phase, and on representative lots of the commercial product. Stability testing must continue for the commercial product as long as it remains on the market because subtle changes in a manufacturing process and/or a raw material can have an impact on the shelf life of a product.

References

1. Urdang G: *What's New*, 1943, pp 5–14; through *J Amer Pharm Assoc 34:* 135, 1945.
2. White RC: *J Amer Pharm Assoc, 11:* 345, 1922.
3. Kremers E, Urdang G: *History of Pharmacy*, Philadelphia, Lippincott, 1940, p 20, 319.
4. Anon: *J Amer Med Assoc, 84:* 829, 1920.
5. Wiegand TS: *Am J Pharm 74:* 33, 1902.
6. Warner WR Jr: *Am J Pharm 74:* 32, 1902.
7. Wurster DE: (Wisconsin Alumni Research Foundations) US Patent 2,648,609 (1953).
8. Signorino CA: US Patents 3,738,952 and 3,741,795 (June, 1973).
9. Tucker SJ *et al:* *J Amer Pharm Assoc 47:* 849–850, 1958.
10. Schwartz JB, Alvino TP: *J Pharm Sci 65:* 572, 1976.
11. Prillig EB: *J Pharm Sci, 50:* 1245–1249, 1969.
12. Porter SC: *Pharm Tech, 4,* 67–75, 1980.
13. Delporte JP, Jaminet F: *J Pharm Belg 31:* 38, 1976.
14. Rowe RC: *J Pharm Pharmacol 33:* 423–426, 1981.
15. Fraade DJ, ed: *Automation of Pharmaceutical Operations*, Pharm Tech Publ, Springfield, OR, 1983.

CHAPTER 92

Sustained-Release Drug Delivery Systems

Mark A Longer

Research Assistant
School of Pharmacy
University of Wisconsin
Madison, WI 53706

Joseph R Robinson, PhD

Professor of Pharmacy
School of Pharmacy
University of Wisconsin
Madison, WI 53706

The goal of any drug delivery system is to provide a therapeutic amount of drug to the proper site in the body to promptly achieve and then maintain the desired drug concentration. This idealized objective points to the two aspects most important to drug delivery, namely, *spatial placement* and *temporal delivery* of a drug. Spatial placement relates to targeting of a drug to a specific organ or tissue, while temporal delivery refers to controlling the rate of drug delivery to the target tissue. An appropriately designed sustained-release drug delivery system can be a major advance toward solving these two problems. It is for this reason that the science and technology responsible for development of sustained-release pharmaceuticals have been and continue to be the focus of a great deal of attention in both industrial and academic laboratories. There currently exist numerous products on the market formulated for both oral and parenteral routes of administration that claim sustained or controlled drug delivery. The bulk of research has been directed at oral dosage forms that satisfy the temporal aspect of drug delivery, but many of the newer approaches under investigation may allow for spatial placement as well. This chapter will define and explain the nature of sustained-release drug therapy, briefly outline relevant physicochemical and biological properties of a drug that affect sustained release performance, and review the more common types of oral and parenteral sustained-release dosage forms. In addition, a brief discussion of some methods currently being used to develop targeted delivery systems will be presented.

Conventional Drug Therapy

To gain an appreciation for the value of sustained drug therapy it is useful to review some fundamental aspects of conventional drug delivery.[1] Consider single dosing of a hypothetical drug that follows a simple one-compartment pharmacokinetic model for disposition. Depending on the route of administration, a conventional dosage form of the drug, eg, a solution, suspension, capsule, tablet, etc, will probably produce a drug blood level versus time profile similar to that shown in Fig 92-1. The term "drug blood level" refers to the concentration of drug in blood or plasma, but the concentration in any tissue could also be plotted on the ordinate. It can be seen from this figure that administration of drug by either intravenous injection or an extravascular route, eg, orally, intramuscularly, rectally, etc, does not maintain drug blood levels within the therapeutic range for extended periods of time. The short duration of action is due to the inability of conventional dosage forms to control temporal delivery. If an attempt is made to maintain drug blood levels in the therapeutic range for longer periods by, for example, increasing the dose of an intravenous injection, as shown by the dotted line in the figure, toxic levels may be produced at early times. This is obviously undesirable and the approach is therefore unsuitable. An alternate approach is to administer the drug repetitively using a constant dosing interval, as in multiple-dose therapy. This is shown in Fig 92-2 for the oral route. In this case the drug blood level reached and the time required to reach that level depend on the dose and the dosing interval. There are several potential problems inherent in multiple-dose therapy[1]:

1. If the dosing interval is not appropriate for the biological half-life of the drug, large "peaks" and "valleys" in the drug

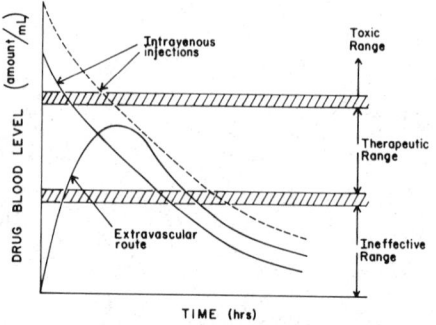

Fig 92-1. Typical drug blood level versus time profiles for intravenous injections and an extravascular route of administration.

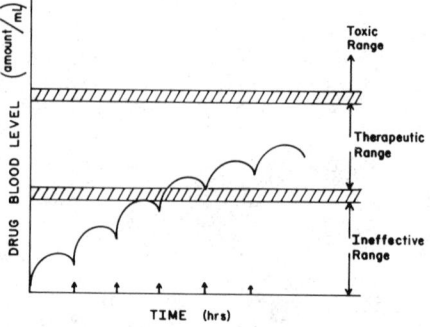

Fig 92-2. Typical drug blood level versus time profile following oral multiple-dose therapy.

blood level may result. For example, drugs with short half-lives require frequent dosings to maintain constant therapeutic levels.

2. The drug blood level may not be within the therapeutic range at sufficiently early times, an important consideration for certain disease states.

3. Patient noncompliance with the multiple-dosing regimen can result in failure of this approach.

In many instances, potential problems associated with conventional drug therapy can be overcome. When this is the case, drugs given in conventional dosage forms by multiple-dosing can produce the desired drug blood level for extended periods of time. Frequently, however, these problems are significant enough to make drug therapy with conventional dosage forms less desirable than sustained-release drug therapy. This fact, coupled with the intrinsic inability of conventional dosage forms to achieve spatial placement, is a compelling motive for investigation of sustained-release drug delivery systems. There are numerous potential advantages of sustained-release drug therapy that will be discussed in the next section.

Sustained-Release Drug Therapy

As already mentioned, conventional dosage forms include solutions, suspensions, capsules, tablets, emulsions, aerosols, foams, ointments, and suppositories. For purposes of this discussion, these dosage forms can be considered to release their active ingredients into an absorption pool immediately. This is illustrated in the following simple kinetic scheme:

$$\text{Dosage Form} \xrightarrow[\substack{\text{drug} \\ \text{release}}]{k_r} \text{Absorption Pool} \xrightarrow[\text{absorption}]{k_a} \text{Target Area} \xrightarrow[\text{elimination}]{k_e}$$

The absorption pool represents a solution the drug at the site of absorption, and the terms k_r, k_a, and k_e are first-order rate constants for drug release, absorption, and overall elimination, respectively. Immediate release from a conventional dosage form implies that $k_r \ggg k_a$ or, alternatively, that absorption of drug across a biological membrane, such as the intestinal epithelium, is the rate-limiting step in delivery of the drug to its target area. For nonimmediate release dosage forms, $k_r \lll k_a$, that is, release of drug from the dosage form is the rate limiting step. This causes the above kinetic scheme to reduce to the following:

$$\text{Dosage Form} \xrightarrow[\substack{\text{drug} \\ \text{release}}]{k_r} \text{Target Area} \xrightarrow[\text{elimination}]{k_e}$$

Essentially, the absorptive phase of the kinetic scheme becomes insignificant compared to the drug release phase. Thus, the effort to develop a nonimmediate release delivery system must be primarily directed at altering the release rate by affecting the value of k_r. The many ways in which this has been attempted will be discussed later in this chapter.

Nonimmediate release delivery systems may be conveniently divided into four categories:

1. Delayed release
2. Sustained release
   a. controlled release
   b. prolonged release
3. Site-specific release
4. Receptor release

Delayed-release systems are those that utilize repetitive, intermittent dosings of a drug from one or more immediate release units incorporated into a single dosage form. Examples of delayed-release systems include repeat action tablets and capsules, and enteric-coated tablets where timed release is achieved by a barrier coating. A delayed-release dosage form does not produce or maintain uniform drug blood levels within the therapeutic range, as shown in Fig 92-3, but nonetheless is more effective for patient compliance than conventional dosage forms.

Sustained-release systems include any drug delivery system that achieves slow release of drug over an extended period of time. If the system is successful at maintaining constant drug levels in the blood or target tissue, it is considered a

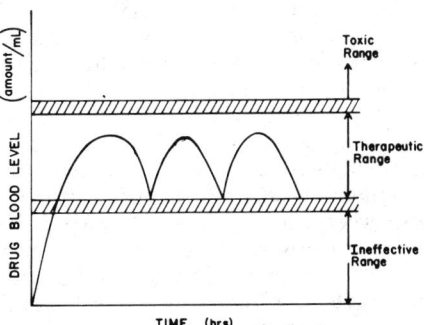

Fig 92-3. Typical drug blood level versus time profiles for delayed release drug delivery by a repeat-action dosage form.

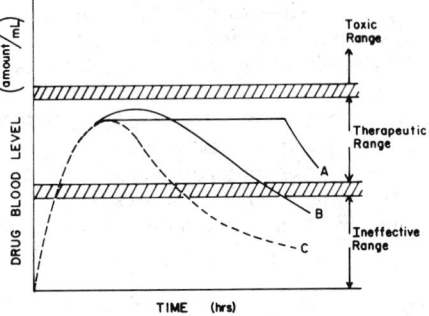

Fig 92-4. Drug blood level versus time profiles showing the relationship between controlled release (A), prolonged release (B), and conventional release (C) drug delivery.

controlled-release system. If it is unsuccessful at this but nevertheless extends the duration of action over that achieved by conventional delivery, it is considered a *prolonged-release* system. This is illustrated in Fig 92-4.

Site-specific and *receptor release* refer to targeting of a drug directly to a certain biological location. In the case of site-specific release, the target is a certain organ or tissue; for receptor release, the target is the particular receptor for a drug within an organ or tissue. Both of these systems satisfy the spatial aspect of drug delivery.

Release Rate and Dose Considerations

Although it is not necessary or desirable to maintain a constant level of drug in the blood or target tissue for all therapeutic cases, this is the ideal goal of a sustained-release delivery system. In fact, in some cases optimum therapy is achieved by oscillating, rather than constant, drug levels. An example of this would be antibiotic therapy, where the activity of the drug is required only during growth phases of the microorganism. A constant drug level will succeed at curing or controlling the condition however, and this is true for most forms of therapy.

The objective in designing a sustained-release system is to deliver drug at a rate necessary to achieve and maintain a constant drug blood level. This rate should be analogous to that achieved by continuous intravenous infusion where drug is provided to the patient at a constant rate just equal to its rate of elimination. This implies that the rate of delivery must be independent of the amount of drug remaining in the dosage form and constant over time. That is, release from the dosage form should follow *zero-order* kinetics, as shown by the following equation,[2]

$$k_r{}^0 = \text{Rate In} = \text{Rate Out} = k_e \cdot C_d \cdot V_d \qquad (1)$$

where $k_r{}^0$ is the zero-order rate constant for drug release (amount/time), k_e is the first-order rate constant for overall drug elimination (time^{-1}), C_d is the desired drug level in the body (amount/volume), and V_d is the volume space in which the drug is distributed. The values of k_e, C_d, and V_d needed to calculate $k_r{}^0$ are obtained from appropriately designed single dose pharmacokinetic studies. Eq 1 provides the method to calculate the zero order release rate constant necessary to maintain a constant drug blood or tissue level for the simplest case where drug is eliminated by first order kinetics. For many drugs, however, more complex elimination kinetics and other factors affecting their disposition are involved. This in turn affects the nature of the release kinetics necessary to maintain a constant drug blood level. It is important to recognize that while zero order release may be theoretically desirable, nonzero order release may be clinically equivalent to constant release in many cases. Aside from the extent of intra- and intersubject variation is the observation that for many drugs, modest changes in drug tissue levels do not result in an improvement in clinical performance. Thus, a non-constant drug level may be clinically indistinguishable from a constant drug level.

To achieve a therapeutic level promptly and sustain the level for a given period of time, the dosage form generally consists of two parts, an initial priming dose, D_i, that releases drug immediately and a maintenance or sustaining dose, D_m. The total dose, W, thus required for the system[2] is,

$$W = D_i + D_m \qquad (2)$$

For a system where the maintenance dose releases drug by a zero order process for a specified period of time, the total dose[2] is

$$W = D_i + k_r{}^0 T_d, \qquad (3)$$

where $k_r{}^0$ is the zero-order rate constant for drug release and T_d is the total time desired for sustained release from one dose. If the maintenance dose begins release of drug at the time of dosing ($t = 0$) it will add to that which is provided by the initial dose, thus increasing the initial drug level. In this case a correction factor is needed to account for the added drug from the maintenance dose[2];

$$W = D_i + k_r{}^0 T_d - k_r{}^0 T_p \qquad (4)$$

The correction factor $k_r{}^0 T_p$ is the amount of drug provided during the period from $t = 0$ to the time of the peak drug level, T_p. No correction factor is needed if the dosage form is constructed in such a fashion that the maintenance dose does not begin to release drug until time T_p.

It has already been mentioned that a perfectly invariant drug blood or tissue level versus time profile is the ideal goal of a sustained-release system. The way to achieve this, in the simplest case, is by use of a maintenance dose that releases its drug by zero order kinetics. However, satisfactory approximations of a constant drug level can be obtained by suitable combinations of the initial dose and a maintenance dose that

releases its drug by a first-order process. The total dose for such a system[2] is,

$$W = D_i + (k_e C_d / k_r) V_d \qquad (5)$$

where k_r is the first-order rate constant for drug release (time^{-1}), and k_e, C_d, and V_d are as previously defined. If the maintenance dose begins releasing drug at $t = 0$, a correction factor is required just as it was in the zero order case. The correct expression in this case[2] is,

$$W = D_i + (k_e C_d / k_r) V_d - D_m k_r T_p \qquad (6)$$

In order to maintain drug blood levels within the therapeutic range over the entire time course of therapy, most sustained-release drug delivery systems are, like conventional dosage forms, administered as multiple rather than single doses. For an ideal sustained-release system that releases drug by zero order kinetics, the multiple dosing regimen is analogous to that used for a constant intravenous infusion, as discussed in Chapter 38. For those sustained release systems utilizing release kinetics other than zero order, the multiple dosing regimen is more complex and its analysis is beyond the scope of this chapter. A more detailed discussion of multiple dosing of sustained-release systems may be found in Reference 3.

Potential Advantages of Sustained Drug Therapy

All sustained-release products share the common goal of improving drug therapy over that achieved with their non-sustained counterparts. This improvement in drug therapy is represented by several potential advantages of the use of sustained-release systems, as shown in Table I.

Patient compliance has been recognized as a necessary and important component in the success of all self-administered drug therapy. Minimizing or eliminating patient compliance problems is an obvious advantage of sustained-release therapy. Because of the nature of its release kinetics, a sustained release system should be able to utilize less total drug over the time course of therapy than a conventional preparation. The advantages of this are a decrease or elimination of both local and systemic side effects, less potentiation or reduction in drug activity with chronic use, and minimization of drug accumulation in body tissues with chronic dosing.

Unquestionably the most important reason for sustained drug therapy is improved efficiency in treatment, ie, optimized therapy. The result of obtaining constant drug blood levels from a sustained-release system is to promptly achieve and maintain the desired effect. Reduction or elimination of fluctuations in the drug blood level allows better disease state management. In addition, the method by which sustained release is achieved can improve the bioavailability of some drugs. For example, drugs susceptible to enzymatic inacti-

Table I—Potential Advantages of Sustained Drug Therapy

1. Avoid patient compliance problems
2. Employ less total drug
   minimize or eliminate local side effects
   minimize or eliminate systemic side effects
   obtain less potentiation or reduction in drug activity with chronic use
   minimize drug accumulation with chronic dosing
3. Improve efficiency in treatment
   cure or control condition more promptly
   improve control of condition, ie, reduce fluctuation in drug level
   improve bioavailability of some drugs
   make use of special effects, eg, sustained release aspirin for morning relief of arthritis by dosing before bedtime
4. Economy

vation or bacterial decomposition can be protected by encapsulation in polymer systems suitable for sustained release. For drugs that have a "specific window" for absorption, increased bioavailability can be attained by localizing the sustained-release delivery system in certain regions of the gastrointestinal tract. Improved efficiency in treatment can also take the form of a special therapeutic effect not possible with a conventional dosage form (see Table I).

The last potential advantage listed in Table I, that of economy, can be examined from two points of view. Although the initial unit cost of most sustained drug delivery systems is usually greater than that of conventional dosage forms because of the special nature of these products, the average cost of treatment over an extended time period may be less. Economy may also result from a decrease in nursing time/hospitalization, less lost work time, etc.

Properties of a Drug Relevant to Sustained-Release Formulation

The design of sustained-release delivery systems is subject to several variables of considerable importance. Among these are the route of drug delivery, the type of delivery system, the disease being treated, the patient, the length of therapy, and the properties of the drug. Each of these variables are interrelated and this imposes certain constraints upon choices for the route of delivery, the design of the delivery system, and the length of therapy. Of particular interest to the scientist designing the system are the constraints imposed by the properties of the drug. It is these properties that have the greatest effect on the behavior of the drug in the delivery system and in the body. For the purpose of discussion, it is convenient to describe the properties of a drug as being either physicochemical or biological. Obviously there is no clearcut distinction between these two categories since the biological properties of a drug are a function of its physicochemical properties. For purposes of this discussion, however, those attributes that can be determined from *in vitro* experiments will be considered as physicochemical properties. Included as biological properties will be those that result from typical pharmacokinetic studies on the absorption, distribution, metabolism, and excretion (ADME) characteristics of a drug, and those resulting from pharmacologic studies.

Physicochemical Properties

Aqueous Solubility and pK_a

It is well known that in order for a drug to be absorbed it must first dissolve in the aqueous phase surrounding the site of administration and then partition into the absorbing membrane. Two of the most important physicochemical properties of a drug that influence its absorptive behavior are its aqueous solubility and, if it is a weak acid or base (as are most drugs), its pK_a. These properties play an influential role in performance of nonsustained release products; their role is even greater in sustained-release systems.

The aqueous solubility of a drug influences its dissolution rate, which in turn establishes its concentration in solution and hence the driving force for diffusion across membranes. Dissolution rate is related to aqueous solubility as shown by the Noyes-Whitney equation which, under sink conditions, is,

$$dC/dt = k_D A C_s \qquad (7)$$

where dC/dt is the dissolution rate, k_D is the dissolution rate constant, A is the total surface area of the drug particles, and C_s is the aqueous saturation solubility of the drug. The dissolution rate is constant only if surface area, A, remains constant, but the important point to note is that the initial rate is directly proportional to aqueous solubility C_s. Therefore, the aqueous solubility of a drug can be used as a first approximation of its dissolution rate. Low solubility limits the dissolution rate and hence the absorption of many drugs.

It will be recalled from Chapter 16 that the aqueous solubility of weak acids and bases is governed by the pK_a of the compound and the pH of the medium. For a weak acid,

$$S_t = S_0(1 + K_a/[H^+]) = S_0(1 + 10^{pH-pK_a}) \qquad (8)$$

where S_t is the total solubility (both the ionized and unionized forms) of the weak acid, S_0 is the solubility of the unionized form, K_a is the acid dissociation constant, and $[H^+]$ is the hydrogen ion concentration of the medium. Eq 8 predicts that the total solubility, S_t, of a weak acid with a given pK_a can be affected by the pH of the medium. Similarly, for a weak base,

$$S_t = S_0(1 + [H^+]/K_a) = S_0(1 + 10^{pK_a-pH}) \qquad (9)$$

where S_t is the total solubility (both the conjugate acid and free base forms) of the weak base, S_0 is the solubility of the free base form, and K_a is the acid dissociation constant of the conjugate acid. Analogous to Eq 8, Eq 9 predicts that the total solubility, S_t, of a weak base whose conjugate acid has a given pK_a can be affected by the pH of the medium. Considering the pH-partition hypothesis, the importance of Eqs 8 and 9 relative to drug absorption is evident. The pH-partition hypothesis simply states that the unionized form of a drug will be preferentially absorbed, in a passive manner, through membranes. Since weakly acidic drugs will exist in the stomach (pH = 1–2) primarily in the unionized form, their absorption will be favored from this acidic environment. On the other hand, weakly basic drugs will exist primarily in the ionized form (conjugate acid) at the same site, and their absorption will be poor. In the upper portion of the small intestine, the pH is more alkaline (pH = 5–7) and the reverse will be expected for weak acids and bases. The ratio of Eq 8 or 9 written for either the pH of the gastric or intestinal fluid and the pH of blood is indicative of the driving force for absorption based on pH gradient. For example, consider the ratio of the total solubility of the weak acid aspirin in the blood and gastric fluid,

$$R = (1 + 10^{pH_b-pK_a})/(1 + 10^{pH_g-pK_a}) \qquad (10)$$

where pH_b is the pH of blood (pH 7.2) pH_g is the pH of the gastric fluid (pH 2) and the pK_a of aspirin is about 3.4. Substituting these values into Eq 10 gives a value for R of $10^{3.8}$ which indicates that aspirin is in a form to be well absorbed from the stomach. The same calculation for intestinal pH (= 7) yields a ratio close to 1, implying a less favorable driving force for absorption at that location. Ideally, release of an ionizable drug from a sustained-release system should be "programmed" in accordance with variation in pH of the different segments of the gastrointestinal (GI) tract so that the amount of preferentially absorbed species, and thus the plasma level of drug, will be approximately constant throughout the time course of drug action.

In general, extremes in the aqueous solubility of a drug are undesirable for formulation into a sustained-release product. A drug with very low solubility and a slow dissolution rate will exhibit dissolution-limited absorption and yield an inherently sustained blood level. In most instances, formulation of such a drug into a sustained-release system is redundant. Even if a poorly soluble drug was considered as a candidate for formulation into a sustained-release system, a restraint would be placed upon the type of delivery system which could be used. For example, any system relying upon diffusion of drug through a polymer as the rate-limiting step in release would be unsuitable for a poorly soluble drug, since the driving force for diffusion is the concentration of drug in the polymer or solution and this concentration would be low. For a drug with very high solubility and a rapid dissolution rate, it is often quite difficult to decrease its dissolution rate and slow its absorption. Preparing a slightly soluble form of a drug with normally high solubility is, however, one possible method for preparing sustained release dosage forms. This will be elaborated upon elsewhere in this chapter.

Partition Coefficient

Between the time that a drug is administered and the time it is eliminated from the body it must diffuse through a variety of biological membranes which act primarily as lipid-like barriers. A major criterion in evaluation of the ability of a drug to penetrate these lipid membranes is its apparent oil/water partition coefficient, defined as

$$K = C_0/C_w \qquad (11)$$

where C_0 is the total concentration of all forms of the drug, eg, ionized and unionized, in some organic phase at equilibrium, and C_w is the total concentration of all forms in an aqueous phase at equilibrium. A frequently used solvent for the organic phase is 1-octanol. Although not always valid, an approximation to the value of K may be obtained by the ratio of the solubility of the drug in 1-octanol to that in water. In general, drugs with extremely large values of K are very oil soluble and will partition into membranes quite readily. The relationship between tissue permeation and partition coefficient for the drug is generally known as the *Hansch correlation*, discussed in Chapter 27. In general, it describes a parabolic relationship between the logarithm of the activity of a drug or its ability to be absorbed and the logarithm of its partition coefficient for a series of drugs as shown in Fig. 92-5. The explanation for this relationship lies in the fact that the activity of a drug is a function of its ability to cross membranes and interact with the receptor; as a first approximation, the more effectively a drug crosses membranes, the greater its activity. There is also an optimum partition coefficient for a drug at which it most effectively permeates membranes and thus shows greatest activity. Values of the partition coefficient below this optimum result in decreased lipid solubility and the drug will remain localized in the first aqueous phase it contacts. Values larger than the optimum result in poorer aqueous solubility but enhanced lipid solubility and the drug will not partition out of the lipid membrane once it gets in, and/or it reaches maximum solubility in the lipid portion of the membrane. The value of K at which optimum activity is observed is approximately 1000/1 in 1-octanol/water. Drugs with a partition coefficient that is either extremely higher or lower than the optimum are, in general, poorer candidates for formulation into sustained-release dosage forms.

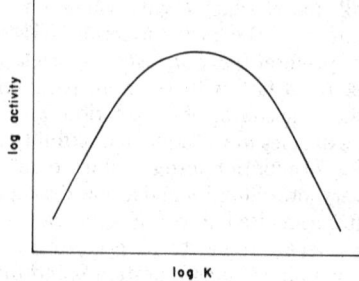

Fig 92-5. Typical relationship between drug activity and partition coefficient, K, generally known as the Hansch correlation.

Drug Stability

Of importance for oral dosage forms is the loss of drug through acid hydrolysis and/or metabolism in the GI tract. Since a drug in the solid state undergoes degradation at a much slower rate than a drug in suspension or solution, it would seem possible to significantly improve the relative bioavailability of a drug, which is unstable in the GI tract, by placing it in a slowly available sustained-release form. For those drugs that are unstable in the stomach, the most appropriate sustaining unit would be one that releases its contents only in the intestine. The reverse is the case for those drugs that are unstable in the environment of the intestine; the most appropriate sustaining unit in this case would be one that releases its contents only in the stomach. However, most sustained-release systems currently in use release their contents over the entire length of the GI tract. Thus, drugs with significant stability problems in any particular area of the GI tract are less suitable for formulation into sustained-release systems that deliver their contents uniformly over the length of the GI tract. Delivery systems that remain localized in a certain area of the GI tract and act as reservoirs for drug release are much more advantageous for drugs that not only suffer from stability problems but have other bioavailability problems as well. Development of this latter type of system is still in its infancy.

The presence of metabolizing enzymes at the site of absorption is not necessarily a negative factor in sustained-release formulation. Indeed, the prodrug approach to drug delivery takes advantage of the presence of these enzymes to regenerate the parent molecule of an inactive drug derivative. This will be amplified upon below.

Protein Binding

Chapters 14 and 39 described the occurrence of drug binding to plasma proteins (eg, albumin) and the resulting retention of drug in the vascular space. Distribution of the drug into the extravascular space is governed by the equilibrium process of dissociation of the drug from the protein. The drug–protein complex can therefore serve as a reservoir in the vascular space for sustained drug release to extravascular tissues, but only for those drugs that exhibit a high degree of binding. Thus, the protein binding characteristics of a drug can play a significant role in its therapeutic effect, regardless of the type of dosage form. Extensive binding to plasma proteins will be evidenced by a long half-life of elimination for the drug, and such drugs generally do not require a sustained-release dosage form. However, drugs that exhibit a high degree of binding to plasma proteins might also bind to biopolymers in the GI tract, which could have an influence on sustained drug delivery.

The main forces of attraction responsible for binding are van der Waals forces, hydrogen bonding, and electrostatic forces. In general, charged compounds have a greater tendency to bind a protein than uncharged compounds, due to electrostatic effects. The presence of a hydrophobic moiety on the drug molecule also increases its binding potential. Some drugs that exhibit greater than 95% binding at therapeutic levels are amitriptyline, bishydroxycoumarin, diazepam, diazoxide, dicumarol, and novobiocin.

Molecular Size and Diffusivity

As previously discussed, a drug must diffuse through a variety of biological membranes during its time course in the body. In addition to diffusion through these biological membranes, drugs in many sustained-release systems must diffuse through a polymeric membrane or matrix that is used to control their release kinetics. The ability of a drug to diffuse through polymeric membranes is a function of its diffusivity (diffusion coefficient). An important influence upon the value of the diffusivity, D, in polymers is the molecular size (or molecular weight) of the diffusing species. In most polymers, it is possible to relate $\log D$ empirically to some function of molecular size, as shown in Eq. 12[4]:

$$\log D = -s_v \log v + k_v = -s_M \log M + k_m \qquad (12)$$

where v is molecular volume, M is molecular weight, and s_v, s_M, k_v, and k_M are constants. This equation is explicable largely on the basis of the free volume theory of diffusion, which considers diffusion of a molecule in a polymer to occur as a series of jumps into preexisting cavities or voids in the polymer. The value of D is thus related to the size and shape of the cavities as well as size and shape of drugs. Generally, values of the diffusion coefficient for intermediate molecular weight drugs, ie, 100–400, through flexible polymers range from 10^{-6} to 10^{-9} cm^2/sec, with values on the order of 10^{-8} being most common.[5] A value of approximately 10^{-6} is typical for these drugs through water as the medium. It is of interest to note that the value of D for one gas in another is on the order of 10^{-1} cm^2/sec, and for one liquid through another, 10^{-5} cm^2/sec. For drugs with a molecular weight greater than 500, the diffusion coefficients in many polymers are frequently so small that they are difficult to quantify, ie, less than 10^{-12} cm^2/sec. Thus, high molecular weight drugs and/or polymeric drugs should be expected to display very slow release kinetics in sustained-release devices utilizing diffusion through polymeric membranes or matrices as the releasing mechanism.

Biological Properties

Absorption

The rate, extent, and uniformity of absorption of a drug are important factors when considering its formulation into a sustained-release system. Since the rate-limiting step in drug delivery from a sustained-release system is release from the dosage form rather than absorption, a rapid rate of absorption of the drug relative to its release is essential if the system is to be successful. As stated previously in discussing terminology, $k_r \lll k_a$. This becomes most critical in the case of oral administration. Assuming that the transit time of a drug through the absorptive area of the GI tract is between 9 and 12 hours, the maximum absorption half life should be 3 to 4 hours.[6] This corresponds to a minimum absorption rate constant k_a of 0.17 hr^{-1} to 0.23 hr^{-1} necessary for about 80 to 95% absorption over a 9 to 12 hour transit time. For a drug with a very rapid rate of absorption (ie, $k_a \gg 0.23$ hr^{-1}) the above discussion implies that a first order release rate constant k_r less than 0.17 hr^{-1} is likely to result in unacceptably poor bioavailability in many patients. Therefore, slowly absorbed drugs will be difficult to formulate into sustained-release systems where the criterion that $k_r \lll k_a$ must be met.

The extent and uniformity of the absorption of a drug, as reflected by its bioavailability and the fraction of the total dose absorbed, may be quite low for a variety of reasons. This is usually not a prohibitive factor in its formulation into a sustained-release system. Some possible reasons for low extent of absorption are poor water solubility, small partition coefficient, acid hydrolysis, and metabolism, or site-specific absorption. The latter reason is also responsible for nonuniformity of absorption. Many of these problems can be overcome by an appropriately designed sustained-release system, as exemplified by the discussion under the potential advantages of sustained drug therapy.

Distribution

For the design of sustained-release systems it is desirable to have as much information as possible regarding drug dis-

position, but in actual practice decisions are usually based on only a few pharmacokinetic parameters, one of which is the volume of distribution as given in Eq. 1. The distribution of a drug into vascular and extravascular spaces in the body is an important factor in its overall elimination kinetics. This in turn influences the formulation of that drug into a sustained-release system, primarily by restricting the magnitude of the release rate and the dose size which can be employed.[5] At present, calculation of these quantities is based primarily on one compartment pharmacokinetic models as described under terminology. A description of the estimation of these quantities based on multicompartment models is beyond the scope of this chapter. However, the main considerations that need to be dealt with if a two compartment model is operative will be presented.

Two parameters that are used to describe the distribution characteristics of a drug are its apparent volume of distribution and the ratio of drug concentration in tissue to that in plasma at the steady state; the so-called T/P ratio. The apparent volume of distribution is merely a proportionality constant which relates drug concentration in the blood or plasma to the total amount of drug in the body. The magnitude of the apparent volume of distribution can be used as a guide for additional studies and as a predictor for a drug dosing regimen and hence the need to employ sustained-release system.[5] For drugs that obey a one-compartment model, the apparent volume of distribution is

$$V = \text{dose}/C_0 \qquad (13)$$

where C_0 is the initial drug concentration immediately after an intravenous bolus injection but before any drug has been eliminated. Application of this equation is based upon the assumption that the distribution of a drug between plasma and tissues takes place instantaneously. This is rarely a good assumption, and it is usually necessary to invoke multicompartment models to account for the finite time required for the drug to distribute fully throughout the available body space. In the case of a two compartment model, it has been shown[7] that the best estimate of total volume of drug distribution is given by the apparent volume of distribution at steady state,

$$V_{ss} = (1 + k_{12}/k_{21})V_1 \qquad (14)$$

where V_1 is the volume of the central compartment, k_{12} is the rate constant for distribution of drug from the central to the peripheral compartment, and k_{21} is that from the peripheral to the central compartment. As its name implies, V_{ss} relates drug concentration in the blood or plasma at the steady state to the total amount of drug in the body during repetitive dosing or constant rate infusion. The use of Eq. 14 is limited to those instances where a steady state drug concentration in both compartments has been reached; at any other time, it tends to overestimate or underestimate the total amount of drug in the body.

To avoid the ambiguity inherent in the apparent volume of distribution as an estimator of the amount of drug in the body, the T/P ratio can also be used. If the amount of drug in the central compartment (P) is known, the amount of drug in the peripheral compartment (T) and hence the total amount of drug in the body can be calculated[5]:

$$T/P = k_{12}/(k_{21} - \beta) \qquad (15)$$

Here, β is the slow disposition rate constant and k_{12} and k_{21} are as previously defined. The important point to note is that the T/P ratio estimates the relative distribution of drug between compartments, whereas V_{ss} estimates the extent of distribution in the body. Both parameters contribute to an estimation of the distribution characteristics of a drug, but their relative importance in this respect is open to debate.

Metabolism

The metabolic conversion of a drug to another chemical form can usually be considered in the design of a sustained-release system for that drug. As long as the location, rate, and extent of metabolism are known and the rate constant(s) for the process(es) are not too large, successful sustained-release products can be developed.[5] There are two factors associated with the metabolism of some drugs, however, that present problems for their use in sustained-release systems. One is the ability of the drug to induce or inhibit enzyme synthesis; this may result in a fluctuating drug blood level with chronic dosing. The other is a fluctuating drug blood level due to intestinal (or other tissue) metabolism or through a hepatic first-pass effect. Examples of drugs that are subject to intestinal metabolism upon oral dosing are hydralazine, salicylamide, nitroglycerin, isoproterenol, chlorpromazine, and levodopa. Examples of drugs that undergo extensive first-pass hepatic metabolism are propoxyphene, nortriptyline, phenacetin, propranolol, and lidocaine.

Elimination and Biological Half-Life

The rate of elimination of a drug is quantitatively described by its biological half-life, $t_{1/2}$. The half-life of a drug is related to its apparent volume of distribution V and its systemic clearance:

$$t_{1/2} = 0.693 \, V/Cl_s = 0.693 \, V \, \text{AUC/dose} \quad (16)$$

The systemic clearance, Cl_s, is equal to the ratio of an intravenously administered dose to the total area under the drug blood level versus time curve, AUC. A drug with a short half-life requires frequent dosing and this makes it a desirable candidate for a sustained-release formulation. On the other hand, a drug with a long half-life is dosed at greater time intervals and thus there is less need for a sustained-release system. It is difficult to define precise upper and lower limits for the value of the half-life of a drug that best suits it for sustained-release formulation. In general, however, a drug with a half-life of less than 2 hours should probably not be used, since such systems will require unacceptably large release rates and large doses. At the other extreme, a drug with a half-life of greater than 8 hours should also probably not be used; in most instances, formulation of such a drug into a sustained-release system is unnecessary. Some examples of drugs with half-lives of less than 2 hours are ampicillin, cephalexin, cloxacillin, furosemide, levodopa, penicillin G, and propylthiouracil. Examples of those with half-lives of greater than 8 hours are dicumarol, diazepam, digitoxin, digoxin, guanethidine, phenytoin, and warfarin.[5]

Side Effects and Safety Considerations

There are very few drugs whose specific therapeutic concentrations are known. Instead, a therapeutic concentration *range* is listed, with increasing toxic effects expected above this range and a fall off in desired therapeutic response observed below the range. For some drugs, the incidence of side effects, in addition to toxicity, is believed to be related to their plasma concentration.[8] As mentioned in the discussion on the potential advantages of sustained drug therapy, a sustained-release system can, at times, minimize side effects for a particular drug by controlling its plasma concentration and utilizing less total drug over the time course of therapy.

The most widely used measure of the margin of safety of a drug is its therapeutic index, TI, discussed in Chapter 37 and defined in the following equation,

$$\text{TI} = \text{TD50/ED50} \quad (17)$$

where TD50 is the median toxic dose and ED50 is the median effective dose. The value of TI varies from as little as one, where the effective dose is also producing toxic symptoms, to several thousand. For very "potent" drugs whose therapeutic concentration range is narrow, the value of TI is small. In general, the larger the value of TI, the safer the drug. Drugs with very small values of TI are usually poor candidates for formulation into sustained-release products primarily because of technological limitations of precise control over release rates. Examples of drugs with values of TI < 10 are aprobarbital, digitoxin, phenobarbital, and digoxin.[5]

Dose Size

Since a sustained-release system is designed to alleviate repetitive dosing, it will naturally contain a greater amount of drug than a corresponding conventional form. The typical administered dose of a drug in the conventional dosage form will give some indication of the total amount needed in the sustained-release preparation. For those drugs requiring large conventional doses, the volume of the sustained dose may be so large as to be impractical or unacceptable, depending on the route of administration. The same may be true of drugs which require a large release rate from the sustained-release system, eg, drugs with short half-lives. For the oral route the volume of the product is limited by patient acceptance. For the intramuscular, intravenous, and subcutaneous routes, the limitation is tolerance of the drug at the injection site. It should also be mentioned that for drugs with a low therapeutic index, incorporation of amounts greater than the TD50 may be potentially dangerous if the system fails.

Oral Dosage Forms

For sustained-release systems, the oral route of administration has by far received the most attention. This is, in part, because there is more flexibility in dosage form design for the oral route than there is for the parenteral route. Patient acceptance of the oral route is quite high. It is a relatively safe route of administration compared to most parenteral routes, and the constraints of sterility and potential damage at the site of administration are minimal. In this section, the more common methods that are used to achieve sustained release of orally administered drugs are discussed.

Diffusional Systems

In diffusional systems, the release rate of drug is determined by its diffusion through a water-insoluble polymer. There are two types of diffusional devices: *reservoir devices*, in which a core of drug is surrounded by a polymeric membrane, and *matrix devices*, in which dissolved or dispersed drug is distributed uniformly throughout an inert polymeric matrix. It should be mentioned that in actual practice many devices that utilize diffusion also rely upon some degree of dissolution to determine the release rate. Systems utilizing dissolution will be discussed later in this section.

Reservoir Devices

The release of drug from a reservoir device is governed by Fick's first law of diffusion,

$$J = -D \, dC_m/dx \quad (18)$$

where J is the flux of drug across a membrane in the direction of decreasing concentration (amount/area-time), D is the

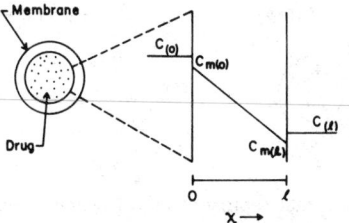

Fig 92-6.   Schematic representation of a reservoir diffusion device. $C_{m(0)}$ and $C_{m(l)}$ represent concentrations of drug at the inside surfaces of the membrane and $C_{(0)}$ and $C_{(l)}$ represent concentrations in the adjacent regions.   (Reproduced with permission from Ref 9.)

diffusion coefficient of the drug in the membrane (area/time), and dC_m/dx is the change in concentration of drug in the membrane over a distance x. If it is assumed that the drug on either side of the membrane is in equilibrium with the respective surface layer of the membrane, as shown in Fig 92-6, then the concentration just inside the membrane surface can be related to the concentration in the adjacent region by the expressions,

$$K = C_{m(0)}/C_{(0)} \text{ at } x = 0 \tag{19}$$

$$K = C_{m(l)}/C_{(l)} \text{ at } x = l \tag{20}$$

where K is a partition coefficient. Assuming that D and K are constant, Eq 18 can be integrated to give,

$$J = DK \, \Delta C/l \tag{21}$$

where ΔC is the concentration difference across the membrane.

If the activity of the drug inside the reservoir is maintained constant and the value of K is less than unity, zero order release can be achieved. This is the case when the drug is present as a solid, ie, its activity is unity. Depending on the shape of the device, the equation describing drug release will vary. Only the simplest geometry, that of a rectangular slab or "sandwich," will be presented here. For the slab geometry, the equation describing release is,

$$dM_t/dt = ADK \, \Delta C/l \tag{22}$$

where M_t is the mass of drug released after time t, dM_t/dt is the steady state release rate at time t, A is the surface area of the device, and D, K, and l are as previously defined. Similar equations can be written for cylindrical or spherical geometric devices. If the terms on the right hand side of Eq 22 are held constant, zero order release will be achieved. This is often not the case in actual practice, however, and nonzero-order release is frequently observed.

Common methods used to develop reservoir type devices include microencapsulation of drug particles and press-coating of whole tablets or particles. In most cases, particles coated by microencapsulation form a system where the drug is contained in the coating film as well as in the core of the microcapsule. Drug release usually involves a combination of dissolution and diffusion, with dissolution being the process that controls the release rate. If the encapsulating material is selected properly, diffusion will be the controlling process. Microencapsulation is discussed further with reference to systems utilizing dissolution. Some materials used as the membrane barrier coat, alone or in combination, are hardened gelatin, methyl and ethylcelluloses, polyhydroxymethacrylate, hydroxypropylcellulose, polyvinylacetate, and various waxes. Examples of some marketed products utilizing an encapsulated reservoir of drug are shown in Table II. Drug release from these products probably is based primarily on diffusion, but dissolution may be occurring as well.

Table II—Reservoir Diffusional Products

Product	Active ingredient(s)	Manufacturer
Plateau CAPS capsules		Marion
Duotrate	pentaerythritol tetranitrate	
Nico-400	nicotinic acid	
Nitro-Bid	nitroglycerin	
Cerespan capsules	papaverine hydrochloride	USV
Histospan capsules	chlorpheniramine maleate, phenylephrine hydrochloride, methscopolamine nitrate	USV
Nitrospan capsules	nitroglycerin	USV
Measurin tablets	acetylsalicylic acid	Breon
Bronkodyl S-R capsules	theophylline	Breon

Matrix Devices

The rate of release of a drug dispersed as a solid in an inert matrix has been described by Higuchi.[10,11] Fig 92-7 depicts the physical model for a planar slab. In this model, it is assumed that solid drug dissolves from the surface layer of the device first; when this layer becomes exhausted of drug, the next layer begins to be depleted by dissolution and diffusion through the matrix to the external solution. In this fashion, the interface between the region containing dissolved drug and that containing dispersed drug moves into the interior as a front. The assumptions made in deriving the mathematical model are as follows:

1. A pseudo-steady state is maintained during release;
2. The total amount of drug present per unit volume in the matrix, C_0, is substantially greater than the saturation solubility of the drug per unit volume in the matrix, C_s;
3. The release medium is a perfect sink at all times;
4. Drug particles are much smaller in diameter than the average distance of diffusion;
5. The diffusion coefficient remains constant;
6. No interaction occurs between the drug and the matrix.

Based on Fig 92-7, the change in amount of drug released per unit area, dM, with a change in the depleted zone thickness, dh, is,

$$dM = C_0 dh - (C_s/2)dh \tag{23}$$

where C_0 and C_s are as defined above. However, based on Fick's first law,

$$dM = (D_m C_s/h)dt \tag{24}$$

where D_m is the diffusion coefficient in the matrix. If Eqs 23 and 24 are equated, solved for h, and that value of h substituted back into the integrated form of Eq 24, an equation for M is obtained;

$$M = [C_s D_m (2C_0 - C_s)t]^{1/2} \tag{25}$$

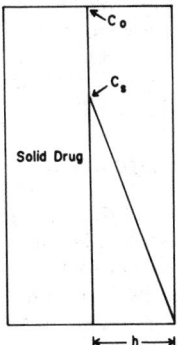

Fig 92-7.   Schematic representation of the physical model used for a planar slab matrix diffusion device.

Table III—Matrix Diffusional Products

Product	Active ingredient(s)	Manufacturer
Gradumet tablets		Abbott
Desoxyn	methamphetamine hydrochloride	
Fero-Gradumet	ferrous sulfate	
Fero-Grad-500	ferrous sulfate, sodium ascorbate	
Tral	hexocyclium methylsulfate	
Lontab tablets		Ciba-Geigy
Forhistal	dimethindone maleate	
Priscoline	tolazoline hydrochloride	
PBZ	tripelennamine	
Procan SR tablets	procainamide hydrochloride	Parke-Davis
Choledyl SA tablets	oxtriphylline	Parke-Davis

Similarly, a drug released from a porous or granular matrix is described by,

$$M = [D_s C_a (\epsilon/T)(2C_0 - \epsilon C_a)t]^{1/2} \qquad (26)$$

where ϵ is porosity of the matrix, T is *tortuosity*, C_a is the solubility of the drug in the release medium, and D_s is the diffusion coefficient in the release medium. In this system, drug is leached from the matrix via channels.

For purposes of data treatment, Eqs 25 and 26 are conveniently reduced to,

$$M = kt^{1/2} \qquad (27)$$

where k is a constant, so that a plot of amount of drug released versus the square root of time should be linear if the release of the drug from the matrix is diffusion controlled. The release rate of drug from such a device is not zero order since it decreases with time but, as previously mentioned, this may be clinically equivalent to constant release for many drugs.

The three major types of materials used in the preparation of matrix devices are insoluble plastics, hydrophilic polymers, and fatty compounds. Plastic matrices which have been investigated include methyl acrylate–methyl methacrylate, polyvinyl chloride, and polyethylene. The Gradumet tablet (*Abbott*) is an example of a dosage form utilizing a plastic matrix. Hydrophilic polymers include methylcellulose, hydroxypropylmethylcellulose, and sodium carboxymethylcellulose. Fatty compounds include various waxes such as carnauba wax, and glyceryl tristearate. An example of a dosage form utilizing a wax matrix is the Lontab tablet (*Ciba-Geigy*).

The most common method of preparation is to mix the drug with the matrix material and then compress the mixture into tablets. In the case of wax matrices, the drug is generally dispersed in molten wax, which is then congealed, granulated, and compressed into cores. In any sustained-release system it is necessary for a portion of the drug to be available immediately as a priming dose and the remainder to be released in a sustained fashion. This is accomplished in a matrix tablet by placing the priming dose in a coat of the tablet. The coat can be applied by press coating or by conventional pan or air suspension coating. Some marketed matrix diffusional products are listed in Table III.

Systems Utilizing Dissolution

As mentioned earlier in the chapter, a drug with a slow dissolution rate will yield an inherently sustained blood level. In principle, then, it would seem possible to prepare sustained-release products by decreasing the dissolution rate of drugs which are highly water soluble. This can be done by preparing an appropriate salt or derivatives, by coating the drug with a slowly dissolving material, or by incorporating it into a tablet with a slowly dissolving carrier. Ideally, the

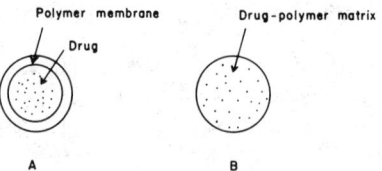

Fig 92-8. Schematic representation of systems utilizing dissolution. A, encapsulated formulation where drug release is determined by thickness and dissolution rate of the polymer membrane; B, matrix formulation where drug release is determined by dissolution rate of the polymer.

surface area available for dissolution must remain constant in order to achieve a constant release rate. This is, however, difficult to achieve in practice.

The dissolution process can be considered diffusion-layer controlled, where the rate of diffusion from the solid surface to the bulk solution through an unstirred liquid film is the rate determining step. In this case the dissolution process at steady state is described by the Noyes-Whitney equation,

$$dC/dt = k_D A (C_s - C) = (D/h)A(C_s - C) \qquad (28)$$

where dC/dt is the dissolution rate, k_D is the dissolution rate constant, A is the total surface area, C_s is the saturation solubility of the solid, and C is the concentration of solute in the bulk solution. The dissolution rate constant k_D is equal to the diffusion coefficient D divided by the thickness of the diffusion layer h. The above equation predicts a constant dissolution rate if the surface area, diffusion coefficient, diffusion layer thickness, and concentration difference are kept constant. However, as dissolution proceeds, all of these parameters may change, especially surface area. For spherical particles, the change in area can be related to the weight of the particle and, under the assumption of sink conditions, Eq 28 becomes the cube-root dissolution equation,

$$w_0^{1/3} - w^{1/3} = k_D' t \qquad (29)$$

where k_D' is the cube-root dissolution rate constant, and w_0 and w are initial weight and weight of the amount remaining at time t, respectively.

Two common formulations relying on dissolution to determine release rate of drug are shown in Fig 92-8. Most of the products fall into two categories; encapsulated dissolution systems and matrix dissolution systems.

Encapsulated dissolution systems can be prepared either by coating particles or granules of drug with varying thicknesses of slowly soluble polymers, or by microencapsulation. The most common method of microencapsulation is *coacervation*, which involves addition of a hydrophilic substance to a colloidal dispersion. The hydrophilic substance, which acts as the coating material, can be selected from a wide variety of natural and synthetic polymers including shellacs, waxes, starches, cellulose acetate phthalate or butyrate, polyvinylpyrrolidone, and polyvinyl chloride. Once the coating material dissolves, all the drug inside the microcapsule is immediately available for dissolution and absorption. Thus, drug release can be controlled by adjusting the thickness and dissolution rate of the coat. The thickness can be varied from less than 1 μm to 200 μm by changing the amount of coating material from 3 to 30% of the total weight. If only a few different thicknesses are used, usually three or four, drugs will be released at different, predetermined times to give a delayed release effect, ie, repeat-action. If a spectrum of different thicknesses is employed, a more uniform blood level of the drug can be obtained. The coated particles can be directly compressed into tablets, or placed in capsules. A partial listing of some marketed sustained-release products relying

Table IV—Encapsulated Dissolution Products

Product	Active ingredient(s)	Manufacturer
Spansule capsules		Smith Kline, & French
Benzedrine	amphetamine sulfate	
Combid	prochlorperazine maleate, isopropamide iodide	
Hispril	diphenylpyraline hydrochloride	
Ornade	phenylpropanolamine hydrochloride, chlorpheniramine maleate	
Thorazine	chlorpromazine hydrochloride	
Contac capsules	phenylpropanolamine hydrochloride, chlorpheniramine maleate, atropine sulfate, scopolamine hydrobromide, hyoscyamine sulfate	Menley & James
Sequel capsules		Lederle
Artane	trihexyphenidyl hydrochloride	
Diamox	acetazolamide	
Ferro-sequels	ferrous fumarate, docusate sodium	

Table V—Matrix Dissolution Products

Product	Active ingredient(s)	Manufacturer
Extentab tablets		Robins
Dimetane	brompheniramine maleate	
Dimetapp	brompheniramine maleate, phenylephrine hydrochloride, phenylpropanolamine hydrochloride	
Donnatal	phenobarbital, hyoscamine sulfate, atropine sulfate, scopolamine hydrobromide	
Quinidex	quinidine sulfate	
Timespan tablets		Hofmann-La Roche
Mestinon	pyridostigmine bromide	
Roniacol	nicotinyl alcohol	
Dospan tablets		Merrell Dow
Tenuate	diethylpropion hydrochloride	
Chronotab tablets		Schering
Disophrol	dexbrompheniramine maleate, pseudoephedrine sulfate	
Tempule capsules		Armour
Nicobid	nicotinic acid	
Pentritol	pentaerythritol tetranitrate	
Repetab tablets		Schering
Chlor-trimeton	chlorpheniramine maleate	
Demazin	chlorpheniramine maleate, phenylephrine hydrochloride	
Polaramine	dexchlorpheniramine maleate	
Trilafon	perphenazine	

primarily on encapsulated dissolution are shown in Table IV.

Matrix dissolution devices are prepared by compressing the drug with a slowly dissolving polymer carrier into a tablet. There are two general methods of preparing drug–polymer particles; congealing and aqueous dispersion methods. In the congealing method, drug is mixed with a polymer or wax material and either cooled and screened or spray-congealed. In the aqueous dispersion method, the drug–polymer mixture is simply sprayed or placed in water and the resulting particles are collected. Examples of marketed products relying primarily on matrix dissolution are listed in Table V.

Osmotic Systems

Osmotic pressure can be employed as the driving force to generate a constant release of drug provided a constant os-

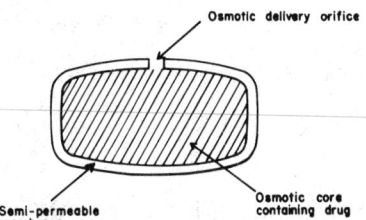

Fig 92-9. Schematic diagram of an osmotic tablet. (Reproduced with permission from Ref 12.)

motic pressure is maintained and a few other features of the physical system are constrained. Consider a tablet consisting of a core of drug surrounded by a semipermeable membrane containing a small orifice, as shown in Fig 92-9. The membrane will allow free diffusion of water, but not drug. When the tablet is exposed to water or any fluid in the body, water will flow into the tablet due to osmotic pressure difference and the volume flow rate, dV/dt, of water into the tablet is,

$$dV/dt = (kA/h)(\Delta\pi - \Delta P) \qquad (30)$$

where k, A, and h are the membrane permeability, area, and thickness, respectively, $\Delta\pi$ is the osmotic pressure difference, and ΔP is the hydrostatic pressure difference. If the orifice is sufficiently large, the hydrostatic pressure difference will be small compared to the osmotic pressure difference, and Eq 30 becomes,

$$dV/dt = (kA/h)\Delta\pi \qquad (31)$$

Thus, the volume flow rate of water into the tablet is determined by permeability, area, and thickness of the membrane. The drug will be pumped out of the tablet through the orifice at a controlled rate, dM/dt, equal to the volume flow rate of water into the tablet multiplied by the drug concentration, C_s;

$$dM/dt = (dV/dt)C_s \qquad (32)$$

The release rate will be constant until the concentration of drug inside the tablet falls below saturation.

The advantage of the osmotic system is that it requires only osmotic pressure to be effective and is essentially independent of the environment. The drug release rate can be predetermined precisely regardless of pH change through the GI tract. Some materials used as the semipermeable membrane include polyvinyl alcohol, polyurethane, cellulose acetate, ethylcellulose, and polyvinyl chloride. Drugs that have demonstrated successful release rates from an osmotic system *in vivo* after oral dosing are potassium chloride and acetazolamide.

Ion Exchange Resins

Ion-exchange resins are water-insoluble crosslinked polymers containing salt forming groups in repeating positions on the polymer chain. Drug is bound to the resin by repeated exposure of the resin to the drug in a chromatographic column, or by prolonged contact of the resin with the drug solution. Drug release from the drug–resin complex depends on the ionic environment, ie, pH and electrolyte concentration, within the GI tract as well as properties of the resin.

Drug molecules attached to the resin are released by exchanging with appropriately charged ions in the GI tract, as shown in Fig 92-10, followed by diffusion of the free drug molecule out of the resin. The rate of diffusion is controlled by the area of diffusion, diffusional pathlength, and extent of crosslinking in the resin. A further modification of the release rate can be made by coating the drug–resin complex.

Most ion-exchange resins currently employed in sustained-release products contain sulfonic acid groups that

$$\text{Resin}^+\text{-Drug}^- + X^- \longrightarrow \text{Resin}^+\text{-}X^- + \text{Drug}^-$$

$$\text{or Resin}^-\text{-Drug}^+ + Y^+ \longrightarrow \text{Resin}^-\text{-}Y^+ + \text{Drug}^+$$

where X^- and Y^+ are ions in the GI tract.

Fig 92-10.

exchange cationic drugs such as those with an amine functionality. Examples of some of these drugs are amphetamine, phenyl t-butylamine (phentermine), phenyltoloxamine, and hydrocodone, as shown in Table VI.

Prodrugs

A prodrug is a compound formed by chemical modification of a biologically active compound which will liberate the active compound *in vivo* by enzymatic or hydrolytic cleavage. The primary purpose of employing a prodrug for oral administration is to increase intestinal absorption or to reduce local side effects, such as GI irritation by aspirin. On this basis, one does not generally classify a prodrug as a sustained-release dosage form. However, the ability to bioreversibly modify the physicochemical properties of a drug allows better intestinal transport properties and hence influences the drug blood level versus time profile. Thus, prodrugs can be used to in-

Table VI—Ion Exchange Products

Product	Active ingredient(s)	Manufacturer
Biphetamine capsules	amphetamine, dextroamphetamine	Pennwalt
Tussionex capsules, tablets, suspension	hydrocodone, phenyltoloxamine	Pennwalt
Ionamin capsules	phentermine	Pennwalt

crease the strategies for sustained release and, in a limited sense, can be sustaining in their own right.

As an example of the use of a prodrug as a sustaining mechanism, consider a water-soluble drug which is modified to a water-insoluble prodrug. The prodrug will have a slower dissolution rate in aqueous fluid than the parent drug and thus the appearance of the parent drug in plasma will be slowed. This is observed with theophylline and its prodrug 7,7′-succinylditheophylline. Alternatively, a water-soluble prodrug of a water-insoluble parent drug can be made to be a substrate for enzymes in the brush border region of the microvilli. The water-soluble prodrug complexes with the enzyme just prior to reaching the membrane surface, is metabolized, and its membrane/water partition coefficient increases. The result is an increase in the blood level of the drug. See Chapter 27.

Parenteral Dosage Forms

The most common types of dosage forms used for parenteral sustained-release drug therapy are intramuscular (IM) injections, implants for subcutaneous tissues and various body cavities, and transdermal devices. Due to physiological and anatomical constraints, many of the other parenteral routes of administration, eg, intravenous, intraarterial, intrathecal, and intraperitoneal, are not as useful in this regard. The application of the former three types of dosage forms to sustained-release drug delivery will be discussed in this section. The final section is devoted to other parenteral dosage forms being developed for targeted drug delivery.

Intramuscular Injections

Complex Formation

The formation of a dissociable complex of a drug with a macromolecule is the same physicochemical phenomenon which occurs when a drug binds to a plasma protein. In this sense, the drug–macromolecule complex can serve as a reservoir at the site of injection for sustained drug release to the surrounding tissues. The macromolecules used are either biological polymers such as antibodies and proteins, or synthetic polymers such as polyvinylpyrrolidone or polyethylene glycol. Drug release from the polymer is governed by the degree of association, as given by the following equation,

$$D + P \underset{}{\overset{K_a}{\rightleftharpoons}} DP \qquad (33)$$

where D, P, and DP represent drug, polymer, and complex, respectively, and K_a is the apparent association constant. Only that fraction of the drug which is free, f, can be absorbed;

$$f = \frac{(D)}{(DP) + (D)} = \frac{1}{1 + K_a(P)} \qquad (34)$$

where (D), (P), and (DP) are equilibrium concentrations of drug, polymer, and complex, respectively. If $K_a(P)$ is much greater than 1, Eq 34 reduces to,

$$f = 1/[K_a(P)] \qquad (35)$$

The rate of absorption of the drug, $d(C)/dt$, is therefore described by,

$$d(C)/dt = k_a f(D_t) = [k_a(D_t)]/[K_a(P)] \qquad (36)$$

where (D_t) is the total drug concentration at the absorption site, ie, $(DP) + (D)$, and k_a is the absorption rate constant. It can be seen from Eq 36 that the rate of absorption can be controlled effectively by the type and concentration of polymer used, assuming that dissociation is instantaneous compared to absorption.

Complexes can also be formed between drugs and small molecules rather than macromolecules. The motive behind formation of a drug–small molecule complex is to alter the physicochemical properties of the drug and thus affect changes in its biological disposition. Unlike macromolecular complexes, drug–small molecule complexes are capable of being absorbed. They usually have very small association constants, however, which means that most of the drug is free. This nullifies any advantage gained from alteration of properties upon complexation. If the drug molecule is large relative to the complexing agent, the association constant will be greater and the complex more stable. This is the approach that has been taken commercially with polypeptide hormones, such as adrenocorticotropic hormone (ACTH) and insulin, and with vitamins such as cyanocobalamin (vitamin B_{12}). The ACTH product, Acthar Gel HP (*Armour*) consists of an ACTH–zinc tannate complex suspended in a gelatin solution. Tannic acid acts as the complexing agent and gelatin inhibits protein binding of ACTH. An analogous product is Depinar (*Armour*), which is a cyanocobalamin–zinc tannate complex suspended in sesame oil. With both of these products, the sustained effect is due to, among other things, a reduction in solubility of the parent drug upon complexation, and not dissociation. In this respect they are much like aqueous suspensions.

Aqueous Suspensions

The rate-limiting step in drug release from an aqueous suspension is dissolution, as given by the Noyes-Whitney equation (Eq 28). The parameters influencing dissolution

Table VII—Effect of Particle Size of Penicillin G Procaine in Aqueous Suspension on the Drug Blood Levels in Rabbits [a]

Particle size [b] (μm)	Average drug blood level (hrs)					
	1	4	24	28	48	72
150–250	1.37	1.29	0.82	0.86	0.31	0.12
105–150	1.24	1.50	0.76	0.28	0.16	0.01
58–105	1.54	1.44	0.47	0.25	0.12	—
35–38	1.64	1.51	0.62	0.33	0.15	—
<35	2.40	2.36	0.33	0.16	0.07	—
1–2	2.14	2.22	0.06	0.02	—	—

[a] Compiled from data by Buckwalter and Dickison, *J Am Pharm Assn 47:* 661, 1958.
[b] Each aqueous suspension contains 300,000 units/mL of penicillin G procaine with the specified particle size range.

rate were shown to be surface area (ie, particle size), diffusion coefficient, and saturation solubility of the drug. Variation in these parameters for an IM injection is limited by the constraints of stability, occlusion of needles, pain upon injection, minimum effective concentration, and other factors. For example, one common approach to decrease dissolution rate is to decrease total surface area by increasing particle size. This generally extends the duration of action of the drug, as illustrated by the data in Table VII. However, increasing the particle size causes an increase in sedimentation rate, as indicated by Stoke's law, resulting in an unstable suspension. In addition, for some drugs there is an upper limit on particle size beyond which therapeutic levels are not attained even though sustained release is achieved. Another approach to decrease dissolution rate is to decrease the diffusion coefficient by increasing the viscosity of the suspension. Recall that diffusion coefficient is inversely related to viscosity by the Stokes-Einstein relation. An increase in viscosity causes a decrease in sedimentation rate (again by Stoke's law), thus countering the effect of increased particle size. By appropriately varying viscosity and particle size, a stable suspension that offers sustained release resulting in therapeutic drug blood levels can be produced.

Probably the most common approach to decrease dissolution rate is to decrease the saturation solubility of the drug. This is accomplished through the formation of less soluble salts and prodrug derivatives and by employing polymorphic crystal forms. A typical example of decreasing dissolution rate through salt formation is provided by penicillin G procaine, a sparingly soluble form of penicillin G. Other examples of marketed aqueous suspensions based upon use of less soluble salts or derivatives of the parent drug are contained in Table VIII.

Solubility varies with polymorphic form because different arrangements of molecules in the solid state give rise to dif-

Table VIII—Aqueous Suspensions

Product	Active ingredient(s)	Manufacturer
Duracillin A.S.	penicillin G procaine	Lilly
Crysticillin A.S.	penicillin G procaine	Squibb
Wycillin	penicillin G procaine	Wyeth
Bicillin L-A	penicillin G benzathine	Wyeth
Bicillin C-R	penicillin G procaine, penicillin G benzathine	Wyeth
Depo-Provera	medroxyprogesterone acetate	Upjohn
Depo-Medrol	methylprednisolone acetate	Upjohn
Percoten Pivalate	desoxycorticosterone pivalate	Ciba-Geigy
Aristospan	triamcinolone hexacetonide	Lederle
Celeston Soluspan	betamethasone sodium phosphate, betamethasone acetate	Schering-Plough

Table IX—Commercial Insulin Zinc Suspensions and their Reported Durations of Action [a]

Product	Manufacturer	Duration of action (hrs)
Semilente Iletin I	Lilly	12–16
Lente Iletin I	Lilly	24
Ultralente Iletin I	Lilly	>36

[a] Compiled from *Physicians' Desk Reference*, 37th ed, Medical Economics Co, Oradell, NJ, 1983.

ferent lattice energies. An example of extending duration of action by use of a crystalline polymorph is insulin zinc suspension. Although insulin is normally administered subcutaneously, it is included here merely to illustrate the principle. Insulin precipitates as an insoluble complex in the presence of zinc chloride and, depending on the pH, either an amorphous or crystalline form results. The crystalline form is less soluble than the amorphous form and will result in a longer duration of action than the amorphous form. The two forms can be mixed in various proportions to generate products offering a wide spectrum of duration of action. A list of these products and their reported durations of action is shown in Table IX.

Oil Solutions and Oil Suspensions

In the case of oil solutions the release rate of a drug is determined by partitioning of the drug out of the oil into the surrounding aqueous medium. The partitioning phenomenon is an equilibrium process described by the apparent oil/water partition coefficient given in Eq 11. Only that fractional concentration of drug in the aqueous phase, f, is available for absorption,

$$f = (1 + \alpha)/(1 + K\alpha) \tag{37}$$

where K is the apparent oil/water partition coefficient and α is the ratio V_0/V_w, the volume of the oil phase to that of the aqueous phase. This equation indicates that the fraction of drug that is available for absorption is controlled by the partition coefficient and the ratio of the volumes of the two phases (α), and that it remains constant as long as α is constant. Since V_w is a physiological parameter it is usually constant, and therefore the value of α is determined solely by the volume of solution injected, V_0. The rate of drug absorption is described by an equation analogous to Eq 36,

$$d(C)/dt = k_a f(D_t) \tag{38}$$

where (D_t) is the total drug concentration in both phases. The success of an oil solution in achieving sustained release is dependent on the magnitude of K, which is a function of the drug involved and the oil selected. Only those drugs which are appreciably oil soluble and have the desired partition characteristics are suitable. Some oils which may be used for intramuscular injection are sesame, olive, arachnis, maize, almond, cottonseed, and castor oil. Table X contains a partial listing of marketed oil solution products.

Drug release from oil suspensions combines the principles involved in aqueous suspensions and oil solutions. Drug particles must first dissolve in the oil phase and then partition into the aqueous medium. The concentration of drug in the oil phase remains close to its equilibrium solubility since excess solid is present, unlike an oil solution, but this has no bearing on the fractional concentration in the aqueous phase as shown in Eq 37. As expected, duration of action obtained from oil suspensions is longer than that from oil solutions. A list of some marketed oil suspension products is shown in Table XI.

Table X—Oil Solutions

Product	Active ingredient(s)	Manufacturer
Prolixin Enanthate	fluphenazine enanthate in sesame oil	Squibb
Prolixin Decanoate	fluphenazine decanoate in sesame oil	Squibb
Deca-Durabolin	nandrolone decanoate in sesame oil	Organon
Depo-Testosterone	testosterone cypionate in cottonseed oil	Upjohn
Ditate-DS	testosterone enanthate, estradiol valerate in sesame oil	Savage
Delatestryl	testosterone enanthate in sesame oil	Squibb

Table XI—Oil Suspensions

Product	Active ingredient(s)	Manufacturer
Solganol	aurothioglucose in sesame oil	Schering
Pitressin Tannate	vasopressin tannate in peanut oil	Parke-Davis

Emulsions

In the case where dissolved drug makes up the entire oil phase in an oil-in-water emulsion, Higuchi[13] showed that the release rate at steady state can be described by,

$$\text{rate} = 4\pi(a_0^2 + 2D \,\Delta Ct/d)^{1/2}D \,\Delta C \qquad (39)$$

where a_0 is the initial radius of the droplet, D is the diffusion coefficient, ΔC is the concentration difference between the surface of the droplet and the bulk phase, d is the density of the solute, and t is time. In the case where solute makes up only part of the oil phase, appropriate corrections for the distribution coefficient of solute between oil and water phases and partial molal volume of the solute in the droplet must be made.

The release rate from water-in-oil emulsions has been treated by Windheuser *et al.*[14] The water-in-oil emulsion is viewed as a uniform dispersion of water droplets containing the drug throughout an external oil phase. Fig 92-11 depicts a simplified model of the system. Drug release is assumed to proceed via diffusion through the external phase rather than by breaking of the emulsion, and the body fluid acts as a perfect sink. The rate of disappearance of drug from the aqueous phase, $d(C)/dt$, is described by,

$$d(C)/dt = -k(C_0)e^{-kt} \qquad (40)$$

where (C_0) is the initial concentration in the aqueous phase and k is the rate constant of disappearance of drug from the aqueous phase. The constant k is given by,

$$k = ADK/Vl \qquad (41)$$

where A is surface area of the droplet, D is the diffusion

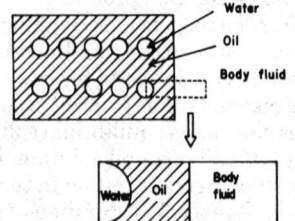

Fig 92-11. Model of a water-in-oil emulsion. (Reproduced with permission from Ref 1.)

coefficient of the drug, K is the partition coefficient of the drug between oil and water, V is the volume of the aqueous phase, and l is the effective thickness of the oil phase. For a given drug, a fast rate of release is favored by a large K, small droplets (ie, large A for a fixed V), and a phase volume ratio favoring the oil phase.

If the body fluid is not a perfect sink, an estimate of the fraction of drug in the body fluid can be made using arguments analogous to those for the oil solution case. Making several simplifying assumptions, an equation identical to Eq 37 is obtained. Based on this argument alone, no apparent advantage is gained by administering a water-in-oil emulsion rather than an oil solution as far as sustained release is concerned. Similar results can be obtained for drug release from oil-in-water emulsions.

Implants

One of the oldest and most highly developed forms of drug delivery is to implant a drug-bearing polymeric device subcutaneously or in various body cavities. This method finds particular applicability to cases where chronic administration of drug over periods ranging from days to years is required. Examples include insulin for diabetes, pilocarpine for glaucoma, immune agents for various diseases and allergies, contraceptive steroids, narcotic antagonists, antibiotics, and anticancer and antihypertensive drugs.

The polymer materials used, which must be biocompatible and nontoxic, are usually chosen from among the following types: hydrogels, silicones, polyethylenes, ethylene–vinyl acetate copolymers, and biodegradable polymers. Each of these will be considered in detail.

A hydrogel is a polymeric material which exhibits the ability to swell in water and retain greater than 20% of that water within its structure, but which will not dissolve in water. These materials resemble living tissue because of their high water content, and are considered very biocompatible because they are soft and rubbery and offer low frictional irritation to surrounding tissue. Structural rigidity is imparted by crosslinking agents. Small molecular weight substances diffuse through hydrogels quickly, however, and this is a significant disadvantage for controlled drug delivery. Examples of hydrogels include polyhydroxyalkyl methacrylates (*p*-HEMA), polyacrylamide and polymethacrylamide, polyvinylpyrrolidone, polyvinyl alcohol, and various polyelectrolyte complexes. The *p*-HEMAs are commonly used for soft contact lenses and surgical implants.

Silicones are a family of polymers that have a backbone structure consisting of alternating silicone and oxygen atoms. The silicone atoms usually have one or more organic side groups which impart various physicochemical properties to the polymer. The most widely used is polydimethylsiloxane, commonly known as silicone rubber:

$$X-\underset{\underset{CH_3}{|}}{\overset{\overset{CH_3}{|}}{Si}}-O-\left[\underset{\underset{CH_3}{|}}{\overset{\overset{CH_3}{|}}{Si}}-O\right]_n\underset{\underset{CH_3}{|}}{\overset{\overset{CH_3}{|}}{Si}}-X$$

Silicones can be fluid, elastomeric, or resinous, depending on molecular weight, extent of crosslinking, and the type of number of organic side groups attached. They are very permeable to lipid-soluble drugs and less permeable to hydrophilic drugs. Silicone rubber is biocompatible and is used in surgical prostheses and devices as well as various types of subcutaneous implants.

Polyethylenes consist of C_2H_4 subunits and the properties are determined by the average molecular weight and degree of crystallinity. Low-density polyethylene has a high degree of side chain branching and a low degree of crystallinity, whereas high-density polyethylene is an almost linear polymer with fewer side chain branches and a high degree of crystallinity. High-density polyethylene is biocompatible and is widely used in contraceptive intrauterine devices.

Ethylene–vinyl acetate (EVA) copolymers are less permeable to lipid-soluble drugs than silicones. Their permeability varies as a function of comonomer ratio. At extremely low vinyl acetate content, EVA copolymer exhibits characteristics similar to low-density polyethylene. Increasing vinyl acetate content causes a decrease in stiffness, tensile strength, and softening point. EVA copolymers are relatively clean, chemically stable, and can be sterilized with heat or radiation. They are used in intrauterine and intraocular devices.

The last type of material used in implants, biodegradable or "erodable" polymers, are unlike the previously discussed materials in that they are consumed or biodegraded during therapy. This usually involves breakdown of the polymer to its monomeric subunits, which must be biocompatible with the surrounding tissue. The life of a biodegradable polymer *in vivo* depends on its molecular weight and degree of crosslinking; the greater the molecular weight and degree of crosslinking, the longer the life. The most highly investigated are polylactic acid (PLA), polyglycolic acid (PGA), copolymers of PLA and PGA, polyamides, and copolymers of polyamides and polyesters. PLA, sometimes referred to as polylactide, undergoes hydrolytic de-esterification to lactic acid, a normal product of muscle metabolism. It loses 12–14% of its mass after 3 months *in vivo* according to Kulkarni,[15] whereas Schindler[16] showed that it takes about 80 days for a PLA composite to halve its molecular weight. PGA is chemically related to PLA and is commonly used for absorbable surgical sutures, as is PLA/PGA copolymer. The use of PGA in sustained-release implants has been limited due to its low solubility in common solvents and subsequent difficulty in fabrication of devices.

In general, the equations describing release rate of drugs from implantable devices, and therefore the factors affecting that rate, are the same as those for oral reservoir and matrix diffusion devices considered in the section on oral dosage forms. The exception is the biodegradable system, which will be considered in detail below.

Subcutaneous Devices

Subcutaneous implantation is currently one of the most popular routes used to investigate the potential of sustained drug delivery. This is partly due to the simplicity of the surgical procedures involved in implantation and removal, and the relatively favorable absorption site offered compared to the oral or percutaneous routes. Surgery could be viewed as a disadvantage, however, depending on the patient and the location and frequency of implantation. It can be avoided in some cases by injecting the implant directly into subcutaneous tissue, provided the implant is capable of being delivered through a syringe. This is the method used for many of the sustained-release insulin products (see Table IX).

The development of subcutaneous implants was initiated by two physicians, Folkman and Long, who discovered that lipid-soluble dyes diffused through silicone rubber tubing. A variety of drugs, including anesthetics, thyroid hormone, and certain cardiovascular agents, were later tested in the system in animals. They found that lipophilic drugs with a molecular weight of less than 1000 diffused through silicone rubber, but that large polar molecules did not. Many experiments with silicone rubber soon followed, with much attention focused on steroid hormones because of their enormous potency and desirability of long-term sustained delivery. Subcutaneous implantation in woman of small capsules of silicone rubber filled with the contraceptive steroid megestrol acetate represented the first effort to reach clinical trial. Other attempts

have included subdermal implants of capsules containing norgestrienone, norethindrone, progestin R2323, and *d*-norgestrel.

Biodegradable polymers that act as a matrix for drug release from subcutaneously implanted devices offer several advantages over silicone devices. The most obvious is that no surgical removal of the device is necessary after it has fulfilled its function. Also, an additional mechanism for release of drug is provided by degradation. Complete delivery and thus maximal absorption occurs after the device has degraded.

The mechanism of release of drugs from erodable slabs, cylinders, and spheres has been described by Hopfenberg.[17] A simple expression describing additive release from these devices is

$$M_t/M_\infty = 1 - [1 - k_0 t/C_0 a]^n \qquad (42)$$

where $n = 3$ for a sphere, $n = 2$ for a cylinder, and $n = 1$ for a slab. The symbol a represents the radius of a sphere or cylinder or the half-thickness of a slab. M_t and M_∞ are the masses of drug released at time t and at infinity, respectively.

Polylactic acid has been applied as a biodegradable subcutaneous implant for the delivery of narcotic antagonists, steroids, and anticancer agents. Narcotic antagonists, such as naltrexone, cyclazocine, and naloxone, are therapeutically useful in the postdetoxification stage of rehabilitation of drug-dependent patients. Steroids investigated include contraceptives (progesterone), anti-inflammatory agents (dexamethasone), and anabolics (estradiol). Anticancer agents investigated include cyclophosphamide, doxorubicin, and cisplatin. A further discussion of the experiments performed and their results can be found in a review by Yolles.[18]

Intravaginal Devices

Intravaginal implants are used for the sustained release of contraceptive steroid hormones due to the more favorable site of absorption offered by the vaginal mucosa relative to the oral route for these drugs. First-pass hepatic metabolism, which inactivates many steroid hormones, and gastrointestinal incompatibility are avoided by using the vaginal route. In addition, the vaginal route allows self-insertion and removal of the device, ensuring better patient compliance.

One of the first applications of intravaginal implants was the medicated vaginal ring, a ring-shaped silicone matrix device containing the contraceptive medroxyprogesterone acetate. Clinical trials of this device in healthy women showed that a contraceptive drug blood level was reached within three days after administration and maintained relatively constant for 3 weeks. This indicated that intravaginal absorption of medroxyprogesterone acetate from the ring provides a constant drug blood level with a total dose that is only one-sixth of the oral dose required.[19] Contraception is reversible after removal of the ring, but one problem is that it may cause bleeding due to irritation and/or epithelial breakthrough in some patients. More recently, a new multilayered vaginal ring was developed that releases a combination of a progestin (eg, d-norgestrel) and an estrogen (eg, estradiol) in order to alleviate this problem.

Intrauterine Devices

The intrauterine device (IUD) is one of the more popular methods of contraception. Initial investigations involving nonmedicated IUDs revealed that the larger the device, the more effective it was in preventing pregnancy. Unfortunately, large devices caused increased incidences of uterine cramps, bleeding, and expulsion. The effort to improve intrauterine contraception and avoid previously demonstrated side effects

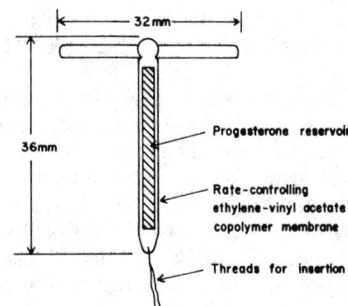

Fig 92-12. Schematic diagram of the Progestasert intrauterine device. (Reproduced with permission from Ref 20.)

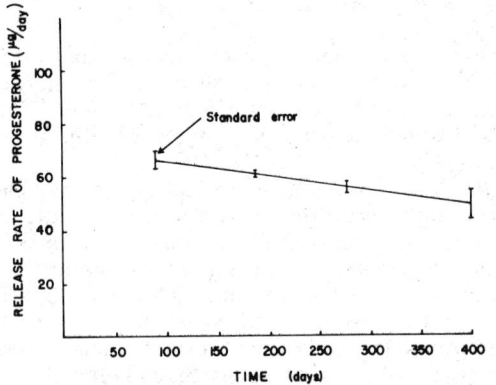

Fig 92-13. In-vivo release rate versus time profile for progesterone from the Progestasert intrauterine device. (Summarized from data by Martinez-Manitou, *J Steroid Biochem 6:* 889, 1975.)

has led to the development of medicated IUDs. Two classes of agents have been used in IUDs of this type: contraceptive metals and steroid hormones.

Examples of commercially available metal-bearing IUDs are the Tatum-T (*Searle*) and the CU-7 (*Searle*). The Tatum-T is a T-shaped polyethylene plastic device wound with 120 mg of copper wire around its vertical stem, providing 210 mm² of exposed copper surface area. The CU-7 contains 89 mg of copper wire wound around the vertical limb of a 7-shaped polypropylene plastic device to give an effective surface area of approximately 200 mm² of copper. A mean dose of 9.87 µg/day of copper is released from this device for up to 40 months. Copper appears to be released by a combination of ionization and chelation.

The hormone-releasing IUD is best exemplified by the Progestasert (*Alza*), a commercially available T-shaped reservoir system composed of ethylene–vinyl acetate copolymer containing progesterone. A schematic diagram of the device is shown in Fig 92-12. The Progestasert does not depend upon physical configuration, size, or presence of a metal to prevent conception. The most common variety releases approximately 65 µg/day of progesterone *in vitro* at a nearly constant rate for over one year, as shown in Fig 92-13. Women wearing the Progestasert ovulate and menstruate regularly due to the small amount of progesterone released.

Intraocular Devices

Chronic open-angle glaucoma usually requires therapy for the lifetime of the patient with a miotic agent such as pilocarpine, for control of intraocular pressure. Conventional pilocarpine therapy requires instillation of eyedrops four times a day. A significant improvement in therapy is offered by the Ocusert (*Ciba-Geigy*), a commercially available reservoir device made of ethylene–vinyl acetate copolymer designed to deliver pilocarpine continuously for 1 week. The implant is a thin, flexible, lamellar ellipse that is placed in the cul-de-sac

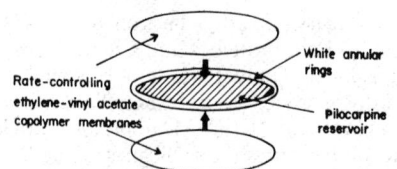

Fig 92-14. Schematic diagram of the Ocusert intraocular device.

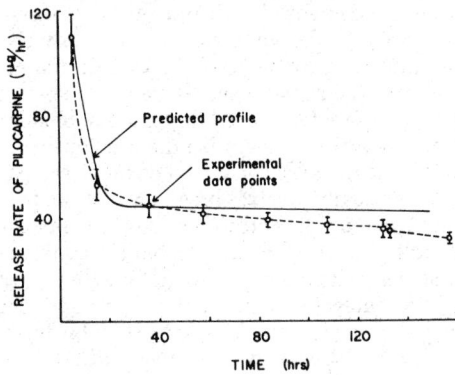

Fig 92-15. In-vitro release rate versus time profile for pilocarpine from the Ocusert intraocular device. (Reproduced with permission from Ref 20.)

of the lower eyelid and floats on the tear film, much like a soft contact lens. Two different varieties are available: one releases 20 µg/hr and the other 40 µg/hr of pilocarpine for up to 1 week. Each measures 6 mm by 13 mm axially and 0.5 mm in thickness. They consist of a pilocarpine-reservoir core laminated between two EVA copolymer membranes and surrounded by an annular ring made of the same copolymer to seal the edges, as shown in Fig 92-14. The drug reservoir is a film of pilocarpine in the natural polymer alginic acid that serves as a carrier medium and allows the reservoir component to be handled as a film during manufacture. The advantages of the Ocusert system over conventional therapy are representative of those discussed in the section on the potential advantages of sustained drug therapy. Fig 92-15 shows a typical *in vitro* release rate versus time profile from an Ocusert designed to release 40 µg/hr. The system has been shown to give *in vivo* release rates of pilocarpine that correlate well with the *in vitro* values over a 7 day period.

Transdermal Systems

Among other things, the skin serves as a barrier against penetration of microorganisms, viruses, and toxic chemicals, and as a restraint against loss of physiologically vital fluids. A discussion of the fundamentals of percutaneous drug absorption, sometimes referred to as transdermal absorption, can be found in Chapter 88. Investigation of mechanisms of transdermal drug absorption has led to new approaches in using this route for systemic drug delivery. One of these is the use of microporous membranes as rate controlling barriers. Microporous membranes are films a few millimeters in thickness and with pore sizes ranging from several micrometers to a few angstroms. Examples of materials from which these membranes are made are regenerated cellulose, cellulose nitrate/acetate, cellulose triacetate, polypropylene, polycarbonate, and polytetrafluoroethylene. The barrier properties of these films depend upon the method of preparation, the medium with which the pores are filled, pore diameter, percent porosity, and tortuosity.

An example of a transdermal delivery system is the Transderm-V (*Ciba-Geigy*) shown in Fig 92-16. This particular system is designed to prevent and treat motion-induced nausea using scopolamine without eliciting the side effects

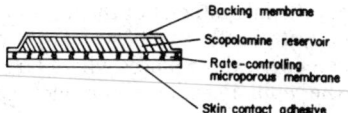

Fig 92-16.   Schematic diagram of a transdermal device for delivery of scopolamine.

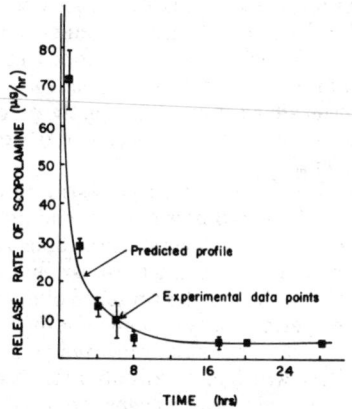

Fig 92-17.   In-vitro release rate versus time profile for scopolamine from a transdermal device.   (Reproduced with permission from Ref 12.)

that normally accompany oral or intramuscular administration of the drug. The system consists of a reservoir containing scopolamine dispersed as a separate phase within a highly permeable matrix, laminated between the rate controlling microporous membrane and an external backing membrane which is impermeable to drug and moisture. The pores of the membrane are filled with a fluid highly permeable to scopolamine. An initial priming dose of drug is contained in a gel on the membrane side of the device. The delivery rate is governed by diffusion through the various lamellae of the device and the skin. At a steady state, the rate-limiting step is diffusion across the microporous membrane. One particular model of the device is 150 μm thick, covers a skin surface area of 2.5 cm^2, and is designed to release 200 μg of scopolamine as a priming dose and 10 μg/hr for 72 hours at steady state. It is generally applied behind the ear. A typical *in vitro* release rate versus time profile from such a system is shown in Fig 92-17.

More recently, transdermal systems have been developed for delivery of nitroglycerin. Nitroglycerin is indicated for treatment of pain caused by angina pectoris. Sublingual dosage forms of nitroglycerin were the first type available for antianginal use, but they suffer from a short duration of action due to rapid metabolism in the liver and other organs by the enzyme glutathione-organic nitrate reductase. This short duration of action is acceptable for treating acute anginal attacks but it is unfavorable when a prophylactic effect is desired. Orally administered nitroglycerin is extensively metabolized during its first pass through the liver and it is

debatable whether sufficient amounts of the drug reach the systemic circulation to elicit the desired response. Topical ointments were developed in an attempt to extend the duration of action but only a 4 to 8 hour effect is achieved and patient compliance is a problem. The fourth generation in nitroglycerin delivery systems is the transdermal device, which offers a significant improvement in sustained-release therapy over its predecessors. There are three different products in several sizes currently on the market that release from 2.5 to 22.4 mg over 24 hours, depending on the drug content and surface area covered. One of the products, Transderm-Nitro (*Ciba-Geigy*), utilizes a microporous membrane similar to that used in the scopolamine device as the rate controlling barrier. The Nitrodisc (*Searle*) uses drug microsealed in a solid silicone polymer, and the Nitro-Dur (*Key*) uses a 2% diffusion matrix. The devices range from 5 to 20 cm^2 in surface area and are generally applied to the upper arm or chest.

Targeted Delivery Systems

Nanoparticles

Nanoparticles are one of several types of systems known collectively as colloidal drug delivery systems. Also included in this group are microcapsules, nanocapsules, macromolecular complexes, polymeric beads, microspheres, and liposomes. A nanoparticle is a particle containing dispersed drug with a diameter of 200–500 nm. The size of a nanoparticle allows it to be administered intravenously via injection, unlike many other colloidal systems which occlude both needles and capillaries. Materials used in the preparation of nanoparticles are sterilizable, nontoxic, and biodegradable; examples are albumin, ethylcellulose, casein, and gelatin. They are usually prepared by a process similar to the coacervation method of microencapsulation.

There have been two main applications of nanoparticles: as carriers of medical diagnostic agents such as radioisotopic technetium-99m and fluorescein isothiocyanate, and for the delivery of liver flukicides in veterinary medicine. Radioisotopes are used to study the morphology, physiology, and blood flow of various organs in the body. The liver is commonly visualized with technetium-99m/sulfur colloid. Preparation of technetium-99m gelatin nanoparticles and subsequent intravenous injection into mice revealed that they are rapidly taken up by the reticuloendothelial system and localized mainly in the liver.[21] The reticuloendothelial system is a system of phagocytic cells designed to cleanse the bloodstream of bacteria, viruses, cell debris, and other unwanted foreign particles. The behavior of nanoparticles *in vivo* is the

same as that exhibited by other colloidal systems of similar size, and points to the possibility of using nanoparticles to target drugs to the liver and phagocytic cells. The use of fluorescein isothiocyanate (FITC) was aimed at determining the availability of surface amino groups on gelatin or albumin nanoparticles. Since FITC is known to bind to amino groups, any such binding on the surface of a nanoparticle would reveal the presence of amino groups and thus their possible use as binding sites for drug molecules as well. Results indicated that free amino groups are indeed present on the surface of the nanoparticle.[21] In addition, preliminary work showed that FITC gelatin nanoparticles incubated with tumor cells *in vitro* are taken up by the tumor cells. This observation implies the possible use of nanoparticles for the targeted delivery of anticancer agents to tumorous tissue.

Liposomes

When phospholipids are gently dispersed in aqueous media, they swell, hydrate, and spontaneously form multilamellar concentric bilayer vesicles with layers of aqueous media separating the lipid bilayers. These systems are commonly referred to as multilamellar liposomes or multilamellar vesicles (MLVs) and have diameters of from 25 nm to 4 μm. Sonication of MLVs results in the formation of small unilamellar vesicles (SUVs) with diameters in the range of 200–500 Å, containing an aqueous solution in the core. Liposomes bear many resemblances to cellular membranes and have been used for over a decade to study membrane behavior and membrane-mediated processes. It is also possible to use liposomes as carriers for drugs and macromolecules since water- or lipid-soluble substances can be entrapped in the aqueous spaces or within the bilayer itself, respectively. More recent studies have been aimed at investigating the potential of these drug-bearing liposomes for site-specific or receptor release of their active agent.

Phospholipids can form a variety of structures other than liposomes when dispersed in water, depending on the molar ratio of lipid to water. At low ratios the liposome is the preferred structure. Physical characteristics of liposomes depend on pH, ionic strength, and the presence of divalent cations. They show low permeability to ionic and polar substances, including many drugs, but at elevated temperatures undergo a phase transition which markedly alters their permeability. The phase transition involves a change from a closely packed, ordered structure known as the gel state to a loosely packed, less ordered structure known as the fluid state. This occurs at a characteristic phase transition temperature and results in an increase in permeability to ions, sugars, and drugs. In addition to temperature, exposure to proteins can alter permeability of liposomes. Certain soluble proteins such as cytochrome-C bind, deform, and penetrate the bilayer, thereby causing changes in permeability. Cholesterol inhibits this penetration of proteins apparently by packing the phospholipids more tightly; most liposome formulations used for drug delivery contain cholesterol to help form a more closely packed bilayer system during preparation. Serum high density lipoproteins cause significant leakage in the membrane, probably due to removal of phospholipid.

The ability to trap solutes varies between different types of liposomes. For example, MLVs are moderately efficient at trapping solutes, but SUVs are extremely inefficient. SUVs offer the advantage of homogeneity and reproducibility in size distribution, however, and a compromise between size and trapping efficiency is offered by large unilamellar vesicles (LUVs). These are prepared by ether evaporation and are three to four times more efficient at solute entrapment than MLVs. In addition to liposome characteristics, an important determinant in drug entrapment is the physicochemical properties of the drug itself. As mentioned previously, polar drugs are trapped in the aqueous spaces and nonpolar drugs bind to the lipid bilayer of the vesicle. Polar drugs are released when the bilayer is broken or by permeation, but nonpolar drugs remain affiliated with the bilayer unless it is disrupted by temperature or exposure to lipoproteins. Both types show maximum efflux rates at the phase transition temperature.

Liposomes can interact with cells by four different mechanisms.[22] These are:

1) Endocytosis by phagocytic cells of the reticuloendothelial system such as macrophages and neutrophils;

2) Adsorption to the cell surface either by nonspecific weak hydrophobic or electrostatic forces, or by specific interactions with cell surface components;

3) Fusion with the plasma cell membrane by insertion of the lipid bilayer of the liposome into the plasma membrane, with simultaneous release of liposomal contents into the cytoplasm;

4) Transfer of liposomal lipids to cellular or subcellular membranes, or *vice versa*, without any association of the liposome contents.

It is often difficult to determine which mechanism is operative and more than one may operate at the same time.

The fate and disposition of intravenously injected liposomes depend on their physical properties, such as size, fluidity, and surface charge. They may persist in tissues for hours or days depending on composition, and half-lives in the blood range from minutes to several hours. Larger liposomes such as MLVs and LUVs are rapidly taken up by phagocytic cells of the reticuloendothelial system, but the physiology of the circulatory system restrains the exit of such large species at most sites. They can only exit in places where large openings or pores exist in the capillary endothelium, such as the sinusoids of the liver or spleen. Thus, these organs are the predominate site of uptake. On the other hand, SUVs show a broader tissue distribution but are still highly sequestered in the liver and spleen. In general, this *in vivo* behavior limits the potential targeting of liposomes to only those organs and tissues accessible to their large size. These include the blood, liver, spleen, bone marrow, and lymphoid organs.

Attempts to overcome the limitation on targeting of liposomes have centered around two approaches. One is the use of antibodies, bound to the liposome surface; to direct the antibody and its drug contents to specific antigenic receptors located on a particular cell-type surface. A second approach is to use carbohydrate determinants as recognition sites. Carbohydrate determinants are glycoprotein or glycolipid cell surface components that play a role in cell–cell recognition, interaction, and adhesion. Although the precise mechanism of their action is still unknown, they show potential in directing liposomes to particular cell types by their inclusion in the liposomal membrane. A discussion of the factors influencing targeting of liposomes has been given by Gregoriadis, *et al.*[23] Potential therapeutic applications of liposomes include their use in treatment of malignant tumors, lysosomal storage diseases, intracellular parasites, metal toxicity, and diabetes. The liposome acts as the carrier of the active agent used in treatment of these conditions. Most of the applications involve intravenous injection of the liposomal preparation, but other routes of administration are conceivable. For example, liposome entrapped insulin may offer some degree of protection of drug from gastric degradation and the possibility of GI absorption by endocytosis. Further details of current applications of liposome-entrapped drugs can be found in References 22 and 23.

Resealed Erythrocytes

When erythrocytes are suspended in a hypotonic medium, they swell to about one and a half times their normal size, and the membrane ruptures resulting in the formation of pores with diameters of 200–500 Å. The pores allow equilibration of the intracellular and extracellular solutions. If the ionic strength of the media is then adjusted to isotonicity and the cells are incubated at 37°, the pores will close and cause the erythrocyte to "reseal." Using this technique with a drug present in the extracellular solution, it is possible to entrap up to 40% of the drug inside the *resealed* erythrocyte and to use this system for targeted delivery via intravenous injection. The advantages to using resealed erythrocytes as drug carriers is that they are biodegradable and nonimmunogenic, they exhibit flexibility in circulation time depending on their physicochemical properties, entrapped drug is shielded from immunologic detection, and chemical modification of drug is not required.

The assessment of resealed erythrocytes for use in targeted delivery has been facilitated by studies on the behavior of normal and modified reinfused erythrocytes. In general, normal aging erythrocytes, slightly damaged erythrocytes, and those lightly coated with antibodies are sequestered in the spleen after intravenous reinfusion, but heavily damaged or modified erythrocytes are removed from the circulation by the liver.[24] This suggests that resealed erythrocytes can be selectively targeted to either the liver or spleen, depending on their membrane characteristics. In addition to coating with antibodies, removal of portions of cell surface carbohydrates reduces the circulating half-life.

The ability of resealed erythrocytes to deliver drug to the

liver or spleen can be viewed as a disadvantage in that other organs and tissues are inaccessible. Thus, the application of this system to targeted delivery has been limited mainly to treatment of lysosomal storage diseases and metal toxicity, where the site of drug action is in the reticuloendothelial system. A more detailed discussion of the application of resealed erythrocytes has been presented by Ihler.[25]

Immunologically Based Systems

As discussed in the section pertaining to intramuscular injections, the formation of dissociable complex of a drug with a macromolecule is a viable method of achieving a sustained-release effect. If the macromolecule used is an antibody, an antigen-specific targeted effect can also be achieved. In addition to complex formation by noncovalent forces, drugs may also be covalently linked to antibodies, provided activity of both drug and antibody is retained or activity of drug is recoverable after release.

Most studies of antibody–drug systems have employed covalent conjugation of the drug to the antibody. Chemical crosslinking agents are commonly used to attach a drug to an antibody by reacting with appropriate groups available on both species. Among the crosslinking agents used are carbodiimide, glutaraldehyde, bisazobenzidine, cyanuric chloride, diethylmalonimidate, and various mixed anhydrides. The reaction should allow effective control of the antibody–drug conjugate size, and the crosslink must be readily broken by available lysosomal hydrolases within the receptor cell if drug release is critical to activity.

Certain specificities expressed on tumor cells, referred to as membrane-bound tumor-associated antigens (TAAs), may be exploited for the purposes of targeting antibody–drug conjugates directly at the malignant tumor by various parenteral routes of administration. Since anticancer drugs are indiscriminate to cell type in their action, a targeted delivery system for these drugs would offer a significant improvement in cancer chemotherapy. A wide variety of antineoplastic drugs has been conjugated to tumor-specific antibodies. Three that have received the most attention are chlorambucil, adriamycin, and methotrexate. The effectiveness of these systems depends on the nature of the cross-linking agent and the method of reaction. The interested reader is directed to two reviews that discuss the use of antibody–drug conjugates for treatment of tumors.[26,27]

References

1. Lee VH, Robinson JR, in Robinson JR, ed: *Sustained and Controlled Release Drug Delivery Systems*, Marcel Dekker, New York, 123–209, 1978.
2. Robinson JR, Eriksen SP. *J Pharm Sci 55:* 1254, 1966.
3. Welling PG, Dobrinska MR, Robinson JR, ed: *Sustained and Controlled Release Drug Delivery Systems*, Marcel Dekker, New York, 631–716, 1978.
4. Flynn GL, Yalkowsky SH, Roseman T. *J Pharm Sci 63:* 479, 1974.
5. Lee VH, Robinson JR, in Robinson JR, ed: *Sustained and Controlled Release Drug Delivery Systems*, Marcel Dekker, New York, 71–121, 1978.
6. Gibaldi M, Perrier D. *Pharmacokinetics*, 2nd ed, Marcel Dekker, New York, 189, 1982.
7. Riegelman S, Loo JCK, Rowland M. *J Pharm Sci 57:* 128, 1968.
8. Wagner JG. *Amer J Pharm 141:* 5, 1969.
9. Park K, Wood RW, Robinson JR, in Langer R, Wise D, eds: *Medical Applications of Controlled Release Technology*, CRC Press, Boca Raton, Florida, in press.
10. Higuchi T. *J Pharm Sci 50:* 874, 1961.
11. Higuchi T. *J Pharm Sci 52:* 1145, 1963.
12. Chandrasekaran SK, Benson H, Urquhart J, in Robinson JR, ed: *Sustained and Controlled Release Drug Delivery Systems*, Marcel Dekker, New York, 557–593, 1978.
13. Higuchi WI. *J Pharm Sci 53:* 405, 1964.
14. Windheuser JL, Best ML, Perrin JH. *Parenteral Drug Assn Bull 24:* 286, 1970.
15. Kulkarni RK, Pani K, Neuman C, Leonard F. *Techn Rep 6608*, Walter Reed Army Medical Center, Washington, DC, 1966.
16. Schindler A, Jeffcoat R, Kimmel GL, Pitt CG, Wall ME, Zweidinger R: *Contemporary Topics in Polymer Sciences*, vol. 11, Plenum Press, New York, 264, 1977.
17. Hopfenberg HB, in Paul DR, Harris FW, eds: *Controlled Release Polymeric Formulations*, American Chemical Society, Washington, DC, 26–32, 1976.
18. Yolles S, Sartori MF, in Juliano RL, ed: *Drug Delivery Systems*, Oxford University Press, New York, 84–111, 1980.
19. Chien YW, in Juliano RL, ed: *Drug Delivery Systems*, Oxford University Press, New York, 42–47, 1980.
20. Heilmann K: *Therapeutic Systems*, Georg Thieme Publishers, Stuttgart, Germany, 1978.
21. Oppenheim RC, in Juliano RL, ed: *Drug Delivery Systems*, Oxford University Press, New York, 182–188, 1980.
22. Juliano RL, Layton D, in Juliano RL, ed: *Drug Delivery Systems*, Oxford University Press, New York, 200–208, 1980.
23. Gregoriadis G, Kirby C, Large P, Meehan A, Senior J, in Gregoriadis G, Senior J, Trout A, eds: *Targeting of Drugs*, Plenum Press, New York, 155–184, 1982.
24. Cooper RA, in Williams WJ, Beutler E, Erslev AJ, Rundles RW, eds: *Hematology*, 2nd ed, McGraw-Hill, New York, 216–229, 1977.
25. Ihler G, in Gregoriadis C, ed: *Drug Carriers in Biology and Medicine*, Academic Press, London, 129–153, 1979.
26. Arnon R, in Spreafico F, Arnon R, eds: *Tumor-Associated Antigens and Their Specific Immune Response*, Academic Press, New York, 287–304, 1979.
27. O'Neill GJ, in Gregoriadis G, ed: *Drug Carriers in Biology and Medicine*, Academic Press, London, 23–41, 1979.

CHAPTER 93

Aerosols

John J Sciarra, PhD
Executive Dean and Professor of Industrial Pharmacy

Anthony J Cutie, PhD
Associate Dean and Professor of Industrial Pharmacy
Arnold & Marie Schwartz College of Pharmacy and Health Sciences

Long Island University
Brooklyn, NY 11201

Many therapeutically active ingredients have been administered or applied to the body by means of the aerosol dosage form. This dosage form has been used both orally and topically to dispense a variety of agents such as epinephrine, isoproterenol, albuterol, antiseptics, beclomethasone, dexamethasone, and ergotamine. Oral aerosols have been used for the symptomatic treatment of asthma as well as for the treatment of migraine headache, while topical aerosols have been used to treat a multitude of dermatological manifestations. From preparations for the treatment of acne to a simple first-aid preparation, aerosols have been readily accepted by both the patient and physician as advantageous dosage forms.

Advantages—One of the main reasons for the rapid and widespread acceptance of the aerosol dosage form for the administration of therapeutically active agents is that it affords many and distinct advantages to the user. These advantages have been described by various investigators.

The pressure package is convenient and easy to use. Medication is dispensed in a ready-to-use form at the push of a button. There is generally no need for further handling of the medication. Since the medication is sealed in a tamper-proof pressure container, there is no danger of contamination of the product with foreign materials, and at the same time the contents can be protected from the deleterious effects of both air and moisture. Easily decomposed drugs, such as epinephrine, lend themselves to this type of package. When one considers the danger of contamination of unused topical, ophthalmic, ear, nose, and throat preparations, the importance of this advantage is obvious. Sterility is always an important consideration with certain pharmaceutical and medicinal preparations. While initial sterility is generally no problem to the manufacturer, there is concern for the maintenance of the sterility of the package during use as, for example, in ophthalmic preparations. When necessary, the aerosol package can be prepared under sterile conditions and sterility can be maintained throughout the life of the product. For those products requiring regulation of dosage, a metered valve can be used. While this is no more accurate than the administration of oral dosage forms, it is advantageous when used with topical preparations since indiscriminate use and overuse of the product can be avoided. In addition, when used with expensive products such as some steroids and antibiotics, savings can be achieved by the user as compared to the use of other topical preparations such as ointments, creams, or lotions. The aerosol dosage form allows for the dispensing of the product in the most desirable form; spray, foam, or semisolid. Depending on the nature of the product, the characteristics of the spray or foam can be changed to insure the proper and most efficient use of the medication.

Topical aerosol preparations have been used over the past 25–30 years as local anesthetics, antiseptics, germicides, first-aid preparations, body rubs, dermatological products, foot preparations, and spray-on protective films. These preparations have met with widespread acceptance, chiefly due to their many advantages over nonaerosol products. In addition to the advantages found in all aerosols, these aerosols possess several distinct advantages of their own.

The irritation produced by the application of an ointment or cream over an abraded area of the skin is reduced and sometimes eliminated by the aerosol. These preparations are more economical since they can be easily applied in a thin layer with no waste due to use of a cotton swab or other applicators. This may result in faster absorption and more efficient use of medications. Since the package is sealed, there is no danger of contamination of the unused portion of the medication. The cooling effect of liquefied-gas aerosols may be desirable in certain skin conditions.

There are many advantages to the administration of medicinal agents by inhalation. Response to drugs administered by inhalation is prompt, often very specific and with minimal side effects, faster in onset of activity compared with response to drugs given orally and with most drugs approaches intravenous therapy in rapidity of action. Drugs that are normally decomposed in the gastrointestinal tract can be safely administered by inhalation. The use of the self-pressurized aerosol package makes inhalation therapy simple, convenient, and acceptable compared to the use of atomizers and nebulizers, which are bulky and require cleaning.

Definitions—The term "aerosol" is used to denote various systems ranging from those of a colloidal nature to systems consisting of "pressurized packages." Aerosols have been defined as colloidal systems consisting of very finely subdivided liquid or solid particles dispersed in and surrounded by a gas. Originally, the term aerosol referred to liquid or solid particles having a specific size range, but this concept is falling into disuse.

An area of development essential to the success of the aerosol package concerned the valve. Various valves were produced that would dispense the product in the form of a fine stream, a fine mist, a coarse spray, or solid stream. Especially important are the metered valves that are essential for medicinal aerosols. These valves make it possible to dispense quantities of aerosol ranging from about 50 mg to 150 mg.

In 1978, the use of certain chlorofluorocarbons was seriously curtailed by the Food and Drug Administration, Environmental Protection Agency, and the Consumer Products Safety Commission. These restrictions applied to the use of Propellants 11, 12, and 114 and will be covered in greater detail in a later section of this chapter. Because of these restrictions, new valve systems and dispensing systems, which allowed greater use of liquefied hydrocarbon gases, were developed.

Mode of Operation

Liquefied-Gas Systems

Liquefied gases have been widely used as propellants for most aerosol products. These compounds are useful for this purpose since they are gases at room temperature and atmospheric pressure. However, they can be easily liquefied by lowering the temperature (below the boiling point) or by increasing the pressure. The compounds chosen generally have boiling points below 70°F (21°C) and vapor pressures between 13.4 and 85 psia at 70°F (21°C). When a liquefied gas propellant is placed into a sealed container, it immediately separates into a liquid and a vapor phase. Since these materials are liquefied gases, some of the molecules will leave the liquid state and enter the vapor state. As molecules enter the vapor state, a pressure gradually develops. As the number of molecules in the vapor state increases, the pressure will also increase. An equilibrium is soon attained between the number of molecules changing from a liquid to a vapor and from a vapor to a liquid. The pressure at this point is referred to as the vapor pressure (expressed as psia*) and is characteristic for each propellant at any given temperature. This vapor pressure is exerted equally in all directions and is independent of the quantity present. The pressure exerted against the liquid phase is sufficient to push the latter up a dip tube and against the valve. When the valve is opened, the liquid phase is emitted and comes into contact with the warm air at atmospheric pressure. The liquid propellant immediately reverts to the vapor state since its boiling point is substantially below room temperature. As the contents of the container are expelled, the volume within the container occupied by the vaporized propellant is increasing causing a temporary fall in pressure. However, as soon as the pressure decreases, a sufficient number of molecules change from the liquid state to the vapor state and restore the original pressure. When a compressed gas is used as the propellant, the relationship is quite different and there is a drop in pressure as the contents are used.

Two-Phase System—This is the simplest of all aerosol systems. It consists of a solution or a suspension of active ingredients in liquid propellant or a mixture of liquid propellant and solvent. Both a liquid and vapor phase are present, and when the valve is depressed, liquid propellant containing dissolved active ingredients and other solvents is released. Depending on the nature of the propellants used, the quantity of propellant present, and the valve mechanism, a fine mist or wet spray is produced due to the large expansion of the propellant at room temperature and atmospheric pressure. This system is used to formulate aerosols for inhalation or nasal application. Fluorocarbon propellants, primarily dichlorodifluoromethane and dichlorotetrafluoroethane, can be used for oral aerosols provided that an exemption is applied for through the filing of a New Drug Application for all new products and a supplemental application for existing products. All other solution- or suspension-type aerosols must utilize a hydrocarbon propellant or a compressed gas.

A *space spray* generally contains from 2 to 20% active ingredients and from 80 to 98% propellant. While the pressure of space sprays is in the range of 30 to 40 psig, the particles which are produced are from less than 1 μm to 50 μm. These particles remain suspended in air for relatively long periods of time. Space insecticides, room deodorants, and vaporizer sprays are examples of this type of system. A *surface-coating spray* (a relatively wet or coarse spray) can be achieved by

---

* The term psig represents the uncorrected gauge pressure and is to be distinguished from psia (pounds per square inch absolute) that is corrected to include atmospheric pressure (0 psig which equals 14.7 psia).

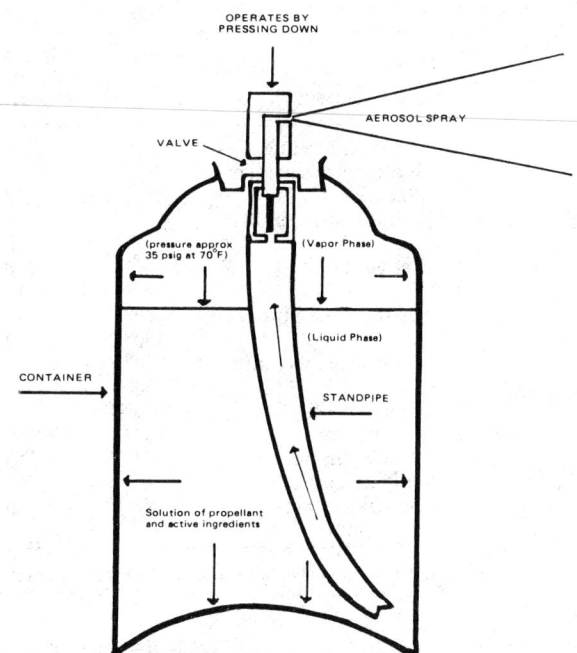

Fig 93-1.   Cross section of a typical space or surface-coating aerosol spray.

decreasing the amount of low-boiling propellants and increasing the ratio of active ingredients and solvents. The product concentrate can vary from 20 to 75% and the propellant from 25 to 80%. Particles are produced ranging in size from 50 μm to 200 μm. Products such as hair sprays, residual insecticides, perfumes, colognes, paints, protective coatings, and topical sprays are formulated in this manner. The pressure of this system is generally lower than the space spray.

Fig 93-1 shows a cross section of a typical space or surface-coating aerosol spray.

The propellants widely used for these aerosol systems consist of Propellants 12 and 114 (Table I), and propane, butane and isobutane (Table II). Combinations of Propellant 12/11 and Propellant 12/114 are used to achieve the desired results as to spray characteristics for inhalation type aerosols. In certain instances the nature of the product will determine the propellant combination. Dispersion or suspension sprays are similar to space and surface coating sprays in that they are two-phase systems where the active ingredients are suspended, rather than dissolved, in the liquid phase.

Three-Phase System—These are useful in that they allow for greater use of liquid components not miscible with the propellants. Water is not miscible with liquefied-gas propellants and in many instances presents a problem since active ingredients are soluble in water. These problems have been overcome to a large extent by use of the three-phase system. Depending on the nature of the formulation, one of the following two systems may be employed.

Two-Layer System—In this system the liquid propellant, the vaporized propellant, and the aqueous solution of active ingredients make up the three phases. Since the liquid propellant and water are not miscible, the liquid propellant will separate as an immiscible layer. When this propellant is of the fluorocarbon type, being denser than water, it will fall to the bottom of the container. Hydrocarbons, on the other hand, are lighter than water, and when used in this manner will float on top of the aqueous layer. A typical three-phase aerosol system is shown in Fig 93-2. A spray is produced by the mechanical action of an exceedingly small valve orifice through which the liquid is forced by the vapor pressure of the

Table I—Properties of Fluorocarbons[a]

Property		Trichloro-monofluoro-methane	Dichloro-difluoro-methane	Dichloro-tetrafluoro-ethane	Difluoro-ethane
Molecular formula		CCl_3F	CCl_2F_2	$CClF_2CClF_2$	CH_3CHF_2
Numerical designation		11	12	114	152a
Molecular weight		137.38	120.93	170.93	66.1
Boiling point (1 atm)	°F	74.7	−21.6	38.39	−12.0
	°C	23.7	−29.8	3.55	−11.0
Freezing point	°F	−168	−252	−137	—
	°C	−111	−158	−94	—
Vapor pressure (psia)	70°F	13.4	84.9	27.6	63.0
	130°F	39.0	196.0	73.5	176.3
Liquid density (g/mL)	70°F	1.485	1.325	1.468	0.91
	130°F	1.403	1.191	1.360	—
Liquid viscosity	70°F	0.439	0.262	0.386	—
(centipoise)	130°F	0.336	0.227	0.296	—
Surface tension (dynes/cm)	77°F	19	9	13	—
Solubility in water (weight %)	77°F	0.11	0.028	0.013	<1.0%

[a] These propellants are available as Freon (DuPont), and Genetron (Allied Chemical Corp.).

Table II—Properties of Hydrocarbons and Ethers

Property	Propane	Isobutane	n-Butane	Dimethyl Ether
Molecular formula	C_3H_8	C_4H_{10}	C_4H_{10}	CH_3OCH_3
Molecular weight	44.1	58.1	58.1	46.1
Boiling point (°F)	−43.7	10.9	31.1	−13
Vapor pressure (psig at 70°F)	110.0	30.4	16.5	63.0
Liquid density (g/mL at 70°F)	0.50	0.56	0.58	0.66
Flash point (°F)	−156	−117	−101	—

propellant. The vapor layer is continuously replaced by vapors from the liquid layer of propellant. None of the liquefied gas propellant is introduced into the aqueous solution while it is being ejected and, therefore, the breakup of the stream

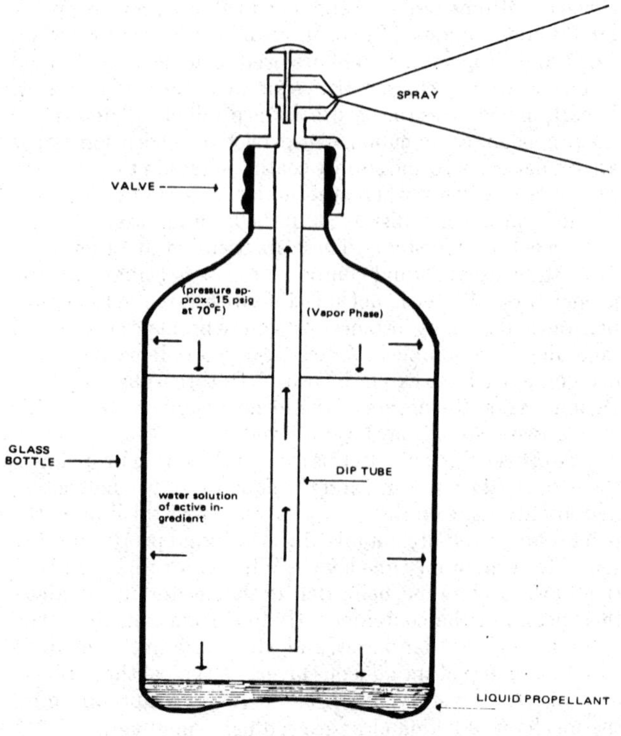

Fig 93-2.   Three-phase glass aerosol.

is due chiefly to the action of the "mechanical breakup actuator." This system generally operates at a pressure of about 15–20 psig and utilizes about 5–10% propellant.

A modification of this system involves replacement of the aqueous solution with a hydroalcoholic component. The propellants used consist of hydrocarbons such as butane, isobutane, and propane. An important characteristic of this system is that the propellant layer can be adjusted by varying the components so its specific gravity almost equals but does not exceed that of the hydroalcoholic phase. The propellant floats on top of the hydroalcoholic phase and, when shaken, is easily dispersed. When the valve is depressed, sprays are produced of varying characteristics depending on the nature of the formulation.

This system is one form of what are generally referred to as "water-based" aerosols. In some cases, water is used as the solvent together with either isobutane, or a mixture of hydrocarbon propellants. Depending on the nature of any surfactants which may be present, the product can be delivered as a spray or foam. While these products tend to produce somewhat larger particles than those produced with solvent-based products, nevertheless they are effective.

A recent development, which is another modification of the three-phase aerosol, is the *Aquasol* system developed by the Precision Valve Corporation. This system provides for the dispensing of a fine mist or spray of active ingredient dissolved in water. This is not possible with the usual three-phase system. Since only active ingredient and water (propellant is in a vapor state and present in only extremely small quantity) are dispensed, there is no problem associated with the use of the propellant.

Fig 93-3 illustrates the Aquasol dispenser system. This system is designed to dispense pressurized products efficiently and economically using relatively small amounts of hydro-

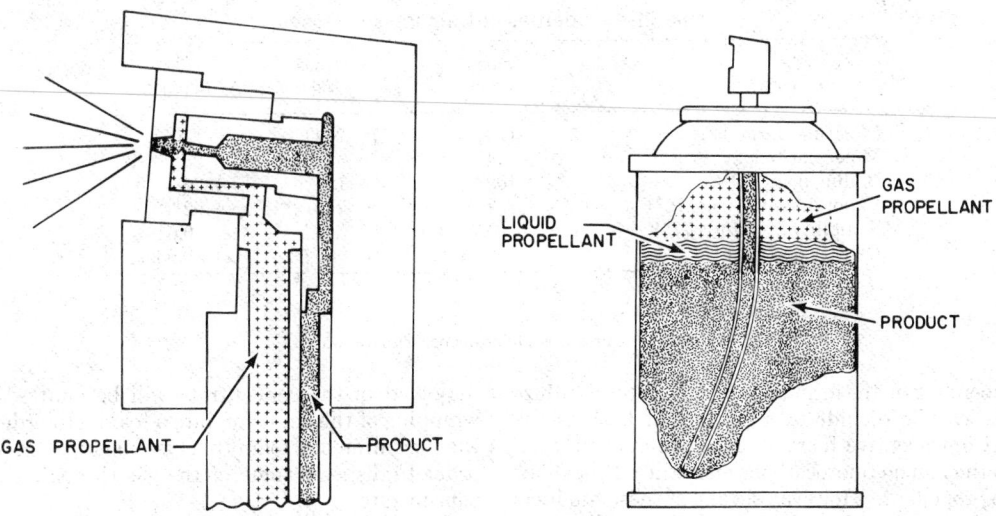

Fig 93-3.   The Aquasol Dispenser System (courtesy, Precision Valve Corporation).

carbon propellant. It should be indicated that the system can also function effectively using fluorocarbon propellant. And fairly large quantities of water may be used in the formulation. The chief difference between this new system and the "three-phase" aerosol system is that the Aquasol will dispense a fairly dry spray of very small particles. While exact measurement of particle-size distribution has not been made, it is believed that the particles are below 10 μm in diameter. This dryness of the particles and their relatively small size is due chiefly to the design of the valve, which dispenses vaporized propellant rather than liquefied propellant. This also contributes to the nonflammability of the stream of product as it is dispensed. For example, a fine, almost dry spray is obtained using six parts of water (or a water/alcohol mixture) with one part of hydrocarbon propellant. The resulting spray is not only nonflammable, but will actually extinguish an open flame.

As one will note from Fig 93-3, the active ingredient is dissolved or suspended in water or a mixture of alcohol and water. The hydrocarbon propellant will float on top of the aqueous layer and will exist as both liquid and vapor. Depending on the amount of alcohol present in the aqueous layer, the propellant and water/alcohol layer may be immiscible. As the amount of alcohol increases, the miscibility of these two layers will be increased. As one approaches a pure alcohol system, complete miscibility will occur, resulting in a two-phase system which can also function satisfactorily. However, flammability will be increased due to the large amount of alcohol present as well as the fact that liquid propellant is now also being dispensed. Fluorocarbon propellants function equally as well as hydrocarbons, since they are heavier than water and will be beneath the water layer. In the Aquasol system the vapor phase of the propellant and the product enter the mixing chamber in the actuator through separate ducts or channels. The vaporized propellant enters, moving at tremendous velocity, while the product is forced into the actuator by the pressure of the propellant. It is at this point that product and vapor are mixed with violent force, resulting in a uniform finely dispersed spray. Depending on the configuration of the valve and actuator either a fine dry or a wet spray can be obtained. Previous studies have shown that a fine dry spray is obtained when one utilizes a system with a ratio of about six parts of product to one part of propellant. Up to thirty parts of product to one part of propellant has also produced a satisfactory spray but then a wetter spray would result. In the Aquasol system it is almost impossible to dispense only the pure propellant.

Water-based aerosols developed for use in this system

would have the advantage that the chilling effect associated with liquefied gas systems is eliminated. Since only vaporized propellant is dispensed, less propellant in the container is required. With greater use of water as a solvent for active ingredients a greater range of products can be developed.

Foam System—Foam aerosols, which are often classified separately, consist of three-phase systems wherein the liquid propellant, which normally does not exceed 10% by weight, is emulsified with the propellant. When the valve is depressed, the emulsion is forced through the nozzle and, in the presence of warm air and at atmospheric pressure, the entrapped propellant reverts to a vapor and whips the emulsion into a foam. The use of a dip tube is optional with this type of system and, when present, the container is designed for upright use. For those containers where the dip tube is omitted, the container must be inverted prior to use. Foam valves have been developed which are applicable to both types of packages. Foam products operate at a pressure of about 35 to 40 psig at 70°F (21°C) and generally contain about 4–7% propellant. A typical foam-type aerosol can be seen in Fig 93-4. Shave creams and shampoos, as well as several topical pharmaceuticals, have been formulated as foam aerosols. Generally, a blend of propane/isobutane is used for foam

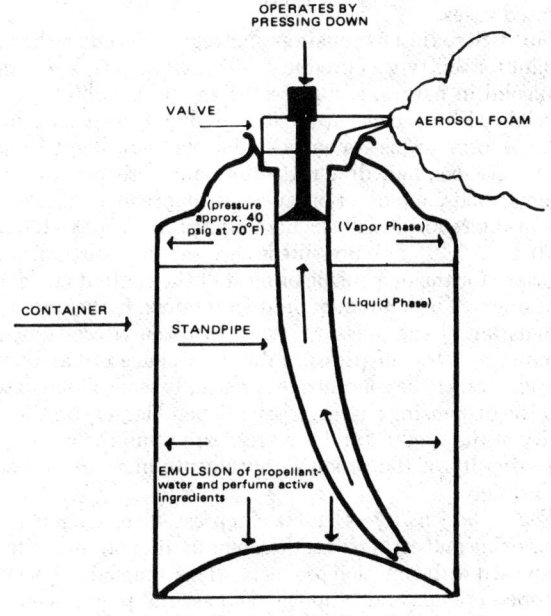

Fig 93-4.   Foam-type aerosol.

Table III—Properties of Compressed Gases

Property	Carbon Dioxide	Nitrous Oxide	Nitrogen
Molecular formula	CO_2	N_2O	N_2
Molecular weight	44	44	28
Boiling point °F	-109^a	-127	-320
Vapor pressure, psia, 70°F	852	735	492^b
Solubility in water,^{c} 77°F	0.7	0.5	0.014
Density (gas) g/mL.	1.53	1.53	0.96699

^{a} Sublimes.

^{b} At Critical Point (−233°F).

^{c} Volume of gas at atmospheric pressure soluble in one volume of water.

aerosols. Depending on the formulation, some aerosols utilize nitrous oxide, carbon dioxide or a mixture of both as the propellant. Contraceptive foam aerosols are currently exempted from the ban on fluorocarbons and utilize Propellant 12/114 as the propellant. However, several of these products have been reformulated using a hydrocarbon propellant.

Several other developments in this area involve the development of the "quick-breaking" foam, nonaqueous foam, and water-based aerosols. These will be covered in a later portion of this chapter.

Compressed-Gas Aerosols

Compressed gases are used to dispense the product as a solid stream, wet spray, or foam. These aerosol products utilize an inert gas such as nitrogen, carbon dioxide, or nitrous oxide as the propellant. The gas is compressed in the container, and it is the expansion of the compressed gas which provides the push or the force necessary to expel the contents from the container. As the contents of the container are expelled, the volume of the gas will increase causing a drop in pressure according to Boyle's law.

$$P = k\frac{1}{V}$$

where P = pressure and V = volume of gas. At constant temperature this law can be expressed as

$$P_1V_1 = P_2V_2$$

This enables one to calculate the drop in pressure as the contents of a compressed-gas aerosol are used. Table III indicates some of the more important properties of these compressed gases.

Solid-Stream Dispensing—Nitrogen is used as the propellant for this type of product. The concentrate is generally semisolid in nature, and since the gas is insoluble and immiscible with the concentrate, the product is dispensed in its original form. This system is applicable to the dispensing of dental creams, hair dressings, ointments, creams, cosmetic creams, foods, and other products. Compressed-gas aerosols operate at a substantially higher initial pressure of 90–100 psig at 70°F (21°C). This pressure is necessary to insure adequate pressure for the dispensing of most of the contents from the container. The amount of product retained in the unit after exhaustion of the pressure varies with the viscosity of the product and loss of pressure due to seepage of gas during storage. Since the concentrate is generally semisolid in nature and the dispensing characteristics depend largely on the viscosity of the product and the pressure within the container, the viscosity of the product concentrate must be adjusted accordingly.

Foam Dispensing—Soluble compressed gases such as nitrous oxide and carbon dioxide can be used to produce a foam when used with emulsion products. This system is typical for whipped creams and toppings, and several pharmaceutical and veterinary products. When this system is used, the gas dissolved in the concentrate will be emitted and cause a whipping of the emulsion into a foam. In order to facilitate the formation of a foam this system is shaken prior to use in order to disperse some of the gas throughout the product concentrate.

Spray Dispensing—This system is similar to a space or surface spray except that a compressed gas is used as the propellant. Since these gases do not possess the dispersing power of the liquefied gases, a mechanical breakup actuator is used. The product is dispensed as a wet spray and is applicable to solutions of medicinal agents in aqueous solvents.

Other Systems

Piston Type—Since it is difficult to completely empty the contents of a semisolid from an aerosol container, a piston-type aerosol system has been developed. This utilizes a polyethylene piston fitted into an aluminum container. The concentrate is placed into the upper portion of the container. The pressure from nitrogen (about 90–100 psig) or a liquefied hydrocarbon gas pushes against the other side of the piston; when the valve is opened, the product is dispensed. The piston scrapes against the sides of the container and dispenses most of the product concentrate.

The piston-type aerosol system, termed "MiraFla" (*Am Can*) is shown in Fig 93-5. This system has been successfully used to package cheese spreads, cake decorating icings, and ointments. Since the products which use this system are semisolid and viscous, they are dispensed as a lazy stream rather than as a foam or spray. This system is limited to

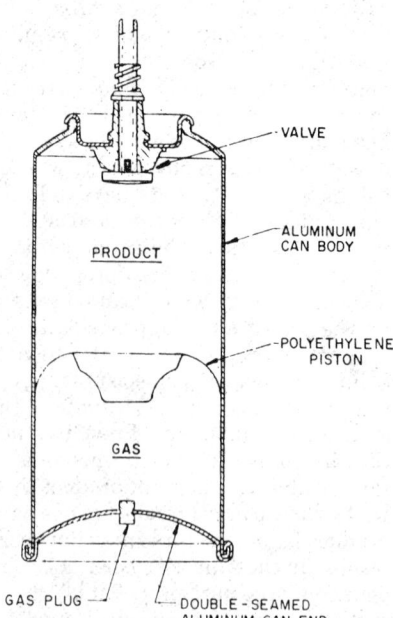

Fig 93-5. Free-piston aerosol system (courtesy, Am Can).

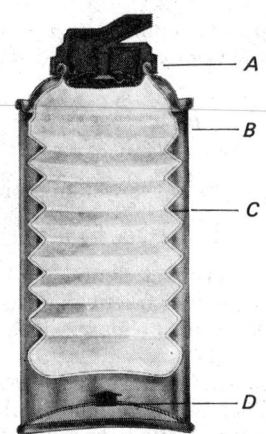

Fig 93-6.   Plastic bag aerosol system (Sepro). *A:* valve; *B:* standard three-piece tin-plate container; *C:* plastic bag; *D:* gas filling port (courtesy, Continental Can).

viscous materials since limpid liquids, such as water, alcohol, etc, will pass between the wall of the container and piston.

Plastic Bag Type—This system consists of a collapsible plastic bag fitted into a standard, three-piece, tinplate container as shown in Fig 93-6. The product is placed within the bag and the propellant is added through the bottom of the container. Since the product is placed into a plastic bag, there is no contact between the product and the container wall except for any product which may escape by permeation through the plastic bag.

Limpid liquids, such as water, can be dispensed either as a stream or fine mist depending on the type of valve used, while semisolid substances are dispensed as a stream. In order to prevent the gas from pinching the bag and preventing the dispensing of product, the inner plastic bag is accordion-pleated. The Sepro container (*Continental Can*), as this system is called, can be used for a variety of different pharmaceutical and nonpharmaceutical systems.

A modification of this system dispenses the product as a gel which will then foam. By dissolving a low-boiling liquid such as pentane in the product, a foam will result when the product is placed on the hands and the warmth of the hands will cause vaporization of the pentane. This system is used to dispense a shaving gel.

Propellants

The propellant is generally regarded as the "heart" of the aerosol package. In addition to supplying the necessary force to expel the product, it must also act as a solvent and diluent and has much to do with determining the characteristics of the product as it leaves the container. Various chemical compounds have been used as aerosol propellants.

Compounds useful as propellants can be classified as follows:

Liquefied gases
    Fluorinated chlorinated hydrocarbons (halocarbons)
    Hydrocarbons
Compressed gases

Liquefied Gases

The liquefied gas compounds have widespread use as propellants since they are extremely effective in dispersing the active ingredients into a fine mist or foam, depending on the form desired. In addition they are relatively inert and nontoxic. They have the added advantage that the pressure within the container remains constant. Prior to the ban on use of fluorocarbons as propellants, two types of liquefied gases were used. The fluorinated hydrocarbons found greater

use since they are nonflammable as contrasted to the flammable hydrocarbons. The hydrocarbons are advantageous since they are less expensive than fluorocarbons. Following the ban on fluorocarbons, hydrocarbon propellants became the propellants of choice for all aerosols except those specifically exempted.

Liquefied gases provide a nearly constant pressure during packaging operations and have a large expansion ratio. Several of the fluorinated hydrocarbons have an expansion ratio of about 240, that is, 1 mL of liquefied gas will occupy a volume of approximately 240 mL if allowed to vaporize. Dimethyl ether has a value of over 350. On the other hand, compressed gases expand only to the extent of 3 to 10 times their original volume.

Fluorinated Hydrocarbons—Several of the fluorocarbons have been used as propellants in the past and since 1978 have been of limited use only in specifically exempted oral aerosols and contraceptive vaginal foams. These propellants are primarily derived from methane, ethane, and cyclobutane and are prepared by replacing one or more of the hydrogens of these compounds with chlorine and/or fluorine.

The physicochemical properties of these compounds are of prime importance in the formulation and manufacture of aerosol products. The solvent power, stability, and reactivity of the propellants must be known and understood. Just as one considers the properties of some of the usually encountered nonaerosol liquids such as ethanol, glycerin, and acetone, so should the propellant be considered.

Nomenclature—In order to refer easily to the fluorinated hydrocarbons a relatively simple system of nomenclature was developed some time ago by the refrigeration industry. A numerical designation is used to identify each propellant.

1. All propellants are designated by three digits. When the first digit is zero, the propellant is designated by two digits.
2. The first digit is one less than the number of carbon atoms in the compound. Where there are only 2 digits, zero is understood to be this figure and indicates a methane derivative (1 + 0). When this digit is 1, the propellant is an ethane derivative.
3. The second digit is one more than the number of hydrogen atoms in the compound.
4. The last digit represents the number of fluorine atoms.
5. The number of chlorine atoms in the compound is found by subtracting the sum of the fluorine and the hydrogen atoms from the total number of atoms which can be added to saturate the carbon chain.
6. In the case of isomers each has the same number and the most symmetric one is indicated by the number alone. As the isomers become more and more asymmetric, the letter a, b, c, etc, follows the number.
7. For cyclic compounds, a C is used before the number.

The use of this system can be exemplified as follows: Propellant 114 is an ethane derivative, has no hydrogens, and contains 4 fluorine atoms. Since 6 atoms are required to saturate the carbon chain, of necessity there must be 2 chlorine atoms. These can be arranged in two different ways; however, since there is no letter following the numerical designation, the symmetrical structure refers to Propellant 114.

$$\begin{array}{cc}
\quad\;\; \mathrm{F}\;\;\;\; \mathrm{F} & \quad\;\; \mathrm{F}\;\;\;\; \mathrm{F}\\
\quad\;\; | \;\;\;\;\; | & \quad\;\; | \;\;\;\;\; |\\
\mathrm{F{-}C{-}C{-}F} & \mathrm{Cl{-}C{-}C{-}F}\\
\quad\;\; | \;\;\;\;\; | & \quad\;\; | \;\;\;\;\; |\\
\quad\;\; \mathrm{Cl}\;\; \mathrm{Cl} & \quad\;\; \mathrm{Cl}\;\; \mathrm{F}\\
\textbf{Propellant 114} & \textbf{Propellant 114a}
\end{array}$$

Physical Properties—Table I shows some of the more useful physicochemical properties of these propellants. Propellants 11, 12, and 114 were admitted to the NF.

From a solubility standpoint, the fluorinated hydrocarbons, which are nonpolar, are miscible with most nonpolar solvents over a wide range of temperature. They also are capable of dissolving many substances. For the most part the propellants are not miscible with water, although the degree of miscibility depends on the individual propellants. A cosolvent such as ethanol, 2-propanol, or acetone must be used with water in order to produce a clear solution. However, when one considers that these propellants can only be used for oral aerosols, the choice of cosolvent is extremely limited, in many cases to the use of ethyl alcohol. The alternative is to form an emulsion.

One of the most important physicochemical properties of a propellant is its vapor pressure, which may be defined as the pressure exerted by a liquid in equilibrium with its vapor. When the vapor pressure exceeds atmospheric pressure, boiling and vaporization take place. However, if the vaporized molecules are prevented from leaving the container (by placing the propellant into a sealed container), they will fill the head space and eventually cause an increase in pressure. The pressure developed at equilibrium is the vapor pressure. The vapor pressure of a liquefied gas is independent of the quantity used but is influenced by temperature changes. Assuming ideal behavior for the liquefied gas, the effect of temperature on the vapor pressure can be calculated from the following equation:

$$\log P = -\frac{\Delta H_{\text{vap}}}{2.303\,RT}$$

where P = vapor pressure, ΔH = heat of vaporization, R = gas constant (generally 1.987 cal deg^{-1} mole^{-1}), and T = absolute temperature.

Since

$$\ln P = -\frac{\Delta H_{\text{vap}}}{RT} + C$$

a plot of the log P vs $1/T$ should yield a straight line and from this the heat of vaporization may be calculated.

$$\Delta H_{\text{vap}} \text{ (cal mole}^{-1}) = -(\text{slope})(2.303\,R)$$

These equations can be used to predict the behavior of pure propellants at elevated temperatures. When one considers that an aerosol preparation consists of a propellant and solvents or mixtures of these, the vapor-pressure considerations are somewhat different. By mixing various propellants such as Propellants 11 and 12 or Propellants 12 and 114, a range of vapor pressures is obtained as seen in Fig 93-7. The vapor pressure of a mixture of propellants may be calculated from Raoult's law, which states that the "vapor pressure of a solution is dependent upon the vapor pressure of the individual components. For ideal solutions, the vapor pressure is equal to the sum of the mole fractions of each component present times the vapor pressure of the pure compound at the desired temperature." Mathematically this law may be expressed as

$$p_A = \frac{n_A}{n_A + n_B}\,p_A{}^\circ = N_A p_A{}^\circ$$

where p_A = partial vapor pressure of Component A, $p_A{}^\circ$ =

vapor pressure of pure Component A, n_A = moles of Component A, n_B = moles of Component B, and N_A = mole fraction of Component A.

$$p_B = \frac{n_B}{n_B + n_A}\,p_B{}^\circ = N_B p_B{}^\circ$$

The total vapor pressure of the system is obtained by

$$P_{\text{total}} = p_A + p_B$$

When the mole fraction of one component is large, the other component has a small mole fraction and as such it does not appreciably affect the vapor pressure. This approaches ideal behavior.

Where the components are of similar physical and chemical nature, the experimentally determined values and the calculated values are approximately the same. In the case of the fluorinated hydrocarbons, the deviation from ideal behavior is not great and the results are approximately equal or within 5%. Where other solvents are present, such as alcohols or acetone, the vapor pressures can be calculated in a similar manner. However, the vapor pressure of mixtures of these solvents and propellants deviates a great deal from ideal behavior and there is significant difference between the actual and theoretical values. The vapor pressure of many systems consisting of mixtures of various propellants and solvents has been determined. Four factors contribute to any positive deviation:

1. Internal pressure of the two components in the propellant-solvent mixture.
2. Polarity.
3. Length of the hydrocarbon chain or analogous grouping.
4. Association in the liquid phase of either component.

For more detailed information concerning the physicochemical aspects of propellants and aerosol systems the references at the end of this chapter should be consulted.

Chemical Properties—The fluorinated hydrocarbons have been widely used as aerosol propellants because they are generally considered to be chemically inert. From the standpoint of formulation, the only chemical property that need be considered is hydrolysis. While addition of fluorine to a carbon atom generally increases stability, a propellant such as trichloromonofluoromethane may undergo hydrolysis with formation of hydrochloric acid. Propellant 11 is not used with aqueous products as hydrolysis will occur; Propellant 114 is generally used instead.

Hydrocarbons—Hydrocarbon propellants have replaced fluorocarbons for pharmaceutical aerosols. Their low-order toxicity makes them suitable for use, while their flammability limits their use. With the development of newer types of dispensing valves, the flammability hazard has been considerably reduced. The advantage of hydrocarbons is their greater range of solubility and lower cost compared to fluorinated hydrocarbons; to date they represent the only suitable replacement for fluorocarbons as propellants.

In addition to having the proper vapor pressure, hydrocarbons have other properties that make them useful as propellants. Thus their density of less than 1, and their immiscibility with water, make them useful in the formulation of three-phase (two-layer) aerosols. Being lighter than water, the hydrocarbon remains on top of the aqueous layer and serves to push the contents out of the container. Not being halogenated, hydrocarbons generally possess better solubility characteristics than the fluorinated hydrocarbons.

As with fluorocarbons, a range of pressures can be obtained by mixing various hydrocarbons in varying proportions. As the composition of the hydrocarbons is likely to vary somewhat, depending on their source, blending of hydrocarbons must be based on the final pressure desired and not on the basis of a stated proportion of each component, the pressure

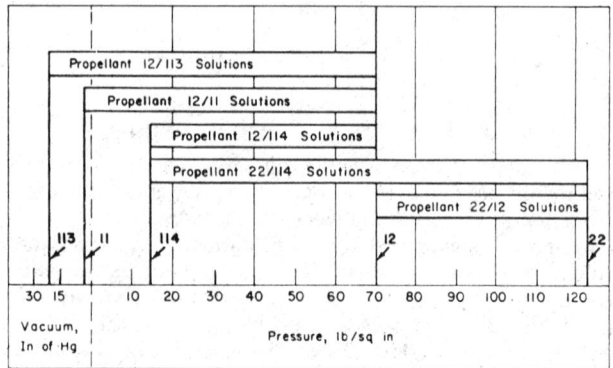

Fig 93-7. Range of pressures obtainable at 70°F with various propellants.

Table IV—Commonly Used Hydrocarbon Blends

Designation[a]	Pressure psig at 70°F	Composition—mole per cent			
		n-Butane	Propane	iso-Butane	Other
A-108	108 ± 4	traces	99	1	traces of ethane
A-31	31 ± 2	3	1	96	
A-17	17 ± 2	98	traces	2	traces of isopentane
A-24	24 ± 2	49.2	0.6	50	0.1 each of *neo*- and *iso*-pentane
A-40	40 ± 2	2	12	86	
A-46	46 ± 2	2	20	78	
A-52	52 ± 2	2	28	70	
A-70	70 ± 2	1	51	48	

[a] Designations used by Phillips Chemical Company, Bartlesville, Oklahoma.

of which will depend on its purity. Table IV lists some commonly used blends that are commercially available.

Finally, it should be indicated that the hydrocarbons are further characterized by their extreme chemical stability. They are not subject to hydrolysis, making them useful with water-based aerosols. They will react with the halogens, but only under severe conditions.

Recently, dimethyl ether (Dymel-*Du Pont*) has become available for use as a propellant. This propellant has been used in combination with other propellants. Dimethyl ether is especially useful due to its high water solubility compared to other propellants.

Compressed Gases

The compressed gases such as nitrogen, nitrous oxide, and carbon dioxide have been used as aerosol propellants. Depending on the nature of the formulation and the valve design, the product can be dispensed as a fine mist, foam, or semisolid. However, unlike the liquefied gases, the compressed gases possess little, if any, expansion power and will produce a fairly wet spray and foams which are not as stable as liquefied-gas foams. This system has been used for the most part to dispense food products and for non-foods to dispense the product in its original form as a semisolid. Compressed gases have been used in products such as dental creams, hair preparations, ointments, and aqueous antiseptic and germicidal aerosols.

Since compressed gases are utilized in the gaseous state and not in the liquid state, a higher initial pressure is required as well as a relatively larger head space than liquefied-gas aerosols. While the pressure of a liquefied-gas aerosol remains constant during use, a drop in pressure is noted during use of a compressed-gas aerosol. This drop in pressure can be calculated by application of the ideal gas laws:

$$PV = nRT$$

where P = pressure in atmosphere, V = volume in L, n = moles of gas (g/mol wt), R = gas constant (0.08205 L atmos deg^{-1} mole^{-1}), and T = absolute temperature.

The initial pressure of a compressed-gas aerosol is usually about 90 psig and occupies a volume of about 15–25% of the container volume. As the contents of the container are expelled, the volume of head space increases with a corresponding decrease in pressure according to Boyle's law.

The physical and chemical properties of the compressed gases are not as vital to formulation as the properties of the liquefied gases. These gases are, for the most part, chemically inert and do not react with the product concentrate. In the case of nitrogen there is no solubility of the gas in the product, whereas nitrous oxide and carbon dioxide are soluble to a certain extent. Table III indicates this solubility. Mixtures of nitrous oxide and carbon dioxide have been used as propellants for whipped creams and toppings and also for several

veterinary emulsion products. The solubility of carbon dioxide in certain beverage food products is advantageous in that a slight degree of carbonation can be obtained. Since these gases are generally inert and replace the air trapped in the head space, the stability of drugs is sometimes increased.

A serious drawback to the use of these gases as propellants is the loss of propellant through product misuse or leakage; once the propellant is lost, the package becomes inoperative.

Flammability and Toxicity Considerations

Aerosol products are intended for spraying into large enclosed areas or application as a foam; as such both flammability and toxicity are important. For pharmaceutical and medicinal aerosols the effects of inhalation or topical application must also be determined.

Fluorinated hydrocarbons do not present any flammability hazards; in fact they will extinguish a flame by excluding oxygen. Hydrocarbons are flammable and will form explosive mixtures with certain concentrations of air. It is for this reason that caution must be exercised during manufacture and packaging of aerosol products containing a hydrocarbon propellant. The compressed gases are not flammable and can be handled safely.

Propellant Toxicity—Ever since the initial reports were issued on the cardiotoxicity of aerosol propellants, a flood of reports have indicated either that the propellants were toxic or safe. Some noted that the fluoroalkane gases used to propel aerosols were toxic to the heart of mice, sensitizing them to asphyxia-induced sinus bradycardia, atrioventricular block, and T-wave depression. The propellants were postulated to possess a spectrum of cardiotoxic effects capable of causing bradyarrhythmias, tachyarrhythmias, or myocardial depression. Others reported that the lack of oxygen, not cardiac toxicity of the fluorocarbon propellants, was the probable cause of death of the mice. The fluorocarbon propellants have very low-order toxicity on the scale of comparative toxicities. The vapors of the fluorocarbon propellants produce narcotic effects if inhaled at a high-enough concentration. Deliberate misuse by collecting and inhaling concentrated vapors of propellants in the absence of oxygen probably causes death. From the practical point of view, it is important to note that the induction of cardiac sensitization or asphyxia requires deliberate inhalation of high concentrations of propellants—much higher concentrations than those generated when aerosol products, including asthma inhalers, are used as directed—and also that there is no evidence of any form of chronic cardiac toxicity.

Product Toxicity—For many years, aerosols containing epinephrine or isoproterenol have been the center of controversy. Restrictions were placed on the labeling of aerosol preparations containing isoproterenol in 1968 when several reports of death through alleged overuse of isoproterenol aerosols came to light. The *Federal Register* of June 18, 1968 indicated that all inhalation preparations containing isoproterenol must bear the following statement:

Occasional patients have been reported to develop severe paradoxical airway resistance with repeated, excessive use of isoproterenol inhalation preparations. The cause of this refractory state is unknown. It is advisable that in such instances the use of this preparation be discontinued immediately and alternative therapy instituted, since in the reported cases the patients did not respond to other forms of therapy until the drug was withdrawn.

Deaths have been reported following excessive use of isoproterenol inhalation preparations, and the exact cause is unknown. Cardiac arrest was noted in several instances.

Since 1968, reports of adverse reaction continued to appear in the medical literature. In addition to isoproterenol preparations, epinephrine aerosols were said to cause similar reactions when overused. The *Federal Register* then published (April 15, 1972) that similar warning statements would be required for epinephrine inhalation preparations. Since the reports showed that severe paradoxical bronchoconstriction episodes, but no deaths, occurred as a result of excessive and repeated use of epinephrine inhalation preparations, only the first warning statement indicated for isoproterenol inhalation preparations must be included and not the statement concerning deaths following excessive use.

From the time the first aerosol product was used commercially in the late 1940s, reports have appeared on the possible hazard of inhaling aerosol particles. Various aerosols have become suspect as to manifestations of toxicity. Feminine hygiene sprays, medicated vaporizer sprays, and adhesive sprays have been subjected to scrutiny by consumer and governmental agencies, often resulting in their withdrawal from the marketplace.

Skin sensitization to the propellants should be considered since many products are applied topically. There have been no reported cases of skin sensitization and rabbit-eye tests have indicated their lack of sensitization. Several investigators reported the possible chilling effect of liquefied gases when applied to the skin.

Containers

Metal

Tin-Plated Steel—In order to produce an aerosol container which was light and relatively inexpensive, tin-plated steel was used for aerosol containers. This resulted in the large scale production of aerosol containers.

Side-Seam—Following this, the beer-can type was developed and finally led to the present-day three-piece container. This container consists of a body and two ends. The body is seamed longitudinally and the bottom is flanged and joined by a double-seaming operation. The top is pressed into shape and curled into a 1-in. opening and attached to the body in a similar manner to the attachment of the bottom. This makes for an exceptionally strong container and is available in sizes varying from 3 to 24 oz.

The tin plate which is used consists of steel base coated with varying thicknesses of tin. For example, a 25 # tin plate indicates that $\frac{1}{4}$ lb of tin has been used to coat both sides of steel in a base box (a base box consists of 112 sheets, 20 × 14 in). A 50 #, 75 #, and 100 # tin plate is available in a hot-dipped plate. In many instances the body of the container is made to have a certain thickness of tin and the ends would have another thickness. This is done in order to obtain increased stability in the container.

For certain products the tin affords sufficient protection so that no further treatment is necessary. Hair lacquers generally can be packaged in this type of container. However, the addition of water and other corrosive ingredients or other

substances which will attack tin requires a container having an additional protective coating. This coating is usually organic in nature and may consist of an oleoresin, phenolic, vinyl, or epoxy coating. The liner (single or double coat) is added to the container prior to fabrication, that is, it is applied to the flat sheets of tin plate.

Two-Piece or Drawn—The body is made of black iron formed from 100-lb deep-drawn sheet stock by a multiple-die drawing process. The bottom is concave and double-seamed into place. The opening is made to hold the standard 1-in. valve. The organic coating is generally applied by a spray process following fabrication. Containers are available in 6- and 12-oz capacity.

Aluminum—These are produced by an impact extrusion process so that the container is seamless. This will give added strength to the container. A variety of different aluminum aerosol containers ranging in size from 15 mL to 45 fl oz is available. While aluminum is less reactive than other metals used in can manufacture, added resistance can be obtained by coating the inside of the container with organic materials such as epoxy, vinyl, and phenolic resins.

Stainless Steel—These containers have been developed mainly for use in perfume and medicinal aerosols. When Propellant 12 is used as the propellant, a stronger than usual container is needed. These containers are relatively expensive and are available in sizes ranging from 5 to 30 mL.

Glass—For pharmaceuticals and medicinals, glass is preferred due to the absence of incompatibilities, as well as for its esthetic value. The use of glass containers is limited to those products having a lower pressure and lower percentage of propellant. Glass aerosols have found use in packaging of many perfumes, colognes, cosmetics, pharmaceuticals, and medicinals. While glass is basically stronger than most metallic containers, a potential hazard is present if, and when, the container is dropped with subsequent breakage. However, the danger involved can be compared somewhat to the hazard involved in the use of carbonated beverages in the home. Two types of glass aerosol containers are available. The uncoated glass container has the advantage of decreased cost and high clarity. The contents can be viewed at all times. The plastic-coated glass containers are protected by a coating which prevents the glass from shattering in the event of breakage. In one type the coating is bonded to the glass and becomes an integral part of the container. In another type, the coating fits over the glass container.

Valves

Probably the most basic part of any aerosol or pressurized package is the valve mechanism through which the content of the package is emitted. Together with the formulation, the valve determines the performance of a pressurized package. The interaction of these two is such that one cannot readily be discussed without reference to the other.

The primary purpose of the valve is to regulate the flow of product from the container. It provides a means of discharging the desired amount when needed and prevents loss at other times. The valve also exerts a major effect on the character of the dispensed product. For example, a product formulated to produce a foam can be dispensed as a spray or as a wet stream by the use of different actuators or push buttons on the valve. The selection of proper propellants also governs whether a foam, spray, or wet stream will be produced.

Spray Valves

Since the spray valve is the most commonly used valve, it will be discussed in detail. A cross-sectional view of one such valve mounted on a glass aerosol bottle is shown in Fig 93-8.

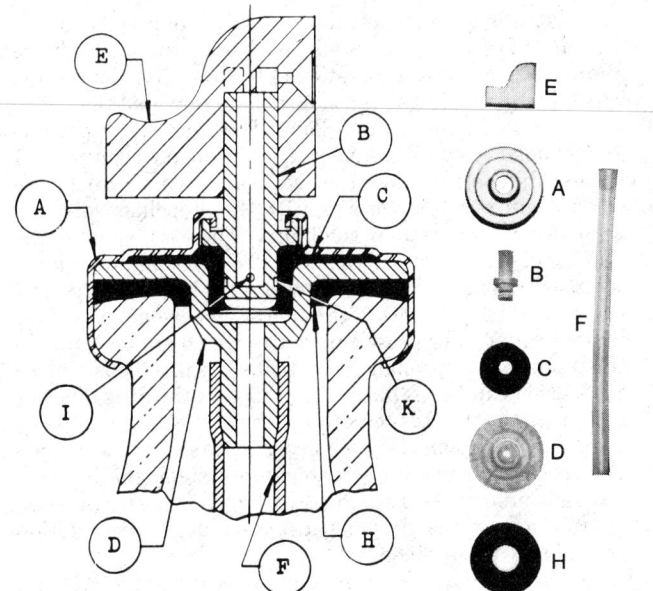

Fig 93-8.   Aerosol valve (courtesy, Risdon).

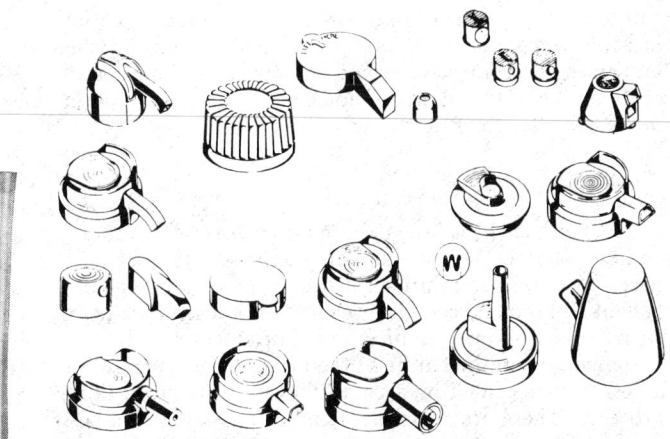

Fig 93-9.   A variety of spray, foam, and solid-stream actuators (courtesy, Precision Valve).

It may be noted that the core, B, is seated in a snugly fitting rubber valve seat, C. The two orifices, I, are 180° apart and extend through the walls of the core into groove K which circles the lower end of the core. Valve seat C is a snug fit in valve cup D to which is attached the dip tube F. Gasket H provides a seal between the valve and the bottle. All of these parts are held together and to the bottle by a ferrule A which has been curled under the lip of the bottle. The actuator, E, carries or has formed in it the spray orifice and also provides a means for operating the valve. If the actuator is pushed at E, the core will be tilted and deflected from the seat at the lower left-hand corner. The groove will be uncovered and will allow the pressurized product to rise through the dip tube, pass through the orifices, rise through the core, and spray out through the terminal orifice. When finger pressure is removed from E, the core snaps back to the closed position due to the elasticity of the rubber seat.

A small hole of about 0.013 to 0.020 in. in diameter is sometimes placed in the valve housing. This allows for the escape of a small quantity of vaporized propellant along with the product. This gives a greater degree of dispersion to the emitted spray as well as cleaning of the valve orifices following discharge. However, since a greater amount of propellant is used as compared to nonvapor tap systems, care must be exercised during formulation of the product to take this into account. One may also note a change in spray pattern from start to finish due to the change in propellant composition which takes place as the contents are used. Vapor tap valves are used with powder aerosols, water-based aerosols and aerosols containing suspended materials and other agents which would tend to clog the valve. They are currently used with hydrocarbon aerosols since the flame extension of the spray can be substantially reduced through use of a vapor tap valve. This is accomplished by balancing the size of the vapor tap opening and the valve orifice.

Foam Valves

Valves for foam or aerated products usually have only one expansion orifice, the one at the seat. Following this is a single expansion chamber which serves as a delivery nozzle or applicator. It is sufficiently large in volume to permit immediate expansion of the pressurized product to form the familiar ball of foam. As demonstrated earlier, the same formulation will be discharged as a solid stream when dispensed with a valve and actuator having small orifices and expansion chambers. Under these latter conditions, the ball of foam will begin to develop where the stream impinges on a surface. This rather interesting performance is utilized in some pressurized surgical soaps on the market.

Because of their large openings foam valves may lend themselves for use with viscous materials such as syrups, creams, and ointments.

After a foam product such as shaving cream has been used a small accumulation of foam often will be seen on the end of the actuator. This buildup is not due either to leakage or slow shutoff of the valve, but rather to the expansion of the residual formulation in the actuator.

Actuators

The actuator provides a rapid and convenient means for releasing the contents from a pressurized container. It provides the additional functional use in allowing the product to be dispensed in the desired form; that is, a fine mist, wet spray, foam, or solid stream. Mechanical breakup actuators are used for three-phase or compressed-gas aerosols. In addition, special actuators are available for use with pharmaceutical and medicinal aerosols which allow for the dispensing of products into the mouth, nose, throat, vagina, and eye. Several of these actuators and applicators are illustrated in Fig 93-9.

Dip Tubes

An additional component which should be considered with the valve is the dip tube. The dip tube serves several purposes:

1. It conveys the liquid from the bottom of the container to the dispensing valve at the top.
2. It prevents the propellant from escaping without dispensing the contents of the package (when used according to directions).

The dip tube comes into intimate contact with both product and propellant and therefore should be resistant to both physical and chemical attack. Polyethylenes and nylon have been found to possess many desirable properties making them useful for this purpose. However, since the dip tube is stretched to fit tightly on the valve housing, it is possible that on standing the polyethylene or nylon will crack or break down at this point, rendering the product useless since it cannot be dispensed. This has been overcome through the use of specially developed polyethylene or polypropylene compounds.

The tube should extend almost to the bottom of the container. If the tube is too short, all the product will not be dispensed, while a tube touching the bottom of the container will tend to block the passage of liquid. In this connection, most of the materials used for dip tubes tend to elongate when immersed in certain solvents and propellants for long periods of time. This elongation should be anticipated when determining the length of the dip tube.

Packaging

Two methods have been used to package aerosol products. Unlike nonaerosol products, part of the manufacturing of necessity takes place during the filling operation. The propellant and product concentrate must be brought together in such a way as to insure uniformity of product.

Depending on the nature of the product concentrate, the aerosol can be filled by a cold-filling or a pressure-filling process. There are advantages and disadvantages to both methods, and there are many factors which must be considered before deciding upon which process to use. Since this is a rather specialized procedure, commercial filling facilities are available.

Applications

Aerosol technology has been applied to the formulation of products containing therapeutically active ingredients.

A pharmaceutical aerosol may be defined as an aerosol product containing therapeutically active ingredients dissolved, suspended, or emulsified in a propellant or a mixture of solvent and propellant and intended for oral or topical administration or for administration into one of the body cavities such as the ear, rectum and vagina.

Oral aerosols are intended for administration as fine, solid particles or as liquid mists via the respiratory system or nasal passages. They are used for their local action in the nasal areas, throat, and lungs, as well as for prompt systemic effect when absorbed from the lungs into the blood stream (inhalation therapy). The particle size must be considerably below 50 μm and, in most instances, should be between 3 and 6 μm for maximum therapeutic response.

According to the USP/NF, "Pharmaceutical aerosols are products that are packaged under pressure and contain therapeutically active ingredients that are released upon activation of an appropriate valve system. They are intended for topical application to the skin as well as local application into various body orifices and local or systemic inhalation into the lungs."

Pharmaceutical Aerosols

Pharmaceuticals may be formulated as aerosols utilizing solutions, suspensions, emulsions, powders, and semisolid preparations. Table V illustrates the basic formulation of aerosol products for oral use.

Solutions Aerosols—These consist of a solution of active

Table V—Pressurized Aerosol Solutions and Suspensions

Prototype Formulation

Solutions
    Active ingredient(s)—solubilized
    Preservatives—cetylpyridinium chloride
    Antioxidants—ascorbic acid
    Solvent blends—water, ethanol, glycols
    Propellants—12/11, 12/114, or 12 alone
Suspensions
    Active ingredient(s)—micronized and suspended
    Dispersing agent(s)—sorbitan oleate, oleyl alcohol, etc
    Density modifers
    Bulking agents
    Propellants—12/11, 12/114, or 12 alone

ingredients in pure propellant or a mixture of propellant and solvents. The solvent is used to dissolve the active ingredients and/or to retard the evaporation of the propellant. Solution aerosols are relatively easy to formulate provided the ingredients are soluble in the propellant. However, the propellants are nonpolar in nature and in most cases are poor solvents for some of the commonly used aerosol ingredients. Through use of a solvent which is miscible with the propellant, one can achieve varying degrees of solubility. There is no limit to the number of solvents which can be used for this purpose except for toxicity considerations. Ethyl alcohol has found greatest use for this purpose although some other solvents may be of limited value. For those substances which are insoluble in the propellant or propellant/solvent system, a dispersion or suspension can be produced. In this case the drug must be micronized so that the majority of the particles are less than 2 μm in average diameter. While it may be easier to formulate a solution system than a suspension system, the latter is generally preferred since a closer control over the particle size distribution of the droplets dispensed from the solution aerosol may be obtained.

The usual fluorocarbon substances of Propellants 11, 12, and 114 are generally blended as indicated in Table V. While Propellant 11 is still employed to a great extent, there are some references in the literature which indicate that it is slightly more toxic than Propellants 12 and 114 when used under conditions of abuse. This is due to the lower vapor pressure of Propellant 11 permitting it to remain in the blood stream longer than the other two propellants.

For the most part, some of the propellant may be inhaled during use but is quickly exhaled. Propellant 11 is often used when solubility of the drug and solvents present a problem as it is a better solvent than either Propellant 12 or 114. Additionally, it may be required to prepare a suitable slurry when preparing a dispersion aerosol. Generally the propellant represents upwards of 60 weight percent of the final formulation and in many cases may be as high as 85–90%.

Propellant 12 may be used alone or in combination as indicated. The proportion of each propellant is varied in order to obtain the desired pressure within the container and the proper particle size distribution.

Dispersions or Suspensions (Powder Aerosols)—These aerosols are similar to solution aerosols except that the active ingredients are suspended or dispersed throughout the propellant or propellant and solvent phase. This system is useful with antibiotics, steroids, and other difficultly soluble compounds. Problems associated with the formulation of this system include agglomeration, caking, particle-size growth, and valve clogging. Some of these problems have been overcome through use of lubricants such as isopropyl myristate, light mineral oil, and other substances which provide slippage between particles of the compound as well as lubricating component parts of the valve. Surfactants have also been used to disperse the particles. The use of dispersing agents such as sorbitan trioleate, oleyl alcohol, and corn oil are useful in keeping the suspended particles from agglomerating. Thought should also be given to the particle size as well as the moisture content of the powder. The moisture content should be kept below 300 ppm and the propellants and solvents must be dried by passing them through a drying agent. The particle size should remain in the micrometer range and should be between 1 and 10 μm.

Emulsions—An emulsion system is useful for a great variety of products. Since it contains a relatively small amount of propellant (4–10%), there is little if any chilling effect. Active ingredients which may be irritating if inhaled can be used as a foam. Depending on the nature of the formulation and the manner in which the product is to be used, the foam is aqueous or nonaqueous and can be stable or quick-breaking.

Emulsions can be dispensed from an aerosol container as a spray, stable foam, or quick-breaking foam depending on the type of valve used and the formulation. Two types of emulsions can be formulated for use in an aerosol. A W/O emulsion is one in which the water phase is dispersed throughout the oil phase; an O/W emulsion is one in which the water is the continuous phase.

If the product concentrate is dispersed throughout a propellant, the system behaves similarly to a W/O emulsion. However, since the propellant is in the external phase, the product is dispersed as a wet stream rather than as a foam. When the propellant is in the internal phase (O/W), a foam will be produced. The consistency and stability of the foam can be modified by choice of surfactants and solvents used.

Many water-based aerosols are of the W/O type where the propellant is in the external phase. Stable shave-cream foams, on the other hand, are produced by keeping the propellant in the internal phase.

The stable foam is similar to a shaving-cream formulation into which therapeutically active ingredients are incorporated. The foam is dispensed and rubbed into the skin or affected area. By substituting glycols and glycol derivatives for the water in an emulsion, a nonaqueous foam is obtained. The foam stability can be varied by the choice of surfactant, solvent, and propellant. It has been suggested that these foams are applicable to ointment bases, rectal and vaginal medication, and burn preparations.

A quick-breaking foam allows for application of medication conveniently and efficiently. In certain instances the product was dispensed as a foam which quickly collapsed. This was useful in covering large areas with no rubbing necessary to disperse the medication. These quick-breaking foams consist of alcohol, surfactant, water, and propellant in the following proportions:

Ethanol	46.0–66.0%
Surfactant	0.5– 5.0%
Water	28.0–42.0%
Propellant	3.0–15.0%

The surfactant can be nonionic, anionic, or cationic and should be soluble in one of the miscible solvents, but not in both. Several of the nonionic emulsifying waxes have been found to be advantageous in this type of formulation.

Topical aerosols now utilize a hydrocarbon propellant. Other than the flammability potential, hydrocarbons produce suitable aerosols. Compressed gases have found limited application. The flammability potential of topical aerosols has been reduced substantially through use of vapor tap valves in which the flame extension can be reduced from over 24 in to less than 18 in and in many instances below 8 in. This is accomplished by using fairly large vapor taps in the valve. The formulator must check to make sure sufficient propellant is present to suitably dispense all of the product. By balancing the vapor tap and dispensing orifices of the valve and by using a capillary dip tube, a satisfactory aerosol system may be formulated.

Semisolid Preparations—These preparations are formulated in the usual manner and depend on nitrogen to push the contents from the package. The piston-type of flexible bag-type systems is used for these products. Creams and ointments are best packaged using these systems.

Container and Valve Components

Pharmaceutical Containers—Various containers have been used for these aerosols. Due to esthetic considerations and excellent compatibility with drugs; glass, stainless steel, and aluminum containers have found widespread use in the pharmaceutical industry. The use of stainless steel containers has been limited primarily due to its costs.

Plastic-coated glass bottles ranging in size from 15 to 30 mL have been employed mainly with solution aerosols although there is no technical or scientific rationale for this use other than one can determine the amount of material left in the container by holding the bottle in the path of a strong light. Glass bottles are not recommended for suspension aerosols due to the visibility of the suspended particles which may present an esthetic problem.

The plastic coating on glass containers serves to protect from flying glass in the event of glass shattering when the container is accidentally broken. Additionally, the plastic coating around the neck of the container serves to absorb some of the shock from the crimping operation and decreases the danger of breaking during this operation.

All commercially available bottles have a 20-mm neck finish and adapt easily to all of the metered aerosol valves presently available. In addition, the plastic coating also serves as an ultraviolet light absorber so that the contents are protected from the deleterious effects of light. These plastic coatings are available in a clear finish or in various colors.

The major drawback to the use of glass bottles is the danger of accidental breakage (although this is remote due to the thick walls of the container and its small size and weight). The latter becomes an important consideration when one is concerned with shipping costs. The advantages of glass lie in its excellent compatibility with pharmaceuticals and its ability to permit one to view the level of contents remaining in the container.

Aluminum is used as the material of construction for most oral aerosols. This material is extremely light weight and also essentially is inert, although aluminum will react with certain solvents and other chemicals. While aluminum can be used without an internal organic coating for certain aerosol formulations (especially those which contain only active ingredient and propellant) many containers are available which have internal coating made from an epon- or epoxy-type resin. The coating formulations are generally manufacturer's secrets, although many of the container producers have a master file with the Food and Drug Administration which contains all pertinent information as to the exact, formulation, safety evaluations, inertness, and other characteristics of the coating material.

Aluminum containers are also made with a 20-mm opening so as to receive the standard metered valves. However, a variety of openings ranging from 15 to 20 mm are also available for special and customized applications. Aluminum containers are manufactured from a "slug" of aluminum and are seamless, therefore, there is virtually no danger of leakage.

Pharmaceutical Valves—Metered valves fitted with a 20-mm ferrule are used with the above containers for all oral aerosols. It is also possible to use these same valves for aerosol nasal preparations.

The metered valve should deliver accurately a measured amount of product and should be reproducible not only for each dose delivered from the same package but from package to package. Two basic types of metered valves are available; one for inverted use and the other for upright use. Generally, valves for upright use contain a thin capillary dip tube and are used with solution type aerosols. On the other hand, suspension or dispersion aerosols utilize a valve for inverted use which does not contain a dip tube. Figures 93-10 and 93-11 illustrate both types of valves and are typical of those commercially available.

An integral part of these valves is the metering chamber which is directly responsible for the delivery of the desired amount of therapeutic agent. The size of the chamber can be varied so that from about 50 to 150 mL of product can be delivered per actuation. Most of the products commercially available utilize dosages in the range of 50–75 μL. The chamber is sealed via the metering and stem gasket. In the

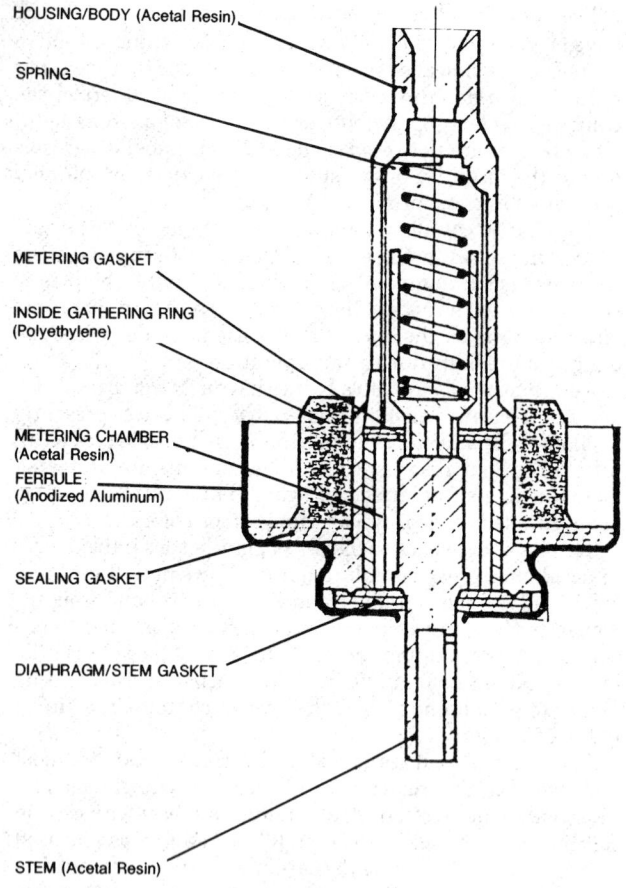

Fig 93-10.   Metering value—inverted (courtesy, Valois).

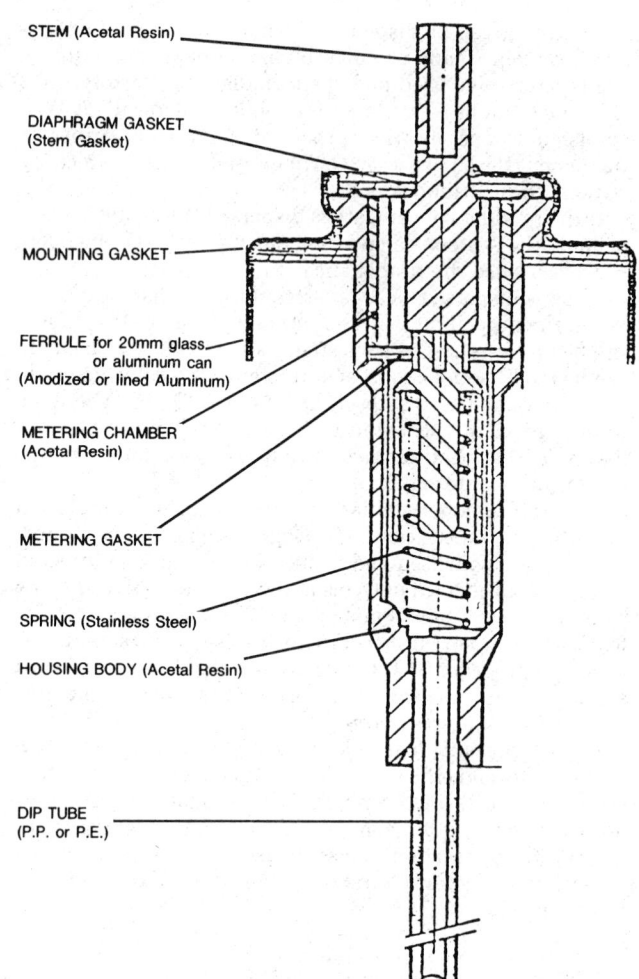

Fig 93-11.   Metering valve—upright (courtesy, Valois).

acutated position, the stem gasket will allow the contents of the metering chamber to be dispensed while the metering gasket will seal off any additional product from entering the chamber. In this manner the chamber is always filled and ready to deliver the desired amount of therapeutic agent.

These valves should retain their prime charge over fairly long periods of time. However, it is possible from the material in the chamber to slowly return to the main body of product in the event the container is stored upright (for those used in the inverted position). The degree to which this can occur varies with the construction of the valve and the length of time between actuations. In normal use this normally does not occur.

Both types of valves are currently used on commercially available oral inhalation aerosols. During the development stage, the compatibility of the valves should be determined with the exact formulation to be used in order to determine the accuracy of the metered dose developed in regard to doses delivered from the same container of product and from different containers. Additionally, one should ensure that there is no interaction between the various valve subcomponents and the formulation. If distortion or elongation of some of the plastic subcomponents occurs, this may result in leakage, inaccurate dosage, and/or decomposition of the active ingredients.

There also have been instances whereby the therapeutic agent was adsorbed or absorbed onto the various plastic components and a lower than normal dose of the active ingredient was dispensed. For these reasons, one must not only determine the total weight of product dispensed per dose but the actual amount of active ingredient in each dose. Some test procedures use the results obtained by taking 10 doses of material and determining the average amount present in one dose. When possible, and where the analytical procedure permits the detecting of fairly small amounts of active ingredient present per dose, multiple single-dose assays should be performed. Using the average of 10 doses may fail to reveal problems of variations in each of the individual doses dispensed.

Metered dose valves suitable for use on oral aerosol products are available from Valois, Riker, Neotectnic, Emson, and Bespak. These valves have been used on most of the aerosol inhalation products either of the solution or dispersion type. They are available in sizes ranging from about 35 µL to about 150 µL.

Particle Size

Up to this point, emphasis has been placed on the reproducibility of drug delivery and on the physicochemical compatibility of inhalation formulations with valve components and containers. Equally important with inhalation aerosol products is the ultimate deposition of materials actuated through the valve into the respiratory passages. Accurate assessment of drug deposition profiles in terms of both the quantity of drug reaching the respiratory airways and its depth of penetration are critical parameters in evaluating the biopharmaceutics of inhalation aerosol products. The major factors influencing the ultimate deposition of inhalation aerosols include the formulation of the product, design of components (specifically the actuators and adaptors), administrative skills and techniques of the product user, and the anatomical and physiological status of the respiratory system.

Although each of these factors will be discussed separately in some detail, the interdependence of one of these factors upon the other cannot be overemphasized.

Formulation Factors—Included among formulation factors are the physicochemical characteristics of the active ingredients, the particle size and shape of the formulation, the type and concentration of surface-active agent used, and to some extent, the vapor pressure and the metered volume of propellants. In terms of physicochemical properties, the lipoidal solubility and pulmonary absorption rates of the active ingredient are of utmost importance. Studies have clearly demonstrated that a more pronounced and rapid pharmacological response is noted when a drug is administered via inhalation as a free base or acid (liquid-soluble form) than as its corresponding water-soluble salt.

The findings are not surprising since they support many of the concepts generally associated with drug transport across other biological membranes. Another physicochemical factor governing the biopharmaceutics of a drug is its dissolution characteristics in pulmonary fluids. Drugs having a rapid dissolution rate in pulmonary fluids predictably produce much more intense and rapid onset of action, having a shorter duration than their less soluble derivatives. Therapeutic agents which exhibit a very poor solubility in pulmonary fluids are to be avoided since they are likely to serve as irritants and precipitate bronchial spasms.

Particle size and shape also play a significant role in the deposition pattern of the drug in the respiratory passageways. It is imperative to keep a minimum of 90% of the particles in inhalation products between 0.5 and 10 μm to maximize their delivery and deposition in respiratory fluids. Most workers agree that particles in the size range from 3–6 μm are most effective. Particles of this size have been demonstrated to deposit in the lung via gravitational sedimentation, inertial impaction, or by diffusion into terminal alveoli via Brownian motion. Particles much greater in size than 10 μm generally deposit in the upper respiratory tract while particles less than 0.5 μm are exhaled or adhere to the walls of the mouth during the exhalation phase.

Table VI indicates some of the methods (with some of their inherent shortcomings) presently employed in the pharmaceutical and cosmetic industries to evaluate particle size distribution. Of those methods listed, the cascade impactor enjoys the greatest popularity with inhalation aerosols. This instrument will classify particles based on inertial impaction which most closely simulates particle collection in the lungs. It should be emphasized, however, that although the *in vitro*

Table VI—Summary of Particle Sizing Methods

Method	Size range, μm	Major problems
Optical microscopy	0.2–300	0.2 μm limit of resolution Spreading of larger droplets
Cascade impactors	0.2–20	Wall losses/disaggregation Rebound/re-entrainment Limited size data
Light scattering counters	0.1–20	Refractive index, shape sensitivity, coincidence, cross-sensitivity, calibration, isokinetic sampling
Holography	3–1000	Lower limit 3 μm Two stages in sizing; formation and reconstruction. Analysis time
Photography	5–1000	Small depth of field Automation difficult but possible. Difficulty in three dimensions

(RW Pengilly, JA Keiner: *J Soc Cosmet Chem* 28: 641, 1977.)

methods listed in Table VI are capable of accurately assessing particles as to size, none of the methods mentioned takes into consideration the shape of the particle or particle growth which may occur when the material is actuated into the high humidity of the respiratory tract. These particle characteristics are presently undergoing careful scrutiny by inhalation aerosol formulators.

The selection of the appropriate surface active agent (required in most pressurized inhalation suspension aerosols) is another important consideration since the surfactant will influence droplet evaporation, particle size, and overall hydrophobicity of the particles reaching the respiratory passageways and pulmonary fluids.

The effects of propellant vapor pressure and the metered volume of propellants on drug deposition in the lungs have recently been studied using rather large specialized plastic adapters. Findings in this area have demonstrated that the amount of material deposited in the mouth, tube and actuator (likely sites of material loss) increased as the vapor pressure was decreased and the metered volume increased.

Component Design—Component design, specifically the actuator and adapter, have also been shown to alter the particle size and the penetration and deposition of drugs into the lungs. Numerous studies have demonstrated a complex set of interactions exist between the actuation type, valve dimensions, distance from actuator, and other component variables and that particle size (mass median diameters) could vary up to 40% by altering one or more of the aforementioned components.

One component that has undergone enormous modification in the last few years to improve drug delivery is the adapter. Up to about the mid 1970's, almost all adapters were short and rather simplistic so as to minimize possible hold-up of material in the adapter. The hold-up in the short stem adapters averages anywhere from 5 to 20%. Recently, however, numerous customized adapters having specific designs and dimensions have entered the marketplace.

Interest in the larger adapters (often referred to as tube spacers) can be attributed to any one or more of the following reasons. The larger adapter designs permit a complete evaporation of propellant reducing initial droplet velocity and particle size. This reduction of particle size improves depth of drug penetration into the lungs while a lower initial velocity decreases product impaction to the back of the esophagus (whiplash effect), common to short stem adapters. The larger adapter designs also permit a decrease in pressure to drop and increased volume flow which has also been reported to increase penetration of particles into the lungs. It should be pointed out that the larger tube spacers are not without problems. They are inconvenient because of their size, they are expensive and are somewhat difficult to clean. They also present the manufacturer with the problem of assessing product hold-up in a rather complex device.

Administrative Techniques—The metered inhalation aerosol dosage form, although popular, is generally considered as one of the most complicated drug delivery systems currently marketed by the pharmaceutical industry. It is viewed by many as being only slightly simpler to use than an injectable, since inhalation products often require up to 10 to 15 maneuvers by the patient during use. Failure of the patient to perform correctly any one of these maneuvers may significantly alter the deposition of the drug into the appropriate portion of the lungs.

Further complicating the problem for the patient is that each inhalation product has considerably different directions for use. For example, many manufacturers require the use of their product in the inverted position and suggest actuating with the lips tightly closed around the actuator while others direct to use their products in the upright position and with the lips open.

Table VII—Relation Between Performance of Maneuvers and Referral Diagnosis

| Maneuver | % of subjects performing maneuver correctly:diagnosis | |
	COPD,[a] n = 51	Asthma, n = 68
Remove cap	100.0	95.6
Shake inhaler	64.7	70.6
Hold inhaler upright	92.2	88.2
Tilt head back	82.4	85.3
Close lips	78.4	86.8
Breathe in and activate inhaler	60.8	66.2
Inhale slowly and deeply	25.5	57.4
Hold breath (10 seconds)	29.4	57.4
Breath out through nose	5.9	25.0
Use one puff	74.5	80.9
Wait 30 seconds	58.8	76.5

[a] Chronic Obstructive Pulmonary Disease.
Epstein SW, *et al: Canadian Med J 120:* 813–824, 1979.

Differences in the directions of use for each inhalation product are a result of the product formulation and actuator design which the manufacturer deemed most appropriate for the particular product. In light of this, it is not surprising to find patients who require two or more aerosol inhalation products or who are constantly changing their medication (such as the asthmatic patient) occasionally experiencing difficulties in complying with the suggested method of application.

A comprehensive study summarized in Table VII conducted in 1979 illustrates the relatively poor compliance of patients to perform the necessary maneuvers so as to ensure maximum deposition of drug into the respiratory airways, even though this study was conducted using a relatively simple oral inhalation aerosol product. In addition, it should be emphasized that each patient employed in this study was briefed concerning the correct use of the inhalation product. Table VII clearly shows that a large percentage of the patients failed to inhale slowly and deeply, hold their breath and breathe out through the nose. All three maneuvers are critical in assuring proper deposition of the drug into the lungs. The pharmaceutical industry, recognizing this problem, has over the last two to three years developed elaborate package inserts to instruct the patient concerning the proper use of their inhalation products.

Other problems associated with the administration of aerosols not listed in Table VII confronting the patient include the cleaning of the device, the occasional loss of prime (charge pressure), and dosage tail-off. Product devices improperly cleaned or not permitted to dry completely can influence drug delivery. The loss of prime charge from the metered valve and dosage tail-off are currently being given considerable attention since they can influence the amount of drug being delivered to the patient.

In spite of the numerous problems associated with this relatively complicated drug delivery system, it is important to emphasize that many inhalation product users often titrate themselves to their own requirements of the drug with their own maneuver characteristics and because of this, the overall success of the inhalation aerosol product is remarkably high.

Anatomical and Physiological Status of the Respiratory System—Many attempts have been made to evaluate the deposition pattern of inhalation aerosols using *in vitro* simulated respiratory designs. Table VIII describes three such methods. Although none of these models describes adequately the complex anatomical and physiological structure of the respiratory airways, they have been used successfully in making product comparisons and formulation as-

Table VIII—Simulated Respiratory Systems for *in vitro* Analysis of Drug Deposition

| Respiratory device | PATTERNS | |
	Functionality & description	Reference
Simulated lung apparatus	A compartmentalized unit based on specific parameters in the human respiratory tract. Compares deposition patterns of soluton and suspension aerosols	Karig A, *et al: J Pharm Sci 62:* 811, 1973.
Simulated respiratory system	Compares macrodeposition patterns of aerosol products. Specifically examines the total amount of drug reaching respiratory airways	Sciarra JJ, Cutie AJ: *J Pharm Sci 67:* 1428, 1978.
Simulated rat lung model	Parameters such as inspired volume, time of inspiration and amount of drug per inspiration are evaluated	Chowdan ZT, Zlinn EE: *Intl J Pharm 3:* 117, 1979.

Table IX—Medicinal Agents Having a High Potential for Use as Aerosol Inhalation Products

Antianginal preparations (nitroglycerin)
Antiasthmatic preparations, steroids (beclomethasone, dexamethasone, triamcinolone, etc), sympathomimetics (isoproterenol, phenylephrine, etc), and anticholinergics (ipratropium bromide)
Antibiotics (kanamycin)
Antivirals (ribavirin)
Ergotamine preparations
Immunizing agents
Insulin
Calcium blockers

sessments. All three models by design have optimum conditions for good deposition and have dealt only modestly with simulating changes in breathing patterns (ie, impaired breathing in asthmatic patients). Related to the latter point concerning breathing patterns, new findings concerning when the drug should be actuated into the respiratory airway are quite thought provoking. More in-depth comparative studies concerning when the product should be administered are on the horizons and currently under study. In either case, whatever the criterion is, pharmaceutical manufacturers are now addressing themselves to the anatomical and physiological status of patients with impaired breathing patterns.

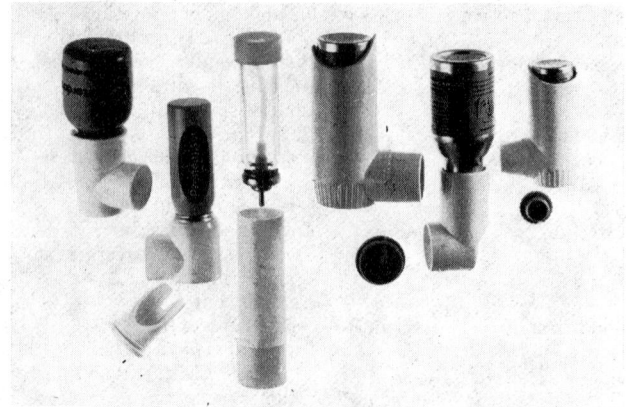

Fig 93-12. Medicinal aerosols with oral applicators.

In spite of the amount of work that remains to be done in the area of pharmaceutical inhalation aerosols, the future is very promising. Table IX lists some therapeutic agents now being considered for use via the inhalation route. Many of these are new drugs while others are being restudied based upon new technology within the industry Several oral aerosols are illustrated in Fig 93-12.

Labeling

In accordance with official regulations, aerosol product labels should include those of the following warning statements that are applicable:

Warning—Avoid inhaling. Keep away from eyes or other mucous membranes.

The statement "avoid inhaling" is not required for preparations intended for use by inhalation, nor is the phrase "or other mucous membranes" required for preparations intended for use on mucous membranes.

Warning—Contents under pressure. Do not puncture or incinerate container. Do not expose to heat or store at temperatures above 120°F (49°C). Keep out of the reach of children.

In addition to the aforementioned warnings, the label of a drug packaged in an aerosol container in which the propellant consists in whole or in part of a halocarbon or hydrocarbon shall, where required under regulations of the Food and Drug Administration, bear the following warning:

Warning—Do not inhale directly; deliberate inhalation of contents can cause death.

or:

Warning—Use only as directed; intentional misuse by deliberately concentrating and inhaling the contents can be harmful or fatal.

Bibliography

Dautrebande L: *Microaerosols*, Academic, New York, 1962.
Goldenberg RL: in *Advances in Cosmetic Technology*, vol I, 97–126, Harcourt Brace Jovanovich, New York, 1978.
Johnsen M, *et al*: *The Aerosol Handbook*, Wayne E Dorland Co, Caldwell, NJ, 1972.
Lachman L, *et al*: *Industrial Pharmacy*, 2nd ed, 270–295, Lea & Febiger, Philadelphia, 1976.
Sanders P: *Handbook of Aerosol Technology*, 2nd ed, Van Nostrand Reinhold, New York, 1979.
Sciarra JJ, Stoller L: *The Science and Technology of Aerosol Packaging*, Wiley, New York, 1974.
Sciarra JJ: Pharmaceutical and Cosmetic Aerosols, *J Pharm Sci 63:* 1815–1836, 1974.
Shepherd HR: *Aerosols: Science and Technology*, 387–408, Interscience, New York, 1961.

PART 9

Pharmaceutical Practice

Melvin R Gibson, PhD

Professor of Pharmacognosy
College of Pharmacy
Washington State University
Pullman, WA 99164

CHAPTER 94

Ambulatory Patient Care

Nicholas G Popovich, PhD
Associate Professor of Pharmacy Practice
School of Pharmacy and Pharmacal Sciences, Purdue University
West Lafayette, IN 47907

Various designations are used to categorize patients, such as institutionalized, noninstitutionalized, inpatient, outpatient, bedridden, and ambulatory.

Strickly speaking, an ambulatory patient is one who is able to walk; that is, one who is not bedridden. Therefore, an ambulatory patient *may* be an inpatient of an institution, such as a hospital or extended-care facility, if he is not confined to bed. However, the term ambulatory patient has become more restrictive in its modern usage to simply mean a noninstitutionalized patient.

The ambulatory patient referred to here is a noninstitutionalized patient who has the responsibility for obtaining his medication, storing it, and taking it. He may or may not be an outpatient, depending upon where he receives his treatment. He may even be in a wheelchair and strictly speaking not ambulatory, but if he is not institutionalized he will have the same basic responsibility for his medication as a "walking patient."

Whether the patient sees a physician who may prescribe medication or whether the patient decides to treat himself, the community pharmacist will more than likely come into contact with the ambulatory patient. It is important, therefore, for the pharmacist to have an understanding of this patient in order that he, as a pharmacist and member of the health care team, can contribute his knowledge and judgment in providing the best possible health care for the ambulatory patient.

Proper Use of Medication

The noted philosopher and educator in medicine, Sir William Osler, in 1891, captured the essence of man and medicine when he stated, "the desire to take medicines is perhaps the greatest feature that distinguishes man from animals." Unfortunately this statement did not capture the mode in which man takes medicine, which is either correct or incorrect. If the patient complies with the instructions from the physician and pharmacist, there is a strong chance that the therapeutic regimen will be successful. However, if the medication is misused through personal ignorance or inadequate information, it could result in either harm to the patient or ineffective treatment.

It is known that the ambulatory patient does not always adhere to the directions for taking medicine. There are a number of reasons for this and the reader is advised to consult Chapter 100 for a thorough and enlightening discussion of patient compliance. Through the decade of the 70's, numerous studies have demonstrated that patients widely misuse medications with frequency ranges between 20 and 82%. This wide variation reflects study differences, medication class differences, and investigator interpretation of patient misuse of medication. Further, it is estimated that at least 30% of patients within the United States do not comply with their therapeutic instructions and one-third of these compliance studies report noncompliance of 50% or higher.[1] Alternatively, other studies have demonstrated the positive impact of pharmacist intervention to encourage patient compliance. As a health care provider, the pharmacist is morally and legally obligated and is perhaps in the best position to provide patients with adequate, understandable information on the drugs they take or use to maximize the therapeutic outcome and prevent conceivable problems during therapy.

To prevent these problems, the pharmacist must first understand how a patient misuses prescribed medications. Latiolais and Berry[2] compiled a number of ways in which a patient can misuse medication. These are outlined below.

1. Overdosage
   a. Taking more than the prescribed dose at any one administration.
   b. Taking more than the prescribed number of doses in any one day.
   c. Taking a dose, prescribed as needed, at a time other than when needed.
   d. Taking the same medication from two or more different bottles simultaneously.
2. Underdosage
   a. Taking less than the prescribed dose at any one administration.
   b. Omitting one or more doses.
   c. Discontinuing the drug before the prescribed time.
   d. Omitting the dose of a medication, prescribed as needed, when it is needed.
3. Taking a dose at a different time if a time has been specified in the directions.
4. Taking a dose in a form other than that specified in the directions.
5. Using the wrong route of administration.
6. Taking medication that has been discontinued.
7. Taking outdated medications.
8. Taking someone else's medications.
9. Taking two or more medications which are therapeutically contraindicated.
10. Failing to get the prescription filled.
11. Failing to understand how to properly use the administration unit (e.g., inhaler).
12. Failing to understand how to properly use or administer the dosage form.

Using the above criteria, they found that 42.8% of the patients sampled were misusing their medications and that 4.4% misused their medicine in such a manner as to pose serious threat to their health. The types of misuse committed most frequently were overdosage and omission of doses. Overdosage represented 41.3% of the total misused prescriptions. Omitting one or more doses occurred in 23.6% of the misused prescriptions. Another result of this study showed that, of the prescriptions being misused, the patients were actually aware they were misusing about half of them. This apparently deliberate misuse is perhaps more understandable when viewed with respect to the second most frequent reason given by the patients for not following directions; they thought they needed another dose. Another frequent reason was that the patient thought he was cured and stopped taking the drug before the prescribed time. The single most often mentioned reason, occurring fully one-third of the time, was that the patient did not understand the instructions.

It is inconceivable that the patient would knowingly misuse medication in a way that would be injurious to his health.

Similarly, with the high cost of health care it is astounding that patients would not maximize the health care they do receive to gain maximum benefit from their expenditures. Thus, an apparent reason for the misuse of medicine by the patient may be a lack of knowledge and understanding of the medication and how it is integrated into a treatment regimen for the disease state of the patient.

Unfortunately, many patients have a preconceived notion that all medication will make one free from disease. Many patients do not realize that medications are often necessary just to maintain one's health at the status quo. This is vividly exemplified by nonsteroidal anti-inflammatory drugs which are intended to provide a level of mobility and relieve the pain, stiffness, and swelling of arthritis. These cannot "cure" the underlying disease but attempt to arrest the disease process and the patient must understand this concept.

A further patient misconception relates to the perception of drug potency. "If one tablet is good, two will be even better," is a philosophy that is fraught with danger. The patient should not be held accountable for a lack of knowledge or understanding of drugs, especially when the most readily available information is found in the lay press and the communication media. The OTC drug industry, comparatively free of restrictions until recent years, has in many instances promoted its products in such a manner that it gives the patient the distinct impression that there are "pills for all ills." Consequently, there is evidence that many people over-medicate themselves and have formed a somewhat distorted or undeserved confidence in all drugs. Pharmacy practice too must accept partial responsibility. Some practitioners have bombarded the public with information that "generic medications are cheaper" or "which pharmacy has the lowest prices," rather than promoting the need for proper compliance and selection of health care providers who, through enhanced professional service, are more cost effective in the long run.

The growing number of published medication guides, directed at the lay person, is a further testimonial to the "drug information gap." But realistically it is difficult to write these at a level to be understood by every person. Out of necessity the scope of these books usually involves only the most frequently prescribed medications. The top 100 most frequently prescribed products in 1982 represented only 48.9% of all prescriptions, down from 55.1% in 1981. What does one do when his medication is not found in the book?

History documents drug use through the ages and it is interesting that only in the last two decades has the problem of patient misuse of medication been identified and demonstrated. This evidence has escalated due to better communication technique, better study design, the fact that more people have access to primary health care, and the use of potent medication. It is estimated that over 75 new drugs were introduced into the marketplace between 1980 and 1983. A high number of these drugs are variations of, or chemically related to, existing drug families/pharmacological classes. Through advances in medicinal chemistry many of these new agents are highly potent, and thus the likelihood that problems will occur is heightened. It is difficult for the medical and the pharmaceutical communities to keep up with the proliferation of new products and rapid therapeutic advancements. Still, however, it is the professional responsibility of the pharmacist to continue to learn about and understand these new chemical entities in the hope of being able to provide necessary and useful information to the patient to ensure these potent medications are used correctly and to their maximal benefit.

Pharmacists Responsibility

The pharmacist must play an active role in the proper use of prescription medication by the patient. The pharmacist is often the last member of the health care team to see the patient before the patient will take the drug without direct medical supervision. Therefore, it is the responsibility of the pharmacist to ensure the safe and appropriate use of the medication by the patient and to answer questions of concern to the patient. This responsibility also encompasses nonprescription (OTC) products (inclusive of health care accessories).

When executing this responsibility, the pharmacist provides certain pharmaceutical services which are as important to the health care of the ambulatory patient as those services provided by the other health practitioners. The pharmaceutical services which contribute to the total health care of the ambulatory patient are summarized below:

1. Counseling the patient concerning the safe and appropriate utilization of medicines.
2. Monitoring the drug utilization of the patient by referring to the patient's medication profile.
3. Serving as a health advisor to the patient by providing advice on nonprescription products and by referring the patient to a physician or an appropriate health agency.
4. Serving as a health educator to the community, particularly in matters relative to medication usage.
5. Serving as a source of drug information to the physician and allied health professionals, thereby influencing directly or indirectly the selection of the drug or drug product or the correct and optional use of the drug or drug product for the patient.

Patient Counseling

It is the responsibility of the pharmacist to counsel the patient before dispensing the medication. During the consultation with the patient, the pharmacist should provide him with sufficient information (eg, how to take it, how long to take it and at what times, proper storage, frequently encountered side effects) to ensure the patient will safely and appropriately use the medication. The amount of information that the pharmacist could conceivably share with the patient is awesome.

Indeed it would be foolhardy to believe that the patient will remember everything. Thus, in addition to verbal information, audiovisual and illustrative materials are beneficial when counseling the patient. This would include appropriate materials provided within the package by the drug manufacturer, or auxiliary, cautionary labels which can be affixed to the dispensed product. More advanced patient counseling systems involve advisory leaflets. Some innovative and creative pharmacists have developed these and provide them for their patients to take home. Others have been developed by local and state pharmacy associations and private enterprise. Further, an interesting new telephone prescription information service (ie, Medi-Message) has been developed as a practical management tool to help satisfy the demand for prescription drug information.[3] The pharmacist may provide access to this communication system through telephones in the pharmacy waiting area, or provide the patient with the toll-free number and access code for the particular medication being taken.

To date (1984) a total of 250 professionally produced "advisories" covering approximately 85% of all prescriptions dispensed have been prepared. For easy identification and selection most drugs are listed by generic name with common brand names mentioned in each message. These advisories last from 2–3 minutes and provide concise, up-to-date information. This is a means to help improve compliance and illustrate the service function of the pharmacist. It must be emphasized, however, that this counseling service does not suffice for the active participation of the pharmacist in patient counseling. The situation for each patient is independent of another person and the pharmacist must provide relevant information specific to that patient. Then, if necessary, the telephone message service is used to reinforce what has been shared with the patient.

The need for pharmacist intervention and counseling the patient about his medication cannot be overemphasized. Historically, pharmacists were taught under the old APhA Code of Ethics adopted in 1921 which discouraged such a discourse with the patient. The new Code of Ethics adopted in 1969 encouraged patient counseling with such statements as the pharmacist "should render to each patient the full measure of his ability as an essential health practitioner," and "he should utilize and make available this (his) knowledge as may be required in accordance with his best professional judgment." The pharmacist may be held liable if harm occurs to the patient as a result of the pharmacist's negligence in counseling the patient. For example, if the pharmacist did not warn the patient that the drug may make him drowsy and the patient harms himself because he was not made aware of this effect, the pharmacist may be held liable. Legislators in at least 12 states (1983) have recognized that there is a void and a potential for problems created when people do not have access to useful information about their prescription medications.[4] These states require pharmacist consultation with the patient at the time the medication is dispensed. A problem with state laws, however, is that some are nebulous while some are specific and pointedly direct the pharmacist to counsel the patient.

Some pharmacists avoid counseling on the premise that it is the responsibility of the physician to provide the information to the patient. The physician does have an obligation to instruct the patient in this regard. However, this environment is not always conducive to counseling. The patient is usually sick, he has probably had to wait a while before seeing the physician, and he will experience anticipation, apprehension, even fear, while waiting. Coupled with the threat of complex instruments and machinery that are not understandable to him, unpleasant thoughts may be developed. After examination there either may be a great deal of relief or the worse as anticipated. The patient may be thinking more about what is wrong with him than concentrating on the instructions of the physician. All of these are barriers to a good counseling environment. Indeed, the American Medical Association also has recognized this and has developed for its members advisory leaflets of the most often prescribed medications so that the physician can distribute these to the patient in the hope of encouraging proper medication use. This recognition is convincing evidence that a lack of communication does exist between the physician and the patient.

A majority of pharmacists are not reimbursed for time spent counseling patients about the proper use of prescription medications, advising patients on the treatment of minor complaints with the most appropriate nonprescription drug product, and monitoring the therapeutic profile of the patient. Indeed, many pharmacists believe that the patient is simply unwilling to pay for counseling. However, the results of a project conducted in community pharmacies in Tucson, AZ, demonstrated that the public will pay for consultation services and at a level that makes the service economically feasible.[5] Further, the American Pharmaceutical Association Academy of Pharmacy Practice Section on Clinical Practice commissioned Louis Harris and Associates, Inc., to conduct a national survey to gauge the willingness of consumers to pay for the clinical services of the pharmacist.[6] A total of 1254 interviews were conducted between March 3rd–13th, 1983. The initial public reaction to the concept of clinical pharmacy reimbursement was positive, and although those consumers saying they were willing to pay for additional services (eg, private consultation, monitoring of patient progress) were almost invariably a minority, it was usually a sizable minority (ie, greater than 31%).

Within the counseling endeavor the pharmacist must remember never to take his impute knowledge to the public. A professional can have a tendency to overlook the fact that things which are commonplace and second nature are not so to others. It must be remembered that although the pharmacist may be counseling the fifth patient of the day on the proper use of penicillin VK, to that patient it is the first time. The patient needs practical, useful information and the pharmacist should share his knowledge. This affords the pharmacist the opportunity to use his knowledge of drugs and dosage forms and provide service to the patient. The following sections exemplify modes of communication between the pharmacist and the patient that should be encouraged within the domain of patient consultation.

How to Remove the Drug from the Package—If, by questioning, it is found that the patient is not familiar with the packaging, the pharmacist should demonstrate how to remove the medicine from the package. In the future, as packaging becomes more sophisticated and tamper resistant, this will become even more important.

Removing medication from its package may seem to be a simple procedure to the pharmacist, but not always to the patient. Most people think eye drops are administered by using a medicine dropper; seeing a container for eye drops which does not contain a dropper (eg, Drop-tainer) may bewilder the patient. Some people may not understand that the dust cap will have to be removed from the aerosol device prior to use. Removing the wrapping from a suppository before insertion is quite obvious to the pharmacist, but not so to some patients; there have been cases of patients who have inserted a wrapped suppository, not realizing that the wrapping must be removed. Opening "safety containers" has presented considerable problems to patients, particularly the arthritic or the elderly patient.

How to Administer—It is important for the pharmacist to tell the patient whether the medicine should be taken by mouth, used in the eye, ear, or nose, inserted rectally or vaginally, or whether it should be used externally. It should not be taken for granted that the patient knows how to use the medicine even though it is obvious to the pharmacist. Some parents have mistakenly introduced oral antibiotic drops into the ears of their children since the child was being treated for an ear infection. The pharmacist should insure that the patient understands the details of using the medicine.

Consider the most common dosage form, the tablet; then consider how many ways it could be used or administered depending upon the medication and the type of tablet.

1. Place on tongue and swallow with water.
2. Warning: Do not chew.
3. Chew and swallow.
4. Let dissolve in mouth; ie, suck on tablet like a "mint."
5. Place under tongue (sublingual) and let dissolve. Do not swallow.
6. Place between gum and cheek (buccal) and let dissolve. Do not swallow.
7. Dissolve in water and swallow.
8. Dissolve in water and use externally.
9. Moisten with water and insert vaginally.

The most common method of administering the tablet is to place on the tongue and swallow with water. Most patients will understand this method of administration. The problem will occur when it should not be taken in this manner, because most patients, if not properly advised, may take all tablets this way, even those which should not be swallowed.

Another service the pharmacist should provide is to ask the patient if he can swallow a tablet since some people are unable to do so. If a person is unable to swallow a tablet the pharmacist has two options to exercise. The first is to suggest a device that assists swallowing a tablet (ie, Drink-A-Pill Drinking Glass) or pursue the second which is to consult the physician and suggest an equivalent liquid dosage form. If a liquid equivalent is not available a convenient option is to place the tablet in a spoon with some water. After the tablet disintegrates, the contents of the spoon should be swallowed. Some drugs which have a disagreeable taste may need to be masked by adding it to some applesauce, syrup, or similar substance to the spoon. Otherwise the pharmacist should consider extemporaneously preparing a liquid dosage form for the patient using a flavored vehicle (eg, Cherry Syrup). Numerous extemporaneous preparations have appeared in the professional literature in recent years and provide a basis for compounding technique and procedure. However, a main concern for the pharmacist is the stability of the drug once it is prepared in liquid form. In some of these instances pharmaceutical information will be required and the pharmacist should use the telephone number of the manufacturer as listed in the "Physicians' Desk Reference." Further, Schneiweiss[7] has surveyed and compiled a list of telephone numbers of drug manufacturers.

Some tablets must be swallowed in their entirety. These tablets are either enteric coated or sustained release. Enteric-coated tablets might contain drugs which are irritating to the stomach or are not stable in gastric juices. Thus, transmitted through the stomach and ultimate release of the contents in the intestines is preferred. Sustained-release medication is intended to provide medication as the dosage form traverses the gastrointestinal tract. Chewing the tablet unknowingly would alter the release characteristics and provide the entire effect of the medication at once. This could be hazardous to the patient and at the same time not afford therapeutic coverage for the patient for the period of time between doses. Lastly, there are a few tableted medications which have the capability to stain teeth and the mouth. The patient should be told to swallow this type, as well as the aforementioned enteric-coated and sustained-release tablets.

The pharmacist should be sure the patient understands how to use ophthalmic preparations. The use of eye drops can easily be demonstrated to the patient by placing a finger below the lower eyelid away from the nose and pulling down. This will form a pocket in the lower lid where the solution should be dropped. For retention in the eye and/or to diminish possible systemic effects of some drugs (eg, timolol maleate), the patient should be told to apply light finger pressure on the lacrimal sac for a minute following administration. Ophthalmic ointments may be used in the eye or on the eyelid depending on the drug and condition of the patient. Therefore, it first should be determined where the ointment should be used. If the ointment is to be used in the eye, pull the lower lid down the same way as when using eye drops; then squeeze a small amount of ointment inside the lower lid. The eye is then closed and the closed eye is gently massaged. If the ointment is to be used on the eyelid, a thin ribbon of ointment is squeezed from the tube directly onto the eyelid.

Currently medications for inhalation are provided to the patient by a variety of means, from the fine mist of a vaporizer to the powder of cromolyn sodium with a *Spinhaler*. There are now dosage forms for oral and nasal inhalation and it is obvious that these products will only be effective when properly used by the patient. The pharmacist must attempt to educate the patient in the use of these products and provide the patient written instruction, usually found within the product carton. It is difficult to predict what percentage of patients will read or even understand the printed instruction. Thus, the pharmacist must verbally transmit instruction for proper use. Using the oral, metered aerosols as a model the pharmacist should demonstrate how the inhaler is to be assembled, stored, and cleaned. The patient should be told if the inhaler requires shaking before use and how to hold between the index finger and thumb so that the aerosol canister is up-side-down. The patient should understand that coordination must be achieved between inhalation (after exhaling as completely as possible) and pressing down the inhaler to

release one dose. The patient should be instructed to hold his breath for several seconds or as long as possible to gain the maximum benefit from the medication. The patient is told to then remove the inhaler from the mouth and exhale slowly through pursed lips.

There are several helpful items of information that the pharmacist should share about the proper use of suppositories. If the suppository must be stored in the refrigerator, it should be allowed to warm to room temperature before insertion. The patient should be advised to rub cocoa butter suppositories gently with the fingers to help melt the surface to provide lubrication for insertion. Glycerinated gelatin or polyethylene glycol suppositories should be moistened with water to enhance lubrication. If the polyethylene glycol suppository formulation does not contain at least 20% water, dipping it in water just prior to insertion prevents moisture from being drawn from rectal tissues after insertion and decreases subsequent irritation. Vaginal inserts (compressed tablets) should also be dipped into water quickly before insertion. This provides lubrication and enhances disintegration. The shape of the suppository determines how it will be inserted. Bullet-shaped rectal suppositories should be inserted pointed-end first. In those instances when the patient is to use one-half suppository, the patient should be told to cut the suppository lengthwise with a clean razor blade.

Whenever the directions for the use of a medication refer to water (eg, dissolve in water, mix with water, take with water), the pharmacist should tell the patient how much water to use and in what manner. For example, one laxative product instructs a patient to place a rounded teaspoonful of granules in the mouth and swallow with a glass of water. Another laxative product instructs the patient to add a teaspoon of powder to the liquid before ingesting it. These are points of clarification that are necessary to ensure correct use by the patient.

Administration Timing—Interpretation of the sig, "one qid" may be variable between the physician, the pharmacist, and the patient. Conceivable interpretations for this might include the following:

One every 6 hours around the clock (6 am, 12 pm, 6 pm, 12 am).
One every 4 hours while awake (8 am, 12 pm, 4 pm, 8 pm).
One before meals and at bedtime.
One after meals and at bedtime.
One with meals and at bedtime.

The pharmacist must use his knowledge of drugs when interpreting the sig and give direction to the patient to ensure that the drug is effective maximally. If the effectiveness of the drug is dependent upon a maintained blood level the patient should be instructed to equally space out through the day appropriate dosing times. If the bioavailability of the drug from oral administration is in doubt when taken with food (eg, antibiotics), it is best to recommend that the drug be taken either one hour before or two hours after meals. The pharmacist cannot lose sight of the fact that some patients do not eat three meals a day and thus if the latter recommendation was made it would be important to emphasize to the patient that even though a meal may not be eaten, the drug should still be taken. Alternatively, the pharmacist should exercise judgment in those instances where the drug that is administered orally causes stomach distress. In these instances the pharmacist should encourage the patient to take the medication with food or milk to prevent this upset. The pharmacist should never assume that the patient knows entirely how to use the medication appropriately. When timing is crucial, the pharmacist should exercise expertise and counsel the patient to exercise good judgement.

The pharmacist should also be extremely wary of "prn" prescriptions. The patient should be told about the correct use of the product. Probably the foremost example is with pain medication. The patient should be told to use the medication only as needed for pain, and not to merely take the medication to prevent pain. At the same time, if the problem persists the patient should be encouraged to take another dose within the prescribed time indicated on the label bearing in mind that the tablet may not work immediately and there will likely be a gap in the relief if the pain is allowed to return before taking the next dose. Another example of difficulty with "prn" use entails the tachyphylaxis that develops with the overuse of aerosol inhalers to treat asthmatic conditions. A pattern of increasing frequency of refills is a signal to the pharmacist that the patient is either overusing the product or simply does not know how to use it in correct fashion. Pharmacist intervention is a necessity in this instance. Another facet with "prn" medication is that patients may not need the medication for a period of time and thus will have to store it. Adequate instructions should accompany the medication that encourage proper storage. Sometimes, however, "prn" instructions are simply inappropriate, eg, medications which accumulate in the system for maximum effectiveness, such as the tricyclic antidepressants.

Dosage regimens are best established when consideration is given to the daily routine of the patient. Dosage regimens can be best developed when these take into account the patient's eating and sleeping habits and work schedule. For instance, a person prescribed hydrochlorothiazide might be hesitant to take the medication in the morning before work simply because it will cause the patient to frequent the bathroom several times during the day. It would be better for the pharmacist to intercede with the recommendation to wait until returning from work at the end of the afternoon, and not later, before taking the tablet. This will allow the patient to benefit from the medication, and not be bothered by frequent trips to the bathroom during the night.

Compliance problems with medications increase as the number of medications a person ingests during the day increases. A medication calendar can prove very useful to a patient and developed almost entirely to the patient's individual needs. The medication calendar should reinforce in the mind of the patient the correct time to take the medication and afford the opportunity for the patient to mark down that the dose was actually taken. This obviates problems of forgetfulness about whether a dose was taken or missed. Numerous calendars have been developed and an exemplary calendar is presented (Fig 94-1). This calendar provides space for writing in *chronic* and *as needed* medications, as well as the administration times within the vertical column. The patient can write in the name and the dosage of the medication (even the prescription number if desired) to be taken at one time. The horizontal column contains the days of the month through day 31. The patient merely checks off the appropriate time slot when a dose of medication has been taken. This helps prevent problems of forgetfulness and avoids unnecessary and dangerous accidental double dosing. Such a calendar can be taped to the refrigerator in the kitchen and encourages the patient to take an active role in the treatment plan by complying with the prescribed medications.

Duration of Use—The pharmacist must ensure that the patient understands clearly the length of time the medication is to be used. Chronic diseases dictate that adequate blood levels of drug be maintained to control the disease process. Thus, emphasis should be toward patient compliance counseling regarding the medication and periodic revisits with the physician to assess the therapeutic regimen. The pharmacist must also emphasize to patients that some medications take longer to see the initial effects of the drug (eg, nonsteroidal anti-inflammatory agents, tricyclic antidepressants) and they should exercise patience. At the same time the pharmacist should provide the patient with a reasonable time period in which the patient should experience the desired effect. After

this time, the patient should be told to contact his physician.

For acute problems the pharmacist must share with the patient the length of time the medication should be taken. This is very important with antibiotic/anti-infective medication which must be taken in its entirety to cure the infection. Early discontinuation of the medication because of feeling better or normal should be discouraged to prevent a relapse of the infection and/or sequelae. The pharmacist must emphasize this fact to patients since some believe that taking a drug is not good for their body and will only take what they think is necessary. This philosophy is particularly dangerous when dealing with parents of young children who do not want to subject their children to more medication than is necessary or, simply because of inconvenience, do not elect to continue the medication once the child feels better. Aside from oral medication, other medication (eg, otic drops, nasal drops, vaginal inserts) might be prescribed for an acute condition. The pharmacist must exercise judgment and instruct the patient on the length of therapy. For example, an infectious otitis externa problem treated with otic drops should be continued for at least two to three days beyond the time the symptoms have abated. It is not necessary to continue using the otic drops until they are finished since the medication could be conceivably used for over twenty days. This information should be told to the patient.

How To Store The Drug—The pharmacist should counsel the patient in the proper storage of the medicine to ensure safety and stability. It is not sufficient to assume the patient will notice, read, or be able to understand an auxiliary label which indicates how to store the medication. Safety is foremost when storing medication, particularly out of the reach of children. Further, medication should be stored in a single area (preferably inside a high cabinet) with external medications separate from internal medications.

Proper storage of the medication also ensures stability of the product. Medications should be stored away from extremes of heat and high humidity. It is difficult to imagine a worse place to store medication than the medicine cabinet in the bathroom. Heat and humidity enhance drug instability and patients should be told to visually inspect the medication before using it. Any color change or odor emanating from the product indicates that the product may be losing its potency. Patients should be instructed to cap the bottle tightly after use, otherwise, environmental humidity could cause stability problems, or the exposure to the atmosphere could promote the evaporation of the vehicle. With topical liquid products (eg, wart removers) this could result in a somewhat more potent and hazardous product. Further, some products may degrade into toxic products, not merely useless products eg, tetracyclines.

When a medication is dispensed to a patient in its original container and still bears the expiration data on its label (eg, ear drops, eye drops) this should be brought to the attention of the patient so that he can exercise judgment to periodically discard old outdated medication. Otherwise, medication not used within one year after it is received by the patient should be discarded.

Side Effects—The instructions about a medication should encourage compliance rather than discourage it, and there is no quicker mechanism to achieve the latter than a hasty, ill-thought presentation by the pharmacist of side effects that might be encountered with a particular medication. The pharmacist should tactfully inform the patient about side effects that could be encountered. If not so instructed the patient might discontinue the use of the product with no benefit. The pharmacist should only share with the patient the most frequently encountered of conceivable side effects and provide the patient a mechanism by which to cope with them. For example, metronidazole is used for trichomonal

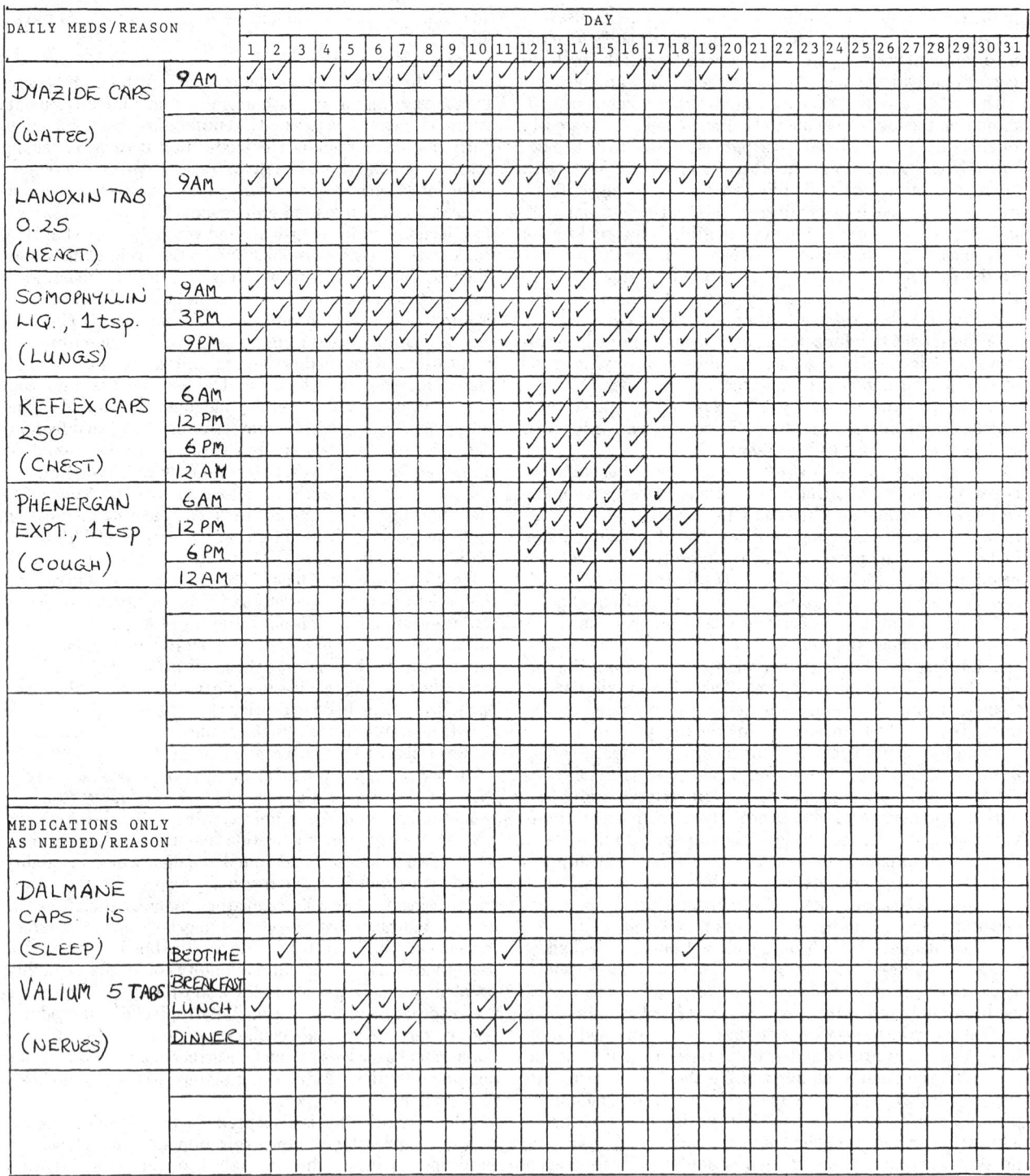

Fig 94-1.   A medication calendar.[3]

infections, and "may cause headaches in some people. If you experience a headache, do not hesitate to take some aspirin or acetaminophen for it. If this does not help, contact your doctor."

The manner in which the patient is told of side effects is crucial. Presentation of the side effect might convince the patient not to take the medication. For example, "Do not drive while taking this medicine; it will make you drowsy." For a person who makes a living traveling this might dictate against taking the medication at all. Thus, the instruction should be, "this medication may make you drowsy and impair your perception. Exercise judgment when doing things that

involve your reflexes or alertness. Thus, use caution when you are driving."

Similarly, patients should be told that some medications cause side effects at first that diminish with continual use. For example, the dizziness or lightheadness with methyldopa should decrease as one adjusts to the medicine. At the same time the patient should be informed if problems persist or get worse the doctor should be consulted.

Auxiliary labels serve a definite purpose to help inform the patient about their prescription medication. These should be used cautiously, and verbally explained by the pharmacist when conveying information about side effects or potential drug interactions. For example, one label that is used cautions patients to avoid excessive exposure to direct sunlight. Unfortunately, without pharmacist explanation this might be construed by the patient to mean avoid going out of doors and keeping the house dark. The word "excessive" is overlooked by the patient, but then again what does the word mean? Obviously, this label needs interpretation by the pharmacist during the counseling encounter. Another label cautions the patient against the concurrent use of alcohol with the medication for fear of an additive depressant effect. Unfortunately, the patient might not read the label or understand that alcohol need not be consumed only from an alcoholic beverage; alcohol is included in a number of liquid medications (eg, cough-cold remedies). Thus, the emphasis should be with good verbal communication with the pharmacist.

Some medications by virtue of their physical-chemical properties could cause compliance problems in some patients. Some medications have the ability to change urine color (eg, phenazopyridine), stool color (eg, ferrous sulfate), and saliva, sweat, and tear color (eg, rifampin). While these are not side effects, these should be brought to the attention of the patient beforehand to allay any encountered fears when these occur.

Drug Interactions—The patient should be forewarned about other drugs (eg, legend, nonprescription) that have the capability to alter the effectiveness of the prescribed medication. Certainly if there is legend medication within the current profile of the patient that conflicts with a newly prescribed medication it is the responsibility of the pharmacist to bring it to the attention of the physician. Unfortunately, however, patients perceive nonprescription drugs as entirely safe and do not realize that these have the ability to aggravate their condition or conflict with prescription medication. Thus, this discussion should also include instruction to carefully read nonprescription drug labels beforehand and if in doubt consult the physician or the pharmacist. Only those drug interactions which are clinically significant (eg, sodium warfarin–aspirin) should be brought to the attention of the patient, and alternative means provided to cope with any problems (eg, use of acetaminophen for headache while maintained on warfarin therapy).

This subject area also encompasses the ingestion of food concurrent with the oral administration of the medication. When a significant alteration in the bioavailability of the drug or the therapeutic effect occurs with the concurrent administration of foods or liquids (eg, tetracycline with milk) the patient should be warned and provided a suitable remedy to ensure that the patient will use the medication. Similarly, if a patient by necessity must ingest food with the medication (e.g., phenytoin, propranolol) to avoid gastrointestinal upset, the patient should be encouraged to maintain this mode of administration whenever possible to avoid fluctuation in the bioavailability of the drug and ultimately the steady state levels of the drug in the blood plasma.

Allergies—Every drug has the capability to effect a hypersensitivity reaction in a patient. However, there are some medications (eg, penicillins, sulfonamides, thiazides) which effect a higher incidence of allergic reactions. When such medications are prescribed, the pharmacist should inquire about the past medication history of the patient and if he is allergic to any medication. In a tactful manner the patient should be told that the prescribed medication has caused a rash or allergic reaction in some people. Thus, in the event the patient experiences a rash, or an itching and burning of the skin, the patient is advised to discontinue the use of the medication and contact the physician.

Refill Information—When presenting the medication to the patient, the pharmacist should verbally indicate whether or not the prescription is refillable, or should be refilled. If the prescription can be refilled, the patient should be informed of this, plus told the number of times it may be refilled and the length of time during which the prescription may be refilled. If the prescription is nonrefillable, the patient should be so instructed, so that if the patient needs additional medication the patient will know to contact the physician. The pharmacist should not, however, give the patient the impression that there is a need to return to the physician's office only for a new prescription, but to have the patient contact the physician by telephone, explain the situation, and then telephone the pharmacist who in turn can contact the physician for the refill authorization.

Whenever possible the pharmacist should encourage those patients who take chronic medications to have them refilled on time. This is a time consuming activity and many pharmacists cannot bring themselves to do it efficiently since they are usually not remunerated for it. A recent pilot study, however, investigated patient willingness to pay for a community pharmacy based medication reminder system.[8] This study blended an initial interview (eg, medication history, counseling session) and follow-up discussions (ie, return visits to the pharmacy) with a medication reminder system for a group of patients who were maintained on at least one regularly scheduled cardiovascular medication (CVM). These patients received a medication reminder card in the mail within three days after the calculated refill date of the CVM was passed. If after 10 days the prescription had not been refilled, the patient was contacted by telephone. The data indicated that nearly 40% of the patients expressed a willingness to pay for the services they received above the cost of the medication. Further, the authors indicated that the reminder system could be maintained in a relatively small amount of time (less than 15 minutes per day) and effort (clerical and pharmacist) and lent itself nicely to a computer function.

Therapeutic Intent of the Medication—It is not advisable for the pharmacist to make reference to the therapeutic use of the medication unless he is absolutely certain of its intended purpose for a particular patient. Rarely does the pharmacist know the diagnosis of the patient, nor the intent of the physician in prescribing a certain drug. Indeed, there are numerous indications for a multitude of drugs which make it difficult to identify the one indication for a specific patient.

When confronted by a patient inquiry about the purpose of the medication the pharmacist should answer a question with a question. A question about the reason the patient consulted a physician and something about their physical health could provide insight for the pharmacist. Careful questioning will usually provide enough information so that the pharmacist can piece together a reasonable response that will answer the patient's question.

Additional Ancillary Information—The therapeutic outcome will only be successful if the patient understands to comply with his medicine. At the same time the pharmacist should bring to the attention of the patient other factors which may embellish or enhance the drug therapy. For instance, patients maintained on oral hypoglycemics should be reminded to maintain their caloric intake and be cognizant of their diet. A patient maintained on daily doses of phenytoin should be advised to exercise good oral hygiene by massaging the gums and brushing the teeth at least on a daily basis. Patients with asthmatic conditions can be advised about things that can be done to relieve asthmatic attacks before these occur. These are all examples of common sense things that are useful to the patient and typify the expertise of the pharmacist as a source of information.

Monitoring Drug Utilization

Pharmacists have always recognized their responsibility to check the safety of the dosage regimen for each medication dispensed. In years past this was an easy task; but recently, with the proliferation of many newer, potent medications this task has become quite formidable. Checking the safety of a dosage regimen is more complex today since, in addition to higher potency, many drugs can be used for more than one clinical indication. Further with the diversification of the medical profession into specialty areas there is a greater chance that patients will consult more than one physician. Thus, the patient of today may be taking a number of drugs simultaneously from more than one physician. Very often these physicians will not be aware that their patient is receiving drugs prescribed by other physicians. This is the perfect avenue by which drug interactions occur. In addition, with greater numbers of patients taking medication there is a greater likelihood of allergic, idiosyncratic, or adverse reactions to occur. When these are manifest it is vital that these be documented to prevent their occurrence in the future. Because of all of these factors it is implicit that the pharmacist be cognizant of each patient as a whole, inclusive of all the medications that the patient may be currently taking when evaluating the safety of a newly prescribed medication about to be dispensed. To effectively do this the pharmacist must keep a record of the past medical history of the patient (eg, chronic disease status, allergic/idiosyncratic/adverse reactions) and medication history. It is inconceivable that the pharmacist could commit to memory the status of each patient and thus the aspect of a patient "profile or record" system looms as a necessity for effective ambulatory pharmacy practice. Integrated into this record system is the ability of the pharmacist to monitor the progress of the patient with the prescribed therapeutic regimen.

Patient (Family) Medication Profiles

Patient Medication Profiles are synonymous with "Family Prescription Records" and "Patient Medication Card." Essentially, these systems are a record of information relative to the drug therapy of a patient or an entire family. Ideally, but not too realistically, it should also include nonprescription drugs/products as well. While the family system allows all the members to be listed on a single card and reduces the number of cards on file, it presents a nightmare when the pharmacist is trying to monitor the therapy for each patient. The individual patient record makes it easier to monitor the patient and is less susceptible to errors and confusion on the part of the pharmacist. This problem may be negated by computer systems which store, a patient record in the family file, but scan only the individual history of the patient and medications when necessary.

Purpose of the Profile—The main purposes of the profile include the documentation of the medication history and the use of medication by the patient (eg, compliance, noncompliance). Further, it provides a data base to facilitate communication and consultation between the pharmacist and other health professionals (eg, drug allergies, idiosyncratic reactions, previous ineffective medication, prevention of potential drug–drug interactions).

Essential Information of the Profile—There are a number of different record systems and cards which are available to the pharmacist. However, because of space limitations the pharmacist might have to design his own and have these duplicated. The essential information that should be included on the patient medication profile is as follows:

1. Name of patient
2. Address of the patient
3. Telephone number of the patient
4. Birth date of the patient
5. Previous drug allergies/idiosyncratic reactions/side effects
6. Diseases/condition of the patient
7. Previous ineffective drug therapy
8. Prescription number
9. Date of prescription
10. Drug product name
11. Dosage form of product
12. Strength of product
13. Quantity dispensed
14. Name of prescriber
15. Identification of pharmacist

Additional information that can prove useful on the profile is the sig of the medication dispensed, refill information, and the charge for the medication. A typical family profile and patient profile is illustrated in Figs 94-2 and 94-3.

The information in the upper left hand corner of the record contains demographic data of the patient(s). The birth date, not the age of the patient should be used since it remains constant. When the family system is utilized, each family member must be identified by a key. In Fig 94-2, the designation (H) is used for the husband, (W) is used for wife, and numbers used to identify the children.

The upper right hand portion of the profile is reserved for necessary information to prevent the dispensing of contraindicated drugs (ie, clinical conditions/problems, allergies/reactions). Further, space should be allotted for notes (eg, past medication failure, inability to use medication) which provide a complete picture of the patient.

The bottom portion of the profile contains relevant information about the dispensed medication.

A color dot or symbol system can be used with a profile system to identify specific pharmacist concerns eg, red dot means to check compliance discrepancy, green dot means to discuss side effects with a particular patient, red star indicates physician contacted and notation of the prescription face. Further, a color code system for a certain sequence of the letters in the alphabet is an effective means to overcome the loss of a patient profile. Every practicing pharmacist who has worked with filed records realizes the danger of "lost records." These records are not lost at all, but are merely misfiled. In a pharmacy where there may be well over a thousand profiles, the file may be misplaced in any part of the system. Thus, searching for the file at the time of prescription dispensing is impractical if not impossible. The pharmacist should follow the example of other professions to help identify a misplaced file. Medical records departments are the prime example. For every 100–200 files, a different color code is used. A misplaced file becomes very obvious under this system if it is in another color space, or if it is to be found among a very small number of similarly coded files. It must also be mentioned that the likelihood of a person replacing a profile incorrectly is less when the color code does not match. In busy pharmacies when a file is pulled for use, a handy ruler, pencil or tongue depressor is usually placed to mark its spot. The system then resembles a porcupine more than a filing system and when the profile is to be refiled, numerous markers may be confusing and lead to misfiling. An effective color code system reduces the incidence of misfiled information.

Implementation and Utilization—The pharmacist must select the medication profile system (family, individual) according to that which best fits his practice. To implement the service the pharmacist must establish a mode to gather and record essential patient information (usually a patient interview). To be effective, the patient medication profile must be used each time a professional service is performed for the patient.

The pharmacist must maintain confidentiality of the profile, consistent with the same accorded a prescription. However, the concept of confidentiality is nebulous since the

Family Name __Public__

Address __123 W. Columbia__

Telephone __555-1212__

(H) John Q.	9-30-44
(W) Mary	3-4-47
(1) Stanley J.	10-11-72
(2) Gabriel N.	1-4-78
(3) Matthew T.	11-2-79

Allergies/Reactions __(H) ALLERGIC TO SULFA__
__(3) ALLERGIC TO PCN__

Clin. Conditions/Problems __(W) GLAUCOMA__
__(H) Migraine__

Notes: (1) CANNOT SWALLOW TABLETS

Date	R$_x$ Number	Price	Physician	Pt.	Prescription	RPh	Ref. Left
1/4/83	224523	10⁰⁰	SMITH	H	100 Inderal 20mg. TAB, i qid	rↄ	5
1/10/83	225221	16⁵⁰	JONES	W	10cc Timoptic 0.25%, i ou bid	rↄ	5
1/29/83	224523	10⁰⁰	SMITH	H	100 Inderal 20mg TAB, i qid	rↄ	4
2/12/83	228461	2⁵⁰	COBB	2	100cc V-CILLIN K ¹²⁵/₅, 5cc q 6°	rↄ	4
2/15/83	231455	5⁵⁰	SMITH	W	24 Dalmane 15mg, 1 hs prn	rↄ	2
2/15/83	231456	12⁰⁰	SMITH	W	20 Keflex 250mg CAP, 1 qid	rↄ	0
3/2/83	224523	10⁰⁰	SMITH	H	100 Inderal 20mg TAB, i qid	rↄ	3
3/2/83	233171	2⁴⁰	COBB	1	120cc DIMETAPP EL., 5cc q 4°	rↄ	3
3/4/83	225221	16⁵⁰	JONES	W	10 cc Timoptic 0.25%, i ou bid	rↄ	4
4/18/83	238901	5⁹⁰	COBB	3	120cc E.E.S. ²⁰⁰/₅, 5cc q 6°	rↄ	0
4/18/83	238902	3⁵⁰	COBB	3	15cc AURALGAN, 2 gtts ear tid	rↄ	0
5/22/83	231455	5⁵⁰	SMITH	W	24 Dalmane 15mg, 1 hs prn	rↄ	1

Fig 94-2.   A family medication record.

patient is not required to provide the information. The pharmacist can usually divulge information (if in good faith) when it is in the best interest of the patient (eg, contact a physician about the past allergic history of the patient). However, the pharmacist should familiarize himself with the state regulations and the state pharmacy practice to know the obligations and responsibilities germane to the dissemination of the information from such a patient profile. Some patient profile systems intentionally have the confidential information on the right-side of the profile (Fig 94-2). Thus, information which might be requested by the patient for the preparation of income tax or insurance purpose is located on the left side (date, medication order number, physician, charge, etc). Thus the right hand side of the card can be covered and a photocopy made of the left hand portion of the profile.

A key problem with confidentiality occurs when the request for information originates outside of the pharmacy. Specifically, when the information is requested by an insurance company. Generally, the pharmacist does not know whether the patient is represented by the company. Perhaps there is a history of patient claims filed for the patient by the pharmacist that gives a clue to the pharmacist about the validity of the request. In those instances when there is no obvious relationship or where there is any question, the pharmacist should respect the privacy of the information and not release it without the express permission either obtained directly from the patient or from a signed statement of waiver presented by the person requesting the information. Clearly, a telephone request is unacceptable. The patient, for example, could be under investigation for fraud. There could be any number of reasons why the patient would want to know of information

Name __Public, Mary__

Address __123 W. Columbia__

Telephone __555-1212__   Sex: M (F)

Birthdate __3-4-47__   Wt. __110__

Allergies/Reactions _____

_____

_____

Clin. Conditions/Problems __GLAUCOMA__

_____

_____

Notes:

Date	R_x Number	Price	Physician	Prescription	RPh	Ref. Left.
1/10/83	225221	16 50	JONES	10cc. Timoptic 0.25%, i ou bid	N	5
2/15/83	231455	5 50	SMITH	24 Dalmane 15mg, i hs prn	N	2
2/15/83	231456	12 00	SMITH	20 Keflex 250mg, i qid	N	0
3/4/83	225221	16 50	JONES	10cc. Timoptic 0.25%, i ou bid	N	4
5/22/83	231455	5 50	SMITH	24 Dalmane 15mg, i hs prn	N	1

Fig 94-3.   An individual patient medication record.

requests and have input into the process. The pharmacist cannot make these decisions.

Finally, the pharmacist should familiarize his patients with the profile system and the need to have continual up-to-date information. Thus, patients realize the value of having a current system and a loyalty is fostered between patient and pharmacist.

Practice Management Aspects—An effective profile system could facilitate additional advantages to the pharmacist that aid in the effective management of his practice. For instance, third party payment information, generation of tax and insurance receipts, and accounting and billing information are just a few examples where the system can be advantageous. Since the first medication profile was introduced into pharmacy practice in 1960, there have been nu-

merous discussions concerning the pros and cons of maintaining such a record. The reasons given by pharmacists for not providing this service are: it is too time consuming, it costs too much, it increases the pharmacist's liability, this is the physician's responsibility, the patient will not like it, and it's an infringement on patient confidentiality. These reasons have been investigated and contested in court with the results in favor of the medication profile. In addition, good managerial procedures diminish the time consuming aspect of the profiles. A good example of this is when a pharmacist deals with one or more members of a family that have different last names. A well-planned and executed cross reference system negates any problems with these blended families. Further, all pharmacists are required by law to file the original prescription by serial number as received. Finding a "lost number" can be frustrating both to the pharmacist and the patient. A cross reference to the patient profile is the best mechanism to solve this universal problem. The pharmacist is now required by statute to renew the safety closure on glass bottles and replace the entire container in the case of plastic vials each time a refill is requested. It would seem that as more patients become familiar with this practice of replacement more of them will return for a prescription refill without the original container. Where then will the pharmacist retrieve the needed prescription number if there is no patient profile system within the pharmacy? Thus, good business practice dictates the use of a patient profile system.

An analysis of the cost and effectiveness of implementing a patient medication record system in one pharmacy was a favorable cost-effectiveness ratio of 1 to 2.54. Another study of 11 pharmacies reported that use of patient medication records does not add more than five cents to the cost of the prescription. Patient acceptance of the medication record was measured by a survey which found that 86% of those responding to a questionnaire felt that the pharmacist should provide this service. A survey of physician's opinions revealed that 60.7% of the respondents stated profiles would be of value to them and 64.3% felt they would be of value to the patient.

In 1972 a regulation was adopted by the New Jersey Board of Pharmacy requiring pharmacies to maintain patient medication profiles. This regulation was contested and on May 8, 1973, the Appellate Division of the Superior Court of New Jersey ruled in favor of the Board of Pharmacy. The court stated in its decision that the regulation would have little economic impact on pharmacies, would not interfere with the physician-patient privilege that protects the confidentiality of medication, and that it would not place an increased liability burden upon the pharmacist.

A majority of states do not mandate pharmacists to keep medication profiles. It is noteworthy to mention, however, that those that have regulations specifying profiles have differing views of how these are to be used. For example, three states in addition to New Jersey require that the pharmacist consult and examine the patient profile for each prescription dispensed. Delaware and New Jersey mandate this through a State Board of Pharmacy Regulation, while Maine and North Dakota mandate this by statute. The State of Kansas requires patient profiles only under special circumstances, eg, if the pharmacist is a consultant to an extended care facility. Virginia and Oregon specify that if profiles are kept in a pharmacy at all, the pharmacist must use patient profiles for professional purposes, and not merely for common business purposes (such as tax or insurance records). The State of Iowa requires patient profiles if pharmacy interns are on the premises. The State of Idaho has requirements which the pharmacist must meet in the eventuality that the pharmacist does not have patient profiles. In actuality, the pharmacist must secure from the patient with each prescription necessary information (allergies, idiosyncratic reactions, chronic conditions, etc). Thus, the pharmacist preferentially opts to maintain profiles in Idaho. The States of Hawaii, Tennessee, and Wisconsin can be classified as "reward" states for the pharmacist to maintain patient profiles. In Hawaii, the pharmacist may advertise the fact that profiles are maintained. In Tennessee and Wisconsin, profiles are allowed as a means for the pharmacist to maintain refill records rather than refer to the original prescription, a process many pharmacists scorn.

When not mandated by law to provide a patient profile system, the pharmacist may be faced with the difficult question of whether or not to provide this service. When faced with "less than ideal conditions," or money to invest in such a system the pharmacist should consider profiles for "at risk" patients only. This group would include the elderly, those

in nursing homes, or patients who have numerous prescription medication therapies. Otherwise, the pharmacist should elect to use the individual prescription to monitor the patient when there is no profile or a limited profile system in use. This offers a means at least to monitor patient drug utilization and compliance. At the same time a portion of the prescription face, usually the lower right hand quadrant, offers space on which to make notations or key words (e.g., counseling, side effects, compliance).

In the event that the pharmacist cannot provide some profile system for his patients it is beneficial for the pharmacist to suggest to or provide for a medication profile card that can be carried on the person of the patient. The patient is then told to present it to the pharmacist whenever a new medication is to be dispensed and also when the patient considers purchasing a nonprescription product for self treatment. Local pharmaceutical associations have disseminated these, also, to provide and enhance better patient care. This system has several benefits in that it identifies those patients who consult more than one physician and pharmacy. Thus, the pharmacist can identify potential problems with prescribed medication from multiple physicians and the physician has, through the card, knowledge of each patient's medication. This avoids potential drug interactions to a degree and duplication of medication. Further, in an emergency situation these cards are useful to everyone since they list the entire medication profile of the patient.

Systematic Profile Review—As mentioned earlier, to be effective the profile system must be up-to-date and used for the benefit of the patient. Pharmacists must develop their skill and method of reviewing patient profiles to improve monitoring and be of service to the patient.

The importance of profile review in ambulatory pharmacy practice cannot be overstated. Effective monitoring requires a systematic approach by the pharmacist. Presented below is the *10 step method* adapted from that developed by Srnka and Self.[9] Each patient, each prescription, and each disease state must be considered separately by the pharmacist. Review of patient profiles will illustrate different types of problems varying greatly in significance, urgency, and complexity. Thus, the pharmacist must develop a plan of action of what to do and how to do it to effect an appropriate solution to the problem. Often a solution will involve the coordination of efforts between various individuals (eg, patient, physician). In this context there are three basic options the pharmacist has available to himself. These are:

1. Dispense the prescription(s) as written.
2. Do not dispense the prescription(s).
3. Dispense the prescription(s) after appropriate action has been taken.

The first two are entirely up to the pharmacist, the third involves resolution after consultation with the prescriber. However, before consultation the pharmacist should have a clear grasp of the problem and be able to provide a concise description of the potential problem. Whenever possible, it is helpful if the pharmacist has a literature reference to substantiate the clinical significance. Realistically, however, this is difficult to attain, but the use of a drug information center might be able to facilitate this. Lastly, the pharmacist should have a suggested solution to the problem, an alternative therapeutic route. Problem resolution depends upon judgment and tact, it is something that is only learned through experience and the willingness to do so by the pharmacist. Through all of this process the pharmacist must keep in mind the patient is always given first priority.[9]

Srnka and Self[9] suggest the following ten elements to look for on a profile.

1. History of adverse effects.
2. Potentially unwarranted/unintended changes in therapeutic regimen.
3. Potential quantitative misuse (noncompliance, misuse, overuse).
4. Duplication of medications.
5. Additive effects from similar medication use.
6. Inappropriate dosage, route of administration, dosing schedule, or dosage form.
7. Potential current adverse effects.
8. Drug-drug interactions.
9. Drug-disease interactions.
10. Irrational therapeutic regimen.

The authors suggest the pharmacist have a pocket card with these elements available to aid the review of the patient profile each time the pharmacist dispenses a prescription. This pocket card provides the pharmacist with a framework to review the profile and with time is ultimately committed to memory and the time necessary to review the process lessened with experience.

Nonprescription Drug Usage

The pharmacist is in a unique position because of his education and training and ready accessibility to the public when it comes to self-medication by the public with nonprescription drug products. It is estimated that there are more than 350,000 nonprescription products available within the United States with more than 8 billion dollars spent for their purchase in 1980. Self medication with these products continues to increase in importance because of spiraling health care costs, as well as a greater awareness and emphasis on the need for more personal involvement and responsibility for health maintenance on the part of the individual. A prime example of this is in dental care where pharmacists today see more persons with dental problems (such as, bleeding gums, broken dentures, toothaches, canker sores) than most dentists. Further, these persons seek out the pharmacist for advice on which toothpaste or dental floss they should purchase.

Nonprescription drug products serve a vital role in health care. Self-medication, already a dominant form of health care, will become even more important in the future. A person may not always desire to seek the advice of a physician each time he becomes ill. Correspondingly, the symptoms of the ailment may be minor enough to treat with a nonprescription product. The decision of the patient concerning which product to purchase is usually based on prior experience with the product, advice received from the pharmacist, neighbor and/or relatives, or commercial advertisements by manufacturers. However, on reflection, the pharmacist is the only expert/specialist in this knowledge area and should make his particular expertise available to the patient.

In the past the pharmacist was not often consulted about nonprescription drugs and/or treatments. Two reasons for this were the fact that the pharmacist was too busy and unavailable for consultation, or when available did not always provide adequate and relevant information. Furthermore, many believe that prior experience with a drug or drug product, or the fact that it is advertised commercially on radio or television is sufficient for their purpose. Others believe that product labels are always clear and answer consumers' questions and they do not need to be counseled with each purchase. However, it is estimated that nearly one-half of all money spent on drugs (prescription and nonprescription) in the United States is wasted because of patient misuse or noncompliance. Also, the availability of a nonprescription drug does not imply a drug which is entirely safe and effective. As an illustration, records maintained by one poison control center for a year indicated that a majority of calls to the center were from consumers and that nearly 40% of these callers requested information about nonprescription drugs.[10]

Consumer trends indicate that the pharmacist is slowly gaining recognition toward providing information to the patient about nonprescription drugs/products. Consumers seek out pharmacists who provide service. The factors (in descending order of importance) germane to the selection of a pharmacist were: (1) the pharmacist discusses instructions for the use of the nonprescription product, including effectiveness, side effects, and ingredients; (2) availability of the pharmacist for consultation; (3) willingness of the pharmacist to offer advice on general health problems; and (4) the pharmacist was more friendly and approachable. One survey indicated that consumers are so intent on having the personal advice of the pharmacist that even when the pharmacist was busy a majority of consumers were willing to wait until he was free. Another study demonstrated that 44% of consumers ask their pharmacist for advice on minor health problems at least once during the year and that people under 40 years of age seek advice more often than people over 40.[11] This is consistent both with the younger group of people having families about which they are concerned and being more attuned to expect information about their health care. This same study demonstrated that 76% of consumers will take the advice of the pharmacist in preference to that of a friend and that 78% of the consumers indicated that they would use the product recommended by the pharmacist. Further, the Food and Drug Administration supports the concepts of self-medication, but unfortunately has not embraced the concept of the pharmacist as the first professional that the patient should consult before using the product. Instead, the FDA has ruled that certain OTC drugs be labelled, "seek the advice of a health professional before using this product." This is unfortunate since "health professional" has a broad definition, sometimes at the exclusion of the pharmacist. However, favorable advertising that suggests people ask their "doctor or pharmacist," helps consumers identify the valuable counsel the pharmacist has to offer.

Only since the 1960s has a concentrated effort been made to educate the pharmacist to provide accurate and useful advice to the patient seeking symptomatic relief with self-medication. Before that, pharmacy was practiced under the influences and restraints of the APhA Code of Ethics adopted in 1921 which deemed it unethical for a pharmacist "to prescribe." This was interpreted to mean that a pharmacist recommending an OTC medication would be committing a violation of ethics because he would be "counter-prescribing" (prescribing over the counter). Pharmacists were taught not to provide this service. Before the adoption of the 1921 Code, and until the 1930s when it began to exert its influence upon the practice of pharmacy, it was common for the patient to seek the advice of a pharmacist for minor ailments and first aid and for the pharmacist to provide this service. Another factor which contributed to isolate the pharmacist from the patient was the increase in prescription volume which occurred in the 1940s. For a period of about 25 years the pharmacist tended to avoid patient contact. During the 1960's pharmacy was rejuvenated with the promotion and gradual introduction of clinical concepts into the practice of pharmacy. Advising the patient on health matters not only became fashionable but was recognized as a responsibility of the pharmacist both ethically and legally. The pharmacist was encouraged to question the patient who had decided to self-medicate and either recommend an OTC medication or recommend that the patient seek medical attention. By 1969 the membership of the APhA voted to adopt a new Code of Ethics which held the health and welfare of the patient to be of first consideration for the pharmacist.

Even though the role of the pharmacist has changed state statutes may not have been updated to reflect this. The pharmacist does walk a very narrow line and paraphrasing the Ohio Revised Code §4731.34 as an example, "a person is regarded as practicing medicine when he/she prescribes, advises, recommends, administers, or dispenses for compensation any kind, direct or indirect, a drug or medicine for the cure or relief of bodily injury, infirmity, or disease." This is provided here not to dissuade the pharmacist from performing this valuable service, but to indicate that these statutes do exist. The pharmacist should be familiar with them as they are written and as they are applied. Frequently, these statutes are not applied, but the pharmacist must keep these in mind when practicing pharmacy.

The above brief historical perspective has been presented in order to explain why the average pharmacist in practice today may not be aware of his responsibility to provide advice to the person who decides to treat himself and why the pharmacist may have neglected to offer this professional service. A number of pharmacists may have to be educated or reeducated on how to counsel the patient who decides upon self-treatment. This is achieved within curriculums of schools and colleges of pharmacy that provide appropriate coursework in the area of nonprescription drug therapy. Furthermore, continuing education providers should strive in part to educate these pharmacists who did not have the benefit of a formal course in nonprescription drug therapy.

Self-medication counseling is a primary-care activity that carries with it a great amount of professional responsibility. Communicating information about OTC products requires the same basic skills used for prescription medication and does not mandate additional specialized training or vast financial expenditures to be done well. In that light, the OTC Drug Review process of the FDA has been a boon to the pharmacist. It has provided the pharmacist a knowledge base which allows him to make sound decisions on comparative product effectiveness and safety. Although the entire review process will not be completed until the late 1980's the process has generated substantial scientific research that has produced impressive amounts of new information and data on nonprescription drugs. At the same time it has placed a burden upon the pharmacist to keep current with new information in this important subject area. A real handicap for the diligent practicing pharmacist is obtaining factual, current information. Few pharmacists realize that they can contact the National Center for Drugs and Biologics, Food and Drug Administration, Rockville, MD 29857, 1-301-443-4960, for appropriate information relative to the review panels.

Usually, it is the patient who will seek assistance and initiate the dialogue when seeking an over-the-counter remedy. Friendliness and courtesy are attributes which facilitate availability and encourage the patient to seek out the pharmacist for advice and counsel. The patient may initiate the conversation with several question types such as:

1. What do you have for diarrhea? (Symptom in the form of a question)
2. What is the best antacid? (Product from a specific class of drug)
3. Do you carry Desenex Powder? (Specific product desired)

Correspondingly, the pharmacist should also recognize that the patient may be deliberating over an awesome number of products in the drug aisle, and offer assistance then or intervene at the time of purchase when the patient has selected a product that is contraindicated based on his medical history or has a significant potential to cause harm to the patient (eg, corn/callus remover for a diabetic patient).

When counseling a patient about nonprescription drugs there are four basic tenets to be followed while getting to the situation at hand. The first of these is to exercise *active listening*. The patient should be allowed to state the problem completely and the pharmacist should provide his undivided attention. Full attention to the patient is necessary to minimize misperception and misunderstanding. The pharmacist must then be able to mentally summarize what the patient has said and provide positive feedback that conveys understanding of the problem, empathy, and concern. Using the words of the patient or paraphrasing what the patient has related indicates understanding the problem. Rewording or having to restate the situation forces the pharmacist to focus on what has been said and indicates to the patient that the pharmacist is actively processing the information and attempting to understand the situation. If the pharmacist can relate to the discomfort of problem the patient is experiencing using his own words, it indicates that the pharmacist has exercised a very important component of communication, active listening. This process also facilitates and enhances personal relations between the pharmacist and patient by the demonstration of a true concern for the patient.

The initial step in deciding whether or not a complaint or condition is amenable to self therapy involves the identification of the problem that the patient is seeking to treat. Quite often patients provide incomplete or conflicting information, much of which is necessarily subjective. Thus, the pharmacist must exercise the second tenet to the basics of counseling, that is *questioning the patient thoroughly*. The object is to elicit specific symptoms from the patient and determine if self-therapy is appropriate (symptom analysis).

Symptom analysis requires that the pharmacist obtain the following information:

1. *Onset of the problem*—When did the symptom(s) start?
2. *Duration of the problem*—How long does it last? Is it continual? Does it come and go away at certain times during the day?
3. *Severity*—How severe is the problem? Is it getting worse each time?
4. *Description of the symptom*—What does it feel like?
5. *Acute versus chronic*—Did it occur suddenly? Or has it occurred before?
6. *Associated symptoms*—Do you have any other symptoms that are occurring?
7. *Exacerbating factors*—Does anything make your symptoms worse or seem to cause the problem?
8. *Relieving factors*—Has anything you tried previously helped your symptoms?
9. *Previous therapy*—Have you tried any products or medications to relieve your symptoms?

The next step in the questioning process is to gather patient-related information. Before an assessment and decision can be made the pharmacist must be cognizant of individual characteristics. The following information should be elicited from the patient:

1. *Patient*—For whom is the request made?
2. *Age of the patient*—Is the patient an infant, a child, an adult, or an elderly patient?
3. *Sex of the patient*—Male or female? If female, is the patient pregnant or nursing a baby?
4. *Prior medical history*—Are there any other diseases or conditions from which the patient suffers?
5. *Prior drug history*—Are there any drugs (ie, prescription/nonprescription) that the patient is taking on a daily basis? Does the patient imbibe social drugs (eg, nicotine, caffeine, alcohol)?
6. *Allergy history*—Is the patient allergic to any drugs, environmental agents, etc?
7. *Adverse drug reaction history*—Has the patient had any bad experiences or side effects from prior use of medication?

The pharmacist must ask a sufficient number of questions to identify and assess the problem before a strategy is conceived. Time constraint necessitates that the pharmacist keep the line of questioning direct and to the point. The pharmacist should exercise judgment relative to the pertinence of the question and not probe on the basis of curiosity. With experience, the pharmacist should develop a style that will gather this information within a period of minutes. If the situation is more complex and time-consuming, the pharmacist can ask the patient to return at a mutually agreeable time, contact the patient by telephone, or refer the patient directly to a physician.

The third tenet in effective counseling is *interpreting verbal and nonverbal communication*. Every question asked of the patient should be carefully phrased by the pharmacist to facilitate interpretation. The patient should be able to understand that the questions the pharmacist asks come from a genuine interest and desire to be of help. The pharmacist may ask two types of questions. The first of these is the open-ended type which are useful to gather information regarding the medical problem. For instance, "can you tell me about the symptoms you have been experiencing?" This question type provides flexibility for patient response and encourages more than a simple yes or no answer. The second, a direct question, is useful when the information is a specific inquiry, eg, "How long have you noticed the burning sensation in your stomach?" It is crucial that these questions be asked one at a time, and not in rapid fashion which only results in confusion and frustration for the patient.

Nonverbal communication skills also serve a vital role in this situation. The body posture, facial expression, and distance of the patient all provide the pharmacist with perception of the patient as a whole. At the same time it is important that the pharmacist be aware of his nonverbal behavior. Physical barriers to communication should be eliminated whenever possible. In fact, anything that impedes the verbal exchange should be eliminated. The pharmacist should make every effort not to talk down to the patient, both verbally (ie, use the vernacular of the patient) and physically (the pharmacist and patient should be at the same eye-level). Patient-pharmacist exchange should be as private and uninterrupted as possible. However, all pharmacies do not have the benefit of a private consultation area or the money to construct one. But privacy can be achieved readily without expense by simply forming a triangle using the patient, the pharmacist, and the wall shelf or gondola as sides. This automatically signals others that the consultation is private and not to be interrupted.

Whenever possible the pharmacist should physically assess the patient through observation or inspection. For example, the skin is easily assessed by inspection and palpation. However, the lung requires percussion and auscultation, not easily attainable for the practicing pharmacist. The clear majority of pharmacists obtain physical data (eg, number of comedones per side of the face) exclusively through the use of observation. Further, there are clues to the overall state of health of the patient and these provide insight into the seriousness of the problem. Facial expressions mirror pain and discomfort; pallor and lethargy may be indicative of an infectious process, while persistent coughing may be a sign of some systemic illness.

After the pharmacist mentally tabulates all the information (verbal, nonverbal, and observation) the pharmacist must then make an assessment to the cause and severity of the condition. These are crucial since it will necessitate a particular treatment path.

Assessment of severity will vary among patient complaints. Some problems may be considered severe only when they accumulate to a certain level, such as persistent vomiting and diarrhea in an infant. The longer these persist, the more severe the problem and the greater the potential for referral to a physician. Further, some patient complaints may be considered severe only when they become symptomatic or the symptoms begin to impair the functional activity of the patient (eg, bleeding, external hemorrhoids). At this point, the fourth tenet of good counseling emerges—*clarifying the facts as needed*.

The plan of action that the pharmacist devises is the most important step in the process of self medication. At this point the pharmacist has three courses of action from which to select. These are referral, drug therapy, or nondrug intervention. Whichever course is chosen the pharmacist must ensure that the patient understands the reasoning behind it and the need to comply with the advice given.

Before the plan is put into effect, additional information may be necessary to enable a thorough assessment of the problem. This may include the consultation with the parent or guardian of the patient, or communication with the patient's physician. In this latter instance, the pharmacist acts as a direct link between the patient and the physician within the referral process. This communication between physician and pharmacist avoids conflict in the overall management of the patient and alleviates patient confusion associated with overlapping responsibilities between the physician and pharmacist. This situation is helpful because it serves a number of purposes. First, it allows for the input of the physician into an evaluation of the problem and determines whether the physician will want to see the patient or deal with the problem over the telephone. In the event that the physician wants to see the patient the pharmacist can provide and share additional information with the physician. Secondly, it serves as a method of obtaining additional data on prior medical conditions that need to be clarified to determine if self-therapy is appropriate or acceptable. Realistically, however, physicians are quite reluctant to give advice on the telephone and to provide service without compensation in the event that the pharmacist cannot handle the question. The pharmacist and the physician may be viewed as "partners" in the health care system but are not so in the business sense. Thus, communication of this type between pharmacist and physician engenders several questions, eg, should the pharmacist bill the patient and then respond in compensation to the physician for his service? Is there a referral fee for the service of the pharmacist when no product is purchased and the patient consults the physician? Will the physician tire of numerous telephone calls?

The first option is to counsel the self-medicating patient to seek the professional care of a physician. This should be executed in a tactful manner not to alarm or frighten the patient, and at the same time consideration should be given by the pharmacist to the treatment center to which the patient should be directed (ie, emergency, private practice) as well as the urgency. Some conditions dictate immediate attention (eg, persistent epigastric pain with bloody vomitus) whereas others do not (eg, mild to severe athlete's foot).

When making a decision to recommend a patient to consult a physician, the following situations support this:

1. Symptoms are too severe to be endured by the patient without definite diagnosis and treatment.
2. The symptoms are minor but have persisted and do not appear to be due to some easily identifiable cause.
3. The symptoms are recurring, more frequently, with no recognizable cause.
4. The pharmacist is in doubt about the condition of the patient.
5. Misuse of the product by the patient could result in harm to the patient.
6. The patient has correctly used (eg, administration, duration) an appropriate nonprescription product with no positive result.

It is important that the pharmacist emphasize to the patient the need for physician consultation. Sometimes patients listen and then purchase a product anyway. This is frustrating to the pharmacist, but sometimes it cannot be avoided. Conversely, there is a danger that when a pharmacist recommends something to hold the patient over until he can schedule an appointment with a physician, some patients simply will not follow through and make the appointment, particularly if the product seems to work for their condition.

When the pharmacist makes the decision that the condition of the person does not warrant physician intervention, a therapeutic endpoint must be identified for the patient and/or the specific condition. This endpoint should be attainable and accessible. At this point the pharmacist can either select a drug or nondrug treatment modality. This decision must be based upon patient variables (eg, age, sex, previous medical and/or drug history, life style) in conjunction with drug variables (dosage regimen, side effects, duration of use, comparable effectiveness to other drugs, etc).

There are instances when nondrug treatment measures are indicated. In this instance, the pharmacist will inform the patient to let the condition run its course (eg, canker sores) or recommend ways to help eliminate the problem (eg, humidification of inspired air to relieve the cough and hoarseness associated with laryngitis). There are, however, instances when the pharmacist must recognize that nondrug measures, although appropriate, might not lend themselves to a particular patient. For example, the standard modality to treat diarrhea in an adult is to encourage a liquid diet for a period of time. However, if the patient is diabetic, caloric intake must be maintained. This example is one where pharmacist consultation with the physician is necessary.

When the pharmacist recommends a drug treatment for a condition amenable to self-therapy, the pharmacist should tell the patient of the condition itself, monitoring guideposts to bear in mind, and the duration of time before the patient should notice the benefit of treatment. Using acne vulgaris as an example, the objective of topical treatment is to control an existing condition, impede acne in the developmental stages, and relieve the discomfort (eg, physical, psychological). The patient should be told to note a decrease in the number of lesions that will occur with the continual, daily application of the medication to the entire face and that it may take approximately 2–3 weeks before the benefits of the medication are observed. Tied into the discussion should be indices that demonstrate the acne condition may be worsening and require medical attention. Lastly, potential toxicity from the treatment selected should be told to the patient. Using benzoyl peroxide as an example for the acne patient, the patient should understand that some skin redness and irritation may develop.

Whenever possible, the pharmacist should follow up with the patient. To facilitate followup the pharmacist should make some notation, perhaps on the patient profile, to document the original problem and reinforce his memory. If the patient does not seem to be responding to the treatment plan, additional information and data assessment (eg, did the patient follow instructions correctly and for a reasonable amount of time?) may determine a new course of action. Frequently, this re-evaluation culminates with the referral of the patient to the physician for further treatment. If at all possible the pharmacist should share information attained from the initial and the followup evaluation with the patient's physician.

In summary, as a drug informational specialist in the area of nonprescription drug products the pharmacist is not displacing the physician when he recommends a nonprescription product. At least in this instance the patient has the benefit of the expertise of the pharmacist whereas, if the product was purchased in a nonpharmacy outlet there would be no chance for a dialogue to occur. In the latter instance there is a great chance for misuse of the product. Given the education of the pharmacist, in conjunction with practical experience, there is no other person who knows the limitations of self-treatment with OTC products and who is in a position to encourage the patient to seek the professional advice of a physician when necessary.

Health Education

A primary concern of the pharmacist should be the welfare of humanity and the relief of human suffering. In fact, one oath of a pharmacist contains the passage, "I will use my knowledge and skills to the best of my ability in serving the public and other health professionals." Today, there is little doubt that the "buzz word" in contemporary pharmacy practice is "information"—specifically, consumer health information.[12]

By virtue of the accessibility of the pharmacist and his familiarity with the community, it is obvious that the pharmacist can exercise a dynamic impact within the community as a whole. This impact can be translated not only into the triage function, deciding whether or not to suggest a patient consult a physician, but the dissemination of effective and useful health education. One study revealed that over 90% of those interviewed visited a pharmacy at least once a month and 60% at least once a week. The hours a pharmacy is open per week greatly exceeds all other health facilities with the possible exception of an emergency room of a hospital. Although many consumers continue to view the pharmacist as, "an invisible man behind a secret counter who delegates responsibility to technicians and clerks to deal directly with the public," this attitude is being changed positively to reflect the pharmacist as a source of health information along with the physician. A vast majority of the public does not hesitate to ask the pharmacist about a health matter and usually the pharmacist is the first person, other than family or friends, who is consulted.

Frequently, the pharmacist is confronted with individual inquiries—a telephone call from a frantic mother whose child has just swallowed a number of chewable vitamin-iron tablets and wants to know what to do. Or a nervous teenage girl who wants to know how to use a home pregnancy kit. Further, the pharmacist may be confronted by a distraught parent who wants to know, "what are these pills that I found in my son's belongings?" The situation may involve an expectant mother who is afraid for her baby since she may have been exposed to a neighborhood child who has since been diagnosed to have German measles. The situations are endless but typify the need for the pharmacist to be approachable and willing to help these people.

To answer these people or synthesize a plan of action the pharmacist must maintain professional competence and keep abreast of developments of drugs and disease states. At the same time the pharmacist should serve as an expeditor to solve patient problems. The familiarity of one pharmacist with the community lends itself to proper referral of patients to physicians in the area (eg, general practitioners, specialists, dentists, podiatrists). Whenever possible, the pharmacist should have available the addresses and telephone numbers for the use of the patient. Indeed, it is the pharmacist who is in a position to form an assessment of a physician by personal communication experience with the physician, the types of prescriptions the physicians writes or telephones for the patient, patient comments about the care they are receiving, and inquiries about physician followup with the patient. Beyond health care assistance the pharmacist should be able also to recommend to a patient nonmedical facilities that provide effective care (eg, a shoe store that exercises judgment and care in fitting a person with a jogging shoe). Further, in the event a patient is indigent and therefore not able to pay for medical care, the pharmacist should know the address and telephone number of the local county assistance office where the patient can initiate steps to ensure proper medical care is attainable.

There are over 600 poison control centers in the United States, and every pharmacy should have the telephone numbers and addresses of those in the local area for quick patient referral. Although unintentional poisonings and deaths have dropped dramatically since child-resistant packaging was introduced, tragedies continue to occur among young children. The pharmacist must be able to deal effectively with these emergencies, exercise judgment, and be decisive with these inquiries.

Another alarming problem that has surfaced within recent years is child and spouse abuse. This of of concern to all communities and the pharmacist, by his involvement, can serve a number of ways to help alleviate the problem. The first of these is to be aware of the warning signs of abuse and neglect from the perspective of the child (eg, seems unduly afraid of his parents, shows evidence of repeated skin or other injuries, shows signs of poor overall care), and the parent (eg, makes no attempt to explain the child's most obvious injuries or offers absurd, contradictory explanations, shows a lack of control, or fear of losing control). Given the warning signs of child abuse and neglect the pharmacist can gently coax information from the parent when either taking the initiative to do so or provided the opportunity. A simple conversation from the pharmacist may be sufficient encouragement for an abusive parent to admit the need for assistance and guidance. At this point the pharmacist must have the name of an individual at the community abuse center with whom the parent can talk both before and during a crisis. Given uncooperative parents the pharmacist must exercise professional judgment and report the matter to local authorities. The pharmacist, like all citizens, is immune from civil and/or criminal liability when reporting any knowledge or suspicion of child abuse. The second mode is participation with local authorities and professionals in information forums conducted by social workers. The pharmacist can provide information to the abusive parent on how drugs, including alcohol, can effect one's behavior, change one's mood, effect depression with long term use, and induce psychotic reactions. When this information is blended with the physician-nurse discussion of physical injury incurred from abuse with teacher awareness of reporting suspicions, it adds immeasurably to the dimension of such a symposium.

The pharmacist should also recognize the need for health education on a broader scale. Many of the health problems encountered by communities can be prevented or alleviated with proper education. But it must be the pharmacist who is willing to share the wealth of knowledge and information he has accrued. All persons are not knowledgable about the extent of the education of a pharmacist and thus do not automatically think of the pharmacist as a source of information. Thus, it is the pharmacist who must provide the impetus to focus attention toward the capability he has relative to health education. There are several ways the pharmacist can achieve this end.

One method is to make the pharmacy the health center of a community. The willingness to participate in "Poison Prevention Week," or "National Diabetes Month," focuses consumer education toward the pharmacy. Coupled with this is the distribution of pamphlets of public interest on health information for the community. A display of free health literature in the pharmacy demonstrates a commitment to effective health care. There are myriads of pamphlets available on a variety of topics (eg, "Diabetes, Dry Skin and You," "The Professional Treatment of Constipation") from drug manufacturers that can be used effectively to promote health care. This encourages inquiries from consumers and if displayed neatly in the prescription waiting area of the pharmacy may afford the opportunity to the patient to read health-related information while waiting for a prescription. The pharmacist should make an effort to question drug company representatives about the availability of such pamphlets for the community. Many times pamphlets are available, but unless requested they remain confined to the box in which they are contained. In the event there is an outbreak of a communicable disease (eg, *Pediculosis capitis* at a local elementary school) the pharmacist should obtain and disseminate useful patient-related information. Disseminated directly at the time of medication purchase for the problem or in conjunction with the local school nurse this mechanism avoids needless worry and confusion on the part of the parents of the affected children.

A key attribute to being a professional in any field is being accessible to those one serves. In this context the role of the pharmacist is aptly illustrated by the dimension encompassed by family planning.[13] By sharing knowledge and information about oral contraceptive therapy, nonprescription modes of contraception control, prevention of venereal disease, and pregnancy testing, and by being of assistance to couples dealing with fertility impairment the pharmacist demonstrates accessibility and increases the awareness of the public that the pharmacy is the place where knowledge and informed advice are available.

Pharmacy school curriculums recognize the need for effective oral communication both on an individual patient basis and to larger numbers of assembled people (eg, civic groups, church groups, clubs) by implementing effective coursework in the undergraduate curriculum. However, if the pharmacist does not accept the challenge and communicate information then other, less qualified persons may be asked by the consuming public to fill this informational void. Sometimes pharmacists are fearful to present talks or discussions with interested groups due to a lack of self confidence in their speaking abilities. At the same time these pharmacists may feel that they do not have the capability to discuss a topic due to a lack of information. As students, pharmacists unfortunately are not taught to develop a framework of library research. At the same time they may not be instructed on whom to ask, or provided with avenues to proceed when in need of information. The pharmacist unfortunately does not always think to contact his alma mater to secure information. Nor do some pharmacists initiate inquiries with local or state pharmacy associations to gain access to meaningful information. It is essential that pharmacists contribute to public informational forums and make the community aware of public health problems related to drugs and their use. A true concern of the pharmacist must center around the casual attitude of the public towards drugs, a concept which unfortunately is reinforced through commercial advertising and communication media. It is bewildering to realize that Americans ingest over 20 billion aspirin tablets a year, 100 for every man, woman, and child in the country.

Whenever possible pharmacists must help restore consumer confidence when it has been put in a position of doubt. The classic example occurred in September, 1982, with the Tylenol tampering incidents in Chicago. Pharmacists responded by displaying posters and informational bulletins that instructed consumers to:

1. Look for signs of tampering, such as broken seals or opened or damaged boxes.
2. Check for loose, torn, or missing wrappings as well as discolored products and unusual odors.
3. If a product does not look right, ask the pharmacist about it.

The FDA has initiated steps to prevent the likelihood of this problem again and by February 1984 no products other than insulin, dermatologicals, and dentrifices will be allowed to be sold without tamper-resistant packaging. However, there are innovative and disturbed individuals still in circulation who may create new problems and the pharmacist must maintain surveillance and be willing to allay consumer fears.

The pharmacist should always remain above reproach in the eye of the public. A pharmacist should avoid even the appearance of professional impropriety and thereby not create questions of ethics within the mind of the patient. A recent failure in this regard involved the so-called starch blockers, which were being sold over-the-counter as a diet aid. The Food and Drug Administration moved to ban the sale of these products on the basis of ineffectiveness and possible harm to consumers, yet some pharmacists continued to stock the products. This attitude does not engender positive feelings of the value of the pharmacist in the minds of some consumers relating to sound health care. The most important means the pharmacist has in educating society on health matters is the personal contact he has with the public in his pharmacy. The pharmacist whenever possible should volunteer health information and encourage people to exercise proper judgment to maintain good health. Some pharmacists have been very creative and have developed and written patient-oriented newsletters on timely subjects that reinforce the attitude that the pharmacist is both a drug information specialist and health care educator and provider. Other pharmacists have achieved this same end by writing health information columns for local newspapers or participation in local media programs to provide health care information.

Finally, by showing a professional interest in and attitude toward the clientele which frequent the pharmacy the pharmacist makes people feel they are important and that they have someone upon whom they can depend for help. A notable example of this is in ostomy care (see Health Care Accessories Chapter 104). There are over 1.1 million ostomates (1983) in the United States with new ostomates numbering 100,000 each year. In the end though, it is the pharmacist who really benefits by the intangible return of fulfillment and enrichment from using skills and information learned through formal and continuing education and practical experience.

New and Expanded Dimensions of Ambulatory Care

Better care of the patient and the public has always been a central goal for the profession of pharmacy. In that context the future direction of the pharmacist in ambulatory care will continue to evolve toward patient-directed services that apply scientific knowledge and clinical skills to the promotion of cost-effective therapy and the prevention and resolution of drug-related needs.

The traditional chain of events in the treatment of the ambulatory patient has been for the physician to make a diagnosis and decide upon a course of treatment. If the treatment required medication the physician would write or telephone a prescription to the pharmacist. The three basic functions involved were diagnosing, prescribing, and dispensing. The physician diagnosed and prescribed and the pharmacist dispensed. These designations have not been directly challenged but there seems to be a trend developing for the pharmacist to have a greater influence in the prescribing function than he has had in the past.

This trend was initiated when the APhA and consumer groups presented a strong case for the repeal of state anti-substitution laws during the 1970's. Since 1972, all states have repealed laws which prohibited the pharmacist from dispensing a generically equivalent drug product may be a different manufacturer from the one prescribed. Gradually, there has been a transition from physician responsibility to pharmacist responsibility for selecting the manufacturer of a drug product. Prescriptions written using generic names for drugs have increased from 6.4% in 1966 to 27.4% in 1982. With this responsibility is also an accountability since the pharmacist must exercise ethical and professional responsibility when selecting generic products which are of quality and approved for marketing by the FDA. Recent surveys indicate that pharmacists have responded favorably and most often opt for branded generic products rather than unbranded products on the basis of past performance and familiarity with the manufacturers. It must be mentioned, however, that typically the preferred source of a generic drug product will demonstrate a brand-name manufacturer in the lead with a long roster of generic company names following.

The second critical incident that shaped a future focus of pharmacy practice evolved with the establishment of the American Board of Family Practice in 1969, as the 20th medical specialty. With its establishment the stage was set for the resurrection of the family doctor and the concept of personal responsibility for the total health care of the patient, including the selection of appropriate allied health professionals to assist in such care. Inclusion of the clinical pharmacist into the family practice health care system has gained acceptance on a continual basis and numerous articles describe this emerging ambulatory role of the pharmacist. Family practice models with clinical pharmacy primary care programs have evolved and have followed one of two paths.

The first, which have been publicly funded, include programs in the Indian Health Service, the Applachian Regional Hospitals, family practice residency programs, and those within colleges of pharmacy. While the success of the first depends to an extent upon the uncertain continuation of government financing, the second type, the private family practice model, depends upon the more traditional marketing pressures.

Within the model of family practice the pharmacist works with physicians and other providers to offer clinical skills and practical experience to current and prospective patients. The pharmacist must demonstrate the value of personalized, comprehensive, continuous, and convenient services (such as medication history, patient education, dispensing function, patient care functions etc) provided to patients to ensure the acutely ill patient gets well, the chronically ill patient gains a better quality of life, and the healthy patient remains healthy.

The success of the pharmacist's role and acceptance by the physician is dependent upon three factors. These are: a contribution to better patient care; increasing the quality of the life of the physician by decreasing patient contact time; and helping the physician market his services to ensure the financial success of the medical practice. An example of this would be the involvement of the pharmacist with postdiagnostic care of hypertension. The physician selects the patients to be monitored under the hypertension protocol and introduces them to the clinical pharmacist. The pharmacist then explains the protocol to the patient, the followup appointment schedule, the fee system for services, and informs the patient when to return to see the physician. Ultimately, pharmacist involvement results in better care and fewer procedures which produces overall patient savings. This is a mode to increase the quality of health care at a reduced cost.

Helling has proposed an excellent listing of the functions of the Family Practice Clinical Pharmacist.[14] These include:

1. Medication History
   a. Drug allergies and sensitivities.
   b. Maintenance prescription medication (current and past).
   c. Nonprescription medication (current and past).
   d. Individual problems associated with the preparation and administration of medication.
   e. Patient symptoms encountered in past (eg, side effects, drug toxicity, incorrect administration).

2. Patient Education
   a. Predictable actions and/or side effects of drugs.
   b. Possible side effects.
   c. Necessity for proper compliance with medication regimens.
   d. Special instructions germane to administration, use, and storage of medication.
   e. Specified disease processes relevant to the patient.
   f. Personal hygiene and health maintenance.
   g. Interactions with other prescription and OTC drugs.
   h. Notification of pharmacist or physician if medication problems develop.
3. Patient Care
   a. Monitor patient drug therapy.
   b. Therapeutic consultations with physicians and other health professionals.
   c. Audit medication orders: chart review/prescription review.
   d. Participate in nursing home visits.
   e. Pharmacokinetic consulting services.
   f. Coordinate follow-up of laboratory results.
   g. Manage selected acute, self-limiting, and chronic disease patients.
   h. Responsible for medication-related inquiries to clinical area.

Clinical pharmacy services will continue to vary in dimension within the framework of pharmacy practice. Some practitioners will participate directly in a number of these activities, while others may only participate from a consulting role (eg, pharmacokinetic consulting service). The fact remains, however, that continued escalation of hospital costs and patient charges will encourage the development and implementation of family practice units and off-site clinical areas for routine screening of patients. Studies have already demonstrated the positive impact that pharmacists have had on these ambulatory health care clinics.

One study analyzed the effectiveness of the clinical pharmacist in improving the accuracy of medical records and increasing patient compliance with outpatient drug regimens in an ambulatory health care rheumatology and renal clinic.[15] A six-month analysis of the data demonstrated that the pharmacist significantly improved drug documentation, decreased duplication of medications, and improved patient compliance with prescribed drugs. Again it highlighted pharmacy involvement as a means to improve health care and reduce overall medical costs. A $31,641 savings was projected as a result of a decrease in drug duplication due to the pharmacist's role during the time the clinic was open. Since there were no other variables introduced into the operation of the clinic during the control and study periods, the data suggested that the presence of the pharmacist within the clinic influenced physician (higher quality drug documentation) and patient (increased drug compliance) behavior. Another study demonstrated that the implementation of pharmacy services in an ambulatory pediatric clinic resulted in a decrease in dispensing medication errors and prescription labelling, as well as an improvement in patient understanding of prescribed therapy.[16]

John S Millis has stated that "wise and forceful action to improve education has resulted directly in higher standards of practice with clearly increased benefits to those who receive professional services." [17] The literature supports this comment and is replete with examples of the impact of clinically-trained pharmacists on the quality of health care. Furthermore, there is testimony to the impact of the pharmacist within the prescribing role. Already there are settings in which pharmacists prescribe medication in cooperation with other health care providers and, as the quality of patient care increases, the cost of the care may well be reduced.

On September 15, 1977, California Assembly Bill 717 was approved allowing two pilot projects for pharmacists to prescribe drugs under the general supervision of a physician when engaged in the experimental health manpower project authorized by the California State Department of Health Services. In one study, Stimmel *et al*, compared the quality of prescribing for psychiatric inpatients by physicians and pharmacists. Statistical analysis of the data revealed no difference in the quality of prescribing anti-Parkinson drugs between pharmacists and physicians, but pharmacists' scores were significantly better than physicians' scores for neuroleptic and antidepressants.[18]

A second report discussed the quality of pharmacists' and physicians' drug prescribing for ambulatory hypertensive patients in a health maintenance organization.[19] Statistical analysis revealed that there was no difference in prescribing between the physician group and the pharmacist group on the scoring for the presence of drug interactions, appropriateness of quantity, dose, and patient directions. The pharmacist group, however, did significantly better than the physician group on choosing the appropriate drug, prescribing for a "positive effect on the patient's health," and overall appropriateness from the combination of all the criteria.

These pilot projects terminated in June 1983, hopefully to be replaced by more permanent and improved legislation. Thirty pharmacists participated in the California study and had to be initially certified as prescribers by successfully completing a course in physical assessment and by a certifying examination. Pharmacists had to meet with their supervising physician once every two weeks, and were restricted to a project formulary of 300 drugs. A variety of health care settings were represented in the project with pharmacists prescribing for ambulatory patients with chronic diseases, geriatric patients in extended care facilities, psychiatric patients, and selected inpatients. While the pharmacists who did participate in this project were not necessarily typical practitioners it did indicate the capability that can be attained and utilized, especially since the education of a pharmacist is targeted toward pharmacology and rational drug prescribing.

In a similar context, the profession of pharmacy has a unique opportunity to contribute effectively to gerontological care. In 1982, approximately 11% (24 million) of the population of the United States was 65 years or older. In 50 years, the percentage of those over 65 is projected to increase to between 17–20%. Thus, community pharmacists can play a vital role in the distribution and maintenance of medical care for the elderly in the community. Indeed the elderly require the attention of the pharmacist since they often have multiple diseases (most often chronic) for which they may take up to a dozen medications or more. By the unique training a pharmacist receives, the pharmacist can play a central role in patient assessment, patient monitoring, and coordinating health care and drug distribution for patients in community and extended health care facilities. The pharmacist should possess an awareness and a sensitivity to an integrated approach to health care that could help to overcome the more traditional limitations in the health care model, such as a lack of attention to the social and emotional aspects of care. This was recently demonstrated in a study where the drug use was greatly reduced and patients' chances for early discharge increased when they were cared for by physician/pharmacist teams (vs physician alone) and patients were encouraged to talk about day-to-day concerns with the pharmacist. Pharmacist intervention under the supervision of physicians in this study effected a decrease in drug use from an average of eight different medications being taken by the patient per month to five and decreased the amount of tranquilizer use.

Under California Assembly Bill 1868 (September, 1981), the California Pharmacy Practice Act has been amended to allow the pharmacist in a licensed health care facility (nursing home) to perform several procedures: adjust the dosage regimen of a patient pursuant to a prescriber order or authorization, order drug-therapy related laboratory tests, and administer drugs and biologicals by parenteral injection pursuant to the orders of the prescriber. These functions are performed under protocol and illustrate the movement and recognition of the pharmacist as a vital member of the health care team. Eventually, legislation could be extended to allow pharmacists this same responsibility in outpatient facilities and community pharmacies, as well. At this point it is relevant to emphasize that when new functions are accepted, such as parenteral administration of drugs, the pharmacist is accountable to the standard by which the person replaced would be judged (eg, nurse, physician). The pharmacist must be cognizant that acceptance of these new roles place additional liability on his practice.

Another area of patient care that will require more pharmacists in the future will be in the interdisciplinary team of hospice care. Hospice care is a program of palliative and supportive services which provides physical, psychological, social, and spiritual care for dying persons and their families. Currently, there are over 800 hospice programs in various stages of development (1983), half of which were not started until after January 1980. Pharmacists today service hospice organizations in functions ranging from dispensing and consulting to administrative and management roles. Aside from the more traditional pharmacy role of compounding and dispensing new roles are emerging for the pharmacist to fulfill. Drug selection and dosing, drug monitoring, drug information and education, and administration of pharmaceuticals are duties which could be performed by the pharmacist within the hospice situation. It is not an easy decision to become involved with hospice care, however, since many pharmacists fear problems with the DEA (a large number of medications are narcotics) or personal jeopardy.

Trends indicate that the number of pharmacists practicing "holistic pharmacy" or participating in "holistic health care" will increase in the future. *Holism* is a model of health care that attempts to direct the efforts of health care providers and patients toward a central goal of meeting all the health needs of the individual. From the standpoint of the patient it is a philosophy that maintains that individuals are responsible for themselves and that they have the capacity for self-healing, usually with the cooperative assistance of a health care provider. This philosophy supports the team concept of providers—physician, nurse, pharmacist, and clergyman—with each contributing an integral component of the total health picture of the patient. There is little doubt that Americans will be handling their health care problems with more knowledge, confidence, and effectiveness in future years. An expanded holistic role for the pharmacist includes the education, screening, and monitoring function. High blood pressure intervention is a classic example of how the pharmacist can practice holistic pharmacy, but another that is worthy of mention is the dynamic movement of men and women toward physical awareness and fitness. An estimated 135 million people exercise on a daily basis, with a notable fitness mode being jogging or running. The pharmacist participates in the aforementioned holistic role by educating the person to prevent foot problems (eg, proper footwear and attire, running environment, running surface, warmup exercises), by screening the patient after an injury has occurred (eg, podiatrist/orthopedist referral, self-medication) and by monitoring the person by periodic inquiry when permissible. Thus, the pharmacist contributes components to the overall health picture of the individual.

Lastly, health care is concerned with the prevention as well as the treatment of disease. It is more difficult to convince a person what he must do to stay well than it is to convince an individual what he must do to get well once he is sick. When a person is ill he will generally seek help. When he is well, he will not as a rule seek help to remain well, yet he must take positive steps to maintain good health. He cannot take these steps unless he is aware of them. Even then, he may not take action unless he is educated in why he must do so and encouraged to take action. Because of the accessibility of the pharmacist to the public and his professional knowledge and training, he is in a premier position to play an important role in maintaining the health of his community by serving as a health educator.

Health-Care Delivery Systems

At present, the United States is in a period of dramatic change toward patterns of health care delivery. Social justice dictates an equal accessibility to good quality health care for all its citizens. Although it has responded in slow incremental steps the government has responded in an attempt to provide health care for all. The goal is a continuing effort to keep people healthy and out of hospitals and thus to contain the high cost of health care.

The major health activities for the United States are consolidated with the Department of Health and Human Services (DHHS). One of the components of this department, the Health Care Financing Administration (HCFA), is gradually assuming a greater role in health care, particularly in the financing of health care services for the elderly, the indigent, and the medically indigent. Further, the HCFA is charged with the responsibility to administer Titles XVIII and XIX (Medicare and Medicaid).

Historically, the original health-care delivery system was the fee-for-service practice rendered by individual practitioners. A problem with this system is that health care delivery is fragmented with little or no continuity. Patients consult various physicians, pharmacists, and clinicians all of whom, after delivering or providing a service to the patient, independently bill the patient for their service. Other fee-for-service practice systems have included group medical practice, prepaid group medical practice, and federally funded neighborhood health centers. Quite commonly within these systems, however, no one takes full responsibility for determining the total appropriate level of care and for managing the patient to assure that quality care is supplied.

In an effort to try to solve this dilemma, and at the same time reduce spiraling medical care costs a form of group practice, the Health Maintenance Organization (HMO), has grown since its inception in the early 1970's. Paraphrasing the official definition, as stated within the Health Maintenance Organization Act of 1973 (Public Law 93-222), an HMO is a private or nonprofit entity which provides basic health care services to enrollees for a fixed amount on a prepayment basis and provides additional supplemental services for additional payments. It is an organized system of health care that is capable of bringing together the necessary components which a defined population might reasonably require. The concept of the HMO was fostered on the basis of prior prepaid group health plans which date back to the late 1920's, eg, Ross-Loss Group Practice Prepayment Plan, Los Angeles, CA; Community Hospital Association Plan, Elk City, OK. There are some who believe that the HMO system will help this country control runaway health costs by basing health care on the premise of prevention as well as treatment. In 1983, there were more than 10 million people enrolled in the approximately 250 HMOs nationwide.[20]

All HMOs have four basic characteristics:

1. The are organized systems of health care in a geographic area, and provide the services of physician and allied health professionals within inpatient and outpatient facilities.
2. They offer a specified set of comprehensive basic and supplemental health maintenance and treatment services.
3. Membership is voluntary.

4.   Reimbursement is through fixed-prenegotiated periodic payments made by, or on behalf of, each person or family unit enrolled in the plan.

The method of paying (capitation payment) for health-care services is the most important of the four characteristics because it dictates the underlying philosophy of this system. This philosophy is to maintain the health of the individual. If the individual becomes sick, it costs the organization money. If the patient is hospitalized, it costs more money. Therefore, to keep the organization solvent, it must practice preventive medicine. The other alternative is to neglect the patient. Therefore, a method to review the quality of patient services is an important element of this system.

Originally, HMOs were federally funded, however, in the early 1980s this funding was terminated. Thus, the system has had to develop new sources of income to continue its growth. Business and labor both have a stake in the success of the HMO concept in view of the current economic climate. Thus, the private sector will have to respond and provide increased financial support to the HMO in the future.

There is no doubt that the development and success of the HMO will have an impact upon the profession of pharmacy. Projections which show potential increases in the numbers of HMOs cause corresponding increases in the interest and activity among allied health professionals and pharmacists are no exceptions. While some pharmacists may perceive the HMO as a threat to their existence, others will seize the opportunity to find rewards in activities other than dispensing medications to patients. Some may actually flourish within the system. Pharmacy as a profession has established its ability in the health care delivery system. Now pharmacists should be encouraged to meet these new challenges presented by the HMOs. The community pharmacists, for example, should investigate the rising volume of prescriptions generated by physicians at HMOs. They will find that a number of these HMOs have in-house pharmacies dispensing a high volume of prescriptions. Further, if the on-site pharmacy participates in the insurance program they may be able to offer prescriptions which are economically attractive to the HMO patient. At the same time, these pharmacies are staffed by other pharmacists who have taken the opportunity to participate in these programs. Given the opportunity, should others follow? Alternatively, should pharmacists contract with the HMO to dispense prescriptions in their traditional pharmacies? In a number of cities, pharmacist foundations have been formed by local pharmacists for this very reason. These foundations are nonprofit corporations of pharmacists who retain their present practices, but collectively contract to provide pharmaceutical services to HMOs. These pharmacists develop standards of practice for their geographic area, negotiate contracts on behalf of the participating member pharmacists, provide all of the pharmaceutical services, and establish peer/utilization review mechanisms for the programs they serve. The method of reimbursement to the individual pharmacies who are under contract to the HMO is usually a fee-for-service. If the HMO contracts with a pharmacy foundation, it will most likely prepay the foundation on a per capita basis. The foundation then reimburses the member pharmacist. Pharmacists who are considering this type of arrangement should, however, obtain competent legal advice. Antitrust laws basically prohibit combined actions which are in restriction of commerce.

"(P)harmacists cannot act collectively in making a decision whether to participate or not participate in a given third-party program. Moreover, it would be unlawful for a representative to negotiate collectively for a number of individually owned pharmacies with a third-party program administrator over fees to be paid in the program. . . . (A)spects of the decision of whether to participate, which are perfectly lawful when conducted by an individual pharmacy owner acting alone and on his or her own initiative, may not be lawful if done by a group of pharmacy owners." [21]

Experience has demonstrated that on-site pharmacies may have some advantages over the off-site counterpart. For example, rapport and open lines of communication can be developed between the pharmacist and the various providers. Since preventive medication is practiced, patient counseling is dictated with each prescription and necessitates the pharmacist to provide concise, clear information to the patient. The pharmacist will have access to the entire record of the patient, including prescribed medications, to encourage monitoring and recognition of potential problems with drug therapy. From the standpoint of the management of an on-site pharmacy, volume purchasing, unit of use packaging, pharmaceutical manufacturing, drug product selection, development of utilization criteria, and a closely controlled formulary system help sustain revenues in excess of expenses and demonstrate the pharmacy as a viable member of the HMO.

Development of an on-site pharmacy takes the innovativeness and creativeness of a skilled pharmacy manager. The HMO pharmacy director should possess good managerial skills and institutional experience. Institutional experience provides a working knowledge of intravenous solution preparation, sterile product preparation, as well as a perspective toward patient monitoring. This person must be clinically adept to identify both acute and preventive health care needs of the ambulatory patient and know the means to develop and implement pharmacy systems and programs that attain these needs. Good management dictates that this person surround himself with competent and dependable colleagues who can deliver effective, clinical pharmacy care. In fact, those pharmacists who practice in on-site situations seem to express a positive feeling toward the practice of pharmacy within an HMO. It rewards the pharmacist for service other than providing a medication or product. For example, the ideal attributes of the HMO pharmacist might include the following:[20]

1.   Team oriented with a commitment toward contributing to and sharing responsibility for patient health care.
2.   Patient oriented with a willingness to provide health information, patient counseling, and problem-solving abilities that enhance preventive patient care.
3.   Learning oriented by exhibiting evidence of maintenance of professional competence through continuing education.
4.   Possession of an ability and aptitude for drug information retrieval and evaluation.
5.   Possession of good communicative abilities at the patient level and the professional level.

All of these embody skills which are truly germane to any effective ambulatory pharmacy practice. Suffice to say, however, the economic incentive serves as a prompter to the pharmacist to carry out all of these functions in behalf of the patient.

The search for new systems of delivering health care will continue until the health needs of all members of society are satisfactorily met. Among these will be systems like the HMO that encourage collegiality among professionals. One relationship which has developed recently is that between pharmacy practice and the Visiting Nurse Home Health Service (VNS). Consultant pharmacy services include regular review of VNS patient charts, providing drug parameters for the nurses on chart drug profiles, and notification of the nurses about suspected or potential drug therapy problems. Also, the pharmacists provide in-service programs on drug therapy for the nurses, answer drug information inquiries from the nurses, and assist in the resolution of patient therapy problems. Resolution of patient problems may encompass home visitation with the nurses, preparation of patient medication-education sheets and patient medication administration schedules, institution of devices for medication set-up, and/or consultation with the prescribing physician. As is obvious from this, as well as the aforementioned responsibilities of the pharmacist in ambulatory care of patients, the role of the pharmacist has evolved from a product-oriented professional to one of a patient-oriented professional. This modification in the role of the pharmacist has been extremely healthy for the patient and the pharmacist. It remains now for pharmacy as a profession and the health care industry to ensure that the pharmacist is justly compensated for all of his services.

References

1. Wuest JR: *Securite et medicaments*, 1982 Pergamon Press, p. 193.
2. Latiolais CJ, Berry CC: *Drug Intell Clin Pharm 3:* 270, 1969.
3. *Medi-Message*, Pharmex Corporation, Willimantic, CT 06226.
4. Valentino JG: *US Pharmacist 3(7):* 24, 1978.
5. Schondelmeyer SW, Trinca CE: *Am Pharm NS23:* 321, 1983.
6. Smith DL: *Am Pharm NS23:* 314, 1983.
7. Schneiweiss F: *Drug Intell Clin Pharm 17:* 27, 1983.
8. Brown GH, Kirking DM, Ascione FJ. *Am Pharm NS23:* 325, 1983.
9. Srnka QM, Self TH: *Systematic Approach to Patient Medication Review*, American College of Apothecaries, Memphis, TN, 1977.
10. Kowolenko M, Campbell B: *Apothecary 94(4):* 51, 1982.
11. *The Pharmacist as an OTC Consultant*, The Schering Report, 1980, Schering Laboratories, Kenilworth, NJ.
12. Gossel TA, Wuest JR: *US Pharmacist 7(8):* 30, 1982.
13. Grindstaff CF: *The Pharmacist and Family Planning: New Roles and Responsibilities*, The Christopher Publishing House, North Quincy, MA, 1980.
14. Helling DK: *Drug Intell Clin Pharm 16:* 35, 1982.
15. Monson R, Bond CA, Schuna A: *Arch Intern Med 141:* 1441, 1981.
16. Edwards R, Adams DW: *Drug Intell Clin Pharm 16:* 939, 1982.
17. *Pharmacists for the Future*, American Association of Colleges of Pharmacy Report of the Study Commission on Pharmacy, Health Administration Press, Ann Arbor, MI, 1975.
18. Stimmel GL, McGhan WF, Wincor M et al: *Am J Hosp Pharm 39:* 1483, 1982.
19. McGhan WF, Stimmel GL, Hall TG et al: *Medical Care 21(4):* 535, 1983.
20. Anon: *Am Pharm NS22:* 252, 1982.
21. Fink JL III, Siecker BR: *Manager's Guide to Third-Party Programs*, Pharmacy Management Institute, American Pharmaceutical Association, Washington, DC, Spring, 1982.

Bibliography

1983 USP DI, Volume I: Drug Information for the Health Care Provider, USP Convention Inc., Rockville, MD, 1982.
1983 USP DI, Volume II: Advice for the Patient, USP Convention Inc., Rockville, MD, 1982.
Pharmacists and Consumers: A Fresh Look From Both Sides of the Counter, The Schering Report, 1979, Schering Laboratories, Kenilworth, NJ.
Smith DL: *Medication Guide for Patient Counseling*, Lea and Febiger, Philadelphia, PA, 1981.
Smith DL: Patient Education—Its Time Has Come. *Am Pharm NS21:* 382, 1981.
Cohen E: What I Expect—What I Get: A Consumer's View. *Am Pharm NS21:* 388, 1981.
Handbook of Nonprescription Drugs, 7th ed., APhA, Washington, DC, 1982.
Curtiss FR: Effective Listening: A Fundamental- and Difficult-Health Care Skill. *Patient Counseling in Community Pharmacy 1(1):* 9, 1982.
Helling DK: Family Practice Pharmacy Service. *Drug Intell Clin Pharm 15:* 971, 1981.
Stimmel GL, McGhan WF: Pharmacist as a Prescriber. *Drug Intell Clin Pharm 15:* 665, 1981.
Quigley JL, Quigley MA, Gumbhir AK: Partners in Patient Care. *Am Pharm NS22:* 420, 1982.
Burton LE, Smith HH, Nichols AW: *Public Health and Community Medicine*, 3rd ed., Williams and Wilkins, Baltimore/London, 1980.

CHAPTER 95

Institutional Patient Care

Harold N Godwin, MS
Professor and Director of Pharmacy
The University of Kansas Medical Center
Kansas City, KS 66103

Historically, health-care services have been provided primarily through physicians' offices and in hospitals. Thus, pharmaceutical services to patients seen in physicians' offices have been provided through community pharmacies while patients in hospitals normally receive pharmaceutical services through the hospital pharmacy.

The changing nature of health-care delivery has expanded the role of the hospital to include ambulatory-care programs and intermediate-care facilities (such as extended-care facilities and nursing homes). Thus, the term "institutional" care has been coined to reflect this broadened role of the hospital. Concurrently, "institutional" pharmacy has also been coined to coincide with this development. Nonetheless, institutional pharmacy is basically hospital pharmacy. The term hospital is really the basis for the designation of the term institutional. Institution, as defined in Webster's Dictionary, is

A significant and persistent element (as a practice, a relationship, an organization) in the life of a culture that centers on a fundamental human need, activity, or value, occupies an enduring and cardinal position within a society, and is usually maintained and stabilized through social regulatory agencies.

Certainly, the hospital and its directly related organizational substructures fit the term institution.

As a corollary, the term "organized health care" setting has been used to refer to the wide gamut of organizational subsystems embracing the total health-care delivery system in America. Hospital or institutional pharmacy should not be confused with the provision of pharmaceutical services to all types of organized health care settings. For example, three physicians practicing in the same office building may have formed a corporation. Thus, they may be properly referred to as a group providing patient-care services in an organized health-care setting because a corporation is an organized structure. Obviously, providing pharmaceutical services to the patients of these three physicians should not properly be referred to as institutional or hospital pharmacy.

Institutional or hospital pharmacy may be defined as the practice of pharmacy in a hospital setting including its organizationally related facilities or services. It may also be defined as that department or division of the hospital wherein the procurement, storage, compounding, manufacturing, packaging, controlling, assaying, dispensing, distribution, and monitoring of medications to hospitalized and ambulatory patients are performed by legally qualified, professionally competent pharmacists. In addition to all these traditional functions, the practice of pharmacy in a hospital also includes broad responsibility for the safe and appropriate use of drugs in patients, which includes among other things, the rational selection, monitoring, dosing and control of the patients overall drug therapy program. This added dimension requires the application of patient-oriented sciences superimposed upon the pharmaceutical sciences—to the subject of rational therapeutics. This approach to pharmacy practice has been referred to as "clinical" pharmacy. Thus, clinical pharmacy is simply good professional patient-oriented pharmaceutical services.

Such practice is a professional goal, not only of institutional or hospital pharmacy but also community pharmacy as well. Essentially, what then makes the practice of pharmacy in a hospital somewhat different from private or community pharmacy?

Uniqueness of Hospital Pharmacy—A major factor is the organizational structure of a hospital or institution: a formalized pattern of authority, responsibility, and coordination which affects every department of the overall health-care team. The administrator implements the policies and philosophies of the governing board; delegates authority and passes on responsibility to department heads to carry out the patient care, teaching, research, and public health objectives of the hospital. Department heads, such as the Director of Pharmacy, are expected to coordinate their services and activities with other department heads; the business and accounting department handles the financial affairs; the building services department provides the essential maintenance, housekeeping, and security functions; the personnel department implements personnel policies; the clinical laboratory department performs a multitude of patient laboratory tests and services; dozens of other departments influence and affect the services of all hospital departments. All of these activities interrelate with the hospital pharmacy.

In addition to the traditional physician–pharmacist–patient relationship which exists in the private practice of medicine and pharmacy, there is a physician–pharmacist–nurse–patient relationship in the hospital. The nurse interjects her professional role in the care of the patient between the traditional physician–pharmacist roles. Thus the hospital pharmacist must work not only with the physician but also very closely with the nurse.

In addition to the internal forces operating within the hospital there are some external forces which affect, in various ways, the practice of pharmacy in the hospital setting. For example, accreditation agencies exert their influence on professional standards of practice as they affect patient care; licensing agencies exert legal influences on hospital operations; the federal government imposes standards and regulations on hospitals, such as the "conditions of Participation for Hospitals" under Medicare; third-party (hospitalization insurance) agencies exert their influence on the methods by which hospitals may be reimbursed for services rendered to patients; social agencies and governmental welfare agencies influence the services provided to medically indigent and totally indigent patients; the governing board and public opinion exert their influences over the policies, objectives, and philosophies of hospital operation and practice. Since the hospital is an institution of and for the community, it is heavily influenced by the needs, expectations, and demands of the members of that community. These are but a few examples of the socio-medico-economic and organizational forces acting on the practice of pharmacy in the institutional setting. These, among many others, are cogent reasons why hospital pharmacy practice differs significantly from community pharmacy practice.

The hospital pharmacy must be considered as one of the many departments of a hospital and as such it has several basic general functions. These functions have been outlined in a document approved by the American Hospital Association, a "Statement on Functions of a Hospital Department."[1] This Statement reads as follows:

A department carries out its functions according to the philosophy and objectives of the hospital. The philosophy and objectives are established by the governing board. Accordingly, the department head is responsible to the administrator of the hospital. Within the organizational pattern, the functions of the department are:
  1. To provide and evaluate service in support of medical care pursuant to the objectives and policies of the hospital.
  2. To implement for departmental services the philosophy, objectives, policies, and standards of the hospital.
  3. To provide and implement a departmental plan of administrative authority which clearly delineates responsibilities and duties of each category of personnel.
  4. To participate in the coordination of the functions of the department with the functions of all other departments and services of the hospital.
  5. To estimate the requirements for the department and to recommend and implement policies and procedures to maintain an adequate and competent staff.
  6. To provide the means and methods by which personnel can work with other groups in interpreting the objectives of the hospital and the department to the patient and community.
  7. To develop and maintain an effective system of clinical and/or administrative records and reports.
  8. To estimate needs for facilities, supplies, and equipment and to implement a system for evaluation, control, and maintenance.
  9. To participate in and adhere to the financial plan of operation for the hospital.
  10. To initiate, utilize and/or participate in studies or research projects designed for the improvement of patient care and the improvement of other administrative and hospital services.
  11. To provide and implement a program of continuing education for all personnel.
  12. To participate in and/or facilitate all educational programs which include student experiences in the department.
  13. To participate in and adhere to the safety program of the hospital.

It is within this framework that the hospital pharmacist practices. The responsibility is to develop a comprehensive pharmaceutical service high in quality, properly coordinated to meet the needs of the numerous diagnostic and therapeutic departments, the nursing service, the medical staff, and the hospital as a whole in the interest of providing better patient care.

Hospital pharmacy has developed so significantly in recent years that there is special education and training at the graduate level; it has its own vigorous professional society—The American Society of Hospital Pharmacists; it has been developing a useful body of specialized knowledge through its documented literature; it has developed a strong corps of well-qualified career hospital practitioners who have adopted a sound philosophy of professional service and have developed high standards of practice.

The setting within which the hospital pharmacist practices requires special education or experience in order to practice with maximum effectiveness. Unlike the pharmacist in community practice, the hospital pharmacist must function within an organization which has additional responsibilities beyond patient care per se. These additional responsibilities include education, research, and public health.

Hospital pharmacists must concern themselves on a daily basis with professional contacts with other highly specialized and skillfully trained professionals. Pharmacists meet with physician specialists on equal grounds in formal pharmacy and therapeutics committee meetings and in medical patient-care rounds in all matters relating to drug therapy; they meet with the nursing profession constantly in their daily practice; they meet with microbiologists, biochemists, and clinical chemists in regard to diagnostic medicine as it relates to drugs; they meet with physicists and radiologists in relation to radioactive pharmaceuticals, diagnostic agents, and contrast media; they meet with clinical pharmacologists and research physicians in matters relating to investigational drugs, drug interactions and reactions; they meet with specialists who have graduate degrees in medical sociology, medical record librarianships, medical dietetics, methods engineering, and hospital administration on a routine basis in the operation of a modern hospital pharmacy.

Hospital pharmacists long recognized the need for additional education and training and developed residency training programs to accomplish these ends. It was also recognized that additional education on a formal basis was desirable and some colleges of pharmacy developed Master of Science degree programs in hospital pharmacy. A number of colleges also offer a professional degree of Doctor of Pharmacy (Pharm D).

The American Association of Colleges of Pharmacy and The American Society of Hospital Pharmacists through a Joint Committee developed *ASHP Guidelines on the Competencies Required in Institutional Pharmacy Practice.*[2] This statement outlines the following seven competencies:

  1. Effective administration and management of a pharmacy department in an institution.
  2. Assimilation and provision of comprehensive information on drugs and their actions.
  3. Development and conduct of a product formulation and packaging program.
  4. Conduct of and participation in research.
  5. Development and conduct of patient-oriented services.
  6. Conduct of and participation in educational activities.
  7. Development and conduct of a quality assurance program for pharmaceutical services.

Colleges of pharmacy have recognized the need for providing an educational program for students interested in hospital pharmacy. Most of the colleges offer an undergraduate course in hospital pharmacy, while a number of colleges offer a graduate educational program leading to a Master of Science degree in hospital pharmacy. Most of the graduate programs are coordinated so that the student serves a residency in a hospital pharmacy concurrently with his graduate work at the university. These combined programs started in 1947 at the Philadelphia College of Pharmacy and Science and the Jefferson Medical College Hospital, and at the University of Maryland and the Johns Hopkins Hospital; the University of Michigan initiated its combined program in 1948. These combined educational and training programs have contributed much to provide career-minded, well-trained hospital pharmacists. Graduates of such programs have gone into hospitals throughout the country and proved their capabilities through the development of comprehensive pharmaceutical services of broad scope and high quality.

There is a trend toward specialization within hospital pharmacy. Hospital pharmacy residency training programs in years past have trained pharmacists primarily as generalists, with a so-called major in administration. While there is a place for the specialty of administration, there is also the need for other specialists. Certainly, the drug-information specialty is critical in the development of comprehensive clinical services. The specialist in drug-distribution systems has emerged. The manufacturing and product development specialist is also needed for investigational-drug studies and for sterile and nonsterile product formulations to meet new medical and surgical techniques, such as kidney, heart, and other organ transplants. There is a need also for a nuclear pharmacy scientist to handle, prepare, and formulate new dosage forms, and to conduct research on the large number of diagnostic and therapeutic radioactive pharmaceutical preparations available today. In some hospitals a pharmacy computer specialist develops systems that improve efficiency in providing better services. There is a need for a research specialist to participate in the wide variety of challenging research opportunities in hospital pharmacy. There is an expanding need for the clinical pharmacy specialist to assist in the rational selection and use of drug therapy. Some of the clinically trained pharmacists are even further specializing their efforts and expertise in specific areas of drug therapy such as in pediatrics, psychopharmacy, geriatrics, pharmacokinetics and other specialty areas.

Thus, we see a healthy trend developing toward so-called "group practice" in hospital pharmacy, analogous to group medical practice. A number of these specialists in different areas of hospital pharmacy practice make up the team of pharmacists in today's progressive hospital. It is the advancement of this concept that will strengthen the professional role of hospital pharmacists and give them entry to the group of professionals who make up the health-care team.

The Hospital

Hospital pharmacists practice within the framework of an organizational structure called a hospital. In order for them to function effectively, it is essential that they understand thoroughly what a hospital is, how it is organized, what its functions are and how the pharmacy service fits into the overall patient-care program.

Definition—Traditionally, a hospital has been defined in terms of its *form;* that is, its physical makeup and the quantitative nature of its services. This definition is best exemplified by the "registration of hospitals program" of the American Hospital Association. In order to be registered under this program an institution must meet certain requirements which constitute the definition of a hospital. Thus, the program differentiates between a hospital and other institutions such as extended-care facilities, convalescent homes, and homes for the aged.

The American Hospital Association has specific definitions for *general* and *special* hospitals in order for these institutions to qualify for the Association's registration program.[3] The AHA's requirements are as follows:

Requirements for Accepting General Hospitals for Registration

1. The institution shall maintain at least six inpatient beds which shall be continuously available for the care of patients who are nonrelated and who stay on the average in excess of 24 hours per admission.
2. The institution shall be constructed, equipped and maintained to ensure the health and safety of patients and to provide uncrowded, sanitary facilities for the treatment of patients.
3. There shall be an identifiable governing authority legally and morally responsible for the conduct of the hospital.
4. There shall be a chief executive to whom the governing authority delegates the continuous responsibility for the operation of the hospital in accordance with established policy.
5. There shall be an organized medical staff of physicians that may include, but shall not be limited to, dentists. The medical staff shall be accountable to the governing authority for maintaining proper standards of medical care, and it shall be governed by bylaws adopted by said staff and approved by the governing authority.
6. Each patient shall be admitted on the authority of a staff member who shall be directly responsible for the patient's diagnosis and treatment. Any graduate of a foreign medical school who is permitted to assume responsibilities for patient care shall possess a valid license to practice medicine, or shall be certified by the Educational Council for Foreign Medical Graduates, or shall have qualified for and have successfully completed an academic year of supervised clinical training under the direction of a medical school approved by the Liaison Committee on Medical Education of the American Medical Association and the Association of American Medical Colleges.
7. Registered nurse supervision and other nursing services are continuous.
8. A current and complete medical record shall be maintained by the institution for each patient and shall be available for reference.
9. Pharmacy service shall be maintained in the institution and shall be supervised by a registered pharmacist.
10. The institution shall provide patients with food service that meets the nutritional and therapeutic requirements; special diets shall also be available.

11. The institution shall maintain diagnostic X-ray service, with facilities and staff for a variety of procedures.
12. The institution shall maintain clinical laboratory service with facilities and staff for a variety of procedures. Anatomical pathology services shall be regularly and conveniently available.
13. The institution shall maintain operating room service with facilities and staff.

Requirements for Accepting Special Hospitals for Registration

1. The institution shall maintain at least six inpatient beds, which shall be continuously available for the care of patients who are nonrelated and who stay on the average in excess of 24 hours per admission.
2. The institution shall be constructed, equipped and maintained to ensure the health and safety of patients and to provide uncrowded, sanitary facilities for the treatment of patients.
3. There shall be an identifiable governing authority legally and morally responsible for the conduct of the hospital.
4. There shall be a chief executive to whom the governing authority delegates the continuous responsibility for the operation of the hospital in accordance with established policy.
5. There shall be an organized medical staff of physicians that may include, but shall not be limited to, dentists. The medical staff shall be accountable to the governing authority for maintaining proper standards of medical care and it shall be governed by bylaws adopted by said staff and approved by the governing authority.
6. Each patient shall be admitted on the authority of a member of the medical staff who shall be directly responsible for the patient's diagnosis and treatment. Any graduate of a foreign medical school who is permitted to assume responsibilities for patient care shall possess a valid license to practice medicine, or shall be certified by the Educational Council for Foreign Medical Graduates, or shall have qualified for and have successfully completed an academic year of supervised clinical training under the direction of a medical school approved by the Liaison Committee on Medical Education of the American Medical Association and the Association of American Medical Colleges.
7. Registered nurse supervision and other nursing services are continuous.
8. A current and complete medical record shall be maintained by the institution for each patient and shall be available for reference.
9. Pharmacy service shall be maintained in the institution and shall be supervised by a registered pharmacist.
10. The institution shall provide patients with food service that meets their nutritional and therapeutic requirements; special diets shall also be available.
11. Such diagnostic and treatment services as may be determined by the Board of Approval of the American Hospital Association to be appropriate for the specified medical conditions for which medical services are provided shall be maintained in the institution, with suitable facilities and staff. If such conditions do not normally require diagnostic X-ray service, laboratory service, or operating room service, and if any such services are therefore not maintained in the institution, there shall be written arrangements to make them available to patients requiring them.
12. When the institution provides pregnancy termination services, clinical laboratory services shall include the capability to provide tissue diagnosis.

On the other hand, a hospital may be defined in terms of its broad *purpose* or *mission* instead of its physical form. The contemporary hospital is a community institution which is an instrument of society. It serves as the focal point for the coordination and delivery of patient care to its community. A hospital may be viewed as an organized structure which pools together all the health professions, the diagnostic and therapeutic facilities, equipment and supplies, and the physical facilities into a coordinated system for delivering health care to the public.

While the hospital was once considered only as a place where patients were treated, today it is considered as a viable institution which extends its services to the patient wherever he may be located. For example, hospitals provide services to patients: within the institution itself (hospitalized patients); in ambulatory-care clinics, emergency rooms, emergency care centers; in physicians' offices at hospitals; in extended-care facilities and nursing homes either affiliated with or owned by the hospital; at home who require home health-care services; at wellness centers; and at community or neighborhood health clinics.

Certain other definitions are required for proper understanding of the differences between hospitals and patient-care institutions other than hospitals. In its accreditation program the Joint Commission on Accreditation of Hospitals (JCAH) divides long-term care facilities into two categories: (1) a Long-Term Health Care Facility, and (2) a Resident-Care Facility.[4] These facilities are defined as follows:

Long-Term Health Care Facility—A facility for inpatient care other than a hospital, with an organized medical staff, medical staff equivalent, or medical director, and with continuous nursing service under professional nurse direction. It is designed to provide, in addition to the medical care dictated by diagnoses, comprehensive preventive, rehabilitative, social, spiritual, and emotional inpatient care to individuals requiring long-term health care and to convalescent patients who have a variety of medical conditions with varying needs.

Resident-Care Facility—A facility providing safe, hygienic living arrangements for residents. Regular and emergency health services are available when needed, and appropriate supportive services, including preventive, rehabilitative, social, spiritual, and emotional, are provided on a regular basis.

* * * *

These two broad categories cover the various types of long-term care designated by governmental agencies for licensure, certification and/or reimbursement purposes, including skilled nursing care and intermediate care. Determination of category for accreditation purposes will be made at the time of survey, based on the primary role of the facility. If identifiable roles in both major areas can be determined, accreditation will be considered in both categories.

A *clinic* is an establishment where ambulatory patients are admitted for special study and treatment by a group of physicians practicing together, and where the patient is not confined as in a hospital. The term *clinic* is also used to indicate the outpatient diagnostic facility operated by a hospital and also facilities operated by other agencies for the care of indigent and medically indigent patients. In the past the term clinic has usually been reserved for facilities of a teaching nature where medical students and resident staff offered treatment to patients unable to afford private practitioners. This concept has changed in recent years with the growing trend of physicians to locate their offices in or adjacent to the hospital, and a so-called private outpatient service has been added to the regular clinic facilities. Essentially these functions are now grouped into a recognized department of ambulatory care at most hospitals.

Development and Expansion—Hospitals had their origin in Indian and Egyptian culture during the sixth century B.C. Evolution of the hospital is related to the sociological development of the individual's expansion of interest beyond himself and his family to the welfare of the community. Although early hospitals were really places to remove people from society to protect society, ie, the insane, the incurables, and the contagious, other hospitals were developed through religious and divine motives. The temples of the gods in early Greek and Roman civilization were used as hospitals where healing was associated with divine powers, while continued illness or death was associated with a lack of purity. Greek temples were forerunners of the modern hospital in the sense that they provided refuge and treatment for the sick and also provided for the teaching of young medical students. Such temples as the Temple of Aesculapius (Greek god of Medicine) existed in 1134 BC, while the temple at Kos, Greece was where Hippocrates (born about 460 BC) practiced.

One of the dominant factors in the development and expansion of hospitals was the religious influence. Prior to the Christian Era, hospitals were temples dedicated to the god of medicine in which care of the sick was accompanied by magical, mystical, and religious ceremonies. The doctrines of Jesus Christ intensified the emotions and virtues of love, pity, and charity. These strong motivating forces toward one's fellow man gave impetus to the expansion of hospitals.

Another major factor in the development and expansion of hospitals devolves from a military influence. Much of the impetus toward medical and surgical progress over the centuries has come from the urgent need for care of the wounded on the battlefield. This was true during the Roman empire; it was also true in the United States before, during, and after the Civil War. The Civil War, however, focused attention on the inadequacy of hospital construction and also on the lack of nursing care. Lincoln requested Catholic Sisters to care for wounded army personnel because hospital care was so poor. The work done in the army set a pattern for improvement in patient care and combined the military and religious influence on hospital development.

Other factors which have influenced the development and expansion of hospitals were: (1) the Flexner report on medical education (1910) which caused revolutionary developments in medical education *per se* and in medical internship training which helped the development of minimum standards for patient care in hospital surroundings, (2) the activities of Florence Nightingale during and after the Crimean War which served as the basis for revolutionizing the quality of nursing care in hospitals and for the development of schools of nursing, and (3) the public interest in hospitals through greater dependence and improved confidence in hospital care. With public dependence and confidence came public support and this support provided the finances for further development, expansion, and improvement in hospital facilities. This public interest extended its influence into private hospitalization insurance and into government participation in health care through social security and other health-related agencies. One of the most significant governmental programs which has affected the development and expansion of hospital facilities in the US was the adoption (in 1946) by the Congress of the Hospital Survey and Construction Act. Commonly known as the Hill–Burton program, this act was passed to provide federal funds for hospital construction on a matching basis with local communities. From 1946 to 1973 hundreds of new hospitals have been built while hundreds of other hospitals have undertaken major expansion programs of existing facilities through the availability of government finances through the Hill–Burton Act.

Since that time a number of legislative amendments have been adopted by the Congress which made funds available for construction and improvement of various health-care facilities, including medical and nursing schools, outpatient facilities, extended-care facilities, and specialized diagnostic and therapeutic facilities in hospitals. In addition, the Social Security Amendments of 1965 (Medicare) will have a long-range impact on the development and expansion of hospitals because funds are made available to pay for services of medically indigent patients lacking means to pay hospitals for services rendered.

The National Planning and Resources Development Act was implemented in 1975 creating the development of Health Systems Agencies (HSAs). These agencies have the responsibility of effective health planning and development of health services, manpower, and facilities in local areas. Each HSA is responsible for (1) improving the health of residents of its health service area; (2) increasing the accessibility, acceptability, continuity, and quality of services provided; (3) restraining increases in the cost of these services; and (4) preventing unnecessary duplication of health resources. In 1983, Congress enacted significant changes in the method by which hospitals are reimbursed for medicare patients in an effort to hold down the escalating hospital costs. A Prospective Payment System was developed to reimburse hospitals at a specific rate based upon the diagnosis of the patient (diagnosis related group (DRG's)). This system of payment may affect other private reimbursement systems.

The first hospital on the American continent was built by the Spaniards (led by Cortez) in 1524—The Hospital of the Immaculate Conception in Mexico City. In 1663 its name was changed to The Hospital of Jesus of Nazareth and it still exists today. In the American colonies a hospital was built in 1663 on Manhattan Island for sick soldiers. The first incorporated hospital in the United States was the Pennsylvania Hospital, established in 1751 through the efforts of Dr Thomas Bond to provide physicians in Philadelphia with a place to treat their private patients. In 1769 New York, with a population of 300,000, had no hospital. Since 1873 the population of the United States has more than doubled but the number of hospitals has increased 44 times—from only 149 to approximately 7000.

Beyond the three basic essentials of human existence (food, clothing, and shelter) the hospital has become a necessary instrument for providing a fourth basic element of survival—health. The hospital serves as a major instrument through which the health professions are able to provide health to the people of the community. It is because of the increasing complexity of health care—diagnostic, preventive, and therapeutic—that the necessary trained personnel, facilities and equipment are consolidated into what is known as the hospital in order to provide the quality of care the public expects, demands, and deserves. Health care has come to be defined as a right for all, rather than a luxury for a few.

Classification—Hospitals may be classified in different ways, by:

1.	Type of service	3.	Ownership
2.	Length of stay	4.	Bed capacity

Hospitals are classified by *type of service* as either general or special hospitals. A general hospital provides care to patients with any type of illness: medical, surgical, pediatric, psychiatric and maternity. On the other hand, special hospitals are those which restrict the care they provide to special conditions, such as cancer, psychiatric, or pediatric cases.

Hospitals are classified by *length of stay* as either short-term or long-term. A short-term hospital is one in which the average length of stay of the patient is less than 30 days. Patients with acute disease conditions and emergency cases are usually hospitalized for less than 30 days. Usually, general hospitals are short-term, since acutely ill patients usually recover in less than 30 days. On the other hand, a long-term hospital is one in which the average length of stay of the patient is 30 days or longer. Such patients have long-term illnesses, such as psychiatric or mental retardation conditions.

Hospitals are classified by *ownership* usually as governmental or nongovernmental. Hospitals falling into these categories of ownership are as follows:

Governmental Hospitals	*Nongovernmental Hospitals*
Federal (Armed Forces, Veterans	Nonprofit
Administration & US Public	Church related or operated
Health Service)	Other nonprofit
State	For profit
County	Individual
City (municipal)	Partnership
City-County	Corporation
Hospital district	

Hospitals are generally classified by *bed capacity* according to the following pattern:

Under 50 beds
50– 99 beds
100–199 beds
200–299 beds
300–399 beds
400–499 beds
500 beds & over

According to these four general classifications, the approximately 7000 hospitals in the US are 80% nongovernmental, short-term, general or special; roughly half are under 100 beds.

The 7000 hospitals represent approximately 1,500,000 beds, admit about 38 million patients annually, and service approximately 266 million outpatient visits per year.

Federal hospitals are owned and operated by various branches of the federal government. The US Army, Air Force, and Navy hospitals are usually general medical and surgical hospitals, provided to care for military personnel, although there are specialized mental institutions within these groups. The Veterans Administration hospitals provide care for additional specialized groups of our population, and operate general medical and surgical hospitals, and also some mental hospitals.

State hospitals are owned by the state and controlled by a board of control or division of the state government, or a similar organization responsible to state government. They are maintained by state appropriations, and consist mainly of psychiatric hospitals. In some instances, state hospitals are general hospitals affiliated with a university involved in the training of physicians and other professional personnel.

County hospitals are owned by the county and are financed and controlled similarly to state hospitals, only on a county level. They are usually general hospitals caring for the indigent.

City hospitals are owned, financed, and controlled by the city government. They are usually general hospitals, caring for the indigent, although there may be a chain of city-owned and operated hospitals as in New York City.

In the nongovernmental hospital group, the majority of institutions are general medical and surgical hospitals, varying only in their control and their eligibility for receipt of state funds for charity or indigent patient care. The *proprietary* or *private hospital organized for profit* is usually a corporation composed of physicians, although other businessmen may be involved in the corporate profit-making structure. In recent years, a number of corporations have been formed whereby they own, operate, and control large chains of hospitals. There has been a great growth recently of "polycorporate" hospital systems in which one hospital manages several other hospitals or there is a multiple hospital grouping. These multiple hospital arrangements will have an influence upon how health care is delivered.

In the *nonprofit*, nongovernmental grouping of hospitals, some are *church hospitals*, supported financially by fees from paying patients or by contributions from the several religious orders or churches. These hospitals are owned and controlled either by the religious order, or diocese, as in the Catholic churches, or by a separate governing board, as in churches of other denominations.

Community hospitals or private nonprofit hospitals are owned and operated by members of the community, but with no relationship to the local government. They are financed by fees from patients and by subscriptions from residents of the community and surrounding area. The cost of providing medical care for the indigent is a problem for the community hospital that is met through local, state, and federal assistance.

Functions—Traditionally, the hospital's basic purpose for existence has been the treatment and care of the sick and injured. In conjunction with this basic function, hospitals have been concerned with teaching, particularly of medical students, ever since the pre-Christian Era of Greek medicine. Research has been another function of the hospital. In modern times a fourth function has been assumed by hospitals, namely, public health (preventive medicine). Thus the four fundamental functions of hospitals are patient care, teaching, research, and public health.

Patient Care—The modern hospital is charged with maintaining and restoring health to the community which it serves. The other three functions are really the handmaidens of patient care since they exist because they contribute either directly or otherwise to the care of the sick and injured. Emergency care of the injured commands prime attention in any hospital—fully as important as the care of the inpatient.

Outpatient care, although becoming more important as a function of the hospital's responsibility to the community, is usually subordinate to inpatient and emergency care. Patient care involves the diagnosis and treatment of illness or injury, preventive medicine, rehabilitation, convalescent care, dental care, and personalized services.

In providing patient care, hospitals usually have two basic types of accommodations based on the patient's ability to pay: namely, the full-pay or private patient and the partially or totally medical indigent (charity) patient. With the marked increase in prepaid hospitalization insurance (through commercial insurance carriers and Blue Cross) there has been a great increase in the number of private (or semiprivate) patients. The federal government's involvement with medical care through Medicare and Medicaid expands coverage for a broad population group who previously were partially or totally medical indigents, including nonindigent groups.

Education—Education is an important function of the modern hospital whether it is or is not affiliated with a university. Education as a hospital function is of two major forms:

1. Education of the medical and allied health professions. This form includes physicians; nurses; medical social service workers; medical record librarians; dietitians; X-ray and laboratory technicians; medical technologists; respiratory, physical and occupational therapists; hospital administrators; pharmacists; and others. The hospital's educational program for these groups includes formal programs (such as medical and nursing schools), in-service training programs for professional personnel such as residencies, and on-the-job training programs for nonprofessional personnel. Such educational programs are essential; it is only in a hospital that such concentrated facilities are available to provide the necessary practical learning experience for dealing with the saving of human lives.
2. Education of the patient. This form is an important hospital function the scope of which is seldom realized by the public. It includes providing general education for children confined to long-term hospitalization; special education in the area of rehabilitation—psychiatrically, socially, physically, and occupationally; and special education in health care, for example, teaching a diabetic or a cardiac patient to care for his ailment or teaching the colostomy patient who requires a reorientation in caring for his personal needs.

Research—Hospitals carry out research as a vital function for two major purposes: the advancement of medical knowledge against disease and the improvement of hospital services. Both purposes are directed toward the basic aim of better health care for the patient. Examples of research activities in the hospital include devising new diagnostic procedures, conducting laboratory and clinical experiments, developing and perfecting new surgical procedures and techniques, and evaluating investigational drugs. Other examples include research to improve administrative procedures for greater efficiency and for lower cost to the patient, improvement of accounting procedures for more equitable cost distribution of services, and designing, developing, and evaluating new equipment and facilities for improving patient care.

Research in hospitals has been carried on primarily by medical staffs in the past. However, in recent years there has been a significant increase in research activities in the various hospital departments by other than medical personnel. Nursing, for example, is now engaged in significant research activities designed to improve patient care. Although pharmacy has played a limited role in hospital research in the past, there is increasing activity in this area. For example, any drug must be tested in a hospital before it can be marketed, and thus the clinical evaluation of investigational drugs presents many opportunities for the hospital pharmacist to participate in research. Pharmacists are involved in many other types of research, such as pharmacokinetic studies involving individualization of drug-dosing in patients, biopharmaceutic studies of drug products, radiopharmaceutical dosage formulations, as well as administrative and professional studies

on drug distribution systems, the effectiveness of clinical roles of pharmacists, and drug utilization review studies.

Public Health—The prime objective of this fourth and relatively new hospital function is to assist the community in reducing the incidence of sickness and to increase the general health of the population. Examples of public health activities are the close working relationships many hospitals have with public health departments of communicable diseases; the participation in disease detection programs as for tuberculosis, diabetes, hypertension, and cancer; the participation in mass public innoculation programs such as against influenza and poliomyelitis; and the participation of hospital ambulatory-care departments in teaching better routine hygienic practices, wellness clinics, exercise and fitness programs, as well as ways in which patients should care for themselves when illness strikes. Hospital pharmacists have an opportunity to contribute to this function by providing health information brochures and services to outpatients and by instructing them on the safe use of drugs and on poison prevention measures.

Standards of Practice—In the United States the public is able to determine whether a hospital provides a minimum quality of patient care through its "accreditation" status. The accreditation program is conducted on a national basis and its purpose is to determine the quality of care rendered to patients. This is achieved through the establishment of minimum standards of quality of patient care and then to invite all hospitals to meet or surpass these standards by improving their services and facilities.

The accreditation program is carried out by the Joint Commission on Accreditation of Hospitals (JCAH).

The Joint Commission is an independent, voluntary agency, and its actions are not subject to ratification by the organizations represented by its component members. One of its objectives is to make known to the public the names of those hospitals which have invited its scrutiny and have been accredited by it through meeting the minimum standards established for good patient care. The net effect of the program is to enable the public to discriminate between hospitals that are accredited and those that are not.

Accreditation of hospitals began in 1918 when The American College of Surgeons initiated its hospital standardization program. The purpose was to elevate the quality of surgical care provided in hospitals. The program involved setting up minimum standards of practice for the operating rooms, but it also pointed up the need for similar standards in all departments of the hospital. The first list of approved hospitals, published in 1919, contained 89 approved hospitals out of 692 surveyed. The American College of Surgeons standardization program was taken over by the Joint Commission on Accreditation of Hospitals in 1953.

During the years the American College of Surgeons carried out the accreditation program, the pharmacy was not included among the essential divisions of the hospital but, rather, was listed as a complementary division. The Joint Commission on Accreditation of Hospitals continued this classification for several years. However, in 1956 the pharmacy department was included among the essential services of the hospital and thus official recognition was given to the importance of the pharmacy. In 1965 the JCAH amended its standards for medical staff functions by requiring a pharmacy and therapeutics committee. Previously, the JCAH had only considered this committee to be a desirable one rather than an essential committee. A more recent development was the inclusion in the requirement for registration by the American Hospital Association that "Pharmacy service shall be maintained in the institution and shall be supervised by a registered pharmacist."

Another major impetus to the development of standards of practice in hospitals came about with the enactment of the

Social Security Amendments of 1965 (Medicare). This law sets forth certain conditions which hospitals are required to meet for purposes of participating as providers of services to recipients of federally financed programs. These requirements are published as a manual entitled, *Conditions of Participation—Hospitals.** This manual includes the conditions of participation for the various departments of the hospital, including the pharmacy department. These conditions have played a major role in challenging small hospitals to consider appointing pharmacists to their staffs, to providing comprehensive pharmacy services, and to establish pharmacy and therapeutics committees.

As the Health Systems Agencies develop in the implementation of their responsibilities, their influence on practice standards and functions will be felt.

Organization and Administration—No matter what the type of organization and control of a hospital there is always a governing body of some sort to which the administrator, director, superintendent, medical director, chief administrative officer, or whatever the individual be titled must report. In the case of the federal hospitals, this is usually not a group on a local area level. In state, county, and city hospitals the governing body is usually from the political subdivision in which the hospital is located, but need not be so where persons of special ability are concerned or in cases where political pressure is applied. In the nonprofit, nongovernmental hospital, there is usually a governing board, board of trustees, board of governors, or other titled group which assumes overall responsibility for the proper operation of the hospital so that adequate service can be rendered to the sick and injured at as low a cost as is compatible with efficiency.

Specifically, the duties of the governing board, performed through the chief administrative officer, are the responsibility for selection of competent personnel including the medical staff, the control of hospital funds, and the supervision of the physical plant. By reason of certain court decisions the responsibility for injury or other act by a member of the hospital staff on the hospital grounds reverts back to the governing board, although the individual hospital personnel is involved.

The governing body, acting on recommendations of the chief administrative officer, must establish the working hours and conditions, salary schedules, and proper checks on personnel. Again, acting on the recommendations of the chief administrative officer, the governing board must establish a schedule of room rates and other charges for hospital inpatient and ambulatory care. The board must devise methods for obtaining endowments and other grants that will supplement income from paying patients and help to balance the hospital budget. The board must wisely invest endowment funds and other grants from which the interest is to be used for operating or other expenses. It must make certain that there is established an adequate accounting system and provide for routine audit of the accounts. This board must determine the needs for additional or replacement construction of the physical plant of the hospital and must contract with the most advantageous bidder.

The governing board has its own internal organization, comprised of a president or chairman, vice-chairman, secretary, and treasurer. On many boards the chief administrative officer of the hospital serves as secretary. There are usually certain standing committees appointed, such as the executive committee; the house or hospital committee dealing with personnel appointments and especially those of the medical staff, and with other activities of departmental nature; the

finance committee which is concerned with the hospital budget, room rates, and other financial matters; and a committee on public relations which is concerned with educating the community on the value of the hospital and with maintaining a desirable relationship with the community. There may be other committees appointed as the need arises such as an expansion and development committee where the hospital is concerned with the need for construction of additional hospital beds.

The chief executive officer (CEO) of the hospital is appointed by the governing board and must produce a two-way channel of communication between the board and the hospital staff and personnel insofar as the needs or desires of both are concerned. The chief executive officer is often the secretary of the governing board, and reports to it all essential facts concerning the operation of the hospital and receives from the board all directives it issues. The hospital administrator must have initiative and leadership as well as executive ability in order to carry out his responsibilities. All functions of professional care of the patient must be carried on within budgetary limitations, and there must be interdepartmental cooperation and harmony.

In order for administrators to carry out the overall responsibilities assigned by the governing board they need assistance. Depending on the size of the hospital there may be one or more associate and several assistant administrators. The administrator also appoints heads of departments. The department heads have the responsibility to operate the departments effectively and properly, within the overall policies and philosophies established by the hospital's governing board.

Among the many departments which make up the modern hospital there are some in which the services involve primarily the *professional care* of the patient while the services of other departments involve mainly the *business management* of the hospital.

Some of the departments which deal with the professional care of the patient (diagnostic or therapeutic) are as follows:

Ambulatory Care	Medical Library
Anesthesia	Medical Records
Blood Bank	Medical Social Service
Central Sterile Supply	Nuclear Medicine
Clinical Laboratories	Nursing Service
Dental Service	Occupational Therapy
Dietary and Nutrition Service	Pharmacy Service
Electrocardiograph Laboratory	Physical Medicine
Electroencephalograph Laboratory	Radiology & X-Ray Therapy
Emergency Room	Respiratory Therapy

Departments which deal with the business management or administrative side of the hospital include:

Accounting	Engineering & Maintenance
Admitting	Housekeeping
Biomedical Engineering	Information Service
Business Office	Personnel & Payroll
Cafeteria & Coffee Shop	Post Office
Central Transportation	Purchase & Store Room
Credit & Collection	Telephone Switchboard
Computer Services	Volunteer Service

The Medical Staff—The medical staff of a hospital falls in a different category organizationally than the departments listed previously. Physicians are independent agents taking care of their patients, and they utilize the hospital, its departments, facilities, and services to care for these patients. The governing board of the hospital and the community which it represents exercise effective control over the medical staff. Although the governing board neither originates nor implements medical policy, it is responsible for it, and while the board members are not competent to pass judgment on the professional care of the patient they are, as representatives of the ownership of the hospital, liable for dereliction of duties

---

* Available from the US Dept of Health and Human Services, Social Security Admin, Washington, DC.

established by law. Thus the board delegates a portion of its duties and responsibilities to its appointed medical staff to originate medical policy honestly and to carry out this policy in good faith. To do this requires that the medical staff be organized to govern itself and appraise its own work, and yet be responsible to the governing board for the details of its work.

In order for a physician to be appointed to the medical staff of a hospital, an application for membership must be made. This application and appropriate credentials are considered by the credentials committee of the medical staff, which determines whether the physician is competent to practice in the claimed specialty. The credentials committee, if favorably impressed, makes its recommendation to the medical staff for appointment. Assuming this is approved, the recommendation goes to the governing board for final approval. Upon approval by the board the physician is designated a member of the medical staff of the hospital for a specified period of time, usually 1 year, subject to renewal.

The organized medical staff of a hospital has certain duties: (1) providing professional care of the sick and injured in the hospital, (2) maintaining its own efficiency, (3) self-government, (4) participating in the educational program of the hospital, (5) auditing its own professional work, and (6) advising and assisting the administrator and the governing board regarding medical policies.

There are two main types of hospital staffs, the *open* and the *closed*. An *open* staff is one in which certain physicians other than those on the attending or active medical staff are allowed to utilize the private room facilities, providing they comply with all rules and regulations of the institution. These physicians are termed members of the "courtesy" medical staff; the hospital is termed an *open staff* hospital.

A *closed* staff is one in which all professional services, private and charity, are provided and controlled by the attending or active medical staff. A hospital with this type of staff is termed a *closed staff* hospital. The closed staff, though it has minor drawbacks, is the more desirable for the average hospital and especially for the teaching hospital, because it allows careful selection of a group of specialists with excellent reputation.

The medical staff consists of the following groups: (1) an honorary staff, (2) a consulting staff, (3) an active staff, (4) an associate staff, (5) a courtesy staff, and (6) a resident staff. The *honorary medical staff* is composed of physicians who have been active in the hospital but who are retired, and of those to whom it is desired to do honor because of outstanding contributions. The *consulting medical staff* consists of specialists who are recognized as such by right of passing specialty boards or belonging to the national organization of their specialty, and who serve as consultants to other members of the medical staff when called upon. The *active* or *attending medical staff* is the group primarily concerned with regular patient care. It is the group most actively involved in the hospital. In internal staff government it is the authoritative body. The *associate medical staff* is composed of junior or less experienced members of the staff. Appointment to this group is the first step toward active or attending staff membership. The *courtesy medical staff* consists of those physicians who desire the privilege of attending private patients but who do not desire active staff membership. The *resident medical staff* is composed of residents, who are full-time employees of the hospital. These persons provide specific services in the care of the patient, for which they receive education and experience.

Financing Hospital Care—The technological developments of our industrialized society and the rapid advances of the medical sciences annually increase the financial burdens of hospitals. Hospitals, in order to provide the best care available, at the insistence of the public must keep up with these advances by obtaining the newest diagnostic and therapeutic equipment, facilities, and products. In addition, the increasing cost of labor is reflected in the increased cost of the personalized services made available in the modern hospital. The cost of hospital care is a direct reflection of these developments. In 1946 the total cost of operating all US hospitals was $1.9 billion; by 1978 the total cost had reached $65.5 billion. By 1983, health care costs approximate $322 billion. This cost is approximately 10.5% of the Gross National Product (GNP).

Perhaps the most widely used statistic to describe hospital costs is the total expense per patient day. In 1946 the average cost per patient day in hospitals was $5.21; in 1974 the cost per patient day averaged $84.00. In 1982 the average cost per patient day is between $200–300. With the trend toward more equitable salaries for hospital personnel, there is every indication that hospital costs will continue to rise dramatically.

For centuries hospitals have struggled with the problem of finances adequate to cover total operating expenses. The fact that, basically, the public does not care to pay for something it does not want has been a major factor in this struggle for financial survival. Individuals resist having to pay hundreds or thousands of dollars for an operation or a long hospital stay which they have not anticipated. At one time hospitals were a place where people went to die; the public cared little about their financial struggles. But as the hospital developed into a place where people went to get well the public took a more positive interest in the financial problems. In other words, the public has come to recognize that although it dislikes paying hospital bills it must do so if the hospital is to continue to exist to protect the public health. Over the last few decades the quality of health and the life span have both increased.

Sources of Income—There are several main sources of income for hospitals: patients, government, third-party hospitalization insurance, voluntary contributions, endowment funds and investments.

Since the majority of hospitals in the US are private, nongovernmentally operated, the bulk of income to these institutions is from the patient, either directly or indirectly. Funds may come from the patient directly or they may come through hospitalization insurance (usually referred to as third-party payments). A large segment of the population is covered by hospitalization insurance.

Another third-party principle involves the workmen's compensation regulations in the various states. These regulations vary among the states but essentially each regulation involves the employer taking out an accident insurance policy which will pay for emergency treatment or hospitalization of the employee in case of accident or injury on the job.

Medically indigent patients are those who do not have sufficient income to pay for their own personal health needs. Although some private organizations provide assistance to this group of patients, the bulk of the financial assistance comes from tax funds through local, state, and federal governmental agencies. The list of public tax-supported programs for health-care assistance is formidable and becomes complex in determining what department, division, or agency of the federal, state, county, or city government is involved. In addition, dependents of members of the Armed Forces, members of the Public Health Service and their families, and the veterans of foreign wars receive health care through public tax funds.

The Social Security Amendments of 1965 and 1972 extend the benefits for hospitalization, physicians services, and outpatient services from the original Social Security Law. A substantial portion of hospital costs is provided under federal government auspices. The total percentage of health-care costs covered by third-party reimbursement of some sort approaches 90%.

Other sources of income to hospitals are the voluntary contributions of individuals, corporations, foundations, and community fund-raising campaigns. Some of these are direct contributions to the hospitals; others are made available in the form of grants for research; still others are given for major expansion or remodeling programs. Private health assistance agencies assist individuals who need help by subsidizing the cost of their hospitalization and other health care needs.

Many hospitals are fortunate in receiving substantial sums for the purpose of setting up endowment trust funds and for use by the hospitals in other ways. In addition some hospitals receive some income through investments, such as in real estate.

Another category of income sources includes the gift shop, small food-service facility, or beauty parlor, many of which are operated by a women's auxiliary on a voluntary basis.

Health Maintenance Organizations—A Health Maintenance Organization (HMO) is a public or private organization which provides comprehensive health services to individuals enrolled with such an organization on a per capita prepayment basis. Such comprehensive or "total" health services include minimum emergency care, inpatient hospital and physician care, ambulatory physician care, and outpatient preventive medical services.

In 1973 Congress passed the "Health Maintenance Organization Act of 1973" (Public Law 93-222) which provided new authority to the Department of Health, Education and Welfare to develop new HMOs. According to the Act an HMO is an organizational entity which includes four essential attributes:

1. An organized system for providing health care in a geographic area, which entity accepts the responsibility to provide or otherwise assure the delivery of
2. an agreed-upon set of basic and supplemental health maintenance and treatment services to
3. a voluntarily enrolled group of persons
4. and for which services the HMO is reimbursed through a predetermined, fixed, periodic prepayment made by or on behalf of each person or family unit enrolled in the HMO without regard to the amounts of actual services provided.

This legislation authorizes, among many other things, an HMO to "maintain, review and evaluate . . . a drug use profile of its members receiving prescription drugs, evaluate patterns of drug utilization to assure optimum drug therapy, and provide for instruction of its members and of health professionals in the use of prescription and nonprescription drugs." Thus, opportunities exist for the development of challenging new roles for pharmacy within HMOs in the broad areas of rational drug therapy including diagnostic and curative, as well as preventive, therapy. Many would agree that pharmacy practice within these organized health care facilities is characteristic of institutional pharmacy practice.

The Hospital Pharmacy

The separation of pharmacy from medicine took place in charitable institutions operated under governmental or ecclesiastic authority. The fact that business interests played no part in the delivery of care to patients in these institutions led to an eventual division of labor in order to improve the quality of care. This division of labor in the physician–apothecary function led to the recognition of pharmacy as a discipline separate from medicine. Since the division occurred in hospitals, the hospital pharmacist was the first recognized practitioner of the profession of pharmacy.

The development of hospital pharmacy in different countries was vitally affected by educational standards and by the caliber of its practitioners. Thus hospital pharmacy as an important professional specialty was virtually neglected in America for almost 168 years, from the time that Jonathan

Roberts became the first hospital pharmacist at the Pennsylvania Hospital (Philadelphia) in 1752, to approximately 1920. After naming Charles Rice (1841–1901) of Bellevue Hospital in New York City, and Martin I Wilbert (1865–1916) of the German Hospital in Philadelphia, it is difficult to recall other equally prominent contemporary hospital pharmacists of the same period.

A National Professional Society—Although the existence of the American hospital covers a span of more than 200 years, only during the past three decades or so have we witnessed the rapid expansion leading to our present vast and complex hospital system. As the movement toward the organization, expansion, and growth of the hospital system in the United States began to take shape, there also developed a movement toward the organization of hospital pharmacists. As Niemeyer, *et al*,[5] point out, the critical years for hospital pharmacy were the two decades from 1920 to 1940. The "awakening in the twenties" came about as a result of a growing realization by hospital pharmacists of the problems, potentialities, and importance of their specialty. The "advances in the thirties" resulted from their determination for organization, recognition, and establishment of higher standards of practice.

The activities of hospital pharmacists during these two critical decades resulted in the formation of The American Society of Hospital Pharmacists in 1942. The development of the Society within the sphere of American pharmacy has been due in large part to the adoption of a philosophy of service by hospital pharmacists which places the patient as the focal point for the existence of pharmacy and which minimizes the professional man's self interests. The unity which binds hospital pharmacists through their national professional society stems from their being a goal-oriented group. The common bond among them is the development of higher standards of professional practice and service, *because the patient needs it*. The membership exceeding 22,000 members represents a significant majority of the pharmacists practicing in the institutional setting. Because of this common goal, the American Society of Hospital Pharmacists has made significant progress during the first 43 years of its existence.

Despite its relative youth, The American Society of Hospital Pharmacists has made significant contributions toward the improvement of hospital pharmacy. The *American Journal of Hospital Pharmacy* is one of the best professional publications in international pharmaceutical circles. The *International Pharmaceutical Abstracts* was introduced by the ASHP because of the need for such a publication. The *American Hospital Formulary Service* is a comprehensive, unbiased source of current information on drugs provided on a supplemented basis annually. It serves as a basis for the pharmacist to extend his role as pharmaceutical consultant to the medical profession. In 1964 the *Mirror to Hospital Pharmacy* provided the findings from an exhaustive study of hospital pharmacy in the United States. The whole basis for this study was to find out existing practices in hospital pharmacy and to determine ways in which to improve the quality and expand the scope of its pharmaceutical service. Continuing education programs, known as "Institutes," have served to help the hospital pharmacy practitioner keep up with current trends of professional practice. Continuing education programs such as this are essential for the practicing pharmacist to maintain his professional competency. Maintaining professional competency is one of the greatest challenges of the profession of pharmacy today, indeed the challenge for all health professions. The success of this program has been the envy of other segments of the profession. The residency training programs in hospital pharmacy are accredited by the Society and serve as a basis for insuring a high quality of training of future practitioners. In addition to general residencies in hospital pharmacy, specialized residencies in nuclear pharmacy, ambulatory care, pediatric pharmacy, psychiatric pharmacy, geriatric pharmacy, drug information pharmacy practice, oncology pharmacy and clinical pharmacy serve to provide a means to develop practitioners with specialized skills to meet future practice needs. The profession as a whole would profit greatly if it were to adopt a similar positive program to insure good residency training. The *Minimum Standard for Pharmacies in Institutions* provides a helpful set of principles on which to develop good professional practices within the hospital. Many other contributions dealing with specific phases of hospital pharmacy have been made by the Society and still others are currently under study. Thus the strengths of a goal-oriented Society are readily apparent in the ASHP's contributions to American hospital pharmacy.

Standards of Practice

The movement to develop standards of practice in the hospital was initiated by the American College of Surgeons during the early 1900s when surgeons recognized the need to standardize and improve on surgical procedures, operating room techniques, and medical records on surgical operations. The College found that to improve the overall care of surgical patients, standards needed to be developed in other departments of the hospital as well as in the operating room. As a result of their initiative, the first Minimum Standard for Pharmacies in Hospitals was presented to the 18th Hospital Standardization Conference of The American College of Surgeons in 1935.[6] In 1942, when The American Society of Hospital Pharmacists was organized, a standing committee on Minimum Standards was appointed for the purpose of maintaining and developing better minimum standards. The original standard of the American College of Surgeons was revised by The American Society of Hospital Pharmacists in 1950. This revised Standard was approved by The American Pharmaceutical Association, American Hospital Association, Catholic Hospital Association, and received editorial endorsement by the American Medical Association. The *Minimum Standard for Pharmacies in Hospitals with Guide to Application** has been revised periodically, resulting in the *Minimum Standard for Pharmacies in Institutions** and the *Statement on the Competencies Required in Institutional Pharmacy Practice.**

To assist hospital administrators and hospital pharmacists to review their pharmacy service in terms of expected qualitative performance, the Joint Commission on Accreditation of Hospitals has revised its standards for a hospital pharmacy. These standards, while not totally inclusive of a broad scope and high quality pharmaceutical service, do challenge the 7000 hospitals to meet at least a respectable basic quality of performance in the pharmacy. The challenge to the profession is to continue to upgrade the basic minimum practices to the point where the Joint Commission on Accreditation of Hospitals will concurrently revise its standards of pharmacy in hospitals to meet this higher quality of service.

Another standard of practice relating to institutional pharmacy is the requirement imposed by the federal government under the Social Security Amendments of 1965 (Medicare) and subsequent amendments.

Organization—Within the organizational structure of the hospital the director of pharmacy, as a department head, reports to the administrator of the hospital on the proper operation and management of the pharmacy. The director of pharmacy formulates and implements departmental administrative and professional policies of the pharmacy subject to

the approval of the administrator. The professional and clinical policies relating to hospital pharmacy practice that have a direct relationship to the medical staff are formulated and developed through the pharmacy and therapeutics committee and are subject to administrative approval (see *Pharmacy and Therapeutics Committee*).

The organizational structure of the hospital pharmacy may be as illustrated in Fig 95-1. This chart attempts to illustrate that coordination and integration of all the technical elements of practice must be effectively implemented into a total pharmaceutical service. For example, there are technical and professional elements of a clinical pharmacy service. On the other hand, there are clinical components of professional, technical, and support services. Likewise, there are educational, technical, and clinical implications to the research and supportive components to a pharmacy service. Therefore, one should look at the organizational structure of a modern hospital pharmacy in terms of the overall elements comprising its services rather than viewing it from a clinical vs an operational standpoint. This philosophical approach to the organizational and operational aspects of hospital pharmacy is essential if one is to effectively utilize all the pharmaceutical sciences which underlie the profession of pharmacy.

A close examination of this organizational chart shows the many ramifications of the practice of pharmacy in today's modern hospital. There follows a comprehensive job description of the pharmacist's responsibilities in general hospital pharmacy activities and in clinical functions and responsibilities.

Pharmacist Responsibilities

I. Inpatient Pharmacist's Responsibilities
  A. Central Dispensing Area
    1. Insures that established policies and procedures are followed.
    2. Checks for accuracy of doses prepared:
      a. Intravenous admixtures
      b. Unit dose
      c. Outpatient pharmacy
    3. Provides for proper drug control:
      a. Insures that drugs are stored and dispensed properly (eg, investigational drugs).
      b. Insures that all state and federal drug laws are followed.
    4. Insures that good techniques are used in compounding intravenous admixtures and extemporaneous preparations.
    5. Provides for proper record keeping and billing:
      a. Patient medication records
      b. Extemporaneous compounding records
      c. Intravenous admixture records and billing
      d. Investigational drug records
      e. Outpatient billings
      f. Reports (eg, monthly workload report)
    6. Maintains professional competence, particularly in knowledge of drug stability and incompatibilities.
    7. Insures that new personnel are properly trained in the policies and procedures of the central dispensing area.
    8. Coordinates the activities of the area with the available staff to make the best possible use of personnel and resources.
    9. Keeps the central dispensing area neat and orderly.
    10. Communicates with all pharmacy staff regarding new developments in the area and assists in employee evaluations.
    11. Provides drug information as necessary to the pharmacy, medical, and nursing staff.
    12. Coordinates the overall pharmaceutical needs of the patient care areas with the central dispensing area (eg delivery schedules).
  B. Patient Care Area
    1. Supervision of drug administration technicians.
      a. Reviews and interprets each unit dose and IV admixture medication order to insure that it is entered accurately into the unit dose or IV admixture system.
      b. Reviews each patient's drug administration form periodically to insure that all doses are being administered and charted correctly.

---

* Available from the American Society of Hospital Pharmacists, 4630 Montgomery Ave, Washington, DC 20014.

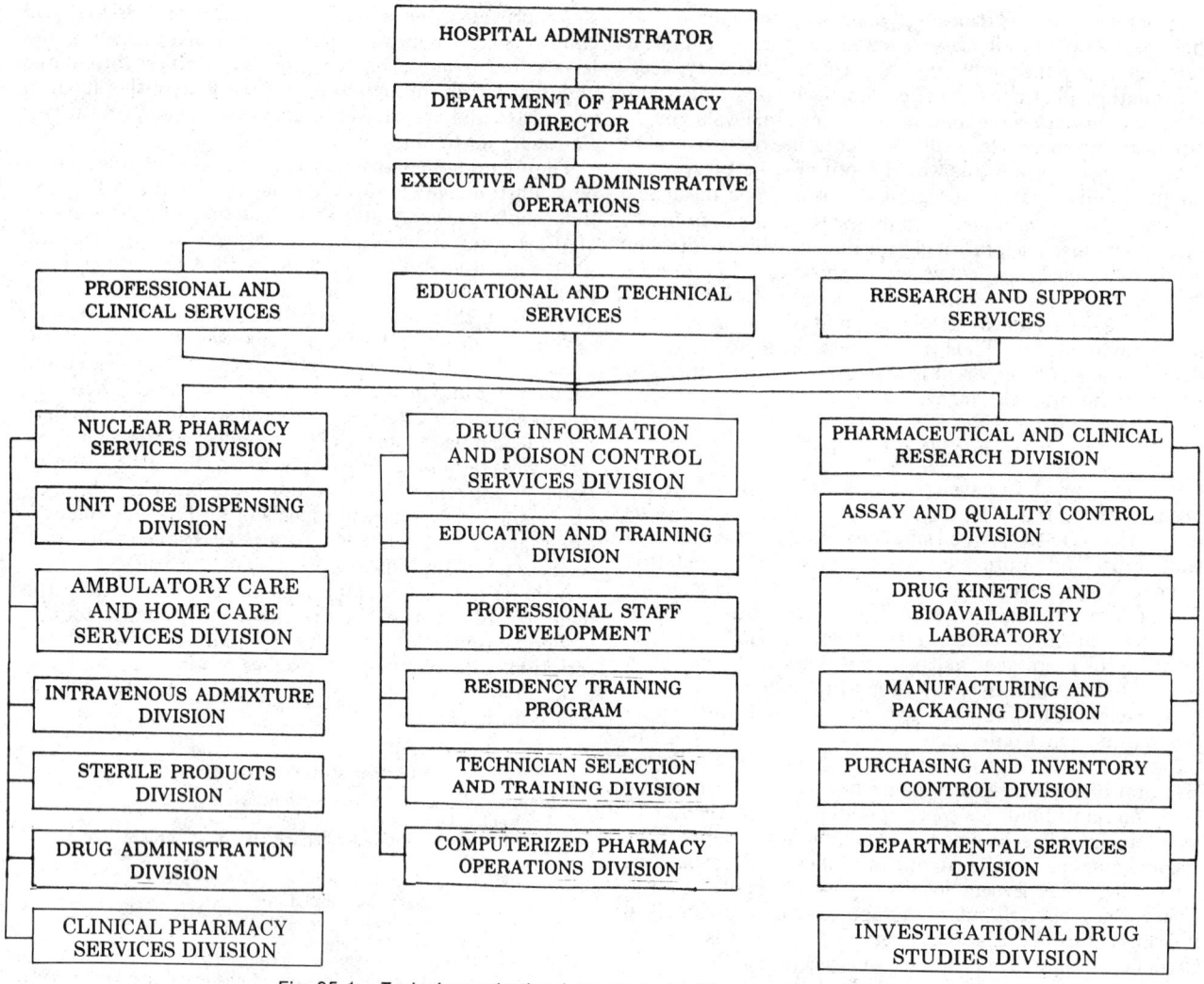

Fig 95-1. Typical organizational structure of a Pharmacy Department.

1. Reviews all doses missed, reschedules the doses as necessary, and signs all "drugs not given" notices.
2. Insures that new drug administration forms are transcribed accurately for continuity of drug therapy and that drug charges are correctly assessed.
   c. Confirms periodically that administered doses are correctly noted on the patient's chart.
   d. Insures that records for administered narcotics are kept correctly and that the physician is informed of all automatic stop orders.
   e. Instructs and assists the technician as needed in dealing with difficult patients.
   f. Assists the technician as needed in dealing with new procedures.
   g. Insures that proper drug administration techniques are used by the technician.
   h. Insures that the technician is communicating with the nurse regarding the need for PRN drugs.
   i. Acts as liaison between the technician and the nursing and medical staff.
   j. Communicates with nurses and physicians concerning medication administration problems.
   k. Periodically inspects the medication areas on the nursing units to insure that adequate levels of floor stock drugs and supplies are maintained.
   l. Insures that drugs and supplies are procured from the central dispensing area as required.
   m. Insures that other supportive services performed by the department of pharmacy are carried out correctly.
   n. Coordinates all pharmacy services on the nursing unit level.
   o. Insures that the technician keeps the medication area neat and orderly.

p. Insures that proper security is maintained in the medication area to prevent pilferage.
q. Insures that technicians understand and follow personnel policies and rules.
r. Insures that adequate technician coverage is provided in the patient-care area (coverage for ill calls, etc).
s. Assists in training new technicians.
2. Direct Patient Care
   a. Identifies drugs brought into the hospital by patients.
   b. Obtains patient medication histories and communicates all pertinent information to the physician.
   c. Assists in drug product and entity selection.
   d. Assists the physician in selecting dosage regimens and schedules, then assigns drug administration times for these schedules.
   e. Monitors patients' total drug therapy for:
      1. Effectiveness/Ineffectiveness
      2. Side effects
      3. Toxicities
      4. Allergic drug reactions
      5. Drug interactions
   f. Counsels patients on:
      1. Medications to be self-administered in the hospital
      2. Discharge medications
   g. Participates in cardiopulmonary emergencies by:
      1. Procurement and preparation of needed drugs
      2. Charting all medications given
      3. Performing cardiopulmonary resuscitation, if necessary
3. General Responsibilities
   a. Provides in-service education to:
      1. Pharmacists, pharmacy interns, residents, and students

2. Nurses and nursing students
3. Physicians and medical students
   b. Provides drug information to physicians, nurses, and other health care personnel.

II. Ambulatory Pharmacist's Responsibilities
  A. Central Dispensing Area
    1. Insures that established policies and procedures are followed.
    2. Checks for accuracy in the work of supportive personnel.
    3. Insures that proper techniques are used in extemporaneous compounding.
    4. Provides for adequate record keeping and billing:
      a. Patient medication records
      b. Investigational drug records
      c. Outpatient billing
      d. Reports
      e. Prescription files
    5. Maintains professional competence.
    6. Insures that new personnel are properly trained in the policies and procedures of the ambulatory pharmacy.
    7. Coordinates the activities of the area with the available staff to make the best use of personnel and resources.
    8. Keeps the ambulatory pharmacy area neat and orderly at all times.
  B. Patient Care Area
    1. Inspects periodically the medication areas on the nursing unit to insure an adequate supply of stock drugs and their proper storage.
    2. Identifies drugs brought into the clinic by patients.
    3. Obtains patient medication histories and communicates pertinent information to the physician.
    4. Assists in drug product and entity selection.
    5. Assists the physician in selecting dosage regimens and schedules.
    6. Monitors the patients' total drug therapy for:
      a. Effectiveness
      b. Side effects
      c. Toxicities
      d. Allergic drug reactions
      e. Drug interactions
    7. Counsels patients on the proper use of their medication.
    8. Prepares medications for intravenous administration.
  C. General Responsibilities
    1. Provides drug information as necessary to pharmacy, medical, and nursing staffs.
    2. Coordinates overall pharmaceutical needs of the ambulatory service area.
    3. Provides adequate drug control:
      a. Insures that drugs are handled properly (eg investigational drug storage).
      b. Insures that all state and federal laws are followed.
    4. Maintains professional competence in area.
    5. Participates in cardiopulmonary emergencies by:
      a. Procurement and preparation of needed drugs
      b. Charting all medications given
      c. Performing cardiopulmonary resuscitation, if necessary
    6. Provides in-service education to:
      a. Pharmacists, pharmacy interns, residents and students
      b. Nurses and nursing students
      c. Physicians and medical students

In a small hospital with only one pharmacist it is a challenge to be knowledgeable in all these activities of hospital pharmacy. In a large hospital with a number of pharmacists who specialize in certain areas of practice each may become expert in one or more fields. The staffing pattern in hospital pharmacy varies, depending on the scope and quality of pharmaceutical service being offered. Some hospitals with less than 100 beds employ a pharmacist on a full-time basis. As the size of the hospital increases, so does the personnel in the pharmacy. For example, in a 300-bed progressive hospital the pharmacy may be staffed with a chief pharmacist, an assistant chief pharmacist, from five to ten staff pharmacists, four to eight nonpharmacists and a full-time department secretary. In the very large hospitals with several hundred beds, one may find the staffing pattern in the hospital pharmacy to consist of a director of pharmacy, an associate director, two or more assistant directors, one or more supervisor pharmacists, as many as 40 to 50 or more staff pharmacists, 10 to 16 pharmacy residents, and about as many nonpharmacist helpers, tech-

nicians, and secretarial personnel as professional personnel.

In order to schedule the workload of the department equitably and to insure that all the functions are carried out, various methods are devised, such as work distribution charts, job descriptions, policy and procedure manuals, and functional organizational charts. These and other management aids are utilized by the director of pharmacy in a large department to insure that all the services and functions are fulfilled adequately.

Facilities—There are great variations in the amount of floor space devoted to the pharmacy in hospitals of the same size and type. Such variations have a direct bearing on the scope of service which can be developed in the pharmacy. A helpful guide for planning hospital pharmacy facilities has been prepared through the cooperative efforts of the Public Health Service and the American Society of Hospital Pharmacists.

In the smaller hospital, with one pharmacist, only one room is usually required for the pharmacy, a combination of dispensing, manufacturing, administrative, and all other features of a complete pharmaceutical service. When sterile products are to be prepared, there should be a separate room or area for such work. An area of this type is required for reconstitution of lyophilized injections, for ophthalmic preparations, for packaging unit-dose injections into syringes, and for the preparation of intravenous admixtures, all of which must remain sterile.

Hospitals of 200 beds and larger provide the opportunity for departmentalization of pharmacy activities. There should be a separate area for inpatient services and unit-dose dispensing, outpatient service, an office for the chief pharmacist, a compounding, prepacking and labeling room, a storeroom, a sterile products and IV admixture room, a room or area for a departmental computer, a separate area for drug information services and space assigned on various nursing units for unit-dose, drug administration, and clinical pharmacy services.

As the hospital size advances to 500, 1000, or more beds, so, of course, will the space requirements of pharmaceutical service increase.

Pharmacy and Therapeutics Committee—The relationship between the community pharmacist and the physicians in the area is a direct person-to-person contact. There is a physician–pharmacist–patient relationship which is uncomplicated by organizational lines. On the other hand, the hospital pharmacist is responsible for maintaining proper relationships with from dozens to a few hundred physicians on the medical staff of one hospital. This is further complicated by the introduction of the nursing profession within the physician–pharmacist–patient relationship. Experience has shown that there is a need for a formal organizational line of communication and liaison between the medical staff and the pharmacy department of a hospital. This was recognized by the American College of Surgeons when it adopted the first Minimum Standard for Pharmacies in Hospitals in 1935. It is also recognized by the Joint Commission on Accreditation of Hospitals as an essential committee of the hospital's medical staff.

The American Society of Hospital Pharmacists has formulated and adopted a statement embodying the definition, purpose, organization, functions, and scope of a pharmacy and therapeutics committee in the hospital. This statement (Fig 95-2), is an effective guide in organizing such a committee within a given hospital.

It has been thought by many that the sole purpose of a pharmacy and therapeutics committee was to develop a formulary and operate a formulary system. It can be seen from the preceding statement that there are many important functions of this committee in addition to the formulary sys-

ASHP Statement on the Pharmacy and Therapeutics Committee

Preamble

The vast majority of hospital patients receive drugs as part of their care. Durg therapy often is the sole treatment modality. The potential and demonstrated benefits of drugs are enormous, as is their potential for harm. Because of the multiplicity of drugs available and the complexities surrounding their effective use, it is necessary that hospitals have an organized, sound program for maximizing rational drug use. The pharmacy and therapeutics committee, or its equivalent, is the organizational keystone of this program.

The Pharmacy and Therapeutics Committee

The pharmacy and therapeutics committee is an advisory group of the medical staff and serves as the organizational line of communication between the medical staff and pharmacy department. This committee is composed of physicians, pharmacists and other health professionals selected with the guidance of the medical staff. It is a policy-recommending body to the medical staff and the administration of the hospital on matters related to the therapeutic use of drugs.

(1) *Purposes.* The primary purposes of the pharmacy and therapeutics committee are:

A. Advisory

The committee recommends the adoption of, or assists in the formulation of, broad professional policies regarding evaluation, selection and therapeutic use of drugs in hospitals.

B. Educational

The committee recommends or assists in the formulation of programs designed to meet the needs of the professional staff (physicians, nurses, pharmacists and other health care practitioners) for complete current knowledge on matters related to drugs and drug use.

Approved by the ASHP House of Delegates, June 7, 1983. Approved by the ASHP Board of Directors, November 18, 1982. Developed by the ASHP Council on Clinical Affairs. Supersedes the "ASHP Statement of Guiding Principles on the Operation of the Hospital Formulary System" approved by the Board of Directors, January 10, 1964. This former ASHP statement had the endorsement of the American Hospital Association, the American Medical Association, and the American Pharmaceutical Association.

(2) *Organization and Operation.* While the composition and operation of the pharmacy and therapeutics committee might vary from hospital to hospital, the following generally will apply:

A. The pharmacy and therapeutics committee should be composed of at least three physicians, a pharmacist and a representative of the nursing staff. Committee members are appointed by a governing unit or elected official of the organized medical staff. The hospital administrator or his/her designee should be an ex officio member of the committee.

B. A chairman from among the physician representatives should be appointed. A pharmacist usually is designated as secretary.

C. The committee should meet regularly, at least six times per year, and when necessary.

D. The committee should invite to its meetings persons within or outside the hospital who can contribute specialized or unique knowledge, skills and judgments.

E. An agenda and supplementary materials (including minutes of the previous meeting) should be prepared by the secretary and submitted to the committee members in sufficient time before the meeting for them to properly review the material.

F. Minutes of the committee meetings should be prepared by the secretary and maintained in the permanent records of the hospital.

G. Recommendations of the committee shall be presented to the medical staff or its appropriate committee for adoption or recommendation.

H. Liaison with other hospital committees concerned with drug use (e.g., infection control, medical audit) shall be maintained.

(3) *Functions and Scope.* The basic organization of the hospital and medical staffs will determine the functions and scope of the pharmacy and therapeutics committee. The following list of committee functions is offered as a guide:

A. To serve in an advisory capacity to the medical staff and hospital administration in all matters pertaining to the use of drugs (including investigational drugs).

B. To develop a formulary of drugs accepted for use in the hospital and provide for its constant revision. The selection of items to be included in the formulary will be based on objective evaluation of their therapeutic merits, safety and cost. The committee should minimize duplication of the same basic drug type, drug entity or drug product.

C. To establish or plan suitable educational programs for the hospital's professional staff on matters related to drug use.

D. To study problems related to the distribution and administration of medications, including medication incidents.

E. To review adverse drug reactions occurring in the hospital.

F. To initiate and/or direct drug use review programs and studies, and review the results of such activities.

G. To advise the pharmacy in the implementation of effective drug distribution and control procedures.

H. To make recommendations concerning drugs to be stocked in hospital patient care areas.

Fig 95-2.

---

tem. A hospital's medical staff could have an effective pharmacy and therapeutics committee without having a formulary system. On the other hand, a hospital could not properly operate a formulary system without a pharmacy and therapeutics committee, unless the medical staff served as a "committee of the whole."

During recent years, with the development of the clinical pharmacy movement, a number of clinical pharmacists on the staff of some departments have developed expertise in specific therapeutic specialty areas. Therefore, it was a logical development that a subcommittee structure could be developed under the Pharmacy and Therapeutics Committee. For example, a cardiologist and a renologist along with a clinical pharmacist who specialized in cardiorenal pharmacology and therapeutics could provide the appropriate expertise to the Pharmacy and Therapeutics Committee in this area of drug therapy. The organizational chart on the Pharmacy and Therapeutics Committee in Fig 95-3 illustrates a more ef-

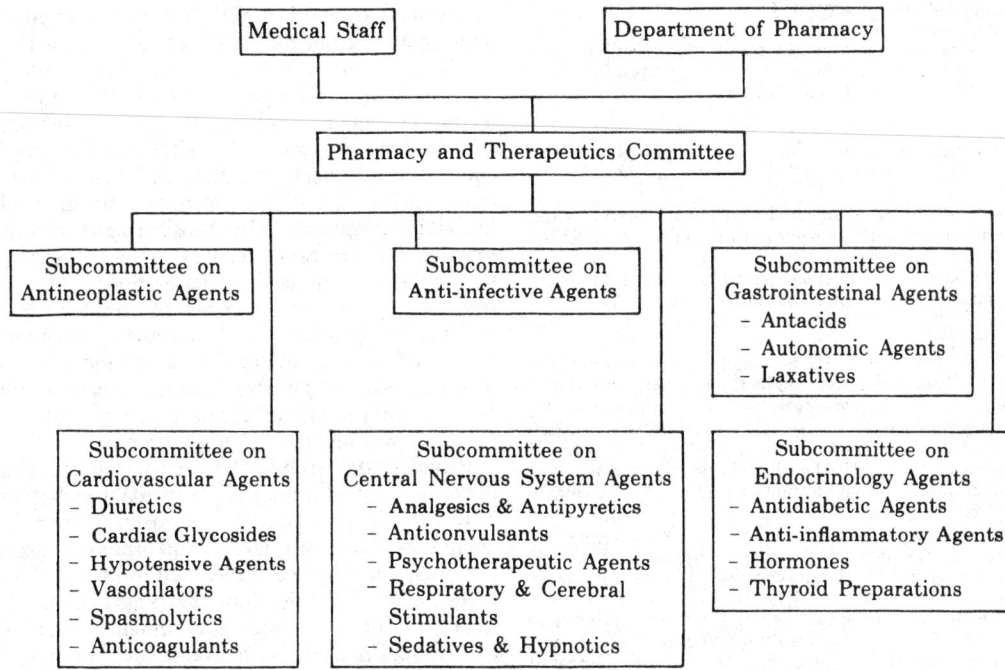

Fig 95-3.   Organization of a Pharmacy and Therapeutics Committee.

fective approach for the medical staff and the pharmacy staff to develop and implement a rational drug therapy program, a subcommittee structure of specialists in defined areas of therapeutics.

In addition, such a structure provides a mechanism for the development of a prospective, on-going, and also a retrospective, drug utilization review program in the hospital.

As hospitals enter the era of cost containment and prospective payment systems, the Pharmacy and Therapeutics Committee assumes added responsibility to promote rational and cost effective drug therapy and procedures. Both the clinical pharmacist and the drug information pharmacist play an ever-increasing role in committee recommendations.

Formulary System—The formulary system and formularies have existed in the United States since the days of the American Revolution; they existed in European hospitals for centuries prior to this. The need for hospital formularies becomes increasingly great because of (1) the increasing number of new drugs being marketed, (2) the increasing influence of biased advertising and unscientific "scientific" drug literature, (3) the increasing complexity of untoward effects of the newer more potent drugs, (4) the highly competitive marketing practices of the pharmaceutical industry and (5) the public's interest in seeing that the health professions are conscientiously providing the best possible care at the lowest possible cost. This is substantiated by the fact that the federal government requires the establishment of Professional Standards Review Organizations (PSROs) whose purpose it is to monitor and control the quality of services rendered to patients. Cost control is also being emphasized by the federal Maximum Allowable Cost (MAC) programs for patients on federally funded programs.

The formulary system—because it has attempted to outline the scientific data on a drug, including its toxicities, untoward side effects, and beneficial effects—has been a controversial method of appraising drug therapy. While the pharmaceutical industry promotes the virtues of a trade-named drug, the formulary system evaluates the virtues and defects of that drug in comparison to other trade-named brands of the same basic drug. While the pharmaceutical industry has sometimes maintained that the formulary system is detrimental to the free enterprise system, the proponents of the formulary

system maintain that it challenges the individual pharmaceutical manufacturers to meet the competition which is the basis of the free enterprise system.

In order to outline precisely what the formulary system is and is not, a *Statement on the Formulary System* was developed and approved by American Society of Hospital Pharmacists. This Statement differentiates between the formulary system and the hospital formulary, and lists a number of guiding principles designed to help physicians, pharmacists, and administrators to operate a hospital formulary system.

ASHP Statement on the Formulary System

Preamble

The care of patients in hospitals and other health-care facilities is often dependent upon the effective use of drugs. The multiplicity of drugs available makes it mandatory that a sound program of drug usage be developed within the institution to ensure that patients receive the best possible care.

In the interest of better patient care, the institution should have a program of objective evaluation, selection, and use of medicinal agents in the facility. This program is the basis of appropriate, economical drug therapy. The formulary concept[a] is a method for providing such a program and has been utilized as such for many years.

To be effective, the formulary system must have the approval of the organized medical staff, the concurrence of individual staff members, and the functioning of a properly organized pharmacy and therapeutics committee[b] of the medical staff. The basic policies and procedures governing the formulary system should be incorporated in the medical staff bylaws, or in the medical staff rules and regulations.

The pharmacy and therapeutics committee represents the official organizational line of communication and liaison between the medical and pharmacy staffs. The committee is responsible to the medical staff as a whole, and its recommendations are subject to approval by the organized medical staff, as well as to the normal administrative approval process.

This committee assists in the formulation of broad professional policies relating to drugs in institutions, including their evaluation or appraisal, selection, procurement, storage, distribution, and safe use.

Definition of Formulary and Formulary System

The *formulary* is a continually revised compilation of pharmaceuticals (plus important ancillary information) that reflects the current clinical judgment of the medical staff.[c]

The *formulary system* is a method whereby the medical staff of an institution, working through the pharmacy and therapeutics committee, evaluates, appraises, and selects from among the numerous available drug entities and drug products those that are considered most useful in patient care. Only those so selected are routinely available from the pharmacy.

The formulary system is thus an important tool for assuring the quality of drug use and controlling its cost.

The formulary system provides for the procuring, prescribing, dispensing, and administering of drugs under either their nonproprietary or proprietary names in instances where drugs have both names.

Guiding Principles

The following principles will serve as a guide to physicians, pharmacists, nurses, and administrators in hospitals and other facilities utilizing the formulary system:

1. The medical staff shall appoint a multidisciplinary pharmacy and therapeutics committee and outline its purposes, organization, function, and scope.

2. The formulary system shall be sponsored by the medical staff based upon the recommendations of the pharmacy and therapeutics committee. The medical staff should adapt the principles of the system to the needs of the particular institution.

3. The medical staff shall adopt written policies and procedures governing the formulary system as developed by the pharmacy and therapeutics committee. Action of the medical staff is subject to the normal administrative approval process. These policies and procedures shall afford guidance in the evaluation or appraisal, selection, procurement, storage, distribution, safe use, and other matters relating to drugs, and shall be published in the institution's formulary or other media available to all members of the medical staff.

4. Drugs should be included in the formulary by their nonproprietary names, even though proprietary names may be in common use in the institution. Prescribers should be strongly encouraged to prescribe drugs by their nonproprietary names.

5. Limiting the number of drug entities and drug products routinely available from the pharmacy can produce substantial patient care and (particularly) financial benefits. These benefits are greatly increased through the use of *generic equivalents* (drug products considered to be identical with respect to their active components; eg, two brands of tetracycline hydrochloride capsules) and *therapeutic equivalents* (drug products differing in composition or in their basic drug entity that are considered to have very similar pharmacologic and therapeutic activities; eg, two different antacid products or two different alkylamine antihistamines.) The pharmacy and therapeutics committee must set forth policies and procedures governing the dispensing of generics and therapeutic equivalents. These policies and procedures should include the following points:

- That the pharmacist is responsible for selecting, from available generic equivalents, those to be dispensed pursuant to a physician's order for a particular drug product.

- That the prescriber has the option, at the time of prescribing, to specify the brand or supplier of drug to be dispensed for that particular medication order/prescription. The prescriber's decision should be based on pharmacologic or therapeutic considerations (or both) relative to that patient.

- That the pharmacy and therapeutics committee is responsible for determining those drug products and entities (if any) that shall be considered therapeutic equivalents. The conditions and procedures for dispensing a therapeutic alternative in place of the prescribed drug shall be clearly delineated.

6. The institution shall make certain that its medical and nursing staffs are informed about the existence of the formulary system, the procedures governing its operation, and any changes in those procedures. Copies of the formulary must be readily available and accessible at all times.

7. Provision shall be made for the appraisal and use of drugs not included in the formulary, by the medical staff.

8. The pharmacist shall be responsible for specifications as to the quality, quantity, and source of supply of all drugs, chemicals, biologicals, and pharmaceutical preparations used in the diagnosis and treatment of patients. When applicable, such products should meet the standards of the *United States Pharmacopeia*.

Recommendation

A formulary system, based upon these guiding principles, is important in drug therapy in institutions. In the interest of better and more economical patient care, its adoption by medical staffs is strongly recommended.

---

[a] The formulary system is adaptable for use in any type of health-care facility and is not limited to hospitals.

[b] For additional information, see the ASHP Statement on the Pharmacy and Therapeutics Committee, *Am J Hosp Pharm.* 1978; 35:813–4.

[c] For additional information, see the ASHP Guidelines for Hospital Formularies, *Am J Hosp Pharm.* 1978; 35:326–8.

Hospital pharmacists have viewed the hospital formulary system as a means for the pharmacist to assume professional responsibilities in drug-product selection. Essentially, the formulary system provided a mechanism to avoid brand duplication, therapeutic duplication, as well as promote rational drug therapy prior to the passage of the new laws.

Many useful reference sources are available to assist Pharmacy and Therapeutics Committees to develop an effective, ongoing rational drug therapy program and formulary system in the hospital. The knowledgeable drug information specialist and the clinical pharmacist can utilize these reference sources effectively to encourage the medical staff of the individual hospital to select those drugs its members consider most effective therapeutically, together with the preparations in which they may be administered most effectively. Such reference sources are described in Chapter 103.

An active Pharmacy and Therapeutics Committee with a well-developed formulary system provides assurance that the medical staff, the pharmacy staff, and the administration of the hospital have taken the necessary steps to assure the patient of a rational drug therapy program.

Purchasing—While the pharmacist may be the actual buyer in a small hospital, the principal function in purchasing is to establish standards and specifications for all drugs, chemicals, diagnostic agents, and other preparations used in patients, and pharmaceutical equipment. The pharmacist is responsible for the quality of drugs dispensed to patients. Especially in the average governmental hospital, the pharmacist does not purchase directly but through a purchasing agent, the hospital's purchase and supply officer. The pharmacist must be prepared to reject purchases not meeting standards acceptable to the pharmacist. The Pharmacy and Therapeutics Committee serves as a potent force in helping the pharmacist to set up adequate specifications for the purchase of quality pharmaceuticals.

Increasing numbers of pharmacists are formalizing standards for purchasing. Such standards are especially necessary in governmental institutions where often the purchasing is not accomplished on the premises but by a central purchasing agent for the state or other governmental agency.

In order to assist practicing pharmacists to properly select drug products, the American Pharmaceutical Association's Academy of Pharmaceutical Sciences in 1969 adopted a *Statement on Drug Product Quality*. This statement was endorsed by the House of Delegates of the American Pharmaceutical Association.[8] Quantity buying is often advantageous from a price or availability standpoint. Before making large purchases, however, the pharmacist should determine the stability of the items and consider the possibility of a change in policy that might render their use obsolete. Many persons feel that a turnover of stock of four to eight times annually is desirable. Turnover, reduction in purchase cost, and storage space must be considered in determining the advisability of large purchases of a drug.

The use of competitive bidding is considered good practice where a drug is used in large amounts and where future continued use seems certain. A quotation request is directed to appropriate manufacturers and the company with the lowest price and yet with standard quality usually receives the order for the material, after which the purchase order is prepared.

Many hospitals have adopted the practice of preparing estimates of drug usage for a given period. Thus, manufacturers are requested to submit their bid quotations on the total quantity of drugs to be used for a 1-year period; or in the case of intravenous solutions, even a 2-year period. The stipulation is that the hospital has the option to determine when and how much will be shipped at any time during the 1- or 2-year period.

Upon review of these bids, the hospital pharmacist determines which vendor will receive the contract and a purchase order is sent to the respective manufacturers. Thus, by issuing an annual purchase order to each of the major pharmaceutical manufacturers, the hospital pharmacist eliminates

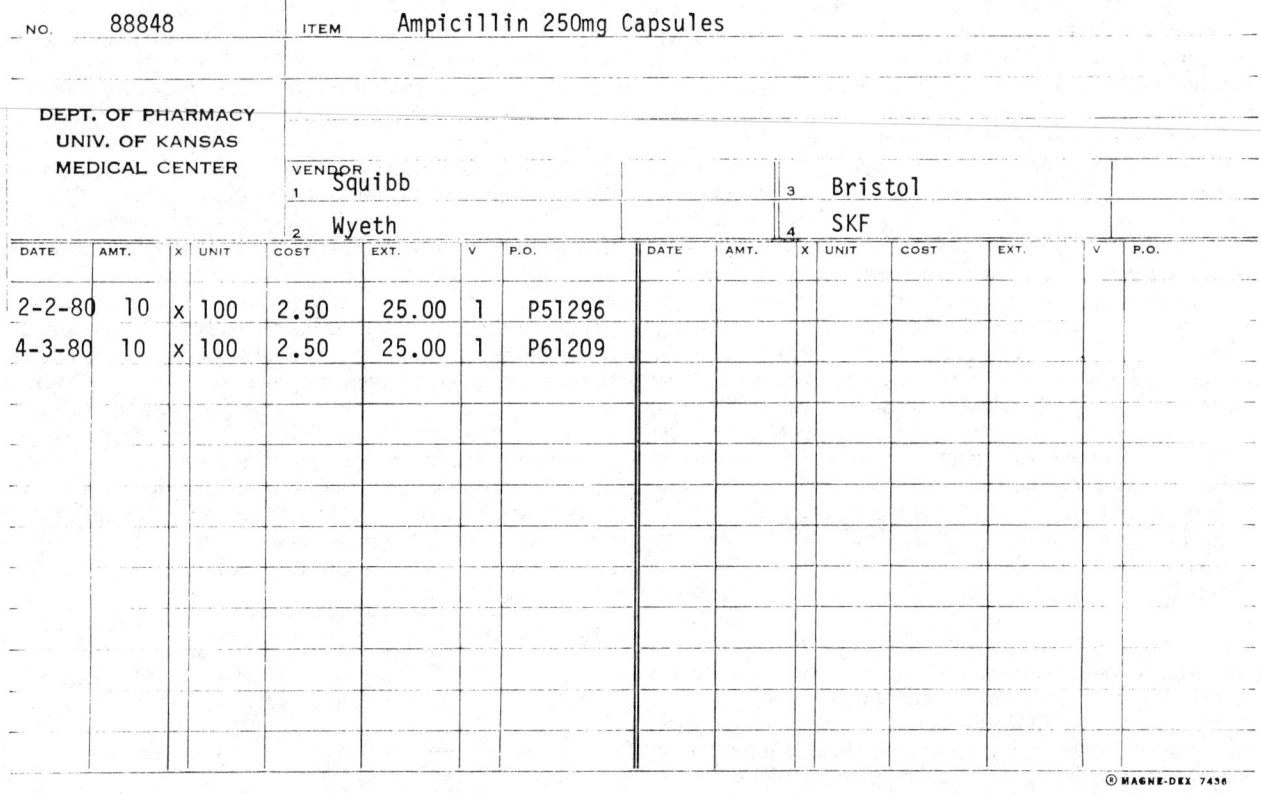

| NO. | 88848 | | ITEM | Ampicillin 250mg Capsules | | | | | | | | | | | | | |

DEPT. OF PHARMACY
UNIV. OF KANSAS
MEDICAL CENTER

VENDOR
1 Squibb   3 Bristol
2 Wyeth   4 SKF

DATE	AMT.	X	UNIT	COST	EXT.	V	P.O.	DATE	AMT.	X	UNIT	COST	EXT.	V	P.O.
2-2-80	10	x	100	2.50	25.00	1	P51296								
4-3-80	10	x	100	2.50	25.00	1	P61209								

® MAGNE-DEX 7456

Fig 95-4.   Purchase record card.

significant amounts of paper work and unnecessary frequent bidding.

Purchase Record—It is desirable that a purchase record be maintained for all items purchased routinely. Each purchase record card should include specifications for the item. With such information at hand, one is at a distinct advantage in obtaining duplicate material on successive purchases.

The purchase record card (Fig 95-4) provides a record of the quantity used over a period of time, a control, and simplification of purchasing procedures. This information is of particular value when the pharmacist is faced with a rising market, as it gives a fairly accurate picture of the immediate future needs and enables purchasing at current prices without overstocking. In addition, such a record furnishes the information necessary so that one purchases only enough of an item for a predetermined time. The purchase record card provides information on quantities purchased in previous months, quarters, or years, and is required for efficient purchasing, whether by contract or otherwise.

Annual inventories should be taken as a check on the theoretical inventory record maintained by either pharmacy or accounting. Various procedures are used to take a drug inventory. Many hospitals are using electronic data processing in inventory value determinations.

In many hospitals it has been observed that proprietary duplications abound and clutter the shelves, increasing inventory and decreasing turnover rate and efficiency. The pharmacist should review such inventory periodically and return outmoded and outdated drugs to the manufacturer for credit. In addition, he should bring this matter to the attention of the Pharmacy and Therapeutics Committee since one of its responsibilities is to delete outmoded drugs from the approved inventory.

The concern for cost containment, better inventory turnover rates, and improved cash flow, has prompted the development of the prime vendor system. In this system contracts for all pharmaceuticals are processed through a local whole-saler. Efficiency is increased with this system yet bid contracts can still be utilized.

Drug Distribution Systems—The organizational structure of the hospital has placed certain constraints on the manner in which hospitalized patients receive their drugs. These constraints revolve around professional prerogatives and traditions, as well as legal responsibilities, established for medicine, nursing, pharmacy, and hospital administration.

Physicians prescribe, pharmacists dispense, and, usually, nurses administer drugs. However, in order to have this simple tripartite order executed, many things must take place. The overall drug distribution and utilization process in the hospital involves an infinite number of procedures, personnel, departments, equipment, and storage. As an illustration, trace the history of a drug from procurement to administration to the patient.

Before a drug can be purchased, specifications must be prepared. This is usually done through the medical staff and the pharmacist by means of a Pharmacy and Therapeutics Committee. Requisitions outlining the specifications for the drugs selected are prepared and processed in the pharmacy and forwarded to the purchasing department for procurement. Drug shipments are received by the receiving department and distributed to the pharmacy. Pharmacy checks these shipments and stores them for future use. Inventory control procedures must be set up. In the meantime, invoicing for payment must be processed through the accounting department through a coordination of efforts among pharmacy, purchasing, receiving, and business offices.

Physicians must prescribe drugs before they can be administered. Nurses must carry out these medication orders and obtain the necessary drugs from the pharmacy. In the pharmacy the drugs are transferred from the storage area to the dispensing area. There they may have to be prepackaged (for future use), may have to be compounded or manufactured and assay and control procedures performed, must be packaged in proper quantities for use by the nurse to administer to the patient, labeled properly, checked for accuracy, and distributed to the nursing unit. At the nursing unit the drugs are stored again for continuous use by the patient according to physicians' orders. The nurse prepares the drug for administration, brings it to the patient, returns to the nursing unit, and records this information on the patient's record.

In the meantime the pharmacy processes these drug orders for billing purposes and sends these charges to the business office. There, they are posted to the patient's account. Then, through coordination between pharmacy and accounting, data are accumulated on the cost of drugs issued, reduction of drug inventory and income received to offset expenses incurred.

While the mechanics of this operation are taking place, other activities must be completed. Problems must be resolved in the procurement phase regarding overshipments or undershipments or other shipping errors; errors in billing may have to be rectified. Outdated or deteriorated drugs may have to be returned to the manufacturer. Further information may be required from the physician or nurse before the prescription can be filled; that is, information as to dosage, toxicity, and side effects. Perhaps the staff physician may cancel the resident's medication order and the nurse must return the drug to the pharmacy for credit. Thus, the cycle starts all over again!

How many people are involved in the medication cycle of one drug from the time of its specification to the time it reaches the patient? They include the pharmacist and five or more physicians on the pharmacy and therapeutics committee in preparing drug specification; the pharmacist in selecting the drug to be ordered; the pharmacy secretary in making out the requisition; the purchasing agent in ordering the drug; the receiving clerk in accepting shipment; the delivery clerk from receiving to pharmacy; the pharmacy stock clerk in checking and storing the drug; the physician in prescribing the drug; the nurse in ordering the drug; the pharmacist in preparing and dispensing the drug; the pharmacy delivery clerk in transporting the drug to the nursing unit; the nursing unit clerk in storing the drug; the nurse in preparing and administering the drug and in charting the data; the pharmacy clerk in recording the charge and sending it to the business office; the account clerk in the receiving and processing of the invoices; the business officer in preparing the check for payment; the posting clerk in posting the charge to the patient's bill; the credit manager in collecting the bill. There must be over 20 people involved in some manner or other with one drug order! One can see why the drug distribution system within a hospital is so complex.

Medication is administered to a hospital patient only upon the written order of a physician. Thus, a prescription order originates in the patient's medical record, where the physician writes out all the orders (prescriptions) he wants carried out on or for the patient. Since the patient's medical record remains at the nursing unit, it is essential that some means be utilized to transmit the prescription order from the nursing unit to the pharmacy. These orders are transmitted to the pharmacy usually in one of four ways: (1) the physician writes the medication order on a separate blank, (2) the medical record has a duplicate copy so that the pharmacy can obtain a carbon copy of the physician's original medication order, (3) the physician's order is transcribed by nursing personnel onto an inpatient prescription or requisition form or (4) the order is transmitted to the pharmacy by the physician inputing the order into a computer terminal. Most hospitals use procedures whereby the pharmacist obtains a direct copy of the physician's medication orders. The transcription method is no longer recognized as an acceptable practice.

Types of Drug Distribution Systems—The pharmacy department makes drugs available at the nursing unit for patient use usually in one of five ways: (1) individual prescription medication for each patient, (2) a complete floor stock system, (3) a combination of numbers 1 and 2, (4) unit-dose dispensing either centralized in the pharmacy or decentralized at the nursing unit level, and (5) a pharmacy-coordinated unit-dose dispensing and drug-administration system. Systems No 1, 2, and 3 are considered poor drug control methods in comparison to No 4 and 5. However, until all hospitals adopt these unit-dose concepts, pharmacists often must operate under these less desirable systems.

Individual patient medications are compounded and dispensed in the usual manner except that the name and strength of the drug are included on the label. In hospital practice all medications are kept in a nursing unit medication cabinet and are under the custody of the nurse in charge. She or her assistant is responsible for administering the appropriate medication to each patient on the nursing unit. Thus it is important for her to know what drug she is administering for it is her professional responsibility to observe the patient for untoward reactions and to report this to the patient's physician. Thus the patient never sees the prescription container dispensed by the pharmacist to the nursing unit nor has the container in his or her possession. A typical inpatient prescription label would contain the following information:

Mr. John Jones		Room 608E
	Tetracycline HCl Capsules, 250 mg	
Quantity #20	Lot #	Exp Date
Doctor's	Pharmacist's	Date
Name	Name	

THE GENERAL HOSPITAL PHARMACY

In order to expedite the dispensing of inpatient prescription medication hospital pharmacists have adopted the practice of prepackaging frequently used drugs in standard dispensing quantities. It is not unusual for a majority of the inpatient prescription medications to be prepackaged. Prepackaging drugs requires accurate procedures, controls, and records in order to trace the identity of the drug at all times. Thus a prepackaging control record form is utilized for documentation of manufacturer's control numbers, expiration date, pharmacy control number which appears on each prepackaged container label, and the pharmacist responsible for the prepackaging operation. In the case of a drug recalled by a manufacturer, the pharmacist can easily trace prepackaged quantities of the drug in question.

Drugs dispensed under a *floor-stock system* are of two classes: free and charge. Free floor stock consists of a predetermined list of medications which are available on every nursing unit of the hospital for use at no specific charge to the patient. Since these drugs are used in large quantities they are prepackaged in standardized containers. Orders are usually received from each nursing unit of the hospital each day of the week. In other hospitals the pharmacy assumes the responsibility for maintaining the proper inventory of free floor stock drugs on each nursing unit through an automatic floor stock replacement system. Under such a system the nurse is relieved of having to maintain an inventory control system, fill out a daily requisition order, and return the drug basket items to the shelves. The pharmacy personnel goes to the nursing unit with an adequate supply of each free floor-stock drug, takes an on-the-spot inventory, brings the inventory to a predetermined level, and records the quantities on a preprinted requisition which lists the drugs in the order in which they are stocked in the drug cabinets. Adequate controls thus can be set up on the basis of usage in relation to number of patient days per given interval of time. Some hospitals have adopted electronic data processing procedures to handle the totaling and cost extension of drugs issued and the preparation of monthly drug usage reports for each nursing unit.

Charge floor stock is medication available at each nursing unit of the hospital and for which a charge is made to the patient. Certain medications are required to be used almost immediately after the physician prescribes them, and it is not practical to go to the pharmacy to obtain them in each instance, yet the cost and the volume of usage necessitates a charge to the patient. Such medications are usually injections or other single-dose forms. A common method of handling charge floor-stock drugs is to attach a small removable label or prestamped pharmacy requisition form bearing the name of the drug to the charge floor-stock drug. When the nurse needs the drug she merely removes the label and affixes it to the usual inpatient prescription or requisition slip. This is then used for charging purposes and for replacement of the drug on the nursing unit.

In hospitals where patients pay for their hospitalization—as compared to military or governmental hospitals—the pharmacy often employs a *combination of the individual inpatient prescription system and the floor-stock drug system.* Drugs which are free floor stock are charged against the nursing service and, in the final analysis, the patient does pay for the drugs since the cost is included as a part of the nursing service portion of the daily room and board rate.

Because of the large number and variety of drugs stored on nursing units—including individual patient prescriptions, free and charge floor stock, narcotics and other controlled drugs, investigational drugs, and emergency drug tray—it is an important responsibility of the pharmacist to inspect these drugs routinely. Proper storage conditions must be adhered to, dated drugs must be checked, narcotic drugs must be safeguarded, and discontinued drugs must be removed from the nursing unit. To insure proper control of a nursing station drug cabinet, the pharmacist prepares a written report to the directors of nursing and of pharmacy. The condition of a nursing unit medication station may warrant remedial attention by personnel from both departments. In some hospitals, the pharmacists are assigned to specific nursing units to coordinate all the drug and drug therapy problems at the nursing unit level. Rather than simply checking drug storage conditions, they are developing new roles which brings them closer to the patient-care team.[9]

A newer trend for dispensing drugs to hospitalized patients, and the most accepted method, is called *unit-dose dispensing.* In this system the pharmacist prepares every dose of medication ready for administration, rather than issuing containers of drugs to nursing units where the nurse must prepare the drug for administration. For example, tablets and capsules are labeled for each patient, liquids are premeasured, lyophilized injections are diluted and accurately measured into sterile syringes, parenteral drug admixtures are added to intravenous solutions prior to use, and oral powders and other unusual dosage forms are measured and mixed appropriately. Most of these procedures involve pharmaceutical techniques which are properly the pharmacist's responsibility. Hospital pharmacists are studying various methods involving centralized pharmacy versus decentralized pharmacies on the nursing units, using automated systems of communication, information scheduling, and retrieval to provide more accurate and effective overall drug distribution and utilization in the hospital.

The unit-dose dispensing concept has changed many of the traditional functions of the hospital pharmacist. For example, the traditional prepackaging system of multiple doses of drugs has been changed to include the use of tablet and capsule strip-packaging and labeling machines and liquid unit-dose packaging equipment. This is necessary since all drugs are not available from the industry in unit-dose packages. The traditional individual inpatient prescription is also eliminated and thereby eliminates prescription label typing. Thus, the unit-dose-dispensing operation enhances the need

for pharmacy technicians to assist in the procedural aspects of this function. Free and charge floor-stock drug activities are essentially eliminated.

Unit-dose dispensing lends itself to certain automation procedures, particularly with electronic data processing and computers. On-line computers are used to program patients' total drug-therapy profile, program the times for administering scheduled doses of drugs, maintain records of drugs administered and initiate the drug charges to patients. This eliminates the traditional nurses' drug Kardex (profile), medication ticket, and record-of-drug-administered-manual-system of keeping track of patients' drug-therapy profiles. Thus, the hourly reports of the on-line computer on patients drug-therapy profiles can be used both by the pharmacy for unit-dose dispensing and by the nurse for drug administration.

There is a developing trend to consider merging drug dispensing and drug administration into a *coordinated system under pharmacy control.* This makes sense particularly when one considers the fact that when a physician writes a medication order for a hospitalized patient, it is essentially a pharmaceutical order and pharmaceutical orders should be carried out under the supervision of pharmacists. This system was initiated at the Providence Hospital in Seattle.[9] Registered nurses have been employed by the Pharmacy Department and in conjunction with a unit-dose dispensing system by the pharmacists and technicians, nurses are responsible for administering all the drugs to hospitalized patients. Thus, such a coordinated system effects certain efficiencies and eliminates many steps from the traditional drug distribution and utilization system.

A pharmacy-coordinated unit-dose dispensing and drug-administration system was initiated at the Ohio State University Hospitals in 1969.[10] This system differs from the Providence Hospital program in that pharmacy technicians have been trained to administer the drugs instead of registered nurses. These pharmacy technicians assist in the unit-dose dispensing phase as well as the drug-administration phase of the coordinated system which is directly controlled and supervised by registered pharmacists. Thus, pharmacists work directly with physicians on the nursing unit to carry out pharmacy's mainstream function of the safe and appropriate use of drugs in patients.

A pharmacy-coordinated unit-dose dispensing and drug administration system requires a complex series of well-integrated procedures in order to administer drugs to patients safely and accurately. A number of studies have shown that uncoordinated drug distribution systems have a high incidence of medication errors. A two-phase comprehensive study of the pharmacy-coordinated unit-dose dispensing and drug administration system showed that it reduced significantly the incidence of medication errors in comparison with the other drug distribution systems in existence.[11]

For effective and efficient functioning, a unit-dose dispensing and drug administration system should include a *procedural manual* which outlines the stepwise procedures for implementing the myriad tasks and the in-process quality control checks required for the safe and accurate handling of drugs in the institutional setting in which the system is used.

The Unit-Dose Drug Distribution System is rapidly becoming the standard of practice in hospitals. The General Accounting Office (GAO) studied several distribution systems in its *Study of Health-Care Facilities Construction Costs* (December, 1972), and reported that in addition to safer and better patient care through minimization of medication errors the unit-dose system was to be recommended also because of its favorable life-cycle cost-to-benefit ratio. The Joint Commission on Accreditation of Hospitals also recommends the unit-dose distribution system. Indeed the unit dose system of drug distribution has become the standard of practice in hospital pharmacy.

Patient Self-Administration of Drugs in Hospitals— Pharmacists generally have considered a unit-dose dispensing system as a panacea for hospital drug problems. However, unit-dose dispensing systems have been primarily "pharmacy-centered" rather than "patient-centered." The new direction in hospital pharmacy is to develop patient-oriented services as the focal point in drug distribution systems.

The self-administration of drugs by patients in the hospital offers many advantages. It allows the patient to assume more responsibility for his direct care and allows him to learn how to use drugs properly, and to be able to anticipate potential side effects and other drug-created problems. It provides a salient opportunity for the pharmacist to help educate patients on the safe and proper use of drugs and thereby alleviates much time spent by nurses and physicians in this essential pharmaceutical function.

Self-administration of drugs by patients can be effectively implemented on numerous hospital services, such as obstetrics, surgery, medicine, physical medicine and rehabilitation and even in psychiatry.[12,13] Again, a procedural manual should be prepared which outlines the methods used to implement a patient self-administration program as part of a unit-dose distribution system. A self-administration medication program gives the patient possession of his medication and makes the patient responsible for its administration. Both the nurse and pharmacist will make rounds to insure that the patient is using his medication properly.

The self-administration medication program enables the nurse to better utilize her time. The patient should become more knowledgeable about his medication, thus enhancing proper and safe use of drugs during hospitalization and after discharge.

A nurse-administered medication program places all responsibility for medication administration on the nurse providing the service. This program is used for patients who are not capable of self-administering their medications or for those medications which the patient cannot administer to himself. This is the interacting role which hospital pharmacists have developed under the umbrella term, "clinical pharmacy."

As the pharmaceutical industry develops the unit-dose-packaging concept and as physicians and the Food and Drug Administration continue their drive to provide patients with drugs labeled with the name of the medication in the original manufacturer's package (to insure stability and identity) this will virtually eliminate the count-and-pour and labeling operations in "filling prescriptions." It substantiates the need to use technicians in the physical handling of drugs. It is obvious that this main purpose of the pharmacist must change if he wants to remain a health professional.

There is, however, a challenging professional role which the pharmacist can assume as a member of the health-care team. This role involves the safe and appropriate use of drugs in patients. Taken in a broad context, this implies a high-level role indeed. This is the mainstream purpose for the existence of pharmacy as a health profession. Thus, the concept behind the clinical pharmacy movement is directed toward the development of this role as the mainstream function of the profession.

Investigational Drugs—The hospital pharmacist is in a strategic position to participate in an evaluation program on investigational drugs because such drugs must be tried in a hospital setting where the necessary laboratory and other medical facilities are available. It is thus a prime responsibility of the pharmacy and therapeutics committee to establish policies and procedures relative to the handling and control of investigational drugs in the hospital. To assist pharmacy and therapeutics committees the American Society

of Hospital Pharmacists developed a statement, entitled *ASHP Guidelines for the Use of Investigational Drugs in Institutions*, embodying basic principles applicable to the safe handling of investigational drugs in the hospital. The ASHP has also provided a manual dealing with pharmacists' responsibilities and opportunities in handling investigational drugs.

There are many problems associated with the use of investigational drugs in the hospital, some of which are:

1. Legal problems may result if a hospital does not exercise due care in the proper handling of investigational drugs in the overall care of the patient.
2. Nurses, as agents of the hospital, are usually responsible for administering investigational drugs to patients. In performing this act it is essential that sufficient information on the proper dosage, route of administration, possible toxic reactions and side effects, precautions, and proper labeling be available to them.
3. Investigational drugs, as they are made available from the manufacturer to the principal investigator, are not labeled sufficiently in many instances to prevent the possibility of error in their administration to patients.
4. Because investigational drugs fall in the area of research in contrast to accepted methods of treatment there are legal implications revolving around the need for written consent by patients.
5. In the case of double-blind studies it is essential that the person holding the code be readily available 24 hours a day, seven days a week, in case the patient's condition warrants a breaking of the code.
6. The legal requirements for proper records on the use of investigational drugs have been delineated by the Food and Drug Administration. In case of a recall because of severe permanent toxicity resulting from an investigational drug, it is essential that records of its use on specific patients in a hospital be readily available. In cases where the lot number of the drug is a significant factor such records should also be available.
7. In cases where investigational drugs are used on outpatients it is essential that such drugs be labeled to conform to legal requirements, such as child-proof packaging requirements and controlled substances requirements. It should be obvious that information must be readily available to assist physicians in other hospitals who may be required to treat patients suffering from accidental overdosage or toxic symptoms.
8. It is essential that the supply of an investigational drug be available during the night and weekends as well as when the principal investigator is at the hospital if nurses are to maintain uninterrupted dosage schedules in the best interest of the patient.

Thus the problems associated with the proper handling of investigational drugs provide ample justification to warrant the establishment of sound policies and procedures governing their use in the hospital. This is a responsibility of the medical staff. The pharmacy and therapeutics committee is a committee of the medical staff and, therefore, it should be the responsibility of this committee to formulate policies and procedures relative to the handling of investigational drugs. The hospital pharmacist as a key member of the pharmacy and therapeutics committee makes a real contribution to better patient care and safety by participating in formulating policies and procedures for handling investigational drugs in the hospital.

It is a common practice for physicians to obtain written consent from the patient prior to use of an investigational drug. A typical form for obtaining patient consent for such special therapy is shown in Fig 95-5.

When the hospital pharmacist is called upon to handle an investigational drug he needs to maintain adequate dispensing records. A typical form which provides the controls necessary for the handling of investigational drugs by the pharmacy is shown in Fig 95-6.

Many hospital pharmacists are involved clinically with oncology-team members in patient monitoring, drug preparation, and drug administration of investigational drugs. Patient consent and patient information are essential in such activity. Pharmacists often provide specific drug information cards to patients so that they may better understand their drug regimen and the various side effects or problems to expect. An example of such a drug information card is shown in Fig 95-7.

A single prescription for a single patient does not raise the

Form 65.4

THE OHIO STATE UNIVERSITY
UNIVERSITY HOSPITAL

CONSENT FOR SPECIAL THERAPY OR PROCEDURE

Date

Room No.

Patient's No.
Name
Address
City

I have been informed by Doctor________________ at University Hospital that my medical condition makes advisable the use of special drugs or procedures and that the expected results of this treatment or these procedures have been explained to me. I hereby give my consent for this treatment or these procedures.

Date________ Patient's Signature________

Witness________

(Place in Patient's Chart When Signed)

I have been informed by Doctor________________ at University Hospital that the medical condition of________________ (Patient's Name).

my________ (relationship), makes advisable the use of special drugs or procedures and that the expected results of this treatment or these procedures have been explained to me. I hereby give my consent for this treatment or these procedures.

Date________ Signature of parent, guardian or responsible relative________

Witness________

(Place in Patient's Chart When Signed)

Fig 95-5.

METHOTREXATE

Methotrexate is used effectively in treating certain cancers through its ability to decrease the growth of tumor cells, as well as normal cells. Methotrexate is available as a yellow liquid given by injection and as a yellow tablet. The prescribed number of tablets are taken orally as <u>ONE DOSE</u> on the same day of every <u>WEEK</u>. Particular care should be taken to notify physicians you are taking Methotrexate in the event they should prescribe certain additional drugs.

Some of the side effects may include:

1. Sores in the mouth or gums (notify your physician).
2. Diarrhea (if bloody or quite frequent notify your physician).
3. Low blood counts which mean one's ability to fight infections is lessened and the blood may clot more slowly possibly allowing some bleeding to occur, and anemia (lack of oxygen to tissues).
4. Nausea and vomiting.
5. Loss of hair temporarily.
6. Weakness, easily become tired, and dizziness.
7. Chills and fever.
8. Various skin rashes.

THE UNIVERSITY OF KANSAS MEDICAL CENTER
DEPARTMENT OF PHARMACY

Fig 95-7. Drug information card for patients.

question of investigational-drug use. The federal law can be violated by preparing large quantities of drugs which have not been approved for human use by the Food and Drug Administration (FDA). To avoid legal violation, a sponsor of a drug investigation must file with the FDA a "Notice of Claimed Investigational Exemption for a New Drug" (IND). Such a form is usually filed by a pharmaceutical manufacturer; however, others may serve as the sponsor, such as a physician, pharmacist, or an institution such as a hospital, or the hospital pharmacy department.

An abbreviated form of IND is acceptable to the FDA where a physician wants to study a drug which no manufacturer wants to sponsor. The physician may serve both as sponsor and investigator; or the hospital pharmacy may serve as sponsor and the physician as investigator. Some hospital pharmacy departments serve as sponsors on many abbreviated INDs for special drug dosage forms that are not available commercially. The required forms for the sponsor and investigator plus the new-drug regulations are available from the FDA in Washington, DC. Additional information is given in Chapter 72.

THE UNIVERSITY OF KANSAS MEDICAL CENTER
PHARMACY DEPARTMENT

INVESTIGATIONAL DRUG DISPENSING RECORD

Name and Synonyms ________

Strength and Dosage Form ________

Manufacturer ________

Principal Investigator ________

Date	Patient Name	Case Number	Physician	Rx # or Location	Lot Number	Amount Dispensed	Amount on Hand

Fig 95-6.

Intravenous Admixtures—The health-care personnel professionally best qualified to prepare intravenous admixtures are hospital pharmacists trained to provide such service. In a number of hospitals pharmacists have successfully organized, developed, and operated a centralized pharmacy intravenous admixture service that:[14]

1. Saves nursing time for other professional nursing roles.
2. Provides a system for screening physical-chemical incompatibilities, and dispensing of stable preparations.
3. Minimizes pharmaceutical calculation errors.
4. Reduces the risk of medication error by providing additional checks.[15]
5. Centralizes responsibility for preparation of parenteral admixtures.
6. Labels admixtures with rate of infusion as prescribed by the physician and provides a standardized label format.
7. Provides an aseptic environment for preparation of admixtures.
8. Conforms to the standards recommended by the Joint Commission on Accreditation of Hospitals.
9. Conforms to the guidelines established by the National Coordinating Committee on Large-Volume Parenterals.

10. Provides a mechanism for charging patients for IV therapy and creating revenue.
11. Insures more effective use of professional personnel in the hospital.
12. Minimizes the potential for medical-legal liability.
13. Provides for the preparation of solutions which are not commercially available.

The Joint Commission on Accreditation of Hospitals wisely promulgated the concept that the pharmacist should be involved in preparing intravenous admixtures. In the Pharmacy Section of its current Standards for Accreditation, the Commission frequently refers to the subject of the safe and accurate handling of all drugs, including intravenous admixtures. One especially relevant statement is:

The compounding and admixture of large-volume parenterals should ordinarily be the responsibility of a qualified pharmacist. Individuals who prepare or administer large-volume parenterals should have special training to do so. When any part of the above functions (preparing, sterilizing, and labeling parenteral medications and solutions) is performed within the hospital but not under direct pharmacy supervision, the director of the pharmaceutical service shall be responsible for providing written guidelines and for approving the procedure to assure that all pharmaceutical requirements are met.

In rising to the challenge posed by the Joint Commission on Accreditation of Hospitals, it is essential that the pharmacist be involved in preparing intravenous admixtures. A pharmacy-controlled intravenous admixture service demonstrates that a hospital is fulfilling its responsibilities to patients. The responsibility for preparing intravenous admixtures is actually the same as assumed for the unit-dose distribution system. An intravenous admixture is a unit dose.

Hospital pharmacists need the support of hospital administrators, directors of nursing, and medical staffs (through their respective pharmacy and therapeutics committees) in order to develop and operate an effective intravenous admixture service. In establishing such a service it is important that specific guidelines for the operation of the service be formulated. The experience of pharmacists who have developed successful intravenous admixture services in hospitals will undoubtedly be helpful in setting up guidelines for the operation of such services in institutions planning to provide them. The intravenous admixture service can serve as a base for other pharmacy services such as chemotherapy compounding, allergy extract preparation, and parenteral home care programs. (See also Chapter 86, on *Intravenous Admixtures*.)

Ambulatory Care Services—As ambulatory care activities continue to increase within the institutional setting, the hospital pharmacist becomes more and more involved in providing services to these patients. While these pharmacy activities parallel community pharmacy practice, hospital pharmacy practitioners have developed many innovative services for the patient. This includes special patient-information brochures, patient-dosing calendars, special packaging, and patient-education audiovisual programs. These activities will continue to increase as more emphasis is placed on ambulatory care as part of the total patient-care program by hospitals.

Clinical Pharmacy—The concept of "clinical or patient-oriented" pharmacy service has gained tremendous acceptance in hospital pharmacy. The hospital environment offers the hospital pharmacist a multitude of opportunities to develop meaningful clinical roles in the safe and rational use of drugs in hospitalized, as well as ambulatory, patients. This chapter does not include a detailed discussion of the hospital pharmacist's clinical roles and responsibilities because they are discussed in Chapters 94, 99, 100 and 102.

It is important to note that significant progress is being made in providing ongoing clinical pharmacy services in hospitals. Various service functions are described in the *ASHP Statement on Clinical Functions in Institutional Practice*. As these roles emerge, various third-party agencies are recognizing the value of the services rendered and are specifically reimbursing the hospital pharmacy department for providing activities not necessarily associated with dispensing a product. Areas of practice in which reimbursement has been made include pharmacokinetic dosing service, patient-education services for home self-administration of growth hormone, total parenteral nutrition solutions service, steroid administration, factor VIII administration, cytarabine administration, and injectable analgesics service.

As increased emphasis is being placed on cost containment in hospitals and improved drug therapy utilization, the clinical pharmacist has been valuable in monitoring patient drug therapy and promoting rational drug therapy. The clinical pharmacist can best carry out the mandates of the Pharmacy and Therapeutics Committee relative to appropriate drug therapy.

Future Practice—In reviewing the activities of hospital pharmacy practice one must conclude that no two hospital practices are alike. Hospital pharmacy practice has made significant strides over the past two decades in changing its practice roles to provide a more patient-oriented pharmacy service. Drug distribution systems have been improved (unit dose and IV admixture services) and patient oriented clinical services have been implemented in large and small hospitals alike. Computerization has increased efficiencies and has provided an improved patient and management data base. Practice in hospitals has adjusted to the changing environment of health care. What the future holds for hospital pharmacy practice in the year 2000 is only speculation.[16] However, with the significant progress in the last few years and the practitioner talent in this area, one can be assured that the role of the hospital pharmacist on the health care team will be significant.

References

1. *Hospitals 38 (Jan 1):* 109, 1964.
2. *Am J Hosp Pharm 32 (Sept):* 917, 1975.
3. *The 1983 AHA Guide to the Health Care Field*, Am Hosp Assoc, Chicago, IL 60611.
4. *Ibid.*
5. Niemeyer GF, et al: *Bull Am Soc Hosp Pharm 9(4):* 287, 1962.
6. Spease E, Porter RM: *J APhA 25:* 65, 1936.
7. *Am J Hosp Pharm 40:* 1384, 1983.
8. *J APhA NS10 (Feb):* 107, 1970.
9. Beste D: *Am J Hosp Pharm 25(8):* 396, 1968.
10. Latiolais CJ, et al: *Am J Hosp Pharm 27 (Nov):* 886, 1970.
11. Shultz SM, et al: *Hospitals 47 (Mar 16):* 106, 1973.
12. Roberts C, et al: *Drug Intel Clin Pharm 6 (Dec):* 408, 1972.
13. Lucarotti RL, et al: *Am J Hosp Pharm 30 (Dec):* 1147, 1973.
14. Shoup LK, Godwin HN: *Implementation Guide for a Centralized Intravenous Admixture Program*, Travenol, 1977.
15. Thur MP, et al: *Am J Hosp Pharm 29 (Apr):* 298, 1972.
16. McConnell WE: *Am J Hosp Pharm 40 (Aug):* 1315, 1983.

CHAPTER 96

Long-Term Care Facilities

Alan Cheung, PharmD, MPH
Deputy Director, Pharmacy Service
Veterans Administration Central Office
Visiting Professor, Howard University, College of Pharmacy and Pharmacal Sciences
Washington, DC 20420

Peter H Vlasses, PharmD
Associate Director, Clinical Pharmacology and Clinical Associate Professor of Medicine
Jefferson Medical College
Clinical Associate Professor of Pharmacy
Philadelphia College of Pharmacy and Science
Philadelphia, PA 19104

Long-term health care has become an important issue in our total health care system. There are more long-term facility beds than acute care beds. Future emphasis will be to increase the number of facilities and beds in long-term care while those of acute care will be reduced.

With advances in medical sciences and technologies, people are living longer. Prolongation of life expectancy has created a totally new set of problems for the health care system. There is a rapid rise of chronic disease conditions, with associated social and emotional problems which require a different approach in their management. Drugs are a key therapeutic modality in the long-term facility care setting.

Health is considered as a microcosm of the broader social system. The growing concern of social obligation and social responsibility in our society has advanced the philosophy that health is a right, a right to have access to quality health care without discrimination. The advent of health insurance and the government involvement in financing health care has greatly changed the practice and reimbursement of health care services. The assurance of payment for health care services has stimulated utilization of new medical technologies, resulting in higher health care cost and more specialization and sub-specialization in medical practice. In addition, most health care providers are acute-care oriented; they are not equipped and trained to render quality long-term care. Long-term care is more than medical intervention and treatment. It requires a multidisciplinary approach to care as well as an array of psychosocial support and services.

The same forces affecting acute care have also impacted on the growth of long-term care. Long-term care facilities have increased in number and sizes. There are a variety of long-term care facilities, with nursing homes, including skilled nursing facilities and intermediate care facilities, among the most common. Many patients in these facilities are treated with long-term and multiple drug therapy. The pharmacist has an important role to play and an opportunity to contribute in the long-term facility care.

Pharmacy services in long-term care facilities are provided by community pharmacist practitioners, who often have little formal institutional care training. Most of them are self-learners. Government is intimately involved in the financing of long-term facility care, and it is not surprising that it has established numerous regulations and requirements governing the provision of long-term care. The pharmacist has to practice within the established rules and guidelines, but compensation for pharmacist services is reimbursed through the facility, which has created the potential for questionable business arrangements between the pharmacist and the facility, especially where the provider of drugs and the pharmacist consultant are one and the same. There is little incentive for the pharmacist to innovate and improve drug utilization and patient care.

Newer standards require the pharmacist to assume greater responsibility and participation in long-term facility care. In addition to maintaining a safe drug distribution and control system, the pharmacist is asked to apply his knowledge, such as reviewing drug regimen, participating in patient-care and related committees, and developing pharmacy policies and procedures. The new requirements are broadly defined and the individual pharmacist has to interpret and apply them according to his own background and experience.

It is impossible to cover the subject of long-term care facilities, pharmacy services in long-term care, and geriatric pharmacology and drug therapy, within the context of a single chapter. Therefore, the approach of this chapter is to outline the important issues and topics relating to the provision of pharmacy services in long-term facility care. The emphasis will be addressed to the activities of drug regimen review, development, and implementation of pharmacy policies and procedures in long-term care facilities. Also, important principles in geriatric pharmacology and major considerations for monitoring geriatric drug therapy are included.

Historical Background

Long-term care is not and should not be construed as an independent segment of total health care. It is a continuum of acute and episodic care integrated closely with rehabilitative, restorative and supportive care. In order to have a greater appreciation of the mission, role and issues of long-term care facilities, it is necessary to review briefly the major developments in public health and medical technologies which shape current health care practice.

Since the beginning of time, good health has been considered one of the more important basic needs of man. What separates the human from other mammalian species is man's ability to maintain a state of physical, social, economic and mental well-being.

In ancient times, disease and sickness were considered afflictions of evil spirits and punishment by God. Those who were sick, weak, poor, and aged were deemed social outcasts and undesirable elements of society. The impoverished aged or elderly who did not have family or relatives to provide for them were often cared for with the sick, the insane, the blind and deaf mutes, and other social destitutes by charitable and religious organizations. The prevailing belief was that institutionalization was an efficient way to manage the dependents of society. The result was a proliferation of public almshouses and church-sponsored institutions whose main services were to provide food, shelter, and medical care. They were the prototypes of today's hospitals and long-term care facilities. The principal care providers were the clergy who functioned both as physicians and pharmacists.

Before the middle of the nineteenth century, communicable and infectious diseases, such as cholera, diphtheria, typhoid, etc., were prevalent in many parts of the world. Little was known about germ theory, public sanitation, personal hygiene, and the cause and control of these diseases. The infant mortality rate was high. People did not live long enough to have chronic diseases or become elderly.

During the same period, the Industrial Revolution was fermenting. There was a general public mood favoring more humanism and social reform. Public health programs were developed and promoted. With the advance of knowledge of bacteriology and immunology, including development of vaccines, the concepts and practices of medical care were greatly altered. Emphasis was placed on prevention and control of epidemic disease. Thus, public health activities were greatly expanded to include not only disease prevention and improvement of environmental and sanitary conditions, but also health promotion and application of social concepts in medical care practice. These public health measures were mostly responsible for the decrease of infant mortality and the increase in the life span of man.

The twentieth century marked the advent of a golden era of medical science and technology. The discovery and development of sulfonamides, penicillin and streptomycin made a spectacular change in the successful management of many common infectious diseases. The isolation and production of insulin revolutionized the treatment and improved the prognosis of patients suffering from diabetes mellitus. Other therapeutic advances in vaccines, antiepileptics, antipsychotics and anesthetics worked wonders in the elimination of some communicable diseases, the management of a substantial number of chronic diseases, and also paved the way for surgical innovations. Progress of medical technologies in devices, equipment, and procedures resulted in major breakthroughs in the diagnosis and treatment of many diseases. The successes of the medical and scientific technologies have prolonged life and improved its quality. But new problems are emerging, such as the increase of chronic diseases which require a new approach and different management.

The Right to Health—Interpreted broadly, the right to good health includes a concomitant right to health care. Even though no one can be guaranteed freedom from sickness, the basic concept of the right to health and to health care can be construed as society having an obligation to provide its citizens equal access to an acceptable level of health care. Health should not have any racial, sexual, economic or age limitation. Health care should not be a commodity available only to those who are fortunate enough to receive it.

Health as a right is established on the same philosophy as a right to an education and to welfare benefits. Because of the emphasis on individual rights, current social philosophy leans increasingly toward emphasis of social obligation to the individual rather than the individual's obligation to society. Acceptance of health as a right has great implications on the financing and delivery of health care services. Health is only one of the components of our social system. Health as a right has more than moral and philosophical implications; it has political, economic and social ramifications as well. It is especially important to the elderly because, while they account for approximately 10% of the total population, they utilize 29% of the national health care expenditures.

Impact of Growing Elderly Population

Since the beginning of the twentieth century, the elderly population in the US has spiraled precipitously. Actually there is no specific physical or physiological basis for defining persons 65 years or over as elderly, aged, or as senior citizens. Rather, the definition reflects the social, political and legislation perception at the time about aging and life span. The chronological number 65 has been determined as a retirement age, and the beginning of the receipt of social security and other public supported and funded programs. In 1978, Congress enacted legislation abolishing mandatory retirement at 65 to eliminate age discrimination in employment, especially when the life span and productive life of an individual have been greatly extended. In 1900, there were approximately 3 million persons 65 and over, representing 4% of the total population. By 1940 the number had tripled to 9 million or 6.8% of US citizens. In 1965, the year when Medicare and Medicaid were instituted, the elderly were 18.5 million or approximately 9.3% of all people. In 1970 the number of the elderly had more than doubled that of 1940 to over 20 million or 9.9% of total population, and the respective figures for 1980 were 25.5 million and over 11%. Projections of the population of the elderly in the year 2000 and in 2030 are 31 million and 46 million persons, or 12% and 17% of total population, respectively.

With the rapid growth of the elderly population, it is important to identify major characteristics and factors of the elderly in order to meet their social and health care needs.

The elderly currently celebrating their 65th birthday will, on the average, live an additional 16 years. There are and will be more elderly women than elderly men. The current ratio at ages 65–74 is 69 elderly men per 100 elderly women and at 85 years and over is 44 elderly men per 100 elderly women.

Up to 95% of the elderly live in their homes or with "relatives." More elderly women than men are likely to be living alone. According to the 1970 census, 5% of people 65 years and over were institutionalized, and by 85 years over 19% were residing in long-term care facilities. The largest number of the elderly live in urban areas. The elderly as a whole are more than twice as likely to be poor.

Economic security is probably the number one issue for a large number of elderly because most of the time they are not employed, are on fixed incomes, and thus are vulnerable to become victims of inflation. Biologically, the elderly are likely to have changes of memory; sensory disturbances in vision, vestibular function and proprioception; loss of muscle strength and decreased joint integrity. They are prone to suffer from falls, incontinence, and mental confusion, especially if they are predisposed to infection, toxins, drugs, and atherosclerosis. They are more prone to contract chronic diseases.

In terms of patterns of medical care utilization, the elderly are two times more vulnerable to hospitalization than those who are under 65. Close to 90% of patients in long-term care facilities are elderly. In 1975, the noninstitutionalized elderly had an average of 6.6 physician visits compared to 5.6 physician visits for persons aged 45–65. The elderly as a whole utilize or consume 25% of prescription drugs.

The estimated per capita personal health care expenditures for the elderly in fiscal 1966 was $445.25, of which 40% was for hospital care, 20% for physician services, 15.4% for nursing home care, 14% for drugs and drug sundries, 3.5% for eye glasses and appliances, 2.9% for dentist service, 2.6% for other professional services, and 1.6% for other health services. In fiscal 1971 the per capita health care expenditures had almost doubled to $877.48, with a distribution of hospital care 43%, physician service 16.7%, nursing home care 23.1%, drugs and drug sundries 10%, eye glasses and appliances 2.2%, dentist service 1.9%, other professional services 1.8%, and other health services 1.3%. In fiscal 1976 the expenditures ($1521.36) again were almost double those of 1971. Hospital care had a net gain of 2.3% to 45.3%, physician services and nursing home care almost maintained the 1971 levels at 16.8% and 23%, respectively. Drugs and drug sundries were further reduced from 10% in 1971 to 8% in 1976. Eye glasses and appliances and other professional services had reductions from 1.8% to 1.5% and from 2.2% to 1.2%, respectively, while other health services increased from 1.3% to 2.1%. Dental services had insignificantly increased from 1.9% to 2.1%. Within this ten-year interval, the greatest percentage increase in health care expenditures for the elderly was nursing home care, followed by hospital care. The greatest percentage reduction was for drugs and drug sundries, and for physician services.

Advent of Health Insurance

The Flexner Report in 1911 not only shaped the trend of today's medical education, but also popularized institutional practice. It was in hospitals that sophisticated knowledge and technologies were available and utilized. The result was a stimulus for proliferation of hospital construction, and the orientation of medical practice was concentrated in acute short-term and highly technological care. Reimbursement for physician services and hospital care was mostly from out-of-pocket and fee-for-service type of payments made by patients. There was no government involvement in financing any aspect of health care.

The depression in the early thirties posed great financial difficulty for many hospitals. A number of hospitals developed a fixed fee contract for delivery of hospital care to those enrolled in the program. This was the beginning of the voluntary hospital or health insurance. Blue Cross was among the first programs established to assure the health and welfare of hospitals as the primary goal.

Voluntary health insurance had significant impact in the promotion of hospital-based practice by the physicians. It was in the hospital that expensive modern equipment, qualified personnel, and appropriate environment were available under one roof. At the time hospitals were competitive and very protective of their patient population; they were not willing to discharge patients to other types of health care facilities, even less sophisticated ones. Furthermore, most health insurance policies covered only medical services provided in the hospital setting.

As the elderly population was increasing and there were drastic changes in social and family structure, more of the elderly found themselves living alone and away from their siblings. Those who could not afford single-unit family dwellings, tended to live in residential or boarding homes. With increasing age, health declined and reduced physical capability. They needed general support and assistance in daily living, as well as some basic forms of health care services. Nurses were eventually hired in these residential institutions and the result was the emergence of the forerunners of nursing homes or long-term care facilities today.

Passage of the Social Security Act in 1935 had great impact on the provision of health care to the elderly. The OASI Program (Old Age Survivors Insurance) which provided monthly payments for the elderly, and the OAA program (Old Age Assistance) which provided financial assistance participated in and administered by the state for needy elderly, for the first time assured the elderly of some forms of continuous economic support. Both of these programs were considered as cash assistance to the elderly, and not as direct payment for medical care programs. Because of federal support for the elderly and their need of long-term care, nursing homes and other related facilities, especially those privately operated, were growing in number.

Other federal programs that directly or indirectly contributed to the increase of long-term care facilities were:

(1) Hospital and Medical Facilities Construction Program (Hill-Burton) which also provided federal matching funds for constructing and equipping of public or nonprofit-operated long-term care facilities;

(2) the Department of Housing and Urban Development, and the Federal Housing Administration also provided mortgage insurance to private lenders to facilitate construction or rehabilitation of qualified proprietary nursing homes, and authority to grant money for loans to nursing homes under the National Housing Act Amendments of 1959, and

(3) the Small Business Administration provided commercial loans to privately owned long-term care facilities for construction of new facilities/expansion of new facilities.

The demand and supply of long-term care facilities were further stimulated by the passage of Medicare and Medicaid in 1965. Medicare is a health insurance program and Medicaid is a welfare program through participation and administration by the state. Both programs are designed to meet the medical needs of high-risk groups, the elderly and the poor. Medicare and Medicaid programs are quite similar to the OASI and OAA of the Social Security Act of 1935 except that the former are vendor programs which provide direct payment to providers of health care services. Medicare signifies the beginning of the federal government's involvement in providing health insurance. Because of the provision in both Medicare and Medicaid to pay for care received in long-term care facilities, these programs sparked continued growth of long-term care facilities.

Definition of Long-Term Care Facilities

In order to define a long-term care facility and its related institutions, it is important to arrive at a common understanding of what is long-term care. The term long-term care has generally been accepted by health care professionals as health care and health-related services provided to individuals who, because of their physical and mental conditions, require medical, nursing, or supportive care for a prolonged period of 30 or more days. The Congressional Discursive Dictionary of Health Care defines long-term care as "health and/or personal care services required by persons who are chronically ill, aged, disabled, or retarded, in an institution or at home on a long term basis. The term is often used more narrowly to refer only to long-term institutional care such as is provided in nursing homes, homes for the retarded and mental hospitals." The APhA publication titled "Pharmaceutical Services in the Long-Term Care Facility" defines a long-term care facility as a facility or unit which is staffed, and equipped to accommodate individuals who do not require hospital care but who are in need of nursing care and related health and social services." Sometimes the term long-term care is used interchangeably with chronic care or care for chronically ill, which describes an impairment of health requiring an extended period of medical supervision. These definitions all connotate care for individuals with a prolonged episode of illness, but they also imply the concept of extended care, continuity of care, and maintenance care which require a wide range of health and social services other than purely medical care.

Long-term care institutions include but are not limited to the following:

1. Nursing homes (including extended care facilities, skilled nursing facilities, and intermediate care facilities.
2. Hospital extended care units.
3. Psychiatric hospitals.
4. Chronic disease hospitals, (eg TB hospitals).
5. Personal care, shelter care, board and care homes.
6. Facilities for mentally retarded.
7. Special facilities for the elderly (eg geriatric centers or institutes, apartments, communities).
8. Half-way houses and other special facilities for alcoholics and drug abusers.
9. Other health and social related institutions (eg detention centers, special residential facilities for children, jail units).

For the purpose of this chapter, the discussion on long-term care facilities will mostly focus on the first category, the nursing homes group. These facilities have the greatest need for quality pharmaceutical services and care because a very large portion of their patient population is elderly who often have a number of chronic disease conditions treated and maintained on pharmacotherapy. The concept, principles, structure and process of pharmaceutical service and care provided in the nursing home setting are applicable to or easily modified for other types of long-term care facilities.

Nursing Homes

Nursing home is a generic term used to describe nonhospital institutions which provide nursing and other health and social related supportive services to the chronically ill and the elderly. The Congressional Discursive Dictionary of Health Care defines nursing homes as "generally, a wide range of institutions, other than hospitals, which provide various levels of maintenance, and personal or nursing care to people who are unable to care for themselves and who may have health problems which range from minimal to very serious. The term includes free-standing institutions, or identifiable components of other health facilities which provide nursing care and related services, personal care, and residential care. Nursing homes include skilled nursing facilities, intermediate care facilities and extended care facilities but not boarding houses."

The major services provided in the nursing homes as defined by the American Health Care Association are:

a. *Nursing Care*—Nursing procedures requiring the professional skills of a registered nurse or a licensed practical nurse. These skills include administering medication, injections, catheterizations, and similar procedures ordered by the physician. Post-hospital stroke, heart, or orthopedic care is available with such related services as physical therapy, occupational therapy, dental services, dietary consultation, laboratory and X-ray services, and a pharmaceutical dispensary.

b. *Personal Care*—Services such as help in walking, getting in and out of bed, bathing, dressing and eating, and the preparation of special diets as prescribed by a physician.

c. *Residential Care*—General supervision in a protective environment, including room and board plus planned programs for the social and spiritual needs of the resident.

The primary goal of long-term care and long-term facility care is to improve and maintain the ability of individuals to function independently and to cope with impairments and disabilities. The professional services and care provided in these settings should then focus on the implementation of this goal with emphasis on rehabilitative, maintenance and psychosocial supports as well as medical and nursing care.

Extended Care Facilities (ECF)

Extended care facility was used in the early years of the Medicare program to designate a nursing home which qualified for participation in Medicare. A nursing home has to meet certain requirements in order to be certified as an extended care facility. While nursing homes that provided a lower level of care and qualified for the Medicaid program were called skilled nursing *homes*, only a relatively small number of nursing homes were certified as extended care facilities. The concept of extended care at the time referred to an extension of care for the original medical condition after hospitalization and not to the duration of long-term facility care required. Medicare covered only up to 100 days of post-hospital extended care services during any spell of illness. Therefore, the extended care facility benefit was limited in duration and must follow a hospital stay and be related to the medical condition being treated in the hospital. If the person exhausted his coverage for extended facility care, he must either finance his own care or resort to seeking eligibility under the Medicaid program. If he was qualified for Medicaid, his

care would be provided in a nursing home that might not be certified or approved by Medicare. In order to establish uniform standards for long-term facility care under Medicare and Medicaid, the term extended care facility was dropped and replaced by the generic definition of skilled nursing *facility* for both Medicare and Medicaid.

Skilled Nursing Facilities (SNF)

A skilled nursing facility is a nursing home that meets requirements for the conditions for participation in both Medicare and Medicaid programs. Some of the major requirements are:

a. Having a transfer agreement with one or more participating hospitals.
b. Primarily engaging in providing skilled nursing care and related services.
c. Having formal policies.
d. Having a physician, a registered professional nurse or a medical staff responsible for the execution of such policies.
e. Requiring the health care of every patient to be under the supervision of a physician and providing for having a physician available to furnish necessary medical care in case of an emergency.
f. Maintaining medical records on all patients.
g. Providing 24-hour nursing services and having at least one registered professional nurse employed full-time.
h. Providing appropriate methods and procedures for dispensing and administering drugs and biologicals.
i. Having in effect a utilization review plan.
j. Meeting licensing standards established by the individual state.
k. Providing a regular program of independent medical review of the patients in the facility.
l. Meeting any conditions relating to the health and safety of individuals.
m. Having the drug regimen of each patient reviewed by the pharmacist at least on a monthly basis.

In addition to providing skilled nursing care, skilled nursing facilities also make available rehabilitative therapy, physical therapy, occupational therapy and other medical services when needed.

Intermediate Care Facilities (ICF)

An intermediate care facility is defined in the Congressional Discursive Dictionary of Health Care as "an institution recognized under the Medicaid program which is licensed under state laws to provide, on a regular basis, health-related care and services to individuals who do not require the degree of care or treatment which a hospital or skilled nursing facility is designed to provide, but who because of their mental or physical condition require care and services (above the level of room and board) which can be made available to them only through institutional facilities."

Many long-term care facilities qualify both as a skilled nursing facility and an intermediate care facility, and both types of facilities are usually licensed by the same state agency.

VA Long-Term Care Programs

By 1990 more than half of US males over the age of 65 years will be veterans, and by 1995 veterans will exceed 60% of the male elderly population. While Medicare adopts a health insurance approach in the provision of medical care to its recipients, the Veterans Administration accepts the responsibility of directly involving the provision of comprehensive and continuous health care to eligible veterans. In the area of long-term care, Medicare sets a limit of institutional benefits to its recipient, but the eligible veteran is assured of all the necessary health care for as long as he needs it. In addition to offering a continuum of hospital care, ambulatory care, and home care, the Veterans Administration offers a variety of forms of long-term care facilities.

VA uses a different terminology in describing its long-term

care programs. The same term in the Medicare and Medicaid programs may mean different things in the VA. The VA offers a full range of long-term care facilities—from hospital-based extended care programs to nursing home care to domiciliary care and to state veterans homes.

Extended Hospital Care

Extended hospital care is a hospital-based program and is defined as care provided to patients who have passed through the acute stage of their illness, but who are still unstable and will require several months of further hospital care before a stable course can be anticipated. The health care and services provided are high-level skilled nursing care, frequent to daily physician supervision, inhalation therapy, physical and other rehabilitative therapy services, speech therapy and other professional services, and the availability of hospital-based laboratory, X-ray, and other diagnostic and therapeutic modalities. In 1977, a total of 10,456 beds were classified as extended hospital care beds.

From the description of services provided, this type of care is quite similar in concept to that required of extended care facility as established by early Medicare program; except the VA program is based in the hospital.

Nursing Home Care

The VA is authorized to provide nursing home care to eligible veterans in VA-operated community and state nursing homes. This type of care is provided to patients, mostly elderly and infirm, who are not acutely ill and not in need of hospital care, but who require much skilled nursing care and a lesser amount of medical and related health services for a protracted period of time.

This may be similar to the type of care provided by the intermediate care facility as defined by the Medicaid program.

In 1977, VA operated a total of 7579 VA nursing home care beds and contracted with community nursing homes for another 7932 beds.

Domiciliary Care

Domiciliary care was originally established as Soldiers Homes for disabled veterans. The domiciliaries are essentially a protected residential program. There are limited medical and psychosocial services. Most of the residents are elderly. The domiciliaries are homes for the aged. These facilities are closely integrated with other VA health care facilities. At present there are a total of 16 domiciliaries with 9897 beds.

State Veterans Homes

The VA is authorized to contract with states to provide care to eligible veterans requiring domiciliary, nursing homes and acute and intermediate hospital care, as well as to assist in the construction of new facilities and expansion and remodeling of existing facilities. Currently, there is a total of 15,815 beds under this program.

As the number of elderly veterans increases, there will be a greater need for this long-term facility care. The VA also has undertaken a number of noninstitutional extended care programs, such as personal care homes, hospital based home care, geriatric day care and senior-citizen centers. VA probably has done more and had more experience in long-term care and long-term facility care than any other federal or private health care agency.

Range and Scope of Patient Care and Services

Long-term care, including both institutional and noninstitutional care, is broadly defined by the Department of Health and Human Services as:

"Long-term care consists of those services designed to provide diagnostic, preventive, therapeutic, rehabilitative, supportive and maintenance services for individuals of all age groups who have chronic physical and/or mental impairments, in a variety of institutional and noninstitutional health care settings, including the home, with the goal of promoting the optimum level of physical, social, and psychological functioning.

"Provisions of care should be the result of assessment and planning by medical, nursing, social work and therapeutic personnel. The plan of care should be based upon the needs of the individual and family/caretaker who participate in decisions regarding the care plan. Program services and facilities serving the individual requiring long-term care must address the needs of the users of the services. Long-term care programs must focus upon appropriate planning and utilization of resources (medical, social, financial, rehabilitative, and supportive) needed by individuals who have continuing care needs."

Most of the patients cared for in the long-term facility setting are generally suffering from some forms of chronic disease conditions, adjusting to changes in institutional living, and experiencing social isolation and individual loneliness. Even though drug therapy is one of the major therapeutic modalities, the patients' needs are often more than medical and physiological, mostly for psychosocial support. Most health professionals are technologically trained and acute-care-oriented and they are not prepared to care for these patients who need more interpersonal care and contact time from health care providers.

Because of his easy accessibility and availability to the long-term care facilities as well as having a vital service role in this setting, the pharmacist can assume a leadership role to improve the quality of care and life in the long-term care facility. Long-term care is broad and diverse and requires the services of a variety of health professionals. The pharmacist must learn to work with other health care professionals as a true member of a realistic multidisciplinary team. The mission of the pharmacist in the long-term care facility should be more than to provide necessary drugs to patients and assure quality of drug used but also to participate with other health care providers in rendering necessary psychosocial support to the patients.

Nursing Care and Services

The core of long-term care is nursing care. Nursing service in the long-term care facility accounts for over 90% of all personnel.

The intensity level of nursing care is generally used to classify and define the type of long-term care facilities, such as skilled nursing facilities and intermediate care facilities. The role as viewed by the nurse in the long-term care facility is to provide and promote the physical, social, emotional, environmental, recreational, spiritual and rehabilitative aspects of care. The emphasis is directed to preventive, therapeutic, and rehabilitative nursing. In addition the nurse has to coordinate all types and levels of care delivered in the long-term care facility. Because of the chronic nature of the diseases suffered by the long-term facility patients, the infrequent physician contact and the age of the patients, nursing care is the key to the long-term care. The quality of the overall long-term care is directly related to the quality of the nursing care.

Medical Services

In long-term facility care, medical care and services are more than the diagnosing and treatment of diseases. Because of the nature of the illnesses, which are mostly chronic, and the altered physiological states as a result of aging, physicians have to acquire an additional biomedical knowledge base to properly manage the medical problems of the long-term care facility patients. In addition, there are social, psychological and economic needs in this population that may have a higher priority in the view of the individual patient.

The traditional medical practice of most physicians is mostly involved in consultation with individual patients and in advising about treatment of acute episodes of diseases. With the increase in the elderly population and the corresponding rise in chronic diseases, geriatric medicine is being developed and promoted in a number of medical schools. Special geriatric residencies are being established. There is an ongoing debate in the medical community whether geriatric medicine should be taught to all practitioners or established as a specialty in medical practice.

Because of current interest in the care of the elderly, concepts of geriatrics and gerontology have been promoted in the education of many health care providers. There is general confusion because these terms have been used interchangeably. Broadly speaking, geriatrics could be considered as a clinical approach to the care and study of the elderly, while gerontology is the basic biological science and psychosocial study and care of the elderly.

The Institute of Medicine, National Academy of Sciences, in its report of a study on "Aging and Medical Education," published in September 1978, includes selected definitions of geriatrics and gerontology:

Geriatrics is the "branch of general medicine concerned with clinical, preventive, remedial, and social aspects of illnesses in the elderly." (British Geriatrics Society.)

Geriatrics is the "clinical side of aging" (Freeman, JT: A Survey of Geriatric Education: Catalogues of US Medical Schools. Journal of the American Geriatrics Society 19: 746–762, 1971).

Gerontology is "a branch of knowledge dealing with aging and the problems of the aged." (Webster's New Collegiate Dictionary.)

Gerontology is "the study of aging process—originating in the biological sciences and expanding more recently into the social and behavioral sciences." (DHEW Publication No HRA 74-3117.)

Gerontology denotes "the scientific study of aging in all its aspects—clinical, biological, historical and social" (American Medical Student Association: Curriculum Development in Geriatric Medicine, January 1976).

Thus, physicians who provide long-term facility care, function more than as experts in clinical medicine in the medical evaluation and problem-identification of the institutionalized elderly, but also as an organizer of a multidisciplinary team of clinical and social professionals to plan and deliver continuous and need-oriented therapeutic and psychosocial care. The American Academy of Family Practice has recently incorporated geriatrics as a formal part of the training of family practice physicians.

Pharmaceutical Services and Care

Since the beginning of long-term facility care, drugs have always been an indispensable therapeutic modality. Most patients in long-term care facilities are elderly and often are afflicted with a number of chronic disease conditions requiring continuous therapeutic treatment. Drugs are used to eliminate symptoms, to reduce suffering, to prevent exacerbation and complications of illness, as well as to maintain a minimal level of health and enhance the quality of life.

The early phase of pharmaceutical services in long-term care facilities was mostly the provision of medication to individual institutionalized patients. The patient or the family of the patient was and still is free to select any community pharmacy to provide prescribed medication. As the facility size and number of patients institutionalized increased, it became clear that there was an urgent need for a specific pharmacy designated to be responsible for coordinating and controlling use of drugs, as well as providing drugs to patients in the facility. Many long-term care facilities were too small to support a pharmacy department of their own, and they negotiated and contracted with specific community pharmacies to provide all pharmaceutical services and needs of the facilities. This marked the advent of the consultant pharmacist in the long-term care setting. The contracted pharmacy was reimbursed for the medications dispensed by submitting bills of services while the facility usually collected payment from patients or third-party payors including Medicare and Medicaid. In return for providing drugs to the patients in the facility, the contracted pharmacy provider was also required to perform certain services in the facility to assure a safe drug-distribution, storage, administration, control and recording system. Some of these services included in-service training, preparation of policy and procedures, and participation in patient-care-related activities.

With the passage of Medicare and Medicaid legislation in the middle sixties, pharmaceutical services to eligible patients in long-term care facilities were guaranteed under the law. It became very attractive for community pharmacies to expand or specialize their services in the long-term care setting because of assured financial rewards. Whenever government pays for services, there are always strings attached to them. Specific conditions are spelled out as to how the services should be provided in order to qualify for reimbursement. Long-term care facility pharmacy services have become complicated and complex, and special knowledge and expertise are required to provide pharmacy services in these types of institutions. Many highly successful long-term care facility pharmacy providers have introduced computer and other technologies in their operations. It is becoming more difficult for a newcomer to enter and compete successfully for the delivery of long-term facility care.

Pharmacist Role and Functions

Needs for Pharmaceutical Care and Services

The profession of pharmacy has a unique body of knowledge and skills to contribute in our health care system. The pharmacist not only dispenses the appropriate drug product but also the knowledge to assure safe and rational use of drugs. Early functions of the pharmacist could be grouped into the following:

a. Assisting in the selection of appropriate drug therapy with physicians and other health care providers on prescription drugs, and with patients on OTC drugs.
b. Preparing, compounding and manufacturing drugs for individualized patients.
c. Dispensing and packaging the prescribed drug products, including proper labeling.
d. Advising and educating patients on proper use of drugs.
e. Monitoring the outcome and responses of patients to the effects of drugs, both beneficial and adverse.
f. Serving as a community resource person on drug and health information.

There is concern among health care providers over the potential abuse, misuse and inappropriate use of drugs, and the resulting increase in health care cost and patient suffering. There is need for professionals who are patient-oriented and able to apply and provide drug knowledge to improve drug use in the health care system. Pharmacy colleges have responded by providing clinical training for their graduates and practitioners. This new breed of pharmacists is more clinically and patient-oriented and better prepared to dispense drug knowledge as well as drug products.

Long-term care patients often have a number of chronic disease conditions requiring multiple and continuous drug therapy. Also, they have less frequent physician contact than do patients in acute care facilities. Furthermore, in most long-term care facilities the staffing pattern usually meets only the minimal requirement as stated by law. In addition to having a greater demand for medical care, long-term care patients often have psychosocial and economic needs. A clinically trained and patient-oriented pharmacist will be in an ideal situation to assist and work with other members of the health care team to provide quality long-term facility care.

Federal Requirements in Skilled Nursing Facilities

The Social Security Act Amendment of 1972 (PL 92-603) has established uniform terminology and requirements for long-term care facilities participating under both Medicare and Medicaid programs. Final regulations for skilled nursing facilities were published in the Federal Register, February 19, 1974 and updated in 1979. These regulations outline the conditions, requirements, and standards for the provision of pharmaceutical services to long-term care facilities (skilled nursing facilities) qualified for the Medicare and Medicaid programs.

a. *Condition of Participation*—Pharmaceutical Services Paragraph 405.1127 of the regulations outlines the condition for participation of pharmaceutical services and states: "The skilled nursing facility provides appropriate methods and procedures for the dispensing and administering of drugs and biologicals. Whether drugs and biologicals are obtained from community or institutional pharmacists or stocked by the facility, the facility is responsible for providing such drugs and biologicals for its patients, insofar as they are covered under the programs, and for pharmaceutical services as provided in accordance with accepted professional principles and appropriate Federal, State, and local laws." This standard designates the skilled nursing facilities rather than the pharmacist as having responsibility to provide drugs and pharmaceutical services to patients in long-term care facilities. The pharmacists are contracted by the facilities to provide pharmaceutical services. Because pharmacists are reimbursed through the facility, some long-term care facility operators have imposed questionable financial arrangements and restraints on the type of pharmaceutical services provided in the facility. This practice has resulted in "kick-back" scandals and limited development of innovative pharmaceutical services to patients.

b. *Supervision of Pharmaceutical Services*—Paragraph 405.1127 (a) of the regulations spells out the standard for supervision of pharmaceutical services: "The pharmaceutical services are under the general supervision of a qualified pharmacist who is responsible to the administrative staff for developing, coordinating, and supervising all pharmaceutical services. The pharmacist (if not a full-time employee) devotes a sufficient number of hours, based upon the needs of the facility, during regularly scheduled visits to carry out these responsibilities. The pharmacist reviews the drug regimen of each patient at least monthly, and reports any irregularities to the medical director and administration. The pharmacist submits a written report at least quarterly to the pharmaceutical services committee on the status of the facility's pharmaceutical service and staff performance." This provision stipulates the responsibilities of the pharmacist. It differs from the previous concept of a "consultant pharmacist" who does not have direct responsibilities in providing long-term facility care. In addition to spending sufficient time in the facility and making appropriate reports, the pharmacist is required to review the drug regimen of each patient at least monthly. This standard has far-reaching implications and has recognized officially the role of the pharmacist more than as a dispenser of drugs.

c. *Review of Drug Regimens*—The intent of this requirement is to improve drug utilization by reducing adverse drug reactions and interactions, duplication and inappropriate concurrent combination of drugs, and medication errors. The pharmacist is asked to deviate from his/her dispensing activities and to apply his/her knowledge in the review of patients' drug regimens. To implement this standard properly, the pharmacist must acquire certain knowledge and skills and undertake some additional activities, such as:

1. To develop, obtain and maintain a valid and comprehensive drug data base (drug profile).
2. To evaluate the drug data base according to predetermined set of guidelines or standards.
3. To establish monitoring criteria for detecting and preventing potential adverse drug reactions and interactions.
4. To detect medication errors and promote compliance.
5. To assimilate and communicate significant findings in an objective and concise manner both verbally and in writing.
6. To apply clinical and interpersonal skills.

Also, the pharmacist should expand and review his/her knowledge base in geriatric drug therapy.

The costs related to the provision of pharmacist consulting services, such as drug regimen review are recognized by most, if not all, the states. The reimbursement of these services are supposedly reflected in the facility's per diem rate in both Medicaid and Medicare programs. The amount of payment is deemed by many pharmacists as grossly inadequate or nonexistent. Some Medicare and Medicaid officials argue that it is difficult to establish an equitable payment system because there are no workable standards for performing and evaluating the regimen review function. But this requirement does open the door for the pharmacist to be reimbursed for dispensing knowledge, in addition to dispensing drug products.

For the past few years, the Department of Health and Human Services has proposed specific outcome measures or indicators to assess the performance of pharmacist's review of drug regimens. The consulting pharmacist in addition to providing written records of the monthly drug regimen review activities, would be expected to prepare necessary documentation for the surveyor to apply the proposed indicator measurements. The data most likely to be requested might include:

1. The total number of drug regimens reviewed each month.
2. The average number of prescriptions utilized per patient each month.
3. The total number of drug-related irregularities discovered each month.
4. The number of drug administration errors discovered and reported to nursing staff each month.
5. The average monthly patient census.

The general areas that might be addressed by the indicator measurements would include:

1. No multiple or duplicative orders for same or similar drugs in the same pharmacological or therapeutic categories (eg multiple antianxiety agents, antidepressants, antipsychotics, laxatives, multivitamins, and sedative-hypnotics).
2. Medication orders on a PRN basis not being given for more than 30 days.
3. Medications being given according to established safe, recommended dosage ranges, especially those requiring reduced dosages in the elderly, such as antianxiety agents, antidepressants, antipsychotics, and sedative-hypnotics.
4. Changes to higher doses or to other drug agents which require extended periods of time to achieve full therapeutic effects, such as antidepressants, antihypertensives, antipsychotics, and some oral hypoglycemics.
5. Drugs requiring periodic or regular laboratory testing (eg anticoagulants, anticonvulsants, digoxin, diuretics, drugs for anemia, hypoglycemics, thyroid preparations, urinary tract bacterial suppressants, and some antirheumatic agents).
6. Monitoring of clinical parameters for efficacy or toxicity of selective drugs such as blood pressures for antihypertensive therapy, daily pulse rate for antiarrhythmics, digoxin, and beta blockers.

d. *Control and Accountability*—Paragraph 405.1127 (b) of the regulations stresses the importance of control and accountability in the provision of pharmacy services in long-term care facility. It states: "The pharmaceutical service has procedures for control and accountability of all drugs and biologicals throughout the facility. Only approved drugs and biologicals are used in the facility, and are dispensed in compliance with Federal and State laws. Records of receipt and disposition of all controlled drugs are maintained in sufficient detail to enable an accurate reconciliation. The pharmacist determines that drug records are in order and that an account of all controlled drugs is maintained and reconciled."

The pharmacist always has the responsibility for drug control and accountability. Very few long-term care facilities have an in-house or on-site pharmacy department, or employ a full-time pharmacist in the facility. The staffing pattern of many of these facilities is barely adequate to meet minimal requirements of regulation and the staff often lacks the training to assure and implement a good drug control and accountability system. There are publications and reports on congressional hearings describing problems of abuse, misuse, and diversion of drugs in long-term care facilities. This statute clearly identifies and emphasizes the role and function of the pharmacist in drug control and accountability.

e. *Pharmaceutical Services Committee*—Paragraph 405.1127 (d) of the regulation stipulates that a pharmacy service committee or similar type of committee is to be developed in the long-term care facility. It reads: "A pharmaceutical services committee (or its equivalent) develops written policies and procedures for safe and effective drug therapy, distribution, control, and use. The committee is comprised of at least the pharmacist, the director of nursing services, the administrator, and one physician. The committee oversees pharmaceutical service in the facility, makes recommendations for improvement, and monitors the service to ensure its accuracy and adequacy. The committee meets at least quarterly and documents its activities, findings, and recommendations."

The concept and intent of this standard can be traced back to the pharmacy services provided in the acute-care inpatient facility. Because drug therapy is becoming complex, and a multiplicity of health care professionals is involved in the delivery of pharmacy and pharmacy-related services, there is general concern about the control and accountability for drug usage, and a need for developing an organized and structured pharmacy services system in the long-term care facility. This statute clearly defines the responsibility of the pharmacy services committee and the membership for development of policy and procedures dealing with pharmacy services and patient care. Some states have expanded this standard to require the participation of the pharmacist in other patient care committees. This increases the pharmacist's role in the long-term care facility from that of a dispenser of drugs to an active participant in the delivery of health care.

f. *Unit-Dose and Unit per Use System*—The unit-dose system is one of the newer medication management techniques originally developed and designed for use in acute patient care settings. In the late 1950s and early 1960s, the traditional ward stock system proved to be inadequate to provide safe and accountable drug distribution. In that period many new drugs were introduced into the health care market, resulting in an increase in drug utilization. With the short length of stay and rapid turnover of patients in acute care hospitals, nursing personnel were overwhelmed with the preparation and administration of multitudes of new drugs and dosage forms. Consequently there emerged a growing problem of medication errors. Leaders in hospital pharmacy proposed the unit-dose system as one solution to improve drug distribution and administration in the hospital setting. Since then, the unit-dose system has been accepted and promoted by agencies such as the General Accounting Office of the Congress, and the Joint Commission on the Accreditation of Hospitals as a safe and effective drug distribution and administration system. The objectives of the unit-dose system of drug distribution to be:

a. To promote safe and effective drug therapy at a reasonable cost.
b. To detect and prevent errors and adverse drug reactions.

c.   To promote efficient utilization of health manpower.
d.   To minimize drug deterioration, obsolescence, pilferage and abuse.
e.   To promote optimum utilization of floor space for medication storage and distribution.
f.   To reduce or simplify medication record-keeping requirements.
g.   To provide greater drug control through accuracy in medication record keeping.

Some of these goals are applicable to long-term care facility settings, while others are not. Long-term care facilities are unique because the drug therapy of most patients is relatively constant and there are few day-to-day changes. Even though the staffing level of nurses in many long-term care facilities is minimal and there is a high turnover rate of staff, the unit-dose system has not yet been justified to be cost-effective. A modified unit-per-use system may be more logical and easier to adopt. Currently, the reimbursement system under Medicare and Medicaid programs is not inducive for long-term care facilities to venture into the unit-dose system. But everyone will agree that there is need for a safe and efficient medication management system in the long-term care facility.

Important Elements of a Pharmacy Policy and Procedures Manual

Generally pharmacists, except those involved in institutional care, do not ordinarily develop formal and written policies and procedures for the provision of their services. Pharmacy services in the long-term care facility began as an extension of pharmacy practice in the community setting. Whatever policies and procedures existed between pharmacists and management in the facility have been based on common understanding and gentlemen's agreement. As long-term care facilities expand responsibility and scope of services, they demand better organization, management control and accountability of all services, including those of pharmacy. Also, Medicare and Medicaid regulations are requiring more documentation and justification of services reimbursed under these laws. The next unavoidable step would be the mandating of written and formal policies and procedures for all long-term care facilities.

A pharmacy policy and procedures manual establishes rules, guidelines, and processes which define and govern how pharmacy services are to be delivered. A well-written and designed manual will clearly identify the responsibilities of and relationship between the pharmacist provider and the facility. In general, pharmacists are inadequately trained in management science and the majority are uncomfortable and lack the necessary competency to develop a structured pharmacy policy and procedures manual. Many pharmacists recognize the value of an organized policy and procedures manual, such as:

a.   providing a uniform standard of practice
b.   defining specific responsibilities and relationships between provider and facility in the provision of services
c.   serving as a teaching guide for in-service training of staff
d.   establishing a foundation for planning, developing and reviewing existing and new services
e.   serving as a management control and assessment tool
f.   providing documentation of services

A number of excellent continuing education programs sponsored by national and state pharmaceutical associations and selected universities are designed to assist the pharmacist in the development of a pharmacy policy and procedures manual. One particular manual developed jointly in the mid-seventies by the staff of the Beverly Enterprises, Inc, faculty from the University of Southern California School of Pharmacy and the staff of the California Pharmacists' Association provided a model workbook for others to adopt, modify and improve their individual manuals. This model manual workbook offers a systematic approach for the development of a pharmacy policy and procedures manual to meet the specific individual facility needs. Such manuals must include and involve input and participation of other health care providers, such as physicians, nurses, and administrators responsible for the delivery of pharmacy and pharmacy-related

services. Also, a good manual must meet requirements and conditions for participation established under federal and state laws. Because of tremendous changes occurring externally as well as internally in long-term facility care, the pharmacy policy and procedures should be periodically updated and reviewed, not less than once a year.

Pharmacy policies and procedures can be grouped into two major categories, administration-related and service or operation-related.

Administration-Related Policies and Procedures

This section describes the arrangement between the pharmacist provider and the facility defining the organization and scope of pharmacy services. It should have a signed and dated agreement or contract outlining responsibilities and activities to be performed and, if possible, should state reimbursement or professional fees.

Major topics should include:

1.   *Those related to the dispensing of drugs and drug products, specifically to:*
a.   Provide drugs and supplies as required for patients and the facility in accordance with state and federal laws.
b.   Furnish and replenish emergency drug supply in acceptable containers and equipment.
c.   Label all medications according to state and federal laws.
d.   Provide pharmacy services to the facility on a 24-hour day, 7-day week basis.
e.   Maintain drug profiles on all active patients.
f.   Provide timely delivery of all medications and supplies.
g.   Apply prudent buyer concepts to all pharmacy charges.
h.   Provide or arrange for pharmacist consultant service.
i.   Develop a drug formulary system and product selection policy.

2.   *Those related to the dispensing of knowledge:*
a.   Review each patient's drug regimen and submit reports at least monthly.
b.   Maintain a log of all visits and activities in the facility.
c.   Review at least quarterly the various aspects of the total drug distribution system.
d.   Provide complete documentation of all professional review activities in accordance with federal and state laws.
e.   Participate as a member of the pharmacy service committee, infection control committee, and patient care committee, and/or other committees, such as utilization review committee.
f.   Assist in establishing policies and procedures governing provision of pharmacy services and supplies in the facility.
g.   Provide ongoing in-service training for the facility staff at least quarterly.
h.   Check emergency drug supply at least monthly.
i.   Inspect each nursing station, its related drug storage area, and the patient's health record, at least quarterly or more often if the need arises.
j.   Make quarterly reports describing problems, solutions, suggestions, and improvements to be submitted to the pharmacy services committee.
k.   Assist in the destruction of unused controlled substances as prescribed by law.

Other information that might be included is the number of hours of services, arrangement for on-call or emergency coverage, current pharmacist license number and renewal date and legal provision for such an agreement.

Service-Related or Operation-Related Policies and Procedures

This section covers policies and procedures related to provision of pharmacy services. It describes processes or methods as to how pharmacy services are to be implemented. The following topics should be considered:

1.   *Medication Procuring Schedules*
a.   A schedule of pharmacy operating hours and drug ordering times should be posted at the nursing station.
b.   The drug delivery schedule and log should be kept.
2.   *Emergency Medication Services*
a.   The 24-hour emergency telephone number of the pharmacist should be posted at the nursing station.
b.   The list of emergency medications should be updated periodically.
c.   An effective and safe exchange system of emergency medication box or cart to avoid misuse of emergency medications.
3.   *Medication Ordering*
a.   All medications should be received by authorized personnel.
b.   Records should be properly kept for ordering medications from the provider pharmacy.

c. Refills of medications, especially maintenance medications, should be ordered appropriately without interruption of therapy.

d. Direct copies of physician orders should be forwarded to the pharmacy provider within 24 hours.

e. Written copies of all telephone medication orders should be promptly sent to the prescribing physician for signature.

f. Signed copies of telephone orders should be included in the patient's chart.

g. Medication orders should be recapped or rewritten monthly, when appropriate and signed by the physician.

h. Medication orders should be properly written, including the drug name, dose, frequency of administration, route (if other than oral), and if PRN, indication for use.

i. Medication orders in the patient's chart should concur with those in the medication administration sheet.

j. Specific nurses should be authorized to transmit medication orders from the patient's chart to the pharmacy.

k. Special provision should be available for patients who wish to obtain drugs from outside pharmacy providers.

l. Outside pharmacy providers should furnish a drug profile of the patient to the pharmacist consultant every 30 days.

4. *Drug Administration*

a. Administration of routine medications should be properly recorded in the patient's health record.

b. Administration of PRN medications should be properly recorded in patient's health record.

c. PRN medications should not be administered on a regular or continuous basis for more than two weeks.

d. All medications should be prepared, dispensed, administered, and charted by the same licensed nurse.

e. Only licensed personnel should administer medications, except for bedside medications when so specifically ordered.

f. Medications should not be borrowed from one patient and administered to another.

g. "Prepouring" of medications should not be allowed. Medications should be administered as soon as possible, but no more than 2 hours after the doses are poured.

1. Dose not administered, for whatever reason, should be documented in the patient's health record.

2. Drugs ordered "STAT" and not in the emergency drug supply should be available and administered within 1 hour of the time ordered during normal pharmacy hours or within 2 hours if the pharmacy is closed. Anti-infectives, pain medications, antiemetics, antianxiety agents, antidiarrheals should be available and administered within 4 hours.

h. When drugs are removed from the original containers they should be maintained in environments insuring purity and potency up to the time of administration.

i. Procedures and equipment used in drug administration should provide for accurate drug dosage, identification, and sanitation.

j. No doses should be charted before administration.

k. There should not be an unusually large amount of doses crushed.

l. The time interval between prescribed doses and actual administration should fall within a range of one hour.

m. The procedure for monitoring and recording medication errors should be implemented and adhered to.

5. *Stop Orders*

a. A stop-order policy should be sent to each physician on the staff.

b. A copy of the stop-order policy should be posted in the medicine room.

c. The stop-order procedures should be followed.

d. Stop orders should be in effect for all categories of drugs.

6. *Drug Returns*

a. Drug returns to the pharmacy should be documented in the facility.

7. *Medication Labels*

a. Medication labels should be clearly and properly prepared.

b. Medication labels should not be altered or reused.

c. Non-legend drugs should be properly labeled and stored in original manufacturer's container.

d. The procedure for updating medication labels should be followed.

8. *Storage of Drugs*

a. Test reagents, germicides, disinfectants, and other household substances which are considered poisons should be stored separately, away from medications.

b. The utility room or cabinet containing commercial poisons and cleaning supplies should be locked.

c. Medications for external use only should be stored separately, away from medications for internal use.

d. The proper temperature (59–80°F) should be maintained in the medication room or drug cabinet.

e. Medications should be stored in a locked cabinet or room that is not accessible to patients or visitors.

f. Keys to the medicine room or drug cabinet should be under the control of the medicine nurse.

g. Unauthorized personnel should not be permitted to enter or use the drug-storage areas.

h. Drug administration areas should be well lighted.

i. Medication counters in the drug room or drug cabinets should be clean and uncluttered.

j. A metric-apothecary conversion chart should be posted in the medication storage area.

k. Discontinued drug containers should be properly marked, stored and appropriately disposed of.

l. Non-drug items should not be stored in the drug storage area.

m. Medications should be stored in the original containers.

n. Amber or glass bottles or other special containers should be used for certain medications to prevent deterioration.

o. Ophthalmic, otic and nasal medications should be stored separately and away from internal medications.

p. Medications for the same patient should be kept together.

q. There should be no excessive quantities of drugs.

r. There should be no prepackaging of bulk or house drug supplies.

s. The emergency medication box should be stored in an area known to all personnel handling medications.

t. No drugs requiring refrigeration should be in the cabinet of the drug room.

u. The proper temperature (36–46°F) for refrigerator items should be maintained.

v. Only drugs requiring refrigeration should be kept in the refrigerator.

w. Outdated drugs should be removed from the refrigerator.

9. *Emergency Drug Supply*

a. A list of the contents of the emergency medication box should be posted near the telephone at the nursing station and on the outside of the box itself.

b. The emergency medication box should be properly sealed.

c. The emergency medication box drugs should not be expired.

d. Use of any emergency medications should be properly recorded in a log book.

e. Staff physician should be informed in writing regarding use of emergency drug supply.

10. *Drug Disposal*

a. Drugs other than controlled substances under Schedules I, II, III, and IV should be destroyed in the facility by the registered nurse in charge of the station and one other licensed nurse or pharmacist.

b. Drug disposal should be properly documented.

c. Discontinued drugs should be properly identified and stored in the medication area.

d. Discontinued drugs not reordered within 90 days should be removed from the cabinet and disposed of.

11. *Discharge Medications*

a. All medications sent with patient on discharge should have been properly ordered by the physician.

b. All medications sent with the patient on discharge should be properly recorded in the patient's health record.

c. All discharge medications should be properly labeled.

12. *"Pass" Medications*

a. All medications sent with the patient on pass should have been properly ordered by the physician.

b. All medications sent with the patient on pass should have been properly recorded in the patient's health record.

c. All medications on pass should be properly labeled.

13. *Controlled Substances*

a. Controlled drugs should not be accessible to non-authorized personnel.

b. Controlled drugs should be stored in a locked cabinet or drawer separate from non-controlled drugs.

c. Separate records should be maintained for controlled drugs.

d. Controlled drugs and records should be reconciled at least every 24 hours.

e. The procedure for discharge drugs should be properly followed and applied to controlled drugs.

f. Controlled drugs should be destroyed in the presence of a registered pharmacist and a registered nurse employed by the facility.

g. Proper records should be kept for controlled drugs destroyed in the facility.

14. *Bedside Medication*

a. The bedside storage of medications should be limited to sublingual or inhalation forms of emergency drugs, unless the item is a non-legend drug.

b. The bedside storage of medications should be specifically ordered by the patient's physician.

c. Medications should be properly labeled for bedside use.

d. The patient should be properly instructed on the use of bedside medications.

e. Use of bedside medication should be properly documented in the patient's health record.

f. The manner of bedside storage should prevent access by other patients.

15. *Physician Drug Samples*

a. Physician drug samples should be properly labeled.

16. *Investigational Drugs*
 a. The procedure for use of investigational drugs should be strictly adhered to.
17. *Reference Sources and Texts*
 a. Each nursing station should have a current edition of Physicians'

Desk Reference, of Facts and Comparisons, and of the ASHP Hospital Formulary or equivalent source material.
18. *Equipment and Supplies*
 a. The nursing station should have adequate supplies for proper storage and administration of medications.

Considerations in Providing Pharmaceutical Care and Services for the Elderly

In order to effectively review patient drug regimens and serve on committees in a long-term care facility, a pharmacist should understand the nature of the geriatric patient. Physiologic changes that commonly occur with age may render the elderly less able to cope with bodily stresses and may affect drug therapy. Various diseases not only occur more frequently in the elderly but the presentation of the disease may be different from that in younger age groups. Pharmacodynamic and pharmacokinetic profiles of agents may be altered; also, drug toxicity, side effects and interactions appear to be more frequent and more severe in the elderly. Thus, the risk-to-benefit relationship of particular therapeutic choices is altered with age in many cases.

Physiologic Variables in the Elderly

Physical Appearance

Most obvious to the pharmacist are physiologic changes in the elderly that alter their appearance. Dehydration of vertebral discs and development of kyphosis result in a loss of height of approximately 2 inches between ages 20 and 70, and a change in posture. A decrease in total body weight usually occurs after age 65 and is accompanied by a marked change in the ratio of lean body mass to fat. A 25 to 30% loss of lean body mass results in changes in body contours and more noticeable bony prominences. The lean body mass loss is replaced by increased fat content of the body, primarily in the area of the hips, pelvis and umbilicus. Loss of subcutaneous supportive tissues with age results in thin, dry skin and ecchymoses with minor trauma; simultaneous loss of cells results in atrophy and wrinkling of the skin. The edentulous state, common in the elderly, may result in resorption of the mandible. Hair patterns change as a result of variations in hormonal and cellular activity and there is generalized thinning and a decreased quantity of hair.

Body Composition

Except for changes in lean body mass and fat, other changes in body composition occurring in the elderly are not obvious. Total body water decreases by approximately 25 to 30%, the majority due to intracellular water loss. However, plasma and extracellular fluid volumes also decrease and these changes may affect distribution of drugs in the body. Cell solids, including elements such as potassium, decrease to the same extent as lean body mass. Hypokalemia is common in the elderly, especially with diuretic therapy. Bone mass decreases approximately 1%, with an accompanying loss of calcium. This loss of calcium predisposes the patient to osteoporosis. With loss of lean body mass, an individual's need for energy-producing food is reduced.

Organ Function

Vital to the understanding of the changes in the elderly that may affect drug therapy is the concept of chronologically altered organ function. These changes, which occur in the absence of disease as it is now understood, are thought to result either from decreases in organ cell populations, oxygen consumption and/or blood flow, or a change in the character of organ tissue, such as that which results from a deposition of collagen fibers.

The eyes undergo many changes with age. Arcus senilis, a yellowish white opaque deposition around the periphery of the iris, is found in approximately 40% of the elderly but does not impair vision. The most common change in vision in the elderly is presbyopia which results from a diminished ability of the lens to focus at different distances and requires approximately 90% of the elderly to wear glasses. Senile cataracts, almost always bilateral, result in opacification. Senile macular degeneration may be due to ischemic changes in the retina and may cause blindness in the elderly. With the increased size of the aged lens, the anterior chamber of the eye becomes smaller and the angle between the root of the iris and the corneoscleral posterior surface becomes more acute and should result in increased pressure in the eye. However, resultant glaucoma occurs only in approximately 5% of the elderly due to the decreased production in aqueous humour that occurs after age 50. Ear function changes also occur in the elderly with presbycusis, a slow, progressive loss of hearing involving various parts of the hearing system, the most common hearing abnormality. Onset of presbycusis is usually in the seventh decade and results in interference with selectivity of hearing and conversation comprehension.

Many changes occur in the cardiovascular system with age. A decrease in the cardiac output of approximately 40% occurs by age 65. Systemic arterial pressure increases, the systolic increasing to a greater extent than the diastolic. These blood pressure changes often result in hypertrophy of the heart secondary to the increased workload placed on it. Atherosclerosis increases with age with an increased collagen and calcium content of blood vessels and a resultant decreased resilience. The increased atherosclerosis contributes to the increase in blood pressure and *vice versa*. Postural hypotension occurs frequently in the elderly. In one survey of elderly ambulant individuals, 24% showed a postural decrease in systolic blood pressure of 20 mm Hg or more and 5% a decrease of 40 mm Hg or more. This altered compensation by the cardiovascular system for postural change is due to impairment of the baroreceptor reflex. The distribution of peripheral blood flow in the elderly favors coronary, cerebral and skeletal circulations at the expense of visceral, hepatic and renal flow.

The respiratory system also undergoes changes with age. An increased lung collagen content results in loss of elasticity and a resultant decrease in vital and total lung capacities. A progressive increase in the number of alveoli supplied with less than an optimal quantity of pulmonary capillary blood flow occurs. The dimensions of the thoracic cage increase, resulting in hyperinflation. A decrease in the number and activity of cilia as well as decreased efficiency of contraction of the expiratory muscles, which makes coughing more difficult, results in decreased ability to clear mucous secretions.

Renal function decreases with age. The number of functioning nephrons decreases but, because of the large reserve in renal function, this within itself does not pose a major problem. However, coupled with decreased renal blood flow of approximately 50 to 60% by age 70, there is a marked decrease in glomerular filtration rate of between 20 and 50%. This drop in glomerular filtration rate may not be mirrored adequately by the creatinine clearance as 24-hour creatinine excretion decreases by 50% from the 3rd to the 9th decade of life. The serum creatinine is thus not a reliable indicator of changes in creatinine clearance across age groups and in the aged. A normal serum creatinine of 1 mg/dL may respond to a creatinine clearance of 120 mL/min at age 20 but only 60 mL/min at age 80. Age adjusted nomograms for estimation of creatinine clearance from serum creatinine have been developed. In addition, alterations in respiratory and renal function in the elderly make them less capable of correcting acid-base insults.

Gastrointestinal changes with age include a decrease in peristaltic activity and a diminished defecation reflex. There is also a decrease in intestinal blood flow, a decrease in the volume and acidity of gastric secretions, and atrophy and deterioration of the colonic musculature with thinning of the intestinal walls. After age 50, pear-shaped diverticula form which, with poor elimination, can become filled with fecal masses and lead to irritation, infection and diverticulitis. Changes in liver anatomy and function occur late in the aging process. A decrease in liver size is noted after the age of 70. Most liver functions, as measured by plasma bilirubin or plasma enzyme concentrations, remain within normal limits and the reserve capacity of the liver is not severely compromised. A notable exception to this, however, might be drug metabolism enzymes due to the postulated decreased activity of the cytochrome P-450 system and the decreased hepatic blood flow with age.

Endocrine changes noted with time include decreases in glucose tolerance, synthesis and release of insulin, and production of thyroid hormone. In addition, there is a change in the anabolic/catabolic ratio of hormones due to a significant decrease in gonadal steroids. Anabolic steroid activity is decreased to 65% with age, while catabolic steroid activity is decreased only 20%. Such changes, in part, account for the osteoporosis seen in the elderly. Loss of calcium is most marked in the postmenopausal female, and resultant fractures may occur spontaneously or with very minor trauma. The activity of the renin-angiotensin-aldosterone system also decreases with age. Also, reduced responsiveness to adrenergic stimuli has been observed in the elderly.

With age, there is a 30% decrease in brain tissue as well as a 30% decrease in nerve conduction velocity. As a result there is a slowing of reflexes and decreased speed of muscle contraction. The central nervous system threshold for excitability and inhibition are reduced, as are perhaps the concentrations of neurotransmitters. Body thermal regulation is impaired. Pain and taste sensations are diminished. In addition, the cardiac conduction system undergoes degeneration.

The immune system responds more slowly and less vigorously in a geriatric patient. Alterations in white blood cell function and reductions in IgG and IgM concentrations have been noted in older individuals.

With all the decreases in organ function occurring over time, the body becomes less able to compensate for stress due to the loss of its reserve capacity. Many of the changes cited predispose the elderly patient to pathologic insults such as infections or fractures which may have devastating results due to the diminished reserve capacity. Drug therapy for these disorders may bear greater risks due to the altered organ function.

Disease Considerations

To perform drug regimen reviews in any setting, the pharmacist must understand the pathophysiology of disease (see Chapter 36). A detailed review of the numerous diseases that may be found in the elderly is beyond the scope of this chapter. However, for the pharmacist monitoring patients in a long-term care facility, it is important to highlight selected aspects of geriatric diseases.

The symptoms and presentation of a myocardial infarction in the elderly may be very different from those in a younger patient. Classical chest-pain syndromes occur in only approximately one-third of patients with otherwise atypical presentations including acute confusion, severe dyspnea, severe hypotension and vomiting, and weakness being the norm. Bradycardias, Adams-Stokes attacks, and cardiac arrhythmias, often asymptomatic, are common. The classical signs and symptoms of congestive heart failure and pulmonary embolism are frequently altered or absent in the elderly and one's index of suspicion must be high.

The management of hypertension in the elderly is a very controversial topic. Patients with diastolic blood pressure greater than 95 mm Hg show mortality rates that increase beyond age 65 for cardiovascular-related death. Thus, classical hypertension is no less a risk factor for those over age 65 and treatment appears effective. Malignant hypertension is rare in the elderly. The bulk of the controversy exists around the management of pure systolic hypertension whose prevalence rises markedly with age. Though systolic hypertension has been related to increased morbidity and mortality, a cause-and-effect relationship has not been established and both may only be a manifestation of severe atherosclerosis. The value of treating systolic hypertension in the elderly is unknown and a large scale, risk-to-benefit evaluation is currently being undertaken by the National Heart, Lung and Blood Institute to better guide treatment decisions. Therefore, the management and investigation of hypertension in the elderly should be flexible and tailored to the individual.

Aged persons with hypertension often manifest diffuse arteriosclerotic disease including the vessels of the head and neck. Treatment of hypertension in such patients may result in sharp reduction in blood pressure which may lead to injurious falls. In such cases, blood pressure should be reduced gradually with cautious initial dosing. The elderly are more susceptible to complications from diuretics, such as hypokalemia and dehydration, especially when intercurrent illness decreases oral intake. The antihypertensive and central nervous system depressant effects of methyldopa, reserpine, and clonidine are greater. Use of beta-blockers is often contraindicated by other concomitant disorders and some investigators report diminished antihypertensive effects in the elderly. Use of reserpine is discouraged in the elderly due to the insidious form of psychic depression which may occur, as is use of guanethidine due to its propensity to cause orthostatic hypotension. Further research is needed to identify the most effective and well-tolerated therapy. It should be recalled that even when diastolic pressure is suitably reduced, a significant systolic elevation may remain. In such cases, a compromise of a slightly higher than desired blood pressure should be accepted.

Peripheral vascular disorders are often seen in the elderly. Peripheral arterial disease is usually unresponsive to vasodilator therapy and, if severe, may lead to gangrene and necessitate amputation. Recent reports indicate that calcium channel blocking agents such as nifedipine may be beneficial medical therapy. Chronic stasis ulcers and deep vein thrombosis also are frequently encountered.

Certain infectious diseases are common and have unique features in the aged. Elderly patients may be predisposed to pneumonias due to decreased immune response, decreased ciliary activity, and potential predisposition to aspiration as a result of concomitant strokes, decreased cough reflex, and impaired swallowing. The classic picture of lobar pneumonia with abrupt onset of fever and signs of lung consolidation is very much the exception. The elderly patient often has an insidious onset of pneumonia which presents as increasing lassitude, apathy, decreased mobility and, thus, no specific localizing symptoms or signs. Confusion may be the key sign in such cases. The advent of pneumococcal vaccine may be of great benefit in the elderly. Influenza, though relatively benign in younger age groups, may cause great morbidity and mortality in the elderly, due to diminished ability to respond to stress. Prophylactic vaccination with influenza vaccine is of great importance in this high-risk group. Incidence of urinary tract infections increases with age in both men and women. Some causes for this include: immobility, which may lead to constipation with resultant contamination of the perineum and urethral orifice in the female; increased residual urine volumes secondary to neurogenic bladder or prostatic hypertrophy changes in men; prostatectomy with loss of the antibacterial prostatic substance; and use of indwelling catheters. Acute infections should be treated as in the younger patient. Catheters should be avoided where possible; if needed due to incontinence, proper care is vital to limit potential infections. Chronic bacteriuria in the elderly appears to be a relatively benign process which does not lead to renal failure.

Disorders of the gastrointestinal tract commonly seen in the elderly include oral moniliasis, dysphagia, hiatal hernia, achlorhydria, peptic ulcer, diverticulosis, ischemic colitis and cancer of the alimentary tract, the latter being one of the commonest causes of death in the very old. Anemia, weight loss, and vague upper abdominal pain is a common presentation of peptic ulcer disease which warrants vigorous evaluation. One-third of all gastric ulcer deaths occur in the elderly; associated perforation and peritonitis may develop in the absence of classical signs and symptoms. Constipation is not a consequence of old age *per se* but is common in the elderly due to decrease in both mobility and dietary fiber consumption.

Evaluation of mental confusion is very important in the elderly. Though senile dementia of the Alzheimer type is common, other causes which must be evaluated before this diagnosis is entertained include depression, drug therapy, infections, cerebral hypoxia, and metabolic disorders. Cerebral arteriosclerosis often leads to dementia, apraxia and parkinsonism though the latter may be due to other causes. Transient ischemic attacks, drop attacks, strokes, and temporal arteritis are common disorders; the drop attacks account for about 20% of fractures of the femur in the aged.

Common bone diseases include osteoporosis, osteomalacia, and Paget's disease. The osteomalacia may be due to poor intake of vitamin D coupled with inadequate exposure to sunlight. Postmenopausal estrogen replacement therapy and dietary calcium and fluoride supplementation have been advocated to prevent development of osteoporosis. Fractures are very slow in healing in the aged. Rheumatoid arthritis can start acutely in the elderly or be present in a "burned out" form. However, osteoarthritis, a degenerative joint disease, is much more common. Use of aspirin can produce tinnitus and further compromise high frequency hearing loss in the elderly.

Thyroid disease is not uncommon in old age. Apathetic thyrotoxicosis, a disease of elderly women is characterized by loss of weight, apathy and depression in the absence of clinical signs of thyroid disorder. Diabetes mellitus is common in the elderly. Diabetic ketoacidosis is uncommon but hyperglycemic hyperosmolar, non-ketotic coma occasionally develops.

Though red-cell life span and morphology do not change with age, iron deficiency anemia, due to blood loss, malabsorption, or malnutrition, megaloblastic anemia due to folate and vitamin B_{12} deficiencies, and the anemia of chronic disease are common in the elderly.

Urinary and fecal incontinence are frequent maladies in the elderly. Causes for urinary incontinence include: stress incontinence in the female, often associated with senile changes in the urethra; benign prostatic hypertrophy in the male; fecal impaction with a low-capacity bladder or chronic retention with outflow incontinence; bladder carcinoma; renal calculi; urinary tract infections; and impaired neurologic control. Management requires correction of the cause, if possible, with anticholinergic agents occasionally providing some relief. Electronic stimulation of the pelvic muscles has been used with some success. Indwelling catheters should be avoided if possible, but are often required. Fecal incontinence may result from constipation, laxative abuse, drug reactions, diseases of the large bowel and impaired neurologic control of defecation. In both types of incontinence, special patient padding should be utilized to minimize irritation and effects of moisture on the surrounding skin as this may predispose to decubitus ulcers.

Many geriatric patients require chronic bedrest. Because of their immobility, these patients are more predisposed to complications such as pneumonia, thrombophlebitis, pulmonary embolism, micturition and defecation problems, muscle wasting, stiffness, contractures, accelerated calcium excretion and decubitus ulcers. Decubitus ulcers are localized areas of cellular necrosis commonly called "bed sores" or pressure sores. It has been estimated that approximately one-third of bedridden geriatric patients have pressure sores. The cause of decubitus ulcers is compression of the skin and subcutaneous tissue severe enough to impair local blood circulation. A pathologic sequence of erythema, induration and necrosis results. Bedridden patients are unable to move and thereby remove pressure from a given area. Certain tissues have enhanced pressure on them, such as those which overlie bony prominences (the sacrum, the heels and buttocks) and those under compressing surfaces (chairs, beds, casts, braces, tight dressings and other factors). Poor hygiene, poor nutrition, edema, fever, and anemia may all enhance decubitus ulcer formation. Moisture secondary to excessive perspiration and incontinence may predispose to tissue breakdown. Good nursing care, utilizing special devices (e.g. water-support mattresses) to relieve the pressure on certain areas of the patient, is vital to prevent tissue breakdown. Excellent reviews on the prevention and treatment of decubitus ulcers have been published.

Geriatric Pharmacology

The vast majority of studies on drug effects, kinetics and other factors have been carried out in young, healthy volunteers. Little research has been done in the field of geriatric clinical pharmacology to date. Currently, the FDA is assessing the need for additional information about the action of a drug in the elderly patient. The New Drug Application process is likely to be modified to require dosing guidelines for the aged. This field offers great opportunity to the clinical pharmacist investigator. Aspects of what is now known about drug therapy changes with age will be reviewed.

Absorption

The increased pH of the gastrointestinal tract with age could alter drug ionization and solubility and the decreased blood flow to the gastrointestinal tract could decrease the rate and extent of drug absorption. Likewise, a decreased absorption surface, the decreased physical activity of the elderly as well as the increased incidence of diverticular disease may predispose to problems in drug absorption. However, little research has been done to document such changes. Decreased absorption has been noted for compounds which undergo active transport, such as iron, thiamine, calcium, galactose, and glucose. However, acidic drugs undergoing passive diffusion, such as acetaminophen, phenylbutazone and sulfamethizole have not been shown to have significant changes in the time to peak plasma levels. Basic drugs such as diazepam, L-dopa, pentazocine, and amitriptyline may undergo gastric absorption and may have decreased absorption as a result of gastric changes. Sustained-release preparations of drugs have not been adequately tested in the geriatric patient and erratic absorption and therapeutic effects may result. Acid-labile compounds, such as potassium penicillin G, may actually reach higher levels in geriatric patients because of increased pH in the gastrointestinal tract. Overall, changes in drug absorption appear to be the least important of age-related changes in pharmacologic action.

Distribution

A drug's distribution in the body is determined by: its binding characteristics to plasma proteins, red blood cells and other body tissues; the distribution of systemic blood flow and microcirculation; and the ability of the drug to pass through various membranes. Serum albumin decreases with age, with a concomitant rise in the globulin-protein fraction. This decrease is more likely the result of disease and immobility, than a function of age *per se;* however, a disturbance in the normal metabolic response to a decreased albumin pool has also been noted. Acidic drugs bind mainly to albumin and decreases in protein binding as a function of age have been reported with warfarin and phenytoin. The character of protein binding seems qualitatively the same as in younger individuals. Basic drugs bind primarily to α_1-acid glycoprotein whose concentration is unchanged by age *per se* but is increased as an acute phase reactant in inflammatory disease or myocardial infarction. Concomitant renal disease and drug interactions may further alter drug-binding capacity in the elderly. Unfortunately, most pharmacokinetic studies evaluate total rather than free drug clearance, but free clearance actually determines the steady-state concentration of pharmacologically active unbound drug.

As body fat content increases with age, if a drug is highly lipid-soluble, it may become localized in body fat. Thus, the volume of distribution of drugs such as diazepam, chlorpromazine, barbiturates, and glutethimide may be increased in the elderly. Drugs distributed mainly in body water and lean body mass might have higher blood levels in the elderly, particularly if the dose is based on total body weight or surface area; examples are ethanol and lidocaine.

The decrease in cardiac output with age results in a decrease in systemic perfusion but, as noted previously, the reduction of blood flow to various organs is not symmetric; redistribution in favor of cerebral and coronary circulations takes place at the expense of flow to the kidney and liver, which are important organs in drug elimination. Likewise, the ability of a drug to pass through various membranes may ultimately affect its drug action. Increased uptake of morphine in the brain of aged rats may reflect increased permeability of the blood-brain barrier. The amount of local anesthetics needed to produce a desired level of segmental anesthesia after injection into the spinal extradural space has been found to be much less in older patients. This may be explained on the basis of age-related changes in connective tissue and increased permeability of the nerve integuments, resulting in greater drug sensitivity.

Metabolism

Animal studies have shown decreased activity in drug metabolizing enzymes which has been associated with increases in the serum levels and the intensity and duration of pharmacologic effect of some drugs. Several drugs which undergo hepatic microsomal oxidation have been reported to exhibit reduced clearances in the elderly; these include antipyrine, chlordiazepoxide, diazepam, quinidine, theophylline and nortriptyline. However, conflicting reports make some of this information difficult to interpret; important factors such as cigarette smoking and nutritional status have not been controlled adequately. A significant prolongation of the $t_{1/2}$ of acetanilid versus no age-related increase in the $t_{1/2}$ of isoniazid suggests that liver function does not decline uniformly with age and that while microsomal enzyme pathways may decrease with time, hepatic acetylation may be unaffected. Likewise, the inducibility of drug metabolizing enzymes declines with age. Thus, the effects of aging on the metabolism of a given drug is complex and difficult to predict.

Hepatic blood flow is decreased secondary to the decreased cardiac output with age. Another important component of the metabolizing capacity of the elderly may be their decreased level of activity. Compounds with high hepatic extraction ratios, such as propranolol and indocyanine green have reduced clearances in the elderly. Four-fold increases in plasma propranolol levels after a single 40 mg dose have been noted in elderly subjects, compared to young individuals.

Excretion

Altered renal function is probably the single most important factor responsible for higher drug levels in an aging population. As noted previously, renal function declines with age; on the average, the decline is approximately 1.5% per year from ages 25 to 65. Also, the serum creatinine level is not a reliable indicator of renal function in the aged. Drugs primarily excreted by the renal route and having a narrow therapeutic index, such as digoxin and the aminoglycoside antibiotics, have been shown to have higher levels in the elderly. The half-life of digoxin has been shown to increase as much as 40% in the elderly, with a decline in creatinine clearance. An important corollary is that many elderly patients are put on digitalis during transient periods of congestive heart failure, secondary to fluid overload and other factors, and then subsequently maintained on digitalis. Studies have shown that such patients can be safely withdrawn from digoxin therapy. Elderly patients are also predisposed to developing alkaline urine. This is due to decreased consumption of protein due to economic factors, with resultant decreased excretion of amino acids, and the catheterizations and other procedures in the elderly which predispose to urinary tract infections with urea-splitting organisms. The end result may be enhanced absorption of basic drugs such as the tricyclic antidepressants.

Alteration in Receptor Site Action

Receptor sites for drugs may also be altered in the elderly. A decrease in the number of CNS receptors has been postulated for some drugs. CNS stimulants show decreased activity in the elderly, while CNS depressants show increased activity. Barbiturates may be more likely to cause paradoxical stimulation in the elderly as a result. Atropine's positive chronotropic activity decreases with increasing age, which is thought to be a result of altered receptor site activity. Propranolol reduces the heart rate and cardiac output during exercise, but to a lesser extent in subjects aged 50 to 65 years, than in subjects aged 20 to 35 years. The sympathetic response of the heart elicited by the stimulus of exercise declines with age. Though the reason for this is not clear, reduced numbers of α_2 receptors on platelets and β-receptors on lymphocytes have been demonstrated in the elderly.

Geriatric Predisposition to Adverse Drug Reactions and Interactions

Various factors predispose the elderly to adverse drug reactions and drug interactions. The age-related changes in organ function previously reviewed may alter drug disposition and activity. In this regard, the side effects of digoxin, lidocaine, propranolol, tricyclic antidepressants, benzodiazepines, sedative-hypnotics, antipsychotics, aminoglycoside antibiotics, meperidine, phenytoin, and heparin have been noted more frequently in the elderly.

In addition, the elderly suffer from numerous diseases. One autopsy study showed that in 40 patients over 90 years of age, 498 pathologic lesions were identified for an average of 12.5 lesions per patient. In many cases, these lesions affected the liver or the kidney and thus had great potential effect on drug elimination. Multiple pathologies may lead to numerous patient complaints. The temptation on the part of the physician is to treat symptomatology with a large number of medications; polypharmacy is very common in the elderly.

As noted previously, patients over age 65 make up 10% of the population in the US, but the same group receives 22% of all prescription medications. Patients in long-term facilities account for the majority of such prescription use. The average nursing home patient may receive 5 to 9 medications, while some have been noted to receive as many as 16 medications concomitantly. As a result, medication errors are more common and the number of errors increases with the number and frequency of medication administration.

Thus, it is no wonder drug reactions and medication errors occur more frequently in the elderly; a 10 to 18% incidence of adverse drug reactions has been estimated in institutionalized patients. Drug-related fatalities have also been noted. The incidence of adverse effects has been correlated with age with an increased incidence in the sixth to eighth decade.

As a result of the number of drugs patients receive, the incidence of drug interactions increases. In one study, 49% of nursing home patients had the potential for at least one drug interaction. In another study of 7 nursing homes, 124 of 130 patients had a potential interaction. Chapter 102 reviews drug interactions and the reader is referred to the combinations which are common in the geriatric patient.

Thus, as general guidelines, pharmacists should try to insure that the minimal number of drugs and the lowest dosage necessary are being employed by long-term facility care prescribers. The doses the elderly require are often lower than those needed by the younger patient.

The authors extend their appreciation to Drs Brad Williams and Richard Ruffalo of the University of Southern California School of Pharmacy, Dr Ronald Kayne of the Beverly Enterprises, Inc, and Dr Samuel Kidder from the Department of Health and Human Services for their contributions, comments and reviews in updating this chapter.

CHAPTER 97

The Pharmacist and Public Health

Frederick J Spencer, MD, BS, MPH

Professor and Chairman, Department of Preventive Medicine
School of Medicine, Medical College of Virginia of the Virginia Commonwealth University
Richmond, VA 23298

Introduction

The role of the pharmacist in public health remains an enigma to many people, lay and professional. This is not surprising as public health workers have only recently welcomed the pharmacist as a colleague. Many pharmacists still fail to perceive their role as members of the community health team although increasing emphasis has been placed on this topic in education and practice.[1]

In today's shrunken world, health services must be viewed on all levels, from international to local. In mid-1984, cholera was occurring in 22 countries in the world; its incubation period is 2–3 days, and the flight time from anywhere in the world to the United States is less than 48 hours. The inference is obvious—the person asking for Kaopectate in the neighborhood pharmacy may be a cholera victim. Insularity is no longer valid in public health—it never was, but today with short travel times and an increasing number of people travelling, it is even more important to be aware of the world picture of health and disease.

Public health concerns remained dormant until cholera struck England and America in 1832, and the response to the urban environment of flies, filth, and feces produced the "Great Sanitary Awakening" of the mid-nineteenth century. The pioneers of this movement were not physicians; they were a lawyer, Edwin Chadwick (1800–1890) in Britain, and a bookseller, Lemuel Shattuck (1793–1859), in America. The "Shattuck Report" to the Massachusetts Legislature in 1850 remains to this day the classic document of American public health;[2] many of its recommendations still await promulgation. By 1900, permanent health agencies had replaced *ad hoc* boards of health on a state and local level until, by World War I, an embryonic network of health departments was in existence throughout the US. Public health programs slowly expanded as funds became available to support them; the unit to administer these programs was the city or county health department with its team of a doctor, a nurse, a sanitarian, and a clerk—still the backbone of the local health department.

Prior to World War II, traditional programs formed the bulk of public health work: disposal of sewage, provision of pure water, communicable disease control, and the care of mothers and infants, with health education as the main weapon of attack. This changed, however, with the advent of antibiotics and the expanded development of vaccines, both of which reduced the danger of infections. Chronic disease began to assume a major role in morbidity and mortality, and hospital care replaced care in the home. Comparable changes in public health accelerated as federal funding increased, until health departments today are providing an increasing amount of direct patient care in the clinic and in the home. Current inflation has reversed this trend to some extent, but all indications point to a planned, organized medical care service with emphasis on keeping people well, perhaps the forerunner of a true national health service.

Epidemiology

Health-care programs must be designed to meet the needs of the communities they serve; to do this, public health officials must know what these needs are—hence the importance of disease reporting and investigation, and the knowledge derived from it. This is epidemiology.

The science of epidemiology is the diagnosis of public health, and all pharmacists should have a knowledge of its rudiments. In essence, epidemiology deals with the determinants and occurrence of disease in defined populations and is based on the interaction of the host and his environment, with attention to those particular agents in the environment that are causal factors of the disease in question; a shorter definition is that epidemiology is medical ecology. Originating in the investigation of outbreaks of communicable disease in the nineteenth century, epidemiology is being applied increasingly to those noncommunicable, chronic diseases which are of the most significance in today's aging population—heart disease, cancer, and stroke, for example. The alert pharmacist who can apply the basic principles of epidemiology in his or her community will become a significant member of the health team as illustrated by this incident.

"On November 11, 1963, a man went into a pharmacy in New York City and asked the pharmacist for something which would relieve his complaints of fatigue and weakness. These symptoms had bothered him for about a month and had been accompanied by disturbances in vision and swallowing. He also had a dry mouth and a sore throat. He had been seen by several physicians and had received an antibiotic for an 'upper respiratory infection.' The pharmacist questioned him about his eating habits and, on learning that the patient had had some liver paste, suspected botulism. Investigation by the New York City Health Department confirmed the pharmacist's suspicion, thereby adding to the epidemiological picture of botulism which emerged into prominence in 1963. The patient recovered." [3]

This incident illustrates perhaps the most vital application of epidemiological principles by the pharmacist. The public seeks medical advice from pharmacists who quite rightly must refuse to diagnose and treat the patient's illness, but who can be of invaluable help in contributing to the knowledge of disease patterns prevalent in the neighborhood. In another field, the pharmacist can contribute extensively to the reporting of accidental poisoning and is, indeed, an expert to be used in any poison control program. It is apparent that the pharmacist should fulfill not only the role of referring the patient to a physician but also the position of collaborating epidemiologist with the local health department. It can be said that anyone can practice epidemiology, a statement illustrated by the part played in New York City in 1946 by a pest-control expert in cracking the riddle of rickettsialpox, at that time a completely new disease.[4]

Communicable Disease Control

The pattern of twentieth century disease has been shaped by the improvements in medical care, diagnosis, treatment,

Table I—Five Leading Causes of Death in 1900 and 1984 in the United States

1900	1984
1. Pneumonia	1. Diseases of the heart
2. Tuberculosis	2. Malignant neoplasms
3. Diarrhea, enteritis and ulceration of intestines	3. Cerebrovascular diseases
4. Diseases of the heart	4. Accidents
5. Intracranial lesions of vascular origin	5. Influenza and pneumonia

and prevention. The control of infectious diseases, brought about first by the environmental control of food, milk, water, and sewage, has resulted in a longer life expectancy and the emergence of the chronic diseases as the main killers in society (Table I). Heart disease, cancer, stroke, and accidents are today's leading causes of death and there is no readily foreseeable solution to their control as there was with the communicable diseases; there is also, of course, still much to be done in the surveillance and control of infections, although they are no longer lethal in most instances.

The common cold is the main cause of absenteeism in the United States, and there is no prospect of a vaccine in the near, or even distant, future; symptomatic, conservative, and common-sense measures remain the best management. The commonest *reported* infection is gonorrhea, which has reached epidemic proportions since World War II, but is only one of the many venereal, or in the current improved terminology, sexually transmitted diseases (STD), rife in society. The pharmacist is in a position to dispel much of the ignorance attached to these diseases.

The classic venereal diseases of syphilis and gonorrhea are similar in their causation but different in their natural history. Both are transmitted by sexual contact, both have causal organisms that disintegrate within seconds outside the human body, and both are susceptible to antibiotic treatment; where they differ is in their natural history. Syphilis, fortunately, remains a latent infection in two-thirds of its victims—usually with a low positive response to a serological test for syphilis, in itself a difficult diagnostic problem; the remaining one-third have systemic lesions, mostly in the cardiovascular and central nervous systems. Gonorrhea, on the other hand, manifests itself mainly in local infections in the genitourinary tract with inflammation, and sometimes abscess formation, and scarring (Table II).

The initial local lesion in syphilis—the hard chancre—will rarely come to the pharmacist's attention but the male urethral discharge produced by "clap" will often require advice. First, many urethral discharges are not gonorrhea—they are nongonococcal urethritis or prostatitis, and can be caused by many organisms and cured by specific, but different, therapies. Diagnosis by culture and microscopic examination is therefore imperative and can best be done in the local health department. A minority of men will have no discharge although infected, in opposition to women in whom 80% will not show the purulent discharge usually associated with gonorrhea. Occasionally, epidemics of venereal disease occur in both heterosexual and homosexual contacts, and the alert

pharmacist can often warn local health officials of this possibility—a sudden run on condoms should indicate the possibility of increased prostitution, or even increased activity of what have been termed "enthusiastic amateurs." This is particularly pertinent when the pharmacy is located near a school or college, or some similar institution.

Not all genital lesions are sexually transmitted, however, and they range from normal skin or mucous membrane variations to trauma, and local nonsexually transmitted infections or infestations such as scabies. In all instances, therefore, an accurate diagnosis must be made; this will be made easier when the stigma of the sexual transmission of disease is removed and public education in venereal disease becomes the same as for any other disease. Again, the pharmacist's role in public education cannot be overemphasized—but it must be by an informed pharmacist who knows the natural history of the sexually transmitted diseases and can therefore judge the efficacy of the advice he offers. It is also ineffective to have a few pamphlets lying in a rack—active distribution to appropriate customers with a few well chosen words will be more telling. One of the best opportunities for health education is when a customer is waiting for a prescription to be filled and has nothing to do but stand, or sit, and wait.

One sexually transmitted disease of current concern is herpes genitalis, which is usually seen as a series of blisters on an inflamed background anywhere in the genital area. In actual fact, the causal virus is closely associated with the cold sore, or oral herpes simplex virus, and treatment is just as ineffective; in itself, herpes genitalis is an unpleasant, innocuous and recurrent nuisance except in those newborn infants infected during delivery—hence the practice of delivering women with active herpes of the genitals by cesarean section. There is also an unproven association of herpes genitalis and cancer of the cervix which has received undue publicity, although it is prudent at present for women with herpes genitalis to have Pap smears more often than those without—six months to a year being a reasonable time interval. The recent use of Acyclovir in treating genital herpes has limited value but the possibility of a vaccine being produced is closer to reality.

Immunization has controlled the childhood infections of measles, mumps, rubella, poliomyelitis, diphtheria, and whooping cough. Pharmacists should obtain immunization schedules from health departments and advise parents of the importance of adhering to the times recommended therein. Where mass community clinics are the accepted and best way of bringing immunization to the public, the pharmacist is the obvious person to bear the responsibility of obtaining, storing, and preparing the vaccine for administration—this method has been most successful in community immunization programs with oral poliomyelitis vaccine. One other practical aspect of cooperation between the pharmacist and the local health department is an agreement to supply vaccine for immediate or urgent administration, with the understanding that it will be replaced as soon as it can be obtained from the central health department supply; this has been particularly effective in administering rabies antiserum and vaccine to individual patients where a delay will occur in receiving the vaccine from the state health department. The pharmacist will often have many vaccines in stock for use by private

Table II—Common Sexually Transmitted Diseases

	Gonorrhea	Syphilis	Herpes Simplex
Causal Organism	*Gonococcus*	*Treponema pallidum*	Herpes simplex virus
Incubation Period (approx)	6 days	3 weeks	10 days
Initial Manifestation	Urethral discharge	Hard chancre (sore)	Blister(s)
Late Manifestations	Local	Systemic	None
Diagnosis	Smear	Microscopic & blood	Clinical & viral studies
Treatment	Penicillin	Penicillin	Acyclovir

physicians which local health departments need only on an occasional basis and, therefore, do not stock routinely.

The control of communicable disease is based on adequate case finding and the supervision and prophylactic treatment of close contacts.

An indispensable reference book should be in each pharmacy—*The Control of Communicable Diseases in Man*, published by the American Public Health Association and frequently revised (the 1981 edition cost $7.50 and is as good as, or even better than, texts costing many times as much). This publication summarizes, in a concise format, all known communicable diseases, and can be referred to if in doubt about the etiology and control of any disease, from the most common to the rarest exotic importation.

In addition, pharmacists who wish to keep abreast of current communicable disease patterns should subscribe to the *Morbidity and Mortality Weekly Report* (*MMWR*) of the Centers for Disease Control (CDC) of the United States Public Health Service (write to US Department of Health and Human Services, Public Health Service, Centers for Disease Control, Atlanta, Georgia 30333). This publication is copied by the publishers of the *New England Journal of Medicine* and may be obtained at a considerably reduced cost by subscribing through the Massachusetts Medical Society, PO Box 9120, Waltham MA 02254-9120. The *MMWR* has epidemiologic notes and reports of outbreaks of disease, and current statistics by disease and geographical location at home and abroad, of which all health professionals should keep informed.

Pharmacists more than any professional group will become aware of epidemic infectious diseases in a community. The arrival of an unusual number of people with diarrheal disease for over-the-counter products may be the result of an outbreak of foodborne disease. The monitoring of numbers and types of prescriptions, even in an unscientific way, often suffices to point to an epidemic, and the interested pharmacist can set up a monitoring system of more scientific validity.

In summary, the role of the pharmacist in the control of communicable diseases consists of an awareness of the natural history of these diseases in both the individual and the community, referral of clients to medical-care facilities where indicated, and public education of an informed type at all times. It is possibly in this aspect of community disease control that the pharmacist can play his or her greatest part.

Global Health

Isolationism was a characteristic American trait until World War II, but today the people of the United States are only too well aware of the shrunken world beyond their shores. Nowadays, the appearance of an exotic disease in any part of this country is a common event and the pharmacist should have an understanding of the complexity of diseases encountered in international travel. This does not mean, of course, that the pharmacist should be concerned with the differential diagnosis and treatment of schistosomiasis or kala azar but he or she should know that both of these diseases have been reported by travellers returning to America and thus be aware of the possibility of their occurrence.

One of the most important questions a pharmacist can ask a client who wants advice about a personal disease is that posed by Roman legionnaires to their colleagues—unde venis? (where have you come from?); certainly a routine question in all suspect illnesses should be to ask whether the client has been abroad in the past two years. By international agreement there are today only three diseases to which quarantine regulations apply—cholera, plague, and yellow fever (Table III)—but during the past 15 years, many exotic diseases have been reported by the Centers for Disease Control (CDC) of the Public Health Service— schistosomiasis, loiasis, malaria, kala azar, dengue, leishmaniasis, giardiasis, trypanosomiasis, and innumerable worm infestations.[5] It is therefore imperative for the pharmacist to ask clients where they have been and to ensure that the information elicited is relayed to the physician if medical consultation is sought. The World Health Organization (WHO) is the only official international health organization, and its 156 member nations, apart from reporting disease trends, control many aspects of international health through an annual budget of some $225,000,000 (25% of which comes from the USA and 13% from the USSR). One WHO program is of particular significance to pharmacy—the international standardization of immunological agents such as measles and other vaccines, and toxoids. Today, the United States does not require any immunizations of persons entering the country, wherever they have been or whatever diseases they have been exposed to. Pharmacists can be of invaluable assistance to international travellers in advising them what to take in the way of medications, especially for malaria and traveller's diarrhea, whose ubiquity is evident from its synonyms of Montezuma's Revenge, the Casablanca Crud, Delhi Belly, and even San Franciscitis!

Information on the traveller's "medical chest" is available in several publications and will generally include a broad-spectrum antibiotic, Bandaids, remedies for travel sickness, aspirin, thermometer, antibiotic cream, etc. Immunizations must be up-to-date and, again, a Public Health Service CDC publication provides this information in *Health Information for International Travel*. Referral to the local health de-

Table III—Global Health

	Quarantinable Diseases		
	Cholera	Plague	Yellow Fever
Causal Organism	*Vibrio cholerae*	*Yersinia pestis*	Yellow fever virus
Incubation Period (approx)	2–3 days	2–6 days	3–6 days
Transmission	Fecal-oral	Flea bite	Mosquito bite
Natural Foci	Asia	Worldwide	Central Africa, South America

This Shrunken World and Wanderlust
Americans Abroad

1950	1960	1970	1975	1980
676,000	1,634,000	5,260,000	6,354,000	8,163,000

Flying Times (Hrs)

New York to		San Francisco to	
London	New Delhi	Tokyo	Hong Kong
3	14	11	14

partment may be easier for those pharmacists who have neither the time nor the interest themselves, and, in any event, it should produce the most recent information; it is wise, however, for pharmacists to retain some degree of interest in travellers' requirements, if only as a public service. Finally, a word about malaria prophylaxis—it is imperative to begin medication 1 week before travel and to continue it for 6 weeks after return from a malarial part of the world if the suppressant (usually chloroquine phosphate) is to be of maximum benefit. A recent increase in strains of *Plasmodia falciparum* resistant to chloroquine phosphate necessitates the addition of other prophylactic drugs such as pyrimethamine–sulfadoxine in some parts of the world.

Disease Prevention

Chronic disease has become the prime target of epidemiological and basic laboratory research. Heart disease has recently and comfortingly shown a slight decrease as a cause of death, the reasons remaining obscure despite claims that it has resulted from a change in diet, more exercise, less smoking, and earlier treatment of hypertension—the last reason being the one with most scientific validity. In all probability, the human machine is beginning to adapt to the change in environmental factors which have come into prominence with modern technology—but proof for this, as with causal factors, remains to be seen. Certainly, man has managed to adapt to disease patterns in previous epochs and it would not be unusual to see history repeating itself in the twentieth century.

Prevention is of three kinds—primary, secondary, and tertiary. Primary prevention is health maintenance—keeping people well. The best example of primary prevention has already been discussed—the control of infections by immunization. Equally important, however, are the many factors of health now generally included under the catchall of "lifestyle," and there is evidence that following certain health practices leads to longevity, eg, not smoking, limiting alcohol consumption, controlling weight, sleeping 7–8 hours a night, being physically active, eating breakfast, and not eating between meals have recently been cited as desirable habits. In summary, the old saw of "moderation in all things" would seem to be a good dictum to observe. The aim of primary prevention is to modify "lifestyles" to the benefit of the individual and, of course, ultimately to the community—a task easier done on paper than in the flesh; time will tell whether the current enthusiasm of the newcomers to this popular way of thinking will be justified.

Secondary prevention is the early diagnosis and treatment of already existing disease and is best illustrated by the use of penicillin in the treatment of streptococcal infections, thereby preventing the occurrence of the much more dangerous rheumatic fever, a disease that "licks the joints but bites the heart." There is no more vital service that a pharmacist can perform than seeing that a child or adolescent receives a complete examination, including a throat culture, if he or she presents with a febrile illness characterized by a sore throat. In no other disease is the old saying that an ounce of prevention is worth a pound of cure more true—although, in this instance, the few cents of prevention by using penicillin is more apropos.

Tertiary prevention is really rehabilitation. Most chronic diseases cannot be cured, but their progress can be retarded with maximum benefit to the patient. Much can be done, for instance, with rheumatoid arthritis to make its victims more comfortable and more productive in their daily lives. It is in these diseases that the challenge to the pharmacist can be taxed to the utmost in his or her knowledge, and use, of individual therapy and community resources.

Chronic Disease Control

The pharmacist can encourage clients to avail themselves of the few proven techniques in chronic disease prevention. Good living habits never did anyone any harm although their degree of positive protective value is still questionable, and they have been recommended as methods of preventing disease, particularly heart disease. Cancer, however is not prevented by these measures and, in general, must be dealt with by early diagnosis and treatment; a few techniques such as the Pap smear serve as specific preventive methods but, in general, secondary prevention is the main point of attack. The pharmacist, therefore, should be acquainted with the warning signals of cancer and advise any client who exhibits them to seek medical advice immediately. Local cancer societies will be only too pleased to provide health education literature for professional and public education.

The prevention of strokes is largely concerned with the control of high blood pressure and the revolution in therapy within the past ten years has probably resulted in the lower death rates from cerebrovascular disease. The pharmacist can, of course, take clients' blood pressure readings, but these may be temporarily high or low, and must, therefore, be followed by at least two more measurements at later dates. The whole question of monitoring the public's blood pressure is fraught with danger, and local medical societies and heart associations should be consulted for advice. Nevertheless, the pharmacist is in an unique position to advise on and, where indicated, measure clients' blood pressure with the added rider that he or she must also educate them about its normal variations. As the basis of hypertensive therapy is with drugs, the pharmacist should be in the forefront of monitoring their application in his clients, especially in encouraging compliance with prescribed regimens.

The many other chronic diseases all require comparable approaches if they are to be controlled. In the main, secondary and tertiary prevention—that is early diagnosis and treatment, and rehabilitation—are the main control measures in chronic disease and the pharmacist should be well acquainted with the services that offer diagnosis, treatment, and rehabilitation in the community.

The fourth most common cause of death in the United States today is accidents. Although there are few specific things that can be done to prevent accidents, such as the use of automobile seat belts, the pharmacist should be the leader in the control of accidental poisoning. In small communities, the pharmacist should be the prime consultant for advice in poisoning cases and should be able to refer the caller to the nearest poison control or information center if unable to deal with the matter personally. In addition, the pharmacist should be the leader in disseminating information about poisoning and other educational services in the community or neighborhood.

Closely allied to accidental poisoning is deliberate poisoning of the body which is so common today—what is called substance abuse. Drugs, including alcohol, have become an everyday topic of conversation and much misinformation has been distributed about them. Again, the expert knowledge of the pharmacist should be used to good advantage in both an individual and community context. Along with the toxins of self-administered drugs go the many industrial toxins now being encountered with new technology. It is imperative that the pharmacist be aware of the dangers arising from industrial toxins and be alert to their manifestations in clients who seek relief in over-the-counter symptomatic medicines.

In summary, the control of chronic disease can range from the support of proven community programs such as screening clinics for cancer to an alertness for the first signs of disease associated with an occupational hazard. The pharmacist is unique in having a basic understanding of disease processes and in being in daily contact with members of the public on an informal, yet professional, basis. His or her ability, therefore, to intervene in the initial stages of illness in chronic disease is unparalleled and should be avidly seized. Another, and perhaps more significant, area of control is in health education.

Health Education

There is perhaps no aspect of public health more praised than health education although concrete proof of its overall effectiveness is singularly lacking. Certainly no other country in the world pays such lip service to health education from the primary school through college into adulthood but, despite this, the American adult is overweight, smokes too many cigarettes, commits too many crimes, drinks too much alcohol, and abuses himself in many other ways. There is currently a popular emphasis on changing what are called "life-styles," but how to do this, and whether the result will be beneficial, is still unclear. Take exercise as an example; the current craze for running and jogging is laudable for those who enjoy it, but there is no proof that it achieves its stated object, ie, to improve the circulatory system with subsequent delay of the pathological variations that lead to disease. No doubt those who run derive considerable virtue from their pastime but whether it will do more for them than this is unproven.

The techniques of health education consist of publicizing health data through the local media, whether spoken or written—a process recently entitled health information to distinguish it from the behavior modification which is the objective of health education proper. The use of illustrative material and catchy phrasing is all part of success, but the presentation of advice does not mean that it will be followed—which is the ultimate and only aim of health education. Pharmacists have unwittingly promoted health education through advertising, some of which was questionable in years gone by when promoted by unscrupulous business enterprises. Today, however, advertising codes have largely eliminated false claims; thus, the pharmacist has a wonderful opportunity to bring correct and valuable information to clients. But more than this can be done—the pharmacist can actively promote good health practices by personal example and by reaching out to impart professional information to the public whom he or she serves. The ideal of public service which is strong at the beginning of a pharmacy student's career unfortunately becomes dulled by time and the demands of work, but if the pharmacist can keep the innate feeling for humans untarnished, more in the way of health education will be done than by all the movies made for that purpose.

Formal methods of health education have their place in public health, but in the pharmacy the informed direction of members of the public is a much more realistic approach. Certainly, participation of pharmacists in community health education programs must be recommended, but it is in the everyday person-to-person contact with people that the pharmacist serves most effectively. To display pamphlets with health information is an admirable move but it is substantially better to add to this verbal instruction and encouragement. This does not mean that every customer needs counselling, but there are always people who can benefit from a few words of advice on health matters. Too often, the pharmacist remains a figure in a white coat occasionally seen behind and above the service counter. The keynote of a pharmacist's health educational service is an informed awareness of the early signs and symptoms of the major diseases of society and a conscientious willingness to pass this information on to those members of the public who require it. Assistance in this matter should be sought from official and voluntary health agencies, remembering that these groups have certain basic differences—of governance, financial support, legal responsibilities, and primary aim. In general, official agencies are governed by appointed officials, supported by taxes to provide direct services to the public, and are somewhat limited by law in what they can do. Voluntary agencies have greater flexibility to experiment with and support new programs, and have no responsibility in law for enforcement (Table IV). The sequence of events has often been that a philanthropic group forms a voluntary agency which demonstrates a need and, once this has been done, transfers the program to an official agency for direct service purposes.[6] One of the best examples of this succession is in the Lung Association as it stands in today's health care program—although there has been some blurring of this distinction recently with federal support of all agencies, voluntary and official. Nevertheless, it is important for the pharmacist to understand the basic origins and differences of these agencies if he or she is to work intelligently with them and the public they serve.

Medical Care

The most pressing matter in medical care today is its high cost. The rapid and alarming increase in costs has become a matter of personal and national concern, and it is the federal government's avowed intent to regulate costs by any means at its disposal.

There are three main methods of payment for physician and other health services: (1) Direct payment, where the physician is paid directly by the patient. (2) Indirect (third-party) payment, where the physician is paid by someone representing the patient (i.e., a third party, the patient and the physician being the first and second parties). (3) Salaried payment, where the physician is a salaried member of the government.

In the United States today, most medical care is provided through third-party indirect payments, usually of a voluntary insurance nature, but with increasing government participation. The trend in the 1960s and 1970s has been towards the federal provision of more and more dollars for direct patient care—possibly a forerunner of some type of national health program. This will, of course, depend upon the prevailing political climate of the electorate. The United States remains the only country in the world in which a government health service is not a reality, and indications point towards a change within the coming years. Most so-called health insurance is sickness insurance, ie, payment is made for treating illness, not for keeping people well. The Blue Cross-Blue Shield, and commercial and government insurance, programs provide limited diagnostic and treatment services for most US citizens, either through group or individual premium payments. In

Table IV—Characteristics of Agencies

	Official	Nonofficial
Basic Financing	Taxes	Donations, gifts, fund drives, endowments
Management	Government bureaucracy	Board of trustees or directors
Legal Status	Law enforcement	No legal responsibility
Program Emphasis	Provision of services	Educational programs
Innovations	Limited by rigidity	Aided by flexibility
Research	Unrestricted	Unrestricted

addition, the federal programs of Medicare and Medicaid pay for elderly and indigent patients respectively. Uniformity, however, is lacking in many of these programs, with local variation being the rule and not the exception.

Recently, a renewed interest has occurred in prepaid health plans from the standpoint of both preventing disease and curtailing costs. The federal government fostered this interest in the 1970's by promoting its version of prepaid medical care through Health Maintenance Organizations (HMOs)—an example now being followed by industry and private enterprise.

The basic principle of a prepaid health plan is that it provides all health services, in or out of hospital, for an annually negotiated premium. The prototype of this method of health care is the Kaiser Permanente program in California.[7] The incentive to keep people well is reflected in the decrease in hospitalization of the prepaid plan members with a consequent increase in money retained by the plan at the end of the fiscal year. Repeated surveys have shown that members of prepaid plans do indeed enter hospital less often and stay less time when they are admitted. Recently, industries have become interested in prepaid plans and indeed have started plans of their own.

The ultimate decision to be reached in the United States today is whether compulsory insurance should replace voluntary insurance, and what proportion of government participation is appropriate to either method. The evolution of health insurance in the United States has seen to it that many citizens already have government-financed medical care: the armed forces and their dependents, veterans, and those covered by Medicare and Medicaid—and the President of the United States! The major component of government medicine is however in two programs—Medicare and Medicaid, which became law in 1965 as Titles XVIII and XIX of the Social Security Act (Table V).

Medicare is designed to pay for costs of medical care in people who are at least 65 years old. The two parts of the program are designed, in the main, to provide institutional and home care, and medical services wherever the patient may be. Everyone is eligible to participate on reaching the age of 65 and the program is financed and administered by the federal government.

Provision for services by all types of health personnel is made, although a monthly premium must be paid by the recipient, and only a percentage of most of the bills will be paid by Medicare. Care in the home is encouraged by paying for skilled nursing visits. Home health services have received much publicity recently, and every indication is that they are becoming an increasingly significant part of health care.

Ill people should be cared for in three, and only three, places—in an institution, in an ambulatory care setting, or at home. Anyone requiring twenty-four hours a day care should be in an institution, usually a hospital or nursing home. The majority of people with disease can, fortunately, be taken care of in an ambulatory care facility—a clinic or office. There is, however, a sizeable group of patients who do not need continuous care and yet who are unable to walk or ride to an outpatient clinic or office; these people need care in the home. There is a lack of awareness and understanding of the avail-

ability and variety of services available for patient care in the home; various estimates have placed from 5%–25% of patients in hospitals and nursing homes as being able to benefit from home care, which has the advantages of economy and familiarity to the patient. One of the greatest contributions pharmacists can make to cost containment is to become acquainted with the home-health services in the community and to promote their use by professional health worker and layman alike.

Medicaid differs from Medicare in that it has no age restriction and is not financed solely by federal funds, each state participating in its support and administration. Medicaid actually has replaced four categorical programs which were operational before 1965—Old Age Assistance, Aid to the Blind, Aid to the Totally and Permanently Disabled, and Aid to Dependent Children. In addition, Medicaid is designed to pay for medical care to the "medically needy"—a group of people who cannot afford to pay for medical care although they may or may not be able to pay for other goods and services. States differ in their eligibility requirements and payments, and also in matters of administration, and pharmacists should obtain information on their state Medicaid program from the appropriate state office.[8]

There has been less talk recently of national health insurance although there will almost certainly be further attempts to introduce some form of this method of care. The form it will take is still debatable—literally debatable—and summaries of proposals may be obtained from government and professional associations. It is unlikely that any drastic change in the current health-care system will ensue unless there is a change in government, which at present leans towards private enterprise and away from government control.

Health Planning

If there is to be a national health insurance program, there must be a national health plan on which it is based. The emphasis on planning for health care is far from new, but it is only within the past 25 years that it has received recognition in this country. The first concerted effort towards planning came with the passage of the federal Comprehensive Health Planning Act (Public Law 89-749) in 1966 which supported national, state, and regional planning bodies. Implementation of the act, however, was difficult because of local differences in enthusiasm and in funding, and in 1974 the National Health Planning and Resources Development Act (Public Law 93-641) replaced it. This legislation has already had a considerable influence on the provision of medical care and was designed to encourage, and indeed enforce, planning for health care at all levels of the nation. Overall, there is a National Health Planning Council appointed by the President which sets the policy through Congress for implementation of local planning in Health Service Areas administered by Health Systems Agencies (HSAs). The HSAs are the fundamental local units for health planning and they advise, direct, and supervise the provision of health services in populations of several hundred thousand people, not necessarily confined by state boundaries. Depending upon their legislative powers, they have the right to review, comment upon, and, in many instances, approve or disapprove new health services or changes in existing health services. HSAs deal with *all* health and medical care services, and it is therefore wise for pharmacists to become acquainted with, and active in, their deliberations. Representation from the pharmacy profession is encouraged, if not required, on the local HSA boards and also on the State Coordinating Councils which act in an advisory capacity in each state. The need for planning to conserve the health resources we have is an obvious move and is echoed by the increasing interest of lay groups in medical care.

Table V—Medicare and Medicaid

	Medicare	Medicaid
Social Security Act	Title XVIII	Title XIX
Age Limit	65 yr or more	None
Eligibility	All if of age	Differs by state
Funding	Federal	Federal & state
Benefits	Uniform	Varies with state
Administration	Federal	State

The HSAs recognize this trend by requiring that a majority of the HSA Board of Directors must be consumers.

Health Services Programs

Health departments in general provide a wide spectrum of services to the public; it must be remembered that the time-honored term for these services is "public health." Too often, public health has the connotation of health care for the poor; in reality, public health services are supported by taxes and are available to, and should be used by, *all* members of the public.

The local health department is a product of the twentieth century. *Ad hoc* local boards of health have existed since the Black Death ravaged Europe in the fourteenth century, but the first permanent county health department in America was not formed until the early years of the twentieth century. The primary aim of public health services at that time was to control communicable disease by enforcing sanitary codes which eliminated contamination of food, water, and milk by human excreta. With the advent of immunization, community programs in disease prevention with immunological agents began and, gradually, more personal health services were added to official health agency programs—maternal and child health, and crippled children, for example. The chief provider of these services was, and still is, the public health nurse—even today in many local areas, the main, and only, focus of personal health services in the community. It is a wise pharmacist who knows the local public health nurses and the multitude of services they can provide his or her clients.

Most local health departments today are affiliated in varying degree with their state health department. In those states with adequate local coverage, the state health department acts in a consultant capacity but in the more sparsely settled states, and in those with weak local services, direct services are often provided by personnel from the state central office. The state may, in turn, call upon federal health consultants for advice and assistance, but the federal government, in general, cannot encroach on the right of the state to determine its own health policies. Interestingly, all federal health legislation is based on the one phrase in the Preamble to the Constitution which says that the federal government has the right to act to "promote the general welfare." It is from these few words that the immense authority of the federal government in health matters is derived.

The state, therefore, has sovereign rights in guarding the health of its inhabitants. Typically, the programs of a local health department are administered by the basic public health team of a physician, a public health nurse, a sanitarian, and a clerk. The physician, who will usually have a higher degree in public health, is responsible for the overall program of the department, with or without the assistance of an administrator. The public health nurse provides the bulk of the personal health services, both in clinics and in the home, and spends her time dealing with the care of people ranging from the newborn infant to the aged chronic invalid—her primary concern being to apply the principles of prevention to her patients and to promote health, or to retard the progress of disease where a return to health is not possible. The sanitarian is responsible for the control of disease by environmental techniques and is following the grand line of the nineteenth century's "Great Sanitary Awakening" in reviewing the environment in its many intricate interrelationships with society and its constituent members. The clerk, of course, remains at the center of the health department's activities, and stores, files and retrieves the ever increasing morass of records required by today's litigious society. Scant justice is accorded to the indispensable clerk and, indeed, to any of the members of the public health team who perform their work unheralded and unsung in most communities. Again, pharmacists should become acquainted with their local health department and its wide range of services and avail themselves of these services whenever the need arises.

Maternal and Child Health

The health of the mother and child—maternal and child health as it is generally called—was the first public health program of the twentieth century. Infant and child mortality rates were exceptionally high, largely because of respiratory and diarrheal diseases; many of the latter were propagated by unclean milk, an ideal medium for bacterial proliferation. The first move to combat this disgrace to the nation came in the form of "milk stations" where clean milk was provided to mothers and their children. Gradually the concept of maternal and child health expanded from this environmental beginning to the formation of programs where direct patient care and advice could be dispensed both in the clinic and at home. No public health program has proved its worth more than the care of the mother and child.

The basic idea behind maternal and child health is to shepherd the mother and her child through the time when they are exposed to the greatest risks of disease and death—during pregnancy, the puerperium, and the first year of life. The early diagnosis of pregnancy, with informed supervision of its progress through delivery and the immediate postpartum period, constitutes the bulwark of care in maternal and child health programs. The earlier that prenatal care is given, the more beneficial is the effect not only to the mother but also to the child, as the health of the infant is directly influenced by its care *in utero*. Consequently, the pharmacist who understands the normal course of pregnancy and infancy is at a distinct advantage to one who does not, as he or she can guide the mother in simple matters of the hygiene and management of her pregnancy, and of her infant. This applies particularly to those women who, through lack of education and other social advantages, have an incomplete understanding of how important it is to have early, professional prenatal care. In addition, the ability of the pharmacist to discuss contraceptive methods intelligently will be a signal service to women in the postpartum phase of their pregnancies or preferably earlier.

Nature has designed the mother to take care of her newborn infant—in many parts of the world she still does this by breast feeding and keeping the baby warm and safe by cuddling it to her body, especially where the climate is tropical. In our society, however, we have produced an artificial environment in which the majority of babies do not receive the food designed for them—that is, their mother's milk. Breast feeding is still the best food for the baby and should be encouraged by the pharmacist whenever possible. One aspect of disease control in the infant, however, which must be supplied by someone other than the mother is protection by immunization, especially in the so-called diseases of childhood; it is paramount that all infants, irrespective of color, creed, or income should be immunized with all the toxoids and vaccines available to help them through the dangerous first few years of childhood. Primary immunization should begin at the age of two months and is not complete until the fourth dose of triple vaccine (diphtheria, tetanus, pertussis) is given at eighteen months (Table VI).

Population Control

In the realm of maternal and child health, no programs have more significance than those pertaining to population control. Worldwide, the alarming increase in population is the most serious public health problem. Although in a land of plenty like the United States it might seem that population control

Table VI—Immunization Schedule

	Age in Months					Age in Years	
	2	4	6	15	18	4–6	14–16
Diphtheria-Tetanus-Pertussis (DTP)	X	X	X		X	X	
Polio (Oral Trivalent)	X	X			X	X	
Measles				X			
Rubella				X			
Mumps				X			
Tetanus-Diphtheria, Adult (Td)							X

is of minor significance, the amount of tax dollars required to support unwanted children is immense. Family planning, as population control is usually called in the western countries, consists not only in spacing births by deliberate contraceptive use but also in helping the few women who cannot conceive to bear children—in proportion, by far the lesser problem of the two except to a barren woman and her consort or spouse. Although abortion is now legal, it is quite obviously the most unsatisfactory way of determining family size—it is far better to prevent conception than to eliminate its products. Contraceptives are obtained from local pharmacies and it is therefore pharmacists who are in the front line of family planning. Whatever they can do to spread the gospel of birth control should be done within the confines of their consciences.

Health Measurement

In general, the pharmacist has been neglected as a dynamic member of the health team, being relegated, in the eyes of many health professionals, to the role of a dispenser of medicines and other products sold in drug stores. The fact that the pharmacist is the health professional in most frequent contact with the general public is often forgotten; it is this propensity and function as a health educator that makes the pharmacist unique.

As that percipient Prime Minister of England, Benjamin Disraeli, is reported to have said, "There are three kinds of lies—lies, damned lies, and statistics." [9] No pharmacist, however, can ignore statistics, particularly those pertaining to health and disease, however formidable or annoying it may be to wrestle with them. In actual fact, a few basic formulae and their application is all that is necessary—but without them, community health services and practice are meaningless.

All events that are measurable must be related to the population in which they occur—usually known as the population at risk; obviously, to compare the actual number of births in Pittsburgh with those in Podunk is valueless, the difference in population being too great. In other words, the events to be measured must be reduced to a common factor of population—usually, for the sake of convenience, a multiple of ten. This device merely produces a manageable number instead of a fraction, or one preceded by a decimal point. As an example, consider live births. Say that, in 1977 there were 50 births in a population of 1000 people; this means that there were 0.05 births per person—which is ridiculous. By saying that there were 5 births per 100 people, or that the birth rate was 5 percent, we come up with a workable figure instead of 0.05 births per person. In actual fact, birth rates usually are computed per thousand of population.

The basic formula for a rate of any type is therefore

$$\text{Rate} = \frac{\text{number of events measured}}{\text{population at risk}} \times k$$

where k is a constant and multiple of ten.

The crude birth rate is what it says—a *crude* measurement of births, as the population at risk includes all the men, women, and children in the geographical area of concern—most of whom are incapable of bearing children. A more accurate measurement would be to confine the population at risk to women—a sex specific rate; but only the women in the child-bearing age group can have babies so a further refinement would be to confine the population at risk to women between the ages of 15 and 44 years—an age/sex specific rate. This is a much more accurate measurement of births and is known as the fertility rate.

Death rates follow the same pattern as birth rates—ranging from the crude death rate to age and sex specific rates; the most commonly used as an indicator of health services being the infant death (or mortality) rate. This age-specific rate measures the number of deaths occurring in infants below the age of one year and is often used as an indicator of the effectiveness of a nation's health services, the implication being that the care of the mother and baby reflects the availability and efficiency of medical care; this use is certainly questionable but it remains the only readily available rate for worldwide comparative purposes.

Earlier in this century the maternal mortality rate—a sex specific rate—was useful for comparative data but it is now so low in the Western World that it has become useless by dint of the small number of deaths that occur in pregnant women because of better medical care.

Further refinement of rates occurs when particular problems become evident in a community and the measurement of trends becomes necessary. The rise in illegitimacy is a case in point, especially as illegitimate infants have a higher mortality rate than babies born in wedlock. The increase in illegitimate births since World War II has been dramatic, with a proportionally greater rise in white than black populations. The stigma which still attaches to illegitimacy casts some doubt on the validity of the figures but the adverse effect on the infant is apparent. As most of the babies at risk are indigent and are therefore cared for by local health departments, it is again imperative for the pharmacist to keep informed of these programs and contribute what he can to them (Table VII).

Nutrition

The outcry against "fast foods" and "junk foods" has brought nutrition into the public eye as no concerted effort on the part of nutritionists and health educators could have done. In actual fact, many "fast foods" have nutritional value—but generally only if supplemented by the elements commonly missing from their composition. In theory, a hamburger with lettuce, tomato, and French fried potatoes contains a balance of protein, fat, and carbohydrate which can be beneficial if the food used in their preparation is nutritious to begin with, ie, if the hamburger is pure lean ground beef and the other foods are of comparable value. In general, however, this type of diet lacks the basic food elements present in fresh fruits and vegetables and, unfortunately, the people to whom "fast foods" appeal seldom bother to obtain these staples. Allied to nutrition is dental health and most health

Table VII—Commonly Used Rates

$$\text{Crude Birth Rate} = \frac{\text{Number of live births}}{\text{Total population}} \times 1,000$$

$$\text{Fertility Rate} = \frac{\text{Number of live births}}{\text{Total number of women aged 15-44 years}} \times 1,000$$

$$\text{Crude Death Rate} = \frac{\text{Number of deaths}}{\text{Total population}} \times 1,000$$

$$\text{Infant Mortality Rate} = \frac{\text{Number of deaths less than one year of age}}{\text{Number of live births}} \times 1,000$$

$$\text{Maternal Mortality Rate} = \frac{\text{Number of deaths associated with pregnancy}}{\text{Number of live births}} \times 10,000$$

$$\text{Illegitimacy Ratio} = \frac{\text{Number of illegitimate births}}{\text{Number of live births}} \times 100$$

departments have access to dental services to which medically needy persons should be referred.

Obesity is the commonest form of malnutrition in this country today. Starvation *per se* is almost nonexistent in the Western World but its corollary of fatness is common; one-third of adults, for instance, are calculated to be at least 15–20% overweight. Despite this, fashion advertising still emphasizes the skeletal, equine figure of the *haute couture* model as its symbol. Unless there is some marked glandular disorder in one of the endocrine organs, people become fat by taking in more calories than they are putting out, although there is no doubt that individual metabolic processes enable some people to deal more efficiently than others with this intake–output system. The prevalence of obesity is evident when the best-seller booklists reveal that, year after year, authors are making money from readers desperately trying to slim; that they don't succeed is also evident by the constant appearance of some new diet fad and book. The correlation of obesity with poor health is well established but, like smoking, it is beyond the power of most fat people to stop eating until some catastrophic event occurs, such as a heart attack, when they will dismally restrict their food intake. There are, of course, many people who voluntarily lose weight when in good health but the trend in these people is to put it on again within a year or two. As a practical point, it has been shown that people lose weight better in groups—when they have encouragement, and also competition, from their peers. The proliferation of "health spas" testifies to this dictum. Hence, the pharmacist can acquaint himself with the local organizations aimed to helping men and women (and children) to lose weight: Weight Watchers, TOPS (Take Off Pounds Safely), and the many other programs such as those offered by the YMCA and the YWCA. In addition to this, the popular notion that there are magic drugs which will control weight may be dispelled with authority by the pharmacist, and nutritional education and guidance offered through the many materials available from voluntary organizations, and local and state health departments.

Environmental Health

Modern society is suffering physically and emotionally from the technology it has created. The four basic necessities of health—air, water, food, and shelter—are all elements of the environment which, in their natural state, have only beneficial effects. To call shelter, whether in the form of personal clothing or housing, an element of nature may seem far-fetched—but the origin of clothes and houses was in skins and wood derived from nature.

Today, society has bent many aspects of nature to its will with harmful results. Air, for instance, now contains noxious substances which are either directly the result of combustion or produced by photochemical change. The classic example of the latter is the famous Los Angeles "smog" (a word first coined from "smoke and fog" in 1905) which results from the interaction of ultraviolet rays in sunshine and unburnt hydrocarbons of automobile engines. The products, when trapped by the thermal inversion engendered by local topography, cause damage to human mucous membranes as well as flowers and many other man-made commodities—nylons, paint, and tires to name three. What the long-term danger is from this intermittent pollution we do not yet know; what we do know is that acute episodes of air pollution cause exacerbation of illness and even death in people who already have diseased respiratory and cardiovascular systems. The most famous of these catastrophes was in Donora, Pennsylvania, in 1948 when there were twenty deaths during a six-day period of air stagnation. The close correlation of disease with age, and in persons whose heart and lungs were already compromised, became immediately evident during the investigation. Similar major episodes have occurred in Belgium and London, and minor disturbances have been reported in several cities in the United States and elsewhere. People with heart or lung disease should stay indoors if air pollution is present or even forecast.

Of more significance than air as a vehicle of disease organisms in this century is food, including milk. Fortunately, pasteurization has virtually eliminated milk as a medium for disease distribution but the same cannot be said for food. Foodborne disease, more commonly but often incorrectly termed food poisoning, is grossly underreported and the four to five hundred outbreaks comprising some five to ten thousand persons per year can probably be multiplied by ten to represent the true magnitude of this common affliction. In most instances the illness produced by contaminated food is mild and of short duration but more severe diseases such as botulism can occur. The central packaging and distribution of food and the enormous increase in the number of people eating away from their homes have both contributed to the renewed interest in this minor but distressing group of diseases. Controls extend from the place of food production to the time of consumption and are, in general, simple, effective, and inexpensive, particularly in the home—"keep hot food hot, and cold food cold" is perhaps the most significant one-liner in the control of foodborne disease. If all food is maintained at temperatures below 45°F or above 140°F, many outbreaks of foodborne disease will be prevented.

Waterborne infectious disease is uncommon today although some 16,000 persons were infected with *Salmonella typhimurium* from a common California water supply.[10] This does not mean, however, that all public water supplies are pure and potable; many complaints about the taste, appearance, and physical qualities of locally supplied water have led to a brisk trade in bottled water. In general, the virtues of bottled water have been inflated as most public supplies are bacteriologically safe, even if some may offend a few persons' esthetic senses. Water pollution is, however, a distinct reality and the pharmacist should keep abreast of events in this field.

Housing codes exist in most communities today either in the form of state law or local ordinance. There is no great contribution to be made by pharmacists in this matter except to lend their weight to logical programs for improving housing in their communities.

In summary, the pharmacist's role in environmental health is mainly one of alertness to the conditions prevailing in his or her community and of working, with others, towards the adequate control of any hazards. This is especially true of air and water pollution which require concerted community action for their control, but pharmacists may play a much more fundamental and personal role in foodborne disease. Often the first indication of an outbreak of foodborne disease is the unusually large number of people seeking relief from nausea, vomiting, and diarrhea, particularly if they are concentrated within a short period of time; a few hours to a day or two. The epidemic pattern of foodborne disease differs completely from the nausea, vomiting, and diarrhea of "intestinal flu"—another common complaint, usually seen in the cooler months of the fall and spring. "Point" epidemics of foodborne disease are dramatic, sudden events with most people becoming sick within 24–48 hours. If this type of epidemic results in an increase in across-the-counter sales of antinauseant and antidiarrheal drugs, the local health department should be notified without delay. This action will not only bring about the rapid investigation of the epidemic but also its control—the ultimate object of any epidemiological investigation.

Recent disclosures of the presence of chemical toxins in our environment is disturbing to say the least. The average citizen confronted by yet another substance that produces cancer in a rat or mouse fed with an inordinate dose of the suspect material will ignore the fact, or defy it by religiously continuing to eat the possible carcinogen to demonstrate his independence. "Moderation in all things" has been a wise edict for centuries; this perhaps should be the attitude of pharmacists whose advice is sought about the need to limit the diet to only those substances pronounced safe by the thousands of scientists who maintain their incomes, and obtain publicity, by performing research into food additives and other possible mutagens in food. There is well documented proof of cancer production by ingested materials in animals but there is also little proof that many of these substances produce human cancer. Certainly host factors must play a significant and vital role in disease of any type—a fact often ignored by the pure environmentalists. Many scientists do not possess the humility to admit to ignorance and to the fact that, in general, we do not know what causes cancer. Certainly the community pharmacist should keep abreast of developments pertaining to toxic and carcinogenic substances but he would do well to maintain a healthy skepticism to the more florid and sweeping statements made today.

Of more real importance are the many diseases resulting from occupation, ranging from the classical lead and mercury poisonings of yesteryear to the lung diseases of today. There is no doubt whatever that occupation may play an immense role in disease occurrence and new occupational hazards emerge every year; one notable example currently in the limelight is asbestos and its relationship to cancer. The pneumoconioses provide another good example of work-related diseases and have been known to occur in miners for hundreds of years in the form of silicosis or "black-lung" disease, but it is only recently that byssinosis or "brown-lung" disease has been demonstrated in textile workers. All occupations in which the participants are exposed to dust are hazardous to a degree, depending on the size of the dust particles, and their consequent ability to penetrate into the lung

substance, combined with their concentration and the length of exposure time in the workers. The pharmacist should, therefore, be aware of local occupations and their dangers and be alert to the first symptoms of disease—the case in point being the pneumoconioses, which first become evident in breathlessness occurring on mild exertion. Again, the emphasis must be on the pharmacist becoming acquainted with the local community and adapting the principles of health and medical care to the particular situations produced therein. The environment is constantly changing—physically, biologically, culturally, socially, and economically. The alert citizen, and even more the pharmacist, should cultivate an informed awareness of these changes and adapt his methods of health education, and disease prevention and control, to the changes in each community in which pharmacy services are provided. The phrase "continuing education" has become associated with professional meetings at which the participants attend meetings lackadaisically between sessions in the dining room and at the bar or on the golf course, whereas the pharmacist's continuing education should include watching the local pattern of society and its diseases, and changing his or her emphasis towards the evolving patterns of disease and its control.

Mental Health

The vast topic of emotional illness and its causation, manifestations, and control remains a puzzle to most people, including many health professionals. Add to this the stigma that still attaches to "crazy" people, and the problem of helping the mentally disturbed person is magnified many times. In some ways, and to some people, society is only now emerging from the era of those unfortunate days when the shackles were struck off in the Bicêtre hospital in Paris by Phillipe Pinel in 1793; in fact there are still too many people who think that mental disease should be treated behind bars and with fetters.

The main trouble with investigating mental disease is that there are few definitive tests on which diagnoses may be based—there is no blood test to measure the occurrence of schizophrenia for instance. In general, pharmacists should be aware of their local community mental health services, especially those catering to ambulatory patients; the timely referral of clients exhibiting bizarre behavior to these facilities may be life-saving, especially in those persons who demonstrate suicidal tendencies.

Suicide is the one manifestation of mental disturbance that can be accurately measured as it results in the death of the person involved. Fortunately, most suicide attempts turn out to be unsuccessful, although this does not negate the importance of prevention whenever possible. The clue to contemplation of suicide may be no more than a solitary phrase expressing disgust with oneself followed by the implication that the best way out is to end it all—comments which should never be ignored. Depression is the forerunner of attempted suicide and its cardinal symptoms are readily recognizable to the observant layman and even more to a health professional—or they should be. There is a distinct epidemiology of suicide; it occurs most commonly in older, reasonably well-off men, especially those who are unmarried. Women attempt to commit suicide more often than men but are not as successful in completing the act. The agents used in suicide vary with their availability; in the United States firearms figure most prominently, as they are readily available; in England drugs are the main agents because of stringent gun-control laws. With these and other epidemiological facts at his disposal, the pharmacist can be alert to potential suicide victims among clients and should do everything possible to bring aid to them. The "cry for help" which may be offered in the form of overt, or covert, references to worthlessness and to the uselessness of life, should never be neglected. The pharmacist should never be reluctant to ask a client directly whether he or she has ever considered, or is now considering, committing suicide—to contradict one of the many myths which pertain to suicide and its prevention. People who say they will kill themselves often do so and repeated suicide attempts are not uncommon, to explode two more myths. In summary, if the pharmacist detects what may be a potentially suicidal client, he or she should talk to the client and seek aid from family and professional contacts in the community; the client's plea for help should not be ignored.

Alcoholism and Drug Abuse

As already pointed out, the diseases of alcoholism and drug abuse (sometimes lumped together in the phrase "substance abuse") are peculiarly within the purview of the pharmacist. No other disease entities, with the possible exception of poison control, lend themselves more readily to intervention by pharmacists; easy as it may seem to advocate the pharmacy as the central point of control, it is far from having become so. The causal factors in these diseases remain obscure and control measures uncertain.

Alcoholism is estimated to affect many millions of men and women in the USA—how many is unimportant, particularly if you are the alcoholic. Society is slowly coming to realize that alcoholism is a biopsychosocial disorder with many causes and many ramifications. The one anchor to which the alcoholic may moor himself is Alcoholics Anonymous (AA)—a voluntary organization founded by an alcoholic for alcoholics, with branches for the spouses of alcoholics (Al-Anon) and their children (Alateen). Branches of AA exist in nearly all cities and many smaller towns, and the AA number is always listed in the local telephone directory; willing workers, all of whom were and, in their parlance, still are alcoholics are ready to help. Apart from AA, various clinics and centers are available through official government agencies such as health and welfare departments, all of which work closely with AA. The pharmacist will have many opportunities to help the unfortunates who become dependent upon alcohol, although many of them will resist the attempt to do so; this, however, should not be a deterrent as one victory is worth countless failures. All community agencies, professional and voluntary, should be called into play, including church, voluntary, and government groups.

Drug abuse is similar to alcoholism yet different in that it has received more acceptance among younger people—especially marihuana, which has been tried at least once by most teenagers, as has alcohol. The trend to accept the smoking of pot as a normal concomitant of growing up is evident and the main concern is that hard drugs may follow use of the milder ones. There is still, too, some concern about the long-term effects of marihuana which will not be resolved for many years. Again, the pharmacist is in the unparalleled position of being professionally the most competent member of the community to advise local agencies about drugs and their effects. The knowledge and participation of the pharmacist will redound to his or her credit both professionally and, to be more mundane, financially, as the contacts and publicity resulting from such interest will be reflected in business returns—a very real, if venal, benefit.

Public Health Research

If the pharmacist evinces a sincere interest in community health programs, there may be opportunities to participate in public health research programs, especially those concerned with drugs and their control. In general, investigation of community disease is based on two methods, known as retrospective and prospective surveys. The retrospective or backward-looking survey is based on past historical data readily obtained by asking questions of the population under investigation. The prospective or forward-looking method actually observes the events that occur in the population as it progresses through time. Obviously, the retrospective method is inexpensive, takes little time, deals with a stable population, and requires a minimum amount of work; its drawbacks, however, are that it relies on memory, is difficult to conduct with a control group, and introduces some observer bias because the surveyor knows what he is looking for. The prospective survey, on the other hand, is the opposite—it may take years to complete, is costly, has to contend with a shifting population, and requires a vast amount of work—but it is easy to use with a control group, does not rely on memory, and observer bias can be reduced to a minimum or eliminated altogether (Table VIII).

The best example of the use of these methods comes from the observation by an Australian ophthalmologist in 1941 that he was seeing an unusually large number of congenital cataracts in infants; investigation revealed that all the women concerned had had rubella (German measles) during their pregnancies—a retrospective discovery. This finding brought about some women obtaining illegal, but medically supervised, abortions when they revealed to their doctors that they had had rubella during their pregnancies and were afraid of having a baby with a congenital deformity. This practice necessitated a prospective survey to determine what the true incidence of rubella-produced congenital deformities was; pregnant women were observed during their pregnancies and their infants followed after birth to determine whether or not the babies developed congenital deformities. This forward-looking survey revealed that the true incidence was somewhere around 20% instead of the 100% thought to occur at first. Today, of course, with more liberal abortion practices, the question is somewhat academic but the original work illustrates the principles involved. Practicing pharmacists should offer their services to surveys of these types in investigating disease patterns in their community, particularly in drug therapy and its abuse.

Summary

Public health practice is influenced by the conservatism or liberalism of government and by the cultural variations of the people it serves. The trend in the United States today is towards private enterprise and away from the paternalism of the liberal administrations of the 1970's. Some aspects of health care now resemble those prior to the introduction of medical insurance in the 1930's—but dependence upon the

Table VIII—Public Health Research Surveys: Advantages (+) and Disadvantages (−)

Type	Time	Cost	Labor	Population Stability	Memory	Control	Observer Bias
Retrospective (Backward)	+	+	+	+	−	−	−
Prospective (Forward)	−	−	−	−	+	+	+

ability to pay a medical bill is sound economy only if charity accepts the burden of the non-paid bill, and increasing avarice may prevent the "old country doctor" approach being accepted today. The value a society places upon the health of its people has always been regarded as a measure of its humanitarianism. The question being posed today is whether the enormous cost of nuclear armament and space exploration is justified at the expense of ill health and disease. How to resolve this dilemma will perhaps never be achieved but an honest attempt will need more than the superficial platitudes often voiced by politicians.

The pharmacist, as an educated observer, should participate in this debate. In particular, he or she has more contact with the general public and, therefore, more opportunity to influence the well-being than other health professionals. In addition to this role, the pharmacist can offer to be a consultant to, or member of, the many official and voluntary health agencies in the community. Obviously, service as a board member of all the health agencies that exist is impossible, but those to which the most can be contributed can be selected. The pharmacist who is a leader, can lead; if not leading, he or she can become a useful member of the group in supporting measures that improve the health of the public.

References

1. American Association of Colleges of Pharmacy: *Public Health in the Curricula of Colleges of Pharmacy*, 1965.
2. Shattuck L: *Report of the Sanitary Commission of Massachusetts, 1850* (reprint), Harvard University Press, Cambridge, 1948.
3. American Association of Colleges of Pharmacy, *op cit.*
4. Roueche B: *Eleven Blue Men*, Berkley, New York, 1965.
5. US Department of Health and Human Services: *Morbidity and Mortality Weekly Report* (selected issues, 1968–1983), Center for Disease Control, Atlanta.
6. Shryock RH: *National Tuberculosis Association, 1904–1954*, National Tuberculosis Association, New York, 1957.
7. Kaiser Foundation Medical Care Program: *Annual Reports, 1960–1983*, Kaiser Center, Oakland, CA.
8. Department of Health, Education and Welfare: *Medicaid, Medicare: Which is Which?* Washington, DC, 1977.
9. Huff D: *How to Lie with Statistics*, Norton, New York, 1954.
10. A Waterborne Epidemic of Salmonellosis in Riverside, California, 1965: Epidemiologic Aspects. *Am J Epidemiology 93:* 33–48, 1971.
11. Farberow NL, Shneidman ES: *The Cry for Help*, McGraw-Hill, New York, 1961.

Bibliography

Public Health and Preventive Medicine

Wilner DM, Walkley RP, O'Neill EJ: *Introduction to Public Health*, 7th ed, Macmillan, New York, 1978.
Last JM, ed: *Preventive Medicine and Public Health* (Maxcy-Rosenau), 11th ed, Appleton-Century-Crofts, New York, 1980.
Shindell S, Salloway JS, Oberembt CM: *A Coursebook in Health Care Delivery*, Appleton-Century-Crofts, New York, 1976.
Preventive Medicine USA, Prodist, New York, 1976.

History

Rosen G: *A History of Public Health*, MD Publications, New York, 1958.
Rosen G: *Preventive Medicine in the United States, 1900–1975: Trends and Interpretations* (*Preventive Medicine USA* offprint), Prodist, New York, 1976.

Epidemiology

Lilienfeld AM: *Foundations of Epidemiology*, 2nd ed., Oxford University Press, New York, 1980.
Mausner JS, Bahn AK: *Epidemiology—An Introductory Text*, Saunders, Philadelphia, 1974.

Public Health and Pharmacy

American Association of Colleges of Pharmacy: *Public Health in the Curricula of Colleges of Pharmacy*, 1965.

International Health

Brockington CF: *World Health*, Penguin, Baltimore, 1958.
Waddell WH, Pierleoni RG, Suter E, eds: *International Health Perspectives*, Springer, New York, 1977.
Basch PF: *International Health*, Oxford University Press, New York, 1978.

Occupational Health

Hunter D: *The Diseases of Occupations*, 6th ed, Hodder and Stoughton, London, 1978.
Levy BS and Wegman DH, eds: *Occupational Health*, Little, Brown, Boston, 1983.

Environmental Health

Karen H: *Handbook of Environmental Health and Safety*. Pergamon Press, New York, 1980.
Purdon PW ed: *Environmental Health*. 2nd ed. Academic Press, New York, 1980.

Mental Health

Allen RD and Cartier MK: *The Mental Health Almanac*. Garland STPM Press, New York, 1978.
Langsley DG, Berlin IN, and Yarvis RM: *Handbook of Community Mental Health*. Medical Examination Publishing Co., New York, 1981.
Stengel E: *Suicide and Attempted Suicide*, Penguin, Baltimore, 1964.

Venereal Disease

Schofield CBS: *Sexually Transmitted Diseases*, 3rd ed, Churchill, Livingstone, Edinburgh, 1979.
King A, Nicol C, and Rodin P: *Venereal Diseases*. 4th ed. Bailliere Tindall, London, 1980.
Morton RS: *Venereal Diseases*, 2nd ed, Penguin, Baltimore, 1972.

Administration

Hanlon J and Picket GE: *Principles of Public Health Administration*, 7th ed, Mosby, St. Louis, 1979.

Bibliography

La Rocco A, Jones B: A Bookshelf in Public Health, Medical Care, and Allied Fields. *Bulletin Medical Library Association 60:* 32–101, 1972.

CHAPTER 98

The Patient: Behavioral Determinants

Albert I Wertheimer, PhD
Professor and Director
Department of Graduate Studies in Social and Administrative Pharmacy
College of Pharmacy, University of Minnesota
Minneapolis, MN 55455

Every man, woman and child fulfills many roles in the course of a single day. The child moves effortlessly from bus passenger to pupil, to playmate, to cub scout, etc. The woman may simultaneously be wife, mother, employee or professional and learn how to juggle her activities to satisfy each role responsibility. The man may be professional, employer, employee, husband, father and son also simultaneously. Most of these roles are voluntary, generally pleasant and controllable by the individual himself/herself. There is one role, though, enjoyed by few people and desired by even fewer persons, and that is being a patient.

Being a patient means yielding responsibility and control of our care to someone else. Someone we may not even know, a perfect stranger sometimes, is then making decisions having important consequences for an individual and his future. The patient role then is an undesirable, unnatural one. The reality, though, is that all of us at one time or another become patients when we, albeit reluctantly, acknowledge that our condition requires care beyond what a layperson might be able to provide.

The pharmacist who wishes to serve his patients to the fullest extent cannot limit his objectives to accurate dispensing based on signs and symptoms. He must consciously address himself to the person in whom the disease process occurs. A totally impersonal approach is not possible in medicine since the pharmacist and the patient react to each other as persons whether they wish to do so or not. Thus, since subjective factors cannot be eliminated, they must be recognized and understood and their therapeutic potentialities used for the patient's benefit. The personality of the patient is the totality of the characteristic ways the individual deals with internal and external stresses. The signs and symptoms are completely bound with different personality traits and, therefore, true communication is impossible unless the pharmacist is vigilant to this implication. What follows in the patient's search for care, reaction to instructions and information, and behaviors in the sick role will be the subject of this chapter.

Illness Behavior

The human psyche is most complex, and many behaviors cannot be predicted with absolute certainty. We can, though, say a few things about the patient. Parsons[1] indicates that we consider a person as ill when he is unable to perform valued tasks. When a sufficient number of tasks cannot be completed so that one's role cannot be fulfilled, that person is generally regarded as too ill to be responsible for the performance of one's normal role responsibilities. Illness is a legitimate excuse for not going to work or school. Illness behavior is a fascinating topic and one that should surely be understood by pharmacy practitioners. There is, though, a caution that must be aired before continuing further. The social sciences have not developed means of calibration sufficiently precise to enable a practitioner to categorize a person solely upon observed behavior. The following material, then,

may serve as a guide but is most certainly not intended to be the basis of a taxonomy.

Mechanic,[2] in discussing illness and illness behavior, indicates that medical care might have maximal effectiveness if the integral importance of the social, psychological and biological factors is understood. We shall concentrate on the social and psychological aspects since the biological domain is well attended-to already.

Illness behavior may be seen as a culturally and socially learned response. Much work has demonstrated that members of various ethnic groups react differently to pain and, moreover, react after different threshold levels are reached. Therefore, we may expect to find members of different societal subcultures behave rather differently in the face of illness. Most of one's ideas regarding normality, illness and health definitions are developed based on one's views of the immediate world surrounding the observer. Were everyone in one's peer group to require a hearing aid, the use of such a device would soon come to be thought of as normal. What this means then is that the practitioner must weigh the response of patients in evaluating their degree of wellness against visible clues of social class level, income level, occupation and likely level of formal education completed.

Countless studies have been performed indicating that views of, reactions to, and concern about health and illness vary according to an individual's age, social class, ethnic origin, knowledge about health and medical care, gender and a number of other sociodemographic variables. Additionally, cultural differences play a major role in determining one's illness behavior. Someone from a remote village who has never seen a physician or nurse or pharmacist will seek aid from an elder in the village who might have some medical experience. So too would be the expectation if a Native American became ill in an area where the power and authority of the medicine man continue and where confidence in his cures and advice endures. There can be little argument that there are links between reaction patterns to pain and illness and physiological response.[3]

Knowing the patient's family is especially important in understanding him. A person who has had a genuinely caring mother usually has a basic feeling of trust in people that helps in coping with an unpredictable and at times unfriendly world. A woman who is inconsistent and emotionally incapable of mothering is apt to send her child out into the world with a wary and hostile attitude. Such a person may misinterpret a friendly and helpful gesture as an attempt to hurt or manipulate him. Siblings usually play an important role in the development of personality. Feelings of jealousy toward other patients and the need to win status in the doctor's eyes may be related to childhood sibling rivalries. A positive and loving father, in addition to helping the mother (directly and indirectly) to fulfill her responsibilities to her children, provides goals, standards, and conditions that help an individual to orient himself realistically to life. Such an individual, when he ventures from home, is prepared to adjust emotionally and socially to his fellow man. Another area or concept that one must bear in mind is the recognition that an emotional component has often been associated with the etiology of illness or with its development. The vast array of disease states associated with psychosomatic implications should be known and appreciated by the pharmacy practitioner. Some social scientists have even argued that the presentation of somatic complaints oftentimes masks an underlying emotional problem which frequently may be the major or compelling reason why the patient has arranged the consultation in the first place.[4,5]

Stress is a variable that has been highly correlated with the use of health services. Yet, both the concept of stress itself as well as the relationship have not been fully elucidated. Even questions dealing with the differential effectiveness of placebos among different patients require greater understanding before definitive or even predictive statements may be made with certainty.

The reactions toward illness may also make illness behavior a candidate as a means to seek secondary advantages. It is universally acknowledged that illness is an acceptable reason for avoidance of some role obligations, social responsibilities and expectations.[6] The problems lie in the widely varying definitions of illness and health seen in various locations, institutions and under differing conditions. To be sure, other factors similarly influence illness behavior. These would include the patient's self-image with reference to an assessment of vulnerability and problem severity, reaction of family or health care providers to the problem, the demands of family or employment, the level of stigmatization of the problem, institutional environment, risks involved in treatment, degree of expected discomfort, expense or disfigurement, and confidence in the provider(s) of care.

The Parsons concept of the sick role explains much of this and should go a long way toward facilitating understanding by the pharmacist of some typical and atypical patient behaviors. It is to be hoped that greater understanding of patient anxiety, placebo effects, compliance research findings, the decision to self-medicate, treatment delay, use of home remedies, reticence to seek professional aid, and other considerations may come about. Briefly stated, Parsons suggested that sickness produces a temporary disturbance in an individual's capacity to fulfill his usual roles. This is a conditionally legitimate state, having the effect of insulating the individual from certain types of mutual influence with other persons, and of alienating him from certain norms accepted in the "well" population.[7] The sick person is not held responsible for having incurred his condition, which is by definition undesirable, and, therefore, one is motivated to "get well." Since the patient is incapable of achieving this goal through self volition, he has an inherent right to receive care, and is, in fact, obligated to seek and accept professional care.

It remained for Suchman, in 1965, to delineate the actual stages of illness and medical care. He took the concept of illness behavior as proposed by Mechanic and Volkart and arrayed some internal sequences.[8] What we see are five stages of medical events and they are examined along four elements. These elements are: content, sequence, spacing, and variability of behavior. The stages are:

1. The symptom experience stage
2. Assumption of the sick-role stage
3. Medical care contact stage
4. Dependent-patient role stage
5. Recovery or rehabilitation stage

In the first stage, the decision that something is wrong is made. This is based on recognition of a pain, or some other discomfort. It is possible that the individual may elect to do nothing, self-medicate, rest, or consult a family member, friend, or even decide to visit a physician if the problem worsens. In the second stage, the decision that one requires professional care is made. One may seek excuse from normal task responsibilities and consult with significant others. In the third stage, the decision to seek professional medical care is made. A scientific diagnosis and treatment regimen are desired and the consulting of the physician legitimizes the abrogation of some role responsibilities. The person may ignore the advice and seek another source of aid more palatable. At the onset of the fourth stage, the person truly becomes a patient and accepts transfer of control for his care to the physician. Here, the patient agrees to be placed in another's hands. At the final stage, a decision is made to relinquish the patient role. Clearly, this is more difficult with some diseases and patients than with others. Now the patient must relearn the full burden of societal responsibilities.

Another system is at work and it oftentimes delivers the would-be patient into the second stage of the Suchman model. This is the Lay Referral System described by Freidson. In this system, one is expected to inquire about a possible medical problem in an ever-widening circle of others. Members of one's nuclear family are queried about the problem, followed by selected persons in the extended family, friends, neighbors, co-workers, etc. In some instances, this search leads to the community pharmacist. Naturally, the search is terminated when an individual indicates knowledge and/or experience with an identical medical problem and offers sensible-sounding advice.

In some cases, the patient will never recover. It is possible that a permanent impairment will exist or that the patient may even die. Two areas of concern for the pharmacist are seen in these situations. The patient who may have a terminal condition might be seen at home or in a community pharmacy as often as he or she may be found within an institution.[9] Contemporary medical-care practices dictate that a dying patient should be able to return to familiar surroundings, and to be enabled to live one's final time with dignity. For example, the cancer patient might be sent home to be with the family until hospitalization might be required at the very end. The response process to the disclosure of the terminal nature of a disease usually follows a now predictable course. The work of Glaser and Kubler-Ross indicates that following disclosure the following steps may be seen.

Depression follows disclosure, yet most patients come to terms with the situation and move on to the next stage. Some do not and withdraw from contact with others. Next, the patient either accepts or denies the forthcoming event. Denial may be seen in patients becoming intensely active, emphasizing a future orientation, forcing reciprocal isolation, comparing oneself with other patients or juggling time. Eventually people overcome the denial stage and accept their fate. Acceptance may be witnessed in one of two forms. The first, active preparation, involves the patient into becoming philosophical, possibly embracing religion, and putting one's social and financial affairs into order. Suicide is a form of active preparation. Here, patients often decide to spare their loved ones protracted grief and expense. Passive preparation for imminent death includes accepting this fate with nonchalance or calm resignation. Accepting the diagnosis but deciding to fight may be seen in this category. A patient may opt for a marginal healer or quack who makes attractive promises. When the patient defines himself as ill, some of the following sociocultural factors influence how one responds: Socioeconomic Class—It is known that business and professional classes respond to illness more so than do persons from blue collar groups. Moreover, poor and less educated persons have greater morbidity, disability and mortality in general, and, ethnicity, which is already discussed.

The other problem mentioned earlier that the pharmacist might encounter is that of the permanently impaired patient. Surely it is obvious to the reader about the possible feelings of an invalid, such as the amputee and others having visible abnormalities. Goffman introduced study of stigma into the health-care milieu. Stigma refers to something deeply discrediting. Diseases and medical problems may be stigmatized. In such cases, shame and guilt are present. Why do people whisper about mental disorders, cancer, epilepsy, venereal diseases and think nothing about discussing colds, flu, headache, etc., with their friends and co-workers? Why is it that people willingly wear eyeglasses, but fight the use of a hearing aid? Is impaired hearing worse than impaired vision? The answer lies in a closer examination of our social morés. Illness had (has?) been closely related to religious beliefs. Many persons believed that illness was a divinely administered punishment and, therefore, were led to accept the concept that ill persons "might have had it coming." Other stigmatized problems include disfigurements, and this becomes the basis for a problem that the pharmacist might be able to alleviate. It is thought that some patients might not be compliant with their medication schedules for fear of having co-workers or others see them swallowing medicine. Others decide not to pursue therapies when they see what visible effects the therapy causes. Examples include loss of hair in chemotherapy against neoplasms, surgery that might leave hideous after-effects or other deviant appearance. Delay in evaluation of breast masses is caused by fear of possible consequences.

Working with Patients—In working with patients a great deal has been written about the therapeutic relationship. Countless commentators tell us that we must project an image or aura of caring, concern, confidence and competency. It is important also, we learn, to make an assessment of the patient at the outset of an interaction.

Studies have reported differential reactions to pain in various *ethnic groups.* In some cultures or subcultures, it is not considered manly for a male to admit illness and require professional care. Here, we can expect male patients to delay seeking care until very threatening or debilitating effects are encountered. On the topic of ethnicity it is important to understand the role of folk healers among Native American, Mexican American and a few other groups. Ridicule of this health-care system will probably do little more than drive away the potential patient.

Rituals for episodic illness occur and are very much a part of folk medicine. The sulfur and molasses in the spring and other home remedies we often hear about, when they cause no harm, should be ignored. Some of the most powerful (and useful) placebo effects are found in this area. Folk cures have a role in the contemporary health-care delivery system and play an important adjunctive role in therapeutics. If the patient is willing to take the penicillin tablet and gargle with dandelion wine concentrate, it makes no difference if the patient elects to credit the dandelion preparation with the cure.

The patient is likely to experience greater illness in the same temporal cluster as stress, family problems, personal problems and other traumatic events. Knowledge about the patient's personal life and *understanding of his/her problems* can be invaluable.

Patient fear/anxiety may be effectively dealt with by the pharmacy practitioner. Blood in the stool, breast masses, and some central nervous system aberrations strike real fear into patients. Knowledge of a friend or relative's unsuccessful bout with the pathology makes the problem even more acute.

Practitioner-patient relationships have been categorized by Szasz and Hollender.[10] In the active-passive mode the practitioner uses the authority inherent in his/her role in which the patient does not participate. The guidance-cooperation mode permits the practitioner considerable authority, but the patient is expected to cooperate. In the mutual participation mode the patient is expected to be actively responsible for treatment. The clinician can decide what might be the optimal strategy for each type of patient.

Interviewing the patient is a delicate and important function. Many complaints can be localized in an area of the body. Quality of the discomfort can be calibrated also, with the aid of the patient. The same holds true for the quantity of the perceived stress. The chronology of the problem can be ferreted out with skill and patience. The time of onset, duration, and frequency of the disease may be sharply defined. Learning of aggravating or alleviating factors may also be of value. Associated symptoms may be a clue to problems. When the responses to these questions have been considered and evaluated, instructions or advice are forthcoming. This communication must be made with due consideration of the person's educational background, intelligence, attitude toward this illness, and financial situation.

One can never afford to ignore the possibility of psychophysiological disorders. For example, marasmus is a term used to describe an infant's failure to grow and develop, where the baby gradually becomes weakened, emaciated, listless and could even die. Asthma is thought to be, at least in part, a psychosomatic disease. Classic physicians since Hippocrates saw emotions as playing a crucial role in asthma. The evidence for psychological factors are that, first, most asthmatics state on report and their physicians note a correlation between their episodes and psychological factors, especially fear or anger.

Fifty to 75 percent of the patients who present gastrointestinal complaints appear to lack a clear pathophysiological basis for their symptoms. The symptom complex presented by such patients has been variously called mucous colitis, spastic colon, functional bowel disorders, nervous diarrhea and, more recently, irritable colon syndrome. In the absence of organic pathology, many physicians ascribe the symptoms presented to emotional factors. In addition, some gastrointestinal diseases, such as peptic ulcer disease and ulcerative colitis, have a history of being regarded as the result of specific psychological conflicts. In fact, gastrointestinal diseases in general have been regarded as having important psychological components. Sexual dysfunction is another problem which appears to be very much related to psychological factors. The pharmacist should not joke during the communication process, should not be interrupted for commercial purposes, and must be willing to answer questions to explain points two or three times, if necessary, to an agitated and confused patient. False assurances or promises do not benefit anyone and must be avoided. The patient often needs and surely deserves support from his/her pharmacist. This empathy may be communicated via verbal and nonverbal means. The encounter may be brought to a close with congruence. Evidence is great that failure to understand or agree with the treatment plan regarding medication and activities may account for much of the high rate of noncompliance.

Dealing with Illness

Defense (or adaptive ego) mechanisms serve as a first line of defense. They may be invoked to keep feelings within bearable limits, to restore psychological homeostasis, and to permit a "time-out" to adjust as well as to deal with unresolvable conflicts. Vaillant's work illuminated this area for us.[11]

Narcissistic defenses are seen in individuals as adult dreams and fantasies, and in healthy people before the age of five. They alter reality for the user.

Delusional projection is a positive delusion about external reality, usually of a persecutory type. Responsibility for feelings is projected to others.

Denial is seen when one insists that a dead person is still alive, or that a disease is not present, etc., in the face of overwhelming contradictory, comprehendable evidence.

Distortion is a gross reshaping of external reality to suit internal needs. It may include hallucinations, megalomanic beliefs and feelings of delusional superiority or entitlement.

Other immature defenses are commonly seen in healthy juveniles, and in adults with some character and affective disorders. They appear as misbehavior and may usually be corrected by improvements in interpersonal relationships (maturation, or in finding a more mature partner or understanding physician).

Projection is found when a person's emotionally unacceptable feelings are unconsciously rejected and attributed to others.

Schizoid fantasy employs the use of fantasy and withdrawal to avoid a conflict or pleasure. It may be associated with an avoidance of intimacy. Here, the patient may not believe the fantasies or even act them out.

Hypochondriasis is thought of as the transfer of feelings toward others resulting from loneliness, bereavement or unacceptable aggressive impulses into complaints of pain, or illness.

Passive-aggressive behavior is aggression expressed indirectly and ineffectively through pouting, negativism, procrastination and illnesses that affect others more than self.

Acting-out is the direct expression of an unconscious wish or impulse in order to avoid being aware of the effect that accompanies it. It may include delinquency, extramarital affairs, exhibitionism, drug use and self-inflicted injury.

Regression is seen as a return to an earlier mode of behavior which was either more successful or pleasant, such as thumb-sucking and baby-talk.

Now to turn from some patient problems and examine the uses of drugs by man. Barber lists some eleven functions of drugs within our society, classifying them as aesthetic, aphrodisiac, ego-disrupting, ideological, political, psychological support, religious, research, social control, therapeutic, and war and other conflict functions.[12] The nature of some of these functions may not be obvious and thus requires some explanation. For example, drugs have been employed in aesthetic functions in the arts for centuries. Ego-disrupting functions are usually caused by hallucinogens, agents taken to cause unpredictable perceptions and experiences.

The exact etiology of visits to health-care providers and the motivation for ingestion of drug substances may remain unknown and may well be due to one of a large number of reasons, as seen in Barber's listing of the functions of drugs. Much of the success of an encounter or treatment regime is determined by the patient's perception of the doctor-patient relationship. This relationship exists today in numerous different surroundings, from the battlefield to the Park Avenue private-practice office. The patient may have selected the practitioner or he or she may have been assigned by some political or administrative organization.

Health care is often carried out by a team, a fact not always understood by the sometimes baffled patient who might not appreciate that personal health services take place in the form of a series of medical events—some diagnostic, others therapeutic—each with one visible member of the team.[13] This form of professional help is only one type of aid. There is the mutual help given one another by friends and lovers or comrades. Entralgo further refines terms in stating that friends or lovers seek communion by forming a single unit for aid—a pair called a diad—while comrades may work toward the external good of the two persons involved, in a duo. There is also unilateral help from one to another that takes three distinct forms: advice, education, medical care.

In medical care, a health-care provider helps a sick person in regaining a state of mental and physical well-being. This requires detachment and objectivity. The union of physicians or other health-service providers and the patient may be visualized as a union between two people called a *quasidiadic* according to Entralgo. The cooperation here between members of the duo is based on their possessing a common purpose. The relationship between a physician and a patient is thought to have four components in its structure.[14]

1. The proper aim of the relationship
2. The proper form of intercourse involved in it
3. The proper link on which this intercourse should depend
4. The proper form of communication between doctor and patient

In an interesting, differing view of the social functions of medical practice, Shuval *et al.* elucidated five latent functions served by providers of medical care. It was postulated that if a latent, rather than manifest, function was provided satisfactorily, such latent needs are being satisfied. Her group identified these as: need for catharsis, coping with failure, status, integration into society, and resolution of a magic-science conflict.[15]

Another cogent passage worthy of notation and consideration is that by Coser: "The sick person who is admitted to the hospital ward is frequently overcome by anxiety to such an extent that he is likely to suffer from a partial blurring of his self-image because of the actual and symbolic threat to his body. His forced passivity, his horizontal pose, the removal of his own clothes and belongings, the fact that doctors and nurses, persons hitherto unknown to him, have full access to his body, and the fact that he cannot anticipate what will happen to him—all these factors contribute to a loss of ego identity."[16]

The idea that mind, body and emotions are not separate entities is no longer subject to question. They are so interrelated that it is now recognized that the cause and treatment of a long list of diseases—bronchial asthma, peptic ulcer, colitis, arterial hypertension, migraine headache and many others—are related to the life history and personality of the patient.[17]

Behavioral Science Concepts—Therefore, treatment of the total patient has come to be viewed as essential by members of all of the health professions. But such treatment, of necessity, requires a knowledge of the patient in his or her psychological and social as well as biological aspects. Mechanic and Newton further the rationale for an understanding of the social and behavioral sciences for health-service practitioners such as the pharmacist by stating that "all medical decisions involve the weighing of probabilities."[18] Here is where behavioral science enters the realm of disease. Failure to utilize sociodemographic data about a patient permits the existence of bias in predictions made in treatment situations. Application of some behavioral science concepts may aid in the reduction of bias or error in prediction. Moreover, a most appropriate regimen may be created. For example, instruction of an elderly patient to take one tablet after meals (where we assume three to be normal) may not be effective if the patient eats only one meal per day.

When the patient learns of a diagnosis, a natural question often arises: that being the etiology of the pathology. Is it genetic or environmental, or is it due to both factors? From numerous studies, one may best respond accurately that both heredity and environment contribute to all behavior traits and that the extent of their respective contributions cannot be specified for any trait.[19]

"Unless the pharmacist strives to achieve a professional standing, he can be caught by the business trends and made an automaton of the manufacturers. The pharmacist must be an able public speaker and writer, able to communicate interprofessionally and to the general public—an active community leader. He must participate more with local school boards, boards of health and other organizations interested in the health of the community. The pharmacist of the future will exist in an environment of rapid transition in the field of medical care, not only scientifically, but socially and economically."[20]

While it probably is unwise for the pharmacist to become involved in behavior modification, a practice which should be left to trained, experienced professionals, the pharmacy practitioner should be aware of techniques and their uses. Natural behaviors include instinct, and imprinting, the name for linkages formed between parents and offspring. Through it, only one or two attempts are needed to "learn," and this learning—very heavily preprogrammed behavior, can take place only during a brief period, the critical period in the life of an individual. Learning is a new behavior being acquired, usually through interaction with one's environment.

In classical conditioning, a person who has learned to avoid bees may extend this avoidance to stimilar insects, such as wasps. In addition, identical elements in a new situation may cause a reactivation of a previously learned response. This occurs in all types of learning. An application of classical conditioning that has gained widespread acceptance is the LaMaze method, which views pain from a Pavlovian view as a response that was unnecessarily conditioned to many stimuli associated with childbirth and furthermore, as an unconditioned response of lower brain centers that could be inhibited or altered by activity of the higher brain centers (an example of classical "reciprocal inhibition").

In operant conditioning, new responses can be acquired and refined. Operant principles may be used to control chronic pain as well as environmental contingencies. This is done by rewarding increases in functioning with praise and by not punishing pain behaviors.

In identification, we see the automatic and largely unconscious process of imitating and copying those who are admired or powerful. It is a continuous process. Persuasion and coercion are practices which can be studied, practiced and learned. We see this with politicians, door-to-door salesmen and others. Such techniques, however, although they produce the desired action or decision, are vulnerable to second thought. Hence they are not particularly effective in inducing changes in ongoing behavior. Peer exploration is the name of Kurt Lewin's method for changing patterns of preference. Small groups that discuss issues openly can change patterns of interpersonal communication. This has been used successfully for post-myocardial infarct and peptic ulcer patients to modify behaviors.

Burlage's list of skills to be required for future pharmacy practice can safely be added to. Surely, the future pharmacist will require an understanding of the concept of society and health, as well as an understanding of the pathology of poverty within our society. She or he will have to have an understanding of the role of the federal government and the reaction to efforts by the government. It is important that an understanding of consumer expectations of health services be inculcated and an idea about the concept of quality and how quality is measured would be needed for a practicing pharmacist. The understanding of medicine in a changing society is an important concept and one which must be mastered by the practitioner. If one is to understand changes by social class as well as by a host of other variables, then an understanding of a vast array of social and behavioral precepts is required. We will turn our attention toward aspects met primarily by the pharmacy practitioner very shortly.

The pharmacist should understand referral behavior, both to and from medical sources as well as nonmedical sources. For example, the pharmacist should ascertain which patients could be referred to a social worker or psychologist or to some other source of aid and which ones might be referred for other formal medical-type care. One must keep in mind that what is oftentimes recommended is a compromise based on the feeling of the recommender as to what is best for the patient,

combined with what the patient might accept as a reasonable referral route. Would it not be pointless to recommend to a patient who has made it clear that he or she has no faith in physicians that he or she go to see a physician? In such a case, it might be wisest to recommend an over-the-counter product or even a self-care book.[21]

Not only is human behavior different amongst different persons in otherwise similar social strata, but differences occur in each of the subcultural groups. Oftentimes men behave differently or react differently than do women to the same event or action and we may see these differences between persons of different education, income, etc. In fact, even behaviors in the health sphere at the national level are different depending on one's national identification. In the classic work by Titmuss, he clearly showed how behavior with reference to the area of voluntary blood donations was different in several nations throughout the world.[22]

In the Millis Commission Report (*Pharmacists for the Future*), recommendation number 11 of the 14 recommendations states: "The Study Commission emphasizes that pharmacy is a knowledge system in which *chemical substances and people called patients interact.* Needed and optimally effective drug therapy results only when drugs and those who consume them are fully understood. We suggest that one of the first steps in reviewing the educational program of a college of pharmacy should be weighing the relative emphasis given to the physical and biological sciences against the behavioral and social sciences in the curriculum for the first professional degree."[23]

"Clearly pharmacists must have ready knowledge about drugs, but they also must have ready knowledge about people, about relationships and communication with them, and about systems and cost service."[24]

As Titmuss quoted, "Two hundred years ago Voltaire defined medical treatment as the art of pouring drugs of which one knew nothing into a patient of whom one knew less."[25] Let us hope that this generation ends the ignorance of the second aspect. The pharmacist is faced with a number of problems beyond the accurate dispensing of the indicated drugs. He or she is at the end point where an item of pharmacological activity has been requested. It has been requested by a physician who must be able to handle ignorance and uncertainty. The patient has described the symptoms as best as possible, and the physician understands that these symptoms could be caused by a number of sources. The physician is constantly reminded of his therapeutic inadequacies due to the ever increasing emphasis on postgraduate medical education, pressure from patients in a science worshiping world, specialization accomplishments, and the proliferation of medical journals which internationally now number over 7000.[26]

The situations which a pharmacist may be expected to face include problems of compliance of prescribed or recommended therapy by patients, the use of the placebo effect, problems in effective communication primarily in the area of patient education, and a number of other issues which hinge on the status and role of the pharmacist. Some of these include the provision of objective advice and counsel. A placebo drug, one used more to please than to benefit the patient has been shown to affect a wide variety of biological and disease processes including fever, headache, cough reflex, common cold, insomnia, mood changes, angina pain, postoperative pain, blood-cell count, vasomotor function and others. Placebo effects are not imaginary and are not necessarily the result of suggestion in the ordinary sense of the term. It is thought that the placebo may result from a patient interaction with health-care personnel or medication and that the patient may be influenced by provider-led expectations. It has been estimated that between 30 and 50% of subjects can be expected to be placebo reactors in any given situation. But, unfortunately, we are unable to predict which patients will react to which placebos during any given situation. When a placebo, either frank—an agent having no pharmacological activity—or a medication—one having some pharmacological activity, but not the one suggested by the practitioner—is used, the placebo response cannot be avoided. It may apply at any part of a therapeutic encounter.

There is also one other factor that must be considered when therapy is being evaluated. If there is a failure in therapeutic situations, personnel must consider whether they may have contributed to it through a negative placebo effect.[27]

It is likely that the pharmacist will be involved often with patients who wish to second-guess or question the information offered by a physician. Pharmacists must be careful, as there is always the possibility that a placebo effect was intended or that an unsure diagnosis was made and various therapies are being tried.

Smith provides interesting orientation when he compares the patient to a hunter in almost the same sense as the early pioneers were hunters. The stakes are just as high—survival. There are dangers—economic and medical—since the patient may be taken advantage of by a pharmacist, physician or may be injured by a drug. Many patients are cautious in their hunt and rightly so. Even for prescribed drugs, the patient has the ultimate choice of where to purchase them. These decisions of whether and where are central to the pharmacist-patient relationship and are subject to two kinds of influence: the basic or patient influences and the external or environmental influences. It is proposed that four basic variables control all patient actions. These would be: needs, motives, perception and attitudes.[28] He continues: Patient behavior with regard to pharmacy in general, or to an individual pharmacy, is shaped by individual encounters with the pharmacist and the historical accumulation of such encounters. Whether pharmacists liked it or not, this is how the process works.

Unfortunately, the field is difficult to understand and it is even more difficult to make definitive statements. For example, in a recent research report, Knapp and others indicated that their observations "led us to serious doubts about the influence pharmacists are having on prescribing decisions despite distinct changes in pharmaceutical education and professed aspiration to more influential, professional roles in drug prescribing control."[29]

Role of Pharmacists

The findings by Knapp *et al.*, just mentioned, must be interpreted with care when one considers the information prepared for and provided to the American Pharmaceutical Association by Ernest Dichter in 1972. It is reported that "despite Medicare and similar organizations, the vast majority of people in this country feel that they are completely isolated and have to face the danger of disease all by themselves. In addition, they expressed that feeling exposed to what I aggressively call biological blackmail on the part of the physician, who apparently does not measure his fee according to the time spent but according to the severity of the case he is treating." Dichter indicates that the ideal doctor is gone and that community doctors, particularly older ones, were inclined to treat the patient as an illiterate. He writes, "The patient doesn't want to be talked down to—he wants at least to be a knowledgeable participant where his own body is concerned. Pharmacists, being a part of the health system, attract a lot of hostility; to a very large extent, without justification. To better understand the source of the hostility, a number of practical measures could be introduced." Dichter continues by informing us that the modern patient-consumer has become much more of an individualist. He does not want to be treated as a case or as a number. The pharmacist, accepting this new role, can do a number of things such as inform each

patient that there is a complete file maintained about him. Modern patients are anti-fatalists, and do not accept getting old. They do not want to suffer pains and they tend to plan much more ahead than people used to. This is a good sign, as they are much more health-conscious and prophylactic-conscious. The pharmacist could provide his patients with pamphlets or even pre-filled medicine chests for emergencies.

"The modern customer and patient wants to be informed. He has unfortunately also become somewhat more suspicious. In contrast to other countries, in America the prescription filled by the pharmacist is not accompanied by a description of any one of the possible negative side effects. The pharmacist should be on the patient's side," said Dichter. The pharmacist may not want to contradict the physician, but he might advise the patient to ask the physician whether he feels that a low-priced cold remedy would not serve just as well.[30]

In another area where the pharmacist has the availability and opportunity to make major contributions toward the effectiveness and quality of patient care, there are few hard and fast rules and guidelines. In patient compliance with therapeutic regimens, enormous variance is indeed the case. To quote Kabat, "Although it is reasonable to assume that patients will follow the physician's directions and benefit from his diagnostic and therapeutic acumen, numerous studies have indicated that alarming rates of medication errors and of noncompliance occur during self-administration of drugs. In reviewing work in the area, he reports that the highest level of patient compliance occurred when the pharmacist verbally reviewed with the patient the directions on the prescription container and provided the patient with a printed data sheet about the drugs. "It would appear that patient education and monitoring by pharmacists can increase patient compliance."[31]

In a study on a related topic, Eshelman and Fitzloff found something of interest. Some 100 patients were randomly assigned to receive a drug (chlorthalidone tablets) in traditional prescription vials or in compliance pack dispensers. Based on thin-layer chromatography assay of urine samples, the commercially marketed convenience package demonstrated an advantageous effect on patient compliance with an antihypertensive medication. Pill counts did not reveal the same significant difference.[32]

Obviously, by knowing the patient and understanding the aspects of the condition and therapy, the pharmacist is in the very best position to be able to assist in the successful therapy for a patient. Critics argue that even if he does, can it have any effect? We know that at New York Hospital, an educational system using patient medication instruction cards and predischarge teaching solves some problems.[33]

Of the literally thousands of studies conducted on the topic of compliance with therapeutic regimens, little emerges as definitive findings. Severity of disease is not conclusively related, much to our surprise. But then sicker patients may have more to do and may be limited in their ability. The demographic characteristics of the patient mean little. While common sense suggests that knowledge about one's illness should be related to compliance, it does not work that way. Patient beliefs about illness and treatment, and the complexity of the regimen as well as the chronic nature of a condition appear to have some relationship. Conflicting evidence indicates that the nature of the physician-patient encounter and patient confidence may play a role.

Ivey *et al.* have reported ways in which the pharmacist can identify the patient's information needs and thereby control communication, timing and define communication objectives. This information should enable the pharmacist to develop methods of communication and to be able to evaluate the effectiveness of his instructions. Since communications exchanges have centered around the concerns of therapists and patients, it is necessary to know some things about the patient's therapy. The pharmacist should attempt to learn the following: (1) the reason or reasons a patient is taking a particular drug; (2) any unpleasant effects produced by the drug that may be self-monitored by the patient; (3) specific instructions on the dosing schedule; (4) interactions with other medications; (5) the diet of the patient; (6) instructions for any monitoring tests to be performed by the patient; (7) a variety of other information expected by the patient.[34]

The pharmacist, partially motivated by a desire to be seen as a mediator and contributory member of the health team, has attempted a number of other prototype demonstrations and experiments. In one such study, 1000 patients who were discharged from a surgery service of the university hospital were studied with the physicians and pharmacists cooperating in an effort to reduce the cost of medications: (1) by substituting less expensive drugs when possible, (2) by relabeling bedside medication, (3) by securing third-party coverage for eligible patients and (4) recommending purchase of nonprescription drugs through an over-the-counter status. Savings of nearly $1700 were realized on 517 out of 1832 prescriptions, which was equal to $9.13 savings to the patients per hour of pharmacists' consultation time.[35]

In a recent study, it was determined that pharmacists can and should play a greater role in developing a consulting program with ambulatory patients. Four basic points were brought out by the survey in the study: (1) no appreciable effect had yet been felt by physicians as a result of a patient information required regulation in that state. (2) There is physician support for pharmacists involved in patient education activities. (3) Physicians did not identify any one method of communicated instructions as the optimal method and indicated that the best policy is to individualize the teaching program to the situation and the patient's ability to understand. (4) Physicians were very supportive of the pharmacist's inclusion of such information as auxiliary directions and common side effects on the medication instructions; mildly supportive of inclusion of indications for use, less commonly occurring side effects and serious side effects; generally opposed to inclusion of self-monitoring techniques.[36]

Some might argue that health education, preventive medicine, and other health services and health educational activities are insufficient and that what is needed, rather, is a health activation or actualization program. It is thought that, in such a program, the patient will come to understand the importance of proper life style, including stress management, diet, use of leisure time, and other factors. It was hoped that the patient would be most interested to exercise and take good care of himself/herself. This then is what is "wellness." This movement is transforming the traditionally passive patient into an active, informed and effective participant in health care and health promotion.[37] Other activities proposed as role responsibilities of the pharmacist would include dealing with the dying patient or the relatives of dying patients, management of a medication refill clinic associated with pharmacist-managed patient assessment. Other studies have shown how the pharmacist is able to make a valuable contribution in a hemodialysis program, in which the involvement of the pharmacist raised patient knowledge and compliance. Some others suggest that the pharmacist be the only person to sell over-the-counter drugs. These data come from a study of over-the-counter drug users where it was learned that heavy users were more likely to be older, female and white and have blue-collar occupations if male, or to be housewives if female. Heavy drug use was associated with greater use of other medical care and was usually a persistent characteristic. Prepayment for drug prescriptions was not associated with heavy use. Among heavy users were found some severely ill individuals and some with emotional problems that appear to contribute to symptoms and requests for drugs. In a 21-month period, adverse drug reactions were experienced by 28% of heavy users, as compared with 8% of light over-the-counter drug users.[38]

Many of the problems encountered by contemporary pharmacy practitioners stem from the perceived level of status or stature held by the pharmacy practitioner. While Dichter found that the pharmacist was one of the very top members of society and that the druggist was somewhat slightly below that level, Knapp and others found that patients use various sources of medical advice for different levels of differently perceived severity of medical problems. The pharmacist was considered an adequate source for problems such as dandruff, etc., while other more credible sources included physicians' columns in newspapers and other such sources.[39]

Shaw analyzed the pharmacist's lack of social acceptance as a true professional. He suggests that retail or community pharmacists are generally alienated from a professional orientation due in part to their training, the structure of interpersonal relationships in the pharmacy, economics, restrictive government laws, lack of egoautonomy, and professional organizations.[40]

According to Stewart *et al.*, progress in this area is being made. Results of his study indicate that pharmacists were able to quite accurately perceive those factors considered important to consumers in their choice of pharmacy. However, pharmacists overestimated the importance of price to consumers and underestimated the importance of location. The pharmacist must, according to Stewart, periodically evaluate such conveniences as charge accounts and delivery to assess whether patrons desire or perceive them as costly extras.[41]

Another area that is worthy of attention is the recently developed popularity of holistic health care. Under this rubric the patient expects the provider or providers to consider the entire person and that individual's normal environment in considering therapy or treatment for the patient. While much is said about holistic health care, there appears to be very little of this type of care, given the very sensitive nature of it. Some have speculated that this is an ideal role for the pharmacist in which to become involved and others have suggested that it is really a fad and that it will pass shortly.

Gable suggests that pharmacists can provide a great deal of worthwhile service to society with a number of innovative roles. Among these would be service in the area of addiction, child abuse, alcoholism, sexuality problems, and contraception.[42] There cannot be any question any longer but that a dynamic relationship exists between human beings and their social environments, which can be the cause of good or poor health. We see these as intangible interactions existing between people modified by the current political, economic and cultural forces and structured by the physical environment.[43] One could continue indefinitely, but perhaps it would be wiser to stop and suggest that for additional information and insight into these areas the books listed in the *Bibliography* should be consulted.

The message and the thesis of this chapter may be simply stated. The patient is the focus for the practice of pharmacy and for all of the activities related to it. Knowledge about therapeutics, no matter in what great depth and quantity, are useless unless they can be translated into specific health-seeking services for patients in need of aid. Also, it must be remembered that illness is a frightening and undesirable state for most patients and that their behaviors and attitudes are very much modified by their state of illness, or well-being.

References

1. Parsons T: *Definitions of Health and Illness in the Light of American Values and Social Structure.* In Jaco EG, ed: *Patients,*

Physicians and Illness, 2nd ed, Free Press, New York, 112, 1972.
2. Mechanic D: Response factors in illness: the study of illness behavior. *Social Psychiatry 1:* 12, 1966.
3. Mechanic D: *Ibid.* p. 18.
4. Mechanic D: *Ibid.* p. 19.
5. Balint M, *et al:* *Treatment or Diagnosis*, Lippincott, Philadelphia, 1970.
6. Mechanic D: *Loc. cit.* p. 19.
7. Kasselbaum GG, Baumann BO: Dimensions of the sick role in chronic illness. *J Health and Human Behavior 6:* 17, 1965 (Spring).
8. Suchman EA: Stages of illness and medical care. *J Health and Human Behavior 6:* 114, 1965 (Fall).
9. Glaser BG: Disclosure of terminal illness. *J Health and Human Behavior 7:* 83, 1966 (Summer).
10. Bowden CL, Burstein AG: *Psychosocial Basis of Medical Practice*, Williams and Wilkins, Baltimore, 32, 1974.
11. Bowden CL, Burstein AG: *Ibid.* p. 40.
12. Barber B: *Drugs and Society*, Russell Sage Foundation, New York, 168, 1967.
13. Entralgo PL: *Doctor and Patient*, World University Library, New York, 150, 1969.
14. Entralgo PL: *Ibid.*, p. 154.
15. Entralgo PL: *Ibid.*, p. 181.
16. Coser RL: A home away from home. *Social Problems 4:* 3, 1956.
17. Brown EL: *Newer Dimensions of Patient Care: Patients as People*, Russell Sage Foundation, New York, 9, 1964.
18. Mechanic D, Newton M: Social considerations in medical education. *J Chronic Disease 18:* 293, 1965.
19. Anastasi A: Heredity, environment and question "how?" *Psychological Review 65:* 198, 1958.
20. Burlage HM, Burlage RK: *The Four Walls of Pharmacy*, Vantage Press, New York, p. xii, 1974.
21. Robinson D: *Patients, Practitioners and Medical Care*, Heinemann Books, London, 142, 1973.
22. Titmuss RM: *The Gift Relationship: From Human Blood to Social Policy*, Allen and Unwin, London, 1970.
23. Millis J, ed: *Pharmacists for the Future: The Report of the Study Commission on Pharmacy*, Health Administration Press, Ann Arbor, 142, 1975.
24. Millis J, ed: *Ibid.*, p. 126.
25. Talalay P, ed: *Drugs in Our Society*, Johns Hopkins Press, Baltimore, 244, 1964.
26. Talalay P, ed: *Ibid.*, p. 245.
27. Bush P: The placebo effect. *J APhA NS14:* 671, 1974.
28. Smith M: Management of the pharmacist-patient relationship: a strategy using sociological concepts. *J APhA NS17:* 761, 1977.
29. Knapp DE, *et al:* Can pharmacists influence drug prescribing? *Am J Hosp Pharm 35:* 594, 1978.
30. Dichter E: Today's patient—friend or foe? *J APhA NS12:* 354, 1972.
31. Kabat H: Pharmacist improvement of patient compliance. *Hospital Formulary 11:* 243, 1976 (May).
32. Eshelman F, Fitzloff J: Effects of packaging on patient compliance with an antihypertensive medication. *Current Therapeutic Research 20:* No. 2, 215, 1976 (August).
33. Romankiewicz J, *et al:* Development of patient medication instruction cards. *Am J Hosp Pharm 33:* 928, 1976.
34. Ivey M, *et al:* Communication techniques for patient instruction. *Am J Hosp Pharm 32:* 828, 1975.
35. Ryan P, *et al:* Economic justification of pharmacist involvement in patient medication consultation. *Am J Hosp Pharm 32:* 389, 1975.
36. Wallace D, Kradjan W: Physicians' opinions of pharmacists as dispensers of patient medication information. *J APhA NS17:* 362, 1977.
37. Shirreffs JH: The relevance of health education to health activation and self care. *J School Health 419*, 1978 (Sept.).
38. Lech S, *et al:* Characteristics of heavy users of outpatient prescription drugs. *Clinical Toxicology 8:* 599, 1975.
39. Knapp DE, *et al:* The pharmacist as perceived by physicians, patrons and other pharmacists. *J APhA NS9:* 80, 1969.
40. Shaw C: Societal sanctioning—the pharmacist's tarnished image. *Social Science and Medicine 6:* 109, 1972.
41. Stewart J, *et al:* Consumer-pharmacist congruence—understanding consumer wants and needs. *J APhA NS17:* 358, 1977.
42. Gable F: *Psychosocial Pharmacy: The Synthetic Society*, Lea and Febiger, Philadelphia, 1974.
43. Hastings A, *et al:* Health for the *Whole Person*, Westview, Boulder 1980.

Bibliography

Bakal D: *Psychology & Medicine*, Springer, New York, 1979.
Blum R, Herxheimer A, Stenzland C, Woodcock J: *Pharmaceuticals and Health Policy*, Holmes & Meier, New York, 1981.
Cassell E: *The Healer's Art*, Penguin, New York, 1971.
Cockerman W: *Medical Sociology*, Prentice-Hall, Englewood Cliffs, NJ, 1978.
Eisenberg L, Kleiman A: *The Relevance of Social Science for Medicine*, Reidel, Dordrecht, Holland, 1981.
Gentry W: *Behavioral Approaches to Medical Treatment*, Ballinger, Cambridge, MA, 1977.
May W: *The Physician's Covenant*, Westminster Press, Philadelphia, 1983.
Maykovich M: *Medical Sociology*, Alfred, Sherman Oaks, CA, 1980.
Mechanic D: *Medical Sociology*, 2nd ed, Free Press, New York, 1978.
Mechanic D: *Politics, Medicine, and Social Science*, John Wiley & Sons, New York, 1974.
Morgan J, Kagan D: *Society and Medication: Conflicting Signals for Prescribers and Patients*, Lexington Books, Lexington, MA, 1983.
Poynter N: *Medicine and Man*, Penguin, New York, 1971.
Wertheimer A, Bush P, eds: *Perspectives on Medicines in Society*, Drug Intelligence Publications, Hamilton, IL, 1977.
Wertheimer A, Smith M, eds: *Pharmacy Practice: Social and Behavioral Aspects*, 2nd ed, University Park Press, Baltimore, 1981.

CHAPTER 99

Patient Communication

Philip P Gerbino, PharmD
Professor of Clinical Pharmacy

Joan M Anderson, MS, EdM
Clinical Assistant Professor of Pharmacy
Philadelphia College of Pharmacy and Science
Philadelphia, PA 19104

Pharmacists Communicating with Patients

Pharmacists today may practice in any of several health care environments. At the community level, pharmacists provide a broad range of pharmaceutical services, including health care information, to a variety of patients. Some patient recipients are not ill, while some are under the care of a physician, receiving drug therapy for a chronic disease. Others are usually well, but currently receiving treatment for a short-term medical condition. There may be some patients who have returned to their homes after a period of hospitalization and may need home health care services before they are ambulatory. Others are either ambulatory or bed-fast residents of a long-term care facility.

Community pharmacists have become the focus and reference source for an increasing volume of information about therapeutic agents and their use. As consumers become more aware of their rights and responsibilities, they seek out not only prescription and non-prescription drug information, but the information important to other components of their own health and well-being, wherever it is offered. They obtain this information from the public media, from their health care providers, including physicians and pharmacists, and through consumer and civic group programs.

Pharmacists who practice in hospitals and other institutions are also expected to be providers of information about the drugs a patient uses while under their care, as well as those agents used before and after the hospitalization. Hospitalized patients are given their medication doses at specific times, but when they are discharged, they are expected to be responsible for managing their own medications and remembering to take them on time. Patients are more likely to follow the instructions of a physician when they understand the therapy prescribed. The hospital pharmacist may be the first pharmacist to establish the patient's understanding of the medication regimen. This drug therapy information is supported and expanded by the community pharmacist.

With greater responsibility being placed on the pharmacist to exercise professional skills and judgment, the necessity for effective communication becomes increasingly compelling. But it is this communications activity that the pharmacist is likely to find the least familiar, and therefore the most difficult. The American Pharmaceutical Association Standards of Practice for the Profession of Pharmacy recognize a number of professional activities in which the pharmacist must communicate effectively with the patient in order to adequately discharge his professional responsibilities:

- Interview the patient or his representative to obtain information for entry into patient record, patient profile, or family health record.
- Confirm and further clarify the patient's understanding of medication dosage, dosage frequency, and correct method of administration.
- Advise the patient of potential drug-related or health-related conditions which may develop from the use of the medication for which patient should seek other medical care.
- Consult with the patient to properly identify symptoms in order to advise for self-medication.
- Refer the patient to other health care providers and/or health resources where indicated.
- Instruct patients in the use of medical or surgical appliances (eg inhalers, colostomy bags, trusses).
- Advise patients on personal health matters (eg smoking, drug abuse).
- Participate in appropriate community educational programs relating to health care and drugs (eg drug abuse, alcoholism, hypertension).

Communication is the act of meaningful exchange of information, ideas, thoughts, and feelings. If it is truly effective, its end result will be to bring about mutual understanding between the pharmacist and his client. Communication involves understanding not just the spoken word, but also what is conveyed through inflection, qualities of voice, facial expression, body posture, and other behavioral responses. The following guidelines are offered to help the pharmacist in his process of learning to communicate with patients.

Communication as a Process

The goal of all communication is understanding. In order for person B to understand a message composed by person A, person B must do more than recognize the words used by person A in the message. Person B will have understood person A if the meaning person B assigns to person A's message is the same meaning person A attached to the message. Thus, it is only when the meaning of a message is held in common by both participants that effective communication has taken place.

The nature of the human organism makes it difficult to attain this point of understanding between two people (the difficulty is multiplied when more than two people are involved). The major obstacle to effective communication is that individuals have their own ways of making sense of their world. Each person's construction of reality is based on his own life experiences and is affected by that person's state of being at any given time.

The perception of an individual about the meaning of a message stems from his or her own view of reality. This individualistic perception will affect both the way in which a message is sent and the way in which it is received. People will select and interpret the messages they send and receive according to their beliefs about the world in which they live.

When person A wishes to share some information with person B, person A must choose a form in which to transmit that message. If person A decides to send the message by the spoken word, as opposed to the written word, or any other form of communication, then person A must choose the words that will best convey the meaning intended for person B to receive. This choice will be determined by person A's construction of reality, his feelings at that time and perception of person B.

Once the information has been encoded and sent, person A loses control of the message. The meaning that person A's message takes on will come from the decoding that takes place at its destination point, person B. Person B's decoding of person A's message will be determined by person B's own construction of reality, his feelings at the moment, and his view of person A. Any response given by person B to person A's message will reflect this evaluation and be the result of the encoding person B does before transmitting a return message.

Once person A has decoded person B's return message he can determine if person B has understood the message. Thus, person B's response to person A acts as feedback to person A. This gives person A the opportunity to correct any misunderstanding that has occurred.

The entire communication sequence can be portrayed diagrammatically as follows:

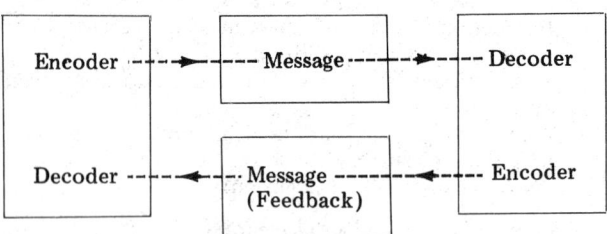

This sequence of encoding, message transmittal, and decoding will continue as long as person A and person B continue to communicate.

An additional factor that must be considered in any discussion of communication is that all communication takes place through multiple channels. At the same time the words of a message are transmitted, facial expressions, gestures, voice quality and other nonverbal cues are being sent. These nonverbal signs can modify a message's meaning. A point can be emphasized or de-emphasized according to how each channel is used in relation to the main channel of the spoken word.

Professional Communications for Pharmacists

Community pharmacists build their practice relationships on good communications and pharmaceutical skills. Few pharmacists, however, have had formal coursework in communication theory or training in communication practice. They may therefore find themselves limited to the casual and/or social conversations and be reluctant to initiate truly professional dialogue with patients.

In order to clearly understand the needs of the patient, pharmacists must learn when and how to use a major communication tool for professionals, the clinical interview. To enable the patient to understand and comply with instructions for appropriate drug use, the pharmacist must be able to convey his message clearly to the patient and to assure that the patient understands other vital prescription and health care information.

To maintain quality and effectiveness in their communications with patients, pharmacists need to understand and appreciate the experiences which may impinge on patient's lives. For any individual, illness almost always represents a crisis. The illness event is filled with stresses which may also impair or interfere with the communications process.

A summary of these patient-illness and adaptive factors, illustrating the opportunities for pharmacist communication with the patient, is shown in Fig 99-1.

Understanding the Patient: The Experience of Illness

A person may be facing separation from family, loss of important social roles, permanent bodily changes, feelings of helplessness, and an uncertain future. For most patients, the strain of illness leads to troubling doubts and common fears associated with illness. It is little wonder that any individual who experiences a serious physical illness faces one or several of the following adaptive tasks.

1. *Dealing with the symptoms of the illness*—A wide range of discomforts may be a continuous problem, eg, pain, weakness, dizziness, incontinence, paralysis.
2. *Dealing with the hospital or physician's office environment*—The bustling environment of the clinic, physician's office or hospital, with its sophisticated equipment, busy practitioners, and expressions of pain, can upset many patients.
3. *Developing adequate relationships with professional staff*—Asking and answering questions, requesting help, advice, information, or additional medication for pain may be difficult for patients unfamiliar with professional communications.
4. *Preserving emotional balance*—Despite the unfamiliarity of the hospital, the brisk office visit, and the pain and uncertainty of illness, the patient must manage feelings of fear, inadequacy and resentment.
5. *Preserving a satisfactory self-image*—Changes in physical functioning and appearance, loss of important social roles, can alter the sense of competence of an individual and greatly affect confidence.
6. *Preserving relationships with family*—Illness can isolate or cause dependency. In either case, relationships with friends and loved ones are often strained.
7. *Preparing for an uncertain future*—Loss of sight, limbs, or life are possibilities that must be faced by sick individuals and their loved ones.

Patients are often aware of these adaptions, fears, and concerns and disguise them with a facade of anger, depression, uncooperativeness, or demanding behavior. The skillful pharmacist, aware of the dynamics of communication and of the stresses imposed on the patient by illness, can help the patient recognize and cope with many of these emotions and fears (See Fig 1).

For the patient in the community or home health care setting, the common fears center around disability and disease severity. Frequently patients do not have a clear understanding of what is wrong with them. Even after repeated discussions with their physicians, many aspects of their illness may remain vague and uncertain. In such instances, fears may arise that could be easily abated by a simple explanations, reassurance and positive reinforcement by primary and supporting health professionals.

For the patient admitted to the hospital, hospitalization can be a terrifying experience. The fear of the unknown can be overwhelming. Busy doctors and nurses, sophisticated instruments, electronic monitors, tubes, IV bottles, laboratory tests, X-ray machines, a dying patient in the next room, a cry of pain, a seriously ill room-mate—all can be quite frightening. Health professionals are usually relaxed in this environment. Crisis occurrences that transpire routinely during the course of the day are commonplace. It is little wonder that anxiety and fears develop in patients while in the hospital. Health professionals may be insensitive to these fears. Awareness

STATE OF HEALTH	HEALTH	ILLNESS	SEVERE ILLNESS
LOCATION OF HEALTH CARE DELIVERY	Home	(ambulatory—acute or chronic)	Institution (hospital or nursing home)
PATIENT EXPERIENCES AND ADAPTIVE TASKS		Dealing with the symptoms of the illness Dealing with the physician's office	Dealing with the hospital environment Developing adequate relationships with professional staff Preserving emotional balance Preserving satisfactory self-image Preserving relationships with family Preparing for an uncertain future
LOCATION OF PHARMACY SERVICE	Community		Institution

PHARMACIST'S HEALTH CARE TASKS	1. Advice on:
	  —self-medication for minor complaints
	  —public health issues
	2. Referrals to other health professionals, when appropriate
		1. Monitoring and advice regarding
		  —OTC and Rx therapy
		  —adverse drug reactions
		2. Instruction, monitoring for compliance
		3. Referrals when appropriate
			1. Monitor medication use during institutionalization
			2. Provide post-discharge drug use education/instruction

PHARMACIST'S COMMUNI-CATION TASKS	1. Establish friendly relationships
	2. Demonstrate professional concern for patient's health
		1. Interview patients regarding:
		  —routine medications
		  —other illnesses
		  —life factors affecting compliance
			1. Establish helping role, "professional personality"
			2. Get information from patient on:
			  —past medication history
			  —life-style factors affecting compliance

COMMUNICATION SKILLS NEEDED	1. Approach to "well" clients	1. Question-asking 2. Sensitivity to patient fears, anxieties, hospital experiences	1. Sensitivity to patient's in-hospital experiences, fears, anxieties

Fig 99-1.   Pharmacists role in the experience of illness.

that patients can develop such fears will facilitate attempts to make them feel more relaxed and remove an important barrier to effective communication.

Many patients fear pain. Always remember this in discussions with a patient prior to a diagnostic or surgical procedure. The anxiety of a patient under these circumstances may be so great that effective communication is virtually impossible. In many cases, reassurance and an explanation of what is to transpire may aid in relieving some of the foreboding and anxiety.

Never underestimate the fear that may arise if there is a possibility of disability. Some patients may have had a serious accident, causing loss of limbs or other permanent impairment. Others may have had severe cardiac damage, leaving them disabled in terms of their usual life styles, activities, or functions. Fears concerning the degree of impairment and how to cope with it are a reality. Nurses, physical therapists, and others play a vital role in restoring confidence and assisting in the adjustment of the patient to such disability. It is important to be aware that such fears exist if effective communication with such patients is to be established.

The fear of death is common in many patients. Some patients subconsciously believe that a hospital is a place where people come to die. Knowing the severity and type of illness will usually be an indication as to which patients are candidates for this type of fear. Some individuals, although having only a relatively minor ailment, will exhibit a fear of dying. Communicating effectively in these cases is a formidable task for both the health professional and the patient. Reassurance within reason when indicated, as well as statements to strengthen confidence in the physician and hospital, are

helpful and recommended. Successful and effective communication with such patients will depend on the degree of genuine concern demonstrated or related in the course of conversations. It is essential to have empathy with such patients, yet it is equally important not to become emotionally involved beyond the scope of one's professional function.

Worries about finance, occupation and family problems will be on the minds of many patients. There should be awareness that they may exist.

Some patients are truly impaired by their disease process or their physical state at the moment, eg, IV's running, a catheter in place, traction or casts. These factors all hinder good communication.

Some patients are embarrassed, self-conscious, modest, or, at the other extreme, even bored while in the hospital. These are additional factors that one must be aware of and consider while communicating with such patients. If the pharmacist can understand how these factors affect the patient, the probability of effective communication with the patient will be increased.

Each patient will react differently to each of these tasks. The way in which the individual reacts will be determined by background and personal characteristics such as age, intelligence, emotional development, religious beliefs, and previous illness experiences. Each of these factors will determine how the crisis will be met.

Astute observation of the adaptive reactions of a patient can yield many clues to a fuller understanding of the patient and, thus, to more effective communication. Certain patients, for example, will be fearful of alienating the health professionals on whom they depend. This behavior is often reinforced by health professionals, by whom they are regarded as "good patients." This is not always beneficial as it can defeat attempts to detect symptoms such as pain and thus may hinder the progress of the patient's treatment. These "noncomplaining" patients can be helped to express themselves by inquiring about their feelings. How? Ask them how they feel and they'll say "fine." Ask them if they have any complaints and they'll say "no." It would probably be more effective to show a genuine interest through conversing with them for a time and then inquiring specifically about any pain or other symptoms that might hinder the treatment process.

Other patients may respond to illness by becoming very helpless and demanding of attention. These patients are often particularly difficult to deal with because they require so much time and patience. In caring for such patients it is essential to encourage them to do as much for themselves as possible; positive recognition should be given when they exhibit independence. A daily schedule of when staff personnel will be available will enable such patients to know that they will be able to depend on someone.

Patients who react by becoming hostile and uncooperative also require patience and understanding. Underlying fears of being helpless and dependent often cause this type of behavior. If these patients can become involved in formulating part of their treatment on a superficial plane and participate in making certain decisions about their care, they may gain assurance of their autonomy. For example, if a patient refuses to take medication, it is important to find out why and then discuss the reason. The task here is not to convince but to motivate. Motivation originates within the person and can seldom be externally controlled. Explain to the patient how the medication can help achieve the end result (recovery from illness) the patient desires—not why the patient should take the medication from the pharmacist's point of view. In other words, shift the center of interest from the pharmacist to the patient in order to motivate him or her. Although at times it is difficult not to become angry and argue with hostile and uncooperative patients, there is a meaning to their behavior that must be understood to establish effective communication.

There are patients who become depressed and withdrawn when confronted with illness. They may be reluctant to discuss their illness and their feelings about it because it is so emotionally painful for them. Short, frequent visits and conversations with such patients will be helpful in letting them know there is genuine interest in them and that someone really cares how they feel. This may eventually encourage them to "open up" and discuss their true feelings. But, as has been noted, the danger in getting the patient to talk about his feelings is the unleashing of excessive anxiety as his defenses are too rapidly dissipated or broken down. When defense mechanisms are threatened without a coordinate strengthening of the ego, where the person becomes aware of unacceptable (to him, at least) feelings, conflicts, or strivings, there is definitely danger of precipitating a crisis. Anxiety may get out of hand and shatter the ego, precipitating a psychosis. Assigning these patients small tasks which they can accomplish will assist them in regaining a sense of self-esteem and confidence.

In recent years, our culture has become increasingly aware of the unique problems of the dying patient. Successive phases of denial or acceptance of death, as well as a changing pattern of behavior, have been identified. Recognizing this behavior will enable comfort and support to be given to a dying patient. Sometimes the professional staff is more uncomfortable and unwilling to talk about death than is the patient. They may unconsciously ignore him because they feel there is little to say. Actually, just someone's general availability to listen to the patient and encourage ventilation of feelings may provide a source of great comfort.

In summary, by responding to patients' questions, clarifying misconceptions, preparing patients for probable feelings or events, the pharmacist can do much to decrease the uncertainties of illness. The pharmacist can also aid the patient by providing emotional support and appropriate reassurance. The emotional needs of the patient may require frequent repetition of such support. The pharmacist who can provide empathic understanding to the patient will be an important source of aid to the patient's attempts to cope with illness.

The Pharmacist as an Interviewer

There are intrinsic anxieties associated with being the pharmacist who must interview a patient to obtain a medication history. Because high levels of anxiety are inimical to good communication, the pharmacist needs to understand the possible causes of the patient's anxieties and how to overcome them.

The first of these anxieties is the "identity crisis." Pharmacists may find themselves in a new role when directly involved in the care of patients. The role of an interviewer has traditionally belonged to the physician. It is not uncommon for the pharmacist, when serving as an interviewer, to be made ill at ease by a patient, or even by other health professionals who ask, "Why does a pharmacist want to interview a patient?" An explanation that establishes the professional expertise of the pharmacist in discussing prescription medications, as well as over-the-counter drug products, should suffice as a valid answer. When placed in this position, it is essential to inform others by a statement of the purpose of the pharmacist's interview. The effectiveness and impact of the interviewer will depend to a great extent on how comfortable he or she is in this role, a quality easily evaluated by all concerned, especially the patient. Discomfort diminishes one's effectiveness and weakens the patient's confidence.

Another anxiety that must be contended with by the pharmacist interviewer is awareness of one's own inexperience. Pharmacists for the most part have not had extensive training as professional interviewers. It should be remembered, however, that very few individuals begin as polished interviewers. Psychiatrists, nurses, and other health professionals make minor errors. At times certain questions are forgotten or important facts are not recorded. Each patient is a unique individual, and different personalities will present an exciting challenge with each new interview. Provided one follows correct interviewing principles, one's proficiency and technique will improve with increasing experience.

The final anxiety that must be confronted is deciding with assurance that all facts have been acquired. At some point in the interview it must be concluded that sufficient information has been obtained to terminate the conversation. The purpose of this scientific inquiry is to obtain a specific and select body of information concerning the patient's medications. When this has been achieved one must not be afraid to terminate the inquiry.

An Approach to the Patient

The manner of the interviewer's approach to the patient determines in large measure the success or failure of the interview. To assure that the interview proceeds smoothly, the interviewer is well advised to spend a few moments in mental preparation for the interchange that is to follow. Being certain of the battery of questions to be used in the actual scientific inquiry and developing an alertness to observe the patient's nonverbal communications will greatly enhance the interpersonal experience and the ultimate quality of the interview.

The interviewer should be prepared to deal with any number of personality or behavioral qualities that are peculiar to patients' reactions to illness. Patients may be know-it-alls, advice seekers, anxious, angry, hostile, guilt-ridden, depressed, suicidal, obnoxious, anti-semitic, complaining, aggressive, provocative, shy, negative, senile, or may display a host of other moods, emotions or behaviors that will affect the interviewer's reaction to the patient and ultimately the quality of the interview.

It is prudent to know something about the patient before entering the room or conducting a less formal consultation or office interview. This objective is easiest to achieve in the hospital setting, but only rarely is it possible in a first-visit office or consultation setting.

In the ideal hospital situation, a medical history has been taken by a physician and recorded on the chart. In addition, nursing personnel have probably had contact with the patient on an interpersonal level. The chart and some prior discussions with other health professionals involved in the care of the patient about to be interviewed are all valuable sources of essential information.

The physical state of the patient should first be determined. Is the patient awake, cooperative, in pain or in distress, lucid or noncommunicative? Was this an emergency or an elective admission? It would be futile to attempt to interview a patient who is in acute pain, uncooperative, moribund, or semicomatose.

If the patient's physical state will allow the interview to be conducted properly, it is helpful to know the probable diagnosis. This information will provide a general index of the possible severity of the disease, the diagnostic procedure that will follow and, often, the prognosis. Earlier in this chapter the emotional and behavioral aspects of disease were mentioned. One can often suspect fear of the unknown, fear of pain, disability, or of dying merely by knowing the nature of the patient's condition.

Finally, the patient's social history and occupational history should be noted, for the content of the discussion will differ considerably depending on whether the patient is the president of a university or a taxicab driver. It is always best to communicate with a patient on his own level. The use of a balanced and understandable vocabulary is critical.

After obtaining this initial information the interviewer is ready to meet the patient and begin the interview. No better rule can be followed in the pharmacist's first contact with the patient than to heed the injunction to be himself/herself. Artificial dignity, practiced pompousness, and professional poise will be readily perceptible to most patients.

After about five minutes it should be possible to determine whether the patient is relaxed, anxious, depressed, unreliable, or uncooperative. One should have an initial index of how the patient will respond to questioning and, in general, what approach should be pursued. If the interviewer has adequately prepared the questions to accumulate a precise data base, the interrogatory phase can begin.

It is important for the interviewer to be observant. Some patients communicate and demonstrate their emotions in a nonverbal way. A blank stare, inattentiveness, lack of concentration, or patient-induced interruptions of the line of questioning, may be quite significant and related to the emotional and behavioral aspects of illness. There are numerous other clues, such as posture, voice tone and inflections, sighs, deep breaths, facial expressions, gestures or silence. Dress may give an indication of mood or emotion, especially if hygiene is poor and the patient is noticeably disheveled. The intensity of light in a patient's room, the presence of cards, flowers, television, radio and visitors may also be helpful nonverbal indicators.

If some of these nonverbal communications are detected, or if it is felt that the interpersonal relationship has not gone well, it is best to relay this impression to other health professionals involved in the patient's care. Their consultation should be solicited to inquire if they have had a similar experience with the patient. This may reveal important data that may prove to be beneficial for everyone's future reference in dealing with this patient.

The Clinical Interview

The clinical interview may be defined as a serious conversation with definite purposes or goals. The goals are to obtain a complete medication history on the patient and to benefit the patient in some way. The primary means to these goals is effective communication. In order to use the interview most effectively, however, one should also understand its dimensions and structure.

The Interview Structure—In discussing a clinical interview, one may take a number of different approaches, but for teaching purposes it is helpful to be somewhat dogmatic and present three basic concepts which are important to the clinical interview.

The first concept is that the clinical interview should function in at least two major dimensions, that of the scientific inquiry and that of the interpersonal experience. Pharmacists are well prepared for the scientific investigation through their years spent in classrooms, laboratories, and in specialized studies. Unfortunately, all too often many are unprepared to function in the dimension described as the interpersonal experience. This is, however, extremely important and will undoubtedly affect the quality of data obtained from the patient. It is possible to be expert in a scientific field, but if the interviewer is insensitive to the human quality of the patient or is unable to deal with this humanely, the scientific inquiry and the collection of data will not reflect scientific expertise. Many have had the experience of "working up a patient" in a hospital and then later, when presenting the patient to a consultant or to a visiting professor, find themselves quite embarassed when the visiting professor is able to elicit a different or at least a more detailed history. Often, of course, this indicates that the patient is unreliable, but on many occasions it represents the response of the patient to the greater expertise of the clinical consultant in the area of interpersonal relationships.

The second concept is that the clinical interview should have at least two major goals, that of the interviewer and the patient. The scientific inquiry should be sufficient to bring to light a specific body of information so that constructive recommendations can be made to the physician and the patient. The second goal is less obvious and is simply that the clinical interview should be made useful to the patient; that is, the patient should feel at the end of the interview that the time has been well spent and that something has been gained from the interview. This point will be discussed in some detail later.

The third concept is that the clinical interview be viewed in a structured way as having an initial phase, a middle phase, and a termination phase.

Beginning the Interview—The first phase of the interview usually involves an initial contact with the patient. In the first contact much can be accomplished. An introduction is made and the patient is told the purpose of the interview and that his physician has asked that it be done. Differences in interests, education and socioeconomic background may make it difficult to explain what the interviewer wants to know and why. Yet it is essential to the success of the interview that the explanation be made in such a way that the patient can understand its purposes. Otherwise, the information obtained is likely to be unreliable. To be frank, the interviewee must feel that his own point of view is respected, that the interviewer has a valid right to the information, and that the questions are relevant and not impertinent.

As the initial phase goes on one should observe the physical status of the patient. Are IV's running? Is there pain? What is the physical condition? In addition, the emotional status of the patient should be evaluated. Much can be learned from observation of the patient's nonverbal communications—facial expression, posture, gestures, and vocal modulations. The tone of voice, for example, may communicate more truly what is felt than what is said ("Speak in order that I may see you," said Socrates). If the interviewer is an astute observer, the hidden messages which reveal the patient's true emotional state will be detected. Is the patient withdrawn? Irritated? Pleased with the interview? Depressed? Anxious? If anxious, a few extra minutes in the initial phase of the interview might be spent to try to undercut this anxiety, because high levels of anxiety will undoubtedly affect the quality of information obtained from the patient. If depressed, it may be advisable to conduct three 10-minute interviews instead of conducting a 30-minute interview. It is a fact that a depressed patient has a difficult time maintaining concentration and attention and if one insists that the interview be a full 30 minutes the quality of information obtained from the patient may deteriorate as the time goes on. In addition, during the initial phase, the intelligence of the patient should be evaluated, and also ability to give a reliable history. Life-style is also important. Is the patient extroverted and verbal or introverted, passive and shy? If introverted, the interviewer must work harder to obtain the kinds of information needed. In summary, the patient's thinking, emotions, and behavior are being judged. In addition, one must be acutely aware of the patient's reactions as related to the interviewer and his emotional reactions to the patient. If a good experience in the past has been had with physicians and other authority figures, the patient will probably relate very positively. If, however, there have been bad experiences in the past, the patient may react in a negative fashion. If the interviewer reminds the patient of someone with whom there has been difficulty in the past, a negative reaction may develop which may interfere with the effort to establish good rapport. By the end of the initial phase of the interview, one should have developed rapport and some awareness of the patient as a human being. At this point one is ready to enter the middle phase of the clinical interview.

The Middle Phase of the Interview—In general, the bulk of the middle phase of the interview involves scientific inquiry. (The substance of the scientific inquiry of the pharmacist will be discussed later.) However, one should continue to evaluate the patient on an interpersonal level and make adjustments as one sees fit in terms of the interview style.

Terminating the Interview—When the inquiry has been completed, the termination phase takes place. This may be introduced by letting the patient know that he has just a few minutes remaining. The patient should now be allowed to comment on anything he thinks might be important that has been omitted in the interview. This can often be the point where very valuable information is obtained. The interviewer who relies entirely on prepared questions and the response of the patient will often miss valuable information.

A few minutes should be spent summarizing impressions and making some recommendations, if possible, to the patient. It is at this point the interview can often be made useful to the patient. If this is done the patient will feel that the time has been well spent and that something has been gained from the interview. If a diagnosis has been presented, the patient should again be allowed to express his concern and feeling about this, and the interviewer should be responsive. Having done this, the interview draws to a close. The only thing that might be added here is that, if possible and if time permits, continuing concern for the patient should be shown at a human level. This may be done by simply saying that a visit will be made at a later time to see how the patient is doing.

Specific Interview Techniques

During the initial or rapport-building phase of the interview it is advisable to begin conversation with simple, nonthreatening remarks. A positive and clear introduction is necessary so that the patient knows the interviewer's name and the purpose of the interview. The interviewer should also know the proper pronunciation of the patient's name. Liberties such as use of nicknames should never be taken unless at the specific request of the patient. Courtesy and respectfulness are always of utmost importance. Telling what you know about the patient often provides convenient entry into discussion of the patient's interests, mutual interests, sports, weather, current events, or other light conversation that facilitates relaxation and rapport.

The middle phase of scientific inquiry requires not only an interrogatory plan, but also the choice of the most effective modes of questioning. Open-ended questions provide the greatest latitude. They enable the patient to do the talking and provide the interviewer an opportunity to listen astutely for critical facts. "Tell me about," "tell me more about," "you mentioned that," "what made you decide," "why do you think," "what was it like," "what can you recall about," "what did you notice about it," are examples of some beginning phrases to open-ended questions.

Facilitating comments by the interviewer may encourage the patient to say more without specifying the area or topic to be discussed. Examples are "what happened then," "what about that," "go on," "I see," "is that so," "what do you mean," "I don't quite understand," "you mentioned . . ." Echo and reflection techniques are also quite useful. They are similar to facilitating comments in that they prompt the patient to continue on the same topic of discussion. Examples include "the pain comes on at night . . . comes on at night," "my nose is always stuffy . . . always stuffy." Direct questions should be used sparingly; however, they are very useful to obtain specific details such as dates, times, and essential patient demography.

In a successful interview, the patient has been the discussant and the interviewer has unbiasedly led the flow of discussion with systematic questioning. At the end of the patient's discussion in the middle phase, there may be some issues which the patient has left unclear. The interviewer should utilize this opportunity to take command in a nonthreatening way and confront the patient on points that were left unclear. It may be useful to repeat to the patient exactly what was said to assist in clarification. Examples are "did you say," "did you mean," "you said that," "I want to make sure I understand you when you say." This type of questioning must proceed in a positive manner or else the patient will sense that there is a problem of reliability or validity.

The terminating and final phase of the interview is important, even though the bulk of the scientific inquiry is completed. It is good practice to summarize aloud, especially highlighting critical points of the interview information. This technique has a high yield since it allows the patient an opportunity to add, delete or clarify items in the conversation. It also provides the patient the courtesy of the last formal words of the scientific inquiry. It is good technique to reestablish rapport with some final non-alarming conversation after the patient has been informed of what will happen with the interview information and the role it will play in the overall scope of care. It may even be prudent to determine if the patient remembers how to pronounce your name and where and how you can be reached. A parting gesture such as a handshake is appropriate, unless the situation is prohibitive.

It is appropriate to take notes during the interview provided they do not become the major focus of attention for either the interviewer or the patient. Excessive note-taking can be distracting to the patient, impair interpersonal dynamics and provide a convenient and absorbing escape for the interviewer. The beginning interviewer should take whatever notes are required to achieve accuracy and strive to gradually decrease this practice over a period of time.

The Pharmacist's Medication History

A medication history is vital to the total patient information accumulation process. All the principles of interviewing patients must be utilized. The scientific inquiry for a medication history is specific since its purpose is to develop a list of the patient's current and past medications, determine if the patient has had drug allergies or symptoms consistent with adverse drug effects. From a well prepared medication history, the interviewer will learn the patient's self-prescribing habits and over-the-counter drug preferences, as well as the patient's ability to follow a prescribed medication regimen and overall compliance.

A mix of direct and indirect questions is most effective for a medication history, for example: Are you able to take aspirin? How often do you take it? What brand did you buy? Does it give you a rash or affect you in any other way? Do you ever get headaches? Do you take medications or do anything to make them go away?

There are numerous question forms and formats available for reference. Any battery of questions deemed fit to obtain comprehensive data may be useful. The interviewer should choose questions and formats that are time-efficient and provide mutual patient/interviewer comfort.

The components of the scientific inquiry include precise patient demography, eg full name, address, age, etc. Very similar to the medical interview, it is essential to construct the past drug history of the patient. Some patients will bring old medications with them; others will only recall whether or not it was the "big white" or "small pink" pill. In indirect questioning on past medications, it is useful to determine if the patient knows why he was taking those medicines and what effects they had. Insertion of a subtle question which gives an indication about compliance is also useful, eg "Did you feel that you took your medicine regularly?"; "How often did you miss doses?"; "What were the reasons?". Among the most important issues to develop in the past medication history are those that relate to effectiveness and side effects. "Did the medicine help you?"; "How?" "Were there any side effects that you can recall?"; "What were they?"

Some patients do not consider over-the-counter medications as drugs and may not consider them during the interview. Pharmacist interviewers may have to ask direct questions such as, "What do you take when you have a cold; fever; constipation; stomach upset?".

Determining if the patient is allergic to medications requires both indirect and direct questioning. After the patient explains in his own words any allergic responses, it is useful to get a full explanation and all the details surrounding the allergic reaction (eg rash, hives, dizziness, chills, difficulty breathing, etc). Sometimes it is necessary to go through the entire list of drugs which have high allergic potential to be certain this area has been adequately explored, eg, penicillins, aspirin, sulfas, vaccines, narcotics, other antibiotics, etc.

Other areas to be explored in the scientific inquiry include exposures to toxins, chemicals, social drugs such as tobacco, alcohol and, finally, questions which may impact on the ability of the patient to take medications. Examples of such questions are: "Have you ever taken someone else's medicine?";

"Have you ever given someone else your medicine to take?"; "Where do you keep your medicine at home?"; "Do you have a system to help you to remember to take your medicine?"; "Do you carry your medicine around with you?"; "Why?"; "Where do you get your medicine?"; "Pharmacy(ies)?"; "Who is your local or regular physician(s)?"; "How often do you see him?"; "When was the last time you saw him?"; "When was the last time you had a blood test?"; "Do you have any trouble getting your medicine? (Distance, transportation)"; "What do you do when you run out of medicine?"; "Do you have or are you on Medical Insurance, Medicare? (Other)".

The interviewer must be flexible enough to obtain information in a variety of situations and environments. Too often in community pharmacy settings the quality of a medication interview is hampered by time factors, lack of privacy, or other adverse situations. Multiple short interviews, a follow-up phone call, or arranging a specific time to conduct an interview are among techniques that are successful in community practice.

The Discharge Interview

Studies continue to indicate that patient compliance with prescribed therapeutic regimens is poor. One of the reasons that patients do not comply is because they lack understanding of their diseases and the beneficial effects that the medications ultimately will have. Pharmacists must strive harder to insure that patients have the understanding they seem to be gravely lacking. The most convenient time for pharmacists to discuss medications and instill importance of compliance is during the discharge interview.

The discharge interview is not confined to a hospital room. It can be held in any ambulatory patient-care setting and on every patient-pharmacist contact within any community pharmacy.

The scope of the discharge interview is one of basic education and instruction. The discharge communication is an opportune time to discuss with the patient what has transpired during the course of his illness. The discussion should include the beneficial effects of the medication and how it will continue to help in the future. The importance of taking the medication as prescribed must be continually stressed and additional care must be taken to explain all special instructions, especially when and how to take the medication, what side effects it might have, what over-the-counter drugs are contraindicated, and so on.

A successful discharge interview should leave the patient with both confidence and trust that the interviewer is genuinely interested in his/her care. The patient should have an understanding of the medication prescribed and its importance. Lines of communication should be established so the patient can be assured that there is a concerned person to turn to in the event something goes wrong or questions arise about present drugs and future medication needs.

Bibliography

Bernstein L, et al, eds: Interviewing: A Guide for Health Professionals, 3rd ed, Appleton-Century-Crofts, New York, 1980.

Froelich RE, Bishop FM: Clinical Interviewing Skills, 3rd ed, C V Mosby Co, St Louis, 1977.

Blackwell B: New Engl J Med 289: 249, 1973.

Kalman SH, Schlegel JF: Standards of Practice for the Profession of Pharmacy, Amer Pharm NS19: 133–137, 1979.

Reisner DE, Schroder AK: Patient Interviewing: The Human Dimension, Williams and Wilkins Co, Baltimore, 1980.

Russell CG, Wilcox EM, Hicks CI: Interpersonal Communication in Pharmacy, Appleton-Century-Crofts, New York, 1982.

CHAPTER 100

Patient Compliance

Daniel A Hussar, PhD

Remington Professor of Pharmacy
Philadelphia College of Pharmacy and Science
Philadelphia, PA 19104

The significant advances that have been made in the understanding of the etiology of many disease states, and the development of new therapeutic agents, have made it possible to cure or provide symptomatic control of many clinical disorders. However, concurrent with the increasing sophistication relative to diagnostic and therapeutic knowledge and skills has been a growing recognition that, in many circumstances, drugs are not being used in a manner conducive to optimal benefit and safety. A need has been identified to ask the most basic questions regarding drug usage—does the patient understand how to take his medication and, if so, is it being taken according to the directions provided? Although problems concerning patient compliance with instructions have been recognized for years, these problems continue to be prevalent and it has only been relatively recently that this issue has begun to receive the attention it deserves.

When the complexity of the patient's illnesses and the actions of potent therapeutic agents are taken into account, the physician and other health professionals can easily become preoccupied with the diagnosis of the disease state as well as the selection and implications of drug therapy and assume that the patient will follow the instructions provided. After all, the medication is being provided to improve and/or maintain the patient's health so why would the patient not cooperate by following instructions? Yet studies continue to show that a large percentage of patients, for a variety of reasons, do not take their medication according to instructions.

Patient Compliance

With regard to the provision of health care the concept of compliance can be broadly viewed, as it relates to instructions concerning diet, exercise, rest, return appointments, etc, in addition to the use of drugs. However, it is in discussions concerning drug therapy that the designation, "patient compliance" is most frequently employed. It is in this context that it will be used in this discussion and compliance can be defined as the extent to which an individual's behavior coincides with medical or health advice. Some have recommended the use of the terms *adherence* or *concordance*, as they are considered to have a less coercive connotation than the designation, *compliance;* however, the latter term continues to be the most widely accepted and utilized.

The term "patient noncompliance" suggests that the patient is at fault for inappropriate use of medication. Although this is often the case, it has become apparent that responsibility for many cases of noncompliance should more appropriately be directed at the physician and/or pharmacist for failing to give the patient adequate instructions or not presenting them in a manner he understands.

The situations most commonly associated with noncompliance with drug therapy include failure to have the prescription filled, omission of doses, errors of dosage, errors in the time of administration of the drug, premature discontinuation of the drug, and taking a drug for the wrong purpose.

Although studies conducted to date reflect a wide variation in the degree of noncompliance, many data indicate that at least a third of the patients failed to comply with instructions, and for patients with chronic illnesses on longterm treatment regimens the results suggest a rate of noncompliance of approximately 50%. To provide a better insight into the extent of the specific problems identified, the results of several studies are reviewed.

In one study[1] of 134 patients who received 380 prescriptions it was judged that errors of major clinical significance were committed on 118 prescriptions (31% of those studied). The most significant type of error was not having the prescription filled, which occurred in 24 cases. The most common error involved use of the medication at improper dosing intervals, although in most cases these occurrences were not considered to be clinically significant. The most frequently occurring error thought to be clinically significant involved premature discontinuation of the drug by the patient.

Another study[2] which showed that 51% of patients in the outpatient setting were noncompliant for written prescriptions prompted an investigation of how patients interpret instructions provided on prescription labels. Sixty-seven patients were asked to interpret instructions on each of ten prescription labels and in not one case was a label uniformly interpreted by all patients. Even when the instructions were not felt by the prescriber to be ambiguous there was frequent misinterpretation with the incidence of interpretive errors ranging from 9 to 64%.

Noncompliance among hypertensive patients is well recognized; in one survey,[3] only 64% of those on medication stated they were taking their medicine all the time as prescribed, while approximately 25% said they never took any.

Problems of compliance have also been frequently noted among elderly patients, many of whom have been prescribed complex therapeutic regimens. In one study[4] of 50 individuals aged 65 years and older who were living independently in the community, it was observed that 66% of the medications were being taken without adequate instructions and 25% of the medications were not being taken as labeled. The challenge of increasing the compliance of elderly patients is the subject of several recent reviews.[5,6]

Similar problems have been reported in pediatric patients. In a study of compliance[7] with treatment of acute otitis media in 300 pediatric outpatients, complete compliance in taking prescribed antibiotics was only about 7%. Parents gave fewer than the prescribed number of doses in 36% of cases and therapy was discontinued early in 37%. Other factors contributing to the noncompliance included incorrect labeling and the use of "teaspoons" having widely varying volumes.

The likelihood of noncompliance is greatest in outpatients since there is a lesser degree of supervision of the therapy and most studies of these problems have been in this group of patients. However, although understandably not as prevalent, noncompliance can also be a problem in patients who are hospitalized or under similar close supervision. The results of one investigation[8] indicate that one in five inpatients did not take the medications given them by the nursing staff as compared to a 48% incidence of noncompliance among outpatients at the same hospitals. The practice of some patients, in particular patients being treated for psychiatric disorders, to "cheek" their medication until the nurse leaves the room is well recognized.

Consequences of Noncompliance

The consequences of noncompliance, although seemingly apparent, are often not fully appreciated. In many cases noncompliance will result in *underutilization* of a drug, thereby depriving the patient of the anticipated therapeutic benefits and possibly resulting in a progressive worsening of the condition being treated.

Several examples of problems can be cited. A patient may discontinue taking an antibiotic for treatment of an infection when the symptoms subside and therefore not use all the prescribed medication. This could result in a recurrence of the infection since the shorter course of therapy was not sufficient to eradicate it. Patients with infections such as tuberculosis have on many occasions been classified as being refractory or developing resistance to agents such as isoniazid when there is a relapse. However, in a number of such cases the relapse has resulted from noncompliance rather than development of resistance to the drugs.

In the management of hypertensive patients, if the physician is unaware that the patient is not taking the medication according to directions and sees that the elevated blood pressure is not well controlled, he may prescribe larger doses of the same agent(s) or prescribe more potent antihypertensive medications. This will expose the patient to a greater risk of adverse effects. Therefore, before a patient is judged to be unresponsive or not optimally controlled with the initial therapy prescribed, it should be ascertained that the medication is being taken according to instructions. True resistance to an antihypertensive regimen is uncommon, and noncompliance and inadequate dosing are the factors most often responsible for the insufficient control of elevated blood pressure. Noncompliance is one of the most commonly missed diagnoses and the manner in which a patient is using his medication should be evaluated before the therapeutic regimen is changed.

There has been considerable discussion about the potential risks associated with the abrupt discontinuation of therapy with antihypertensive drugs, in particular clonidine (*Catapres*) and propranolol (*Inderal*). Opinions differ as to the incidence and severity of the problems which could result. However, there have been reports of rebound hypertension and ventricular arrhythmias when antihypertensive agents have been suddenly withdrawn and additional complications such as worsening of angina may be associated with propranolol withdrawal. Patients should be advised of the risks of missing doses, and when it is desired to discontinue the drug(s), the dosage should be gradually reduced over a period of several days.

One report[9] has called attention to the hazards of noncompliance with anticonvulsant drug regimens. In examining autopsy records pertaining to 11 cases of unattended, unexpected deaths of epileptic patients, no anticonvulsant drugs were found in four patients and subtherapeutic levels were noted in six others. It is suggested that a number of these deaths may have been preventable had there been better compliance with the instructions for using the medication(s).

The underutilization of one drug may actually result in an excessive response to other agents being employed concurrently. Agents such as digoxin and hydrochlorothiazide (*HydroDiuril*) are frequently used together in patients with congestive heart failure, and potassium chloride is also often administered to replace the potassium that is excreted as a result of the action of the diuretic. If the patient were to stop taking the potassium chloride, potassium depletion could result, making the heart more sensitive to the effect of digoxin. That this type of a problem is a definite possibility is borne out by the results of a study[10] in which the compliance rate for potassium chloride was only 60% as compared to 92% for digoxin and 83% for hydrochlorothiazide. Therefore, noncompliance is a contributing factor to the rather large number of cases of potassium depletion and toxicity of cardiac glycosides that continue to occur with frequency.

Noncompliance may also result in the *overutilization* of a drug. When excessive doses are employed or when the medication is given more frequently than intended there is an increased risk of adverse reactions. These problems may develop rather innocently, as in the case where a patient recognizes that he has forgotten a dose of medication and doubles the next dose to make up for it. Some other patients apparently subscribe to a philosophy that if the one-tablet dose that has been prescribed provides some relief of symptoms, two or three tablets will be even more effective.

The problems associated with noncompliance may be serious enough to require hospitalization. Although estimates vary, one commentary[11] suggests that noncompliance may be a contributing factor in approximately one in 20 hospital admissions.

Noncompliance may also take other forms. The problems associated with drug misuse and abuse, whether unintentional or deliberate, are well recognized. Although usually not thought of in terms of noncompliance, drug abuse problems sometimes result from excessive use of medications which have been prescribed for existing clinical disorders.

Another implication relates to the storage of drugs that are not completely utilized during the intended period of treatment. Keeping these drugs may result in their inappropriate use at some later time. Accidental poisonings have resulted, and stockpiled medications have been used to commit suicide.

It should also be recognized that some individuals use medication that has been prescribed for relatives or friends, and this practice also reflects an attitude toward the use of drugs that can result in problems. In one study[12] of 75 patients it was found that 9 were using drugs that had been prescribed for other individuals.

The recognition that noncompliance is so prevalent has raised questions regarding the attention this variable has received in clinical trials of new therapeutic agents. Although numerous controls are built into these studies, the difficulty in assuring compliance and the potential changes in therapeutic response resulting from noncompliance dictate that close attention be given to this aspect of the study of the action of therapeutic agents.

Although the consideration of the consequences of noncompliance should focus primarily on the problems that may develop, there also should be an awareness of situations in which some patients may benefit from being noncompliant. Designated by one investigator[13] as *intelligent noncompliance*, it is noted that certain individuals have a rational basis (eg, avoiding adverse effects) for altering the dosage of their medication and that good treatment outcomes are still attained. In one study[14] of patients treated with digoxin, it was observed that patients identified as being noncompliant were considered to be under adequate therapeutic control. This study suggests that certain patients could be successfully treated with dosages of digoxin that were less than those initially prescribed and that some patients did not need the digoxin at all.

It would be hoped that those patients who do have a valid basis for noncompliance would discuss this matter with the practitioners responsible for their treatment program so that the clinical disorder(s) and therapeutic regimen may be re-evaluated.

The fact that selected patients may benefit from not adhering to a treatment regimen must not be considered a reason for health professionals being less diligent in detecting noncompliance and initiating the appropriate corrective measures, as any situation in which noncompliance occurs requires careful evaluation.

Detection of Noncompliance

Studies of noncompliance have employed a number of methods to obtain data. Direct methods in which the medication can be detected in the patient most frequently involve a determination of the presence, absence, or actual levels of the drug, or an added marker substance (eg, riboflavin in urine measurements), in the urine or blood. Although the absence of drug in the body fluid being analyzed is indicative of noncompliance, these methods are less definitive in patients who are taking some of their medication but not in the prescribed manner. Other limitations of these methods include variations in serum or urine concentrations based on pharmacokinetic factors, as well as the patient inconvenience and expense associated with obtaining and analyzing the sample of fluid.

The efficacy and safety of certain medications are monitored, in part, by the determination of serum levels on a periodic basis, and this information will also be useful in assessing compliance. However, there are few situations in which the routine monitoring of serum levels primarily for the evaluation of compliance can be justified.

The indirect methods of identifying noncompliance involve an assessment by the patient or another individual of the extent to which the patient has taken the medication. These methods include *pill counts*, interviews of the patient (ie, self-reporting), evaluation of the outcome of therapy, and physician estimates of compliance. The pill count method (in which the patient is asked to return the medication container at regular intervals so that the remaining dosage units may be counted) has limitations but is considered more reliable than patient interviews.

The effectiveness of interviews of patients in assessing compliance depends, to a large extent, on the skill of the interviewer. However, noncompliance may not be detected when even the best interviewing technique is used as patients will often overstate compliance because of forgetfulness, embarrassment, or fear. In spite of the limitations of this method, asking carefully constructed questions (eg, "Most people have trouble remembering to take their medicine. Do you have trouble remembering to take yours?")[15] in a non-threatening manner will be helpful in identifying some noncompliant patients.

In some conditions (eg, convulsive disorders) the treatment outcome (ie, reduced incidence and/or severity of seizures) usually reflects the level of compliance. However, in a number of other conditions, treatment outcome cannot be considered a reliable measure of compliance as some highly compliant patients may fail to show significant clinical improvement, and some poorly compliant patients may improve without having taken the full treatment regimen or for reasons other than the use of medication.

In several studies in which physicians were asked to predict their patients' compliance, compliance was overestimated and the results were little better than could be obtained by chance. In one study,[16] physicians overestimated their patients' compliance with an antacid regimen by about 50% and patients overstated their compliance with the regimen by about 100%.

The challenge of assessing compliance is further complicated by the fact that it is difficult to observe compliance without affecting it.[17] Nevertheless, in spite of the limitations noted, it is important that health professionals persist in efforts to identify noncompliance with treatment regimens. Several have suggested an approach of asking the patient about compliance while also making the patient aware that other methods might be used to confirm the claimed level of compliance.

The Noncompliant Patient

Efforts have been made to demonstrate the relationship of noncompliance to a number of variables such as age, education, occupation, socioeconomic status, personality factors, physiologic variables, and the number, types, and severity of illnesses. Although certain patterns have been noted in some studies, the results, in general, have been inconsistent and it continues to be difficult to identify which patients are most likely to be noncompliant.

A distinction has been made between attitudinal and behavioral compliance, since often the attitude and behavior of a patient may be incongruent. For example, a patient may fully intend to take the medication according to instructions but actually not do so because he is forgetful or does not really understand the instructions. On the other hand, some patients may have no intention of complying but nevertheless do so.

Some individuals are intentionally noncompliant. In one study[18] of elderly patients, almost three-quarters of the individuals observed to be noncompliant intentionally did not take their medication(s) according to instructions. The reason most frequently provided was that the patient did not believe the drug was needed in the dosage prescribed by the physician. It was noted that intentional noncompliance was more likely to occur in patients who used two or more pharmacies and two or more physicians.

The recognition that noncompliance may be intentional as well as unintentional underscores the complexity of the challenge to develop strategies to improve compliance. Although considerable progress has been made in recognizing and addressing the problems associated with noncompliance, an observation made in an early discussion[19] of this subject continues to be valid today—"It has not proved possible to identify an uncooperative type. Every patient is a potential defaulter; compliance can never be assumed."

Considerable attention has been directed toward the sociobehavioral determinants of compliance and a number of models based on behavioral principles have been described.[20,21] Of primary interest is a *health belief* model initially developed[22] to explain preventive health behaviors such as obtaining immunizations and prophylactic dental care. This model was subsequently revised[23] to apply to compliance with prescribed medical regimens and, most recently, a *third-generation* model has been proposed[24] which focuses more specifically on health decisions. This *health decision* model combines decision analysis, behavioral decision theory, and health beliefs to yield a model of health decisions and resultant behavior. The components of this model and the manner in which they are inter-related are outlined in Fig 1.

With respect to the relationship between health beliefs and compliance, if compliance is to be achieved, the patient must believe (1) that he actually has the illness which has been diagnosed, (2) that the illness could cause severe consequences with regard to his health and daily functioning, (3) that the treatment prescribed will reduce the present or future severity of the condition, and (4) that the benefits of the regimen prescribed outweigh the perceived disadvantages and costs of following the recommended action. In addition, there must

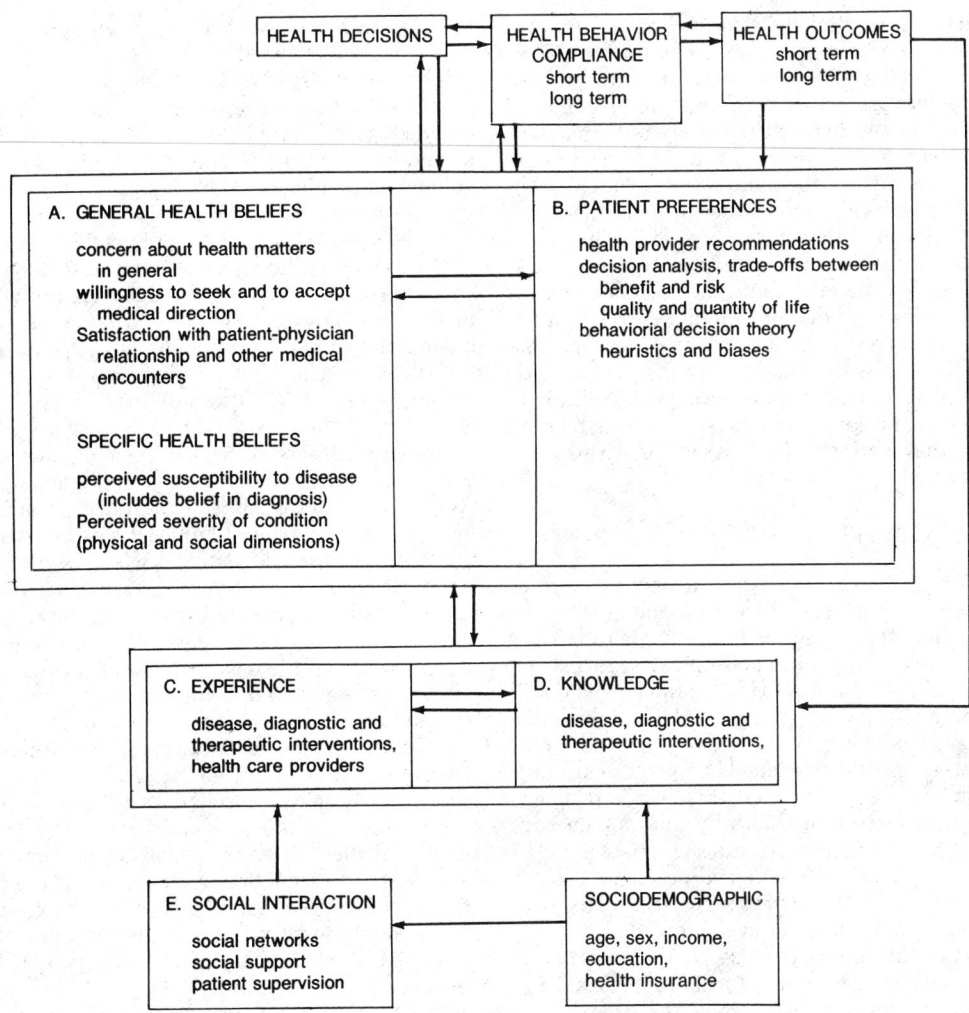

Fig 100-1. The health decision model, combining the health belief model and patient preferences, including decision analysis and behavioral decision theory, (reprinted with permission from *Ann Intern Med 100:* 261, 1984.   Eraker SA, *et al.   Understanding and Improving Patient Compliance.*)

be a stimulus to trigger the advocated health behavior, which can be either internal (eg, concern about the disease) or external (eg, interaction with the physician or pharmacist).

There are also other "patient factors" which may result in noncompliance. Patients who live alone are less likely to comply than those who live with another family member who can take an interest in and/or supervise their therapy. The increasing problems of drug abuse and addiction have increased the awareness and concern about becoming dependent on agents that are prescribed for legitimate medical reasons.

Although drugs that carry a potential for abuse and development of dependence are often prescribed and utilized too casually, some patients develop a fear of dependence regarding use of any drug that is to be employed for a prolonged period. To avoid such a possibility or to prove to themselves that they are not dependent, they may interrupt or stop therapy, or use the medication in smaller amounts.

Numerous other factors have been suggested to contribute to patient noncompliance and the more important of these are considered in the following discussion.

Factors Associated with Noncompliance

In addition to the patient factors previously considered, a number of other determinants of patient compliance have been cited. These have been carefully analyzed by Haynes,[25] who has identified determinants whose association with noncompliance has been confirmed by research studies, and has also discussed other factors which have been suggested, but not conclusively documented, to contribute to noncompliance.

Some of the more important and/or commonly considered factors are discussed below. Although the relationship of some of these factors to the occurrence of noncompliance has not been proven, there should be an awareness of the potential implications in selected patients.

Disease Factors

The nature of the patient's illness may, in some circumstances, contribute to noncompliance. In patients with psychiatric disorders, the ability to cooperate as well as the attitude toward treatment may be compromised by the illness, and these individuals may be more likely than other patients to be noncompliant. Several studies of patients with conditions like schizophrenia have shown a high incidence of noncompliance. However, others have questioned[17] whether psychiatric patients are any less compliant than other patients.

Patients with chronic illnesses, particularly conditions such as hypertension which are often not associated with significant symptomatology, are also more likely to be noncompliers. Patients understandably tend to become discouraged with extended therapeutic programs that do not produce "cures" of the conditions. Even when "cures" can be anticipated as a result of long-term therapy, problems can still occur, as exemplified by patients with tuberculosis who frequently become noncompliant as the treatment period continues.

It might be anticipated that if a patient experiences significant symptoms if the therapy is prematurely discontinued that he will be more attentive to taking medication correctly. However, few studies have demonstrated a correlation between disease severity and compliance, and it cannot be assumed that these patients will comply with their therapeutic regimens. The relationship between the degree of disability caused by a disease and compliance is better defined, and it can be expected that increased disability will motivate compliance in most patients.

Therapeutic Regimen Factors

Multiple Drug Therapy—Although several studies suggest otherwise, it is generally felt that the greater the number of drugs a patient is taking the higher is the risk of noncompliance. Even when rather specific dosage instructions for the medications are provided, problems can still occur. For example, many geriatric patients are taking five or six or more medications several times a day at different times. It becomes easier to understand how geriatric patients can become confused regarding their therapeutic regimens when one considers how often healthy young women have difficulty in taking oral contraceptives according to a simple dosage schedule using specially designed packages. In addition, some geriatric patients may experience lapses of memory that make noncompliance even more likely.

The similarity of appearance (eg, size, color, shape) of certain drugs may contribute to the confusion that can exist in the use of multiple drugs. It is desirable that there be an awareness of the physical characteristics of the drugs utilized so that the patient will not be taking, for example, only small white tablets. In one report,[26] serious complications experienced by two patients are described, which were apparently attributable to the patients' confusing digoxin, 0.25 mg, with furosemide (*Lasix*), 40 mg, another small white tablet.

Although combination drug products have a number of disadvantages and have received quite a bit of negative publicity in recent years, their use may help improve compliance with therapy since only one tablet need be administered rather than several. The issue of compliance provides a reasonable argument for the use of combination products although some have raised questions as to whether the available evidence supports claims of improved compliance. Therapy should not be initiated with a combination product but rather with the individual agents. Once the optimal dosages of the individual drugs have been determined, if they correspond to the amounts included in the combination, these products can be used to advantage.

Frequency of Administration—The administration of medication at frequent intervals makes it more likely that the patient's normal routine or work schedule will have to be interrupted to take a dose of medication and in many cases the patient will forget, not want to be inconvenienced, or even be embarrassed to do so. Although it would seem likely that the administration of individual drugs at less frequent intervals would enhance compliance, multiple dosage with a single drug appears to have less of an influence on compliance than the use of multiple drugs.

Many drugs must be given at frequent intervals to maintain desired blood and tissue levels. However, some drugs (eg, tricyclic antidepressants) that were traditionally administered three or four times daily are usually just as efficacious when administered once daily.

The use of drugs at less frequent intervals will only be successful with those agents having long half-lives as well as an adequate interval between the blood levels that produce a therapeutic response and those that can result in the development of adverse effects. If the latter situation was not the case, the use of larger doses at less frequent intervals could provide blood levels that result in adverse effects.

Duration of Therapy—Several studies have shown that the rate of noncompliance becomes greater when the treatment period is long. As noted earlier, a greater risk of noncompliance should be anticipated in patients having chronic disorders, especially if discontinuation of therapy is not likely to be associated with prompt recurrence of symptoms or worsening of the illness.

Adverse Effects—The development of unpleasant effects of a drug is a likely deterrent to compliance although several studies suggest that this is not as important a factor as might be expected. In some situations it may be possible to change the dosage or use alternative drugs to minimize adverse effects. However, in other cases these alternatives may not exist and the benefits expected from therapy must be weighed against the risks. Particularly disconcerting are those situations in which the development of side effects makes the patient feel worse than he did before therapy was initiated, as often occurs in hypertensive patients.

In a recent survey[27] of oncologists, over 60 percent identified noncompliance as a problem. The adverse effects (eg, nausea, vomiting, hair loss) associated with the use of many antineoplastic drugs, are sufficiently distressing to a number of patients that they do not take their medication in the manner intended. The reduction in the quality of life resulting from effects such as severe nausea and vomiting, may be of such importance to some individuals that they do not comply with a regimen which, in some cases, may even offer the hope of being curative.

The ability of certain drugs to cause sexual dysfunction has been cited[28] as a reason for noncompliance by some patients, with the antipsychotic and antihypertensive agents being implicated most frequently.

Even a warning about possible adverse reactions may result in some individuals not complying with instructions. It is inadvisable for patients being treated with sedatives or other agents having a central nervous system depressant effect to consume alcoholic beverages because of the possibility of an excessive depressant response. However, there should be a realistic recognition that many patients, if faced with a mandate not to drink while on drug therapy, will choose not to take their prescribed medication. Although problems of combined alcohol-drug usage are well known, this situation continues to present a challenge of effectively communicating with the patient so that optimal benefit can be achieved at minimal risk. Every patient for whom a depressant drug has been prescribed should be alerted to the fact that this effect may be enhanced by alcohol. If it is anticipated that the patient will not cooperate in completely avoiding alcoholic beverages, he should be urged to use them in moderation, particularly when therapy is initiated, and cautioned to observe his own tolerance when they are employed in combination. However, the fact that many individuals can take depressant drugs and consume relatively large amounts of alcoholic beverages with no apparent difficulty should not be cause to forget that such combinations have proven lethal in some individuals.

Patients May be Asymptomatic or Symptoms Subside—It is understandably difficult to convince a patient of the value of drug therapy when the patient has not experienced symptoms prior to initiation of therapy. Such is often the case in the treatment of hypertension, and the lack of previous symptoms coupled with the probable lack of appearance of symptoms if therapy is discontinued contributes to the high rate of noncompliance in these patients.

Other situations in which the benefits of drug therapy are not directly apparent include circumstances in which a drug is used on a prophylactic basis. Noncompliance is often seen in children for whom penicillin has been prescribed prophylactically to prevent recurrence of rheumatic fever. Since compliance in administering penicillin orally on a continuing basis is often difficult to achieve, many physicians prefer to give monthly injections of benzathine penicillin G (*Bicillin*).

In other circumstances the patient may feel better after taking the drug and feel that he no longer needs to take it once the symptoms subside. Situations frequently occur where a patient does not complete a full course of antibiotic therapy once he feels that the infection has been controlled. This practice increases the likelihood of a relapse of the infection.

Cost of Medication—Although noncompliance does frequently exist with the use of drugs that are relatively inexpensive, it might be anticipated that patients will be even more reluctant to comply with instructions for the use of more expensive agents.

The expense involved has been cited by some patients as the reason for not having prescriptions filled at all, whereas in other cases the medication is taken less frequently than intended or prematurely discontinued because of the cost. Antibiotics are among the higher priced drugs, and it is recognized that some patients will discontinue taking the drug as soon as symptoms subside so that they can save the balance of the medication for similar problems they may encounter in the future.

One observer has noted[29] that psychiatrists often prescribe expensive medication that some patients cannot afford. He goes on to state that "many people would rather be sick than poor or at least they would be willing to be less than healthy if they could remain relatively wealthy—something doctors seldom understand."

In a recent study[30] of patient behavior patterns regarding prescription refills, it was observed that the refill ratio for the highest-priced prescriptions was greater than the refill ratio for the lower-priced prescriptions. This finding differs from the general perception that there is a lower rate of compliance with higher-priced medications, and the authors offer a possible explanation that these patients are truly compliant and might be requesting larger quantities when the prescriptions are refilled for the purpose of obtaining a lower per unit price through quantity purchase.

Administration of Medication—Although a patient may fully intend to comply with instructions, he may inadvertently receive the wrong quantity of medication due to incorrect measurement of medication or use of inappropriate measuring devices. In one study[7] of the use of antibiotics in pediatric patients, the volume of 130 "teaspoons" was measured and found to vary from 2 to 9 mL. The inaccuracy of using teaspoons to administer liquid medications is compounded by the possibility of spillage and when the patient is called on to measure a fraction of a teaspoonful. Although this problem has been long recognized, it has still not been effectively addressed and the importance of providing the patient with measuring cups, oral syringes, or calibrated droppers for the use of oral liquids is evident.

The techniques for administering medication to infants and young children, as well as the appropriate use of oral dosing devices, are the subject of a recent review.[31] Although in one study[32] it is observed that the dosage range of certain pediatric oral medicines is quite broad and extreme accuracy may not be critical, accuracy in measuring medications should be emphasized, and the pharmacist has an important responsibility in providing information and, if necessary, the appropriate devices to assure the administration of the intended amount of medication.

It has been noted[33] that some patients do not use metered-dose aerosol inhalation devices correctly and this could result in inadequate control of the conditions (eg, asthma) for which their use are intended. In this study, the provision of verbal instruction by the pharmacist regarding the correct use of the inhaler, significantly increased compliance.

Unpleasant Taste of Medication—Taste problems of medications are most commonly encountered with the use of oral liquids by children. Getting a child to take a dose of medication may be such a difficult task for a parent that noncompliance may result or administration of the drug discontinued as soon as the parent sees any sign of improvement. However, compliance problems relating to the taste of medication are not limited to children. Objections to the taste of liquid potassium chloride preparations are often raised; a number of patients discontinue taking the medication for this reason. This is borne out, in part, by a study[10] cited earlier in which it was noted that compliance in taking potassium chloride was less than with digoxin or hydrochlorothiazide. For patients who object to the taste of the available liquid potassium chloride preparations, the use of sustained-release potassium chloride tablets might be considered.

Patient/Health Professional Interaction Factors

The circumstances surrounding the visit of a patient with a physician and/or pharmacist, and the quality and effectiveness of the interaction and communication of these health professionals with the patient, are major determinants of the patient's understanding of and attitude toward his or her illness and therapeutic regimen. One of the patient's greatest needs is psychological support provided in a compassionate manner and it has been observed that patients are more inclined to comply with the instructions of a physician they know well and respect, and from whom they receive information and assurance about their illnesses and medications.

One group of investigators[34] has viewed the patient-physician interaction as a negotiation among two active and equal participants with a strategy which includes the elements of "putting the ill at ease," respect, positive attitude, information, translation, feedback, patient response, and negotiation. Respect for the patient and a realistic appraisal of the circumstances of the individual patient are essential if therapeutic goals are to be achieved. One observer[35] has called attention to the difference between rational prescribing on a clinical pharmacological basis and realistic prescribing for the individual patient. The former approach represents a narrow concept which regards the patient as an object of therapeutic decisions, whereas the latter recognizes the patient as an individual with personal characteristics who must cooperate and share in the responsibilities pertaining to his therapy.

In one commentary,[36] a patient calls on physicians to be consistent and respectful in the manner in which they address their patients. Specifically, the author notes that if physicians address their patients by first names, they should also introduce themselves by their first names, and if they wish to be addressed more formally, they should extend the same courtesy to their patients.

The following factors are among those which could adversely influence compliance if there is inadequate attention to the considerations discussed above.

Waiting to See the Physician or Pharmacist—When a patient experiences a significant wait in getting to see his physician or having his prescription filled, the annoyance may contribute to poorer compliance with the instructions provided. In one study[37] it was noted that only 31% of the patients who usually wait more than 60 minutes to see their physicians are full compliers as opposed to 67% of the patients who see the physician within 30 minutes of the time they arrive. In another investigation[38] designed to determine why about one-half of the patients had dropped out of a hypertension clinic, it was noted that about two-thirds of the patients complained about the time it took to see the physician, with the average waiting time being 2½ hours. In addition, the patients waited an average of 1¾ hours to obtain their prescriptions at the pharmacy. By comparison, the actual time spent with the physician and pharmacist was almost negligible. Efforts to reduce these delays have resulted in a more favorable patient response and a lower dropout rate.

Failure to Comprehend the Importance of Therapy—A major reason for noncompliance is that the importance of the drug therapy and the potential consequences if the medication is not used according to instructions have not been impressed upon the patient. Patients usually know relatively little about their illnesses, let alone the therapeutic benefits and problems that could result from drug therapy. Therefore, they establish their own ideas regarding their conditions and their own expectations of the effect of drug therapy. If the therapy does not then meet these expectations they are more inclined to become noncompliant. Greater attention to educating the patient regarding his condition as well as the benefits and limitations of drug therapy will contribute to a more cooperative attitude on the part of the patient.

Poor Understanding of the Instructions—Numerous investigations have described problems of this type. In one study[39] of approximately 6000 prescriptions, 4% were written with the designation for patient instructions being "as directed." In following up on 151 of these prescriptions it was found that in 36 cases the patients had received auxiliary written instructions from the prescriber. Of the other 115 prescriptions the patient gave the same instructions that the physician intended (as determined by contacting the physician) in 71 cases but in 44 cases the understanding of the directions on the part of the patient was different than that intended by the prescriber. The possible consequences of some of these misunderstandings could be serious. For example, one patient was going to take two phenytoin capsules (100 mg) three times daily rather than one capsule three times daily as the physician intended. Another patient would have used oral contraceptive tablets incorrectly, and it is of interest to note that the patient had become pregnant once before while taking oral contraceptives.

The rationale for use by some physicians of the instruction "Take as directed" has been examined in a recent study.[40] Although the use of this designation in selected situations has been defended, the potential for confusion and resulting difficulty documented in other studies speaks to the need for making the instructions as specific as possible.

Even when directions to the patients are more specific than "as directed," confusion can still occur. In a study[2] of interpretation of prescription instructions it was shown that there were frequent errors of interpretation even when the instructions were not thought by the prescriber to be ambiguous. For example, in interpreting a prescription that read "Tetracycline, 250 mg every six hours," only 36% of the 67 patients in the study indicated they would take the drug every six hours around the clock for a total of four doses each day. About 25% of the patients would not take a night-time dose since they divided the time that they were awake into three six-hour periods.

A prescription for chlorpropamide (*Diabinese*) was written with instructions to take the drug "every twelve hours" but 36% of the patients would not have taken the drug at this interval. A particularly interesting response was seen with a prescription designated "Furosemide, 40 mg as needed for

fluid retention." The patients were asked whether the medication allowed one to keep the fluid inside the body or helped to eliminate fluid from the body and more than half the patients felt that the drug would cause one to retain fluid. In this case the confusion involved the use of the word "for," as many interpreted it as *causing* the circumstances designated rather than *preventing* or *correcting* them.

The designation "as needed" in the instructions is also subject to varying interpretations.[41] Patients shown a label for a prescription for propoxyphene (*Darvon*) with the directions "every 4 hours as needed," were asked to indicate the maximum number of capsules permitted in 24 hours. Approximately one-half responded incorrectly, with the responses ranging from two to eight capsules.

In another study[42] of 451 outpatient prescriptions it was found that in 70 cases the patients were unable to interpret a dosage schedule from the instructions provided or only had a vague idea of how to use the drug. In 161 cases the instructions were to administer the medication two, three, or four times daily (bid, tid, or qid). When the patients were asked the specific times they would take the medication the responses varied greatly. The following are cited as examples of individual problems. One patient who was to take two doses of sulfamethoxazole (*Gantanol*) a day scheduled the doses within four hours of each other. Another patient would have taken four tetracycline doses per day at two-hour intervals.

These studies point out the confusion that may exist on the part of the patient even when instructions are seemingly clear. However, many prescriptions are written and labeled to indicate how many doses are to be taken each day with no additional clarification as to how the doses are to be scheduled. For example, how should instructions to take one tablet three times daily be interpreted? Does this mean every eight hours, or with meals, or possibly some other schedule? If the drug is to be given with meals or at a specified time before or after meals, it is usually assumed that the patient eats three meals a day. Yet this is not always the case. Some drugs that are given several times a day include a bedtime dose. However, there can be a wide variation among patients in the time that this dose would be administered. In a recent study,[43] patients being treated with hydralazine (*Apresoline*), verapamil (*Calan, Isoptin*), or slow-release potassium chloride, with instructions to take the medications three times daily, were interviewed with respect to the times at which they administered the individual doses of medication. Of 137 patients, only one was administering the medication at regular eight-hour intervals between doses, and 79 percent of the patients reported taking all three doses within 12 hours, leaving a dosage interval of 12 hours or more.

A patient may be knowledgeable about the dosage and the specific times at which the medication is to be administered but not recognize the importance of *auxiliary* instructions. In one study,[44] compliance with the use of topical ophthalmic corticosteroid suspensions was evaluated. The containers were labeled, "Instill one drop in each eye four times daily. "Shake well" with the instruction to "shake well" being typed in red. It was observed that 63 of the 100 patients in the study did not shake the bottle at all after reading the label and the authors estimate that these patients would have administered 29% or less of the maximum concentration of the corticosteroid.

Nothing should be taken for granted regarding the patient's understanding of how to use medication. Not only are there reports of medications being used according to wrong dosage schedules, but in some cases the uncertainty or confusion on the part of the patient is such that medications are given by the wrong route of administration (eg, instilling oral pediatric antibiotic drops into the ear for an ear infection or administering suppositories by the oral route).

Although not a complete listing of all factors that result in noncompliance, those discussed give an indication of the difficult challenge of assuring optimal drug therapy. Inherent in many of the factors considered is the matter of communication of the physician and pharmacist with the patient. This communication is in many cases not only incomplete and ineffective but often there is the impression that physicians and pharmacists are too busy or not interested in talking with the patient. Improving communications must be considered the key to increasing compliance and some of the approaches and recommendations directed toward this goal are reviewed in the following discussion.

Improving Compliance

A number of strategies to enhance compliance have been proposed and there has been increasing documentation of the effectiveness of certain of these methods. Although increased compliance is the desired outcome of these efforts, one observer has cautioned[45] about the possible negative effects of increased compliance such as an increase in dose-related adverse effects which result from greater compliance with the prescribed regimen. It is further noted[45] that "At a minimum we must aspire to improve adherence only with those treatments or actions for which we have reasonable evidence of efficacy, and we must maintain contant vigilance for any harmful results of our interventions, however well intentioned."

In most situations both the physician and the pharmacist have the opportunity to talk directly with the patient about the drugs that have been prescribed; the effectiveness of this communication will be a major determinant of patient compliance. Not to be overlooked is the desirability of also having effective communication between the physician and the pharmacist so that their efforts in the patient's behalf are consistent.

The pharmacist has a particularly valuable opportunity to encourage compliance since his advice accompanies the actual dispensing of the medication and he is usually the last health professional to see the patient prior to the time the medication is to be used. In addition, the patient may find it easier to establish rapport with the pharmacist, and this is reflected by the many occasions in which a patient asks a pharmacist about his or her illness or medications because of reluctance to discuss these matters with the physician. In the following discussion particular emphasis is placed on the pharmacist's role in addressing the problem of noncompliance.

Identification of Risk Factors

All patients should be viewed as potential noncompliers. However, a first step in efforts to improve compliance should be to recognize individuals who are most likely to be noncompliant, as judged by a consideration of the risk factors noted earlier. These factors should be taken into account in planning the patient's therapy so that the simplest regimen which is, to the extent possible, compatible with the patient's normal activities can be developed.

Development of Treatment Plan

The more complex the treatment regimen, the greater is the risk of noncompliance, and this must be recognized in the development of the treatment plan. A patient must not be deprived of needed medication; however, there should be a valid indication for each of the medications in the regimen and the use of any nonessential drugs should be avoided. The use of longer-acting drugs in a therapeutic class, or dosage forms that are administered less frequently, may also simplify the regimen. The use of a once-daily regimen (eg, at bedtime) with agents such as the tricyclic antidepressants may help enhance compliance in a number of individuals. However, it should be recognized that such an approach also has some disadvantages (eg, certain side effects may be more pro-nounced with the use of large single doses; a patient on a once-daily regimen who misses a single dose loses more of the therapeutic effect than a patient who misses a single dose of a regimen in which the daily dose is divided), and the benefits of a less-frequently administered regimen should be evaluated on an individual basis.

The treatment plan should be individualized based on the patient's needs and, when possible, the patient should be a participant in decisions regarding the therapeutic regimen. To help reduce inconvenience and forgetfulness, the regimen should be *tailored* so that the doses of medication are administered at times which correspond to some regular activities in the patient's daily schedule.

When prescriptions are written, the instructions should be as specific as possible. Instructions such as "as directed" or other directions that are subject to misinterpretation should be avoided. Even such seemingly specific instructions as "one tablet three times daily" are often misinterpreted, as discussed previously. Where possible, and with a recognition of the patient's normal routine, the specific times of day at which the patient is to take the medication should be indicated. In all cases the pharmacist should ascertain that the patient understands how to use the medication.

The American Pharmaceutical Association and the American Society of Internal Medicine have developed a statement on prescription writing and prescription labeling (Appendix A). Not only do the guidelines provide important information and suggestions but the statement reflects the type of interdisciplinary cooperation which must also be achieved in practice if patient needs are to be best served.

It has been noted[46] that the prescription can be used as the organizing instrument of instruction; however, "most often the prescription slip is simply handed over as the closing act of the encounter, while the patient or parent is outward bound." The prescription should signal the start of an alliance, and it behooves the physician to appropriately emphasize its importance.

So that one important aspect of noncompliance is not overlooked it should be noted that many prescriptions that patients receive from their physicians are never filled. In one study[47] involving 2000 prescriptions, 3% were not filled within 10 days and, in another investigation,[48] the rate of noncompliance in initially having the prescription filled was found to be 6%. Little progress has been made in detecting and correcting these occurrences, further emphasizing the need for more effective communication and a closer working relationship between physicians and pharmacists.

Patient Education

Decisions must be made as to what information should be provided to patients with regard to their disease states and drug therapy, and the importance of exercising careful judgment in making these decisions should be recognized. This matter has been the subject of considerable controversy with respect to the development of patient package inserts as a number feel that the provision of information that is very comprehensive and highly specific relative to the occurrence of adverse effects, etc, may actually discourage the patient from taking his medication. However comprehensive written patient information may be, it must be recognized that this represents a supplement to, and does not take the place of, the consultation of the physician and the pharmacist with the patient.

In discussing an illness or drug therapy with a patient a distinction should be made between "information" and "education." Patients may receive information but not understand it and utilize it correctly, whereas education implies understanding and behavioral change. Patients should be encouraged to participate in the discussion and where possible they should be brought in on the decision-making process. They should also be encouraged to ask questions, and it is desirable for the pharmacist, after he has explained the directions for using a drug, to ask the patient if he has any questions as to how the drug is to be used.

To provide the degree of understanding which will lead to favorable therapeutic outcomes, patients should be knowledgeable concerning a number of aspects of their drug therapy. These factors are identified in the "Statement of Pharmacist-Conducted Patient Counseling" developed by the American Society of Hospital Pharmacists (Appendix B). In certain cases some of the factors identified may not be applicable. However, presently, many patients are receiving minimal information and greater attention must be directed to the provision of all the pertinent information to the patient.

The goal of communications with the patient is to provide information that the patient is able to understand and utilize. The approach should be one that will be reassuring to the patient and will not unnecessarily cause alarm, as may occur when an over-zealous discussion of adverse effects makes the patient afraid to use the drug. Thus, the provision of too much information, or an inappropriate approach in presenting it, can actually contribute to noncompliance rather than prevent it.

Verbal Communication/Counseling—Communication between the pharmacist and patient regarding the use of medication can be both verbal and written. Although it may be supplemented and reinforced by written instructions, verbal communication is a very important aspect of patient education since it directly involves both the patient and the pharmacist in a two-way exchange and provides the opportunity for the patient to raise questions. For such communication to be most effective it should be conducted in a setting that provides privacy and is free of distractions.

Although most pharmacies do not presently have a separate patient consultation area, this is a desirable goal. Not only will this emphasize to the patient the importance the pharmacist attaches to the information being discussed, but it will also further strengthen the recognition of the pharmacist as one who is contributing to the patient's health care. Even in the absence of such a separate area, however, there must be an awareness of the need for a setting that is conducive to effective communication.

Medication is often obtained in a manner that does not lend itself to verbal communication. For example, the pharmacist may receive a telephoned prescription from a physician that is to be delivered to the patient's home or picked up at the pharmacy by a relative or friend. In these circumstances, when appropriate, the pharmacist might call the patient to discuss the use of the medication.

The effect of pharmacist counseling on patient compliance has been evaluated in a number of studies. In an early investigation[49] of patients being discharged from the hospital, it was found that 90 percent of the patients who had been counseled by the pharmacist at the time of discharge were compliant with the prescription instructions, whereas only 24 percent of the patients who received no consultation prior to discharge were compliant.

In another study,[50] the effect of pharmacist counseling of patients with hypertension was assessed. The results of this study reflect a significant increase in the patients' knowledge of hypertension and its treatment, their compliance with prescribed therapy, and the number of patients whose blood pressures were maintained in the normal range.

One evaluation[51] of the use of antibiotic and decongestant preparations in pediatric patients revealed a high rate of noncompliance, as well as errors in labeling and the amount of medication dispensed. In the second phase of this investigation, the patients in one group were counseled by a pharmacist and it was observed that the rate of compliance was considerably greater than in the group of patients not receiving counseling. These authors also emphasize the importance of providing supplemental written information and a device in which liquid medications may be accurately measured.

Other investigators[52] have also demonstrated the value of pharmacist counseling in increasing compliance and further note the contribution the pharmacist makes in the clinic setting in documenting the drug therapy on the medical record and in decreasing the duplication of prescriptions.

A *compliance clinic* has been described[53] in which pharmacists endeavored to improve the compliance of patients referred to the clinic by physicians. Six of the 14 patients seen on a regular basis demonstrated a significant reduction in emergency room visits and eight patients exhibited reduced hospitalizations, as determined by a comparison of pre- and postclinic records. In addition to the therapeutic benefits most patients will experience as a result of improved compliance, there is a considerable cost savings to be achieved as a result of the reduced hospitalization.

Written Communication—The emphasis on verbal communication should not be interpreted to indicate that written communication is not important. Although at the time of the visit to the physician or pharmacist the patient may understand how the medication is to be used, he may not later remember the details relating to administration of the drug. Therefore, specific instructions for use should be placed on the prescription label. The importance of accurately designating the intended instructions on the prescription label is obvious. In one study[54] of prescription labeling, however, it was found that the directions for use were grossly incorrect on 2.6% of the labels, with some of the errors attributable to the pharmacist and others to the physician. Additional labels were deficient in other respects. It would seem that some pharmacists do not place enough emphasis on the accuracy, completeness, and neatness of the label. If this is evident to the patient it could reduce their respect for the therapy as well as the pharmacist.

Several approaches have been taken to modify the prescription label in such a manner to call greater attention to the times at which the medication is to be administered. In one study[55] compliance was improved by using labels on which a clock face was imprinted and on which the pharmacist circled the times at which the drug was to be administered. However, in another investigation[41] it is noted that one group of patients who understood the verbal instructions were confused by the clock.

It is often desirable to provide supplementary written instructions or other information pertaining to the patient's illness or drug therapy, and many pharmacists are now giving patients medication instruction cards or inserts. The provision of supplementary written information appears to be most effective in improving compliance with short-term therapeutic regimens (eg, antibiotic therapy) and, in a review[56] of compliance studies, it is noted that, for drugs used on a long-term basis, written information as a sole intervention has not been shown to be sufficient for improving patient compliance.

As excellent as the labeling and supplemental written instructions may be, they must be viewed as one-way communication unless provision is also made to permit the patient to discuss and ask questions about his therapy. Therefore, verbal and written communication should be used to complement each other and both should be viewed as important components of the effort to educate the patient regarding his drug therapy.

Audiovisual Materials—The use of audiovisual aids may be particularly valuable in certain situations since the patient may be better able to visualize the nature of his illness, or how his medication acts or is to be administered (eg, the administration of insulin). An increasing number of pharmacists have made good use of such aids by making them available for viewing in a patient waiting area or consultation room while the prescription is being prepared, and then answering questions the patient may have.

Controlled Therapy—It has been proposed[57] that hospitalized patients be given the responsibility for self-medication prior to discharge. Usually, patients go from a complete dependence on others for the administration of their medication while hospitalized to a situation where they are given the full responsibility when discharged, with the assumption often made that the patient knows about his drugs because he was taking them in the hospital. Similar situations are encountered by many ambulatory patients who are expected to be responsible for their treatment, yet have not been provided with adequate information and encouragement.

The suggested arrangement would permit the patient to start using the medication on his own in a setting in which health professionals are available to answer questions and identify problems. It may also be possible at this early stage in the patient's therapy to identify situations that could eventually result in noncompliance.

It has been assumed by many that patients who are knowledgeable about their illness and therapeutic regimen are more likely to be compliant. Although this premise may be valid for many individual patients, several studies suggest that increased patient knowledge does not necessarily alter patient behavior and compliance. In one of these studies,[58] it was noted that some of the most flagrant noncompliers could identify their drugs by name and correctly recite the instructions for use.

The fact that such observations have been made must not detract from patient education efforts and, indeed, there must be a commitment to further enhance these programs. However, there must be an awareness of the need to motivate the patient to use the knowledge that has been acquired for the purpose of achieving optimum benefit from his therapy.

Patient Motivation—Information must be provided to patients in a manner that is not coercive, threatening, or demeaning. The best-intentioned, most comprehensive educational efforts will not be effective if the patient cannot be motivated to comply with the instructions for taking the medication(s). In addition to providing specific written instructions, supplying cues for appropriate behavior (*prompting*) may be of value in motivating the patient to be compliant. Cues may be verbal or nonverbal with examples of the latter including the use of special packaging or reminder systems.

In one discussion[24] it is suggested that compliance with a complex regimen might be increased by *prioritizing* the regimen (ie, emphasizing the most important aspects of the treatment), and/or by dividing the treatment plan into less complex stages that can be implemented sequentially. Although these approaches may be effective in some patients, the patient may gain an impression that certain components of the treatment are *less important* and not be compliant with respect to these medications and/or instructions.

Reference has been made previously to the consideration of the physician-patient interaction as a *negotiation*. Some have extended this concept further in the development of *contracts* between patients and health care providers in which the agreed upon treatment goals and responsibilities are outlined. As summarized in a recent review,[24] contracts offer "a written outline of expected behavior, the involvement of the patient in the decision-making process concerning the regimen and the opportunity to discuss potential problems and solutions with the physician, a formal commitment to the program from the patient, and rewards . . . which create incentives for achieving compliance goals." Although such a formalized approach will not be needed in most individuals, it may be effective in patients who have not responded to other initiatives to assure compliance, as the reinforcement and "reward" might provide the necessary incentive to comply.

Compliance Aids

Labeling—The importance of the accuracy and specificity of the information on the label of the prescription container has already been noted. Auxiliary labels which provide additional information regarding the use, precautions, and/or storage of the medication will also contribute to the attainment of compliance.

Recognition should be taken of any limitations a patient is experiencing which might compromise his ability to read and understand the information on the label. For example, patients with poor eyesight may have difficulty reading the prescription labels, and the use of upper case or larger type in preparing the label and/or supplementary written information can be important.

Medication Calendars and Drug Reminder Charts—Various forms, of which a patient calendar sheet[59] is an example, have been developed and are designed to assist the patient in self-administration of drugs. In addition to their use in helping the patient understand which medication to take and when to take it, the forms, on which the patient is to check the appropriate area for each dose of medication he takes, can be evaluated by the pharmacist or physician when the patient returns for more medication or has his next appointment.

In one study[60] of patients with hypertension, patient knowledge of drug use, dose, and frequency of administration was significantly improved with the use of a daily drug reminder chart. The pharmacist spent an equivalent amount of time discussing the use and administration of each drug with those patients receiving the chart and those not receiving the chart. There were fewer errors due to forgetfulness and an overall lower number of deviations from the prescribed regimen in the group of patients receiving the chart, and it is concluded that the chart is an effective means of visual reinforcement of verbal instructions.

Others have described[61] a color-keyed system in which a self-adhesive colored dot is placed on each medication container and corresponding dots of the same color and size are placed on an appropriate medication calendar to designate the times at which the medication is to be administered. It is noted that this method may be an effective alternative in patient-education systems in which communication and language barriers exist.

The concept of color coding has been extended further in another study[62] in which color-coded tablet bottles are matched to a color-coded weekly pill tray. Colored labels are affixed to the tablet bottles with each color corresponding to a particular time of day (eg, red for morning or breakfast). A weekly color-coded tray is used and patients are taught to load the trays by matching the colors on the medication bottle with the colors on the tray. Individuals using this strategy had only a 1.7% deviation from their ideal pill count compared to a 17% deviation for the patients in the control group.

Special Medication Containers—Several types of medication containers have been developed for the purpose of helping patients organize their medications and to monitor self-administration of the drugs on a daily and weekly basis. As an example, the MEDISET device contains 28 compartments, representing four compartments for different time periods (ie, 7–9 AM, 11 AM–1 PM, 4–6 PM, 8–10 PM) for each day of the week).

The effects of counseling and the use of MEDISET containers on compliance among hypertensive patients has been evaluated[63] and both approaches were noted to improve compliance. Patients observed that it was easier to take their medications when using the MEDISET container although the bulkiness of the containers is an inconvenience.

Other special medication containers/caps have also been described. One individual[64] has developed a vial cap into which is built a digital timepiece [Compliance Aid for Pharmaceuticals (CAP)]. The timepiece is modified so as not to advance the display of the time while the cap is on the vial. Thus, the patient can look at the vial and see displayed on it the time of his last dose. At the next time of the cap's removal, the time displayed catches up to the correct time.

Rather than displaying a particular time, the *Med-Tymer* caps[65] are pre-programmed to flash a small red light and sound an alarm whenever it is time to take medication. The caps are pre-programmed using four common medication schedules and a tab attached to the cap is pulled to set the time for the first dose.

It appears that the special prescription containers will be most effective in achieving compliance with short-term treatment regimens; their use in conjunction with long-term therapy is not likely to be as beneficial.

Packaging—The manner in which medication is packaged may also have an influence on patient compliance. Specially designed packaging for oral contraceptives has been valuable in increasing patient understanding of how these agents are to be taken. Special packages of certain steroids to be used for a treatment period of six days (*Medrol Dosepak*, *Aristo-Pak*) or in an alternate-day regimen (*Medrol ADT Pak*) have been designed to facilitate use of steroids in dosage regimens that may be difficult to understand or remember. Other agents, such as certain diuretics and antibiotics are now also marketed in "compliance packages." In a study of the effect of packaging and instruction on outpatient compliance, it is noted[66] that special packaging of penicillin V potassium tablets complemented the pharmacist's instructions to the patient in achieving increased compliance.

One observer[67] has reviewed the potential advantages of giving more attention to packaging considerations in efforts to enhance compliance. It is noted that the "ideal packaging solution should include six component functions: storage, education, cueing, monitoring, dispensing, and reinforcement." The interrelationships of these components necessitate some trade-offs and the package becomes more expensive and less portable as functions are combined. However, the potential exists for designing additional packages that will improve compliance and also contribute to a more efficient use of the time of the health professionals in addressing this challenge.

A possible negative effect of drug packaging on patient compliance is seen with the use of the child-resistant containers. Some patients, particularly the elderly and those with conditions like arthritis and parkinsonism, have difficulty in opening some of these containers and may not persist in their efforts to do so. There also may be difficulty in opening some foil-packed drugs. Pharmacists should be alert to problems of this type and, where appropriate, suggest use of standard containers.

Dosage Forms—New dosage forms of certain drugs have also been developed in large part as a recognition of problems of noncompliance. The increasing practice of using tricyclic antidepressants in larger single evening doses to increase compliance and minimize certain adverse effects has led to the introduction of higher potency formulations. The use of transdermal drug delivery systems permits less frequent administration of the drugs (eg, nitroglycerin) given by this route.

Monitoring Therapy

Self-Monitoring—The patient should be apprised of the importance of monitoring his own treatment regimen and, in some situations, the response parameters. In using certain of the medication calendars and drug reminder charts described earlier, the patient maintains a continuing record of the use of the prescribed medication.

Several studies have suggested that the compliance with antihypertensive regimens may be increased when patients take their own blood pressures or have a member of the family do it. In this manner they become more involved in monitoring the outcome of the therapy as well as the progress of treatment. This approach may be highly effective in patients who can accurately record and interpret the blood pressure measurements; however, patients to whom this additional responsibility is given should be selected carefully as some patients may make decisions regarding the adjustment of their therapeutic regimen on their own. Although decisions based on the results of self-monitoring may be valid in some cases, changes in the therapeutic regimen should be made only after consultation with the health professional having the responsibility for the treatment program.

Pharmacist Monitoring—The pharmacist's role in minimizing noncompliance does not end when the prescription is dispensed. If he becomes aware that the patient is not using the drug as intended, he should endeavor to determine the reason and resolve any problem that may exist. The pharmacist is in an excellent position to detect noncompliance pertaining to the use of drugs used in the management of chronic conditions such as hypertension and diabetes by paying close attention to the frequency with which a patient has his prescription refilled. For example, if a 30-day supply of medication has been dispensed to a patient and he does not return for a refill until 45 days later it may be that the medication is not being taken according to directions. The physician may have told the patient to take the medication less frequently, but more probably the patient did not understand or decided not to follow the instructions; thus the pharmacist should be alert to situations in which the refill frequency is not consistent with the directions for use.

It is highly desirable that pharmacists utilize systems by which the refill frequency for chronic medications may be quickly checked so that potential problems can be identified early. If there is one tool that is essential in addressing the challenge of noncompliance as well as other drug-related problems, it is the patient medication record. It is not enough to just maintain these records—they must be used to identify potential problems and to enhance consultation with patients.

A "tickler" file system has been employed successfully in minimizing noncompliance. The tickler is a clip-on attachment which can be affixed to the top of the patient medication record. Self-adhesive colored dots indicate the month the patient should return and a number written on the dot indicates the day of the month.

Once the tickler system is set up, the medication records can be monitored on a daily, or once-a-week, basis. When the pharmacist identifies that a patient has not had his medication refilled by the time that his supply should have been exhausted, he can contact the patient regarding it. It may be found that there is a valid reason for the patient not refilling the prescription at the expected time. Nevertheless, the awareness of the patient that the pharmacist is paying attention to his therapy and has taken a personal interest in contacting him should not only contribute to compliance but also increase the respect of the patient for the pharmacist.

Situations in which drug usage would seem to be excessive, as evidenced by the patient desiring to refill his prescription more frequently than the directions suggest, represent equally important problems that are easier to detect. Again the pharmacist should attempt to identify the reason for the inconsistency and any problem that may exist.

Pharmacist Follow-up—Several studies have evaluated the influence of follow-up efforts on the part of pharmacists in enhancing compliance. In one investigation[68] in patients receiving a 10–14 day course of antibiotic therapy, patients were randomly assigned to four groups; a control group, a group receiving a follow-up telephone call on the fourth or fifth day of treatment, a group receiving written and oral consultation, and a group receiving written and oral consultation plus a telephone call. It was found that the compliance in the control group was less than for each of the study groups but that the three study groups were not significantly different with respect to the rate of compliance. It was concluded that a follow-up telephone call was equal to, but did not enhance, written and oral consultation in improving compliance.

In another study,[69] pharmacists anticipated the dates that compliant patients would exhaust their supply of medications and mailed postcard refill reminders to the individuals who had not obtained refills by the anticipated dates. Patients who did not respond to the reminder cards within 5 days were contacted by telephone. Of 121 anticipated refill visits, only 49 patients refilled their medications on or before the anticipated dates. Forty-six of the 72 patients receiving postcard reminders responded within 5 days and telephone calls were placed to 24 out of the remaining 26 patients. It was determined that 25 of the patients receiving the refill reminders accumulated a 1- to 30-day excess medication supply because of omitted doses. The system described represents an effective approach in identifying patients who are noncompliant although, in view of the personal and confidential nature of the matters pertaining to an individual's health, it would be preferable to mail refill reminders in a letter rather than a postcard.

The programs designed to improve compliance which are discussed in this review are primarily those in which pharmacists have been involved. Additional information regarding these and other compliance strategies may be found in more comprehensive references on this subject.[70]

Conclusion

Considerable time, effort, and expense have often gone into the diagnosis of a patient's illnesses and the development of his treatment program. Yet the goals of therapy will not be reached unless the patient understands and follows the instructions for use of the drugs prescribed. One cannot also help but wonder how often patients have been categorized as treatment failures and have had their therapy changed, possibly to more potent and toxic agents, when the reason for the lack of response or an unanticipated altered response has been noncompliance.

Despite the increasing attention directed to the matter of noncompliance, the problem is still not accorded the attention it deserves and continues to be prevalent. Although the approaches taken and suggestions advanced in an effort to decrease noncompliance have met with varying success, they have significantly contributed to recognition of the problem and provided a valuable base on which to develop modified or new approaches to the problem. Certain approaches that involve a significantly increased commitment of time on the part of physicians and pharmacists may be viewed by some as impractical. Yet can this compare with the commitment of time and expense that is presently wasted as a result of noncompliance?

The pharmacist is in an excellent position to assume a major responsibility in minimizing noncompliance. Of priority importance is the need to strengthen communications with patients and physicians. Yet many pharmacists are reluctant to accept, and sometimes even resist, opportunities to become more involved in advising patients or contributing to decisions regarding drug therapy because they do not feel adequately prepared. The desirability of pharmacists increasing their knowledge about disease states and the properties of drugs cannot be too strongly emphasized. However, there is no reason why every pharmacist cannot have at least some initial involvement in decreasing the problem of noncompliance even if it is limited to reviewing the directions with the patient or determining the frequency of refill of chronic medications. The satisfaction that this contribution to patient care can bring will serve as a challenge to further increase one's knowledge and professional involvement.

The problem of noncompliance has been identified and is receiving increasing attention. Patients for too long have been deprived of a close attention to and monitoring of their drug therapy. An excuse that pharmacists are too busy to advise patients regarding their drug therapy cannot be accepted; the highest priority must be assigned to taking the steps to ensure that patients will use their medications in the appropriate manner. If pharmacists do not assume the responsibility for decreasing noncompliance, someone else will. The profession cannot afford to default on this valuable opportunity to enhance its contribution to patient care.

References

1. Boyd JR, *et al*: Drug Defaulting (Part II): Analysis of Noncompliance Factors. *Am J Hosp Pharm 31*: 485, 1974.
2. Mazzullo JM III, *et al*: Variations in Interpretation of Prescription Instructions: *J Am Med Assoc 227*: 929, 1974.
3. 1974 Health Interview Survey Data—Hypertension Supplement, National Heart, Lung and Blood Institute.
4. Lundin DV: Medication-Taking Behavior of the Elderly: *Drug Intell Clin Pharm 12*: 518, 1978.
5. Fedder DO: Drug Use in the Elderly: Issues of Noncompliance. *Drug Intell Clin Pharm 18*: 158, 1984.
6. Bootman JL: Maximizing Compliance in the Elderly: Chapter 14, Geriatrics Curriculum Project of the American Association of Colleges of Pharmacy, 1984.
7. Mattar ME, *et al*: Inadequacies in the Pharmacologic Management of Ambulatory Children. *J Pediatr 87*: 137, 1975.
8. Hare EH, Willcox DC: Do Psychiatric In-patients Take Their Pills? *Brit J Psychiatry 113*: 1435, 1967.
9. Bowerman DL, *et al*: Premature Deaths in Persons with Seizure Disorders. *J Forensic Sci 23*: 522, 1978.
10. Brook RH, *et al*: Effectiveness of Inpatient Follow-up Care. *New Engl J Med 285*: 1509, 1971.
11. Noncompliance: About your Medicines Newsletter, United States Pharmacopeial Conv: 3 July/August, 1983.
12. Stewart RB: A Study of Outpatients' Use of Medication. *Hosp Pharm 7*: 108, 1972.
13. Weintraub M: Intelligent Noncompliance with Special Emphasis on the Elderly. *Contemp Pharm Pract 4*: 8, 1981.
14. Weintraub M, *et al*: Compliance as a Determinant of Serum Digoxin Concentration. *J Am Med Assoc 224*: 481, 1973.
15. Sackett DL: A Compliance Practicum for the Busy Practitioner. In *Compliance in Health Care*, Haynes RB, Taylor DW, and Sackett DL, eds, Johns Hopkins University Press, Baltimore, 286, 1979.
16. Roth RP, Caron HS: Accuracy of Doctors' Estimates and Patients' Statements on Adherence to a Drug Regimen. *Clin Pharmacol Ther 23*: 361, 1978.
17. Blackwell B: Antidepressant Drugs: Side Effects and Compliance. *J Clin Psychiatry 43*: 14, Nov, 1982.

18. Cooper JK, *et al:* Intentional Prescription Nonadherence (Noncompliance) by the Elderly. *J Am Geriatr Soc 30:* 329, 1982.

19. Porter AMW: Drug Defaulting in a General Practice. *Brit Med J 1:* 218, 1969.

20. McKenney JM: Methods of Modifying Compliance Behavior in Hypertensive Patients. *Drug Intell Clin Pharm 15:* 8, 1981.

21. McKenney JM: A Behavioral Approach to Patient Compliance. *US Pharmacist 6:* 58, Feb, 1981.

22. Rosenstock IM: Why People Use Health Services. *Milbank Mem Fund Q 55:* 94, July, 1966.

23. Becker MH, *et al:* Selected Psychosocial Models and Correlates of Individual Health-Related Behaviors. *Med Care 15 (Suppl 5):* 27, 1977.

24. Eraker SA, *et al:* Understanding and Improving Patient Compliance. *Ann Intern Med 100:* 258, 1984.

25. Haynes RB: Determinants of Compliance: The Disease and the Mechanics of Treatment. In *Compliance in Health Care*, Haynes RB, Taylor DW, and Sackett DL, eds, Johns Hopkins University Press, Baltimore, 49, 1979.

26. Feder R: Small White Pills (Letter). *New Engl J Med 298:* 463, 1978.

27. Hoagland AC, *et al:* Oncologists' Views of Cancer Patient Noncompliance. *Am J Clin Oncol 6:* 239, 1983.

28. Aldridge SA: Drug-Induced Sexual Dysfunction. *Clin Pharm 1:* 141, 1982.

29. Havens LL: Some Difficulties in Giving Schizophrenic and Borderline Patients Medication. *Psychiatry 31:* 44, 1968.

30. Schulz RM, *et al:* Patient Behavior Patterns Regarding Prescription Refills. *Contemp Pharm Pract 5:* 150, 1982.

31. McKenzie MW: Administration of Oral Medications to Infants and Young Children. *US Pharmacist 6:* 55, June/July, 1981.

32. Ellison RS, *et al:* Effect of Use of a Measured Dispensing Device on Oral Antibiotic Compliance. *Clin Pediatr 21:* 668, 1982.

33. Roberts RJ, *et al:* A Comparison of Various Types of Patient Instruction in the Proper Administratioin of Metered Inhalers. *Drug Intell Clin Pharm 16:* 53, 1982.

34. Benarde MA, Mayerson EW: Patient-Physician Negotiation. *J Am Med Assoc 239:* 1413, 1978.

35. Frolund F: Better Prescribing. *Brit Med J 2:* 741, 1978.

36. Natkins LG: "Hi, Lucille, This is Dr. Gold." *J Amer Med Assoc 247:* 2415, 1982.

37. Geertsen HR, *et al:* Patient Non-Compliance Within the Context of Seeking Medical Care for Arthritis. *J Chron Dis 26:* 689, 1973.

38. Long Waits are Trying for Patients: *Med World News 14:* 60, Feb 23, 1973.

39. Powell JR, *et al:* Inadequately Written Prescriptions. *J Amer Med Assoc 226:* 999, 1973.

40. Cirn JT, *et al:* Inadequately Written Prescriptions: Prescriber Rationales for "Take as Needed" and "Take as Directed." *Contemp Pharm Pract 5:* 85, 1982.

41. Mazzullo JM: Methods of Improving Patient Compliance. *Drug Therapy 6:* 148, Mar, 1976.

42. Hermann F: The Outpatient Prescription Label as a Source of Medication Errors. *Am J Hosp Pharm 30:* 155, 1973.

43. Norell SE, *et al:* Spacing of Medications Scheduled t i d *Am J Hosp Pharm 41:* 1183, 1984.

44. Apt L, *et al:* Patient Compliance with use of Topical Ophthalmic Corticosteroid Suspension. *Amer J Ophthalmol 87:* 210, 1979.

45. Haynes RB: Strategies to Improve Compliance with Referrals, Appointments, and Prescribed Medical Regimens. In *Compliance in Health Care*, Haynes RB, Taylor DW, and Sackett DL, eds, Johns Hopkins University Press, Baltimore, 121, 1979.

46. Yaffe SJ, *et al:* Pediatric Compliance: The Physician's Responsibilities. *Drug Therapy 7:* 64, Nov, 1977.

47. Hammel RW, Williams PO: Do Patients Receive Prescribed Medication? *J APhA NS4:* 331, 1964.

48. Taubman AH, *et al:* Noncompliance in Initial Prescription Filling. *Apothecary 9:* 14, Oct, 1975.

49. Cole P, *et al:* Drug Consultation: Its Significance to the Discharged Hospital Patient and its Relevance as a Role for the Pharmacist. *Am J Hosp Pharm 28:* 954, 1971.

50. McKenney JM, *et al:* The Effect of Clinical Pharmacy Services on Patients with Essential Hypertension. *Circulation 48:* 1104, 1973.

51. Dickey FF, *et al:* Pharmacist Counseling Increases Drug Regimen Compliance. *J Am Hosp Assoc 49:* 85, May 1, 1975.

52. Monson R, *et al:* Role of the Clinical Pharmacist in Improving Drug Therapy. *Arch Intern Med 141:* 1441, 1981.

53. Cable GL, *et al:* Experiences with the Compliance Clinic: Assessment of the Effect. *Contemp Pharm Pract 5:* 38, 1982.

54. Fleckenstein L, *et al:* Prescription Labeling as a Factor in Patients Compliance. *Drug Therapy 6:* 81, May, 1976.

55. Lima J, *et al:* Compliance with Short-Term Antimicrobial Therapy: Some Techniques that Help. *Pediatrics 57:* 383, 1976.

56. Morris LA, *et al:* Effects of Written Drug Information on Patient Knowledge and Compliance: A Literature Review. *Am J Public Health 69:* 47, 1979.

57. Stewart RB, Cluff LE: A Review of Medication Errors and Compliance in Ambulant Patients. *Clin Pharmacol Ther 13:* 463, 1972.

58. McKercher PL, Rucker TD: Patient Knowledge and Compliance with Medication Instructions. *J APhA NS17:* 283, 1977.

59. Liberman P: A Guide to Help Patients Keep Track of Their Drugs. *Am J Hosp Pharm 29:* 507, 1972.

60. Gabriel M, *et al:* Improved Patient Compliance through use of a Daily Drug Reminder Chart. *Am J Public Health 67:* 968, 1977.

61. Abel SR, *et al:* Color-Keyed Patient Medication Counseling System. *Am J Hosp Pharm 38:* 704, 1981.

62. Martin DC, *et al:* Reducing Mediation Errors in a Geriatric Population. *J Am Geriatr Soc 30:* 258, 1982.

63. Rehder TC, *et al:* Improving Medication Compliance by Counseling and Special Prescription Container. *Am J Hosp Pharm 37:* 379, 1980.

64. Micro-Electronics: An Aid to Patient Drug Compliance. *Amer Druggist 187:* 106, February, 1983.

65. The Cap Reminds You: Take your Medicine. *The Philadelphia Inquirer*, 10-D, March 10, 1984.

66. Linkewich JA, *et al:* The Effect of Packaging and Instruction on Outpatient Compliance with Medication Regimens. *Drug Intell Clin Pharm 8:* 10, 1974.

67. Rudd P. Medication Packaging: Simple Solutions to Nonadherence Problems? *Clin Pharmacol Ther 25:* 257, 1979.

68. Garnett WR, *et al:* Effect of Telephone Follow-up on Patient Compliance. *Am J Hosp Pharm 38:* 676, 1981.

69. Brown DJ, *et al:* Identification of Potentially Noncompliant Patients with a Mailed Medication Refill Reminder System. *Contemp Pharm Pract 3:* 244, 1980.

70. *Compliance in Health Care*, Haynes RB, Taylor DW, Sackett DL, eds: Johns Hopkins University Press, Baltimore, 1979.

Selected Additional References

Books

Barofsky I, ed: *Medication Compliance: A Behavioral Management Approach*, Charles B. Slack, Thorofare, NJ, 1977.

Cohen SJ, ed: *New Directions in Patient Compliance*, Lexington, Mass 1979.

Sackett DL, Haynes RB, eds: *Compliance with Therapeutic Regimens;* Johns Hopkins University Press, Baltimore, 1976.

Lasagna L, ed: *Patient Compliance*, Futura Publishing Co, Mount Kisco, NY, 1976.

Papers

Blackwell B: Patient Compliance. *New Engl J Med 289:* 249, 1973.

Chrischilles EA, *et al:* Clinical Pharmacy Services in Family Practice. *Drug Intell Clin Pharm 18:* 436, 1984.

Dirks JF, *et al:* Nondichotomous Patterns of Medication Usage: The Yes-No Fallacy. *Clin Pharmacol Ther 31:* 413, 1982.

Evans L, *et al:* The Problem of Non-compliance with Drug Therapy. *Drugs 25:* 63, 1983.

Haynes RB: Strategies for Enhancing Patient Compliance. *Drug Ther 12:* 147, Jan, 1982.

Hershey JC, *et al:* Patient Compliance with Antihypertensive Medication. *Am J Pub Health 70:* 1081, 1980.

Hulka BS, *et al:* Communication, Compliance, and Concordance Between Physicians and Patients with Prescribed Mediations. *Am J Public Health 66:* 847, 1976.

Inui TS, *et al:* Variations in Patient Compliance with Common Long-Term Drugs. *Med Care 18:* 986, 1980.

Litt IF, *et al:* Compliance with Medical Regimens During Adolescence. *Ped Clin North Amer 27:* 3, Feb, 1980.

Matthew D, Hingson R: Improving Patient Compliance. *Med Clin North America 61:* 879, 1977.

Moore SR, *et al:* Receipt of Prescription Drug Information by the Elderly. *Drug Intell Clin Pharm 17:* 920, 1983.

Peck CL, *et al:* Increasing Patient Compliance with Prescriptions. *JAMA 248:* 2874, 1982.

Shope JT: Medication Compliance. *Ped Clin North Amer 28:* 5, Feb, 1981.

Smith DL: Patient Compliance with Medication Regimens. *Drug Intell Clin Pharm 10:* 386, 1976.

Taubman A, *et al:* Prescriber, Pharmacist, and Patient Interpretation of Commonly Used Prescription Directions. *Contemp Pharm Pract 5:* 10, 1982.

Veatch RM: Pharmacist's Role in Enlisting Drug Compliance. *US Pharmacist 7:* 90, Nov, 1982.

Appendix A—Statement on Prescription Writing and Prescription Labeling*

Introduction

Historically, the pharmaceutical and medical professions have devoted considerable time and effort to the development and rational utilization of safe and effective drugs for the treatment and prevention of illness. Today, that successful effort continues, helping to achieve the highest standards of health in the world for the American people. But in order to gain maximum benefit from the use of drugs while minimizing their adverse side effects, prescribers and pharmacists must maintain effective communications not only among themselves, but with their patients as well. The directions for drug use and other information which prescribers indicate on prescription orders and which pharmacists transfer to prescription labels are critical to safe and effective drug therapy. In order to assure that this information is conveyed clearly and effectively to patients, the following guidelines have been developed by the American Pharmaceutical Association and the American Society of Internal Medicine.

Guidelines for Prescribers

The following guidelines are recommended for prescribers when writing directions for drug use on their prescription orders.

1. The name and strength of the drug dispensed will be recorded on the prescription label by the pharmacist unless otherwise directed by the prescriber.
2. Whenever possible, specific times of the day for drug administration should be indicated. (For example, *Take one capsule at 8:00 am, 12:00 noon, and 8:00 pm* is preferable to *Take one capsule three times daily*. Likewise, *Take one tablet two hours after meals* is preferable to *Take one tablet after meals*.)
3. The use of potentially confusing abbreviations, ie, *qid*, *qod*, *qd*, etc, is discouraged.
4. Vague instructions such as *Take as necessary* or *Take as directed* which are confusing to the patient are to be avoided.
5. If dosing at specific intervals around-the-clock is therapeutically important, this should specifically be stated on the prescription by indicating appropriate times for drug administration.
6. The symptom, indication, or the intended effect for which the drug is being used should be included in the instructions whenever possible. (For example, *Take one tablet at 8:00 am and 8:00 pm for high blood pressure*, or *Take one teaspoonful at 8:00 am, 11:00 am, 3:00 pm, and 6:00 pm for cough*.)
7. The Metric System of weights and measures should be used.
8. The prescription order should indicate whether or not the prescription should be renewed and, if so, the number of times and the period of time such renewal is authorized. Statements such as *Refill prn* or *Refill ad lib* are discouraged.
9. Either single or multi-drug prescription forms may be used when appropriately designed, and pursuant to the desires of local medical and pharmaceutical societies.
10. When institutional prescription blanks are used, the prescriber should print his/her name, telephone number, and registration number on the prescription blank.

Guidelines for Pharmacists

1. Pharmacists should include the following information on the prescription label: name, address, and telephone number of pharmacy; name of prescriber; name, strength, and quantity of drug dispensed (unless otherwise directed by the prescriber); directions for use; prescription number; date on which prescription is dispensed; full name of patient; and any other information required by law.
2. Instructions to the patient regarding directions for use of medication should be concise and precise, but readily understandable to the patient. Where the pharmacist feels that the prescription order does not meet these criteria, he should attempt to clarify the order with the prescriber in order to prevent confusion. Verbal reinforcement and/or clarification of instructions should be given to the patient by the pharmacist when appropriate.
3. For those dosage forms where confusion may develop as to how the medication is to be administered (for example, oral drops which may be mistakenly instilled in the ear or suppositories which may be mistakenly administered orally), the pharmacist should clearly indicate the intended route of administration on the prescription label.
4. The pharmacist should include an expiration date on the prescription label when appropriate.
5. Where special storage conditions are required, the pharmacist should indicate appropriate instructions for storage on the prescription label.

Conclusion

Communicating effective dosage instructions to patients clearly and succinctly is a responsibility of both the medical and pharmaceutical professions. Recent studies documenting the low order of compliance with prescription instructions indicate that poor communication between the medical and pharmaceutical professions and poor comprehension by the public may be causative factors.

The American Pharmaceutical Association and the American Society of Internal Medicine believe that the guidelines as stated above will serve as an initial step toward patients achieving a better understanding of their medication and dosing instructions. The two associations urge state and local societies representing pharmacists and prescribers to appoint joint committees for the purpose of refining these guidelines further as local desires and conditions warrant. The associations believe that such cooperative efforts between the professions are essential to good patient care and that significant progress can be made in other areas by initiating discussions between the two professions concerning common interests and goals.

* By American Pharmaceutical Association/American Society of Internal Medicine (revised March 1976).

Appendix B—Statement on Pharmacist-Conducted Patient Counseling*

It is well documented that safe and effective drug therapy most frequently occurs when patients are well informed about medications and their use. Knowledgeable patients exhibit increased compliance with drug regimens, resulting in improved therapeutic outcomes. Therefore, pharmacists, as well as other health professionals, have a responsibility to properly inform patients about their drug therapy.

Pharmacists' drug consultations with patients should be aimed at improving therapeutic outcomes by maximizing proper use of medications. Pharmacists, in conjunction with other health team members whenever possible, must make appropriate value judgements to determine the specific information and counseling required in each patient care situation.

Using suitable verbal, written or audio-visual communication techniques and methods, the pharmacist should inform, educate and counsel patients (or their representative or guardian) about the following items for each medication in the patient's drug regimen:

1. Name (trademark, generic, common synonym, or other descriptive name(s))
2. Intended use and expected action
3. Route, dosage form, dosage, and administration schedule
4. Special directions for preparation
5. Special directions for administration
6. Precautions to be observed during administration
7. Common side effects that may be encountered including their avoidance and action required if they occur
8. Techniques for self-monitoring of drug therapy
9. Proper storage
10. Potential drug-drug or drug-food interactions or other therapeutic contraindications
11. Prescription refill information
12. Action to be taken in the event of a missed dose
13. Any other information peculiar to the specific patient or drug

These thirteen points are applicable to non-prescription drugs as well as those ordered by a physician or other prescriber. In addition, pharmacists must counsel patients in the proper selection of non-prescription drugs as well as when and if they should be used.

* Approved by the Board of Directors, American Society of Hospital Pharmacists (November 17–18, 1975).

CHAPTER 101

The Prescription

Howard C Ansel, PhD

Professor of Pharmacy and Dean, College of Pharmacy
University of Georgia
Athens, GA 30602

A *prescription* is an order for medication issued by a physician, dentist, veterinarian, or other properly licensed medical practitioner. Prescriptions designate a specific medication and dosage to be administered to a particular patient at a specified time. Commonly, the prescribed medication also is referred to as the "prescription" by the patient.

The prescription order is a part of the professional relationship between the prescriber, pharmacist, and patient. It is the pharmacist's responsibility in this relationship to provide the medication needs of the patient. The pharmacist must be precise, not only in the manual aspects of filling the prescription order, but must provide the patient with the necessary information and guidance to assure the patient's compliance in taking the medication properly. It is also the pharmacist's responsibility to advise the prescriber of drug sensitivities the patient may have, or other medications that the patient may be taking which may limit the effectiveness of the newly prescribed medication. To meet these responsibilities it is essential that the pharmacist maintains a high level of practice competence, keeps appropriate records on the health status and medication history of his patients, and develops professional working relationships with other health professionals.

In this role the pharmacist must maintain the trust of the prescriber and patient. This trust includes maintaining confidentiality. The medication being taken by a patient and the nature of his illness is a private matter which must be respected.

There are two broad legal classifications of medications: (1) those which can be obtained only by prescription, and (2) those which may be purchased without a prescription. The latter are termed *nonprescription* drugs or *over-the-counter* (OTC) drugs. Medications which may be dispensed legally only upon prescription are referred to as *prescription* drugs or *legend* drugs. The latter term refers to the "legend" that must appear on the label of the product as it is provided to the pharmacist by the manufacturer—"Caution: Federal Law Prohibits Dispensing without Prescription." Occasionally, physicians may issue prescriptions for non-legend drugs which they desire the patient to receive.

Prescriptions may be written by the prescriber and given to the patient for presentation at the pharmacy, or they may be telephoned or communicated directly to the pharmacist. Prescription orders received by oral communication should be immediately reduced to proper written form by the pharmacist.

Form of the Prescription Order

Prescriptions are usually written on printed forms that contain blank spaces for the required information. These forms are called *prescription blanks* and are supplied in the form of a pad. Prescription blanks that are utilized in the physician's office practice are imprinted with the name, address, telephone number, and other pertinent information of the physician or other prescriber (Fig 101-1). Prescription blanks that are utilized by the pharmacist in his transposition of orally received prescriptions are commonly imprinted with the name, address, and telephone number of the pharmacy (Fig 101-2). These blanks also may be used by physicians to write prescriptions when visiting the pharmacy. Specially imprinted prescription blanks are not required legally for prescriptions; any paper or other writing material may be used.

For the purpose of study, the component parts of a prescription may be identified as follows:

1. Patient information
2. Date
3. ℞ symbol or *superscription*
4. Medication prescribed or *inscription*
5. Dispensing directions to pharmacist or *subscription*
6. Directions for patient or *signa* (to be placed on label)
7. Refill, special labeling, and/or other instructions
8. Prescriber's signature, address, and other pertinent information

A model prescription showing these various parts is shown below:

(1) Mary Jones
1114 Grady Avenue
Athens, Georgia
(2) Date: 5-16-84
(3) ℞
(4) Codeine Phosphate Tabs 30 mg
(5) Dispense tabs No 12
(6) Sig: tab i q 6 h prn pain
(7) Refills: 0 Label: yes
(8) John Brown, M.D. (Signature)
1600 Main Street
Atlanta, Georgia
DEA No AS11192498

In practice some of the above information (as the patient's address) may be absent when the prescription is received by the pharmacist. In these instances the pharmacist obtains

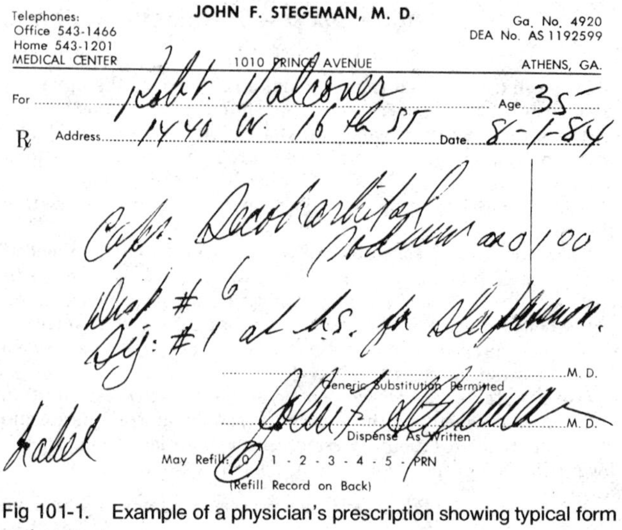

Telephones:
Office 543-1466
Home 543-1201
MEDICAL CENTER

JOHN F. STEGEMAN, M. D.

1010 PRINCE AVENUE

Ga. No. 4920
DEA No. AS 1192599
ATHENS, GA.

For .... Age ....

℞ Address .... Date ....

.... M. D.
Generic Substitution Permitted

.... M. D.
Dispense As Written

May Refill: 0 · 1 · 2 · 3 · 4 · 5 · PRN
(Refill Record on Back)

Fig 101-1. Example of a physician's prescription showing typical form and content.

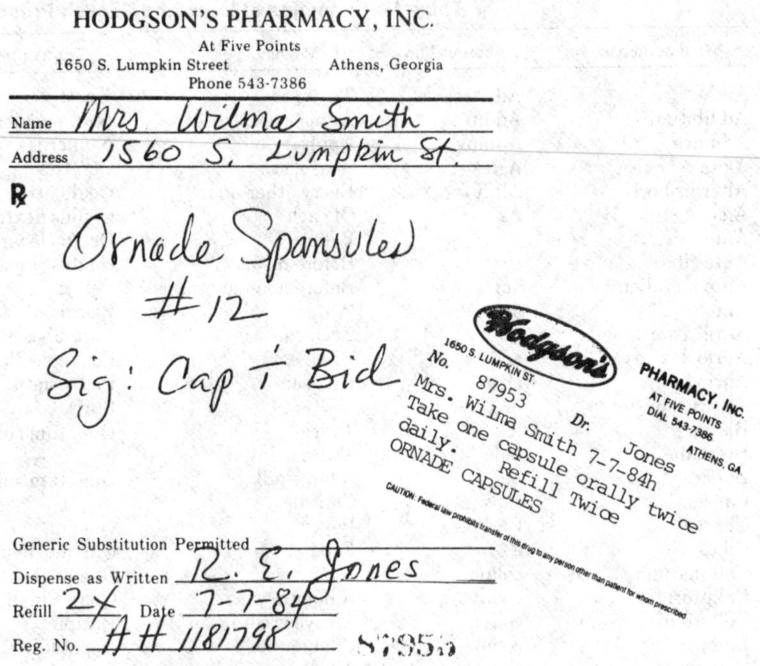

HODGSON'S PHARMACY, INC.
At Five Points
1650 S. Lumpkin Street Athens, Georgia
Phone 543-7386

Name Mrs Wilma Smith
Address 1560 S. Lumpkin St.

℞

Ornade Spansules
#12
Sig: Cap i Bid

Hodgson's 1650 S. LUMPKIN ST. PHARMACY, INC. AT FIVE POINTS DIAL 543-7386 ATHENS, GA
No. 87953 Dr. Jones
Mrs. Wilma Smith 7-7-84h
Take one capsule orally twice
daily. Refill Twice
ORNADE CAPSULES
CAUTION: Federal law prohibits transfer of this drug to any person other than patient for whom prescribed

Generic Substitution Permitted
Dispense as Written R. E. Jones
Refill 2X Date 7-7-84
Reg. No. AH 1181798 87953

Fig 101-2. Example of a prescription written on a community pharmacy prescription blank and associated prescription label.

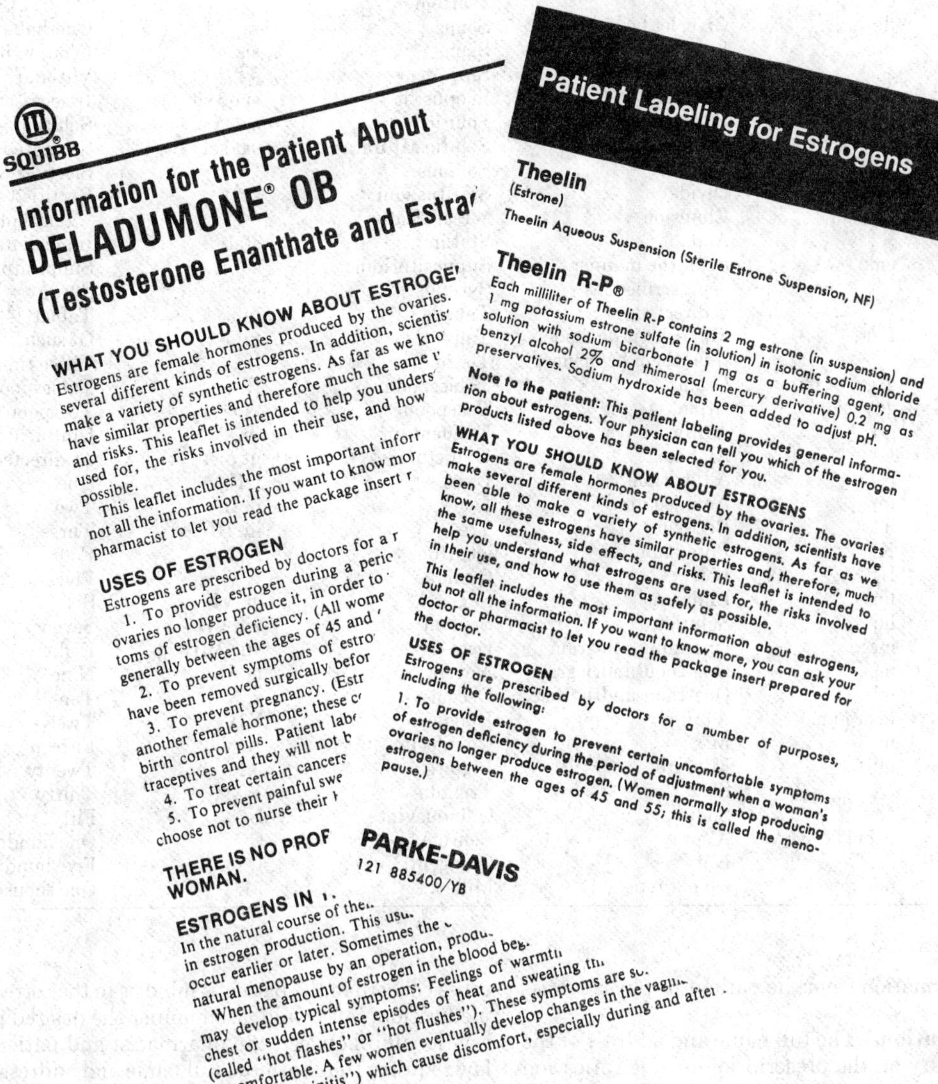

SQUIBB

Information for the Patient About
DELADUMONE® OB
(Testosterone Enanthate and Estra

WHAT YOU SHOULD KNOW ABOUT ESTROGE
Estrogens are female hormones produced by the ovaries. several different kinds of estrogens. In addition, scientis make a variety of synthetic estrogens. As far as we kno have similar properties and therefore much the same u and risks. This leaflet is intended to help you unders used for, the risks involved in their use, and how possible.
This leaflet includes the most important infor not all the information. If you want to know mor pharmacist to let you read the package insert r

USES OF ESTROGEN
Estrogens are prescribed by doctors for a r
1. To provide estrogen during a perio ovaries no longer produce it, in order to toms of estrogen deficiency. (All wome generally between the ages of 45 and
2. To prevent symptoms of estro have been removed surgically befor
3. To prevent pregnancy. (Estr another female hormone; these c birth control pills. Patient labe traceptives and they will not b
4. To treat certain cancers
5. To prevent painful swe choose not to nurse their b

THERE IS NO PROF WOMAN.

ESTROGENS IN
In the natural course of thei in estrogen production. This usu occur earlier or later. Sometimes the natural menopause by an operation, produ
When the amount of estrogen in the blood beg may develop typical symptoms: Feelings of warmth chest or sudden intense episodes of heat and sweating th (called "hot flashes" or "hot flushes"). These symptoms are so uncomfortable. A few women eventually develop changes in the vagin "atrophic vaginitis") which cause discomfort, especially during and afte tercourse.

Patient Labeling for Estrogens

Theelin
(Estrone)
Theelin Aqueous Suspension (Sterile Estrone Suspension, NF)

Theelin R-P®
Each milliliter of Theelin R-P contains 2 mg estrone (in suspension) and 1 mg potassium estrone sulfate (in solution) in isotonic sodium chloride solution with sodium bicarbonate 1 mg as a buffering agent, and benzyl alcohol 2% and thimerosal (mercury derivative) 0.2 mg as preservatives. Sodium hydroxide has been added to adjust pH.
Note to the patient: This patient labeling provides general information about estrogens. Your physician can tell you which of the estrogen products listed above has been selected for you.

WHAT YOU SHOULD KNOW ABOUT ESTROGENS
Estrogens are female hormones produced by the ovaries. The ovaries make several different kinds of estrogens. In addition, scientists have been able to make a variety of synthetic estrogens. As far as we know, all these estrogens have similar properties and, therefore, much the same usefulness, side effects, and risks. This leaflet is intended to help you understand what estrogens are used for, the risks involved in their use, and how to use them as safely as possible.
This leaflet includes the most important information about estrogens, but not all the information. If you want to know more, you can ask your doctor or pharmacist to let you read the package insert prepared for the doctor.

USES OF ESTROGEN
Estrogens are prescribed by doctors for a number of purposes, including the following:
1. To provide estrogen to prevent certain uncomfortable symptoms of estrogen deficiency during the period of adjustment when a woman's ovaries no longer produce estrogen. (Women normally stop producing estrogens between the ages of 45 and 55; this is called the menopause.)

PARKE-DAVIS
121 885400/YB

Fig 101-3. Examples of manufacturer's patient package inserts intended to enhance patient's understanding of the medication taken.

Table I—Examples of Latin and English Prescription Abbreviations

Word or phrase	Abbreviation	Meaning	Word or phrase	Abbreviation	Meaning
Ad	Ad	To, up to	Nocte	noct	At night
Ad libitum	Ad lib	At pleasure, freely	Nox, noctis	. . .	Night
Admove	Admov	Apply	Numerus	no	Number
Agita	Agit	Shake, stir	Octarius	o	A pint
Alternis horis	Alt h	Every other hour	Oculo utro	ou	Each eye
Ana	Aa	Of each	Oculus dexter	od	Right eye
Ante	A	Before	Oculus lævus	ol	Left eye
Ante cibos	ac	Before meals	Oculus sinister	os	Left eye
Ante meridien	am	Before noon, morning	Per os	po	By mouth
Aqua	aq	Water	Placebo	. . .	To please, satisfy
Auris utræ	au	Each ear	Post cibos	pc	After eating
Aurio dextra	ad	Right ear	Post meridiem	pm	Afternoon, evening
Aurio læva aurio sinister	al, as	Left ear	Pro re nata	prn	When necessary
			Pulvis	pulv	A powder
Bis	. . .	Twice	Quantum sufficiat	qs	As much as is sufficient
Bis in die	bid	Twice a day			
Bolus	bol	A large pill	Quantum sufficiat ad	qs ad	A sufficient quantity to (prepare)
Capsula	caps	Capsule			
Charta	Chart	Paper	Quaque	q	Each, every
Cibus	c	Food	Quaque diem	qd	Everyday
Collunarium	collun	A nose wash	Quaque hora	qh	Every hour
Collutorium	collut	A mouth wash	Quater in die	qid	Four times a day
Collyrium	collyr	An eye wash	Recipe	R_x	(You) Take
Compositus	comp	Compounded	Repetatur	rept	Let it be repeated
Congius	cong, C	A gallon	Secundum artem	sa	According to art
Cum	$\bar{c}$	With			
Da, detur, dentur	d	Give, let be given	Semis	ss	One-half
Dentur tales doses	dtd	Let four such doses be given	Signa	sig	(You) write
			Sine	$\bar{s}$	Without
Dexter, dextra	d	The right	Si opus sit	si op sit	If necessary
Diebus alternis	dieb alt	Every other day	Solutio	sol	Solution
Dilutus	dil	Dilute, diluted	Solutio saturata	sat sol	Saturated solution
Dispense	disp	Dispense	Somnus	. . .	Sleep
Divided	div	Divide	Spiritus vini rectificatus	svr	Rectified spirit of wine (alcohol)
Emulsum	emuls	Emulsion			
Et	. . .	And	Statim	stat	Immediately
Ex modo prescipto	emp	After the manner prescribed, as directed	Suppositorium	supp	Suppository
			Syrupus	syr	Syrup
			Tabella	tab	Tablet
Fac, fiat, fiant	F, Ft	Make, let it be made, let them be made	Talis	t	Of such
			Ter in die	tid	Three times a day
Gram	g, gm or Gm	Gram	Tablespoon	tbsp	Tablespoon
Granum	gr	Grain	Teaspoon	tsp	Teaspoon
Gutta	gtt	A drop	Unguentum	ung	Ointment
Hora	h	An hour	Ut dictum	ut dict	As directed
Hora somni	hs	At bedtime	Unus	i, I	One
Injectio	inj	An injection	Duo	ii, II	Two
Inter	int	Between	Tres	iii, III	Three
Kalium	K	Potassium	Quattour	iv, IV	Four
Lævo	L	Left	Quinque	v, V	Five
Linimentum	lin	Liniment	Sex	vi, VI	Six
Liquor	liq	Solution	Septem	vii, VII	Seven
Microgram	mcg	One-millionth gram	Octo	viii, VIII	Eight
Milligram	mg	One-thousandth gram	Novem	ix, IX	Nine
Milliliter	ml	One-thousandth liter	Decem	x, X	Ten
Minimum	m or min	A minim	Duodecim	XII	Twelve
Misce	m	Mix	Quindecim	XV	Fifteen
Mistura	mist	Mixture	Viginti	XX	Twenty
Mitte	. . .	Send	Triginta	XXX	Thirty
Natrium	Na	Sodium	Quinquaginta	L	Fifty
Nebula	nebul	A spray	Centum	C	One hundred
Non	. . .	Not	Quingenti	D	Five hundred
Non repetatur	non rep	Do not repeat	Mille	M	One thousand

the necessary information from the patient or physician, as is required.

Patient Information—The full name and address of the patient are necessary on the prescription for identification purposes. Names and addresses written illegibly should be clarified on acceptance of the prescription. Incorrect spelling of a patient's name on a prescription label might not only cause concern in the patient's mind as to the correctness of the medication, but would also hamper the desired professional relationship between the pharmacist and patient. Federal law requires that both the full name and address of both the prescriber and the patient be included on prescriptions for certain controlled drugs. Controlled drugs are legend drugs which, because of their potential for abuse, are controlled

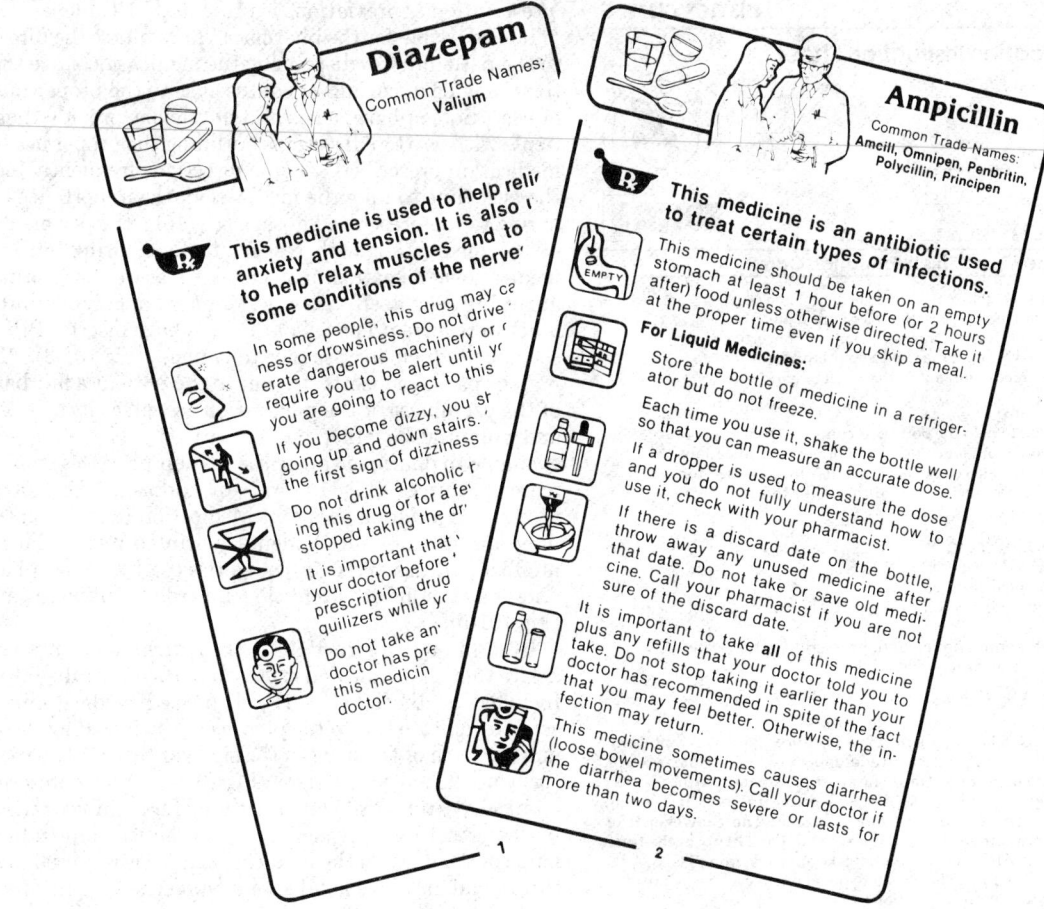

Fig 101-4. Examples of commercially available Patient Advisory Leaflet (Reproduced with the permission of the PHARMEX division of Automated Business Products Co, Inc, Box 57, Willimantic, CT 06226).

under special regulations by the federal government. The address of the patient is useful for identification purposes as well as for delivery of medication to the patient's home.

Some prescription blanks utilized by medical specialists, particularly pediatricians, include a space for insertion of the patient's age and/or weight. This information is placed on the prescription by the physician when medication dosage is an important function of age or weight. This information assists the pharmacist in interpreting the prescription, and is particularly useful when a child has the same name as one of his parents.

Date—Prescriptions should be dated at the time they are written and also when they are received and filled in the pharmacy. The date is important in establishing the medication record of the patient. A lapse of time of more than a couple of days between the date a prescription was written and the date it is brought to the pharmacy may be questioned by a pharmacist to determine if the intent of the physician and the needs of the patient can still be met. The date prescribed is also important to a pharmacist in filling prescriptions for controlled substances. The Drug Abuse Control Amendments specify that no prescription order for controlled drugs may be dispensed or renewed more than six months after the date prescribed.

R Symbol or Superscription—The R symbol is generally understood to be a contraction of the Latin verb *recipe*, meaning "take thou" or "you take." Some historians believe this symbol originated from the sign of jupiter, ♃, employed by the ancients in requesting aid in healing. Gradual distortion through the years has led to the symbol currently used.

Today, the symbol is representative both the prescription and pharmacy itself.

Medication Prescribed or Inscription—This is the body or principal part of the prescription order. It contains the names and quantities of the prescribed ingredients.

Today, the majority of prescriptions are written for medications already prepared or prefabricated into dosage forms by industrial manufacturers. The medications may be prescribed under their trademarked or manufacturer's name or by their nonproprietary or *generic* names. Pharmacists are required to dispense the trademarked product as prescribed, unless substitution of an equivalent product is permitted by the prescribing physician or by state law. Some states which permit substitution require the utilization of prescription blanks as shown in Fig 101-1, which allows a physician to authorize substitution by the placement of his signature on the appropriate line.

Prescription orders requiring the pharmacist to mix ingredients are termed *compounded* prescriptions. Prescriptions requiring compounding contain the names and quantities of each ingredient required. The names of the ingredients are generally written using the nonproprietary names of the materials, although occasionally proprietary names may be employed. Quantities of ingredients to be used may be indicated in the metric or apothecary system of weights and measures; however, the use of the apothecary system is diminishing. These systems are described in Chapter 9.

In the use of the metric system, the decimal is often replaced by a vertical line that may be imprinted on the prescription blank or drawn by the prescriber. The symbols g or mL are

PMI 008   **Tetracyclines**

Patient Medication Instruction Sheet

For: _____

Drug Prescribed: _____

Directions for Use: _____

_____

Special Instructions: _____

Please Read This Information Carefully

This sheet tells you about the medicine your
doctor has just prescribed for you. If any of
this information causes you special concern,
check with your doctor. **Keep this and all
other medicines out of the reach of children.**

Uses of This Medicine

Tetracyclines are used to help the body overcome bacterial infections.
However, they will not work for colds, flu, or other virus infections.
Some tetracyclines may help control acne and also may be used for
other conditions as determined by your doctor. Take this medicine
only as directed by your doctor.

Before Using This Medicine

BE SURE TO TELL YOUR DOCTOR IF YOU . . .
• are allergic to any medicine;
• are pregnant or intend to become pregnant while using this medicine;
• are breast-feeding;
• are taking any other prescription or nonprescription medications, or if
  you have any other medical problems.

Proper Use of This Medicine

DOSAGE
Tetracyclines should be taken with a full glass (8 ounces) of water to prevent
irritation of the esophagus or stomach. In addition, most tetracyclines (except
doxycyline or minocycline) are best taken on an empty stomach (either 1 hour
before or 2 hours after meals). However, if this medicine upsets your stomach,
your doctor may want you to take it with food. **You should not, however, take
milk, milk formulas, or other dairy products within 1 or 2 hours of the time
you take tetracyclines.** Also, you should not take antacids, iron pills, or
vitamins with minerals within 2 hours after you take tetracyclines. Consult
with your doctor if you have any questions.

To help clear up your infection completely, **keep taking this medicine for the
full time of treatment** even if you begin to feel better after a few days; **do not
miss any doses.**

Fig 101-5. Example of a Patient Medication Instruction Sheet (Courtesy, the American Medical Association).

often eliminated, as it is understood that solids are dispensed
by weight and liquids by volume.

**Dispensing Directions to Pharmacist or Subscrip-
tion**—This part of the prescription consists of directions to
the pharmacist for preparing the prescription. With diminished frequency of compounded prescriptions, such directions are likewise less frequent. In a large majority of prescriptions, the subscription serves merely to designate the
dosage form (as tablets, capsules, etc) and the number of
dosage units to be supplied. Examples of prescription directions to the pharmacist are:

M ft caps dtd no xxiv (Mix and make capsules. Dispense
24 such doses) *Ft sup No xii* (Make 12 suppositories) *M ft ung*
(Mix and make an ointment) *Disp tabs No c* (Dispense 100
tablets).

Directions for Patient or Signa—The prescriber indicates the directions for the patient's use of the medication in
the portion of the prescription called the *Signatura*. The
word signatura, usually abbreviated "Signa" or "Sig" means
"mark thou." The directions in the signa are commonly
written using abbreviated forms of English or Latin terms or
a combination of each. Examples are:

Tabs ii q4h (Take two tablets every four hours)
Caps i 4xd pc & hs (Take one capsule four times a day
   after meals and at bedtime)
Instill gtts ii od prn pain (Instill two drops into the right
   eye as needed for pain)

The directions are transcribed by the pharmacist onto the
label of the container of dispensed medication. A list of some

prescription abbreviations is presented in Table I.

It is advisable for the pharmacist to reinforce the directions
to the patient upon dispensing the medication since the patient may be uncertain or confused as to the proper method
of use. Some pharmacists and physicians provide their patients with written directions outlining the proper use of the
medication prescribed. These directions frequently include
the best time to take the medication, the importance of adhering to the prescribed dosage schedule, the permitted use
of the medication with respect to food, drink, and other
medications the patient may be taking, as well as information
about the drug itself. As a requirement of law, certain manufacturers have prepared patient package inserts (PPIs) for
specific products for issuance to patients (Fig 101-3). These
patient package inserts present to the patient a fair balance
of the usefulness of the medication as well as its side effects
and potential hazards. Other patient package inserts are
available to pharmacists for use in their practices from commercial sources (Fig 101-4). In addition, the American
Medical Association's Patient Medication Instruction (PMI)
program provides supplementary printed instructions on a
number of drugs and drug categories to physicians, pharmacists and other health professionals for distribution to patients
(Fig 101-5).

In addition to instructions to the patient, many prescribers
desire that the name and strength of the prescribed drug be
included on the label of the dispensed medication. Prescribers indicate this to the pharmacist by including the name
and strength of the drug in the signa or by simply writing in
the word "label" in the signa (Fig 101-1). Some prescription
blanks have the word "label" printed for circling or checking
by the prescribing physician. The practice of including the
name of the drug on the medication label is required in some
states, and may be excluded only upon the specific direction
of the prescriber. The advantages to having the name and
strength of the drug identified on the prescription label include: (1) facilitation of communication between the patient
and the pharmacist and/or physician; and (2) rapid identification of the medication in times of accidental or purposeful
overdose. One criticism of labeling often cited is the over-
zealous and sometimes troublesome pursuit of information
about the medication and the diseases for which it is prescribed by some patients when they know the names of medications they are taking.

The expiration date of the medication is also placed on the
label when such information is included on the original
manufacturer's package. This precaution is important for
certain drugs that rapidly deteriorate and lose their potency.
For example, many oral liquid formulations of antibiotics
remain stable for only a period of 14 days under refrigeration,
and half that time when non-refrigerated following their
preparation by the pharmacist. Physicians do not generally
specify that expiration dates be noted on the label since they
recognize that the pharmacist should provide this information
when dispensing such preparations. Statements on auxiliary
labels such as "do not use after ___ days" or "discard after
___ days" serve this purpose.

Special Labeling and Other Instructions—The number
of authorized refills should be indicated on each prescription
by the prescriber. In case no refill information is provided,
it is understood that no refills have been authorized. Most
prescription blanks include a section where this information
may be indicated (see Fig 101-1). No refills are permitted for
certain controlled substances.

Federal law requires that prescriptions for certain controlled drugs be validated by the full signature of the prescriber.

In most cases, the prescriber's name, address, telephone
number, and DEA Registry Number (the number assigned to
the medical practitioner by the Drug Enforcement Adminis-

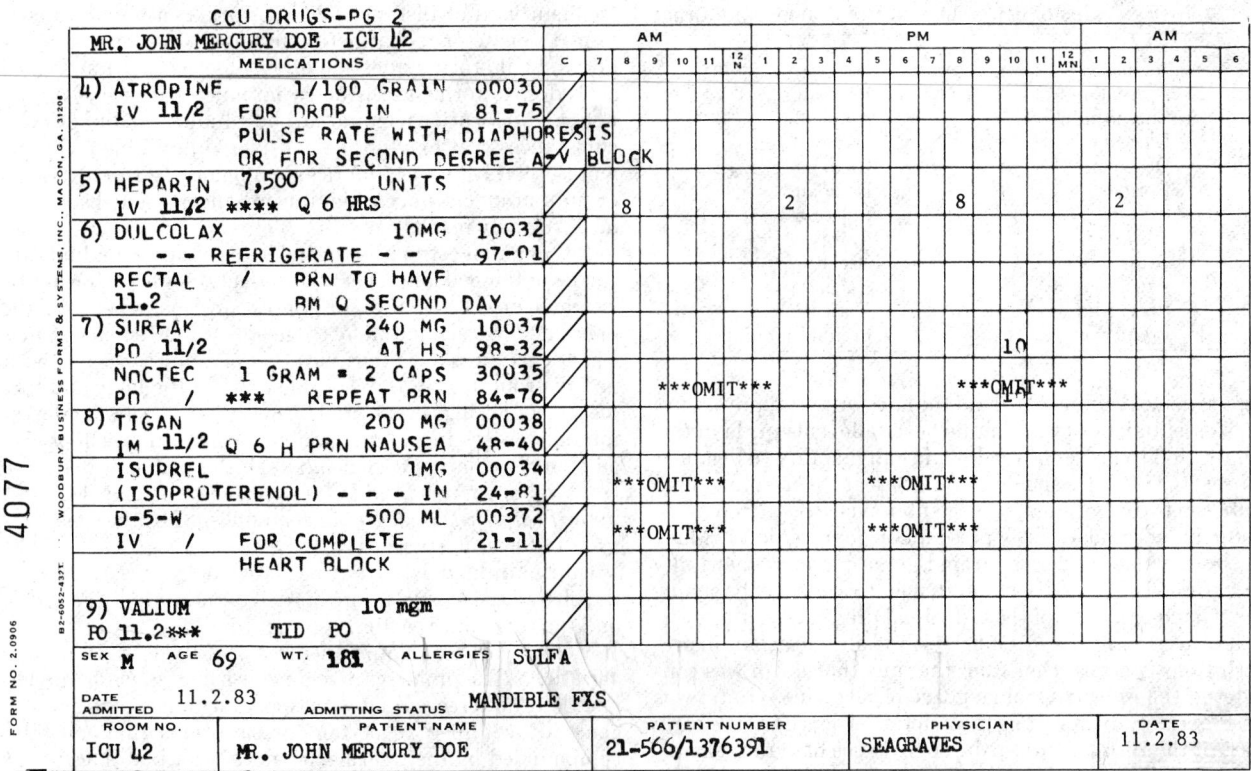

Fig 101-6.   Hospital form used in the scheduling of medication and recording of doses administered.

tration) are printed on his prescription blanks. The state license number of the prescriber may also be included. The printed name serves to clarify the prescriber's name when it is signed illegibly. On occasion the pharmacist may wish to telephone the prescriber's office to verify the authenticity of the prescription or to check an unclearly written drug name, dose, or direction.

Hospital Medication Orders

Medication orders for in-patients in hospitals and other institutions are written by the physician on forms called the "Physician's Order Sheet." The type of form utilized varies between institutions and even within the institution depending upon the unit rendering the care. For example, some physician's order sheets are essentially blank forms with each item to be ordered written in by the prescriber, whereas other forms, as those used in specialized areas such as Cardiac Care Units (CCU) may utilize a checklist of commonly employed drugs and procedures. Physician order sheets are prepared in multiple copies for utilization in the pharmacy as well as in the nursing station and in patient records. Additional forms are utilized in recording the scheduling and administration of the medications prescribed, as shown in Fig 101-6.

Processing the Prescription Order

The manner in which a pharmacist processes a prescription order is important in fulfilling his professional responsibilities, and can enhance his image with both the physician and patient. Proper procedures are given below for receiving, reading and checking, numbering and dating, labeling, preparing, packaging, rechecking, delivering, recording and filing, and pricing the prescriptions.

Receiving the Prescription—It is desirable that the patient hand the prescription order directly to the pharmacist since this enhances the pharmacist-patient relationship. In situations where this is not practical, the individual receiving the prescription should be trained to accept it in a professional manner and obtain the correct name, address, and, if necessary, the age of the patient. It is also important to determine if the patient's medications are provided through insurance coverage and whether the patient wishes to wait, call back, or have the medication delivered. If the pharmacist is unable to receive the prescription order personally, he should be available to provide an estimate of the length of time required to fill the prescription and to price it if requested by the pa-

tient. Many pharmacists make it a practice to price prescriptions before dispensing, especially in the case of unusually expensive medication, to avoid subsequent questions concerning the charge.

In order to identify the filled prescription properly some busy pharmacies employ a prescription claim check. A typical check is divided into three parts, each part bearing an identical number. One part is given to the patient, the second is attached to the prescription order, and the third is attached to the final container. In many community pharmacies, identification is made by personal recognition or by means of the patient's name and address; this tends to give a more personal touch to the service.

Reading and Checking the Prescription—The prescription order first should be completely and carefully read in the privacy of the prescription department. There should be no doubt as to the ingredients or quantities prescribed. If something is illegible or if it appears that an error has been made, the pharmacist should consult another pharmacist or the prescriber. The pharmacist has justifiably earned the

Table II—Examples of Look-alike and/or Sound-alike Drugs

Ananase	Orinase
Apresoline	Priscoline
Compocillin	Ampicillin
Daricon	Darvon
Digitoxin	Digoxin
Doriden	Doxidan
Indocin	Lincocin
Marax	Atarax
Orinase	Ornade
Pabalate	Robalate
Persantine	Trasentine
Prednisone	Prednisolone

reputation of being able to read the handwriting of physicians. It is essential, however, that he never allow his pride in this reputation to prevent his admitting an inability to decipher a prescription. He should never guess at the meaning of an indistinct word or unrecognized abbreviation. There is no "official" or standard list of prescription abbreviations. Many of them in use are derived from the Latin and are generally recognized (see Table I); however, many others may be simply shorthand creations of the individual prescriber.

The use of Latin words, phrases, and abbreviations in prescriptions is a carryover from the time that Latin was considered the international language of medicine. Latin was used extensively in writing prescription orders until the early part of the 20th century. Although its use has gradually diminished, it is still widely used, in the form of abbreviations, in the subscription and signa portions of prescriptions.

The pharmacist is frequently confronted in his interpretation of the prescription order with the names of drugs which look alike or sound alike. Examples of such drugs are listed in Table II.

The pharmacist must take great care and use his broad knowledge of drug products to prevent dispensing errors. A call to the physician, made so as not to alarm the patient, will serve to verify the meaning of a prescription that is unclear and at the same time bolster the professional reputation of the pharmacist as a careful practitioner and valuable member of the health team.

Omissions, such as failure to specify the desired strength of a medication or its dosage form, should be corrected. In such a case, the pharmacist should never elect to dispense the usual dose or dosage form, but should consult the prescriber. The pharmacist must be familiar with available strengths and dosage forms of prefabricated drug products in order to detect such omissions and provide the physician with the necessary information.

Amount and frequency of dose must be carefully noted and checked. In determining the safety of the dose of a medicinal agent, the age, weight, and condition of the patient, dosage form prescribed, possible influence of other drugs being taken, and the frequency of administration must all be considered. Because of the many factors involved in the calculation of an individual dose, there are no hard and fast rules on which the pharmacist can rely. However, a number of guides are available to the pharmacist in evaluating the safety of a prescribed dose. The publication *USP Dispensing Information* (published by The United States Pharmacopeial Convention, Inc) provides usual doses and dosage ranges for many drugs in use. Manufacturers' catalogs, file cards, and package inserts provide dosage information on their products. References such as *Physicians' Desk Reference*, *AMA Drug Evaluations*, and *United States Dispensatory* are useful general sources of such information. In the case of a suspected error in dose, appropriate references should be checked prior to consulting the physician.

Problems may arise when a usual dose is administered too frequently. For instance, a prescription calling for a sustained-release or repeat-action product to be given every 4 hours should raise a question in the pharmacist's mind since such dosage forms are usually administered every 8 to 12 hours. Medications should not be administered under circumstances that may not be considered desirable. For example, tetracycline antibiotics should not be given with milk or milk products since a significantly decreased absorption of a drug may result.

Although an estimation of doses for children and infants can be obtained from several empirical rules based on age or weight, a dose is not always a simple function of body weight or age and its calculation by these means is often inaccurate. Experience has shown that the doses of many drugs are more nearly proportional to the surface area of the body and this method of dosing is preferred by many as the basis for determining dosages for infants and children. An excellent discussion of pediatric dosage and a table of pediatric doses related to body weight and to body surface area may be found in the *Pediatric Dosage Handbook* published by the American Pharmaceutical Association.

Unusually high doses may be occasionally prescribed, and the pharmacist should assure himself of the prescriber's intent and the therapeutic rationale.

Measurement of liquid medication may lead to dosage variation. The problems associated with teaspoonful dosage have long been recognized. Teaspoonful dosage problems are generally confined to certain prescriptions that must be compounded by the pharmacist since most pharmaceutical manufacturers base their formulations for oral liquids on 5-mL doses.

A compounding and dispensing problem may arise because of the use of the fluid dram symbol (f$\mathfrak{z}$) in certain prescriptions. The fluid dram represents one-eighth of an apothecary fluid ounce, but is commonly interpreted as one teaspoonful when the physician uses this designation in the signa.

A standard teaspoon has been established by the American National Standards Institute as containing 4.93 ± 0.24 mL. For practical purposes, the standard teaspoonful is considered to be equivalent to 5 mL, although different household teaspoons vary widely in capacity. Thus, one fluid ounce (29.57 mL) of a medicated liquid is considered to provide approximately six standard teaspoonful doses. The difficulty occurs in compounding a prescription as written below:

> R Atropine sulfate   gr 1/250
>   Flavored vehicle qs ad   f$\mathfrak{z}$i
> Disp f$\mathfrak{z}$ii
> Sig f$\mathfrak{z}$i tid

The physician may intend to give his patient 16 doses of medication (16 fluid drams). However, if an ordinary household teaspoon is used to measure each dose, only 12 doses will be obtained. It is obvious that if the prescription were compounded to provide 16 doses and the instructions to the patient were to administer one teaspoonful, a significant dosage error would occur. One method of handling this prescription is to compound on the basis of twelve 5-mL doses, each containing $\frac{1}{250}$ gr of atropine sulfate, and instruct the patient to use a medicinal teaspoon or other device calibrated to measure 5 mL. An alternative would be to compound on the basis of 16 one-fluid-dram doses, each containing $\frac{1}{250}$ gr of atropine sulfate, and supply the patient with a dramspoon to measure accurately one fluid dram. Figs 101-7 and 101-8 show some available measuring devices for liquid medications.

Numbering and Dating—It is universal practice to number the prescription order and to place the same number on the label. This serves to identify the bottle or package and to connect it with the original order for reference or to renew the prescription. Consecutive numbers may be assigned by

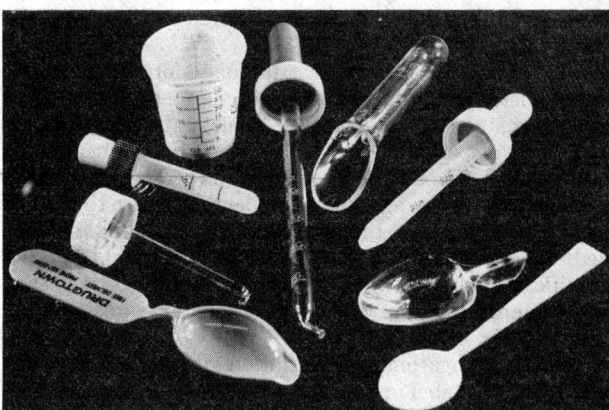

Fig 101-7. Examples of medicinal spoons of various capacities, calibrated medicine droppers, an oral medication tube, and a disposable medication cup (courtesy, Lea & Febiger, Publisher, "Introduction to Pharmaceutical Dosage Forms, 3rd edition, 1981, by Howard C Ansel).

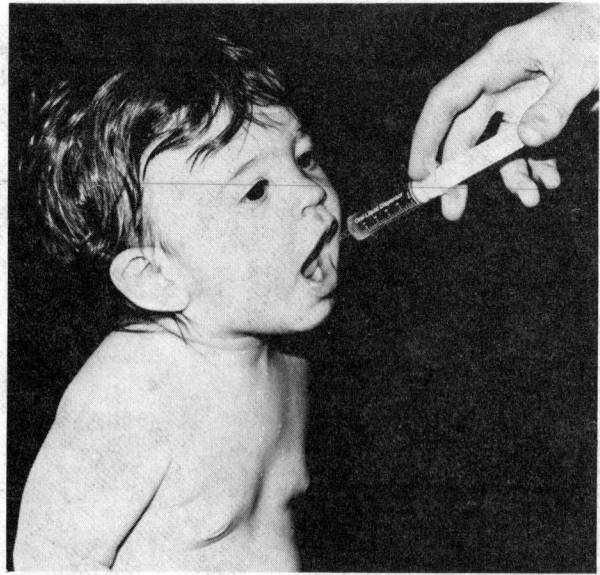

Fig 101-8. An oral liquid dispenser for the accurate delivery of small doses of liquid medication to infants (courtesy, Baxa Corporation).

use of a numbering machine. These machines can be set to number consecutively in duplicate or triplicate, so that the same number can be clearly and neatly stamped on the prescription order, label, and record book as desired. Some pharmacies utilize labels that are prenumbered. One such system is shown in Fig 101-9. In this example, the prenumbered form is perforated to enable easy separation into four parts; one part is a preglued label to be placed on the container of medication, another portion is placed on the prescription as the numbering and pricing record, the third part becomes the patient's receipt, and the fourth portion is utilized with the patient's medication record card as a record of refills.

Prescription computers also are being utilized to assign prescription numbers to prescriptions as described later in this chapter.

Dating of the prescription on the date filled also helps to establish its identity and should never be omitted. This in-

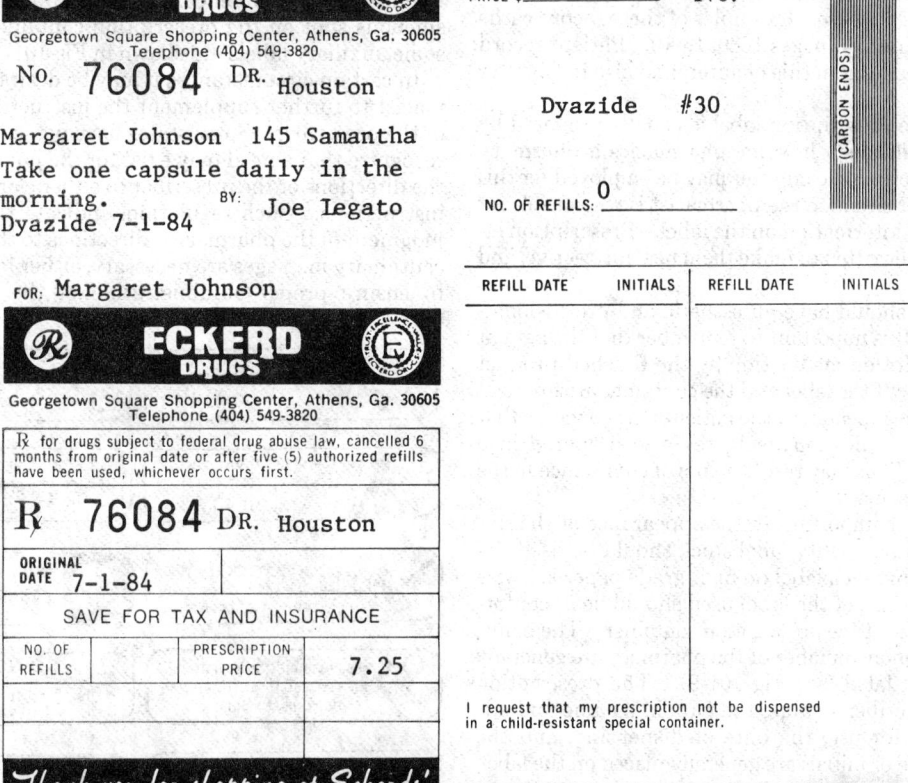

Fig 101-9. Example of prenumbered prescription label with multiple function. Upper left portion is the prescription container label; lower left portion is the patient's receipt; upper right portion is attached to the back of the prescription for its identification; and, lower right portion is for the refill record, placed in the patient's medication profile record in the pharmacy file.

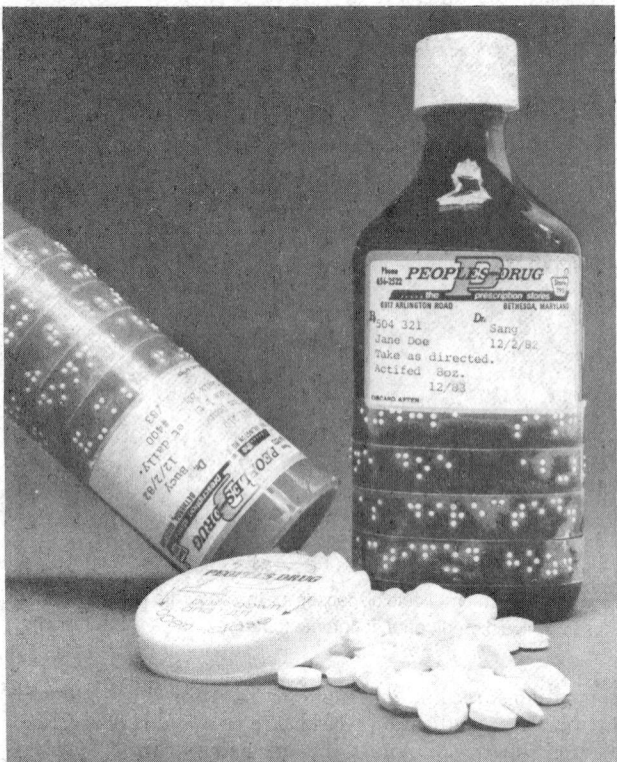

Fig 101-10. Example of a prescription label including directions in Braille. (Courtesy, People's Drug Stores, Inc, Alexandria, Virginia.)

formation may prove important as an alternate means of locating the prescription order if the number is lost by a patient. The use of patient record cards by the pharmacy can be similarly used for this purpose. Examples of these record cards are shown in Chapter 94 (pages 1689, 1690). Patient record cards are discussed later in this chapter, and also in Chapter 99.

Labeling—The prescription label is usually prepared by the pharmacist, although in some pharmacies a pharmacy assistant or a prescription computer may be employed for this purpose. In either situation the pharmacist is responsible for the correctness of information on the label. Prescription labels should be typewritten to make them neat, attractive, and legible.

A prescription should have an esthetic and professional-appearing label. It is important to remember that the patient judges his prescription medication by the finished product presented to him. If the label and the container are not neat and professional in appearance, the patient may conclude that the prescription medication itself was also prepared in a careless manner. This may result in loss of confidence in the pharmacist or pharmacy.

Since the label is important in the appearance of the finished prescription, a quality label stock should be used. A lithographed or engraved label on high-grade paper is a wise investment. The size of the label used should be in conformance with the size of the prescription container. The name, address, and telephone number of the pharmacy are generally imprinted on the label (see Fig 101-9). The prescription number, the prescriber's name, the patient's name and address, directions for use, the date of dispensing, and the pharmacist's name or initials are generally placed on the label. As indicated earlier, the name of the medication may also be placed on the label as requested by the prescriber. The pharmacist should make the directions to the patient for taking the medication as clear and complete as possible. For example, "Take one (1) tablet four (4) times a day before

meals and at bedtime" would be preferred to "One 4 times a day."

Some state laws require that the name or initials of the pharmacist dispensing the medication appear on the label. Also some states require that the name and strength of the medication dispensed appear on the label. Some pharmacists indicate the refill or renewal status of the prescription on the primary label or use an auxiliary label to indicate this information. Occasionally, the manufacturer's lot number for the medication dispensed is entered on the label to aid in rapid identification of medication that might be recalled. Labeling requirements for controlled substances are presented in Chapter 107.

A recent innovation in prescription labeling has been the placement of a label in braille along side of the regular typewritten label for blind or vision-impaired patients. The presence of the typewritten label allows sighted family members to assist in the proper administration of the medication (see Fig 101-10).

Auxiliary labels are used to emphasize a number of important aspects of the dispensed medication, including its proper use, handling, storage, refill status, and necessary warnings or precautions. A "shake-well" label is indicated for a prescription containing material that may separate on standing, such as mixtures, lotions, and emulsions. Use of labels such as "For the Ear," "For the Eye," and "External Use" is recommended because of the added safety they offer, even when the primary directions indicate proper use. The use of a "poison" label is rarely indicated since it may cause the patient to become unduly alarmed or fearful of using the medication; instead other precautionary labels may be used to warn that the medication should not be swallowed or used internally or should be kept out of reach of children and others for whom it is not intended.

Auxiliary labels are available in a variety of colors to give them special prominence. They should be placed in a conspicuous spot on the prescription container. Examples of some auxiliary labels are shown in Fig 101-11.

In certain circumstances it may be desirable for the pharmacist to further supplement the instructions or directions of the prescriber. Some states have passed regulations that recognize that a need may exist for the pharmacist to add to the directions of the prescriber to either clarify or expand his instructions. Such regulations indicate that when, in the judgment of the pharmacist, directions to the patient and/or cautionary messages are necessary, either for clarification or to ensure proper administration of the medication, the

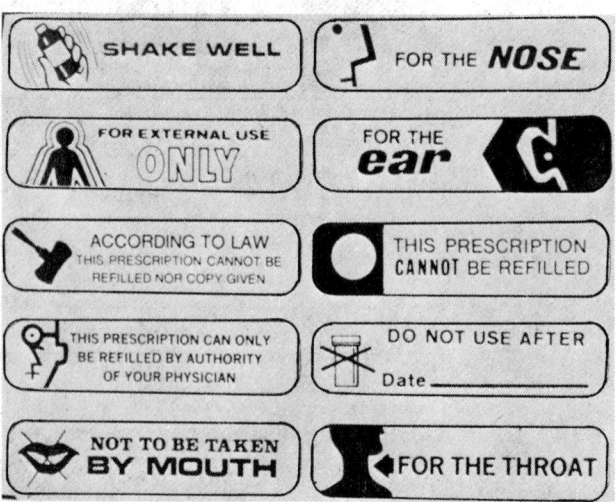

Fig 101-11. Examples of pharmacy auxiliary labels. Actual labels are available in color (courtesy, PHARMEX Division, Automated Business Products Co, Inc).

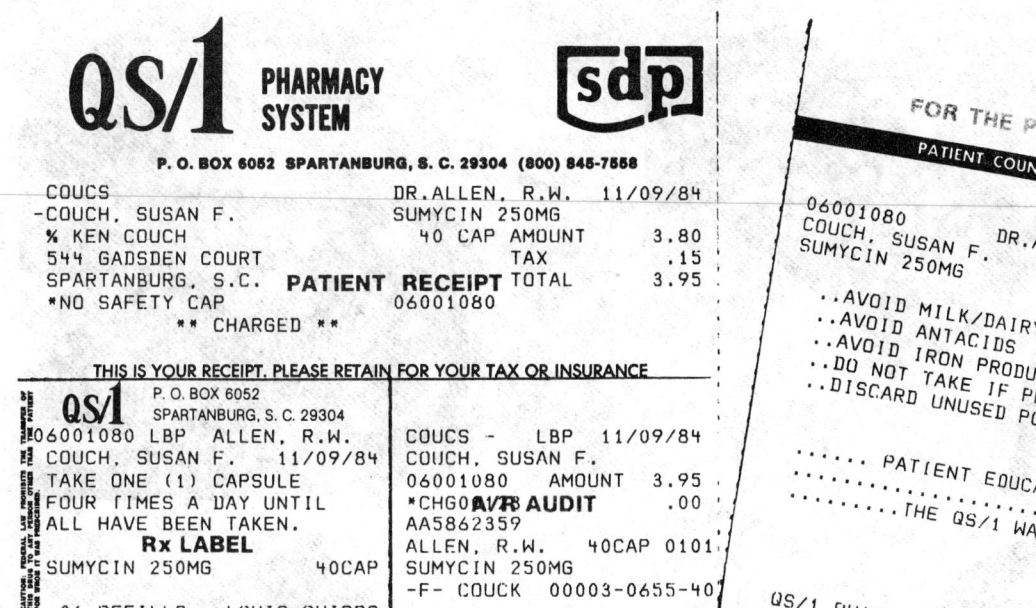

Fig 101-12.   Example of computer-prepared prescription label, patient receipt, and patient counseling information.   (Courtesy, Smith Data Processing, Spartanburg, SC).

pharmacist may add such directions or cautionary messages to those indicated by the prescriber on the original prescription.   For example, a pharmacist might advise that a medication be taken with a large volume of water or that certain foods or activities are to be avoided when taking the medication.

The federal government has required that patient product information be provided with the dispensing of certain drugs to ensure that the patient is apprised of proper use of the medication, its benefits and risks, and signs of adverse reaction.   Examples of these are shown in Fig 101-3.   Other types of patient information sheets have been noted earlier in this chapter and may be utilized by pharmacists in their practice.   Some prescription computers are programmed to provide supplemental instructions to patients (see Fig 101-12).   These printed instructions may be used by the pharmacist to reinforce his personal efforts in patient counseling.

Preparing the Prescription—After reading and checking the prescription order the pharmacist should decide on the exact procedure to be followed in dispensing or compounding the ingredients.

Most prescriptions call for the dispensing of medications already prefabricated into dosage forms by pharmaceutical manufacturers.   Care must be exercised by the pharmacist in making certain that the product dispensed is of the prescribed dosage, form, strength, and number of dosage units.   As noted previously, when substitution is permitted, the pharmacist is responsible for the selection of the manufacturer's product to use in filling the prescription.   He performs this responsibility on the basis of his knowledge of the quality, effectiveness, and cost to the patient of the selected product.   In filling prescriptions with prefabricated products, the pharmacist should check the manufacturer's label, comparing it to the prescription order, before and after filling the order to make certain of its correctness.   Products which show signs of poor manufacture or which look deteriorated or are past the stated expiration date on the label should never be dispensed.

Although the number of prescriptions that now require compounding represents only a very small percentage of the total, the pharmacist must acquire and maintain the knowledge and skills necessary to prepare them accurately.   When a prescription requiring compounding is received, the phar-

macist should take into consideration the chemical and physical compatibility of the ingredients, the proper order of mixing, the need for special adjuvants or techniques, and the mathematical calculations required.   Once he has decided on the procedure, he assembles the necessary materials in a single location on the prescription counter.   As he uses each ingredient, he moves it to some other established location on the counter (transfer from the left side of the balance to the right side is often suggested).   The use of this technique provides the pharmacist with a mechanical check on the introduction of each ingredient.   If he is interrupted during the process, there is then no doubt as to which ingredients have already been used.   When he has finished with all ingredients, he returns them to their proper location.   He has, therefore, had the opportunity to read the label of each ingredient three times: once when the container is removed from the shelf, again when the contents are weighed and measured, and finally when the container is returned to the shelf.

Any calculations or compounding information that would be useful in refilling the prescription at a later date should be noted on the face or on the back of the prescription order.   Adjuvants used, order of mixing, amount of each ingredient, capsule size used, type and size of the container, name and product identification number of the manufacturer, auxiliary labels used, clarification of illegible words or numbers, the price charged, and any special notations should be recorded.   Failure to do this may result in differences in the appearance of the prescription when refilled and possibly create doubt and apprehension in the mind of the patient.   Solid prefabricated dosage forms are generally counted in the pharmacy using a device such as that shown in Fig 101-13.   Such a device enables the rapid and sanitary counting and transferring of medication from the stock package to the prescription container.   To prevent contamination of tablets and capsules, the counting tray should be wiped clean after each counting, as powder tends to get on the tray, especially when uncoated tablets are counted.

The term *incompatibility* may be applied to prescriptions when certain problems arise during their compounding, dispensing, or administration.   Incompatibilities are categorized as being physical, chemical, or therapeutic.   The problems usually develop as a result of using two or more drug substances but problems involving the use of a single drug may

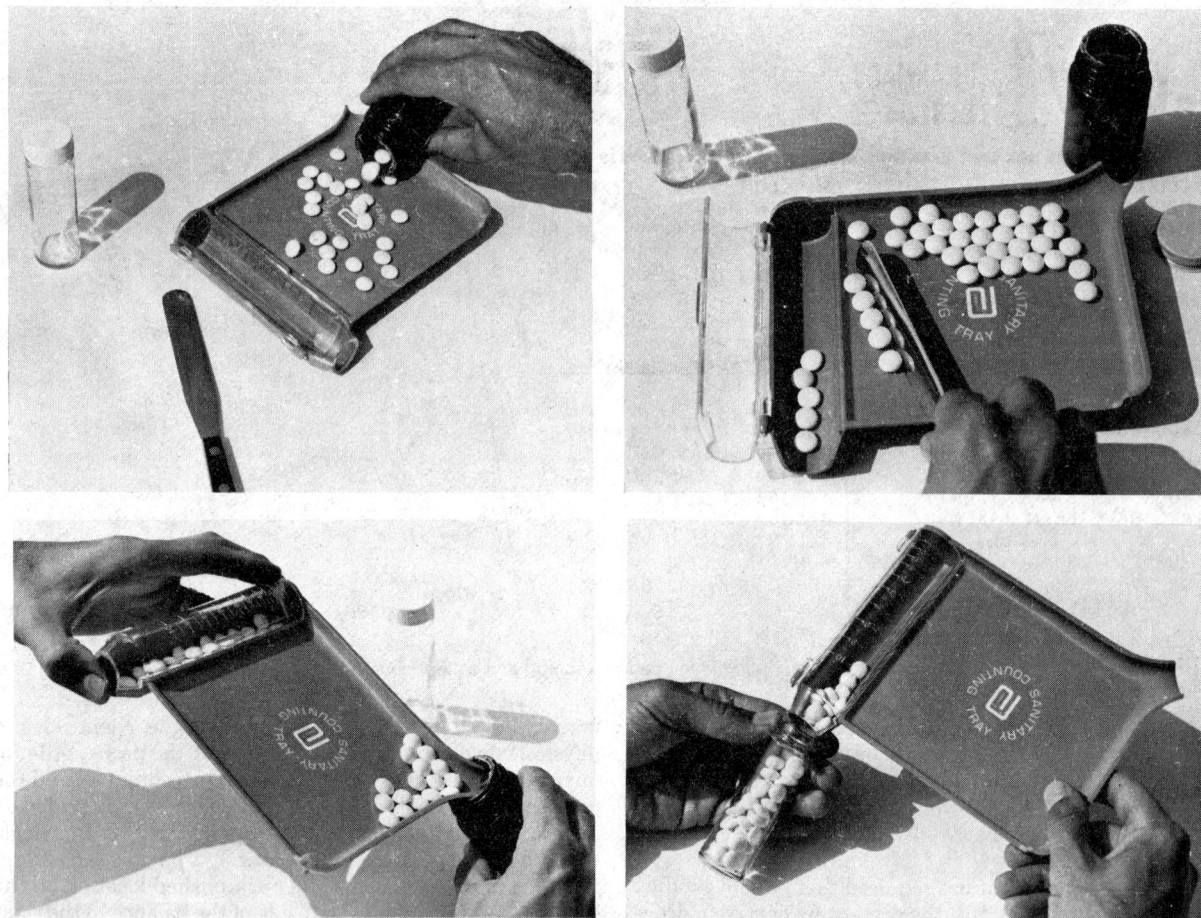

Fig 101-13.   Steps in the hygienic counting of solid dosage units with the Abbott Sanitary Counting Tray: (1) placing units from stock package onto tray, (2) counting and transferring units to trough, (3) returning excess units to stock container, and (4) transferring counted units into prescription container (courtesy, Lea & Febiger, Publisher, "Introduction to Pharmaceutical Dosage Forms," 3rd edition, 1981, by Howard C Ansel).

also occur. *Physical incompatibility* is usually the result of drug insolubility, liquefaction, or physical complexation. *Chemical incompatibility* may be the result of oxidation-reduction, acid-base, hydrolysis, or combination reactions. The occurrence of physical and chemical incompatibilities generally results in drug deterioration, discoloration, precipitation, or other effects which render the product unsatisfactory. These incompatibilities are overcome by the pharmacist through his knowledge of chemistry, physical pharmacy, and compounding techniques. The chemical and physical stability of dry substances and their reactions and interactions are covered in Chapter 102.

A *therapeutic incompatibility* exists when the response to one or more drugs administered to a patient is different in nature or intensity than that intended. Therapeutic effectiveness may be reduced or delayed as the result of a physical or chemical reaction. The taking of multiple drugs by a patient can result in drug interactions, which in turn may result in altered drug response. These effects may accentuate or diminish the activity of one or more of the drug substances or may produce synergistic or antagonistic effects. Adverse drug reactions may also be considered as therapeutic incompatibilities.

The alteration of a prescription order to correct or prevent a therapeutic incompatibility generally requires permission of the prescriber. Before contact is made, however, the pharmacist should be certain of the potential incompatibility and its therapeutic significance and should be prepared to make the appropriate recommendation to the prescriber to overcome the problem.

The areas of drug interactions and adverse drug effects are covered in Chapter 102.

Packaging—In filling a prescription, pharmacists may select a container from among various shapes, sizes, mouth openings, colors, and composition. Selection is based primarily upon the type and quantity of medication to be dispensed and the method of its use.

Among the types of containers generally utilized in the pharmacy are: *round vials*, used primarily for solid dosage forms as capsules and tablets; *prescription bottles*, used for dispensing liquids of low viscosity; *wide-mouth bottles*, used for bulk powders, large quantities of tablets or capsules, and viscous liquids that cannot be poured readily from the narrow-necked standard prescription bottles; *dropper bottles*, used for dispensing ophthalmic, nasal, otic (ear), or oral liquids to be administered by drop; *applicator bottles*, used for applying medication to a wound or skin surface; *ointment jars* and *collapsible tubes*, used to dispense semisolid dosage forms, as ointments and creams; *sifter top containers*, used for powders to be applied by sprinkling; and *hinged-lid* or *slide boxes*, used for dispensing suppositories and powders prepared in packets.

Most of the prescription containers are usually available in colorless, amber- or green-colored glass or plastic. Amber-colored glass containers are most widely used since they provide maximum protection of their contents against photochemical deterioration. In most instances a container made of good quality amber glass will reduce light transmission sufficiently to protect light-sensitive pharmaceuticals. The containers shown in Fig 101-14 are examples of such

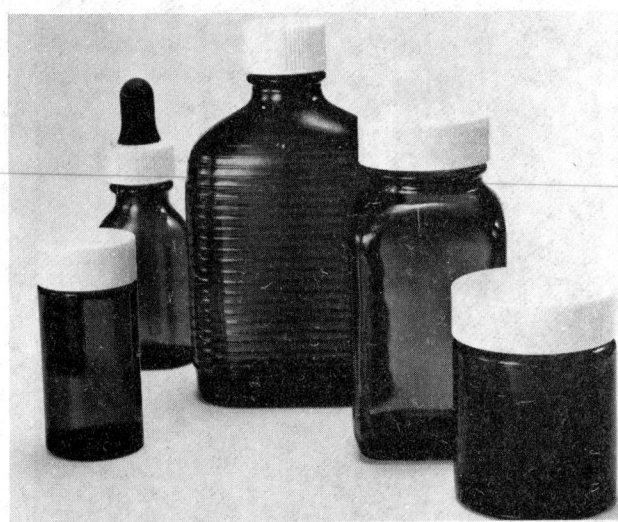

Fig 101-14. Examples of light-protective amber prescription containers for, from left to right: small numbers of solid dosage forms, as tablets and capsules; liquid preparations administered by drops; liquid preparations; powders, or large numbers of solid dosage forms; and semi-solid preparations, as ointments and creams (courtesy, Armstrong Cork Company).

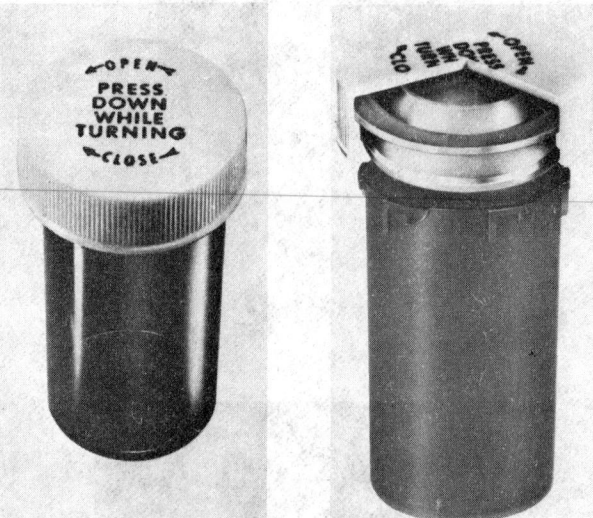

Fig 101-15. Gross and cut-away views of moisture-tight prescription container (courtesy, Kerr Glass Manufacturing Corporation).

containers. For total light restriction, opaque glass or glass rendered opaque by special coating may be employed. The use of outer wrappings or cartons also may be used to protect light-sensitive pharmaceuticals. A good-quality glass container will also be resistant toward the leaching of alkali from the glass into a liquid pharmaceutical preparation. Standards for the constitution of official glass types are provided by the USP. Pharmaceutical manufacturers select and utilize containers which do not adversely affect the composition or stability of their products. Similar types of containers should be used by the pharmacist in dispensing the medication to the patient. FDA regulations require pharmaceutical manufacturers to include in their prescription product labeling the type of container to be utilized by the pharmacist when dispensing the prescription drug to preserve its "identity, strength, quality and purity." The regulation does not apply to products intended to be dispensed in the manufacturer's original container.

The closure on a prescription container is as important as the container itself. By law, prescription containers must be moisture-proof and thus the ability of the closure to restrict entrance of moisture into the container is of prime importance. Moisture has a deteriorating effect on many dosage forms, especially capsules, tablets, and powders. For example, aspirin tablets will be hydrolyzed in the presence of moisture and broken down into acetic acid and salicylic acid. Plastic closures are most frequently used since they are durable and less reactive than other types of closures. Many pharmacies utilize screw-cap glass or tight-fitting closures to reduce moisture penetration (see Fig 101-15).

Plastic containers have widespread use in the pharmaceutical industry and in prescription practice. The advantages of plastic over glass containers include lightness of weight, resistance to breakage upon impact, and greater versatility in container design. Flexible polyethylene is widely utilized in the packaging of squeeze bottles for medication to be administered as drops or as a spray. Nose drops and throat sprays, as well as oral medication to be administered dropwise, are frequently packaged and dispensed in these containers. Lotions, shampoos, and creams are also conveniently packaged in flexible polyethylene containers. Pliable ointment tubes and flexible plastic containers for intravenous fluids are also widely used.

Rigid polystyrene vials are commonly employed by pharmacists to dispense capsules and tablets. This type of plastic is also widely utilized in ointment jars and box packages for suppositories. The modern compact-type container used for oral contraceptives, which contain sufficient tablets for a monthly cycle of administration and permit scheduled removal of one tablet at a time, is a prime example of the imaginative packaging possible with plastic. Examples of these containers are shown in Fig 101-16. These prepackaged containers, as obtained from the manufacturer, are properly labeled by the pharmacist and dispensed in the original container to the patient.

The increased responsibilities of pharmacists in drug distribution and inventory control in hospitals, nursing homes, and other patient-care facilities have had an impact on the development of the single-unit drug package, such as the strip-package, blister-package, and plastic disposable syringe. These single-unit packages are termed *unit-dose* packages at the time of administration to a specific patient. Examples of such packaging are shown in Fig 101-17.

The use of plastics in packaging pharmaceuticals is not without problems. Among problems found with the use of some plastics are: (1) permeability of containers to atmospheric gases and to moisture vapor; (2) leaching of constituents of the container to the internal content; (3) absorption of drugs from the contents to the container; (4) transmission of light through the container; and (5) alteration of the container on storage, particularly at extremes in temperatures.

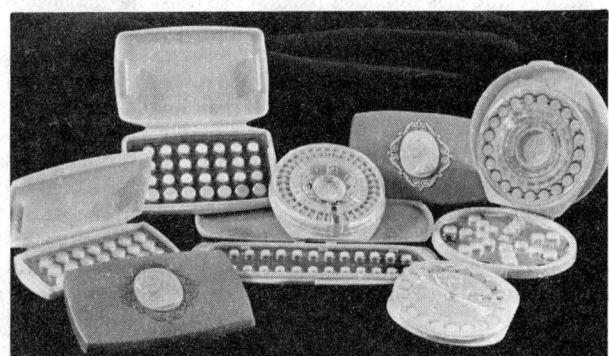

Fig 101-16. Examples of plastic packaging used for oral contraceptive products (courtesy, Lea & Febiger, Publisher, "Introduction to Pharmaceutical Dosage Forms," 3rd edition, 1981, by Howard C Ansel).

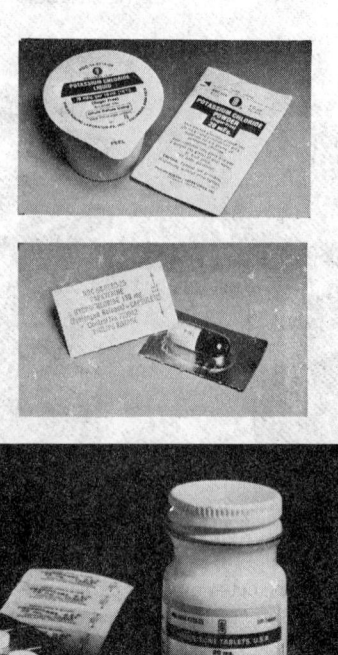

Fig 101-17.   Examples of multiple-unit and single-unit packaging, including patient cup, unit dose of powder, blister packaging of single capsule, and strip packaging of tablets (courtesy, Philips Roxane Laboratories).

Child-Resistant Containers—The high number of accidental poisonings following ingestion of medication and other household chemicals by children led to the passage of the Poison Prevention Packaging Act in 1970. The initial regulation called for use of "child-proof" closures for aspirin products and certain household chemical products shown to have significant potential for causing accidental poisoning in youngsters. As the technical capability in producing effective closures was developed, the regulations were extended to include the use of such safety closures in the packaging of both legend and over-the-counter medications. The Consumer Product Safety Commission has ruled that manufacturers must place prescription drugs in child-resistant packages if the original package is intended to go directly from the pharmacist to the patient. However, manufacturers need not place drugs in safety packaging if the drugs are intended to be repackaged by pharmacists.

All legend drugs intended for oral use must be dispensed by the pharmacist to the patient in containers having safety closures unless the prescribing physician or the patient specifically requests otherwise. There are some exceptions, as oral contraceptive packages because of their unique and useful design, and certain cardiac drugs (as nitroglycerin) because of the importance to the patient for direct and immediate access to his medication. Exemptions are also permitted in the case of over-the-counter medication for one-package size or specially marked packages to be available to consumers for whom safety closures might be unnecessary or too difficult to manipulate. These consumers include childless persons, arthritic patients, and the debilitated. Further, drugs which are utilized or dispensed in in-patient institutions, as hospitals, nursing homes, and extended care facilities, need not be dispensed with safety closures unless they are intended for patients who are leaving the confines of the institution. Ex-

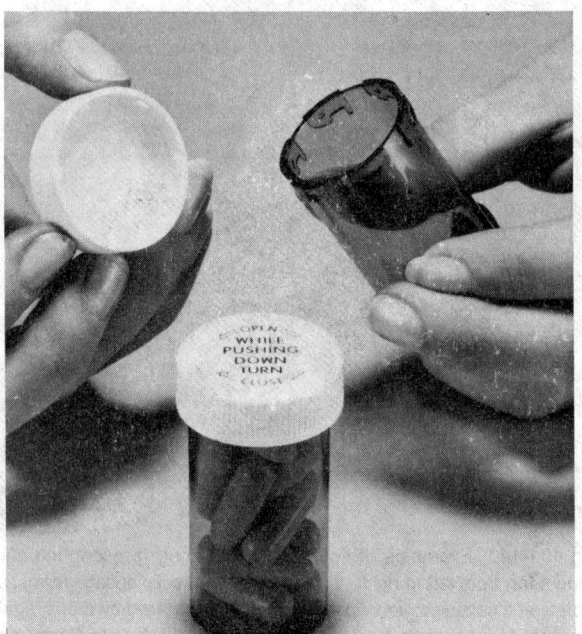

Fig 101-18.   Example of child-resistant safety closure on a prescription container (courtesy, Owens-Illinois).

amples of child-resistant containers are shown in Figs 101-15 and 101-18.

Rechecking—The importance of this step cannot be overemphasized. Every prescription should be rechecked and the ingredients and amounts used verified by the pharmacist. All details of the label should be rechecked against the prescription order to verify directions, patient's name, prescription number, date, and prescriber's name.

Delivering the Prescription—The pharmacist should personally present the prescription medication to the patient (or family member) unless it is to be delivered to the patient's home or workplace. This gives the pharmacist assurance that the patient knows how to use the medication properly. When presenting the medication to the patient, the pharmacist should also call attention to any auxiliary labeling instructions and provide further information regarding the medication as may be desirable. When personal delivery of the prescription is not possible, the pharmacist should make certain that the appropriate instructions are provided to the patient and that the patient be encouraged to phone should there be any questions.

The prescription medication is frequently placed in specially designed and imprinted prescription bags. Some pharmacists place the patient's name, address, prescription number, and price on the package to identify the prescription. Many patients retain the prescription label or bag for purposes of tax records, although an increasing number of pharmacies have computerized statements or other means of providing patients with this information.

Recording and Filing—A record of the prescriptions dispensed is maintained in the pharmacy through the use of prescription files.

A variety of prescription file types are available to maintain original prescription orders. Metal or cardboard units, which conveniently store about 1,000 prescriptions are the most common. In using these files, holes are punched in the prescription orders, they are then slipped onto two metal rods firmly attached to the file and placed in a designated compartment in numerical order for safe storage and rapid retrieval.

Suitably partitioned drawers are sometimes used for filing. The partitions may be placed between every 200 or 300 prescriptions, plainly marked with the numbers of the prescriptions filed in that section. This method permits removal of a single prescription without preventing ready access to others, as normally occurs when metal rod files are used. Some pharmacies utilize file folders alphabetically arranged by patient name to maintain patient medication record cards and the individual prescriptions. Prescription computers are also used for recording and storing prescription orders. Microfilming of prescriptions for purposes of filing and retrieving is an available but little used method.

Special regulations govern the manner in which prescriptions of controlled substances must be filed. These are discussed in Chapter 107. The patient or family record card method is frequently used to provide prescription record and patient information. A file card, as shown in Chapter 94, pages 1689, 1690, may be used for each patient or family. The patient's name is typed at the top of the card and as each prescription is dispensed, the prescription number, date, name and amount of medication, prescribing physician's name, and the fee for the medication are placed on the card. The purchase of OTC medications may also be noted on the card; thus, the card may serve as a complete record of medication obtained by the patient. Special information concerning the patient, such as drug allergies or a particular disease state (eg, diabetes, glaucoma), are also recorded. With this information available, the pharmacist is better able to detect potential problems related to drug therapy. For example, a problem may arise when a patient is taking a number of medications which may have the potential for interacting in a counterproductive manner. These medications may be solely legend drugs or combinations of OTC and legend drugs prescribed by a single physician or several that a patient may be seeing. The use of such record cards permits rapid location of prescription records without the need of prescription number or date, and enables the pharmacist to provide rapidly and completely a listing of all medications dispensed to a patient upon the inquiry of the physician. The information also may be useful to the patient for income tax purposes. Additional information on patient medication record systems may be found in Chapter 94.

Pricing the Prescription

In order for a pharmacist's prescription practice to be successful, he must be an effective manager of the financial aspects of his practice. To maintain the types of pharmaceutical services desired by his community, the pharmacist must make a fair and equitable profit.

Each pharmacy should have a method for pricing prescriptions which is applied consistently by each pharmacist practicing in that pharmacy. The pricing method should be established to ensure a profitable operation of the prescription department. A uniform and consistently applied system is beneficial to the pharmacists and helps to avoid misunderstandings from patrons.

The charge applied to a prescription should cover the costs of the ingredients, including the container and label, the time of the pharmacist and auxiliary personnel involved, the cost of inventory maintenance and other operational costs of the department, as well as providing a reasonable margin of profit on investment.

Although many methods of pricing prescriptions have been utilized through the years, the most commonly used are:

1. *% Markup*
   Cost of ingredients + (cost of ingredients × % markup) = dispensing price.
2. *% Markup + Minimum Fee*
   Cost of ingredients + (cost of ingredients × % markup) + minimum fee = dispensing price.
3. *Professional Fee*
   Cost of ingredients + professional fee = dispensing price.

% Markup—This method and the % markup plus minimum fee method are commonly utilized in prescription practice. In utilizing the straight markup method, the desired percentage markup is taken of the cost of the ingredients and added to the cost of the ingredients to obtain the dispensing price. For example, if the ingredients in a prescription cost the pharmacist $4.00 and he wishes to apply an 80% markup on cost, he would add $3.20 to the cost of the ingredients and arrive at a dispensing price of $7.20. The percentage markup applied may be varied depending upon the cost of the ingredients, with a lower percent markup generally utilized for prescription items of higher cost and a higher percent markup applied for prescription items of a lower cost.

In order to obtain price consistency many multiple-pharmacy operations, as chain-store pharmacies, provide each pharmacy with a pricing schedule for prescription items. These pricing schedules are frequently provided on microfiche or affixed directly to the bulk container of prescription products by chain-store warehouses; the schedules are updated on a regular basis to account for changes in costs of ingredients or in percent markup desired.

Markup Plus Minimum Fee—In this method, a minimum fee is added to the cost of ingredients plus a percent markup. The percent markup in this method is usually lower than the one utilized in the method described above. The minimum fee is usually established to recover the combined cost of the container, label, overhead, and professional services. This method is applied as follows: if the cost of the prescription ingredients is $4.00, and a 40% markup on cost is applied, the charge to that point would be $5.60. Then, a minimum fee is added and the final dispensing price determined. If, for example, a minimum fee of $2.25 is added, the final prescription price would be $7.85. To achieve the desired profit, the percent markup utilized in this method may be adjusted upward or downward depending upon the minimum fee established.

Professional Fee—This method involves the addition of a specified professional fee to the cost of the ingredients used in filling a prescription. The professional fee includes all the dispensing costs and professional remuneration. A true professional fee is independent of the cost of the ingredients and thus, does not vary from one prescription to another. Some pharmacists utilize a variable or sliding professional fee method, whereby the magnitude of the fee is varied somewhat on the cost of the ingredients. By this method, the greater the cost of prescription ingredients, the greater is the fee; the rationale being that the cost of inventory maintenance must be recovered in this manner. However, a single fee for all prescriptions is the true basis of the professional fee method. The fee represents payment for professional service rendered in the filling of a prescription and is the same without regard to the cost of ingredients.

In practice, the professional fee may vary widely between pharmacies depending on the cost and types of pharmaceutical services rendered (eg, family record systems, delivery service, home health-care needs, etc) and the professional desires of the pharmacist. A pharmacy may determine its professional fee by (1) averaging the amount previously charged, above ingredient cost, for prescriptions dispensed over a specified period of time or (2) using a more exacting cost analysis method in which *all* costs attributed to the prescription department are divided by the prescription volume in determining the actual cost of filling a prescription, with the profit and desired fee then determined. Pharmacies utilizing the professional fee commonly make adjustments for prescriptions requiring compounding to compensate for the extra time, materials, and equipment utilized.

Many governmental units, such as state human services agencies, and many insurance companies, have adopted the professional fee method for the reimbursement of pharmacists in filling prescriptions covered under their programs. Such third-party payers negotiate the professional fee to be utilized with pharmacists interested in participating in the programs. Many of these programs have a "copayment" provision which requires the patient to pay a part of the charge for each prescription he has filled.

After pricing a prescription, pharmacists place the price, or sometimes a code, on the prescription for future reference should the prescription later be renewed. In using codes, some word or combination of characters is generally selected and utilized in the pharmacy. The word selected should have ten letters with no duplicate letters. For example, the following code has been used by some pharmacists:

REPUBLICAN
1 2 3 4 5 6 7 8 9 0

In utilizing this code, a price of $7.85 would be indicated by the letters "ICB." Such a coding method can be used also to indicate the cost of items in the pharmacy for inventory purposes.

Prescription Refilling

Instructions for refilling of a prescription are provided by the prescriber, on the original prescription or by verbal communication. Although prescriptions for non-controlled substances have no limitation according to federal law as to the number of refills permitted or the date of expiration, state laws may impose such limits. The refilling of prescriptions for controlled substances is limited as described later in Chapter 107. Physicians and pharmacists should work together so that prescriptions are renewed only with the frequency consistent with directions for use and the pharmacist should check with the prescriber after a reasonable time to assure himself that his intent is being met. No prescription should be renewed indefinitely without the patient being reevaluated by the prescriber to assure that the medication as originally prescribed remains the medication of choice.

Renewals should be noted on the reverse side of the prescription order with the date, the quantity dispensed, if different from the original, and the name or initials of the pharmacist dispensing the medication. If verbal authorization has been obtained from the prescriber, this should be noted.

The maintenance of accurate records of renewals is not only important to follow federal and state laws, but is also to provide information on the patient's medication history.

Copies of Prescription Orders—These are occasionally requested by the patient or a pharmacist in behalf of the patient. In some instances, the intention is to provide information, and in other instances the patient is desirous of having the copy refilled at another pharmacy.

Although the Food and Drug Administration maintains that a copy of a prescription order has no legal status and should not be honored, the agency has opened the door for honoring copies under certain circumstances. The FDA does not object to the exchange of prescription copies between pharmacies

for the purpose of renewal, provided that certain safeguards are taken: (1) the original order is voided and marked to indicate that a copy has been issued, to whom, and the date of issuance; (2) the copy should be so marked and the location and number of original noted; and (3) the copy shows the date of original dispensing, the date of the last renewal, and the number of renewals remaining.* This procedure does not apply to Schedule II controlled drugs or if individual states prohibit such a procedure. In instances in which copies of prescriptions are provided by the pharmacist and in which the copy may not be legally refilled, the pharmacist supplying the copy should write "Copy—Not to be Dispensed" or a similar designation across the top. A copy should be made exactly like the original including all pertinent information that a pharmacist might require in dispensing the medication as originally provided. The copy preferably should be written or typed on a preprinted form identifying the pharmacy.

The Drug Enforcement Administration amended the Code of Federal Regulations in 1981 to permit the transfer of prescription orders between two pharmacies for controlled substance prescriptions which may be lawfully renewed.

The amendment allows for the transfer of an original prescription order for controlled substances listed in Schedules III, IV, or V between pharmacies on a *one-time basis only*.

To comply with the new regulations, pharmacists must first ascertain if the transfer of a prescription order for renewal dispensing purposes is permissible under state or other applicable law.

When a prescription order is transferred, it must be communicated directly between two licensed pharmacists, and the transferring pharmacist must record the following information: (1) write "VOID" on the face of the invalidated prescription order; (2) on the back of the invalidated prescription order, the name, address, and DEA registration number of the pharmacy it was transferred to and the name of the pharmacist who received the information; and (3) the date of transfer and the transferring pharmacist's name.

The pharmacist receiving the transferred prescription order must reduce to writing the following: (1) the word "transfer" on the face of the transferred prescription order; (2) all information required on a controlled substance prescription order as it appears on the original prescription order; (3) date of issuance of original prescription order; (4) original number of renewals authorized on the original prescription order; (5) the date of the original prescription order; (6) number of valid renewals remaining and the date of the last renewal; (7) pharmacy's name, address, DEA registration number, and original prescription number for which the prescripton order was transferred; and (8) the name of the transferring pharmacist.

DEA requires that the original and transferred prescription orders must be maintained for a period of two years from the date of last renewal.

---

* Pharmacy Practice, American Pharmaceutical Association, Academy of Pharmacy Practice, Volume 13, No 3, March, 1978, p 18.

Patient Counseling Information

There is an increased awareness that labeling instructions are frequently inadequate to ensure patient understanding of his medication and his adherence or compliance with recommended instructions. The responsibility that the patient receive specific instructions, precautions, and warnings for safe and effective use of prescribed drugs is the shared responsibility of the prescriber and the pharmacist. Reinforcement of the labeled instructions are through verbal

communication between the prescriber, pharmacist, and patient, or as supplemental printed instructions, as noted previously.

To assist the pharmacist in having up-to-date and pertinent information available for the counseling of his patients, a number of organized and conveniently arranged sources of dispensing information for patients are available. For example, *USP Dispensing Information*, Vol II, *Advice for the*

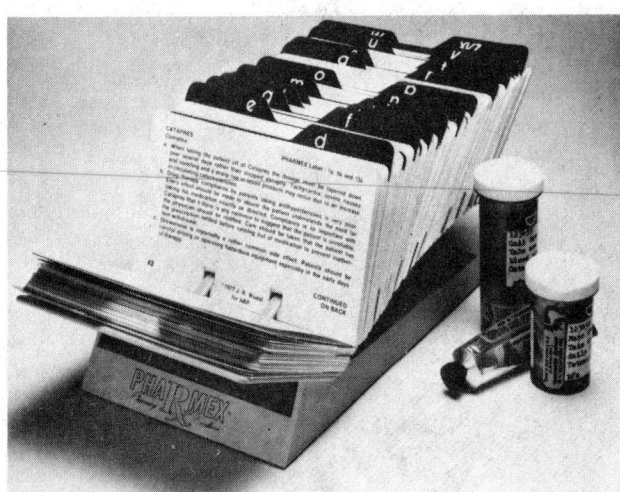

Fig 101-19. Example of drug information and consultation guide for pharmacist's use in reinforcing labeled instructions to his patients (courtesy, PHARMEX Division, Automatic Business Products Co, Inc).

Patient, provides useful information on officially recognized medications for use by pharmacists in counseling of their patients. Patient counseling information is also available from a number of sources on handy, alphabetically arranged file cards (see Fig 101-19). These reference units usually provide the pharmacist with resource information including: clinical indications and applications; adverse drug reactions; drug interactions; interference with diagnostic tests; known effects on the fetus and newborn; relevant biopharmaceutics and pharmacokinetics; excretion of the drug through breast milk; sugar and/or content of the medication; and other in-

formation deemed important. The cards also provide suggested patient information that may be conveyed by the pharmacist to the patient in an easily presented and understood manner. See also Chapter 99.

Patient Compliance with Prescribed Medication

When a prescriber writes a prescription, he intends the patient to have the prescription filled immediately and to begin utilizing the medication according to directions. Patient adherence or compliance with the prescribed medication schedule has been a source of concern to both the physician and the pharmacist.

Patients may delay unnecessarily initiation of drug therapy or may wait to see if they "feel better" before having the prescription filled. Some patients discontinue their medication prematurely because they are feeling better and see no particular need to continue taking the medication. Other patients may take excessive doses of the medication believing that they will get better faster, while others take their medication at incorrect intervals or whenever they remember.

On refilling a prescription, a pharmacist can generally determine the compliance of the patient in taking his medication by comparing the dosage units dispensed vs the dosage units apparently taken over the treatment period. Pharmacy computer systems have recently been utilized in determining patient compliance (see Fig 101-20).

Specially designed medication containers have shown usefulness in assisting a patient to adhere to his medication schedule. These containers have individual compartments for daily medication and generally hold a week's supply (see Fig 101-21). Containers for oral contraceptive medication, previously discussed in this chapter and shown in Fig 101-16, have proven to be effective in patient compliance during the monthly medication cycle. See also Chapter 100.

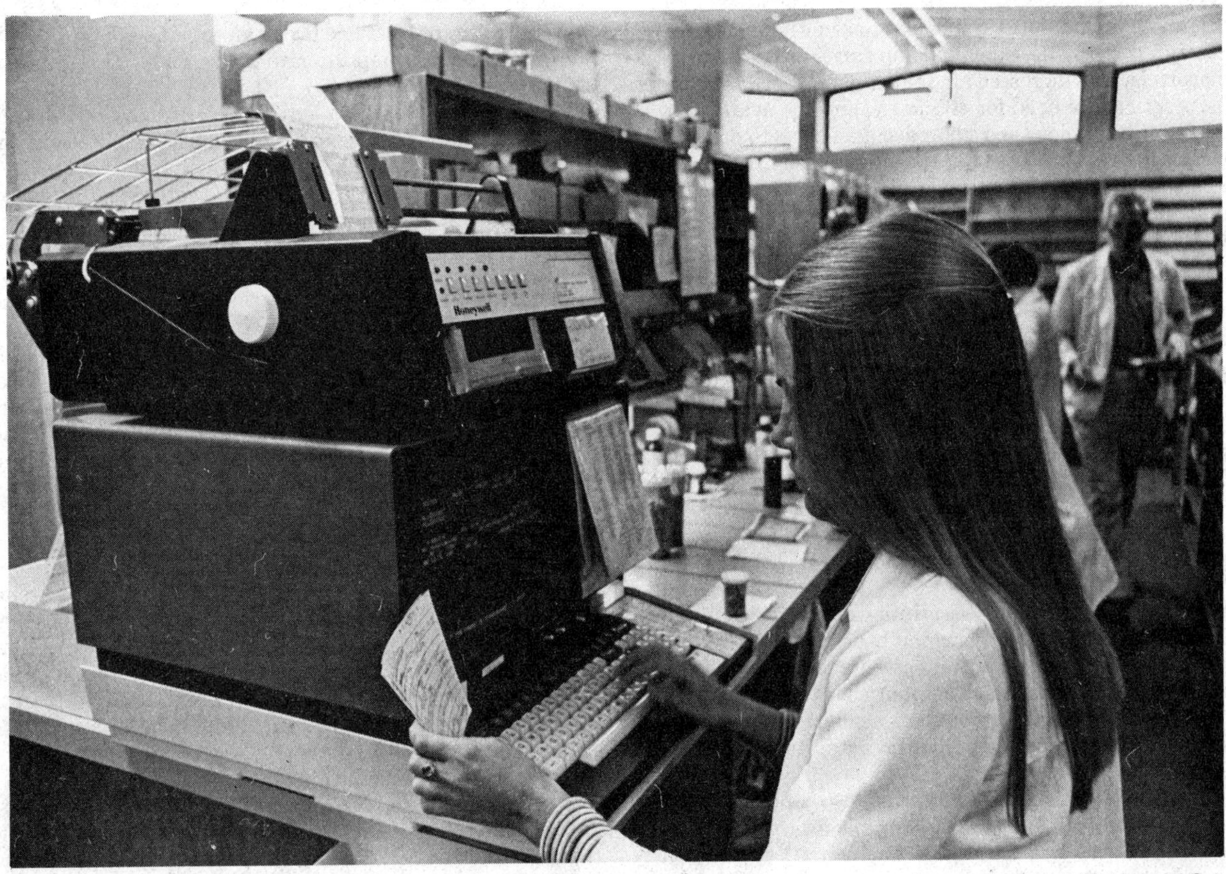

Fig 101-20. Pharmacist monitoring patient utilization of prescribed medication utilizing computer technology (courtesy, Eli Lilly and Co).

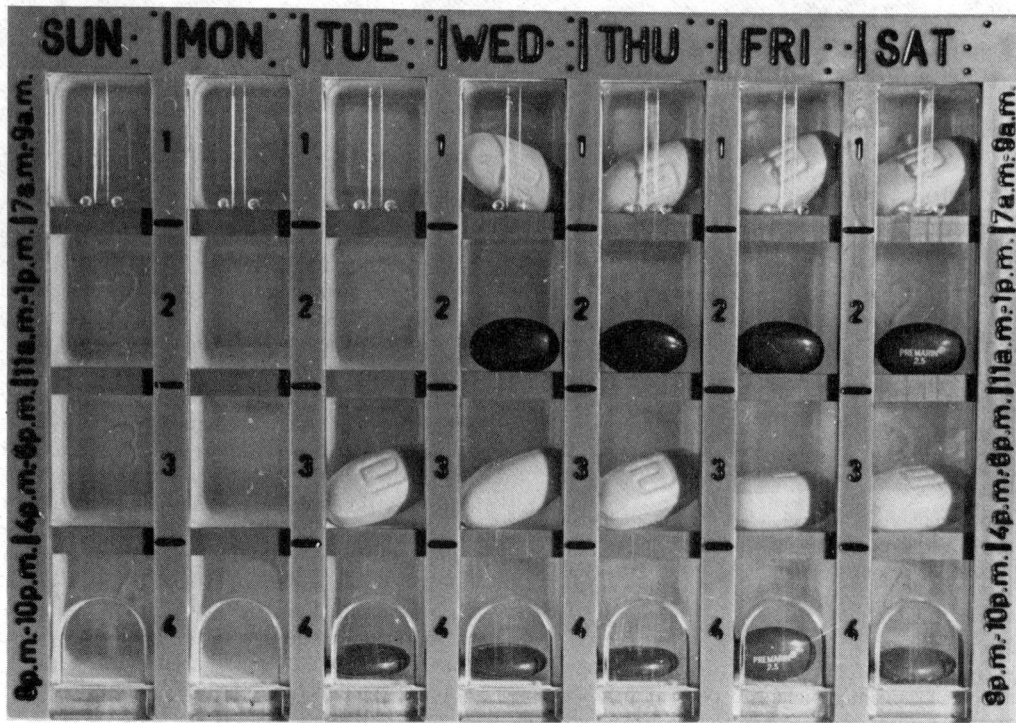

Fig 101-21. Example of MEDISET medication container designed to assist patient compliance with prescribed medication schedule (courtesy, Drug Intelligence Publications, Inc).

Pharmacy Computer Systems

The use of computer systems in pharmacy practice is increasing due to the expanded informational needs of the pharmacist, the increased amount of paper work required in the practice, the need for efficiency, and the availability of computer technology and expanded data bases to provide the necessary support. (See Fig 101-22 and also Chapter 11.)

In general, computerized systems in pharmacy are utilized in three areas: (1) prescription dispensing and associated record maintenance; (2) clinical support; and (3) accounting and business management. Computer utilization in these areas will be briefly outlined below.

Prescription Dispensing and Associated Record Maintenance

Label Preparation—Upon entry of the basic prescription information, the computer produces an error-free label or multiple labels if required.

Prescription Number Assignment—Consecutive numbers are assigned to prescriptions by the computer, and the problem of lost and duplicate numbers is virtually eliminated.

Price Calculations—Prescription computer systems can accommodate multiple pricing methods including: cost plus a professional fee, cost plus a percentage markup, or other more complex formulas. The pharmacist specifies the formula desired and the computer calculates the dispensing charge based upon drug cost information contained in its files.

Receipt Preparation—Prescription computers calculate and store information; thus, it is simple for the computer to automatically prepare a receipt for the patient which may include the amount paid for an individual prescription or for the total prescriptions filled over a given period of time. This information may be important to the patient for insurance or tax purposes.

Prescription Notation—As a prescription order is processed, the pharmacist typically makes several notations, including: the initials of the dispensing pharmacist, the drug cost and product dispensed, and special entries as "dispensed only one-half at patient request." This information may be retained by the computer and utilized in renewal processing.

Renewal Processing—The computer-assisted renewal processing of prescriptions is almost automatic. If the computerized records indicate that the prescription renewal is allowable, the computer automatically prepares the new label and receipt, updates the renewal status of the prescription, recalculates the price based on current cost information, and adds the entire transaction to the patient's medication profile.

Clinical Support

Patient Medication Profiles—On command, the computer presents on its monitor the most recent medications that have been dispensed to the individual patient. This information is utilized by the pharmacist in ascertaining potential drug-drug interactions. Information pertaining to the patient's drug allergies and primary illnesses also permits the pharmacist to assess the drug therapy and dispense only rational and effective medications.

Drug Utilization Monitoring—By tracking the dispensing dates and quantities dispensed, a pharmacist is able to determine a patient's compliance in taking the prescribed medication properly.

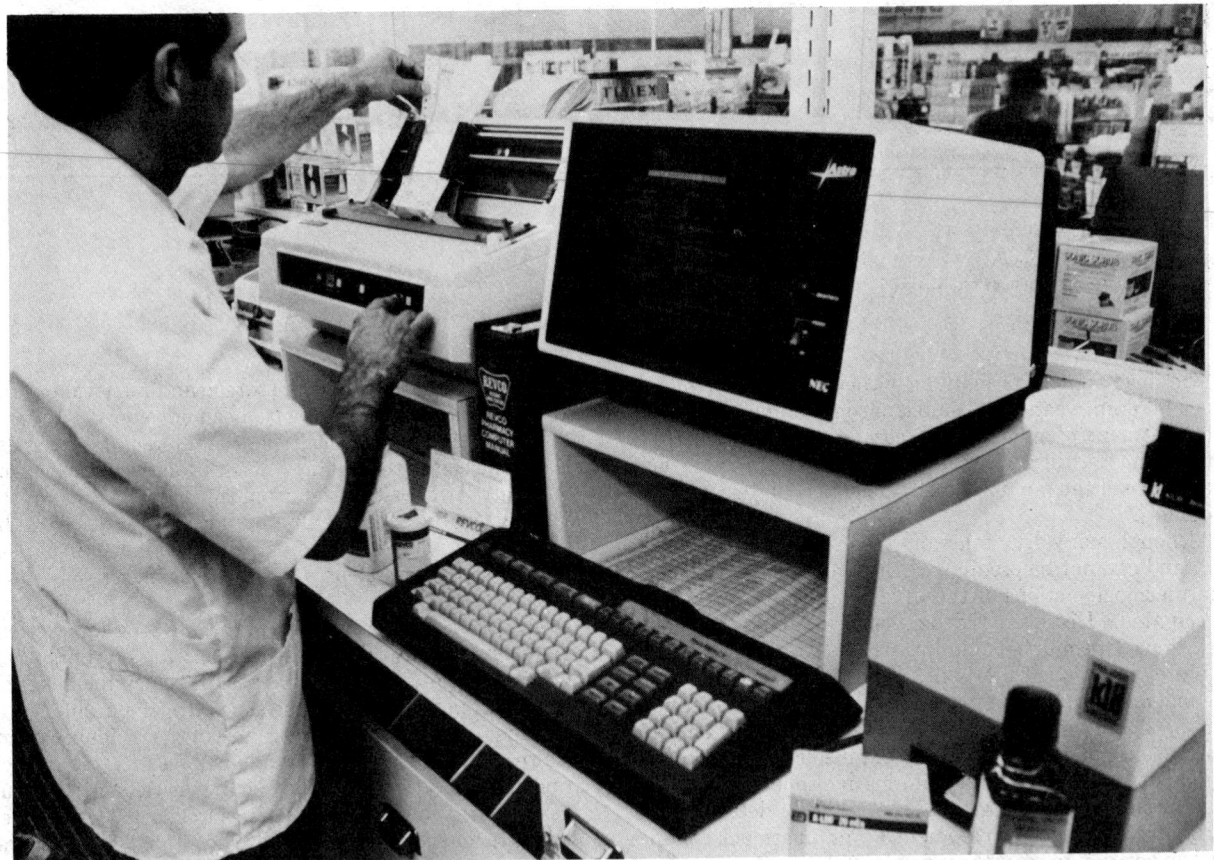

Fig 101-22.   A pharmacist utilizing a prescription computer system in his professional practice (courtesy, General Computer Corporation).

Accounting and Business Management

Business Record Keeping—The computer may be programmed to provide: accounts receivable, payroll, general ledger, accounts payable, third-party claims processing and records, inventory control and ordering, sales analysis functions, and daily summary of business.

Prescription Analysis—The computer provides retrievable information on daily, monthly, yearly prescription totals, new vs refilled prescriptions, medication costs per prescription filled, and profit per prescription filled.

Legal Considerations

All aspects of manufacture, distribution, and possession of drugs are controlled by both state and federal laws. State laws governing the practice of pharmacy are generally administered by state boards of pharmacy comprised of varying numbers of pharmacy practitioners and in some instances by consumer representation. These boards generally regulate the licensing of pharmacy interns, pharmacists, and pharmacies, and enforce rules and regulations pertaining to the legal and ethical practice of pharmacy within the state. State regulations regarding drugs frequently include and extend the federal law. Federal laws are administered by various federal agencies and pertain primarily to products considered to be in interstate commerce.

The laws governing the practice of pharmacy are presented in Chapter 107.

Bibliography

Liguori S: *Patient Package Inserts: An Overview, The Apothecary 89:22*, November/December 1977.

Lauer JE, ed: *Computers for Pharmacy*, APhA, Washington, DC, 1978.

Siecker BR: *Computers for Pharmacy, JApHA NS 20:* 19–47, March 1980.

CHAPTER 102

Drug Interactions

Daniel A Hussar, PhD
Remington Professor of Pharmacy
Philadelphia College of Pharmacy and Science
Philadelphia, PA 19104

The development of many new therapeutically effective drugs in recent years has resulted in considerable progress in the treatment of numerous disease states. However, accompanying the therapeutic benefits derived from use of these agents has been an increased incidence of drug-related problems.

Although many drug-related problems develop unexpectedly and can not be predicted, others are related to known pharmacologic actions of the drugs and can reasonably be anticipated. However, as drug therapy becomes more complex, and as the number of individuals being treated with two or more drugs concurrently increases, the ability to predict the magnitude of a specific action of any given drug diminishes. These circumstances point to a need not only for maintenance of complete and current medication records for patients but also for closer monitoring and supervision of drug therapy so that problems can be prevented, or detected at an early stage in their development. The pharmacist is in a unique position to meet these needs, and opportunities exist for greater involvement in and contribution to provision of drug therapy that is both efficacious and safe.

An increasing number of drug-related problems are caused by drug interactions. As a basis for this discussion a drug interaction may be considered a situation in which the effects of one drug are altered by prior or concurrent administration of another drug (ie, drug-drug interactions). The concept of drug interaction is often extended to include situations in which

1. food or certain dietary items influence the activity of a drug (ie, drug-nutrient interactions) or
2. environmental chemicals or smoking influences the activity of a drug or
3. a drug causes alterations of diagnostic laboratory test results (ie, drug-laboratory test interactions) or
4. a drug causes undesired effects in patients with certain disease states (ie, drug-disease interactions).

Considerable attention has been focused on the subject of drug interaction in recent years and information pertaining to these occurrences has been widely publicized. Several comprehensive references, such as *Drug Interactions* and *Drug Interaction Facts*, deal exclusively with this subject, while other references give extensive attention to it. Computer systems that provide for storage and retrieval of drug interaction information have also been developed.

Problems that may result from drug interactions have also been publicized to the public. In addition to cautions given to patients by physicians and pharmacists, articles on the subject have appeared in many publications widely read by the public. In some of these articles the value of patient medication records kept by the pharmacist has been stressed.

Even with the extensive publicity that drug interactions have received, it is still usually difficult to determine their incidence or clinical significance because often there is little information pertaining to these aspects of the problem. In one of the few comprehensive studies of the incidence of adverse reactions and drug interactions, investigators participating in the Boston Collaborative Drug Surveillance Program have noted that of 83,200 drug exposures in 9900 monitored patients (primarily in acute disease hospitals), 3600 adverse reactions were reported. A total of 234 (6.9%) of the adverse reactions were attributed to a drug interaction. In almost all cases the interaction resulted from cumulative pharmacologic effects, the most common problem being excessive central nervous system depression resulting from administration of two or more CNS depressants. Nine deaths were believed to have resulted from the combined effects of two or more drugs.

Some drug interactions continue to occur even though they are well documented and recognized. Cardiac glycosides (eg, digoxin) and diuretics are often given concurrently, and rationally so, in treating patients with congestive heart failure. It is well known that most diuretics can cause potassium depletion which, if uncorrected, could become excessive and lead to adverse effects of the cardiac glycoside. Yet toxicity continues to occur for this reason.

Numerous studies have demonstrated that many patients receive multiple drug therapy with agents of recognized potential for interaction. As the number of drugs in a patient's therapeutic regimen increases, the greater is the risk of occurrence of a drug interaction. Although there are only limited data regarding many of the potential drug interactions which have been suggested, considerable progress has been made in defining the incidence and level of risk attending the use of a number of combinations of drugs.

Factors Contributing to the Occurrence of Drug Interactions

A number of factors contribute to the occurrence of drug interactions.

Multiple Pharmacologic Effects—Most drugs used in current therapy do not possess only one specific type of activity but have the capacity to influence many physiologic systems. Therefore, there is an increased possibility that two concomitantly administered drugs will affect some of the same systems. When considering the potential for interactions between drugs there is often a tendency only to be concerned with the primary effects of the drugs involved and to overlook the secondary activities they possess. Combined therapy with a phenothiazine antipsychotic [eg, chlorpromazine (*Thorazine*)], a tricyclic antidepressant [eg, amitriptyline (*Elavil*)], and an antiparkinson agent [eg, trihexyphenidyl (*Artane*)] is frequently employed. Each of these agents has a considerably different primary effect; however, all of them possess anticholinergic activity, characterized by such symptoms as dryness of the mouth and blurring of vision. Even though the anticholinergic effect of any one of the drugs may be slight, the additive effects of the three agents may be significant.

As the number of drugs a patient takes increases, it is obvious that the monitoring of the drug therapy as well as the keeping of accurate patient medication records becomes more complex.

Multiple Physicians—It is necessary for some individuals to go to more than one physician and it is not uncommon for a patient to be seeing one or more specialists in addition to a family physician. It is frequently difficult for one physician to learn completely what medications have been prescribed for a patient by another physician and many difficulties could arise from such situations. For example, one physician may prescribe an antihistamine for a patient for whom another physician has prescribed an antianxiety agent, with the possible consequence of an excessive depressant effect.

Even though the patient is seeing different physicians, he will usually have the prescriptions dispensed by the same pharmacy. Therefore, the pharmacist, by maintaining patient medication records, can play an important role in the detection and prevention of drug-related problems.

Concurrent Use of Prescription and Nonprescription Drugs—Many reports of drug interactions have involved the concurrent use of a prescription drug with a nonprescription drug (eg, aspirin, antacids, decongestants). When a physician questions a patient about medications that he is taking, the patient will often neglect to mention the nonprescription medications that he has purchased. Many patients have been taking preparations such as antacids, analgesics, and iron preparations for such long periods or in such a routine manner that they do not consider them to be drugs. This information can easily be missed in casually questioning a patient and some prefer to utilize a list of symptoms that might ordinarily be treated with nonprescription drugs in trying to obtain this information from the patient.

Although many individuals will have their prescriptions filled in their local pharmacy, they often purchase nonprescription drugs in a supermarket or department store, thus making identification of potential problems extremely difficult for the pharmacist as well as the physician. For this reason, patients should be encouraged to obtain both their prescription and nonprescription medications at a pharmacy. Such advice is justified, however, only when the pharmacist personally supervises the sale of nonprescription medications with which problems may develop.

Patient Noncompliance—For a variety of reasons many patients do not take medication according to directions. Some have not received adequate instructions from the physician and pharmacist as to how and when to take their medication. In other situations, particularly involving patients who are taking several medications, confusion about the instructions may develop even though the patient may have understood them initially. It is easy to understand how the geriatric patient who may be taking five or six medications several times a day at different times can become confused or forget to take his medication, although these occurrences are by no means unique to the geriatric population.

Although the situations involving noncompliance would usually result in a patient not taking enough medication, some circumstances could lead to excessive use of certain medications, thereby increasing the possibility of drug interaction. For example, some patients if they realize they have forgotten a dose of medication, double the next dose to make up for it. Some other patients apparently subscribe to a philosophy that if the one-tablet-dose that has been prescribed provides some relief of symptoms, two or three tablets will be even more effective.

Drug Abuse—The tendencies of some individuals to abuse or deliberately misuse drugs may also lead to an increased incidence of drug interactions. One study of 332 young hospitalized psychiatric patients revealed that at least 60% of these patients employed nonprescribed abusable drugs while hospitalized. The use of these drugs was on an occasional basis and did not represent a persistent practice. However, the drugs involved included barbiturates, narcotics, and amphetamines whose use, if not recognized, might cause alterations in the patient's psychiatric state and also problems in interpreting treatment results. An increased potential for drug interaction also exists.

In one study theophylline was cleared from the blood more rapidly in both marihuana and tobacco smokers, with an additive increase in those who smoked both substances. It has been suggested that these agents increase the rate of metabolism of theophylline; similar effects may be seen with other drugs.

Problems have also been reported in drug abusers contemplating surgery. These individuals may swallow or inject their drug prior to going to surgery because of fear of withdrawal during surgery or the recovery period. Serious consequences could result following administration of anesthetics, analgesics, and CNS depressants used prior to, and during, surgery.

Many interactions that occur are undetected or unreported. Koch-Weser (*Drug Inform J*, *6:* 42, 1972) observed that detection of drug interactions by clinicians is inefficient and cited six reasons for existence of this situation. Although initially noted in 1972, the observations are just as valid today.

1. In most cases the clinical situation is too complex to allow recognition of an unexpected event in a patient's course as related to his drug therapy.
2. With few exceptions, the intensity of action of drugs in the therapeutic setting cannot be accurately quantitated.

One reason for the many reports of interactions involving anticoagulants, hypoglycemic agents, and antihypertensive agents is that there are specific parameters such as prothrombin time, blood glucose levels, and blood pressure that can be measured and provide a quantitative indication of drug activity. Therefore, any change in these values that may be caused by introducing another drug into therapy can be measured with relative ease. In contrast, when one considers drugs like the tranquilizers and analgesics with which it is far more difficult to measure degree of activity, it becomes increasingly difficult to observe and measure the effect of other drugs on their activity.

3. Even when a deficient, excessive, or abnormal response to one or both drugs is clearly recognized during concomitant administration, it is usually attributed to factors other than drug interaction.

When an unexpected response to a drug develops, it is usually attributed to something other than a drug interaction, such as patient idiosyncrasy in the case of an excessive response, or tolerance in the case of a deficient response.

4. The index of suspicion of most clinicians concerning drug interactions is quite low and many practicing physicians are hardly aware of the phenomenon.
5. Practicing physicians tend to doubt their observations concerning drug interactions unless the same interaction has been previously reported.

In many situations in which a drug interaction may be occurring there are often other factors that also could contribute to the altered response noted. Therefore, the physician often accepts a reasonable explanation, albeit incomplete, based on information that he is familiar with, rather than suspects a possibility that has not been previously reported. Although many interactions that have been reported via case reports have not been confirmed by other observations or additional study, many single-case reports have served as the stimulus for additional study that has resulted in warnings about potentially dangerous interactions.

6. Physicians frequently fail to report drug interactions even when they have unequivocally recognized them.

Several factors, no doubt, contribute to this situation. The time it would take to write up a case report to submit to a journal is a deterrent to many physicians and pharmacists.

Also, since drug interactions often represent an undesirable experience for the patient, a health professional is often reluctant to expose himself to possible criticism, or even liability, regarding the therapy. Even when therapy may not be the most appropriate, there should be a mechanism whereby health professionals can communicate information that will be useful to others or will help others to avoid the same problems, without fear of criticism or liability.

Using Drug Interaction Information

The extensive publicity that certain drug interactions have received and the large number of case reports, charts, tables, editorials, and studies that have been published would give the impression that there has been considerable progress in identifying and correcting the problems that may develop. Although this may be true in certain circumstances, a careful analysis of the literature reveals that some of the information is conflicting, incomplete, and misleading. Too frequently, the suggested clinical importance of an alleged drug interaction which is based more on theory than on clinical data is greatly overstated and publicized.

The use of some of this information has unfortunately led, in a number of situations, to an undue degree of alarm characterized by some observers as "drug interaction hysteria" or a "drug interaction anxiety syndrome." Caution is needed, therefore, in evaluating and using the information available because by misusing it or by over-reacting to a possible problem, a more difficult situation may result than might have occurred if nothing were done. In some situations patients have been deprived of therapy from which they could benefit as a result of concern about a potential interaction with other medication they are taking. Conversely, some health-care practitioners who have critically evaluated drug interaction literature have found so much of it lacking in clinical relevance that their skepticism regarding the exaggerations and extrapolations precludes adequate attention to those interactions that are clinically important. Recognition of the importance of exercising the appropriate clinical perspective is essential if optimal therapy is to be achieved.

In studying the literature on drug interactions and deciding what action is appropriate, a number of factors should be kept in mind.

Interacting Drugs Can Usually Be Used Together—In most cases, two drugs that are known to interact can be administered concurrently as long as adequate precautions are taken (eg, closer monitoring of therapy, dosage adjustments to compensate for the altered response). Although there are situations where the use of one drug is usually contraindicated while another is being given, such combinations are not likely to be employed frequently and there may be exceptions to the contraindication under certain circumstances. In those situations though where another agent with similar therapeutic properties and a lesser risk of interacting could be used, such a course of action would be preferable.

Serious reactions have been reported to occur following the concurrent use of a monoamine oxidase inhibitor [eg, tranylcypromine (*Parnate*)] with a tricyclic antidepressant (eg, amitriptyline), and the literature for these products warns that use of such combinations is contraindicated. However, it has been indicated by some that such reactions do not occur commonly and that these combinations, when very cautiously used, may be of benefit in some patients when conventional drug therapy has failed. The fact that these combinations may be used beneficially in some patients does not excuse the pharmacist from his responsibility in checking the therapy with the physician. However, he should be aware that certain circumstances may justify the concomitant use of even "contraindicated" drugs.

Beneficial Interactions—It should be recognized that sometimes a second drug is prescribed deliberately to modify the effects of another. Such an approach might be utilized in an effort to enhance the effectiveness or to reduce the adverse effects of the primary agent. In these situations the efficacy and/or safety of a drug is increased indicating that interactions are not always harmful as frequently thought, but can also be beneficial.

The ability of probenecid (*Benemid*) to increase the serum levels and prolong the activity of penicillin derivatives has been known for many years and this interaction can be used to therapeutic advantage. In the treatment of sexually-transmitted diseases, it has been noted that many patients cannot be depended upon to take a 5- to 10-day course of antibiotic therapy when they are not supervised. Therefore, when possible, it is often preferable to give the antibiotic in a large single dose to assure that the patient receives all the drug intended. Several studies have noted improved results when probenecid was given concurrently with ampicillin, amoxicillin, or procaine penicillin G in the treatment of gonorrhea. Current recommendations for the treatment of uncomplicated gonorrhea indicate that procaine penicillin G (4.8 million units intramuscularly divided into at least two doses and injected at different sites at one visit), ampicillin (3.5 g orally), or amoxicillin (3 g orally) are among the preferred treatments. It is also recommended that 1 g of probenecid be given, being administered simultaneously with ampicillin and amoxicillin or just before an injection of procaine penicillin G.

An example of a situation where one drug is given to minimize the undesirable effects of another is seen with the use of an antiparkinson drug with an antipsychotic agent in an effort to reduce the extrapyramidal effects of the latter.

Animal Studies—Some reports of drug interactions are based on animal studies. Although such data may be of value in anticipating potential problems in humans, there is no guarantee that the results seen in animals can be extrapolated to the clinical situation. It is known that a number of drugs are handled differently (eg, metabolism, excretion) and can produce a different type and intensity of effect in animals than they will in man. Thus, one must be aware of the source of the data.

Nature of Reports—Reports and reviews of interactions often attach importance to isolated observations of problems in one patient or a limited number of patients. On several occasions a suspected interaction that was observed in a single patient has been reported in a number of reviews and tables without qualification as to the nature of the report or the possible significance of the interaction. The fact that such an interaction is now included in a number of publications can result in an impression that the problem is well documented and clinically significant.

Depth of Information—Most of the charts and tables of drug interactions do not provide enough information about specific situations. The mere mention of an increased or decreased effect of one drug in the presence of another is not enough to form a judgment as to the clinical importance and potential severity of the situation. Because of this, most references of this type should be used only to initially screen for possible interactions and more comprehensive reference sources should be consulted for further information.

Documentation—One of the shortcomings of many of the charts, tables, and reviews of drug interactions that have appeared is that no reference to the original source of the information is included. This can place the pharmacist at a disadvantage when the physician whom he has contacted requests further information or wishes to know the source of the information that has prompted the pharmacist to contact him.

Although these publications may be helpful in reviewing the subject of drug interaction or in initially identifying a drug interaction, their limitations should be recognized.

Current Literature—It is important to constantly review the current literature since new evidence may change the significance of earlier reports. The existence of conflicting reports will also become evident as the literature is carefully searched.

The chloral hydrate–anticoagulant interaction provides an example. Early reports indicated that chloral hydrate could decrease the activity of anticoagulants such as warfarin, whereas subsequent investigations indicated that just the opposite effect, an increased anticoagulant effect, could result. Still other investigators suggested that an interaction is not likely to occur. Although conclusive answers cannot always be obtained, there should be an awareness of the various results that have been reported. In this particular situation, if an interaction does develop, an increase in the action of the anticoagulant is the most likely result.

Although there is no assurance that more recent information is more accurate or pertinent, the date of publication of a particular reference should be noted and, when appropriate, more current references consulted.

Recommendations and Therapeutic Alternatives—There is not enough information available on many reported interactions to permit the development of specific guidelines to govern such combination therapy. When such guidelines are presented they can be extremely helpful and the increasing number of such statements in the literature for various products serves as evidence that pharmaceutical manufacturers are trying to make such information available when possible. Where possible, the pharmacist should not only identify a potential problem but also be prepared to make a recommendation to the physician and/or patient as to how problems can best be avoided or minimized.

For example, it is known that aspirin may enhance the anticoagulant activity of warfarin (*Coumadin*). Although all patients taking the two drugs concurrently will not experience such a response, it would seem preferable to use acetaminophen (*Tylenol*) in patients on anticoagulant therapy. However, before making a recommendation that a patient on anticoagulant therapy use acetaminophen instead of aspirin, there should be an awareness of the purpose for which the aspirin is to be used. Although acetaminophen is comparable to aspirin with regard to analgesic and antipyretic activity, it does not possess anti-inflammatory activity and could not be used as an alternative to aspirin in most conditions where such an action is needed.

The use of tetracycline by a patient also taking antacids provides an example of a situation where a specific recommendation can be made to avoid difficulty. If taken at the same time, the antacid can decrease the absorption of the tetracycline. However, if the two agents are given at least one hour apart, difficulty should be avoided.

Viewing Interactions in Perspective—Even after the previously discussed factors have been considered and the data have been critically analyzed, the possibility of interactions developing must be viewed in perspective. Although an altered response appears likely, it might not be clinically significant in many patients. In these situations a patient should not be deprived of needed therapy because of the possibility of an interaction, but such therapy should be closely monitored.

In addition to using the primary literature, use of an authoritative and comprehensive reference source such as *Drug Interactions*, by Philip D Hansten, and *Drug Interaction Facts*, published by Facts and Comparisons, is recommended and can be very helpful in identifying potential problems and in making judgments as to their clinical importance and therapeutic alternatives. However, even though certain interactions are well documented, it is often difficult, if not impossible, to predict the severity of an interaction, if indeed it does develop. The many variables, usually of unknown degree, that may influence the activity of a drug and its ability to interact with other agents, contribute to the existing uncertainty. Many of these variables pertain to the drugs being used and include dosage, route of administration, time of administration, sequence of administration, and duration of therapy, whereas other variables, which are considered in the following discussion, pertain to the patient.

Patient Variables

There are many factors that will influence, either favorably or unfavorably, the response to a drug in man. A number of reports have indicated how these factors may predispose a patient to the development of adverse effects to a drug and it can be anticipated that many of these considerations also will apply to the development of drug interactions.

Age—When considering the risk of drug-related problems, age is a particularly important factor. Studies indicate that there is an increased incidence of adverse drug reactions in pediatric and geriatric patients and it is reasonable to expect that the occurrence of drug interactions is also highest in these patient groups.

Drug-related problems in young patients are most frequently encountered in newborn infants. The blood-brain barrier in the newborn, particularly in premature infants, is more permeable to bilirubin than it is in older children and adults. Under certain circumstances excessive amounts of bilirubin in the brain could result, leading to kernicterus. Since bilirubin is bound to albumin-binding sites, administration of a sulfonamide, salicylate or other agent that could displace bilirubin from these binding sites should be avoided since it may precipitate or aggravate this condition.

A number of factors point to an increased risk of interactions in the elderly. Most elderly patients have at least one chronic illness (eg, hypertension, diabetes) and this is reflected in the prescribing of a larger number of medications for this patient group. The types of diseases more frequently experienced by geriatric patients (eg, renal disorders) may contribute to an altered drug response, and there appears to be an increased sensitivity to the action of certain drugs with advancing age. In addition, there may be age-related changes in the absorption, distribution, metabolism, and excretion of certain drugs which increase the possibility of adverse drug reactions and drug interactions. Accordingly, drug therapy in geriatric patients must be monitored especially closely.

Genetic Factors—Genetic factors may be responsible for development of an unexpected drug response in a particular patient. Isoniazid is metabolized by an acetylation process, the rate of which appears to be under genetic control. Some individuals metabolize isoniazid rapidly, whereas others metabolize it slowly, thus necessitating careful dosage adjustment as the dose which provides satisfactory levels in rapid acetylators may cause toxicity in slow acetylators. For example, isoniazid causes peripheral neuritis in a number of patients and this effect has been most frequently noted in slow acetylators.

It has been observed that isoniazid may inhibit the metabolism of phenytoin (*Dilantin*), possibly resulting in development of toxic effects (nystagmus, ataxia, lethargy) of the latter. However, studies have indicated that those patients who developed phenytoin toxicity when also receiving isoniazid were slow acetylators of isoniazid. It is likely that this interaction will be of significance only in patients who metabolize isoniazid at a very slow rate.

Disease States—A number of disease states, other than the one for which a particular drug is being used, may influence patient response to a drug. Impaired renal and hepatic function are the most important conditions that may alter drug activity; however, other disorders may also bring about a change in the activity of a drug. Since many drugs are extensively bound to plasma proteins and only the unbound fraction of the drug is active, a decreased concentration or amount of protein could conceivably change the availability of drugs and, thus, their activity. This possibility must be recognized in patients with conditions that may be associated with hypoalbuminemia.

Renal Function—Renal function is one of the most important determinants of drug activity. The patient's renal status should be known, particularly when drugs that are primarily excreted in an active form by the kidney are to be used for long periods of time. If there is renal impairment and the usual dose of a drug that is excreted by the kidney is given, there can be a prolonged effect since it is not being excreted at the normal rate. As additional doses are given, blood levels will build up, possibly resulting in toxicity. Therefore, a need exists for careful dosage adjustment and particular caution when other potentially interacting drugs are added to the therapeutic regimen.

The alteration of renal excretion as a mechanism by which a number of drug interactions develop is considered later, and the status of the patient's renal function is an obvious determinant of the rate of excretion of the drugs involved and the occurrence of interactions.

Hepatic Function—Many drugs are metabolized in the liver by a number of mechanisms. Therefore, when there is hepatic damage, these drugs may be metabolized at a slower rate and exhibit a prolonged effect. Although each situation should be evaluated to determine whether a reduction in dosage is necessary, it should be recognized that some drugs will be metabolized at the normal rate even though hepatic function is impaired. A number of studies of drug metabolism in patients with liver disease have been conducted; however, the results vary considerably and it is difficult to predict with certainty whether the rate of metabolism will be altered in a given patient.

Many therapeutic agents are metabolized by liver microsomal enzymes. If other drugs alter the amount or activity of these enzymes, a modified response to the drugs that depend on these enzymes for their metabolism might occur. For example, many substances (eg, barbiturates) are known to stimulate the activity of liver microsomal enzymes (enzyme induction). The result would be a more rapid metabolism and excretion of concurrently administered agents that are metabolized by these enzymes. This mechanism of drug interaction is discussed in greater detail later as are the situations in which the action of hepatic enzymes is inhibited.

Alcohol Consumption—Several studies have shown that chronic use of alcoholic beverages may increase the rate of metabolism of drugs such as warfarin, phenytoin, and tolbutamide (*Orinase*), probably by increasing the activity of liver enzymes. However, in contrast, acute use of alcohol by nonalcoholic individuals may cause an inhibition of hepatic enzymes.

Concurrent use of alcoholic beverages with sedatives and other depressant drugs could result in an excessive depressant response. The fact that use of such combinations is commonplace cannot be cause for failing to exercise the caution that must be observed if problems are to be averted.

Smoking—Several investigations have suggested that smoking increases the activity of drug-metabolizing enzymes in the liver with the result that certain therapeutic agents are metabolized more rapidly and their effect is decreased.

The activity of chlordiazepoxide (*Librium*), diazepam (*Valium*), and phenobarbital has been compared in nonsmokers, light smokers (20 cigarettes per day or less) and heavy smokers. With chlordiazepoxide and diazepam it was noted that central nervous system depression, as evidenced by drowsiness, was less common the greater the number of cigarettes smoked. However, an altered response was not seen with phenobarbital. It is suggested that metabolism of benzodiazepines may be increased in smokers. It was also observed that the CNS depression attributed to benzodiazepines was more common in older patients. The frequency of drowsiness was almost twice as high in patients over 70 years of age as it was in patients aged 40 years or less.

Diet—Food may often affect the rate and extent of absorption of drugs from the gastrointestinal tract. For example, many penicillin and tetracycline derivatives should be given preferably one hour before or two hours after meals to achieve optimal absorption.

The type of food may be important with regard to the absorption of concurrently administered drugs. For example, dietary items such as milk and other dairy products that contain calcium may decrease absorption of tetracycline derivatives by forming a complex with them in the gastrointestinal tract that is poorly absorbed.

Some dietary items, such as certain cheeses and alcoholic beverages, have a relatively high content of the pressor amine tyramine. Tyramine is metabolized by monoamine oxidase and normally these enzymes in the intestinal wall and liver protect against the pressor actions of amines in foods. However, if these enzymes were to be inhibited by a monoamine oxidase inhibitor, large quantities of unmetabolized tyramine could accumulate which could lead to the development of a severe hypertensive reaction.

Some individuals may regard vitamin preparations and nutritional supplements as dietary items rather than drugs. However, some of the agents included in these preparations could cause problems in certain circumstances. Pyridoxine, for example, which is present in most multivitamin mixtures, may antagonize the effects of levodopa (*Dopar, Larodopa*).

Certain dietary items contain an appreciable amount of vitamin K. A change in dietary habits that would significantly alter the intake of these materials could cause problems in patients on anticoagulant therapy.

Diet may also influence urinary pH values. One study has compared the excretion of amphetamine in two groups of patients maintained on different diets. One group was placed on a balanced protein diet that provided an acidic urine (average pH of 5.9) whereas the other group was put on a low-protein diet that provided an alkaline urine (average pH of 7.5). Each group was given a dose of amphetamine and those with the acidic urine excreted 23–56% of unchanged amphetamine in the first eight hours and 5–13% in the next eight hours. In comparison, in those with an alkalinized urine, there was a 2–6% excretion in the first eight hours, followed by an 0.5–3% excretion in the next eight hours.

Environmental Factors—There have been suggestions that DDT and related materials can increase the activity of liver enzymes and thereby increase the rate of metabolism of other agents. Although this possibility has not been well confirmed, individuals whose jobs necessitate intensive exposure to these materials should be observed more closely for altered metabolic responses.

Individual Variation—Even after the preceding factors have been considered, wide variations in the response of patients to drugs will be seen that are often difficult to explain. As an example, it has been noted that plasma levels of tricyclic antidepressants vary widely among individuals using the same dosage regimen over the same time period. When recognition is taken of the difficulty in predicting the response to many therapeutic agents when they are given alone, the challenge and limitations in endeavoring to anticipate the response with a multiple-drug regimen become clearly apparent.

Mechanisms of Drug Interaction

The list of reported drug interactions has become too long to try to commit them all to memory. However, an understanding of the mechanisms by which these interactions develop will be valuable in anticipating such situations and dealing with problems that do develop. Although the circumstances surrounding the development of some drug interactions are complex and poorly understood, the mechanisms by which most interactions develop are well documented and relate to the basic processes by which a drug acts and is acted upon in the body.

These mechanisms are often generally categorized as being pharmacokinetic or pharmacodynamic types. *Pharmaco-* *kinetic interactions* are those in which the absorption, distribution, metabolism, or excretion (ADME) of a drug is altered. Included among the *pharmacodynamic interactions* are those in which drugs having similar (or opposing) pharmacological effects are administered concurrently, and situations in which the sensitivity or responsiveness of the tissues to one drug is altered by another. Although the pharmacokinetic interactions often present challenging clinical problems which have been widely publicized, the pharmacodynamic interactions are more frequently encountered. It should also be recognized that several mechanisms may be involved in the development of certain interactions.

Pharmacokinetic Interactions

Alteration of Gastrointestinal Absorption

Interactions that involve a change in the absorption of a drug from the gastrointestinal tract may develop through different mechanisms and be of varying clinical importance. In some situations the absorption of the drug may be reduced and its therapeutic activity compromised. In others, absorption may be delayed but the same amount of drug is eventually absorbed. A delay in drug absorption can be undesirable when a rapid effect is needed to relieve acute symptoms such as pain. The slower absorption rate may also prolong the effects of a drug, which could also present difficulty. For example, if the effects of a hypnotic agent are prolonged, the patient may experience excessive residual sedation or "hangover" in the morning. A slower rate of absorption may preclude achievement of effective plasma and tissue concentrations of drugs that are rapidly metabolized and excreted.

Conversely, a delay in drug absorption may not be clinically significant and this is usually the case when a drug is being used on a continual basis and therapeutic concentrations in the body have already been achieved.

As a general guideline, it is the drugs that are not completely absorbed under "normal" circumstances that are most susceptible to alterations of gastrointestinal absorption.

Alteration of pH

Since many drugs are weak acids or weak bases, the pH of the gastrointestinal contents may influence the extent of absorption. It is recognized that the nonionized form of a drug (the more lipid-soluble form) will be more readily absorbed than the ionized form. Acidic drugs primarily exist in the nonionized form in the upper region of the gastrointestinal tract (having a lower pH). If a drug such as an antacid is ingested which will raise the pH of the gastrointestinal contents, it is possible that the absorption of such acidic drugs can be delayed and/or partially inhibited.

Although changes in absorption might be predicted for many acidic and basic drugs on a theoretical basis, it would appear that clinically important interactions are likely to occur in only a few situations. A number of reviews of drug interaction literature contain lengthy lists of acidic and basic drugs with the implication that administration of an antacid will influence their absorption. However, only a few of these interactions have been documented in humans and factors other than pH seem to be more important determinants of gastrointestinal absorption.

Aspirin—Antacids—The situation seen with aspirin is an interesting one. As a weak acid it might be anticipated that aspirin would be primarily absorbed from the upper region of the gastrointestinal tract and that antacids would decrease its absorption. Since aspirin produces gastrointestinal side effects in many patients, various efforts including concurrent use of an antacid have been employed to minimize these problems. Use of an antacid does apparently improve gastrointestinal tolerance to aspirin, and combination products such as *Bufferin*, *Ascriptin*, and *Alka-Seltzer* have been marketed. Although some studies suggest that absorption of aspirin from buffered products is decreased, other investigations indicate that absorption is not altered or may even be increased. Drugs such as aspirin that are administered orally in solid dosage forms must first dissolve in the gastrointestinal fluids before they can be absorbed. The fact that aspirin dissolves faster in an alkaline medium, even though it is predominantly in the ionized form, is the probable explanation for successful use of aspirin products that also contain antacids.

Ketoconazole—Antacids—An acidic medium is required to achieve adequate dissolution of ketoconazole (*Nizoral*) following oral administration. Therefore, an antacid, anticholinergic agent, or a histamine H_2 receptor antagonist [ie, cimetidine (*Tagamet*), ranitidine (*Zantac*)] should not be given simultaneously; if one or more of these agents is needed, it should be given at least two hours after ketoconazole is administered.

Bisacodyl—Antacids—A change in the pH of the gastrointestinal contents may also cause another type of problem. For example, oral dosage forms of the laxative bisacodyl (*Dulcolax*) are enteric-coated because the drug can be extremely irritating. It has been suggested that this agent should not be given orally within an hour of antacid therapy or milk because an increase in the pH of the gastrointestinal contents may cause disintegration of the enteric coating in the stomach, resulting in release of the drug in this area which could cause irritation and vomiting.

Antacids may also alter the gastrointestinal absorption of drugs through other mechanisms and additional examples are considered in the following discussion.

Complexation and Adsorption

Tetracycline—Metals—The interaction between tetracycline derivatives and certain metal ions is well known. Tetracycline can combine with metal ions such as calcium, magnesium, aluminum, and iron in the gastrointestinal tract to form complexes that are poorly absorbed. Thus, administration of certain dietary items (eg, milk, containing calcium) or drugs (eg, antacids, iron preparations, products containing calcium salts) to patients on tetracycline therapy could cause a significant decrease in the amount of tetracycline absorbed.

It appears that the absorption of doxycycline (*Vibramycin*) and minocycline (*Minocin*) is not markedly influenced by simultaneous ingestion of food or milk and one of these agents may be preferred to tetracycline when gastric irritation occurs or appears likely. It should be recognized, however, that concurrent administration of aluminum hydroxide gel will decrease absorption of these analogs, as is seen with other tetracyclines.

When two drugs are recognized as being capable of interacting there is often a tendency to believe that one of them should be discontinued. In the case of the antacid–tetracycline interaction, problems can be avoided by allowing an appropriate interval of time to separate administration of the two agents. This interval should be as long as possible but a minimum period of one to two hours should elapse between administration of the drugs.

Several authors have called attention to problems that may result if iron salts, such as ferrous sulfate, are given concurrently with tetracyclines. Subsequent investigation has revealed that if iron is given not less than three hours before or two hours after administration of tetracycline, significant interference with absorption does not occur. It has been suggested that a non-enteric coated, non-sustained release dosage form of iron be used in patients also receiving a tetracycline.

The interaction between doxycycline and iron salts calls attention to another factor that must be considered as the results of one study suggest that the interaction cannot be completely avoided by allowing an interval of three hours (or even a longer period) to separate administration of the two drugs. It is noted that a significant amount of doxycycline is transported back to the gastrointestinal tract via the enterohepatic circulation, and the unabsorbed iron still present in the tract prevents reabsorption of the antibiotic.

Cholestyramine and Colestipol—Other interactions involving complexation might be anticipated when the drugs cholestyramine (*Questran*) and colestipol (*Colestid*) are used. These resinous materials, which are not absorbed from the gastrointestinal tract, bind with bile acids and prevent their reabsorption. In addition to binding with bile acids, cholestyramine and colestipol can bind with drugs that are present in the gastrointestinal tract, and reports suggest that these agents may reduce the absorption of thyroid hormone, warfarin, cardiac glycosides, and thiazide diuretics. To minimize the possibility of an interaction, the interval between the administration of cholestyramine or colestipol and another drug should be as long as possible.

It should also be recognized that prolonged administration of cholestyramine can decrease the absorption of fat-soluble vitamins such as vitamin K. This could lead to increased bleeding tendencies in some patients if the vitamin K intake is not increased. When cholestyramine is administered to a patient on warfarin therapy, it is understandably difficult to predict the eventual response since conceivably the absorption of both the anticoagulant and its antagonist, vitamin K, could be reduced.

Reports suggest that cholestyramine and colestipol may be effective in the management of toxic reactions with certain drugs and industrial toxins. They have been used successfully in the treatment of digitoxin and digoxin intoxication, presumably by interrupting their enterohepatic recycling and hastening their elimination. As a result of this same action, cholestyramine has been found to be of value in treating industrial workers who experienced toxicity following exposure to the organo-chlorine pesticide chlordecone (*Kepone*).

Antidiarrheal Mixtures—Antacids—It has been suggested that since antidiarrheal mixtures can adsorb toxic substances responsible for causing diarrhea, they might also be capable of adsorbing certain medications that are administered concurrently, resulting in a decrease in their absorption. Several studies have noted that administration of antidiarrheal preparations can decrease the bioavailability of tetracycline, digoxin, and lincomycin (*Lincocin*).

Absorption of digoxin may be significantly reduced by simultaneous use of kaolin-pectin mixtures or antacids. Although physical adsorption of digoxin to the other agents represents the most probable explanation of the interaction, it is likely that other mechanisms may also be involved. In one study, coadministration of a kaolin-pectin suspension and digoxin delayed absorption of the latter and decreased by 62% the amount absorbed. When the antidiarrheal preparation was given two hours before the digoxin, the absorption rate was not affected although the extent of absorption was reduced by about 20%. When the antidiarrheal was given two hours after the digoxin, neither the rate nor the extent of absorption was altered.

It has been reported that concomitant use of a magnesium trisilicate–aluminum hydroxide type of antacid resulted in a significant lowering of plasma levels of chlorpromazine, and this has been attributed to decreased absorption resulting from adsorption of the phenothiazine into the gel structure of the antacid. The change in pH produced by the antacid is believed not to be involved in this reaction since, theoretically at least, increased pH should favor absorption of chlorpromazine. Administration of the antacid at least one hour before or two hours after the phenothiazine is a likely solution to the problem. Further studies suggest that only certain types of antacids are likely to alter chlorpromazine absorption. The decreased absorption of chlorpromazine was associated with use of a trisilicate-containing antacid that appears to be capable of adsorbing the phenothiazine; hydroxide (eg, aluminum and magnesium hydroxides) and ionic (eg, calcium carbonate) antacids apparently do not exhibit this action.

Penicillamine—Metals—Aluminum and iron salts have been reported to significantly reduce the absorption of penicillamine (*Cuprimine*), probably through chelation and/or adsorption mechanisms. An interval of at least two hours should separate the administration of an antacid or iron salt and penicillamine. Food will also decrease the absorption of penicillamine and the drug should be administered apart from meals.

Alteration of Motility/Rate of Gastric Emptying

Cathartics—A cathartic, by increasing gastrointestinal motility, may increase the rate at which another drug passes through the gastrointestinal tract. This could result in a decreased absorption of drugs, particularly those that are normally slowly absorbed and require prolonged contact with the absorbing surface or those that are absorbed only at a particular site along the gastrointestinal tract. Similar problems might be noted with enteric-coated and sustained-release formulations.

Anticholinergics—Anticholinergics, by decreasing gastrointestinal motility, may also influence drug absorption. The effect may be one of decreased absorption since the reduced peristalsis may retard dissolution and the slowing of gastric emptying may delay absorption from the small intestine, or increased absorption if a drug is retained for a longer period of time in the area from which it is optimally absorbed.

Acetaminophen—Propantheline—Studies have demonstrated that the rate of acetaminophen absorption depends on the rate of gastric emptying. In one study it has been shown that propantheline (Pro-Banthine), by reducing the rate of gastric emptying, causes a significant delay in absorption of acetaminophen even though it does not apparently alter the total amount of the analgesic that is eventually absorbed. This interaction may not be of significance in patients taking acetaminophen over an extended period of time. However, when the analgesic is taken to relieve acute symptoms, the onset of activity could be delayed. More study is needed to determine whether a variation of the time interval between administration of the two drugs will minimize the possibility of interaction.

Metoclopramide—Since metoclopramide (*Reglan*) stimulates motility of the upper gastrointestinal tract, it should be anticipated that it may influence the absorption of other drugs administered concurrently; however, conclusive documentation of such interactions is not yet available. It has been reported that metoclopramide may increase the rate of absorption of acetaminophen, ethanol, levodopa, and tetracycline but significant changes in the activity of these agents do not appear likely. Anticholinergic drugs will antagonize the effects of metoclopramide on gastrointestinal motility.

The combined use of metoclopramide and cimetidine in the treatment of esophageal reflux disease was evaluated in a recent study. The combination was found to offer no therapeutic advantage over cimetidine alone and caused a significantly higher incidence of adverse effects.

Griseofulvin—Phenobarbital—Phenobarbital has been reported to decrease the effect of griseofulvin, an action initially attributed to enzyme induction caused by phenobarbital. Subsequent studies, however, indicate that phenobarbital reduces absorption of griseofulvin from the gastrointestinal tract. One proposed explanation for this effect is that phenobarbital stimulates secretion of bile, which in turn stimulates peristalsis. The resultant increase in motility would decrease transit time in the upper portion of the intestinal tract, from which griseofulvin is absorbed most efficiently.

Antacids—There have been a number of reports of interactions attributed to antacid-induced alteration of absorption. For example, administration of aluminum hydroxide gel has been reported to decrease absorption of isoniazid. Studies suggest that aluminum hydroxide gel will delay gastric emptying time although the mechanisms of adsorption/complexation and elevation of gastric pH cannot be excluded as contributing factors. In what manner and to what extent magnesium and calcium salts which are commonly used in antacids influence gastric emptying has not been adequately studied and it should be anticipated that different antacid preparations may exhibit varying effects relative to the absorption of another drug administered simultaneously. Unless there is a specific reason for administering the two agents simultaneously, a general guideline for concurrent use would be to give the antacid separately from any other agents in the patient's therapeutic regimen, allowing as long an interval as possible—but at least one hour—to elapse between the administration of the two agents.

Food—It is well known that food can influence absorption of a number of drugs. In some cases absorption may be delayed but not reduced, while in others the total amount of drug absorbed may be reduced. The effect of food in influencing drug absorption is often due to its action in slowing gastric emptying. Food may, however, also affect absorption by binding with drugs, by decreasing access of drugs to sites of absorption, or by decreasing the dissolution rate of solid dosage forms.

The presence of food in the gastrointestinal tract will adversely affect absorption of many anti-infective agents. Although there are some exceptions, it generally can be recommended that penicillin derivatives, tetracyclines, rifampin (Rimactane), and lincomycin be given at least one hour before or two hours after meals to achieve maximal absorption. In many hospitals drug administration time schedules may closely correspond to times at which meals are served. It is important that a proper dosage schedule for these antibiotics, and other drugs that should be administered apart from meals, be established.

The absorption of captopril (*Capoten*) has been reduced 30–40% by food and it is recommended that the drug be administered one hour before meals.

Although situations in which food reduces drug absorption are the best recognized, an increasing number of reports have noted that food may enhance absorption of selected drugs. Many of these reports have been based primarily on single-meal, single-dose studies; however, the findings could also be of importance when these agents are used for extended periods. Absorption of hydrochlorothiazide (*HydroDiuril*) and nitrofurantoin (*Furadantin*, *Macrodantin*) has been reported to be enhanced in the presence of food, probably as a result of the delay in gastric emptying.

With few exceptions, little is known about the influence of different types of foods on the absorption of drugs whose action is known to be affected by food. Griseofulvin is more rapidly absorbed when taken with a meal having a high fat content; however, it is not necessary to institute dietary changes when using this drug.

Inhibition of Gastrointestinal Enzymes

Folic Acid—Phenytoin—Folic acid is generally present in dietary sources in the form of poorly absorbed polyglutamates; to be efficiently absorbed it must be converted to the readily absorbed monoglutamate by action of an intestinal conjugase enzyme. Folic acid deficiency anemias have been reported in a number of patients receiving phenytoin and it has been suggested that this effect results, in part, from the ability of the anticonvulsant to inhibit this enzyme. Although this is an attractive explanation, it has not been conclusively documented, and it is possible that other mechanisms are more important in the development of phenytoin-induced folic acid deficiency. The problem arises most often in patients who already have reduced folate stores although it is not limited to these individuals.

In using folic acid to correct the deficiency, some investigators have noted an increased frequency of seizures and it has been suggested that folic acid may increase the rate of metabolism of phenytoin, resulting in a reduction in blood levels of anticonvulsant.

Disagreement still exists as to the relationship between phenytoin and folic acid and many questions remain to be answered concerning the use of these agents in combination.

Vitamins—Oral Contraceptives—Various studies have suggested that use of oral contraceptives may result in deficiencies of folic acid, cyanocobalamin, pyridoxine, and ascorbic acid, and several vitamin-mineral preparations have been specifically promoted as supplements for women taking oral contraceptives. The folic acid deficiencies have received the most attention, and it is suggested that the contraceptive may interfere with deconjugation of polyglutamate forms of folic acid.

Although the evidence is clear that women taking oral contraceptives have a higher folate requirement than other women, clinical and hematologic signs of folic acid deficiency are not common. When such signs are present, other contributory factors such as a low dietary intake of folate, malabsorption, liver disease, and use of other drugs that can cause a folate deficiency should be evaluated. In the absence of these other factors, it is not likely that women eating a well-balanced diet will experience folic acid or other vitamin deficiencies as a result of using oral contraceptives. However, if it is anticipated that the patient will not utilize a balanced diet or if other factors are present that may contribute to a deficiency, use of a vitamin-mineral supplement is advisable.

Malabsorption States

Certain drugs, such as laxatives, colchicine, cholestyramine, and colestipol, have been reported to cause malabsorption problems that result in decreased absorption of vitamins and nutrients from the gastrointestinal tract. It should be recognized that these agents could alter absorption of other drugs that are administered simultaneously and several examples with cholestyramine have already been considered.

Alteration of Distribution

Displacement from Protein Binding Sites

An interaction of this type may occur when two drugs that are capable of binding to proteins are administered concurrently. Although they may bind at different sites on the protein, the binding characteristics of one of the drugs may be altered (noncompetitive displacement). Probably more significant are situations in which two drugs are capable of binding to the same sites on the protein (competitive displacement). Since there are only a limited number of protein binding sites, competition will exist and the drug that has the greater affinity for the binding sites will displace the other from plasma or tissue proteins. It is recognized that the protein-bound fraction of a drug in the body is not pharmacologically active. However, an equilibrium exists between bound and unbound fractions, and as the unbound or "free" form of the drug is metabolized and excreted, bound drug is gradually released to maintain the equilibrium and pharmacologic response.

The binding of acidic drugs to serum albumin represents the type of drug-protein binding which has been most extensively studied. The binding to albumin is readily reversible and the albumin-drug complex essentially serves as a reservoir that releases more drug as the free drug is metabolized and/or excreted. More recently, the importance of the binding of basic drugs [eg, propranolol (*Inderal*), lidocaine (*Xylocaine*)] to α_1-acid glycoprotein (AAG) has been recognized. Even small increases in the reactant protein concentration, such as might be associated with infection and inflammation, can result in significant changes in the concentration of free drug.

The risk of an interaction occurring is greatest with drugs that are highly protein-bound (more than 90%) and that also have a small apparent volume of distribution. Since only a small fraction of the drug would ordinarily be available in the "free" form, the displacement of even a small percentage of the amount that is bound to proteins could produce a considerable increase in activity.

Warfarin—Phenylbutazone—Both phenylbutazone (*Butazolidin*) and warfarin are extensively bound to plasma proteins, in particular to albumin. Phenylbutazone, however, apparently has a greater affinity for the binding sites, resulting in displacement of warfarin and making increased quantities of the "free" drug available. In this situation the activity of the anticoagulant is increased, and risk of hemorrhaging exists. This interaction is highly significant and potentially dangerous and concurrent therapy should be avoided.

The risk of interactions resulting from protein displacement appears to be greatest during the first several days of concurrent therapy. It has been suggested that drugs having the greatest capability of displacing warfarin can increase the anticoagulant response within 24 hours and exhibit maximum potentiation in three to five days. After this period the effect levels off since the drug, as a result of greater amounts being available in the unbound form, is also being more rapidly metabolized and excreted. Therefore, the anticoagulant usually has a shorter half-life when a displacing agent is given concurrently.

In the case of the warfarin–phenylbutazone interaction, it has been noted that the enhancement of anticoagulant activity persisted beyond the time which could be explained by the mechanism of drug displacement alone. Subsequent studies have shown that phenylbutazone also inhibits the metabolism of warfarin resulting in an increased anticoagulant response, which represents a second important mechanism contributing to the occurrence of the interaction and provides the explanation for the continued enhancement of the anticoagulant effect.

It would be expected that oxyphenbutazone (*Tandearil*), a metabolite of phenylbutazone, and its analog sulfinpyrazone (*Anturane*), would show similar effects and various studies have suggested this to be the case.

Warfarin—Chloral Hydrate—The first report of a chloral hydrate–anticoagulant interaction suggested that the former drug could *decrease* the effect of dicumarol. It was presumed that chloral hydrate could act similarly to phenobarbital and stimulate the activity of liver microsomal enzymes involved in the metabolism of anticoagulants. Subsequent investigation indicated that chloral hydrate may *potentiate* the response to warfarin. It is suggested that trichloroacetic acid, a major metabolite of chloral hydrate that is highly bound to protein, can displace warfarin from protein-binding sites, thus increasing anticoagulant response. Several studies designed to assess the risk of an interaction between chloral hydrate and warfarin have found either no evidence of an interaction or a moderate increase in anticoagulant response. Although the risk of a serious interaction may be low, the possibility cannot be excluded, and it would seem preferable to use an alternate hypnotic agent such as a benzodiazepine, which is not likely to interact.

The fact that reports differ on this interaction emphasizes the importance of keeping current in the literature so that all evidence can be considered in evaluating a potential problem. Whereas the most recent studies indicate the likelihood of an increased anticoagulant effect in patients in whom the interaction develops, many early tables and charts of drug interactions indicate that chloral hydrate decreases anticoagulant activity.

The precautions noted for concurrent chloral hydrate-anticoagulant therapy should also be observed when triclofos (*Triclos*)—an analog of chloral hydrate—is administered with an anticoagulant.

Warfarin—*In vitro* reports and several case studies have indicated that ethacrynic acid (*Edecrin*), mefenamic acid (*Ponstel*), nalidixic acid (*NegGram*), miconazole (*Monistat*), and diazoxide (*Hyperstat, Proglycem*) can displace warfarin from albumin. Although these results are not conclusive, caution should be exercised in administering any of these drugs to a patient on anticoagulant therapy.

Methotrexate—Methotrexate is highly bound to plasma

proteins, and it has been suggested that agents such as the salicylates may be capable of displacing it from binding sites. Studies also indicate that salicylates may increase the action of methotrexate by inhibiting its renal excretion. Although data pertaining to this interaction are limited, the potential for toxicity with methotrexate dictates extreme caution in any situation in which it is used.

Bilirubin—Sulfonamides—The presence of excessive amounts of unconjugated bilirubin, particularly in premature infants, may lead to development of kernicterus. Bilirubin is bound to albumin binding sites and a number of drugs have been shown to be capable of *in vitro* displacement of bilirubin from albumin. Although clinical problems of this type have not been noted with most of these agents, it has been reported that sulfisoxazole (*Gantrisin*) can precipitate or aggravate kernicterus, presumably by displacing bilirubin from albumin. It has been suggested that other sulfonamides and possibly salicylates may cause a similar effect.

Reduced Albumin Levels—Since many drugs are extensively bound to plasma proteins, a decreased concentration or amount of protein could theoretically change the availability of drugs, and thus their activity. Although the type and incidence of clinical problems have not been conclusively determined, several reports suggest that the incidence of adverse effects with certain drugs may be higher in patients with conditions associated with hypoalbuminemia (eg, renal, hepatic, and gastrointestinal diseases).

A relationship between prednisone dosage, frequency of side effects, and serum albumin levels has been shown in one study. When the serum albumin concentration is less than 2.5 g/100 mL, the frequency of prednisone side effects is almost doubled, and this is attributed to an increased level of prednisolone, an active metabolite of prednisone.

In another study it was noted that the incidence of adverse reactions to phenytoin was greater in patients with low serum albumin levels. It is suggested that the higher incidence of adverse effects in the hypoalbuminemic patients is probably due to increased circulating levels of unbound phenytoin.

Protein Binding in Disease States—It has been noted in an increasing number of reports that the response to a particular drug was altered in the presence of a certain pathologic state. Most studies have evaluated the action of drugs in the presence of impaired renal function. In one study the binding of phenytoin to plasma proteins was found to be decreased in patients with poor renal function, this being attributed to a qualitative change in the drug-binding proteins rather than to a decrease in serum albumin or total protein concentrations. Since this results in a greater amount of the drug being available in the "free" or active form, it is likely that favorable clinical responses with phenytoin will be noted at relatively low total plasma levels ordinarily considered to be nontoxic. This must be considered when total plasma concentration values of protein-bound drugs are used to establish or monitor dosage regimens.

Stimulation of Metabolism

Many drug interactions have resulted from the ability of one drug to stimulate the metabolism of another, most often by increasing the activity of hepatic enzymes that are involved in the metabolism of numerous therapeutic agents. The increased activity is probably due to enhanced enzyme synthesis, resulting in increased amounts of drug-metabolizing enzymes, an effect frequently referred to as *enzyme induction*. These situations have been well documented and several comprehensive reviews of enzyme induction and its therapeutic implications have been published (see *Bibliography*).

Drug metabolism most commonly involves oxidation, reduction, hydrolysis, or conjugation (eg, with glucuronic acid)

reactions. Quantitatively, the most important enzymes are the hepatic microsomal P-450 mixed-function oxidases. In most situations, drugs are converted to less active, water-soluble metabolites, and enzyme induction will usually result in an increased metabolism and excretion, and a reduced pharmacologic action of the agent being metabolized by hepatic enzymes. Less frequently, a drug may be converted to a metabolite that is more active than the parent compound and there may be an enhanced response. However, the increased effect may be somewhat offset since the drug will be more rapidly excreted and have a shorter duration of action.

The stimulation of hepatic enzyme activity is not only a factor in the development of drug interactions, but may also be responsible for the development of tolerance to certain drugs that are given for prolonged periods. For example, it has been suggested that tolerance may develop to glutethimide (Doriden) as a result of the ability of this agent to stimulate its own metabolism. This type of tolerance should be distinguished from the type that develops to the use of narcotics, the latter apparently being due to decreased tissue sensitivity to the drug and not associated with decreased blood levels.

Warfarin—Phenobarbital—It has been demonstrated by a number of investigators that phenobarbital, by causing enzyme induction, can increase the rate of metabolism of coumarin anticoagulants such as warfarin. The result of this interaction would be a decreased response to the anticoagulant since it is being more rapidly metabolized and excreted, possibly leading to an increased risk of thrombus formation if the interaction is not recognized. To compensate for this loss of effect, the dose of the anticoagulant would have to be increased until the desired activity was obtained. Again, a potentially dangerous situation could arise if the patient was to discontinue taking the phenobarbital and the dose of the anticoagulant was not then appropriately reduced.

Although it is well recognized that barbiturate–anticoagulant interactions can result with the use of usual therapeutic doses of these agents, problems continue to occur. If the dose of warfarin has been increased to compensate for loss of activity, it will probably have to be reduced when phenobarbital is discontinued. Otherwise, the readjusted higher dosage that was necessary when phenobarbital was given concurrently may be excessive when it is withdrawn and possibly result in hemorrhaging. Situations where such a potential exists probably occur commonly.

It is probable that all barbiturates have the ability to cause enzyme induction although it has been suggested that phenobarbital is a more potent inducing agent than analogs having a shorter duration of action. Evidence also indicates that the degree of enzyme induction is related to the dosage of the agent employed. It is difficult to anticipate the rate of onset and the extent of enzyme induction, as well as how rapidly the enzyme activity will return to normal levels when the barbiturate is discontinued. These factors vary with the individual and also depend on the dosage and the duration of treatment with the barbiturate. Several studies indicate that the effect of barbiturates in decreasing anticoagulant activity is evident within two to five days and it is suggested that the administration of a barbiturate for a week or longer is likely to produce this effect in most patients. There have been varying reports as to how rapidly enzyme activity returns to pretreatment levels when the barbiturate is discontinued. However, it is probable that in most situations normal enzyme activity will be restored in two to three weeks.

Although close monitoring of combined barbiturate–anticoagulant therapy will usually prevent problems from developing, it would seem unwise to expose the patient unnecessarily to the risk of an interaction when therapeutic alternatives are available. The benzodiazepines [eg, chlordiazepoxide, flurazepam (*Dalmane*)] are not likely to interact with anticoagulants and one of these agents might be useful as an alternative to a barbiturate. These alternatives apply to the use of a barbiturate as a sedative-hypnotic. Although some benzodiazepines have been used in certain types of convulsive disorders they would not be adequate alternatives to phenobarbital when the latter is used in the treatment of these conditions.

Phenytoin—Phenobarbital—Several studies have suggested that phenobarbital, by stimulating liver microsomal enzymes, may increase the rate of metabolism of phenytoin, resulting in a reduction of the blood levels and activity of the latter. However, there is some evidence that, under certain circumstances, the action of phenytoin may be increased by phenobarbital. Even though the rate of metabolism of phenytoin may be altered, the effect is probably of little clinical significance in most patients since both drugs possess anticonvulsant activity. In the few patients in whom there is difficulty in achieving anticonvulsant control with usual doses of these drugs, the interaction might be suspected to be a factor. For the majority of patients, however, this combination, successfully used for many years, represents rational and effective therapy and there is little need for concern about an alteration in effectiveness as long as appropriate attention has been given to the establishment of the dosage levels for both agents that will provide optimal anticonvulsant action.

Anticonvulsants in Combination—As exemplified by the concurrent use of phenobarbital and phenytoin, the most effective therapy for management of many convulsive disorders involves the use of two anticonvulsant drugs. Frequently, however, these agents are capable of interacting with each other and particular care must be exercised in initial dosage determinations and subsequent monitoring of therapy. Phenobarbital, phenytoin, and carbamazepine (*Tegretol*) are recognized as being enzyme inducers. Although not likely to be used in the same anticonvulsant regimen, one report indicates that carbamazepine reduces the plasma levels of clonazepam (*Clonopin*) by increasing its rate of metabolism. Valproic acid (*Depakene*) may increase serum phenobarbital levels but decrease phenytoin concentrations by mechanisms that have not yet been fully clarified.

Meperidine—Phenytoin—The results of a recent study suggest that phenytoin, by increasing the activity of hepatic enzymes, may increase the rate and extent to which meperidine (*Demerol*) is metabolized to normeperidine, a derivative which possesses only weak analgesic activity. Since the level of analgesia relates to blood concentrations of meperidine, it may be necessary to administer more frequent than usual parenteral doses, and larger and more frequent oral doses of the analgesic, in patients also being treated with phenytoin. Therapy must be monitored especially closely, as the resulting higher concentrations of normeperidine may increase the risk of toxicity, since it is eliminated at a slower rate than meperidine.

Phenytoin may also increase the rate of metabolism and reduce the activity of a number of other agents and there have been reports of such interactions with glucocorticoids, warfarin, carbamazepine, quinidine, disopyramide (*Norpace*), theophylline, and methadone.

Oral Contraceptives—Phenobarbital and other drugs are known to increase the metabolism of steroid hormones, including estrogens and progestogens that are used in oral contraceptive combinations. The high rate of effectiveness of oral contraceptives may suggest that other agents are not likely to significantly reduce their effect. However, there has been increasing concern that agents capable of causing enzyme induction may indeed reduce the effectiveness of oral contraceptives. This possibility takes on increased significance in view of the fact that the dosages of the hormones included in these products have been continually decreased in the in-

terest of minimizing the risk of adverse effects. It is possible that the lower dosages of the hormones used in certain products could be approaching the minimum effective level and that addition of another agent which can reduce their action is sufficient to compromise their effectiveness.

It has been reported that women taking other drugs in addition to an oral contraceptive experience more spotting and breakthrough bleeding. It is suggested that enzyme-inducing agents cause a decrease in hormonal levels which results in withdrawal bleeding and, that when such disturbances occur in women who have not previously experienced such a response with the use of oral contraceptives, the method should be regarded as no longer reliable.

Several investigators have noted a decrease in effectiveness of oral contraceptives when rifampin was administered concurrently. Rifampin is a potent inducer of hepatic enzymes and it is apparently through this mechanism that the altered effect developed. An alternative method of contraception should be employed when it is necessary to use rifampin.

Rifampin has also been reported to decrease the activity of warfarin, theophylline, prednisolone, digitoxin, methadone, quinidine, and the sulfonylurea hypoglycemic agents and appropriate dosage adjustments should be made.

Glucocorticoids—One study of patients with bronchial asthma noted increased bronchospasm and pulmonary function deterioration when phenobarbital therapy (120 mg daily in four divided doses) was initiated in three prednisone-dependent patients. Withdrawal of phenobarbital reversed these changes. Further investigation revealed that phenobarbital causes a significant decrease in the half-life of dexamethasone (*Decadron*). It is likely that the ability of phenobarbital to increase the rate of metabolism of these steroids is responsible for these effects.

Other studies have shown phenytoin to increase the rate of metabolism of prednisolone and dexamethasone, and similar caution should be exercised when phenytoin or other agents capable of causing enzyme induction are given concurrently with steroid hormones.

Vitamin D—Phenytoin and Phenobarbital—The chemical similarity of vitamin D and the steroid hormones makes it reasonable to believe that the metabolism of this vitamin may also be influenced by the same agents that are known to affect steroid metabolism. A number of studies have associated disturbances of calcium metabolism and development of rickets and osteomalacia with use of anticonvulsants such as phenobarbital and phenytoin. Reduced serum-calcium levels have been noted in a number of patients on long-term anticonvulsant therapy, evidence indicating that this is the result of vitamin D deficiency. Although other factors may also be involved, most reports indicate that anticonvulsants, by causing enzyme induction, increase the rate of metabolism of vitamin D, thereby causing the deficiency. Some evidence suggests that the anticonvulsants may also exhibit a direct effect on mineral and bone metabolism which is independent of their effects on vitamin D.

The possibility of deficiency developing is greater in individuals whose dietary intake of this vitamin is low or borderline. The incidence and severity of the clinical problems are increased with use of multiple-drug regimens and appear to be directly proportional to the total daily dose of anticonvulsant drugs. Limited exposure to sunlight has also been identified as a contributing factor and the risk of difficulty has been noted to be greater in black patients.

Doxycycline—It has been reported that phenobarbital, phenytoin, and carbamazepine can decrease the half-life of doxycycline by increasing the rate at which it is metabolized by hepatic enzymes. To date, studies have not been carried out to determine whether similar interactions occur with other tetracycline derivatives. Although interactions involving doxycycline may be more likely because of its pharmacokinetic properties, the possibility of an interaction involving any of the tetracyclines cannot be excluded.

Propranolol—It has been reported that there is a higher plasma clearance of propranolol in patients receiving phenobarbital, phenytoin, or rifampin, presumably as a result of the ability of the latter agents to cause enzyme induction. Although the data are insufficient to reach a conclusion regarding the clinical importance of this interaction, it may be necessary to increase the dosage of propranolol when administered concurrently.

Environmental Chemicals—Several studies have indicated that phenobarbital and phenytoin can decrease levels of DDT and its metabolites in individuals exposed to this agent and enzyme induction is suggested as the mechanism by which these agents reduce the storage of DDT. Other investigations have also shown that environmental chemicals such as DDT, chlorinated organic pesticides, and polycyclic hydrocarbons can increase the activity of hepatic microsomal enzymes. As a result, individuals exposed to these chemicals may experience a decreased response to therapeutic agents which are metabolized by these enzymes. In one report a decreased response to warfarin is noted following occupational insecticide exposure.

Smoking—A number of studies have indicated that the effects of certain drugs may be decreased in individuals who are heavy smokers, presumably due to increased hepatic enzyme activity resulting from the action of polycyclic hydrocarbons, such as 3,4-benzpyrene, which are present in cigarette smoke. Among the drugs whose metabolism is increased and therapeutic activity likely to be reduced are chlorpromazine, chlordiazepoxide, diazepam, propoxyphene (*Darvon*), theophylline, pentazocine (*Talwin*), and tricyclic antidepressants. Smoking may also reduce serum propranolol levels although it has been observed that this response is more likely in younger patients. In addition to carefully monitoring therapy with drugs that are metabolized by hepatic enzyme systems in patients who are moderate or heavy smokers, attention has also been called to the need to ascertain the level of smoking when drugs are initially evaluated in clinical trials.

In the examples noted, the effect of smoking is to increase the rate of metabolism of other agents being utilized, and a decreased response to these agents can be anticipated. In contrast, a significant risk of toxicity exists when oral contraceptives are used by women who smoke as it has been noted that smoking markedly increases the risk of serious cardiovascular effects (eg, myocardial infarction), especially in women over 35 years of age.

Some of the polycyclic hydrocarbons in cigarette smoke are also found in certain foods such as charcoal broiled beef. It has been reported that the rate of metabolism of theophylline is increased in individuals consuming large amounts of charcoal-broiled beef and this has been attributed to the enzyme induction effect of the polycyclic hydrocarbons introduced in this cooking process.

Alcohol—Certain agents, such as alcohol, can either stimulate or inhibit the activity of hepatic enzymes, depending on the circumstances of use. Decreased sensitivity to sedative drugs, as well as to the effects of alcohol, has been observed in chronic alcoholics. In one investigation an increased rate of metabolism of tolbutamide, warfarin, and phenytoin was found in alcoholic patients and this was attributed to increased liver enzyme activity caused by chronic administration of alcohol.

In contrast, acute use of alcohol by nonalcoholic individuals may cause inhibition of hepatic enzymes. This may decrease the rate of metabolism, and thereby increase the effect of other agents administered concurrently, and may be responsible, at least in part, for the enhanced sedation experienced when alcoholic beverages and sedative drugs are taken together by individuals who are not alcoholics. The extent to which the mechanism of enzyme inhibition and central nervous system summation or synergism are involved in this interaction remains to be clarified.

Acetaminophen—Although acetaminophen is well tolerated when used as indicated, acute hepatic necrosis can be a complication of overdosage. Animal studies have suggested that enzyme induction may be a factor in the development of hepatic toxicity following overdosage since metabolites of acetaminophen can be bound to liver-cell proteins. A retrospective analysis in patients taking overdoses of acetaminophen provides further evidence in this direction since patients taking drugs known to cause enzyme induction during the three weeks prior to taking the overdosage of acetaminophen developed significantly more severe hepatic necrosis than "non-induced" patients.

Enzyme inducing agents may increase the formation of hepatotoxic reactive metabolites of acetaminophen. It has been observed that chronic alcohol abuse may increase the risk of hepatotoxicity with acetaminophen, presumably by enhancing the oxidative metabolism of acetaminophen to toxic metabolites.

Levodopa—Pyridoxine—Pyridoxine has been shown to antagonize the action of levodopa, presumably by accelerating its decarboxylation to dopamine in the peripheral tissues. Consequently, less levodopa reaches and crosses the blood-brain barrier, with the result that less dopamine is formed in the brain and the therapeutic effect is diminished. The labeling for levodopa formulations notes that pyridoxine, in doses of 10 to 25 mg, rapidly reverses the effect of the antiparkinson drug and it would seem advisable for patients on levodopa therapy to avoid using preparations containing pyridoxine in quantities greater than the recommended daily dietary allowance of 2 mg per day.

The combination product, *Sinemet*, contains both levodopa and carbidopa, the latter agent acting as an inhibitor of decarboxylase enzymes. When administered with levodopa, carbidopa permits the use of significantly lower doses of the former since it is now metabolized to a lesser extent in the peripheral tissues. The decrease in dosage is often accompanied by a decreased incidence of adverse effects. Since carbidopa does not cross the blood-brain barrier, it will not hinder the conversion of levodopa to dopamine in the brain.

The use of carbidopa with levodopa intially raised questions because of the awareness that agents which are similar chemically to carbidopa can induce pyridoxine deficiency. Therefore, it was anticipated that if such a deficiency did develop, the need to give pyridoxine to overcome the deficiency would result in an antagonism of the effects of levodopa. However, in studies of patients receiving levodopa and carbidopa, the addition of pyridoxine did not result in a reappearance of parkinsonian symptoms; indeed, in some investigations there appeared to be an enhancement of the effect of levodopa.

The apparent explanation for this paradoxical effect of pyridoxine is that carbidopa, which does not enter the brain, blocks the action of pyridoxine in the peripheral tissues, thereby inhibiting the action of decarboxylase enzymes. This permits passage of greater amounts of levodopa to the brain. The pyridoxine that is not blocked enters the brain and activates the decarboxylase enzymes, thereby facilitating the conversion of levodopa to dopamine.

Inhibition of Metabolism

Although interactions involving stimulation of metabolism have received more attention, a number of situations have been reported in which one drug has inhibited the metabolism of a second agent, usually resulting in a prolonged and intensified activity of the latter.

Alcohol—Disulfiram—A well-known example of inhibition of metabolism that has been used to advantage is the use of disulfiram (Antabuse) in the treatment of alcoholism. Evidence indicates that disulfiram inhibits the activity of aldehyde dehydrogenase, thus inhibiting oxidation of acetaldehyde, an oxidation product of alcohol. This results in accumulation of excessive quantities of acetaldehyde and development of the unpleasant effects characteristic of the disulfiram reaction.

Further study has shown that disulfiram is not a selective inhibitor of aldehyde dehydrogenase but exhibits several inhibitory actions that can result in the development of drug interactions. It has been reported that it can enhance the activity of warfarin and phenytoin, presumably by inhibiting their metabolism. In one report it is noted that disulfiram decreases the metabolism of chlordiazepoxide and diazepam, and also their active metabolites. In contrast, the disposition of oxazepam (*Serax*), which has no important metabolites, is minimally affected and dosing adjustments will usually be unnecessary when this benzodiazepine is used in patients receiving disulfiram.

Alcohol—Metronidazole—Some patients being treated with metronidazole (*Flagyl*) have developed a disulfiram-like reaction following the consumption of alcoholic beverages. The mechanism has not yet been identified and not all patients using these agents in combination experience this response. The use of alcoholic beverages is best avoided by patients taking metronidazole.

Alcohol—Cephalosporins—Disulfiram-like reactions have been observed in patients receiving cefamandole (*Mandol*), cefoperazone (*Cefobid*), and moxalactam (*Moxam*), following the consumption of alcoholic beverages. The interaction is likely to occur only when the alcohol ingestion follows the administration of the antibiotic and the reaction may be observed as late as 72 hours after the last dose of antibiotic.

The three cephalosporins implicated in these interactions contain a methylthiotetrazole substituent and this structural characteristic is considered to be responsible for these interactions.

Mercaptopurine and Azathioprine—Allopurinol—Allopurinol (*Zyloprim*), by inhibiting the enzyme xanthine oxidase, reduces production of uric acid and has proven to be very useful in treating gout. It is important to recognize, however, that xanthine oxidase is involved also in the metabolism of such potentially toxic drugs as mercaptopurine (*Purinethol*) and azathioprine (*Imuran*) and when this enzyme is inhibited the effect of the latter agents can be markedly increased. When allopurinol is given in doses of 300–600 mg/day concurrently with either of these drugs, it is advised that the dose of mercaptopurine or azathioprine be reduced to about ⅓ to ¼ the usual dose.

In a recent report it is noted that although allopurinol pretreatment results in a significant increase in the peak plasma concentration of orally administered mercaptopurine, allopurinol did not affect the concentration of mercaptopurine when the latter agent was administered intravenously (a parenteral dosage form of mercaptopurine is not marketed in the US). This difference in response is attributed to the extensive first-pass metabolism of mercaptopurine following oral administration, and the action of allopurinol to inhibit the action of liver and intestinal xanthine oxidase, thereby substantially reducing the initial metabolism of mercaptopurine.

It is interesting that the metabolism of thioguanine, which is closely related both chemically and pharmacologically to mercaptopurine and azathioprine, apparently is not influenced by allopurinol and thus might be used as an alternative to mercaptopurine in treating leukemia when it is desired to avoid interactions with allopurinol. Although it may

seem more logical to avoid using allopurinol, use of this agent is often necessary to prevent severe hyperuricemia and subsequent complications in patients with leukemia when rapid destruction of cells by antineoplastic agents or radiation has caused a marked rise in uric acid production.

Phenytoin—Isoniazid—Isoniazid is metabolized by an acetylation process, the rate of which is under genetic control. It has been noted that isoniazid may inhibit the metabolism of phenytoin, possibly resulting in development of toxic effects of the latter. Studies have shown, however, that patients who developed phenytoin toxicity when also receiving isoniazid were slow inactivators of isoniazid. Even within this group it is likely that this interaction will be of significance only in the slowest inactivators.

Benzodiazepines—Cimetidine—The inhibition of oxidative metabolic pathways by cimetidine has been demonstrated in a number of investigations, and it should be anticipated that the action of concurrently administered drugs which are metabolized via these pathways will be increased. Cimetidine has been reported to inhibit the metabolism of chlordiazepoxide, diazepam, and desmethyldiazepam, an active metabolite of diazepam; it is also likely to interact in a similar manner with alprazolam (*Xanax*), clorazepate (*Tranxene*), flurazepam (*Dalmane*), halazepam (*Paxipam*), prazepam (*Centrax*), and triazolam (*Halcion*). The sedative effect of the benzodiazepine is likely to be enhanced as a result of the interaction and particular caution is necessary in elderly patients who often exhibit an increased sensitivity to the depressant effects of the benzodiazepines, even when one of these agents is given alone. One group of investigators has speculated that some of the adverse effects (eg, mental confusion) which have been attributed to cimetidine, may be due in part not only to the central effects of cimetidine, but also to the inhibition of metabolism of other drugs which are administered concomitantly. The metabolism of lorazepam (*Ativan*), oxazepam (*Serax*), and temazepam (*Restoril*) is not likely to be affected, since cimetidine does not alter the glucuronide conjugation of these agents and one of these agents may be preferred when a benzodiazepine is indicated in a patient being treated with cimetidine. The recent introduction of ranitidine provides another alternative to minimize the risk of an interaction. Unlike cimetidine, ranitidine does not significantly inhibit oxidative enzyme systems and interaction with any of the benzodiazepines is unlikely.

Cimetidine—Since cimetidine is known to inhibit hepatic oxidative enzyme systems, it should be anticipated that the action of other agents which are extensively metabolized via this pathway will be increased. There have been reports of such interactions with carbamazepine, phenytoin, theophylline, quinidine, warfarin, metronidazole, and the tricyclic antidepressants [eg, imipramine (*Tofranil*)] and it will often be necessary to reduce the dosage of these agents when cimetidine is included in the therapeutic regimen. Although ranitidine also binds to a limited extent to the cytochrome P-450 enzyme complex involved in the metabolism of these agents, it does so in a different manner and has a much lower affinity for the enzyme complex than cimetidine. Consequently, clinically significant interactions are not likely to occur with ranitidine via this mechanism.

Propranolol—Cimetidine—In addition to inhibiting oxidative pathways, cimetidine also reduces hepatic blood flow and the combination of these factors has been reported to reduce the clearance of propranolol. Pulse rates at rest were noted to be markedly lower when the two agents were given concurrently than when propranolol was administered alone. It is probable that cimetidine interacts with metoprolol (*Lopressor*) in a similar manner; however, interactions are unlikely with the beta-adrenergic blocking agents which are largely excreted unchanged in the urine [eg, atenolol (*Te-*

normin), nadolol (*Corgard*), pindolol (*Visken*), and timolol (*Blocadren*)].

It has been estimated that ranitidine reduces hepatic blood flow by about 20%; however, interactions have not been reported in patients receiving propranolol concurrently and this has raised a question whether the reduction of hepatic blood flow is sufficient to cause clinically important interactions. Ranitidine has, however, been reported to increase plasma levels of metoprolol and concurrent therapy with either metoprolol or propranolol should be closely monitored.

The reduction of hepatic blood flow by cimetidine has important implications when other agents having a high hepatic extraction ratio (eg, lidocaine, morphine) are administered concurrently, since the metabolism of these agents is highly dependent on hepatic blood flow. Although there have only been several reports of interactions, it should be anticipated that cimetidine might potentiate the antiarrhythmic effects or toxicity of lidocaine, and the analgesic and respiratory depressant actions of morphine and certain other analgesics.

Propranolol—Food—Observations of an enhanced bioavailability of propranolol and metoprolol in the presence of food, present interesting implications. Both drugs are subject to considerable first-pass metabolism in the liver after oral administration and it is suggested that the transient increase in hepatic blood flow associated with the ingestion of food may reduce hepatic extraction of the drugs and first-pass metabolism, resulting in increased bioavailability. The increase in bioavailability appears to be related to the protein content of the meal and a minimum amount of protein must be present in the meal to induce an effect. In contrast to propranolol and metoprolol, the other beta-adrenergic blocking agents are not significantly metabolized and it is unlikely that the bioavailability of these agents would be appreciably altered by food.

Propranolol—Hydralazine—Hydralazine (*Apresoline*) exhibits a vasodilating effect which may influence hepatic blood flow, and it is often given concurrently with propranolol in the management of hypertension. Several studies have suggested that hydralazine may increase the availability of propranolol by reducing first-pass hepatic clearance. Further study is necessary to clarify the interrelationships of these agents as well as the effect of the simultaneous administration of food on their activity. In the meantime, it is recommended that these agents be administered in a standardized relation to each other, as well as to meals, so as to minimize effect variations within a patient.

Theophylline—Erythromycin—Erythromycin has been reported to increase significantly serum theophylline concentrations by inhibiting its hepatic metabolism. Patients receiving high doses of theophylline or who are otherwise predisposed to theophylline toxicity, should be closely monitored when erythromycin is administered concurrently.

Carbamazepine—Erythromycin—The hepatic metabolism of carbamazepine may be inhibited by erythromycin and the less commonly used macrolide antibiotic, troleandomycin (*TAO*). The metabolism of both carbamazepine and erythromycin involves cytochrome P-450 and erythromycin appears to interfere with carbamazepine metabolism, thereby increasing its effect and the risk of toxicity.

Carbamazepine—Propoxyphene—Increases in serum carbamazepine levels have been reported in patients also receiving propoxyphene, and it is suggested that the hepatic metabolism of carbamazepine is inhibited. It has generally been felt that propoxyphene is not likely to influence the action of agents such as warfarin, which are metabolized in the liver. However, in the light of the findings of the study with carbamazepine, as well as several other reports, propoxyphene should be viewed as possessing a potential to inhibit the metabolism of certain other drugs, and further studies should be conducted to determine the significance of this possibility.

Carbamazepine—Isoniazid—The development of adverse effects with carbamazepine has been associated with the concurrent use of isoniazid and it has been suggested that the latter agent may inhibit the hepatic metabolism of carbamazepine. It has also been noted that the ability of carbamazepine to cause enzyme induction may increase the formation of a metabolite of isoniazid which is hepatotoxic; thus, concurrent therapy may increase the risk of toxicity with both agents.

Benzodiazepines—Oral Contraceptives—The oral contraceptives have been reported to inhibit the metabolism of drugs such as diazepam which are oxidatively metabolized and the effects of the latter agents may be increased. A similar response is not likely with the benzodiazepines such as lorazepam which are primarily metabolized via glucuronidation. In one report, the clearance of lorazepam was not significantly affected by the use of oral contraceptives whereas in another report the contraceptive appeared to enhance the rate of elimination of lorazepam.

Chloramphenicol—Reports indicate that chloramphenicol (*Chloromycetin*) can inhibit the metabolism of tolbutamide, chlorpropamide (*Diabinese*), phenytoin, phenobarbital, and dicumarol in man. One case of hypoglycemic coma is attributed to combined use of chloramphenicol and tolbutamide, and other studies describe the development of chloramphenicol-induced phenytoin toxicity.

Tolbutamide—Dicumarol—A significant increase in the half-life of tolbutamide in patients taking dicumarol has been reported, and it is suggested that dicumarol inhibits conversion of tolbutamide to carboxytolbutamide (an inactive metabolite) in the liver. The effect of phenindione (*Hedulin*) was also investigated but this agent was shown not to have a similar effect on the metabolism of tolbutamide.

Monoamine Oxidase Inhibitors—There have been many reports of drug interactions involving use of a monoamine oxidase inhibitor with another drug or with certain dietary items. It is likely that MAO inhibitors enhance the effect of drugs like the barbiturates and narcotics by inhibiting hepatic enzyme systems involved in their metabolism. However, other mechanisms are involved in some of the more publicized problems with these compounds and will be considered later.

Theophylline—Influenza Virus Vaccine—There have been several reports of theophylline toxicity following use of influenza virus vaccine, presumably as a result of an inhibition of the hepatic metabolism of theophylline. Although this interaction may be clinically important, it probably will not occur in most patients and the potential problem should not limit the use of the vaccine in patients who are appropriate candidates for its use.

Alteration of Excretion

Alteration of Urinary pH

Alteration of urinary pH, either done intentionally or occurring unknowingly, can influence the activity of certain drugs. For example, acidifying agents are administered with methenamine to enhance its antibacterial activity. Methenamine must be converted to formaldehyde, which is the active antibacterial substance, and for this conversion to take place so that an adequate concentration of formaldehyde is achieved, the urinary pH should be 5.5 or less. Even when methenamine is combined with acidifying agents such as mandelic acid (*Mandelamine*) and hippuric acid (*Hiprex*) or other acidifying agents such as ascorbic acid, it is often difficult to decrease the urinary pH sufficiently when urea-splitting strains of organisms such as *Pseudomonas* and *Proteus* are responsible for the infection.

It should be noted that the most important clinical implications of altering urinary pH involve the use of drugs that are excreted in unchanged form or in the form of an active metabolite. Thus, substances with therapeutic activity are either being reabsorbed or excreted to a greater extent when the urinary pH is changed. In contrast, when only inactive metabolites are being excreted, changes in therapeutic activity are less likely to be associated with changes in urinary pH.

Salicylates—Acidifying and Alkalinizing Agents—Urinary pH will influence ionization of weak acids and weak bases and thus affect the extent to which these agents are reabsorbed and excreted. When a drug is in its nonionized form it will more readily diffuse from urine back into blood. Therefore, for an acidic drug, there will be a larger proportion of drug in the nonionized form in an acid urine than in an alkaline urine—where it will exist primarily as an ionized salt. The result is that from an acid urine more of an acidic drug will diffuse back into the blood and produce a prolonged, and perhaps intensified, activity. In one study it was noted that a salicylate dosage regimen that provided a serum concentration of 20–30 mg% in a patient when the urinary pH was approximately 6.5, produced serum concentrations that were approximately twice as high when the urinary pH was decreased to 5.5. As this could result in salicylate toxicity it is advisable that patients using large doses of salicylates for conditions such as arthritis should monitor urinary pH, with serum concentrations being determined at appropriate intervals.

The ability of "systemic" antacids such as sodium bicarbonate to increase urinary pH is well known. Not as well recognized, however, are the circumstances in which "nonsystemic" antacids may increase urinary pH. In one study, an aluminum and magnesium hydroxide antacid (*Maalox*) was administered concomitantly with aspirin to three children with rheumatic fever. In each case the urinary pH was increased, and serum salicylate concentrations decreased by 30 to 70%. The effect of an antacid on urinary pH depends on the kind of antacid, the dose, and the pH before antacid administration. In patients on salicylate therapy (especially when the maximum recommended dosage level is approached), the initiation or discontinuation of antacid administration, or switching of antacid products, is cause to monitor serum salicylate concentrations and patient response.

Amphetamines—Alkalinizing Agents—Converse effects will be seen for a basic drug like dextroamphetamine (*Dexedrine*). In one investigation the excretion of a dose of dextroamphetamine at urinary pH values of approximately 5 and 8 was studied. When the urinary pH was maintained at approximately 5, 54.5% of the dose of dextroamphetamine was excreted within 16 hours, as compared to a 2.9% excretion in the same period when the urinary pH was maintained at approximately 8.

Similar observations have been made with other basic drugs. One report calls attention to the possible development of quinidine toxicity when urine becomes alkaline, since excretion of quinidine was shown to decrease considerably as urinary pH was raised. In another investigation, when the urinary pH was increased to about 8 with sodium bicarbonate, the plasma half-life of pseudoephedrine (*Sudafed*) was approximately double that in normal subjects. When urinary pH in the same subjects was decreased to 5.2, using ammonium chloride, the plasma half-life decreased markedly from control values.

Interference with Urinary Excretion

Penicillins—Probenecid—It is well recognized that probenecid can increase serum levels and prolong activity of penicillin derivatives by blocking their tubular secretion, and this interaction has been used to therapeutic advantage. Often there will be a twofold to fourfold elevation of serum penicillin levels, although the degree to which these levels is increased and the duration activity is prolonged depend on a number of factors.

Probenecid has also been reported to decrease renal excretion of other agents, including methotrexate, and clofibrate (*Atromid-S*).

Acetohexamide—Phenylbutazone—Potentiation of acetohexamide (*Dymelor*) hypoglycemia by phenylbutazone has been described and it is suggested that phenylbutazone produces this response, in part, by interfering with the renal excretion of hydroxyhexamide, the active metabolite of acetohexamide.

Digoxin—Quinidine—A number of reports have noted significantly greater serum digoxin levels when quinidine was administered concurrently than when digoxin was given alone. A primary cause of the quinidine-induced increase in serum digoxin levels appears to be a reduction in the renal clearance of digoxin; however, other mechanisms are probably also involved. It has been suggested that quinidine may also reduce the nonrenal clearance of digoxin and reduce the volume of distribution by displacing digoxin from tissue binding sites.

In one study, a rise in the serum digoxin levels was observed within two to three days following the addition of quinidine to the regimen. A new plateau was reached in approximately five days and, when quinidine was discontinued, an average of five days passed before the serum digoxin concentrations returned to the prequinidine levels. These findings are of particular importance with respect to the high incidence of adverse effects associated with the cardiac glycosides and a reduction in the maintenance dose of digoxin will often be necessary when quinidine therapy is initiated.

It is surprising that an interaction involving agents which have been so frequently used together for such a long period of time would not have been recognized earlier. The fact that adverse effects often occur with each drug when given individually has sufficed as an explanation for problems that have developed during concurrent use. However, the opportunity acquired relatively recently to monitor serum digoxin levels on a routine basis has resulted in the recognition of the changes in these levels and activity which can be induced by other agents in the therapeutic regimen.

In some patients, it may be advantageous to use therapeutic alternatives to quinidine or digoxin for the purpose of reducing the risk of an interaction. Procainamide (*Pronestyl*) and disopyramide (*Norpace*) do not appear to influence serum digoxin concentrations, and one of these agents might be used instead of quinidine in selected patients. A recent study of the effect of quinidine on the action of digitoxin showed that the serum digitoxin concentrations were elevated. Although the mechanism(s) responsible for this interaction may be different, the clinical implications are similar to those for the digoxin-quinidine interaction, and digitoxin would probably not be a safer alternative to digoxin.

Digoxin—Calcium Channel Blockers—Verapamil (*Calan, Isoptin*) has been reported to increase serum digoxin levels by 50% to 70% during the first week in which the agents are administered concurrently and it will usually be necessary to reduce the dose of the cardiac glycoside. It has been suggested that verapamil may inhibit both the renal and nonrenal elimination of digoxin, resulting in the increase in the serum levels of the latter.

Nifedipine (*Procardia*) may act through similar mechanisms to increase digoxin levels. Although the interaction involving nifedipine is not as pronounced or as well documented as the digoxin-verapamil interaction, it should be anticipated that it will probably be necessary to reduce the dosage of digoxin when nifedipine is administered concomitantly.

Lithium—Antiinflammatory Agents—The serum levels and incidence of adverse effects of lithium salts have been reported to be increased by the concurrent administration of selected antiinflammatory agents such as indomethacin (*Indocin*) and piroxicam (*Feldene*). It is suggested that the renal clearance of lithium is reduced as a result of the action of these antiinflammatory agents to inhibit prostaglandin synthesis.

This interaction should probably be anticipated when any antiinflammatory agent is administered concurrently with a lithium salt. However, it has been noted that aspirin and sulindac (*Clinoril*) do not appear to reduce lithium clearance, presumably due to a lesser effect on renal prostaglandins. Therefore, one of these agents would be preferred in patients receiving a lithium salt who also require treatment with an antiinflammatory agent.

Pharmacodynamic Interactions

Drugs Having Opposing Pharmacological Effects

Interactions resulting from the use of two drugs that have opposing pharmacological effects should be among the easiest to detect. There may, however, be factors that could preclude early identification of such an antagonism. For example, an ophthalmologist may prescribe a cholinergic drug such as pilocarpine for a patient who is also taking an anticholinergic preparation prescribed by his family physician for a gastrointestinal condition. Although in many patients the anticholinergic agent will not alter intraocular pressure or the action of a drug like pilocarpine, some individuals may experience difficulty as a result of concurrent use of these drugs. Particular caution is indicated in patients with angle-closure (narrow-angle) glaucoma.

The tendency of the thiazide and certain other diuretics to elevate blood glucose levels is well known. When the diuretic is prescribed for a diabetic patient being treated with insulin or one of the sulfonylureas (eg, tolbutamide), this diabetogenic effect may partially counteract the hypoglycemic action of the antidiabetic drug, necessitating an adjustment in dosage.

Drugs Having Similar Pharmacological Effects

An excessive central nervous system depressant effect, resulting from the concurrent use of two or more drugs exhibiting a depressant action, represents one of the most frequently encountered drug-related problems. In considering multiple drug regimens, recognition must be taken of the large number of agents (eg, sedative-hypnotics, antipsychotics, tricyclic antidepressants, analgesics, antihistamines) which can exhibit a depressant effect that will be at least additive to the effect contributed by other drugs. At the minimum, the dosages of the drugs having a depressant effect should be reduced from the "usual" dose, and consideration should be also given as to whether it is necessary to utilize all the drugs concurrently.

Alcohol—Sedatives—The increased central nervous system depressant effect that is experienced by individuals being treated with sedatives or other depressant drugs when they consume alcoholic beverages provides an example of this type of situation. Although this interaction is among the best known and has been recognized for years, it serves to point out the difficulties in trying to predict what response will develop in a particular patient. The response will depend on many variables, including the patient's tolerance to alcohol. How then should the patient be instructed when he is to take a depressant medication? Certainly it would be most desirable not to consume alcoholic beverages during the period the medication is being taken. However, there should be a realistic recognition that many patients if faced with a mandate not to drink while on drug therapy, will decide not to take their drug. Every patient should be alerted to the fact that the depressant effect of the drug prescribed may be enhanced by alcohol. If it is anticipated that the patient would not cooperate in completely avoiding alcoholic beverages, he should be urged to use them in moderation, particularly when therapy

is initiated, and cautioned to observe his own tolerance when they are employed in combination. However, the fact that many individuals can take depressant drugs and consume relatively large amounts of alcoholic beverages with no apparent difficulty should not be cause to forget that such combinations have proven lethal in some individuals and that there is an important need to caution all patients for whom such drugs are prescribed.

The effect of combined alcohol-drug usage on driving skills has also been a matter for concern. It has been suggested that the phenothiazines, tricyclic antidepressants, and the benzodiazepines may increase the effect of alcohol in inhibiting motor skills. One study of blood samples taken from drivers suspected of being drunk because of erratic driving indicated that many of those individuals with low blood-alcohol levels had significant levels of barbiturates or other sedatives. In addition, a number of individuals with high blood-alcohol levels also had detectable levels of a sedative in their blood.

In another study of cases involving propoxyphene intoxication, it is noted that 12 deaths were apparently attributed to alcohol-propoxyphene combinations and the authors recommend that patients should be warned not to drink alcoholic beverages when taking propoxyphene.

Antipsychotic Agents—Antiparkinson Drugs—Antidepressants—Drugs that differ considerably in their primary pharmacological activities may exhibit the same adverse effects. Many patients being treated with antipsychotic agents such as chlorpromazine are also given an antiparkinson agent such as trihexyphenidyl to control the extrapyramidal effects of the former. In addition, a number of patients experience depressive symptoms and a tricyclic antidepressant such as amitriptyline might be added to the therapy. Each of these three agents possesses anticholinergic activity and the additive effect could lead to the development of side effects such as dryness of the mouth, blurred vision, urinary retention, constipation, and elevation of intraocular pressure.

Even an effect such as dryness of the mouth, which most health professionals would consider as a minor problem, could be troublesome in certain patients. For example, persistent dryness of the mouth could make the use of dentures more difficult and also cause other dental complications. In addition, there would be increased difficulty in chewing and swallowing, an important factor with respect to the problem of malnutrition in many elderly individuals. See also Chapter 109.

It has been observed that an excessive anticholinergic effect can cause an atropine-like delirium, particularly in geriatric patients. This effect could be mistaken as an increase in psychiatric symptoms which might be treated by increasing the dosage of the offending therapeutic agents. This example points out the difficulty that can often exist in distinguishing between the symptoms of the condition(s) being treated and the effect of the drug(s) being employed as therapy.

A recent case report describes another potential problem attributable to the anticholinergic side effects of commonly used drugs. A patient being treated with imipramine experienced persistent dryness of the mouth. When the patient utilized sublingual nitroglycerin tablets for the management of exertional angina, the relief of the symptoms was delayed because of the slower dissolution of the sublingual tablets.

Additional observations concerning the development of extrapyramidal effects with antipsychotic agents and the treatment of these symptoms with antiparkinson agents merit further study. Several reports have described the development of severe hyperpyrexia in patients taking phenothiazine–antiparkinson combinations who were exposed to high environmental temperature and humidity. These investigators call attention to the ability of these combinations to interfere with the thermoregulatory system of the body and recommend that physicians treating patients in hot and humid climates should minimize outdoor exposure of patients receiving high doses of these agents.

Diazoxide—Diuretics—Although the potent antihypertensive agent diazoxide is closely related chemically to the thiazide diuretics, it can cause sodium and water retention. Therefore, it will frequently be necessary to administer a diuretic to patients being treated with diazoxide to minimize these effects. Diazoxide will often cause hyperglycemia and can also increase blood levels of uric acid. It should be kept in mind that the additional use of an agent such as a thiazide diuretic will enhance the hyperglycemic and hyperuricemic, as well as the antihypertensive, actions of diazoxide.

Aminoglycoside Antibiotics—Diuretics—There have been occasional reports of ototoxicity, including deafness, associated with the use of ethacrynic acid and furosemide (*Lasix*). In most cases in which these problems developed, the drug was given intravenously in high doses to patients with impaired renal function. The aminoglycoside antibiotics [eg, gentamicin (*Garamycin*), tobramycin (*Nebcin*), netilmicin (*Netromycin*), amikacin (*Amikin*)] have a well recognized potential to cause ototoxicity and reports have appeared that indicate that ototoxicity can develop rapidly when diuretics are also administered intravenously to patients being treated with an aminoglycoside even when the usual doses of these agents are employed. The mechanism by which diuretics may cause ototoxicity has not been fully clarified. The rapid diuresis that results from intravenous use may be a major factor and the literature for the parenteral formulations of aminoglycosides cautions against concurrent use with any rapid-acting diuretic [eg, ethacrynic acid, furosemide, bumetanide (*Bumex*)] because of the possibility of irreversible deafness. It is possible that intravenously administered diuretics may cause a rapid rise in the serum level of the antibiotic, thereby potentiating its neurotoxicity.

Isotretinoin—Vitamin A—Isotretinoin (*Accutane*) has proven to be a highly effective agent in the treatment of severe cystic acne but the frequency of adverse effects with its use is high. Since isotretinoin is so closely related to Vitamin A, patients should be advised against taking vitamin supplements that contain Vitamin A, since the severity of adverse effects may be increased.

Alteration of Electrolyte Levels

Cardiac Glycosides—Diuretics—One of the problems associated with use of most of the commonly employed diuretics, including the thiazide derivatives, bumetanide, chlorthalidone (*Hygroton*), ethacrynic acid, furosemide, indapamide (*Lozol*), metolazone (*Zaroxolyn*), and quinethazone (*Hydromox*), is that they can cause an excessive loss of potassium; in some patients this effect may occur within the first two weeks of diuretic therapy. Excessive loss of potassium induced by a diuretic can cause problems; it has been suggested that there may be an association between hypokalemia and occurrence of certain cardiovascular complications. Particular caution is necessary in patients also being treated with a cardiac glycoside (eg, digoxin), many of whom would be candidates for diuretic therapy since edema is often troublesome in patients with congestive heart failure. If potassium depletion remains uncorrected the heart may become more sensitive to the effects of the cardiac glycoside and arrhythmia may result.

Although this interaction is well recognized, there have been a number of questions as to the circumstances under which it occurs. For example, in some studies of patients with cardiac glycoside-induced arrhythmias, only a small fraction were hypokalemic, leading some to suggest that potassium depletion may not often be associated with digitalis-induced arrhythmias. However, it is recognized that such a conclusion does not correspond to observations that administration of potassium is usually beneficial in the treatment of most of these arrhythmias.

Recent studies have provided a greater insight into the relationship between potassium levels and action of cardiac glycosides. The importance of the relative concentrations of intracellular and extracellular potassium has been observed in man and it has been noted that depletion of intracellular potassium may occur in the presence of normokalemia and even hyperkalemia. Attention is also called to the fact that the level of potassium in serum is an unreliable index of intracellular concentrations of potassium. Although serum-potassium levels provide information that will be useful in monitoring therapy, there should be an awareness that significant problems can occur in normokalemic patients. Since intracellular concentrations of potassium cannot be readily determined, it is suggested that electrocardiograms provide the best guide for management of therapy.

Although potassium supplementation will be necessary in many individuals being treated with a potassium-depleting diuretic, the initiation of therapy with such a diuretic must not be viewed as an automatic indication for also providing potassium supplementation. This decision should be based on a consideration of the individual patient situation, and the appropriate parameters should be periodically monitored. It must be recognized that dangers also exist if hyperkalemia occurs as a result of excessive supplementation. This risk of such complications is greatest in patients with diminished renal function.

In those situations in which potassium supplementation is considered necessary, the patient could be advised to increase his intake of potassium-rich foods (eg, bananas, orange and tomato juices), or pharmaceutical formulations containing a potassium salt such as potassium chloride could be prescribed. Another measure would be to use a potassium-sparing diuretic like amiloride (*Midamor*), spironolactone (*Aldactone*), or triamterene (*Dyrenium*) in combination with the potassium-depleting agent.

In addition to the diuretics, other agents also can cause potassium depletion. Prolonged therapy with cathartics and corticosteroids may cause potassium depletion although this is not likely to occur as quickly or to the same extent as with diuretics. A number of antibiotics (eg, carbenicillin) are also capable of lowering potassium levels, particularly when therapy is prolonged.

In patients in whom potassium depletion has been identified it is sometimes difficult to determine the cause of the condition. One report comments on the surreptitious self-administration by three patients of large amounts of diuretics that resulted in hypokalemia. The desire for a slim figure was regarded as being one of the motivations that resulted in use of these agents.

Considerable interest has developed in the clinical implications of magnesium depletion. Concern has been expressed that this condition occurs much more commonly than is recognized and that some clinical problems may continue or worsen despite seemingly adequate electrolyte therapy because magnesium deficiency has not been identified and corrected.

Diuretic therapy may lead to development of magnesium depletion and, as observed when potassium is depleted, the activity of cardiac glycosides may be enhanced and possibly result in toxicity. In some patients with cardiac glycoside toxicity, low serum-magnesium concentrations may coexist with normal potassium values. However, it has also been suggested that hypomagnesemia may decrease intracellular potassium and that if adequate potassium levels are maintained the increased response to digitalis will be nullified in spite of the hypomagnesemia.

Cardiac Glycosides—Calcium—The action of cardiac glycosides is also influenced by calcium. In contrast to the effect of potassium and magnesium, however, it is an increase in the level of calcium that can enhance the sensitivity of the heart to cardiac glycosides since the myocardial actions of these two agents are in certain respects similar. Usually problems will be encountered only when calcium salts are given parenterally to patients receiving a cardiac glycoside. Although the possibility has not received as much attention, at least one case has been reported in which a decrease in the response to digoxin was attributed to hypocalcemia.

Lithium—Diuretics—Sodium depletion is known to enhance lithium toxicity, for which reason it has been generally recommended that lithium salts should not be used in patients on diuretic therapy or on a sodium-restricted diet. Even protracted sweating or diarrhea can cause sufficient depletion of sodium to result in decreased tolerance to lithium.

The sodium depletion caused by diuretics reduces the renal clearance and increases the activity of lithium. However, it has been noted by some that, if preferable therapeutic alternatives are not available, concurrent therapy need not be contraindicated as long as the interaction is recognized and steps are taken to monitor therapy and adjust dosage. Indeed, in several situations concomitant use of a lithium salt and a diuretic may be beneficial and represents the best therapy available. For example, a thiazide diuretic may be very useful in the management of lithium-induced nephrogenic diabetes insipidus and may permit the continued use of lithium which might otherwise have to be discontinued.

Interactions at Receptor Sites

Monoamine Oxidase Inhibitors—Sympathomimetic Agents—Monoamine oxidase (MAO) functions to break down catecholamines such as norepinephrine. When the enzyme is inhibited increased levels of norepinephrine, within adrenergic neurons, result. Production of norepinephrine continues without the usual rate of destruction. Since greater-than-usual amounts of norepinephrine are now being stored, any drug that might release these stores can bring about exaggerated responses. It is by this mechanism that interactions between monoamine oxidase inhibitors [isocarboxazid (*Marplan*), phenelzine (*Nardil*), tranylcypromine (*Parnate*), and pargyline (*Eutonyl*)] and indirectly acting sympathomimetic amines (eg, amphetamine) develop. Thus, if amphetamine is administered to a patient whose stores of norepinephrine have been increased by MAO inhibition, he may experience severe headache, hypertension (possibly a hypertensive crisis), and cardiac arrhythmias. The serious consequences associated with these interactions contraindicate use of these agents in combination.

Although most sympathomimetic amines, such as amphetamine, are available only by prescription, others such as ephedrine, phenylephrine, and phenylpropanolamine, which also have been reported to interact similarly with MAO inhibitors, are found in most of the popular nonprescription cold and allergy preparations, as well as many of the over-the-counter "weight-reducing" products. Certainly it is impor-

tant that patients being treated with MAO inhibitors avoid using products containing these agents.

MAO Inhibitors—Tyramine—There have also been reports of serious reactions (hypertensive crisis) occurring in people being treated with MAO inhibitors following ingestion of certain foods having a high content of pressor substances such as tyramine. These foods include certain cheeses (eg, Cheddar, Camembert and Stilton, but not cream cheese, cottage cheese or ricotta), certain alcoholic beverages (eg, Chianti wine), chocolate, pickled herring, yeast extract, avocado, and liver.

Tyramine is metabolized by MAO (in contrast to amphetamine, which is not a substrate for MAO) and normally these enzymes in the intestinal wall and in the liver protect against the pressor actions of amines in foods. However, when these enzymes are inhibited, large quantities of unmetabolized tyramine can accumulate, resulting in the release of norepinephrine from adrenergic neurons.

MAO Inhibitors—Tricyclic Antidepressants—Cautions in the product literature as well as case reports warn against concurrent use of an MAO inhibitor with a tricyclic antidepressant (eg, amitriptyline, imipramine) because severe atropine-like reactions, tremors, convulsions, hyperthermia, and vascular collapse have been reported to result from such use. It is recommended in the product literature that therapy with an MAO inhibitor or a tricyclic antidepressant should not be initiated until at least 7 to 14 days after therapy with the other has been discontinued.

Although the approved labeling for MAO inhibitors and tricyclic antidepressants notes that concurrent use is contraindicated, there is controversy as to the degree of risk involved. Several studies of the combined use of these agents have revealed little evidence of interaction and the growing impression that serious interactions are uncommon, coupled with the reports of favorable results with such combinations in selected patients who did not respond to either agent given alone, have led many to conclude that these combinations can be cautiously employed. In patients who are refractory to single antidepressants and who are not candidates for alternative therapeutic approaches, the potential benefits of combination therapy may outweigh the risks. However, such therapy should be undertaken only by those who are thoroughly familiar with the risks involved and under circumstances in which therapy can be closely monitored.

It should be noted that the antineoplastic, procarbazine (*Matulane*), and the anti-infective, furazolidone (*Furoxone*) or probably its metabolite, can also inhibit monoamine oxidase enzymes and warnings applying to the use of other MAO inhibitors should be heeded for these drugs also. With furazolidone, however, it is not likely that enzyme inhibition will occur within the first five days of therapy and usually the course of treatment will be completed within that time.

Several recent case reports describe the development of vascular reactions in patients taking isoniazid, following the ingestion of cheese. Although these reactions have not been commonly encountered, patients receiving isoniazid should be cautioned about the ingestion of cheeses and other dietary items known to interact with MAO inhibitors.

Guanethidine—Tricyclic Antidepressants—Guanethidine (*Ismelin*) is transported to its site of action within adrenergic neurons by a transport system that is also responsible for uptake of norepinephrine as well as several indirectly acting sympathomimetic amines such as ephedrine and the amphetamines. Concentration of guanethidine in these neurons is necessary for its hypotensive effect. It is suggested that tricyclic antidepressants can inhibit uptake of guanethidine into the neuron terminal, thereby preventing its concentration at these sites and reducing its activity. It should also be anticipated that the tricyclic antidepressants will also reduce the antihypertensive action of guanadrel

(Hylorel), a more recently introduced analog of guanethidine.

If it is necessary to administer a tricyclic antidepressant to a patient receiving guanethidine, doxepin (*Adapin*, *Sinequan*) may be preferred since the available data indicates that it is less likely (in the dosage range of 75–150 mg daily) to alter the effects of guanethidine. However, since these antidepressants have similar pharmacological properties, the possibility of an interaction involving even low doses of doxepin cannot be excluded.

Guanethidine—Sympathomimetic Agents—The effect of guanethidine is also antagonized by amines such as amphetamine and by ephedrine and methylphenidate (*Ritalin*). It is suggested that amphetamine probably acts similarly to the tricyclic antidepressants in producing this response but, in addition, it may also cause release of guanethidine from its storage sites in neurons.

Since nasal congestion is a side effect that can be associated with use of guanethidine it should be anticipated that patients may wish to obtain products that will relieve these symptoms. Ephedrine is commonly included as a decongestant in both prescription and nonprescription cold and allergy products and could inhibit the antihypertensive effect of guanethidine. It is probable that phenylephrine and phenylpropanolamine, which are comparable to ephedrine in many respects, will have a similar effect.

Guanethidine—Antipsychotic Agents—Several studies have indicated that chlorpromazine can reverse the antihypertensive effects of guanethidine, probably in a manner similar to that seen with tricyclic antidepressants. Significant but less dramatic reversals of guanethidine activity also occurred with haloperidol (*Haldol*) and thiothixene (*Navane*). Since these three agents are representative of the classes of antipsychotic agents that are most frequently prescribed, it is likely that the other agents in these classes are also capable of producing this response.

Although similar pharmacologically to the above-mentioned classes of antipsychotic agents, the new agents molindone (*Moban*) and loxapine (*Loxitane*) differ from a chemical standpoint. At this time data to evaluate their potential to interact with guanethidine are inadequate, although one study in rats noted that molindone did not interact, in contrast to the results with chlorpromazine in the same investigation.

Alteration of Gastrointestinal Flora

Anticoagulants—Antibiotics—A number of anti-infective agents have been reported to enhance the effect of simultaneously administered anticoagulants. It has been suggested that this effect develops, in part, as a result of interference by the anti-infective agent with production of vitamin K by microorganisms in the gastrointestinal tract. Broad-spectrum antibiotics, such as the tetracyclines and cephalosporins, are most likely to cause problems of this type. Although similar effects may also be seen with other antibiotics, the significance of this mechanism has been questioned; if it is a factor, it is likely that problems will occur only in patients who have a low dietary intake of vitamin K.

It is also probable that other mechanisms may be involved in some of these interactions. For example, the increased anticoagulant effect noted when sulfonamides and anticoagulants are given concurrently may be due, in part, to displacement from protein-binding sites.

Digoxin—Antibiotics—It is estimated that approximately 10% of patients being treated with digoxin convert a significant portion of the parent compound to inactive reduction metabolites in the gastrointestinal tract. The bacterial flora of the intestine contributes to this metabolic process. Elevated serum digoxin levels have been observed in patients receiving erythromycin or tetracycline concurrently and it is suggested that these antibiotics, by reducing the bacterial flora, decrease the extent to which digoxin is metabolized in the gastrointestinal tract, resulting in the higher serum levels of the cardiac glycoside.

Oral Contraceptives—Ampicillin—Several antibiotics have been suggested to decrease the effectiveness of oral contraceptives. The estrogen component of the contraceptive formulation is conjugated to a large extent in the liver and excreted in the bile. Bacteria in the intestine hydrolyze the conjugated form of the estrogen, permitting the free drug to be reabsorbed and to contribute to the serum level of the estrogen. Ampicillin, by reducing the bacterial flora, interrupts the enterohepatic circulation with a resultant reduction in serum estrogen levels.

Although a question has been raised regarding the significance of this interaction, it would be desirable for patients to use supplementary contraceptive measures in addition to the oral contraceptive, during cycles in which ampicillin is used.

Antibiotic Combinations

The use of antibiotics in combination has been the subject of considerable discussion. Although many believe that antibiotic combinations are overused, there is agreement that situations exist in which therapy with two or more agents is superior to use of one drug alone. Such situations include the following:

1. *Treatment of mixed infections*—In some infections two or more microorganisms that are not susceptible to the same antibiotic are responsible for causing infection. For example, intraabdominal sepsis secondary to intestinal perforation is often caused by anaerobic organisms (eg, *Bacteroides fragilis*) and aerobic Gram-negative bacilli (*Enterobacteriaceae*).

2. *Treatment of severe infections in which the causative organism(s) has not been identified*—Therapy must be initiated promptly in treating severe infections and the use of several antibiotics that provide a broader spectrum of activity than one agent alone is often appropriate.

3. *Enhancement or synergy of antibacterial action*—The penicillins and aminoglycosides exhibit a synergistic action against enterococci and combination therapy is recommended for infections such as enterococcal endocarditis. Sulfamethoxazole and trimethoprim (*Bactrim*, *Septra*) have been used in combination to advantage because each of these agents blocks a different step in the metabolism of folate. Each of these agents usually exhibits a bacteriostatic action when used alone but the combination is bactericidal against many organisms.

4. *Prevention of emergence of resistant organisms*—Resistance will often develop rapidly when an antitubercular agent is used by itself. The use of two or three antitubercular drugs in combination will prevent or significantly delay the development of resistant organisms.

5. *Reduction of adverse effects*—The use of flucytosine (*Ancobon*) in conjunction with amphotericin B (*Fungizone*) in the treatment of meningitis due to *Cryptococcus neoformans* has permitted a reduction in the length of the treatment period (from 10 weeks with amphotericin B alone to 6 weeks with the combination). The shorter duration of amphotericin B administration resulted in a decrease in the toxicity with this agent.

Most of the discussion concerning interactions of antibiotics relates to the concept of antibiotic antagonism. Antagonism between antibiotics has been reported to occur when a bacteriostatic antibiotic, such as tetracycline, is administered in combination with a bactericidal agent such as a penicillin derivative. Penicillin derivatives inhibit cell-wall synthesis and must act on multiplying bacteria that are making new cell walls to exert a lethal effect. If a bacteriostatic agent that stops cell multiplication by another mechanism that does not lead to cell death is given concurrently, the penicillin derivative cannot exert a bactericidal effect because the cells are no longer multiplying.

Penicillin—Tetracycline—One study compared the use of penicillin alone with the use of penicillin and chlortetracycline (*Aureomycin*) in combination in the treatment of pneumococcal meningitis. The results showed a 79% mortality rate in patients treated with penicillin and chlortetracycline as compared to a 30% mortality rate in the patients treated with penicillin alone.

In another study of children with bacterial meningitis it was noted that the mortality was greater (10.5%) when various combinations of ampicillin, chloramphenicol, and streptomycin were administered than when ampicillin was given alone (4.3%). The difference was less pronounced in adults.

Although the possibility of antibiotic antagonism may exist under certain circumstances, there is a question as to whether it is often of clinical significance in man since in the treatment of most infections all that is necessary is to stop multiplication of the organism causing the infection. Some antibiotics can be either bacteriostatic or bactericidal, depending on the concentrations achieved in a particular tissue and the susceptibility of the organism causing the infection. It should also be recognized that there are several exceptions to the rule against concurrent use of bactericidal and bacteriostatic antibiotics.

Aminoglycosides—Penicillins—Aminoglycosides (eg, gentamicin) have often been used in combination with penicillin analogs such as carbenicillin in the treatment of *Pseudomonas* infections and excellent results have been achieved. Therefore, there was considerable concern when a report appeared suggesting that the antimicrobial activity of gentamicin may be antagonized by carbenicillin and that, in certain circumstances, the combination may be less effective than one of the agents alone.

Further study demonstrated that the loss of gentamicin activity in the presence of carbenicillin can probably be attributed to a physicochemical interaction which would be most likely to occur if the two antibiotics were physically mixed, as in a solution intended for intravenous administration. Hence the recommendation that gentamicin should not be mixed with other agents but should be given separately. When it is given in such manner to patients with normal renal function who are also receiving carbenicillin, antagonism is not likely to occur and use of these two agents continues to be regarded as a therapy of choice in the treatment of severe *Pseudomonas* infections.

Although the problem described might better be categorized as a "pharmaceutical" interaction than as a pharmacodynamic interaction, there are special implications for patients with impaired renal function. In these patients, gentamicin is given less frequently or in lower doses and a single dose remains in the blood and tissues for a prolonged period of time. Even when the two antibiotics are administered separately, the possibility exists that the prolonged period during which gentamicin remains in the body may provide adequate time for high doses of carbenicillin to inactivate gentamicin. The significance of this possibility is not clear but, as is the case with any patient with renal impairment, the therapy and dosages must be closely monitored. Cephalosporins should be expected to interact with the aminoglycosides in the same manner as the penicillins.

Although other mechanisms may be involved in the development of drug interactions, the ones cited appear to be the most important. As often stated, more than one mechanism may be responsible for certain interactions; these mechanisms may work in concert or in opposition as determinants of the resulting effect. Still other drug interactions develop by mechanisms yet to be identified.

Even though the discussion of some interactions has raised more questions than have been answered, it is anticipated that an awareness of the factors predisposing to development of drug interactions, as well as the mechanisms by which they occur, will be of value in the identification and prevention of potential problems.

It is evident that much remains to be learned about drug interactions and that significant limitations still exist in trying to predict the results of combination therapy. In the following section, guidelines are provided to minimize the risk of the occurrence of drug interactions.

Minimizing the Risk of Drug Interaction

The reduction of the risk of drug interactions is a challenge that embraces a number of considerations. Although they could be applied to drug therapy in general, the following principles are offered as guidelines for health professionals having the responsibility for the decisions regarding the selection and monitoring of the therapeutic regimen.

1. *Identify the patient risk factors*—Factors such as age, the nature of the patient's medical problems (eg, impaired renal function), dietary habits, smoking, and problems like alcoholism will influence the effect of certain drugs and should be considered during the initial patient interview.

2. *Take a thorough drug history*—An accurate and complete record of both the prescription and nonprescription medications a patient is taking must be obtained. Numerous interactions have resulted from a lack of awareness of prescription medications prescribed by another physician, or nonprescription medications the patient did not consider important enough to mention.

3. *Be knowledgeable about all the drugs being utilized*—The knowledge of the properties and the primary and secondary pharmacologic actions of each of the agents used, or being considered for use, is essential if the interaction potential is to be accurately assessed. Therapeutic alternatives that are less likely to interact should be considered.

4. *Keep the potential for interaction in perspective.*

5. *Avoid complex therapeutic regimens where possible*—The number of medications utilized should be kept to a minimum. In some patients, combination products may be used to advantage if the quantities of the individual medications included in the formulations correspond to the dosage levels considered to be most appropriate. The use of medications or dosage regimens that permit less-frequent administration may help avoid interactions that result from an alteration of absorption (eg, when a drug is administered in close proximity to meals).

6. *Educate the patient*—Patients often know little about their illnesses, let alone the benefits and problems that could result from drug therapy. Individuals who are aware of, and understand, this information can be expected to be in greater compliance with the instructions for administering medications and more attentive to the development of symptoms which could be early indicators of drug-related problems. Patients should be encouraged to ask questions about their therapy and to report any excessive or unexpected responses. There should be no uncertainty on the part of the patient as to the manner in which medications should be used to obtain optimum effectiveness and safety.

7. *Therapy should be frequently monitored*—The risk of drug-related problems warrants close monitoring, not only for the possible occurrence of drug interactions but also for adverse effects occurring with individual agents and noncompliance. Any change in patient behavior should be suspected as being drug-related until that possibility is excluded.

8. *Therapy must be individualized*—Although the development of a therapeutic regimen that meets the specific needs of individual patients is inherent in many of the above guidelines, the importance of this consideration cannot be emphasized too strongly. Wide variations in the response of patients to the same dose of certain individual drugs is well recognized. When recognition is taken of the difficulty in predicting the response of many therapeutic agents when they are given alone, the challenge and limitations in endeavoring to anticipate the response with a multiple-drug regimen become apparent. Therefore, priority should be assigned to the needs and clinical response of the individual patient, rather than usual dosage recommendations and standard treatment and monitoring guidelines.

The pharmacist will be actively involved in the observance of the guidelines described above. In addition, the need to not only maintain complete and current patient medication records, but also to supervise and monitor drug therapy more closely, places the pharmacist in a strategic position to detect and prevent drug interactions. By observing the preceding guidelines and recommendations, and by strengthening communication with patients and other health professionals, the pharmacist has a valuable opportunity to make a significant contribution toward the further enhancement of the efficacy and safety of drug therapy.

Bibliography

Books

Drug Interaction Facts, Facts and Comparisons, St Louis, 1983.
Evaluations of Drug Interactions, 3rd ed, CV Mosby, St Louis, 1984.
The Medical Letter Handbook of Drug Interactions, The Medical Letter, New Rochelle, New York, 1983.
Hansten PD, ed: Drug Interactions, 4th ed, Lea and Febiger, Philadelphia, 1979.
Hansten PD, ed: Drug Interactions Newsletter, Applied Therapeutics, San Francisco.
Lerman F, Weibert RT, ed: Drug Interactions Index, Medical Economic Books, Oradell, NJ, 1982.
Stockley IH, ed: Drug Interactions. A Source Book of Adverse Interactions, Their Clinical Importance, Mechanisms and Management. Blackwell Publications, St Louis, 1981.

Papers

Interactions of drugs with alcohol. Med Letter 23: 33–34, 1981.
Drug interactions update. Med Letter 26: 11–14, 1984.
Back DJ, et al: Interindividual variation and drug interactions with hormonal steroid contraceptives. Drugs 21: 46–61, 1981.
Bell JE: Comparative evaluation of drug interaction publications—1976. Am J Hosp Pharm 33: 1299–1303, 1976.
Brater DC, Morrelli HF: Digoxin toxicity in patients with normokalemic potassium depletion. Clin Pharmacol Ther 22: 21–33, 1977.
D'Arcy PF, McElnay JC: Drug interactions involving the displacement of drugs from plasma protein and tissue binding sites. Pharmac Ther 17: 211–220, 1982.
Doering W: Quinidine-digoxin interaction. New Engl J Med 301: 400–404, 1979.

Feely J, et al: Reduction of liver blood flow and propranolol metabolism by cimetidine. New Engl J Med 304: 692–695, 1981.
Gelehrter TD: Enzyme induction. Parts I, II, and III. New Engl J Med 294: 522–526, 589–595, 646–651, 1976.
Griffin JP: Drug interactions occurring during absorption from the gastrointestinal tract. Pharmac Ther 15: 79–88, 1981.
Hansten J, et al: Smoking and drug interactions. Amer Pharm NS 22: 492–494, 1982.
Klein HO et al: The influence of verapamil on serum digoxin concentration. Circulation 65: 998–1003, 1982.
Koch-Weser J, Greenblatt DJ: Drug interactions in clinical perspective. Europ J Clin Pharmacol 11: 405–408, 1977.
Koch-Weser J, Sellers EM: Binding of drugs to serum albumin. Parts I and II. New Engl J Med 294: 311–315 and 526–531, 1976.
Kristensen MB: Drug interactions and clinical pharmacokinetics. Clin Pharmacokin 1: 351–372, 1976.
Lindenbaum J, et al: Inactivation of digoxin by the gut flora: reversal by antibiotic therapy. New Engl J Med 305: 789–794, 1981.
McElnay JC, et al: A practical guide to interactions involving theophylline kinetics. Drug Intell Clin Pharm 16: 533–542, 1982.
McLean AM, et al: Food, splanchnic blood flow, and bioavailability of drugs subject to first-pass metabolism. Clin Pharmacol Ther 24: 5–10, 1978.
Melander A: Influence of food on the bioavailability of drugs. Clin Pharmacokin 3: 337–351, 1978.
Melmon KL, Nierenberg DW: Drug interactions and the prepared observer. New Engl J Med 304: 723–725, 1981.
Miller RR: Effects of smoking on drug action. Clin Pharmacol Ther 22: 749–756, 1977.
Nimmo WS: Drugs, diseases and altered gastric emptying. Clin Pharmacokin 1: 189–203, 1976.
Offerhaus L: Drug interactions as excretory mechanisms. Pharmac Ther 15: 69–78, 1981.
Park BK, Breckenridge AM: Clinical implications of enzyme induction and enzyme inhibition. Clin Pharmacokin 6: 1–24, 1981.
Perucca E, Richens A: Drug interactions with phenytoin. Drugs 21: 120–137, 1981.
Ponto LB, et al: Tricyclic antidepressant and monoamine oxidase inhibitor combination therapy. Am J Hosp Pharm 34: 954–961, 1977.
Schou JS: Drug interactions at (pharmacodynamically active) receptor sites. Pharmac Ther 17: 199–210, 1982.
Sorkin EM, Darvey DL: Review of cimetidine drug interactions. Drug Intell Clin Pharm 17: 110–120, 1983.
Vesell ES: Genetic and environmental factors affecting drug disposition in man. Clin Pharmacol Ther 22: 659–679, 1977.
Vesell ES: On the significance of host factors that affect drug disposition. Clin Pharmacol Ther 31: 1–7, 1982.

CHAPTER 103

Utilization and Evaluation of Clinical Drug Literature

Donald G Fraser, PharmD
Director—Medical & Clinical Affairs
Reid-Provident Labs Inc
Atlanta, GA 30308

When the Study Commission on Pharmacy was published in 1975, a major finding was that "the system of pharmacy cannot be described as either effective or efficient in developing, organizing and distributing knowledge and information about drugs."[1] The Study Commission recommended "that major attention be given to the problems of drug information to find who needs to know, what he needs to know, and how these problems can best be met with speed and economy."[1]

Some progress has been made since the Study Commission Report was published. We know that consumers and health care professionals pose most of the questions to which pharmacists are asked to respond. The majority of the questions fall into the following categories:[2]

Category

(a) Availability
Prescription, OTC, investigational and foreign drugs
(b) Compounding
Questions concerning the extemporaneous preparation of medication
(c) Dosage
Adult, pediatric or neonatal dosage of a drug
(d) Identification
Identification of foreign and domestic prescription, and OTC drugs
(e) Injectables
Questions on compatibility and stability
(f) Interaction
Drug-drug, Drug-food, Drug-lab test interactions
(g) OTC Products
Any question on OTC drugs or devices
(h) Patient Instructions
Any question concerning instructions a pharmacist would impart to a patient prior to dispensing a product
(i) R or OTC
A question referring to the legal status of a product
(j) Therapeutic Use
Questions regarding drugs of choice for a disease state
(k) Toxicity
Side effects and adverse reactions
(l) Use in Pregnancy or Breast-Feeding Mothers
Teratogenic potential of a drug; excretion of a drug in breast milk.

We now know the questions to which we must respond, but how effective have we become in developing, organizing and distributing knowledge and information about drugs to health care professionals and consumers?

The increase in the number of drug information centers[3,4] and clinically trained pharmacists through degree programs and on-the-job training[5,6] has enhanced significantly the ability of pharmacists to respond to questions posed by health care professionals in the university and community hospital setting. Another major factor is that the hospital pharmacist is becoming more accessible to the physicians and nurses in

the patient care areas[7,8] and more influential on various committees eg, the Pharmacy and Therapeutics Committee and Drug Utilization Review Committee. The publication of original research and review articles in the medical literature by clinically trained pharmacists with academic and/or hospital appointments has helped physicians realize that pharmacists can be good sources of drug information. If this is the case, then why have a number of studies over the last three decades continually ranked pharmacists as poor sources of drug information?[8-11] Eckel suggests that pharmacists have been ranked low as drug information sources in previous studies because physicians generally associate the term pharmacist with community pharmacists.[8] The survey by Eckel ranks clinical and hospital pharmacists much higher than peer physicians, the PDR (Physician's Drug Reference—see Table I), community pharmacists and pharmaceutical representatives as sources of drug information for physicians.[8]

A large number (64%) of community pharmacists in Miller's survey indicated that they felt they were being well utilized as a drug information resource.[9] The community pharmacists who felt they were poorly utilized cited physician's pride or lack of knowledge by the public and health professionals as the reason; almost none recognized himself as being in any way inadequate.[9] When pharmacists were then asked what personal factors could be preventing their development as an information source, 48% indicated a lack of clinical experience, 21% a lack of knowledge, 16% a lack of reference material, 24% a lack of confidence, 13% a lack of training in using information resources, 4% specified a lack of time, and 4% lack of questions.[9]

Which came first, the chicken or the egg? That may seem like a strange question to ask, but how are pharmacists going to be reliable sources of drug information when certain state boards of pharmacy may only require two reference texts in each pharmacy, ie, USP/NF and the AMA Drug Evaluations, or Facts and Comparisons, or the Pharmacological Basis of Therapeutics by Goodman and Gilman? Several surveys indicate that most community pharmacies do not have basic text and journal resources which could be consulted to answer questions on drug interactions, adverse drug reactions, etc.[9,10] It is no wonder then, that the primary sources of drug information for physicians are the medical literature, professional colleagues, association meetings, continuing education courses, and pharmaceutical representatives.[12,13]

Consumer satisfaction is one of the major factors in developing a successful community pharmacy. Consumers want not only quality medication at a reasonable price, but also drug information from a pharmacist who is accessible and can supply up-to-date and accurate drug information. Evidence of consumer interest in drug information can be found in bookstores where best seller lists recently have included drug information guides written for the general public; even the relatively technical PDR has been among the top ten on several best seller lists.[14]   Tax dollars or independent funding has been used to support active consumer drug information centers in several states.[15-18]   Nevertheless, the majority of questions posed by the consumer are answered from the community pharmacist's own knowledge or available reference texts.[16]   The number, variety and sophistication of the questions consumers ask may increase if pharmacists make themselves more available to the consumer.   Unfortunately, many patients feel the pharmacist is too busy to discuss the use of their medications with them.[10]

Within the next ten years, we may find most pharmacists dispensing medications in unit of use containers (ie, no more "count and pour"), and using computers to manage patient medication records, print labels for prescriptions, check for drug interactions, and do all the billing.[19]   The technology to do all these functions is available now.   Hopefully, this will allow pharmacists to devote more time and financial resources to develop, organize and distribute information about drugs to consumers and health care professionals.[20,21,33]

The list of references in Table 1 depicts a reasonable variety of resources which would allow community and hospital pharmacists to answer many drug information questions. Backup drug information support services also must be developed, but questions remain as to the scope of such drug information centers.[22]   Should regional drug information centers answer questions from both health professionals and consumers, or just health professionals?[22,23]   If drug information centers encourage consumers to bypass their community or hospital pharmacist, will the role of the pharmacist as a provider of drug information simply be diminished further?   Funding is also a key question.   In the past, regional drug information programs have been established with federal and/or state funding, however, drug information centers traditionally have not been revenue producers and many have failed to survive after grant funds have been spent.[16,22-24]   If regional drug information centers are to become a viable information source for health professionals, each center must become self-sufficient.[16,22-24]   This could be accomplished by charging for services rendered, a concept advocated by a number of drug information specialists.[22-24]   The most feasible idea may be the development of combination drug information/poison control centers.   The advantages of such a program have recently been described by Troutman and Wanke.[30]

Computerized medical information data bases have provided pharmacists in academic institutions and hospitals with drug information for many years.   Extensive training is required before one can utilize many of these data bases effectively.   In the future, user-friendly computerized medical information data bases may be able to provide drug information on demand to health care practitioners with access to computer terminals.   The success or failure of data bases such as the *Formulary Service* (by the Am Soc Hosp Pharm) and *AMA/NET* (by the AMA) will depend upon factors such as: cost; ability to provide current therapeutic information in the form of an on-line, searchable, full text data base; and ease plus speed of use by the health care practitioner in his office, home or hospital.[23,32]

Regional drug information/poison control centers, carefully selected references (see Table I) and computer databases can provide pharmacists with an effective communication link to the clinical literature.   Whether one decides to maintain the *status quo* or use the drug information resources available to him is a personal decision, however, the best interests of the public and the pharmacy profession would be served if more pharmacists became drug-information-conscious pharmacists.

The following information will provide some of the basics necessary to utilize and evaluate the clinical drug literature effectively.

Organization and Use of the Literature

The scientific literature can be divided into three broad categories: *primary*, *secondary*, and *tertiary* references.

Primary literature is composed of all original contributions to the published record.   The major components of the primary literature are journals and books.   Government reports, conference proceedings and graduate theses also may be useful sources of information on drugs.

Secondary references consist of a group of information sources which serve to guide or direct the inquirer to the primary literature.   They are available in a variety of forms, eg, abstracting services, bibliographic listings, specialized microfilm and microfiche systems, as well as a variety of computerized data bases.   Examples of secondary resources are *Index Medicus*, *International Pharmaceutical Abstracts* (IPA), *Inpharma*, *Reactions*, the *de Haen Information Systems*, *Iowa System*, *Drugdex*, *Excerpta Medica*, *Science Citation Index*, *Current Contents—Clinical Practice*, *Clin-Alert*, *Pharmaceutical News Index* (PNI), *Biological Abstracts*, *Chemical Abstracts*, etc.   Refer to Chapter 7 or your reference librarian for further information.

The term *tertiary reference* usually refers to publications in the form of texts.

The pharmacist who seeks to be an expert in drug therapy will learn to use the clinical literature to: (1) keep abreast of new developments in drug therapy and (2) to answer questions from consumers, physicians, nurses and other health care professionals.   A pharmacist who keeps up with current developments by actively perusing a large number of journals and abstracting services inevitably has a better comprehension of the current optimal approaches to drug therapy than those who do not.   The list of journals and newsletters listed in Appendix A contains most of the important contributions to the clinical drug literature.   From the journals listed in Appendix A, one may select 20 or 30 titles which will be most helpful in a practice situation.   Regular examination of these publications will be possible only for those pharmacists who have a large medical or hospital library close by.   If one does not have convenient access to such a facility, then one must rely on the core collection of texts, newsletters, journals and current awareness publications, such as *Inpharma*, listed in Table I.   *Inpharma* is a weekly publication that reviews approximately 1500 medical/pharmacy journals for articles relevant to drug therapy.   It has a short lag time (1 to 3 months) and informative abstracts; useful bibliographies on selected topics also are included.   A copy of the cited journal articles often may be obtained from the local medical or hospital library.   If the local library does not subscribe to the journal, a copy of the article usually can be obtained on interlibrary loan from a Regional Medical Library in the US.

By reviewing Current Contents in Clinical Practice and Current Contents in Life Sciences, pharmacists can request reprints of articles of interest.   A preprinted postcard provides a convenient way to do this.   One must keep in mind that it is expensive for authors to purchase and mail reprints of their articles, and some may refuse to do so.   A procedure which many pharmacists have found useful is to file reprints and photocopies of articles under the drug categories of the American Hospital Formulary Service.

As noted above, a second major use of the drug literature is in answering questions on drugs and drug therapy.   A knowledge of the current literature and a file of journal reprints or photocopies often are useful, but reference books are indispensable for the majority of questions.   A core collection of reference books is included in Table I.   For a more complete listing of information sources on drug and pharmaceutical information, the following two publications are recommended: (1) *Concepts in Clinical Pharmacology—Information*

Table I—Core Collection of Clinical Drug Literature

Reference Books

Applied Therapeutics (Katcher BS, Young LY, Koda-Kimble M), Applied Therapeutics, Inc, San Francisco, California.

Manual of Medical Therapeutics (Freitag JJ, Miller LW), Little Brown and Co, Boston.

Manual of Pediatric Therapeutics (Graef JW, Cone TE, Jr), Little Brown and Co, Boston.

Handbook of Clinical Drug Data (Knoben JE, Anderson PO), Drug Intelligence Publications, Hamilton, Illinois.

Clinical Use of Drugs in Patients with Kidney and Liver Disease (Anderson RJ, Schrier RW), W.B. Saunders Co, Philadelphia, PA.

Textbook of Medicine (Wyngaarden JB, Smith LH, Jr), W.B. Saunders Co, Philadelphia or *Harrison's Principles of Internal Medicine* (Petersdorf RG, Adams RD, Braunwald E et al), McGraw-Hill, New York.

Martindale: The Extra Pharmacopoeia (Reynolds JEF, Prasad AB), The Pharmaceutical Press, London, England.

Facts and Comparisons, Facts and Comparisons Division, JB Lippincott Co, St Louis, MO.

Handbook of Non-prescription Drugs, American Pharmaceutical Association, Washington, DC.

AMA Drug Evaluations, American Medical Association, Chicago, Illinois.

Physicians Desk Reference, Medical Economics Co, Oradell, NJ.

USAN—Dictionary of Drug Names (Griffiths MC), United States Pharmacopeial Convention, Inc, Rockville, MD.

National Drug Code Directory, US Dept Health and Human Services, Food and Drug Administration, Drug Listing Branch, Rockville, MD.

Merck Index, Merck and Co Inc, Rahway, NJ.

USP—Drug Information, United States Pharmacopeial Convention, Inc, Rockville, MD.

Medication Guide for Patient Counseling (Smith DL), Lea and Febiger, Philadelphia, PA.

Drug Interactions (Hansten PD), Lea and Febiger, Philadelphia, PA.

Evaluations of Drug Interactions, American Pharmaceutical Association, Washington, DC.

Applied Biopharmaceutics and Pharmacokinetics (Shargel L, Yu ABC), Appleton-Century Crofts, New York, NY.

Applied Pharmacokinetics: Principles of Therapeutic Drug Monitoring (Evans WE, Schentag JJ, Jusko WJ), Applied Therapeutics Inc, San Francisco.

Handbook of Injectable Drugs (Trissel LA), American Society of Hospital Pharmacists, Bethesda, MD.

Principles of Drug Information Services (Watanabe AS, Conner CS), Drug Intelligence Publications, Inc, Hamilton, IL.

Journals

Pharmacotherapy (Pharmacotherapy Publications, Inc., Carlisle, MA).

Clinical Pharmacy (American Society of Hospital Pharmacists, Bethesda, MD).

Drug Intelligence and Clinical Pharmacy (Drug Intelligence and Clinical Pharmacy Inc, Cincinnati, OH).

American Journal of Hospital Pharmacy (American Society of Hospital Pharmacists, Bethesda, MD).

New England Journal of Medicine (Massachusetts Medical Society, Boston, MA).

Annals of Internal Medicine (American College of Physicians, Philadelphia, PA).

Journal of American Medical Association (American Medical Association, Chicago, IL).

Clinical Pharmacology and Therapeutics, (CV Mosby Co, St Louis, MO).

British Medical Journal (British Medical Association, London, England).

Drug Therapy (BMI, New York, NY).

Newsletters

The Medical Letter on Drugs and Therapeutics, New Rochelle, NY.

Drug Interaction Newsletter, Applied Therapeutics Inc, Spokane, WA.

Current Awareness Services

Inpharma, ADIS Press International Inc, Newtown, PA.

Clin-Alert, Science Editors Inc, Louisville, KY.

Reactions, ADIS Press International Inc, Newtown, PA.

Current Contents in Clinical Practice, Institute for Scientific Information, Philadelphia.

(The total cost of the core collection is approximately $2000.00 per year.)

Sources in Pharmacy and Pharmacology[29] (this Scope® publication is available from the Upjohn Company and is updated at frequent intervals and reviews the content of texts, journals and indexing systems which can be used to answer a wide variety of questions posed to pharmacists), and (2) *Drug and Pharmaceutical Information Resources*[26]. This publication is produced by the Medical Library Association as part of its continuing education program. Both publications are excellent and should be part of the library of every pharmacist.

Answering Drug and Drug Therapy Questions

When a health practitioner or a patient asks a question concerning a drug, the pharmacist must be sure he understands what information is being sought. Questions often are improperly or incompletely framed. If an answer is supplied on the basis of insufficient information, the answer may be totally inaccurate or inappropriate.

As an aid to pharmacy students and pharmacists with little clinical experience, the following suggestions for obtaining background information and answers for a variety of questions are offered.[27] These suggestions are far from being compulsory rules. Through experience, each pharmacist learns what information to gather on the question being asked and which literature sources are most useful in answering different types of questions in his particular practice.

Drug Identification/Availability/Market Status— Prescription and OTC Drugs

The following questions will be of assistance in obtaining background information:[25-27] (A) what is the trade, generic, chemical, numerical or code name of the drug? Try to obtain the source of this information ie, prescription, prescription label, manufacturer's label, patient, physician, etc. Obviously, the source can help to determine the accuracy of the information. (B) what is the drug used for therapeutically? Two drugs may be spelled similarly but may be differentiated if their therapeutic use is known. Also, it is helpful to know the disease states of the patient. (C) what is the country of origin of the drug? An answer to this question will help to determine if domestic or foreign reference sources will be of the most assistance. (D) who is the drug manufacturer? (E) what dosage form of the drug is available or requested? ie, tablet, capsule, parenteral. (F) what is the reason for the inquiry? Determine whether an American equivalent may be necessary if the inquiry concerns a foreign drug. If the patient has ingested a large amount of the drug, poison information may be required.

One of the problems in identifying drugs is the fact that multiple research numbers, generic names, and trade names may refer to the same product.

Standards for generic names of drugs include: BAN (British Approved Name), INN (International Nonproprietary Name), USAN (US Adopted Name), NFN (Nordiska Farmacopenamden), and DCF (Denomination Commune Francaise). Different drug forms (eg, salts, isomers) often are not distinguished in nomenclature systems used abroad.[25]

Investigation numbers, or company research codes assigned to drugs in their early stages of development may be identified by using a variety of resources. The *USAN and the USP Dictionary of Drug Names* is published annually by the USP Pharmacopeial Convention and is an excellent source to find investigational numbers, company research codes, chemical names, manufacturer and structure of the compound in question. *Unlisted Drugs* arranges these codes in numerical order, ignoring the alphabetical portion; it also supplies information on the manufacturer, source of the information, and structure of the compound, is updated monthly and can identify compounds back to 1949. The *Merck Index* contains a list of company code letters in the miscellaneous tables. One then can contact the manufacturer to identify the compound. The *de Haen System* (Drugs in Use, Drugs in Research) also contains a list of investigation numbers and company research codes, as do *Pharmaprojects* and *Pharmacast*. Keep in mind that a variety of research codes may refer to the same product.

Many references can be used to identify foreign drug products.[25-27] *Martindale: The Extra Pharmacopeia* and *Unlisted Drugs* often are the most useful sources of information, however, a variety of foreign and domestic publications also may prove to be of use: *Rote List* (German), *Index Nominum* (Swiss), *Compendium of Pharmaceutical Sciences* (Canada), *Dictionnaire Vidal* (French), *Diccionario De Especialidades Farmaceuticas* (Mexican), *Organisch— Chemische Arzneimittel und ihre Synomyma* (German), *L'Informatore Farmaceutico* (Italian), and the *de Haen Drugs in Use/Drugs in Research. Pharmaprojects, Pharmacast, Inpharma, SCRIP,* and *Pharmascope* may be useful.

Domestic drug identification sources include: *Facts and Comparisons, Physician's Desk Reference, Pharm Index, American Drug Index, USAN, Merck Index, Red Book* (Drug Topics), *Blue Book* (American Druggist), *Martindale's, Unlisted Drugs,* the *APhA's Handbook of Nonprescription Drugs,* the *PDR for Nonprescription Drugs, AMA Drug Nomenclature,* and *Chem Sources USA* etc.[25-27]

The identification of drug products from a description of the dosage form and manufacturer markings can be aided by a variety of resources. Pictorial inserts are included in the *PDR, Drug Topics Red Book,* and *Veterinary Pharmaceuticals and Biologicals.* Tablet or capsule imprints also are indexed in the *Chemist and Druggist Directory, MIMS, Imprex, Poisindex,* and the *National Drug Code Directory* (published every two years with quarterly updates).[25] The Drug Listing Branch of the FDA maintains an up-to-date list of NDC codes and can provide invaluable assistance in identifying drug products. They can be contacted currently at the following phone number: (301) 443-7259.

Computer searching may prove to be extremely valuable in identifying new or investigational drugs. Data bases available include SCISEARCH, CAS ONLINE, MEDLINE, TOXLINE, BIOSIS PREVIEWS, INTERNATIONAL PHARMACEUTICAL ABSTRACTS, CHEMLINE, SDC ORBIT'S CHEMDEX, DIALOG'S CHEMNAME, CHEMSIS and CHEMSEARCH, and EXCERPTA MEDICA.[25,28]

Drug Dosing

Drug dosing questions often are answered without sufficient patient information. The following questions are structured to solicit this information:[27] (A) what is the diagnosis or indication for which the drug is prescribed? Although the indication may appear to be obvious, new indications for drugs

are being discovered all the time and may require different dosing regimens. Old dosing regimens constantly are being re-evaluated and changed as well. (B) what is the status of the kidney, liver and cardiac function of the patient (recent specific laboratory levels are required)? (C) what other medications (prescription and OTC) is the patient now taking and during the past 6 months? Does the patient have any known allergies? (D) what is the age of the patient? (E) what is the weight and nutritional status of the patient?

There are numerous texts that will provide information on drug dosing. Some of the most useful general references are: *Applied Therapeutics, Facts and Comparisons, Manual of Medical Therapeutics,* the *PDR,* the *American Hospital Formulary Service, AMA Drug Evaluations, Handbook of Drug Therapy, Handbook of Clinical Drug Data, Clinical Use of Drugs in Patients with Kidney and Liver Disease,* Conn: *Current Therapy,* Krupp: *Current Medical Diagnosis and Therapy,* and the *Handbook of Non-Prescription Drugs.* Numerous specialty texts are also available, eg, *Bugs and Drugs, The Use of Antibiotics* by Kucer and Bennett etc.

For information on pediatric doses, refer to the following references: *Manual of Pediatric Therapeutics, The Harriet Lane Handbook, Current Pediatric Therapy,* or the *Pediatric Drug Handbook.*

Texts rapidly become out of date, therefore indices and abstracts such as *Inpharma* and *Index Medicus* should be consulted for the most current information.

Drug Interactions

Charts, tables and reference texts often are used to answer questions on this topic. Drug interactions may or may not occur, depending on the clinical circumstances. The following background questions apply to drug-drug and drug-lab test interaction questions:[27] (A) what is the patient's prescription and OTC drug history? ie doses, duration of therapy and time course of administration. If the question concerns a laboratory test modification, the specific laboratory test method must be obtained. (B) what are the clinical symptoms or manifestations of the drug interaction? Pertinent laboratory values and the time sequence of events as related to the drug administration also must be noted. (C) what is the current medical status of the patient. (D) what has been done to date in the management of this drug interaction?

Texts such as *Evaluations of Drug Interactions* by the APhA, and *Drug Interactions* by Hansten should be consulted initially. Abstract/indexing sources such as *Inpharma, Reactions, de Haen Drug Interactions* and the *Drug Interactions Newsletter* by Hansten also *must* be consulted to insure that the information in accurate and up-to-date. Other indexing sources such as *Index Medicus, Excerpta Medica, Science Citation Index* and *IPA* often provide additional information.

Laboratory Test Modification

The effects of drugs on lab tests are reviewed by Hansten in *Drug Interactions,* and in *Clinical Chemistry 21:* 1–432 D, 1975, and *Drugs 24:* 24–63, 1982. More current information may be obtained by examining appropriate indexing/abstracting services such as *Index Medicus, IPA, de Haen,* etc. The effects of disease states on clinical lab tests are reviewed in *Clinical Chemistry 26:* 1–476 D, 1980.

Adverse Drug Reactions

The following questions can assist in determining whether a cause/effect relationship exists between administration of a drug and the development of an adverse drug reaction;[27] (A) what are the signs and symptoms of the possible adverse reaction? (B) how severe is the reaction? ie anaphylaxis, rash, etc. (C) when did the reaction first become apparent? (D) what medications (prescription and OTC) is the patient taking now and has he taken in the past 6 months? Obtain information on the dose, duration, route of administration, and indication for each drug. (E) has the patient or any family member experienced any allergic or adverse reactions to medications in the past? (F) what is the current medical status of the patient? (G) what has been done in the management of the patient to date?

There are a number of quality resources which can provide information on the adverse effects of drugs. *Side Effects of Drugs* is one of the most useful texts. Each volume of this text is produced every 4 or 5 years; supplements are produced annually. Other texts of value include the *Textbook of Adverse Drug Reactions* by Davies, *Drugs, Chemicals and Blood Dyscrasias* by Swanson and Cook, *Martindale: The Extra Pharmacopeia*, *Drug Induced Ocular Side Effects and Drug Interactions* by Fraunfelder, *Non-prescription Drugs and Their Side Effects* by Benowicz and *Drug Effects in Hospitalized Patients* by Miller and Greenblatt. A number of publications also *must* be consulted to provide up-to-date information on the adverse effects of drugs. Abstracting services such as *Inpharma, Reactions, de Haen—Adverse Drug Reactions, Clin-Alert* and *Drugdex* prove to be invaluable. Computer or hand searching of *Index Medicus, IPA, Science Citation Index*, and *Excerpta Medica* also can prove to be extremely valuable as can pharmaceutical companies which maintain accurate records of published and unpublished data on adverse reactions produced by products they manufacture.

Biopharmaceutics/Pharmacokinetics

Current bioavailability/pharmacokinetic data must be found by searching the primary journal literature. The individual pharmaceutical companies also should be consulted for in depth information about products they produce. The following references may be of value in interpreting data in this specialized area: *Applied Pharmacokinetics* by Evans, Schentag and Jusko, *Applied Clinical Pharmacokinetics* by Mungall, *The Effect of Disease on Drug Pharmacokinetics* by Benet, *Basic Clinical Pharmacokinetics* by Winter et al, *Handbook of Clinical Pharmacokinetics* by Gibaldi and Prescott, and *Applied Biopharmaceutics and Pharmacokinetics* by Shargel and Yu.

Physical and Chemical Compatibilities

Remington's Pharmaceutical Sciences, the *American Hospital Formulary Service*, *Merck Index* and package inserts are useful for answering questions concerning incompatibilities which may occur when two or more drugs are mixed together. Questions on incompatibilities encountered in preparing parenteral admixtures may be answered by referring to the most recent issue of *Handbook on Injectable Drugs* by Trissel. The current journal literature and manufacturer also may provide valuable information.

Nonapproved Indications

A significant number of drugs are used for indications not formally approved by the FDA; only approved indications are discussed in the manufacturer's package inserts. The most useful sources of information are abstracts/indexes such as *Inpharma, Index Medicus, Science Citation Index*, and *Excerpta Medica*. The pharmaceutical manufacturer also can provide pertinent information on this topic.

Investigational Drugs

A wide variety of references supply information on investigational drugs. Some of the most accessible resources include *Martindale—The Extra Pharmacopeia*, the *USAN—Dictionary of Drug Names*, *Unlisted Drugs* and the Products Pending section of *PharmIndex*. If more indepth information is required, the following indexes/abstracting services should be consulted: *Inpharma, deHaen Drugs in Use and Drugs in Research, Pharmaceutical News Index, Pharmaprojects, Pharmacast, Pharmascope, Science Citation Index, Excerpta Medica, Iowa System*, and *Index Medicus*. The pharmaceutical manufacturer also can provide pertinent information on this topic.

Drug Evaluations

A wealth of resources is available to help the practitioner evaluate drugs. The most valuable publications in this field include *Pharmacotherapy, Drug Intelligence and Clinical Pharmacy, Clinical Pharmacy, Drugs*, and *The Medical Letter*. Review articles also can be found in a number of other journals and can be obtained by reviewing *Current Contents—Clinical Practice* every week and requesting reprints. A review of the index/abstracting services such as *Inpharma, Index Medicus*, as well as *Drugdex* and *AMA Drug Evaluations* also will prove to be of value.

Therapy

Drug therapy questions cover a variety of topics ranging from drug of choice questions to comparative therapeutic efficacy. A particular patient may or may not be involved, but when the question concerns a specific patient, the following background information must be solicited:[27] (A) what is the age, sex, weight and race of the patient? (B) what is (are) the indication(s) and/or diagnosis in this patient? What other disease states does the patient have? (C) what are the current renal and liver functions of the patient? (D) what medications (prescription and OTC) is the patient taking currently or has he taken in the recent past? (E) has the patient experienced any allergic and/or adverse reactions to medications in the past?

If one is not acquainted with the disease process in question, a general reference such as *Harrison's Principles of Internal Medicine, Textbook of Medicine, Textbook of Pediatrics*, or a specialty reference will be of value in reviewing the disease state prior to reviewing the therapy. The following texts often prove useful in answering this type of question: *Applied Therapeutics, Manual of Medical Therapeutics, Manual of Pediatric Therapeutics, Conn: Current Therapy, Krupp: Current Medical Diagnosis and Treatment, AMA Drug Evaluations, Handbook of OTC Drugs, Drugdex*, and a variety of other publications.[26,27,29] Textbooks become out of date very quickly, thus indexes/abstracts such as *Inpharma, Index Medicus*, etc are recommended to obtain the most current information.

Government and Industry Activity

The *Pharmaceutical News Index* (PNI) is one of the most useful resources to find information on controversial health care issues, major health bills, drug recalls, legislation and regulation of drugs, trade and professional association activities, marketing trends, joint ventures, drug approvals, etc. PNI source publications include the following: *FDC Reports, Drug Research Reports, Medical Devices, Diagnostics, and Instrumentation Reports, Weekly Pharmacy Reports, SCRIP, World Pharmaceutical News, Quality Control Reports, Clinical World Medical Device News*, and *Pharma*.

The *Federal Register* and *Code of Federal Regulations* also provide a useful means of accessing federal government regulations regarding food and drugs.

Patient Instructions

A number of publications are available which may assist the pharmacist in providing instructions for the patient. The USP publishes a two-part annual publication entitled *USP DI—Advice for the Patient and Drug Information for the Health Care Provider* which provides current up-to-date information. Other very useful publications include the *Medication Guide for Patient Counseling* by D. Smith, and the *Handbook of Nonprescription Drugs* by the APhA.

Toxicology and Poisoning

Poisindex is the most complete single source of poison identification and management information available with emphasis on specific symptoms and step-by-step treatment. Data are gathered from pharmaceutical, commercial, chemical, cosmetic and OTC industries. It also contains information on plants and has an index which lists commercial name, generic name, slang term, botanical and zoological common and scientific names. The information is updated 4 times a year. Text references of value include: *Handbook of Poisoning* by Dreisbach, Casarett and Doull's *Toxicology*, and *Clinical Management of Drug Overdoses* by Haddad and Winchester. Various other publications are available.[26,27,29] Indexes/abstracts such as *Toxicology Abstracts* which review referred toxicology and therapeutic journals are also very valuable sources of information.

Evaluation

Pharmacists must develop the ability to evaluate critically the drug literature. Far too often we are guilty of reading the abstract and conclusion of journal articles without critically examining the article. A procedure for evaluating the medical and pharmacy literature must be developed by reviewing text and journal articles on the design and evaluation of clinical trials. Invaluable experience also can be obtained by working on clinical research projects with experienced clinical researchers, taking courses in Drug Literature Evaluation, and working in a drug information/poison control service. Although a detailed discussion of literature evaluation is beyond the scope of this chapter, the following considerations will be helpful in assessing the usefulness of a given journal article:[27]

1. Is the article in a reputable journal? In general, the best, most critically analyzed drug articles are found in refereed pharmacy, pharmacology and medical journals.

2. Is the objective of the study clearly defined? Ideally, all subjectivity and bias on the part of the investigator should be absent or negated in the study. If the objectives of the study indicate a preconceived bias, then the results of the study are questionable.

3. Is the patient population appropriate? The patient population must be carefully described since the study drugs may produce different therapeutic responses in patients with different diseases or different stages of a disease. The results of a study may not necessarily be extrapolated to another patient population. For example, if a researcher wants to determine if benzodiazepine accumulates with repetitive dosing, the study should be done initially in the patient population who will be at the greatest risk of drug accumulation: eg the elderly patient, not a young healthy male or female. How large was the patient population? A large study population is desirable, but is not always possible, especially if one is studying a rare disease. A single case of an adverse reaction can be significant if an adequate cause/effect relationship can be established.

4. Was the study prospective or retrospective? A prospective design permits advance planning to study experimental groups before the group is exposed to the drug being studied. This study design allows the investigator to establish better methods for control, randomization, and data collection. In retrospective trials, the researcher usually collects data by chart reviews. Unfortunately, much of the pertinent data may be missing, or subject to bias.

5. Were adequate controls established? Control groups should be comparable to the treatment group except for the factor being tested. Controls should also be concurrent in time and place with respect to the subjects receiving the treatment. In some cases, historical controls may be satisfactory; eg a disease which is universally or rapidly fatal.

6. Was subject or patient allocation based upon a random selection method? This must de done to assure that the study is free of unconscious or conscious selection bias on the part of the investigator.

7. Were adequate blinding techniques used in the study? In a double-blind study, neither the patient nor the investigator is aware of which medication the patient is receiving. Identical medications must therefore be used. If the side effects of each medication are different, the patients and investigator will soon realize which medication is being used unless appropriate precautions are taken.

8. Were the study medications used appropriately? The following factors must be considered. The dose of the study medication must not be subtherapeutic or excessive; the dosage interval and route of administration must be appropriate. The duration of the trial must be adequate. Concomitant drug administration may influence the results of the study and must therefore be accounted for.

9. Were the methods of data collection appropriate? Were standard measurements used and are they reproducible? What factors may influence the parameters being measured?

10. Were the results reported accurately? Were the nature and incidence of side effects documented? Were dropouts reported along with specific reasons for their non-participation in the study?

11. Were appropriate statistical methods used? Are the results clinically significant?

12. Were valid conclusions made which can be supported by the results of the study? Extrapolation of data and conclusions beyond the conditions of the study must be avoided.

13. Does the author(s) provide appropriate references to support statements made in the article?

Conclusion

There is no doubt that pharmacists can make a significant contribution to health care by providing clinical services such as therapeutic monitoring and patient counseling services. A recent survey conducted by the APhA (American Pharmacy, *23:* 58–64, 1983) indicates that consumers are willing to pay for clinical services provided by pharmacists. If we are to meet this challenge we must develop and continue to refine our knowledge about drugs. It is hoped that the information provided in this chapter will help us to accomplish this task.

References

1. American Association of Colleges of Pharmacy: Pharmacists for the Future—The Report of the Study Commission of Pharmacy. Health Administration Press, Ann Arbor, 1975.
2. Schneiweiss F: *Drug Info J 14:* 7–9, 1980.
3. Rosenberg JM, Kirschenbaum HL, Labella NA Jr: *Am J Hosp Pharm 39:* 94–8, 1982.
4. Rosenberg JM: *Am J Hosp Pharm 39:* 1157, 1982.
5. Dukes GE, Rubin H: *Am J Hosp Pharm 40:* 810–2, 1983.
6. Appleby DH, Russillo NJ, Edgerton WL: *Am J Hosp Pharm 40:* 807–10, 1983.
7. Nelson AA Jr, Meinhold JM, Hutchinson RA: *Am J Hosp Pharm 35:* 1201–6, 1978.
8. Eckel FM: *Drug Info J 13:* 15–20, 1979.
9. Miller DR: *Drug Info J 14:* 186–90, 1980.
10. Fink JL, Stern AR: *Pharmacy Management 152:* 210–8, 1980.
11. Cardoni AA, Palmer HA, Grover R: *J Am Pharm Assoc 17:* 680–4, 1979.
12. Meadows RJ: *Drug Info J 15:* 11–5, 1981.
13. Stinson ER, Mueller DA: *JAMA 243:* 140–3, 1980.
14. Talley CR: *Am J Hosp Pharm 37:* 1195, 1980.

15. Sigell LT, Piascik MF, Parker RE et al: Am J Hosp Pharm 37: 1206–10, 1980.

16. Montagne M, Clute SS, McKennell T: Am J Hosp Pharm 37: 1211–5, 1980.

17. Conner CS, Murphrey KJ, Sawyer D et al: Am J Hosp Pharm 37: 1215–9, 1980.

18. Lee B, Gumpert NF, Oksas RM: Am J Hosp Pharm 37: 1176, 1980.

19. Archambault GF: Medical Marketing Media 18: 26–30, 1983.

20. Rolfe E, Cyr JG: Can Pharm J 116: 83–8, 1983.

21. Anon: NARD, 104: 18–21, 1982.

22. Cardoni AA: Am J Hosp Pharm 40: 1215–7, 1983.

23. Rosenberg JM: Am J Hosp Pharm 40: 1213–5, 1983.

24. Amerson AB, Wallingford DM: Am J Hosp Pharm 40: 1172–8, 1983.

25. Snow B: Medical Reference Services Quarterly 1 No 3 (Fall): 37–52, 1982.

26. Snow B: Drug and Pharmaceutical Information Resources, Medical Library Assoc., 1981.

27. Watanabe AS, Conner CS: Principles of Drug Information Services, Drug Intelligence Publications, 1978.

28. Heymen JJ, Karasinska EH, Giles PM Jr: Drug Info J 17: 185–90, 1982.

29. Cohon MS, Rice BS, Noble V: Information Sources in Pharmacy and Pharmacology, Upjohn Co. Kalamazoo. 1983.

30. Troutman WG, Wanke LA: Am J Hosp Pharm 40: 1219–22, 1983.

31. Anon: Medical Marketing Media 18: No 3. 21–7, 1983.

32. Anon: Am J Hosp Pharm 40: 1035–7, 1983.

33. Avorn J, Soumerai SB: N Engl J Med 308: 1457–63, 1983.

Appendix A—Journals and Serials that Publish a Significant Number of Articles Relevant to the Clinical Use of Drugs

Acta Medica Scandinavica
Adverse Drug Reaction Bulletin
Adverse Drug Reactions and Acute Poisoning Reviews
American Journal of Cardiology
American Journal of Digestive Diseases
American Journal of Diseases of Children
American Journal of Gastroenterology
* American Journal of Hospital Pharmacy
* American Journal of Intravenous Therapy and Clinical Nutrition
American Journal of Medicine
American Journal of Obstetrics and Gynecology
* Annals of Internal Medicine
Antimicrobial Agents and Chemotherapy
Archives of Dermatology
Archives of Disease in Childhood
Archives of General Psychiatry
* Archives of Internal Medicine
Archives of Neurology
Biopharmaceutics and Drug Disposition
* British Journal of Clinical Pharmacology
British Journal of Pharmacology
* British Medical Journal
Canadian Journal of Hospital Pharmacy
Canadian Medical Association Journal
Circulation
Clinical Neuropharmacology
Clinical Pediatrics
* Clinical Pharmacokinetics
* Clinical Pharmacology and Therapeutics
* Clinical Pharmacy
Clinical Therapeutics
Clinical Toxicology
Controlled Clinical Trials, Design and Methods
* Current Therapeutic Research
Drug Information Journal
* Drug Intelligence and Clinical Pharmacy
* Drug Interaction Newsletter
Drug Metabolism and Disposition
Drug Metabolism Reviews
Drug-Nutrient Interactions

* Drug and Therapeutics Bulletin
* Drug Therapy
Drug Therapy Bulletin
Drugs
* European Journal of Clinical Pharmacology
European Journal of Drug Metabolism and Pharmacokinetics
* FDA Bulletin
FDC Reports
Gastroenterology
Geriatrics
Journal of the American Geriatrics Society
* Journal of the American Medical Association
Journal of Clinical and Hospital Pharmacy
* Journal of Clinical Pharmacology
Journal of Clinical Psychopharmacology
Journal of Infectious Diseases
Journal of Parenteral and Enteral Nutrition
* Journal of Pediatrics
Journal of Pharmaceutical Sciences
Journal of Pharmacokinetics and Biopharmaceutics
Kidney International
* Lancet
Medical Clinics of North America
* Medical Letter on Drugs and Therapeutics
* Morbidity and Mortality Weekly Report
Nephron
Neurology
* New England Journal of Medicine
Obstetrics and Gynecology
* Parenterals
Pediatric Clinics of North America
Pediatric Pharmacology
* Pediatrics
* Pharmacotherapy
Postgraduate Medicine
* Rational Drug Therapy
SCRIP
Therapeutic Drug Monitoring
US Pharmacist

* An asterisk denotes those publications which are recommended for subscription by large pharmacies.

CHAPTER 104

Health Accessories

Barry N Eigen, MBA

President, Sickroom Service, Inc
Milwaukee, WI 53233

For too long, many pharmacists treated health accessories as merely a convenience for their prescription patients. Physicians and other health professionals were convinced that the pharmacist had neither the necessary expertise nor equipment and sent their patients elsewhere for such services. In recent years, however, few aspects of professional practice have changed as much or grown as rapidly as the pharmacy's health accessory department. The specially trained pharmacist is becoming more widely recognized as an expert in this area by other health professionals and can provide a professional and profitable adjunct to the pharmacy's other services.

A comprehensive health accessory department includes a wide variety of surgical supplies and convalescent aids including wheelchairs, walkers, hospital beds, hydraulic patient lifters, urology supplies, ostomy appliances, elastic supports, and orthopedic braces. In addition, many pharmacies specialize in home health-care equipment such as traction devices, suction machines, respiratory therapy equipment, paraffin baths, parallel bars, muscle stimulators, and quadriceps boots.

Even more important than merely providing large varieties of health accessories is the pharmacist's growing involvement in selecting and fitting them and also in instructing the patient in their proper use and maintenance.

To provide these services the pharmacist must acquire new skills and expertise which can be obtained through special courses given by several health accessory manufacturers, and some wholesale distributors.

The initial step in selecting the appropriate health accessory is a thorough evaluation of both the patient and the available accessories including;

Age	Prognosis
Disability-related factors	Areas of activity
Patient and equipment measurements	Financial resources

Each of these factors should be considered when selecting the correct health accessory for the patient.

Other steps may include consulting with the patient, his physician, and his family; preparing a prescription, when applicable, as a recommendation to the physician; selecting the accessory from stock or ordering it from the manufacturer or distributor; and checking the accessory to insure that it meets the appropriate specifications. Followup adjustments or modifications may also be necessary.

Useful forms—eg, disability analysis, measurement, prescription, and ordering forms—are usually available from health accessory manufacturers.

Wheelchairs

There are literally hundreds of different wheelchairs to serve the patient's different needs. Fig 104-1 shows one ex-

ample. The importance of an individualized prescription cannot be overemphasized. A carefully prescribed chair has a prolonged and useful life and promotes the patient's maximal physical independence.

Age—The general loss of body functions in the aged patient serves as a guide to providing the best chair for his needs. Thus he may have less strength and endurance than a younger person and therefore requires safety and convenience features. This reemphasizes the general rule when fitting any wheelchair: the primary consideration in fitting is the user's physical limitations.

Disability-Related Factors—A comprehensive disability analysis should be undertaken including a detailed examination of specific disabilities and a comparison of chair equipment relative to each type of disability.

Paraplegia and Quadriplegia—Two main factors influence chair requirements for these patients—loss of both function and sensation below the lesion. The paraplegic has the advantage of functioning upper extremities and needs no wheeling adaptations. Some paraplegics or quadriplegics have the physical abilities to handle light frames or sports chairs enabling them to participate in activities too restrictive for a standard wheelchair. The quadriplegic is, in varying degrees, without hand function and such provisions as vertical handrim projections aid him in wheeling the chair: if severely disabled, he may need a motorized chair. The quadriplegic may also require a special release mechanism on swinging, detachable footrests; brake lever extensions may be added to improve the patient's independence, and the need for special environmental control systems or respiratory equipment requiring special frame adjustments.

Amputations (particularly bilateral above the knee)—To compensate for absence of leg weight and change in center of gravity, the chair should have the axle set back; sandbags on the footrests help if an "amputee frame" chair is unavailable. Unilateral amputation of the arm, or single-arm dysfunction, may require use of a wheelchair with a one-arm drive mechanism to enable operation of a manual wheelchair.

Hemiplegia—The stroke patient generally wheels the chair with one hand and one foot, so he must be able to reach the floor; the seat height must be low enough to allow this. The footrest on that side of the chair should be removed. Patients unable to manipulate in this way can be accommodated with a "one-arm drive" chair which has, by means of a special axle, both handrims on the same side. Brake lever extensions allow the operation of both brakes with one hand. Hemiplegics and patients with edema in the upper extremities may require a lap board or tray to keep their arms high and out of danger.

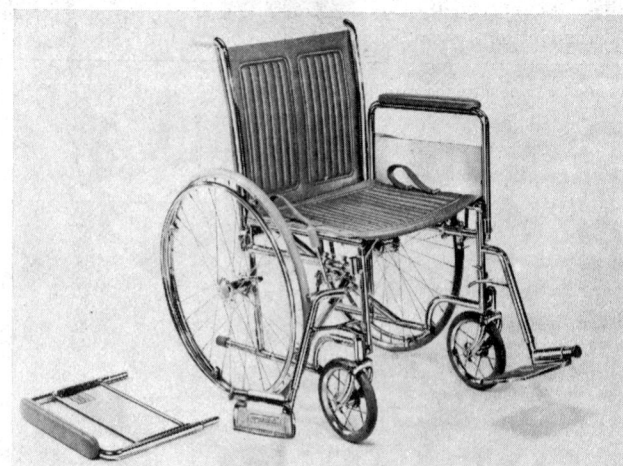

Fig 104-1. Adult wheelchair with full-length, removable arms and swing-away, detachable footrests (courtesy, Everest & Jennings).

The author acknowledges the contributions of Thomas J Smith, RPh, and David F Eigen, MS, of Sickroom Service, Inc, in the preparation of this chapter.

Arthritis—These patients have limited physical activity due to pain, muscular atrophy, and joint destruction. Of great benefit is a lightweight chair. Poor hand function is aided by vertical handrim projections, and an elevating legrest is helpful in preventing lower extremity contractures. Arthritics require a greater than standard seat height to allow them to come to a standing position with more ease.

Braces—If braces are worn, it may be necessary to reconsider the seat width as well as the possible need for heavy-duty seat upholstery and offset or detachable armrests. When the patient's weight exceeds 180 lb, a heavy-duty chair with heavy-duty upholstery should definitely be considered. Additional factors may indicate heavy-duty or reinforced chairs even if the patient weighs less than 180 lb.

Stiff, Weak, Contracted, or Painful Joints—Elevating (fracture type) legrests and other footrest accessories should be considered as well as various arm support devices used for temporarily incapacitated persons.

Respiratory Difficulties, Lack of Sitting Tolerance, and Limitation of Hip Range—These patients may require either a semireclining (to 30° from vertical) or a fully reclining (to 90° from vertical) chair.

Leg Spasms—Patients with occasional leg spasms may require heel loops, ankle straps, toe loops, calf straps, pneumatic ties, or legrest panels to insure that their feet stay safely on the foot plates.

Cerebral Palsy and Multiple Sclerosis—The patients may require a safety belt or vest to keep them from sliding out of the chair and other special positioning adaptations. Some manufacturers provide a modular wheelchair back with adjustable body side supports.

Measurements—Following the disability analysis, the measurements of both the patient and the chair should be considered when preparing a prescription for the proper chair.

The Patient—Ideally, the patient should be sitting when measured, preferably in a chair that allows good body alignment.

Floor-to-Head—Relates to the overall height of the reclining back chairs after adding all other height modifications.

Floor-to-Knee—Used to determine footrest adjustments from seat level and/or special seat height. The minimum footrest adjustment should be at least 2″ less than this measurement in order to avoid pressure against the underside of the legs. A good visual guide for proper footrest adjustment (especially when using a standard chair) is to make sure that the tops of the patient's thighs are horizontal and parallel to the floor. To obtain greater-than-standard maximum footrest adjustment, a special seat height must be considered. Sometimes the use of a solid insert seat and/or seat cushion will solve this problem, although it should be remembered that optimum seat height allows the patient to place his feet on the floor without excessive pressure behind the knees.

Knee-to-Hip—Critical in determining the actual chair seat depth. Normally the seat depth will be approximately 2 to 3″ less than this measurement in order to provide adequate support, yet avoid pressure behind the knee. If a back panel or back cushion is to be inserted, its thickness must be considered.

Seat-to-Elbow—Serves as an indicator for armrest height. Depending on seating posture, armrest height should provide proper body support. *Danger signals:* drooping or hunched up shoulders when the patient's elbows are resting on the armrests. It should be noted that an armrest height one inch more than the patient's seat-to-elbow measurement will force the patient's elbows slightly forward, providing a natural brace against forward body slumping, especially when descending ramps.

Seat-to-Armpit—Used to determine back upholstery height on standard back chairs; this is important because many patients must be able to put their arms over the back upholstery and hook their elbows under the push handle to achieve leverage when reaching for things.

Seat-to-Top-of-Head—Used to confirm the height of the head support when a headrest extension is indicated or a reclining back is required.

Wrist-to-Elbow—Indicates requirements in the consideration of various arm styles, arm slings, brake locations, etc.

Wrist-to-Shoulder-Joint—In conjunction with the wrist to elbow measurement, may suggest the relocation of or special-sized wheels, and brake lever extensions to accommodate the short-armed patients.

Side-to-Side (widest area of hips while sitting)—Important in determining the chair seat width. In order to avoid pressure on the hips or thighs, yet help maintain good seating posture and stability, the chair seat width should be 2″ more than the width straight across the hips.

Total Height Standing (or prone, if the patient cannot stand)—Confirms certain of the measurements and better visualizes the overall size of the patient.

The Chair—Certain wheelchair dimensions (see Fig 104-2) are important in preparing an individualized prescription.

Seat Height—Should be high enough to allow maximum distal thigh support at the front edge of the seat panel so the patient's heels are barely touching the foot pedals. With this adjustment, the seat must be high enough so the foot pedals are at least 2″ from the floor. *Common error:* when the seat is too low, the footrests hit the ground over uneven surfaces, or hit a ramp during ascent or the level ground following descent.

Seat Depth—Should be deep enough to not allow more than the width of the hand between the front edge of the seat and the back of the calf (approximately 4 to 5″ for an adult), and proportionately smaller for a child. *Common error:* when too shallow, excess pressure is placed on the ischii increasing the danger of pressure sores.

Seat Width—Should be as narrow as possible and still allow the thickness of an extended hand between the skirt guard and the widest part of the hips. *Common error:* excess width inhibits reaching the handrims and propelling the chair with ease. It also frequently results in a chair which is too wide for typical doorways in the home.

Back Height—For patients with fair or better trunk muscles the back height should be 2″ below the inferior angle of the scapula; with no trunk musculature, but good shoulders and elbow flexors: 1″ below; with no trunk musculature, fair to good shoulders, and trace to fair elbow flexors: 1″ above; and with no trunk musculature and upper extremity muscle power: even with or above. The seat back may also have to be reclined 15°. *Common errors:* in patients with some ability to propel a chair, a back which is too high interferes with shoulder mobility and decreases the ability to maneuver the chair; a back which is too low does not give upper trunk stability. The rule, however, is to make the back as low as possible within the limitations imposed by the patient's trunk control.

Armrests—Should support elbows and forearms with shoulders in a relaxed position. *Common error:* when too low, patients complain of shoulder discomfort from upper extremity weight drag on the shoulders.

Overall Width—Should be compared with the width of the narrowest doorway through which the chair must pass. Width of the chair can be estimated by adding 6½″ to the seat width when standard or offset armrests are used; add 7¾″ if detachable armrests are used. If the overall width is the critical factor in using the chair, subtract this difference from the width of the open door to determine usable seat width. If it is not possible to meet both seat and overall width requirements, wrap around armrests to decrease the overall width should be used or a chair-narrowing device fastened to the seat rail should be considered.

Miscellaneous Assessories—

Detachable Back Upholsteries—May be just the answer where small bathrooms make front and side transfers from the chair nearly impossible.

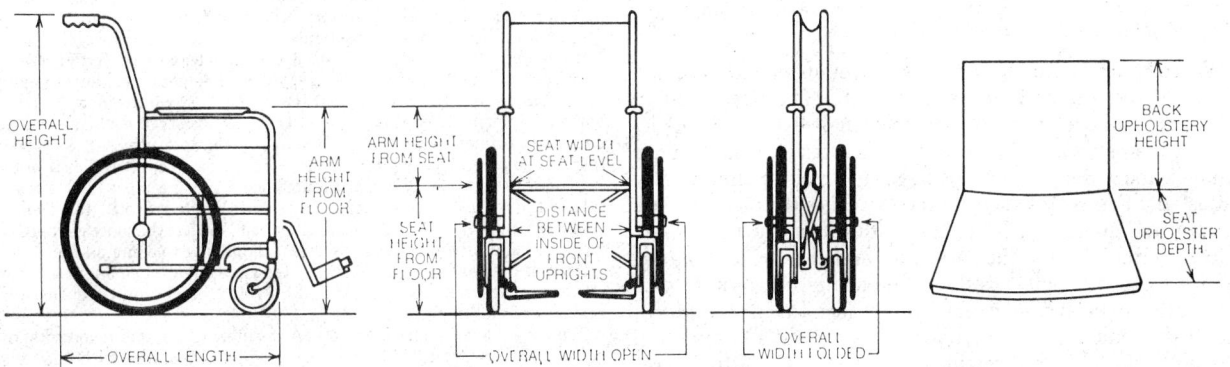

Fig 104-2. Key to wheelchair dimensions (courtesy, Everest & Jennings).

Desk-Style Armrests—Enable any patient to wheel up comfortably close to tables and desks, and should always be considered; these are most important to patients with limited trunk control.

Solid Insert Seats—Can often remedy rotation sometimes caused by the folding chair's hammock seat. *Danger signal:* pressure sores developing between the knees; an aware observer will notice this potential long before it develops.

Push-Type Brakes—Aids the patient who cannot pull the brakes; in the final check, the brakes may have to be adjusted for tension.

Removable Armrests—Facilitate difficult transfers. Standard removable armrests add 1½″ to seat width; however, wrap around armrests will not increase chair width.

Seat Cushions—Prevent skin breakdown from sitting pressure.

Reclining Feature—For support and comfort of patients with poor trunk balance.

Cushions and Supplies for Pressure Sores

Many types of cushions are available for a variety of purposes. Some are used to simulate a hospital bed's gatch spring, thus enabling the patient to eat and work in bed in relative comfort, while others are used to bolster the patient's legs to achieve flexion of the lumbar spine during traction. The most important use is to protect the patient from bruises and prevent the occurrence of pressure sores (decubitus ulcers, bed sores).

Pressure sores result from pressure at the thinly covered bony prominences of the body such as the sacrum, tuberosities of the ischium (below the buttocks), heels, elbows, shoulder blades, and ears and back of the head in children. When pressure interferes with the normal circulation of capillary blood in the tissues, it causes localized ulceration and gangrene.

A pressure sore begins as a reddened area which, if left untreated, will develop into an open sore; if not corrected early, surgery may be the only feasible remedy. The best cure is prevention. According to Richard M Meer, Founder and Executive Director of the Center for Tissue Trauma Research and Education (Jensen Beach, Florida), "all pressure sores are preventable," a notion which unfortunately is still denied by some health professionals in institutions where pressure sores continue to occur. As health-care consultant to his or her customers, the community pharmacist is in a unique position to facilitate an understanding of pressure sore prevention techniques which can be used in the home-care environment.

Pressure sores most commonly occur after long-term confinement in either a bed or a wheelchair. If institutions where nursing services are provided or at home where family members are available, the following measures will prevent their occurrence:

1. Keep the bed dry and clean.
2. Thoroughly pat dry the skin after baths.
3. To increase circulation, regularly and gently massage the skin.
4. Change the position of the patient in bed as frequently as possible, at least a minimum of every two hours.
5. Relieve pressure as soon as the first signs of redness appear.
6. Expose the reddened area to the air and reduce pressure by using commercially available items (ie, cushions) to increase circulation.
7. Maintain proper nutrition.

Wheelchairs should never be used over an extended period of time without some kind of seat cushion. The most frequent occurrence of pressure sores in wheelchair users is at the ischial tuberosities. Pressure sores also result from a chair which is too wide, too small, or whose footrests are improperly adjusted. Footrests which are too low cause the patient's legs to hang off the front edge of the seat upholstery, thus interrupting circulation to the lower legs, and also cause some patient's knees to come together, increasing the possibility of pressure sores between the knees (see *Ring Cushion*). Footrests which are too high force the patient's knees up in the air and take body weight off the back of the thighs, re-

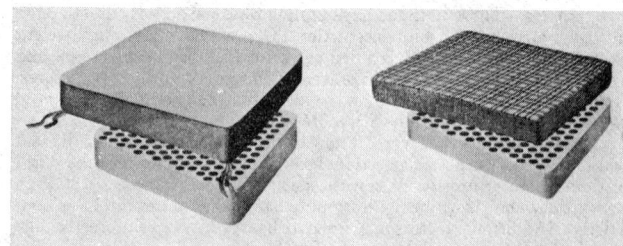

Fig 104-3. *Left:* 3″ latex foam rubber wheelchair cushion with seat ties; *right:* 2″ latex foam rubber wheelchair cushion in washable cover (courtesy, Guardian Products).

sulting in all of the patient's body weight being focused directly on the ischial tuberosities.

There are literally scores of wheelchair cushions on the market, ranging in price from under $10 to more than $350. The most commonly used types are:

Ring Cushion—When pressure sores begin to develop between the patient's knees, perhaps the best cushion to relieve the pressure is the ring cushion (doughnut cushion). It has a relatively small inside and outside diameter and is made of either foam rubber or inflatable rubber; both work equally well.

Sheepskin Cushion (or Pad)—A standard cushion used in hospitals for decades, in wheelchairs and in the hospital bed, is the natural sheepskin cushion. Its fluffy thick hair provides a good relief from pressure. While it is still used in bed, by itself it is inadequate for the wheelchair. Today, there are several manufacturers of synthetic sheepskins which are superior to natural sheepskin because their polyester fibers will not support bacterial growth and their porous back permits adequate drainage and air flow. The synthetic sheepskin is helpful to the wheelchair user if placed on top of another cushion and works best when in direct contact with the skin.

The usual solution for pressure sores occurring on the elbows and heels is either a large synthetic sheepskin or individual heel and elbow protectors. They incorporate the sheepskin in a plastic holder that straps to the foot or elbow.

Foam Cushion—The most common wheelchair cushions are made of polyfoam or latex foam rubber (see Fig 104-3). They come in a variety of seat sizes and in 1″, 2″, 3″, and 4″ thicknesses. A study conducted by the Rancho Los Amigos Hospital in Downey, CA, compared these and other wheelchair cushions. The study showed that the best for the money was the 3″ cushion and, further, that dense latex foam rubber was superior to polyfoam. The pharmacist should recommend a cushion with a removable cloth cover that has ties, thus enabling the cushion to be secured to the wheelchair seat back.

Horseshoe Cushion—This is an effective modification of the foam cushion with its cut-out in one side. It usually comes with a board insert which provides stability in an inherently unstable cushion. This cushion is ideal when pressure sores exist or are anticipated at the base of the patient's spine, and is also used postsurgically for hemorrhoidectomies and patients who have suffered a fracture of the coccyx.

Inflatable Ring Cushion—The wheelchair size inflatable ring cushion can also be effective providing it is neither underinflated (permitting the patient to bottom out) nor overinflated (making it hard and nonresilient). Circular air cushions vary in outside diameter from 12 to 17″ The ischial tuberosities in the adult are customarily 4 to 6″ apart. The inside diameter of a ring cushion used in a wheelchair should parallel these bones, or not be more than 2″ wider. The hole in the center of the circular air cushion is generally slightly more than one-third the outside diameter. Air cushions that are too small force the bones apart and cause rectal and anal discomfort; too large, the bones are forced together, closing the rectum and anus and causing pain, particularly when hemorrhoids are present. For most adults a 16″ cushion with a 4½″ id is usually preferred.

Silicone Gel Cushion—In recent years wheelchair cushions of many types have appeared on the market. The first of the new breed of wheelchair cushions, developed by Stryker, consists of a silicone gel enclosed in a rubber bladder. The idea was to simulate adipose tissue (body fat) and so perfectly distribute body weight that decubitus ulcers would be nearly impossible. This cushion, which sells for almost $400, was the talk of the industry for a number of years. While it is still an excellent cushion for many patients, it has a drawback in that the loose gel permits some roll and creates a shearing effect damaging to some patients with tendencies toward pressure sores. Less expensive gel cushions are now on the market, some selling for under $100. The boron gel cushion by Spenco sells for about $100.

Water-Filled Foam Cushion—A cushion which has received some acclaim is the water-filled foam cushion, which when filled with water and all the air is expelled, conforms to the body contours to provide almost even pressure throughout. While it is an excellent cushion, it is extremely heavy and, like the silicone gel cushion, is hard to carry. Wheelchair users who drive their own cars with the aid of hand controls, and must transfer to their cars independently, find this type of cushion most difficult to handle. The water makes it sloppy and hard to hold onto even with its carrying straps.

Resin-Filled Cushion—This cushion received one of the highest ratings in the Rancho Los Amigos study. It is considerably lighter than the silicone or water cushions, yet also conforms to the body contours. It does so more slowly, due to its nature, and maintains a "memory" enabling the patient to jostle and move a bit while in his chair without the roll typical of the water and gel cushions.

Alternating Pressure Pad—An old standby both in wheelchair cushions and hospital bed mattresses is the alternating pressure pad (APP). The pad is an air mattress arranged in longitudinal tubes and connected to an air pump which alternately inflates and deflates alternate rows of tubes every 60 to 120 sec. To eliminate counter pressure sometimes created by the smooth long tubes in earlier APP pads, newer configurations include small pillows arranged longitudinally, in lieu of straight tubes. It works on the principle that circulation in the tissues occurs in the absence of pressure. The pad is very effective in preventing and treating pressure sores in hospital beds but is less effective in wheelchairs. The pads, either permanent or the newer disposable type, present problems with respect to punctures and care should be exercised with sharp objects. The pad is placed beneath the bottom bed sheet and, with connectors, most machines can operate two pads simultaneously.

Convoluted Foam Cushion—The top surface of this foam cushion consists of rows of cones, giving it an egg-crate appearance. It remains popular in retail stores and many nursing homes, but has yet to be utilized extensively in the rehabilitation setting.

Roho Balloon Cushion—Rows of inflatable balloons make up the surface of this cushion. A pressure gauge is used to adjust the pressure in each balloon. After a tenuous beginning, this cushion is enjoying increasing popularity. It sells for about $250.

Newer Cushions on the market include a beanbag type filled with polyethylene beads and, in competition with the large and expensive hospital-style water bed, there is a complete water mattress for any bed at home or in the hospital.

All the wheelchair seat cushions described above may be used on the bed, but they are usually inserted in a foam mattress designed to admit the wheelchair seat-size cushion and provide a full level surface.

Canes and Crutches

Canes

Although walking canes are very simple devices, they are frequently misused and misfitted. The problem stems from a lack of basic knowledge as to what a walking cane is supposed to do and how it should be properly used.

A walking cane serves two important functions: weight transfer and balance.

Weight Transfer—It provides a means to transfer weight off the weak limb. To accomplish this weight must be put on the cane. If the patient carries the cane on the side of his weak limb and puts 50 lb of weight on it, he transfers 50 lb off his weak limb. The same is true if the cane is carried on the strong side. While the choice of carrying hand has nothing to do with weight transfer, it is crucial for proper balance.

Balance—Good balance in walking is no more than keeping one's center of gravity over the supporting limbs. If you suddenly lift one of your feet off the floor, you would reduce your base of support to one foot, your center of gravity would be outside the base of your support, and you would fall. People who walk with legs apart tend to waddle as they must move their centers of gravity from one foot to the other to avoid falling. Fashion models avoid waddling by learning to place one foot directly in front of the other so their centers of gravity move forward rather than side to side.

If the patient carries his cane on the same side as his weak limb, his base of support will be narrow (ie, the distance between the cane tip and his weak limb is small) and he will have to transfer his weight from side to side, increasing the possibility of falling. A narrow base of support makes it difficult for the patient to keep his center of gravity over that base. If he is instructed to carry his walking cane on the side opposite his weak limb, his base of support will be wide and his center of gravity can move primarily forward rather than side to side. He uses the cane together with his weak limb, alternately swinging his strong limb through for the next step.

Unless specifically instructed by the patient's physician or physical therapist to the contrary, always instruct the patient to carry his walking cane on his strong side.

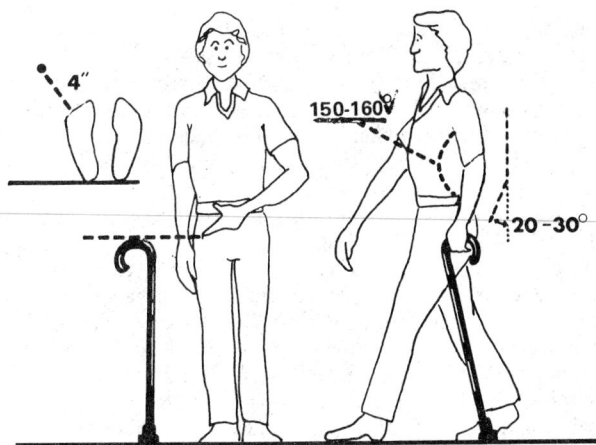

Fig 104-4.   Proper fitting for canes, walkers, and crutches.

Fitting—A cane should be neither too long nor too short. Each one must be adjusted or cut to fit the patient. Fitting a cane is quite simple. Most schools of physical therapy recommend that a walking cane should fit so that the patient's arm makes a 150–160° (from vertical) bend at the elbow; this places the muscle groups in the arm in the best position for firm support. The cane tip should be placed 4″ in front of the toe at an approximate 45° angle; angle the cane back to the hanging arm and the handle of the cane should be at the crease in the wrist. Then, when the patient lifts his hand up to the cane handle, his elbow will form the desired 20–30° bend automatically. See Fig 104-4.

If the patient normally has one shoulder higher than the other, as in cases where the patients has scoliosis (an S-shaped curvature of the spine), no effort should be made to straighten them for the fitting. One cannot measure one side of the patient and then use that measurement for the other side. Each side must be measured separately. His arms should be made to hang normally. If the patient has trouble standing without support, he should be backed up against a wall during the fitting. The back of a chair can be used effectively for support. Rather than measuring at the top of the cane for an indication of where to cut it, turn the cane upside down for the fitting.

These rules apply in the fitting and use of all ambulatory aids including forearm crutches, axillary crutches, and walkers.

Walkers

The most common walker in terms of sales and rentals continues to be the adult adjustable walker. A basic inventory of walkers in any pharmacy should include:

1. Adult adjustable walker
2. Adult nonadjustable walker
3. Child's adjustable walker
4. Adult folding, adjustable walker
5. Adult reciprocating, adjustable walker
6. Hemiplegic walker
7. Walkane

Except for the reciprocating walker, proper use is the same for all nonwheeled walkers. The patient is instructed to lift the walker, place it in front of him, and walk to it. With this method, the walker is firmly on the floor when the patient is moving. A walker should never be carried by a walking patient; if he is able to do this with relative security, a cane would probably suffice.

A frequent problem encountered is that patients tend to lean into the walker while walking up to it. The danger is that they may lose their balance and push the walker over as it is relatively light. This tendency can be overcome by lengthening the front two legs of the walker by one adjustment making the walker tilt back. This should not be a routine adjustment for all walkers, however; rather, it should be a response to a specific tendency of the patient to lean into the walker.

The reciprocating walker is used differently than the typical nonwheeled walker. It is hinged so that the right side can be swung forward independently of the left so that the walker is actually made to walk. As though the patient were using two walking canes, he is instructed to use the side of the walker opposite the leg getting his body weight. It may take some practice but the patient should learn to develop the necessary two-point gait (see next page). This walker was designed for a fairly agile and relatively strong patient. It should not be used for very infirm patients.

The only safe wheeled walker is one with a braking mechanism that will stop it if the patient trips or loses his balance. The braking mechanism should work when the patient's weight is increased on the normal hand holds.

As in the case of walking canes, all walkers should be adjusted for each user. Nonadjustable walkers should also be cut to size with an ordinary tubing cutter. For this reason, nonadjustable walkers should be sold, not rented.

To properly fit a walker, the patient should stand normally against a wall if necessary. The legs of the walker are adjusted or cut off so that the top of the handgrips come to the patient's wrist. On raising his hands to the walker handgrips, the patient's elbows will form the proper bend. See Fig 104-4. When it is also necessary to lengthen the front legs of a nonwheeled walker, the wrist-crease length should be accurate for the walker's rear legs. The front legs of the walker will then be 1 to 2" longer depending on the extent to which the patient leans into the walker.

In terms of support, a walker can best be compared to the simple cane. While a walker does provide a steadier support for the patient, like the cane, it requires reasonably good arms, wrists, and hands.

Crutches

Forearm Crutches—Neither walking canes nor walkers provide support to the patient's wrists and elbows. The forearm crutch, however, is designed specifically to provide such support in that it has a vertical member which extends above the wrist and is secured reasonably well to the fleshy part of the forearm by a collar or cuff.

The term forearm crutch is generic. They are commonly referred to as Canadian crutches, Lofstrand crutches, cuff crutches, or Kenny sticks. All can be recognized by the collar or cuff which encircles the patient's forearm. With the exception of the Kenny stick, the cuff is usually open and the opening may either face the side or front. It is important that the cuff is open so the crutches may be thrown out of the way if the patient falls. The handgrip projects from the main shaft and, unless specifically instructed by the physician or physical therapist to the contrary, the patient should be instructed to hold the handgrip so that it points forward.

If only one crutch is used, it should be used on the side opposite the weak leg. When two crutches are used, the patient should be instructed to step forward with his right leg and his left crutch, followed by his left leg and right crutch, and so on. Commonly known as the two-point gait, it is recommended for persons using forearm crutches, unless of course, the physician or physical therapist suggests a different gait.

In fitting the forearm crutch, the patient should stand normally erect, with arms at his sides. The forearm cuff is

flipped back out of the way, and the handgrip is brought to the crease in his wrists by adjusting or cutting the main shaft. The length of the vertical member between the handgrip and the forearm cuff should also be adjusted so that the cuff comes to the middle of the patient's forearm, usually over the fleshiest part. Care should be taken to see that the cuff doesn't interfere with the elbow when it is fully bent. The cuff can be opened or closed by bending and shaping by hand with very little effort. The patient should be shown how to do this as he may want the cuff larger or tighter depending on his clothing.

Axillary Crutches—More common than the forearm crutch is the ordinary wooden or aluminum underarm crutch—the axillary crutch. It provides more support than the forearm crutch because it braces both wrist and elbow.

Adjustable crutches are preferred as they offer better and easier fitting. First, the patient should stand normally erect with arms at his sides. The crutch is placed under the arms with the crutch tip on the floor at a point approximately 6 to 8" ahead of his toes and 6 to 8" to the side. The main shaft is lengthened or shortened so that the top of the crutch is about 1½" (two finger-widths) from the armpit. This fitting should be done with crutch tips and axillary cushions in place on the crutch.

The second step is to adjust the position of the handgrip on the crutch so that it comes to the crease in the wrist. The crutch should be in the same position for this handgrip adjustment as it was during the fitting of its entire length. The arm is then brought out alongside the crutch for the handgrip adjustment.

A flexed elbow is important when using an axillary crutch. If the handgrip is not positioned at the wrist so that the elbow bends when he takes hold of the handgrip, the tops of the crutches would push up into his armpits with each swing. But with his elbows bent initially, the crutch tops are safely below the armpits since the patient must straighten his arms on the swing through. When axillary crutches are properly fitted, there is little or no danger of injury to the lymph glands, blood vessels or radial nerves in the armpits which can lead to "crutch paralysis". The primary danger signal is an elevation in the patient's shoulders with each swing through his crutches. When that happens it is clear that the patient's weight is bearing on the crutch tops and not on the hand grips as it should be.

There are several axillary crutch gaits; the safest, most stable, and most common is the four-point gait. The patient begins by moving his left crutch forward. Next, he moves his right leg forward. His right crutch is then brought up to his right foot, and, finally, his left leg is brought up to his left crutch.

The two-point gait, the principal gait used when two canes are employed, is also commonly used with forearm and axillary crutches. Simply, both the left crutch and right leg are brought forward; then the right crutch and left leg are brought forward.

The three-point gait has two variations: the swing-to gait and the swing-through gait. In either form, the patient begins by moving both crutches forward simultaneously. In the swing-to gait, both feet (or one foot for an amputee or when one leg is in a non-weight-bearing cast) are swung to a point between the two crutches. In the swing-through gait, the feet (or foot) are swung through the crutches to a point ahead of the two crutches—it helps to visualize a triangle made by the two crutch tips and foot, and flipping that triangle end-over-end.

Another common crutch gait is the hemiplegic gait. It is nothing more than the use of a single axillary crutch in exactly the same manner as one would use a single cane. The crutch is carried on the strong side and is moved forward together with the weak limb alternating with the good leg.

Accessories

Tips—The most important accessory is the tip which makes contact with the floor. No cane or crutch should ever be sold or rented without a good tip. Safety requires that cane and crutch tips have the following minimum characteristics: they must fit the cane or crutch shaft snugly, have a suction-grip bottom, and have a flexible neck so the bottom of the tip will stay in complete contact with the floor when the cane or crutch rocks through a gait. The suction-grip bottom of a crutch or cane tip should be as large as possible—the more rubber in contact with the floor, the less chance of slippage.

Axillary cushions are available in two basic styles—one with a powdery finish and the other without a powdery finish in almost a translucent, amber-colored rubber—and a variety of sizes. The powdery one doesn't last as long as the amber one, but the amber one is rougher on clothing. Both types adequately protect the underarm from bruises and inhibit slippage of the crutch top from under the arm.

Handgrips are more varied in type and style, however, as they are designed for various purposes. The most common kinds are dense foam rubber sleeves which fit over the standard crutch grip. The split handgrips should be used for nonadjustable crutches only, as they tend to slip around the handgrip. Taping them tightly will secure them somewhat. The nonsplit, often called closed, handgrip is better for the patient but it requires removal of the crutch's handgrip to put it on.

Other contoured handgrips and "palmgrips" are available. Since the natural palm line is not horizontal, they are designed to alleviate problems such as hand discomfort and wrist soreness associated with the traditional horizontal crutch handgrip. Many walking canes are now manufactured with handles that solve this problem, but few crutches are.

Commodes

A commode is little more than a portable toilet and yet there are a variety of different types. More than a convenience, a commode can mean the difference between coming home and staying in the hospital. Whenever the patient is unable to ambulate from his bed to the bathroom, there is a need for a commode.

Perhaps the most common type is the steel or aluminum frame commode with a toilet seat and cover plus a removable plastic pail and cover. It adequately serves its intended purpose though it may look like a commode and be undesirable for that reason. This type comes with either nonadjustable or adjustable legs. The latter is most desirable since some patients need a rather tall one to aid them both in sitting and getting up more easily. The "Drop-arm" steel commode enables easier transfer to and from the commode seat. Some patients also find this innovation helpful where there is a need to insert suppositories. Depending upon the attitude of the patient and, more often, that of his family, an aluminum folding commode can be removed from view when it is not in use.

The common aluminum and steel frame commode uses its uplifted toilet seat cover as a backrest. Commodes are available with padded and nonpadded backs, an upholstered seat and armrests, and casters for moving about easily (see Fig 104-5); others are made of wood and resemble furniture—eg, the disguised, Danish Modern commode. Many wheelchairs provide a commode insert in place of the regular seat upholstery. They are difficult to use, however, as the toilet seat cover cannot be removed when the patient is sitting in the chair.

Although commodes may be rented in most states, it is unwise to reuse the commode pail; it should be sold to the customer during the first month's rental. It is also helpful to

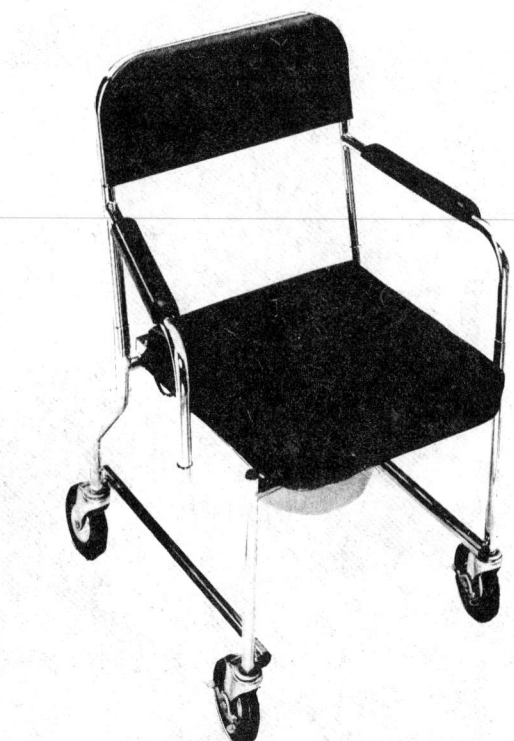

Fig 104-5.   Padded commode on casters with pivot arms (courtesy, Lumex).

advise the patient's family that a pail filled to one-third with water will be easier to keep clean. Deodorant tablets and drops are also appropriate as an accessory to any commode rental or sale.

Bathroom Safety Aids

Safety in the bathroom primarily means safety in the tub or at the toilet. An elevated toilet seat makes it easier for patients to sit or stand and suggests the need for some kind of toilet guard rail (see Fig 104-6); they are available in both aluminum and steel and are either free-standing or attaching. Attaching-type toilet rails either attach to the wall behind the toilet or to the bowl with the regular toilet seat bolts. Some attaching types are designed with detachable sides permitting the use of one side only, as well as easier cleaning of the rail in general.

Elevated toilet seats vary considerably with respect to the materials from which they are fabricated, whether or not they have full or partial splash guards, to what extent they are adjustable in height, and whether or not they are padded for softness or, like any normal toilet seat, quite hard. The full splash guard may be preferred by many people, but the pharmacist should keep in mind that persons without good legs and body control (paraplegics and quadriplegics particularly) need the open sides which only the elevated toilet seat with the partial splash guard has in order to administer to their personal cleanliness independently and to insert suppositories without assistance.

Other safety aids for the bathtub include adhesive strips and spots for the tub bottom and mats for the prevention of slips and a variety of tub seats and safety grab bars. Tub seats are either bench types with legs, or seats that straddle the tub sides (Fig 104-7). One of the more popular bath seats is a bench-type seat that hangs from the tub sides by means of wing-like extensions. A variation of this seat has a round swivel seat at the side which enables a person to sit and swing his legs into the tub before sliding down onto the tub seat.

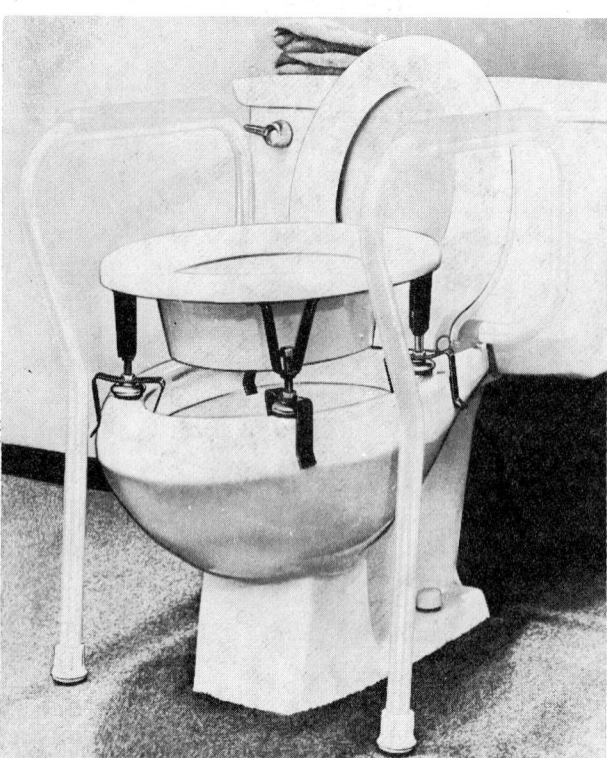

Fig 104-6.   Elevated toilet seat with continuous splash guard (courtesy, Lumex).

The other bathtub benches are waterproof stools with suction cupped legs that grip the tub floor, some of which have backs. They vary in height from 5″ to 22″. One bath seat has a hose which attaches to the water faucet and, powered by water pressure, actually raises and lowers from the height of the tub side to near the bottom. This seat can also be classified as a bath lift.

Bathtub grab bars range from those which attach to the side of the bathtub to wall-mounted grab bars. Perhaps the most frequently used type is one that extends high enough for a person standing outside the tub to get a firm support before stepping into the tub. Wall grab bars take a variety of shapes

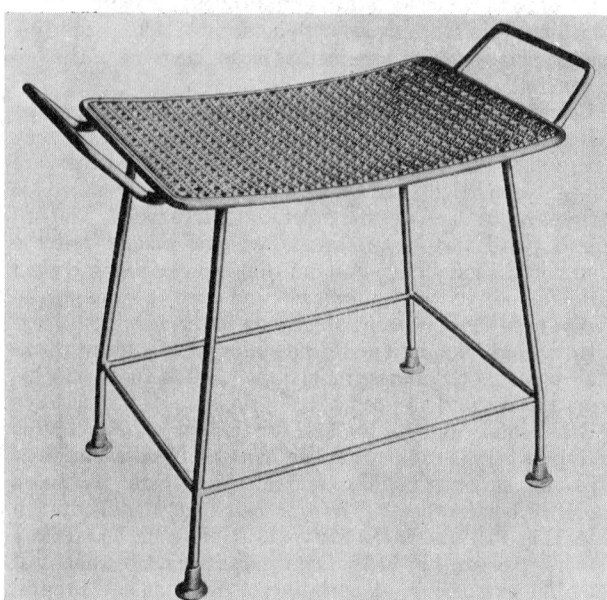

Fig 104-7.   Waterproof bathtub bench (courtesy, Edco).

and angles. The most important difference is whether they are resting bars or arm-hooking bars. Resting bars have their hand-holds approximately $1\frac{1}{2}$″ from the wall, enabling the patient to rest his forearm against both the bar and the wall. True grab bars extend from the wall at least 4 to 5″, enabling a falling person to slip his forearm behind the bar and hook his elbow over it. There is considerable controversy over which type is superior. The pharmacist should be familiar with both types and determine which certain doctors and physical therapists prefer.

Another important consideration is how the various bars are attached to the wall. Whatever the method, the pharmacist should know how the bars he stocks are best mounted for safety and either be able to instruct the customer in mounting procedure, provide such service, or have someone who will provide installation services on call and also be aware of liability when providing installation services.

Hospital Beds

The health accessories department of a pharmacy may also have hospital beds for sale or rental, including a manually operated and an electrically operated bed. The former may have a split gatch spring that allows the bed to be separated into the headboard, the footboard, and the two halves of the gatch spring. The bed should be variable in height, and its gatch spring should have an adjustable head section and also an adjustable foot section that raises the patient's knees as well as permits the feet to be elevated.

The electrically operated bed may be either the 6-way or 4-way type. The height of the 6-way bed is adjustable from the floor, and it has a gatch spring which permits positioning of both the head and foot sections. The 4-way bed has the adjustable gatch spring but its height from the floor must be adjusted manually.

Mattresses—Polyfoam mattresses are excellent for rental purposes, especially with split-spring hospital beds, as one man can handle them easily. An innerspring mattress should be used with an electrically operated bed, or when the heavier mattress is preferred; however not every innerspring mattress will work well on a hospital bed, since the springs must be hinged in order to have the mattress flex properly when the gatch spring is adjusted.

Any mattress used for rental purposes should be covered with a plastic-impregnated mattress ticking and it is well also to provide plastic mattress covers. Some states have laws regulating the sanitizing of rental mattresses. The pharmacist should be aware of the local laws in his community.

Bedside Safety Rails—It is recommended to stock two types of bedside safety rails, one for use on a hospital bed, and the other for use on any kind of bed normally used in the home. Rails for use with a hospital bed have clamps which attach to the steel parts of the gatch spring. Rails used on home-type beds are attached by connecting rods placed between the regular mattress and box spring. This "any-bed" type of safety rail is usually made of aluminum with cross-members of steel (Fig 104-8). Hospital bed rails may be constructed of aluminum or steel.

Trapeze Bars—The typical over-bed trapeze bar is used by the patient as an assist in sitting up and getting into and out of bed. It is usually made of steel and by means of clamps is attached to the headboard of a hospital bed. A trapeze-bar floor-stand, which enables the trapeze to be used over any bed, is also available (Fig 104-9).

Trapeze bars are adjustable in height, and some models also provide adjustability in the position of the bar over the bed. A special clamp permits the bar to be swung to various positions and locked for security. A pivoting trapeze bar should never be used with the floor stand, as accidents may occur unless the bar is suspended properly.

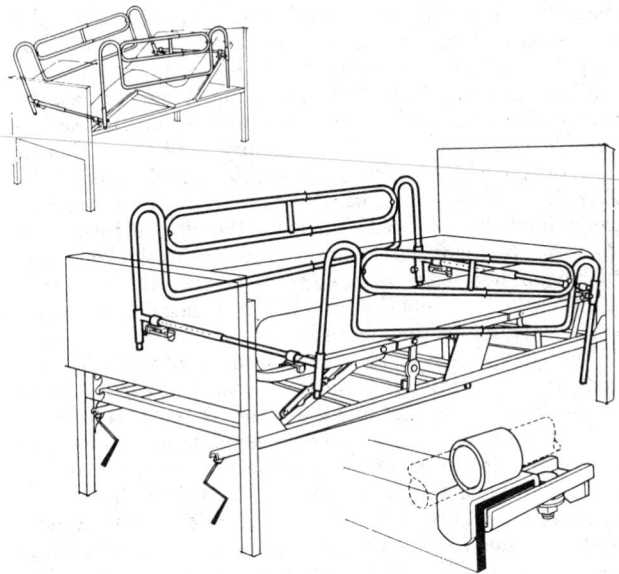

Fig 104-8.   Any-bed model safety rails showing connecting cross bar (courtesy, Edco).

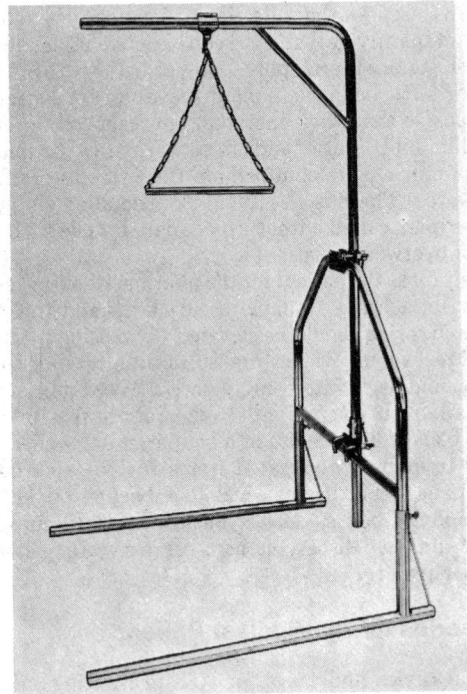

Fig 104-9.   Overbed trapeze bar with floor stand (courtesy, Invacare).

Traction

Overdoor traction sets provide for cervical traction at home using any open door for the purpose of mounting the traction pulleys. Weight is applied to the cervical spine by a rope running over the pulleys and attaching to a halter which fits over the patient's head and applies pressure to the patient's mandible and occiput. The weights may be cast-iron traction weights suspended on a traction-weight hanger, or a graduated water-weight bag containing tap water in accordance with the weight-of-water markings on the plastic bag, or a cloth bag containing weighed articles (cans of soup, etc). An additional item in most overdoor traction sets is a metal or wooden

spreader bar which spreads the top of the head halter in order to avoid pressure against the patient's ears.

Unless specifically instructed by the patient's physician to the contrary, the pharmacist should tell the patient to use the overdoor traction set while sitting in a chair facing the door. When doing so, the patient's head will be pulled toward the front, bending his chin down and flexing his cervical spine. Flexion is generally preferred over hyperextension in any type of traction. If the patient were to sit with his back to the door, as has been illustrated on the covers of overdoor traction sets for many years, his chin would be pulled up and his cervical spine would be hyperextended—usually an undesirable attitude during cervical traction.

Approximately 95% of patients who require traction will need it in a flexion posture, the remaining 5% needing hyperextension. It may be dangerous to use flexion on patients who require hyperextension.

Any traction set—even the ordinary overdoor traction set—should be sold or rented only on the written prescription of a physician who specifies the frequency of treatment, the length of each treatment, the weight to be applied, whether the traction is to be static or intermittent, and special instructions as to positioning of the patient with respect to flexion and hyperextension.

Traction in Bed—While cervical traction may be given either while the patient is sitting in a chair or reclining in bed, pelvic traction is administered to a patient at home only when he is in prone position. There are two basic types of applied-in-bed traction sets; one is for use with a hospital bed and the other for use with any bed. The any-bed traction device has the typical vertical adjustments and pulleys and is mounted on a floor-stand. Buck's extension traction device requires a sturdy headboard or footboard as it has no floorstand. Either type of traction unit is used for both pelvic and cervical traction.

When applying cervical traction to a patient lying in bed, unless specifically instructed by the patient's physician to the contrary, traction pulleys are usually mounted quite high so as to develop flexion of the cervical spine and mildly depress the patient's chin.

When pelvic traction is applied, flexion is also important, and the pulleys should be mounted quite high to produce flexion of the lumbar spine. It may also be helpful to raise the head section of the hospital bed or bolster the ordinary bed with a wedge cushion or mattress elevator. Additionally, the patient's knees should be elevated either with the knee adjustments of the hospital gatch spring or ordinary pillows placed under the patient's knees. These recommendations must have the approval of the patient's physician.

A complete traction department will also have pelvic traction belts in a variety of sizes, without which pelvic traction cannot be applied. If overstock is a concern, it should be noted that a universal traction device fits "all", therefore reducing inventory for pelvic traction devices. In addition, a variety of traction leggings and anklets are necessary accessories, as is a wide assortment of cast-iron and aluminum traction weights and weight hangers.

An intermittent traction machine that electrically sets pounds of pull, number of seconds of pull, and number of seconds of rest during the treatment is available. Some machines can also be set for length of the entire traction treatment. Intermittent traction machines, used in physical therapy departments of hospitals, may be attached to wall brackets, where they are used for vertical applications of cervical traction, or clamped to special tables which wheel up to the hospital bed for horizontal applications of cervical and pelvic traction. Such tables are also appropriate for use in the patient's home when intermittent traction is prescribed.

Sometimes special types of traction are prescribed for patients at home. Many of these require use of a variety of over-the-bed fracture frames and clamp-on pulleys which are connected to provide traction longitudinally and laterally to arms and legs; their setup and application require the expertise of a physical therapist or doctor of physical medicine. Where this kind of traction may be prescribed, the pharmacist should arrange to meet the physical therapist at the patient's home to be certain that the equipment the therapist will need is procured.

Traction accessories include various sizes of bed blocks, slatted bedboards, and adjustable footboards.

Patient Lifters

Among a wide range of hydraulic and screw-type patient lifters, the floor-model hydraulic patient lifter is the most commonly used (Fig 104-10). All lifters have an adjustable boom to which a patient-carrying sling or seat is attached. Lifter bases differ though they are typically U-shaped and may be either adjustable or nonadjustable in width. The adjustable base can be spread wide and moved around almost any chair or commode so the patient sling is suspended directly over the seat to which the patient will transfer.

Sling design is an important consideration when choosing a patient lifter. Slings in all fabrics come as one- or two-piece units, with and without head supports; they may also be had with a commode opening.

Positioning the sling under the patient while he is in bed is accomplished in much the same way that bed linens are changed under a patient. He is rolled to his side while half the sling is folded in accordion fashion and tucked up against the patient. The sling should be so positioned that on rolling the patient back his spine will rest on the middle of the sling. The patient is rolled back over the folded portion of the sling and to his other side while the folded part of the sling is unfolded; then the patient is returned to his back. Attention

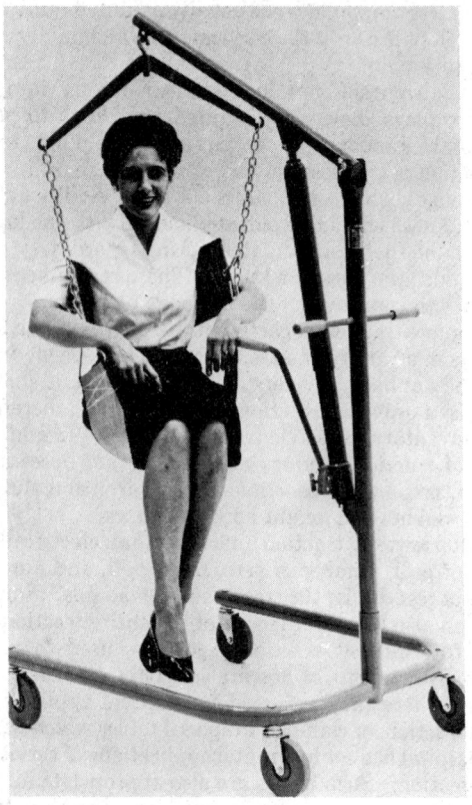

Fig 104-10. Painted hydraulic patient lifter with nonadjustable base and two-piece canvas patient sling (courtesy, Ted Hoyer & Co.).

should be paid to the vertical positioning of the sling also—the bottom edge of the sling should not extend to the middle of the patient's knee, but rather should just come to the knee.

When the sling is properly placed under the patient, the lifter is brought to the bed, the chains or straps are hooked up and the boom raised slowly and gently until the patient is lifted off the mattress. The patient should take hold of the lifter chains if he is able, otherwise his arms should be safely inside the sling. To avoid swinging of the sling on moving the lifter, the attendant should cross the patient's ankles and hold the bottom heel with one hand while he pulls the lifter with the other. The patient should always be facing the lifter when he is suspended by the lifter sling.

When the patient is ready to be lowered into a chair, commode or tub, the attendant should release the hydraulic valve carefully and slowly, guiding the patient into position by his heel. A common mistake is to remove the sling from beneath the patient after transferring him to a chair or commode. It is considerably easier, and safer too, to let the patient sit on his sling, and remove only the chains and lifter from his view. When it's time to pick him up again, the lifter need only be brought into position, the chains hooked up, and the patient lifted slowly out of his chair.

Bedpans

Bedpans, used for the collection of feces, may be round but are predominantly oval and are constructed of plastic, stainless steel, enamelware, porcelain, or rubber. Single-patient-use plastic bedpans (nonautoclavable) are considerably less expensive than their metal and porcelain counterparts. Plastic, like rubber, also tends to be warmer to the touch and therefore much more comfortable than steel, porcelain, or enamelware. There is also available a smaller, sloping and flatter bedpan, called a fracture bedpan, for use with immobilized or overweight patients.

It is helpful to the patient for the pharmacist to suggest that, when a hospital bed is available, the back rest and knee section of the gatch spring should be elevated when using the bedpan. The backrest should be elevated substantially while the knee section should be elevated only slightly. When a hospital bed is not available in the patient's home, four or five pillows behind his back will make use of a bedpan much easier.

Other frequently requested items for the sickroom are douche pans, wash basins, oval foot basins, buckets with covers, sponge bowls, emesis basins, sputum cups, thermometer jars, soap dishes, pitchers, carafes, water glasses, and medicine cups.

Accessories for the Bedfast Patient

Special tables and trays for spill-preventing safety and patient comfort are near-essentials in any sickroom (Fig 104-11). The common overbed table is an ideal accessory whether or not the patient has a hospital bed. Some overbed tables have a center section that can be raised to a slanted position for the support of a book or magazine; others have a vanity tray and mirror which slide out from beneath the table top for use by the bedfast patient. Sturdy breakfast trays that straddle the patient's hips while he is in bed, special folding tables and trays with contoured fronts which enable the wheelchair user to get comfortably close, and even a special lounge chair with its own adjustable and self-storing table contribute to the nonambulatory patient's comfort and convenience in the sickroom at home.

Easy-reachers are devices that enable the bedfast patient to reach out and pick up things normally beyond his reach. A whistle switch permits a light or television set to be turned on and off from a distance. The patient merely squeezes a rubber syringe bulb with a high frequency whistle; the whistle is

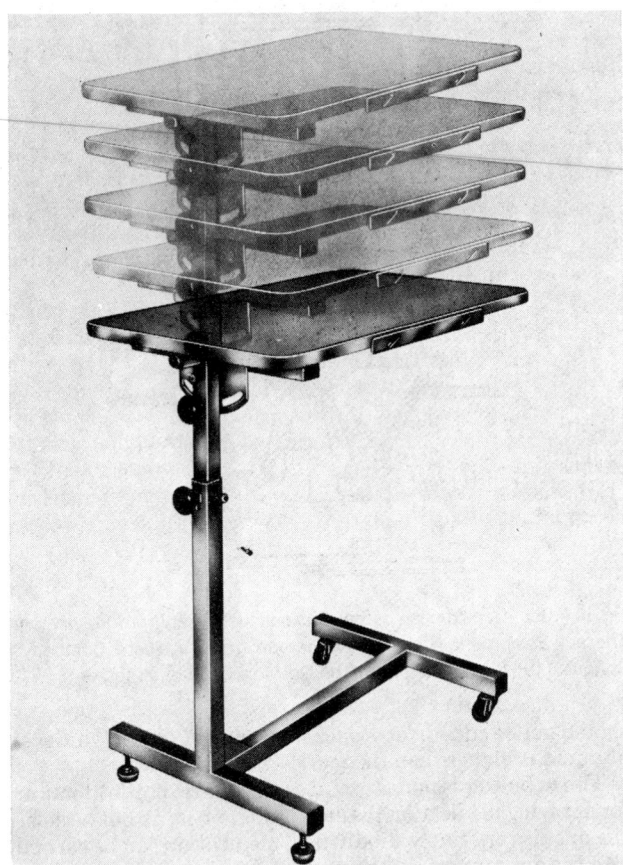

Fig 104-11.   Adjustable overbed table with tilt-top for books or magazines (courtesy, Lumex).

picked up by a control device at the wall socket into which the lamp, TV set, or other electrical appliance is plugged. Simple Environmental Control Units also allow the patient to control the TV, lights, etc by the touch of a button or the use of a *joystick*. BSR brand is common. Electric timers are also useful in enabling the bedfast patient to maintain some degree of independence at home.

A plastic shampoo tray facilitates shampooing for patients who cannot leave their beds. The tray fits across the mattress where a pillow normally goes, and is designed to carry shampoo water to a drain at the side of the bed where it may be collected in a plastic bucket. The patient's head rests in the shampoo tray which, though it has quite high sides, has a depression for the back of the patient's neck.

Folding backrests with or without arms, mattress elevators which are placed between an ordinary mattress and the boxspring, wedge-shaped foam cushions, bedboards, and footboards with adjustable cushions for the prevention of foot rotation are additional articles for the comfort and convenience of the bedfast patient. When it is necessary to keep bed linens and blankets off the patient's feet and legs, a blanket support, sometimes referred to as a leg or body cradle, is desirable. Holding mitts, built-up forks and swivel spoons, food-guards, feeding-cups, pencil and cigarette holders, and simple drinking straws with accordion hinges that bend without collapsing, are some of the devices which make patient home-care effective.

Folding patient-privacy screens are a frequently requested sickroom accessory, especially when the patient will be using a bedside commode.

Finally, a health accessories department will also stock a modest assortment of safety vests and belts, crib nets, and restraints for use by nursing homes and extended-care facilities, as well as by the patient at home.

Respiratory Therapy

Steam Vaporizers—The modern steam inhaler is essentially the same as the now nearly forgotten croup kettle, except that it uses electricity to generate heat and steam. The advantage of this more modern adaptation lies in the attainment of a constant temperature. Also most forms of this apparatus are equipped with a regulator so that when they run dry, the heating unit shuts off simultaneously. These are also easier to handle in the home, especially at night.

The familiar vaporizer provides the conventional hot-steam therapy for the relief of upper respiratory illnesses. Physicians recommend it for colds, sinusitis, and similar ailments.

The portable room humidifier, on the other hand, provides a cool mist to compensate for the lack of sufficient moisture in the air in dry, steam-heated rooms, and occasionally for its expectorant effect in liquefying tenacious mucus in the airway. An additional advantage is that, since no heater is used, it is entirely safe for small children.

Some vaporizers are used solely for their warm, moist spray while others are provided with a chamber or cup in which a volatile medication can be placed in liquid form or on cotton. The steam passes over this material, as in Bergson's original vaporizer, causing the medication to volatilize and pass out of the spray.

Steam inhalers do not deliver a spray and can carry medication in their vapors only when such medication is volatile at the temperature of boiling water. However, steam vaporizers are valuable for ordinary home treatment of colds, coughs, and other respiratory diseases.

In the electrode-type vaporizer, two electrodes are separated from contact by an insulating nonconductor. When mineral-containing water is added to the reservoir, an electric current passes between the electrodes and heats the water to boiling. The mineral content is necessary to permit the passage of electricity. The content of minerals should be kept to a minimum, however, as an excess of dissolved material will cause foaming, frothing, and spilling over. Distilled water, to which a small quantity of salt has been added, is preferable. Hard water is usually not satisfactory. Electrode-type vaporizers should be cleaned periodically.

In heater-type vaporizers, an ordinary heating element connected to ordinary house current is immersed in a reservoir of water. Many heater-type vaporizers now have thermostatic controls. A cup or chamber is provided for volatile medication. Any kind of water is satisfactory and the reservoir can be replenished at will. The value of this type of vaporizer rests almost entirely with its warmth and moist spray.

Vaporizers are used extensively in the home today to humidify bedrooms or chambers where patients suffering from various bronchial conditions may rest. Cool-vapor humidifiers provide effective high-humidity inhalation therapy for respiratory patients, and can be used as well to restore proper humidity to rooms dried out by winter heating. They are of breakproof metal or plastic, in modern colorful designs. Prominent among such humidifiers is the versatile heat, moisture and medication vaporizer, *Croupaire* (produced by Air-Shields), and those supplied by Hankscraft, Northern Electric, and others.

Types of electrode and heater vaporizers are shown in Figs 104-12 and 104-13.

Plastic Bottle Atomizers—Several firms are now offering solutions, intended for the treatment of the nasal passages, in plastic containers or accompanied with plastic atomizers. These bottle-like containers are flexible and when pressed produce an atomized spray or, when inverted and pressed, force out the solution in drops. Where a very potent drug is to be employed infrequently, with a single inhalation generally affording control of an acute attack, as in bronchial asthma,

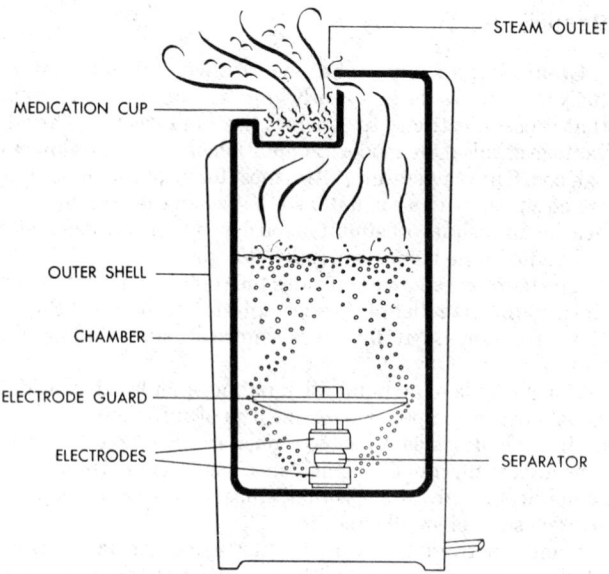

Fig 104-12.   Electrode-type vaporizer.

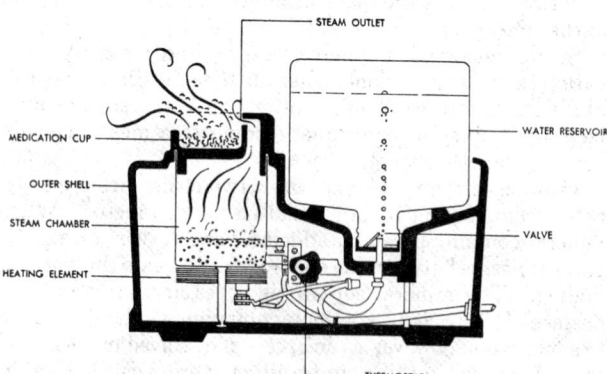

Fig 104-13.   Heater-type vaporizer.

emphysema, or bronchitis, a modified form of aerosol device may be employed. Typical of these are the *Mistometer* (Winthrop) or *Medihaler* (Riker). The *Mistometer* and *Medihaler* are similar in construction and the former is shown as assembled for use (Fig 104-14).

Nebulizers—Instruments that generate very fine particles of liquid in a gas of uniform particle size are called nebulizers. Within the container of the nebulizer apparatus is a small atomizing unit that produces atomization inside the flask. The wall of the flask acts as a baffle, removing large droplets from the mist which run down the wall and drop back into the reservoir, and producing a mist of small droplets that penetrate further into the lung. A current of air or oxygen carries the fine mist through the large outlet tube of the nebulizer. The flask of the nebulizer has a mark beyond which fluid

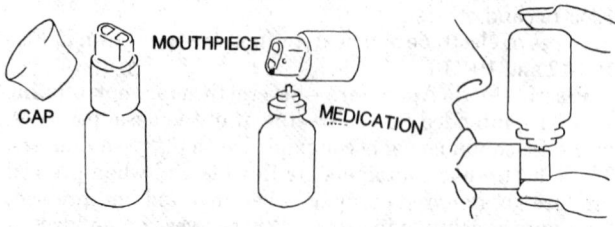

Fig 104-14.   "Mistometer" type of inhaler, used by Isuprel (courtesy, Winthrop).

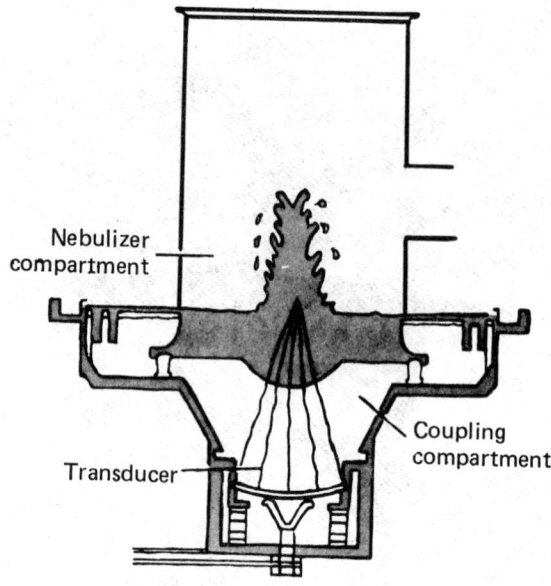

Fig 104-15.   Construction of the ultrasonic nebulizer (from *Respiratory Therapy Equipment*, Steven P McPherson; The CV Mosby Company: St Louis (1981); modified from The DeVilbis Co, Somerset, Pa).

should not be added, for atomization will not occur if the level of liquid is higher than the mark.

The nebulizer is not as useful as the plastic bottle atomizer for applying medication to the nose and pharynx but because the mist is very finely subdivided, medication can be carried into the deeper parts of the respiratory tract. The nebulizer is especially valuable for diseases of the larynx and trachea as well as various kinds of obstructive airway disease and accompanying conditions which inhibit efficient ventilation.

Within the past decade, the ultrasonic nebulizer (Fig 104-15) has gained widespread application in respiratory therapy. The ultrasonic nebulizer produces sound waves by electric current causing vibrations that are utilized to break up water into aerosol particles. The resulting aerosol is a very dense mist with a water content in excess of 100 mg/L. The ultrasonic nebulizer is regarded as the most efficient of nebulizers since it is claimed to create better than 90% of its particles within the "effective" range of 0.5 to 3 μm.

The transducer of the ultrasonic nebulizer often is placed in a coupling chamber filled with water. Water helps absorb mechanically produced heat and acts as a transfer medium for sound waves to the nebulizer chamber.

Aerosol Therapy—A common use of the term *aerosol* is to describe a nebulized solution consisting of very fine particles carried by a propellent gas under pressure to a site of therapeutic application. The principal purpose of the use of an aerosol in respiratory therapy is the topical administration of medication and/or water or saline solution to the mucosal linings of the tracheobronchial tree. See Fig 104-16. To accomplish this the liquid has to be dispersed as droplets 5 μm or less in diameter. Various medications are used to treat a variety of conditions that accompany respiratory disease. Conditions requiring aerosol therapy, particularly when such therapy can be administered to a patient on a program of home care, include: (1) infection, (2) mucosal edema, (3) tenacious secretions, (4) foam buildup, (5) bronchospasms, and (6) loss of compliance.

Aerosol therapy provides an efficient means of administering an antibiotic directly to the infection and generally requires a smaller dosage than would be necessary if the drug were given systemically. Infection is often accompanied by one or more of the five other conditions cited above.

Edema of the mucous membrane which lines the interior

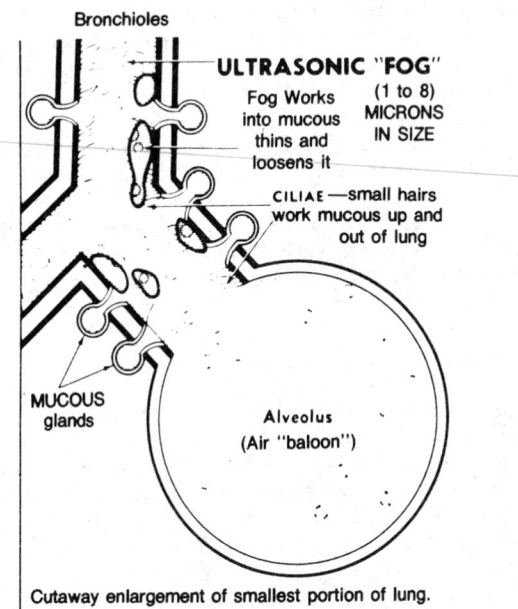

ULTRASONIC "FOG"
Fog Works into mucous thins and loosens it   **(1 to 8) MICRONS IN SIZE**

CILIAE—small hairs work mucous up and out of lung

Bronchioles

MUCOUS glands

Alveolus (Air "baloon")

Cutaway enlargement of smallest portion of lung.

Fig 104-16.   Ultrasonic aerosol is the most efficient at penetrating the terminal bronchioles and alveoli (courtesy, Wisconsin Lung Assoc).

walls of the tracheobronchial tree may seriously affect ventilation in the alveoli. Any swelling of the linings of the airways, especially in the terminal bronchioles and respiratory bronchioles, may severely impede the flow of air to alveoli, making breathing difficult and reducing efficiency of oxygen pickup.

When the mucosa becomes edematous the serous fluid it excretes may be profuse and thickened. Cold dry air or a compressed gas when used without adequate humidification will draw moisture out of the mucus, leaving it sludgelike and tenacious. Such mucus resists movement up the walls of the tracheobronchial tree normally accomplished with efficiency by the cilia throughout the airways and, instead, becomes gradually more viscous and forms mucus plugs which can shut off alveoli and, for that matter, entire airways, depriving whole sections of the lung of oxygen-rich air. Medications that help to loosen these plugs of mucus include wetting agents and a variety of proteolytic enzymes. Distilled water and normal saline solution are also effective in dissolving tenacious secretions.

Plugs of mucus in the tracheobronchial tree which only partially block the flow of air through an airway can cause other problems. Unobstructed passageways are said to exhibit laminar flow, but when smoothly flowing air moves over such plugs it becomes turbulent—a sound one hears as wheezing. The turbulent air then agitates the liquid on the surface of the mucosa and creates bubbles. When there are enough bubbles, they become foam—foam which can clog bronchioles and alveoli and dramatically diminish respiration at the capillaries. Alcohol, administered as an aerosol, will effectively break up foam and clear the airways. One pulmonary physiologist has been reported to prescribe vodka for use in the nebulizer by his home-care patient with admirable success.

Bronchospasms are contractions of the smooth, involuntary muscle surrounding the bronchioles. Bronchospasms severely constrict the bronchioles and, for obvious reasons, dangerously inhibit fluid ventilation of the lung. Bronchodilators are medications of choice in these cases, but care should be taken when the patient has a history of coronary problems.

When, due to tissue damage, edema, or simply lack of use, the lung's interstitial tissues lose their elasticity, the patient is said to have a loss of compliance of the lung. An inelastic lung works against the efforts of the rib cage and diaphragm, making lung ventilation extremely difficult. This condition is typical in the patient who has chronic emphysema, but also occurs in varying degree with other respiratory diseases. Exercise, not aerosol, is the method by which some compliance may be returned—and in those persons who suffer from a loss of compliance, an intermittent positive-pressure breathing machine may be necessary. Loss of compliance is included in the section, because it will affect the usefulness of aerosol in administration of a medication. Where lung compliance is a factor, the aerosol should be given under pressure.

Aerosol may be given using either a mask or mouthpiece. Short delivery tubes from the aerosol generator will provide optimum density of aerosol; long and bending main tubes should be avoided as they reduce the concentration of particles in the aerosol which "rain out" on their way to the patient. Warm aerosols tend to carry more moisture into the lung, thereby reducing evaporation from the mucous membrane. Warm aerosols also tend to be more soothing to the patient. If aerosol generators are cleaned scrupulously after each treatment, their effectiveness will be maintained.

Other medicinal and pharmaceutical uses of aerosols are discussed in Chapter 93.

Intermittent Positive Pressure Breathing Machines—Intermittent positive pressure breathing (IPPB) machines for patient treatment at home have been available for many years. IPPB is a technique in which the lungs are actively inflated by means of regulated positive pressure during inspiration. Positive pressure on inspiration enables a patient with chronic obstructive airway disease to inhale deeply when conditions within his lungs make full ventilation impossible on his own. The technique is called intermittent because the positive pressure is cut off when the lung is adequately filled, permitting the patient to exhale without assistance. While negative pressure is sometimes used to assist the patient during exhalation, its use is extremely infrequent outside the critical-care hospital or medical treatment center.

IPPB is used to accomplish several things. Pressure is needed in some patients in order to get air into blocked areas of the lungs. In those instances, forcing air into an area of the lung which was previously blocked or which was not ventilated due to lung tissues having become rigid, allows an aerosol to be delivered to that part of the lung. And with air behind a plug of mucus the patient is able to expel the plug by coughing. IPPB therapy may provide a significantly deeper breath than the patient can produce with spontaneous ventilation. Positive pressure also aids in relief of bronchospasms through delivered medication, helps to improve drainage, and provides exercise for stiff lung tissues, by far the most important way to return compliance to the lung.

IPPB machines operate using either the force of compressed gas from a cylinder at home or in the hospital or a hospital in-wall system, or, as is the case with most home models, by means of self-contained compression using ordinary room air.

IPPB machines may be either automatic cycling, manually operated, or entirely responsive to the patient's breathing. Machines that operate automatically, beginning and ending each inspiration and expiration regardless of what the patient has in mind, are really respirators designed for unconscious patients and are not well-suited for therapy treatments. While there are some manually operated IPPB machines, the much preferred models are responsive to the patient's breathing.

The latter machines begin the inspiration cycle the instant the patient begins to inhale. The cycling valve responds to the slightest negative pressure and begins the positive flow of air immediately. Machines that have this capability are said to have a "patient-demand" inspiration cycle. These IPPB machines also end the inspiration cycle in response to the patient's breathing. The cycling valve reacts to a predetermined positive pressure. On these machines, a pressure gauge is set by adjusting a dial on the front of the machine. Pressure in all IPPB machines is measured in centimeters of water, a uniform standard in all makes and models. Once set, the machine will automatically shut off flow of air when the patient's pulmonary pressure reaches the preset level. Theoretically, because there is a closed system between the machine's cycling valve and the patient's lung via the main IPPB tube, mouthpiece and trachea, the pressure at the cycling valve is equal to the pressure inside the patient's lung. The cycling pressure can then be set so air will continue to flow into the patient's lung—opening airways and ventilating alveoli in the process, until the preset pressure is reached.

The difficulty frequently encountered with persons just beginning to use an IPPB machine is that they feel uncomfortable having air forced into their lungs, though there is rarely any pain. There is a tendency in these persons to want to stop the flow of air into their lungs. Almost involuntarily, the glottis is closed and the accessory muscles of expiration are brought into action causing back-pressure against the inflow of air and registering an immediate high pressure at the sensitive cycling valve. When that back pressure is equal to the preset cycling pressure in the machine, it does indeed cycle, permitting exhalation. It takes practice and time for most new patients to feel comfortable with an IPPB machine. Part of the responsibility of the pharmacist who sets up such a machine in the patient's home is to guide him in the use of his machine and help him get over any initial uneasiness.

During the first few treatments, many patients tend to overdo it, especially soon after they have become used to the machine. Because they may be breathing much deeper than usual while they are using the machine, they may easily become hyperventilated. Oxygen intoxication, as the condition is sometimes called, may leave the patient feeling dizzy. He should be counseled to take his time and after a couple of breaths on the IPPB machine, alternate with several normal breaths. At signs of dizziness, he should breathe normally until his dizziness disappears. Breathing with an IPPB machine should be a comfortable and relaxing experience.

Among specifications which the physician will include in his prescription for IPPB therapy at home are:

1. The level of positive pressure in centimeters of water, and further instructions as to when, and if, and to what extent, the pressure should be increased.
2. The duration of each treatment.
3. The number of treatments per day and/or week, and at what times during the day those treatments should be taken.
4. The specific medication or medications for each treatment, including concentration and dosage. If the physician does not want to administer medication with each treatment, he should specify whether the nebulizer should contain distilled water or normal saline solution—an IPPB machine must never be run dry.

On the average, the prescription for IPPB therapy at home requires a pressure setting of between 10 and 20 cm of water pressure and treatment duration of between 10 and 20 min. The number of treatments varies greatly, from two to three/week, to three to four times/day. Sometimes the prescription merely suggests "As needed." But under no circumstances should an intermittent positive pressure breathing machine be rented or sold without a doctor's prescription!

During equipment setup, the pharmacist should teach the patient how to adjust the pressure dial on the face of the machine and how to read the pressure gauges. IPPB therapy is not without its potential risks, due mainly to overuse. Potential hazards of significant frequency are: excessive ventilation; excessive oxygenation; decreased cardiac output; increased intracranial pressure; pneumothorax; and hemoptysis. The pharmacist should be aware of these potential risk hazards and work closely with the respiratory therapist and the physician, following prescription orders precisely. It is generally advisable to type the complete prescription on a gummed label, and paste the label on the face of the machine where the patient can see it.

An IPPB setup is never complete until the pharmacist has reviewed with the patient details of the doctor's prescription, how the medication is measured and the nebulizer prepared, how the pressure is adjusted, how the gauges are read, how to clean the nebulizer jets and main tube accessories after each treatment, and where to reach the pharmacist during and after working hours in the event of an emergency.

Hypodermic Equipment

Syringes are instruments intended for the injection of water or other liquids into the body or its cavities. They are classified according to differences in principle of action into three categories: (1) *plunger syringes*, such as the hypodermic syringes; (2) *bulb syringes*, of which the ear and ulcer syringes are a type; and (3) *gravity syringes*, characterized by the fountain syringes.

On the basis of capacity, syringes may also be classified into three groups: (1) *small*, those of 10 mL or less capacity, such as the hypodermic type; (2) *medium*, those from 10 mL to 100 mL in volume, of which the ear and ulcer syringes are examples (although some special hypodermic syringes are available in sizes up to 500-mL capacity); and (3) *large*, such as enema or vaginal syringes.

Hypodermic Syringes—These syringes are used to administer medication *subcutaneously* (under the skin) or *intradermally, intravenously* (into a vein or artery), or *intramuscularly* (into the muscle).

Hypodermic syringes are seldom used by the average patient, with the exception of diabetics. Because of their illicit application in the administration of narcotics, in some states it is illegal for hypodermic syringes to be found in the possession of laymen.

Parenteral therapy or injection of medication under the skin and through tissues dates from the beginning of the 19th century. The first crude instrument of this type was a needle trocar, developed to deposit morphine in paste form. The principle of introducing medication under the skin, however, became popular in the first half of the 20th century.

The basic principle of the *hypodermic syringe* uses a combination of a glass barrel through which a carefully fitted glass plunger passes and a needle attachment which pierces the skin. Two developments led to the basic principle of hypodermic medication. At first, glass syringes were merely drawn to a glass needle point, a dangerous device due to breakage. The application by Pravaz in 1853 of a separate needle and a separate syringe led to the later development of the all-glass syringe and metal needle. Screw-joint connections of needle and syringe did not prove satisfactory. These required washers to prevent leakage and their attachment was time-consuming. The familiar friction connection of metal on ground glass was later developed and proved safer, more practical, and provided a secure fastening.

Luer Syringes—The inventor of this type of apparatus, Dr Luer, patented his syringe; the letters patent have long since expired but today most hypodermic syringes of this style bear his name. The outstanding feature of the Luer syringe was its ground-glass surfaces. In many instances, the inside of the glass barrel and the outside of the glass plunger were ground individually. Later, they were ground together so that they will provide a perfect fit and prevent back leakage. The plunger must accurately fit and securely close the barrel or cylinder. The latest type of Luer syringe has an unground glass barrel with a fitted ground glass plunger. The clear glass barrel is tougher, stronger, more resistant to breakage, and

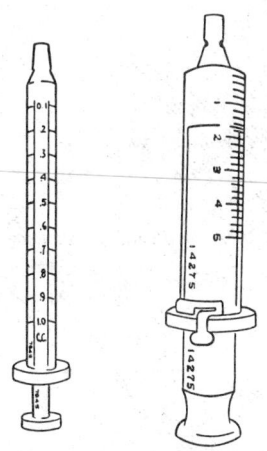

Fig 104-17. Hypodermic syringes. Left, tuberculin or vaccine syringe, graduated in 10ths or 100ths of a mL; right, Luer-type syringe 1 mL to 50 mL capacity.

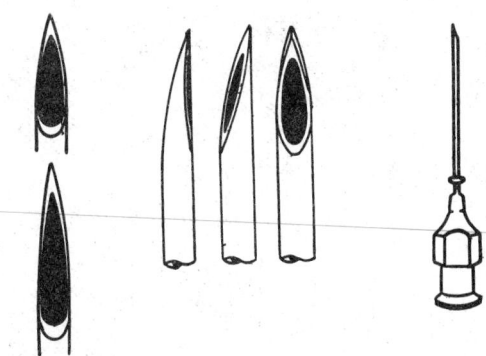

Fig 104-18. Hypodermic needles. Left, short-bevel and long-bevel needle points; left center, the Huber point with closed bevel and side opening to avoid producing tissue plugs; right center, regular point showing features which insure less cutting, more distention of tissue, reduced trauma, seepage, and after-pain; *right*, needle with security button which prevents a broken cannula from becoming lost in the tissues.

eliminates the loss from friction or erosion that occurs with the ground-glass barrel. Although Luer syringes are comparatively expensive and easily broken, they have many superior qualities. They are accurate in measuring medication for administration, they can be sterilized readily by boiling the pieces separately, and they may be adapted to many purposes and needs.

Luer syringes are customarily prepared of *resistance* or *Pyrex glass*. The latter is more fragile. Shock-resistant glass can withstand rapid temperature changes from freezing to boiling. Manufacturers customarily place identical matching numbers on each paired plunger and cylinder to insure that the user will properly match or "pair" the parts. It is not always necessary to "pair" the plunger and barrel. Several manufacturers are now making syringes with interchangeable barrels and plungers. See Fig 104-17.

Hypodermic syringes are always of the plunger type, characterized by the type of piston and difference of size or capacity. The *tuberculin syringe* is a small syringe not exceeding 1 mL in capacity, and graduated in 0.1- or 0.01-mL divisions. The *hypodermic syringe* is usually of 2-mL to 50-mL capacity. There are larger piston syringes, ranging up to 200 mL, for various purposes such as transfusions and veterinary medicine. Graduations may be in fractions of a mL or in *minims*. Syringes may also be prepared with special graduations, such as *units* of insulin.

To test the efficiency of a hypodermic syringe, close the tip with the finger and attempt to withdraw the plunger. If the plunger and barrel fit perfectly the vacuum created in the cylinder will prevent withdrawal of the plunger.

Disposable Hypodermic Syringes—Various types of disposable hypodermic syringes, each carrying a single dose of sterile medication, are now supplied as a standard dosage container by many pharmaceutical manufacturers. They have become popular for the administration of penicillin, and other antibiotics, antihistamines, tranquilizers, heparin, narcotics, biologicals, and the vitamins.

Disposable hypodermic syringes—empty, without medication—are available from several sources. See Appendices A and B for a complete listing of suppliers; some are plastic, others glass. Separate disposable needles, packed sterile in envelopes, are also available.

Hypodermic Needles—Hypodermic needles used with Luer syringes are of metal, and consist of a hub, which locks to the ground-glass tip by friction, and a needle point which varies in diameter and length. Needles are also called *cannulas*. Hypodermic needles may be made of stainless steel, hyperchrome steel, carbon steel, chromium, nickeloid, platinum, platinum-iridium, silver, or gold.

Hypodermic needles are characterized by their different points, which have a long, tapering reinforced point and beveled cutting edges of varying degree. A *long-bevel* or

long-taper needle is used for local anesthesia, aspirating, hypodermoclysis, and subcutaneous administration. A *short-bevel* needle is used for intravenous administration, infusions, and transfusions. A *special short-bevel* needle is employed for intradermal and spinal administration (Fig 104-18).

Size of Hypodermic Needles—Selection of a size is governed by four factors—safety, rate of flow, comfort of patient, and depth of penetration. There are three standard dimensions—length, outside diameter of the cannula and wall thickness. Regular needles are measured for length from where the cannula joins the hub to the tip of the point (hub not included). Special needles that have a "bead" or stop on the cannula (such as the B-D "Security") are measured from the "bead" to the tip of the point; always the working part of the cannula.

The gauge of a needle is measured by the outside diameter of the cannula or needle shaft. The usual range of diameter for needles is from 13-gauge (largest diameter) to 27-gauge. Needles seldom are less than $\frac{1}{4}''$ in length or longer than $3\frac{1}{2}''$.

There are many special needles, designed for a variety of purposes. Various *biopsy* and *bone-marrow transfusion* needles range from 16-gauge to 19-gauge and $\frac{1}{2}''$ to $3\frac{1}{2}''$ in size. They are characterized by their heavy shaped hubs.

Needles for *local anesthesia* range from 26-gauge $\frac{1}{2}''$ to 20-gauge 6″. *Intravenous*, *blood transfusion* needles, some with fitted cannulae, range from 19-gauge $1\frac{1}{4}''$ to 15-gauge $2\frac{1}{2}''$.

There are also special needles and cannulae for *abscess*, *eye*, *hemorrhoidal*, *tonsil*, *laryngeal*, and *pneumothorax* use.

These many types of special purpose hypodermic needles are of varying sizes in diameter, and varying lengths. Some of these are shown in Fig 104-19. These are intended for single-shot anesthesia, epidural; long-needle and short-bevel needles for *intravenous anesthesia; caudal* needles; *blood transfusion* needles; short-bevel beaded needles for *local anesthesia; biopsy* needle for bone-marrow aspirations; *infusion* needle, with female Luer slip; *hemorrhoidal injection* needle, with threaded adjustable gauge to adjust depth of puncture; *cerebral angiography* needle with thin-walled outer cannula, corrugated shield, and inner cannula. There are many others, such as specially shaped needles for pneumothorax, electroencephalography, aortography, arteriography, cholangiography, discography, lymphangiography, myelography, ventriculography, and tracheotomy.

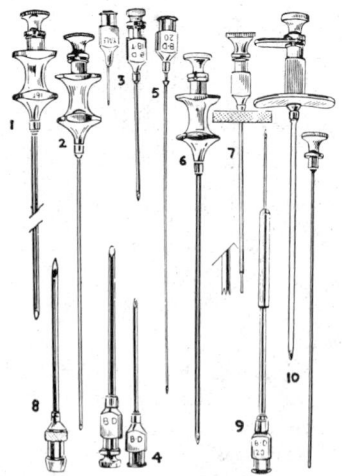

Fig 104-19. Special hypodermic needles—1: caudal needle; 2: epidural needle for single-shot anesthesia; 3: intravenous anesthesia short-bevel and long needles (with vinyl tubing); 4: blood transfusion needles (with vinyl tubing); 5: short-bevel beaded local anesthesia needles; 6: spinal needle with large spool hub; 7: biopsy needle for bone marrow aspirations; 8: infusion needle, with female luer slip; 9: hemorrhoidal needle with threaded adjustable gauge to adjust depth of puncture; 10: cerebral angiography needle with thin-walled outer cannula, corrugated shield, and inner cannula (courtesy, Becton-Dickinson).

Bulb Syringes

Bulb syringes are frequently preferred for use where sterility is not necessary or where plunger-type syringes, because of their force, would be dangerous to use. Bulb syringes are of particular value in the nose and ear.

The Asepto Syringe—This type, modifications of which are produced by several firms, consists of a glass barrel with a tip shaped to meet a particular need, with a small rubber bulb whose compression provides the necessary force. The rubber bulb is fitted inside one end of the barrel, instead of outside as is usually the case in bulb syringes. The rubber does not stretch and the syringe is less likely to get out of shape. The size of the bulb is gauged to the capacity of the barrel, so that the fluid is not drawn into the rubber bulb. The bulb is readily removable and the barrel can be easily cleansed and sterilized. Various modifications of this type of syringe are available for bladder, urethra, cervix, ear, nose, and larynx treatment (Fig 104-20).

A sterile, disposable syringe with finger grips and printed calibrations on the shatterproof polypropylene barrel is the *Medaseptic D* unit with catheter tip and tip protector, packed in peel-pack envelope (Baxter—Canada). See Fig 104-21.

Other Bulb Syringes—These syringes are customarily known by the name of the part of the body for which they are intended.

Nasal syringes or *nasal aspirators* are soft rubber bulbs of about 1 ounce capacity, with an acorn-shaped nasal tip to fit the nostril. The tip may be either glass or hard rubber. Glass is more popular as the transparency allows visual examination of the mucous removed from the nostril (Fig 104-22).

Ear syringes and *ulcer syringes* are one-piece molded bulbs of soft, flexible rubber, with long, narrow nozzles and are

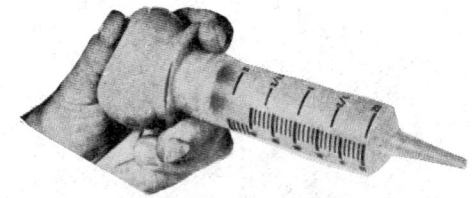

Fig 104-21. Special disposable formed bulb with printed polyethylene barrel and catheter point.

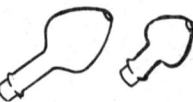

Fig 104-22. Nasal aspirator tips (either glass or hard rubber).

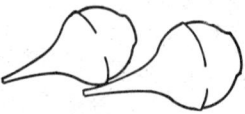

Fig 104-23. Infant's and adult's soft rubber ear and ulcer syringes.

employed in treating the eye, ear, and nose, and for irrigation of any open cavity or ulcer. See Fig 104-23.

If necessary, bulb syringes should be sterilized with germicidal solutions. Prolonged boiling will injure the rubber.

Nasal douches as the "Birmingham douche" are now only infrequently employed, and their use should be discouraged. Tilting the head backward forces the irrigating fluid and any infectious material into the Eustachian tubes connecting the nasal cavity and the ear. This spreads the infection. If a nasal syringe must be used, then the head should be bent forward and the nose washed out, allowing the liquid to flow out of the nose freely by gravity. For administration of medication into the nose, an atomizer is preferably employed.

Rectal syringes are customarily of the bulb type, with a long narrow nozzle. They are frequently employed in the administration of enemas to infants. These are the safest and least expensive of syringes requiring minimal maintenance. Such syringes customarily are of 1- to 4-oz capacity. Although many syringes provide hard rubber or vulcanite tips, the use of hard tips should be discouraged because of occasional injury to the soft tissues from their use (Fig 104-24).

Vaginal syringes, used for irrigation of the vagina, are 8- to 10-oz capacity bulb syringes with a large vulcanite or rubber spray tube. Pressure on the bulb forces the medicated or irrigating liquid through the tip of the syringe either in a direct stream or with a "whirling" motion. These syringes in white or various colors are provided with rubber sleeve-shaped round or oval shields to prevent leakage when in use. Caps sealing the nozzles are provided to avoid leakage or loss of the contents before use (Fig 104-25). One model has a convenient plastic stopper at the bottom of the bulb opening with a removable strainer, which permits mixing of medications.

Enema Syringes—*Enema syringes* are of two types, the more popular and preferable *fountain syringe*, and the other, the *valve syringe*. The latter has a rubber bulb with two

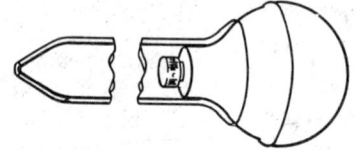

Fig 104-20. The Asepto syringe with improved bulb and plastic plug for easy cleaning.

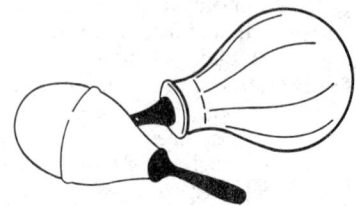

Fig 104-24. Infant's and adult's rectal syringes; soft rubber bulb and hard tip.

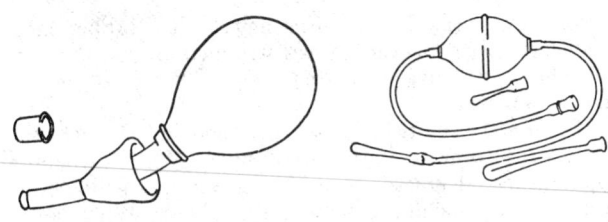

Fig 104-25.   Vaginal syringe

Fig 104-26.   Valve syringe for giving enemas or for vaginal irrigation; convenient for travelers.

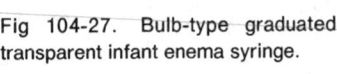

Fig 104-27.   Bulb-type graduated transparent infant enema syringe.

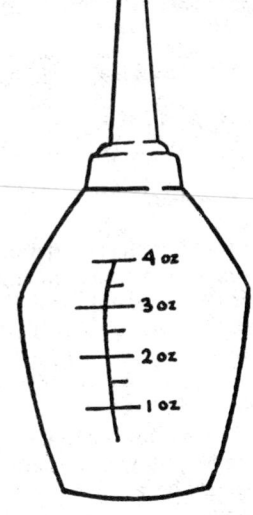

openings to which are connected flexible rubber tubes, one leading to the reservoir and the other to the spray tip. Alternate constriction of the bulb creates vacuum to draw up the irrigant from the reservoir into the bulb and then forces the liquid through the tube to the nozzle and the process is repeated. The intermittent flow of the latter may provide too great a force. This type is inferior to the fountain syringe although it is convenient for traveler's use (Fig 104-26).

Fountain syringes consist of a reservoir with a capacity of 1 to 3 qt, a 5-ft rubber tube, and a vaginal or rectal nozzle. These are used for irrigation with water, salt solution, soap suds, or special medications. The reservoir may be of rubber, which requires little storage space, and some grades are guaranteed to last a long time. Previously, glass or enamelware reservoirs were also employed. These proved to be readily cleaned and more sanitary.

Precautions to be observed by pharmacists in cautioning users of enema syringes are: the "drop" must not exceed 4 feet, to prevent excessive gravity pressure; the fluid should be maintained at body temperature to avoid chills or burns; and the tube is customarily closed with a mechanical metal pinchcock. Before using the syringe, the cut-off should be released for a moment until some liquid issues from the nozzle. The user must be certain that no air remains which might be forced from the tube into the body cavity. Hard rubber nozzles are frequently supplied with enema syringes but as they may cause damage to the rectum they are preferably replaced by catheters or tubes of soft rubber, about $3/16''$ in diameter by $15''$ in length.

Enemas—In simple constipation, whenever evacuation of the lower bowel is indicated, and when proctologic examination or surgery is indicated, an enema is customarily given because of its local, comfortable, and safe action in a relatively short period time. Castile soapsuds and other similar evacuants have long been employed but are now partially replaced by preparations whose hypertonic and surfactant properties insure rectal peristalsis and softening of impacted feces. Some aqueous solutions, 4 to 6 oz in quantity, contain sodium phosphate and biphosphate or sodium citrate and laurylsulfoacetate, sorbitol and sorbic acid, and glycerin. Liquid petrolatum is also employed. Either an unbreakable vinyl plastic squeeze bottle, or a plastic container and 30 to 60″ of tubing, each with a smooth 2-inch rectal tip, is provided. Enemas should not be used when nausea, vomiting, or abdominal pain is present, nor more often than necessary, to avoid dependence. Available as well are transparent, plastic, graduated (in half-ounces), 4-oz transparent or opaque infant enema syringes which allow accurate filling, mixing and use of the physician's prescribed formulas. See Fig 104-27. Prepared enemas are available for use in simple constipation or whenever evacuation of the lower bowel is indicated, such as in proctologic or sigmoidoscopic examinations; small, disposable units comprising flexible plastic bottles of 6 to 50 mL aqueous or oil solutions, with self-fitted comfortable plastic or rubber tip are available.

Dressings and First-Aid Supplies

The pharmacist is the proper distributor of sterile materials for treating wounds. His training enables him to appreciate the care necessary in their handling and storage, and he is often called upon for advice, or instruction as to their use. The following items fall in this class: absorbent cotton, cotton balls and buds, sterile rolls and pads of gauze, muslin and elastic bandages, disposable fabric tissues and underpads, eye pads, sponges, tissues and towels, plaster of Paris, adhesive plaster, adhesive elastic bandages, aerosol adherent, spray dressings, first-aid kits, scissors, tweezers, and applicators.

The pharmacy with a comprehensive health accessories department will stock bulk packages of these items for use by nursing homes, visiting nurses services, and patients who consume quantities sufficient to warrant their making larger purchases, in addition to the smaller packages for the pharmacy's usual customers.

The Family Medicine Cabinet—There is a place in every home where medicines are kept. The medicine cabinet should be either locked or completely out of the reach of children. Every bottle or box should be clearly labeled. Unused prescription medications, outdated over-the-counter drugs and empty bottles do not belong in the medicine cabinet and should be removed. Some community pharmacists provide folders containing information on first-aid, poison antidotes, and simple home medication for use by their customers so that the pharmacy's name is always in view in the medicine cabinet. This is also accomplished by providing a gummed "family prescription record" for the inside of the cabinet door, or an "emergency label" bearing space for entry of telephone numbers for doctor, pharmacy, hospital, fire and police departments, to be attached to the telephone or telephone book.

The following items for a family medicine cabinet were suggested in *Non-Prescription Drugs*, by the Editors of *Consumer Guide*, Beekman House, New York, 1979 (See Table I).

These items may be replaced by any others intended for the same purpose as may be selected by the pharmacist. In addition, in this age of interstate highways and greater leisure time the pharmacist should urge that every family car, camper, and boat be equipped with an adequate first-aid kit, in addition to a flashlight, flares, and a hand fire extinguisher.

Snake-Bite Kits—Anyone in snake, bee, or wasp country should carry a snake-bite kit (Fig 104-28). Usually available in a compact plastic or metal case are a tourniquet rubber or

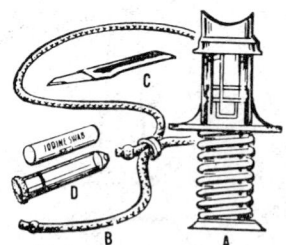

Fig 104-28. Pocket snake bite kit contains (A) suction device, (B) tourniquet, (C) incision blade, and (D) antiseptic swab.

other lymph constrictor, antiseptic, razor blade or knife, and one or more suction cups or syringes. These are available from Cutter or Becton-Dickinson. Many lives are saved each year by prompt action at the spot where the snake attacks, and relief from the pain and swelling of severe insect stings is also important. Snake bites are medical emergencies that require immediate treatment.

Every hospital pharmacist should have a chart of disaster unit equipment required for a hospital and all pharmacists should be familiar with the requirements and needs of disaster units.

Hot-Water Bottles—The best instruments for applying dry heat are the hot-water bottle and the electric heating pad. Made of rubber, hot-water bottles may be of the usual 2-qt size, or of the 1 pt capacity in the form of a "face bottle" for neuralgia of the head and for infant conditions. Each hot-water bottle has an opening through which warm water is added and a stopper securely sealed with a washer. It is more convenient to permanently attach the stopper to the bottle to prevent its loss. Some have screw stopper attachments, which permit conversion of the bottle into a fountain syringe.

Leakage must be guarded against. If customers are not familiar with the use of hot-water bottles they should be directed to fill the bottle with water to not more than one-half of its capacity. After the hot water is poured into the bottle, the bottle should be compressed to remove the remaining air, and then securely closed. This removal of excess air provides a more flexible bottle, one which shapes well to the contours of the body.

When filling a hot-water bottle, it should be held against the back of the hand or forearm to insure that the temperature is not too high. Bare rubber should never be allowed to come

Table I—The Home Medicine Cabinet

Medication	Purpose
Emetrol antinauseant	Nausea, vomiting
Antihistamine (oral)	Colds and allergy
Decongestant	Colds and allergy
Cough syrup	Coughs of colds
Aspirin, acetaminophen	Pain and fever
Activated charcoal	Poisoning
Syrup of ipecac	Poisoning
Rubbing alcohol	Mild antiseptic
Anti-infective cream	Minor cuts
Anesthetic cream	Burns, insect bites, etc
Antihistamine cream	Insect bites, minor skin allergies
Hydrocortisone cream	Insect bites, minor skin allergies

Supplies	
Adhesive tape (½″ wide)	Tweezers
Sterile bandages (2″ × 2″ and 4″ × 4″)	Thermometer (oral and rectal)
	Wooden tongue depressors
Cotton-tipped swabs	Flashlight
Gauze bandage rolls (1″ wide and 4″ wide)	Stethoscope
	Sphygmomanometer
Adhesive bandages (assorted sizes)	First aid manual
Scissors	

in contact with the skin, or burns may result. Rubber pads, flannelette bags, or even a towel wrapped around the hot-water bottle will give adequate passage of heat and comfort and convenience.

After use, the empty hot-water bottle should be hung by the tap at its bottom for thorough draining. Water of boiling temperature, oil, grease, alcohol, or turpentine should not be permitted to come in contact with the rubber. When not in use, all rubber devices should be protected from direct light to avoid hardening of the rubber.

Steam Packs—The hot-water bottle can also be used to apply moist heat by soaking a Turkish towel in hot water, squeezing out excess water, and wrapping the wet towel around the bottle. The use of a hot-water bottle in this fashion will maintain the temperature of the hot compress longer than is possible with the compress alone.

Various commercial steam packs are now in common use in hospitals and nursing homes, and are also available for use at home. These steam packs appear as compartmented, cloth bean bags when new, and are filled with tiny beads. When boiled in water, however, the beads become hydrated and combine into a gelatinous substance which has the unique property of holding its temperature far longer than any other steam pack—about 30 to 40 min.

Steam packs such as these must be wrapped in at least six layers of Turkish towel to prevent burns, and should never be used directly in contact with the skin. They are available in a variety of sizes, including a contoured pack designed specifically for neck and shoulders. The neck-contour steam pack, as well as others, also have optional terry-cloth covers, lined with foam rubber which takes the place of layers of toweling. Heating units are also available, but the patient at home can prepare a steam pack in an ordinary pot of boiling water. They can be used over and over again without loss of effectiveness if care is taken to avoid dehydration—easily accomplished by wrapping the steam pack in plastic kitchen-wrap and storing it in the refrigerator.

Electric Heating Pads—The advantage of the electric heating pad over the hot-water bottle lies in the fact that there is no possibility of leakage or spilling, and the temperature is constantly and indefinitely controlled. Most are wet-proof for wet or dry application, have soft foam padding and washable flannel covers. Some have adjustable heating elements which permit the temperature to be set at the desired level, and an illuminated temperature-control panel. One of the more popular electric, moist-heating pads is manufactured by Battle Creek under the trade name *Thermophore*. These heating pads are controlled by means of a handheld switch which automatically turns the unit off when released, eliminating the possibility of burns due to a patient's falling asleep. The Thermophore heating pad creates moist heat without pre-boiling or use of large amounts of water, hence its desirability in the home environment. The unit's flannel cover is dipped into water and then wrung dry. Intermittent applications of heat create "fomentation" or intense moist heat. The manufacturer recommends that treatments not exceed 30 minutes in length. All such electrical devices customarily are inspected to insure safe operation; however, short circuits and breakage of the heating element may result from constant use.

Automatic heat bonnets for scalp treatments; heat bandages for sprains, bursitis, arthritis; neck and throat heating pads for stiff neck or whiplash cases; sinus masks for heat therapy of sinus areas; and even thermal massagers are available.

Cold Application—In deep inflammation the effects of external application of either heat or cold are essentially similar, due to reflexes arising from the stimulation of the nerves conducting temperature sensation. Experience has shown that there are some conditions (such as appendicitis) where the application of cold is the more desirable.

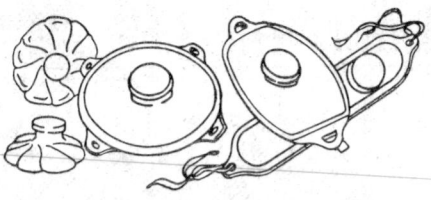

Fig 104-29.   Ice caps and bags.   Left, mackintosh cloth and rubber collapsible ice cap; center, ice bags; right, spinal and throat ice bags.

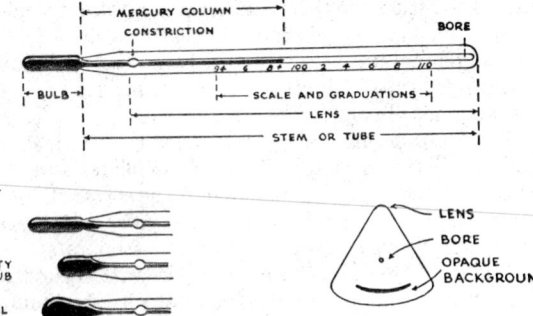

Fig 104-30.   Diagram of thermometer construction.

Appliances for local application of cold are: reusable cold packs and the familiar ice bag or ice cap. See Fig 104-29. The latter is usually a circular rubber or rubberized mackintosh cloth bag, circular in shape, with a large opening to admit cracked ice. Occasionally thick rubber, similar to that used in hot water bottles, is employed. Ice caps usually require a cover of some type to protect the skin. The contents of an ice cap are less flaccid than the liquid in hot-water bottles. Therefore, thin rubber or cloth construction is preferable in order to insure better conformation with the body. The pleated shape common to many ice caps avoids the bulginess and allows introduction of large amounts of ice.

An adaptation of the ice cap is used for throat inflammation. It is the collar-shaped rubber bag known as a tonsillectomy bag. It fits snugly around the neck, holding the ice on the parts. There are two styles, one with a spring clip and the other tying into place with strings or laces. Ice bags are also made in a long narrow shape for use around the throat and along the spine.

Cold Packs—Instead of using ice, some hospitals keep their ice bags filled with glycerin or an isopropyl alcohol-water mixture. These *redi-freeze ice packs* are stored in refrigerators until needed and are exchanged in the wards for bags which have become warm in use. Thus cold packs are immediately available at all times, and the liquid contents conform more readily to the contours of the body.

Ice packs of soft rubber or plastic, filled with a nontoxic solution of 10% propylene glycol and water are available in the usual designs. When stored in the freezing compartment or in the deep-freeze compartment of the refrigerator, the contents freeze to a semisolid or slush which provides greater comfort in use and longer retention of cold temperature than ice cubes. Fitted with tabs and tie-tapes, they are available in throat and body shapes.

In addition, instant hot and cold packs are available which provide a portable modality for heat and cold therapy ideal in situations where refrigeration or heating units are not accessible. To activate, the packs are struck firmly, which breaks an inner packet containing an activating fluid. This fluid comes into contact with the base chemical and the resulting chemical reaction is either endothermic producing cold, or exothermic producing heat. They maintain heat or cold for about 30 min, and then must be discarded.

Thermometers

Hippocrates in 460 BC recognized that abnormal human temperature was a disease symptom. In 1610 AD Sanctorius developed the first clumsy oral thermometer. The thermometer was unreliable until 1714, when Fahrenheit developed the first dependable scale and instrument. It had standard graduations and mercury was used as the heat-measuring liquid. In 1835, two Frenchmen, Becquerel and Breschet, established the mean, or average, temperature of a healthy man as 98.6° on the scale devised by Fahrenheit. A Hollander, Antoon Van Haen, in 1754 developed the first practical clinical thermometer. Thermometers were seldom depended on in medical practice until about 1865, when a

Scottish physician named Aitken invented a self-registering thermometer.

Thermometers for Home Use—The various types of thermometers usually employed in the home are: (1) the *household thermometer* or common type for reading interior or outside air temperature, (2) *bath thermometers* for recording the temperature of bath water, and (3) *clinical* or *fever thermometers* (Fig 104-30). The temperature of the atmosphere at the surface of the earth varies more than 200°F, but man's body temperature rarely varies beyond 97° to 104°F, with the portent of danger at either extreme.

The change in temperature of the patient is one of the important symptoms upon which the physician bases his diagnosis and treatment. The instrument employed for body temperature determination is the *clinical* or more popularly called *fever thermometer.*

An abnormal temperature is nature's warning that something is wrong. Rapid rise or fall and substantial deviations from normal are danger signals. Every home should have a fever thermometer available at all times.

The essential difference between an ordinary thermometer and one designed for determining body temperature is the self-registering feature of the fever thermometer. When the mercury column has risen to the maximum temperature, it remains until shaken back into the reservoir at the bottom of the instrument. This is due to a constriction which acts as a tiny check valve in the thermometer bore, just above the bulb, and permits passage of the mercury on expansion but does not permit return on contraction.

Clinical or Fever Thermometers—Three bulb types of fever thermometers are available: (1) the *oral type*, characterized by the slender mercury reservoir, most sensitive for mouth use; (2) the *rectal*, with a blunt, strong, pear-shaped bulb for safety and to insure retention in the rectum; and (3) a small, sturdy "universal," "security," "snub," or "stubby" type with a short stubby bulb, for oral or rectal use, and safer for babies or irrational patients. See Fig 104-30.

All fever thermometers have a magnifying lens front which renders the mercury column visible against an opaque background. Some have a colored line which by reflection helps detect the mercury column, or guide lines which center the eye on the image of the column. Others are flat in shape so that the markings are on the same plane as the mercury when the thermometer is held in normal reading position.

Taking Body Temperature—Fever thermometers should always be sterilized and shaken down below 97° before taking a reading. For *oral* temperatures, the thermometer should be placed in the mouth with the bulb under the rear edge of the tongue and rotated once or twice to assure complete contact. Transfer of body heat to the thermometer is speeded by then shifting the bulb to the opposite rear edge of the tongue. The lips should be kept closed and the thermometer left in the mouth for at least three minutes. Regardless of length of initial oral exposure, it is always well after the initial reading to return the thermometer to the patient's mouth for another minute, to provide a check or verification of the original temperature reading. Oral temperatures should not be taken for thirty minutes after exercising, smoking, eating, or taking hot or cold drinks.

Rectal temperature should be taken only with a rectal or stubby bulb thermometer. The bulb should be lubricated and gently inserted deeply enough to pass the constricting muscle, leaving about half the thermometer exposed. Babies should be held firmly face down, their buttocks separated with one hand and the thermometer held in place with the other. The thermometer should be left in place at least four minutes.

A longer time may be necessary for temperature readings if the thermometer is cold or if the patient is anemic or aged, with poor blood circulation. Axillary (under-arm) temperature is not recommended except when all other methods are impossible.

Normal Temperatures—The average normal mouth temperature is 98.6°F but some variations are natural. Healthy persons may have temperatures as much as 1°F above or below the average normal temperature. One's temperature may range from about 97.3°F at 2 to 5 am to about 98°F in the morning and to about 99°F in the late afternoon. One should determine his normal temperature by a series of readings while in good health for comparison as a personal standard when one is ill.

Normal rectal temperatures are usually 1°F higher, or 99.6°F, though the "normal" mark on all types of fever thermometers, including the rectal type, is at 98.6°.

Basal Temperature Graph—A woman who wishes to become pregnant may increase her chances of conception greatly by having intercourse at the time of ovulation, or she may decrease the chance of contraception by avoiding intercourse then. And one may use her knowledge of the fertile interval for avoidance of conception for some time by natural means, then use it for a planned pregnancy (*natural child spacing*).

Basal temperature graphs are helpful in determining whether and when ovulation occurs. Ovulation, the release of an egg (ovum) from the ovary, ordinarily happens only once in each menstrual cycle. Conception can take place only if intercourse takes place at or near this time, during the interval of transition between low and high temperature levels.

The basal temperature graph* reflects slight body changes taking place during the menstrual cycle. The "basal" *resting* temperature in the first part of the cycle is usually well below normal; in the last 2 weeks or so of the cycle the basal temperature is closer to 98.6. Most important, *the shift from the lower to the higher temperature level occurs about the time of ovulation.* See Fig 104-31.

The variations in the temperature before and after ovulation are slight, often only a few tenths to a half degree, so it is important that the temperature be taken carefully and recorded accurately. Special thermometers are available for this purpose. They record temperatures within the usual range of cyclic variations (from 96° to 100° only) and are graduated in tenths of a degree and are easier to read than the ordinary fever thermometers, although the latter may be used.

Temperature Comparisons—Throughout the United States the Fahrenheit scale is still employed, although use of the Centigrade scale is rapidly increasing in medical circles. Some hospitals and physicians prefer the latter scale, and clinical thermometers graduated in Centigrade degrees are available. Normal body temperature on the Centigrade scale

---

* Charts for plotting the daily temperatures are available from Schering, Becton-Dickinson, and elsewhere.

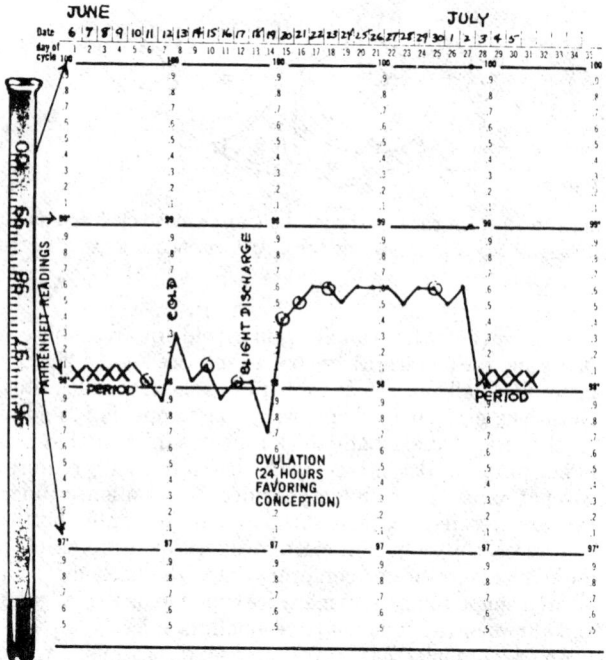

Fig 104-31.   Basal temperature graph for determination of ovulation period in the female.

is 37°. A comparison of temperature equivalents of the two scales, in the range of body temperatures below and above normal, is given in Table II.

Accuracy—The critical factors in obtaining maximum accuracy are: the thermometer must be properly designed, it must be sufficiently accurate to meet each specific requirement, and it must be properly used.

In general, the accuracy of fever thermometers is established either by federal standards, or by states, local authorities, and sometimes private institutions, usually operating for hospital groups. The national standard is known as CS1-52 (Commercial Standard No 1, 1952 revision). Special "state seal" standard requirements for thermometers are required in Connecticut, Massachusetts, and Michigan for thermometers sold in these states. Since issuance of CS1-52, state requirements have been modified to be in close conformity with the commercial standard.

Thermometers are offered for sale which exceed the standards, and usually bear specific information on the certificate indicating special accuracy or selection for other factors beyond the minimum requirements. They are valuable for critical temperature use, such as in diagnosis of certain pulmonary diseases and infectious cases, both surgical and medical, also for basal temperature studies, now being used

Table II—Temperature Comparison

Fahrenheit	Centigrade
96.0°	35.55°
97.0	36.11
97.5	36.38
98.0	36.65
98.6	37.0
99.0	37.22
99.5	37.50
100.0	37.77
101.0	38.33
102.0	38.88
103.0	39.44
104.0	40.0

widely in the study of human fertility. For ordinary use the CS1-52 *certified thermometer* is entirely adequate.

It must be realized that even the most carefully made thermometer is subject to normal hazards after it leaves the factory. It may be overheated or dropped, and while not externally damaged the constriction inside may have been shattered. A minute break in the constricted area may block the capillary tube or the contraction to develop a "hard shaker" or produce a "retreater."

Few actual hard-shaking or retreating thermometers escape from the rigid inspection guards of reputable manufacturers. The retreaters are more serious because they may endanger human life. Such dangerous thermometers are destroyed by reliable manufacturers when detected and should be disposed of immediately if the condition develops in use.

All well-made fever thermometers are "aged" before certification to remove most of the strains in the glass which would cause later shrinkage and errors in readings. This is done by laying the unfinished thermometers away for several months or by an accelerated heat-treating method which removes stress in the whole instrument, and anneals the constriction as well as the bulb.

Reading the Thermometer—Next to accuracy, the most important feature of a fever thermometer is its ease of reading. This is especially true for the inexperienced home user, who will appreciate being shown thermometers with easy-reading features, as offered by many manufacturers. Always demonstrate how to hold the thermometer for reading, which should be done with the back to good light and the instrument held horizontally in the right hand, about 12″ from the eyes. The bulb should never be held while reading, but the thermometer may be steadied by the left-hand index finger placed behind it. With the markings to the front, the thermometer should be rotated slowly until the mercury is visible.

Care of the Thermometer—After the thermometer has been read and the temperature recorded, it should always be shaken down so that it is ready for use the next time it is needed. In shaking down the mercury column, the thermometer should be grasped firmly between the thumb and the forefinger at the scale end and shaken vigorously by several snaps of the wrist until the reading is below 97°. This is effective and a good way to describe this method is to liken it to shaking water off the bulb, which the customer can visualize. The thermometer should *never* be held in the fingers while the hand is struck upon a solid surface to jar down the mercury column. Such rough handling is almost certain to cause breakage or a rupture of the constriction, even though it may appear unbroken. If dropped, even though apparently unbroken, the thermometer should be tested before using. Fever thermometers should never be exposed to heat, to the sun's rays, or to a heat unit, or be displayed in a shop window.

Disinfection of Thermometers—After using, and before re-use, thermometers should be carefully cleansed to avoid the possibility of carrying infection from one patient to another. They must never be washed in hot water. Sommermeyer and Carroll, who studied the disinfection of oral thermometers, recommended the following procedure:

1. Wipe the contaminated oral thermometer with a cotton ball moistened with a solution of equal parts of 95% ethyl alcohol and tincture of green soap.
2. Rinse the soap from the thermometer with cold running water.
3. Place the thermometer in a solution containing 0.5 to 1% iodine in either 70% ethyl alcohol or 70% isopropyl alcohol.

In 1972, the single-use thermometer cover was introduced, providing sterility without the need to actually clean the thermometer. This disposable sleeve encloses any oral thermometer in a sterile sheath of plastic thin enough not to interfere with its accuracy. Each sleeve is discarded after a single use.

Thermometers should never be placed on a hard surface but are preferably stored at the bedside, placed upright and resting on a pad of absorbent cotton in a sterilizer jar or in a tumbler. A plastic thermometer holder with a wide base is perfect for the bedside table. It is highly desirable to clean them immediately after use and, if possible, restore them to their cases. A thermometer which has not been thoroughly cleansed should never be used.*

Special Types of Thermometers—A number of special types of fever thermometers are available, including one intended for dermatologic use and having a special, flat-bladed, thin-glass, mercury reservoir for contact with the skin surface.† Other types have been developed for special uses, including remote-reading dial and recording instruments for continuous records. Thermocouples are employed extensively in some biological testing.

A disposable, economical thermometer system has been developed for taking and reading human temperatures, replacing routine use of conventional glass thermometers. The *Steridyne*, "stick-on" fever thermometer utilizes a liquid crystal display. It is placed on the skin of the patient, reads the surface temperature and calculates the body core temperature, which is then displayed, once the unit is activated. It is reusable and can be left on the skin for continuous monitoring.

Currently there are also available a variety of low-cost, battery-operated electronic fever thermometers, with visible gauge, that sell for around $30 and up. The most popular is the digital type, however, models with analog indicators are available. This type of thermometer gives precise temperature readings within a minute and are safe to use. Most have a "peak hold" feature so that the maximum temperature attained can be read and use disposable probe covers for sanitation.

A thermometer, designed to make quantitative temperature measurements directly from the surface of the skin, has been developed at the University of Colorado, Craig Rehabilitation Hospital. The instrument is accurate to within one-tenth of a degree when measuring the difference in heat generated by an arthritic joint and that generated by a healthy tissue. Its probe is about 6″ long and about $5/8$″ in diameter. Its hollow aluminum barrel holds a spring mechanism—like a ballpoint pen—that permits the user to exert uniform pressure when measuring skin temperatures.

Ostomy Appliances and Supplies

Understanding the Ostomy—An ostomy is a surgical procedure whereby parts of the intestinal and/or urinary tract are removed from the patient, the remaining end(s) are then brought to the abdominal wall and a stoma, or artificial opening, is surgically constructed through which urine or feces will pass from then on.

It is estimated that more than 50,000 such operations are performed annually in the US, most resulting in the saving of the patients' lives. There are approximately a million Americans now living who have had such surgery, and each one of them is buying appliances and supplies on a regular basis, primarily from the community pharmacy.

Since the pharmacist will be called on to offer advice to the ostomy patient as to the kind of ostomy appliance that will best serve his needs, and since there are many different kinds of ostomy surgery, each of which has its own special requirements as to the fitting and type of appliance best suited to it,

---

* Instructional, professional, or consumer literature on the products mentioned herein are generally available from the supplier or manufacturer.

† Becton-Dickinson, Steridyne, and Medisco-Federal are some of the major manufacturers of thermometers in the US.

it behooves the pharmacist who wishes to develop a successful ostomy section in his or her health-accessories department to become familiar with every type of surgery and the idiosyncrasies of each.

One could develop three basic classifications of ostomy surgery: those surgeries which involve the intestinal tract, those which involve the urinary tract, and those which involve both.

Among the surgeries that involve the intestinal tract, there are two types. If the ostomy results from part of the colon being brought to the abdominal wall for the surgical construction of a stoma, the operation is called a *colostomy*. If, on the other hand, the ostomy results from part of the ileum (the most distal third of the small intestine, between the jejunum and the colon) being brought to the abdominal wall for the construction of a stoma, the operation is referred to as an *ileostomy*. The differences in the appearance of these two categories of intestinal ostomies consist primarily in the sizes and locations of their stomas.

Stoma (Gk, mouth) is the name given to the artificial anus on the abdominal wall; it has the appearance of a small bud, normally flush though sometimes protruding up to about $\frac{1}{2}''$, and usually pink to bright red though stomas vary in color and sometimes appear darker. While most stomas do not protrude more than about $\frac{1}{2}''$, there are some which may have been constructed so that they protrude an inch or more. But when the pharmacist sees a stoma which protrudes more than $1\frac{1}{2}''$ (this author has seen one over $3''$ long) he should question the patient as to whether it was that long shortly following his surgery. In cases where the length of the stoma has changed drastically since the patient's surgery, the chances are that the stoma has become distended and the patient should be advised to see his physician for possible corrective surgery to avoid the potentiality of strangulation of the intestine.

Stomas appear red because the surgeon inverts the end of the intestine slightly when he brings it to the outside of the abdominal wall. After suturing the intestine to the abdominal skin, it becomes an integral part of the body wall, and all tissues live normally. The red surface of an ostomy stoma is actually the intestinal capillary bed; it stays red because blood continues to flow through it. As it is also a mucous membrane, it will continue to stay wet.

As most ileostomies result in the entire colon being separated from the small intestine at a point just behind the ileocecal valve (where the ileum joins the cecum), that is usually where the incision is made in the abdominal wall and where the ileum is brought to the outside of the body. The location of the ileocecal valve is near the appendix in the abdomen's lower right quadrant, and where an ileostomy stoma is typically located. And since the stoma in an ileostomy is constructed from the small intestine, it will be smaller in size than the colostomy stoma, which is made from the colon. However, it is important to note that the location of stomas on the outside of the body cannot be standardized as colostomy on the left side and ileostomy on the right side. Complications may occur or problems existing unique to the patient obstructing typical stoma placement—eg, kidney transplant, requiring the surgeon to place the stoma in an unobstructive location. The fecal matter or output indicates what type of surgery was performed.

In a colostomy only part of the colon is removed from the body. The types of colostomies depend upon where the diseased part of the colon is separated from the healthy part of the colon. When only the juncture of the sigmoid colon with the rectum and anus is involved, the surgeon brings the sigmoid colon to the surface of the abdomen and the surgery is termed a *sigmoid colostomy*. When the separation occurs along the length of the descending colon, anywhere between the splenic flexure (the bend where the transverse colon meets the descending colon) and the sigmoid flexure, the operation is called a *descending colostomy*. Accordingly, when the surgeon makes the separation along the length of the transverse colon anywhere between the splenic flexure and the hepatic flexure (where the transverse and ascending colon meet), the surgery is termed a *transverse colostomy;* an *ascending colostomy* occurs between the hepatic flexure and the cecum. Finally, when the stoma is constructed with that part of the colon called the cecum, the surgery is simply called a *cecostomy*.

These five surgeries, while they are all colostomies, are distinctly different from each other in that different lengths of colon remain in patients having different types of colostomies. Since a primary function of the colon is the removal of water from the feces as it passes through it, it is understandable that the feces produced at a cecostomy stoma will be quite loose and watery while the feces produced at a sigmoid colostomy stoma are generally quite solid. Likewise, the ascending, transverse, and descending colostomies produce feces, within the extremes just described, of varying degrees of consistency. The additional fact that all colostomies, because of the reservoir effect of the colon still remaining, can be managed better than ileostomies in which there is no reservoir remaining, has implications for the pharmacist with regard to the types of appliances that are best suited for each type of ostomy.

The implications are that different colostomies in particular, and intestinal ostomies in general, because of differences in fecal products, create nonidentical problems for the patient, ie, not all colostomies can successfully be irrigated, they require different types of appliances, and they utilize different kinds of accessories. There is very little difference in the size of the stomas of each of the five colostomies, but they may be located on the abdominal wall differently. Colostomy stomas which are usually located in the lower left quadrant of the patient's abdomen tend toward more solid feces, while those usually located in the lower right quadrant tend toward feces which contain more water and are, therefore, of looser consistency. Most colostomies are performed as the result of cancer of the lower bowel and occur in persons over the age of 60.

When the entire colon must be removed, the surgeon performs an *ileostomy* by separating the colon from the small intestine behind the ileocecal valve. The result is a stoma much smaller than any colostomy stoma, located in the lower right quadrant, and producing fecal material which is always loose and watery. The majority of ileostomies are performed on people between the ages of 18 and 40, and are usually the result of an ulceration of the inner lining of the colon which is called ulcerative colitis.

There are several types of urinary diversions, the most common of which are those in which the patient's bladder must be removed. Then the two tubes which connect and carry urine from the kidneys to the bladder are brought forward to the abdominal wall where two tiny stomas, totally unlike intestinal stomas, are constructed above the navel line on either side of the body. The two tubes are called ureters and so the operation is referred to as a *ureterostomy* or *cutaneous ureterostomy*. The product of this kind of ostomy is, obviously, only urine.

Patients with bilateral cutaneous ureterostomies are forced to manage two separate stomas and wear two separate appliances. Because of the difficulties associated with the cutaneous ureterostomy in terms of postoperative management and because of the availability of an ingenious alternative surgical procedure, very few cutaneous ureterostomies are still being performed. The preferred alternative is a surgical procedure which brings the two ureters together, implants them in an artificial bladder and enables the patient to have but one stoma to manage and one appliance to wear instead of the usual two.

This innovative operation is called a *Bricker's loop*, after the surgeon who perfected it, but it is also frequently referred to as an *ileal bladder*, *ileal conduit*, or urinary diversion. All four names indicate the same operation, however.

During this operation, the surgeon removes a piece of the healthy small intestine at the ileum, after which he performs a resection of the two ends of the ileum, joining them together again. The missing piece is usually between 6 and 8 in., and is a relatively insignificant loss to the small intestine, which measures nearly 24 ft in the average adult. One end of the piece of ileum is closed and the other is brought to the outside of the body to become the single stoma. Once the two ureters are implanted in the closed end of the piece of ileum, that piece becomes a conduit for the urine—actually a substitute bladder. Since this conduit or bladder is made from a piece of the ileum, it has gotten the names ileal conduit and ileal bladder.

The stoma has the appearance of an ileostomy stoma and is usually located within the same quadrant, the lower right, but its product is only urine. While most ileostomy stomas are located in the lower half of the lower right quadrant of the abdomen, most ileal conduit stomas are located in the upper half of the lower right quadrant. The only way to be sure which ostomy is which, is to determine the nature of the waste product.

Sometimes patients who have colostomies also must have their bladders removed. In these cases, rather than create an ileal conduit which would result in a second stoma for the patient to manage so that he would ultimately have two, his old colostomy stoma and now his new ileal conduit stoma, the surgeon merely implants the two ureters in the active colon. The result is a single stoma (the original colostomy stoma) which produces both solid and semi-solid feces as well as urine. This surgery is called a *wet colostomy* though it is rarely done today due to the high probability of genitourinary tract infection.

When the two ureters are severed or cannot be brought forward to the abdominal wall for any reason, the surgeon is forced to bring the ureters to the nearest outside surface—the patient's back. Stomas appearing on the dorsal side of the patient or openings through which renal catheters lead directly to the kidneys, indicate an operation called a *nephrostomy*. Persons with bilateral nephrostomies wear two appliances.

Openings directly into the bladder, just above the pubic bone (the symphysis pubis) are the result of a urinary diversion made necessary by involvement of the urethra which normally carries urine from the bladder to the outside. Called *vesicotomies*, these are often temporary operations and are rarely of concern to the pharmacist.

All of the surgeries described above, with the exception of the last, are irreversible and permanent. A patient with an ileostomy will always have an ileostomy, for example. But there are two other ostomies which are temporary and with which the pharmacist should be familiar. One is a modified kind of descending colostomy in which the lower portion of the descending colon, sigmoid colon, and rectum are not removed from the patient. After the surgical separation is made, both ends of the colon are brought to the outside and two stomas are constructed, one active and the other inactive.

This operation, the *double-barrel colostomy*, results in two stomas, side-by-side, normally located in the lower left quadrant and producing solid fecal material exactly like the ordinary descending colostomy. This condition may last from one month to a year or longer, depending entirely on when the surgeon is satisfied that a resection can be performed without further complication. Sometimes the double-barrel colostomy is performed in the hope that the lower bowel can be brought back to normal with treatment and rest. On occasion,

a patient with a double-barrel colostomy must return to the hospital for a permanent colostomy.

The second kind of temporary colostomy is called a *decompression colostomy* or *loop colostomy*, and is done as an emergency procedure to relieve a bowel impaction and avoid an intestinal rupture. Normally, the patient who has a loop colostomy performed will have his colon repaired and back to normal within a few weeks and before he leaves the hospital. Loop colostomy appliances are applied during surgery by the physician, and the only ostomy appliances which are packaged sterile besides the common postoperative drain. This kind of ostomy gets its name from the fact that, unlike the double-barrel colostomy, the loop colostomy doesn't result in the complete separation of the intestine, but rather, a loop of intestine is brought through an incision and is temporarily secured to the abdominal wall by means of a glass rod which is slipped under the loop and across the incision; the loop is then perforated surgically to relieve the impaction. The wound stays open and the loop remains visible until the perforation in the intestine is closed and the loop is returned to its normal position within the visceral cavity. It is highly unlikely that the pharmacist will ever be called upon to fit a loop colostomy appliance though he may still want to stock the appliances for use by the hospital.

Choosing the Right Appliance—The various ostomies described above can be grouped into three major categories for the purpose of understanding which kinds of appliances are most appropriate for each. First, there are those ostomies which only produce solid waste at their stomas. They include the sigmoid colostomy, descending colostomy, transverse colostomy, double-barrel colostomy, and often the loop colostomy. Second, there are those ostomies which only produce urine at their stomas. They include the cutaneous ureterostomy, nephrostomy, vesicotomy and Bricker's loop or ileal conduit. And third, there are those ostomies which, for one reason or another, produce liquid or semisolid fecal matter at their stomas. They include the ileostomy, cecostomy, ascending colostomy, wet colostomy, and sometimes the loop colostomy.

In real life, neat and perfectly reliable categories such as the ones just described do not exist. People are different from each other; their digestive processes are different, and their diets are different. The consistency of the waste matter in any one individual also varies from day to day. Yet these categories are useful generally, and in addition, they point up the fact that an appliance should be chosen primarily for the nature of the waste matter it will have to collect.

Further, the groupings do indicate that among a host of ostomy appliances presently on the market from numerous manufacturers, there are just three basic types, categorized primarily by the nature of the waste material for which they are intended. There are appliances designed for pure urine, appliances designed for semisolids, and appliances designed for solid waste matter. Other considerations in choosing the right appliance for each patient include size of gasket openings which fit around the stoma, method of attaching the appliance around the stoma, the patient's financial resources, and activities in which the patient engages at work or at play, during the day or at night. See Fig 104-32.

Ostomy Appliances for Solid Wastes—The colostomy appliance, so-called because the majority of colostomies are solid-waste-producing, is the appliance used for most colostomies. There are many types of colostomy appliances on the market, recognizable by larger size gasket openings to accommodate the larger stomas characteristic of all colostomies, and by detachable, throw-away pouches made of thin polyethylene plastic and most are sealed at their bottoms. However, some colostomates do use open-ended pouches. The fact that these pouches are sealed at the bottom and disposable indicates the impracticability of bottom drains for

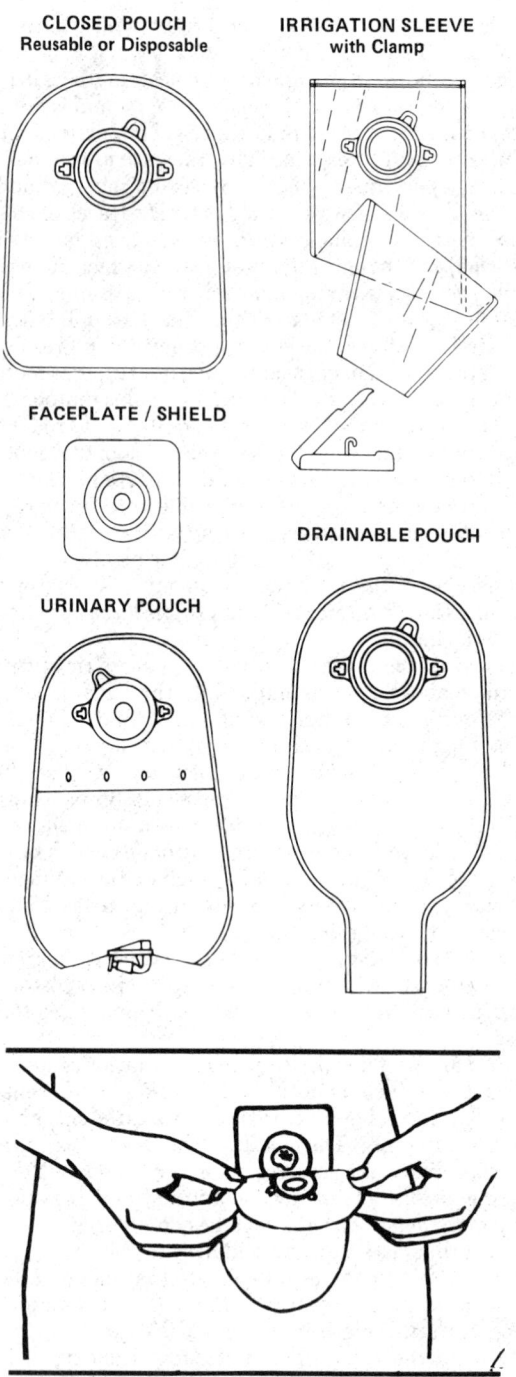

CLOSED POUCH
Reusable or Disposable

IRRIGATION SLEEVE
with Clamp

FACEPLATE / SHIELD

DRAINABLE POUCH

URINARY POUCH

ATTACHING THE POUCH TO THE FACEPLATE

Fig 104-32.   Ostomy appliances (courtesy, Convatec).

solid wastes generally. By and large, colostomy appliances are not the permanent, cement-on type since those ostomies which produce solid wastes do not cause the problems with skin excoriation typical of the wetter ostomies. These appliances are either worn with an elastic waist belt or are the self-adhesive, no-belt types.

The self-adhesive colostomy appliance is more of a collection bag with adhesive around the stoma opening than it is an appliance. The openings may be cut with a scissors to fit the stoma precisely though most manufacturers provide several sizes. Advantages with this type of appliance are that it is light-weight and quite flat against the body so it is less likely to show through clothing. Those colostomates who irrigate regularly find this type of appliance perfect for safety's sake.

Those colostomy appliances worn with an elastic waist belt typically consist of a rubber or plastic gasket to which the elastic waist belt clips, disposable pouches which snap on the gasket or are fastened to it with rubber bands and, like the adhesive type colostomy pouches, are sealed at the bottom. These appliances either come with gaskets of varying sizes or have adaptor face plates which enable the appliance to fit properly. While this appliance is usually worn without any adhesive, many patients prefer to use double-sized adhesive gaskets between the regular gasket and their skin, or a washer-type gasket made of a combination of karaya gum and gelatin for added security. While most colostomy appliances of this type use disposable polyethylene pouches, some patients still prefer the cheaper-in-the-long-run, but more troublesome to clean, reuseable rubber pouch. Appliances are usually chosen according to control or lack of control in the fecal output.

Many colostomates are urged by their doctors to irrigate on a regular basis. Irrigation is the process of administering an enema to the colon via the stoma for the purpose of establishing regular, conveniently-timed evacuation of the bowel—in other words to become relatively stool-free. Irrigation is necessary just once per day at the most, and may be scheduled in the morning before dressing or in the evening before retiring. Irrigation is a highly individual thing and some persons need irrigate only every other day or two to three times per week. And there are some people who have quite irritable bowels and cannot remain stool-free.

After irrigation, the colostomate can expect to have no bowel activity until the next irrigation, except perhaps for slight dripping now and then. Many ostomates, after irrigation, wear only a gauze pad over the stoma for safety and psychological confidence. The pad can be taped over the stoma or secured with a two-way stretch wrap-around.

The irrigation process is quite simple and takes between 30 to 45 min for completion. Important steps are these: The stoma should be dilated with a gloved finger (finger cot) and a bit of lubricating jelly prior to insertion of the colon tube. About one quart of tepid water (some patients add a couple of tablespoons of salt) is placed in the irrigating bag—never hung more than head high. Care should be taken on insertion of the colon tube that risk of perforating the colon is absolutely minimal. Rarely will the colon tube be inserted more than 3 to 4″. About 15 min should be allowed before permitting evacuation; after the initial gush it normally takes another 20 to 25 min before the colon is really empty. Most people close the end of the irrigating sleeve with a rubber band and then shower or shave during this period. Sometimes drinking a cup of strong black coffee or a glass of ice cold water will start the intestinal peristalsis necessary for complete evacuation.

Irrigation is a technique for accomplishing regularity and security throughout the day, but is only useful in those ostomies which produce solid wastes. Many physicians and enterostomal therapists are now recognizing the importance of diet in gaining control and regularity of bowel movements and irrigation. The question of whether or not a particular colostomy patient should irrigate should be answered only by the patient's physician.

Appliances for Urine—Ostomies which produce only urine at their stomas typically require a permanent type appliance which is usually cemented directly to the skin. These appliances are usually made of rubber and have at their bottoms a nylon screw-type drain which need only be twisted a half turn to empty. The tops of these appliances typically have a detachable plastic gasket over which a rubber cover or face plate is stretched to facilitate sizing, or plastic inserts are utilized to accomplish appropriate-sized openings.

Most urinary appliances are permanent in that they employ a high quality skin bond cement to make a leakproof seal between the appliance's face plate and the skin immediately around the stoma. Close fit and leakproof seal are the necessary requirements of an adequate urinary appliance since a leaking seal around the stoma will surely lead to serious problems with skin breakdown later.

Cement is applied in a very thin layer to both the face plate and the skin around the stoma, and after waiting about 60 seconds for the cemented surfaces to get tacky, the cemented face plate is pressed against the cemented skin and held there for a moment or two until the bond is quite secure. The appliance may then be worn with or without a security waist belt. When the appliance is changed, in two or three days on the average, a specially prepared cement solvent (purchased with the cement) is carefully squirted between the face plate and the skin until the bond begins to loosen, then the face plate is carefully pulled off. The remaining cement on the skin and on the appliance will come off easily with a bit more solvent.

Appliances for Semisolids—The typical ileostomy or colostomy appliance looks very much like the top of the urinary appliance as both are normally cemented to the skin. But in addition to skin cement-on appliances, a number of ileostomy appliances are now on the market which use only karaya-gum washers to maintain a waterproof seal. These appliances are almost always worn with an elastic waist belt, however. Another innovation in the ileostomy appliance is the combination of skin bond cement and the use of half-moon-shaped skin tapes. The tapes are used to provide added security to a *base plate* which is cemented to the skin over the stoma. The appliance then clips onto the face plate and may easily be removed for cleaning without disturbing the base plate. But this type of appliance requires skin in good condition, free of excoriation.

The real difference between a urinary appliance and an appliance for semisolids is in their bottoms, however. Where the urinary appliance has a nylon twist-drain plug in the bottom, the "ileostomy" appliance merely narrows down to between 1½ to 2½" and is just open. The bottom is either closed by folding and wrapping with a rubber band or folding and securing with a clip. To drain, the clip or rubber band is removed and the bottom of the appliance unfolded.

Different manufacturers—and there are scores—make appliances which, though basically similar in design or function, differ with respect to method of securing to the skin, type of rubber, ease with which the appliance can be turned inside out for cleaning and drying, type of drain closure, and method of sizing the stoma opening for proper fit. One manufacturer even makes an interchangeable face plate which can be flat, concave, or convex—a helpful advantage with some patients, especially those who are obese.

Ostomy Appliance Accessories—Most popular among a host of accessories for ostomy appliances of all kinds are karaya gum powder and karaya gum washers. Already indicated as a standard part of some brands of appliances, karaya gum washers are available in a variety of sizes packaged separately. Pliable and flexible as they are, they are almost indispensable in providing a leakproof seal around the stoma when the patient's stoma has been constructed by the surgeon so it is right next to the iliac crest of his pelvis, or when scar tissue near the stoma forms hills and valleys impossible to seal in any other way. Foam rubber pads are sometimes used with success in those cases.

Karaya gum powder is quite useful in preparing the skin prior to fitting any appliance with or without skin cement. The powder's ability to absorb moisture and protect the skin from excoriation makes it an asked-for item. It usually comes in small plastic "poof" bottles and bigger, large-mouth jars. The technique for applying karaya gum powder is quite simple: the skin around the stoma, after being thoroughly cleaned, is dampened with plain water; the powder is dusted or "poofed" on over the moistened skin; and the excess is

blown or dusted off leaving a thin, dry covering around the stoma. If a cement-on appliance is used, the cement is simply brushed on right over the coating of powder; a colostomy appliance is merely pressed in place and secured with a waist belt.

Varieties of deodorant drops, tablets, and sprays are available; some are applied to the outside of the appliance while others are dropped into the bag prior to applying it. Silicone and benzoin tincture sprays are also used to prepare the skin around the stoma. In addition, racks for drying an appliance after washing, abdominal dressings and cover sponges, gloves and wipes, and even zippered, purse-size pouches for supplies are available to make things easier for the ostomate. Some manufacturers now offer new easy-to-apply appliances featuring synthetic materials to reduce skin irritation and prevent leakage.

But perhaps the most helpful things which the pharmacist can provide his customers who have ostomies are suggestions and ideas on how to get along with a minimum of difficulty. Knowledge of these things will come from the ostomates themselves, and it is therefore wise to spend some time asking them questions. Examples of some suggestions are: (1) it is possible to prevent urine in the urinary appliance from running back up over the stoma, when reclining, by folding a piece of tissue into a small rectangle and inserting it into the appliance before putting on the appliance; the tissue will soak up the liquid as it enters the appliance and effectively convert that liquid into a solid that won't run. (2) A pin-prick and a piece of tape will provide an excellent outlet port for release of gas that tends to build up inside a cement-on appliance; the tape can be removed in a convenient bathroom. (3) Since gas develops mostly from some foods, the ostomate can eliminate some of the problem by avoiding such foods as cabbage and beans; however, foods react differently in different persons and each must develop his own list of food taboos.

Urology and Incontinence Supplies

Urinals—These containers are employed to collect urine. They differ in shape according to male or female use. They are ordinarily made of glass, white enamelware, or plastic which is by far the most common especially for use at home. Plastic urinals may be had in two basic types: single-patient use or autoclavable. Rubber urinals designed to be worn by the patient are also available. This type of urinal is becoming more widely used and is available in a number of different styles. The selection of style is usually a matter of personal preference and of size and capacity requirements. See Figs 104-33 to 104-36.

The complete rubber urinal consists of two parts, the top portion, fitted by means of a penal sheath in the male urinal and a vaginal cup in the female urinal and worn utilizing an adjustable waist strap and leg straps, and the lower collection bag. Urinal bags come in different capacities, and two styles, long and oval-short. The bag may be drained by turning the outlet plug at its bottom. Adjustable elastic leg straps hold the bag against the inside of the thigh or leg where it is not conspicuous. A common error is to fasten the leg straps so that they encircle the bag, thereby restricting its volume. Special drip urinals consist of the top only with an outlet drain plug at its bottom.

Urinals for males are for wear during the day or night, while standing erect or reclining during sleep. The penal sheath, if properly fitted, will prevent any back flow of urine from the collection bag. When fitting a male rubber urinal, the penal sheath should be pulled inside out. The sheath can be stretched for insertion of the penis. It should fit snugly but not constrict. If it is necessary to enlarge the sheath opening, it can be cut with a small scissors by starting at one edge and cutting around. The sheath, should never be cut with one

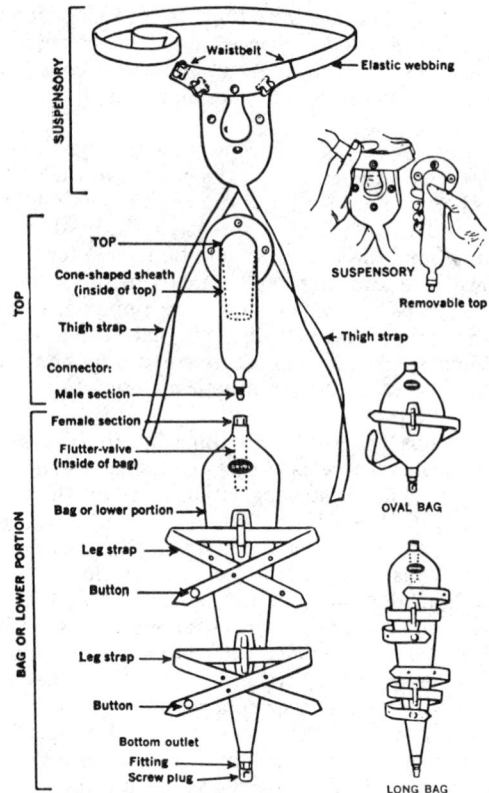

Fig 104-33. Nomenclature of urinal components (Bard Home Health)

slice using a large scissors, as that usually results in an uneven opening which will surely leak. Because the sheath is conical, it is necessary that only a tiny bit of rubber be removed between each try for a good fit.

Female rubber urinals are useful only when the user is standing erect and cannot be used successfully when reclining. The incontinent female patient may have to resort to wearing incontinence pants or an indwelling retention catheter, as there is still no adequate method for providing a good seal with an external female urinary appliance.

Incontinence Pants—A variety of body-contoured incontinence pants are available for both men and women. Most are of soft, flexible fabric with plastic or rubber coating inside. They are made to remain soft and pliable even after repeated washing and boiling. Children's sizes are also available.

Incontinence pants are typically made with elastic tops and legs, snaps at the sides for ease in putting them on when the

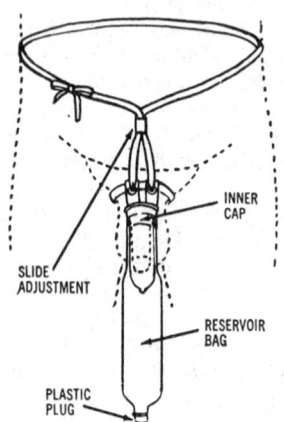

Fig 104-34. Belt type adjustable, leakproof, male urinal.

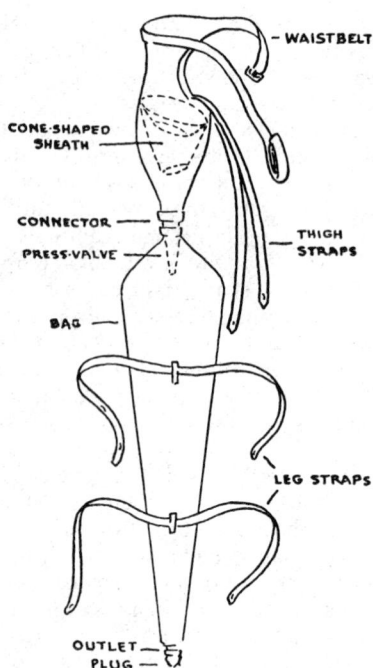

Fig 104-35. Male suspensory urinary, Bard Home Health type.

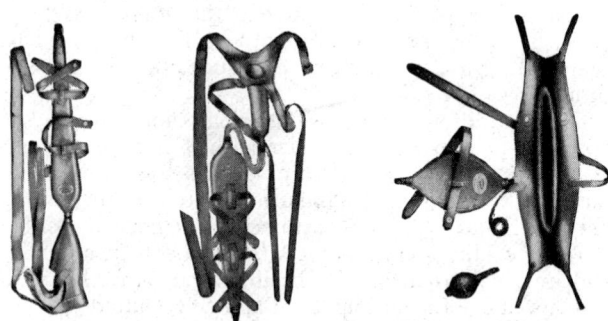

Fig 104-36. Types of urinals for ambulatory patients. Male urinals (left and center) and female urinal (right).

patient is bedfast, and either a disposable or snap-in absorbent liner which can be removed for washing. Often, these liners consist of several separate layers, with one made of a material called Olefin. The Olefin fabric permits liquids to permeate into the absorbent layers beneath, maintaining a feeling of being comfortably dry. Newer models of pants for the incontinent patient consist of an incontinence pouch with waist and leg straps. These briefs are generally more comfortable to wear as they are much less bulky beneath the clothing.

Other products helpful where there is an incontinent patient include disposable underpads, rubber sheeting, silicone skin sprays and body lotions, and deodorants.

Catheters—To collect urine from the patient unable to void naturally or where incontinence pants and urinals are inadequate, catheters are employed (Fig 104-37). Nonflexible

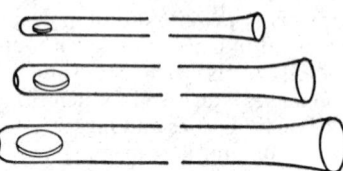

Fig 104-37. Rubber catheter (above); rubber rectal tube (center); rubber colon tube (bottom).

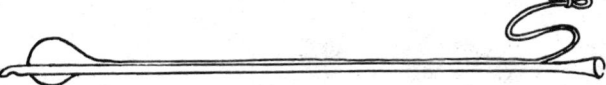

Fig 104-38. Balloon catheter, for prolonged insertion through the urethra into the bladder.

Fig 104-39. Cross-section views of colon tubes (above) with dual-spaced openings, and rectal tubes (below).

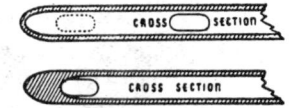

catheters of glass, or of metals such as silver, are used for females but are rarely employed in males except for special diseases or where constriction of the urethra has occurred requiring a rather stiff catheter for insertion. They are very narrowly limited in use, however. Rather, the flexible soft-rubber type of catheter is commonly preferred for both male and female patients.

The insertion of catheters is a dangerous procedure customarily handled by physicians or trained nurses and orderlies. Serious infections of the bladder and damage to the urethral and bladder tissues may result from improper insertion.

Flexible soft rubber catheters consist of small rubber tubes with a closed solid tip. At one end is a flaring funnel-shaped opening to facilitate attachment of the catheter to a glass junction or another tube leading to a collection unit. At the inserted end is a wide opening which leads to the channel through which urine flows to the collection unit. This type of catheter is referred to as a straight catheter, in contrast to the retention catheter which is designed to remain in the urethra for long periods of time.

The indwelling retention catheter, or Foley catheter as it is commonly known, is characterized by a balloon at its insertion end (Fig 104-38). The balloon is designed to secure the catheter tip within the patient's bladder to keep it from slipping or being pulled out. There are two channels which run from the insertion tip to the end of the Foley catheter—one for the passing of urine and the other for the injection of sterile water which inflates the balloon.

Foley catheters are available with either 5-mL balloons or 30-mL balloons. The 30-mL balloon catheter, which is also known as a hemostatic catheter, is commonly used in nursing homes for patients whose urethras have become dilated or for those patients who have pulled the 5-mL balloon catheter out. A common mistake in filling a balloon catheter is to use too little water. It takes about 10 mL of water to inflate a 5-mL Foley balloon because nearly 5 mL is held in the filling lumen that runs the length of the catheter. Diameters of the catheter also vary in size. Though their usage is somewhat limited, 75-mL balloon retention catheters are also available. The three chief scales used for catheters have been named from their respective countries of origin. They are compared in Table III. The French scale is the most commonly employed, although catheters may bear imprinted on their sides one or another, or even all three, scale readings.

Other innovations in the urinary catheter include a Foley catheter with its own supply of sterile water for balloon inflation. With these catheters, a valve is released following insertion of the catheter, and the sterile water, which is under pressure, runs up its channel and inflates the balloon. They are especially convenient, as there is no need to prepare a syringe for balloon inflation, but they are considerably more expensive than the typical Foley catheter. Another improvement is the silicone and Teflon coatings on the outside and inside of Foley catheters. Such coatings not only cut

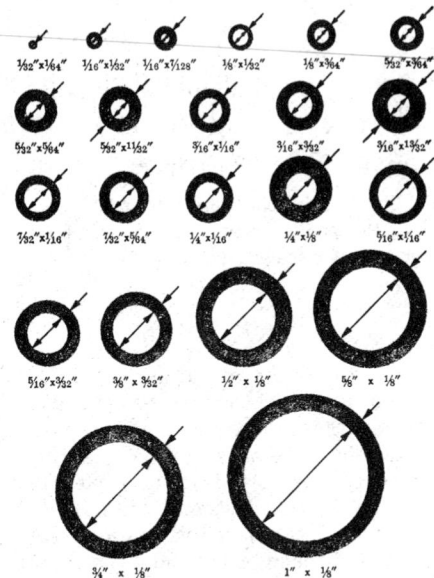

Fig 104-40. Actual diameter and thickness of standard medical tubing.

down friction during insertion and removal of the catheter, but also inhibit buildup of deposits on catheter walls, thus extending the time-period between catheter changes. The newest improvement is the all-silicone catheter, now manufactured by Kendall, CR Bard, and others.

The pharmacy may also stock a variety of urine collection units and catheter administration trays. The bladder-care tray, sometimes called a *cathtray*, is a sterile package containing the items required during the administration of a Foley catheter, and packed sequentially with those things needed first on top.

Administration trays are also available for catheter irrigation, pulmonary and gastric suction, and IV placement.

Rectal Tubes—Rectal tubes are merely larger catheters intended for rectal use in removal of feces. They are straight catheters and differ somewhat in construction in that the flexible rubber tube has an opening on the tip rather than on the side only. Three scales of diameters are employed (Table IV). These are the tubes commonly used by persons with colostomies in performing regular irrigation, sometimes referred to as colon tubes (Fig 104-39). See Table V.

Hospital Tubing—Other disposable plastic tubing includes sterile feeding tubes, French size 5 to 8 and from 15 to 42"; urinary drainage tubes with $3/16$ or $9/32$" lumen; stomach tubes for aspiration of the stomach content and for feeding, French scale 12 to 18 and 50" in length; rectal or enema tubes for gas expulsion (French 24, 20") or colonic evacuation (French 24, 60"); and sterile suction tubes (French 10 to 18, 22") with nylon adapters. In addition there are oxygen, sterile extension, and connecting tubes.

Table III—Catheter Scales

French (Nos)	10	12	14	16	18	20	22
American (Nos)	7	8	10	11	12	14	15
English (Nos)	4	5	6	7	9	11	12
Size (in)	$13/100$	$15/100$	$18/100$	$20/100$	$23/100$	$26/100$	$29/100$

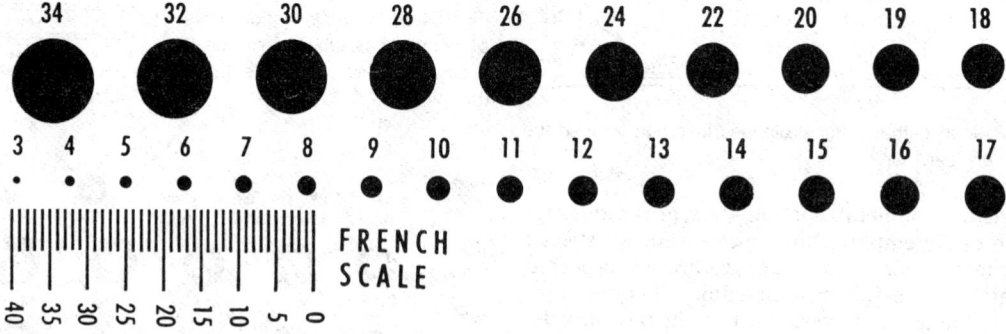

Fig 104-41.   Standard French Scale for hospital tubing, catheters, rectal and colon, stomach feeding, suction, urinary drainage and oxygen tubes (courtesy, Becton-Dickinson).   To determine French size if instruments are oval or other shape, use strip of paper to measure the periphery—then lay on the scale at the left.

Trusses

Hernias and trusses are as old as mankind. The first trusses were nothing more than a rope or strap and a rock. Celsus developed the use of a plate and in medieval times a form of plaster and plate were used. The spring-and-belt-type truss, practically as it is today in principle, was developed by the Netherlands physician Camper in 1785.

True hernias are not the same as ruptures. A true hernia is the protrusion of the intestine and its surrounding membrane, the peritoneum, through a natural opening in the abdominal wall, whereas a rupture is such a protrusion through the muscles of the abdomen usually occurring at a point previously weakened. A rupture occurring at the site of a previous surgical incision is sometimes referred to as an incisional hernia. The natural openings in the abdominal musculature through which a true hernia may occur include the umbilical opening; the inguinal openings, through which, in the male, the spermatic cord passes, and in the female, the round ligament passes; and the openings for the femoral arteries. See Fig 104-42.

Abdominal or umbilical hernias are exceedingly common. Infants in the first year of life show an incidence of 19.6/1000. Between ages 20 and 24, the incidence is lowest, rising to 24.2/1000 in the 70- to 74-age group.

Of all males afflicted with hernias, 96% suffer from the inguinal type, often showing up as scrotal hernias. The corresponding incidence of inguinal hernias among females is just 44.3%. A hernia may undergo a spontaneous cure, but on the other hand, strangulation is a frequent occurrence and one which requires quick and forceful surgical action. While surgery is becoming the preferred treatment for all hernias, it is not always the best solution for all patients. Some will require trusses in lieu of surgery. In addition, trusses are often recommended for support immediately following surgery.

Inguinal and umbilical trusses for infants, of gum rubber, are occasionally called for. Inguinal devices, with button fasteners for adjustment, are available in single right or left, or double in three sizes, 10 to 12″, 14 to 16″, and 18 to 22″. Umbilical trusses are also available in three sizes.

Hernia trusses of all kinds vary from soft fabric supports to heavier models requiring experienced judgment on the part of the fitter. Type and location of truss pads, and the weight and build of the patient are all important considerations in truss fitting. All trusses must be fitted while the patient is lying down and the hernia is reduced (the protruding intestine has been returned to the abdominal cavity) or the truss itself may cause strangulation.

A well-fitted truss, appropriate to the specific patient and his specific type of hernia, may be tested by having the patient bend, stoop and squat. If the patient can do those things without having a protrusion of the intestine past the truss pad, it is likely that the truss is properly fitted. Finally, it is important for the pharmacist to teach the patient how to properly put on his truss and test its security while he is in the fitting room, so he can remove it with confidence when he is on his own.

Fitting Schools—The pharmacist who will be in charge of the truss service and orthopedic department should attend a fitting school. This may require time and travel, but it basically trains the pharmacist in the anatomy involved, and appliance selection and fitting skills which are absolutely necessary. Several good schools are conducted by surgical appliance manufacturers and typically run 3 to 5 days consecutively. Such schools are given by OTC, Camp, Sickroom Service, and others.

Attendance at one of these schools provides background on the definition, location, varieties, frequency, symptoms,

Table IV—Rectal Tube Scales

French (Nos)	22	24	26	28	30	32
American (Nos)	15	16	17	19	20	21
English (Nos)	12	14	15	17	18	20
Size (in)	$9/32$	$10/32$	$10.5/32$	$11/32$	$12/32$	$13/32$

Table V—Colon Tube Scales

French (Nos)	30	32	34
American (Nos)	20	21	22
English (Nos)	18	20	21
Size (in)	$12/32$	$13/32$	$14/32$

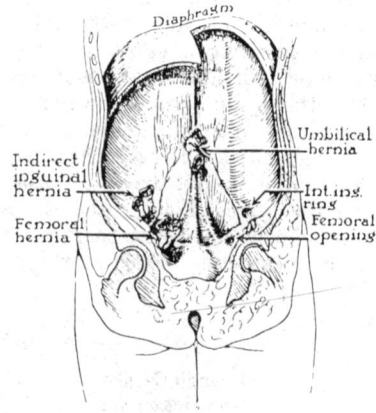

Fig 104-42.   Looking toward the front of the abdominal wall, from within the cavity, showing the five congenitally weak points.

causes, complications, treatment and anticipated results in the following conditions and appliances:

1. Trusses for inguinal, scrotal, femoral, and umbilical hernias; and incisional ruptures
2. Postoperative supports
3. Ptosis, uterine supports
4. Obesity supports
5. Postnatal supports
6. Sacroiliac supports and braces
7. Sacrolumbar supports and braces
8. Dorsolumbar supports and braces
9. Cervical supports and braces
10. Varicocele, hydrocele supports
11. Varicosity and lymphedema supports
12. Wrist, ankle, and knee supports and braces
13. Appliances for traction
14. Mastectomy prostheses

Reference should be made by the interested pharmacist to literature available from appliance manufacturers.

Orthopedic Supports and Braces

The spinal column can be divided into five major sections: the cervical spine, consisting of seven vertebrae, supports the head and is characterized by an anterior curve; the thoracic spine, consisting of 12 vertebrae to each of which a pair of ribs is attached, is characterized by a posterior curve; the lumbar spine, consisting of five vertebrae and characterized by an anterior curve; the sacrum, consisting of five vertebrae which are so tightly joined as to appear as one bone, is situated beneath the fifth lumbar vertebra and between the two innominate bones of the pelvis forming the sacroiliac joints, and is characterized by a posterior curve; and finally, the coccyx, consisting of three to five vertebrae immediately beneath the sacrum and continuing its posterior curve. See Fig 104-43A.

Apart from the cervical spine, anomalies of the spinal column include: Lordosis, a hyperextension of the lumbar spine, recognizable as sway-back; kyphosis, a flexion of the lumbar spine and/or hyperextension of the thoracic spine, often appearing as hunch-back; and scoliosis, an S-shaped lateral curve of the spine. See Fig 104-43B, C, and D. Each of these conditions, in varying degree, often requires use of supportive garments or braces. Sometimes ruptures of the intervertebral discs, the cartilaginous shock-absorbing cushions between separate vertebrae, interfere with the spinal cord or the nerves leading from it. An example is sciatica, in which a ruptured intervertebral disc causes compression or trauma at the base of the sciatic nerve resulting in extreme pain at the back of the thigh and running down the inside of the leg along the course of the sciatic nerve. This condition may also require use of a spinal garment or brace. And occasionally, the occurrence of spondylolisthesis, the slippage of lower vertebrae usually against the sacrum, will bring the patient to the pharmacy with a prescription for a garment or brace-fitting.

These and other conditions create a need for spinal braces and orthopedic garments to limit motion in the spine and permit healing. And while the pharmacist should be knowledgeable about them, he should never diagnose such conditions or prescribe the wearing of an orthopedic appliance. That should be left entirely to the physician. Unhappy consequences can be avoided and the surgical appliance business strengthened if the pharmacist will adhere to the simple rule never to fit any brace or support except on the prescription of a physician.

In addition to trusses and orthopedic supports for anomalies of the spine, the surgical appliance department should include elastic supports for ankle, knee, and wrist; support hosiery and elastic stockings; rib belts, arm slings, cervical collars, and shoulder braces. A complete department for the mastectomy patient is a suitable adjunct also. It will require a varied selection of breast prostheses, specialized brassieres and even swimwear, but most important, a trained woman fitter. Custom-fitted gradient pressure sleeves and pneumatic appliances for the reduction of postoperative edema which frequently accompanies radical mastectomy are also very important. Space does not permit a more detailed discussion. See Appendixes A and B.

The Fitting Room—For such a department, an adequate, private fitting room and stock space nearby are an absolute necessity. The fitting room need be no more than 8 ft × 8 ft, but should be clean, free of any stock or display, and have an inward swinging door to shield the fitting table from view. The fitting room should also be sound-treated to provide privacy and enable the patient to feel comfortable discussing his or her condition. As most fittings are done with the patient in a horizontal position, a table 72″ by 26″ and 30″ high, padded with moistureproof vinyl and a pillow are needed. Also needed are a chair, coat hooks and clothes hangers, four-legged stool, small dressing table, and a full-length mirror. Professional simplicity and cleanliness are exceedingly important. The use of rolled paper on the table and floor is practical and economical. If the pharmacy also has a comprehensive ostomy center a second chair, so both the patient and the pharmacist can sit, is recommended.

Conveniently near the fitting room should be the orthopedic inventory. The inventory depends on volume of sales, types and number of physicians prescribing appliances, and the extent of the pharmacy's promotion. An estimate of the required stock space is about 30 to 40 square feet. Also near the fitting room should be a sink with disposable paper toweling for use by the pharmacist before and after each fitting. Where ostomy fittings are concerned, it is advisable to have such a sink inside the fitting room.

Fitting orthopedic and ostomy appliances is a professional service. While it is well to have a trained woman to fit women, with the exception of mastectomies and ostomies the fitting of both sexes can be done by men. Male pharmacists fitting appliances today in a proper environment almost never experience a complaint or unpleasant occurrence with female patients.

Finally, each pharmacy should keep a service record for each patient, with data on physician's instructions, appliances fitted, and any reorders.

What to Stock

There are perhaps as many opinions as to which items should be represented within the pharmacy's surgical supplies and convalescent aids department as there are pharmacies and

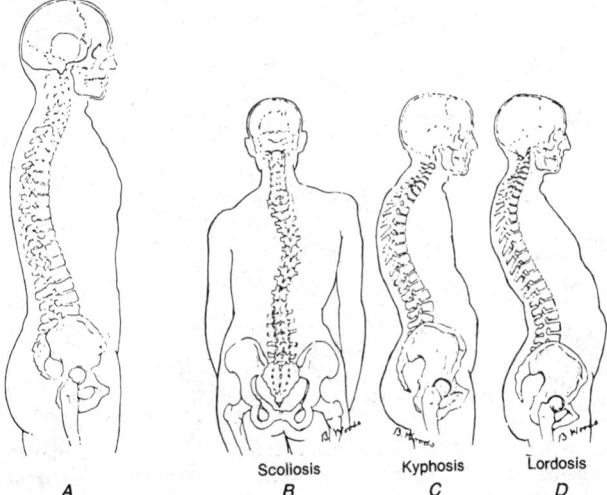

Fig 104-43. A: Curves of the normal spine; B, C, D: abnormal curves of the spine.

Scoliosis   Kyphosis   Lordosis
A   B   C   D

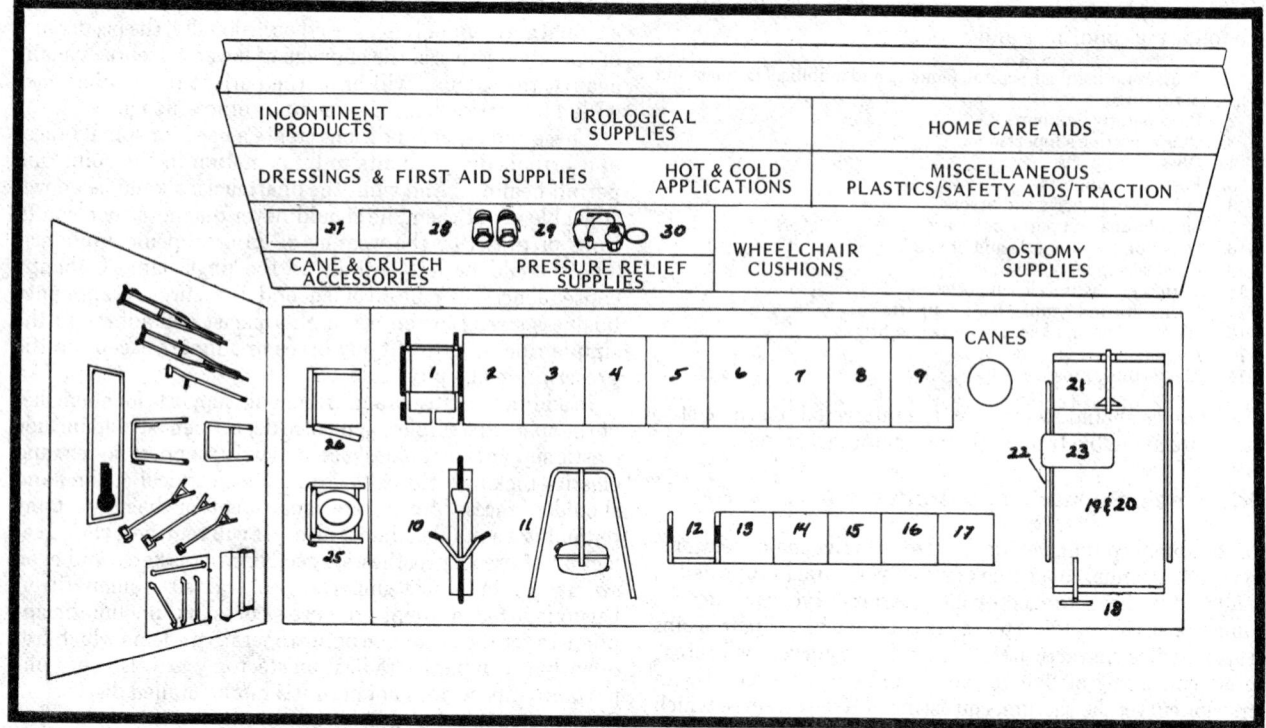

Fig 104-44.   Durable medical equipment and consumable merchandise display.

wholesale distributors with experience in this field. Suggestions for the level and depth of inventory range from as little as a selection which requires a total investment of only $5,000, to one which requires more than $15,000 in initial investment. Some national wholesalers have developed standardized packages requiring a beginning investment of under $1,000, and while that inventory may be adequate for many pharmacies there are other pharmacies that should have inventories which represent larger variety and greater depth in their health accessories departments.

But certainly, standardized inventory packages cannot be right for all pharmacies, for all pharmacies are simply not the same. Pharmacies differ, one from the other, in a multitude of ways. They face different limitations with regard to the available space within their pharmacies for the establishment of health accessories departments. Their financial resources are different. The markets they purport to serve are different, both with respect to size and demographics. With regard to

their drawing areas, differences exist due to various, specific economic factors reflecting distinctively different kinds of demand: in an area with a heavy coal-mining industry, the market demand for respiratory therapy equipment might be very high relative to that in a rural farming community. And further, the extent to which hospital outpatient departments and homecare-oriented health agencies provide the thrust for a viable home health care market within the community is vastly different from one town to another. And not the least important, different pharmacies in different communities face widely divergent forms of competition, both in degree and kind.

All these considerations affect different pharmacies differently. Each pharmacist who contemplates the development of a surgical supplies and convalescent aids department must take these considerations into account when making decisions about what to stock. These are the issues which ultimately determine the optimum variety and depth of in-stock inventory for any given pharmacy.

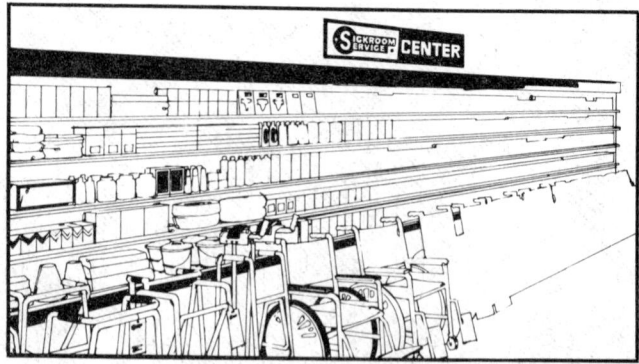

Fig 104-45.   Corner display with window: This arrangement can be extremely beneficial. When placed properly, it is an advertising tool in itself. Its visability to everyone who walks by, drives past or comes into your store makes this a superb choice.

Fig 104-46.   Floor display and wall space: This very common arrangement can be most productive. With the advantage of being able to display all the wheelchairs and walkers open, it gives the consumer a total and comprehensive picture of your Home Care Department, at once.

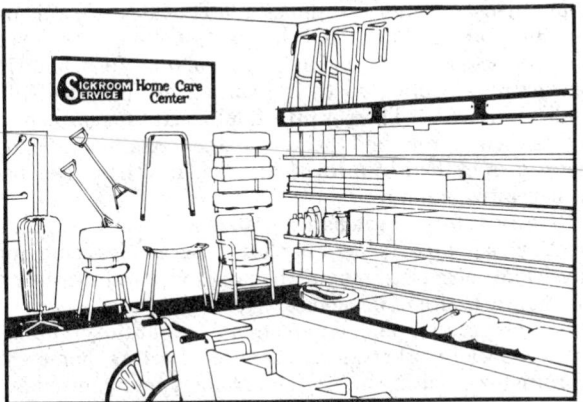

Fig 104-47. Corner display without window: This display can be a very productive one, especially when located next to your prescription department. Its proximity to you and other pharmacist staff members, adds to your professional image. It is also convenient and will be noticed by every one waiting for their prescription.

In many pharmacies it is the actual experience of having capital tied up in inventory that does not turn over that has led many owners to the unfortunate practice of choosing a stocking inventory for health accessories departments solely on the basis of the kind and number of requests received for various types of medical equipment in the past.

Thus begins a vicious circle: The pharmacist has no calls for specialized kinds of wheelchairs, for example; therefore he stocks only four or five basic wheelchair types. Then, when someone comes into the pharmacy for a wheelchair, because of a lack of wheelchair expertise and because more specialized types of wheelchairs are not immediately available, he buys one of the wheelchairs that happens to be in stock. Sometime in the future, if that person visits his physician or physical therapist, he reports, often without realizing it, that the pharmacy was unable to meet his wheelchair needs. The result is that the physician or therapist will not send patients to the pharmacy for further wheelchair fittings.

From then on, the only persons who come to the pharmacy for wheelchairs are those who are either that pharmacy's regular customers or those who are largely uncounseled and self-initiate their visits to the pharmacy. And so, based on his past experience of not having had calls for specialized types of wheelchairs, the pharmacist concludes there is not much demand for them.

Without question, the pharmacist who is interested in developing a successful surgical supplies and convalescent aids department within his pharmacy faces a very serious dilemma. Either he plays it safe, and continues to stock those things he knows he will have calls for, or he decides to expand his inventory and his expertise in an effort to become relatively sophisticated and, by so doing, run the risk of raising his operating costs in an industry about which, at the very least, he is uncertain.

What many pharmacists who are successfully involved in providing a comprehensive health accessories service are finding is that when they give better service with the more specialized kinds of equipment, they also do better with ordinary kinds of equipment. That is because their pharmacies become recognized as *the* places where patients should be sent for a wheelchair, a walker, and other kinds of durable medical equipment and surgical supplies. It is also true that improvement in health accessories service tends to boost a pharmacy's prescription volume as well.

In preparation for the development of a list of inventory items for a pharmacy's health accessories department, the pharmacist should formulate guidelines for himself which incorporate those variables discussed previously regarding space available within the pharmacy for a health accessories department, financial resources, etc. It is also helpful to categorize the kinds of equipment and merchandise he might want to stock, and then rank the various articles within each category as to the relative importance of each in meeting the health needs of his community.

Examples of some of these categories are:

1. Ambulatory aids and accessories
2. Aspirators
3. Bathroom safety aids
4. Commodes
5. Exercise equipment
6. Hospital beds and bed accessories
7. Hot and cold packs, and units
8. Respiratory therapy equipment
9. Patient lifters and accessories
10. Traction equipment and accessories
11. Wheelchairs and accessories
12. Bandages, dressings, and tapes
13. Cushions and pillows
14. Elastic stockings and supports
15. Lymphedema appliances
16. Mastectomy prostheses and accessories
17. Needles and syringes
18. Orthopedic braces and supports
19. Ostomy appliances and accessories
20. Plastic patient care accessories
21. Restraints and safety garments
22. Pressure sore supplies
23. Trusses
24. Urological and incontinence supplies
25. Transcutaneous electrical nerve stimulators

While the above list of product categories could certainly be expanded, it does represent the preponderance of surgical supplies and convalescent aids in the comprehensive health accessories department.

Sample Inventory for a Complete Convalescent Aids Department and Floor Plan Layout

As an example, Sickroom Service Agency pharmacies begin their convalescent aids departments with the following minimum assortment of durable medical equipment items:

1. Mobile Lounge Geriatric Chair
2. Standard Adult Wheelchair with Fixed Footrests
3. Standard Adult Wheelchair with Swinging Detachable Footrests
4. Standard Adult Wheelchair with Swinging Detachable Legrests
5. Standard Adult Wheelchair with Desk Removable Armrests
6. Narrow Adult Wheelchair with Desk Removable Armrests
7. Tiny Tot Wheelchair with Swinging Detachable Legrests
8. Universal Adult Wheelchair with Detachable Desk Arms & Footrests
9. Full Reclining Back Wheelchair with Desk Removable Armrests
10. Exercise Bicycle with Tension Control, Odometer & Timer
11. Economy Exercise Bike with Tension Control & Odometer
12. Chrome Hydraulic Patient Lifter with One Piece Nylon Sling
13. Adjustable Adult Walker
14. Adjustable Adult Walker with Lower Brace
15. Adjustable Swing-Folding Adult Walker
16. Adjustable Reciprocal Adult Walker
17. Adjustable Adult Walkane
18. Manual Variable Height Hospital Bed
19. 80" Polyfoam Mattress with Patient-Proof Ticking
20. 80" Innerspring Mattress with Patient-Proof Ticking
21. Trapeze Bar
22. ¾ to Full Length Telescoping Bed Safety Rails
23. Overbed Table with Glides
24. Floor Standing Traction Unit
25. Adjustable Steel Commode with Pail
26. Pivot Arm Commode on Casters with Pail

27. Alternating Pressure Pump and APP Pad
28. Tempump Control Unit and Pad
29. Adult Quadriceps Boot Assembly and Assorted Cast Iron Weights
30. Portable Aspirator
31. Standard Elevated Toilet Seat with Splash Guard
32. Doughnut-type Elevated Toilet Seat
33. Adjustable Toilet Guard Rail
34. Bathtub Grab Bar—8″ × 11″
35. Bathtub Grab Bar—7″ × 18″
36. Bathroom Wall Grab Bar—Straight 12″
37. Bathroom Wall Grab Bar—Straight 18″
38. Bathroom Wall Grab Bar—Straight 24″
39. Versaguard Bathtub Grab Bar
40. 15″ Bathtub Bench
41. 15″ Bathtub Bench with Back
42. Folding Bed Table
43. Adjustable Blanket Support
44. Easy Read Bed Tray
45. Assorted Wood Walking Canes
46. Small Base Adult Quad Cane
47. Large Base Adult Quad Cane
48. Large Base Adult Quad Cane with Tilt Handle
49. Adult Regular Forearm Crutches
50. Two Intensity Vibrator
51. Foot Whirlpool Unit
52. Infra-Red Heat Massager
53. Aneroid Sphygmomanometer
54. Blood Pressure Monitoring Kit
55. Assorted Stethoscopes

The above list of durable medical equipment items totals approximately $6,000 at normal dealer net cost, and requires about 300 square feet of floor space with accompanying wall shelving units to display a complimentary assortment of consumable products.

It is extremely important that the pharmacy's convalescent aids and surgical supplies department not be too crowded. These products should be displayed in a manner which promotes the pharmacy's professional image. The following sample floorplan layout and sketches illustrate effective merchandising in the health accessories department.

One of the very first things the pharmacist must do is to familiarize himself with the industry's manufacturers and become knowledgeable about the products they manufacture. While his local wholesaler may have many of the items he will need in his health accessories department, he will have to establish direct-buying relationships in order that he be able to obtain the scores of things his wholesaler does not stock. He should begin an alphabetical file of manufacturers' catalogs and price lists, and develop an index which cross-references products with their manufacturers. An index of this type will save hours of time and possible embarrassment before his customers as well by enabling him to go quickly to appropriate information when faced with questions for which he doesn't have ready answers. Questions of this type will not come infrequently, and the pharmacist will realize it as he becomes aware of how broad this field really is.

Appendix A is a list of some of the manufacturers of convalescent aids and surgical supplies, and is presented here as a tool for the beginner. While this list has many of the important manufacturers in which the community pharmacist should have an interest, it should be understood that there are literally hundreds more, and as the pharmacist becomes familiar with them, they, too, should be incorporated in the list.

Promotion

Prior to deciding on the kind of promotion to undertake, the community pharmacist must first determine where the majority of his health accessories volume is most likely to come from. What pharmacists who are successfully involved in comprehensive surgical supplies and convalescent aids departments are finding is that the greatest share of their surgical business is not done with their regular patrons, but with new patrons coming to their pharmacies specifically for medical supplies. There is little doubt that the reason most of these new patrons find their way to these pharmacies is that they were sent there by medical and allied health professionals in their own communities.

Referrals for wheelchairs, walkers, ostomy supplies, breathing equipment, and other health accessories come from physicians, hospitals, nursing homes, and a wide variety of community health professionals, among whom are: therapists (physical, occupational, enterostomal, respiratory), nurses, medical social workers, social service directors, home-care coordinators, visiting nurses, and trainers in organized athletics. Physicians in most major specialties will make referrals. It is important that each health professional be approached about *products or services relevant to his or her specific discipline*. Organizations in which these and other health professionals can be found include: hospitals and nursing homes, visiting nurse associations, private physical therapy associations, state departments of vocational rehabilitation, insurance companies, athletic departments in schools, commercial and manufacturing plants, rehabilitation centers, home health agencies, and clinics; also agencies such as Easter Seal Society, American Cancer Society, Multiple Sclerosis Association, Muscular Dystrophy Foundation, National Paraplegia Foundation, United Cerebral Palsy, United Ostomy Association, and many others. These, then, are the people and the organizations at which the pharmacy's principal promotional programs must be aimed. And while promotion to the general public is still very important, it is crucial that the pharmacist develop effective promotional programs aimed at the professional community.

Because it is quite common for many of these "new" patrons to begin to patronize their "new" pharmacy for other health needs, it is not surprising that the very existence of a comprehensive health accessories department is regarded by the pharmacies who operate them as an excellent means for promoting the pharmacy as a whole.

Since the largest part of surgical supplies and health accessories volume originates with medical and allied health professionals within the community, the question must be asked: What prompts these professionals to recommend one dealer over another?

Aspects about the retail distribution of medical equipment and supplies, which most concerns a community's medical and allied health professionals, are:

1. That the supplier have the academic background and practical know-how to recommend the right equipment for each patient need, and be able to show the patient correctly how the equipment should be used.
2. That the supplier not practice medicine, physical therapy, etc., but call on practitioners of these professions for consultation and guidance when appropriate.
3. That the supplier have in stock an adequate inventory, in kind and quantity, to meet the immediate needs of his patients.
4. That the supplier, in addition to having ample stock, have access to wide varieties of medical equipment and supplies from numerous manufacturers, to service the special and unique needs of patients.
5. That the supplier distribute only merchandise of good quality and stand behind what he rents and sells. Many medical professionals are name-brand conscious also.
6. That the supplier have the capability of providing basic maintenance and repair services for what he sells and rents.
7. That the suppliers' equipment be competitively priced in both rentals and sales.
8. That the supplier operate his business in an immaculate, well-organized, efficient and thoroughly professional manner.

Advertising in professional journals, direct mail campaigns, and face-to-face detailing are all effective and commonly used methods of proclaiming that a pharmacy has the attributes which the professional community expects. But perhaps the most effective way to communicate the fact that the pharmacy has the expertise and inventory to meet the community's health-care needs is by a program of regular hospital displays and in-service training classes for the staffs in hospitals and nursing homes.

The "hospital display" is a productive way to meet the doctor and have him see the kinds of medical equipment and supplies a pharmacy has available. The hospital display usually runs from about 7:30 am to noon, and is set up in or near the physician's lounge or primary entrance through which the physicians arrive each morning. Permission to set up a display must be obtained a month or two beforehand, most often from the hospital administrator though sometimes from the director of purchasing, the head of central-supply, or the manager of the hospital pharmacy. Some hospitals do not allow hospital displays as a general rule, but may permit one to introduce a new service to the community.

There should be plenty of equipment for display, also a small sign which gives the name of the pharmacy and lists the kinds of articles available. It is also helpful to have business cards and a variety of catalogs handy. Even those physicians who do not stop by to visit will note the availability of a new service and also the variety of equipment supplied. Depending on the size of the hospital, from a half dozen to 70 or more physicians may see the display in the course of the morning—that makes a hospital display worthwhile by any standard.

How better to demonstrate one's expertise in selecting, and when necessary measuring and fitting, health accessories than by providing instruction to groups of health professionals in a hospital or nursing home in the basic principles and proper use of the accessories, particularly those that serve as aids in convalescence or home care of the patient. Thus, for example, the important subject of walking aids—canes, forearm crutches, axillary crutches, walkers—should include discussion of the physiological factors of ambulation; the selection, measurement, and fitting of the devices to provide maximum leverage and comfort; and the manner of their use in walking on level areas as well as ascending or descending stairs. Many other subjects can be similarly presented by community pharmacists knowledgeable in the use of convalescent aids and other health accessories.

Various equipment manufacturers offer in-service training programs which may be used as a guide to developing training programs for hospitals, nursing homes, visiting nurse associations, and schools.

The Future

Increased life expectancy has produced an increase in the number of aged persons and a corresponding increase in the number of ill and infirm persons in this segment of our population. The growing number of aged persons, the trend toward their greater subsidization, and the rapid increase in services from home health-care agencies and hospital-out-patient departments portends an ever-increasing number of potential candidates for surgical supplies and convalescent aids in the future. This is also true of many persons who are not aged but still are ill or infirm.

Though nursing homes do care for a substantial number of such patients, more patients want to remain at home and avoid the spiraling costs of institutional care. Hospitals are reluctant to provide services to persons not in need of acute care facilities, except on an outpatient basis, as it is too costly for both the patient and the hospital. As a result, the trend is to transfer the patient to home care as soon as possible. Encouraged to do so by the principal health insurance companies such as Blue Cross and by developing home-health-care agencies, the demand for surgical appliances and medical equipment for use in the patient's home is growing daily.

Professional Approach

Not every pharmacist should hastily conclude that he will be successful in this field, regardless of his estimate of the local market, his inventory, and his display facilities. Unless the pharmacist is willing to devote time and intelligent effort to the venture, he will fail. He must be interested in helping the aged, the infirm, and the sick. His attitude must be professional and his approach to prospective referring physicians and the public must be made on that basis, not on mere availability or price. And most important, he must have developed the expertise to recommend the right equipment and supplies and instruct his patrons in their proper use.

The pharmacist who is seriously considering developing this specialty will need to expand his reading list of relevant professional journals and periodicals. In addition to the major pharmacy journals, the following publications will broaden his knowledge and perspective concerning convalescent aids and surgical supplies: *Health Industry Today; Ostomy Quarterly; Home Healthcare Business; Medical Products Salesman; Respiratory Therapy; Progress Report, American Physical Therapy Association; American Journal of Occupational Therapy; Homecare Rentals/Sales.*

The surgical supply department of the modern community pharmacy is recognized by physician and layman alike as a proper extension of the pharmacist's professional service. Physicians and allied health professionals quickly assess this new service as an important contribution to the health-team concept.

Appendix A—Manufacturers of Medical Equipment and Supplies

1. A-Bec, Torrance, CA
2. Accu-Back, Inc, Carson, CA
3. Acme Cotton Prod Co, Inc, Dayville, CT
4. Acme United Corp, Bridgeport, CT
5. Action Products, Inc, Hagerstown, MD
6. Activeaid, Inc, Redwood Falls, MN
7. Adaptive Therapeutic, Hemden, CT
8. ADC-Automatic Devices, Allentown, PA
9. ADCO Hearing Conservation, Denver, CO
10. Adjustable Fixture Co, Milwaukee, WI
11. Aerobics, Inc, Clifton, NJ
12. Aeroceuticals, Inc, (ATI), Southport, CT
13. Aircast, Inc, Summit, NJ
14. All Orthopedic Appliances, Miami, FL
15. Allied Healthcare Prod Inc, Buffalo, NY
16. Alsons Corporation, Hillsdale, MI
17. AM Fab, Inc, Kalamazoo, MI
18. Ambiomed, International, Lake Park, FL
19. American Gen'l Health Care, Glendale, CA
20. American Health Products, Elgin, IL
21. American Hospital Supply, Brown Deer, WI
22. American Medical Products, Evansville, IL
23. American Stair-Glide Corp, Grandview, MO
24. American Thermometer Co, Dayton, OH
25. American Walker, Inc, Oregon, WI
26. AMF Inc-Whitely, Div, Maywood, NJ
27. AMF Wheel Goods, Chicago, IL
28. AMI Medical Electronics, Ronkonkoma, NY
29. Angelica Uniforms, St Louis, MO
30. Ansell, S H & Son, Inc, Boston, MA
31. Aquatherm Products Corp, Rahway, NJ
32. Arcoa Industries, Santee, CA
33. Armstrong Premier Prod Co, Grand Rapids, MI
34. Arrco Playing Card Co, Chicago, IL
35. Atco Surgical, Cuyahoga Falls, OH
36. Attwood Corporation, Lowell, MI
37. Averill Equipment Co, Troy, MI

38. B & F Medical Products Inc, Toledo, OH
39. Bailey Mfg Co, Lodi, OH
40. Baka Mfg Co, Plainville, MA
41. Banyan International, Abilene, TX
42. Bard Home Health Division, Berkeley Height, NJ
43. Bard Urological Division, Murray Hill, NJ
44. Barns-Ely Co, Englewood, FL
45. Basic Telecommunications, Fort Collins, CO
46. Battle Creek Equipment, Battle Creek, MI

47. Becton Dickinson & Co, Rutherford, NJ
48. Beecham Laboratories, Bristol, TN
49. Beemak Plastics, Los Angeles, CA
50. Beiersdorf, Inc, South Norwalk, CT
51. Belvedere Inc, Belvidere, IL
52. Bemis Health Care, Sheboygan Falls, WI
53. Bennett Brothers, Inc, Chicago, IL
54. Better Sleep Inc, Berkeley Height, NJ
55. Bio Clinic Co, San Bernardino, CA
56. Bio-Dynamics, Indianapolis, IN
57. Bio-Medical Sciences, Inc, Fairfield, NJ
58. Bird Corporation (3M), Palm Springs, CA
59. Body Care, Inc, New York, NY
60. Brandt Industries, Inc, Bronx, NY
61. Brewer, E F, Company, Menomonee Falls, WI
62. Briox Technologies, Inc, Worcester, MA
63. Brockway Glass Co, Inc, St Louis, MO
64. Brown, I, of Hartley Inc, Hartley, IA
65. Bunn Company, The John, Tonawanda, NY
66. Burr Engineering Co, Battle Creek, MI

67. C & H Distributors, Inc, Milwaukee, WI
68. Camp International Inc, Jackson, MI
69. Care Medical Equip Inc, Portland, OR
70. Carex Products, Newark, NJ
71. Caring International, Northbrook, IL
72. Carpenter Company, Inc, E R, Russellville, KY
73. Carstens Health Industries, Chicago, IL
74. Central States Diversified, St Louis, MO
75. Chair Concern, The, South Gate, CA
76. Char-Mag Co of Glendale, Milwaukee, WI
77. Chattanooga Pharmacal Co, Chattanooga, TN
78. Chec Portable Bath Lift, Boonton, NJ
79. Chesebrough Ponds, Inc, Monticello, IN
80. Classique Inc, Miami, FL
81. Clearco-Reibman Mfg, Chicago, IL
82. Cleo Living Aids, Cleveland, OH
83. Clinipad Corp, The, Caruthersville, MO
84. Cloud 9, Bensenville, IL
85. Colgate-Palmolive Co, New York, NY
86. Colson Company, Chicago, IL
87. Columbia Vital Systems, Inc, Westmont, IL
88. Commander-Omni, Garden City, NY
89. Conmed Equipment Corp, Westfield, NJ
90. Consumer Care Products Inc, Sheboygan Falls, WI
91. Continental Scale Corp, Bridgeview, IL
92. Creative Rehabilitation, Portland, OR
93. Cryogenic Associates, Indianapolis, IN
94. Curmed Inc, Arcadia, CA

95. Davol Inc, Providence, RI
96. Detecto Scale Company, Webb City, MO
97. Detroit First Aid, Southgate, MI
98. DeVilbis Company, Somerset, PA
99. Dexon Inc, Minneapolis, MN
100. Diamond Match Company, The, Waukesha, WI
101. Diana Manufacturing Co, Green Bay, WI
102. Dome Lab, Div of Miles, West Haven, CT
103. Donley Battery, Los Angeles, CA
104. Dow Corning Corporation, Midland, MI
105. Doyle Pharmaceutical Corp, Minneapolis, MN
106. Dralle Paper Company, Waukesha, WI
107. Du-It Control Systems GRP, Shreve, OH
108. Duro-Med Industries, Hackensack, NJ
109. Dwyer Medical Supply, Arroyo Grande, CA
110. Dyna Industries Inc, Carlsbad, CA
111. Dynamed Corporation, Elmsford, NY

112. EAR Division, Indianapolis, IN
113. Eagle Plastics Inc, Oak Creek, WI
114. Elder Pharmaceuticals, Inc, Bryan, OH
115. Electronic Monitors, Inc, Euless, TX
116. Elgin Exercise Equip Co, Sandwich, IL
117. Elgin Medical Corp, Elgin, IL
118. Ellisco Inc, Philadelphia, PA
119. Elmed Incorporated, Addison, IL
120. Elmer's Weights, Inc, Walfforth, TX
121. Erie Controls, Milwaukee, WI
122. Ethox Corp, Buffalo, NY
123. Everest & Jennings Inc, Cararillo, CA
124. Exercycle Corp, Woonsocket, RI

125. Fabrication Enterprises, Irvington, NY
126. Fairhope Fabrics, Inc, Fall River, MA
127. Falcon Research & Dev, Englewood, CO
128. Ferno-Washington Inc, Wilmington, OH
129. Fesco Plastics Corp, Kankakee, IL
130. Flat Free (Evergreen Med), Evergreen, CO
131. Foam Rubber Products, Milwaukee, WI
132. Fox Converting Inc, De Pere, WI

133. Freedom Designs, Inc, Ventura, CA
134. Frohock-Stewart Inc, Northboro, MA
135. Frye Electronics Inc, Tigard, OR
136. Futuro Company, The (Jung), Cincinnati, OH

137. G & W Healthcare, Inc, Atlanta, GA
138. GAM Industries, Stoughton, MA
139. Garelick Mfg Co, St Paul Park, MN
140. Garelick Mfg Co, St Paul Park, MN
141. Gaymar Industries, Inc, Orchard Park, NY
142. Gen'l Physiotherapy Inc, St Louis, MO
143. Genac Inc, Lafayette, CO
144. Gendron, Inc, Archbold, OH
145. General Bandages, Inc, Morton Grove, IL
146. George Glove Company, Inc, Englewood, NJ
147. Gerber Products Co, Chicago, IL
148. Gilbert Surgical Instr, Bellmawr, NJ
149. Glenwood Inc, Tenafly, NJ
150. Goss, R E, Inc, Alsip, IL
151. Graham-Field Surgical Co, New Hyde Park, NY
152. Grant Airmass Corp, Stamford, CT
153. Greer Company, John F, Oakland, CA
154. Guardian Products Co, Inc, Memphis, TN

155. HMC Products, New Hudson, MI
156. Halbrand Inc, Willoughby, OH
157. Hamilton Industries Inc, Two Rivers, WI
158. Handi-Ramp Inc, Mundelein, IL
159. Hard Manufacturing Co, Inc, Buffalo, NY
160. Harvey Surgical Supply Corp, Flushing, NY
161. Hausmann Industries Inc, Northvale, NJ
162. Hawk Enterprises, Inc, Oakland, CA
163. Healthdyne, Inc, Marietta, GA
164. Healthscan Inc, Upper Montclair, NJ
165. Heelbo Corporation, Niles, IL
166. Helena Laboratories, Beaumont, TX
167. Hendrickson Inc, Minneapolis, MN
168. Hi-Trac Industries Inc, So Lyon, MI
169. Hill-Rom Co, Inc, Batesville, IN
170. Hollister, Inc, Chicago, IL
171. Hospal Medical Products, Littleton, CO
172. Hoyer & Company, Ted, Oshkosh, WI
173. Hudson Oxygen Therapy Sale, Wadsworth, OH
174. Humanicare International, E Brunswick, NJ
175. Hygienic Dental Mfg Co, Akron, OH
176. Hyman Products Co, Inc, Maryland Hghts, MD

177. Ille, Ferno, Williamsport, PA
178. Infawatch, Newport Beach, CA
179. Inspiron Division, Rancho Cucamong, CA
180. Instrumentation Industries, Bethel Park, PA
181. Intermed, Inc, Sparta, NJ
182. International Therapeutics, Dallas, TX
183. Invacare Corporation, Elyria, OH
184. Isramed, Inc, Fairfield, NJ

185. Jacuzzi Whirlpool Bath, Walnut Creek, CA
186. Jobst Institute, Inc, Toledo, OH
187. Johnson & Johnson, Braintree, MA
188. Johnson & Johnson Prod, Inc, New Brunswick, NJ
189. Jones-Zylon Inc, W Lafayette, OH

190. Kadan Company, Inc, DA, Mt Vernon, NY
191. Kees Goebel Medical, Cincinnati, OH
192. Ken Mcright Supplies, Tulsa, OK
193. Kendall Company, Boston, MA
194. Kenrich Supply Co, Milwaukee, WI
195. Key Ros Corp, Lower Falls, MA
196. KGB Research & Development, Punta Gorda, FL
197. Kimberly-Clark Corp, Neenah, WI
198. Kinetics Measurement Co, Tuxedo, NY
199. Kleen Test Products, Inc, Milwaukee, WI
200. Korex Corporation, Downers Grove, IL

201. Laberne Mfg Co, Columbia, SC
202. Labtron Sci Corp, Hauppauge, NY
203. Lakeside Manufacturing, Milwaukee, WI
204. Lamico Inc, Oshkosh, WI
205. Latimer Rubber Co, J R, Cuyahoga Falls, OH
206. Lenanco Products, Virginia Beach, VA
207. Lif-O-Gen, St Louis, MO
208. Life Products Inc, Boulder, CO
209. Ling Products, Inc, Neenah, WI
210. Little & Company, Laguna Hills, CA
211. Logan Inc, Santa Ana, CA
212. Lopuco, Ltd, Woodbine, MD
213. Lotus Health Care Products, Naugatuck, CT
214. Lumex Inc, Bay Shore, NY
215. Luminaud Inc, Mentor, OH
216. Lumiscope Company, Inc, Edison, NJ

217. M & R Industries Inc, Redmond, WA
218. Macbick Div of C R Bard, Murray Hill, NJ
219. Maclevy Products Corp, Elmhurst, NY
220. Mada Medical Products Inc, Carlstadt, NJ
221. Maddak Inc, Pequannock, NJ
222. Mallard Inc, Detroit, MI
223. Marathon Medical Equipment, Denver, CO
224. Mark-Clark Products, Topeka, KS
225. Marshall Electronics, Inc, Skokie, IL
226. Mason Laboratories, Horsham, PA
227. McCarty's Inc, Coeur d'Alene, ID
228. Mead Johnson & Co, Evansville, IN
229. Med Labs, Goleta, CA
230. Medela Inc, Crystal Lake, IL
231. Medi, Inc, Holbrook, MA
232. Medical Devices, Inc, St Paul, MN
233. Medical Disposables Co, Inc, Dyersburg, TN
234. Medical Marketing Group, Atlanta, GA
235. Medisco-Federal, Garnerville, NY
236. Medline Industries, Inc, Chicago, IL
237. Medtronic-Neuro Div, Minneapolis, MN
238. Menda Scientific Products, Santa Barbara, CA
239. Mentor Corporation, Minneapolis, MN
240. Mettler Electronics Corp, Anaheim, CA
241. Miltex Instrument, Lake Success, NY
242. Milwaukee Mattress &, Milwaukee, WI
243. Minn. Mining & Mfg (3M), St Paul, MN
244. Minnesota Chemical Co, St Paul, MN
245. Mintron, Inc, Erie, PA
246. Misdom Frank Corp, New York, NY
247. Modular Medical Corp, Bronx, NY
248. Monogram Mfg Co, Chicago, IL
249. Monterey Laboratories, Inc, Las Vegas, NV
250. Monterey Mills, Inc, Janesville, WI
251. Mor-Loc Corporation, Claremont, NC
252. Motion Designs Inc, Clovis, CA
253. MSE Corporation, Sacramento, CA
254. Mutronic Products, Englewood, CO

255. N-K Products Co, Inc, Soquel, CA
256. Nageldinger, Inc, John & Son, Westbury, NY
257. National Chemsearch, Dallas, TX
258. Natural Health Research, Sausalito, CA
259. Nelkin/Piper International, Kansas City, MO
260. Neuromedics, Inc, Clute, TX
261. Newark Electronics, Brookfield, WI
262. Nidco of Colorado Inc, Denver, CO
263. Nilodor Inc, No Canton, OH
264. Nolan & Son, J E, Louisville, KY
265. Northern Electric Co, Chicago, IL
266. Norwich-Eaton, Norwich, NY
267. Nu-Hope Laboratories, Los Angeles, CA
268. Nurse-Dri Breast Shield Co, Mill Valley, CA
269. Nytone Medical Products, Salt Lake City, UT

270. Oak Medical Supply Co, Ravenna, OH
271. Obus Forme Ltd, Canada M5R 2MB
272. Ocelco, Inc, Minneapolis, MN
273. Ohio Medical Products, Madison, WI
274. Orthomedics Inc, Brea, CA
275. Orthopedic Splints, Inc, Lindenhurst, NY
276. Oster, Div of Sunbeam Corp, Milwaukee, WI
277. OTC Professional Appliance, Cincinnati, OH

278. P A Medical Corporation, Columbia, TN
279. Parker Laboratories, Orange, NJ
280. PCP-Champion, Ripley, OH
281. Pelouze Scale Co, Evanston, IL
282. Peters Mfg Co, Inc, Pelham, AL
283. Pharmaceutical Innovations, Newark, NJ
284. Phoenix Glove Company, Waynesville, OH
285. Plymouth Rubber Co, Kansas City, MO
286. Posey Company, J T, Chicago, IL
287. Precision Plastics Corp, Northglenn, CO
288. Prentke Romich Company, Shreve, OH
289. Presto Galaxy, Inc, Greenpoint, NY
290. Principle Business, Dunbridge, OH
291. Procter & Gamble Distr Co, Oakbrook, IL
292. Production Research Corp, Beltsville, MD
293. Professional Specialties, St Louis, MO
294. Protech Pacific, Larkspur, CA
295. Purdue Frederick Co, Norwalk, CT
296. Puritan-Bennett Corp, Westmont, IL
297. Pymah Corporation, Somerville, NJ
298. Pymm Thermometer Corp, Brooklyn, NY

299. Quadra Productions, Inc, New York, NY
300. Quadra Wheelchairs, Inc, Westlake Vlge, CA

301. R & J Medical Supply, Milwaukee, WI
302. Rajowalt/Carters, Elkhart, IN
303. Ranco Products, Battle Creek, MI
304. Raymo Products Inc, Olathe, KS

305. Replogle Globes, Chicago, IL
306. Repro Corporation, Chattanooga, TN
307. Rival Manufacturing Co, Kansas City, MO
308. Rocket, Branford, CT
309. Roho Research, E St Louis, IL
310. Rok-A-Chair Mfg, Coffeyville, KS
311. Roloke Company, Beverly Hills, CA
312. Rolyan Mfg Co, Inc, Menomonee Falls, WI
313. Ross Laboratories, Columbus, OH

314. S & W Enterprises Inc, Blaine, MN
315. Safety Travel Chairs, Inc, Elyria, OH
316. Salk, Inc, Murray, Boston, MA
317. Sammons, Inc, Fred, Brookfield, IL
318. Schell Leather Co, Cincinnati, OH
319. Schinner Company, A D, Milwaukee, WI
320. Scholl, Inc, Memphis, TN
321. Schuco, Williston Park, NY
322. Sci-O-Tech/Goodman, Lancaster, PA
323. Scimedics, Inc, Corona, CA
324. Scott Specialties, Inc, Belleville, KS
325. Shelton Company, Richard C, Dayton, OH
326. Shurtleff, Inc, Codman &, Randolph, MA
327. Sickroom Service, Inc, Milwaukee, WI
328. Siebe Norton, Inc, Cranston, RI
329. Skil-Care Corp, Yonkers, NY
330. Slip-X-Safety Treads, Grand Rapids, MI
331. Smalley & Bates, Inc, Cedar Grove, NJ
332. Smith & Davis, St Louis, MO
333. Solo Products, W Sacramento, CA
334. Spectrum Diagnostics, Inc, Glenwood, IL
335. Spenco Medical Corp, Waco, TX
336. Sperti Sun Lamp Div, Erlenger, NY
337. Sports Supports Inc, Dallas, TX
338. Squibb, E R & Sons, Rolling Meadows, IL
339. Stainless Medical Products, San Diego, CA
340. Stall & Dean, Brockton, MA
341. Standard Lamp Co, Milwaukee, WI
342. Staodynamics, Inc, Longmont, CO
343. Steelcraft Inc, Millbury, MA
344. Steridyne Corporation, Riviera Beach, FL
345. Stokely-Van Camp, Inc, Cincinnati, OH
346. Stryker Corporation, Kalamazoo, MI
347. Superior Specialties, Inc, Appleton, WI
348. Sween Corporation, Lake Crystal, MN

349. T I C, New York, NY
350. Tafco Mfg Co, Portland, OR
351. Talcott Laboratories, Inc, Houston, PA
352. Tasch, Canada M4N 3M5
353. Temco Healthcare Ind, Inc, Passaic, NJ
354. Theradyne Corp, Lakeville, MN
355. Therapeutic Equipment Corp, Clifton, NJ
356. Theratech Inc, Colorado Springs, CO
357. Thompson Medical Special, Minneapolis, MN
358. Thompson Respiration, Boulder, CO
359. TIDI Products, Troy, MI
360. Timex Medical Prod Corp, Waterbury, CT
361. Trail Ridge Products Inc, Castle Rock, CO
362. Trans Medical, Inc, Bloomington, MN
363. Trans-Aid Corporation, Carson, CA
364. Tru-Eze Mfg Co, Temecula, CA
365. TSM Safety Products, Inc, Los Angeles, CA
366. Twenty-First Century, Van Nuys, CA

367. Ulico, Inc, Dearborn, MI
368. Ulster Scientific, Inc, Highland, NY
369. Uni-Patch Inc, Wabasha, MN
370. Union Carbide Corp, Itasca, IL
371. United Metal Fabricators, Johnstown, PA
372. United, Div of Howmedica, Largo, FL
373. Urocare Products Inc, S El Monte, CA

374. Vestal Laboratories, St Louis, MO
375. Vitaire Corporation, Queens, NY
376. Vital Signs Inc, E Rutherford, NJ
377. Vollrath Co, Sheboygan, WI

378. WR Medical Electronics Co, St Paul, MN
379. Walker Seat Co, Inc, Canada K1G3H8
380. Walton Mfg Co, Dallas, TX
381. Weyerhaeuser Co, Freemont, MI
382. White Cap Enterprises Corp, Hull, MA
383. Whitehall Electro Medical, Hackensack, NJ
384. Whitehall Laboratories, St Louis, MO
385. Whitestone Products, Piscataway, NJ
386. Winco Incorporated, St Petersburg, FL
387. Woodlets, Inc, Buffalo, NY

388. Xttrium Laboratories, Inc, Chicago, IL

389. Zeus Industries Intl, Buena Park, CA
390. Zygo Industries, Inc, Portland, OR

CHAPTER 105

Surgical Supplies

Richard L Kronenthal, PhD
Director of Research
Ethicon, Inc
Somerville, NJ 08876

A professional service rendered by many pharmacists consists of supplying surgical instruments, sutures, surgical dressings, and other equipment employed by the surgeon prior to, during, and after a surgical operation. Some pharmacists, who have obtained the necessary background of information, carry a complete line of such supplies, and are even able to provide operating tables and other heavy equipment.

There are comparatively few such completely equipped pharmacies; the major outlet is through surgical supply houses. Every pharmacist, however, should be familiar with two of the products mentioned above, namely, *Surgical Dressings* and *Sutures*, which are discussed in detail below. The selection of the correct type of surgical dressing or suture is a critical factor in safeguarding the welfare of the patient undergoing surgery. Many items belonging in these categories are handled routinely by the pharmacist and all of these items come within the purview of his professional responsibility.

Surgical Dressings

Definition—*Surgical dressing* or *curatio* is a term applied to a wide range of materials used for the dressing of wounds. They are employed as coverings, absorbents, protectives, or supports for injured or diseased tissues.

Classification—Dressings may be classified as:

1. Primary wound dressings
2. Absorbents
3. Bandages
4. Adhesive tapes
5. Protectives

Specifications—Surgical dressings and sutures are required to meet specific requirements of the USP for many characteristics. For these specific requirements and the performance of several of the official tests, eg, *Absorbency test* and *Fiber length* of cotton, the *Diameter* of sutures and the *Tensile strength* of sutures, textile fabrics, and films, the reader is directed to the detailed instructions provided in the USP.

Primary Wound Dressings

This term refers to dressings that are designed to be placed next to a wound surface and are usually reinforced by materials of various types to absorb the wound secretion and minimize maceration.

Gauze compresses of suitable mesh and thickness have long been widely used as primary wound dressings, but they have the drawback of adherence to other than clean, incised wound surfaces. To minimize this difficulty, various types of dressings have been designed to avoid the pain and trauma caused when a dressing which is adhered to a wound surface is removed.

Petrolatum-impregnated gauze has been widely used for this purpose on the theory that since it possesses hydrophobic characteristics it should not adhere. However, this often does not prove to be the case, and, in addition, this material very frequently causes maceration and is difficult to sterilize.

In an effort to eliminate these problems, a special type of gauze, knitted from pure, regenerated cellulose and impregnated with a bland, hydrophilic, oil-in-water emulsion in such a way that all pores remain open, has proved to have an ex-tremely low degree of adherence to all types of wounds. It is known as Adaptic Non-Adhering Dressing (*J&J*). Each dressing is packaged sterile in a unique envelope that guarantees sterility and, at the same time, can be opened easily under sterile conditions.

The weave is tight enough so that buds of new skin can not grow through the dressing and become entangled in the filaments. The dressing has a sidewise stretch which allows conformability without wrinkling.

The versatility of this dressing makes it excellent for all types of wounds such as burns, skin grafts, colostomies, ileostomies, open ulcers, and cases where packing is needed.

Another type of nonadhering dressing consists of an absorbent pad faced with a soft plastic film having openings. These are large enough to allow fluids to pass through, but too small to allow adhesion of the wound to take place. This dressing is available both in the form of pads of many sizes with various backings, including perforated adhesive tape. Still another nonadhering dressing consists of nonadherent-coated, open-structured, nonwoven facing fabric which is used over various absorbent filler materials.

It is important to use a nonadherent dressing next to any wound surface wherever possible, both as a matter of patient comfort and to minimize interference with wound healing when the dressing is removed.

Absorbents

Surgical Cotton—Cotton is the basic surgical absorbent. It is an official USP listing under *Purified Cotton.*

Domestic cotton grown in the Southern United States is suitable for surgical purposes. The domestic cotton plant reaches a height of from 2 to 4 ft. Growing from the seeds is a pod or boll which bursts open upon ripening, exposing a mass of white cotton fibers. Each of these fibers is a minute, hair-like tube, the outer wall being pure cellulose, the opening filled with plant fluids. When the boll bursts open, the fiber collapses into a flat ribbon-like form, twisted and doubled upon itself more than a hundred times from end to end.

The picking season for cotton begins in the late summer.

Most cotton is now picked by machine. The cotton, after the seeds have been removed by the gin, is compressed into bales weighing about 500 lb.

All cotton grades are standardized by the US Department of Agriculture. Samples of each bale are classified into one of six color groups, then given a "staple length" according to the length of the average fibers, and finally graded as to the amount of foreign matter present and the condition and ripeness of the fibers. From these hundreds of possible grading combinations, each bale is given a "quality rating" which determines its price.

The raw cotton fiber, mechanically cleaned of dirt and carded into layers, but not otherwise treated, has a limited use for paddings and coverings of unbroken surfaces. This form is supplied under the name of *nonabsorbent cotton*. It is also frequently used as cotton plugs in the bacteriological laboratory because of its nonabsorbency.

Absorbent Cotton is prepared from the raw cotton fiber by a series of processes which remove the natural waxes and all impurities and foreign substances and render the fibers absorbent. Briefly summarized the processes may be described as follows. Each cotton bale goes through a mechanical cleaning process. Foreign matter, dust, seed hulls, and soil, etc, are removed by means of "openers," "pickers," etc. From the mechanical cleaners, the cotton is blown through large pipes to the boiling kier and the bleaching tub where it is made absorbent and bleached. In these processes it is freed from the waxes, resins, fats, and coloring matter normally present in the raw fiber.

During the chemical treatment, all surgical cotton is thoroughly washed using a fresh supply of water for each washing. A practically pure, white cellulose fiber is the result.

Cotton thus treated is dried by being passed, on a moving screen, through long drying ovens. The dried cotton is then ready for the "lapping" process. This process is similar to the cleaning process. The beaters tear the tufts of cotton to smaller pieces. The grid bars eliminate the short fibers and foreign matter. The rollers press the cotton into a continuous lap in which form it passes through the carding machine. There, thousands of wire needles remove the short fibers and straighten out the longer cotton fibers, forming a thin web. This is the familiar roll cotton. Other cards fold the web which is then cut into uniform strips and automatically rolled into cotton balls.

Besides the familiar roll form, Purified Cotton may be obtained in various prepared forms such as cotton balls, cotton-tipped applicators, etc.

Cotton Balls can be prepared by hand but they are more advantageously made on special machines. Machine-made balls are firm, compact, and uniform in size, shape, and weight. They are produced in several sizes. The larger size balls are made for obstetrical uses, in the delivery room, or when changing perineal pads. The medium cotton ball is particularly useful for applying antiseptics or medication locally, cleansing the skin, and in the nursery where manifold uses are apparent. The small cotton ball is often used for skin cleansing before hypodermic or intravenous injections, and in applying local medications to small areas.

Absorbent balls made of a uniform surgical viscose-rayon fiber are also available. These absorbent balls absorb fluids faster and retain their shape better than cotton balls.

Nonabsorbent Bleached Cotton, prepared by a modified bleaching process, wherein the water-repellent natural oils and waxes are retained, is also available. This cotton is easily identified by its silky feel. Because it is repellent to water, it does not become matted or inelastic. Consequently it is well adapted to packing, padding, and cushioning of dressings over traumatized areas and as nonabsorbent backing on sanitary napkins, combines, and drainage dressings.

Surgical Gauzes—The function of surgical gauze is to provide an absorbent material of sufficient tensile strength for surgical dressings. It is listed in the USP under *Absorbent Gauze*.

In the process of making surgical gauze, the raw cotton fiber is mechanically cleaned and then spun or twisted into a thread, and the thread, in turn, woven into an open-mesh cloth. This cloth is gray in appearance and nonabsorbent. It is bleached white and rendered absorbent by much the same processes as those used in the preparation of surgical cotton.

The gauze thus treated is dried by passing in a continuous length through a tentering machine. Tenterhooks straighten, stretch, and hold the gauze taut as it is dried. When it leaves this apparatus, the dried gauze is cut into lengths, folded, rolled, and packaged.

Gauze is classified according to its mesh or number of threads per inch. Some types of surgical dressing require a close-meshed gauze for extra strength and greater protection, while other uses such as primary wound dressings, absorbent secondary dressings, and larger dressings to absorb purulent matter or other drainage require softer, more absorbent gauzes, having a more open structure.

Various forms of pads, compresses, and dressings are made from surgical gauze, alone or in conjunction with absorbent cotton, tissue paper, and other materials.

Filmated Gauze is a folded absorbent gauze with a thin, even film of cotton or rayon distributed over each layer. This filmation fluffs up and gives ample dressing volume, yet costs less than gauze alone of equivalent volume. It possesses quick absorption and unusual softness.

Non-Woven Surgical Sponges. During the past decade, non-woven fabrics have been developed which are suitable alternatives to woven cotton gauze for use in wound cleaning, wound dressing, and tissue handling sponges. These non-woven fabrics depend on dense entanglement of their synthetic fibers (Dacron, Rayon, etc) to provide the fabric with an acceptable tensile strength approaching that of woven cotton gauze. They typically offer greater absorbent capacity than cotton gauze sponges of comparable bulk while generating less lint. Specialty versions of the non-woven sponges are available pre-fenestrated for IV tubing or drain dressing procedures. One manufacturer (*J&J*) provides both a non-woven sponge for wound dressing (SOF-WICK; very soft texture, very absorbent) and a non-woven general purpose cleansing/prep sponge (NU GAUZE; gauze-like texture, more absorbent than gauze).

Antiseptic or *Medicated Surgical Gauze* originated in the Listerian era of surgery, and it is still used to some extent but with the advent of antibiotics and other therapeutic agents, its popularity is decreasing. Most commonly used is iodoform gauze, which contains 5% iodoform and is largely used as a packing or drainage material. The so-called *Penrose drain*, commonly used for draining surgical wounds, is made by drawing a piece of plain or iodoform gauze through a thin-walled tube of latex and cutting to the desired length.

Selvage-Edge Gauze Strips in widths of $1/4$ to 2 in are specially designed and woven for use both as packing strips in surgery of the nose and sinuses, nasal hemostasis, etc, and as drainage wicks in the treatment of boils, abscesses, fistulas, and other draining wounds. The ravel-proof, selvage edges on both sides eliminate all loose threads. These selvage edge gauzes are available unmedicated, or medicated with iodoform 5%. These gauze strips are obtainable in sterile form packed in sealed glass jars.

Gauze Pads or *Sponges* are folded squares of surgical gauze. These pads are so folded that no cut gauze edges or loose threads are exposed. This prevents loose fibers from entering the wound. The edges are so folded that each size may be unfolded to larger sizes without exposing cut edges or loose threads. Most popular sizes are:

2 × 2-in—12-ply
3 × 3-in—12-ply
4 × 4-in— 8-ply
4 × 4-in—16-ply
8 × 4-in—12-ply
8 × 4-in—24-ply

Sterilized packages of these frequently used all-gauze sponges are available in tamper-proof packages of 2's. Such sterile units are particularly well suited to the numerous tray sets prepared in hospitals.

X-ray Detectable Gauze pads are similar to all-gauze pads but contain inserts treated with barium sulfate. They are nontoxic, soft, and nonabrasive. They remain permanently detectable because they do not deteriorate in the body nor are they affected by either sterilization or time. Ray-Tec X-Ray Detectable Sponges (*J&J*) contain a nonabrasive vinyl plastic monofilament which gives a characteristic pattern in the X-ray.

Composite absorbent dressings have been developed for specific purposes. They usually consist of layers of absorbent gauze or nonwoven fabric with fillers of cotton, rayon, nonwoven fabric, or tissue paper in suitable arrangements. Composite sponges have gauze or nonwoven fabric surfaces with fillers of cotton, rayon, nonwoven fabric, or absorbent tissue.

Dressing Combines are designed to provide warmth and protection and to absorb large quantities of fluid that may drain from an incision or wound. Each combine consists of a nonwoven fabric cover enclosing fiber with or without absorbent tissue. They may also incorporate a nonabsorbent layer of cotton, tissue, or plastic film to prevent fluid from coming through to soil liners and bedding, though some combined dressings are entirely absorbent.

Laparotomy Sponges, also known as *Abdominal Packs, Tape Pads* or *Packs, Walling-Off Mops, Stitched Pads, Quilted Pads, Gauze Mops,* etc, are used to form a nonabrasive wall that will prevent abdominal or other organs from escaping into the field of operation and to help maintain body temperature during exposure. They are made of four layers of 28 × 24-mesh gauze. The edges are folded in and hemmed. The entire pack is cross-stitched and a looped tape ½ in wide and 20 in long is attached to one corner of it. A desirable feature of one type is an X-ray detectable insert, so firmly incorporated into the gauze that it cannot become detached. Treated with barium sulfate, the monofilament is nontoxic and, were it to be left inadvertently *in situ*, would cause no more foreign body reaction than an ordinary dressing.

Sanitary Napkins, intended for special hospital use, otherwise known as *V-Pads, Obstetrical (OB) Pads, Perineal Pads, Maternity Pads,* etc, are used in obstetrical, gynecological, or maternity cases. Napkins which have repellent tissue on the side and back surfaces of the napkin are usually preferred because of their greater fluid-holding capacity. Sanitary napkins generally come with two sizes of filler, 3 × 9 or 3 × 11 in. The napkin cover is generally made from a nonwoven fabric or a nonwoven fabric supported with an open mesh scrim. Packaged, sterilized napkins are available and generally used to reduce cross-contamination possibilities.

Disposable Cleaners made from various types of nonwoven fabrics are available, and generally offer advantages over paper of wet strength, abrasion resistance, as well as better cleaning ability, and advantages over cloth of reduced laundry expense and cross-contamination possibilities.

Eye Pads are scientifically shaped to fit comfortably and to completely cover the eye, thus protecting the eyebrow when taped. These pads are made using nonwoven fabric. Two sides are enclosed to prevent the cotton from escaping and the pad from distorting. Where desired the pad may be folded and used as a pressure dressing. Eye pads are especially useful in the outpatient clinic of the hospital, the industrial medical department, and the physician's office. They are sealed in individual sterile envelopes.

Nursing Pads are designed in a contour shape to fit comfortably under the nursing brassiere or breast binder.

Disposable Underpads are used for incontinent patients, maternity patients, and other cases where there is severe drainage. Such pads cost less than the average hospital-made product and provide a neat, clean, easy-to-handle pad that is quickly changed and easily disposed.

Cotton Tipped Applicators are used to apply medications or cleanse an area. Machine-made cotton-tipped applicators are uniform in size, resulting in no waste of cotton or medications. The cotton is firmly attached to the stick and may be readily sterilized without affecting the anchorage of the cotton. These applicators are available in 3- or 6-in lengths.

Bandages

The function of bandages is to hold dressings in place to provide pressure or support. They may be inelastic, elastic, or become rigid after shaping for immobilization.

Common Gauze Roller Bandage is listed in the USP as a form in which *Absorbent Gauze* may be provided. It is prepared from *Type I Absorbent Gauze* in various widths and lengths. Each bandage is in one continuous piece, tightly rolled, and substantially free from loose threads and ravelings.

Muslin Bandage Rolls are made of heavier unbleached material (56 × 60 mesh). They are supplied in the same widths as the regular gauze bandage. Muslin bandages are very strong and are used wherever gauze bandages do not provide sufficient strength or support. They are frequently used to hold splints or bulky compression dressings in place.

Elastic Bandages are made in several types:

1. Woven Elastic Bandage is made of heavy elastic webbing containing rubber threads. Good support and pressure are provided by this type of rubber elastic bandage.

2. Crepe Bandage is elastic, but contains no rubber. Its elasticity is due to a special weave that allows it to stretch to practically twice its length, even after repeated launderings. This elasticity makes the crepe bandage especially serviceable in bandaging varicose veins, sprains, etc, because it conforms closely to the skin or joint surfaces, lies flat and secure, yet allows limited motion and stretches in case of swelling so that circulation is not impaired.

3. Conforming Bandage is a new type of readily conforming bandage made from two plies of specially processed, high quality, 14 × 8 cotton gauze folded to the center. This type of bandage is much easier to use and apply than ordinary roller bandage since it tends to cling to itself during application, thus preventing slipping. It readily conforms to all body contours without the necessity of "reversing" or twisting. A further advantage is the fact that there can be no rough or frayed edge. Kling Conforming Gauze Bandage (*J&J*) is a conforming bandage available in a variety of sizes up to 6 in wide. This Gauze is widely used to hold dressings or splints firmly in place and is used occasionally as a primary dressing when sticking to the wound is not a problem. A mercerized cotton Conforming Gauze Bandage clings to itself and thus remains in place better than gauze made of other materials.

4. High Bulk Bandage is made of multiple layers of typically 6 layers of crimped cotton gauze. The high bulk of this bandage type is designed to provide padding protection in wound dressing applications. It also provides the absorbent capacity of a cotton dressing component. One version (*J&J* SOF-BAND High Bulk) is made of mercerized cotton to help the bandage to cling to itself which facilitates application and improves dressing stability.

Triangular Bandages are usually made by cutting a square of bleached muslin diagonally from corner to corner, forming two right triangles of equal size and shape. The length of the base is approximately 54 in. These bandages were brought into prominence by Esmarch and still bear his name. They are used in first-aid work for head dressings, binders, arm slings, and as temporary splints for broken bones.

Orthopedic Bandages are used to provide immobilization and support in treatment of broken bones and in certain conditions of bones and joints. Plaster of Paris-impregnated gauze has been the standard material for this purpose. Newly introduced are synthetic cast materials made of polyester cotton or fiberglass. Various types of plastic sheets are also offered which can be shaped easily and harden to a rigid form by cooling or chemical reaction. These are chiefly useful for splints and corrective braces.

Individually packaged plaster of Paris bandages and splints are available in a wide variety of sizes. The Specialist (*J&J*) brand is made from specially treated plaster, uniformly spread and firmly bonded to the fabric. This results in a high strength-to-weight ratio in casts made from such bandages. Synthetic casts are applied like Plaster of Paris. The Delta-Lite Synthetic Casting System (*J&J*) offers both polyester/cotton and fiberglass casting materials. The casts are water resistant, light weight, and durable.

Orthoflex Elastic Plaster Bandages (*J&J*) are plaster of Paris bandages containing elastic threads in the fabric and are intended for specialized prosthetic usages.

Stockinette Bandages are made of stockinette material knitted or woven in tubular form without seams. Surgical stockinette is unbleached. Because it is soft and will stretch readily to conform comfortably to the arm, leg, or body, it is used to cover the skin prior to the application of a plaster of Paris or synthetic cast.

Cast Paddings are soft, absorbent, protective paddings, applied like a bandage to the areas affected before application of a cast. They are composed of various fiber constructions which conform and cling, absorb moisture, and allow the skin to breathe.

Adhesive Tape

Surgical adhesive tapes are made in many different forms, varying both in the type of backing and in the formulation of the adhesive mass according to specific needs and requirements. The tapes available today may be divided into two broad categories: those with a rubber-based adhesive and those with an acrylate adhesive. Both types have a variety of uses. Where strength of backing, superior adhesion, and economy are required (eg, athletic strapping), rubber adhesives are commonly used. Acrylate adhesives on a variety of backing materials are used widely in surgical dressing applications, where reduced skin trauma is required as in operative and postoperative procedures; they are supplied in various strength and adhesion levels.

Acrylate Adhesives—Acrylate adhesives on a nonwoven or fabric backing have been widely accepted for use as surgical tapes, owing largely to what may be termed their hypoallergenic nature. Because acrylate adhesives are basically a unipolymeric system, they eliminate the use of a large number of components in rubber-based adhesives. In poly(alkylacrylate) adhesives, the desired balance between adhesion, cohesion, and flow properties is determined by the choice of monomers and the control of the polymerization reactions. Once the polymer is made, no other formulating or compounding is needed. In addition, the acrylics have excellent shelf-life because they are not readily affected by heat, light, or air, factors which tend to degrade rubber-based adhesives.

Acrylate adhesives combine the proper balance of tack and long-term adhesion. Their molecular structure permits the passage of water vapor so they are nonocclusive, and thus, when coated on a porous backing material, do not cause overhydration in the stratum corneum. Traumatic response to surgical tapes is substantially minimized when tapes are constructed to allow normal skin moisture to pass through adhesive and backing material. With this construction, the

moisture content and strength of the horny cell layers remain relatively normal. When a porous tape is removed, the planes of separation develop near the surface of the stratum corneum, in the region of the naturally desquamating cells. This allows for repeated use of tape over the same site with minimal damage to the skin.

Hypoallergenic Surgical Tapes with acrylate adhesive are available with a variety of porous backing materials. Rayon taffeta cloth backing provides a high strength tape well suited for affixing heavy dressings. Lighter dressing applications can be accomplished with lower strength, economical paper backed surgical tapes. A new knitted backing tape (dermiform, *J&J*) provides some of the economies of paper surgical tape with the strength and conformability of a cloth backing. Other tapes feature elastic cloth or foam backing materials for special taping need.

Rubber-Based Adhesives—A second group of surgical adhesive tapes is the cloth-backed and plastic-backed rubber adhesives. These are used principally where heavy support and a high level of adhesion are required. Modern rubber-based adhesive tape masses consist of varying mixtures of several classes of substances and are composed of an elastomer (para or pale crepe rubber in the case of natural rubber tapes, and synthetic elastomers made from polymers of isobutylene, alkylacrylate, and similar materials); one of several types of rosin or modified rosin; antioxidants; plasticizers; and fillers and coloring agents to give the tape the desired tint or whiteness.

Adhesive Tape Reactions—While skin reactions were formerly accepted by the medical profession as almost predictable sequelae to the use of adhesive tape, with better understanding of the mechanisms of such reactions and progress in research and technology, the long-sought-for objective of hyporeactivity has in large degree been attained.

Because adhesive tape masses have historically consisted of heterogeneous and complex mixtures of organic compounds, it is not surprising that many workers have ascribed adhesive tape reaction to allergy. More recent work, however, has shown that a true allergic response to the modern adhesive tape mass or to its components is a factor in only a small proportion of clinical reactions and that the majority of observed reactions are properly ascribed to other factors, mainly mechanical irritation and to a lesser degree chemical irritation. There is apparently no significant difference in reaction between patients with or without a history of allergy, but true specific dermatitis may occur more readily in persons who have manifested some other form of contact dermatitis.

Adverse manifestations produced by adhesive tape are characterized by erythema, edema, papules, vesicles, and, in severe cases, desquamation. Itching may be intense, or it may be absent. The reaction may readily be demonstrated by patch testing, and usually manifests itself early—within 24 to 48 hours. Characteristically, the reaction becomes more severe the longer the tape is left in place and continues to increase in intensity for some time after the tape is removed. This type of reaction is long-lasting and requires days for its complete subsidence.

Two distinct types of irritation can result from the mechanical dynamics of removing tape from the skin. One response—induced vasodilatation—is a relatively nontraumatic, transitory effect in which no actual damage to the skin occurs. A second type of mechanical irritation—skin stripping—is a traumatic response in which skin is removed with the tape and actual damage to the epidermal layers results. Such mechanical skin removal is possibly the dominant cause of clinical reactions seen with the use of adhesive tape.

Chemical irritation from adhesive tape results when irritating components in the mass or backing of the tape permeate the underlying tissues of the skin. The tape construction can substantially influence the reactivity of such ingredients. For example, many compounds that normally do not penetrate intact stratum corneum can penetrate overhydrated corneum.

When portions of the stratum corneum are removed, the barrier capacity of the skin is substantially damaged. In this situation, any irritating components of the tape have ready access to underlying tissues. These substances can then cause a degree of irritation that is far greater than would be observed on intact skin.

Protectives

Until recently, protectives included only the various impermeable materials intended to be used adjunctively with other dressing components to prevent the loss of moisture or heat from a wound site or to protect clothing or bed liners from wound exudate. The recent introduction of adhesive film dressings adds a significant new dimension to the concept of protectives.

Film Dressings—Acrylate adhesive coated on a transparent, moisture vapor permeable plastic film applied directly onto a wound surface represents a new approach for dressing selected wounds. This type of dressing system helps protect the wound site because it is impervious to liquid water and bacteria yet will allow the passage of moisture vapor from the wound site. While film dressings are not recommended for infected or profusely exudative wounds, they do represent an alternative for dressing many clean, scantly draining wounds of various types in which epithelial regeneration is occurring. Dressing removal without disruption of healing tissues is accomplished because the acrylate adhesive, which holds well to intact skin, will not adhere to set wound surfaces.

Traditional Protectives—Protectives are employed to cover wet dressings and hot or cold compresses. In common use as protectives are plastic sheeting, and waxed or plastic-coated paper to prevent escape of moisture or heat from dressing or compress and to protect clothing or bed linens. Rubber sheeting is a rubber-coated cloth, waterproof and flexible, in various lengths and widths for use as a covering for bedding. A so-called "nursery sheeting" is supplied, coated only on one side.

Operating Room Supplies

Oxidized Regenerated Cellulose Hemostat—Oxidized regenerated cellulose is an absorbable hemostatic agent the action of which depends on the formation of a coagulum consisting of salts of polyanhydroglucuronic acid and hemoglobin. When applied to a bleeding surface, it swells to form a brown gelatinous mass that is gradually absorbed by the tissues, usually within 7 to 14 days. Oxidized regenerated cellulose is employed in surgery for the control of moderate bleeding where suturing or ligation is impractical or ineffective.

Disposable Sterile OR and OB Packs are prepared, packaged and sterilized assemblies of diapering and gown units, designed to fulfill the operating and delivery room needs. They eliminate the hospital problems of laundering, storage, assembly and sterilization of muslin drapes and gowns. They introduce many special materials with particular properties of porosity, repellency to water, alcohol, blood and other fluids, abrasion resistance, and other desirable attributes.

Double packages of contamination-resistant paper have been developed to permit opening and use without compromise of sterility. Retention of sterile characteristics until used eliminates the need for resterilization.

Face masks for use in the operating room and where contamination must be controlled are generally made of plied, fine-mesh gauze, shaped to cover the nose, mouth, and chin. They are laundered and autoclaved. Disposable face masks with special filtration material giving high retention of particulate matter, and designed for more effective fitting are available from several manufacturers. Surgine Face Mask (*J&J*) claims a 94% filtration efficiency with high user comfort.

Surgical Dressings

Adhesive Bandage

Adhesive Absorbent Bandage USP XVI; Adhesive Absorbent Compress; Adhesive Absorbent Gauze.

A compress of four layers of Type I absorbent gauze, or other suitable material, affixed to a film or fabric coated with a pressure-sensitive adhesive substance. It is sterile. The compress may contain a suitable antimicrobial agent and may contain one or more suitable colors. The adhesive surface is protected by a suitable removable covering.

Description—The compress is substantially free from loose threads or ravelings; the adhesive strip may be perforated, and the back may be coated with a water-repellent film.

Gauze Bandage

Type I absorbent gauze; contains no dye or other additives.

Description—One continuous piece, tightly rolled, in various widths and lengths and substantially free from loose threads and ravelings.

Oxidized Cellulose

Absorbable Cellulose; Absorbable Cotton; Cellulosic Acid; Oxycel (*Parke-Davis*)

Sterile gauze or cotton which has been chemically oxidized to make it both hemostatic and absorbable; contains 16–24% of carboxyl (COOH) groups.

Description—In the form of gauze or lint. Is slightly off-white in color, is acid to the taste, and has a slight, charred odor.

Solubility—Insoluble in water and in acids; soluble in dilute alkalies.

Uses—The value of oxidized cellulose in various surgical procedures is based upon its properties of absorbability when buried in tissues and its remarkable hemostatic effect. Absorption occurs between the second and seventh day following implantation of the dry material, depending on the adequacy of the blood supplied to the area and the degree of chemical degradation of the implanted material. Complete absorption of large amounts of blood-soaked gauze may take 6 weeks or longer and serious surgical complications have been reported as the result of failure to absorb, and also cyst formation. Hemostasis depends upon the marked affinity of *cellulosic acid* for hemoglobin. When exposed to blood, either *in vitro* or in surgical conditions, the oxidized gauze or cotton turns very dark brown or black and forms a soft gelatinous mass which readily molds itself to the contours of irregular surfaces and controls surgical hemorrhage by providing an artificially induced clot. Pressure should be exerted on the gauze or cotton for about 2 min in order to facilitate the sealing off of the mouths of the bleeding vessels.

Two factors require emphasis: (1) cellulosic acid does not enter the physiological clotting mechanism *per se* but forms what might be termed an "artificial clot," as described and, therefore, is effective in controlling the bleeding hemophiliac, and (2) the hemostatic action of cellulosic acid is not enhanced by the addition of other hemostatic agents, such as thrombin (which in any case would be destroyed by the pH of the gauze unless some means of neutralization were practicable). The hemostatic effect of either one alone is greater than the combination.

Oxidized cellulose is useful as a temporary packing for the control of capillary, venous, or small arterial *hemorrhage*, but since it inhibits epithelialization, it should be used only for the immediate control of hemorrhage and not as a surface dressing. Recently a purer and more uniform product prepared from oxidized regenerated cellulose has been developed and is available as Surgicel Absorbable Hemostat. This product offers many advantages over the older, less uniform oxidized cellulose derived from cotton and, because of its chemical uniformity, assures dependable performance and overcomes many of the difficulties encountered with the older type of cotton product. The knitted fabric strips do not fragment, may easily be sutured in place if necessary, and provide prompt and complete absorption with minimum tissue reaction.

Application—*Topical*, as necessary, to control hemorrhage.
Forms Available—Sterile Pads; Sterile Pledgets; Sterile Strips.

Purified Cotton

Gossypium Purificatum; Absorbent Cotton

The hair of the seed of cultivated varieties of *Gossypium hirsutum* Linné, or of other species of *Gossypium* (Fam *Malvaceae*), freed from adhering impurities, deprived of fatty matter, bleached, and sterilized in its final container.

Description—White, soft, fine, filament-like hairs appearing under the microscope as hollow, flattened, and twisted bands, striate and slightly thickened at the edges; practically odorless and practically tasteless.
Solubility—Insoluble in ordinary solvents; soluble in ammoniated cupric oxide TS.

Dextranomer

Debrisan (*Pharmacia*)

Dextranomer is a three-dimensional cross-linked dextran polymer prepared by interaction of dextran with epichlorohydrin.

Description—White, spherical beads, 0.1 to 0.3 mm in diameter; hydrophilic.
Solubility—Insoluble in water and in alcohol. Each g absorbs about 4 ml of aqueous fluid, the beads swelling and forming a gel.

Uses—Dextranomer is used topically to cleanse secreting lesions such as venous stasis ulcers, decubitus ulcers, infected traumatic and surgical wounds, and infected burns. It absorbs the exudates, including the components that tend to impede tissue repair, and thereby retards eschar formation and keeps lesions soft and pliable.

Application—Sufficient dextranomer is applied to cover the cleansed lesion (1/8 to 1/4 inch) and a bandage is applied lightly to keep the beads in place. When saturated with exudate the beads become greyish-yellow, and should be removed by irrigation with water, saline solution, or other cleansing solution. Dextranomer dressings are usually changed once or twice daily, but 3 or 4 changes may be required if draining is profuse.
Packaging—Sterile beads, in containers of 60 and 120 g, and in 4-g packets.

Absorbable Dusting Powder

Starch-derivative Dusting Powder

An absorbable powder prepared by processing cornstarch and intended for use as a lubricant for surgical gloves; contains not more than 2% of magnesium oxide.

Description—White, odorless powder; pH (1 in 10 suspension) between 10 and 10.8.

Absorbent Gauze

Carbasus Absorbens; Gauze

Cotton, or a mixture of cotton and not more than 53.0%, by weight, of purified rayon, in the form of a plain woven cloth. If rendered sterile, it is packaged to protect it from contamination.

Description—White cotton cloth of various thread counts and weights; may be supplied in various lengths and widths, and in the form of rolls and folds.

Adhesive Tape

Adhesive Plaster USP XVI; Sterile Adhesive Tape

Fabric and/or film evenly coated on one side with a pressure-sensitive, adhesive mixture. If rendered sterile, it is protected from contamination by appropriate packaging.

Other Surgical Dressings

Purified Rayon—A fibrous form of bleached, regenerated cellulose. It may contain not more than 1.25% of titanium dioxide. *Description* and *Solubility:* White, lustrous or dull, fine, soft, filamentous fibers, appearing under the microscope as round, oval, or slightly flattened, translucent rods, straight or crimped, striate, and with serrate cross-sectional edges; practically odorless and practically tasteless. Very soluble in ammoniated cupric oxide TS and dilute H_2SO_4 (3 in 5); insoluble in ordinary solvents.

Sutures and Suture Materials

A surgical suture is a strand or fiber used to hold wound edges in apposition during healing, and the process of applying such a strand is called *suturing*. When such material, without a needle, is used to stop bleeding by tying off severed blood vessels, the strand is called a *ligature*, and the process is known as *ligating*. Suture materials, however, have uses beyond those involved in the repair of wounds in that they are often used in reconstructive procedures.

Surgical sutures were first listed in the second supplement of USP XI in a monograph on catgut sutures, which were then officially designated, "Surgical Gut." USP XII carried a similar monograph on surgical silk. USP XVI contained, in addition to surgical gut, a generalized monograph designed to cover all sutures in addition to catgut, and this is also true of USP XX. These monographs have the force of law, establish the standards by which acceptability of sutures is judged, and are the final reference in cases of complaint and dispute concerning properties defined by them.

Since there are many available histories on the development and use of sutures, no attempt will be made to review the subject. At one time or another, nearly every form of fibrous material or wire that offered any promise at all has been used as a suture, and, indeed, many materials which, by present standards offer no promise at all, have been evaluated.

Cotton and linen were among the earliest suture materials, but the use of animal intestines and sinews also claims great antiquity. As in many other fields of science, there have been fads, and numerous materials have enjoyed varying favor through the centuries. Frequently, the acceptance of a given suture material depended on its successful use by an eminent surgeon whose authority encouraged emulation and in many cases, there appeared to be legitimate scientific justification for such use. Possibly the most important factor in the acceptance of suture materials has been their characteristics in the presence of infection. As knowledge of bacteriology increased and methods of sterilization improved, the earlier disadvantages of certain sutures have been overcome, so that currently a wide variety of surgical suture materials may be conveniently and effectively sterilized. Among the widely accepted methods for the sterilization of sutures are: autoclave sterilization with free access of water vapor, applicable only for those sutures which are not harmed by this process; dry heat at 310°F; ethylene oxide; and irradiation sterilization using either beta or gamma rays. Irradiation sterilization has many advantages over the older methods insofar as commercial production is concerned. The sutures are sterilized in their final sealed packages, eliminating any danger of recontamination. The radiation dose is greater than necessary to kill even the most resistant spore-forming organisms. One great advantage of this method lies in the relative lack of deteriorating effect upon the suture. Irradiation-sterilized surgical gut is stronger, more pliable and easier to handle than dry-heat-sterilized surgical gut sutures.

Suture materials may be divided into two principal classes, *absorbable* and *nonabsorbable*. In the first class are found those materials which are capable of being broken down or digested in animal tissues. Catgut, the classical absorbable suture derived from collagen-rich animal tissue, is proteinaceous in nature and it appears that certain proteolytic enzymes in tissues are responsible for the digestion of catgut and its disappearance from the wound area.

New forms of absorbable sutures based upon synthetic polyesters such as polyglycolic acid, copolymers of lactide and glycolide, and polydioxanone have been introduced as alternative absorbable materials.

Absorbable Sutures

Surgical Gut—Catgut is probably still the most widely used suture material and is, therefore, of great importance to surgery generally.

The basic constituent of surgical catgut is collagen derived from connective tissue obtained from healthy animals, usually sheep and cattle.

In the older and still widely used method, the catgut is obtained from the submucosal layer of the small intestine of sheep. The intestines from the freshly killed animal are cleaned of their contents and split longitudinally into ribbons. Mechanical processes remove the innermost mucosa and the outer muscularis and serosal layers, leaving essentially only the submucosa. This appears as a thin, strong network consisting chiefly of collagen, whose orientation and strength are increased markedly by subsequent processing. From one to five or six such ribbons are stretched, spun or twisted under tension, and dried under tension to form a uniform strand. These strands are polished and cut into appropriate lengths for packaging and sterilization. Intestines from cattle may also be used to prepare catgut but, in this case, it is the serosal layer that is isolated and used.

In another method collagen sutures are produced from collagen derived from beef tendon. The tendons are suitably treated and dispersed. The dispersed collagen is extruded, precipitated, and reconstituted as fine strands which are then twisted, stretched, tanned, and otherwise treated to give absorbable sutures with the desired characteristics.

In the US, practically no unsterilized surgical gut is sold, although in certain other countries this is a more common practice.

Diameter and strength requirements for absorbable surgical suture (surgical gut) are specified in the USP. In the USP will be found descriptions of the suture as well as the apparatus and methods for measuring diameter, tensile strength and sterility, and other tests.

Plain and Chromicized Surgical Gut—Two varieties of catgut, as distinguished by their resistance to absorptive action by tissue enzymes, are described in the USP as *Type A*, plain or untreated, and *Type C*, medium treatment. The availability of both types of catgut reflects the surgeon's requirements for catgut that will retain its tensile strength for varying periods of time, or that will show an increased resistance to the proteolytic substances found in certain body tissues. This is accomplished by the incorporation of chromium salts or other chemicals to prolong its survival in tissues. Such products were formerly designated as 10-, 20-, or 40-day catgut, on the assumption that these sutures would remain for such periods in normal tissue. The variations in catgut as a natural product, variations in patients, and in sites of implantations make such designations qualitative, so that they were replaced by the more general statement of type. While many tests for the expected duration of resistance have been proposed, none is fully accepted as being comparable to digestion in animal tissues, and none has been included in the USP.

Approximately half the surgical gut used in the US has been either chromicized or otherwise treated. Raw catgut is analogous to rawhide, while chromicized catgut is comparable to chrome-tanned leather. The tanning process is applied either to the ribbons before they have been twisted into the strand form or to the finished twisted strand. Treatment in the ribbon form is reported to result in a more uniform deposition of chromium salts throughout the entire cross section of the suture, while string chromicization sometimes causes the deposition of relatively heavier concentrations of the tanning agent near the periphery of the strand, with less penetration to its center. Deficient tanning of catgut may result in its premature absorption with possible wound disruption, although such incidents are now often recognized as effects of nutritional or other inadequacies with resultant weakness of the tissues themselves. Excessive chrome concentration in surgical gut may produce sutures that are slow to digest. Since they survive in normal tissues for a long time, they may occasionally extrude through the skin some months following surgery. The mechanism of such extrusion by highly tanned catgut or by nonabsorbable sutures is not clear, although it probably reflects the natural tendency of the body to eliminate or reject foreign material.

Tissue Reaction to Catgut—Following any surgical incision, there is an outpouring of blood and lymph into and through the wound. These fluids coagulate or clot, forming a network upon which new cells may build. The capillaries in the area dilate, and the blood supply in the vicinity of the wound is increased. Leukocytes in the area also increase in number.

The absorption of surgical gut takes place along with the tissue repair processes. The leukocytes, which appear early in any wound, produce proteolytic enzymes which, among other functions, carry out the digestion of absorbable catgut sutures. After this process is well along, fibroblasts appear and begin to lay down the collagen fibers essential for the increasing strength and healing of the wound. In the first phase of wound healing, the number and character of the debriding cells, together with such secondary effects as swelling, pain and redness constitute "tissue reaction." Chromic catgut elicits a less intense tissue reaction of a leukocytic or exudative type than does the plain variety.

Plain gut is digested by enzymes at a faster rate than is chromic gut. The surgeon chooses either plain or chromic gut, depending on the type of tissue involved, the condition of the patient and the estimated healing time of the wound. Small sizes of surgical gut cause less tissue reaction and irritation than large sizes. There is less digestive work for the enzymes to do. For this reason surgeons try never to use a suture that is stronger than the tissue in which it is to be used. The larger sutures merely add to tissue irritation without supplying any needed strength to the wound.

Sterilization and Packaging of Surgical Gut—Disappointing experiences with many attempts to sterilize gut by means of chemicals have created widespread distrust of the effectiveness of most chemicals. The exception has been the use of ethylene oxide which has provided an effective means for the sterilization of sutures. The more common methods are dry-heat sterilization (after first dehydrating the catgut) and irradiation sterilization in the final sealed packet.

At one time most surgical gut was produced and labeled as *boilable*. It was packaged in glass tubes with the strands immersed in a water-free high-boiling tubing fluid—usually xylol. Exteriors of the tubes could be sterilized at the hospital by autoclaving—hence, the term *boilable*.

The disadvantage of boilable catgut has been that the drying necessary to permit high-temperature sterilization produces a stiff strand, which is still stiff as removed from the tube, and which requires soaking for several minutes in sterile water before surgeons find it pliable enough to use. This process is no longer used (with isolated exceptions).

The present method of packaging catgut provides sutures ready for use as removed from the packet. The catgut, designated *nonboilable*, is contained in either a foil or plastic packet, immersed in a pliabilizing fluid which generally consists of an alcohol or mixtures of an alcohol with a small percentage of water. The water has a pliabilizing effect on the catgut, but would ruin the gut if the latter is subjected to high temperatures—therefore, the designation *nonboilable*. New irradiation and ethylene oxide sterilization techniques as described in the USP have largely replaced the older accepted method of dry-heat sterilization. These methods have permitted the development of more convenient packaging innovations which were not practical with the older methods.

For even greater convenience, all foil or plastic packets are now overwrapped in a secondary package. Both the contents and the outside of the inner packet are rendered sterile. By peeling open the overwrap package, the inner packet can be delivered ready for use in a sterile condition on the operating table.

Sterility Testing—Freedom from contamination is the most important property of any suture. Every lot of sutures furnished by reputable manufacturers is subjected to a series of physical and chemical tests, as well as to complete bacteriological examination in accordance with prescribed USP sterility test procedures. No lot of sutures is released until all of these tests have been successfully passed; hence, the surgeon has come to have justified confidence in the adequacy and sterility of these products. Because of the extraordinary reliability of radiation sterilization, acceptance of product sterility based on measurement and control of the radiation dose is becoming more widespread.

Operating Room Procedures with Sutures—Before a scheduled operation, the nurse usually selects the necessary types of sutures designated by the operating surgeon. The required number of overwrapped packages is opened by peeling apart the outer package and flipping or otherwise removing in an aseptic manner the inner sterile packets and placing them on the Mayo stand. The packets are opened by tearing if foil and by cutting with sterile scissors if plastic. Straightening the nonboilable suture is accomplished by a gentle pull. Nonboilable sutures are commonly used as removed from the packet. Abuse of catgut sutures may lead to their failure in tissues, with possible serious consequences to the patient.

Synthetic Absorbable Sutures—The combination of high tensile strength and absorbability that makes catgut so useful as a suture has been incorporated into synthetic fibers. Polymers derived from condensing the cyclic derivative of glycolic acid (glycolide) and mixtures of glycolide and lactide (derived by cyclicizing lactic acid) polydioxanone have been shown to possess properties which make them suitable for many surgical procedures. The first two polyesters mentioned are melt-extruded into multifilament yarns which are then braided into various sizes of sutures. Such braids have high tensile strength and, unlike catgut, must be packaged without fluid to avoid degradation. Synthetic absorbable sutures do not undergo the enzymically mediated absorption process that is well-known for catgut. Rather, the suture is completely broken down by simple hydrolysis as it resides in the tissue.

Cargile Membrane—This is a thin sheet of pliable tissue obtained from the appendix ("blind gut") of the steer or ox. It is designed primarily to cover surfaces from which the peritoneum has been removed, especially where a sterile membrane would lessen the formation of adhesions. The membrane is available in sterile sheets of approximately 4 ×

6 in and is sometimes used as a packing or protective sheath. At the present time use of such material is limited.

Fascia Lata—This is obtained from ox fascia and is designed for use as a heavy suture or repair in hernia or similar cases. It is usually attached firmly to a strong structure by means of a nonabsorbable suture. Fascia lata is supplied in the form of sterile strips approximately $\frac{1}{2}$ in wide and 8 in long and also in sheets about 3 × 5 in.

It should be emphasized, in connection with the above, that catgut strands and ribbons are the only ones which are completely and readily absorbable. The other materials may be absorbed very slowly or may be incorporated in the tissues by invasion of fibroblasts and a kind of replacement process.

Nonabsorbable Sutures

The second principal class of suture consists of natural and synthetic nonabsorbable suture materials which are relatively resistant to attack by normal tissue fluids. Several of these sutures survive, apparently unchanged, for many years in tissue and will usually be found encapsulated in a thin sheath of fibrous tissue. When nonabsorbable sutures are used for skin closure, they are usually removed after the incision or wound has healed to the point where suture support is no longer necessary.

Silk is an important nonabsorbable surgical suture. Selected grades of degummed commercial silk fibers are utilized, and consist chiefly of the protein fibroin as extruded by the silkworm. Many such fibers are twisted into a single strand of various diameters as specified in the USP, and sold in the natural color or after dyeing. By far the most popular construction is braided silk in which several twisted yarns are braided into a compact structure favored for its firmness and strength. Most braided silk is dyed and also given a treatment to render it noncapillary. In use as a skin suture this minimizes the rise of tissue fluids to the surface and thus the counterpassage inward of organisms from the surface. Further objects of such treatments are to impart a degree of stiffness to improve the handling and tying properties, to minimize attachment of tissue cells that would cause pain on removal of the suture and to lubricate the implantation and removal of the silk. When silk or any other suture is dyed, the USP requires that such dyeing be done with a color additive approved by the Food and Drug Administration.

Specifications—The USP describes in the monograph for Nonabsorbable Surgical Suture (which now includes cotton, linen, metallic wire, nylon, rayon, dacron, and silk) the respective sizes, diameters, and tensile strengths.

Uses of Silk—Silk sutures are easily handled, and well tolerated by body tissue. In the presence of infection, however, the interstices of silk strands protect organisms from antimicrobial agents and from the body's defense mechanisms, so that chronic sinuses may form which do not heal until the silk is removed or is sloughed by the tissues. Silk, as well as any other nonabsorbable suture, occasionally migrates from the site of implantation and comes to the surface to be extruded months after the operation. In certain sites, the suture knots or ends may serve as centers for the formation of concretions or for other irritating action. Silk usually becomes encapsulated and remains permanently in the tissues. Silk sutures are used in a wide variety of surgical procedures, as in the brain, eye, gastrointestinal tract, nerves, blood vessels, or in general in any wound which is not infected. Many surgeons, using catgut or other materials in tissues, employ silk for skin closure, either braided or as the artificial silkworm gut or dermal sutures described below.

Dermal Silk Sutures—These sutures consist of natural twisted silk encased in an insoluble coating of tanned gelatin or other protein. This coating must withstand autoclaving without stripping, and its purpose is to prevent the ingrowth of tissue cells which would interfere with its removal after use as a skin or dermal suture.

Cotton and Linen—Sutures derived from cellulose are among the oldest known but are currently used to a limited extent. Such sutures are twisted from fiber staple, have moderately high tensile strength, and are stable to heat sterilization. Cotton sutures prepared by suture manufacturers are uniform and have reproducible strength and have largely replaced the household sewing cotton used by many surgeons years ago. These sutures are desirable because of their handling properties and low order of tissue reactivity but are not widely used in critical areas where strength must be maintained for long periods of time because they slowly degrade.

Synthetic Nonabsorbable Sutures

Nylon—Nylon, the first modern synthetic fiber, came into use as a suture partly as a result of World War II shortages of high-grade silk and partly because of its own merits. It is a synthetic polyamide obtained from the condensation of adipic acid and hexamethylenediamine or from condensing caprolactam. It is available in the form of monofilaments in the useful range of sizes, as well as in the form of multifilament fibers braided into strands of comparable diameter. It is strong and water-resistant, and has come into some use for all suturing or ligating. Monofilament nylon is used as a skin or stay suture or for plastic surgery. Braided nylon is more often buried in tissues and is subject to the same limitations as braided silk in the presence of infection.

Polyester Fiber—Of the numerous multifilament synthetic fibers introduced after the success of nylon, only polyester has been accepted as a suitable braided nonabsorbable suture while polypropylene has enjoyed increasing popularity as a nonabsorbable monofilament suture. Polyester suture is prepared by melt-extruding polyethylene terephthalate into fine filaments which are then braided into the various sizes of sutures. In general, the tensile strength of polyester braided sutures is superior to that of braided silk and nylon and twisted cotton.

The polyester sutures, in contrast with most other materials except polypropylene and stainless steel, do not lose significant strength when in contact with water or body fluids. For this reason, they have become a suture of choice when there is a critical need for permanent reinforcement as in, for example, the installation of artificial heart valves. Polyester sutures contain no wax or other additives and have the advantage of excellent knot-holding characteristics. They are available in the natural color or dyed to enhance visibility in the surgical field.

Recent developments have seen the commercialization of braided polyester fiber sutures coated or impregnated with nontoxic lubricants such as polytetrafluoroethylene or silicone resins. Recently, polybutilate, a lubricant especially designed for polyester suture use, has been derived from a condensation polymer of butanediol and adipic acid. These sutures present the advantage of a smoother surface which gives the suture improved handling properties and permits an easier and more gentle passage through tissue.

Polyolefin Fibers—Of increasing interest in the nonabsorbable suture field is the development of fibers based on polyolefins. Although polyethylene sutures have been available, the use of polypropylene monofilament has greatly increased during recent years. Polypropylene sutures withstand autoclaving sterilization and, compared to monofilament nylon tie more secure knots and have a very low order of tissue reactivity. Because of the smoothness of polypropylene sutures, they slip through tissue easily and, because there is no tissue ingrowth, they may be easily removed when necessary. These sutures have found wide application in cardiovascular and other surgical specialties.

Metallic Sutures

For some years increased attention has been paid to the use of various metal wire sutures and other metallic devices to assist surgical repair.

Silver—Among the older materials which are still used to some extent are silver wire, foil, and other forms. Relatively little work has been reported recently on these items. Silver is readily available and is alleged to have some antiseptic action, but in some tissues is definitely irritating. Irritation has been shown by a great many metals and alloys, and is now regarded as a controlling consideration in the choice of substances for implantation in tissues.

Stainless Steel—This ferrous alloy, which has so long been usefully employed in industrial and other applications where resistance to chemical attack is essential, has been used widely in the form of wire sutures, fixation plates, screws, and other items. Stainless steel is a rather general term covering a wide variety of materials, and many of the early alloys were attacked by body fluids. The proper selection of stainless steel compositions seems to provide a material essentially inert in tissues and free from the earlier disadvantages. Stainless steel sutures are available as both twisted and monofilament strands and represent the strongest available material. However, it is relatively difficult to use and it is most commonly employed in areas where great strength is required such as the repair of the sternum after chest surgery.

Surgical Needles—Suture materials may be threaded on eyed needles for suturing. While formerly only eyed needles were available, there is an overwhelming trend to the use of eyeless needles, one or two being attached to each individual strand. One such needle is manufactured with an open channel into which the suture can be placed, and the channel is then swaged around the strand. Another type, known as "seamless," has a very delicate hole drilled in the shank. To prevent pull-out, the shank is pressed firmly about the suture. These sutures offer great advantage in minimizing trauma. With an eyed needle an opening in tissue must be made large enough to accommodate the needle and two thicknesses of suture, but with the eyeless needle, the opening need only accommodate the needle, slightly larger than the single suture which follows. This is greatly esteemed in fine surgery such as plastic and eye work. Suitable eyeless needles on catgut and other materials are now available to meet most of the demands of the modern surgeon. By a recent innovation, it has been possible to control the release of a suture from an eyeless needle by a gentle tug so that the surgeon need not take the time to cut the needle from the suture when it is no longer required.

Vitallium—This metal, which is an alloy of cobalt, chromium and molybdenum, has been applied to many surgical problems in various forms since 1937, although not in the form of sutures or ligatures. The alloy has shown some variability in strength and stiffness and is incapable of much modification at the time of operation, but generally shows negligible tissue reactions. In addition to some use for dentures, surgical forms of vitallium include: fracture plates, screws, bolts, nails and appliances, orbital implants, nasal skeletal supports, tendon rods, tubes for blood vessel anastomosis and for bile duct repair, and skull plates.

Other Suturing Techniques

Although sutures and ligatures have remained the most effective and popular devices for closing wounds and hemostasis, other techniques are being used with increasing frequency. Surgical stapling devices are available which automatically approximate tissue with rows of steel staples which remain permanently. Such devices exist for closing skin, anastomosing blood vessels as well as for reconstructing other organs such as stomach and intestines.

During the last several years, V-shaped steel clips have been used to clamp small blood vessels and this alternative to ligation is becoming increasingly popular as the applying-instruments become more convenient and easy to use. Stainless steel clips or staples have been used frequently to coapt skin incisions. More recently strips of fabric or plastic material coated with a suitable adhesive have been used for the same application.

New approaches to ligating clips are represented by absorbable materials, polydioxanone and lactomer. Ligating clips made from these substances absorb after their function is completed and do not remain in the patient permanently as do the metallic clips. Thus, interference with diagnostic imaging techniques such as X-ray and CAT scans is avoided.

Sutures

Absorbable Surgical Suture

Surgical Catgut; Catgut Suture; Surgical Gut; Sterilized Surgical Catgut BP; Sterilized Surgical Ligature

A sterile strand prepared from collagen derived from healthy mammals, or from a synthetic polymer. It is capable of being absorbed by living mammalian tissue, but may be treated to modify its resistance to absorption. It may be modified with respect to body or texture. It may be impregnated or coated with a suitable antimicrobial agent. It may be colored by a color additive approved by the Federal Food and Drug Administration.

Description—Flexible strand varying in treatment, color, size, packaging, and resistance to absorption, according to the intended purpose. The collagen suture is either *Type A* Suture or *Type C* Suture. Both types consist of processed strands of collagen, but *Type C* Suture is processed by physical or chemical means so as to provide greater resistance to absorption in living mammalian tissue.

Nonabsorbable Surgical Suture

Surgical Sutures; Surgical Silk; Sterile Surgical Silk

A strand of material that is suitably resistant to the action of living mammalian tissue. It may be non-sterile or sterile. It may be impregnated or coated with a suitable antimicrobial agent.

Nonabsorbable Surgical Suture may be modified with respect to body or texture, or to reduce capillarity, and may be suitably bleached. It may be colored by a color additive approved by the Federal Food and Drug Administration.

Description—Flexible, monofilament, or multifilament, continuous strand, placed in an envelope, tube or other suitable container or wound on a reel or spool. If it is a multifilament strand, the individual filaments may be combined by spinning, twisting, braiding, or any combination thereof.

Nonabsorbable Surgical Suture is classed and typed as follows: *Class I* Suture is composed of silk or synthetic fibers of monofilament, twisted, or braided construction. *Class II* Suture is composed of cotton or linen fibers or coated natural or synthetic fibers where the coating forms a casing of significant thickness but does not contribute appreciably to strength. *Class III* Suture is composed of monofilament or multifilament metal wire.

CHAPTER 106

Poison Control

Anthony R Temple, MD

Medical Director, McNeil Consumer Products Co
Adjunct Associate Professor, Department of Pediatrics
University of Pennsylvania School of Medicine
Lecturer, Philadelphia College of Pharmacy and Science
Ft Washington, PA 19034

It is estimated that there are between five and ten millions of toxic exposures annually in the United States. Among children beyond the first year of life, accidents cause more deaths than do the five leading fatal diseases combined. Also among the most common causes of death of preadolescents, adolescents, and adults is suicide. Both accidents and suicides frequently involve poisons. Another important cause of morbidity and mortality, especially among the young, is the deliberate abuse of drugs and chemicals for their effects on the central nervous system. Even though the reporting, especially of suicides and abuses, undoubtedly is incomplete, there are known to be over 10,000 deaths in the United States each year attributable to poisoning.

In addition to the fatalities due to poisoning, there are staggering numbers of nonfatal cases requiring treatment. The toll in terms of manpower, expense, and occupation of medical facilities cannot be estimated, but must be tremendous.

Accidental poisonings should be preventable in most instances. Especially is this true of accidental poisonings of young children by drugs and chemicals in the home. This is a problem of great public-health significance the solution of which will require efforts of individuals in many disciplines. Among these are pharmacists, who can play a key role in preventing or mitigating the consequences of accidental poisonings, especially those due to drugs.

Epidemiology

Effective preventive measures require a knowledge of who and what are involved, how it happened and what are any predisposing or contributory factors. In order to delineate some of these factors, a description of the experience of a poison control center may be instructive. The Intermountain Regional Poison Control Center (IRPCC) was established in 1971. At that time, initial staffing of the IRPCC telephone was initiated using pharmacists, pharmacy students, and a physician consultant. With the eventual growth of the program, the IRPCC was then staffed with full-time clinical pharmacists with training in clinical toxicology, under the supervision of a physician-medical toxicologist. The IRPCC provided services to the State of Utah, with some back-up and consulting services to adjacent states.

The increase in the center's call frequency paralleled the provision of more sophisticated services. As a regional center, during the initial full year of operation, 1972, the IRPCC handled 5673 cases. By 1975, this figure had almost tripled, and in 1977 25,600 calls were received. A growth pattern similar to this has occurred in essentially every instance where regionalization has occurred. A detailed analysis of case experience for the year 1975 is reported.

Table I summarizes the classification of calls by type. Poisoning calls made up 79.8% of all calls, while 20.2% were informational in nature in which no poisoning victim was involved. The majority of the information calls were toxicology or drug information requests, but the IRPCC also received requests for medical information and veterinary information. Of the poisoning cases, 87.2% were accidental in nature. Suicidal or intentional poisonings made up 8.1%, while poisonings involving drug abuse amounted to 4.6%. Environ-

Table I—Typical Call Pattern Received by a Regional Poison Control Center (IRPCC, 1975)

Type	Number of cases	Total	Percent
Poisoning		12,663	79.8
Accidental	10,485		
Suicidal	1,022		
Drug abuse	581		
Environmental	430		
Other	142		
Not recorded	13		
Information		3,203	20.2
Toxicology	1,394		
Drug	927		
Medical	522		
Veterinary	153		
Other	200		
Not recorded	7		
Not recorded		2	0.0

Table II—Typical Distribution of Poisoning Cases by Mode of Exposure (IRPCC, 1975)

Mode	Number of cases	Percent
Ingestion	10,772	85.0
Ocular	581	4.6
Inhalation	446	3.5
Topical	415	3.3
Envenomation	363	2.9
Other	92	0.7
Not recorded	4	0.0

Table III—Typical Distribution of Poisoning Cases by Age of Victim (IRPCC, 1975)

Age in Years	Number of cases	Percent
Under 1	805	6.4
1	2153	17.0
2	2661	21.0
3	1827	14.4
4	690	5.4
5	344	2.7
6	178	1.4
7–17	1121	8.8
18 and over	2598	20.5
Not recorded	298	2.3

Table IV—Characteristics of Poisoning Severity as Characterized by an Assessment by Type of Agent and Amount Involved at Initial IRPCC Contact

Assessed Toxicity	Number of Cases	Total	Percent
Nontoxic agent		505	4.0
Known toxic agent		11,065	87.3
Amount insignificant	3819		
Mild to moderate toxicity	6278		
Serious toxicity	956		
Not recorded	12		
Toxicity of agent unknown		596	4.7
Amount insignificant	171		
Mild to moderate toxicity	410		
Serious toxicity	11		
Not recorded	4		
Agent unknown		492	3.9
Not recorded		15	0.1

mental or industrial exposures accounted for 3.4% of the poisoning cases.

Of the 12,663 poisoning cases, 85.0% involved ingestions as the mode of exposure (Table II). The next most frequent mode of exposure was that of ocular exposure, 4.6%, while inhalation exposures, 3.5%, topical exposures, 3.3%, and envenomations, 2.9%, made up the remainder of the cases.

Children five years of age and under were involved in 66.9% of the cases (Table III). Ages 6 through 17 were involved in 10.2%, while 20.5% involved adults aged 18 and above. In our overall experience, 50.7% of the victims were males, while 48.5% were females.

In terms of the severity of the exposures handled by poison control centers (Table IV), 4.0% of the calls involved nontoxic agents, and 4.7% of the calls involved cases where the toxicity of the agent was unknown. In another 3.9% of the cases, an apparent poisoning had occurred, but the agent was unknown or unidentifiable. Altogether, in 87.3% of the cases a toxic agent could be identified by the poison control center staff. Of these, in 31.5% of the cases the amount of agent involved in the exposure was considered to be too small to produce any toxic manifestations, which meant that 35.5% of the cases could be considered to be nontoxic exposures. At the time of the initial contact with the poison center, 38.7% of the victims reported symptoms that could be related to their toxic exposure, while 60.0% of the victims were asymptomatic. In cases where a poisoning was suspected, 79.6% were managed at home, 25.4% receiving no therapy, while 74.6% were given some form of treatment (Table V). As a general rule, this treatment consisted of simple administration of demulcents, dilution, or irrigation, but in 7.9% of the cases emesis was induced. Of those cases where ipecac was to be used, 44.1% of the time it was available in the home. The remainder of the time ipecac had to be obtained from a nearby pharmacy. Another 16.1% of the total poisoning cases were managed in an emergency care facility and released. Only 4.3% of the total poisonings were hospitalized. Less than 0.05% of the cases proved to be fatal.

At the IRPCC, the most frequently encountered agents were psychopharmacologic agents, which make up 10.0% of the cases seen (Table VI). The next most frequent group of agents include soaps, detergents, and household cleaning products, followed by petroleum distillates and related polishes and waxes, aspirin products, vitamins and minerals, and plants. A wide variety of agents made up the remaining cases. In contrast to the overall center experience, the most frequent category of toxic substances in children's exposures was the analgesic/anti-inflammatory/antipyretic class of agents, which includes both aspirin and acetaminophen. The next most common category was petroleum distillates, followed by soaps, detergents, and other household cleaning agents, plants, and

vitamin- and mineral-containing products. A similar pattern is seen in data reported by the National Clearinghouse for Poison Control Centers (Table VII). With increased use of child-resistant packaging and increased awareness of the hazards of aspirin, aspirin has fallen from the top of the list of substances most frequently ingested by children to be replaced by plants, vitamins, and household cleaning agents.

Of continued importance, however, is therapeutic overdosage with aspirin, a fact which has important preventive implications for the pharmacist. It is not at all uncommon for a parent who has never been told of the toxic potential of such a commonplace item to administer several times the safe dose of aspirin to a small infant over a period of several days. In fact, such unintentional overdoses are responsible for many of the most serious cases of aspirin poisoning.

Particularly tragic are accidental poisonings due to materials which are either outmoded, excessively toxic for their intended use, or for which there is only questionable rationale. Oil of wintergreen (methyl salicylate) and camphorated oil lead the list. Also, household chemicals, solvents, cleaners, some pesticides, while valuable to the professional user, are excessively toxic for routine household use. There is little reason for employing highly dangerous inorganic materials such as arsenic, phosphorus, and thallium as rodenticides when warfarin, practically devoid of acute human toxicity, will do the job.

Influential Factors

A number of factors seem to be important in the consideration of poisoning risk and in poison prevention. The following is a brief discussion of some of those factors.

Age—Approximately two-thirds of poisonings occur in children and are accidental, while a majority of the poisonings in adolescents and adults represent suicide attempts. Poisonings do occur in adults from the inadvertent taking of some material other than intended medication or accidental overdosage of proper medication. While such accidents are rather rare, people should nonetheless be cautioned to read labels

Table V—Level of Care Required for IRPCC Poisoning Cases

Management Site	Number of Cases	Percent
At home	10,067	79.6
Ipecac emesis	796	
Other treatment	6,721	
No treatment	2,550	
Emergency room or doctor's office	2,042	16.1
Hospitalized	550	4.3

Table VI—Typical Distribution of Poison Center Calls by Category of Toxic Agent Involved in the Exposure (IRPCC, 1975)

Category of agent[a]	Number of cases	Percent
Psychopharmacologic agents	1592	10.0
Soaps, detergents, cleansers	1139	7.2
Miscellaneous petroleum products, polishes, wax	891	5.6
Aspirin	808	5.1
Vitamins, minerals	789	5.0
Plants (excluding mushrooms)	673	4.2
Miscellaneous internal medicines	647	4.1
Miscellaneous analgesics	640	4.0
Narcotic	385	2.4
Nonnarcotic	255	1.6
Cosmetics (fingernail polish/perfume/cologne)	624	3.9
Pesticides (insecticides, rodenticides, and herbicides)	507	3.2
Antihistamines, cold medicine	498	3.1
Alcohols/glycols	451	2.8
Bites/stings	406	2.6
Household disinfectants/deodorizers	374	2.4
Glues, adhesives	269	1.7
Bleach	252	1.6
Miscellaneous external medicines/liniments	234	1.5
Corrosive acids/alkalies	241	1.5
Hormones	224	1.4
Paint/art supplies	159	1.0
Fertilizers	163	1.0
Food	111	0.6
Solvents	74	0.5
Hallucinogens	69	0.4
Local anesthetics	63	0.4
Cough medicines	54	0.3

[a] Categories based on those published in annual statistics by the National Clearinghouse for Poison Control Centers.

carefully before taking medications, not to take medications in the dark, not to transfer materials from their original containers, to protect medication labels against destruction, and to follow recommended dosage schedules carefully.

Accidental poisoning is less common under the age of 1 year or beyond 5 or 6 years of age. The most critical age period is between 1 and 3 years, where one-half of the accidental poisonings occur and the poisoning is more likely to bring a child to the hospital for emergency treatment than any other single cause. The reasons for the high incidence in that age range relate to certain characteristics of child development. During these early years the youngster is inquisitive and accustomed to mouthing everything within reach. By 1 year of age he is also usually able either to creep or to walk, yet he is too young to recognize danger. It is to be expected that he will attempt to mouth or ingest any substance left within reach.

No matter how distasteful a product may be, a child will still make an initial attempt to eat or taste it. While pleasant flavoring may be influential in a child's ingesting a larger dose, it has little bearing on the likelihood that he initially will attempt to ingest the material. During the first 2 to 3 years of life, texture is at least as important as flavor in determining acceptability of something to be eaten. Materials that would gag or dissuade an older individual may be ingested readily by the young child. Obviously, even highly caustic substances such as lye are ingested without hesitation by children at this age.

Among children less than 1 year old, an infant may be given a toxic material by an older sibling. Thus, it is important to keep potentially toxic materials inaccessible not only to very young children but to their older brothers and sisters as well. In addition, children should be educated not to give things to the baby without a parent's permission. Pre-school education programs are potential times to teach children these principles, and they should be a standard part of parenting in every household.

It is of interest also that among children older than 3 years of age ingestions often occur as group activities. Occasionally two or more children will share the material in some form of play, where they might otherwise be unlikely to ingest it by themselves. Again at this age, children are more educable than earlier, so that instruction in avoidance of potentially toxic non-food substances should be given in the home and educational environment.

Some of the supposedly accidental poisonings in teenage and younger children are actually suicide attempts or gestures or attempts at drug abuse. It is important to realize that serious suicide attempts may occur at 9 or 10 years of age. Suicidal attempts or gestures are, of course, quite common among adolescents and in the few years immediately before and for many years after this important transitional stage of life.

"Accident Proneness"—Only a small number of patients treated for poisoning have had a previous history of having been involved in similar accidents. Thus, while some children may be involved in repetitive episodes, they account for a small percentage of such cases. Nonetheless, a child who has ingested something once, especially if some effort was required in the act, may be at greater future risk and should be treated accordingly. The idea that there are accident-prone children is probably less valid than that there are accident-prone situations and surroundings. Parental education about poison prevention techniques and what to do in case of a poisoning should be considered as part of the routine follow-up in all childhood poisoning episodes.

Location—The vast majority of childhood accidental poisonings occur in the home. As is pointed out below, materials which become involved in childhood accidental poisoning usually have been left out of place while in use, rather than being in their usual place of storage at the time they were taken. The most common areas for poisoning within the home are the kitchen, bathroom, and bedroom.

The highest incidence of accidental childhood poisoning is in the late afternoon and around the dinner hour or in the

Table VII—Categories of Substances Most Frequently Ingested by Children Under 5 Years of Age Reported by Poison Control Centers, 1972-1974-1976-1978.

	Type of Substance	1978		1976		1974		1972	
		No	%	No	%	No	%	No	%
1.	Plants	11010	11.7	9085	10.1	6483	6.9	4759	4.5
2.	Soaps, detergents, cleansers	5836	6.2	5323	5.9	5474	5.8	5940	5.7
3.	Vitamins, minerals	3677	3.9	3801	4.2	4577	4.8	5320	5.1
4.	Aspirin	3557	3.8	3652	4.1	4837	5.1	8146	7.8
	Baby	2557	3.7	2373	2.6	3195	3.4	5305	5.1
	Adult	380	0.4	609	0.7	750	0.8	1322	1.3
	Unspecified	640	0.7	670	0.8	892	0.9	1519	1.4
5.	Antihistamines, cold medications	4003	4.3	3492	3.9	3783	4.0	4355	4.1
6.	Perfume, cologne, toilet water	3748	4.0	3398	3.8	3385	3.6	3108	3.0
7.	Insecticides (excluding mothballs)	2675	2.9	2749	3.1	2879	3.0	2306	2.2
8.	Household disinfectants, deodorizers	2752	2.9	2664	3.0	2944	3.1	3301	3.1
9.	Miscellaneous analgesics	2752	2.9	2532	2.8	2095	2.2	2220	2.1
10.	Miscellaneous internal medicines	2303	2.5	2215	2.5	2761	2.9	3186	3.0
11.	Household bleach	1863	2.0	2197	2.4	2361	2.5	2794	2.7
12.	Liniments	2016	2.2	2061	2.3	2045	2.2	2133	2.0
13.	Fingernail preparations	2270	2.4	1931	2.2	1632	1.7	1191	1.1
14.	Psychopharmacologic agents	1463	1.6	1779	2.0	2237	2.4	2998	2.9
15.	Cosmetic lotions, creams	1625	1.7	1721	1.9	1844	1.9	1783	1.7
16.	Miscellaneous external medicines	2151	2.3	1660	1.8	1602	1.7	1587	1.5
17.	Hormones	1386	1.5	1514	1.7	1811	1.9	1970	1.9
18.	Antiseptic medications	1603	1.7	1432	1.6	1316	1.4	1346	1.3
19.	Rodenticides	1347	1.4	1410	1.6	1378	1.5	1508	1.4
20.	Liquid polish or wax	—	—	1369	1.5	1620	1.7	1872	1.8
21.	Glues, adhesives	1384	1.5	1343	1.5	1680	1.8	1866	1.8
22.	Fertilizers, plant foods	—	—	1292	1.4	917	1.0	577	0.5
23.	Corrosive acids, alkalies	1204	1.3	1232	1.4	1543	1.6	1815	1.7
24.	Paint	1204	1.3	1203	1.3	1350	1.4	1633	1.6
25.	Cough medicines	1443	1.5	1175	1.3	1235	1.3	1279	1.2

Source: Individual poison reports (phone inquiries and treated cases) submitted to the National Clearinghouse for Poison Control Centers from poison control centers in the United States, Canal Zone, Virgin Island, and military bases abroad.

early morning hours, but poisonings occur with regular consistency during a child's waking hours. Poisonings in the late morning hours occur in the kitchen and the substances most frequently involved are common household products such as cleaning agents, polishes, and other materials commonly kept in the kitchen. In the early afternoon poisonings often occur in the bedroom and may involve cosmetics and, to a lesser extent, medications. In the early evening the kitchen is again a common site. Bathroom incidents are scattered throughout the day and tend usually to involve either medications or cosmetics.

Among cases that occur outside the home, the garage and the family automobile are common sites of accidental poisoning in young children. Involved most frequently in the automobile are medications left either in the glove compartment or in mother's purse. In the garage, pesticides, petroleum products, cleaning agents, and paint products are often stored and thus involved in poisoning. An increasing percentage of cases occurring inside or outside the home involve plants kept for decorative purposes or which are growing either in the yard or wild in the fields. Parents should be reminded that children may be poisoned when they visit the homes of others (especially grandparents) who leave things within reach because they are not accustomed to having children about.

Accessibility—Poison prevention campaigns often focus on the provision of a locked medicine cabinet. The availability of such a place for safe storage of medicines is desirable, but it should be recognized that this would likely prevent less than half the cases of accidental childhood poisoning unless the materials will be replaced there, something which is not often done.

In as many as three-fourths of the cases, the materials involved in childhood accidental poisoning have been left within reach of a child. In many instances, ingestion occurs when the individual responsible for the care of a child is interrupted during his or her use of the material in question.

People must be instructed not only to provide a storage place for potentially toxic materials, but also to return these materials immediately thereto and not to let them out of their sight even for a moment until so secured.

The Container—Removal of potentially toxic materials from their original containers is a significant factor in increasing risk of accidental poisoning, especially with certain compounds. The common practice, for example, of storing a small quantity of gasoline or solvents in a soft-drink bottle is especially hazardous, for obvious reasons. Other hazardous materials with which this is frequently done are cleaning solutions, paint products, turpentine, and pesticides. Sometimes the container to which they are transferred is a drinking glass or dish. In all such instances, a material may be made to seem more attractive to the child because of resemblance to food or other ingestable items.

In addition to the foregoing, transfer of materials from their original containers creates problems of accurate identification if and when poisoning does occur. A similar problem exists when materials, particularly medications, are not properly identified in their original containers. Obviously, all prescription vials should identify accurately the contents on the label.

Occasionally there are poisonings that result from placing of containers of smaller size, shape, and/or color in proximity, either in medicine cabinets, on pharmacy shelves or nursing stations. This invites errors and should be discouraged. One common problem occurs by mistaking camphorated oil for castor oil, although the former is disappearing from store shelves.

Supervision—Most children are considered to be under the supervision of one or both of their parents at the time an accidental poisoning occurs, but usual adult supervision is not adequate to prevent poisoning accidents in young children. This may be due in part to the fact that parents underestimate the ability of the child to obtain and to ingest a potentially toxic material. A common error is to leave medications on a bedside stand after administering them to a young child, so that the child for whom it was intended or a sibling may ingest the entire contents.

A significant number of childhood poisonings occur when there is a disruption in normal household routine. Times of moving or painting, holidays, visits by friends or relatives, or death or illness in the family are occasions when increased caution should be exercised. Other circumstances that invite unsupervised access of children to potentially toxic materials are when items are sent through the mail or after being discarded into a refuse container.

When deteriorated or unwanted materials are to be discarded, the safest procedure for potentially toxic liquids or powders is either to pour them down a drain or flush them down a toilet. With some highly concentrated and highly toxic materials, such as pesticide concentrates, even the amount left remaining in an "empty" bottle may be sufficient to cause serious poisoning. Such containers should be thoroughly rinsed before being discarded and placed carefully in closed refuse containers as far from normal access by children as possible.

Optimal supervision of self or others also involves attention to detail in the legitimate use of potentially hazardous materials. As previously noted, drug labels always should be examined carefully to ensure accurate identification before a medication is administered or taken. Self-medication, use of another individual's medications for the "same problem," and unsupervised self-diagnosis and prescription of a child's treatment by the parents should be encouraged only with appropriate education and potential for consumer understanding.

There is a tendency for many to believe that if a material were significantly hazardous it would not be available for over-the-counter sales, but obviously this is not true. Frequently, parents may overmedicate a child, either because they underestimate the potential hazard or are given inadequate instructions. It is important that physicians who order medications, and pharmacists who dispense them, provide and emphasize specific instructions concerning proper use. The pharmacist can play a key role in this, even if only a minute or two is spent in appropriate patient education.

Although seemingly unlikely, it is not at all uncommon for a patient who has been advised to take or administer "some aspirin every once in a while" to use two or three times the safe dose every few hours for several days or to take concurrent medications containing salicylates until serious intoxication occurs. Instructions on the label are meaningful to the cautious and the concerned, but these are rarely the people who become poisoned. Person-to-person conversation is far more effective and can well take place at the time a material is prescribed or dispensed.

Treatment

The most important treatment measure for poisoning is prevention. Of course, once a poisoning occurs, it is important to be able to provide highly skilled supportive medical care. It is not sufficient to focus only on simple first-aid measures and antidotal therapy or home remedies.

Actually, there are very few poisons for which there are effective antidotes; for most cases of poisoning, good supportive care is all that can be offered and all that is needed. Even in those instances where antidotes are available, supportive care is at least as important; indeed, the best antidote in the world is of little value without good supportive care. Most of the home remedies which have been recommended from time to time actually are of little value, and most tend to waste valuable time that could better be devoted to proper treatment under adequate medical supervision.

Unfortunately, many lay publications, including first-aid texts, are outmoded in this respect and continue to recommend all sorts of elaborate but ineffective procedures to be carried out in the home. The same criticism can be leveled at the instructions provided on the many rather complicated antidote lists and first-aid treatment charts that are disseminated for use of the public, often by well-meaning professional organizations.

"First-Aid Principles"

The cardinal rule for first-aid treatment of poisoning is to remove the poison from contact with the patient (unless such removal is contraindicated) and to obtain further definitive medical care at the earliest possible moment if warranted.

The more simplified one can make any instructions for home treatment, the more likely they are to be followed and the less likely they are to either delay or be substituted for proper care by a physician. Thus, general procedures that can be carried out simply and are applicable almost irrespective of the nature of the poison are to be recommended until medical help can be obtained.

Recommended procedures for lay use in the first-aid treatment of poisoning are outlined in Table VIII. The principal elements are (1) knowing what to do before you call someone, (2) obtaining medical advice immediately to determine what to do next, and (3) terminating the exposure of the victim by removal of the poison usually through induction of vomiting. In regard to the latter point, it should be noted that induction of vomiting has been shown to be superior to gastric lavage in the removal of ingested poisons in small children, while the two procedures may be comparable in adults. Many measures recommended in the past for induction of vomiting, such as mechanical stimulation of the posterior pharynx or giving mustard water or salt water, are usually not effective and may be dangerous. The most serviceable emetic for first-aid use is ipecac syrup, which is highly effective if used in the doses recommended here. Up to 1 oz can now be dispensed without a prescription. Patients who will not cooperate by taking ipecac syrup can be induced to vomit by parenteral use of apomorphine.

Activated charcoal is a highly effective adsorbent of a large number of poisons. Most organic and inorganic materials are adsorbed to a greater or lesser extent by this material and so its use more or less routinely in cases of poisoning by ingestion is worthwhile. It should be remembered, however, that if activated charcoal is given before syrup of ipecac, it will inactivate the latter; consequently, it is advisable to induce vomiting first before administering charcoal. Activated charcoal is worthwhile as a nonspecific antidote not only for home use but also for use in hospitals and in poison treatment centers. It is best given as a slurry in water, to which flavorings, sweeteners or thickeners can be added, but adding other materials to enhance palatability may result in a decrease in adsorptive capacity.

In recent years parents have been encouraged to keep ipecac syrup and activated charcoal in homes where there are children of poisoning-prone age. If such items are to be used, it is important that a prominent part of the instruction on the label is to call the local poison control center or a doctor before administering either.

Antidotes—Before discussing specific antidotes, it should be emphasized that while activated charcoal is an effective, nonspecific adsorbent of a large number of materials, there is no true "universal antidote." The classical universal antidote which was in use for a long period of time consisted of activated charcoal, tannic acid, and magnesium oxide (or,

Table VIII—First-Aid Treatment for Poisoning

I. DO THESE THINGS BEFORE YOU CALL SOMEONE
    A. Remove poisons from contact with eyes, skin or mouth.
        1. Eyes: Gently wash eyes with plenty of water (or milk) for 10 to 15 minutes with the eyelids held open.   Remove contact lenses and again wash the eyes.   Do not allow victims to rub their eyes.
        2. Skin: Wash poisons off the skin with large amounts of plain water.   Then wash the skin with a detergent if it is possible.   Remove and discard all contaminated clothing.
        3. Mouth: Look into victim's mouth and remove all tablets, powder, plants, or any other material that you find.   Also examine for cuts, burns, or any unusual coloring.   Wipe out mouth with a cloth and wash thoroughly with water.
    B. Remove victim from contact with poisonous fumes or gases.
        Get the victim into fresh air.
        Loosen all tight-fitting clothing.
        If the victim is not breathing, you should start artificial respiration immediately.   Do not stop until the victim is either breathing well or help arrives.   Use oxygen if available.   Send someone else to call for help.
    C. If a caustic poison has been swallowed, you should dilute it by giving 1 or 2 glassfuls of milk or water.
II. CALL FOR INFORMATION ABOUT WHAT TO DO NEXT:
    A. Call your doctor, or call the poison control center.
        1. Identify yourself and your relationship to the victim.
        2. Describe the victim by name, age and sex.
        3. Have the package or poison in your hand and identify exactly (as best as you can) what the victim took and how much he took.
    B. Call for information even if you are not sure.   Keep calm.   You have enough time to act, but don't delay unnecessarily.
III. IF YOU ARE INSTRUCTED TO INDUCE VOMITING
    Never induce vomiting until you are instructed to do so.
    A. Have syrup of ipecac available to induce vomiting.   Purchase one ounce of ipecac syrup from your pharmacist.   You may do this without a prescription.   It will keep stored at room temperature for several years.
    B. To use ipecac:
        In an adult give 2 tablespoons (30 mL), in a child over one year give one tablespoon (15 mL), and in a child less than one year (10 mL), of ipecac syrup followed by a glass (8 oz) of liquid (water, juices, etc).   Then give additional liquid as tolerated.   If patient hasn't vomited within 15 to 20 minutes, repeat the dose of ipecac and give more water.
    C. Don't waste time trying other ways to make the victim vomit.
        Tickling the back of the throat with your fingers, a spoon, or some other object is not very effective.   Do not use salt water.   It is potentially dangerous.
    D. Never induce vomiting if the patient:
        Is unconscious.
        Is having convulsions (fits).
        Has swallowed strong caustics or corrosives.
        And induce vomiting only if instructed, if the patient:
        Has swallowed petroleum products, cleaning fluids, gasoline, lighter fluid, etc.
IV. IF YOU GO TO THE HOSPITAL:
    A. Take or send the poison container, poisonous plant, etc, with you.
    B. Take any vomitus you collect.
    C. Don't give substances like coffee, alcohol, stimulants, or drugs to the victim.

in the home: burnt toast, strong tea, and milk of magnesia). It now has been well established that the last two constituents have no significant efficacy and may actually impede the one active ingredient, activated charcoal. The long-advocated preparation of burnt toast and strong tea in the home has no merit; the materials do not have significant therapeutic properties.

Because they are not often used, it is important for information to be available readily concerning antidotes; not only so that they can be used properly and at the earliest possible moment, but also so that time is not wasted in searching for nonexistent antidotes. For a few poisons, there are chemical antidotes that react with the poison in the stomach either to inactivate it or to retard its absorption. Such local antidotes are sufficiently innocuous that they can be administered safely.

The most useful antidotes are those available for systemic administration to counteract the effects of poisons which have already been absorbed. Table IX summarizes the local and systemic antidotes that are currently available and how they

are administered. Information is given concerning doses or other details of administration as a reference.

Other Measures—Aside from removal or inactivation of the poison and use of antidotes when available, the treatment of poisoning is supportive. The symptomatic or supportive approach to treatment does not differ significantly from that encountered in other medical problems. Common problems requiring supportive care include coma, respiratory insufficiency, convulsions, shock, vomiting, diarrhea, fluid and electrolyte disturbances, cerebral edema, kidney failure, and damage to other organs.

Additionally there are a number of procedures that may be utilized to hasten elimination of a poison. In some instances drugs can be eliminated more rapidly by using diuresis induced by use of pharmacologic or osmotic diuretics along with alkalinization of the urine. With poisons that are dialyzable, extracorporeal hemodialysis (use of artificial kidney) is preferred. A newer procedure, sorbent hemoperfusion is also effective with many agents. These procedures are indicated when normal excretory processes fail or prove to be inade-

Table IX—Summary of Local and Systemic Antidotes

Poison	Local Antidote	Systemic Antidote
Acetaminophen	activated charcoal (not to be used if *N*-acetylcysteine is to be given)	*N*-acetylcysteine (Mucomist) initial dose of 140 mg/kg orally in soft drinks, fruit juice, or water; then, 70 mg/kg every 4 hr for 68 hr (17 doses)
Acids, corrosive	dilute with water or milk, then give a nonabsorbable antacid	
Alkali, caustic	dilute with water or milk, then give demulcent	
Alkaloids coniine, quinine, strychnine, etc	activated charcoal	
Amphetamines	activated charcoal	chlorpromazine, 1 mg/kg IM or IV (administered slowly if given IV); may repeat in 15 min; reduce to 0.5 mg/kg if other CNS depressants involved.
Anticholinergics	activated charcoal	physostigmine, adult: 2 mg; child: 0.5 mg; may be given slowly IV; may repeat in 15 min until desired effect is achieved; subsequent doses may be given q 2–3 hr prn. Use only for specific indications associated with severe toxicity.
Anticholinesterases organophosphates neostigmine physostigmine pyridostigmine carbamates	activated charcoal	atropine, 1–2 mg (for children under 2 yr, 1 mg or 0.05 mg/kg) IV repeated every few min until atropinization is evident; then give pralidoxime chloride 25–50 mg/kg (1 gm in adults) IV; repeat in 8–12 hr prn. atropine as above, but *do not* use pralidoxime
Antihistamines	(see Anticholinergics)	
Arsenic	(see Heavy metals)	
Atropine	(see Anticholinergics)	
Barium salts	sodium sulfate, 300 mg/kg	sodium or magnesium sulfate, 10 mL of 10% solution IV q 15 min until symptoms stop
Belladonna alkaloids	(see Anticholinergics)	
Bromides		sodium or ammonium chloride, 6–12 gm/day PO, or the equivalent as normal saline, q 6 hr IV
Cadmium	(see Heavy metals)	
Carbon monoxide		100% oxygen by inhalation hyperbaric oxygen is a recommended alternative in comatose patients.)
Cholinergic compounds	(see Anticholinesterases)	
Copper	(see Heavy metals)	
Cyanide		Adult: amyl nitrite inhalation (inhale for 15–30 sec q 60 sec) pending administration of 300 mg sodium nitrite (10 mL of a 3% solution) IV slowly (over 2–4 min); follow immediately with 12.5 gm sodium thiosulfate (2.5–5 mL/min of 25% solution) IV slowly (over 10 min) Children: (sodium nitrite should not exceed recommended dose as fatal methemoglobinemia may result). Use the following table as a guide:

Hemoglobin	Initial dose 3% Na nitrite IV	Initial dose 25% Na thiosulfate IV
8 gm	0.22 mL (6.6 mg/kg)	1.10 mL/kg
10 gm	0.27 mL (8.7 mg/kg)	1.35 mL/kg
12 gm	0.33 mL (10. mg/kg)	1.65 mL/kg
14 gm	0.39 mL (11.6 mg/kg)	1.95 mL/kg

Poison	Local Antidote	Systemic Antidote
Ethylene glycol	(see Methanol)	
Fluoride	calcium gluconate or lactate, 150 mg/kg, or milk	calcium gluconate, 10 mL of 10% solution, given slowly IV until symptoms abate; may be repeated prn.
Gold	(see Heavy metals)	
Heavy metals	Milk or egg whites	BAL (dimercaprol): 3–5 mg/kg/dose deep IM q 4 hr for 2 days, q 4–6 hr for an additional 2 days, then q 4–12 hr for up to 7 additional days

Table IX—Continued

Poison	Local Antidote	Systemic Antidote
metal	usual chelators used	EDTA: 75 mg/kg 24 hr deep IM
arsenic	BAL	or slow IV infusion given in 3–6 divided
cadmium	satisfactory use not demonstrated	doses for up to 5 days; may be repeated
copper	BAL, penicillamine	for a second course after a minimum of 2
gold	BAL	days; each course should not exceed a
lead	BAL, EDTA, penicillamine	total of 500 mg/kg body weight
mercury	BAL, penicillamine	
silver	satisfactory use not demonstrated	penicillamine: 100 mg/kg/day (max 1 gm) PO
thallium	Prussian blue	in divided doses for up to 5 days; for long-term
Hypochlorites	(see Alkali, caustic)	therapy do not exceed 40 mg/kg/day
Iron	sodium bicarbonate, 1–5% solution, preferably by lavage	deferoxamine, 20–40 mg/kg IV given as slow drip
		over 4 hr period not to exceed 15 mg/kg/hr;
		followed by 20 mg/kg every 4–8 hrs until urine
		color normal or iron level normal. (Can give 20
		mg/kg IM every 4–12 hr if no IV sites
		available)
Isoniazid	activated charcoal	pyridoxine (vitamin B_6) 1 mg per gm of INH
		ingested in divided doses given slow IV push (5
		mg/50 mL each bolus). If seizures, initially
		give 5 mg IV over 3–5 min. May repeat dose at
		5–15 intervals until seizures stop of
		consciousness regained.
Lead	(see Heavy metals)	
Mercury	(see Heavy metals)	
Methanol		ethanol, loading dose to achieve blood level of 100
		mg/dL. Adult: 0.6 gm/kg body weight + 7–10
		gm to be infused IV over 1 hr. Child: 0.6
		gm/kg body weight + 4–5 gm to be infused IV
		over 1 hr. Maintenance doses should
		approximate 10 gm/hr in adults and 5 gm/hr in
		children, to be adjusted according to measured
		blood ethanol levels
Methemoglobinemic		methylene blue, 1–2 mg (0.1–0.2 mL/kg) of a 1%
agents		solution IV slowly over 5–10 min if cyanosis is
nitrites		severe (or methemoglobin level is greater than
chlorates		40%)
nitrobenzene		
Narcotics	activated charcoal	naloxone, 0.005–0.01 mg/kg (adult 0.4 mg) IV; if
		no response, give 0.1 mg/kg (adult 4.0 mg) IV.
		Alternate schedule is to give 0.03 mg/kg (adult
		1.2 mg) IV, repeated once or twice.
Nitrites	(see Methemoglobinemic agents)	
Oxalate	dilute with water or milk, then give calcium gluconate or lactate, 150 mg/kg	calcium gluconate, 10 mL of 10% solution, given slowly IV until symptoms abate; may be repeated prn
Phenothiazines (neuromuscular reaction only)		diphenhydramine, 0.5–1.0 mg/kg IM or IV; or benztropine, 2 mg IM or IV
Phosgene		methenamine, 20 mL of 20% solution (4 gm) IV. Probably ineffective after full development of pulmonary edema
Physostigmine	(see Anticholinesterases)	
Quaternary ammonium compounds	(see Detergents, cationic)	
Silver	(see Heavy metals)	
Thallium	(see Heavy metals)	
Tricyclic antidepressants	(see Anticholinergics)	
Warfarin		Vitamin K_1, 0.5–1.0 mg/kg IM or IV
		adults: 10 mg IM or IV
		children: 1–5 mg IM or IV

For Envenomation

Animals	Antivenin*
Snake, Crotalidae (all North American rattlers and moccasins)	Antivenin (Crotalidae) Polyvalent (Wyeth)
Snake, Coral	Antivenin (Microcrurus fulvius, monovalent (Wyeth)
Spider, Black Widow	Antivenin, Latrodectus mactans (Merck, Sharp & Dohme)

NOTE: All antisera should be tested for sensitivity to horse serum.
* See package insert for dosage and administration

of this period. Special displays in pharmacies have been one type of effective weapon. Other worthwhile activities have included television or radio messages, special meetings, and newspaper articles, all of which can be made more effective by interested pharmacists. By joing forces with the regional or local poison control centers, this week can be used to highlight the year-round educational activities of the center and the community.

Role of the Pharmacist—There is much that the pharmacist can do to help prevent poisoning and to improve the treatment thereof. While he may or may not become involved in the therapy of poisoning except for necessary first-aid, he plays a key role in ensuring that adequate equipment and information are available. Indeed, it is often the pharmacist of a hospital or medical group who initiates the development of adequate facilities and materials for the treatment of cases.

Undoubtedly the most important role can be played by the pharmacist in the area of prevention. This role relative to poison prevention packaging of prescription drugs was mentioned above. However, the role of the pharmacist is particularly critical with regard to nonprescription items. With prescription medications there is involvement of a physician who may provide instructions and precautionary advice. However, with over-the-counter materials, the pharmacist is often the only person who is in a position to serve these functions.

The pharmacist can and should provide, explain and amplify directions for proper use of potentially toxic materials, bearing in mind that the concern is not only for the safety of the patient but also for other individuals in the household. Thus, the dispensing of a toxic medication provides an opportunity to warn the buyer about the hazards of leaving the material within reach of children.

In some instances it is desirable to affix warning labels on the products that a pharmacist dispenses or to hand out patient information materials. The dispensing of a drug also provides an opportunity also to inquire and to give advice about facilities for safe storage. Because of this contact with his patrons the pharmacist can play a personalized role in cautioning about many prescription drugs and a host of commercial products.

The pharmacist can do much to reduce the aforementioned limitations of labeling. While the public often may not read or appreciate precautions on labels, the effectiveness of the latter are increased significantly if they are explained by a pharmacist. The pharmacist also has a unique role to play in detecting product or labeling defects. He has an obligation to call to the attention of appropriate manufacturers or regulatory agencies potential labeling or product defects.

When the pharmacist is consulted about a poisoning, he can advise the individual to contact a physician or poison control center immediately. In the meantime, he can help to ensure proper first-aid treatment and, more importantly, help to prevent injurious maltreatment by disseminating appropriate advice. He can be most effective in his advisory capacity if he has acquainted himself thoroughly with the existing poison information and treatment facilities of his area.

As indicated, there has been a tendency in the past for the development of too many small and ineffectual poison centers the activities of which could be carried out more effectively and efficiently if they were amalgamated with others in the same area. A trend toward centralization and regionalization of poison information and treatment facilities should be encouraged by local pharmacy associations.

Finally, pharmacists can assist greatly in the educational efforts of a community by distributing literature provided by himself or by the local medical or pharmaceutical societies, and by providing space for displays related to poisoning prevention.

Bibliography

Arena JM: *Poisoning*, 3rd ed, Thomas, Springfield, IL, 1976.

Dreisbach RH: *Handbook of Poisoning*, 10th ed, Lange, Los Altos, CA, 1980.

Gillman AG, Goodman LS, Gilman A: *The Pharmacological Basis of Therapeutics*, 6th ed, Macmillan, New York, 1980.

Gosselin RE, *et al: Clinical Toxicology of Commercial Products*, 4th ed, Williams & Wilkins, Baltimore, 1976.

Grant WM: *Toxicology of the Eye*, 2nd ed, Charles C Thomas, Springfield, IL, 1974.

Haddad LM and Winchester JF (eds): *Clinical Management of Poisoning and Drug Overdose*, WB Saunders Co, Philadelphia, 1983.

Hardin JW, Arena JM: *Human Poisoning from Native and Cultivated Plants*, 2nd ed, Duke Univ Press, Durham, NC, 1974.

Henretig FM, Cupit GC, Temple AR: "Toxicologic Emergencies" in Fleisher G, Ludwig S, (eds): *Textbook of Pediatric Emergency Medicine*, Williams & Wilkins, Baltimore, 1983.

Lampe KF, Fagerstrom R: *Plant Toxicity and Dermatitis*, Williams & Wilkins, Baltimore, 1968.

Morgan DP: *Recognition and Management of Pesticide Poisonings*, 2nd ed, USEPA, Office of Pesticide Programs, EPA-540/9-77-013, Washington, DC, 1977.

Physicians' Desk Reference, 37th ed, Medical Economics, Oradell, NJ, 1983.

PDR For Nonprescription Drugs, 4th ed Medical Economics, Oradell, NJ, 1983.

Rumack BH, Temple AR: *Management of the Poisoned Patient*, Science Press, Princeton, NJ, 1977.

Temple AR: Poison Control Centers: Prospects and Capabilities, *Ann Rev Pharmacol Toxicol 17:* 215–22, 1977.

Temple AR, Done AK: in Oats WW, Spitzer S, eds: *Emergency Room Care*, Grune & Stratton, New York, 107, 1972.

Temple AR, Mancini RE: "Management of Poisoning" in Yaffe SJ, (ed) *Pediatric Pharmacology*, Grune & Stratton, New York, 1980.

Temple AR, ed: American Poison Control Centers, *Clin Toxicol 8:* No 3, 1978.

Temple AR, Woolley BW: *Toxicology and Poison Prevention*, University of Southern California School of Pharmacy, 1977.

Acknowledgment

The author wishes to thank Alan K Done, MD, for his previous contribution to this chapter and for his personal contribution to the author's training and interest in poison control. Also, the author wishes to thank the staff of the Intermountain Regional Poison Control Center for their support and contribution of previously published materials from which portions of this chapter were derived.

In addition, if the corporation distributes profits to its shareholders, the profit is again taxed as personal income to the shareholder. This gives rise to the concept of "double taxation." This scheme can be a distinct disadvantage to the corporate entity. Many larger companies simply accept the disadvantage, but smaller closely held corporations must minimize the tax liability.

To reduce taxes the corporation could pay salaries to the shareholder-officers rather than distribute dividends. Reasonable salaries paid to corporate officials may be deducted in computing the taxable income of the business, but dividends may not. The corporation might choose to accumulate earnings rather than distribute them to the shareholders. The Internal Revenue Service permits the accumulation of earnings up to certain levels.

Another alternative for the small, closely held corporation is to take advantage of special provisions in the Internal Revenue Code which allows such corporations to be treated as partnerships for income-tax purposes and thereby avoid having a tax assessed on the corporate income itself. This is termed a Subchapter S election. This procedure allows the company earnings to be passed directly to the shareholder where the earnings are taxed for the first time as part of the shareholder's personal income. A Subchapter S corporation cannot have over ten shareholders, and a number of other restrictions exist as to its formulation. Legal assistance should be acquired to facilitate the procedure.

Pension Plans—The corporate structure has been attractive to many individuals because it permits the corporation to offer certain benefit plans to its employees. The corporation may establish more favorable qualified pension and profit-sharing plans for its employees, including the shareholder employees, than those allowed to partnerships and sole proprietorships. Following these plans, the corporation is entitled to deduct as expenses all payments made to a qualified pension or profit-sharing plan, and the income is not taxable to the employee until the time it is actually distributed.

The Tax Equity and Fiscal Responsibility Act of 1982 generally eliminated distinctions in the tax law between qualified plans of corporations and those of self-employed individuals (Keogh plans). The special deduction limits for contributions on behalf of a self-employed individual under a Keogh plan have been repealed. In addition, individuals may now establish individual retirement accounts (IRAs) even if they are also participants in qualified employer pension plans. The annual ceiling on deductible IRA contributions has been increased to the smaller of $2,000 or 100% of annual earned income.

Many professionals have desired to obtain the more favorable deferment of income which has been available to the corporate entity through use of pension plans, profit-sharing plans, and stock bonus plans. However, because a corporation could possess no conscience, nor could it take an examination, it could not meet the requirement for professional licensure. During the 1960s state legislatures responded to lobbying efforts by the various professions by enacting legislation which will permit corporations to practice a profession. The laws regarding professional service corporations will vary from state to state. In some states the legislation will apply to all professions, while in other instances the law will apply only to certain designated professions. The statutes are rather specific as to the purpose of a corporation, and in many cases there will be no choice as to whether to incorporate as a professional service corporation or as a business corporation. The statutes regarding professional corporations do not alter the relationship between the professional person and the patient. As a general rule, the statutes preserve the personal liability of the professional individual and will not provide a corporate shield for the professional's negligent acts.

Contract Law

A contract may be defined as a promise or set of promises for the breach of which the law provides a remedy, or the performance of which the law in some way recognizes as a duty. Yet the law requires much more for a contract to result than a mere exchange of promises. Perhaps a more complete definition of a contract is an agreement between legally competent individuals based on genuine assent of the parties and supported by consideration, made for a lawful purpose and in the form required by law, if any. This definition provides a framework for discussion of these elements of a contract.

The agreement between the parties which forms a basis for the contract is composed of both an offer and an acceptance. In order for an offer to be legally sufficient the party making it must have the intention of entering into an agreement with the other party. For example, an offer made in jest would not indicate the required contractual intent. Moreover, an invitation to make an offer or an offer to negotiate is not a legally cognizable offer for it, too, lacks contractual intent. Advertisements are not an offer of sale but rather an indication of willingness to consider an offer made by the potential purchaser. The offer must be communicated to the other party prior to acceptance for an agreement to result.

An additional requirement for an offer is that it be definite. This means that the offer must be sufficiently detailed to provide a basis for the agreement. Courts will not add an essential element to an offer, agreement or contract. At the time of acceptance the offer must still be viable. An offer may be withdrawn prior to acceptance, in the absence of an option having been granted. An option is a binding promise to keep an offer open for a stated period of time. If an option exists the person making the offer may not withdraw it until the option period has expired. An offer may also be terminated by rejection or by lapse of a period of time stated in the offer.

Acceptance is assent by the recipient of the offer to the terms of the offer. No particular form of acceptance is required, eg, in writing, unless specified in the offer. However, the acceptance must be absolute and unconditional. Any variation of the terms or conditions in the acceptance will result in rejection of the offer.

The parties entering into a contract must be legally competent to do so. This means that each party must have contractual capacity. Minors generally lack contractual capacity and contracts they enter into are subject to their avoidance. The other party may not be able to enforce the contract against a minor because the contract can be voided by the minor due to his lack of contractual capacity. However, parents may be liable under contract theory for "necessaries" provided to their minor dependents. "Necessaries" are those things relating to the health, education or comfort of the minor. Prescription drugs probably would fall within the category of "necessaries" and a pharmacist providing them to a minor would in all likelihood be able to collect the reasonable value of the medication from the parents.

Insane persons may also be under a contractual incapacity. If a person is so mentally deranged as not to know that a contract is being made or does not understand the consequences of what he/she is doing, the contract may be voided on recovering sanity. The same is true of a person who is so intoxicated as to be unaware that he/she was making a contract.

The requirement of genuineness of assent relates to mistake, misrepresentation, concealment, fraud, or exercise of undue influence or duress over one of the parties. Each of these activities has a different effect on the enforceability of the contract, and a full discussion of each is beyond the scope of this discussion. Nonetheless, the pharmacist should be aware that each bears a possibility for interference with the enforceability of the contract.

Consideration is essential for a contract to be enforceable. It may be defined as an act or forbearance, or the promise of either, which is offered by one party to an agreement and accepted by the other as an inducement to the other's act or promise. When you have given consideration you have agreed to do something that you were not bound to do or you have agreed to refrain from doing that which you have the right to do.

Consideration must be provided by both parties to the contract. If only one is providing consideration, no contract results. It is a mere gift and not legally enforceable.

Ordinarily courts will not inquire into the adequacy of the consideration exchanged by the parties. The fact that the amount of consideration may appear to be small in the eyes of one person does not necessarily mean that the amount is inadequate or inappropriate. Hence, if some consideration is provided the contract will be enforceable. One sometimes hears of employment contracts for "a dollar-a-year man," as in the case of a wealthy individual working for the government or a charity. Such an employment contract will be enforceable even though the value of a person's services will be much greater than the amount of compensation provided.

In order for a contract to be enforceable it must be made for a lawful purpose, and this purpose must be achieved in a lawful manner. If this were not so the courts might be placed in the uncomfortable situation of compelling one party to a contract to commit a crime in order to have the contract performed. An example of this doctrine is the rule that contracts of an unlicensed operator cannot be enforced. Hence, one who practices pharmacy without being licensed to do so not only is likely to be charged with the crime of violating the state pharmacy practice act but will also be unable to enforce the contracts he made while "practicing" pharmacy, ie, he will be unable to sue to collect for his services.

Contracts for the sale of prohibited articles are also unenforceable. Sale of a federal legend drug without a valid prescription would fall in this category. Contracts which unreasonably restrain trade are also unlawful and, consequently, unenforceable. When a pharmacist sells a pharmacy it is customary for the purchaser to request that the contract contain a "non-competition" clause which bans the seller from owning a pharmacy within certain geographic and time limits. The purpose is to prevent the seller from selling and immediately opening up a pharmacy, attracting away all his prior patients. If such a clause is drafted to include too large a geographic area or for too long a time it will be unenforceable due to its restraint on trade. However, note that only contracts which "unreasonably" restrain trade are unlawful. Consequently, if the "non-competition" clause is carefully drafted it will be enforceable.

Most contracts are not required to be in writing to be enforceable. Obviously though, it is much easier to prove the existence of and enforce one that is written. Each state has a Statute of Frauds which dictates which types of contracts must be in writing to be enforceable. Generally, contracts for creation of an interest in land which run for more than one year must be in writing, those that involve employment for more than one year and those which are for sale of goods of a value of $500 or more must be in writing, among others. Each state may have additional categories, and the minimum limits just mentioned may vary from state to state.

When a contract is breached, the non-breaching party has the right to bring legal action against the breaching party to recover that sum of money that will place him in the same position as he would have been had the contract been performed. There are a number of types of damages which may be assessed against the breaching party. Nominal damages are awarded when the injured party did not suffer an actual loss. They usually are of minimal magnitude. Compensatory damages are those which are designed to compensate the injured party for his loss. Liquidated damages may also be encountered. Liquidated damages are those for which provision was made in the contract itself by the contracting parties when they entered into the agreement. Liquidated damages clauses generally will be enforced if the amount specified is not excessive and if the contract is of such a nature that it would be difficult to determine the actual amount of damages.

The Uniform Commercial Code addresses a special category of contracts known as "sales." A sale may be defined as a transaction wherein a seller transfers title for personal property to a buyer for a price (consideration). Article 2 of the UCC addresses the law of sales in great detail and the interested readers may wish to refer to that source for information beyond the scope of this discussion.

Of particular interest to pharmacists is the law applicable to warranties in sales transactions. A warranty is an assurance or guarantee by a seller that the goods sold are, or will be, as represented. Warranties may be divided into two general categories, express and implied. Express warranties are those based on an affirmation of fact or promise relating to the goods, whereas an implied warranty is one that exists by virtue of law, not because of an express statement by the seller. Express warranties may be made about nearly any attribute of the goods, but the warranties implied by law are more limited in scope. One such implied warranty is the implied warranty of merchantability. It is seen only with sellers who usually deal in goods of that type and means that the goods provided must be fit for the ordinary purposes for which such goods are used. The implied warranty of fitness for a particular purpose is present when the seller knows the use to which the goods will be put and has reason to know that the buyer is relying on the seller's skill and judgment to select suitable goods for the purpose. These implied warranties are automatically present in a transaction without any action on the part of the seller to place them there. They can be removed from the sale but require a specific type of action. Goods sold "as is" are sold with no implied warranties. To remove the implied warranty of "merchantability" those specific words must be used, but the disclaimer can be made orally. Removal of the implied warranty of fitness for a particular purpose can only be done by written words, but no special language is required. However, the statement that the warranty is absent must be conspicuous. Naturally, express warranties can be kept out of a transaction merely by not making an express statement about the goods.

The Magnuson-Moss Warranty Act went into effect during 1975 and requires that a firm offering a warranty must state the warranty in simple language and must clearly state what the warranty covers. Under this statute the implied warranty cannot be disclaimed or modified in a written warranty; however, the duration of the implied warranties can be limited. The Act also requires that warranty statements be made available to the public in a form to which they can obtain easy access.

Commercial Paper

Commercial paper is a specialized branch of contract law and is governed in most states by Article 3 of the Uniform Commercial Code. The three basic kinds of commercial paper are the promissory note, the draft, and the check.

Commercial paper or negotiable instruments are substitutes for money and are negotiable by endorsement or delivery. In order to be negotiable the written instrument must be signed by the maker and must contain an unconditional promise or order to pay a sum certain in money, be payable on demand or at a definite time, and be payable to order or to bearer.

Writing—The UCC provides that a negotiable instrument may be handwritten in ink, pencil or blood, or it may be typed, printed or stamped. However, most banks will refuse instruments unless written in a commercially acceptable manner. In case of ambiguity handwritten terms will control over typewritten and printed terms, and typewritten terms control printed terms. If there is an inconsistency between words and figures, the words will control.

Signature—A person is not liable on a negotiable instrument unless his signature appears thereon. The signature may be written, printed, typed, or stamped. As a general rule a signature made by an agent will bind the principal. However, if the instrument does not show the representative capacity of the agent, he may be personally bound in such an instance, even though authorized. By signing a check in payment for goods, the drawer suspends his obligation on the underlying contract. However, it is revived again if the check is dishonored.

Payable on Demand—A negotiable instrument is payable on demand when the holder can collect it at any time he pleases. This would be the case with the typical check. If no time is stated, the instrument is deemed payable on demand. If the instrument is not payable on demand, it must be payable at a definite time. The fact that the instrument is undated or postdated does not affect the negotiability of the document. Postdated instruments simply put the payee on notice that the maker of the instrument does not have sufficient funds at the present time but will at the future date. An instrument is payable to order when by its terms it is payable to the order of any person specified with reasonable certainty. An instrument is payable to bearer when by its terms it is payable to the bearer, or cash, or any other indication which does not purport to designate a specific payee. If negotiable paper is payable to bearer it may be transferred simply by delivery. However, if the paper is payable to the order of a designated person it may be transferred only by the endorsement of that person followed by delivery.

Endorsement—An endorsement is a written signature usually found on the back of a commercial instrument or a paper attached to it. An endorsement may be special, in blank, or restrictive. A blank endorsement occurs when the payee simply signs his name on the back, while in a special endorsement the payee endorses to the order of a specific person. An instrument with a blank endorsement becomes a bearer instrument and may be transferred by delivery, but an instrument with a special endorsement requires the signature of the specified person in order to further the negotiation of the instrument. Endorsements are restrictive when they are conditional or when they include words such as "for collection," "for deposit," or "pay any bank." If the payee's name is misspelled, he may endorse in that name, his own name, or both, but the person paying the instrument may require that he sign both names.

Liability of Endorsers—Rather complex rules exist under the UCC regarding the liabilities and responsibilities of the parties to a negotiable instrument. Endorsers of checks or notes are liable in the order in which they endorse the instrument. However, they are not liable until presentation for payment, dishonor, and notice of dishonor have occurred. If one desires to endorse commercial paper without incurring any liability, he should place over his signature the words "without recourse."

Forgery—Forgeries may occur either in the signature of the maker or drawer, or the endorsee's signature may be forged. If the signature of the drawer of the check has been forged and the bank on which the check is drawn proceeds to pay the check before discovery of the forgery, the bank cannot recover payment and must assume the loss. An unauthorized or forged signature is wholly inoperative as the signature of the person whose name is forged. The bank's only recourse would be to collect from the forger.

If the payee's endorsement has been forged, the loss will land on the party who first took the forged instrument. A party cashing an endorsed check does so at his own risk because there is an obligation to pay the document by the drawee bank only upon the genuineness of the payee's endorsement. If several successive parties have negotiated the instrument following a forgery, each party can demand repayment from an earlier holder until the instrument is back in the hands of the party who took it from the forger. This individual could only demand repayment from the forger. This legal theory gives rise to the adage, "Know your endorser." Many exceptions exist to these general rules and local statutes should be consulted.

The UCC provides that the customer has the right to stop payment if a check has not been paid, but the bank must have a reasonable opportunity to act on the stop-payment order. A stop-payment order given verbally is effective for 14 days and a written order is effective for six months.

Holder in Due Course—Commercial paper is intended to circulate freely, and one of the basic principles in this area of law is that a holder in due course of a negotiable instrument takes the document free from all of the personal defenses of the maker or the drawer. In order to be a holder in due course, a holder of a negotiable instrument must take the document for value, in good faith, and without notice that it is overdue or has been dishonored or of any defense against it. Any party who takes the document which meets these requirements is free from any claims which are personal in nature, such as breach of warranty, breach of contract, fraud in the inducement, or nondelivery of the goods. But the holder in due course does not take the instrument free from all defenses. He is subject to the so-called real defenses such as incapacity of a party to make a contract, duress, bankruptcy, or forged signatures. If a party cannot qualify as a holder in due course, he takes the instrument subject to all conflicting claims of ownership including real and personal defenses.

The holder in due course doctrine has come under severe criticism by both state legislatures and the federal government. This is particularly true in the area of consumer transactions, because oftentimes the holder in due course is a third-party financer. States which have adopted the Uniform Consumer Credit Code have limited this doctrine in consumer installment sale arrangements. The Federal Trade Commission has gone even further and has declared it to be an unfair or deceptive act for any retail seller to cut off the consumer's defenses against the seller when commercial paper is transferred on to a third-party financer. Essentially, this rule means that the consumer will not have to continue to pay third parties for goods which were defective or never delivered. It must be emphasized that this new application of the rule does not apply to transactions between business people or to credit card transactions.

Agency

Agency is a consensual relationship between at least two parties involving both contractual and tort responsibilities and liabilities between the two parties and to third parties. While it is true that a person is accountable for his own actions, the reverse is also true that an individual, without any wrongful conduct himself, may be held liable in certain instances for the acts of others.

The terminology in this area can be confusing. One who performs physical services for another, but who has no power to bind the other contractually with a third party is known as a servant. The person for whom the servant is performing the task is known as the master. Those who represent others, most often for the purpose of making contracts, are known as agents, and the individual being represented is known as the principal. A master has the right to control his servant's physical activities, but this is not true in the principal-agent relationship.

In the past these legal characteristics were much easier to distinguish than in today's employer-employee relationship. It is highly likely now that the same person may act as both agent and servant depending on the functions which have been delegated to him. An employee pharmacist may be an agent of the pharmacy owner with respect to his duties to purchase inventory, but the individual may also be a servant of the pharmacy owner with respect to duties such as dispensing prescriptions and record-keeping chores. Tort and contractual liability will turn upon which roles are being performed by the servant/agent.

It must be remembered that not everyone who performs work for another will be a servant. An individual who contracts with an employer to accomplish a specific objective is an independent contractor. An independent contractor is not an agent, and the employer has no right of control as to the means of accomplishing the objective. Distinguishing between an independent contractor and a servant will be important in determining rights under vicarious liability doctrines, workmen's compensation statutes, and unemployment insurance statutes.

The agency relationship is simply founded upon consent between the parties, but in most cases the relationship will actually be based upon a contract although this is not necessary. Many of these contracts will be oral in nature.

Operation of the Agency—A principal has a number of duties to his agent: compensation for services, reimbursement for authorized payments which the agent has made out of his own pocket, and performing in accordance with the terms of the agency. By the same token, the agent has a number of duties to his principal. The agent must be loyal to the principal. He may not make a secret profit out of his employment nor may he compete with his principal. The agent must also exercise reasonable care in performing the agency and to account to the principal for what he has received under the agency.

Tort Liability—An innocent master may be held vicariously liable for the harm caused to third persons by the tortious acts of his servants while they are acting within the scope of their employment. Such a theory is based on the legal maxim that "he who acts through another acts himself." This is often referred to as the doctrine of "respondeat superior," ie, let the master answer. Because the master/employer has the right to control the acts of his servant/employee, he may be held financially responsible for the outcome of those acts. In some states, the master has a right to be indemnified by his servant for any damages he has paid to third parties because of the servant's tortious acts. Because of the doctrine of vicarious liability, a pharmacy owner will want to make sure that his insurance policy covers not only his own negligent acts, but also shelters him for the negligent acts of his employee pharmacists, supportive personnel, and other employees.

The master will not always be liable for all the wrongful acts of his servant, and the determination of whether or not the servant was acting within the scope of his employment will become a question of fact. One of the most important factors in determining whether or not the act was performed within the scope of employment is whether the servant's activities were done with the purpose of benefiting the master. If the facts indicate that the servant was off on a "frolic of his own," he will be held to be acting outside the scope of his authority.

It is important to remember that under the doctrine of vicarious liability, the employee is still personally liable for his own torts. In addition, the master may also be held liable pursuant to conventional tort theories if he was guilty of aiding in the commission of the tort, directed his servant to commit the tortious act, or was guilty of employing an incompetent servant.

Because the principal has no right of control over the physical acts of non-servant agents, the principal will not be liable for damages caused by the tortious physical acts of such agents unless they were acting as authorized by the principal. An employer is also generally not liable for the torts of an independent contractor. Thus, it becomes important to determine which functions the employee may be performing.

Contractual Liability—In somewhat the same manner that a master may be found liable for the acts of the servant, the principal may be held bound to contracts made by his agent. Generally, a principal may be held to a contract so long as the agent making the contract was acting within the scope of authority given to him by his principal. As is true with most legal theories, the general rule is not without its exceptions. In order to appreciate these exceptions it becomes necessary to elaborate on the types of principals, agents, and authority.

Principals may be disclosed, partially disclosed, or undisclosed. A disclosed principal is one whose existence and identity are known to the third party, but the existence and identity of an undisclosed principal are totally unknown to the third party. A principal whose existence, but not whose identity is known to the third party, is termed a partially disclosed principal.

Three varieties of agents also exist. A universal agent is one who has been delegated power to do all acts which can be lawfully delegated to another person. A general agent is one who is usually authorized to do all the acts connected with a particular trade or business. A special agent is one who is authorized to perform a single transaction or one who is authorized to do some specific act pursuant to particular instructions. Stock brokers, real estate agents, and attorneys often fall within the category of special agents.

It is also important to distinguish the type of authority which the agent may hold. Actual or real authority is the agent's power to accomplish whatever his principal has expressly or implicitly assigned him to do. The principal may by means of written or oral communication expressly direct the agent, or the principal by his conduct or by the general circumstances may imply his intention to confer actual authority upon the agent.

Even though an agent has never received actual authority to bind his principal, the principal will be held liable for "apparent authority" if the principal gives the appearance that his agent has a certain measure of authority. The principal will be held liable to a third party who relies on this sort of manifestation of authority. If a person without any authority whatever claims to be an agent of a certain principal, it is the duty of that principal to speak out and deny the agency so as to put all other persons on notice. If the so-called principal remains silent, and third parties are by his silence deceived into thinking that the person claiming to be such agent is telling the truth, then there is danger that the principal will become liable "by estoppel" for any loss suffered by such third party. Estoppel is a principle of law which prevents a person from asserting the reverse of what he has represented previously if the other party has changed his position in reasonable reliance on the previous representation. Thus, manifestations created or tolerated by the principal may be relied upon, but not those given by the agent. In the latter case, if an individual convinces a third party that he is an agent and arranges a contract when in reality there is no authority, the imposter himself is the only party who can be held to the contract.

In those situations in which the principal has been disclosed, the agent is not a party to the contract and the third party is liable directly to the principal and vice versa. If the principal is partially disclosed, then he is liable for the performance of the contract, but the agent may also be held a surety for the performance. At all times, the agent will be liable on the contract if he pledges his own personal liability. If the principal has not been disclosed to the third party, the agent will be liable as a party to the contract. However, in such a case the agent would have a right of indemnification against the undisclosed principal. In those instances in which the agent does possess some type of authority, the principal will usually be liable for the agent's misrepresentations.

If an agent is not authorized or exceeds his authorization, only the agent is bound to the contract because he has breached his authority to bind his principal. This would be true only in those situations where the principal cannot be inculpated under a doctrine such as apparent authority or authority by estoppel.

These preceding concepts of agency law are very relevant to the various forms of business organization. Every member of a partnership is an agent of the partnership and the other partners. The act of every partner in carrying on the business, therefore, will bind the partnership unless the act falls in an area where the partner has no authority at all. The partnership and each individual partner can be held liable for the tortious acts, including malpractice, of the other partners. By the same token, a corporation will be liable for the acts of its agents, although it must be remembered that the shareholder-owners of the corporation are not personally liable for the wrong-doings of the corporation's agents.

Termination of an Agency Relationship—Because an agency relationship is based upon the consent of the individuals, that relationship may be terminated when either or both parties withdraw consent. The agency may also terminate upon expiration of a specified term originally agreed upon. Naturally, the relationship would terminate upon the death of either the principal or the agent. Bankruptcy or insanity of the principal or agent will also act to terminate the agency relationship. The agent's authority will continue until the agent knows, or has reason to know, of a change in circumstances to terminate the agency. Further notice to third parties may also be necessary. An agent's apparent authority may continue despite the principal's termination of the relationship unless the third party receives notice from some source that the agent's authority has been cancelled.

Ownership of Prescriptions

A question arises from time to time regarding ownership of the prescription. When the prescription is issued by the prescriber, the patient gains ownership of the document. When that document is transferred to the pharmacist for purposes of dispensing the medication, ownership then passes to the pharmacist, pursuant to the contract between the pharmacist and the patient. However, the patient retains certain rights with regard to the document.

While the document itself is the property of the pharmacist and must be retained by law by him for record-keeping purposes, the patient has the legal right to refills which the law and the prescriber have authorized. Moreover, the patient may have a right to obtain a copy of the prescription, except in those cases where the giving of a copy is prohibited or limited. For example, in some states copies provided to patients must be marked with a statement indicating that the prescription copy is provided for informational use only and cannot serve as the basis for dispensing medication.

In some situations, such as prescriptions which are suspected to be forgeries or those which bear the potential for a harmful drug interaction, the pharmacist may wish to retain or deface the document even though he will not be dispensing the medication. The pharmacist who does so is running the risk that the prescription might be legitimate or that the drug

interaction would not result. In such a case the pharmacist could be sued for any damages which resulted from his action, for he does not own the document. Should the pharmacist receive a prescription which he does not intend to follow, the problem should be handled through communication with either the patient or the prescriber, not by defacing the document which he does not own.

Because the pharmacist owns the prescription records reflecting medication which he has dispensed, the prescription files are assets of the pharmacy which may be transferred on cessation of practice. Prescription records should be maintained for a minimum of five years, the statute of limitations of the federal Food Drug and Cosmetic Act.

Insurance Plans and Antitrust

Third-party prescription plans have burgeoned in the United States in recent years, and a substantial portion of Americans now have insurance coverage for their medication expenditures. This brief discussion shall center on legal problems associated with private third-party prescription plans, not those administered by governmental agencies.

In the typical third-party plan, the pharmacy owner receives an offer to participate in the insurance plan and a contract to be signed. The contract usually provides for reimbursement of the pharmacist's cost in acquiring the drug product dispensed and the addition of a dispensing fee of fixed magnitude. Other provisions in the contract may relate to what products are compensable, eg, many plans will not pay for non-prescription medication, or limit quantities which may be dispensed. Provisions are also seen dealing with claims submission, services the pharmacist is required to provide, and access to the pharmacist's financial records for purposes of program accountability. Often the offer to participate in such plans is distributed to many pharmacies in an area in order for the insurer to offer the subscriber maximum flexibility in selecting a pharmacist with whom to deal.

When such offers to participate are widely disseminated, the possibility of the offers being discussed collectively arises. This may run afoul of the Sherman Antitrust Act of 1890, which provides that:

"Every contract, combination . . . or conspiracy, in restraint of trade or commerce among the several States . . . is declared to be illegal."

Thus, collective action by pharmacists to withhold entering into contracts with the insurer because the professional fee is too low or because other provisions of the contract are objectionable may violate this federal statute. Individual penalties may be assessed under this statute:

"Every person who shall monopolize, or attempt to monopolize, or combine or conspire with any other person or persons, to monopolize any part of the trade or commerce among the several States . . . shall be deemed guilty of a misdemeanor, and, on conviction thereof, shall be punished by fine not exceeding fifty thousand dollars, or by imprisonment not exceeding one year or both."

Applicability of this statute to pharmacy was affirmed by the United States Supreme Court in the 1962 case of *United States v Utah Pharmaceutical Association*. In that case the activity which brought federal sanctions was publication of a recommended fee schedule in an attempt to encourage the adoption of a uniform professional fee.

With third-party prescription plans, the activity which may violate the statute is collective action by pharmacists ("combination . . . or conspiracy") to withhold their participation ("restrain trade") in the insurance plan until the contract is worded in terms acceptable to them as a group. While such action is legally permissible if done by an individual acting alone, collective action toward the same end would not be legally permissible.

In addition to the criminal penalties outlined above, the

customers who are injured by such unlawful activity may bring a civil suit to recover damages. Of importance is the fact that in an antitrust claim, the award is for treble damages, ie, the amount of damages is calculated and then multiplied by three to yield the amount the party engaging in the unlawful activity must pay.

A federal court is currently considering a case which raises the issue of whether the offering of a uniform professional fee to all pharmacies by insurers is violative of the antitrust laws.

Advertising

The regulation of the advertising and promotion of drugs on an interstate commerce basis is a shared commitment of numerous federal agencies, including the Postal Service, Federal Communications Commission, Federal Trade Commission, and Food and Drug Administration. The latter two bear the brunt of the responsibility. The FTC is actively involved in the regulation of over-the-counter drug advertising while the FDA exercises its jurisdiction primarily over matters involving the labeling and advertising of prescription drugs. There is, however, considerable overlap between the two agencies because of statutory definitions and by mutual agreement.

In intrastate commerce, analogous controls often exist both in terms of substantive law and enforcement apparatus. However, state limitations imposed primarily by budget give these controls much less effect in comparison to federal activities. The pharmacist, therefore, will be bound primarily by federal restrictions in the area of advertising.

Federal Trade Commission—The FTC derives its authority over advertising in general and drug advertising in particular from the Federal Trade Commission Act. Section 5 of that statute provides:

"Unfair methods of competition in commerce and unfair or deceptive acts or practices in commerce are hereby declared unlawful."

In addition, Section 12 of the Federal Trade Commission Act makes it unlawful to disseminate a false advertisement for the purpose of inducing, or which is likely to induce, the purchase of food, drugs, devices, or cosmetics. The Wheeler-Lea Amendment to the Federal Trade Commission Act defines "false advertising" as follows:

"The term "false advertisement" means an advertisement, other than labeling, which is misleading in a material respect; and in determining whether any advertisement is misleading, there shall be taken into account (among other things) not only representations made or suggested by statement, word, design, device, sound, or any combination thereof, but also the extent to which the advertisement fails to reveal facts material in the light of such representations or material with respect to consequences which may result from the use of the commodity to which the advertisement relates under the conditions prescribed in said advertisement, or under such conditions as are customary or usual."

Based on the above provision, the FTC has authority to move against not only false advertisements for OTC drug products, but also advertisements which operate in an unfair or deceptive way. The Commission can use its powers by either promulgating a Trade Regulation Rule (TRR) or by issuing a complaint against an advertiser when there is reason to believe that the law has been violated.

In most cases in which a complaint is issued by the FTC, the advertiser is willing to enter into an agreement to cease and desist from the use of the acts and practices being investigated. Such an agreement is for settlement purposes only, and it does not constitute an admission by the advertiser that the law has been violated. The FTC has been successful in obtaining consent agreements from a number of corporations, including those practicing pharmacy, which require all items advertised to be readily available for sale at or below the advertised price. Displays of advertised items must be conspicuously marked

by a sign or other means disclosing that the item is "as advertised" or "on sale." In addition, many of the consent orders provide that if the advertised item is unavailable, the consumer may either be given a rain-check or be allowed to purchase a similar product of equal or better quality at or below the advertised price. Phrases such as "regular price" or "manufacturer's suggested list price" and words of similar import should not be used unless they can be documented. Whenever a "free," "2-for-1," "half price sale," "1¢ sale" or similar type of offer is made, all the terms and conditions of the offer to the consumer should be made clear at the outset.

If the parties are unable to agree to a consent order, a FTC complaint will result in a trial before an administrative law judge who will determine if a violation has occurred and, if so, the appropriate remedies. This decision may be appealed by either party to the full Commission sitting as an appellate body. Thereafter, review can be pursued to a US Court of Appeals and possibly to the United States Supreme Court. A case involving a well-known mouthwash followed just such a procedure. An administrative law judge ruled that the advertisements for the mouthwash had made claims which were false, misleading and deceptive. Under the administrative ruling, the manufacturer was ordered not only to stop making such claims, but also to institute corrective advertising to inform consumers that the product would not help prevent colds or sore throats or lessen their severity. This ruling was upheld by the full Commission and by a federal appeals court, and the US Supreme Court rejected the manufacturer's petition for further review.

In another action, a 1975 FTC complaint alleging false and misleading advertising included a pharmacy retailer as a defendant even though the ads were prepared by the manufacturer's advertising agency. The administrative law judge held that although the retailer did not know whether the ad claims were true or false, it was not relieved of responsibility simply because the ad copy and content were prepared by others. The full FTC bench ruled that the Federal Trade Commission Act does not exempt the seller of a product from investigating the truthfulness of claims set forth over the retailer's own name. The lack of knowledge of the falsity of the ad was found not to be a defense.

Food and Drug Administration—Prior to 1962 the FTC was vested with sole authority for regulating the advertising of drugs. The Kefauver-Harris Amendments of 1962 to the Food, Drug and Cosmetic Act gave the FDA control over prescription drug advertising. Thus, the FDA regulates not only the labeling of prescription drugs but their advertising as well. All advertisements and other descriptive printed matter issued by the manufacturer must include a statement of the established name, quantitative formula, and other information such as side effects, contraindications, and effectiveness.

The FDA's authority over the regulation of prescription drug advertising extends not only over ads to professionals, but also to that advertising presented to the lay public. By regulation, the FDA has determined that any pharmacy which posts or advertises the price of prescription drugs must include the following information: brand name, if any; generic name, if any; the drug's strength, if the product contains a single active ingredient; dosage form; and the price charged for a specific quantity of the drug. Optional information such as delivery service, charge account service, senior citizen's discount, etc. may be included if such information is not false or misleading. The regulations do not require any pharmacy to post or advertise prescription drug prices, but pharmacies which do so must follow the FDA format.

State Regulation of Drug Advertising—For some time, many states had pharmacy act provisions or pharmacy board regulations which prohibited prescription drug advertising.

Numerous state court decisions had been handed down regarding the permissibility of such prohibitions, but their dictate was anything but clear. In order to obtain an ultimate decision on this controversy, a group of consumers filed suit against the Virginia State Board of Pharmacy alleging a First Amendment right to receive prescription price information. The case of *Virginia State Board of Pharmacy v Virginia Citizens Consumer Council, Inc* eventually reached the US Supreme Court. The court, basing its decision on the First Amendment to the Constitution, held that even speech which is primarily commercial in nature is protected by the First Amendment. The consumer should have the freedom to obtain the price information necessary to make a choice regarding prescription drugs. The Federal Trade Commission had previously proposed a Trade Regulation Rule which would preempt and override all state statutes and regulations which prohibited prescription drug advertising, but with the advent of the *Virginia* case the FTC did not feel it was necessary to move further in this area.

A number of states have also maintained restrictions against the advertisement or display of contraceptives. Such a provision of New York law came under judicial attack, and this case also reached the US Supreme Court. The Court relied heavily on its decision in the *Virginia* prescription price advertising case in holding that the prohibition of any advertisement or display of contraceptives is unconstitutional. All total bans on the advertising of such products were struck down, but the states would still be allowed to regulate against obscene ads. The case of *Carey v Population Services International* also held that the limiting of retail sales of nonmedical contraceptives by licensed pharmacists only clearly imposed a significant burden upon the right of individuals to use contraceptives. The state of New York could demonstrate no compelling reason for such a limitation, and thus the Supreme Court found it unconstitutional.

Credit

In recent years major changes in the practice of extending credit have been required by the Truth-in-Lending Act of 1968. The Act primarily deals with divulgence of information by the potential creditor.

The Truth-in-Lending Act requires that lenders detail their finance charges to the consumer so that he may engage in comparison shopping for credit. However, it goes even further than would appear on the face of its title for it requires disclosure even by those who offer credit free of charge, if the amount is to be repaid in more than four installments. Hence, the pharmacist who offers charge privileges to his patients and does not charge interest on the unpaid balance may still be subject to the provision of the Act if the amount owed is to be paid in more than four installments.

Where credit is offered in such a way that it falls under this statute, the potential debtor must be informed in writing of the finance charge and the annual percentage rate which the opportunity to pay over time will cost him. The finance charge is the amount the total cost the credit customer must pay either directly or indirectly for obtaining the credit. The annual percentage rate is the cost of credit expressed in percentage terms. The finance charge must be clearly stated in dollars and cents and the annual percentage rate must be accurately stated to the nearest 0.25 percent.

When a credit sale is made, the following information must also be provided:

1. the cash price
2. the down payment
3. the difference between the two
4. an itemization of all other charges included in the amount financed but not part of the finance charge, eg, sales tax
5. the unpaid balance
6. the amount deducted as prepaid finance charges
7. the amount financed
8. the total cash price, finance charge and all other charges.

One who fails to make the disclosures required by this statute may be sued by the credit customer for twice the amount of the finance charge, with a minimum of $100 and a maximum of $1000, plus court costs and attorney's fees. Criminal conviction for violation of the requirements of the statute may result in a fine of up to $5000, imprisonment for one year, or both.

Tort Law

Tort law is that subdivision of the civil law which deals with relationships between individuals created by law rather than by the parties themselves. A tort is a private injury or wrong arising from a breach of a duty created by law. A tort may involve harm to a person, as well as damage to property, caused negligently or intentionally.

Negligent torts are those which arise because the tort-feasor (the person doing the act) breached a duty or level of care expected of him. Intentional torts are those which the actor does purposefully or with an intention of achieving the desired result. In this section a number of miscellaneous torts will also be discussed. These are torts which do not fall clearly into either of the prior categories. Finally, liability of the owner or occupier of land or business premises will be discussed, for there are some special rules applicable in that area.

Negligence

Negligence has been defined as the omission to do something that a reasonable man, guided by those ordinary considerations which ordinarily regulate human affairs, would do, or the doing of something which a reasonable and prudent man would not do. As is obvious from this statement, one can be negligent either by doing something or by failing to do something. A more direct description of negligence is that negligence occurs when a person under a duty to another to use due care breaches that duty, resulting in the other party suffering damages as a direct result of that breach. Using this statement as a point of departure, we shall consider each element of negligence in order.

In the normal situation, the existence of a legal duty will be created by the activities of other persons. The jury will be charged with determining what the fictional reasonable and prudent man mentioned above would have done under the circumstances. To do this, the jurors receive testimony from a number of people to determine what they would have done. The jury then determines what the reasonable and prudent man would have done, and that creates the existence of a legal duty. In the ordinary circumstance, the duty will be created by the actions of laymen. Yet, when the pharmacist is acting within the scope of his professional calling, his performance will be evaluated in light of what his professional peers would have done. Generally, a pharmacist will be held liable for negligence only if he departed from the practice of other reputable practitioners of pharmacy. For the general practitioner of pharmacy, the reference standard to be used is other general practitioners of pharmacy. While there may be individuals within the profession with greater knowledge or skill in a particular area, eg, detection of drug interactions, the general practitioner of pharmacy will be required to discharge only that amount of skill exhibited by his peers, not the experts.

Nonetheless, this does not mean that the members of a profession can unduly lag in adoption of new methods or procedures. A number of courts have ruled that while in the usual case the law will recognize the standard of care established by the members of the trade, industry or profession, the entire group may have lagged in adopting an innovation. In such cases, the courts will not be bound by the standards used by the profession, but rather the court will establish the standard of care to be exercised under the circumstance.

The concept of duty is not fixed but rather constantly evolving and changing. An example of this is the doctrine of the pharmacist's duty to consult with patients about proper drug use. Through a number of cases decided during the past twenty years, various courts have ruled that the pharmacist does have the legal duty to instruct the patient about safe and proper use of medication. This duty is owed the patient, and should a pharmacist fail to fulfill this responsibility he may be held answerable in court.

A second requirement for the existence of negligence is damage. The party who is alleging negligence must prove that he suffered legally sufficient damages. Generally, these damages must be substantial, not slight, eg, a temporary skin rash would be insufficient.

The party bringing the suit must next prove that the damages were the direct result of the pharmacist's breach of a legal duty. This may be quite difficult. In some cases it is known that the patient suffered legally cognizable damages but it cannot be established by a preponderance of the evidence that damages flowed directly from breach of duty.

The plaintiff has the burden of establishing those first three elements. Once they have been shown in a legally sufficient manner, the pharmacist has a number of defenses which may be available to result in his being held not liable. One such defense may be contributory negligence. That is, the rule that a party which has in some way contributed to his own injury will not be entitled to recover. In some states the rule is one of comparative negligence. While contributory negligence is a total bar to recovery by the plaintiff, in states which follow the comparative negligence rule the jury engages in an allocation of responsibility and bases the amount of damages awarded on the parties' relative contributions to the injury.

Another defense which the pharmacist has is known as voluntary assumption of the risk. This is the doctrine that a patient who understands the risk inherent in a transaction or procedure and who voluntarily gives his informed consent to assume the risk cannot sue to recover for damages which occur from the defined risk. An unresolved issue is whether presenting a patient with a patient package insert which outlines the potential hazards of use of a certain medication results in informed consent and, consequently, voluntary assumption of the risk. Generally the procedure required for informed consent is a lengthy discussion covering the alternatives and the relative incidence of the various risks. This point will probably be litigated in the future.

Another defense which may be available to the pharmacist is the statute of limitations. The legislature imposes a time limit on filing of suits for negligence. Generally, the statute of limitations in this area is two years, meaning that the suit must be filed within two years of the time of reasonable discovery of the damage. Note, however, that a person may suffer some damage and not be able to discover it until some time long after the incident, as in the diethylstilbestrol cases which are being litigated. In those cases, the injured parties, daughters of women who took the drug during pregnancy, developed precancerous lesions 15–20 years after the drug was consumed. The statute of limitations would not start to run until the time of reasonable discovery, not the time when the drug was dispensed.

The issue of liability of the pharmacist for negligence has been raised in conjunction with a number of developments and innovations in pharmacy practice in recent years. Consideration of application of the above discussion to these developments is in order. Of necessity, a detailed discussion of these areas is impossible in this space. The professional literature contains a number of articles which address these issues in detail, and the interested reader may wish to refer to those.

Patient medication records (PMRs) have been widely adopted in pharmacy practice. There are data from some states which indicate that a majority of the pharmacists maintain such records. In such cases, it may be possible for the attorney representing a party injured due to a pharmacist's failure to detect a drug interaction to establish that the standard of due care is maintenance and proper use of PMRs. Even without such data it may be possible for the attorney to establish that the pharmacist has a duty to detect potentially serious drug interactions. This may well have become part of the pharmacist's standard of due care just as is detecting other prescribing errors. The PMR should probably be viewed as a tool to assist in discharging the responsibility. It does not create the responsibility. The responsibility has its origins in the activities of other practicing pharmacists.

Even if the majority of pharmacists do not maintain PMRs, the skillful attorney may make the argument that the entire profession has delayed in implementing an innovation.

Some states have mandated by statute that the pharmacist maintain PMRs. In such a case, special rules of negligence would apply. The doctrine of negligence *per se* is that where a criminal statute mandates that a certain activity be performed to protect an identifiable group of people from an identifiable type of harm and one does not do it, that fact and the statute may be introduced into evidence at trial to establish the duty and breach of it. This facilitates the case of the plaintiff. Consequently, pharmacists practicing in states where maintenance and use of PMRs has been dictated by statute should be especially careful to comply with the law. Note that this rule of negligence *per se* is applicable only in the case where the activity is required by a statute. A regulation of a board of pharmacy, for example, would not suffice to establish the duty in and of itself. Nonetheless, such a regulation could be introduced into evidence to buttress the testimony of pharmacists on this point.

The vast majority of states have now enacted drug product selection legislation which frees the pharmacist from the restrictions of the antisubstitution laws, enabling him to use his professional judgment in selecting products to be dispensed on certain prescriptions. Naturally, because these statutes give the pharmacist greater responsibility, they increase his potential liability. However, so long as the pharmacist discharges this responsibility in a prudent fashion, the potential for legal entanglements will be minimal. In some states the government has provided guidance for the pharmacist in the form of a positive formulary, designating those drugs for which interchange is permissible. The Food and Drug Administration has also published such a list. In the case of a pharmacist who selects a product from the formulary for brand interchange, he should have a fairly good defense based on his reliance on such governmental lists.

There has not been a successful law suit based on negligence in drug product selection. This is even more significant in light of the fact that pharmacists have been selecting the brand of product to be dispensed extensively for years pursuant to prescriptions written using generic terminology.

Pharmacists should not be unduly concerned with their potential liability exposure as they move into new areas of practice. So long as they are competent to assume the new responsibility and perform the task in a diligent fashion, their liability problems should continue to be minimal.

Intentional Torts

The law distinguishes intentional acts from those which are negligent or careless in nature. Intentional wrongs to persons or property involve such torts as assault, battery, and false imprisonment. At the onset, it is important for one to distinguish between a tort and a crime. The same act may give rise, but not necessarily, to both a tort and a crime. The criminal violation will be prosecuted in the name of the state, but the same act may also result in a separate civil lawsuit between individuals involved. Quite naturally, intentional torts require a showing of the element of intent, but it is not necessary to demonstrate harmful or hostile design.

Assault—An intentional act, other than the mere speaking of words, which places another individual in apprehension of harmful or offensive contact is an assault. The danger must be of an immediate nature and the individual must be aware of the defendant's apparent intent. Bodily contact is not necessary to establish a claim for relief and, thus, damages for an assault alone are likely to be nominal.

Battery—A battery is defined as an intentional act which directly or indirectly is the cause of harmful or offensive contact with another's person or something the person is touching. Assault and battery are separate torts but very often will go hand in hand. A person may be liable for battery even though he intended only to play a practical joke or intended to confer a benefit on the other party.

In patient-care settings it is possible for a cause of action based upon battery to rise during unauthorized surgical operations. Assault and battery offenses may also occur when a pharmacist attempts to control the conduct of patrons of the pharmacy. The case law in some states will permit the owner of a place of business to which the public is invited to request that individuals who are causing a disturbance leave the premises. Upon non-compliance, the owner may use such force as is necessary to eject the disturber.

A number of defenses exist for the torts of assault and battery. If an individual inflicts an injury in self-defense, he would not be liable if he believes that the other person intended to cause him harm and that the injury could be prevented only by infliction of injury on the other person. However, excessive force is not permissible in the exercise of self-defense.

Some parties are privileged to touch others without fear of claims of assault and battery. Police officers may touch an arrested party without fear as long as reasonable force is used. In some states store owners also are privileged to remove boisterous patrons with reasonable force.

An individual who consents to physical contact may not successfully claim a battery. Consent to physical contact may be expressed or implied in nature. Consent to surgical procedures will also negate an action based upon assault and battery, but the consent obtained from the patient should be an informed consent, ie, the patient must have a sufficient understanding of what he is consenting to. The use of investigational drugs will also require an informed consent.

False Imprisonment—The unlawful detention of another person for any length of time may result in an action for false imprisonment. The elements of this tort require the intentional confinement of a person so as to deprive him of his liberty to move about. Negligent imprisonment is not actionable as false imprisonment. A confinement does not have to be by means of physical barriers but may be created by threats of physical force.

This tort may pose a real dilemma for the pharmacy owner who has problems with shoplifters. Many states have enacted laws to aid in this situation. These statutes often provide that the owner of a store or his employee may detain and question an individual in a reasonable manner to determine whether a theft has been committed. The detainment must be for a reasonable time and there must be good cause to believe that the person has committed the act of shoplifting.

An illegal confinement caused by the assertion of legal authority where there is none may result in a false arrest situation. Mere words asserting legal authority without acquiescence do not constitute an arrest. The arrestor should have some element of control if the person acted upon does not acquiesce voluntarily. The law does not require the victim to resist the arrest before he has the cause of action for wrongful arrest. In most states an arrest can be made by a police officer or a private party for a crime committed in his presence.

Miscellaneous Torts

Some torts are not easily pigeon-holed into either the negligent or the intentional tort categories. These miscellaneous torts may require some showing of the element of intent, but it is often more subtle in nature than in the previous section on intentional torts.

Malicious Prosecution—Traditionally, this tort was defined as the unjustifiable instigation of criminal prosecution. However, the tort now also applies to the field of wrongful civil suits. Lawsuits based upon malicious prosecution have not been favored by the courts because instead of terminating litigation, the malicious prosecution case simply continues an action, and the plaintiff in one case becomes the defendant in the new case. Malicious prosecution actions have become particularly attractive to health-care professionals who wish to file counter-suits against parties who had originally filed frivolous malpractice claims.

A number of elements are essential in order to establish a case based on malicious prosecution. The defendant in the first action now becomes the plaintiff in the second suit. The original proceedings must have terminated in favor of the defendant. In addition, the first suit must have been lacking in probable cause. If there were no reasonable grounds to warrant an ordinarily prudent man to believe the defendant was guilty of the alleged claims, then probable cause is undoubtedly lacking. If a case is instigated simply for its nuisance value or for harrassment, probable cause will also be found missing. The third element is that the original suit must have been filed with malice. This can be a very difficult element to prove. If an individual knowingly withholds information which may be harmful to his claim, this could be construed as evidence of bad faith or malice. Lastly, it must be shown that the defendant was damaged as a result of the original lawsuit. Some states will require that the damages be more than the mere expense and annoyance of defending the civil lawsuit.

Malicious prosecution actions may also be the response against individuals who falsely instigate disciplinary proceedings before an administrative board or agency, ie, the original proceeding does not have to be a court action but may be an administrative legal proceeding instead.

Defamation—Defamation is a communication which injures the good name or reputation of another. Defamatory statements which are communicated in a permanent form such as the written word, pictures, statues, etc, are libelous in nature. Communications which are more transient in nature such as the spoken word or a gesture are termed slander.

A defamatory statement, either libel or slander, must be communicated to a third person, ie, one other than the person defamed. The statement will be deemed defamatory if it harms the reputation of another or exposes an individual to scorn, ridicule, or contempt.

Because of its historical background, special rules have been developed regarding the showing of actual damages in a case of defamation. Almost any action based upon libel will be able to proceed regardless of whether actual monetary damages have been suffered by the plaintiff. Most courts have held that special harm or actual dollar loss must be shown in cases of slander unless the slander fits into one of four established exceptions.

As is true with the other tort situations, several defenses exist to actions for libel and slander. Truth is always a defense to actions based upon defamation of character. The burden is on the defendant in a defamation action to prove that the statement was true.

Certain individuals are said to be privileged to defame, or free from liability for slander or libel. An absolute privilege exists for defamatory remarks made during the course of judicial, legislative or executive proceedings. Many states have enacted statutes which provide immunity from civil lawsuits for pharmacists and other health-care professionals who file charges or present evidence against another member of their profession regarding alleged incompetency or gross misconduct. The immunity is often extended to claims filed with a board of pharmacy or with the regularly constituted review committee of a pharmaceutical society or hospital. In addition, most states will also provide immunity for those individuals, including pharmacists, who are required to report suspected cases of child abuse.

Privilege to defame may also exist in a variety of other situations. Comments made during the course of a business relationship are protected by a qualified privilege. A qualified privilege also exists as to defamatory remarks made about public officials or public figures. However, the defense of qualified or conditional privilege is forfeited if the publication is malicious in nature. Malice means that the defamation was published with improper motive or for an improper purpose.

Pharmacists may subject themselves to litigation for careless remarks made about their patients or other health-care professionals in the community. Oral statements which accuse another of improper conduct of a business or unprofessionalism are slanderous *per se*, and subject the maker to liability without the necessity of showing actual damages. A pharmacist's untrue accusations of unchastity or infidelity or imputation of certain loathsome diseases could also result in litigation based upon slander *per se*.

Right to Privacy—More and more states are recognizing a new tort for the invasion of another's privacy. The oral or written publication of private information about an individual, even if true, may give rise to an action based on invasion of privacy. Information contained in patient medication records or prescriptions is confidential in nature and should be released only on the consent of the patient or pursuant to other statutory authority. The admission of nonessential persons during medical treatment or taking medical photographs without the consent of the patient constitutes an invasion of privacy. The invasion must be objectionable and not too trifling. Truth is not a defense to this type of action nor is the absence of malice.

The right to privacy often conflicts with the state's exercise of its power to protect the public's health, safety and welfare. Certain individuals in the state of New York filed a lawsuit against that state for the inclusion of prescription information in a computerized data bank. The plaintiffs alleged that the inclusion of the names of patients who receive Schedule II prescription drugs in a centralized computer file violated their rights to privacy. The case was eventually decided by the US Supreme Court which held that the New York statute did not impair any privacy interest. The court found that the requirement was a reasonable exercise of the state's police powers:

> Disclosures of private medical information to physicians, hospital personnel, to insurance companies, and to public health agencies are often an essential part of modern practice even when the disclosures may reflect unfavorably on the character of the patient. Requiring such disclosures to representatives of the state having responsibility for the health of the community, does not automatically amount to an impermissible invasion of privacy. *Whalen v Roe*, 97 S Ct 869 (1977).

Liability based upon the tortious invasion of privacy should not be confused with the constitutional right of privacy which protects an individual from unconstitutional intrusions by government. The constitutional right of privacy is being increasingly used by courts as the basis for allowing medical decisions to be made not by health-care professionals but by the patients themselves. A number of recent cases have relied on this right of privacy doctrine to knock down regulations curbing the use of laetrile by cancer patients. A series of convictions of physicians who have used unapproved drugs or unconventional therapy in such cases have been overturned. These cases show the attempts by courts to balance the possible medical treatment against the right of privacy, but a key element in each of these cases has been the uncertainty of the success of any known therapy or alternative.

Business Premises Liability

The liability for injuries which occur on the real property of another will most often be imposed upon the individual in possession of the property. The determination of liability of owners and occupiers of land is primarily based on principles of negligence, but the law has created varying duties on the part of the occupier depending on the category of the injured party. Those who enter on another's property are classified as either trespassers, licensees or invitees, and the category into which the plaintiff falls will be a major determinant in developing a successful case.

Trespasser—A trespasser is an individual who comes onto the land of another without permission, even though the trespass may be innocent or by mistake. The possessor of real property is not liable for harm to trespassers caused by the occupier's failure to put the property in a safe condition. In most states the occupier is entitled to use reasonable force to remove a trespasser from the premises. A narrow exception to this rule exists in the case of trespassing children. The exception is termed the "attractive nuisance doctrine," and it imposes liability upon the occupier of land for injuries sustained by trespassing children when the occupier knew or should have known that children were likely to be attracted on the premises and be injured. The occupier of the land is not an absolute insurer in these cases, and a court must balance a number of factors in determining liability.

Licensees—A licensee is one who comes onto the land of another for his own purposes, but with the occupier's consent. The licensee enters another's property for other than business reasons. The possessor of the land is under no duty to maintain reasonably safe premises for the licensee, but does owe a duty to warn the individual of dangerous conditions.

Invitee—The highest duty of care goes to the business invitee, ie, the individual who enters the property of another for business reasons. The customer in a retail establishment would be the most common example of business invitee. Not only does the occupier owe a duty to maintain safe premises but also owes a duty to warn the business guest of dangerous conditions of which the occupier knows or should have known and has reason to believe the invitee will not discover. However, the occupier is not held absolutely responsible for every injury which occurs in the premises. If another customer or patient has created a dangerous condition which the occupier of the premises has had no reasonable opportunity to discover, there is no basis of liability. In addition, the format and location of merchandise displays should be carefully considered, as the owner of the premises may be bound to anticipate the actions of his customers.

A number of jurisdictions have rejected the common-law classification of trespassers, licensees and invitees. These jurisdictions have declared that they will no longer predicate the liability of a landowner on the status of the person entering the property, but will instead apply ordinary principles of negligence to govern the conduct of a landowner. This new approach holds that one's status is not the sole determinant of the duty of care, and that the landowner must act as a reasonable person in maintaining his property in a safe condition. Under this approach, other circumstances such as the probability of injuries to others and the burden on the parties to avoid the risk must also be considered.

Laws Governing the Practice of Pharmacy

State Laws

The regulation of the practice of pharmacy is primarily a function of the states and not of the federal government. It rests upon the power vested in the state to protect the health, safety, and welfare of its citizens.

Like every profession, the practice of pharmacy is a privilege bestowed by the state under the constitutional reservation of "police powers." However, this is a privilege available to a class of persons who satisfy stated minimal qualifications. No one may practice pharmacy without a license, except for those exempted by specification within the act. However, anyone may achieve such licensure by successfully completing the statutory pattern of qualification which the state has established and administered by an agency generally termed a board of pharmacy. In some instances the board of pharmacy is a subagency in that it exists as part of a larger state agency, such as a department of health or licensing.

Once licensure is gained it may not be taken lightly by either the state or the licentiate. The former may suspend, revoke, or terminate it after due process and for just cause as set out in the act. At the same time, the state undertakes to protect the public and the licensed members of the pharmacy profession from practice by unlicensed (hence, unqualified) parties in its jurisdiction.

As to the licensed pharmacist, he has gained a profession the practice of which is safeguarded by the federal and state constitutions as a property right. While he must abide by the act to preserve it, must pay fees required to accomplish initial and continuing registration, must satisfy the legal, moral, and ethical standards of his peers as set out in law and regulations, he does have the right to legal redress against any who would seek to unjustifiably deprive him of the benefits and prerogatives of licensure. Pharmacy practice acts must specifically identify the conduct for which sanctions can be imposed.

While pharmacy laws of the different states may vary among themselves, they are in agreement with respect to the fundamental principles, purposes, aims, and objectives of pharmaceutical practice.

Pharmacy laws generally provide for:

1. The educational and experience qualifications which pharmacists must meet at the time of examination or registration.
2. The agency, usually known as the State Board of Pharmacy, charged with enforcement and administration of the law.
3. The granting of permits for the conduct of a community pharmacy. In most states permits are issued for one year and application must be made for their renewal.
4. The minimum of professional and technical equipment and apparatus which the pharmacy must, at all times, possess.
5. Periodic re-registration of pharmacists. In most states, certificates of registration are granted for the period of one year.
6. The conditions under which certificates of registration or pharmacy licenses may be canceled or revoked.
7. The prominent display of the certificate of registration in the pharmacy in which the holder is employed.
8. Penalties for violations. Infractions of pharmacy laws are punishable by fines or the revocation or suspension of a license. Some state laws specify that violations of the pharmacy act are punishable as a misdemeanor.
9. Reciprocal registration. A pharmacist licensed by examination in one state may, by conforming to more or less nominal rules, become registered in another state, the latter registration being without full examination.
10. The discretion vested in boards of pharmacy. While the board is authorized to make rules and regulations for the enforcement and administration of the pharmacy law, such rules and regulations must be strictly in accord with the expressed or implied purposes of the law. The board is an administrative, not legislative, agency. It may not exercise any power or authority not clearly delegated to it.

Every state has a pharmacy practice act which regulates the profession, but there is significant variation in the detail of these acts from state to state. Many of the states' statutes are antiquated, with amendments being added in a haphazard manner. Many of these early acts regulated a profession which was primarily product-oriented and involved in the preparation of dosage forms.

Nuclear pharmacy, clinical pharmacy and drug product selection are just some of the more recent developments to have an impact upon the regulation of the profession. These developments, along with the need to provide more uniformity among the states, caused the National Association of Boards of Pharmacy to develop a Model State Pharmacy Act. This Act is intended to provide a greater degree of uniformity but still offer flexibility to the states which adopt it. The Model Act has been adopted by at least one state and other states are considering either the Act or variations of it.

The NABP's Model State Pharmacy Act will be reviewed here to afford the reader an example of the overall objectives and purposes of state pharmacy acts. Although the format will be similar to the laws of many states, the pharmacist must be versed in the statutory and regulatory requirements of his own state.

The quoted paragraphs set forth below are taken verbatim either from the Model State Pharmacy Act (MSPA) or from various state pharmacy acts. The source of the quoted paragraph is given in each instance.

Title

The title is an important part of all bills submitted to the legislature. The title must, in a very precise sense, give the purpose of the measure.

"An Act relating to the regulation of the practice of pharmacy, including the sales, use and distribution of drugs and devices at retail; and amending, revising, consolidating and repealing certain laws relating thereto." (*Pennsylvania Pharmacy Act*)

Many acts will also designate a "short title" which is a convenient device by which the legislation may be referred to in a brief, concise manner.

"This Act shall be known as the (name of state) Pharmacy Act." (*MSPA*)

Declaration of Policy and Purpose

While it is not necessary that a legislative act, such as the state pharmacy law, include a declaration of policy and purpose, such declaration often proves advantageous. It is of aid to the court when the constitutionality of the measure is questioned, and also throws much light upon the meaning of the various provisions of the law. Also, it serves to inform the members of the legislature having the measure under consideration the objectives sought by the passage of the law.

"The Practice of Pharmacy in the State of _____ is declared a professional practice affecting the public health, safety and welfare and is subject to regulation and control in the public interest. It is further declared to be a matter of public interest and concern that the Practice of Pharmacy, as defined in this Act, merit and receive the confidence of the public and that only qualified persons be permitted to engage in the Practice of Pharmacy in the State of _____. This Act shall be liberally construed to carry out these objects and purposes . . . .

"It is the purpose of this Act to promote, preserve and protect the public health, safety and welfare by and through the effective control and regulation of the Practice of Pharmacy and of the registration of Drug Outlets engaged in the manufacture, production, sale and distribution of drugs, medications, devices and such other materials as may be used in the diagnosis and treatment of injury, illness and disease." (MSPA)

Definitions

Basic definitions are essential to the clarity, administration and enforcement of any law. The comments to the NABP Model Act indicate that the writers of that act felt that the definition of the "practice of pharmacy" was one of the most important clauses. Although every state has found it necessary to define a "pharmacy," a number of states have not defined what activities fall within the scope of the practice of pharmacy.

Many state statutes have become dated in that they limit the practice of pharmacy to the preparation and distribution of a dosage form. The NABP Model Act includes very broad language to allow boards of pharmacy to promulgate rules and regulations with considerable flexibility as the profession changes to meet future needs.

"The 'Practice of Pharmacy' shall mean the interpretation and evaluation of prescription orders; the compounding, dispensing, labeling of drugs and devices (except labeling by a manufacturer, packer or distributor of Non-Prescription Drugs and commercially packaged legend drugs and devices); the participation in drug selection and drug utilization reviews; the proper and safe storage of drugs and devices and the maintenance of proper records therefore; the responsibility for advising, where necessary or where regulated, of therapeutic values, content, hazards and use of drugs and devices; and the offering or performing of those acts, services, operations or transactions necessary in the conduct, operation, management and control of pharmacy." (MSPA)

Although one might interpret some of the provisions of the above Model Act as authorizing drug product selection, the comments to the Act indicate that the language is to apply to the selection of drug therapy in a clinical setting and does not cover the question of drug substitution by a pharmacist. Each state should specifically cover this latter situation by another statutory provision.

Other selected definitions from the Model State Pharmacy Act of the NABP are:

" 'Deliver' or 'Delivery' means the actual, constructive or attempted transfer of a drug or device from one person to another, whether or not for a consideration.

" 'Device' means an instrument, apparatus, implement, machine, contrivance, implant, in vitro reagent or other similar or related article, including any component part or accessory, which is required under federal or state law to be prescribed by a Practitioner and dispensed by a Pharmacist.

" 'Dispense' or 'Dispensing' shall mean the preparation and delivery of a prescription drug pursuant to a lawful order of a Practitioner in a suitable container appropriately labeled for subsequent administration to or use by a patient or other individual entitled to receive the prescription drug.

" 'Drug' means: (i) Articles recognized as drugs in the official *United States Pharmacopeia*, official *National Formulary*, official *Homeopathic Pharmacopeia*, other drug compendium or any supplement to any of them; (ii) Articles intended for use in the diagnosis, cure, mitigation, treatment or prevention of disease in man or other animal; (iii) Articles (other than food) intended to affect the structure or any function of the body of man or other animals; and (iv) Articles intended for use as a component of any articles specified in clause (i), (ii) or (iii) of this subsection." (MSPA)

The definitions of a device or a drug are similar to those included in the Federal Food, Drug and Cosmetic Act, but their application will often be different under state law as the board of pharmacy is primarily interested in the dispensing aspects of such drugs or devices.

" 'Manufacture' shall mean the production, preparation, propagation, compounding, conversion, or processing of a Device or a Drug, either directly or indirectly by extraction from substances of natural origin or independently by means of chemical synthesis or by a combination of extraction and chemical synthesis and includes any packaging or repackaging of the substances or labeling or relabeling of its container, except that this term does not include the preparation or compounding of a drug by an individual for his own use or the preparation, compounding, packaging or labeling of a drug (i) by a pharmacist or practitioner as an incident to his administering or dispensing of a drug in the course of his professional practice or (ii) by a practitioner or by his authorization under his supervision for the purpose of or as an incident to research, teaching, or chemical analysis and not for sale." (MSPA)

It is often difficult to determine what constitutes manufacturing. Such a determination is often necessary for purposes of licensing, inspection and other board procedures. The Model Act has attempted to clarify the definition of manufacturer by excluding those acts by which a pharmacist prepares a preparation in the course of his professional practice.

" 'Person' shall mean an individual, corporation, partnership, association or any other legal entity." (MSPA)

This definition of a person is customary as it provides broad coverage without undue repetition and confusing language throughout the Act.

" 'Pharmacist' shall mean an individual licensed by this State to engage in the Practice of Pharmacy.

" 'Practitioner' shall mean a physician, dentist, veterinarian, scientific investigator or other person (other than pharmacists) licensed by this State and permitted by such license to dispense, conduct research with respect to or administer drugs in the course of professional practice or research in this state." (MSPA)

The various states may include other individuals within the definition of a practitioner, such as a podiatrist. Such practitioners may either be explicitly set forth in the statute or be covered by the language "or other person licensed by this state."

Each state pharmacy practice act as well as state controlled substances legislation must be carefully examined to determine the legality of pharmacists filling prescription orders written by prescribers in other states. The majority of the states do not prohibit the dispensing of prescription orders which originate out-of-state, but some states prohibit the dispensing of prescriptions from all out-of-state prescribers except those living in "border states." Pharmacists should carefully consult state statutes and with the board of pharmacy to determine the legal status of prescription orders originating in another state.

" 'Prescription Drug or Legend Drug' shall mean a drug which, under Federal Law is required, prior to being dispensed or delivered, to be labeled with either of the following statements: (1) 'Caution: Federal law prohibits dispensing without prescription' (2) 'Caution: Federal law restricts this drug to use by or on the order of a licensed veterinarian; or a drug which is required by any applicable Federal or State law or regulation to be dispensed on prescription only or is restricted to use by practitioners only.

" 'Non Prescription Drugs' shall mean non-narcotic medicines or drugs which may be sold without a prescription and which are prepackaged for use by the consumer and labeled in accordance with the requirements of the statutes and regulations of this State and the federal government." (MSPA)

Board of Pharmacy

"The responsibility for enforcement of the provisions of this Act is hereby vested in the Board of Pharmacy. The Board shall have all of the duties, powers and authority specifically granted by and necessary to the enforcement of this Act, as well as such other duties, powers and authority as it may be granted from time to time by appropriate statute.

"The Board of Pharmacy shall consist of (_____) members . . . (each) of whom shall be licensed pharmacists who possess the qualifications specified . . . ."   (*MSPA*)

The numerical strength of the board varies greatly, and the number of board members will be determined by each individual state according to its particular requirements. In most states, the total number of board members selected is an odd number. The Model Act offers an optional provision by which states may elect to include public member(s). Many state agencies which are responsible for the protection of the public's health, safety and welfare have included public members to assist in the regulatory process. The US Department of Justice and the Federal Trade Commission are investigating state regulatory agencies which are composed entirely of members of the profession to be regulated. The antitrust implications of such boards will undoubtedly continue to be explored.

"The licensed pharmacist members of the Board of Pharmacy shall at the time of their appointment: (1) Be residents of this State; (2) Be licensed and in good standing to engage in the Practice of Pharmacy in this State; (3) Be engaged in the Practice of Pharmacy in this State; (4) Have five (5) years of experience in the Practice of Pharmacy in this State after licensure."   (*MSPA*)

Because one of the duties of the board of pharmacy is to pass upon the fitness of applicants to engage in the practice of pharmacy, it is generally required that the board members shall have been actively engaged in pharmacy practice for a designated period of years. The NABP Model Act contains very broad language to allow a pharmacist involved in almost any area of practice eligible for appointment.

Appointment and Removal

"The Governor shall appoint the members of the Board of Pharmacy, subject to the advice and consent of the Senate, and in accordance with the other provisions of this Section."   (*MSPA*)

The state pharmacy acts customarily provide for the submittal of a list of nominees by the state pharmaceutical association to the governor from which he may select with the advice and consent of the state senate, the persons to constitute the board of pharmacy. In most states nominations may also be received from any other interested party.

Board of pharmacy members most often serve in staggered terms to provide continuity. Many state provisions prevent a member of the board from serving more than two consecutive full terms. The governor will have the authority to fill any vacancies which might arise and also to remove a member of the board pursuant to specified procedures.

"The Governor may remove a member of the Board, pursuant to the procedures set forth in subsection (b) hereinbelow, upon one or more of the following grounds. (1) The refusal or inability for any reason of a Board Member to perform his duties as a member of the Board in an efficient, responsible and professional manner; (2) The misuse of office by a member of the Board to obtain personal, pecuniary or material gain or advantage for himself or another through such office; (3) The violation by any member of this Act or any of the rules and regulations adopted hereunder."   (*MSPA*)

Executive Director

"The Board shall employ a licensed pharmacist who shall be an *ex officio* member of the Board without vote to serve as a full-time employee of the Board in the position of Executive Director. The Executive Director shall be responsible for the performance of the regular administrative functions of the Board and such other duties as the Board may direct. The Executive Director shall not perform any discretionary or decision-making functions for which the Board is solely responsible."   (*MSPA*)

As the board is a functioning agency, it must be organized so as to conform to parliamentary usage. Most states will require that the secretary or executive director of the board be a registered pharmacist, but in most instances he will not be a voting member of the board. It is also necessary that the executive officer of the board has his duties defined and his specific responsibilities fixed insofar as these can be done by the legislative act.

Meetings

"The Board of Pharmacy shall meet at least once every (_____) months to transact its business. One such meeting held during each fiscal year of the State shall be designated as the annual meeting and shall be for the purpose of electing officers and for the reorganization of the Board. The Board shall meet at such additional times as it may determine. Such additional meetings may be called by the President of the Board or by two-thirds (2/3) of the members of the Board . . . . Notice of all meetings of the Board shall be given in the manner and pursuant to requirements prescribed by the State's applicable statutes, rules and regulations . . . . All Board meetings and hearings shall be open to the public. The Board may, in its discretion and according to law, conduct any portion of its meeting in executive session closed to the public."   (*MSPA*)

As a general rule, meetings of a public agency must be open to all parties. The people of the states do not yield their sovereignty to an agency, and thus, the people have the right to be informed of public business. The open meetings statutes of most states do provide exceptions in which public agencies may meet in closed sessions such as those which involve the suspension or revocation of a license.

Rules and Regulations

"The Board of Pharmacy shall make, adopt, amend and repeal such rules and regulations as may be deemed necessary by the Board, from time to time, for the proper administration and enforcement of this Act. Such rules and regulations shall be promulgated in accordance with the procedures specified in the Administrative Procedures Act of this State."   (*MSPA*)

It is virtually impossible for the state legislature to clearly detail all the aspects of regulation of the practice of pharmacy. Therefore, administrative agencies are given the power to make rules and regulations which may modify or interpret the legislative mandate. In promulgating rules and regulations, it is vitally important that the board of pharmacy does not exceed its statutory authority. The power to make rules and regulations must not be used to accomplish that which the legislature has not specifically sanctioned. Most states will have adopted some sort of Administrative Procedure Act which will specify the appropriate constitutionally required procedures for rule-making, conduct of hearings, and other board functions. It is vital that the board rely upon the provisions of the Administrative Procedure Act so that it can insure that the public and any affected individuals are provided due process of law in the promulgation of rules and in the conduct of hearings.

Duties and Powers

The enabling legislation should also set forth the duties and powers of the board of pharmacy. Specifically, the state board of pharmacy has the power to do the following:

"The licensing by examination or by reciprocity of applicants who are qualified to engage in the Practice of Pharmacy under the provisions of this Act; The renewal of licenses to engage in the Practice of Pharmacy; The determination and issuance of standards for recognition and approval of schools and colleges of pharmacy whose graduates shall be eligible for licensure in this State, and the specification and enforcement of requirements for practical training, including internship; . . . The enforcement of those provisions of this Act relating to the conduct or competence of pharmacists practicing in this State, and the suspension, revocation or restriction of licenses to engage in the Practice of Pharmacy; The regulation of the training, qualifications and employment of pharmacy interns; . . . The regulation of the sale at retail and the dispensing of medications, drugs, devices and other materials including the right to seize any such drugs, devices and other materials found to be detrimental to the public health and welfare by the Board after appropriate hearing as required under the Administrative Procedures Act; The specifications of minimum professional and technical equipment, environment, supplies and procedures for the compounding and/or dispensing of such medications, drugs, devices and other materials within the Practice of Pharmacy; The control of the purity and quality of such medications, drugs, devices and other materials within the Practice of Pharmacy; The issuance and renewal of certificates of registration of Drug Outlets for purposes of ascertaining those persons engaged in the manufacture and distribution of drugs . . . . The Board or its authorized representatives shall also have power to investigate and gather evidence concerning alleged violations of the provisions of this Act or of the rules and regulations of the Board." (*MSPA*)

Licensing

Qualifications for Licensure

"To obtain a license to engage in the Practice of Pharmacy, an applicant for licensure by examination shall: (1) Have submitted a written application in the form prescribed by the Board of Pharmacy; (2) Have attained the age of majority; (3) Be of good moral character and temperate habits; . . . (4) Have graduated and received the first professional undergraduate degree from a school or college of pharmacy which has been approved by the Board of Pharmacy; . . . (5) Have completed an internship or other program which has been approved by the Board of Pharmacy, or demonstrated to the Board's satisfaction experience in the Practice of Pharmacy which meets or exceeds the minimum internship requirements of the Board; (6) Have successfully passed an examination given by the Board of Pharmacy; (7) Paid the fees specified by the Board of Pharmacy for examination and issuance of license." (*MSPA*)

Each state may exercise its police powers by determining the qualifications necessary for an individual to obtain a pharmacy license. It is likely that there will be a substantial degree of similarity among the various state laws regarding qualifications, but each act should be examined by the applicant.

Most states will require that the applicant be 21 years of age, but with the increasing trend to lower the age of majority it is likely that many states will simply require the applicant be 18. Those individuals who apply for a pharmacy license must be of good moral character. The case law in this area indicates a tremendous variation by the courts as to what constitutes "good moral character." Although it is expected that professional boards will continue to have the authority to inquire as to moral character of the applicant, the boards must be careful that their inquiry is reasonably related to the protection of the public's health and safety.

One could expect that an applicant for pharmacy licensure must be a graduate of an accredited college of pharmacy. Although the programs of United States pharmacy schools are accredited by the American Council on Pharmaceutical Education (ACPE), the board may not delegate the accrediting function to this private organization. The comments to the NABP Model Act indicate that it is contemplated that boards will accredit those schools with programs whose standards are at least equivalent to the minimum standards required by the ACPE, but it is important that the government agency make its own determinations regarding accreditation rather than direct reliance upon the private organization.

A requirement that the applicant be a citizen of the United States is unconstitutional under existing case law. Such a requirement would deprive non-citizens of the equal protection of the law under the US Constitution.

A variety of internship, externship, and clinical clerkship programs have developed in the various states. While the states generally require some sort of internship training, the programs and duration of experience vary among the states. Six-months or one-year experiences are common. There is an increasing emphasis by the ACPE for colleges of pharmacy to include a substantial portion of the required internship hours within the curriculum of the school.

An examination is also a necessary prerequisite prior to licensure. All but a few states administer the NABPLEX Standard Examination which was developed through the auspices of the National Association of Boards of Pharmacy. The NABPLEX exam consists of sections on chemistry, pharmacology, practice of pharmacy, pharmacy, and calculations. A national jurisprudence exam has also been introduced, but its use is optional.

Licensure by Reciprocity

As an alternative to licensure by examination, some applicants may also seek licensure by the reciprocal process. Such an applicant must:

"Have possessed at the time of initial licensure as a pharmacist such other qualifications necessary to have been eligible for licensure at that time in this State; Have engaged in the Practice of Pharmacy for a period of at least one (1) year or have met the internship requirements of this State within the one (1) year period immediately previous to the date of such application; Have presented to the Board proof of initial licensure by examination and proof that such license and any other license or licenses granted to the applicant by any other state or states have not been suspended, revoked, cancelled or otherwise restricted for any reason except non-renewal or the failure to obtain required continuing education credits in any state where the applicant is licensed but not engaged in the Practice of Pharmacy." (*MSPA*)

At the present time, not all states require one year of licensure in order to be eligible to be licensed by reciprocity. However, an applicant will not be eligible for licensure by reciprocity unless the state in which the applicant was initially licensed also grants reciprocal licensure to those from the state wherein the applicant seeks to be registered. At the present time, reciprocity is available from all boards of pharmacy except California, Florida and Hawaii.

The National Association of Boards of Pharmacy acts as a clearinghouse for the reciprocal process. The applicant provides information to the NABP which in turn verifies these facts relating to licensure and provides that information to the reciprocating state. The reciprocating state reviews the application, and it is highly likely that before it will issue a license it will require the applicant to pass an examination on state and local laws.

Renewal of License

In the majority of the states, certificates of licensure expire annually, but may be renewed upon the payment of a specific fee. An increasing number of states require proof that the pharmacist has satisfactorily completed an accredited program of continuing education prior to the issuance of the renewal certificate. It is beneficial if the legislature mandates a continuing education requirement by statute. The board of pharmacy may then adopt rules and regulations to carry out the objectives and purposes of the statute.

Discipline

As one would expect, the board of pharmacy is also endowed with the power to refuse or revoke the license of those individuals who have failed to exhibit fitness to practice the profession of pharmacy. In order to safeguard the public's health and safety, the board of pharmacy may find it necessary to permanently or temporarily discipline unfit practitioners. The board of pharmacy also has an important role to assist and educate wrong-doers to prevent recurrences of the errant behavior.

"Refusal to Issue or Renew. The Board of Pharmacy may refuse to issue or renew, or may suspend, revoke or restrict the licenses of any person, pursuant to the procedures set forth in Section 402 herein below, upon one or more of the following grounds: (1) Unprofessional conduct as that term is defined by the rules and regulations of the Board; (2) Incapacity of a nature that prevents a pharmacist from engaging in the Practice of Pharmacy with reasonable skill, competence and safety to the public; (3) Being found guilty by a court of competent jurisdiction of one (1) or more of the following: (i) A felony, as defined by the statutes of this State; (ii) Any act involving moral turpitude or gross immorality; or (iii) Violations of the pharmacy or drug laws of this State or rules and regulations of any other state, or of the federal government; (4) Fraud or intentional misrepresentation by a licensee in securing the issuance or renewal of a license; (5) Engaging or aiding and abetting an individual to engage in the Practice of Pharmacy without a license, or falsely using the title of pharmacist; (6) Being found by the Board to be in violation of any of the provisions of this Act or rules and regulations adopted pursuant to this Act." (*MSPA*)

Moral turpitude, unprofessional conduct, and gross immorality may be terms which defy definition. However, the board of pharmacy must make every attempt to set forth by rule and regulation that which is being legislated against. The pharmacist should be able to reasonably understand the type of conduct which is being discouraged. The board of pharmacy will have at its disposal, as per the legislative enactment, the authority to suspend, revoke or restrict the offender's license. In addition, the board may be able to impose a fine for each offense. The board may also place the offender on probation for a stated period of time. None of these board imposed penalties would bar a criminal prosecution on behalf of the state for the violations of the Pharmacy Practice Act if the violations were criminal in nature.

Registration of Facilities

In most states retail pharmacies, as well as institutional pharmacies, may be operated only under permits issued by the board of pharmacy. State law will normally require an annual fee, provisions for inspection of the premises, proper maintenance of prescription records, and the maintenance of certain minimums of equipment or stock. Nonprescription or proprietary medicines may usually be sold in any establishment, and the sale need not be made by licensed pharmacists. However, some states do require such a nonpharmacy outlet to obtain a permit from the state board of pharmacy in order to sell over-the-counter preparations.

Most state pharmacy statutes or regulations will provide for certain specified equipment for dispensing and compounding such as mortars and pestles, spatulas, weights, Class A balances, etc. In addition, certain minimal library references may also be specified. The statutes or regulations are also likely to set forth certain standards for the pharmacy area such as ventilation, lighting, and sanitary conditions.

Few states have ownership restrictions on pharmacies. Some states have attempted to legislate against physician-owned pharmacies or any other type of non-pharmacist-owned pharmacies. The United States Supreme Court in 1928 held that laws restricting pharmacy ownership only to pharmacists violated the Fourteenth Amendment of the United States Constitution. Forty-four years later, the same issue was again raised in the North Dakota courts. The North Dakota Pharmacy Act required that the majority of stock of a pharmacy corporation be owned by registered pharmacists in good standing in North Dakota. The statute was challenged by an out-of-state chain operation, and the case eventually was appealed to the US Supreme Court. The nation's highest court reversed its earlier decision and held that pharmacy-ownership laws were constitutionally sound if such a requirement could be reasonably related to the public's health and welfare. The case was returned to the North Dakota Supreme Court and that court identified seven possible reasons for ownership restrictions:

1. The professional and ethical standards of pharmacy demand the pharmacist's concern for the quantity and quality of stock and equipment. A drug which has deteriorated because of improper storage facilities can be a detriment to public health. A drug not in stock poses a threat to the individual who needs it now. Decisions made in conjunction with the quantity and quality of stock and equipment by non-registered-pharmacist-owners could be detrimental to the public health and welfare.
2. Supervision of hired pharmacists by registered-pharmacist-owners would be in the best interests of public health and safety.

3. Responsibility for improper action could be more readily pinpointed when supervision is in registered-pharmacist-owners.
4. The dignity of a profession and the morale and proficiency of those licensed to engage therein is enhanced by prohibiting the practitioner from subordinating himself to the direction of untrained supervisors.
5. If control and management is vested in laymen unacquainted with pharmaceutical service, who are untrained and unlicensed, the risk is that social accountability will be subordinated to the profit motive.
6. The term "pharmacy" was intended to identify a particular type of establishment within which a health profession is practiced, and thus was intended to be more than a mere means of making a profit. He who holds the purse strings controls the policy.
7. Doctor-owned pharmacies with built-in conflict-of-interest problems could be restricted.

Although this case cleared the way for state legislatures to develop restrictions on the ownership of pharmacies, there has not been a great deal of momentum in this area. Consumer groups and large national pharmacy operations have successfully lobbied against such proposals.

Miscellaneous State Provisions

Poisons

State law will also provide for restrictions on the sale of poisons. The statutes will likely set forth the labeling and packaging requirements for the sale of poisons such as the requirement that the word "POISON" and other label material be printed in red ink. The maintenance of a poison register in which all retail sales must be logged is also required. The register must include such entries as date, name and address of purchaser, name and quantity of poison, purpose, and the name of the dispenser. Sales of poisons are as a general rule prohibited to minors, intoxicated persons, or those known to be of unsound mind. The pharmacist must satisfy himself that the purchaser is aware of the poisonous nature of the substance and that the poison is to be used for a legitimate purpose (see also page 1916).

Prophylactics

It is also likely that the states will have regulated the sale of prophylactics. Special retail permits will often be required. There is a wide variance among the states as to the type of outlet licensed to sell prophylactics. As was previously discussed in the section on "Advertising," it is highly likely that statutes which restrict the sale to pharmacies will be found unconstitutional unless the state can support such a limitation. With an increase in the number of cases of venereal disease being reported, many states are expanding the categories of those who may hold a permit to sell prophylactics to pharmacies, hospitals, family-planning programs, venereal disease prevention and treatment programs, and to vending-machine operations. The First Amendment to the U.S. Constitution has been interpreted to permit the advertising and display of prophylactic devices.

Hypodermic Needles and Syringes

Some states permit the sale of hypodermic needles and syringes by the pharmacist on an over-the-counter basis. The pharmacist of course must use good professional discretion to insure that the devices are not to be used illegally. Other states will require that these devices be sold only upon a physician's order. This provision has been modified in some states to permit the sale of hypodermic needles and syringes without a prescription order when they are to be used by diabetics, for the administration of adrenalin, or for veterinary use. In these latter cases a registry is often required as evidence of the OTC sale.

The Federal Food, Drug and Cosmetic Act

The first attempt by the United States government to regulate the quality of drugs occurred during 1848. The government had discovered that adulterated quinine was being supplied for use by American troops in Mexico. In 1906, Congress enacted the first federal statute designed to regulate drug products manufactured domestically. The Food and Drug Act of 1906 required that drugs marketed in interstate commerce meet their professed minimal standards of strength, purity and quality. This law did not attempt to regulate therapeutic claims for medication. Labeling was first regulated by the Sherley Amendment to the Food and Drug Act, which Congress enacted during 1912. Here the term "misbranded" was first used in drug regulation to refer to fraudulent or false claims of therapeutic effects. A deficiency in this revision of the Act was that to establish a violation the enforcement agency was required to show deliberate fraud.

In 1938, further amendments were made as result of a firm's marketing a product using diethylene glycol as a vehicle for sulfanilamide. Approximately forty people were killed by the formulation, so Congress acted to require that a product be shown to be safe before it could be distributed in interstate commerce. However, there was a grandfather clause included in the revision which provided that anything that was on the market prior to enactment of the amendment could continue to be marketed, unless challenged by the Food and Drug Administration.

During the 1940s the FDA began to use internal regulations to establish categories of prescription and nonprescription drugs. The process did not work very well, so in 1951, Senator Hubert Humphrey, a pharmacist from Minnesota, and Congressman Carl Durham, a pharmacist from North Carolina, sponsored legislation to establish clear criteria for such decisions.

In 1962, the Act was again amended to require that drug products, both prescription and nonprescription, be shown to be effective as well as safe. Once again a grandfather clause was included, covering drugs marketed prior to 1938. However, every product marketed between 1938 and 1962 was now subject to the safety and efficacy requirements. At this time provisions were added to the Act concerning factory inspections and investigational drugs and responsibility for regulating drug advertising was shifted from the Federal Trade Commission to the Food and Drug Administration.

In 1976, the Medical Device Amendments were enacted, representing the first major change in this area since 1938. This amendment substantially increased the regulation of these products.

A complete discussion of the provisions of the federal Food Drug and Cosmetic Act and the regulations promulgated by FDA for enforcement of the statute would likely be longer than this entire chapter. Consequently, this discussion shall focus primarily upon those sections of the Act that are of primary importance to practitioners of pharmacy. Interested readers may wish to obtain an up-to-date copy of the Act and its effectuating regulations—21 CFR, parts 1-end. These may be obtained from the Government Printing Office, Washington, DC 20402.

A drug is defined in Section 201(g) of the Act to be an article recognized in the official compendia (*United States Pharmacopeia, National Formulary* or *Homeopathic Pharmacopeia of the United States*), or intended for use in the diagnosis, cure, mitigation, prevention or treatment of disease in man or other animals, or intended to alter a bodily function or structure of man or other animal. For purposes of determining the intended use of the drug, reference must be made to the intention of the person labeling the drugs, not the intentions of the purchaser. The same is true in the case of a device, which is an instrument, apparatus, implement or contrivance intended for the same use as a drug. An article may be classified as both a drug and a cosmetic under the Act. Moreover, the distinction between a drug and device under the Act may not be clearcut. For example, is a soft contact lens a drug or a device?

A cosmetic is an item intended to be rubbed, poured, sprinkled, or sprayed on, introduced into, or otherwise applied to the human body or any part thereof for cleansing, beautifying, promoting attractiveness, or altering the appearance. However, the Act specifically excludes soap from the definition of cosmetics. Note that a deodorant would be a cosmetic whereas an antiperspirant may be a drug because it is intended to alter a bodily function.

An important distinction is made in the Act between a label and labeling. A label is a display of written, printed, or graphic matter upon the immediate container of the item. Labeling includes the label as well as other written, printed or graphic matter upon the article or any of its containers or wrappers or accompanying the item. If information is required to appear on the label, it must also appear on the outside container or wrapper or be easily legible through the container or wrapper. In the case of labeling, it is not necessary that the printed matter directly accompany the item. Literature may be shipped separately and still constitute part of the labeling.

A "new drug" as defined in the Act is one which is not yet generally recognized by medical experts as being safe and effective for the intended use. This might be by virtue of its having a new drug entity as an ingredient, or by having an older chemical ingredient for which a new use, new dosage level, or new period of usage is proposed. Sometimes a combination of old drugs in a new dosage form with claims for use extending beyond those for each ingredient individually is considered a new drug. Such agents may not be shipped in interstate commerce unless the FDA has approved a New Drug Application (NDA) or Abbreviated New Drug Application (ANDA) for the drug.

However, this provision poses a problem for if the drug cannot be shipped in interstate commerce without being approved by FDA, how can the drug be tested for safety and efficacy? The Act contains an exemption from the interstate shipment ban for drugs undergoing clinical trials. In order to secure exemption from that provision of the Act, the individual or firm sponsoring the research must apply to the FDA for an exemption by filing an Investigational New Drug (IND) application. Once approved, the drug can be shipped in interstate commerce for testing purposes only. The detailed regulations adopted by FDA on this topic can be found at 21 CFR part 312.

Once the clinical trials have been completed the sponsor may submit an NDA to FDA. Section 505 of the Act specifies what information must be provided by the sponsor and the basis on which the agency may disapprove the application. At the time of approving the NDA, FDA determines whether the drug should be available to the public as a nonprescription medication or restricted to prescription-only status. Guidance for this decision can be found in the Durham-Humphrey Amendment of 1951. The applicability of this provision of the Act is restricted to drugs for human use, the standard for restriction of a drug to prescription-only status are:

1. the drug is habit-forming;
2. the drug is not safe for self medication because of its toxicity or other potentiality for harmful effect, or the method of its use or the collateral measures necessary to its use;
3. the drug is a "new drug" which has not been shown to be safe and is restricted to prescription-only distribution by FDA when it issues the NDA.

FDA has taken the position that drugs may also be restricted to prescription distribution if a layman would not know how to use them properly or because the conditions for which they are used and the diagnostic techniques and collateral therapeutic measures necessary to their use make it necessary. If a drug is to be restricted to prescription-only distribution, the Act requires that its label bear the statement, "Caution—Federal Law Prohibits Dispensing Without Prescription." This phrase is known as the prescription legend and, hence, prescription drugs are sometimes referred to as legend drugs.

Section 301 of the Act sets forth the acts which are prohibited. First, introduction or delivery for introduction into interstate commerce of any food, drug, device or cosmetic that is adulterated or misbranded is prohibited. Second, adulteration or misbranding of any food, drug, device or cosmetic in interstate commerce is violative of the Act. Third, receipt in interstate commerce of any food, drug, device or cosmetic that is adulterated or misbranded may also subject the individual to the penalties under the Act. In the landmark case of *United States v Sullivan*, the United States Supreme Court stated that under the Act, once something has been in interstate commerce it is considered to always be subject to the interstate jurisdiction of the FDA. Indeed, the Act specifically provides that an article in violation of the Act may be seized at any time while the drug is in interstate commerce or at any time thereafter.

One section of the Act that is of particular interest to pharmacy practitioners prohibits alteration, mutilation, destruction, obliteration or removal of the whole or any part of the labeling or the doing of any other act after shipment in interstate commerce which results in the article being adulterated or misbranded. Consequently, the pharmacist may not remove or destroy the label or labeling of a drug product, eg, the package insert.

Refusal to permit entry to an FDA inspector is also a violation of the Act.

The Act is designed to prevent two evils—adulteration and misbranding of products. Adulteration relates to the composition of the product. A drug is deemed to be adulterated if among other reasons:

1. it consists in whole or in part of any filthy, putrid, or decomposed substance;
2. it has been prepared, packed, or held under insanitary conditions whereby it may have become contaminated with filth or may have been rendered injurious to health;
3. it was manufactured, processed, packed, or held under conditions which do not comply with FDA's current good manufacturing practice (GMP) regulations;
4. its container is composed of any poisonous or deleterious substance which may render the drug injurious to health.

A drug will also be considered to be adulterated if it purports to meet compendial standards and does not, or if its strength differs from labeled strength.

Misbranding deals primarily with labeling violations, not the composition of the drug. A drug will be considered to be misbranded if among other reasons:

1. its labeling is false or misleading in any particular;
2. its label does not bear the name and address of the manufacturer, packer or distributor as well as an accurate statement of the quantity of the contents;
3. it contains a habit-forming substance specified in the Act or regulations and does not bear the statement "Warning—May Be Habit Forming" directly adjacent to the name of the agent;
4. it does not bear the established name of the agent and, in the case of legend drugs only, the quantity of ingredients;
5. its labeling bears adequate directions for use, unless exempted by FDA, and adequate warnings against use in situations where it may be dangerous to health;
6. it purports to be a drug which meets compendial standards and is not labeled in accordance with compendial standards;
7. its container is so made, formed or filled as to be misleading;
8. it is an antibiotic or insulin which has not been certified;
9. its advertising does not meet the standards contained in FDA regulations;
10. it was manufactured or processed in a plant which was not registered with FDA;
11. its packaging and labeling are not in conformity with the Poison Prevention Packaging Act of 1970.

Recently the packaging standards for drug products have been revised. Some drugs must be distributed in containers with "tight" closures and others with "well closed" caps.

An exemption exists under the Act for the generally applicable labeling requirements when a drug is dispensed pursuant to a prescription. The label of a drug dispensed pursuant to a prescription is required to bear:

1. name and address of the dispenser;
2. the serial number of the prescription and date of its dispensing;
3. the name of the prescriber;
4. the name of the patient, if stated in the prescription;
5. the directions for use and cautionary statements contained in the prescription.

This list in the Act is not intended to be all inclusive and the pharmacist may add other truthful information, eg, additional warnings or auxiliary labels bearing messages directed to the patient. It should be emphasized that the requirement that the container "bear" a label has been interpreted to mean that the label be affixed to the outside of the container, not inserted inside the container.

Also of note is the point that the labeling and packaging requirements of the Act apply to all who dispense medication, eg, pharmacists, physicans, or others.

As noted above, the Food and Drug Administration has responsibility for enforcement of the federal Food, Drug and Cosmetic Act. Drugs or other articles which violate the Act are subject to seizure by FDA and individuals who cause a violation are subject to criminal penalties. Conviction of the first offense under the Act holds the possibility of a fine of up to $1,000 and imprisonment for up to one year. Subsequent violations or violations involving an intent to defraud or mislead are punishable by a fine of up to $10,000 and incarceration for up to three years for each offense. Note that each act would constitute a separate violation.

Nonprescription Medication

As mentioned above, the Durham-Humphrey Amendment to the Food, Drug and Cosmetic Act embodies the criteria for determining whether a given drug is to be restricted to prescription distribution. If a drug does not fall within at least one of those three categories, it is available to the public without a prescription.

Drugs which may legally be sold without a prescription must bear a "7-point label." The elements which must be borne on the label, and the sections of the FDA regulations in which discussion of the requirements can be found, are:

1. the name of the product.
2. the name and address of the manufacturer, packer or distributor (21 CFR §201.1).
3. the net contents of the package (21 CFR §201.62).
4. the established name of all active ingredients, and the quantity of certain other ingredients whether active or not, eg, alcohol, potent alkaloids, etc (21 CFR §201.10).
5. the name of any habit-forming drug contained in the preparation (21 CFR §201.10).
6. cautions and warnings needed for protection of the user (21 CFR §201.300 et seq).
7. adequate directions for safe and effective use (21 CFR §201.5).

The most important distinction between nonprescription and prescription medication is based on the availability of "adequate directions for use" under which a layman can use the drug safely and for the purposes for which it is intended.

One issue related to labeling of nonprescription medication

is whether a pharmacist must relabel a product which has just been changed from legend to non-legend status. FDA has ruled that former legend drugs which may now lawfully be distributed without a prescription must be relabeled prior to dispensing. The reason for this is that if the drug is still in a package bearing the federal prescription legend but is lawfully sold without a prescription, the drug is misbranded. Moreover, the labeling requirements which apply to prescription drugs are not the same as those which apply to nonprescription products. Consequently, the former legend drug probably does not bear all the information required to be on the "7-point label." That, too, would render the drug misbranded. Hence, should a pharmacist wish to distribute a former legend drug without a prescription, relabeling must occur. The same requirement of relabeling is seen when the pharmacist purchases a large quantity of nonprescription medication and then repackages it in smaller quantities for distribution to the public. All seven points must be included on the label of the repackaged drug.

In 1972, the FDA initiated the Over-the-Counter Drug Review. Nonprescription drugs marketed before 1962 were not required to be shown to be both safe and effective. Rather than review the contents of each of the estimated 100,000 to 500,000 nonprescription products on the market, the agency decided to proceed in a rule-making fashion. FDA selected panels of experts who are reviewing nonprescription drug therapy of 27 categories of drug use, eg, antirheumatics, laxatives, antiemetics, etc. When the panel has completed its review, it prepares a monograph setting forth the drugs that have been found to be safe and effective for nonprescription use in that area of therapy. Following a period for public comment the monograph is finalized and any product in that therapeutic category which does not meet the standards established in the monograph will be subject to FDA sanctions. The Federal Trade Commission is attempting to carry this activity one step further by considering a trade regulation rule which would prohibit manufacturers or distributors of non-prescription drugs from using any terminology other than that specifically approved in the FDA monograph in its advertising to the public. The OTC Review concluded during the 1980s and it may be several years before the action by the FTC in this area is finalized.

During recent years a number of pharmacy organizations have proposed that a third and fourth class of drug products be established in addition to the currently existing classes of legend and non-legend drugs. The third class of drugs would be those which would be available only from a pharmacist and the fourth class of drugs would include those for which a prescription from a licensed prescriber would be required for initiation of therapy but which could be refilled at the professional discretion of the pharmacist.

One additional question which frequently arises is the legal status of refilling a prescription written for a nonprescription medication when no refills have been authorized by the prescriber. The answer turns on the definition of a "prescription" under state law. If it is described as an order for drugs authorized by a licensed practitioner and the statute further states that the pharmacist must have the prescriber's authorization to dispense a prescription, then refilling the prescription probably would not be lawful. Note that this is so even though the patient could merely pick up the same drug from a counter display. On the other hand, if the state statute is phrased differently, then it may be lawful for a pharmacist to refill the prescription because under the federal scheme of regulation the drug may be distributed without a prescription.

The Comprehensive Drug Abuse Prevention and Control Act of 1970

The federal Comprehensive Drug Abuse Prevention and Control Act (Public Law 91-513) became effective on May 1, 1971. Title II of that Act is known as the "Controlled Substances Act" (CSA) and it regulates the manufacture, distribution and dispensing of controlled substances. This law supersedes most previous narcotic and drug-abuse control laws, and places the enforcement of this Act with the Drug Enforcement Administration (DEA), which is part of the US Department of Justice. The DEA has promulgated extensive regulations to implement the Act, and these regulations appear in Title 21 of the Code of Federal Regulations, Part 1300 to the end.

The statute provides a "closed" system for virtually every person who legitimately handles controlled substances other than the ultimate user. Over 500,000 individuals and institutions, such as hospitals, pharmacies, researchers, drug manufacturers, physicians, and others are included in the class of persons subject to direct regulation through registration by the Drug Enforcement Administration. In addition to replacing or amending the numerous federal laws relating to the control of drugs, the Controlled Substances Act is intended to aid in reducing the widespread diversion of these substances from legitimate channels.

When enacting the Controlled Substances Act Congress no longer relied upon the tax clause of the US Constitution as had been done in the past. The authority for Congress to enact this legislation was derived from the interstate commerce clause of the Constitution. The power to regulate the health, safety and welfare of the American people has been left primarily within the jurisdiction of the individual states through the "police powers" which were reserved to the states via the Tenth Amendment of the US Constitution. However, Congress determined that the federal control of intrastate incidents of the traffic in controlled substances is essential to the effective control of the interstate incidents of such traffic, and it thereby felt compelled to enter into the regulation of subject matter which had previously been left to the states. It must be remembered that if a provision of state or local law is inconsistent or conflicts with a provision of the federal Controlled Substances Act, then the state or local law must yield to the federal provision. However, if the state or local law augments or strengthens the federal act, then the more stringent provision must be followed. In order to provide uniformity with the federal government, the majority of the states have adopted a Uniform Controlled Substances Act.

Important Definitions

The following selected definitions are derived from the Controlled Substances Act or from the DEA regulations. These definitions must be read carefully for their language will greatly affect the use of the words within the Act. The following definitions are those which bear most heavily upon pharmacy practice:

The term *administer* refers to the direct application of a controlled substance to the body of a patient or research subject.

The term *dispenser* means an individual practitioner, an institutional practitioner, pharmacy or pharmacist who dispenses a controlled substance.

The term *individual practitioner* means a physician, dentist, veterinarian, or other individual licensed, registered, or otherwise permitted, by the United States or the jurisdiction in which he practices, to dispense a controlled substance in the course of professional practice, but does not include a pharmacist, a pharmacy, or an institutional practitioner.

The term *institutional practitioner* means a hospital or other person (other than an individual) licensed, registered, or otherwise permitted, by the United States or the jurisdiction in which it practices, to dispense a controlled substance in the course of professional practice, but does not include a pharmacy.

The term *narcotic drug* means any of the following, whether produced directly or indirectly by extraction from substances of vegetable origin, or independently by means of chemical synthesis: (a) opium, coca leaves, and opiates; (b) a compound, manufacture, salt, derivative, or preparation of opium, coca leaves, or opiates; (c) a substance which is chemically identical with any of the substances referred to in a or b.

The term *person* includes any individual, corporation, government or governmental subdivision or agency, business trust, partnership, association, or other legal entity.

The term *pharmacist* means any pharmacist licensed by a State to dispense controlled substances, and shall include any other person (eg, pharmacist-intern) authorized by a State to dispense controlled substances under the supervision of a pharmacist licensed by such State.

The term *prescription* means an order for medication which is dispensed to or for an ultimate user but does not include an order for medication which is dispensed for immediate administration to the ultimate user (eg, an order to dispense a drug to a bed patient for immediate administration in a hospital is not a prescription).

The term *readily retrievable* means that certain records are kept by automatic data processing systems or other electronic or mechanized recording systems in such a manner that they can be separated out from all other records in a reasonable time and/or records are kept on which certain items are asterisked, redlined, or in some other manner visually identifiable apart from other items appearing on the records.

Schedules

The drugs that come under the jurisdiction of the Controlled Substances Act have been categorized according to their potential for abuse and are divided into five schedules. Procedures for controlling a substance under the CSA are set forth in Section 201 of the Act. Proceedings may be initiated by the Department of Health and Human Services, by the DEA, or by petition of a manufacturer, medical society, pharmaceutical association, public interest group, or an individual citizen.

Once the DEA receives a request to control a drug or remove a substance entirely from the schedules, the agency must request the Department of Health and Human Services to conduct a scientific and medical evaluation. The Secretary of Health and Human Services then consults with the Food and Drug Administration and the other affected agencies regarding recommendations whether the drug or other substance should be controlled or removed from control. The medical and scientific evaluations are binding on the DEA with respect to scientific and medical matters, and if HHS recommends that a drug not be controlled, the DEA may not control the substance.

After the DEA receives the HHS report, it will then proceed to make a final decision. If it has determined to control the drug, a proposal will be published in the *Federal Register* setting forth the proposed schedule and inviting all interested parties to file comments. At this point the affected parties may request a hearing before an administrative law judge. If no hearing is requested, the DEA will evaluate all the comments received and publish a final order in the *Federal Register*.

In reaching a final decision, the Drug Enforcement Administration is required by the statute to consider a number of factors with respect to each drug proposed to be controlled or removed from the schedules. These factors include such things as potential for abuse, pharmacological effects, risk to public health, the history, scope, duration, and significance of the abuse, and the potential for psychic or physiological dependence.

The drugs that come under the jurisdiction of the Controlled Substances Act are divided into five schedules based upon their potential for abuse. Those schedules are as follows:

Schedule I

The drugs in Schedule I have a high potential for abuse and no accepted medical use in the United States. The three broad categories of substances found in this schedule are the opiates, opium derivatives, and hallucinogens. Some examples are heroin, marihuana, LSD, peyote, mescaline, psilocybin, tetrahydrocannabinols, dihydromorphine, and others.

Properly registered persons may use Schedule I substances for research purposes. Some states and the FDA have begun to authorize the use of marihuana or its active ingredient, tetrahydrocannabinol (THC), for treatment of glaucoma and the alleviation of the nausea and vomiting associated with cancer chemotherapy.

Schedule II

Drugs included in this schedule also have a high potential for abuse, but do have a currently accepted medical use in treatment in the United States. It has been determined that the abuse of a drug or other substances included in this schedule may lead to severe psychological or physical dependence. The broad categories of Schedule II drugs include opiates and opium derivatives, derivatives of coca leaves, and certain central nervous system stimulants and depressants. Some examples of Schedule II controlled narcotic substances are: opium, morphine, codeine, hydromorphone (Dilaudid), methadone (Dolophine), pantopon, meperidine (Demerol), cocaine, oxycodone (Percodan), anileridine (Leritine), and oxymorphone (Numorphan). Also in Schedule II are amphetamine (Benzedrine, Dexedrine) and methamphetamine (Desoxyn), phenmetrazine (Preludin), methylphenidate (Ritalin), amobarbital, pentobarbital, secobarbital, methaqualone, etorphine hydrochloride, diphenoxylate, and phencyclidine.

The quantity of the substance in a drug often determines under which schedule it will be controlled. For example, amphetamines and codeine generally are included in Schedule II. However, certain products containing smaller quantities, most often in combination with a noncontrolled substance, are controlled in Schedules III and V.

Schedule III

The drugs in this Schedule have accepted medical use in the United States, but they have a lower potential for abuse than Schedule I and II drugs. Schedule III includes compounds containing limited quantities of certain narcotic drugs, and non-narcotic drugs such as: derivatives of barbituric acid except those that are listed in another schedule, glutethimide (Doriden), methyprylon (Noludar), chlorhexadol, sulfondiethylmethane, sulfonmethane, nalorphine, benzphetamine, chlorphentermine, clortermine, mazindol, phendimetrazine, and paregoric.

Schedule IV

The drugs included in this schedule have a low potential for abuse relative to those in Schedule III. Abuse of Schedule IV drugs or substances may lead to limited physical dependence or psychological dependence as compared to those included in Schedule III. Schedule IV drugs are generally the long-acting barbiturates, certain hypnotics, and the minor tranquilizers. For all practical purposes there are no regulatory differences between Schedule III and IV. Some of the more common drugs found in Schedule IV are: barbital, phenobarbital, methylphenobarbital, chloral betaine (Beta Chlor), chloral hydrate, ethchlorvynol (Placidyl), ethinamate (Valmid), meprobamate (Equanil, Miltown), paraldehyde, methohexital, fenfluramine, diethylpropion, phentermine, chlordiazepoxide (Librium), diazepam (Valium), oxazepam (Serax), clorazepate (Tranxene), flurazepam (Dalmane), clonazepam (Clonopin), prazepam (Verstran), lorazepam (Ativan), mebutamate, and dextropropoxyphene (Darvon).

Schedule V

Drugs in this schedule have the lowest abuse potential of the controlled substances and consist of preparations containing limited quantities of certain narcotic drugs generally for antitussive and antidiarrheal purposes. As a general rule Schedule V items are over-the-counter preparations that might be sold without a prescription. There are notable exceptions, and the pharmacist should always check the label to see if the Food and Drug Administration has determined the item to be an Ŗ-only item. For example, Lomotil is a Schedule V item, but it is prescription only. Paregoric is now restricted to prescription sales and included in Schedule III.

Manufacturers of nonnarcotic substances that may be sold over-the-counter under the terms of the federal Food, Drug, and Cosmetic Act may apply to the DEA to have their product excluded from any schedule. Phenobarbital is the most common substance found in those products which are excluded from the scheduling process. One of the prime factors considered in determining whether to exclude a product would be the amount of the controlled substance involved. Once a product is excluded under Section 201 (g)(1) of the CSA it is no longer subject to DEA control. Examples of excluded nonnarcotic over-the-counter products are Amodrine, Bronkotabs, Primatene P, Tedral, and Verequad. However, the pharmacist should always consult with state and local law to determine if these products have been given more restrictive controls under state law.

Schedule V Retail Distribution Restrictions

Controlled substances listed in Schedule V which are not legend drugs, may be dispensed without a prescription by a pharmacist to a purchaser at retail, provided that the following conditions are met:

a. Such dispensing is made only by a pharmacist (which by definition also includes a pharmacist intern). However, after the pharmacist has fulfilled his professional and legal responsibilities, the actual cash, credit transaction, or delivery, may be completed by a nonpharmacist.
b. Not more than 240 mL (8 oz) or 48 solid dosage units of any substance containing opium, nor more than 120 mL (4 oz) or 24 solid dosage units of any other controlled substance may be dispensed at retail to the same purchaser in any given 48 hour period without a prescription.
c. The purchaser at retail is at least 18 years of age.
d. The pharmacist requires every purchaser at retail of a controlled substance not known to him to furnish suitable identification (including proof of age where appropriate).
e. A bound record book is maintained which contains the name and address of the purchaser, name and quantity of controlled substance purchased, date of each sale and initials of the selling pharmacist. This record book shall be maintained for a period of two years from the date of the last transaction entered in the record book, and it must be made available for inspection and copying by officers of the United States, authorized by the Attorney General.
f. Other federal, state or local law does not require a prescription.

The pharmacist must be cautioned that in some states certain or all Schedule V substances have been placed on prescription-only status. In these states the more restrictive state law would apply and prohibit the over-the-counter sale of Schedule V items.

Symbols and Labeling

Each commercial container of controlled substances will have on its label a symbol designating to which schedule it belongs. The symbol for Schedule I through V controlled substances will be as follows: Ⓒ I or C-I; Ⓒ II or C-II; Ⓒ III or C-III; Ⓒ IV or C-IV; and Ⓒ V or C-V. The symbols will be at least twice as large as the largest letter printed on the label. Controlled substances symbols will be located in the upper right corner of the principal panel of the label of the commercial container.

There are exceptions to the preceding commercial labeling requirements. In those cases where the commercial container is too small to accommodate the label, only the box and the package insert must contain the "C" symbol.

As a general rule, these symbols are not required on prescription containers dispensed by a pharmacist to a patient in the course of his professional practice, although laws of some states may require such symbols on prescriptions dispensed to extended care facilities.

Registration

Every person who manufacturers, distributes or dispenses any controlled substance or who proposes to engage in the manufacture, distribution or dispensing of any controlled substance shall obtain annually a registration unless exempted. A unique DEA number is assigned to those who must register under the law including manufacturers, distributors, wholesalers, and practitioners such as physicians, dentists, veterinarians, scientists, pharmacies, podiatrists, and hospitals. There are, however, seven general categories of persons who are exempt from registration under the statute

or the regulations. Some of those exempted from registration are civil defense officials, law enforcement officials, certain government employees, practitioners affiliated with registered institutions, and agents or employees of registrants. It is this latter exemption which permits individual pharmacists to not register with the Drug Enforcement Administration since such pharmacists serve as agents of the registered pharmacies.

Every pharmacy engaged in distributing or dispensing any controlled substance must register with the DEA. The registration must be renewed annually and a certificate of registration must be maintained at the registered location and kept available for official inspections. The fee for each registration or re-registration is $5. If an individual owns and operates more than one pharmacy, he must register each place of business separately.

Applications for re-registration will be mailed by the DEA to each registered person approximately 60 days before the expiration date of the registration. If a registered pharmacy does not receive such forms within 45 days before the expiration date of the registration, it must give notice of such fact and request the re-registration forms by writing to the Registration Section of the Drug Enforcement Administration, PO Box 28083, Central Station, Washington, DC 20005.

New Registrations

Pharmacies that seek to become registered for the first time must request a registration application from the Drug Enforcement Administration, PO Box 28083, Central Station, Washington, DC 20005, or from any DEA Regional Office. No pharmacy may engage in any activity for which registration is required until its application for registration has been granted and a certificate has been beeen issued to it by the DEA. However, a pharmacy may not dispense controlled substances if it has not been issued a valid state license even though the DEA may have already registered the pharmacy and authorized it to obtain controlled substances.

Modifications such as change of address, location or name by existing registrants may be made without going through the new registration process. To make such a modification, the registrant should submit a letter to the DEA requesting the modification. No fee is required to be paid for the modification. A registrant may also apply to modify his registration to authorize the handling of additional schedules of controlled substances, but may not modify his registration to transfer it to another party.

Termination of Registration

The DEA has the authority under the Controlled Substances Act to suspend or revoke a registration where the registrant has falsified his application, or has been convicted of a felony under the federal or state Controlled Substances Act, or has had his state license or registration suspended and is no longer authorized by state law to dispense controlled substances. Except in emergency situations, registrants are assured of a hearing and due process of law prior to suspension or revocation of registration. In addition, the registration of any person terminates if and when such a person dies, ceases legal existence, or discontinues business or professional practice.

Distribution by a Pharmacy

As a general rule a separate DEA registration is required for each activity a registrant wishes to engage in such as manufacturing, distributing, dispensing, conducting research, etc. However, a pharmacy registered to dispense a controlled substance may distribute (without being registered as a distributor) a quantity of controlled substances to a physician or to another pharmacy, hospital, or nursing home for the purpose of general dispensing by that practitioner provided that the following conditions are met:

   a. The pharmacy or practitioner to which the controlled substance is being distributed is registered under the Act to dispense that controlled substance.

   b. The distribution is recorded as being distributed by the pharmacy and the pharmacy or practitioner records the substance being received. The pharmacy distributing a controlled substance must record the name of the substance, the dosage form, the quantity and the name, address and DEA registration number of the pharmacy or practitioner to whom it is distributed as well as the date of distribution.

   c. If the substance is listed in Schedule I or II, the transfer must be made on an official order form.

   d. The total number of dosage units of controlled substances distributed by a pharmacy may not exceed five percent of all controlled substances dispensed by the pharmacy during the 12-month period in which the pharmacy is registered. If at any time it does exceed five percent the pharmacy is required to register as a distributor as well as being registered as a pharmacy.

As an incident to the distribution as stated above, a pharmacist may manufacture (without being registered to manufacture) an aqueous or oleaginous solution or solid dosage form containing a narcotic controlled substance in a proportion not exceeding 20% of the complete solution, compound or mixture.

The regulations also permit a person lawfully in possession of controlled substances to return them to the supplier without registering as a distributor. Registrants would have to use official order forms for the return of Schedule I and II substances to a supplier.

Records and Reports

Every pharmacy engaged in the handling of controlled substances must keep complete and accurate records of all receiving and dispensing transactions. All such records shall be maintained for a period of two years. Many states require that the records be kept for as long as five years.

All inventories and records of controlled substances in Schedule II must be maintained separately from all other records of the registrant. All inventories and records of controlled substances in Schedules III, IV, and V must be maintained separately or must be in such form that they are readily retrievable from the ordinary professional and business records of the pharmacy.

All records pertaining to controlled substances shall be made available for inspection and copying by duly authorized officials of the Drug Enforcement Administration.

When a registrant first engages in business, and every two years thereafter, he must make a complete and accurate inventory of all stocks of controlled substances on hand. This inventory record shall be kept by the registrant for a period of two years. Pharmacies are not required to submit a copy of the inventory to the Drug Enforcement Administration.

Continuing Records Kept by a Pharmacist

Every pharmacy must maintain on a current basis a complete and accurate record of each controlled substance received. Copy 3 of executed order forms retained by the pharmacy which have been completed as described under the section entitled "Order Forms" will constitute a pharmacy's receiving records for Schedule II controlled substances. Invoices for Schedule III, IV, and V controlled substances will be considered as complete receiving records if the actual date of receipt is clearly recorded on the invoices by the pharmacist or other responsible individual. He may add other details on such invoices as would help reconcile his figures.

Filing Prescriptions

Prescription orders for controlled substances must be filed in one of the following three ways:

   a. A pharmacy can maintain three separate files—a file for Schedule II drugs dispensed, a file for Schedules III, IV, and V drugs dispensed, and a file for prescription orders for all other drugs dispensed.

   b. A pharmacy can maintain two files—a file for all Schedule II drugs dispensed and another file for all other drugs dispensed including those in Schedules III, IV, and V. If this method is used, the prescription orders in the file for Schedules III, IV, and V must be stamped with the letter "C" in red ink, not less than one inch high, in the lower right corner. This distinctive marking makes the records "readily retrievable" for inspection.

   c. A pharmacy can maintain two files—one file for all controlled drugs in all schedules and a second file for all prescription orders for non-controlled drugs dispensed. If this method is used, the prescription orders for drugs in Schedules III, IV, and V in the controlled drug prescription file must be stamped with the red letter "C" not less than one inch high in the lower right corner, as previously mentioned.

In states where the Uniform Narcotic Act (or other state law) requires all narcotic prescription records be kept together, DEA is of the opinion that a positive conflict exists between federal and state law and, under Section 708 of the Controlled Substances Act, federal requirements prevail.

Inventory Requirements

The Controlled Substances Act (Public Law 91-513) requires each registrant to make a complete and accurate record of all stocks of controlled substances on hand every two years. The biennial inventory date of May 1, may be changed by the registrant to fit his regular general physical inventory date, if any, so long as the date is not more than six months from the biennial date that would otherwise apply. The actual taking of the inventory should not vary more than four days from the biennial inventory date. The inventory record must:

   a. List the name, address, and DEA registration number of the registrant.

   b. Indicate the date and the time the inventory is taken, ie, opening or close of business.

   c. Be signed by the person or persons responsible for taking the inventory.

   d. Be maintained at the location appearing on the registration certificate for at least two years.

   e. Keep records of Schedule II drugs separate from all other controlled substances.

When taking the inventory of Schedule II controlled substances, an exact count or measure must be made. When taking the inventory of Schedules III, IV, and V controlled substances, an estimated count may be made unless the container holds more than 1,000 dosage units, in which case an exact count must be made if the container has been opened.

Newly controlled substances—occasionally a drug that has not been previously controlled will be placed in one of the drug schedules or a controlled substance will be moved into a higher or lower schedule. In either of the cases, the drug must be inventoried as of the effective date of transfer, and this inventory should be added to the biennial inventory.

Order Forms

The order form system developed by the DEA is a completely closed system of drug distribution. The DEA permits only authorized persons to obtain or distribute Schedule I or II controlled substances and only pursuant to official order forms. The regulations set forth those instances where official order forms are not required to transfer Schedule I or II controlled substances, ie, transfer to a patient pursuant to a written prescription, administration to a patient by a registered practitioner, procurement by civil defense officials, delivery by a common carrier to a warehouse, etc.

A pharmacy desiring DEA forms may requisition the appropriate order forms from the DEA. Such order forms are serially numbered, and issued with the name, address and registration number of the pharmacy, the authorized activity and authorized schedules with respect to that pharmacy. Each triplicate order form is contained in a book of seven forms. Up to six books may be ordered at one time unless the pharmacy can show that it needs to exceed this limit. There is no charge for the order forms.

The pharmacist must prepare and execute the order form in triplicate through the use of a typewriter, pen or indelible pencil. One must enter on the form the name and address of the supplier from whom the controlled substances are being ordered. Only one supplier may be listed on any one form. There are ten lines on the "item" section of each order form. The regulations require that each of the ten lines contain a different drug or "item." The number of lines completed must be totaled at the bottom of the form. This is the total number of lines or items and not the total number of commercial containers ordered. The order form must be completed properly and have no material alterations or erasures. In these latter instances a distributor will be obligated to refuse the form and may elect to do so in other cases as well if the order form is not completed correctly.

The purchaser must sign his name and date the order form on the day he places the order. If his name is different from the authorized registrant, ie, if he has been given a power of attorney to complete order forms, he must also include the name of the authorized registrant in the signature space. When the form is completed, the purchaser separates the three copies of the triplicate form in the following manner: Copy 1 and Copy 2 must be kept intact with the carbon in between them. These copies are sent in with the registrant's order to his supplier. Copy 3 is retained by the purchaser separately from other records. When the registrant receives the items ordered he must record, on this retained Copy 3, the number of packages and the date such packages were received. A space is provided for this on the DEA order form.

Power of Attorney

Any registered pharmacy may authorize one or more individuals, whether or not located at the registered location of the pharmacy, to obtain and execute order forms on its behalf by executing a power of attorney for each such individual. The power of attorney must be signed by the same person who signed the most recent application for registration or re-registration and must contain the signature of the individual being authorized to obtain and execute order forms. The power of attorney is not submitted to the DEA but must be retained by the pharmacy with the executed order forms. The power of attorney must be available for inspection together with the order form records. A power of attorney may be revoked at any time by filing a notice of revocation, signed by the individual who signed the most recent application for registration or re-registration, and by filing with the DEA the revocation of the power of attorney.

Lost or Stolen Order Forms

When unfilled order forms are lost, the pharmacy must execute a new form in triplicate. The pharmacy must also execute a statement containing the serial number and date of the lost form, stating that the drugs in the lost form were never received, and attach a copy of that statement to Copy 3 of the lost form. A copy of that statement should also be attached to Copies 1 and 2 of the newly executed order form.

Whenever any used or unused order forms are stolen or lost, the pharmacy must immediately, upon discovery of such theft or loss, report this to the Drug Enforcement Administration, Compliance Division, Investigations Section, 1405 I Street, NW, Washington, DC 20537, stating the serial numbers of each form lost or stolen. If an entire book or books of order forms are lost or stolen, and the pharmacist is unable to state

the serial numbers, he shall report, in lieu of the serial numbers, the date or approximate date of issuance. Lost or stolen order forms should also be reported to the State Board of Pharmacy or other state controlled substance agency.

Prescriptions

Who May Issue

In order to issue a prescription an individual practitioner must be both (1) authorized to prescribe controlled substances by the jurisdiction in which he is licensed to practice his profession and (2) either registered or exempted from registration by the Drug Enforcement Administration.

Purpose of Issue

A prescription for a controlled substance to be effective must be issued for a legitimate medical purpose by a practitioner acting in the usual course of his professional practice. The responsibility for the proper prescribing and dispensing of controlled substances is upon the prescribing practitioner, but a corresponding liability rests with the pharmacist who dispenses the prescription. An order purporting to be a prescription issued not in the usual course of professional treatment or in legitimate and authorized research is not a prescription within the meaning and intent of Section 309 of the Controlled Substances Act, and the person knowingly dispensing such a purported prescription, as well as the person issuing it, will be subject to the penalties provided for violations of the provisions of law relating to controlled substances.

A prescription by which a practitioner attempts to resupply his office stock or to maintain drug dependent individuals is not a valid prescription and is therefore void.

Execution of Prescriptions by Practitioner

All prescriptions for controlled substances shall be dated as of, and signed on, the day when issued and shall bear the full name and address of the patient and the name, address and registration number of the practitioner. A practitioner may sign a prescription in the same manner as he would sign a check or legal document; for instance, JH Smith or John H Smith. Where an oral order is not permitted, prescriptions must be written with ink or indelible pencil or typewriter and must be manually signed by the practitioner. The prescription may be prepared by a secretary or agent for the signature of a practitioner, but the prescribing practitioner is responsible in case the prescription does not conform in all essential respects to the law and regulations.

Prescription orders that are written for controlled substances in Schedule II must be typewritten or written in ink or indelible pencil and must be signed by the practitioner issuing such prescription orders. In emergency situations, defined and set forth in the section below, Schedule II drugs may be dispensed upon an oral authorization. Prescription orders for controlled substances in Schedules III, IV, or V may be issued either orally or in writing by a practitioner or his authorized agent.

Emergency Dispensing—Schedule II

In the case of a bona fide emergency situation, as defined by the Secretary of Health and Human Services a pharmacist may dispense a Schedule II controlled substance upon receiving oral authorization of a prescribing practitioner provided that:

a. The quantity prescribed and dispensed is limited to the amount adequate to treat the patient during the emergency period. Prescribing or dispensing beyond the emergency period must be pursuant to a written prescription order.

b. The prescription order shall be immediately reduced to writing by the pharmacist and shall contain all information, except for the prescribing practitioner's signature.

c. If the prescribing practitioner is not known to the pharmacist, he must make a reasonable effort to determine that the oral authorization came from a practitioner, by verifying his telephone number against that listed in the directory and other good faith efforts to insure his identity.

d. Within 72 hours after authorizing an emergency oral prescription order, the prescribing practitioner must cause a written prescription order for the emergency quantity prescribed to be delivered to the dispensing pharmacist. The prescription order shall have written on its face "Authorization for Emergency Dispensing." The written prescription order may be delivered in person or by mail, but if delivered by mail it must be postmarked within the 72 hour period. Upon receipt, the dispensing pharmacist shall attach this prescription order to the oral emergency prescription order which had earlier been reduced to writing. The pharmacist shall notify the nearest office of DEA if the prescribing practitioner fails to deliver a written prescription order to him; failure of the pharmacist to do so shall void the authority conferred by the subsection to dispense without a written prescription order of a prescribing practitioner.

Definition of Emergency

For the purpose of authorizing an oral prescription order of a controlled substance listed in Schedule II of the Controlled Substances Act, the term "emergency situation" means those situations in which the prescribing practitioner determines that:

a. Immediate administration of the controlled substance is necessary for the proper treatment of the intended ultimate user.

b. No appropriate alternative treatment is available, including administration of a drug which is not a controlled substance under Schedule II of the Act.

c. It is not reasonably possible for the prescribing practitioner to provide a written prescription order to be presented to the person dispensing the substance, prior to the dispensing.

Refills and Renewals

No prescription for a controlled substance in Schedule II may be refilled, and such prescriptions must be kept in a separate file.

Prescriptions for controlled substances in Schedule III or IV may be issued either orally or in writing by a practitioner and may be refilled if so authorized. The prescriptions may not be filled or refilled more than six months after the date issued or be refilled more than five times after the date issued. After five refills or after six months, the practitioner may renew the prescription. A renewal of any such prescription shall be recorded on a new prescription blank and a new prescription number assigned to the prescription. Oral prescriptions must be committed to writing and filed by the pharmacist.

A prescription for a controlled substance listed in Schedule V may be refilled only as authorized by the prescribing practitioner on the prescription. If no such authorization is given, the prescription may not be refilled. However, if the item may be legally sold over-the-counter, the burden of determining the propriety of the sale will be upon the pharmacist.

Recording Refills

A pharmacist after refilling a prescription for any controlled substance in Schedules III, IV, or V must enter on the back of that prescription his initials, the date the prescription was refilled, and the amount of drug dispensed on such refill. If the pharmacist merely initials and dates the back of the prescription, he shall be deemed to have dispensed a refill for the full face amount of the prescription.

Computerization of Refill Information

A pharmacy is permitted to use a data processing system as an alternative method for the storage and retrieval of prescription order refill information for controlled substances in Schedules III and IV.

The computerized system must provide immediate retrieval (via CRT display or hard-copy printout) of original prescription order information for those prescription orders which are currently authorized for refilling. The information which must be readily retrievable from this type of system must include, but is not limited to, data such as the original prescription number, date of issuance of the prescription order by the practitioner, full name and address of the patient, the practitioner's name and DEA registration number, the name, strength, dosage form, quantity of the controlled substance prescribed, the quantity dispensed if different from the quantity prescribed, and the total number of refills authorized by the prescribing practitioner.

In addition, the system must provide immediate retrieval of the current refill history for Schedule III or IV controlled substance prescription orders that have been authorized for refills during the past six months and backup documentation to show that the refill information is correct. The backup documentation must be stored in a separate file at the pharmacy and be maintained for a two year period from the dispensing date.

Transmittal of Oral Authorization for Renewal

A practitioner's nurse or other member of his staff cannot authorize the renewal of a prescription for a controlled substance that has been refilled five times or is six months old. The authority for prescribing controlled substances is vested only with the practitioner, and he cannot delegate this function to anyone else. However, nurses or staff members receiving calls from pharmacies regarding renewals may act as the practitioner's agent and transmit the practitioner's order.

Practitioners' Office Stock

A pharmacist may not dispense a controlled substance on the order of a prescription which is issued by a practitioner and is intended for office use or bag use of the practitioner. Distribution must be made on invoice and/or order form, if required.

Prescription Label Requirements

The pharmacist filling a prescription for controlled substances listed in Schedules II, III, IV, or V must affix to the package a label showing the pharmacy name and address, the serial number and date of initial filling, the name of the patient, the name of the practitioner issuing the prescription, directions for use, and cautionary statements, if any.

The label of any drug listed as a controlled substance in Schedules II, III, or IV of the Controlled Substances Act shall, when dispensed to a patient, contain the following warning:

CAUTION: Federal law prohibits the transfer of this drug to any person other than the patient for whom it was prescribed.

Partial Filling-Schedule II

The partial filling of a Schedule II controlled substance prescription is permissible, if the pharmacist is unable to supply the full quantity called for in a written or emergency oral prescription. He may supply a portion of the quantity called for provided he makes a notation of the quantity supplied on the face of the written prescription (or written record of the emergency oral prescription). The remaining portion may be filled within 72 hours of the first dispensing, however, if the remaining portion is not, or cannot be filled within the 72-hour period, the pharmacist must notify the prescribing practitioner. No further quantity may be supplied beyond the 72 hours except on a new prescription.

CHAPTER 108

Pharmaceutical Economics and Management

James W Richards, MBA

Professor of Pharmacy Administration
College of Pharmacy, University of Michigan
Ann Arbor, MI 48109

The economic impact of the health care industry on our society is difficult to evaluate. It is accepted that advances made by the industry during the past few decades have reduced morbidity and mortality rates which, in turn, have increased productivity and added to the gross national product.

At the same time, the cost of health care is rising at a faster rate than is the consumer price index for all items, and this cost continues to represent an increasingly larger share of the gross national product.

Economics of Health Care

Total US expenditures for health services, facilities, products, administration, and research were estimated to be $286.6 billion in fiscal year 1981. The total expenditures represented about 9.8% of the gross national product, at a per capita cost of $1225.[1]

Health expenditures rose between 1971 and 1981 from a per capita cost of $358 to the $1225 figure. Total expenditures are influenced by a variety of factors, including the following:

Population increases and aging of the population
Inflation (general and medical)
Increased utilization of facilities and services
Increased governmental involvement in health care
Increased quality of care from new techniques, equipment, and drugs

Further analysis of national health expenditures reveals a continuing upward trend in the portion of total health expenditures paid with public funds. In 1981, governmental outlays represented almost 43% of all health care expenditures. Medicare payments accounted for a major portion of governmental health care expenditures. However, state Medicaid programs and other social welfare programs also contributed to the $122.5 billion public expenditure for health care.[2]

The magnitude of health care expenditures in the US and the growing governmental involvement as a third-party payer of health care costs are evidence of our society's commitment to providing the best care possible for all citizens. Those involved in the delivery of health care share society's commitment and, therefore, must be concerned with the economics of the delivery system.

The pharmaceutical segment of the health care industry entails a significant expenditure. In 1981 $21 billion was spent at the retail level for drugs and drug sundries in the US. The 1981 expenditure for drugs and pharmaceutical services represented 7.5% of the nation's health bill.[3]

In view of the level of expenditures for drugs and pharmaceutical services and given the trend of health care costs, it is apparent that those involved in the delivery of pharmaceutical services must be aware of their responsibility to provide high-quality services in the most economical way. Although some experts look on third-party payment as a mechanism for solving the high cost of health care, including the drug-cost segment, it should be understood that third-party payment

does not reduce the cost. It simply spreads it over a larger population.

Actually, third-party payment may increase the total cost of health care as additional administrative costs and increased utilization of services are inherent in third-party payment programs. It follows that third-party payers, whether governmental or private, have an obligation to their constituents to ensure the delivery of quality services at reasonable prices. In this regard, health professionals will find their services under scrutiny by a sophisticated group of agencies representing a large portion of the general public.

In the past the economics of health care was given little attention by the providers of health services. It was assumed that the primary obligation of the provider was to ensure the physical well being of the patient, without regard to cost. It is now apparent that it does little good to develop a level of health care which is unsurpassed in the world if a sizable segment of the population cannot afford to pay for it.

The obligation of health professionals to consider the economic dimensions of health care is now recognized. For example, pharmacy practice laws in most states have been amended to allow pharmacists to practice drug product selection. These amendments allow the pharmacist, under specified conditions, to choose drug products with due regard for both the physical and the economic well-being of the patient. The drug product selection amendments are tangible evidence of societal concern with the cost of health care.

The concern of health professionals with the cost of health care now reinforces the efforts of consumer groups, government, and others involved in financing health care, to the end of providing the best care for all, regardless of economic status.

According to the Health Insurance Council, comprehensive health service planning and delivery should be based upon the following guidelines.[4]

Health services cost money, and good health service costs a good deal of money. Agencies which spend money on behalf of others have a responsibility to get their money's worth for their beneficiaries.

Financing methods for health service should encourage efficient organization and management of the professional personnel and institutions.

Financing methods should distribute the burden of medical care costs in the way which best assures proper care of the entire population.

Health personnel and institutions must be reimbursed in amounts and by methods which permit them to maintain standards and achieve efficiency.

Although the guidelines of the Health Insurance Council are intended for the total health care system, they may be applied to any segment of the system. The guidelines include concepts which are applicable to pharmacy practice. The guidelines suggest that health insurers promote efficient organization and management of personnel and facilities. It follows that pharmacists should promote efficient organization and management. With the utilization of carefully developed organizational plans and modern management techniques, pharmacists in community practice can contribute to the efforts being made to contain health care costs.

The Community Pharmacy

The majority of consumer expenditures for prescription drugs, proprietary medicines, and health appliances are channeled through the approximately 50,000 community pharmacies in the US. Although heterogeneous in some respects, as in type of ownership and type of goods and services offered, community pharmacies are generally recognized by the public as the most accessible source of drugs and of information about drugs.

Community pharmacy, as used here, is defined broadly to include all of those establishments that are privately owned and whose function, in varying degrees, is to serve society's need for drug products and for pharmaceutical services. It is difficult to characterize or describe the typical pharmacy because of the great variance among pharmacies. They range from the corporately-owned chain pharmacy, resembling a small department store, to the independently owned pharmaceutical center, providing prescription service along with a relatively few lines of health-related products.

According to the operating data submitted to the *Lilly Digest* by over 1700 community pharmacy owners, the average independent community pharmacy generated sales of $439,133 in 1981.[5] The data reported represent a summary of individual pharmacy operating figures which were supplied voluntarily by pharmacy managers and owners.

It should be noted that the editors of the *Lilly Digest* make no attempt to structure the sample that comprises the data input and, therefore, citations therefrom are subject to the statistical limitations inherent in the collection of unstructured voluntary data. It appears, however, that the figures reported serve to describe fairly accurately the economics of the independent community pharmacy.

The data from the *Lilly Digest* indicate that approximately 55% of the revenues of the independent pharmacy are derived from prescription medication. Over a recent 20-year period the average annual number of prescription medication orders dispensed from the typical independent community pharmacy has increased by about 75%. During the same period the average prescription charge has risen from $3.32 in 1962 to $8.80 in 1981.[6]

It should be noted that the average prescription charge is not an accurate measure of the price changes for prescription drugs. Over a period of years the mix of drugs dispensed changes as do the prescribing habits of physicians for quantities of drugs ordered. Therefore, the average prescription charge in 1981 was for a different kind of medication and for a different quantity than was the average charge in 1962.

Trends in the data related to prescription activity in *Lilly Digest* pharmacies are given in Table I. Increased per capita utilization of prescription drugs and availability of more efficacious drugs with higher costs have contributed to the growing importance of prescription medication revenues in the economics of community pharmacy practice.

Chain Pharmacies

The foregoing discussion has dealt mainly with the independent community pharmacies which represent about 70% of the total number of pharmacies in the US. Chain pharmacies are also an important factor in the delivery of pharmaceutical services and products to the public.

A universal definition for a chain pharmacy is not available, as there appears to be a question as to what criteria are ap-

Table I—Prescription Trends in *Lilly Digest* Pharmacies: 1962–1981 (Averages per Pharmacy)[6]

Year	Prescription Sales	Percentage of Prescription Sales to Total Sales	Number of Prescriptions	Percent Renewals	Prescription Charge	Prescription Inventory	Prescription Sales per Dollar of Prescription Inventory
1962	$ 52,578	36.0%	15,817	52.1%	$3.32	$ 8,620	$6.10
1963	58,688	38.3%	17,320	52.0%	3.39	9,270	6.33
1964	63,157	39.0%	18,532	53.7%	3.41	9,495	6.65
1965	68,587	40.9%	19,708	53.7%	3.48	9,928	6.91
1966	71,586	41.0%	19,962	53.6%	3.59	10,235	6.99
1967	78,789	41.8%	21,544	54.5%	3.66	10,881	7.24
1968	85,953	43.2%	22,848	54.8%	3.76	11,478	7.49
1969	93,299	43.7%	23,951	54.5%	3.90	12,220	7.63
1970	98,445	44.5%	24,243	54.8%	4.06	12,592	7.82
1971	105,875	44.7%	25,122	54.9%	4.21	13,268	7.98
1972	112,777	46.6%	25,743	54.1%	4.38	13,969	8.07
1973	122,615	47.3%	27,019	54.5%	4.54	14,827	8.27
1974	130,384	47.9%	27,089	53.7%	4.81	15,925	8.19
1975	142,915	48.6%	27,572	53.0%	5.18	17,342	8.24
1976	153,735	49.6%	27,163	52.7%	5.66	18,554	8.29
1977	162,631	50.4%	26,649	51.5%	6.10	19,471	8.35
1978	176,705	51.2%	26,913	51.6%	6.57	21,133	8.36
1979	195,159	49.8%	27,187	50.3%	7.18	22,941	8.51
1980	212,949	51.2%	27,126	50.4%	7.85	24,639	8.64
1981	239,561	54.6%	27,225	51.4%	8.80	26,854	8.92

propriate for classifying a group of centrally owned pharmacies as chain pharmacies. To some, the matter of central ownership is itself sufficient to classify the individual units as chain pharmacies. Another approach is to classify individual units which are centrally owned as chain pharmacies only when there is also centralized organization and management.

The number of centrally owned units has also been used as a method of defining chain pharmacies. However, this criterion does not provide a satisfactory answer to the question; many multiple units are centrally owned and yet each unit functions independently from the central ownership. In mode of operation these pharmacies are more similar to individually owned community pharmacies. On the other hand, as the number of units under a central ownership increases, at some point there must be some coordination of policies and activities which results in more central management.

Although it is not possible to establish an exact number of units as the point where all units assume the characteristics of a true chain pharmacy operation, it appears that there is some relationship between the number of units owned and the definition of a pharmacy chain. The US Department of Commerce defines a pharmacy chain as those units with prescription departments which are centrally owned by individuals or organizations who own four or more units.

Although chain pharmacies represent about 30% of the community pharmacies in the US, they generated approximately 56% of the total sales volume reported for all community pharmacies in 1982.[7] Over the past decade, chain pharmacies have demonstrated a much larger growth rate in sales volume than independently owned community pharmacies.

The typical chain pharmacy operates from a broader base in the variety of goods offered for sale than does the independent pharmacy. The kinds of goods offered for sale in chain pharmacies are almost limitless, and include innumerable durable consumer goods in addition to health-related products.

In this regard it may be somewhat misleading to compare sales in the chain pharmacy with sales in the independent community pharmacy. However, when trends over the past few years are studied, it is apparent that the chain pharmacies are also improving their relative position in such areas as income from prescription medications and from nonprescription drugs.

Establishment of a Community Pharmacy

The pharmacist considering the establishment of a new pharmacy should subject the basic decision to an objective analysis. The analysis should include a consideration of community needs—does the community really need another facility for pharmaceutical services?

The question may have both a quantitative and a qualitative dimension. Perhaps a given community has a sufficient number of pharmacies and yet none of them is providing the full scope of modern services. If a community need is identified, the analysis should continue in terms of evaluating the various alternatives that are available for satisfying the need. Perhaps an existing pharmacy could be purchased and made to provide more extensive pharmaceutical services. There may be an opportunity to join with another pharmacist in the ownership of an existing pharmacy and to establish a group practice.

Such alternatives provide the opportunity for improving services to the community while promoting the most efficient use of professional personnel and facilities.

If the analysis indicates that a new pharmacy should be established, the pharmacist must then consider a number of questions, some of them simultaneously; eg, What is the appropriate legal organization for the enterprise? What specific location should be chosen? How may the necessary capital be obtained? Although each of the foregoing questions is related to the others and cannot be isolated in a practical situation, for purposes of this discussion each will be treated by itself.

Organization

The pharmacist may choose from three widely recognized forms of legal organization for the community pharmacy enterprise. Traditionally, the majority of pharmacies have been organized as individual or sole proprietorships, with relatively little governmental control applied to the organizational structure.

In recent years, because of the increase in the joint ownership of pharmacies by two or more individuals, the partnership and corporate forms of organization have become more significant. The partnership as a form of business organization enjoys relative independence from governmental control. The corporation, as a creation of the state government, is subject to rather strict governmental regulation. Each form of organization presents advantages that must be weighed against the advantages, disadvantages, and limitations that become apparent when comparison is made with the alternative forms of organization.

The business enterprise owned and managed by an unincorporated sole proprietor is not considered in law to be a separate legal entity; rather, the owner and the enterprise are considered as one. It follows, then, that the risk inherent in establishing a business enterprise in this way has implications for the nonbusiness assets of the proprietor.

The unincorporated sole proprietor has unlimited personal liability. Personal assets are available to satisfy business obligations and business assets may be used to satisfy personal debts. In return for assuming unlimited liability, the sole proprietor enjoys the freedom to conduct the enterprise in any lawful manner he or she deems appropriate.

Further, except for required licenses, the sole proprietor may begin or quit operations without legal formality or governmental permission. Some states do require that a statement of ownership be filed with a designated office when the owner's name is not indicated in the name of the enterprise. The sole proprietor receives all profits from the enterprise and as a general rule income taxes are at a minimum level for this form of business organization.

Size or scope of operation is not necessarily a determining factor in the decision to organize as a sole proprietorship as opposed to one of the other forms of organization. However, due to the risks involved and to the fact that few persons possess all of the abilities and capacities necessary for carrying on a large complex enterprise, the sole proprietorship is most often associated with smaller, less complex, operations.

Historically, the majority of community pharmacists are independent by nature, and have chosen this rather informal form of organization. Further, the typical community pharmacy being geographically local and only moderately complex in scope of operation generally succeeds under the unincorporated sole-ownership system.

When the resources of one individual are not sufficient to provide a proper base for establishing a pharmacy or when the individual does not wish to assume the entire risk associated with the entrepreneurial function, joint ownership may be considered. Partnership arrangements and incorporation are mechanisms that may be utilized to broaden the financial or talent base for an enterprise and may also serve to spread the risk involved. The partnership may be described as an association of two or more individuals based on an expressed or implied contract. They combine their resources as co-owners of an enterprise for their mutual profit. This provides a way for the individuals to do jointly what they could not do separately.

As to liability, a partnership may be described as an association of sole proprietors, because at law the partnership is not considered separate from those who compose it. As with the sole proprietorship, each partner is liable for all debts of the partnership, even to the extent of personal assets. Within the scope of partnership activities, each general partner is considered an agent of the other general partners and as such each has the right to bind or commit the partnership in business affairs. Because of the mutual agency concept and the unlimited liability inherent in partnership associations, it is especially important that the full implications of such an arrangement be understood before adopting this form of organization.

Although it is a contractual arrangement, there are relatively few legal restrictions or regulations applied to the partnership association. No expressed governmental consent is required to establish or to dissolve a partnership, and the contract may be written or simply based on a handshake, as long as the elements of a valid contract are present. This is not to imply that the partnership should be consummated on the basis of an informal verbal agreement. The contractual relationship between partners should be attested by a written document, drafted with the assistance of a lawyer.

The close personal relationship among partners tends to foster a disregard for formalized written documents relating to the operation of the partnership. In the interest of producing a smoothly functioning organization and to help prevent disagreements among the partners, it is most important that a written partnership agreement be prepared at the outset.

Such matters as the investment of each partner, duties, responsibilities, and division of profits and losses should be considered and incorporated into the partnership agreement. The agreement not only provides a reference for solving future misunderstanding but also serves to compel the partners, at the inception of the agreement, to consider matters that might otherwise remain hidden until a specific problem arises.

The partnership as a form of business organization provides a mechanism for joint ownership of an enterprise which is relatively free of governmental regulation and which embodies the same flexibility of operation enjoyed by the sole proprietorship. As the partnership is not considered a legal entity, it is not required to pay income taxes on profits; rather, the individual partners are assigned their share of profits and pay income taxes on them as individuals.

When compared to the corporate form of joint ownership, the partnership usually presents an advantage to the co-owners with regard to income tax liability. The partnership has been a popular form of organization for the co-ownership of community pharmacies.

Co-ownership may also be effected through a more formal type of organization known as the corporation. The corporation is a separate legal entity, created by the expressed authority of the state. A properly constituted corporation offers the stockholders the advantage of limited liability.

In contrast to the sole proprietorship and the partnership, the incorporated business enterprise is considered as separate from the persons who own it. Consequently, in the absence of a statute to the contrary, corporate stockholders are liable only to the extent of their contributions to the capital of the enterprise. As a general rule, creditors of the corporation cannot proceed against the individual stockholders for debts of the corporation.

As a legal entity created by the state, the corporation enjoys continuity of life subject only to limitation included in its charter. The death or incapacity of a stockholder or the transfer of ownership in no way affects the corporate existence.

The corporation provides a way for individuals to invest in a business venture without placing their personal assets in jeopardy. It also provides a convenient, highly organized mechanism for accumulating a large amount of capital from several individuals in order to establish a business enterprise.

In terms of initial organization, the formation of a corporation is more complex and formal than other types of ownership. Each state has a required procedure to be followed in the creation of a corporation, and once franchised, the corporation is subject to regulation and control by the state.

By definition, the corporation has only those powers and can do only those things that are authorized by the state, in contrast to the partnership, which may do any lawful thing agreed to by the partners. The corporation may be dissolved only by or with the expressed consent of the state.

Further, the status of the corporate enterprise as a legal person makes it subject to local, state, and federal income taxes upon its earnings. When the earnings after corporate income taxes are distributed to the stockholders as dividends, the individual stockholders are required to pay personal income taxes upon them. As a result, owners of corporations are said to be subject to double taxation, a factor which in many cases has deterred sole proprietorships and partnerships from adopting the corporate form of organization.

In the field of community pharmacy, the majority of chain pharmacy organizations are corporations. The corporate form provides the protection of limited liability, which is especially important for larger multiunit operations. In addition, a fair number of the larger nonchain pharmacies are also incorporated, although it should be noted that neither size nor scope of operation is necessarily the only determinant in the decision to incorporate.

In establishing a new pharmacy, the prospective owner or owners must decide at the outset which form of organization to follow. The factors of liability, flexibility of operations, governmental regulation, continuity of life, and income taxes should be considered in relationship to the scope of the operation and the personal circumstances of the organizers. It is especially important to seek legal counsel in arriving at a decision.

Site Selection

Much has been written on the criteria that should be employed in choosing a specific community as the site for a new pharmacy. Such factors as population in the trading area, distribution of income among the population, type of industry, and the competitive climate have been cited as being important in site selection.

Sometimes a pharmacy is established in a community because the pharmacist-owner is determined to own a pharmacy in a specific community because of personal factors such as family ties, climate, or other appeals of the community. In such cases, the decision is often made without regard to the key issue of whether or not the community needs another facility for pharmaceutical services. As stated previously, the selection of a community as a site for a new pharmacy should turn on an objective analysis of community need.

If a need is identified in a given town or city, the selection of a specific site within the community will require careful consideration. The degree of success of a community pharmacy may depend on the choice of the location most suitable among those available. In some cases, the choice of a specific site is extremely limited; the pharmacist must choose from what is available rather than that which is most desirable.

The majority of consumers choose the pharmacy they will patronize on the basis of convenience and accessibility, as long as the pharmacy offers adequate service and fair prices.

Therefore, the primary emphasis in site selection should be on obtaining a location that is central to the population to be served. Further, the modern pharmacy must provide easy access and adequate parking for a motorized society. The growth of shopping centers may be cited as evidence of the importance of these factors.

As a general rule, shopping centers are located centrally in relation to the neighborhood, community, or region they serve and they provide easy access and adequate free parking. Interestingly, the growth in prescription volume is greater among neighborhood and community shopping centers than in the larger regional centers. This tends to substantiate the impression that consumers wish to obtain professional pharmacy services near home.

Although a site in a neighborhood or community shopping center may be considered to be a choice location for a new pharmacy, as a practical matter few independent community pharmacists are able to obtain such locations. Because of the nature of the system used to finance new shopping centers, preference is given by the developers of the centers to large well-established chain pharmacies.

However, it appears that there are other suitable locations for a traditional pharmacy that emphasizes professional services rather than the sale of nonhealth-related merchandise.

The island type of location, where the pharmacy sits by itself on a main traffic artery into a suburb and surrounded by adequate parking facilities, has proven to be attractive to consumers. A location within a large medical clinic may also prove to be valuable, although, because of the tendency of patients to obtain prescription service near home, the clinic location may not be so significant as some believe it to be. The selection of a site solely because it is readily or inexpensively available should be avoided. Usually a bargain location in terms of rent proves in the long run to be a liability rather than an asset.

The selection of the proper site for a new pharmacy is especially important because it is a decision that the phar-

macist may have to live with for 5, 10, or more years, depending on the terms of the lease if the pharmacy is operated in a rented facility. Whenever possible, advice should be obtained from others regarding site selection. Some wholesale drug firms provide counsel in this regard, or a business consulting firm may be engaged to assist in making an objective evaluation of alternatives.

Capital Requirements

Planning and assembling the capital requirements for a new pharmacy are predicated on careful evaluation of projected sales volume, breadth and depth of inventory requirements, and estimated operating expenses. The amount of capital required for the operation of a successful pharmacy is a function of the productivity of the pharmacy.

Although certain of the assets required represent a fixed core necessary for any pharmacy, regardless of sales volume, beyond these the amount of assets required depends, in large measure, upon the scope of operation and the volume anticipated. As illustrated in Table II, as sales volume increases, investment in inventory, fixtures and other assets also increases.

Other factors also have an impact on capital requirements. For example, the policy of the pharmacy owner toward offering credit may require more or less working capital. The mix of sales volume may also affect capital requirements. As a general rule, prescription revenues can be generated with a lower inventory investment than can revenues from other sources.

The problem of determining capital requirements for a new pharmacy is difficult. Most of the underlying factors are based on conjecture and forecasts regarding the future, for which there is no reliable basis at the outset. However, some judgment must be made as to what assets are required for a specific venture so that the pharmacist may explore the feasibility of assembling a definite amount of capital.

When making the forecasts and estimates needed to es-

Table II—Balance Sheets for *Lilly Digest* Pharmacies under 5 Years Old: 1981 (Averages per Pharmacy)[8]

	Sales under $200,000 (118 Pharmacies)	Sales $200,000 to $400,000 (199 Pharmacies)	Sales $400,000 to $600,000 (53 Pharmacies)
ASSETS			
Current assets			
Cash	$ 5,856— 11.5%	$ 8,507— 10.2%	$ 14,459— 10.9%
Accounts receivable	4,694— 9.2%	8,997— 10.8%	18,029— 13.6%
Inventory	28,656— 56.3%	47,304— 56.8%	71,653— 53.8%
Total current assets	$ 39,206— 77.0%	$ 64,808— 77.8%	$104,141— 78.3%
Fixed assets			
Fixtures and equipment and leasehold improvements (net after reserve for depreciation)	9,946— 19.5%	15,052— 18.1%	21,240— 16.0%
Other assets			
Prepaid expenses, deposits, etc.	1,773— 3.5%	3,428— 4.1%	7,622— 5.7%
Total assets[a]	$ 50,925—100.0%	$ 83,288—100.0%	$133,003—100.0%
LIABILITIES			
Current and accrued liabilities			
Accounts payable	$ 6,229— 12.2%	$ 12,901— 15.5%	$ 22,485— 16.9%
Notes payable (within one year)	3,079— 6.0%	6,624— 8.0%	8,494— 6.4%
Accrued expenses and other liabilities	1,673— 3.3%	3,584— 4.3%	5,896— 4.4%
Total current and accrued liabilities	$ 10,981— 21.5%	$ 23,109— 27.8%	$ 36,875— 27.7%
Long-term liabilities			
Notes payable (due more than one year later)	16,487— 32.4%	25,531— 30.7%	38,630— 29.0%
Total liabilities	$ 27,468— 53.9%	$ 48,640— 58.5%	$ 75,505— 56.7%
NET WORTH	23,457— 46.1%	34,648— 41.5%	57,498— 43.3%
Total liabilities and net worth[a]	$ 50,925—100.0%	$ 83,288—100.0%	$133,003—100.0%
Net working capital	$ 28,225	$ 41,699	$ 67,266
Sales	$148,243	$279,615	$470,542
Purchases	$ 95,908	$188,034	$310,393
Net profit (before taxes)	$ 6,148	$ 13,257	$ 24,814

[a] Excludes land, buildings, investments, and goodwill and corresponding liabilities.

tablish the basis from which to estimate capital requirements, a sense of conservatism should prevail. The projected sales volume should be estimated in terms of minimum level, while operating expenses should be projected at maximum level. It is usually easier to add new capital if sales exceed expectation than it is to recall committed capital if sales are less than anticipated. When operating expenses are estimated on the high side and planned for accordingly with adequate capital, a margin of safety is provided. If expenses are estimated at a level lower than is actually realized, financial difficulty may be encountered.

The method of estimating the capital requirements for a new pharmacy can be described by example. Assume that a conservative estimate indicates that a new pharmacy can produce $300,000 in sales volume during the first year of operation. The question becomes: What kinds of capital will be necessary to support the estimated volume and in what amounts? The kinds of capital are as follows: cash, inventory, fixtures, and equipment. The assumption made here is that the pharmacy owner will not own the building or land used for the pharmacy. The amount of capital required in each category is in varying degrees related to the anticipated sales volume, and may be estimated as follows.

Cash—Sufficient cash is required to pay preopening expenses, operating expenses for a stated period of time, and some excess for emergency use. Preopening expenses include license fees, legal fees, utility deposits, and advertising. These expenses, with the possible exception of advertising, are relatively fixed for any new pharmacy and are not related to sales volume. They are easily determined and usually total $1,000 to $2,000. Let us here assume the higher figure.

It is considered good practice to start a new business venture with sufficient cash to pay the first 2- to 3-months operating expenses, on the theory that the first months of operation may be extremely slow. For a new pharmacy, the amount required may be determined by relating estimated monthly sales volume to operating expense statistics, available from such sources as the *Lilly Digest*. Only cash expense items are used in the calculation. Such noncash expenses as depreciation and bad debt losses are not considered.

For a pharmacy in the volume category of our example, the *Lilly Digest* indicates that approximately 30% of sales go to cover cash operating expenses, including a salary for the pharmacy owner. Applying this percentage to 3-months sales of a pharmacy with annual sales of $300,000 gives a figure of $22,500 needed to pay operating expenses for a 3-month period. There are no guidelines in regard to emergency requirements. However, we will arbitrarily set aside $1,000 for this purpose. The total amount of cash required equals $25,500. In addition, cash will be needed to provide the other kinds of capital described below.

Inventory—The amount of inventory necessary to support a $300,000 sales volume may be determined by referring to data that give averages for cost of goods sold and annual stock-turnover rates. Again referring to the *Lilly Digest*, the cost of goods sold for a pharmacy with sales of $300,000 is about 66%, or $198,000. The average annual stock-turnover rate is given as 4.2, and is determined by dividing cost of goods sold by average inventory at cost. Knowing the cost of goods sold and the stock-turnover rate, it is possible to estimate the average inventory; in this case, approximately $47,000.

Fixtures and Equipment—The fixtures and equipment necessary for a new pharmacy are also related to estimated volume. Larger volume means more inventory, which in turn requires more fixtures and equipment to facilitate storage and display. The size of the building to be furnished and the quality of fixtures chosen will also affect the total expended. On occasion, savings may be realized by purchasing good used fixtures and equipment, usually available at a fraction of the cost of new fixtures and equipment. A reasonable expenditure for these items for a pharmacy properly equipped to generate annual sales of $300,000 would be about $18,000.

Total Investment and Sources of Capital

The total investment required for a new pharmacy with estimated sales per year of $300,000 would be approximately $90,500, broken down as follows:

Cash (for preopening and operating expenses)	$25,500
Inventory	47,000
Fixtures and equipment	18,000
Total investment	$90,500

The total represents the cash value of the assets required to establish the new pharmacy in this example. However, the amount of actual cash needed will be somewhat less than the total amount stated. In most cases, the pharmacy owner will be able to assemble the required assets by utilizing a combination of equity capital, borrowed capital, and credit.

Equity capital consists of the investment of the owner or owners, and comes from personal savings or from other sources that require no security and no commitment as to date of repayment. Relatives may be a source of equity capital, either on a co-ownership basis or simply by providing unsecured undated loans. It is thought that at least one-half to two-thirds of the total requirement should be equity capital, although many successful pharmacies have been established with lower equity investments. The amount of equity capital provided will influence the availability of borrowed capital and the level of credit that may be obtained by the pharmacy owner.

Commercial lending institutions, such as banks and savings and loan associations, usually require a substantial equity interest in a new business venture before they will consider lending the funds necessary to supplement the owner's contribution. As a general rule, commercial lending institutions should not be depended upon for a significant portion of initial capital needs. Such institutions are limited in the amount of risk they are willing to assume, especially for new ventures.

Trade sources, such as suppliers of fixtures and wholesale drug firms, present the best opportunity for obtaining non-equity capital for the new pharmacy. It is common for wholesalers to supply the opening inventory requirements for a new pharmacy on the basis of approximately 50% of the total cost as a down-payment, with the balance to be paid over an extended period of time. The period of time allowed varies with the individual circumstances. Usually, if the time exceeds 90 to 180 days, the supplier will attach an interest charge to the unpaid balance.

The amount of cash required for inventory may be further reduced by cutting back the level of inventory at the outset and then building it up to the required level as operations continue and sales volume increases. Two cautions should be considered in obtaining any significant amount of capital through the use of trade credit: (1) the interest factor should be studied; depending upon the rate and the method of calculation, interest charges can be surprisingly high; (2) the use of credit simply postpones the underlying obligation to some future date or dates. Repayment of credit obligations should be considered in terms of the practical feasibility of meeting the obligations when they are due.

Fixtures and equipment may be obtained by relatively long-term financing through suppliers, or in some cases through finance companies by a mechanism similar to the one used to finance a personal automobile. Underlying this form of financing is a chattel mortgage which places title to the fixtures and equipment in the hands of the lender as security.

The interest charges from this type of financing may be especially significant, often reaching an effective rate of 15%

or more annually. Usually a down-payment of one-quarter to one-third of the value of the fixtures is required, with the balance to be paid in installments over as many as 5 years. The scheduled installment payments should be included in long-range financial budgeting and planning.

After the potential sources of capital have been carefully evaluated, it may be necessary to make compromises or adjustments regarding the amounts estimated originally. In some cases the pharmacist-owner will reduce his withdrawals or salary during early operations to reduce the amount of cash needed for operating expenses. Inventories may also be reduced at the outset. In fact, it is considered good practice to hold about 20% of the amount budgeted for inventory in abeyance until the needs of the particular community are identified.

The amount required for fixtures and equipment may be reduced by purchasing some used fixtures and equipment. It is also possible to obtain fixtures and equipment on a lease basis. Lease arrangements may increase the cost of fixtures and equipment over the long term. However, such arrangements will also reduce initial capital requirements. By these means, and through the judicious use of borrowed funds and credit, a new pharmacy may be established with less cash than is indicated by the figure for the total investment.

Pharmacy Management

In an era of increasing specialization, the owner of the typical community pharmacy continues to function as a generalist, in both professional and business activities. More often than not the pharmacy owner is also manager, staff pharmacist, and salesperson. As a result, the management function, by practical necessity, is relegated to a part-time activity. Under such circumstances, it becomes especially important for the pharmacist to make the best use of the time and energy that he or she is able to devote to the management function.

In general terms, the management function may be described as all those activities involved in the organization and direction of the elements of an economically productive enterprise. Money, material, equipment, and people must be brought together in the proper relationships to one another to achieve the objectives and goals that management has identified. Management practices predicated on predetermined goals and objectives provide for more efficient operation and provide a basis for measuring the effectiveness of management activities.

The management activities of the pharmacist too often consist of handling day-to-day problems and crises. Much of the activity labeled management in the typical community pharmacy is actually routine administrative work that can and should be delegated to nonmanagement personnel. Perhaps this point is best illustrated by the axiom "management's job is not to do, but to get others to do."

The traditional casual approach to community pharmacy management consisting of the *ad hoc* handling of problems as they arise is not consistent with the nature or responsibilities of modern practice. The sum total of all activities in a pharmacy is becoming increasingly complex, due to increased volume of operations and to outside pressures for more effective delivery of pharmaceutical services and products.

All health workers are being called on to develop a social conscience, and to assume more responsibility for the economic impact of their activities. Although technological changes may relieve some of the pressure on health-care costs, better management and administrative techniques can also contribute significantly to solving the problem.

The impact of more effective management may also be reflected in improved professional services to the public. For example, a management decision to assign certain record-keeping functions in the prescription department to non-professional personnel allows a more economical use of professional staff. At the same time, it provides the pharmacist with more time for consultation with the patient.

The Role of Management

The first role of management for any business enterprise should be to establish the objectives and goals for the organization. Concurrently, management must provide the policies which will serve as the framework for accomplishing the stated objectives. For example, an atmosphere of patient orientation might be stated as one of the objectives for a given community pharmacy. The elements of patient orientation would need to be identified: proper record-keeping procedures, facilities for consultation with patients, and patient-oriented personnel would be prerequisite for carrying out the stated objective.

Working with predetermined objectives provides the manager with a basis for establishing policy and assists in decision making. As in the example cited, the objective of patient orientation has implications in the area of personnel policies and practices. Recruitment and selection techniques geared toward obtaining professional and supporting staff who can function effectively in a patient-oriented environment would have to be developed by the manager.

The kinds of objectives to be established by management might be divided into two categories: (1) a set of rather basic, almost philosophical objectives need to be developed; for example, will the pharmacy stress low prices rather than full service? (2) objectives concerned with more specific operational matters are needed, as meeting a projected sales volume level during a given year. In either case, it is management's responsibility to provide a sense of direction by setting forth both basic and specific objectives as guidelines for current and future activities.

Objectives lie in the future and, therefore, are subject to adjustments dictated by forces outside the control of management. Management personnel should keep abreast of those technological, economic, and social changes that relate to stated organizational objectives. In this regard the role of management in establishing objectives and goals must include a mechanism for continuing re-evaluation and updating of objectives.

Organization of the material and human resources necessary to pursue the objectives of the enterprise represents the second management function. The kinds and amounts of resources required are dictated in large measure by the nature of the organizational objectives. The ability to obtain capital, generally considered to be an entrepreneurial rather than a managerial function, may also influence this management responsibility.

For the typical community pharmacy, it is neither possible nor practical to divorce acquisition of capital from its application and management. In most cases, the same person is charged with both functions. Assuming that the required inventories, equipment, and people can be assembled, it remains for management to provide the organizational structure and the coordination necessary to mold these resources into an efficiently functioning community pharmacy.

The third management function is that of planning. Although a major share of the manager's time must be devoted to the fourth function (controlling day-to-day operations), he or she must maintain a balance between the present and the future. Control of current operations far too often becomes the sole management function of many pharmacy managers, who devote little or no time to planning for future operations.

Lack of planning often compounds the problems associated with day-to-day operations, resulting in a situation where the controlling function requires all of the management effort. For example, many pharmacy managers spend a disproportionate amount of time ordering merchandise and maintaining inventory when, through a properly planned inventory-control program, this routine activity could be delegated to others.

The brief and simplistic description of management functions given here tends to understate the complexity and significance of these functions. Management may be considered an art rather than a science. There are few established laws or formulas for solving the problems inherent in conducting an economically productive enterprise. It is especially difficult to make the numerous and varied decisions required in exercising the management functions. Although there have been attempts to quantify management decisions through the use of mathematics and mathematical models, in the last analysis the human element still dominates the management decision-making process.

As management decisions are made and implemented by human beings to affect human beings, it is apparent that those who manage need to consider and study the behavioral and social sciences in order to function effectively. For the community pharmacist who performs the dual role of health professional and manager, such a background is especially appropriate.

Essentially, management is an excercise in group dynamics. The manager must be able to organize, direct, and control a group of individuals toward the stated objectives of the organization. The manager who is unable to get the cooperation of his subordinates or who fails to delegate the responsibility for routine operational matters to others is not functioning effectively.

In the community pharmacy setting the human dimension of management practice is especially crucial. The nature of the typical community pharmacy is such that the manager is constantly in close personal contact with his employees, suppliers, and patrons.

In such an environment it is difficult to make consistently objective management decisions. Further, the dual role of the pharmacist–manager tends to create situations involving conflicts between sound management decisions and professional responsibilities. For example, in the management role the pharmacist establishes policies regarding the extension of credit to patrons. Yet when a patron with a poor credit rating has an immediate need for prescription medication, the established policies may be waived or adjusted to satisfy the professional obligation of the pharmacist to the patron.

These rather unique characteristics, and the need for the pharmacist–manager to be more flexible than those performing the management function in other types of organizations, should not be construed to minimize the importance of effective management in community pharmacy practice. In the current socioeconomic climate, with increasing costs of operation and pressures to reduce the costs of health care, the management function takes on greater rather than lesser significance.

The functions of management provide a somewhat theoretical basis for understanding the overall role of management in the continuing operation of an economically viable enterprise. For practical purposes, however, it may be more valuable to examine the role of management as it relates to the various resources and activities which go to comprise the business entity.

In the community pharmacy the following items require effective management: money, inventory, facilities, personnel, credit, and risk. The management functions of establishing objectives, organization, planning, and control apply to each of these items as well as to the pharmacy as a unit. At this level the objectives will be more specific, and the organization, planning, and control more definitive.

Consideration of the management of the specific elements that in total represent the community pharmacy does not imply that each element is managed in isolation from the others. There are many interrelationships among the various elements, and a management decision regarding one element often has an impact on one or more of the others. For example, the decision to expand the inventory of the pharmacy may have implications to the management of money, facilities, personnel, and risk.

Money Management

To a large extent, success of the community pharmacy depends on ability to obtain money from a variety of sources in sufficient quantity to acquire and to support the resources necessary for operation. Once the money is obtained it becomes management's function to employ it in the most appropriate way to achieve the objectives of the pharmacy.

In its simplest and most pragmatic form the objective of money management is to maximize the rate of return on investment. Such an objective may appear inconsistent with the responsibilities of professionals engaged in providing health services, yet in the long run the economical use of money is beneficial to society.

In theory, money is in limited supply and demand exceeds supply. In the competition for the limited supply, only the most efficient users of money will be able to obtain it. Applying this concept to community pharmacy practice would suggest that only those pharmacy owners who can effectively manage money in all its forms will succeed. In a sense the foregoing concept is simply a statement of the basis of our economic system, where efficiency is rewarded and inefficiency is not.

In the broad sense money management applies not only to cash but to all those materials and services which are utilized in the operation of a pharmacy and are purchased with money. Given a limited amount of money, the pharmacy manager must make judgments and decisions about the use of the money in terms of the stated objectives.

In this regard conflicts may develop between basic objectives. For example, the objective of maximizing return on investment may conflict with the objective of offering full services, as in the case where a decision must be made regarding the purchase of a delivery vehicle. The money invested in a delivery vehicle represents an inefficient use of money for many pharmacies and thus is contrary to the objective of maximizing return on investment. Yet, in order to meet the goal of providing full services to the patrons of the pharmacy, such an investment may be necessary.

The effectiveness of money management may be measured to some extent by the progress made toward meeting noneconomic objectives. For the most part, however, the most meaningful measure of effectiveness is in economic terms, specifically, by the return on investment. The return on investment for a pharmacy may be expressed in two ways:

1. *Return on Total Assets*—The rate of return on total assets is determined by dividing the sum total of all assets employed in the pharmacy into the net profit. No distinction is made between owner's equity and borrowed capital in this calculation. This ratio describes the productivity of the total asset investment.

2. *Return on Owner's Equity*—The rate of return realized on the owner's investment in the pharmacy is determined by dividing the difference between total assets and total liabilities (owner's equity) into the

net profit. This ratio describes how well the funds provided by the owners are being utilized.

The pharmacy manager may calculate these rates for his or her pharmacy and compare them with national data to obtain some idea of the effectiveness of the money management policies. Rates below the national averages, such as those reported in the *Lilly Digest*, may indicate too much investment for the level of operation or inefficient management of other operational features of the pharmacy.

In either event, by utilizing the return on investment concept and analyzing the operation of the pharmacy, the pharmacy manager is able to identify a problem requiring attention and can take appropriate steps to correct the problem.

The management of money in terms of the total commitment of capital and in terms of the application of the owner's equity represents only one dimension of the management function in this area. In a narrower sense, money management is also concerned with day-to-day inflow and outflow of cash from operations. Maintenance of balanced cash flow requires application of the management function of planning and control.

Advance planning through the budgeting mechanism is necessary in order to assure that sufficient cash will be available to meet such obligations as accounts payable, wages, and taxes. To a large extent, cash needs can be anticipated in advance by an analysis of past experiences combined with projections regarding the level of operations in the future.

The inflow of cash may be estimated in the same way. Matching of cash revenues with cash expenditures is of more than academic significance: both excessive and deficient cash balances may prove to be uneconomical. In the case where more cash is maintained than is necessary for normal operations, the excess amount represents earning power which is not being utilized.

For the pharmacy that consistently maintains a balance of several thousand dollars in the firm's checking account, it may be possible to transfer some of the cash to a savings account or to convert the cash into high-quality marketable securities. In this way, excess cash will be earning interest or otherwise appreciating and yet still will be easily available for emergency use. A deficient cash position presents some obvious problems, including possible impairment of the firm's credit rating which may have long-term implications.

One specific problem associated with an unfavorable cash position is inability to pay bills on time. In many cases this results in a loss of cash discounts. It is common practice for suppliers to allow a 1 or 2% discount for payment of invoices within a given time. The usual terms allow the discount to be taken if the amount is paid within 10 days of a specified date; otherwise the full amount is due in 30 days. The buyer is offered what appears to be a small discount for paying the bill 20 days early. In terms of interest rates, however, the 2% cash discount for paying 20 days early represents an annual interest rate of 36%.

For the typical pharmacy, cash discounts can amount to $1,000 or more each year. Too often, pharmacy managers do not recognize the significance of taking advantage of all cash discounts, and consequently they do not devote sufficient thought to alternative courses of action when faced with an unfavorable cash position. It may be possible to borrow money on a short-term basis at a relatively low annual interest in order to take advantage of a 2% cash discount representing an effective annual interest rate of 36%.

To some extent, the manager is able to control the cash flow in the pharmacy. Although certain obligations such as payrolls and taxes are relatively fixed as to time of payment, the manager may be able to influence other aspects of cash flow. Good management of credit and collection procedures, for example, can increase cash inflow. Proper scheduling of purchases of inventory can effect a degree of control over the timing of the outflow of cash for such purposes.

The manager makes the decisions regarding acquisition of new fixtures and equipment that requires outflows of cash either in a lump sum or in installments. Depending on future prospects for cash inflow, the manager can decide whether or not to proceed with such acquisitions.

In actual practice, cash inflow for a given period should be estimated and known fixed obligations for the same period should be deducted. If a balance remains, this represents discretionary cash available for expenditure. If a negative figure results, it is management's responsibility to attempt to increase the inflow or decrease the outflow of cash in order to achieve a balance. During periods of temporary cash deficiencies, management may be required to obtain additional funds through borrowing. Knowledge of the sources of funds and the cost of such funds is a prerequisite for the effective management of money.

Inventory Management

The merchandise inventory represents the largest single asset on the balance sheet for the typical community pharmacy. About 57% of all assets excluding real estate holdings were reported as merchandise inventory for *Lilly Digest* pharmacies in 1981. The extent of this investment plus the fact that the inventory requirements for a given pharmacy are in a constant state of flux forces a need for continuing management attention to this area of operation.

It has been stated that the community pharmacist is the buying agent in the community for health-related products. The community pharmacist must provide the right products in the right quantities at the right time at the right prices to serve the needs of patrons.

Due to varying consumer preferences and geographical differences in prescribing habits of physicians, management of inventory becomes a highly individualized management function in each community pharmacy. Given a limited amount of capital and the responsibility to utilize the capital economically, the pharmacy manager must develop systems and policies that will ensure a continuous flow of needed goods while avoiding the problems of excessive inventory levels.

Although the objective of effective inventory management is simply stated here, in practice it represents one of the most challenging responsibilities of management.

In the community pharmacy the management of inventory is complicated by the fact that a major portion of the inventory consists of prescription legend drugs. This factor makes the problem of inventory control in the pharmacy unique in comparison with control in other enterprises that distribute products at the retail level.

The demand for prescription drugs is generated by physicians and other health practitioners rather than by the ultimate consumer. When dealing directly with the consumer, it is easier to manage inventory. Excessive inventory levels can be reduced by special sales and markdowns. These techniques cannot be utilized to effect reduction in overstock of prescription drugs.

On the other hand, the successful pharmacy depends on maintaining a breadth and depth of prescription drug inventory which is adequate to handle all prescription orders received. Usually the need for a prescription drug is immediate. The patient cannot wait until the drug is ordered, to be delivered in a few days. The dilemma of the manager in this situation is apparent: that of providing a continuous supply of products that are characterized by an unpredictable and uncontrollable demand.

The management of other segments of the merchandise

inventory such as proprietary drugs, cosmetics, and sundry items, while not subject to the limitations inherent in the prescription drug segment, present no less a problem to the manager. Changing consumer preferences and pressures by suppliers to buy greater quantities and greater assortments of nonprescription drugs and nondrug items increase the need for careful attention to this area of management.

Three basic decisions are required for the effective management of inventory: the specific items to be included in the inventory, the quantity of each item required, and the best source of supply.

The specific items included in the inventory should be chosen according to the needs of the community served by the pharmacy. Although there is a core of items common to every pharmacy, a significant portion of the inventory will be dictated by local demand. In this regard the pharmacy manager must be objective in the selection of goods. The manager must ignore those personal preferences that might influence purchasing decisions. For the newly established pharmacy it is important that a portion of the capital budgeted for the initial inventory be held in reserve until the preferences of the local community are identified. As operations continue, the manager will constantly be faced with decisions on additions to the original selection.

Some managers adopt the policy of stocking all new items immediately, as long as the items are related to current merchandise assortments. Other managers adopt the wait-and-see policy, stocking new items only when a local demand is definitely established. Both approaches have advantages and drawbacks.

The wait-and-see manager runs the risk of losing considerable sales volume and perhaps, more importantly, the pharmacy develops a reputation for not having in stock what the patrons desire. On the other hand, the manager who indiscriminately adds all new items to the inventory runs the risk of an overcommitment of capital to inventory, with its serious economic implications. Striking a balance between these two extremes presents a challenge to the manager.

Perhaps as important as the specific items to be included in the inventory is the quantity of each item carried in stock. Assuming that a given item should be stocked, the manager must decide what quantity is necessary. At this point, a number of decisions must be made, based on a consideration of sources of supply, extent of demand for the products, and such financial factors as quantity discounts and buying terms.

In most instances the pharmacy manager may choose from alternative sources of supply. Most manufacturers of prescription drugs and many producers of the other goods distributed through pharmacies will sell directly to the pharmacy. The pharmacist may also obtain a majority of inventory needs from indirect sources, such as drug wholesale companies.

Direct sources offer the advantage of lower prices while indirect sources offer the advantage of faster delivery. As a general rule, direct purchasing requires a larger commitment to inventory investment because of minimum order requirements established by the manufacturer and increased delivery time.

Indirect sellers, such as wholesale drug firms, do not usually establish a minimum order level and emphasize rapid and frequent delivery service. The quantity of a given item carried in the pharmacy's stock, therefore, will be influenced to some degree by the source of supply.

Quantity-purchase discounts play an important role in decisions regarding inventory levels. As a general rule, the purchase of larger numbers or larger sizes of the items stocked in the pharmacy will effect lower cost per item or unit. Such cost savings can be beneficial to both the owner of the pharmacy and to the public being served. It should be noted, however, that cost savings on the purchase of goods in larger quantities can be offset by additional expenses that accrue from excessive inventory levels.

The costs associated with maintaining a merchandise inventory include implicit and explicit interest, obsolescence, deterioration, storage, property taxes, and insurance. Generally these costs increase in direct proportion to the level of inventory.

The capital invested in inventory represents money that could be utilized in other ways to earn a return. To the extent that such an investment is necessary to generate sales and to earn a profit, it may be said that the investment is economically sound. However, when the investment in inventory exceeds what is actually required for the level of operation realized, the excess represents an uneconomical use of capital.

For example, assume that a pharmacy has $40,000 invested in inventory. The safest alternative use of this capital might be to buy time savings certificates at an effective annual rate of 10%. At this rate, the $40,000 would earn $4,000/year and it can be said that this inventory investment has an implicit interest cost of $4,000. To the extent that the inventory produces net profit in excess of $4,000, the capital represented is being used economically.

Assume further that it can be shown that the $40,000 inventory could be reduced to $35,000 without adversely affecting sales or net profit. In terms of the safest alternative use of funds, the excess inventory of $5,000 is costing $500/year in interest that could be earned and added to net profit.

An explicit interest cost may also result from excess inventory levels if the capital tied up in inventory is needed to pay other operational expenses. The pharmacy owner may be forced to borrow money at current interest rates in order to support current activities. To the extent that the need to borrow is caused by excessive inventory investment, the cost of borrowing should be considered as a cost of the excess inventory.

The possibility of obsolescence and deterioration are risks associated with the maintenance of an inventory, and although such risks may result in some unavoidable losses, these losses are minimized at optimum inventory levels. When the costs of storage, insurance, and taxes are added to the interest factors and to the risk of obsolescence and deterioration, the cost of each dollar invested in inventory can be significant. An awareness of the costs associated with inventory investment will prove useful to the pharmacy manager as he or she makes decisions regarding the types and quantities of goods to be included in the merchandise inventory.

The effectiveness of inventory management has traditionally been measured by the stock-turnover rate (the annual rate of turnover for the inventory). The rate is calculated using the following formula:

$$\frac{\text{cost of goods sold for the year}}{\text{average inventory at cost}} = \text{stock-turnover rate}$$

The stock-turnover rate denotes the number of times, on the average, that the inventory has been sold and replaced during a given year. It represents the turnover of dollars invested in inventory, but tells nothing of the turnover of specific items or units that go to make up the inventory. As presented here, the stock-turnover rate relates to the entire inventory of the pharmacy. However, the same concept may be applied to departments if appropriate data are available.

The stock-turnover rate may be calculated for a specific pharmacy and then compared with national averages such as those reported in the *Lilly Digest*. The average stock-turnover rate reported by the *Lilly Digest* pharmacies for the past several years has been about 4 times/year. It is generally assumed that a stock-turnover rate of approximately 4 times/year is indicative of adequate management of inventory.

Rates considerably below this level may indicate an overinvestment in inventory.

It should be noted that pharmacies with rather low sales volumes typically have stock-turnover rates much lower than the average. For these pharmacies, increased sales represent the only real opportunity for improving their position in this area.

The typical community pharmacy with a sales volume near the national average should show an annual stock-turnover rate of about 4 times/year. If the rate falls significantly below the average, the management of inventory should be reexamined.

The rate may be improved in two ways. Attempts can be made to increase sales while the inventory level is held constant. Generating more sales with the same inventory increases the rate. In the event it is not possible to increase sales, the alternative is to reduce the inventory level. With constant sales, this will produce a faster rate of turnover.

A combination of the two alternatives, increasing sales while reducing inventory levels, can have a profound effect on stock-turnover rate. As a practical matter, the manager may be best able to work toward a reduction of the inventory level as an immediate means of improving the rate. Certain items in the inventory may be returned to suppliers for refunds or credit. Items that cannot be returned may be sold at reduced prices. Most importantly, buying practices should be reviewed with the objective of reducing purchases until a more favorable rate is achieved.

If a stock-turnover rate of 4 is adequate, a rate of 7 or 8 might appear to be excellent. In some cases this is a valid assumption. However, unless the merchandise inventory is managed carefully, high rates may cause problems that are as serious as those resulting from low rates. An extremely high rate may be achieved by ultraconservative buying policies. Conservative buying will better the rate for capital invested in inventory, but the improvement may prove to be uneconomical in the long run.

When undue emphasis is placed on maintaining a high stock-turnover rate, quantity discounts may be lost, resulting in an increase in cost of goods sold. As a general rule, a pharmacy can afford to do at least some quantity buying, thus realizing the benefits accruing from quantity discounts. Frequently, buying in small quantities increases the time and effort involved in the buying process. More orders must be submitted and checked in, and more accounting time is required to process several small orders as compared with a few large ones.

Finally, and perhaps most importantly, the pharmacy manager who attempts to control the inventory level too closely runs the risk of frequently being out of items called for by patrons. The disadvantages of being out of goods requested by patrons include a reduced sales volume and accompanying gross margin. Further, a reputation for being out of stock may result in loss of patrons to other pharmacies where their needs will be met more consistently.

Through good management, however, it is possible to realize an annual stock-turnover rate higher than the accepted norm without creating the problems described here, and many successful pharmacies do this. However, unusually high rates reduce the likelihood of meeting the objective of having on hand the right goods at the right time in the right quantity at the right price.

In the final analysis the key to effective management of merchandise is stock control on a day-to-day basis. The manager is responsible for designing policies, procedures, and systems for controlling and maintaining the proper selection and level of goods carried in stock. Proper training of employees in the importance of stock control and proper use of established control systems in the pharmacy is the responsibility of management.

The pharmacy manager must take the time to impress on the employee the need to maintain a continuous supply of goods. Otherwise, the employee may be careless or apathetic about following the established inventory control systems. Most pharmacies use the want-list or want-book system for recording those items that need to be reordered. Unless each employee is made aware of the importance of recording items on the list or in the book, the system will fail to serve its purpose.

There are a number of fairly sophisticated formal systems that may be employed to assist in inventory control. Many larger pharmacies, for example, maintain and control stock by using computer-based reorder systems. Other firms utilize the perpetual inventory method of stock control. At the present time, however, most of these formal systems may not be cost-effective for the average community pharmacy. This is not to imply that a system of inventory control cannot or should not be utilized in the community pharmacy.

The pharmacy manager can effect a reasonable control over inventory by implementing a well-organized visual stock-control system. By predetermining the number of units of each item to be carried in stock, based on estimated sales and adequate turnover, the manager can establish minimum and maximum stock levels for each item. The indicated levels for each item are recorded in an inventory control book or on the shelf where the item is stored. It becomes a simple task for an employee to check the stock on a regularly scheduled basis and to note those items that should be reordered.

There is nothing profound about such a system, but it does formalize an important function and provides a mechanism for maintenance of inventory levels. Such a system also forces the manager to think in terms of minimum and maximum stock levels for each item. This in itself effects a degree of control over the total inventory.

Very often, overcommitment of capital to inventory is not apparent until the end of an accounting period, when a physical inventory is made. In many cases the inventory level creeps upward without a corresponding increase in sales. When little attention is given to a comparison of the inflow of goods against the outflow, it is easy to accumulate excessive inventory.

One mechanism that may be used to combat this problem is the buying budget. In its simplest form the buying budget provides a means of dollar control of inventory based upon matching purchases with sales. In a pharmacy, each dollar of sales generally represents about 65 cents in inventory at cost prices. Assuming a balanced inventory level at the outset, about $650 would be required to restore the inventory level after $1,000 worth of goods had been sold at retail.

The buying budget concept is most effective when used to plan purchases in the near future. A budget is determined by estimating sales for a future period, as for the next month, then calculating the amount of new inventory that will be necessary to support the anticipated sales. The resulting figure becomes the merchandise or buying budget for the period involved.

As purchases of inventory items are made during the period, they are subtracted from the budgeted amount. The balance is termed the open-to-buy allowance for the remainder of the period. Although the budgeted figure represents neither an absolute minimum nor maximum, it does provide a guide for management control of the dollars invested in inventory. The real advantage of the buying budget lies in the fact that continuing management attention is directed toward an important operating problem.

Facilities Management

On the average approximately 15% of the capital required for a typical community pharmacy is invested in fixtures, equipment, and leasehold improvements. Charges for housing the pharmacy are second only to wages among the costs of operation. Expressed as a percentage of annual net sales, rent represents about 2.5%.[9]

Overall, the cost of facilities necessary to operate a pharmacy represents a significant portion of total costs. Management of these costs is especially difficult, because they are based on long-term commitments from which there is little opportunity for retreat. Rent, for example, is most often agreed on in advance for a 5- to 10-year period. The lease that establishes the level of rent to be paid is a legal contract which, once agreed to, is enforceable for its term. Fixtures and equipment, once purchased, represent costs that can only be recovered by long-time use.

Management's main role in the effective and economical utilization of facilities lies in a careful consideration of the original commitment to these assets. In a sense, facilities must be managed in advance.

Rental Agreements

As is the case in most areas of management, decisions regarding the types and amounts of facilities depend in large measure on projections and forecasts of future operations. Basic decisions on size of building and quantities of fixtures and equipment are intimately related to anticipated sales volume. The nature of the pharmacy also plays a role in these decisions. An exclusively prescription pharmacy usually requires less space than does a pharmacy that emphasizes general merchandise.

In negotiating the rental agreement the manager must have some notion of anticipated sales and the relationship of rent to sales. Although such information may be useful as a guideline for negotiating with potential landlords, as a general rule landlords refuse to be bound by statistics.

In many cases rental figures for two or more pharmacies are difficult to compare because the services provided by landlords may vary. A pharmacy located in a medical clinic may pay rent considerably in excess of the average figure for a pharmacy doing a similar volume in another location. However, it may be that the rent includes janitorial services, centralized heating, air conditioning, or other services not normally provided.

When negotiating a rental agreement or renewing a lease, the manager may be able to get a stabilization of the rental charge as a percentage of sales by obtaining a percentage lease arrangement. The percentage lease provides that the landlord will receive rent based on a percentage of net sales. Such an arrangement is especially attractive for a new pharmacy where there is doubt about the level of sales volume that may be realized.

Landlords are increasingly receptive to percentage lease arrangements. In most cases, however, they will insist on a guaranteed minimum rent, with a percentage to be added after a specified sales volume has been realized. If the guaranteed minimum rent is set at a modest figure, this arrangement may prove to be advantageous for the community pharmacy.

It would be inaccurate to infer that the pharmacy manager has significant command of the alternatives and terms of the rental agreement. More often than not, the landlord dictates the terms of the lease. Management's main role is to avoid gross errors in judgment, resulting in long-term overcommitments for space and rent.

Fixtures and Equipment

To a greater extent than with the rental agreement, the manager is able to "manage" problems of fixtures and equipment. The original commitment for these items should be made only after careful analysis of requirements, and after searching the market for the most economical and suitable

fixtures and equipment. The pharmacy manager has options regarding quantity, quality, and sources of supply for these facilities. It is good practice to secure bids from several sources before making the final decision on purchase of fixtures and equipment. Further, many suppliers will provide counsel and advice.

Once acquired, the problem of proper arrangement of fixtures and equipment requires additional management decisions. For example, should the prescription laboratory be located in the front or the rear of the pharmacy? When located in the front, it is visible from the street and tends to emphasize prescription service to passers-by. When located in the rear of the pharmacy, the prescription laboratory provides a private atmosphere, free from congestion and activity.

Numerous other decisions regarding layout must be made, and the pharmacy manager is well advised to utilize the services of experts in store design before making these decisions. Studies have demonstrated that arrangement of fixtures and proper departmentalization of goods can help increase sales volume, promote employee efficiency, and make the pharmacy more pleasant and convenient for the patrons. With modern fixtures designed for flexibility, the manager is able to experiment with various arrangements and layouts until the most efficient combination is achieved. Proper management of facilities can play a significant role in the efficient and profitable operation of a community pharmacy.

Personnel Management

One of the most important aspects of developing an efficiently operating community pharmacy is a well-conceived program of personnel administration. The uniquely personal nature of the atmosphere in the typical community pharmacy dictates that the proper selection, training, and maintenance of employees be given top priority as management functions. Each employee represents the pharmacy in daily interaction with patrons, physicians, and suppliers. The ability of employees to reflect and to carry out the objectives of the pharmacy may mean the difference between financial success and failure.

In view of the obvious benefits of sound personnel management, it is surprising to observe that many pharmacy managers look upon good personnel administration as an area for which they have neither inclination nor time. Deficiencies in this area arise in part from the numerous and diverse responsibilities assumed by most pharmacy managers. Yet, time and attention devoted to personnel administration would, in the long run, free more time for other management functions. The properly selected and well-trained employee can assume many duties that may otherwise be the responsibility of the manager.

The nature of retail employment also contributes to the complexity of personnel management in the pharmacy. In general, retail concerns experience significant variations in the demand for employees. Seasonal variations in sales during certain periods of the year require adjustments in staff needs. Further, retail activity is often concentrated during certain days of the week and certain hours of the day. Under such conditions, it is difficult to manage payroll costs without extensive use of part-time help.

Due to the extensive use of part-time employees, many of the people employed by retail firms are young people without previous work experience. Quite often they have little understanding of the economic value of the services they are expected to render. Personnel of this type present special problems in training and orientation, not only to a specific job but also to the general obligation of an employee to an employer.

Attracting competent employees is further made difficult

by the need for the owners of retail stores to cater to the desires of the public regarding store hours. Modern consumers expect to shop 7 days a week and into the late evening hours. The retail employee, therefore, is expected to work during hours and on days when others in society are free to shop and play.

Other problems associated with obtaining good employees are inherent in the nature of retailing. Retail employees are continually meeting the public, so these employees must be of at least average intelligence, present a good appearance, and have an acceptable personality. Add to these factors the fact that wages paid to retail employees are ordinarily well below those paid in other industries and it becomes apparent that the effective management of retail personnel requires devotion and imagination.

Selection

Although the nature of retail employment is unique in many respects, the basic principles of personnel administration may be applied in the development of a program for selecting, training, and maintaining employees for the retail field and specifically for the community pharmacy. Proper selection techniques must be developed in order to ensure that employees will be compatible with the job to be done and with the objectives of the pharmacy.

A high rate of turnover in a pharmacy often makes the attitude of management towards selection of employees rather casual. Managers rationalize that the employee will not be staying very long; therefore, why worry about selectivity. Further, the manager is frequently faced with the problem of replacing employees on relatively short notice. In such emergencies selectivity is often ignored.

Improper selection of employees has the effect of perpetuating and intensifying the turnover problem, and the employee who is not suited to his job can be detrimental to the operation of the pharmacy. Two general rules should be incorporated into the personnel policies regarding selection.

First, minimum standards for qualifications of employees should not be allowed to fall below the minimum standards for service established for the pharmacy. To "underhire" for a given position can only serve to undermine the reputation of the pharmacy. Second, "overhiring" should be avoided: obviously superior people should not be hired for inferior jobs. Such personnel rapidly become discontented and may have an adverse effect on staff morale and efficiency.

Proper selection of personnel for a specific job is predicated on an understanding of the duties and responsibilities involved and on knowledge of the individual characteristics required for efficient performance. The manager should develop a job description and a job specification for each position in the pharmacy.

The job description is a brief summary of the scope of the job, its relationship to other jobs, and such details as working hours and pay scales. The job description also serves to prevent misunderstandings about the nature or duties of a particular job. The job specification sets forth the characteristics and competencies required in the individual who fills the position.

With these materials the manager is in a position objectively to evaluate the candidates who apply for the position. Selection also requires a knowledge of the sources of potential employees. For some jobs, promotion from within the pharmacy staff may be appropriate. In most cases external sources must be used, such as employment agencies, placement offices of schools and universities, or classified newspaper advertising.

A growing source of part-time employees are the co-op work–study programs being instituted in many high schools. An availability file should be established in the pharmacy—a record of qualified people who applied for jobs when no openings existed.

The pharmacy manager should develop an application blank to assist in the selection process. Although the application blank serves basically to provide information about the applicant, it can serve other purposes as well. For example, it provides a means for observing the applicant's ability to follow simple written instructions.

The application blank also serves as a guide in the employment interview. If no openings are currently available, it can go into the availability file. Finally, the application blank serves a practical purpose as a part of the employee's permanent record, and as a source of information for social security and withholding tax reports.

A properly designed application form can serve as an effective screening device for prospective employees. The information supplied on the application form will often indicate that the applicant does not meet the job specifications and thus should not be considered further. If the information supplied suggests that the applicant is a good prospect, the selection procedure should continue with an interview.

Often the employment interview is the sole selection procedure used by pharmacy managers, and this is not advisable. At the very least, the references provided by the applicant should be checked thoroughly to substantiate the impressions generated by the interview. The interview, however, is a key step in most selections. It should be conducted in an unhurried manner, in privacy, and in a relatively informal atmosphere. Much can be learned about the prospective employee through a properly conducted interview.

The pharmacy manager might also consider developing some simple tests to be utilized in the selection process. Testing is used as a selection technique by many larger firms and it can be most useful. In the pharmacy, simple arithmetic tests can be utilized in selecting personnel for sales or clerking positions. These positions require that the person be able to handle the simple problems involved in making change and computing sales taxes.

It should be noted that all employment policies and procedures should be consistent with applicable federal and state laws governing equal employment opportunity. In general such laws prohibit discrimination in selection and hiring practices.

Orientation and Training

Proper selection needs to be followed by adequate orientation and training of the employee. Proper orientation and training can serve to increase productivity and reduce employee turnover. The orientation process should include a give-and-take discussion with the employee on the following questions:

What are the basic philosophies of the pharmacy (toward patrons, toward other health professionals, toward employees)?
What hours will the employee be expected to work (evenings, weekends, holidays)?
How long is the lunch hour?
How is overtime handled?
What is the policy regarding coffee breaks?
What are the regulations about smoking?
What are the rules regarding punctuality?
Are uniforms required? If so, who buys them and who pays for laundering?
What are the safety and security regulations?
May this employee answer the telephone? If so what information is he or she authorized to give?
Can the telephone be used for personal calls?
What is the vacation policy?
What is the policy regarding leave (sick, personal business)?
What are the opportunities and procedures for advancement?
What are the policies on employee purchases and discounts?

The preceding questions are by no means all-inclusive on those matters that might be of concern to both the employer and the employee, but the use of such a list will provide a basis for posing additional specific questions. Although some of the questions may appear to be trivial, studies show that these are the kinds of matters that often cause problems between employers and employees.

In an extreme case disagreements over such matters may lead to termination of employment. In other cases employee resentment may be reflected in attitudes toward and dealings with patrons of the pharmacy. This could be the most serious consequence of such disagreement. If these matters are discussed in advance, misunderstandings may be minimized, to the mutual benefit of both parties.

After a general orientation to the pharmacy the employee needs specific training in the duties and responsibilities of the job. Too often the new pharmacy employee is trained by the sink-or-swim method. The new employee is simply put to work and is expected to pick up knowledge about the job as best he or she can. Obviously such a method of training is inefficient and in the long run costly, although it does offer the advantage of requiring little or no management time or effort.

Even though the typical community pharmacy has neither staff nor facilities for sophisticated training programs, there are effective simple training methods that can be used. For example, the sponsor system of training is most appropriate for a pharmacy. A new employee is assigned to a capable experienced employee who explains and demonstrates the job in question.

The conference method also may be used, by itself or to supplement the sponsor system. Here, the new employee meets privately with the pharmacy manager or a designated employee to discuss the techniques of the job. In either case the management responsibility lies in organizing and structuring the training so that all aspects of the employee's duties are considered.

Compensation

Retaining good employees is one of the most difficult problems faced by the community pharmacy manager. There are many elements in the employment environment that may help in keeping employees, but most important among them is the compensation program. Adequate compensation is necessary not only to retain employees but also to encourage them to work toward the overall goals and objectives of the pharmacy. The basic elements of a sound compensation plan are as follows:

Adequacy—The amount of compensation should be commensurate with the responsibility of the job and sufficient to provide the employee with a reasonable standard of living. Adequacy also may be viewed in a legal sense in terms of state and federal minimum wage laws.

Simplicity—Compensation plans that are uncomplicated are easily understood by the employee and have the further advantage of being easy to administer.

Progressiveness—A compensation plan should recognize and reward initiative, productivity, and increasing value of the employee to the pharmacy. The plan should provide incentive for doing a better job. Periodic review of performance and salary should be provided for in the compensation program.

Patron Protection—The plan should not encourage acts that are detrimental to the best interests of the patrons of the pharmacy. For example, it is inappropriate to offer extra commission for promoting the sale of nonprescription drugs. If commissions are paid on these drugs, the employee may be tempted to place personal economic gain ahead of the real needs of the patron.

Traditionally, the compensation program for pharmacy employees has consisted of an hourly or weekly salary plus the employers legally required social security contribution for each employee. Modern personnel management calls for a broader compensation program in order to compete effectively for the limited number of good employees.

Increasingly, even small pharmacies are offering compen-sation programs that include not only salary but such fringe benefits as health insurance, life insurance, paid vacation and sick days, and supplemental retirement benefits. When such benefits are provided, the employer should calculate the value of the benefits in terms of pre-income tax dollars in order to demonstrate to the employee the real economic value of the benefits.

Although pharmacists have been slow in general to recognize the benefits of effective personnel management, recent evidence indicates improvement in this area. Social pressures resulting in labor legislation and increased union activities have drawn attention to this aspect of management. Given the importance of the human element in community pharmacy practice, it is apparent that continued attention to the management of personnel will be required.

Credit Management

The need for credit is especially apparent when health products and services are involved. The need for drugs and pharmaceutical services is often immediate and independent of the cash position of the patient. Further, a charge account statement provides the patient with a mechanism for keeping track of expenditures for drugs for insurance and income tax purposes.

These factors suggest that the community pharmacy will be increasingly involved in the delivery of goods and services on a credit basis. Further evidence of this trend is shown by the fact that chain pharmacies, traditionally operated on a cash-and-carry basis, are now investigating methods of providing credit to their patrons.

Credit management in the community pharmacy, on occasion, presents a conflict between sound business practice and professional responsibility. Sound business practice may indicate that credit should not be given to a particular patron, while professional responsibility may dictate that credit must be given. It is not possible to develop inflexible credit policies that will solve such problems. However, it is possible to develop policies and procedures that will be effective in a majority of situations. There are two general areas that require attention in credit management.

The first general area of concern is that policies and procedures must be established for granting credit. Included here are the matters of eligibility, limits on credit, credit terms, maintaining accurate records, and identification of credit patrons. Deciding which patrons are eligible for credit is the most troublesome problem for the pharmacy manager.

It is difficult to make a decision without knowing the credit history of the patron. Data on past credit experiences must be obtained and should be checked. The patron can be asked to supply the necessary information and usually will do so. However, verification presents a serious practical problem. Some managers attempt to verify the information personally by contacting each credit reference. Such a procedure is time-consuming and the information received is often incomplete.

A better approach appears to lie in the use of professional credit bureaus. Most localities are now served by such bureaus; agencies which, for a fee, will investigate prospective credit customers and supply a report on their ratings. With this information the manager is able to make better decisions and minimize the problems associated with the granting of credit.

The second general area is that of collection. The best policies can be thwarted by careless collection procedures. The terms of credit granted should be made clear to the grantee at the outset. If the terms are not complied with, appropriate and prompt action should be taken. The manager is responsible for establishing the guidelines and procedures necessary to ensure prompt payment of credit accounts.

Collection policies that result in prompt payment offer a number of advantages.

Prompt payment means rapid turnover of capital invested in accounts receivable; this permits a given level of operations to be supported with less capital. Operating expenses are lower when accounts are paid on time; delinquent accounts cost money in terms of employee time and supplies required for follow-ups.

Finally, there is a definite relationship between the length of time accounts are outstanding and bad debt losses; as a general rule the longer an account is outstanding, the less likely it is to be collected.

Although guidelines and procedures should be established for collecting past-due accounts, rarely is the same procedure appropriate for all such accounts. New accounts, for example, should be handled firmly in order to impress the patron with the importance of prompt payment. Casual handling or lack of follow-up of delinquent new accounts sets a precedent that may be hard to overcome.

For established accounts, more individualized treatment is indicated. Some patrons fail to pay promptly simply out of negligence. Usually a simple reminder will stimulate payment. Other patrons may be willing to pay their debts but for reasons beyond their control are unable to do so. The pharmacy manager may be able to work out a budget plan for those in this category to help solve their problems.

A small group of patrons may fall into the category of those who simply do not wish to pay. Outside collection agencies or legal action may be the only alternative for this group. In any event, policies and procedures for collection should be included as part of the credit management function.

Credit may also be provided to patrons via a variety of charge-card systems operated by banks. The charge-card system involves the establishment of a line of credit for an individual with a participating bank or group of banks. The individual is issued a charge card which will be honored by participating businesses for goods or services. The participating business then forwards the receipts for sales of goods or services to the bank and receives immediate payment, less a service charge of between 2 and 5% of the sales amount.

The advantages of this system lie in the fact that bad-debt losses are reduced almost to zero; the cost of billing is assumed by the bank. Even though the amount realized from the sales transaction is reduced by the amount of the service charge, some pharmacy owners view the bank charge-card system as the answer to problems associated with credit transactions. In fact many pharmacies use such systems as their only credit program.

As a practical matter, however, many people who require drugs and pharmaceutical services cannot qualify, and some people refuse to participate in this type of charge-account system. As a result, most pharmacies use such systems simply as a supplement to their own charge-account system. In addition, increasing numbers of pharmacies are accepting nationally recognized credit cards such as Carte Blanche, American Express, and Diners' Club.

In order to measure the effectiveness of management control over credit sales, it is useful to calculate the average collection period of customers' accounts receivable. Average daily credit sales are divided into the total of accounts receivable at the end of a period, giving the average collection period for accounts receivable. In theory this figure should be about 40 days if all accounts are paid on time. Figures in excess of 60 days indicate deficiencies in credit policies and credit management, and call for prompt action.

Risk Management

As a commercial enterprise, a community pharmacy presents numerous risks in terms of economic gain or loss. Certain of the risks inherent in the operation are speculative in nature. For example, will operations produce a profit or a loss? With this type of risk there is an uncertainty that may work to the detriment or to the benefit of the pharmacy owner. Such risks can only be managed indirectly by careful attention to the management of all of the elements comprising the pharmacy. Even then there is no guarantee of success.

Other risks associated with the operation of a pharmacy may be termed pure risks. Pure risk involves uncertainty and chance of loss but does not directly provide a gain if the loss is not realized. Tangible destructible property is subject to pure risk; its destruction is always possible but not certain. For example, there is a risk that the merchandise inventory owned by the pharmacy may be destroyed by fire. If a fire occurs a loss will surely be suffered, but if a fire does not occur no direct increase in value or profit is realized. Pure risk may be controlled or protected against by appropriate direct management action.

Types

The first function of management related to controlling pure risk is to identify and analyze the several perils to which business assets are subject. Some perils are common to all pharmacies while others are unique to specific situations. It is important, therefore, that the analysis of risk be individualized. There are four common categories of perils to be considered.

Actual Loss of Property—All tangible property is subject to being lost. For the pharmacy most such losses are due to dishonesty such as shoplifting, burglary, robbery, or embezzlement.

Damage or Destruction of Property—Most tangible property is exposed to possible destruction or damage by fire, the elements, civil commotion, and a variety of other causes.

Civil Liability—Every pharmacy is subject to a variety of risks associated with dealing with the public and with employing people. Negligence or breach of responsibility, alleged or proven, can cause financial losses to the pharmacy. Injuries to individuals in the pharmacy, malpractice by pharmacists, and product liability are examples of these perils.

Contractual Liability—Legal liability beyond that imposed by the law may be assumed in a contractual relationship between a pharmacist and other persons. The lease signed by the pharmacist to obtain the building for the pharmacy is an example of contractual liability.

Methods of Handling Risks

Each peril identified by the pharmacy manager must be further analyzed to determine the probability of occurrence of an actual loss as follows: the loss must be quantified in terms of its impact on the total assets of the pharmacy and the ability to handle the loss; the manager must decide which of the alternative methods or combination of methods should be utilized to protect against each peril or loss. The three commonly recognized ways to handle risks are as follows:

Self-Insurance—Self-insurance may be utilized to protect against relatively small losses with a low probability of occurrence. A reserve is established and in the event such losses occur they are paid for out of the reserve. The reserve is created by systematically setting aside money for this purpose. A major danger is that a large loss may occur before a sufficient reserve has been established. Except for large multiunit pharmacies, self-insurance is not practical for community pharmacies.

Assumption of Risk—When the probability of loss is low and the loss is of small magnitude, it may be economically advantageous for the owner to assume the risk. For example, when the cost of insuring plate glass against perils other than fire and the elements is compared with the probability of loss from these perils, most pharmacy owners decide to assume the risk involved. Assumption of risk differs from self-insurance in that no reserve is established. Obviously, this method of risk management must be used carefully.

Insurance through Others—The majority of pure risks associated with community pharmacy practice are of sufficient magnitude to dictate the placement of risks with other parties such as insurance companies. Insurance companies offer service to the insured and provide indemnity in the event a loss is suffered. Such firms provide the technical knowledge and the legal experience required to settle losses quickly and efficiently. Often the services of insurance companies are as important as the indemnification they provide, as is the case in liability suits.

Too often the management of risk is considered to be adequate when proper provision has been made to insure indemnification in the event of a loss. A complete-risk management program should include a consideration of loss prevention as well as protection. An attempt to prevent losses can be beneficial in many ways.

Insurance companies are beginning to recognize clients with good records and to reward them by reductions in premiums. A direct cash savings is thus effected by reducing or preventing losses. More importantly, most tangible losses result in other losses that cannot be handled by insurance. For example, when an error is made in dispensing prescription medication and a malpractice suit is brought, the tangible dollar cost of such a suit may be paid by the insurance company.

The intangible loss due to damage to the reputation of the pharmacy can not be alleviated by cash payment. Prevention of such occurrences is the best way to avoid all of the losses involved. Loss prevention, both philosophically and practically, should be an integral part of risk management programs.

The services of an insurance counselor may prove valuable to the manager of a pharmacy in developing a risk management program. The complexities involved in evaluating risks and in understanding the various types of insurance policies and terminology call for expert advice. The insurance counselor is generally the best source of unbiased information.

The insurance counselor does not usually order policies. The counselor's function is to evaluate the risks of a specific individual or firm and to make recommendations regarding the best way to deal with them. The insurance counselor receives his or her fee from the insured rather than the insurer. Expenditures of money for this service may prove to be extremely economical in the long run.

Insurance

Among the types of insurance coverage required for the community pharmacy are:

Fire insurance
Malpractice insurance
General public liability insurance
Products liability insurance
Employer's liability or worker's compensation
Crime insurance
Business interruption insurance

The specific coverages described above may be acquired separately, or a number of them may be included in a package policy, similar to the well-known homeowner's policy. Package policies have the advantage of offering broader coverage at the same or even at lower cost than do the individual policies purchased separately. Such policies should be evaluated carefully; the multiple coverage involved may leave gaps in protection that are not readily apparent until a loss occurs. It is often difficult to know exactly what is covered, and to what extent, under package "all risks" policies.

Perhaps the most important coverage for the tangible assets of the pharmacy is fire insurance. Although most pharmacies are protected to some degree, often the amount of the fire insurance falls below the actual value of the property.

This is particularly important because most fire insurance policies contain a co-insurance clause. This clause requires that insurance equal to a specified percentage of the value of the property be carried at all times. A common requirement is 80% of the value.

Under co-insurance, if at the time of a loss the amount of insurance carried is below the required amount, the insured will have to bear part of the loss. For example, if the insurable value of the property owned by a pharmacist is $50,000 and the fire insurance policy has an 80% co-insurance clause, the pharmacist must carry $40,000 worth of insurance on the property. If only $30,000 is carried and a $10,000 loss is suffered, the insurer is required to pay only $7,500. The pharmacist must assume the balance of the loss because only 75% of the required amount of insurance was maintained.

The standard fire insurance policy should be supplemented by an extended coverage endorsement. For a small additional fee this endorsement has the effect of extending protection to cover damage by windstorm, hail, explosion, riot, smoke, and from land vehicles and aircraft. It should be noted that usually neither the standard fire insurance policy nor the extended coverage endorsement covers losses of documents, accounts receivable, prescription files, or currency.

Several types of liability insurance are becoming increasingly important in modern practice. The pharmacy owner may be required to answer a suit arising out of the negligence or alleged negligence of the owner or of his or her employees. In addition, the pharmacy is a public facility where there are innumerable opportunities for injury to patrons.

Product liability may arise out of claims of patrons that they have suffered injuries from products purchased in the pharmacy. Although the pharmacist may be able to fall back on the manufacturer under the concept of implied warranty, such claims must be answered by the pharmacist. Insurance can provide the financial and legal resources necessary to answer suits of this type.

The pharmacy owner must obtain coverage of sufficient scope and of dollar amounts adequate to protect against liability claims. It is not unusual for such claims to result in awards of $50,000 or more. Without insurance coverage, an unfavorable judgment from one such claim may be sufficient to bankrupt the owner.

Insurance coverage against dishonesty and criminal acts also should be obtained. In addition, the pharmacy manager is in an excellent position to utilize loss prevention as a means of minimizing these risks. Minimizing the amount of cash carried on the premises, installation of burglar alarm systems, and carefully observed security measures can greatly reduce losses in this area.

The dishonesty of employees can be controlled best by adequate systems and policies regarding handling of cash and other assets of the pharmacy. Shoplifting losses can be reduced by proper surveillance and proper training of employees; as a rule, insurance is not available to cover these losses.

When a pharmacy suffers losses because of fire or other causes that interrupt operations, the actual loss goes beyond the property that is damaged or destroyed. Profits will be lost during the period when the pharmacy is closed. Certain business expenses continue, even during interrupted operations. Key employees may be forced to seek other employment. Such losses may be covered by business interruption insurance. This insurance is designed to indemnify the pharmacy owner for lost profits, continuing expenses, and salaries of key employees during a reasonable period of interrupted operations.

Life insurance may also have a role in a comprehensive risk-management program for a community pharmacy. If a pharmacist is the sole owner of a pharmacy, insurance on his or her life can provide funds to take care of the debts of the pharmacy in the event of the owner's death. If the pharmacist is the co-owner of the pharmacy as a partner, arrangements should be made for life insurance on each partner with the other partner or partners named as beneficiaries. The amount of such insurance should be sufficient to pay for each partner's equity in the enterprise.

In the event of the death of a partner, the surviving partner or partners can use the proceeds from the insurance to buy a deceased partner's interest in the pharmacy from the heirs. Such an arrangement reduces the possibility that the enterprise would be dissolved in order to settle the estate of a deceased partner. The premium payments made for partnership life insurance policies are regarded as a business expense.

There are a variety of other risks that may be covered effectively by insurance. Some of these are peculiar to individual circumstances and must be analyzed and managed in terms of the specific pharmacy. Effective management of all the insurable risks associated with modern community pharmacy practice must be combined with effective management of the uninsurable speculative risks inherent in entrepreneurial activity.

Records

For a variety of reasons—some legal, some financial and some professional—the maintenance of records in the pharmacy is becoming increasingly important. The types of records required may be classified as follows:

Records required by law regarding the acquisition and disposition of drugs
Records regarding patient utilization of drugs
Records regarding the past and present financial status of the pharmacy

Management's role in the record-keeping function is to identify the specific records required, to develop systems for keeping them, and to delegate the responsibility for day-to-day record keeping to capable personnel.

Legal Records

According to federal and state law, the pharmacy owner or manager is charged with maintaining accurate up-to-date records on specific classes of drugs and poisons. Under the provisions of the Federal Controlled Substances Act of 1970, the pharmacist is charged with maintaining accurate records related to the acquisition and disposition of certain drugs that are deemed to be subject to possible misuse or abuse. Several states have enacted legislation that requires accurate records on the distribution of poisons and other hazardous substances.

The legal implications of record keeping as it relates to these drugs are serious. Improperly maintained or incomplete records can bring legal action and penalties. For further details regarding the legal record-keeping requirements see Chapter 107.

Patient Records

In recent years many pharmacists have broadened their record-keeping activities to include patient drug histories. Although the form of patient record varies, the basic idea is to establish a record, usually on a family-unit basis, that will allow the pharmacist to monitor the drug usage of each member of the family. It is increasingly apparent that, because of the kinds and amounts of drugs being taken by the average patient, there is need for a drug history for each individual.

In order to reduce the problems associated with drug interactions and individual idiosyncrasies to drugs, the pharmacist has a professional obligation to maintain records of this type. In addition, patient records may also serve economic purposes, as sources of information for insurance claims and for income tax deductions of the patient.

Financial Records

Financial records derived from properly collected and organized accounting data serve a variety of important uses in the community pharmacy. Such records are of value to the pharmacy owner in measuring return on investment. Management personnel require financial records to evaluate past operations and to plan for the future. Potential granters of credit and loans to the pharmacy base their decisions upon the financial records of the pharmacy. Federal, state and local governmental agencies may be interested in certain financial records as they relate to income and personal property tax levies.

Accountability through adequate financial records is an increasingly important management responsibility in current pharmacy practice. Accounting data and the statements that summarize such data provide basic tools for efficient management. Sound decisions regarding future cash needs, inventory requirements, personnel matters, and expansion of facilities can be made only if adequate financial records are available.

Future planning and forecasting by management is based upon accounting data. Effective control of current operations also may be expedited by proper financial records. Such records provide a basis for analyzing revenues and expenses to the end of maintaining a balance that will ensure a profitable operation. Finally, adequate financial records provide the main criteria for measuring the effectiveness of community pharmacy management.

As a general rule, the manager no longer acts as bookkeeper in the community pharmacy. Although some pharmacists themselves continue to maintain an outmoded single-entry accounting system, modern managers for the most part delegate the responsibility for accounting either to a qualified employee or to an outside public accounting firm.

Considering the complexities of contemporary business practice and the importance of good financial records, the pharmacist is well advised to employ experts to assist in the development and maintenance of his or her accounting system. The experts can help to develop an individualized system that meets the accepted criteria for good financial records: objectivity, conservatism, consistency, and comparability.

Financial records should reflect insofar as is possible an objective evaluation of the transactions and data on which they are based. Personal opinion and judgment should not be allowed to prevail over an objective analysis of financial data. For example, the cost of fixtures in the pharmacy should be reported in the financial statement on the basis of acquisition cost as evidenced by a bill of sale or an invoice.

The value of these fixtures should not be increased on the statements simply because management feels they are worth more than the original cost because of increasing price levels. Convincing objective evidence of the dollar amounts reported on the financial statement is a prerequisite to maintaining the integrity of such statements.

The generally optimistic attitude of many owners and managers of business enterprises may be in conflict with the principle of conservatism as it relates to financial records. A moderately conservative approach should be employed in reporting financial data; otherwise, the data may tend to overstate earnings and assets and to understate liabilities. The consequences of overstated earnings include the possibility of excess income tax liability in a given year.

If a choice must be made between understatement or overstatement of income or assets, the principle of conservatism would dictate understatement. This does not imply that earnings or assets should be deliberately understated. However, when estimates or opinions must be utilized in making decisions regarding financial records, a conservative attitude should prevail. For example, many pharmacy managers are reluctant to admit that a certain percentage of accounts receivable will prove to be uncollectable.

They are inclined to report accounts receivable in the financial records without a realistic reduction for bad debts. To report accounts receivable without adjustment based on

Dermatologic diseases including erythema multiforme, Stevens-Johnson syndrome, Behcet's syndrome, lichen planus, scleroderma, pemphigus, systemic lupus erythematosus, psoriasis

Malnutritional deficiency diseases including (in addition to vitamin deficiencies) celiac disease, sprue, and cystic fibrosis

Hematologic disorders including anemia, polycythemia, leukemia, leukopenia, purpura, hemophilia

Infectious diseases of a systemic nature including syphilis, tuberculosis, acute primary herpes, herpangina, infectious mononucleosis

Recurrent ulcerative stomatitis (systemic background)

Secondary Herpes (*Herpes labialis*)

Serum and infectious hepatitis

Keratotic diseases including hyperkeratosis and leukoplakia

Toxic lesions (bismuth, gold, etc)

Osteoradionecrosis

Neurological disturbances including Bell's palsy, Parkinson's disease, trigeminal neuralgia, atypical neuralgia, convulsive disorders

Maxillary sinusitis

Tonsilitis

Laryngitis

Angular stomatitis (systemic background)

Denture stomatitis (systemic background)

Hypo- and hypersalivation

Sialoliths

Glossodynia

Halitosis

Oral Disturbances Directly Related to Drugs

Dryness of mouth related to intake of drugs, including major tranquilizers among others

Fluorine intoxication (endemic or iatrogenically induced fluorosis of teeth)

Mucosal lesions following therapy with cancer chemotherapeutic agents, such as aminopterin

Phenytoin fibromatosis

Tetracycline discoloration of teeth

Toxic lesions resulting from therapy with bismuth, gold, etc

Systemic Diseases Which May Influence Dental Care

Cardiovascular diseases including those requiring anticoagulant therapy, rheumatic heart disease, subacute bacterial endocarditis

Respiratory tract disease

Urinary tract disease

Central nervous system disease

Hematopoietic disturbances

Gastrointestinal disease

Skin diseases

Neuromuscular disturbances

Malignancies

Serum and infectious hepatitis

Pregnancy

Pharmacist–Dentist Relationship

Restrictions of space prohibit other than a partial listing for illustrative purposes of the various diseases which are of interest and concern to the dentist with regard to therapeutics. Also, it must be assumed that the pharmacist has access to descriptions concerning the nature of these many disease processes when a knowledge of them appears to be pertinent.

It is of particular importance, insofar as the pharmacist—dentist relationship is concerned, that the pharmacist be thoroughly familiar with the vastly expanded responsibilities of the dentist for the diagnosis and treatment of diseases affecting the tissues of the mouth and jaws.

Numerous cooperative relationships have arisen over the years between the pharmacist and the dentist. For example, dentists have found that pharmacists can best prepare many of the dental products which are commonly used either at the dental chair or in the dental laboratory. It is also of interest to mention that in recent years prescription writing on the part of the dentist has increased markedly, undoubtedly because of the introduction of such useful drugs as the antibiotics, corticosteroids, and tranquilizers.

Pharmacists frequently render invaluable service to the dental profession by cooperating in matters pertaining to the dental education of the public. The dissemination of infor-mation concerning the values of fluoridation of public water supplies, the usefulness of dentifrices employed to combat dental caries, the effectiveness of oral hygienic measures as these relate to periodontal disease as well as to caries, and the dental implications of halitosis are but a few of the benefits to the dental profession obtainable through the aid of the pharmacist. The introduction of the electric toothbrush and water propellant mechanical devices has further enhanced the interprofessional bond.

To play the proper role in advising patrons, the pharmacist must keep in touch with sources of information relating to dental drugs and adjuncts. His best sources of such information are, in general, the *Journal of the American Dental Association* and *Accepted Dental Therapeutics* (*ADT*). The latter is published every other year and incorporates the deliberations of the Council on Dental Therapeutics of the Association, as well as information about various kinds of dental products (the book is available through the Association's office, at 211 E Chicago Avenue, Chicago, IL 60611).

It seems to be almost axiomatic that people develop toothache only after the dentist's office is closed. They then obtain from the pharmacist toothache drops and similar preparations. Once relief is obtained, many afflicted people fail to seek the requisite dental treatment. The pharmacist should encourage such persons to consult the dentist promptly, for early treatment is nearly always simpler and less painful, and in the best interests of the patient's general health.

Pharmacology and Therapeutics

This section deals with a *few* of the many broad generalizations which are possible concerning the pharmacology of drugs and their applications in the treatment of diseases of the mouth and jaws. Of particular interest in this respect, from the viewpoint of the pharmacist, are considerations pertinent to the following classes of drugs: antibiotics, other antibacterial agents, antihistaminics, corticosteroids, hemostatics, local anesthetics (topical and injectable), protectant-vehicles, sedatives and hypnotics, tranquilizers, and vitamins.

Although the basic course in pharmacology as taught to dental students is similar in most respects to that taught to medical students, the clinical applications of drugs and the art of therapeutics are often markedly different in dentistry in comparison with medicine.

For instance, the therapeutic index of drugs becomes of particular significance when concerned with drugs employed in dentistry since safety *per se* usually must be of paramount importance in dental practice. This aspect assumes even greater significance when it is realized that the clinical training and experience of the dentist in the management of acute allergic or toxic drug reactions are considerably less than in the situation of the physician.

As another example, although the oral route of drug administration is generally the most convenient and economical for both physician and dentist, it is particularly suited to dental practice as often being the safest from the standpoint of severe allergic and toxic reactions to drugs. Furthermore, the oral route of administration more suitably fits the pattern of dental practice, the parenteral routes being generally avoided for one reason or another, such as lack of training in the necessary techniques, lack of suitable office facilities, or lack of office nursing care.

The distribution, fate, and elimination of drugs are of as much interest to dentists as to members of the medical profession. But again, there are areas in these fields which are of specific interest to dentistry, such as the evaluation of the advantages and hazards of drugs excreted into the saliva. For example, the presence of broad-spectrum antibiotics in the saliva undoubtedly exerts a considerable influence on the oral microbial flora. This influence may affect caries incidence or calculus formation, or may predispose to or trigger the onset of oral diseases such as moniliasis.

Drug synergism, addition, and potentiation, as well as chemical, physiological, and specific competitive antagonism are also of interest to dentists, but the areas of application of these concepts are less frequently encountered because of the nature of the usual general dental practice. Nevertheless, certain combinations of drugs are commonly and even routinely utilized, but these combinations more often involve pairing of a local anesthetic with a vasoconstrictor (e.g., lidocaine with epinephrine) or groups of analgesics (e.g., acetaminophen with codeine). Furthermore, the specific competitive antagonists that are more often encountered in practice by the dentist are not those agents he prescribes but those administered by medical practitioners.

Until recent years little attention has been directed toward improvement of vehicles which might afford a more effective medium for application of drugs topically to surface tissues of the mouth—an approach that might be useful in the treatment of mouth diseases or that might serve as another means of administering systemic therapy. An adhesive paste, *Orabase*, has been introduced as a vehicle for oral topical administration of active agents, with the result that a wholly new and potentially valuable technique has been made available for applying drugs to the oral mucous membranes. Nearly any drug available as a powder can be mixed with almost any adhesive (denture) powder and the resulting formulation can be applied with a cotton applicator or powder spray atomizer for highly effective topical usage. Adhesive denture pastes can be utilized as vehicles with similar advantageous effects. It is hoped that, these as well as other special vehicles (such as long-lasting lozenges, formulations that have been under definitive investigative study), may assume a useful place in the pharmaceutical armamentarium for the treatment of certain mouth diseases.

The introduction of the sweetener *aspartame* throughout the food and drug scene will likely have no greater impact anywhere than in oral pharmacotherapeutics. Nearly every formulation OTC, on prescription, or extemporaneously conceived which presently incorporates saccharin, innumerable others containing sugars not considered sugar substitutes, and indeed all formulations of a topical nature will doubtlessly be scrutinized for appropriate use of aspartame—assuming its record (including dental caries aspects) continues unblemished.

In summary, although no attempt has been made to present a comprehensive comparative concept of dentistry as it resembles and as it differs from medicine in regard to principles of pharmacology and therapeutics, it is hoped that on the basis of the above discussion the pharmacist will recognize and understand the meaningful differences which do exist.

Drugs Used for Oral Lesions and in Routine Practice

Although the topical application of drugs continues to be the favored route of therapy, both in the dental office and in prescriptions written by dentists, in recent years there has been a marked increase in the systemic use of drugs by dental practitioners.

The following discussion of the various classes of drugs is by no means intended to circumvent the need for reading and understanding classical concepts of pharmacology and therapeutics. It is offered, rather, to place proper emphasis and perspective on specific therapeutic agents as they relate to the practice of dentistry.

Although new drugs or analogues of old ones have been marketed, there appear to be few specifically designed for use by dentists or indicated for differential dental use, and not many which would preempt the use of carefully selected agents available for some time.

Analgesics

Dentistry utilizes nearly all of the various techniques available for relieving pain associated with the oral structures. In addition, the dentist concerns himself as often as possible with the removal of the cause of the pain, namely the excavation of dental caries, the extirpation of a diseased pulp, or the extraction of an infected tooth. In other words, the dentist frequently resorts to an instrumental or surgical approach to the relief of pain, in addition to employing drug therapy.

Of the analgesics, reliance is placed on aspirin, acetaminophen, APC formulations, codeine, propoxyphene, pentazocine, meperidine, and morphine; codeine with aspirin, Tylenol formulations, and *Darvon Compound* are frequently prescribed in dental practice.

The entire group of nonsteroidal anti-inflammatory agents having well established analgesic properties is available for use in dental care and has been widely employed. For a detailed discussion of these newer agents, see Chapter 60. The precipitous side effects encountered with zomepirac sodium (*Zomax*) in general usage remain of equal concern for future dental usage. Diflunisal (*Dolobid*) is finding increasing use in dental practice, as are other agents of this type.

Meperidine (*Demerol*), a drug highly effective in controlling many and severe types of dental pain, remains a very popular prescription analgesic. Levorphanol, which is reliably absorbed by the oral route, perhaps deserves more usage than it has at present in dentistry.

Any potent nonaddictive analgesic that can be administered orally will substantially influence dental practice, since its use will not so largely depend on whether or not the dentist has an aversion to such agents because they must often be administered by parenteral injection.

For a detailed discussion of analgesics see Chapter 60 on that subject.

Antibacterial Agents Other than Antibiotics and Sulfonamides

Antibacterial agents are frequently used in dental practice:

1. To disinfect penetrating and nonpenetrating instruments,
2. To control superficial infections of the skin, mucous membranes, or bone either for prophylactic purposes or as a distinct therapeutic procedure, and
3. To disinfect tooth cavities prior to the insertion of a filling material in routine tooth preparations, pulp capping, pulpotomy, or endodontic (root canal) procedures.

A brief discussion of the role and efficacy of the more commonly used antibacterial agents as they pertain to dental practice is in order.

Ethyl alcohol as an intraoral antibacterial agent is seldom used. Boric acid and boric acid formulations are far less frequently employed today than heretofore. The dyes, such as gentian violet and methylene blue, are still widely used antiseptic agents for the treatment of mouth infections and lesions in spite of the fact that their clinical efficacy leaves much to be desired.

Formaldehyde finds its most effective role in dental therapeutics as the active component of a desensitizing toothpaste prescribed for relief of pain and discomfort associated with sensitive necks of teeth. A 10% solution is also employed in dental offices as a fixative of surgical biopsies and excised specimens.

Weak solutions of sodium hypochlorite are often used as effective antibacterial agents in combatting organisms adherent to denture appliances and causing denture stomatitis.

Iodine is widely used as a prophylactic agent for preoperative use on intraoral injection sites and as an antiseptic following a dental prophylaxis. Iodoform-impregnated gauze drains continue to enjoy widespread usage in oral surgical procedures despite the fact that the clinical effectiveness of the iodoform *per se* is open to question.

Hydrogen peroxide is frequently used. A 1–3% solution is often employed in combatting mouth infections (used as a mouth wash as well as by topical application) although its effectiveness has been found to result more from its cleansing action than from its germicidal potency. Hydrogen peroxide (30%) is employed as a tooth-bleaching agent.

Chromic acid and silver nitrate are used much less frequently today as antibacterial agents since their detrimental caustic actions far outweigh their beneficial values and since safer and more effective antibacterial agents are presently available. Zinc chloride and aluminum acetate, astringents with some antibacterial action, are seldom used as such.

Phenol is infrequently used since it possesses only a weak antiseptic action, is not self-limiting, and possesses a high tissue toxicity potential. However, a number of chemically related compounds are widely employed, including thymol, the cresols, guaiacol, creosote, and particularly eugenol. Eugenol, a constituent of essential oils, has been found to be highly effective not only as an antiseptic but also as a topical analgesic and as a substance which possesses desirable counterirritant properties. It is of particular benefit as a component of temporary dressing formulations, e.g., zinc oxide and eugenol, which is commonly employed as a temporary filling material for one or more of the above reasons.

Hexachlorophene is also used in dentistry, as it is in medicine.

Wide use is made of anionic and cationic surfactants, particularly benzalkonium (*Zephiran*) chloride. Cetylpyridinium chloride (*Ceepryn*), as *Cepacol* mouthwash and *Cepacol* lozenges, are other surfactants quite commonly used in dental practice. However, it is essential to note that cold sterilization is ineffective for eradication of the viruses of serum and infectious hepatitis, as well as many other organisms.

The reader is referred to the current edition of ADT for a discussion of numerous substances of consequence to dentistry, and to Chapter 64 for a more complete discussion of antibacterial agents.

Antibiotics

Perhaps even more so than in medicine, the frequency of penicillin reactions, particularly those which are life endangering, has often compelled dentists to resort to the use of antibiotics other than the penicillins. The frequency of penicillin reactions has been such that many dentists will use penicillin only when this agent is the antibiotic of choice (mandatory) or when it can be employed in hospital environments where resuscitative equipment is instantly available to treat emergency situations. Nevertheless, practically all of the available penicillins find some use in dental practice. Penicillin G Benzathine (*Bicillin*), however, is used only rarely. Oxacillin and other penicillins which can be given by mouth are being used by increasing numbers of dentists to manage resistant staphylococcus infections. Methicillin, used for similar purposes, has a substantial drawback in dental practice since it must be administered parenterally. Ampicillin and related agents are now more often prescribed because of their broader spectrum of action. Cephalexin (*Keflex*) and other cephalosporins, including second and third generation agents in this group (see Chapter 64), are increasingly finding beneficial use in dentistry, as in medicine.

Broad-spectrum antibiotics, particularly those that can be administered orally with full assurance of effectiveness, namely, chlortetracycline, oxytetracycline, tetracycline, and other newer agents, are extensively used by dentists.

Chloramphenicol and streptomycin are rarely employed in dental practice, in accord with officially stated positions of the American Dental Association and the American Medical Association.

Nystatin (*Mycostatin*) is widely used as an antifungal agent and is particularly effective in the management of oral and circumoral monilial infections.

Dentists frequently use erythromycins, prescribing erythromycin base rather than the estolate because of the potential hazards of hepatic damage associated with the latter derivative in some patients.

Antibiotics of "last resort," although well known to dentists, are usually employed only by physicians.

Topical applications of antibiotics intraorally should be restricted to those antibiotics (bacitracin, neomycin, polymyxin B, etc) that lack hazardous local and/or systemic side effects. Development of resistance to these agents by microorganisms is of substantially less consequence since they are not used for systemic effect. It is to be noted, however, that all topical formulations of antibiotics are severely restricted in efficacy of action in the management of oral lesions. Deep-seated, well-entrenched oral infections nearly always require systemically administered agents, with or without supplemental topical antibacterial medication.

Dentists are well aware of the importance of prophylactic administration of antibiotics (penicillin, wherever possible) to patients with a history of rheumatic fever, rheumatic heart disease, congenital heart defects, or subacute bacterial endocarditis and prosthetic joint replacement. However, as stated above, erythromycins or tetracyclines are employed whenever a history of allergy to penicillin is uncovered. A full and authoritative discussion of the usage of antibiotics in dentistry under these circumstances is found in Chapter 3, Section I of ADT.

The dentist is called upon occasionally to prescribe for the treatment of an iatrogenic oral allergic or toxic reaction resulting from the use of antibiotics. A variety of therapeutic approaches may be employed. Mouthwashes of antihistamines, such as elixir of Tripelennamine, may be used. After being distributed throughout the mouth, these may be swallowed for systemic action also. Nystatin is used for combatting monilial superinfections. Multivitamin formulations are frequently employed to overcome any deficiency aspects of the problem. Topical protectants are also often used. When indicated, a corticosteroid eg, prednisone (*Kenalog*) may be employed, preferably in an adhesive vehicle such as *Orabase* or a bland adhesive denture powder.

The reader is referred to the current edition of ADT for a discussion of antibiotics used in dentistry, and also to Chapter 64 for additional information concerning antibiotics.

Antihistamines

Antihistamines are commonly employed in dental practice although some of their proposed merits have not been realized. They are most often used in controlling allergic reactions involving the oral tissues and structures. Tripelennamine (*Pyribenzamine*) elixir and other similar formulations have been found to be beneficial in providing a means of obtaining a mild topical anesthetic action in addition to local and systemic antiallergic effects.

Chlorpheniramine (*Chlor-Trimeton*) and diphenhydramine (*Benadryl*) are other commonly employed antihistaminic drugs. Promethazine (*Phenergan*) is valued not only as an antihistaminic but also as an antiemetic, antisialagogue, sedative, and tranquilizer. Benadryl has some use as a hypnotic in the enlarging elderly population which the dental profession serves.

The use of antihistaminics in the management of postoperative sequelae associated with oral surgical procedures (edema, facial swelling, trismus, etc.) has been highly disappointing.

Information concerning antihistamines used in dentistry is included in the current edition of ADT.

Consult also Chapter 61 for a more complete discussion of antihistamines.

Corticosteroids

No group of drugs has changed the pattern of drug therapy of noninfectious diseases of the mouth more remarkably than the corticosteroids. These agents have been found to be highly effective in the management of a large number of acute and chronic lesions of the oral mucosae.

Perhaps one of the more efficacious corticosteroids and one which is enjoying widespread intraoral use is Kenalog (triamcinolone acetonide). One of the more important reasons for its popularity is that it is the only corticosteroid marketed in an adhesive vehicle (Orabase), thus assuring more adequate adherence to moistened oral mucosal lesions. Some dentists, unfortunately, are reluctant to prescribe corticosteroids, even as topical agents, for fear of their side effects. It should be borne in mind, however, that the employment of corticosteroids should be restricted to those patients who do not exhibit or give a history of contraindications to their use. It should also be emphasized that the local or systemic side effects from the use of topically applied corticosteroids, administered in proper dosages, are essentially nil, at most minimal.

Systemically administered corticosteroids are, however, relatively seldom prescribed by dentists without a medical consultation, the exceptions being in severe allergic reactions. They are far more often used when the patient is attended by both a physician and a dentist.

As with the treatment of other diseases, so, too, in corticosteroid therapy of acute and chronic oral mucosal disease states, such agents are primarily ameliorative or suppressant in their actions.

Consult also Chapter 52 for a more complete discussion of corticosteroids.

Hemostatic Agents

There are many approaches, exclusive of drugs, which are employed by dentists for controlling bleeding episodes within the mouth. For example, various pressure-packing techniques, sutures, and refrigerants are utilized frequently and are commonly found to be effective.

However, on occasion, drugs must be utilized in controlling oral bleeding. Those that are more commonly used are Gelfoam, oxidized cellulose, carboxymethylcellulose, epinephrine, and thrombin. These are employed as topical agents for promoting blood coagulation. They are contraindicated when the bleeding is due to the rupture of a larger blood vessel or when the coagulating agent may lead to the formation of a thrombus.

Epinephrine is a particularly effective agent in controlling the ooze associated with capillary bleeding; for instance, to eliminate oozing of blood during dental operative procedures such as the insertion of a filling material at the gum line.

Systemic approaches for control of oral bleeding are seldom employed by the dentist if he is not in close consultation with a physician. Such approaches are frequently used in the hospital as prophylactic or therapeutic measures for controlling oral hemorrhagic incidents, such as may occur in hemophiliacs who are to undergo or have undergone extraction of teeth or other oral surgical procedures.

In the management of patients who are on anticoagulant therapy, dentists often seek the aid of, and collaborate closely with, the physician prior to dental intervention.

A discussion of hemostatic agents used in dentistry is included in the current edition of ADT. Consult also Chapter 42 for a more complete discussion of hemostatic agents.

Local Anesthetics

There are many local anesthetic agents and formulations at the disposal of the dentist (a number of which are used almost exclusively in dentistry), which will be found to be suitable for practically every conceivable situation. Almost invariably the therapeutic index of these agents is extremely high.

The desirability of including a vasoconstrictor in all local anesthetic solutions for intraoral use, even for patients with cardiovascular disease, is now well established and has the endorsement of the American Heart Association. There appears to be no specific superiority amongst the various available vasoconstrictors. Those most customarily employed include epinephrine, levoarterenol and levonordefrin.

Although procaine long enjoyed widespread popularity, in the past decade dentists have turned to other local anesthetics, such as lidocaine and mepivacaine, which have been found to be far more effective in anesthetic action and, in general, at least as nontoxic as procaine. Prilocaine and propoxycaine are still utilized, but minimally.

Carbocaine, in a 3% solution without epinephrine, has been found to be an effective injectable local anesthetic which satisfactorily avoids the necessity for the use of a vasoconstrictor.

Recent reports, concerned with a hazard (cardiac arrest) associated with the use of bupivicaine in obstetrical procedures serve as a reminder of the possible side effects of local anesthetics wherever they are employed.

Allergic reactions in dentists resulting from the constant handling of local anesthetics are not rare. These generally are local inflammatory reactions of the fingers or face. Allergic reactions are usually avoided when anesthetics of a chemical family other than that causing the reaction are substituted. The dentist enjoys a high degree of flexibility in the general use of injectable local anesthetics.

A wide variety of topical anesthetic formulations is also available for dental practice. It includes such agents as tetracaine, dibucaine, benzocaine, butacaine, dyclonine, and tripelennamine. Adequate and sometimes profound topical anesthesia can be obtained, particularly through the use of tetracaine and dibucaine, but these agents will not produce sufficient depth of anesthesia to permit the painless entry of a hypodermic needle past the superficial epithelial structures. Overdosage of tetracaine and dibucaine may cause hazardous consequences following systemic absorption through the mucosae. Spray formulations of tetracaine have been advocated, but such use intraorally should be discouraged. Benzocaine in high concentrations may produce an oral mucosal slough.

Ethyl chloride is occasionally employed as a spray, particularly for obtaining anesthesia prior to lancing a fluctuant and superficially located abscess. Ethyl chloride is also used in certain temporomandibular joint dysfunction states.

Benzocaine Solution

Ethyl Aminobenzoate	3 g
Propylene Glycol,	
To make	$\overline{30\text{ mL}}$

Warm slightly if desired to hasten solution of the ethyl aminobenzoate. The solution may be colored if desired.

A topical anesthetic for application to the mucous membrane before inserting the needle. Apply and wait for 2 min.

Butacaine Sulfate Solution

Butacaine Sulfate	1.5 g
Purified Water, a sufficient quantity,	
To make	30 mL

Benzocaine Troches

Ethyl Aminobenzoate	0.75 g
Vanillin	0.03 g
Sucrose	8 g
Tragacanth	0.25 g
Carmine	0.01 g
Purified Water,	
To make	12 troches

A troche dissolved on the tongue is very useful in preventing gagging when impressions are being taken and similar operations are being performed.

A variety of benzocaine formulation troches are available over the counter.

The current edition of ADT includes information concerning numerous local anesthetics used in dentistry. For a more complete discussion of these agents see also Chapter 56.

Vehicle-Protectants

Attempts to treat acute and chronic lesions of the oral mucous membranes (including chronic marginal gingivitis, the keratoses, desquamative stomatitis, recurrent ulcerative stomatitis, pemphigus, erythema multiforme, and drug eruptions) with topical medications have in the past been severely hampered by the difficulty in maintaining a medication at the site of application.

Orabase, an adhesive-vehicle protectant preparation, was designed especially for the purpose of retaining topically applied drugs on the oral mucous membranes. Studies with this preparation have indicated that it adheres to oral mucosal sites for periods varying from 15 min to 2 hours or longer, the duration depending on the degree of mobility of the oral tissues, the "washing action" of saliva, and the amount of vehicle applied.

Orabase, gelatin, pectin, carboxymethylcellulose, a mineral oil–polyethylene base—and the combination of these drugs, have been found to be free of deleterious, toxic, or allergenic properties.

Owing to its physical properties, which favor prolonged adherence, Orabase offers the following potential advantages over previously used vehicles: (1) increased contact–duration time of the tissues with the active component, (2) increased effectiveness of the active component by maintenance of higher concentration at the desired site, (3) decreased amount of an active material which need be applied at any one time, (4) decreased total dosage of active medication—highly desirable in many instances from a systemic-activity point of view, and (5) marked protective action.

Approximately 60 to 250 mg of the adhesive vehicle, with or without a therapeutic agent incorporated therein, is usually applied to the lesion site, in the form of a thin film, after meals and before retiring.

Further study of Orabase, however, has shown that its efficacy as a vehicle or protectant is somewhat limited. For example, erosions or ulcerations which are more than 2 cm in diameter cannot be easily or effectively coated with this vehicle. Still another problem is the inability to apply the paste to lesions in the less accessible areas of the mouth, such as the uvula, soft palate, anterior pillars, and the posterior tongue.

In an effort to overcome these problems, powder-form adhesive vehicle formulations, using almost any powder denture adhesive as the vehicle, have been prepared. Formulations of this type containing medication may be applied by a spray insufflator, such as the No 119 DeVilbiss spray atomizer. Adhesion of the powder vehicle to the oral mucosae has been found to be very satisfactory, and it has proved to be more effective than the paste for reaching less accessible oral lesions, since by properly manipulating the spray dispenser nearly every specific site of the oral cavity can be reached. The powder vehicle has proved to be advantageous in still another respect; ie, it can be applied evenly to as large an area as is indicated. Furthermore, the thinness of the film which is applied is easily controlled, of particular importance when the total dosage of active drug incorporated in the vehicle is best kept at minimal levels.

The therapeutic results obtained through the use of active drugs incorporated in an adhesive powder vehicle (employing nearly any denture adhesive powder as the base) parallel closely the results obtained from the use of the same drugs in equal concentrations prepared in the paste (Orabase).

Long-lasting lozenges, having dissolution-duration times in the mouth of several hours, have been studied; while they appear to be suitable for topical and transmucosal administration of drugs, therapeutic formulations of such a dosage form have not yet been marketed.

Black currant glycerin pastilles are also used as a surface protectant. Compound benzoin tincture, when properly applied by the dentist, also provides a soothing although transient coating.

Consult also Chapter 68 for a more complete discussion of vehicle-protectants.

Sedatives and Hypnotics

Sedatives and hypnotics are widely employed in dental practice for purposes of decreasing anxiety, improving patient cooperation, lowering the level of reflex excitability, and facilitating postoperative sleep.

Barbiturates are frequently used for these purposes. The most commonly employed members of this family are sodium secobarbital, sodium pentobarbital, sodium amobarbital, and phenobarbital.

These are usually administered by mouth, but on occasion the dentist employs the intramuscular route. Intoxication with barbiturates is seldom a problem in dental practice, since the dosage prescribed and the period of administration are generally restricted.

Chloral hydrate is an excellent sedative–hypnotic but has not achieved widespread popularity in dentistry. Paraldehyde is rarely if ever used.

Dalmane is increasingly prescribed by dentists, and various minor tranquilizers are among drugs in this category that may be used by dental practitioners.

The reader is referred to the current edition of ADT for a discussion of sedatives and hypnotics used in dentistry, and also to Chapter 57 for a more complete discussion of these substances.

Stimulants

The dentist usually administers aromatic ammonia spirit by inhalation for the initial treatment of syncope. In severe cases of shock where collapse occurs, a differential diagnosis is obviously the essential initial procedure. Thereafter, management follows accepted medical emergency therapeutic techniques—matters beyond the scope of this section.

A discussion of stimulants used in dentistry is included in the current edition of ADT. Consult also Chapter 62 for a more complete discussion of stimulants.

Tranquilizers

Although the administration of a tranquilizer is most often under the direction of the physician, occasionally the dentist will prescribe one or another member of this group.

The overall usefulness of promethazine, both as an anti-histaminic and tranquilizer, has been previously noted. In dentistry, meprobamate is one of the most widely utilized of the antianxiety agents, and has been described as being effective for dental and oral indications when employed in adequate dosages for suitable periods of time. Both Librium and Valium are worthy of equivalent if not greater usage in these areas when employed in proper dosages.

Chlorpromazine is rarely administered by dentists. Promazine, prochlorperazine, perphenazine, and triflupromazine are even less frequently employed. The prolonged time required for the onset of action of the rauwolfia alkaloids has made their role in dental therapeutics of minimal importance.

When considering the overall usefulness and applicability of tranquilizers to oral pharmacotherapeutics, the dentist must consider the following questions: (1) are tranquilizers really effective for office use, (2) when indicated, how reliable are they, (3) from a time standpoint, are they practical, (4) how long does the tranquilizer remain effective, and what are the hazards to the patient after leaving the office, (5) are changes required in the choice or dosage of agents which are concomitantly employed for the management of oral and allied disease states, (6) does a useful response necessitate a large dose?

Antidepressants and other psychopharmacologic agents have been studied and are appropriately employed in the practice of dentistry; however, the interest of most dentists in these agents is related more to the care of patients who are known to be receiving these drugs than to the prescribing of them. This stance may change in the future.

Nitrous oxide-oxygen psychosedation is widely employed in dentistry. Intravenous diazepam (*Valium*) is widely employed in oral surgical procedures.

Consult also Chapter 59 for a more complete discussion of tranquilizers.

Dentists necessarily are concerned with the nature, effects of, and relief of dryness of the mouth resulting from the use of psychoactive agents. Several *artificial salivas* have been approved by The American Dental Association: *X-ero-Lube*, and *Moi-Stir* artificial salivas and *Salivart* synthetic saliva.

Vitamins

Dentists frequently prescribe vitamins. The mouth may be the initial site of signs of vitamin deficiency. Since the clinical features are nonspecific, the dentist may even prescribe vitamins as a diagnostic procedure.

Although the multivitamin approach to deficiency states is usually favored, there are instances wherein single vitamins or restricted vitamin formulations are utilized in dentistry. For example, high dosages of vitamin A have been employed in the treatment of certain keratotic diseases of oral mucosal surfaces with some therapeutic success. *Vi-Dom-A* lozenges in dosages of up to 600,000 units per day have been found to be of some value when allowed to dissolve at the site of the oral lesion, followed by swallowing of the resultant "solution." Such therapy is *never* employed where the possibility of a true leukoplakia or malignancy has not been ruled out conclusively by a suitable biopsy procedure except when the patient refuses *all* other forms of therapy (including the biopsy). It is conjectured that the vitamin A in such instances may manifest a pharmacodynamic action other than that attributable to its being a vitamin.

Vitamins used in dentistry are discussed in the current edition of ADT. For a more complete discussion of vitamins see Chapter 53.

Other Remedies for Local Application

While the consultative function of the pharmacist is important, it is his ability to undertake the formulation of individualized dental preparations that particularly distinguishes his service. Many sources of formulas are available. A number of articles on dental formulas have been published in the *Journal of the American Pharmaceutical Association* by various authors. *Accepted Dental Therapeutics* is another good source and one which has official backing. Standard texts in dental pharmacology and operative dentistry and reference books in dental materials also frequently contain formulas. Lastly, professional and research periodicals in dentistry and pharmacy may be consulted.

The more frequently used dental preparations can often be supplied by dental supply houses at less cost than the pharmacist can make them. Nevertheless, the pharmacist can still provide a real service by compounding those preparations which are less readily available. Furthermore, the dentist, upon consultation, often may wish a modified preparation which gives better penetration, is more adhesive, has greater stability, or possesses some other property not available in the original product to the desired degree.

Many of the medicines used in dental practice, especially those dissolved in volatile solvents, should be dispensed in quantities not greater than one ounce, since they are used in very small amounts.

A statement concerning the use of aspartame in the place of saccharin appears elsewhere in this chapter and in more depth in Chapter 68.

The formulas which follow are not to be considered the ideal, necessarily. Rather they are to be considered prototypes and representative of dental preparations which have been and are used in practice.

Dental Caries Prophylactic Materials

Topical Fluoride Solution

Sodium Fluoride	2 g
Purified Water,	
To make	100 mL

It is important to use a good quality of sodium fluoride. In general the USP grade is satisfactory. ADT lists acceptable brands. The solution should be stored in plastic, paraffin-lined, or pyrex bottles. It may be supplied to dentists in quantities of 100 mL or less in ordinary pharmaceutical glass bottles, since such amounts will be used up within a few months in the ordinary course of dental practice. The sodium fluoride reacts with ordinary glass at a slow but appreciable rate. The reaction may result in the formation of sediment, but does not decrease the sodium fluoride content of the solution significantly. The preparation should be dispensed for office use only, and should bear a "poison" label.

Tablets, each consisting of pure sodium fluoride in quantity sufficient to make 2 mL of topical fluoride solution, are available commercially. Their use permits the extemporaneous preparation of fresh solution.

An 8% solution of stannous fluoride, freshly prepared, is frequently employed by dentists as a locally applied prophylactic to reduce incidence of dental caries in children.

Fluoride gels, applied in specially constructed appliances that fit over the teeth and adjacent sensitive areas, are being used with considerable success in combating radiation-therapy-induced caries and in other situations where extreme dryness of the mouth may lead to rampant decay.

Desensitizers for Dentin

The following preparations tend to decrease hypersensitivity of teeth when applied to their outer surface, especially where erosion has occurred near the gum line:

Ammoniacal Silver Nitrate Solution
Formaldehyde Solution
Liquefied Phenol
Zinc Chloride, 80% Solution

Sodium Fluoride Paste

Sodium Fluoride Powder	10 g
Kaolin	10 g
Glycerin	10 g

To make a paste.

Add more or less glycerin as needed to make a smooth but rather stiff paste.

Thermodent toothpaste is not infrequently prescribed.
Sensodyne toothpaste, including 10% strontium chloride, is likewise occasionally prescribed.

Cavity Liners (Varnishes)

Cavity liners or varnishes are used in the dental office to seal the dental tubuli in deep-seated cavities so as to protect the pulp from acid-containing dental cements. Cavity-lining preparations which depend solely upon the development of a film intended to be impervious to aqueous acid are believed to be inadequate because of the difficulty in maintaining the integrity of the film under filling conditions. Cavity liner preparations should be kept in a tightly stoppered bottle to prevent undue evaporation of solvent. The following preparations may be of limited usefulness:

Copal Varnish

Copal	5 g
Chloroform	100 mL

Powder the copal mix with 5 g of dry washed sand, place in a flask, add the chloroform, and shake occasionally during at least 24 hours, frequently breaking up the gummy mass to facilitate extraction. Filter, and add chloroform to make 100 mL. If necessary, add 5 g of purified talc and again filter.

Mastic Varnish

Mastic	30 g
Peruvian Balsam	30 mL
Chloroform,	
To make	100 mL

Dissolve the mastic and Peruvian balsam in about 50 mL of chloroform and add sufficient chloroform to make 100 mL.

Rosin Varnish

I

Rosin, fragments	7 g
Chloroform	100 mL

Make a solution.

II

Rosin	6.7 g
Sodium Carbonate, Monohydrate	1.7 g
Acetone	100 mL

Mix. Do not filter.

Several commercial preparations are available which utilize the chemical effect of calcium hydroxide for neutralizing the acid derived from acid dental cements. These are stated to contain various percentages of calcium hydroxide suspended in aqueous methylcellulose solution. A brand of calcium hydroxide paste produced by Rower Dental Mfg Co, Boston, MA, is called *Pulpdent Paste* and is stated to contain 48.6% calcium hydroxide suspended in an aqueous methylcellulose solution. *Pulpdent Liquid* contains 8.7% calcium hydroxide in the same vehicle.

Other useful commercially marketed cavity liners are available especially from dental supply houses.

Pulp Cappings or Temporary Cements

Zinc Oxide and Eugenol Cement

Make a thick, putty-like paste of zinc oxide and eugenol. Protect from air and moisture. The zinc oxide and eugenol are supplied separately.

Zinc Oxide and Thymol Cement

Zinc Oxide	67 g
Thymol	33 g

Melt the thymol in a porcelain evaporating dish on a water bath. Add the zinc oxide and rub the mixture to a smooth paste. Spread in a thin layer over the dish and cool. Break into small pieces and keep in a well-closed container.

Calcium Hydroxide Paste

Disinfectants for Root Canals

Chloroazodin Solution
Creosote
Formocresol
Camphorated Parachlorophenol

Disinfectants for Instruments

Chemical disinfectants which are safe and practical for use on dental instruments will usually not kill all bacterial spores, including those of pathogens. Many of them will not kill *Mycobacterium tuberculosis*. In addition, chemical agents may in one concentration kill bacteria and in another dilution, or under a different set of conditions, merely inhibit or perhaps even stimulate bacterial growth. The Council on Dental Therapeutics of the American Dental Association strongly discourages the use of chemical solutions for the disinfection of dental instruments which might be contaminated with a *hepatitis virus* since there have been reports of many well-documented cases of *viral hepatitis* following the use of nonsterile injection needles or syringes, or other instruments contaminated with blood containing the virus of serum or infectious hepatitis. There is no evidence that chemical solutions will destroy these viruses.

Recognizing these and numerous other limitations of chemical solutions, the following are presented for limited use:

Benzalkonium Chloride Solution 1:1000
Benzethonium Chloride Solution 1:1000
Metaphen Disinfecting Solution
Saponated Cresol Solution

Denture Preparations

Denture Adherent Powder

Tragacanth, fine powder	75 g
Karaya Gum, fine powder	25 g
Sassafras Oil	1.5 mL

Mix. To be sprinkled sparingly on the denture before placing it in the mouth. Powdered gum tragacanth alone will serve as well, but its flavor may not be as pleasant.

Adherent powders which are used in connection with denture service are made from finely powdered gums such as karaya, acacia or tragacanth as well as other newly introduced materials. These materials swell to many times their original volume on the addition of water and assume mucilaginous or gelatinous properties. The powders are prepared by mixing several of the gums or by the use of one alone. They may be flavored with suitable volatile oils and may contain antiseptic agents as well.

Denture Cleanser

Trisodium Phosphate	120	g
Cinnamon Oil	0.3	mL
Coloring Solution	qs*	

* A suitable, approved coloring material may be used in this and succeeding formulations, primarily for asthetic purposes, but is not necessary.

Mix. Dissolve ¼ teaspoonful in half a glass of water and use with a brush.

Note—The cellulose acetate type of denture is decomposed by alkaline substances. Phenol-formaldehyde and acrylic types withstand most chemical agents.

Formulas Used in General Practice

Abrasives

These preparations are used by the dentist in cleaning and polishing teeth. They are not suitable for use by the laity, since they may be entirely too harsh for continued or unsupervised use.

Paste Abrasive

I

Pumice, in very fine powder	40 g
Methyl Salicylate	1 mL
Coloring Solution	qs
Starch Glycerite	60 g
To make about	100 g

The coloring agent should provide a pink color which disguises the color of blood, and the starch glycerite base gives a product which clings well to the brush.

II

Pumice, in very fine powder	61.8 g
Sodium Borate	10.8 g
Coloring Agent	qs
Glycerin	27.2 mL
Spearmint Oil	0.1 mL
To make about	100 g

Mix the glycerin and coloring agent with the sodium borate and add the pumice a little at a time. The final consistency may be adjusted by the addition of further amounts of pumice or glycerin.

Powder Abrasive

Pumice, in very fine powder	80	g
Starch	16	g
Methyl Salicylate	4	mL
Coloring Agent	qs	
To make about	100	g

For office use only. May be dispensed in capsules, each to contain about 1.5 g for convenience in the treatment of the individual patient. Contents of one or more capsules used as an *abrasive*. After removing contents of capsule, add a small quantity of water or glycerin to powder before use.

Dentifrices

A dentifrice is a substance used with a toothbrush for the purpose of cleaning the accessible surfaces of the teeth. Commercial dentifrices are available in the form of pastes and powders.

Many dentifrices contain flavors and soap or synthetic detergents. The powders and pastes contain abrasives such as calcium carbonate, one or more of the calcium phosphates, calcium sulfate, insoluble sodium metaphosphate, hydrated aluminum oxide, magnesium carbonates and phosphates, sodium bicarbonate and sodium chloride. Tooth pastes contain liquids such as glycerin, propylene glycol, sorbitol solution, water, and alcohol, and thickeners such as starch, tragacanth, algin, and cellulose derivatives. Dentifrices usually contain noncarbohydrate sweetening agents, but a few contain sugar.

It has been shown that individuals vary markedly in their need for an abrasive in dentifrices. Generally speaking, commercial dentifrice powders are more abrasive than pastes.

Some individuals who require only a slight degree of abrasion to keep the teeth from staining may find that a mixture of baking soda and finely powdered table salt is satisfactory. Others may require a more abrasive substance, but the Council on Dental Therapeutics of the American Dental Association maintains that there is no valid reason for the use of a dentifrice with a greater abrasiveness than necessary to prevent residual accumulations on the teeth.

The primary purpose of a dentifrice is to assist the toothbrush in cleaning the teeth. This cleansing process of brushing *per se*, with or without a dentifrice, is beneficial to dental health.

There is a continuing effort to obtain additional dental benefits from dentifrices through the inclusion of agents designed to have some specific biological or therapeutic action. For the most part, when such dentifrices are employed as adjuncts to supervised toothbrushing in controlled clinical investigations, their superiority over conventional dentifrices has not been clearly established. Among such dentifrices are those which are claimed to "remineralize" the tooth substance, those which include urea and dibasic ammonium phosphate in their formulas, penicillin dentifrices, foaming agents, and others which have been promoted as "antienzyme" and "antibacterial" agents. In many cases the Council has indicated that more extensive evidence is required for an accurate evaluation of the claims made by various manufacturers.

In 1960 a dentifrice containing stannous fluoride was approved by the Council as a result of controlled studies in which its usefulness as an anticaries agent was demonstrated. This dentifrice is said to contain 0.4% stannous fluoride, 39% calcium pyrophosphate, 30% glycerin, 1.0% stannous pyrophosphate, 4.63% miscellaneous agents, and 24.97% water. It is marketed under the trade name Crest (*Proctor & Gamble*). More recently, a number of manufacturers have marketed fluoride dentifrices and many have been granted Council acceptance.

Liquid Dentifrice

Hard Soap, powdered	60 g
Saccharin	2 g
Coloring Solution	qs
Cinnamon Oil	5 mL
Peppermint Oil	5 mL
Clove Oil	10 mL
Alcohol	750 mL
Purified Water,	
To make	1000 mL

Dissolve the soap, the saccharin, and the oils in the alcohol; add the coloring solution and sufficient water to make 1000 mL. Sprinkle on the moistened toothbrush and use as a dentifrice.

Dentifrice NF XI

Hard Soap, in fine powder	50 g
Precipitated Calcium Carbonate	935 g
Saccharin Sodium	2 g
Peppermint Oil	4 mL
Cinnamon Oil	2 mL
Methyl Salicylate	8 mL
To make about	1000 g

Thoroughly triturate the saccharin sodium, the oils, and the methyl salicylate with about one-half of the precipitated calcium carbonate, and mix the soap with the remainder of the precipitated calcium carbonate. Mix the two powders thoroughly, and pass through a fine sieve.

Uses—This is a basic powder used only as a general cleanser. It is not medicated but it forms a splendid vehicle for medication, eg, with sodium perborate or astringent substances.

Oxidizing, astringent, and alkaline qualities may be provided by additions as may be indicated. Only ingredients listed in ADT should be used. In selecting abrasives, eg, calcium carbonate or calcium phosphate, it is safer to use brands and grades listed in ADT since others may be unduly harsh.

Paste Dentifrice

CMC 120 H	0.9 g
Glycerin	1 g
Propylene Glycol	18.0 g
Purified Water	13.5 g
Methylparaben	0.1 g
Saccharin Sodium Solution 50%	0.1 g
Peppermint Oil	0.3 g
Mineral Oil	1 g
Sodium Lauryl Sulfate	2.5 g
Dicalcium Phosphate, in very fine powder	54 g

The fluoride compounds most often used in toothpastes are sodium fluoride (*Crest, Aim* and *Gleam II*) and sodium monofluorophosphate (*Colgate with MFP*). See Chapter 40.

Mouthwashes

Dental and medical dictionaries in general define a mouthwash as a medicated liquid used for cleansing the mouth or treating diseased states of the oral mucous membranes. Unfortunately, advertisers attempt to imply wider uses for many such products. *Accepted Dental Therapeutics* questions the use of the term "antiseptic" in connection with mouthwashes and states that the only legitimate use of a mouthwash for the general public is an adjunct in the toilet of the mouth. Claims that certain mouthwashes overcome mouth odors should be viewed with reserve. Most persistent abnormal mouth odors must be recognized as symptoms of diseases or detritus in the mouth, nose, sinuses, chest, or intestinal tract. The elimination of these symptoms cannot be accomplished by the use of a mouthwash. Neither does it appear that odors arising from certain ingested foods can be eliminated by this means. In dental practice mouthwashes may be employed as a part of postoperative treatment, and during the course of certain operative procedures—when such use adds to the comfort or oral hygiene of the patient.

Because of their effervescence, oxygenating preparations are effective debriding agents when used as oral rinses or sprays. Included in this group are hydrogen peroxide, carbamide (urea) peroxide, metallic peroxides, perborates, and permanganates. Hydrogen peroxide, USP, diluted with water can be used as a rinse. Two commercial perborate preparations also used are *Vince* and *Amosan*. The carbamide peroxides (*Gly-oxide*), a complex of urea and hydrogen peroxide, are viscous rather than aqueous solutions and, therefore, are not technically mouthwashes. Phenol and its derivatives, although used for their antibacterial and anodyne effects in mouthwash preparations, have limited value because of their toxicity, objectionable taste, sensitization properties, and decreased activity in the presence of organic matter. Phenol is an active ingredient in *Chloraseptic* solution and *Cepastat*. Cetylpyridinum chloride, studied as an antiplaque agent with mixed results, is the active ingredient contained in *Cepacol* mouthwash.

In addition to the preparations formulated as below, the following solutions are frequently employed as mouth rinses: Sodium Chloride Irrigation USP, Mouthwash NF XII, Antiseptic Solution NF XII, Compound Sodium Borate Solution NF XI, and sodium bicarbonate solution (2%).

Peppermint Mouth Rinse

Peppermint Spirit	43.2 mL
Saccharin Sodium	0.07 g
Purified Water,	
To make	240 mL

Hypertonic Saline Mouth Rinse

Sodium Chloride	2 g
Purified Water,	
To make	100 mL

Alkaline Saline Mouth Rinse

Sodium Chloride	2 g
Sodium Bicarbonate	1 g
Coloring Solution	qs
Peppermint Water,	
To make	240 mL

Saline Mouth Rinse Powder

Calcium Oxide	2 g
Phenolphthalein	0.1 g
Saccharin Sodium	0.3 g
Cinnamon Oil	0.5 g
Sodium Chloride,	
To make	100 g

Mix thoroughly. The calcium oxide and the phenolphthalein produce a pink color in the product. Use ¼ teaspoonful to a cup of warm water as a mouthwash.

Irrigation Solution for Exodontia

The dental surgeon employs Sodium Chloride Irrigation USP as an irrigating solution.

Alveolar Analgesics

Several formulas are given below for liquids and pastes to be employed by the dental surgeon for the symptomatic relief of pain arising from postextraction alveolitis, commonly called "dry socket."

Benzocaine Ointment
Benzocaine Paste

Benzocaine	3 g
Clove Oil	3 g
Hydrous Wool Fat	12 g
Yellow Wax	15 g
Petrolatum	15 g

Mix the last three ingredients together on a water bath, and then add the benzocaine and clove oil with stirring.

Benzocaine–Guaiacol Solution

Benzocaine	3 g
Guaiacol	3 g
Peruvian Balsam	9 g

Triturate the benzocaine with the guaiacol to form a smooth paste and then incorporate the Peruvian balsam.

Other formulations include:
Liquids

1. Guaiacol and glycerin, equal parts
2. Chlorobutanol, 25 g
   Clove oil to make 100 mL

Pastes

1. Benzocaine, 750 mg
   Petrolatum to make 15 g
2. Benzocaine, 1.5 g
   Chlorobutanol, 1.5 g
   Methyl salicylate, 5 drops
   Petrolatum or lanolin to make 30 g

Bibliography

Kutscher AH, *et al: Pharmacotherapeutics of Oral Disease*, McGraw-Hill New York, 1964.

Kutscher AH, *et al: Pharmacology for the Dental Hygienist*, 2nd ed, Lea and Febiger, Philadelphia, 1982.

AMA Drug Evaluations, 3rd ed, AMA, Chicago, IL, 1977.

The Medical Letter (a periodical), Drug and Therapeutic Information, Inc, New York.

Physicians' Desk Reference, Medical Economics, Oradell, NJ.

Accepted Dental Therapeutics, ADA, Chicago. 38th ed, 1979.

---

* Entries in this index follow one another in alphabetic order of the complete entry, letter by letter, and regardless of spaces between words in entries of two or more words. Exceptions to this rule are pH and Rh, for which all indented entries are grouped under the single main heading. Italicized prefixes (*sec-*, *para-*, etc), which are not part of an official drug monograph title, and numbers or Greek letters used as locant (1-Propenol, -Blockers, etc) are disregarded in determining alphabetical sequence. All official names of drugs will appear in the uninverted form (Diluted Acidic Acid) as a minimum but also may be found in the inverted form if this is deemed more descriptive (Acidic acid, diluted).

PERIODIC CHART

METALS

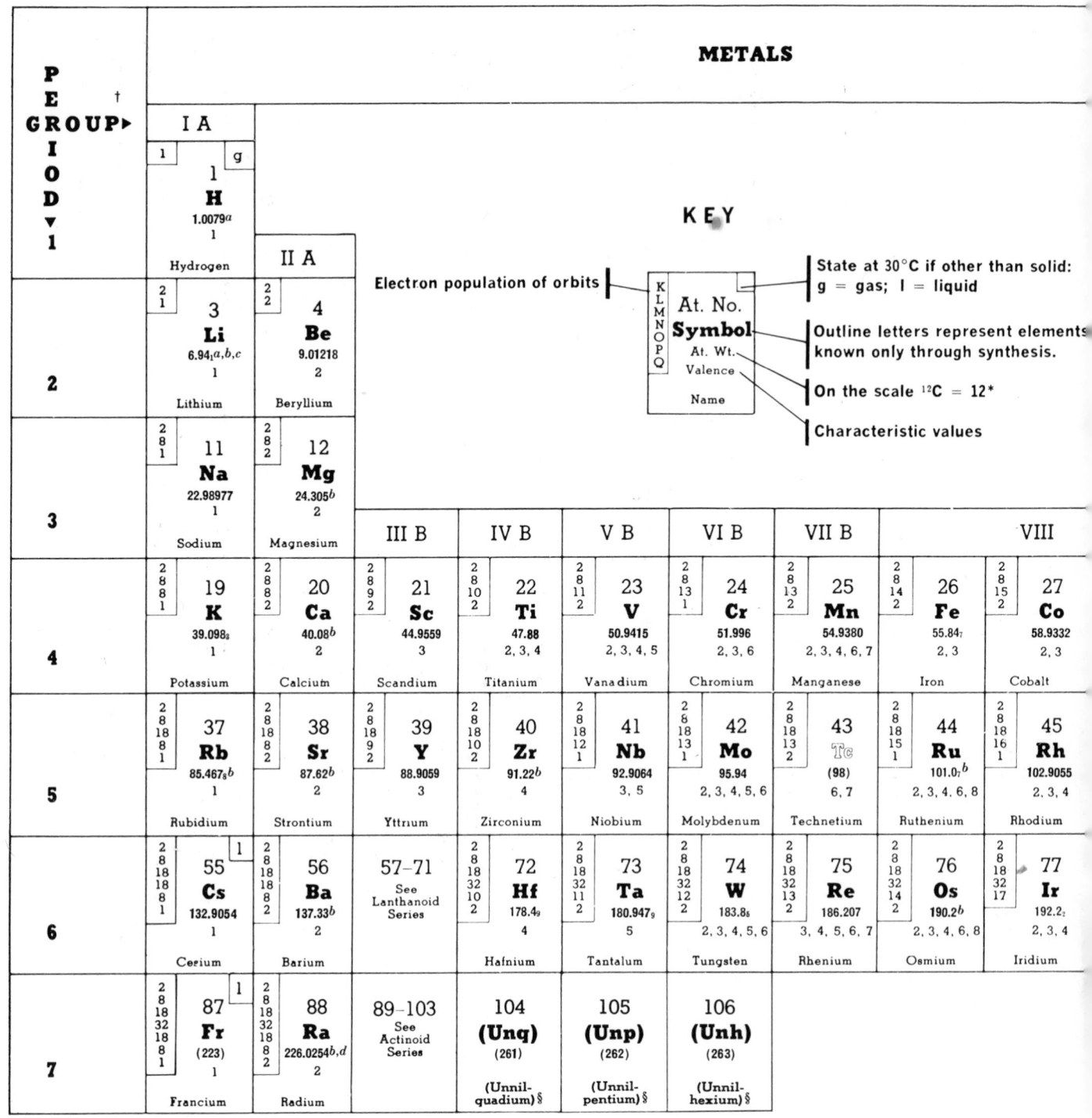

KEY

Electron population of orbits

K L M N O P Q | At. No. / Symbol / At. Wt. / Valence / Name

State at 30°C if other than solid: g = gas; l = liquid

Outline letters represent elements known only through synthesis.

On the scale $^{12}C = 12$*

Characteristic values

PERIOD	IA	IIA	IIIB	IVB	VB	VIB	VIIB		VIII	
1	1 H 1.0079ᵃ Hydrogen (g)									
2	3 Li 6.941ᵃ,ᵇ,ᶜ Lithium	4 Be 9.01218 Beryllium								
3	11 Na 22.98977 Sodium	12 Mg 24.305ᵇ Magnesium								
4	19 K 39.098₃ 1 Potassium	20 Ca 40.08ᵇ 2 Calcium	21 Sc 44.9559 3 Scandium	22 Ti 47.88 2,3,4 Titanium	23 V 50.9415 2,3,4,5 Vanadium	24 Cr 51.996 2,3,6 Chromium	25 Mn 54.9380 2,3,4,6,7 Manganese	26 Fe 55.84₇ 2,3 Iron	27 Co 58.9332 2,3 Cobalt	
5	37 Rb 85.467₈ᵇ 1 Rubidium	38 Sr 87.62ᵇ 2 Strontium	39 Y 88.9059 3 Yttrium	40 Zr 91.22ᵇ 4 Zirconium	41 Nb 92.9064 3,5 Niobium	42 Mo 95.94 2,3,4,5,6 Molybdenum	43 Tc (98) 6,7 Technetium	44 Ru 101.0₇ᵇ 2,3,4,6,8 Ruthenium	45 Rh 102.9055 2,3,4 Rhodium	
6	55 Cs 132.9054 1 (l) Cesium	56 Ba 137.33ᵇ 2 Barium	57–71 See Lanthanoid Series	72 Hf 178.4₉ 4 Hafnium	73 Ta 180.947₉ 5 Tantalum	74 W 183.8₅ 2,3,4,5,6 Tungsten	75 Re 186.207 3,4,5,6,7 Rhenium	76 Os 190.2ᵇ 2,3,4,6,8 Osmium	77 Ir 192.2₂ 2,3,4 Iridium	
7	87 Fr (223) 1 (l) Francium	88 Ra 226.0254ᵇ,ᵈ 2 Radium	89–103 See Actinoid Series	104 (Unq) (261) (Unnilquadium)§	105 (Unp) (262) (Unnilpentium)§	106 (Unh) (263) (Unnilhexium)§				

Lanthanoid Series (Rare Earth Elements)

57 La 138.905₅ᵇ 3 Lanthanum	58 Ce 140.12ᵇ 3,4 Cerium	59 Pr 140.9077 3,4 Praseodymium	60 Nd 144.2₄ᵇ 3 Neodymium	61 Pm (145) 3 Promethium	62 Sm 150.36 2,3 Samarium	63 Eu 151.96ᵇ 2,3 Europium

Actinoid Series

89 Ac 227.0278ᵈ 3 Actinium	90 Th 232.0381ᵇ,ᵈ 4 Thorium	91 Pa 231.0359ᵈ 5 Protactinium	92 U 238.0289ᵇ,ᶜ 3,4,5,6 Uranium	93 Np 237.0482ᵈ 3,4,5,6 Neptunium	94 Pu (244) 3,4,5,6 Plutonium	95 Am (243) 3,4,5,6 Americium

* Atomic weight is an alternative term for 'relative atomic mass of an element', A_r (E). The IUPAC values given here are scaled to A_r (^{12}C) = 12 and apply to elements as they exist in materials of terrestrial origin and to certain artificial elements. When used with due regard to the footnotes they are considered reliable to ±1 in the last digit or ±3 if that digit is subscript. Values in parentheses are for radioactive elements whose atomic weights cannot be quoted precisely without knowledge of the origin of the elements; the value given is the atomic mass number of the isotope of that element of longest known half-life.
† Beginning with Group III, authors differ in their presentation of the "A" and "B" groups of elements.
‡ Expected value from theoretical considerations. § Names and symbols provisionally suggested by IUPAC.